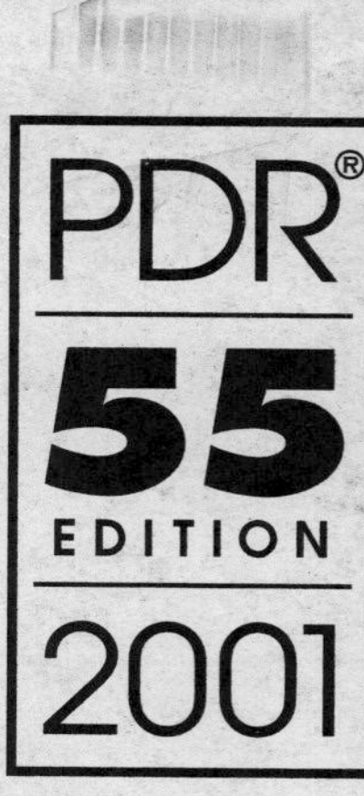

PDR®

55

EDITION

2001

PHYSICIANS' DESK REFERENCE®

Senior Vice President, Directory Services: Paul Walsh

Vice President, Sales and Marketing: Dikran N. Barsamian
National Sales Manager, Custom Sales: Anthony Sorce
Senior Account Manager: Frank Karkowsky
Account Managers:
Marion Gray, RPh
Lawrence C. Keary
Suzanne E. Yarrow, RN
National Sales Manager, Medical Economics Trade Sales:
Bill Gaffney
Senior Business Manager: Mark S. Ritchin
Financial Analyst: Wayne M. Soltis
Vice President, Clinical Communications and New Business Development: Mukesh Mehta, RPh
New Business Development Manager: Jeffrey D. Dubin
Manager, Drug Information Services: Thomas Fleming, RPh
Drug Information Specialists: Maria Deutsch, MS, PharmD, CDE; Christine Wyble, PharmD
Editor, Directory Services: David W. Sifton
Project Manager: Edward P. Connor
Senior Associate Editor: Lori Murray
Assistant Editor: Gwynned L. Kelly
Director of Direct Marketing: Michael Bennett
Direct Mail Manager: Lorraine M. Loening
Senior Marketing Analyst: Dina A. Maeder
Director of Production: Carrie Williams
Data Manager: Jeffrey D. Schaefer
Production Manager: Amy Brooks
Production Coordinators: Gianna Caradonna, Dee Ann DeRuvo, Melissa Katz
Index Supervisor: Johanna M. Mazur
Index Editor: Shannon Reilly
Art Associate: Joan K. Akerlind
Digital Imaging Supervisor: Shawn W. Cahill
Digital Imaging Coordinator: Frank J. McElroy, III
Pharmaceutical Coordinator: Mary Kaadan
Electronic Publishing Designer: Livio Udina
Fulfillment Managers: Louis J. Bolcik, Stephanie DeNardi

MEDICAL ECONOMICS
THOMSON HEALTHCARE™

Officers of Medical Economics Company: *President and Chief Executive Officer:* Curtis B. Allen; *Vice President, New Media:* L. Suzanne BeDell; *Vice President, Corporate Human Resources:* Pamela M. Bilash; *Chief Financial Officer:* Christopher Caridi; *Vice President and Controller:* Barry Gray; *Vice President, Finance:* Donna Santarpia; *Senior Vice President, Directory Services:* Paul Walsh; *Senior Vice President, Operations:* John R. Ware

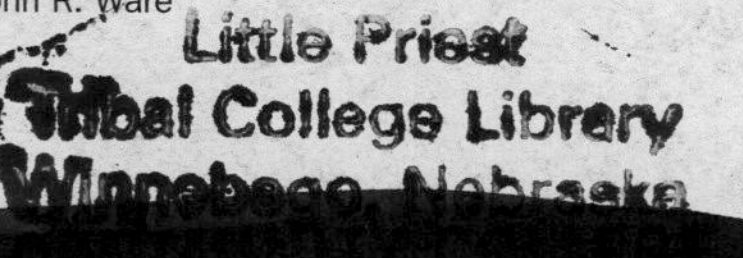

ISBN: 1-56363-330-2

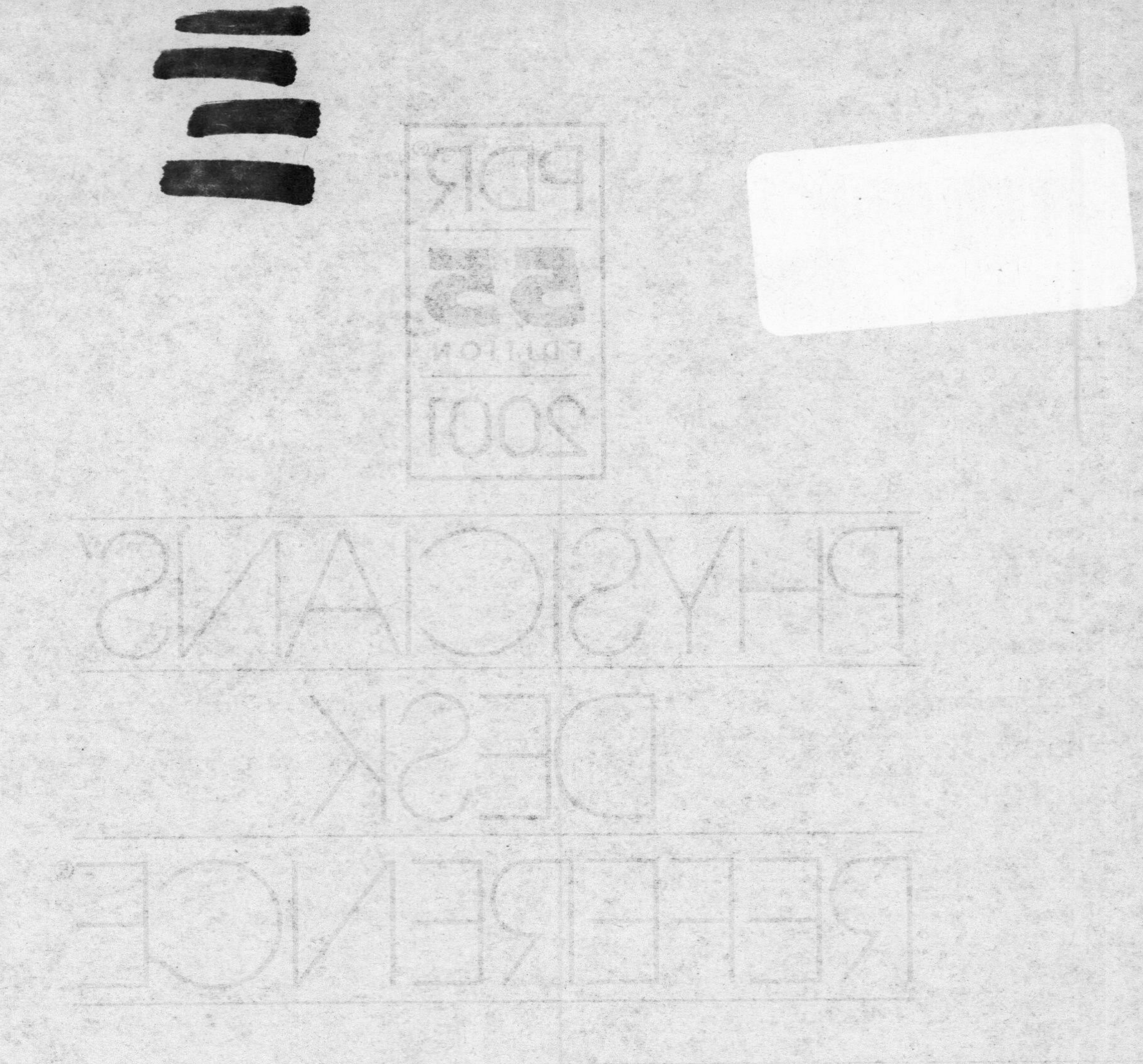

FOREWORD TO THE FIFTY-FIFTH EDITION

Once again you're looking at *PDR's* biggest edition ever. The 2001 edition outstrips last year's by some 100 pages. It's so big, in fact, that we've launched a new companion reference that makes *PDR* information easier to access if you're simply double-checking a dose.

Entitled the *PDR Pharmacopoeia™ Pocket Edition*, this little handbook accompanies you wherever you need to go, around the office or on rounds. Only slightly larger than an index card, and a quarter of an inch thick, it fits easily into any pocket, while providing you with FDA-approved dosing recommendations for over 1,500 drugs.

For complicated cases, patients on multi-drug regimens, those with hepatic or renal conditions, and members of special populations, there's still no substitute for the detailed guidelines found in *Physicians' Desk Reference* itself. But if all you're looking for is quick confirmation of a form, strength, or dose, the new *PDR Pharmacopoeia* is just what you need.

Unlike other condensed drug references, this new handbook is drawn almost exclusively from the FDA-approved drug labeling published in *Physicians' Desk Reference*, so you can rely on it for authoritative, official dosage guidelines. Its tabular presentation makes lookups a breeze. And to expedite comparisons, it lists drugs by major category and specific indication. At $9.95 a copy, it's a tool you really can't afford to be without.

If portability is your goal, we have two other intriguing new options for you. Now you can get the full text of six key topics for every fully-described prescription drug in *PDR* and load it into your Palm®, Visor™, or other handheld organizer. Or if you prefer, you can get a brand new Franklin eBookman unit loaded with the same information.

Whether you have a Palm, Visor, or eBookman, you'll get the complete, FDA-approved text of six crucial topics: Indications and Usage, Contraindications, Warnings, Adverse Reactions, How Supplied, and Dosage and Administration. (These topics are also available on a traditional *Pocket PDR*® DataCard.) No matter how you choose to view it, you'll have a complete databank of prescribing information at your fingertips wherever you go!

If you're looking to expand your library of traditional printed medical references, we have still more good news. The second edition of our phenomenally popular *PDR® for Herbal Medicines™* is now available for immediate shipment. Enhanced and expanded with over 100 additional botanicals (now totaling more than 700 in all), the new edition supplies you with important new information on the latest clinical studies, plus new indices of Asian and homeopathic indications, and a new Safety Guide that lists herbs to be avoided during pregnancy and nursing, and herbs to be used only under professional supervision.

Although botanical products are not officially regulated or monitored in the United States, *PDR for Herbal Medicines* provides you the closest analog to FDA-approved labeling—the findings of the German Regulatory Authority's herbal watchdog agency, Commission E—augmented with exhaustive literature reviews from the PhytoPharm U.S. Institute for Phytopharmaceuticals. These reports represent the most accurate, impartial, and reliable assessment of a botanical agent's safety and effectiveness currently available in medicine.

Also coming in 2001 is the brand new *PDR for Nutritional Supplements™*, a compendium of the latest consensus on some 300 popular supplement products, including an array of amino acids, co-factors, fatty acids, probiotics, phytoestrogens, phytosterols, over-the-counter hormones, hormonal precursors, and much more. Focused on the scientific evidence (or lack of evidence) for each supplement's claims, this unique new reference offers you today's most detailed, informed, and objective overview of a burgeoning new area in the field of self-treatment. To protect your patients from bogus remedies and steer them towards truly beneficial products, this book is a must.

And as always, to maximize the value of your *PDR*, there's the 2001 edition of the *PDR Companion Guide™*, an 1,800-page reference that augments *PDR* with a total of 10 unique decision-making tools:

- **Interactions Index** identifies all pharmaceuticals and foods capable of interacting with a chosen medication.
- **Food Interactions Cross-Reference** lists the drugs that may interact with a given dietary item.
- **Side Effects Index** pinpoints the pharmaceuticals associated with each of 3,600 distinct adverse reactions.
- **Indications Index** presents the full range of therapeutic options for any given diagnosis.
- **Off-Label Treatment Guide** lists medications routinely used—but never officially approved—for treatment of nearly 1,000 specific disorders.
- **Contraindications Index** lists all drugs to avoid in the presence of any given medical condition.
- **International Drug Index** names the U.S. equivalents of some 15,000 foreign medications.
- **Generic Availability Guide** shows which forms and strengths of a brand-name drug are also available generically.
- **Cost of Therapy Guide** provides a quick overview of the relative expense of the leading therapeutic options for a variety of common indications.

- **Imprint Identification Guide** enables you to establish the nature of any unknown tablet or capsule by matching its imprint against an exhaustive catalog of identifying codes.

The PDR Companion Guide includes all drugs described in *PDR, PDR For Nonprescription Drugs and Dietary Supplements™*, and *PDR For Ophthalmic Medicines™*. We're certain that you'll find it makes safe, appropriate selection of drugs faster and easier than ever before.

PDR and its major companion volumes are also found in the *PDR® Electronic Library™* on CD-ROM, now used in over 100,000 practices. This Windows-compatible disc provides users with a complete database of *PDR* prescribing information, electronically searchable for instant retrieval. A standard subscription includes *PDR*'s sophisticated search software and an extensive file of chemical structures, illustrations, and full-color product photographs. Optional enhancements include the complete contents of *The Merck Manual Seventeenth Edition*, *Stedman's Medical Dictionary*, and *Stedman's Spellchecker*. For anyone who wants to run a fast double check on a proposed prescription, there's also the *PDR® Drug Interactions and Side Effects System™* — sophisticated software capable of automatically screening a 20-drug regimen for conflicts, then proposing alternatives for any problematic medication. This unique decision-making tool now comes free with the *PDR Electronic Library.*

Remember, too, that the contents of *PDR* and its main companion volumes can always be found on the Internet at **www.pdr.net.** For more information on these products, please call, toll-free, 1-800-232-7379 or fax 201-573-4956. For corporate users of the electronic *PDR* products, please call 1-800-446-8380.

Physicians' Desk Reference is published by Medical Economics Company in cooperation with participating manufacturers. Each full-length entry provides you with an exact copy of the product's FDA-approved labeling. Under the federal Food, Drug and Cosmetics (FD&C) Act, a drug approved for marketing may be labeled, promoted, and advertised by the manufacturer for only those uses for which the drug's safety and effectiveness have been established. The Code of Federal Regulations 201.100(d)(1) pertaining to labeling for prescription products requires that for *PDR* content "indications, effects, dosages, routes, methods, and frequency and duration of administration and any relevant warnings, hazards, contraindications, side effects, and precautions" must be *"same in language and emphasis"* as the approved labeling for the products. The Food and Drug Administration (FDA) regards the words *same in language and emphasis* as requiring VERBATIM use of the approved labeling providing such information. Furthermore, information that is emphasized in the approved labeling by the use of type set in a box, or in capitals, boldface, or italics, must be given the same emphasis in *PDR*.

The FDA has also recognized that the FD&C Act does not, however, limit the manner in which a physician may use an approved drug. Once a product has been approved for marketing, a physician may choose to prescribe it for uses or in treatment regimens or patient populations that are not included in approved labeling. The FDA also observes that accepted medical practice includes drug use that is not reflected in approved drug labeling. For products that do not have official package circulars, the publisher has emphasized the necessity of describing such products comprehensively, so that physicians can have access to all information essential for intelligent and informed decision-making. Particularly in the case of over-the-counter dietary supplements, it should be remembered that this information has not been evaluated by the Food and Drug Administration, and that such products are not intended to diagnose, treat, cure, or prevent any disease.

The function of the publisher is the compilation, organization, and distribution of this information. Each product description has been prepared by the manufacturer, and edited and approved by the manufacturer's medical department, medical director, and/or medical consultant. In organizing and presenting the material in *Physicians' Desk Reference*, the publisher does not warrant or guarantee any of the products described, or perform any independent analysis in connection with any of the product information contained herein. *Physicians' Desk Reference* does not assume, and expressly disclaims, any obligation to obtain and include any information other than that provided to it by the manufacturer. It should be understood that by making this material available, the publisher is not advocating the use of any product described herein, nor is the publisher responsible for misuse of a product due to typographical error. Additional information on any product may be obtained from the manufacturer.

CONTENTS

MANUFACTURERS' INDEX

Listed in this index are all manufacturers participating in PHYSICIANS' DESK REFERENCE®. It is through their courtesy that PDR® is brought to the medical profession.

Each company's entry includes the address, phone, and fax number of its headquarters and regional offices, as well as contacts for inquiries, orders, and medical emergency information. Products with entries in the Product Information or Diagnostic Product Information sections are listed with their page numbers. Other products available from the manufacturer are listed following the described products.

If an entry in the index lists multiple page numbers, the first ones shown refer to photographs of the product, the last one to its prescribing information.

- **Bold page numbers** indicate full prescribing information.
- *Italic page numbers* signify partial information.
- The ◆ symbol marks drugs shown in the Product Identification Guide.
- The ▣ symbol means product information is located in *PDR For Nonprescription Drugs and Dietary Supplements*™.
- The ⊙ symbol means product information is located in *PDR For Ophthalmic Medicines*™.

100 Abbott Park Rd.
Abbott Park, IL 60064

Pharmaceutical Products Division--
Direct Inquiries to:
Customer Service:
(800) 255-5162
Technical Services:
(800) 441-4987
For Medical Information Contact:
Generally:
(800) 633-9110
Adverse Drug Experiences:
(800) 633-9110
Sales and Ordering:
(800) 255-5162

Hospital Products Division--
Direct Inquiries to:
Customer Service
(800) 222-6883
For Medical Information Contact:
(800) 615-0187
Sales and Ordering:
(800) 222-6883

Products Described:

Other Products Available:

0.25% Acetic Acid Irrigation, USP (Aqualite)
5% Alcohol & 5% Dextrose Injection
Amidate (Etomidate Injection) Ampul, Abboject
Aminophylline 250 mg, 10 mL, Ampul & Vial
Aminophylline 500 mg, 20 mL, Ampul & Vial
Aminosyn 3.5% M
Aminosyn 5%
Aminosyn 7%
Aminosyn 7% TPN Kit
Aminosyn 7% with Electrolytes
Aminosyn 7% with Electrolytes TPN Kit
Aminosyn 8.5%
Aminosyn 8.5% TPN Kit
Aminosyn 8.5% with Electrolytes
Aminosyn 10%
Aminosyn 10% TPN Kit
Aminosyn-HBC 7%
Aminosyn II 7%
Aminosyn II 8.5%
Aminosyn II 10%
Aminosyn II in Dextrose, Nutrimix Dual Chamber
Aminosyn-PF 7% and 10%
Aminosyn with Dextrose, Nutrimix Dual Chamber
Ammonium Chloride
Anticoagulant Citrate Phosphate Dextrose Solution, USP
Atropine 0.05 mg/mL, 5 mL, Abboject Syringe
Atropine 0.1 mg/mL, 5 mL, 10 mL, Abboject Syringe
Balanced Salt Solution
Bretylium Tosylate in 5% Dextrose Injection (50 mg/mL)
Bupivacaine Hydrochloride Injection, USP, 0.25%, 0.5%, 0.75%, Ampul, Abboject Syringe
Calcium Acetate 0.5 mEq/mL Injection
Calcium Chloride 10%, (1.4 mEq/mL) Abboject
Calcium Gluceptate Injection Ampul & Abboject (0.9 mEq/mL)
Cecon Solution
Cenolate Ampules (500 mg/mL)
Chromium 10 mL (4 mcg/mL)
Colchicine Tablets
Copper 10 mL (0.4 mg/mL)
Cysteine Hydrochloride Injection
Dayalets Filmtab
Dayalets Plus Iron Filmtab
Dehydrated Alcohol Injection, USP
6% Dextran 70 w/v & 5% Dextrose Injection
6% Dextran 70 w/v & 0.9% Sodium Chloride Injection
2.5% Dextrose & 1/2 Str Lactated Ringer's Injection
2.5% Dextrose & 0.45% Sodium Chloride Injection, USP
5% Dextrose & Lactated Ringer's Injection
5% Dextrose & 0.224% Pot Chl Injection (30 mEq)
5% Dextrose & 0.3% Pot Chl Injection (40 mEq)
5% Dextrose & Ringer's Injection
5% Dextrose & 0.225% Sodium Chloride with 0.075% Potassium Chloride Injection (10 mEq)
5% Dextrose & 0.225% Sodium Chloride with 0.15% Potassium Chloride Injection (20 mEq)
5% Dextrose & 0.225% Sodium Chloride with 0.224% Potassium Chloride Injection (30 mEq)
5% Dextrose & 0.225% Sodium Chloride with 0.3% Potassium Chloride Injection (40 mEq)
5% Dextrose & 0.3% Sodium Chloride with 0.075% Potassium Chloride Injection (10 mEq)
5% Dextrose & 0.3% Sodium Chloride with 0.15% Potassium Chloride Injection (20 mEq)
5% Dextrose & 0.3% Sodium Chloride with 0.224% Potassium Chloride Injection (30 mEq)
5% Dextrose & 0.45% Sodium Chloride with 0.075% Potassium Chloride Injection (10 mEq)
5% Dextrose & 0.45% Sodium Chloride with 0.15% Potassium Chloride Injection (20 mEq)
5% Dextrose & 0.45% Sodium Chloride with 0.224% Potassium Chloride Injection (30 mEq)
5% Dextrose & 0.45% Sodium Chloride with 0.3% Potassium Chloride Injection (40 mEq)
5% Dextrose & 0.225% Sodium Chloride Injection, USP
5% Dextrose & 0.3% Sodium Chloride Injection, USP
5% Dextrose & 0.45% Sodium Chloride Injection, USP
5% Dextrose & 0.9% Sodium Chloride Injection, USP
10% Dextrose & 0.9% Sodium Chloride Injection, USP
2.5% Dextrose Injection, USP
5% Dextrose Injection, USP
5% Dextrose Injection, USP (ADD-Vantage)
5% Dextrose Injection, USP (Partial fill)
10% Dextrose Injection, USP
20% Dextrose Injection, USP
30% Dextrose Injection, USP
40% Dextrose Injection, USP
50% Dextrose Injection, USP
60% Dextrose Injection, USP
70% Dextrose Injection, USP
Dical-D Tablets
Dopamine Hydrochloride in 5% Dextrose Injection (800, 1600, 3200 mcg/mL)
Empty Evacuated Container
Endrate Solution, Ampules (150 mg/mL)
Enduronyl Forte Tablets
Enduronyl Tablets
Ephedrine Sulfate, Injection (50 mg/mL)
Epinephrine 1:10,000, 10 mL, Abboject
EryDerm Topical Solution
Erythrocin ADD-Vantage Kits
Erythrocin Lactobionate-I.V.
Erythrocin Piggyback
Fentanyl Injection, Ampul, Vial
Fentanyl Oralet (oral transmucosal fentanyl citrate) CII
Gentamicin Premix ADD-Vantage Products
Gentamicin Sulfate in 0.9% Sodium Chloride Injection (0.8, 0.9, 1.0, 1.2, 1.4 mg/mL)
1.5% Glycine Irrigation, USP (Flex & Aqualite)
1.5% Glycine Irrigation/Aqualite
Heparin Sodium in 0.45% Sodium Chloride Injection (50 & 100 Units/mL)
Heparin Sodium in 5% Dextrose Injection (50 & 100 Units/mL)
A-hydroCort
Hydroxyzine HCl Injection, Abbojects, Ampuls, Vials, Syringes
Isoproterenol HCl 1:5,000 5 mL, Universal Add Syringe
Isoproterenol HCl 1:5,000 10 mL, Universal Add Syringe
Isoproterenol HCl 1:50,000, 10 mL, Abboject
Lactated Ringer's Injection, USP
Lactated Ringers for Irrigation (Flex)
Lidocaine HCl Injection, 0.2% in 5% Dextrose
Lidocaine HCl Injection, 0.4% in 5% Dextrose
Lidocaine HCl Injection, 0.8% in 5% Dextrose
Lidocaine HCl Injection, USP, 1%, 5 mL, Abboject
Lidocaine HCl Injection, USP, 1%, 5 mL, Sterile Pack Abboject
Lidocaine HCl Injection, USP, 2%, 5 mL, Abboject
Lidocaine HCl Injection, USP, 2%, 5 mL, Sterile Pack Abboject
Lidocaine HCl Injection, USP, 5% with 7.5% Dextrose
Lidocaine HCl Injection, USP, 20%, 5 mL, 1 gram-Pintop, U.A.S.
Lidocaine HCl Injection, USP, 20%, 10 mL, 2 gram-Pintop, U.A.S.
Liposyn II 10% and 20%
10% LMD w/v and 5% Dextrose Injection
10% LMD w/v and 0.9% Sodium Chloride Injection
LTA II Kit
LTA Kit, Preattached
LTA Pediatric Kit
Magnesium Sulfate 12.5%, 8 mL, Pintop
Magnesium Sulfate 50% w/v Ampoules, Vials & Abboject
Manganese 10 mL (1 mg/mL)
5% Mannitol Injection, USP
10% Mannitol Injection, USP
15% Mannitol Injection, USP
20% Mannitol Injection, USP
25% Mannitol Injection, USP
Meperidine HCl Injection (10 mg/mL, PCA Vials)
A-methaPred
Metronidazole Injection, USP (5 mg/mL)
Morphine Sulfate Injection, USP (1 & 5 mg/mL, PCA Vials)
Nalbuphine Hydrochloride Injection
Neut Abbo-Vial & Pintop
Nitropress
Normosol-M & 5% Dextrose Injection
Normosol-R
Normosol-R & 5% Dextrose Injection
Normosol-R pH 7.4
Optilets-500 Filmtab
Optilets-M-500 Filmtab
Oretic Tablets
Peganone Tablets
Pentothal (Thiopental Sodium for Injection)
Pentothal Kit
Pentothal RTM Syringe
Physiosol Irrigation (Aqualite)
Plegisol
Potassium Acetate 40 mEq Vial, Pintop & Fliptop
Potassium Chloride Injection Ampoules & Vials, Pintop & Universal Additive Syringe
Potassium Phosphate 15 mM Vial & Fliptop
Potassium Phosphate 45 mM Vial
Procainamide Hydrochloride Injection, USP
Procaine Hydrochloride Injection 1% & 2% Vial
Quelicin (Succinylcholine Chloride Injection) Ampul & Vial, Pintop
Ringer's Injection, USP
Ringer's Irrigation, USP (Aqualite)
Sodium Acetate 40 mEq, 100 mEq and 200 mEq Vials
4.2% Sodium Bicarbonate Injection, 10 mEq in 10 mL Abboject (Neonatal)
5% Sodium Bicarbonate Injection, USP
7.5% Sodium Bicarbonate Injection, 44.6 mEq in 50 mL ampul or Abboject
8.4% Sodium Bicarbonate Injection, 10 mEq in 10 mL Abboject (Pediatric)
8.4% Sodium Bicarbonate Injection, 50 mEq in 50 mL Abboject or Fliptop Vial
5% Sodium Chloride
0.45% Sodium Chloride Injection, USP
0.9% Sodium Chloride Injection
0.9% Sodium Chloride Injection, USP (ADD-Vantage)
0.9% Sodium Chloride Injection, USP (Partial Fill)
0.45% Sodium Chloride Irrigation, USP (Aqualite)

0.9% Sodium Chloride Irrigation, USP (Flex and Aqualite)
Sodium Lactate Injection, USP, 1/6 Molar
Sodium Phosphate 45 mMoL
Sorbitol-Mannitol Irrigation (Flex & Aqualite)
Surbex 750 with Zinc Filmtab
Surbex with C Filmtab
Surbex-T Filmtab
Tham Solution
Theophylline in 5% Dextrose Injection (0.4, 0.8, 1.6, 2, 3.2, 4 mg/mL)
TPN Electrolytes
Tridione Dulcet Tablets
Tronothane Hydrochloride Cream
Tubocurarine Chloride Injection, USP
Ultane (Sevoflurane)
Ureaphil
Urologic G Irrigation (Aqualite)
Water for Injection Bacteriostatic 30 mL Fliptop
Water for Injection, Sterile, USP, Amps, Vial
Water for Irrigation, Sterile, USP (Flex and Aqualite)
Water for Respiratory Therapy, Sterile (Flex)
Zinc 10 mL (1 mg/1 mL)

ADVANCED NUTRITIONAL TECHNOLOGY, INC. **495**
6988 Sierra Ct.
Dublin, CA 94568

Direct Inquiries to:
(925) 828-2128
FAX: (925) 828-6848

Products Described:
Nutr-E-Sol Liquid.................... **495**
SuperEPA Softgels.................... **496**
Ultra Zn Tablets.................... **496**

AGOURON PHARMACEUTICALS, INC. **303, 496**
10350 North Torrey Pines Road
La Jolla, CA 92037-1020

Direct Inquiries to:
Customer Communications
(888) 847-2237
FAX: (858) 678-8266

For Medical Emergencies Contact:
Medical Affairs
(888) 847-2237

Products Described:
◆Rescriptor Tablets.................... **303, 496**
◆Viracept Oral Powder.................... **303, 499**
◆Viracept Tablets.................... **303, 499**

ALCON LABORATORIES, INC. **303, 503**
Alcon Laboratories, Inc.
And its affiliates
Corporate Headquarters
6201 South Freeway
Fort Worth, TX 76134

Direct Inquiries to:
Pharmaceuticals/Consumer: (800) 451-3937 (Therapeutic Drugs/Lens Care)
Surgical: (800) 862-5266 (Instrumentation/Surgical Meds)

Products Described:
Azopt Ophthalmic Suspension.......... **503**
Betaxon Ophthalmic Suspension.......... **504**
Betoptic S Ophthalmic Suspension.......... **505**
Bion Tears Lubricant Eye Drops.......... **506**
Ciloxan Ophthalmic Ointment.......... **506**
Ciloxan Ophthalmic Solution.......... **506**
◆Cipro HC Otic Suspension.......... **303, 507**
Naphcon-A Ophthalmic Solution.......... **508**
Patanol Ophthalmic Solution.......... **508**
Tears Naturale Free Lubricant Eye Drops.......... **508**
Tears Naturale II Lubricant Eye Drops.......... **508**
TobraDex Ophthalmic Ointment.......... **509**
TobraDex Ophthalmic Suspension.......... **508**

Other Products Available:
A.C.S. Closure System Needles and Sutures
Alcon Surgical System (Irrigation/Aspiration Kits; Phacoemulsification Kits)
Alomide Ophthalmic Solution
A-OK Ophthalmic Knives
BSS and BSS Plus Irrigation Solution Administration Set
BSS Irrigation Solution (15 mL, 30 mL, 250 mL, 500 mL)
BSS Plus Irrigation Solution (250 mL, 500 mL)
Cetamide Ointment
Cetapred Ointment
Cyclogyl Ophthalmic Solution
Cystitomes & Cannulas
DuoVisc Viscoelastic System
Duratears Naturale Lubricant Eye Ointment
Econopred Plus Ophthalmic Suspension
Emadine Ophthalmic Solution
Enuclene Cleaning/Lubricating Solution for Artificial Eyes
Epinal Ophthalmic Solution
Eye Pak Surgical Drapes
Eye Stream Eye Irrigating Solution
Flarex Ophthalmic Suspension
Fluorescite Injection
Gonioscopic Prism Solution
I-Knife Ophthalmic Knife
Intraocular Lenses
Iopidine Ophthalmic Solution
Ismotic Isosorbide Solution
I-Spear Surgical Eye Sponge
Maxidex Ointment
Maxitrol Ointment
Microsponge Surgical Eye Sponge
Miostat Intraocular Miotic Solution
Natacyn Ophthalmic Suspension
Ocucel Lint-Free Surgical Products
Optemp Sterile Disposable Cautery
Osmoglyn Oral Osmotic Agent
Pilopine HS Gel
Post-Operative Kits
Procedure Packs
Profenal Ophthalmic Solution
ProShield Corneal Collagen Shield
ProVisc Ophthalmic Viscosurgical Device
PTG, Alcon Applanation Pneumatonograph
SofGuard Flexible Eye Shield
Steri-Units Single Dose Surgical Drops
Vexol Ophthalmic Suspension
Viscoat Ophthalmic Viscosurgical Device

ALLERGAN, INC. **303, 510**
2525 Dupont Drive
P.O. Box 19534
Irvine, CA 92623-9534

Direct Inquiries to:
(714) 246-4500

Products Described:
◆Acular Ophthalmic Solution.......... **303, 510**
◆Acular PF Ophthalmic Solution.......... **303, 511**
◆Alocril Ophthalmic Solution.......... **303, 511**
◆Alphagan Ophthalmic Solution.......... **304, 512**
Azelex Cream.......... **512**
◆Blephamide Ophthalmic Ointment.......... **304, 513**
◆Blephamide Ophthalmic Suspension.......... **304, 514**
Botox Purified Neurotoxin Complex.......... **515**
Elimite Cream.......... **516**
Exsel Lotion/Shampoo.......... *517*
Fluoroplex Topical Cream.......... **517**
Fluoroplex Topical Solution.......... **517**
Maxiflor Cream.......... *517*
Maxiflor Ointment.......... *517*
◆Ocuflox Ophthalmic Solution.......... **304, 517**
Opticrom Ophthalmic Solution.......... **518**
Polytrim Ophthalmic Solution.......... **519**
Tazorac Gel.......... **520**

Other Products Available:
Albalon Ophthalmic Solution
Betagan Ophthalmic Solution with C Cap Compliance Cap Q.D. and B.I.D.
Bleph-10 Ophthalmic Ointment
Bleph-10 Ophthalmic Solution
Celluvisc Lubricant Eye Drops
Chloroptic Ophthalmic Ointment
Chloroptic Ophthalmic Solution
Epifrin Sterile Ophthalmic Solution
FML Forte Ophthalmic Suspension
FML Ophthalmic Suspension
FML S.O.P. Ophthalmic Ointment
FML-S Ophthalmic Suspension
Genoptic Ophthalmic Ointment
Genoptic Ophthalmic Solution
HMS Ophthalmic Suspension
Ocufen Ophthalmic Solution
Ophthetic Ophthalmic Solution
Poly-Pred Ophthalmic Suspension
Pred Forte Ophthalmic Suspension
Pred-G Ophthalmic Ointment
Pred-G Ophthalmic Suspension
Pred Mild Ophthalmic Suspension
Propine Ophthalmic Solution
Refresh Plus Lubricant Eye Drops
Refresh P.M. Lubricant Eye Ointment
Refresh Tears Lubricant Eye Drops

ALLERGAN SKIN CARE
(See ALLERGAN, INC.)

ALPHA THERAPEUTIC CORPORATION **521**
5555 Valley Boulevard
Los Angeles, CA 90032
Internet: www.alphather.com

Contacts:
Medical Director: (323) 227-7077
Professional Services: (800) 292-6118
After Hours Emergency Orders: (800) 421-0008
Direct Inquiries: (323) 225-2221
Customer Service: (800) 421-0008
FAX: (323) 227-7027

Products Described:
Albutein 5% Solution.......... *521*
Albutein 25% Solution.......... *521*
Alphanate Solvent Detergent/Heat Treated.......... *521*
AlphaNine SD Solvent Detergent Treated/Virus Filtered.......... *522*
Profilnine SD Solvent Detergent Treated.......... *522*
Venoglobulin-S 5% Solution Solvent Detergent Treated.......... *522*
Venoglobulin-S 10% Solution Solvent Detergent Treated.......... *522*

ALPHARMA **522**
U.S. Pharmaceuticals Division
7205 Windsor Blvd.
Baltimore, MD 21244

Direct Inquiries to:
Customer Service
(800) 638-9096

Products Described:
Lindane Lotion USP 1%.......... **522**
Lindane Shampoo USP 1%.......... **523**

ALZA PHARMACEUTICALS **304, 524**
A Division of ALZA Corporation
1900 Charleston Road
Mountain View, California 94043

Direct Inquiries to:
Customer Service
(800) 227-9953
FAX: (888) 261-8045

For Medical Information or Emergencies Contact:
Medical Communications
(800) 634-8977 or (800) 506-4959
FAX: (650) 962-2488

Products Described:
Bicitra Oral Solution.......... *524*
◆Concerta Tablets.......... **342, 3474**
Ditropan Tablets and Syrup.......... *524*
◆Ditropan XL Extended Release Tablets.......... **304, 525**
◆Doxil Injection.......... **304, 526**
◆Elmiron Capsules.......... **304, 531**
◆Ethyol for Injection.......... **304, 532**
◆Mycelex Troche.......... **304, 534**
Polycitra Syrup and Polycitra-LC Oral Solution.......... *535*
Polycitra-K Crystals.......... *535*
Polycitra-K Oral Solution.......... *535*
◆Testoderm Transdermal Systems.......... **304, 535**
Urispas Tablets.......... *538*

AMARIN PHARMACEUTICALS **538**
25 Independence Blvd.
Warren, NJ 07059

Direct Inquiries to:
For Medical Information Contact:
(888) 952-7462
To Report Adverse Events Contact:
(888) 952-7462

Products Described:
Bontril PDM Tablets.......... *538*
Bontril Slow-Release Capsules.......... **538**
Capital and Codeine Oral Suspension.......... *539*
Exgest LA Tablets.......... *539*
Hydrocet Capsules.......... *539*
Motofen Tablets.......... **539**
Nolamine Timed-Release Tablets.......... *540*
Phrenilin Forte Capsules.......... **540**
Phrenilin Tablets.......... **540**
Salflex Tablets.......... *541*

AMERICAN LECITHIN COMPANY **541**
115 Hurley Rd.
Unit 2 B
Oxford, CT 06478

Direct Inquiries to:
Randall E. Zigmont
(203) 262-7100
FAX: (203) 262-7101

For Medical Information Contact:
Randall E. Zigmont
(203) 262-7100
FAX: (203) 262-7101

Products Described:
PhosChol Concentrate.......... **541**
PhosChol 900 Softgels.......... **541**

Other Products Available:
PhosChol Gold

AMERICAN RED CROSS **541**
National Headquarters
Biomedical Services
1616 Ft. Myer Dr., 17th Floor
Arlington, VA 22209-3100

Direct Inquiries to:
Professional Services Department:
(800) 293-5023
FAX: (703) 312-8742
Customer Service Department:
(800) 446-8883
FAX: (703) 312-8746

Products Described:
Albumarc 5% Solution.......... *541*
Albumarc 25% Solution.......... *541*
Monarc-M.......... *541*
Panglobulin.......... *542*
Polygam S/D.......... *542*

AMGEN INC. **304, 542**
One Amgen Center Drive
Thousand Oaks, CA 91320-1799

Direct Inquiries to:
Customer Service Department
(800) 282-6436
FAX: (800) 292-6436

For Medical Information Contact:
Generally:
Professional Services Department
(800) 772-6436
FAX: (805) 376-8550
In Emergencies:
(800) 772-6436
After Hours and Weekends:
(800) 772-6436

Sales and Ordering:
Customer Service Department
(800) 282-6436
FAX: (800) 292-6436

Products Described:
◆Epogen for Injection.......... **304, 542**
◆Infergen.......... **304, 548**
◆Neupogen for Injection.......... **304, 551**

ANESTA CORP. **304, 556**
4745 Wiley Post Way
Salt Lake City, UT 84116

Direct Inquiries to:
(801) 595-1405
FAX: (801) 595-1406
Internet: www.anesta.com

Products Described:
◆Actiq.......... **304, 556**

APOTHECON **561**
A Bristol-Myers Squibb Company
General Offices
P.O. Box 4500
Princeton, NJ 08543-4500

For Medical Information Contact:
Generally:
Bristol-Myers Squibb Drug Information Department
P.O. Box 4500
Princeton, NJ 08543-4500
(800) 321-1335
Adverse Drug Experiences
and Product Defects Reporting call between 8:30 AM-4:30 PM EST:
(609) 818-3737

Sales and Ordering:
Orders for Apothecon Products may be placed by:

1. Calling toll-free between 8:30 AM - 6:00 PM EST: (800) 631-5244

2. Mailing your purchase orders to:
Apothecon
Attn: Customer Service Department
P.O. Box 5250
Princeton, NJ 08543-5250

3. Faxing your purchase orders to:
Customer Service Department
(800) 523-2965

For listing of standard, purified, and human insulins, see NOVO NORDISK PHARMACEUTICALS, INC.

Products Described:
Acyclovir Capsules.......... *561*
Acyclovir Tablets.......... *561*
Amantadine Hydrochloride Capsules, USP.......... *561*
Atenolol and Chlorthalidone Tablets.......... *561*
Atenolol Tablets.......... *561*
Benztropine Mesylate Tablets, USP.......... *561*
Buspirone HCl Tablets, USP.......... *561*
Captopril and Hydrochlorothiazide Tablets, USP.......... *561*
Captopril Tablets, USP.......... *561*
Cefaclor Capsules, USP.......... *561*
Cefadroxil Capsules, USP.......... *561*
Cephalexin Capsules USP.......... *561*
Clomipramine HCl Capsules.......... *561*
Clonazepam Tablets, USP.......... *561*
Cyclobenzaprine Hydrochloride Tablets, USP.......... *561*
Desyrel Dividose Tablets.......... *561*
Desyrel Tablets.......... *561*
Diclofenac Potassium Tablets.......... *561*
Dicloxacillin Sodium Capsules.......... *561*
Dynapen Capsules.......... *561*
Estradiol Tablets, USP.......... *561*
Etodolac Capsules.......... *561*
Florinef Tablets.......... *561*
Hydroxychloroquine Sulfate Tablets, USP.......... *561*
Indapamide Tablets, USP.......... *561*
Kantrex Capsules.......... *561*
Klotrix Tablets.......... *561*
Methylphenidate Hydrochloride Tablets, USP.......... *561*
Methylprednisolone Tablets, USP.......... *561*
Metoclopramide Tablets, USP.......... *561*
Metoprolol Tartrate Tablets, USP.......... *561*
Mycostatin Oral Tablets.......... *561*
Nadolol Tablets, USP.......... *561*
Naldecon Tablets.......... *561*
Naproxen Sodium Delayed Release Tablets, USP.......... *561*
Naturetin Tablets.......... *561*
Niacin Tablets USP.......... *561*
Orphenadrine Citrate Extended Release Tablets.......... *561*

Orphenadrine Citrate/Aspirin/Caffeine Tablets *561*
Potassium Chloride Extended Release Tablets *561*
Principen Capsules *561*
Prochlorperazine Maleate Tablets, USP *561*
Prolixin Tablets *561*
Pronestyl Capsules *561*
Pronestyl Tablets *561*
Pronestyl-SR Tablets *561*
Rauzide Tablets *561*
Sumycin Capsules *561*
Sumycin Tablets *561*
Theragran Hematinic Tablets *561*
Trazodone Hydrochloride Tablets, USP *561*
Trimox Capsules and Chewable Tablets *561*
Vasodilan Tablets *561*
Veetids Tablets *561*
Velosef '250' Capsules *561*
Velosef '500' Capsules *561*

Other Products Available:
Albuterol Inhalation Aerosol
Amikin Injection
Amoxicillin Oral Suspension
Ampicillin for Injection USP and in ADD-Vantage Vials
Ampicillin Oral Suspension
Cefaclor for Oral Suspension, USP
Cefazolin for Injection USP
Cholestyramine for Oral Suspension Light, USP
Cholestyramine for Oral Suspension, USP
Corzide (See Bristol-Myers Squibb Company)
Cromolyn Sodium Inhalation Solution, USP
Delestrogen (Estradiol Valerate Injection, USP)
Dicloxacillin Sodium Oral Suspension USP
Dynapen (Dicloxacillin Sodium) Oral Suspension
Fungizone for Tissue Culture
Fungizone Intravenous
Hydrocortisone Valerate Cream and Ointment
Kantrex Pediatric Injection
Kenalog Cream, Lotion, and Ointment
Kenalog in Orabase
Kenalog Spray Aerosol
Kenalog-10 and Kenalog-40 Injectable Suspension
K-Lyte Effervescent Tablets
K-Lyte DS Effervescent Tablets
K-Lyte/Cl Tablets
K-Lyte/Cl 50 Effervescent Tablets
Labetalol Hydrochloride Injection
Mucomyst-10 and Mucomyst-20
Mycolog-II Cream and Ointment
Mycostatin Oral Suspension
Nafcillin for Injection USP and in ADD-Vantage Vials
Nitrazine Paper
Nydrazid Injection
Oxacillin for Injection USP and in ADD-Vantage Vials
Oxacillin for Oral Solution
Prolixin Decanoate Injection
Prolixin Elixir
Prolixin Enanthate Injection
Prolixin Injection
Prolixin Oral Concentrate
Questran for Oral Suspension
Questran Light for Oral Suspension
Ranitidine Tablets
Tobramycin Sulfate Injection USP
Trifluoperazine Hydrochloride Tablets, USP
Tubocurarine Chloride Injection USP
Vesprin Injection

ARCO PHARMACEUTICALS, INC. **561**
105 Orville Drive
Bohemia, NY 11716

Direct Inquiries to:
Professional Service Department
(631) 567-9500

Products Described:
Arco-Lase Tablets **561**
Arco-Lase Plus Tablets **561**
Mega-B Tablets **562**
Megadose Tablets **562**

Other Products Available:
Arcoret Tablets
Arcoret w/Iron Tablets
Arcotinic Liquid
Arcotinic Tablets
C-B Time Capsules
C-B Time Liquid
Co-Gel Tablets
Spantuss Liquid

ASTRA MERCK INC.
(See ASTRAZENECA LP)

ASTRA PHARMACEUTICALS, L.P.
(See ASTRAZENECA LP)

ASTRAZENECA LP **304, 562**
Wilmington, DE 19850-5437

For Product and Business Information, and Adverse Drug Experiences:
Information Center
(800) 236-9933

For Product Ordering:
Trade Customer Service
(800) 842-9920
Internet: www.astrazeneca-us.com

Products Described:
Aquasol A Parenteral **562**
Astramorph/PF Injection, USP (Preservative-Free) **563**
◆Atacand Tablets **304, 564**
Calcitonin-Salmon Injection, Synthetic *566*
Duranest Injections **566**
◆EMLA Cream **304, 568**
◆EMLA Anesthetic Disc **304, 568**
Foscavir Injection **571**
◆Lexxel Tablets **304, 575**
M.V.I. Pediatric for Infusion *579*
M.V.I.-12 Multi-Vitamin Infusion *578*
Nalbuphine Hydrochloride Injection *579*
◆Naropin Injection **304, 579**
Nesacaine Injection **583**
Nesacaine-MPF Injection **583**
◆Plendil Extended-Release Tablets **304, 585**
Polocaine Injection, USP *587*
Polocaine-MPF Injection, USP *587*
◆Prilosec Delayed-Release Capsules **305, 587**
◆Pulmicort Turbuhaler Inhalation Powder **305, 591**
◆Rhinocort Aqua Nasal Spray **305, 597**
◆Rhinocort Nasal Inhaler **305, 595**
Sensorcaine Injection **599**
Sensorcaine with Epinephrine Injection **599**
◆Sensorcaine-MPF Injection **305, 599**
Sensorcaine-MPF Spinal Injection *602*
◆Sensorcaine-MPF with Epinephrine Injection **305, 599**
Streptase for Infusion **602**
◆Tonocard Tablets **305, 604**
◆Toprol-XL Tablets **305, 606**
◆Xylocaine Injection **305, 607**
Xylocaine Injection for Ventricular Arrhythmias *610*
◆Xylocaine 2% Jelly *305, 610*
Xylocaine 2.5% Ointment .... ⊙
Xylocaine 5% Ointment *610*
Xylocaine 4% Topical Solution *610*
Xylocaine 2% Viscous Solution *611*
◆Xylocaine with Epinephrine Injection **305, 607**
Xylocaine-MPF 1.5% Solution with Dextrose 7.5% *610*
Xylocaine-MPF 4% Sterile Solution *610*
Xylocaine-MPF 5% with Glucose 7.5% *610*

Other Products Available:
Aquasol E
Citanest Solutions

ASTRAZENECA PHARMACEUTICALS LP **305, 611**
1800 Concord Pike
Wilmington, DE 19850-5437 USA

For Product and Business Information, and Adverse Drug Experiences:
Information Center
(800) 236-9933

For Product Ordering:
Trade Customer Service
(800) 842-9920
Internet: www.astrazeneca-us.com

Products Described:
◆Accolate Tablets **305, 611**
◆Arimidex Tablets **305, 613**
◆Casodex Tablets **305, 615**
◆Cefotan for Injection **305, 617**
Cefotan Injection **617**
◆Diprivan Injectable Emulsion **305, 620**
Elavil Injection **626**
◆Elavil Tablets **305, 626**
◆Hibiclens Antimicrobial Skin Cleanser **305, 628**
◆Hibiclens Packettes *305*
◆Hibiclens Sponge/Brush with Nail Cleaner *305*
Hibistat Germicidal Hand Rinse **629**
◆Hibistat Towelette **305, 629**
◆Merrem I.V. **305, 629**
◆Nolvadex Tablets **306, 633**
◆Seroquel Tablets **306, 639**
◆Sorbitrate Chewable Tablets **306, 643**
◆Sorbitrate Oral Tablets **306, 643**
◆Sular Tablets **306, 645**
◆Tenoretic Tablets **306, 647**
◆Tenormin I.V. Injection **306, 649**
◆Tenormin Tablets **306, 649**
◆Zestoretic Tablets **306, 652**
◆Zestril Tablets **306, 655**
◆Zoladex **306, 659**
Zoladex 3-month **662**
◆Zomig Tablets **306, 665**

ATHENA NEUROSCIENCES **306, 668**
800 Gateway Boulevard
South San Francisco, CA 94080

For Medical Information Contact:
(888) NEURO-05
(888) 638-7605

To Report Adverse Events Contact:
(877) ELAN GSS
(877) 352-6477

Products described below are distributed by Athena Neurosciences, a business unit of Elan Pharmaceuticals, Inc.

Products Described:
Atamet Tablets *668*
◆Permax Tablets **306, 668**
◆Zanaflex Tablets **306, 670**

AVENTIS BEHRING **754**
1020 First Avenue
P.O. Box 61501
King of Prussia, PA 19406-0901

Direct Inquiries to:
(610) 878-4000

For Medical Information Contact:
(800) 504-5434

Sales and Ordering:
Customer Support Center
(800) 683-1288
FAX: (610) 878-4888

Products Described:
Albuminar-5, U.S.P. **754**
Albuminar-25, U.S.P. **755**
Gammar-P I.V. **756**
Helixate Concentrate **758**
Humate-P Concentrate **760**
Monoclate-P Concentrate **762**
Mononine Concentrate **764**
Stimate Nasal Spray **766**

AVENTIS PASTEUR INC. **767**
Swiftwater, PA 18370

For Medical Information Contact:
Generally:
Medical Affairs
(800) VACCINE
(800) 822-2463
Adverse Drug Experiences:
Medical Director
(570) 839-7187
(800) 822-2463

Sales and Ordering:
Aventis Pasteur Inc.
Customer Service
(800) VACCINE
(800) 822-2463
(570) 839-7187

Products Described:
ActHIB **767**
Fluzone **771**
Imogam Rabies - HT **774**
Imovax Rabies Vaccine **776**
IPOL **778**
JE-VAX **781**
Menomune-A/C/Y/W-135 .... **783**
MSTA Mumps Skin Test Antigen **3498**
ProHIBiT *792*
Tetanus and Diphtheria Toxoids Adsorbed For Adult Use **785**
TheraCys **792**
TriHIBit (see ActHIB and Tripedia)
Tripedia **787**
Tubersol **3498**
TYPHIM Vi **794**
YF-VAX **796**

Other Products Available:
Diphtheria & Tetanus Toxoids Adsorbed USP (For Pediatric Use) (DT)
Tetanus Toxoid Adsorbed USP
Tetanus Toxoid USP

AVENTIS PHARMACEUTICALS **306, 673**
399 Interpace Parkway
P.O. Box 663
Parsippany, NJ 07054

Direct Inquiries to:
Customer Service
399 Interpace Parkway
P.O. Box 663
Parsippany, NJ 07054
(800) 207-8049

For Medical Information Contact:
Generally:
Medical Informatics
399 Interpace Parkway
Parsippany, NJ 07054
(800) 633-1610

Products Described:
◆Allegra Capsules **306, 673**
◆Allegra Tablets **306, 673**
◆Allegra-D Extended-Release Tablets **306, 675**
◆Amaryl Tablets **306, 678**
◆Anzemet Injection **306, 680**
◆Anzemet Tablets **306, 683**
◆Arava Tablets **306, 685**
◆Azmacort Inhalation Aerosol **306, 689**
Carafate Suspension **692**
◆Carafate Tablets **306, 691**
◆Cardizem CD Capsules **306, 693**
◆Cardizem Injectable **306, 695**
Cardizem Lyo-Ject Syringe **695**
Cardizem Monovial **695**
◆Claforan **306, 697**
◆Clomid Tablets **306, 700**
◆DDAVP Injection 4 mcg/mL **306, 702**
◆DDAVP Nasal Spray **307, 703**
DDAVP Rhinal Tube *673*
◆DDAVP Tablets **307, 704**
◆DiaBeta Tablets **307, 706**
◆Gliadel Wafer **307, 707**
Lantus Injection **709**
◆Lovenox Injection **307, 713**
◆Nasacort AQ Nasal Spray **307, 719**
◆Nasacort Nasal Inhaler **307, 717**
◆Nilandron Tablets **307, 720**
◆Norpramin Tablets **307, 722**
Oncaspar **724**
Penetrex Tablets **725**
Priftin Tablets **728**
Refludan **731**
◆Rifadin Capsules **307, 734**
Rifadin IV **734**
◆Rifamate Capsules **307, 737**
◆Rifater **307, 738**
◆Rilutek Tablets **307, 742**
Slo-Phyllin 80 Syrup *673*
Slo-Phyllin GG Capsules *673*
Slo-Phyllin GG Syrup *673*
Slo-Phyllin Tablets *673*
◆Synercid I.V. **307, 744**
◆Taxotere for Injection Concentrate **307, 748**
◆Trental Tablets **307, 753**

Other Products Available:
Bentyl Capsules, Tablets, Injection, Syrup
Cantil Tablets
Cardizem SR Capsules
Cardizem Tablets
Cephulac Solution
Chronulac Solution
Hiprex
Lasix Tablets
Novafed A Capsules
Tenuate Tablets/Dospan

AXCAN PHARMA U.S. INC.
(See AXCAN SCANDIPHARM INC.)

AXCAN SCANDIPHARM INC. **307, 798**
22 Inverness Parkway
Birmingham, AL 35242

Direct Inquiries to:
Customer Service
(800) 950-8085
FAX: (205) 991-8426

For Medical Information Contact:
John S. Cipriano, M.S., R.Ph.
(205) 991-8085
FAX: (205) 991-8047

Products Described:
Photofrin for Injection **798**
◆Ultrase Capsules **307, 802**
◆Ultrase MT Capsules **307, 803**
◆Urso Tablets 250 mg **307, 804**
Viokase Powder **805**
◆Viokase Tablets **307, 805**

Other Products Available:
ADEKs Multivitamin Supplement
ADEKs Pediatric Drops
FLUTTER
SCANDICAL
SCANDISHAKE
SCANDISHAKE -- Lactose Free
SCANDISHAKE -- Sweetened with Aspartame

AYERST LABORATORIES INC. **805**
A Wyeth-Ayerst Company
(See listing under WYETH-AYERST PHARMACEUTICALS for prescription products and WHITEHALL-ROBINS LABORATORIES INC. in PDR for Nonprescription Drugs and Dietary Supplements for nonprescription products)

BAXTER HEALTHCARE CORPORATION **805**
Hyland Division
550 North Brand Boulevard
Glendale, CA 91203

Direct Inquiries to:
Product Management
(800) 423-2090

For Medical Emergencies Contact:
Edward Gomperts, M.D.
Medical Director,
Baxter Healthcare Corporation:
(818) 956-3200

Manufacturing and Distribution:
Coagulation Products Distributed By:
Baxter Healthcare Corporation,
Hyland Division
Glendale, CA 91203
(800) 423-2090

Plasma Expanders & Gamma Globulin Products Distributed By:
Baxter Healthcare Corporation,
Hyland Division
Glendale, CA 91203
(800) 423-2090

Products Described:
Albumin (Human) 5% **805**
Albumin (Human) 25% **806**
Bebulin VH Immuno **807**
Buminate 5% Solution, USP **809**
Buminate 25% Solution, USP **810**
Feiba VH Immuno **810**
Gammagard S/D **812**
Hemofil M **814**
Iveegam EN IGIV **816**
Proplex T **818**
Recombinate **820**

BAXTER PHARMACEUTICAL PRODUCTS INC. 821
95 Spring Street
New Providence, NJ 07974

Direct Inquiries to:
Professional Services Department
(800) ANA-DRUG
(800) 262-3784

For Medical Emergencies Contact:
Kent Allenby
VP Clinical Research & Medical Affairs
(800) ANA-DRUG
(800) 262-3784

Sales and Ordering:
To place an order call or fax:
(800) 667-0959
FAX: (877) 702-3580

Products Described:
Alfentanil HCl Injection *821*
Ativan Injection *821*
Atracurium Besylate Injection *821*
Atropine Sulfate Injection, USP *822*
Brevibloc Injection **822**
Bumetanide Injection, USP *824*
Butorphanol Tartrate Injection, USP *824*
CISplatin Injection *824*
Diazepam Injection, USP *825*
Diltiazem Hydrochloride Injection *825*
Dobutamine Hydrochloride Injection *825*
Doxorubicin Hydrochloride for Injection, USP *825*
Duramorph Injection *825*
Enlon Injection *826*
Enlon-Plus Injection *826*
Ethrane Liquid for Inhalation *826*
Etoposide Injection *826*
Fentanyl Citrate Injection, USP *826*
Fluorouracil Injection, USP *826*
Forane Liquid for Inhalation *826*
Furosemide Injection, USP *827*
6% Hetastarch in 0.9% Sodium Chloride Injection *827*
Ketorolac Tromethamine Injection, USP *827*
Labetalol Hydrochloride Injection, USP *828*
Lidocaine HCl Injection, USP *828*
Meperidine Hydrochloride Injection, USP - Dosette *828*
Meperidine Hydrochloride Injection, USP - Tubex *828*
Methotrexate Injection, USP *828*
Metoclopramide Injection, USP *829*
Midazolam HCl Injection *829*
Morphine Sulfate Injection, USP - Dosette *830*
Morphine Sulfate Injection, USP - Tubex *830*
Naloxone HCl Injection, USP *830*
Neostigmine Methylsulfate Injection, USP *830*
Pancuronium Bromide Injection *830*
Phenylephrine Hydrochloride Injection, USP *830*
Propofol Injectable Emulsion 1% **831**
Revex Injection *831*
Robinul Injectable *831*
Sodium Nitroprusside Injection *831*
Sufentanil Citrate Injection, USP *831*
Suprane Liquid for Inhalation **832**
Thiopental Sodium for Injection, USP *835*
Vecuronium Bromide for Injection *835*

BAYER CORPORATION PHARMACEUTICAL DIVISION 307, 342, 836
400 Morgan Lane
West Haven, CT 06516

For Medical Information Contact:
Director, Clinical Services
(800) 288-8371
(203) 812-2000

Adverse Drug Experiences:
(888) 765-3203

Products Described:
◆Adalat Capsules **307, 836**
◆Adalat CC Tablets **307, 837**
◆Avelox Tablets **342, 839**
◆Baycol Tablets **307, 843**
◆Biltricide Tablets **307, 846**
◆Cipro I.V. **307, 852**
◆Cipro I.V. Pharmacy Bulk Package **307, 856**
◆Cipro Oral Suspension **307, 847**
◆Cipro Tablets **307, 847**
DTIC-Dome **860**
Mithracin for Intravenous Use **861**
Mycelex-G 500 mg Vaginal Tablets **863**
◆Nimotop Capsules **308, 863**
Otic Domeboro Solution **865**
◆Precose Tablets **308, 865**
Trasylol Injection **868**

Other Products Available:
Dome-Paste Bandage (Unna's Boot)

BAYER CORPORATION PHARMACEUTICAL DIVISION BIOLOGICAL PRODUCTS 308, 871
400 Morgan Lane
West Haven, CT 06516

For Medical Information Contact:
Director, Clinical Services
(800) 468-0894
(203) 812-2000

Adverse Drug Experiences:
(888) 765-3203

Products Described:
BayGam **871**
BayHep B **872**
BayRab **874**
BayRho-D Full Dose **876**
BayRho-D Mini-Dose **876**
BayTet **878**
◆Gamimune N, 5% Solvent/Detergent Treated **308, 879**
◆Gamimune N, 10% Solvent/Detergent Treated **308, 882**
Koāte-DVI **885**
Koāte-HP **887**
Kogenate **888**
Kogenate FS **890**
Konȳne 80 .... **892**
Plasbumin-5 .... **893**
Plasbumin-20 .... **894**
Plasbumin-25 .... **895**
Plasmanate **896**
Prolastin **897**
Thrombate III **899**

BEACH PHARMACEUTICALS 308, 900
Division of Beach Products, Inc.
5220 S. Manhattan Avenue
Tampa, FL 33611

Direct Inquiries to:
Richard Stephen Jenkins
(813) 839-6565
FAX: (813) 837-2511

Manufacturing and Distribution:
201 Delaware Street
Greenville, SC 29605
(800) 845-8210

Products Described:
◆Beelith Tablets **308, 900**
◆K-Phos M.F. Tablets *308, 900*
◆K-Phos Neutral Tablets **308, 900**
◆K-Phos No. 2 Tablets *308, 900*
◆K-Phos Original (Sodium Free) Tablets **308, 901**
◆Uroqid-Acid No. 2 Tablets **308, 901**

BEDFORD LABORATORIES 902
A Division of Ben Venue Laboratories, Inc.
300 Northfield Road
Bedford, OH 44146

Direct Inquiries to:
Customer Service
(800) 562-4797
FAX: (440) 232-6264

For Medical Emergencies Contact:
Professional Services
(800) 521-5169

Products Described:
Cerubidine for Injection **902**
GlucaGen for Injection Diagnostic Kit **903**

Other Products Available:
Acetazolamide for Injection USP
Acetylcysteine Solution, USP (not for injection)
Acyclovir for Injection USP
Alprostadil Injection, USP
Amikacin Sulfate Injection, USP
Atracurium Besylate Injection
Azathioprine Sodium for Injection, USP
Bumetanide Injection, USP
Butorphanol Tartrate Injection, USP CIV
Caffeine and Sodium Benzoate Injection USP
Chloroprocaine Hydrochloride Injection, USP
Cladribine Injection
Colchicine Injection, USP
Cyclosporine Injection, USP
Cytarabine for Injection USP
Daunorubicin Hydrochloride Injection (Solution)
Desmopressin Acetate Injection
Diltiazem Hydrochloride Injection
Dipyridamole Injection
Dobutamine Injection USP
Doxorubicin Hydrochloride for Injection, USP
Doxorubicin Hydrochloride Injection, USP
Enaliprilat Injection
Ephedrine Sulfate Injection, USP
Ergotrate Maleate
Etomidate Injection
Etoposide Injection
Floxuridine for Injection USP
Fluphenazine Decanoate Injection, USP
Folic Acid Injection, USP
Haloperidol Decanoate Injection
Inamrinone Injection, USP
Ketamine Hydrochloride Injection, USP CIII
Ketorolac Tromethamine Injection USP
Labetalol Hydrochloride Injection USP
Leucovorin Calcium for Injection
Levothyroxine Sodium for Injection
Methotrexate Injection USP
Midazolam Hydrochloride Injection
Mitomycin for Injection, USP
Papaverine Hydrochloride Injection, USP
Phentolamine Mesylate for Injection, USP
Polymyxin B for Injection
Propranolol Hydrochloride Injection USP
Rifampin for Injection, USP
Vecuronium Bromide for Injection
Vinblastine Sulfate for Injection, USP

BERLEX LABORATORIES 308, 905
300 Fairfield Road
Wayne, NJ 07470

Direct Inquiries to:
(973) 694-4100

For Medical Information and to Report Drug Adverse Events Contact:
Department of Epidemiology and Medical Affairs
300 Fairfield Road
Wayne, NJ 07470
(888) BERLEX-4

Products Described:
◆Betapace Tablets **308, 905**
◆Betapace AF Tablets **308, 908**
◆Climara Transdermal System **308, 912**
Levlen 21 Tablets **916**
◆Levlen 28 Tablets **308, 916**
Levlite 21 Tablets **916**
◆Levlite 28 Tablets **308, 916**
◆Quinaglute Dura-Tabs Tablets **308, 924**
Tri-Levlen 21 Tablets **916**
◆Tri-Levlen 28 Tablets **308, 916**

BERLEX LABORATORIES 308, 927
15049 San Pablo Avenue
P.O. Box 4099
Richmond, CA 94804-0099

Direct Inquiries to:
(888) BERLEX-4

Products Described:
◆Betaseron for SC Injection **308, 927**
◆Fludara for Injection **308, 931**

BERNA PRODUCTS, CORP. 308, 933
4216 Ponce de Leon Boulevard
Coral Gables, FL 33146

Direct Inquiries to:
Myrtha Entrialgo
(305) 443-2900, Ext. 221
(800) 533-5899

For Medical Information Contact:
Generally:
Andres Murai, Jr.
(305) 443-2900
(800) 533-5899
In Emergencies:
Andres Murai, Jr.
(305) 443-2900
(800) 533-5899

Products Described:
◆Vivotif Berna **308, 933**

BERTEK PHARMACEUTICALS INC. 308, 935
781 Chestnut Road
Morgantown, WV 26505

For Medical Information Contact:
Clinical Affairs Department
3711 Collins Ferry Road
Morgantown, WV 26504
(888) 823-7835
FAX: (304) 285-6453

Products Described:
◆Acticin Cream **308, 935**
◆Avita Cream **308, 935**
◆Avita Gel **308, 937**
◆Clorpres Tablets **308, 938**
Digitek Tablets **940**
Granulex Aerosol **943**
Kristalose for Oral Solution **943**
◆Maxzide Tablets **308, 943**
◆Maxzide-25 mg Tablets **308, 943**
◆Mentax Cream **308, 945**
Sulfamylon Cream **947**
Sulfamylon Topical Solution **947**
◆Zagam Tablets **308, 948**

Other Products Available:
Biobrane Temporary Burn Dressing
Flexderm Hydrogel Wound Dressing
Flexzan Wound Dressing
Hydrocol Hydrocolloid Wound Dressing
Sorbsan Wound Dressing

BEUTLICH LP PHARMACEUTICALS 952
1541 Shields Drive
Waukegan, IL 60085-8304

Direct Inquiries to:
(847) 473-1100
(800) 238-8542 (in U.S. and Canada)
FAX: (847) 473-1122
E-mail: fjb1541@worldnet.att.net
Internet: http://www.beutlich.com

Products Described:
Ceo-Two Evacuant Suppository *952*
Hurricaine Topical Anesthetic Aerosol Spray, 2 oz. Wild Cherry *952*
Hurricaine Topical Anesthetic Gel: 1 oz. Wild Cherry, Fresh Mint, Pina Colada, Watermelon, 1/6 oz. Wild Cherry, Watermelon *952*
Hurricaine Topical Anesthetic Liquid: 1 oz. Wild Cherry and Pina Colada .25 ml Dry Handle Swab Wild Cherry, 1/6 oz. Wild Cherry *952*
Hurricaine Topical Anesthetic Spray Extension Tubes (200) *952*
Hurricaine Topical Anesthetic Spray Kit *952*
Peridin-C Tablets *952*

BIOGEN, INC. 952
14 Cambridge Center
Cambridge, MA 02142

Direct Inquiries to:
Customer Service
(800) 456-2255
FAX: (617) 679-3100

For Medical Emergencies Contact:
Customer Service
(800) 456-2255
FAX: (617) 679-3100

Products Described:
Avonex **952**

BIOGLAN PHARMA, INC. 956
7 Great Valley Parkway
Suite 301
Malvern, PA 19355

Direct Inquiries to:
(610) 232-2000
FAX: (610) 232-2020

Products Described:
Micanol 1% Cream *956*
Theramycin Z Topical Solution *956*
Zonalon Cream *956*

BIO-TECHNOLOGY GENERAL CORP. 310, 1075
BTG Pharmaceuticals
70 Wood Avenue South
Iselin, N.J. 08830

Direct Inquiries to:
(732) 632-8800

For Medical Information or Emergencies Contact:
(800) 741-2698

For Customer Service and Ordering:
(800) 741-2698
FAX: (800) 741-2696

Products Described:
◆Delatestryl Injection **310, 1075**
◆Oxandrin Tablets **310, 1076**

BLAINE PHARMACEUTICALS 956
1515 Production Drive
Burlington, KY 41005

For Inquiries or Medical Information Contact:
(859) 283-9437
(800) 633-9353
FAX: (859) 283-9460
E-mail: blainepharma.com

Products Described:
Mag-Ox 400 Tablets **956**
Uro-Mag Capsules **956**

BLANSETT PHARMACAL CO., INC. 956
P.O. Box 638
North Little Rock, AR 72115

Direct Inquiries to:
Customer Service
(501) 758-8635
FAX: (501) 758-5369

Products Described:
Anolor 300 Capsules *956*
Cortane-B Aqueous Ear Drops *956*
Cortane-B Otic Drops *956*
Nalex-A Liquid *956*
Nalex-A Tablets *956*

Other Products Available:
Cortane-B Otic Lotion
Nalex Expectorant
Prolex DH Liquid
Prolex DM Liquid
Prolex-D Tablets
Relagard

BLOCK DRUG COMPANY, INC. 957
257 Cornelison Avenue
Jersey City, NJ 07302

Direct Inquiries to:
Consumer Affairs
(201) 434-3000, Ext. 1308
FAX: (201) 432-6183

For Medical Information Contact:
Consumer Affairs
(800) 365-6500, Ext. 1308
FAX: (201) 432-6183

Products Described:
Aphthasol Oral Paste 957

BOEHRINGER INGELHEIM PHARMACEUTICALS, INC. 308, 957
A subsidiary of Boehringer Ingelheim Corporation
900 Ridgebury Road
P.O. Box 368
Ridgefield, CT 06877-0368
(203) 798-9988

For Medical Information Contact:
(800) 542-6257
E-mail:
druginfo@rdg.boehringer-ingelheim.com

Products Described:
◆Aggrenox Capsules 308, 957
◆Alupent Inhalation Aerosol 308, 960
◆Alupent Inhalation Solution 308, 960
Alupent Syrup 960
Alupent Tablets 960
◆Atrovent Inhalation Aerosol 308, 962
◆Atrovent Inhalation Solution 308, 963
◆Atrovent Nasal Spray 0.03% 308, 964
◆Atrovent Nasal Spray 0.06% 308, 966
◆Catapres Tablets 309, 967
◆Catapres-TTS 309, 968
◆Combipres Tablets 309, 970
◆Combivent Inhalation Aerosol 309, 972
◆Flomax Capsules 309, 974
◆Mexitil Capsules 309, 977
◆Micardis Tablets 309, 979
◆Mobic Tablets 309, 981
◆Persantine Tablets 309, 984
Serentil Ampuls 984
Serentil Concentrate 984
◆Serentil Tablets 309, 984

BOEHRINGER MANNHEIM THERAPEUTICS
(See ROCHE LABORATORIES INC.)

BONE CARE INTERNATIONAL 986
One Science Court
Madison, WI 53711

Direct Inquiries to:
Professional Services Department
(888) 389-4242 Ext. 554
FAX: (608) 236-0313

Products Described:
Hectorol Capsules 986
Hectorol Injection 988

BRAINTREE LABORATORIES, INC. 309, 990
P.O. Box 850929
Braintree, MA 02185-0929

Direct Inquiries to:
Harry P. Keegan, President
(781) 843-2202

For Medical Information or Emergencies Contact:
Jack DiPalma, M.D.
(800) 874-6756

Products Described:
◆GoLYTELY and Pineapple Flavor GoLYTELY for Oral Solution 309, 990
◆MiraLax Powder for Oral Solution 309, 991
◆NuLYTELY, Cherry Flavor, Lemon-Lime Flavor, and Orange Flavor NuLYTELY for Oral Solution 309, 990
◆PhosLo Tablets 309, 991

BRISTOL-MYERS PRODUCTS 309, 992
A Bristol-Myers Squibb Company
345 Park Avenue
New York, NY 10154

Direct Inquiries to:
Products Division
Consumer Affairs Department
1350 Liberty Avenue
Hillside, NJ 07207
(800) 468-7746

Products Described:
◆Excedrin Migraine Caplets 309, 992
◆Excedrin Migraine Geltabs 309, 992
◆Excedrin Migraine Tablets 309, 992

Other Products Available:
Alpha Keri Moisture Rich Cleansing Bar
Alpha Keri Moisture Rich Shower and Bath Oil
Bufferin Tablets
Arthritis Strength Bufferin Caplets
Extra Strength Bufferin Tablets
Comtrex Acute Head Cold & Sinus Relief
Comtrex Allergy-Sinus Treatment, Maximum Strength
Comtrex Deep Chest Cold & Congestion Relief Non-Drowsy
Comtrex Maximum Strength Multi-Symptom Cold & Flu Relief
Comtrex Maximum Strength Multi-Symptom Day/Night
Comtrex Maximum Strength Multi-Symptom Non-Drowsy
Aspirin Free Excedrin Caplets
Aspirin Free Excedrin Geltabs
Excedrin P.M. Caplets
Excedrin P.M. Geltabs
Excedrin P.M. Tablets
Fostex 10% Benzoyl Peroxide Bar
Fostex 10% Benzoyl Peroxide (Vanish) Gel
Fostex 10% Benzoyl Peroxide Wash
Fostex Medicated Cleansing Bar
Fostex Medicated Cleansing Cream
4-Way Fast Acting Nasal Spray - Regular & Mentholated Formulas
4-Way Long Lasting Nasal Spray
4-Way Nasal Moisturizing Saline Mist
Keri Anti-bacterial Hand Lotion
Keri Lotion Fast Absorbing
Keri Lotion - Original Formula, Sensitive Skin Fragrance - Free, and Silky Smooth
Keri Skin Renewal
No Doz Maximum Strength Caplets
Nuprin Tablets and Caplets
Nuprin Backache
Pazo Hemorrhoid Ointment
Tempra 1 Infant Drops
Theragran Heart Right
Theragran-M, High Potency Multivitamins
Therapeutic Mineral Ice
Vagistat-1

BRISTOL-MYERS SQUIBB COMPANY 309, 993
P.O. Box 4500
Princeton, NJ 08543-4500
(609) 897-2000

For Medical Information Contact:
Generally:
Bristol-Myers Squibb Drug Information Department
P.O. Box 4500
Princeton, NJ 08543-4500
(800) 321-1335
Adverse Drug Experiences
and Product Defects Reporting call between 8:30 AM-4:30 PM EST:
(609) 818-3737

Sales and Ordering:
Orders may be placed by:

1. Calling your purchase orders toll-free between 8:30 AM-5:00 PM EST: (800) 631-5244
2. Mailing your purchase orders to: Bristol-Myers Squibb U.S. Pharmaceuticals Attn: Customer Service P.O. Box 5250 Princeton, NJ 08543-5250
3. Faxing your purchase orders to: (800) 523-2965
4. Transmitting computer-to-computer on the NWDA and UCS formats through Ordernet Services use: DEA # PE0048579

Products Described:
◆Avalide Tablets 309, 993
◆Avapro Tablets 309, 996
Cefzil for Oral Suspension 998
◆Cefzil Tablets 309, 998
Corzide 40/5 Tablets 1001
Corzide 80/5 Tablets 1001
◆Duricef Capsules 309, 1003
Duricef Oral Suspension 1003
◆Duricef Tablets 309, 1003
◆Glucophage Tablets 309, 1005
Glucovance Tablets 3477
◆Monopril Tablets 309, 1009
◆Plavix Tablets 309, 1012
◆Pravachol Tablets 309, 1014
◆Serzone Tablets 309, 1018
◆Stadol NS Nasal Spray 309, 1023
◆Tequin Injection 309, 1025
◆Tequin Tablets 309, 1025

BRISTOL-MYERS SQUIBB DERMATOLOGY 1031
A Bristol-Myers Squibb Company
P.O. Box 4500
Princeton, NJ 08543-4500

For Medical Information Contact:
Generally:
Bristol-Myers Squibb Drug Information Department
P.O. Box 4500
Princeton, NJ 08543-4500
(800) 321-1335
Adverse Drug Experiences
and Product Defects Reporting call between 8:30 AM-4:30 PM EST:
(609) 818-3737

Sales and Ordering:
Orders may be placed by:

1. Calling your purchase orders toll-free between 8:30 AM-5:00 PM EST: (800) 631-5244
2. Mailing your purchase orders to: Bristol-Myers Squibb U.S. Pharmaceuticals Attn: Customer Service P.O. Box 5250 Princeton, NJ 08543-5250
3. Faxing your purchase orders to: (800) 523-2965
4. Transmitting computer-to-computer on the NWDA and UCS formats through Ordernet Services use DEA: # PE0048579

Products Described:
Vaniqa Cream 1031

Other Products Available:
For information on the following products, see listing under WESTWOOD-SQUIBB PHARMACEUTICALS, INC.:

Dovonex Cream
Dovonex Ointment
Dovonex Scalp Solution
Lac-Hydrin Cream
Lac-Hydrin Lotion
Ultravate Cream
Ultravate Ointment

BRISTOL-MYERS SQUIBB ONCOLOGY/ IMMUNOLOGY DIVISION 310, 1033
A Bristol-Myers Squibb Company
P.O. Box 4500
Princeton, NJ 08543-4500
(609) 897-2000

For Medical Information Contact:
Generally:
Bristol-Myers Squibb Drug Information Department
P.O. Box 4500
Princeton, NJ 08543-4500
(800) 426-7644
Adverse Drug Experiences
and Product Defects Reporting call between 8:30 AM-4:30 PM EST:
(609) 818-3737

Sales and Ordering:
Orders may be placed by:

1. Calling the following toll-free number between 8:30 AM-5:00 PM EST: (800) 631-5244
2. Mail orders and all inquiries should be sent to: Bristol-Myers Squibb Oncology Division Attn: Customer Service P.O. Box 5250 Princeton, NJ 08543-5250
3. Faxing your purchase orders to: (800) 523-2965
4. Transmitting computer-to-computer on the NWDA and UCS formats through Ordernet Services use: DEA # PE0048579

Products Described:
BiCNU 1033
◆Blenoxane 310, 1034
CeeNU Capsules 1036
◆Cytoxan for Injection 310, 1037
◆Cytoxan Tablets 310, 1037
◆Droxia Capsules 310, 1039
◆Etopophos for Injection 310, 1041
Hydrea Capsules 1043
◆Ifex for Injection 310, 1044
Lysodren Tablets 1046
◆Megace Oral Suspension 310, 1047
◆Megace Tablets 310, 1048
◆Mesnex Injection 310, 1049
◆Mutamycin for Injection 310, 1050
Mycostatin Pastilles 1051
◆Paraplatin for Injection 310, 1052
◆Platinol-AQ Injection 310, 1055
Rubex for Injection 1057
◆Taxol Injection 310, 1059
Teslac Tablets 1067
◆VePesid Capsules 310, 1068
◆VePesid for Injection 310, 1068
Videx Powder for Oral Solution 3482
Videx Pediatric Powder for Oral Solution 3482
◆Videx Chewable Tablets 310, 3482
Vumon for Injection 1070
◆Zerit Capsules 310, 1072
◆Zerit for Oral Solution 310, 1072

J. R. CARLSON LABORATORIES, INC. 1077
15 College Drive
Arlington Heights, IL 60004-1985

Direct Inquiries to:
Customer Service
(847) 255-1600
FAX: (847) 255-1605

For Medical Emergencies Contact:
Customer Service
(847) 255-1600
FAX: (847) 255-1605

Products Described:
ACES Antioxidant Soft Gels *1077*
E-Gems Soft Gels *1077*

CARNRICK LABORATORIES 310, 1077
A Business Unit of Elan Pharmaceuticals
45 Horse Hill Road
Cedar Knolls, NJ 07927

Direct Inquiries to:
For Customer Service Contact:
(877) CARNRICK
(877) 227-6742
For Medical Information Contact:
(888) NEURO-05
(888) 638-7605
To Report Adverse Events Contact:
(877) ELAN GSS
(877) 352-6477

Products Described:
◆Midrin Capsules 310, 1077
◆Naprelan Tablets 310, 1078
◆Skelaxin Tablets 310, 1080

CELGENE CORPORATION 310, 1081
7 Powder Horn Drive
Warren, NJ 07059
(732) 271-1001
(800) 890-4619

Direct Inquiries to:
Customer Service:
(888) 4-CELGENE
(888) 423-5436
Medical Services:
(732) 805-3905
FAX: (732) 805-3671
Drug Safety:
(732) 805-3667
FAX: (732) 271-4115

Products Described:
◆Thalomid Capsules 310, 1081

CENTEON L.L.C.
(See AVENTIS BEHRING)

CENTOCOR, INC. 310, 1085
200 Great Valley Parkway
Malvern, PA 19355

Direct General Inquiries to:
(610) 651-6000
(888) 874-3083
FAX: (610) 651-6100

For Medical Emergencies Contact:
(800) 457-6399

For Medical Information/Adverse Experience Reporting Contact:
Medical Information and Product Surveillance
(800) 457-6399
FAX: (610) 651-6197

Branch Office:
Centocor B.V.
Einsteinweg 101
2333 CB Leiden, The Netherlands

Products Described:
◆Remicade for IV Injection 310, 1085
◆Retavase Vials 310, 1088

Other Products Available:
Fragmin Injection
ReoPro Vials

CEPHALON, INC. 310, 1090
145 Brandywine Parkway
West Chester, PA 19380

For Medical Information Contact:
(800) 896-5855

Adverse Drug Experiences:
(800) 896-5855

Customer Service:
(888) 535-2374

Products Described:
◆Provigil Tablets 310, 1090

CETYLITE INDUSTRIES, INC. 310, 1093
9051 River Road
Pennsauken, NJ 08110-3293
Mailing Address:
P.O. Box 90006
Pennsauken, NJ 08110-0700

Direct Inquiries to:
Mr. Stanley L. Wachman, President
(856) 665-6111
(800) 257-7740
FAX: (856) 665-5408

Products Described:
◆Cetacaine Topical Anesthetic 310, 1093

Other Products Available:
Cetylcide G Sterilant
Cetylcide II Germicidal Concentrate
Cetylite Airfresh Deodorizer

Cetylite Skin Screen Protective Skin Lotion
Protexin Oral Breath Spray
Release Antiadhesive
Ultrasonic Cleaner
Varnal Cavity Varnish
Zarosen Desensitizer

CHIRON CORPORATION **311, 1094**
4560 Horton Street
Emeryville, CA 94608-2916

For Medical Information Contact:
Generally:
Professional Services (7:00 AM to 5:00 PM PST):
(800) CHIRON-8 selection #2
(800) 244-7668 selection #2
FAX: (510) 923-3435
E-mail: drug_info@cc.chiron.com
In Emergencies:
(7:00 AM to 5:00 PM PST):
(800) CHIRON-8 selection #3
(800) 244-7668 selection #3
After Hours & Weekend Emergencies:
(415) 487-8335

Sales and Ordering:
(800) CHIRON-8 selection #1
(800) 244-7668 selection #1
FAX: (510) 923-3434

Products Described:
DepoCyt Injection.................. **1094**
Proleukin for Injection.............. **1096**
◆Rabies Vaccine RabAvert....... **311, 1100**

CIBAGENEVA PHARMACEUTICALS
(See NOVARTIS PHARMACEUTICALS CORPORATION for branded products)
(See GENEVA PHARMACEUTICALS, INC. for branded generic products)

COLGATE ORAL PHARMACEUTICALS, INC. **1103**
A subsidiary of Colgate-Palmolive Company
One Colgate Way
Canton, MA 02021 USA

Direct Inquiries to:
Professional Services Department
(800) 226-5428

For Medical Emergencies Contact:
Pittsburgh Poison Control
(412) 692-5596

Products Described:
Luride Drops 50 ml.................. *1103*
Luride Lozi-Tabs Tablets............ *1103*
Periogard Oral Rinse................ *1103*
PreviDent 5000 Plus Dental Cream... *1103*

COLLAGENEX PHARMACEUTICALS, INC. **1103**
41 University Drive, Ste. 200
Newtown, PA 18940

Direct Inquiries to:
(888) 339-5678

Products Described:
Periostat Capsules.................. **1103**

CONNETICS CORPORATION **311, 1104**
3400 West Bayshore Road
Palo Alto, CA 94303

Direct Inquiries to:
(650) 843-2800
FAX: (650) 843-2899
Internet: www.connetics.com

For Medical Information Contact:
Medical Information Department
(650) 843-2800
FAX: (650) 843-2898
E-mail: medicalaffairs@connetics.com

Products Described:
◆Luxíq Foam..................... **311, 1104**

COOKE PHARMA **311, 1106**
1404 Old County Road
Belmont, CA 94002

Direct Inquiries to:
Customer Service Dept.
(888) 808-6838

Products Described:
◆HeartBar...................... **311, 1106**

COR THERAPEUTICS, INC. **311, 1106**
256 East Grand Avenue
South San Francisco, CA 94080

Direct Inquiries to:
(888) 267-4-MED

Products Described:
◆Integrilin Injection............. **311, 1106**

CYPROS PHARMACEUTICAL CORPORATION
(See QUESTCOR PHARMACEUTICALS, INC.)

DAIICHI PHARMACEUTICAL CORPORATION **311, 1110**
11 Philips Parkway
Montvale, NJ 07645

Direct Inquiries to:
Medical Services Department
(877) 324-4244 (877-DAIICHI)
FAX: (888) 727-5666

For Medical Emergencies and Product Information Contact:
Medical Services Department
(888) 727-2500
FAX: (888) 272-7979

Products Described:
◆Evoxac Capsules............... **311, 1110**
◆Floxin Otic Solution............ **311, 1112**

DERMIK LABORATORIES, INC. **1113**
1050 Westlakes Drive
Berwyn, PA 19312

Direct Inquiries to:
Customer Service
399 Interpace Parkway
P.O. Box 663
Parsippany, NJ 07054
(800) 207-8049

For Medical Information Contact:
Generally:
Medical Informatics
399 Interpace Parkway
Parsippany, NJ 07054
(800) 633-1610

Products Described:
5 Benzagel Acne Gel................ *1114*
10 Benzagel Acne Gel............... *1114*
Benzamycin Topical Gel............. **1114**
Drithocreme 0.1%, 0.25%, 0.5%, 1.0% (HP) Cream............... *1114*
Dritho-Scalp 0.25%, 0.5% Cream..... *1114*
Hytone Cream 2½%.................. *1115*
Hytone Lotion 2½%................. *1115*
Hytone Ointment 2½%............... *1115*
Klaron Lotion 10%.................. **1115**
Noritate Cream..................... **1115**
Penlac Topical Solution............ **1116**
Psorcon Cream 0.05%............... *1118*
Psorcon E Cream.................... **1118**
Psorcon E Ointment................. **1119**
Psorcon Ointment 0.05%............ *1118*
Sulfacet-R Lotion.................. **1119**
Sulfacet-R Tint Free Lotion........ *1120*
Vanoxide-HC Acne Lotion........... *1120*
Vytone Cream 1%................... *1120*
Zetar Emulsion..................... *1120*

Other Products Available:
Anthra-Derm Ointment 1%, 1/2%, 1/4%, 1/10%
Shepard's Cream Lotion
Shepard's Skin Cream
Vanoxide Acne Lotion
Zetar Shampoo

DEY **311, 1120**
2751 Napa Valley Corporate Drive
Napa, CA 94558
(800) 755-5560
Internet: www.deyinc.com

Direct Inquiries to:
Alan Witten
(800) 755-5560
FAX: (707) 224-8918

For Medical Emergencies Contact:
Mary Lou Freathy
(707) 224-3200
FAX: (707) 224-1415

Products Described:
Acetylcysteine Solution USP, Mucosil.......................... *1120*
◆Albuterol Inhalation Aerosol.... *311, 1120*
◆Albuterol Sulfate Inhalation Solutions....................... *311, 1120*
◆Cromolyn Sodium Inhalation Solution USP.................. *311, 1120*
◆Curosurf Intratracheal Suspension..................... **311, 1120**
◆EasiVent Valved Holding Chamber....................... *311, 1122*
◆EpiPen Auto-Injector............ **311, 1122**
◆EpiPen Jr. Auto-Injector......... **311, 1122**
◆EpiPen Trainer....................... *311*
◆Ipratropium Bromide Inhalation Solution............. *311, 1120*
Metaproterenol Sulfate Inhalation Solution USP..................... *1120*
Sodium Chloride Inhalation Solutions USP.................... *1120*

DISTA PRODUCTS COMPANY **311, 1123**
Division of Eli Lilly and Company

For Medical Information Contact:
Customer Services
Lilly Corporate Center
Indianapolis, IN 46285
(800) 545-5979

Direct Inquiries to:
Lilly Corporate Center
Indianapolis, IN 46285
(317) 276-2000

AREA SALES OFFICES:
Atlanta, GA 30328
North Park Town Center
Building 500, Suite 1200
1100 Abernathy Road, NE
(770) 551-5360
Bala Cynwyd, PA 19004
401 City Avenue
Suite 400
(610) 617-1157
Birmingham, AL 35243
3800 Colonnade Parkway
Suite 250
(205) 969-4556
Anaheim, CA 92806
2400 East Katella Avenue
Suite 530
(714) 940-0800
Chicago, IL 60631
Suite 810, O'Hare Plaza
8725 West Higgins Road
(773) 693-8740
Addison, TX 75001
15305 Dallas Parkway
Suite 840
(972) 960-9372
Indianapolis, IN 46268
Suite 200, Parkwood Five
510 E. 96th 46240
(317) 277-6583
Stamford, CT 06902
300 First Stamford Place
(203) 357-1422

Products Described:
Ilotycin Ophthalmic Ointment........ **1123**
Keflex Oral Suspension............. **1124**
Keflex Pulvules.................... **1124**
Nalfon Capsules.................... **1125**
◆Prozac Pulvules & Liquid, Oral Solution................. **311, 1127**

DJ PHARMA INC. **342, 1132**
12730 High Bluff Blvd.
Suite 160
San Diego, CA 92130

Direct Inquiries to:
(877) DJ Pharm
(877) 357-4276

Products Described:
Cedax Capsules..................... **1132**
Cedax Oral Suspension.............. **1132**
D.A. Chewable Tablets.............. *1135*
D.A. II Tablets.................... *1135*
Dura-Vent Tablets.................. *1135*
Dura-Vent/DA Tablets............... *1135*
Fenesin Tablets.................... *1135*
Fenesin DM Tablets................. *1136*
Guai-Vent/PSE Tablets.............. *1136*
◆Keftab Tablets................. **342, 1136**
Rondec Oral Drops.................. *1137*
Rondec Syrup....................... *1137*
Rondec Tablet...................... *1137*
Rondec-DM Oral Drops............... *1137*
Rondec-DM Syrup.................... *1137*
Rondec-TR Tablet................... *1137*

DOW HICKAM PHARMACEUTICALS
(See BERTEK PHARMACEUTICALS INC.)

DUPONT PHARMACEUTICALS COMPANY **311, 1137**
Chestnut Run Plaza
Hickory Run
P.O. Box 80723
Wilmington, DE 19880-0723
(302) 992-5000

Direct All Product-Related Inquiries to:
Medical Affairs Department

For Product Information/Adverse Drug Experience Reporting Contact:
Product Information
(302) 992-4240 or (800) 474-2762

Products Described:
Coumadin for Injection.............. **1137**
◆Coumadin Tablets.............. **311, 1137**
Innohep Injection.................. **1141**
Lodosyn Tablets.................... **1145**
◆ReVia Tablets.................. **311, 1146**
◆Sinemet Tablets................ **311, 1149**
◆Sinemet CR Tablets............. **311, 1151**
◆Sustiva Capsules............... **311, 1154**

DURA PHARMACEUTICALS **311, 1159**
7475 Lusk Boulevard
San Diego, CA 92121

For Medical Information and Adverse Drug Experiences Contact:
Medical Affairs Department
(888) 859-8583
FAX: (858) 657-0977

For Sales Representatives Requests Contact:
(800) 859-8586

Products Described:
◆Azactam for Injection........... **311, 1159**
◆Ceclor CD Tablets.............. **311, 1163**
Entex Capsules..................... *1165*
Entex LA Tablets................... **1165**
Entex Liquid....................... *1165*
Entex PSE Tablets.................. **1166**
◆Maxipime for Injection.......... **311, 1167**
Myambutol Tablets.................. **1166**
◆Nasalide Nasal Spray........... **311, 1172**
◆Nasarel Nasal Solution 0.025%......................... **311, 1173**

DURAMED PHARMACEUTICALS, INC. **1174**
5040 Duramed Dr.
Cincinnati, OH 45213

Direct Inquiries to:
Customer Service
(513) 731-9900
(800) 543-3763
FAX: (513) 247-9621

For Medical Emergencies Contact:
Duramed Medical Response Line
(800) 859-3347

Products Described:
Cenestin Tablets................... **1174**

Other Products Available:
APAP & Codeine Tablets, #2, #3 and #4
Duradrin Capsules
Estradiol Tablets
Methylprednisolone Tablets
Oxycodone & APAP Capsules
Triamterene/HCTZ Capsules
Verapamil HCl Extended Release Tablets

ECR PHARMACEUTICALS **1177**
Distributor of ECR Pharmaceuticals & Wm. P. Poythress Products
3969 Deep Rock Road
P.O. Box 71600
Richmond, VA 23255

Direct Inquiries to:
Professional Services Department
(804) 527-1950
FAX: (804) 527-1959

For Medical Emergencies Contact:
Professional Services Department
(804) 527-1950
FAX: (804) 527-1959

Products Described:
Anaplex DM Cough Syrup............. *1177*
Anaplex HD Cough Syrup............. *1177*
Bensulfoid Cream................... *1177*
Bupap Tablets...................... *1177*
DEXPAK Taperpak Tablets............ *1177*
Lodrane Allergy Capsules........... *1177*
Lodrane LD Capsules................ *1177*
Lodrane Liquid..................... *1177*
Nasatab LA Tablets................. *1177*
Panalgesic Gold Cream.............. *1177*
Panalgesic Gold Topical Liquid..... *1177*
Pneumotussin 2.5 Cough Syrup....... *1177*
Pneumotussin Tablets............... *1177*

EDWARDS LIFESCIENCES RESEARCH MEDICAL, INC. **3487**
One Edwards Way
Irvine, CA 92614

Direct Inquiries to:
Customer Service
(800) 453-8432
FAX: (801) 565-6209
Internet: www.edwards.com

Products Described:
Rimso-50 Solution.................. **3487**

EISAI INC. **311, 1178**
500 Frank W. Burr Boulevard
Teaneck, NJ 07666

Direct Inquiries to:
Eisai Medical Services
(888) 422-4743
888-4ACIPHEX
FAX: (201) 287-9744

For Medical Emergencies Contact:
(888) 422-4743 (888-4ACIPHEX)
(24 hours/day, 7 days/week)

Products Described:
◆Aciphex Tablets................ **311, 1178**
◆Aricept Tablets................ **312, 1181**

ELAN PHARMA **312, 1184**
800 Gateway Boulevard
South San Francisco, CA 94080

For Medical Information Contact:
(888) NEURO-05
(888) 638-7605

To Report Adverse Events Contact:
(877) ELAN GSS
(877) 352-6477

Products described below are distributed by Elan Pharma, a business unit of Elan Pharmaceuticals, Inc.

Products Described:
◆Diastat Rectal Delivery System ... **312, 1184**
Mysoline Suspension ... **1188**
◆Mysoline Tablets ... **312, 1188**
◆Zonegran Capsules ... **312, 1189**

ELKINS-SINN, INC. 1193
2 Esterbrook Lane
Cherry Hill, NJ 08003-4099

Direct General Inquiries to:
(610) 688-4400

For Emergency Medical Information Contact:
Day: (800) 934-5556 (8:30 AM to 4:30 PM, Eastern Standard Time, Weekdays only)
Night: (610) 688-4400 (Emergencies only; non-emergencies should wait until the next day)

For Medical/Pharmacy Inquiries on Marketed Products Contact:
(800) 934-5556 (8:30 AM to 4:30 PM, Eastern Standard Time, Weekdays only)

Products Described:
Amikacin Sulfate Injection, USP ... **1193**
Atropine Sulfate Injection ... *1193*
Chlorpromazine Hydrochloride Injection ... *1193*
Cyanocobalamin (Vit. B_{12}) Injection ... *1193*
Dexamethasone Sodium Phosphate Injection ... *1193*
Diazepam Injection ... *1193*
Digoxin Injection ... *1193*
Diphenhydramine Hydrochloride Injection ... *1193*
Dipyridamole Injection ... *1193*
Duramorph Injection ... **1195**
Epinephrine Injection ... *1193*
Fentanyl Citrate Injection (Preservative-Free) ... *1193*
Gentamicin Sulfate Injection ... *1193*
Heparin Sodium Injection ... *1193*
Hep-Lock (Heparin Lock Flush Solution) ... *1193*
Hep-Lock (Preservative-Free Heparin Lock Flush Solution) ... *1193*
Hydromorphone Hydrochloride Injection ... *1193*
Hydroxyzine Hydrochloride Injection ... *1193*
Infumorph 200 and Infumorph 500 Sterile Solutions ... **1197**
Isoproterenol Hydrochloride Injection ... *1193*
Leucovorin Calcium for Injection ... *1193*
Lidocaine Hydrochloride Injection ... *1193*
Lidocaine Hydrochloride Injection (Preservative-Free) ... *1193*
Lidocaine Hydrochloride & Epinephrine Injection ... *1193*
Lorazepam Injection ... *1193*
Meperidine Hydrochloride Injection ... *1193*
Morphine Sulfate Injection ... *1193*
Naloxone Hydrochloride Injection ... *1193*
Neostigmine Methylsulfate Injection ... *1193*
Pancuronium Bromide Injection ... *1193*
Phenobarbital Sodium Injection ... *1193*
Phenylephrine Hydrochloride Injection ... *1193*
Phenytoin Sodium Injection ... *1193*
Procainamide Hydrochloride Injection ... *1193*
Prochlorperazine Edisylate Injection ... *1193*
Promethazine Hydrochloride Injection ... *1193*
Protamine Sulfate Injection (Preservative-Free) ... *1193*
Sodium Chloride Injection, Bacteriostatic ... *1193*
Sodium Chloride Injection (Preservative-Free) ... *1193*
Sotradecol Injection ... **1199**
Sufentanil Citrate Injection ... *1193*
Sulfamethoxazole & Trimethoprim Concentrate for Injection ... *1193*
Thiamine Hydrochloride Injection ... *1193*

Other Products Available:
Dobutamine Hydrochloride Injection

ENDO PHARMACEUTICALS INC. 312, 1200
223 Wilmington West Chester Pike
Chadds Ford, PA 19317
(800) 462-3636

Direct Inquiries to:
Customer Service
(800) 462-3636
FAX: (877) 329-3636

For Medical Information/Adverse Drug Experience Reporting Contact:
Product Information:
(800) 462-3636

ENDO LABORATORIES

Products Described:
Hycodan Syrup ... **1200**
◆Hycodan Tablets ... **312, 1200**
◆Hycomine Compound Tablets ... **312, 1201**
Hycomine Syrup ... **1202**
Hycomine Pediatric Syrup ... **1202**
Hycotuss Expectorant Syrup ... **1203**
Lidoderm Patch ... **1204**
Moban Oral Concentrate ... **1205**
◆Moban Tablets ... **312, 1205**
Narcan Injection ... **1206**
Nubain Injection ... **1208**
Numorphan Injection ... **1209**
Numorphan Suppositories ... **1209**
◆Percocet Tablets ... **312, 1211**
◆Percodan Tablets ... **312, 1211**
◆Percodan-Demi Tablets ... **312, 1212**
◆Percolone Tablets ... **312, 1213**
Symmetrel Syrup ... **1213**
◆Symmetrel Tablets ... **312, 1213**
◆Zydone Tablets ... **312, 1215**

ENDO PHARMACEUTICALS INC.
223 Wilmington West Chester Pike
Chadds Ford, PA 19317
(800) 462-3636

Direct Inquiries to:
Customer Service
(800) 462-3636
FAX: (877) 329-3636

For Medical Information/Adverse Drug Experience Reporting Contact:
Product Information:
(800) 462-3636

ENDO GENERIC PRODUCTS

Products Described:
Amantadine Hydrochloride Syrup, USP ... *1200*
Amiloride Hydrochloride and Hydrochlorothiazide Tablets, USP ... *1200*
Butalbital, Aspirin, Caffeine, and Codeine Phosphate Capsules, USP ... *1200*
Captopril and Hydrochlorothiazide Tablets, USP ... *1200*
Carbidopa and Levodopa Tablets, USP ... *1200*
Cimetidine Hydrochloride Injection ... *1200*
Cimetidine Hydrochloride Oral Solution ... *1200*
Cimetidine Tablets, USP ... *1200*
Dicyclomine Hydrochloride Capsules, USP ... *1200*
Dicyclomine Hydrochloride Tablets, USP ... *1200*
Endocet Tablets, USP CII ... *1200*
Endocodone, USP CII ... *1200*
Endodan Tablets, USP CII ... *1200*
Glipizide Tablets, USP ... *1200*
Indomethacin Extended-Release Capsules, USP ... *1200*
Morphine Sulfate Extended-Release Tablets CII ... *1200*
Nitroglycerin Tablets, USP ... *1200*
Oxycodone/Acetaminophen Capsules ... *1200*
Selegiline Hydrochloride Tablets, USP ... *1200*

ENZON, INC. 1217
20 Kingsbridge Road
Piscataway, NJ 08854

Direct Inquiries to:
Toni L. Klich
(732) 980-4619
FAX: (732) 980-5911

For Medical Emergencies Contact:
(732) 980-4560
FAX: (732) 980-4566

Products Described:
Adagen Injection ... **1217**

ESI LEDERLE INC. 312, 1218
P.O. Box 41502
Philadelphia, PA 19101

Direct General Inquiries to:
(610) 688-4400

For Emergency Medical Information Contact:
Medical Affairs
Day: (800) 934-5556 (8:30 AM to 4:30 PM, Eastern Standard Time, Weekdays only)
Night: (610) 688-4400 (Emergencies only; non-emergencies should wait until the next day)

For Medical/Pharmacy Inquiries on Marketed Products Contact:
(800) 934-5556 (8:30 AM to 4:30 PM, Eastern Standard Time, Weekdays only)

Products Described:
◆Aygestin Tablets ... **312, 1218**

Other Products Available:
Acebutolol Hydrochloride Capsules
Acyclovir Capsules
Acyclovir Injection
Acyclovir Tablets
Atracurium Besylate Injection
Captopril Tablets
Cephalexin Capsules
Cephalexin Oral Suspension
Estradiol Tablets
Etodolac Capsules
Etodolac Tablets
Griseofulvin
Guaifenesin AC
Guaifenesin DAC
Guanfacine Hydrochloride Tablets
Hydrocodone Bitartrate and Acetaminophen Tablets
Ketoprofen ER Capsules
Ketoprofen SR Capsules
Lorazepam Cartridge
Lorazepam Tablets
Metoclopramide Tablets
Minocycline HCl Capsules
Oxazepam Capsules
Pentoxifylline ER Tablets
Promethazine HCl and Codeine Phosphate Syrup
Promethazine HCl and Dextromethorphan Hydrobromide Syrup
Promethazine HCl and Phenylephrine HCl Syrup
Promethazine HCl, Phenylephrine HCl and Codeine Phosphate Syrup
Propanolol HCl Long-Acting Capsules
Quinidine Sulfate E-R
Selegiline HCl Tablets
Vancomycin HCl Injection

ESI PHARMA, INC.
(See ESI LEDERLE INC.)

EVERETT LABORATORIES, INC. 1219
29 Spring Street
West Orange, NJ 07052

Direct Inquiries to:
Professional Service Department
(973) 324-0200
FAX: (973) 324-0795

Products Described:
Cortic Ear Drops ... *1219*
Renax Caplets ... *1219*
Strovite Forte Caplets ... *1220*
Strovite Forte Syrup ... *1220*
Tussafed-EX Drops ... *1220*
Tussafed-EX Syrup ... *1220*
Tussafed-HC Syrup ... *1220*
Tussafed-LA Caplets ... *1220*
Vitafol Caplets ... *1220*
Vitafol Syrup ... *1220*
Vitafol-PN Caplets ... *1220*

Other Products Available:
Repan-CF Tablets
Repan Tablets
Strovite Plus Caplets
Strovite Tablets
Tussafed Syrup

FARO PHARMACEUTICALS, INC. 312, 1220
135 Route 202/206
Bedminster, NJ 07921

Direct Inquiries to:
Customer Service
(877) 994-3276
FAX: (877) 280-6677

Products Described:
◆Imuran Injection ... **312, 1220**
◆Imuran Tablets ... **312, 1220**
◆Trandate Injection ... *312, 1222*
◆Trandate Tablets ... *312, 1222*
Zyloprim Tablets ... *1224*

FAULDING LABORATORIES INC. 312, 1227
5511 Capital Center Drive
Suite 550
Raleigh, NC 27606

Direct Inquiries to:
Customer Service
(800) 432-8534
FAX: (908) 820-0142

Products Described:
◆Kadian Capsules ... **312, 1227**

FERNDALE LABORATORIES, INC. 1230
780 West Eight Mile Road
Ferndale, MI 48220

Direct Inquiries to:
Mr. Thayer McMillan
(248) 548-0900
FAX: (248) 548-8427

For Medical Emergencies Contact:
Mr. Pravin M. Patel
(248) 548-0900
FAX: (248) 548-0708

Products Described:
Analpram HC Lotion 2.5% ... **1230**
Analpram-HC Rectal Cream 1% and 2.5% ... **1230**
Decubitene Oxygenated Oil ... *1231*
Dermamist Spray ... *1231*
ELA-Max Cream ... **1231**
ELA-Max 5 Cream ... **1232**
Kronofed-A Kronocaps ... **1233**
Kronofed-A-Jr. Kronocaps ... **1233**
Locoid Cream ... **1233**
Locoid Lipocream Cream ... **1234**
Locoid Ointment ... **1233**
Locoid Topical Solution ... **1233**
Pramosone Cream ... **1235**
Pramosone Lotion ... **1235**
Pramosone Ointment ... **1235**
Prax Lotion ... *1235*
Pro-Q Skin Protectant ... *1235*
SBR-Lipocream ... *1235*

Other Products Available:
Detachol Adhesive Remover
Liqui-Doss
Mastisol Liquid Adhesive
Tin-Ben Dispenser
Tin-Co-Ben Dispenser
Topiclude Occlusive Dressing

FERRING PHARMACEUTICALS INC. 1235
120 White Plains Road
Suite 400
Tarrytown, NY 10591

Direct Inquiries to:
Ferring Pharmaceuticals Inc.
Customer Service Department
120 White Plains Road
Suite 400
Tarrytown, NY 10591
(888) FERRING (337-7464)

For Medical Emergencies Contact:
Ferring Pharmaceuticals Inc.
Professional Services Department
120 White Plains Road
Suite 400
Tarrytown, NY 10591
(888) 793-6367

Products Described:
Acthrel for Injection ... **3499**
Desmopressin Acetate Injection ... **1236**
Desmopressin Acetate Rhinal Tube ... **1237**
Novarel for Injection ... **1238**
Repronex for Intramuscular and Subcutaneous Injection ... **1239**
Thyrel TRH for Injection ... **3501**

FIELDING PHARMACEUTICAL COMPANY 1242
P.O. Box 2186
11551 Adie Road
Maryland Heights, MO 63043

Direct Inquiries to:
Professional Services Department
(314) 567-5462

For Medical Emergencies Contact:
(314) 567-5462

Products Described:
Gynodiol Tablets ... *1242*
Nestabs CBF Tablets ... **1242**
Nestabs RX Tablets ... **1242**

Other Products Available:
Nestabs FA Tablets
Vitelle Irospan Capsules
Vitelle Irospan Tablets
Vitelle Lurline PMS Tablets
Vitelle Nesentials Tablets (formerly Gerimed)
Vitelle Nestabs OTC Tablets
Vitelle Nestrex Tablets

FIRST HORIZON PHARMACEUTICAL CORPORATION 312, 1242
660 Hembree Parkway
Suite 106
Roswell, GA 30076

Direct Inquiries to:
Alan Roberts
(770) 442-9707
FAX: (770) 442-9594

For Medical Emergencies Contact:
(800) 849-9707
FAX: (770) 442-9594

Products Described:
Cognex Capsules ... **1242**
Defen-L.A. Tablets ... *1246*
Mescolor Tablets ... *1246*
◆Nitrolingual Pumpspray ... **312, 1246**
Ponstel Kapseals ... **1247**
Protuss Liquid ... *1249*
Protuss-D Liquid ... *1249*
Protuss-DM Tablets ... *1249*
Robinul Forte Tablets ... **1249**
Robinul Tablets ... **1249**
Tanafed Suspension ... *1250*
Zebutal Capsules ... *1250*
Zoto-HC Ear Drops ... *1250*

C. B. FLEET CO., INC. 1250
4615 Murray Place
Lynchburg, VA 24506-1349

Direct Inquiries to:
David Vaughan
Director of Quality Assurance
(804) 528-4000
FAX: (804) 847-4219

Products Described:
Fleet Bisacodyl Laxatives............ **1250**
Fleet Enema.............................. **1251**
Fleet Enema for Children.............. **1251**
Fleet Glycerin Laxatives................ **1250**
Fleet Mineral Oil Enema................ **1251**
Fleet Phospho-Soda..................... **1251**
Fleet Prep Kits.......................... **1252**

FLEMING & COMPANY 1252
1600 Fenpark Dr.
Fenton, MO 63026

Direct Inquiries to:
H.C. Mansmann, Jr. M.D.
(636) 343-8200
FAX: (636) 343-5322
Internet: www.flemingcompany.com
For product orders, call (800) 343-0164

Products Described:
Aerolate Liquid........................ **1252**
Aerolate Jr. T.D. Capsules........... **1252**
Aerolate Sr. T.D. Capsules........... **1252**
Alumadrine Tablets.................... **1253**
Chlor-3.................................. **1253**
Extendryl Chewable Tablets.......... **1253**
Extendryl Sr. & Jr. Capsules........ **1253**
Extendryl Syrup........................ **1253**
Magonate Natal Liquid................ **1253**
Magonate Tablets and Liquid......... **1253**
Marblen Antacid......................... ■
Nephrocaps.............................. **1253**
Nicotinex Elixir.......................... ■
Obegyn Prenatal Supplement......... **1254**
Ocean Nasal Mist......................... ■
Pima Syrup.............................. **1254**
Purge...................................... ■
Rum-K.................................... **1254**

FOREST PHARMACEUTICALS, INC. 312, 1254
Subsidiary of FOREST LABORATORIES, INC.
13600 Shoreline Drive
St. Louis, MO 63045

Direct Inquiries to:
Professional Affairs Department
13600 Shoreline Drive
St. Louis, MO 63045
(800) 678-1605

Products Described:
◆Aerobid Inhaler System......... **312, 1254**
◆Aerobid-M Inhaler System...... **312, 1254**
◆AeroChamber and AeroChamber with Mask..... *312, 1256*
◆Armour Thyroid Tablets........ *312, 1257*
Celexa Oral Suspension.............. **1258**
◆Celexa Tablets.................... **312, 1258**
◆Cervidil Vaginal Insert.......... **312, 1261**
Endal-HD Liquid........................ *1263*
Esgic Capsules.......................... *1263*
Esgic Tablets............................ *1263*
◆Esgic-Plus Tablets................. *312, 1263*
Flumadine Syrup........................ **1263**
◆Flumadine Tablets................. **312, 1263**
◆Infasurf Intratracheal Suspension.................. **312, 1264**
◆Levothroid Tablets................ **312, 1266**
◆Lorcet 10/650 Tablets............ *313, 1268*
◆Lorcet Plus Tablets............... *312, 1268*
Lorcet-HD Capsules.................... *1268*
◆Monurol Sachet.................... **313, 1268**
◆Tessalon Capsules................. **313, 1270**
◆Tessalon Perles..................... *313, 1270*
◆Thyrolar Tablets.................... *313, 1270*
◆Tiazac Capsules..................... **313, 1270**

Other Products Available:
Ambenyl D Syrup
Banalg Hospital Strength Arthritic Pain Reliever
Banalg Liniment
Cebocap Capsules
Elixophyllin Elixir
Elixophyllin-GG Oral Solution
Elixophyllin-KI Elixir
Endal Expectorant
Endal Tablets
Endal-HD Plus Liquid
Enzone Cream
Eudal SR Tablets
Feostat Drops
Feostat Suspension
Feostat Tablets
Kay Ciel Oral Solution
Kay Ciel Powder Packets
Nitrogard Tablets
Pedameth Liquid
Theochron Tablets
Triad Capsules
Zone A Forte Lotion
Zone A Lotion 1%

FUJISAWA HEALTHCARE, INC. 313, 1273
Parkway North Center
Three Parkway North
Deerfield, IL 60015-2548

For Medical Information Contact:
Generally:
Medical and Scientific Information
(800) 727-7003
In Emergencies:
Medical and Scientific Information
(800) 727-7003

Products Described:
◆Adenocard Injection............ **313, 1273**
◆Adenoscan........................ **313, 1274**
◆AmBisome for Injection........ **313, 1275**
Aristocort A 0.025% Cream.......... *1280*
Aristocort A 0.1% Cream............. *1281*
Aristocort A 0.5% Cream............. *1281*
Aristocort A 0.1% Ointment......... *1280*
Aristocort Suspension (Forte Parenteral)........................ *1280*
Aristocort Suspension (Intralesional)....................... *1280*
Aristospan Suspension (Intra-articular)..................... *1281*
Aristospan Suspension (Intralesional)....................... *1281*
Cefizox for Intramuscular or Intravenous Use.................... **1281**
Cefizox for Intramuscular or Intravenous Use Pharmacy Bulk Package........................... *1283*
Cefizox for Intravenous Infusion..... *1284*
Cefizox for Intravenous Use in Galaxy Plastic Container.......... *1284*
Cyclocort Topical Cream 0.1%....... *1284*
Cyclocort Topical Lotion 0.1%....... *1284*
Cyclocort Topical Ointment 0.1%..... *1284*
◆Prograf........................... **313, 1284**

GALDERMA LABORATORIES, L.P. 1289
P.O. Box 331329
Fort Worth, TX 76163

Direct Inquiries to:
(800) 582-8225
8 a.m. to 5 p.m. Central (Monday through Friday)

Products Described:
Benzac AC 2½, 5 & 10 Gel **1289**
Benzac AC Wash 2½, 5 & 10 ...... **1289**
DesOwen Cream........................ **1289**
DesOwen Lotion....................... **1289**
DesOwen Ointment.................... **1289**
Differin Gel............................. **1290**
Differin Solution/Pledgets........... **1290**
MetroCream............................. **1291**
MetroGel................................ **1291**
MetroLotion............................ **1292**

GATE PHARMACEUTICALS 313, 1293
A Division of TEVA PHARMACEUTICALS USA
1090 Horsham Road
P.O. Box 1090
North Wales, PA 19454

Direct Inquiries to:
(800) 292-4283
FAX: (215) 653-0839

Products Described:
Adipex-P Capsules..................... **1293**
◆Adipex-P Tablets.................. **313, 1293**
◆Orap Tablets....................... **313, 1294**

GEBAUER COMPANY 1296
9410 St. Catherine Avenue
Cleveland, OH 44104

Direct Inquiries to:
(800) 321-9348
(216) 271-5252
Internet: www.gebauerco.com

For Medical Emergencies Contact:
(800) 321-9348
(216) 271-5252

After Hours and Weekend Emergencies:
Chemtrec:
(800) 424-9300

Products Described:
Gebauer's Ethyl Chloride........... **1296**
Gebauer's Fluori-Methane.......... **1296**

Other Products Available:
Dr's. Cream
Fluori-Methane
Salivart

GENENTECH, INC. 313, 1297
1 DNA Way
South San Francisco, CA 94080-4990
(650) 225-1000

For Medical Information Contact:
Medical Information or Drug Safety Departments (24 hours):
(800) 821-8590
(650) 225-1000
E-mail: medinfo@gene.com
Or write:
Medical Information or Drug Safety Departments:
Genentech, Inc.
1 DNA Way
South San Francisco, CA 94080-4990

Products Described:
◆Activase I.V....................... **313, 1297**
◆Herceptin I.V...................... **313, 1301**
◆Nutropin AQ Injection.......... **313, 1307**
◆Nutropin Depot for Injectable Suspension...................... **313, 1310**
◆Nutropin for Injection........... **313, 1304**
◆Protropin for Injection.......... *313, 1312*
◆Pulmozyme Inhalation Solution......................... **313, 1312**
◆Rituxan I.V........................ **313, 1314**
◆TNKase I.V........................ **313, 1316**

GENETICS INSTITUTE 313, 1318
87 Cambridge Park Drive
Cambridge, MA 02140

Direct Inquiries to:
(888) 237-3200

Products Described:
◆BeneFix for Injection........... **313, 1318**
◆Neumega for Injection.......... **313, 1320**
ReFacto Vials........................... **1323**

GENEVA PHARMACEUTICALS, INC. 1324
2655 West Midway Boulevard
P.O. Box 446
Broomfield, CO 80038-0446

Direct Inquiries to:
Customer Support Department
(800) 525-8747
(303) 466-2400
FAX: (303) 727-4656

Products Described:
Albuterol Tablets....................... *1324*
Alprazolam Tablets..................... *1324*
Amitriptyline HCl Tablets............. *1324*
Amoxapine Tablets..................... *1324*
Atenolol Tablets........................ *1324*
Bromocriptine Mesylate Capsules.... *1324*
Bromocriptine Mesylate Tablets...... *1324*
Bupropion HCl Tablets................. *1324*
Carisoprodol Tablets................... *1324*
Chlorpromazine HCl Tablets.......... *1324*
Cimetidine Tablets...................... *1324*
Clemastine Fumarate Syrup........... *1324*
Clemastine Fumarate Tablets......... *1324*
Clomipramine HCl Capsules.......... *1324*
Cyclobenzaprine HCl Tablets......... *1324*
Desipramine HCl Tablets.............. *1324*
Diclofenac Potassium Immediate Release Tablets..................... *1324*
Diclofenac Sodium Delayed-Release Tablets........... *1324*
Diclofenac Sodium Extended Release Tablets..................... *1324*
Fiortal Capsules......................... *1324*
Fiortal w/Codeine Capsules........... *1324*
Fluphenazine HCl Tablets............. *1324*
Flurbiprofen Tablets................... *1324*
Furosemide Tablets.................... *1324*
Glipizide Tablets........................ *1324*
Haloperidol Tablets..................... *1324*
Hydroxychloroquine Sulfate Tablets................................... *1324*
Imipramine HCl Tablets................ *1324*
Isosorbide Dinitrate Tablets.......... *1324*
Isoxsuprine HCl Tablets............... *1324*
Lonox Tablets............................ *1324*
Loperamide HCl Capsules............. *1324*
Lorazepam Tablets...................... *1324*
Meclizine HCl Tablets.................. *1324*
Methazolamide Tablets................ *1324*
Methocarbamol Tablets............... *1324*
Methylphenidate HCl Tablets......... *1324*
Methylphenidate Sustained Release Tablets................................... *1324*
Metoprolol Injectable.................. *1324*
Metoprolol Tartrate Tablets........... *1324*
Mexiletine HCl Capsules.............. *1324*
Naproxen Tablets....................... *1324*
Naproxen Sodium Tablets............. *1324*
Nortriptyline HCl Capsules........... *1324*
Orphenadrine Citrate Extended Release Tablets...................... *1324*
Oxazepam Capsules................... *1324*
Pemoline Tablets....................... *1324*
Perphenazine Tablets.................. *1324*
Perphenazine/Amitriptyline HCl Tablets................................... *1324*
Pindolol Tablets......................... *1324*
Promethazine HCl Tablets............. *1324*
Pseudoephedrine HCl Tablets......... *1324*
Ranitidine HCl Capsules............... *1324*
Ranitidine HCl Tablets................. *1324*
Rimactane Capsules.................... *1324*
Spironolactone Tablets................ *1324*
Sulindac Tablets........................ *1324*
Temazepam Capsules.................. *1324*
Terazosin Capsules.................... *1324*
Terazosin Tablets....................... *1324*
Thioridazine HCl Tablets.............. *1324*
Thiothixene Capsules.................. *1324*
Trazodone HCl Tablets................. *1324*
Tretinoin Cream........................ *1324*
Tretinoin Gel............................ *1324*
Triamterene/HCTZ 50mg/25mg Capsules................................. *1324*
Triamterene/HCTZ (Dyazide) 37.5mg/25mg Capsules.............. *1324*
Triamterene/HCTZ (mini-Maxzide) 37.5mg/25mg Tablets............... *1324*
Triamterene/HCTZ (Maxzide) 75mg/50mg Tablets................... *1324*
Trifluoperazine HCl Tablets........... *1324*
Verapamil HCl Tablets.................. *1324*

GENZYME CORPORATION 314, 1325
One Kendall Square
Cambridge, MA 02139

Direct Inquiries to:
Clinical Services
(800) 745-4447
FAX: (617) 252-7700

For Medical Emergencies Contact:
(800) 745-4447

Products Described:
Cerezyme for Injection................. **1325**
◆Renagel Capsules................. **314, 1326**
◆Renagel Tablets.................... **314, 1326**
Thyrogen for Injection................ **1328**

GILEAD SCIENCES, INC. 1329
333 Lakeside Drive
Foster City, CA 94404

Direct Inquiries to:
Customer Service
(800) GILEAD5

For Medical Information or to Report an Adverse Event Contact:
Medical Information/Safety Surveillance
(800) GILEAD5
FAX: (650) 522-5477

Products Described:
DaunoXome Injection.................. **1329**
Vistide Injection........................ **1332**

GLAXO WELLCOME INC. 314, 1335
Five Moore Drive
Research Triangle Park
North Carolina 27709
(919) 483-2100

For Medical Information for Healthcare Professionals Contact:
(888) 825-5249

For Medical Emergencies Contact:
Medical Information:
(800) 334-0089

For Consumer Inquiries Contact:
(888) 825-5249

Products Described:
◆Aclovate Cream................... **314, 1335**
◆Aclovate Ointment............... **312, 1335**
◆Agenerase Capsules.............. **314, 1336**
◆Agenerase Oral Solution........ **314, 1341**
◆Alkeran for Injection............. **314, 1346**
◆Alkeran Tablets................... **314, 1348**
◆Amerge Tablets................... **314, 1349**
◆Anectine Injection................ **314, 1352**
◆Beclovent Inhalation Aerosol and Refill.......................... **314, 1354**
◆Beconase Inhalation Aerosol.... **314, 1356**
◆Beconase AQ Nasal Spray....... **314, 1357**
◆Ceftin for Oral Suspension...... **314, 1358**
◆Ceftin Tablets..................... **314, 1358**
◆Ceptaz............................. **314, 1362**
◆Combivir Tablets.................. **314, 1365**
◆Cutivate Cream.................... **314, 1368**
◆Cutivate Ointment................ **314, 1370**
◆Daraprim Tablets................. **314, 1371**
◆Digibind........................... **314, 1372**
◆Emgel 2% Topical Gel............ **314, 1373**
◆Epivir Oral Solution.............. **314, 1374**
◆Epivir Tablets..................... **314, 1374**
◆Epivir-HBV Oral Solution........ **314, 1377**
◆Epivir-HBV Tablets............... **314, 1377**
◆Exosurf Neonatal for Intratracheal Suspension...... **314, 1380**
◆Flolan for Injection.............. **315, 1384**
◆Flonase Nasal Spray.............. **315, 1388**
◆Flovent 44 mcg Inhalation Aerosol........................... **315, 1390**
◆Flovent 110 mcg Inhalation Aerosol........................... **315, 1390**
◆Flovent 220 mcg Inhalation Aerosol........................... **315, 1390**
◆Flovent Rotadisk 50 mcg........ **315, 1393**
◆Flovent Rotadisk 100 mcg....... **315, 1393**
◆Flovent Rotadisk 250 mcg....... **315, 1393**
◆Fortaz............................. **315, 1396**
◆Imitrex Injection................. **315, 1399**
◆Imitrex Nasal Spray.............. **315, 1403**
◆Imitrex Tablets................... **315, 1407**
◆Lamictal Tablets.................. **315, 1412**
◆Lamictal Chewable Dispersible Tablets................ **315, 1412**
◆Lanoxicaps........................ **315, 1418**
◆Lanoxin Elixir Pediatric.......... **315, 1422**
◆Lanoxin Injection................. **315, 1425**
◆Lanoxin Injection Pediatric...... **315, 1429**
◆Lanoxin Tablets................... **315, 1432**
◆Leukeran Tablets................. **315, 1435**
◆Lotronex Tablets.................. **315, 1437**
Malarone Tablets....................... **1439**
Malarone Pediatric Tablets........... **1439**
◆Mepron Suspension.............. **315, 1442**
◆Myleran Tablets.................. **316, 1446**
◆Navelbine Injection.............. **316, 1448**
◆Oxistat Cream..................... **316, 1451**
◆Oxistat Lotion..................... **316, 1451**
◆Purinethol Tablets................ **316, 1452**
◆Relenza Rotadisk................. **316, 1454**
◆Retrovir Capsules................ **316, 1456**
◆Retrovir IV Infusion............. **316, 1460**
◆Retrovir Syrup.................... **316, 1456**
◆Retrovir Tablets.................. **316, 1456**
◆Serevent Diskus.................. **316, 1468**
◆Serevent Inhalation Aerosol..... **316, 1464**
◆Temovate Cream.................. **316, 1473**
◆Temovate E Emollient............ **316, 1475**
◆Temovate Gel..................... **316, 1474**
◆Temovate Ointment.............. **316, 1473**
◆Temovate Scalp Application..... **316, 1474**
◆Thioguanine Tablets, Tabloid Brand.............................. **316, 1471**
◆Valtrex Caplets................... **316, 1476**
◆Ventolin Inhalation Aerosol and Refill.......................... **316, 1478**
◆Ventolin Inhalation Solution.... **316, 1480**
◆Ventolin Rotacaps for Inhalation....................... **316, 1482**
◆Ventolin Syrup.................... **316, 1484**

◆Fast-Acting Mylanta Liquid Antacid........318, 1594
◆Extra Strength Fast-Acting Mylanta Liquid........318, 1594
◆Fast-Acting Mylanta Ultra Tabs........318, 1595
◆Maximum Strength Mylanta Gas Relief Softgels........318, 1595
Mylanta Gas Relief Tablets........1595
Maximum Strength Mylanta Gas Relief Tablets........1595
◆Mylanta Night Time Strength Liquid........318, 1596
◆Mylanta Supreme Liquid........318, 1595
◆Mylicon Infants' Drops........318, 1594
◆Pepcid AC Chewable Tablets........318, 1596
◆Pepcid AC Gelcaps........318, 1596
◆Pepcid AC Tablets........318, 1596

JONES PHARMA INCORPORATED 319, 1597
1945 Craig Road
P.O. Box 46903
St. Louis, MO 63146

Direct Inquiries to:
Customer Service
(314) 576-6100
FAX: (314) 469-5749
Internet: www.jmedpharma.com

Products Described:
Brevital Sodium for Injection, USP........*1597*
Cytomel Tablets........*1597*
◆Levoxyl Tablets........*319, 1597*
Tapazole Tablets........*1597*
Thrombin-JMI........*1597*
Triostat Injection........*1597*

KEY PHARMACEUTICALS, INC. 319, 1597
Galloping Hill Road
Kenilworth, NJ 07033
(908) 298-4000

For Medical Information Contact:
Generally:
Drug Information Services
(800) 526-4099
(9:00 AM to 5:00 PM EST)
After Hours and Weekends:
(908) 298-4000

Products Described:
◆Imdur Tablets........319, 1597
Integrilin Injection........1599
◆K-Dur Microburst Release System ER Tablets........319, 1603
◆Nitro-Dur Transdermal Infusion System........319, 1604
◆Theo-Dur Extended-Release Tablets........319, 1605
◆Trinalin Repetabs Tablets........*319*
◆Uni-Dur Extended-Release Tablets........319, 1611

KNOLL LABORATORIES 319, 1617
A Division of
Knoll Pharmaceutical Company
3000 Continental Drive North
Mount Olive, NJ 07828-1234

Direct Inquiries to:
BASF Group
Customer Information Center:
General Information (800) 240-3820
Customer Operations Department:
Orders, Credits/Returns, Wholesaler and Hospital Inquiries, Deductions, New Accounts
(800) 526-0710

For Medical Information Contact:
(800) 526-0221

Products Described:
Akineton Injection........1617
◆Akineton Tablets........319, 1617
◆Dilaudid Ampules........319, 1618
Dilaudid Injection........1618
◆Dilaudid Multiple Dose Vials (Sterile Solution)........319, 1618
◆Dilaudid Oral Liquid........319, 1621
Dilaudid Powder........1618
◆Dilaudid Rectal Suppositories........319, 1618
◆Dilaudid Tablets 2 mg and 4 mg........319, 1618
◆Dilaudid Tablets - 8 mg........319, 1621
◆Dilaudid-HP Injection........319, 1619
◆Dilaudid-HP Lyophilized Powder 250mg........319, 1619
◆Isoptin SR Tablets........319, 1623
◆Rythmol Tablets -- 150mg, 225mg, 300mg........319, 1625
◆Vicodin Tablets........319, 1629
◆Vicodin ES Tablets........319, 1630
◆Vicodin HP Tablets........319, 1628
◆Vicodin Tuss Expectorant........319, 1632
◆Vicoprofen Tablets........319, 1632

KNOLL PHARMACEUTICAL COMPANY 319, 1635
3000 Continental Drive North
Mount Olive, NJ 07828

Direct Inquiries to:
BASF Group
Customer Information Center:
General Information (800) 240-3820
Customer Operations Department:
Orders, Credits/Returns, Wholesaler and Hospital Inquiries, Deductions, New Accounts
(800) 526-0710

For Medical Information Contact:
(800) 526-0221

Products Described:
◆Mavik Tablets........319, 1635
◆Meridia Capsules........319, 1637
◆Synthroid Injection........320, 1641
◆Synthroid Tablets........319, 1641
◆Tarka Tablets........320, 1644

KOS PHARMACEUTICALS, INC. 320, 1648
1001 Brickell Bay Drive
25th Floor
Miami, FL 33131

For Medical Information Contact:
Drug Information Services
(888) 4-LIPIDS
(888) 454-7437

Products Described:
◆Niaspan Extended-Release Tablets........320, 1648

KRAMER LABORATORIES INC. 1651
8778 S.W. 8th Street
Miami, FL 33174
Internet: www.kramerlabs.com

Direct Inquiries to:
8778 S.W. 8th Street
Miami, FL 33174
(800) 824-4894

For Medical Emergencies Contact:
Professional Director
(800) 824-4894

Products Described:
Halfprin Tablets........1651

LASER, INC. 1652
2200 W. 97th Place, P.O. Box 905
Crown Point, IN 46308

Direct Inquiries to:
Joseph N. Allegretti, R.Ph., President & C.O.O.
(219) 663-1165

Products Described:
Dallergy Caplets, Syrup, Tablets........*1652*
Dallergy-JR Capsules........*1652*
Donatussin Drops........*1652*
Donatussin Syrup........*1652*
Donatussin DC Syrup........*1652*
Fumatinic Capsules........*1652*
Kie Syrup........*1652*
Lactocal-F Tablets........*1652*
Respaire-SR Capsules 60, 120........*1652*

LAYTON BIOSCIENCE, INC. 1652
709 East Evelyn Avenue
Sunnyvale, CA 94086

Direct Inquiries to:
Robert Alonso, Vice President, Marketing
(610) 975-9290

Products Described:
Inversine Tablets........1652

LEDERLE PHARMACEUTICAL 320, 1653
Division of American Cyanamid Company
Pearl River, NY 10965

LEDERLE PARENTERALS, INC.
Carolina, Puerto Rico 00987

LEDERLE PIPERACILLIN, INC.
Carolina, Puerto Rico 00987

(For oncology products, please see IMMUNEX CORPORATION)

For Medical Information Contact:
MARKETED ONCOLOGY PRODUCTS:
Immunex Corporation
Professional Services Department
51 University Street
Seattle, WA 98101
(800) IMMUNEX

OTHER MARKETED DRUG AND BIOLOGICAL PRODUCTS:
Lederle Pharmaceutical / Wyeth-Ayerst Pharmaceuticals
Medical Affairs Department
P.O. Box 8299
Philadelphia, PA 19101
Day: (800) 934-5556 (8:30 AM to 4:30 PM, Eastern Standard Time, Weekdays only)
Night: (610) 688-4400 (Emergencies only; non-emergencies should wait until the next day)
Distribution: See Wyeth-Ayerst Pharmaceuticals' listing

Products Described:
◆Acel-Imune........320, 1653
Achromycin V Capsules........1657
◆Artane Elixir........320, 1658
◆Artane Tablets........320, 1658
◆Declomycin Tablets........320, 1658
Diamox Intravenous........⊙
Diamox Sequels (Sustained Release)........⊙
Diamox Tablets........⊙
Diphtheria & Tetanus Toxoids Adsorbed Purogenated for Pediatric Use........1659
◆HibTITER........320, 1662
◆Materna Tablets........320, 1664
◆Methotrexate Tablets........*320*
◆Minocin Intravenous........320, 1665
◆Minocin Oral Suspension........320, 1667
◆Minocin Pellet-Filled Capsules........320, 1666
Neptazane Tablets........⊙
◆Pipracil........320, 1669
◆Pnu-Imune 23........320, 1671
◆Prevnar for Injection........320, 1673
Pyrazinamide Tablets........1679
◆Suprax for Oral Suspension........320, 1680
◆Suprax Tablets........320, 1680
Tetanus & Diphtheria Toxoids Adsorbed for Adult Use........1682
Tetanus Toxoid Adsorbed Purogenated........1685
◆Tine Test PPD........320, 3502
◆Tuberculin, Old, Tine Test........320, 3504
◆Zebeta Tablets........320, 1686
◆Ziac Tablets........320, 1688
◆Zosyn........321, 1692
Zosyn in Galaxy Containers........1695
◆Zosyn Pharmacy Bulk Package........*321, 1699*

LEDERLE STANDARD PRODUCTS 321, 1699
P.O. Box 41502
Philadelphia, PA 19101

Direct General Inquiries to:
(610) 688-4400

For Medical Information Contact:
Medical Affairs
Day: (800) 934-5556 (8:30 AM to 4:30 PM, Eastern Standard Time, Weekdays only)
Night: (610) 688-4400 (Emergencies only; non-emergencies should wait until the next day)

Products Described:
Albuterol Sulfate Tablets........*1699*
◆Alprazolam Tablets........*321, 1699*
Atenolol Tablets........*1699*
Cimetidine Tablets........*1699*
Clonidine HCl Tablets........*1699*
Diazepam Tablets........*1699*
Diltiazem Hydrochloride Tablets........*1699*
Dipyridamole Tablets........*1699*
Erythromycin Ethylsuccinate/ Sulfisoxazole Acetyl Oral Suspension........*1699*
Sterile Erythromycin Lactobionate for Injection........*1699*
Fenoprofen Calcium Tablets........*1699*
Folic Acid Injection........*1699*
Hydralazine HCl Tablets........*1699*
Hydrochlorothiazide Tablets........*1699*
Ketoprofen Capsules........*1699*
Methazolamide Tablets........*1699*
Methocarbamol Tablets........*1699*
Methyldopa Tablets........*1699*
◆Naproxen Tablets........*321, 1699*
◆Nystatin Oral Suspension........*321, 1699*
Prazosin HCl Capsules........*1699*
Propylthiouracil Tablets........*1699*
◆Pyrazinamide Tablets........*321, 1699*
Quinidine Sulfate Tablets........*1699*
Sulfamethoxazole & Trimethoprim Tablets........*1699*
Sulindac Tablets........*1699*
◆Tetracycline HCl Capsules........*321, 1699*
Tobramycin Sulfate Injection........*1699*
Vancomycin HCl Injection........*1699*

Other Products Available:
Furosemide Tablets
Indomethacin Capsules
Tetracycline Ointment 3%

LIGAND PHARMACEUTICALS INCORPORATED 1699
10275 Science Center Drive
San Diego, CA 92121

Direct Inquiries to:
(858) 550-7500
Customer Service:
(877) 454-4263
Medical Information:
(800) 964-5836
Reimbursement Support:
(877) 654-4263

Products Described:
Ontak Vials........1699
Panretin Gel........1701
Targretin Capsules........3487

ELI LILLY AND COMPANY 321, 1704

For Medical Information Contact:
Customer Services
Lilly Corporate Center
Indianapolis, IN 46285
(800) 545-5979

Direct Inquiries to:
Lilly Corporate Center
Indianapolis, IN 46285
(317) 276-2000

AREA SALES OFFICES:
Atlanta, GA 30328
North Park Town Center
Building 500, Suite 1200
1100 Abernathy Road, NE
(770) 551-5360
Bala Cynwyd, PA 19004
401 City Avenue
Suite 400
(610) 617-1157
Birmingham, AL 35243
3800 Colonnade Parkway
Suite 250
(205) 969-4556
Anaheim, CA 92806
2400 East Katella Avenue
Suite 530
(714) 940-0800
Chicago, IL 60631
Suite 810, O'Hare Plaza
8725 West Higgins Road
(773) 693-8740
Addison, TX 75001
15305 Dallas Parkway
(972) 960-7637
Indianapolis, IN 46268
Suite 200, Parkwood Five
510 E. 96th 46240
(317) 277-6583
Stamford, CT 06902
300 First Stamford Place
(203) 357-1422

Products Described:
◆Axid Pulvules........321, 1704
Ceclor Pulvules........1706
Ceclor Suspension........1706
Darvocet-N 50 Tablets........1708
◆Darvocet-N 100 Tablets........321, 1708
Darvon Compound-65 Pulvules........1712
Darvon Pulvules........1710
Darvon-N Tablets........1713
Dobutrex Solution Vials........1715
◆Evista Tablets........321, 1717
Gemzar for Injection........1721
Glucagon for Injection Vials and Emergency Kit........1725
Heparin Sodium Vials........1727
Humalog........1729
Humalog Mix75/25 Pen........1731
Humatrope Vials and Cartridges........1733
Humulin 50/50, 100 Units........1736
Humulin 70/30, 100 Units........1737
Humulin 70/30 Cartridge........1739
Humulin 70/30 Pen........1740
Humulin L, 100 Units........1742
Humulin N, 100 Units........1743
Humulin R Regular (U-500)........1751
Humulin R, 100 Units........1748
Humulin U, 100 Units........1751
Humulin N NPH Cartridge........1745
Humulin N NPH Pen........1747
Humulin R Regular Cartridge........1749
Iletin II, Lente (Pork), 100 Units........1753
Iletin II, NPH (Pork), 100 Units........1754
Iletin II, Regular (Pork), 100 Units........1755
Kefurox Vials, ADD-Vantage........1756
Kefzol Vials, ADD-Vantage........1759
Mandol Vials........1761
Nebcin Vials, Hyporets & ADD-Vantage........1763
Oncovin Solution Vials........1766
Protamine Sulfate Vials........1768
◆Prozac Scored Tablets........*321*
Quinidine Gluconate Injection, USP........1768
◆ReoPro Vials........321, 1771
◆Sarafem Pulvules........321, 1774
Tazidime Vials, Faspak & ADD-Vantage........1779
Vancocin HCl Capsules & Pulvules........1785
Vancocin HCl Oral Solution........1784
Vancocin HCl, Vials & ADD-Vantage........1782
Velban Vials........1786
◆Zyprexa Tablets........321, 1788
Zyprexa ZYDIS Orally Disintegrating Tablets........1788

Other Products Available:
Amytal Sodium Vials
Atropine Sulfate Vials
Aventyl HCl Liquid
Aventyl Pulvules
Calcium Carbonate, USP
Methenamine, for Timed Burning
Morphine Sulfate Vials & Soluble Tablets
Opium Tincture, USP
Phenobarbital, USP
Seconal Sodium
Sodium Bicarbonate Tablets
Sodium Chloride, USP
Tuinal Pulvules

THE LIPOSOME COMPANY, INC. 321, 1793
One Research Way
Princeton, NJ 08540-6619

MERICON INDUSTRIES, INC. **2058**
8819 N. Pioneer Road
Peoria, IL 61615

Direct Inquiries to:
William R. Connelly
(309) 693-2150
E-mail: MONOCAL@aol.com
FAX: (309) 693-2158

Sales & Ordering:
(800) 242-6464

Products Described:

Other Products Available:
Chromium Picolinate 1.6 mg
Ginkgo Biloba Extract 60 mg
Glucosamine Sulfate 500 mg
Hydrocortisone Cream 1%
Hydrocortisone Lotion 1%
Ipriflavone 200 mg
St. John's Wort 150 mg
Zinc Gluconate Lozenges
Zinc Oxide Ointment
Zinc Sulfate Tabs & Caps

MERZ PHARMACEUTICALS **2059**
Division of Merz, Inc.
4215 Tudor Lane (27410)
P.O. Box 18806
Greensboro, NC 27419

Direct Inquiries to:
Director of Technical Operations
(336) 856-2003
FAX: (336) 856-0107

For Medical Emergencies Contact:
Director of Technical Operations
(336) 856-2003
FAX: (336) 856-0107

Products Described:

Other Products Available:
Anamine Syrup
Anatuss Syrup

METHAPHARM, INC. **2061**
2825 University Drive
Suite 240
Coral Springs, Florida 33065

Direct Inquiries to:
(800) 287-7686
FAX: (877) 718-9222
E-mail: sales@methapharm.com
Internet: www.methapharm.com

Products Described:

MGI PHARMA, INC. **324, 2061**
6300 West Old Shakopee Road
Suite 110
Bloomington, MN 55438-2318

For Medical Information or to Report Adverse Drug Experiences Contact:
(800) 644-4811
FAX: (952) 346-4800
Customer Service
(800) 562-4531
FAX: (952) 346-4800

Products Described:

MILEX PRODUCTS, INC. **2063**
4311 N. Normandy
Chicago, IL 60634-1403

Direct Inquiries to:
(800) 621-1278
FAX: (800) 972-0696

Manufacturing and Distribution:
SHIPPING OFFICES:
Milex Carolinas
4409 Lebanon Road
Post Office Box 23060
Charlotte, NC 28227
(704) 545-4567
Milex Puerto Rico
Post Office Box 360554
San Juan, PR 00936-0554
(787) 767-7358
Milex Southern
1001 Palo Pinto Street
Weatherford, TX 76086
(817) 599-7604
Milex Western
Post Office Box 46305
639 N. Fairfax
Los Angeles, CA 90046
(213) 651-4301
Milex Hawaii
Box 6337
Honolulu, HI 96818
(808) 422-9581

Products Described:

MISSION PHARMACAL COMPANY **2063**
10999 IH 10 West, Suite 1000
San Antonio, TX 78230-1355

Direct Inquiries to:
P.O. Box 786099
San Antonio, TX 78278-6099
Toll Free: (800) 292-7364
(210) 696-8400
FAX: (210) 696-6010

For Medical Emergencies Contact:
George Alexandrides
(830) 249-9822
FAX: (830) 816-2545

Products Described:

Other Products Available:
Compete

MONARCH PHARMACEUTICALS **324, 2066**
501 Fifth Street
Bristol, TN 37620

Direct Inquiries to:
(800) 776-3637
FAX: (423) 989-6279

For Medical Emergencies Contact:
Kathy Montgomery
(800) 546-4906
FAX: (248) 650-6407

Products Described:

Other Products Available:
Chloromycetin Ophthalmic
Chloromycetin Ophthalmic Ointment, 1%
Chloromycetin Otic
Chloromycetin Sodium Succinate
Cortisporin Ophthalmic Ointment Sterile
Cortisporin Otic Solution Sterile
Cortisporin Otic Suspension Sterile
Histoplasmin
Humatin
Ketalar
Nucofed Capsules CIII
Nucofed Expectorant Syrup CIII
Nucofed Pediatric Expectorant Syrup CV
Nucofed Syrup CIII
Pitocin
Pitressin
Polysporin Ophthalmic Ointment Sterile
Proloprim Tablets
Quibron
Quibron-T
Quibron-T/SR
Tussend Expectorant Syrup CIII
Vira-A

MURO PHARMACEUTICAL, INC. **2105**
an ASTA Medica company
890 East Street
Tewksbury, MA 01876-1496

Direct Inquiries to:
Professional Service Department
(800) 225-0974
(978) 851-5981

Products Described:

MYLAN PHARMACEUTICALS INC. **2115**
781 Chestnut Ridge Road
P.O. Box 4310
Morgantown, WV 26504-4310
(304) 599-2595

Direct Inquiries to:
(304) 599-2595

For Medical Information Contact:
Clinical Research Department
(877) 446-3679
(877) 4INFO-RX

Sales and Ordering:
Sales Department
(800) RX-MYLAN

Products Described:

NABI **325, 2128**

5800 Park of Commerce Blvd., NW
Boca Raton, FL 33487

For Medical Information Contact:

Generally:
Immunotherapy Customer Service
(800) 458-4244
(305) 625-5303
(800) 4-WINRHO (494-6746)
(800) 327-7106 - AUTOPLEX
(800) 685-5579 - Medical
FAX: (305) 625-0925

In Emergencies:
Immunotherapy Customer Service
(800) 458-4244
(800) 4-WINRHO (494-6746)
(800) 327-7106 - AUTOPLEX
FAX: (305) 625-0925

Products Described:

NEUTROGENA DERMATOLOGICS **325, 2136**

5760 West 96th Street
Los Angeles, CA 90045

Direct Inquiries to:
Diane Foster
(310) 642-1150
FAX: (310) 337-2156

For Medical Emergencies Contact:
Kamran Mather, Ph.D.
(310) 642-1150
FAX: (310) 216-5399

Products Described:

Other Products Available:

Acne Mask
Instant Bronzer Tinted Sunless Tanner
Neutrogena Clean Shampoo
Neutrogena Cleansing Bar for Acne-prone Skin
Neutrogena Cleansing Bar for Dry Skin
Neutrogena Cleansing Bar for Dry Skin fragrance-free
Neutrogena Cleansing Bar for Oily Skin
Neutrogena Cleansing Bar Original Formula
Neutrogena Cleansing Bar Original Formula fragrance-free
Neutrogena Cleansing Wash
Neutrogena Cosmetics
Neutrogena Extra Gentle Cleanser
Neutrogena Extra Gentle Cleansing Bar
Neutrogena Healthy Skin Anti-Wrinkle Cream with Stabilized Retinol
Neutrogena Healthy Skin Face Lotion with SPF 15
Neutrogena Lip Moisturizer
Liquid Neutrogena
Liquid Neutrogena, fragrance free
Neutrogena Moisture
Neutrogena Moisture SPF 15 Untinted
Neutrogena Moisture SPF 15 with Sheer Tint
Neutrogena Norwegian Formula Body Moisturizer
Neutrogena Norwegian Formula Emulsion
Neutrogena Norwegian Formula Hand Cream
Neutrogena Oil-Free Sunblock SPF 30
Neutrogena Rainbath
Neutrogena Sensitive Skin Sunblock SPF 30
Neutrogena Sunblock SPF 15
Neutrogena Sunblock SPF 30
Neutrogena Sunblock SPF 45
Neutrogena T/Derm Tar Emollient
Oil-Free Acne Wash
On-the-Spot Acne Treatment
Sunblock Stick SPF25
Sunless Tanning Foam
Sunless Tanning Lotion
Sunless Tanning Spray
T/Gel Extra Strength Therapeutic Shampoo (4% Neutar)
T/Gel Intensive Anti-Flake Treatment
T/Gel Therapeutic Conditioner
Maximum Strength T/Sal Therapeutic Shampoo (3% salicylic acid)

NORTH AMERICAN BIOLOGICALS, INC.

(See NABI)

NOVARTIS CONSUMER HEALTH, INC. **325, 2136**

560 Morris Avenue
Summit, NJ 07901-1312

Direct Product Inquiries to:
Consumer & Professional Affairs
(800) 452-0051
FAX: (800) 635-2801
or write to:
445 State Street
Fremont, MI 49423

Products Described:

Other Products Available:

Arthritis Pain Ascriptin
Enteric Ascriptin
Maximum Strength Ascriptin
Regular Strength Ascriptin
Prescription Strength Cruex Cream
Cruex Spray Powder
Prescription Strength Cruex Spray Powder
Cruex Squeeze Powder
Desenex Foot and Sneaker Shake Powder
Desenex Foot and Sneaker Spray Powder
Desenex Ointment
Desenex Shake Powder
Desenex Spray Powder
Prescription Strength Desenex Spray Powder
Doan's Extra Strength Analgesic
Extra Strength Doan's P.M.
Doan's Regular Strength Analgesic
Maalox Anti-Gas Tablets, Regular Strength and Extra Strength
Nupercainal Hemorrhoidal and Anesthetic Ointment
Nupercainal Suppositories
Otrivin Nasal Drops
Otrivin Pediatric Nasal Drops
Otrivin Nasal Spray
Sunkist Children's Chewable Multivitamins - Complete
Sunkist Children's Chewable Multivitamins - Plus Extra C
Sunkist Vitamin C - Chewable
Sunkist Vitamin C Rolls

NOVARTIS PHARMACEUTICALS CORPORATION **325, 2141**

Novartis Pharmaceuticals Corporation
59 Route 10
East Hanover, NJ 07936
(for branded products)

For Information Contact:
Customer Response Department
(888) NOW-NOVARTIS (888-669-6682)
Internet: http://www.novartis.com

Geneva Pharmaceuticals, Inc.
A Novartis Company
2655 West Midway Boulevard
P.O. Box 446
Broomfield, CO 80038-0446
(for branded generic products refer to Geneva Pharmaceuticals, Inc.)

For Information Contact:
Customer Support Department
(800) 525-8747
(303) 466-2400
FAX: (303) 727-4656

Products Described:

Other Products Available:

Anturane Capsules
Anturane Tablets
Apresazide Capsules
Cafergot Suppositories
Esidrix Tablets
Hydergine Liquid
Hydergine LC Liquid Capsules
Hydergine Oral Tablets
Ismelin Tablets
Klorvess Effervescent Granules
Lamprene Capsules
Lioresal Tablets
Ludiomil Tablets
Mellaril Concentrate
Mellaril Tablets
Mellaril-S Oral Suspension
Mesantoin Tablets
Methergine Injection
Methergine Tablets
Metopirone Capsules
Neo-Calglucon Syrup
Priscoline Hydrochloride Ampuls
Rimactane Capsules
Sansert Tablets
Ser-Ap-Es Tablets
Slow-K Extended-Release Tablets
Tavist Syrup
Tavist Tablets
Tofranil Tablets
Visken Tablets

NOVO NORDISK PHARMACEUTICALS, INC. **326, 2235**

100 College Road West
Princeton, NJ 08540

Direct Inquiries to:
Novo Nordisk Pharmaceuticals, Inc.
(800) 727-6500

In Emergencies After Hours & Weekends:
(609) 987-5800

Products Described:

NOVOGYNE PHARMACEUTICALS
A joint venture between
Novartis Pharmaceuticals Corporation
East Hanover, New Jersey 07936
and
Noven Pharmaceuticals, Inc.
Miami, Florida 33186

For Information Contact:
Customer Response Department
(888) NOW-NOVARTIS (888-669-6682)

[See NOVARTIS PHARMACEUTICALS CORPORATION, the distributor of **Vivelle** (estradiol transdermal system) and **Vivelle-Dot** (estradiol transdermal system)]

NUTRACEUTICS CORPORATION **2248**
4100 Laclede Avenue
Suite 112
St. Louis, MO 63108

Direct Inquiries to:
(800) 391-0114

Products Described:
Cardiotropin........................*2248*
Osteo I.P.........................*2248*
Osteomax.........................*2248*
Pro Endorphin.........................*2248*
Q-Bid.........................*2248*
Redox.........................*2248*
SAMe Plus.........................*2248*
Symbiotropin.........................*2248*

OCLASSEN DERMATOLOGICS **327, 2248**
A Division of Watson Pharma, Inc.
311 Bonnie Circle
P.O. Box 1900
Corona, CA 92878-1900

Direct Inquiries to:
Customer Service Department
(800) 272-5525
FAX: (909) 735-2871

For Medical Information Contact:
Customer Service Department
(800) 272-5525
FAX: (909) 737-8540

Products Described:
◆Condylox Gel.................**327, 2248**
◆Condylox Topical Solution......**327, 2249**
◆Cordran Lotion.................**327, 2250**
◆Cordran Tape.................**327, 2251**
◆Cormax Cream.................**327, 2252**
◆Cormax Ointment.................**327, 2252**
◆Cormax Scalp Application......**327, 2253**
◆Monodox Capsules.............**327, 2254**

Other Products Available:
Cinobac Capsules, 250mg, 500mg
Cordran Ointment 0.025%, 30g, 60g
Cordran Ointment 0.05%, 15g, 30g, 60g
Cordran SP Cream 0.025%, 30g, 60g
Cordran SP Cream 0.05%, 15g, 30g, 60g

ODYSSEY PHARMACEUTICALS, INC. **2256**
72 DeForest Ave.
East Hanover, NJ 07936

Direct Inquiries to:
(877) 427-9068

Products Described:
Nystatin Vaginal Tablets, USP.......*2256*
Urecholine Tablets.................**2256**

ORGANON INC. **327, 2256**
375 Mt. Pleasant Ave.
West Orange, NJ 07052

Direct Inquiries to:
(973) 325-4500

For Medical Inquiries Contact:
(800) 631-1253
FAX: (973) 325-4699

Products Described:
Antagon Injection.....................**2257**
◆Calderol Capsules.............*327, 2259*
Cortrosyn for Injection.................**2259**
◆Cotazym Capsules.............**327, 2259**
◆Cotazym-S Capsules.............*327, 2261*
Deca-Durabolin Injection.............*2261*
◆Desogen Tablets.................**327, 2261**
◆Follistim for Injection.............**327, 2267**
◆Follistim/Antagon Kit.................*327*
◆Humegon for Injection.............**327, 2270**
◆Mircette Tablets.................**327, 2272**
Norcuron for Injection.................**2279**
◆Organan Injection.................**327, 2282**
Pavulon Injection.................*2284*
Pregnyl for Injection.................**2284**
◆Raplon for Injection.............**327, 2284**
Regonol Injection.................*2290*
◆Remeron Tablets.................**327, 2290**
Reversol Injection.................*2293*
Succinylcholine Chloride Injection....*2293*
◆Tice BCG, BCG Live.............**327, 2293**
◆Wigraine Tablets.................**327, 2295**
◆Zemuron Injection.................**327, 2296**
◆Zymase Capsules.................**327, 2300**

ORTHO BIOTECH PRODUCTS, L.P. **327, 2300**
P.O. Box 670
Raritan, NJ 08869-0670

Direct Inquiries to:
(800) 325-7504
Prompt #1, Customer Service
Prompt #2, Medical Information
FAX: (908) 526-9230
FAX: (908) 526-6457

Products Described:
◆Leustatin Injection.............**327, 2300**
Orthoclone OKT3 Sterile Solution....**2303**
◆Procrit for Injection.........**327, 328, 2307**
◆Sporanox Capsules.............*328, 2313*
◆Sporanox Injection.............**328, 2314**
◆Sporanox Oral Solution.........**328, 2317**

ORTHO DERMATOLOGICAL **328, 2320**
199 Grandview Road
Skillman, NJ 08558

For Medical Information Contact:
Dermatological Medical Information
(800) 426-7762

Products Described:
◆Dermatop Emollient Cream......**328, 2320**
◆Grifulvin V Tablets
Microsize and Oral
Suspension Microsize.........**328, 2321**
◆Renova Cream.................**328, 2322**
◆Retin-A Micro Microsphere, 0.1%.........................**328, 2323**

ORTHO DIAGNOSTIC SYSTEMS INC.
(See ORTHO-CLINICAL DIAGNOSTICS, INC.)

ORTHO-CLINICAL DIAGNOSTICS, INC. **2325**
A Johnson & Johnson Company
1001 U.S. Hwy 202
Raritan, NJ 08869-0606

Direct Inquiries to:
Customer Service
(800) 828-6316

Products Described:
MICRhoGAM.........................**2325**
RhoGAM.........................**2325**

ORTHO-McNEIL PHARMACEUTICAL, INC. **328, 2326**
1000 Route 202, P.O. Box 300
Raritan, NJ 08869-0602

For Medical Information/Emergencies Contact:
Generally:
(800) 682-6532
In Emergencies:
(908) 218-7325

Products Described:
Aci-Jel Therapeutic Vaginal Jelly.....**2326**
◆All-Flex Arcing Spring Diaphragm
(See Ortho Diaphragm Kits).........*328*
◆Floxin I.V.....................**328, 2327**
◆Floxin Tablets.................**328, 2330**
◆Haldol Decanoate 50
Injection.....................**328, 2336**
◆Haldol Decanoate 100
Injection.....................**328, 2336**
◆Haldol Injection, Tablets and
Concentrate.....................**328, 2334**
◆Levaquin Injection.............**328, 2338**
◆Levaquin Tablets.................**328, 2338**
◆Micronor Tablets.................**328, 2344**
Modicon 21 Tablets.....................**2363**
◆Modicon 28 Tablets.............**328, 2363**
Ortho Coil Spring Diaphragm (See Ortho Diaphragm Kits)
Ortho Diaphragm Kits -- All-Flex
Arcing Spring; Ortho Coil Spring..**2353**
Ortho Dienestrol Cream.................**2355**
Ortho Tri-Cyclen 21 Tablets.............**2374**
◆Ortho Tri-Cyclen 28 Tablets.....**328, 2374**
Ortho-Cept 21 Tablets.................**2346**
◆Ortho-Cept 28 Tablets.............**328, 2346**
Ortho-Cyclen 21 Tablets.................**2374**
◆Ortho-Cyclen 28 Tablets.........**328, 2374**
Ortho-Novum 1/35 □ 21 Tablets......**2363**
◆Ortho-Novum 1/35 □ 28
Tablets.........................**328, 2363**
◆Ortho-Novum 1/50 □ 28
Tablets.........................**328, 2357**
Ortho-Novum 7/7/7 □ 21 Tablets......**2363**
◆Ortho-Novum 7/7/7 □ 28
Tablets.........................**328, 2363**
Ortho-Novum 10/11 □ 21 Tablets......**2363**
◆Ortho-Novum 10/11 □ 28
Tablets.........................**328, 2363**
◆Ortho-Prefest Tablets.............**328, 2370**
◆Pancrease Capsules.............**328, 2381**
◆Pancrease MT Capsules.........**329, 2382**
◆Parafon Forte DSC Caplets......**329, 2383**
◆ParaGard T 380A Intrauterine
Copper Contraceptive.........**329, 2383**
◆Regranex Gel.....................**329, 2387**
Sultrin Triple Sulfa Cream.............**2388**
◆Terazol 3 Vaginal Cream.........**329, 2388**
◆Terazol 3 Vaginal
Suppositories.....................**329, 2389**
◆Terazol 7 Vaginal Cream.........**329, 2389**
◆Tolectin 200 Tablets.............**329, 2390**
◆Tolectin 400 Tablets.....................*329*
◆Tolectin 600 Tablets.............**329, 2390**
◆Tolectin DS Capsules.............**329, 2390**
◆Topamax Sprinkle Capsules......**329, 2391**
◆Topamax Tablets.................**329, 2391**
◆Tylenol with Codeine Elixir......**329, 2397**
◆Tylenol with Codeine Tablets.....**329, 2397**
◆Tylox Capsules.................**329, 2398**
◆Ultram Tablets.................**329, 2398**
◆Vascor Tablets.................**329, 2401**

OTSUKA AMERICA PHARMA, INC. **329, 2404**
2440 Research Boulevard
Rockville, MD 20850

Direct Inquiries to:
Medical Affairs, Otsuka America
Pharma, Inc.
(800) 441-6763
FAX: (301) 212-5577

To Request Routine or Emergency Medical Information, or to Report an Adverse Experience:
(800) 441-6771

Products Described:
◆Pletal Tablets.....................**329, 2404**

PADDOCK LABORATORIES, INC. **2406**
3940 Quebec Avenue North
Minneapolis, MN 55427

Direct Inquiries to:
David Chinnock, R.Ph.
(612) 546-4676
FAX: (612) 546-4842

For Medical Emergencies Contact:
Carol Anding, Regulatory Affairs
(800) 328-5113
FAX: (612) 546-4842

Products Described:
Actidose with Sorbitol Suspension....*2406*
Actidose-Aqua Suspension.............*2406*
Colocort Enema, USP (Retention)
100 mg/60 mL.....................**2406**
Compro Suppositories, USP 25 mg....**2407**
Glutose 15, Glutose 45 (Oral
Glucose Gel).....................*2408*
Kionex Powder.........................**2408**
Paddock Nystatin USP for
Extemporaneous Preparation of
Oral Suspension.....................*2409*
Nystop Topical Powder USP.........**2409**
Podocon-25 Liquid.....................**2409**

Other Products Available:
Acetaminophen Tablets 325 mg
Aluminum Paste
Aquabase
Aspirin Suppositories 300 mg, 600 mg
Aspirin Tablets, Enteric-Coated 325 mg
Belladonna and Opium Suppositories
16.2 mg/30 mg and 16.2 mg/60 mg CII
Benzoin Compound Tincture USP
Bisacodyl Suppositories 10 mg
Bisacodyl Tablets 5 mg
Castor Oil USP
Colistin Sulfate USP Powder
Dermabase
Dexamethasone Sodium Phosphate USP
Powder
Docusate Sodium Capsules 100 mg,
250 mg
Docusate Sodium Capsules w/Casanthranol
100 mg/30 mg
Emulsoil (Self-Emulsifying Castor Oil)
Erythra-Derm Solution
Erythromycin USP Powder
Fattibase
Ferrous Gluconate Tablets 324 mg
Ferrous Sulfate Tablets 324 mg
Glutol
Hydrocortisone USP Micronized Powder
Hydrocortisone Acetate USP Micronized
Powder
Hydrocortisone Acetate Suppositories
25 mg
Hydrocream Base
Hydromorphone HCl USP non-sterile
Powder CII
Hydromorphone HCl Suppositories 3 mg
CII
Ipecac Syrup USP
Liqua-Gel
Milk of Magnesia USP
Morphine Sulfate USP Powder CII
Morphine Sulfate Suppositories 5 mg,
10 mg, 20 mg, 30 mg CII
Ora-Plus
Ora-Sweet
Ora-Sweet SF
Polybase
Progesterone USP Micronized Powder
Progesterone USP Wettable
Microcrystalline Powder
Sorbitol Solution USP 70%
Suspendol-S
Testosterone USP Micronized non-sterile
Powder CIII
Testosterone Propionate USP Micronized
non-sterile Powder CIII
Triamcinolone Acetonide USP Micronized
Powder
Trimethobenzamide HCl Suppositories
100 mg, 200 mg
Zincate Capsules 220 mg

PAR PHARMACEUTICAL, INC. **2410**
One Ram Ridge Road
Spring Valley, NY 10977

Direct Inquiries to:
Customer Service
(800) 828-9393
(845) 425-7100

Products Described:
Acebutolol Capsules.................*2410*
Acyclovir Capsules.................*2410*
Allopurinol Tablets.................*2410*
Alprazolam Tablets.................*2410*
Amiloride HCl Tablets.................*2410*
Amiodarone HCl Tablets.................*2410*
Amoxicillin Capsules.................*2410*
Amoxicillin Oral Suspension.........*2410*
Ampicillin Capsules.................*2410*
Ampicillin Oral Suspension.........*2410*
Benztropine Mesylate Tablets.........*2410*
Captopril Tablets.................*2410*
Carisoprodol and Aspirin Tablets.....*2410*
Clomiphene Tablets.................*2410*
Clonazepam Tablets.................*2410*
Cyproheptadine Tablets.................*2410*
Dexamethasone Tablets.................*2410*
Diphenoxylate with Atropine
Sulfate Tablets.....................*2410*
Doxepin HCl Capsules.................*2410*
Etodolac Tablets.................*2410*
Fluphenazine HCl Tablets.............*2410*
Flurazepam HCl Capsules.............*2410*
Guanfacine Tablets.................*2410*
Hydralazine HCl Tablets.............*2410*
Hydra-Zide Capsules.................*2410*
Hydroxyurea Capsules.................*2410*
IBU Tablets.........................*2410*
Ibuprofen Capsules.................*2410*
Ibuprofen Suspension.................*2410*
Ibuprofen Tablets.................*2410*
Imipramine HCl Tablets.............*2410*
Indapamide Tablets.................*2410*
Isosorbide Dinitrate Tablets.........*2410*
Meclizine HCl Tablets.................*2410*
Megestrol Acetate Tablets.............*2410*
Methimazole Tablets.................*2410*
Methocarbamol and Aspirin Tablets..*2410*
Methylprednisolone Tablets.........*2410*
Minocycline Capsules.................*2410*
Minoxidil Tablets.................*2410*
Naproxen Sodium Tablets.............*2410*
Nicardipine Capsules.................*2410*
Orphengesic Tablets.................*2410*
Orphengesic Forte Tablets.............*2410*
Penicillin V Potassium Suspension....*2410*
Penicillin V Potassium Tablets........*2410*
Prochlorperazine Tablets.............*2410*
Ranitidine Tablets.................*2410*
Selegiline Tablets.................*2410*
Sotalol Tablets.................*2410*
SSD Cream.........................*2410*
SSD AF Cream.....................*2410*
Temazepam Capsules.................*2410*
Ticlopidine HCl Tablets.............*2410*
Triazolam Tablets.................*2410*
Zorprin Tablets.................*2410*

PARKEDALE PHARMACEUTICALS **329, 2410**
870 Parkdale Road
Rochester, MI 48307

Direct Inquiries to:
(888) 401-2879
FAX: (423) 989-6279

For Medical Emergencies Contact:
Kathy Montgomery
(800) 546-4906
FAX: (248) 650-6407

Products Described:
◆Aplisol Injection.................**329, 2410**
◆Fluogen Injection.................**329, 2412**

PARKE-DAVIS **329, 2414**
A Warner-Lambert Division
A Pfizer Company
201 Tabor Rd.
Morris Plains, NJ 07950

For Medical Information Contact:
During working hours:
Customer Service
Product/Medical Information
(800) 223-0432
FAX: (973) 385-2248
After Hours and Weekend Emergencies:
(973) 385-6089

Distribution:
1855 Shelby Oaks Drive North
Memphis, TN 38134
(901) 387-5200
Customer Service
(800) 533-4535

EXPORT INQUIRIES:
Pfizer International Inc.
(212) 573-2323

Products Described:
◆Accupril Tablets.................**329, 2414**
◆Accuretic Tablets.................**329, 2417**
Benadryl Parenteral.....................**2420**
◆Celontin Capsules.................**329, 2421**
Cerebyx Injection.....................**2422**

◆Dilantin Infatabs ... 329, 2427
◆Dilantin Kapseals ... 329, 2425
Dilantin-125 Suspension ... 2428
Estrostep 21 Tablets ... 2430
◆Estrostep Fe Tablets ... 329, 2430
◆femhrt Tablets ... 329, 2438
◆Lipitor Tablets ... 329, 2442
Loestrin 21 Tablets ... 2445
Loestrin Fe Tablets ... 2445
◆Lopid Tablets ... 329, 2453
◆Nardil Tablets ... 329, 2456
◆Neurontin Capsules ... 329, 2458
Neurontin Tablets ... 2458
◆Nitrostat Tablets ... 330, 2461
Parcode Product List ... *2414*
◆Zarontin Capsules ... 330, 2462
Zarontin Syrup ... 2463

PASTEUR MÉRIEUX CONNAUGHT
(See AVENTIS PASTEUR INC.)

PATHOGENESIS CORPORATION 330, 2463
201 Elliott Avenue West
Seattle, WA 98119

Direct Inquiries to:
(888) 508-TOBI (8624)

Products Described:
◆TOBI Solution for Inhalation ... 330, 2463

PEDINOL PHARMACAL INC. 2466
30 Banfi Plaza North
Farmingdale, NY 11735

Direct Inquiries to:
Director of Professional Services
(631) 293-9500

Products Described:
Castellani Paint Modified ... *2466*
Formalyde-10 Spray ... *2466*
Fungoid Solution ... *2466*
Fungoid Tincture ... *2466*
Gris-PEG Tablets ... 2466
Lactinol Lotion ... *2467*
Lactinol-E Creme ... *2467*
Lazerformalyde Solution ... *2467*
Pedi-Boro Soak Paks ... *2467*
Pedi-Dri Topical Powder ... *2467*
TI-Screen Sunscreens, Sunblock, Sportsgel, and Lip Protectant ... *2467*
Ureacin-10 Lotion ... *2467*
Ureacin-20 Creme ... *2467*

Other Products Available:
Alginate Styptic Gauze
Breezee Mist Foot Powder
CitraDerm Facial Complex Cream
Fungoid Tincture Topical Antifungal Treatment Kit
Hydrisalic Gel
Hydrisinol Creme
Hydrisinol Lotion
LazerCreme
Nail Scrub with Brush
Ony-Clear Solution
Ostiderm
Ostiderm Roll-On
Pedi-Pro Foot Powder
PNS Unna Boot
Sal-Acid Plasters
Salactic Film
Sal-Plant Gel
Totéphan Creme

PENEDERM INCORPORATED
(See BERTEK PHARMACEUTICALS INC.)

PERSŌN & COVEY, INC. 2467
616 Allen Avenue
P.O. Box 25018
Glendale, CA 91221-5018

Direct Inquiries to:
Frank Brisben, C.O.O.
(818) 240-1030
(800) 423-2341
FAX: (818) 547-9821
E-mail: helpdesk@personandcovey.com

Products Described:
Aquanil Lotion ... *2467*
Aquanil HC Lotion ... *2467*
DHS Shampoo ... *2467*
DHS Clear Shampoo ... *2467*
DHS Sal Shampoo ... *2467*
DHS Tar Shampoo ... *2467*
DHS Tar Gel Shampoo ... *2467*
DHS Zinc Shampoo ... *2467*
DML Facial Moisturizer with Sunscreen ... *2467*
DML-Forte Cream ... *2467*
DML-Lotion ... *2467*
Drysol Solution ... 2467
Solbar AVO Lotion SPF 32 ... 2468
Solbar PF Cream SPF 50 (PABA Free) ... 2468
Solbar PF Liquid SPF 30 ... 2468
Xerac AC Solution ... 2468

PFIZER INC. 330, 2468
235 East 42nd Street
New York, NY 10017-5755

For Medical Information Contact:
24 hours a day, seven days a week:
(800) 438-1985

Distribution:
1855 Shelby Oaks Drive North
Memphis, TN 38134
(901) 387-5200
Customer Service:
(800) 533-4535

EXPORT INQUIRIES:
Pfizer International Inc.
(212) 573-2323

Products Described:
Antivert, Antivert/25, & Antivert/50 Tablets ... 2469
◆Aricept Tablets ... 330, 2469
Atarax Tablets & Syrup ... 2472
◆Cardura Tablets ... 330, 2473
Cefobid Intravenous/Intramuscular ... 2477
Cefobid Pharmacy Bulk Package - Not for Direct Infusion ... 2479
◆Celebrex Capsules ... 330, 2482
Diabinese Tablets ... 2485
◆Diflucan Tablets, Injection, and Oral Suspension ... 330, 2487
◆Feldene Capsules ... 330, 2491
Geocillin Tablets ... 2493
◆Glucotrol Tablets ... 330, 2494
◆Glucotrol XL Extended Release Tablets ... 330, 2495
◆Lipitor Tablets ... 330, 2498
Minipress Capsules ... 2501
Minizide Capsules ... 2502
◆Navane Capsules ... 330, 2503
Navane Concentrate ... 2503
Navane Intramuscular ... 2504
◆Norvasc Tablets ... 330, 2506
Permapen Isoject ... 2508
Pfizerpen for Injection ... 2508
◆Procardia Capsules ... 330, 2510
◆Procardia XL Extended Release Tablets ... 330, 2512
Product Identification Codes ... *2468*
Renese Tablets ... 2514
◆Sinequan Capsules ... 330, 2515
Sinequan Oral Concentrate ... 2515
Streptomycin Sulfate Injection ... 2516
Tao Capsules ... 2518
Terra-Cortril Ophthalmic Suspension ... 2518
Terramycin Intramuscular Solution ... 2518
Terramycin with Polymyxin B Sulfate Ophthalmic Ointment ... 2520
◆Tikosyn Capsules ... 330, 2520
◆Trovan I.V. ... 330, 2525
◆Trovan Tablets ... 330, 2525
◆Unasyn for Injection ... 330, 2531
Urobiotic-250 Capsules ... 2534
◆Viagra Tablets ... 330, 2534
Vibramycin Calcium Oral Suspension Syrup ... 2537
Vibramycin Hyclate Capsules ... 2537
Vibramycin Hyclate Intravenous ... 2539
Vibramycin Monohydrate for Oral Suspension ... 2537
Vibra-Tabs Film Coated Tablets ... 2537
Vistaril Capsules ... 2541
Vistaril Intramuscular Solution ... 2541
Vistaril Oral Suspension ... 2541
Zithromax Capsules, 250 mg ... 2546
◆Zithromax for IV Infusion ... 331, 2550
◆Zithromax for Oral Suspension, 1 g ... 331, 2546
◆Zithromax for Oral Suspension, 300 mg, 600 mg, 900 mg, 1200 mg ... 330, 2542
◆Zithromax Tablets, 250 mg ... 330, 2542
◆Zithromax Tablets, 600 mg ... 330, 2546
◆Zithromax Z-Pak ... *330*
Zoloft Oral Concentrate ... 2553
◆Zoloft Tablets ... 331, 2553
◆Zyrtec Syrup ... 331, 2558
◆Zyrtec Tablets ... 331, 2558

PFIZER INC. CONSUMER HEALTH CARE GROUP
(See WARNER-LAMBERT CONSUMER GROUP OF PFIZER INC.)

PFIZER LABS DIVISION
235 East 42nd Street
New York, NY 10017-5755

For Medical Information Contact:
24 hours a day, seven days a week:
(800) 438-1985

Distribution:
1855 Shelby Oaks Drive North
Memphis, TN 38134
(901) 387-5200
Customer Service:
(800) 533-4535

EXPORT INQUIRIES:
Pfizer International Inc.
(212) 573-2323
(See PFIZER INC.)

PHARMACEUTICAL ASSOCIATES, INC. 2560
A Subsidiary of Beach Products, Inc.
201 Delaware Street
Greenville, SC 29605

Direct Inquiries to:
Clete Harmon, Director of Q.A.
(800) 845-8210
(864) 277-7282
FAX: (864) 277-8045

Products Described:
Acetaminophen Oral Solution USP ... *2560*
Acetaminophen and Codeine Phosphate Oral Solution USP ... *2560*
Aluminum Hydroxide Gel USP ... *2560*
Aluminum Hydroxide Gel Concentrate ... *2560*
Amantadine Hydrochloride Syrup USP ... *2560*
Aromatic Cascara Fluidextract USP ... *2560*
Chloral Hydrate Syrup USP ... *2560*
Cimetidine Hydrochloride Oral Solution ... *2560*
Diphenhydramine Hydrochloride Elixir USP ... *2560*
Docusate Sodium Liquid ... *2560*
Docusate Sodium Syrup USP ... *2560*
Docusate Sodium with Casanthranol ... *2560*
Ferrous Sulfate Liquid ... *2560*
Fluphenazine Hydrochloride Elixir USP ... *2560*
Fluphenazine Hydrochloride Oral Solution USP (Concentrate) ... *2560*
Guaifenesin Syrup USP ... *2560*
Guaifenesin Syrup with Codeine ... *2560*
Guaifenesin Syrup and Dextromethorphan ... *2560*
Haloperidol Oral Solution USP (Concentrate) ... *2560*
Hydrocodone Bitartrate and Acetaminophen Elixir ... *2560*
Hydrocodone Bitartrate and Guaifenesin Expectorant ... *2560*
Lactulose Solution USP ... *2560*
Metoclopramide Oral Solution USP ... *2560*
Milk of Magnesia USP ... *2560*
Milk of Magnesia Concentrate ... *2560*
Milk of Magnesia Cascara Suspension ... *2560*
Mineral Oil ... *2560*
Oxybutynin Chloride Syrup USP ... *2560*
Phenobarbital Elixir ... *2560*
Potassium Chloride Oral Solution USP 10% ... *2560*
Potassium Chloride Oral Solution USP 20% ... *2560*
Potassium Citrate and Citric Acid Oral Solution USP ... *2560*
Promethazine Hydrochloride and Codeine Phosphate Syrup ... *2560*
Pseudoephedrine Hydrochloride Syrup USP ... *2560*
Sodium Citrate and Citric Acid Oral Solution USP ... *2560*
Sorbitol Solution USP ... *2560*
Sore Throat Spray ... *2560*
Thioridazine Hydrochloride Oral Solution USP (Concentrate) ... *2560*
Tricitrates Oral Solution ... *2560*
Trihexyphenidyl Hydrochloride Elixir USP ... *2560*

Other Products Available:
Nortriptyline Hydrochloride Oral Solution USP

PHARMACIA
(See PHARMACIA & UPJOHN)

PHARMACIA & UPJOHN 331, 2561
100 Route 206 North
Peapack, NJ 07977

Direct Inquiries to:
(888) 768-5501

For Medical and Pharmaceutical Information, Including Emergencies, Contact:
(616) 833-8244

Pharmacia & Upjohn Customer Service:
(800) 821-7000

Products Described:
Activella Tablets ... 2561
Adriamycin PFS/RDF Injection ... 2565
Aromasin Tablets ... 2567
◆Azulfidine EN-tabs Tablets ... 331, 2569
Camptosar Injection ... 2571
◆Caverject Sterile Powder ... 331, 2579
Cleocin HCl Capsules ... 2583
Cleocin Phosphate Sterile Solution ... 2584
◆Cleocin T Topical Gel ... 331, 2589
◆Cleocin T Topical Lotion ... 331, 2589
◆Cleocin T Topical Solution ... 331, 2589
Cleocin Vaginal Cream ... 2586
Cleocin Vaginal Ovules ... 2588
Colestid Tablets ... 2590
Corvert Injection ... 2592
Depo-Medrol Injectable Suspension ... 2594
◆Depo-Provera Contraceptive Injection ... 331, 2596
◆Detrol Tablets ... 331, 2600
Dipentum Capsules ... 2602
Dostinex Tablets ... 2603
Ellence Injection ... 2605
Emcyt Capsules ... 2609
Estring Vaginal Ring ... 2610
Fragmin Injection ... 2613
◆Genotropin Lyophilized Powder ... 331, 2616
Glyset Tablets ... 2619
◆Halcion Tablets ... 331, 2621
Idamycin PFS Injection ... 2624
◆Mirapex Tablets ... 331, 2626
◆Mycobutin Capsules ... 331, 2630
Ogen Tablets ... 2632
◆Pletal Tablets ... 331, 2634
Prepidil Gel ... 2637
Prostin E2 Suppositories ... 2638
◆Provera Tablets ... 331, 2639
Solu-Medrol Sterile Powder ... 2641
Vagifem Tablets ... 2643
◆Vantin Tablets and Oral Suspension ... 331, 2646
◆Xanax Tablets ... 331, 2650
Zinecard for Injection ... 2654
Zyvox Injection ... 2656
Zyvox for Oral Suspension ... 2656
Zyvox Tablets ... 2656

Other Products Available:
Adrucil Injection
Albamycin Capsules
Amphocin Injection
Ansaid Tablets
Atgam Sterile Solution
Azulfidine Tablets
Bacitracin Sterile Powder, USP
Cleocin Pediatric Flavored Granules
Colestid/Flavored Colestid for Oral Suspension
Cortef Oral Suspension
Cortef Tablets
Cortisone Acetate Tablets, USP
Cyklokapron Ampoule
Cytosar-U Sterile Powder
Deltasone Tablets
Depo-Estradiol Sterile Solution
Depo-Medrol Sterile Aqueous Suspension and Single-Dose Vial
Depo-Provera Sterile Aqueous Suspension
Depo-Testadiol Sterile Solution
Depo-Testosterone Sterile Solution
Gelfilm Sterile Film
Gelfilm Sterile Ophthalmic Film
Gelfoam Dental Packs
Gelfoam Sterile Powder
Gelfoam Sterile Sponge
Gelfoam Sterile Compressed Sponge
Glynase PresTab Tablets
Hemabate Sterile Solution (Sales restricted to hospitals only)
Idamycin Injection
Lincocin Capsules
Lincocin Sterile Solution
Maolate Tablets
Medrol Tablets
Medrol Tablets and Dosepak
Micronase Tablets
Motrin Tablets
Neosar Injection
Orinase Tablets
Prostin VR Pediatric Sterile Solution
R-Gene 10 Injection
Solu-Cortef Sterile Powder
Tolinase Tablets
Trobicin Sterile Powder
Vincasar Injection
Zanosar Sterile Powder

POLYMEDICA PHARMACEUTICALS (U.S.A.), INC. 2660
11 State Street
Woburn, MA 01801

Direct Inquiries to:
Peter M. Etzel
(781) 933-2020
FAX: (781) 933-7992

For Medical Emergencies Contact:
Peter M. Etzel or Arthur Siciliano
(781) 933-2020
FAX: (781) 933-7992

Products Described:
Anestacon Jelly ... *2660*
B & O Supprettes No. 15A & No. 16A ... *2660*
Cystospaz Tablets ... 2661
Cystospaz-M Capsules ... 2661
Urised Tablets ... 2661

WILLIAM P. POYTHRESS COMPANY
(See ECR PHARMACEUTICALS)

PROCTER & GAMBLE 2662
(For Rx products, see Procter & Gamble Pharmaceuticals
or call 1-800-836-0658)
P.O. Box 5516
Cincinnati, OH 45201
Charles E. Lambert
(800) 358-8707

For Medical Information Contact:
In Emergencies, call collect:
(513) 558-4422

Products Described:
Head & Shoulders Dandruff Shampoo ... 2662
Head & Shoulders Dandruff Shampoo Dry Scalp ... 2662
Head & Shoulders Intensive Treatment Dandruff and Seborrheic Dermatitis Shampoo ... 2662

Metamucil Original Texture Powder, Orange Flavor ... **2662**
Metamucil Original Texture Powder, Regular Flavor ... **2662**
Metamucil Smooth Texture Powder, Orange Flavor ... **2662**
Metamucil Smooth Texture Powder, Sugar-Free, Orange Flavor ... **2662**
Metamucil Smooth Texture Powder, Sugar-Free, Regular Flavor ... **2662**
Metamucil Wafers, Apple Crisp and Cinnamon Spice Flavors ... **2662**
Pepto-Bismol Maximum Strength Liquid ... **2663**
Pepto-Bismol Original Liquid, Original and Cherry Tablets and Easy-To-Swallow Caplets ... **2663**
Vicks 44 Cough Relief ... ▣
Vicks 44D Cough & Head Congestion Relief ... ▣
Vicks 44E Cough & Chest Congestion Relief ... ▣
Pediatric Vicks 44e Cough & Chest Congestion Relief ... ▣
Vicks 44M Cough, Cold & Flu Relief ... ▣
Pediatric Vicks 44m Cough & Cold Relief ... ▣
Vicks Cough Drops, Menthol & Cherry Flavors ... ▣
Vicks DayQuil Multi-Symptom Cold/Flu Relief Liquid & LiquiCaps ... ▣
Vicks DayQuil Sinus Pressure & Pain Relief with Ibuprofen ... ▣
Children's Vicks NyQuil Cold/Cough Relief ... ▣
Vicks NyQuil LiquiCaps ... ▣
Vicks NyQuil Liquid ... ▣
Vicks Sinex 12-Hour Nasal Spray and Ultra Fine Mist for Sinus Relief ... ▣
Vicks Sinex Nasal Spray and Ultra Fine Mist for Sinus Relief ... ▣
Vicks Vapor Inhaler ... ▣
Vicks VapoRub Cream ... ▣
Vicks VapoRub Ointment ... ▣
Vicks VapoSteam ... ▣

PROCTER & GAMBLE PHARMACEUTICALS, INC. **331, 2664**
Health Care Research Center
8700 Mason Montgomery Road
Mason, OH 45040

Direct Inquiries to:
Customer Service
(800) 448-4878

For Medical Information Contact:
Generally:
Medical Communications
(800) 836-0658
FAX: (800) 438-0138
Or Write:
Procter & Gamble Company
Medical Communications Department
Health Care Research Center
P.O. Box 8006
Mason, OH 45040-8006
In Emergencies:
Medical Communications
(800) 836-0658

Products Described:
◆Actonel Tablets ... **331, 2664**
◆Asacol Delayed-Release Tablets ... **331, 2669**
Dantrium Capsules ... **2671**
Dantrium Intravenous ... **2672**
◆Didronel Tablets ... **331, 2673**
◆Macrobid Capsules ... **331, 2675**
◆Macrodantin Capsules ... **331, 2676**

THE PURDUE FREDERICK COMPANY **331, 2678**
One Stamford Forum
Stamford, CT 06901-3431

For Medical Information Contact:
(888) 726-7535
Adverse Drug Experiences:
(888) 726-7535
Customer Service:
(800) 877-5666
FAX: (800) 877-3210

Products Described:
Betadine Brand First Aid Antibiotics & Moisturizer Ointment ... **2678**
Betadine Brand Plus First Aid Antibiotics & Pain Reliever Ointment ... **2678**
Betadine Medicated Douche ... **2678**
Betadine Ointment ... **2679**
Betadine PrepStick Applicator ... **2679**
Betadine PrepStick Plus Applicator ... **2679**
Betadine Skin Cleanser ... **2679**
Betadine Solution ... **2679**
Betadine Surgical Scrub ... **2679**
Betasept Surgical Scrub ... **2679**
Cerumenex Eardrops ... **2680**
◆MS Contin Tablets ... **331, 2680**
◆MSIR Oral Capsules ... **331, 2683**
◆MSIR Oral Solution ... **332, 2683**
◆MSIR Oral Solution Concentrate ... **332, 2683**
◆MSIR Oral Tablets ... **331, 2683**
Senokot Granules ... **2685**
Senokot Children's Syrup ... **2685**
Senokot Tablets ... **2685**
Senokot-S Tablets ... **2685**
SenokotXTRA Tablets ... **2685**
◆Trilisate Liquid ... **332, 2686**
◆Trilisate Tablets ... **332, 2686**
◆Uniphyl 400 mg and 600 mg Tablets ... **332, 2687**
X-Prep Liquid ... **2685**

Other Products Available:
Arthropan Liquid
Betadine Aerosol Spray
Betadine Medicated Disposable Douche
Betadine Pre-Mixed Medicated Disposable Douche
Betadine Mouthwash/Gargle
Betadine Perineal Wash Concentrate Kit
Betadine Shampoo
Betadine Solution Swab Aid
Betadine Solution Swabsticks
Betadine Surgi-Prep Sponge-Brush
Senokot Syrup
T-Phyl Tablets
X-Prep Kit 1
X-Prep Kit 2

PURDUE PHARMA L.P. **332, 2693**
One Stamford Forum
Stamford, CT 06901-3431

For Medical Information Contact:
(888) 726-7535
Adverse Drug Experiences:
(888) 726-7535
Customer Service:
(800) 877-5666
FAX: (800) 877-3210

Products Described:
◆Chirocaine Injection ... **332, 2693**
◆OxyContin Tablets ... **332, 2697**
◆OxyFast Oral Concentrate Solution ... **332, 2701**
◆OxyIR Capsules ... **332, 2701**

QUESTCOR PHARMACEUTICALS, INC. **2703**
26118 Research Road
Hayward, CA 94545

Direct Inquiries to:
(510) 732-5551
FAX: (510) 732-7741

Products Described:
Ethamolin Injection, 5% ... *2703*
Glofil-125 Injection ... *2703*
Inulin and Sodium Chloride Injection ... *2703*

R&D LABORATORIES, INC. **2703**
4640 Admiralty Way, Suite 710
Marina del Rey, CA 90292

Direct Inquiries to:
Gregory Little
(310) 305-8053, ext.227
(800) 338-9066
FAX: (310) 305-8103

For Medical Emergencies Contact:
Jur Strobos, M.D.
(310) 345-6370

Products Described:
Calci-Chew Tablets ... **2703**
Calci-Mix Capsules ... **2703**
L-Carnitine Capsules ... *2703*
Mag-Carb Capsules ... **2703**
NephrAmine Injection ... **2703**
Nephro-Calci Tablets ... **2703**
Nephro-Fer Tablets ... **2703**
Nephro-Fer Rx Tablets ... **2703**
Nephro-Vite Tablets ... *2705*
Nephro-Vite + Fe Tablets ... **2705**
Nephro-Vite Rx Tablets ... **2705**

RECKITT BENCKISER PHARMACEUTICALS INC. **332, 2705**
1909 Huguenot Road
Richmond, VA 23235

Direct Inquiries to:
Professional Services
(804) 379-1090
FAX: (804) 379-1215

For Medical Emergencies Contact:
Medical Department
(804) 379-1090
FAX: (804) 379-1215

Manufacturing and Distribution:
Distribution Center
220 Lake Drive
Newark, DE 19702
(800) 627-7413
FAX: (302) 323-3222

Products Described:
◆Buprenex Injectable ... **332, 2705**

REID-ROWELL
(See SOLVAY PHARMACEUTICALS, INC.)

RESPA PHARMACEUTICALS, INC. **2706**
P.O. Box 88222
Carol Stream, IL 60188

Direct Inquiries to:
(630) 462-9986
FAX: (630) 462-9934

Products Described:
Respa-1st Tablets ... *2706*
Respa-A.R.M. Tablets ... *2706*
Respa-DM Tablets ... *2706*
Respa-GF Tablets ... *2706*
Respahist Capsules ... *2706*
Trikof-D Tablets ... *2706*

RHÔNE-POULENC RORER PHARMACEUTICALS INC.
(Due to the merger of HOECHST MARION ROUSSEL and RHÔNE-POULENC RORER, please refer to AVENTIS PHARMACEUTICALS for product information)

RICHARDSON-VICKS INC
(See PROCTER & GAMBLE)

RICHWOOD PHARMACEUTICAL COMPANY INC.
(See SHIRE US INC.)

RIKER LABORATORIES, INC.
(See 3M PHARMACEUTICALS)

ROBERTS PHARMACEUTICAL CORPORATION
(See SHIRE US INC.)

A. H. ROBINS COMPANY, INC. **332, 2707**
1407 Cummings Drive
Richmond, VA 23220

Direct General Inquiries to:
(610) 688-4400

For Emergency Medical Information Contact:
Medical Affairs
Day: (800) 934-5556 (8:30 AM to 4:30 PM, Eastern Standard Time, Weekdays only)
Night: (610) 688-4400 (Emergencies only; non-emergencies should wait until the next day)

For Medical/Pharmacy Inquiries on Marketed Products Contact:
(800) 934-5556 (8:30 AM to 4:30 PM, Eastern Standard Time, Weekdays only)

Products Described:
Dimetane-DX Cough Syrup ... **2707**
◆Donnatal Capsules ... **332, 2708**
Donnatal Elixir ... **2708**
◆Donnatal Extentabs ... **332, 2708**
◆Donnatal Tablets ... **332, 2708**
◆Donnazyme Tablets ... **332, 2709**
Dopram Injectable ... **2709**
Phenaphen with Codeine Capsules ... *2710*
◆Quinidex Extentabs ... **332, 2711**
◆Reglan Injectable ... **332, 2713**
Reglan Syrup ... **2713**
◆Reglan Tablets ... **332, 2713**
◆Robaxin Injectable ... **332, 2716**
◆Robaxin Tablets ... **332, 2716**
◆Robaxin-750 Tablets ... **332, 2716**
◆Robaxisal Tablets ... **332, 2717**
◆Robinul Injectable ... **332, 2717**
Robitussin A-C Syrup ... **2718**
Robitussin-DAC Syrup ... **2718**
◆Tenex Tablets ... **332, 2719**

Other Products Available:
Mitrolan Tablets

ROCHE PHARMACEUTICALS **332, 2721**
Roche Laboratories Inc.
340 Kingsland Street
Nutley, New Jersey 07110-1199

For Medical Information:
(including routine inquiries, adverse drug events and product complaints)
Call: (800) 526-6367
For the Medical Needs Program
Call: (800) 285-4487
Write: Professional Product Information

Order Fulfillment:
(800) 526-0625

Products Described:
◆Accutane Capsules ... **332, 2721**
◆Anaprox Tablets ... **332, 2744**
◆Anaprox DS Tablets ... **332, 2744**
Bactrim I.V. Infusion ... **2724**
Bactrim Pediatric Suspension ... **2725**
◆Bactrim Tablets ... **332, 2725**
◆Bactrim DS Tablets ... **332, 2725**
◆CellCept Capsules ... **332, 2728**
CellCept Intravenous ... **2728**
CellCept Oral Suspension ... **2728**
◆CellCept Tablets ... **332, 2728**
◆Cytovene Capsules ... **332, 2736**
Cytovene-IV ... **2736**
◆Demadex Tablets and Injection ... **332, 2742**
◆EC-Naprosyn Delayed-Release Tablets ... **332, 2744**
◆Fortovase Capsules ... **332, 2747**
Sterile FUDR ... **2751**
◆Hivid Tablets ... **332, 2752**
◆Invirase Capsules ... **333, 2756**
◆Klonopin Tablets ... **333, 2759**
◆Lariam Tablets ... **333, 2762**
Naprosyn Suspension ... **2744**
◆Naprosyn Tablets ... **333, 2744**
◆Rocaltrol Capsules ... **333, 2763**
Rocaltrol Oral Solution ... **2763**
Rocephin Injectable Vials, ADD-Vantage, Galaxy, Bulk ... **2765**
Roferon-A Injection ... **2768**
Romazicon Injection ... **2772**
◆Soriatane Capsules ... **333, 2775**
◆Tamiflu Capsules ... **333, 2780**
◆Tasmar Tablets ... **333, 2782**
◆Ticlid Tablets ... **333, 2786**
Toradol IM Injection, IV Injection ... **2789**
◆Toradol Tablets ... **333, 2789**
Valium Injectable ... **2793**
Versed Injection ... **2794**
Versed Syrup ... **2800**
◆Vesanoid Capsules ... **333, 2804**
◆Xeloda Tablets ... **333, 2806**
◆Xenical Capsules ... **333, 2809**
Zenapax for Injection ... **2813**

Other Products Available:
Berocca Tablets
Berocca Plus Tablets
Bumex Injection
Bumex Tablets
Cardene Capsules
Cardene SR Capsules
Fansidar Tablets
Gantanol Tablets
Gantrisin Pediatric Suspension
Larodopa Tablets
Trimpex Tablets

ROCHE PHARMACEUTICALS **332, 2814**
Roche Products Inc.

For Medical Information Contact:
Roche Laboratories Inc.
(800) 526-6367

Order Fulfillment:
Roche Laboratories Inc.
(800) 526-0625

Products Described:
◆Valium Tablets ... **333, 2814**

ROERIG DIVISION
235 East 42nd Street
New York, NY 10017-5755

For Medical Information Contact:
24 hours a day, seven days a week:
(800) 438-1985

Distribution:
1855 Shelby Oaks Drive North
Memphis, TN 38134
(901) 387-5200
Customer Service:
(800) 533-4535

EXPORT INQUIRIES:
Pfizer International Inc.
(212) 573-2323
(See PFIZER INC.)

ROSS PRODUCTS DIVISION **2815**
Abbott Laboratories USA
Columbus, OH 43215-1724

Direct Inquiries to:
(800) 227-5767

Products Described:
Clear Eyes ACR Astringent/Lubricant Redness Reliever Eye Drops ... ⊙
Clear Eyes CLR Soothing Drops ... ⊙
Clear Eyes Lubricant Eye Redness Reliever Drops ... ⊙
Elecare Powder ... **2815**
Murine Ear Wax Removal System/Murine Ear Drops ... *2816*
Murine Tears Lubricant Eye Drops ... ⊙
Murine Tears Plus Lubricant Redness Reliever Eye Drops ... ⊙
Pediaflor Drops ... *2822*
Pedialyte Oral Electrolyte Maintenance Solution ... **2816**
PediaSure Complete Liquid Nutrition ... **2818**
Pediazole Suspension ... **2816**
Rehydralyte Oral Electrolyte Rehydration Solution ... **2819**
Ross Metabolic Formula System ... *2819*
Calcilo XD Low-Calcium/Vitamin D-Free Infant Formula With Iron ... *2819*
Cyclinex-1 Amino Acid-Modified Medical Food With Iron ... *2819*
Cyclinex-2 Amino Acid-Modified Medical Food ... *2819*
Flavonex Flavored Energy Supplement ... *2819*

Lotrimin Topical Solution 1% 2912
Lotrisone Cream 2912
◆Nasonex Nasal Spray 334, 2914
Nitro-Dur Transdermal Infusion
System 2916
◆Normodyne Injection 334, 2917
◆Normodyne Tablets 334, 2920
Proventil Inhalation Aerosol 2922
◆Proventil HFA Inhalation
Aerosol 334, 2929
Proventil Inhalation Solution
0.083% 2926
◆Proventil Repetabs Tablets 334, 2928
Proventil Solution for Inhalation
0.5% 2924
◆Proventil Tablets 334, 2928
Rebetron Combination Therapy 2932
Temodar Capsules 2936
Trilafon Injection 2939
◆Trilafon Tablets 334, 2939
◆Vancenase AQ Double
Strength Nasal Spray
0.084% 334, 2942
◆Vancenase PocketHaler Nasal
Inhaler 334, 2941
Vanceril Inhalation Aerosol 2944
◆Vanceril Double Strength
Inhalation Aerosol 334, 2945

Other Products Available:
Celestone Phosphate Injection
Celestone Syrup
Celestone Tablets
Chlor-Trimeton Injection
Diprosone Cream 0.05%
Diprosone Lotion 0.05%
Diprosone Ointment 0.05%
Estinyl Tablets
Fulvicin-U/F Tablets
Meticorten Tablets
Metimyd Ophthalmic Ointment--Sterile
Metimyd Ophthalmic Suspension--Sterile
Miradon Tablets
Naqua Tablets
Optimine Tablets
Oreton Methyl Buccal Tablets
Oreton Methyl Tablets
Otobiotic Otic Solution
Paxipam Tablets
Permitil Oral Concentrate
Permitil Tablets
Polaramine Expectorant
Polaramine Syrup
Polaramine Tablets
Polarmine Repetabs Tablets
Sebizon Lotion
Valisone Lotion 0.1%
Valisone Reduced Strength Cream .01%

SCHWARZ PHARMA, INC. 334, 2948

6140 W. Executive Drive
Mequon, WI 53092

For Medical Information Contact:
Professional Services
(262) 238-9994
(800) 558-5114

Products Described:
Calciferol Drops *2948*
Calciferol in Oil Injection *2948*
Colyte for Oral Solution *2948*
Colyte - Flavored for Oral Solution *2948*
◆Colyte with Flavor Packs for
Oral Solution 334, 2948
◆Cortifoam 335, 2949
Dilatrate-SR Capsules *2949*
◆Edex for Injection *335, 2950*
◆Epifoam *335, 2950*
Kutrase Capsules *2950*
Ku-Zyme Capsules *2950*
Ku-Zyme HP Capsules *2950*
Levatol Tablets *2950*
◆Levbid Extended-Release
Tablets 335, 2951
Levsin Drops 2951
Levsin Elixir 2951
Levsin Injection 2951
Levsin Tablets 2951
◆Levsin/SL Tablets 335, 2951
Levsinex Timecaps 2951
◆Monoket Tablets *335, 2952*
◆Nascobal Gel 335, 2952
Niferex Elixir 2954
Niferex Tablets 2954
◆Niferex-150 Capsules 335, 2954
◆Niferex-150 Forte Capsules 335, 2954
◆Niferex-PN Tablets 335, 2955
◆Niferex-PN Forte Tablets 335, 2955
◆proctoCream-HC 2.5% *335, 2955*
◆ProctoFoam-HC 335, 2955
◆Uniretic Tablets 335, 2956
◆Univasc Tablets 335, 2960
◆Verelan Capsules 335, 2962
◆Verelan PM Capsules 335, 2964

Other Products Available:
Codiclear DH Syrup
Codimal DH Syrup
Codimal DM Syrup
Codimal PH Syrup
Co-Gesic Tablets
Guaimax-D Extended-Release Tablets
Kudrox Suspension
Kutapressin Injection
Lactrase Capsules
Mono-Gesic Tablets
ProctoFoam-NS (Non-Steroid)

SCS PHARMACEUTICALS 2967

Box 5110
Chicago, IL 60680-5110

Direct Inquiries to:
(800) 821-7000

For Medical Information Contact:
Generally:
G.D. Searle & Co.
Healthcare Information Services
5200 Old Orchard Road
Skokie, IL 60077
In Emergencies:
Outside IL:
(800) 323-4204 (business hours)
(847) 982-7000 (at other times)
Within IL:
(847) 982-7000

Sales and Ordering:
(800) 821-7000

Products Described:
Flagyl I.V. 2967

Other Products Available:
Piroxicam Capsules USP

G.D. SEARLE & CO. 335, 2969

Box 5110
Chicago, IL 60680-5110

Direct Inquiries to:
(800) 821-7000

For Medical Information Contact:
Generally:
G.D. Searle & Co.
Healthcare Information Services
5200 Old Orchard Road
Skokie, IL 60077
In Emergencies:
Outside IL:
(800) 323-4204 (business hours)
(847) 982-7000 (at other times)
Within IL:
(847) 982-7000

Sales and Ordering:
(800) 821-7000

Products Described:
◆Aldactazide Tablets 335, 2969
◆Aldactone Tablets 335, 2971
◆Ambien Tablets 335, 2973
◆Arthrotec Tablets 335, 2977
◆Calan Tablets 335, 2981
◆Calan SR Caplets 335, 2983
◆Celebrex Capsules 335, 2985
◆Covera-HS Tablets 335, 2989
◆Cytotec Tablets 335, 2991
◆Daypro Caplets 335, 2993
◆Demulen 1/35-21 Tablets 335, 2995
◆Demulen 1/35-28 Tablets 335, 2995
◆Demulen 1/50-21 Tablets 335, 2995
◆Demulen 1/50-28 Tablets 335, 2995
◆Flagyl 375 Capsules 336, 3002
◆Flagyl ER Tablets 336, 3004
◆Kerlone Tablets 336, 3006
Lomotil Liquid 3008
◆Lomotil Tablets 336, 3008
◆Norpace Capsules 336, 3009
◆Norpace CR Capsules 336, 3009
Synarel Nasal Solution for Central
Precocious Puberty 3012
Synarel Nasal Solution for
Endometriosis 3013

Other Products Available:
Flagyl Tablets

SEPRACOR INC. 3493

111 Locke Drive
Marlborough, MA 01752

Direct Inquiries to:
Customer Service
877-SEPRACOR
FAX: (508) 357-7589

Products Described:
Xopenex Inhalation Solution 3493

SERONO LABORATORIES, INC. 336, 3015

100 Longwater Circle
Norwell, MA 02061
Internet: www.seronousa.com

Direct Inquiries to:
Customer Service, Sales and Ordering
(888) 398-4567
(781) 982-9000

For Medical Information or to Report Adverse Drug Experiences Contact:
Product Information and Surveillance
(888) 275-7376
(781) 982-9000 ext. 5562

Products Described:
Cetrotide for Injection 3015
Crinone 4% Gel 3018
◆Crinone 8% Gel 336, 3018
Fertinex for Injection 3020
Geref for Injection 3022
Gonal-F for Injection 3023
Pergonal for Injection 3027
Profasi for Injection 3028
Saizen for Injection 3029
Serophene Tablets 3030
Serostim for Injection 3032

Other Products Available:
Geref Diagnostic for Injection

SHIRE RICHWOOD INC.

(See SHIRE US INC.)

SHIRE US INC. 336, 3034

7900 Tanners Gate Drive
Suite 200
Florence, KY 41042

Direct Inquiries to:
Customer Service
(800) 536-7878
(859) 282-2100
FAX: (859) 282-2118

For Medical Information Contact:
(800) 536-7878

Products Described:
◆Adderall Tablets 336, 3034
◆Agrylin Capsules 336, 3035
◆Carbatrol Capsules 336, 3037
Colace Capsules, Syrup, Liquid 3039
◆DextroStat Tablets 336, 3039
◆Fareston Tablets 336, 3040
◆Pentasa Capsules 336, 3042
Peri-Colace Capsules and Syrup 3044
◆ProAmatine Tablets 336, 3044
Slow-Mag Tablets *3045*

SIGMA-TAU PHARMACEUTICALS, INC. 3045

800 South Frederick Avenue, Suite 300
Gaithersburg, MD 20877

Direct Inquiries to:
(301) 948-1041
(800) 447-0169
FAX: (301) 948-3194

Products Described:
Carnitor Injection 3045
Carnitor Tablets and Oral Solution 3048
Matulane Capsules 3049

SMITH & NEPHEW, INC. 336, 3050

11775 Starkey Road
Largo, FL 33773

Direct Inquiries to:
(800) 3-SANTYL
(800) 372-6895
(800) 876-1261
(727) 392-1261

Products Described:
◆Collagenase Santyl Ointment 336, 3050

SMITHKLINE BEECHAM CONSUMER HEALTHCARE, L.P. 3051

Unit of SmithKline Beecham Inc.
P.O. Box 1467
Pittsburgh, PA 15230

Direct Inquiries to:
Professional Services Department
(800) BEECHAM
PA Residents: (800) 242-1718

Products Described:
Debrox Drops .... ▣
Denavir Cream 3051
Ecotrin Enteric Coated Aspirin
Low, Regular and Maximum
Strength Tablets 3052
Feosol Caplets 3053
Feosol Tablets 3053
Gaviscon Regular Strength Antacid
Tablets .... ▣
Gaviscon Extra Strength Antacid
Tablets .... ▣
Gaviscon Regular Strength Liquid
Antacid .... ▣
Gaviscon Extra Strength Liquid
Antacid .... ▣
Gly-Oxide Liquid .... ▣
Massengill Douches, Towelettes and
Cleansing Wash .... ▣
Nicoderm CQ Patch 3054
Nicorette Gum 3056
Os-Cal 250 + D, 500, 500 + D, and 500
Chewable Tablets .... ▣
Singlet Tablets .... ▣
Tagamet HB 200 Liquid .... ▣
Tagamet HB 200 Tablets .... ▣
Tums Regular, Tums EX, and Tums
ULTRA Antacid/Calcium
Supplement Tablets .... ▣

SMITHKLINE BEECHAM PHARMACEUTICALS 336, 3058

One Franklin Plaza
P.O. Box 7929
Philadelphia, PA 19101

For Medical Information Contact:
Medical Department
(800) 366-8900, Ext. 5231

Products Described:
◆Albenza Tablets 336, 3058
◆Amoxil Capsules, Tablets and
Chewable Tablets 336, 3059
Amoxil Pediatric Drops, Powder
for Oral Suspension 3059
◆Ancef for Injection 336, 3063
◆Augmentin Powder for Oral
Suspension and Chewable
Tablets 336, 3065
◆Augmentin Tablets 336, 3068
◆Avandia Tablets 336, 3071
Bactroban Cream 3076
Bactroban Nasal 3076
Bactroban Ointment 3075
◆Compazine Multi-dose Vials 337, 3077
◆Compazine Spansule
Capsules 337, 3077
◆Compazine Suppositories 337, 3077
◆Compazine Syrup 337, 3077
◆Compazine Tablets 337, 3077
◆Compazine Vials 337, 3077
◆Coreg Tablets 337, 3080
◆Dexedrine Spansule Capsules 337, 3083
◆Dexedrine Tablets 337, 3083
◆Dyazide Capsules 337, 3085
◆Engerix-B 337, 3087
◆Eskalith Capsules 337, 3090
◆Eskalith CR Controlled
Release Tablets 337, 3090
◆Famvir Tablets 337, 3091
◆Havrix 337, 3094
◆Hycamtin for Injection 337, 3096
◆Infanrix 337, 3100
◆Kytril Injection 337, 3104
◆Kytril Tablets 337, 3106
◆LYMErix 337, 3108
◆Ornade Spansule Capsules 337, 3112
◆Parnate Tablets 337, 3113
Paxil Oral Suspension 3114
◆Paxil Tablets 337, 3114
◆Relafen Tablets 337, 3120
◆Requip Tablets 337, 3122
◆Stelazine Concentrate 337, 3127
◆Stelazine Multi-dose Vials 337, 3127
◆Stelazine Tablets 337, 3127
Tagamet Injection 3129
Tagamet Liquid 3129
◆Tagamet Tablets 337, 3129
Tazicef for Injection 3132
◆Thorazine Ampuls 337, 3135
◆Thorazine Multi-dose Vials 337, 3135
◆Thorazine Spansule Capsules 338, 3135
◆Thorazine Suppositories 338, 3135
◆Thorazine Syrup 338, 3135
◆Thorazine Tablets 337, 3135
◆Timentin for Injection 338, 3138

SMITHKLINE CONSUMER PRODUCTS

(See SMITHKLINE BEECHAM CONSUMER HEALTHCARE, L.P.)

SOLVAY PHARMACEUTICALS, INC. 338, 3141

901 Sawyer Road
Marietta, GA 30062
(770) 578-9000

For Medical Information Contact:
Generally:
Medical Information Department
(800) 241-1643
In Emergencies:
(770) 429-7110

Sales and Ordering:
Orders may be placed by calling this toll free number:
(800) 241-1643
FAX: (770) 578-5901
Ordernet access is available.
Mail orders should be sent to:
Solvay Pharmaceuticals
Order Entry Department
901 Sawyer Road
Marietta, GA 30062

Products Described:
◆Aceon Tablets (2 mg, 4 mg,
8 mg) 338, 3141
Cortenema 3143
◆Creon 5 Capsules 338, 3144
◆Creon 10 Capsules 338, 3144
◆Creon 20 Capsules 338, 3144
◆Estratab Tablets (0.3, 0.625,
2.5 mg) 338, 3145
◆Estratest Tablets 338, 3148
◆Estratest H.S. Tablets 338, 3148
◆Lithobid Slow-Release
Tablets 338, 3151
◆Luvox Tablets (25, 50,
100 mg) 338, 3153
◆Prometrium Capsules
(100 mg, 200 mg) 338, 3157
◆Rowasa Rectal Suspension
Enema 4.0 grams/unit
(60 mL) 338, 3160

Other Products Available:
Rowasa Suppository (500 mg)

SOMERSET PHARMACEUTICALS, INC. 338, 3162

2202 North Westshore Boulevard
Suite 450
Tampa, FL 33607

For Medical Information Contact:
Generally:
Professional Services Department
(813) 288-0040
FAX: (813) 282-0287
In Emergencies:
(800) 892-8889
FAX: (813) 282-0287

Products Described:
◆Eldepryl Capsules **338, 3162**

STAR PHARMACEUTICALS, INC. **3164**
1990 N.W. 44th Street
Pompano Beach, FL 33064-8712

Direct Inquiries to:
Scott L. Davidson, President
(954) 971-9704

Sales and Ordering:
(800) 845-7827
FAX: (954) 971-7718
Internet: http://www.starpharm.com

Products Described:
Aphrodyne Caplets **3164**
Prosed/DS Tablets **3164**
Uro-KP-Neutral Tablets **3165**
Urolene Blue Tablets *3165*
Virilon Capsules *3165*
Virilon IM Injection *3165*

STIEFEL LABORATORIES, INC. **3165**
255 Alhambra Circle
Coral Gables, FL 33134

BRANCH OFFICES:
Georgia
500 Satellite Blvd.
Suwanee, GA 30024
(770) 945-0101
Nevada
605 Boxington Way, Suite 107
Sparks, NV 89434
New York
Route 145
Oak Hill, NY 12460
(518) 239-6901

Direct Inquiries to:
Professional Services Department
(305) 443-3800

Products Described:
Brevoxyl-4 Cleansing Lotion **3166**
Brevoxyl-8 Cleansing Lotion **3166**
Brevoxyl-4 Creamy Wash **3166**
Brevoxyl-8 Creamy Wash **3166**
Brevoxyl-4 Gel **3165**
Brevoxyl-8 Gel **3165**
Clindets Pledgets **3166**
Clobevate Gel **3167**
LactiCare-HC Lotion, 1% *3168*
LactiCare-HC Lotion, 2½% *3168*
PanOxyl 5 Acne Gel *3168*
PanOxyl 10 Acne Gel *3168*
PanOxyl AQ 2½ Acne Gel *3168*
PanOxyl AQ 5 Acne Gel *3168*
PanOxyl AQ 10 Acne Gel *3168*
Sulfoxyl Lotion Regular *3168*
Sulfoxyl Lotion Strong *3168*

Other Products Available:
Benoxyl-10 Lotion
Brasivol Base
Brasivol Medium
Brasivol Rough
Epilyt Lotion
LactiCare Lotion
Oilatum-AD Soap Free Cleanser
Oilatum Cleansing Bar (Scented)
Oilatum Cleansing Bar (Unscented)
PanOxyl Bar 10
Polytar Shampoo
Polytar Soap
Salicylic Acid & Sulfur Soap
Salicylic Acid Cleansing Bar
Sarna Lotion
SAStid Soap
SFC Lotion
Sulfur Soap
Zeasorb Powder
Zeasorb-AF Lotion/Powder
Zeasorb-AF Powder
ZNP Bar

SUPERGEN, INC. **3168**
1059 Serpentine Lane
Pleasanton, CA 94566

Direct Inquiries to:
Corporate Headquarters
(800) 353-1075
FAX: (925) 327-7347

For Medical Information Contact:
Generally:
Medical Affairs Department
(888) 43-SUPER
(888) 437-8737
FAX: (888) 437-8454
In Emergencies:
(415) 487-8441

Sales and Ordering:
Nipent: (800) 222-6883
Mitomycin: (800) 905-5474

Products Described:
Mitomycin for Injection, USP *3168*
Nipent for Injection **3168**

SWISS BIOCEUTICAL INTERNATIONAL, LTD. **3171**
2533 No. Carson Street, Suite 3573
Carson City, NV 89706

Direct Inquiries to:
Executive Director
(775) 841-7020
FAX: (775) 883-2384
Internet: www.imuplus.com

Products Described:
IMUPlus Formula **3171**

TAKEDA PHARMACEUTICALS AMERICA, INC. **338, 3171**
475 Half Day Road, Suite 500
Lincolnshire, IL 60069

Direct Inquiries to:
Sales and Ordering:
Customer Service
(877) 5 TAKEDA
(877) 582-5332

For Medical Information Contact:
Generally:
(877) TAKEDA 7
(877) 825-3327
Adverse Drug Experiences:
(877) TAKEDA 7
(877) 825-3327

Products Described:
◆Actos Tablets **338, 3171**

TAP PHARMACEUTICALS INC. **338, 3175**
675 N. Field Drive
Lake Forest, IL 60045

Direct Inquiries to:
Customer Service
(800) 621-1020

For Medical Information Contact:
Medical Department:
(800) 622-2011 (LUPRON)
(800) 478-9526 (PREVACID)
In Emergencies:
(800) 622-2011 (LUPRON)
(800) 478-9526 (PREVACID)

Products Described:
◆Lupron Depot 3.75 mg **338, 3178**
◆Lupron Depot 7.5 mg **338, 3180**
◆Lupron Depot--3 Month 11.25 mg **338, 3182**
◆Lupron Depot--3 Month 22.5 mg **338, 3184**
◆Lupron Depot--4 Month 30 mg **338, 3186**
Lupron Depot-PED 7.5 mg, 11.25 mg and 15 mg **3187**
◆Lupron Injection **338, 3175**
Lupron Injection Pediatric **3177**
◆Prevacid Delayed-Release Capsules **338, 3189**
◆PREVPAC **338, 3194**

TEVA MARION PARTNERS **338, 3198**
10450 B. Hickman Mills Dr.
Kansas City, MO 64137

Direct Inquiries to:
(816) 966-3977

Products Described:
◆Copaxone for Injection **338, 3198**

THER-Rx CORPORATION **338, 3202**
13622 Lakefront Drive
St. Louis, MO 63045

Direct Inquiries to:
(314) 209-1517
FAX: (314) 770-0371

Products Described:
◆Gynazole-1 Vaginal Cream **338, 3202**
◆Micro-K Extencaps **338, 3203**
◆Micro-K 10 Extencaps **338, 3203**
◆PreCare Chewable Tablets **338, 3204**
◆PreCare Conceive Tablets **338, 3205**
◆PreCare Prenatal Caplets **338, 3204**
◆PremesisRx Tablets **338, 3205**

UAD LABORATORIES
(See FOREST PHARMACEUTICALS, INC.)

UCB PHARMA, INC. **338, 3205**
1950 Lake Park Drive
Smyrna, GA 30080

Direct Inquiries to:
(800) 477-7877

For Medical Information Contact:
Medical Affairs Department
24 hours a day, seven days a week:
(800) 477-7877

Products Described:
◆Duratuss DM Elixir *338, 3206*
◆Duratuss G Tablets *338, 3205*
◆Duratuss HD Elixir *338, 3206*
◆Duratuss Tablets *338, 3205*
◆Duratuss GP Tablets **338, 3205**
◆Keppra Tablets **339, 3206**
◆Lortab 2.5/500 Tablets **339, 3209**
◆Lortab 5/500 Tablets **339, 3209**
◆Lortab 7.5/500 Tablets **339, 3209**
◆Lortab 10/500 Tablets **339, 3209**
◆Lortab Elixir **339, 3209**
◆Theo-24 Extended Release Capsules **339, 3211**
◆Trinsicon Capsules *339, 3216*
◆Vicon Forte Capsules *339, 3217*

Other Products Available:
Corticaine Cream
Vicon-C Capsules
Vi-Zac Capsules

UNIMED PHARMACEUTICALS, INC. **339, 3217**
A Solvay Pharmaceuticals, Inc. Company
4 Parkway North
Deerfield, IL 60015

Direct Inquiries to:
(847) 282-5400
(800) 541-3492
FAX: (847) 374-8480

Products Described:
◆Anadrol-50 Tablets **339, 3217**
◆AndroGel **339, 3218**
◆Marinol Capsules **339, 3220**
◆Maxaquin Tablets **339, 3222**
◆Teveten Tablets **339, 3225**

THE UPJOHN COMPANY
(See PHARMACIA & UPJOHN)

UPSHER-SMITH LABORATORIES, INC. **339, 3228**
14905 23rd Avenue North
Minneapolis, MN 55447

For Medical Information Contact:
Write: Professional Services Department
or call: (800) 654-2299
(during business hours-8 a.m. to 5 p.m. CST)

Products Described:
Altinac Cream *3228*
Folgard Tablets *3228*
Klor-Con/EF Tablets *3228*
◆Klor-Con 8/Klor-Con 10 Tablets *339, 3228*
Klor-Con Powder *3228*
Klor-Con/25 Powder *3228*
Niacor Tablets *3228*
◆Pacerone Tablets **339, 3228**
Pentoxil Tablets *3232*
Prevalite Powder *3232*
RMS Suppositories CII *3232*
◆Slo-Niacin Tablets *339, 3232*
SSKI Solution *3232*

Other Products Available:
Alterra (St. John's Wort) Tablets
Bisacodyl Uniserts Suppositories
Feratab Tablets
Ferrous Gluconate Tablets
Hemorrhoidal-HC Uniserts Suppositories (Hemril-HC)
Hemril-30
Provol (pygeum africanum) Capsules
Sorbitol Solution
Stress-600 with Zinc Tablets
Therapeutic B Complex with Vitamin C Capsules
Therapeutic Multivitamin Tablets
Therapeutic Multivitamin with Minerals Tablets
Zinc Sulfate Capsules

U.S. PHARMACEUTICAL CORPORATION **3232**
2401-C Mellon Court
Decatur, GA 30035
(800) 330-3040
FAX: (404) 987-4806

MAILING ADDRESS:
2401-C Mellon Court
Decatur, GA 30035

Direct Inquiries to:
Peter J. Krebs, Ph.D.
CEO, Management Unit
(800) 330-3040, or
Clayton W. Bishop
National Sales Manager
(512) 847-3357 or
(800) 330-3040

Products Described:
Cenogen-OB Capsules *3232*
Hemocyte Tablets *3232*
Hemocyte Plus Tabules *3232*
Hemocyte-F Elixir *3232*
Hemocyte-F Tablets *3232*
Magsal Tablets *3232*
Medigesic Capsules *3233*
Mediplex Ultra Tabules *3233*
Norel DM Liquid *3233*
Norel Plus Capsules *3233*

USANA, INCORPORATED **339, 3233**
3838 West Parkway Boulevard
Salt Lake City, UT 84120-6336

Direct Inquiries to:
Technical Services Department
(801) 954-7860
FAX: (801) 954-7658

Products Described:
◆Active Calcium Tablets **339, 3233**
◆Chelated Mineral Tablets **339, 3233**
◆CoQuinone Capsules **339, 3233**
◆Mega Antioxidant Tablets **339, 3233**
◆Proflavanol Tablets **339, 3233**

VITALINE CORPORATION **3234**
385 Williamson Way
Ashland, OR 97520

Direct Inquiries to:
Jed D. Meese, Technical Director
(800) 648-4755
(541) 482-9231
FAX: (541) 482-9112
E-mail: jmeese@vitaline.com

Products Described:
Coenzyme Q10 200mg, 100mg & 60mg Chewable Wafers, 200mg, 60mg and 25mg Tablets, and 60mg Softgels **3234**
L-Carnitine USP 500mg Chewable Wafers, 250mg Tablets, 500mg Caplets, and 500mg Capsules **3234**

Other Products Available:
Alka-Aid (antacid)
Antioxidant Formula (Advanced)
B-Complex "50" Regular and Controlled Time Release
B-Complex "100" Regular and Controlled Time Release
Betazyme (Betaine HCl)
Biotin Forte 3mg
Biotin Forte 5mg
Boron 6mg
Bromelain 500mg
Cal-Carb Forte (500mg elemental calcium)
Calcium Citrate 250mg
Cal-Mag Aspartate
Catalytic Formula (proteolytic enzymes)
Cellasorb
Chromium GTF 1mg
Chromium Picolinate 200 and 500mcg
CV Co-Factors
Digestive Enzymes
E-Pherol (d-alpha tocopherol) 400 I.U.
Echinacea 125mg/Goldenseal 125mg
Enviro-Stress
Folic Acid/B12 Powder
Free Form Amino Acid Complex
Garlic Forte 3
Ginkgo Biloba Plus
Glucosamine Sulfate 500mg with Chondroitin Sulfate 200mg
Herbal Antioxidant Formula with Pycnogenol
Herbal-Boost
K-Mag Aspartate (potassium & magnesium)
L-Glutamine with Choline and Inositol
L-Lysine HCl 1000mg
Manganese 15mg
Marine Lipid Concentrate 1200mg
Maximum Formula Red, Blue and Green (multivitamin-multimineral)
Melatonin Forte 3mg with Kava Kava
Multimineral Plus Advanced Formula
N-Acetylcysteine 500mg
Neuro-Essentials
Ox-Absorb
Pancreatin 4X 600mg
Pancreatin 8X 900mg
Pantothenic Acid 500mg
Pros-Forte
Proteolytic Formula (proteolytic enzymes)
Renal Multivitamin Formula
Renal Multivitamin Formula plus Iron
Renal Multivitamin Formula with Zinc
Resveratrol Forte (grape seed and grape skin extracts)
SAMe 200mg (S-Adenosyl L-Methionine)
Selenium 200mcg
Sharper Focus
St. John's Wort 300mg
Superoxide Dismutase
Thymus 200
Total Formula 1, 2 and 3 (multivitamin-multimineral)
Veg-Pancreatin 4X (vegetarian pancreatin)
Vita-Calcium (calcium and vitamin D)
Vita-Mag (magnesium 400mg)
Vitamin A 10,000 I.U.
Vitamin B-6 Controlled Time Release 200mg
Vitamin B-12 2500mcg Sublingual Tablets
Vitamin C 1000mg Controlled Time Release
Vitamin C 1000mg with Citrus Bioflavonoids
Vitamin C Buffered Powder
Vitamin D3 400 I.U.
Vitamin E 400 I.U. Softgels
Zinc-220 (50mg elemental zinc)

VIVUS, INC. **339, 3234**
1172 Castro Street
Mountain View, CA 94040

Direct Inquiries to:
(888) 345-6873

For Medical Information or Emergencies Contact:
Medical Services Department @ VIVUS:
(650) 934-5200
FAX: (650) 934-5389

Products Described:
◆MUSE Urethral Suppository ... **339, 3234**

WAKEFIELD PHARMACEUTICALS, INC. 3237

310 Maxwell Road, Suite 100
Alpharetta, GA 30004

Direct Inquiries to:
(770) 664-1661
FAX: (770) 664-1126

Products Described:
Biohist LA Tablets ... *3237*
Muco-fen 800 Tablets ... *3237*
Muco-fen 800 DM Tablets ... *3237*
Profen II Tablets ... *3237*
Profen II DM Liquid ... *3237*
Profen II DM Tablets ... *3238*
Profen Forte Tablets ... *3238*
Profen Forte DM Tablets ... *3238*

Other Products Available:
Muco-fen 1200 Tablets
Muco-fen DM Tablets
Muco-fen LA Tablets
Profen LA Tablets

WAKUNAGA CONSUMER PRODUCTS 343, 3238

23501 Madero
Mission Viejo, CA 92691

Direct Inquiries to:
(800) 527-5200

Products Described:
◆Kyolic Caplets ... **343, 3238**
◆Probiata Tablets ... **343, 3238**

WALLACE LABORATORIES 339, 3238

P.O. Box 1001
Cranbury, NJ 08512

For Medical Information Contact:
Generally:
Professional Services
(800) 526-3840
After Hours and Weekend Emergencies:
(609) 655-6474

Sales and Ordering:
Wallace Laboratories
Div. of Carter-Wallace, Inc.
P.O. Box 1001
Cranbury, NJ 08512

Products Described:
Aquatensen Tablets ... *3238*
◆Astelin Nasal Spray ... **339, 3238**
Depen Titratable Tablets ... **3239**
Diutensen-R Tablets ... *3242*
◆Felbatol Oral Suspension ... **339, 3242**
◆Felbatol Tablets ... **339, 3242**
Lufyllin Elixir ... *3246*
Lufyllin Tablets ... **3246**
Lufyllin-400 Tablets ... **3246**
Lufyllin-GG Elixir ... **3246**
Lufyllin-GG Tablets ... **3246**
Maltsupex Powder, Liquid, Tablets ... ▣
Miltown Tablets ... **3247**
◆Organidin NR Liquid ... **339, 3248**
◆Organidin NR Tablets ... **339, 3248**
Ryna Liquid ... ▣
Ryna-C Liquid ... ▣
◆Ryna-12 S Suspension ... **339, 3249**
◆Rynatan Tablets ... **339, 3249**
◆Rynatan-P Pediatric Suspension ... **339, 3251**
◆Rynatuss Tablets ... **339, 3251**
◆Rynatuss Pediatric Suspension ... **339, 3251**
◆Soma Tablets ... **339, 3252**
◆Soma Compound Tablets ... **339, 3252**
◆Soma Compound w/Codeine Tablets ... **339, 3253**
◆Tussi-12 Suspension ... **339, 3254**
◆Tussi-12 Tablets ... **339, 3254**
Tussi-Organidin NR Liquid ... **3248**
Tussi-Organidin DM NR Liquid ... **3248**
◆Tussi-Organidin DM-S NR Liquid ... **340, 3248**
◆Tussi-Organidin-S NR Liquid ... **340, 3248**
VōSoL HC Otic Solution ... **3255**

Other Products Available:
Barbidonna Tablets
Butibel Elixir & Tablets
Butisol Sodium Elixir
Butisol Sodium Tablets
Doral Tablets
Lufyllin-EPG Tablets
Micrainin Tablets
Syllact Powder
Vascor Tablets (See Ortho-McNeil Pharmaceutical, Inc.)
VōSoL Otic Solution

WARNER CHILCOTT LABORATORIES 3255

Rockaway 80 Corporate Center
100 Enterprise Drive
Suite 280
Rockaway, NJ 07866

Direct Inquiries to:
(800) 521-8813

For Product or Medical Information Contact:
(800) 521-8813
(973) 442-3236

For After Hours and Weekend Emergencies Contact:
(303) 739-1110

Products Described:
Choledyl SA Extended-Release Tablets ... *3255*
Doryx Coated Pellet Filled Capsules ... **3255**
Eryc Delayed-Release Capsules ... *3255*
Estrace Vaginal Cream ... **3256**
Mandelamine Tablets ... *3255*
NataChew Tablets ... **3259**
NataFort Tablets ... *3255*
Ovcon 35 Tablets ... **3259**
Ovcon 50 Tablets ... **3259**
Pyridium Tablets ... *3255*
Pyridium Plus Tablets ... *3255*

WARNER-LAMBERT CONSUMER GROUP OF PFIZER INC. 3265

182 Tabor Road
Morris Plains, NJ 07950

For Medical Information and Emergencies Contact:
Consumer Relations Group
(800) 723-7529
FAX: (973) 385-6667

Products Described:
Bonine Chewable Tablets ... **3265**
Maximum Strength Unisom SleepGels ... **3265**
Unisom SleepTabs ... **3265**

WARNER-LAMBERT CONSUMER HEALTHCARE 3265

201 Tabor Road
Morris Plains, NJ 07950

Direct Inquiries and For Medical Information Contact:
Consumer Affairs
1-(800) 223-0182

Products Described:
Actifed Cold & Allergy Tablets ... *3265*
Actifed Cold & Sinus Caplets ... *3265*
Anusol HC-1 Ointment ... *3265*
Anusol Hemorrhoidal Ointment ... *3265*
Anusol Hemorrhoidal Suppositories ... *3265*
Benadryl Allergy Chewables ... *3265*
Benadryl Allergy Kapseal Capsules ... *3265*
Benadryl Allergy Liquid Medication ... *3266*
Benadryl Allergy Ultratab Tablets ... *3265*
Benadryl Allergy/Cold Tablets ... *3265*
Benadryl Allergy/Congestion Liquid Medication ... *3265*
Benadryl Allergy/Congestion Tablets ... *3265*
Benadryl Allergy/Sinus Headache Caplets & Gelcaps ... *3266*
Benadryl Dye-Free Allergy Liquid Medication ... *3266*
Benadryl Dye-Free Allergy Liqui-gels Softgel ... *3266*
Benadryl Itch Relief Stick Extra Strength ... *3266*
Benadryl Itch Stopping Cream Original and Extra Strength ... *3266*
Benadryl Itch Stopping Gel Original and Extra Strength ... *3266*
Benadryl Itch Stopping Spray Original and Extra Strength ... *3266*
Benylin Adult Formula ... *3266*
Benylin Expectorant ... *3266*
Benylin Multi Symptom ... *3266*
Benylin Pediatric ... *3266*
Caladryl Clear Lotion ... *3266*
Caladryl Cream For Kids ... *3266*
Caladryl Lotion ... *3266*
Listerine Antiseptic ... *3266*
Tartar Control Listerine Antiseptic ... *3266*
Cool Mint Listerine ... *3266*
FreshBurst Listerine ... *3266*
Listermint Alcohol-Free Mouthwash ... *3266*
Lubriderm Daily UV Lotion with Sunscreen ... *3266*
Neosporin + Pain Relief Maximum Strength Cream ... *3266*
Neosporin + Pain Relief Maximum Strength Ointment ... *3266*
Neosporin Ointment ... *3266*
Nix Creme Rinse ... *3266*
Nix Lice Control Spray ... *3266*
Polysporin Ointment ... *3266*
Polysporin Powder ... *3266*
Sinutab Sinus Allergy Medication MS Tablets and Caplets ... *3266*
Sinutab Sinus Medication MS Without Drowsiness Tablets and Caplets ... *3266*
Sinutab Non-Drying Liquid Caps ... *3266*
Sudafed 12 Hour Tablets ... *3266*
Sudafed 24 Hour Tablets ... *3266*
Children's Sudafed Cough & Cold Liquid ... *3267*
Children's Sudafed Nasal Decongestant Chewables ... *3267*
Children's Sudafed Nasal Decongestant Liquid ... *3267*
Sudafed Cold & Allergy Tablets ... *3266*
Sudafed Cold & Cough Liquid Caps ... *3266*
Sudafed Cold & Sinus Liquid Caps ... *3267*
Sudafed Nasal Decongestant 30 mg Tablets ... *3267*
Sudafed Non-Drying Sinus Liquid Caps ... *3267*
Sudafed Severe Cold Formula MS Caplets and Tablets ... *3267*
Sudafed Sinus MS Caplets and Tablets ... *3267*
Tucks Pre-moistened Hemorrhoidal/Vaginal Pads ... *3267*
Tucks Take Alongs Towelettes ... *3267*
Zantac 75 ... *3267*

WATSON LABORATORIES, INC. 340, 3267

311 Bonnie Circle
Corona, CA 92880

Direct Inquiries to:
Customer Service Department
(800) 272-5525
FAX: (909) 735-2871

For Medical Information Contact:
(800) 272-5525
FAX: (909) 737-8540

Products Described:
Acebutolol Hydrochloride Capsules ... *3267*
Acetaminophen and Codeine Phosphate Tablets, USP CIII ... *3267*
Acyclovir Tablets, USP ... *3267*
Alora Transdermal System ... **3269**
Alprazolam Tablets, USP CIV ... *3267*
Amiloride HCl and HCTZ Tablets, USP ... *3267*
Amoxapine Tablets, USP ... *3267*
Androderm Transdermal System CIII ... **3274**
Baclofen Tablets, USP ... *3267*
◆Brevicon 28-Day Tablets ... **340, 3276**
Butalbital, Aspirin, Caffeine, and Codeine Phosphate Capsules, USP CIII ... *3267*
Butalbital, Acetaminophen, and Caffeine Tablets, USP ... *3267*
Captopril Tablets, USP ... *3267*
Carisoprodol Tablets ... *3267*
Chlordiazepoxide Hydrochloride Capsules CIV ... *3267*
Chlorzoxazone Tablets, USP ... *3267*
Clomiphene Citrate Tablets ... *3267*
Clomipramine Hydrochloride Capsules ... *3267*
Clonazepam Tablets, USP CIV ... *3267*
Clorazepate Dipotassium Tablets CIV ... *3267*
Cyclobenzaprine Hydrochloride Tablets, USP ... *3267*
Desipramine Hydrochloride Tablets ... *3267*
Diclofenac Potassium Tablets ... *3267*
Diclofenac Sodium Delayed Release Tablets, USP ... *3267*
Dicyclomine Hydrochloride Capsules ... *3267*
Dicyclomine Hydrochloride Tablets ... *3267*
Diethylpropion Hydrochloride Tablets CIV ... *3267*
Diethylpropion Hydrochloride Extended Release Tablets CIV ... *3267*
Diltiazem Extended Release Capsules ... *3267*
Diltiazem Hydrochloride Tablets ... *3267*
Doxepin Hydrochloride Capsules, USP ... *3267*
Estazolam Tablets CIV ... *3267*
Estradiol Tablets, USP ... *3267*
Estropipate Tablets, USP ... *3267*
Ethynodiol Diacetate and Ethinyl Estradiol Tablets, USP (ZOVIA) ... *3269*
Etodolac Capsules ... *3267*
Etodolac Tablets ... *3267*
Furosemide Tablets, USP ... *3267*
Glipizide Tablets, USP ... *3267*
Guanabenz Acetate Tablets, USP ... *3267*
Guanfacine Hydrochloride Tablets, USP ... *3267*
Hydrocodone Bitartrate and APAP Tablets, USP CIII ... *3267*
Hydroxychloroquine Sulfate Tablets, USP ... *3267*
Hydroxyzine Hydrochloride Tablets, USP ... *3267*
Hydroxyzine Pamoate Capsules ... *3267*
Indapamide Tablets, USP ... *3267*
Ketorolac Tromethamine Tablets, USP ... *3267*
Labetalol HCl Tablets ... *3267*
◆Levora Tablets ... **340, 3282**
Lorazepam Tablets, USP CIV ... *3267*
◆Low-Ogestrel-28 Tablets ... **340, 3285**
Loxapine Capsules, USP ... *3267*
◆Loxitane Capsules ... **340, 3291**
Loxitane C Oral Concentrate ... **3291**
Loxitane IM ... **3291**
Maprotiline Hydrochloride Tablets, USP ... *3267*
Meclizine Hydrochloride Tablets ... *3267*
Meperidine Hydrochloride Tablets, USP CII ... *3267*
Meprobamate Tablets CIV ... *3267*
Methocarbamol Tablets ... *3267*
Methylprednisolone Tablets ... *3267*
Metoprolol Tartrate Tablets, USP ... *3267*
Mexiletine Hydrochloride Capsules, USP ... *3267*
◆Microzide Capsules ... **340, 3292**
Naproxen Sodium Tablets ... *3267*
Naproxen Tablets ... *3267*
◆Necon 0.5/35 Tablets ... **340, 3294**
◆Necon 1/35 Tablets ... **340, 3294**
◆Necon 1/50 Tablets ... **340, 3294**
◆Necon 10/11 Tablets ... **340, 3294**
◆Norco Tablets CIII ... **340, 3303**
◆Norinyl 1 + 35 28-Day Tablets ... **340, 3276**
◆Norinyl 1 + 50 28-Day Tablets ... **340, 3276**
◆Nor-QD Tablets ... **340, 3301**
Ogestrel 0.5/50-28 Tablets ... **3304**
Oxybutynin Chloride Tablets ... *3267*
Oxycodone and Acetaminophen Capsules, USP CII ... *3267*
Oxycodone and Acetaminophen Tablets, USP CII ... *3267*
Oxycodone and Aspirin Tablets, USP CII ... *3267*
Oxycodone Hydrochloride Tablets, USP CII ... *3267*
Pentazocine and Naloxone HCl Tablets, USP CIV ... *3267*
Perphenazine/Amitriptyline Hydrochloride Tablets, USP ... *3267*
Piroxicam Capsules, USP ... *3267*
Prednisone Tablets ... *3267*
Propoxyphene Hydrochloride and Acetaminophen Tablets, USP CIV ... *3267*
Propranolol Hydrochloride Tablets, USP ... *3267*
Quinine Sulfate Capsules, USP ... *3267*
Quinine Sulfate Tablets, USP ... *3267*
Ranitidine Tablets ... *3267*
Selegiline HCl Capsules ... *3267*
Selegiline HCl Tablets ... *3267*
Silver Sulfadiazine Cream ... *3267*
Sucralfate Tablets ... *3267*
Sulfasalazine Tablets ... *3267*
Triamterene and Hydrochlorothiazide Tablets, USP ... *3267*
Trihexyphenidyl HCl Tablets, USP ... *3267*
◆Tri-Norinyl-28 Tablets ... **340, 3309**
◆Trivora Tablets ... **340, 3315**
Valproic Acid Syrup ... *3267*
Verapamil Hydrochloride Tablets, USP ... *3267*
Yohimbine Hydrochloride Tablets ... *3267*
◆Zovia 1/35E Tablets ... **340, 3318**
◆Zovia 1/50E Tablets ... **340, 3318**

Other Products Available:
Sotalol Hydrochloride Tablets

WE PHARMACEUTICALS, INC. 3322

P.O. Box 1142
Ramona, CA 92065

Direct Inquiries to:
(760) 788-9155

For Medical Emergencies Contact:
(760) 788-9155

Products Described:
Ah-Chew Chewable Tablets ... *3322*
Ah-Chew D Chewable Tablets ... *3322*
D-Feda II Tablets ... *3322*
E-Z Spacer ... *3322*
E-Z Spacer and Mask ... *3322*
E-Z Spacer Mask ... *3322*
Omnihist L.A. Tablets ... *3322*
Prednisolone Syrup, USP ... *3322*
Sinuvent Tablets ... *3322*
Ultrabrom Capsules ... *3322*
Ultrabrom PD Capsules ... *3322*

WELLSPRING PHARMACEUTICAL CORPORATION 3322

172 County Route 537 E
Colts Neck, NJ 07722

Direct Inquiries to:
(732) 460-9788

Products Described

Products Described:
Dibenzyline Capsules ... **3322**
Dyrenium Capsules ... **3323**

WESTLAKE LABORATORIES, INC. 3324

24700 Center Ridge Road
Cleveland, OH 44145
Internet: www.westlake-labs.com

Direct Inquiries to:
Customer Service
(888) WSTLAKE (978-5253)
FAX: (440) 835-2177

For Medical Information Contact:
Customer Service
(888) WSTLAKE (978-5253)
FAX: (440) 835-2177

Products Described:
Bevitamel Tablets ... **3324**

Other Products Available:
Bona-Bacillus Capsules
Coenzyme Q-10 Chewable Tablets
GFS-2000 Capsules
Glutanac Capsules
Nutrision Capsules
Nutrisure OTC Tablets
Pantethine Capsules

Phosphatidyl-Serine Capsules
Total-E Softgels
Ultra G.I. Capsules
Ultra-Carotenoids Capsules
Ultra-Lipoic Forte Capsules
Uro-Pro Capsules

WESTWOOD-SQUIBB PHARMACEUTICALS, INC. 3324
A Bristol-Myers Squibb Company
100 Forest Avenue
Buffalo, NY 14213
(716) 887-3400

For Medical Information Contact:
Generally:
Consumer Affairs Department
1-(800) 494-7258
Adverse Drug Experiences
and Product Defects Reporting
call during business hours only:
1-(800) 494-7258

Products Described:
Dovonex Cream 0.005%.......... **3324**
Dovonex Ointment 0.005%.......... **3325**
Dovonex Scalp Solution 0.005%..... **3326**
Lac-Hydrin 12% Cream.......... **3326**
Lac-Hydrin 12% Lotion.......... **3327**
Ultravate Cream 0.05%.......... **3327**
Ultravate Ointment 0.05%.......... **3328**

Other Products Available:
Balnetar
Capitrol Shampoo
Desquam-E 2.5 Emollient Gel
Desquam-E 5 Emollient Gel
Desquam-E 10 Emollient Gel
Desquam-X 10 Bar
Desquam-X 5 Gel
Desquam-X 10 Gel
Desquam-X 5 Wash
Desquam-X 10 Wash
Estar Gel
Eurax Cream
Eurax Lotion
Exelderm Cream 1.0%
Exelderm Solution 1.0%
Fostril
Halog Cream 0.1%
Halog Ointment 0.1%
Halog Solution 0.1%
Halog-E Cream 0.1%
Lac-Hydrin Five Lotion
Lowila Cake
Maxivate Cream, Lotion & Ointment 0.05%
Moisturel Cream
Moisturel Lotion
Moisturel Sensitive Skin Cleanser
Mycostatin Cream
Mycostatin Topical Powder
Pernox Scrub Cleanser
PreSun Sensitive Sunblock 28
PreSun Ultra Cream 15
PreSun Ultra Gel 15
PreSun Ultra Gel 30
PreSun Ultra Spray 27
Sebulex Dandruff Shampoo
Sebulex Dandruff Shampoo with Conditioners
Sebulon Shampoo
Sebutone Tar Shampoo
T-Stat 2.0% Topical Solution and Pads
Westcort Cream 0.2%
Westcort Ointment 0.2%

WOMEN FIRST HEALTHCARE, INC. 341, 3329
12220 El Camino Real
Suite 400
San Diego, CA 92130

Direct Inquiries to:
(888) 796-6361
FAX: (888) 509-0853

Products Described:
Esclim Transdermal System.......... **3329**
◆Ortho-Est Tablets.......... **341, 3333**

WYETH-AYERST PHARMACEUTICALS 341, 3336
Division of American Home Products Corporation
P.O. Box 8299
Philadelphia, PA 19101

Direct Inquiries to:
(610) 688-4400

For Medical Information Contact:
Medical Affairs
Day: (800) 934-5556 (8:30 AM to 4:30 PM, Eastern Standard Time, Weekdays only)
In Emergencies:
Day: (800) 934-5556 (8:30 AM to 4:30 PM, Eastern Standard Time, Weekdays only)
Night: (610) 688-4400 (Emergencies only; non-emergencies should wait until the next day)

Manufacturing and Distribution:
(Do not use freight addresses for mailing of orders.)

Atlanta, GA--
P.O. Box 1773
Paoli, PA 19301-1773
(800) 666-7248
Freight address:
1000 Union Court
Kennesaw, GA 30144
Mail DEA order forms to:
P.O. Box 4365
Atlanta, GA 30302-4365
Chicago, IL--
P.O. Box 1773
Paoli, PA 19301-1773
(800) 666-7248
Freight address:
248 Lies Road
Carol Stream, IL 60188
Mail DEA order forms to:
P.O. Box 140
Wheaton, IL 60189-0140
Dallas, TX--
P.O. Box 1773
Paoli, PA 19301-1773
(800) 666-7248
Freight address:
11240 Petal Street
Dallas, TX 75238
Mail DEA order forms to:
P.O. Box 650231
Dallas, TX 75265-0231
Philadelphia, PA--
P.O. Box 1773
Paoli, PA 19301-1773
(800) 666-7248
Freight address:
31 Morehall Road
Frazer, PA 19355
Mail DEA order forms to:
P.O. Box 61
Paoli, PA 19301
Sparks, NV--
P.O. Box 1773
Paoli, PA 19301-1773
(800) 666-7248
Freight address:
1802 Brierley Way
Sparks, NV 89434
Mail DEA order forms to:
1802 Brierley Way
Sparks, NV 89434
San Juan, Puerto Rico--
GPO Box 362917
San Juan, PR 00936
(800) 462-4748
Freight address:
Wyeth-Ayerst Laboratories P.R. Inc.
Amelia Industrial Center
Street D
Lots 32-35
Guaynabo, Puerto Rico 00968
Mail DEA order forms to:
GPO Box 362917
San Juan, PR 00936-2917

Products Described:
◆Alesse-21 Tablets.......... **341, 3337**
◆Alesse-28 Tablets.......... **341, 3342**
◆Amphojel Suspension.......... **341, 3342**
◆Antabuse Tablets.......... **341, 3343**
Antivenin (Micrurus fulvius).......... *3344*
A.P.L.......... *3344*
Ativan Injection.......... **3344**
◆Ativan Tablets.......... **341, 3348**
Ativan in Tubex.......... *3465*
◆Atromid-S Capsules.......... **341, 3349**
Auralgan Otic Solution.......... **3351**
Bicillin C-R 900/300 in Tubex.......... *3465*
Bicillin C-R in Tubex.......... *3465*
Bicillin L-A in Tubex.......... *3465*
Cardene I.V.......... **3351**
Cholera Vaccine.......... **3353**
Codeine Phosphate in Tubex.......... *3465*
Cordarone Intravenous.......... **3357**
◆Cordarone Tablets.......... **341, 3354**
Digoxin in Tubex.......... *3465*
Dimenhydrinate in Tubex.......... *3465*
Diphenhydramine Hydrochloride in Tubex.......... *3465*
◆Diucardin Tablets.......... **341, 3360**
◆Effexor Tablets.......... **341, 3361**
◆Effexor XR Capsules.......... **341, 3365**
Enbrel for Injection.......... **3370**
Epinephrine in Tubex.......... *3465*
Equagesic Tablets.......... *3373*
Equanil Tablets.......... *3373*
Factrel.......... **3505**
Fluothane.......... **3374**
◆Grisactin Capsules.......... *341, 3374*
◆Grisactin Tablets.......... *341, 3374*
Heparin Lock Flush Solution.......... **3375**
Heparin Lock Flush Solution in Tubex.......... *3465*
Heparin Sodium Injection.......... **3376**
Heparin Sodium in Tubex.......... *3465*
Hydromorphone Hydrochloride in Tubex.......... *3465*
◆Inderal Injectable.......... **341, 3377**
◆Inderal LA Long-Acting Capsules.......... **341, 3380**
◆Inderal Tablets.......... **341, 3377**
◆Inderide LA Long-Acting Capsules.......... **341, 3383**
◆Inderide Tablets.......... **341, 3381**
Influenza Virus Vaccine, Trivalent, Types A & B, FluShield, 2000-2001 Formula.......... **3385**
Influenza Virus Vaccine, Trivalent, Types A & B, FluShield, 2000-2001 Formula, in Tubex.......... *3465*
◆Ismo Tablets.......... **341, 3388**
◆Isordil Sublingual Tablets.......... **341, 3389**
◆Isordil Titradose Tablets.......... **341, 3390**
◆Lodine Capsules.......... **341, 3392**
◆Lodine Tablets.......... **341, 3392**
◆Lodine XL Extended-Release Tablets.......... **341, 3394**
◆Lo/Ovral Tablets.......... **341, 3397**
◆Lo/Ovral-28 Tablets.......... **341, 3402**
Mepergan Injection.......... **3403**
Mepergan in Tubex.......... *3465*
Meperidine Hydrochloride in Tubex.......... *3465*
Morphine Sulfate in Tubex.......... *3465*
Mylotarg for Injection.......... **3404**
◆Norplant System.......... **341, 3407**
◆Orudis Capsules.......... **341, 3411**
◆Oruvail Capsules.......... **342, 3411**
◆Ovral Tablets.......... **342, 3414**
◆Ovral-28 Tablets.......... **342, 3415**
Ovrette Tablets.......... **3415**
Pentobarbital Sodium in Tubex.......... *3465*
Phenergan Injection.......... **3416**
◆Phenergan Suppositories.......... **342, 3419**
Phenergan Syrup Fortis.......... **3418**
Phenergan Syrup Plain.......... **3418**
◆Phenergan Tablets.......... **342, 3419**
Phenergan in Tubex.......... *3465*
Phenergan VC Syrup.......... **3423**
Phenergan VC with Codeine Syrup... **3424**
Phenergan with Codeine Syrup.......... **3420**
Phenergan with Dextromethorphan Syrup.......... **3422**
Phenobarbital Sodium in Tubex.......... *3465*
Premarin Intravenous.......... **3426**
◆Premarin Tablets.......... **342, 3429**
◆Premarin Vaginal Cream.......... **342, 3432**
◆Premphase Tablets.......... **342, 3434**
◆Prempro Tablets.......... **342, 3434**
Protonix Tablets.......... **3439**
Protopam Chloride for Injection.......... **3442**
Rapamune Oral Solution.......... **3443**
◆Sectral Capsules.......... **342, 3448**
Sodium Chloride, Bacteriostatic in Tubex.......... *3465*
◆Sonata Capsules.......... **342, 3450**
◆Surmontil Capsules.......... **342, 3454**
Synalgos-DC Capsules.......... *3455*
Synvisc.......... **3455**
Trecator-SC Tablets.......... **3457**
◆Triphasil-21 Tablets.......... **342, 3459**
◆Triphasil-28 Tablets.......... **342, 3464**
◆Tubex Closed Injection System Products.......... *342, 3465*
◆Tubex Injector.......... *342, 3465*
Typhoid Vaccine.......... **3467**
Wycillin in Tubex.......... *3465*
Wydase, Lyophilized.......... *3468*
◆Wygesic Tablets.......... **342, 3468**
Wytensin Tablets.......... *3469*

Other Products Available:
Codeine Phosphate Injection
Cordarone Tablets, 200 mg
Digoxin Injection
Diphenhydramine HCl Injection
Effexor Tablets, 25 mg
Effexor Tablets, 37.5 mg
Effexor Tablets, 50 mg
Effexor Tablets, 75 mg
Effexor Tablets, 100 mg
Effexor XR Capsules, 150 mg
Effexor XR Capsules, 37.5 mg
Effexor XR Capsules, 75 mg
Epinephrine Injection (1:1000)
Hydromorphone HCl Injection
Isordil Sublingual Tablets, 2.5 mg
Isordil Sublingual Tablets, 5 mg
Isordil 5 Titradose Tablets, 5 mg
Isordil 20 Titradose Tablets, 20 mg
Isordil 30 Titradose Tablets, 30 mg
Lodine Capsules, 300 mg
Lodine Tablets, 200 mg
Lodine Tablets, 400 mg
Mepergan Fortis Capsules
Meperidine HCl Injection
Morphine Sulfate Injection
Opium & Belladonna Rectal Suppositories
Orudis Capsules, 75 mg
Pentobarbital Sodium Injection
Phenergan Tablets, 25 mg
Phenobarbital Sodium Injection
Redipak (Respiratory Therapy Unit) Products:
Sodium Chloride 0.9%
Redipak Unit Dose Medications
Redipak Unit Dose Medications (Strip Pack and/or Individually Wrapped) Products:
Saline Solution (see Sodium Chloride Injection)
Sectral Capsules, 200 mg
Sodium Chloride Injection, Bacteriostatic
Sodium Chloride Solution, 0.9%
Testuria
Wyamine Sulfate Injection
Wydase, Stabilized Solution

ZENECA PHARMACEUTICALS
(See ASTRAZENECA PHARMACEUTICALS LP)

HOW TO USE THE BRAND AND GENERIC NAME INDEX

This index lists every product alphabetically by both brand and generic name. Generic names are underlined; brand names are not.

Under each generic name, you will find a list of the brands that contain it. This enables you to find a particular product by either of its names. For example, "Ativan Injection" is listed once alphabetically and again under its generic name, lorazepam.

Each time a brand name appears, it is followed by the manufacturer's name and the page to consult for further information. Under a generic heading, all fully described brands are listed first, followed by those with only partial information. In each case, the brands are listed alphabetically.

Brand name — **ATIVAN INJECTION**
(Wyeth-Ayerst) **3344**

◆ **ATIVAN TABLETS**
(Wyeth-Ayerst) **341, 3348**

ATIVAN IN TUBEX
(Wyeth-Ayerst) *3465*

Generic name — **LORAZEPAM**

Brands of lorazepam:

Ativan Injection
(Wyeth-Ayerst) .... **3344** (Manufacturer; Bold page number Indicates complete prescribing information)

Ativan Tablets
(Wyeth-Ayerst) **341, 3348**

Ativan in Tubex
(Wyeth-Ayerst) .... *3465* (Italic page number Indicates partial prescribing information)

Lorazepam Intensol *(Roxane)* ... *2822*

Lorazepam Tablets *(Geneva)* *1324*

Lorazepam Tablets *(Mylan)* *2115*

Lorazepam Tablets, USP CIV
(Watson) *3265*

Indicates photo in Product Identification Guide — ◆ **LORCET 10/650 TABLETS**
(Forest) *313, 1268*

◆ **LORCET PLUS TABLETS**
(Forest) *312, 1268*

◆ **LORCET-HD CAPSULES**
(Forest) *1268*

BRAND AND GENERIC NAME INDEX

This index includes all entries in the Product Information and Diagnostic Product Information sections. Products are listed alphabetically by both brand and generic name. Generic names are underlined; brand names are not. Under each generic name, you will find a list of the brands that contain it. This enables you to find a product by either of its names. For example, the brand Ativan appears once in the A's, and again under its generic name, lorazepam.

Each time a brand name appears, it is followed by the manufacturer's name and the page number to consult for further information. If multiple page numbers appear, the first ones refer to photos of the product, the last one to its prescribing information. Under a generic heading, all fully described brands are listed first, followed by those with only partial information.

- **Bold page numbers** indicate full prescribing information.
- *Italic page numbers* signify partial information.
- The ◆ symbol marks drugs shown in the Product Identification Guide.
- The ◘ symbol means product information is located in *PDR For Nonprescription Drugs and Dietary Supplements*™.
- The ⊙ symbol means product information is located in *PDR For Ophthalmic Medicines*™.

A

F

I

J

K

L

◆ Shown in Product Identification Guide

Underline Denotes Generic Name

Italic Page Number Indicates Brief Listing

N

SECTION 3

PRODUCT CATEGORY INDEX

This index lists products by prescribing category, allowing you to quickly and easily identify all agents with a given therapeutic use or mechanism of action. Categories are based on the latest medical terminology and are comprehensively cross-referenced. Included are all fully described products in both the Product Information and Diagnostic Product Information sections of PDR®.

If an entry in the index lists multiple page numbers, the first ones shown refer to photographs of the product, the last one to its prescribing information. The Quick-Reference Guide below gives you an overview of the categories.

PRODUCT CATEGORY QUICK-REFERENCE GUIDE

PRODUCT CATEGORY INDEX

F

FERTILITY AGENTS

Antagon Injection *(Organon)* 2257
Cetrotide for Injection *(Serono)* 3015
Clomid Tablets *(Aventis)* 306, 700
Crinone 4% Gel *(Serono)* 3018
Crinone 8% Gel *(Serono)* 336, 3018
Fertinex for Injection *(Serono)* 3020
Follistim for Injection *(Organon)* 327, 2267
Gonal-F for Injection *(Serono)* 3023
Humegon for Injection *(Organon)* 327, 2270
Novarel for Injection *(Ferring)* 1238
Pergonal for Injection *(Serono)* 3027
Profasi for Injection *(Serono)* 3028
Repronex for Intramuscular and Subcutaneous Injection *(Ferring)* 1239
Serophene Tablets *(Serono)* 3030

FEVER PREPARATIONS

(see under:
ANALGESICS
ACETAMINOPHEN & COMBINATIONS
NONSTEROIDAL ANTI-INFLAMMATORY AGENTS (NSAIDS)
SALICYLATES)

FIBROTICS

(see under:
ANTIFIBROSIS THERAPY, SYSTEMIC)

FLUORIDE PREPARATIONS

(see under:
DIETARY SUPPLEMENTS
MINERALS & ELECTROLYTES
FLUORIDE & COMBINATIONS)

FLUOROQUINOLONES

(see under:
ANTI-INFECTIVE AGENTS, SYSTEMIC
QUINOLONES
OPHTHALMIC PREPARATIONS
ANTI-INFECTIVES
QUINOLONES)

FOODS

(see under:
DIETARY SUPPLEMENTS
NUTRITIONAL THERAPY, ENTERAL)

FOOT CARE PRODUCTS

Penlac Topical Solution *(Dermik)* 1116

FUNGAL MEDICATIONS

(see under:
ANTI-INFECTIVE AGENTS, SYSTEMIC
ANTIFUNGALS
SKIN & MUCOUS MEMBRANE AGENTS
ANTI-INFECTIVES
ANTIFUNGALS & COMBINATIONS
VAGINAL PREPARATIONS
ANTI-INFECTIVES
ANTIFUNGALS & COMBINATIONS)

G

GASTROINTESTINAL AGENTS

ANTACID & ANTIFLATULENT COMBINATIONS

Maximum Strength Maalox Antacid/Anti-Gas Liquid *(Novartis Consumer)* 2137
Fast-Acting Mylanta Liquid Antacid *(J&J • Merck)* 318, 1594
Extra Strength Fast-Acting Mylanta Liquid *(J&J • Merck)* 318, 1594

ANTACIDS

ALUMINUM ANTACIDS & COMBINATIONS

Amphojel Suspension *(Wyeth-Ayerst)* 341, 3342
Mylanta Night Time Strength Liquid *(J&J • Merck)* 318, 1596

CALCIUM ANTACIDS & COMBINATIONS

Extra Strength Mylanta Calci Tabs *(J&J • Merck)* 318, 1596
Ultra Mylanta Calci Tabs *(J&J • Merck)* 318, 1596
Children's Mylanta Upset Stomach Relief Liquid *(J&J • Merck)* 318, 1594
Children's Mylanta Upset Stomach Relief Tablets *(J&J • Merck)* 318, 1594

COMBINATION ANTACIDS

Maalox Magnesia and Alumina Oral Suspension *(Novartis Consumer)* 2136
Fast-Acting Mylanta Antacid Gelcaps *(J&J • Merck)* 318, 1595
Fast-Acting Mylanta Ultra Tabs *(J&J • Merck)* 318, 1595
Mylanta Supreme Liquid *(J&J • Merck)* 318, 1595

MAGNESIUM ANTACIDS & COMBINATIONS

Mag-Ox 400 Tablets *(Blaine)* 956
Mylanta Night Time Strength Liquid *(J&J • Merck)* 318, 1596
Uro-Mag Capsules *(Blaine)* 956

MISCELLANEOUS ANTACID PREPARATIONS

Quick Dissolve Maalox Antacid Tablets, Maximum Strength *(Novartis Consumer)* 2137
Quick Dissolve Maalox Antacid Tablets, Regular Strength *(Novartis Consumer)* .. 2137

ANTICHOLINERGIC AGENTS

Robinul Forte Tablets *(First Horizon)* 1249
Robinul Tablets *(First Horizon)* 1249

ANTIDIARRHEALS

Arco-Lase Plus Tablets *(Arco)* 561
Imodium A-D Caplets and Liquid *(McNeil Consumer)* 321, 1817
Imodium Advanced Chewable Tablets *(McNeil Consumer)* 321, 1818
Lomotil Liquid *(Searle)* 3008
Lomotil Tablets *(Searle)* 336, 3008
Lotronex Tablets *(Glaxo Wellcome)* ... 315, 1437
Motofen Tablets *(Amarin)* 539
Pepto-Bismol Maximum Strength Liquid *(Procter & Gamble)* 2663
Pepto-Bismol Original Liquid, Original and Cherry Tablets and Easy-To-Swallow Caplets *(Procter & Gamble)* 2663
Sandostatin Injection *(Novartis)* 326, 2213
Sandostatin LAR Depot *(Novartis)* 326, 2215

ANTIEMETICS

Antivert, Antivert/25, & Antivert/50 Tablets *(Pfizer)* 2469
Anzemet Injection *(Aventis)* 306, 680
Anzemet Tablets *(Aventis)* 306, 683
Atarax Tablets & Syrup *(Pfizer)* 2472
Benadryl Parenteral *(Parke-Davis)* 2420
Bonine Chewable Tablets *(Warner-Lambert/Pfizer)* 3265
Compazine Multi-dose Vials *(SmithKline Beecham)* 337, 3077
Compazine Spansule Capsules *(SmithKline Beecham)* 337, 3077
Compazine Suppositories *(SmithKline Beecham)* 337, 3077
Compazine Syrup *(SmithKline Beecham)* 337, 3077
Compazine Tablets *(SmithKline Beecham)* 337, 3077
Compazine Vials *(SmithKline Beecham)* 337, 3077
Compro Suppositories, USP 25 mg *(Paddock)* 2407
Kytril Injection *(SmithKline Beecham)* 337, 3104
Kytril Tablets *(SmithKline Beecham)* .. 337, 3106
Marinol Capsules *(Roxane)* 333, 2828
Marinol Capsules *(Unimed)* 339, 3220
Pepto-Bismol Maximum Strength Liquid *(Procter & Gamble)* 2663
Pepto-Bismol Original Liquid, Original and Cherry Tablets and Easy-To-Swallow Caplets *(Procter & Gamble)* 2663
Phenergan Injection *(Wyeth-Ayerst)* 3416
Phenergan Suppositories *(Wyeth-Ayerst)* 342, 3419
Phenergan Syrup Fortis *(Wyeth-Ayerst)* 3418
Phenergan Syrup Plain *(Wyeth-Ayerst)* 3418
Phenergan Tablets *(Wyeth-Ayerst)* 342, 3419
Reglan Injectable *(Robins)* 332, 2713
Reglan Syrup *(Robins)* 2713
Reglan Tablets *(Robins)* 332, 2713
Thorazine Ampuls *(SmithKline Beecham)* 337, 3135
Thorazine Multi-dose Vials *(SmithKline Beecham)* 337, 3135
Thorazine Spansule Capsules *(SmithKline Beecham)* 338, 3135
Thorazine Suppositories *(SmithKline Beecham)* 338, 3135
Thorazine Syrup *(SmithKline Beecham)* 338, 3135
Thorazine Tablets *(SmithKline Beecham)* 337, 3135
Tigan Capsules *(Monarch)* 2102
Tigan Injectable *(Monarch)* 2102
Tigan Suppositories *(Monarch)* 2102
Transderm Scōp Transdermal Therapeutic System *(Novartis Consumer)* 325, 2138
Trilafon Injection *(Schering)* 2939
Trilafon Tablets *(Schering)* 334, 2939
Vistaril Capsules *(Pfizer)* 2541
Vistaril Oral Suspension *(Pfizer)* 2541
Zofran Injection *(Glaxo Wellcome)* 317, 1503
Zofran Injection Premixed *(Glaxo Wellcome)* 317, 1503
Zofran Oral Solution *(Glaxo Wellcome)* 317, 1507
Zofran Tablets *(Glaxo Wellcome)* 317, 1507
Zofran ODT Orally Disintegrating Tablets *(Glaxo Wellcome)* 317, 1507

ANTIFLATULENTS

Imodium Advanced Chewable Tablets *(McNeil Consumer)* 321, 1818
Maximum Strength Mylanta Gas Relief Softgels *(J&J • Merck)* 318, 1595
Mylanta Gas Relief Tablets *(J&J • Merck)* ... 1595
Maximum Strength Mylanta Gas Relief Tablets *(J&J • Merck)* 1595
Mylicon Infants' Drops *(J&J • Merck)* 318, 1594

ANTI-INFLAMMATORY AGENTS

Asacol Delayed-Release Tablets *(Procter & Gamble Pharmaceuticals)* 331, 2669
Azulfidine EN-tabs Tablets *(Pharmacia & Upjohn)* 331, 2569
Colazal Capsules *(Salix)* 333, 2842
Colocort Enema, USP (Retention) 100 mg/60 mL *(Paddock)* 2406
Dipentum Capsules *(Pharmacia & Upjohn)* .. 2602
Pentasa Capsules *(Shire US)* 336, 3042
Rowasa Rectal Suspension Enema 4.0 grams/unit (60 mL) *(Solvay)* ... 338, 3160

ANTISPASMODICS & ANTICHOLINERGICS

Arco-Lase Plus Tablets *(Arco)* 561
Cystospaz Tablets *(PolyMedica)* 2661
Cystospaz-M Capsules *(PolyMedica)* 2661
Donnatal Capsules *(Robins)* 332, 2708
Donnatal Elixir *(Robins)* 2708
Donnatal Extentabs *(Robins)* 332, 2708
Donnatal Tablets *(Robins)* 332, 2708
Levbid Extended-Release Tablets *(Schwarz)* 335, 2951
Levsin Drops *(Schwarz)* 2951
Levsin Elixir *(Schwarz)* 2951
Levsin Injection *(Schwarz)* 2951
Levsin Tablets *(Schwarz)* 2951
Levsin/SL Tablets *(Schwarz)* 335, 2951
Levsinex Timecaps *(Schwarz)* 2951
Robinul Injectable *(Robins)* 332, 2717

BOWEL EVACUANTS

Colyte with Flavor Packs for Oral Solution *(Schwarz)* 334, 2948
Fleet Bisacodyl Laxatives *(Fleet)* 1250
Fleet Enema *(Fleet)* 1251
Fleet Enema for Children *(Fleet)* 1251
Fleet Mineral Oil Enema *(Fleet)* 1251
Fleet Phospho-Soda *(Fleet)* 1251
Fleet Prep Kits *(Fleet)* 1252
GoLYTELY and Pineapple Flavor GoLYTELY for Oral Solution *(Braintree)* 309, 990
NuLYTELY, Cherry Flavor, Lemon-Lime Flavor, and Orange Flavor NuLYTELY for Oral Solution *(Braintree)* 309, 990
X-Prep Liquid *(Purdue Frederick)* 2685

CYTOPROTECTIVE AGENTS

Arthrotec Tablets *(Searle)* 335, 2977
Cytotec Tablets *(Searle)* 335, 2991

DIGESTIVE ENZYMES

Arco-Lase Tablets *(Arco)* 561
Arco-Lase Plus Tablets *(Arco)* 561
Cotazym Capsules *(Organon)* 327, 2259
Creon 5 Capsules *(Solvay)* 338, 3144
Creon 10 Capsules *(Solvay)* 338, 3144
Creon 20 Capsules *(Solvay)* 338, 3144
Donnazyme Tablets *(Robins)* 332, 2709
Lactaid Original Strength Caplets *(McNeil Consumer)* 321, 1821
Lactaid Extra Strength Caplets *(McNeil Consumer)* 321, 1821
Lactaid Ultra Caplets and Chewable Tablets *(McNeil Consumer)* 321, 1821
Lactaid Drops *(McNeil Consumer)* 321, 1820
Pancrease Capsules *(Ortho-McNeil)* ... 328, 2381
Pancrease MT Capsules *(Ortho-McNeil)* 329, 2382
Ultrase Capsules *(Axcan Scandipharm)* 307, 802
Ultrase MT Capsules *(Axcan Scandipharm)* 307, 803
Viokase Powder *(Axcan Scandipharm)* 805
Viokase Tablets *(Axcan Scandipharm)* .. 307, 805
Zymase Capsules *(Organon)* 327, 2300

DUODENAL ULCER ADHERENT COMPLEX

Carafate Suspension *(Aventis)* 692
Carafate Tablets *(Aventis)* 306, 691

GASTROINTESTINAL STIMULANTS

Reglan Injectable *(Robins)* 332, 2713
Reglan Syrup *(Robins)* 2713
Reglan Tablets *(Robins)* 332, 2713

HISTAMINE (H_2) RECEPTOR ANTAGONISTS

Axid Pulvules *(Lilly)* 321, 1704
Pepcid AC Chewable Tablets *(J&J • Merck)* 318, 1596
Pepcid AC Gelcaps *(J&J • Merck)* 318, 1596
Pepcid AC Tablets *(J&J • Merck)* 318, 1596
Pepcid Injection *(Merck)* 1990
Pepcid Injection Premixed *(Merck)* 1990
Pepcid for Oral Suspension *(Merck)* 1988
Pepcid RPD Orally Disintegrating Tablets *(Merck)* 324, 1988
Pepcid Tablets *(Merck)* 324, 1988
Tagamet Injection *(SmithKline Beecham)* 3129
Tagamet Liquid *(SmithKline Beecham)* 3129
Tagamet Tablets *(SmithKline Beecham)* 337, 3129
Zantac 150 EFFERdose Granules *(Glaxo Wellcome)* 316, 1495
Zantac 150 EFFERdose Tablets *(Glaxo Wellcome)* 316, 1495
Zantac 150 Tablets *(Glaxo Wellcome)* 316, 1495
Zantac 300 Tablets *(Glaxo Wellcome)* 316, 1495
Zantac Injection *(Glaxo Wellcome)* 317, 1493
Zantac Injection Premixed *(Glaxo Wellcome)* 316, 1493
Zantac Syrup *(Glaxo Wellcome)* 316, 1495

LAXATIVES

BULK-PRODUCING LAXATIVES

Metamucil Original Texture Powder, Orange Flavor *(Procter & Gamble)* 2662
Metamucil Original Texture Powder, Regular Flavor *(Procter & Gamble)* 2662
Metamucil Smooth Texture Powder, Orange Flavor *(Procter & Gamble)* 2662
Metamucil Smooth Texture Powder, Sugar-Free, Orange Flavor *(Procter & Gamble)* 2662
Metamucil Smooth Texture Powder, Sugar-Free, Regular Flavor *(Procter & Gamble)* 2662
Metamucil Wafers, Apple Crisp and Cinnamon Spice Flavors *(Procter & Gamble)* 2662
Perdiem Fiber Therapy *(Novartis Consumer)* 2137
Perdiem Overnight Relief *(Novartis Consumer)* 2138

EMOLLIENT LAXATIVES

Fleet Mineral Oil Enema *(Fleet)* 1251

ENEMAS

Fleet Enema *(Fleet)* 1251
Fleet Enema for Children *(Fleet)* 1251
Fleet Mineral Oil Enema *(Fleet)* 1251

FECAL SOFTENERS & COMBINATIONS

Colace Capsules, Syrup, Liquid *(Shire US)* 3039
Senokot-S Tablets *(Purdue Frederick)* 2685

HYPEROSMOLAR AGENTS

MiraLax Powder for Oral Solution *(Braintree)* 309, 991

LAXATIVE COMBINATIONS

Peri-Colace Capsules and Syrup *(Shire US)* 3044
Senokot-S Tablets *(Purdue Frederick)* 2685

MISCELLANEOUS LAXATIVES

Fleet Glycerin Laxatives *(Fleet)* 1250
Kristalose for Oral Solution *(Bertek)* 943

SALINE LAXATIVES

Fleet Phospho-Soda *(Fleet)* 1251

STIMULANT LAXATIVES & COMBINATIONS

Fleet Bisacodyl Laxatives *(Fleet)* 1250
Fleet Prep Kits *(Fleet)* 1252
Perdiem Overnight Relief *(Novartis Consumer)* 2138
Senokot Granules *(Purdue Frederick)* 2685
Senokot Children's Syrup *(Purdue Frederick)* 2685
Senokot Tablets *(Purdue Frederick)* 2685
Senokot-S Tablets *(Purdue Frederick)* 2685
SenokotXTRA Tablets *(Purdue Frederick)* 2685

MISCELLANEOUS GASTROINTESTINAL AGENTS

Calm Colon Capsules *(Samra)* 2843
Celebrex Capsules *(Pfizer)* 330, 2482
Celebrex Capsules *(Searle)* 335, 2985
Elecare Powder *(Ross)* 2815
PREVPAC *(TAP)* 338, 3194
Remicade for IV Injection *(Centocor)* 310, 1085
Urso Tablets 250 mg *(Axcan Scandipharm)* 307, 804

PROSTAGLANDINS

Cytotec Tablets *(Searle)* 335, 2991

PROTON PUMP INHIBITORS

Aciphex Tablets *(Eisai)* 311, 1178
Aciphex Tablets *(Janssen)* 318, 1570
Prevacid Delayed-Release Capsules *(TAP)* 338, 3189
PREVPAC *(TAP)* 338, 3194
Prilosec Delayed-Release Capsules *(AstraZeneca LP)* 305, 587
Protonix Tablets *(Wyeth-Ayerst)* 3439

GASTROINTESTINAL ANTIGRANULOMATOUS DISEASE

(see under:
GASTROINTESTINAL AGENTS
ANTI-INFLAMMATORY AGENTS)

GASTROINTESTINAL PROKINETIC AGENTS

(see under:
GASTROINTESTINAL AGENTS
GASTROINTESTINAL STIMULANTS)

GAUCHER'S DISEASE MANAGEMENT

Cerezyme for Injection *(Genzyme)* 1325

GENITAL WART PREPARATIONS

(see under:
SKIN & MUCOUS MEMBRANE AGENTS
WART PREPARATIONS)

GLAUCOMA PREPARATIONS

(see under:
OPHTHALMIC PREPARATIONS
BETA ADRENERGIC BLOCKING AGENTS
CARBONIC ANHYDRASE INHIBITORS
MIOTICS
SYMPATHOMIMETICS & COMBINATIONS)

GLUCOSE ELEVATING AGENTS

(see under:
HORMONES
GLUCOSE ELEVATING AGENTS)

GONADOTROPIN INHIBITORS

(see under:
HORMONES
GONADOTROPIN INHIBITORS)

PSYCHOTHERAPEUTIC AGENTS—*cont.*

ANTIPSYCHOTIC AGENTS—*cont.*

PHENOTHIAZINES & COMBINATIONS—*cont.*

Thorazine Spansule Capsules *(SmithKline Beecham)*.......... **338, 3135**
Thorazine Suppositories *(SmithKline Beecham)*.......... **338, 3135**
Thorazine Syrup *(SmithKline Beecham)*.................... **338, 3135**
Thorazine Tablets *(SmithKline Beecham)*.................... **337, 3135**
Trilafon Injection *(Schering)*............ **2939**
Trilafon Tablets *(Schering)*........ **334, 2939**

MISCELLANEOUS PSYCHOTHERAPEUTIC AGENTS

Sarafem Pulvules *(Lilly)*............ **321, 1774**

OBSESSIVE-COMPULSIVE DISORDER MANAGEMENT

SELECTIVE SEROTONIN REUPTAKE INHIBITORS (SSRI)

Luvox Tablets (25, 50, 100 mg) *(Solvay)*.................... **338, 3153**
Paxil Oral Suspension *(SmithKline Beecham)*...................... **3114**
Paxil Tablets *(SmithKline Beecham)*...................... **337, 3114**
Prozac Pulvules & Liquid, Oral Solution *(Dista)*............... **311, 1127**
Zoloft Oral Concentrate *(Pfizer)*......... **2553**
Zoloft Tablets *(Pfizer)*............ **331, 2553**

PSYCHOSTIMULANTS

(see under:
CENTRAL NERVOUS SYSTEM STIMULANTS)

PSYCHOTROPICS

(see under:
PSYCHOTHERAPEUTIC AGENTS)

Q

QUINOLONES

(see under:
ANTI-INFECTIVE AGENTS, SYSTEMIC
QUINOLONES
OPHTHALMIC PREPARATIONS
ANTI-INFECTIVES
QUINOLONES)

R

RADIOPAQUE AGENTS

Ethiodol Injection *(Savage)*............... **2874**

RENAL STONE PREVENTION

(see under:
URINARY TRACT AGENTS
CALCIUM OXALATE STONE PREVENTION)

RESINS, ION EXCHANGE

(see also under:
CARDIOVASCULAR AGENTS
ANTILIPEMIC AGENTS
BILE ACID SEQUESTRANTS)

Kayexalate Powder *(Sanofi-Synthelabo)*..... **2855**
Kionex Powder *(Paddock)*............... **2408**

RESPIRATORY AGENTS

(see also under:
ANTIHISTAMINES & COMBINATIONS
NASAL PREPARATIONS)

ANTI-INFECTIVE AGENTS

CYSTIC FIBROSIS MANAGEMENT

(see also under:
CYSTIC FIBROSIS MANAGEMENT)

ANTI-INFLAMMATORY AGENTS

STEROIDAL ANTI-INFLAMMATORY AGENTS

Aerobid Inhaler System *(Forest)*.... **312, 1254**
Aerobid-M Inhaler System *(Forest)*..................... **312, 1254**
Azmacort Inhalation Aerosol *(Aventis)*..................... **306, 689**
Beclovent Inhalation Aerosol and Refill *(Glaxo Wellcome)*......... **314, 1354**
Flovent 44 mcg Inhalation Aerosol *(Glaxo Wellcome)*.............. **315, 1390**
Flovent 110 mcg Inhalation Aerosol *(Glaxo Wellcome)*....... **315, 1390**
Flovent 220 mcg Inhalation Aerosol *(Glaxo Wellcome)*....... **315, 1390**
Flovent Rotadisk 50 mcg *(Glaxo Wellcome)*................... **315, 1393**
Flovent Rotadisk 100 mcg *(Glaxo Wellcome)*................... **315, 1393**
Flovent Rotadisk 250 mcg *(Glaxo Wellcome)*................... **315, 1393**
Pulmicort Turbuhaler Inhalation Powder *(AstraZeneca LP)*........ **305, 591**
Vanceril Inhalation Aerosol *(Schering)*.... **2944**
Vanceril Double Strength Inhalation Aerosol *(Schering)*.... **334, 2945**

ANTITUSSIVES

NARCOTIC ANTITUSSIVES & COMBINATIONS

Hycodan Syrup *(Endo Labs)*............ **1200**
Hycodan Tablets *(Endo Labs)*...... **312, 1200**
Hycomine Compound Tablets *(Endo Labs)*.................. **312, 1201**
Hycomine Syrup *(Endo Labs)*........... **1202**
Hycomine Pediatric Syrup *(Endo Labs)*... **1202**
Hycotuss Expectorant Syrup *(Endo Labs)*............................. **1203**
Phenergan VC with Codeine Syrup *(Wyeth-Ayerst)*...................... **3424**
Phenergan with Codeine Syrup *(Wyeth-Ayerst)*.......................... **3420**
Robitussin A-C Syrup *(Robins)*.......... **2718**
Robitussin-DAC Syrup *(Robins)*......... **2718**
Tussend Syrup *(Monarch)*............... **2103**
Tussend Tablets *(Monarch)*............. **2103**
Tussionex Pennkinetic Extended-Release Suspension *(Medeva)*............... **1849**
Tussi-Organidin NR Liquid *(Wallace)*.... **3248**
Tussi-Organidin-S NR Liquid *(Wallace)*.................... **340, 3248**
Vicodin Tuss Expectorant *(Knoll Labs)*......................... **319, 1632**

NON-NARCOTIC ANTITUSSIVES & COMBINATIONS

Phenergan with Dextromethorphan Syrup *(Wyeth-Ayerst)*....................... **3422**
Rynatuss Tablets *(Wallace)*........ **339, 3251**
Rynatuss Pediatric Suspension *(Wallace)*.......................... **339, 3251**
Tessalon Capsules *(Forest)*......... **313, 1270**
Tussi-12 Suspension *(Wallace)*...... **339, 3254**
Tussi-12 Tablets *(Wallace)*.......... **339, 3254**
Tussi-Organidin DM NR Liquid *(Wallace)*............................. **3248**
Tussi-Organidin DM-S NR Liquid *(Wallace)*...................... **340, 3248**
Children's Tylenol Cold Plus Cough Suspension Liquid and Chewable Tablets *(McNeil Consumer)*................... **322, 1816**
Children's Tylenol Flu Suspension Liquid *(McNeil Consumer)*...... **322, 1816**
Tylenol Cold Complete Formula, Multi-Symptom Caplets *(McNeil Consumer)*............ **322, 1834**
Tylenol Cold Non-Drowsy, Multi-Symptom Caplets and Gelcaps *(McNeil Consumer)*..... **322, 1834**
Tylenol Cold Severe Congestion Non-Drowsy, Multi-Symptom Caplets *(McNeil Consumer)*...... **323, 1835**
Tylenol Flu NightTime, Maximum Strength Liquid *(McNeil Consumer)*..................... **323, 1836**
Tylenol Flu Non-Drowsy, Maximum Strength Gelcaps *(McNeil Consumer)*............ **323, 1836**
Infants' Tylenol Cold Decongestant and Fever Reducer Concentrated Drops Plus Cough *(McNeil Consumer)*.. **322, 1819**

BRONCHODILATORS

ANTICHOLINERGICS

Atrovent Inhalation Aerosol *(Boehringer Ingelheim)*.......... **308, 962**
Atrovent Inhalation Solution *(Boehringer Ingelheim)*.......... **309, 963**

ANTICHOLINERGICS WITH SYMPATHOMIMETICS

Combivent Inhalation Aerosol *(Boehringer Ingelheim)*.......... **309, 972**

SYMPATHOMIMETICS & COMBINATIONS

Adrenalin Chloride Inhalation Solution *(Monarch)*.......................... **2066**
Adrenalin Chloride Injection *(Monarch)*... **2066**
Alupent Inhalation Aerosol *(Boehringer Ingelheim)*.......... **308, 960**
Alupent Inhalation Solution *(Boehringer Ingelheim)*.......... **308, 960**
Alupent Syrup *(Boehringer Ingelheim)*..... **960**
Alupent Tablets *(Boehringer Ingelheim)*.... **960**
Brethine Ampuls *(Novartis)*......... **325, 2150**
Brethine Tablets *(Novartis)*......... **325, 2149**
Maxair Autohaler *(3M)*............ **321, 1800**
Maxair Inhaler *(3M)*................ **321, 1803**
Proventil Inhalation Aerosol *(Schering)*... **2922**
Proventil HFA Inhalation Aerosol *(Schering)*.................... **334, 2929**
Proventil Inhalation Solution 0.083% *(Schering)*.......................... **2926**
Proventil Repetabs Tablets *(Schering)*.................... **334, 2928**
Proventil Solution for Inhalation 0.5% *(Schering)*.......................... **2924**
Proventil Tablets *(Schering)*........ **334, 2928**
Rynatuss Tablets *(Wallace)*........ **339, 3251**
Rynatuss Pediatric Suspension *(Wallace)*......................... **339, 3251**
Serevent Diskus *(Glaxo Wellcome)*.. **316, 1468**
Serevent Inhalation Aerosol *(Glaxo Wellcome)*.............. **316, 1464**
Ventolin Inhalation Aerosol and Refill *(Glaxo Wellcome)*......... **316, 1478**
Ventolin Inhalation Solution *(Glaxo Wellcome)*.............. **316, 1480**
Ventolin Rotacaps for Inhalation *(Glaxo Wellcome)*.............. **316, 1482**
Ventolin Syrup *(Glaxo Wellcome)*.... **316, 1484**
Volmax Extended-Release Tablets *(Muro)*.............................. **2113**
Xopenex Inhalation Solution *(Sepracor)*... **3493**

XANTHINE DERIVATIVES & COMBINATIONS

Aerolate Liquid *(Fleming)*............. **1252**
Aerolate Jr. T.D. Capsules *(Fleming)*..... **1252**
Aerolate Sr. T.D. Capsules *(Fleming)*..... **1252**
Cafcit Injection *(Roxane)*.............. **2823**
Cafcit Oral Solution *(Roxane)*.......... **2823**
Lufyllin Tablets *(Wallace)*.............. **3246**
Lufyllin-400 Tablets *(Wallace)*.......... **3246**
Lufyllin-GG Elixir *(Wallace)*........... **3246**
Lufyllin-GG Tablets *(Wallace)*.......... **3246**
Theo-24 Extended Release Capsules *(UCB)*.............. **339, 3211**
Theo-Dur Extended-Release Tablets *(Key)*.............. **319, 1605**
Uni-Dur Extended-Release Tablets *(Key)*........................ **319, 1611**
Uniphyl 400 mg and 600 mg Tablets *(Purdue Frederick)*...... **332, 2687**

DECONGESTANTS & COMBINATIONS

Allegra-D Extended-Release Tablets *(Aventis)*.......................... **306, 675**
Alumadrine Tablets *(Fleming)*............ **1253**
Bromfed Capsules (Extended-Release) *(Muro)*.............................. **2105**
Bromfed-PD Capsules (Extended-Release) *(Muro)*.............................. **2105**
Claritin-D 12 Hour Extended Release Tablets *(Schering)*........ **334, 2885**
Claritin-D 24 Hour Extended Release Tablets *(Schering)*........ **334, 2887**
Dimetane-DX Cough Syrup *(Robins)*...... **2707**
Extendryl Chewable Tablets *(Fleming)*..... **1253**
Extendryl Sr. & Jr. Capsules *(Fleming)*..... **1253**
Extendryl Syrup *(Fleming)*.............. **1253**
Hycomine Pediatric Syrup *(Endo Labs)*...... **1202**
Kronofed-A Kronocaps *(Ferndale)*........ **1233**
Kronofed-A-Jr. Kronocaps *(Ferndale)*...... **1233**
Motrin Cold & Flu Caplets *(McNeil Consumer)*..................... **322, 1821**
Motrin Sinus Headache Caplets *(McNeil Consumer)*............... **322, 1822**
Phenergan VC Syrup *(Wyeth-Ayerst)*........ **3423**
Ryna-12 S Suspension *(Wallace)*...... **339, 3249**
Rynatan Tablets *(Wallace)*........... **339, 3249**
Rynatan-P Pediatric Suspension *(Wallace)*..................... **339, 3251**
Rynatuss Tablets *(Wallace)*.......... **339, 3251**
Rynatuss Pediatric Suspension *(Wallace)*..................... **339, 3251**
Semprex-D Capsules *(Medeva)*........... **1847**
Tussend Syrup *(Monarch)*................. **2103**
Tussend Tablets *(Monarch)*............... **2103**
Tussi-12 Suspension *(Wallace)*....... **339, 3254**
Tussi-12 Tablets *(Wallace)*........... **339, 3254**
Tylenol Allergy Sinus, Maximum Strength Caplets, Gelcaps, and Geltabs *(McNeil Consumer)*....... **323, 1833**
Tylenol Allergy Sinus NightTime, Maximum Strength Caplets *(McNeil Consumer)*............... **323, 1833**
Children's Tylenol Allergy-D Liquid and Chewable Tablets *(McNeil Consumer)*..................... **322, 1814**
Children's Tylenol Cold Suspension Liquid and Chewable Tablets *(McNeil Consumer)*............. **322, 1815**
Children's Tylenol Cold Plus Cough Suspension Liquid and Chewable Tablets *(McNeil Consumer)*....... **322, 1816**
Children's Tylenol Flu Suspension Liquid *(McNeil Consumer)*......... **322, 1816**
Children's Tylenol Sinus Suspension Liquid and Chewable Tablets *(McNeil Consumer)*............ **322, 1817**
Tylenol Cold Complete Formula, Multi-Symptom Caplets *(McNeil Consumer)*..................... **322, 1834**
Tylenol Cold Non-Drowsy, Multi-Symptom Caplets and Gelcaps *(McNeil Consumer)*...... **322, 1834**
Tylenol Flu NightTime, Maximum Strength Gelcaps *(McNeil Consumer)*..................... **323, 1836**
Tylenol Flu NightTime, Maximum Strength Liquid *(McNeil Consumer)*..................... **323, 1836**
Tylenol Flu Non-Drowsy, Maximum Strength Gelcaps *(McNeil Consumer)*..................... **323, 1836**
Infants' Tylenol Cold Decongestant and Fever Reducer Concentrated Drops *(McNeil Consumer)*......... **322, 1818**
Infants' Tylenol Cold Decongestant and Fever Reducer Concentrated Drops Plus Cough *(McNeil Consumer)*..................... **322, 1819**
Tylenol Sinus NightTime, Maximum Strength Caplets *(McNeil Consumer)*..................... **323, 1838**
Tylenol Sinus Non-Drowsy, Maximum Strength Geltabs, Gelcaps, Caplets, and Tablets *(McNeil Consumer)*........... **323, 1838**

DECONGESTANTS, EXPECTORANTS & COMBINATIONS

Duratuss GP Tablets *(UCB)*.......... **338, 3205**
Entex LA Tablets *(Dura)*............... **1165**
Entex PSE Tablets *(Dura)*.............. **1166**
Guaifed Capsules *(Muro)*................ **2109**
Guaifed-PD Capsules *(Muro)*............ **2109**
Ornade Spansule Capsules *(SmithKline Beecham)*.......... **337, 3112**
Tylenol Cold Severe Congestion Non-Drowsy, Multi-Symptom Caplets *(McNeil Consumer)*....... **323, 1835**

ENZYMES

Pulmozyme Inhalation Solution *(Genentech)*.................. **313, 1312**

EXPECTORANTS & COMBINATIONS

Lufyllin-GG Elixir *(Wallace)*............. **3246**
Lufyllin-GG Tablets *(Wallace)*........... **3246**
Organidin NR Liquid *(Wallace)*...... **339, 3248**
Organidin NR Tablets *(Wallace)*...... **339, 3248**
Pima Syrup *(Fleming)*.................. **1254**
Tussi-Organidin NR Liquid *(Wallace)*...... **3248**
Tussi-Organidin DM NR Liquid *(Wallace)*... **3248**
Tussi-Organidin DM-S NR Liquid *(Wallace)*...................... **340, 3248**
Tussi-Organidin-S NR Liquid *(Wallace)*...................... **340, 3248**
Vicodin Tuss Expectorant *(Knoll Labs)*......................... **319, 1632**

LEUKOTRIENE ANTAGONISTS

Accolate Tablets *(AstraZeneca)*........ **305, 611**
Singulair Tablets *(Merck)*........... **324, 2018**
Singulair Chewable Tablets *(Merck)*... **324, 2018**

LEUKOTRIENE FORMATION INHIBITORS

Zyflo Filmtab Tablets *(Abbott)*......... **303, 493**

LUNG SURFACTANTS

Curosurf Intratracheal Suspension *(Dey)*......................... **311, 1120**
Exosurf Neonatal for Intratracheal Suspension *(Glaxo Wellcome)*..... **314, 1380**
Infasurf Intratracheal Suspension *(Forest)*.................... **312, 1264**
Survanta Intratracheal Suspension *(Ross)*.... **2820**

MISCELLANEOUS COLD & COUGH PRODUCTS WITH ANALGESICS

Children's Tylenol Cold Plus Cough Suspension Liquid and Chewable Tablets *(McNeil Consumer)*....... **322, 1816**
Children's Tylenol Flu Suspension Liquid *(McNeil Consumer)*........ **322, 1816**
Tylenol Cold Complete Formula, Multi-Symptom Caplets *(McNeil Consumer)*..................... **322, 1834**
Tylenol Cold Non-Drowsy, Multi-Symptom Caplets and Gelcaps *(McNeil Consumer)*...... **322, 1834**
Tylenol Cold Severe Congestion Non-Drowsy, Multi-Symptom Caplets *(McNeil Consumer)*....... **323, 1835**
Tylenol Flu NightTime, Maximum Strength Liquid *(McNeil Consumer)*..................... **323, 1836**
Tylenol Flu Non-Drowsy, Maximum Strength Gelcaps *(McNeil Consumer)*..................... **323, 1836**
Infants' Tylenol Cold Decongestant and Fever Reducer Concentrated Drops Plus Cough *(McNeil Consumer)*..................... **322, 1819**

MISCELLANEOUS COUGH & COLD PRODUCTS

Tussi-12 Suspension *(Wallace)*....... **339, 3254**
Tussi-12 Tablets *(Wallace)*........... **339, 3254**

MISCELLANEOUS RESPIRATORY AGENTS

Synagis Intramuscular *(MedImmune)*.. **323, 1863**

RESPIRATORY STIMULANTS

Dopram Injectable *(Robins)*.............. **2709**

REVERSE TRANSCRIPTASE INHIBITORS

(see under:
ANTI-INFECTIVE AGENTS, SYSTEMIC
AIDS CHEMOTHERAPEUTIC AGENTS
NON-NUCLEOSIDE REVERSE TRANSCRIPTASE INHIBITORS
NUCLEOSIDE REVERSE TRANSCRIPTASE INHIBITORS)

S

SALIVA STIMULANTS

(see under:
SKIN & MUCOUS MEMBRANE AGENTS
MOUTH & THROAT PRODUCTS
SALIVA PRODUCTS)

SALT SUBSTITUTES

Chlor-3 *(Fleming)*...................... **1253**

SCABICIDES

(see under:
SKIN & MUCOUS MEMBRANE AGENTS
ANTI-INFECTIVES
SCABICIDES & PEDICULICIDES)

SCLEROSING AGENTS

Sotradecol Injection *(Elkins-Sinn)*.......... **1199**

SEBORRHEA TREATMENT

(see under:
SKIN & MUCOUS MEMBRANE AGENTS
ANTISEBORRHEIC AGENTS)

SEDATIVES & HYPNOTICS

BARBITURATES

Mebaral Tablets *(Sanofi-Synthelabo)*........ **2855**
Nembutal Sodium Capsules *(Abbott)*.... **303, 466**
Nembutal Sodium Solution *(Abbott)*......... **468**
Nembutal Sodium Suppositories *(Abbott)*..... **470**

BENZODIAZEPINES

Ativan Injection *(Wyeth-Ayerst)*........... **3344**
Halcion Tablets *(Pharmacia & Upjohn)*..................... **331, 2621**
ProSom Tablets *(Abbott)*.................. **485**
Valium Injectable *(Roche Labs)*........... **2793**
Versed Injection *(Roche Labs)*............ **2794**
Versed Syrup *(Roche Labs)*............... **2800**

MISCELLANEOUS SEDATIVES & HYPNOTICS

Ambien Tablets *(Searle)*............ **335, 2973**
Bevitamel Tablets *(Westlake)*............ **3324**
Diprivan Injectable Emulsion *(AstraZeneca)*................... **305, 620**
Mepergan Injection *(Wyeth-Ayerst)*......... **3403**
Phenergan Injection *(Wyeth-Ayerst)*........ **3416**

SECTION 4

PRODUCT IDENTIFICATION GUIDE

To aid in quick identification, this section provides full-color, actual-size photographs of tablets and capsules. A variety of other dosage forms and packages are shown at less than actual size. In all, the guide contains more than 2,400 photos.

Products in this section are arranged alphabetically by manufacturer. In some instances, not all dosage forms and sizes are pictured. If others are available, a † symbol precedes the product's name. Letters or numbers representing the manufacturer's identification code are followed by an asterisk.

For more information on any of the products in this section, please turn to the Product Information Section, or check directly with the manufacturer. The page number of each product's text entry appears with its photographs.

While every effort has been made to guarantee faithful reproduction of the photos in this section, changes in size, color, and design are always a possibility. Be sure to confirm a product's identity with the manufacturer or your pharmacist.

INDEX BY MANUFACTURER

This section is made possible through the courtesy of the manufacturers whose products appear on the following pages.

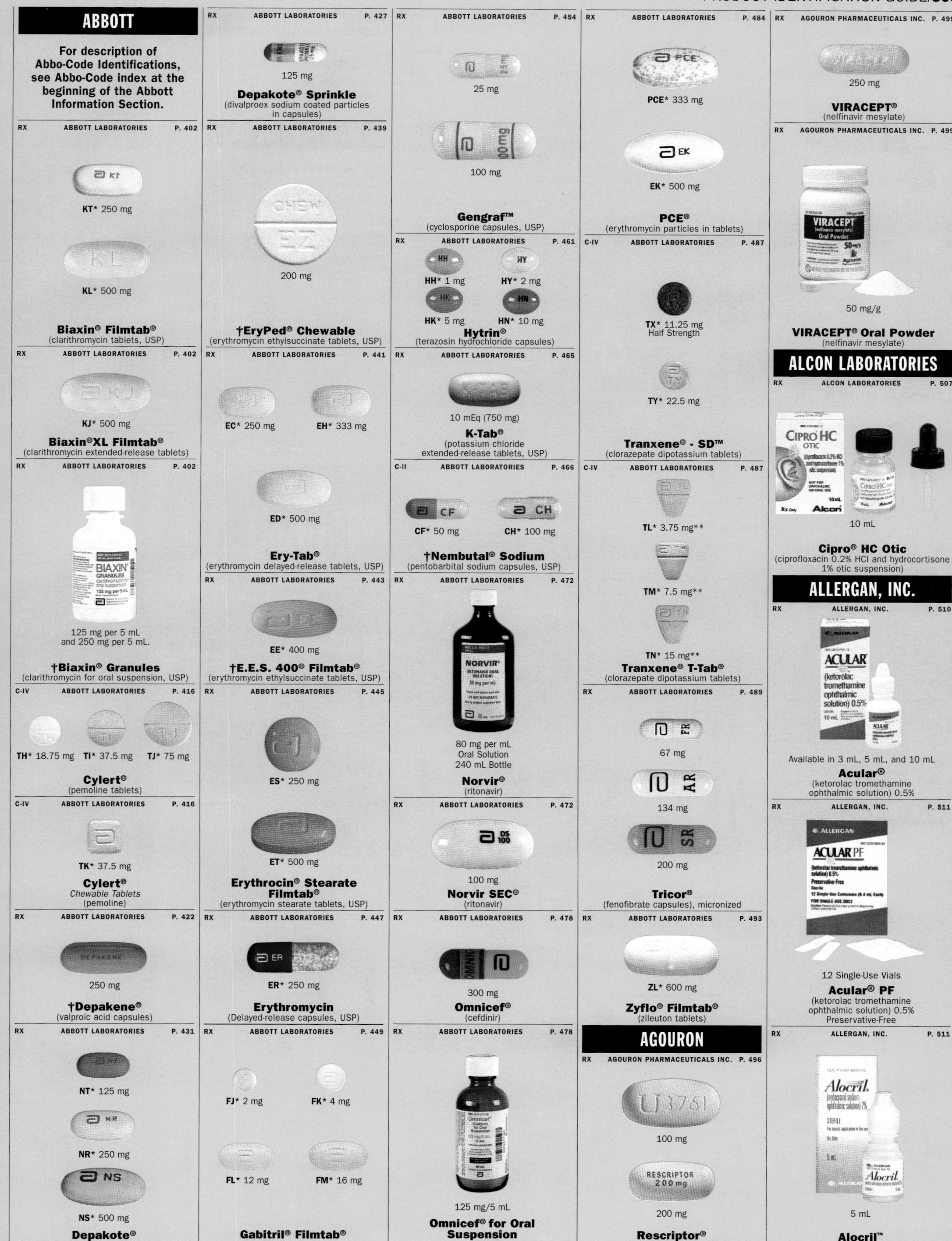

ABBOTT

For description of Abbo-Code Identifications, see Abbo-Code index at the beginning of the Abbott Information Section.

RX ABBOTT LABORATORIES P. 402

KT* 250 mg

KL* 500 mg

Biaxin® Filmtab®
(clarithromycin tablets, USP)

RX ABBOTT LABORATORIES P. 402

KJ* 500 mg

Biaxin®XL Filmtab®
(clarithromycin extended-release tablets)

RX ABBOTT LABORATORIES P. 402

125 mg per 5 mL and 250 mg per 5 mL.

†Biaxin® Granules
(clarithromycin for oral suspension, USP)

C-IV ABBOTT LABORATORIES P. 416

TH* 18.75 mg TI* 37.5 mg TJ* 75 mg

Cylert®
(pemoline tablets)

C-IV ABBOTT LABORATORIES P. 416

TK* 37.5 mg

Cylert®
Chewable Tablets
(pemoline)

RX ABBOTT LABORATORIES P. 422

250 mg

†Depakene®
(valproic acid capsules)

RX ABBOTT LABORATORIES P. 431

NT* 125 mg

NR* 250 mg

NS* 500 mg

Depakote®
(divalproex sodium delayed-release tablets)

RX ABBOTT LABORATORIES P. 427

125 mg

Depakote® Sprinkle
(divalproex sodium coated particles in capsules)

RX ABBOTT LABORATORIES P. 439

200 mg

†EryPed® Chewable
(erythromycin ethylsuccinate tablets, USP)

RX ABBOTT LABORATORIES P. 441

EC* 250 mg EH* 333 mg

ED* 500 mg

Ery-Tab®
(erythromycin delayed-release tablets, USP)

RX ABBOTT LABORATORIES P. 443

EE* 400 mg

†E.E.S. 400® Filmtab®
(erythromycin ethylsuccinate tablets, USP)

RX ABBOTT LABORATORIES P. 445

ES* 250 mg

ET* 500 mg

Erythrocin® Stearate Filmtab®
(erythromycin stearate tablets, USP)

RX ABBOTT LABORATORIES P. 447

ER* 250 mg

Erythromycin
(Delayed-release capsules, USP)

RX ABBOTT LABORATORIES P. 449

FJ* 2 mg FK* 4 mg

FL* 12 mg FM* 16 mg

Gabitril® Filmtab®
(tiagabine hydrochloride tablets)

RX ABBOTT LABORATORIES P. 454

25 mg

100 mg

Gengraf™
(cyclosporine capsules, USP)

RX ABBOTT LABORATORIES P. 461

HH* 1 mg HY* 2 mg

HK* 5 mg HN* 10 mg

Hytrin®
(terazosin hydrochloride capsules)

RX ABBOTT LABORATORIES P. 465

10 mEq (750 mg)

K-Tab®
(potassium chloride extended-release tablets, USP)

C-II ABBOTT LABORATORIES P. 466

CF* 50 mg CH* 100 mg

†Nembutal® Sodium
(pentobarbital sodium capsules, USP)

RX ABBOTT LABORATORIES P. 472

80 mg per mL
Oral Solution
240 mL Bottle

Norvir®
(ritonavir)

RX ABBOTT LABORATORIES P. 472

100 mg

Norvir SEC®
(ritonavir)

RX ABBOTT LABORATORIES P. 478

300 mg

Omnicef®
(cefdinir)

RX ABBOTT LABORATORIES P. 478

125 mg/5 mL

Omnicef® for Oral Suspension
(cefdinir)

RX ABBOTT LABORATORIES P. 484

PCE* 333 mg

EK* 500 mg

PCE®
(erythromycin particles in tablets)

C-IV ABBOTT LABORATORIES P. 487

TX* 11.25 mg
Half Strength

TY* 22.5 mg

Tranxene® - SD™
(clorazepate dipotassium tablets)

C-IV ABBOTT LABORATORIES P. 487

TL* 3.75 mg**

TM* 7.5 mg**

TN* 15 mg**

Tranxene® T-Tab®
(clorazepate dipotassium tablets)

RX ABBOTT LABORATORIES P. 489

67 mg

134 mg

200 mg

Tricor®
(fenofibrate capsules), micronized

RX ABBOTT LABORATORIES P. 493

ZL* 600 mg

Zyflo® Filmtab®
(zileuton tablets)

AGOURON

RX AGOURON PHARMACEUTICALS INC. P. 496

100 mg

200 mg

Rescriptor®
(delavirdine mesylate)

RX AGOURON PHARMACEUTICALS INC. P. 499

250 mg

VIRACEPT®
(nelfinavir mesylate)

RX AGOURON PHARMACEUTICALS INC. P. 499

50 mg/g

VIRACEPT® Oral Powder
(nelfinavir mesylate)

ALCON LABORATORIES

RX ALCON LABORATORIES P. 507

10 mL

Cipro® HC Otic
(ciprofloxacin 0.2% HCl and hydrocortisone 1% otic suspension)

ALLERGAN, INC.

RX ALLERGAN, INC. P. 510

Available in 3 mL, 5 mL, and 10 mL

Acular®
(ketorolac tromethamine ophthalmic solution) 0.5%

RX ALLERGAN, INC. P. 511

12 Single-Use Vials

Acular® PF
(ketorolac tromethamine ophthalmic solution) 0.5%
Preservative-Free

RX ALLERGAN, INC. P. 511

5 mL

Alocril™
(nedocromil sodium ophthalmic solution) 2%

*Abbott Abbo-Code identification letters. Filmtab® – Film sealed tablets, Abbott. **Grooved tablets.

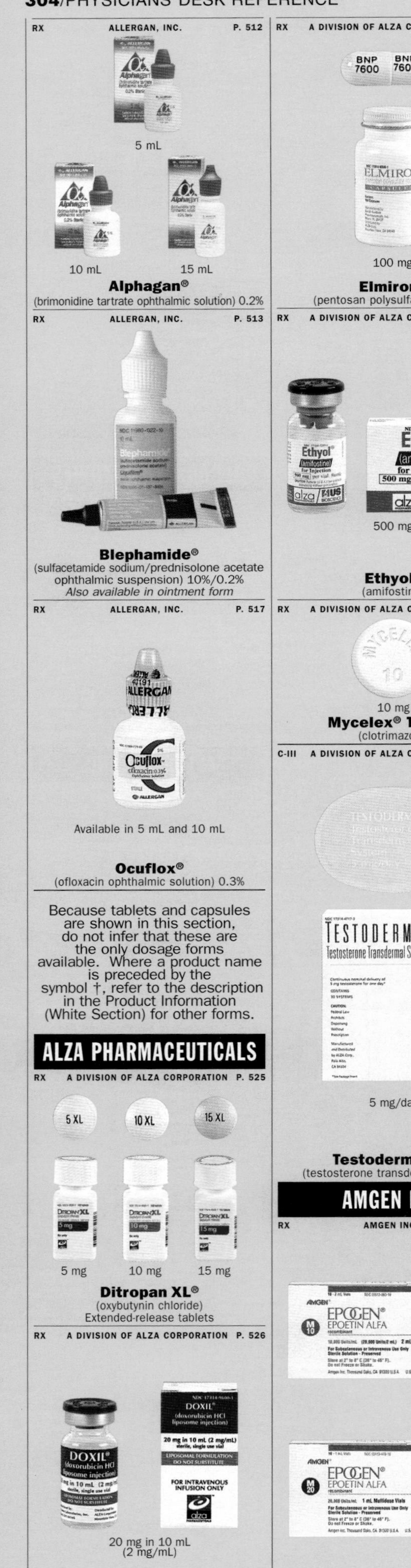

RX ALLERGAN, INC. P. 512

5 mL

10 mL 15 mL

Alphagan®
(brimonidine tartrate ophthalmic solution) 0.2%

RX ALLERGAN, INC. P. 513

Blephamide®
(sulfacetamide sodium/prednisolone acetate ophthalmic suspension) 10%/0.2%
Also available in ointment form

RX ALLERGAN, INC. P. 517

Available in 5 mL and 10 mL

Ocuflox®
(ofloxacin ophthalmic solution) 0.3%

Because tablets and capsules are shown in this section, do not infer that these are the only dosage forms available. Where a product name is preceded by the symbol †, refer to the description in the Product Information (White Section) for other forms.

ALZA PHARMACEUTICALS

RX A DIVISION OF ALZA CORPORATION P. 525

5 mg 10 mg 15 mg

Ditropan XL®
(oxybutynin chloride)
Extended-release tablets

RX A DIVISION OF ALZA CORPORATION P. 526

20 mg in 10 mL (2 mg/mL)

Doxil®
(doxorubicin HCl liposome injection)

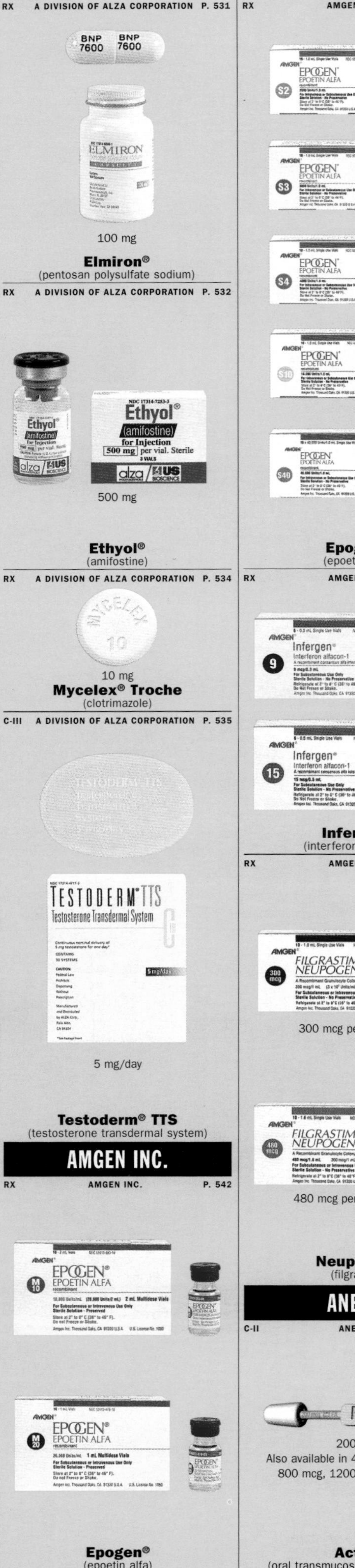

RX A DIVISION OF ALZA CORPORATION P. 531

100 mg

Elmiron®
(pentosan polysulfate sodium)

RX A DIVISION OF ALZA CORPORATION P. 532

500 mg

Ethyol®
(amifostine)

RX A DIVISION OF ALZA CORPORATION P. 534

10 mg

Mycelex® Troche
(clotrimazole)

C-III A DIVISION OF ALZA CORPORATION P. 535

5 mg/day

Testoderm® TTS
(testosterone transdermal system)

AMGEN INC.

RX AMGEN INC. P. 542

Epogen®
(epoetin alfa)

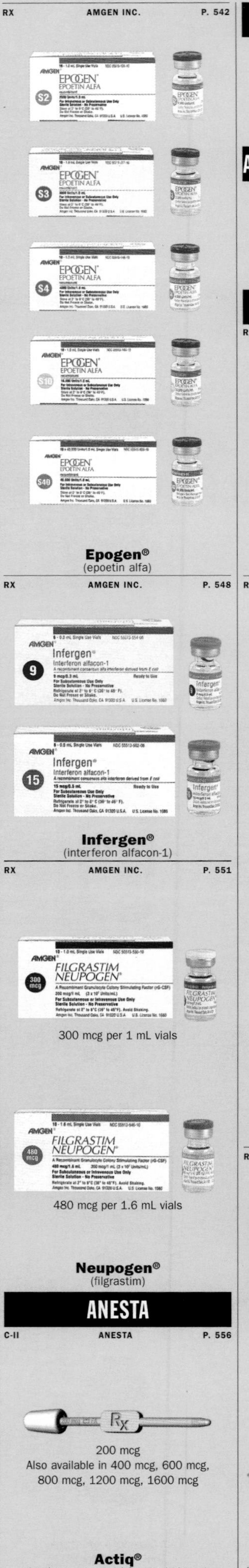

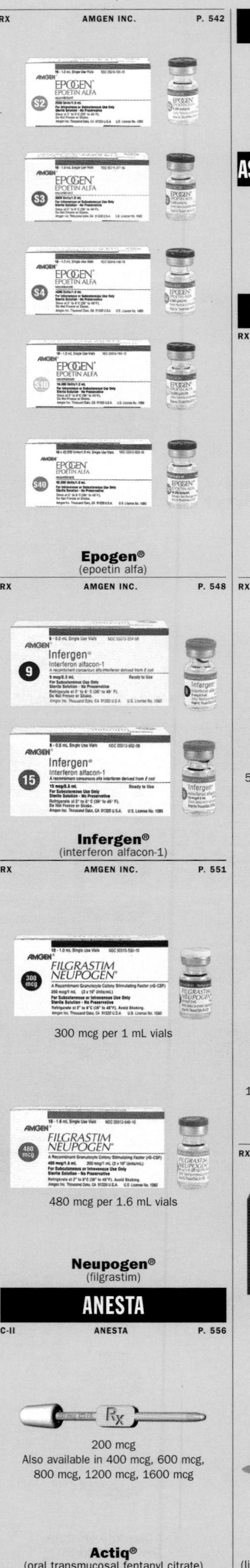

RX AMGEN INC. P. 542

Epogen®
(epoetin alfa)

RX AMGEN INC. P. 548

Infergen®
(interferon alfacon-1)

RX AMGEN INC. P. 551

300 mcg per 1 mL vials

480 mcg per 1.6 mL vials

Neupogen®
(filgrastim)

ANESTA

C-II ANESTA P. 556

200 mcg
Also available in 400 mcg, 600 mcg, 800 mcg, 1200 mcg, 1600 mcg

Actiq®
(oral transmucosal fentanyl citrate)

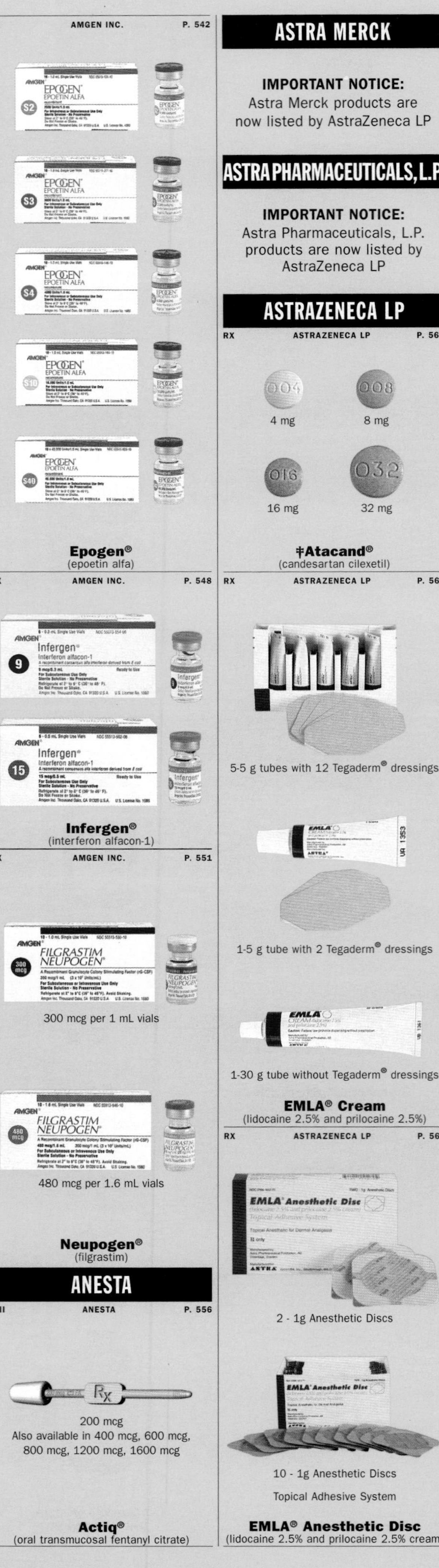

ASTRA MERCK

IMPORTANT NOTICE:
Astra Merck products are now listed by AstraZeneca LP

ASTRA PHARMACEUTICALS, L.P.

IMPORTANT NOTICE:
Astra Pharmaceuticals, L.P. products are now listed by AstraZeneca LP

ASTRAZENECA LP

RX ASTRAZENECA LP P. 564

4 mg 8 mg

16 mg 32 mg

†Atacand®
(candesartan cilexetil)

RX ASTRAZENECA LP P. 568

5-5 g tubes with 12 Tegaderm® dressings

1-5 g tube with 2 Tegaderm® dressings

1-30 g tube without Tegaderm® dressings

EMLA® Cream
(lidocaine 2.5% and prilocaine 2.5%)

RX ASTRAZENECA LP P. 568

2 - 1g Anesthetic Discs

10 - 1g Anesthetic Discs

Topical Adhesive System

EMLA® Anesthetic Disc
(lidocaine 2.5% and prilocaine 2.5% cream)

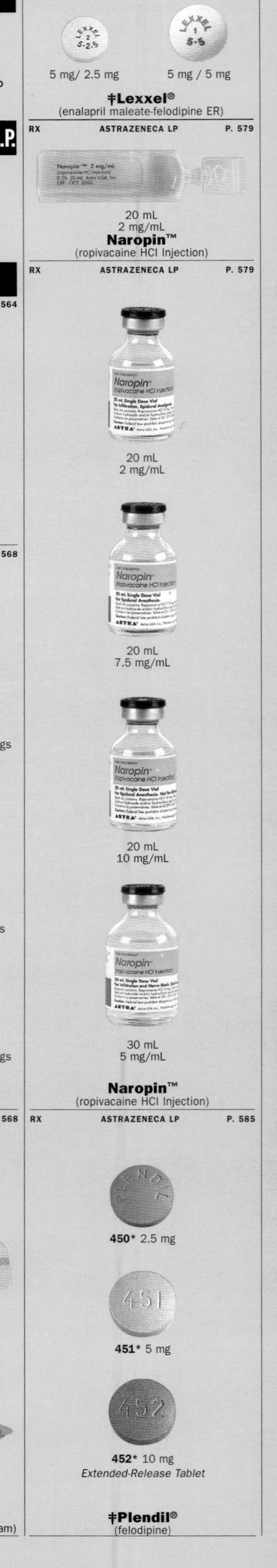

RX ASTRAZENECA LP P. 575

5 mg/ 2.5 mg 5 mg / 5 mg

†Lexxel®
(enalapril maleate-felodipine ER)

RX ASTRAZENECA LP P. 579

20 mL
2 mg/mL

Naropin™
(ropivacaine HCl Injection)

RX ASTRAZENECA LP P. 579

20 mL
2 mg/mL

20 mL
7.5 mg/mL

20 mL
10 mg/mL

30 mL
5 mg/mL

Naropin™
(ropivacaine HCl Injection)

RX ASTRAZENECA LP P. 585

450* 2.5 mg

451* 5 mg

452* 10 mg
Extended-Release Tablet

†Plendil®
(felodipine)

†Registered trademark of the AstraZeneca group of companies.

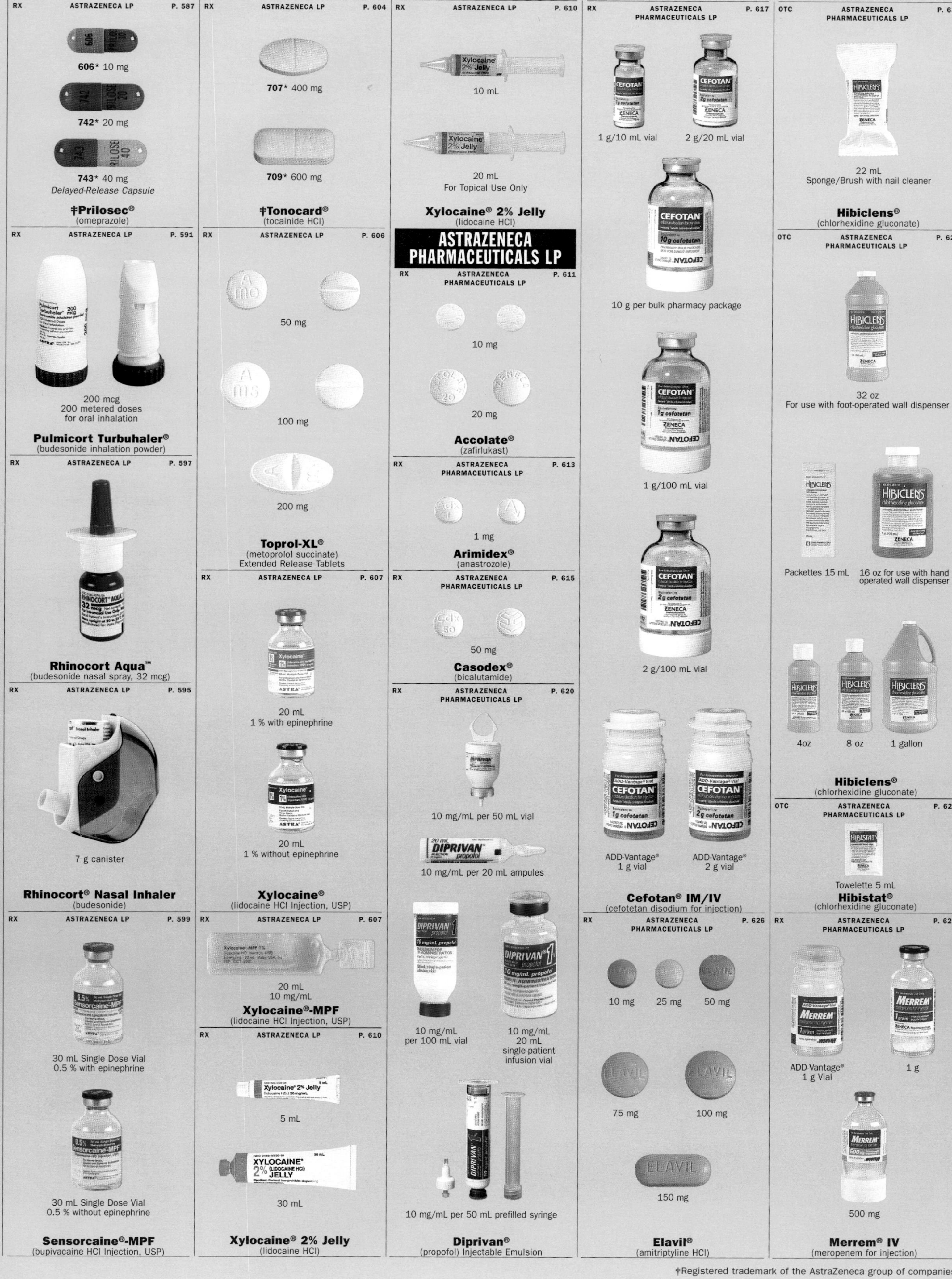
RX ASTRAZENECA LP P. 587
606* 10 mg
742* 20 mg
743* 40 mg
Delayed-Release Capsule
‡Prilosec®
(omeprazole)
RX ASTRAZENECA LP P. 591
200 mcg
200 metered doses
for oral inhalation
Pulmicort Turbuhaler®
(budesonide inhalation powder)
RX ASTRAZENECA LP P. 597
Rhinocort Aqua™
(budesonide nasal spray, 32 mcg)
RX ASTRAZENECA LP P. 595
7 g canister
Rhinocort® Nasal Inhaler
(budesonide)
RX ASTRAZENECA LP P. 599
30 mL Single Dose Vial
0.5 % with epinephrine
30 mL Single Dose Vial
0.5 % without epinephrine
Sensorcaine®-MPF
(bupivacaine HCl Injection, USP)
RX ASTRAZENECA LP P. 604
707* 400 mg
709* 600 mg
‡Tonocard®
(tocainide HCl)
RX ASTRAZENECA LP P. 606
50 mg
100 mg
200 mg
Toprol-XL®
(metoprolol succinate)
Extended Release Tablets
RX ASTRAZENECA LP P. 607
20 mL
1 % with epinephrine
20 mL
1 % without epinephrine
Xylocaine®
(lidocaine HCl Injection, USP)
RX ASTRAZENECA LP P. 607
20 mL
10 mg/mL
Xylocaine®-MPF
(lidocaine HCl Injection, USP)
RX ASTRAZENECA LP P. 610
5 mL
30 mL
Xylocaine® 2% Jelly
(lidocaine HCl)
RX ASTRAZENECA LP P. 610
10 mL
20 mL
For Topical Use Only
Xylocaine® 2% Jelly
(lidocaine HCl)
ASTRAZENECA
PHARMACEUTICALS LP
RX ASTRAZENECA PHARMACEUTICALS LP P. 611
10 mg
20 mg
Accolate®
(zafirlukast)
RX ASTRAZENECA PHARMACEUTICALS LP P. 613
1 mg
Arimidex®
(anastrozole)
RX ASTRAZENECA PHARMACEUTICALS LP P. 615
50 mg
Casodex®
(bicalutamide)
RX ASTRAZENECA PHARMACEUTICALS LP P. 620
10 mg/mL per 50 mL vial
10 mg/mL per 20 mL ampules
10 mg/mL
per 100 mL vial
10 mg/mL
20 mL
single-patient
infusion vial
10 mg/mL per 50 mL prefilled syringe
Diprivan®
(propofol) Injectable Emulsion
RX ASTRAZENECA PHARMACEUTICALS LP P. 617
1 g/10 mL vial
2 g/20 mL vial
10 g per bulk pharmacy package
1 g/100 mL vial
2 g/100 mL vial
ADD-Vantage®
1 g vial
ADD-Vantage®
2 g vial
Cefotan® IM/IV
(cefotetan disodium for injection)
RX ASTRAZENECA PHARMACEUTICALS LP P. 626
10 mg
25 mg
50 mg
75 mg
100 mg
150 mg
Elavil®
(amitriptyline HCl)
OTC ASTRAZENECA PHARMACEUTICALS LP P. 628
22 mL
Sponge/Brush with nail cleaner
Hibiclens®
(chlorhexidine gluconate)
OTC ASTRAZENECA PHARMACEUTICALS LP P. 628
32 oz
For use with foot-operated wall dispenser
Packettes 15 mL
16 oz for use with hand
operated wall dispenser
4oz
8 oz
1 gallon
Hibiclens®
(chlorhexidine gluconate)
OTC ASTRAZENECA PHARMACEUTICALS LP P. 629
Towelette 5 mL
Hibistat®
(chlorhexidine gluconate)
RX ASTRAZENECA PHARMACEUTICALS LP P. 629
ADD-Vantage®
1 g Vial
1 g
500 mg
Merrem® IV
(meropenem for injection)

‡Registered trademark of the AstraZeneca group of companies.

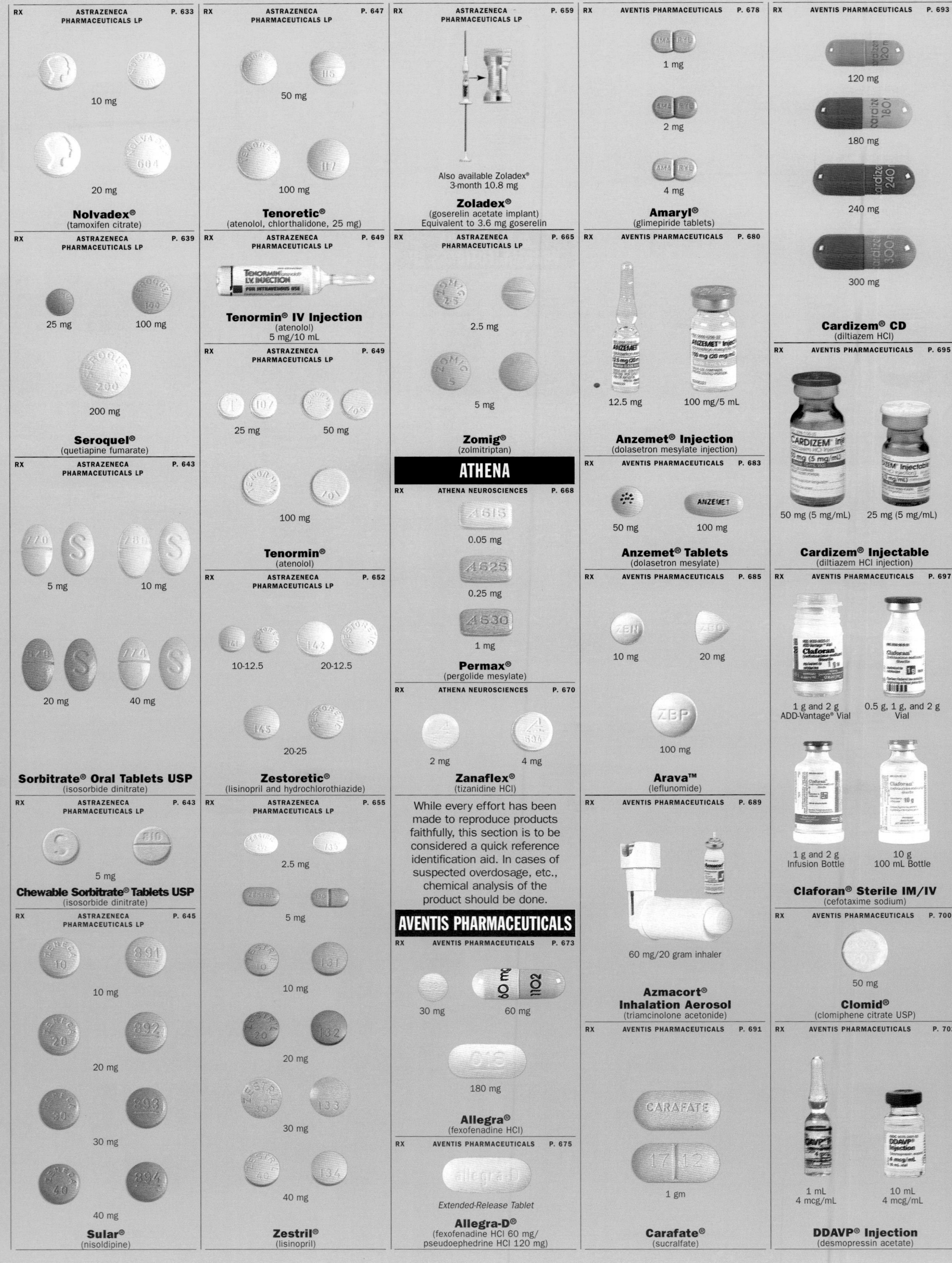
RX ASTRAZENECA PHARMACEUTICALS LP P. 633
10 mg
20 mg
Nolvadex®
(tamoxifen citrate)
RX ASTRAZENECA PHARMACEUTICALS LP P. 639
25 mg
100 mg
200 mg
Seroquel®
(quetiapine fumarate)
RX ASTRAZENECA PHARMACEUTICALS LP P. 643
5 mg
10 mg
20 mg
40 mg
Sorbitrate® Oral Tablets USP
(isosorbide dinitrate)
RX ASTRAZENECA PHARMACEUTICALS LP P. 643
5 mg
Chewable Sorbitrate® Tablets USP
(isosorbide dinitrate)
RX ASTRAZENECA PHARMACEUTICALS LP P. 645
10 mg
20 mg
30 mg
40 mg
Sular®
(nisoldipine)
RX ASTRAZENECA PHARMACEUTICALS LP P. 647
50 mg
100 mg
Tenoretic®
(atenolol, chlorthalidone, 25 mg)
RX ASTRAZENECA PHARMACEUTICALS LP P. 649
Tenormin® IV Injection
(atenolol)
5 mg/10 mL
RX ASTRAZENECA PHARMACEUTICALS LP P. 649
25 mg
50 mg
100 mg
Tenormin®
(atenolol)
RX ASTRAZENECA PHARMACEUTICALS LP P. 652
10-12.5
20-12.5
20-25
Zestoretic®
(lisinopril and hydrochlorothiazide)
RX ASTRAZENECA PHARMACEUTICALS LP P. 655
2.5 mg
5 mg
10 mg
20 mg
30 mg
40 mg
Zestril®
(lisinopril)
RX ASTRAZENECA PHARMACEUTICALS LP P. 659
Also available Zoladex® 3-month 10.8 mg
Zoladex®
(goserelin acetate implant)
Equivalent to 3.6 mg goserelin
RX ASTRAZENECA PHARMACEUTICALS LP P. 665
2.5 mg
5 mg
Zomig®
(zolmitriptan)
ATHENA
RX ATHENA NEUROSCIENCES P. 668
0.05 mg
0.25 mg
1 mg
Permax®
(pergolide mesylate)
RX ATHENA NEUROSCIENCES P. 670
2 mg
4 mg
Zanaflex®
(tizanidine HCl)
While every effort has been made to reproduce products faithfully, this section is to be considered a quick reference identification aid. In cases of suspected overdosage, etc., chemical analysis of the product should be done.
AVENTIS PHARMACEUTICALS
RX AVENTIS PHARMACEUTICALS P. 673
30 mg
60 mg
180 mg
Allegra®
(fexofenadine HCl)
RX AVENTIS PHARMACEUTICALS P. 675
Extended-Release Tablet
Allegra-D®
(fexofenadine HCl 60 mg/ pseudoephedrine HCl 120 mg)
RX AVENTIS PHARMACEUTICALS P. 678
1 mg
2 mg
4 mg
Amaryl®
(glimepiride tablets)
RX AVENTIS PHARMACEUTICALS P. 680
12.5 mg
100 mg/5 mL
Anzemet® Injection
(dolasetron mesylate injection)
RX AVENTIS PHARMACEUTICALS P. 683
50 mg
100 mg
Anzemet® Tablets
(dolasetron mesylate)
RX AVENTIS PHARMACEUTICALS P. 685
10 mg
20 mg
100 mg
Arava™
(leflunomide)
RX AVENTIS PHARMACEUTICALS P. 689
60 mg/20 gram inhaler
Azmacort®
Inhalation Aerosol
(triamcinolone acetonide)
RX AVENTIS PHARMACEUTICALS P. 691
1 gm
Carafate®
(sucralfate)
RX AVENTIS PHARMACEUTICALS P. 693
120 mg
180 mg
240 mg
300 mg
Cardizem® CD
(diltiazem HCl)
RX AVENTIS PHARMACEUTICALS P. 695
50 mg (5 mg/mL)
25 mg (5 mg/mL)
Cardizem® Injectable
(diltiazem HCl injection)
RX AVENTIS PHARMACEUTICALS P. 697
1 g and 2 g
ADD-Vantage® Vial
0.5 g, 1 g, and 2 g
Vial
1 g and 2 g
Infusion Bottle
10 g
100 mL Bottle
Claforan® Sterile IM/IV
(cefotaxime sodium)
RX AVENTIS PHARMACEUTICALS P. 700
50 mg
Clomid®
(clomiphene citrate USP)
RX AVENTIS PHARMACEUTICALS P. 702
1 mL
4 mcg/mL
10 mL
4 mcg/mL
DDAVP® Injection
(desmopressin acetate)

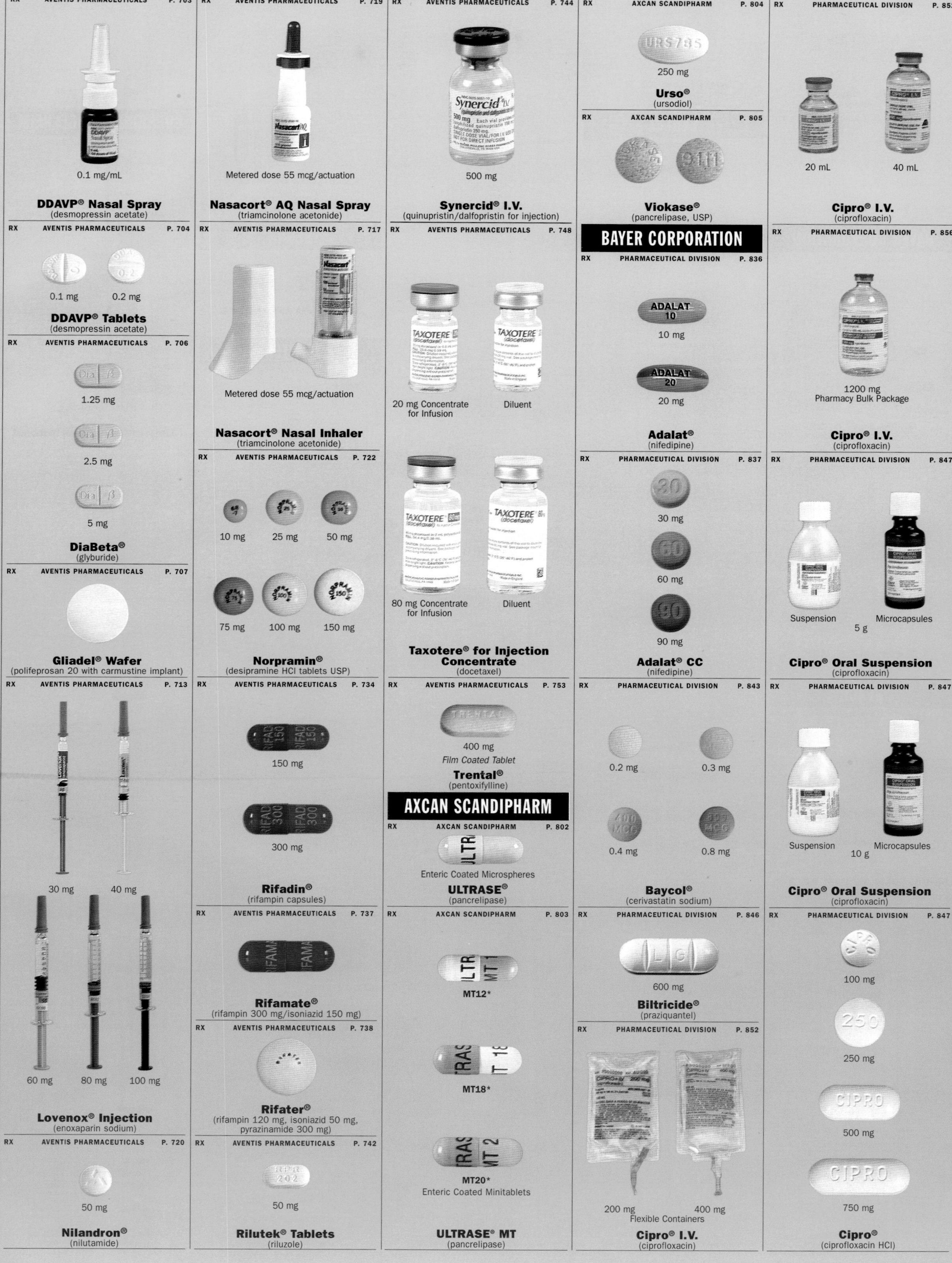

RX AVENTIS PHARMACEUTICALS P. 703
0.1 mg/mL
DDAVP® Nasal Spray
(desmopressin acetate)
RX AVENTIS PHARMACEUTICALS P. 704
0.1 mg 0.2 mg
DDAVP® Tablets
(desmopressin acetate)
RX AVENTIS PHARMACEUTICALS P. 706
1.25 mg
2.5 mg
5 mg
DiaBeta®
(glyburide)
RX AVENTIS PHARMACEUTICALS P. 707
Gliadel® Wafer
(polifeprosan 20 with carmustine implant)
RX AVENTIS PHARMACEUTICALS P. 713
30 mg 40 mg
60 mg 80 mg 100 mg
Lovenox® Injection
(enoxaparin sodium)
RX AVENTIS PHARMACEUTICALS P. 720
50 mg
Nilandron®
(nilutamide)
RX AVENTIS PHARMACEUTICALS P. 719
Metered dose 55 mcg/actuation
Nasacort® AQ Nasal Spray
(triamcinolone acetonide)
RX AVENTIS PHARMACEUTICALS P. 717
Metered dose 55 mcg/actuation
Nasacort® Nasal Inhaler
(triamcinolone acetonide)
RX AVENTIS PHARMACEUTICALS P. 722
10 mg 25 mg 50 mg
75 mg 100 mg 150 mg
Norpramin®
(desipramine HCl tablets USP)
RX AVENTIS PHARMACEUTICALS P. 734
150 mg
300 mg
Rifadin®
(rifampin capsules)
RX AVENTIS PHARMACEUTICALS P. 737
Rifamate®
(rifampin 300 mg/isoniazid 150 mg)
RX AVENTIS PHARMACEUTICALS P. 738
Rifater®
(rifampin 120 mg, isoniazid 50 mg, pyrazinamide 300 mg)
RX AVENTIS PHARMACEUTICALS P. 742
50 mg
Rilutek® Tablets
(riluzole)
RX AVENTIS PHARMACEUTICALS P. 744
500 mg
Synercid® I.V.
(quinupristin/dalfopristin for injection)
RX AVENTIS PHARMACEUTICALS P. 748
20 mg Concentrate for Infusion
Diluent
80 mg Concentrate for Infusion
Diluent
Taxotere® for Injection Concentrate
(docetaxel)
RX AVENTIS PHARMACEUTICALS P. 753
400 mg
Film Coated Tablet
Trental®
(pentoxifylline)
AXCAN SCANDIPHARM
RX AXCAN SCANDIPHARM P. 802
Enteric Coated Microspheres
ULTRASE®
(pancrelipase)
RX AXCAN SCANDIPHARM P. 803
MT12*
MT18*
MT20*
Enteric Coated Minitablets
ULTRASE® MT
(pancrelipase)
RX AXCAN SCANDIPHARM P. 804
250 mg
Urso®
(ursodiol)
RX AXCAN SCANDIPHARM P. 805
Viokase®
(pancrelipase, USP)
BAYER CORPORATION
RX PHARMACEUTICAL DIVISION P. 836
10 mg
20 mg
Adalat®
(nifedipine)
RX PHARMACEUTICAL DIVISION P. 837
30 mg
60 mg
90 mg
Adalat® CC
(nifedipine)
RX PHARMACEUTICAL DIVISION P. 843
0.2 mg 0.3 mg
0.4 mg 0.8 mg
Baycol®
(cerivastatin sodium)
RX PHARMACEUTICAL DIVISION P. 846
600 mg
Biltricide®
(praziquantel)
RX PHARMACEUTICAL DIVISION P. 852
200 mg 400 mg
Flexible Containers
Cipro® I.V.
(ciprofloxacin)
RX PHARMACEUTICAL DIVISION P. 852
20 mL 40 mL
Cipro® I.V.
(ciprofloxacin)
RX PHARMACEUTICAL DIVISION P. 856
1200 mg
Pharmacy Bulk Package
Cipro® I.V.
(ciprofloxacin)
RX PHARMACEUTICAL DIVISION P. 847
Suspension Microcapsules
5 g
Cipro® Oral Suspension
(ciprofloxacin)
RX PHARMACEUTICAL DIVISION P. 847
Suspension Microcapsules
10 g
Cipro® Oral Suspension
(ciprofloxacin)
RX PHARMACEUTICAL DIVISION P. 847
100 mg
250 mg
500 mg
750 mg
Cipro®
(ciprofloxacin HCl)

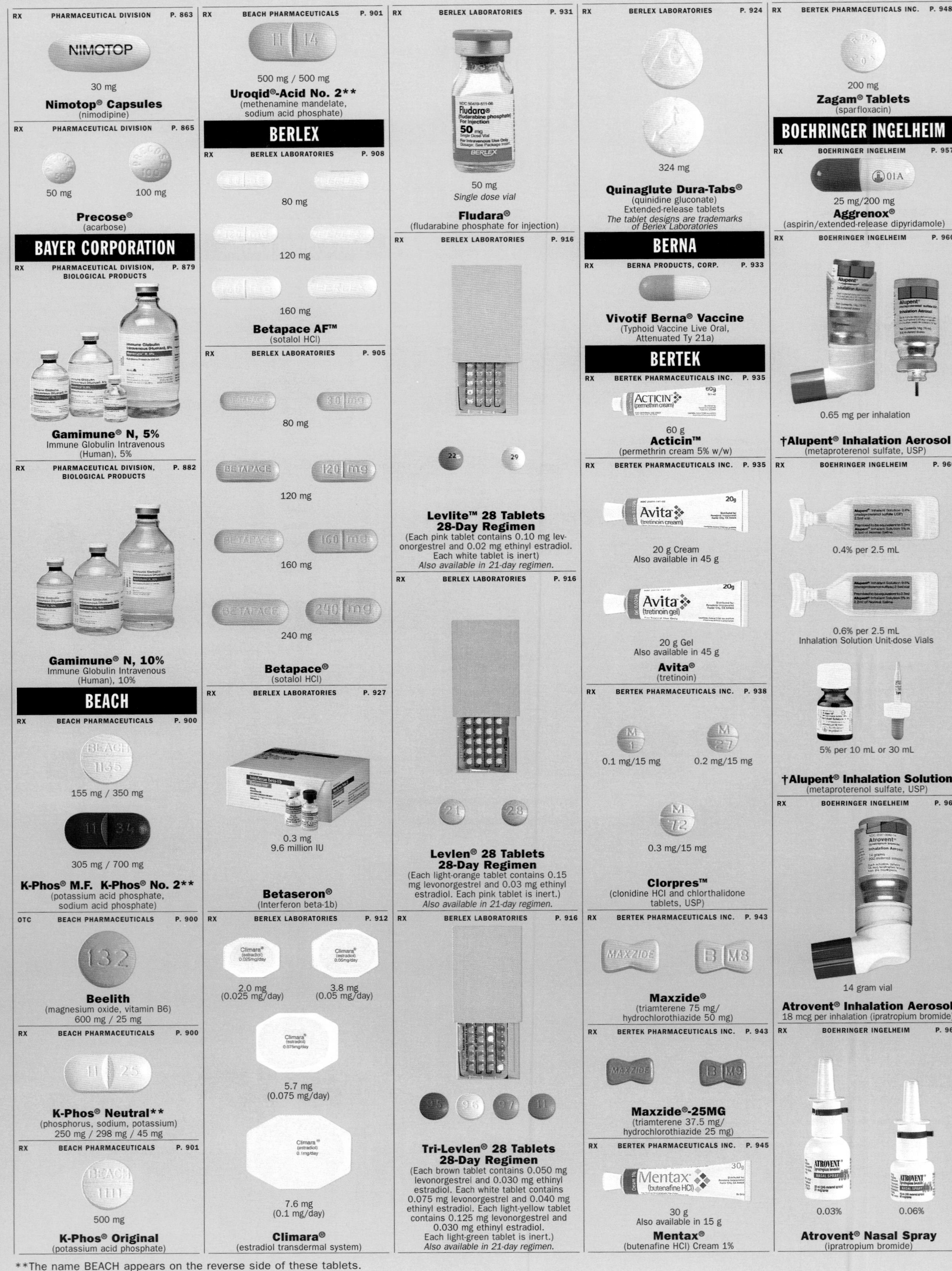

RX PHARMACEUTICAL DIVISION P. 863
NIMOTOP
30 mg
Nimotop® Capsules
(nimodipine)

RX PHARMACEUTICAL DIVISION P. 865
50 mg 100 mg
Precose®
(acarbose)

BAYER CORPORATION

RX PHARMACEUTICAL DIVISION, BIOLOGICAL PRODUCTS P. 879
Gamimune® N, 5%
Immune Globulin Intravenous (Human), 5%

RX PHARMACEUTICAL DIVISION, BIOLOGICAL PRODUCTS P. 882
Gamimune® N, 10%
Immune Globulin Intravenous (Human), 10%

BEACH

RX BEACH PHARMACEUTICALS P. 900
155 mg / 350 mg
305 mg / 700 mg
K-Phos® M.F. K-Phos® No. 2**
(potassium acid phosphate, sodium acid phosphate)

OTC BEACH PHARMACEUTICALS P. 900
Beelith
(magnesium oxide, vitamin B6)
600 mg / 25 mg

RX BEACH PHARMACEUTICALS P. 900
K-Phos® Neutral**
(phosphorus, sodium, potassium)
250 mg / 298 mg / 45 mg

RX BEACH PHARMACEUTICALS P. 901
500 mg
K-Phos® Original
(potassium acid phosphate)

RX BEACH PHARMACEUTICALS P. 901
500 mg / 500 mg
Uroqid®-Acid No. 2**
(methenamine mandelate, sodium acid phosphate)

BERLEX

RX BERLEX LABORATORIES P. 908
80 mg
120 mg
160 mg
Betapace AF™
(sotalol HCl)

RX BERLEX LABORATORIES P. 905
80 mg
120 mg
160 mg
240 mg
Betapace®
(sotalol HCl)

RX BERLEX LABORATORIES P. 927
0.3 mg
9.6 million IU
Betaseron®
(Interferon beta-1b)

RX BERLEX LABORATORIES P. 912
2.0 mg (0.025 mg/day)
3.8 mg (0.05 mg/day)
5.7 mg (0.075 mg/day)
7.6 mg (0.1 mg/day)
Climara®
(estradiol transdermal system)

RX BERLEX LABORATORIES P. 931
50 mg
Single dose vial
Fludara®
(fludarabine phosphate for injection)

RX BERLEX LABORATORIES P. 916
Levlite™ 28 Tablets 28-Day Regimen
(Each pink tablet contains 0.10 mg levonorgestrel and 0.02 mg ethinyl estradiol. Each white tablet is inert)
Also available in 21-day regimen.

RX BERLEX LABORATORIES P. 916
Levlen® 28 Tablets 28-Day Regimen
(Each light-orange tablet contains 0.15 mg levonorgestrel and 0.03 mg ethinyl estradiol. Each pink tablet is inert.)
Also available in 21-day regimen.

RX BERLEX LABORATORIES P. 916
Tri-Levlen® 28 Tablets 28-Day Regimen
(Each brown tablet contains 0.050 mg levonorgestrel and 0.030 mg ethinyl estradiol. Each white tablet contains 0.075 mg levonorgestrel and 0.040 mg ethinyl estradiol. Each light-yellow tablet contains 0.125 mg levonorgestrel and 0.030 mg ethinyl estradiol. Each light-green tablet is inert.)
Also available in 21-day regimen.

RX BERLEX LABORATORIES P. 924
324 mg
Quinaglute Dura-Tabs®
(quinidine gluconate)
Extended-release tablets
The tablet designs are trademarks of Berlex Laboratories

BERNA

RX BERNA PRODUCTS, CORP. P. 933
Vivotif Berna® Vaccine
(Typhoid Vaccine Live Oral, Attenuated Ty 21a)

BERTEK

RX BERTEK PHARMACEUTICALS INC. P. 935
60 g
Acticin™
(permethrin cream 5% w/w)

RX BERTEK PHARMACEUTICALS INC. P. 935
20 g Cream
Also available in 45 g
20 g Gel
Also available in 45 g
Avita®
(tretinoin)

RX BERTEK PHARMACEUTICALS INC. P. 938
0.1 mg/15 mg 0.2 mg/15 mg
0.3 mg/15 mg
Clorpres™
(clonidine HCl and chlorthalidone tablets, USP)

RX BERTEK PHARMACEUTICALS INC. P. 943
Maxzide®
(triamterene 75 mg/ hydrochlorothiazide 50 mg)

RX BERTEK PHARMACEUTICALS INC. P. 943
Maxzide®-25MG
(triamterene 37.5 mg/ hydrochlorothiazide 25 mg)

RX BERTEK PHARMACEUTICALS INC. P. 945
30 g
Also available in 15 g
Mentax®
(butenafine HCl) Cream 1%

RX BERTEK PHARMACEUTICALS INC. P. 948
200 mg
Zagam® Tablets
(sparfloxacin)

BOEHRINGER INGELHEIM

RX BOEHRINGER INGELHEIM P. 957
25 mg/200 mg
Aggrenox®
(aspirin/extended-release dipyridamole)

RX BOEHRINGER INGELHEIM P. 960
0.65 mg per inhalation
†Alupent® Inhalation Aerosol
(metaproterenol sulfate, USP)

RX BOEHRINGER INGELHEIM P. 960
0.4% per 2.5 mL
0.6% per 2.5 mL
Inhalation Solution Unit-dose Vials
5% per 10 mL or 30 mL
†Alupent® Inhalation Solution
(metaproterenol sulfate, USP)

RX BOEHRINGER INGELHEIM P. 962
14 gram vial
Atrovent® Inhalation Aerosol
18 mcg per inhalation (ipratropium bromide)

RX BOEHRINGER INGELHEIM P. 964
0.03% 0.06%
Atrovent® Nasal Spray
(ipratropium bromide)

**The name BEACH appears on the reverse side of these tablets.

RX BOEHRINGER INGELHEIM P. 963

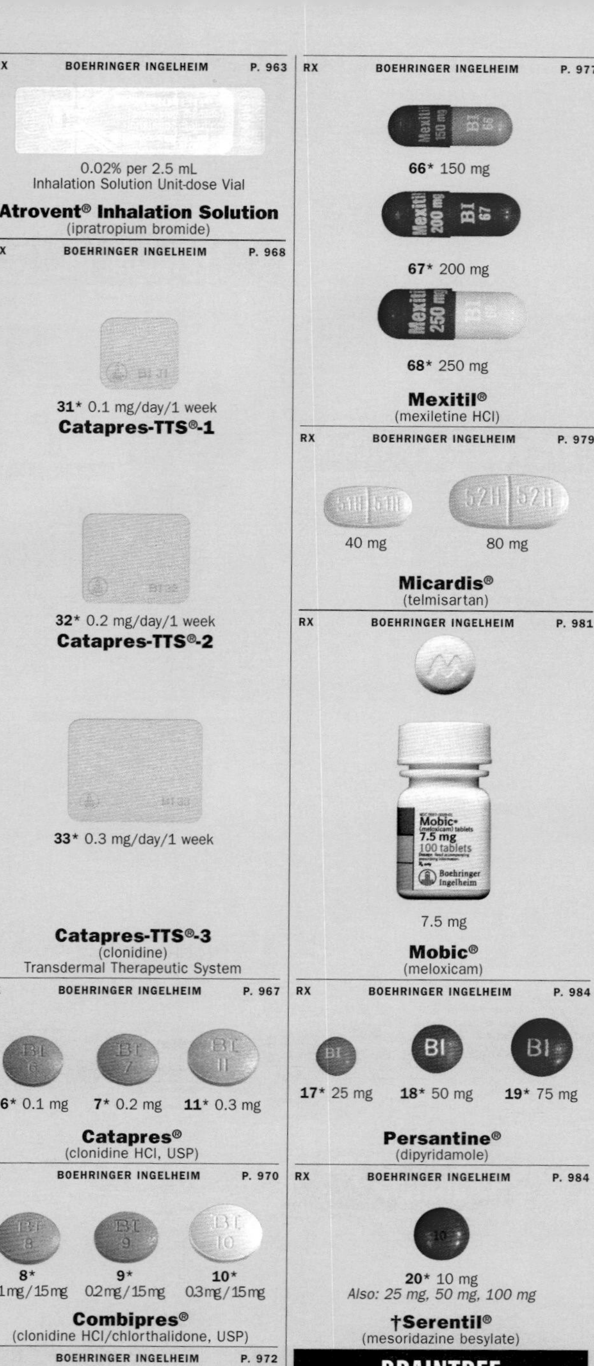

0.02% per 2.5 mL
Inhalation Solution Unit-dose Vial

Atrovent® Inhalation Solution
(ipratropium bromide)

RX BOEHRINGER INGELHEIM P. 968

31* 0.1 mg/day/1 week
Catapres-TTS®-1

32* 0.2 mg/day/1 week
Catapres-TTS®-2

33* 0.3 mg/day/1 week

Catapres-TTS®-3
(clonidine)
Transdermal Therapeutic System

RX BOEHRINGER INGELHEIM P. 967

6* 0.1 mg 7* 0.2 mg 11* 0.3 mg

Catapres®
(clonidine HCl, USP)

RX BOEHRINGER INGELHEIM P. 970

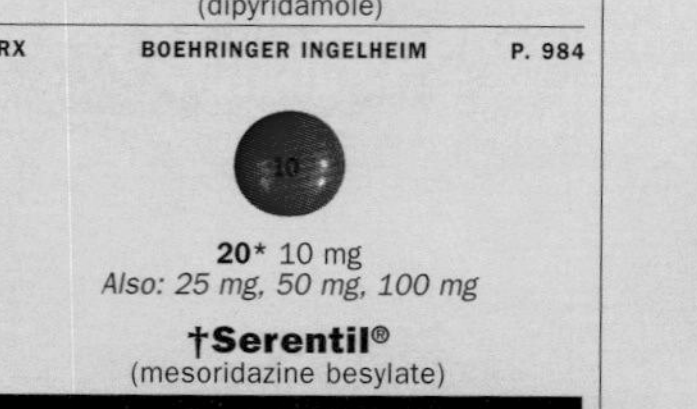

8* 0.1mg/15mg 9* 0.2mg/15mg 10* 0.3mg/15mg

Combipres®
(clonidine HCl/chlorthalidone, USP)

RX BOEHRINGER INGELHEIM P. 972

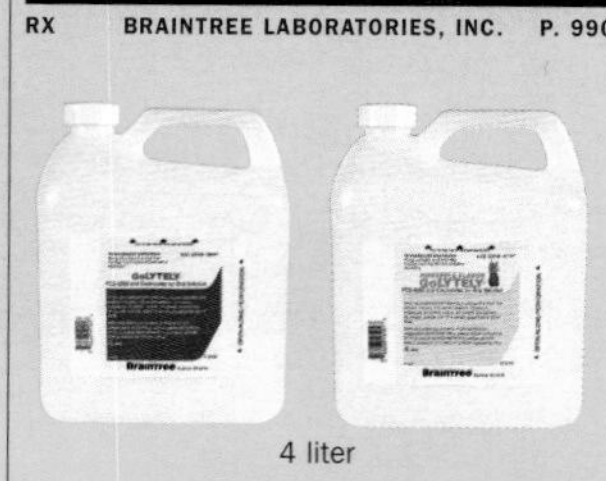

Combivent® Inhalation Aerosol
(ipratropium bromide and albuterol sulfate)

RX BOEHRINGER INGELHEIM P. 974

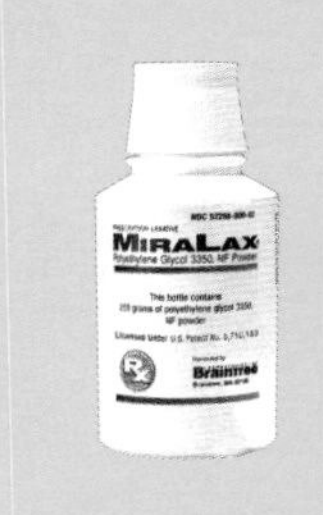

0.4 mg

Flomax®
(tamsulosin HCl)

RX BOEHRINGER INGELHEIM P. 977

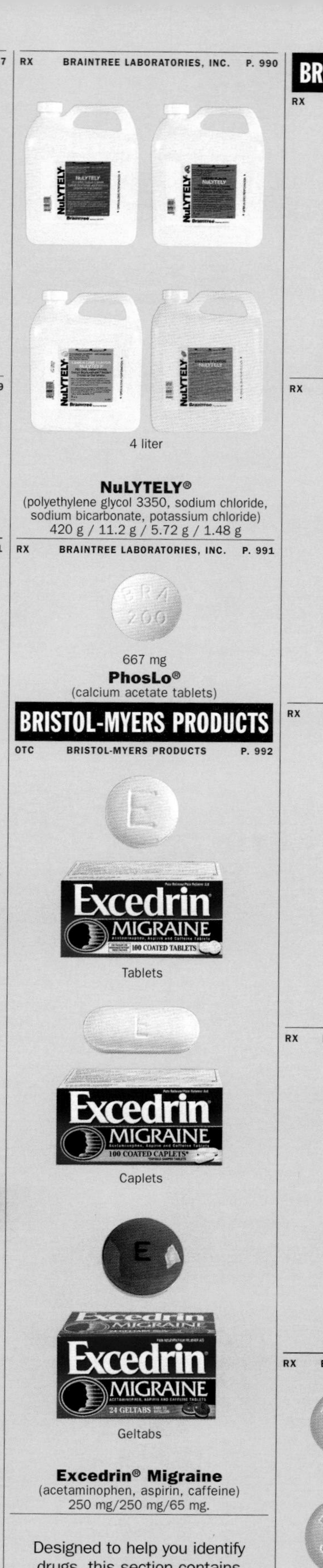

66* 150 mg

67* 200 mg

68* 250 mg

Mexitil®
(mexiletine HCl)

RX BOEHRINGER INGELHEIM P. 979

40 mg 80 mg

Micardis®
(telmisartan)

RX BOEHRINGER INGELHEIM P. 981

7.5 mg

Mobic®
(meloxicam)

RX BOEHRINGER INGELHEIM P. 984

17* 25 mg 18* 50 mg 19* 75 mg

Persantine®
(dipyridamole)

RX BOEHRINGER INGELHEIM P. 984

20* 10 mg
Also: 25 mg, 50 mg, 100 mg

†Serentil®
(mesoridazine besylate)

BRAINTREE

RX BRAINTREE LABORATORIES, INC. P. 990

4 liter

GoLYTELY®
(polyethylene glycol 3350, sodium sulfate (anhydrous), sodium bicarbonate, sodium chloride, potassium chloride)
236 g / 22.74 g / 6.74 g / 5.86 g / 2.97 g

RX BRAINTREE LABORATORIES, INC. P. 991

MiraLax™
(polyethylene glycol 3350, NF Powder)

RX BRAINTREE LABORATORIES, INC. P. 990

4 liter

NuLYTELY®
(polyethylene glycol 3350, sodium chloride, sodium bicarbonate, potassium chloride)
420 g / 11.2 g / 5.72 g / 1.48 g

RX BRAINTREE LABORATORIES, INC. P. 991

667 mg
PhosLo®
(calcium acetate tablets)

BRISTOL-MYERS PRODUCTS

OTC BRISTOL-MYERS PRODUCTS P. 992

Tablets

Caplets

Geltabs

Excedrin® Migraine
(acetaminophen, aspirin, caffeine)
250 mg/250 mg/65 mg.

Designed to help you identify drugs, this section contains actual size pills and full color reproduction of products selected for inclusion by participating manufacturers.

Because tablets and capsules are shown in this section, do not infer that these are the only dosage forms available. Where a product name is preceded by the symbol †, refer to the description in the Product Information (White Section) for other forms.

BRISTOL-MYERS SQUIBB CO.

RX BRISTOL-MYERS SQUIBB COMPANY P. 993

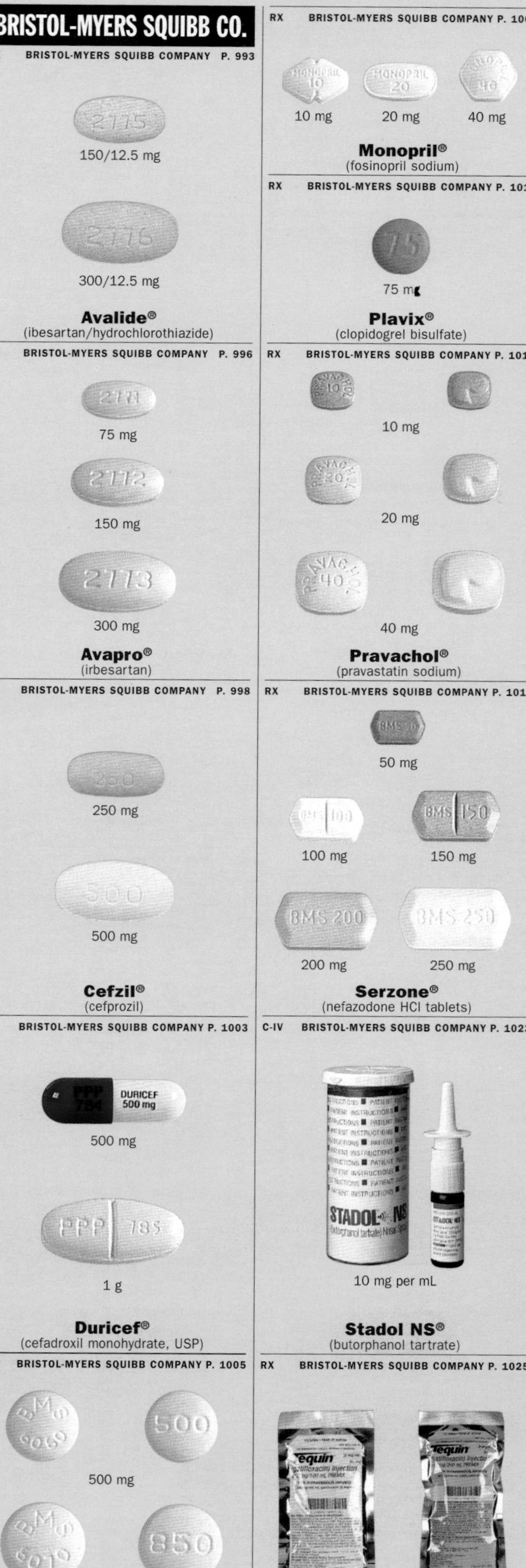

150/12.5 mg

300/12.5 mg

Avalide®
(ibesartan/hydrochlorothiazide)

RX BRISTOL-MYERS SQUIBB COMPANY P. 996

75 mg

150 mg

300 mg

Avapro®
(irbesartan)

RX BRISTOL-MYERS SQUIBB COMPANY P. 998

250 mg

500 mg

Cefzil®
(cefprozil)

RX BRISTOL-MYERS SQUIBB COMPANY P. 1003

500 mg

1 g

Duricef®
(cefadroxil monohydrate, USP)

RX BRISTOL-MYERS SQUIBB COMPANY P. 1005

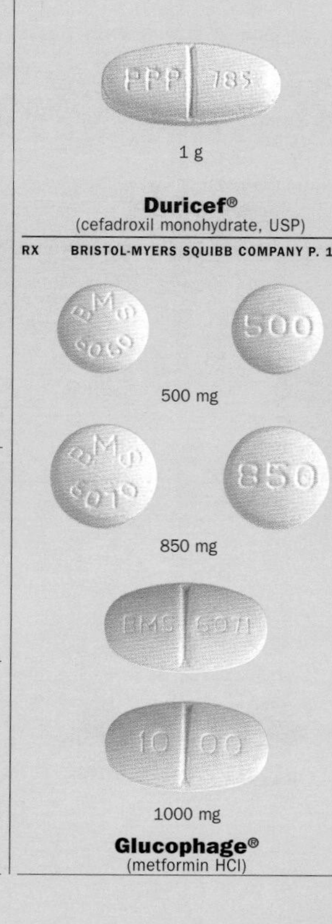

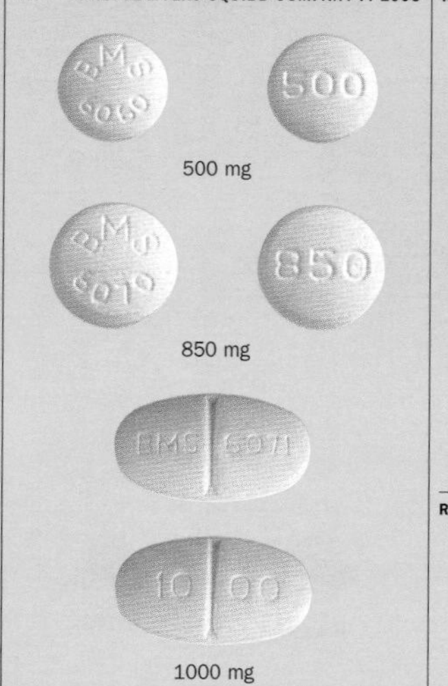

500 mg

850 mg

1000 mg

Glucophage®
(metformin HCl)

RX BRISTOL-MYERS SQUIBB COMPANY P. 1009

10 mg 20 mg 40 mg

Monopril®
(fosinopril sodium)

RX BRISTOL-MYERS SQUIBB COMPANY P. 1012

75 mg

Plavix®
(clopidogrel bisulfate)

RX BRISTOL-MYERS SQUIBB COMPANY P. 1014

10 mg

20 mg

40 mg

Pravachol®
(pravastatin sodium)

RX BRISTOL-MYERS SQUIBB COMPANY P. 1018

50 mg

100 mg 150 mg

200 mg 250 mg

Serzone®
(nefazodone HCl tablets)

C-IV BRISTOL-MYERS SQUIBB COMPANY P. 1023

10 mg per mL

Stadol NS®
(butorphanol tartrate)

RX BRISTOL-MYERS SQUIBB COMPANY P. 1025

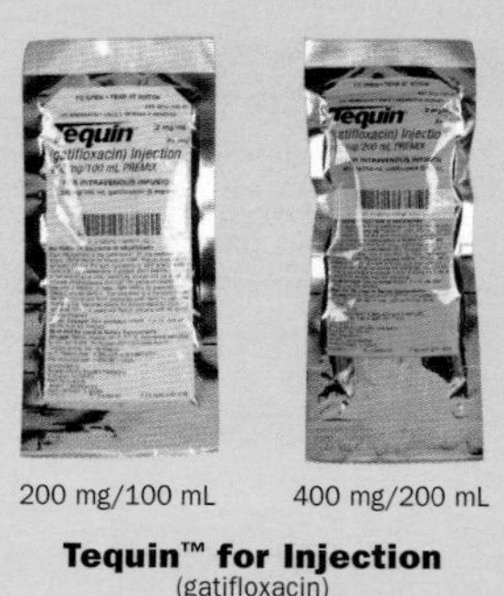

200 mg/100 mL 400 mg/200 mL

Tequin™ for Injection
(gatifloxacin)

RX BRISTOL-MYERS SQUIBB COMPANY P. 1025

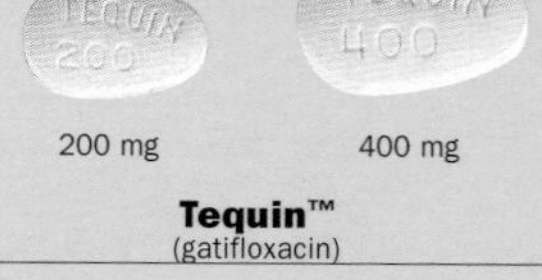

200 mg 400 mg

Tequin™
(gatifloxacin)

While every effort has been made to reproduce products faithfully, this section is to be considered a quick reference identification aid. In cases of suspected overdosage, etc., chemical analysis of the product should be done.

BRISTOL-MYERS SQUIBB ONC.

RX BRISTOL-MYERS SQUIBB ONCOLOGY P. 1034

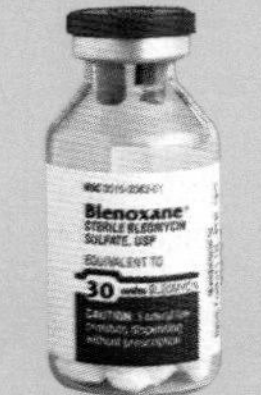

30 units per vial
Also available in 15 units per vial.

Blenoxane®
(sterile bleomycin sulfate, USP)

RX BRISTOL-MYERS SQUIBB ONCOLOGY P. 1037

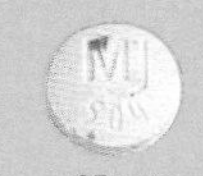
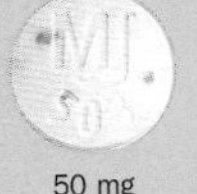

25 mg 50 mg

Cytoxan®
(cyclophosphamide tablets, USP)

RX BRISTOL-MYERS SQUIBB ONCOLOGY P. 1037

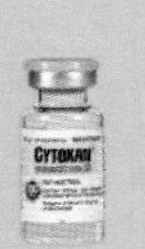
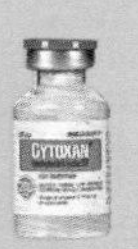
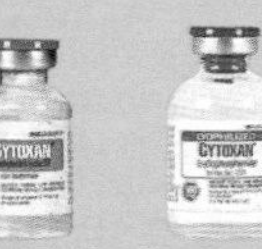

100 mg 200 mg 500 mg

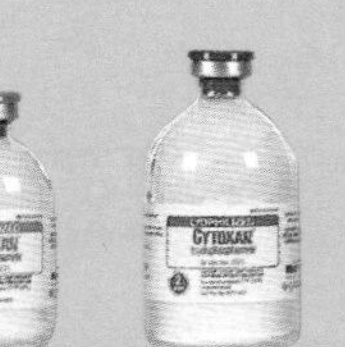

1 g 2 g
For injection

Lyophilized Cytoxan®
(cyclophosphamide for injection, USP)

RX BRISTOL-MYERS SQUIBB ONCOLOGY P. 1039

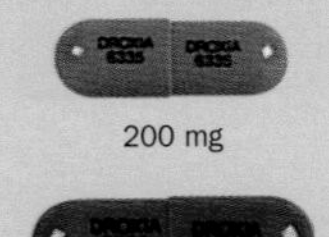

200 mg

300 mg

400 mg

Droxia™
(hydroxyurea capsules, USP)

RX BRISTOL-MYERS SQUIBB ONCOLOGY P. 1041

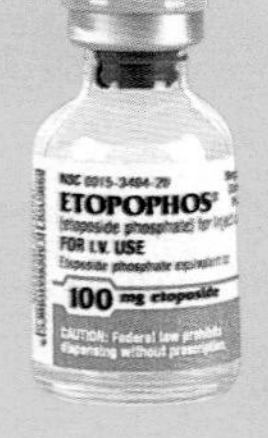

100 mg
Single-dose vial

Etopophos®
(etoposide phosphate) for Injection

RX BRISTOL-MYERS SQUIBB ONCOLOGY P. 1044

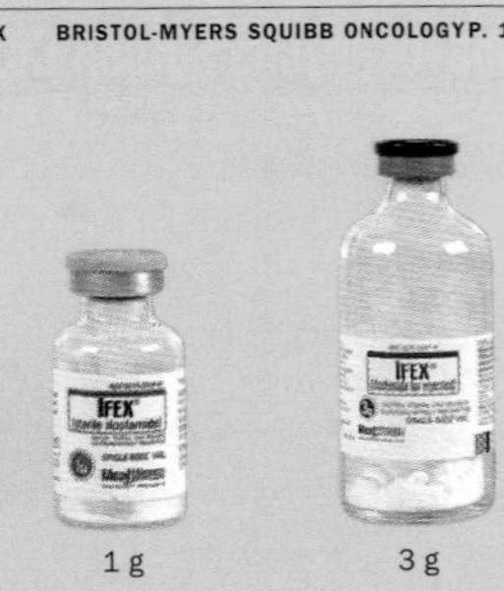

1 g 3 g

Ifex®
(ifosfamide for injection)

RX BRISTOL-MYERS SQUIBB ONCOLOGY P. 1047

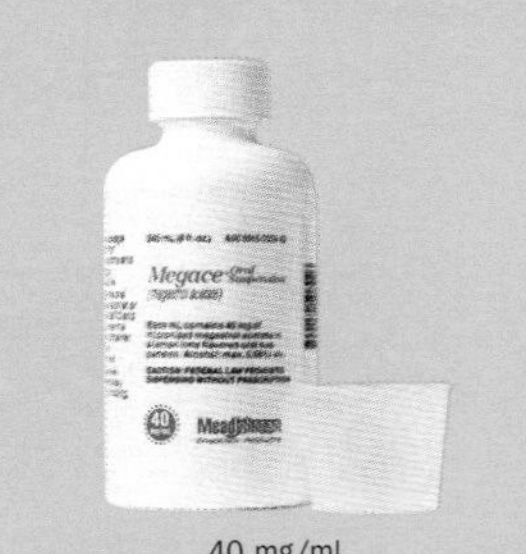

40 mg/mL

Megace® Oral Suspension
(megestrol acetate)

RX BRISTOL-MYERS SQUIBB ONCOLOGY P. 1048

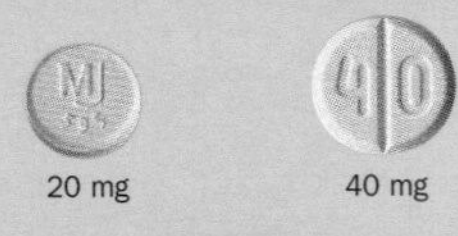

20 mg 40 mg

Megace®
(megestrol acetate tablets, USP)

RX BRISTOL-MYERS SQUIBB ONCOLOGY P. 1049

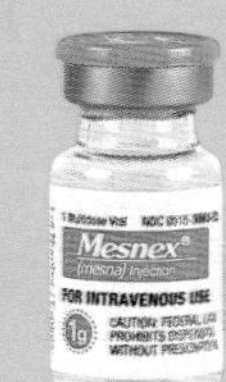

1-gm Multi-dose vial

Mesnex®
(mesna) Injection

RX BRISTOL-MYERS SQUIBB ONCOLOGY P. 1050

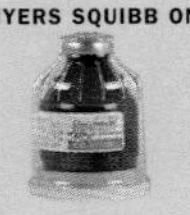

40 mg
Also available in 5 mg and 20 mg

Mutamycin®
(mitomycin for injection, USP)

RX BRISTOL-MYERS SQUIBB ONCOLOGY P. 1052

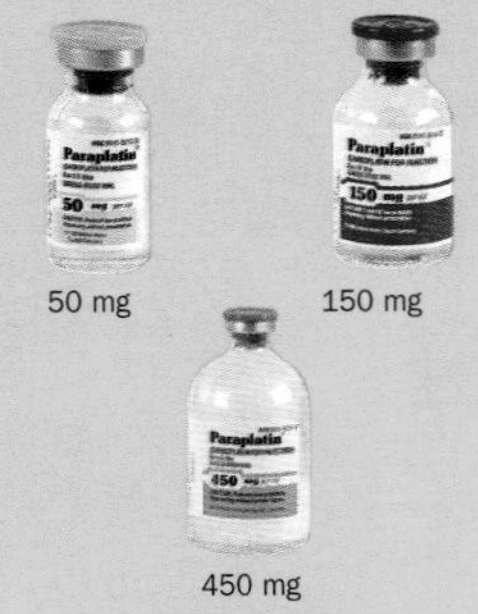

50 mg 150 mg

450 mg

Paraplatin®
(carboplatin for injection)

RX BRISTOL-MYERS SQUIBB ONCOLOGY P. 1055

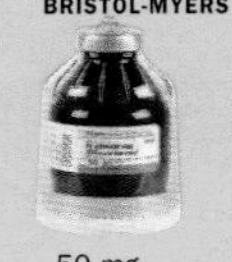
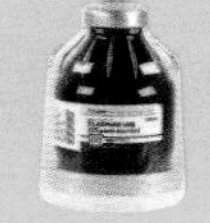

50 mg 100 mg

Platinol®-AQ
(cisplatin injection)

RX BRISTOL-MYERS SQUIBB ONCOLOGY P. 1059

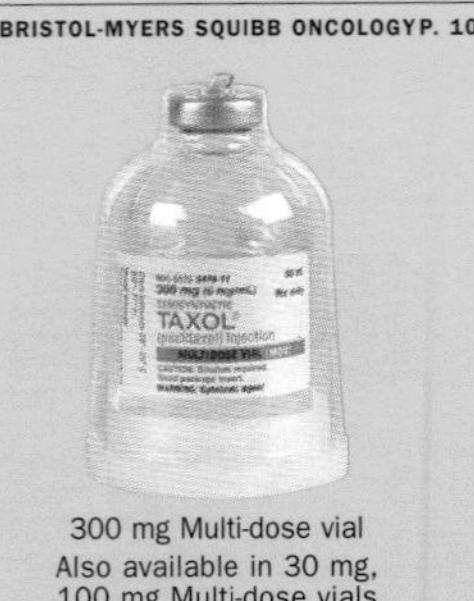

300 mg Multi-dose vial
Also available in 30 mg,
100 mg Multi-dose vials

TAXOL®
(paclitaxel) Injection
6 mg/mL

RX BRISTOL-MYERS SQUIBB ONCOLOGY P. 1068

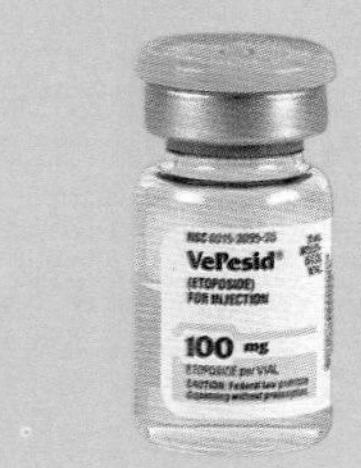

100 mg
Also available in 150 mg, 500 mg, 1 g

VePesid®
(etoposide) for Injection

RX BRISTOL-MYERS SQUIBB ONCOLOGY P. 1068

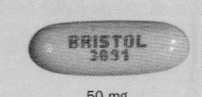

50 mg

VePesid®
(etoposide) Capsules

RX BRISTOL-MYERS SQUIBB ONCOLOGY P. 1070

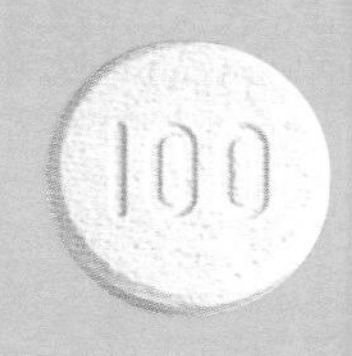

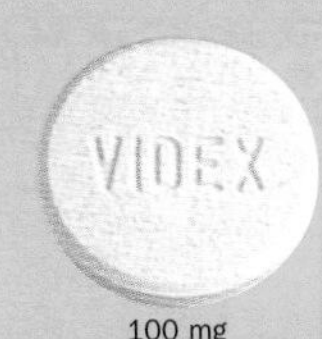

100 mg
Also available in 200 mg
tablets for once a day dosing

Videx®
(didanosine)
Chewable/Dispersible Buffered Tablets

RX BRISTOL-MYERS SQUIBB ONCOLOGY P. 1072

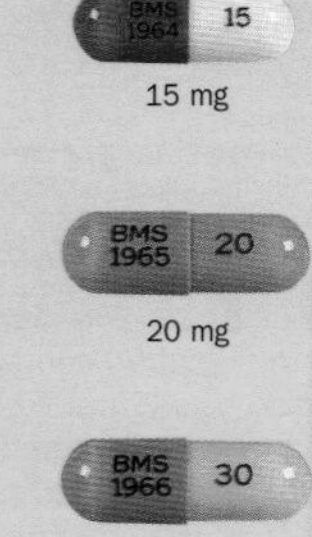

15 mg

20 mg

30 mg

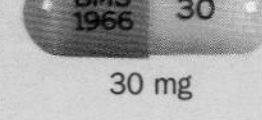

40 mg

Zerit®
(stavudine) Capsules

RX BRISTOL-MYERS SQUIBB ONCOLOGY P. 1072

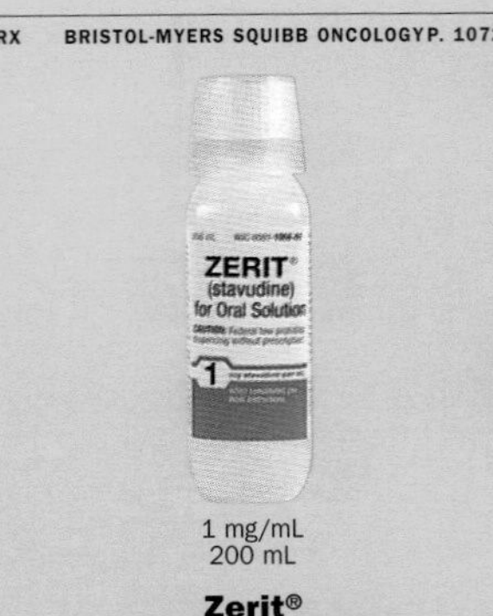

1 mg/mL
200 mL

Zerit®
(stavudine) for Oral Solution

BTG PHARMACEUTICALS

C-III BTG PHARMACEUTICALS P. 1076

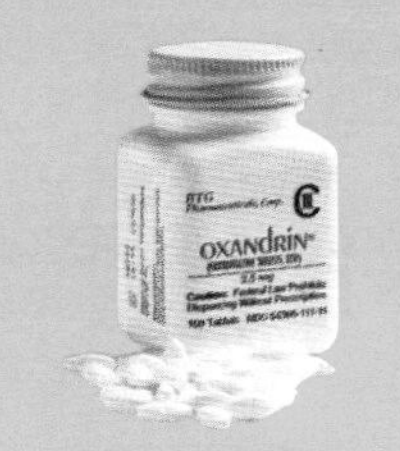

2.5 mg tablets

Oxandrin®
(oxandrolone tablets, USP)

RX BTG PHARMACEUTICALS P. 1075

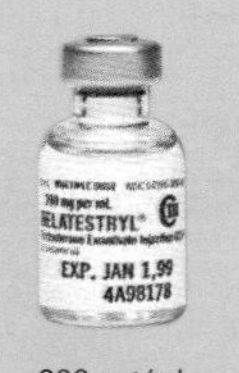

200 mg/mL
5 mL multiple
dose vial

200 mg/mL
1 mL unimatic
single dose syringe

Delatestryl®
(testosterone enanthate injection, USP)

CARNRICK

RX CARNRICK P. 1077

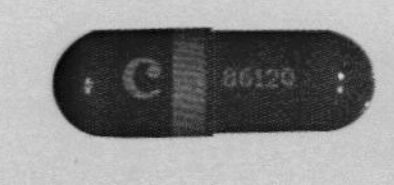

Midrin®
(isometheptene mucate, USP,
dichloralphenazone, USP,
acetaminophen, USP)
65 mg / 100 mg / 325 mg

RX CARNRICK P. 1078

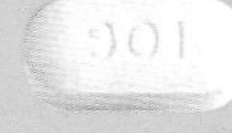

375 mg

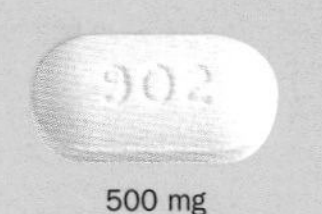

500 mg

Naprelan®
(naproxen sodium
controlled-release tablets)

RX CARNRICK P. 1080

400 mg

Skelaxin®
(metaxalone)

CELGENE

RX CELGENE CORPORATION P. 1081

50 mg

THALOMID®
(thalidomide) Capsules

CENTOCOR, INC.

RX CENTOCOR, INC. P. 1085

100 mg
Lyophilized Concentrate For IV Injection

Remicade®
(infliximab recombinant)

RX CENTOCOR, INC. P. 1088

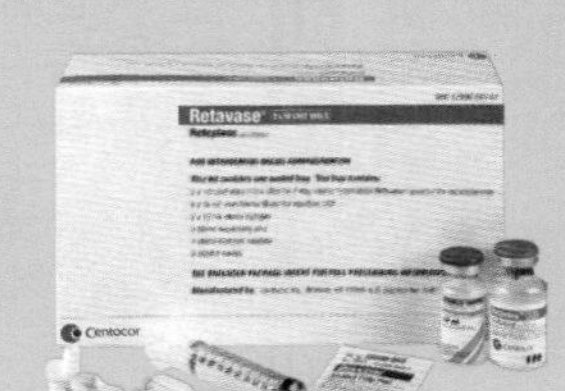

Retavase® Full-Kit
(reteplase recombinant)

RX CENTOCOR, INC. P. 1088

Retavase® Half-Kit
(reteplase recombinant)

CEPHALON, INC.

C-IV CEPHALON, INC. P. 1090

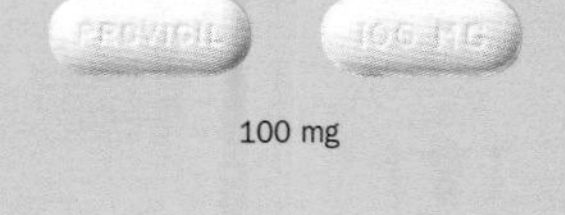

100 mg

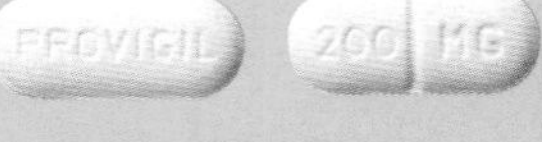

200 mg

Provigil®
(modafinil)

CETYLITE

RX CETYLITE INDUSTRIES INC. P. 1093

Topical Anesthetic Spray

Cetacaine®
(benzocaine, butamben & tetracaine HCl)

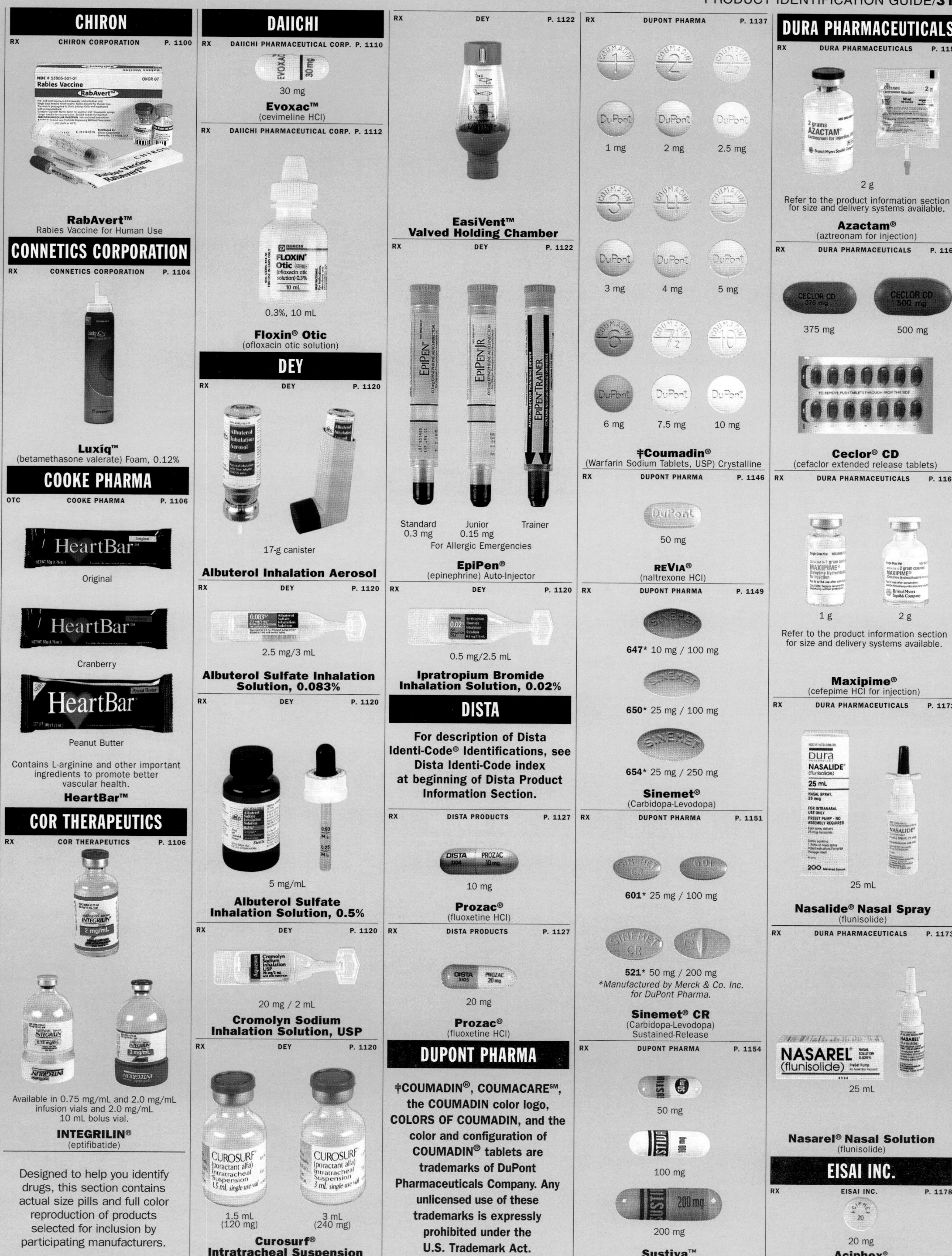

CHIRON

RX CHIRON CORPORATION P. 1100

RabAvert™
Rabies Vaccine for Human Use

CONNETICS CORPORATION

RX CONNETICS CORPORATION P. 1104

Luxíq™
(betamethasone valerate) Foam, 0.12%

COOKE PHARMA

OTC COOKE PHARMA P. 1106

Original

Cranberry

Peanut Butter

Contains L-arginine and other important ingredients to promote better vascular health.
HeartBar™

COR THERAPEUTICS

RX COR THERAPEUTICS P. 1106

Available in 0.75 mg/mL and 2.0 mg/mL infusion vials and 2.0 mg/mL 10 mL bolus vial.
INTEGRILIN®
(eptifibatide)

Designed to help you identify drugs, this section contains actual size pills and full color reproduction of products selected for inclusion by participating manufacturers.

DAIICHI

RX DAIICHI PHARMACEUTICAL CORP. P. 1110

30 mg
Evoxac™
(cevimeline HCl)

RX DAIICHI PHARMACEUTICAL CORP. P. 1112

0.3%, 10 mL
Floxin® Otic
(ofloxacin otic solution)

DEY

RX DEY P. 1120

17-g canister
Albuterol Inhalation Aerosol

RX DEY P. 1120

2.5 mg/3 mL
Albuterol Sulfate Inhalation Solution, 0.083%

RX DEY P. 1120

5 mg/mL
Albuterol Sulfate Inhalation Solution, 0.5%

RX DEY P. 1120

20 mg / 2 mL
Cromolyn Sodium Inhalation Solution, USP

RX DEY P. 1120

1.5 mL (120 mg)
3 mL (240 mg)
Curosurf®
Intratracheal Suspension
(poractant alpha)

RX DEY P. 1122

EasiVent™
Valved Holding Chamber

RX DEY P. 1122

Standard 0.3 mg
Junior 0.15 mg
Trainer
For Allergic Emergencies
EpiPen®
(epinephrine) Auto-Injector

RX DEY P. 1120

0.5 mg/2.5 mL
Ipratropium Bromide Inhalation Solution, 0.02%

DISTA

For description of Dista Identi-Code® Identifications, see Dista Identi-Code index at beginning of Dista Product Information Section.

RX DISTA PRODUCTS P. 1127

10 mg
Prozac®
(fluoxetine HCl)

RX DISTA PRODUCTS P. 1127

20 mg
Prozac®
(fluoxetine HCl)

DUPONT PHARMA

†COUMADIN®, COUMACARE℠, the COUMADIN color logo, COLORS OF COUMADIN, and the color and configuration of COUMADIN® tablets are trademarks of DuPont Pharmaceuticals Company. Any unlicensed use of these trademarks is expressly prohibited under the U.S. Trademark Act.

RX DUPONT PHARMA P. 1137

1 mg 2 mg 2.5 mg

3 mg 4 mg 5 mg

6 mg 7.5 mg 10 mg

†Coumadin®
(Warfarin Sodium Tablets, USP) Crystalline

RX DUPONT PHARMA P. 1146

50 mg
REVIA®
(naltrexone HCl)

RX DUPONT PHARMA P. 1149

647* 10 mg / 100 mg

650* 25 mg / 100 mg

654* 25 mg / 250 mg

Sinemet®
(Carbidopa-Levodopa)

RX DUPONT PHARMA P. 1151

601* 25 mg / 100 mg

521* 50 mg / 200 mg
Manufactured by Merck & Co. Inc. for DuPont Pharma.

Sinemet® CR
(Carbidopa-Levodopa)
Sustained-Release

RX DUPONT PHARMA P. 1154

50 mg

100 mg

200 mg

Sustiva™
(efavirenz)

DURA PHARMACEUTICALS

RX DURA PHARMACEUTICALS P. 1159

2 g
Refer to the product information section for size and delivery systems available.
Azactam®
(aztreonam for injection)

RX DURA PHARMACEUTICALS P. 1163

375 mg 500 mg

Ceclor® CD
(cefaclor extended release tablets)

RX DURA PHARMACEUTICALS P. 1167

1 g 2 g
Refer to the product information section for size and delivery systems available.

Maxipime®
(cefepime HCl for injection)

RX DURA PHARMACEUTICALS P. 1172

25 mL
Nasalide® Nasal Spray
(flunisolide)

RX DURA PHARMACEUTICALS P. 1173

25 mL
Nasarel® Nasal Solution
(flunisolide)

EISAI INC.

RX EISAI INC. P. 1178

20 mg
Aciphex®
(rabeprazole sodium)

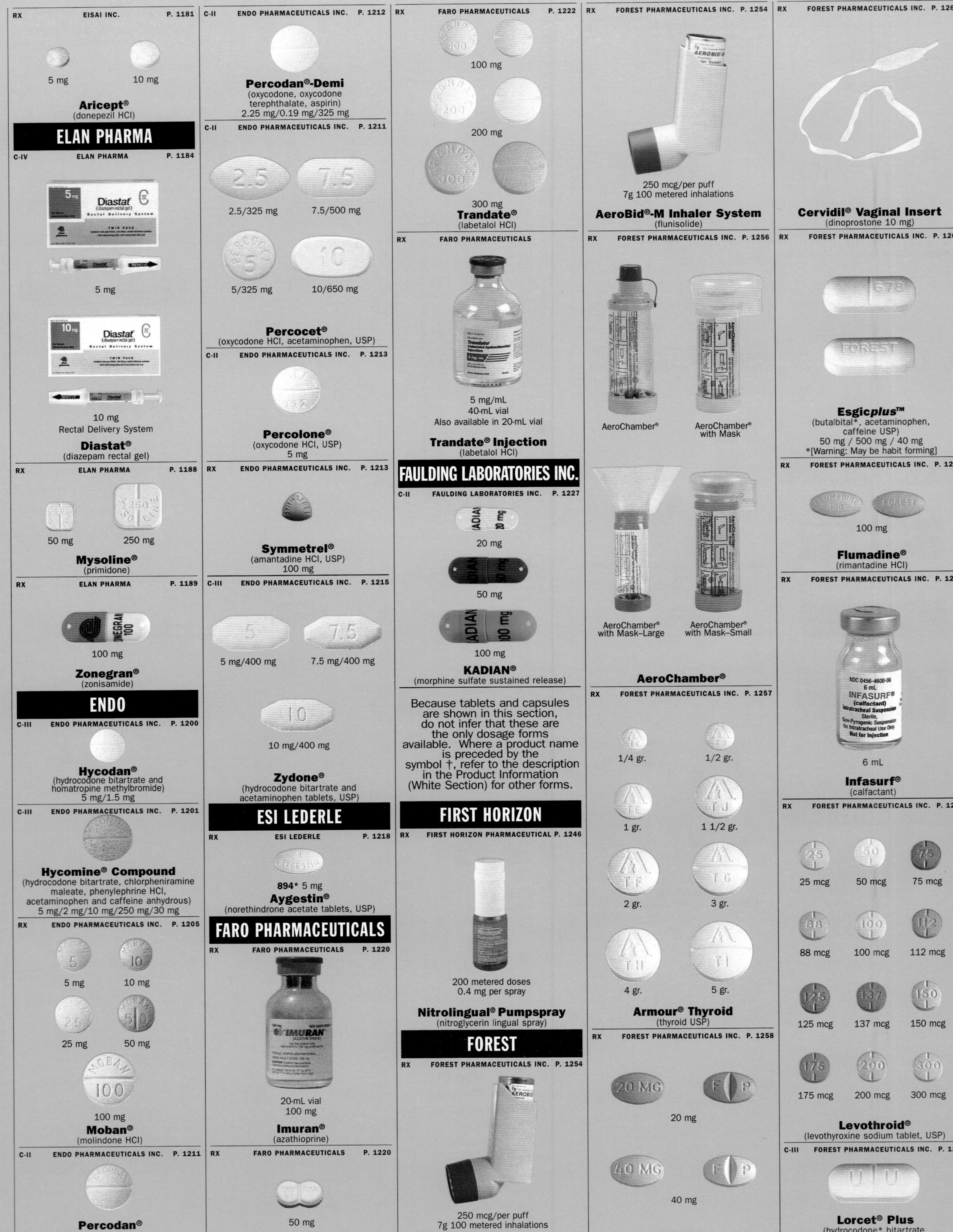
RX EISAI INC. P. 1181
5 mg
10 mg
Aricept®
(donepezil HCl)
ELAN PHARMA
C-IV ELAN PHARMA P. 1184
5 mg
10 mg
Rectal Delivery System
Diastat®
(diazepam rectal gel)
RX ELAN PHARMA P. 1188
50 mg
250 mg
Mysoline®
(primidone)
RX ELAN PHARMA P. 1189
100 mg
Zonegran®
(zonisamide)
ENDO
C-III ENDO PHARMACEUTICALS INC. P. 1200
Hycodan®
(hydrocodone bitartrate and homatropine methylbromide)
5 mg/1.5 mg
C-III ENDO PHARMACEUTICALS INC. P. 1201
Hycomine® Compound
(hydrocodone bitartrate, chlorpheniramine maleate, phenylephrine HCl, acetaminophen and caffeine anhydrous)
5 mg/2 mg/10 mg/250 mg/30 mg
RX ENDO PHARMACEUTICALS INC. P. 1205
5 mg
10 mg
25 mg
50 mg
100 mg
Moban®
(molindone HCl)
C-II ENDO PHARMACEUTICALS INC. P. 1211
Percodan®
(oxycodone, oxycodone terephthalate, aspirin, USP)
4.5 mg/0.38 mg/325 mg
C-II ENDO PHARMACEUTICALS INC. P. 1212
Percodan®-Demi
(oxycodone, oxycodone terephthalate, aspirin)
2.25 mg/0.19 mg/325 mg
C-II ENDO PHARMACEUTICALS INC. P. 1211
2.5/325 mg
7.5/500 mg
5/325 mg
10/650 mg
Percocet®
(oxycodone HCl, acetaminophen, USP)
C-II ENDO PHARMACEUTICALS INC. P. 1213
Percolone®
(oxycodone HCl, USP)
5 mg
RX ENDO PHARMACEUTICALS INC. P. 1213
Symmetrel®
(amantadine HCl, USP)
100 mg
C-III ENDO PHARMACEUTICALS INC. P. 1215
5 mg/400 mg
7.5 mg/400 mg
10 mg/400 mg
Zydone®
(hydrocodone bitartrate and acetaminophen tablets, USP)
ESI LEDERLE
RX ESI LEDERLE P. 1218
894* 5 mg
Aygestin®
(norethindrone acetate tablets, USP)
FARO PHARMACEUTICALS
RX FARO PHARMACEUTICALS P. 1220
20-mL vial
100 mg
Imuran®
(azathioprine)
RX FARO PHARMACEUTICALS P. 1220
50 mg
Imuran®
(azathioprine)
RX FARO PHARMACEUTICALS P. 1222
100 mg
200 mg
300 mg
Trandate®
(labetalol HCl)
RX FARO PHARMACEUTICALS
5 mg/mL
40-mL vial
Also available in 20-mL vial
Trandate® Injection
(labetalol HCl)
FAULDING LABORATORIES INC.
C-II FAULDING LABORATORIES INC. P. 1227
20 mg
50 mg
100 mg
KADIAN®
(morphine sulfate sustained release)
Because tablets and capsules are shown in this section, do not infer that these are the only dosage forms available. Where a product name is preceded by the symbol †, refer to the description in the Product Information (White Section) for other forms.
FIRST HORIZON
RX FIRST HORIZON PHARMACEUTICAL P. 1246
200 metered doses
0.4 mg per spray
Nitrolingual® Pumpspray
(nitroglycerin lingual spray)
FOREST
RX FOREST PHARMACEUTICALS INC. P. 1254
250 mcg/per puff
7g 100 metered inhalations
Aerobid® Inhaler System
(flunisolide)
RX FOREST PHARMACEUTICALS INC. P. 1254
250 mcg/per puff
7g 100 metered inhalations
AeroBid®-M Inhaler System
(flunisolide)
RX FOREST PHARMACEUTICALS INC. P. 1256
AeroChamber®
AeroChamber® with Mask
AeroChamber® with Mask–Large
AeroChamber® with Mask–Small
AeroChamber®
RX FOREST PHARMACEUTICALS INC. P. 1257
1/4 gr.
1/2 gr.
1 gr.
1 1/2 gr.
2 gr.
3 gr.
4 gr.
5 gr.
Armour® Thyroid
(thyroid USP)
RX FOREST PHARMACEUTICALS INC. P. 1258
20 mg
40 mg
Celexa™
(citalopram hydrobromide)
RX FOREST PHARMACEUTICALS INC. P. 1261
Cervidil® Vaginal Insert
(dinoprostone 10 mg)
RX FOREST PHARMACEUTICALS INC. P. 1263
Esgicplus™
(butalbital*, acetaminophen, caffeine USP)
50 mg / 500 mg / 40 mg
*[Warning: May be habit forming]
RX FOREST PHARMACEUTICALS INC. P. 1263
100 mg
Flumadine®
(rimantadine HCl)
RX FOREST PHARMACEUTICALS INC. P. 1264
6 mL
Infasurf®
(calfactant)
RX FOREST PHARMACEUTICALS INC. P. 1266
25 mcg
50 mcg
75 mcg
88 mcg
100 mcg
112 mcg
125 mcg
137 mcg
150 mcg
175 mcg
200 mcg
300 mcg
Levothroid®
(levothyroxine sodium tablet, USP)
C-III FOREST PHARMACEUTICALS INC. P. 1268
Lorcet® Plus
(hydrocodone* bitartrate, acetaminophen USP)
7.5 mg/650 mg *[Warning: May be habit forming]

C-III FOREST PHARMACEUTICALS INC. P. 1268

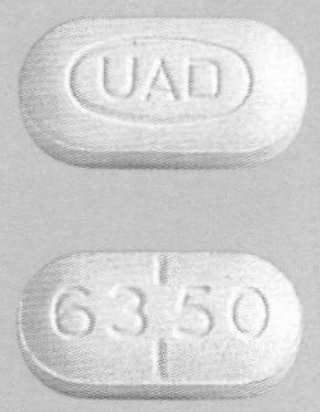

Lorcet® 10/650
(hydrocodone* bitartrate, acetaminophen USP)
10 mg/650 mg *[Warning: May be habit forming]

RX FOREST PHARMACEUTICALS INC. P. 1268

NDC 0456-4300-08
MONUROL™
(fosfomycin tromethamine)
(equivalent to 3 grams of fosfomycin)
Dissolve contents in 3 to 4 ounces of water. Drink immediately.
CAUTION: Federal law prohibits dispensing without prescription

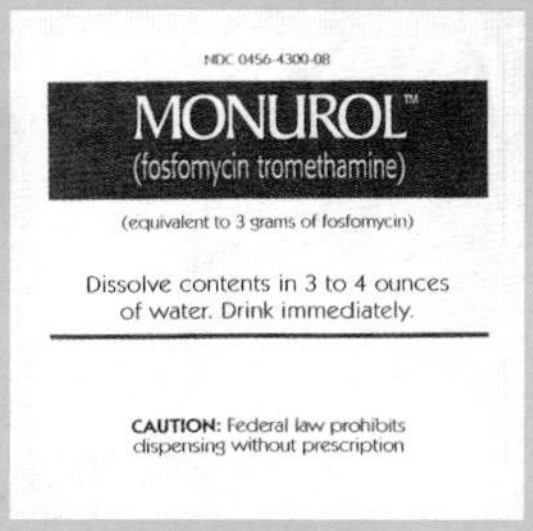

Monurol®
(fosfomycin tromethamine)

RX FOREST PHARMACEUTICALS INC. P. 1270

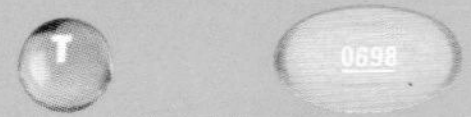

100 mg 200 mg

Tessalon®
(benzonatate USP)

RX FOREST PHARMACEUTICALS INC. P. 1270

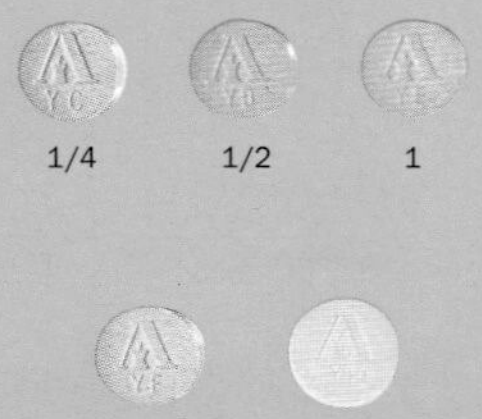

1/4 1/2 1

2 3

Thyrolar®
(liotrix)

RX FOREST PHARMACEUTICALS INC. P. 1270

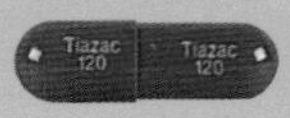

120 mg

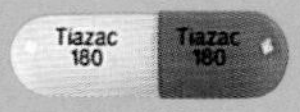

180 mg

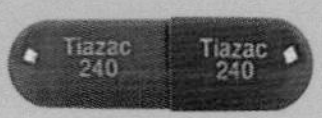

240 mg

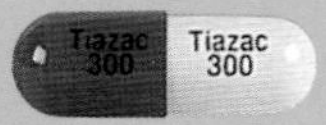

300 mg

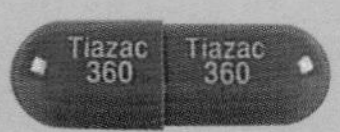

360 mg

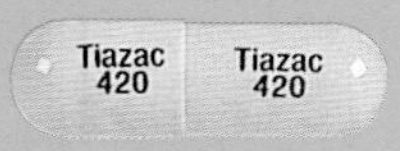

420 mg

Tiazac™
(diltiazem HCl)
Extended-Release Capsules

FUJISAWA HEALTHCARE, INC.

RX FUJISAWA HEALTHCARE, INC. P. 1273

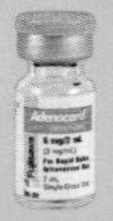

6 mg/2 mL 2 mL Single-Dose Vial

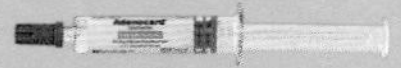

6 mg/2 mL 2 mL Disposable Syringe

12 mg/4 mL 5 mL Disposable Syringe

Adenocard®
(adenosine injection)

RX FUJISAWA HEALTHCARE, INC. P. 1274

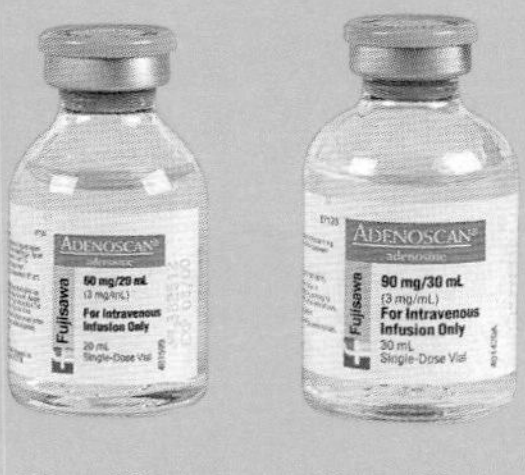

60 mg/20 mL 90 mg/30 mL
3 mg/mL
Single-Dose Vials

Adenoscan®
(adenosine injection)

RX FUJISAWA HEALTHCARE, INC. P. 1275

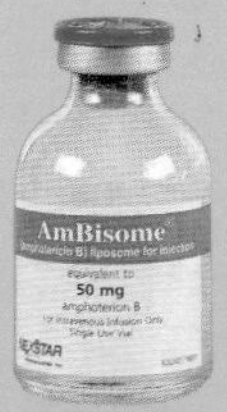

50 mg

AmBisome®
(amphotericin B) liposome for injection

RX FUJISAWA HEALTHCARE, INC. P. 1284

0.5 mg 1 mg

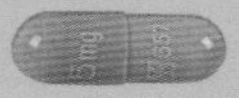

5 mg

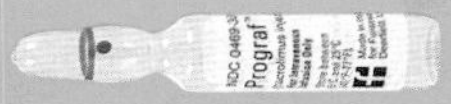

5 mg/mL
1 mL ampule

Prograf®
(tacrolimus)

GATE PHARMACEUTICALS

C-IV GATE PHARMACEUTICALS P. 1293

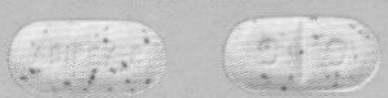

37.5 mg

†Adipex-P®
(phentermine HCl)

RX GATE PHARMACEUTICALS P. 1294

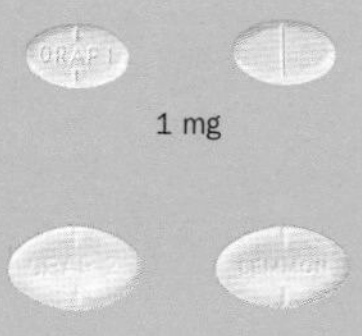

1 mg

2 mg

Orap®
(pimozide)

GENENTECH, INC.

RX GENENTECH, INC. P. 1297

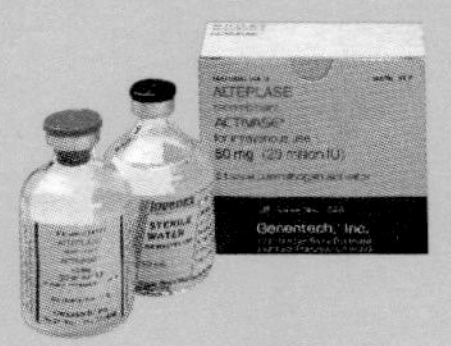

50 mg
29 million IU
Packaged with diluent

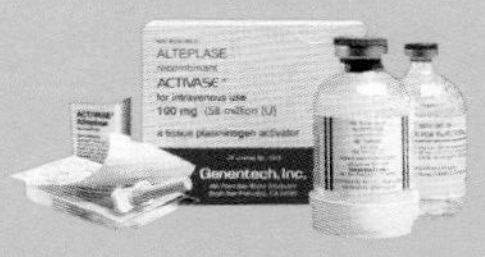

100 mg
58 million IU
Packaged with diluent and double-sided sterile, siliconized transfer device

Activase®
(Alteplase, recombinant)

RX GENENTECH, INC. P. 1301

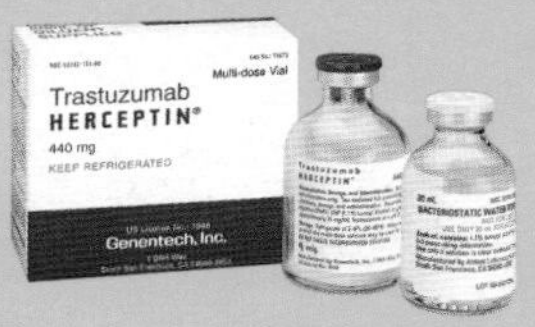

440 mg
Multi-dose vial

Herceptin®
(Trastuzumab)

RX GENENTECH, INC. P. 1304

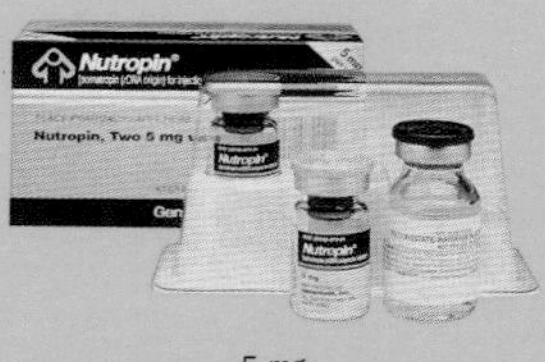

5 mg
approx. 15 IU
Packaged with 10 mL multi-dose vial of bacteriostatic water
(benzyl alcohol preserved)

10 mg
approx. 30 IU
Packaged with 10 mL multi-dose vial of bacteriostatic water
(benzyl alcohol preserved)

Nutropin®
(somatropin [rDNA origin] for injection)

RX GENENTECH, INC. P. 1307

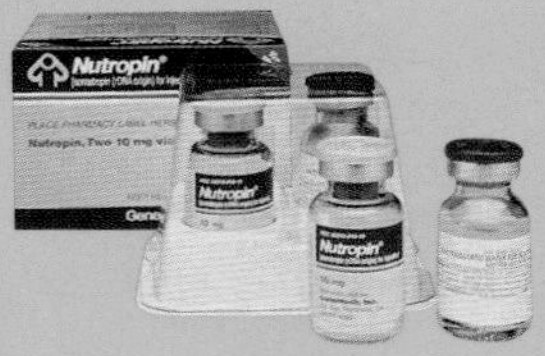

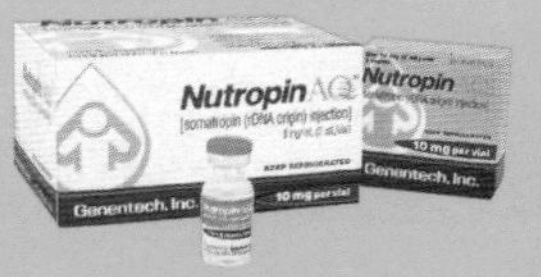

10 mg (5mg/mL)
approx. 30 IU
Each carton contains six (2 mL) vials

Nutropin AQ®
(somatropin [rDNA origin] injection)

RX GENENTECH, INC. P. 1310

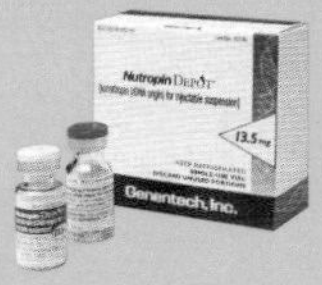

13.5 mg

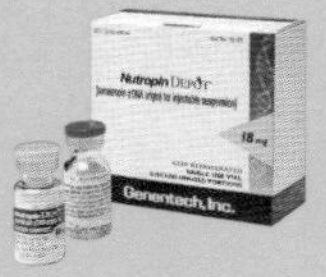

18 mg

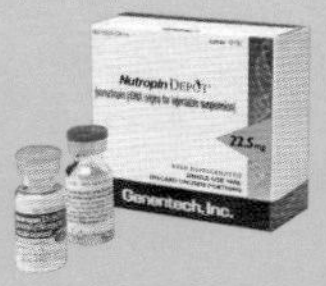

22.5 mg

Nutropin Depot®
(somatropin)

RX GENENTECH, INC. P. 1312

5 mg
approx. 15 IU
Packaged with 10 mL multi-dose vial of bacteriostatic water
(benzyl alcohol preserved)

10 mg
approx. 30 IU
Packaged with 10 mL multi-dose vial of bacteriostatic water
(benzyl alcohol preserved)

Protropin®
(somatrem for injection)

RX GENENTECH, INC. P. 1312

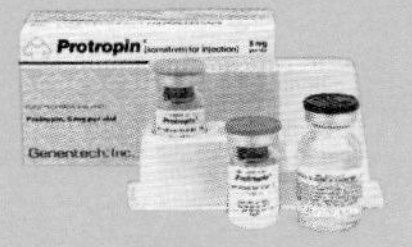

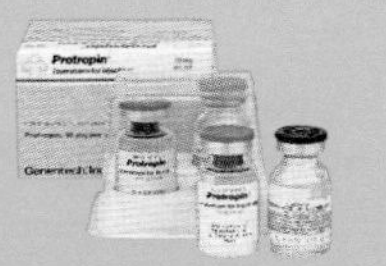

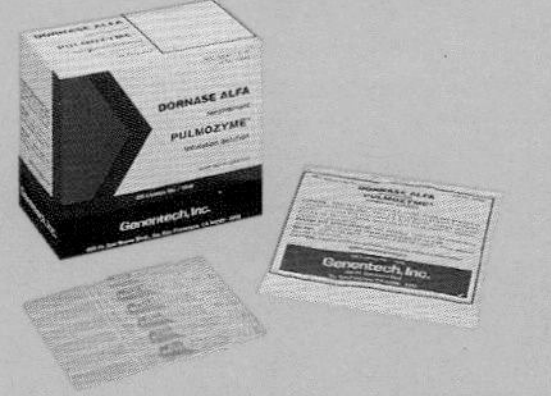

2.5 mL
(1.0 mg/mL dornase alfa)
Each carton contains 30 single-use ampules

Pulmozyme®
(dornase alfa) recombinant,
Inhalation Solution

RX GENENTECH, INC. P. 1314

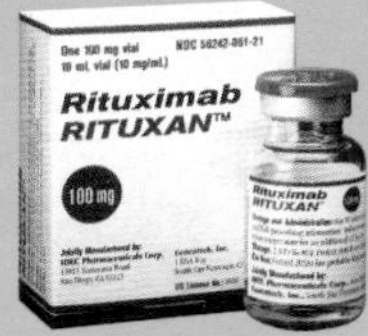

100 mg (10mg/mL)

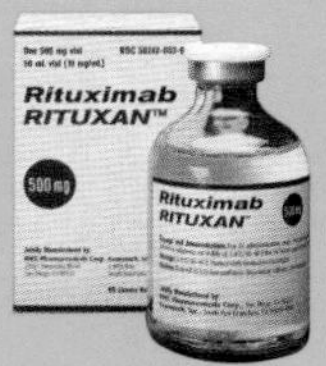

500 mg (10mg/mL)

Rituxan®
(Rituximab)
*Jointly marketed by IDEC Pharmaceuticals Corp. and Genentech, Inc.

RX GENENTECH, INC. P. 1316

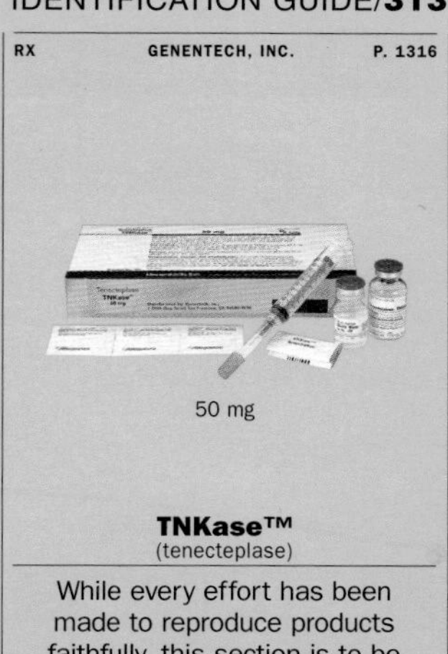

50 mg

TNKase™
(tenecteplase)

While every effort has been made to reproduce products faithfully, this section is to be considered a quick reference identification aid. In cases of suspected overdosage, etc., chemical analysis of the product should be done.

GENETICS INSTITUTE

RX GENETICS INSTITUTE P. 1318

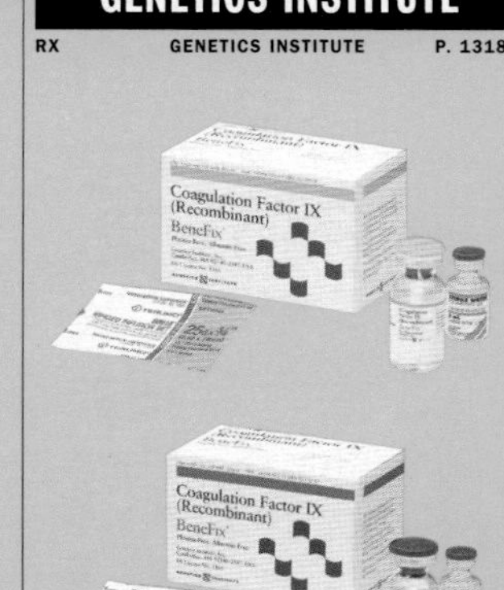

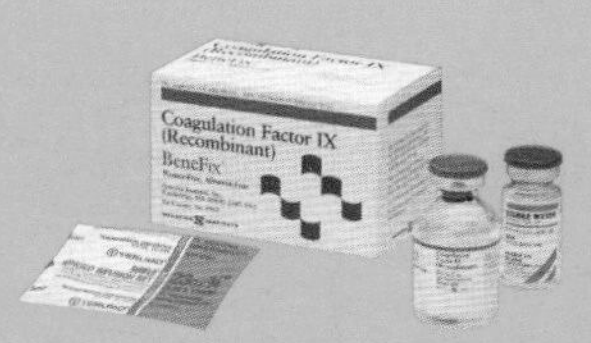

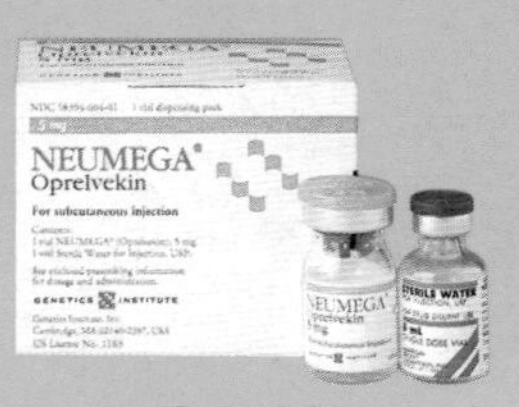

BeneFix®
(coagulation factor IX [recombinant])

RX GENETICS INSTITUTE P. 1320

5 mg per vial
1 vial dispensing pack

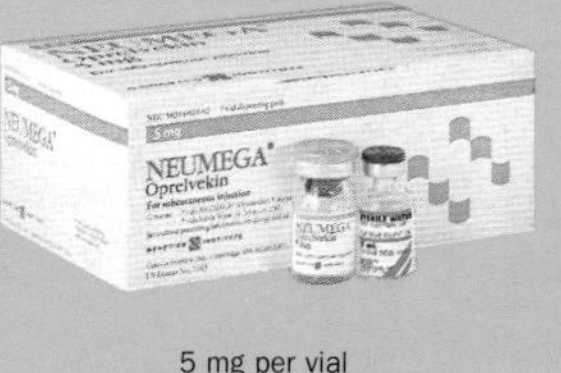

5 mg per vial
7 vial dispensing pack

Neumega®
(Oprelvekin)

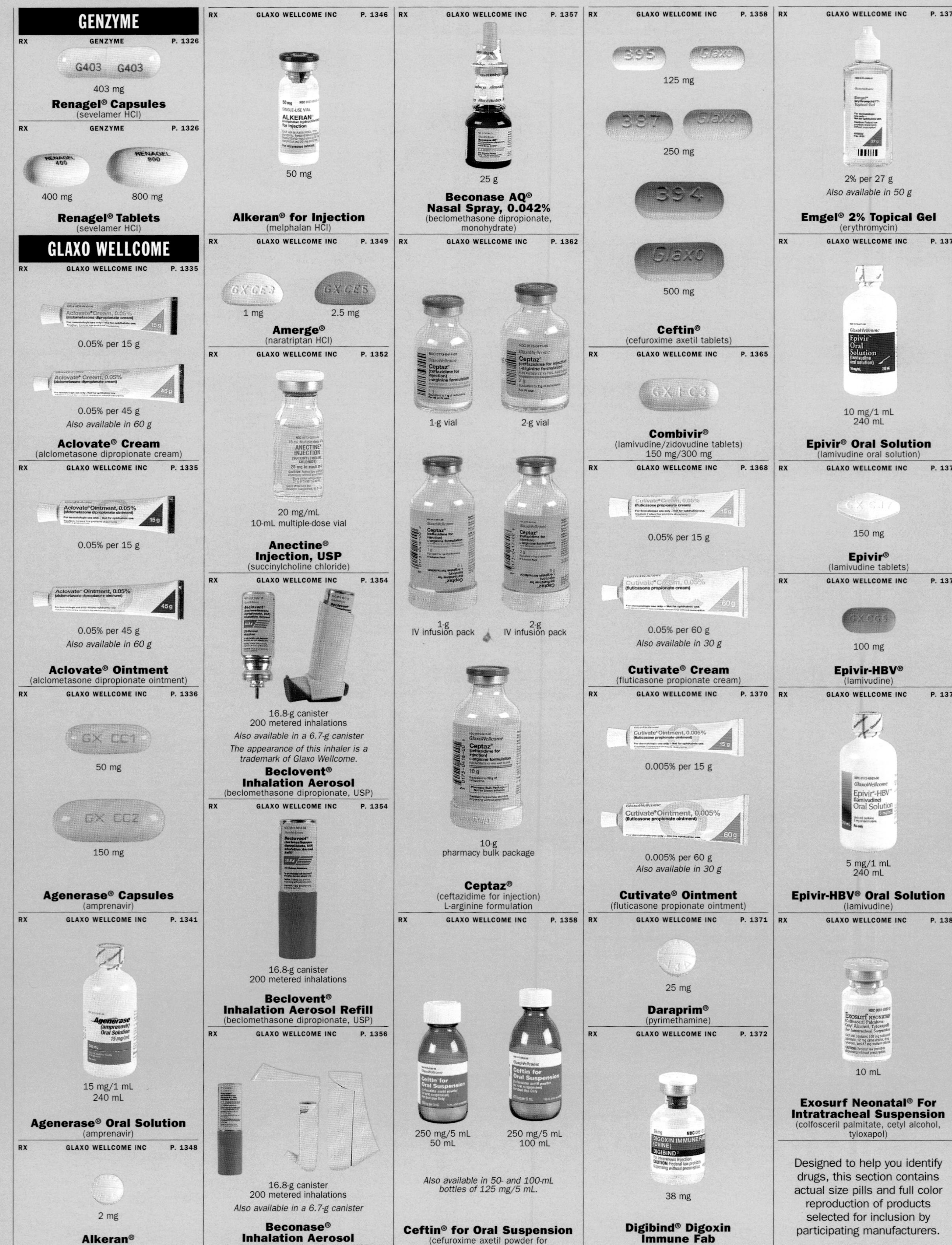

GENZYME

RX GENZYME P. 1326

403 mg

Renagel® Capsules
(sevelamer HCl)

RX GENZYME P. 1326

400 mg 800 mg

Renagel® Tablets
(sevelamer HCl)

GLAXO WELLCOME

RX GLAXO WELLCOME INC P. 1335

0.05% per 15 g

0.05% per 45 g
Also available in 60 g

Aclovate® Cream
(alclometasone dipropionate cream)

RX GLAXO WELLCOME INC P. 1335

0.05% per 15 g

0.05% per 45 g
Also available in 60 g

Aclovate® Ointment
(alclometasone dipropionate ointment)

RX GLAXO WELLCOME INC P. 1336

50 mg

150 mg

Agenerase® Capsules
(amprenavir)

RX GLAXO WELLCOME INC P. 1341

15 mg/1 mL
240 mL

Agenerase® Oral Solution
(amprenavir)

RX GLAXO WELLCOME INC P. 1348

2 mg

Alkeran®
(melphalan)

RX GLAXO WELLCOME INC P. 1346

50 mg

Alkeran® for Injection
(melphalan HCl)

RX GLAXO WELLCOME INC P. 1349

1 mg 2.5 mg

Amerge®
(naratriptan HCl)

RX GLAXO WELLCOME INC P. 1352

20 mg/mL
10-mL multiple-dose vial

Anectine® Injection, USP
(succinylcholine chloride)

RX GLAXO WELLCOME INC P. 1354

16.8-g canister
200 metered inhalations
Also available in a 6.7-g canister
The appearance of this inhaler is a trademark of Glaxo Wellcome.

Beclovent® Inhalation Aerosol
(beclomethasone dipropionate, USP)

RX GLAXO WELLCOME INC P. 1354

16.8-g canister
200 metered inhalations

Beclovent® Inhalation Aerosol Refill
(beclomethasone dipropionate, USP)

RX GLAXO WELLCOME INC P. 1356

16.8-g canister
200 metered inhalations
Also available in a 6.7-g canister

Beconase® Inhalation Aerosol
(beclomethasone dipropionate, USP)

RX GLAXO WELLCOME INC P. 1357

25 g

Beconase AQ® Nasal Spray, 0.042%
(beclomethasone dipropionate, monohydrate)

RX GLAXO WELLCOME INC P. 1362

1-g vial 2-g vial

1-g IV infusion pack 2-g IV infusion pack

10-g
pharmacy bulk package

Ceptaz®
(ceftazidime for injection)
L-arginine formulation

RX GLAXO WELLCOME INC P. 1358

250 mg/5 mL
50 mL

250 mg/5 mL
100 mL

Also available in 50- and 100-mL bottles of 125 mg/5 mL.

Ceftin® for Oral Suspension
(cefuroxime axetil powder for oral suspension)

RX GLAXO WELLCOME INC P. 1358

125 mg

250 mg

500 mg

Ceftin®
(cefuroxime axetil tablets)

RX GLAXO WELLCOME INC P. 1365

Combivir®
(lamivudine/zidovudine tablets)
150 mg/300 mg

RX GLAXO WELLCOME INC P. 1368

0.05% per 15 g

0.05% per 60 g
Also available in 30 g

Cutivate® Cream
(fluticasone propionate cream)

RX GLAXO WELLCOME INC P. 1370

0.005% per 15 g

0.005% per 60 g
Also available in 30 g

Cutivate® Ointment
(fluticasone propionate ointment)

RX GLAXO WELLCOME INC P. 1371

25 mg

Daraprim®
(pyrimethamine)

RX GLAXO WELLCOME INC P. 1372

38 mg

Digibind® Digoxin Immune Fab
(Ovine)

RX GLAXO WELLCOME INC P. 1373

2% per 27 g
Also available in 50 g

Emgel® 2% Topical Gel
(erythromycin)

RX GLAXO WELLCOME INC P. 1374

10 mg/1 mL
240 mL

Epivir® Oral Solution
(lamivudine oral solution)

RX GLAXO WELLCOME INC P. 1374

150 mg

Epivir®
(lamivudine tablets)

RX GLAXO WELLCOME INC P. 1377

100 mg

Epivir-HBV®
(lamivudine)

RX GLAXO WELLCOME INC P. 1377

5 mg/1 mL
240 mL

Epivir-HBV® Oral Solution
(lamivudine)

RX GLAXO WELLCOME INC P. 1380

10 mL

Exosurf Neonatal® For Intratracheal Suspension
(colfosceril palmitate, cetyl alcohol, tyloxapol)

Designed to help you identify drugs, this section contains actual size pills and full color reproduction of products selected for inclusion by participating manufacturers.

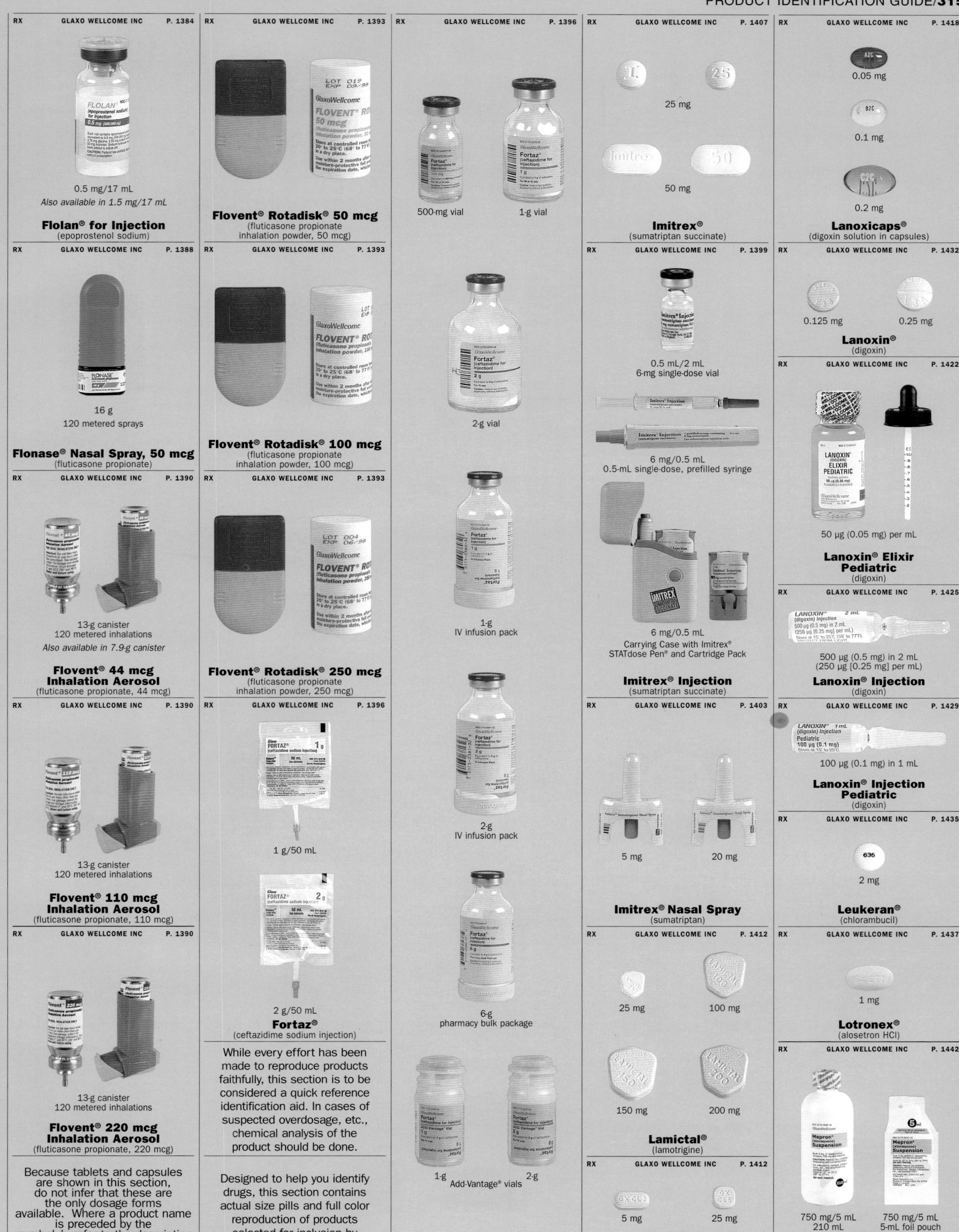

RX GLAXO WELLCOME INC P. 1384

0.5 mg/17 mL
Also available in 1.5 mg/17 mL

Flolan® for Injection
(epoprostenol sodium)

RX GLAXO WELLCOME INC P. 1388

16 g
120 metered sprays

Flonase® Nasal Spray, 50 mcg
(fluticasone propionate)

RX GLAXO WELLCOME INC P. 1390

13-g canister
120 metered inhalations
Also available in 7.9-g canister

Flovent® 44 mcg Inhalation Aerosol
(fluticasone propionate, 44 mcg)

RX GLAXO WELLCOME INC P. 1390

13-g canister
120 metered inhalations

Flovent® 110 mcg Inhalation Aerosol
(fluticasone propionate, 110 mcg)

RX GLAXO WELLCOME INC P. 1390

13-g canister
120 metered inhalations

Flovent® 220 mcg Inhalation Aerosol
(fluticasone propionate, 220 mcg)

Because tablets and capsules are shown in this section, do not infer that these are the only dosage forms available. Where a product name is preceded by the symbol †, refer to the description in the Product Information (White Section) for other forms.

RX GLAXO WELLCOME INC P. 1393

Flovent® Rotadisk® 50 mcg
(fluticasone propionate inhalation powder, 50 mcg)

RX GLAXO WELLCOME INC P. 1393

Flovent® Rotadisk® 100 mcg
(fluticasone propionate inhalation powder, 100 mcg)

RX GLAXO WELLCOME INC P. 1393

Flovent® Rotadisk® 250 mcg
(fluticasone propionate inhalation powder, 250 mcg)

RX GLAXO WELLCOME INC P. 1396

1 g/50 mL

2 g/50 mL

Fortaz®
(ceftazidime sodium injection)

While every effort has been made to reproduce products faithfully, this section is to be considered a quick reference identification aid. In cases of suspected overdosage, etc., chemical analysis of the product should be done.

Designed to help you identify drugs, this section contains actual size pills and full color reproduction of products selected for inclusion by participating manufacturers.

RX GLAXO WELLCOME INC P. 1396

500-mg vial 1-g vial

2-g vial

1-g
IV infusion pack

2-g
IV infusion pack

6-g
pharmacy bulk package

1-g Add-Vantage® vials 2-g

Fortaz®
(ceftazidime for injection)

RX GLAXO WELLCOME INC P. 1407

25 mg

50 mg

Imitrex®
(sumatriptan succinate)

RX GLAXO WELLCOME INC P. 1399

0.5 mL/2 mL
6-mg single-dose vial

6 mg/0.5 mL
0.5-mL single-dose, prefilled syringe

6 mg/0.5 mL
Carrying Case with Imitrex® STATdose Pen® and Cartridge Pack

Imitrex® Injection
(sumatriptan succinate)

RX GLAXO WELLCOME INC P. 1403

5 mg 20 mg

Imitrex® Nasal Spray
(sumatriptan)

RX GLAXO WELLCOME INC P. 1412

25 mg 100 mg

150 mg 200 mg

Lamictal®
(lamotrigine)

RX GLAXO WELLCOME INC P. 1412

5 mg 25 mg

Lamictal® Chewable Dispersible Tablets
(lamotrigine)

RX GLAXO WELLCOME INC P. 1418

0.05 mg

0.1 mg

0.2 mg

Lanoxicaps®
(digoxin solution in capsules)

RX GLAXO WELLCOME INC P. 1432

0.125 mg 0.25 mg

Lanoxin®
(digoxin)

RX GLAXO WELLCOME INC P. 1422

50 µg (0.05 mg) per mL

Lanoxin® Elixir Pediatric
(digoxin)

RX GLAXO WELLCOME INC P. 1425

500 µg (0.5 mg) in 2 mL
(250 µg [0.25 mg] per mL)

Lanoxin® Injection
(digoxin)

RX GLAXO WELLCOME INC P. 1429

100 µg (0.1 mg) in 1 mL

Lanoxin® Injection Pediatric
(digoxin)

RX GLAXO WELLCOME INC P. 1435

2 mg

Leukeran®
(chlorambucil)

RX GLAXO WELLCOME INC P. 1437

1 mg

Lotronex®
(alosetron HCl)

RX GLAXO WELLCOME INC P. 1442

750 mg/5 mL
210 mL

750 mg/5 mL
5-mL foil pouch

Mepron® Suspension
(atovaquone)

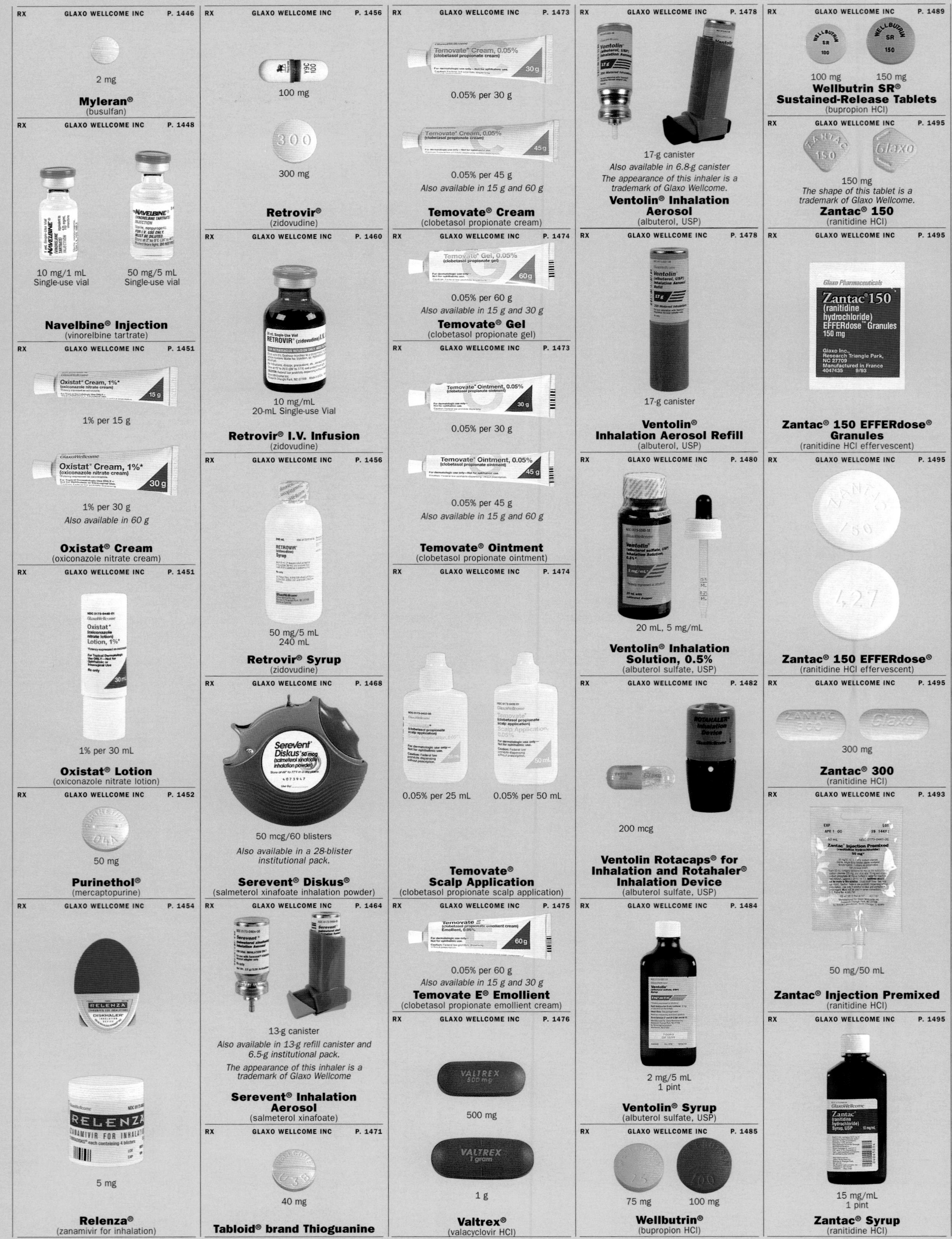

RX GLAXO WELLCOME INC P. 1446

2 mg

Myleran®
(busulfan)

RX GLAXO WELLCOME INC P. 1448

10 mg/1 mL
Single-use vial

50 mg/5 mL
Single-use vial

Navelbine® Injection
(vinorelbine tartrate)

RX GLAXO WELLCOME INC P. 1451

1% per 15 g

1% per 30 g
Also available in 60 g

Oxistat® Cream
(oxiconazole nitrate cream)

RX GLAXO WELLCOME INC P. 1451

1% per 30 mL

Oxistat® Lotion
(oxiconazole nitrate lotion)

RX GLAXO WELLCOME INC P. 1452

50 mg

Purinethol®
(mercaptopurine)

RX GLAXO WELLCOME INC P. 1454

5 mg

Relenza®
(zanamivir for inhalation)

RX GLAXO WELLCOME INC P. 1456

100 mg

300 mg

Retrovir®
(zidovudine)

RX GLAXO WELLCOME INC P. 1460

10 mg/mL
20-mL Single-use Vial

Retrovir® I.V. Infusion
(zidovudine)

RX GLAXO WELLCOME INC P. 1456

50 mg/5 mL
240 mL

Retrovir® Syrup
(zidovudine)

RX GLAXO WELLCOME INC P. 1468

50 mcg/60 blisters
Also available in a 28-blister institutional pack.

Serevent® Diskus®
(salmeterol xinafoate inhalation powder)

RX GLAXO WELLCOME INC P. 1464

13-g canister
Also available in 13-g refill canister and 6.5-g institutional pack.
The appearance of this inhaler is a trademark of Glaxo Wellcome

Serevent® Inhalation Aerosol
(salmeterol xinafoate)

RX GLAXO WELLCOME INC P. 1471

40 mg

Tabloid® brand Thioguanine

RX GLAXO WELLCOME INC P. 1473

0.05% per 30 g

0.05% per 45 g
Also available in 15 g and 60 g

Temovate® Cream
(clobetasol propionate cream)

RX GLAXO WELLCOME INC P. 1474

0.05% per 60 g
Also available in 15 g and 30 g

Temovate® Gel
(clobetasol propionate gel)

RX GLAXO WELLCOME INC P. 1473

0.05% per 30 g

0.05% per 45 g
Also available in 15 g and 60 g

Temovate® Ointment
(clobetasol propionate ointment)

RX GLAXO WELLCOME INC P. 1474

0.05% per 25 mL

0.05% per 50 mL

Temovate® Scalp Application
(clobetasol propionate scalp application)

RX GLAXO WELLCOME INC P. 1475

0.05% per 60 g
Also available in 15 g and 30 g

Temovate E® Emollient
(clobetasol propionate emollient cream)

RX GLAXO WELLCOME INC P. 1476

500 mg

1 g

Valtrex®
(valacyclovir HCl)

RX GLAXO WELLCOME INC P. 1478

17-g canister
Also available in 6.8-g canister
The appearance of this inhaler is a trademark of Glaxo Wellcome.

Ventolin® Inhalation Aerosol
(albuterol, USP)

RX GLAXO WELLCOME INC P. 1478

17-g canister

Ventolin® Inhalation Aerosol Refill
(albuterol, USP)

RX GLAXO WELLCOME INC P. 1480

20 mL, 5 mg/mL

Ventolin® Inhalation Solution, 0.5%
(albuterol sulfate, USP)

RX GLAXO WELLCOME INC P. 1482

200 mcg

Ventolin Rotacaps® for Inhalation and Rotahaler® Inhalation Device
(albuterol sulfate, USP)

RX GLAXO WELLCOME INC P. 1484

2 mg/5 mL
1 pint

Ventolin® Syrup
(albuterol sulfate, USP)

RX GLAXO WELLCOME INC P. 1485

75 mg

100 mg

Wellbutrin®
(bupropion HCl)

RX GLAXO WELLCOME INC P. 1489

100 mg

150 mg

Wellbutrin SR® Sustained-Release Tablets
(bupropion HCl)

RX GLAXO WELLCOME INC P. 1495

150 mg
The shape of this tablet is a trademark of Glaxo Wellcome.

Zantac® 150
(ranitidine HCl)

RX GLAXO WELLCOME INC P. 1495

Zantac® 150 EFFERdose® Granules
(ranitidine HCl effervescent)

RX GLAXO WELLCOME INC P. 1495

Zantac® 150 EFFERdose®
(ranitidine HCl effervescent)

RX GLAXO WELLCOME INC P. 1495

300 mg

Zantac® 300
(ranitidine HCl)

RX GLAXO WELLCOME INC P. 1493

50 mg/50 mL

Zantac® Injection Premixed
(ranitidine HCl)

RX GLAXO WELLCOME INC P. 1495

15 mg/mL
1 pint

Zantac® Syrup
(ranitidine HCl)

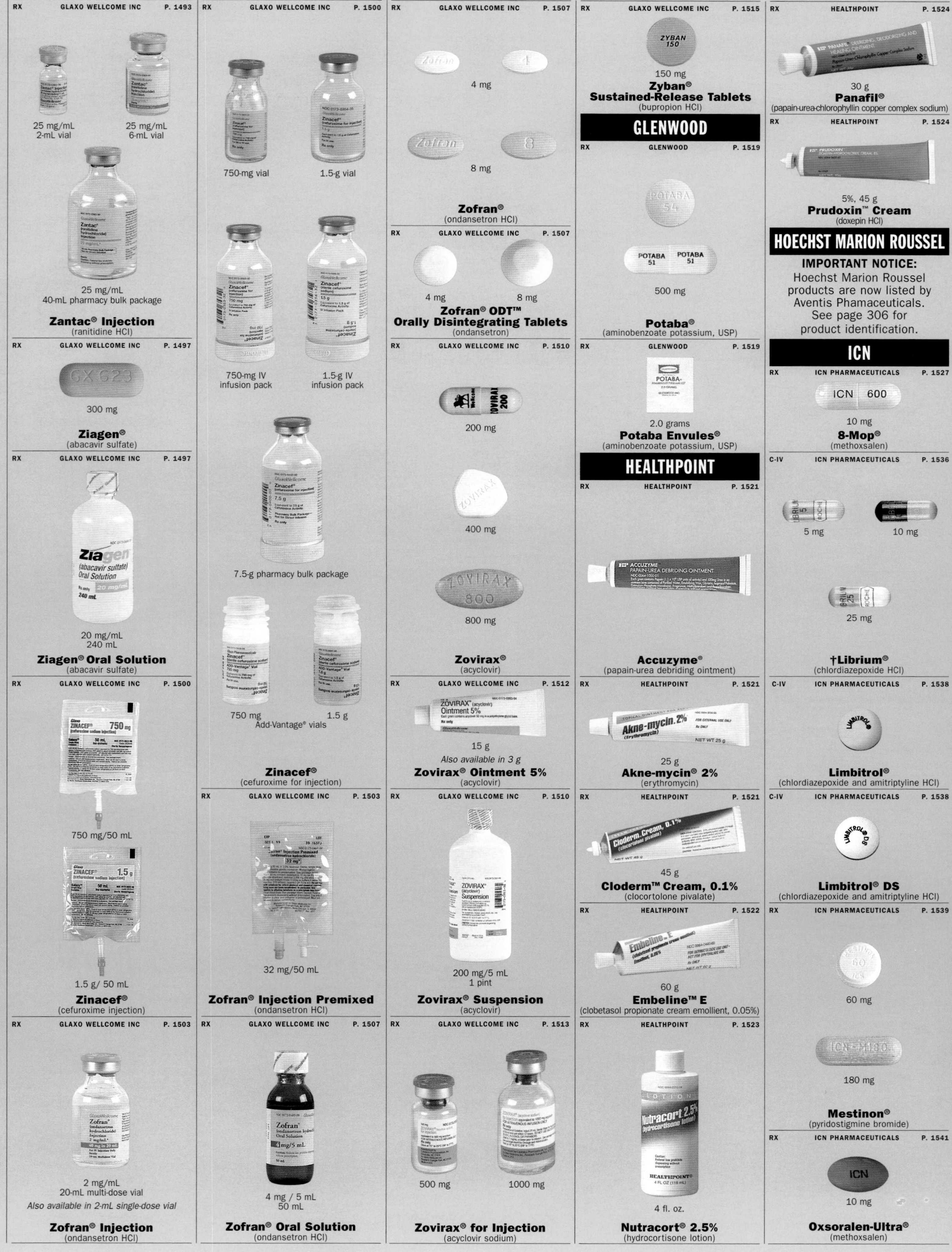
RX GLAXO WELLCOME INC P. 1493
25 mg/mL 2-mL vial
25 mg/mL 6-mL vial
25 mg/mL 40-mL pharmacy bulk package
Zantac® Injection
(ranitidine HCl)
RX GLAXO WELLCOME INC P. 1497
GX 623
300 mg
Ziagen®
(abacavir sulfate)
RX GLAXO WELLCOME INC P. 1497
Ziagen
(abacavir sulfate)
Oral Solution
20 mg/mL
240 mL
Ziagen® Oral Solution
(abacavir sulfate)
RX GLAXO WELLCOME INC P. 1500
750 mg/50 mL
1.5 g/ 50 mL
Zinacef®
(cefuroxime injection)
RX GLAXO WELLCOME INC P. 1503
2 mg/mL
20-mL multi-dose vial
Also available in 2-mL single-dose vial
Zofran® Injection
(ondansetron HCl)
RX GLAXO WELLCOME INC P. 1500
750-mg vial
1.5-g vial
750-mg IV infusion pack
1.5-g IV infusion pack
7.5-g pharmacy bulk package
750 mg
1.5 g
Add-Vantage® vials
Zinacef®
(cefuroxime for injection)
RX GLAXO WELLCOME INC P. 1503
32 mg/50 mL
Zofran® Injection Premixed
(ondansetron HCl)
RX GLAXO WELLCOME INC P. 1507
4 mg / 5 mL
50 mL
Zofran® Oral Solution
(ondansetron HCl)
RX GLAXO WELLCOME INC P. 1507
4 mg
8 mg
Zofran®
(ondansetron HCl)
RX GLAXO WELLCOME INC P. 1507
4 mg
8 mg
Zofran® ODT™
Orally Disintegrating Tablets
(ondansetron)
RX GLAXO WELLCOME INC P. 1510
200 mg
400 mg
ZOVIRAX 800
800 mg
Zovirax®
(acyclovir)
RX GLAXO WELLCOME INC P. 1512
15 g
Also available in 3 g
Zovirax® Ointment 5%
(acyclovir)
RX GLAXO WELLCOME INC P. 1510
200 mg/5 mL
1 pint
Zovirax® Suspension
(acyclovir)
RX GLAXO WELLCOME INC P. 1513
500 mg
1000 mg
Zovirax® for Injection
(acyclovir sodium)
RX GLAXO WELLCOME INC P. 1515
ZYBAN 150
150 mg
Zyban®
Sustained-Release Tablets
(bupropion HCl)
GLENWOOD
RX GLENWOOD P. 1519
POTABA 54
POTABA 51
500 mg
Potaba®
(aminobenzoate potassium, USP)
RX GLENWOOD P. 1519
2.0 grams
Potaba Envules®
(aminobenzoate potassium, USP)
HEALTHPOINT
RX HEALTHPOINT P. 1521
Accuzyme®
(papain-urea debriding ointment)
RX HEALTHPOINT P. 1521
25 g
Akne-mycin® 2%
(erythromycin)
RX HEALTHPOINT P. 1521
45 g
Cloderm™ Cream, 0.1%
(clocortolone pivalate)
RX HEALTHPOINT P. 1522
60 g
Embeline™ E
(clobetasol propionate cream emollient, 0.05%)
RX HEALTHPOINT P. 1523
4 fl. oz.
Nutracort® 2.5%
(hydrocortisone lotion)
RX HEALTHPOINT P. 1524
30 g
Panafil®
(papain-urea-chlorophyllin copper complex sodium)
RX HEALTHPOINT P. 1524
5%, 45 g
Prudoxin™ Cream
(doxepin HCl)
HOECHST MARION ROUSSEL
IMPORTANT NOTICE:
Hoechst Marion Roussel products are now listed by Aventis Phamaceuticals. See page 306 for product identification.
ICN
RX ICN PHARMACEUTICALS P. 1527
ICN 600
10 mg
8-Mop®
(methoxsalen)
C-IV ICN PHARMACEUTICALS P. 1536
5 mg
10 mg
25 mg
†Librium®
(chlordiazepoxide HCl)
C-IV ICN PHARMACEUTICALS P. 1538
Limbitrol®
(chlordiazepoxide and amitriptyline HCl)
C-IV ICN PHARMACEUTICALS P. 1538
Limbitrol® DS
(chlordiazepoxide and amitriptyline HCl)
RX ICN PHARMACEUTICALS P. 1539
60 mg
180 mg
Mestinon®
(pyridostigmine bromide)
RX ICN PHARMACEUTICALS P. 1541
ICN
10 mg
Oxsoralen-Ultra®
(methoxsalen)

RX ICN PHARMACEUTICALS P. 1544

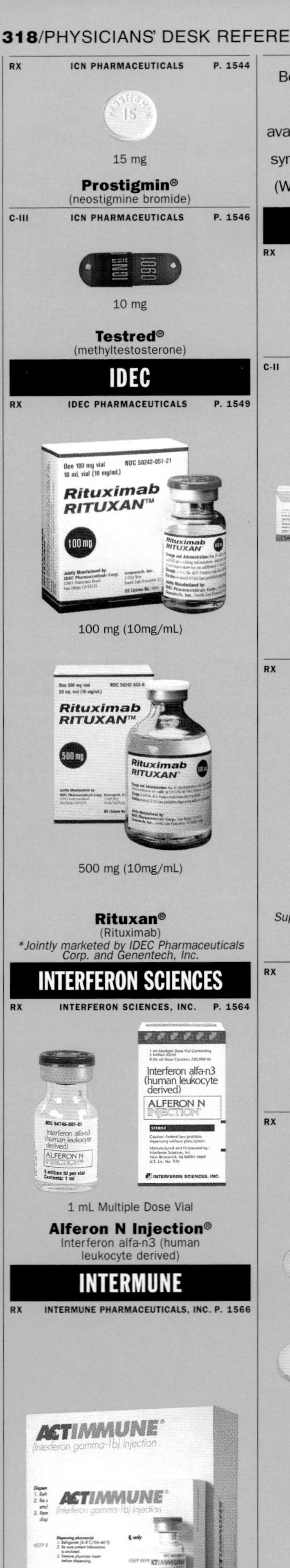

15 mg

Prostigmin®
(neostigmine bromide)

C-III ICN PHARMACEUTICALS P. 1546

10 mg

Testred®
(methyltestosterone)

IDEC

RX IDEC PHARMACEUTICALS P. 1549

100 mg (10mg/mL)

500 mg (10mg/mL)

Rituxan®
(Rituximab)
*Jointly marketed by IDEC Pharmaceuticals Corp. and Genentech, Inc.

INTERFERON SCIENCES

RX INTERFERON SCIENCES, INC. P. 1564

1 mL Multiple Dose Vial

Alferon N Injection®
Interferon alfa-n3 (human leukocyte derived)

INTERMUNE

RX INTERMUNE PHARMACEUTICALS, INC. P. 1566

100 mcg

Actimmune®
(Interferon gamma-1b) Injection

Because tablets and capsules are shown in this section, do not infer that these are the only dosage forms available. Where a product name is preceded by the symbol †, refer to the description in the Product Information (White Section) for other forms.

JANSSEN

RX JANSSEN PHARMACEUTICA P. 1570

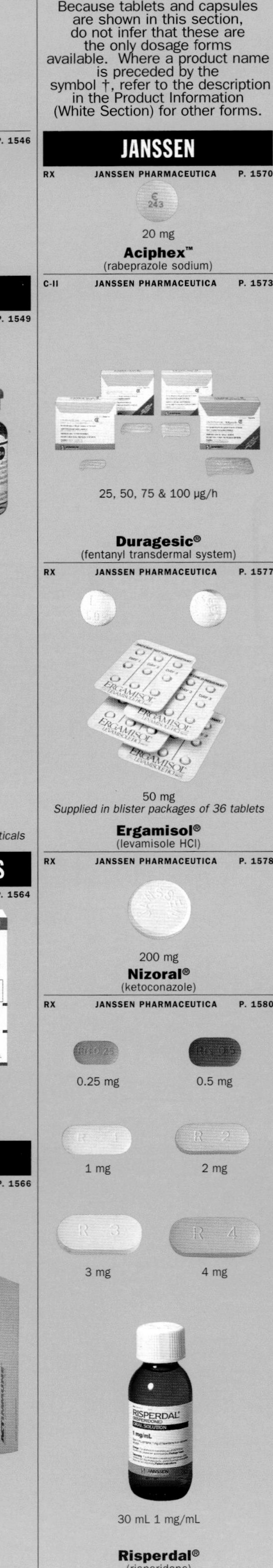

20 mg

Aciphex™
(rabeprazole sodium)

C-II JANSSEN PHARMACEUTICA P. 1573

25, 50, 75 & 100 µg/h

Duragesic®
(fentanyl transdermal system)

RX JANSSEN PHARMACEUTICA P. 1577

50 mg
Supplied in blister packages of 36 tablets

Ergamisol®
(levamisole HCl)

RX JANSSEN PHARMACEUTICA P. 1578

200 mg

Nizoral®
(ketoconazole)

RX JANSSEN PHARMACEUTICA P. 1580

0.25 mg 0.5 mg

1 mg 2 mg

3 mg 4 mg

30 mL 1 mg/mL

Risperdal®
(risperidone)

RX JANSSEN PHARMACEUTICA P. 1584

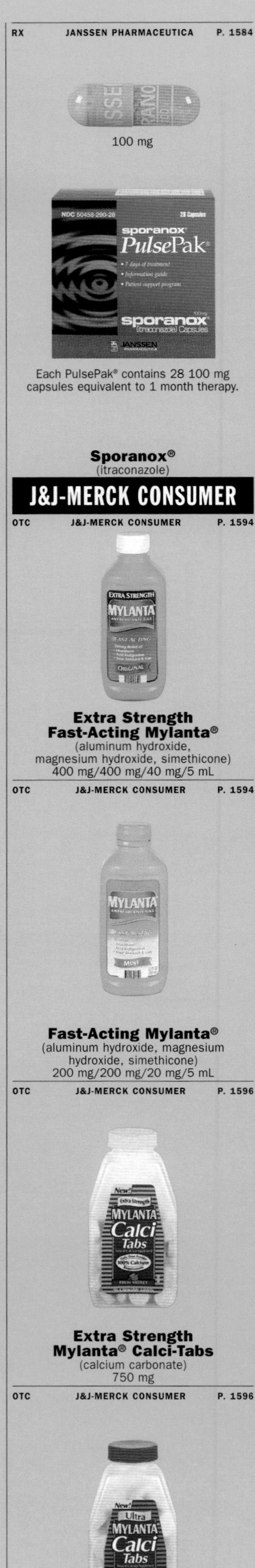

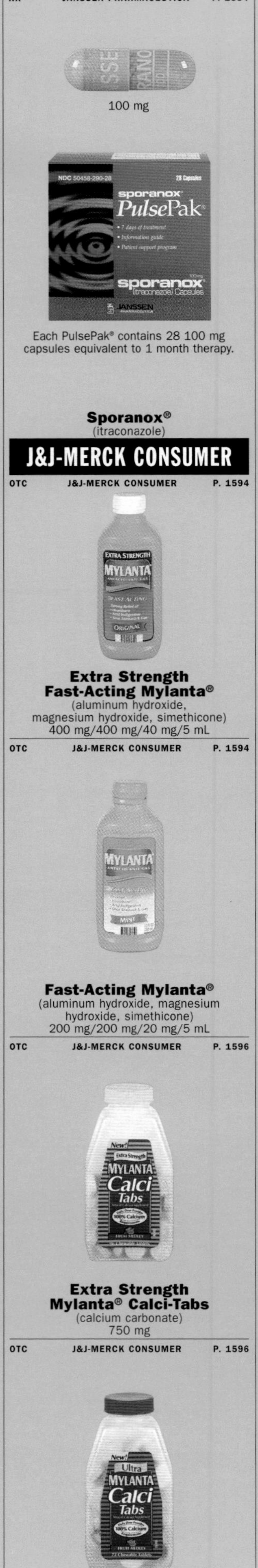

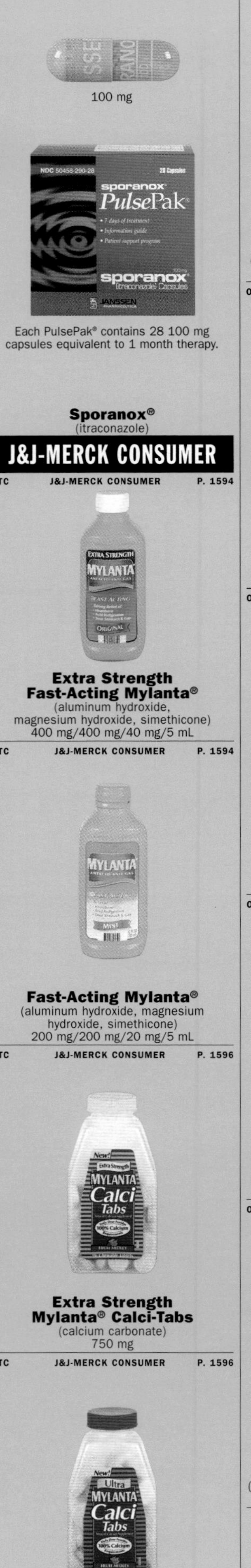

100 mg

Each PulsePak® contains 28 100 mg capsules equivalent to 1 month therapy.

Sporanox®
(itraconazole)

J&J-MERCK CONSUMER

OTC J&J-MERCK CONSUMER P. 1594

Extra Strength Fast-Acting Mylanta®
(aluminum hydroxide, magnesium hydroxide, simethicone)
400 mg/400 mg/40 mg/5 mL

OTC J&J-MERCK CONSUMER P. 1594

Fast-Acting Mylanta®
(aluminum hydroxide, magnesium hydroxide, simethicone)
200 mg/200 mg/20 mg/5 mL

OTC J&J-MERCK CONSUMER P. 1596

Extra Strength Mylanta® Calci-Tabs
(calcium carbonate)
750 mg

OTC J&J-MERCK CONSUMER P. 1596

Ultra Mylanta® Calci-Tabs
(calcium carbonate)
1000 mg

OTC J&J-MERCK CONSUMER P. 1595

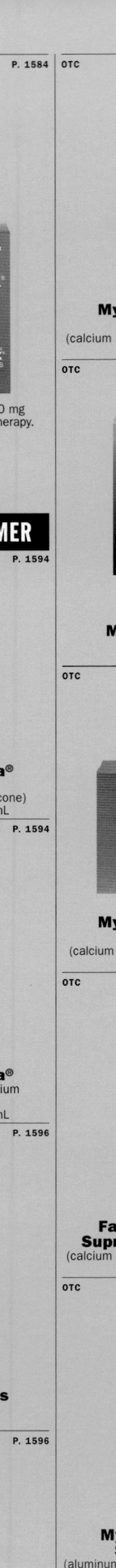

Mylanta® Fast-Acting Ultra Tabs
(calcium carbonate, magnesium hydroxide)
700 mg/300 mg

OTC J&J-MERCK CONSUMER P. 1595

Mylanta® Gas Maximum Strength
(simethicone)
125 mg

OTC J&J-MERCK CONSUMER P. 1595

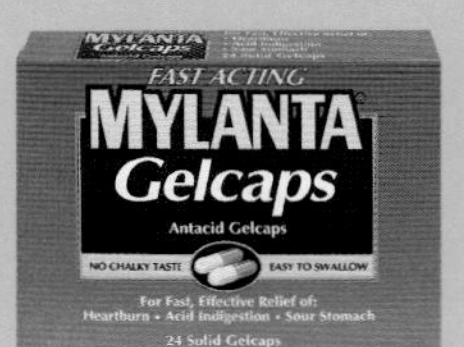

Mylanta® Fast Acting Gelcaps Antacid
(calcium carbonate, magnesium hydroxide)
550 mg/125 mg

OTC J&J-MERCK CONSUMER P. 1595

Fast-Acting Mylanta® Supreme Tasting Antacid
(calcium carbonate, magnesium hydroxide)
400 mg/135 mg/5 mL

OTC J&J-MERCK CONSUMER P. 1596

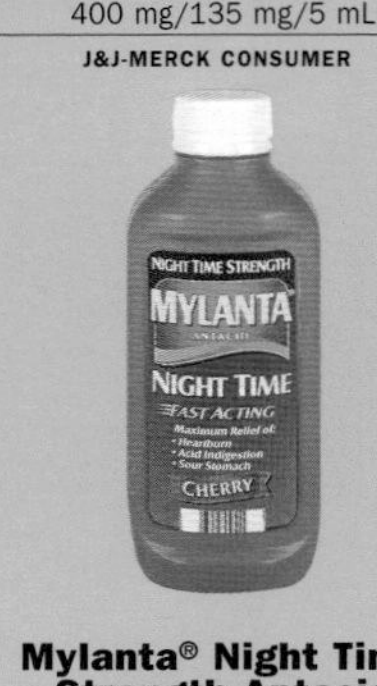

Mylanta® Night Time Strength Antacid
(aluminum hydroxide, magnesium hydroxide)
500 mg/500 mg/5 mL

While every effort has been made to reproduce products faithfully, this section is to be considered a quick reference identification aid. In cases of suspected overdosage, etc., chemical analysis of the product should be done.

OTC J&J-MERCK CONSUMER P. 1594

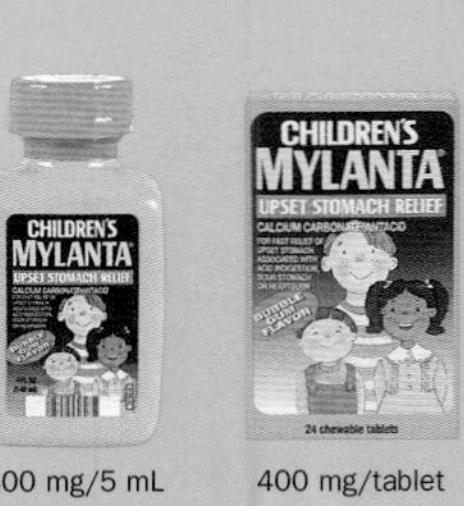

400 mg/5 mL 400 mg/tablet

Children's Mylanta® Upset Stomach Relief Liquid and Tablets
(calcium carbonate)

OTC J&J-MERCK CONSUMER P. 1594

Infants Mylicon® Drops
(simethicone)
40 mg/0.6 mL

OTC J&J-MERCK CONSUMER P. 1596

Pepcid AC®
(famotidine)
10 mg

OTC J&J-MERCK CONSUMER P. 1596

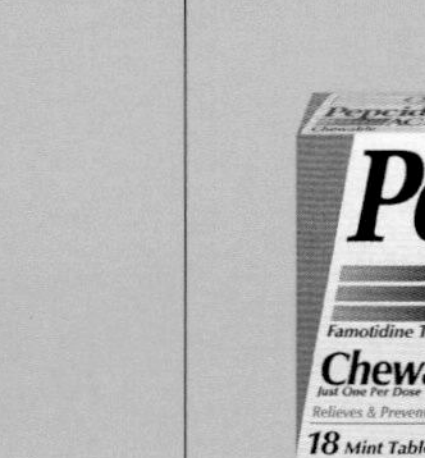

Pepcid AC® Chewable Tablets
(famotidine)
10 mg

OTC J&J-MERCK CONSUMER P. 1596

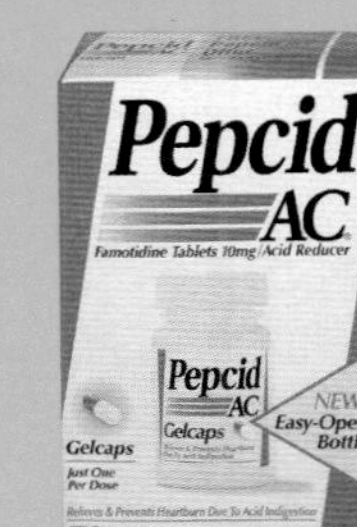

Pepcid AC® Gelcaps
(famotidine)
10 mg

Designed to help you identify drugs, this section contains actual size pills and full color reproduction of products selected for inclusion by participating manufacturers.

JONES PHARMA

RX JONES PHARMA INCORPORATED P. 1597

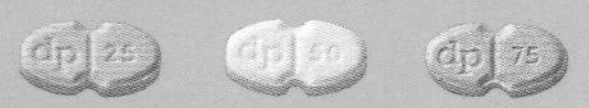

25 mcg (0.025 mg) | 50 mcg (0.05 mg) | 75 mcg (0.075 mg)
88 mcg (0.088 mg) | 100 mcg (0.1 mg) | 112 mcg (0.112 mg)
125 mcg (0.125 mg) | 137 mcg (0.137 mg) | 150 mcg (0.15 mg)
175 mcg (0.175 mg) | 200 mcg (0.2 mg) | 300 mcg (0.3 mg)

Levoxyl®
(levothyroxine sodium tablets, USP)

Because tablets and capsules are shown in this section, do not infer that these are the only dosage forms available. Where a product name is preceded by the symbol †, refer to the description in the Product Information (White Section) for other forms.

KEY

RX KEY PHARMACEUTICALS P. 1597

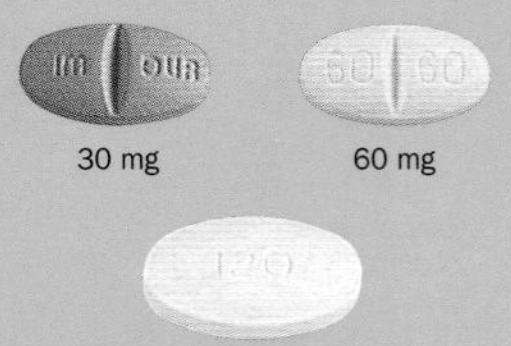

30 mg | 60 mg
120 mg
Extended release tablets

Imdur®
(isosorbide mononitrate)

RX KEY PHARMACEUTICALS P. 1603

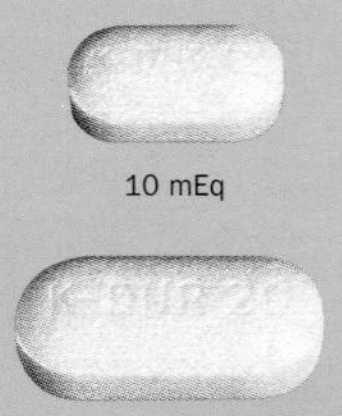

10 mEq
20 mEq
Microburst Release System®

K-Dur®
(potassium chloride USP)

RX KEY PHARMACEUTICALS P. 1604

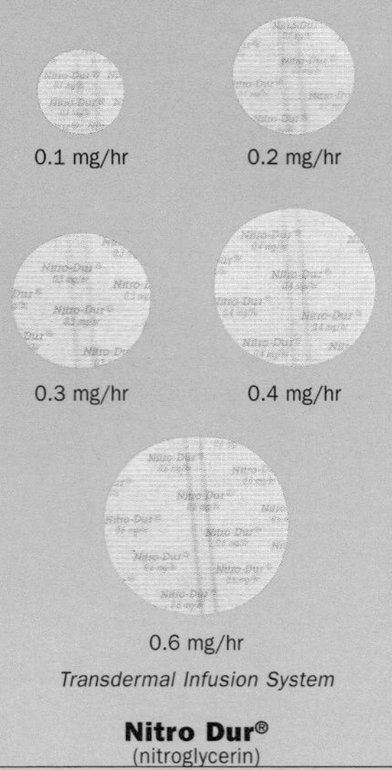

0.1 mg/hr | 0.2 mg/hr
0.3 mg/hr | 0.4 mg/hr
0.6 mg/hr
Transdermal Infusion System

Nitro Dur®
(nitroglycerin)

RX KEY PHARMACEUTICALS P. 1605

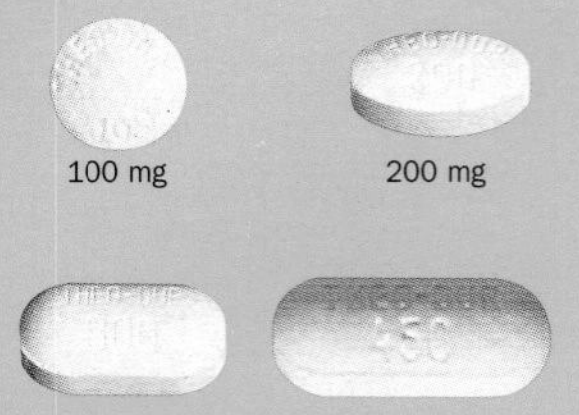

100 mg | 200 mg
300 mg | 450 mg
Extended release tablets

Theo-Dur®
(theophylline anhydrous)

RX KEY PHARMACEUTICALS

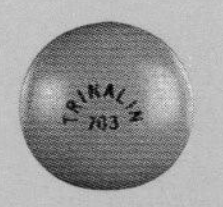

703* 1 mg / 120 mg
Long acting antihistamine/decongestant

Trinalin® Repetabs®
(azatadine maleate USP, pseudoephedrine sulfate USP)

RX KEY PHARMACEUTICALS P. 1611

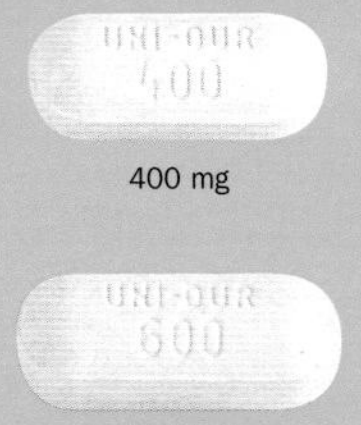

400 mg
600 mg

Uni-Dur®
(theophylline)

KNOLL LABORATORIES

RX KNOLL LABORATORIES P. 1617

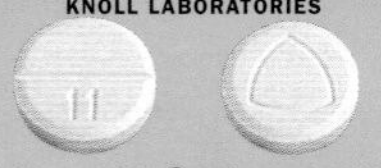

2 mg

†Akineton®
(biperiden HCl)

C-II KNOLL LABORATORIES P. 1618

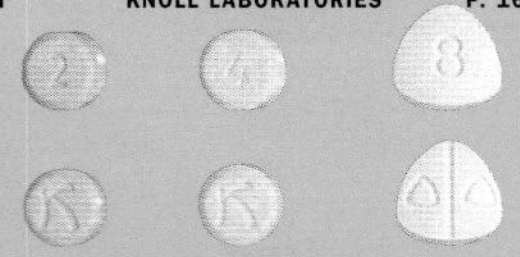

2 mg | 4 mg | 8 mg

†Dilaudid®
(hydromorphone HCl)

C-II KNOLL LABORATORIES P. 1618

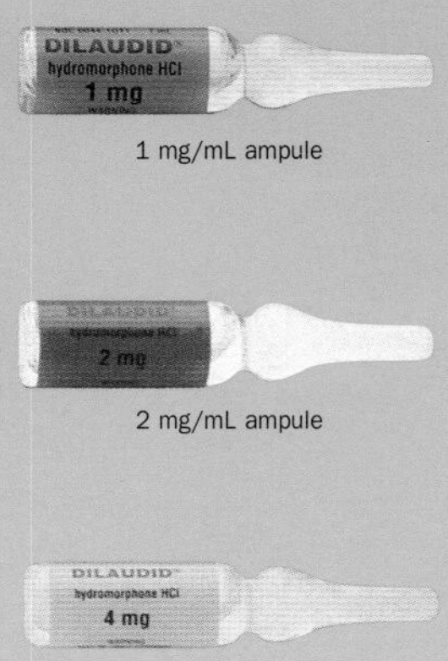

1 mg/mL ampule
2 mg/mL ampule
4 mg/mL ampule

Dilaudid®
(hydromorphone HCl)

C-II KNOLL LABORATORIES P. 1618

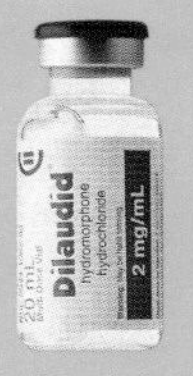

2 mg/mL
Multi dose vial

Dilaudid®
(hydromorphone HCl)

C-II KNOLL LABORATORIES P. 1618

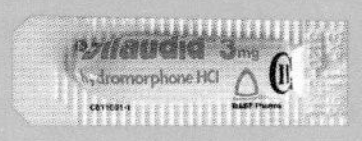

3 mg Suppository

Dilaudid®
(hydromorphone HCl)

C-II KNOLL LABORATORIES P. 1621

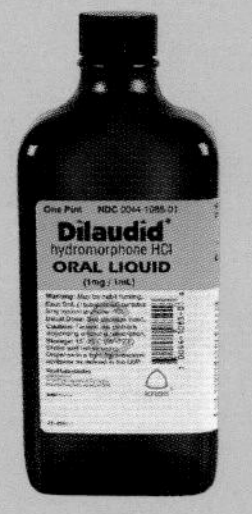

5 mg/5 mL

Dilaudid® Oral Liquid
(hydromorphone HCl)

C-II KNOLL LABORATORIES P. 1619

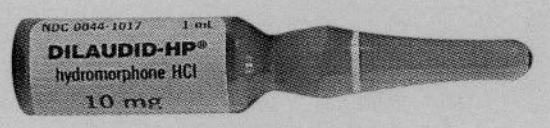

10 mg/mL

Dilaudid-HP®
(hydromorphone HCl)

C-II KNOLL LABORATORIES P. 1619

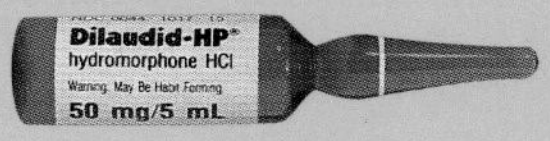

50 mg/5 mL

Dilaudid-HP®
(hydromorphone HCl)

C-II KNOLL LABORATORIES P. 1619

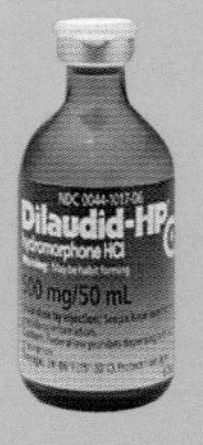

500 mg/50 mL

Dilaudid-HP®
(hydromorphone HCl)

C-II KNOLL LABORATORIES P. 1619

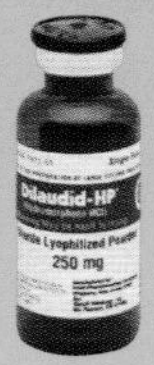

250 mg
Sterile Lyophilized Powder

Dilaudid-HP®
(hydromorphone HCl)

RX KNOLL LABORATORIES P. 1623

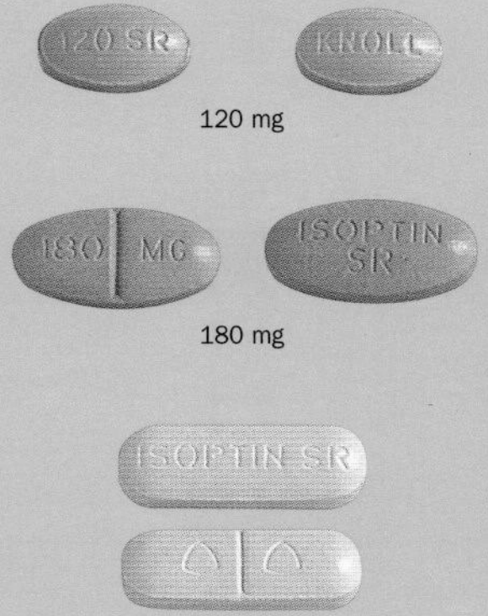

120 mg
180 mg
240 mg
Film-coated sustained release oral tablets

Isoptin® SR
(verapamil HCl)

RX KNOLL LABORATORIES P. 1625

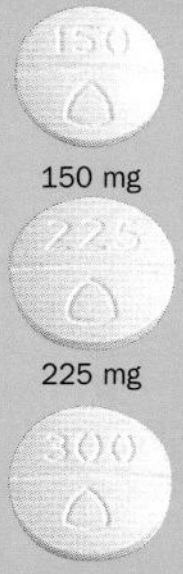

150 mg
225 mg
300 mg

Rythmol®
(propafenone HCl)

C-III KNOLL LABORATORIES P. 1629

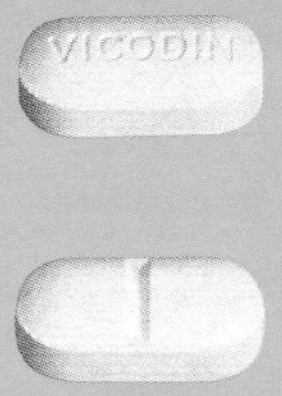

Vicodin®
(hydrocodone bitartrate, acetaminophen)
5 mg/500 mg

C-III KNOLL LABORATORIES P. 1630

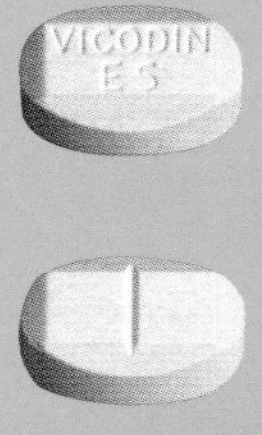

Vicodin ES®
(hydrocodone bitartrate, acetaminophen)
7.5 mg / 750 mg

C-III KNOLL LABORATORIES P. 1628

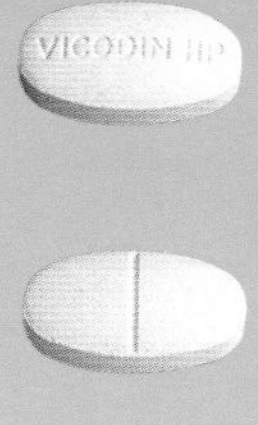

Vicodin HP™
(hydrocodone bitartrate, acetaminophen)
10 mg/660 mg

C-III KNOLL LABORATORIES P. 1632

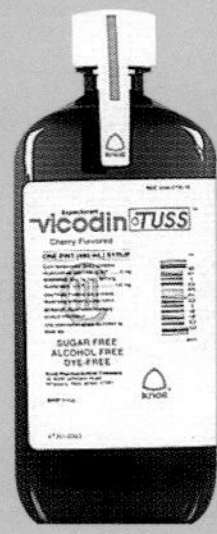

480 mL

Vicodin Tuss™
(hydrocodone bitartrate, guaifenesin)
5 mg/100 mg per 5 mL

C-III KNOLL LABORATORIES P. 1632

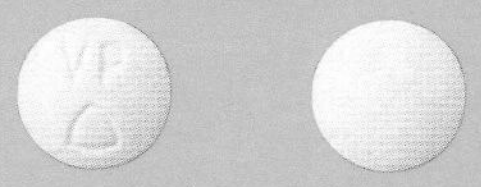

Vicoprofen®
(hydrocodone bitartrate, ibuprofen)
7.5 mg/200 mg

While every effort has been made to reproduce products faithfully, this section is to be considered a quick reference identification aid. In cases of suspected overdosage, etc., chemical analysis of the product should be done.

KNOLL PHARM. COMPANY

RX KNOLL PHARMACEUTICAL COMPANY P .1635

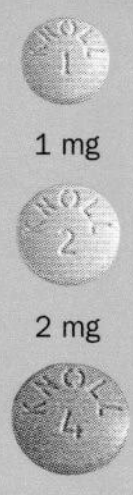

1 mg
2 mg
4 mg

Mavik®
(trandolapril)

C-IV KNOLL PHARMACEUTICAL COMPANY P. 1637

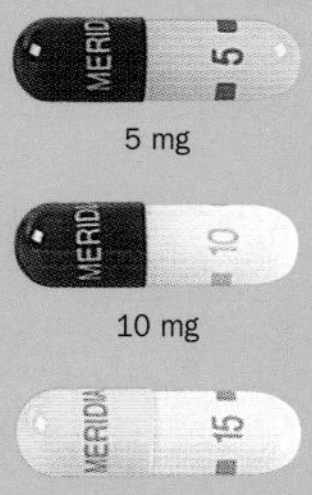

5 mg
10 mg
15 mg

Meridia®
(sibutramine HCl monohydrate)

RX KNOLL PHARMACEUTICAL COMPANY P. 1641

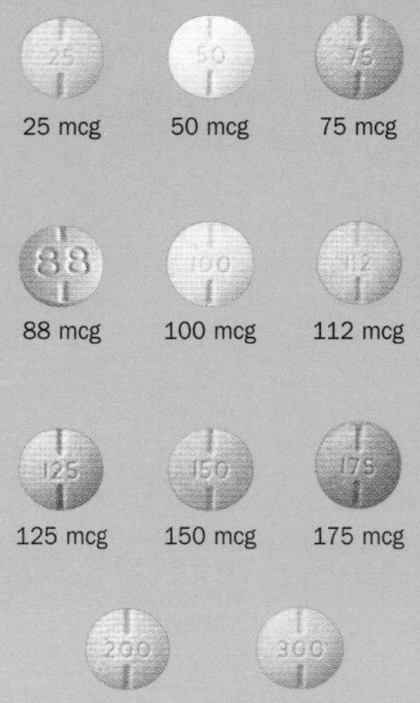

25 mcg | 50 mcg | 75 mcg
88 mcg | 100 mcg | 112 mcg
125 mcg | 150 mcg | 175 mcg
200 mcg | 300 mcg

Synthroid®
(levothyroxine sodium tablets, USP)

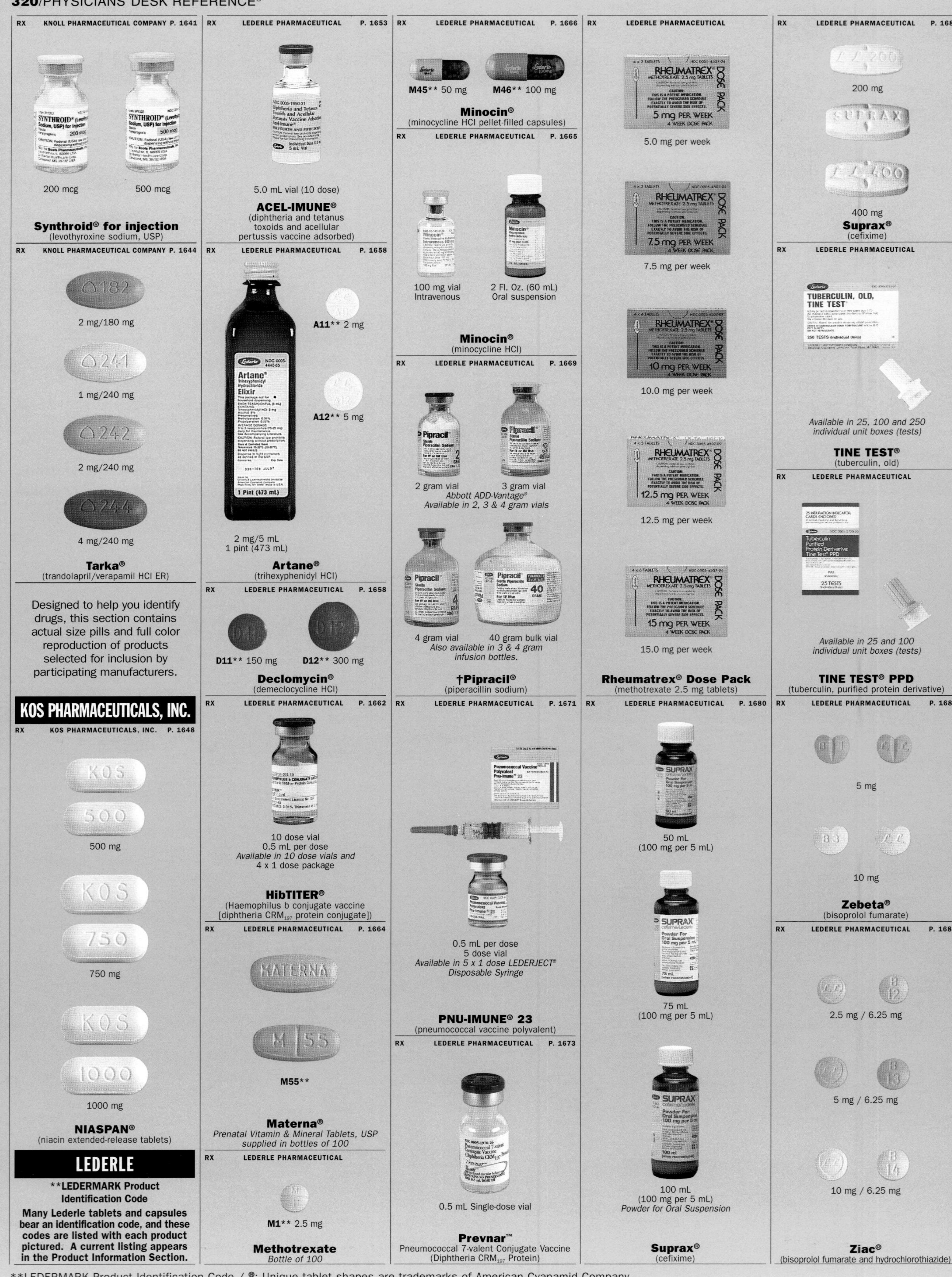

RX KNOLL PHARMACEUTICAL COMPANY P. 1641

200 mcg 500 mcg

Synthroid® for injection
(levothyroxine sodium, USP)

RX KNOLL PHARMACEUTICAL COMPANY P. 1644

2 mg/180 mg

1 mg/240 mg

2 mg/240 mg

4 mg/240 mg

Tarka®
(trandolapril/verapamil HCl ER)

Designed to help you identify drugs, this section contains actual size pills and full color reproduction of products selected for inclusion by participating manufacturers.

KOS PHARMACEUTICALS, INC.

RX KOS PHARMACEUTICALS, INC. P. 1648

500 mg

750 mg

1000 mg

NIASPAN®
(niacin extended-release tablets)

LEDERLE

****LEDERMARK Product Identification Code**

Many Lederle tablets and capsules bear an identification code, and these codes are listed with each product pictured. A current listing appears in the Product Information Section.

RX LEDERLE PHARMACEUTICAL P. 1653

5.0 mL vial (10 dose)

ACEL-IMUNE®
(diphtheria and tetanus toxoids and acellular pertussis vaccine adsorbed)

RX LEDERLE PHARMACEUTICAL P. 1658

A11** 2 mg

A12** 5 mg

2 mg/5 mL
1 pint (473 mL)

Artane®
(trihexyphenidyl HCl)

RX LEDERLE PHARMACEUTICAL P. 1658

D11** 150 mg D12** 300 mg

Declomycin®
(demeclocycline HCl)

RX LEDERLE PHARMACEUTICAL P. 1662

10 dose vial
0.5 mL per dose
Available in 10 dose vials and 4 x 1 dose package

HibTITER®
(Haemophilus b conjugate vaccine [diphtheria CRM_{197} protein conjugate])

RX LEDERLE PHARMACEUTICAL P. 1664

M55**

Materna®
Prenatal Vitamin & Mineral Tablets, USP supplied in bottles of 100

RX LEDERLE PHARMACEUTICAL

M1** 2.5 mg

Methotrexate
Bottle of 100

RX LEDERLE PHARMACEUTICAL P. 1666

M45** 50 mg M46** 100 mg

Minocin®
(minocycline HCl pellet-filled capsules)

RX LEDERLE PHARMACEUTICAL P. 1665

100 mg vial
Intravenous

2 Fl. Oz. (60 mL)
Oral suspension

Minocin®
(minocycline HCl)

RX LEDERLE PHARMACEUTICAL P. 1669

2 gram vial 3 gram vial
Abbott ADD-Vantage®
Available in 2, 3 & 4 gram vials

4 gram vial 40 gram bulk vial
Also available in 3 & 4 gram infusion bottles.

†Pipracil®
(piperacillin sodium)

RX LEDERLE PHARMACEUTICAL P. 1671

0.5 mL per dose
5 dose vial
Available in 5 x 1 dose LEDERJECT® Disposable Syringe

PNU-IMUNE® 23
(pneumococcal vaccine polyvalent)

RX LEDERLE PHARMACEUTICAL P. 1673

0.5 mL Single-dose vial

Prevnar™
Pneumococcal 7-valent Conjugate Vaccine
(Diphtheria CRM_{197} Protein)

RX LEDERLE PHARMACEUTICAL

5.0 mg per week

7.5 mg per week

10.0 mg per week

12.5 mg per week

15.0 mg per week

Rheumatrex® Dose Pack
(methotrexate 2.5 mg tablets)

RX LEDERLE PHARMACEUTICAL P. 1680

50 mL
(100 mg per 5 mL)

75 mL
(100 mg per 5 mL)

100 mL
(100 mg per 5 mL)
Powder for Oral Suspension

Suprax®
(cefixime)

RX LEDERLE PHARMACEUTICAL P. 1680

200 mg

400 mg

Suprax®
(cefixime)

RX LEDERLE PHARMACEUTICAL

Available in 25, 100 and 250 individual unit boxes (tests)

TINE TEST®
(tuberculin, old)

RX LEDERLE PHARMACEUTICAL

Available in 25 and 100 individual unit boxes (tests)

TINE TEST® PPD
(tuberculin, purified protein derivative)

RX LEDERLE PHARMACEUTICAL P. 1686

5 mg

10 mg

Zebeta®
(bisoprolol fumarate)

RX LEDERLE PHARMACEUTICAL P. 1688

2.5 mg / 6.25 mg

5 mg / 6.25 mg

10 mg / 6.25 mg

Ziac®
(bisoprolol fumarate and hydrochlorothiazide)

**LEDERMARK Product Identification Code / ®: Unique tablet shapes are trademarks of American Cyanamid Company.

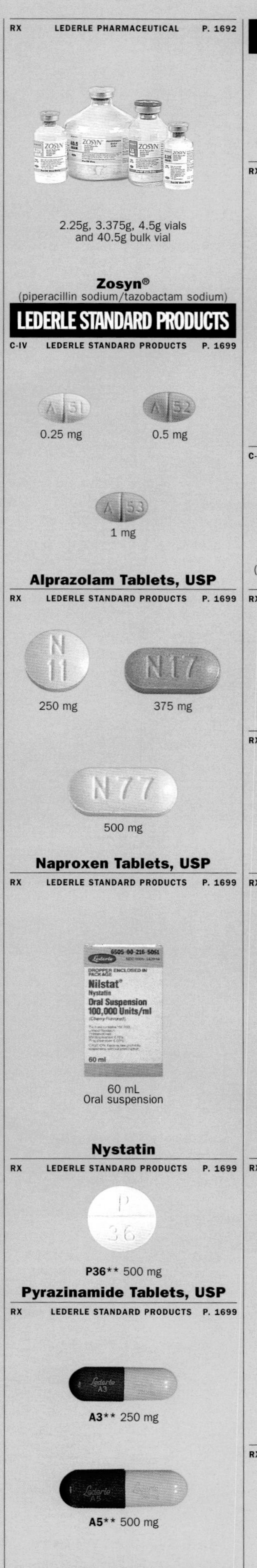

RX LEDERLE PHARMACEUTICAL P. 1692

2.25g, 3.375g, 4.5g vials and 40.5g bulk vial

Zosyn®
(piperacillin sodium/tazobactam sodium)

LEDERLE STANDARD PRODUCTS

C-IV LEDERLE STANDARD PRODUCTS P. 1699

0.25 mg 0.5 mg

1 mg

Alprazolam Tablets, USP

RX LEDERLE STANDARD PRODUCTS P. 1699

250 mg 375 mg

500 mg

Naproxen Tablets, USP

RX LEDERLE STANDARD PRODUCTS P. 1699

60 mL
Oral suspension

Nystatin

RX LEDERLE STANDARD PRODUCTS P. 1699

P36** 500 mg

Pyrazinamide Tablets, USP

RX LEDERLE STANDARD PRODUCTS P. 1699

A3** 250 mg

A5** 500 mg

†Tetracycline HCl Capsules

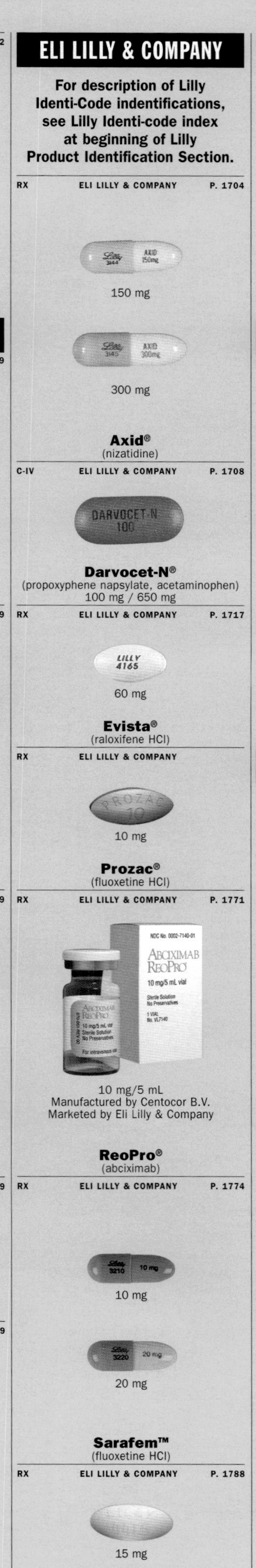

ELI LILLY & COMPANY

For description of Lilly Identi-Code indentifications, see Lilly Identi-code index at beginning of Lilly Product Identification Section.

RX ELI LILLY & COMPANY P. 1704

150 mg

300 mg

Axid®
(nizatidine)

C-IV ELI LILLY & COMPANY P. 1708

Darvocet-N®
(propoxyphene napsylate, acetaminophen)
100 mg / 650 mg

RX ELI LILLY & COMPANY P. 1717

60 mg

Evista®
(raloxifene HCl)

RX ELI LILLY & COMPANY

10 mg

Prozac®
(fluoxetine HCl)

RX ELI LILLY & COMPANY P. 1771

10 mg/5 mL
Manufactured by Centocor B.V.
Marketed by Eli Lilly & Company

ReoPro®
(abciximab)

RX ELI LILLY & COMPANY P. 1774

10 mg

20 mg

Sarafem™
(fluoxetine HCl)

RX ELI LILLY & COMPANY P. 1788

15 mg

Zyprexa®
(olanzapine)

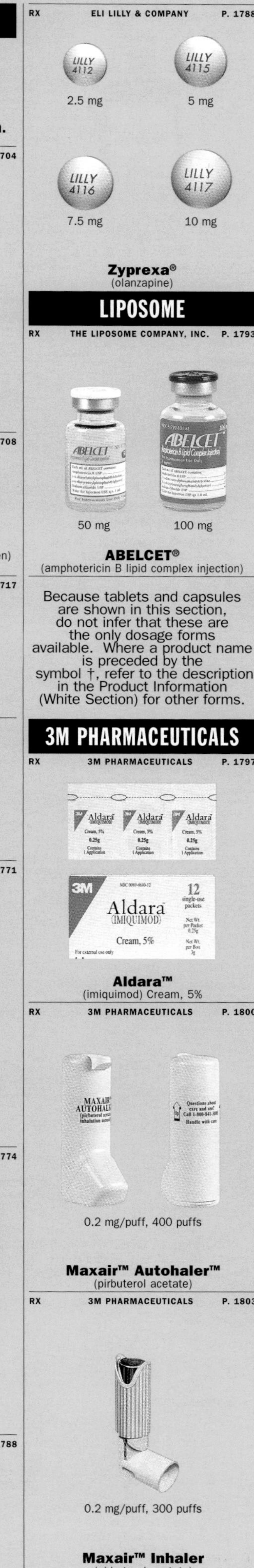

RX ELI LILLY & COMPANY P. 1788

2.5 mg 5 mg

7.5 mg 10 mg

Zyprexa®
(olanzapine)

LIPOSOME

RX THE LIPOSOME COMPANY, INC. P. 1793

50 mg 100 mg

ABELCET®
(amphotericin B lipid complex injection)

Because tablets and capsules are shown in this section, do not infer that these are the only dosage forms available. Where a product name is preceded by the symbol †, refer to the description in the Product Information (White Section) for other forms.

3M PHARMACEUTICALS

RX 3M PHARMACEUTICALS P. 1797

Aldara™
(imiquimod) Cream, 5%

RX 3M PHARMACEUTICALS P. 1800

0.2 mg/puff, 400 puffs

Maxair™ Autohaler™
(pirbuterol acetate)

RX 3M PHARMACEUTICALS P. 1803

0.2 mg/puff, 300 puffs

Maxair™ Inhaler
(pirbuterol acetate)

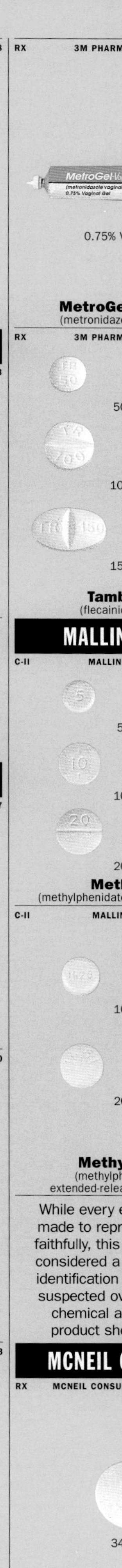

RX 3M PHARMACEUTICALS P. 1804

0.75% Vaginal Gel

MetroGel-Vaginal®
(metronidazole vaginal gel)

RX 3M PHARMACEUTICALS P. 1806

50 mg

100 mg

150 mg

Tambocor™
(flecainide acetate)

MALLINCKRODT

C-II MALLINCKRODT P. 1810

5 mg

10 mg

20 mg

Methylin™
(methylphenidate HCl tablets, USP)

C-II MALLINCKRODT P. 1810

10 mg

20 mg

Methylin ER™
(methylphenidate HCl extended-release tablets, USP)

While every effort has been made to reproduce products faithfully, this section is to be considered a quick reference identification aid. In cases of suspected overdosage, etc., chemical analysis of the product should be done.

MCNEIL CONSUMER

RX MCNEIL CONSUMER HEALTHCARE P. 1813

340 mg

Aflexa™
(glucosamine)

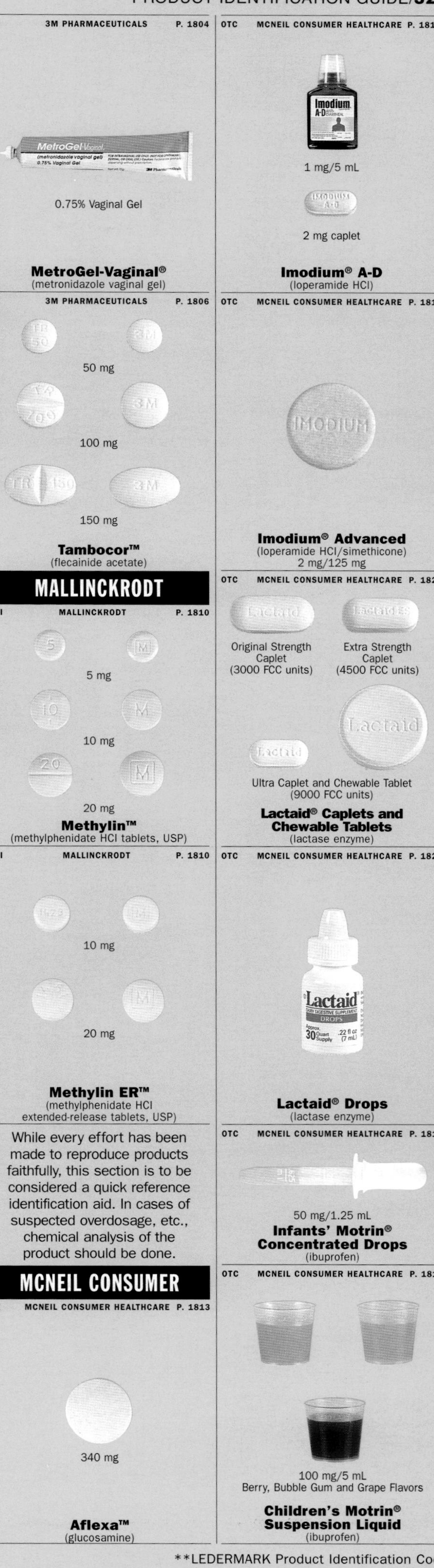

OTC MCNEIL CONSUMER HEALTHCARE P. 1817

1 mg/5 mL

2 mg caplet

Imodium® A-D
(loperamide HCl)

OTC MCNEIL CONSUMER HEALTHCARE P. 1818

Imodium® Advanced
(loperamide HCl/simethicone)
2 mg/125 mg

OTC MCNEIL CONSUMER HEALTHCARE P. 1821

Original Strength Caplet (3000 FCC units) Extra Strength Caplet (4500 FCC units)

Ultra Caplet and Chewable Tablet (9000 FCC units)

Lactaid® Caplets and Chewable Tablets
(lactase enzyme)

OTC MCNEIL CONSUMER HEALTHCARE P. 1820

Lactaid® Drops
(lactase enzyme)

OTC MCNEIL CONSUMER HEALTHCARE P. 1818

50 mg/1.25 mL

Infants' Motrin® Concentrated Drops
(ibuprofen)

OTC MCNEIL CONSUMER HEALTHCARE P. 1813

100 mg/5 mL
Berry, Bubble Gum and Grape Flavors

Children's Motrin® Suspension Liquid
(ibuprofen)

**LEDERMARK Product Identification Code

OTC MCNEIL CONSUMER HEALTHCARE P. 1813

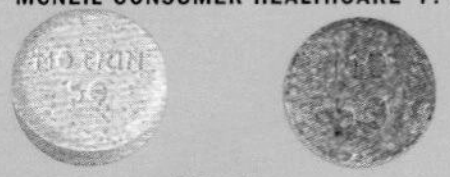

50 mg
Orange and Grape Flavors
Children's Motrin® Chewable Tablets
(ibuprofen)

OTC MCNEIL CONSUMER HEALTHCARE P. 1819

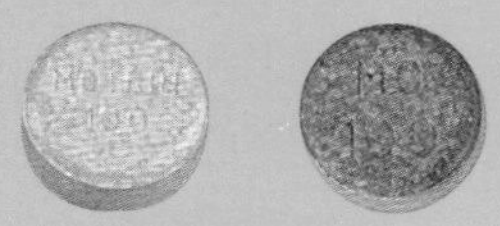

100 mg
Chewable Tablet
Orange and Grape Flavors

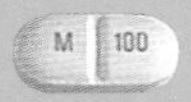

100 mg
Caplet

Junior Strength Motrin®
(ibuprofen)

RX MCNEIL CONSUMER HEALTHCARE P. 1823

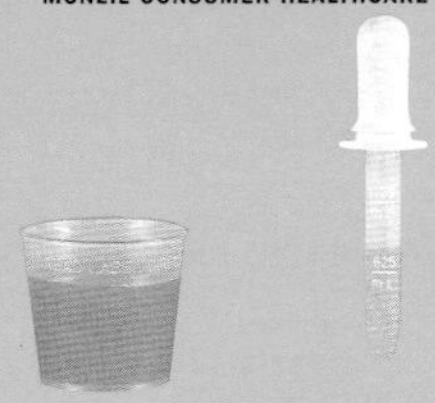

100 mg/5 mL
Suspension

40 mg/mL
Oral Drops

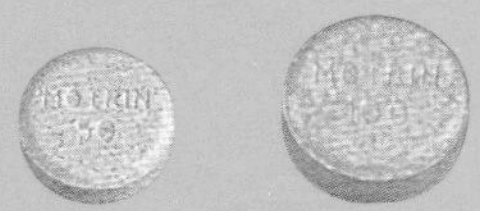

50 mg
100 mg
Chewable Tablets

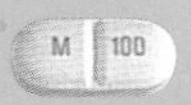

100 mg Caplets
Motrin®
(ibuprofen)

OTC MCNEIL CONSUMER HEALTHCARE P. 1822

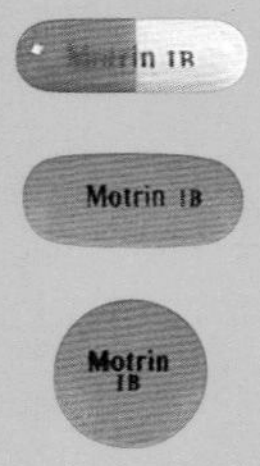

200 mg
Gelcaps, Caplets and Tablets

Motrin® IB
(ibuprofen)

OTC MCNEIL CONSUMER HEALTHCARE P. 1821

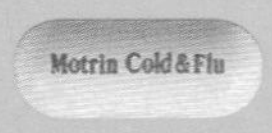

Motrin® Cold & Flu
(ibuprofen, pseudoephedrine HCl)

OTC MCNEIL CONSUMER HEALTHCARE P. 1821

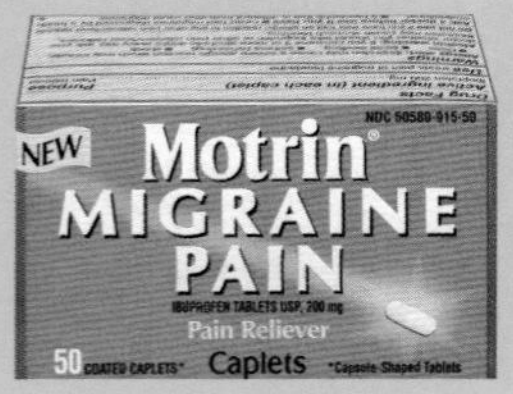

Motrin® Migraine Pain
(ibuprofen)

OTC MCNEIL CONSUMER HEALTHCARE P. 1822

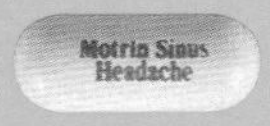

Motrin® Sinus Headache
(ibuprofen, pseudoephedrine HCl)

RX MCNEIL CONSUMER HEALTHCARE P. 1825

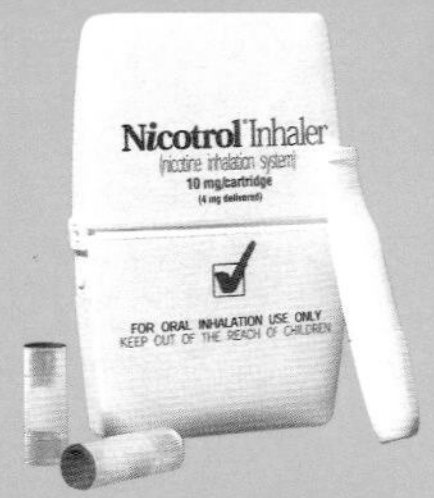

10 mg per cartridge
(4 mg delivered)

Nicotrol® Inhaler
(nicotine inhalation system)

RX MCNEIL CONSUMER HEALTHCARE P. 1831

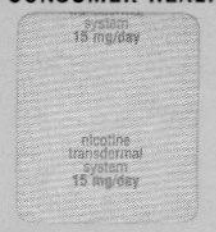

15 mg/day
Nicotrol®
(nicotine transdermal system)

RX MCNEIL CONSUMER HEALTHCARE P. 1828

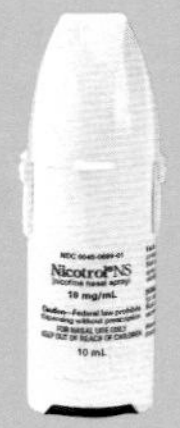

10 mg/mL

Nicotrol®NS
(nicotine nasal spray)

RX MCNEIL CONSUMER HEALTHCARE P. 1831

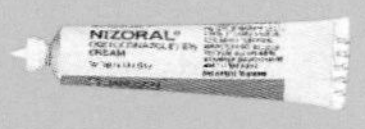

15 gm

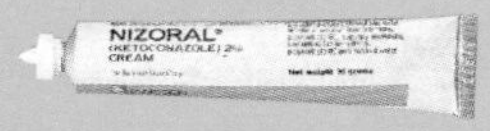

30 gm

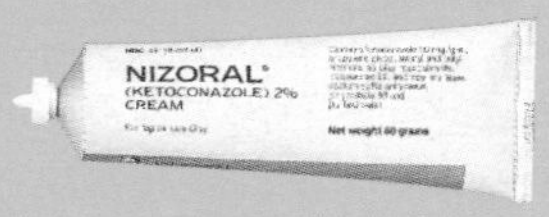

60 gm

Nizoral® 2% Cream
(ketoconazole)

RX MCNEIL CONSUMER HEALTHCARE P. 1832

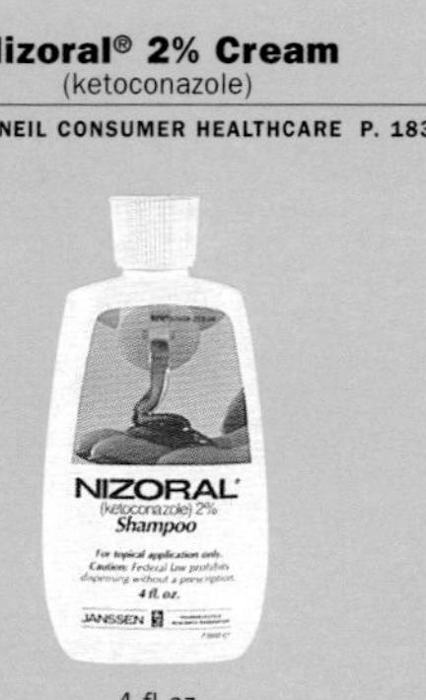

4 fl oz

Nizoral® 2% Shampoo
(ketoconazole)

OTC MCNEIL CONSUMER HEALTHCARE P. 1831

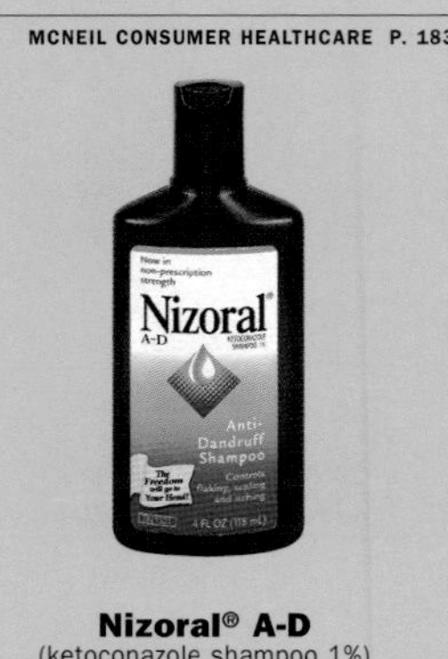

Nizoral® A-D
(ketoconazole shampoo 1%)

OTC MCNEIL CONSUMER HEALTHCARE P. 1832

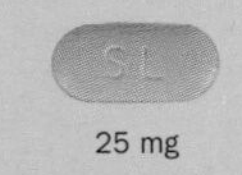

25 mg

Simply Sleep™
(diphenhydramine HCl)

OTC MCNEIL CONSUMER HEALTHCARE P. 1832

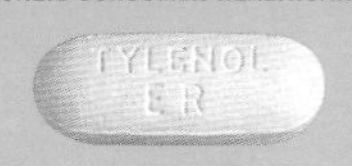

650 mg Caplet

TYLENOL® Arthritis Pain Extended Relief
(acetaminophen extended release)

OTC MCNEIL CONSUMER HEALTHCARE P. 1832

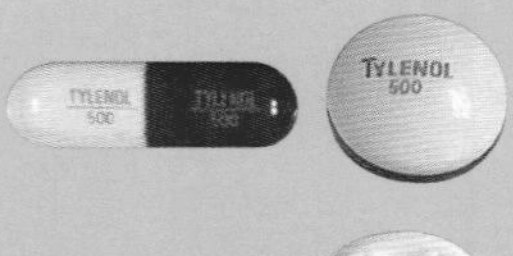

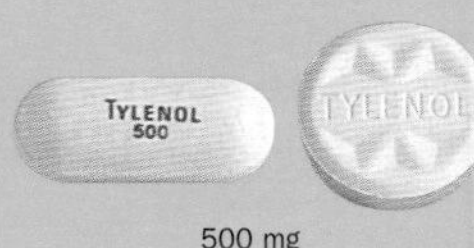

500 mg
Gelcaps, Geltabs, Caplets, and Tablets
Also Available: Extra Strength
Tylenol® Adult Liquid
Extra Strength TYLENOL®
(acetaminophen)

OTC MCNEIL CONSUMER HEALTHCARE P. 1832

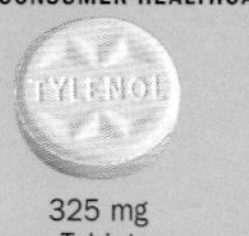

325 mg
Tablet
Regular Strength TYLENOL®
(acetaminophen)

OTC MCNEIL CONSUMER HEALTHCARE P. 1818

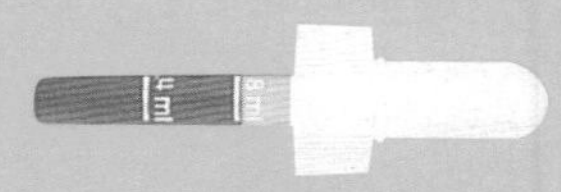

Infants' TYLENOL® Cold Decongestant and Fever Reducer Concentrated Drops
(acetaminophen, pseudoephedrine HCl)

OTC MCNEIL CONSUMER HEALTHCARE P. 1819

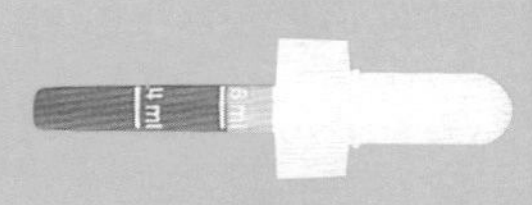

Infants' TYLENOL® Cold Decongestant and Fever Reducer Concentrated Drops Plus Cough
(acetaminophen, pseudoephedrine HCl, dextromethorphan HBr)

OTC MCNEIL CONSUMER HEALTHCARE P. 1814

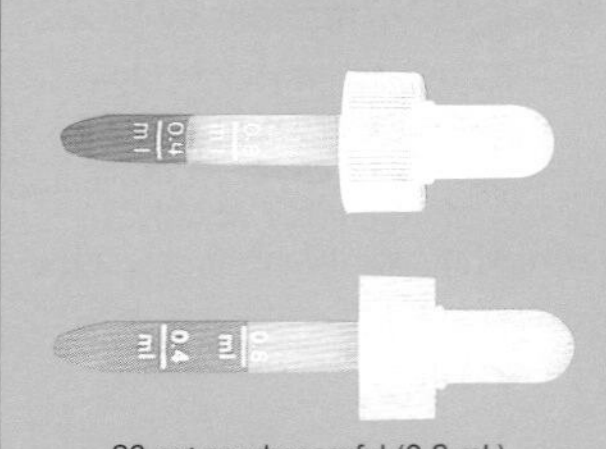

80 mg per dropperful (0.8 mL)
Rich Cherry Flavor
and Rich Grape Flavor

Infants' TYLENOL® Concentrated Drops
(acetaminophen)

OTC MCNEIL CONSUMER HEALTHCARE P. 1814

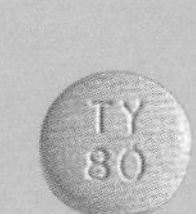

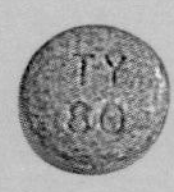

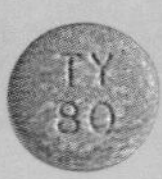

80 mg
Fruit, Grape and
Bubble Gum Flavors

Children's TYLENOL® Soft-Chews Chewable Tablets
(acetaminophen)

OTC MCNEIL CONSUMER HEALTHCARE P. 1814

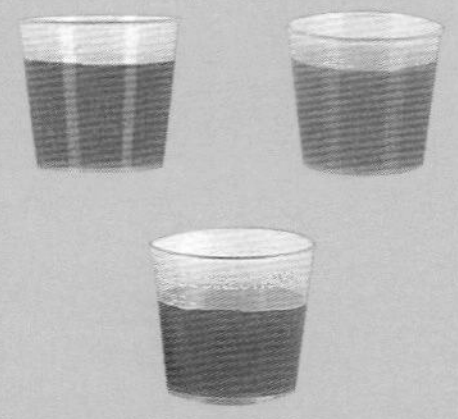

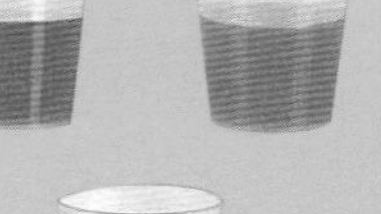

80 mg per 1/2 tsp. (160 mg per 5 mL)
Rich Cherry, Bubble
Gum and Grape Flavors.
Children's TYLENOL® Suspension Liquid
(acetaminophen)

OTC MCNEIL CONSUMER HEALTHCARE P. 1820

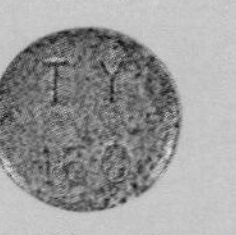

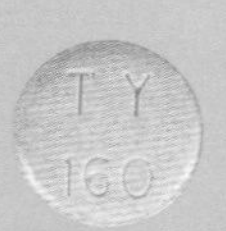

160 mg Grape and Fruit Flavor
Soft-Chews Chewable Tablets

Junior Strength TYLENOL® Soft-Chews Chewable Tablets
(acetaminophen)

OTC MCNEIL CONSUMER HEALTHCARE P. 1815

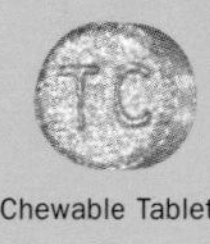

Chewable Tablets

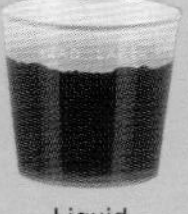

Liquid
Great Grape Flavor
Children's TYLENOL® Cold
(acetaminophen, chlorpheniramine maleate, pseudoephedrine HCl)

OTC MCNEIL CONSUMER HEALTHCARE P. 1816

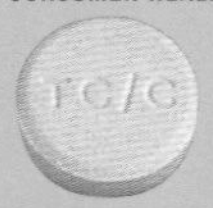

Chewable Tablets

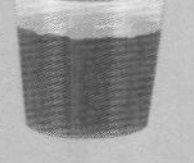

Suspension Liquid
Wild Cherry Flavor
Children's TYLENOL® Cold Plus Cough
(acetaminophen, dextromethorphan HBr, chlorpheniramine maleate, pseudoephedrine HCl)

OTC MCNEIL CONSUMER HEALTHCARE P. 1816

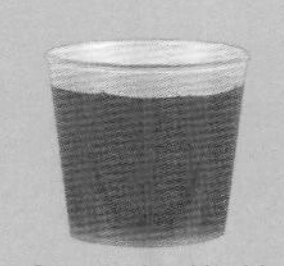

Suspension Liquid
Bubble Gum Blast Flavor

Children's TYLENOL® FLU
(acetaminophen, pseudoephedrine HCl, dextromethorphan HBr, chlorpheniramine maleate)

OTC MCNEIL CONSUMER HEALTHCARE P. 1814

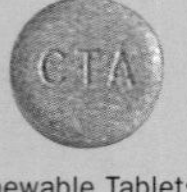

Chewable Tablets

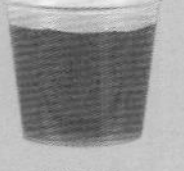

Liquid
Bubble Gum Blast Flavor

Children's TYLENOL® ALLERGY-D
(acetaminophen, diphenhydramine HCl, pseudoephedrine HCl)

OTC MCNEIL CONSUMER HEALTHCARE P. 1817

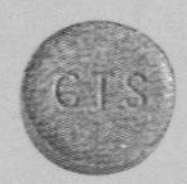

Chewable Tablets

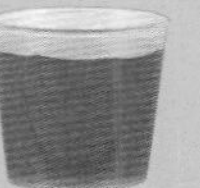

Liquid
Fruit Burst Flavor
Children's TYLENOL® SINUS
(acetaminophen, pseudoephedrine HCl)

OTC MCNEIL CONSUMER HEALTHCARE P. 1834

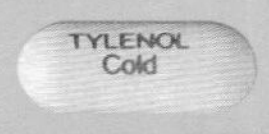

Multi-Symptom TYLENOL® COLD Complete Formula
(acetaminophen, chlorpheniramine maleate, pseudophedrine HCl, dextromethorphan HBr)

OTC MCNEIL CONSUMER HEALTHCARE P. 1834

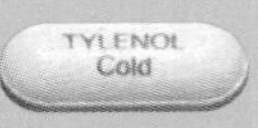

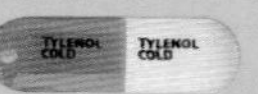

Multi-Symptom TYLENOL® COLD Non-Drowsy
(acetaminophen, pseudoephedrine HCl, dextromethorphan HBr)

OTC MCNEIL CONSUMER HEALTHCARE P. 1835

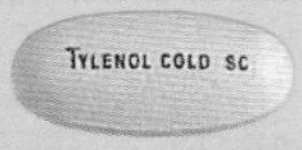

TYLENOL COLD SC

Multi-Symptom TYLENOL® COLD SEVERE CONGESTION Non-Drowsy
(acetaminophen, pseudoephedrine HCl, guaifenesin, dextromethorphan HBr)

OTC MCNEIL CONSUMER HEALTHCARE P. 1836

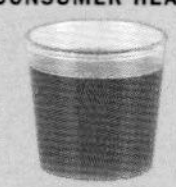

Maximum Strength TYLENOL® FLU NightTime Liquid
(acetaminophen, dextromethorphan HBr, doxylamine succinate, pseudoephedrine HCl)

OTC MCNEIL CONSUMER HEALTHCARE P. 1836

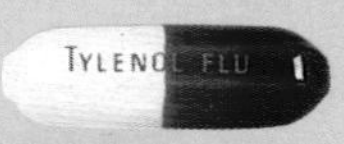

TYLENOL FLU

Maximum Strength TYLENOL® FLU Non-Drowsy
(acetaminophen, dextromethorphan HBr, pseudoephedrine HCl)

OTC MCNEIL CONSUMER HEALTHCARE P. 1836

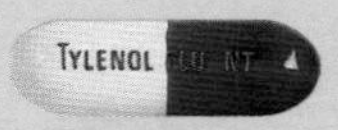

TYLENOL FLU NT

Maximum Strength TYLENOL® FLU NightTime
(acetaminophen, diphenhydramine HCl, pseudoephedrine HCl)

OTC MCNEIL CONSUMER HEALTHCARE P. 1837

Maximum Strength TYLENOL NEW! SORE THROAT Fast Acting 4 Hour Relief

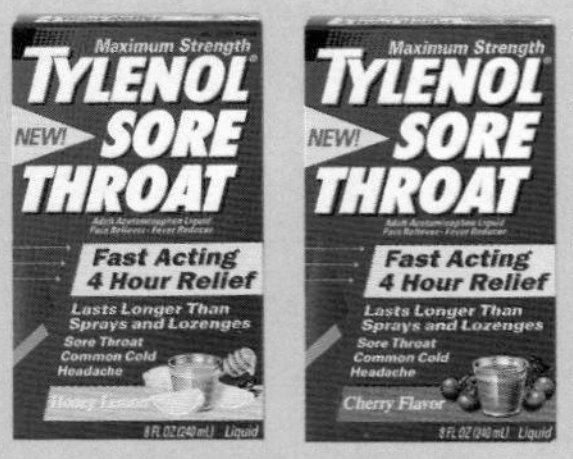

Honey-Lemon Flavor — Cherry Flavor

Maximum Strength TYLENOL® SORE THROAT
(acetaminophen)

OTC MCNEIL CONSUMER HEALTHCARE P. 1837

TYLENOL PM

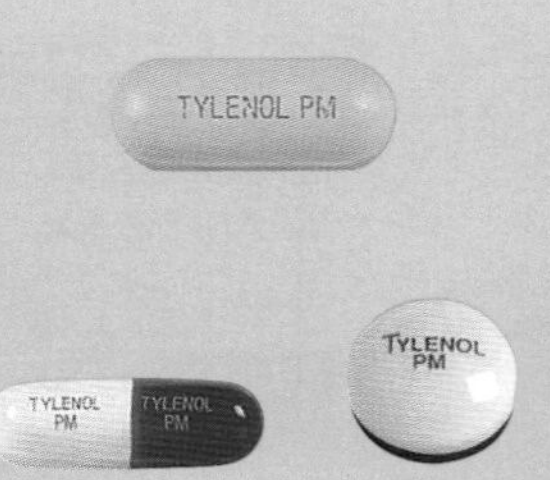

Extra Strength TYLENOL® PM
(acetaminophen, diphenhydramine HCl)

OTC MCNEIL CONSUMER HEALTHCARE P. 1833

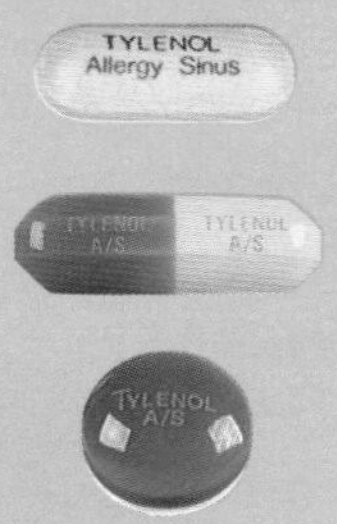

TYLENOL Allergy Sinus

TYLENOL A/S

Maximum Strength TYLENOL® ALLERGY SINUS
(acetaminophen, chlorpheniramine maleate, pseudoephedrine HCl)

OTC MCNEIL CONSUMER HEALTHCARE P. 1833

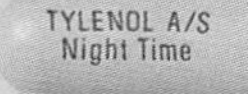

Maximum Strength TYLENOL® ALLERGY SINUS NightTime
(acetaminophen, diphenhydramine HCl, pseudoephedrine HCl)

OTC MCNEIL CONSUMER HEALTHCARE P. 1833

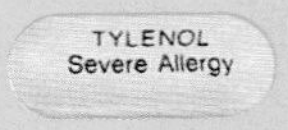

TYLENOL Severe Allergy

TYLENOL® SEVERE ALLERGY
(acetaminophen, diphenhydramine HCl)

OTC MCNEIL CONSUMER HEALTHCARE P. 1838

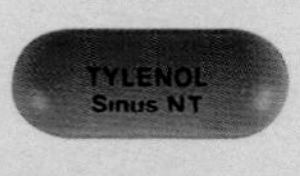

TYLENOL Sinus NT

Maximum Strength TYLENOL® SINUS NightTime
(acetaminophen, doxylamine succinate, pseudoephedrine HCl)

OTC MCNEIL CONSUMER HEALTHCARE P. 1838

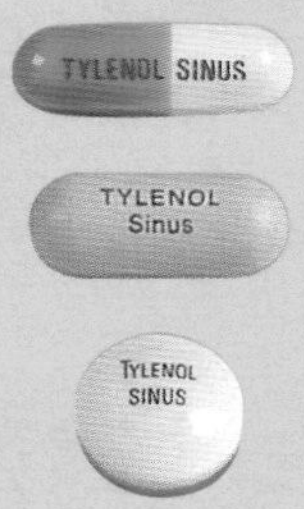

TYLENOL SINUS

Maximum Strength TYLENOL® SINUS Non-Drowsy
(acetaminophen, pseudoephedrine HCl)

RX MCNEIL CONSUMER HEALTHCARE P. 1838

Women's TYLENOL Multi-Symptom MENSTRUAL RELIEF 40 Caplets

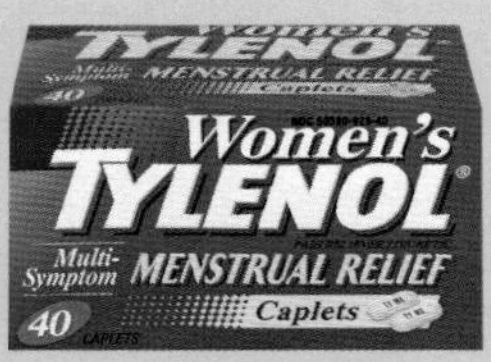

Women's TYLENOL®
(acetaminophen, pamabrom)

RX MCNEIL CONSUMER HEALTHCARE P. 1839

100 mg
Chewable Tablets
Vermox®
(mebendazole)

MEDIMMUNE

RX MEDIMMUNE, INC. P. 1861

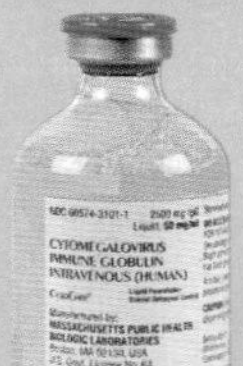

2500 mg IgG Liquid
50 mg/mL
CytoGam®
(cytomegalovirus immune globulin intravenous (human) CMV-IGIV)

RX MEDIMMUNE, INC. P. 1863

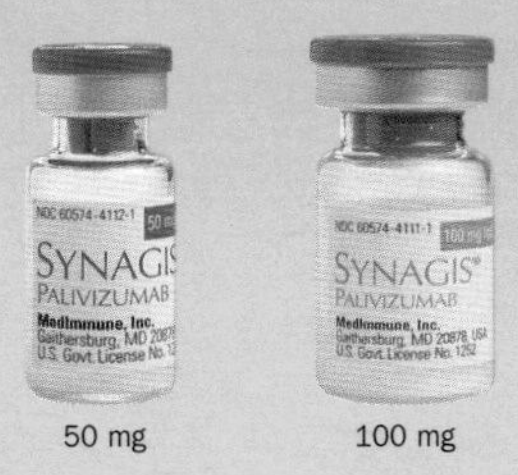

50 mg — 100 mg

Synagis®
(palivizumab)

MEDIMMUNE ONCOLOGY INC.

RX MEDIMMUNE ONCOLOGY INC. P. 1864

50 mg
Hexalen®
(altretamine)

RX MEDIMMUNE ONCOLOGY INC. P. 1865

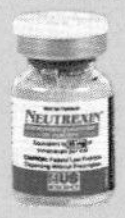

25 mg and 200 mg
Neutrexin®
(trimetrexate glucuronate for injection)

MERCK & CO., INC.

RX MERCK & CO., INC. P. 1872

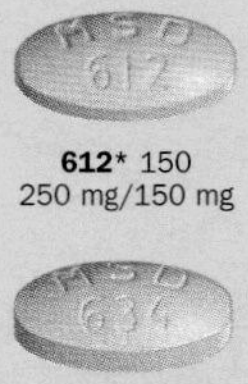

612* 150
250 mg/150 mg

634* 250
250 mg/250 mg

Aldoclor®
(methyldopa, chlorothiazide)

RX MERCK & CO., INC. P. 1874

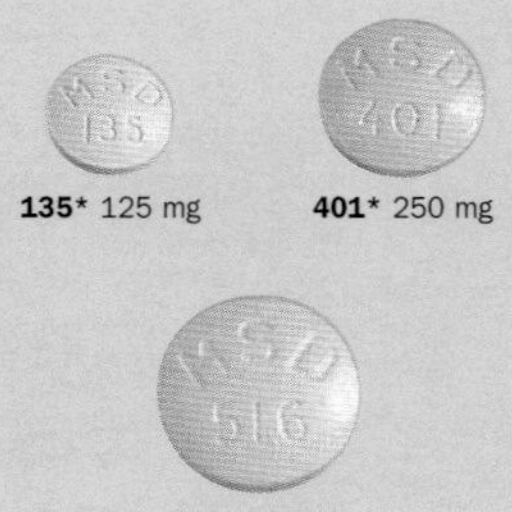

135* 125 mg — **401*** 250 mg

516* 500 mg

†Aldomet®
(methyldopa)

RX MERCK & CO., INC. P. 1877

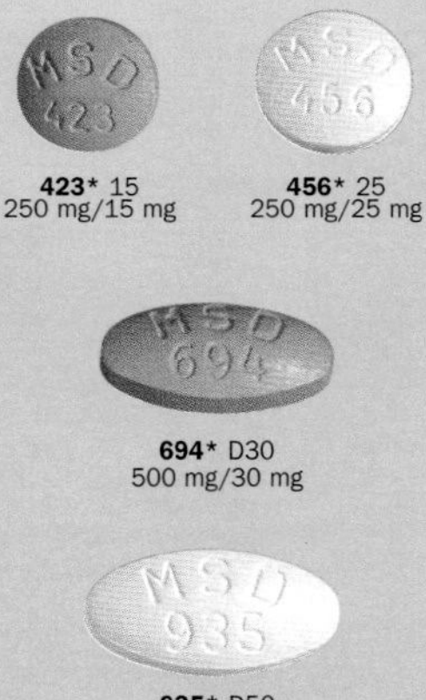

423* 15
250 mg/15 mg — **456*** 25
250 mg/25 mg

694* D30
500 mg/30 mg

935* D50
500 mg/50 mg

Aldoril®
(methyldopa, hydrochlorothiazide)

RX MERCK & CO., INC. P. 1886

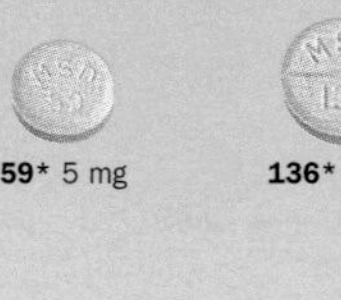

59* 5 mg — **136*** 10 mg

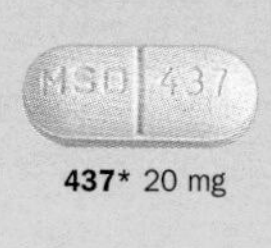

437* 20 mg

Blocadren®
(timolol maleate)

RX MERCK & CO., INC. P. 1888

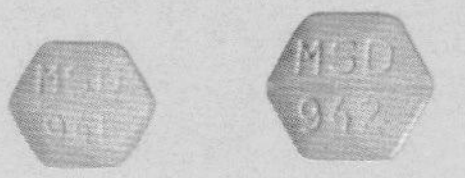

941* 150 mg — **942*** 200 mg

Clinoril®
(sulindac)

RX MERCK & CO., INC. P. 1892

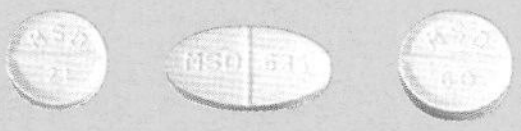

21* 0.5 mg — **635*** 1 mg — **60*** 2 mg

†Cogentin®
(benztropine mesylate)

RX MERCK & CO., INC. P. 1897

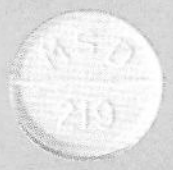

219* 25 mg
†Cortone®
(cortisone acetate)

RX MERCK & CO., INC. P. 1902

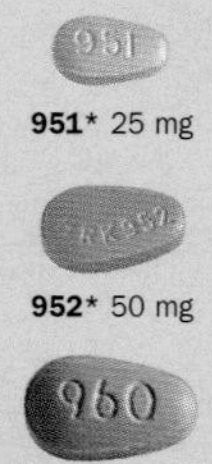

951* 25 mg

952* 50 mg

960* 100 mg
Cozaar®
(losartan potassium tablets)
Registered trademark of E.I. du Pont de Nemours and Company.

RX MERCK & CO., INC. P. 1904

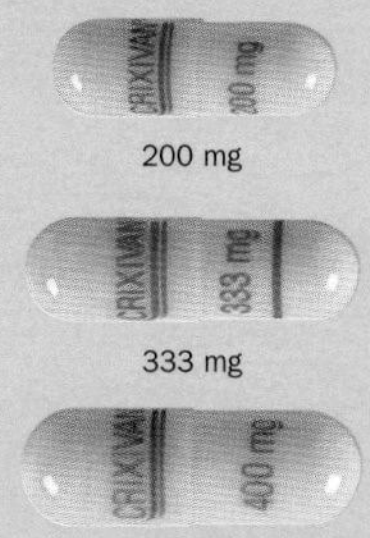

200 mg

333 mg

400 mg

Crixivan®
(indinavir sulfate)

RX MERCK & CO., INC. P. 1909

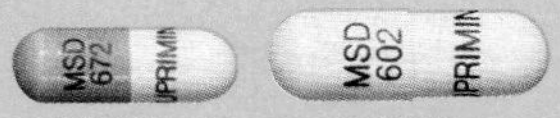

672* 125 mg — **602*** 250 mg

Cuprimine®
(penicillamine)

RX MERCK & CO., INC. P. 1914

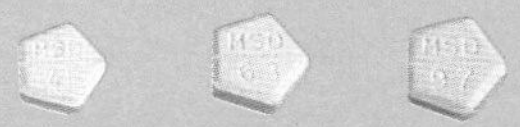

41* 0.5 mg — **63*** 0.75 mg — **97*** 4 mg

†Decadron®
(dexamethasone)

RX MERCK & CO., INC. P. 1919

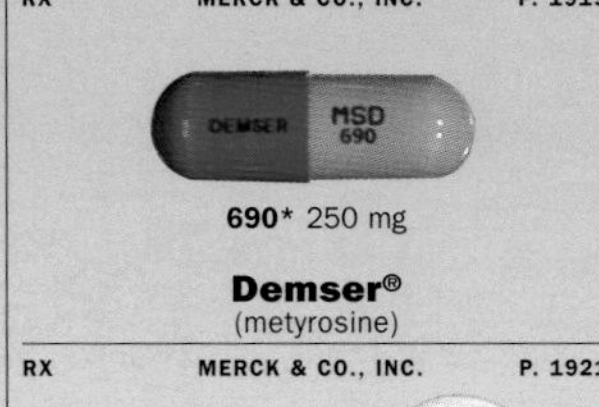

690* 250 mg

Demser®
(metyrosine)

RX MERCK & CO., INC. P. 1921

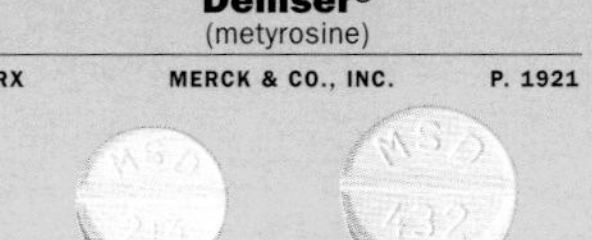

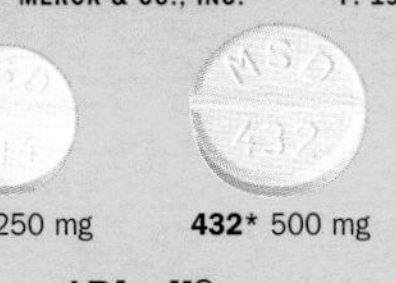

214* 250 mg — **432*** 500 mg

†Diuril®
(chlorothiazide)

RX MERCK & CO., INC. P. 1923

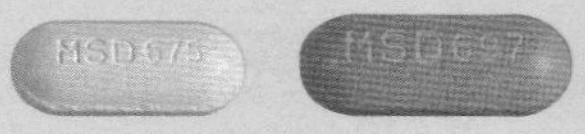

675* 250 mg — **697*** 500 mg

Dolobid®
(diflunisal)

RX MERCK & CO., INC. P. 1925

65* 25 mg — **90*** 50 mg

†Edecrin®
(ethacrynic acid)

RX MERCK & CO., INC. P. 1929

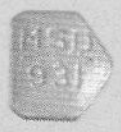

931* 10 mg
Flexeril®
(cyclobenzaprine HCl)

RX MERCK & CO., INC. P. 1930

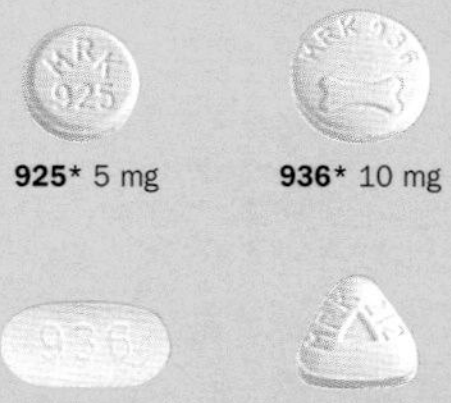

925* 5 mg — **936*** 10 mg

936* 10 mg — **212*** 40 mg

Fosamax®
(alendronate sodium tablets)

RX MERCK & CO., INC. P. 1940

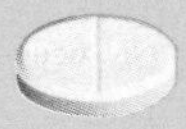

619* 10 mg

†Hydrocortone®
(hydrocortisone)

RX MERCK & CO., INC. P. 1941

42* 25 mg — **105*** 50 mg

HydroDIURIL®
(hydrochlorothiazide)

RX MERCK & CO., INC. P. 1942

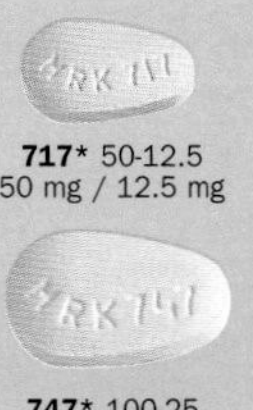

717* 50-12.5
50 mg / 12.5 mg

747* 100-25
100 mg / 25 mg

Hyzaar®
(losartan potassium, hydrochlorothiazide tablets)
Registered trademark of E.I. du Pont de Nemours and Company.

RX MERCK & CO., INC. P. 1946

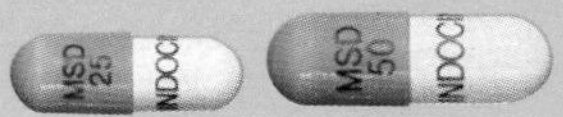

25* 25 mg — **50*** 50 mg

†Indocin®
(indomethacin)

RX MERCK & CO., INC. P. 1946

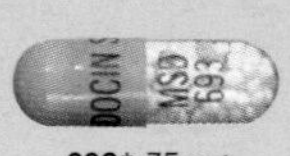

693* 75 mg

†Indocin® SR
(indomethacin)

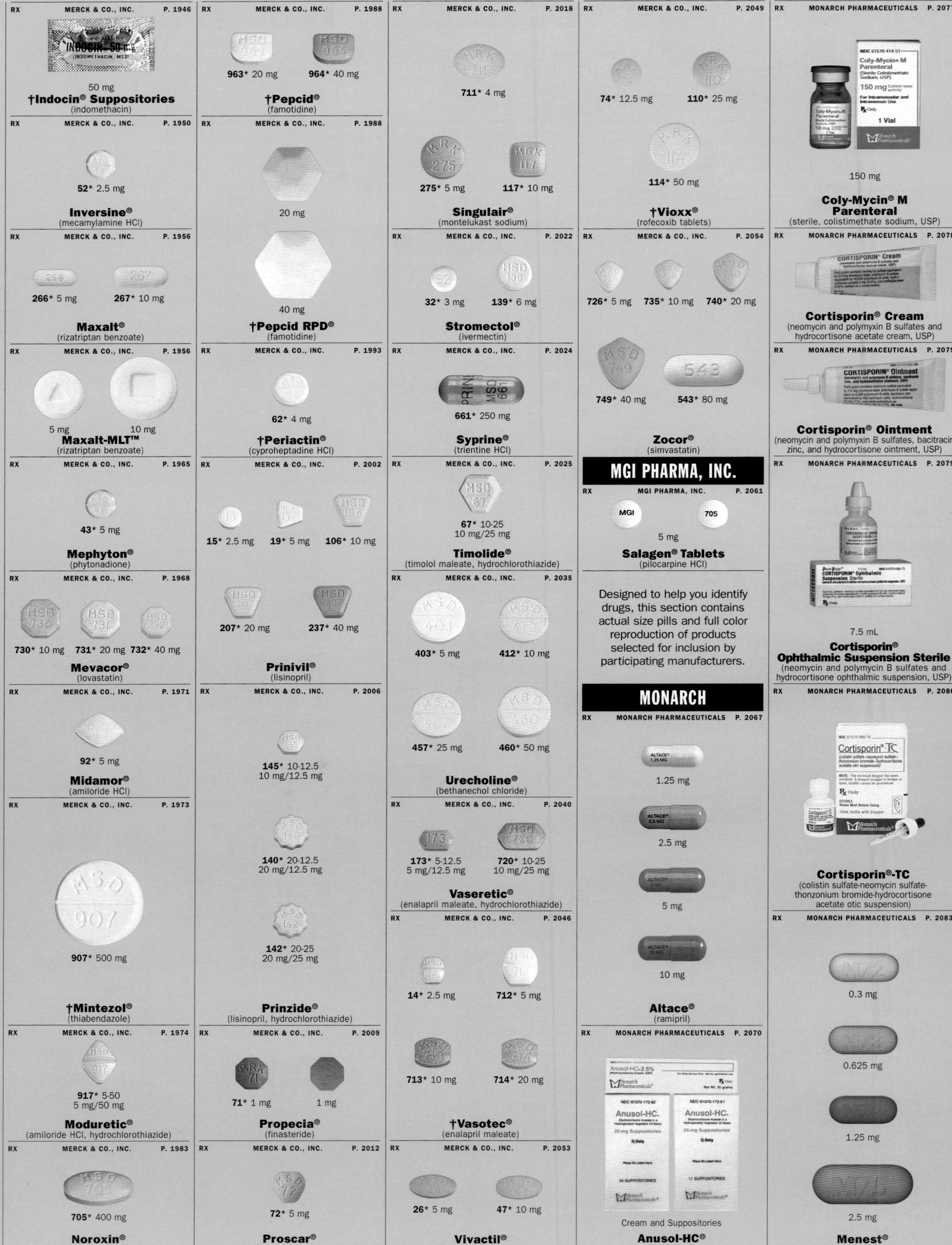

RX MERCK & CO., INC. P. 1946
50 mg
†Indocin® Suppositories
(indomethacin)

RX MERCK & CO., INC. P. 1950
52* 2.5 mg
Inversine®
(mecamylamine HCl)

RX MERCK & CO., INC. P. 1956
266* 5 mg 267* 10 mg
Maxalt®
(rizatriptan benzoate)

RX MERCK & CO., INC. P. 1956
5 mg 10 mg
Maxalt-MLT™
(rizatriptan benzoate)

RX MERCK & CO., INC. P. 1965
43* 5 mg
Mephyton®
(phytonadione)

RX MERCK & CO., INC. P. 1968
730* 10 mg 731* 20 mg 732* 40 mg
Mevacor®
(lovastatin)

RX MERCK & CO., INC. P. 1971
92* 5 mg
Midamor®
(amiloride HCl)

RX MERCK & CO., INC. P. 1973
907* 500 mg
†Mintezol®
(thiabendazole)

RX MERCK & CO., INC. P. 1974
917* 5-50
5 mg/50 mg
Moduretic®
(amiloride HCl, hydrochlorothiazide)

RX MERCK & CO., INC. P. 1983
705* 400 mg
Noroxin®
(norfloxacin)

RX MERCK & CO., INC. P. 1988
963* 20 mg 964* 40 mg
†Pepcid®
(famotidine)

RX MERCK & CO., INC. P. 1988
20 mg
40 mg
†Pepcid RPD®
(famotidine)

RX MERCK & CO., INC. P. 1993
62* 4 mg
†Periactin®
(cyproheptadine HCl)

RX MERCK & CO., INC. P. 2002
15* 2.5 mg 19* 5 mg 106* 10 mg
207* 20 mg 237* 40 mg
Prinivil®
(lisinopril)

RX MERCK & CO., INC. P. 2006
145* 10-12.5
10 mg/12.5 mg
140* 20-12.5
20 mg/12.5 mg
142* 20-25
20 mg/25 mg
Prinzide®
(lisinopril, hydrochlorothiazide)

RX MERCK & CO., INC. P. 2009
71* 1 mg 1 mg
Propecia®
(finasteride)

RX MERCK & CO., INC. P. 2012
72* 5 mg
Proscar®
(finasteride)

RX MERCK & CO., INC. P. 2018
711* 4 mg
275* 5 mg 117* 10 mg
Singulair®
(montelukast sodium)

RX MERCK & CO., INC. P. 2022
32* 3 mg 139* 6 mg
Stromectol®
(ivermectin)

RX MERCK & CO., INC. P. 2024
661* 250 mg
Syprine®
(trientine HCl)

RX MERCK & CO., INC. P. 2025
67* 10-25
10 mg/25 mg
Timolide®
(timolol maleate, hydrochlorothiazide)

RX MERCK & CO., INC. P. 2035
403* 5 mg 412* 10 mg
457* 25 mg 460* 50 mg
Urecholine®
(bethanechol chloride)

RX MERCK & CO., INC. P. 2040
173* 5-12.5
5 mg/12.5 mg
720* 10-25
10 mg/25 mg
Vaseretic®
(enalapril maleate, hydrochlorothiazide)

RX MERCK & CO., INC. P. 2046
14* 2.5 mg 712* 5 mg
713* 10 mg 714* 20 mg
†Vasotec®
(enalapril maleate)

RX MERCK & CO., INC. P. 2053
26* 5 mg 47* 10 mg
Vivactil®
(protriptyline HCl)

RX MERCK & CO., INC. P. 2049
74* 12.5 mg 110* 25 mg
114* 50 mg
†Vioxx®
(rofecoxib tablets)

RX MERCK & CO., INC. P. 2054
726* 5 mg 735* 10 mg 740* 20 mg
749* 40 mg 543* 80 mg
Zocor®
(simvastatin)

MGI PHARMA, INC.

RX MGI PHARMA, INC. P. 2061
5 mg
Salagen® Tablets
(pilocarpine HCl)

Designed to help you identify drugs, this section contains actual size pills and full color reproduction of products selected for inclusion by participating manufacturers.

MONARCH

RX MONARCH PHARMACEUTICALS P. 2067
1.25 mg
2.5 mg
5 mg
10 mg
Altace®
(ramipril)

RX MONARCH PHARMACEUTICALS P. 2070
Cream and Suppositories
Anusol-HC®
(hydrocortisone)

RX MONARCH PHARMACEUTICALS P. 2077
150 mg
Coly-Mycin® M Parenteral
(sterile, colistimethate sodium, USP)

RX MONARCH PHARMACEUTICALS P. 2078
Cortisporin® Cream
(neomycin and polymyxin B sulfates and hydrocortisone acetate cream, USP)

RX MONARCH PHARMACEUTICALS P. 2079
Cortisporin® Ointment
(neomycin and polymyxin B sulfates, bacitracin zinc, and hydrocortisone ointment, USP)

RX MONARCH PHARMACEUTICALS P. 2079
7.5 mL
Cortisporin® Ophthalmic Suspension Sterile
(neomycin and polymycin B sulfates and hydrocortisone ophthalmic suspension, USP)

RX MONARCH PHARMACEUTICALS P. 2080
Cortisporin®-TC
(colistin sulfate-neomycin sulfate-thonzonium bromide-hydrocortisone acetate otic suspension)

RX MONARCH PHARMACEUTICALS P. 2083
0.3 mg
0.625 mg
1.25 mg
2.5 mg
Menest®
(esterified estrogens tablets, USP)

RX MONARCH PHARMACEUTICALS P. 2086

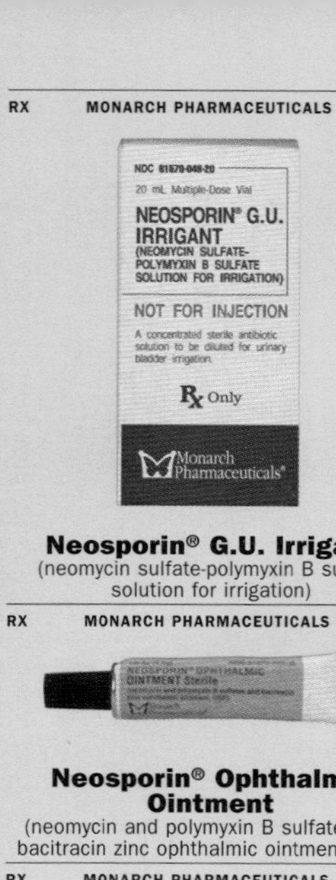

Neosporin® G.U. Irrigant
(neomycin sulfate-polymyxin B sulfate solution for irrigation)

RX MONARCH PHARMACEUTICALS P. 2087

Neosporin® Ophthalmic Ointment
(neomycin and polymyxin B sulfates and bacitracin zinc ophthalmic ointment, USP)

RX MONARCH PHARMACEUTICALS P. 2087

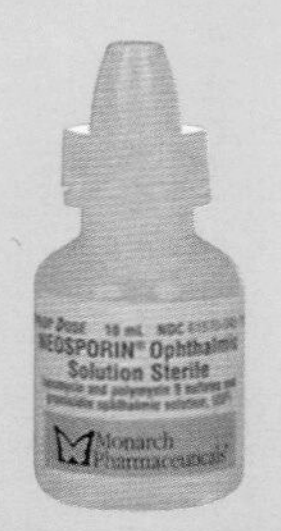

Neosporin® Ophthalmic Solution
(neomycin and polymyxin B sulfates and gramicidin ophthalmic solution, USP)

RX MONARCH PHARMACEUTICALS P. 2092

Pediotic® Suspension Sterile
(neomycin and polymyxin B sulfates and hydrocortisone otic suspension, USP)

RX MONARCH PHARMACEUTICALS P. 2093

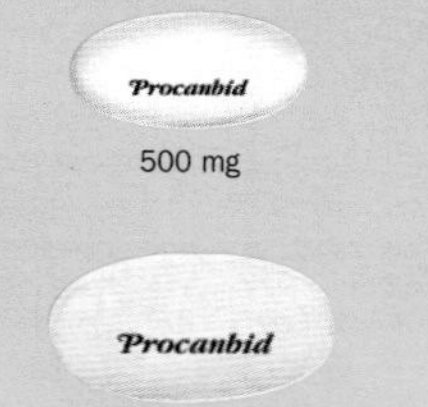

500 mg

1000 mg

Procanbid®
(procainamide HCl extended-release tablets)

RX MONARCH PHARMACEUTICALS P. 2095

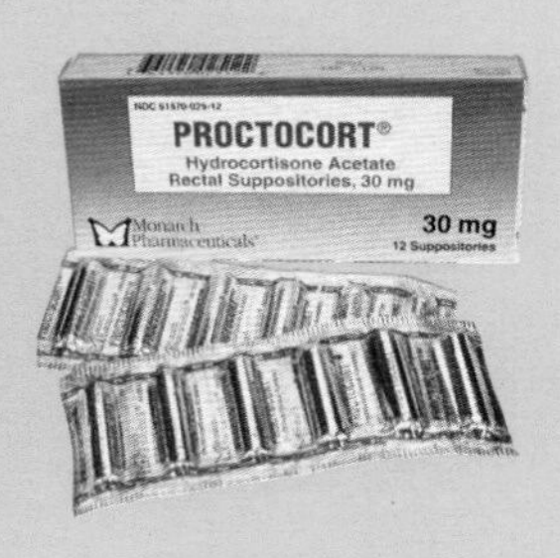

Proctocort®
(hydrocortisone acetate rectal suppositories, 30 mg)

RX MONARCH PHARMACEUTICALS P. 2100

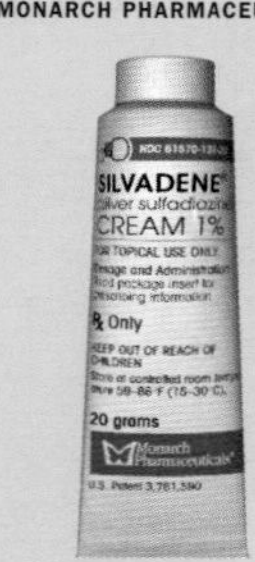

Silvadene® Cream 1%
(silver sulfadiazine)

RX MONARCH PHARMACEUTICALS P. 2101

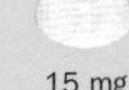

15 mg

Thalitone®
(chlorthalidone, USP)

RX MONARCH PHARMACEUTICALS P. 2104

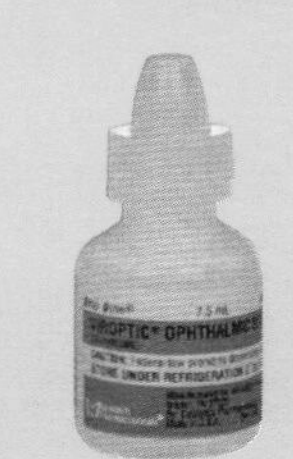

Viroptic® Ophthalmic Solution
(trifluridine ophthalmic solution)

NABI

RX NABI P. 2128

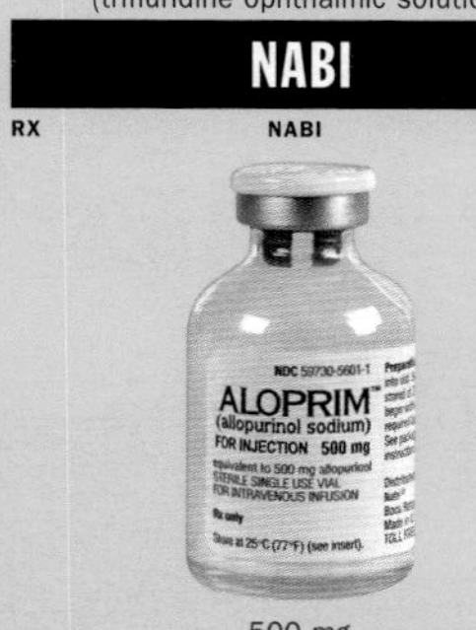

500 mg

Aloprim™
(allopurinol sodium)

RX NABI P. 2130

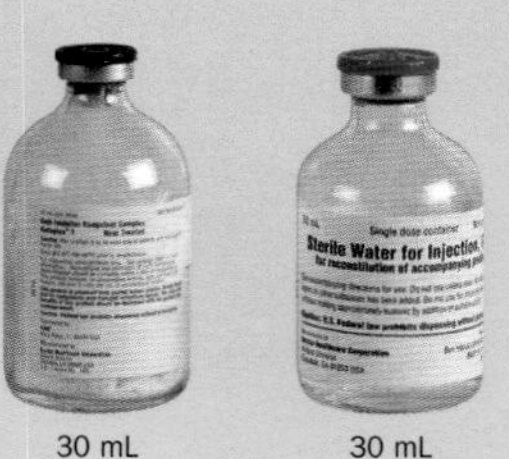

30 mL

30 mL Sterile Water

Autoplex® T
(anti-inhibitor coagulant complex)

RX NABI P. 2132

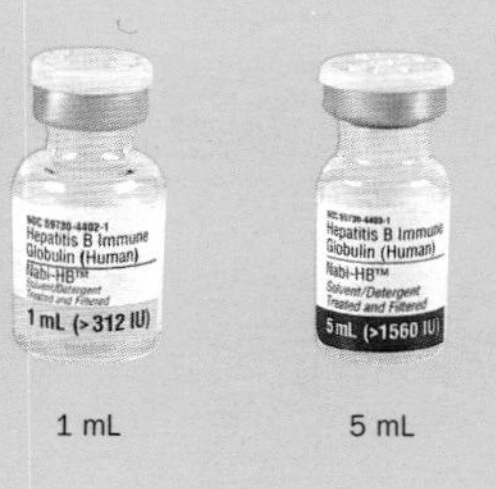

1 mL

5 mL

Nabi-HB™
(Hepatitis B Immune Globulin (Human))

RX NABI P. 2133

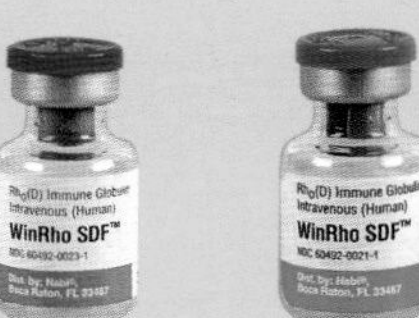

600 IU

1500 IU

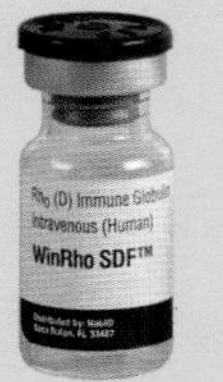

5000 IU

WinRho SDF™
(Rh_0(D) Immune Globulin Intravenous (Human))

NEUTROGENA

RX NEUTROGENA DERMATOLOGICS P. 2136

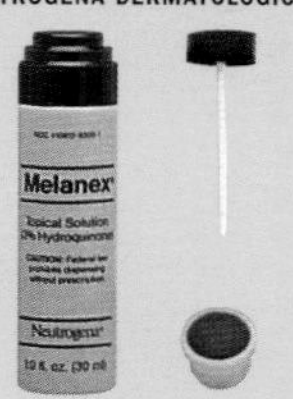

Available with broad sponge and pin-point rod applicator

Neutrogena® Melanex® Topical Solution
(hydroquinone USP, 3.0%)

Because tablets and capsules are shown in this section, do not infer that these are the only dosage forms available. Where a product name is preceded by the symbol †, refer to the description in the Product Information (White Section) for other forms.

NOVARTIS CONSUMER HEALTH

RX NOVARTIS CONSUMER HEALTH INC. P. 2138

4345* 1.0 mg/3 days
Transdermal Therapeutic System

Transderm Scop®
(scopolamine)

NOVARTIS

RX NOVARTIS PHARMACEUTICALS P. 2141

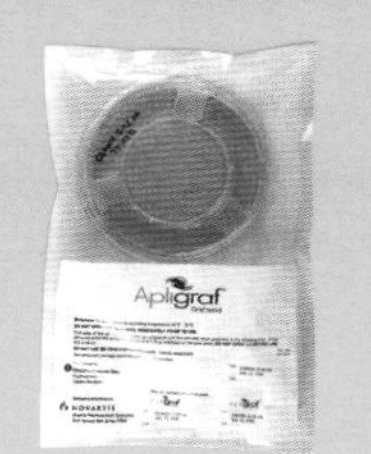

Apligraf®
(graftskin)

RX NOVARTIS PHARMACEUTICALS P. 2145

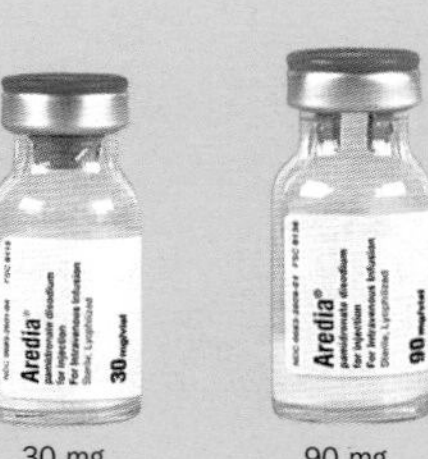

30 mg

90 mg

Aredia®
(pamidronate disodium for injection)

RX NOVARTIS PHARMACEUTICALS P. 2149

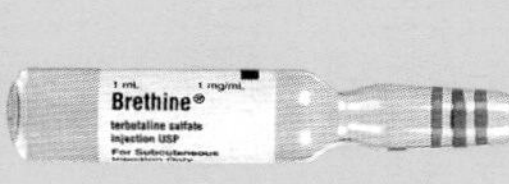

7507* 1 mg/mL per Ampul-1 mL

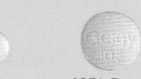

72* 2.5 mg

105* 5 mg

Brethine®
(terbutaline sulfate)

RX NOVARTIS PHARMACEUTICALS P. 2151

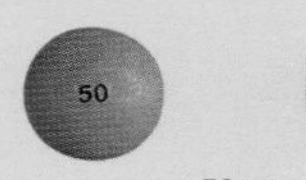

50 mg

Cataflam®
(diclofenac potassium)

RX NOVARTIS PHARMACEUTICALS P. 2155

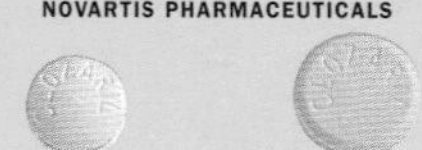

25 mg

100 mg

Other side: engraved with a facilitated score and the dosage strength.

Clozaril® Tablets
(clozapine)

RX NOVARTIS PHARMACEUTICALS P. 2159

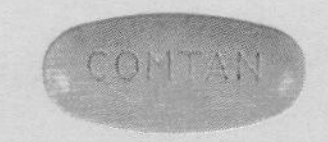

200 mg

Comtan®
(entacapone)

RX NOVARTIS PHARMACEUTICALS P. 2164

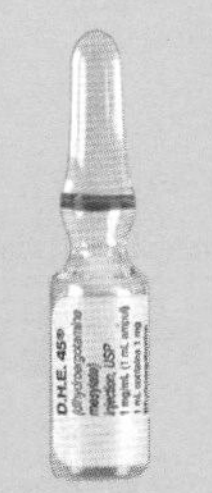

1 mg/mL

DHE 45® Injection
(dihydroergotamine mesylate)

RX NOVARTIS PHARMACEUTICALS P. 2166

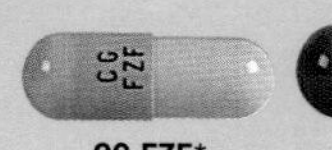

CG FZF* 80 mg

CG GOG* 160 mg

Diovan®
(valsartan)

RX NOVARTIS PHARMACEUTICALS P. 2168

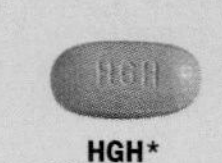

HGH* 80/12.5 mg

HHH* 160/12.5 mg

Other side: engraved with "CG".

Diovan HCT®
(valsartan and hydrochlorothiazide)

RX NOVARTIS PHARMACEUTICALS

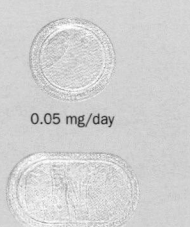

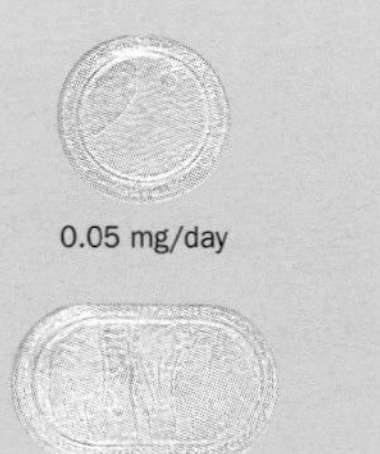

0.05 mg/day

0.1 mg/day

Estraderm®
(estradiol transdermal system)

RX NOVARTIS PHARMACEUTICALS P. 2171

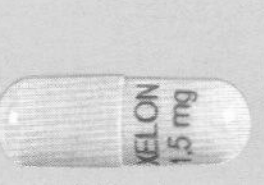

1.5 mg

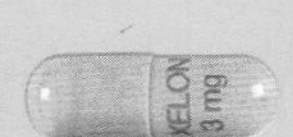

3.0 mg

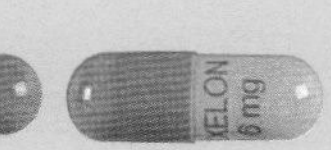

4.5 mg

6.0 mg

Exelon®
(rivastigmine tartrate)

RX NOVARTIS PHARMACEUTICALS P. 2177

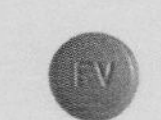

FV* 2.5 mg
Other side: imprinted "CG"

Femara®
(letrozole tablets)

RX NOVARTIS PHARMACEUTICALS P. 2179

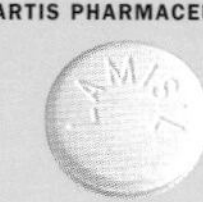

250 mg
Other side: imprinted "250"

Lamisil®
(terbinafine HCl tablets) Tablets

RX NOVARTIS PHARMACEUTICALS P. 2181

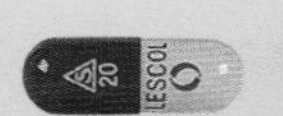

20 mg

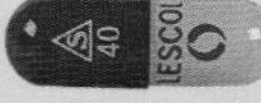

40 mg

Lescol®
(fluvastatin sodium) Capsules

RX NOVARTIS PHARMACEUTICALS

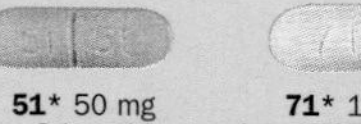

51* 50 mg

71* 100 mg

Other side: imprinted "GEIGY".

†Lopressor®
(metoprolol tartrate tablets, USP)

RX NOVARTIS PHARMACEUTICALS

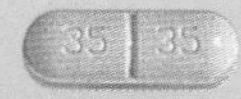

35* 50 mg/25 mg

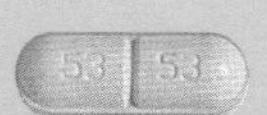

53* 100 mg/25 mg

73* 100 mg/50 mg

Other side: imprinted "GEIGY".

Lopressor HCT®
(metoprolol tartrate USP and hydrochlorothiazide USP)

RX NOVARTIS PHARMACEUTICALS P. 2184

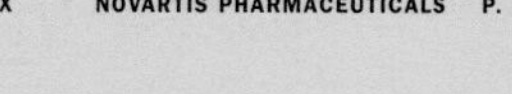

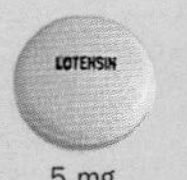

5 mg

10 mg

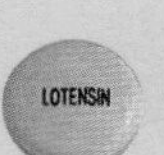

20 mg

40 mg

Lotensin®
(benazepril HCl)

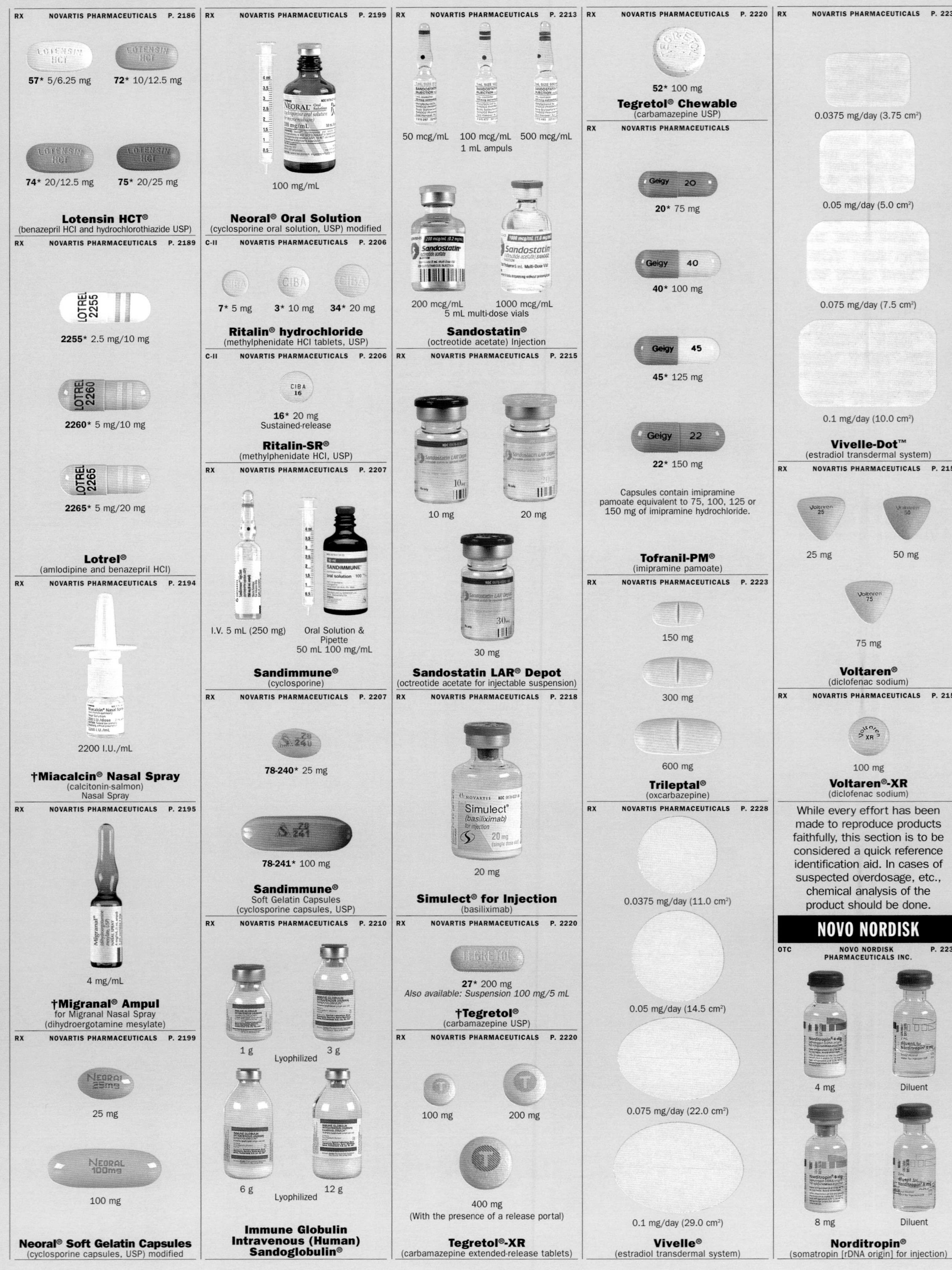
RX NOVARTIS PHARMACEUTICALS P. 2186
57* 5/6.25 mg
72* 10/12.5 mg
74* 20/12.5 mg
75* 20/25 mg
Lotensin HCT®
(benazepril HCl and hydrochlorothiazide USP)
RX NOVARTIS PHARMACEUTICALS P. 2189
2255* 2.5 mg/10 mg
2260* 5 mg/10 mg
2265* 5 mg/20 mg
Lotrel®
(amlodipine and benazepril HCl)
RX NOVARTIS PHARMACEUTICALS P. 2194
2200 I.U./mL
†Miacalcin® Nasal Spray
(calcitonin-salmon)
Nasal Spray
RX NOVARTIS PHARMACEUTICALS P. 2195
4 mg/mL
†Migranal® Ampul
for Migranal Nasal Spray
(dihydroergotamine mesylate)
RX NOVARTIS PHARMACEUTICALS P. 2199
25 mg
100 mg
Neoral® Soft Gelatin Capsules
(cyclosporine capsules, USP) modified
RX NOVARTIS PHARMACEUTICALS P. 2199
100 mg/mL
Neoral® Oral Solution
(cyclosporine oral solution, USP) modified
C-II NOVARTIS PHARMACEUTICALS P. 2206
7* 5 mg
3* 10 mg
34* 20 mg
Ritalin® hydrochloride
(methylphenidate HCl tablets, USP)
C-II NOVARTIS PHARMACEUTICALS P. 2206
16* 20 mg
Sustained-release
Ritalin-SR®
(methylphenidate HCl, USP)
RX NOVARTIS PHARMACEUTICALS P. 2207
I.V. 5 mL (250 mg)
Oral Solution & Pipette
50 mL 100 mg/mL
Sandimmune®
(cyclosporine)
RX NOVARTIS PHARMACEUTICALS P. 2207
78-240* 25 mg
78-241* 100 mg
Sandimmune®
Soft Gelatin Capsules
(cyclosporine capsules, USP)
RX NOVARTIS PHARMACEUTICALS P. 2210
1 g
3 g
Lyophilized
6 g
12 g
Lyophilized
Immune Globulin
Intravenous (Human)
Sandoglobulin®
RX NOVARTIS PHARMACEUTICALS P. 2213
50 mcg/mL
100 mcg/mL
500 mcg/mL
1 mL ampuls
200 mcg/mL
1000 mcg/mL
5 mL multi-dose vials
Sandostatin®
(octreotide acetate) Injection
RX NOVARTIS PHARMACEUTICALS P. 2215
10 mg
20 mg
30 mg
Sandostatin LAR® Depot
(octreotide acetate for injectable suspension)
RX NOVARTIS PHARMACEUTICALS P. 2218
20 mg
Simulect® for Injection
(basiliximab)
RX NOVARTIS PHARMACEUTICALS P. 2220
27* 200 mg
Also available: Suspension 100 mg/5 mL
†Tegretol®
(carbamazepine USP)
RX NOVARTIS PHARMACEUTICALS P. 2220
100 mg
200 mg
400 mg
(With the presence of a release portal)
Tegretol®-XR
(carbamazepine extended-release tablets)
RX NOVARTIS PHARMACEUTICALS P. 2220
52* 100 mg
Tegretol® Chewable
(carbamazepine USP)
RX NOVARTIS PHARMACEUTICALS
20* 75 mg
40* 100 mg
45* 125 mg
22* 150 mg
Capsules contain imipramine pamoate equivalent to 75, 100, 125 or 150 mg of imipramine hydrochloride.
Tofranil-PM®
(imipramine pamoate)
RX NOVARTIS PHARMACEUTICALS P. 2223
150 mg
300 mg
600 mg
Trileptal®
(oxcarbazepine)
RX NOVARTIS PHARMACEUTICALS P. 2228
0.0375 mg/day (11.0 cm²)
0.05 mg/day (14.5 cm²)
0.075 mg/day (22.0 cm²)
0.1 mg/day (29.0 cm²)
Vivelle®
(estradiol transdermal system)
RX NOVARTIS PHARMACEUTICALS P. 2231
0.0375 mg/day (3.75 cm²)
0.05 mg/day (5.0 cm²)
0.075 mg/day (7.5 cm²)
0.1 mg/day (10.0 cm²)
Vivelle-Dot™
(estradiol transdermal system)
RX NOVARTIS PHARMACEUTICALS P. 2151
25 mg
50 mg
75 mg
Voltaren®
(diclofenac sodium)
RX NOVARTIS PHARMACEUTICALS P. 2151
100 mg
Voltaren®-XR
(diclofenac sodium)
While every effort has been made to reproduce products faithfully, this section is to be considered a quick reference identification aid. In cases of suspected overdosage, etc., chemical analysis of the product should be done.
NOVO NORDISK
OTC NOVO NORDISK PHARMACEUTICALS INC. P. 2235
4 mg
Diluent
8 mg
Diluent
Norditropin®
(somatropin [rDNA origin] for injection)

OTC NOVO NORDISK PHARMACEUTICALS INC. P. 2238

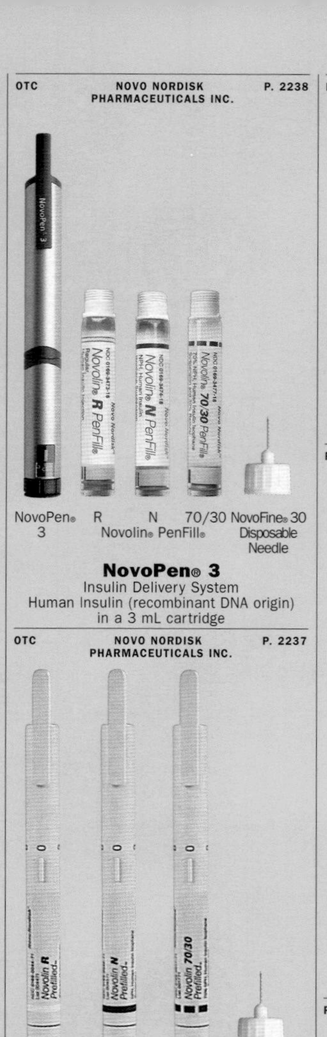

NovoPen® 3 R N 70/30 Novolin® PenFill® NovoFine® 30 Disposable Needle

NovoPen® 3
Insulin Delivery System
Human Insulin (recombinant DNA origin) in a 3 mL cartridge

OTC NOVO NORDISK PHARMACEUTICALS INC. P. 2237

Novolin® R Novolin® N Novolin® 70/30 NovoFine® 30 Disposable Needle

Novolin Prefilled®
Insulin Delivery System
Human Insulin (recombinant DNA origin) in a 1.5 mL prefilled syringe

NOVOGYNE

IMPORTANT NOTICE:
For product identification of Vivelle® and Vivelle-Dot™, please refer to Novartis Pharmaceuticals Corp. See page 326.

Designed to help you identify drugs, this section contains actual size pills and full color reproduction of products selected for inclusion by participating manufacturers.

OCLASSEN DERMATOLOGICS

RX OCLASSEN DERMATOLOGICS P. 2248

3.5 g
Condylox® Gel 0.5%
(podofilox gel)

RX OCLASSEN DERMATOLOGICS P. 2249

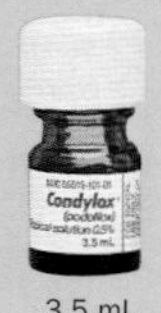

3.5 mL

Condylox® Topical Solution 0.5%
(podofilox)

RX OCLASSEN DERMATOLOGICS P. 2250

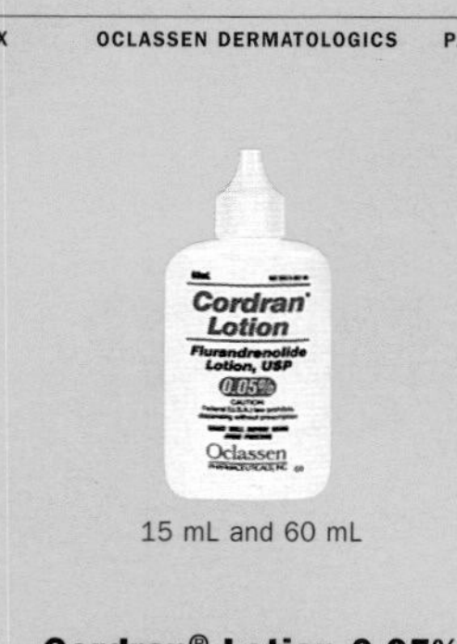

15 mL and 60 mL

Cordran® Lotion 0.05%
(flurandrenolide lotion, USP)

RX OCLASSEN DERMATOLOGICS P. 2251

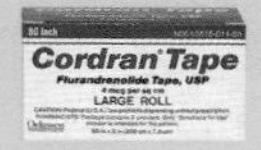

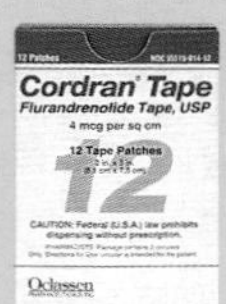

4 mcg per sq cm, 24 inch x 3 inch roll

4 mcg per sq cm, 80 inch x 3 inch roll

4 mcg per sq cm, (12) 2 inch x 3 inch patches

Cordran® Tape
(flurandrenolide tape, USP)

RX OCLASSEN DERMATOLOGICS P. 2252

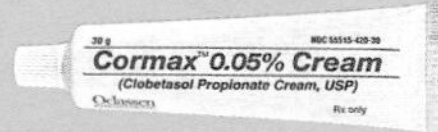

15 g, 30 g and 45 g

Cormax® 0.05% Cream
(clobetasol propionate cream, USP)

RX OCLASSEN DERMATOLOGICS P. 2252

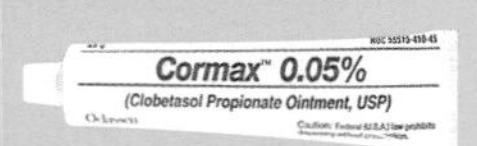

15 g and 45 g

Cormax® Ointment 0.05%
(clobetasol propionate ointment, USP)

RX OCLASSEN DERMATOLOGICS P. 2253

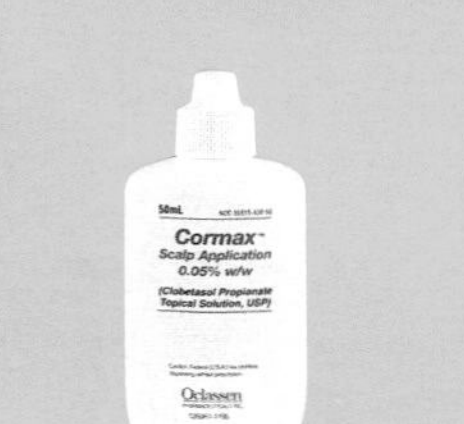

25 mL and 50 mL

Cormax® Scalp Application 0.05% w/w
(clobetasol propionate topical solution, USP)

RX OCLASSEN DERMATOLOGICS P. 2254

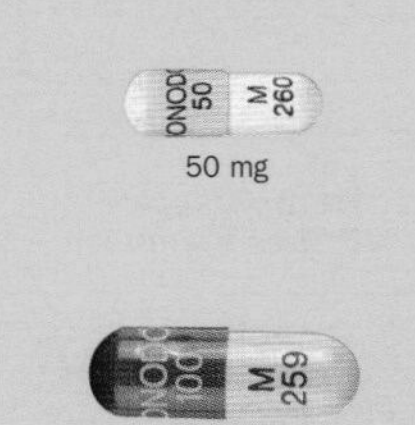

50 mg

100 mg

Monodox®
(doxycycline monohydrate)

Because tablets and capsules are shown in this section, do not infer that these are the only dosage forms available. Where a product name is preceded by the symbol †, refer to the description in the Product Information (White Section) for other forms.

ORGANON INC.

RX ORGANON INC. P. 2259

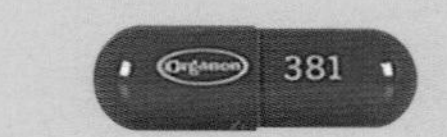

20 mcg

50 mcg

Calderol®
(calcifediol capsules, USP)

RX ORGANON INC. P. 2259

381*

†Cotazym®
(pancrelipase, USP)

RX ORGANON INC. P. 2261

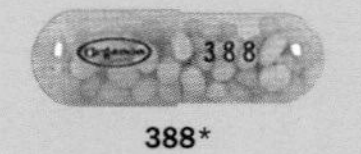

388*

Cotazym®-S
(pancrelipase, USP)
enteric coated spheres

RX ORGANON INC. P. 2261

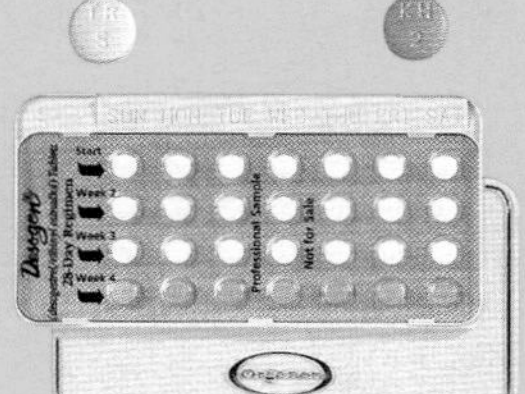

Desogen®
(desogestrel and ethinyl estradiol) Tablets

RX ORGANON INC. P. 2267

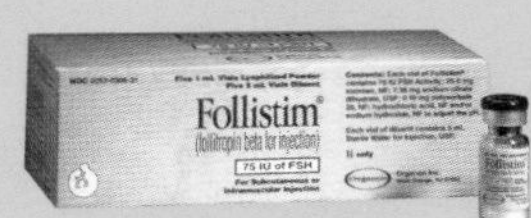

Follistim®
(follitropin beta for injection)

RX ORGANON INC. P. 2256

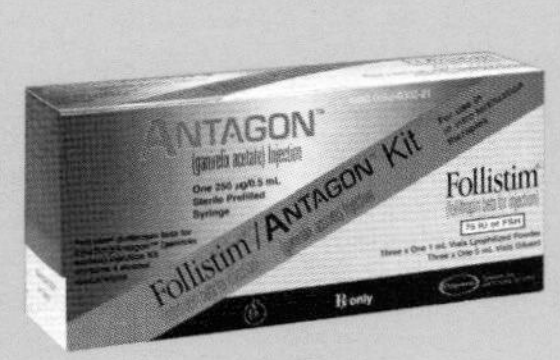

250 µg/0.5 mL
ganirelix acetate

Follistim®/Antagon™ Kit
(follitropin beta for injection/ ganirelix acetate injection)

RX ORGANON INC. P. 2272

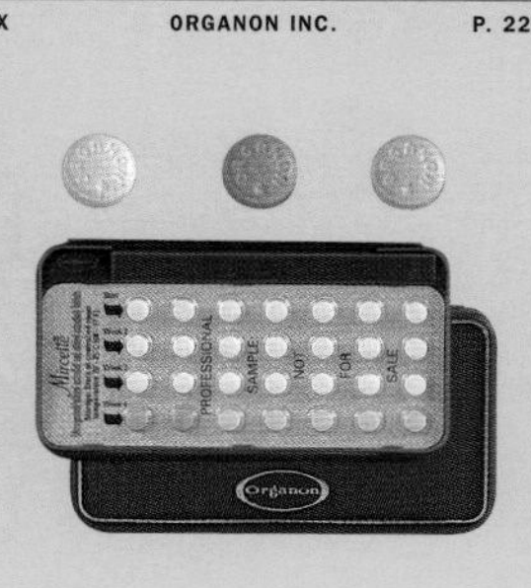

Mircette®
(desogestrel/ethinyl estradiol and ethinyl estradiol) Tablets

RX ORGANON INC. P. 2282

750 anti-Xa units

Orgaran®
(danaparoid sodium) Injection

RX ORGANON INC. P. 2284

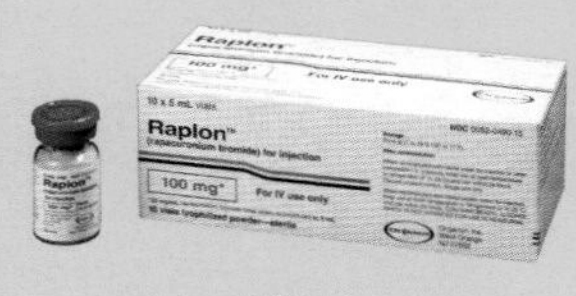

100 mg
(20 mg/mL)

Raplon™
(rapacuronium bromide) for injection

RX ORGANON INC. P. 2290

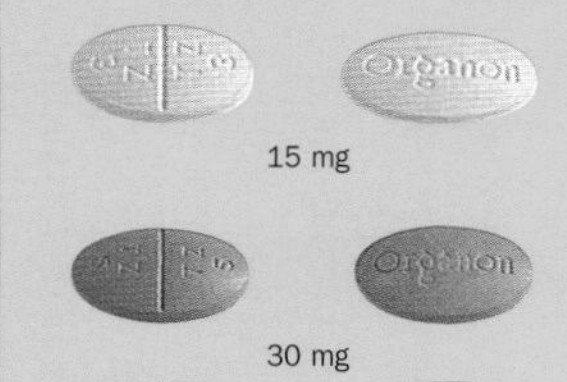

15 mg

30 mg

45 mg

Remeron®
(mirtazapine) Tablets

RX ORGANON INC. P. 2293

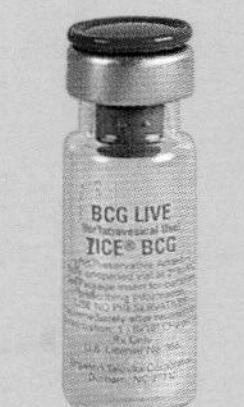

BCG LIVE TICE® BCG
(for Intravesical use)

RX ORGANON INC. P. 2295

542*

Wigraine®
(ergotamine tartrate and caffeine tablets, USP)
1 mg / 100 mg

RX ORGANON INC. P. 2296

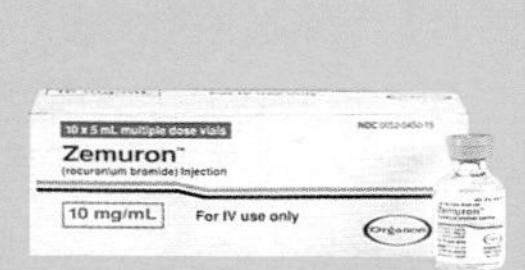

10 mg/mL per 5 mL vials

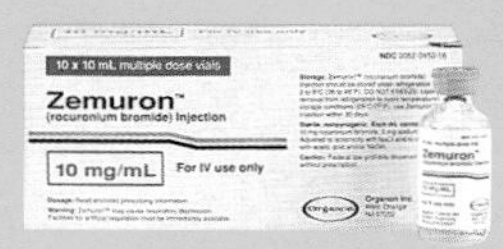

10 mg/mL per 10 mL vials

Zemuron®
(rocuronium bromide)
Injection

RX ORGANON INC. P. 2300

393*

Zymase®
(pancrelipase, USP)
enteric coated spheres

ORTHO BIOTECH

RX ORTHO BIOTECH PRODUCTS, L.P.. P. 2300

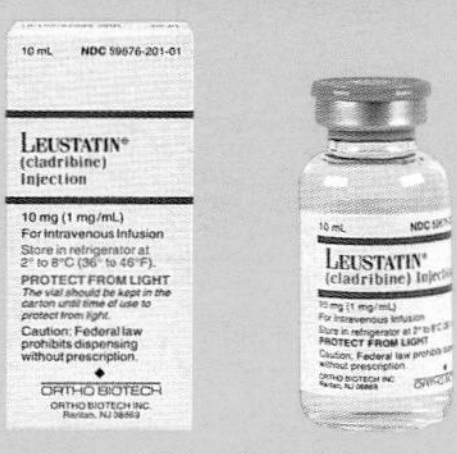

10 mg (1 mg/mL)
Available in 7-vial case

LEUSTATIN®
(cladribine) Injection

RX ORTHO BIOTECH PRODUCTS, L.P.. P. 2307

2,000 units/mL x 1 mL

3,000 units/mL x 1 mL

4,000 units/mL x 1 mL

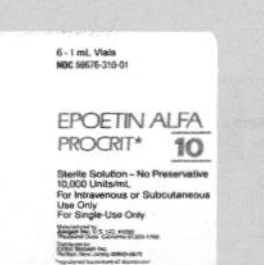

10,000 units/mL x 1 mL

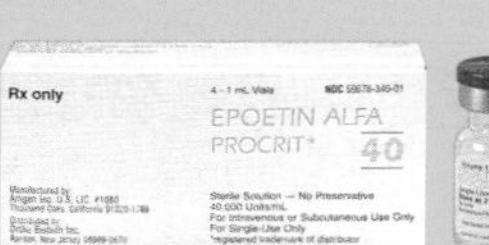

40,000 units/mL x 1 mL

PROCRIT®
(Epoetin alfa)

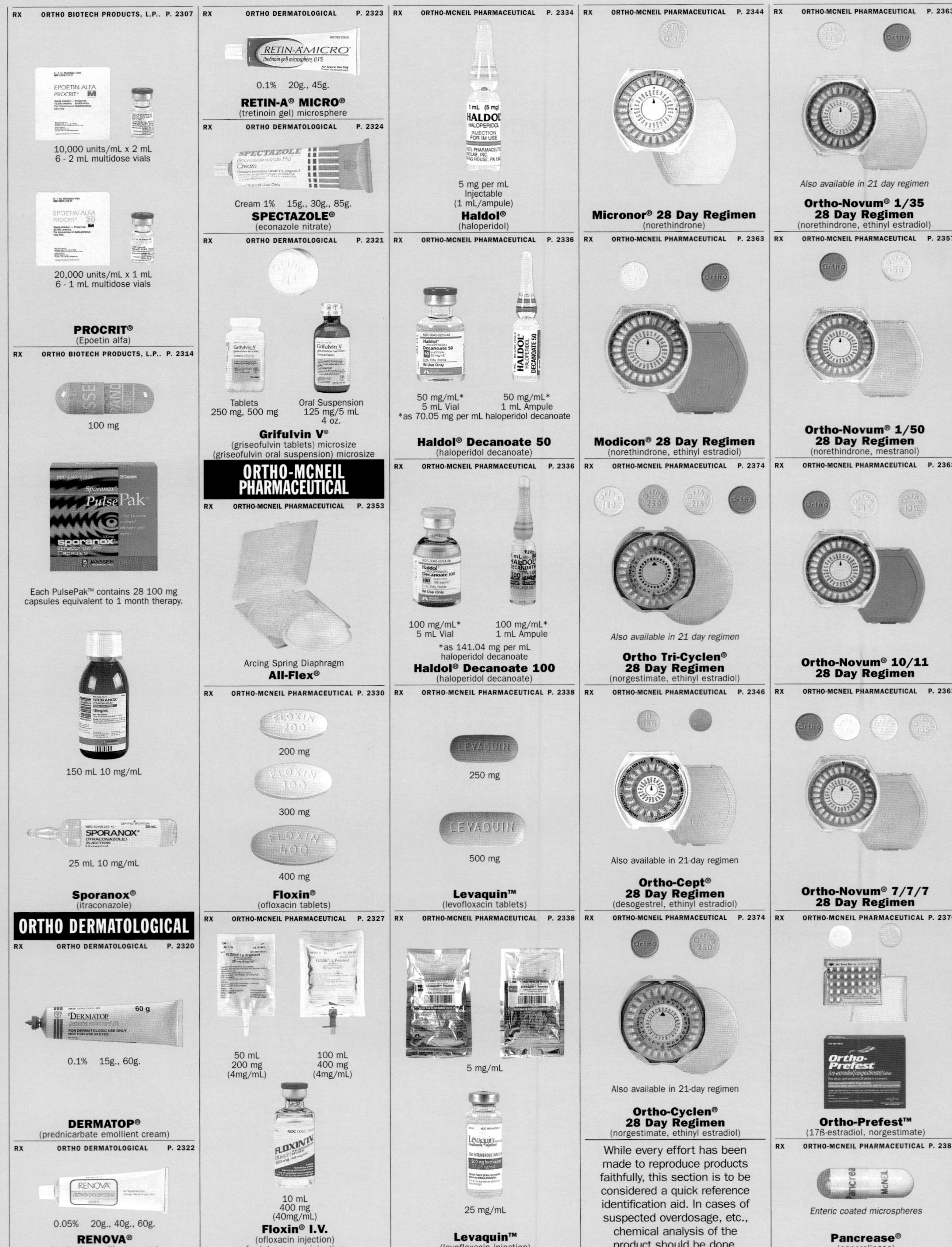

RX ORTHO BIOTECH PRODUCTS, L.P.. P. 2307
10,000 units/mL x 2 mL
6 - 2 mL multidose vials
20,000 units/mL x 1 mL
6 - 1 mL multidose vials
PROCRIT®
(Epoetin alfa)
RX ORTHO BIOTECH PRODUCTS, L.P.. P. 2314
100 mg
Each PulsePak™ contains 28 100 mg capsules equivalent to 1 month therapy.
150 mL 10 mg/mL
25 mL 10 mg/mL
Sporanox®
(itraconazole)
ORTHO DERMATOLOGICAL
RX ORTHO DERMATOLOGICAL P. 2320
0.1% 15g., 60g.
DERMATOP®
(prednicarbate emollient cream)
RX ORTHO DERMATOLOGICAL P. 2322
0.05% 20g., 40g., 60g.
RENOVA®
(tretinoin emollient cream)
RX ORTHO DERMATOLOGICAL P. 2323
0.1% 20g., 45g.
RETIN-A® MICRO®
(tretinoin gel) microsphere
RX ORTHO DERMATOLOGICAL P. 2324
Cream 1% 15g., 30g., 85g.
SPECTAZOLE®
(econazole nitrate)
RX ORTHO DERMATOLOGICAL P. 2321
Tablets
250 mg, 500 mg
Oral Suspension
125 mg/5 mL
4 oz.
Grifulvin V®
(griseofulvin tablets) microsize
(griseofulvin oral suspension) microsize
ORTHO-MCNEIL PHARMACEUTICAL
RX ORTHO-MCNEIL PHARMACEUTICAL P. 2353
Arcing Spring Diaphragm
All-Flex®
RX ORTHO-MCNEIL PHARMACEUTICAL P. 2330
200 mg
300 mg
400 mg
Floxin®
(ofloxacin tablets)
RX ORTHO-MCNEIL PHARMACEUTICAL P. 2327
50 mL
200 mg
(4mg/mL)
100 mL
400 mg
(4mg/mL)
10 mL
400 mg
(40mg/mL)
Floxin® I.V.
(ofloxacin injection)
for intravenous injection
RX ORTHO-MCNEIL PHARMACEUTICAL P. 2334
5 mg per mL
Injectable
(1 mL/ampule)
Haldol®
(haloperidol)
RX ORTHO-MCNEIL PHARMACEUTICAL P. 2336
50 mg/mL*
5 mL Vial
50 mg/mL*
1 mL Ampule
*as 70.05 mg per mL haloperidol decanoate
Haldol® Decanoate 50
(haloperidol decanoate)
RX ORTHO-MCNEIL PHARMACEUTICAL P. 2336
100 mg/mL*
5 mL Vial
100 mg/mL*
1 mL Ampule
*as 141.04 mg per mL
haloperidol decanoate
Haldol® Decanoate 100
(haloperidol decanoate)
RX ORTHO-MCNEIL PHARMACEUTICAL P. 2338
250 mg
500 mg
Levaquin™
(levofloxacin tablets)
RX ORTHO-MCNEIL PHARMACEUTICAL P. 2338
5 mg/mL
25 mg/mL
Levaquin™
(levofloxacin injection)
RX ORTHO-MCNEIL PHARMACEUTICAL P. 2344
Micronor® 28 Day Regimen
(norethindrone)
RX ORTHO-MCNEIL PHARMACEUTICAL P. 2363
Modicon® 28 Day Regimen
(norethindrone, ethinyl estradiol)
RX ORTHO-MCNEIL PHARMACEUTICAL P. 2374
Also available in 21 day regimen
Ortho Tri-Cyclen®
28 Day Regimen
(norgestimate, ethinyl estradiol)
RX ORTHO-MCNEIL PHARMACEUTICAL P. 2346
Also available in 21-day regimen
Ortho-Cept®
28 Day Regimen
(desogestrel, ethinyl estradiol)
RX ORTHO-MCNEIL PHARMACEUTICAL P. 2374
Also available in 21-day regimen
Ortho-Cyclen®
28 Day Regimen
(norgestimate, ethinyl estradiol)
While every effort has been made to reproduce products faithfully, this section is to be considered a quick reference identification aid. In cases of suspected overdosage, etc., chemical analysis of the product should be done.
RX ORTHO-MCNEIL PHARMACEUTICAL P. 2363
Also available in 21 day regimen
Ortho-Novum® 1/35
28 Day Regimen
(norethindrone, ethinyl estradiol)
RX ORTHO-MCNEIL PHARMACEUTICAL P. 2357
Ortho-Novum® 1/50
28 Day Regimen
(norethindrone, mestranol)
RX ORTHO-MCNEIL PHARMACEUTICAL P. 2363
Ortho-Novum® 10/11
28 Day Regimen
RX ORTHO-MCNEIL PHARMACEUTICAL P. 2363
Ortho-Novum® 7/7/7
28 Day Regimen
RX ORTHO-MCNEIL PHARMACEUTICAL P. 2370
Ortho-Prefest™
(17ß-estradiol, norgestimate)
RX ORTHO-MCNEIL PHARMACEUTICAL P. 2381
Enteric coated microspheres
Pancrease®
(pancrelipase)

RX ORTHO-MCNEIL PHARMACEUTICAL P. 2382

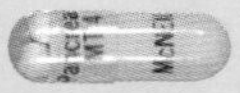

Enteric coated microtablets

Pancrease® MT 4
(pancrelipase)

RX ORTHO-MCNEIL PHARMACEUTICAL P. 2382

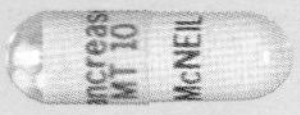

Enteric coated microtablets

Pancrease® MT 10
(pancrelipase)

RX ORTHO-MCNEIL PHARMACEUTICAL P. 2382

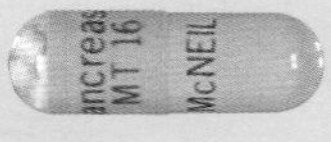

Enteric coated microtablets

Pancrease® MT 16
(pancrelipase)

RX ORTHO-MCNEIL PHARMACEUTICAL P. 2382

Enteric coated microtablets

Pancrease® MT 20
(pancrelipase)

RX ORTHO-MCNEIL PHARMACEUTICAL P. 2383

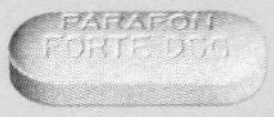

500 mg

Parafon Forte® DSC
(chlorzoxazone)

RX ORTHO-MCNEIL PHARMACEUTICAL P. 2383

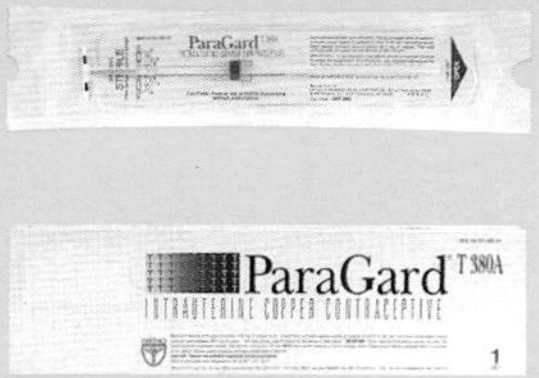

Intrauterine Copper Contraceptive

ParaGard® T 380A

RX ORTHO-MCNEIL PHARMACEUTICAL P. 2387

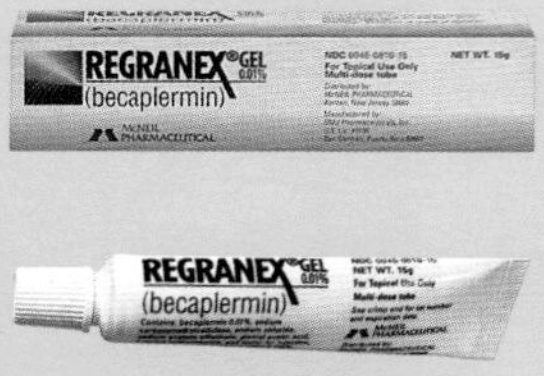

15 g

Regranex® Gel 0.01%
(becaplermin)

RX ORTHO-MCNEIL PHARMACEUTICAL P. 2388

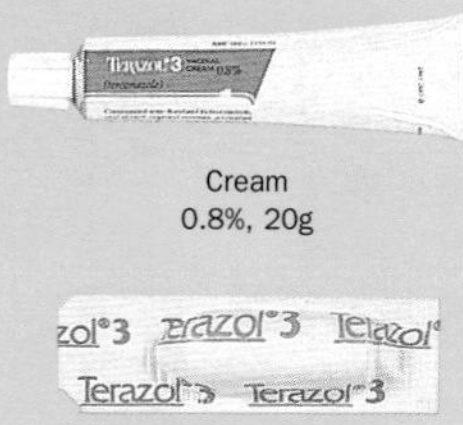

Cream
0.8%, 20g

Vaginal Suppository
80 mg

Terazol® 3
(terconazole)

RX ORTHO-MCNEIL PHARMACEUTICAL P. 2389

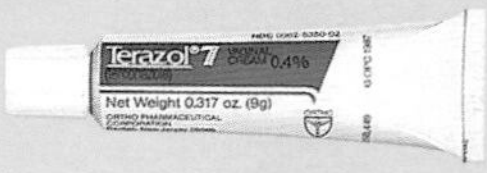

Terazol® 7
(terconazole)

RX ORTHO-MCNEIL PHARMACEUTICAL P. 2390

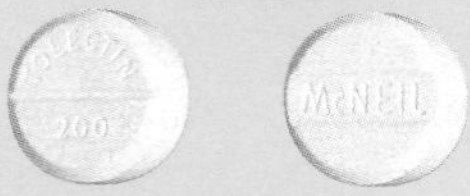

200 mg

Tolectin® 200
(tolmetin sodium)

RX ORTHO-MCNEIL PHARMACEUTICAL P. 2390

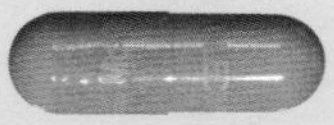

400 mg

Tolectin® 400
(tolmetin sodium)

RX ORTHO-MCNEIL PHARMACEUTICAL P. 2390

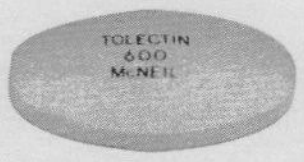

600 mg

Tolectin® 600
(tolmetin sodium)

RX ORTHO-MCNEIL PHARMACEUTICAL P. 2391

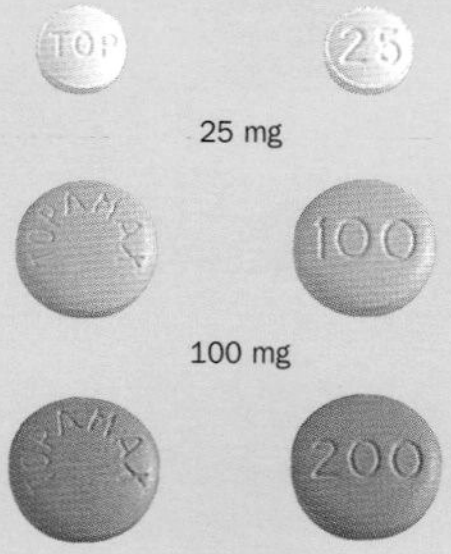

25 mg

100 mg

200 mg

Topamax®
(topiramate tablets)

RX ORTHO-MCNEIL PHARMACEUTICAL P. 2391

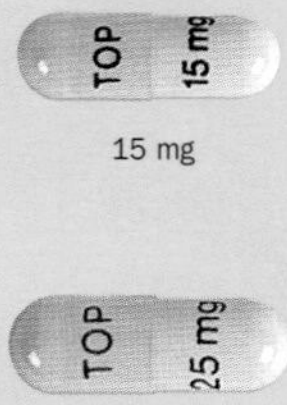

15 mg

25 mg

Topamax® Sprinkle
(topiramate capsules)

C-V ORTHO-MCNEIL PHARMACEUTICAL P. 2397

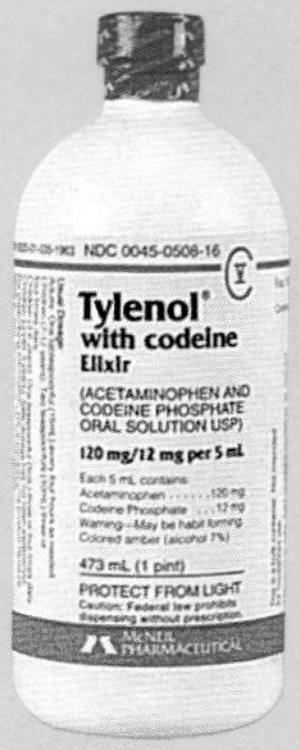

Tylenol® with Codeine Elixir
(acetaminophen and codeine phosphate oral solution USP)
120 mg / 12 mg per 5 mL

C-III ORTHO-MCNEIL PHARMACEUTICAL P. 2397

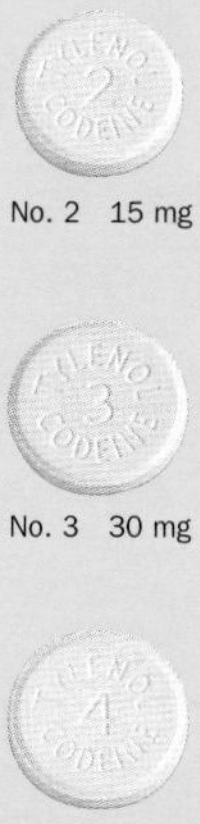

No. 2 15 mg

No. 3 30 mg

No. 4 60 mg

Tylenol® w/Codeine
(acetaminophen and codeine phosphate tablets)

C-II ORTHO-MCNEIL PHARMACEUTICAL P. 2398

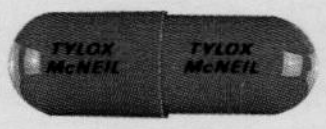

Tylox®
(oxycodone and acetaminophen capsules USP)
5 mg / 500 mg

RX ORTHO-MCNEIL PHARMACEUTICAL P. 2398

50 mg

Ultram®
(tramadol HCl tablets)

RX ORTHO-MCNEIL PHARMACEUTICAL P. 2401

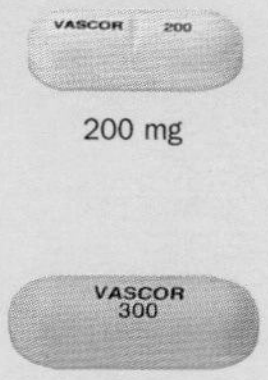

200 mg

300 mg

Vascor®
(bepridil HCl)

Designed to help you identify drugs, this section contains actual size pills and full color reproduction of products selected for inclusion by participating manufacturers.

OTSUKA

RX OTSUKA AMERICA PHARMACEUTICAL P. 2404

50 mg 100 mg

Pletal®
(cilostazol)

PARKEDALE

RX PARKEDALE P. 2410

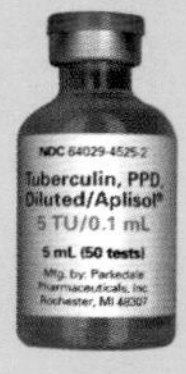

5 mL
50 tests

Aplisol®
Tuberculin, PPD, Diluted

PARKE-DAVIS

PARCODE®
(Parke-Davis Accurate Recognition Code)
For prompt, accurate product identification

The imprinted P-D identifies the product as manufactured by Parke-Davis. The imprinted number designates the particular Parke-Davis product.

A complete listing of PARCODE numbers appears at the beginning of Parke-Davis product monographs in the white section.

RX PARKE-DAVIS P. 2414
A WARNER-LAMBERT DIVISION
A PFIZER COMPANY

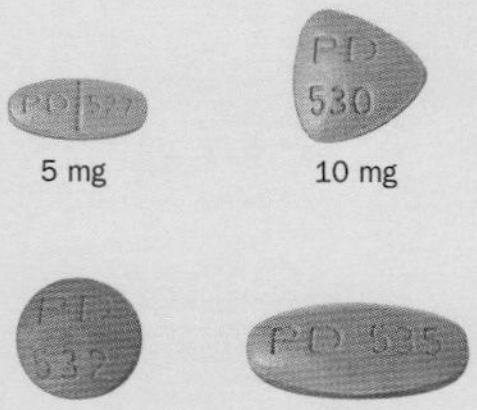

5 mg 10 mg

20 mg 40 mg

Accupril®
(quinapril HCl tablets)

RX PARKE-DAVIS P. 2417
A WARNER-LAMBERT DIVISION
A PFIZER COMPANY

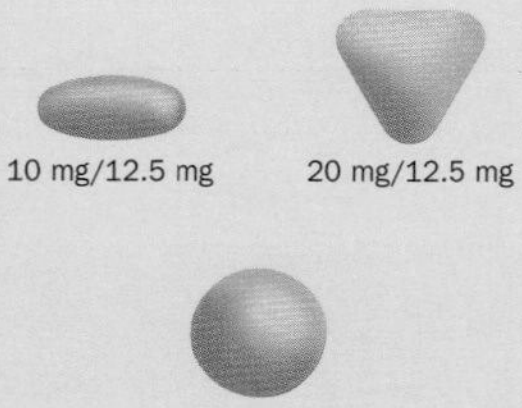

10 mg/12.5 mg 20 mg/12.5 mg

20 mg/25 mg

Accuretic®
(quinapril HCl/hydrochlorothiazide)

RX PARKE-DAVIS P. 2421
A WARNER-LAMBERT DIVISION
A PFIZER COMPANY

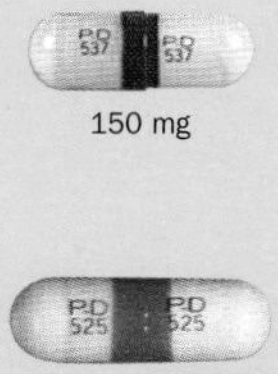

150 mg

300 mg

Celontin® Kapseals®
(methsuximide capsules, USP)

RX PARKE-DAVIS P. 2427
A WARNER-LAMBERT DIVISION
A PFIZER COMPANY

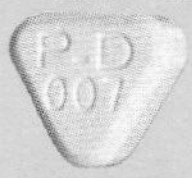

50 mg

†Dilantin® Infatabs®
(phenytoin tablets, USP)

RX PARKE-DAVIS P. 2425
A WARNER-LAMBERT DIVISION
A PFIZER COMPANY

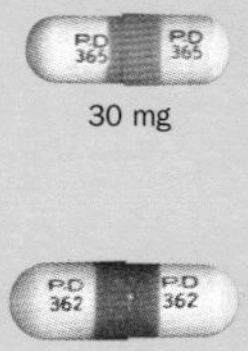

30 mg

100 mg

†Dilantin® Kapseals®
(extended phenytoin sodium capsules, USP)

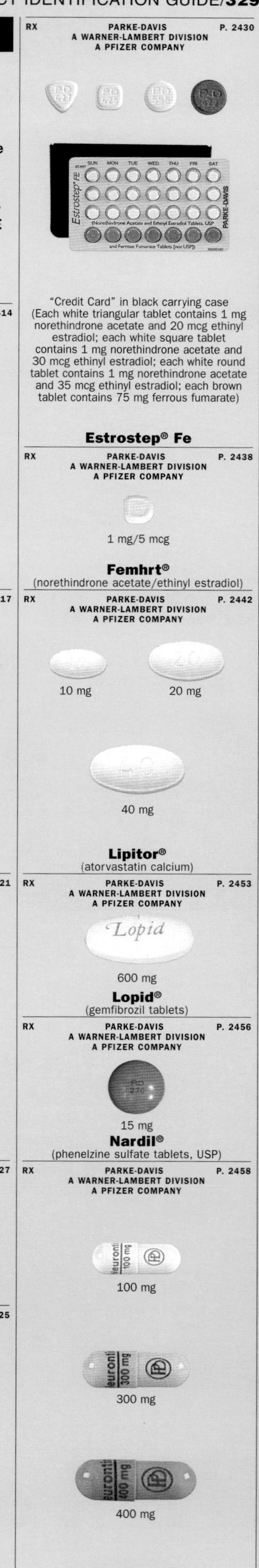

RX PARKE-DAVIS P. 2430
A WARNER-LAMBERT DIVISION
A PFIZER COMPANY

"Credit Card" in black carrying case (Each white triangular tablet contains 1 mg norethindrone acetate and 20 mcg ethinyl estradiol; each white square tablet contains 1 mg norethindrone acetate and 30 mcg ethinyl estradiol; each white round tablet contains 1 mg norethindrone acetate and 35 mcg ethinyl estradiol; each brown tablet contains 75 mg ferrous fumarate)

Estrostep® Fe

RX PARKE-DAVIS P. 2438
A WARNER-LAMBERT DIVISION
A PFIZER COMPANY

1 mg/5 mcg

Femhrt®
(norethindrone acetate/ethinyl estradiol)

RX PARKE-DAVIS P. 2442
A WARNER-LAMBERT DIVISION
A PFIZER COMPANY

10 mg 20 mg

40 mg

Lipitor®
(atorvastatin calcium)

RX PARKE-DAVIS P. 2453
A WARNER-LAMBERT DIVISION
A PFIZER COMPANY

600 mg

Lopid®
(gemfibrozil tablets)

RX PARKE-DAVIS P. 2456
A WARNER-LAMBERT DIVISION
A PFIZER COMPANY

15 mg

Nardil®
(phenelzine sulfate tablets, USP)

RX PARKE-DAVIS P. 2458
A WARNER-LAMBERT DIVISION
A PFIZER COMPANY

100 mg

300 mg

400 mg

Neurontin®
(gabapentin capsules)

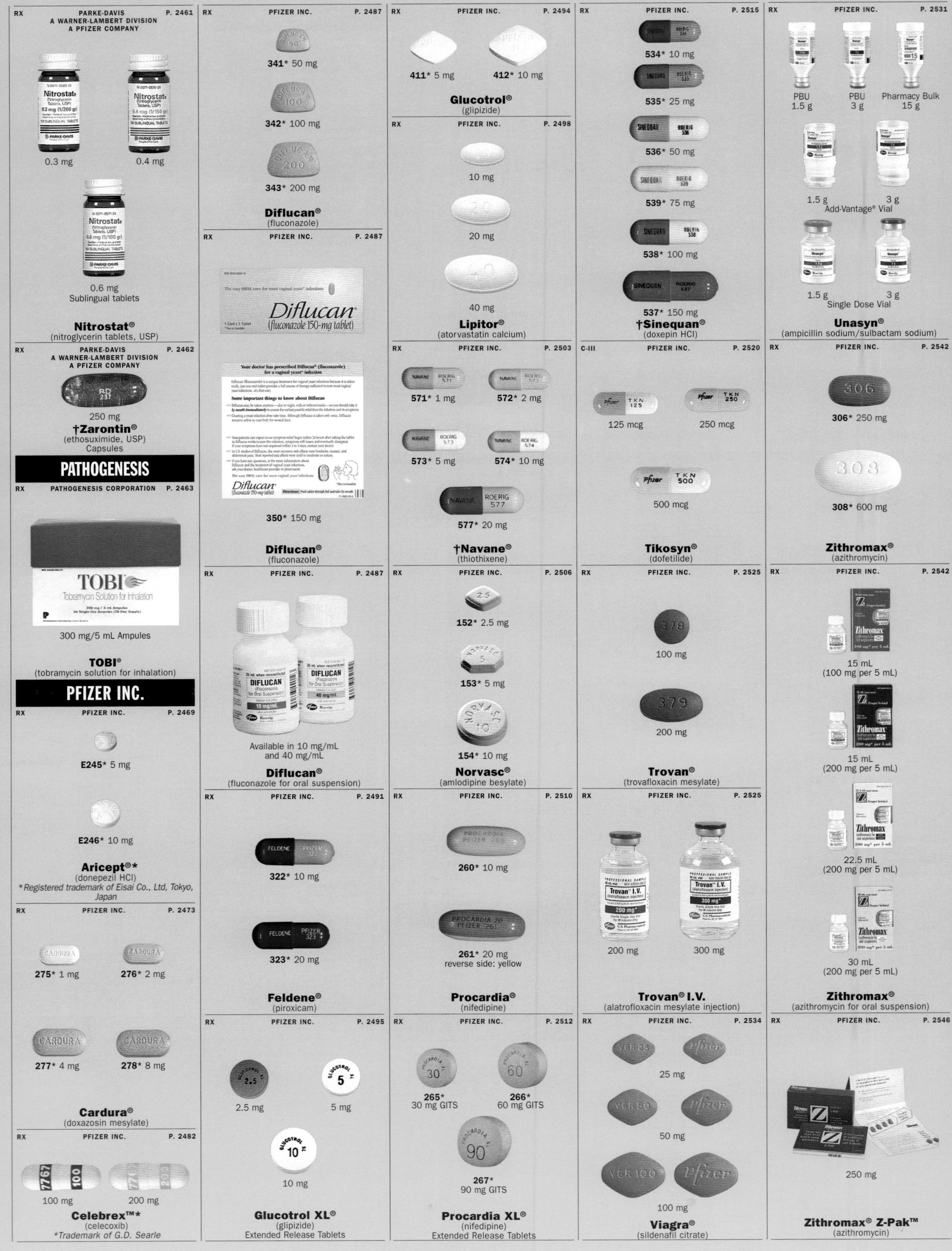
RX PARKE-DAVIS A WARNER-LAMBERT DIVISION A PFIZER COMPANY P. 2461
0.3 mg
0.4 mg
0.6 mg
Sublingual tablets
Nitrostat®
(nitroglycerin tablets, USP)
RX PARKE-DAVIS A WARNER-LAMBERT DIVISION A PFIZER COMPANY P. 2462
250 mg
†Zarontin®
(ethosuximide, USP)
Capsules
PATHOGENESIS
RX PATHOGENESIS CORPORATION P. 2463
TOBI
Tobramycin Solution for Inhalation
300 mg/5 mL Ampules
TOBI®
(tobramycin solution for inhalation)
PFIZER INC.
RX PFIZER INC. P. 2469
E245* 5 mg
E246* 10 mg
Aricept®*
(donepezil HCl)
*Registered trademark of Eisai Co., Ltd, Tokyo, Japan
RX PFIZER INC. P. 2473
275* 1 mg
276* 2 mg
277* 4 mg
278* 8 mg
Cardura®
(doxazosin mesylate)
RX PFIZER INC. P. 2482
100 mg
200 mg
Celebrex™*
(celecoxib)
*Trademark of G.D. Searle
RX PFIZER INC. P. 2487
341* 50 mg
342* 100 mg
343* 200 mg
Diflucan®
(fluconazole)
RX PFIZER INC. P. 2487
Diflucan
(fluconazole 150-mg tablet)
Your doctor has prescribed Diflucan® (fluconazole) for a vaginal yeast* infection
Some important things to know about Diflucan
350* 150 mg
Diflucan®
(fluconazole)
RX PFIZER INC. P. 2487
DIFLUCAN
10 mg/mL
40 mg/mL
Available in 10 mg/mL and 40 mg/mL
Diflucan®
(fluconazole for oral suspension)
RX PFIZER INC. P. 2491
322* 10 mg
323* 20 mg
Feldene®
(piroxicam)
RX PFIZER INC. P. 2495
2.5 mg
5 mg
10 mg
Glucotrol XL®
(glipizide)
Extended Release Tablets
RX PFIZER INC. P. 2494
411* 5 mg
412* 10 mg
Glucotrol®
(glipizide)
RX PFIZER INC. P. 2498
10 mg
20 mg
40 mg
Lipitor®
(atorvastatin calcium)
RX PFIZER INC. P. 2503
571* 1 mg
572* 2 mg
573* 5 mg
574* 10 mg
577* 20 mg
†Navane®
(thiothixene)
RX PFIZER INC. P. 2506
152* 2.5 mg
153* 5 mg
154* 10 mg
Norvasc®
(amlodipine besylate)
RX PFIZER INC. P. 2510
260* 10 mg
261* 20 mg
reverse side: yellow
Procardia®
(nifedipine)
RX PFIZER INC. P. 2512
265*
30 mg GITS
266*
60 mg GITS
267*
90 mg GITS
Procardia XL®
(nifedipine)
Extended Release Tablets
RX PFIZER INC. P. 2515
534* 10 mg
535* 25 mg
536* 50 mg
539* 75 mg
538* 100 mg
537* 150 mg
†Sinequan®
(doxepin HCl)
C-III PFIZER INC. P. 2520
125 mcg
250 mcg
500 mcg
Tikosyn®
(dofetilide)
RX PFIZER INC. P. 2525
100 mg
200 mg
Trovan®
(trovafloxacin mesylate)
RX PFIZER INC. P. 2525
200 mg
300 mg
Trovan® I.V.
(alatrofloxacin mesylate injection)
RX PFIZER INC. P. 2534
25 mg
50 mg
100 mg
Viagra®
(sildenafil citrate)
RX PFIZER INC. P. 2531
PBU
1.5 g
PBU
3 g
Pharmacy Bulk
15 g
1.5 g
3 g
Add-Vantage® Vial
1.5 g
3 g
Single Dose Vial
Unasyn®
(ampicillin sodium/sulbactam sodium)
RX PFIZER INC. P. 2542
306* 250 mg
308* 600 mg
Zithromax®
(azithromycin)
RX PFIZER INC. P. 2542
15 mL
(100 mg per 5 mL)
15 mL
(200 mg per 5 mL)
22.5 mL
(200 mg per 5 mL)
30 mL
(200 mg per 5 mL)
Zithromax®
(azithromycin for oral suspension)
RX PFIZER INC. P. 2546
250 mg
Zithromax® Z-Pak™
(azithromycin)

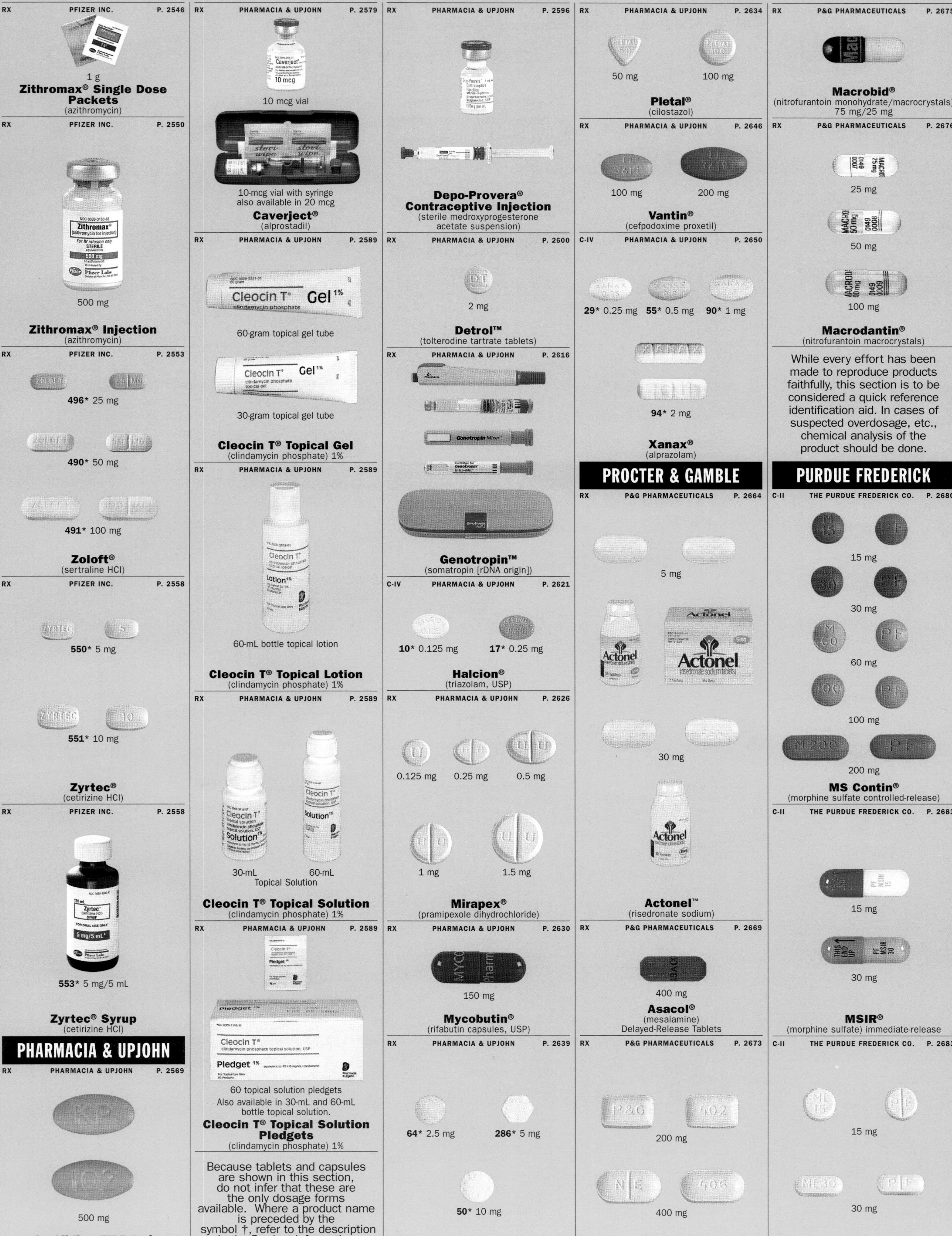
RX PFIZER INC. P. 2546
1 g
Zithromax® Single Dose Packets
(azithromycin)
RX PFIZER INC. P. 2550
500 mg
Zithromax® Injection
(azithromycin)
RX PFIZER INC. P. 2553
496* 25 mg
490* 50 mg
491* 100 mg
Zoloft®
(sertraline HCl)
RX PFIZER INC. P. 2558
550* 5 mg
551* 10 mg
Zyrtec®
(cetirizine HCl)
RX PFIZER INC. P. 2558
553* 5 mg/5 mL
Zyrtec® Syrup
(cetirizine HCl)
PHARMACIA & UPJOHN
RX PHARMACIA & UPJOHN P. 2569
500 mg
Azulfidine EN-Tabs®
(sulfasalazine delayed release tablets, USP)
Enteric-coated
RX PHARMACIA & UPJOHN P. 2579
10 mcg vial
10-mcg vial with syringe
also available in 20 mcg
Caverject®
(alprostadil)
RX PHARMACIA & UPJOHN P. 2589
60-gram topical gel tube
30-gram topical gel tube
Cleocin T® Topical Gel
(clindamycin phosphate) 1%
RX PHARMACIA & UPJOHN P. 2589
60-mL bottle topical lotion
Cleocin T® Topical Lotion
(clindamycin phosphate) 1%
RX PHARMACIA & UPJOHN P. 2589
30-mL
60-mL
Topical Solution
Cleocin T® Topical Solution
(clindamycin phosphate) 1%
RX PHARMACIA & UPJOHN P. 2589
60 topical solution pledgets
Also available in 30-mL and 60-mL
bottle topical solution.
Cleocin T® Topical Solution Pledgets
(clindamycin phosphate) 1%
Because tablets and capsules are shown in this section, do not infer that these are the only dosage forms available. Where a product name is preceded by the symbol †, refer to the description in the Product Information (White Section) for other forms.
RX PHARMACIA & UPJOHN P. 2596
Depo-Provera®
Contraceptive Injection
(sterile medroxyprogesterone
acetate suspension)
RX PHARMACIA & UPJOHN P. 2600
2 mg
Detrol™
(tolterodine tartrate tablets)
RX PHARMACIA & UPJOHN P. 2616
Genotropin™
(somatropin [rDNA origin])
C-IV PHARMACIA & UPJOHN P. 2621
10* 0.125 mg
17* 0.25 mg
Halcion®
(triazolam, USP)
RX PHARMACIA & UPJOHN P. 2626
0.125 mg
0.25 mg
0.5 mg
1 mg
1.5 mg
Mirapex®
(pramipexole dihydrochloride)
RX PHARMACIA & UPJOHN P. 2630
150 mg
Mycobutin®
(rifabutin capsules, USP)
RX PHARMACIA & UPJOHN P. 2639
64* 2.5 mg
286* 5 mg
50* 10 mg
Provera®
(medroxyprogesterone acetate)
RX PHARMACIA & UPJOHN P. 2634
50 mg
100 mg
Pletal®
(cilostazol)
RX PHARMACIA & UPJOHN P. 2646
100 mg
200 mg
Vantin®
(cefpodoxime proxetil)
C-IV PHARMACIA & UPJOHN P. 2650
29* 0.25 mg
55* 0.5 mg
90* 1 mg
94* 2 mg
Xanax®
(alprazolam)
PROCTER & GAMBLE
RX P&G PHARMACEUTICALS P. 2664
5 mg
30 mg
Actonel™
(risedronate sodium)
RX P&G PHARMACEUTICALS P. 2669
400 mg
Asacol®
(mesalamine)
Delayed-Release Tablets
RX P&G PHARMACEUTICALS P. 2673
200 mg
400 mg
Didronel®
(etidronate disodium)
RX P&G PHARMACEUTICALS P. 2675
Macrobid®
(nitrofurantoin monohydrate/macrocrystals)
75 mg/25 mg
RX P&G PHARMACEUTICALS P. 2676
25 mg
50 mg
100 mg
Macrodantin®
(nitrofurantoin macrocrystals)
While every effort has been made to reproduce products faithfully, this section is to be considered a quick reference identification aid. In cases of suspected overdosage, etc., chemical analysis of the product should be done.
PURDUE FREDERICK
C-II THE PURDUE FREDERICK CO. P. 2680
15 mg
30 mg
60 mg
100 mg
200 mg
MS Contin®
(morphine sulfate controlled-release)
C-II THE PURDUE FREDERICK CO. P. 2683
15 mg
30 mg
MSIR®
(morphine sulfate) immediate-release
C-II THE PURDUE FREDERICK CO. P. 2683
15 mg
30 mg
MSIR®
(morphine sulfate) immediate-release

C-II THE PURDUE FREDERICK CO. P. 2683

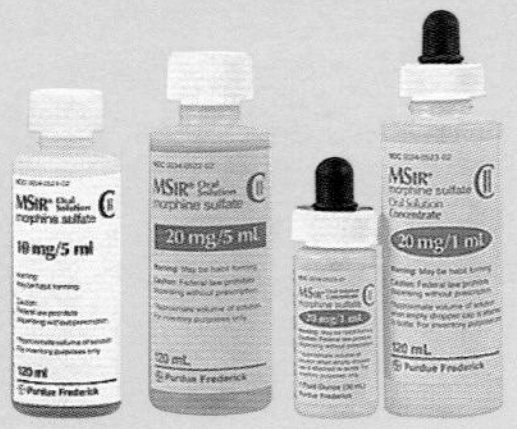

MSIR Oral Solution 10 mg/5 mL and 20 mg/5 mL in plastic bottles of 120 mL. MSIR Oral Solution Concentrate 20 mg/1 mL child-resistant plastic bottles of 30 mL and 120 mL with child-resistant droppers

MSIR® Oral Solution
(morphine sulfate) immediate-release

RX THE PURDUE FREDERICK CO. P. 2686

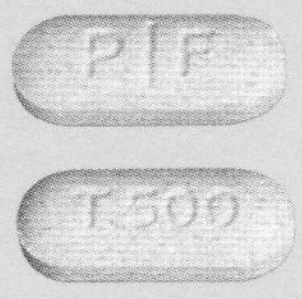

500 mg

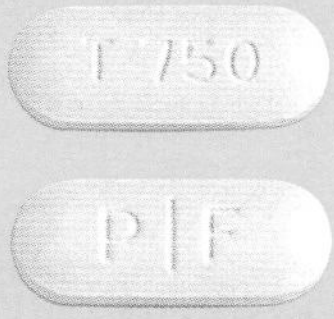

750 mg

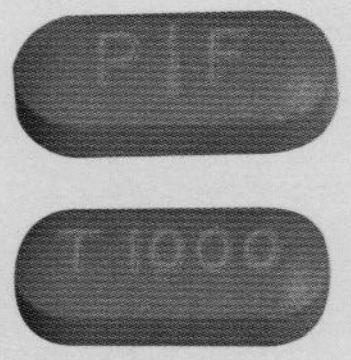

1000 mg

Trilisate®
(choline magnesium trisalicylate)

RX THE PURDUE FREDERICK CO. P. 2686

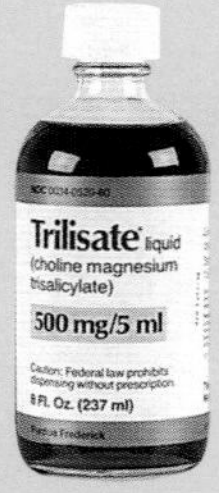

500 mg / 5 mL

Trilisate®
(choline magnesium trisalicylate)

RX THE PURDUE FREDERICK CO. P. 2687

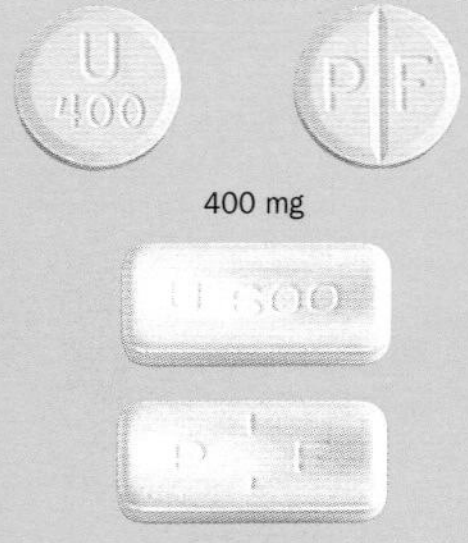

400 mg

600 mg
Controlled-release tablets

Uniphyl®
(theophylline, anhydrous)

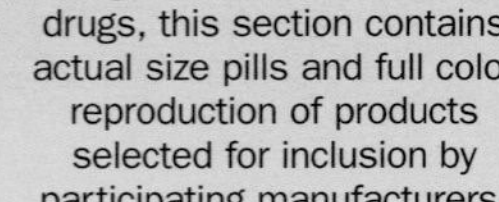

Designed to help you identify drugs, this section contains actual size pills and full color reproduction of products selected for inclusion by participating manufacturers.

PURDUE PHARMA L.P.

RX PURDUE PHARMA L.P. P. 2693

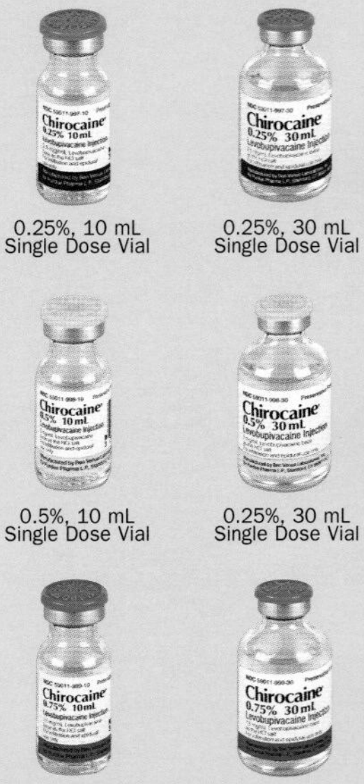

0.25%, 10 mL Single Dose Vial

0.25%, 30 mL Single Dose Vial

0.5%, 10 mL Single Dose Vial

0.25%, 30 mL Single Dose Vial

0.75%, 10 mL Single Dose Vial

0.75%, 30 mL Single Dose Vial

Chirocaine®
(levobupivicaine injection)

C-II PURDUE PHARMA L.P. P. 2697

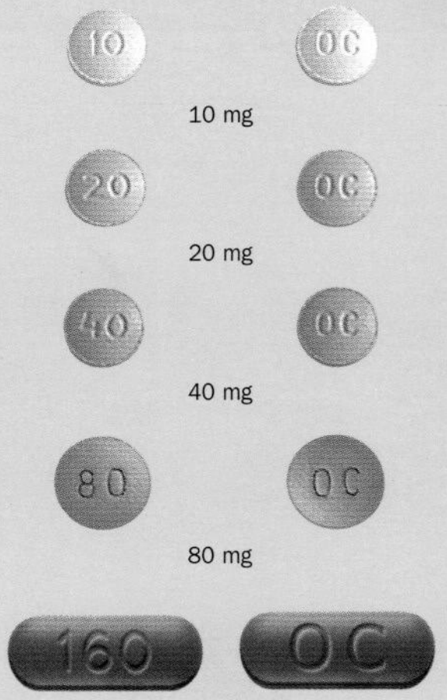

10 mg

20 mg

40 mg

80 mg

160 mg

OxyContin®
(oxycodone HCl controlled-release)

C-II PURDUE PHARMA L.P. P. 2701

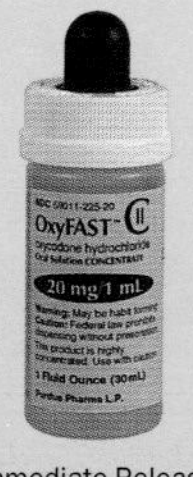

Immediate-Release Oral CONCENTRATE Solution 20 mg/1 mL in plastic bottle of 30 mL with child-resistant dropper

OxyFAST™
(oxycodone HCl)

C-II PURDUE PHARMA L.P. P. 2701

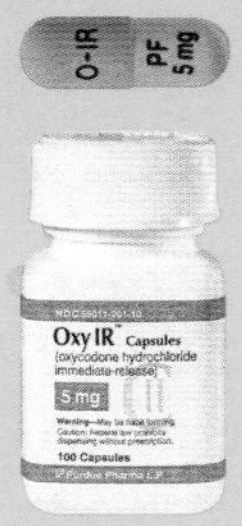

5 mg

OxyIR®
(oxycodone HCl immediate-release)

RECKITT BENCKISER

C-V RECKITT BENCKISER P. 2705

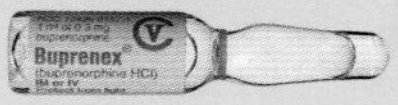

0.3 mg per 1 mL ampul

Buprenex® Injectable
(buprenorphine HCl)

RHONE-POULENC RORER

IMPORTANT NOTICE:
Rhone-Poulenc Rorer products are now listed by Aventis Phamaceuticals. See page 306 for product identification.

RICHWOOD

IMPORTANT NOTICE:
Richwood Pharmaceutical products are now listed by Shire US Inc. Please see page 336 for product identification.

ROBERTS

IMPORTANT NOTICE:
Roberts Pharmaceutical products are now listed by Shire US Inc. Please see page 336 for product identification.

A. H. ROBINS

RX A. H. ROBINS COMPANY P. 2708

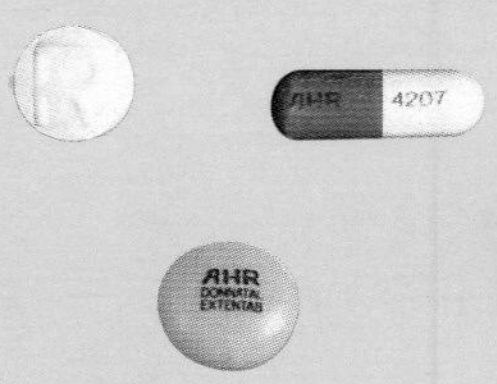

Extentabs®

†Donnatal®

RX A. H. ROBINS COMPANY P. 2709

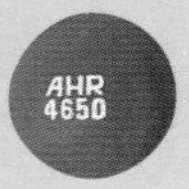

500 mg

Donnazyme®
(pancreatin)

RX A. H. ROBINS COMPANY P. 2711

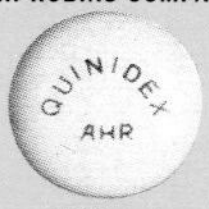

300 mg
Extended-Release Tablets

Quinidex Extentabs®
(quinidine sulfate, USP)

RX A. H. ROBINS COMPANY P. 2713

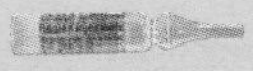

2 mL ampul

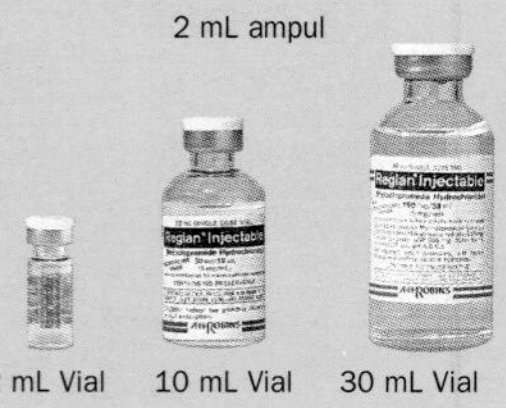

2 mL Vial 10 mL Vial 30 mL Vial

Reglan® Injectable
(metoclopramide, USP)
5 mg/mL

RX A. H. ROBINS COMPANY P. 2713

5 mg 10 mg

†Reglan®
(metoclopramide, USP)

RX A. H. ROBINS COMPANY P. 2716

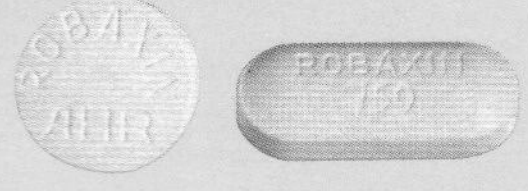

500 mg 750 mg

Robaxin®/Robaxin®-750
(methocarbamol tablets, USP)

RX A. H. ROBINS COMPANY P. 2716

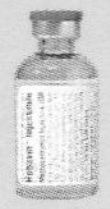

Robaxin® Injectable
(methocarbamol injection, USP)
100 mg/mL

RX A. H. ROBINS COMPANY P. 2717

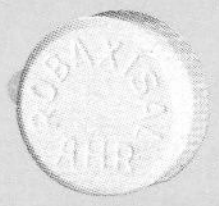

Robaxisal®
(methocarbamol, USP/aspirin, USP)
400 mg / 325 mg

RX A. H. ROBINS COMPANY P. 2717

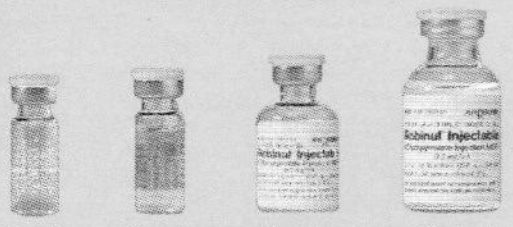

1 mL 2 mL 5 mL 20 mL

Robinul® Injectable
(glycopyrrolate injection, USP)

RX A. H. ROBINS COMPANY P. 2719

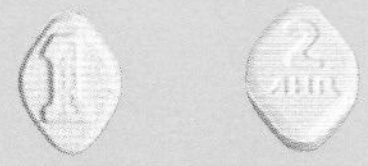

1 mg 2 mg

Tenex®
(guanfacine HCl)

ROCHE

RX ROCHE P. 2721

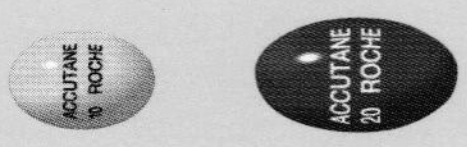

10 mg 20 mg

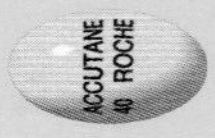

40 mg

Accutane®
(isotretinoin)

RX ROCHE P. 2744

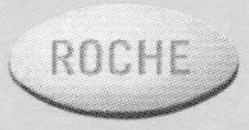

275 mg

Anaprox®
(naproxen sodium)

RX ROCHE P. 2744

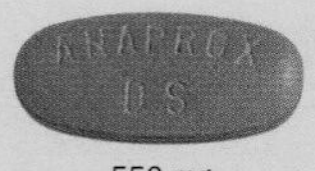

550 mg

Anaprox® DS
(naproxen sodium)

RX ROCHE P. 2725

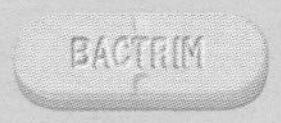

†Bactrim™
(trimethoprim and sulfamethoxazole)
80 mg / 400 mg

RX ROCHE P. 2725

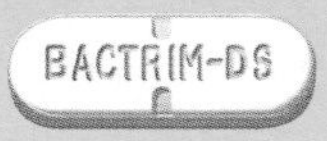

†Bactrim™ DS
(trimethoprim and sulfamethoxazole)
160 mg / 800 mg

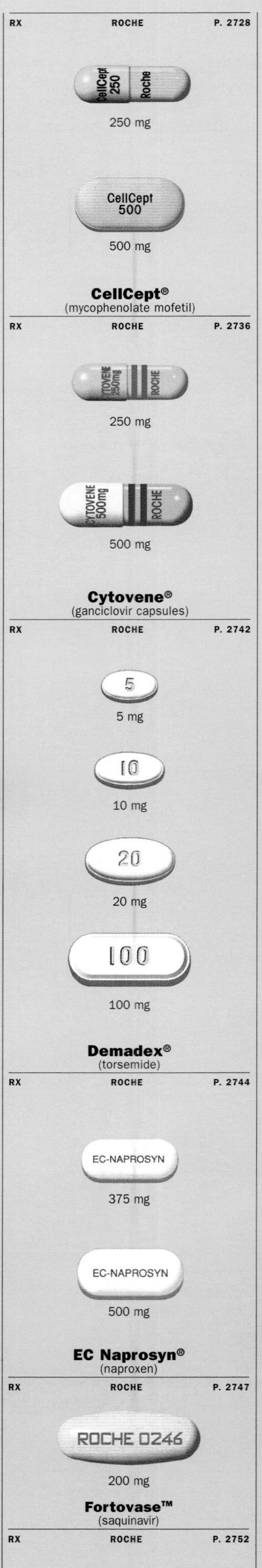

RX ROCHE P. 2728

250 mg

500 mg

CellCept®
(mycophenolate mofetil)

RX ROCHE P. 2736

250 mg

500 mg

Cytovene®
(ganciclovir capsules)

RX ROCHE P. 2742

5 mg

10 mg

20 mg

100 mg

Demadex®
(torsemide)

RX ROCHE P. 2744

375 mg

500 mg

EC Naprosyn®
(naproxen)

RX ROCHE P. 2747

200 mg

Fortovase™
(saquinavir)

RX ROCHE P. 2752

0.375 mg 0.750 mg

Hivid®
(zalcitabine)

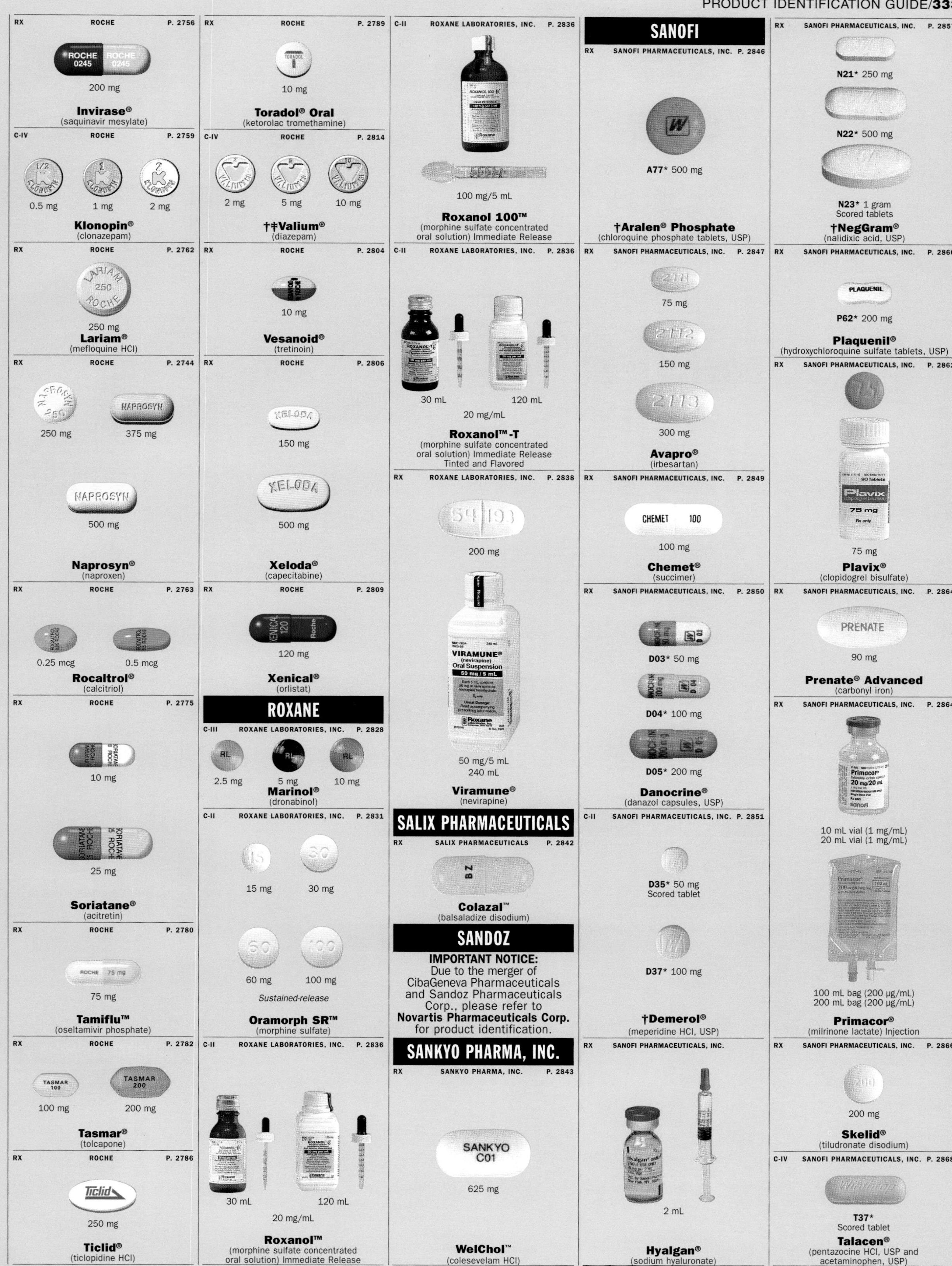
RX ROCHE P. 2756
ROCHE 0245 ROCHE 0245
200 mg
Invirase®
(saquinavir mesylate)
C-IV ROCHE P. 2759
0.5 mg 1 mg 2 mg
Klonopin®
(clonazepam)
RX ROCHE P. 2762
LARIAM 250 ROCHE
250 mg
Lariam®
(mefloquine HCl)
RX ROCHE P. 2744
NAPROSYN 250
NAPROSYN
250 mg 375 mg
NAPROSYN
500 mg
Naprosyn®
(naproxen)
RX ROCHE P. 2763
0.25 mcg 0.5 mcg
Rocaltrol®
(calcitriol)
RX ROCHE P. 2775
10 mg
25 mg
Soriatane®
(acitretin)
RX ROCHE P. 2780
ROCHE 75 mg
75 mg
Tamiflu™
(oseltamivir phosphate)
RX ROCHE P. 2782
TASMAR 100
TASMAR 200
100 mg 200 mg
Tasmar®
(tolcapone)
RX ROCHE P. 2786
Ticlid
250 mg
Ticlid®
(ticlopidine HCl)
RX ROCHE P. 2789
TORADOL
10 mg
Toradol® Oral
(ketorolac tromethamine)
C-IV ROCHE P. 2814
2 mg 5 mg 10 mg
†‡Valium®
(diazepam)
RX ROCHE P. 2804
10 mg
Vesanoid®
(tretinoin)
RX ROCHE P. 2806
XELODA
150 mg
XELODA
500 mg
Xeloda®
(capecitabine)
RX ROCHE P. 2809
XENICAL 120 Roche
120 mg
Xenical®
(orlistat)
ROXANE
C-III ROXANE LABORATORIES, INC. P. 2828
RL RL RL
2.5 mg 5 mg 10 mg
Marinol®
(dronabinol)
C-II ROXANE LABORATORIES, INC. P. 2831
15 30
15 mg 30 mg
60 100
60 mg 100 mg
Sustained-release
Oramorph SR™
(morphine sulfate)
C-II ROXANE LABORATORIES, INC. P. 2836
30 mL 120 mL
20 mg/mL
Roxanol™
(morphine sulfate concentrated oral solution) Immediate Release
C-II ROXANE LABORATORIES, INC. P. 2836
100 mg/5 mL
Roxanol 100™
(morphine sulfate concentrated oral solution) Immediate Release
C-II ROXANE LABORATORIES, INC. P. 2836
30 mL 120 mL
20 mg/mL
Roxanol™-T
(morphine sulfate concentrated oral solution) Immediate Release Tinted and Flavored
RX ROXANE LABORATORIES, INC. P. 2838
54 193
200 mg
VIRAMUNE® (nevirapine) Oral Suspension 50 mg / 5 mL
50 mg/5 mL
240 mL
Viramune®
(nevirapine)
SALIX PHARMACEUTICALS
RX SALIX PHARMACEUTICALS P. 2842
BZ
Colazal™
(balsalazide disodium)
SANDOZ
IMPORTANT NOTICE:
Due to the merger of CibaGeneva Pharmaceuticals and Sandoz Pharmaceuticals Corp., please refer to Novartis Pharmaceuticals Corp. for product identification.
SANKYO PHARMA, INC.
RX SANKYO PHARMA, INC. P. 2843
SANKYO C01
625 mg
WelChol™
(colesevelam HCl)
SANOFI
RX SANOFI PHARMACEUTICALS, INC. P. 2846
W
A77* 500 mg
†Aralen® Phosphate
(chloroquine phosphate tablets, USP)
RX SANOFI PHARMACEUTICALS, INC. P. 2847
2771
75 mg
2772
150 mg
2773
300 mg
Avapro®
(irbesartan)
RX SANOFI PHARMACEUTICALS, INC. P. 2849
CHEMET 100
100 mg
Chemet®
(succimer)
RX SANOFI PHARMACEUTICALS, INC. P. 2850
D03* 50 mg
D04* 100 mg
D05* 200 mg
Danocrine®
(danazol capsules, USP)
C-II SANOFI PHARMACEUTICALS, INC. P. 2851
D35* 50 mg
Scored tablet
D37* 100 mg
†Demerol®
(meperidine HCl, USP)
RX SANOFI PHARMACEUTICALS, INC.
2 mL
Hyalgan®
(sodium hyaluronate)
RX SANOFI PHARMACEUTICALS, INC. P. 2857
N21* 250 mg
N22* 500 mg
N23* 1 gram
Scored tablets
†NegGram®
(nalidixic acid, USP)
RX SANOFI PHARMACEUTICALS, INC. P. 2860
PLAQUENIL
P62* 200 mg
Plaquenil®
(hydroxychloroquine sulfate tablets, USP)
RX SANOFI PHARMACEUTICALS, INC. P. 2862
75
Plavix 75 mg
75 mg
Plavix®
(clopidogrel bisulfate)
RX SANOFI PHARMACEUTICALS, INC. P. 2864
PRENATE
90 mg
Prenate® Advanced
(carbonyl iron)
RX SANOFI PHARMACEUTICALS, INC. P. 2864
Primacor® 20 mg/20 mL
10 mL vial (1 mg/mL)
20 mL vial (1 mg/mL)
100 mL bag (200 µg/mL)
200 mL bag (200 µg/mL)
Primacor®
(milrinone lactate) Injection
RX SANOFI PHARMACEUTICALS, INC. P. 2866
200
200 mg
Skelid®
(tiludronate disodium)
C-IV SANOFI PHARMACEUTICALS, INC. P. 2868
Winthrop
T37*
Scored tablet
Talacen®
(pentazocine HCl, USP and acetaminophen, USP)

†Roche Products Inc., Humaco, PR 00791

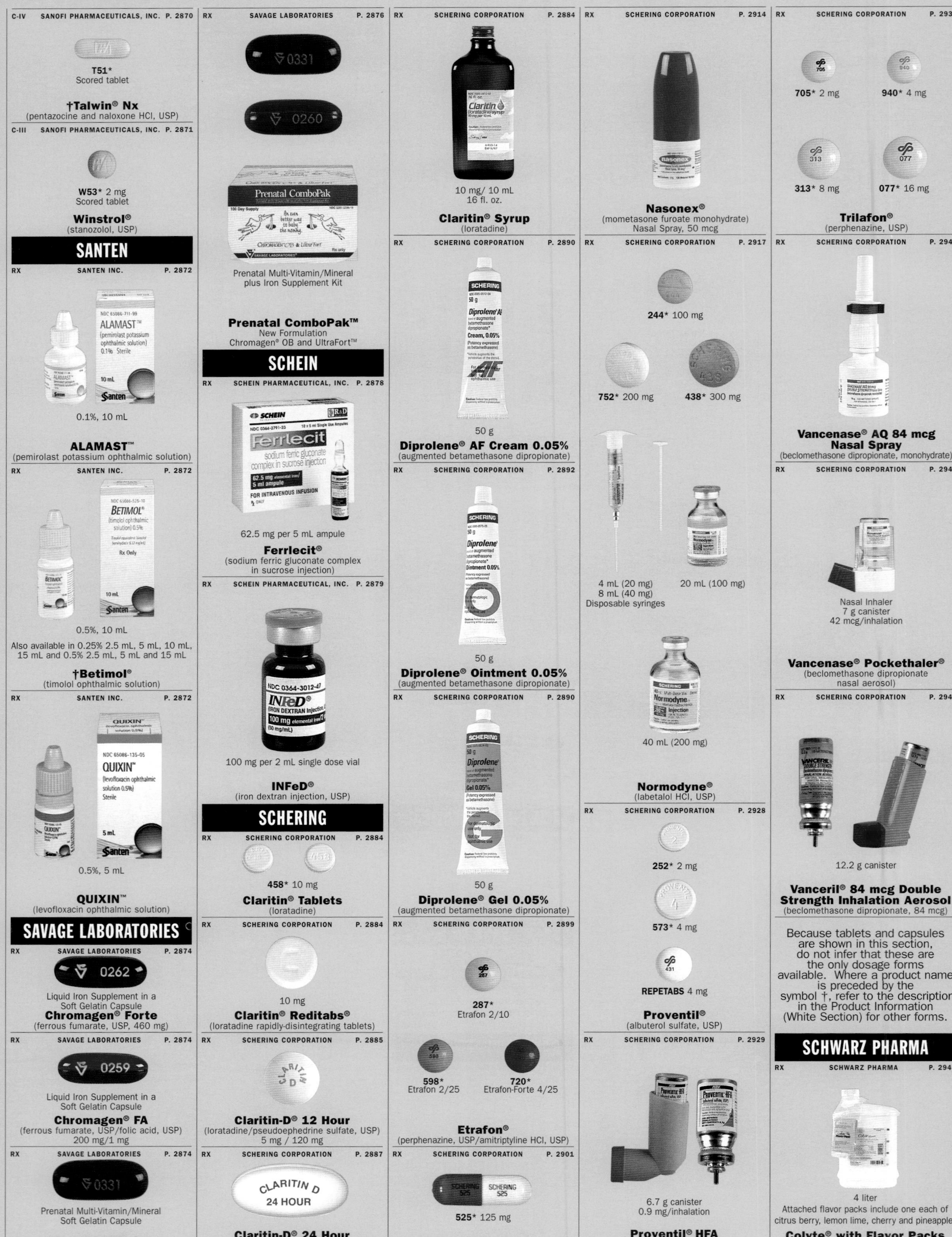

C-IV SANOFI PHARMACEUTICALS, INC. P. 2870

T51* Scored tablet

†Talwin® Nx
(pentazocine and naloxone HCl, USP)

C-III SANOFI PHARMACEUTICALS, INC. P. 2871

W53* 2 mg Scored tablet

Winstrol®
(stanozolol, USP)

SANTEN

RX SANTEN INC. P. 2872

0.1%, 10 mL

ALAMAST™
(pemirolast potassium ophthalmic solution)

RX SANTEN INC. P. 2872

0.5%, 10 mL

Also available in 0.25% 2.5 mL, 5 mL, 10 mL, 15 mL and 0.5% 2.5 mL, 5 mL and 15 mL

†Betimol®
(timolol ophthalmic solution)

RX SANTEN INC. P. 2872

0.5%, 5 mL

QUIXIN™
(levofloxacin ophthalmic solution)

SAVAGE LABORATORIES

RX SAVAGE LABORATORIES P. 2874

Liquid Iron Supplement in a Soft Gelatin Capsule

Chromagen® Forte
(ferrous fumarate, USP, 460 mg)

RX SAVAGE LABORATORIES P. 2874

Liquid Iron Supplement in a Soft Gelatin Capsule

Chromagen® FA
(ferrous fumarate, USP/folic acid, USP)
200 mg/1 mg

RX SAVAGE LABORATORIES P. 2874

Prenatal Multi-Vitamin/Mineral Soft Gelatin Capsule

New Formulation Chromagen® OB

RX SAVAGE LABORATORIES P. 2876

Prenatal Multi-Vitamin/Mineral plus Iron Supplement Kit

Prenatal ComboPak™
New Formulation
Chromagen® OB and UltraFort™

SCHEIN

RX SCHEIN PHARMACEUTICAL, INC. P. 2878

62.5 mg per 5 mL ampule

Ferrlecit®
(sodium ferric gluconate complex in sucrose injection)

RX SCHEIN PHARMACEUTICAL, INC. P. 2879

100 mg per 2 mL single dose vial

INFeD®
(iron dextran injection, USP)

SCHERING

RX SCHERING CORPORATION P. 2884

458* 10 mg

Claritin® Tablets
(loratadine)

RX SCHERING CORPORATION P. 2884

10 mg

Claritin® Reditabs®
(loratadine rapidly-disintegrating tablets)

RX SCHERING CORPORATION P. 2885

Claritin-D® 12 Hour
(loratadine/pseudoephedrine sulfate, USP)
5 mg / 120 mg

RX SCHERING CORPORATION P. 2887

Claritin-D® 24 Hour
(loratadine/pseudoephedrine sulfate, USP)
10 mg / 240 mg

RX SCHERING CORPORATION P. 2884

10 mg/ 10 mL
16 fl. oz.

Claritin® Syrup
(loratadine)

RX SCHERING CORPORATION P. 2890

50 g

Diprolene® AF Cream 0.05%
(augmented betamethasone dipropionate)

RX SCHERING CORPORATION P. 2892

50 g

Diprolene® Ointment 0.05%
(augmented betamethasone dipropionate)

RX SCHERING CORPORATION P. 2890

50 g

Diprolene® Gel 0.05%
(augmented betamethasone dipropionate)

RX SCHERING CORPORATION P. 2899

287* Etrafon 2/10

598* Etrafon 2/25

720* Etrafon-Forte 4/25

Etrafon®
(perphenazine, USP/amitriptyline HCl, USP)

RX SCHERING CORPORATION P. 2901

525* 125 mg

Eulexin® Capsules
(flutamide, USP)

RX SCHERING CORPORATION P. 2914

Nasonex®
(mometasone furoate monohydrate)
Nasal Spray, 50 mcg

RX SCHERING CORPORATION P. 2917

244* 100 mg

752* 200 mg

438* 300 mg

4 mL (20 mg)
8 mL (40 mg)
Disposable syringes

20 mL (100 mg)

40 mL (200 mg)

Normodyne®
(labetalol HCl, USP)

RX SCHERING CORPORATION P. 2928

252* 2 mg

573* 4 mg

REPETABS 4 mg

Proventil®
(albuterol sulfate, USP)

RX SCHERING CORPORATION P. 2929

6.7 g canister
0.9 mg/inhalation

Proventil® HFA Inhalation Aerosol
(albuterol sulfate)

RX SCHERING CORPORATION P. 2939

705* 2 mg

940* 4 mg

313* 8 mg

077* 16 mg

Trilafon®
(perphenazine, USP)

RX SCHERING CORPORATION P. 2942

Vancenase® AQ 84 mcg Nasal Spray
(beclomethasone dipropionate, monohydrate)

RX SCHERING CORPORATION P. 2941

Nasal Inhaler
7 g canister
42 mcg/inhalation

Vancenase® Pockethaler®
(beclomethasone dipropionate nasal aerosol)

RX SCHERING CORPORATION P. 2945

12.2 g canister

Vanceril® 84 mcg Double Strength Inhalation Aerosol
(beclomethasone dipropionate, 84 mcg)

Because tablets and capsules are shown in this section, do not infer that these are the only dosage forms available. Where a product name is preceded by the symbol †, refer to the description in the Product Information (White Section) for other forms.

SCHWARZ PHARMA

RX SCHWARZ PHARMA P. 2948

4 liter
Attached flavor packs include one each of citrus berry, lemon lime, cherry and pineapple.

Colyte® with Flavor Packs
(PEG-3350 & Electrolytes)
For Oral Solution

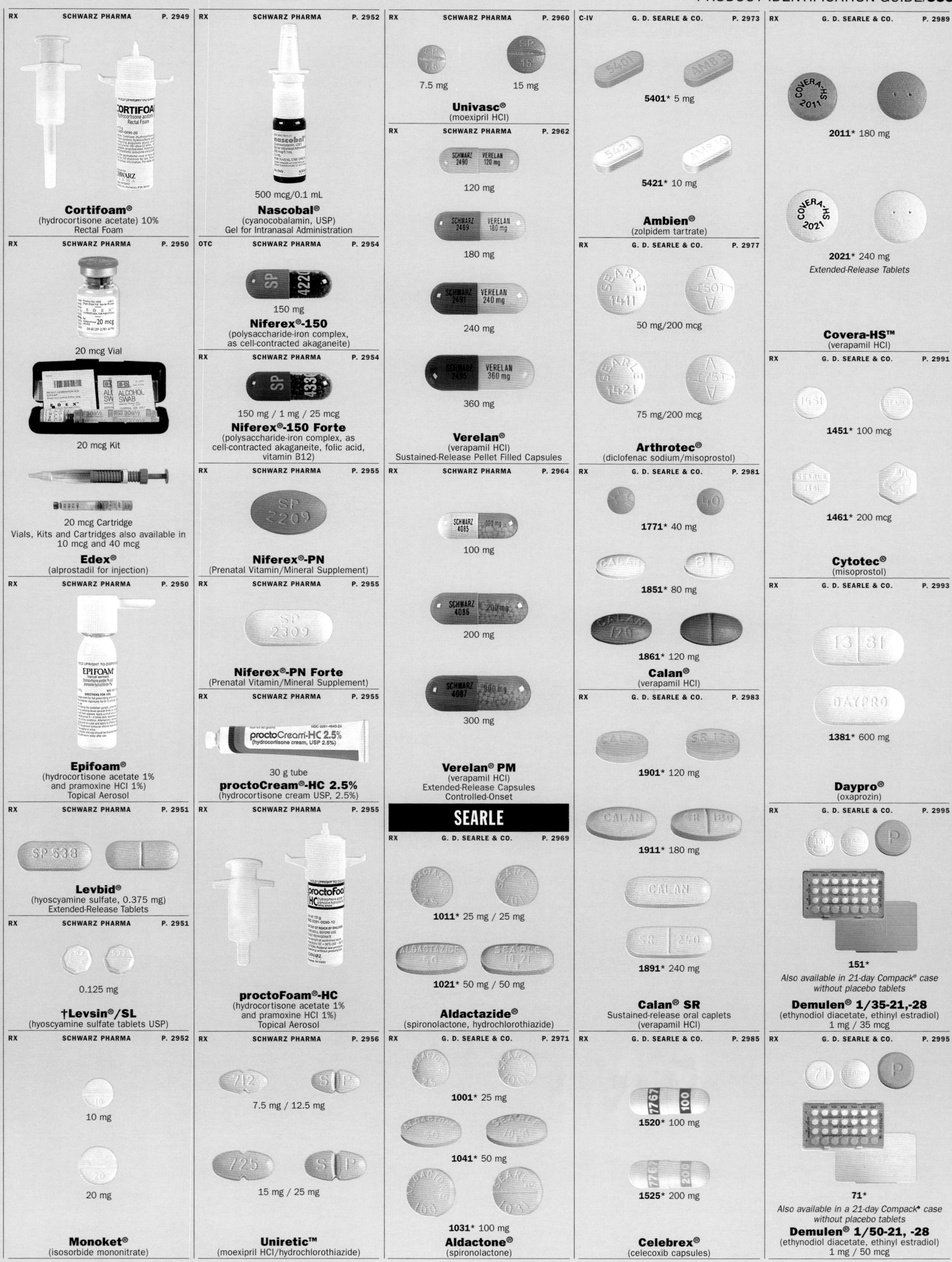

RX SCHWARZ PHARMA P. 2949
Cortifoam®
(hydrocortisone acetate) 10%
Rectal Foam
RX SCHWARZ PHARMA P. 2950
20 mcg Vial
20 mcg Kit
20 mcg Cartridge
Vials, Kits and Cartridges also available in 10 mcg and 40 mcg
Edex®
(alprostadil for injection)
RX SCHWARZ PHARMA P. 2950
Epifoam®
(hydrocortisone acetate 1% and pramoxine HCl 1%)
Topical Aerosol
RX SCHWARZ PHARMA P. 2951
Levbid®
(hyoscyamine sulfate, 0.375 mg)
Extended-Release Tablets
RX SCHWARZ PHARMA P. 2951
0.125 mg
†Levsin®/SL
(hyoscyamine sulfate tablets USP)
RX SCHWARZ PHARMA P. 2952
10 mg
20 mg
Monoket®
(isosorbide mononitrate)
RX SCHWARZ PHARMA P. 2952
500 mcg/0.1 mL
Nascobal®
(cyanocobalamin, USP)
Gel for Intranasal Administration
OTC SCHWARZ PHARMA P. 2954
150 mg
Niferex®-150
(polysaccharide-iron complex, as cell-contracted akaganeite)
RX SCHWARZ PHARMA P. 2954
150 mg / 1 mg / 25 mcg
Niferex®-150 Forte
(polysaccharide-iron complex, as cell-contracted akaganeite, folic acid, vitamin B12)
RX SCHWARZ PHARMA P. 2955
Niferex®-PN
(Prenatal Vitamin/Mineral Supplement)
RX SCHWARZ PHARMA P. 2955
Niferex®-PN Forte
(Prenatal Vitamin/Mineral Supplement)
RX SCHWARZ PHARMA P. 2955
procto Cream-HC 2.5%
30 g tube
proctoCream®-HC 2.5%
(hydrocortisone cream USP, 2.5%)
RX SCHWARZ PHARMA P. 2955
proctoFoam®-HC
(hydrocortisone acetate 1% and pramoxine HCl 1%)
Topical Aerosol
RX SCHWARZ PHARMA P. 2956
7.5 mg / 12.5 mg
15 mg / 25 mg
Uniretic™
(moexipril HCl/hydrochlorothiazide)
RX SCHWARZ PHARMA P. 2960
7.5 mg
15 mg
Univasc®
(moexipril HCl)
RX SCHWARZ PHARMA P. 2962
120 mg
180 mg
240 mg
360 mg
Verelan®
(verapamil HCl)
Sustained-Release Pellet Filled Capsules
RX SCHWARZ PHARMA P. 2964
100 mg
200 mg
300 mg
Verelan® PM
(verapamil HCl)
Extended-Release Capsules
Controlled-Onset
SEARLE
RX G. D. SEARLE & CO. P. 2969
1011* 25 mg / 25 mg
1021* 50 mg / 50 mg
Aldactazide®
(spironolactone, hydrochlorothiazide)
RX G. D. SEARLE & CO. P. 2971
1001* 25 mg
1041* 50 mg
1031* 100 mg
Aldactone®
(spironolactone)
C-IV G. D. SEARLE & CO. P. 2973
5401* 5 mg
5421* 10 mg
Ambien®
(zolpidem tartrate)
RX G. D. SEARLE & CO. P. 2977
50 mg/200 mcg
75 mg/200 mcg
Arthrotec®
(diclofenac sodium/misoprostol)
RX G. D. SEARLE & CO. P. 2981
1771* 40 mg
1851* 80 mg
1861* 120 mg
Calan®
(verapamil HCl)
RX G. D. SEARLE & CO. P. 2983
1901* 120 mg
1911* 180 mg
1891* 240 mg
Calan® SR
Sustained-release oral caplets
(verapamil HCl)
RX G. D. SEARLE & CO. P. 2985
1520* 100 mg
1525* 200 mg
Celebrex®
(celecoxib capsules)
RX G. D. SEARLE & CO. P. 2989
2011* 180 mg
2021* 240 mg
Extended-Release Tablets
Covera-HS™
(verapamil HCl)
RX G. D. SEARLE & CO. P. 2991
1451* 100 mcg
1461* 200 mcg
Cytotec®
(misoprostol)
RX G. D. SEARLE & CO. P. 2993
1381* 600 mg
Daypro®
(oxaprozin)
RX G. D. SEARLE & CO. P. 2995
151*
Also available in 21-day Compack® case without placebo tablets
Demulen® 1/35-21,-28
(ethynodiol diacetate, ethinyl estradiol)
1 mg / 35 mcg
RX G. D. SEARLE & CO. P. 2995
71*
Also available in a 21-day Compack* case without placebo tablets
Demulen® 1/50-21, -28
(ethynodiol diacetate, ethinyl estradiol)
1 mg / 50 mcg

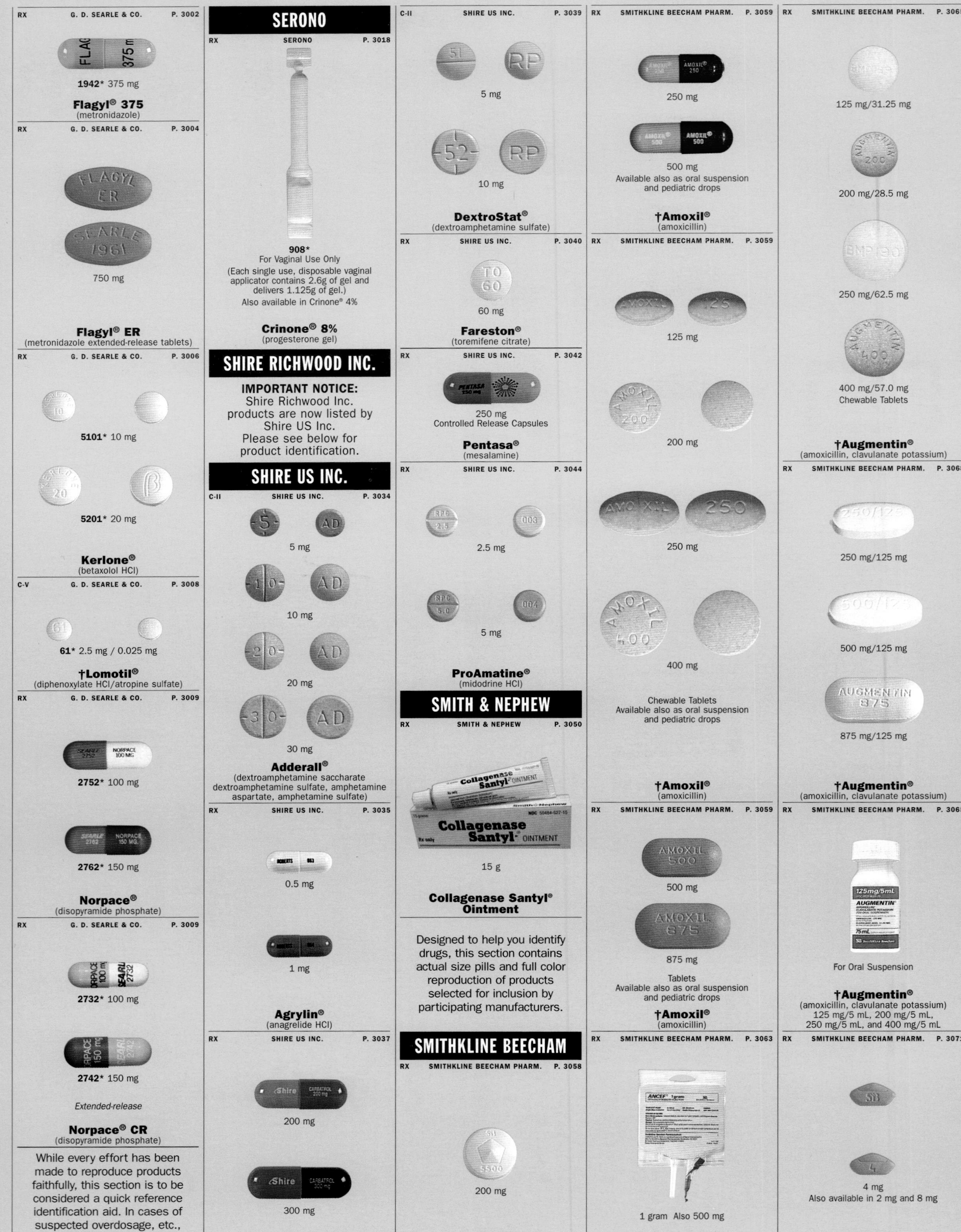
RX G. D. SEARLE & CO. P. 3002
1942* 375 mg
Flagyl® 375
(metronidazole)
RX G. D. SEARLE & CO. P. 3004
750 mg
Flagyl® ER
(metronidazole extended-release tablets)
RX G. D. SEARLE & CO. P. 3006
5101* 10 mg
5201* 20 mg
Kerlone®
(betaxolol HCl)
C-V G. D. SEARLE & CO. P. 3008
61* 2.5 mg / 0.025 mg
†Lomotil®
(diphenoxylate HCl/atropine sulfate)
RX G. D. SEARLE & CO. P. 3009
2752* 100 mg
2762* 150 mg
Norpace®
(disopyramide phosphate)
RX G. D. SEARLE & CO. P. 3009
2732* 100 mg
2742* 150 mg
Extended-release
Norpace® CR
(disopyramide phosphate)
While every effort has been made to reproduce products faithfully, this section is to be considered a quick reference identification aid. In cases of suspected overdosage, etc., chemical analysis of the product should be done.
SERONO
RX SERONO P. 3018
908*
For Vaginal Use Only
(Each single use, disposable vaginal applicator contains 2.6g of gel and delivers 1.125g of gel.)
Also available in Crinone® 4%
Crinone® 8%
(progesterone gel)
SHIRE RICHWOOD INC.
IMPORTANT NOTICE:
Shire Richwood Inc. products are now listed by Shire US Inc.
Please see below for product identification.
SHIRE US INC.
C-II SHIRE US INC. P. 3034
5 mg
10 mg
20 mg
30 mg
Adderall®
(dextroamphetamine saccharate dextroamphetamine sulfate, amphetamine aspartate, amphetamine sulfate)
RX SHIRE US INC. P. 3035
0.5 mg
1 mg
Agrylin®
(anagrelide HCl)
RX SHIRE US INC. P. 3037
200 mg
300 mg
Carbatrol®
(carbamazepine extended-release capsules)
C-II SHIRE US INC. P. 3039
5 mg
10 mg
DextroStat®
(dextroamphetamine sulfate)
RX SHIRE US INC. P. 3040
60 mg
Fareston®
(toremifene citrate)
RX SHIRE US INC. P. 3042
250 mg
Controlled Release Capsules
Pentasa®
(mesalamine)
RX SHIRE US INC. P. 3044
2.5 mg
5 mg
ProAmatine®
(midodrine HCl)
SMITH & NEPHEW
RX SMITH & NEPHEW P. 3050
Collagenase Santyl® Ointment
15 g
Collagenase Santyl® Ointment
Designed to help you identify drugs, this section contains actual size pills and full color reproduction of products selected for inclusion by participating manufacturers.
SMITHKLINE BEECHAM
RX SMITHKLINE BEECHAM PHARM. P. 3058
200 mg
Albenza™ Tiltab®
(albendazole)
RX SMITHKLINE BEECHAM PHARM. P. 3059
250 mg
500 mg
Available also as oral suspension and pediatric drops
†Amoxil®
(amoxicillin)
RX SMITHKLINE BEECHAM PHARM. P. 3059
125 mg
200 mg
250 mg
400 mg
Chewable Tablets
Available also as oral suspension and pediatric drops
†Amoxil®
(amoxicillin)
RX SMITHKLINE BEECHAM PHARM. P. 3059
500 mg
875 mg
Tablets
Available also as oral suspension and pediatric drops
†Amoxil®
(amoxicillin)
RX SMITHKLINE BEECHAM PHARM. P. 3063
1 gram Also 500 mg
Ancef®
(cefazolin for injection)
RX SMITHKLINE BEECHAM PHARM. P. 3065
125 mg/31.25 mg
200 mg/28.5 mg
250 mg/62.5 mg
400 mg/57.0 mg
Chewable Tablets
†Augmentin®
(amoxicillin, clavulanate potassium)
RX SMITHKLINE BEECHAM PHARM. P. 3068
250 mg/125 mg
500 mg/125 mg
875 mg/125 mg
†Augmentin®
(amoxicillin, clavulanate potassium)
RX SMITHKLINE BEECHAM PHARM. P. 3065
For Oral Suspension
†Augmentin®
(amoxicillin, clavulanate potassium)
125 mg/5 mL, 200 mg/5 mL, 250 mg/5 mL, and 400 mg/5 mL
RX SMITHKLINE BEECHAM PHARM. P. 3071
4 mg
Also available in 2 mg and 8 mg
Avandia®
(rosiglitazone maleate)

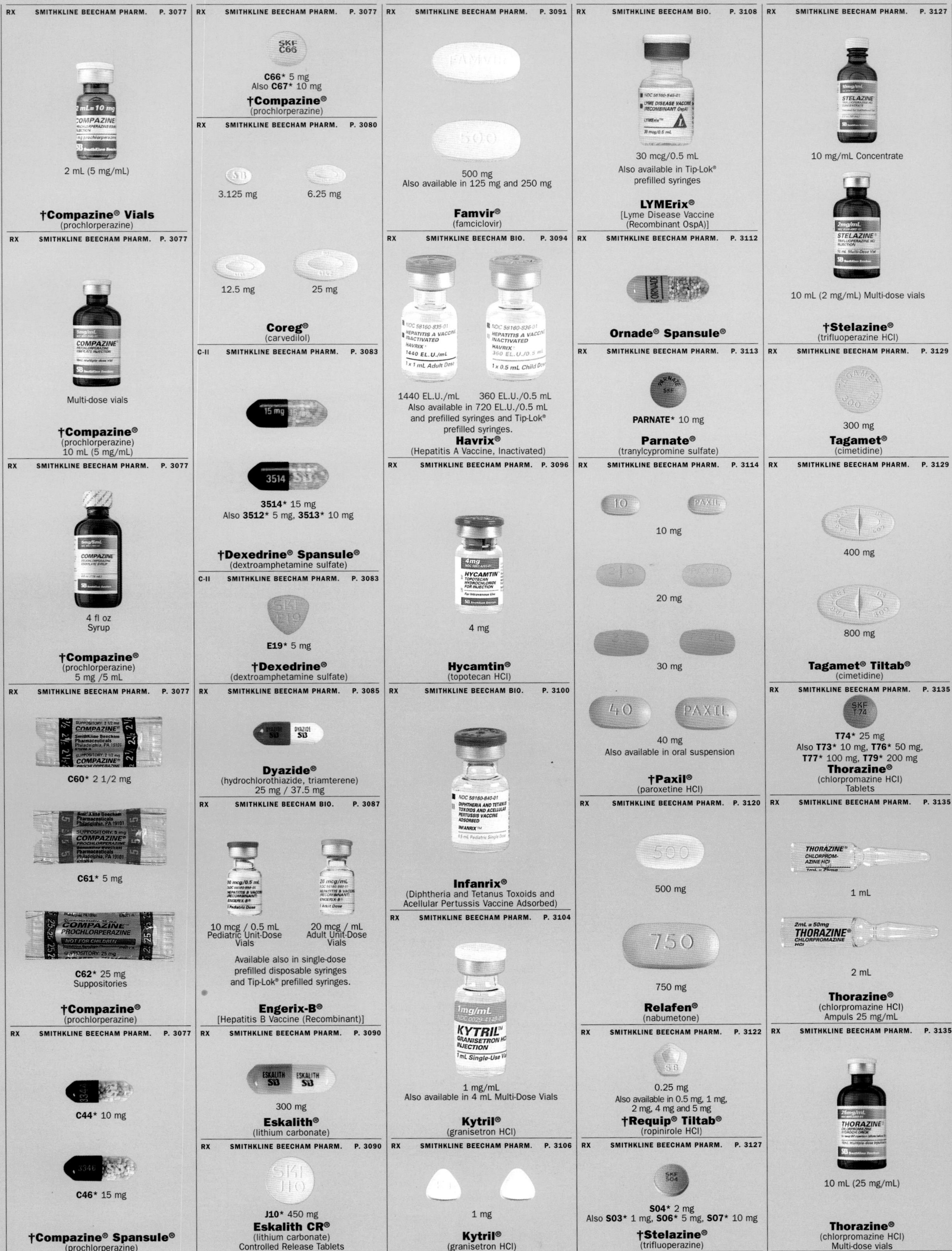
RX SMITHKLINE BEECHAM PHARM. P. 3077
2 mL (5 mg/mL)
†Compazine® Vials
(prochlorperazine)
RX SMITHKLINE BEECHAM PHARM. P. 3077
Multi-dose vials
†Compazine®
(prochlorperazine)
10 mL (5 mg/mL)
RX SMITHKLINE BEECHAM PHARM. P. 3077
4 fl oz
Syrup
†Compazine®
(prochlorperazine)
5 mg /5 mL
RX SMITHKLINE BEECHAM PHARM. P. 3077
C60* 2 1/2 mg
C61* 5 mg
C62* 25 mg
Suppositories
†Compazine®
(prochlorperazine)
RX SMITHKLINE BEECHAM PHARM. P. 3077
C44* 10 mg
C46* 15 mg
†Compazine® Spansule®
(prochlorperazine)
RX SMITHKLINE BEECHAM PHARM. P. 3077
C66* 5 mg
Also C67* 10 mg
†Compazine®
(prochlorperazine)
RX SMITHKLINE BEECHAM PHARM. P. 3080
3.125 mg
6.25 mg
12.5 mg
25 mg
Coreg®
(carvedilol)
C-II SMITHKLINE BEECHAM PHARM. P. 3083
3514* 15 mg
Also 3512* 5 mg, 3513* 10 mg
†Dexedrine® Spansule®
(dextroamphetamine sulfate)
C-II SMITHKLINE BEECHAM PHARM. P. 3083
E19* 5 mg
†Dexedrine®
(dextroamphetamine sulfate)
RX SMITHKLINE BEECHAM PHARM. P. 3085
Dyazide®
(hydrochlorothiazide, triamterene)
25 mg / 37.5 mg
RX SMITHKLINE BEECHAM BIO. P. 3087
10 mcg / 0.5 mL
Pediatric Unit-Dose
Vials
20 mcg / mL
Adult Unit-Dose
Vials
Available also in single-dose
prefilled disposable syringes
and Tip-Lok® prefilled syringes.
Engerix-B®
[Hepatitis B Vaccine (Recombinant)]
RX SMITHKLINE BEECHAM PHARM. P. 3090
300 mg
Eskalith®
(lithium carbonate)
RX SMITHKLINE BEECHAM PHARM. P. 3090
J10* 450 mg
Eskalith CR®
(lithium carbonate)
Controlled Release Tablets
RX SMITHKLINE BEECHAM PHARM. P. 3091
500 mg
Also available in 125 mg and 250 mg
Famvir®
(famciclovir)
RX SMITHKLINE BEECHAM BIO. P. 3094
1440 EL.U./mL
360 EL.U./0.5 mL
Also available in 720 EL.U./0.5 mL
and prefilled syringes and Tip-Lok®
prefilled syringes.
Havrix®
(Hepatitis A Vaccine, Inactivated)
RX SMITHKLINE BEECHAM PHARM. P. 3096
4 mg
Hycamtin®
(topotecan HCl)
RX SMITHKLINE BEECHAM BIO. P. 3100
Infanrix®
(Diphtheria and Tetanus Toxoids and
Acellular Pertussis Vaccine Adsorbed)
RX SMITHKLINE BEECHAM PHARM. P. 3104
1 mg/mL
Also available in 4 mL Multi-Dose Vials
Kytril®
(granisetron HCl)
RX SMITHKLINE BEECHAM PHARM. P. 3106
1 mg
Kytril®
(granisetron HCl)
RX SMITHKLINE BEECHAM BIO. P. 3108
30 mcg/0.5 mL
Also available in Tip-Lok®
prefilled syringes
LYMErix®
[Lyme Disease Vaccine
(Recombinant OspA)]
RX SMITHKLINE BEECHAM PHARM. P. 3112
Ornade® Spansule®
RX SMITHKLINE BEECHAM PHARM. P. 3113
PARNATE* 10 mg
Parnate®
(tranylcypromine sulfate)
RX SMITHKLINE BEECHAM PHARM. P. 3114
10 mg
20 mg
30 mg
40 mg
Also available in oral suspension
†Paxil®
(paroxetine HCl)
RX SMITHKLINE BEECHAM PHARM. P. 3120
500 mg
750 mg
Relafen®
(nabumetone)
RX SMITHKLINE BEECHAM PHARM. P. 3122
0.25 mg
Also available in 0.5 mg, 1 mg,
2 mg, 4 mg and 5 mg
†Requip® Tiltab®
(ropinirole HCl)
RX SMITHKLINE BEECHAM PHARM. P. 3127
S04* 2 mg
Also S03* 1 mg, S06* 5 mg, S07* 10 mg
†Stelazine®
(trifluoperazine)
RX SMITHKLINE BEECHAM PHARM. P. 3127
10 mg/mL Concentrate
10 mL (2 mg/mL) Multi-dose vials
†Stelazine®
(trifluoperazine HCl)
RX SMITHKLINE BEECHAM PHARM. P. 3129
300 mg
Tagamet®
(cimetidine)
RX SMITHKLINE BEECHAM PHARM. P. 3129
400 mg
800 mg
Tagamet® Tiltab®
(cimetidine)
RX SMITHKLINE BEECHAM PHARM. P. 3135
T74* 25 mg
Also T73* 10 mg, T76* 50 mg,
T77* 100 mg, T79* 200 mg
Thorazine®
(chlorpromazine HCl)
Tablets
RX SMITHKLINE BEECHAM PHARM. P. 3135
1 mL
2 mL
Thorazine®
(chlorpromazine HCl)
Ampuls 25 mg/mL
RX SMITHKLINE BEECHAM PHARM. P. 3135
10 mL (25 mg/mL)
Thorazine®
(chlorpromazine HCl)
Multi-dose vials

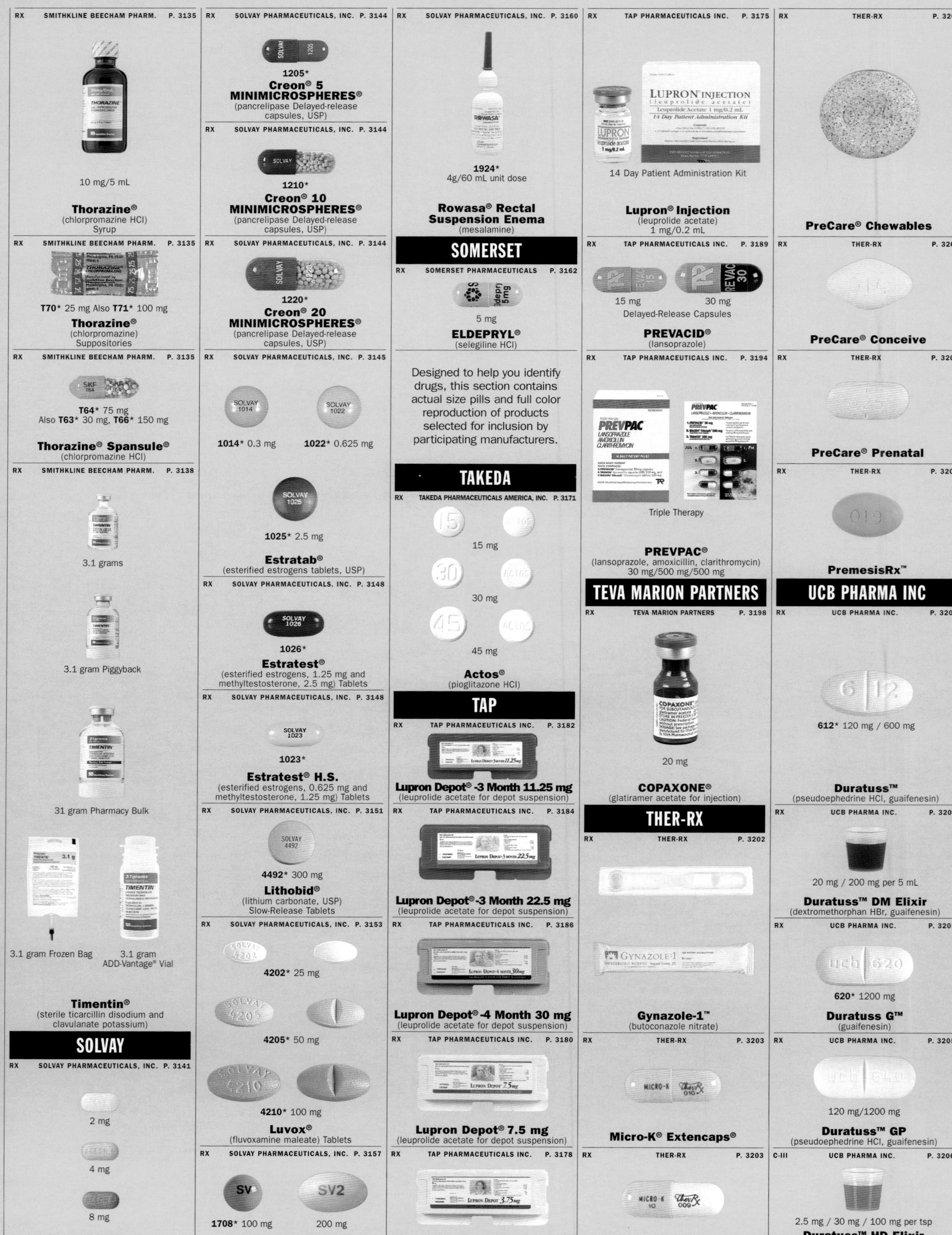
RX SMITHKLINE BEECHAM PHARM. P. 3135
10 mg/5 mL
Thorazine®
(chlorpromazine HCl)
Syrup
RX SMITHKLINE BEECHAM PHARM. P. 3135
T70* 25 mg Also T71* 100 mg
Thorazine®
(chlorpromazine)
Suppositories
RX SMITHKLINE BEECHAM PHARM. P. 3135
T64* 75 mg
Also T63* 30 mg, T66* 150 mg
Thorazine® Spansule®
(chlorpromazine HCl)
RX SMITHKLINE BEECHAM PHARM. P. 3138
3.1 grams
3.1 gram Piggyback
31 gram Pharmacy Bulk
3.1 gram Frozen Bag
3.1 gram ADD-Vantage® Vial
Timentin®
(sterile ticarcillin disodium and clavulanate potassium)
SOLVAY
RX SOLVAY PHARMACEUTICALS, INC. P. 3141
2 mg
4 mg
8 mg
Aceon®
(perindopril erbumine)
RX SOLVAY PHARMACEUTICALS, INC. P. 3144
1205*
Creon® 5 MINIMICROSPHERES®
(pancrelipase Delayed-release capsules, USP)
RX SOLVAY PHARMACEUTICALS, INC. P. 3144
1210*
Creon® 10 MINIMICROSPHERES®
(pancrelipase Delayed-release capsules, USP)
RX SOLVAY PHARMACEUTICALS, INC. P. 3144
1220*
Creon® 20 MINIMICROSPHERES®
(pancrelipase Delayed-release capsules, USP)
RX SOLVAY PHARMACEUTICALS, INC. P. 3145
1014* 0.3 mg
1022* 0.625 mg
1025* 2.5 mg
Estratab®
(esterified estrogens tablets, USP)
RX SOLVAY PHARMACEUTICALS, INC. P. 3148
1026*
Estratest®
(esterified estrogens, 1.25 mg and methyltestosterone, 2.5 mg) Tablets
RX SOLVAY PHARMACEUTICALS, INC. P. 3148
1023*
Estratest® H.S.
(esterified estrogens, 0.625 mg and methyltestosterone, 1.25 mg) Tablets
RX SOLVAY PHARMACEUTICALS, INC. P. 3151
4492* 300 mg
Lithobid®
(lithium carbonate, USP)
Slow-Release Tablets
RX SOLVAY PHARMACEUTICALS, INC. P. 3153
4202* 25 mg
4205* 50 mg
4210* 100 mg
Luvox®
(fluvoxamine maleate) Tablets
RX SOLVAY PHARMACEUTICALS, INC. P. 3157
1708* 100 mg
200 mg
Prometrium®
(progesterone, USP) Capsules
RX SOLVAY PHARMACEUTICALS, INC. P. 3160
1924*
4g/60 mL unit dose
Rowasa® Rectal Suspension Enema
(mesalamine)
SOMERSET
RX SOMERSET PHARMACEUTICALS P. 3162
5 mg
ELDEPRYL®
(selegiline HCl)
Designed to help you identify drugs, this section contains actual size pills and full color reproduction of products selected for inclusion by participating manufacturers.
TAKEDA
RX TAKEDA PHARMACEUTICALS AMERICA, INC. P. 3171
15 mg
30 mg
45 mg
Actos®
(pioglitazone HCl)
TAP
RX TAP PHARMACEUTICALS INC. P. 3182
Lupron Depot® -3 Month 11.25 mg
(leuprolide acetate for depot suspension)
RX TAP PHARMACEUTICALS INC. P. 3184
Lupron Depot®-3 Month 22.5 mg
(leuprolide acetate for depot suspension)
RX TAP PHARMACEUTICALS INC. P. 3186
Lupron Depot®-4 Month 30 mg
(leuprolide acetate for depot suspension)
RX TAP PHARMACEUTICALS INC. P. 3180
Lupron Depot® 7.5 mg
(leuprolide acetate for depot suspension)
RX TAP PHARMACEUTICALS INC. P. 3178
Lupron Depot® 3.75 mg
(leuprolide acetate for depot suspension)
RX TAP PHARMACEUTICALS INC. P. 3175
14 Day Patient Administration Kit
Lupron® Injection
(leuprolide acetate)
1 mg/0.2 mL
RX TAP PHARMACEUTICALS INC. P. 3189
15 mg
30 mg
Delayed-Release Capsules
PREVACID®
(lansoprazole)
RX TAP PHARMACEUTICALS INC. P. 3194
Triple Therapy
PREVPAC®
(lansoprazole, amoxicillin, clarithromycin)
30 mg/500 mg/500 mg
TEVA MARION PARTNERS
RX TEVA MARION PARTNERS P. 3198
20 mg
COPAXONE®
(glatiramer acetate for injection)
THER-RX
RX THER-RX P. 3202
Gynazole-1™
(butoconazole nitrate)
RX THER-RX P. 3203
Micro-K® Extencaps®
RX THER-RX P. 3203
Micro-K® 10 Extencaps®
RX THER-RX P. 3204
PreCare® Chewables
RX THER-RX P. 3204
PreCare® Conceive
RX THER-RX P. 3204
PreCare® Prenatal
RX THER-RX P. 3205
PremesisRx™
UCB PHARMA INC
RX UCB PHARMA INC. P. 3205
612* 120 mg / 600 mg
Duratuss™
(pseudoephedrine HCl, guaifenesin)
RX UCB PHARMA INC. P. 3206
20 mg / 200 mg per 5 mL
Duratuss™ DM Elixir
(dextromethorphan HBr, guaifenesin)
RX UCB PHARMA INC. P. 3205
620* 1200 mg
Duratuss G™
(guaifenesin)
RX UCB PHARMA INC. P. 3205
120 mg/1200 mg
Duratuss™ GP
(pseudoephedrine HCl, guaifenesin)
C-III UCB PHARMA INC. P. 3206
2.5 mg / 30 mg / 100 mg per tsp
Duratuss™ HD Elixir
(hydrocodone bitartrate, pseudoephedrine HCl, guaifenesin)

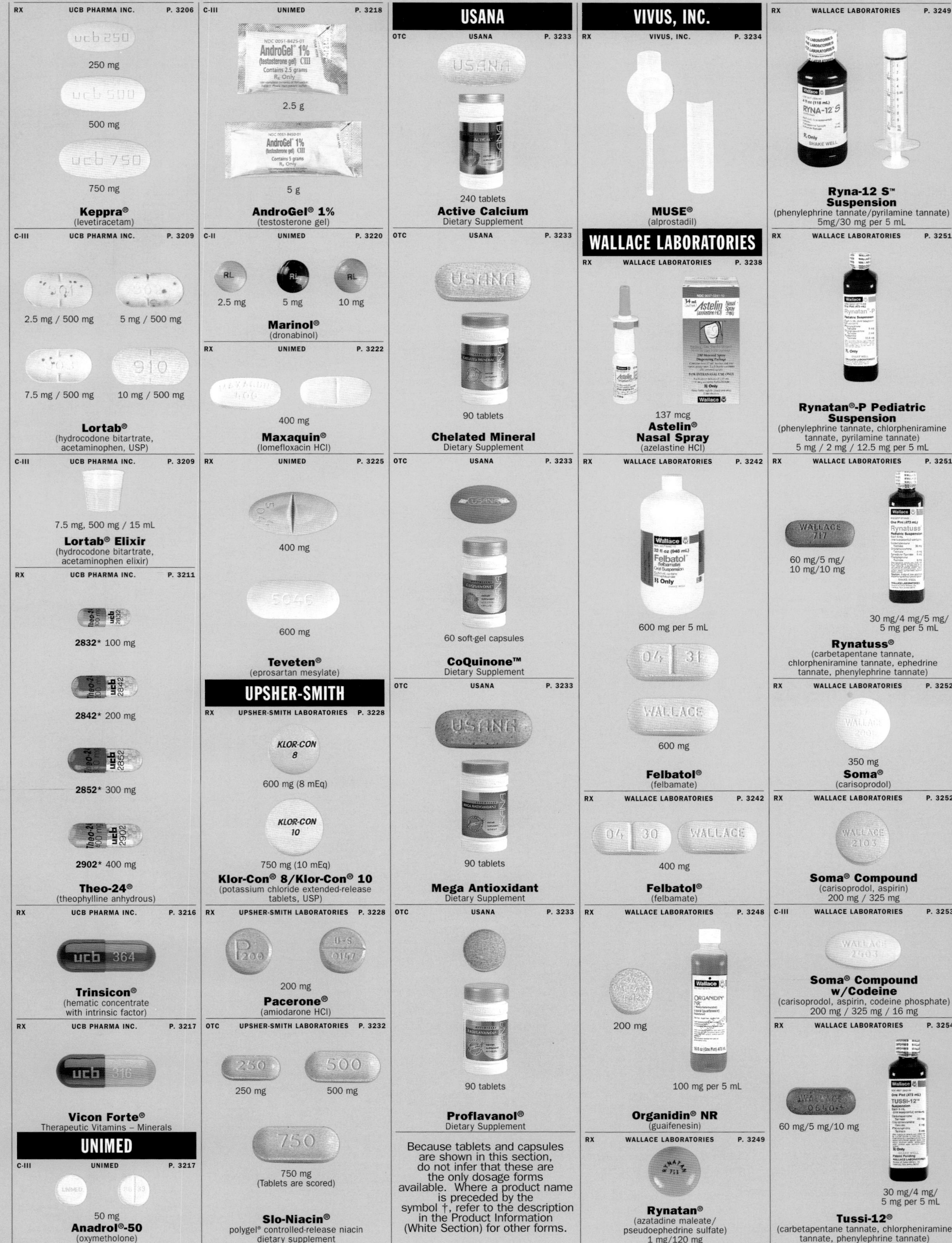

RX UCB PHARMA INC. P. 3206

250 mg

500 mg

750 mg

Keppra®
(levetiracetam)

C-III UCB PHARMA INC. P. 3209

2.5 mg / 500 mg
5 mg / 500 mg
7.5 mg / 500 mg
10 mg / 500 mg

Lortab®
(hydrocodone bitartrate, acetaminophen, USP)

C-III UCB PHARMA INC. P. 3209

7.5 mg, 500 mg / 15 mL

Lortab® Elixir
(hydrocodone bitartrate, acetaminophen elixir)

RX UCB PHARMA INC. P. 3211

2832* 100 mg

2842* 200 mg

2852* 300 mg

2902* 400 mg

Theo-24®
(theophylline anhydrous)

RX UCB PHARMA INC. P. 3216

Trinsicon®
(hematic concentrate with intrinsic factor)

RX UCB PHARMA INC. P. 3217

Vicon Forte®
Therapeutic Vitamins – Minerals

UNIMED

C-III UNIMED P. 3217

50 mg

Anadrol®-50
(oxymetholone)

C-III UNIMED P. 3218

2.5 g

5 g

AndroGel® 1%
(testosterone gel)

C-II UNIMED P. 3220

2.5 mg
5 mg
10 mg

Marinol®
(dronabinol)

RX UNIMED P. 3222

400 mg

Maxaquin®
(lomefloxacin HCl)

RX UNIMED P. 3225

400 mg

600 mg

Teveten®
(eprosartan mesylate)

UPSHER-SMITH

RX UPSHER-SMITH LABORATORIES P. 3228

600 mg (8 mEq)

750 mg (10 mEq)

Klor-Con® 8/Klor-Con® 10
(potassium chloride extended-release tablets, USP)

RX UPSHER-SMITH LABORATORIES P. 3228

200 mg

Pacerone®
(amiodarone HCl)

OTC UPSHER-SMITH LABORATORIES P. 3232

250 mg
500 mg

750 mg
(Tablets are scored)

Slo-Niacin®
polygel® controlled-release niacin dietary supplement

USANA

OTC USANA P. 3233

240 tablets

Active Calcium
Dietary Supplement

OTC USANA P. 3233

90 tablets

Chelated Mineral
Dietary Supplement

OTC USANA P. 3233

60 soft-gel capsules

CoQuinone™
Dietary Supplement

OTC USANA P. 3233

90 tablets

Mega Antioxidant
Dietary Supplement

OTC USANA P. 3233

90 tablets

Proflavanol®
Dietary Supplement

Because tablets and capsules are shown in this section, do not infer that these are the only dosage forms available. Where a product name is preceded by the symbol †, refer to the description in the Product Information (White Section) for other forms.

VIVUS, INC.

RX VIVUS, INC. P. 3234

MUSE®
(alprostadil)

WALLACE LABORATORIES

RX WALLACE LABORATORIES P. 3238

137 mcg

Astelin®
Nasal Spray
(azelastine HCl)

RX WALLACE LABORATORIES P. 3242

600 mg per 5 mL

600 mg

Felbatol®
(felbamate)

RX WALLACE LABORATORIES P. 3242

400 mg

Felbatol®
(felbamate)

RX WALLACE LABORATORIES P. 3248

200 mg

100 mg per 5 mL

Organidin® NR
(guaifenesin)

RX WALLACE LABORATORIES P. 3249

Rynatan®
(azatadine maleate/pseudoephedrine sulfate)
1 mg/120 mg

RX WALLACE LABORATORIES P. 3249

Ryna-12 S™
Suspension
(phenylephrine tannate/pyrilamine tannate)
5mg/30 mg per 5 mL

RX WALLACE LABORATORIES P. 3251

Rynatan®-P Pediatric Suspension
(phenylephrine tannate, chlorpheniramine tannate, pyrilamine tannate)
5 mg / 2 mg / 12.5 mg per 5 mL

RX WALLACE LABORATORIES P. 3251

60 mg/5 mg/
10 mg/10 mg

30 mg/4 mg/5 mg/
5 mg per 5 mL

Rynatuss®
(carbetapentane tannate, chlorpheniramine tannate, ephedrine tannate, phenylephrine tannate)

RX WALLACE LABORATORIES P. 3252

350 mg

Soma®
(carisoprodol)

RX WALLACE LABORATORIES P. 3252

Soma® Compound
(carisoprodol, aspirin)
200 mg / 325 mg

C-III WALLACE LABORATORIES P. 3253

Soma® Compound w/Codeine
(carisoprodol, aspirin, codeine phosphate)
200 mg / 325 mg / 16 mg

RX WALLACE LABORATORIES P. 3254

60 mg/5 mg/10 mg

30 mg/4 mg/
5 mg per 5 mL

Tussi-12®
(carbetapentane tannate, chlorpheniramine tannate, phenylephrine tannate)

C-V WALLACE LABORATORIES P. 3248

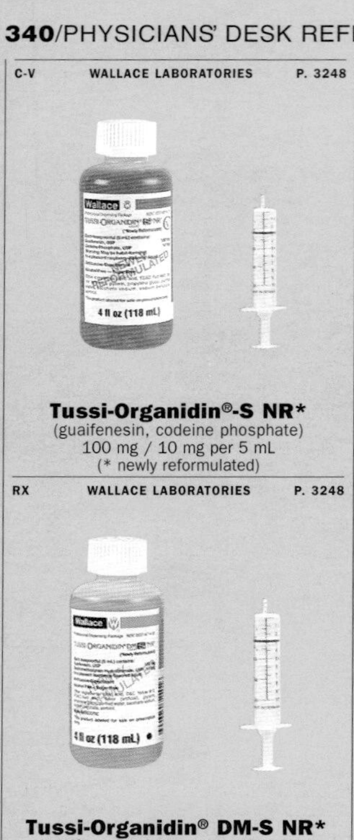

Tussi-Organidin®-S NR*
(guaifenesin, codeine phosphate)
100 mg / 10 mg per 5 mL
(* newly reformulated)

RX WALLACE LABORATORIES P. 3248

Tussi-Organidin® DM-S NR*
(guaifenesin, dextromethorphan HBr)
100 mg / 10 mg per 5 mL
(* newly reformulated)

While every effort has been made to reproduce products faithfully, this section is to be considered a quick reference identification aid. In cases of suspected overdosage, etc., chemical analysis of the product should be done.

WATSON

RX WATSON LABORATORIES INC. P. 3276

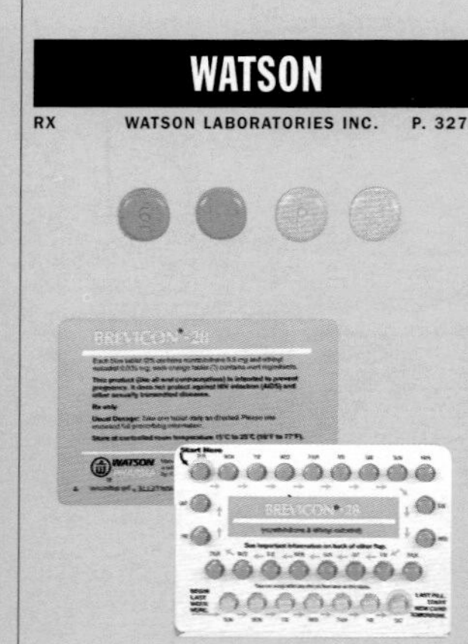

Each blue tablet (21) contains norethindrone 0.5 mg and ethinyl estradiol 0.035 mg; each orange tablet (7) contains inert ingredients

Brevicon® - 28

RX WATSON LABORATORIES INC. P. 3282

Also available in a 21 day unit without placebo tablets.

Levora®
(levonorgestrel 0.15 mg and ethinyl estradiol 0.03 mg)

RX WATSON LABORATORIES INC. P. 3285

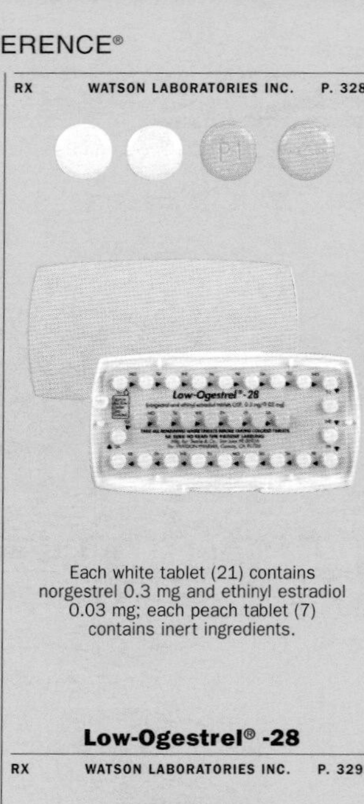

Each white tablet (21) contains norgestrel 0.3 mg and ethinyl estradiol 0.03 mg; each peach tablet (7) contains inert ingredients.

Low-Ogestrel® -28

RX WATSON LABORATORIES INC. P. 3291

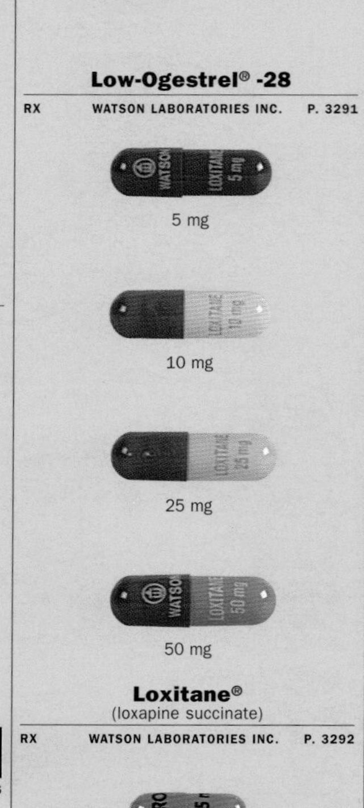

5 mg

10 mg

25 mg

50 mg

Loxitane®
(loxapine succinate)

RX WATSON LABORATORIES INC. P. 3292

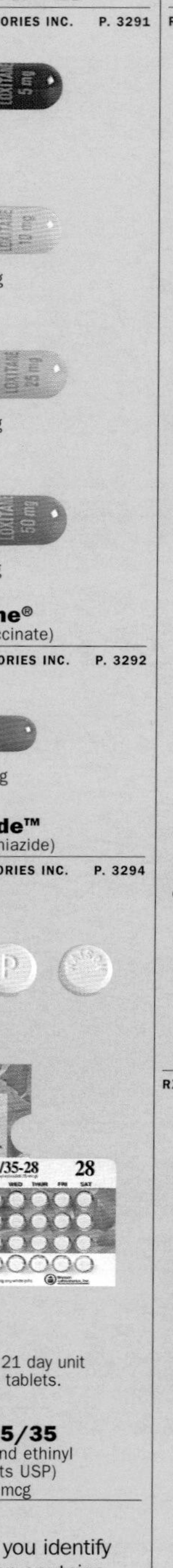

12.5 mg

Microzide™
(hydrochlorothiazide)

RX WATSON LABORATORIES INC. P. 3294

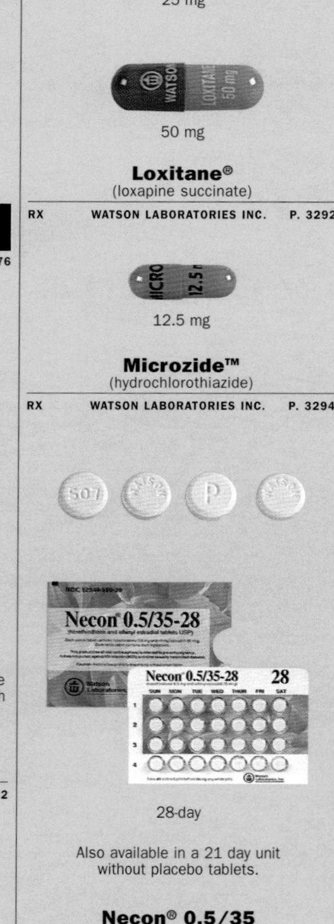

28-day

Also available in a 21 day unit without placebo tablets.

Necon® 0.5/35
(norethindrone and ethinyl estradiol tablets USP)
0.5 mg/35 mcg

Designed to help you identify drugs, this section contains actual size pills and full color reproduction of products selected for inclusion by participating manufacturers.

RX WATSON LABORATORIES INC. P. 3294

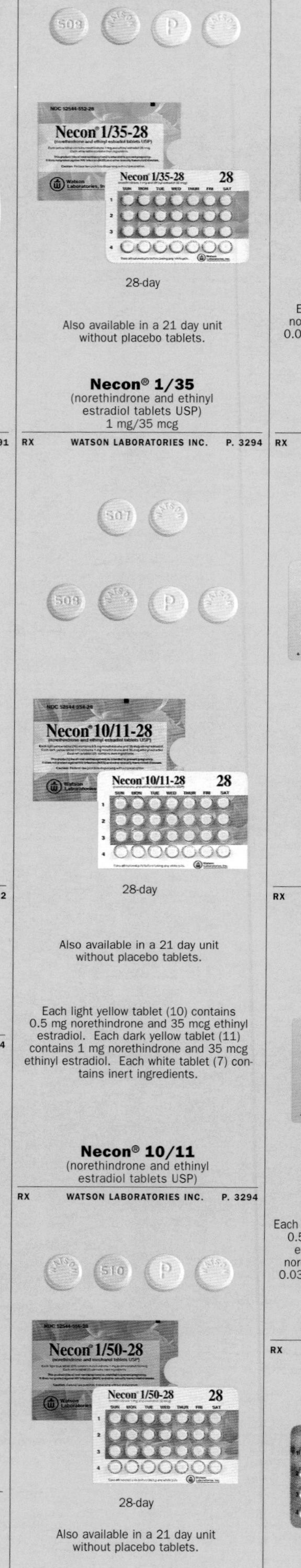

28-day

Also available in a 21 day unit without placebo tablets.

Necon® 1/35
(norethindrone and ethinyl estradiol tablets USP)
1 mg/35 mcg

RX WATSON LABORATORIES INC. P. 3294

28-day

Also available in a 21 day unit without placebo tablets.

Each light yellow tablet (10) contains 0.5 mg norethindrone and 35 mcg ethinyl estradiol. Each dark yellow tablet (11) contains 1 mg norethindrone and 35 mcg ethinyl estradiol. Each white tablet (7) contains inert ingredients.

Necon® 10/11
(norethindrone and ethinyl estradiol tablets USP)

RX WATSON LABORATORIES INC. P. 3294

28-day

Also available in a 21 day unit without placebo tablets.

Necon® 1/50
(norethindrone and mestranol tablets USP)
1 mg/50 mcg

RX WATSON LABORATORIES INC. P. 3276

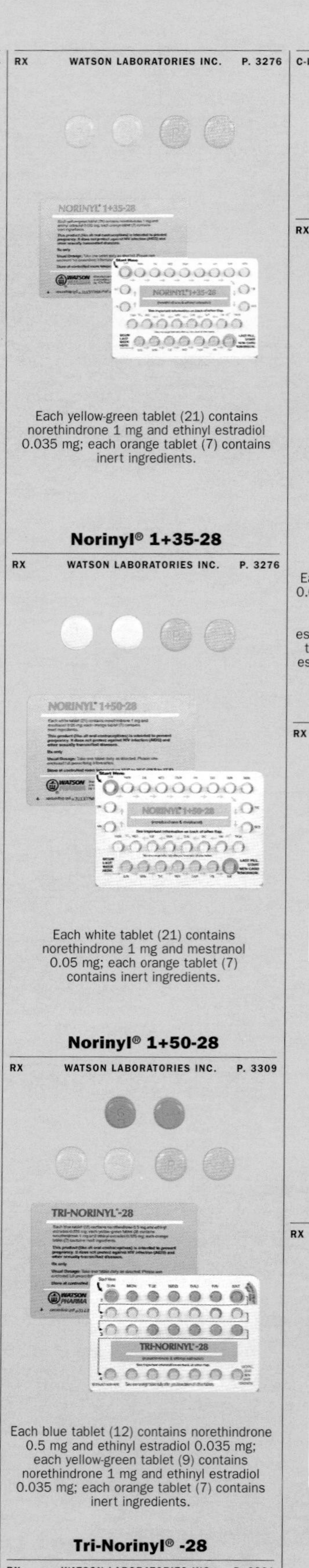

Each yellow-green tablet (21) contains norethindrone 1 mg and ethinyl estradiol 0.035 mg; each orange tablet (7) contains inert ingredients.

Norinyl® 1+35-28

RX WATSON LABORATORIES INC. P. 3276

Each white tablet (21) contains norethindrone 1 mg and mestranol 0.05 mg; each orange tablet (7) contains inert ingredients.

Norinyl® 1+50-28

RX WATSON LABORATORIES INC. P. 3309

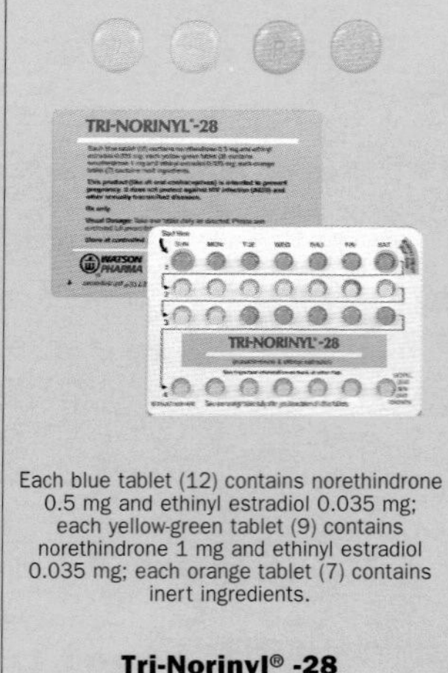

Each blue tablet (12) contains norethindrone 0.5 mg and ethinyl estradiol 0.035 mg; each yellow-green tablet (9) contains norethindrone 1 mg and ethinyl estradiol 0.035 mg; each orange tablet (7) contains inert ingredients.

Tri-Norinyl® -28

RX WATSON LABORATORIES INC. P. 3301

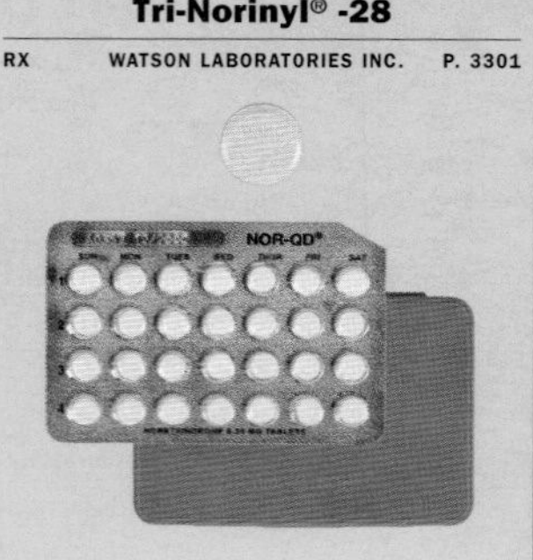

Nor-QD®
(norethindrone)
0.35 mg

C-III WATSON LABORATORIES INC. P. 3303

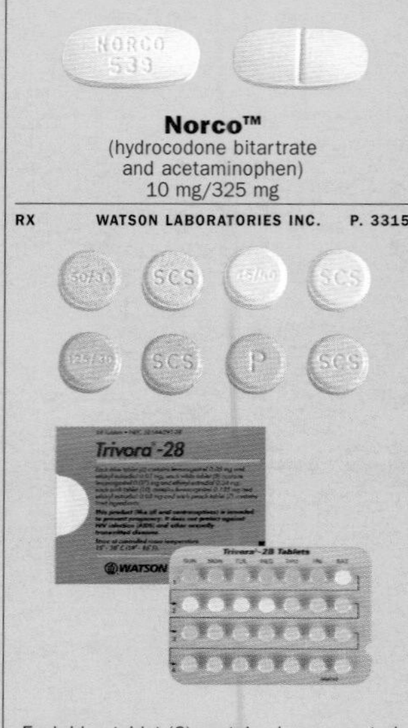

Norco™
(hydrocodone bitartrate and acetaminophen)
10 mg/325 mg

RX WATSON LABORATORIES INC. P. 3315

Each blue tablet (6) contains levonorgestrel 0.05 mg and ethinyl estradiol 0.03 mg, each white tablet (5) contains levonorgestrel 0.075 mg and ethinyl estradiol 0.04 mg, each pink tablet (10) contains levonorgestrel 0.125 mg and ethinyl estradiol 0.03 mg and each peach tablet (7) contains inert ingredients.

Trivora® -28
(levonorgestrel and ethinyl estradiol)

RX WATSON LABORATORIES INC. P. 3318

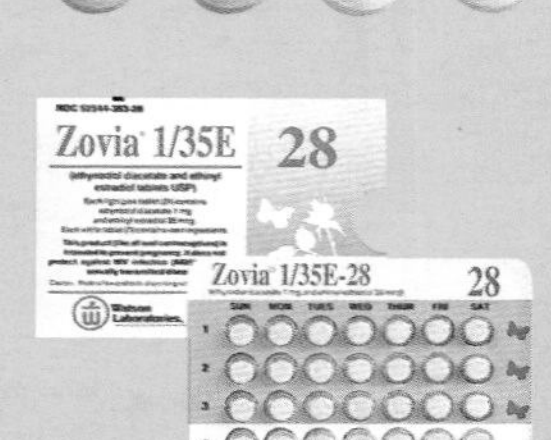

28-day

Also available in a 21 day unit without placebo tablets.

Zovia™ 1/35E
(ethynodiol diacetate and ethinyl estradiol tablets USP)
1 mg/35 mcg

RX WATSON LABORATORIES INC. P. 3318

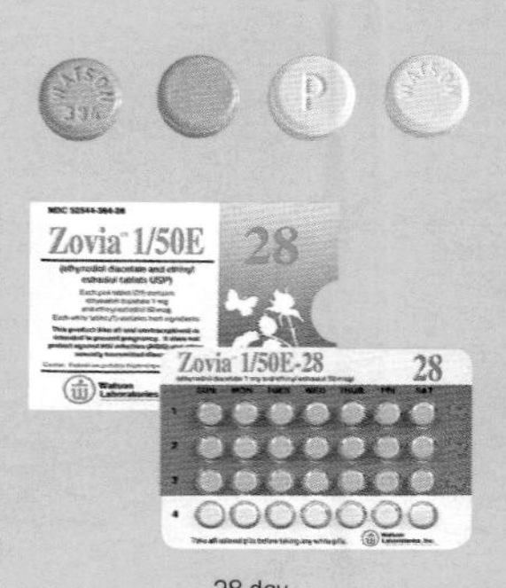

28-day

Also available in a 21 day unit without placebo tablets.

Zovia™ 1/50E
(ethynodiol diacetate and ethinyl estradiol tablets USP)

Because tablets and capsules are shown in this section, do not infer that these are the only dosage forms available. Where a product name is preceded by the symbol †, refer to the description in the Product Information (White Section) for other forms.

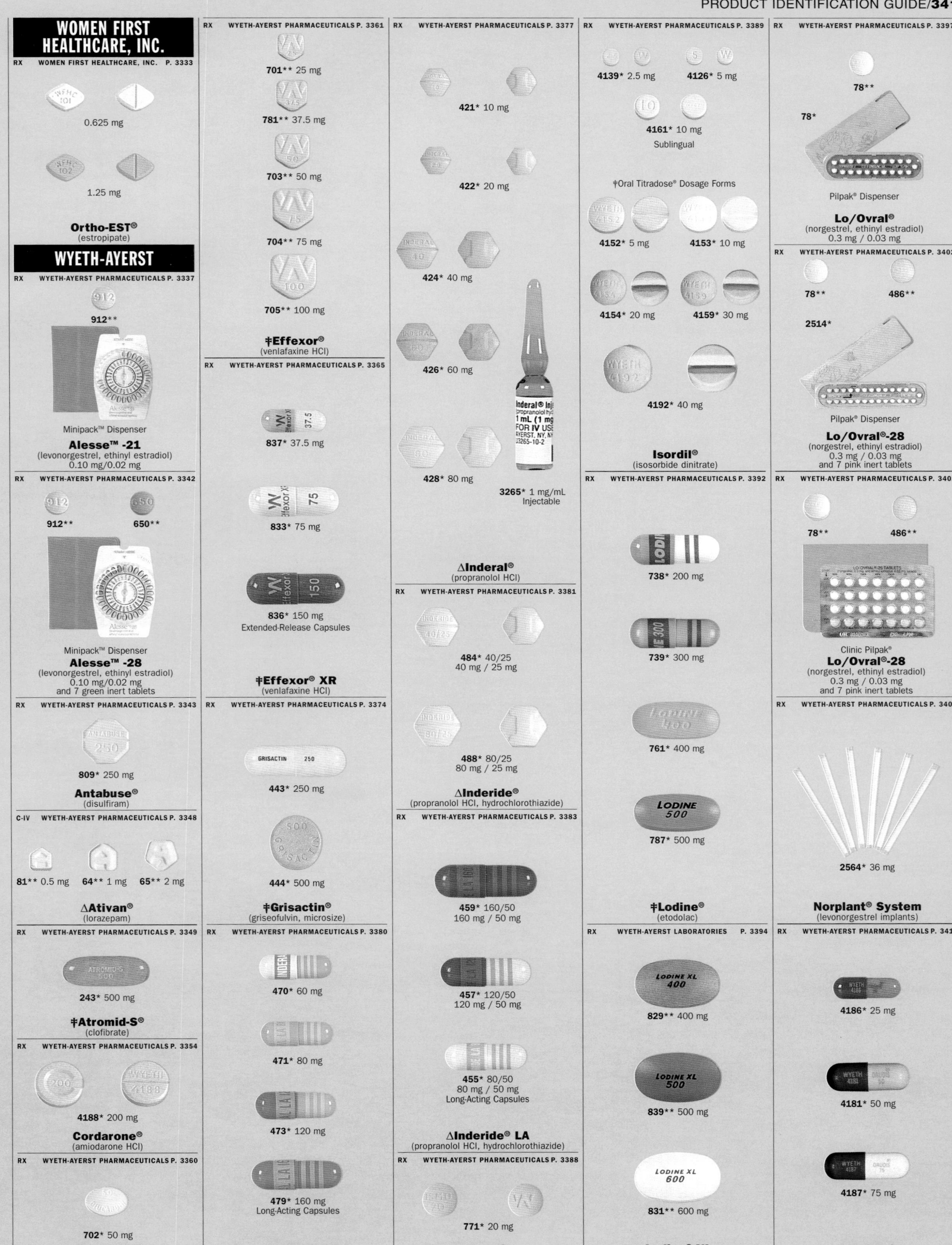
WOMEN FIRST HEALTHCARE, INC.
RX WOMEN FIRST HEALTHCARE, INC. P. 3333
0.625 mg
1.25 mg
Ortho-EST®
(estropipate)
WYETH-AYERST
RX WYETH-AYERST PHARMACEUTICALS P. 3337
912**
Minipack™ Dispenser
Alesse™ -21
(levonorgestrel, ethinyl estradiol)
0.10 mg/0.02 mg
RX WYETH-AYERST PHARMACEUTICALS P. 3342
912**
650**
Minipack™ Dispenser
Alesse™ -28
(levonorgestrel, ethinyl estradiol)
0.10 mg/0.02 mg
and 7 green inert tablets
RX WYETH-AYERST PHARMACEUTICALS P. 3343
809* 250 mg
Antabuse®
(disulfiram)
C-IV WYETH-AYERST PHARMACEUTICALS P. 3348
81** 0.5 mg
64** 1 mg
65** 2 mg
ΔAtivan®
(lorazepam)
RX WYETH-AYERST PHARMACEUTICALS P. 3349
243* 500 mg
†Atromid-S®
(clofibrate)
RX WYETH-AYERST PHARMACEUTICALS P. 3354
4188* 200 mg
Cordarone®
(amiodarone HCl)
RX WYETH-AYERST PHARMACEUTICALS P. 3360
702* 50 mg
Diucardin®
(hydroflumethiazide)
RX WYETH-AYERST PHARMACEUTICALS P. 3361
701** 25 mg
781** 37.5 mg
703** 50 mg
704** 75 mg
705** 100 mg
†Effexor®
(venlafaxine HCl)
RX WYETH-AYERST PHARMACEUTICALS P. 3365
837* 37.5 mg
833* 75 mg
836* 150 mg
Extended-Release Capsules
†Effexor® XR
(venlafaxine HCl)
RX WYETH-AYERST PHARMACEUTICALS P. 3374
443* 250 mg
444* 500 mg
†Grisactin®
(griseofulvin, microsize)
RX WYETH-AYERST PHARMACEUTICALS P. 3380
470* 60 mg
471* 80 mg
473* 120 mg
479* 160 mg
Long-Acting Capsules
ΔInderal® LA
(propranolol HCl)
RX WYETH-AYERST PHARMACEUTICALS P. 3377
421* 10 mg
422* 20 mg
424* 40 mg
426* 60 mg
428* 80 mg
3265* 1 mg/mL
Injectable
ΔInderal®
(propranolol HCl)
RX WYETH-AYERST PHARMACEUTICALS P. 3381
484* 40/25
40 mg / 25 mg
488* 80/25
80 mg / 25 mg
ΔInderide®
(propranolol HCl, hydrochlorothiazide)
RX WYETH-AYERST PHARMACEUTICALS P. 3383
459* 160/50
160 mg / 50 mg
457* 120/50
120 mg / 50 mg
455* 80/50
80 mg / 50 mg
Long-Acting Capsules
ΔInderide® LA
(propranolol HCl, hydrochlorothiazide)
RX WYETH-AYERST PHARMACEUTICALS P. 3388
771* 20 mg
Ismo®
(isosorbide mononitrate)
RX WYETH-AYERST PHARMACEUTICALS P. 3389
4139* 2.5 mg
4126* 5 mg
4161* 10 mg
Sublingual
†Oral Titradose® Dosage Forms
4152* 5 mg
4153* 10 mg
4154* 20 mg
4159* 30 mg
4192* 40 mg
Isordil®
(isosorbide dinitrate)
RX WYETH-AYERST PHARMACEUTICALS P. 3392
738* 200 mg
739* 300 mg
761* 400 mg
787* 500 mg
†Lodine®
(etodolac)
RX WYETH-AYERST LABORATORIES P. 3394
829** 400 mg
839** 500 mg
831** 600 mg
Lodine® XL
(etodolac extended-release tablets)
RX WYETH-AYERST PHARMACEUTICALS P. 3397
78**
78*
Pilpak® Dispenser
Lo/Ovral®
(norgestrel, ethinyl estradiol)
0.3 mg / 0.03 mg
RX WYETH-AYERST PHARMACEUTICALS P. 3402
78**
486**
2514*
Pilpak® Dispenser
Lo/Ovral®-28
(norgestrel, ethinyl estradiol)
0.3 mg / 0.03 mg
and 7 pink inert tablets
RX WYETH-AYERST PHARMACEUTICALS P. 3402
78**
486**
Clinic Pilpak®
Lo/Ovral®-28
(norgestrel, ethinyl estradiol)
0.3 mg / 0.03 mg
and 7 pink inert tablets
RX WYETH-AYERST PHARMACEUTICALS P. 3407
2564* 36 mg
Norplant® System
(levonorgestrel implants)
RX WYETH-AYERST PHARMACEUTICALS P. 3411
4186* 25 mg
4181* 50 mg
4187* 75 mg
†Orudis®
(ketoprofen)

† The appearance of these tablets and capsules is a trademark of Wyeth-Ayerst Laboratories.
**Product identification number on reverse side

Δ The appearance of these tablets and capsules is a registered trademark of Wyeth-Ayerst Laboratories.

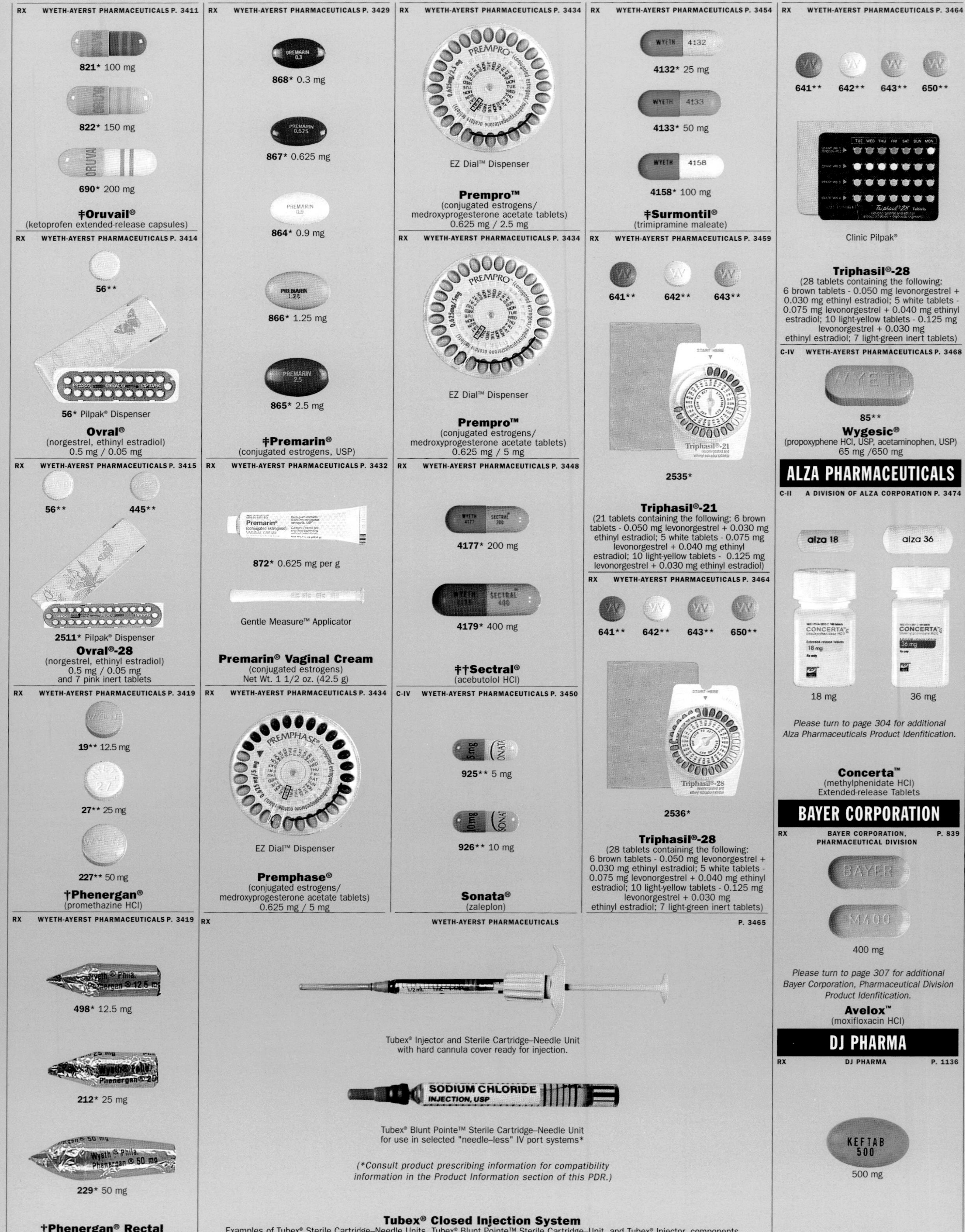

RX WYETH-AYERST PHARMACEUTICALS P. 3411

821* 100 mg

822* 150 mg

690* 200 mg

†Oruvail®
(ketoprofen extended-release capsules)

RX WYETH-AYERST PHARMACEUTICALS P. 3414

56**

56* Pilpak® Dispenser

Ovral®
(norgestrel, ethinyl estradiol)
0.5 mg / 0.05 mg

RX WYETH-AYERST PHARMACEUTICALS P. 3415

56** 445**

2511* Pilpak® Dispenser

Ovral®-28
(norgestrel, ethinyl estradiol)
0.5 mg / 0.05 mg
and 7 pink inert tablets

RX WYETH-AYERST PHARMACEUTICALS P. 3419

19** 12.5 mg

27** 25 mg

227** 50 mg

†Phenergan®
(promethazine HCl)

RX WYETH-AYERST PHARMACEUTICALS P. 3419

498* 12.5 mg

212* 25 mg

229* 50 mg

†Phenergan® Rectal Suppositories
(promethazine HCl)

RX WYETH-AYERST PHARMACEUTICALS P. 3429

868* 0.3 mg

867* 0.625 mg

864* 0.9 mg

866* 1.25 mg

865* 2.5 mg

†Premarin®
(conjugated estrogens, USP)

RX WYETH-AYERST PHARMACEUTICALS P. 3432

872* 0.625 mg per g

Gentle Measure™ Applicator

Premarin® Vaginal Cream
(conjugated estrogens)
Net Wt. 1 1/2 oz. (42.5 g)

RX WYETH-AYERST PHARMACEUTICALS P. 3434

EZ Dial™ Dispenser

Premphase®
(conjugated estrogens/
medroxyprogesterone acetate tablets)
0.625 mg / 5 mg

RX WYETH-AYERST PHARMACEUTICALS P. 3434

EZ Dial™ Dispenser

Prempro™
(conjugated estrogens/
medroxyprogesterone acetate tablets)
0.625 mg / 2.5 mg

RX WYETH-AYERST PHARMACEUTICALS P. 3434

EZ Dial™ Dispenser

Prempro™
(conjugated estrogens/
medroxyprogesterone acetate tablets)
0.625 mg / 5 mg

RX WYETH-AYERST PHARMACEUTICALS P. 3448

4177* 200 mg

4179* 400 mg

†‡Sectral®
(acebutolol HCl)

C-IV WYETH-AYERST PHARMACEUTICALS P. 3450

925** 5 mg

926** 10 mg

Sonata®
(zaleplon)

RX WYETH-AYERST PHARMACEUTICALS P. 3454

4132* 25 mg

4133* 50 mg

4158* 100 mg

‡Surmontil®
(trimipramine maleate)

RX WYETH-AYERST PHARMACEUTICALS P. 3459

641** 642** 643**

2535*

Triphasil®-21
(21 tablets containing the following: 6 brown tablets - 0.050 mg levonorgestrel + 0.030 mg ethinyl estradiol; 5 white tablets - 0.075 mg levonorgestrel + 0.040 mg ethinyl estradiol; 10 light-yellow tablets - 0.125 mg levonorgestrel + 0.030 mg ethinyl estradiol)

RX WYETH-AYERST PHARMACEUTICALS P. 3464

641** 642** 643** 650**

2536*

Triphasil®-28
(28 tablets containing the following:
6 brown tablets - 0.050 mg levonorgestrel + 0.030 mg ethinyl estradiol; 5 white tablets - 0.075 mg levonorgestrel + 0.040 mg ethinyl estradiol; 10 light-yellow tablets - 0.125 mg levonorgestrel + 0.030 mg ethinyl estradiol; 7 light-green inert tablets)

RX WYETH-AYERST PHARMACEUTICALS P. 3464

641** 642** 643** 650**

Clinic Pilpak®

Triphasil®-28
(28 tablets containing the following:
6 brown tablets - 0.050 mg levonorgestrel + 0.030 mg ethinyl estradiol; 5 white tablets - 0.075 mg levonorgestrel + 0.040 mg ethinyl estradiol; 10 light-yellow tablets - 0.125 mg levonorgestrel + 0.030 mg ethinyl estradiol; 7 light-green inert tablets)

C-IV WYETH-AYERST PHARMACEUTICALS P. 3468

85**

Wygesic®
(propoxyphene HCl, USP, acetaminophen, USP)
65 mg /650 mg

RX WYETH-AYERST PHARMACEUTICALS P. 3465

Tubex® Injector and Sterile Cartridge–Needle Unit
with hard cannula cover ready for injection.

Tubex® Blunt Pointe™ Sterile Cartridge–Needle Unit
for use in selected "needle–less" IV port systems*

*(*Consult product prescribing information for compatibility information in the Product Information section of this PDR.)*

Tubex® Closed Injection System
Examples of Tubex® Sterile Cartridge–Needle Units, Tubex® Blunt Pointe™ Sterile Cartridge–Unit, and Tubex® Injector, components of the Tubex Closed Injection System, the most comprehensive line of small–volume unit–dose prefilled syringe injectables.
For complete list of products available, consult Tubex listing in the Product Information Section.

ALZA PHARMACEUTICALS

C-II A DIVISION OF ALZA CORPORATION P. 3474

18 mg 36 mg

Please turn to page 304 for additional Alza Pharmaceuticals Product Idenfitication.

Concerta™
(methylphenidate HCl)
Extended-release Tablets

BAYER CORPORATION

RX BAYER CORPORATION, PHARMACEUTICAL DIVISION P. 839

400 mg

Please turn to page 307 for additional Bayer Corporation, Pharmaceutical Division Product Idenfitication.

Avelox™
(moxifloxacin HCl)

DJ PHARMA

RX DJ PHARMA P. 1136

500 mg

Keftab®
(cephalexin HCl)

‡ The appearance of these tablets and capsules is a trademark of Wyeth-Ayerst Laboratories.

Δ The appearance of these tablets and capsules is a registered trademark of Wyeth-Ayerst Laboratories.

**Product identification number on reverse side

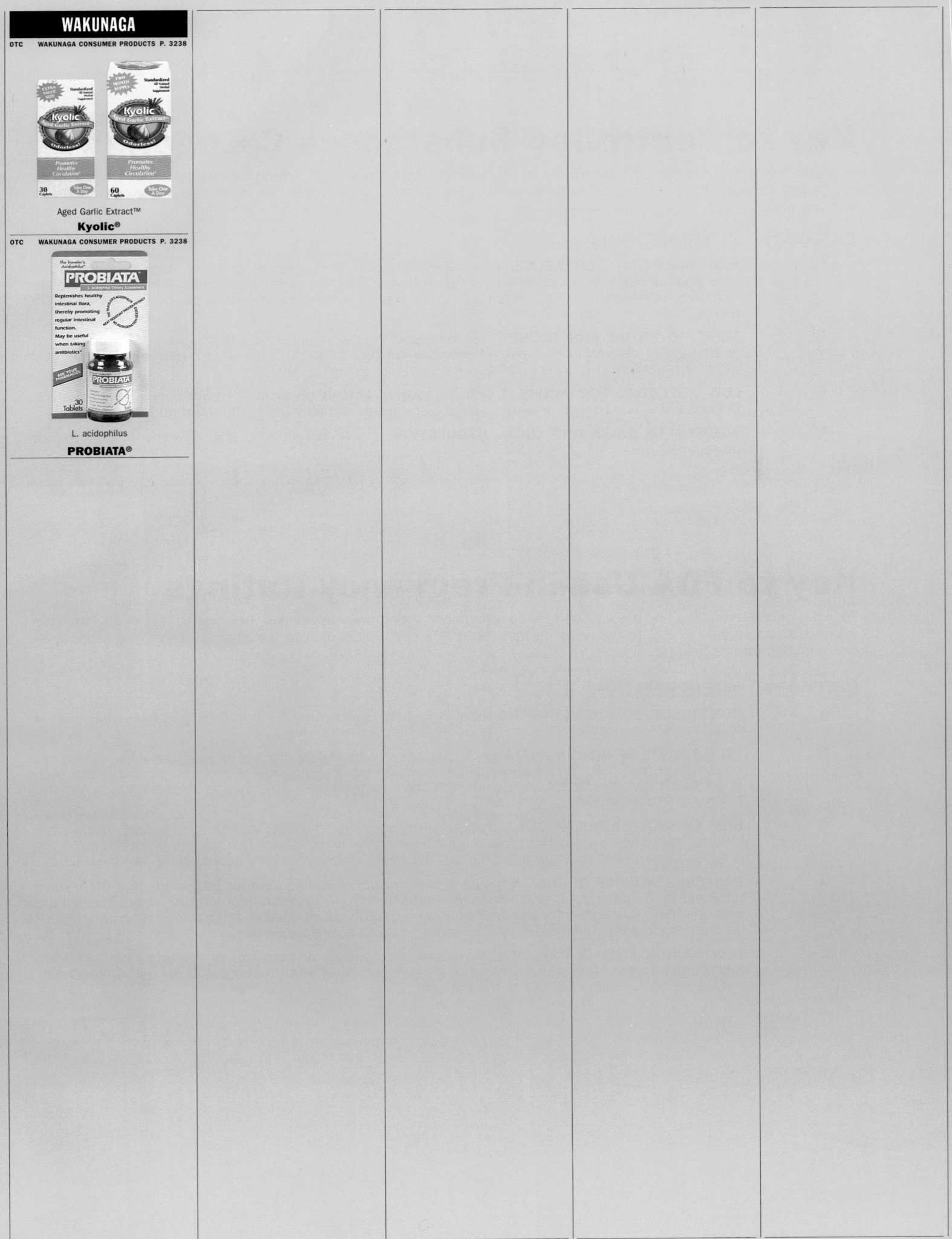

WAKUNAGA

OTC WAKUNAGA CONSUMER PRODUCTS P. 3238

Aged Garlic Extract™

Kyolic®

OTC WAKUNAGA CONSUMER PRODUCTS P. 3238

L. acidophilus

PROBIATA®

Key to Controlled Substances Categories

Products listed with the symbols shown below are subject to the Controlled Substances Act of 1970. These drugs are categorized according to their potential for abuse. The greater the potential, the more severe the limitations on their prescription.

CATEGORY	INTERPRETATION
CII	**HIGH POTENTIAL FOR ABUSE.** Use may lead to severe physical or psychological dependence. Prescriptions must be written in ink, or typewritten and signed by the practitioner. Verbal prescriptions must be confirmed in writing within 72 hours, and may be given only in a genuine emergency. No renewals are permitted.
CIII	**SOME POTENTIAL FOR ABUSE.** Use may lead to low-to-moderate physical dependence or high psychological dependence. Prescriptions may be oral or written. Up to 5 renewals are permitted within 6 months.
CIV	**LOW POTENTIAL FOR ABUSE.** Use may lead to limited physical or psychological dependence. Prescriptions may be oral or written. Up to 5 renewals are permitted within 6 months.
CV	**SUBJECT TO STATE AND LOCAL REGULATION.** Abuse potential is low; a prescription may not be required.

Key to FDA Use-in-Pregnancy Ratings

The U.S. Food and Drug Administration's use-in-pregnancy rating system weighs the degree to which available information has ruled out risk to the fetus against the drug's potential benefit to the patient. The ratings, and their interpretation, are as follows:

CATEGORY	INTERPRETATION
A	**CONTROLLED STUDIES SHOW NO RISK.** Adequate, well-controlled studies in pregnant women have failed to demonstrate a risk to the fetus in any trimester of pregnancy.
B	**NO EVIDENCE OF RISK IN HUMANS.** Adequate, well-controlled studies in pregnant women have not shown increased risk of fetal abnormalities despite adverse findings in animals, or, in the absence of adequate human studies, animal studies show no fetal risk. The chance of fetal harm is remote, but remains a possibility.
C	**RISK CANNOT BE RULED OUT.** Adequate, well-controlled human studies are lacking, and animal studies have shown a risk to the fetus or are lacking as well. There is a chance of fetal harm if the drug is administered during pregnancy; but the potential benefits may outweigh the potential risk.
D	**POSITIVE EVIDENCE OF RISK.** Studies in humans, or investigational or post-marketing data, have demonstrated fetal risk. Nevertheless, potential benefits from the use of the drug may outweigh the potential risk. For example, the drug may be acceptable if needed in a life-threatening situation or serious disease for which safer drugs cannot be used or are ineffective.
X	**CONTRAINDICATED IN PREGNANCY.** Studies in animals or humans, or investigational or post-marketing reports, have demonstrated positive evidence of fetal abnormalities or risk which clearly outweighs any possible benefit to the patient.

POISON CONTROL CENTERS

Many of the centers listed below are certified by the American Association of Poison Control Centers. Certified centers are marked by an asterisk after the name. Each has to meet certain criteria. It must, for example, serve a large geographic area; it must be open 24 hours a day and provide direct-dial or toll-free access; it must be supervised by a medical director; and it must have registered pharmacists or nurses available to answer questions from the public.

The centers have a wide variety of toxicology resources, including a computerized database of some 750,000 substances maintained by MICROMEDEX, INC., an affiliate of *Physicians' Desk Reference.* Staff members are trained to resolve toxic situations in the home of the caller, though hospital referrals are given in some instances. The centers also offer a range of educational services to both the public and healthcare professionals. In some states, these larger centers exist side by side with smaller centers offering a more limited range of services.

Within each state, centers are listed alphabetically by city. Telephone numbers designated "TTY" are teletype lines for the hearing-impaired. "TDD" numbers reach a telecommunication device for the deaf.

ALABAMA

BIRMINGHAM

Regional Poison Control Center, The Children's Hospital of Alabama (*)

1600 7th Ave. South
Birmingham, AL 35233-1711
Business: 205-939-9720
Emergency: 205-933-4050
205-939-9201
800-292-6678(AL)
Fax: 205-939-9245

TUSCALOOSA

Alabama Poison Center (*)

2503 Phoenix Dr.
Tuscaloosa, AL 35405
Business: 205-345-0600
Emergency: 205-345-0600
800-462-0800(AL)
Fax: 205-343-7410

ALASKA

ANCHORAGE

Anchorage Poison Control Center, Providence Hospital

P.O. Box 196604
3200 Providence Dr.
Anchorage, AK 99519-6604
Business: 907-562-2211
ext. 3193
Emergency: 907-261-3193
800-478-3193(AK)
Fax: 907-261-3684

FAIRBANKS

Fairbanks Poison Control Center

1650 Cowles St.
Fairbanks, AK 99701
Business and Emergency:
907-456-7182
Fax: 907-458-5553

ARIZONA

PHOENIX

**Samaritan Regional Poison Center (*)
Good Samaritan Regional Medical Center**

Ancillary-1
1111 East McDowell Rd.
Phoenix, AZ 85006
Business: 602-495-4884
Emergency: 602-253-3334
800-362-0101(AZ)
Fax: 602-256-7579

TUCSON

**Arizona Poison and Drug Information Center (*)
Arizona Health Sciences Center**

1501 North Campbell Ave.
Room. 1156
Tucson, AZ 85724
Emergency: 520-626-6016
800-362-0101(AZ)
Fax: 520-626-2720

ARKANSAS

LITTLE ROCK

**Arkansas Poison
College of Pharmacy - UAMS**

4301 West Markham St.
Mail Slot 522/2
Little Rock, AR 72205-7122
Business: 501-686-6161
Emergency: 800-376-4766
TDD/TTY: 800-641-3805

CALIFORNIA

FRESNO

**California Poison Control System-Fresno/Madera (*)
Valley Children's Hospital**

9300 Valley Children's Place
Madera, CA 93638-8762
Business: 559-353-3000
Emergency: 800-876-4766(CA)

SACRAMENTO

California Poison Control System-Sacramento (*)

UCDMC-HSF Room 1024
2315 Stockton Blvd.
Sacramento, CA 95817
Business: 916-227-1400
Emergency: 800-876-4766(CA)
TDD/TTY: 800-972-3323
Fax: 916-227-1414

SAN DIEGO

**California Poison Control System-San Diego (*)
UCSD Medical Center**

200 West Arbor Dr.
San Diego, CA 92103-8925
Emergency: 800-876-4766(CA)
TDD/TTY: 800-972-3323

SAN FRANCISCO

**California Poison Control System-San Francisco
San Francisco General Hospital**

1001 Potrero Ave., Room 1E86
San Francisco, CA 94110
Emergency: 800-876-4766(CA)
TDD/TTY: 800-876-4766

COLORADO

DENVER

Rocky Mountain Poison and Drug Center (*)

1010 Yosemite Circle,
Bldg 752, Suite B
Denver, CO 80230-6800
Business: 303-739-1100
Emergency: 303-739-1123
800-332-3073(CO)
TTY: 303-739-1127(CO)
Fax: 303-739-1119

CONNECTICUT

FARMINGTON

**Connecticut Regional Poison Control Center (*)
University of Connecticut Health Center**

263 Farmington Ave.
Farmington, CT 06030-5365
Business: 860-679-3056
Emergency: 800-343-2722(CT)
TDD/TTY: 860-679-4346
Fax: 860-679-1623

DELAWARE

PHILADELPHIA, PA

The Poison Control Center of Philadelphia(*)

3535 Market St.
Suite 985
Philadelphia, PA 19104-3309
Business: 215-590-2003
Emergency: 800-722-7112
215-386-2100
Fax: 215-590-4419

DISTRICT OF COLUMBIA

WASHINGTON, DC

National Capital Poison Center (*)

3201 New Mexico Ave., NW
Suite 310
Washington, DC 20016
Business: 202-362-3867
Emergency: 202-625-3333
TTY: 202-362-8563
Fax: 202-362-8377

FLORIDA

JACKSONVILLE

**Florida Poison Information Center-Jacksonville (*)
SHANDS Jacksonville Medical Center**

655 W. 8th St.
Jacksonville, FL 32209
Emergency: 904-244-4480
800-282-3171(FL)
TDD/TTY: 800-282-3171(FL)
Fax: 904-244-4063

MIAMI

**Florida Poison Information Center-Miami (*)
University of Miami, School of Medicine
Department of Pediatrics**

P.O. Box 016960 (R-131)
Miami, FL 33101
Business: 305-585-5253
Emergency: 305-585-8417
800-282-3171(FL)
Fax: 305-545-9762

TAMPA

Florida Poison Information Center-Tampa (*) Tampa General Hospital

P.O. Box 1289
Tampa, FL 33601
Emergency: 813-253-4444
800-282-3171(FL)
Fax: 813-253-4443

GEORGIA

ATLANTA

Georgia Poison Center (*) Hughes Spalding Children's Hospital, Grady Health System

80 Butler St., SE
P.O. Box 26066
Atlanta, GA 30335-3801
Emergency: 404-616-9000
800-282-5846(GA)
TDD: 404-616-9287
Fax: 404-616-6657

HAWAII

HONOLULU

Hawaii Poison Center

1319 Punahou St.
Honolulu, HI 96826
Emergency: 808-941-4411
800-362-3585
(outer islands only)
Fax: 808-535-7922

IDAHO

(DENVER, CO)

Rocky Mountain Poison & Drug Center (*)

1010 Yosemite Circle,
Bldg 752, Suite B
Denver, CO 80230-6800
Emergency: 800-860-0620(ID)
208-334-4570
TTY: 303-739-1127(ID)
Fax: 303-739-1119

ILLINOIS

CHICAGO

Illinois Poison Center (*)

222 South Riverside Plaza
Suite 1900
Chicago, IL 60606
Business: 312-906-6136
Emergency: 800-942-5969(IL)
TDD/TTY: 312-906-6185
Fax: 312-803-5400

URBANA

ASPCA/National Animal Poison Control Center (*)

1717 S. Philo Rd., Suite 36
Urbana, IL 61802
Business: 217-337-5030
Emergency: 888-426-4435
Fax: 217-337-0599

INDIANA

INDIANAPOLIS

Indiana Poison Center (*)

I-65 at 21st St.
P.O. Box 1367
Indianapolis, IN 46206-1367
Emergency: 317-929-2323
800-382-9097(IN)
TTY: 317-929-2336
Fax: 317-929-2337

IOWA

SIOUX CITY

Iowa Statewide Poison Control Center

2720 Stone Park Blvd.
Sioux City, IA 51104
Business: 712-279-3710
Emergency: 800-352-2222(IA)
712-277-2222
Fax: 712-234-8775

KANSAS

KANSAS CITY

Mid-America Poison Control Center, University of Kansas Medical Center

3901 Rainbow Blvd.
Room B-400
Kansas City, KS 66160-7231
Business & 913-588-6638
Emergency: 800-332-6633(KS)
TDD/TTY: 913-588-6639
Fax: 913-588-2350

TOPEKA

Stormont-Vail Regional Medical Center Emergency Department

1500 S.W. 10th
Topeka, KS 66604-1353
Business: 785-354-6000
Emergency: 785-354-6100
Fax: 785-354-5004

KENTUCKY

LOUISVILLE

Kentucky Regional Poison Center (*)

Medical Towers South
Suite 572
234 E. Gray St.
Louisville, KY 40202
Business: 502-629-7264
Emergency: 502-589-8222
800-722-5725
(Louisville only)
Fax: 502-629-7277

LOUISIANA

MONROE

Louisiana Drug and Poison Information Center (*) University of Louisiana at Monroe College of Pharmacy

Sugar Hall
Monroe, LA 71209-6430
Business: 318-342-1710
Emergency: 800-256-9822(LA)
Fax: 318-342-1744

MAINE

PORTLAND

Maine Poison Center Maine Medical Center

22 Bramhall St.
Portland, ME 04102
Emergency: 207-871-2950
800-442-6305(ME)
TDD/TTY: 207-871-2879
Fax: 207-871-6226

MARYLAND

BALTIMORE

Maryland Poison Center (*) University of Maryland at Baltimore School of Pharmacy

20 North Pine St., PH 230
Baltimore, MD 21201
Business: 410-706-7604
Emergency: 410-706-7701
800-492-2414(MD)
TDD: 410-706-1858
Fax: 410-706-7184

MASSACHUSETTS

BOSTON

Regional Center for Poison Control and Prevention (*)

300 Longwood Ave.
Boston, MA 02115
Emergency: 617-232-2120
800-682-9211
(MA, RI)
TDD/TTY: 888-244-5313
Fax: 617-738-0032

MICHIGAN

DETROIT

Regional Poison Control Center (*) Children's Hospital of Michigan

4160 John R. Harper Prof. Office Bldg.
Suite 616
Detroit, MI 48201
Business: 313-745-5335
Emergency: 313-745-5711
800-764-7661(MI)
TDD/TTY: 800-356-3232
Fax: 313-745-5493

GRAND RAPIDS

Spectrum Health Regional Poison Center (*)

1840 Wealthy SE
Grand Rapids, MI 49506-2968
Business: 616-774-7851
Emergency: 800-764-7661(MI)
TDD/TTY: 800-356-3232
Fax: 616-774-7204

MINNESOTA

MINNEAPOLIS

Hennepin Regional Poison Center (*) Hennepin County Medical Center

701 Park Ave.
Minneapolis, MN 55415
Business: 612-347-3144
Emergency: 800-764-7661
(MN, SD)
612-347-3141
TTY: 612-904-4691
Fax: 612-904-4289

ST.PAUL

PROSAR International Poison Center

1295 Bandana Blvd.
Suite 335
St.Paul, MN 55108
Business: 651-917-6100
Emergency: 888-779-7921
Fax: 651-641-0341

MISSISSIPPI

HATTIESBURG

Poison Center, Forrest General Hospital

P. O. Box 16389
400 South 28th Ave.
Hattiesburg, MS 39404
Emergency: 601-288-2100
601-288-2197
601-288-2199
Fax: 601-288-2125

JACKSON

Mississippi Regional Poison Control Center, University of Mississippi Medical Center

2500 North State St.
Jackson, MS 39216
Business: 601-984-1675
Emergency: 601-354-7660
Fax: 601-984-1676

MISSOURI

ST. LOUIS

Cardinal Glennon Children's Hospital Regional Poison Center (*)

1465 South Grand Blvd.
St. Louis, MO 63104
Emergency: 800-366-8888(MO)
314-772-5200
TTY: 314-577-5336
Fax: 314-577-5355

MONTANA

(DENVER, CO)

Rocky Mountain Poison and Drug Center (*)

1010 Yosemite Circle,
Bldg 752, Suite B
Denver, CO 80230-6800
Emergency: 800-525-5042(MT)
303-739-1123
Fax: 303-739-1119

NEBRASKA

OMAHA

The Poison Center (*) Children's Hospital

8301 Dodge St.
Omaha, NE 68114
Emergency: 402-354-5555
(Omaha)
800-955-9119
(NE, WY)

NEVADA

(DENVER, CO)

Rocky Mountain Poison and Drug Center (*)

1010 Yosemite Circle,
Bldg 752, Suite B
Denver, CO 80230-6800
Emergency: 800-446-6179(NV)
303-739-1123
Fax: 303-739-1119

(PORTLAND, OR)

Oregon Poison Center (*) Oregon Health Sciences University

3181 SW Sam Jackson Park Rd, CB550
Portland, OR 97201
Emergency: 503-494-8968
Fax: 503-494-4980

NEW HAMPSHIRE

LEBANON

New Hampshire Poison Information Center, Dartmouth-Hitchcock Medical Center

1 Medical Center Dr.
Lebanon, NH 03756
Emergency: 603-650-8000
800-562-8236(NH)
Fax: 603-650-8986

NEW JERSEY

NEWARK

New Jersey Poison Information and Education System (*)

201 Lyons Ave.
Newark, NJ 07112
Business: 973-926-7443
Emergency: 800-764-7661(NJ)
TDD/TTY: 973-926-8008
Fax: 973-926-0013

NEW MEXICO

ALBUQUERQUE

New Mexico Poison and Drug Information Center (*) University of New Mexico

Health Science Center Library,
Room 130
Albuquerque, NM 87131-1076
Emergency: 505-272-2222
800-432-6866(NM)
Fax: 505-272-5892

NEW YORK

BUFFALO

Western New York Regional Poison Control Center (*) Children's Hospital of Buffalo

219 Bryant St.
Buffalo, NY 14222
Business: 716-878-7657
Emergency: 716-878-7654
800-888-7655
(NY Western Regions Only)

MINEOLA

Long Island Regional Poison and Drug Information Center (*) Winthrop University Hospital

259 First St.
Mineola, NY 11501
Emergency: 516-542-2323
516-663-2650
TDD: 516-747-3323
(Nassau)
516-924-8811
(Suffolk)
Fax: 516-739-2070

NEW YORK CITY

New York City Poison Control Center (*) NYC Dept. of Health

455 First Ave., Room 123
New York, NY 10016
Business: 212-447-8152
Emergency: 800-210-3985
212-340-4494
212-POISONS
(212-764-7667)
212-VENENOS
(212-836-3667)
(Spanish)
TDD: 212-689-9014
Fax: 212-447-8223

ROCHESTER

Finger Lakes Regional Poison and Drug Information Center (*) University of Rochester Medical Center

601 Elmwood Ave.
Box 321
Rochester, NY 14642
Business: 716-273-4155
Emergency: 716-275-3232
800-333-0542(NY)
TTY: 716-273-3854
Fax: 716-244-1677

SLEEPY HOLLOW

Hudson Valley Regional Poison Center (*) Phelps Memorial Hospital Center

701 N. Broadway
Sleepy Hollow, NY 10591
Emergency: 914-366-3030
800-336-6997(NY)
Fax: 914-366-1400

SYRACUSE

Central New York Poison Center (*) SUNY Health Science Center

750 East Adams St.
Syracuse, NY 13210
Business: 315-464-7078
Emergency: 315-476-4766
800-252-5655(NY)
Fax: 315-464-7077

NORTH CAROLINA

CHARLOTTE

Carolinas Poison Center (*) Carolinas Medical Center

5000 Airport Center Pkwy.
Suite B
P.O. Box 32861
Charlotte, NC 28232
Business: 704-395-3795
Emergency: 704-355-4000
800-848-6946

NORTH DAKOTA

FARGO

North Dakota Poison Information Center, Meritcare Medical Center

720 4th St. North
Fargo, ND 58122
Business: 701-234-6062
Emergency: 701-234-5575
800-732-2200
(ND, MN, SD)
Fax: 701-234-5090

OHIO

CINCINNATI

Cincinnati Drug & Poison Information Center and Regional Poison Control System (*)

3333 Burnet Ave.
Vernon Place, 3rd floor
Cincinnati, OH 45229
Emergency: 513-558-5111
800-872-5111(OH)
TDD/TTY: 800-253-7955
Fax: 513-636-5069

CLEVELAND

Greater Cleveland Poison Control Center

11100 Euclid Ave.
Cleveland, OH 44106-6010
Emergency: 216-231-4455
888-231-4455(OH)
Fax: 216-844-3242

COLUMBUS

Central Ohio Poison Center (*)

700 Children's Dr.
Room L032
Columbus, OH 43205-2696
Business: 614-722-2635
Emergency: 614-228-1323
800-682-7625(OH)
800-762-0727(OH)
937-222-2227
(Dayton Region)
TTY: 614-222-2272
Fax: 614-221-2672

TOLEDO

Poison Information Center of NW Ohio, Medical College of Ohio Hospital

3000 Arlington Ave.
Toledo, OH 43614
Emergency: 419-383-3897
800-589-3897(OH)
Fax: 419-383-6066

OKLAHOMA

OKLAHOMA CITY

Oklahoma Poison Control Center, University of Oklahoma

940 Northeast 13th St.
Room 3512
Oklahoma City, OK 73104
Business: 405-271-5062
Emergency: 800-764-7661(OK)
405-271-5454
TDD: 405-271-1122
Fax: 405-271-1816

OREGON

PORTLAND

Oregon Poison Center, CB 550(*) Oregon Health Sciences University

3181 S.W. Sam Jackson Park Rd.
Portland, OR 97201
Emergency: 503-494-8968
800-452-7165(OR)
Fax: 503-494-4980

PENNSYLVANIA

HERSHEY

Central Pennsylvania Poison Center (*) Pennsylvania State University Milton S. Hershey Medical Center

MC H043, P.O. Box 850
500 University Dr.
Hershey, PA 17033-0850
Emergency: 800-521-6110
717-531-6111
TTY: 717-531-8335
Fax: 717-531-6932

PHILADELPHIA

The Poison Control Center (*)

3535 Market St., Suite 985
Philadelphia, PA 19104-3309
Business: 215-590-2003
Emergency: 215-386-2100
800-722-7112
Fax: 215-590-4419

PITTSBURGH

Pittsburgh Poison Center (*)
Children's Hospital of Pittsburgh

3705 Fifth Ave.
Pittsburgh, PA 15213
Business: 412-692-5600
Emergency: 412-681-6669
Fax: 412-692-7497

PUERTO RICO

SANTURCE

San Jorge Children's Hospital Poison Center

258 San Jorge St.
Santurce, PR 00912
Emergency: 787-726-5674

RHODE ISLAND

(BOSTON, MA)

Regional Center for Poison Control and Prevention Serving Massachusetts and Rhode Island(*)

300 Longwood Ave.
Boston, MA 02115
Emergency: 800-682-9211
(MA, RI)
617-232-2120
TTD/TTY: 888-244-5313

SOUTH CAROLINA

COLUMBIA

Palmetto Poison Center,
College of Pharmacy,
University of South Carolina

Columbia, SC 29208
Business: 803-777-7909
Emergency: 803-777-1117
800-922-1117(SC)
Fax: 803-777-6127

SOUTH DAKOTA

(FARGO, ND)

North Dakota Poison Information Center
Meritcare Medical Center

720 4th St. North
Fargo, ND 58122
Business: 701-234-6062
Emergency: 701-234-5575
800-732-2200
(SD, MN, ND)
Fax: 701-234-5090

(MINNEAPOLIS, MN)

Hennepin Regional Poison Center (*) Hennepin County Medical Center

701 Park Ave.
Minneapolis, MN 55415
Business: 612-347-3144
Emergency: 800-764-7661
(MN, SD)
612-904-4691
TTY: 612-904-4289

TENNESSEE

MEMPHIS

Southern Poison Center

875 Monroe Ave.
Suite 104
Memphis, TN 38163
Business: 901-448-6800
Emergency: 901-528-6048
800-288-9999(TN)
Fax: 901-448-5419

NASHVILLE

Middle Tennessee Poison Center (*)

1161 21st Ave. South
501 Oxford House
Nashville, TN 37232-4632
Business: 615-936-0760
Emergency: 615-936-2034
(Greater Nashville)
800-288-9999(TN)
Fax: 615-936-0756

TEXAS

AMARILLO

Texas Panhandle Poison Center
Northwest Texas Hospital

1501 S. Coulter Dr.
Amarillo, TX 79106
Emergency: 806-354-1100
800-764-7661(TX)

DALLAS

North Texas Poison Center (*)
Texas Poison Center Network
Parkland Health and Hospital System

5201 Harry Hines Blvd.
P.O. Box 35926
Dallas, TX 75235
Business: 214-589-0911
Emergency: 800-764-7661(TX)
Fax: 214-590-5008

EL PASO

West Texas Regional Poison Center (*)

4815 Alameda Ave.
El Paso, TX 79905
Business 915-534-3800
Emergency: 800-764-7661(TX)

GALVESTON

Southeast Texas Poison Center (*)
The University of Texas Medical Branch

3112 Trauma Bldg.
301 University Ave.
Galveston, TX 77555-1175
Business: 409-766-4403
Emergency: 800-764-7661(TX)
409-765-1420
Fax: 409-772-3917

SAN ANTONIO

South Texas Poison Center(*)
The University of Texas Health Science Center–San Antonio

7703 Floyd Curl Dr., MC 7849
San Antonio, TX 78229-3900
Emergency: 210-567-5762
800-764-7661(TX)
TDD/TTY: 800-764-7661(TX)
Fax: 210-567-5718

TEMPLE

Central Texas Poison Center (*)
Scott & White Memorial Hospital

2401 South 31st St.
Temple, TX 76508
Emergency: 800-764-7661(TX)
254-724-7401
Fax: 254-724-1731

UTAH

SALT LAKE CITY

Utah Poison Control Center (*)

410 Chipeta Way
Suite 230
Salt Lake City, UT 84108
Emergency: 801-581-2151
800-456-7707(UT)
Fax: 801-581-4199

VERMONT

BURLINGTON

Vermont Poison Center,
Fletcher Allen Health Care

111 Colchester Ave.
Burlington, VT 05401
Business: 802-847-2721
Emergency: 802-658-3456
877-658-3456
(toll-free)
Fax: 802-847-4802

VIRGINIA

CHARLOTTESVILLE

Blue Ridge Poison Center (*)
University of Virginia Health System

PO Box 800774
Charlottesville, VA 22908-0774
Emergency: 804-924-5543
800-451-1428(VA)
Fax: 804-971-8657

RICHMOND

Virginia Poison Center (*)
Virginia Commonwealth University

P.O. Box 980522
Richmond, VA 23298-0522
Emergency: 800-552-6337(VA)
804-828-9123
TDD/TTY: 800-828-1120
Fax: 804-828-5291

WASHINGTON

SEATTLE

Washington Poison Center (*)

155 NE 100th St.
Suite 400
Seattle, WA 98125-8012
Business: 206-517-2351
Emergency: 206-526-2121
800-732-6985(WA)
TDD: 800-572-0638(WA)
206-517-2394
Fax: 206-526-8490

WEST VIRGINIA

CHARLESTON

West Virginia Poison Center (*)

3110 MacCorkle Ave. SE
Charleston, WV 25304
Business: 304-347-1212
Emergency: 304-348-4211
800-642-3625(WV)
Fax: 304-348-9560

WISCONSIN

MADISON

Poison Control Center,
University of Wisconsin Hospital and Clinics

600 Highland Ave.
F6-133
Madison, WI 53792
Business: 608-262-7537
Emergency: 800-815-8855(WI)

MILWAUKEE

Children's Hospital of Wisconsin Poison Center

9000 W. Wisconsin Ave.
P.O. Box 1997
Milwaukee, WI 53201
Business: 414-266-2000
Emergency: 414-266-2222
800-815-8855(WI)
Fax: 414-266-2820

WYOMING

(OMAHA, NE)

The Poison Center (*)
Children's Hospital

8301 Dodge St.
Omaha, NE 68114
Emergency: 800-955-9119
(WY, NE)

SECTION 5

PRODUCT INFORMATION

This section is made possible through the courtesy of the manufacturers whose products appear in it. The information concerning each product has been prepared, edited, and approved by the medical department, medical director, and/or medical counsel of its manufacturer.

When a product appearing in *Physicians' Desk Reference* has an official package circular, its description must be in full compliance with Food and Drug Administration (FDA) regulations pertaining to labeling for prescription drugs. These regulations require that in *PDR* "indications, effects, dosages, routes, methods, and frequency and duration of administration, and any relevant warnings, hazards, contraindications, side effects, and precautions" must be "*same in language and emphasis*" as those in the approved labeling for the product. The FDA regards the words "*same in language and emphasis*" as requiring VERBATIM use of the approved labeling providing such information. Furthermore, information in the approved labeling that is emphasized by the use of type set in a box or in capitals, boldface, or italics must be given the same emphasis in *PDR*.

For products that do not have official package circulars, the publisher has emphasized the necessity of describing such products comprehensively, so that physicians have access to all information essential for intelligent and informed decision making.

The product descriptions in *Physicians' Desk Reference* include all information made available to *PDR* by the manufacturer. The publisher does not warrant or guarantee any product, and does not perform any independent analysis of the information provided. Inclusion of a product in *PDR* does not represent an endorsement, and the publisher does not necessarily advocate the use of any product listed.

This edition of *Physicians' Desk Reference* contains the latest information available when the book went to press. As new drugs are released, and new research data and clinical findings become available throughout the year, the information in the *PDR* database is revised accordingly. These revisions are published twice annually in the *PDR* Supplements. To be certain that you have the most current data, always consult the supplements before prescribing or administering any product described in the following pages.

Abbott Laboratories Inc.

Pharmaceutical Products Division
NORTH CHICAGO, IL 60064, U.S.A.

Pharmaceutical Products Division—
Direct Inquiries to:
Customer Service:
(800) 255-5162
Technical Services:
(800) 441-4987
For Medical Information Contact:
Generally:
(800) 633-9110
Adverse Drug Experiences:
(800) 633-9110
Sales and Ordering:
(800) 255-5162

Hospital Products Division—
Direct Inquiries to:
Customer Service
(800) 222-6883
For Medical Information Contact:
(800) 615–0187
Sales and Ordering:
(800) 222-6883

ABBO–CODE™ INDEX

The Abbo-Code identification system provides positive identification of a drug and dosage strength. The following Abbott products are imprinted or debossed with an Abbo-Code designation:

PRODUCT	*ABBO-CODE*
Biaxin® Filmtab® Tablets (clarithromycin tablets, USP)	
250 mg	KT
500 mg	KL
Biaxin® XL Filmtab® Tablets (clarithromycin extended-release tablets)	
500 mg	KJ
Cartrol® (carteolol hydrochloride) Filmtab® Tablets	
2.5 mg	IA
5 mg	IC
Cefol® Filmtab® Tablets B-complex vitamins with folic acid, vitamin E, and vitamin C	NJ
Colchicine Tablets, USP	
0.6 mg	AF
Cylert® Tablets (C-IV) (pemoline)	
18.75 mg	TH
37.5 mg	TI
75 mg	TJ
37.5 mg Chewable	TK
Depakene® Capsules (valproic acid capsules, USP)	
250 mg	DEPAKENE
Depakote® Sprinkle Capsules (divalproex sodium coated particles in capsules)	
125 mg	DEPAKOTE SPRINKLE
Depakote® Tablets (divalproex sodium delayed-release tablets)	
125 mg	NT
250 mg	NR
500 mg	NS
E.E.S. 400® Filmtab® Tablets (erythromycin ethylsuccinate tablets, USP)	
400 mg erythromycin activity	EE
EryPed® Chewable Tablets (erythromycin ethylsuccinate tablets, USP)	
200 mg erythromycin activity	EZ
Enduron® Tablets (methyclothiazide tablets, USP)	
2.5 mg	ENDURON
5 mg	ENDURON
Enduronyl® Tablets	
5 mg methyclothiazide and 0.25 mg deserpidine	LS
Enduronyl® Forte Tablets	
5 mg methyclothiazide and 0.5 mg deserpidine	LT
Ery-Tab® Enteric-Coated Tablets (erythromycin delayed-release tablets, USP)	
250 mg	EC
333 mg	EH
500 mg	ED
Erythrocin® Stearate Filmtab® Tablets (erythromycin stearate tablets, USP)	
250 mg erythromycin activity	ES
500 mg erythromycin activity	ET
Erythromycin Base Filmtab® Tablets (erythromycin tablets, USP)	
250 mg	EB
500 mg	EA
Erythromycin Delayed-release Capsules, USP	
250 mg	ER
Fero-Folic-500® Filmtab® Tablets controlled-release iron, folic acid, and vitamin C	AJ
Gabitril® Filmtab® Tablets (tiagabine HCl tablets)	
2 mg	FJ
4 mg	FK
12 mg	FL
16 mg	FM
20 mg	FN
Gengraf™ Capsules (cyclosporine capsules, USP [MODIFIED])	
25 mg	OR
100 mg	OT
Iberet-Folic-500® Filmtab® Tablets controlled-release iron with vitamin C and B-complex including folic acid	AK
Hytrin® Capsules (terazosin hydrochloride capsules)	
1 mg	HH
2 mg	HY
5 mg	HK
10 mg	HN
K-Tab® Filmtab® Tablets (potassium chloride extended-release tablets, USP)	
10 mEq (750 mg)	K-TAB
Nembutal® Sodium Capsules (C-II) (pentobarbital sodium capsules, USP)	
50 mg	CF
100 mg	CH
Norvir® (ritonavir capsules) soft gelatin	
100 mg	DS
Omnicef® Capsules (cefdinir) capsules	
300 mg	OMNICEF
Oretic® Tablets (hydrochlorothiazide tablets, USP)	
25 mg	ORETIC
50 mg	ORETIC
PCE® Dispertab® Tablets (erythromycin particles in tablets)	
333 mg	PCE
500 mg	EK
Peganone® Tablets (ethotoin tablets, USP)	
250 mg	AE
Placidyl® Capsules (C-IV) (ethchlorvynol capsules, USP)	
500 mg	PLACIDYL 500
750 mg	PLACIDYL 750
ProSom™ Tablets (C-IV) (estazolam tablets)	
1 mg	UC
2 mg	UD
Tranxene® T-Tab® Tablets (C-IV) (clorazepate dipotassium)	
3.75 mg Tablet	TL
7.5 mg Tablet	TM
15 mg Tablet	TN
Tranxene-SD™ (C-IV) (clorazepate dipotassium) Single Dose Tablets	
11.25 mg Half Strength	TX
22.5 mg	TY
Tricor® (fenofibrate capsules), micronized	
67 mg	FR
134 mg	AR
200 mg	SR
Tridione® Dulcet® Tablets	
150 mg	LE
Zyflo® Filmtab® Tablets (zileuton tablets)	
600 mg	ZL

BIAXIN® Filmtab® ℞
(clarithromycin tablets, USP)
BIAXIN® XL Filmtab®
(clarithromycin extended-release tablets)
BIAXIN® Granules
(clarithromycin for oral suspension, USP)
℞ only

DESCRIPTION

Clarithromycin is a semi-synthetic macrolide antibiotic. Chemically, it is 6-*0*-methylerythromycin. The molecular formula is $C_{38}H_{69}NO_{13}$, and the molecular weight is 747.96. The structural formula is:

[See chemical structure at top of next column]

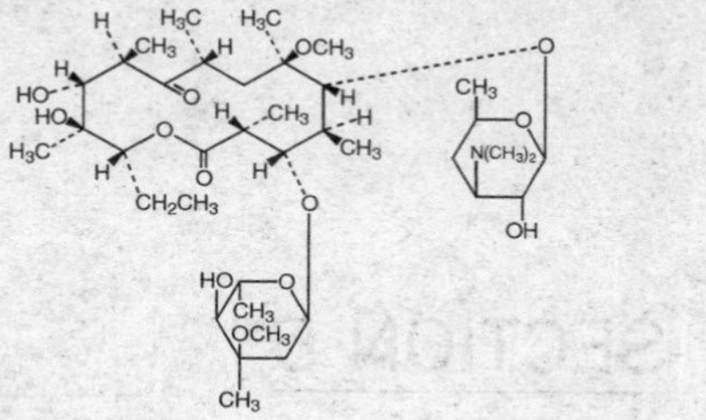

Clarithromycin is a white to off-white crystalline powder. It is soluble in acetone, slightly soluble in methanol, ethanol, and acetonitrile, and practically insoluble in water.

BIAXIN is available as immediate-release tablets, extended-release tablets, and granules for oral suspension.

Each yellow oval film-coated immediate-release BIAXIN tablet contains 250 mg or 500 mg of clarithromycin and the following inactive ingredients:

250 mg tablets: hydroxypropyl methylcellulose, hydroxypropyl cellulose, croscarmellose sodium, D&C Yellow No. 10, FD&C Blue No. 1, magnesium stearate, microcrystalline cellulose, povidone, pregelatinized starch, propylene glycol, silicon dioxide, sorbic acid, sorbitan monooleate, stearic acid, talc, titanium dioxide, and vanillin.

500 mg tablets: hydroxypropyl methylcellulose, hydroxypropyl cellulose, colloidal silicon dioxide, croscarmellose sodium, D&C Yellow No. 10, magnesium stearate, microcrystalline cellulose, povidone, propylene glycol, sorbic acid, sorbitan monooleate, titanium dioxide, and vanillin.

Each yellow oval film-coated BIAXIN XL tablet contains 500 mg of clarithromycin and the following inactive ingredients: cellulosic polymers, D&C Yellow No. 10, lactose monohydrate, magnesium stearate, propylene glycol, sorbic acid, sorbitan monooleate, talc, titanium dioxide, and vanillin.

After constitution, each 5 mL of BIAXIN suspension contains 125 mg, 187.5 mg or 250 mg of clarithromycin. Each bottle of BIAXIN granules contains 1250 mg (50 mL size), 2500 mg (50 and 100 mL sizes), 3750 mg (100 mL size) or 5000 mg (100 mL size) of clarithromycin and the following inactive ingredients: carbomer, castor oil, citric acid, hypromellose phthalate, maltodextrin, potassium sorbate, povidone, silicon dioxide, sucrose, xanthan gum, titanium dioxide and fruit punch flavor.

CLINICAL PHARMACOLOGY

Pharmacokinetics:

Clarithromycin is rapidly absorbed from the gastrointestinal tract after oral administration. The absolute bioavailability of 250-mg clarithromycin tablets was approximately 50%. For a single 500-mg dose of clarithromycin, food slightly delays the onset of clarithromycin absorption, increasing the peak time from approximately 2 to 2.5 hours. Food also increases the clarithromycin peak plasma concentration by about 24%, but does not affect the extent of clarithromycin bioavailability. Food does not affect the onset of formation of the antimicrobially active metabolite, 14-OH clarithromycin or its peak plasma concentration but does slightly decrease the extent of metabolite formation, indicated by an 11% decrease in area under the plasma concentration-time curve (AUC). Therefore, BIAXIN tablets may be given without regard to food.

In nonfasting healthy human subjects (males and females), peak plasma concentrations were attained within 2 to 3 hours after oral dosing. Steady-state peak plasma clarithromycin concentrations were attained within 3 days and were approximately 1 to 2 µg/mL with a 250-mg dose administered every 12 hours and 3 to 4 µg/mL with a 500-mg dose administered every 8 to 12 hours. The elimination half-life of clarithromycin was about 3 to 4 hours with 250 mg administered every 12 hours but increased to 5 to 7 hours with 500 mg administered every 8 to 12 hours. The nonlinearity of clarithromycin pharmacokinetics is slight at the recommended doses of 250 mg and 500 mg administered every 8 to 12 hours. With a 250 mg every 12 hours dosing, the principal metabolite, 14-OH clarithromycin, attains a peak steady-state concentration of about 0.6 µg/mL and has an elimination half-life of 5 to 6 hours. With a 500 mg every 8 to 12 hours dosing, the peak steady-state concentration of 14-OH clarithromycin is slightly higher (up to 1 µg/mL), and its elimination half-life is about 7 to 9 hours. With any of these dosing regimens, the steady-state concentration of this metabolite is generally attained within 3 to 4 days.

After a 250-mg tablet every 12 hours, approximately 20% of the dose is excreted in the urine as clarithromycin, while after a 500-mg tablet every 12 hours, the urinary excretion of clarithromycin is somewhat greater, approximately 30%. In comparison, after an oral dose of 250 mg (125 mg/5 mL) suspension every 12 hours, approximately 40% is excreted in urine as clarithromycin. The renal clearance of clarithromycin is, however, relatively independent of the dose size and approximates the normal glomerular filtration rate. The major metabolite found in urine is 14-OH clarithromycin, which accounts for an additional 10% to 15% of the dose with either a 250-mg or a 500-mg tablet administered every 12 hours.

Steady-state concentrations of clarithromycin and 14-OH clarithromycin observed following administration of 500-mg doses of clarithromycin every 12 hours to adult patients with HIV infection were similar to those observed in healthy volunteers. In adult HIV-infected patients taking 500- or 1000-mg doses of clarithromycin every 12 hours, steady-state clarithromycin C_{max} values ranged from 2 to 4 µg/mL and 5 to 10 µg/mL, respectively.

The steady-state concentrations of clarithromycin in subjects with impaired hepatic function did not differ from those in normal subjects; however, the 14-OH clarithromycin concentrations were lower in the hepatically impaired subjects. The decreased formation of 14-OH clarithromycin was at least partially offset by an increase in renal clearance of clarithromycin in the subjects with impaired hepatic function when compared to healthy subjects.

The pharmacokinetics of clarithromycin was also altered in subjects with impaired renal function. (See **PRECAUTIONS** and **DOSAGE AND ADMINISTRATION**.)
Clarithromycin and the 14-OH clarithromycin metabolite distribute readily into body tissues and fluids. There are no data available on cerebrospinal fluid penetration. Because of high intracellular concentrations, tissue concentrations are higher than serum concentrations. Examples of tissue and serum concentrations are presented below.

CONCENTRATION
(after 250 mg q12h)

Tissue Type	Tissue (µg/g)	Serum (µg/mL)
Tonsil	1.6	0.8
Lung	8.8	1.7

Clarithromycin extended-release tablets provide extended absorption of clarithromycin from the gastrointestinal tract after oral administration. Relative to an equal total daily dose of immediate-release clarithromycin tablets, clarithromycin extended-release tablets provide lower and later steady-state peak plasma concentrations but equivalent 24-hour AUC's for both clarithromycin and its microbiologically-active metabolite, 14-OH clarithromycin. While the extent of formation of 14-OH clarithromycin following administration of BIAXIN XL tablets (2 × 500 mg once daily) is not affected by food, administration under fasting conditions is associated with approximately 30% lower clarithromycin AUC relative to administration with food. Therefore, BIAXIN XL tablets should be taken with food.

Steady-State Clarithromycin Plasma Concentration-Time Profiles

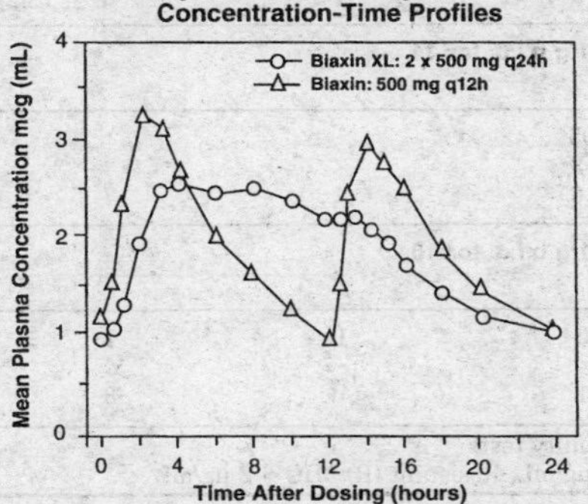

In healthy human subjects, steady-state peak plasma clarithromycin concentrations of approximately 2 to 3 µg/mL were achieved about 5 to 8 hours after oral administration of 2 × 500 mg BIAXIN XL tablets once daily; for 14-OH clarithromycin, steady-state peak plasma concentrations of approximately 0.8 µg/mL were attained about 6 to 9 hours after dosing. Steady-state peak plasma clarithromycin concentrations of approximately 1 to 2 µg/mL were achieved about 5 to 6 hours after oral administration of a single 500 mg BIAXIN XL tablet once daily; for 14-OH clarithromycin, steady-state peak plasma concentrations of approximately 0.6 µg/mL were attained about 6 hours after dosing.
When 250-mg doses of clarithromycin as BIAXIN suspension were administered to fasting healthy adult subjects, peak plasma concentrations were attained around 3 hours after dosing. Steady-state peak plasma concentrations were attained in 2 to 3 days and were approximately 2 µg/mL for clarithromycin and 0.7 µg/mL for 14-OH clarithromycin when 250-mg doses of the clarithromycin suspension were administered every 12 hours. Elimination half-life of clarithromycin (3 to 4 hours) and that of 14-OH clarithromycin (5 to 7 hours) were similar to those observed at steady state following administration of equivalent doses of BIAXIN tablets.
For adult patients, the bioavailability of 10 mL of the 125-mg/5 mL suspension or 10 mL of the 250-mg/5 mL suspension is similar to a 250-mg or 500-mg tablet, respectively.
In children requiring antibiotic therapy, administration of 7.5 mg/kg q12h doses of clarithromycin as the suspension generally resulted in steady-state peak plasma concentrations of 3 to 7 µg/mL for clarithromycin and 1 to 2 µg/mL for 14-OH clarithromycin.
In HIV-infected children taking 15 mg/kg every 12 hours, steady-state clarithromycin peak concentrations generally ranged from 6 to 15 µg/mL.
Clarithromycin penetrates into the middle ear fluid of children with secretory otitis media.

CONCENTRATION
(after 7.5 mg/kg q12h for 5 doses)

Analyte	Middle Ear Fluid (µg/mL)	Serum (µg/mL)
Clarithromycin	2.5	1.7
14-OH Clarithromycin	1.3	0.8

In adults given 250 mg clarithromycin as suspension (n=22), food appeared to decrease mean peak plasma clarithromycin concentrations from 1.2 (± 0.4) µg/mL to 1.0 (± 0.4) µg/mL and the extent of absorption from 7.2 (± 2.5) hr•µg/mL to 6.5 (± 3.7) hr•µg/mL.
When children (n=10) were administered a single oral dose of 7.5 mg/kg suspension, food increased mean peak plasma clarithromycin concentrations from 3.6 (± 1.5) µg/mL to 4.6 (± 2.8) µg/mL and the extent of absorption from 10.0 (± 5.5) hr•µg/mL to 14.2 (± 9.4) hr•µg/mL.
Clarithromycin 500 mg every 8 hours was given in combination with omeprazole 40 mg daily to healthy adult males. The plasma levels of clarithromycin and 14-hydroxy-clarithromycin were increased by the concomitant administration of omeprazole. For clarithromycin, the mean C_{max} was 10% greater, the mean C_{min} was 27% greater, and the mean AUC_{0-8} was 15% greater when clarithromycin was administered with omeprazole than when clarithromycin was administered alone. Similar results were seen for 14-hydroxy-clarithromycin, the mean C_{max} was 45% greater, the mean C_{min} was 57% greater, and the mean AUC_{0-8} was 45% greater. Clarithromycin concentrations in the gastric tissue and mucus were also increased by concomitant administration of omeprazole.
[See table above]

Clarithromycin Tissue Concentrations 2 hours after Dose (µg/mL)/(µg/g)

Treatment	N	antrum	fundus	N	mucus
Clarithromycin	5	10.48 ± 2.01	20.81 ± 7.64	4	4.15 ± 7.74
Clarithromycin + Omeprazole	5	19.96 ± 4.71	24.25 ± 6.37	4	39.29 ± 32.79

For information about other drugs indicated in combination with BIAXIN, refer to the CLINICAL PHARMACOLOGY section of their package inserts.

Microbiology:
Clarithromycin exerts its antibacterial action by binding to the 50S ribosomal subunit of susceptible microorganisms resulting in inhibition of protein synthesis.
Clarithromycin is active *in vitro* against a variety of aerobic and anaerobic gram-positive and gram-negative microorganisms as well as most *Mycobacterium avium* complex (MAC) microorganisms.
Additionally, the 14-OH clarithromycin metabolite also has clinically significant antimicrobial activity. The 14-OH clarithromycin is twice as active against *Haemophilus influenzae* microorganisms as the parent compound. However, for *Mycobacterium avium* complex (MAC) isolates the 14-OH metabolite is 4 to 7 times less active than clarithromycin. The clinical significance of this activity against *Mycobacterium avium* complex is unknown.
Clarithromycin has been shown to be active against most strains of the following microorganisms both *in vitro* and in clinical infections as described in the **INDICATIONS AND USAGE** section:

Aerobic Gram-positive microorganisms
Staphylococcus aureus
Streptococcus pneumoniae
Streptococcus pyogenes

Aerobic Gram-negative microorganisms
Haemophilus influenzae
Haemophilus parainfluenzae
Moraxella catarrhalis

Other microorganisms
Mycoplasma pneumoniae
Chlamydia pneumoniae (TWAR)

Mycobacteria
Mycobacterium avium complex (MAC) consisting of:
Mycobacterium avium
Mycobacterium intracellulare

Beta-lactamase production should have no effect on clarithromycin activity.
NOTE: Most strains of methicillin-resistant and oxacillin-resistant staphylococci are resistant to clarithromycin.
Omeprazole/clarithromycin dual therapy; ranitidine bismuth citrate/clarithromycin dual therapy; omeprazole/clarithromycin/amoxicillin triple therapy; and lansoprazole/clarithromycin/amoxicillin triple therapy have been shown to be active against most strains of *Helicobacter pylori in vitro* and in clinical infections as described in the **INDICATIONS AND USAGE** section.

Helicobacter
Helicobacter pylori

Pretreatment Resistance
Clarithromycin pretreatment resistance rates were 3.5% (4/113) in the omeprazole/clarithromycin dual-therapy studies (M93-067, M93-100) and 9.3% (41/439) in the omeprazole/clarithromycin/amoxicillin triple-therapy studies (126, 127, M96-446). Clarithromycin pretreatment resistance was 12.6% (44/348) in the ranitidine bismuth citrate/clarithromycin b.i.d. versus t.i.d. clinical study (H2BA3001). Clarithromycin pretreatment resistance rates were 9.5% (91/960) by E-test and 11.3% (12/106) by agar dilution in the lansoprazole/clarithromycin/amoxicillin triple therapy clinical trials (M93-125, M93-130, M93-131, M95-392, and M95-399).
Amoxicillin pretreatment susceptible isolates (< 0.25 µg/mL) were found in 99.3% (436/439) of the patients in the omeprazole/clarithromycin/amoxicillin clinical studies (126, 127, M96-446). Amoxicillin pretreatment minimum inhibitory concentrations (MICs) > 0.25 µg/mL occurred in 0.7% (3/439) of the patients, all of whom were in the clarithromycin/amoxicillin study arm. Amoxicillin pretreatment susceptible isolates (< 0.25 µg/mL) occurred in 97.8% (936/957) and 98.0% (98/100) of the patients in the lansoprazole/clarithromycin/amoxicillin triple-therapy clinical trials by E-test and agar dilution, respectively. Twenty-one of the 957 patients (2.2%) by E-test and 2 of 100 patients (2.0%) by agar dilution had amoxicillin pretreatment MICs of > 0.25 µg/mL. Two patients had an unconfirmed pretreatment amoxicillin minimum inhibitory concentration (MIC) of > 256 µg/mL by E-test.
[See table at top of next page]
Patients not eradicated of *H. pylori* following omeprazole/clarithromycin, ranitidine bismuth citrate/clarithromycin, omeprazole/clarithromycin/amoxicillin, or lansoprazole/clarithromycin/amoxicillin therapy would likely have clarithromycin resistant *H. pylori* isolates. Therefore, for patients who fail therapy, clarithromycin susceptibility testing should be done, if possible. Patients with clarithromycin resistant *H. pylori* should not be treated with any of the following: omeprazole/clarithromycin dual therapy; ranitidine bismuth citrate/clarithromycin dual therapy; omeprazole/clarithromycin/amoxicillin triple therapy; lansoprazole/clarithromycin/amoxicillin triple therapy; or other regimens which include clarithromycin as the sole antimicrobial agent.

Amoxicillin Susceptibility Test Results and Clinical/Bacteriological Outcomes
In the omeprazole/clarithromycin/amoxicillin triple-therapy clinical trials, 84.9% (157/185) of the patients who had pretreatment amoxicillin susceptible MICs (< 0.25 µg/mL) were eradicated of *H. pylori* and 15.1% (28/185) failed therapy. Of the 28 patients who failed triple therapy, 11 had no post-treatment susceptibility test results, and 17 had post-treatment *H. pylori* isolates with amoxicillin susceptible MICs. Eleven of the patients who failed triple therapy also had post-treatment *H. pylori* isolates with clarithromycin resistant MICs.
In the lansoprazole/clarithromycin/amoxicillin triple-therapy clinical trials, 82.6% (195/236) of the patients that had pretreatment amoxicillin susceptible MICs (< 0.25 µg/mL) were eradicated of *H. pylori*. Of those with pretreatment amoxicillin MICs of > 0.25 µg/mL, three of six had the *H. pylori* eradicated. A total of 12.8% (22/172) of the patients failed the 10- and 14-day triple-therapy regimens. Post-treatment susceptibility results were not obtained on 11 of the patients who failed therapy. Nine of the 11 patients with amoxicillin post-treatment MICs that failed the triple-therapy regimen also had clarithromycin resistant *H. pylori* isolates.
The following *in vitro* data are available, **but their clinical significance is unknown**. Clarithromycin exhibits *in vitro* activity against most strains of the following microorganisms; however, the safety and effectiveness of clarithromycin in treating clinical infections due to these microorganisms have not been established in adequate and well-controlled clinical trials.

Aerobic Gram-positive microorganisms
Streptococcus agalactiae
Streptococci (Groups C, F, G)
Viridans group streptococci

Aerobic Gram-negative microorganisms
Bordetella pertussis
Legionella pneumophila
Pasteurella multocida

Anaerobic Gram-positive microorganisms
Clostridium perfringens
Peptococcus niger
Propionibacterium acnes

Anaerobic Gram-negative microorganisms
Prevotella melaninogenica (formerly *Bacteriodes melaninogenicus*)

Susceptibility Testing Excluding Mycobacteria and Helicobacter:
Dilution Techniques:
Quantitative methods are used to determine antimicrobial minimum inhibitory concentrations (MICs). These MICs provide estimates of the susceptibility of bacteria to antimicrobial compounds. The MICs should be determined using a standardized procedure. Standardized procedures are based on a dilution method[1] (broth or agar) or equivalent with standardized inoculum concentrations and standardized concentrations of clarithromycin powder. The MIC values should be interpreted according to the following criteria:

MIC (µg/mL)	Interpretation
≤ 2.0	Susceptible (S)
4.0	Intermediate (I)
≥ 8.0	Resistant (R)

A report of "Susceptible" indicates that the pathogen is likely to be inhibited if the antimicrobial compound in the blood reaches the concentrations usually achievable.
A report of "Intermediate" indicates that the result should be considered equivocal, and, if the microorganism is not fully susceptible to alternative, clinically feasible drugs, the test should be repeated. This category implies possible clinical applicability in body sites where the drug is physiologically concentrated or in situations where high dosage of

Continued on next page

Biaxin—Cont.

drug can be used. This category also provides a buffer zone which prevents small uncontrolled technical factors from causing major discrepancies in interpretation.
A report of "Resistant" indicates that the pathogen is not likely to be inhibited if the antimicrobial compound in the blood reaches the concentrations usually achievable; other therapy should be selected.
Standardized susceptibility test procedures require the use of laboratory control microorganisms to control the technical aspects of the laboratory procedures. Standard clarithromycin powder should provide the following MIC values:

Microorganism		MIC (µg/mL)
S. aureus	ATCC 29213	0.12 to 0.5

Diffusion Techniques:
Quantitative methods that require measurement of zone diameters also provide reproducible estimates of the susceptibility of bacteria to antimicrobial compounds. One such standardized procedure[2] requires the use of standardized inoculum concentrations. This procedure uses paper disks impregnated with 15-µg clarithromycin to test the susceptibility of microorganisms to clarithromycin.
Reports from the laboratory providing results of the standard single-disk susceptibility test with a 15-µg clarithromycin disk should be interpreted according to the following criteria:

Zone diameter (mm)	Interpretation
≥ 18	Susceptible (S)
14 to 17	Intermediate (I)
≤ 13	Resistant (R)

Interpretation should be as stated above for results using dilution techniques. Interpretation involves correlation of the diameter obtained in the disk test with the MIC for clarithromycin. However, standardized diffusion methods for routine *in vitro* susceptibility testing, using the 15-µg clarithromycin disk, do not measure the additive antimicrobial activity of the 14-OH metabolite and, thus, may underestimate the drug's potential activity against *Haemophilus influenzae. Haemophilus influenzae* isolates falling into the "Intermediate" category often respond to treatment.
As with standardized dilution techniques, diffusion methods require the use of laboratory control microorganisms that are used to control the technical aspects of the laboratory procedures. For the diffusion technique, the 15-µg clarithromycin disk should provide the following zone diameters in this laboratory test quality control strain:

Microorganism		Zone diameter (mm)
S. aureus	ATCC 25923	26 to 32

***In vitro* Activity of Clarithromycin against Mycobacteria:**
Clarithromycin has demonstrated *in vitro* activity against *Mycobacterium avium* complex (MAC) microorganisms isolated from both AIDS and non-AIDS patients. While gene probe techniques may be used to distinguish *M. avium* species from *M. intracellulare*, many studies only reported results on *M. avium* complex (MAC) isolates.
Various *in vitro* methodologies employing broth or solid media at different pH's, with and without oleic acid-albumin-dextrose-catalase (OADC), have been used to determine clarithromycin MIC values for mycobacterial species. In general, MIC values decrease more than 16-fold as the pH of Middlebrook 7H12 broth media increases from 5.0 to 7.4. At pH 7.4, MIC values determined with Mueller-Hinton agar were 4- to 8-fold higher than those observed with Middlebrook 7H12 media. Utilization of oleic acid-albumin-dextrose-catalase (OADC) in these assays has been shown to further alter MIC values.
Clarithromycin activity against 80 MAC isolates from AIDS patients and 211 MAC isolates from non-AIDS patients was evaluated using a microdilution method with Middlebrook 7H9 broth. Results showed an MIC value of ≤ 4.0 µg/mL in 81% and 89% of the AIDS and non-AIDS MAC isolates, respectively. Twelve percent of the non-AIDS isolates had an MIC value ≤ 0.5 µg/mL. Clarithromycin was also shown to be active against phagocytized *M. avium* complex (MAC) in mouse and human macrophage cell cultures as well as in the beige mouse infection model.
Clarithromycin activity was evaluated against *Mycobacterium tuberculosis* microorganisms. In one study utilizing the agar dilution method with Middlebrook 7H10 media, 3 of 30 clinical isolates had an MIC of 2.5 µg/mL. Clarithromycin inhibited all isolates at > 10.0 µg/mL.
Susceptibility Testing for *Mycobacterium avium* Complex (MAC):
The disk diffusion and dilution techniques for susceptibility testing against gram-positive and gram-negative bacteria should not be used for determining clarithromycin MIC values against mycobacteria. *In vitro* susceptibility testing methods and diagnostic products currently available for determining minimum inhibitory concentration (MIC) values against *Mycobacterium avium* complex (MAC) organisms have not been standardized or validated. Clarithromycin MIC values will vary depending on the susceptibility testing method employed, composition and pH of the media, and the utilization of nutritional supplements. Breakpoints to determine whether clinical isolates of *M. avium* or *M. intracellulare* are susceptible or resistant to clarithromycin have not been established.

Clarithromycin Susceptibility Test Results and Clinical/Bacteriological Outcomes[a]

Clarithromycin Pretreatment Results		Clarithromycin Post-treatment Results: *H. pylori* negative - eradicated	*H. pylori* positive - not eradicated, Post-treatment susceptibility results: S[b]	I[b]	R[b]	No MIC
Omeprazole 40 mg q.d./clarithromycin 500 mg t.i.d. for 14 days followed by omeprazole 20 mg q.d. for another 14 days (M93-067, M93-100)						
Susceptible[b]	108	72	1		26	9
Intermediate[b]	1				1	
Resistant[b]	4				4	
Ranitidine bismuth citrate 400 mg b.i.d./clarithromycin 500 mg t.i.d. for 14 days followed by ranitidine bismuth citrate 400 mg b.i.d. for another 14 days (H2BA3001)						
Susceptible[b]	124	98	4		14	8
Intermediate[b]	3	2				1
Resistant[b]	17	1			15	1
Ranitidine bismuth citrate 400 mg b.i.d./clarithromycin 500 mg b.i.d. for 14 days followed by ranitidine bismuth citrate 400 mg b.i.d. for another 14 days (H2BA3001)						
Susceptible[b]	125	106	1	1	12	5
Intermediate[b]	2	2				
Resistant[b]	20	1			19	
Omeprazole 20 mg b.i.d./clarithromycin 500 mg b.i.d./amoxicillin 1 g b.i.d. for 10 days (126, 127, M96-446)						
Susceptible[b]	171	153	7		3	8
Intermediate[b]						
Resistant[b]	14	4	1		6	3
Lansoprazole 30 mg b.i.d./clarithromycin 500 mg b.i.d./amoxicillin 1 g b.i.d. for 14 days (M95-399, M93-131, M95-392)						
Susceptible[b]	112	105				7
Intermediate[b]	3	3				
Resistant[b]	17	6			7	4
Lansoprazole 30 mg b.i.d./clarithromycin 500 mg b.i.d./amoxicillin 1 g b.i.d. for 10 days (M95-399)						
Susceptible[b]	42	40	1		1	
Intermediate[b]						
Resistant[b]	4	1			3	

[a] Includes only patients with pretreatment clarithromycin susceptibility tests
[b] Susceptible (S) MIC < 0.25 µg/mL, Intermediate (I) MIC 0.5–1.0 µg/mL, Resistant (R) MIC > 2 µg/mL

Microorganisms	Antimicrobial Agent	MIC (µg/mL)[c]
H. pylori ATCC 43504	Clarithromycin	0.015 – 0.12 µg/mL
H. pylori ATCC 43504	Amoxicillin	0.015 – 0.12 µg/mL

[c] These are quality control ranges for the agar dilution methodology and they should not be used to control test results obtained using alternative methods.

Susceptibility Test for *Helicobacter pylori*
The reference methodology for susceptibility testing of *H. pylori* is agar dilution MICs.[3] One to three microliters of an inoculum equivalent to a No. 2 McFarland standard ($1 \times 10^7 - 1 \times 10^8$ CFU/mL for *H. pylori*) are inoculated directly onto freshly prepared antimicrobial containing Mueller-Hinton agar plates with 5% aged defibrinated sheep blood (> 2-weeks old). The agar dilution plates are incubated at 35°C in a microaerobic environment produced by a gas generating system suitable for *Campylobacter* species. After 3 days of incubation, the MICs are recorded as the lowest concentration of antimicrobial agent required to inhibit growth of the organism. The clarithromycin and amoxicillin MIC values should be interpreted according to the following criteria:

Clarithromycin MIC (µg/mL)[a]	Interpretation
< 0.25	Susceptible (S)
0.5 – 1.0	Intermediate (I)
> 2.0	Resistant (R)

Amoxicillin MIC (µg/mL)[a,b]	Interpretation
< 0.25	Susceptible (S)

[a] These are tentative breakpoints for the agar dilution methodology, and they should not be used to interpret results obtained using alternative methods.
[b] There were not enough organisms with MICs > 0.25 µg/mL to determine a resistance breakpoint.

Standardized susceptibility test procedures require the use of laboratory control microorganisms to control the technical aspects of the laboratory procedures. Standard clarithromycin and amoxicillin powders should provide the following MIC values:
[See table at top of page]

INDICATIONS AND USAGE

BIAXIN Filmtab tablets and BIAXIN Granules for oral suspension are indicated for the treatment of mild to moderate infections caused by susceptible strains of the designated microorganisms in the conditions as listed below:
Adults (BIAXIN Filmtab tablets and Granules for oral suspension):
Pharyngitis/Tonsillitis due to *Streptococcus pyogenes* (The usual drug of choice in the treatment and prevention of streptococcal infections and the prophylaxis of rheumatic fever is penicillin administered by either the intramuscular or the oral route. Clarithromycin is generally effective in the eradication of *S. pyogenes* from the nasopharynx; however, data establishing the efficacy of clarithromycin in the subsequent prevention of rheumatic fever are not available at present.)
Acute maxillary sinusitis due to *Haemophilus influenzae, Moraxella catarrhalis,* or *Streptococcus pneumoniae*
Acute bacterial exacerbation of chronic bronchitis due to *Haemophilus influenzae, Haemophilus parainfluenzae, Moraxella catarrhalis,* or *Streptococcus pneumoniae*
Pneumonia due to *Mycoplasma pneumoniae, Streptococcus pneumoniae,* or *Chlamydia pneumoniae* (TWAR)
Uncomplicated skin and skin structure infections due to *Staphylococcus aureus,* or *Streptococcus pyogenes* (Abscesses usually require surgical drainage.)
Disseminated mycobacterial infections due to *Mycobacterium avium,* or *Mycobacterium intracellulare*
BIAXIN (clarithromycin) Filmtab tablets in combination with amoxicillin and PREVACID (lansoprazole) or PRILOSEC (omeprazole) Delayed-Release Capsules, as triple therapy, are indicated for the treatment of patients with *H. pylori* infection and duodenal ulcer disease (active or five-year history of duodenal ulcer) to eradicate *H. pylori.*
BIAXIN Filmtab tablets in combination with PRILOSEC (omeprazole) capsules or TRITEC (ranitidine bismuth citrate) tablets are also indicated for the treatment of patients with an active duodenal ulcer associated with *H. pylori* infection. However, regimens which contain clarithromycin as the single antimicrobial agent are more likely to be associated with the development of clarithromycin resistance among patients who fail therapy. Clarithromycin-containing regimens should not be used in patients with

known or suspected clarithromycin resistant isolates because the efficacy of treatment is reduced in this setting.
In patients who fail therapy, susceptibility testing should be done if possible. If resistance to clarithromycin is demonstrated, a non-clarithromycin-containing therapy is recommended. (For information on development of resistance see **Microbiology** section.) The eradication of *H. pylori* has been demonstrated to reduce the risk of duodenal ulcer recurrence.

Children (BIAXIN Filmtabs and Granules for oral suspension):

Pharyngitis/Tonsillitis due to *Streptococcus pyogenes*
Pneumonia due to *Mycoplasma pneumoniae, Streptococcus pneumoniae,* or *Chlamydia pneumoniae* (TWAR)
Acute maxillary sinusitis due to *Haemophilus influenzae, Moraxella catarrhalis,* or *Streptococcus pneumoniae*
Acute otitis media due to *Haemophilus influenzae, Moraxella catarrhalis,* or *Streptococcus pneumoniae*

NOTE: For information on otitis media, see **CLINICAL STUDIES: Otitis Media.**

Uncomplicated skin and skin structure infections due to *Staphylococcus aureus,* or *Streptococcus pyogenes* (Abscesses usually require surgical drainage.)
Disseminated mycobacterial infections due to *Mycobacterium avium,* or *Mycobacterium intracellulare*

Adults (BIAXIN XL Filmtab tablets):

BIAXIN XL Filmtab tablets are indicated for the treatment of adults with mild to moderate infection caused by susceptible strains of the designated microorganisms in the conditions listed below:
Acute maxillary sinusitis due to *Haemophilus influenzae, Moraxella catarrhalis,* or *Streptococcus pneumoniae*
Acute bacterial exacerbation of chronic bronchitis due to *Haemophilus influenzae, Haemophilus parainfluenzae, Moraxella catarrhalis,* or *Streptococcus pneumoniae*

THE EFFICACY AND SAFETY OF BIAXIN XL IN TREATING OTHER INFECTIONS FOR WHICH OTHER FORMULATIONS OF BIAXIN ARE APPROVED HAVE NOT BEEN ESTABLISHED.

Prophylaxis:

BIAXIN Filmtab tablets and BIAXIN Granules for oral suspension are indicated for the prevention of disseminated *Mycobacterium avium* complex (MAC) disease in patients with advanced HIV infection.

CONTRAINDICATIONS

Clarithromycin is contraindicated in patients with a known hypersensitivity to clarithromycin, erythromycin, or any of the macrolide antibiotics.
Concomitant administration of clarithromycin with cisapride, pimozide, or terfenadine is contraindicated. There have been post-marketing reports of drug interactions when clarithromycin and/or erythromycin are co-administered with cisapride, pimozide, or terfenadine resulting in cardiac arrhythmias (QT prolongation, ventricular tachycardia, ventricular fibrillation, and torsades de pointes) most likely due to inhibition of hepatic metabolism of these drugs by erythromycin and clarithromycin. Fatalities have been reported.
For information about contraindications of other drugs indicated in combination with BIAXIN, refer to the CONTRAINDICATIONS section of their package inserts.

WARNINGS

CLARITHROMYCIN SHOULD NOT BE USED IN PREGNANT WOMEN EXCEPT IN CLINICAL CIRCUMSTANCES WHERE NO ALTERNATIVE THERAPY IS APPROPRIATE. IF PREGNANCY OCCURS WHILE TAKING THIS DRUG, THE PATIENT SHOULD BE APPRISED OF THE POTENTIAL HAZARD TO THE FETUS. CLARITHROMYCIN HAS DEMONSTRATED ADVERSE EFFECTS OF PREGNANCY OUTCOME AND/OR EMBRYO-FETAL DEVELOPMENT IN MONKEYS, RATS, MICE, AND RABBITS AT DOSES THAT PRODUCED PLASMA LEVELS 2 TO 17 TIMES THE SERUM LEVELS ACHIEVED IN HUMANS TREATED AT THE MAXIMUM RECOMMENDED HUMAN DOSES. (See PRECAUTIONS – *Pregnancy.*)

Pseudomembranous colitis has been reported with nearly all antibacterial agents, including clarithromycin, and may range in severity from mild to life threatening. Therefore, it is important to consider this diagnosis in patients who present with diarrhea subsequent to the administration of antibacterial agents.

Treatment with antibacterial agents alters the normal flora of the colon and may permit overgrowth of clostridia. Studies indicate that a toxin produced by *Clostridium difficile* is a primary cause of "antibiotic-associated colitis".
After the diagnosis of pseudomembranous colitis has been established, therapeutic measures should be initiated. Mild cases of pseudomembranous colitis usually respond to discontinuation of the drug alone. In moderate to severe cases, consideration should be given to management with fluids and electrolytes, protein supplementation, and treatment with an antibacterial drug clinically effective against *Clostridium difficile* colitis.
For information about warnings of other drugs indicated in combination with BIAXIN, refer to the WARNINGS section of their package inserts.

PRECAUTIONS

General: Clarithromycin is principally excreted via the liver and kidney. Clarithromycin may be administered without dosage adjustment to patients with hepatic impairment and normal renal function. However, in the presence of severe renal impairment with or without coexisting hepatic impairment, decreased dosage or prolonged dosing intervals may be appropriate.
Clarithromycin in combination with ranitidine bismuth citrate therapy is not recommended in patients with creatinine clearance less than 25 mL/min. (See **DOSAGE AND ADMINISTRATION.**)
Clarithromycin in combination with ranitidine bismuth citrate should not be used in patients with a history of acute porphyria.
For information about precautions of other drugs indicated in combination with BIAXIN, refer to the PRECAUTIONS section of their package inserts.

Information to Patients: BIAXIN tablets and oral suspension can be taken with or without food and can be taken with milk; however, BIAXIN XL tablets should be taken with food. Do **NOT** refrigerate the suspension.

Drug Interactions: Clarithromycin use in patients who are receiving theophylline may be associated with an increase of serum theophylline concentrations. Monitoring of serum theophylline concentrations should be considered for patients receiving high doses of theophylline or with baseline concentrations in the upper therapeutic range. In two studies in which theophylline was administered with clarithromycin (a theophylline sustained-release formulation was dosed at either 6.5 mg/kg or 12 mg/kg together with 250 or 500 mg q12h clarithromycin), the steady-state levels of C_{max}, C_{min}, and the area under the serum concentration time curve (AUC) of theophylline increased about 20%.
Concomitant administration of single doses of clarithromycin and carbamazepine has been shown to result in increased plasma concentrations of carbamazepine. Blood level monitoring of carbamazepine may be considered.
When clarithromycin and terfenadine were coadministered, plasma concentrations of the active acid metabolite of terfenadine were threefold higher, on average, than the values observed when terfenadine was administered alone. The pharmacokinetics of clarithromycin and the 14-hydroxy-clarithromycin were not significantly affected by coadministration of terfenadine once clarithromycin reached steady-state conditions. Concomitant administration of clarithromycin with terfenadine is contraindicated. (See **CONTRAINDICATIONS.**)
Clarithromycin 500 mg every 8 hours was given in combination with omeprazole 40 mg daily to healthy adult subjects. The steady-state plasma concentrations of omeprazole were increased (C_{max}, AUC_{0-24}, and $T_{1/2}$ increases of 30%, 89%, and 34%, respectively), by the concomitant administration of clarithromycin. The mean 24-hour gastric pH value was 5.2 when omeprazole was administered alone and 5.7 when co-administered with clarithromycin.
Co-administration of clarithromycin with ranitidine bismuth citrate resulted in increased plasma ranitidine concentrations (57%), increased plasma bismuth trough concentrations (48%), and increased 14-hydroxy-clarithromycin plasma concentrations (31%). These effects are clinically insignificant.
Simultaneous oral administration of BIAXIN tablets and zidovudine to HIV-infected adult patients resulted in decreased steady-state zidovudine concentrations. When 500 mg of clarithromycin were administered twice daily, steady-state zidovudine AUC was reduced by a mean of 12% (n=4). Individual values ranged from a decrease of 34% to an increase of 14%. Based on limited data in 24 patients, when BIAXIN tablets were administered two to four hours prior to oral zidovudine, the steady-state zidovudine C_{max} was increased by approximately 2-fold, whereas the AUC was unaffected.
Simultaneous administration of BIAXIN tablets and didanosine to 12 HIV-infected adult patients resulted in no statistically significant change in didanosine pharmacokinetics.
Concomitant administration of fluconazole 200 mg daily and clarithromycin 500 mg twice daily to 21 healthy volunteers led to increases in the mean steady-state clarithromycin C_{min} and AUC of 33% and 18%, respectively. Steady-state concentrations of 14-OH clarithromycin were not significantly affected by concomitant administration of fluconazole.
Concomitant administration of clarithromycin and ritonavir (n=22) resulted in a 77% increase in clarithromycin AUC and a 100% decrease in the AUC of 14-OH clarithromycin. Clarithromycin may be administered without dosage adjustment to patients with normal renal function taking ritonavir. However, for patients with renal impairment, the following dosage adjustments should be considered. For patients with CL_{CR} 30 to 60 mL/min, the dose of clarithromycin should be reduced by 50%. For patients with CL_{CR} < 30 mL/min, the dose of clarithromycin should be decreased by 75%.
Spontaneous reports in the post-marketing period suggest that concomitant administration of clarithromycin and oral anticoagulants may potentiate the effects of the oral anticoagulants. Prothrombin times should be carefully monitored while patients are receiving clarithromycin and oral anticoagulants simultaneously.
Elevated digoxin serum concentrations in patients receiving clarithromycin and digoxin concomitantly have also been reported in post-marketing surveillance. Some patients have shown clinical signs consistent with digoxin toxicity, including potentially fatal arrhythmias. Serum digoxin levels should be carefully monitored while patients are receiving digoxin and clarithromycin simultaneously.
The following drug interactions, other than increased serum concentrations of carbamazepine and active acid metabolite of terfenadine, have not been reported in clinical trials with clarithromycin; however, they have been observed with erythromycin products and/or with clarithromycin in post-marketing experience.
Concurrent use of erythromycin or clarithromycin and ergotamine or dihydroergotamine has been associated in some patients with acute ergot toxicity characterized by severe peripheral vasospasm and dysesthesia.
Erythromycin has been reported to decrease the clearance of triazolam and, thus, may increase the pharmacologic effect of triazolam. There have been post-marketing reports of drug interactions and CNS effects (e.g., somnolence and confusion) with the concomitant use of clarithromycin and triazolam.
There have been reports of an interaction between erythromycin and astemizole resulting in QT prolongation and torsades de pointes. Concomitant administration of erythromycin and astemizole is contraindicated. Because clarithromycin is also metabolized by cytochrome P450, concomitant administration of clarithromycin with astemizole is not recommended.
As with other macrolides, clarithromycin has been reported to increase concentrations of HMG-CoA reductase inhibitors (e.g., lovastatin and simvastatin), through inhibition of cytochrome P450 metabolism of these drugs. Rare reports of rhabdomyolysis have been reported in patients taking these drugs concomitantly.
The use of erythromycin and clarithromycin in patients concurrently taking drugs metabolized by the cytochrome P450 system may be associated with elevations in serum levels of these other drugs. There have been reports of interactions of erythromycin and/or clarithromycin with carbamazepine, cyclosporine, tacrolimus, hexobarbital, phenytoin, alfentanil, disopyramide, lovastatin, bromocriptine, valproate, terfenadine, cisapride, pimozide, rifabutin, and astemizole. Serum concentrations of drugs metabolized by the cytochrome P450 system should be monitored closely in patients concurrently receiving these drugs.

Carcinogenesis, Mutagenesis, Impairment of Fertility:
The following *in vitro* mutagenicity tests have been conducted with clarithromycin:
Salmonella/Mammalian Microsomes Test
Bacterial Induced Mutation Frequency Test
In Vitro Chromosome Aberration Test
Rat Hepatocyte DNA Synthesis Assay
Mouse Lymphoma Assay
Mouse Dominant Lethal Study
Mouse Micronucleus Test
All tests had negative results except the *In Vitro* Chromosome Aberration Test which was weakly positive in one test and negative in another.
In addition, a Bacterial Reverse-Mutation Test (Ames Test) has been performed on clarithromycin metabolites with negative results.
Fertility and reproduction studies have shown that daily doses of up to 160 mg/kg/day (1.3 times the recommended maximum human dose based on mg/m^2) to male and female rats caused no adverse effects on the estrous cycle, fertility, parturition, or number and viability of offspring. Plasma levels in rats after 150 mg/kg/day were 2 times the human serum levels.
In the 150 mg/kg/day monkey studies, plasma levels were 3 times the human serum levels. When given orally at 150 mg/kg/day (2.4 times the recommended maximum human dose based on mg/m^2), clarithromycin was shown to produce embryonic loss in monkeys. This effect has been attributed to marked maternal toxicity of the drug at this high dose.
In rabbits, *in utero* fetal loss occurred at an intravenous dose of 33 mg/m^2, which is 17 times less than the maximum proposed human oral daily dose of 618 mg/m^2.
Long-term studies in animals have not been performed to evaluate the carcinogenic potential of clarithromycin.

Pregnancy: Teratogenic Effects. Pregnancy Category C.
Four teratogenicity studies in rats (three with oral doses and one with intravenous doses up to 160 mg/kg/day administered during the period of major organogenesis) and two in rabbits at oral doses up to 125 mg/kg/day (approximately 2 times the recommended maximum human dose based on mg/m^2) or intravenous doses of 30 mg/kg/day administered during gestation days 6 to 18 failed to demonstrate any teratogenicity from clarithromycin. Two additional oral studies in a different rat strain at similar doses and similar conditions demonstrated a low incidence of cardiovascular anomalies at doses of 150 mg/kg/day administered during gestation days 6 to 15. Plasma levels after 150 mg/kg/day were 2 times the human serum levels. Four studies in mice revealed a variable incidence of cleft palate following oral doses of 1000 mg/kg/day (2 and 4 times the recommended maximum human dose based on mg/m^2, respectively) during gestation days 6 to 15. Cleft palate was also seen at 500 mg/kg/day. The 1000 mg/kg/day exposure resulted in plasma levels 17 times the human serum levels. In monkeys, an oral dose of 70 mg/kg/day (an approximate equidose of the recommended maximum human dose based on mg/m^2) produced fetal growth retardation at plasma levels that were 2 times the human serum levels.
There are no adequate and well-controlled studies in pregnant women. Clarithromycin should be used during pregnancy only if the potential benefit justifies the potential risk to the fetus. (See **WARNINGS.**)

Continued on next page

Biaxin—Cont.

Nursing Mothers: It is not known whether clarithromycin is excreted in human milk. Because many drugs are excreted in human milk, caution should be exercised when clarithromycin is administered to a nursing woman. It is known that clarithromycin is excreted in the milk of lactating animals and that other drugs of this class are excreted in human milk. Preweaned rats, exposed indirectly via consumption of milk from dams treated with 150 mg/kg/day for 3 weeks, were not adversely affected, despite data indicating higher drug levels in milk than in plasma.
Pediatric Use: Safety and effectiveness of clarithromycin in pediatric patients under 6 months of age have not been established. The safety of clarithromycin has not been studied in MAC patients under the age of 20 months. Neonatal and juvenile animals tolerated clarithromycin in a manner similar to adult animals. Young animals were slightly more intolerant to acute overdosage and to subtle reductions in erythrocytes, platelets and leukocytes but were less sensitive to toxicity in the liver, kidney, thymus, and genitalia.
Geriatric Use: In a steady-state study in which healthy elderly subjects (age 65 to 81 years old) were given 500 mg every 12 hours, the maximum serum concentrations and area under the curves of clarithromycin and 14-OH clarithromycin were increased compared to those achieved in healthy young adults. These changes in pharmacokinetics parallel known age-related decreases in renal function. In clinical trials, elderly patients did not have an increased incidence of adverse events when compared to younger patients. Dosage adjustment should be considered in elderly patients with severe renal impairment.

ADVERSE REACTIONS

The majority of side effects observed in clinical trials were of a mild and transient nature. Fewer than 3% of adult patients without mycobacterial infections and fewer than 2% of pediatric patients without mycobacterial infections discontinued therapy because of drug-related side effects. Fewer than 3% of adult patients taking BIAXIN XL tablets discontinued therapy because of drug-related side effects.
The most frequently reported events in adults taking BIAXIN tablets were diarrhea (3%), nausea (3%), abnormal taste (3%), dyspepsia (2%), abdominal pain/discomfort (2%), and headache (2%). In pediatric patients, the most frequently reported events were diarrhea (6%), vomiting (6%), abdominal pain (3%), rash (3%), and headache (2%). Most of these events were described as mild or moderate in severity. Of the reported adverse events, only 1% was described as severe.
The most frequently reported events in adults taking BIAXIN XL were diarrhea (6%), abnormal taste (6%), and nausea (3%). Most of these events were described as mild or moderate in severity. Of the reported adverse events, less than 2% were described as severe.
In the acute exacerbation of chronic bronchitis and acute maxillary sinusitis studies overall gastrointestinal adverse events were reported by a similar proportion of patients taking either BIAXIN tablets or BIAXIN XL tablets; however, patients taking BIAXIN XL tablets reported significantly less severe gastrointestinal symptoms compared to patients taking BIAXIN tablets. In addition, patients taking BIAXIN XL tablets had significantly fewer premature discontinuations for drug-related gastrointestinal or abnormal taste adverse events compared to BIAXIN tablets.
In pneumonia studies conducted in adults comparing clarithromycin to erythromycin base or erythromycin stearate, there were fewer adverse events involving the digestive system in clarithromycin-treated patients compared to erythromycin-treated patients (13% vs 32%; p<0.01). Twenty percent of erythromycin-treated patients discontinued therapy due to adverse events compared to 4% of clarithromycin-treated patients.
In two U.S. studies of acute otitis media comparing clarithromycin to amoxicillin/potassium clavulanate in pediatric patients, there were fewer adverse events involving the digestive system in clarithromycin-treated patients compared to amoxicillin/potassium clavulanate-treated patients (21% vs 40%, p<0.001). One-third as many clarithromycin-treated patients reported diarrhea as did amoxicillin/potassium clavulanate-treated patients.
Post-Marketing Experience:
Allergic reactions ranging from urticaria and mild skin eruptions to rare cases of anaphylaxis, Stevens-Johnson syndrome, and toxic epidermal necrolysis have occurred. Other spontaneously reported adverse events include glossitis, stomatitis, oral moniliasis, anorexia, vomiting, tongue discoloration, thrombocytopenia, leukopenia, neutropenia, and dizziness. There have been reports of tooth discoloration in patients treated with BIAXIN. Tooth discoloration is usually reversible with professional dental cleaning. There have been isolated reports of hearing loss, which is usually reversible, occurring chiefly in elderly women. Reports of alterations of the sense of smell, usually in conjunction with taste perversion or taste loss have also been reported.
Transient CNS events including anxiety, behavioral changes, confusional states, depersonalization, disorientation, hallucinations, insomnia, manic behavior, nightmares, psychosis, tinnitus, tremor, and vertigo have been reported during post-marketing surveillance. Events usually resolve with discontinuation of the drug.

ADULT DOSAGE GUIDELINES

Infection	BIAXIN Tablets Dosage (q12H)	BIAXIN Tablets Duration (days)	BIAXIN XL Tablets Dosage (q24h)	BIAXIN XL Tablets Duration (days)
Pharyngitis/Tonsillitis due to				
S. pyogenes	250 mg	10	—	—
Acute maxillary sinusitis due to	500 mg	14	2 × 500 mg	14
H. influenzae				
M. catarrhalis				
S. pneumoniae				
Acute exacerbation of chronic bronchitis due to				
H. influenzae	500 mg	7–14	2 × 500 mg	7
H. parainfluenzae	500 mg	7	2 × 500 mg	7
M. catarrhalis	250 mg	7–14	2 × 500 mg	7
S. pneumoniae	250 mg	7–14	2 × 500 mg	7
Pneumonia due to				
C. pneumoniae	250 mg	7–14	—	—
M. pneumoniae	250 mg	7–14	—	—
S. pneumoniae	250 mg	7–14	—	—
Uncomplicated skin and skin structure	250 mg	7–14	—	—
S. aureus				
S. pyogenes				

PEDIATRIC DOSAGE GUIDELINES

Based on Body Weight

Weight kg	Weight lbs	Dose (q12h)	Dosing Calculated on 7.5 mg/kg q12h: 125 mg/5 mL	187.5 mg/5 mL	250 mg/5 mL
9	20	62.5 mg	2.5 mL q12h	1.67 mL q12h	1.25 mL q12h
17	37	125 mg	5 mL q12h	3.33 mL q12h	2.5 mL q12h
25	55	187.5 mg	7.5 mL q12h	5.0 mL q12h	3.75 mL q12h
33	73	250 mg	10 mL q12h	6.67 mL q12h	5 mL q12h

Total volume after constitution	Clarithromycin concentration after constitution	Amount of water to be added*
50 mL	125 mg/5 mL	27 mL
100 mL	125 mg/5 mL	55 mL
100 mL	187.5 mg/5 mL	55 mL
50 mL	250 mg/5 mL	27 mL
100 mL	250 mg/5 mL	55 mL

* see instructions below.

Hepatic dysfunction, including increased liver enzymes, and hepatocellular and/or cholestatic hepatitis, with or without jaundice, has been infrequently reported with clarithromycin. This hepatic dysfunction may be severe and is usually reversible. In very rare instances, hepatic failure with fatal outcome has been reported and generally has been associated with serious underlying diseases and/or concomitant medications.
There have been rare reports of hypoglycemia, some of which have occurred in patients taking oral hypoglycemic agents or insulin.
As with other macrolides, clarithromycin has been associated with QT prolongation and ventricular arrhythmias, including ventricular tachycardia and torsades de pointes.
Changes in Laboratory Values: Changes in laboratory values with possible clinical significance were as follows:
Hepatic – elevated SGPT (ALT) < 1%; SGOT (AST) < 1%; GGT <1%; alkaline phosphatase <1%; LDH < 1%; total bilirubin < 1%
Hematologic – decreased WBC < 1%; elevated prothrombin time 1%
Renal – elevated BUN 4%; elevated serum creatinine < 1%
GGT, alkaline phosphatase, and prothrombin time data are from adult studies only.

DOSAGE AND ADMINISTRATION

BIAXIN® Filmtab® (clarithromycin tablets) and BIAXIN® Granules (clarithromycin for oral suspension) may be given with or without food. BIAXIN® XL Filmtab® (clarithromycin extended-release tablets) should be taken with food.
[See first table above]
H. pylori Eradication to Reduce the Risk of Duodenal Ulcer Recurrence
Triple therapy: BIAXIN/lansoprazole/amoxicillin
The recommended adult dose is 500 mg BIAXIN, 30 mg lansoprazole, and 1 gram amoxicillin, all given twice daily (q12h) for 10 or 14 days. (See **INDICATIONS AND USAGE** and **CLINICAL STUDIES** sections.)
Triple therapy: Biaxin/omeprazole/amoxicillin
The recommended adult dose is 500 mg BIAXIN, 20 mg omeprazole, and 1 gram amoxicillin, all given twice daily (q12h) for 10 days. (See **INDICATIONS AND USAGE** and **CLINICAL STUDIES** sections.) In patients with an ulcer present at the time of initiation of therapy, an additional 18 days of omeprazole 20 mg once daily is recommended for ulcer healing and symptom relief.
Dual therapy: BIAXIN/omeprazole
The recommended adult dose is 500 mg BIAXIN given three times daily (q8h) and 40 mg omeprazole given once daily (qAM) for 14 days. (See **INDICATIONS AND USAGE** and **CLINICAL STUDIES** sections.) An additional 14 days of omeprazole 20 mg once daily is recommended for ulcer healing and symptom relief.
Dual therapy: BIAXIN/ranitidine bismuth citrate
The recommended adult dose is 500 mg BIAXIN given twice daily (q12h) or three times daily (q8h) and 400 mg ranitidine bismuth citrate given twice daily (q12h) for 14 days. An additional 14 days of 400 mg twice daily is recommended for ulcer healing and symptom relief. BIAXIN and ranitidine bismuth citrate combination therapy is not recommended in patients with creatinine clearance less than 25 mL/min. (See **INDICATIONS AND USAGE** and **CLINICAL STUDIES** sections.)
Children – The usual recommended daily dosage is 15 mg/kg/day divided q12h for 10 days.
[See second table above]
Clarithromycin may be administered without dosage adjustment in the presence of hepatic impairment if there is normal renal function. However, in the presence of severe renal impairment (CR_{CL} < 30 mL/min), with or without coexisting hepatic impairment, the dose should be halved or the dosing interval doubled.
Mycobacterial infections:
Prophylaxis: The recommended dose of BIAXIN for the prevention of disseminated *Mycobacterium avium* disease is 500 mg b.i.d. In children, the recommended dose is 7.5 mg/kg b.i.d. up to 500 mg b.i.d. No studies of clarithromycin for MAC prophylaxis have been performed in pediatric populations and the doses recommended for prophylaxis are derived from MAC treatment studies in children. Dosing recommendations for children are in the table above.
Treatment: Clarithromycin is recommended as the primary agent for the treatment of disseminated infection due to *Mycobacterium avium* complex. Clarithromycin should be used in combination with other antimycobacterial drugs that have shown *in vitro* activity against MAC or clinical benefit in MAC treatment. (See **CLINICAL STUDIES**.) The recommended dose for mycobacterial infections in adults is 500 mg b.i.d. In children, the recommended dose is 7.5 mg/kg b.i.d. up to 500 mg b.i.d. Dosing recommendations for children are in the table above.
Clarithromycin therapy should continue for life if clinical and mycobacterial improvements are observed.
Constituting Instructions
The table below indicates the volume of water to be added when constituting:
[See third table above]

Total volume after constitution	Clarithromycin concentration after constitution	Clarithromycin contents per bottle	NDC
50 mL	125 mg/5 mL	1250 mg	0074-3163-50
100 mL	125 mg/5 mL	2500 mg	0074-3163-13
100 mL	187.5 mg/5 mL	3750 mg	0074-3494-13
50 mL	250 mg/5 mL	2500 mg	0074-3188-50
100 mL	250 mg/5 mL	5000 mg	0074-3188-13

	Mortality		Reduction in
	Placebo	Clarithromycin	Mortality on Clarithromycin
6 month	9.4%	6.5%	31%
12 month	29.7%	20.5%	31%
18 month	46.4%	37.5%	20%

Treatment-related* Adverse Event Incidence Rates (%) in Immunocompromised Adult Patients Receiving Prophylaxis Against *M. avium* Complex

Body System‡ Adverse Event	Clarithromycin (n = 339) %	Placebo (n = 339) %
Body as a Whole		
Abdominal pain	5.0%	3.5%
Headache	2.7%	0.9%
Digestive		
Diarrhea	7.7%	4.1%
Dyspepsia	3.8%	2.7%
Flatulence	2.4%	0.9%
Nausea	11.2%	7.1%
Vomiting	5.9%	3.2%
Skin & Appendages		
Rash	3.2%	3.5%
Special Senses		
Taste Perversion	8.0%	0.3%

* Includes those events possibly or probably related to study drug and excludes concurrent conditions.
‡ >2% Adverse Event Incidence Rates for either treatment group.

Percentage of Patients[(a)] Exceeding Extreme Laboratory Value in Patients Receiving Prophylaxis Against *M. avium* Complex

		Clarithromycin 500 mg b.i.d.		Placebo	
Hemoglobin	< 8 g/dL	4/118	3%	5/103	5%
Platelet Count	< 50 × 10^9/L	11/249	4%	12/250	5%
WBC Count	< 1 × 10^9/L	2/103	4%	0/95	0%
SGOT	> 5 × ULN[b]	7/196	4%	5/208	2%
SGPT	> 5 × ULN[b]	6/217	3%	4/232	2%
Alk. Phos.	> 5 × ULN[b]	5/220	2%	5/218	2%

(a) Includes only patients with baseline values within the normal range or borderline high (hematology variables) and within the normal range or borderline low (chemistry variables).
(b) ULN = Upper Limit of Normal

Add half the volume of water to the bottle and shake vigorously. Add the remainder of water to the bottle and shake. Shake well before each use. Oversize bottle provides shake space. Keep tightly closed. Do not refrigerate. After mixing, store at 15° to 30°C (59° to 86°F) and use within 14 days.

HOW SUPPLIED

BIAXIN® Filmtab® (clarithromycin tablets, USP) are supplied as yellow oval film-coated tablets in the following packaging sizes:

250 mg tablets: (imprinted in blue with the Abbott logo and Abbo-Code KT)

Bottles of 60 (**NDC** 0074-3368-60) and ABBO-PAC unit dose strip packages of 100 (**NDC** 0074-3368-11).

Store BIAXIN 250 mg tablets at controlled room temperature 15° to 30°C (59° to 86°F) in a well-closed container. Protect from light.

500 mg tablets: (debossed with the Abbott logo on one side and Abbo-Code KL on the opposite side)

Bottles of 60 (**NDC** 0074-2586-60), ABBO-PAC unit dose strip packages of 100 (**NDC** 0074-2586-11) and BIAXIN 7-PAK® carton of 2 blister packages of 14 tablets (**NDC** 0074-2586-41).

Store BIAXIN 500 mg tablets at controlled room temperature 20° to 25°C (68° to 77°F) in a well-closed container.

BIAXIN® XL Filmtab® (clarithromycin extended-release tablets) are supplied as yellow oval film-coated 500 mg tablets debossed (on one side) with the Abbott logo and a two-letter Abbo-Code designation, KJ in the following packaging sizes:

500 mg tablets:

Bottles of 60 (**NDC** 0074-3165-60) and BIAXIN XL-PAC® carton of 4 blister packages 14 tablets each (**NDC** 0074-3165-41).

Store BIAXIN XL tablets at 20° to 25°C (68° to 77°F). Excursions permitted to 15° to 30°C (59° to 86°F). [See USP Controlled Room Temperature.]

BIAXIN® Granules (clarithromycin for oral suspension, USP) is supplied in the following strengths and sizes:

[See first table above]

Store BIAXIN granules for oral suspension at controlled room temperature 15° to 30°C (59° to 86°F) in a well-closed container. Do not refrigerate BIAXIN suspension.

CLINICAL STUDIES

Mycobacterial Infections

Prophylaxis:

A randomized, double-blind study (561) compared clarithromycin 500 mg b.i.d. to placebo in patients with CDC-defined AIDS and CD_4 counts <100 cells/µL. This study accrued 682 patients from November 1992 to January 1994, with a median CD_4 cell count at study entry of 30 cells/µL. Median duration of clarithromycin was 10.6 months vs. 8.2 months for placebo. More patients in the placebo arm than the clarithromycin arm discontinued prematurely from the study (75.6% and 67.4%, respectively). However, if premature discontinuations due to MAC or death are excluded, approximately equal percentages of patients on each arm (54.8% on clarithromycin and 52.5% on placebo) discontinued study drug early for other reasons. The study was designed to evaluate the following endpoints:

1. MAC bacteremia, defined as at least one positive culture for *M. avium* complex bacteria from blood or another normally sterile site.
2. Survival.
3. Clinically significant disseminated MAC disease, defined as MAC bacteremia accompanied by signs or symptoms of serious MAC infection, including fever, night sweats, weight loss, anemia, or elevations in liver function tests.

MAC bacteremia:

In patients randomized to clarithromycin, the risk of MAC bacteremia was reduced by 69% compared to placebo. The difference between groups was statistically significant (p<0.001). On an intent-to-treat basis, the one-year cumulative incidence of MAC bacteremia was 5.0% for patients randomized to clarithromycin and 19.4% for patients randomized to placebo. While only 19 of the 341 patients randomized to clarithromycin developed MAC, 11 of these cases were resistant to clarithromycin. The patients with resistant MAC bacteremia had a median baseline CD_4 count of 10 cells/mm³ (range 2 to 25 cells/mm³). Information regarding the clinical course and response to treatment of the patients with resistant MAC bacteremia is limited. The 8 patients who received clarithromycin and developed susceptible MAC bacteremia had a median baseline CD_4 count of 25 cells/mm³ (range 10 to 80 cells/mm³). Comparatively, 53 of the 341 placebo patients developed MAC; none of these isolates were resistant to clarithromycin. The median baseline CD_4 count was 15 cells/mm³ (range 2 to 130 cells/mm³) for placebo patients that developed MAC.

Survival:

A statistically significant survival benefit was observed.

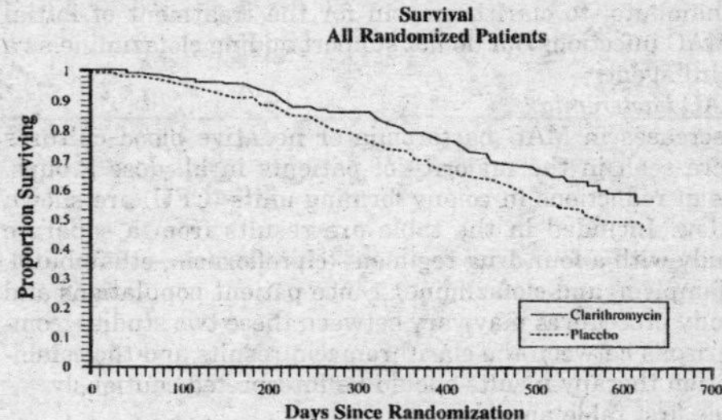

[See second table at left]

Since the analysis at 18 months includes patients no longer receiving prophylaxis the survival benefit of clarithromycin may be underestimated.

Clinically significant disseminated MAC disease:

In association with the decreased incidence of bacteremia, patients in the group randomized to clarithromycin showed reductions in the signs and symptoms of disseminated MAC disease, including fever, night sweats, weight loss, and anemia.

Safety:

In AIDS patients treated with clarithromycin over long periods of time for prophylaxis against *M. avium*, it was often difficult to distinguish adverse events possibly associated with clarithromycin administration from underlying HIV disease or intercurrent illness. Median duration of treatment was 10.6 months for the clarithromycin group and 8.2 months for the placebo group.

[See third table at left]

Among these events, taste perversion was the only event that had significantly higher incidence in the clarithromycin-treated group compared to the placebo-treated group.

Discontinuation due to adverse events was required in 18% of patients receiving clarithromycin compared to 17% of patients receiving placebo in this trial. Primary reasons for discontinuation in clarithromycin treated patients include headache, nausea, vomiting, depression and taste perversion.

Changes in Laboratory Values of Potential Clinical Importance:

In immunocompromised patients receiving prophylaxis against *M. avium*, evaluations of laboratory values were made by analyzing those values outside the seriously abnormal value (i.e., the extreme high or low limit) for the specified test.

[See fourth table at left]

Treatment:

Three randomized studies (500, 577, and 521) compared different dosages of clarithromycin in patients with CDC-defined AIDS and CD_4 counts <100 cells/µL. These studies accrued patients from May 1991 to March 1992. Study 500 was randomized, double-blind; Study 577 was open-label compassionate use. Both studies used 500 and 1000 mg b.i.d. doses; Study 500 also had a 2000 mg b.i.d. group. Study 521 was a pediatric study at 3.75, 7.5, and 15 mg/kg b.i.d. Study 500 enrolled 154 adult patients, Study 577 enrolled 469 adult patients, and Study 521 enrolled 25 patients between the ages of 1 to 20. The majority of patients had CD_4 cell counts <50/µL at study entry. The studies were designed to evaluate the following end points:

1. Change in MAC bacteremia or blood cultures negative for *M. avium.*
2. Change in clinical signs and symptoms of MAC infection including one or more of the following: fever, night sweats, weight loss, diarrhea, splenomegaly, and hepatomegaly.

The results for the 500 study are described below. The 577 study results were similar to the results of the 500 study. Results with the 7.5 mg/kg b.i.d. dose in the pediatric study were comparable to those for the 500 mg b.i.d. regimen in the adult studies.

Study 069 compared the safety and efficacy of clarithromycin in combination with ethambutol versus clarithromycin in combination with ethambutol and clofazimine for the treatment of disseminated MAC (dMAC) infection[4]. This 24-week study enrolled 106 patients with AIDS and dMAC, with 55 patients randomized to receive clarithromycin and ethambutol, and 51 patients randomized to receive clarithromycin, ethambutol, and clofazimine. Baseline characteristics between study arms were similar with the exception of median CFU counts being at least 1 log higher in the clarithromycin, ethambutol, and clofazimine arm.

Compared to prior experience with clarithromycin monotherapy, the two-drug regimen of clarithromycin and ethambutol was well tolerated and extended the time to microbiologic relapse, largely through suppressing the emergence of clarithromycin resistant strains. However, the addition of clofazimine to the regimen added no additional microbiologic or clinical benefit. Tolerability of both multidrug regimens was comparable with the most common adverse events being gastrointestinal in nature. Patients receiving

Continued on next page

Biaxin—Cont.

the clofazimine-containing regimen had reduced survival rates; however, their baseline mycobacterial colony counts were higher. The results of this trial support the addition of ethambutol to clarithromycin for the treatment of initial dMAC infections but do not support adding clofazimine as a third agent.

MAC bacteremia:

Decreases in MAC bacteremia or negative blood cultures were seen in the majority of patients in all dose groups. Mean reductions in colony forming units (CFU) are shown below. Included in the table are results from a separate study with a four drug regimen[5] (ciprofloxacin, ethambutol, rifampicin, and clofazimine). Since patient populations and study procedures may vary between these two studies, comparisons between the clarithromycin results and the combination therapy results should be interpreted cautiously.

[See first table above]

Although the 1000 mg and 2000 mg b.i.d. doses showed significantly better control of bacteremia during the first four weeks of therapy, no significant differences were seen beyond that point. The percent of patients whose blood was sterilized as shown by one or more negative cultures at any time during acute therapy was 61% (30/49) for the 500 mg b.i.d. group and 59% (29/49) and 52% (25/48) for the 1000 and 2000 mg b.i.d. groups, respectively. The percent of patients who had 2 or more negative cultures during acute therapy that were sustained through study Day 84 was 25% (12/49) in both the 500 and 1000 mg b.i.d. groups and 8% (4/48) for the 2000 mg b.i.d. group. By Day 84, 23% (11/49), 37% (18/49), and 56% (27/48) of patients had died or discontinued from the study, and 14% (7/49), 12% (6/49), and 13% (6/48) of patients had relapsed in the 500, 1000, and 2000 mg b.i.d. dose groups, respectively. All of the isolates had an MIC < 8 µg/mL at pre-treatment. Relapse was almost always accompanied by an increase in MIC. The median time to first negative culture was 54, 41, and 29 days for the 500, 1000, and 2000 mg b.i.d. groups, respectively. The time to first decrease of at least 1 log in CFU count was significantly shorter with the 1000 and 2000 mg b.i.d. doses (median equal to 16 and 15 days, respectively) in comparison to the 500 mg b.i.d. group (median equal to 29 days). The median time to first positive culture or study discontinuation following the first negative culture was 43, 59 and 43 days for the 500, 1000, and 2000 mg b.i.d. groups, respectively.

Clinically significant disseminated MAC Disease:

Among patients experiencing night sweats prior to therapy, 84% showed resolution or improvement at some point during the 12 weeks of clarithromycin at 500 to 2000 mg b.i.d. doses. Similarly, 77% of patients reported resolution or improvement in fevers at some point. Response rates for clinical signs of MAC are given below:

[See second table above]

The median duration of response, defined as improvement or resolution of clinical signs and symptoms, was 2 to 6 weeks.

Since the study was not designed to determine the benefit of monotherapy beyond 12 weeks, the duration of response may be underestimated for the 25 to 33% of patients who continued to show clinical response after 12 weeks.

Survival:

Median survival time from study entry (Study 500) was 249 days at the 500 mg b.i.d. dose compared to 215 days with the 1000 mg b.i.d. dose. However, during the first 12 weeks of therapy, there were 2 deaths in 53 patients in the 500 mg b.i.d. group versus 13 deaths in 51 patients in the 1000 mg b.i.d. group. The reason for this apparent mortality difference is not known. Survival in the two groups was similar beyond 12 weeks. The median survival times for these dosages were similar to recent historical controls with MAC when treated with combination therapies.[5]

Median survival time from study entry in Study 577 was 199 days for the 500 mg b.i.d. dose and 179 days for the 1000 mg b.i.d. dose. During the first four weeks of therapy, while patients were maintained on their originally assigned dose, there were 11 deaths in 255 patients taking 500 mg b.i.d. and 18 deaths in 214 patients taking 1000 mg b.i.d.

Safety:

The adverse event profiles showed that both the 500 and 1000 mg b.i.d. doses were well tolerated. The 2000 mg b.i.d. dose was poorly tolerated and resulted in a higher proportion of premature discontinuations.

In AIDS patients and other immunocompromised patients treated with the higher doses of clarithromycin over long periods of time for mycobacterial infections, it was often difficult to distinguish adverse events possibly associated with clarithromycin administration from underlying signs of HIV disease or intercurrent illness.

The following analyses summarize experience during the first 12 weeks of therapy with clarithromycin. Data are reported separately for Study 500 (randomized, double-blind) and Study 577 (open-label, compassionate use) and also combined. Adverse events were reported less frequently in Study 577, which may be due in part to differences in monitoring between the two studies. In adult patients receiving clarithromycin 500 mg b.i.d., the most frequently reported adverse events, considered possibly or probably related to study drug, with an incidence of 5% or greater, are listed below. Most of these events were mild to moderate in severity, although 5% (Study 500: 8%; Study 577: 4%) of patients receiving 500 mg b.i.d. and 5% (Study 500: 4%; Study 577: 6%) of patients receiving 1000 mg b.i.d. reported severe adverse events. Excluding those patients who discontinued therapy or died due to complications of their underlying non-mycobacterial disease, approximately 8% (Study 500: 15%; Study 577: 7%) of the patients who received 500 mg b.i.d. and 12% (Study 500: 14%; Study 577: 12%) of the patients who received 1000 mg b.i.d. discontinued therapy due to drug-related events during the first 12 weeks of therapy.

Overall, the 500 and 1000 mg b.i.d. doses had similar adverse event profiles.

[See third table above]

A limited number of pediatric AIDS patients have been treated with clarithromycin suspension for mycobacterial infections. The most frequently reported adverse events, excluding those due to the patient's concurrent condition, were consistent with those observed in adult patients.

Mean Reductions in Log CFU from Baseline (After 4 Weeks of Therapy)

500 mg b.i.d. (N=35)	1000 mg b.i.d. (N=32)	2000 mg b.i.d. (N=26)	Four Drug Regimen (N=24)
1.5	2.3	2.3	1.4

Resolution of Fever			Resolution of Night Sweats		
b.i.d. dose (mg)	% ever afebrile	% afebrile ≥6 weeks	b.i.d. dose (mg)	% ever resolving	% resolving ≥6 weeks
500	67%	23%	500	85%	42%
1000	67%	12%	1000	70%	33%
2000	62%	22%	2000	72%	36%

Weight Gain >3%			Hemoglobin Increase >1 gm		
b.i.d. dose (mg)	% ever gaining	% gaining ≥6 weeks	b.i.d. dose (mg)	% ever increasing	% increasing ≥6 weeks
500	33%	14%	500	58%	26%
1000	26%	17%	1000	37%	6%
2000	26%	12%	2000	62%	18%

Treatment-related* Adverse Event Incidence Rates (%) in Immunocompromised Adult Patients During the First 12 Weeks of Therapy with 500 mg b.i.d. Clarithromycin Dose

Adverse Event	Study 500 (n=53)	Study 577 (n=255)	Combined (n=308)
Abdominal Pain	7.5	2.4	3.2
Diarrhea	9.4	1.6	2.9
Flatulence	7.5	0.0	1.3
Headache	7.5	0.4	1.6
Nausea	28.3	9.0	12.3
Rash	9.4	2.0	3.2
Taste Perversion	18.9	0.4	3.6
Vomiting	24.5	3.9	7.5

* Includes those events possibly or probably related to study drug and excludes concurrent conditions.

Percentage of Patients[(a)] Exceeding Extreme Laboratory Value Limits During First 12 Weeks of Treatment 500 mg b.i.d. Dose[(b)]

		Study 500	Study 577	Combined
BUN	>50 mg/dL	0%	<1%	<1%
Platelet Count	$<50 \times 10^9$/L	0%	<1%	<1%
SGOT	>5 × ULN[c]	0%	3%	2%
SGPT	>5 × ULN[c]	0%	2%	1%
WBC	$<1 \times 10^9$/L	0%	1%	1%

(a) Includes only patients with baseline values within the normal range or borderline high (hematology variables) and within the normal range or borderline low (chemistry variables)
(b) Includes all values within the first 12 weeks for patients who start on 500 mg b.i.d.
(c) ULN = Upper Limit of Normal

H. pylori **Eradication Rates-Triple Therapy (BIAXIN/lansoprazole/amoxicillin) Percent of Patients Cured [95% Confidence Interval] (number of patients)**

Study	Duration	Triple Therapy Evaluable Analysis*	Triple Therapy Intent-to-Treat Analysis#
M93–131	14 days	92† [80.0 – 97.7] (n = 48)	86† [73.3 – 93.5] (n = 55)
M95–392	14 days	86‡ [75.7 – 93.6] (n = 66)	83‡ [72.0 – 90.8] (n = 70)
M95–399¶	14 days	85 [77.0 – 91.0] (N = 113)	82 [73.9 – 88.1] (N = 126)
	10 days	84 [76.0 – 89.8] (N = 123)	81 [73.9 – 87.6] (N = 135)

* Based on evaluable patients with confirmed duodenal ulcer (active or within one year) and *H. pylori* infection at baseline defined as at least two of three positive endoscopic tests from CLOtest (Delta West LTD., Bentley, Australia), histology, and/or culture. Patients were included in the analysis if they completed the study. Additionally, if patients were dropped out of the study due to an adverse event related to the study drug, they were included in the analysis as evaluable failures of therapy.
\# Patients were included in the analysis if they had documented *H. pylori* infection at baseline as defined above and had a confirmed duodenal ulcer (active or within one year). All dropouts were included as failures of therapy.
† ($p<0.05$) versus BIAXIN/lansoprazole and lansoprazole/amoxicillin dual therapy.
‡ ($p<0.05$) versus BIAXIN/amoxicillin dual therapy.
¶ The 95% confidence interval for the difference in eradication rates, 10-day minus 14-day, is (−10.5, 8.1) in the evaluable analysis and (−9.7, 9.1) in the intent-to-treat analysis.

Changes in Laboratory Values:
In immunocompromised patients treated with clarithromycin for mycobacterial infections, evaluations of laboratory values were made by analyzing those values outside the seriously abnormal level (i.e., the extreme high or low limit) for the specified test.
[See fourth table on previous page]

Otitis Media

In a controlled clinical study of acute otitis media performed in the United States, where significant rates of beta-lactamase producing organisms were found, clarithromycin was compared to an oral cephalosporin. In this study, very strict evaluability criteria were used to determine clinical response. For the 223 patients who were evaluated for clinical efficacy, the clinical success rate (i.e., cure plus improvement) at the post-therapy visit was 88% for clarithromycin and 91% for the cephalosporin.
In a smaller number of patients, microbiologic determinations were made at the pre-treatment visit. The following presumptive bacterial eradication/clinical cure outcomes (i.e., clinical success) were obtained:

U.S. Acute Otitis Media Study
Clarithromycin vs. Oral Cephalosporin
EFFICACY RESULTS

PATHOGEN	OUTCOME
S. pneumoniae	clarithromycin success rate, 13/15 (87%), control 4/5
*H. influenzae**	clarithromycin success rate, 10/14 (71%), control 3/4
M. catarrhalis	clarithromycin success rate, 4/5, control 1/1
S. pyogenes	clarithromycin success rate, 3/3, control 0/1
Overall	clarithromycin success rate, 30/37 (81%), control 8/11 (73%)

* None of the *H. influenzae* isolated pre-treatment was resistant to clarithromycin; 6% were resistant to the control agent.

Safety:
The incidence of adverse events in all patients treated, primarily diarrhea and vomiting, did not differ clinically or statistically for the two agents.
In two other controlled clinical trials of acute otitis media performed in the United States, where significant rates of beta-lactamase producing organisms were found, clarithromycin was compared to an oral antimicrobial agent that contained a specific beta-lactamase inhibitor. In these studies, very strict evaluability criteria were used to determine the clinical responses. In the 233 patients who were evaluated for clinical efficacy, the combined clinical success rate (i.e., cure and improvement) at the post-therapy visit was 91% for both clarithromycin and the control.
For the patients who had microbiologic determinations at the pre-treatment visit, the following presumptive bacterial eradication/clinical cure outcomes (i.e., clinical success) were obtained:

Two U.S. Acute Otitis Media Studies Clarithromycin vs. Antimicrobial/Beta-lactamase Inhibitor
EFFICACY RESULTS

PATHOGEN	OUTCOME
S. pneumoniae	clarithromycin success rate, 43/51 (84%), control 55/56 (98%)
*H. influenzae**	clarithromycin success rate, 36/45 (80%), control 31/33 (94%)
M. catarrhalis	clarithromycin success rate, 9/10 (90%), control 6/6
S. pyogenes	clarithromycin success rate, 3/3, control 5/5
Overall	clarithromycin success rate, 91/109 (83%), control 97/100 (97%)

* Of the *H. influenzae* isolated pre-treatment, 3% were resistant to clarithromycin and 10% were resistant to the control agent.

Safety:
The incidence of adverse events in all patients treated, primarily diarrhea (15% vs. 38%) and diaper rash (3% vs. 11%) in young children, was clinically and statistically lower in the clarithromycin arm versus the control arm.

Duodenal Ulcer Associated with *H. pylori* Infection

Clarithromycin + Lansoprazole and Amoxicillin

H. pylori Eradication for Reducing the Risk of Duodenal Ulcer Recurrence:
Two U.S. randomized, double-blind clinical studies in patients with *H. pylori* and duodenal ulcer disease (defined as an active ulcer or history of an active ulcer within one year) evaluated the efficacy of clarithromycin in combination with lansoprazole and amoxicillin capsules as triple 14-day therapy for eradication of *H. pylori*. Based on the results of these studies, the safety and efficacy of the following eradication regimen were established:
Triple therapy: BIAXIN 500 mg b.i.d. + lansoprazole 30 mg b.i.d. + amoxicillin 1 gm b.i.d.
Treatment was for 14 days. *H. pylori* eradication was defined as two negative tests (culture and histology) at 4 to 6 weeks following the end of treatment.

Per-Protocol and Intent-To-Treat *H. pylori* Eradication Rates
% of Patients Cured [95% Confidence Interval]

	Clarithromycin + omeprazole + amoxicillin		Clarithromycin + amoxicillin	
	Per-Protocol†	Intent-To-Treat‡	Per-Protocol†	Intent-To-Treat‡
Study 126	*77 [64, 86] (n = 64)	69 [57, 79] (n = 80)	43 [31, 56] (n = 67)	37 [27, 48] (n = 84)
Study 127	*78 [67, 88] (n = 65)	73 [61, 82] (n = 77)	41 [29, 54] (n = 68)	36 [26, 47] (n = 84)
Study M96–446	*90 [80, 96] (n = 69)	83 [74, 91] (n = 84)	32 [24, 44] (n = 93)	32 [23, 42] (n = 99)

† Patients were included in the analysis if they had confirmed duodenal ulcer disease (active ulcer studies 126 and 127; history of ulcer within 5 years, study M96–446) and *H. pylori* infection at baseline defined as at least two of three positive endoscopic tests from CLOtest®, histology, and/or culture. Patients were included in the analysis if they completed the study. Additionally, if patients dropped out of the study due to an adverse event related to the study drug, they were included in the analysis as failures of therapy. The impact of eradication on ulcer recurrence has not been assessed in patients with a past history of ulcer.
‡ Patients were included in the analysis if they had documented *H. pylori* infection at baseline and had confirmed duodenal ulcer disease. All dropouts were included as failures of therapy.
* $p < 0.05$ versus clarithromycin plus amoxicillin.

End-of-Treatment Ulcer Healing Rates
Percent of Patients Healed (n/N)

Study	Clarithromycin + Omeprazole	Omeprazole	Clarithromycin
U.S. Studies			
Study 100	94% (58/62)†	88% (60/68)	71% (49/69)
Study 067	88% (56/64)†	85% (55/65)	64% (44/69)
Non-U.S. Studies			
Study 058	99% (84/85)	95% (82/86)	N/A
Study 812b[1]	100% (64/64)	99% (71/72)	N/A

† $p<0.05$ for clarithromycin + omeprazole versus clarithromycin monotherapy.
[1] In Study 812b patients received omeprazole 40 mg daily for days 15 to 28.

***H. pylori* Eradication Rates (Per-Protocol Analysis) at 4 to 6 weeks**
Percent of Patients Cured (n/N)

Study	Clarithromycin + Omeprazole	Omeprazole	Clarithromycin
U.S. Studies			
Study 100	64% (39/61)†‡	0% (0/59)	39% (17/44)
Study 067	74% (39/53)†‡	0% (0/54)	31% (13/42)
Non-U.S. Studies			
Study 058	74% (64/86)‡	1% (1/90)	N/A
Study 812b	83% (50/60)‡	1% (1/74)	N/A

† Statistically significantly higher than clarithromycin monotherapy ($p<0.05$).
‡ Statistically significantly higher than omeprazole monotherapy ($p<0.05$).

Ulcer Recurrence at 6 months by *H. pylori* Status at 4–6 Weeks

	H. pylori Negative	*H. pylori* Positive
U.S. Studies		
Study 100		
Clarithromycin + Omeprazole	6% (2/34)	56% (9/16)
Omeprazole	(0/0)	71% (35/49)
Clarithromycin	12% (2/17)	32% (7/22)
Study 067		
Clarithromycin + Omeprazole	38% (11/29)	50% (6/12)
Omeprazole	- (0/0)	67% (31/46)
Clarithromycin	18% (2/11)	52% (14/27)
Non-U.S. Studies		
Study 058		
Clarithromycin + Omeprazole	6% (3/53)	24% (4/17)
Omeprazole	0% (0/3)	55% (39/71)
Study 812b*		
Clarithromycin + Omeprazole	5% (2/42)	0% (0/7)
Omeprazole	0% (0/1)	54% (32/59)
***12-month recurrence rates:**		
Clarithromycin + Omeprazole	3% (1/40)	0% (0/6)
Omeprazole	0% (0/1)	67% (29/43)

The combination of BIAXIN plus lansoprazole and amoxicillin as triple therapy was effective in eradicating *H. pylori*. Eradication of *H. pylori* has been shown to reduce the risk of duodenal ulcer recurrence.
A randomized, double-blind clinical study performed in the U.S. in patients with *H. pylori* and duodenal ulcer disease (defined as an active ulcer or history of an ulcer within one year) compared the efficacy of clarithromycin in combination with lansoprazole and amoxicillin as triple therapy for 10 and 14 days. This study established that the 10-day triple therapy was equivalent to the 14-day triple therapy in eradicating *H. pylori*.
[See fifth table on previous page]

Clarithromycin + Omeprazole and Amoxicillin Therapy

H. pylori Eradication for Reducing the Risk of Duodenal Ulcer Recurrence:
Three U.S., randomized, double-blind clinical studies in patients with *H. pylori* infection and duodenal ulcer disease (n = 558) compared clarithromycin plus omeprazole and amoxicillin to clarithromycin plus amoxicillin. Two studies (Studies 126 and 127) were conducted in patients with an active duodenal ulcer, and the third study (Study 446) was conducted in patients with a duodenal ulcer in the past 5 years, but without an ulcer present at the time of enrollment. The dosage regimen in the studies was clarithromycin 500 mg b.i.d. plus omeprazole 20 mg b.i.d. plus amoxicillin 1 gram b.i.d. for 10 days. In Studies 126 and 127, patients who took the omeprazole regimen also received an additional 18 days of omeprazole 20 mg q.d. Endpoints studied were eradication of *H. pylori* and duodenal ulcer healing (studies 126 and 127 only). *H. pylori* status was determined by CLOtest®, histology, and culture in all three studies. For a given patient, *H. pylori* was considered eradicated if at

Continued on next page

Biaxin—Cont.

least two of these tests were negative, and none was positive. The combination of clarithromycin plus omeprazole and amoxicillin was effective in eradicating *H. pylori.*
[See first table at top of previous page]
Safety:
In clinical trials using combination therapy with clarithromycin plus omeprazole and amoxicillin, no adverse reactions peculiar to the combination of these drugs have been observed. Adverse reactions that have occurred have been limited to those that have been previously reported with clarithromycin, omeprazole, or amoxicillin.
The most frequent adverse experiences observed in clinical trials using combination therapy with clarithromycin plus omeprazole and amoxicillin (n=274) were diarrhea (14%), taste perversion (10%), and headache (7%).
For information about adverse reactions with omeprazole or amoxicillin, refer to the ADVERSE REACTIONS section of their package inserts.

Clarithromycin + Omeprazole Therapy
Four randomized, double-blind, multi-center studies (067, 100, 812b, and 058) evaluated clarithromycin 500 mg t.i.d. plus omeprazole 40 mg q.d. for 14 days, followed by omeprazole 20 mg q.d. (067, 100, and 058) or by omeprazole 40 mg q.d. (812b) for an additional 14 days in patients with active duodenal ulcer associated with *H. pylori.* Studies 067 and 100 were conducted in the U.S. and Canada and enrolled 242 and 256 patients, respectively. *H. pylori* infection and duodenal ulcer were confirmed in 219 patients in Study 067 and 228 patients in Study 100. These studies compared the combination regimen to omeprazole and clarithromycin monotherapies. Studies 812b and 058 were conducted in Europe and enrolled 154 and 215 patients, respectively. *H. pylori* infection and duodenal ulcer were confirmed in 148 patients in Study 812b and 208 patients in Study 058. These studies compared the combination regimen to omeprazole monotherapy. The results for the efficacy analyses for these studies are described below.
Duodenal Ulcer Healing:
The combination of clarithromycin and omeprazole was as effective as omeprazole alone for healing duodenal ulcer.
[See second table on previous page]
Eradication of H. pylori Associated with Duodenal Ulcer:
The combination of clarithromycin and omeprazole was effective in eradicating *H. pylori.*
[See third table on previous page]
H. pylori eradication was defined as no positive test (culture or histology) at 4 weeks following the end of treatment, and two negative tests were required to be considered eradicated. In the per-protocol analysis, the following patients were excluded: dropouts, patients with major protocol violations, patients with missing *H. pylori* tests post-treatment, and patients that were not assessed for *H. pylori* eradication at 4 weeks after the end of treatment because they were found to have an unhealed ulcer at the end of treatment.
Ulcer recurrence at 6-months following the end of treatment was assessed for patients in whom ulcers were healed post-treatment.
[See fourth table on previous page]
Thus, in patients with duodenal ulcer associated with *H. pylori* infection, eradication of *H. pylori* reduced ulcer recurrence.
Safety:
The adverse event profiles for the four studies showed that the combination of clarithromycin 500 mg t.i.d. and omeprazole 40 mg q.d. for 14 days, followed by omeprazole 20 mg q.d. (067, 100, and 058) or 40 mg q.d. (812b) for an additional 14 days was well tolerated. Of the 346 patients who received the combination, 12 (3.5%) patients discontinued study drug due to adverse events.
[See first table above]

Adverse Events with an Incidence of 3% or Greater

Adverse Event	Clarithromycin + Omeprazole (N = 346) % of Patients	Omeprazole (N = 355) % of Patients	Clarithromycin (N = 166) % of Patients*
Taste Perversion	15%	1%	16%
Nausea	5%	1%	3%
Headache	5%	6%	9%
Diarrhea	4%	3%	7%
Vomiting	4%	<1%	1%
Abdominal Pain	3%	2%	1%
Infection	3%	4%	2%

* Studies 067 and 100, only

Most of these events were mild to moderate in severity.
Changes in Laboratory Values:
Changes in laboratory values with possible clinical significance in patients taking clarithromycin and omeprazole were as follows:
Hepatic – elevated direct bilirubin <1%; GGT <1%; SGOT (AST) <1%; SGPT (ALT) <1%.
Renal – elevated serum creatinine <1%.
For information on omeprazole, refer to the ADVERSE REACTIONS section of the PRILOSEC package insert.

Clarithromycin + Ranitidine Bismuth Citrate Therapy
In a U.S. double-blind, randomized, multicenter, dose-comparison trial, ranitidine bismuth citrate 400 mg b.i.d. for 4 weeks plus clarithromycin 500 mg b.i.d. for the first 2 weeks was found to have an equivalent *H. pylori* eradication rate (based on culture and histology) when compared to ranitidine bismuth citrate 400 mg b.i.d. for 4 weeks plus clarithromycin 500 mg t.i.d. for the first 2 weeks. The intent-to-treat *H. pylori* eradication rates are shown below:
[See second table above]

***H. pylori* Eradication Rates in Study H2BA-3001**

Analysis	RBC 400 mg + Clarithromycin 500 mg b.i.d.	RBC 400 mg + Clarithromycin 500 mg t.i.d.	95% CI Rate Difference
ITT	65% (122/188) [58%, 72%]	63% (122/195) [55%, 69%]	(-8%, 12%)
Per-Protocol	72% (117/162) [65%, 79%]	71% (120/170) [63%,77%]	(-9%, 12%)

H. pylori eradication was defined as no positive test at 4 weeks following the end of treatment. Patients must have had two tests performed, and these must have been negative to be considered eradicated of *H. pylori.* The following patients were excluded from the per-protocol analysis: patients not infected with *H. pylori* prestudy, dropouts, patients with major protocol violations, patients with missing *H. pylori* tests. Patients excluded from the intent-to-treat analysis included those not infected with *H. pylori* prestudy and those with missing *H. pylori* tests prestudy. Patients were assessed for *H. pylori* eradication (4 weeks following treatment) regardless of their healing status (at the end of treatment).
The relationship between *H. pylori* eradication and duodenal ulcer recurrence was assessed in a combined analysis of six U.S. randomized, double-blind, multicenter, placebo-controlled trials using ranitidine bismuth citrate with or without antibiotics. The results from approximately 650 U.S. patients showed that the risk of ulcer recurrence within 6 months of completing treatment was two times less likely in patients whose *H. pylori* infection was eradicated compared to patients in whom *H. pylori* infection was not eradicated.
Safety:
In clinical trials using combination therapy with clarithromycin plus ranitidine bismuth citrate, no adverse reactions peculiar to the combination of these drugs (using clarithromycin twice daily or three times a day) were observed. Adverse reactions that have occurred have been limited to those reported with clarithromycin or ranitidine bismuth citrate. (See **ADVERSE REACTIONS** section of the Tritec package insert.) The most frequent adverse experiences observed in clinical trials using combination therapy with clarithromycin (500 mg three times a day) with ranitidine bismuth citrate (n = 329) were taste disturbance (11%), diarrhea (5%), nausea and vomiting (3%). The most frequent adverse experiences observed in clinical trials using combination therapy with clarithromycin (500 mg twice daily) with ranitidine bismuth citrate (n = 196) were taste disturbance (8%), nausea and vomiting (5%), and diarrhea (4%).

ANIMAL PHARMACOLOGY AND TOXICOLOGY

Clarithromycin is rapidly and well-absorbed with dose-linear kinetics, low protein binding, and a high volume of distribution. Plasma half-life ranged from 1 to 6 hours and was species dependent. High tissue concentrations were achieved, but negligible accumulation was observed. Fecal clearance predominated. Hepatotoxicity occurred in all species tested (i.e., in rats and monkeys at doses 2 times greater than and in dogs at doses comparable to the maximum human daily dose, based on mg/m^2). Renal tubular degeneration (calculated on a mg/m^2 basis) occurred in rats at doses 2 times, in monkeys at doses 8 times, and in dogs at doses 12 times greater than the maximum human daily dose. Testicular atrophy (on a mg/m^2 basis) occurred in rats at doses 7 times, in dogs at doses 3 times, and in monkeys at doses 8 times greater than the maximum human daily dose. Corneal opacity (on a mg/m^2 basis) occurred in dogs at doses 12 times and in monkeys at doses 8 times greater than the maximum human daily dose. Lymphoid depletion (on a mg/m^2 basis) occurred in dogs at doses 3 times greater than and in monkeys at doses 2 times greater than the maximum human daily dose. These adverse events were absent during clinical trials.

REFERENCES

1. National Committee for Clinical Laboratory Standards, Methods for Dilution Antimicrobial Susceptibility Tests for Bacteria that Grow Aerobically – Fourth Edition. Approved Standard NCCLS Document M7-A4, Vol. 17, No. 2, NCCLS, Wayne, PA, January, 1997.
2. National Committee for Clinical Laboratory Standards, Performance Standards for Antimicrobial Disk Susceptibility Tests – Sixth Edition. Approved Standard NCCLS Document M2-A6, Vol. 17, No. 1, NCCLS, Wayne, PA, January, 1997.
3. National Committee for Clinical Laboratory Standards. Summary Minutes, Subcommittee on Antimicrobial Susceptibility Testing, Tampa, FL. January 11–13, 1998.
4. Chaisson RE, et al. Clarithromycin and Ethambutol with or without Clofazimine for the Treatment of Bacteremic *Mycobacterium avium* Complex Disease in Patients with HIV Infection. *AIDS.* 1997;11:311-317.
5. Kemper CA, et al. Treatment of *Mycobacterium avium* Complex Bacteremia in AIDS with a Four-Drug Oral Regimen. *Ann Intern Med.* 1992;116:466–472.

Filmtab – Film-sealed tablets, Abbott
Revised: April, 2000
Ref.: 03-5049
ABBOTT LABORATORIES
NORTH CHICAGO, IL 60064, U.S.A.
Shown in Product Identification Guide, page 303

CALCIJEX® ℞
CALCITRIOL
INJECTION
1 mcg and 2 mcg/mL

DESCRIPTION

Calcijex® (calcitriol injection) is synthetically manufactured calcitriol and is available as a sterile, isotonic, clear, colorless to yellow, aqueous solution for intravenous injection. Calcijex® is available in 1 mL ampuls. Each 1 mL contains calcitriol, 1 or 2 mcg; Polysorbate 20, 4 mg; sodium ascorbate 2.5 mg added. May contain hydrochloric acid and/or sodium hydroxide for pH adjustment. pH is 6.5 (5.9 to 7.0). Contains no more than 1 mcg/mL of aluminum.
Calcitriol is a crystalline compound which occurs naturally in humans. It is soluble in organic solvents but relatively insoluble in water.
Calcitriol is chemically designated (5Z,7E)-9, 10-secocholesta-5,7,10(19)-triene-1α,3β,25-triol and has the following structural formula:

Molecular Formula: $C_{27}H_{44}O_3$
The other names frequently used for calcitriol are 1α,25-dihydroxycholecalciferol, 1α,25-dihydroxyvitamin D_3, 1,25-DHCC, 1,25$(OH)_2D_3$ and 1,25-diOHC.

CLINICAL PHARMACOLOGY

Calcitriol is the active form of vitamin D_3 (cholecalciferol). The natural or endogenous supply of vitamin D in man mainly depends on ultraviolet light for conversion of 7-dehydrocholesterol to vitamin D_3 in the skin. Vitamin D_3 must be metabolically activated in the liver and the kidney before it is fully active on its target tissues. The initial transformation is catalyzed by a vitamin D_3-25-hydroxylase enzyme present in the liver, and the product of this reaction is 25-$(OH)D_3$ (calcifediol). The latter undergoes hydroxylation in the mitochondria of kidney tissue, and this reaction is activated by the renal 25-hydroxyvitamin D_3-1-α-hydroxylase to produce 1,25-$(OH)_2D_3$ (calcitriol), the active form of vitamin D_3.
The known sites of action of calcitriol are intestine, bone, kidney and parathyroid gland. Calcitriol is the most active known form of vitamin D_3 in stimulating intestinal calcium transport. In acutely uremic rats, calcitriol has been shown to stimulate intestinal calcium absorption. In bone, calcitriol, in conjunction with parathyroid hormone, stimulates resorption of calcium; and in the kidney, calcitriol increases the tubular reabsorption of calcium. *In vitro* and *in vivo* studies have shown that calcitriol directly suppresses secretion and synthesis of PTH. A vitamin D-resistant state may exist in uremic patients because of the failure of the kidney to adequately convert precursors to the active compound, calcitriol.

Calcitriol when administered by bolus injection is rapidly available in the blood stream. Vitamin D metabolites are known to be transported in blood, bound to specific plasma proteins. The pharmacologic activity of an administered dose of calcitriol is about 3 to 5 days. Two metabolic pathways for calcitriol have been identified, conversion to 1,24,25-$(OH)_3D_3$ and to calcitroic acid.

INDICATIONS AND USAGE

Calcijex® (calcitriol injection) is indicated in the management of hypocalcemia in patients undergoing chronic renal dialysis. It has been shown to significantly reduce elevated parathyroid hormone levels. Reduction of PTH has been shown to result in an improvement in renal osteodystrophy.

CONTRAINDICATIONS

Calcijex® (calcitriol injection) should not be given to patients with hypercalcemia or evidence of vitamin D toxicity.

WARNINGS

Since calcitriol is the most potent metabolite of vitamin D available, vitamin D and its derivatives should be withheld during treatment.

A non-aluminum phosphate-binding compound should be used to control serum phosphorus levels in patients undergoing dialysis.

Overdosage of any form of vitamin D is dangerous (see also OVERDOSAGE). Progressive hypercalcemia due to overdosage of vitamin D and its metabolites may be so severe as to require emergency attention. Chronic hypercalcemia can lead to generalized vascular calcification, nephrocalcinosis and other soft-tissue calcification. The serum calcium times phosphate (Ca x P) product should not be allowed to exceed 70. Radiographic evaluation of suspect anatomical regions may be useful in the early detection of this condition.

PRECAUTIONS

1. General

Excessive dosage of Calcijex® (calcitriol injection) induces hypercalcemia and in some instances hypercalciuria; therefore, early in treatment during dosage adjustment, serum calcium and phosphorus should be determined at least twice weekly. Should hypercalcemia develop, the drug should be discontinued immediately.

Calcijex® should be given cautiously to patients on digitalis, because hypercalcemia in such patients may precipitate cardiac arrhythmias.

2. Information for the Patient

The patient and his or her parents should be informed about adherence to instructions about diet and calcium supplementation and avoidance of the use of unapproved non-prescription drugs, including magnesium-containing antacids. Patients should also be carefully informed about the symptoms of hypercalcemia (see ADVERSE REACTIONS).

3. Essential Laboratory Tests

Serum calcium, phosphorus, magnesium and alkaline phosphatase and 24-hour urinary calcium and phosphorus should be determined periodically. During the initial phase of the medication, serum calcium and phosphorus should be determined more frequently (twice weekly).

Adynamic bone disease may develop if PTH levels are suppressed to abnormal levels. If biopsy is not being done for other (diagnostic) reasons, PTH levels may be used to indicate the rate of bone turnover. If PTH levels fall below recommended trarget range (1.5 to 3 times the upper limit of normal), in patients treated with Calcijex®, the Calcijex® dose should be reduced or therapy discontinued. Discontinuation of Calcijex® therapy may result in rebound effect, therefore, appropriate titration downward to a maintenance dose is recommended.

4. Drug Interactions

Magnesium-containing antacid and Calcijex® should not be used concomitantly, because such use may lead to the development of hypermagnesemia.

5. Carcinogenesis, Mutagenesis, Impairment of Fertility

Long-term studies in animals have not been conducted to evaluate the carcinogenic potential of Calcijex® (calcitriol injection). Calcitriol was not mutagenic *in vitro* in the Ames Test nor was oral calcitriol genotoxic *in vivo* in the Mouse Micronucleus Test. No significant effects on fertility and/or general reproductive performances were observed in a Segment I study in rats using oral calcitriol at doses of up to 0.3 mcg/kg.

6. Pregnancy: *Teratogenic Effects: Pregnancy Category C:* Calcitriol has been found to be teratogenic in rabbits when given orally at doses of 0.08 and 0.3 mcg/kg. All 15 fetuses in 3 litters at these doses showed external and skeletal abnormalities. However, none of the other 23 litters (156 fetuses) showed external and skeletal abnormalities compared with controls. Teratogenicity studies in rats at doses up to 0.45 mcg/kg orally showed no evidence of teratogenic potential. There are no adequate and well-controlled studies in pregnant women. Calcijex® should be used during pregnancy only if the potential benefit justifies the potential risk to the fetus.

Nonteratogenic Effects: In the rabbit, oral dosages of 0.3 mcg/kg/day administered on days 7 to 18 of gestation resulted in 19% maternal mortality, a decrease in mean fetal body weight and a reduced number of newborns surviving to 24 hours. A study of the effects on orally administered calcitriol on peri- and postnatal development in rats resulted in hypercalcemia in the offspring of dams given calcitriol at doses of 0.08 or 0.3 mcg/kg/day, hypercalcemia and hypophosphatemia in dams given calcitriol at a dose of 0.08 or 0.3 mcg/kg/day and increased serum urea nitrogen in dams given calcitriol at a dose of 0.3 mcg/kg/day. In another study in rats, maternal weight gain was slightly reduced at an oral dose of 0.3 mcg/kg/day administered on days 7 to 15 of gestation.

The offspring of a woman administered oral calcitriol at 17 to 36 mcg/day during pregnancy manifested mild hypercalcemia in the first 2 days of life which returned to normal at day 3.

7. Nursing Mothers

It is not known whether this drug is excreted in human milk. Because many drugs are excreted in human milk and because of the potential for serious adverse reactions in nursing infants from calcitriol, a decision should be made whether to discontinue nursing or to discontinue the drug, taking into account the importance of the drug to the mother.

8. Pediatric Use

Safety and efficacy of Calcijex® in pediatric patients have not been established.

ADVERSE REACTIONS

Adverse effects of Calcijex® (calcitriol injection) are, in general, similar to those encountered with excessive vitamin D intake. The early and late signs and symptoms of vitamin D intoxication associated with hypercalcemia include:

1. Early

Weakness, headache, somnolence, nausea, vomiting, dry mouth, constipation, muscle pain, bone pain and metallic taste.

2. Late

Polyuria, polydipsia, anorexia, weight loss, nocturia, conjunctivitis (calcific), pancreatitis, photophobia, rhinorrhea, pruritus, hyperthermia, decreased libido, elevated BUN, albuminuria, hypercholesterolemia, elevated SGOT and SGPT, ectopic calcification, hypertension, cardiac arrhythmias and, rarely, overt psychosis.

Occasional mild pain on injection has been observed.

OVERDOSAGE

Administration of Calcijex® (calcitriol injection) to patients in excess of their requirements can cause hypercalcemia, hypercalciuria and hyperphosphatemia. High intake of calcium and phosphate concomitant with Calcijex® may lead to similar abnormalities.

1. Treatment of Hypercalcemia and Overdosage in Patients on Hemodialysis

General treatment of hypercalcemia (greater than 1 mg/dL above the upper limit of normal range) consists of immediate discontinuation of Calcijex® therapy, institution of a low calcium diet and withdrawal of calcium supplements. Serum calcium levels should be determined daily until normocalcemia ensues. Hypercalcemia usually resolves in two to seven days. When serum calcium levels have returned to within normal limits, Calcijex® therapy may be reinstituted at a dose 0.5 mcg less than prior therapy. Serum calcium levels should be obtained at least twice weekly after all dosage changes.

Persistent or markedly elevated serum calcium levels may be corrected by dialysis against a calcium-free dialysate.

2. Treatment of Accidental Overdosage of Calcitriol Injection

The treatment of acute accidental overdosage of Calcijex® should consist of general supportive measures. Serial serum electrolyte determinations (especially calcium), rate of urinary calcium excretion and assessment of electrocardiographic abnormalities due to hypercalcemia should be obtained. Such monitoring is critical in patients receiving digitalis. Discontinuation of supplemental calcium and low calcium diet are also indicated in accidental overdosage. Due to the relatively short duration of the pharmacological action of calcitriol, further measures are probably unnecessary. Should, however, persistent and markedly elevated serum calcium levels occur, there are a variety of therapeutic alternatives which may be considered, depending on the patients' underlying condition. These include the use of drugs such as phosphates and corticosteroids as well as measures to induce an appropriate forced diuresis. The use of peritoneal dialysis against a calcium-free dialysate has also been reported.

DOSAGE AND ADMINISTRATION

The optimal dose of Calcijex® (calcitriol injection) must be carefully determined for each patient.

The effectiveness of Calcijex® therapy is predicated on the assumption that each patient is receiving an adequate and appropriate daily intake of calcium. The RDA for calcium in adults is 800 mg. To ensure that each patient receives an adequate daily intake of calcium, the physician should either prescribe a calcium supplement or instruct the patient in proper dietary measures.

The recommended initial dose of Calcijex®, depending on the severity of the hypocalcemia and/or secondary hyperparathyroidism, is 1 mcg (0.02 mcg/kg) to 2 mcg administered three times weekly, approximately every other day. Doses as small as 0.5 mcg and as large as 4 mcg three times weekly have been used as an initial dose. If a satisfactory response is not observed, the dose may be increased by 0.5 to 1 mcg at two to four week intervals. During this titration period, serum calcium and phosphorus levels should be obtained at least twice weekly. If hypercalcemia or a serum calcium times phosphate product greater than 70 is noted, the drug should be immediately discontinued until these parameters are appropriate. Then, the Calcijex® dose should be reinitiated at a lower dose. Doses may need to be reduced as the PTH levels decrease in response to the therapy. Thus, incremental dosing must be individualized and commensurate with PTH, serum calcium and phosphorus levels. The following is a suggested approach in dose titration:

PTH Levels	Calcijex® Dose
the same or inceasing	increase
decreasing by <30%	increase
decreasing by >30%, <60%	maintain
decreasing by >60%	decrease
one and one-half to three times the upper limit of normal	maintain

Parenteral drug products should be inspected visually for particulate matter and discoloration prior to administration, whenever solution and container permit.

Discard unused portion.

HOW SUPPLIED

Calcijex® (calcitriol injection) is supplied as follows:

List	Container	Concentration	Fill
8110	Ampul	1 mcg/mL	1 mL
8131	Ampul	2 mcg/mL	1 mL

Protect from light.

Store at controlled room temperature 15° to 30°C (59° to 86°F).

Patent Pending.

Reference 58-6003-R3 Rev. February, 2000

ABBOTT LABORATORIES, NORTH CHICAGO, IL 60064, USA

CARTROL® ℞

[*kär 'trōl*]

(Carteolol Hydrochloride)

Filmtab® Tablets

DESCRIPTION

CARTROL (carteolol hydrochloride) is a synthetic, nonselective, beta-adrenergic receptor blocking agent with intrinsic sympathomimetic activity. It is chemically described as 5-[3-[(1,1-dimethylethyl)amino]-2-hydroxypropoxy]-3,4-dihydro-2(1H)-quinolinone monohydrochloride. The structural formula is:

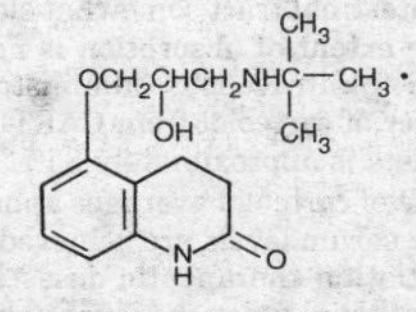

Carteolol hydrochloride is a stable, white crystalline powder which is soluble in water and slightly soluble in ethanol. The molecular weight is 328.84 and $C_{16}H_{24}N_2O_3 \cdot HCl$ is the empirical formula.

CARTROL (carteolol hydrochloride) is available as tablets containing either 2.5 mg or 5 mg of carteolol hydrochloride for oral administration.

INACTIVE INGREDIENTS

2.5 mg Tablet: Cellulosic polymers, corn starch, iron oxide, lactose, magnesium stearate, microcrystalline cellulose, polyethylene glycol, propylene glycol, and titanium dioxide.

5 mg Tablet: Cellulosic polymers, corn starch, lactose, magnesium stearate, microcrystalline cellulose, polyethylene glycol, propylene glycol, and titanium dioxide.

CLINICAL PHARMACOLOGY

CARTROL (carteolol hydrochloride) is a long-acting, nonselective, beta-adrenergic receptor blocking agent with intrinsic sympathomimetic activity (ISA) and without significant membrane stabilizing (local anesthetic) activity.

Pharmacodynamics:

Carteolol specifically competes with beta-adrenergic receptor agonists for both $beta_1$-receptors located principally in cardiac muscle and $beta_2$-receptors located in the bronchial and vascular musculature, blocking the chronotropic, inotropic, and vasodilator responses to beta-adrenergic stimulation proportionately. Because of its partial agonist activity, however, carteolol does not reduce resting beta-agonist activity as much as beta-adrenergic blockers lacking this activity. Thus, in clinical trials in man, the decreases in resting pulse rate produced by carteolol (2–5 beats per minute in various studies) were less than those produced by beta-blockers (nadolol and propranolol) without ISA (10–12 beats per minute). There are also equivocal effects on renin secretion, in contrast to beta-blockers without ISA, which inhibit renin secretion.

Continued on next page

Cartrol—Cont.

In controlled clinical trials carteolol, at doses up to 20 mg as monotherapy or in combination with thiazide type diuretics, produced significantly greater reductions in blood pressure than did placebo, with the full effect seen between two and four weeks. The observed differences from placebo ranged from 3.1 to 6.7 mmHg for supine diastolic blood pressure. The antihypertensive effects of carteolol are smaller in black populations but do not seem to be affected by age or sex. Doses of carteolol greater than 10 mg once a day did not produce greater reductions in blood pressure. In fact, doses of 20 mg and above appeared to produce blood pressure reductions less than those produced by 10 mg and below. When carteolol was compared to nadolol and propranolol, although the differences were not statistically significant in relatively small studies, carteolol at doses up to 20 mg produced supine diastolic blood pressure changes consistently 2 mmHg less than that produced by either nadolol or propranolol.

Although the mechanism of the antihypertensive effect of beta-adrenergic blocking agents has not been established, multiple factors are thought to contribute to the lowering of blood pressure, including diminished response to sympathetic nerve outflow from vasomotor centers in the brain, diminished release of renin from the kidneys, and decreased cardiac output. Carteolol does not have a consistent effect on renin and other agents with ISA have been shown to have less effect than other beta-blockers on resting cardiac output (although they cause the usual decrease in exercise cardiac output so that the difference is of uncertain clinical importance), so that the mechanism of its action is particularly uncertain.

Beta-blockade interferes with endogenous adrenergic bronchodilator activity and diminishes the response to exogenous bronchodilators. This is especially important in patients subject to bronchospasm.

Single intravenous doses of carteolol (0.5 mg, 1 mg, 2.5 mg and 5 mg) produced statistically, but not clinically, significant increases from baseline in AV node conduction time and RR and PR intervals.

CARTROL (carteolol hydrochloride) induced no significant alteration in total serum cholesterol and triglycerides.

Following discontinuation of carteolol treatment in man, pharmacologic activity (evaluated by blockade of the tachycardia induced by isoproterenol or postural changes) is present for 2 to 21 days (median 14 days) after the last dose of carteolol. Following administration of recommended doses of CARTROL (carteolol hydrochloride), both beta-blocking and antihypertensive effects persist for at least 24 hours.

Pharmacokinetics and Metabolism:

Following oral administration in man, peak plasma concentrations of carteolol usually occur within one to three hours. Carteolol is well absorbed when administered orally as CARTROL (carteolol hydrochloride) tablets. The presence of food in the gastrointestinal tract somewhat slows the rate of absorption, but the extent of absorption is not appreciably affected. Compared to intravenous administration, the absolute bioavailability of carteolol from CARTROL (carteolol hydrochloride) tablets is approximately 85%.

The plasma half-life of carteolol averages approximately six hours. Steady-state serum levels are achieved within one to two days after initiating therapeutic doses of carteolol in persons with normal renal function. Since approximately 50 to 70% of a carteolol dose is eliminated unchanged by the kidneys, the half-life is increased in patients with impaired renal function. Significant reductions in the rate of carteolol elimination (and prolongations of the half-life) occur in patients as creatinine clearance decreases. Therefore, a reduction in maintenance dose and/or prolongation in dosing interval is appropriate (see DOSAGE and ADMINISTRATION).

Carteolol is 23–30% bound to plasma proteins in humans. The major metabolites of carteolol are 8-hydroxycarteolol and the glucuronic acid conjugates of both carteolol and 8-hydroxycarteolol. In man, 8-hydroxycarteolol is an active metabolite with a half-life of approximately 8 to 12 hours and represents approximately 5% of the administered dose excreted in the urine.

INDICATIONS AND USAGE

CARTROL (carteolol hydrochloride) is indicated in the management of hypertension. It may be used alone or in combination with other antihypertensive agents, especially thiazide diuretics. Preliminary data indicate that carteolol does not have a favorable effect on arrhythmias.

CONTRAINDICATIONS

CARTROL (carteolol hydrochloride) is contraindicated in patients with: 1) bronchial asthma, 2) severe bradycardia, 3) greater than first degree heart block, 4) cardiogenic shock, and 5) clinically evident congestive heart failure (see WARNINGS).

WARNINGS

Congestive Heart Failure:

Sympathetic stimulation may be a vital component supporting circulatory function in patients with congestive heart failure, and impairing that support by beta-blockade may precipitate more severe decompensation. Although CARTROL (carteolol hydrochloride) should be avoided in clinically evident congestive heart failure, it can be used with caution, if necessary, in patients with a history of failure who are well-compensated and are receiving digitalis and diuretics. Beta-adrenergic blocking agents do not abolish the inotropic action of digitalis on heart muscle.

IN PATIENTS WITHOUT A HISTORY OF CONGESTIVE HEART FAILURE, the use of beta-blockers can, in some instances, lead to congestive heart failure. Therefore, at the first sign or symptom of cardiac decompensation, discontinuation of beta-blocker therapy should be considered. The patient should be closely observed and treatment should include a diuretic and/or digitalization as necessary.

Exacerbation of Angina Pectoris Upon Withdrawal:

In patients with angina pectoris, exacerbation of angina and, in some cases, myocardial infarction have been reported following abrupt discontinuation of therapy with some beta-blockers. Therefore such patients should be cautioned against interruption of therapy without a physician's advice. The long persistence of beta-adrenergic blockade following abrupt discontinuation of CARTROL (carteolol hydrochloride), however, might be expected to minimize the possibility of this complication. When discontinuation of CARTROL (carteolol hydrochloride) is planned, dosage should be tapered gradually, as it is with other beta-blockers. If exacerbation of angina occurs when CARTROL (carteolol hydrochloride) therapy is interrupted, it is advisable to reinstitute CARTROL (carteolol hydrochloride) or other beta-blocker therapy, at least temporarily, and to take other measures appropriate for the management of unstable angina pectoris.

PATIENTS WITHOUT CLINICALLY RECOGNIZED ANGINA PECTORIS should be carefully monitored after withdrawal of CARTROL (carteolol hydrochloride) therapy, since coronary artery disease may be unrecognized.

Nonallergic Bronchospasm (e.g., chronic bronchitis, emphysema):

Patients with bronchospastic disease generally should not receive beta-blocker therapy and carteolol is contraindicated in patients with bronchial asthma. If use of CARTROL (carteolol hydrochloride) is essential, it should be administered with caution since it may block bronchodilation produced by endogenous catecholamine stimulation of $beta_2$-receptors or diminish response to therapy with a beta-receptor agonist.

Major Surgery:

The necessity, or desirability, of withdrawal of beta-blocking therapy prior to major surgery is controversial. Because beta-blockade impairs the ability of the heart to respond to reflex stimuli and may increase risks of general anesthesia and surgical procedures resulting in protracted hypotension or low cardiac output, and difficulty in restarting or maintaining a heartbeat, it has been suggested that beta-blocker therapy should be withdrawn several days prior to surgery. It is also recognized, however, that increased sensitivity to catecholamines of patients recently withdrawn from beta-blocker therapy could increase certain risks. Given the persistence of the beta-blocking activity of CARTROL (carteolol hydrochloride), effective withdrawal would take several weeks and would ordinarily be impractical. When beta-blocker therapy is not discontinued, anesthetic agents that depress the myocardium should be avoided. In one study using intravenous carteolol during surgery, recovery from anesthesia was somewhat delayed in three patients who received carteolol near the end of anesthesia, and respiratory arrest occurred in one of these patients immediately following administration of intravenous carteolol.

In the event that CARTROL (carteolol hydrochloride) treatment is not discontinued before surgery, the anesthesiologist should be informed that the patient is receiving CARTROL (carteolol hydrochloride). The effects on the heart of beta-adrenergic blocking agents, such as CARTROL (carteolol hydrochloride), may be reversed by cautious administration of isoproterenol or dobutamine.

Diabetes Mellitus and Hypoglycemia:

Beta-adrenergic blockade may prevent the appearance of premonitory signs and symptoms (e.g., tachycardia and blood pressure changes) of acute hypoglycemia, and it inhibits glycogenolysis, a normal compensatory mechanism for hypoglycemia. This is especially important for patients with labile diabetes mellitus. Beta-blockade also reduces the release of insulin in response to hyperglycemia; therefore, it may be necessary to adjust the dose of antidiabetic agents used to treat hyperglycemia.

Thyrotoxicosis:

Beta-adrenergic blockade may mask certain clinical signs of hyperthyroidism such as tachycardia. Patients suspected of having thyrotoxicosis should be managed carefully to avoid abrupt withdrawal of beta-adrenergic blockade which might precipitate a thyroid storm.

PRECAUTIONS

General:

Impaired Renal Function:

CARTROL (carteolol hydrochloride) should be used with caution in patients with impaired renal function. Patients with impaired renal function clear carteolol at a reduced rate, and dosage should be reduced accordingly (see Dosage and Administration).

Beta-adrenoreceptor blockade can cause reduction in intraocular pressure. Therefore, CARTROL (carteolol hydrochloride) may interfere with glaucoma testing. Withdrawal may lead to a return of increased intraocular pressure.

Information for Patients:

Patients, especially those with evidence of coronary artery insufficiency, should be warned against interruption or discontinuation of CARTROL (carteolol hydrochloride) therapy without the physician's advice. Although cardiac failure rarely occurs in properly selected patients, patients being treated with beta-adrenergic blocking agents should be advised to consult the physician at the first sign or symptom of impending failure (i.e., fatigue with exertion, difficulty breathing, cough or unusually fast heartbeat).

Drug Interactions:

Catecholamine-depleting drugs (e.g., reserpine) may have an additive effect when given with beta-blocking agents. Therefore, patients treated with CARTROL (carteolol hydrochloride) plus a catecholamine-depleting agent must be observed carefully for evidence of hypotension and/or excessive bradycardia, which may produce syncope or postural hypotension.

Risk of Anaphylactic Reaction: While taking beta-blockers, patients with a history of severe anaphylactic reaction to a variety of allergens may be more reactive to repeated challenge, either accidental, diagnostic, or therapeutic. Such patients may be unresponsive to the usual doses of epinephrine used to treat allergic reaction.

Concurrent administration of *general anesthetics* and beta-blocking agents may result in exaggeration of the hypotension induced by general anesthetics (see WARNINGS, Major Surgery).

Blunting of the antihypertensive effect of beta-adrenoreceptor blocking agents by *non-steroidal anti-inflammatory drugs* has been reported. When using these agents concomitantly, patients should be observed carefully to confirm that the desired therapeutic effect has been obtained.

Literature reports suggest that *oral calcium antagonists* may be used in combination with beta-adrenergic blocking agents when heart function is normal, but should be avoided in patients with impaired cardiac function. Hypotension, AV conduction disturbances, and left ventricular failure have been reported in some patients receiving beta-adrenergic blocking agents when an oral calcium antagonist was added to the treatment regimen. Hypotension was more likely to occur if the calcium antagonist were a dihydropyridine derivative, e.g., nifedipine, while left ventricular failure and AV conduction disturbances were more likely to occur with either verapamil or diltiazem.

Intravenous calcium antagonists should be used with caution in patients receiving beta-adrenergic blocking agents. The concomitant use of beta-adrenergic blocking agents with digitalis and either diltiazem or verapamil may have additive effects in prolonging AV conduction time.

Concomitant use of oral antidiabetic agents or *insulin* with beta-blocking agents may be associated with hypoglycemia or possibly hyperglycemia. Dosage of the antidiabetic agent should be adjusted accordingly (see WARNINGS, Diabetes Mellitus and Hypoglycemia).

Carcinogenesis, Mutagenesis, Impairment of Fertility:

CARTROL (carteolol hydrochloride) did not produce carcinogenic effects at doses 280 times the maximum recommended human dose (10 mg/70 kg/day) in two-year oral rat and mouse studies.

Tests of mutagenicity, including the Ames Test, recombinant (rec)-assay, *in vivo* cytogenetics and dominant lethal assay demonstrated no evidence for mutagenic potential.

Fertility of male and female rats and male and female mice was unaffected by administration of CARTROL (carteolol hydrochloride) at dosages up to 150 mg/kg/day. This dosage is approximately 1052 times the maximum recommended human dose.

Pregnancy:

Teratogenic Effects: Pregnancy Category C. CARTROL (carteolol hydrochloride) increased resorptions and decreased fetal weights in rabbits and rats at maternally toxic doses approximately 1052 and 5264 times the maximum recommended human dose (10 mg/70 kg/day), respectively. A dose-related increase in wavy ribs was noted in the developing rat fetus when pregnant females received daily doses of approximately 212 times the maximum recommended human dose. No such effects were noted in pregnant mice subjected to up to 1052 times the maximum recommended human dose. There are no adequate and well-controlled studies in pregnant women. CARTROL (carteolol hydrochloride) should be used during pregnancy only if the potential benefit justifies the potential risk to the fetus.

Nursing Mothers:

Studies have not been conducted in lactating humans and, therefore, it is not known whether carteolol is excreted in human milk. Studies in lactating rats indicate that CARTROL (carteolol hydrochloride) is excreted in milk. Because many drugs are excreted in human milk, caution should be exercised when CARTROL (carteolol hydrochloride) is administered to a nursing woman.

Pediatric Use:

Safety and effectiveness in children have not been established.

ADVERSE REACTIONS

The prevalence of adverse reactions has been ascertained from clinical studies conducted primarily in the United States. All adverse experiences (events) reported during these studies were recorded as adverse reactions. The prevalence rates presented below are based on combined data from nineteen placebo-controlled studies of patients with hypertension, angina or dysrhythmias, using once-daily carteolol at doses up to 60 mg. Table 1 summarizes those adverse experiences reported for patients in these studies where the prevalence in the carteolol group is 1% or greater and exceeds the prevalence in the placebo group. Asthenia and muscle cramps were the only symptoms that were significantly more common in patients receiving carteolol than in patients receiving placebo. Patients in clinical trials were carefully selected to exclude those, such as patients with asthma or known bronchospasm, or congestive heart failure, who would be at high risk of experiencing beta-adrenergic blocker adverse effect (See WARNINGS and CONTRAINDICATIONS):

TABLE 1
Adverse Reactions During
Placebo-Controlled Studies

	Placebo (n=448) %	Carteolol (n=761) %
Body as a Whole		
†Asthenia	4.0	7.1*
Abdominal Pain	0.4	1.3
Back Pain	1.6	2.1
Chest Pain	1.8	2.2
Digestive System		
Diarrhea	2.0	2.1
Nausea	1.8	2.1
Metabolic/Nutritional Disorders		
Abnormal Lab Test	1.1	1.2
Peripheral Edema	1.1	1.7
Musculoskeletal System		
Arthralgia	1.1	1.2
Muscle Cramps	0.2	2.6*
Lower Extremity Pain	0.2	1.2
Nervous System		
Insomnia	0.7	1.7
Paresthesia	1.1	2.0
Respiratory System		
Nasal Congestion	0.9	1.1
Pharyngitis	0.9	1.1
Skin and Appendages		
Rash	1.1	1.3

† Includes weakness, tiredness, lassitude and fatigue.
* Statistically significant at p=0.05 level.

The adverse experiences were usually mild or moderate in intensity and transient, but sometimes were serious enough to interrupt treatment. The adverse reactions that were most bothersome, as judged by their being reported as reasons for discontinuation of therapy by at least 0.4% of the carteolol group are shown in Table 2.

TABLE 2
Discontinuations During
Placebo-Controlled Studies

	Placebo (n=448) %	Carteolol (n=761) %
Body as a Whole		
Asthenia	0.2	0.5
Headache	0.7	0.7
Chest Pain	0.2	0.4
Skin and Appendages		
Rash	0.0	0.4
Sweating	0.2	0.4
Digestive System		
Nausea	0.0	0.4
Overall Adverse Reactions	4.2	3.3

Additional adverse reactions have been reported, but these are, in general, not distinguishable from symptoms that might have occurred in the absence of exposure to carteolol. The following additional adverse reactions were reported by at least 1% of 1568 patients who received carteolol in controlled or open, short- or long-term clinical studies, or represent less common, but potentially important, reactions reported in clinical studies or marketing experience (these rarer reactions are shown in italics): *Body as a Whole:* fever, infection, injury, malaise, pain, neck pain, shoulder pain; *Cardiovascular System:* angina pectoris, arrhythmia, *heart failure,* palpitations, *second degree heart block,* vasodilation; *Digestive System: acute hepatitis with jaundice,* constipation, dyspepsia, flatulence, gastrointestinal disorder; *Metabolic/Nutritional Disorder:* gout; *Musculoskeletal System:* pain in extremity, joint disorder, arthritis; *Nervous System: abnormal dreams,* anxiety, depression, dizziness, nervousness, somnolence; *Respiratory System:* bronchitis, *bronchospasm,* cold symptoms, cough, dyspnea, flu symptoms, lung disorder, rhinitis, sinusitis, *wheezing; Skin and Appendages:* sweating; *Special Senses:* blurred vision, conjunctivitis, eye disorder, tinnitus; *Urogenital:* impotence, urinary frequency, urinary tract infection.

In studies of patients with hypertension or angina pectoris where carteolol and positive reference beta-adrenergic blocking agents [nadolol (n=82) and propranolol (n=50)] have been compared, the differences in prevalence rates between the carteolol group and the reference agent group were statistically significant (p≤0.05) for the adverse reactions listed in Table 3.

TABLE 3
Adverse Reactions During
Positive-Controlled Studies

	Reference Agents (n=132) %	Carteolol (n=135) %
Body as a Whole		
Chest Pain	5.3	0.7
Cardiovascular System		
Bradycardia	4.5	0.0
Digestive System		
Diarrhea	11.4	4.4
Nervous System		
Somnolence	0.8	7.4
Skin and Appendages		
Sweating	5.3	0.7

POTENTIAL ADVERSE REACTIONS

In addition, other adverse reactions not listed above have been reported with other beta-adrenergic blocking agents and should be considered potential adverse reactions of CARTROL (carteolol hydrochloride).

Body as a Whole:
Fever combined with aching and sore throat.
Cardiovascular System:
Intensification of AV block. (See *CONTRAINDICATIONS*).
Digestive System:
Mesenteric arterial thrombosis, ischemic colitis.
Hemic/Lymphatic System:
Agranulocytosis, thrombocytopenic and nonthrombocytopenic purpura.
Nervous System:
Reversible mental depression progressing to catatonia; an acute reversible syndrome characterized by disorientation to time and place, short-term memory loss, emotional lability, slightly clouded sensorium, and decreased performance on neuropsychometric testing.
Respiratory System: Laryngospasm, respiratory distress.
Skin and Appendages: Erythematous rash, reversible alopecia.
Urogenital System: Peyronie's disease.
The oculomucocutaneous syndrome associated with the beta-adrenergic blocking agent practolol has not been reported with carteolol.

OVERDOSAGE

No specific information on emergency treatment of overdosage in humans is available. The most common effects expected with overdosage of a beta-adrenergic blocking agent are bradycardia, bronchospasm, congestive heart failure and hypotension.

In case of overdosage, treatment with CARTROL (carteolol hydrochloride) should be discontinued and gastric lavage considered. The patient should be closely observed and vital signs carefully monitored. The prolonged effects of carteolol must be considered when determining the duration of corrective therapy. On the basis of the pharmacologic profile, the following additional measures should be considered as appropriate.

Symptomatic Bradycardia:
Administer atropine. If there is no response to vagal blockade, administer isoproterenol cautiously.
Bronchospasm:
Administer a $beta_2$-stimulating agent such as isoproterenol and/or a theophylline derivative.
Congestive Heart Failure:
Administer diuretics and digitalis glycosides as necessary.
Hypotension:
Administer vasopressors such as intravenous dopamine, epinephrine or norepinephrine bitartrate.

DOSAGE AND ADMINISTRATION

Dosage must be individualized. The initial dose of CARTROL (carteolol hydrochloride) is 2.5 mg given as a single daily oral dose either alone or added to diuretic therapy. If an adequate response is not achieved, the dose can be gradually increased to 5 mg and 10 mg as single daily doses. Increasing the dose above 10 mg per day is unlikely to produce further substantial benefits and, in fact, may decrease the response. The usual maintenance dose of carteolol is 2.5 or 5 mg once daily.

Dosage Adjustment in Renal Impairment:
Carteolol is excreted principally by the kidneys. When administering CARTROL (carteolol hydrochloride) to patients with renal impairment, the dosage regimen should be adjusted individually by the physician. Guidelines for dose interval adjustment are shown below:

Creatinine Clearance (mL/min)	Dosage Interval (hours)
>60	24
20–60	48
<20	72

HOW SUPPLIED

CARTROL (carteolol hydrochloride) is supplied as:
2.5 mg gray tablets:
Bottles of 100 .... (**NDC** 0074-1664-13).
5 mg white tablets:
Bottles of 100 .... (**NDC** 0074-1665-13).

Recommended storage: Store under controlled room temperature, 59°–86°F (15°–30°C).
Revised: February, 1992
Ref. 01-2531-R3

CEFOL® Filmtab® Tablets ℞

[*c 'full*]
(B-Complex, Folic Acid, Vitamin E with 750 mg Vitamin C)

DESCRIPTION

Each oral tablet provides:
Ascorbic Acid (C) (as sodium ascorbate) .... 750 mg
Niacinamide .... 100 mg
Calcium Pantothenate .... 20 mg
Thiamine Mononitrate (B_1) .... 15 mg
Riboflavin (B_2) .... 10 mg
Pyridoxine Hydrochloride (B_6) .... 5 mg
Folic Acid .... 500 mcg
Cyanocobalamin (B_{12}) .... 6 mcg
Vitamin E (as dl-alpha tocopheryl acetate) .... 30 IU

Inactive Ingredients: Cellulosic polymers, colloidal silicon dioxide, corn starch, D&C Yellow No. 10, FD&C Blue No. 1, magnesium stearate, microcrystalline cellulose, polyethylene glycol, povidone, titanium dioxide, and vanillin.

CLINICAL PHARMACOLOGY

The vitamin components of Cefol are absorbed by the active transport process. All but Vitamin E are rapidly eliminated and not stored in the body. Vitamin E is stored in body tissues.

INDICATIONS AND USAGE

Indicated in non-pregnant* adults for treatment of Vitamin C deficiency states with associated deficient intake or increased need for Vitamin B-Complex, Folic Acid, and Vitamin E.

*Pregnancy may require greater Folic Acid intake.

CONTRAINDICATIONS

Rare hypersensitivity to Folic Acid.

WARNINGS

Folic Acid alone is improper treatment of pernicious anemia and other megaloblastic anemias where Vitamin B_{12} is deficient.

PRECAUTIONS

Folic Acid above 0.1 mg daily may obscure pernicious anemia (hematologic remission may occur while neurological manifestations remain progressive).

ADVERSE REACTIONS

Allergic sensitization has been reported following oral and parenteral administration of Folic Acid.

DOSAGE

Usual adult dose is one tablet daily.

HOW SUPPLIED

Green tablets in bottles of 100.
Filmtab—Film-sealed tablets, Abbott.
Store below 77°F (25°C).
Ref. 03-2285-3/R26

CORLOPAM® ℞

[*cŏr-lō-pam*]
brand of (fenoldopam mesylate) Injection

DESCRIPTION

CORLOPAM (fenoldopam mesylate) is a dopamine D_1-like receptor agonist. The product is formulated as a solution to be diluted for intravenous infusion. Chemically it is 6-chloro-2,3,4,5-tetrahydro-1-(4-hydroxyphenyl)-[1*H*]-3-benzazepine-7,8-diol methanesulfonate with the following structure:

Cl
HO
NH • CH_3SO_3H
HO
OH
fenoldopam mesylate

Fenoldopam mesylate is a white to off-white powder with a molecular weight of 401.87 and a molecular formula of $C_{16}H_{16}ClNO_3 \cdot CH_3SO_3H$. It is sparingly soluble in water, ethanol and methanol, and is soluble in propylene glycol.

Ampules: Each 1 mL contains, in sterile aqueous solution, citric acid 3.44 mg; fenoldopam mesylate equivalent to fenoldopam 10 mg; propylene glycol 518 mg; sodium citrate dihydrate 0.61 mg; sodium metabisulfite 1 mg.

CLINICAL PHARMACOLOGY

Mechanism of Action

Fenoldopam is a rapid-acting vasodilator. It is an agonist for D_1-like dopamine receptors and binds with moderate affin-

Continued on next page

Corlopam—Cont.

Table 1
CORLOPAM Plasma Concentrations in Normotensive, Mild to Moderate and Malignant Hypertensive Patients
CORLOPAM PLASMA CONCENTRATION (ng/mL)

CORLOPAM Infusion Rate (µg/kg/min)	Patient Populations		
	Normotensive Subjects n=10	Mild to Moderate Hypertensive Patients n=7	Malignant Hypertension Patients n=20
0.1	3.2	4.0	3.3

Table 2
PHARMACODYNAMIC EFFECTS OF FENOLDOPAM IN MILD TO MODERATE HYPERTENSIVE PATIENTS

	Infusion Rate (µg/kg/min)				
Time Point and Mean Change From Time Zero ± SE	**Placebo n = 7**	**0.04 n = 7**	**0.1 n = 7**	**0.4 n = 5**	**0.8 n = 6**
15 Minutes of Infusion*					
Systolic BP	0 ± 6	−15 ± 6	−19 ± 8	−14 ± 4	−24 ± 6
Diastolic BP	0 ± 2	−5 ± 3	−12 ± 4	−15 ± 3	−20 ± 4
Heart rate	+2 ± 2	+3 ± 2	+5 ± 1	+16 ± 3	+19 ± 3
30 Minutes of Infusion*					
Systolic BP	−6 ± 5	−17 ± 6	−18 ± 6	−14 ± 8	−26 ± 6
Diastolic BP	−6 ± 3	−7 ± 3	−16 ± 4	−14 ± 3	−20 ± 2
Heart rate	+2 ± 2	+3 ± 2	+10 ± 2	+18 ± 3	+23 ± 3
1 Hour of Infusion*					
Systolic BP	−15 ± 4	−22 ± 7	−22 ± 7	−26 ± 9	−22 ± 9
Diastolic BP	−5 ± 3	−9 ± 2	−18 ± 4	−19 ± 4	−21± 1
Heart rate	+1 ± 3	+5 ± 2	+12 ± 3	+19 ± 4	+25 ± 4
4 Hours of Infusion*					
Systolic BP	−14 ± 5	−16 ± 9	−31± 15	−22 ± 11	−25 ± 7
Diastolic BP	−14 ± 8	−8 ± 4	−19 ± 9	−25 ± 3	−20 ± 1
Heart rate	+5 ± 3	+6 ± 3	+10 ± 4	+21 ± 2	+27 ± 7
24 Hours of Infusion*					
Systolic BP	−20 ± 6	−23 ± 8	−35 ± 7	−22 ± 6	−23 ± 11
Diastolic BP	−11 ± 6	−11 ± 5	−23 ± 10	−22 ± 5	−13 ± 3
Heart rate	+6 ± 3	+5 ± 3	+13 ± 2	+17 ± 4	+15 ± 3
48 Hours of Infusion*					
Systolic BP	−12± 8	−31± 6	−22 ± 8	−9 ± 6	−14 ± 10
Diastolic BP	−9 ± 5	−10 ± 6	−9 ± 7	−9 ± 2	−9 ± 3
Heart rate	+1 ± 2	0 ± 4	+1 ± 4	+12 ± 3	+8 ± 3

* Mean change from time zero ± S.E.

Table 3
PHARMACODYNAMIC EFFECTS OF FENOLDOPAM IN HYPERTENSIVE EMERGENCY PATIENTS

	Infusion Rate µg/kg/min			
Time Point and Pharmacodynamic Parameters	**0.01 n = 25**	**0.03 n = 24**	**0.1 n = 22**	**0.3 n = 23**
Pre-Infusion Baseline				
Systolic BP—mean ± SE	210 ± 21	208 ± 26	205 ± 24	211 ± 17
Diastolic BP—mean ± SE	136 ± 16	135 ± 11	133 ± 14	136 ± 15
Heart rate—mean ± SE	87 ± 20	84 ± 14	81 ± 19	80 ± 14
15 Minutes of Infusion*				
Systolic BP	−5 ± 4	−7 ± 4	−16 ± 4	−19± 4
Diastolic BP	−5 ± 3	−8 ± 3	−12 ± 2	−21 ± 2
Heart rate	−2 ± 3	+1 ± 1	+2 ± 1	+11 ± 2
30 Minutes of Infusion*				
Systolic BP	−6 ± 4	−11 ± 4	−21 ± 3	−16 ± 4
Diastolic BP	−10 ± 3	−12 ± 3	−17 ± 3	−20 ± 2
Heart rate	−2 ± 3	−1 ± 1	+3 ± 2	+12 ± 3
1 Hour of Infusion*				
Systolic BP	−5 ± 3	−9 ± 4	−19 ± 4	−22 ± 4
Diastolic BP	−8 ± 3	−13 ± 3	−18 ± 2	−23 ± 2
Heart rate	−1 ± 3	0 ± 2	+3 ± 2	+11 ± 3
4 Hours of Infusion*				
Systolic BP	−14 ± 4	−20 ± 5	−23± 4	−37 ± 4
Diastolic BP	−12 ± 3	−18 ± 3	−21 ± 3	−29 ± 3
Heart rate	−2 ± 4	0 ± 2	+4 ± 2	+11 ± 2

* Mean change from baseline ± S.E.

ity to α_2-adrenoceptors. It has no significant affinity for D_2-like receptors, α_1 and β adrenoceptors, $5HT_1$ and $5HT_2$ receptors, or muscarinic receptors. Fenoldopam is a racemic mixture with the R-isomer responsible for the biological activity. The R-isomer has approximately 250-fold higher affinity for D_1-like receptors than does the S-isomer. In nonclinical studies, fenoldopam had no agonist effect on presynaptic D_2-like dopamine receptors, or α- or β-adrenoceptors, nor did it affect angiotensin-converting enzyme activity. Fenoldopam may increase norepinephrine plasma concentration.

In animals, fenoldopam has vasodilating effects in coronary, renal, mesenteric and peripheral arteries. All vascular beds, however, do not respond uniformly to fenoldopam. Vasodilating effects have been demonstrated in renal efferent and afferent arterioles. In humans, increases in renal blood flow were demonstrated in hypertensive and normal subjects treated with intravenous fenoldopam in two small controlled trials. No beneficial clinical effect on renal function has been shown in patients with heart failure or hepatic or severe renal disease.

Pharmacokinetics

Administered as a constant infusion at rates of 0.01 to 1.6 µg/kg/min, fenoldopam produced steady-state plasma concentrations that were proportional to infusion rates. The elimination half-life was about 5 minutes in mild to moderate hypertensives, with little difference between the R (active) and S isomers. Steady state concentrations are attained in about 20 minutes (4 half-lives). The steady state plasma concentrations of fenoldopam, at comparable infusion rates, were similar in normotensive subjects and in patients with mild to moderate hypertension or hypertensive emergencies (Table 1).

[See table 1 above]

Clearance of parent (active) fenoldopam is not altered in patients with end-stage renal disease on continuous ambulatory peritoneal dialysis (CAPD) and is not affected on average, in severe hepatic failure. The effects of hemodialysis on the pharmacokinetics of fenoldopam have not been evaluated.

In radiolabeled studies in rats, no more than 0.005% of fenoldopam crossed the blood-brain barrier.

Excretion and Metabolism

Radiolabeled studies show that about 90% of infused fenoldopam is eliminated in urine, 10% in feces. Elimination is largely by conjugation, without participation of cytochrome P-450 enzymes. The principal routes of conjugation are methylation, glucuronidation, and sulfation. Only 4% of the administered dose is excreted unchanged. Animal data indicate that the metabolites are inactive.

Special Population: The pharmacokinetics of fenoldopam were not influenced by age, gender, or race in hypertensive emergency patients. Effects of renal and hepatic dysfunction are described above. There have been no formal drug-drug interaction studies using intravenous fenoldopam.

Pharmacodynamics and Clinical Studies

In a randomized double-blind, placebo-controlled, 5-group study in 32 patients with mild to moderate essential hypertension (diastolic blood pressure between 95 and 119 mm Hg), and a mean baseline pressure of about 154/98 mm Hg, and heart rate of about 75 bpm, fixed-rate IV infusions of CORLOPAM produced dose-related reductions in systolic and diastolic blood pressure. Infusions were maintained at a fixed rate for 48 hours. Table 2 shows the results of the study. The onset of response was rapid at all infusion rates, with the 15-minute response representing 50–100% of the one-hour response in all groups. There was some suggestion of partial tolerance at 48 hours in the two higher dose infusions, but a substantial effect persisted through 48 hours. When infusions were stopped, blood pressure gradually returned to pretreatment values with no evidence of rebound. This study suggests that there is no greater response to 0.8 µg/kg/min than to 0.4 µg/kg/min.

[See table 2 above]

In a multicenter, randomized, double-blind comparison of four infusion rates, CORLOPAM was administered as constant rate infusions of 0.01, 0.03, 0.1 and 0.3 µg/kg/min for up to 24 hours to 94 patients experiencing hypertensive emergencies (defined as diastolic blood pressure ≥ 120 mm Hg with evidence of compromise of end-organ function involving the cardiovascular, renal, cerebral or retinal systems). Infusion rates could be doubled after one hour if clinically indicated. There were dose-related, rapid-onset, decreases in systolic and diastolic blood pressures and increases in heart rate (Table 3).

[See table 3 above]

Two hundred and thirty six severely hypertensive patients (DBP ≥ 120 mm Hg), with or without end-organ compromise, were randomized to receive in two open-label studies either fenoldopam or nitroprusside. The response rate was 79% (92/117) in the fenoldopam group and 77% (90/119) in the nitroprusside group. Response required a decline in supine diastolic blood pressure to less than 110 mm Hg if the baseline were between 120 and 150 mm Hg, inclusive, or by ≥ 40 mm Hg if the baseline were ≥ 150 mm Hg. Patients were titrated to the desired effect. For fenoldopam, the dose ranged from 0.1 to 1.5 µg/kg/min; for nitroprusside, the dose ranged from 1.0 to 8.0 µg/kg/min. As in the study in mild to moderate hypertensives, most of the effect seen at one hour is present at 15 minutes. The additional effect seen after 1 hour occurs in all groups and may not be drug-related (there was no placebo group to evaluate this).

INDICATIONS AND USAGE

CORLOPAM is indicated for the in-hospital, short-term (up to 48 hours) management of severe hypertension when rapid, but quickly reversible, emergency reduction of blood pressure is clinically indicated, including malignant hypertension with deteriorating end-organ function. Transition to oral therapy with another agent can begin at any time after blood pressure is stable during CORLOPAM infusion.

CONTRAINDICATIONS

None known.

WARNINGS

Contains sodium metabisulfite, a sulfite that may cause allergic-type reactions including anaphylactic symptoms and life-threatening or less severe asthmatic episodes in certain susceptible people. The overall prevalence of sulfite sensitivity in the general population is unknown and probably low. Sulfite sensitivity is seen more frequently in asthmatic than in nonasthmatic people.

PRECAUTIONS

Intraocular Pressure: In a clinical study of 12 patients with open-angle glaucoma or ocular hypertension (mean baseline intraocular pressure was 29.2 mm Hg with a range of 22.0–33.0 mm Hg), infusion of CORLOPAM at escalating doses ranging from 0.05–0.5 μg/kg/min over a 3.5 hour period caused a dose-dependent increase in intraocular pressure (IOP). At the peak effect, the intraocular pressure was raised by a mean of 6.5 mm Hg (range −2.0 to +8.5 mm Hg, corrected for placebo effect). Upon discontinuation of the CORLOPAM infusion, the IOP returned to baseline values within 2 hours. CORLOPAM administration to patients with glaucoma or intraocular hypertension should be undertaken with caution.

Tachycardia: CORLOPAM causes a dose-related tachycardia (Table 2 and Table 3), particularly with infusion rates above 0.1 μg/kg/min. Tachycardia diminishes over time but remains substantial at higher doses.

Hypotension: CORLOPAM may occasionally produce symptomatic hypotension and close monitoring of blood pressure during administration is essential. (See Adverse Reactions.) It is particularly important to avoid systemic hypotension when administering the drug to patients who have sustained an acute cerebral infarction or hemorrhage.

Hypokalemia: Decreases in serum potassium occasionally to values below 3.0 meq/L were observed after less than 6 hours of fenoldopam infusion. It is not clear if the hypokalemia reflects a pressure natriuresis with enhanced potassium-sodium exchange or a direct drug effect. During clinical trials, electrolytes were monitored at intervals of 6 hours. Hypokalemia was treated with either oral or intravenous potassium supplementation. Patient management should include appropriate attention to serum electrolytes.

Drug Interactions: Although there have been no formal interaction studies, intravenous CORLOPAM has been administered safely with drugs such as digitalis and sublingual nitroglycerin. There is limited experience with concomitant antihypertensive agents such as beta-blockers, alpha-blockers, calcium channel-blockers, ACE inhibitors, and diuretics (both thiazide-like and loop).

Carcinogenesis, Mutagenesis, Impairment of Fertility: In a 24-month study, mice treated orally with fenoldopam at 12.5, 25, or 50 mg/kg/day, reduced to 25 mg/kg/day on day 209 of study, showed no increase above controls in the incidence of neoplasms. Female mice in the highest dose group had an increased incidence and degree of severity of a fibro-osseous lesion of the sternum compared with control or low-dose animals. Compared to controls, female mice in the middle- and upper-dose groups had a higher incidence and degree of severity of chronic nephritis. These pathologic lesions were not seen in male mice treated with fenoldopam. In a 24-month study, rats treated orally with fenoldopam at 5, 10 or 20 mg/kg/day, with the mid- and high-dose groups increased to 15 or 25 mg/kg/day, respectively, on day 372 of the study, showed no increase above controls in the incidence or type of neoplasms. Compared with the controls, rats in the mid- and high-dose groups had a higher incidence of hyperplasia of collecting duct epithelium at the tip of the renal papilla.

In *in vitro* assays, fenoldopam did not induce bacterial gene mutation in the Ames test or mammalian gene mutation in the Chinese hamster ovary (CHO) cell assay. In the *in vitro* chromosomal aberration assay with CHO cells, fenoldopam was associated with statistically significant and dose-dependent increases in chromosomal aberrations, and in the proportion of aberrant metaphases. However, no chromosomal damage was seen in the *in vivo* mice micronucleus or bone marrow assays. The data support the conclusion that fenoldopam is not genotoxic or clastogenic.

Oral fertility and general reproduction performance studies in male and female rats at 12.5, 37.5 or 75 mg/kg/day revealed no impairment of fertility or reproduction performance due to fenoldopam.

Pregnancy: *Pregnancy Category B.* Oral reproduction studies have been performed in rats and rabbits at doses of 12.5 to 200 mg/kg/day and 6.25 to 25 mg/kg/day, respectively. Studies have revealed maternal toxicity at the highest doses tested but no evidence of impaired fertility or harm to the fetus due to fenoldopam. However, there are no adequate and well-controlled studies in pregnant women. Since animal reproduction studies are not always predictive of human response, fenoldopam should be used in pregnancy only if clearly needed.

Nursing Mothers: Fenoldopam is excreted in milk in rats. It is not known whether this drug is excreted in human milk. Because many drugs are excreted in human milk, caution should be exercised when CORLOPAM is administered to a nursing woman.

Pediatric Use: Safety and effectiveness in children have not been established.

ADVERSE REACTIONS

CORLOPAM causes a dose-related fall in blood pressure and increase in heart rate (see Precautions, Tachycardia, and Hypotension). In controlled clinical studies of severe hypertension in patients with end-organ damage, 3% (4/137) of patients withdrew because of excessive falls in blood pressure. Increased heart rate could, in theory, lead to ischemic cardiac events or worsened heart failure, although these events have not been observed. The most common events reported as associated with CORLOPAM use are headache, cutaneous dilation (flushing), nausea, and hypotension, each reported in more than 5% of patients.

Table 4
ADVERSE EVENTS* FROM FIXED-DOSE INFUSION STUDIES BY DOSE GROUP

		CORLOPAM Doses (μg/kg/min)					
Body System	**Event**	**Placebo (n = 7)**	**0.01 (n = 26)**	**0.03–0.04 (n = 31)**	**0.1 (n = 28)**	**0.3–0.4 (n = 29)**	**0.6 –0.8 (n = 11)**
Body, General	Headache	1	5	4	7	8	6
	Injection site reaction	0	1	3	0	3	2
Cardiovascular	ST-T abnormalities (primarily T-wave inversion)	0	2	4	0	1	0
	Flushing	0	0	0	0	1	3
	Hypotension**	0	0	0	2	0	2
	Postural hypotension	0	2	0	0	0	0
	Tachycardia**	0	0	0	0	0	2
Digestive	Nausea	0	3	0	3	5	4
	Vomiting	0	2	0	2	1	2
	Abdominal pain/ fullness	0	2	0	0	2	1
	Constipation	0	0	0	0	0	2
	Diarrhea	0	0	0	0	2	0
Metabolic and Nutritional	Increased creatinine**	0	0	2	0	0	0
	Hypokalemia**	0	2	2	0	1	0
Nervous	Nervousness/ anxiety	0	0	1	0	0	2
	Insomnia	0	2	0	0	0	0
	Dizziness	0	1	1	2	2	0
Respiratory	Nasal congestion	0	0	0	0	0	2
Skin and Appendages	Sweating	0	0	0	1	1	2
Urogenital	Urinary tract infection	0	2	0	1	0	0
Musculoskeletal	Back pain	0	1	0	1	2	2

*Includes events reported by 2 or more patients receiving CORLOPAM treatment across all dose groups.
**Investigator defined; no protocol definition.

Table 5
INFUSION RATES (mL/min) TO ACHIEVE A GIVEN DRUG DOSE RATE (μg//kg/min)

	Drug Dose Rate				
Body Weiight (kg)	**0.025 μg/kg/min**	**0.05 μg/kg/min**	**0.1 μg/kg/min**	**0.2 μg/kg/min**	**0.3 μg/kg/min**
	Infusion Rates (mL/min)				
40	0.025	0.05	0.10	0.20	0.30
50	0.031	0.06	0.13	0.25	0.38
60	0.038	0.08	0.15	0.30	0.45
70	0.044	0.09	0.18	0.35	0.53
80	0.050	0.10	0.20	0.40	0.60
90	0.056	0.11	0.23	0.45	0.68
100	0.063	0.13	0.25	0.50	0.75
110	0.069	0.14	0.28	0.55	0.83
120	0.075	0.15	0.30	0.60	0.90
130	0.081	0.16	0.33	0.65	0.98
140	0.088	0.18	0.35	0.70	1.05
150	0.094	0.19	0.38	0.75	1.13

Adverse reactions in controlled trials in hypertension

Adverse events occurring more than once in any dosing group (once if potentially important or plausibly drug-related) in the fixed-dose constant-infusion studies are presented in the following Table by infusion-rate group. There was no clear dose relationship, except possibly for headache, nausea, flushing.

[See table 4 above]

Adverse effects in overall data base

The adverse event incidences listed below are based on observations of over 1,000 CORLOPAM treated patients and not listed in the Table above.

Events reported with a frequency between 0.5-5% in patients treated with IV CORLOPAM

Cardiovascular:	extrasystoles, palpitations, bradycardia, heart failure, ischemic heart disease, myocardial infarction, angina pectoris
Metabolic:	elevated BUN, elevated serum glucose, elevated transaminase, elevated LDH
General Body:	non-specific chest pain, pyrexia
Hematologic / Lymphatic:	leukocytosis, bleeding
Respiratory:	dyspnea, upper respiratory disorder

Corlopam—Cont.

Genitourinary: oliguria
Musculoskeletal: limb cramp

ANIMAL TOXICOLOGY

Unusual toxicologic findings (arterial lesions in the rat) with fenoldopam are summarized below. These findings have not been observed in mice or dogs. No evidence of a similar lesion in humans has been observed.

Arterial lesions characterized by medial necrosis and hemorrhage have been seen in renal and splanchnic arteries of rats given fenoldopam mesylate by continuous intravenous infusion at doses of 1 to 100 μg/kg/min for 24 hours. The incidence of these lesions is dose related. Arterial lesions morphologically identical to those observed with fenoldopam have been reported in rats infused with dopamine. Data suggest that the mechanism for this injury involves activation of D_1-like dopaminergic receptors. Such lesions have not been seen in dogs given doses up to 100 μg/kg/min by continuous intravenous infusion for 24 hours, nor were they seen in dogs infused at the same dose for 6 hours daily for 24 days. The clinical significance of this finding is not known.

Oral administration of fenoldopam doses of 10 to 15 mg/kg/day or 20 to 25 mg/kg/day to rats for 24 months induced a higher incidence of polyarteritis nodosa compared to controls. Such lesions were not seen in rats given 5 mg/kg/day of fenoldopam or in mice given the drug at doses up to 50 mg/kg/day for 24 months.

OVERDOSAGE

Intentional CORLOPAM overdosage has not been reported. The most likely reaction would be excessive hypotension which should be treated with drug discontinuation and appropriate supportive measures.

DOSAGE AND ADMINISTRATION

The optimal magnitude and rate of blood pressure reduction in acutely hypertensive patients have not been rigorously determined, but, in general, both delay and too rapid decreases appear undesirable in sick patients. An initial CORLOPAM dose may be chosen from Tables 2 and 3 in the Clinical Pharmacology Section that produces the desired magnitude and rate of blood pressure reduction in a given clinical situation. Doses below 0.1 μg/kg/min have very modest effects and appear only marginally useful in this population. In general, as the initial dose increases, there is a greater and more rapid blood pressure reduction. However, lower initial doses (0.03–0.1 μg/kg/min) titrated slowly have been associated with less reflex tachycardia than have higher initial doses (≥ 0.3 μg/kg/min). In clinical trials, doses from 0.01–1.6 μg/kg/min have been studied. Most of the effect of a given infusion rate is attained in 15 minutes. CORLOPAM should be administered by continuous intravenous infusion. **A bolus dose should not be used.** Hypotension and rapid decreases of blood pressure should be avoided. The initial dose should be titrated upward or downward, no more frequently than every 15 minutes (and less frequently as goal pressure is approached) to achieve the desired therapeutic effect. The recommended increments for titration are 0.05–0.1 μg/kg/min.

Use of a calibrated, mechanical infusion pump is recommended for proper control of infusion rate during CORLOPAM infusion. In clinical trials, CORLOPAM treatment was safely performed **without** the need for intra-arterial blood pressure monitoring; blood pressure and heart rate were monitored at frequent intervals, typically every 15 minutes. Frequent blood pressure monitoring is recommended.

Use of beta-blockers in conjunction with CORLOPAM has not been studied in hypertensive patients and, if possible, concomitant use should be avoided. If the drugs are used together, caution should be exercised because unexpected hypotension could result from beta-blocker inhibition of the reflex response to fenoldopam.

The CORLOPAM infusion can be abruptly discontinued or gradually tapered prior to discontinuation. Oral antihypertensive agents can be added during CORLOPAM infusion or following its discontinuation. Patients in controlled clinical trials have received intravenous CORLOPAM for as long as 48 hours.

PREPARATION OF INFUSION SOLUTION

WARNING: CONTENTS OF AMPULES MUST BE DILUTED BEFORE INFUSION. EACH AMPULE IS FOR SINGLE USE ONLY.

Dilution:

The CORLOPAM Injection ampule concentrate must be diluted in 0.9% Sodium Chloride Injection USP or 5% Dextrose Injection USP using the following dilution schedule:

mL of Concentrate (mg of drug)	Added to	Final Concentration
4 mL (40 mg)	1000 mL	40 μg/mL
2 mL (20 mg)	500 mL	40 μg/mL
1 mL (10 mg)	250 mL	40 μg/mL

The drug dose rate must be individualized according to body weight and according to the desired rapidity and extent of pharmacodynamic effect. The following Table provides the calculated infusion volume in mL/min for a range of drug doses and body weights. The infusion should be administered using a calibrated mechanical infusion pump that can accurately and reliably deliver the desired infusion rate.

[See table 5 on previous page]

The diluted solution is stable under normal ambient light and temperature conditions for at least 24 hours. Diluted solution that is not used within 24 hours of preparation should be discarded. Parenteral products should be inspected visually. If particulate matter or cloudiness is observed, the drug should be discarded.

HOW SUPPLIED

List	Container	Concentration	Fill	Quantity
2304	Single-dose ampule	10 mg/mL	1 mL	one per carton
2304	Single-dose ampule	10 mg/mL	2 mL	one per carton

Store at 2 to 30°C.

Reference 58-6048-R1-Rev., March 2000

 Printed in USA

ABBOTT LABORATORIES, NORTH CHICAGO, IL 60064, USA

CYLERT® Ⓒ℞

[*cī'lert*]

(Pemoline)

CYLERT SHOULD NOT BE USED BY PATIENTS UNTIL THERE HAS BEEN A COMPLETE DISCUSSION OF THE RISKS AND BENEFITS OF CYLERT THERAPY AND WRITTEN INFORMED CONSENT HAS BEEN OBTAINED (SEE **PATIENT INFORMATION/CONSENT FORM**). A SUPPLY OF PATIENT INFORMATION/CONSENT FORMS AS PRINTED AT THE END OF THIS INSERT IS AVAILABLE, FREE OF CHARGE, BY CALLING (847) 937-7302. PERMISSION TO USE THE PATIENT INFORMATION/ CONSENT FORM BY PHOTOCOPY REPRODUCTION IS HEREBY GRANTED BY ABBOTT LABORATORIES.

Because of its association with life threatening hepatic failure, CYLERT should not ordinarily be considered as first line drug therapy for ADHD (see INDICATIONS AND USAGE). Because CYLERT provides an observable symptomatic benefit, patients who fail to show substantial clinical benefit within 3 weeks of completing dose titration, should be withdrawn from CYLERT therapy.

Since CYLERT's marketing in 1975, 15 cases of acute hepatic failure have been reported to the FDA. While the absolute number of reported cases is not large, the rate of reporting ranges from 4 to 17 times the rate expected in the general population. This estimate may be conservative because of under reporting and because the long latency between initiation of CYLERT treatment and the occurrence of hepatic failure may limit recognition of the association. If only a portion of actual cases were recognized and reported, the risk could be substantially higher.

Of the 15 cases reported as of December 1998, 12 resulted in death or liver transplantation, usually within four weeks of the onset of signs and symptoms of liver failure. The earliest onset of hepatic abnormalities occurred six months after initiation of CYLERT. Although some reports described dark urine and nonspecific prodromal symptoms (e.g., anorexia, malaise, and gastrointestinal symptoms), in other reports it was not clear if any prodromal symptoms preceded the onset of jaundice.

Treatment with CYLERT should be initiated only in individuals without liver disease and with normal baseline liver function tests. It is not clear if baseline and periodic liver function testing are predictive of these instances of acute liver failure; however it is generally believed that early detection of drug-induced hepatic injury along with immediate withdrawal of the suspect drug enhances the likelihood for recovery. Accordingly, the following liver monitoring program is recommended: Serum ALT (SGPT) levels should be determined at baseline, and every two weeks thereafter. If CYLERT therapy is discontinued and then restarted, liver function test monitoring should be done at baseline and reinitiated at the frequency above.

CYLERT should be discontinued if serum ALT (SGPT) is increased to a clinically significant level, or any increase ≥ 2 times the upper limit of normal, or if clinical signs and symptoms suggest liver failure (see PRECAUTIONS).

The physician who elects to use CYLERT should obtain written informed consent from the patient prior to initiation of CYLERT therapy (see PATIENT INFORMATION/CONSENT FORM).

DESCRIPTION

CYLERT (pemoline) is a central nervous system stimulant. Pemoline is structurally dissimilar to the amphetamines and methylphenidate.

It is an oxazolidine compound and is chemically identified as 2-amino-5-phenyl-2-oxazolin-4-one. Pemoline has the following structural formula:

Pemoline is a white, tasteless, odorless powder, relatively insoluble (less than 1 mg/mL) in water, chloroform, ether, acetone, and benzene; its solubility in 95% ethyl alcohol is 2.2 mg/mL.

CYLERT (pemoline) is supplied as tablets containing 18.75 mg, 37.5 mg or 75 mg of pemoline for oral administration. CYLERT is also available as chewable tablets containing 37.5 mg of pemoline.

Inactive Ingredients

18.75 mg tablet: corn starch, gelatin, lactose, magnesium hydroxide, polyethylene glycol and talc.

37.5 mg tablet: corn starch, FD&C Yellow No. 6, gelatin, lactose, magnesium hydroxide, polyethylene glycol and talc.

37.5 mg chewable tablet: corn starch, FD&C Yellow No. 6, magnesium hydroxide, magnesium stearate, mannitol, polyethylene glycol, povidone, talc and artificial flavor.

75 mg tablet: corn starch, gelatin, iron oxide, lactose, magnesium hydroxide, polyethylene glycol and talc.

CLINICAL PHARMACOLOGY

CYLERT (pemoline) has a pharmacological activity similar to that of other known central nervous system stimulants; however, it has minimal sympathomimetic effects. Although studies indicate that pemoline may act in animals through dopaminergic mechanisms, the exact mechanism and site of action of the drug in man is not known.

There is neither specific evidence which clearly establishes the mechanism whereby CYLERT produces its mental and behavioral effects in children, nor conclusive evidence regarding how these effects relate to the condition of the central nervous system.

Pemoline is rapidly absorbed from the gastrointestinal tract. Approximately 50% is bound to plasma proteins. The serum half-life of pemoline is approximately 12 hours. Peak serum levels of the drug occur within 2 to 4 hours after ingestion of a single dose. Multiple dose studies in adults at several dose levels indicate that steady state is reached in approximately 2 to 3 days. In animals given radiolabeled pemoline, the drug was widely and uniformly distributed throughout the tissues, including the brain.

Pemoline is metabolized by the liver. Metabolites of pemoline include pemoline conjugate, pemoline dione, mandelic acid, and unidentified polar compounds. CYLERT is excreted primarily by the kidneys with approximately 50% excreted unchanged and only minor fractions present as metabolites.

CYLERT (pemoline) has a gradual onset of action. Using the recommended schedule of dosage titration, significant clinical benefit may not be evident until the third or fourth week of drug administration.

INDICATIONS AND USAGE

CYLERT (pemoline) is indicated in Attention Deficit Hyperactivity Disorder (ADHD). Because of its association with life threatening hepatic failure, CYLERT should not ordinarily be considered as first line therapy for ADHD (see **BOXED WARNING**).

CYLERT (pemoline) therapy should be part of a total treatment program which typically includes other remedial measures (psychological, educational, social) for a stabilizing effect in children with a behavioral syndrome characterized by the following group of developmentally inappropriate symptoms: moderate to severe distractibility, short attention span, hyperactivity, emotional lability, and impulsivity. The diagnosis of this syndrome should not be made with finality when these symptoms are only of comparatively recent origin. Nonlocalizing (soft) neurological signs, learning disability, and abnormal EEG may or may not be present, and a diagnosis of central nervous system dysfunction may or may not be warranted.

CONTRAINDICATIONS

CYLERT (pemoline) is contraindicated in patients with known hypersensitivity or idiosyncrasy to the drug. CYLERT should not be administered to patients with impaired hepatic function (see **BOXED WARNING** and **ADVERSE REACTIONS**).

WARNINGS

Decrements in the predicted growth (i.e., weight gain and/or height) rate have been reported with the long-term use of stimulants in children. Therefore, patients requiring long-term therapy should be carefully monitored.

PRECAUTIONS

General:

Clinical experience suggests that in psychotic children, administration of CYLERT may exacerbate symptoms of behavior disturbance and thought disorder.

CYLERT should be administered with caution to patients with significantly impaired renal function.

Information for Patients:

Patients should be informed that CYLERT therapy has been associated with liver abnormalities ranging from reversible liver function test increases that do not cause any symptoms to liver failure, which may result in death. Patients should be informed that the risk of liver failure in the general population is relatively rare; however patients taking CYLERT are at a greater risk of developing liver failure than that expected in the general population. At present, there is no way to predict who is likely to develop liver failure; however only patients without liver disease and with normal baseline liver function tests should initiate CYLERT therapy. Patients should be advised to follow their doctors directives for liver function tests prior to and during CYLERT therapy. Patients should be advised to be alert for signs of liver dysfunction (jaundice, anorexia, gastrointestinal complaints, malaise, etc.) and to report them to their doctor immediately if they should occur.

The physician who elects to use CYLERT should obtain written informed consent from patients prior to initiation of CYLERT therapy (see **PATIENT INFORMATION/CONSENT FORM**.)

Laboratory Tests:

Since CYLERT's market introduction, there have been reports of elevated liver enzymes associated with its use. Many of these patients had this increase detected several months after starting CYLERT. Most patients were asymptomatic, with the increase in liver enzymes returning to normal after CYLERT was discontinued.

Treatment with CYLERT should be initiated only in individuals without liver disease and with normal baseline liver function tests. It is not clear if baseline and periodic liver function testing are predictive of these instances of acute liver failure; however it is generally believed that early detection of drug-induced hepatic injury along with immediate withdrawal of the suspect drug enhances the likelihood for recovery. Accordingly, the following liver monitoring program is recommended.

Serum ALT (SGPT) levels should be determined at baseline, and every two weeks thereafter. If CYLERT therapy is discontinued and then restarted, liver function test monitoring should be done at baseline and reinitiated at the frequency above. CYLERT should be discontinued if serum ALT (SGPT) is increased to a clinically significant level, or any increase ≥ 2 times the upper limit of normal, or if clinical signs and symptoms suggest liver failure (see **BOXED WARNING**).

Drug Interactions:

The interaction of CYLERT (pemoline) with other drugs has not been studied in humans. Patients who are receiving CYLERT concurrently with other drugs, especially drugs with CNS activity, should be monitored carefully.

Decreased seizure threshold has been reported in patients receiving CYLERT concomitantly with *antiepileptic medications.*

Carcinogenesis:

Long-term studies have been conducted in rats with doses as high as 150 mg/kg/day for eighteen months. There was no significant difference in the incidence of any neoplasm between treated and control animals.

Mutagenesis:

Data are not available concerning long-term effects on mutagenicity in animals or humans.

Impairment of Fertility:

The results of studies in which rats were given 18.75 and 37.5 mg/kg/day indicated that pemoline did not affect fertility in males or females at those doses.

Pregnancy:

Teratogenic effects: Pregnancy Category B. Reproduction studies have been performed in rats and rabbits at doses of 18.75 and 37.5 mg/kg/day and have revealed no evidence of impaired fertility or harm to the fetus. There are, however, no adequate and well-controlled studies in pregnant women. Because animal reproduction studies are not always predictive of human response, this drug should be used during pregnancy only if clearly needed.

Nonteratogenic effects:

Studies in rats have shown an increased incidence of stillbirths and cannibalization when pemoline was administered at a dose of 37.5 mg/kg/day. Postnatal survival of offspring was reduced at doses of 18.75 and 37.5 mg/kg/day.

Nursing Mothers:

It is not known whether this drug is excreted in human milk. Because many drugs are excreted in human milk, caution should be exercised when CYLERT is administered to a nursing woman.

Pediatric Use:

Safety and effectiveness in children below the age of 6 years have not been established.

Long-term effects of CYLERT in children have not been established (see **WARNINGS**).

CNS stimulants, including pemoline, have been reported to precipitate motor and phonic tics and Tourette's syndrome. Therefore, clinical evaluation for tics and Tourette's syndrome in children and their families should precede use of stimulant medications.

Drug treatment is not indicated in all cases of ADHD and should be considered only in light of complete history and evaluation of the child. The decision to prescribe CYLERT (pemoline) should depend on the physician's assessment of the chronicity and severity of the child's symptoms and their appropriateness for his/her age.

Prescription should not depend solely on the presence of one or more of the behavioral characteristics.

ADVERSE REACTIONS

The following are adverse reactions in decreasing order of severity within each category associated with CYLERT:

Hepatic: There have been reports of hepatic dysfunction, ranging from asymptomatic reversible increases in liver enzymes to hepatitis, jaundice and fatal hepatic failure, in patients taking CYLERT (see **BOXED WARNING** and **PRECAUTIONS**).

Hematopoietic: There have been isolated reports of aplastic anemia.

Central Nervous System: The following CNS effects have been reported with the use of CYLERT: convulsive seizures; literature reports indicate that CYLERT may precipitate attacks of Gilles de la Tourette syndrome; hallucinations; dyskinetic movements of the tongue, lips, face and extremities; abnormal oculomotor function including nystagmus and oculogyric crisis; mild depression; dizziness; increased irritability; headache; and drowsiness.

Insomnia is the most frequently reported side effect of CYLERT; it usually occurs early in therapy prior to an optimum therapeutic response. In the majority of cases it is transient in nature or responds to a reduction in dosage.

Gastrointestinal: Anorexia and weight loss may occur during the first weeks of therapy. In the majority of cases it is transient in nature; weight gain usually resumes within three to six months.

Nausea and stomach ache have also been reported.

Genitourinary: A case of elevated acid phosphatase in association with prostatic enlargement has been reported in a 63 year old male who was treated with CYLERT for sleepiness. The acid phosphatase normalized with discontinuation of CYLERT and was again elevated with rechallenge.

Miscellaneous: Suppression of growth has been reported with the long-term use of stimulants in children. (See **WARNINGS**.) Skin rash has been reported with CYLERT.

If adverse reactions are of a significant or protracted nature, dosage should be reduced or the drug discontinued.

DRUG ABUSE AND DEPENDENCE

Controlled Substance: CYLERT is subject to control under DEA schedule IV.

Abuse: CYLERT failed to demonstrate a potential for self-administration in primates. However, the pharmacologic similarity of pemoline to other psychostimulants with known dependence liability suggests that psychological and/or physical dependence might also occur with CYLERT. There have been isolated reports of transient psychotic symptoms occurring in adults following the long-term misuse of excessive oral doses of pemoline. CYLERT should be given with caution to emotionally unstable patients who may increase the dosage on their own initiative.

OVERDOSAGE

Signs and symptoms of acute overdosage, resulting principally from overstimulation of the central nervous system and from excessive sympathomimetic effects, may include the following: vomiting, agitation, tremors, hyperreflexia, muscle twitching, convulsions (may be followed by coma), euphoria, confusion, hallucinations, delirium, sweating, flushing, headache, hyperpyrexia, tachycardia, hypertension and mydriasis. Consult with a Certified Poison Control Center regarding treatment for up-to-date guidance and advice. Treatment consists of appropriate supportive measures. The patient must be protected against self-injury and against external stimuli that would aggravate overstimulation already present. Gastric contents may be evacuated by gastric lavage. Other measures to detoxify the gut include administration of activated charcoal and a cathartic. Chlorpromazine has been reported in the literature to be useful in decreasing CNS stimulation and sympathomimetic effects. Efficacy of peritoneal dialysis or extracorporeal hemodialysis for CYLERT overdosage has not been established.

DOSAGE AND ADMINISTRATION

CYLERT (pemoline) is administered as a single oral dose each morning. The recommended starting dose is 37.5 mg/day. This daily dose should be gradually increased by 18.75 mg at one week intervals until the desired clinical response is obtained. The effective daily dose for most patients will range from 56.25 to 75 mg. The maximum recommended daily dose of pemoline is 112.5 mg.

Clinical improvement with CYLERT is gradual. Using the recommended schedule of dosage titration, significant benefit may not be evident until the third or fourth week of drug administration. Because CYLERT provides an observable symptomatic benefit, patients who fail to show substantial clinical benefit within 3 weeks of completing dose titration, should be withdrawn from CYLERT therapy.

Where possible, drug administration should be interrupted occasionally to determine if there is a recurrence of behavioral symptoms sufficient to require continued therapy.

HOW SUPPLIED

CYLERT (pemoline) is supplied as monogrammed, grooved tablets in three dosage strengths:

18.75 mg tablets (white) in bottles of 100 (**NDC** 0074-6025-13);

37.5 mg tablets (orange-colored) in bottles of 100 (**NDC** 0074-6057-13);

75 mg tablets (tan-colored) in bottles of 100 (**NDC** 0074-6073-13).

CYLERT (pemoline) Chewable is supplied as 37.5 mg monogrammed, grooved tablets (orange-colored) in bottles of 100 (**NDC** 0074-6088-13).

Recommended Storage: Store below 86°F (30°C).

PATIENT INFORMATION/CONSENT FORM

Cylert® (pemoline) should not be used by patients until there has been a complete discussion of the risks and benefits of Cylert therapy and written informed consent has been obtained.

IMPORTANT INFORMATION:

Cylert therapy has been associated with liver abnormalities ranging from reversible liver function test increases that do not cause any symptoms to liver failure, which may result in death. Therefore, you should have a full discussion of the risks and benefits of Cylert before beginning therapy.

PATIENT CONSENT:

My (son, daughter, ward) ______________'s treatment with Cylert has been explained to me by Dr. ______________.

The following points of information, among others, have been specifically discussed and explained and I have had the opportunity to ask any questions concerning this information.

1. I, ______________ (Patient/Parent/Guardian's name), understand that Cylert is used to treat certain types of patients with the behavioral syndrome called attention deficit hyperactivity disorder (ADHD) and that I (my son/daugher/ward) am that type of patient.
   Initials: ______________
2. I understand that there is a risk that I (my son/daughter/ward) might develop liver failure, which may result in death, while taking Cylert. I understand that this could occur even after long-term therapy.
   Initials: ______________
3. I understand that I (my son/daughter/ward) should have blood taken to test liver function before Cylert is begun, and every two weeks from then on while taking Cylert. I understand that although the liver function tests may help detect if I (my son/daughter/ward) develop liver damage, it may do so only after significant, irreversible and potentially fatal damage has already occurred.
   Initials: ______________
4. I understand that if I (my son/daughter/ward) stop taking Cylert and then restart it at a later time (e.g., after summer vacation), I (my son/daughter/ward) should again have blood taken to test liver function before Cylert is restarted, and every two weeks from then on while taking Cylert.
   Initials: ______________
5. I understand that I should immediately report any unusual symptoms to the doctor and should be especially aware of persistent nausea, vomiting, fatigue, lethargy, loss of appetite, abdominal pain, dark urine, or yellowing of the skin or eyes.
   Initials: ______________

I now authorize Dr. ______________ to begin my (son/daughter/ward's) treatment with Cylert, or if treatment with Cylert has already begun, to continue this treatment.

____
Signature Date

____
Address

____
Telephone

PHYSICIAN STATEMENT:

I have fully explained to the patient (parent/guardian), ______________ the nature and purpose of treatment with Cylert and the potential risks associated with Cylert and the potential risks associated with that treatment. I have asked if he/she has any questions regarding this treatment or the associated risks and have answered these questions to the best of my ability.

____
Physician Signature

____
Date

NOTE TO PHYSICIAN: It is strongly recommended that you retain a completed copy of this informed consent form in your patient's records.

SUPPLY OF PATIENT INFORMATION/CONSENT FORMS: A supply of Patient Information/Consent Forms as printed above is available, free of charge, by calling (847) 937-7302. Permission to use the above Patient Information/Consent Form by photocopy reproduction is hereby granted by Abbott Laboratories.

ABBOTT LABORATORIES
NORTH CHICAGO, IL 60064, U.S.A.
(Nos. 6025, 6057, 6073, and 6088)
03-4964-R19-Rev. June, 1999

Shown in Product Identification Guide, page 303

DEPACON® ℞

[*dəp' ā-con*]

VALPROATE SODIUM INJECTION

BOX WARNING:

HEPATOTOXICITY:

HEPATIC FAILURE RESULTING IN FATALITIES HAS OCCURRED IN PATIENTS RECEIVING VALPROIC ACID AND ITS DERIVATIVES. EXPERIENCE HAS INDICATED THAT CHILDREN UNDER THE AGE OF TWO YEARS ARE AT A CONSIDERABLY INCREASED RISK OF DEVELOPING FATAL HEPATO-

Continued on next page

Depacon—Cont.

TOXICITY, ESPECIALLY THOSE ON MULTIPLE ANTICONVULSANTS, THOSE WITH CONGENITAL METABOLIC DISORDERS, THOSE WITH SEVERE SEIZURE DISORDERS ACCOMPANIED BY MENTAL RETARDATION, AND THOSE WITH ORGANIC BRAIN DISEASE. WHEN DEPACON IS USED IN THIS PATIENT GROUP, IT SHOULD BE USED WITH EXTREME CAUTION AND AS A SOLE AGENT. THE BENEFITS OF THERAPY SHOULD BE WEIGHED AGAINST THE RISKS. ABOVE THIS AGE GROUP, EXPERIENCE IN EPILEPSY HAS INDICATED THAT THE INCIDENCE OF FATAL HEPATOTOXICITY DECREASES CONSIDERABLY IN PROGRESSIVELY OLDER PATIENT GROUPS.

THESE INCIDENTS USUALLY HAVE OCCURRED DURING THE FIRST SIX MONTHS OF TREATMENT. SERIOUS OR FATAL HEPATOTOXICITY MAY BE PRECEDED BY NON-SPECIFIC SYMPTOMS SUCH AS MALAISE, WEAKNESS, LETHARGY, FACIAL EDEMA, ANOREXIA, AND VOMITING. IN PATIENTS WITH EPILEPSY, A LOSS OF SEIZURE CONTROL MAY ALSO OCCUR. PATIENTS SHOULD BE MONITORED CLOSELY FOR APPEARANCE OF THESE SYMPTOMS. LIVER FUNCTION TESTS SHOULD BE PERFORMED PRIOR TO THERAPY AND AT FREQUENT INTERVALS THEREAFTER, ESPECIALLY DURING THE FIRST SIX MONTHS.

TERATOGENICITY:

VALPROATE CAN PRODUCE TERATOGENIC EFFECTS SUCH AS NEURAL TUBE DEFECTS (E.G., SPINA BIFIDA). ACCORDINGLY, THE USE OF VALPROATE PRODUCTS IN WOMEN OF CHILDBEARING POTENTIAL REQUIRES THAT THE BENEFITS OF ITS USE BE WEIGHED AGAINST THE RISK OF INJURY TO THE FETUS.

PANCREATITIS:

CASES OF LIFE-THREATENING PANCREATITIS HAVE BEEN REPORTED IN BOTH CHILDREN AND ADULTS RECEIVING VALPROATE. SOME OF THE CASES HAVE BEEN DESCRIBED AS HEMORRHAGIC WITH A RAPID PROGRESSION FROM INITIAL SYMPTOMS TO DEATH. CASES HAVE BEEN REPORTED SHORTLY AFTER INITIAL USE AS WELL AS AFTER SEVERAL YEARS OF USE. PATIENTS AND GUARDIANS SHOULD BE WARNED THAT ABDOMINAL PAIN, NAUSEA, VOMITING, AND/OR ANOREXIA CAN BE SYMPTOMS OF PANCREATITIS THAT REQUIRE PROMPT MEDICAL EVALUATION. IF PANCREATITIS IS DIAGNOSED, VALPROATE SHOULD ORDINARILY BE DISCONTINUED. ALTERNATIVE TREATMENT FOR THE UNDERLYING MEDICAL CONDITION SHOULD BE INITIATED AS CLINICALLY INDICATED. (See **WARNINGS** and **PRECAUTIONS**.)

DESCRIPTION

Valproate sodium is the sodium salt of valproic acid designated as sodium 2-propylpentanoate. Valproate sodium has the following structure:

$$\mathrm{(CH_3{-}CH_2{-}CH_2)_2CH{-}COO^{\ominus}\ Na^{\oplus}}$$

Valproate sodium has a molecular weight of 166.2. It occurs as an essentially white and odorless, crystalline, deliquescent powder.

DEPACON solution is available in 5 mL single-dose vials for intravenous injection. Each mL contains valproate sodium equivalent to 100 mg valproic acid, edetate disodium 0.40 mg, and water for injection to volume. The pH is adjusted to 7.6 with sodium hydroxide and/or hydrochloric acid. The solution is clear and colorless.

CLINICAL PHARMACOLOGY

DEPACON exists as the valproate ion in the blood. The mechanisms by which valproate exerts its therapeutic effects have not been established. It has been suggested that its activity in epilepsy is related to increased brain concentrations of gamma-aminobutyric acid (GABA).

Pharmacokinetics

Bioavailability

Equivalent doses of intravenous (IV) valproate and oral valproate products are expected to result in equivalent C_{max}, C_{min}, and total systemic exposure to the valproate ion. However, the rate of valproate ion absorption may vary with the formulation used. These differences should be of minor clinical importance under the steady state conditions achieved in chronic use in the treatment of epilepsy.

Administration of DEPAKOTE (divalproex sodium) tablets and IV valproate (given as a one hour infusion), 250 mg every 6 hours for 4 days to 18 healthy male volunteers resulted in equivalent AUC, C_{max}, C_{min} at steady state, as well as after the first dose. The T_{max} after IV DEPACON occurs at the end of the one hour infusion, while the T_{max} after oral dosing with DEPAKOTE occurs at approximately 4 hours. Because the kinetics of unbound valproate are linear, bioequivalence between DEPACON and DEPAKOTE up to the maximum recommended dose of 60 mg/kg/day can be assumed. The AUC and C_{max} resulting from administration of IV valproate 500 mg as a single one hour infusion and a single 500 mg dose of DEPAKENE syrup to 17 healthy male volunteers were also equivalent.

Patients maintained on valproic acid doses of 750 mg to 4250 mg daily (given in divided doses every 6 hours) as oral DEPAKOTE (divalproex sodium) alone (n=24) or with another stabilized antiepileptic drug [carbamazepine (n=15), phenytoin (n=11), or phenobarbital (n=1)], showed comparable plasma levels for valproic acid when switching from oral DEPAKOTE to IV valproate (1-hour infusion).

Distribution

Protein Binding:

The plasma protein binding of valproate is concentration dependent and the free fraction increases from approximately 10% at 40 µg/mL to 18.5% at 130 µg/mL. Protein binding of valproate is reduced in the elderly, in patients with chronic hepatic diseases, in patients with renal impairment, and in the presence of other drugs (e.g., aspirin). Conversely, valproate may displace certain protein-bound drugs (e.g., phenytoin, carbamazepine, warfarin, and tolbutamide). (See **PRECAUTIONS, Drug Interactions** for more detailed information on the pharmacokinetic interactions of valproate with other drugs.)

CNS Distribution:

Valproate concentrations in cerebrospinal fluid (CSF) approximate unbound concentrations in plasma (about 10% of total concentration).

Metabolism

Valproate is metabolized almost entirely by the liver. In adult patients on monotherapy, 30–50% of an administered dose appears in urine as a glucuronide conjugate. Mitochondrial β-oxidation is the other major metabolic pathway, typically accounting for over 40% of the dose. Usually, less than 15–20% of the dose is eliminated by other oxidative mechanisms. Less than 3% of an administered dose is excreted unchanged in urine.

The relationship between dose and total valproate concentration is nonlinear; concentration does not increase proportionally with the dose, but rather, increases to a lesser extent due to saturable plasma protein binding. The kinetics of unbound drug are linear.

Elimination

Mean plasma clearance and volume of distribution for total valproate are 0.56 L/hr/1.73 m^2 and 11 L/1.73 m^2, respectively. Mean terminal half-life for valproate monotherapy after a 60 minute intravenous infusion of 1000 mg was 16 ± 3.0 hours.

The estimates cited apply primarily to patients who are not taking drugs that affect hepatic metabolizing enzyme systems. For example, patients taking enzyme-inducing antiepileptic drugs (carbamazepine, phenytoin, and phenobarbital) will clear valproate more rapidly. Because of these changes in valproate clearance, monitoring of antiepileptic concentrations should be intensified whenever concomitant antiepileptics are introduced or withdrawn.

Special Populations

Effect of Age:

Neonates—Children within the first two months of life have a markedly decreased ability to eliminate valproate compared to older children and adults. This is a result of reduced clearance (perhaps due to delay in development of glucuronosyltransferase and other enzyme systems involved in valproate elimination) as well as increased volume of distribution (in part due to decreased plasma protein binding). For example, in one study, the half-life in children under 10 days ranged from 10 to 67 hours compared to a range of 7 to 13 hours in children greater than 2 months.

Children - Pediatric patients (i.e., between 3 months and 10 years) have 50% higher clearances expressed on weight (i.e., mL/min/kg) than do adults. Over the age of 10 years, children have pharmacokinetic parameters that approximate those of adults.

Elderly—The capacity of elderly patients (age range: 68 to 89 years) to eliminate valproate has been shown to be reduced compared to younger adults (age range: 22 to 26). Intrinsic clearance is reduced by 39%; the free fraction is increased by 44%. Accordingly, the initial dosage should be reduced in the elderly. (See **DOSAGE AND ADMINISTRATION**).

Effect of Gender:

There are no differences in the body surface area adjusted unbound clearance between males and females (4.8±0.17 and 4.7±0.07 L/hr per 1.73 m^2, respectively).

Effect of Race:

The effects of race on the kinetics of valproate have not been studied.

Effect of Disease:

Liver Disease—(See **BOXED WARNING, CONTRAINDICATIONS**, and **WARNINGS**). Liver disease impairs the capacity to eliminate valproate. In one study, the clearance of free valproate was decreased by 50% in 7 patients with cirrhosis and by 16% in 4 patients with acute hepatitis, compared with 6 healthy subjects. In that study, the half-life of valproate was increased from 12 to 18 hours. Liver disease is also associated with decreased albumin concentrations and larger unbound fractions (2 to 2.6 fold increase) of valproate. Accordingly, monitoring of total concentrations may be misleading since free concentrations may be substantially elevated in patients with hepatic disease whereas total concentrations may appear to be normal.

Renal Disease—A slight reduction (27%) in the unbound clearance of valproate has been reported in patients with renal failure (creatinine clearance < 10 mL/minute); however, hemodialysis typically reduces valproate concentrations by about 20%. Therefore, no dosage adjustment appears to be necessary in patients with renal failure. Protein binding in these patients is substantially reduced; thus, monitoring total concentrations may be misleading.

Plasma Levels and Clinical Effect

The relationship between plasma concentration and clinical response is not well documented. One contributing factor is the nonlinear, concentration dependent protein binding of valproate which affects the clearance of the drug. Thus, monitoring of total serum valproate cannot provide a reliable index of the bioactive valproate species.

For example, because the plasma protein binding of valproate is concentration dependent, the free fraction increases from approximately 10% at 40 µg/mL to 18.5% at 130 µg/mL. Higher than expected free fractions occur in the elderly, in hyperlipidemic patients, and in patients with hepatic and renal diseases.

Epilepsy:

The therapeutic range in epilepsy is commonly considered to be 50 to 100 µg/mL of total valproate, although some patients may be controlled with lower or higher plasma concentrations.

Equivalent doses of DEPACON and DEPAKOTE (divalproex sodium) yield equivalent plasma levels of the valproate ion (see **CLINICAL PHARMACOLOGY, Pharmacokinetics**).

Clinical Studies

The studies described in the following section were conducted with oral divalproex sodium products.

Epilepsy

The efficacy of DEPAKOTE (divalproex sodium) in reducing the incidence of complex partial seizures (CPS) that occur in isolation or in association with other seizure types was established in two controlled trials.

In one, multiclinic, placebo controlled study employing an add-on design (adjunctive therapy), 144 patients who continued to suffer eight or more CPS per 8 weeks during an 8 week period of monotherapy with doses of either carbamazepine or phenytoin sufficient to assure plasma concentrations within the "therapeutic range" were randomized to receive, in addition to their original antiepilepsy drug (AED), either DEPAKOTE or placebo. Randomized patients were to be followed for a total of 16 weeks. The following table presents the findings.

Adjunctive Therapy Study
Median Incidence of CPS per 8 Weeks

Add-on Treatment	Number of Patients	Baseline Incidence	Experimental Incidence
DEPAKOTE	75	16.0	8.9*
Placebo	69	14.5	11.5

*Reduction from baseline statistically significantly greater for DEPAKOTE than placebo at p ≤ 0.05 level.

Figure 1 presents the proportion of patients (X axis) whose percentage reduction from baseline in complex partial seizure rates was at least as great as that indicated on the Y axis in the adjunctive therapy study. A positive percent reduction indicates an improvement (i.e., a decrease in seizure frequency), while a negative percent reduction indicates worsening. Thus, in a display of this type, the curve for an effective treatment is shifted to the left of the curve for placebo. This figure shows that the proportion of patients achieving any particular level of improvement was consistently higher for DEPAKOTE than for placebo. For example, 45% of patients treated with DEPAKOTE had a ≥ 50% reduction in complex partial seizure rate compared to 23% of patients treated with placebo.

Figure 1

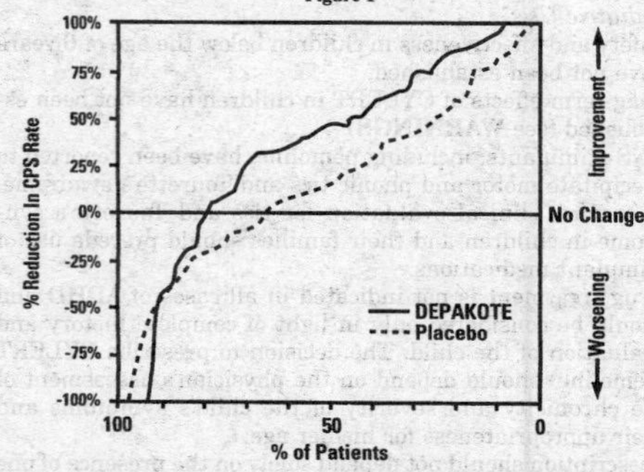

The second study assessed the capacity of DEPAKOTE to reduce the incidence of CPS when administered as the sole AED. The study compared the incidence of CPS among patients randomized to either a high or low dose treatment arm. Patients qualified for entry into the randomized comparison phase of this study only if 1) they continued to experience 2 or more CPS per 4 weeks during an 8 to 12 week long period of monotherapy with adequate doses of an AED (i.e., phenytoin, carbamazepine, phenobarbital, or primidone) and 2) they made a successful transition over a two week interval to DEPAKOTE. Patients entering the randomized phase were then brought to their assigned target dose, gradually tapered off their concomitant AED and followed for an interval as long as 22 weeks. Less than 50% of

the patients randomized, however, completed the study. In patients converted to DEPAKOTE monotherapy, the mean total valproate concentrations during monotherapy were 71 and 123 µg/mL in the low dose and high dose groups, respectively.
The following table presents the findings for all patients randomized who had at least one post-randomization assessment.

Monotherapy Study
Median Incidence of CPS per 8 Weeks

Treatment	Number of Patients	Baseline Incidence	Randomized Phase Incidence
High dose DEPAKOTE	131	13.2	10.7*
Low dose DEPAKOTE	134	14.2	13.8

*Reduction from baseline statistically significantly greater for high dose than low dose at $p \leq 0.05$ level.

Figure 2 presents the proportion of patients (X axis) whose percentage reduction from baseline in complex partial seizure rates was at least as great as that indicated on the Y axis in the monotherapy study. A positive percent reduction indicates an improvement (i.e., a decrease in seizure frequency), while a negative percent reduction indicates worsening. Thus, in a display of this type, the curve for a more effective treatment is shifted to the left of the curve for a less effective treatment. This figure shows that the proportion of patients achieving any particular level of reduction was consistently higher for high dose DEPAKOTE than for low dose DEPAKOTE. For example, when switching from carbamazepine, phenytoin, phenobarbital or primidone monotherapy to high dose DEPAKOTE monotherapy, 63% of patients experienced no change or a reduction in complex partial seizure rates compared to 54% of patients receiving low dose DEPAKOTE.

Figure 2

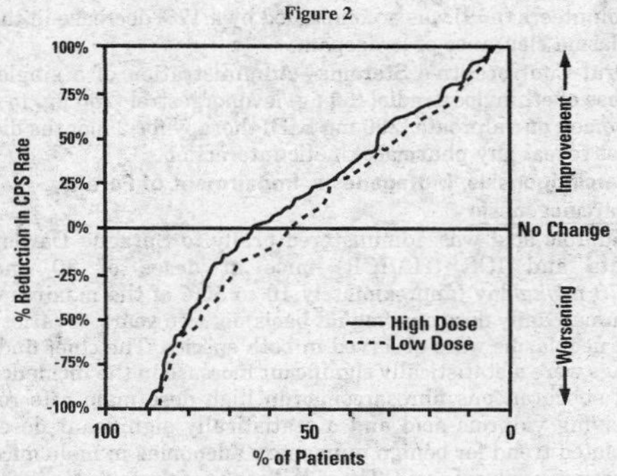

INDICATIONS AND USAGE

DEPACON is indicated as an intravenous alternative in patients for whom oral administration of valproate products is temporarily not feasible in the following conditions:
DEPACON is indicated as monotherapy and adjunctive therapy in the treatment of patients with complex partial seizures that occur either in isolation or in association with other types of seizures. DEPACON is also indicated for use as sole and adjunctive therapy in the treatment of patients with simple and complex absence seizures, and adjunctively in patients with multiple seizure types that include absence seizures.
Simple absence is defined as very brief clouding of the sensorium or loss of consciousness accompanied by certain generalized epileptic discharges without other detectable clinical signs. Complex absence is the term used when other signs are also present.
SEE **WARNINGS** FOR STATEMENT REGARDING FATAL HEPATIC DYSFUNCTION.

CONTRAINDICATIONS

VALPROATE SODIUM INJECTION SHOULD NOT BE ADMINISTERED TO PATIENTS WITH HEPATIC DISEASE OR SIGNIFICANT HEPATIC DYSFUNCTION.
Valproate sodium injection is contraindicated in patients with known hypersensitivity to the drug.

WARNINGS

Hepatotoxicity

Hepatic failure resulting in fatalities has occurred in patients receiving valproic acid. These incidents usually have occurred during the first six months of treatment. Serious or fatal hepatotoxicity may be preceded by non-specific symptoms such as malaise, weakness, lethargy, facial edema, anorexia, and vomiting. In patients with epilepsy, a loss of seizure control may also occur. Patients should be monitored closely for appearance of these symptoms. Liver function tests should be performed prior to therapy and at frequent intervals thereafter, especially during the first six months of valproate therapy. However, physicians should not rely totally on serum biochemistry since these tests may not be abnormal in all instances, but should also consider the results of careful interim medical history and physical examination.
Caution should be observed when administering valproate products to patients with a prior history of hepatic disease. Patients on multiple anticonvulsants, children, those with congenital metabolic disorders, those with severe seizure disorders accompanied by mental retardation, and those with organic brain disease may be at particular risk. Experience has indicated that children under the age of two years are at a considerably increased risk of developing fatal hepatotoxicity, especially those with the aforementioned conditions. When DEPACON is used in this patient group, it should be used with extreme caution and as a sole agent. The benefits of therapy should be weighed against the risks. Use of DEPACON has not been studied in children below the age of 2 years. Above this age group, experience with valproate products in epilepsy has indicated that the incidence of fatal hepatotoxicity decreases considerably in progressively older patient groups.
The drug should be discontinued immediately in the presence of significant hepatic dysfunction, suspected or apparent. In some cases, hepatic dysfunction has progressed in spite of discontinuation of drug.

Pancreatitis

Cases of life-threatening pancreatitis have been reported in both children and adults receiving valproate. Some of the cases have been described as hemorrhagic with rapid progression from initial symptoms to death. Some cases have occurred shortly after initial use as well as after several years of use. The rate based upon the reported cases exceeds that expected in the general population and there have been cases in which pancreatitis recurred after rechallenge with valproate. In clinical trials, there were 2 cases of pancreatitis without alternative etiology in 2416 patients, representing 1044 patient-years experience. Patients and guardians should be warned that abdominal pain, nausea, vomiting, and/or anorexia can be symptoms of pancreatitis that require prompt medical evaluation. If pancreatitis is diagnosed, valproate should ordinarily be discontinued. Alternative treatment for the underlying medical condition should be initiated as clinically indicated (see **BOXED WARNING**).

Somnolence in the Elderly

In a double-blind, multicenter trial of valproate in elderly patients with dementia (mean age = 83 years), doses were increased by 125 mg/day to a target dose of 20 mg/kg/day. A significantly higher proportion of valproate patients had somnolence compared to placebo, and although not statistically significant, there was a higher proportion of patients with dehydration. Discontinuations for somnolence were also significantly higher than with placebo. In some patients with somnolence (approximately one-half), there was associated reduced nutritional intake and weight loss. There was a trend for the patients who experienced these events to have a lower baseline albumin concentration, lower valproate clearance, and a higher BUN. In elderly patients, dosage should be increased more slowly and with regular monitoring for fluid and nutritional intake, dehydration, somnolence, and other adverse events. Dose reductions or discontinuation of valproate should be considered in patients with decreased food or fluid intake and in patients with excessive somnolence (see **DOSAGE AND ADMINISTRATION**).

Thrombocytopenia

The frequency of adverse effects (particularly elevated liver enzymes and thrombocytopenia [see **PRECAUTIONS**]) may be dose-related. In a clinical trial of DEPAKOTE as monotherapy in patients with epilepsy, 34/126 patients (27%) receiving approximately 50 mg/kg/day on average, had at least one value of platelets $\leq 75 \times 10^9$/L. Approximately half of these patients had treatment discontinued, with return of platelet counts to normal. In the remaining patients, platelet counts normalized with continued treatment. In this study, the probability of thrombocytopenia appeared to increase significantly at total valproate concentrations of ≥ 110 µg/mL (females) or ≥ 135 µg/mL (males). The therapeutic benefit which may accompany the higher doses should therefore be weighed against the possibility of a greater incidence of adverse effects.

Post-traumatic Seizures

A study was conducted to evaluate the effect of IV valproate in the prevention of post-traumatic seizures in patients with acute head injuries. Patients were randomly assigned to receive either IV valproate given for one week (followed by oral valproate products for either one or six months per random treatment assignment) or IV phenytoin given for one week (followed by placebo). In this study, the incidence of death was found to be higher in the two groups assigned to valproate treatment compared to the rate in those assigned to the IV phenytoin treatment group (13% vs 8.5%, respectively). Many of these patients were critically ill with multiple and/or severe injuries, and evaluation of the causes of death did not suggest any specific drug-related causation. Further, in the absence of a concurrent placebo control during the initial week of intravenous therapy, it is impossible to determine if the mortality rate in the patients treated with valproate was greater or less than that expected in a similar group not treated with valproate, or whether the rate seen in the IV phenytoin treated patients was lower than would be expected. Nonetheless, until further information is available, it seems prudent not to use DEPACON in patients with acute head trauma for the prophylaxis of post-traumatic seizures.

Usage In Pregnancy

ACCORDING TO PUBLISHED AND UNPUBLISHED REPORTS, VALPROIC ACID MAY PRODUCE TERATOGENIC EFFECTS IN THE OFFSPRING OF HUMAN FEMALES RECEIVING THE DRUG DURING PREGNANCY.
THERE ARE MULTIPLE REPORTS IN THE CLINICAL LITERATURE WHICH INDICATE THAT THE USE OF ANTIEPILEPSY DRUGS DURING PREGNANCY RESULTS IN AN INCREASED INCIDENCE OF BIRTH DEFECTS IN THE OFFSPRING. ALTHOUGH DATA ARE MORE EXTENSIVE WITH RESPECT TO TRIMETHADIONE, PARAMETHADIONE, PHENYTOIN, AND PHENOBARBITAL, REPORTS INDICATE A POSSIBLE SIMILAR ASSOCIATION WITH THE USE OF OTHER ANTIEPILEPSY DRUGS. THEREFORE, ANTIEPILEPSY DRUGS SHOULD BE ADMINISTERED TO WOMEN OF CHILDBEARING POTENTIAL ONLY IF THEY ARE CLEARLY SHOWN TO BE ESSENTIAL IN THE MANAGEMENT OF THEIR SEIZURES.
THE INCIDENCE OF NEURAL TUBE DEFECTS IN THE FETUS MAY BE INCREASED IN MOTHERS RECEIVING VALPROATE DURING THE FIRST TRIMESTER OF PREGNANCY. THE CENTERS FOR DISEASE CONTROL (CDC) HAS ESTIMATED THE RISK OF VALPROIC ACID EXPOSED WOMEN HAVING CHILDREN WITH SPINA BIFIDA TO BE APPROXIMATELY 1 TO 2%.
OTHER CONGENITAL ANOMALIES (E.G., CRANIOFACIAL DEFECTS, CARDIOVASCULAR MALFORMATIONS AND ANOMALIES INVOLVING VARIOUS BODY SYSTEMS), COMPATIBLE AND INCOMPATIBLE WITH LIFE, HAVE BEEN REPORTED. SUFFICIENT DATA TO DETERMINE THE INCIDENCE OF THESE CONGENITAL ANOMALIES IS NOT AVAILABLE.
THE HIGHER INCIDENCE OF CONGENITAL ANOMALIES IN ANTIEPILEPSY DRUG-TREATED WOMEN WITH SEIZURE DISORDERS CANNOT BE REGARDED AS A CAUSE AND EFFECT RELATIONSHIP. THERE ARE INTRINSIC METHODOLOGIC PROBLEMS IN OBTAINING ADEQUATE DATA ON DRUG TERATOGENICITY IN HUMANS; GENETIC FACTORS OR THE EPILEPTIC CONDITION ITSELF, MAY BE MORE IMPORTANT THAN DRUG THERAPY IN CONTRIBUTING TO CONGENITAL ANOMALIES.
PATIENTS TAKING VALPROATE MAY DEVELOP CLOTTING ABNORMALITIES. A PATIENT WHO HAD LOW FIBRINOGEN WHEN TAKING MULTIPLE ANTICONVULSANTS INCLUDING VALPROATE GAVE BIRTH TO AN INFANT WITH AFIBRINOGENEMIA WHO SUBSEQUENTLY DIED OF HEMORRHAGE. IF VALPROATE IS USED IN PREGNANCY, THE CLOTTING PARAMETERS SHOULD BE MONITORED CAREFULLY.
HEPATIC FAILURE, RESULTING IN THE DEATH OF A NEWBORN AND OF AN INFANT, HAVE BEEN REPORTED FOLLOWING THE USE OF VALPROATE DURING PREGNANCY.
Animal studies have demonstrated valproate-induced teratogenicity. Increased frequencies of malformations, as well as intrauterine growth retardation and death, have been observed in mice, rats, rabbits, and monkeys following prenatal exposure to valproate. Malformations of the skeletal system are the most common structural abnormalities produced in experimental animals, but neural tube closure defects have been seen in mice exposed to maternal plasma valproate concentrations exceeding 230 µg/mL (2.3 times the upper limit of the human therapeutic range) during susceptible periods of embryonic development. Administration of an oral dose of 200 mg/kg/day or greater (50% of the maximum human daily dose or greater on a mg/m^2 basis) to pregnant rats during organogenesis produced malformations (skeletal, cardiac, and urogenital) and growth retardation in the offspring. These doses resulted in peak maternal plasma valproate levels of approximately 340 µg/mL or greater (3.4 times the upper limit of the human therapeutic range or greater). Behavioral deficits have been reported in the offspring of rats given a dose of 200 mg/kg/day throughout most of pregnancy. An oral dose of 350 mg/kg/day (2 times the maximum human daily dose on a mg/m^2 basis) produced skeletal and visceral malformations in rabbits exposed during organogenesis. Skeletal malformations, growth retardation, and death were observed in rhesus monkeys following administration of an oral dose of 200 mg/kg/day (equal to the maximum human daily dose on a mg/m^2 basis) during organogenesis. This dose resulted in peak maternal plasma valproate levels of approximately 280 µg/mL (2.8 times the upper limit of the human therapeutic range).
The prescribing physician will wish to weigh the benefits of therapy against the risks in treating or counseling women of childbearing potential. If this drug is used during pregnancy, or if the patient becomes pregnant while taking this drug, the patient should be apprised of the potential hazard to the fetus.
Antiepilepsy drugs should not be discontinued abruptly in patients in whom the drug is administered to prevent major seizures because of the strong possibility of precipitating status epilepticus with attendant hypoxia and threat to life. In individual cases where the severity and frequency of the seizure disorder are such that the removal of medication does not pose a serious threat to the patient, discontinuation of the drug may be considered prior to and during pregnancy, although it cannot be said with any confidence that even minor seizures do not pose some hazard to the developing embryo or fetus.
Tests to detect neural tube and other defects using current accepted procedures should be considered a part of routine prenatal care in childbearing women receiving valproate.

Continued on next page

Depacon—Cont.

PRECAUTIONS

Hepatic Dysfunction

See **BOXED WARNING, CONTRAINDICATIONS** and **WARNINGS.**

Pancreatitis

See **BOXED WARNING** and **WARNINGS.**

General

Because of reports of thrombocytopenia (See **WARNINGS**), inhibition of the secondary phase of platelet aggregation, and abnormal coagulation parameters, (e.g., low fibrinogen), platelet counts and coagulation tests are recommended before initiating therapy and at periodic intervals. It is recommended that patients receiving DEPACON be monitored for platelet count and coagulation parameters prior to planned surgery. In a clinical trial of DEPAKOTE (divalproex sodium) as monotherapy in patients with epilepsy, 34/126 patients (27%) receiving approximately 50 mg/kg/day on average, had at least one value of platelets $\leq$ 75 x 10^9/L. Approximately half of these patients had treatment discontinued, with return of platelet counts to normal. In the remaining patients, platelet counts normalized with continued treatment. In this study, the probability of thrombocytopenia appeared to increase significantly at total valproate concentrations of $\geq$ 110 µg/mL (females) or $\geq$ 135 µg/mL (males). Evidence of hemorrhage, bruising, or a disorder of hemostasis/coagulation is an indication for reduction of the dosage or withdrawal of therapy.

Hyperammonemia with or without lethargy or coma has been reported and may be present in the absence of abnormal liver function tests. Asymptomatic elevations of ammonia are more common and when present require more frequent monitoring. If clinically significant symptoms occur, DEPACON therapy should be modified or discontinued.

Since DEPACON may interact with concurrently administered drugs which are capable of enzyme induction, periodic plasma concentration determinations of valproate and concomitant drugs are recommended during the early course of therapy. (See **PRECAUTIONS—Drug Interactions.**)

Valproate is partially eliminated in the urine as a keto-metabolite which may lead to a false interpretation of the urine ketone test.

There have been reports of altered thyroid function tests associated with valproate. The clinical significance of these is unknown.

There are *in vitro* studies that suggest valproate stimulates the replication of the HIV and CMV viruses under certain experimental conditions. The clinical consequence, if any, is not known. Additionally, the relevance of these *in vitro* findings is uncertain for patients receiving maximally suppressive antiretroviral therapy. Nevertheless, these data should be borne in mind when interpreting the results from regular monitoring of the viral load in HIV infected patients receiving valproate or when following CMV infected patients clinically.

Information for Patients

Patients and guardians should be warned that abdominal pain, nausea, vomiting, and/or anorexia can be symptoms of pancreatitis and, therefore, require further medical evaluation promptly.

Since DEPACON may produce CNS depression, especially when combined with another CNS depressant (e.g., alcohol), patients should be advised not to engage in hazardous activities, such as driving an automobile or operating dangerous machinery, until it is known that they do not become drowsy from the drug.

Drug Interactions

Effects of Co-Administered Drugs on Valproate Clearance

Drugs that affect the level of expression of hepatic enzymes, particularly those that elevate levels of glucuronosyltransferases, may increase the clearance of valproate. For example, phenytoin, carbamazepine, and phenobarbital (or primidone) can double the clearance of valproate. Thus, patients on monotherapy will generally have longer half-lives and higher concentrations than patients receiving polytherapy with antiepilepsy drugs.

In contrast, drugs that are inhibitors of cytochrome P450 isozymes, e.g., antidepressants, may be expected to have little effect on valproate clearance because cytochrome P450 microsomal mediated oxidation is a relatively minor secondary metabolic pathway compared to glucuronidation and beta-oxidation.

Because of these changes in valproate clearance, monitoring of valproate and concomitant drug concentrations should be increased whenever enzyme inducing drugs are introduced or withdrawn.

The following list provides information about the potential for an influence of several commonly prescribed medications on valproate pharmacokinetics. The list is not exhaustive nor could it be, since new interactions are continuously being reported.

Drugs for which a potentially important interaction has been observed:

Aspirin—A study involving the co-administration of aspirin at antipyretic doses (11 to 16 mg/kg) with valproate to pediatric patients (n=6) revealed a decrease in protein binding and an inhibition of metabolism of valproate. Valproate free fraction was increased 4-fold in the presence of aspirin compared to valproate alone. The β-oxidation pathway consisting of 2-E-valproic acid, 3-OH-valproic acid, and 3-keto valproic acid was decreased from 25% of total metabolites excreted on valproate alone to 8.3% in the presence of aspirin. Caution should be observed if valproate and aspirin are to be co-administered.

Felbamate—A study involving the co-administration of 1200 mg/day of felbamate with valproate to patients with epilepsy (n=10) revealed an increase in mean valproate peak concentration by 35% (from 86 to 115 µg/mL) compared to valproate alone. Increasing the felbamate dose to 2400 mg/day increased the mean valproate peak concentration to 133 µg/mL (another 16% increase). A decrease in valproate dosage may be necessary when felbamate therapy is initiated.

Rifampin—A study involving the administration of a single dose of valproate (7 mg/kg) 36 hours after 5 nights of daily dosing with rifampin (600 mg) revealed a 40% increase in the oral clearance of valproate. Valproate dosage adjustment may be necessary when it is co-administered with rifampin.

Drugs for which either no interaction or a likely clinically unimportant interaction has been observed:

Antacids—A study involving the co-administration of valproate 500 mg with commonly administered antacids (Maalox, Trisogel, and Titralac—160 mEq doses) did not reveal any effect on the extent of absorption of valproate.

Chlorpromazine—A study involving the administration of 100 to 300 mg/day of chlorpromazine to schizophrenic patients already receiving valproate (200 mg BID) revealed a 15% increase in trough plasma levels of valproate.

Haloperidol—A study involving the administration of 6 to 10 mg/day of haloperidol to schizophrenic patients already receiving valproate (200 mg BID) revealed no significant changes in valproate trough plasma levels.

Cimetidine and Ranitidine—Cimetidine and ranitidine do not affect the clearance of valproate.

Effects of Valproate on Other Drugs

Valproate has been found to be a weak inhibitor of some P450 isozymes, epoxide hydrase, and glucuronyl transferases.

The following list provides information about the potential for an influence of valproate co-administration on the pharmacokinetics or pharmacodynamics of several commonly prescribed medications. The list is not exhaustive, since new interactions are continuously being reported.

Drugs for which a potentially important valproate interaction has been observed:

Amitriptyline/Nortriptyline—Administration of a single oral 50 mg dose of amitriptyline to 15 normal volunteers (10 males and 5 females) who received valproate (500 mg BID) resulted in a 21% decrease in plasma clearance of amitriptyline and a 34% decrease in the net clearance of nortriptyline. Rare postmarketing reports of concurrent use of valproate and amitriptyline resulting in an increased amitriptyline level have been received. Concurrent use of valproate and amitriptyline has rarely been associated with toxicity. Monitoring of amitriptyline levels should be considered for patients taking valproate concomitantly with amitriptyline. Consideration should be given to lowering the dose of amitriptyline/nortriptyline in the presence of valproate.

Carbamazepine/carbamazepine-10,11-Epoxide—Serum levels of carbamazepine (CBZ) decreased 17% while that of carbamazepine-10,11-epoxide (CBZ-E) increased by 45% upon co-administration of valproate and CBZ to epileptic patients.

Clonazepam—The concomitant use of valproic acid and clonazepam may induce absence status in patients with a history of absence type seizures.

Diazepam—Valproate displaces diazepam from its plasma albumin binding sites and inhibits its metabolism. Co-administration of valproate (1500 mg daily) increased the free fraction of diazepam (10 mg) by 90% in healthy volunteers (n=6). Plasma clearance and volume of distribution for free diazepam were reduced by 25% and 20%, respectively, in the presence of valproate. The elimination half-life of diazepam remained unchanged upon addition of valproate.

Ethosuximide—Valproate inhibits the metabolism of ethosuximide. Administration of a single ethosuximide dose of 500 mg with valproate (800 to 1600 mg/day) to healthy volunteers (n=6) was accompanied by a 25% increase in elimination half-life of ethosuximide and a 15% decrease in its total clearance as compared to ethosuximide alone. Patients receiving valproate and ethosuximide, especially along with other anticonvulsants, should be monitored for alterations in serum concentrations of both drugs.

Lamotrigine—In a steady-state study involving 10 healthy volunteers, the elimination half-life of lamotrigine increased from 26 to 70 hours with valproate co-administration (a 165% increase). The dose of lamotrigine should be reduced when co-administered with valproate.

Phenobarbital—Valproate was found to inhibit the metabolism of phenobarbital. Co-administration of valproate (250 mg BID for 14 days) with phenobarbital to normal subjects (n=6) resulted in a 50% increase in half-life and a 30% decrease in plasma clearance of phenobarbital (60 mg single-dose). The fraction of phenobarbital dose excreted unchanged increased by 50% in presence of valproate.

There is evidence for severe CNS depression, with or without significant elevations of barbiturate or valproate serum concentrations. All patients receiving concomitant barbiturate therapy should be closely monitored for neurological toxicity. Serum barbiturate concentrations should be obtained, if possible, and the barbiturate dosage decreased, if appropriate.

Primidone, which is metabolized to a barbiturate, may be involved in a similar interaction with valproate.

Phenytoin—Valproate displaces phenytoin from its plasma albumin binding sites and inhibits its hepatic metabolism. Co-administration of valproate (400 mg TID) with phenytoin (250 mg) in normal volunteers (n=7) was associated with a 60% increase in the free fraction of phenytoin. Total plasma clearance and apparent volume of distribution of phenytoin increased 30% in the presence of valproate. Both the clearance and apparent volume of distribution of free phenytoin were reduced by 25%.

In patients with epilepsy, there have been reports of breakthrough seizures occurring with the combination of valproate and phenytoin. The dosage of phenytoin should be adjusted as required by the clinical situation.

Tolbutamide—From *in vitro* experiments, the unbound fraction of tolbutamide was increased from 20% to 50% when added to plasma samples taken from patients treated with valproate. The clinical relevance of this displacement is unknown.

Warfarin—In an *in vitro* study, valproate increased the unbound fraction of warfarin by up to 32.6%. The therapeutic relevance of this is unknown; however, coagulation tests should be monitored if valproate therapy is instituted in patients taking anticoagulants.

Zidovudine—In six patients who were seropositive for HIV, the clearance of zidovudine (100 mg q8h) was decreased by 38% after administration of valproate (250 or 500 mg q8h); the half-life of zidovudine was unaffected.

Drugs for which either no interaction or a likely clinically unimportant interaction has been observed:

Acetaminophen—Valproate had no effect on any of the pharmacokinetic parameters of acetaminophen when it was concurrently administered to three epileptic patients.

Clozapine—In psychotic patients (n=11), no interaction was observed when valproate was co-administered with clozapine.

Lithium—Co-administration of valproate (500 mg BID) and lithium carbonate (300 mg TID) to normal male volunteers (n=16) had no effect on the steady-state kinetics of lithium.

Lorazepam—Concomitant administration of valproate (500 mg BID) and lorazepam (1 mg BID) in normal male volunteers (n=9) was accompanied by a 17% decrease in the plasma clearance of lorazepam.

Oral Contraceptive Steroids—Administration of a single-dose of ethinyloestradiol (50 µg)/levonorgestrel (250 µg) to 6 women on valproate (200 mg BID) therapy for 2 months did not reveal any pharmacokinetic interaction.

Carcinogenesis, Mutagenesis, Impairment of Fertility

Carcinogenesis

Valproic acid was administered orally to Sprague Dawley rats and ICR (HA/ICR) mice at doses of 80 and 170 mg/kg/day (approximately 10 to 50% of the maximum human daily dose on a mg/m^2 basis) for two years. A variety of neoplasms were observed in both species. The chief findings were a statistically significant increase in the incidence of subcutaneous fibrosarcomas in high dose male rats receiving valproic acid and a statistically significant dose-related trend for benign pulmonary adenomas in male mice receiving valproic acid. The significance of these findings for humans is unknown.

Mutagenesis

Valproate was not mutagenic in an *in vitro* bacterial assay (Ames test), did not produce dominant lethal effects in mice, and did not increase chromosome aberration frequency in an *in vivo* cytogenetic study in rats. Increased frequencies of sister chromatid exchange (SCE) have been reported in a study of epileptic children taking valproate, but this association was not observed in another study conducted in adults. There is some evidence that increased SCE frequencies may be associated with epilepsy. The biological significance of an increase in SCE frequency is not known.

Fertility

Chronic toxicity studies in juvenile and adult rats and dogs demonstrated reduced spermatogenesis and testicular atrophy at oral doses of 400 mg/kg/day or greater in rats (approximately equivalent to or greater than the maximum human daily dose on a mg/m^2 basis) and 150 mg/kg/day or greater in dogs (approximately 1.4 times the maximum human daily dose or greater on a mg/m^2 basis). Segment I fertility studies in rats have shown oral doses up to 350 mg/kg/day (approximately equal to the maximum human daily dose on a mg/m^2 basis) for 60 days to have no effect on fertility. THE EFFECT OF VALPROATE ON TESTICULAR DEVELOPMENT AND ON SPERM PRODUCTION AND FERTILITY IN HUMANS IS UNKNOWN.

Pregnancy

Pregnancy Category D: See **WARNINGS.**

Nursing Mothers

Valproate is excreted in breast milk. Concentrations in breast milk have been reported to be 1–10% of serum concentrations. It is not known what effect this would have on a nursing infant. Consideration should be given to discontinuing nursing when valproate is administered to a nursing woman.

Pediatric Use

Experience with oral valproate has indicated that pediatric patients under the age of two years are at a considerably increased risk of developing fatal hepatotoxicity, especially those with the aforementioned conditions (see **BOXED WARNING**). The safety of DEPACON has not been studied in individuals below the age of 2 years. If a decision is made to use DEPACON in this age group, it should be used with extreme caution and as a sole agent. The benefits of therapy should be weighed against the risks. Above the age of 2

years, experience in epilepsy has indicated that the incidence of fatal hepatotoxicity decreases considerably in progressively older patient groups.
Younger children, especially those receiving enzyme-inducing drugs, will require larger maintenance doses to attain targeted total and unbound valproic acid concentrations.
The variability in free fraction limits the clinical usefulness of monitoring total serum valproic acid concentrations. Interpretation of valproic acid concentrations in children should include consideration of factors that affect hepatic metabolism and protein binding.
No unique safety concerns were identified in the 24 patients age 2 to 17 years who received DEPACON in clinical trials.
The basic toxicology and pathologic manifestations of valproate sodium in neonatal (4-day old) and juvenile (14-day old) rats are similar to those seen in young adult rats. However, additional findings, including renal alterations in juvenile rats and renal alterations and retinal dysplasia in neonatal rats, have been reported. These findings occurred at 240 mg/kg/day, a dosage approximately equivalent to the human maximum recommended daily dose on a mg/m^2 basis. They were not seen at 90 mg/kg, or 40% of the maximum human daily dose on a mg/m^2 basis.

Geriatric Use

No patients above the age of 65 years were enrolled in double-blind prospective clinical trials of mania associated with bipolar illness. In a case review study of 583 patients, 72 patients (12%) were greater than 65 years of age. A higher percentage of patients above 65 years of age reported accidental injury, infection, pain, somnolence, and tremor. Discontinuation of valproate was occasionally associated with the latter two events. It is not clear whether these events indicate additional risk or whether they result from preexisting medical illness and concomitant medication use among these patients.
A study of elderly patients with dementia revealed drug related somnolence and discontinuation for somnolence (see **WARNINGS—Somnolence in the Elderly**). The starting dose should be reduced in these patients, and dosage reductions or discontinuation should be considered in patients with excessive somnolence (see **DOSAGE AND ADMINISTRATION**).
No unique safety concerns were identified in the 19 patients > 65 years of age receiving DEPACON in clinical trials.

ADVERSE REACTIONS

The adverse events that can result from DEPACON use include all of those associated with oral forms of valproate. The following describes experience specifically with DEPACON. DEPACON has been generally well tolerated in clinical trials involving 111 healthy adult male volunteers and 352 patients with epilepsy, given at doses of 125 to 6000 mg (total daily dose). A total of 2% of patients discontinued treatment with DEPACON due to adverse events. The most common adverse events leading to discontinuation were 2 cases each of nausea/vomiting and elevated amylase. Other adverse events leading to discontinuation were hallucinations, pneumonia, headache, injection site reaction, and abnormal gait. Dizziness and injection site pain were observed more frequently at a 100 mg/min infusion rate than at rates up to 33 mg/min. At a 200 mg/min rate, dizziness and taste perversion occurred more frequently than at a 100 mg/min rate. The maximum rate of infusion studied was 200 mg/min.
Adverse events reported by at least 0.5% of all subjects/patients in clinical trials of DEPACON are summarized in Table 1.

Table 1
Adverse Events Reported During Studies of DEPACON

Body System/Event	N = 463
Body as a Whole	
Chest Pain	1.7%
Headache	4.3%
Injection Site Inflammation	0.6%
Injection Site Pain	2.6%
Injection Site Reaction	2.4%
Pain (unspecified)	1.3%
Cardiovascular	
Vasodilation	0.9%
Dermatologic	
Sweating	0.9%
Digestive System	
Abdominal Pain	1.1%
Diarrhea	0.9%
Nausea	3.2%
Vomiting	1.3%
Nervous System	
Dizziness	5.2%
Euphoria	0.9%
Hypesthesia	0.6%
Nervousness	0.9%
Paresthesia	0.9%
Somnolence	1.7%
Tremor	0.6%
Respiratory	
Pharyngitis	0.6%
Special Senses	
Taste Perversion	1.9%

Epilepsy

Based on a placebo-controlled trial of adjunctive therapy for treatment of complex partial seizures, DEPAKOTE (divalproex sodium) was generally well tolerated with most adverse events rated as mild to moderate in severity. Intolerance was the primary reason for discontinuation in the DEPAKOTE-treated patients (6%), compared to 1% of placebo-treated patients.
Table 2 lists treatment-emergent adverse events which were reported by ≥ 5% of DEPAKOTE-treated patients and for which the incidence was greater than in the placebo group, in the placebo-controlled trial of adjunctive therapy for treatment of complex partial seizures. Since patients were also treated with other antiepilepsy drugs, it is not possible, in most cases, to determine whether the following adverse events can be ascribed to DEPAKOTE alone, or the combination of DEPAKOTE and other antiepilepsy drugs.

Table 2
Adverse Events Reported by ≥ 5% of Patients Treated with DEPAKOTE During Placebo-Controlled Trial of Adjunctive Therapy for Complex Partial Seizures

Body System/Event	Depakote (%) (n = 77)	Placebo (%) (n = 70)
Body as a Whole		
Headache	31	21
Asthenia	27	7
Fever	6	4
Gastrointestinal System		
Nausea	48	14
Vomiting	27	7
Abdominal Pain	23	6
Diarrhea	13	6
Anorexia	12	0
Dyspepsia	8	4
Constipation	5	1
Nervous System		
Somnolence	27	11
Tremor	25	6
Dizziness	25	13
Diplopia	16	9
Amblyopia/Blurred Vision	12	9
Ataxia	8	1
Nystagmus	8	1
Emotional Lability	6	4
Thinking Abnormal	6	0
Amnesia	5	1
Respiratory System		
Flu Syndrome	12	9
Infection	12	6
Bronchitis	5	1
Rhinitis	5	4
Other		
Alopecia	6	1
Weight Loss	6	0

Table 3 lists treatment-emergent adverse events which were reported by ≥ 5% of patients in the high dose DEPAKOTE group, and for which the incidence was greater than in the low dose group, in a controlled trial of DEPAKOTE monotherapy treatment of complex partial seizures. Since patients were being titrated off another antiepilepsy drug during the first portion of the trial, it is not possible, in many cases, to determine whether the following adverse events can be ascribed to DEPAKOTE alone, or the combination of DEPAKOTE and other antiepilepsy drugs.

Table 3
Adverse Events Reported by ≥ 5% of Patients in the High Dose Group in the Controlled Trial of DEPAKOTE Monotherapy for Complex Partial Seizures[1]

Body System/Event	High Dose (%) (n = 131)	Low Dose (%) (n = 134)
Body as a Whole		
Asthenia	21	10
Digestive System		
Nausea	34	26
Diarrhea	23	19
Vomiting	23	15
Abdominal Pain	12	9
Anorexia	11	4
Dyspepsia	11	10
Hemic/Lymphatic System		
Thrombocytopenia	24	1
Ecchymosis	5	4
Metabolic/Nutritional		
Weight Gain	9	4
Peripheral Edema	8	3
Nervous System		
Tremor	57	19
Somnolence	30	18
Dizziness	18	13
Insomnia	15	9
Nervousness	11	7
Amnesia	7	4
Nystagmus	7	1
Depression	5	4
Respiratory System		
Infection	20	13
Pharyngitis	8	2
Dyspnea	5	1
Skin and Appendages		
Alopecia	24	13
Special Senses		
Amblyopia/Blurred Vision	8	4
Tinnitus	7	1

[1] Headache was the only adverse event that occurred in ≥ 5% of patients in the high dose group and at an equal or greater incidence in the low dose group.

The following additional adverse events were reported by greater than 1% but less than 5% of the 358 patients treated with DEPAKOTE in the controlled trials of complex partial seizures:
Body as a Whole: Back pain, chest pain, malaise.
Cardiovascular System: Tachycardia, hypertension, palpitation.
Digestive System: Increased appetite, flatulence, hematemesis, eructation, pancreatitis, periodontal abscess.
Hemic and Lymphatic System: Petechia.
Metabolic and Nutritional Disorders: SGOT increased, SGPT increased.
Musculoskeletal System: Myalgia, twitching, arthralgia, leg cramps, myasthenia.
Nervous System: Anxiety, confusion, abnormal gait, paresthesia, hypertonia, incoordination, abnormal dreams, personality disorder.
Respiratory System: Sinusitis, cough increased, pneumonia, epistaxis.
Skin and Appendages: Rash, pruritus, dry skin.
Special Senses: Taste perversion, abnormal vision, deafness, otitis media.
Urogenital System: Urinary incontinence, vaginitis, dysmenorrhea, amenorrhea, urinary frequency.

Other Patient Populations

Adverse events that have been reported with all dosage forms of valproate from epilepsy trials, spontaneous reports, and other sources are listed below by body system.
Gastrointestinal: The most commonly reported side effects at the initiation of therapy are nausea, vomiting, and indigestion. These effects are usually transient and rarely require discontinuation of therapy. Diarrhea, abdominal cramps, and constipation have been reported. Both anorexia with some weight loss and increased appetite with weight gain have also been reported. The administration of delayed-release divalproex sodium may result in reduction of gastrointestinal side effects in some patients using oral therapy.
CNS Effects: Sedative effects have occurred in patients receiving valproate alone but occur most often in patients receiving combination therapy. Sedation usually abates upon reduction of other antiepileptic medication. Tremor (may be dose-related), hallucinations, ataxia, headache, nystagmus, diplopia, asterixis, "spots before eyes", dysarthria, dizziness, confusion, hypesthesia, vertigo, incoordination, and parkinsonism. Rare cases of coma have occurred in patients receiving valproate alone or in conjunction with phenobarbital. In rare instances encephalopathy with fever has developed shortly after the introduction of valproate monotherapy without evidence of hepatic dysfunction or inappropriate plasma levels; all patients recovered after the drug was withdrawn.
Several reports have noted reversible cerebral atrophy and dementia in association with valproate therapy.
Dermatologic: Transient hair loss, skin rash, photosensitivity, generalized pruritus, erythema multiforme, and Stevens-Johnson syndrome. Rare cases of toxic epidermal necrolysis have been reported including a fatal case in a 6 month old infant taking valproate and several other concomitant medications. An additional case of toxic epidermal necrosis resulting in death was reported in a 35 year old patient with AIDS taking several concomitant medications and with a history of multiple cutaneous drug reactions.
Psychiatric: Emotional upset, depression, psychosis, aggression, hyperactivity, hostility, and behavioral deterioration.
Musculoskeletal: Weakness.
Hematologic: Thrombocytopenia and inhibition of the secondary phase of platelet aggregation may be reflected in altered bleeding time, petechiae, bruising, hematoma formation, epistaxis, and frank hemorrhage (see **PRECAUTIONS—General** and **Drug Interactions**). Relative lymphocytosis, macrocytosis, hypofibrinogenemia, leukopenia, eosinophilia, anemia including macrocytic with or without folate deficiency, bone marrow suppression, pancytopenia, aplastic anemia, and acute intermittent porphyria.
Hepatic: Minor elevations of transaminases (e.g., SGOT and SGPT) and LDH are frequent and appear to be dose-related. Occasionally, laboratory test results include increases in serum bilirubin and abnormal changes in other liver function tests. These results may reflect potentially serious hepatotoxicity (see **WARNINGS**).
Endocrine: Irregular menses, secondary amenorrhea, breast enlargement, galactorrhea, and parotid gland swelling. Abnormal thyroid function tests (see **PRECAUTIONS**).
There have been rare spontaneous reports of polycystic ovary disease. A cause and effect relationship has not been established.
Pancreatic: Acute pancreatitis including fatalities (see **WARNINGS**).

Continued on next page

Depacon—Cont.

Metabolic: Hyperammonemia (see **PRECAUTIONS**), hyponatremia, and inappropriate ADH secretion.
There have been rare reports of Fanconi's syndrome occurring chiefly in children.
Decreased carnitine concentrations have been reported although the clinical relevance is undetermined.
Hyperglycinemia has occurred and was associated with a fatal outcome in a patient with preexistent nonketotic hyperglycinemia.
Genitourinary: Enuresis and urinary tract infection.
Special Senses: Hearing loss, either reversible or irreversible, has been reported; however, a cause and effect relationship has not been established. Ear pain has also been reported.
Other: Anaphylaxis, edema of the extremities, lupus erythematosus, bone pain, cough increased, pneumonia, otitis media, bradycardia, cutaneous vasculitis, and fever.

Mania

Although DEPACON has not been evaluated for safety and efficacy in the treatment of manic episodes associated with bipolar disorder, the following adverse events not listed above were reported by 1% or more of patients from two placebo-controlled clinical trials of DEPAKOTE (DIVALPROEX SODIUM) tablets.
Body as a Whole: Chills, neck pain, neck rigidity.
Cardiovascular System: Hypotension, postural hypotension, vasodilation.
Digestive System: Fecal incontinence, gastroenteritis, glossitis.
Musculoskeletal System: Arthrosis.
Nervous System: Agitation, catatonic reaction, hypokinesia, reflexes increased, tardive dyskinesia, vertigo.
Skin and Appendages: Furunculosis, maculopapular rash, seborrhea.
Special Senses: Conjunctivitis, dry eyes, eye pain.
Urogenital: Dysuria.

Migraine

Although DEPACON has not been evaluated for safety and efficacy in the prophylactic treatment of migraine headaches, the following adverse events not listed above were reported by 1% or more of patients from two placebo-controlled clinical trials of DEPAKOTE (DIVALPROEX SODIUM) tablets.
Body as a Whole: Face edema.
Digestive System: Dry mouth, stomatitis.
Urogenital System: Cystitis, metrorrhagia, and vaginal hemorrhage.

OVERDOSAGE

Overdosage with valproate may result in somnolence, heart block, and deep coma. Fatalities have been reported; however patients have recovered from valproate serum concentrations as high as 2120 µg/mL.
In overdose situations, the fraction of drug not bound to protein is high and hemodialysis or tandem hemodialysis plus hemoperfusion may result in significant removal of drug. General supportive measures should be applied with particular attention to the maintenance of adequate urinary output.
Naloxone has been reported to reverse the CNS depressant effects of valproate overdosage. Because naloxone could theoretically also reverse the antiepilepsy effects of valproate, it should be used with caution in patients with epilepsy.

DOSAGE AND ADMINISTRATION

DEPACON IS FOR INTRAVENOUS USE ONLY.
Use of DEPACON for periods of more than 14 days has not been studied. Patients should be switched to oral valproate products as soon as it is clinically feasible.
DEPACON should be administered as a 60 minute infusion (but not more than 20 mg/min) with the same frequency as the oral products, although plasma concentration monitoring and dosage adjustments may be necessary.

Initial Exposure to Valproate:

The following dosage recommendations were obtained from studies utilizing oral divalproex sodium products.
Complex Partial Seizures: For adults and children 10 years of age or older.
Monotherapy (Initial Therapy): DEPACON has not been systematically studied as initial therapy. Patients should initiate therapy at 10 to 15 mg/kg/day. The dosage should be increased by 5 to 10 mg/kg/week to achieve optimal clinical response. Ordinarily, optimal clinical response is achieved at daily doses below 60 mg/kg/day. If satisfactory clinical response has not been achieved, plasma levels should be measured to determine whether or not they are in the usually accepted therapeutic range (50 to 100 µg/mL). No recommendation regarding the safety of valproate for use at doses above 60 mg/kg/day can be made.
The probability of thrombocytopenia increases significantly at total trough valproate plasma concentrations above 110 µg/mL in females and 135 µg/mL in males. The benefit of improved seizure control with higher doses should be weighed against the possibility of a greater incidence of adverse reactions.
Conversion to Monotherapy: Patients should initiate therapy at 10 to 15 mg/kg/day. The dosage should be increased by 5 to 10 mg/kg/week to achieve optimal clinical response. Ordinarily, optimal clinical response is achieved at daily doses below 60 mg/kg/day. If satisfactory clinical response has not been achieved, plasma levels should be measured to determine whether or not they are in the usually accepted therapeutic range (50–100 µg/mL). No recommendation regarding the safety of valproate for use at doses above 60 mg/kg/day can be made. Concomitant antiepilepsy drug (AED) dosage can ordinarily be reduced by approximately 25% every 2 weeks. This reduction may be started at initiation of DEPACON therapy, or delayed by 1 to 2 weeks if there is a concern that seizures are likely to occur with a reduction. The speed and duration of withdrawal of the concomitant AED can be highly variable, and patients should be monitored closely during this period for increased seizure frequency.
Adjunctive Therapy: DEPACON may be added to the patient's regimen at a dosage of 10 to 15 mg/kg/day. The dosage may be increased by 5 to 10 mg/kg/week to achieve optimal clinical response. Ordinarily, optimal clinical response is achieved at daily doses below 60 mg/kg/day. If satisfactory clinical response has not been achieved, plasma levels should be measured to determine whether or not they are in the usually accepted therapeutic range (50 to 100 µg/mL). No recommendation regarding the safety of valproate for use at doses above 60 mg/kg/day can be made. If the total daily dose exceeds 250 mg, it should be given in divided doses.
In a study of adjunctive therapy for complex partial seizures in which patients were receiving either carbamazepine or phenytoin in addition to DEPAKOTE (divalproex sodium), no adjustment of carbamazepine or phenytoin dosage was needed (see **CLINICAL STUDIES**). However, since valproate may interact with these or other concurrently administered AEDs as well as other drugs (see **Drug Interactions**), periodic plasma concentration determinations of concomitant AEDs are recommended during the early course of therapy (see **PRECAUTIONS—Drug Interactions**).
Simple and Complex Absence Seizures: The recommended initial dose is 15 mg/kg/day, increasing at one week intervals by 5 to 10 mg/kg/day until seizures are controlled or side effects preclude further increases. The maximum recommended dosage is 60 mg/kg/day. If the total daily dose exceeds 250 mg, it should be given in divided doses.
A good correlation has not been established between daily dose, serum concentrations, and therapeutic effect. However, therapeutic valproate serum concentrations for most patients with absence seizures is considered to range from 50 to 100 µg/mL. Some patients may be controlled with lower or higher serum concentrations (see **CLINICAL PHARMACOLOGY**).
As the DEPACON dosage is titrated upward, blood concentrations of phenobarbital and/or phenytoin may be affected (see **PRECAUTIONS**).
Antiepilepsy drugs should not be abruptly discontinued in patients in whom the drug is administered to prevent major seizures because of the strong possibility of precipitating status epilepticus with attendant hypoxia and threat to life.

Replacement Therapy:

When switching from oral valproate products, the total daily dose of DEPACON should be equivalent to the total daily dose of the oral valproate product (see **CLINICAL PHARMACOLOGY**), and should be administered as a 60 minute infusion (but not more than 20 mg/min) with the same frequency as the oral products, although plasma concentration monitoring and dosage adjustments may be necessary. Patients receiving doses near the maximum recommended daily dose of 60 mg/kg/day, particularly those not receiving enzyme-inducing drugs, should be monitored more closely. If the total daily dose exceeds 250 mg, it should be given in a divided regimen. However, the equivalence shown between DEPACON and oral valproate products (DEPAKOTE) at steady state was only evaluated in an every 6 hour regimen. Whether, when DEPACON is given less frequently (i.e., twice or three times a day), trough levels fall below those that result from an oral dosage form given via the same regimen, is unknown. For this reason, when DEPACON is given twice or three times a day, close monitoring of trough plasma levels may be needed.

General Dosing Advice

Dosing in Elderly Patients—Due to a decrease in unbound clearance of valproate and possibly a greater sensitivity to somnolence in the elderly, the starting dose should be reduced in these patients. Dosage should be increased more slowly and with regular monitoring for fluid and nutritional intake, dehydration, somnolence, and other adverse events. Dose reductions or discontinuation of valproate should be considered in patients with decreased food or fluid intake and in patients with excessive somnolence. The ultimate therapeutic dose should be achieved on the basis of both tolerability and clinical response (see **WARNINGS**).
Dose-Related Adverse Events—The frequency of adverse effects (particularly elevated liver enzymes and thrombocytopenia) may be dose-related. The probability of thrombocytopenia appears to increase significantly at total valproate concentrations of ≥ 110 µg/mL (females) or ≥ 135 µg/mL (males) (see **PRECAUTIONS**). The benefit of improved therapeutic effect with higher doses should be weighed against the possibility of a greater incidence of adverse reactions.

Administration

Rapid infusion of DEPACON has been associated with an increase in adverse events. Infusion times of less than 60 minutes or rates of infusion > 20 mg/min have not been studied in patients with epilepsy (see **ADVERSE REACTIONS**).
DEPACON should be administered intravenously as a 60 minute infusion, as noted above. It should be diluted with at least 50 mL of a compatible diluent. Any unused portion of the vial contents should be discarded.
Parenteral drug products should be inspected visually for particulate matter and discoloration prior to administration whenever solution and container permit.

Compatibility and Stability

DEPACON was found to be physically compatible and chemically stable in the following parenteral solutions for at least 24 hours when stored in glass or polyvinyl chloride (PVC) bags at controlled room temperature 15–30°C (59–86°F).

- dextrose (5%) injection, USP
- sodium chloride (0.9%) injection, USP
- lactated ringer's injection, USP

HOW SUPPLIED

DEPACON (valproate sodium injection), equivalent to 100 mg of valproic acid per mL, is a clear, colorless solution in 5 mL single-dose vials, available in trays of 10 vials (**NDC** 0074-1564-10).
Recommended storage: Store vials at controlled room temperature 15–30°C (59–86°F). No preservatives have been added. Unused portion of container should be discarded.
Revised: June, 2000
ABBOTT LABORATORIES
NORTH CHICAGO, IL 60064, U.S.A.

DEPAKENE® ℞

[dep 'a-kāne]
VALPROIC ACID
CAPSULES and SYRUP
℞ only

> **BOX WARNING:**
>
> **HEPATOTOXICITY:**
>
> HEPATIC FAILURE RESULTING IN FATALITIES HAS OCCURRED IN PATIENTS RECEIVING VALPROIC ACID. EXPERIENCE HAS INDICATED THAT CHILDREN UNDER THE AGE OF TWO YEARS ARE AT A CONSIDERABLY INCREASED RISK OF DEVELOPING FATAL HEPATOTOXICITY, ESPECIALLY THOSE ON MULTIPLE ANTICONVULSANTS, THOSE WITH CONGENITAL METABOLIC DISORDERS, THOSE WITH SEVERE SEIZURE DISORDERS ACCOMPANIED BY MENTAL RETARDATION, AND THOSE WITH ORGANIC BRAIN DISEASE. WHEN DEPAKENE PRODUCTS ARE USED IN THIS PATIENT GROUP, THEY SHOULD BE USED WITH EXTREME CAUTION AND AS A SOLE AGENT. THE BENEFITS OF THERAPY SHOULD BE WEIGHED AGAINST THE RISKS. ABOVE THIS AGE GROUP, EXPERIENCE IN EPILEPSY HAS INDICATED THAT THE INCIDENCE OF FATAL HEPATOTOXICITY DECREASES CONSIDERABLY IN PROGRESSIVELY OLDER PATIENT GROUPS.
> THESE INCIDENTS USUALLY HAVE OCCURRED DURING THE FIRST SIX MONTHS OF TREATMENT. SERIOUS OR FATAL HEPATOTOXICITY MAY BE PRECEDED BY NON-SPECIFIC SYMPTOMS SUCH AS MALAISE, WEAKNESS, LETHARGY, FACIAL EDEMA, ANOREXIA, AND VOMITING. IN PATIENTS WITH EPILEPSY, A LOSS OF SEIZURE CONTROL MAY ALSO OCCUR. PATIENTS SHOULD BE MONITORED CLOSELY FOR APPEARANCE OF THESE SYMPTOMS. LIVER FUNCTION TESTS SHOULD BE PERFORMED PRIOR TO THERAPY AND AT FREQUENT INTERVALS THEREAFTER, ESPECIALLY DURING THE FIRST SIX MONTHS.
>
> **TERATOGENICITY:**
>
> VALPROATE CAN PRODUCE TERATOGENIC EFFECTS SUCH AS NEURAL TUBE DEFECTS (E.G., SPINA BIFIDA). ACCORDINGLY, THE USE OF VALPROATE PRODUCTS IN WOMEN OF CHILDBEARING POTENTIAL REQUIRES THAT THE BENEFITS OF ITS USE BE WEIGHED AGAINST THE RISK OF INJURY TO THE FETUS.
>
> **PANCREATITIS:**
>
> CASES OF LIFE-THREATENING PANCREATITIS HAVE BEEN REPORTED IN BOTH CHILDREN AND ADULTS RECEIVING VALPROATE. SOME OF THE CASES HAVE BEEN DESCRIBED AS HEMORRHAGIC WITH A RAPID PROGRESSION FROM INITIAL SYMPTOMS TO DEATH. CASES HAVE BEEN REPORTED SHORTLY AFTER INITIAL USE AS WELL AS AFTER SEVERAL YEARS OF USE. PATIENTS AND GUARDIANS SHOULD BE WARNED THAT ABDOMINAL PAIN, NAUSEA, VOMITING, AND/OR ANOREXIA CAN BE SYMPTOMS OF PANCREATITIS THAT REQUIRE PROMPT MEDICAL EVALUATION. IF PANCREATITIS IS DIAGNOSED, VALPROATE SHOULD ORDINARILY BE DISCONTINUED. ALTERNATIVE TREATMENT FOR THE UNDERLYING MEDICAL CONDITION SHOULD BE INITIATED AS CLINICALLY INDICATED. (See **WARNINGS** and **PRECAUTIONS**.)

DESCRIPTION

DEPAKENE (valproic acid) is a carboxylic acid designated as 2-propylpentanoic acid. It is also known as dipropylacetic acid. Valproic acid has the following structure:
[See chemical structure at top of next column]

$$\begin{array}{l} CH_3-CH_2-CH_2 \\ \quad\quad\quad\quad\quad\quad\; CH-C(=O)OH \\ CH_3-CH_2-CH_2 \end{array}$$

Valproic acid (pKa 4.8) has a molecular weight of 144 and occurs as a colorless liquid with a characteristic odor. It is slightly soluble in water (1.3 mg/mL) and very soluble in organic solvents.

DEPAKENE capsules and syrup are antiepileptics for oral administration. Each soft elastic capsule contains 250 mg valproic acid. The syrup contains the equivalent of 250 mg valproic acid per 5 mL as the sodium salt.

Inactive Ingredients

250 mg capsules: corn oil, FD&C Yellow No. 6, gelatin, glycerin, iron oxide, methylparaben, propylparaben, and titanium dioxide.

Syrup: FD&C Red No. 40, glycerin, methylparaben, propylparaben, sorbitol, sucrose, water, and natural and artificial flavors.

CLINICAL PHARMACOLOGY

Pharmacodynamics

Valproic acid dissociates to the valproate ion in the gastrointestinal tract. The mechanisms by which valproate exerts its antiepileptic effects have not been established. It has been suggested that its activity in epilepsy is related to increased brain concentrations of gamma-aminobutyric acid (GABA).

Pharmacokinetics

Absorption/Bioavailability

Equivalent oral doses of DEPAKOTE (divalproex sodium) products and DEPAKENE (valproic acid) capsules deliver equivalent quantities of valproate ion systemically. Although the rate of valproate ion absorption may vary with the formulation administered (liquid, solid, or sprinkle), conditions of use (e.g., fasting or postprandial) and the method of administration (e.g., whether the contents of the capsule are sprinkled on food or the capsule is taken intact), these differences should be of minor clinical importance under the steady state conditions achieved in chronic use in the treatment of epilepsy.

However, it is possible that differences among the various valproate products in T_{max} and C_{max} could be important upon initiation of treatment. For example, in single dose studies, the effect of feeding had a greater influence on the rate of absorption of the DEPAKOTE tablet (increase in T_{max} from 4 to 8 hours) than on the absorption of the DEPAKOTE sprinkle capsules (increase in T_{max} from 3.3 to 4.8 hours).

While the absorption rate from the G.I. tract and fluctuation in valproate plasma concentrations vary with dosing regimen and formulation, the efficacy of valproate as an anticonvulsant in chronic use is unlikely to be affected. Experience employing dosing regimens from once-a-day to four-times-a-day, as well as studies in primate epilepsy models involving constant rate infusion, indicate that total daily systemic bioavailability (extent of absorption) is the primary determinant of seizure control and that differences in the ratios of plasma peak to trough concentrations between valproate formulations are inconsequential from a practical clinical standpoint.

Co-administration of oral valproate products with food and substitution among the various DEPAKOTE and DEPAKENE formulations should cause no clinical problems in the management of patients with epilepsy (see **DOSAGE AND ADMINISTRATION**). Nonetheless, any changes in dosage administration, or the addition or discontinuance of concomitant drugs should ordinarily be accompanied by close monitoring of clinical status and valproate plasma concentrations.

Distribution

Protein Binding:

The plasma protein binding of valproate is concentration dependent and the free fraction increases from approximately 10% at 40 µg/mL to 18.5% at 130 µg/mL. Protein binding of valproate is reduced in the elderly, in patients with chronic hepatic diseases, in patients with renal impairment, and in the presence of other drugs (e.g., aspirin). Conversely, valproate may displace certain protein-bound drugs (e.g., phenytoin, carbamazepine, warfarin, and tolbutamide). (See **PRECAUTIONS, Drug Interactions** for more detailed information on the pharmacokinetic interactions of valproate with other drugs.)

CNS Distribution:

Valproate concentrations in cerebrospinal fluid (CSF) approximate unbound concentrations in plasma (about 10% of total concentration).

Metabolism

Valproate is metabolized almost entirely by the liver. In adult patients on monotherapy, 30–50% of an administered dose appears in urine as a glucuronide conjugate. Mitochondrial β-oxidation is the other major metabolic pathway, typically accounting for over 40% of the dose. Usually, less than 15–20% of the dose is eliminated by other oxidative mechanisms. Less than 3% of an administered dose is excreted unchanged in urine.

The relationship between dose and total valproate concentration is nonlinear; concentration does not increase proportionally with the dose, but rather, increases to a lesser extent due to saturable plasma protein binding. The kinetics of unbound drug are linear.

Elimination

Mean plasma clearance and volume of distribution for total valproate are 0.56 L/hr/1.73 m^2 and 11 L/1.73 m^2, respectively. Mean plasma clearance and volume of distribution for free valproate are 4.6 L/hr/1.73 m^2 and 92 L/1.73 m^2. Mean terminal half-life for valproate monotherapy ranged from 9 to 16 hours following oral dosing regimens of 250 to 1000 mg.

The estimates cited apply primarily to patients who are not taking drugs that affect hepatic metabolizing enzyme systems. For example, patients taking enzyme-inducing antiepileptic drugs (carbamazepine, phenytoin, and phenobarbital) will clear valproate more rapidly. Because of these changes in valproate clearance, monitoring of antiepileptic concentrations should be intensified whenever concomitant antiepileptics are introduced or withdrawn.

Special Populations

Effect of Age:

Neonates—Children within the first two months of life have a markedly decreased ability to eliminate valproate compared to older children and adults. This is a result of reduced clearance (perhaps due to delay in development of glucuronosyltransferase and other enzyme systems involved in valproate elimination) as well as increased volume of distribution (in part due to decreased plasma protein binding). For example, in one study, the half-life in children under 10 days ranged from 10 to 67 hours compared to a range of 7 to 13 hours in children greater than 2 months.

Children—Pediatric patients (i.e., between 3 months and 10 years) have 50% higher clearances expressed on weight (i.e., mL/min/kg) than do adults. Over the age of 10 years, children have pharmacokinetic parameters that approximate those of adults.

Elderly—The capacity of elderly patients (age range: 68 to 89 years) to eliminate valproate has been shown to be reduced compared to younger adults (age range: 22 to 26). Intrinsic clearance is reduced by 39%; the free fraction is increased by 44%. Accordingly, the initial dosage should be reduced in the elderly. (See **DOSAGE AND ADMINISTRATION**).

Effect of Gender:

There are no differences in the body surface area adjusted unbound clearance between males and females (4.8±0.17 and 4.7±0.07 L/hr per 1.73 m^2, respectively).

Effect of Race:

The effects of race on the kinetics of valproate have not been studied.

Effect of Disease:

Liver Disease—(See **BOXED WARNING, CONTRAINDICATIONS,** and **WARNINGS**). Liver disease impairs the capacity to eliminate valproate. In one study, the clearance of free valproate was decreased by 50% in 7 patients with cirrhosis and by 16% in 4 patients with acute hepatitis, compared with 6 healthy subjects. In that study, the half-life of valproate was increased from 12 to 18 hours. Liver disease is also associated with decreased albumin concentrations and larger unbound fractions (2 to 2.6 fold increase) of valproate. Accordingly, monitoring of total concentrations may be misleading since free concentrations may be substantially elevated in patients with hepatic disease whereas total concentrations may appear to be normal.

Renal Disease—A slight reduction (27%) in the unbound clearance of valproate has been reported in patients with renal failure (creatinine clearance < 10 mL/minute); however, hemodialysis typically reduces valproate concentrations by about 20%. Therefore, no dosage adjustment appears to be necessary in patients with renal failure. Protein binding in these patients is substantially reduced; thus, monitoring total concentrations may be misleading.

Plasma Levels and Clinical Effect

The relationship between plasma concentration and clinical response is not well documented. One contributing factor is the nonlinear, concentration dependent protein binding of valproate which affects the clearance of the drug. Thus, monitoring of total serum valproate cannot provide a reliable index of the bioactive valproate species.

For example, because the plasma protein binding of valproate is concentration dependent, the free fraction increases from approximately 10% at 40 µg/mL to 18.5% at 130 µg/mL. Higher than expected free fractions occur in the elderly, in hyperlipidemic patients, and in patients with hepatic and renal diseases.

Epilepsy:

The therapeutic range is commonly considered to be 50 to 100 µg/mL of total valproate, although some patients may be controlled with lower or higher plasma concentrations.

Clinical Trials

The studies described in the following section were conducted using DEPAKOTE (divalproex sodium) tablets.

Epilepsy

The efficacy of DEPAKOTE in reducing the incidence of complex partial seizures (CPS) that occur in isolation or in association with other seizure types was established in two controlled trials.

In one, multiclinic, placebo controlled study employing an add-on design (adjunctive therapy), 144 patients who continued to suffer eight or more CPS per 8 weeks during an 8 week period of monotherapy with doses of either carbamazepine or phenytoin sufficient to assure plasma concentrations within the "therapeutic range" were randomized to receive, in addition to their original antiepilepsy drug (AED), either DEPAKOTE or placebo. Randomized patients were to be followed for a total of 16 weeks. The following table presents the findings.

Adjunctive Therapy Study
Median Incidence of CPS per 8 Weeks

Add-on Treatment	Number of Patients	Baseline Incidence	Experimental Incidence
DEPAKOTE	75	16.0	8.9*
Placebo	69	14.5	11.5

* Reduction from baseline statistically significantly greater for DEPAKOTE than placebo at $p \leq 0.05$ level.

Figure 1 presents the proportion of patients (X axis) whose percentage reduction from baseline in complex partial seizure rates was at least as great as that indicated on the Y axis in the adjunctive therapy study. A positive percent reduction indicates an improvement (i.e., a decrease in seizure frequency), while a negative percent reduction indicates worsening. Thus, in a display of this type, the curve for an effective treatment is shifted to the left of the curve for placebo. This figure shows that the proportion of patients achieving any particular level of improvement was consistently higher for DEPAKOTE than for placebo. For example, 45% of patients treated with DEPAKOTE had a ≥50% reduction in complex partial seizure rate compared to 23% of patients treated with placebo.

Figure 1

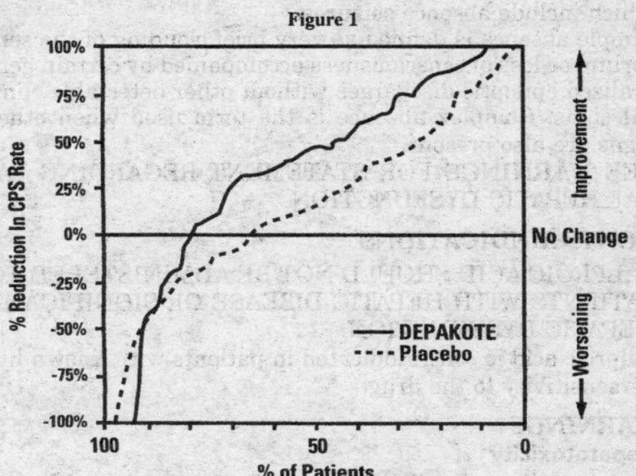

The second study assessed the capacity of DEPAKOTE to reduce the incidence of CPS when administered as the sole AED. The study compared the incidence of CPS among patients randomized to either a high or low dose treatment arm. Patients qualified for entry into the randomized comparison phase of this study only if 1) they continued to experience 2 or more CPS per 4 weeks during an 8 to 12 week long period of monotherapy with adequate doses of an AED (i.e., phenytoin, carbamazepine, phenobarbital, or primidone) and 2) they made a successful transition over a two week interval to DEPAKOTE. Patients entering the randomized phase were then brought to their assigned target dose, gradually tapered off their concomitant AED and followed for an interval as long as 22 weeks. Less than 50% of the patients randomized, however, completed the study. In patients converted to DEPAKOTE monotherapy, the mean total valproate concentrations during monotherapy were 71 and 123 µg/mL in the low dose and high dose groups, respectively.

The following table presents the findings for all patients randomized who had at least one post-randomization assessment.

Monotherapy Study
Median Incidence of CPS per 8 Weeks

Treatment	Number of Patients	Baseline Incidence	Randomized Phase Incidence
High dose DEPAKOTE	131	13.2	10.7*
Low dose DEPAKOTE	134	14.2	13.8

*Reduction from baseline statistically significantly greater for high dose than low dose at $p \leq 0.05$ level.

Figure 2 presents the proportion of patients (X axis) whose percentage reduction from baseline in complex partial seizure rates was at least as great as that indicated on the Y axis in the monotherapy study. A positive percent reduction indicates an improvement (i.e., a decrease in seizure frequency), while a negative percent reduction indicates worsening. Thus, in a display of this type, the curve for a more effective treatment is shifted to the left of the curve for a less effective treatment. This figure shows that the proportion of patients achieving any particular level of reduction was consistently higher for high dose DEPAKOTE than for low dose DEPAKOTE. For example, when switching from carbamazepine, phenytoin, phenobarbital or primidone monotherapy to high dose DEPAKOTE monotherapy, 63% of patients experienced no change or a reduction in complex partial seizure rates compared to 54% of patients receiving low dose DEPAKOTE.

[See figure 2 at top of next page]

Continued on next page

Depakene—Cont.

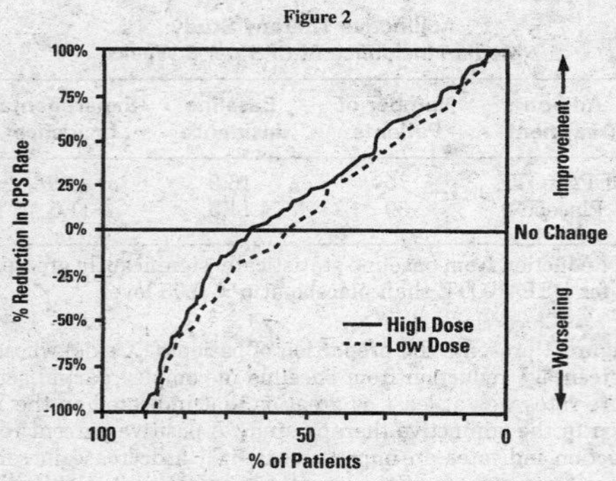

INDICATIONS AND USAGE

DEPAKENE (valproic acid) is indicated as monotherapy and adjunctive therapy in the treatment of patients with complex partial seizures that occur either in isolation or in association with other types of seizures. DEPAKENE (valproic acid) is indicated for use as sole and adjunctive therapy in the treatment of simple and complex absence seizures, and adjunctively in patients with multiple seizure types which include absence seizures.

Simple absence is defined as very brief clouding of the sensorium or loss of consciousness accompanied by certain generalized epileptic discharges without other detectable clinical signs. Complex absence is the term used when other signs are also present.

SEE **WARNINGS** FOR STATEMENT REGARDING FATAL HEPATIC DYSFUNCTION.

CONTRAINDICATIONS

VALPROIC ACID SHOULD NOT BE ADMINISTERED TO PATIENTS WITH HEPATIC DISEASE OR SIGNIFICANT HEPATIC DYSFUNCTION.

Valproic acid is contraindicated in patients with known hypersensitivity to the drug.

WARNINGS

Hepatotoxicity

Hepatic failure resulting in fatalities has occurred in patients receiving valproic acid. These incidents usually have occurred during the first six months of treatment. Serious or fatal hepatotoxicity may be preceded by non-specific symptoms such as malaise, weakness, lethargy, facial edema, anorexia, and vomiting. In patients with epilepsy, a loss of seizure control may also occur. Patients should be monitored closely for appearance of these symptoms. Liver function tests should be performed prior to therapy and at frequent intervals thereafter, especially during the first six months. However, physicians should not rely totally on serum biochemistry since these tests may not be abnormal in all instances, but should also consider the results of careful interim medical history and physical examination. Caution should be observed when administering DEPAKENE (valproic acid) to patients with a prior history of hepatic disease. Patients on multiple anticonvulsants, children, those with congenital metabolic disorders, those with severe seizure disorders accompanied by mental retardation, and those with organic brain disease may be at particular risk. Experience has indicated that children under the age of two years are at a considerably increased risk of developing fatal hepatotoxicity, especially those with the aforementioned conditions. When DEPAKENE products are used in this patient group, they should be used with extreme caution and as a sole agent. The benefits of therapy should be weighed against the risks. Above this age group, experience has indicated that the incidence of fatal hepatotoxicity decreases considerably in progressively older patient groups.

The drug should be discontinued immediately in the presence of significant hepatic dysfunction, suspected or apparent. In some cases, hepatic dysfunction has progressed in spite of discontinuation of drug.

Pancreatitis

Cases of life-threatening pancreatitis have been reported in both children and adults receiving valproate. Some of the cases have been described as hemorrhagic with rapid progression from initial symptoms to death. Some cases have occurred shortly after initial use as well as after several years of use. The rate based upon the reported cases exceeds that expected in the general population and there have been cases in which pancreatitis recurred after rechallenge with valproate. In clinical trials, there were 2 cases of pancreatitis without alternative etiology in 2416 patients, representing 1044 patient-years experience. Patients and guardians should be warned that abdominal pain, nausea, vomiting, and/or anorexia can be symptoms of pancreatitis that require prompt medical evaluation. If pancreatitis is diagnosed, valproate should ordinarily be discontinued. Alternative treatment for the underlying medical condition should be initiated as clinically indicated (see **BOXED WARNING**).

Somnolence in the Elderly

In a double-blind, multicenter trial of valproate in elderly patients with dementia (mean age = 83 years), doses were increased by 125 mg/day to a target dose of 20 mg/kg/day. A significantly higher proportion of valproate patients had somnolence compared to placebo, and although not statistically significant, there was a higher proportion of patients with dehydration. Discontinuations for somnolence were also significantly higher than with placebo. In some patients with somnolence (approximately one-half), there was associated reduced nutritional intake and weight loss. There was a trend for the patients who experienced these events to have a lower baseline albumin concentration, lower valproate clearance, and a higher BUN. In elderly patients, dosage should be increased more slowly and with regular monitoring for fluid and nutritional intake, dehydration, somnolence, and other adverse events. Dose reductions or discontinuation of valproate should be considered in patients with decreased food or fluid intake and in patients with excessive somnolence (see **DOSAGE AND ADMINISTRATION**).

Thrombocytopenia

The frequency of adverse effects (particularly elevated liver enzymes and thrombocytopenia [see **PRECAUTIONS**]) may be dose-related. In a clinical trial of DEPAKOTE (divalproex sodium) as monotherapy in patients with epilepsy, 34/126 patients (27%) receiving approximately 50 mg/kg/day on average, had at least one value of platelets $\leq 75 \times 10^9$/L. Approximately half of these patients had treatment discontinued, with return of platelet counts to normal. In the remaining patients, platelet counts normalized with continued treatment. In this study, the probability of thrombocytopenia appeared to increase significantly at total valproate concentrations of $\geq$110 µg/mL (females) or $\geq$135 µg/mL (males). The therapeutic benefit which may accompany the higher doses should therefore be weighed against the possibility of a greater incidence of adverse effects.

Usage In Pregnancy

ACCORDING TO PUBLISHED AND UNPUBLISHED REPORTS, VALPROIC ACID MAY PRODUCE TERATOGENIC EFFECTS IN THE OFFSPRING OF HUMAN FEMALES RECEIVING THE DRUG DURING PREGNANCY. THERE ARE MULTIPLE REPORTS IN THE CLINICAL LITERATURE WHICH INDICATE THAT THE USE OF ANTIEPILEPTIC DRUGS DURING PREGNANCY RESULTS IN AN INCREASED INCIDENCE OF BIRTH DEFECTS IN THE OFFSPRING. ALTHOUGH DATA ARE MORE EXTENSIVE WITH RESPECT TO TRIMETHADIONE, PARAMETHADIONE, PHENYTOIN, AND PHENOBARBITAL, REPORTS INDICATE A POSSIBLE SIMILAR ASSOCIATION WITH THE USE OF OTHER ANTIEPILEPTIC DRUGS. THEREFORE, ANTIEPILEPSY DRUGS SHOULD BE ADMINISTERED TO WOMEN OF CHILDBEARING POTENTIAL ONLY IF THEY ARE CLEARLY SHOWN TO BE ESSENTIAL IN THE MANAGEMENT OF THEIR SEIZURES.

THE INCIDENCE OF NEURAL TUBE DEFECTS IN THE FETUS MAY BE INCREASED IN MOTHERS RECEIVING VALPROATE DURING THE FIRST TRIMESTER OF PREGNANCY. THE CENTERS FOR DISEASE CONTROL (CDC) HAS ESTIMATED THE RISK OF VALPROIC ACID EXPOSED WOMEN HAVING CHILDREN WITH SPINA BIFIDA TO BE APPROXIMATELY 1 TO 2%.

OTHER CONGENITAL ANOMALIES (E.G., CRANIOFACIAL DEFECTS, CARDIOVASCULAR MALFORMATIONS AND ANOMALIES INVOLVING VARIOUS BODY SYSTEMS), COMPATIBLE AND INCOMPATIBLE WITH LIFE, HAVE BEEN REPORTED. SUFFICIENT DATA TO DETERMINE THE INCIDENCE OF THESE CONGENITAL ANOMALIES IS NOT AVAILABLE.

THE HIGHER INCIDENCE OF CONGENITAL ANOMALIES IN ANTIEPILEPTIC DRUG-TREATED WOMEN WITH SEIZURE DISORDERS CANNOT BE REGARDED AS A CAUSE AND EFFECT RELATIONSHIP. THERE ARE INTRINSIC METHODOLOGIC PROBLEMS IN OBTAINING ADEQUATE DATA ON DRUG TERATOGENICITY IN HUMANS; GENETIC FACTORS OR THE EPILEPTIC CONDITION ITSELF, MAY BE MORE IMPORTANT THAN DRUG THERAPY IN CONTRIBUTING TO CONGENITAL ANOMALIES.

PATIENTS TAKING VALPROATE MAY DEVELOP CLOTTING ABNORMALITIES. A PATIENT WHO HAD LOW FIBRINOGEN WHEN TAKING MULTIPLE ANTICONVULSANTS INCLUDING VALPROATE GAVE BIRTH TO AN INFANT WITH AFIBRINOGENEMIA WHO SUBSEQUENTLY DIED OF HEMORRHAGE. IF VALPROATE IS USED IN PREGNANCY, THE CLOTTING PARAMETERS SHOULD BE MONITORED CAREFULLY.

HEPATIC FAILURE, RESULTING IN THE DEATH OF A NEWBORN AND OF AN INFANT, HAVE BEEN REPORTED FOLLOWING THE USE OF VALPROATE DURING PREGNANCY.

Animal studies have demonstrated valproate-induced teratogenicity. Increased frequencies of malformations, as well as intrauterine growth retardation and death, have been observed in mice, rats, rabbits, and monkeys following prenatal exposure to valproate. Malformations of the skeletal system are the most common structural abnormalities produced in experimental animals, but neural tube closure defects have been seen in mice exposed to maternal plasma valproate concentrations exceeding 230 µg/mL (2.3 times the upper limit of the human therapeutic range) during susceptible periods of embryonic development. Administration of an oral dose of 200 mg/kg/day or greater (50% of the maximum human daily dose or greater on a mg/m^2 basis) to pregnant rats during organogenesis produced malformations (skeletal, cardiac, and urogenital) and growth retardation in the offspring. These doses resulted in peak maternal plasma valproate levels of approximately 340 µg/mL or greater (3.4 times the upper limit of the human therapeutic range or greater). Behavioral deficits have been reported in the offspring of rats given a dose of 200 mg/kg/day throughout most of pregnancy. An oral dose of 350 mg/kg/day (approximately 2 times the maximum human daily dose on a mg/m^2 basis) produced skeletal and visceral malformations in rabbits exposed during organogenesis. Skeletal malformations, growth retardation, and death were observed in rhesus monkeys following administration of an oral dose of 200 mg/kg/day (equal to the maximum human daily dose on a mg/m^2 basis) during organogenesis. This dose resulted in peak maternal plasma valproate levels of approximately 280 µg/mL (2.8 times the upper limit of the human therapeutic range).

The prescribing physician will wish to weigh the benefits of therapy against the risks in treating or counseling women of childbearing potential. If this drug is used during pregnancy, or if the patient becomes pregnant while taking this drug, the patient should be apprised of the potential hazard to the fetus.

Antiepileptic drugs should not be discontinued abruptly in patients in whom the drug is administered to prevent major seizures because of the strong possibility of precipitating status epilepticus with attendant hypoxia and threat to life. In individual cases where the severity and frequency of the seizure disorder are such that the removal of medication does not pose a serious threat to the patient, discontinuation of the drug may be considered prior to and during pregnancy, although it cannot be said with any confidence that even minor seizures do not pose some hazard to the developing embryo or fetus.

Tests to detect neural tube and other defects using current accepted procedures should be considered a part of routine prenatal care in childbearing women receiving valproate.

PRECAUTIONS

Hepatic Dysfunction

See **BOXED WARNING**, **CONTRAINDICATIONS**, and **WARNINGS**.

Pancreatitis

See **BOXED WARNING** and **WARNINGS**.

General

Because of reports of thrombocytopenia (see **WARNINGS**), inhibition of the secondary phase of platelet aggregation, and abnormal coagulation parameters, (e.g., low fibrinogen), platelet counts and coagulation tests are recommended before initiating therapy and at periodic intervals. It is recommended that patients receiving DEPAKENE (valproic acid) be monitored for platelet count and coagulation parameters prior to planned surgery. In a clinical trial of DEPAKOTE (divalproex sodium) as monotherapy in patients with epilepsy, 34/126 patients (27%) receiving approximately 50 mg/kg/day on average, had at least one value of platelets $\leq 75 \times 10^9$/L. Approximately half of these patients had treatment discontinued, with return of platelet counts to normal. In the remaining patients, platelet counts normalized with continued treatment. In this study, the probability of thrombocytopenia appeared to increase significantly at total valproate concentrations of $\geq$ 110 µg/mL (females) or $\geq$ 135 µg/mL (males). Evidence of hemorrhage, bruising, or a disorder of hemostasis/coagulation is an indication for reduction of the dosage or withdrawal of therapy.

Hyperammonemia with or without lethargy or coma has been reported and may be present in the absence of abnormal liver function tests. Asymptomatic elevations of ammonia are more common and when present require more frequent monitoring. If clinically significant symptoms occur, DEPAKENE therapy should be modified or discontinued.

Since valproate may interact with concurrently administered drugs which are capable of enzyme induction, periodic plasma concentration determinations of valproate and concomitant drugs are recommended during the early course of therapy (see **PRECAUTIONS—Drug Interactions**).

Valproate is partially eliminated in the urine as a keto-metabolite which may lead to a false interpretation of the urine ketone test.

There have been reports of altered thyroid function tests associated with valproate. The clinical significance of these is unknown.

There are *in vitro* studies that suggest valproate stimulates the replication of the HIV and CMV viruses under certain experimental conditions. The clinical consequence, if any, is not known. Additionally, the relevance of these *in vitro* findings is uncertain for patients receiving maximally suppressive antiretroviral therapy. Nevertheless, these data should be borne in mind when interpreting the results from regular monitoring of the viral load in HIV infected patients receiving valproate or when following CMV infected patients clinically.

Information for Patients

Patients and guardians should be warned that abdominal pain, nausea, vomiting, and/or anorexia can be symptoms of pancreatitis and, therefore, require further medical evaluation promptly.

Since DEPAKENE products may produce CNS depression, especially when combined with another CNS depressant (e.g., alcohol), patients should be advised not to engage in hazardous activities, such as driving an automobile or operating dangerous machinery, until it is known that they do not become drowsy from the drug.

Drug Interactions

Effects of Co-Administered Drugs on Valproate Clearance

Drugs that affect the level of expression of hepatic enzymes, particularly those that elevate levels of glucuronosyltransferases, may increase the clearance of valproate. For example, phenytoin, carbamazepine, and phenobarbital (or primidone) can double the clearance of valproate. Thus, patients on monotherapy will generally have longer half-lives and higher concentrations than patients receiving polytherapy with antiepilepsy drugs.

In contrast, drugs that are inhibitors of cytochrome P450 isozymes, e.g., antidepressants, may be expected to have little effect on valproate clearance because cytochrome P450 microsomal mediated oxidation is a relatively minor secondary metabolic pathway compared to glucuronidation and beta-oxidation.

Because of these changes in valproate clearance, monitoring of valproate and concomitant drug concentrations should be increased whenever enzyme inducing drugs are introduced or withdrawn.

The following list provides information about the potential for an influence of several commonly prescribed medications on valproate pharmacokinetics. The list is not exhaustive nor could it be, since new interactions are continuously being reported.

Drugs for which a potentially important interaction has been observed:

Aspirin—A study involving the co-administration of aspirin at antipyretic doses (11 to 16 mg/kg) with valproate to pediatric patients (n=6) revealed a decrease in protein binding and an inhibition of metabolism of valproate. Valproate free fraction was increased 4-fold in the presence of aspirin compared to valproate alone. The β-oxidation pathway consisting of 2-E-valproic acid, 3-OH-valproic acid, and 3-keto valproic acid was decreased from 25% of total metabolites excreted on valproate alone to 8.3% in the presence of aspirin. Caution should be observed if valproate and aspirin are to be co-administered.

Felbamate—A study involving the co-administration of 1200 mg/day of felbamate with valproate to patients with epilepsy (n=10) revealed an increase in mean valproate peak concentration by 35% (from 86 to 115 μg/mL) compared to valproate alone. Increasing the felbamate dose to 2400 mg/day increased the mean valproate peak concentration to 133 μg/mL (another 16% increase). A decrease in valproate dosage may be necessary when felbamate therapy is initiated.

Rifampin—A study involving the administration of a single dose of valproate (7 mg/kg) 36 hours after 5 nights of daily dosing with rifampin (600 mg) revealed a 40% increase in the oral clearance of valproate. Valproate dosage adjustment may be necessary when it is co-administered with rifampin.

Drugs for which either no interaction or a likely clinically unimportant interaction has been observed:

Antacids—A study involving the co-administration of valproate 500 mg with commonly administered antacids (Maalox, Trisogel, and Titralac—160 mEq doses) did not reveal any effect on the extent of absorption of valproate.

Chlorpromazine—A study involving the administration of 100 to 300 mg/day of chlorpromazine to schizophrenic patients already receiving valproate (200 mg BID) revealed a 15% increase in trough plasma levels of valproate.

Haloperidol—A study involving the administration of 6 to 10 mg/day of haloperidol to schizophrenic patients already receiving valproate (200 mg BID) revealed no significant changes in valproate trough plasma levels.

Cimetidine and Ranitidine—Cimetidine and ranitidine do not affect the clearance of valproate.

Effects of Valproate on Other Drugs

Valproate has been found to be a weak inhibitor of some P450 isozymes, epoxide hydrase, and glucuronyltransferases.

The following list provides information about the potential for an influence of valproate co-administration on the pharmacokinetics or pharmacodynamics of several commonly prescribed medications. The list is not exhaustive, since new interactions are continuously being reported.

Drugs for which a potentially important valproate interaction has been observed:

Amitriptyline/Nortriptyline—Administration of a single oral 50 mg dose of amitriptyline to 15 normal volunteers (10 males and 5 females) who received valproate (500 mg BID) resulted in a 21% decrease in plasma clearance of amitriptyline and a 34% decrease in the net clearance of nortriptyline. Rare postmarketing reports of concurrent use of valproate and amitriptyline resulting in an increased amitriptyline level have been received. Concurrent use of valproate and amitriptyline has rarely been associated with toxicity. Monitoring of amitriptyline levels should be considered for patients taking valproate concomitantly with amitriptyline. Consideration should be given to lowering the dose of amitriptyline/nortriptyline in the presence of valproate.

Carbamazepine/carbamazepine-10,11-Epoxide—Serum levels of carbamazepine (CBZ) decreased 17% while that of carbamazepine-10,11-epoxide (CBZ-E) increased by 45% upon co-administration of valproate and CBZ to epileptic patients.

Clonazepam—The concomitant use of valproic acid and clonazepam may induce absence status in patients with a history of absence type seizures.

Diazepam—Valproate displaces diazepam from its plasma albumin binding sites and inhibits its metabolism. Co-administration of valproate (1500 mg daily) increased the free fraction of diazepam (10 mg) by 90% in healthy volunteers (n=6). Plasma clearance and volume of distribution for free diazepam were reduced by 25% and 20%, respectively, in the presence of valproate. The elimination half-life of diazepam remained unchanged upon addition of valproate.

Ethosuximide—Valproate inhibits the metabolism of ethosuximide. Administration of a single ethosuximide dose of 500 mg with valproate (800 to 1600 mg/day) to healthy volunteers (n=6) was accompanied by a 25% increase in elimination half-life of ethosuximide and a 15% decrease in its total clearance as compared to ethosuximide alone. Patients receiving valproate and ethosuximide, especially along with other anticonvulsants, should be monitored for alterations in serum concentrations of both drugs.

Lamotrigine—In a steady-state study involving 10 healthy volunteers, the elimination half-life of lamotrigine increased from 26 to 70 hours with valproate co-administration (a 165% increase). The dose of lamotrigine should be reduced when co-administered with valproate.

Phenobarbital—Valproate was found to inhibit the metabolism of phenobarbital. Co-administration of valproate (250 mg BID for 14 days) with phenobarbital to normal subjects (n=6) resulted in a 50% increase in half-life and a 30% decrease in plasma clearance of phenobarbital (60 mg single-dose). The fraction of phenobarbital dose excreted unchanged increased by 50% in presence of valproate.

There is evidence for severe CNS depression, with or without significant elevations of barbiturate or valproate serum concentrations. All patients receiving concomitant barbiturate therapy should be closely monitored for neurological toxicity. Serum barbiturate concentrations should be obtained, if possible, and the barbiturate dosage decreased, if appropriate.

Primidone, which is metabolized to a barbiturate, may be involved in a similar interaction with valproate.

Phenytoin—Valproate displaces phenytoin from its plasma albumin binding sites and inhibits its hepatic metabolism. Co-administration of valproate (400 mg TID) with phenytoin (250 mg) in normal volunteers (n=7) was associated with a 60% increase in the free fraction of phenytoin. Total plasma clearance and apparent volume of distribution of phenytoin increased 30% in the presence of valproate. Both the clearance and apparent volume of distribution of free phenytoin were reduced by 25%.

In patients with epilepsy, there have been reports of breakthrough seizures occurring with the combination of valproate and phenytoin. The dosage of phenytoin should be adjusted as required by the clinical situation.

Tolbutamide—From *in vitro* experiments, the unbound fraction of tolbutamide was increased from 20% to 50% when added to plasma samples taken from patients treated with valproate. The clinical relevance of this displacement is unknown.

Warfarin—In an *in vitro* study, valproate increased the unbound fraction of warfarin by up to 32.6%. The therapeutic relevance of this is unknown; however, coagulation tests should be monitored if DEPAKENE therapy is instituted in patients taking anticoagulants.

Zidovudine—In six patients who were seropositive for HIV, the clearance of zidovudine (100 mg q8h) was decreased by 38% after administration of valproate (250 or 500 mg q8h); the half-life of zidovudine was unaffected.

Drugs for which either no interaction or a likely clinically unimportant interaction has been observed:

Acetaminophen—Valproate had no effect on any of the pharmacokinetic parameters of acetaminophen when it was concurrently administered to three epileptic patients.

Clozapine—In psychotic patients (n=11), no interaction was observed when valproate was co-administered with clozapine.

Lithium—Co-administration of valproate (500 mg BID) and lithium carbonate (300 mg TID) to normal male volunteers (n=16) had no effect on the steady-state kinetics of lithium.

Lorazepam—Concomitant administration of valproate (500 mg BID) and lorazepam (1 mg BID) in normal male volunteers (n=9) was accompanied by a 17% decrease in the plasma clearance of lorazepam.

Oral Contraceptive Steroids—Administration of a single-dose of ethinyloestradiol (50 μg)/levonorgestrel (250 μg) to 6 women on valproate (200 mg BID) therapy for 2 months did not reveal any pharmacokinetic interaction.

Carcinogenesis, Mutagenesis, Impairment of Fertility

Carcinogenesis

Valproic acid was administered orally to Sprague Dawley rats and ICR (HA/ICR) mice at doses of 80 and 170 mg/kg/day (approximately 10 to 50% of the maximum human daily dose on a mg/m^2 basis) for two years. A variety of neoplasms were observed in both species. The chief findings were a statistically significant increase in the incidence of subcutaneous fibrosarcomas in high dose male rats receiving valproic acid and a statistically significant dose-related trend for benign pulmonary adenomas in male mice receiving valproic acid. The significance of these findings for humans is unknown.

Mutagenesis

Valproate was not mutagenic in an *in vitro* bacterial assay (Ames test), did not produce dominant lethal effects in mice, and did not increase chromosome aberration frequency in an *in vivo* cytogenetic study in rats. Increased frequencies of sister chromatid exchange (SCE) have been reported in a study of epileptic children taking valproate, but this association was not observed in another study conducted in adults. There is some evidence that increased SCE frequencies may be associated with epilepsy. The biological significance of an increase in SCE frequency is not known.

Fertility

Chronic toxicity studies in juvenile and adult rats and dogs demonstrated reduced spermatogenesis and testicular atrophy at oral doses of 400 mg/kg/day or greater in rats (approximately equivalent to or greater than the maximum human daily dose on a mg/m^2 basis) and 150 mg/kg/day or greater in dogs (approximately 1.4 times the maximum human daily dose or greater on a mg/m^2 basis). Segment I fertility studies in rats have shown oral doses up to 350 mg/kg/day (approximately equal to the maximum human daily dose on a mg/m^2 basis) for 60 days to have no effect on fertility. THE EFFECT OF VALPROATE ON TESTICULAR DEVELOPMENT AND ON SPERM PRODUCTION AND FERTILITY IN HUMANS IS UNKNOWN.

Pregnancy

Pregnancy Category D: See **WARNINGS**.

Nursing Mothers

Valproate is excreted in breast milk. Concentrations in breast milk have been reported to be 1–10% of serum concentrations. It is not known what effect this would have on a nursing infant. Consideration should be given to discontinuing nursing when valproic acid is administered to a nursing woman.

Pediatric Use

Experience has indicated that pediatric patients under the age of two years are at a considerably increased risk of developing fatal hepatotoxicity, especially those with the aforementioned conditions (see **BOXED WARNING**). When DEPAKENE is used in this patient group, it should be used with extreme caution and as a sole agent. The benefits of therapy should be weighed against the risks. Above the age of 2 years, experience in epilepsy has indicated that the incidence of fatal hepatotoxicity decreases considerably in progressively older patient groups.

Younger children, especially those receiving enzyme-inducing drugs, will require larger maintenance doses to attain targeted total and unbound valproic acid concentrations.

The variability in free fraction limits the clinical usefulness of monitoring total serum valproic acid concentrations. Interpretation of valproic acid concentrations in children should include consideration of factors that affect hepatic metabolism and protein binding.

The basic toxicology and pathologic manifestations of valproate sodium in neonatal (4-day old) and juvenile (14-day old) rats are similar to those seen in young adult rats. However, additional findings, including renal alterations in juvenile rats and renal alterations and retinal dysplasia in neonatal rats, have been reported. These findings occurred at 240 mg/kg/day, a dosage approximately equivalent to the human maximum recommended daily dose on a mg/m^2 basis. They were not seen at 90 mg/kg, or 40% of the maximum human daily dose on a mg/m^2 basis.

Geriatric Use

No patients above the age of 65 years were enrolled in double-blind prospective clinical trials of mania associated with bipolar illness. In a case review study of 583 patients, 72 patients (12%) were greater than 65 years of age. A higher percentage of patients above 65 years of age reported accidental injury, infection, pain, somnolence, and tremor. Discontinuation of valproate was occasionally associated with the latter two events. It is not clear whether these events indicate additional risk or whether they result from preexisting medical illness and concomitant medication use among these patients.

A study of elderly patients with dementia revealed drug related somnolence and discontinuation for somnolence (see **WARNINGS—Somnolence in the Elderly**). The starting dose should be reduced in these patients, and dosage reductions or discontinuation should be considered in patients with excessive somnolence (see **DOSAGE AND ADMINISTRATION**).

ADVERSE REACTIONS

Epilepsy

The data described in the following section were obtained using DEPAKOTE (divalproex sodium) tablets.

Based on a placebo-controlled trial of adjunctive therapy for treatment of complex partial seizures, DEPAKOTE was generally well tolerated with most adverse events rated as mild to moderate in severity. Intolerance was the primary reason for discontinuation in the DEPAKOTE-treated patients (6%), compared to 1% of placebo-treated patients.

Table 1 lists treatment-emergent adverse events which were reported by ≥ 5% of DEPAKOTE-treated patients and for which the incidence was greater than in the placebo group, in a placebo-controlled trial of adjunctive therapy for the treatment of complex partial seizures. Since patients were also treated with other antiepilepsy drugs, it is not possible, in most cases, to determine whether the following adverse events can be ascribed to DEPAKOTE alone, or the combination of DEPAKOTE and other antiepilepsy drugs.

Table 1
Adverse Events Reported by ≥ 5% of Patients Treated with DEPAKOTE During Placebo-Controlled Trial of Adjunctive Therapy for Complex Partial Seizures

Body System/Event	Depakote (%) (n = 77)	Placebo (%) (n = 70)
Body as a Whole		
Headache	31	21
Asthenia	27	7
Fever	6	4

Continued on next page

Depakene—Cont.

Gastrointestinal System		
Nausea	48	14
Vomiting	27	7
Abdominal Pain	23	6
Diarrhea	13	6
Anorexia	12	0
Dyspepsia	8	4
Constipation	5	1
Nervous System		
Somnolence	27	11
Tremor	25	6
Dizziness	25	13
Diplopia	16	9
Amblyopia/Blurred Vision	12	9
Ataxia	8	1
Nystagmus	8	1
Emotional Lability	6	4
Thinking Abnormal	6	0
Amnesia	5	1
Respiratory System		
Flu Syndrome	12	9
Infection	12	6
Bronchitis	5	1
Rhinitis	5	4
Other		
Alopecia	6	1
Weight Loss	6	0

Table 2 lists treatment-emergent adverse events which were reported by ≥ 5% of patients in the high dose DEPAKOTE group, and for which the incidence was greater than in the low dose group, in a controlled trial of DEPAKOTE monotherapy treatment of complex partial seizures. Since patients were being titrated off another antiepilepsy drug during the first portion of the trial, it is not possible, in many cases, to determine whether the following adverse events can be ascribed to DEPAKOTE alone, or the combination of DEPAKOTE and other antiepilepsy drugs.

Table 2
Adverse Events Reported by ≥ 5% of Patients in the High Dose Group in the Controlled Trial of DEPAKOTE Monotherapy for Complex Partial Seizures[1]

Body System/Event	High Dose (%) (n = 131)	Low Dose (%) (n = 134)
Body as a Whole		
Asthenia	21	10
Digestive System		
Nausea	34	26
Diarrhea	23	19
Vomiting	23	15
Abdominal Pain	12	9
Anorexia	11	4
Dyspepsia	11	10
Hemic/Lymphatic System		
Thrombocytopenia	24	1
Ecchymosis	5	4
Metabolic/Nutritional		
Weight Gain	9	4
Peripheral Edema	8	3
Nervous System		
Tremor	57	19
Somnolence	30	18
Dizziness	18	13
Insomnia	15	9
Nervousness	11	7
Amnesia	7	4
Nystagmus	7	1
Depression	5	4
Respiratory System		
Infection	20	13
Pharyngitis	8	2
Dyspnea	5	1
Skin and Appendages		
Alopecia	24	13
Special Senses		
Amblyopia/Blurred Vision	8	4
Tinnitus	7	1

[1] Headache was the only adverse event that occurred in ≥ 5% of patients in the high dose group and at an equal or greater incidence in the low dose group.

The following additional adverse events were reported by greater than 1% but less than 5% of the 358 patients treated with DEPAKOTE in the controlled trials of complex partial seizures:

Body as a Whole: Back pain, chest pain, malaise.

Cardiovascular System: Tachycardia, hypertension, palpitation.

Digestive System: Increased appetite, flatulence, hematemesis, eructation, pancreatitis, periodontal abscess.

Hemic and Lymphatic System: Petechia.

Metabolic and Nutritional Disorders: SGOT increased, SGPT increased.

Musculoskeletal System: Myalgia, twitching, arthralgia, leg cramps, myasthenia.

Weight (Kg)	Weight (Lb)	Total Daily Dose (mg)	Number of Capsules or Teaspoonfuls of Syrup: Dose 1	Dose 2	Dose 3
10–24.9	22–54.9	250	0	0	1
25–39.9	55–87.9	500	1	0	1
40–59.9	88–131.9	750	1	1	1
60–74.9	132–164.9	1,000	1	1	2
75–89.9	165–197.9	1,250	2	1	2

Nervous System: Anxiety, confusion, abnormal gait, paresthesia, hypertonia, incoordination, abnormal dreams, personality disorder.

Respiratory System: Sinusitis, cough increased, pneumonia, epistaxis.

Skin and Appendages: Rash, pruritus, dry skin.

Special Senses: Taste perversion, abnormal vision, deafness, otitis media.

Urogenital System: Urinary incontinence, vaginitis, dysmenorrhea, amenorrhea, urinary frequency.

Other Patient Populations

Adverse events that have been reported with all dosage forms of valproate from epilepsy trials, spontaneous reports, and other sources are listed below by body system.

Gastrointestinal: The most commonly reported side effects at the initiation of therapy are nausea, vomiting, and indigestion. These effects are usually transient and rarely require discontinuation of therapy. Diarrhea, abdominal cramps, and constipation have been reported. Both anorexia with some weight loss and increased appetite with weight gain have also been reported. The administration of delayed-release divalproex sodium may result in reduction of gastrointestinal side effects in some patients.

CNS Effects: Sedative effects have occurred in patients receiving valproate alone but occur most often in patients receiving combination therapy. Sedation usually abates upon reduction of other antiepileptic medication. Tremor (may be dose-related), hallucinations, ataxia, headache, nystagmus, diplopia, asterixis, "spots before eyes", dysarthria, dizziness, confusion, hypesthesia, vertigo, incoordination, and parkinsonism. Rare cases of coma have occurred in patients receiving valproic acid alone or in conjunction with phenobarbital. In rare instances encephalopathy with fever has developed shortly after the introduction of valproate monotherapy without evidence of hepatic dysfunction or inappropriate plasma levels; all patients recovered after the drug was withdrawn.

Several reports have noted reversible cerebral atrophy and dementia in association with valproate therapy.

Dermatologic: Transient hair loss, skin rash, photosensitivity, generalized pruritus, erythema multiforme, and Stevens-Johnson syndrome. Rare cases of toxic epidermal necrolysis have been reported including a fatal case in a 6 month old infant taking valproate and several other concomitant medications. An additional case of toxic epidermal necrosis resulting in death was reported in a 35 year old patient with AIDS taking several concomitant medications and with a history of multiple cutaneous drug reactions.

Psychiatric: Emotional upset, depression, psychosis, aggression, hyperactivity, hostility, and behavioral deterioration.

Musculoskeletal: Weakness.

Hematologic: Thrombocytopenia and inhibition of the secondary phase of platelet aggregation may be reflected in altered bleeding time, petechiae, bruising, hematoma formation, epistaxis, and frank hemorrhage (see **PRECAUTIONS—General** and **Drug Interactions**). Relative lymphocytosis, macrocytosis, hypofibrinogenemia, leukopenia, eosinophilia, anemia including macrocytic with or without folate deficiency, bone marrow suppression, pancytopenia, aplastic anemia, and acute intermittent porphyria.

Hepatic: Minor elevations of transaminases (e.g., SGOT and SGPT) and LDH are frequent and appear to be dose-related. Occasionally, laboratory test results include increases in serum bilirubin and abnormal changes in other liver function tests. These results may reflect potentially serious hepatotoxicity (see **WARNINGS**).

Endocrine: Irregular menses, secondary amenorrhea, breast enlargement, galactorrhea, and parotid gland swelling. Abnormal thyroid function tests (see **PRECAUTIONS**).

There have been rare spontaneous reports of polycystic ovary disease. A cause and effect relationship has not been established.

Pancreatic: Acute pancreatitis, including fatalities (see **WARNINGS**).

Metabolic: Hyperammonemia (see **PRECAUTIONS**), hyponatremia, and inappropriate ADH secretion.

There have been rare reports of Fanconi's syndrome occurring chiefly in children.

Decreased carnitine concentrations have been reported although the clinical relevance is undetermined.

Hyperglycinemia has occurred and was associated with a fatal outcome in a patient with preexistent nonketotic hyperglycinemia.

Genitourinary: Enuresis and urinary tract infection.

Special Senses: Hearing loss, either reversible or irreversible, has been reported; however, a cause and effect relationship has not been established. Ear pain has also been reported.

Other: Anaphylaxis, edema of the extremities, lupus erythematosus, bone pain, cough increased, pneumonia, otitis media, bradycardia, cutaneous vasculitis, and fever.

Mania

Although DEPAKENE has not been evaluated for safety and efficacy in the treatment of manic episodes associated with bipolar disorder, the following adverse events not listed above were reported by 1% or more of patients from two placebo-controlled clinical trials of DEPAKOTE tablets.

Body as a Whole: Chills, neck pain, neck rigidity.

Cardiovascular System: Hypotension, postural hypotension, vasodilation.

Digestive System: Fecal incontinence, gastroenteritis, glossitis.

Musculoskeletal System: Arthrosis.

Nervous System: Agitation, catatonic reaction, hypokinesia, reflexes increased, tardive dyskinesia, vertigo.

Skin and Appendages: Furunculosis, maculopapular rash, seborrhea.

Special Senses: Conjunctivitis, dry eyes, eye pain.

Urogenital System: Dysuria.

Migraine

Although DEPAKENE has not been evaluated for safety and efficacy in the treatment of prophylaxis of migraine headaches, the following adverse events not listed above were reported by 1% or more of patients from two placebo-controlled clinical trials of DEPAKOTE tablets.

Body as a Whole: Face edema.

Digestive System: Dry mouth, stomatitis.

Urogenital System: Cystitis, metrorrhagia, and vaginal hemorrhage.

OVERDOSAGE

Overdosage with valproate may result in somnolence, heart block, and deep coma. Fatalities have been reported; however, patients have recovered from valproate levels as high as 2120 μg/mL.

In overdose situations, the fraction of drug not bound to protein is high and hemodialysis or tandem hemodialysis plus hemoperfusion may result in significant removal of drug. The benefit of gastric lavage or emesis will vary with the time since ingestion. General supportive measures should be applied with particular attention to the maintenance of adequate urinary output.

Naloxone has been reported to reverse the CNS depressant effects of valproate overdosage. Because naloxone could theoretically also reverse the antiepileptic effects of valproate, it should be used with caution in patients with epilepsy.

DOSAGE AND ADMINISTRATION

THE CAPSULES SHOULD BE SWALLOWED WITHOUT CHEWING TO AVOID LOCAL IRRITATION OF THE MOUTH AND THROAT.

DEPAKENE (valproic acid) is administered orally. DEPAKENE is indicated as monotherapy and adjunctive therapy in complex partial seizures in adults and pediatric patients down to the age of 10 years, and in simple and complex absence seizures. As the DEPAKENE dosage is titrated upward, concentrations of phenobarbital, carbamazepine, and/or phenytoin may be affected (see **PRECAUTIONS-Drug Interactions**).

Complex Partial Seizures: For adults and children 10 years of age or older.

Monotherapy (Initial Therapy): DEPAKENE has not been systematically studied as initial therapy. Patients should initiate therapy at 10 to 15 mg/kg/day. The dosage should be increased by 5 to 10 mg/kg/week to achieve optimal clinical response. Ordinarily, optimal clinical response is achieved at daily doses below 60 mg/kg/day. If satisfactory clinical response has not been achieved, plasma levels should be measured to determine whether or not they are in the usually accepted therapeutic range (50 to 100 μg/mL). No recommendation regarding the safety of valproate for use at doses above 60 mg/kg/day can be made.

The probability of thrombocytopenia increases significantly at total trough valproate plasma concentrations above 110 μg/mL in females and 135 μg/mL in males. The benefit of improved seizure control with higher doses should be weighed against the possibility of a greater incidence of adverse reactions.

Conversion to Monotherapy: Patients should initiate therapy at 10 to 15 mg/kg/day. The dosage should be increased by 5 to 10 mg/kg/week to achieve optimal clinical response. Ordinarily, optimal clinical response is achieved at daily doses below 60 mg/kg/day. If satisfactory clinical response has not been achieved, plasma levels should be measured to determine whether or not they are in the usually accepted therapeutic range (50–100 μg/mL). No recommendation regarding the safety of valproate for use at doses above 60 mg/kg/day can be made. Concomitant antiepilepsy drug (AED) dosage can ordinarily be reduced by approximately 25% every 2 weeks. This reduction may be started at initiation of DEPAKENE therapy, or delayed by 1 to 2 weeks if there is a concern that seizures are likely to occur with a reduction. The speed and duration of withdrawal of the concomitant AED can be highly variable, and patients should be monitored closely during this period for increased seizure frequency.

Adjunctive Therapy: DEPAKENE may be added to the patient's regimen at a dosage of 10 to 15 mg/kg/day. The dosage may be increased by 5 to 10 mg/kg/week to achieve optimal clinical response. Ordinarily, optimal clinical response is achieved at daily doses below 60 mg/kg/day. If satisfactory clinical response has not been achieved, plasma levels should be measured to determine whether or not they are in the usually accepted therapeutic range (50 to 100 µg/mL). No recommendation regarding the safety of valproate for use at doses above 60 mg/kg/day can be made. If the total daily dose exceeds 250 mg, it should be given in divided doses.

In a study of adjunctive therapy for complex partial seizures in which patients were receiving either carbamazepine or phenytoin in addition to DEPAKOTE tablets, no adjustment of carbamazepine or phenytoin dosage was needed (see **CLINICAL STUDIES**). However, since valproate may interact with these or other concurrently administered AEDs as well as other drugs (see **Drug Interactions**), periodic plasma concentration determinations of concomitant AEDs are recommended during the early course of therapy (see **PRECAUTIONS-Drug Interactions**).

Simple and Complex Absence Seizures: The recommended initial dose is 15 mg/kg/day, increasing at one week intervals by 5 to 10 mg/kg/day until seizures are controlled or side effects preclude further increases. The maximum recommended dosage is 60 mg/kg/day. If the total daily dose exceeds 250 mg, it should be given in divided doses.

A good correlation has not been established between daily dose, serum concentrations, and therapeutic effect. However, therapeutic valproate serum concentrations for most patients with absence seizures is considered to range from 50 to 100 µg/mL. Some patients may be controlled with lower or higher serum concentrations (see **CLINICAL PHARMACOLOGY**).

As the DEPAKENE dosage is titrated upward, blood concentrations of phenobarbital and/or phenytoin may be affected (see **PRECAUTIONS**).

Antiepilepsy drugs should not be abruptly discontinued in patients in whom the drug is administered to prevent major seizures because of the strong possibility of precipitating status epilepticus with attendant hypoxia and threat to life.

The following table is a guide for the initial daily dose of DEPAKENE (valproic acid) (15 mg/kg/day):

[See table at top right of previous page]

General Dosing Advice

Dosing in Elderly Patients—Due to a decrease in unbound clearance of valproate and possibly a greater sensitivity to somnolence in the elderly, the starting dose should be reduced in these patients. Dosage should be increased more slowly and with regular monitoring for fluid and nutritional intake, dehydration, somnolence, and other adverse events. Dose reductions or discontinuation of valproate should be considered in patients with decreased food or fluid intake and in patients with excessive somnolence. The ultimate therapeutic dose should be achieved on the basis of both tolerability and clinical response (see **WARNINGS**).

Dose-Related Adverse Events—The frequency of adverse effects (particularly elevated liver enzymes and thrombocytopenia) may be dose-related. The probability of thrombocytopenia appears to increase significantly at total valproate concentrations of ≥ 110 µg/mL (females) or ≥ 135 µg/mL (males) (see **PRECAUTIONS**). The benefit of improved therapeutic effect with higher doses should be weighed against the possibility of a greater incidence of adverse reactions.

G.I. Irritation—Patients who experience G.I. irritation may benefit from administration of the drug with food or by slowly building up the dose from an initial low level.

HOW SUPPLIED

DEPAKENE (valproic acid) is available as orange-colored soft gelatin capsules of 250 mg valproic acid, bearing the trademark DEPAKENE for product identification, in bottles of 100 capsules (**NDC** 0074-5681-13), and as a red syrup containing the equivalent of 250 mg valproic acid per 5 mL as the sodium salt in bottles of 16 ounces (**NDC** 0074-5682-16).

Store capsules at 59–77°F (15–25°C). Store syrup below 86°F (30°C).

Revised: June, 2000

ABBOTT LABORATORIES

NORTH CHICAGO, IL 60064, U.S.A.

Shown in Product Identification Guide, page 303

DEPAKOTE® Sprinkle Capsules ℞

[dəp' ā-coat]

DIVALPROEX SODIUM

COATED PARTICLES IN CAPSULES

BOX WARNING:

HEPATOTOXICITY:

HEPATIC FAILURE RESULTING IN FATALITIES HAS OCCURRED IN PATIENTS RECEIVING VALPROIC ACID AND ITS DERIVATIVES. EXPERIENCE HAS INDICATED THAT CHILDREN UNDER THE AGE OF TWO YEARS ARE AT A CONSIDERABLY INCREASED RISK OF DEVELOPING FATAL HEPATOTOXICITY, ESPECIALLY THOSE ON MULTIPLE ANTICONVULSANTS, THOSE WITH CONGENITAL METABOLIC DISORDERS, THOSE WITH SEVERE SEIZURE DISORDERS ACCOMPANIED BY MENTAL RETARDATION, AND THOSE WITH ORGANIC BRAIN DISEASE. WHEN DEPAKOTE IS USED IN THIS PATIENT GROUP, IT SHOULD BE USED WITH EXTREME CAUTION AND AS A SOLE AGENT. THE BENEFITS OF THERAPY SHOULD BE WEIGHED AGAINST THE RISKS. ABOVE THIS AGE GROUP, EXPERIENCE IN EPILEPSY HAS INDICATED THAT THE INCIDENCE OF FATAL HEPATOTOXICITY DECREASES CONSIDERABLY IN PROGRESSIVELY OLDER PATIENT GROUPS.

THESE INCIDENTS USUALLY HAVE OCCURRED DURING THE FIRST SIX MONTHS OF TREATMENT. SERIOUS OR FATAL HEPATOTOXICITY MAY BE PRECEDED BY NON-SPECIFIC SYMPTOMS SUCH AS MALAISE, WEAKNESS, LETHARGY, FACIAL EDEMA, ANOREXIA, AND VOMITING. IN PATIENTS WITH EPILEPSY, A LOSS OF SEIZURE CONTROL MAY ALSO OCCUR. PATIENTS SHOULD BE MONITORED CLOSELY FOR APPEARANCE OF THESE SYMPTOMS. LIVER FUNCTION TESTS SHOULD BE PERFORMED PRIOR TO THERAPY AND AT FREQUENT INTERVALS THEREAFTER, ESPECIALLY DURING THE FIRST SIX MONTHS.

TERATOGENICITY:

VALPROATE CAN PRODUCE TERATOGENIC EFFECTS SUCH AS NEURAL TUBE DEFECTS (E.G., SPINA BIFIDA). ACCORDINGLY, THE USE OF VALPROATE PRODUCTS IN WOMEN OF CHILDBEARING POTENTIAL REQUIRES THAT THE BENEFITS OF ITS USE BE WEIGHED AGAINST THE RISK OF INJURY TO THE FETUS.

PANCREATITIS:

CASES OF LIFE-THREATENING PANCREATITIS HAVE BEEN REPORTED IN BOTH CHILDREN AND ADULTS RECEIVING VALPROATE. SOME OF THE CASES HAVE BEEN DESCRIBED AS HEMORRHAGIC WITH A RAPID PROGRESSION FROM INITIAL SYMPTOMS TO DEATH. CASES HAVE BEEN REPORTED SHORTLY AFTER INITIAL USE AS WELL AS AFTER SEVERAL YEARS OF USE. PATIENTS AND GUARDIANS SHOULD BE WARNED THAT ABDOMINAL PAIN, NAUSEA, VOMITING, AND/OR ANOREXIA CAN BE SYMPTOMS OF PANCREATITIS THAT REQUIRE PROMPT MEDICAL EVALUATION. IF PANCREATITIS IS DIAGNOSED, VALPROATE SHOULD ORDINARILY BE DISCONTINUED. ALTERNATIVE TREATMENT FOR THE UNDERLYING MEDICAL CONDITION SHOULD BE INITIATED AS CLINICALLY INDICATED. (See **WARNINGS** and **PRECAUTIONS**.)

DESCRIPTION

Divalproex sodium is a stable co-ordination compound comprised of sodium valproate and valproic acid in a 1:1 molar relationship and formed during the partial neutralization of valproic acid with 0.5 equivalent of sodium hydroxide. Chemically it is designated as sodium hydrogen bis (2-propylpentanoate). Divalproex sodium has the following structure:

$CH_3CH_2CH_2$—CH—$CH_2CH_2CH_3$
HO—C=O Na⊕
O=C—O⊖
$CH_3CH_2CH_2$—CH—$CH_2CH_2CH_3$
n

Divalproex sodium occurs as a white powder with a characteristic odor.

DEPAKOTE Sprinkle Capsules are for oral administration. DEPAKOTE Sprinkle Capsules contain specially coated particles of divalproex sodium equivalent to 125 mg of valproic acid in a hard gelatin capsule.

Inactive Ingredients

125 mg DEPAKOTE Sprinkle Capsules: cellulosic polymers, D&C Red No. 28, FD&C Blue No. 1, gelatin, iron oxide, magnesium stearate, silica gel, titanium dioxide, and triethyl citrate.

CLINICAL PHARMACOLOGY

Pharmacodynamics

Divalproex sodium dissociates to the valproate ion in the gastrointestinal tract. The mechanisms by which valproate exerts its therapeutic effects have not been established. It has been suggested that its activity in epilepsy is related to increased brain concentrations of gamma-aminobutyric acid (GABA).

Pharmacokinetics

Absorption/Bioavailability

Equivalent oral doses of DEPAKOTE (divalproex sodium) products and DEPAKENE (valproic acid) capsules deliver equivalent quantities of valproate ion systemically. Although the rate of valproate ion absorption may vary with the formulation administered (liquid, solid, or sprinkle), conditions of use (e.g., fasting or postprandial) and the method of administration (e.g., whether the contents of the capsule are sprinkled on food or the capsule is taken intact), these differences should be of minor clinical importance under the steady state conditions achieved in chronic use in the treatment of epilepsy.

However, it is possible that differences among the various valproate products in T_{max} and C_{max} could be important upon initiation of treatment. For example, in single dose studies, the effect of feeding had a greater influence on the rate of absorption of the tablet (increase in T_{max} from 4 to 8 hours) than on the absorption of the sprinkle capsules (increase in T_{max} from 3.3 to 4.8 hours).

While the absorption rate from the G.I. tract and fluctuation in valproate plasma concentrations vary with dosing regimen and formulation, the efficacy of valproate as an anticonvulsant in chronic use is unlikely to be affected. Experience employing dosing regimens from once-a-day to four-times-a-day, as well as studies in primate epilepsy models involving constant rate infusion, indicate that total daily systemic bioavailability (extent of absorption) is the primary determinant of seizure control and that differences in the ratios of plasma peak to trough concentrations between valproate formulations are inconsequential from a practical clinical standpoint.

Co-administration of oral valproate products with food and substitution among the various DEPAKOTE and DEPAKENE formulations should cause no clinical problems in the management of patients with epilepsy (see **DOSAGE AND ADMINISTRATION**). Nonetheless, any changes in dosage administration, or the addition or discontinuance of concomitant drugs should ordinarily be accompanied by close monitoring of clinical status and valproate plasma concentrations.

Distribution

Protein Binding:

The plasma protein binding of valproate is concentration dependent and the free fraction increases from approximately 10% at 40 µg/mL to 18.5% at 130 µg/mL. Protein binding of valproate is reduced in the elderly, in patients with chronic hepatic diseases, in patients with renal impairment, and in the presence of other drugs (e.g., aspirin). Conversely, valproate may displace certain protein-bound drugs (e.g., phenytoin, carbamazepine, warfarin, and tolbutamide). (See **PRECAUTIONS, Drug Interactions** for more detailed information on the pharmacokinetic interactions of valproate with other drugs.)

CNS Distribution:

Valproate concentrations in cerebrospinal fluid (CSF) approximate unbound concentrations in plasma (about 10% of total concentration).

Metabolism

Valproate is metabolized almost entirely by the liver. In adult patients on monotherapy, 30–50% of an administered dose appears in urine as a glucuronide conjugate. Mitochondrial β-oxidation is the other major metabolic pathway, typically accounting for over 40% of the dose. Usually, less than 15–20% of the dose is eliminated by other oxidative mechanisms. Less than 3% of an administered dose is excreted unchanged in urine.

The relationship between dose and total valproate concentration is nonlinear; concentration does not increase proportionally with the dose, but rather, increases to a lesser extent due to saturable plasma protein binding. The kinetics of unbound drug are linear.

Elimination

Mean plasma clearance and volume of distribution for total valproate are 0.56 L/hr/1.73 m^2 and 11 L/1.73 m^2, respectively. Mean plasma clearance and volume of distribution for free valproate are 4.6 L/hr/1.73 m^2 and 92 L/1.73 m^2. Mean terminal half-life for valproate monotherapy ranged from 9 to 16 hours following oral dosing regimens of 250 to 1000 mg.

The estimates cited apply primarily to patients who are not taking drugs that affect hepatic metabolizing enzyme systems. For example, patients taking enzyme-inducing antiepileptic drugs (carbamazepine, phenytoin, and phenobarbital) will clear valproate more rapidly. Because of these changes in valproate clearance, monitoring of antiepileptic concentrations should be intensified whenever concomitant antiepileptics are introduced or withdrawn.

Special Populations

Effect of Age:

Neonates—Children within the first two months of life have a markedly decreased ability to eliminate valproate compared to older children and adults. This is a result of reduced clearance (perhaps due to delay in development of glucuronosyltransferase and other enzyme systems involved in valproate elimination) as well as increased volume of distribution (in part due to decreased plasma protein binding). For example, in one study, the half-life in children under 10 days ranged from 10 to 67 hours compared to a range of 7 to 13 hours in children greater than 2 months.

Children—Pediatric patients (i.e., between 3 months and 10 years) have 50% higher clearances expressed on weight (i.e., mL/min/kg) than do adults. Over the age of 10 years, children have pharmacokinetic parameters that approximate those of adults.

Elderly—The capacity of elderly patients (age range: 68 to 89 years) to eliminate valproate has been shown to be reduced compared to younger adults (age range: 22 to 26). Intrinsic clearance is reduced by 39%; the free fraction is increased by 44%. Accordingly, the initial dosage should be reduced in the elderly. (See **DOSAGE AND ADMINISTRATION**).

Effect of Gender:

There are no differences in the body surface area adjusted unbound clearance between males and females (4.8±0.17 and 4.7±0.07 L/hr per 1.73 m^2, respectively).

Effect of Race: The effects of race on the kinetics of valproate have not been studied.

Continued on next page

Depakote Sprinkle—Cont.

Effect of Disease:
Liver Disease—(See **BOXED WARNING, CONTRAINDICATIONS**, and **WARNINGS**). Liver disease impairs the capacity to eliminate valproate. In one study, the clearance of free valproate was decreased by 50% in 7 patients with cirrhosis and by 16% in 4 patients with acute hepatitis, compared with 6 healthy subjects. In that study, the half-life of valproate was increased from 12 to 18 hours. Liver disease is also associated with decreased albumin concentrations and larger unbound fractions (2 to 2.6 fold increase) of valproate. Accordingly, monitoring of total concentrations may be misleading since free concentrations may be substantially elevated in patients with hepatic disease whereas total concentrations may appear to be normal.
Renal Disease—A slight reduction (27%) in the unbound clearance of valproate has been reported in patients with renal failure (creatinine clearance < 10 mL/minute); however, hemodialysis typically reduces valproate concentrations by about 20%. Therefore, no dosage adjustment appears to be necessary in patients with renal failure. Protein binding in these patients is substantially reduced; thus, monitoring total concentrations may be misleading.

Plasma Levels and Clinical Effect
The relationship between plasma concentration and clinical response is not well documented. One contributing factor is the nonlinear, concentration dependent protein binding of valproate which affects the clearance of the drug. Thus, monitoring of total serum valproate cannot provide a reliable index of the bioactive valproate species.
For example, because the plasma protein binding of valproate is concentration dependent, the free fraction increases from approximately 10% at 40 µg/mL to 18.5% at 130 µg/mL. Higher than expected free fractions occur in the elderly, in hyperlipidemic patients, and in patients with hepatic and renal diseases.
Epilepsy:
The therapeutic range in epilepsy is commonly considered to be 50 to 100 µg/mL of total valproate, although some patients may be controlled with lower or higher plasma concentrations.

CLINICAL STUDIES

Epilepsy
The efficacy of DEPAKOTE in reducing the incidence of complex partial seizures (CPS) that occur in isolation or in association with other seizure types was established in two controlled trials.
In one, multiclinic, placebo controlled study employing an add-on design (adjunctive therapy), 144 patients who continued to suffer eight or more CPS per 8 weeks during an 8 week period of monotherapy with doses of either carbamazepine or phenytoin sufficient to assure plasma concentrations within the "therapeutic range" were randomized to receive, in addition to their original antiepilepsy drug (AED), either DEPAKOTE or placebo. Randomized patients were to be followed for a total of 16 weeks. The following table presents the findings.

Adjunctive Therapy Study
Median Incidence of CPS per 8 Weeks

Add-on Treatment	Number of Patients	Baseline Incidence	Experimental Incidence
DEPAKOTE	75	16.0	8.9*
Placebo	69	14.5	11.5

* Reduction from baseline statistically significantly greater for DEPAKOTE than placebo at $p \leq 0.05$ level.

Figure 1 presents the proportion of patients (X axis) whose percentage reduction from baseline in complex partial seizure rates was at least as great as that indicated on the Y axis in the adjunctive therapy study. A positive percent reduction indicates an improvement (i.e., a decrease in seizure frequency), while a negative percent reduction indicates worsening. Thus, in a display of this type, the curve for an effective treatment is shifted to the left of the curve for placebo. This figure shows that the proportion of patients achieving any particular level of improvement was consistently higher for DEPAKOTE than for placebo. For example, 45% of patients treated with DEPAKOTE had a ≥ 50% reduction in complex partial seizure rate compared to 23% of patients treated with placebo.

Figure 1

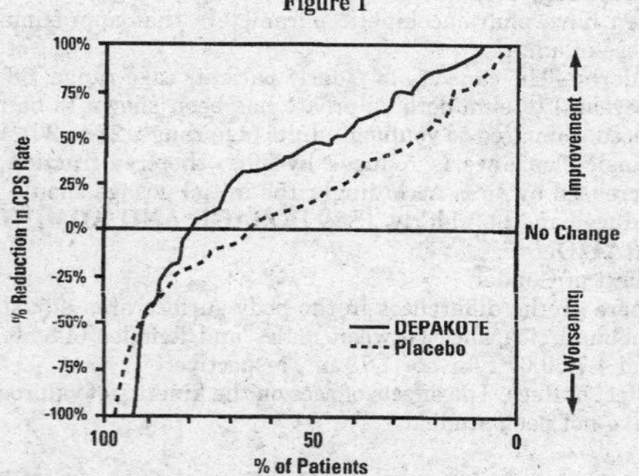

The second study assessed the capacity of DEPAKOTE to reduce the incidence of CPS when administered as the sole AED. The study compared the incidence of CPS among patients randomized to either a high or low dose treatment arm. Patients qualified for entry into the randomized comparison phase of this study only if 1) they continued to experience 2 or more CPS per 4 weeks during an 8 to 12 week long period of monotherapy with adequate doses of an AED (i.e., phenytoin, carbamazepine, phenobarbital, or primidone) and 2) they made a successful transition over a two week interval to DEPAKOTE. Patients entering the randomized phase were then brought to their assigned target dose, gradually tapered off their concomitant AED and followed for an interval as long as 22 weeks. Less than 50% of the patients randomized, however, completed the study. In patients converted to DEPAKOTE monotherapy, the mean total valproate concentrations during monotherapy were 71 and 123 µg/mL in the low dose and high dose groups, respectively.
The following table presents the findings for all patients randomized who had at least one post-randomization assessment.

Monotherapy Study
Median Incidence of CPS per 8 Weeks

Treatment	Number of Patients	Baseline Incidence	Randomized Phase Incidence
High dose DEPAKOTE	131	13.2	10.7*
Low dose DEPAKOTE	134	14.2	13.8

* Reduction from baseline statistically significantly greater for high dose than low dose at $p \leq 0.05$ level.

Figure 2 presents the proportion of patients (X axis) whose percentage reduction from baseline in complex partial seizure rates was at least as great as that indicated on the Y axis in the monotherapy study. A positive percent reduction indicates an improvement (i.e., a decrease in seizure frequency), while a negative percent reduction indicates worsening. Thus, in a display of this type, the curve for a more effective treatment is shifted to the left of the curve for a less effective treatment. This figure shows that the proportion of patients achieving any particular level of reduction was consistently higher for high dose DEPAKOTE than for low dose DEPAKOTE. For example, when switching from carbamazepine, phenytoin, phenobarbital or primidone monotherapy to high dose DEPAKOTE monotherapy, 63% of patients experienced no change or a reduction in complex partial seizure rates compared to 54% of patients receiving low dose DEPAKOTE.

Figure 2

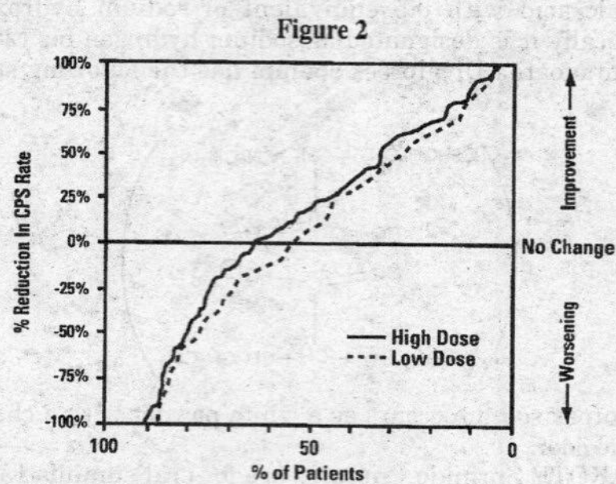

INDICATIONS AND USAGE

DEPAKOTE Sprinkle Capsules are indicated as monotherapy and adjunctive therapy in the treatment of patients with complex partial seizures that occur either in isolation or in association with other types of seizure. DEPAKOTE Sprinkle Capsules are also indicated for use as sole and adjunctive therapy in the treatment of simple and complex absence seizures, and adjunctively in patients with multiple seizure types that include absence seizures.
Simple absence is defined as very brief clouding of the sensorium or loss of consciousness accompanied by certain generalized epileptic discharges without other detectable clinical signs. Complex absence is the term used when other signs are also present.
SEE **WARNINGS** FOR STATEMENT REGARDING FATAL HEPATIC DYSFUNCTION.

CONTRAINDICATIONS

DIVALPROEX SODIUM SHOULD NOT BE ADMINISTERED TO PATIENTS WITH HEPATIC DISEASE OR SIGNIFICANT HEPATIC DYSFUNCTION.
Divalproex sodium is contraindicated in patients with known hypersensitivity to the drug.

WARNINGS

Hepatotoxicity
Hepatic failure resulting in fatalities has occurred in patients receiving valproic acid. These incidents usually have occurred during the first six months of treatment. Serious or fatal hepatotoxicity may be preceded by non-specific symptoms such as malaise, weakness, lethargy, facial edema, anorexia, and vomiting. In patients with epilepsy, a loss of seizure control may also occur. Patients should be monitored closely for appearance of these symptoms. Liver function tests should be performed prior to therapy and at frequent intervals thereafter, especially during the first six months. However, physicians should not rely totally on serum biochemistry since these tests may not be abnormal in all instances, but should also consider the results of careful interim medical history and physical examination.
Caution should be observed when administering DEPAKOTE products to patients with a prior history of hepatic disease. Patients on multiple anticonvulsants, children, those with congenital metabolic disorders, those with severe seizure disorders accompanied by mental retardation, and those with organic brain disease may be at particular risk. Experience has indicated that children under the age of two years are at a considerably increased risk of developing fatal hepatotoxicity, especially those with the aforementioned conditions. When DEPAKOTE is used in this patient group, it should be used with extreme caution and as a sole agent. The benefits of therapy should be weighed against the risks. Above this age group, experience in epilepsy has indicated that the incidence of fatal hepatotoxicity decreases considerably in progressively older patient groups.
The drug should be discontinued immediately in the presence of significant hepatic dysfunction, suspected or apparent. In some cases, hepatic dysfunction has progressed in spite of discontinuation of drug.

Pancreatitis
Cases of life-threatening pancreatitis have been reported in both children and adults receiving valproate. Some of the cases have been described as hemorrhagic with rapid progression from initial symptoms to death. Some cases have occurred shortly after initial use as well as after several years of use. The rate based upon the reported cases exceeds that expected in the general population and there have been cases in which pancreatitis recurred after rechallenge with valproate. In clinical trials, there were 2 cases of pancreatitis without alternative etiology in 2416 patients, representing 1044 patient-years experience. Patients and guardians should be warned that abdominal pain, nausea, vomiting, and/or anorexia can be symptoms of pancreatitis that require prompt medical evaluation. If pancreatitis is diagnosed, valproate should ordinarily be discontinued. Alternative treatment for the underlying medical condition should be initiated as clinically indicated (see **BOXED WARNING**).

Somnolence in the Elderly
In a double-blind, multicenter trial of valproate in elderly patients with dementia (mean age = 83 years), doses were increased by 125 mg/day to a target dose of 20 mg/kg/day. A significantly higher proportion of valproate patients had somnolence compared to placebo, and although not statistically significant, there was a higher proportion of patients with dehydration. Discontinuations for somnolence were also significantly higher than with placebo. In some patients with somnolence (approximately one-half), there was associated reduced nutritional intake and weight loss. There was a trend for the patients who experienced these events to have a lower baseline albumin concentration, lower valproate clearance, and a higher BUN. In elderly patients, dosage should be increased more slowly and with regular monitoring for fluid and nutritional intake, dehydration, somnolence, and other adverse events. Dose reductions or discontinuation of valproate should be considered in patients with decreased food or fluid intake and in patients with excessive somnolence (see **DOSAGE AND ADMINISTRATION**).

Thrombocytopenia
The frequency of adverse effects (particularly elevated liver enzymes and thrombocytopenia [see **PRECAUTIONS**]) may be dose-related. In a clinical trial of DEPAKOTE (divalproex sodium) as monotherapy in patients with epilepsy, 34/126 patients (27%) receiving approximately 50 mg/kg/day on average, had at least one value of platelets $\leq 75 \times 10^9$/L. Approximately half of these patients had treatment discontinued, with return of platelet counts to normal. In the remaining patients, platelet counts normalized with continued treatment. In this study, the probability of thrombocytopenia appeared to increase significantly at total valproate concentrations of ≥ 110 µg/mL (females) or ≥ 135 µg/mL (males). The therapeutic benefit which may accompany the higher doses should therefore be weighed against the possibility of a greater incidence of adverse effects.

Usage In Pregnancy
ACCORDING TO PUBLISHED AND UNPUBLISHED REPORTS, VALPROIC ACID MAY PRODUCE TERATOGENIC EFFECTS IN THE OFFSPRING OF HUMAN FEMALES RECEIVING THE DRUG DURING PREGNANCY.
THERE ARE MULTIPLE REPORTS IN THE CLINICAL LITERATURE WHICH INDICATE THAT THE USE OF ANTIEPILEPTIC DRUGS DURING PREGNANCY RESULTS IN AN INCREASED INCIDENCE OF BIRTH DEFECTS IN THE OFFSPRING. ALTHOUGH DATA ARE MORE EXTENSIVE WITH RESPECT TO TRIMETHADIONE, PARAMETHADIONE, PHENYTOIN, AND PHENOBARBITAL, REPORTS INDICATE A POSSIBLE SIMILAR ASSOCIATION WITH THE USE OF OTHER ANTIEPILEPTIC DRUGS. THEREFORE, ANTIEPILEPSY DRUGS SHOULD BE ADMINISTERED TO WOMEN OF CHILD-

BEARING POTENTIAL ONLY IF THEY ARE CLEARLY SHOWN TO BE ESSENTIAL IN THE MANAGEMENT OF THEIR SEIZURES.
THE INCIDENCE OF NEURAL TUBE DEFECTS IN THE FETUS MAY BE INCREASED IN MOTHERS RECEIVING VALPROATE DURING THE FIRST TRIMESTER OF PREGNANCY. THE CENTERS FOR DISEASE CONTROL (CDC) HAS ESTIMATED THE RISK OF VALPROIC ACID EXPOSED WOMEN HAVING CHILDREN WITH SPINA BIFIDA TO BE APPROXIMATELY 1 TO 2%.
OTHER CONGENITAL ANOMALIES (E.G., CRANIOFACIAL DEFECTS, CARDIOVASCULAR MALFORMATIONS AND ANOMALIES INVOLVING VARIOUS BODY SYSTEMS), COMPATIBLE AND INCOMPATIBLE WITH LIFE, HAVE BEEN REPORTED. SUFFICIENT DATA TO DETERMINE THE INCIDENCE OF THESE CONGENITAL ANOMALIES IS NOT AVAILABLE.
THE HIGHER INCIDENCE OF CONGENITAL ANOMALIES IN ANTIEPILEPTIC DRUG-TREATED WOMEN WITH SEIZURE DISORDERS CANNOT BE REGARDED AS A CAUSE AND EFFECT RELATIONSHIP. THERE ARE INTRINSIC METHODOLOGIC PROBLEMS IN OBTAINING ADEQUATE DATA ON DRUG TERATOGENICITY IN HUMANS; GENETIC FACTORS OR THE EPILEPTIC CONDITION ITSELF, MAY BE MORE IMPORTANT THAN DRUG THERAPY IN CONTRIBUTING TO CONGENITAL ANOMALIES.
PATIENTS TAKING VALPROATE MAY DEVELOP CLOTTING ABNORMALITIES. A PATIENT WHO HAD LOW FIBRINOGEN WHEN TAKING MULTIPLE ANTICONVULSANTS INCLUDING VALPROATE GAVE BIRTH TO AN INFANT WITH AFIBRINOGENEMIA WHO SUBSEQUENTLY DIED OF HEMORRHAGE. IF VALPROATE IS USED IN PREGNANCY, THE CLOTTING PARAMETERS SHOULD BE MONITORED CAREFULLY.
HEPATIC FAILURE, RESULTING IN THE DEATH OF A NEWBORN AND OF AN INFANT, HAVE BEEN REPORTED FOLLOWING THE USE OF VALPROATE DURING PREGNANCY.
Animal studies have demonstrated valproate-induced teratogenicity. Increased frequencies of malformations, as well as intrauterine growth retardation and death, have been observed in mice, rats, rabbits, and monkeys following prenatal exposure to valproate. Malformations of the skeletal system are the most common structural abnormalities produced in experimental animals, but neural tube closure defects have been seen in mice exposed to maternal plasma valproate concentrations exceeding 230 µg/mL (2.3 times the upper limit of the human therapeutic range) during susceptible periods of embryonic development. Administration of an oral dose of 200 mg/kg/day or greater (50% of the maximum human daily dose or greater on a mg/m^2 basis) to pregnant rats during organogenesis produced malformations (skeletal, cardiac, and urogenital) and growth retardation in the offspring. These doses resulted in peak maternal plasma valproate levels of approximately 340 µg/mL or greater (3.4 times the upper limit of the human therapeutic range or greater). Behavioral deficits have been reported in the offspring of rats given a dose of 200 mg/kg/day throughout most of pregnancy. An oral dose of 350 mg/kg/day (approximately 2 times the maximum human daily dose on a mg/m^2 basis) produced skeletal and visceral malformations in rabbits exposed during organogenesis. Skeletal malformations, growth retardation, and death were observed in rhesus monkeys following administration of an oral dose of 200 mg/kg/day (equal to the maximum human daily dose on a mg/m^2 basis) during organogenesis. This dose resulted in peak maternal plasma valproate levels of approximately 280 µg/mL (2.8 times the upper limit of the human therapeutic range).
The prescribing physician will wish to weigh the benefits of therapy against the risks in treating or counseling women of childbearing potential. If this drug is used during pregnancy, or if the patient becomes pregnant while taking this drug, the patient should be apprised of the potential hazard to the fetus.
Antiepileptic drugs should not be discontinued abruptly in patients in whom the drug is administered to prevent major seizures because of the strong possibility of precipitating status epilepticus with attendant hypoxia and threat to life. In individual cases where the severity and frequency of the seizure disorder are such that the removal of medication does not pose a serious threat to the patient, discontinuation of the drug may be considered prior to and during pregnancy, although it cannot be said with any confidence that even minor seizures do not pose some hazard to the developing embryo or fetus.
Tests to detect neural tube and other defects using current accepted procedures should be considered a part of routine prenatal care in childbearing women receiving valproate.

PRECAUTIONS

Hepatic Dysfunction

See **BOXED WARNING**, **CONTRAINDICATIONS** and **WARNINGS**.

Pancreatitis

See **BOXED WARNING** and **WARNINGS**.

General

Because of reports of thrombocytopenia (see **WARNINGS**), inhibition of the secondary phase of platelet aggregation, and abnormal coagulation parameters, (e.g., low fibrinogen), platelet counts and coagulation tests are recommended before initiating therapy and at periodic intervals. It is recommended that patients receiving DEPAKOTE be monitored for platelet count and coagulation parameters prior to planned surgery. In a clinical trial of DEPAKOTE as monotherapy in patients with epilepsy, 34/126 patients (27%) receiving approximately 50 mg/kg/day on average, had at least one value of platelets $\leq 75 \times 10^9$/L. Approximately half of these patients had treatment discontinued, with return of platelet counts to normal. In the remaining patients, platelet counts normalized with continued treatment. In this study, the probability of thrombocytopenia appeared to increase significantly at total valproate concentrations of ≥ 110 µg/mL (females) or ≥ 135 µg/mL (males). Evidence of hemorrhage, bruising, or a disorder of hemostasis/coagulation is an indication for reduction of the dosage or withdrawal of therapy.
Hyperammonemia with or without lethargy or coma has been reported and may be present in the absence of abnormal liver function tests. Asymptomatic elevations of ammonia are more common and when present require more frequent monitoring. If clinically significant symptoms occur, DEPAKOTE therapy should be modified or discontinued.
Since DEPAKOTE may interact with concurrently administered drugs which are capable of enzyme induction, periodic plasma concentration determinations of valproate and concomitant drugs are recommended during the early course of therapy. (See **PRECAUTIONS - Drug Interactions.**)
Valproate is partially eliminated in the urine as a keto-metabolite which may lead to a false interpretation of the urine ketone test.
There have been reports of altered thyroid function tests associated with valproate. The clinical significance of these is unknown.
There are *in vitro* studies that suggest valproate stimulates the replication of the HIV and CMV viruses under certain experimental conditions. The clinical consequence, if any, is not known. Additionally, the relevance of these *in vitro* findings is uncertain for patients receiving maximally suppressive antiretroviral therapy. Nevertheless, these data should be borne in mind when interpreting the results from regular monitoring of the viral load in HIV infected patients receiving valproate or when following CMV infected patients clinically.

Information for Patients

Patients and guardians should be warned that abdominal pain, nausea, vomiting, and/or anorexia can be symptoms of pancreatitis and, therefore, require further medical evaluation promptly.
Since DEPAKOTE products may produce CNS depression, especially when combined with another CNS depressant (e.g., alcohol), patients should be advised not to engage in hazardous activities, such as driving an automobile or operating dangerous machinery, until it is known that they do not become drowsy from the drug.
The specially coated particles in DEPAKOTE Sprinkle Capsules have been observed in the stool, but this occurrence has not been associated with clinically significant effects.

Drug Interactions

Effects of Co-Administered Drugs on Valproate Clearance

Drugs that affect the level of expression of hepatic enzymes, particularly those that elevate levels of glucuronosyltransferases, may increase the clearance of valproate. For example, phenytoin, carbamazepine, and phenobarbital (or primidone) can double the clearance of valproate. Thus, patients on monotherapy will generally have longer half-lives and higher concentrations than patients receiving polytherapy with antiepilepsy drugs.
In contrast, drugs that are inhibitors of cytochrome P450 isozymes, e.g., antidepressants, may be expected to have little effect on valproate clearance because cytochrome P450 microsomal mediated oxidation is a relatively minor secondary metabolic pathway compared to glucuronidation and beta-oxidation.
Because of these changes in valproate clearance, monitoring of valproate and concomitant drug concentrations should be increased whenever enzyme inducing drugs are introduced or withdrawn.
The following list provides information about the potential for an influence of several commonly prescribed medications on valproate pharmacokinetics. The list is not exhaustive nor could it be, since new interactions are continuously being reported.

Drugs for which a potentially important interaction has been observed:

Aspirin—A study involving the co-administration of aspirin at antipyretic doses (11 to 16 mg/kg) with valproate to pediatric patients (n=6) revealed a decrease in protein binding and an inhibition of metabolism of valproate. Valproate free fraction was increased 4-fold in the presence of aspirin compared to valproate alone. The β-oxidation pathway consisting of 2-E-valproic acid, 3-OH-valproic acid, and 3-keto valproic acid was decreased from 25% of total metabolites excreted on valproate alone to 8.3% in the presence of aspirin. Caution should be observed if valproate and aspirin are to be co-administered.
Felbamate—A study involving the co-administration of 1200 mg/day of felbamate with valproate to patients with epilepsy (n=10) revealed an increase in mean valproate peak concentration by 35% (from 86 to 115 µg/mL) compared to valproate alone. Increasing the felbamate dose to 2400 mg/day increased the mean valproate peak concentration to 133 µg/mL (another 16% increase). A decrease in valproate dosage may be necessary when felbamate therapy is initiated.
Rifampin—A study involving the administration of a single dose of valproate (7 mg/kg) 36 hours after 5 nights of daily dosing with rifampin (600 mg) revealed a 40% increase in the oral clearance of valproate. Valproate dosage adjustment may be necessary when it is co-administered with rifampin.

Drugs for which either no interaction or a likely clinically unimportant interaction has been observed:

Antacids—A study involving the co-administration of valproate 500 mg with commonly administered antacids (Maalox, Trisogel, and Titralac—160 mEq doses) did not reveal any effect on the extent of absorption of valproate.
Chlorpromazine—A study involving the administration of 100 to 300 mg/day of chlorpromazine to schizophrenic patients already receiving valproate (200 mg BID) revealed a 15% increase in trough plasma levels of valproate.
Haloperidol—A study involving the administration of 6 to 10 mg/day of haloperidol to schizophrenic patients already receiving valproate (200 mg BID) revealed no significant changes in valproate trough plasma levels.
Cimetidine and Ranitidine—Cimetidine and ranitidine do not affect the clearance of valproate.

Effects of Valproate on Other Drugs

Valproate has been found to be a weak inhibitor of some P450 isozymes, epoxide hydrase, and glucuronosyltransferases.
The following list provides information about the potential for an influence of valproate co-administration on the pharmacokinetics or pharmacodynamics of several commonly prescribed medications. The list is not exhaustive, since new interactions are continuously being reported.

Drugs for which a potentially important valproate interaction has been observed: Amitriptyline/Nortriptyline—Administration of a single oral 50 mg dose of amitriptyline to 15 normal volunteers (10 males and 5 females) who received valproate (500 mg BID) resulted in a 21% decrease in plasma clearance of amitriptyline and a 34% decrease in the net clearance of nortriptyline. Rare postmarketing reports of concurrent use of valproate and amitriptyline resulting in an increased amitriptyline level have been received. Concurrent use of valproate and amitriptyline has rarely been associated with toxicity. Monitoring of amitriptyline levels should be considered for patients taking valproate concomitantly with amitriptyline. Consideration should be given to lowering the dose of amitriptyline/nortriptyline in the presence of valproate.
Carbamazepine/carbamazepine-10,11-Epoxide—Serum levels of carbamazepine (CBZ) decreased 17% while that of carbamazepine-10,11-epoxide (CBZ-E) increased by 45% upon co-administration of valproate and CBZ to epileptic patients.
Clonazepam—The concomitant use of valproic acid and clonazepam may induce absence status in patients with a history of absence type seizures.
Diazepam—Valproate displaces diazepam from its plasma albumin binding sites and inhibits its metabolism. Co-administration of valproate (1500 mg daily) increased the free fraction of diazepam (10 mg) by 90% in healthy volunteers (n=6). Plasma clearance and volume of distribution for free diazepam were reduced by 25% and 20%, respectively, in the presence of valproate. The elimination half-life of diazepam remained unchanged upon addition of valproate.
Ethosuximide—Valproate inhibits the metabolism of ethosuximide. Administration of a single ethosuximide dose of 500 mg with valproate (800 to 1600 mg/day) to healthy volunteers (n=6) was accompanied by a 25% increase in elimination half-life of ethosuximide and a 15% decrease in its total clearance as compared to ethosuximide alone. Patients receiving valproate and ethosuximide, especially along with other anticonvulsants, should be monitored for alterations in serum concentrations of both drugs.
Lamotrigine—In a steady-state study involving 10 healthy volunteers, the elimination half-life of lamotrigine increased from 26 to 70 hours with valproate co-administration (a 165% increase). The dose of lamotrigine should be reduced when co-administered with valproate.
Phenobarbital—Valproate was found to inhibit the metabolism of phenobarbital. Co-administration of valproate (250 mg BID for 14 days) with phenobarbital to normal subjects (n=6) resulted in a 50% increase in half-life and a 30% decrease in plasma clearance of phenobarbital (60 mg single-dose). The fraction of phenobarbital dose excreted unchanged increased by 50% in presence of valproate.
There is evidence for severe CNS depression, with or without significant elevations of barbiturate or valproate serum concentrations. All patients receiving concomitant barbiturate therapy should be closely monitored for neurological toxicity. Serum barbiturate concentrations should be obtained, if possible, and the barbiturate dosage decreased, if appropriate.
Primidone, which is metabolized to a barbiturate, may be involved in a similar interaction with valproate.
Phenytoin—Valproate displaces phenytoin from its plasma albumin binding sites and inhibits its hepatic metabolism. Co-administration of valproate (400 mg TID) with phenytoin (250 mg) in normal volunteers (n=7) was associated with a 60% increase in the free fraction of phenytoin. Total plasma clearance and apparent volume of distribution of phenytoin increased 30% in the presence of valproate. Both the clearance and apparent volume of distribution of free phenytoin were reduced by 25%.
In patients with epilepsy, there have been reports of breakthrough seizures occurring with the combination of valproate and phenytoin. The dosage of phenytoin should be adjusted as required by the clinical situation.

Continued on next page

Depakote Sprinkle—Cont.

Tolbutamide—From *in vitro* experiments, the unbound fraction of tolbutamide was increased from 20% to 50% when added to plasma samples taken from patients treated with valproate. The clinical relevance of this displacement is unknown.
Warfarin—In an *in vitro* study, valproate increased the unbound fraction of warfarin by up to 32.6%. The therapeutic relevance of this is unknown; however, coagulation tests should be monitored if DEPAKOTE therapy is instituted in patients taking anticoagulants.
Zidovudine—In six patients who were seropositive for HIV, the clearance of zidovudine (100 mg q8h) was decreased by 38% after administration of valproate (250 or 500 mg q8h); the half-life of zidovudine was unaffected.
Drugs for which either no interaction or a likely clinically unimportant interaction has been observed:
Acetaminophen—Valproate had no effect on any of the pharmacokinetic parameters of acetaminophen when it was concurrently administered to three epileptic patients.
Clozapine—In psychotic patients (n=11), no interaction was observed when valproate was co-administered with clozapine.
Lithium—Co-administration of valproate (500 mg BID) and lithium carbonate (300 mg TID) to normal male volunteers (n=16) had no effect on the steady-state kinetics of lithium.
Lorazepam—Concomitant administration of valproate (500 mg BID) and lorazepam (1 mg BID) in normal male volunteers (n=9) was accompanied by a 17% decrease in the plasma clearance of lorazepam.
Oral Contraceptive Steroids—Administration of a single-dose of ethinyloestradiol (50 µg)/levonorgestrel (250 µg) to 6 women on valproate (200 mg BID) therapy for 2 months did not reveal any pharmacokinetic interaction.

Carcinogenesis, Mutagenesis, Impairment of Fertility

Carcinogenesis

Valproic acid was administered orally to Sprague Dawley rats and ICR (HA/ICR) mice at doses of 80 and 170 mg/kg/day (approximately 10 to 50% of the maximum human daily dose on a mg/m^2 basis) for two years. A variety of neoplasms were observed in both species. The chief findings were a statistically significant increase in the incidence of subcutaneous fibrosarcomas in high dose male rats receiving valproic acid and a statistically significant dose-related trend for benign pulmonary adenomas in male mice receiving valproic acid. The significance of these findings for humans is unknown.

Mutagenesis

Valproate was not mutagenic in an *in vitro* bacterial assay (Ames test), did not produce dominant lethal effects in mice, and did not increase chromosome aberration frequency in an *in vivo* cytogenetic study in rats. Increased frequencies of sister chromatid exchange (SCE) have been reported in a study of epileptic children taking valproate, but this association was not observed in another study conducted in adults. There is some evidence that increased SCE frequencies may be associated with epilepsy. The biological significance of an increase in SCE frequency is not known.

Fertility

Chronic toxicity studies in juvenile and adult rats and dogs demonstrated reduced spermatogenesis and testicular atrophy at oral doses of 400 mg/kg/day or greater in rats (approximately equivalent to or greater than the maximum human daily dose on a mg/m^2 basis) and 150 mg/kg/day or greater in dogs (approximately 1.4 times the maximum human daily dose or greater on a mg/m^2 basis). Segment I fertility studies in rats have shown oral doses up to 350 mg/kg/day (approximately equal to the maximum human daily dose on a mg/m^2 basis) for 60 days to have no effect on fertility. THE EFFECT OF VALPROATE ON TESTICULAR DEVELOPMENT AND ON SPERM PRODUCTION AND FERTILITY IN HUMANS IS UNKNOWN.

Pregnancy

Pregnancy Category D: See **WARNINGS**.

Nursing Mothers

Valproate is excreted in breast milk. Concentrations in breast milk have been reported to be 1–10% of serum concentrations. It is not known what effect this would have on a nursing infant. Consideration should be given to discontinuing nursing when divalproex sodium is administered to a nursing woman.

Pediatric Use

Experience has indicated that pediatric patients under the age of two years are at a considerably increased risk of developing fatal hepatotoxicity, especially those with the aforementioned conditions (see **BOXED WARNING**). When DEPAKOTE is used in this patient group, it should be used with extreme caution and as a sole agent. The benefits of therapy should be weighed against the risks. Above the age of 2 years, experience in epilepsy has indicated that the incidence of fatal hepatotoxicity decreases considerably in progressively older patient groups.
Younger children, especially those receiving enzyme-inducing drugs, will require larger maintenance doses to attain targeted total and unbound valproic acid concentrations.
The variability in free fraction limits the clinical usefulness of monitoring total serum valproic acid concentrations. Interpretation of valproic acid concentrations in children should include consideration of factors that affect hepatic metabolism and protein binding.
The basic toxicology and pathologic manifestations of valproate sodium in neonatal (4-day old) and juvenile (14-day old) rats are similar to those seen in young adult rats. However, additional findings, including renal alterations in juvenile rats and renal alterations and retinal dysplasia in neonatal rats, have been reported. These findings occurred at 240 mg/kg/day, a dosage approximately equivalent to the human maximum recommended daily dose on a mg/m^2 basis. They were not seen at 90 mg/kg, or 40% of the maximum human daily dose on a mg/m^2 basis.

Geriatric Use

No patients above the age of 65 years were enrolled in double-blind prospective clinical trials of mania associated with bipolar illness. In a case review study of 583 patients, 72 patients (12%) were greater than 65 years of age. A higher percentage of patients above 65 years of age reported accidental injury, infection, pain, somnolence, and tremor. Discontinuation of valproate was occasionally associated with the latter two events. It is not clear whether these events indicate additional risk or whether they result from preexisting medical illness and concomitant medication use among these patients.
A study of elderly patients with dementia revealed drug related somnolence and discontinuation for somnolence (see **WARNINGS—Somnolence in the Elderly**). The starting dose should be reduced in these patients, and dosage reductions or discontinuation should be considered in patients with excessive somnolence (see **DOSAGE AND ADMINISTRATION**).

ADVERSE REACTIONS

Epilepsy

Based on a placebo-controlled trial of adjunctive therapy for treatment of complex partial seizures, DEPAKOTE was generally well tolerated with most adverse events rated as mild to moderate in severity. Intolerance was the primary reason for discontinuation in the DEPAKOTE-treated patients (6%), compared to 1% of placebo-treated patients.
Table 1 lists treatment-emergent adverse events which were reported by ≥ 5% of DEPAKOTE-treated patients and for which the incidence was greater than in the placebo group, in the placebo-controlled trial of adjunctive therapy for treatment of complex partial seizures. Since patients were also treated with other antiepilepsy drugs, it is not possible, in most cases, to determine whether the following adverse events can be ascribed to DEPAKOTE alone, or the combination of DEPAKOTE and other antiepilepsy drugs.

Table 1
Adverse Events Reported by ≥5% of Patients Treated with DEPAKOTE During Placebo-Controlled Trial of Adjunctive Therapy for Complex Partial Seizures

Body System/Event	Depakote (%) (n=77)	Placebo (%) (n=70)
Body as a Whole		
Headache	31	21
Asthenia	27	7
Fever	6	4
Gastrointestinal System		
Nausea	48	14
Vomiting	27	7
Abdominal Pain	23	6
Diarrhea	13	6
Anorexia	12	0
Dyspepsia	8	4
Constipation	5	1
Nervous System		
Somnolence	27	11
Tremor	25	6
Dizziness	25	13
Diplopia	16	9
Amblyopia/Blurred Vision	12	9
Ataxia	8	1
Nystagmus	8	1
Emotional Lability	6	4
Thinking Abnormal	6	0
Amnesia	5	1
Respiratory System		
Flu Syndrome	12	9
Infection	12	6
Bronchitis	5	1
Rhinitis	5	4
Other		
Alopecia	6	1
Weight Loss	6	0

Table 2 lists treatment-emergent adverse events which were reported by ≥ 5% of patients in the high dose DEPAKOTE group, and for which the incidence was greater than in the low dose group, in a controlled trial of DEPAKOTE monotherapy treatment of complex partial seizures. Since patients were being titrated off another antiepilepsy drug during the first portion of the trial, it is not possible, in many cases, to determine whether the following adverse events can be ascribed to DEPAKOTE alone, or the combination of DEPAKOTE and other antiepilepsy drugs.

Table 2
Adverse Events Reported by ≥5% of Patients in the High Dose Group in the Controlled Trial of DEPAKOTE Monotherapy for Complex Partial Seizures[1]

Body System/Event	High Dose (%) (n=131)	Low Dose (%) (n=134)
Body as a Whole		
Asthenia	21	10
Digestive System		
Nausea	34	26
Diarrhea	23	19
Vomiting	23	15
Abdominal Pain	12	9
Anorexia	11	4
Dyspepsia	11	10
Hemic/Lymphatic System		
Thrombocytopenia	24	1
Ecchymosis	5	4
Metabolic/Nutritional		
Weight Gain	9	4
Peripheral Edema	8	3
Nervous System		
Tremor	57	19
Somnolence	30	18
Dizziness	18	13
Insomnia	15	9
Nervousness	11	7
Amnesia	7	4
Nystagmus	7	1
Depression	5	4
Respiratory System		
Infection	20	13
Pharyngitis	8	2
Dyspnea	5	1
Skin and Appendages		
Alopecia	24	13
Special Senses		
Amblyopia/Blurred Vision	8	4
Tinnitus	7	1

[1] Headache was the only adverse event that occurred in ≥ 5% of patients in the high dose group and at an equal or greater incidence in the low dose group.

The following additional adverse events were reported by greater than 1% but less than 5% of the 358 patients treated with DEPAKOTE in the controlled trials of complex partial seizures:
Body as a Whole: Back pain, chest pain, malaise.
Cardiovascular System: Tachycardia, hypertension, palpitation.
Digestive System: Increased appetite, flatulence, hematemesis, eructation, pancreatitis, periodontal abscess.
Hemic and Lymphatic System: Petechia.
Metabolic and Nutritional Disorders: SGOT increased, SGPT increased.
Musculoskeletal System: Myalgia, twitching, arthralgia, leg cramps, myasthenia.
Nervous System: Anxiety, confusion, abnormal gait, paresthesia, hypertonia, incoordination, abnormal dreams, personality disorder.
Respiratory System: Sinusitis, cough increased, pneumonia, epistaxis.
Skin and Appendages: Rash, pruritus, dry skin.
Special Senses: Taste perversion, abnormal vision, deafness, otitis media.
Urogenital System: Urinary incontinence, vaginitis, dysmenorrhea, amenorrhea, urinary frequency.

Other Patient Populations

Adverse events that have been reported with all dosage forms of valproate from epilepsy trials, spontaneous reports, and other sources are listed below by body system.
Gastrointestinal: The most commonly reported side effects at the initiation of therapy are nausea, vomiting, and indigestion. These effects are usually transient and rarely require discontinuation of therapy. Diarrhea, abdominal cramps, and constipation have been reported. Both anorexia with some weight loss and increased appetite with weight gain have also been reported. The administration of delayed-release divalproex sodium may result in reduction of gastrointestinal side effects in some patients.
CNS Effects: Sedative effects have occurred in patients receiving valproate alone but occur most often in patients receiving combination therapy. Sedation usually abates upon reduction of other antiepileptic medication. Tremor (may be dose-related), hallucinations, ataxia, headache, nystagmus, diplopia, asterixis, "spots before eyes", dysarthria, dizziness, confusion, hypesthesia, vertigo, incoordination, and parkinsonism. Rare cases of coma have occurred in patients receiving valproate alone or in conjunction with phenobarbital. In rare instances encephalopathy with fever has developed shortly after the introduction of valproate monotherapy without evidence of hepatic dysfunction or inappropriate plasma levels; all patients recovered after the drug was withdrawn.
Several reports have noted reversible cerebral atrophy and dementia in association with valproate therapy.
Dermatologic: Transient hair loss, skin rash, photosensitivity, generalized pruritus, erythema multiforme, and Stevens-Johnson syndrome. Rare cases of toxic epidermal

necrolysis have been reported including a fatal case in a 6 month old infant taking valproate and several other concomitant medications. An additional case of toxic epidermal necrosis resulting in death was reported in a 35 year old patient with AIDS taking several concomitant medications and with a history of multiple cutaneous drug reactions.
Psychiatric: Emotional upset, depression, psychosis, aggression, hyperactivity, hostility, and behavioral deterioration.
Musculoskeletal: Weakness.
Hematologic: Thrombocytopenia and inhibition of the secondary phase of platelet aggregation may be reflected in altered bleeding time, petechia, bruising, hematoma formation, epistaxis, and frank hemorrhage (see **PRECAUTIONS—General** and **Drug Interactions**). Relative lymphocytosis, macrocytosis, hypofibrinogenemia, leukopenia, eosinophilia, anemia including macrocytic with or without folate deficiency, bone marrow suppression, pancytopenia, aplastic anemia, and acute intermittent porphyria.
Hepatic: Minor elevations of transaminases (eg, SGOT and SGPT) and LDH are frequent and appear to be dose-related. Occasionally, laboratory test results include increases in serum bilirubin and abnormal changes in other liver function tests. These results may reflect potentially serious hepatotoxicity (see **WARNINGS**).
Endocrine: Irregular menses, secondary amenorrhea, breast enlargement, galactorrhea, and parotid gland swelling. Abnormal thyroid function tests (see **PRECAUTIONS**).
There have been rare spontaneous reports of polycystic ovary disease. A cause and effect relationship has not been established.
Pancreatic: Acute pancreatitis including fatalities (see **WARNINGS**).
Metabolic: Hyperammonemia (see **PRECAUTIONS**), hyponatremia, and inappropriate ADH secretion.
There have been rare reports of Fanconi's syndrome occurring chiefly in children.
Decreased carnitine concentrations have been reported although the clinical relevance is undetermined.
Hyperglycinemia has occurred and was associated with a fatal outcome in a patient with preexistent nonketotic hyperglycinemia.
Genitourinary: Enuresis and urinary tract infection.
Special Senses: Hearing loss, either reversible or irreversible, has been reported; however, a cause and effect relationship has not been established. Ear pain has also been reported.
Other: Anaphylaxis, edema of the extremities, lupus erythematosus, bone pain, cough increased, pneumonia, otitis media, bradycardia, cutaneous vasculitis, and fever.

Mania
Although DEPAKOTE Sprinkle Capsules have not been evaluated for safety and efficacy in the treatment of manic episodes associated with bipolar disorder, the following adverse events not listed above were reported by 1% or more of patients from two placebo-controlled clinical trials of DEPAKOTE tablets.
Body as a Whole: Chills, neck pain, neck rigidity.
Cardiovascular System: Hypotension, postural hypotension, vasodilation.
Digestive System: Fecal incontinence, gastroenteritis, glossitis.
Musculoskeletal System: Arthrosis.
Nervous System: Agitation, catatonic reaction, hypokinesia, reflexes increased, tardive dyskinesia, vertigo.
Skin and Appendages: Furunculosis, maculopapular rash, seborrhea.
Special Senses: Conjunctivitis, dry eyes, eye pain.
Urogenital System: Dysuria.

Migraine
Although DEPAKOTE Sprinkle Capsules have not been evaluated for safety and efficacy in the treatment of prophylaxis of migraine headaches, the following adverse events not listed above were reported by 1% or more of patients from two placebo-controlled clinical trials of DEPAKOTE tablets.
Body as a Whole: Face edema.
Digestive System: Dry mouth, stomatitis.
Urogenital System: Cystitis, metrorrhagia, and vaginal hemorrhage.

OVERDOSAGE

Overdosage with valproate may result in somnolence, heart block, and deep coma. Fatalities have been reported; however patients have recovered from valproate levels as high as 2120 µg/mL.
In overdose situations, the fraction of drug not bound to protein is high and hemodialysis or tandem hemodialysis plus hemoperfusion may result in significant removal of drug. The benefit of gastric lavage or emesis will vary with the time since ingestion. General supportive measures should be applied with particular attention to the maintenance of adequate urinary output.
Naloxone has been reported to reverse the CNS depressant effects of valproate overdosage. Because naloxone could theoretically also reverse the antiepileptic effects of valproate, it should be used with caution in patients with epilepsy.

DOSAGE AND ADMINISTRATION

Epilepsy
DEPAKOTE Sprinkle Capsules are administered orally. DEPAKOTE is indicated as monotherapy and adjunctive therapy in complex partial seizures in adults and pediatric patients down to the age of 10 years, and in simple and complex absence seizures. As the DEPAKOTE dosage is titrated upward, concentrations of phenobarbital, carbamazepine, and/or phenytoin may be affected (see **PRECAUTIONS—Drug Interactions**).
Complex Partial Seizures: For adults and children 10 years of age or older.
Monotherapy (Initial Therapy): DEPAKOTE has not been systematically studied as initial therapy. Patients should initiate therapy at 10 to 15 mg/kg/day. The dosage should be increased by 5 to 10 mg/kg/week to achieve optimal clinical response. Ordinarily, optimal clinical response is achieved at daily doses below 60 mg/kg/day. If satisfactory clinical response has not been achieved, plasma levels should be measured to determine whether or not they are in the usually accepted therapeutic range (50 to 100 µg/mL). No recommendation regarding the safety of valproate for use at doses above 60 mg/kg/day can be made.
The probability of thrombocytopenia increases significantly at total trough valproate plasma concentrations above 110 µg/mL in females and 135 µg/mL in males. The benefit of improved seizure control with higher doses should be weighed against the possibility of a greater incidence of adverse reactions.
Conversion to Monotherapy: Patients should initiate therapy at 10 to 15 mg/kg/day. The dosage should be increased by 5 to 10 mg/kg/week to achieve optimal clinical response. Ordinarily, optimal clinical response is achieved at daily doses below 60 mg/kg/day. If satisfactory clinical response has not been achieved, plasma levels should be measured to determine whether or not they are in the usually accepted therapeutic range (50–100 µg/mL). No recommendation regarding the safety of valproate for use at doses above 60 mg/kg/day can be made. Concomitant antiepilepsy drug (AED) dosage can ordinarily be reduced by approximately 25% every 2 weeks. This reduction may be started at initiation of DEPAKOTE therapy, or delayed by 1 to 2 weeks if there is a concern that seizures are likely to occur with a reduction. The speed and duration of withdrawal of the concomitant AED can be highly variable, and patients should be monitored closely during this period for increased seizure frequency.
Adjunctive Therapy: DEPAKOTE may be added to the patient's regimen at a dosage of 10 to 15 mg/kg/day. The dosage may be increased by 5 to 10 mg/kg/week to achieve optimal clinical response. Ordinarily, optimal clinical response is achieved at daily doses below 60 mg/kg/day. If satisfactory clinical response has not been achieved, plasma levels should be measured to determine whether or not they are in the usually accepted therapeutic range (50 to 100 µg/mL). No recommendation regarding the safety of valproate for use at doses above 60 mg/kg/day can be made. If the total daily dose exceeds 250 mg, it should be given in divided doses.
In a study of adjunctive therapy for complex partial seizures in which patients were receiving either carbamazepine or phenytoin in addition to DEPAKOTE, no adjustment of carbamazepine or phenytoin dosage was needed (see **CLINICAL STUDIES**). However, since valproate may interact with these or other concurrently administered AEDs as well as other drugs (see **Drug Interactions**), periodic plasma concentration determinations of concomitant AEDs are recommended during the early course of therapy (see **PRECAUTIONS—Drug Interactions**).
Simple and Complex Absence Seizures: The recommended initial dose is 15 mg/kg/day, increasing at one week intervals by 5 to 10 mg/kg/day until seizures are controlled or side effects preclude further increases. The maximum recommended dosage is 60 mg/kg/day. If the total daily dose exceeds 250 mg, it should be given in divided doses.
A good correlation has not been established between daily dose, serum concentrations, and therapeutic effect. However, therapeutic valproate serum concentrations for most patients with absence seizures is considered to range from 50 to 100 µg/mL. Some patients may be controlled with lower or higher serum concentrations (see **CLINICAL PHARMACOLOGY**).
As the DEPAKOTE dosage is titrated upward, blood concentrations of phenobarbital and/or phenytoin may be affected (see **PRECAUTIONS**).
Antiepilepsy drugs should not be abruptly discontinued in patients in whom the drug is administered to prevent major seizures because of the strong possibility of precipitating status epilepticus with attendant hypoxia and threat to life.
In epileptic patients previously receiving DEPAKENE (valproic acid) therapy, DEPAKOTE Sprinkle Capsules should be initiated at the same daily dose and dosing schedule. After the patient is stabilized on DEPAKOTE Sprinkle Capsules, a dosing schedule of two or three times a day may be elected in selected patients.

General Dosing Advice
Dosing in Elderly Patients—Due to a decrease in unbound clearance of valproate and possibly a greater sensitivity to somnolence in the elderly, the starting dose should be reduced in these patients. Dosage should be increased more slowly and with regular monitoring for fluid and nutritional intake, dehydration, somnolence, and other adverse events. Dose reductions or discontinuation of valproate should be considered in patients with decreased food or fluid intake and in patients with excessive somnolence. The ultimate therapeutic dose should be achieved on the basis of both tolerability and clinical response (see **WARNINGS**).
Dose-Related Adverse Events—The frequency of adverse effects (particularly elevated liver enzymes and thrombocytopenia) may be dose-related. The probability of thrombocytopenia appears to increase significantly at total valproate concentrations of ≥ 110 µg/mL (females) or ≥ 135 µg/mL (males) (see **PRECAUTIONS**). The benefit of improved therapeutic effect with higher doses should be weighed against the possibility of a greater incidence of adverse reactions.
G.I. Irritation—Patients who experience G.I. irritation may benefit from administration of the drug with food or by slowly building up the dose from an initial low level.
Administration of Sprinkle Capsules—DEPAKOTE Sprinkle Capsules may be swallowed whole or may be administered by carefully opening the capsule and sprinkling the entire contents on a small amount (teaspoonful) of soft food such as applesauce or pudding. The drug/food mixture should be swallowed immediately (avoid chewing) and not stored for future use. Each capsule is oversized to allow ease of opening.

HOW SUPPLIED

DEPAKOTE Sprinkle Capsules (divalproex sodium coated particles in capsules), 125 mg, are white opaque and blue, and are supplied in bottles of 100 (**NDC** 0074-6114-13) and Abbo-Pac® unit dose packages of 100 (**NDC** 0074-6114-11).
Recommended storage: Store capsules below 77°F (25°C).
Revised: June, 2000
ABBOTT LABORATORIES
NORTH CHICAGO, IL 60064, U.S.A.
Shown in Product Identification Guide, page 303

DEPAKOTE® Tablets ℞
[*dəp 'ā-coat*]
DIVALPROEX SODIUM
DELAYED-RELEASE TABLETS

BOX WARNING:

HEPATOTOXICITY:
HEPATIC FAILURE RESULTING IN FATALITIES HAS OCCURRED IN PATIENTS RECEIVING VALPROIC ACID AND ITS DERIVATIVES. EXPERIENCE HAS INDICATED THAT CHILDREN UNDER THE AGE OF TWO YEARS ARE AT A CONSIDERABLY INCREASED RISK OF DEVELOPING FATAL HEPATOTOXICITY, ESPECIALLY THOSE ON MULTIPLE ANTICONVULSANTS, THOSE WITH CONGENITAL METABOLIC DISORDERS, THOSE WITH SEVERE SEIZURE DISORDERS ACCOMPANIED BY MENTAL RETARDATION, AND THOSE WITH ORGANIC BRAIN DISEASE. WHEN DEPAKOTE IS USED IN THIS PATIENT GROUP, IT SHOULD BE USED WITH EXTREME CAUTION AND AS A SOLE AGENT. THE BENEFITS OF THERAPY SHOULD BE WEIGHED AGAINST THE RISKS. ABOVE THIS AGE GROUP, EXPERIENCE IN EPILEPSY HAS INDICATED THAT THE INCIDENCE OF FATAL HEPATOTOXICITY DECREASES CONSIDERABLY IN PROGRESSIVELY OLDER PATIENT GROUPS.
THESE INCIDENTS USUALLY HAVE OCCURRED DURING THE FIRST SIX MONTHS OF TREATMENT. SERIOUS OR FATAL HEPATOTOXICITY MAY BE PRECEDED BY NON-SPECIFIC SYMPTOMS SUCH AS MALAISE, WEAKNESS, LETHARGY, FACIAL EDEMA, ANOREXIA, AND VOMITING. IN PATIENTS WITH EPILEPSY, A LOSS OF SEIZURE CONTROL MAY ALSO OCCUR. PATIENTS SHOULD BE MONITORED CLOSELY FOR APPEARANCE OF THESE SYMPTOMS. LIVER FUNCTION TESTS SHOULD BE PERFORMED PRIOR TO THERAPY AND AT FREQUENT INTERVALS THEREAFTER, ESPECIALLY DURING THE FIRST SIX MONTHS.

TERATOGENICITY:
VALPROATE CAN PRODUCE TERATOGENIC EFFECTS SUCH AS NEURAL TUBE DEFECTS (E.G., SPINA BIFIDA). ACCORDINGLY, THE USE OF DEPAKOTE TABLETS IN WOMEN OF CHILDBEARING POTENTIAL REQUIRES THAT THE BENEFITS OF ITS USE BE WEIGHED AGAINST THE RISK OF INJURY TO THE FETUS. THIS IS ESPECIALLY IMPORTANT WHEN THE TREATMENT OF A SPONTANEOUSLY REVERSIBLE CONDITION NOT ORDINARILY ASSOCIATED WITH PERMANENT INJURY OR RISK OF DEATH (E.G., MIGRAINE) IS CONTEMPLATED. SEE WARNINGS, INFORMATION FOR PATIENTS.
AN INFORMATION SHEET DESCRIBING THE TERATOGENIC POTENTIAL OF VALPROATE IS AVAILABLE FOR PATIENTS.

PANCREATITIS:
CASES OF LIFE-THREATENING PANCREATITIS HAVE BEEN REPORTED IN BOTH CHILDREN AND ADULTS RECEIVING VALPROATE. SOME OF THE CASES HAVE BEEN DESCRIBED AS HEMORRHAGIC WITH A RAPID PROGRESSION FROM INITIAL SYMPTOMS TO DEATH. CASES HAVE BEEN REPORTED SHORTLY AFTER INITIAL USE AS WELL AS AFTER SEVERAL YEARS OF USE. PATIENTS AND GUARDIANS SHOULD BE WARNED THAT ABDOMINAL PAIN, NAUSEA, VOMITING,

Continued on next page

Depakote—Cont.

AND/OR ANOREXIA CAN BE SYMPTOMS OF PANCREATITIS THAT REQUIRE PROMPT MEDICAL EVALUATION. IF PANCREATITIS IS DIAGNOSED, VALPROATE SHOULD ORDINARILY BE DISCONTINUED. ALTERNATIVE TREATMENT FOR THE UNDERLYING MEDICAL CONDITION SHOULD BE INITIATED AS CLINICALLY INDICATED. (See **WARNINGS** and **PRECAUTIONS**.)

DESCRIPTION

Divalproex sodium is a stable co-ordination compound comprised of sodium valproate and valproic acid in a 1:1 molar relationship and formed during the partial neutralization of valproic acid with 0.5 equivalent of sodium hydroxide. Chemically it is designated as sodium hydrogen bis(2-propylpentanoate). Divalproex sodium has the following structure:

$CH_3CH_2CH_2 - CH - CH_2CH_2CH_3$
HO—C=O Na⊕
O=C—O⊖
$CH_3CH_2CH_2 - CH - CH_2CH_2CH_3$
n

Divalproex sodium occurs as a white powder with a characteristic odor.

DEPAKOTE tablets are for oral administration. DEPAKOTE tablets are supplied in three dosage strengths containing divalproex sodium equivalent to 125 mg, 250 mg, or 500 mg of valproic acid.

Inactive Ingredients

DEPAKOTE tablets: cellulosic polymers, diacetylated monoglycerides, povidone, pregelatinized starch (contains corn starch), silica gel, talc, titanium dioxide, and vanillin.

In addition, individual tablets contain:

125 mg tablets: FD&C Blue No. 1 and FD&C Red No. 40.
250 mg tablets: FD&C Yellow No. 6 and iron oxide.
500 mg tablets: D&C Red No. 30, FD&C Blue No. 2, and iron oxide.

CLINICAL PHARMACOLOGY

Pharmacodynamics

Divalproex sodium dissociates to the valproate ion in the gastrointestinal tract. The mechanisms by which valproate exerts its therapeutic effects have not been established. It has been suggested that its activity in epilepsy is related to increased brain concentrations of gamma-aminobutyric acid (GABA).

Pharmacokinetics

Absorption/Bioavailability

Equivalent oral doses of DEPAKOTE (divalproex sodium) products and DEPAKENE (valproic acid) capsules deliver equivalent quantities of valproate ion systemically. Although the rate of valproate ion absorption may vary with the formulation administered (liquid, solid, or sprinkle), conditions of use (e.g., fasting or postprandial) and the method of administration (e.g., whether the contents of the capsule are sprinkled on food or the capsule is taken intact), these differences should be of minor clinical importance under the steady state conditions achieved in chronic use in the treatment of epilepsy.

However, it is possible that differences among the various valproate products in T_{max} and C_{max} could be important upon initiation of treatment. For example, in single dose studies, the effect of feeding had a greater influence on the rate of absorption of the tablet (increase in T_{max} from 4 to 8 hours) than on the absorption of the sprinkle capsules (increase in T_{max} from 3.3 to 4.8 hours).

While the absorption rate from the G.I. tract and fluctuation in valproate plasma concentrations vary with dosing regimen and formulation, the efficacy of valproate as an anticonvulsant in chronic use is unlikely to be affected. Experience employing dosing regimens from once-a-day to four-times-a-day, as well as studies in primate epilepsy models involving constant rate infusion, indicate that total daily systemic bioavailability (extent of absorption) is the primary determinant of seizure control and that differences in the ratios of plasma peak to trough concentrations between valproate formulations are inconsequential from a practical clinical standpoint. Whether or not rate of absorption influences the efficacy of valproate as an antimanic or antimigraine agent is unknown.

Co-administration of oral valproate products with food and substitution among the various DEPAKOTE and DEPAKENE formulations should cause no clinical problems in the management of patients with epilepsy (see **DOSAGE AND ADMINISTRATION**). Nonetheless, any changes in dosage administration, or the addition or discontinuance of concomitant drugs should ordinarily be accompanied by close monitoring of clinical status and valproate plasma concentrations.

Distribution

Protein Binding:

The plasma protein binding of valproate is concentration dependent and the free fraction increases from approximately 10% at 40 μg/mL to 18.5% at 130 μg/mL. Protein binding of valproate is reduced in the elderly, in patients with chronic hepatic diseases, in patients with renal impairment, and in the presence of other drugs (e.g., aspirin). Conversely, valproate may displace certain protein-bound drugs (e.g., phenytoin, carbamazepine, warfarin, and tolbutamide). (See **PRECAUTIONS, Drug Interactions** for more detailed information on the pharmacokinetic interactions of valproate with other drugs.)

CNS Distribution:

Valproate concentrations in cerebrospinal fluid (CSF) approximate unbound concentrations in plasma (about 10% of total concentration).

Metabolism

Valproate is metabolized almost entirely by the liver. In adult patients on monotherapy, 30–50% of an administered dose appears in urine as a glucuronide conjugate. Mitochondrial β-oxidation is the other major metabolic pathway, typically accounting for over 40% of the dose. Usually, less than 15–20% of the dose is eliminated by other oxidative mechanisms. Less than 3% of an administered dose is excreted unchanged in urine.

The relationship between dose and total valproate concentration is nonlinear; concentration does not increase proportionally with the dose, but rather, increases to a lesser extent due to saturable plasma protein binding. The kinetics of unbound drug are linear.

Elimination

Mean plasma clearance and volume of distribution for total valproate are 0.56 L/hr/1.73 m^2 and 11 L/1.73 m^2, respectively. Mean plasma clearance and volume of distribution for free valproate are 4.6 L/hr/1.73 m^2 and 92 L/1.73 m^2. Mean terminal half-life for valproate monotherapy ranged from 9 to 16 hours following oral dosing regimens of 250 to 1000 mg.

The estimates cited apply primarily to patients who are not taking drugs that affect hepatic metabolizing enzyme systems. For example, patients taking enzyme-inducing antiepileptic drugs (carbamazepine, phenytoin, and phenobarbital) will clear valproate more rapidly. Because of these changes in valproate clearance, monitoring of antiepileptic concentrations should be intensified whenever concomitant antiepileptics are introduced or withdrawn.

Special Populations

Effect of Age:

Neonates - Children within the first two months of life have a markedly decreased ability to eliminate valproate compared to older children and adults. This is a result of reduced clearance (perhaps due to delay in development of glucuronosyltransferase and other enzyme systems involved in valproate elimination) as well as increased volume of distribution (in part due to decreased plasma protein binding). For example, in one study, the half-life in children under 10 days ranged from 10 to 67 hours compared to a range of 7 to 13 hours in children greater than 2 months.

Children - Pediatric patients (i.e., between 3 months and 10 years) have 50% higher clearances expressed on weight (i.e., mL/min/kg) than do adults. Over the age of 10 years, children have pharmacokinetic parameters that approximate those of adults.

Elderly - The capacity of elderly patients (age range: 68 to 89 years) to eliminate valproate has been shown to be reduced compared to younger adults (age range: 22 to 26). Intrinsic clearance is reduced by 39%; the free fraction is increased by 44%. Accordingly, the initial dosage should be reduced in the elderly. (See **DOSAGE AND ADMINISTRATION**).

Effect of Gender:

There are no differences in the body surface area adjusted unbound clearance between males and females (4.8±0.17 and 4.7±0.07 L/hr per 1.73 m^2, respectively).

Effect of Race:

The effects of race on the kinetics of valproate have not been studied.

Effect of Disease:

Liver Disease—(See **BOXED WARNING, CONTRAINDICATIONS**, and **WARNINGS**). Liver disease impairs the capacity to eliminate valproate. In one study, the clearance of free valproate was decreased by 50% in 7 patients with cirrhosis and by 16% in 4 patients with acute hepatitis, compared with 6 healthy subjects. In that study, the half-life of valproate was increased from 12 to 18 hours. Liver disease is also associated with decreased albumin concentrations and larger unbound fractions (2 to 2.6 fold increase) of valproate. Accordingly, monitoring of total concentrations may be misleading since free concentrations may be substantially elevated in patients with hepatic disease whereas total concentrations may appear to be normal.

Renal Disease—A slight reduction (27%) in the unbound clearance of valproate has been reported in patients with renal failure (creatinine clearance < 10 mL/minute); however, hemodialysis typically reduces valproate concentrations by about 20%. Therefore, no dosage adjustment appears to be necessary in patients with renal failure. Protein binding in these patients is substantially reduced; thus, monitoring total concentrations may be misleading.

Plasma Levels and Clinical Effect

The relationship between plasma concentration and clinical response is not well documented. One contributing factor is the nonlinear, concentration dependent protein binding of valproate which affects the clearance of the drug. Thus, monitoring of total serum valproate cannot provide a reliable index of the bioactive valproate species.

For example, because the plasma protein binding of valproate is concentration dependent, the free fraction increases from approximately 10% at 40 μg/mL to 18.5% at 130 μg/mL. Higher than expected free fractions occur in the elderly, in hyperlipidemic patients, and in patients with hepatic and renal diseases.

Epilepsy:

The therapeutic range in epilepsy is commonly considered to be 50 to 100 μg/mL of total valproate, although some patients may be controlled with lower or higher plasma concentrations.

Mania:

In placebo-controlled clinical trials of acute mania, patients were dosed to clinical response with trough plasma concentrations between 50 and 125 μg/mL (See **DOSAGE AND ADMINISTRATION**).

Clinical Trials

Mania

The effectiveness of DEPAKOTE for the treatment of acute mania was demonstrated in two 3-week, placebo controlled, parallel group studies.

(1) Study 1: The first study enrolled adult patients who met DSM-III-R criteria for Bipolar Disorder and who were hospitalized for acute mania. In addition, they had a history of failing to respond to or not tolerating previous lithium carbonate treatment. DEPAKOTE was initiated at a dose of 250 mg tid and adjusted to achieve serum valproate concentrations in a range of 50–100 μg/mL by day 7. Mean DEPAKOTE doses for completers in this study were 1118, 1525, and 2402 mg/day at days 7, 14, and 21, respectively. Patients were assessed on the Young Mania Rating Scale (YMRS; score ranges from 0–60), an augmented Brief Psychiatric Rating Scale (BPRS-A), and the Global Assessment Scale (GAS). Baseline scores and change from baseline in the week 3 endpoint (last-observation-carry-forward) analysis were as follows:

Study 1

YMRS Total Score

Group	Baseline[1]	BL to Wk 3[2]	Difference[3]
Placebo	28.8	+ 0.2	
DEPAKOTE	28.5	− 9.5	9.7

BPRS-A Total Score

Group	Baseline[1]	BL to Wk 3[2]	Difference[3]
Placebo	76.2	+ 1.8	
DEPAKOTE	76.4	− 17.0	18.8

GAS Score

Group	Baseline[1]	BL to Wk 3[2]	Difference[3]
Placebo	31.8	0.0	
DEPAKOTE	30.3	+ 18.1	18.1

1 Mean score at baseline
2 Change from baseline to week 3 (LOCF)
3 Difference in change from baseline to week 3 endpoint (LOCF) between DEPAKOTE and placebo

DEPAKOTE was statistically significantly superior to placebo on all three measures of outcome.

(2) Study 2: The second study enrolled adult patients who met Research Diagnostic Criteria for manic disorder and who were hospitalized for acute mania. DEPAKOTE was initiated at a dose of 250 mg tid and adjusted within a dose range of 750–2500 mg/day to achieve serum valproate concentrations in a range of 40–150 μg/mL. Mean DEPAKOTE doses for completers in this study were 1116, 1683, and 2006 mg/day at days 7, 14, and 21, respectively. Study 2 also included a lithium group for which lithium doses for completers were 1312, 1869, and 1984 mg/day at days 7, 14, and 21, respectively. Patients were assessed on the Manic Rating Scale (MRS; score ranges from 11–63), and the primary outcome measures were the total MRS score, and scores for two subscales of the MRS, i.e., the Manic Syndrome Scale (MSS) and the Behavior and Ideation Scale (BIS). Baseline scores and change from baseline in the week 3 endpoint (last-observation-carry-forward) analysis were as follows:

Study 2

MRS Total Score

Group	Baseline[1]	BL to Day 21[2]	Difference[3]
Placebo	38.9	−4.4	
Lithium	37.9	−10.5	6.1
DEPAKOTE	38.1	−9.5	5.1

MSS Total Score

Group	Baseline[1]	BL to Day 21[2]	Difference[3]
Placebo	18.9	−2.5	
Lithium	18.5	−6.2	3.7
DEPAKOTE	18.9	−6.0	3.5

BIS Total Score

Group	Baseline[1]	BL to Day 21[2]	Difference[3]
Placebo	16.4	−1.4	
Lithium	16.0	−3.8	2.4
DEPAKOTE	15.7	−3.2	1.8

1 Mean score at baseline
2 Change from baseline to day 21 (LOCF)

3 Difference in change from baseline to day 21 endpoint (LOCF) between DEPAKOTE and placebo and lithium and placebo

DEPAKOTE was statistically significantly superior to placebo on all three measures of outcome. An exploratory analysis for age and gender effects on outcome did not suggest any differential responsiveness on the basis of age or gender.

A comparison of the percentage of patients showing ≥ 30% reduction in the symptom score from baseline in each treatment group, separated by study, is shown in Figure 1.

Figure 1
Percentage of Patients Achieving ≥ 30% Reduction in Symptom Score From Baseline

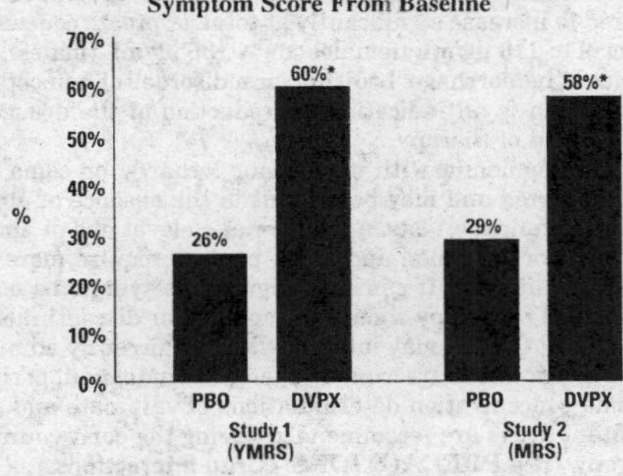

* $p < 0.05$
PBO = placebo, DVPX = DEPAKOTE

Migraine

The results of two multicenter, randomized, double-blind, placebo-controlled clinical trials established the effectiveness of DEPAKOTE in the prophylactic treatment of migraine headache.

Both studies employed essentially identical designs and recruited patients with a history of migraine with or without aura (of at least 6 months in duration) who were experiencing at least 2 migraine headaches a month during the 3 months prior to enrollment. Patients with cluster headaches were excluded. Women of childbearing potential were excluded entirely from one study, but were permitted in the other if they were deemed to be practicing an effective method of contraception.

In each study following a 4-week single-blind placebo baseline period, patients were randomized, under double blind conditions, to DEPAKOTE or placebo for a 12-week treatment phase, comprised of a 4-week dose titration period followed by an 8-week maintenance period. Treatment outcome was assessed on the basis of 4-week migraine headache rates during the treatment phase.

In the first study, a total of 107 patients (24 M, 83 F), ranging in age from 26 to 73 were randomized 2:1, DEPAKOTE to placebo. Ninety patients completed the 8-week maintenance period. Drug dose titration, using 250 mg tablets, was individualized at the investigator's discretion. Adjustments were guided by actual/sham trough total serum valproate levels in order to maintain the study blind. In patients on DEPAKOTE doses ranged from 500 to 2500 mg a day. Doses over 500 mg were given in three divided doses (TID). The mean dose during the treatment phase was 1087 mg/day resulting in a mean trough total valproate level of 72.5 µg/mL, with a range of 31 to 133 µg/mL.

The mean 4-week migraine headache rate during the treatment phase was 5.7 in the placebo group compared to 3.5 in the DEPAKOTE group (see Figure 2). These rates were significantly different.

In the second study, a total of 176 patients (19 males and 157 females), ranging in age from 17 to 76 years, were randomized equally to one of three DEPAKOTE dose groups (500, 1000, or 1500 mg/day) or placebo. The treatments were given in two divided doses (BID). One hundred thirty-seven patients completed the 8-week maintenance period. Efficacy was to be determined by a comparison of the 4-week migraine headache rate in the combined 1000/1500 mg/day group and placebo group.

The initial dose was 250 mg daily. The regimen was advanced by 250 mg every 4 days (8 days for 500 mg/day group), until the randomized dose was achieved. The mean trough total valproate levels during the treatment phase were 39.6, 62.5, and 72.5 µg/mL in the DEPAKOTE 500, 1000, and 1500 mg/day groups, respectively.

The mean 4-week migraine headache rates during the treatment phase, adjusted for differences in baseline rates, were 4.5 in the placebo group, compared to 3.3, 3.0, and 3.3 in the DEPAKOTE 500, 1000, and 1500 mg/day groups, respectively, based on intent-to-treat results (see Figure 2). Migraine headache rates in the combined DEPAKOTE 1000/1500 mg group were significantly lower than in the placebo group.

[See figure 2 at top of next column]

Figure 2
Mean 4-week Migraine Rates

1 Mean dose of DEPAKOTE was 1087 mg/day.
2 Dose of DEPAKOTE was 500 or 1000 mg/day.

Epilepsy

The efficacy of DEPAKOTE in reducing the incidence of complex partial seizures (CPS) that occur in isolation or in association with other seizure types was established in two controlled trials.

In one, multiclinic, placebo controlled study employing an add-on design, (adjunctive therapy) 144 patients who continued to suffer eight or more CPS per 8 weeks during an 8 week period of monotherapy with doses of either carbamazepine or phenytoin sufficient to assure plasma concentrations within the "therapeutic range" were randomized to receive, in addition to their original antiepilepsy drug (AED), either DEPAKOTE or placebo. Randomized patients were to be followed for a total of 16 weeks. The following table presents the findings.

Adjunctive Therapy Study
Median Incidence of CPS per 8 Weeks

Add-on Treatment	Number of Patients	Baseline Incidence	Experimental Incidence
DEPAKOTE	75	16.0	8.9*
Placebo	69	14.5	11.5

*Reduction from baseline statistically signficantly greater for DEPAKOTE than placebo at $p \leq 0.05$ level.

Figure 3 presents the proportion of patients (X axis) whose percentage reduction from baseline in complex partial seizure rates was at least as great as that indicated on the Y axis in the adjunctive therapy study. A positive percent reduction indicates an improvement (i.e., a decrease in seizure frequency), while a negative percent reduction indicates worsening. Thus, in a display of this type, the curve for an effective treatment is shifted to the left of the curve for placebo. This figure shows that the proportion of patients achieving any particular level of improvement was consistently higher for DEPAKOTE than for placebo. For example, 45% of patients treated with DEPAKOTE had a ≥ 50% reduction in complex partial seizure rate compared to 23% of patients treated with placebo.

Figure 3

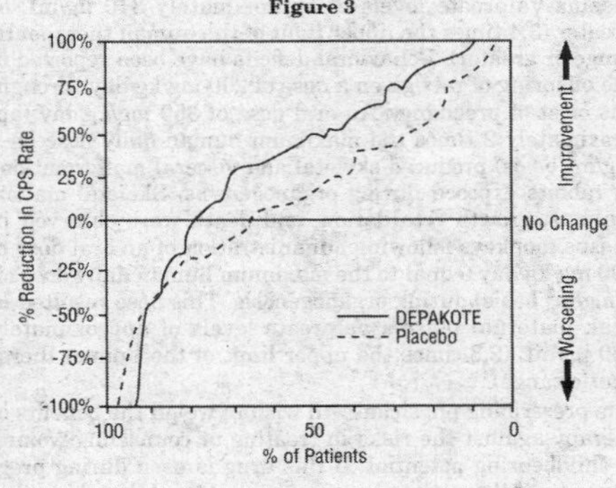

The second study assessed the capacity of DEPAKOTE to reduce the incidence of CPS when administered as the sole AED. The study compared the incidence of CPS among patients randomized to either a high or low dose treatment arm. Patients qualified for entry into the randomized comparison phase of this study only if 1) they continued to experience 2 or more CPS per 4 weeks during an 8 to 12 week long period of monotherapy with adequate doses of an AED (i.e., phenytoin, carbamazepine, phenobarbital, or primidone) and 2) they made a successful transition over a two week interval to DEPAKOTE. Patients entering the randomized phase were then brought to their assigned target dose, gradually tapered off their concomitant AED and followed for an interval as long as 22 weeks. Less than 50% of the patients randomized, however, completed the study. In patients converted to DEPAKOTE monotherapy, the mean total valproate concentrations during monotherapy were 71 and 123 µg/mL in the low dose and high dose groups, respectively.

The following table presents the findings for all patients randomized who had at least one post-randomization assessment.

Monotherapy Study
Median Incidence of CPS per 8 Weeks

Treatment	Number of Patients	Baseline Incidence	Randomized Phase Incidence
High dose			
DEPAKOTE	131	13.2	10.7*
Low dose			
DEPAKOTE	134	14.2	13.8

*Reduction from baseline statistically significantly greater for high dose than low dose at $p \leq 0.05$ level.

Figure 4 presents the proportion of patients (X axis) whose percentage reduction from baseline in complex partial seizure rates was at least as great as that indicated on the Y axis in the monotherapy study. A positive percent reduction indicates an improvement (i.e., a decrease in seizure frequency), while a negative percent reduction indicates worsening. Thus, in a display of this type, the curve for a more effective treatment is shifted to the left of the curve for a less effective treatment. This figure shows that the proportion of patients achieving any particular level of reduction was consistently higher for high dose DEPAKOTE than for low dose DEPAKOTE. For example, when switching from carbamazepine, phenytoin, phenobarbital or primidone monotherapy to high dose DEPAKOTE monotherapy, 63% of patients experienced no change or a reduction in complex partial seizure rates compared to 54% of patients receiving low dose DEPAKOTE.

Figure 4

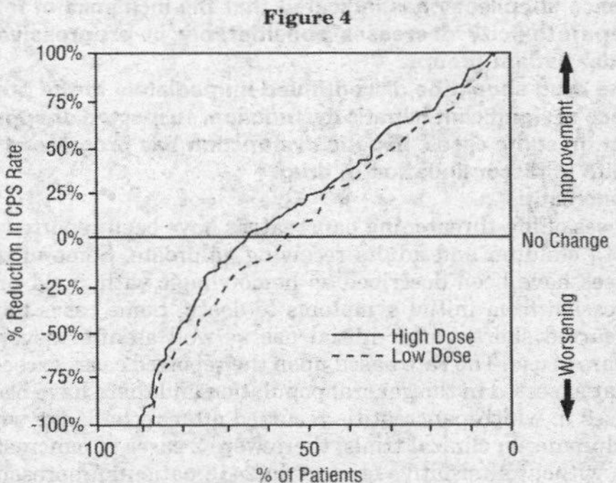

INDICATIONS AND USAGE

Mania

DEPAKOTE (divalproex sodium) is indicated for the treatment of the manic episodes associated with bipolar disorder. A manic episode is a distinct period of abnormally and persistently elevated, expansive, or irritable mood. Typical symptoms of mania include pressure of speech, motor hyperactivity, reduced need for sleep, flight of ideas, grandiosity, poor judgement, aggressiveness, and possible hostility. The efficacy of DEPAKOTE was established in 3-week trials with patients meeting DSM-III-R criteria for bipolar disorder who were hospitalized for acute mania (See **Clinical Trials** under **CLINICAL PHARMACOLOGY**).

The safety and effectiveness of DEPAKOTE for long-term use in mania, i.e., more than 3 weeks, has not been systematically evaluated in controlled clinical trials. Therefore, physicians who elect to use DEPAKOTE for extended periods should continually reevaluate the long-term usefulness of the drug for the individual patient.

Epilepsy

DEPAKOTE (divalproex sodium) is indicated as monotherapy and adjunctive therapy in the treatment of patients with complex partial seizures that occur either in isolation or in association with other types of seizures. DEPAKOTE (divalproex sodium) is also indicated for use as sole and adjunctive therapy in the treatment of simple and complex absence seizures, and adjunctively in patients with multiple seizure types that include absence seizures.

Simple absence is defined as very brief clouding of the sensorium or loss of consciousness accompanied by certain generalized epileptic discharges without other detectable clinical signs. Complex absence is the term used when other signs are also present.

Migraine

DEPAKOTE is indicated for prophylaxis of migraine headaches. There is no evidence that DEPAKOTE is useful in the acute treatment of migraine headaches. Because valproic acid may be a hazard to the fetus, DEPAKOTE should be considered for women of childbearing potential only after this risk has been thoroughly discussed with the patient and weighed against the potential benefits of treatment (see **WARNINGS - Usage In Pregnancy, PRECAUTIONS - Information for Patients**).

SEE **WARNINGS** FOR STATEMENT REGARDING FATAL HEPATIC DYSFUNCTION.

CONTRAINDICATIONS

DIVALPROEX SODIUM SHOULD NOT BE ADMINISTERED TO PATIENTS WITH HEPATIC DISEASE OR SIGNIFICANT HEPATIC DYSFUNCTION.

Divalproex sodium is contraindicated in patients with known hypersensitivity to the drug.

Continued on next page

Depakote—Cont.

WARNINGS

Hepatotoxicity

Hepatic failure resulting in fatalities has occurred in patients receiving valproic acid. These incidents usually have occurred during the first six months of treatment. Serious or fatal hepatotoxicity may be preceded by non-specific symptoms such as malaise, weakness, lethargy, facial edema, anorexia, and vomiting. In patients with epilepsy, a loss of seizure control may also occur. Patients should be monitored closely for appearance of these symptoms. Liver function tests should be performed prior to therapy and at frequent intervals thereafter, especially during the first six months. However, physicians should not rely totally on serum biochemistry since these tests may not be abnormal in all instances, but should also consider the results of careful interim medical history and physical examination. Caution should be observed when administering DEPAKOTE products to patients with a prior history of hepatic disease. Patients on multiple anticonvulsants, children, those with congenital metabolic disorders, those with severe seizure disorders accompanied by mental retardation, and those with organic brain disease may be at particular risk. Experience has indicated that children under the age of two years are at a considerably increased risk of developing fatal hepatotoxicity, especially those with the aforementioned conditions. When DEPAKOTE is used in this patient group, it should be used with extreme caution and as a sole agent. The benefits of therapy should be weighed against the risks. Above this age group, experience in epilepsy has indicated that the incidence of fatal hepatotoxicity decreases considerably in progressively older patient groups.

The drug should be discontinued immediately in the presence of significant hepatic dysfunction, suspected or apparent. In some cases, hepatic dysfunction has progressed in spite of discontinuation of drug.

Pancreatitis

Cases of life-threatening pancreatitis have been reported in both children and adults receiving valproate. Some of the cases have been described as hemorrhagic with rapid progression from initial symptoms to death. Some cases have occurred shortly after initial use as well as after several years of use. The rate based upon the reported cases exceeds that expected in the general population and there have been cases in which pancreatitis recurred after rechallenge with valproate. In clinical trials, there were 2 cases of pancreatitis without alternative etiology in 2416 patients, representing 1044 patient-years experience. Patients and guardians should be warned that abdominal pain, nausea, vomiting, and/or anorexia can be symptoms of pancreatitis that require prompt medical evaluation. If pancreatitis is diagnosed, valproate should ordinarily be discontinued. Alternative treatment for the underlying medical condition should be initiated as clinically indicated (see **BOXED WARNING**).

Somnolence in the Elderly

In a double-blind, multicenter trial of valproate in elderly patients with dementia (mean age = 83 years), doses were increased by 125 mg/day to a target dose of 20 mg/kg/day. A significantly higher proportion of valproate patients had somnolence compared to placebo, and although not statistically significant, there was a higher proportion of patients with dehydration. Discontinuations for somnolence were also significantly higher than with placebo. In some patients with somnolence (approximately one-half), there was associated reduced nutritional intake and weight loss. There was a trend for the patients who experienced these events to have a lower baseline albumin concentration, lower valproate clearance, and a higher BUN. In elderly patients, dosage should be increased more slowly and with regular monitoring for fluid and nutritional intake, dehydration, somnolence, and other adverse events. Dose reductions or discontinuation of valproate should be considered in patients with decreased food or fluid intake and in patients with excessive somnolence (see **DOSAGE AND ADMINISTRATION**).

Thrombocytopenia

The frequency of adverse effects (particularly elevated liver enzymes and thrombocytopenia [see **PRECAUTIONS**]) may be dose-related. In a clinical trial of DEPAKOTE as monotherapy in patients with epilepsy, 34/126 patients (27%) receiving approximately 50 mg/kg/day on average, had at least one value of platelets $\leq 75 \times 10^9$/L. Approximately half of these patients had treatment discontinued, with return of platelet counts to normal. In the remaining patients, platelet counts normalized with continued treatment. In this study, the probability of thrombocytopenia appeared to increase significantly at total valproate concentrations of ≥ 110 µg/mL (females) or ≥ 135 µg/mL (males). The therapeutic benefit which may accompany the higher doses should therefore be weighed against the possibility of a greater incidence of adverse effects.

Usage In Pregnancy

ACCORDING TO PUBLISHED AND UNPUBLISHED REPORTS, VALPROIC ACID MAY PRODUCE TERATOGENIC EFFECTS IN THE OFFSPRING OF HUMAN FEMALES RECEIVING THE DRUG DURING PREGNANCY. THERE ARE MULTIPLE REPORTS IN THE CLINICAL LITERATURE WHICH INDICATE THAT THE USE OF ANTIEPILEPTIC DRUGS DURING PREGNANCY RESULTS IN AN INCREASED INCIDENCE OF BIRTH DEFECTS IN THE OFFSPRING. ALTHOUGH DATA ARE MORE EXTENSIVE WITH RESPECT TO TRIMETHADIONE, PARAMETHADIONE, PHENYTOIN, AND PHENOBARBITAL, REPORTS INDICATE A POSSIBLE SIMILAR ASSOCIATION WITH THE USE OF OTHER ANTIEPILEPTIC DRUGS. THEREFORE, ANTIEPILEPSY DRUGS SHOULD BE ADMINISTERED TO WOMEN OF CHILDBEARING POTENTIAL ONLY IF THEY ARE CLEARLY SHOWN TO BE ESSENTIAL IN THE MANAGEMENT OF THEIR SEIZURES.

THE INCIDENCE OF NEURAL TUBE DEFECTS IN THE FETUS MAY BE INCREASED IN MOTHERS RECEIVING VALPROATE DURING THE FIRST TRIMESTER OF PREGNANCY. THE CENTERS FOR DISEASE CONTROL (CDC) HAS ESTIMATED THE RISK OF VALPROIC ACID EXPOSED WOMEN HAVING CHILDREN WITH SPINA BIFIDA TO BE APPROXIMATELY 1 TO 2%.

OTHER CONGENITAL ANOMALIES (EG, CRANIOFACIAL DEFECTS, CARDIOVASCULAR MALFORMATIONS AND ANOMALIES INVOLVING VARIOUS BODY SYSTEMS), COMPATIBLE AND INCOMPATIBLE WITH LIFE, HAVE BEEN REPORTED. SUFFICIENT DATA TO DETERMINE THE INCIDENCE OF THESE CONGENITAL ANOMALIES IS NOT AVAILABLE.

THE HIGHER INCIDENCE OF CONGENITAL ANOMALIES IN ANTIEPILEPTIC DRUG-TREATED WOMEN WITH SEIZURE DISORDERS CANNOT BE REGARDED AS A CAUSE AND EFFECT RELATIONSHIP. THERE ARE INTRINSIC METHODOLOGIC PROBLEMS IN OBTAINING ADEQUATE DATA ON DRUG TERATOGENICITY IN HUMANS; GENETIC FACTORS OR THE EPILEPTIC CONDITION ITSELF, MAY BE MORE IMPORTANT THAN DRUG THERAPY IN CONTRIBUTING TO CONGENITAL ANOMALIES.

PATIENTS TAKING VALPROATE MAY DEVELOP CLOTTING ABNORMALITIES. A PATIENT WHO HAD LOW FIBRINOGEN WHEN TAKING MULTIPLE ANTICONVULSANTS INCLUDING VALPROATE GAVE BIRTH TO AN INFANT WITH AFIBRINOGENEMIA WHO SUBSEQUENTLY DIED OF HEMORRHAGE. IF VALPROATE IS USED IN PREGNANCY, THE CLOTTING PARAMETERS SHOULD BE MONITORED CAREFULLY.

HEPATIC FAILURE, RESULTING IN THE DEATH OF A NEWBORN AND OF AN INFANT, HAVE BEEN REPORTED FOLLOWING THE USE OF VALPROATE DURING PREGNANCY.

Animal studies have demonstrated valproate-induced teratogenicity. Increased frequencies of malformations, as well as intrauterine growth retardation and death, have been observed in mice, rats, rabbits, and monkeys following prenatal exposure to valproate. Malformations of the skeletal system are the most common structural abnormalities produced in experimental animals, but neural tube closure defects have been seen in mice exposed to maternal plasma valproate concentrations exceeding 230 µg/mL (2.3 times the upper limit of the human therapeutic range) during susceptible periods of embryonic development. Administration of an oral dose of 200 mg/kg/day or greater (50% of the maximum human daily dose or greater on a mg/m^2 basis) to pregnant rats during organogenesis produced malformations (skeletal, cardiac, and urogenital) and growth retardation in the offspring. These doses resulted in peak maternal plasma valproate levels of approximately 340 µg/mL or greater (3.4 times the upper limit of the human therapeutic range or greater). Behavioral deficits have been reported in the offspring of rats given a dose of 200 mg/kg/day throughout most of pregnancy. An oral dose of 350 mg/kg/day (approximately 2 times the maximum human daily dose on a mg/m^2 basis) produced skeletal and visceral malformations in rabbits exposed during organogenesis. Skeletal malformations, growth retardation, and death were observed in rhesus monkeys following administration of an oral dose of 200 mg/kg/day (equal to the maximum human daily dose on a mg/m^2 basis) during organogenesis. This dose resulted in peak maternal plasma valproate levels of approximately 280 µg/mL (2.8 times the upper limit of the human therapeutic range).

The prescribing physician will wish to weigh the benefits of therapy against the risks in treating or counseling women of childbearing potential. If this drug is used during pregnancy, or if the patient becomes pregnant while taking this drug, the patient should be apprised of the potential hazard to the fetus.

Antiepileptic drugs should not be discontinued abruptly in patients in whom the drug is administered to prevent major seizures because of the strong possibility of precipitating status epilepticus with attendant hypoxia and threat to life. In individual cases where the severity and frequency of the seizure disorder are such that the removal of medication does not pose a serious threat to the patient, discontinuation of the drug may be considered prior to and during pregnancy, although it cannot be said with any confidence that even minor seizures do not pose some hazard to the developing embryo or fetus.

Tests to detect neural tube and other defects using current accepted procedures should be considered a part of routine prenatal care in childbearing women receiving valproate.

PRECAUTIONS

Hepatic Dysfunction

See **BOXED WARNING, CONTRAINDICATIONS** and **WARNINGS.**

Pancreatitis

See **BOXED WARNING** and **WARNINGS**.

General

Because of reports of thrombocytopenia (see **WARNINGS**), inhibition of the secondary phase of platelet aggregation, and abnormal coagulation parameters, (e.g., low fibrinogen), platelet counts and coagulation tests are recommended before initiating therapy and at periodic intervals. It is recommended that patients receiving DEPAKOTE be monitored for platelet count and coagulation parameters prior to planned surgery. In a clinical trial of DEPAKOTE as monotherapy in patients with epilepsy, 34/126 patients (27%) receiving approximately 50 mg/kg/day on average, had at least one value of platelets $\leq 75 \times 10^9$/L. Approximately half of these patients had treatment discontinued, with return of platelet counts to normal. In the remaining patients, platelet counts normalized with continued treatment. In this study, the probability of thrombocytopenia appeared to increase significantly at total valproate concentrations of ≥ 110 µg/mL (females) or ≥ 135 µg/mL (males). Evidence of hemorrhage, bruising, or a disorder of hemostasis/coagulation is an indication for reduction of the dosage or withdrawal of therapy.

Hyperammonemia with or without lethargy or coma has been reported and may be present in the absence of abnormal liver function tests. Asymptomatic elevations of ammonia are more common and when present require more frequent monitoring. If clinically significant symptoms occur, DEPAKOTE therapy should be modified or discontinued.

Since DEPAKOTE may interact with concurrently administered drugs which are capable of enzyme induction, periodic plasma concentration determinations of valproate and concomitant drugs are recommended during the early course of therapy. (See **PRECAUTIONS - Drug Interactions**.)

Valproate is partially eliminated in the urine as a keto-metabolite which may lead to a false interpretation of the urine ketone test.

There have been reports of altered thyroid function tests associated with valproate. The clinical significance of these is unknown.

Suicidal ideation may be a manifestation of certain psychiatric disorders, and may persist until significant remission of symptoms occurs. Close supervision of high risk patients should accompany initial drug therapy.

There are *in vitro* studies that suggest valproate stimulates the replication of the HIV and CMV viruses under certain experimental conditions. The clinical consequence, if any, is not known. Additionally, the relevance of these *in vitro* findings is uncertain for patients receiving maximally suppressive antiretroviral therapy. Nevertheless, these data should be borne in mind when interpreting the results from regular monitoring of the viral load in HIV infected patients receiving valproate or when following CMV infected patients clinically.

Information for Patients

Patients and guardians should be warned that abdominal pain, nausea, vomiting, and/or anorexia can be symptoms of pancreatitis and, therefore, require further medical evaluation promptly.

Since DEPAKOTE products may produce CNS depression, especially when combined with another CNS depressant (eg, alcohol), patients should be advised not to engage in hazardous activities, such as driving an automobile or operating dangerous machinery, until it is known that they do not become drowsy from the drug.

Migraine Patients: Since DEPAKOTE has been associated with certain types of birth defects, female patients of child-bearing age considering the use of DEPAKOTE for the prevention of migraine should be advised to read the **Patient Information Leaflet**, which appears as the last section of the labeling.

Drug Interactions

Effects of Co-Administered Drugs on Valproate Clearance

Drugs that affect the level of expression of hepatic enzymes, particularly those that elevate levels of glucuronosyltransferases, may increase the clearance of valproate. For example, phenytoin, carbamazepine, and phenobarbital (or primidone) can double the clearance of valproate. Thus, patients on monotherapy will generally have longer half-lives and higher concentrations than patients receiving polytherapy with antiepilepsy drugs.

In contrast, drugs that are inhibitors of cytochrome P450 isozymes, e.g., antidepressants, may be expected to have little effect on valproate clearance because cytochrome P450 microsomal mediated oxidation is a relatively minor secondary metabolic pathway compared to glucuronidation and β-oxidation.

Because of these changes in valproate clearance, monitoring of valproate and concomitant drug concentrations should be increased whenever enzyme inducing drugs are introduced or withdrawn.

The following list provides information about the potential for an influence of several commonly prescribed medications on valproate pharmacokinetics. The list is not exhaustive nor could it be, since new interactions are continuously being reported.

Drugs for which a potentially important interaction has been observed:

Aspirin—A study involving the co-administration of aspirin at antipyretic doses (11 to 16 mg/kg) with valproate to pediatric patients (n=6) revealed a decrease in protein binding and an inhibition of metabolism of valproate. Valproate free fraction was increased 4-fold in the presence of aspirin compared to valproate alone. The β-oxidation pathway consisting of 2-E-valproic acid, 3-OH-valproic acid, and 3-keto valproic acid was decreased from 25% of total metabolites excreted on valproate alone to 8.3% in the presence of aspirin. Caution should be observed if valproate and aspirin are to be co-administered.

Felbamate—A study involving the co-administration of 1200 mg/day of felbamate with valproate to patients with epilepsy (n=10) revealed an increase in mean valproate peak concentration by 35% (from 86 to 115 μg/mL) compared to valproate alone. Increasing the felbamate dose to 2400 mg/day increased the mean valproate peak concentration to 133 μg/mL (another 16% increase). A decrease in valproate dosage may be necessary when felbamate therapy is initiated.

Rifampin—A study involving the administration of a single dose of valproate (7 mg/kg) 36 hours after 5 nights of daily dosing with rifampin (600 mg) revealed a 40% increase in the oral clearance of valproate. Valproate dosage adjustment may be necessary when it is co-administered with rifampin.

Drugs for which either no interaction or a likely clinically unimportant interaction has been observed:

Antacids—A study involving the co-administration of valproate 500 mg with commonly administered antacids (Maalox, Trisogel, and Titralac—160 mEq doses) did not reveal any effect on the extent of absorption of valproate.

Chlorpromazine—A study involving the administration of 100 to 300 mg/day of chlorpromazine to schizophrenic patients already receiving valproate (200 mg BID) revealed a 15% increase in trough plasma levels of valproate.

Haloperidol—A study involving the administration of 6 to 10 mg/day of haloperidol to schizophrenic patients already receiving valproate (200 mg BID) revealed no significant changes in valproate trough plasma levels.

Cimetidine and Ranitidine—Cimetidine and ranitidine do not affect the clearance of valproate.

Effects of Valproate on Other Drugs

Valproate has been found to be a weak inhibitor of some P450 isozymes, epoxide hydrase, and glucuronosyltransferases.

The following list provides information about the potential for an influence of valproate co-administration on the pharmacokinetics or pharmacodynamics of several commonly prescribed medications. The list is not exhaustive, since new interactions are continuously being reported.

Drugs for which a potentially important valproate interaction has been observed:

Amitriptyline/Nortriptyline—Administration of a single oral 50 mg dose of amitriptyline to 15 normal volunteers (10 males and 5 females) who received valproate (500 mg BID) resulted in a 21% decrease in plasma clearance of amitriptyline and a 34% decrease in the net clearance of nortriptyline. Rare postmarketing reports of concurrent use of valproate and amitriptyline resulting in an increased amitriptyline level have been received. Concurrent use of valproate and amitriptyline has rarely been associated with toxicity. Monitoring of amitriptyline levels should be considered for patients taking valproate concomitantly with amitriptyline. Consideration should be given to lowering the dose of amitriptyline/nortriptyline in the presence of valproate.

Carbamazepine/carbamazepine-10,11-Epoxide—Serum levels of carbamazepine (CBZ) decreased 17% while that of carbamazepine-10,11-epoxide (CBZ-E) increased by 45% upon co-administration of valproate and CBZ to epileptic patients.

Clonazepam—The concomitant use of valproic acid and clonazepam may induce absence status in patients with a history of absence type seizures.

Diazepam—Valproate displaces diazepam from its plasma albumin binding sites and inhibits its metabolism. Co-administration of valproate (1500 mg daily) increased the free fraction of diazepam (10 mg) by 90% in healthy volunteers (n=6). Plasma clearance and volume of distribution for free diazepam were reduced by 25% and 20%, respectively, in the presence of valproate. The elimination half-life of diazepam remained unchanged upon addition of valproate.

Ethosuximide—Valproate inhibits the metabolism of ethosuximide. Administration of a single ethosuximide dose of 500 mg with valproate (800 to 1600 mg/day) to healthy volunteers (n=6) was accompanied by a 25% increase in elimination half-life of ethosuximide and a 15% decrease in its total clearance as compared to ethosuximide alone. Patients receiving valproate and ethosuximide, especially along with other anticonvulsants, should be monitored for alterations in serum concentrations of both drugs.

Lamotrigine—In a steady-state study involving 10 healthy volunteers, the elimination half-life of lamotrigine increased from 26 to 70 hours with valproate co-administration (a 165% increase). The dose of lamotrigine should be reduced when co-administered with valproate.

Phenobarbital—Valproate was found to inhibit the metabolism of phenobarbital. Co-administration of valproate (250 mg BID for 14 days) with phenobarbital to normal subjects (n=6) resulted in a 50% increase in half-life and a 30% decrease in plasma clearance of phenobarbital (60 mg single-dose). The fraction of phenobarbital dose excreted unchanged increased by 50% in presence of valproate.

There is evidence for severe CNS depression, with or without significant elevations of barbiturate or valproate serum concentrations. All patients receiving concomitant barbiturate therapy should be closely monitored for neurological toxicity. Serum barbiturate concentrations should be obtained, if possible, and the barbiturate dosage decreased, if appropriate.

Primidone, which is metabolized to a barbiturate, may be involved in a similar interaction with valproate.

Phenytoin—Valproate displaces phenytoin from its plasma albumin binding sites and inhibits its hepatic metabolism. Co-administration of valproate (400 mg TID) with phenytoin (250 mg) in normal volunteers (n=7) was associated with a 60% increase in the free fraction of phenytoin. Total plasma clearance and apparent volume of distribution of phenytoin increased 30% in the presence of valproate. Both the clearance and apparent volume of distribution of free phenytoin were reduced by 25%.

In patients with epilepsy, there have been reports of breakthrough seizures occurring with the combination of valproate and phenytoin. The dosage of phenytoin should be adjusted as required by the clinical situation.

Tolbutamide—From *in vitro* experiments, the unbound fraction of tolbutamide was increased from 20% to 50% when added to plasma samples taken from patients treated with valproate. The clinical relevance of this displacement is unknown.

Warfarin—In an *in vitro* study, valproate increased the unbound fraction of warfarin by up to 32.6%. The therapeutic relevance of this is unknown; however, coagulation tests should be monitored if DEPAKOTE therapy is instituted in patients taking anticoagulants.

Zidovudine—In six patients who were seropositive for HIV, the clearance of zidovudine (100 mg q8h) was decreased by 38% after administration of valproate (250 or 500 mg q8h); the half-life of zidovudine was unaffected.

Drugs for which either no interaction or a likely clinically unimportant interaction has been observed:

Acetaminophen—Valproate had no effect on any of the pharmacokinetic parameters of acetaminophen when it was concurrently administered to three epileptic patients.

Clozapine—In psychotic patients (n=11), no interaction was observed when valproate was co-administered with clozapine.

Lithium—Co-administration of valproate (500 mg BID) and lithium carbonate (300 mg TID) to normal male volunteers (n=16) had no effect on the steady-state kinetics of lithium.

Lorazepam—Concomitant administration of valproate (500 mg BID) and lorazepam (1 mg BID) in normal male volunteers (n=9) was accompanied by a 17% decrease in the plasma clearance of lorazepam.

Oral Contraceptive Steroids—Administration of a single-dose of ethinyloestradiol (50 μg)/levonorgestrel (250 μg) to 6 women on valproate (200 mg BID) therapy for 2 months did not reveal any pharmacokinetic interaction.

Carcinogenesis, Mutagenesis, Impairment of Fertility

Carcinogenesis

Valproic acid was administered orally to Sprague Dawley rats and ICR (HA/ICR) mice at doses of 80 and 170 mg/kg/day (approximately 10 to 50% of the maximum human daily dose on a mg/m^2 basis) for two years. A variety of neoplasms were observed in both species. The chief findings were a statistically significant increase in the incidence of subcutaneous fibrosarcomas in high dose male rats receiving valproic acid and a statistically significant dose-related trend for benign pulmonary adenomas in male mice receiving valproic acid. The significance of these findings for humans is unknown.

Mutagenesis

Valproate was not mutagenic in an *in vitro* bacterial assay (Ames test), did not produce dominant lethal effects in mice, and did not increase chromosome aberration frequency in an *in vivo* cytogenetic study in rats. Increased frequencies of sister chromatid exchange (SCE) have been reported in a study of epileptic children taking valproate, but this association was not observed in another study conducted in adults. There is some evidence that increased SCE frequencies may be associated with epilepsy. The biological significance of an increase in SCE frequency is not known.

Fertility

Chronic toxicity studies in juvenile and adult rats and dogs demonstrated reduced spermatogenesis and testicular atrophy at oral doses of 400 mg/kg/day or greater in rats (approximately equivalent to or greater than the maximum human daily dose on a mg/m^2 basis) and 150 mg/kg/day or greater in dogs (approximately 1.4 times the maximum human daily dose or greater on a mg/m^2 basis). Segment I fertility studies in rats have shown doses up to 350 mg/kg/day (approximately equal to the maximum human daily dose on a mg/m^2 basis) for 60 days to have no effect on fertility. THE EFFECT OF VALPROATE ON TESTICULAR DEVELOPMENT AND ON SPERM PRODUCTION AND FERTILITY IN HUMANS IS UNKNOWN.

Pregnancy

Pregnancy Category D: See **WARNINGS**.

Nursing Mothers

Valproate is excreted in breast milk. Concentrations in breast milk have been reported to be 1–10% of serum concentrations. It is not known what effect this would have on a nursing infant. Consideration should be given to discontinuing nursing when divalproex sodium is administered to a nursing woman.

Pediatric Use

Experience has indicated that pediatric patients under the age of two years are at a considerably increased risk of developing fatal hepatotoxicity, especially those with the aforementioned conditions (see **BOXED WARNING**). When DEPAKOTE is used in this patient group, it should be used with extreme caution and as a sole agent. The benefits of therapy should be weighed against the risks. Above the age of 2 years, experience in epilepsy has indicated that the incidence of fatal hepatotoxicity decreases considerably in progressively older patient groups.

Younger children, especially those receiving enzyme-inducing drugs, will require larger maintenance doses to attain targeted total and unbound valproic acid concentrations.

The variability in free fraction limits the clinical usefulness of monitoring total serum valproic acid concentrations. Interpretation of valproic acid concentrations in children should include consideration of factors that affect hepatic metabolism and protein binding.

The safety and effectiveness of DEPAKOTE for the treatment of acute mania has not been studied in individuals below the age of 18 years.

The safety and effectiveness of DEPAKOTE for the prophylaxis of migraines has not been studied in individuals below the age of 16 years.

The basic toxicology and pathologic manifestations of valproate sodium in neonatal (4-day old) and juvenile (14-day old) rats are similar to those seen in young adult rats. However, additional findings, including renal alterations in juvenile rats and renal alterations and retinal dysplasia in neonatal rats, have been reported. These findings occurred at 240 mg/kg/day, a dosage approximately equivalent to the human maximum recommended daily dose on a mg/m^2 basis. They were not seen at 90 mg/kg, or 40% of the maximum human daily dose on a mg/m^2 basis.

Geriatric Use

No patients above the age of 65 years were enrolled in double-blind prospective clinical trials of mania associated with bipolar illness. In a case review study of 583 patients, 72 patients (12%) were greater than 65 years of age. A higher percentage of patients above 65 years of age reported accidental injury, infection, pain, somnolence, and tremor. Discontinuation of valproate was occasionally associated with the latter two events. It is not clear whether these events indicate additional risk or whether they result from preexisting medical illness and concomitant medication use among these patients.

A study of elderly patients with dementia revealed drug related somnolence and discontinuation for somnolence (see **WARNINGS—Somnolence in the Elderly**). The starting dose should be reduced in these patients, and dosage reductions or discontinuation should be considered in patients with excessive somnolence (see **DOSAGE AND ADMINISTRATION**).

There is insufficient information available to discern the safety and effectiveness of DEPAKOTE for the prophylaxis of migraines in patients over 65.

ADVERSE REACTIONS

Mania

The incidence of treatment-emergent events has been ascertained based on combined data from two placebo-controlled clinical trials of DEPAKOTE in the treatment of manic episodes associated with bipolar disorder. The adverse events were usually mild or moderate in intensity, but sometimes were serious enough to interrupt treatment. In clinical trials, the rates of premature termination due to intolerance were not statistically different between placebo, DEPAKOTE, and lithium carbonate. A total of 4%, 8% and 11% of patients discontinued therapy due to intolerance in the placebo, DEPAKOTE, and lithium carbonate groups, respectively.

Table 1 summarizes those adverse events reported for patients in these trials where the incidence rate in the DEPAKOTE-treated group was greater than 5% and greater than the placebo incidence, or where the incidence in the DEPAKOTE-treated group was statistically significantly greater than the placebo group. Vomiting was the only event that was reported by significantly ($p \leq 0.05$) more patients receiving DEPAKOTE compared to placebo.

Table 1
Adverse Events Reported by > 5% of DEPAKOTE-Treated Patients During Placebo-Controlled Trials of Acute Mania[1]

Adverse Event	DEPAKOTE (n=89)	Placebo (n=97)
Nausea	22%	15%
Somnolence	19%	12%
Dizziness	12%	4%
Vomiting	12%	3%
Asthenia	10%	7%
Abdominal Pain	9%	8%
Dyspepsia	9%	8%
Rash	6%	3%

[1] The following adverse events occurred at an equal or greater incidence for placebo than for DEPAKOTE: back pain, headache, constipation, diarrhea, tremor, and pharyngitis.

The following additional adverse events were reported by greater than 1% but not more than 5% of the 89 divalproex sodium-treated patients in controlled clinical trials:

Body as a Whole: Chest pain, chills, chills and fever, fever, neck pain, neck rigidity.

Cardiovascular System: Hypertension, hypotension, palpitations, postural hypotension, tachycardia, vasodilation.

Digestive System: Anorexia, fecal incontinence, flatulence, gastroenteritis, glossitis, periodontal abscess.

Hemic and Lymphatic System: Ecchymosis.

Metabolic and Nutritional Disorders: Edema, peripheral edema.

Continued on next page

Depakote—Cont.

Musculoskeletal System: Arthralgia, arthrosis, leg cramps, twitching.
Nervous System: Abnormal dreams, abnormal gait, agitation, ataxia, catatonic reaction, confusion, depression, diplopia, dysarthria, hallucinations, hypertonia, hypokinesia, insomnia, paresthesia, reflexes increased, tardive dyskinesia, thinking abnormalities, vertigo.
Respiratory System: Dyspnea, rhinitis.
Skin and Appendages: Alopecia, discoid lupus erythematosis, dry skin, furunculosis, maculopapular rash, seborrhea.
Special Senses: Amblyopia, conjunctivitis, deafness, dry eyes, ear pain, eye pain, tinnitus.
Urogenital System: Dysmenorrhea, dysuria, urinary incontinence.

Migraine

Based on two placebo-controlled clinical trials and their long term extension, DEPAKOTE was generally well tolerated with most adverse events rated as mild to moderate in severity. Of the 202 patients exposed to DEPAKOTE in the placebo-controlled trials, 17% discontinued for intolerance. This is compared to a rate of 5% for the 81 placebo patients. Including the long term extension study, the adverse events reported as the primary reason for discontinuation by ≥1% of 248 DEPAKOTE-treated patients were alopecia (6%), nausea and/or vomiting (5%), weight gain (2%), tremor (2%), somnolence (1%), elevated SGOT and/or SGPT (1%), and depression (1%).

Table 2 includes those adverse events reported for patients in the placebo-controlled trials where the incidence rate in the DEPAKOTE-treated group was greater than 5% and was greater than that for placebo patients.

Table 2
Adverse Events Reported by >5% of DEPAKOTE-Treated Patients During Migraine Placebo-Controlled Trails with a Greater Incidence Than Patients Taking Placebo[1]

Body System Event	Depakote (N = 202)	Placebo (N= 81)
Gastrointestinal System		
Nausea	31%	10%
Dyspepsia	13%	9%
Diarrhea	12%	7%
Vomiting	11%	1%
Abdominal pain	9%	4%
Increased appetite	6%	4%
Nervous System		
Asthenia	20%	9%
Somnolence	17%	5%
Dizziness	12%	6%
Tremor	9%	0%
Other		
Weight gain	8%	2%
Back pain	8%	6%
Alopecia	7%	1%

[1] The following adverse events occurred in at least 5% of DEPAKOTE-treated patients and at an equal or greater incidence for placebo than for DEPAKOTE: flu syndrome and pharyngitis.

The following additional adverse events were reported by greater than 1% but not more than 5% of the 202 divalproex sodium-treated patients in the controlled clinical trials:
Body as a Whole: Chest pain, chills, face edema, fever and malaise.
Cardiovascular System: Vasodilatation.
Digestive System: Anorexia, constipation, dry mouth, flatulence, gastrointestinal disorder (unspecified), and stomatitis.
Hemic and Lymphatic System: Ecchymosis.
Metabolic and Nutritional Disorders: Peripheral edema, SGOT increase, and SGPT increase.
Musculoskeletal System: Leg cramps and myalgia.
Nervous System: Abnormal dreams, amnesia, confusion, depression, emotional lability, insomnia, nervousness, paresthesia, speech disorder, thinking abnormalities, and vertigo.
Respiratory System: Cough increased, dyspnea, rhinitis, and sinusitis.
Skin and Appendages: Pruritus and rash.
Special Senses: Conjunctivitis, ear disorder, taste perversion, and tinnitus.
Urogenital System: Cystitis, metrorrhagia, and vaginal hemorrhage.

Epilepsy

Based on a placebo-controlled trial of adjunctive therapy for treatment of complex partial seizures, DEPAKOTE was generally well tolerated with most adverse events rated as mild to moderate in severity. Intolerance was the primary reason for discontinuation in the DEPAKOTE-treated patients (6%), compared to 1% of placebo-treated patients.

Table 3 lists treatment-emergent adverse events which were reported by ≥ 5% of DEPAKOTE-treated patients and for which the incidence was greater than in the placebo group, in the placebo-controlled trial of adjunctive therapy for treatment of complex partial seizures. Since patients were also treated with other antiepilepsy drugs, it is not possible, in most cases, to determine whether the following adverse events can be ascribed to DEPAKOTE alone, or the combination of DEPAKOTE and other antiepilepsy drugs.

Table 3
Adverse Events Reported by ≥ 5% of Patients Treated with DEPAKOTE During Placebo-Controlled Trial of Adjunctive Therapy for Complex Partial Seizures

Body System/Event	Depokote (%) (n = 77)	Placebo (%) (n = 70)
Body as a Whole		
Headache	31	21
Asthenia	27	7
Fever	6	4
Gastrointestinal System		
Nausea	48	14
Vomiting	27	7
Abdominal Pain	23	6
Diarrhea	13	6
Anorexia	12	0
Dyspepsia	8	4
Constipation	5	1
Nervous System		
Somnolence	27	11
Tremor	25	6
Dizziness	25	13
Diplopia	16	9
Ambylopia/Blurred Vision	12	9
Ataxia	8	1
Nystagmus	8	1
Emotional Lability	6	4
Thinking Abnormal	6	0
Amnesia	5	1
Respiratory System		
Flu Syndrome	12	9
Infection	12	6
Bronchitis	5	1
Rhinitis	5	4
Other		
Alopecia	6	1
Weight Loss	6	0

Table 4 lists treatment-emergent adverse events which were reported by ≥ 5% of patients in the high dose DEPAKOTE group, and for which the incidence was greater than in the low dose group, in a controlled trial of DEPAKOTE monotherapy treatment of complex partial seizures. Since patients were being titrated off another antiepilepsy drug during the first portion of the trial, it is not possible, in many cases, to determine whether the following adverse events can be ascribed to DEPAKOTE alone, or the combination of DEPAKOTE and other antiepilepsy drugs.

Table 4
Adverse Events Reported by ≥ 5% of Patients Treated in the High Dose Group in the Controlled Trial of DEPAKOTE Monotherapy for Complex Partial Seizures[1]

Body System/Event	High Dose (%) (n = 131)	Low Dose (%) (n = 134)
Body as a Whole		
Asthenia	21	10
Digestive System		
Nausea	34	26
Diarrhea	23	19
Vomiting	23	15
Abdominal Pain	12	9
Anorexia	11	4
Dyspepsia	11	10
Hemic/Lymphatic System		
Thrombocytopenia	24	1
Ecchymosis	5	4
Metabolic/Nutritional		
Weight Gain	9	4
Peripheral Edema	8	3
Nervous System		
Tremor	57	19
Somnolence	30	18
Dizziness	18	13
Insomnia	15	9
Nervousness	11	7
Amnesia	7	4
Nystagmus	7	1
Depression	5	4
Respiratory System		
Infection	20	13
Pharyngitis	8	2
Dyspnea	5	1
Skin and Appendages		
Alopecia	24	13
Special Senses		
Amblyopia/Blurred Vision	8	4
Tinnitus	7	1

[1] Headache was the only adverse event that occurred in ≥ 5% of patients in the high dose group and at an equal or greater incidence in the low dose group.

The following additional adverse events were reported by greater than 1% but less than 5% of the 358 patients treated with DEPAKOTE in the controlled trials of complex partial seizures:
Body as a Whole: Back pain, chest pain, malaise.
Cardiovascular System: Tachycardia, hypertension, palpitation.
Digestive System: Increased appetite, flatulence, hematemesis, eructation, pancreatitis, periodontal abscess.
Hemic and Lymphatic System: Petechia.
Metabolic and Nutritional Disorders: SGOT increased, SGPT increased.
Musculoskeletal System: Myalgia, twitching, arthralgia, leg cramps, myasthenia.
Nervous System: Anxiety, confusion, abnormal gait, paresthesia, hypertonia, incoordination, abnormal dreams, personality disorder.
Respiratory System: Sinusitis, cough increased, pneumonia, epistaxis.
Skin and Appendages: Rash, pruritus, dry skin.
Special Senses: Taste perversion, abnormal vision, deafness, otitis media.
Urogenital System: Urinary incontinence, vaginitis, dysmenorrhea, amenorrhea, urinary frequency.

Other Patient Populations

Adverse events that have been reported with all dosage forms of valproate from epilepsy trials, spontaneous reports, and other sources are listed below by body system.

Gastrointestinal: The most commonly reported side effects at the initiation of therapy are nausea, vomiting, and indigestion. These effects are usually transient and rarely require discontinuation of therapy. Diarrhea, abdominal cramps, and constipation have been reported. Both anorexia with some weight loss and increased appetite with weight gain have also been reported. The administration of delayed-release divalproex sodium may result in reduction of gastrointestinal side effects in some patients.

CNS Effects: Sedative effects have occurred in patients receiving valproate alone but occur most often in patients receiving combination therapy. Sedation usually abates upon reduction of other antiepileptic medication. Tremor (may be dose-related), hallucinations, ataxia, headache, nystagmus, diplopia, asterixis, "spots before eyes", dysarthria, dizziness, confusion, hypesthesia, vertigo, incoordination, and parkinsonism. Rare cases of coma have occurred in patients receiving valproate alone or in conjunction with phenobarbital. In rare instances encephalopathy with fever has developed shortly after the introduction of valproate monotherapy without evidence of hepatic dysfunction or inappropriate plasma levels; all patients recovered after the drug was withdrawn.

Several reports have noted reversible cerebral atrophy and dementia in association with valproate therapy.

Dermatologic: Transient hair loss, skin rash, photosensitivity, generalized pruritus, erythema multiforme, and Stevens-Johnson syndrome. Rare cases of toxic epidermal necrolysis have been reported including a fatal case in a 6 month old infant taking valproate and several other concomitant medications. An additional case of toxic epidermal necrosis resulting in death was reported in a 35 year old patient with AIDS taking several concomitant medications and had with a history of multiple cutaneous drug reactions.

Psychiatric: Emotional upset, depression, psychosis, aggression, hyperactivity, hostility, and behavioral deterioration.

Musculoskeletal: Weakness.

Hematologic: Thrombocytopenia and inhibition of the secondary phase of platelet aggregation may be reflected in altered bleeding time, petechiae, bruising, hematoma formation, epistaxis, and frank hemorrhage (see **PRECAUTIONS—General** and **Drug Interactions**). Relative lymphocytosis, macrocytosis, hypofibrinogenemia, leukopenia, eosinophilia, anemia including macrocytic with or without folate deficiency, bone marrow suppression, pancytopenia, aplastic anemia, and acute intermittent porphyria.

Hepatic: Minor elevations of transaminases (eg, SGOT and SGPT) and LDH are frequent and appear to be dose-related. Occasionally, laboratory test results include increases in serum bilirubin and abnormal changes in other liver function tests. These results may reflect potentially serious hepatotoxicity (see **WARNINGS**).

Endocrine: Irregular menses, secondary amenorrhea, breast enlargement, galactorrhea, and parotid gland swelling. Abnormal thyroid function tests (see **PRECAUTIONS**).

There have been rare spontaneous reports of polycystic ovary disease. A cause and effect relationship has not been established.

Pancreatic: Acute pancreatitis including fatalities (see **WARNINGS**).

Metabolic: Hyperammonemia (see **PRECAUTIONS**), hyponatremia, and inappropriate ADH secretion.

There have been rare reports of Fanconi's syndrome occurring chiefly in children.

Decreased carnitine concentrations have been reported although the clinical relevance is undetermined.

Hyperglycinemia has occurred and was associated with a fatal outcome in a patient with preexistent nonketotic hyperglycinemia.

Genitourinary: Enuresis and urinary tract infection.

Special Senses: Hearing loss, either reversible or irreversible, has been reported; however, a cause and effect relationship has not been established. Ear pain has also been reported.

Other: Anaphylaxis, edema of the extremities, lupus erythematosus, bone pain, cough increased, pneumonia, otitis media, bradycardia, cutaneous vasculitis, and fever.

OVERDOSAGE

Overdosage with valproate may result in somnolence, heart block, and deep coma. Fatalities have been reported; however patients have recovered from valproate levels as high as 2120 µg/mL.

In overdose situations, the fraction of drug not bound to protein is high and hemodialysis or tandem hemodialysis plus hemoperfusion may result in significant removal of drug. The benefit of gastric lavage or emesis will vary with the time since ingestion. General supportive measures should be applied with particular attention to the maintenance of adequate urinary output.

Naloxone has been reported to reverse the CNS depressant effects of valproate overdosage. Because naloxone could theoretically also reverse the antiepileptic effects of valproate, it should be used with caution in patients with epilepsy.

DOSAGE AND ADMINISTRATION

Mania

DEPAKOTE tablets are administered orally. The recommended initial dose is 750 mg daily in divided doses. The dose should be increased as rapidly as possible to achieve the lowest therapeutic dose which produces the desired clinical effect or the desired range of plasma concentrations. In placebo-controlled clinical trials of acute mania, patients were dosed to a clinical response with a trough plasma concentration between 50 and 125 µg/mL. Maximum concentrations were generally achieved within 14 days. The maximum recommended dosage is 60 mg/kg/day.

There is no body of evidence available from controlled trials to guide a clinician in the longer term management of a patient who improves during DEPAKOTE treatment of an acute manic episode. While it is generally agreed that pharmacological treatment beyond an acute response in mania is desirable, both for maintenance of the initial response and for prevention of new manic episodes, there are no systematically obtained data to support the benefits of DEPAKOTE in such longer-term treatment. Although there are no efficacy data that specifically address longer-term antimanic treatment with DEPAKOTE, the safety of DEPAKOTE in long-term use is supported by data from record reviews involving approximately 360 patients treated with DEPAKOTE for greater than 3 months.

Epilepsy

DEPAKOTE tablets are administered orally. DEPAKOTE is indicated as monotherapy and adjunctive therapy in complex partial seizures in adults and pediatric patients down to the age of 10 years, and in simple and complex absence seizures. As the DEPAKOTE dosage is titrated upward, concentrations of phenobarbital, carbamazepine, and/or phenytoin may be affected (see **PRECAUTIONS—Drug Interactions**).

Complex Partial Seizures: For adults and children 10 years of age or older.

Monotherapy (Initial Therapy): DEPAKOTE has not been systematically studied as initial therapy. Patients should initiate therapy at 10 to 15 mg/kg/day. The dosage should be increased by 5 to 10 mg/kg/week to achieve optimal clinical response. Ordinarily, optimal clinical response is achieved at daily doses below 60 mg/kg/day. If satisfactory clinical response has not been achieved, plasma levels should be measured to determine whether or not they are in the usually accepted therapeutic range (50 to 100 µg/mL). No recommendation regarding the safety of valproate for use at doses above 60 mg/kg/day can be made.

The probability of thrombocytopenia increases significantly at total trough valproate plasma concentrations above 110 µg/mL in females and 135 µg/mL in males. The benefit of improved seizure control with higher doses should be weighed against the possibility of a greater incidence of adverse reactions.

Conversion to Monotherapy: Patients should initiate therapy at 10 to 15 mg/kg/day. The dosage should be increased by 5 to 10 mg/kg/week to achieve optimal clinical response. Ordinarily, optimal clinical response is achieved at daily doses below 60 mg/kg/day. If satisfactory clinical response has not been achieved, plasma levels should be measured to determine whether or not they are in the usually accepted therapeutic range (50–100 µg/mL). No recommendation regarding the safety of valproate for use at doses above 60 mg/kg/day can be made. Concomitant antiepilepsy drug (AED) dosage can ordinarily be reduced by approximately 25% every 2 weeks. This reduction may be started at initiation of DEPAKOTE therapy, or delayed by 1 to 2 weeks if there is a concern that seizures are likely to occur with a reduction. The speed and duration of withdrawal of the concomitant AED can be highly variable, and patients should be monitored closely during this period for increased seizure frequency.

Adjunctive Therapy: DEPAKOTE may be added to the patient's regimen at a dosage of 10 to 15 mg/kg/day. The dosage may be increased by 5 to 10 mg/kg/week to achieve optimal clinical response. Ordinarily, optimal clinical response is achieved at daily doses below 60 mg/kg/day. If satisfactory clinical response has not been achieved, plasma levels should be measured to determine whether or not they are in the usually accepted therapeutic range (50 to 100 µg/mL). No recommendation regarding the safety of valproate for use at doses above 60 mg/kg/day can be made. If the total daily dose exceeds 250 mg, it should be given in divided doses.

In a study of adjunctive therapy for complex partial seizures in which patients were receiving either carbamazepine or phenytoin in addition to DEPAKOTE, no adjustment of carbamazepine or phenytoin dosage was needed (see **CLINICAL STUDIES**). However, since valproate may interact with these or other concurrently administered AEDs as well as other drugs (see **Drug Interactions**), periodic plasma concentration determinations of concomitant AEDs are recommended during the early course of therapy (see **PRECAUTIONS—Drug Interactions**).

Simple and Complex Absence Seizures: The recommended initial dose is 15 mg/kg/day, increasing at one week intervals by 5 to 10 mg/kg/day until seizures are controlled or side effects preclude further increases. The maximum recommended dosage is 60 mg/kg/day. If the total daily dose exceeds 250 mg, it should be given in divided doses.

A good correlation has not been established between daily dose, serum concentrations, and therapeutic effect. However, therapeutic valproate serum concentrations for most patients with absence seizures is considered to range from 50 to 100 µg/mL. Some patients may be controlled with lower or higher serum concentrations (see **CLINICAL PHARMACOLOGY**).

As the DEPAKOTE dosage is titrated upward, blood concentrations of phenobarbital and/or phenytoin may be affected (see **PRECAUTIONS**).

Antiepilepsy drugs should not be abruptly discontinued in patients in whom the drug is administered to prevent major seizures because of the strong possibility of precipitating status epilepticus with attendant hypoxia and threat to life.

In epileptic patients previously receiving DEPAKENE (valproic acid) therapy, DEPAKOTE tablets should be initiated at the same daily dose and dosing schedule. After the patient is stabilized on DEPAKOTE tablets, a dosing schedule of two or three times a day may be elected in selected patients.

Migraine

DEPAKOTE tablets are administered orally. The recommended starting dose is 250 mg twice daily. Some patients may benefit from doses up to 1000 mg/day. In the clinical trials, there was no evidence that higher doses led to greater efficacy.

General Dosing Advice

Dosing in Elderly Patients—Due to a decrease in unbound clearance of valproate and possibly a greater sensitivity to somnolence in the elderly, the starting dose should be reduced in these patients. Dosage should be increased more slowly and with regular monitoring for fluid and nutritional intake, dehydration, somnolence, and other adverse events. Dose reductions or discontinuation of valproate should be considered in patients with decreased food or fluid intake and in patients with excessive somnolence. The ultimate therapeutic dose should be achieved on the basis of both tolerability and clinical response (see **WARNINGS**).

Dose-Related Adverse Events—The frequency of adverse effects (particularly elevated liver enzymes and thrombocytopenia) may be dose-related. The probability of thrombocytopenia appears to increase significantly at total valproate concentrations of ≥ 110 µg/mL (females) or ≥ 135 µg/mL (males) (see **PRECAUTIONS**). The benefit of improved therapeutic effect with higher doses should be weighed against the possibility of a greater incidence of adverse reactions.

G.I. Irritation—Patients who experience G.I. irritation may benefit from administration of the drug with food or by slowly building up the dose from an initial low level.

HOW SUPPLIED

DEPAKOTE tablets (divalproex sodium delayed-release tablets) are supplied as:

125 mg salmon pink-colored tablets:

Bottles of 100 .... (**NDC** 0074-6212-13)

Abbo-Pac® unit dose packages of
100 .... (**NDC** 0074-6212-11).

250 mg peach-colored tablets:

Bottles of 100 .... (**NDC** 0074-6214-13)

Bottles of 500 .... (**NDC** 0074-6214-53)

Abbo-Pac® unit dose packages of
100 .... (**NDC** 0074-6214-11).

500 mg lavender-colored tablets:

Bottles of 100 .... (**NDC** 0074-6215-13)

Bottles of 500 .... (**NDC** 0074-6215-53)

Abbo-Pac® unit dose packages of
100 .... (**NDC** 0074-6215-11).

Recommended storage: Store tablets below 86°F (30°C).

Patient Information Leaflet

Important Information for Women Who Could Become Pregnant

About the Use of Depakote® (divalproex sodium) Tablets for Migraine

Please read this leaflet carefully before you take Depakote® (divalproex sodium) tablets. This leaflet provides a summary of important information about taking Depakote for migraine to women who could become pregnant. Depakote is also prescribed for uses other than those discussed in this leaflet. If you have any questions or concerns, or want more information about Depakote, contact your doctor or pharmacist.

Information For Women Who Could Become Pregnant

Depakote is used to prevent or reduce the number of migraines you experience. Depakote can be obtained only by prescription from your doctor. The decision to use Depakote for the prevention of migraine is one that you and your doctor should make together, taking into account your individual needs and medical condition.

Before using Depakote, women who can become pregnant should consider the fact that **Depakote has been associated with birth defects, in particular, with spina bifida and other defects related to failure of the spinal canal to close normally. Although the incidence is unknown in migraine patients treated with Depakote, approximately 1 to 2% of children born to women with epilepsy taking Depakote in the first 12 weeks of pregnancy had these defects (based on data from the Centers for Disease Control, a U.S. agency based in Atlanta). The incidence in the general population is 0.1 to 0.2%.**

Information For Women Who Are Planning to Get Pregnant

- Women taking Depakote for the prevention of migraine who are planning to get pregnant should discuss with their doctor temporarily stopping Depakote, before and during their pregnancy.

Information For Women Who Become Pregnant While Taking Depakote

- If you become pregnant while taking Depakote for the prevention of migraine, you should contact your doctor immediately.

Other Important Information About Depakote Tablets

- Depakote tablets should be taken exactly as it is prescribed by your doctor to get the most benefits from Depakote and reduce the risk of side effects.
- If you have taken more than the prescribed dose of Depakote, contact your hospital emergency room or local poison center immediately.
- This medication was prescribed for your particular condition. Do not use it for another condition or give the drug to others.

Facts About Birth Defects

It is important to know that birth defects may occur even in children of individuals not taking any medications or without any additional risk factors.

Facts About Migraine

About 23 million Americans suffer from migraine headaches. About 75% of migraine sufferers are women. A migraine is described as a throbbing headache that gets worse with activity. Migraine may also include nausea and/or vomiting as well as sensitivity to light and sound. Migraine usually happens about once a month, but some people may have them as often as once or twice a week. Often, the symptoms from a migraine can cause people to miss work or school. If you have frequent migraines, or if acute treatment is not working for you, your doctor may prescribe a preventative therapy. Preventative (prophylactic) treatment is used to prevent attacks and reduce the frequency and severity of headache events.

This summary provides important information about the use of Depakote for migraine to women who could become pregnant. If you would like more information about the other potential risks and benefits of Depakote, ask your doctor or pharmacist to let you read the professional labeling and then discuss it with them. If you have any questions or concerns about taking Depakote, you should discuss them with your doctor.

Revised: June, 2000

Ref.: 03-5012

ABBOTT LABORATORIES

NORTH CHICAGO, IL 60064, USA

Shown in Product Identification Guide, page 303

DESOXYN® Ⓒ℞
METHAMPHETAMINE HYDROCHLORIDE TABLETS, USP

METHAMPHETAMINE HAS A HIGH POTENTIAL FOR ABUSE. IT SHOULD THUS BE TRIED ONLY IN WEIGHT REDUCTION PROGRAMS FOR PATIENTS IN WHOM ALTERNATIVE THERAPY HAS BEEN INEFFECTIVE. ADMINISTRATION OF METHAMPHETAMINE FOR PROLONGED PERIODS OF TIME IN OBESITY MAY LEAD TO DRUG DEPENDENCE AND MUST BE AVOIDED. PARTICULAR ATTENTION SHOULD BE PAID TO THE POSSIBILITY OF SUBJECTS OBTAINING METHAMPHETAMINE FOR NON-THERAPEUTIC USE OR DISTRIBUTION TO OTHERS, AND THE DRUG SHOULD BE PRESCRIBED OR DISPENSED SPARINGLY.

DESCRIPTION

DESOXYN (methamphetamine hydrochloride tablets, USP), chemically known as (S)-N, α-dimethylbenzeneethanamine hydrochloride, is a member of the amphetamine group of sympathomimetic amines. It has the following structural formula:

$$\left[C_6H_5-CH_2-\underset{\displaystyle CH_3}{\underset{|}{CH}}-\overset{+}{N}H_2CH_3 \right] Cl^-$$

DESOXYN tablets contain 5 mg of methamphetamine hydrochloride for oral administration.

Continued on next page

Desoxyn—Cont.

Inactive Ingredients:

Corn starch, lactose, sodium paraminobenzoate, stearic acid and talc.

CLINICAL PHARMACOLOGY

Methamphetamine is a sympathomimetic amine with CNS stimulant activity. Peripheral actions include elevation of systolic and diastolic blood pressures and weak bronchodilator and respiratory stimulant action. Drugs of this class used in obesity are commonly known as "anorectics" or "anorexigenics". It has not been established, however, that the action of such drugs in treating obesity is primarily one of appetite suppression. Other central nervous system actions, or metabolic effects, may be involved, for example.

Adult obese subjects instructed in dietary management and treated with "anorectic" drugs, lose more weight on the average than those treated with placebo and diet, as determined in relatively short-term clinical trials.

The magnitude of increased weight loss of drug-treated patients over placebo-treated patients is only a fraction of a pound a week. The rate of weight loss is greatest in the first weeks of therapy for both drug and placebo subjects and tends to decrease in succeeding weeks. The origins of the increased weight loss due to the various possible drug effects are not established. The amount of weight loss associated with the use of an "anorectic" drug varies from trial to trial, and the increased weight loss appears to be related in part to variables other than the drug prescribed, such as the physician-investigator, the population treated, and the diet prescribed. Studies do not permit conclusions as to the relative importance of the drug and non-drug factors on weight loss.

The natural history of obesity is measured in years, whereas the studies cited are restricted to a few weeks duration; thus, the total impact of drug-induced weight loss over that of diet alone must be considered clinically limited.

The mechanism of action involved in producing the beneficial behavioral changes seen in hyperkinetic children receiving methamphetamine is unknown.

In humans, methamphetamine is rapidly absorbed from the gastrointestinal tract. The primary site of metabolism is in the liver by aromatic hydroxylation, N-dealkylation and deamination. At least seven metabolites have been identified in the urine. The biological half-life has been reported in the range of 4 to 5 hours. Excretion occurs primarily in the urine and is dependent on urine pH. Alkaline urine will significantly increase the drug half-life. Approximately 62% of an oral dose is eliminated in the urine within the first 24 hours with about one-third as intact drug and the remainder as metabolites.

INDICATIONS AND USAGE

Attention Deficit Disorder with Hyperactivity—DESOXYN tablets are indicated as an integral part of a total treatment program which typically includes other remedial measures (psychological, educational, social) for a stabilizing effect in children over 6 years of age with a behavioral syndrome characterized by the following group of developmentally inappropriate symptoms: moderate to severe distractibility, short attention span, hyperactivity, emotional lability, and impulsivity. The diagnosis of this syndrome should not be made with finality when these symptoms are only of comparatively recent origin. Nonlocalizing (soft) neurological signs, learning disability, and abnormal EEG may or may not be present, and a diagnosis of central nervous system dysfunction may or may not be warranted.

Exogenous Obesity—as a short-term (i.e., a few weeks) adjunct in a regimen of weight reduction based on caloric restriction, for patients in whom obesity is refractory to alternative therapy, e.g., repeated diets, group programs, and other drugs. The limited usefulness of DESOXYN tablets (see **CLINICAL PHARMACOLOGY**) should be weighed against possible risks inherent in use of the drug, such as those described below.

CONTRAINDICATIONS

DESOXYN tablets are contraindicated during or within 14 days following the administration of monoamine oxidase inhibitors; hypertensive crisis may result. It is also contraindicated in patients with glaucoma, advanced arteriosclerosis, symptomatic cardiovascular disease, moderate to severe hypertension, hyperthyroidism or known hypersensitivity or idiosyncrasy to sympathomimetic amines. Methamphetamine should not be given to patients who are in an agitated state or who have a history of drug abuse.

WARNINGS

Tolerance to the anorectic effect usually develops within a few weeks. When this occurs, the recommended dose should not be exceeded in an attempt to increase the effect; rather, the drug should be discontinued (see **DRUG ABUSE AND DEPENDENCE**).

Decrements in the predicted growth (i.e., weight gain and/or height) rate have been reported with the long-term use of stimulants in children. Therefore, patients requiring long-term therapy should be carefully monitored.

Usage in Nursing Mothers: Amphetamines are excreted in human milk. Mothers taking amphetamines should be advised to refrain from nursing.

PRECAUTIONS

General:

DESOXYN tablets should be used with caution in patients with even mild hypertension.

Methamphetamine should not be used to combat fatigue or to replace rest in normal persons.

Prescribing and dispensing of methamphetamine should be limited to the smallest amount that is feasible at one time in order to minimize the possibility of overdosage.

Information for Patients:

The patient should be informed that methamphetamine may impair the ability to engage in potentially hazardous activities, such as, operating machinery or driving a motor vehicle.

The patient should be cautioned not to increase dosage, except on advice of the physician.

Drug Interactions:

Insulin requirements in diabetes mellitus may be altered in association with the use of methamphetamine and the concomitant dietary regimen.

Methamphetamine may decrease the hypotensive effect of *guanethidine*.

DESOXYN should not be used concurrently with *monoamine oxidase inhibitors* (see **CONTRAINDICATIONS**).

Concurrent administration of *tricyclic antidepressants* and indirect-acting sympathomimetic amines such as the amphetamines, should be closely supervised and dosage carefully adjusted.

Phenothiazines are reported in the literature to antagonize the CNS stimulant action of the amphetamines.

Drug/Laboratory Test Interactions:

Literature reports suggest that amphetamines may be associated with significant elevation of plasma corticosteroids. This should be considered if determination of plasma corticosteroid levels is desired in a person receiving amphetamines.

Carcinogenesis, Mutagenesis, Impairment of Fertility:

Data are not available on long-term potential for carcinogenicity, mutagenicity, or impairment of fertility.

Pregnancy:

Teratogenic effects: Pregnancy Category C. Methamphetamine has been shown to have teratogenic and embryocidal effects in mammals given high multiples of the human dose. There are no adequate and well-controlled studies in pregnant women. DESOXYN tablets should not be used during pregnancy unless the potential benefit justifies the potential risk to the fetus.

Nonteratogenic effects: Infants born to mothers dependent on amphetamines have an increased risk of premature delivery and low birth weight. Also, these infants may experience symptoms of withdrawal as demonstrated by dysphoria, including agitation and significant lassitude.

Nursing Mothers:

See **WARNINGS**.

Pediatric Use:

Safety and effectiveness for use as an anorectic agent in children below the age of 12 years have not been established.

Long-term effects of methamphetamine in children have not been established (see **WARNINGS**).

Drug treatment is not indicated in all cases of the behavioral syndrome characterized by moderate to severe distractibility, short attention span, hyperactivity, emotional lability and impulsivity. It should be considered only in light of the complete history and evaluation of the child. The decision to prescribe DESOXYN tablets should depend on the physician's assessment of the chronicity and severity of the child's symptoms and their appropriateness for his/her age. Prescription should not depend solely on the presence of one or more of the behavioral characteristics.

When these symptoms are associated with acute stress reactions, treatment with DESOXYN tablets is usually not indicated.

Clinical experience suggests that in psychotic children, administration of DESOXYN tablets may exacerbate symptoms of behavior disturbance and thought disorder.

Amphetamines have been reported to exacerbate motor and phonic tics and Tourette's syndrome. Therefore, clinical evaluation for tics and Tourette's syndrome in children and their families should precede use of stimulant medications.

ADVERSE REACTIONS

The following are adverse reactions in decreasing order of severity within each category that have been reported:

Cardiovascular: Elevation of blood pressure, tachycardia and palpitation.

Central Nervous System: Psychotic episodes have been rarely reported at recommended doses. Dizziness, dysphoria, overstimulation, euphoria, insomnia, tremor, restlessness and headache. Exacerbation of motor and phonic tics and Tourette's syndrome.

Gastrointestinal: Diarrhea, constipation, dryness of mouth, unpleasant taste and other gastrointestinal disturbances.

Hypersensitivity: Urticaria.

Endocrine: Impotence and changes in libido.

Miscellaneous: Suppression of growth has been reported with the long-term use of stimulants in children (see **WARNINGS**).

DRUG ABUSE AND DEPENDENCE

Controlled Substance: DESOXYN tablets are subject to control under DEA schedule II.

Abuse: Methamphetamine has been extensively abused. Tolerance, extreme psychological dependence, and severe social disability have occurred. There are reports of patients who have increased the dosage to many times that recommended. Abrupt cessation following prolonged high dosage administration results in extreme fatigue and mental depression; changes are also noted on the sleep EEG. Manifestations of chronic intoxication with methamphetamine include severe dermatoses, marked insomnia, irritability, hyperactivity, and personality changes. The most severe manifestation of chronic intoxication is psychosis often clinically indistinguishable from schizophrenia.

OVERDOSAGE

Manifestations of acute overdosage with methamphetamine include restlessness, tremor, hyperreflexia, rapid respiration, confusion, assaultiveness, hallucinations, panic states, hyperpyrexia, and rhabdomyolysis. Fatigue and depression usually follow the central stimulation. Cardiovascular effects include arrhythmias, hypertension or hypotension, and circulatory collapse. Gastrointestinal symptoms include nausea, vomiting, diarrhea, and abdominal cramps. Fatal poisoning usually terminates in convulsions and coma.

Consult with a Certified Poison Control Center regarding treatment for up to date guidance and advice. Management of acute methamphetamine intoxication is largely symptomatic and includes gastric evacuation, administration of activated charcoal, and sedation. Experience with hemodialysis or peritoneal dialysis is inadequate to permit recommendations in this regard.

Acidification of urine increases methamphetamine excretion, but is believed to increase risk of acute renal failure if myoglobinuria is present. Intravenous phentolamine (Regitine®) has been suggested for possible acute, severe hypertension, if this complicates methamphetamine overdosage. Usually a gradual drop in blood pressure will result when sufficient sedation has been achieved. Chlorpromazine has been reported to be useful in decreasing CNS stimulation and sympathomimetic effects.

DOSAGE AND ADMINISTRATION

DESOXYN tablets are given orally.

Methamphetamine should be administered at the lowest effective dosage, and dosage should be individually adjusted. Late evening medication should be avoided because of the resulting insomnia.

Attention Deficit Disorder with Hyperactivity: For treatment of children 6 years or older with a behavioral syndrome characterized by moderate to severe distractibility, short attention span, hyperactivity, emotional lability and impulsivity: an initial dose of 5 mg DESOXYN once or twice a day is recommended. Daily dosage may be raised in increments of 5 mg at weekly intervals until an optimum clinical response is achieved. The usual effective dose is 20 to 25 mg daily. The total daily dose may be given in two divided doses daily. Where possible, drug administration should be interrupted occasionally to determine if there is a recurrence of behavioral symptoms sufficient to require continued therapy.

For Obesity: One 5 mg tablet should be taken one-half hour before each meal. Treatment should not exceed a few weeks in duration. Methamphetamine is not recommended for use as an anorectic agent in children under 12 years of age.

HOW SUPPLIED

DESOXYN (methamphetamine hydrochloride tablets, USP) is supplied as white tablets imprinted with the Abbott logo, a, and two letter Abbo-Code designation, TE, containing 5 mg methamphetamine hydrochloride in bottles of 100 (**NDC** 0074-3377-04).

Recommended Storage: Store below 86°F (30°C).

Revised: December, 1995

ABBOTT LABORATORIES
NORTH CHICAGO, IL 60064, U.S.A.

ENDURON® ℞

[en 'de-ron]

METHYCLOTHIAZIDE TABLETS, USP

DESCRIPTION

Methyclothiazide is a member of the benzothiadiazine (thiazide) class of drugs. It is an analogue of hydrochlorothiazide and occurs as a white to practically white crystalline powder which is basically odorless. Methyclothiazide is very slightly soluble in water and chloroform, and slightly soluble in alcohol. Chemically, methyclothiazide is represented as 6-chloro-3-(chloromethyl)-3,4-dihydro-2-methyl-2H-1,2,4-benzothiadiazine-7-sulfonamide 1,1-dioxide. The structural formula is:

Clinically, ENDURON (methyclothiazide) is an oral diuretic-antihypertensive agent. ENDURON tablets are available in two dosage strengths containing 2.5 mg and 5 mg of methyclothiazide.

Inactive Ingredients

2.5 mg tablets: corn starch, FD&C Yellow No. 6, lactose, magnesium stearate and talc.

5 mg tablets: corn starch, D&C Red No. 36, lactose, magnesium stearate and talc.

CLINICAL PHARMACOLOGY

The diuretic and saluretic effects of methyclothiazide result from a drug-induced inhibition of the renal tubular reab-

sorption of electrolytes. The excretion of sodium and chloride is greatly enhanced. Potassium excretion is also enhanced to a variable degree, as it is with the other thiazides. Although urinary excretion of bicarbonate is increased slightly, there is usually no significant change in urinary pH. Methyclothiazide has a per mg natriuretic activity approximately 100 times that of the prototype thiazide, chlorothiazide. At maximal therapeutic dosages, all thiazides are approximately equal in their diuretic/natriuretic effects. There is significant natriuresis and diuresis within two hours after administration of a single dose of methyclothiazide. These effects reach a peak in about six hours and persist for 24 hours following oral administration of a single dose.
Like other benzothiadiazines, methyclothiazide also has antihypertensive properties, and may be used for this purpose either alone or to enhance the antihypertensive action of other drugs. The mechanism by which the benzothiadiazines, including methyclothiazide, produce a reduction of elevated blood pressure is not known. However, sodium depletion appears to be involved.
Methyclothiazide is rapidly absorbed and slowly eliminated by the kidneys as intact drug but primarily as an inactive metabolite. Additional information on the pharmacokinetics is not known at this time.

INDICATIONS AND USAGE

ENDURON (methyclothiazide) is indicated in the management of hypertension either as the sole therapeutic agent or to enhance the effect of other antihypertensive drugs in the more severe forms of hypertension.
ENDURON tablets are indicated as adjunctive therapy in edema associated with congestive heart failure, hepatic cirrhosis, and corticosteroid and estrogen therapy.
ENDURON tablets have also been found useful in edema due to various forms of renal dysfunction such as the nephrotic syndrome, acute glomerulonephritis, and chronic renal failure.
Usage in Pregnancy: The routine use of diuretics in an otherwise healthy pregnant woman is inappropriate and exposes mother and fetus to unnecessary hazard. Diuretics do not prevent development of toxemia of pregnancy, and there is no satisfactory evidence that they are useful in the treatment of developed toxemia.
Edema during pregnancy may arise from pathological causes or from the physiological and mechanical consequences of pregnancy. Thiazides are indicated in pregnancy when edema is due to pathological causes, just as they are in the absence of pregnancy (see PRECAUTIONS—Pregnancy). Dependent edema in pregnancy, resulting from restriction of venous return by the expanded uterus, is properly treated through elevation of the lower extremities and use of support hose; use of diuretics to lower intravascular volume in this case is illogical and unnecessary. There is hypervolemia during normal pregnancy that is harmful to neither the fetus nor the mother (in the absence of cardiovascular disease), but that is associated with edema, including generalized edema, in the majority of pregnant women. If this edema produces discomfort, increased recumbency will often provide relief. In rare instances, this edema may cause extreme discomfort that is not relieved by rest. In these cases, a short course of diuretics may provide relief and may be appropriate.

CONTRAINDICATIONS

Methyclothiazide is contraindicated in patients with anuria and in patients with a history of hypersensitivity to this compound or other sulfonamide-derived drugs.

WARNINGS

Methyclothiazide shares with other thiazides the propensity to deplete potassium reserves to an unpredictable degree.
There have been isolated reports that certain nonedematous individuals developed severe fluid and electrolyte derangements after only brief exposure to normal doses of thiazide and non-thiazide diuretics.
Thiazides should be used with caution in patients with renal disease or significant impairment of renal function, since azotemia may be precipitated and cumulative drug effects may occur.
Thiazides should be used with caution in patients with impaired hepatic function or progressive liver disease, since minor alterations of fluid and electrolyte balance may precipitate hepatic coma.
Sensitivity reactions may occur in patients with a history of allergy or bronchial asthma.
The possibility of exacerbation or activation of systemic lupus erythematosus has been reported.
Hyperuricemia may occur or frank gout may be precipitated in certain patients receiving thiazide therapy.

PRECAUTIONS

Laboratory Tests: Initial and periodic determinations of serum electrolytes should be performed at appropriate intervals for the purpose of detecting possible electrolyte imbalances such as hyponatremia, hypochloremic alkalosis, and hypokalemia. Serum and urine electrolyte determinations are particularly important when a patient is vomiting excessively or receiving parenteral fluids.
General: All patients should be observed for clinical signs of electrolyte imbalances such as dryness of mouth, thirst, weakness, lethargy, drowsiness, restlessness, muscle pains or cramps, muscular fatigue, hypotension, oliguria, tachycardia, and gastrointestinal disturbances such as nausea and vomiting.
Hypokalemia may develop, especially with brisk diuresis, when severe cirrhosis is present, during concomitant use of corticosteroids or ACTH, or after prolonged therapy.
Interference with adequate oral electrolyte intake will also contribute to hypokalemia. Hypokalemia may be avoided or treated by use of potassium supplements or foods with a high potassium content.
Any chloride deficit is generally mild and usually does not require specific treatment except under extraordinary circumstances (as in liver disease or renal disease). Dilutional hyponatremia may occur in edematous patients in hot weather; appropriate therapy is water restriction rather than administration of salt, except in rare instances when the hyponatremia is life threatening. In actual salt depletion, appropriate replacement is the therapy of choice.
Latent diabetes mellitus may become manifest during thiazide administration.
The antihypertensive effects of the drug may be enhanced in the postsympathectomy patient.
If progressive renal impairment becomes evident as indicated by a rising nonprotein nitrogen or blood urea nitrogen, a careful reappraisal of therapy is necessary with consideration given to withholding or discontinuing diuretic therapy.
Thiazides may decrease urinary calcium excretion. Thiazides may cause intermittent and slight elevation of serum calcium in the absence of known disorders of calcium metabolism. Marked hypercalcemia may be evidence of hidden hyperparathyroidism.
Thiazides should be discontinued before carrying out tests for parathyroid function.
Thiazides may cause increased concentrations of total serum cholesterol, total triglycerides, and low-density lipoproteins in some patients. Use thiazides with caution in patients with moderate or high cholesterol concentrations and in patients with elevated triglyceride levels.
Information for Patients: Patients should inform their doctor if they have: 1) had an allergic reaction to methyclothiazide or other diuretics 2) asthma 3) kidney disease 4) liver disease 5) gout 6) systemic lupus erythematosus, or 7) been taking other drugs such as cortisone, digitalis, lithium carbonate, or drugs for diabetes.
The physician should inform patients of possible side effects and caution the patient to report any of the following symptoms of electrolyte imbalance; dryness of mouth, thirst, weakness, tiredness, drowsiness, restlessness, muscle pains or cramps, nausea, vomiting or increased heart rate.
The physician should advise the patient to take this medication every day as directed. Physicians should also caution patients that drinking alcohol can increase the chance of dizziness.
Drug Interactions: Hypokalemia can sensitize or exaggerate the response of the heart to the toxic effects of *digitalis* (e.g., increased ventricular irritability).
Hypokalemia may develop during concomitant use of *steroids* or *ACTH*.
Insulin requirements in diabetic patients may be increased, decreased, or unchanged.
Thiazides may decrease arterial responsiveness to *norepinephrine*. This diminution is not sufficient to preclude effectiveness of the pressor agent for therapeutic use.
Thiazide drugs may increase the responsiveness to *tubocurarine*.
Lithium renal clearance is reduced by thiazides, increasing the risk of lithium toxicity.
Thiazides may add to or potentiate the action of *other antihypertensive drugs*. Potentiation occurs with ganglionic or peripheral adrenergic blocking drugs.
Drug/Laboratory Test Interactions: Thiazides may decrease serum PBI levels without signs of thyroid disturbance.
Thiazides should be discontinued before carrying out tests for parathyroid function.
Carcinogenesis, Mutagenesis, Impairment of Fertility: No data are available concerning the potential for carcinogenicity or mutagenicity in animals or humans. Methyclothiazide did not impair fertility in rats receiving up to 4 mg/kg/day (at least 20 times the maximum recommended human dose of 10 mg, assuming patient weight equal to or greater than 50 kg).
Pregnancy—Teratogenic Effects: Pregnancy Category B. Reproduction studies performed in rats and rabbits at doses up to 4 mg/kg/day have revealed no evidence of harm to the fetus due to methyclothiazide. There are, however, no adequate and well-controlled studies in pregnant women. Because animal reproduction studies are not always predictive of human response, this drug should be used during pregnancy only if clearly needed.
Nonteratogenic Effects: Thiazides cross the placental barrier and appear in cord blood. The use of thiazides in pregnant women requires that the anticipated benefit be weighed against possible hazards to the fetus. These hazards include fetal or neonatal jaundice, thrombocytopenia and possible other adverse reactions that have occurred in the adult.
Nursing Mothers: Thiazides are excreted in breast milk. Because of the potential for serious adverse reactions in nursing infants, a decision should be made whether to discontinue nursing or to discontinue the drug taking into account the importance of the drug to the mother.
Pediatric Use: Safety and effectiveness in children have not been established.

ADVERSE REACTIONS

Adverse reactions are usually reversible upon reduction of dosage or discontinuation of ENDURON tablets. Whenever adverse reactions are moderate or severe, it may be necessary to discontinue the drug.
The following adverse reactions have been observed, but there has not been enough systematic collection of data to support an estimate of their frequency. Consequently the reactions are categorized by organ system and are listed in decreasing order of severity and not frequency.
Body as a Whole: Headache, cramping, weakness.
Cardiovascular System: Orthostatic hypotension (may be potentiated by alcohol, barbiturates, or narcotics).
Digestive System: Pancreatitis, jaundice (intrahepatic cholestatic), sialadenitis, vomiting, diarrhea, nausea, gastric irritation, constipation, anorexia.
Hemic and Lymphatic System: Aplastic anemia, hemolytic anemia, agranulocytosis, leukopenia, thrombocytopenia.
Hypersensitivity Reactions: Anaphylactic reactions, necrotizing angiitis (vasculitis, cutaneous vasculitis), Stevens-Johnson syndrome, respiratory distress including pneumonitis and pulmonary edema, fever, purpura, urticaria, rash, photosensitivity.
Metabolic and Nutritional Disorders: Hyperglycemia, hyperuricemia, electrolyte imbalance (see PRECAUTIONS section), hypercalcemia.
Nervous System: Vertigo, dizziness, paresthesias, muscle spasms, restlessness.
Special Senses: Transient blurred vision, xanthopsia.
Urogenital System: Glycosuria.

OVERDOSAGE

Symptoms of overdosage include electrolyte imbalance and signs of potassium deficiency such as confusion, dizziness, muscular weakness, and gastrointestinal disturbances. General supportive measures including replacement of fluids and electrolytes may be indicated in treatment of overdosage.

DOSAGE AND ADMINISTRATION

ENDURON (methyclothiazide) is administered orally. Therapy should be individualized according to patient response. This therapy should be titrated to gain maximal therapeutic response as well as the minimal dose possible to maintain that therapeutic response.
For edematous conditions: The usual adult dose ranges from 2.5 to 10 mg once daily. Maximum effective single dose is 10 mg; larger single doses do not accomplish greater diuresis, and are not recommended.
For the treatment of hypertension: The usual Adult dose ranges from 2.5 to 5 mg once daily.
If control of blood pressure is not satisfactory after 8 to 12 weeks of therapy with 5 mg once daily, another antihypertensive drug should be added. Increasing the dosage of methyclothiazide will usually not result in further lowering of blood pressure.
Methyclothiazide may be either employed alone for mild to moderate hypertension or concurrently with other antihypertensive drugs in the management of more severe forms of hypertension. Combined therapy may provide adequate control of hypertension with lower dosage of the component drugs and fewer or less severe side effects. An enhanced response frequently follows its concurrent administration with Harmonyl® (deserpidine) so that dosage of both drugs may be reduced.
When other antihypertensive agents are to be added to the regimen, this should be accomplished gradually. Ganglionic blocking agents should be given at only half the usual dose since their effect is potentiated by pretreatment with ENDURON tablets.

HOW SUPPLIED

ENDURON (methyclothiazide tablets, USP) is provided in two dosage sizes as monogrammed, grooved, square-shaped tablets:
2.5 mg, orange-colored tablets bearing the ⊐ and the trademark **ENDURON** for product identification:
bottles of 100 (**NDC** 0074-6827-01).
5 mg, salmon-colored tablets bearing the ⊐ and the trademark **ENDURON** for product identification:
bottles of 100 (**NDC** 0074-6812-01).
Dispense in a USP tight container.
Recommended storage: Store below 86° F (30° C).
Revised: October, 1998
Ref. 03-4913-R10
ABBOTT LABORATORIES
NORTH CHICAGO, IL 60064, U.S.A.
PRINTED IN U.S.A.

ERY-PED® ℞

[erē ' ped]
(ERYTHROMYCIN ETHYLSUCCINATE, USP)

DESCRIPTION

Erythromycin is produced by a strain of *Saccharopolyspora erythraea* (formerly *Streptomyces erythraeus*) and belongs to the macrolide group of antibiotics. It is basic and readily forms salts with acids. The base, the stearate salt, and the esters are poorly soluble in water. Erythromycin ethylsuccinate is an ester of erythromycin suitable for oral adminis-

Continued on next page

Ery-Ped—Cont.

tration. Erythromycin ethylsuccinate is known chemically as erythromycin 2′-(ethyl succinate). The molecular formula is $C_{43}H_{75}NO_{16}$ and the molecular weight is 862.06. The structural formula is:

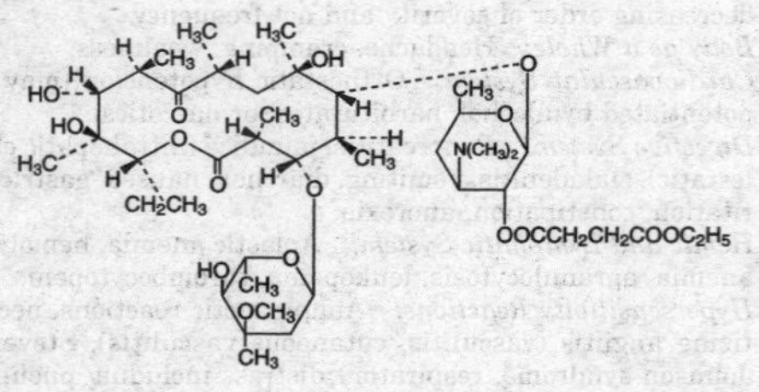

EryPed 200 and EryPed Drops (erythromycin ethylsuccinate for oral suspension) when reconstituted with water, forms a suspension containing erythromycin ethylsuccinate equivalent to 200 mg erythromycin per 5 mL (teaspoonful) or 100 mg per 2.5 mL (dropperful) with an appealing fruit flavor. EryPed 400 when reconstituted with water, forms a suspension containing erythromycin ethylsuccinate equivalent to 400 mg of erythromycin per 5 mL (teaspoonful) with an appealing banana flavor.

Fruit-flavored EryPed Chewable tablets are easily ingested and are particularly acceptable for the administration of antibiotic medication to young children who are unable to swallow regular tablets or in whom persuasion of a pleasant taste insures cooperation.

Each chewable tablet contains erythromycin ethylsuccinate equivalent to 200 mg of erythromycin and is scored for division into half-dose (100 mg) portions.

These products are intended primarily for pediatric use but can also be used in adults.

Inactive Ingredients:

EryPed 200, EryPed 400 and EryPed Drops: Caramel, polysorbate, sodium citrate, sucrose, xanthan gum and artificial flavors.

EryPed Chewable Tablets: Citric acid, confectioner's sugar (contains corn starch), magnesium aluminum silicate, magnesium stearate, sodium carboxymethylcellulose, sodium citrate and artificial flavor.

CLINICAL PHARMACOLOGY

Orally administered erythromycin ethylsuccinate suspension is readily and reliably absorbed under both fasting and nonfasting conditions.

Erythromycin diffuses readily into most body fluids. Only low concentrations are normally achieved in the spinal fluid, but passage of the drug across the blood-brain barrier increases in meningitis. In the presence of normal hepatic function, erythromycin is concentrated in the liver and excreted in the bile; the effect of hepatic dysfunction on excretion of erythromycin by the liver into the bile is not known. Less than 5 percent of the orally administered dose of erythromycin is excreted in active form in the urine.

Erythromycin crosses the placental barrier, but fetal plasma levels are low. The drug is excreted in human milk.

Microbiology:

Erythromycin acts by inhibition of protein synthesis by binding 50 *S* ribosomal subunits of susceptible organisms. It does not affect nucleic acid synthesis. Antagonism has been demonstrated *in vitro* between erythromycin and clindamycin, lincomycin, and chloramphenicol.

Many strains of *Haemophilus influenzae* are resistant to erythromycin alone but are susceptible to erythromycin and sulfonamides used concomitantly.

Staphylococci resistant to erythromycin may emerge during a course of therapy.

Erythromycin has been shown to be active against most strains of the following microorganisms, both *in vitro* and in clinical infections as described in the **INDICATIONS AND USAGE** section.

Gram-positive Organisms:

Corynebacterium diphtheriae
Corynebacterium minutissimum
Listeria monocytogenes
Staphylococcus aureus (resistant organisms may emerge during treatment)
Streptococcus pneumoniae
Streptococcus pyogenes

Gram-negative Organisms:

Bordetella pertussis
Legionella pneumophila
Neisseria gonorrhoeae

Other Microorganisms:

Chlamydia trachomatis
Entamoeba histolytica
Mycoplasma pneumoniae
Treponema pallidum
Ureaplasma urealyticum

The following *in vitro* data are available, **but their clinical significance is unknown.**

Erythromycin exhibits *in vitro* minimal inhibitory concentrations (MIC's) of 0.5 μg/mL or less against most (≥ 90%) strains of the following microorganisms; however, the safety and effectiveness of erythromycin in treating clinical infections due to these microorganisms have not been established in adequate and well-controlled clinical trials.

Gram-positive Organisms:

Viridans group streptococci

Gram-negative Organisms:

Moraxella catarrhalis

Susceptibility Tests:

Dilution Techniques:

Quantitative methods are used to determine antimicrobial minimum inhibitory concentrations (MIC's). These MIC's provide estimates of the susceptibility of bacteria to antimicrobial compounds. The MIC's should be determined using a standardized procedure. Standardized procedures are based on a dilution method[1] (broth or agar) or equivalent with standardized inoculum concentrations and standardized concentrations of erythromycin powder. The MIC values should be interpreted according to the following criteria:

MIC (μg/mL)	Interpretation
≤0.5	Susceptible (S)
1–4	Intermediate (I)
≥8	Resistant (R)

A report of "Susceptible" indicates that the pathogen is likely to be inhibited if the antimicrobial compound in the blood reaches the concentrations usually achievable. A report of "Intermediate" indicates that the result should be considered equivocal, and, if the microorganism is not fully susceptible to alternative, clinically feasible drugs, the test should be repeated. This category implies possible clinical applicability in body sites where the drug is physiologically concentrated or in situations where high dosage of drug can be used. This category also provides a buffer zone which prevents small uncontrolled technical factors from causing major discrepancies in interpretation. A report of "Resistant" indicates that the pathogen is not likely to be inhibited if the antimicrobial compound in the blood reaches the concentrations usually achievable; other therapy should be selected.

Standardized susceptibility test procedures require the use of laboratory control microorganisms to control the technical aspects of the laboratory procedures. Standard erythromycin powder should provide the following MIC values:

Microorganism	MIC (μg/mL)
S. aureus ATCC 29213	0.12-0.5
*E. faecalis*ATCC 22912	1–4

Diffusion Techniques:

Quantitative methods that require measurement of zone diameters also provide reproducible estimates of the susceptibility of bacteria to antimicrobial compounds. One such standardized procedure[2] requires the use of standardized inoculum concentrations. This procedure uses paper disks impregnated with 15-μg erythromycin to test the susceptibility of microorganisms to erythromycin.

Reports from the laboratory providing results of the standard single-disk susceptibility test with a 15-μg erythromycin disk should be interpreted according to the following criteria:

Zone Diameter (mm)	Interpretation
≥23	Susceptible (S)
14–22	Intermediate (I)
≤13	Resistant (R)

Interpretation should be as stated above for results using dilution techniques. Interpretation involves correlation of the diameter obtained in the disk test with the MIC for erythromycin.

As with standardized dilution techniques, diffusion methods require the use of laboratory control microorganisms that are used to control the technical aspects of the laboratory procedures. For the diffusion technique, the 15-μg erythromycin disk should provide the following zone diameters in these laboratory test quality control strains:

Microorganism	Zone Diameter (mm)
S. aureus ATCC 25923	22–30

INDICATIONS AND USAGE

Ery-Ped is indicated in the treatment of infections caused by susceptible strains of the designated organisms in the diseases listed below:

Upper respiratory tract infections of mild to moderate degree caused by *Streptococcus pyogenes, Streptococcus pneumoniae*, or *Haemophilus influenzae* (when used concomitantly with adequate doses of sulfonamides, since many strains of *H. influenzae* are not susceptible to the erythromycin concentrations ordinarily achieved). (See appropriate sulfonamide labeling for prescribing information.)

Lower-respiratory tract infections of mild to moderate severity caused by *Streptococcus pneumoniae* or *Streptococcus pyogenes*.

Listeriosis caused by *Listeria monocytogenes*.

Pertussis (whooping cough) caused by *Bordetella pertussis*. Erythromycin is effective in eliminating the organism from the nasopharynx of infected individuals rendering them noninfectious. Some clinical studies suggest that erythromycin may be helpful in the prophylaxis of pertussis in exposed susceptible individuals.

Respiratory tract infections due to *Mycoplasma pneumoniae*.

Skin and skin structure infections of mild to moderate severity caused by *Streptococcus pyogenes* or *Staphylococcus aureus* (resistant staphylococci may emerge during treatment).

Diphtheria: Infections due to *Corynebacterium diphtheriae*, as an adjunct to antitoxin, to prevent establishment of carriers and to eradicate the organism in carriers.

Erythrasma: In the treatment of infections due to *Corynebacterium minutissimum*.

Intestinal amebiasis caused by *Entamoeba histolytica* (oral erythromycins only). Extraenteric amebiasis requires treatment with other agents.

Acute pelvic inflammatory disease caused by *Neisseria gonorrhoeae*: As an alternative drug in treatment of acute pelvic inflammatory disease caused by *N. gonorrhoeae* in female patients with a history of sensitivity to penicillin. Patients should have a serologic test for syphilis before receiving erythromycin as treatment of gonorrhea and a follow-up serologic test for syphilis after 3 months.

Syphilis caused by *Treponema pallidum*: Erythromycin is an alternate choice of treatment for primary syphilis in penicillin-allergic patients. In primary syphilis, spinal fluid examinations should be done before treatment and as part of follow-up after therapy.

Erythromycins are indicated for the treatment of the following infections caused by *Chlamydia trachomatis*: conjunctivitis of the newborn, pneumonia of infancy, and urogenital infections during pregnancy. When tetracyclines are contraindicated or not tolerated, erythromycin is indicated for the treatment of uncomplicated urethral, endocervical, or rectal infections in adults due to *Chlamydia trachomatis*.

When tetracyclines are contraindicated or not tolerated, erythromycin is indicated for the treatment of nongonococcal urethritis caused by *Ureaplasma urealyticum*.

Legionnaires' Disease caused by *Legionella pneumophila*. Although no controlled clinical efficacy studies have been conducted, *in vitro* and limited preliminary clinical data suggest that erythromycin may be effective in treating Legionnaires' Disease.

Prophylaxis:

Prevention of Initial Attacks of Rheumatic Fever: Penicillin is considered by the American Heart Association to be the drug of choice in the prevention of initial attacks of rheumatic fever (treatment of *Streptococcus pyogenes* infections of the upper respiratory tract, e.g., tonsillitis or pharyngitis). Erythromycin is indicated for the treatment of penicillin-allergic patients.[3] The therapeutic dose should be administered for 10 days.

Prevention of Recurrent Attacks of Rheumatic Fever: Penicillin or sulfonamides are considered by the American Heart Association to be the drugs of choice in the prevention of recurrent attacks of rheumatic fever. In patients who are allergic to penicillin and sulfonamides, oral erythromycin is recommended by the American Heart Association in the long-term prophylaxis of streptococcal pharyngitis (for the prevention of recurrent attacks of rheumatic fever).[3]

CONTRAINDICATIONS

Erythromycin is contraindicated in patients with known hypersensitivity to this antibiotic.

Erythromycin is contraindicated in patients taking terfenadine, astemizole, or cisapride. (See **PRECAUTIONS** - *Drug Interactions*.)

WARNINGS

There have been reports of hepatic dysfunction, including increased liver enzymes, and hepatocellular and/or cholestatic hepatitis, with or without jaundice, occurring in patients receiving oral erythromycin products.

There have been reports suggesting that erythromycin does not reach the fetus in adequate concentration to prevent congenital syphilis. Infants born to women treated during pregnancy with oral erythromycin for early syphilis should be treated with an appropriate penicillin regimen.

Pseudomembranous colitis has been reported with nearly all antibacterial agents, including erythromycin, and may range in severity from mild to life threatening. Therefore, it is important to consider this diagnosis in patients who present with diarrhea subsequent to the administration of antibacterial agents.

Treatment with antibacterial agents alters the normal flora of the colon and may permit overgrowth of clostridia. Studies indicate that a toxin produced by *Clostridium difficile* is a primary cause of "antibiotic-associated colitis".

After the diagnosis of pseudomembranous colitis has been established, therapeutic measures should be initiated. Mild cases of pseudomembranous colitis usually respond to discontinuation of the drug alone. In moderate to severe cases, consideration should be given to management with fluids and electrolytes, protein supplementation, and treatment with an antibacterial drug clinically effective against *Clostridium difficile* colitis.

Rhabdomyolysis with or without renal impairment has been reported in seriously ill patients receiving erythromycin concomitantly with lovastatin. Therefore, patients receiving concomitant lovastatin and erythromycin should be carefully monitored for creatine kinase (CK) and serum transaminase levels. (See package insert for lovastatin.)

PRECAUTIONS

General: Since erythromycin is principally excreted by the liver, caution should be exercised when erythromycin is administered to patients with impaired hepatic function. (See **CLINICAL PHARMACOLOGY** and **WARNINGS** sections.)

There have been reports that erythromycin may aggravate the weakness of patients with myasthenia gravis.

Prolonged or repeated use of erythromycin may result in an overgrowth of nonsusceptible bacteria or fungi. If superinfection occurs, erythromycin should be discontinued and appropriate therapy instituted.

When indicated, incision and drainage or other surgical procedures should be performed in conjunction with antibiotic therapy.

Drug Interactions: Erythromycin use in patients who are receiving high doses of theophylline may be associated with an increase in serum theophylline levels and potential theophylline toxicity. In case of theophylline toxicity and/or elevated serum theophylline levels, the dose of theophylline should be reduced while the patient is receiving concomitant erythromycin therapy.

Concomitant administration of erythromycin and digoxin has been reported to result in elevated digoxin serum levels.

There have been reports of increased anticoagulant effects when erythromycin and oral anticoagulants were used concomitantly. Increased anticoagulation effects due to interactions of erythromycin with various oral anticoagulants may be more pronounced in the elderly.

Concurrent use of erythromycin and ergotamine or dihydroergotamine has been associated in some patients with acute ergot toxicity characterized by severe peripheral vasospasm and dysesthesia.

Erythromycin has been reported to decrease the clearance of triazolam and midazolam and, thus, may increase the pharmacologic effect of these benzodiazepines.

The use of erythromycin in patients concurrently taking drugs metabolized by the cytochrome P450 system may be associated with elevations in serum levels of these other drugs. There have been reports of interactions of erythromycin with carbamazepine, cyclosporine, tacrolimus, hexobarbital, phenytoin, alfentanil, cisapride, disopyramide, lovastatin, bromocriptine, valproate, terfenadine, and astemizole. Serum concentrations of drugs metabolized by the cytochrome P450 system should be monitored closely in patients concurrently receiving erythromycin.

Erythromycin has been reported to significantly alter the metabolism of the nonsedating antihistamines terfenadine and astemizole when taken concomitantly. Rare cases of serious cardiovascular adverse events, including electrocardiographic QT/QT_c interval prolongation, cardiac arrest, torsades de pointes, and other ventricular arrhythmias have been observed. (See **CONTRAINDICATIONS.**) In addition, deaths have been reported rarely with concomitant administration of terfenadine and erythromycin.

There have been post-marketing reports of drug interactions when erythromycin was coadministered with cisapride, resulting in QT prolongation, cardiac arrhythmias, ventricular tachycardia, ventricular fibrillation, and torsades de pointes most likely due to the inhibition of hepatic metabolism of cisapride by erythromycin. Fatalities have been reported. (See **CONTRAINDICATIONS.**)

Drug/Laboratory Test Interactions: Erythromycin interferes with the fluorometric determination of urinary catecholamines.

Carcinogenesis, Mutagenesis, Impairment of Fertility: Long-term (2-year) oral studies in rats with erythromycin ethylsuccinate and erythromycin base did not provide evidence of tumorigenicity. Mutagenicity studies have not been conducted. There was no apparent effect on male or female fertility in rats fed erythromycin (base) at levels up to 0.25% of diet.

Pregnancy: Teratogenic Effects. Pregnancy Category B: There is no evidence of teratogenicity or any other adverse effect on reproduction in female rats fed erythromycin base (up to 0.25% of diet) prior to and during mating, during gestation, and through weaning of two successive litters. There are, however, no adequate and well-controlled studies in pregnant women. Because animal reproduction studies are not always predictive of human response, this drug should be used during pregnancy only if clearly needed.

Labor and Delivery: The effect of erythromycin on labor and delivery is unknown.

Nursing Mothers: Erythromycin is excreted in human milk. Caution should be exercised when erythromycin is administered to a nursing woman.

Pediatric Use: See **INDICATIONS AND USAGE** and **DOSAGE AND ADMINISTRATION** sections.

ADVERSE REACTIONS

The most frequent side effects of oral erythromycin preparations are gastrointestinal and are dose-related. They include nausea, vomiting, abdominal pain, diarrhea and anorexia. Symptoms of hepatitis, hepatic dysfunction and/or abnormal liver function test results may occur. (See **WARNINGS** section.)

Onset of pseudomembranous colitis symptoms may occur during or after antibacterial treatment. (See **WARNINGS.**)

Rarely, erythromycin has been associated with the production of ventricular arrhythmias, including ventricular tachycardia and torsades de pointes, in individuals with prolonged QT intervals.

Allergic reactions ranging from urticaria to anaphylaxis have occurred. Skin reactions ranging from mild eruptions to erythema multiforme, Stevens-Johnson syndrome, and toxic epidermal necrolysis have been reported rarely.

There have been isolated reports of reversible hearing loss occurring chiefly in patients with renal insufficiency and in patients receiving high doses of erythromycin.

OVERDOSAGE

In case of overdosage, erythromycin should be discontinued. Overdosage should be handled with the prompt elimination of unabsorbed drug and all other appropriate measures should be instituted.

Erythromycin is not removed by peritoneal dialysis or hemodialysis.

DOSAGE AND ADMINISTRATION

EryPed (erythromycin ethylsuccinate) oral suspensions and chewable tablets may be administered without regard to meals.

Children: Age, weight, and severity of the infection are important factors in determining the proper dosage. In mild to moderate infections, the usual dosage of erythromycin ethylsuccinate for children is 30 to 50 mg/kg/day in equally divided doses every 6 hours. For more severe infections this dosage may be doubled. If twice-a-day dosage is desired, one-half of the total daily dose may be given every 12 hours. Doses may also be given three times daily by administering one-third of the total daily dose every 8 hours.

The following dosage schedule is suggested for mild to moderate infections:

Body Weight	Total Daily Dose
Under 10 lbs	30–50 mg/kg/day 15–25 mg/lb/day
10 to 15 lbs	200 mg
16 to 25 lbs	400 mg
26 to 50 lbs	800 mg
51 to 100 lbs	1200 mg
over 100 lbs	1600 mg

Adults: 400 mg erythromycin ethylsuccinate every 6 hours is the usual dose. Dosage may be increased up to 4 g per day according to the severity of the infection. If twice-a-day dosage is desired, one-half of the total daily dose may be given every 12 hours. Doses may also be given three times daily by administering one-third of the total daily dose every 8 hours.

For adult dosage calculation, use a ratio of 400 mg of erythromycin activity as the ethylsuccinate to 250 mg of erythromycin activity as the stearate, base or estolate.

In the treatment of streptococcal infections, a therapeutic dosage of erythromycin ethylsuccinate should be administered for at least 10 days. In continuous prophylaxis against recurrences of streptococcal infections in persons with a history of rheumatic heart disease, the usual dosage is 400 mg twice a day.

For treatment of urethritis due to *C. trachomatis* or *U. urealyticum:* 800 mg three times a day for 7 days.

For treatment of primary syphilis: Adults: 48 to 64 g given in divided doses over a period of 10 to 15 days.

For intestinal amebiasis: Adults: 400 mg four times daily for 10 to 14 days. Children: 30 to 50 mg/kg/day in divided doses for 10 to 14 days.

For use in pertussis: Although optimal dosage and duration have not been established, doses of erythromycin utilized in reported clinical studies were 40 to 50 mg/kg/day, given in divided doses for 5 to 14 days.

For treatment of Legionnaires' Disease: Although optimal doses have not been established, doses utilized in reported clinical data were 1.6 to 4 g daily in divided doses.

For the EryPed 200 unit dose, reconstitute with 2.9 mL of water. For the EryPed 400 unit dose, reconstitute with 2.7 mL of water.

HOW SUPPLIED

EryPed 200 (erythromycin ethylsuccinate for oral suspension, USP) is supplied in bottles of 100 mL (**NDC** 0074-6302-13), 200 mL (**NDC** 0074-6302-53), and 5 mL unit dose ABBO-PAC® packages of 100 bottles (**NDC** 0074-6302-05).

EryPed 400 (erythromycin ethylsuccinate for oral suspension, USP) is supplied in bottles of 60 mL (**NDC** 0074-6305-60), 100 mL (**NDC** 0074-6305-13), 200 mL (**NDC** 0074-6305-53), and 5 mL unit dose ABBO-PAC packages of 100 bottles (**NDC** 0074-6305-05).

EryPed Drops (erythromycin ethylsuccinate for oral suspension) is supplied in 50 mL bottles (**NDC** 0074-6303-50).

EryPed Chewable (erythromycin ethylsuccinate tablets, USP) are fruit-flavored wafers containing activity equivalent to 200 mg of erythromycin and are available in packages of 40 (**NDC** 0074-6314-40). Each wafer is individually sealed in a blister package.

Recommended storage: Store EryPed Chewable below 86°F (30°C). Store EryPed 200, EryPed 400, and EryPed Drops, prior to mixing, below 86°F (30°C). After reconstitution, EryPed 200, EryPed 400, and EryPed Drops must be stored at or below 77°F (25°C) and used within 35 days; refrigeration is not required.

REFERENCES

1. National Committee for Clinical Laboratory Standards, *Method for Dilution Antimicrobial Susceptibility Tests for Bacteria that Grow Aerobically*, Third Edition. Approved Standard NCCLS Document M7-A3, Vol. 13, No. 25. NCCLS, Villanova, PA, December 1993.
2. National Committee for Clinical Laboratory Standards, *Performance Standards for Antimicrobial Disk Susceptibility Tests*, Fifth Edition. Approved Standard NCCLS Document M2-A5, Vol. 13, No. 24. NCCLS, Villanova, PA, December 1993.
3. Committee on Rheumatic Fever, Endocarditis, and Kawasaki Disease of the Council on Cardiovascular Disease in the Young, the American Heart Association: Prevention of Rheumatic Fever. *Circulation.* 78(4):1082-1086, October 1988.

Ref. 03-5041-R10

Revised: April, 2000

ABBOTT LABORATORIES

NORTH CHICAGO, IL 60064, U.S.A.

Shown in Product Identification Guide, page 303

ERY-TAB® ℞

[*ē rē 'tab*]

(ERYTHROMYCIN DELAYED-RELEASE TABLETS, USP) ENTERIC-COATED

℞ only

DESCRIPTION

ERY-TAB (erythromycin delayed-release tablets) is an antibacterial product containing erythromycin base in a specially enteric-coated tablet to protect it from the inactivating effects of gastric acidity and to permit efficient absorption of the antibiotic in the small intestine. ERY-TAB tablets for oral administration are available in three dosage strengths, each white oval tablet containing either 250 mg, 333 mg, or 500 mg of erythromycin as the free base. ERY-TAB tablets comply with *USP Drug Release Test 1.*

Erythromycin is produced by a strain of *Saccharopolyspora erythraea* (formerly *Streptomyces erythraeus*) and belongs to the macrolide group of antibiotics. It is basic and readily forms salts with acids. Erythromycin is a white to off-white powder, slightly soluble in water, and soluble in alcohol, chloroform, and ether. Erythromycin is known chemically as (3R*, 4S*, 5S*, 6R*, 7R*, 9R*, 11R*, 12R*, 13S*, 14R*)-4-[(2,6-dideoxy-3-C-methyl-3-O-methyl-α-L-*ribo*-hexopyranosyl)oxy]-14-ethyl-7,12,13-trihydroxy-3,5,7,9,11,13-hexamethyl-6-[[3,4,6-trideoxy-3-(dimethylamino)-β-D-*xylo*-hexopyranosyl]oxy]oxacyclotetradecane-2,10-dione. The molecular formula is $C_{37}H_{67}NO_{13}$, and the molecular weight is 733.94. The structural formula is:

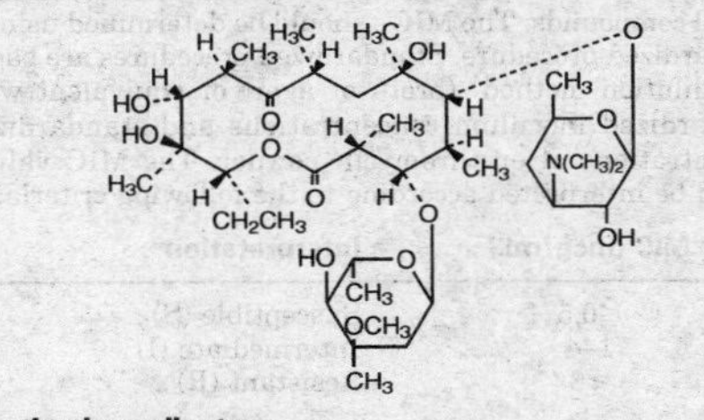

Inactive Ingredients

Ammonium hydroxide, colloidal silicon dioxide, croscarmellose sodium, crospovidone, diacetylated monoglycerides, hydroxypropyl cellulose, hydroxypropyl methylcellulose, hypromellose phthalate, magnesium stearate, microcrystalline cellulose, povidone, propylene glycol, sodium citrate, sorbitan monooleate, talc, and titanium dioxide.

CLINICAL PHARMACOLOGY

Orally administered erythromycin base and its salts are readily absorbed in the microbiologically active form. Interindividual variations in the absorption of erythromycin are, however, observed, and some patients do not achieve optimal serum levels. Erythromycin is largely bound to plasma proteins. After absorption, erythromycin diffuses readily into most body fluids. In the absence of meningeal inflammation, low concentrations are normally achieved in the spinal fluid but the passage of the drug across the blood-brain barrier increases in meningitis. Erythromycin crosses the placental barrier, but fetal plasma levels are low. The drug is excreted in human milk. Erythromycin is not removed by peritoneal dialysis or hemodialysis.

In the presence of normal hepatic function, erythromycin is concentrated in the liver and is excreted in the bile; the effect of hepatic dysfunction on biliary excretion of erythromycin is not known. After oral administration, less than 5% of the administered dose can be recovered in the active form in the urine.

ERY-TAB tablets are coated with a polymer whose dissolution is pH dependent. This coating allows for minimal release of erythromycin in acidic environments, e.g. stomach. The tablets are designed for optimal drug release and absorption in the small intestine. In multiple-dose, steady-state studies, ERY-TAB tablets have demonstrated adequate drug delivery in both fasting and non-fasting conditions. Bioavailability data are available from Abbott Laboratories, Dept. 422.

Continued on next page

Ery-Tab—Cont.

Microbiology:
Erythromycin acts by inhibition of protein synthesis by binding 50 S ribosomal subunits of susceptible organisms. It does not affect nucleic acid synthesis. Antagonism has been demonstrated *in vitro* between erythromycin and clindamycin, lincomycin, and chloramphenicol.
Many strains of *Haemophilus influenzae* are resistant to erythromycin alone, but are susceptible to erythromycin and sulfonamides used concomitantly.
Staphylococci resistant to erythromycin may emerge during a course of erythromycin therapy.
Erythromycin has been shown to be active against most strains of the following microorganisms, both *in vitro* and in clinical infections as described in the **INDICATIONS AND USAGE** section.

Gram-positive organisms:
Corynebacterium diphtheriae
Corynebacterium minutissimum
Listeria monocytogenes
Staphylococcus aureus (resistant organisms may emerge during treatment)
Streptococcus pneumoniae
Streptococcus pyogenes

Gram-negative organisms:
Bordetella pertussis
Legionella pneumophila
Neisseria gonorrhoeae

Other microorganisms:
Chlamydia trachomatis
Entamoeba histolytica
Mycoplasma pneumoniae
Treponema pallidum
Ureaplasma urealyticum

The following *in vitro* data are available, **but their clinical significance is unknown.**
Erythromycin exhibits *in vitro* minimal inhibitory concentrations (MIC's) of 0.5 mcg/mL or less against most (≥ 90%) strains of the following microorganisms; however, the safety and effectiveness of erythromycin in treating clinical infections due to these microorganisms have not been established in adequate and well-controlled clinical trials.

Gram-positive organisms:
Viridans group streptococci

Gram-negative organisms:
Moraxella catarrhalis

Susceptibility Tests:

Dilution Techniques:
Quantitative methods are used to determine antimicrobial minimum inhibitory concentrations (MIC's). These MIC's provide estimates of the susceptibility of bacteria to antimicrobial compounds. The MIC's should be determined using a standardized procedure. Standardized procedures are based on a dilution method[1] (broth or agar) or equivalent with standardized inoculum concentrations and standardized concentrations of erythromycin powder. The MIC values should be interpreted according to the following criteria:

MIC (mcg/mL)	Interpretation
≤0.5	Susceptible (S)
1–4	Intermediate (I)
≥8	Resistant (R)

A report of "Susceptible" indicates that the pathogen is likely to be inhibited if the antimicrobial compound in the blood reaches the concentrations usually achievable. A report of "Intermediate" indicates that the result should be considered equivocal, and, if the microorganism is not fully susceptible to alternative, clinically feasible drugs, the test should be repeated. This category implies possible clinical applicability in body sites where the drug is physiologically concentrated or in situations where high dosage of drug can be used. This category also provides a buffer zone which prevents small uncontrolled technical factors from causing major discrepancies in interpretation. A report of "Resistant" indicates that the pathogen is not likely to be inhibited if the antimicrobial compound in the blood reaches the concentrations usually achievable; other therapy should be selected.
Standardized susceptibility test procedures require the use of laboratory control microorganisms to control the technical aspects of the laboratory procedures. Standard erythromycin powder should provide the following MIC values:

Microorganism	MIC (mcg/mL)
S. aureus ATCC 29213	0.12–0.5
E. faecalis ATCC 29212	1–4

Diffusion Techniques:
Quantitative methods that require measurement of zone diameters also provide reproducible estimates of the susceptibility of bacteria to antimicrobial compounds. One such standardized procedure[2] requires the use of standardized inoculum concentrations. This procedure uses paper disks impregnated with 15-mcg erythromycin to test the susceptibility of microorganisms to erythromycin.
Reports from the laboratory providing results of the standard single-disk susceptibility test with a 15-mcg erythromycin disk should be interpreted according to the following criteria:

Zone Diameter (mm)	Interpretation
≥23	Susceptible (S)
14–22	Intermediate (I)
≤13	Resistant (R)

Interpretation should be as stated above for results using dilution techniques. Interpretation involves correlation of the diameter obtained in the disk test with the MIC for erythromycin.
As with standardized dilution techniques, diffusion methods require the use of laboratory control microorganisms that are used to control the technical aspects of the laboratory procedures. For the diffusion technique, the 15-mcg erythromycin disk should provide the following zone diameters in these laboratory test quality control strains:

Microorganism	Zone Diameter (mm)
S. aureus ATCC 25923	22–30

INDICATIONS AND USAGE

ERY-TAB tablets are indicated in the treatment of infections caused by susceptible strains of the designated microorganisms in the diseases listed below:
Upper respiratory tract infections of mild to moderate degree caused by *Streptococcus pyogenes; Streptococcus pneumoniae; Haemophilus influenzae* (when used concomitantly with adequate doses of sulfonamides, since many strains of *H. influenzae* are not susceptible to the erythromycin concentrations ordinarily achieved). (See appropriate sulfonamide labeling for prescribing information.)
Lower respiratory tract infections of mild to moderate severity caused by *Streptococcus pyogenes* or *Streptococcus pneumoniae*.
Listeriosis caused by *Listeria monocytogenes*.
Respiratory tract infections due to *Mycoplasma pneumoniae*.
Skin and skin structure infections of mild to moderate severity caused by *Streptococcus pyogenes* or *Staphylococcus aureus* (resistant staphylococci may emerge during treatment).
Pertussis (whooping cough) caused by *Bordetella pertussis*. Erythromycin is effective in eliminating the organism from the nasopharynx of infected individuals, rendering them noninfectious. Some clinical studies suggest that erythromycin may be helpful in the prophylaxis of pertussis in exposed susceptible individuals.
Diphtheria: Infections due to *Corynebacterium diphtheriae*, as an adjunct to antitoxin, to prevent establishment of carriers and to eradicate the organism in carriers.
Erythrasma—In the treatment of infections due to *Corynebacterium minutissimum*.
Intestinal amebiasis caused by *Entamoeba histolytica* (oral erythromycins only). Extraenteric amebiasis requires treatment with other agents.
Acute pelvic inflammatory disease caused by *Neisseria gonorrhoeae:* Erythrocin® Lactobionate-I.V. (erythromycin lactobionate for injection, USP) followed by erythromycin base orally, as an alternative drug in treatment of acute pelvic inflammatory disease caused by *N. gonorrhoeae* in female patients with a history of sensitivity to penicillin. Patients should have a serologic test for syphilis before receiving erythromycin as treatment of gonorrhea and a follow-up serologic test for syphilis after 3 months.
Erythromycins are indicated for treatment of the following infections caused by *Chlamydia trachomatis*: conjunctivitis of the newborn, pneumonia of infancy, and urogenital infections during pregnancy. When tetracyclines are contraindicated or not tolerated, erythromycin is indicated for the treatment of uncomplicated urethral, endocervical, or rectal infections in adults due to *Chlamydia trachomatis*.
When tetracyclines are contraindicated or not tolerated, erythromycin is indicated for the treatment of nongonococcal urethritis caused by *Ureaplasma urealyticum*.
Primary syphilis caused by *Treponema pallidum*. Erythromycin (oral forms only) is an alternative choice of treatment for primary syphilis in patients allergic to the penicillins. In treatment of primary syphilis, spinal fluid should be examined before treatment and as part of the follow-up after therapy.
Legionnaires' Disease caused by *Legionella pneumophila*. Although no controlled clinical efficacy studies have been conducted, *in vitro* and limited preliminary clinical data suggest that erythromycin may be effective in treating Legionnaires' Disease.

Prophylaxis
Prevention of Initial Attacks of Rheumatic Fever—Penicillin is considered by the American Heart Association to be the drug of choice in the prevention of initial attacks of rheumatic fever (treatment of *Streptococcus pyogenes* infections of the upper respiratory tract e.g., tonsillitis, or pharyngitis).[3] Erythromycin is indicated for the treatment of penicillin-allergic patients. The therapeutic dose should be administered for ten days.
Prevention of Recurrent Attacks of Rheumatic Fever—Penicillin or sulfonamides are considered by the American Heart Association to be the drugs of choice in the prevention of recurrent attacks of rheumatic fever. In patients who are allergic to penicillin and sulfonamides, oral erythromycin is recommended by the American Heart Association in the long-term prophylaxis of streptococcal pharyngitis (for the prevention of recurrent attacks of rheumatic fever).[3]
Prevention of Bacterial Endocarditis—Although no controlled clinical efficacy trials have been conducted, oral erythromycin has been recommended by the American Heart Association for prevention of bacterial endocarditis in penicillin-allergic patients with prosthetic cardiac valves, most congenital cardiac malformations, surgically constructed systemic pulmonary shunts, rheumatic or other acquired valvular dysfunction, idiopathic hypertrophic subaortic stenosis (IHSS), previous history of bacterial endocarditis or mitral valve prolapse with insufficiency when they undergo dental procedures or surgical procedures of the upper respiratory tract.[4]

CONTRAINDICATIONS

Erythromycin is contraindicated in patients with known hypersensitivity to this antibiotic.
Erythromycin is contraindicated in patients taking terfenadine, astemizole, or cisapride. (See **PRECAUTIONS**—*Drug Interactions.*)

WARNINGS

There have been reports of hepatic dysfunction, including increased liver enzymes, and hepatocellular and/or cholestatic hepatitis, with or without jaundice, occurring in patients receiving oral erythromycin products.
There have been reports suggesting that erythromycin does not reach the fetus in adequate concentration to prevent congenital syphilis. Infants born to women treated during pregnancy with oral erythromycin for early syphilis should be treated with an appropriate penicillin regimen.
Rhabdomyolysis with or without renal impairment has been reported in seriously ill patients receiving erythromycin concomitantly with lovastatin. Therefore, patients receiving concomitant lovastatin and erythromycin should be carefully monitored for creatine kinase (CK) and serum transaminase levels. (See package insert for lovastatin.)
Pseudomembranous colitis has been reported with nearly all antibacterial agents, including erythromycin, and may range in severity from mild to life threatening. Therefore, it is important to consider this diagnosis in patients who present with diarrhea subsequent to the administration of antibacterial agents.
Treatment with antibacterial agents alters the normal flora of the colon and may permit overgrowth of clostridia. Studies indicate that a toxin produced by *Clostridium difficile* is a primary cause of "antibiotic-associated colitis".
After the diagnosis of pseudomembranous colitis has been established, therapeutic measures should be initiated. Mild cases of pseudomembranous colitis usually respond to discontinuation of the drug alone. In moderate to severe cases, consideration should be given to management with fluids and electrolytes, protein supplementation, and treatment with an antibacterial drug clinically effective against *Clostridium difficile* colitis.

PRECAUTIONS

General: Since erythromycin is principally excreted by the liver, caution should be exercised when erythromycin is administered to patients with impaired hepatic function. (See **CLINICAL PHARMACOLOGY** and **WARNINGS**.)
There have been reports that erythromycin may aggravate the weakness of patients with myasthenia gravis.
Prolonged or repeated use of erythromycin may result in an overgrowth of nonsusceptible bacteria or fungi. If superinfection occurs, erythromycin should be discontinued and appropriate therapy instituted.
When indicated, incision and drainage or other surgical procedures should be performed in conjunction with antibiotic therapy.
Drug Interactions: Erythromycin use in patients who are receiving high doses of theophylline may be associated with an increase in serum theophylline levels and potential theophylline toxicity. In case of theophylline toxicity and/or elevated serum theophylline levels, the dose of theophylline should be reduced while the patient is receiving concomitant erythromycin therapy.
Concomitant administration of erythromycin and digoxin has been reported to result in elevated digoxin serum levels.
There have been reports of increased anticoagulant effects when erythromycin and oral anticoagulants were used concomitantly. Increased anticoagulation effects due to interactions of erythromycin with oral anticoagulants may be more pronounced in the elderly.
Concurrent use of erythromycin and ergotamine or dihydroergotamine has been associated in some patients with acute ergot toxicity characterized by severe peripheral vasospasm and dysesthesia.
Erythromycin has been reported to decrease the clearance of triazolam and midazolam and, thus, may increase the pharmacologic effect of these benzodiazepines.
The use of erythromycin in patients concurrently taking drugs metabolized by the cytochrome P450 system may be associated with elevations in serum levels of these other drugs. There have been reports of interactions of erythromycin with carbamazepine, cyclosporine, tacrolimus, hexobarbital, phenytoin, alfentanil, cisapride, disopyramide, lovastatin, bromocriptine, valproate, terfenadine, and astemizole. Serum concentrations of drugs metabolized by the cytochrome P450 system should be monitored closely in patients concurrently receiving erythromycin.
Erythromycin has been reported to significantly alter the metabolism of the nonsedating antihistamines terfenadine

and astemizole when taken concomitantly. Rare cases of serious cardiovascular adverse events, including electrocardiographic QT/QT_c interval prolongation, cardiac arrest, torsades de pointes, and other ventricular arrhythmias, have been observed. (See **CONTRAINDICATIONS**.) In addition, deaths have been reported rarely with concomitant administration of terfenadine and erythromycin.

There have been post-marketing reports of drug interactions when erythromycin was coadministered with cisapride, resulting in QT prolongation, cardiac arrhythmias, ventricular tachycardia, ventricular fibrillation, and torsades de pointes, most likely due to the inhibition of hepatic metabolism of cisapride by erythromycin. Fatalities have been reported. (See **CONTRAINDICATIONS**).

Drug/Laboratory Test interactions: Erythromycin interferes with the fluorometric determination of urinary catecholamines.

Carcinogenesis, Mutagenesis, Impairment of Fertility: Long-term (2-year) oral studies conducted in rats with erythromycin base did not provide evidence of tumorigenicity. Mutagenicity studies have not been conducted. There was no apparent effect on male or female fertility in rats fed erythromycin (base) at levels up to 0.25 percent of diet.

Pregnancy: Teratogenic effects. Pregnancy Category B: There is no evidence of teratogenicity or any other adverse effect on reproduction in female rats fed erythromycin base (up to 0.25 percent of diet) prior to and during mating, during gestation, and through weaning of two successive litters. There are, however, no adequate and well-controlled studies in pregnant women. Because animal reproduction studies are not always predictive of human response, this drug should be used during pregnancy only if clearly needed.

Labor and Delivery: The effect of erythromycin on labor and delivery is unknown.

Nursing Mothers: Erythromycin is excreted in human milk. Caution should be exercised when erythromycin is administered to a nursing woman.

Pediatric Use: See **INDICATIONS AND USAGE** and **DOSAGE AND ADMINISTRATION**.

ADVERSE REACTIONS

The most frequent side effects of oral erythromycin preparations are gastrointestinal and are dose-related. They include nausea, vomiting, abdominal pain, diarrhea and anorexia. Symptoms of hepatitis, hepatic dysfunction and/or abnormal liver function test results may occur. (See **WARNINGS**.)

Onset of pseudomembranous colitis symptoms may occur during or after antibacterial treatment. (See **WARNINGS**.)

Rarely, erythromycin has been associated with the production of ventricular arrhythmias, including ventricular tachycardia and torsades de pointes, in individuals with prolonged QT interval.

Allergic reactions ranging from urticaria to anaphylaxis have occurred. Skin reactions ranging from mild eruptions to erythema multiforme, Stevens-Johnson syndrome, and toxic epidermal necrolysis have been reported rarely.

There have been isolated reports of reversible hearing loss occurring chiefly in patients with renal insufficiency and in patients receiving high doses of erythromycin.

OVERDOSAGE

In case of overdosage, erythromycin should be discontinued. Overdosage should be handled with the prompt elimination of unabsorbed drug and all other appropriate measures should be instituted.

Erythromycin is not removed by peritoneal dialysis or hemodialysis.

DOSAGE AND ADMINISTRATION

In most patients, ERY-TAB (erythromycin delayed-release tablets) are well absorbed and may be given without regard to meals.

Adults: The usual dose is 250 mg four times daily in equally spaced doses. The 333 mg tablet is recommended if dosage is desired every 8 hours. If twice-a-day dosage is desired, the recommended dose is 500 mg every 12 hours. Dosage may be increased up to 4 g per day according to the severity of the infection. However, twice-a-day dosing is not recommended when doses larger than 1 g daily are administered.

Children: Age, weight, and severity of the infection are important factors in determining the proper dosage. The usual dosage is 30 to 50 mg/kg/day, in equally divided doses. For more severe infections, this dose may be doubled but should not exceed 4 g per day.

In the treatment of streptococcal infections of the upper respiratory tract (e.g., tonsillitis or pharyngitis), the therapeutic dosage of erythromycin should be administered for at least ten days.

The American Heart Association suggests a dosage of 250 mg of erythromycin orally, twice a day in long-term prophylaxis of streptococcal upper respiratory tract infections for the prevention of recurring attacks of rheumatic fever in patients allergic to penicillin and sulfonamides.[3]

In prophylaxis against bacterial endocarditis (See **INDICATIONS AND USAGE**) the oral regimen for penicillin allergic patients is erythromycin 1 gram, 1 hour before the procedure followed by 500 mg six hours later.[4]

Conjunctivitis of the newborn caused by *Chlamydia trachomatis:* Oral erythromycin suspension 50 mg/kg/day in 4 divided doses for at least 2 weeks.[3]

Pneumonia of infancy caused by *Chlamydia trachomatis:* Although the optimal duration of therapy has not been established, the recommended therapy is oral erythromycin suspension 50 mg/kg/day in 4 divided doses for at least 3 weeks.

Urogenital infections during pregnancy due to *Chlamydia trachomatis:* Although the optimal dose and duration of therapy have not been established, the suggested treatment is 500 mg of erythromycin by mouth four times a day or two erythromycin 333 mg tablets orally every 8 hours on an empty stomach for at least 7 days. For women who cannot tolerate this regimen, a decreased dose of one erythromycin 500 mg tablet orally every 12 hours, one 333 mg tablet orally every 8 hours or 250 mg by mouth four times a day should be used for at least 14 days.[5]

For adults with uncomplicated urethral, endocervical, or rectal infections caused by *Chlamydia trachomatis,* when tetracycline is contraindicated or not tolerated: 500 mg of erythromycin by mouth four times a day or two 333 mg tablets orally every 8 hours for at least 7 days.[5]

For patients with nongonococcal urethritis caused by *Ureaplasma urealyticum* when tetracycline is contraindicated or not tolerated: 500 mg of erythromycin by mouth four times a day or two 333 mg tablets orally every 8 hours for at least seven days.[5]

Primary syphilis: 30 to 40 g given in divided doses over a period of 10 to 15 days.

Acute pelvic inflammatory disease caused by *N. gonorrhoeae:* 500 mg Erythrocin Lactobionate-I.V. (erythromycin lactobionate for injection, USP) every 6 hours for 3 days, followed by 500 mg of erythromycin base orally every 12 hours, or 333 mg of erythromycin base orally every 8 hours for 7 days.

Intestinal amebiasis: Adults: 500 mg every 12 hours, 333 mg every 8 hours or 250 mg every 6 hours for 10 to 14 days. Children: 30 to 50 mg/kg/day in divided doses for 10 to 14 days.

Pertussis: Although optimal dosage and duration have not been established, doses of erythromycin utilized in reported clinical studies were 40 to 50 mg/kg/day, given in divided doses for 5 to 14 days.

Legionnaires' Disease: Although optimal dosage has not been established, doses utilized in reported clinical data were 1 to 4 grams daily in divided doses.

Preoperative Prophylaxis for Elective Colorectal Surgery: Listed below is an example of a recommended bowel preparation regimen. A proposed surgery time of 8:00 a.m. has been used.

Pre-op Day 3: Minimum residue or clear liquid diet. Bisacodyl, 1 tablet orally at 6:00 p.m.

Pre-op Day 2: Minimum residue or clear liquid diet. Magnesium sulfate, 30 mL, 50% solution (15g) orally at 10:00 a.m., 2:00 p.m. and 6:00 p.m. Enema at 7:00 p.m. and 8:00 p.m.

Pre-op Day 1: Clear liquid diet. Supplemental (IV) fluids as needed. Magnesium sulfate, 30 mL, 50% solution (15g) orally at 10:00 a.m. and 2:00 p.m. Neomycin sulfate (1.0g) and erythromycin base (two 500 mg tablets, three 333 mg tablets or four 250 mg tablets) orally at 1:00 p.m., 2:00 p.m. and 11:00 p.m. No enema.

Day of operation: Patient evacuates rectum at 6:30 a.m. for scheduled operation at 8:00 a.m.

HOW SUPPLIED

ERY-TAB (erythromycin delayed-release tablets, USP) are supplied as white oval enteric-coated tablets debossed on one side with the Abbott logo, and on the other side with a two letter Abbo-Code designation, EC for the 250 mg tablets, EH for the 333 mg tablets, and ED for the 500 mg tablets, in the following package sizes:

250 mg tablets: bottles of 100 (**NDC** 0074-6304-13), bottles of 500 (**NDC** 0074-6304-53), and Abbo-Pac® unit dose packages of 100 (**NDC** 0074-6304-11).

333 mg tablets: bottles of 100 (**NDC** 0074-6320-13), and bottles of 500 (**NDC** 0074-6320-53), and Abbo-Pac® unit dose packages of 100 (**NDC** 0074-6320-11).

500 mg tablets: bottles of 100 (**NDC** 0074-6321-13) and Abbo-Pac® unit dose packages of 100 (**NDC** 0074-6321-11).

Recommended Storage: Store below 86°F (30°C).

REFERENCES

1. National Committee for Clinical Laboratory Standards. *Methods for Dilution Antimicrobial Susceptibility Tests for Bacteria that Grow Aerobically,* Third Edition. Approved Standard NCCLS Document M7-A3, Vol. 13, No. 25 NCCLS, Villanova, PA, December 1993.
2. National Committee for Clinical Laboratory Standards, *Performance Standards for Antimicrobial Disk Susceptibility Tests,* Fifth Edition. Approved Standard NCCLS Document M2-A5, Vol. 13, No. 24 NCCLS, Villanova, PA, December 1993.
3. Committee on Rheumatic Fever, Endocarditis, and Kawasaki Disease of the Council on Cardiovascular Disease in the Young, the American Heart Association: Prevention of Rheumatic Fever. *Circulation.* 78(4):1082-1086, October 1988.
4. Dajani, Adnan S.,M.D., et al.: Prevention of Bacterial Endocarditis Recommendations by the American Heart Association. *JAMA.* 264(22):2919-2922, December 1990.
5. Data on file, Abbott Laboratories.

333 mg and 500 mg tablets—U.S. Pat. No. 4,340,582

Revised: September, 1999

Ref. 03-4954-R3

ABBOTT LABORATORIES

NORTH CHICAGO, IL 60064, U.S.A.

Shown in Product Identification Guide, page 303

E.E.S.® ℞

[ē-ē-s]

(ERYTHROMYCIN ETHYLSUCCINATE)

Rx only

DESCRIPTION

Erythromycin is produced by a strain of *Saccharopolyspora erythraea* (formerly *Streptomyces erythraeus*) and belongs to the macrolide group of antibiotics. It is basic and readily forms salts with acids. The base, the stearate salt, and the esters are poorly soluble in water. Erythromycin ethylsuccinate is an ester of erythromycin suitable for oral administration. Erythromycin ethylsuccinate is known chemically as erythromycin 2′-(ethylsuccinate). The molecular formula is $C_{43}H_{75}NO_{16}$ and the molecular weight is 862.06. The structural formula is:

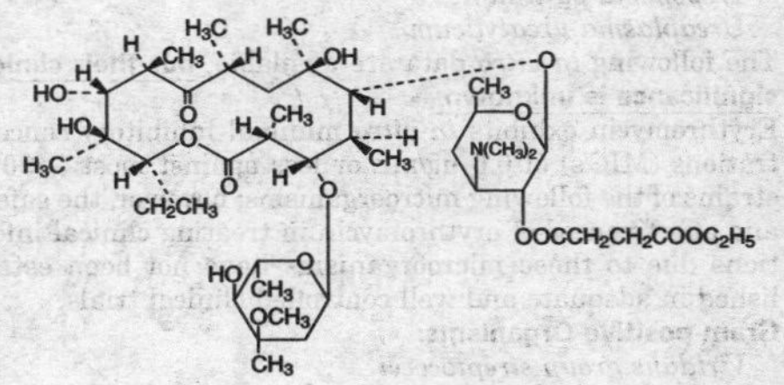

E.E.S. Granules are intended for reconstitution with water. Each 5-mL teaspoonful of reconstituted cherry-flavored suspension contains erythromycin ethylsuccinate equivalent to 200 mg of erythromycin.

The pleasant tasting, fruit-flavored liquids are supplied ready for oral administration.

E.E.S. 200 Liquid: Each 5-mL teaspoonful of fruit-flavored suspension contains erythromycin ethylsuccinate equivalent to 200 mg of erythromycin.

E.E.S. 400 Liquid: Each 5-mL teaspoonful of orange-flavored suspension contains erythromycin ethylsuccinate equivalent to 400 mg of erythromycin.

Granules and ready-made suspensions are intended primarily for pediatric use but can also be used in adults.

E.E.S. 400® Filmtab® Tablets: Each tablet contains erythromycin ethylsuccinate equivalent to 400 mg of erythromycin.

The Filmtab® tablets are intended primarily for adults or older children.

Inactive Ingredients:

E.E.S. 200 Liquid: FD&C Red No. 40, methylparaben, polysorbate 60, propylparaben, sodium citrate, sucrose, water, xanthan gum and natural and artificial flavors.

E.E.S. 400 Liquid: D&C Yellow No. 10, FD&C Yellow No. 6, methylparaben, polysorbate 60, propylparaben, sodium citrate, sucrose, water, xanthan gum and natural and artificial flavors.

E.E.S. Granules: Citric acid, FD&C Red No. 3, magnesium aluminum silicate, sodium carboxymethylcellulose, sodium citrate, sucrose and artificial flavor.

E.E.S. 400 Filmtab Tablets: Cellulosic polymers, confectioner's sugar (contains corn starch), corn starch, D&C Red No. 30, D&C Yellow No. 10, FD&C Red No. 40, magnesium stearate, polacrilin potassium, polyethylene glycol, propylene glycol, sodium citrate, sorbic acid, and titanium dioxide.

CLINICAL PHARMACOLOGY

Orally administered erythromycin ethylsuccinate suspensions and Filmtab tablets are readily and reliably absorbed. Comparable serum levels of erythromycin are achieved in the fasting and nonfasting states.

Erythromycin diffuses readily into most body fluids. Only low concentrations are normally achieved in the spinal fluid, but passage of the drug across the blood-brain barrier increases in meningitis. In the presence of normal hepatic function, erythromycin is concentrated in the liver and excreted in the bile; the effect of hepatic dysfunction on excretion of erythromycin by the liver into the bile is not known. Less than 5 percent of the orally administered dose of erythromycin is excreted in active form in the urine.

Erythromycin crosses the placental barrier, but fetal plasma levels are low. The drug is excreted in human milk.

Microbiology:

Erythromycin acts by inhibition of protein synthesis by binding 50 *S* ribosomal subunits of susceptible organisms. It does not affect nucleic acid synthesis. Antagonism has been demonstrated *in vitro* between erythromycin and clindamycin, lincomycin, and chloramphenicol.

Many strains of *Haemophilus influenzae* are resistant to erythromycin alone but are susceptible to erythromycin and sulfonamides used concomitantly.

Staphylococci resistant to erythromycin may emerge during a course of therapy.

Erythromycin has been shown to be active against most strains of the following microorganisms, both *in vitro* and in clinical infections as described in the **INDICATIONS AND USAGE** section.

Continued on next page

E.E.S.—Cont.

Gram-positive Organisms:
Corynebacterium diphtheriae
Corynebacterium minutissimum
Listeria monocytogenes
Staphylococcus aureus (resistant organisms may emerge during treatment)
Streptococcus pneumoniae
Streptococcus pyogenes
Gram-negative Organisms:
Bordetella pertussis
Legionella pneumophila
Neisseria gonorrhoeae
Other Microorganisms:
Chlamydia trachomatis
Entamoeba histolytica
Mycoplasma pneumoniae
Treponema pallidum
Ureaplasma urealyticum

The following *in vitro* data are available, **but their clinical significance is unknown.**

Erythromycin exhibits *in vitro* minimal inhibitory concentrations (MIC's) of 0.5 μg/mL or less against most (≥90%) strains of the following microorganisms; however, the safety and effectiveness of erythromycin in treating clinical infections due to these microorganisms have not been established in adequate and well controlled clinical trials.

Gram-positive Organisms:
Viridans group streptococci
Gram-negative Organisms:
Moraxella catarrhalis

Susceptibility Tests:
Dilution Techniques:
Quantitative methods are used to determine antimicrobial minimum inhibitory concentrations (MIC's). These MIC's provide estimates of the susceptibility of bacteria to antimicrobial compounds. The MIC's should be determined using a standardized procedure. Standardized procedures are based on a dilution method[1] (broth or agar) or equivalent with standardized inoculum concentrations and standardized concentrations of erythromycin powder. The MIC values should be interpreted according to the following criteria:

MIC (μg/mL)	Interpretation
≤0.5	Susceptible (S)
1–4	Intermediate (I)
≥8	Resistant (R)

A report of "Susceptible" indicates that the pathogen is likely to be inhibited if the antimicrobial compound in the blood reaches the concentrations usually achievable. A report of "Intermediate" indicates that the result should be considered equivocal, and, if the microorganism is not fully susceptible to alternative, clinically feasible drugs, the test should be repeated. This category implies possible clinical applicability in body sites where the drug is physiologically concentrated or in situations where high dosage of drug can be used. This category also provides a buffer zone which prevents small uncontrolled technical factors from causing major discrepancies in interpretation. A report of "Resistant" indicates that the pathogen is not likely to be inhibited if the antimicrobial compound in the blood reaches the concentrations usually achievable; other therapy should be selected.

Standardized susceptibility test procedures require the use of laboratory control microorganisms to control the technical aspects of the laboratory procedures. Standard erythromycin powder should provide the following MIC values:

Microorganism	MIC (μg/mL)
S. aureus ATCC 25923	0.12–0.5
E. faecalis ATCC 29212	1–4

Diffusion Techniques:
Quantitative methods that require measurement of zone diameters also provide reproducible estimates of the susceptibility of bacteria to antimicrobial compounds. One such standardized procedure[2] requires the use of standardized inoculum concentrations. This procedure uses paper disks impregnated with 15-μg erythromycin to test the susceptibility of microorganisms to erythromycin.

Reports from the laboratory providing results of the standard single-disk susceptibility test with a 15-μg erythromycin disk should be interpreted according to the following criteria:

Zone Diameter (mm)	Interpretation
≥23	Susceptible (S)
14–22	Intermediate (I)
≤13	Resistant (R)

Interpretation should be as stated above for results using dilution techniques. Interpretation involves correlation of the diameter obtained in the disk test with the MIC for erythromycin.

As with standardized dilution techniques, diffusion methods require the use of laboratory control microorganisms that are used to control the technical aspects of the laboratory procedures. For the diffusion technique, the 15-μg erythromycin disk should provide the following zone diameters in these laboratory test quality control strains:

Microorganism	Zone Diameter (mm)
S. aureus ATCC 25923	22–30

INDICATIONS AND USAGE

E.E.S. is indicated in the treatment of infections caused by susceptible strains of the designated organisms in the diseases listed below:

Upper respiratory tract infections of mild to moderate degree caused by *Streptococcus pyogenes, Streptococcus pneumoniae*, or *Haemophilus influenzae* (when used concomitantly with adequate doses of sulfonamides, since many strains of *H. influenzae* are not susceptible to the erythromycin concentrations ordinarily achieved). (See appropriate sulfonamide labeling for prescribing information.)

Lower-respiratory tract infections of mild to moderate severity caused by *Streptococcus pneumoniae* or *Streptococcus pyogenes.*

Listeriosis caused by *Listeria monocytogenes.*

Pertussis (whooping cough) caused by *Bordetella pertussis.* Erythromycin is effective in eliminating the organism from the nasopharynx of infected individuals rendering them noninfectious. Some clinical studies suggest that erythromycin may be helpful in the prophylaxis of pertussis in exposed susceptible individuals.

Respiratory tract infections due to *Mycoplasma pneumoniae.*

Skin and skin structure infections of mild to moderate severity caused by *Streptococcus pyogenes* or *Staphylococcus aureus* (resistant staphylococci may emerge during treatment).

Diphtheria: Infections due to *Corynebacterium diphtheriae*, as an adjunct to antitoxin, to prevent establishment of carriers and to eradicate the organism in carriers.

Erythrasma: In the treatment of infections due to *Corynebacterium minutissimum.*

Intestinal amebiasis caused by *Entamoeba histolytica* (oral erythromycins only). Extraenteric amebiasis requires treatment with other agents.

Acute pelvic inflammatory disease caused by *Neisseria gonorrhoeae*: As an alternative drug in treatment of acute pelvic inflammatory disease caused by *N. gonorrhoeae* in female patients with a history of sensitivity to penicillin. Patients should have a serologic test for syphilis before receiving erythromycin as treatment of gonorrhea and a follow-up serologic test for syphilis after 3 months.

Syphilis caused by *Treponema pallidum*: Erythromycin is an alternate choice of treatment for primary syphilis in patients allergic to the penicillins. In treatment of primary syphilis, spinal fluid examinations should be done before treatment and as part of follow-up after therapy.

Erythromycins are indicated for the treatment of the following infections caused by *Chlamydia trachomatis*: conjunctivitis of the newborn, pneumonia of infancy, and urogenital infections during pregnancy. When tetracyclines are contraindicated or not tolerated, erythromycin is indicated for the treatment of uncomplicated urethral, endocervical, or rectal infections in adults due to *Chlamydia trachomatis.*

When tetracyclines are contraindicated or not tolerated, erythromycin is indicated for the treatment of nongonococcal urethritis caused by *Ureaplasma urealyticum.*

Legionnaires' Disease caused by *Legionella pneumophila.* Although no controlled clinical efficacy studies have been conducted, *in vitro* and limited preliminary clinical data suggest that erythromycin may be effective in treating Legionnaires' Disease.

Prophylaxis:

Prevention of Initial Attacks of Rheumatic Fever: Penicillin is considered by the American Heart Association to be the drug of choice in the prevention of initial attacks of rheumatic fever (treatment of *Streptococcus pyogenes* infections of the upper respiratory tract, e.g., tonsillitis or pharyngitis). Erythromycin is indicated for the treatment of penicillin-allergic patients.[3] The therapeutic dose should be administered for 10 days.

Prevention of Recurrent Attacks of Rheumatic Fever: Penicillin or sulfonamides are considered by the American Heart Association to be the drugs of choice in the prevention of recurrent attacks of rheumatic fever. In patients who are allergic to penicillin and sulfonamides, oral erythromycin is recommended by the American Heart Association in the long-term prophylaxis of streptococcal pharyngitis (for the prevention of recurrent attacks of rheumatic fever).[3]

CONTRAINDICATIONS

Erythromycin is contraindicated in patients with known hypersensitivity to this antibiotic.

Erythromycin is contraindicated in patients taking terfenadine, astemizole, or cisapride. (See **PRECAUTIONS** - *Drug Interactions.*)

WARNINGS

There have been reports of hepatic dysfunction, including increased liver enzymes, and hepatocellular and/or cholestatic hepatitis, with or without jaundice, occurring in patients receiving oral erythromycin products.

There have been reports suggesting that erythromycin does not reach the fetus in adequate concentration to prevent congenital syphilis. Infants born to women treated during pregnancy with oral erythromycin for early syphilis should be treated with an appropriate penicillin regimen.

Pseudomembranous colitis has been reported with nearly all antibacterial agents, including erythromycin, and may range in severity from mild to life threatening. Therefore, it is important to consider this diagnosis in patients who present with diarrhea subsequent to the administration of antibacterial agents.

Treatment with antibacterial agents alters the normal flora of the colon and may permit overgrowth of clostridia. Studies indicate that a toxin produced by *Clostridium difficile* is a primary cause of "antibiotic-associated colitis".

After the diagnosis of pseudomembranous colitis has been established, therapeutic measures should be initiated. Mild cases of pseudomembranous colitis usually respond to discontinuation of the drug alone. In moderate to severe cases, consideration should be given to management with fluids and electrolytes, protein supplementation, and treatment with an antibacterial drug clinically effective against *Clostridium difficile* colitis.

Rhabdomyolysis with or without renal impairment has been reported in seriously ill patients receiving erythromycin concomitantly with lovastatin. Therefore, patients receiving concomitant lovastatin and erythromycin should be carefully monitored for creatine kinase (CK) and serum transaminase levels. (See package insert for lovastatin.)

PRECAUTIONS

General: Since erythromycin is principally excreted by the liver, caution should be exercised when erythromycin is administered to patients with impaired hepatic function. (See **CLINICAL PHARMACOLOGY** and **WARNINGS** sections.)

There have been reports that erythromycin may aggravate the weakness of patients with myasthenia gravis.

Prolonged or repeated use of erythromycin may result in an overgrowth of nonsusceptible bacteria or fungi. If superinfection occurs, erythromycin should be discontinued and appropriate therapy instituted.

When indicated, incision and drainage or other surgical procedures should be performed in conjunction with antibiotic therapy.

Drug Interactions: Erythromycin use in patients who are receiving high doses of theophylline may be associated with an increase in serum theophylline levels and potential theophylline toxicity. In case of theophylline toxicity and/or elevated serum theophylline levels, the dose of theophylline should be reduced while the patient is receiving concomitant erythromycin therapy.

Concomitant administration of erythromycin and digoxin has been reported to result in elevated digoxin serum levels.

There have been reports of increased anticoagulant effects when erythromycin and oral anticoagulants were used concomitantly. Increased anticoagulation effects due to interactions of erythromycin with various oral anticoagulants may be more pronounced in the elderly.

Concurrent use of erythromycin and ergotamine or dihydroergotamine has been associated in some patients with acute ergot toxicity characterized by severe peripheral vasospasm and dysesthesia.

Erythromycin has been reported to decrease the clearance of triazolam and midazolam and, thus, may increase the pharmacologic effect of these benzodiazepines.

The use of erythromycin in patients concurrently taking drugs metabolized by the cytochrome P450 system may be associated with elevations in serum levels of these other drugs. There have been reports of interactions of erythromycin with carbamazepine, cyclosporine, tacrolimus, hexobarbital, phenytoin, alfentanil, cisapride, disopyramide, lovastatin, bromocriptine, valproate, terfenadine, and astemizole. Serum concentrations of drugs metabolized by the cytochrome P450 system should be monitored closely in patients concurrently receiving erythromycin.

Erythromycin has been reported to significantly alter the metabolism of the nonsedating antihistamines terfenadine and astemizole when taken concomitantly. Rare cases of serious cardiovascular adverse events, including electrocardiographic QT/QT_c interval prolongation, cardiac arrest, torsades de pointes, and other ventricular arrhythmias have been observed. (See **CONTRAINDICATIONS.**) In addition, deaths have been reported rarely with concomitant administration of terfenadine and erythromycin.

There have been post-marketing reports of drug interactions when erythromycin is coadministered with cisapride, resulting in QT prolongation, cardiac arrhythmias, ventricular tachycardia, ventricular fibrillation, and torsades de pointes, most likely due to inhibition of hepatic metabolism of cisapride by erythromycin. Fatalities have been reported. (See **CONTRAINDICATIONS.**)

Drug/Laboratory Test Interactions: Erythromycin interferes with the fluorometric determination of urinary catecholamines.

Carcinogenesis, Mutagenesis, Impairment of Fertility: Long-term (2-year) oral studies in rats with erythromycin ethylsuccinate and erythromycin base did not provide evidence of tumorigenicity. Mutagenicity studies have not been conducted. There was no apparent effect on male or female fertility in rats fed erythromycin (base) at levels up to 0.25% of diet.

Pregnancy: Teratogenic Effects. Pregnancy Category B: There is no evidence of teratogenicity or any other adverse effect on reproduction in female rats fed erythromycin base (up to 0.25% of diet) prior to and during mating, during gestation, and through weaning of two successive litters. There are, however, no adequate and well-controlled studies in pregnant women. Because animal reproduction studies are

not always predictive of human response, this drug should be used during pregnancy only if clearly needed.
Labor and Delivery: The effect of erythromycin on labor and delivery is unknown.
Nursing Mothers: Erythromycin is excreted in human milk. Caution should be exercised when erythromycin is administered to a nursing woman.
Pediatric Use: See **INDICATIONS AND USAGE** and **DOSAGE AND ADMINISTRATION** sections.

ADVERSE REACTIONS

The most frequent side effects of oral erythromycin preparations are gastrointestinal and are dose-related. They include nausea, vomiting, abdominal pain, diarrhea and anorexia. Symptoms of hepatitis, hepatic dysfunction and/or abnormal liver function test results may occur. (See **WARNINGS.**)
Onset of pseudomembranous colitis symptoms may occur during or after antibiotic treatment. (See **WARNINGS.**)
Rarely, erythromycin has been associated with the production of ventricular arrhythmias, including ventricular tachycardia and torsades de pointes, in individuals with prolonged QT intervals.
Allergic reactions ranging from urticaria to anaphylaxis have occurred. Skin reactions ranging from mild eruptions to erythema multiforme, Stevens-Johnson syndrome, and toxic epidermal necrolysis have been reported rarely.
There have been isolated reports of reversible hearing loss occurring chiefly in patients with renal insufficiency and in patients receiving high doses of erythromycin.

OVERDOSAGE

In case of overdosage, erythromycin should be discontinued. Overdosage should be handled with the prompt elimination of unabsorbed drug and all other appropriate measures should be instituted.
Erythromycin is not removed by peritoneal dialysis or hemodialysis.

DOSAGE AND ADMINISTRATION

Erythromycin ethylsuccinate suspensions and Filmtab tablets may be administered without regard to meals.
Children: Age, weight, and severity of the infection are important factors in determining the proper dosage. In mild to moderate infections the usual dosage of erythromycin ethylsuccinate for children is 30 to 50 mg/kg/day in equally divided doses every 6 hours. For more severe infections this dosage may be doubled. If twice-a-day dosage is desired, one-half of the total daily dose may be given every 12 hours. Doses may also be given three times daily by administering one-third of the total daily dose every 8 hours.
The following dosage schedule is suggested for mild to moderate infections:

Body Weight	Total Daily Dose
Under 10 lbs	30–50 mg/kg/day 15–25 mg/kg/q 12 h
10 to 15 lbs	200 mg
16 to 25 lbs	400 mg
26 to 50 lbs	800 mg
51 to 100 lbs	1200 mg
over 100 lbs	1600 mg

Adults: 400 mg erythromycin ethylsuccinate every 6 hours is the usual dose. Dosage may be increased up to 4 g per day according to the severity of the infection. If twice-a-day dosage is desired, one-half of the total daily dose may be given every 12 hours. Doses may also be given three times daily by administering one-third of the total daily dose every 8 hours.
For adult dosage calculation, use a ratio of 400 mg of erythromycin activity as the ethylsuccinate to 250 mg of erythromycin activity as the stearate, base or estolate.
In the treatment of streptococcal infections, a therapeutic dosage of erythromycin ethylsuccinate should be administered for at least 10 days. In continuous prophylaxis against recurrences of streptococcal infections in persons with a history of rheumatic heart disease, the usual dosage is 400 mg twice a day.
For treatment of urethritis due to *C. trachomatis* or *U. urealyticum*: 800 mg three times a day for 7 days.
For treatment of primary syphilis: Adults: 48 to 64 g given in divided doses over a period of 10 to 15 days.
For intestinal amebiasis: Adults: 400 mg four times daily for 10 to 14 days. Children: 30 to 50 mg/kg/day in divided doses for 10 to 14 days.
For use in pertussis: Although optimal dosage and duration have not been established, doses of erythromycin utilized in reported clinical studies were 40 to 50 mg/kg/day, given in divided doses for 5 to 14 days.
For treatment of Legionnaires' Disease: Although optimal doses have not been established, doses utilized in reported clinical data were those recommended above (1.6 to 4 g daily in divided doses.)

HOW SUPPLIED

E.E.S. 200 LIQUID (erythromycin ethylsuccinate oral suspension, USP) is supplied in 1 pint bottles (**NDC** 0074-6306-16) and in packages of six 100-mL bottles (**NDC** 0074-6306-13).
E.E.S. 400® LIQUID (erythromycin ethylsuccinate oral suspension, USP) is supplied in 1 pint bottles (**NDC** 0074-6373-16) and in packages of six 100-mL bottles (**NDC** 0074-6373-13).
Both liquid products require refrigeration to preserve taste until dispensed. Refrigeration by patient is not required if used within 14 days.
E.E.S. GRANULES (erythromycin ethylsuccinate for oral suspension, USP) is supplied in 100-mL (**NDC** 0074-6369-02) and 200-mL (**NDC** 0074-6369-10) size bottles.
E.E.S. 400 Filmtab tablets (erythromycin ethylsuccinate tablets, USP) 400 mg, are supplied as pink tablets imprinted with the Abbott logo, , and two letter Abbo-Code designation, EE, in bottles of 100 (**NDC** 0074-5729-13), 500 (**NDC** 0074-5729-53) and 1000 (**NDC** 0074-5729-19) and in ABBO-PAC unit dose strip packages of 100 (**NDC** 0074-5729-11).
Recommended storage: Store tablets below 86°F (30°C). Store granules, prior to mixing, below 86°F (30°C). After mixing, refrigerate and use within 10 days.

REFERENCES

1. National Committee for Clinical Laboratory Standards, *Methods for Dilution Antimicrobial Susceptibility Tests for Bacteria that Grow Aerobically*, Third Edition. Approved Standard NCCLS Document M7-A3, Vol. 13, No. 25. NCCLS, Villanova, PA, December 1993.
2. National Committee for Clinical Laboratory Standards, *Performance Standards for Antimicrobial Disk Susceptibility Tests*, Fifth Edition. Approved Standard NCCLS Document M2-A5, Vol. 13, No. 24. NCCLS, Villanova, PA, December 1993.
3. Committee on Rheumatic Fever, Endocarditis, and Kawasaki Disease of the Council on Cardiovascular Disease in the Young, the American Heart Association: Prevention of Rheumatic Fever. *Circulation*. 78(4): 1082-1086, October 1988.

Filmtab—Film-sealed tablets, Abbott.
Ref. 03-5016-R20
Revised: February, 2000
ABBOTT LABORATORIES
NORTH CHICAGO, IL 60064, U.S.A.
Shown in Product Identification Guide, page 303

ERYTHROCIN® STEARATE ℞

[e-ry 'thrō-sin]
(erythromycin stearate tablets, USP)
Filmtab® Tablets

DESCRIPTION

Erythromycin is produced by a strain of *Streptomyces erythraeus* and belongs to the macrolide group of antibiotics. It is basic and readily forms salts with acids. The base, the stearate salt, and the esters are poorly soluble in water, and are suitable for oral administration.
ERYTHROCIN STEARATE Filmtab tablets (erythromycin stearate tablets, USP) contain the stearate salt of the antibiotic in a unique film coating.
Inactive Ingredients: 250 mg tablet: Cellulosic polymers, corn starch, D&C Red No. 7, polacrilin potassium, polyethylene glycol, povidone, propylene glycol, sodium carboxymethylcellulose, sodium citrate, sorbic acid, sorbitan monooleate and titanium dioxide.
500 mg tablet: Cellulosic polymers, corn starch, FD&C Red No. 3, magnesium hydroxide, polacrilin potassium, povidone, propylene glycol, sorbitan monooleate, titanium dioxide and vanillin.

ACTIONS

Microbiology
Biochemical tests demonstrate that erythromycin inhibits protein synthesis of the pathogen without directly affecting nucleic acid synthesis. Antagonism has been demonstrated between clindamycin and erythromycin.
NOTE: Many strains of *Hemophilus influenzae* are resistant to erythromycin alone, but are susceptible to erythromycin and sulfonamides together. Staphylococci resistant to erythromycin may emerge during a course of erythromycin therapy. Culture and susceptibility testing should be performed.
Disc Susceptibility Tests:
Quantitative methods that require measurement of zone diameters give the most precise estimates of antibiotic susceptibility. One recommended procedure (21 CFR section 460.1) uses erythromycin class discs for testing susceptibility; interpretations correlate zone diameters of this disc test with MIC values for erythromycin. With this procedure, a report from the laboratory of "susceptible" indicates that the infecting organism is likely to respond to therapy. A report of "resistant" indicates that the infective organism is not likely to respond to therapy. A report of "intermediate susceptibility" suggests that the organism would be susceptible if higher doses were used.
Clinical Pharmacology
Erythromycin binds to the 50 S ribosomal subunits of susceptible bacteria and suppresses protein synthesis.
Orally administered ERYTHROCIN STEARATE tablets are readily and reliably absorbed. Optimal serum levels of erythromycin are reached when the drug is taken in the fasting state or immediately before meals.
Erythromycin diffuses readily into most body fluids. Only low concentrations are normally achieved in the spinal fluid, but passage of the drug across the blood-brain barrier increases in meningitis. In the presence of normal hepatic function, erythromycin is concentrated in the liver and excreted in the bile; the effect of hepatic dysfunction on excretion of erythromycin by the liver into the bile is not known. Less than 5 percent of the orally administered dose of erythromycin is excreted in active form in the urine.
Erythromycin crosses the placental barrier and is excreted in breast milk.

INDICATIONS

Streptococcus pyogenes (Group A beta hemolytic streptococcus): Upper and lower respiratory tract, skin, and soft tissue infections of mild to moderate severity.
Injectable benzathine penicillin G is considered by the American Heart Association to be the drug of choice in the treatment and prevention of streptococcal pharyngitis and in long-term prophylaxis of rheumatic fever.
When oral medication is preferred for treatment of the above conditions, penicillin G, V, or erythromycin are alternate drugs of choice.
When oral medication is given, the importance of strict adherence by the patient to the prescribed dosage regimen must be stressed. A therapeutic dose should be administered for at least 10 days.
Alpha-hemolytic streptococci (viridans group):
Although no controlled clinical efficacy trials have been conducted, oral erythromycin has been suggested by the American Heart Association and American Dental Association for use in a regimen for prophylaxis against bacterial endocarditis in patients hypersensitive to penicillin who have congenital heart disease, or rheumatic or other acquired valvular heart disease when they undergo dental procedures and surgical procedures of the upper respiratory tract.[1] Erythromycin is not suitable prior to genitourinary or gastrointestinal tract surgery. NOTE: When selecting antibiotics for the prevention of bacterial endocarditis the physician or dentist should read the full joint statement of the American Heart Association and the American Dental Association.[1]
Staphylococcus aureus: Acute infections of skin and soft tissue of mild to moderate severity. Resistant organisms may emerge during treatment.
Streptococcus pneumoniae (Diplococcus pneumoniae): Upper respiratory tract infections (e.g., otitis media, pharyngitis) and lower respiratory tract infections (e.g., pneumonia) of mild to moderate degree.
Mycoplasma pneumoniae (Eaton agent, PPLO): For respiratory infections due to this organism.
Hemophilus influenzae: For upper respiratory tract infections of mild to moderate severity when used concomitantly with adequate doses of sulfonamides. (See sulfonamide labeling for appropriate prescribing information.) The concomitant use of the sulfonamides is necessary since not all strains of *Hemophilus influenzae* are susceptible to erythromycin at the concentrations of the antibiotic achieved with usual therapeutic doses.
Chlamydia trachomatis: Erythromycin is indicated for treatment of the following infections caused by *Chlamydia trachomatis:* conjunctivitis of the newborn, pneumonia of infancy and urogenital infections during pregnancy. When tetracyclines are contraindicated or not tolerated, erythromycin is indicated for the treatment of uncomplicated urethral, endocervical, or rectal infections in adults due to *Chlamydia trachomatis.*[2]
Treponema pallidum: Erythromycin is an alternate choice of treatment for primary syphilis in patients allergic to the penicillins. In treatment of primary syphilis, spinal fluid examinations should be done before treatment and as part of follow-up after therapy.
Corynebacterium diphtheriae: As an adjunct to antitoxin, to prevent establishment of carriers, and to eradicate the organism in carriers.
Corynebacterium minutissimum: For the treatment of erythrasma.
Entamoeba histolytica: In the treatment of intestinal amebiasis only. Extra-enteric amebiasis requires treatment with other agents.
Listeria monocytogenes: Infections due to this organism.
Neisseria gonorrhoeae: Erythrocin Lactobionate-I.V. (erythromycin lactobionate for injection) in conjunction with erythromycin stearate orally, as an alternative drug in treatment of acute pelvic inflammatory disease caused by *N. gonorrhoeae* in female patients with a history of sensitivity to penicillin. Before treatment of gonorrhea, patients who are suspected of also having syphilis should have a microscopic examination for *T. pallidum* (by immunofluorescence or darkfield) before receiving erythromycin, and monthly serologic tests for a minimum of 4 months.
Bordetella pertussis: Erythromycin is effective in eliminating the organism from the nasopharynx of infected individuals, rendering them non-infectious. Some clinical studies suggest that erythromycin may be helpful in the prophylaxis of pertussis in exposed susceptible individuals.
Legionnaires' Disease: Although no controlled clinical efficacy studies have been conducted, *in vitro* and limited preliminary clinical data suggest that erythromycin may be effective in treating Legionnaires' Disease.

CONTRAINDICATIONS

Erythromycin is contraindicated in patients with known hypersensitivity to this antibiotic.

WARNINGS

There have been reports of hepatic dysfunction with or without jaundice, occurring in patients receiving oral erythromycin products.

Continued on next page

Erythrocin Stearate—Cont.

PRECAUTIONS

General: Erythromycin is principally excreted by the liver. Caution should be exercised when erythromycin is administered to patients with impaired hepatic function. (See "Clinical Pharmacology" and "Warnings" sections.)
Prolonged or repeated use of erythromycin may result in an overgrowth of nonsusceptible bacteria or fungi. If superinfection occurs, erythromycin should be discontinued and appropriate therapy instituted.
When indicated, incision and drainage or other surgical procedures should be performed in conjunction with antibiotic therapy.
Laboratory Tests: Erythromycin interferes with the fluorometric determination of urinary catecholamines.
Drug Interactions: Erythromycin use in patients who are receiving high doses of theophylline may be associated with an increase in serum theophylline levels and potential theophylline toxicity. In case of theophylline toxicity and/or elevated serum theophylline levels, the dose of theophylline should be reduced while the patient is receiving concomitant erythromycin therapy.
Concomitant administration of erythromycin and digoxin has been reported to result in elevated digoxin serum levels.
There have been reports of increased anticoagulant effects when erythromycin and oral anticoagulants were used concomitantly.
Concurrent use of erythromycin and ergotamine or dihydroergotamine has been associated in some patients with acute ergot toxicity characterized by severe peripheral vasospasm and dysesthesia.
Erythromycin has been reported to decrease the clearance of triazolam and thus may increase the pharmacologic effect of triazolam.
The use of erythromycin in patients concurrently taking drugs metabolized by the cytochrome P450 system may be associated with elevations in serum erythromycin with carbamazepine, cyclosporine, hexobarbital and phenytoin. Serum concentrations of drugs metabolized by the cytochrome P450 system should be monitored closely in patients concurrently receiving erythromycin.
Troleandomycin significantly alters the metabolism of terfenadine when taken concomitantly; therefore, observe caution when erythromycin and terfenadine are used concurrently.
Patients receiving concomitant lovastatin and erythromycin should be carefully monitored; cases of rhabdomyolysis have been reported in seriously ill patients.
Carcinogenesis, Mutagenesis, Impairment of Fertility: Long-term (2-year) oral studies conducted in rats with erythromycin base did not provide evidence of tumorigenicity. Mutagenicity studies have not been conducted. There was no apparent effect on male or female fertility in rats fed erythromycin (base) at levels up to 0.25 percent of diet.
Pregnancy: Pregnancy Category B: There is no evidence of teratogenicity or any other adverse effect on reproduction in female rats fed erythromycin base (up to 0.25 percent of diet) prior to and during mating, during gestation, and through weaning of two successive litters. There are, however, no adequate and well-controlled studies in pregnant women. Because animal reproduction studies are not always predictive of human response, this drug should be used during pregnancy only if clearly needed. Erythromycin has been reported to cross the placental barrier in humans, but fetal plasma levels are generally low.
Labor and Delivery: The effect of erythromycin on labor and delivery is unknown.
Nursing Mothers: Erythromycin is excreted in breast milk, therefore, caution should be exercised when erythromycin is administered to a nursing woman.
Pediatric Use: See "Indications and Usage" and "Dosage and Administration" sections.

ADVERSE REACTIONS

The most frequent side effects of oral erythromycin preparations are gastrointestinal and are dose-related. They include nausea, vomiting, abdominal pain, diarrhea and anorexia. Symptoms of hepatic dysfunction and/or abnormal liver function test results may occur (see "Warnings" section). Pseudomembranous colitis has been rarely reported in association with erythromycin therapy.
There have been isolated reports of transient central nervous system side effects including confusion, hallucinations, seizures, and vertigo; however, a cause and effect relationship has not been established.
Occasional case reports of cardiac arrhythmias such as ventricular tachycardia have been documented in patients receiving erythromycin therapy. There have been isolated reports of other cardiovascular symptoms such as chest pain, dizziness, and palpitations; however, a cause and effect relationship has not been established.
Allergic reactions ranging from urticaria and mild skin eruptions to anaphylaxis have occurred.
There have been isolated reports of reversible hearing loss occurring chiefly in patients with renal insufficiency and in patients receiving high doses of erythromycin.

OVERDOSAGE

In case of overdosage, erythromycin should be discontinued. Overdosage should be handled with the prompt elimination of unabsorbed drug and all other appropriate measures.
Erythromycin is not removed by peritoneal dialysis or hemodialysis.

DOSAGE AND ADMINISTRATION

Optimal serum levels of erythromycin are reached when ERYTHROCIN STEARATE (erythromycin stearate) is taken in the fasting state or immediately before meals.
Adults: The usual dosage is 250 mg every 6 hours; or 500 mg every 12 hours, taken in the fasting state or immediately before meals. Up to 4 g per day may be administered, depending upon the severity of the infection.
Children: Age, weight, and severity of the infection are important factors in determining the proper dosage. For the treatment of mild to moderate infections, the usual dosage is 30 to 50 mg/kg/day in 3 or 4 divided doses. When dosage is desired on a twice-a-day schedule, one-half of the total daily dose may be taken every 12 hours in the fasting state or immediately before meals. For the treatment of more severe infections the total daily dose may be doubled.
In the treatment of streptococcal infections, a therapeutic dosage of erythromycin should be administered for at least 10 days. In continuous prophylaxis of streptococcal infections in persons with a history of rheumatic heart disease, the dose is 250 mg twice a day.
For prophylaxis against bacterial endocarditis[1] in patients with congenital heart disease, or rheumatic or other acquired valvular heart disease when undergoing dental procedures or surgical procedures of the upper respiratory tract, give 1 g (20 mg/kg for children) orally 1½ to 2 hours before the procedure, and then, 500 mg (10 mg/kg for children) orally every 6 hours for 8 doses.
For conjunctivitis of the newborn caused by *Chlamydia trachomatis:* Oral erythromycin suspension 50 mg/kg/day in 4 divided doses for at least 2 weeks.[2]
For pneumonia of infancy caused by *Chlamydia trachomatis.* Although the optimal duration of therapy has not been established, the recommended therapy is oral erythromycin suspension 50 mg/kg/day in 4 divided doses for at least 3 weeks.[2]
For urogenital infections during pregnancy due to *Chlamydia trachomatis:* Although the optimal dose and duration of therapy have not been established, the suggested treatment is erythromycin 500 mg, by mouth, 4 times a day on an empty stomach for at least 7 days. For women who cannot tolerate this regimen, a decreased dose of 250 mg, by mouth, 4 times a day should be used for at least 14 days.[2]
For adults with uncomplicated urethral, endocervical, or rectal infections caused by *Chlamydia trachomatis* in whom tetracyclines are contraindicated or not tolerated: 500 mg, by mouth, 4 times a day for at least 7 days.[2]
For treatment of primary syphilis: 30 to 40 g given in divided doses over a period of 10 to 15 days.
For treatment of acute pelvic inflammatory disease caused by *N. gonorrhoeae:* 500 mg Erythrocin Lactobionate-I.V. (erythromycin lactobionate for injection) every 6 hours for 3 days, followed by 250 mg ERYTHROCIN STEARATE every 6 hours for 7 days.
For intestinal amebiasis: Adults: 250 mg four times daily for 10 to 14 days. Children: 30 to 50 mg/kg/day in divided doses for 10 to 14 days.
For use in pertussis: Although optimal dosage and duration have not been established, doses of erythromycin utilized in reported clinical studies were 40 to 50 mg/kg/day, given in divided doses for 5 to 14 days.
For treatment of Legionnaires' Disease: Although optimal doses have not been established, doses utilized in reported clinical data were 1 to 4 g daily in divided doses.

HOW SUPPLIED

ERYTHROCIN STEARATE Filmtab Tablets (erythromycin stearate tablets, USP) are supplied as:
ERYTHROCIN STEARATE Filmtab, 250 mg
Bottles of 100 .... (**NDC** 0074-6346-20)
Bottles of 500 .... (**NDC** 0074-6346-53)
Bottles of 1000 .... (**NDC** 0074-6346-19)
ABBO-PAC® unit dose strip packages of
100 tablets .... (**NDC** 0074-6346-38)
ERYTHROCIN STEARATE Filmtab, 500 mg
Bottles of 100 .... (**NDC** 0074-6316-13)
Recommended storage: Store below 86°F (30°C).

REFERENCES

1. American Heart Association. 1977. Prevention of bacterial endocarditis. Circulation 56: 139A-143A.
2. CDC Sexually Transmitted Diseases Treatment Guidelines 1982.

FILMTAB—Film-sealed tablets, Abbott
Ref. 01-2538-R13

Shown in Product Identification Guide, page 303

ERYTHROMYCIN Base Filmtab® ℞

[*e-ri-thrō-mī 'sin*]
(erythromycin tablets, USP)

DESCRIPTION

Erythromycin is produced by a strain of *Streptomyces erythraeus* and belongs to the macrolide group of antibiotics. It is basic and readily forms salts with acids. The base, the stearate salt, and the esters are poorly soluble in water, and are suitable for oral administration.
ERYTHROMYCIN Base Filmtab tablets contain erythromycin, USP, in a unique, nonenteric film coating.
Inactive Ingredients: 250 mg tablet: Cellulosic polymers, corn starch, D&C Red No. 30, iron oxide, magnesium hydroxide, magnesium stearate, polyethylene glycol, propylene glycol, sodium starch glycolate, sorbic acid, sorbitan monooleate and titanium dioxide.
500 mg tablet: Cellulosic polymers, corn starch, D&C Red No. 30, magnesium hydroxide, magnesium stearate, microcrystalline cellulose, polyethylene glycol, propylene glycol, sodium starch glycolate, sorbic acid, sorbitan monooleate and titanium dioxide.

ACTIONS

Microbiology: Biochemical tests demonstrate that erythromycin inhibits protein synthesis of the pathogen without directly affecting nucleic acid synthesis. Antagonism has been demonstrated between clindamycin and erythromycin.
NOTE: Many strains of *Hemophilus influenzae* are resistant to erythromycin alone, but are susceptible to erythromycin and sulfonamides together. Staphylococci resistant to erythromycin may emerge during a course of erythromycin therapy. Culture and susceptibility testing should be performed.
Disc Susceptibility Tests: Quantitative methods that require measurement of zone diameters give the most precise estimates of antibiotic susceptibility. One recommended procedure (21 CFR section 460.1) uses erythromycin class discs for testing susceptibility; interpretations correlate zone diameters of this disc test with MIC values for erythromycin. With this procedure, a report from the laboratory of "susceptible" indicates that the infecting organism is likely to respond to therapy. A report of "resistant" indicates that the infective organism is not likely to respond to therapy. A report of "intermediate susceptibility" suggests that the organism would be susceptible if higher doses were used.
Clinical Pharmacology: Erythromycin binds to the 50 S ribosomal subunits of susceptible bacteria and suppresses protein synthesis.
Orally administered erythromycin is readily absorbed by most patients, especially on an empty stomach, but patient variation is observed. Due to its formulation and nonenteric coating, this erythromycin tablet gives reliable blood levels in the average subject; however, the levels may vary with the individual.
Erythromycin diffuses readily into most body fluids. Only low concentrations are normally achieved in the spinal fluid, but passage of the drug across the blood-brain barrier increases in meningitis. In the presence of normal hepatic function, erythromycin is concentrated in the liver and excreted in the bile; the effect of hepatic dysfunction on excretion of erythromycin by the liver into the bile is not known. Less than 5 percent of the orally administered dose of erythromycin is excreted in active form in the urine.
Erythromycin crosses the placental barrier and is excreted in breast milk.

INDICATIONS

Streptococcus pyogenes (Group A beta-hemolytic streptococcus): Upper and lower respiratory tract, skin, and soft tissue infections of mild to moderate severity.
Injectable benzathine penicillin G is considered by the American Heart Association to be the drug of choice in the treatment and prevention of streptococcal pharyngitis and in long-term prophylaxis of rheumatic fever.
When oral medication is preferred for treatment of the above conditions, penicillin G, V, or erythromycin are alternate drugs of choice.
When oral medication is given, the importance of strict adherence by the patient to the prescribed dosage regimen must be stressed. A therapeutic dose should be administered for at least 10 days.
Alpha-hemolytic streptococci (viridans group): Although no controlled clinical efficacy trials have been conducted, oral erythromycin has been suggested by the American Heart Association and American Dental Association for use in a regimen for prophylaxis against bacterial endocarditis in patients hypersensitive to penicillin who have congenital heart disease, or rheumatic or other acquired valvular heart disease when they undergo dental procedures and surgical procedures of the upper respiratory tract.[1] Erythromycin is not suitable prior to genitourinary or gastrointestinal tract surgery. NOTE: When selecting antibiotics for the prevention of bacterial endocarditis the physician or dentist should read the full joint statement of the American Heart Association and the American Dental Association.[1]
Staphylococcus aureus: Acute infections of skin and soft tissue of mild to moderate severity. Resistant organisms may emerge during treatment.
Streptococcus pneumoniae (Diplococcus pneumoniae): Upper respiratory tract infections (e.g., otitis media, pharyngitis) and lower respiratory tract infections (e.g., pneumonia) of mild to moderate degree.
Mycoplasma pneumoniae (Eaton agent, PPLO): For respiratory infections due to this organism.
Hemophilus influenzae: For upper respiratory tract infections of mild to moderate severity when used concomitantly with adequate doses of sulfonamides. (See sulfonamide labeling for appropriate prescribing information). The concomitant use of the sulfonamides is necessary since not all strains of *Hemophilus influenzae* are susceptible to erythromycin at the concentrations of the antibiotic achieved with usual therapeutic doses.
Chlamydia trachomatis: Erythromycin is indicated for treatment of the following infections caused by *Chlamydia trachomatis:* conjunctivitis of the newborn, pneumonia of infancy and urogenital infections during pregnancy. When tet-

racyclines are contraindicated or not tolerated, erythromycin is indicated for the treatment of uncomplicated urethral, endocervical, or rectal infections in adults due to *Chlamydia trachomatis*.[2]
Treponema pallidum: Erythromycin is an alternate choice of treatment for primary syphilis in patients allergic to the penicillins. In treatment of primary syphilis, spinal fluid examinations should be done before treatment and as part of follow-up after therapy.
Corynebacterium diphtheriae: As an adjunct to antitoxin, to prevent establishment of carriers, and to eradicate the organism in carriers.
Corynebacterium minutissimum: For the treatment of erythrasma.
Entamoeba histolytica: In the treatment of intestinal amebiasis only. Extra-enteric amebiasis requires treatment with other agents.
Listeria monocytogenes: Infections due to this organism.
Neisseria gonorrhoeae: Erythrocin® Lactobionate-I.V. (erythromycin lactobionate for injection) in conjunction with erythromycin base orally, as an alternative drug in treatment of acute pelvic inflammatory disease caused by *N. gonorrhoeae* in female patients with a history of sensitivity to penicillin. Before treatment of gonorrhea, patients who are suspected of also having syphilis should have a microscopic examination for *T. pallidum* (by immunofluorescence or darkfield) before receiving erythromycin, and monthly serologic tests for a minimum of 4 months.
Bordetella pertussis: Erythromycin is effective in eliminating the organism from the nasopharynx of infected individuals, rendering them non-infectious. Some clinical studies suggest that erythromycin may be helpful in the prophylaxis of pertussis in exposed susceptible individuals.
Legionnaires' Disease: Although no controlled clinical efficacy studies have been conducted, *in vitro* and limited preliminary clinical data suggest that erythromycin may be effective in treating Legionnaires' Disease.

CONTRAINDICATIONS

Erythromycin is contraindicated in patients with known hypersensitivity to this antibiotic.

WARNINGS

There have been reports of hepatic dysfunction with or without jaundice, occurring in patients receiving oral erythromycin products.

PRECAUTIONS

General: Erythromycin is principally excreted by the liver. Caution should be exercised when erythromycin is administered to patients with impaired hepatic function. (See "Clinical Pharmacology" and "Warnings" sections).
Prolonged or repeated use of erythromycin may result in an overgrowth of nonsusceptible bacteria or fungi. If superinfection occurs, erythromycin should be discontinued and appropriate therapy instituted.
When indicated, incision and drainage or other surgical procedures should be performed in conjunction with antibiotic therapy.
Laboratory Tests: Erythromycin interferes with the fluorometric determination of urinary catecholamines.
Drug Interactions: Erythromycin use in patients who are receiving high doses of theophylline may be associated with an increase in serum theophylline levels and potential theophylline toxicity. In case of theophylline toxicity and/or elevated serum theophylline levels, the dose of theophylline should be reduced while the patient is receiving concomitant erythromycin therapy.
Concomitant administration of erythromycin and digoxin has been reported to result in elevated digoxin serum levels.
There have been reports of increased anticoagulant effects when erythromycin and oral anticoagulants were used concomitantly.
Concurrent use of erythromycin and ergotamine or dihydroergotamine has been associated in some patients with acute ergot toxicity characterized by severe peripheral vasospasm and dysethesia.
Erythromycin has been reported to decrease the clearance of triazolam and thus may increase the pharmacologic effect of triazolam.
The use of erythromycin in patients concurrently taking drugs metabolized by the cytochrome P450 system may be associated with elevations in serum erythromycin with carbamazepine, cyclosporine, hexobarbital and phenytoin. Serum concentrations of drugs metabolized by the cytochrome P450 system should be monitored closely in patients concurrently receiving erythromycin.
Troleandomycin significantly alters the metabolism of terfenadine when taken concomitantly; therefore, observe caution when erythromycin and terfenadine are used concurrently.
Patients receiving concomitant lovastatin and erythromycin should be carefully monitored; cases of rhabdomyolysis have been reported in seriously ill patients.
Carcinogenesis, Mutagenesis, Impairment of Fertility: Long-term (2-year) oral studies conducted in rats with erythromycin base did not provide evidence of tumorigenicity. Mutagenicity studies have not been conducted. There was no apparent effect on male or female fertility in rats fed erythromycin (base) at levels up to 0.25 percent of diet.
Pregnancy: Pregnancy Category B: There is no evidence of teratogenicity or any other adverse effect on reproduction in female rats fed erythromycin base (up to 0.25 percent of diet) prior to and during mating, during gestation, and through weaning of two successive litters. There are, however, no adequate and well-controlled studies in pregnant women. Because animal reproduction studies are not always predictive of human response, this drug should be used during pregnancy only if clearly needed. Erythromycin has been reported to cross the placental barrier in humans, but fetal plasma levels are generally low.
Labor and Delivery: The effect of erythromycin on labor and delivery is unknown.
Nursing Mothers: Erythromycin is excreted in breast milk, therefore, caution should be exercised when erythromycin is administered to a nursing woman.
Pediatric Use: See "Indications and Usage" and "Dosage and Administration" sections.

ADVERSE REACTIONS

The most frequent side effects of oral erythromycin preparations are gastrointestinal and are dose-related. They include nausea, vomiting, abdominal pain, diarrhea and anorexia. Symptoms of hepatic dysfunction and/or abnormal liver function test results may occur (see "Warnings" section). Pseudomembranous colitis has been rarely reported in association with erythromycin therapy.
There have been isolated reports of transient central nervous system side effects including confusion, hallucinations, seizures, and vertigo; however, a cause and effect relationship has not been established.
Occasional case reports of cardiac arrhythmias such as ventricular tachycardia have been documented in patients receiving erythromycin therapy. There have been isolated reports of other cardiovascular symptoms such as chest pain, dizziness, and palpitations; however a cause and effect relationship has not been established.
Allergic reactions ranging from urticaria and mild skin eruptions to anaphylaxis have occurred.
There have been isolated reports of reversible hearing loss occurring chiefly in patients with renal insufficiency and in patients receiving high doses of erythromycin.

OVERDOSAGE

In case of overdosage, erythromycin should be discontinued. Overdosage should be handled with the prompt elimination of unabsorbed drug and all other appropriate measures.
Erythromycin is not removed by peritoneal dialysis or hemodialysis.

DOSAGE AND ADMINISTRATION

Optimum blood levels are obtained when doses are given on an empty stomach.
Adults: 250 mg every 6 hours is the usual dose; or 500 mg every 12 hours one hour before meals. Dosage may be increased up to 4 g per day according to the severity of the infection.
Children: Age, weight, and severity of the infection are important factors in determining the proper dosage. 30 to 50 mg/kg/day, in divided doses, is the usual dose. For more severe infections this dose may be doubled. If dosage is desired on a twice-a-day schedule, one-half of the total daily dose may be given every 12 hours, one hour before meals.
For treatment of streptococcal infections: a therapeutic dosage should be administered for at least 10 days. In continuous prophylaxis of streptococcal infections in persons with rheumatic heart disease history, the dose is 250 mg twice a day.
For prophylaxis against bacterial endocarditis[1] in patients with congenital heart disease, or rheumatic or other acquired valvular heart disease when undergoing dental procedures or surgical procedures of the upper respiratory tract, give 1 g (20 mg/kg for children) orally $1^1/_2$ to 2 hours before the procedure, and then, 500 mg (10 mg/kg for children) orally every 6 hours for 8 doses.
For conjunctivitis of the newborn caused by *Chlamydia trachomatis:* Oral erythromycin suspension 50 mg/kg/day in 4 divided doses for at least 2 weeks.[2]
For pneumonia of infancy caused by *Chlamydia trachomatis:* Although the optimal duration of therapy has not been established, the recommended therapy is oral erythromycin suspension 50 mg/kg/day in 4 divided doses for at least 3 weeks.[2]
For urogenital infections during pregnancy due to *Chlamydia trachomatis:* Although the optimal dose and duration of therapy have not been established, the suggested treatment is erythromycin 500 mg, by mouth, 4 times a day on an empty stomach for at least 7 days. For women who cannot tolerate this regimen, a decreased dose of 250 mg, by mouth, 4 times a day should be used for at least 14 days.[2]
For adults with uncomplicated urethral, endocervical, or rectal infections caused by *Chlamydia trachomatis* in whom tetracyclines are contraindicated or not tolerated: 500 mg, by mouth, 4 times a day for at least 7 days.[2]
For treatment of primary syphilis: 30 to 40 g given in divided doses over a period of 10 to 15 days.
For treatment of acute pelvic inflammatory disease caused by *N. gonorrhoeae:* 500 mg Erythrocin® Lactobionate-I.V. (erythromycin lactobionate for injection) every 6 hours for 3 days, followed by 250 mg erythromycin base every 6 hours for 7 days.
For intestinal amebiasis: Adults: 250 mg four times daily for 10 to 14 days. Children: 30 to 50 mg/kg/day in divided doses for 10 to 14 days.
For use in pertussis: Although optimal dosage and duration have not been established, doses of erythromycin utilized in reported clinical studies were 40 to 50 mg/kg/day, given in divided doses for 5 to 14 days.
For treatment of Legionnaires' Disease: Although optimal doses have not been established, doses utilized in reported clinical data were 1 to 4 g daily in divided doses.

HOW SUPPLIED

ERYTHROMYCIN Base Filmtab tablets (erythromycin tablets, USP) are supplied as pink, capsule-shaped tablets in two dosage strengths:
250 mg tablets:
Bottles of 100 .... (**NDC** 0074-6326-13);
Bottles of 500 .... (**NDC** 0074-6326-53);
ABBO-PAC® unit dose strip packages of
100 tablets .... (**NDC** 0074-6326-11).
500 mg tablets:
Bottles of 100 .... (**NDC** 0074-6227-13).
Recommended storage: Store below 86°F (30°C).

REFERENCES

1. American Heart Association. 1977. Prevention of bacterial endocarditis. Circulation. 56: 139A-143A.
2. CDC Sexually Transmitted Diseases Treatment Guidelines 1982.

FILMTAB—Film-sealed tablets, Abbott.
Revised: October, 1991
Ref. 01-2541-R3

ERYTHROMYCIN DELAYED-RELEASE CAPSULES, USP ℞

DESCRIPTION

Erythromycin Delayed-release Capsules contain enteric-coated pellets of erythromycin base for oral administration. Erythromycin is produced by a strain of *Streptomyces erythraeus* and belongs to the macrolide group of antibiotics. It is basic and readily forms salts with acids, but it is the base which is microbiologically active. Each Erythromycin Delayed-release Capsule contains 250 milligrams of erythromycin base.
Inactive Ingredients: Cellulosic polymers, citrate ester, D&C Red No. 30, D&C Yellow No. 10, magnesium stearate and povidone. The capsule shell contains FD&C Blue No. 1, FD&C Red No. 3, gelatin, and titanium dioxide.
Erythromycin base is (3R*, 4S*, 5S*, 6R*, 7R*, 9R*, 11R*, 12R*, 13S*, 14R*)-4-[(2,6-Dideoxy-3-C-methyl-3-0-methyl-α-L-*ribo*-hexopyranosyl)oxy]-14-ethyl-7,12,13-trihydroxy-3,5,7,9,11,13-hexamethyl-6-[[3,4,6-trideoxy-3-(dimethylamino)-β-D-*xylo*-hexopyranosyl]oxy]oxacyclotetradecane-2,10-dione. The structural formula is:

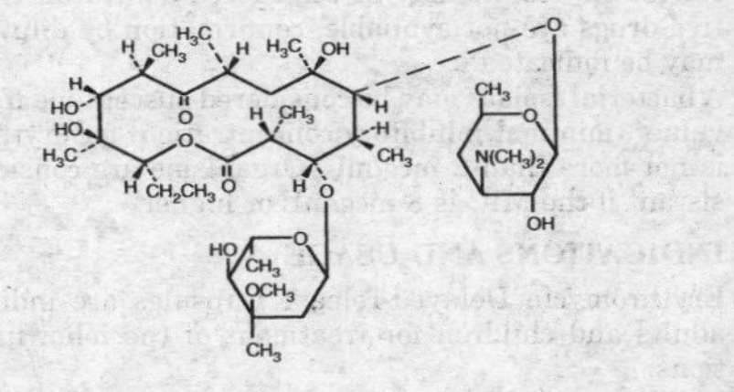

$C_{37}H_{67}NO_{13}$ MW 734

CLINICAL PHARMACOLOGY

Orally administered erythromycin base and its salts are readily absorbed in the microbiologically active form. Interindividual variations in the absorption of erythromycin are, however, observed, and some patients do not achieve acceptable serum levels. Erythromycin is largely bound to plasma proteins, and the freely dissociating bound fraction after administration of erythromycin base represents 90% of the total erythromycin absorbed. After absorption, erythromycin diffuses readily into most body fluids. In the absence of meningeal inflammation, low concentrations are normally achieved in the spinal fluid, but the passage of the drug across the blood-brain barrier increases in meningitis.
Erythromycin is excreted in breast milk. The drug crosses the placental barrier but plasma levels are low.
In the presence of normal hepatic function, erythromycin is concentrated in the liver and is excreted in the bile; the effect of hepatic dysfunction on biliary excretion of erythromycin is not known. After oral administration, less than 5% of the administered dose can be recovered in the active form in the urine.
The enteric coating of pellets in Erythromycin Delayed-release Capsules protects the erythromycin base from inactivation by gastric acidity. Because of their small size and enteric coating, the pellets readily pass intact from the stomach to the small intestine and dissolve efficiently to allow absorption of erythromycin in a uniform manner. After administration of a single dose of a 250 mg Erythromycin Delayed-release Capsule, peak serum levels in the range of 1.13 to 1.68 mcg/mL are attained in approximately 3 hours and decline to 0.30-0.42 mcg/mL in 6 hours. Optimal conditions for stability in the presence of gastric secretion and for complete absorption are attained when Erythromycin Delayed-release Capsules are taken on an empty stomach.
Microbiology:
Erythromycin acts by inhibition of protein synthesis by binding 50 S ribosomal subunits of susceptible organisms. It

Continued on next page

Erythromycin Delayed-Rel.—Cont.

does not affect nucleic acid synthesis. Antagonism has been demonstrated between clindamycin and erythromycin. Resistance to erythromycin of many strains of *Haemophilus influenzae* and some strains of staphylococci has been demonstrated. Specimens should be obtained for culture and susceptibility testing.

Erythromycin is usually active against the following organisms *in vitro* and in clinical infections:

Streptococcus pyogenes
Alpha-hemolytic streptococci (viridans group)
Staphylococcus aureus (Resistant organisms may emerge during treatment.)
Streptococcus pneumoniae
Mycoplasma pneumoniae (Eaton's Agent)
Haemophilus influenzae (Many strains are resistant to erythromycin alone, but are susceptible to erythromycin and sulfonamides together.)
Treponema pallidum
Corynebacterium diphtheriae
Corynebacterium minutissimum
Entamoeba histolytica
Listeria monocytogenes
Neisseria gonorrhoeae
Bordetella pertussis
Legionella pneumophila (agent of Legionnaires' disease)

Susceptibility Testing

Quantitative methods that require measurement of zone diameters give the most precise estimates of antibiotic susceptibility. One such standardized single-disc procedure has been recommended for use with discs to test susceptibility to erythromycin.[1] Interpretation involves correlation of the zone diameters obtained in the disc test with minimal inhibitory concentration (MIC) values for erythromycin.

Reports from the laboratory giving results of the standardized single-disc susceptibility test using a 15 mcg erythromycin disc should be interpreted according to the following criteria:

Susceptible organisms produce zones of 18 mm or greater, indicating that the tested organism is likely to respond to therapy.

Resistant organisms produce zones of 13 mm or less, indicating that other therapy should be selected.

Organisms of intermediate susceptibility produce zones of 14 to 17 mm. The "intermediate" category provides a "buffer zone" which should prevent small, uncontrolled technical factors from causing major discrepancies in interpretations; thus, when a zone diameter falls within the "intermediate" range, the results may be considered equivocal. If alternative drugs are not available, confirmation by dilution tests may be indicated.

A bacterial isolate may be considered susceptible if the MIC value[2] (minimal inhibitory concentration) for erythromycin is not more than 2 mcg/mL. Organisms are considered resistant if the MIC is 8 mcg/mL or higher.

INDICATIONS AND USAGE

Erythromycin Delayed-release Capsules are indicated in adults and children for treatment of the following conditions:

Upper respiratory tract infections of mild to moderate degree caused by *Streptococcus pyogenes* (Group A beta-hemolytic streptococci); *Streptococcus pneumoniae (Diplococcus pneumoniae); Haemophilus influenzae* (when used concomitantly with adequate doses of sulfonamides, since many strains of *H. influenzae* are not susceptible to the erythromycin concentrations ordinarily achieved). (See appropriate sulfonamide labeling for prescribing information.)

Lower respiratory tract infections of mild to moderate severity caused by *Streptococcus pyogenes* (Group A beta-hemolytic streptococci); *Streptococcus pneumoniae (Diplococcus pneumoniae).*

Respiratory tract infections due to *Mycoplasma pneumoniae* (Eaton's agent).

Pertussis (whooping cough) caused by *Bordetella pertussis.* Erythromycin is effective in eliminating the organism from the nasopharynx of infected individuals, rendering them noninfectious. Some clinical studies suggest that erythromycin may be helpful in the prophylaxis of pertussis in exposed susceptible individuals.

Diphtheria—As an adjunct to antitoxin in infections due to *Corynebacterium diphtheriae,* to prevent establishment of carriers and to eradicate the organism in carriers.

Erythrasma—In the treatment of infections due to *Corynebacterium minutissimum.*

Intestinal amebiasis caused by *Entamoeba histolytica* (oral erythromycins only). Extraenteric amebiasis requires treatment with other agents.

Infections due to *Listeria monocytogenes.*

Skin and soft tissue infections of mild to moderate severity caused by *Streptococcus pyogenes* and *Staphylococcus aureus* (resistant staphylococci may emerge during treatment).

Primary syphilis caused by *Treponema pallidum.* Erythromycin (oral forms only) is an alternate choice of treatment for primary syphilis in patients allergic to the penicillins. In treatment of primary syphilis, spinal fluid should be examined before treatment and as part of the follow-up after therapy. The use of erythromycin for the treatment of *in utero* syphilis is not recommended. (See "CLINICAL PHARMACOLOGY" section.)

Erythromycins are indicated for treatment of the following infections caused by *Chlamydia trachomatis:* conjunctivitis of the newborn, pneumonia of infancy, and urogenital infections during pregnancy. When tetracyclines are contraindicated or not tolerated, erythromycin is indicated for the treatment of uncomplicated urethral, endocervical, or rectal infections in adults due to *Chlamydia trachomatis.*[3]

Legionnaires' Disease caused by *Legionella pneumophila.* Although no controlled clinical efficacy studies have been conducted, *in vitro* and limited preliminary clinical data suggest that erythromycin may be effective in treating Legionnaires' Disease.

Therapy with erythromycin should be monitored by bacteriological studies and by clinical response. (See "CLINICAL PHARMACOLOGY—Microbiology" section.)

Injectable benzathine penicillin G is considered by the American Heart Association to be the drug of choice in the treatment and prevention of streptococcal pharyngitis and in long-term prophylaxis of rheumatic fever. When oral medication is preferred for treatment of the above conditions, penicillin G, V or erythromycin are alternate drugs of choice.

Although no controlled clinical efficacy trials have been conducted, erythromycin has been suggested by the American Heart Association and the American Dental Association for use in a regimen for prophylaxis against bacterial endocarditis in patients allergic to penicillin who have congenital and/or rheumatic or other acquired valvular heart disease when they undergo dental procedures and surgical procedures of the upper respiratory tract.[3] (Erythromycin is not suitable prior to genitourinary surgery where the organisms likely to lead to bacteremia are gram-negative bacilli or the enterococcal group of streptococci.)

NOTE: When selecting antibiotics for the prevention of bacterial endocarditis the physician or dentist should read the full joint 1984 statement of the American Heart Association and the American Dental Association.[3]

CONTRAINDICATION

Erythromycin is contraindicated in patients with known hypersensitivity to this antibiotic.

WARNINGS

There have been a few reports of hepatic dysfunction, with or without jaundice, occurring in patients receiving oral erythromycin products.

PRECAUTIONS

General: Erythromycin is principally excreted by the liver. Caution should be exercised when erythromycin is administered to patients with impaired hepatic function. (See "Clinical Pharmacology" and "Warnings" sections).

Prolonged or repeated use of erythromycin may result in an overgrowth of nonsusceptible bacteria or fungi. If superinfection occurs, erythromycin should be discontinued and appropriate therapy instituted.

When indicated, incision and drainage or other surgical procedures should be performed in conjunction with antibiotic therapy.

Laboratory Tests: Erythromycin interferes with the fluorometric determination of urinary catecholamines.

Drug Interactions: Erythromycin use in patients who are receiving high doses of theophylline may be associated with an increase in serum theophylline levels and potential theophylline toxicity. In case of theophylline toxicity and/or elevated serum theophylline levels, the dose of theophylline should be reduced while the patient is receiving concomitant erythromycin therapy.

Concomitant administration of erythromycin and digoxin has been reported to result in elevated digoxin serum levels.

There have been reports of increased anticoagulant effects when erythromycin and oral anticoagulants were used concomitantly.

Concurrent use of erythromycin and ergotamine or dihydroergotamine has been associated in some patients with acute ergot toxicity characterized by severe peripheral vasospasm and dysesthesia.

Erythromycin has been reported to decrease the clearance of triazolam and thus may increase the pharmacologic effect of triazolam.

The use of erythromycin in patients concurrently taking drugs metabolized by the cytochrome P450 system may be associated with elevations in serum erythromycin with carbamazepine, cyclosporine, hexobarbital and phenytoin. Serum concentrations of drugs metabolized by the cytochrome P450 system should be monitored closely in patients concurrently receiving erythromycin.

Troleandomycin significantly alters the metabolism of terfenadine when taken concomitantly; therefore, observe caution when erythromycin and terfenadine are used concurrently.

Patients receiving concomitant lovastatin and erythromycin should be carefully monitored; cases of rhabdomyolysis have been reported in seriously ill patients.

Carcinogenesis, Mutagenesis, Impairment of Fertility: Long-term (2-year) oral studies conducted in rats with erythromycin base did not provide evidence of tumorigenicity. Mutagenicity studies have not been conducted. There was no apparent effect on male or female fertility in rats fed erythromycin (base) at levels up to 0.25 percent of diet.

Pregnancy: Pregnancy Category B: There is no evidence of teratogenicity or any other adverse effect on reproduction in female rats fed erythromycin base (up to 0.25 percent of diet) prior to and during mating, during gestation, and through weaning of two successive litters. There are, however, no adequate and well-controlled studies in pregnant women. Because animal reproduction studies are not always predictive of human response, this drug should be used during pregnancy only if clearly needed. Erythromycin has been reported to cross the placental barrier in humans, but fetal plasma levels are generally low.

Labor and Delivery: The effect of erythromycin on labor and delivery is unknown.

Nursing Mothers: Erythromycin is excreted in breast milk, therefore, caution should be exercised when erythromycin is administered to a nursing woman.

Pediatric Use: See "Indications and Usage" and "Dosage and Administration" sections.

ADVERSE REACTIONS

The most frequent side effects of oral erythromycin preparations are gastrointestinal and are dose-related. They include nausea, vomiting, abdominal pain, diarrhea and anorexia. Symptoms of hepatic dysfunction and/or abnormal liver function test results may occur (see "Warnings" section). Pseudomembranous colitis has been rarely reported in association with erythromycin therapy.

There have been isolated reports of transient central nervous system side effects including confusion, hallucinations, seizures, and vertigo; however, a cause and effect relationship has not been established.

Occasional case reports of cardiac arrhythmias such as ventricular tachycardia have been documented in patients receiving erythromycin therapy. There have been isolated reports of other cardiovascular symptoms such as chest pain, dizziness, and palpitations; however, a cause and effect relationship has not been established.

Allergic reactions ranging from urticaria and mild skin eruptions to anaphylaxis have occurred.

There have been isolated reports of reversible hearing loss occurring chiefly in patients with renal insufficiency and in patients receiving high doses of erythromycin.

OVERDOSAGE

In case of overdosage, erythromycin should be discontinued. Overdosage should be handled with the prompt elimination of unabsorbed drug and all other appropriate measures.

Erythromycin is not removed by peritoneal dialysis or hemodialysis.

DOSAGE AND ADMINISTRATION

Administration of a dose of Erythromycin Delayed-release Capsules in the presence of food lowers the blood levels of systemically available erythromycin. Although the blood levels obtained upon administration of enteric-coated erythromycin products in the presence of food are still above minimum inhibitory concentrations (MICs) of most organisms for which erythromycin is indicated, optimum blood levels are obtained on a fasting stomach (administration at least 1/2 hour and preferably two hours before or after a meal).

Adults: The usual dose is 250 mg every 6 hours taken one hour before meals. If twice-a-day dosage is desired, the recommended dose is 500 mg every 12 hours. Dosage may be increased up to 4 grams per day, according to the severity of infection. Twice-a-day dosing is not recommended when doses larger than 1 gram daily are administered.

Children: Age, weight, and severity of the infection are important factors in determining the proper dosage. The usual dosage is 30 to 50 mg/kg/day, in divided doses. For the treatment of more severe infections this dosage may be doubled.

Streptococcal infections: A therapeutic dosage of oral erythromycin should be administered for at least ten days. For continuous prophylaxis against recurrences of streptococcal infections in persons with a history of rheumatic heart disease, the dose is 250 mg twice a day.

For the prevention of bacterial endocarditis in penicillin-allergic patients with valvular heart disease who are to undergo dental procedures or surgical procedures of the upper respiratory tract, the adult dose is 1 gram orally (20 mg/kg for children) one hour prior to the procedure and then 500 mg (10 mg/kg for children) orally 6 hours later.[3] (See "INDICATIONS AND USAGE" section.)

Primary syphilis: 30 to 40 g given in divided doses over a period of 10 to 15 days.

Intestinal amebiasis: 250 mg every 6 hours for 10 to 14 days for adults; 30 to 50 mg/kg/day in divided doses for 10 to 14 days for children.

Legionnaires' disease: Although optimal doses have not been established, doses utilized in reported clinical data were those recommended above (1 to 4 g daily in divided doses).

Urogenital infections during pregnancy due to *Chlamydia trachomatis:* Although the optimal dose and duration of therapy have not been established, the suggested treatment is 500 mg by mouth four times a day on an empty stomach for at least 7 days. For women who cannot tolerate this regimen, a decreased dose of 250 mg by mouth four times a day should be used for at least 14 days.[4]

For adults with uncomplicated urethral, endocervical, or rectal infections caused by *Chlamydia trachomatis,* when tetracycline is contrainidicated or not tolerated, 500 mg of erythromycin by mouth four times a day for at least 7 days.[4]

Pertussis: Although optimum dosage and duration of therapy have not been established, doses of erythromycin utilized in reported clinical studies were 40 to 50 mg/kg/day, given in divided doses for 5 to 14 days.

HOW SUPPLIED

Erythromycin Delayed-release Capsules, USP, are clear and opaque maroon capsules with pink and yellow particles containing 250 mg of erythromycin supplied in bottles of 100 (**NDC** 0074-6301-13) and 500 (**NDC** 0074-6301-53).

Storage Conditions: Protect from moisture and excessive heat. **Store below 86°F (30°C).**

REFERENCES

1. Approved Standard ASM-2 "Performance Standards for Antimicrobial Disc Susceptibility Test." National Committee for Clinical Laboratory Standards, 771 East Lancaster Avenue, Villanova, PA 19085.
2. Ericson, H.M., Sherris, J.C.: "Antibiotic Sensitivity Testing Report of an International Collaborative Study." *Acta Pathologica et Microbiologica Scandinavica,* Section B, Supp. 217, 1971.
3. American Heart Assoc. and American Dental Assoc. "Prevention of Bacterial Endocarditis," *Circulation:* Vol. 70, No. 6, December, 1984, 1123A-1127A.
4. CDC Sexually Transmitted Diseases Treatment Guidelines 1982.

Revised: September, 1991
Ref. 01-2563-R4

Shown in Product Identification Guide, page 303

FERO–FOLIC–500® Filmtab® Tablets ℞
[fe 'ro fo-lic]
Controlled-Release Iron with Folic Acid and Vitamin C

IBERET–FOLIC–500® Filmtab® Tablets ℞
Controlled-Release Iron with Vitamin C, and B-Complex including Folic Acid

> **WARNING:** Accidental overdose of iron-containing products is a leading cause of fatal poisoning in children under 6. Keep this product out of reach of children. In case of accidental overdose, call doctor or poison control center immediately.

DESCRIPTION

FERO-FOLIC-500 Filmtab tablets are a hematinic for oral administration containing iron in the Gradumet controlled-release vehicle; Vitamin C for enhancement of iron absorption; and folic acid. Each tablet provides 525 mg of ferrous sulfate (equivalent to 105 mg of elemental iron), 800 mcg of folic acid and 500 mg of ascorbic acid present as sodium ascorbate.

Inactive Ingredients: Castor oil, cellulosic polymers, D&C Red No. 30, magnesium stearate, methyl acrylate-methyl methacrylate copolymer, pregelatinized starch (contains corn starch), polyethylene glycol, povidone, propylene glycol, talc, titanium dioxide and vanillin.

IBERET-FOLIC-500 tablets are a hematinic for oral administration containing iron in the Gradumet® controlled-release vehicle; vitamin C for enhancement of iron absorption; and the B-Complex vitamins including folic acid.

Each Filmtab tablet provides:

*Ferrous Sulfate (equivalent to 105 mg of elemental iron)	525 mg
Ascorbic Acid (present as sodium ascorbate) (C)	500 mg
Niacinamide	30 mg
Calcium Pantothenate	10 mg
Thiamine Mononitrate (B_1)	6 mg
Riboflavin (B_2)	6 mg
Pyridoxine Hydrochloride (B_6)	5 mg
Folic Acid	800 mcg
Cyanocobalamin (B_{12})	25 mcg

*In controlled-release form (Gradumet)
Filmtab®-Film—Film-sealed tablets, Abbott

Inactive Ingredients: Castor oil, cellulosic polymers, corn starch, D&C Red No. 7, FD&C Blue No. 1, FD&C Blue No. 2, magnesium stearate, methyl acrylate-methyl methacrylate copolymer, polyethylene glycol, povidone, propylene glycol, stearic acid, talc, titanium dioxide and vanillin.

Controlled-release of iron from the Gradumet protects against gastric side effects. The Gradumet is an inert, porous, plastic matrix impregnated with ferrous sulfate. Iron is leached from the Gradumet as it passes through the gastrointestinal tract, and the expended matrix is excreted harmlessly in the stool. Controlled-release iron is particularly helpful in patients who have demonstrated intolerance to oral iron preparations.

CLINICAL PHARMACOLOGY

Oral iron is absorbed most efficiently when administered between meals. Conventional iron preparations frequently cause gastric irritation when taken on an empty stomach. Studies with iron in the Gradumet have indicated that relatively little of the iron is released in the stomach, gastric intolerance is seldom encountered, and hematologic response ranks with that obtained from plain ferrous sulfate.

Iron is found in the body principally as hemoglobin. Storage in the form of ferritin occurs in the liver, spleen, and bone marrow. Concentrations of plasma iron and the total iron-binding capacity of plasma vary greatly in different physiological conditions and disease states.

Large amounts of ascorbic acid administered orally with ferrous sulfate have been shown to enhance iron absorption. Apparently this is due to the ability of ascorbic acid to prevent the oxidation of ferrous iron to the less effectively absorbed ferric form.

Folic acid and iron are absorbed in the proximal small intestine, particularly the duodenum. Folic acid is absorbed maximally and rapidly at this site, and iron is absorbed in a descending gradient from the duodenum distally.

After absorption folic acid is rapidly converted into its metabolically active forms. Approximately two-thirds is bound to plasma protein. Half of the folic acid stored in the body is found in the liver. Folic acid is also concentrated in spinal fluid.

Except for the folates ingested in liver, yeast, and egg yolk, the percentage of absorption of food folates averages about 10%.

The B-complex vitamins in IBERET-FOLIC-500 are absorbed by the active transport process. B-complex vitamins are rapidly eliminated and therefore are not stored in the body. Calcium pantothenate is absorbed readily from the gastrointestinal tract and distributed to all body tissues.

INDICATIONS AND USAGE

FERO-FOLIC-500 is indicated for the treatment of iron deficiency and prevention of concomitant folic acid deficiency in non-pregnant adults. FERO-FOLIC-500 is also indicated in pregnancy for the prevention and treatment of iron deficiency and to supply a maintenance dosage of folic acid.

IBERET-FOLIC-500 is indicated in non-pregnant adults for the treatment of iron deficiency and prevention of concomitant folic acid deficiency with an associated deficient intake or increased need for the B-complex vitamins. IBERET-FOLIC-500 is also indicated in pregnancy for the prevention and treatment of iron deficiency with a concomitant deficient intake or increased need for the B-complex vitamins (including folic acid).

CONTRAINDICATIONS

FERO-FOLIC-500 and IBERET-FOLIC-500 are contraindicated in patients with pernicious anemia.

FERO-FOLIC-500 and IBERET-FOLIC-500 are also contraindicated in the rare instance of hypersensitivity to folic acid.

WARNINGS

Folic acid alone is improper therapy in the treatment of pernicious anemia and other megaloblastic anemias where vitamin B_{12} is deficient. See **boxed WARNING** regarding overdose in children.

PRECAUTIONS

Where anemia exists, its nature should be established and underlying causes determined.

FERO-FOLIC-500 and IBERET-FOLIC-500 contain 800 mcg of folic acid per tablet. Folic acid especially in doses above 0.1 mg daily may obscure pernicious anemia, in that hematologic remission may occur while neurological manifestations remain progresssive. Concomitant parenteral therapy with vitamin B_{12} may be necessary in patients with deficiency of vitamin B_{12}. Pernicious anemia is rare in women of childbearing age, and the likelihood of its occurrence along with pregnancy is reduced by the impairment of fertility associated with vitamin B_{12} deficiency.

Laboratory Tests: In older patients and those with conditions tending to lead to vitamin B_{12} depletion, serum B_{12} levels should be regularly assessed during treatment with FERO-FOLIC-500 or IBERET-FOLIC-500.

Drug Interactions: Absorption of iron is inhibited by *magnesium trisilicate* and *antacids containing carbonates.*

Ferrous sulfate may interfere with the absorption of *tetracyclines.*

The antiparkinsonism effects of *levodopa* may be reversed by pyridoxine.

Iron absorption is inhibited by the ingestion of eggs or milk.

Carcinogenesis: Adequate data are not available on long-term potential for carcinogenesis in animals or humans.

Pregnancy: Pregnancy Category A. Studies in pregnant women have not shown that FERO-FOLIC-500 or IBERET-FOLIC-500 increase the risk of fetal abnormalities if administered during pregnancy. If either of these drugs is used during pregnancy, the possibility of fetal harm appears remote. Because studies cannot rule out the possibility of harm, however, FERO-FOLIC-500 or IBERET-FOLIC-500 should be used during pregnancy only if clearly needed.

Nursing Mothers: Folic acid, ascorbic acid, and B-complex vitamins are excreted in breast milk.

ADVERSE REACTIONS

The likelihood of gastric intolerance to iron in the controlled-release Gradumet vehicle is remote. If such should occur, the tablet may be taken after a meal. Allergic sensitization has been reported following both oral and parenteral administration of folic acid.

OVERDOSAGE

Signs of serious toxicity may be delayed because the iron is in a controlled-release dose form. Increased capillary permeability, reduced plasma volume, increased cardiac output, and sudden cardiovascular collapse may occur in acute iron intoxication. In overdosage, efforts should be made to hasten the elimination of the Gradumet tablets ingested. An emetic should be administered as soon as possible, followed by gastric lavage if indicated. Immediately following emesis, a large dose of a saline cathartic should be used to speed passage through the intestinal tract. X-ray examination may then be considered to determine the position and number of Gradumet tablets remaining in the gastrointestinal tract.

DOSAGE AND ADMINISTRATION

Adults, including Pregnant Females: The recommended dose is one Fero-Folic-500 or one Iberet-Folic-500 tablet daily on an empty stomach.

HOW SUPPLIED

FERO-FOLIC-500 red Filmtab tablets, imprinted with the Abbott logo and Abbo-Code identification letters AJ, are supplied in packages of 30 tablets (**NDC** 0074-7079-30) each containing 5 child-resistant blisters of 6 tablets.

IBERET-FOLIC-500 red Filmtab tablets, imprinted with the Abbott logo and Abbo-Code identification letters AK, are supplied in packaes of 30 tablets (**NDC** 0074-7125-30) each containing 5 child-resistant blisters of 6 tablets.

FILMTAB—Film-sealed tablets, Abbott.
GRADUMET—Controlled-release dose form, Abbott.

Recommended Storage: Store below 77°F (25°C). Protect from light to avoid tablet color changes.
Ref. 13-1743-8/R1 and 13-1746-7/R1

FERO–GRAD–500® Filmtab® tablets OTC
[fe 'ro-grad]
High Potency Dietary Supplement
CONTROLLED-RELEASE IRON, plus Vitamin C
Well-tolerated once-daily iron supplement

> **WARNING:** Accidental overdose of iron-containing products is a leading cause of fatal poisoning in children under 6. Keep this product out of reach of children. In case of accidental overdose, call doctor or poison control center immediately.

DESCRIPTION

Each Fero-Grad-500 tablet provides the equivalent of 95 mg of elemental iron in a unique controlled-release vehicle, the Gradumet® and 500 mg of vitamin C (as sodium ascorbate).

Supplement Facts
Serving Size 1 Tablet

Amount Per Tablet		%Daily Value
Vitamin C	500 mg	833%
Iron	95 mg	528%
Sodium	65 mg	3%

Ingredients: Sodium ascorbate, ferrous sulfate, povidone, methyl acrylate-methyl methacrylate copolymer, polyethylene glycol, hydroxypropyl methylcellulose, pregelatinized starch (contains corn starch), talc, D&C Red No. 7, titanium dioxide, hydroxypropyl cellulose, magnesium stearate, ethylcellulose, propylene glycol, castor oil and vanillin.

DOSAGE AND ADMINISTRATION

Usual dose for adults and children 4 or more years of age: One tablet daily, or as directed by the physician.

TO OPEN CHILD-RESISTANT BLISTER PACKAGE:

1. Tear from bottom edge on perforations at START TEAR arrows.
2. Fold back and peel paper from corner marked PEEL.
3. Push tablet through foil.

HOW SUPPLIED

Fero-Grad-500 is supplied as red tablets in reclosable cartons of 30 tablets (5 child-resistant blister packages of 6 tablets) list no. 0074-7238-30. Do not accept if blister unit has been opened or seal has been broken. The ingredients of these products are listed in one or more of the Medicare designated compendia.

Recommended storage: Store below 77°F (25°C). Protect from light to avoid tablet color changes.
Ref. 13-1928-9/R2
ABBOTT LABORATORIES
NORTH CHICAGO, IL 60064, U.S.A.

GABITRIL® Filmtab® ℞
[găb-ĭ-trĭll]
(tiagabine hydrochloride)
Tablets

DESCRIPTION

GABITRIL (tiagabine HCl) is an antiepilepsy drug available as 2 mg, 4 mg, 12 mg, 16 mg, and 20 mg tablets for oral administration. Its chemical name is (-)-(R)-1-[4,4-Bis(3-methyl-2-thienyl)-3-butenyl]nipecotic acid hydrochloride, its molecular formula is $C_{20}H_{25}NO_2S_2$ HCl, and its molecular weight is 412.0. Tiagabine HCl is a white to off-white,

Continued on next page

Gabitril—Cont.

odorless, crystalline powder. It is insoluble in heptane, sparingly soluble in water, and soluble in aqueous base. The structural formula is:

CH_3 H COOH •HCl
C=CH–CH_2–CH_2–N
CH_3

Inactive Ingredients
GABITRIL tablets contain the following inactive ingredients: Ascorbic acid, colloidal silicon dioxide, crospovidone, hydrogenated vegetable oil wax, hydroxypropyl cellulose, hydroxypropyl methylcellulose, lactose, magnesium stearate, microcrystalline cellulose, pregelatinized starch, stearic acid, and titanium dioxide.
In addition, individual tablets contain:
2 mg tablets: FD&C Yellow No. 6.
4 mg tablets: D&C Yellow No. 10.
12 mg tablets: D&C Yellow No. 10 and FD&C Blue No. 1.
16 mg tablets: FD&C Blue No. 2.
20 mg tablets: D&C Red No. 30.

CLINICAL PHARMACOLOGY

Mechanism of Action
The precise mechanism by which tiagabine exerts its antiseizure effect is unknown, although it is believed to be related to its ability, documented in *in vitro* experiments, to enhance the activity of gamma aminobutyric acid (GABA), the major inhibitory neurotransmitter in the central nervous system. These experiments have shown that tiagabine binds to recognition sites associated with the GABA uptake carrier. It is thought that, by this action, tiagabine blocks GABA uptake into presynaptic neurons, permitting more GABA to be available for receptor binding on the surfaces of post-synaptic cells. Inhibition of GABA uptake has been shown for synaptosomes, neuronal cell cultures, and glial cell cultures. In rat-derived hippocampal slices, tiagabine has been shown to prolong GABA-mediated inhibitory postsynaptic potentials. Tiagabine increases the amount of GABA available in the extracellular space of the globus pallidus, ventral palladum, and substantia nigra in rats at the ED_{50} and ED_{85} doses for inhibition of pentylenetetrazol (PTZ)-induced tonic seizures. This suggests that tiagabine prevents the propagation of neural impulses that contribute to seizures by a GABA-ergic action.
Tiagabine has shown efficacy in several animal models of seizures. It is effective against the tonic phase of subcutaneous PTZ-induced seizures in mice and rats, seizures induced by the proconvulsant DMCM in mice, audiogenic seizures in genetically epilepsy-prone rats (GEPR), and amygdala-kindled seizures in rats. Tiagabine has little efficacy against maximal electroshock seizures in rats and is only partially effective against subcutaneous PTZ-induced clonic seizures in mice, picrotoxin-induced tonic seizures in the mouse, bicuculline-induced seizures in the rat, and photic seizures in photosensitive baboons. Tiagabine produces a biphasic dose-response curve against PTZ- and DMCM-induced convulsions, with attenuated effectiveness at higher doses.
Based on *in vitro* binding studies, tiagabine does not significantly inhibit the uptake of dopamine, norepinephrine, serotonin, glutamate, or choline and shows little or no binding to dopamine D1 and D2, muscarinic, serotonin $5HT_{1A}$, $5HT_2$, and $5HT_3$, beta-1 and 2 adrenergic, alpha-1 and alpha-2 adrenergic, histamine H2 and H3, adenosine A_1 and A_2, opiate μ and K_1, NMDA glutamate, and $GABA_A$ receptors at 100 μM. It also lacks significant affinity for sodium or calcium channels. Tiagabine binds to histamine H1, serotonin $5HT_{1B}$, benzodiazepine, and chloride channel receptors at concentrations 20 to 400 times those inhibiting the uptake of GABA.

PHARMACOKINETICS

Tiagabine is well absorbed, with food slowing absorption rate but not altering the extent of absorption. Although its elimination half-life is 7 to 9 hours in normal volunteers, it is only 4 to 7 hours in patients receiving hepatic enzyme-inducing drugs (carbamazepine, phenytoin, primidone, and phenobarbital). In clinical trials, most patients were induced.
Absorption and Distribution: Absorption of tiagabine is rapid, with peak plasma concentrations occurring at approximately 45 minutes following an oral dose in the fasting state. Tiagabine is nearly completely absorbed (>95%), with an absolute oral bioavailability of about 90%. A high fat meal decreases the rate (mean T_{max} was prolonged to 2.5 hours, and mean C_{max} was reduced by about 40%) but not the extent (AUC) of tiagabine absorption. In all clinical trials, tiagabine was given with meals.
The pharmacokinetics of tiagabine are linear over the single dose range of 2 to 24 mg. Following multiple dosing, steady state is achieved within 2 days.
Tiagabine is 96% bound to human plasma proteins, mainly to serum albumin and α1-acid glycoprotein over the concentration range of 10 ng/mL to 10,000 ng/mL. While the relationship between tiagabine plasma concentrations and clinical response is not currently understood, trough plasma concentrations observed in controlled clinical trials at doses from 30 to 56 mg/day ranged from <1 ng/mL to 234 ng/mL.

Table 1
Median Reduction and Median Percent Reduction from Baseline in 4-Week Seizure Rates in Study 1

		Placebo (N=91)	GABITRIL 16 mg/day (N=61)	GABITRIL 32 mg/day (N=87)	GABITRIL 56 mg/day (N=56)	Combined 32 + 56 mg/day (N=143)
Complex Partial	Median Reduction	0.6	0.8	2.2*	2.9*	2.6*
	Median % Reduction†	9%	13%	25%	32%	29%
All Partial	Median Reduction	0.2	1.2	2.7*	3.5*	2.9*
	Median % Reduction†	3%	12%	24%	36%	27%

* p<0.05
† Statistical significance was not assessed for median % reduction.

Table 2
Median Reduction and Median Percent Reduction from Baseline in 4-Week Seizure Rates in Study 2

		Placebo (N=107)	GABITRIL 16 mg BID (N=106)	GABITRIL 8 mg QID (N=104)
Complex Partial	Median Reduction	0.3	1.6	1.3*
	Median % Reduction†	4%	22%	15%
All Partial	Median Reduction	0.5	1.6	1.3
	Median % Reduction†	5%	19%	13%

* p < 0.027, necessary for statistical significance due to multiple comparisons.
† Statistical significance was not assessed for median % reduction.

Metabolism and Elimination: Although the metabolism of tiagabine has not been fully elucidated, *in vivo* and *in vitro* studies suggest that at least two metabolic pathways for tiagabine have been identified in humans: 1) thiophene ring oxidation leading to the formation of 5-oxo-tiagabine; and 2) glucuronidation. The 5-oxo-tiagabine metabolite does not contribute to the pharmacologic activity of tiagabine.
Based on *in vitro* data, tiagabine is likely to be metabolized primarily by the 3A isoform subfamily of hepatic cytochrome P450 (CYP 3A), although contributions to the metabolism of tiagabine from CYP 1A2, CYP 2D6 or CYP 2C19 have not been excluded.
Approximately 2% of an oral dose of tiagabine is excreted unchanged, with 25% and 63% of the remaining dose excreted into the urine and feces, respectively, primarily as metabolites, at least 2 of which have not been identified. The mean systemic plasma clearance is 109 mL/min (CV = 23%) and the average elimination half-life for tiagabine in healthy subjects ranged from 7 to 9 hours. The elimination half-life decreased by 50 to 65% in hepatic enzyme-induced patients with epilepsy compared to uninduced patients with epilepsy.
A diurnal effect on the pharmacokinetics of tiagabine was observed. Mean steady-state C_{min} values were 40% lower in the evening than in the morning. Tiagabine steady-state AUC values were also found to be 15% lower following the evening tiagabine dose compared to the AUC following the morning dose.

SPECIAL POPULATIONS

Renal Insufficiency: The pharmacokinetics of total and unbound tiagabine were similar in subjects with normal renal function (creatinine clearance >80 mL/min) and in subjects with mild (creatinine clearance 40 to 80 mL/min), moderate (creatinine clearance 20 to 39 mL/min), or severe (creatinine clearance 5 to 19 mL/min) renal impairment. The pharmacokinetics of total and unbound tiagabine were also unaffected in subjects with renal failure requiring hemodialysis.
Hepatic Insufficiency: In patients with moderate hepatic impairment (Child-Pugh Class B), clearance of unbound tiagabine was reduced by about 60%. Patients with impaired liver function may require reduced initial and maintenance doses of tiagabine and/or longer dosing intervals compared to patients with normal hepatic function (see **PRECAUTIONS**).
Geriatric: The pharmacokinetic profile of tiagabine was similar in healthy elderly and healthy young adults.
Pediatric: Tiagabine has not been investigated in adequate and well-controlled clinical trials in patients below the age of 12. The apparent clearance and volume of distribution of tiagabine per unit body surface area or per kg were fairly similar in 25 children (age: 3 to 10 years) and in adults taking enzyme-inducing antiepilepsy drugs ([AEDs] e.g., carbamazepine or phenytoin). In children who were taking a non-inducing AED (e.g., valproate), the clearance of tiagabine based upon body weight and body surface area was 2 and 1.5-fold higher, respectively, than in uninduced adults with epilepsy.
Gender, Race and Cigarette Smoking: No specific pharmacokinetic studies were conducted to investigate the effect of gender, race and cigarette smoking on the disposition of tiagabine. Retrospective pharmacokinetic analyses, however, suggest that there is no clinically important difference between the clearance of tiagabine in males and females, when adjusted for body weight. Population pharmacokinetic analyses indicated that tiagabine clearance values were not significantly different in Caucasian (N=463), Black (N=23), or Hispanic (N=17) patients with epilepsy, and that tiagabine clearance values were not significantly affected by tobacco use.
Interactions with other Antiepilepsy Drugs: The clearance of tiagabine is affected by the co-administration of hepatic enzyme-inducing antiepilepsy drugs. Tiagabine is eliminated more rapidly in patients who have been taking hepatic enzyme-inducing drugs, e.g. carbamazepine, phenytoin, primidone and phenobarbital than in patients not receiving such treatment (see **PRECAUTIONS, Drug Interactions**).
Interactions with Other Drugs: See **PRECAUTIONS, Drug Interactions.**

CLINICAL STUDIES

The effectiveness of GABITRIL as adjunctive therapy (added to other antiepilepsy drugs) was examined in three multi-center, double-blind, placebo-controlled, parallel-group, clinical trials in 769 patients with refractory partial seizures who were taking at least one hepatic enzyme-inducing antiepilepsy drug (AED), and two placebo-controlled cross-over studies in 90 patients. In the parallel-group trials, patients had a history of at least six complex partial seizures (Study 1 and Study 2, U.S. studies), or six partial seizures of any type (Study 3, European study), occurring alone or in combination with any other seizure type within the 8-week period preceding the first study visit in spite of receiving one or more AEDs at therapeutic concentrations.
In the first two studies, the primary protocol-specified outcome measure was the median reduction from baseline in the 4-week complex partial seizure (CPS) rates during treatment. In the third study, the protocol-specified primary outcome measure was the proportion of patients achieving a 50% or greater reduction from baseline in the 4-week seizure rate of all partial seizures during treatment. The results given below include data for complex partial seizures and all partial seizures for the intent-to-treat population (all patients who received at least one dose of treatment and at least one seizure evaluation) in each study.
Study 1 was a double-blind, placebo-controlled, parallel-group trial comparing GABITRIL 16 mg/day, GABITRIL 32 mg/day, GABITRIL 56 mg/day, and placebo. Study drug was given as a four times a day regimen. After a prospective Baseline Phase of 12 weeks, patients were randomized to one of the four treatment groups described above. The 16-week Treatment Phase consisted of a 4-week Titration Period, followed by a 12-week Fixed-Dose Period, during which concomitant AED doses were held constant. The primary outcome was assessed for the combined 32 and 56 mg/day groups compared to placebo.
Study 2 was a double-blind, placebo-controlled, parallel-group trial consisting of an 8-week Baseline Phase and a 12-week Treatment Phase, the first 4 weeks of which constituted a Titration Period and the last 8 weeks a Fixed-Dose Period. This study compared GABITRIL 16 mg BID and 8 mg QID to placebo. The protocol-specified primary outcome measure was assessed separately for each group treated with GABITRIL.
The following tables display the results of the analyses of these two trials.
[See table 1 above]
[See table 2 above]

Figures 1 to 4 present the proportion of patients (X-axis) whose percent reduction from baseline in the all partial seizure rate was at least as great as that indicated on the Y axis in the three placebo-controlled adjunctive studies (Studies 1, 2, and 3). A positive value on the Y axis indicates an improvement from baseline (i.e., a decrease in seizure rate), while a negative value indicates a worsening from baseline (i.e., an increase in seizure rate). Thus, in a display of this type, the curve for an effective treatment is shifted to the left of the curve for placebo.

Figure 1 indicates that the proportion of patients achieving any particular level of reduction in seizure rate was consistently higher for the combined GABITRIL 32 mg and 56 mg groups compared to the placebo group in Study 1. For example, Figure 1 indicates that approximately 24% of patients treated with GABITRIL experienced a 50% or greater reduction, compared to 4% in the placebo group.

Figure 1
Study 1

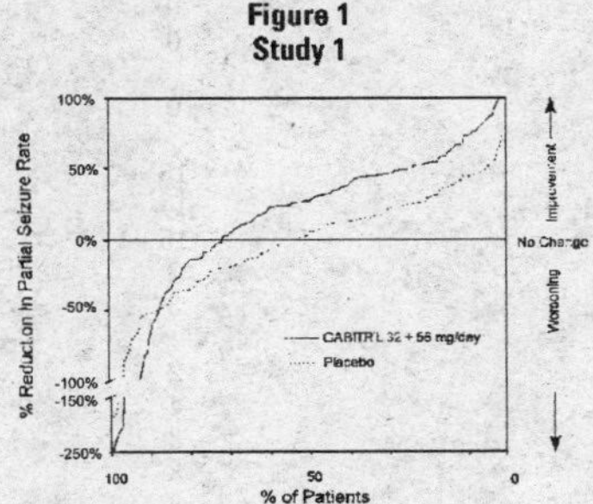

Figure 2 also displays the results for Study 1, which was a dose-response study, by treatment group, without combining GABITRIL dosage groups. Figure 2 indicates a dose-response relationship across the three GABITRIL groups. The proportion of patients achieving any particular level of reduction in all partial seizure rates was consistently higher as the dose of GABITRIL was increased. For example, Figure 2 indicates that approximately 4% of patients in the placebo group experienced a 50% or greater reduction in all partial seizure rate, compared to approximately 10% of the GABITRIL 16 mg/day group, 21% of the GABITRIL 32 mg/day group, and 30% of the GABITRIL 56 mg/day group.

Figure 2
Study 1

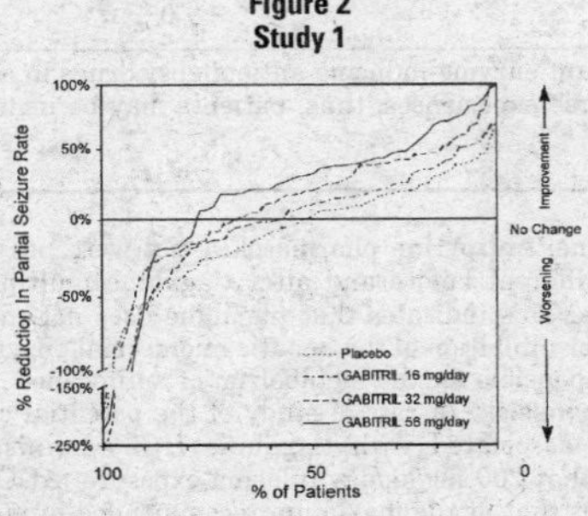

Figure 3 indicates that the proportion of patients achieving any particular level of reduction in partial seizure rate was consistently greater in patients taking GABITRIL than in those taking placebo in Study 2. (Study 2 compared placebo to GABITRIL 32 mg/day; one of the GABITRIL groups received 8 mg QID, while the other GABITRIL group received 16 mg BID). For example, Figure 3 indicates that approximately 7% of patients in the placebo group experienced a 50% or greater reduction in their partial seizure rate, compared to approximately 23% of patients in the GABITRIL 8 mg QID group and 28% of patients in the GABITRIL 16 mg BID group.

Figure 3
Study 2

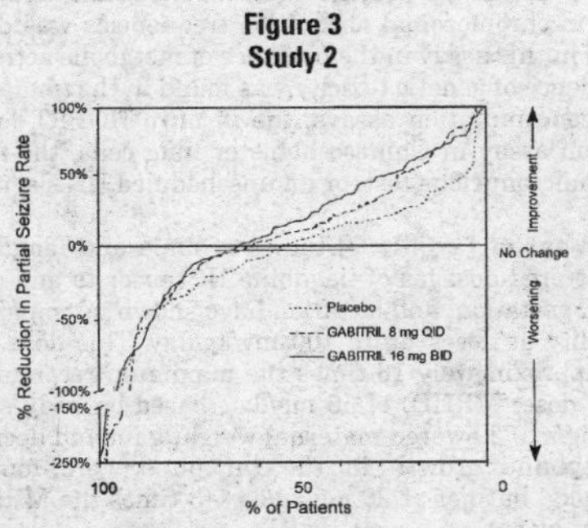

Study 3 was a double-blind, placebo-controlled, parallel-group trial that compared GABITRIL 10 mg TID (N=77) with placebo (N=77). In this trial, patients were followed prospectively during a 12-week Baseline Phase and then randomized to receive study drug during an 18-week Treatment Phase. During the first 6 weeks of treatment (Titration Period), patients were titrated to 30 mg/day, after which they were maintained on this dose during the 12-week Fixed-Dose Period. The protocol-specified primary outcome measure (proportion of patients who achieved at least a 50% reduction from baseline in partial seizure rate) did not reach statistical significance. However, analyses of the median reduction from baseline in 4-week partial seizure rate (the analyses presented above for Study 1 and Study 2) were performed and showed a statistically significant improvement compared to placebo in all partial and complex partial seizure rates (Table 3):

[See table 3 above]

Table 3
Median Reduction and Median Percent Reduction from Baseline in 4-Week Seizure Rates in Study 3

		Placebo (N=77)	GABITRIL 30 mg/day (N=77)
Complex Partial‡	Median Reduction	-0.1	1.3*
	Median % Reduction†	-1%	14%
All Partial	Median Reduction	-0.5	1.1*
	Median % Reduction†	-7%	11%

* p <0.05
† Statistical significance was not assessed for median % reduction.
‡ N=72 and 75 for placebo and GABITRIL, respectively.

Figure 4 indicates that the proportion of patients achieving any particular level of reduction in seizure activity was consistently higher in those taking GABITRIL than those taking placebo in Study 3. For example, Figure 4 indicates that approximately 5% of patients in the placebo group experienced a 50% or greater reduction in their partial seizure rate compared to approximately 10% of patients in the GABITRIL group.

Figure 4
Study 3

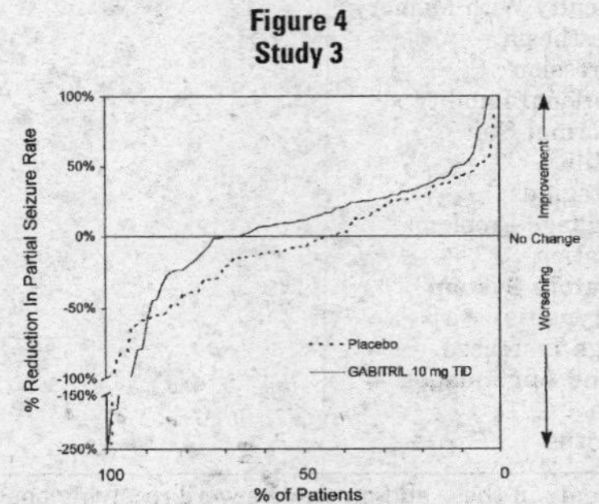

The two other placebo-controlled trials that examined the effectiveness of GABITRIL were small cross-over trials (N=46 and 44). Both trials included an open Screening Phase during which patients were titrated to an optimal dose and then treated with this dose for an additional 4 weeks. After this Open Phase, patients were randomized to one of two blinded treatment sequences (GABITRIL followed by placebo or placebo followed by GABITRIL). The Double-Blind Phase consisted of two Treatment Periods, each lasting 7 weeks (with a 3 week washout between periods). The outcome measures were median with-in patient differences between placebo and GABITRIL Treatment Periods in 4-week complex partial and all partial seizure rates. The reductions in seizure rates were statistically significant in both studies.

INDICATIONS AND USAGE

GABITRIL (tiagabine hydrochloride) is indicated as adjunctive therapy in adults and children 12 years and older in the treatment of partial seizures.

CONTRAINDICATIONS

GABITRIL is contraindicated in patients who have demonstrated hypersensitivity to the drug or its ingredients.

WARNINGS

Withdrawal Seizures: As a rule, antiepilepsy drugs should not be abruptly discontinued because of the possibility of increasing seizure frequency. In a placebo-controlled, double-blind, dose-response study (Study 1 described in **CLINICAL STUDIES**) designed, in part, to investigate the capacity of GABITRIL to induce withdrawal seizures, study drug was tapered over a 4-week period after 16 weeks of treatment. Patients' seizure frequency during this 4-week withdrawal period was compared to their baseline seizure frequency (before study drug). For each partial seizure type, for all partial seizure types combined, and for secondarily generalized tonic-clonic seizures, more patients experienced increases in their seizure frequencies during the withdrawal period in the three GABITRIL groups than in the placebo group. The increase in seizure frequency was not affected by dose. GABITRIL should be withdrawn gradually to minimize the potential of increased seizure frequency, unless safety concerns require a more rapid withdrawal.

Cognitive/Neuropsychiatric Adverse Events: Adverse events most often associated with the use of GABITRIL were related to the central nervous system. The most significant of these can be classified into 2 general categories: 1) impaired concentration, speech or language problems, and confusion (effects on thought processes); and 2) somnolence and fatigue (effects on level of consciousness). The majority of these events were mild to moderate. In controlled clinical trials, these events led to discontinuation of treatment with GABITRIL in 6% (31 of 494) of patients compared to 2% (5 of 275) of the placebo-treated patients. A total of 1.6% (8 of 494) of the GABITRIL treated patients in the controlled trials were hospitalized secondary to the occurrence of these events compared to 0% of the placebo treated patients. Some of these events were dose related and usually began during initial titration.

Patients with a history of spike and wave discharges on EEG have been reported to have exacerbations of their EEG abnormalities associated with these cognitive/neuropsychiatric events. This raises the possibility that these clinical events may, in some cases, be a manifestation of underlying seizure activity (see **PRECAUTIONS, EEG**). In the documented cases of spike and wave discharges on EEG with cognitive/neuropsychiatric events, patients usually continued tiagabine, but required dosage adjustment.

Additionally, there have been postmarketing reports of patients who have experienced cognitive/neuropsychiatric symptoms, some accompanied by EEG abnormalities such as generalized spike and wave activity, that have been reported as nonconvulsant status epilepticus. Some reports describe recovery following reduction of dose or discontinuation of GABITRIL.

Status Epilepticus: In the three double-blind, placebo-controlled, parallel-group studies (Studies 1, 2, and 3), the incidence of any type of status epilepticus (simple, complex, or generalized tonic-clonic) in patients receiving GABITRIL was 0.8% (4 of 494 patients) versus 0.7% (2 of 275 patients) receiving placebo. Among the patients treated with GABITRIL across all epilepsy studies (controlled and uncontrolled), 5% had some form of status epilepticus. Of the 5%, 57% of patients experienced complex partial status epilepticus. A critical risk factor for status epilepticus was the presence of a previous history; 33% of patients with a history of status epilepticus had recurrence during GABITRIL treatment. Because adequate information about the incidence of status epilepticus in a similar population of patients with epilepsy who have not received treatment with GABITRIL is not available, it is impossible to state whether or not treatment with GABITRIL is associated with a higher or lower rate of status epilepticus than would be expected to occur in a similar population not treated with GABITRIL.

Sudden Unexpected Death In Epilepsy (SUDEP): There have been as many as 10 cases of sudden unexpected deaths during the clinical development of tiagabine among 2531 patients with epilepsy (3831 patient-years of exposure).

This represents an estimated incidence of 0.0026 deaths per patient-year. This rate is within the range of estimates for the incidence of sudden and unexpected deaths in patients with epilepsy not receiving GABITRIL (ranging from 0.0005 for the general population with epilepsy, 0.003 to 0.004 for clinical trial populations similar to that in the clinical development program for GABITRIL, to 0.005 for patients with refractory epilepsy). The estimated SUDEP rates in patients receiving GABITRIL are also similar to those observed in patients receiving other antiepilepsy drugs, chemically unrelated to GABITRIL, that underwent clinical testing in similar populations at about the same time. This evidence suggests that the SUDEP rates reflect population rates, not a drug effect.

PRECAUTIONS

General

Use in Non-Induced Patients: Virtually all experience with GABITRIL has been obtained in patients receiving at least one concomitant enzyme-inducing antiepilepsy drug (AED). Use in non-induced patients (e.g., patients receiving valproate monotherapy) may require lower doses or a slower dose titration of GABITRIL for clinical response. Patients taking a combination of inducing and non-inducing drugs (e.g., carbamazepine and valproate) should be considered to be induced.

Generalized Weakness: Moderately severe to incapacitating generalized weakness has been reported following administration of GABITRIL in 28 of 2531 (approximately 1%) patients with epilepsy. The weakness resolved in all cases after a reduction in dose or discontinuation of GABITRIL.

Binding in the Eye and Other Melanin-Containing Tissues: When dogs received a single dose of radiolabeled tiagabine, there was evidence of residual binding in the retina and uvea after 3 weeks (the latest time point measured). Al-

Continued on next page

Gabitril—Cont.

though not directly measured, melanin binding is suggested. The ability of available tests to detect potentially adverse consequences, if any, of the binding of tiagabine to melanin-containing tissue is unknown and there was no systematic monitoring for relevant ophthalmological changes during the clinical development of GABITRIL. However, long term (up to one year) toxicological studies of tiagabine in dogs showed no treatment-related ophthalmoscopic changes and macro- and microscopic examinations of the eye were unremarkable. Accordingly, although there are no specific recommendations for periodic ophthalmologic monitoring, prescribers should be aware of the possibility of long-term ophthalmologic effects.

Use in Hepatically-Impaired Patients: Because the clearance of tiagabine is reduced in patients with liver disease, dosage reduction may be necessary in these patients.

Serious Rash: Four patients treated with tiagabine during the product's premarketing clinical testing developed what were considered to be serious rashes. In two patients, the rash was described as maculopapular; in one it was described as vesiculobullous; and in the 4th case, a diagnosis of Stevens Johnson Syndrome was made. In none of the 4 cases is it certain that tiagabine was the primary, or even a contributory, cause of the rash. Nevertheless, drug associated rash can, if extensive and serious, cause irreversible morbidity, even death.

Information for Patients: Patients should be instructed to take GABITRIL only as prescribed.

Patients should be advised that GABITRIL may cause dizziness, somnolence, and other symptoms and signs of CNS depression. Accordingly, they should be advised neither to drive nor to operate other complex machinery until they have gained sufficient experience on GABITRIL to gauge whether or not it affects their mental and/or motor performance adversely.

Because of the possible additive depressive effects, caution should also be used when patients are taking other CNS depressants in combination with GABITRIL.

Because teratogenic effects were seen in the offspring of rats exposed to maternally toxic doses of tiagabine and because experience in humans is limited, patients should be advised to notify their physicians if they become pregnant or intend to become pregnant during therapy.

Because of the possibility that tiagabine may be excreted in breast milk, patients should be advised to notify those providing care to themselves and their children if they intend to breast-feed or are breast-feeding an infant.

Laboratory Tests

Therapeutic Monitoring of Plasma Concentrations of Tiagabine: A therapeutic range for tiagabine plasma concentrations has not been established. In controlled trials, trough plasma concentrations observed among patients randomized to doses of tiagabine that were statistically significantly more effective than placebo ranged from <1 ng/mL to 234 ng/mL (median, 10th and 90th percentiles are 23.7 ng/mL, 5.4 ng/mL, and 69.8 ng/mL, respectively). Because of the potential for pharmacokinetic interactions between GABITRIL and drugs that induce or inhibit hepatic metabolizing enzymes, it may be useful to obtain plasma levels of tiagabine before and after changes are made in the therapeutic regimen.

Clinical Chemistry and Hematology: During the development of GABITRIL, no systematic abnormalities on routine laboratory testing were noted. Therefore, no specific guidance is offered regarding routine monitoring; the practitioner retains responsibility for determining how best to monitor the patient in his/her care.

EEG: Patients with a history of spike and wave discharges on EEG have been reported to have exacerbations of their EEG abnormalities associated with cognitive/neuropsychiatric events. This raises the possibility that these clinical events may, in some cases, be a manifestation of underlying seizure activity (see **WARNINGS, Cognitive/Neuropsychiatric Adverse Events**). In the documented cases of spike and wave discharges on EEG with cognitive/neuropsychiatric events, patients usually continued tiagabine, but required dosage adjustment.

Drug Interactions

In evaluating the potential for interactions among co-administered antiepilepsy drugs (AEDs), whether or not an AED induces or does not induce metabolic enzymes is an important consideration. Phenytoin, phenobarbital and carbamazepine are generally classified as enzyme inducers; valproate and gabapentin are not. GABITRIL is considered to be a non-enzyme inducing AED.

The drug interaction data described in this section were obtained from studies involving either healthy subjects or patients with epilepsy.

Effects of GABITRIL on other Antiepilepsy Drugs (AEDs):

Phenytoin: Tiagabine had no effect on the steady-state plasma concentrations of phenytoin in patients with epilepsy.

Carbamazepine: Tiagabine had no effect on the steady-state plasma concentrations of carbamazepine or its epoxide metabolite in patients with epilepsy.

Valproate: Tiagabine causes a slight decrease (about 10%) in steady-state valproate concentrations.

Phenobarbital or Primidone: No formal pharmacokinetic studies have been performed examining the addition of tiagabine to regimens containing phenobarbital or primidone. The addition of tiagabine in a limited number of patients in

Table 4
Treatment-Emergent Adverse Event[1] Incidence in Parallel-Group, Placebo-Controlled, Add-On Trials (events in at least 1% of patients treated with GABITRIL and numerically more frequent than in the placebo group)

Body System/ COSTART	GABITRIL N=494 %	Placebo N=275 %
Body as a Whole		
Abdominal Pain	7	3
Pain (unspecified)	5	3
Cardiovascular		
Vasodilation	2	1
Digestive		
Nausea	11	9
Diarrhea	7	3
Vomiting	7	4
Increased Appetite	2	0
Mouth Ulceration	1	0
Musculoskeletal		
Myasthenia	1	0
Nervous System		
Dizziness	27	15
Asthenia	20	14
Somnolence	18	15
Nervousness	10	3
Tremor	9	3
Difficulty With Concentration/ Attention*	6	2
Insomnia	6	4
Ataxia	5	3
Confusion	5	3
Speech Disorder	4	2
Difficulty With Memory*	4	3
Paresthesia	4	2
Depression	3	1
Emotional Lability	3	2
Abnormal Gait	3	2
Hostility	2	1
Nystagmus	2	1
Language Problems*	2	0
Agitation	1	0
Respiratory System		
Pharyngitis	7	4
Cough Increased	4	3
Skin and Appendages		
Rash	5	4
Pruritus	2	0

[1] Patients in these add-on studies were receiving one to three concomitant enzyme-inducing antiepilepsy drugs in addition to GABITRIL or placebo. Patients may have reported multiple adverse experiences; thus, patients may be included in more than one category.

* COSTART term substituted with a more clinically descriptive term.

three well-controlled studies caused no systematic changes in phenobarbital or primidone concentrations when compared to placebo.

Effects of other Antiepilepsy Drugs (AEDs) on GABITRIL:

Carbamazepine: Population pharmacokinetic analyses indicate that tiagabine clearance is 60% greater in patients taking carbamazepine with or without other enzyme-inducing AEDs.

Phenytoin: Population pharmacokinetic analyses indicate that tiagabine clearance is 60% greater in patients taking phenytoin with or without other enzyme-inducing AEDs.

Phenobarbital (Primidone): Population pharmacokinetic analyses indicate that tiagabine clearance is 60% greater in patients taking phenobarbital (primidone) with or without other enzyme-inducing AEDs.

Valproate: The addition of tiagabine to patients taking valproate chronically had no effect on tiagabine pharmacokinetics, but valproate significantly decreased tiagabine binding *in vitro* from 96.3 to 94.8%, which resulted in an increase of approximately 40% in the free tiagabine concentration. The clinical relevance of this *in vitro* finding is unknown.

Interaction of GABITRIL with Other Drugs:

Cimetidine: Co-administration of cimetidine (800 mg/day) to patients taking tiagabine chronically had no effect on tiagabine pharmacokinetics.

Theophylline: A single 10 mg dose of tiagabine did not affect the pharmacokinetics of theophylline at steady state.

Warfarin: No significant differences were observed in the steady-state pharmacokinetics of R-warfarin or S-warfarin with the addition of tiagabine given as a single dose. Prothrombin times were not affected by tiagabine.

Digoxin: Concomitant administration of tiagabine did not affect the steady-state pharmacokinetics of digoxin or the mean daily trough serum level of digoxin.

Ethanol or Triazolam: No significant differences were observed in the pharmacokinetics of triazolam (0.125 mg) and tiagabine (10 mg) when given together as a single dose. The pharmacokinetics of ethanol were not affected by multiple-dose administration of tiagabine. Tiagabine has shown no clinically important potentiation of the pharmacodynamic effects of triazolam or alcohol. Because of the possible additive effects of drugs that may depress the nervous system, ethanol or triazolam should be used cautiously in combination with tiagabine.

Oral Contraceptives: Multiple dose administration of tiagabine (8 mg/day monotherapy) did not alter the pharmacokinetics of oral contraceptives in healthy women of child-bearing age.

Antipyrine: Antipyrine pharmacokinetics were not significantly different before and after tiagabine multiple-dose regimens. This indicates that tiagabine does not cause induction or inhibition of the hepatic microsomal enzyme systems responsible for the metabolism of antipyrine.

Carcinogenesis: In rats, a study of the potential carcinogenicity associated with tiagabine HCl administration showed that 200 mg/kg/day (plasma exposure [AUC] 36 to 100 times that at the maximum recommended human dosage [MRHD] of 56 mg/day) for 2 years resulted in small, but statistically significant increases in the incidences of hepatocellular adenomas in females and Leydig cell tumors of the testis in males. The significance of these findings relative to the use of GABITRIL in humans is unknown. The no effect dosage for induction of tumors in this study was 100 mg/kg/day (17 to 50 times the exposure at the MRHD). No statistically significant increases in tumor formation were noted in mice at dosages up to 250 mg/kg/day (20 times the MRHD on a mg/m^2 basis).

Mutagenesis: Tiagabine produced an increase in structural chromosome aberration frequency in human lymphocytes *in vitro* in the absence of metabolic activation. No increase in chromosomal aberration frequencies was demonstrated in this assay in the presence of metabolic activation. No evidence of genetic toxicity was found in the *in vitro* bacterial gene mutation assays, the *in vitro* HGPRT forward mutation assay in Chinese hamster lung cells, the *in vivo* mouse micronucleus test, or an unscheduled DNA synthesis assay.

Impairment of Fertility: Studies of male and female rats administered dosages of tiagabine HCl prior to and during mating, gestation, and lactation have shown no impairment of fertility at doses up to 100 mg/kg/day. This dose represents approximately 16 times the maximum recommended human dose (MRHD) of 56 mg/day, based on body surface area (mg/m^2). Lowered maternal weight gain and decreased viability and growth in the rat pups were found at 100 mg/kg, but not at 20 mg/kg/day (3 times the MRHD on a mg/m^2 basis).

Pregnancy: Pregnancy Category C: Tiagabine has been shown to have adverse effects on embryo-fetal development, including teratogenic effects, when administered to pregnant rats and rabbits at doses greater than the human therapeutic dose.

An increased incidence of malformed fetuses (various craniofacial, appendicular, and visceral defects) and decreased fetal weights were observed following oral administration of 100 mg/kg/day to pregnant rats during the period of organogenesis. This dose is approximately 16 times the maximum recommended human dose (MRHD) of 56 mg/day, based on body surface area (mg/m^2). Maternal toxicity (transient weight loss/reduced maternal weight gain during gestation) was associated with this dose, but there is no evidence to suggest that the teratogenic effects were secondary to the maternal effects. No adverse maternal or embryo-fetal effects were seen at a dose of 20 mg/kg/day (3 times the MRHD on a mg/m^2 basis).

Decreased maternal weight gain, increased resorption of embryos and increased incidences of fetal variations, but not malformations, were observed when pregnant rabbits were given 25 mg/kg/day (8 times the MRHD on a mg/m^2 basis) during organogenesis. The no effect level for maternal and embryo-fetal toxicity in rabbits was 5 mg/kg/day (equivalent to the MRHD on a mg/m^2 basis).

When female rats were given tiagabine 100 mg/kg/day during late gestation and throughout parturition and lactation, decreased maternal weight gain during gestation, an increase in stillbirths, and decreased postnatal offspring viability and growth were found. There are no adequate and well-controlled studies in pregnant women. Tiagabine should be used during pregnancy only if clearly needed.

Use in Nursing Mothers: Studies in rats have shown that tiagabine HCl and/or its metabolites are excreted in the milk of that species. Levels of excretion of tiagabine and/or its metabolites in human milk have not been determined and effects on the nursing infant are unknown. GABITRIL should be used in women who are nursing only if the benefits clearly outweigh the risks.

Pediatric Use: Safety and effectiveness in pediatric patients below the age of 12 have not been established. The pharmacokinetics of tiagabine were evaluated in pediatric patients age 3 to 10 years (see **CLINICAL PHARMACOLOGY** - Pediatric).

Geriatric Use: Because few patients over the age of 65 (approximately 20) were exposed to GABITRIL during its clinical evaluation, no specific statements about the safety or effectiveness of GABITRIL in this age group could be made.

ADVERSE REACTIONS

The most commonly observed adverse events in placebo-controlled, parallel-group, add-on epilepsy trials associated with the use of GABITRIL in combination with other antiepilepsy drugs not seen at an equivalent frequency among placebo-treated patients were dizziness/light-headedness, asthenia/lack of energy, somnolence, nausea, nervousness/irritability, tremor, abdominal pain, and thinking abnormal/difficulty with concentration or attention.

Approximately 21% of the 2531 patients who received GABITRIL in clinical trials of epilepsy discontinued treatment because of an adverse event. The adverse events most commonly associated with discontinuation were dizziness (1.7%), somnolence (1.6%), depression (1.3%), confusion (1.1%), and asthenia (1.1%).

In Studies 1 and 2 (U.S. studies), the double-blind, placebo-controlled, parallel-group, add-on studies, the proportion of patients who discontinued treatment because of adverse events was 11% for the group treated with GABITRIL and 6% for the placebo group. The most common adverse events considered the primary reason for discontinuation were confusion (1.2%), somnolence (1.0%), and ataxia (1.0%).

Adverse Event Incidence in Controlled Clinical Trials: Table 4 lists treatment-emergent signs and symptoms that occurred in at least 1% of patients treated with GABITRIL for epilepsy participating in parallel-group, placebo-controlled trials and were numerically more common in the GABITRIL group. In these studies, either GABITRIL or placebo was added to the patient's current antiepilepsy drug therapy. Adverse events were usually mild or moderate in intensity. The prescriber should be aware that these figures, obtained when GABITRIL was added to concurrent antiepilepsy drug therapy, cannot be used to predict the frequency of adverse events in the course of usual medical practice when patient characteristics and other factors may differ from those prevailing during clinical studies. Similarly, the cited frequencies cannot be directly compared with figures obtained from other clinical investigations involving different treatments, uses, or investigators. An inspection of these frequencies, however, does provide the prescribing physician with one basis to estimate the relative contribution of drug and nondrug factors to the adverse event incidences in the population studied.

[See table 4 at top of previous page]

Other events reported by 1% or more of patients treated with GABITRIL but equally or more frequent in the placebo group were: accidental injury, chest pain, constipation, flu syndrome, rhinitis, anorexia, back pain, dry mouth, flatulence, ecchymosis, twitching, fever, amblyopia, conjunctivitis, urinary tract infection, urinary frequency, infection, dyspepsia, gastroenteritis, nausea and vomiting, myalgia, diplopia, headache, anxiety, acne, sinusitis, and incoordination.

Study 1 was a dose-response study including doses of 32 mg and 56 mg. Table 5 shows adverse events reported at a rate of ≥ 5% in at least one GABITRIL group and more frequent than in the placebo group. Among these events, tremor, difficulty with concentration/attention, and perhaps asthenia exhibited a positive relationship to dose.

[See table 5 above]

The effects of GABITRIL in relation to those of placebo on the incidence of adverse events and the types of adverse events reported were independent of age, weight, and gender. Because only 10% of patients were non-Caucasian in parallel-group, placebo-controlled trials, there is insufficient data to support a statement regarding the distribution of adverse experience reports by race.

Table 5
Treatment-Emergent Adverse Event Incidence in Study 1†
(events in at least 5% of patients treated with GABITRIL 32 or 56 mg and numerically more frequent than in the placebo group)

Body System/ COSTART Term	GABITRIL 56 mg (N=57) %	GABITRIL 32 mg (N=88) %	Placebo (N=91) %
Body as a Whole			
Accidental Injury	21	15	20
Infection	19	10	12
Flu Syndrome	9	6	3
Pain	7	2	3
Abdominal Pain	5	7	4
Digestive System			
Diarrhea	2	10	6
Hemic and Lymphatic System			
Ecchymosis	0	6	1
Musculoskeletal System			
Myalgia	5	2	3
Nervous System			
Dizziness	28	31	12
Asthenia	23	18	15
Tremor	21	14	1
Somnolence	19	21	17
Nervousness	14	11	6
Difficulty With Concentration/Attention*	14	7	3
Ataxia	9	6	6
Depression	7	1	0
Insomnia	5	6	3
Abnormal Gait	5	5	3
Hostility	5	5	2
Respiratory System			
Pharyngitis	7	8	6
Special Senses			
Amblyopia	4	9	8
Urogenital System			
Urinary Tract Infection	5	0	2

† Patients in this study were receiving one to three concomitant enzyme-inducing antiepilepsy drugs in addition to GABITRIL or placebo. Patients may have reported multiple adverse experiences; thus, patients may be included in more than one category.
* COSTART term substituted with a more clinically descriptive term.

Table 6
Typical Dosing Titration Regimen for Patients Taking Enzyme-Inducing AEDs

	Initiation and Titration Schedule	Total Daily Dose
Week 1	Initiate at 4 mg once daily	4 mg/day
Week 2	Increase total daily dose by 4 mg	8 mg/day (in two divided doses)
Week 3	Increase total daily dose by 4 mg	12 mg/day (in three divided doses)
Week 4	Increase total daily dose by 4 mg	16 mg/day (in two to four divided doses)
Week 5	Increase total daily dose by 4 to 8 mg	20 to 24 mg/day (in two to four divided doses)
Week 6	Increase total daily dose by 4 to 8 mg	24 to 32 mg/day (in two to four divided doses)
Usual Adult Maintenance Dose:	32 to 56 mg/day in two to four divided doses	

Other Adverse Events Observed During All Clinical Trials: GABITRIL has been administered to 2531 patients during all phase 2/3 clinical trials, only some of which were placebo-controlled. During these trials, all adverse events were recorded by the clinical investigators using terminology of their own choosing. To provide a meaningful estimate of the proportion of individuals having adverse events, similar types of events were grouped into a smaller number of standardized categories using modified COSTART dictionary terminology. These categories are used in the listing below. The frequencies presented represent the proportion of the 2531 patients exposed to GABITRIL who experienced events of the type cited on at least one occasion while receiving GABITRIL. All reported events are included except those already listed above, events seen only three times or fewer (unless potentially important), events very unlikely to be drug-related, and those too general to be informative. Events are included without regard to determination of a causal relationship to tiagabine.

Events are further classified within body system categories and enumerated in order of decreasing frequency using the following definitions: frequent adverse events are defined as those occurring in at least 1/100 patients; infrequent adverse events are those occurring in 1/100 to 1/1000 patients; rare events are those occurring in fewer than 1/1000 patients.

Body as a Whole: *Frequent:* Allergic reaction, chest pain, chills, cyst, neck pain, and malaise. *Infrequent:* Abscess, cellulitis, facial edema, halitosis, hernia, neck rigidity, neoplasm, pelvic pain, photosensitivity reaction, sepsis, sudden death, and suicide attempt.

Cardiovascular System: *Frequent:* Hypertension, palpitation, syncope, and tachycardia. *Infrequent:* Angina pectoris, cerebral ischemia, electrocardiogram abnormal, hemorrhage, hypotension, myocardial infarct, pallor, peripheral vascular disorder, phlebitis, postural hypotension, and thrombophlebitis.

Digestive System: *Frequent:* Gingivitis and stomatitis. *Infrequent:* Abnormal stools, cholecystitis, cholelithiasis, dysphagia, eructation, esophagitis, fecal incontinence, gastritis, gastrointestinal hemorrhage, glossitis, gum hyperplasia, hepatomegaly, increased salivation, liver function tests abnormal, melena, periodontal abscess, rectal hemorrhage, thirst, tooth caries, and ulcerative stomatitis.

Endocrine System: *Infrequent:* Goiter and hypothyroidism.

Hemic and Lymphatic System: *Frequent:* Lymphadenopathy. *Infrequent:* Anemia, erythrocytes abnormal, leukopenia, petechia, and thrombocytopenia.

Metabolic and Nutritional: *Frequent:* Edema, peripheral edema, weight gain, and weight loss. *Infrequent:* Dehydration, hypercholesteremia, hyperglycemia, hyperlipemia, hypoglycemia, hypokalemia, and hyponatremia.

Musculoskeletal System: *Frequent:* Arthralgia. *Infrequent:* Arthritis, arthrosis, bursitis, generalized spasm, and tendinous contracture.

Nervous System: *Frequent:* Depersonalization, dysarthria, euphoria, hallucination, hyperkinesia, hypertonia, hypesthesia, hypokinesia, hypotonia, migraine, myoclonus, paranoid reaction, personality disorder, reflexes decreased, stupor, twitching, and vertigo. *Infrequent:* Abnormal dreams,

Continued on next page

Gabitril—Cont.

apathy, choreoathetosis, circumoral paresthesia, CNS neoplasm, coma, delusions, dry mouth, dystonia, encephalopathy, hemiplegia, leg cramps, libido increased, libido decreased, movement disorder, neuritis, neurosis, paralysis, peripheral neuritis, psychosis, reflexes increased, and urinary retention.

Respiratory System: *Frequent:* Bronchitis, dyspnea, epistaxis, and pneumonia. *Infrequent:* Apnea, asthma, hemoptysis, hiccups, hyperventilation, laryngitis, respiratory disorder, and voice alteration.

Skin and Appendages: *Frequent:* Alopecia, dry skin, and sweating. *Infrequent:* Contact dermatitis, eczema, exfoliative dermatitis, furunculosis, herpes simplex, herpes zoster, hirsutism, maculopapular rash, psoriasis, skin benign neoplasm, skin carcinoma, skin discolorations, skin nodules, skin ulcer, subcutaneous nodule, urticaria, and vesiculobullous rash.

Special Senses: *Frequent:* Abnormal vision, ear pain, otitis media, and tinnitus. *Infrequent:* Blepharitis, blindness, deafness, eye pain, hyperacusis, keratoconjunctivitis, otitis externa, parosmia, photophobia, taste loss, taste perversion, and visual field defect.

Urogenital System: *Frequent:* Dysmenorrhea, dysuria, metrorrhagia, urinary incontinence, and vaginitis. *Infrequent:* Abortion, amenorrhea, breast enlargement, breast pain, cystitis, fibrocystic breast, hematuria, impotence, kidney failure, menorrhagia, nocturia, papanicolaou smear suspicious, polyuria, pyelonephritis, salpingitis, urethritis, urinary urgency, and vaginal hemorrhage.

DRUG ABUSE AND DEPENDENCE

The abuse and dependence potential of GABITRIL have not been evaluated in human studies.

OVERDOSAGE

Human Overdose Experience: Human experience of acute overdose with GABITRIL is limited. Eleven patients in clinical trials took single doses of GABITRIL up to 800 mg. All patients fully recovered, usually within one day. The most common symptoms reported after overdose included somnolence, impaired consciousness, agitation, confusion, speech difficulty, hostility, depression, weakness, and myoclonus. One patient who ingested a single dose of 400 mg experienced generalized tonic-clonic status epilepticus, which responded to intravenous phenobarbital.

Eleven individuals (including five children <7 years old) not in tiagabine clinical trials accidentally ingested tiagabine in single doses up to 20 mg. These individuals were asymptomatic in six cases. Symptoms exhibited in at least one of the other five individuals included ataxia, confusion, somnolence, impaired consciousness, impaired speech, agitation, lethargy, drowsiness, and myoclonus. One individual experienced a tonic-clonic seizure but was taking other agents which may be associated with seizures. All individuals recovered, usually within one day.

Management of Overdose: There is no specific antidote for overdose with GABITRIL. If indicated, elimination of unabsorbed drug should be achieved by emesis or gastric lavage; usual precautions should be observed to maintain the airway. General supportive care of the patient is indicated including monitoring of vital signs and observation of clinical status of the patient. Since tiagabine is mostly metabolized by the liver and is highly protein bound, dialysis is unlikely to be beneficial. A Certified Poison Control Center should be consulted for up to date information on the management of overdose with GABITRIL.

DOSAGE AND ADMINISTRATION

GABITRIL (tiagabine HCl) is recommended as adjunctive therapy in patients 12 years and older. GABITRIL is given orally and should be taken with food.

Adequate and controlled clinical studies with GABITRIL were conducted in patients taking enzyme-inducing AEDs (e.g., phenytoin, carbamazepine, and barbiturates). Patients taking only non-enzyme-inducing AEDs (e.g., valproate, gabapentin, and lamotrigine) may require lower doses or a slower titration of GABITRIL for clinical response.

Adults and Adolescents 12 Years or Older: In adolescents 12 to 18 years old, GABITRIL should be initiated at 4 mg once daily. Modification of concomitant antiepilepsy drugs is not necessary, unless clinically indicated. The total daily dose of GABITRIL may be increased by 4 mg at the beginning of Week 2. Thereafter, the total daily dose may be increased by 4 to 8 mg at weekly intervals until clinical response is achieved or up to 32 mg/day. The total daily dose should be given in divided doses two to four times daily. Doses above 32 mg/day have been tolerated in a small number of adolescent patients for a relatively short duration.

In adults, GABITRIL should be initiated at 4 mg once daily. Modification of concomitant antiepilepsy drugs is not necessary, unless clinically indicated. The total daily dose of GABITRIL may be increased by 4 to 8 mg at weekly intervals until clinical response is achieved or, up to 56 mg/day. The total daily dose should be given in divided doses two to four times daily. Doses above 56 mg/day have not been systematically evaluated in adequate well-controlled trials.

Experience is limited in patients taking total daily doses above 32 mg/day using twice daily dosing. A typical dosing titration regimen for patients taking enzyme-inducing AEDs is provided in Table 6.

[See table 6 on previous page]

HOW SUPPLIED

GABITRIL Filmtab tablets are available in five dosage strengths.

2 mg orange-peach, round tablets, debossed with on one side and the Abbo-Code FJ on the opposite side, are available in bottles of 100 (**NDC** 0074-3963-13).

4 mg yellow, round tablets, debossed with on one side and the Abbo-Code FK on the opposite side, are available in bottles of 100 (**NDC** 0074-3904-13).

12 mg green, ovaloid tablets, debossed with on one side and the Abbo-Code FL on the opposite side, are available in bottles of 100 (**NDC** 0074-3910-13).

16 mg blue, ovaloid tablets, debossed with on one side and the Abbo-Code FM on the opposite side, are available in bottles of 100 (**NDC** 0074-3960-13).

20 mg pink, ovaloid tablets, debossed with on one side and the Abbo-Code FN on the opposite side, are available in bottles of 100 (**NDC** 0074-3982-13).

Recommended Storage: Store tablets at controlled room temperature, between 20–25°C (68–77°F). See USP. Protect from light and moisture.

ANIMAL TOXICOLOGY

In repeat dose toxicology studies, dogs receiving daily oral doses of 5 mg/kg/day or greater experienced unexpected CNS effects throughout the study. These effects occurred acutely and included marked sedation and apparent visual impairment which was characterized by a lack of awareness of objects, failure to fix on and follow moving objects, and absence of a blink reaction. Plasma exposures (AUCs) at 5 mg/kg/day were equal to those in humans receiving the maximum recommended daily human dose of 56 mg/day. The effects were reversible upon cessation of treatment and were not associated with any observed structural abnormality. The implications of these findings for humans are unknown.

Filmtab® - Film-sealed tablets, Abbott
Revised: August, 1999
Ref. 03-4957-R5
ABBOTT LABORATORIES
NORTH CHICAGO, IL 60064, U.S.A.
Shown in Product Identification Guide, page 303

GENGRAF™ Capsules ℞

[*gĕn-grăf*]
(cyclosporine capsules, USP [MODIFIED])
Rx only

WARNING

Only physicians experienced in the management of systemic immunosuppressive therapy for the indicated disease should prescribe Gengraf™ (cyclosporine capsules, USP **[MODIFIED]**). At doses used in solid organ transplantation, only physicians experienced in immunosuppressive therapy and management of organ transplant recipients should prescribe Gengraf™. Patients receiving the drug should be managed in facilities equipped and staffed with adequate laboratory and supportive medical resources. The physician responsible for maintenance therapy should have complete information requisite for the follow-up of the patient.

Gengraf™, a systemic immunosuppressant, may increase the susceptibility to infection and the development of neoplasia. In kidney, liver, and heart transplant patients Gengraf™ may be administered with other immunosuppressive agents. Increased susceptibility to infection and the possible development of lymphoma and other neoplasms may result from the increase in the degree of immunosuppression in transplant patients.

Gengraf™ (cyclosporine capsules, USP **[MODIFIED]**) has increased bioavailability in comparison to Sandimmune®* (cyclosporine capsules, USP **[NON-MODIFIED]**). Gengraf™ and Sandimmune®* are not bioequivalent and cannot be used interchangeably without physician supervision. For a given trough concentration, cyclosporine exposure will be greater with Gengraf™ than with Sandimmune®*. If a patient who is receiving exceptionally high doses of Sandimmune®* is converted to Gengraf™, particular caution should be exercised. Cyclosporine blood concentrations should be monitored in transplant and rheumatoid arthritis patients taking Gengraf™ to avoid toxicity due to high concentrations. Dose adjustments should be made in transplant patients to minimize possible organ rejection due to low concentrations. Comparison of blood concentrations in the published literature with blood concentrations obtained using current assays must be done with detailed knowledge of the assay methods employed.

For Psoriasis Patients (*see also Boxed WARNINGS above*)

Psoriasis patients previously treated with PUVA and to a lesser extent, methotrexate or other immunosuppressive agents, UVB, coal tar, or radiation therapy, are at an increased risk of developing skin malignancies when taking Gengraf™ (cyclosporine capsules, USP **[MODIFIED]**). Cyclosporine, the active ingredient in Gengraf™, in recommended dosages, can cause systemic hypertension and nephrotoxicity. The risk increases with increasing dose and duration of cyclosporine therapy. Renal dysfunction, including structural kidney damage, is a potential consequence of cyclosporine, and therefore, renal function must be monitored during therapy.

DESCRIPTION

Gengraf™ (cyclosporine capsules, USP **[MODIFIED]**) is a modified oral formulation of cyclosporine that forms an aqueous dispersion in an aqueous environment.

NOTE: The nomenclature "Cyclosporine Capsules for Microemulsion" has been changed throughout the insert to read "Cyclosporine, Capsules USP **(MODIFIED)**".

Cyclosporine, the active principle in Gengraf™ Capsules, is a cyclic polypeptide immunosuppressant agent consisting of 11 amino acids. It is produced as a metabolite by the fungus species *Aphanocladium album*.

Chemically, cyclosporine is designated as [R-[R*, R*-(E)]]-cyclic-(L-alanyl-D-alanyl-*N*-methyl-L-leucyl-*N*-methyl-L-leucyl-*N*-methyl-L-valyl-3-hydroxy-*N*,4-dimethyl-L-2-amino-6-octenoyl-L-α-amino-butyryl-*N*-methylglycyl-*N*-methyl-L-leucyl-L-valyl-*N*-methyl-L-leucyl).

Gengraf™ Capsules (cyclosporine capsules, USP **[MODIFIED]**) are available in 25 mg and 100 mg strengths.

Each 25 mg capsule contains: cyclosporine, 25 mg, alcohol, USP, absolute, 12.8% v/v (10.1% wt/vol.).

Each 100 mg capsule contains: cyclosporine, 100 mg, alcohol, USP, absolute, 12.8% v/v (10.1% wt/vol.).

Inactive Ingredients: FD&C Blue No. 2, gelatin NF, polyethylene glycol NF, polyoxyl 35 castor oil NF, polysorbate 80 NF, propylene glycol USP, sorbitan monooleate NF, titanium dioxide.

The chemical structure for cyclosporine USP is:

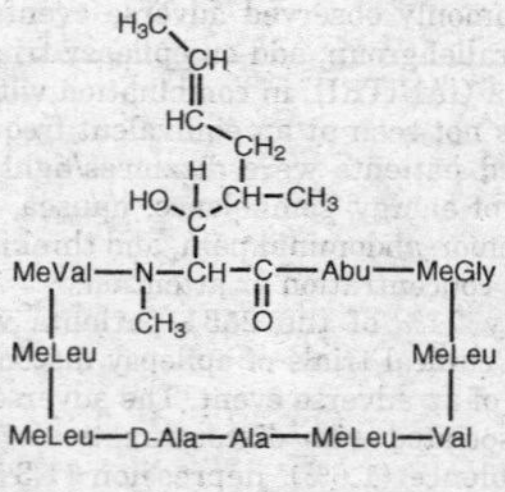

$C_{62}H_{111}N_{11}O_{12}$ Mol. Wt. 1202.64

CLINICAL PHARMACOLOGY:

Cyclosporine is a potent immunosuppressive agent that in animals prolongs survival of allogeneic transplants involving skin, kidney, liver, heart, pancreas, bone marrow, small intestine, and lung. Cyclosporine has been demonstrated to suppress some humoral immunity and to a greater extent, cell-mediated immune reactions such as allograft rejection, delayed hypersensitivity, experimental allergic encephalomyelitis, Freund's adjuvant arthritis, and graft vs. host disease in many animal species for a variety of organs.

The effectiveness of cyclosporine results from specific and reversible inhibition of immunocompetent lymphocytes in the G_0- and G_1-phase of the cell cycle. T-lymphocytes are preferentially inhibited. The T-helper cell is the main target, although the T-suppressor cell may also be suppressed. Cyclosporine also inhibits lymphokine production and release including interleukin-2.

No effects on phagocytic function (changes in enzyme secretions, chemotactic migration of granulocytes, macrophage migration, carbon clearance *in vivo*) have been detected in animals. Cyclosporine does not cause bone marrow suppression in animal models or man.

Pharmacokinetics: The immunosuppressive activity of cyclosporine is primarily due to parent drug. Following oral administration, absorption of cyclosporine is incomplete. The extent of absorption of cyclosporine is dependent on the individual patient, the patient population, and the formulation. Elimination of cyclosporine is primarily biliary with only 6% of the dose (parent drug and metabolites) excreted in urine. The disposition of cyclosporine from blood is generally biphasic, with a terminal half-life of approximately 8.4 hours (range 5 to 18 hours). Following intravenous administration, the blood clearance of cyclosporine (assay: HPLC) is approximately 5 to 7 mL/min/kg in adult recipients of renal or liver allografts. Blood cyclosporine clearance appears to be slightly slower in cardiac transplant patients.

The relationship between administered dose and exposure (area under the concentration versus time curve, AUC) is linear within the therapeutic dose range. The intersubject variability (total, % CV) of cyclosporine exposure (AUC) when cyclosporine **(MODIFIED)** or cyclosporine **(NON-MODIFIED)** is administered ranges from approximately 20% to 50% in renal transplant patients. This intersubject variability contributes to the need for individualization of the dosing regimen for optimal therapy (*see DOSAGE AND ADMINISTRATION*). Intrasubject variability of AUC in renal transplant recipients (% CV) was 9%–21% for cyclosporine

(MODIFIED) and 19%–26% for cyclosporine **(NON-MODIFIED)**. In the same studies, intrasubject variability of trough concentrations (% CV) was 17%–30% for cyclosporine **(MODIFIED)** and 16%-38% for cyclosporine **(NON-MODIFIED)**.

Absorption: Cyclosporine **(MODIFIED)** has increased bioavailability compared to cyclosporine **(NON-MODIFIED)**. The absolute bioavailability of cyclosporine administered as Sandimmune®* (cyclosporine **[NON-MODIFIED]**) is dependent on the patient population, estimated to be less than 10% in liver transplant patients and as great as 89% in some renal transplant patients. The absolute bioavailability of cyclosporine administered as cyclosporine **(MODIFIED)** has not been determined in adults. In studies of renal transplant, rheumatoid arthritis and psoriasis patients, the mean cyclosporine AUC was approximately 20% to 50% greater and the peak blood cyclosporine concentration (C_{max}) was approximately 40% to 106% greater following administration of cyclosporine **(MODIFIED)** compared to following administration of cyclosporine **(NON-MODIFIED)**. The dose normalized AUC in *de novo* liver transplant patients administered cyclosporine **(MODIFIED)** 28 days after transplantation was 50% greater and C_{max} was 90% greater than in those patients administered cyclosporine **(NON-MODIFIED)**. AUC and C_{max} are also increased cyclosporine **(MODIFIED)** relative to cyclosporine **(NON-MODIFIED)** in heart transplant patients, but data are very limited. Although the AUC and C_{max} values are higher on cyclosporine **(MODIFIED)** relative to cyclosporine **(NON-MODIFIED)**, the pre-dose trough concentrations (dose-normalized) are similar for the two formulations.

Following oral administration of cyclosporine **(MODIFIED)**, the time to peak blood cyclosporine concentration (T_{max}) ranged from 1.5 to 2.0 hours. The administration of food with cyclosporine **(MODIFIED)** decreases the cyclosporine AUC and C_{max}. A high fat meal (669 kcal, 45 grams fat) consumed within one-half hour before cyclosporine **(MODIFIED)** administration decreased the AUC by 13% and C_{max} by 33%. The effects of a low fat meal (667 kcal, 15 grams fat) were similar.

The effect of T-tube diversion of bile on the absorption of cyclosporine from cyclosporine **(MODIFIED)** was investigated in eleven *de novo* liver transplant patients. When the patients were administered cyclosporine **(MODIFIED)** with and without T-tube diversion of bile, very little difference in absorption was observed, as measured by the change in maximal cyclosporine blood concentrations from pre-dose values with the T-tube closed relative to when it was open: 6.9±41% (range –55% to 68%).

[See first table above]

Pharmacokinetic Parameters (mean ± SD)

Patient Population	Dose/day[1] (mg/d)	Dose/weight (mg/kg/d)	AUC[2] (ng•hr/mL)	C_{max} (ng/mL)	Trough[3] (ng/mL)	CL/F (mL/min)	CL/F (mL/min/kg)
De novo renal transplant[4] Week 4 (N=37)	597±174	7.95±2.81	8772±2089	1802±428	361±129	593±204	7.8±2.9
Stable renal transplant[4] (N=55)	344±122	4.10±1.58	6035±2194	1333±469	251±116	492±140	5.9±2.1
De novo liver transplant[5] Week 4 (N=18)	458±190	6.89±3.68	7187±2816	1555±740	268±101	577±309	8.6±5.7
De novo rheumatoid arthritis[6] (N=23)	182±55.6	2.37±0.36	2641±877	728±263	96.4±37.7	613±196	8.3±2.8
De novo psoriasis[6] Week 4 (N=18)	189±69.8	2.48±0.65	2324±1048	655±186	74.9±46.7	723±186	10.2±3.9

[1]Total daily dose was divided into two doses administered every 12 hours.
[2]AUC was measured over one dosing interval.
[3]Trough concentration was measured just prior to the morning cyclosporine (**MODIFIED**) dose, approximately 12 hours after the previous dose.
[4]Assay: TDx specific monoclonal fluorescence polarization immunoassay.
[5]Assay: Cyclo-trac specific monoclonal radioimmunoassay.
[6]Assay: INCSTAR specific monoclonal radioimmunoassay.

Distribution: Cyclosporine is distributed largely outside the blood volume. The steady state volume of distribution during intravenous dosing has been reported as 3–5 L/kg in solid organ transplant recipients. In blood, the distribution is concentration dependent. Approximately 33%–47% is in plasma, 4%–9% in lymphocytes, 5%–12% in granulocytes, and 41%–58% in erythrocytes. At high concentrations, the binding capacity of leukocytes and erythrocytes becomes saturated. In plasma, approximately 90% is bound to proteins, primarily lipoproteins. Cyclosporine is excreted in human milk (*see PRECAUTIONS, Nursing Mothers*).

Metabolism: Cyclosporine is extensively metabolized by the cytochrome P-450 III-A enzyme system in the liver, and to a lesser degree in the gastrointestinal tract, and the kidney. The metabolism of cyclosporine can be altered by the coadministration of a variety of agents (*see PRECAUTIONS, Drug Interactions*). At least 25 metabolites have been identified from human bile, feces, blood, and urine. The biological activity of the metabolites and their contributions to toxicity are considerably less than those of the parent compound. The major metabolites (M1, M9, and M4N) result from oxidation at the 1-beta, 9-gamma, and 4-N-demethylated positions, respectively. At steady state following the oral administration of cyclosporine **(NON-MODIFIED)**, the mean AUCs for blood concentrations of M1, M9 and M4N are about 70%, 21%, and 7.5% of the AUC for blood cyclosporine concentrations, respectively. Based on blood concentration data from stable renal transplant patients (13 patients administered cyclosporine **(MODIFIED)** and cyclosporine **(NON-MODIFIED)** in a crossover study), and bile concentration data from *de novo* liver transplant patients (4 administered cyclosporine **(MODIFIED)**, 3 administered cyclosporine **(NON-MODIFIED)**, the percentage of dose present as M1, M9, and M4N metabolites is similar when either cyclosporine **(MODIFIED)** or cyclosporine **(NON-MODIFIED)** is administered.

Excretion: Only 0.1% of a cyclosporine dose is excreted unchanged in the urine. Elimination is primarily biliary with only 6% of the dose (parent drug and metabolites) excreted in the urine. Neither dialysis nor renal failure alter cyclosporine clearance significantly.

Drug Interactions: (*see PRECAUTIONS, Drug Interactions*). When diclofenac or methotrexate was co-administered with cyclosporine in rheumatoid arthritis patients, the AUC of diclofenac and methotrexate, each was significantly increased (*see PRECAUTIONS, Drug Interactions*). No clinically significant pharmacokinetic interactions occurred between cyclosporine and aspirin, ketoprofen, piroxicam, or indomethacin.

Special Population: ***Pediatric Population:*** Pharmacokinetic data from pediatric patients administered cyclosporine **(MODIFIED)** or cyclosporine **(NON-MODIFIED)** are very limited. In 15 renal transplant patients aged 3-16 years, cyclosporine whole blood clearance after IV administration of cyclosporine **(NON-MODIFIED)** was 10.6±3.7 mL/min/kg (assay: Cyclo-trac specific RIA). In a study of 7 renal transplant patients aged 2–16, the cyclosporine clearance ranged from 9.8 to 15.5 mL/min/kg. In 9 liver transplant patients aged 0.6 to 5.6 years, clearance was 9.3±5.4 mL/min/kg (assay: HPLC).

In the pediatric population, cyclosporine **(MODIFIED)** also demonstrates an increased bioavailability as compared to cyclosporine **(NON-MODIFIED)**. In 7 liver *de novo* transplant patients aged 1.4 to 10 years, the absolute bioavailability of cyclosporine **(MODIFIED)** was 43% (range 30% to 68%) and for cyclosporine **(NON-MODIFIED)** in the same individuals absolute bioavailability was 28% (range 17% to 42%).

[See second table above]

Pediatric Pharmacokinetic Parameters (mean ± SD)

Patient Population	Dose/day (mg/d)	Dose/weight (mg/kg/d)	AUC[1] (ng•hr/mL)	C_{max} (ng/mL)	CL/F (mL/min)	CL/F (mL/min/kg)
Stable liver transplant[2]						
Age 2–8, Dosed TID (N=9)	101±25	5.95±1.32	2163±801	629±219	285±94	16.6±4.3
Age 8–15, Dosed BID (N=8)	188±55	4.96±2.09	4272±1462	975±281	378±80	10.2±4.0
Stable liver transplant[3]						
Age 3, Dosed BID (N=1)	120	8.33	5832	1050	171	11.9
Age 8–15, Dosed BID (N=5)	158±55	5.51±1.91	4452±2475	1013±635	328±121	11.0±1.9
Stable renal transplant[3]						
Age 7–15, Dosed BID (N=5)	328±83	7.37±4.11	6922±1988	1827±487	418±143	8.7±2.9

[1]AUC was measured over one dosing interval.
[2]Assay: Cyclo-trac specific monoclonal radioimmunoassay.
[3]Assay: TDx specific monoclonal fluorescence polarization immunoassay.

Geriatric Population: Comparison of single dose data from both normal elderly volunteers (N=18, mean age 69 years) and elderly rheumatoid arthritis patients (N=16, mean age 68 years) to single dose data in young adult volunteers (N=16, mean age 26 years) showed no significant difference in the pharmacokinetic parameters.

CLINICAL TRIALS

Rheumatoid Arthritis: The effectiveness of cyclosporine **(NON-MODIFIED)** and cyclosporine **(MODIFIED)** in the treatment of severe rheumatoid arthritis was evaluated in five clinical studies involving a total of 728 cyclosporine treated patients and 273 placebo treated patients.

A summary of the results is presented for the "responder" rates per treatment group, with a responder being defined as a patient having *completed* the trial with a 20% improvement in the tender and the swollen joint count and a 20% improvement in 2 of 4 of investigator global, patient global, disability, and erythrocyte sedimentation rates (ESR) for the Studies 651 and 652 and 3 of 5 of investigator global, patient global, disability, visual analog pain, and ESR for Studies 2008, 654, and 302.

Study 651 enrolled 264 patients with active rheumatoid arthritis with at least 20 involved joints, who had failed at least one major RA drug, using a 3:3:2 randomization to one of the following three groups: (1) cyclosporine dosed at 2.5–5 mg/kg/day, (2) methotrexate at 7.5–15 mg/week, or (3) placebo. Treatment duration was 24 weeks. The mean cyclosporine dose at the last visit was 3.1 mg/kg/day. See Graph below.

Study 652 enrolled 250 patients with active RA with >6 active painful or tender joints who had failed at least one major RA drug. Patients were randomized using a 3:3:2 randomization to 1 of 3 treatment arms: (1) 1.5–5 mg/kg/day of cyclosporine, (2) 2.5–5 mg/kg/day of cyclosporine, and (3) placebo. Treatment duration was 16 weeks. The mean cyclosporine dose for group 2 at the last visit was 2.92 mg/kg/day. See Graph below.

Study 2008 enrolled 144 patients with active RA and >6 active joints who had unsuccessful treatment courses of aspirin and gold or Penicillamine. Patients were randomized to one of two treatment groups: (1) cyclosporine 2.5–5 mg/kg/day with adjustments after the first month to achieve a target trough level and (2) placebo. Treatment duration was 24 weeks. The mean cyclosporine dose at the last visit was 3.63 mg/kg/day. See Graph below.

Study 654 enrolled 148 patients who remained with active joint counts of 6 or more despite treatment with maximally tolerated methotrexate doses for at least three months. Patients continued to take their current dose of methotrexate and were randomized to receive, in addition, one of the following medications: (1) cyclosporine 2.5 mg/kg/day with dose increases of 0.5 mg/kg/day at weeks 2 and 4 if there was no evidence of toxicity and further increases of 0.5 mg/kg/day at weeks 8 and 16 if a <30% decrease in active joint count occurred without any significant toxicity; dose decreases could be made at any time for toxicity or (2) placebo. Treatment duration was 24 weeks. The mean cyclosporine dose at the last visit was 2.8 mg/kg/day (range: 1.3-4.1). See Graph below.

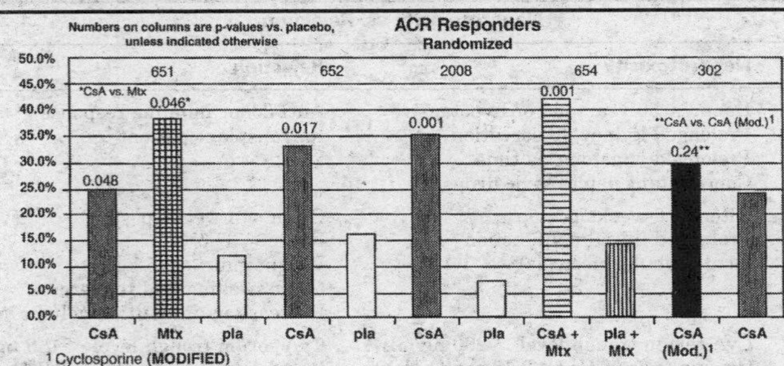

Continued on next page

Gengraf—Cont.

Study 302 enrolled 299 patients with severe active RA, 99% of whom were unresponsive or intolerant to at least one prior major RA drug. Patients were randomized to 1 of 2 treatment groups (1) cyclosporine **(MODIFIED)** and (2) cyclosporine **(NON-MODIFIED)**, both of which were started at 2.5 mg/kg/day and increased after 4 weeks for inefficacy in increments of 0.5 mg/kg/day to a maximum of 5 mg/kg/day and decreased at any time for toxicity. Treatment duration was 24 weeks. The mean cyclosporine dose at the last visit was 2.91 mg/kg/day (range: 0.72-5.17) for cyclosporine **(MODIFIED)** and 3.27 mg/kg/day (range: 0.73-5.68) for cyclosporine **(NON-MODIFIED)**. See Graph below.
[See graphic on previous page third from top]

INDICATIONS AND USAGE

Kidney, Liver and Heart Transplantation: Gengraf™ (cyclosporine capsules, USP **[MODIFIED]**) is indicated for the prophylaxis of organ rejection in kidney, liver, and heart allogeneic transplants. Cyclosporine **(MODIFIED)** has been used in combination with azathioprine and corticosteroids.
Rheumatoid Arthritis: Gengraf™ (cyclosporine capsules, USP **[MODIFIED]**) is indicated for the treatment of patients with severe active, rheumatoid arthritis where the disease has not adequately responded to methotrexate. Gengraf™ can be used in combination with methotrexate in rheumatoid arthritis patients who do not respond adequately to methotrexate alone.
Psoriasis: Gengraf™ (cyclosporine capsules, USP **[MODIFIED]**) is indicated for the treatment of *adult, nonimmunocompromised* patients with severe (i.e., extensive and/or disabling), recalcitrant, plaque psoriasis who have failed to respond to at least one systemic therapy (e.g., PUVA, retinoids, or methotrexate) or in patients for whom other systemic therapies are contraindicated, or cannot be tolerated.
While rebound rarely occurs, most patients will experience relapse with Gengraf™ as with other therapies upon cessation of treatment.

CONTRAINDICATIONS

General: Gengraf™ (cyclosporine capsules, USP **[MODIFIED]**) is contraindicated in patients with a hypersensitivity to cyclosporine or to any of the ingredients of the formulation.
Rheumatoid Arthritis: Rheumatoid arthritis patients with abnormal renal function, uncontrolled hypertension or malignancies should not receive Gengraf™ (cyclosporine capsules, USP **[MODIFIED]**).
Psoriasis: Psoriasis patients who are treated with Gengraf™ (cyclosporine capsules, USP **[MODIFIED]**) should not receive concomitant PUVA or UVB therapy, methotrexate or other immunosuppressive agents, coal tar or radiation therapy. Psoriasis patients with abnormal renal function, uncontrolled hypertension, or malignancies should not receive Gengraf™.

WARNINGS

(*see also Boxed WARNINGS*). **All Patients:** Cyclosporine, the active ingredient of Gengraf™ (cyclosporine capsules, USP **[MODIFIED]**), can cause nephrotoxicity and hepatotoxicity. The risk increases with increasing doses of cyclosporine. Renal dysfunction including structural kidney damage is a potential consequence of Gengraf™ and therefore renal function must be monitored during therapy. **Care should be taken in using cyclosporine with nephrotoxic drugs (see *PRECAUTIONS*).**
Patients receiving Gengraf™ require frequent monitoring of serum creatinine (*see Special Monitoring under DOSAGE AND ADMINISTRATION*). Elderly patients should be monitored with particular care, since decreases in renal function also occur with age. If patients are not properly monitored and doses are not properly adjusted, cyclosporine therapy can be associated with the occurrence of structural kidney damage and persistent renal dysfunction.
An increase in serum creatinine and BUN may occur during Gengraf™ therapy and reflect a reduction in the glomerular filtration rate. Impaired renal function at any time requires close monitoring, and frequent dosage adjustment may be indicated. The frequency and severity of serum creatinine elevations increase with dose and duration of cyclosporine therapy. These elevations are likely to become more pronounced without dose reduction or discontinuation.
Because Gengraf™ (cyclosporine capsules, USP [MODIFIED]) is not bioequivalent to Sandimmune®* (cyclosporine [NON-MODIFIED]), conversion from Gengraf™ to Sandimmune®* (cyclosporine [NON-MODIFIED]) using a 1:1 ratio (mg/kg/day) may result in lower cyclosporine blood concentrations. Conversion from Gengraf™ to Sandimmune®* (cyclosporine [NON-MODIFIED]) should be made with increased monitoring to avoid the potential of underdosing.
Kidney, Liver, and Heart Transplant: Cyclosporine, the active ingredient of Gengraf™ (cyclosporine capsules, USP **[MODIFIED]**), can cause nephrotoxicity and hepatotoxicity when used in high doses. It is not unusual for serum creatinine and BUN levels to be elevated during cyclosporine therapy. These elevations in renal transplant patients do not necessarily indicate rejection, and each patient must be fully evaluated before dosage adjustment is initiated.
Based on the historical cyclosporine **(NON-MODIFIED)** experience with oral solution, nephrotoxicity associated with cyclosporine had been noted in 25% of cases of renal transplantation, 38% of cases of cardiac transplantation, and 37% of cases of liver transplantation. Mild nephrotoxicity was generally noted 2–3 months after renal transplant and consisted of an arrest in the fall of the pre-operative elevations of BUN and creatinine at a range of 35–45 mg/dL and 2.0–2.5 mg/dL respectively. These elevations were often responsive to cyclosporine dosage reduction.
More overt nephrotoxicity was seen early after transplantation and was characterized by a rapidly rising BUN and creatinine. Since these events are similar to renal rejection episodes, care must be taken to differentiate between them. This form of nephrotoxicity is usually responsive to cyclosporine dosage reduction.
Although specific diagnostic criteria which reliably differentiate renal graft rejection from drug toxicity have not been found, a number of parameters have been significantly associated with one or the other. It should be noted however, that up to 20% of patients may have simultaneous nephrotoxicity and rejection.
[See table below]

Nephrotoxicity vs. Rejection

Parameter	Nephrotoxicity	Rejection
History	Donor > 50 years old or hypotensive Prolonged kidney preservation Prolonged anastomosis time Concomitant nephrotoxic drugs	Anti-donor immune response Retransplant patient
Clinical	Often > 6 weeks postop[b] Prolonged initial nonfunction (acute tubular necrosis)	Often < 4 weeks postop[b] Fever > 37.5°C Weight gain > 0.5 kg Graft swelling and tenderness Decrease in daily urine volume > 500 mL (or 50%)
Laboratory	CyA serum trough level > 200 ng/mL Gradual rise in Cr (< 0.15 mg/dL/day)[a] Cr plateau < 25% above baseline BUN/Cr ≥ 20	CyA serum trough level < 150 ng/mL Rapid rise in Cr (> 0.3 mg/dL/day)[a] Cr > 25% above baseline BUN/Cr < 20
Biopsy	Arteriolopathy (medial hypertrophy[a], hyalinosis, nodular deposits, intimal thickening, endothelial vacuolization, progressive scarring) Tubular atrophy, isometric vacuolization, isolated calcifications Minimal edema Mild focal infiltrates[c] Diffuse interstitial fibrosis, often striped form	Endovasculitis[c] (proliferation[a], intimal arteritis[b], necrosis, sclerosis) Tubulitis with RBC[b] and WBC[b] casts, some irregular vacuolization Interstitial edema[c] and hemorrhage[b] Diffuse moderate to severe mononuclear infiltrates[d] Glomerulitis (mononuclear cells)[c]
Aspiration Cytology	CyA deposits in tubular and endothelial cells Fine isometric vacuolization of tubular cells	Inflammatory infiltrate with mononuclear phagocytes, macrophages, lymphoblastoid cells, and activated T-cells These strongly express HLA-DR antigens
Urine Cytology	Tubular cells with vacuolization and granularization	Degenerative tubular cells, plasma cells, and lymphocyturia > 20% of sediment
Manometry Ultrasonography	Intracapsular pressure < 40 mm Hg[b] Unchanged graft cross sectional area	Intracapsular pressure > 40 mm Hg[b] Increase in graft cross sectional area AP diameter ≥ Transverse diameter
Magnetic Resonance Imagery	Normal appearance	Loss of distinct corticomedullary junction, swelling image intensity of parachyma approaching that of psoas, loss of hilar fat
Radionuclide Scan	Normal or generally decreased perfusion Decrease in tubular function (^{131}I-hippuran) > decrease in perfusion (^{99m}Tc DTPA)	Patchy arterial flow Decrease in perfusion > decrease in tubular function Increased uptake of Indium 111 labeled platelets or Tc-99m in colloid
Therapy	Responds to decreased cyclosporine	Responds to increased steroids or antilymphocyte globulin

[a]$p < 0.05$, [b]$p < 0.01$, [c]$p < 0.001$, [d]$p < 0.0001$

A form of a cyclosporine-associated nephropathy is characterized by serial deterioration in renal function and morphologic changes in the kidneys. From 5% to 15% of transplant recipients who have received cyclosporine will fail to show a reduction in rising serum creatinine despite a decrease or discontinuation of cyclosporine therapy. Renal biopsies from these patients will demonstrate one or several of the following alterations: tubular vacuolization, tubular microcalcifications, peritubular capillary congestion, arteriolopathy, and a striped form of interstitial fibrosis with tubular atrophy. Though none of these morphologic changes is entirely specific, a diagnosis of cyclosporine-associated structural nephrotoxicity requires evidence of these findings.
When considering the development of cyclosporine-associated nephropathy, it is noteworthy that several authors have reported an association between the appearance of interstitial fibrosis and higher cumulative doses or persistently high circulating trough levels of cyclosporine. This is particularly true during the first 6 post-transplant months when the dosage tends to be highest and when, in kidney recipients, the organ appears to be most vulnerable to the toxic effects of cyclosporine. Among other contributing factors to the development of interstitial fibrosis in these patients are prolonged perfusion time, warm ischemia time, as well as episodes of acute toxicity, and acute and chronic rejection. The reversibility of interstitial fibrosis and its correlation to renal function have not yet been determined. Reversibility of arteriolopathy has been reported after stopping cyclosporine or lowering the dosage.
Impaired renal function at any time requires close monitoring, and frequent dosage adjustment may be indicated.
In the event of severe and unremitting rejection, when rescue therapy with pulse steroids and monoclonal antibodies fail to reverse the rejection episode, it may be preferable to switch to alternative immunosuppressive therapy rather than increase the Gengraf™ dose to excessive levels.
Occasionally patients have developed a syndrome of thrombocytopenia and microangiopathic hemolytic anemia which may result in graft failure. The vasculopathy can occur in the absence of rejection and is accompanied by avid platelet consumption within the graft as demonstrated by Indium 111 labeled platelet studies. Neither the pathogenesis nor the management of this syndrome is clear. Though resolution has occurred after reduction or discontinuation of cyclosporine and 1) administration of streptokinase and heparin or 2) plasmapheresis, this appears to depend upon early detection with Indium 111 labeled platelet scans (*see ADVERSE REACTIONS*).
Significant hyperkalemia (sometimes associated with hyperchloremic metabolic acidosis) and hyperuricemia have been seen occasionally in individual patients.
Hepatotoxicity associated with cyclosporine use had been noted in 4% of cases of renal transplantation, 7% of cases of cardiac transplantation, and 4% of cases of liver transplantation. This was usually noted during the first month of therapy when high doses of cyclosporine were used and consisted of elevations of hepatic enzymes and bilirubin. The chemistry elevations usually decreased with a reduction in dosage.
As in patients receiving other immunosuppressants, those patients receiving cyclosporine are at increased risk for development of lymphomas and other malignancies, particularly those of the skin. The increased risk appears related to the intensity and duration of immunosuppression rather than to the use of specific agents. Because of the danger of oversuppression of the immune system resulting in increased risk of infection or malignancy, a treatment regimen containing multiple immunosuppressants should be used with caution.
There have been reports of convulsions in adult and pediatric patients receiving cyclosporine, particularly in combination with high dose methylprednisolone.
Care should be taken in using cyclosporine with nephrotoxic drugs (*see PRECAUTIONS*).
Rheumatoid Arthritis: Cyclosporine nephropathy was detected in renal biopsies of six out of 60 (10%) rheumatoid arthritis patients after the average treatment duration of 19

months. Only one patient, out of these 6 patients, was treated with a dose ≤4 mg/kg/day. Serum creatinine improved in all but one patient after discontinuation of cyclosporine. The "maximal creatinine increase" appears to be a factor in predicting cyclosporine nephropathy.

There is a potential, as with other immunosuppressive agents, for an increase in the occurrence of malignant lymphomas with cyclosporine. It is not clear whether the risk with cyclosporine is greater than that in Rheumatoid Arthritis patients or in Rheumatoid Arthritis patients on cytotoxic treatment for this indication. Five cases of lymphoma were detected: four in a survey of approximately 2,300 patients treated with cyclosporine for rheumatoid arthritis, and another case of lymphoma was reported in a clinical trial. Although other tumors (12 skin cancers, 24 solid tumors of diverse types, and 1 multiple myeloma) were also reported in this survey, epidemiologic analyses did not support a relationship to cyclosporine other than for malignant lymphomas.

Patients should be thoroughly evaluated before and during Gengraf™ (cyclosporine capsules, USP **[MODIFIED]**) treatment for the development of malignancies. Moreover, use of Gengraf™ therapy with other immunosuppressive agents may induce an excessive immunosuppression which is known to increase the risk of malignancy.

Psoriasis: (*see also Boxed WARNINGS for Psoriasis*). Since cyclosporine is a potent immunosuppressive agent with a number of potentially serious side effects, the risks and benefits of using Gengraf™ (cyclosporine capsules, USP **[MODIFIED]**) should be considered before treatment of patients with psoriasis. Cyclosporine, the active ingredient in Gengraf™, can cause nephrotoxicity and hypertension (*see PRECAUTIONS*) and the risk increases with increasing dose and duration of therapy. Patients who may be at increased risk such as those with abnormal renal function, uncontrolled hypertension or malignancies, should not receive Gengraf™.

Renal dysfunction is a potential consequence of Gengraf™, therefore renal function must be monitored during therapy. Patients receiving Gengraf™ require frequent monitoring of serum creatinine (*see Special Monitoring under DOSAGE AND ADMINISTRATION*). Elderly patients should be monitored with particular care, since decreases in renal function also occur with age. If patients are not properly monitored and doses are not properly adjusted, cyclosporine therapy can cause structural kidney damage and persistent renal dysfunction.

An increase in serum creatinine and BUN may occur during Gengraf™ therapy and reflects a reduction in the glomerular filtration rate.

Kidney biopsies from 86 psoriasis patients treated for a mean duration of 23 months with 1.2–7.6 mg/kg/day of cyclosporine showed evidence of cyclosporine nephropathy in 18/86 (21%) of the patients. The pathology consisted of renal tubular atrophy and interstitial fibrosis. On repeat biopsy of 13 of these patients maintained on various dosages of cyclosporine for a mean of 2 additional years, the number with cyclosporine induced nephropathy rose to 26/86 (30%). The majority of patients (19/26) were on a dose of ≥5.0 mg/kg/day (the highest recommended dose is 4 mg/kg/day). The patients were also on cyclosporine for greater than 15 months (18/26) and/or had a clinically significant increase in serum creatinine for greater than 1 month (21/26). Creatinine levels returned to normal range in 7 of 11 patients in whom cyclosporine therapy was discontinued.

There is an increased risk for the development of skin and lymphoproliferative malignancies in cyclosporine-treated psoriasis patients. The relative risk of malignancies is comparable to that observed in psoriasis patients treated with other immunosuppressive agents.

Tumors were reported in 32 (2.2%) of 1439 psoriasis patients treated with cyclosporine worldwide from clinical trials. Additional tumors have been reported in 7 patients in cyclosporine postmarketing experience. Skin malignancies were reported in 16 (1.1%) of these patients; all but 2 of them had previously received PUVA therapy. Methotrexate was received by 7 patients. UVB and coal tar have been used by 2 and 3 patients, respectively. Seven patients had either a history of previous skin cancer or a potentially predisposing lesion was present prior to cyclosporine exposure. Of the 16 patients with skin cancer, 11 patients had 18 squamous cell carcinomas and 7 patients had 10 basal cell carcinomas.

There were two lymphoproliferative malignancies; one case of non-Hodgkin's lymphoma which required chemotherapy, and one case of mycosis fungoides which regressed spontaneously upon discontinuation of cyclosporine. There were four cases of benign lymphocytic infiltration: 3 regressed spontaneously upon discontinuation of cyclosporine, while the fourth regressed despite continuation of the drug. The remainder of the malignancies, 13 cases (0.9%), involved various organs.

Patients should not be treated concurrently with cyclosporine and PUVA or UVB, other radiation therapy, or other immunosuppressive agents, because of the possibility of excessive immunosuppression and the subsequent risk of malignancies (*see CONTRAINDICATIONS*). Patients should also be warned to protect themselves appropriately when in the sun, and to avoid excessive sun exposure. Patients should be thoroughly evaluated before and during treatment for the presence of malignancies remembering that malignant lesions may be hidden by psoriatic plaques. Skin lesions not typical of psoriasis should be biopsied before

Antibiotics	*Antineoplastics*	*Anti-inflammatory Drugs*	*Gastrointestinal Agents*
gentamicin	melphalan	azapropazon	cimetidine
tobramycin		diclofenac	ranitidine
vancomycin	*Antifungals*	naproxen	
trimethoprim with sulfamethoxazole	amphotericin B	sulindac	*Immunosuppressives*
	ketoconazole		tacrolimus

starting treatment. Patients should be treated with Gengraf™ (cyclosporine capsules, USP **[MODIFIED]**) only after complete resolution of suspicious lesions, and only if there are no other treatment options (*see Special Monitoring for Psoriasis Patients*).

PRECAUTIONS

General: ***Hypertension:*** Cyclosporine is the active ingredient of Gengraf™ (cyclosporine capsules, USP **[MODIFIED]**). Hypertension is a common side effect of cyclosporine therapy which may persist (*see ADVERSE REACTIONS and DOSAGE AND ADMINISTRATION for monitoring recommendations*). Mild or moderate hypertension is encountered more frequently than severe hypertension and the incidence decreases over time. In recipients of kidney, liver, and heart allografts treated with cyclosporine, antihypertensive therapy may be required (*see Special Monitoring of Rheumatoid Arthritis and Psoriasis Patients*). However, since cyclosporine may cause hyperkalemia, potassium-sparing diuretics should not be used. While calcium antagonists can be effective agents in treating cyclosporine-associated hypertension, they can interfere with cyclosporine metabolism (*see PRECAUTIONS, Drug Interactions*).

Vaccination: During treatment with cyclosporine, vaccination may be less effective; and the use of live attenuated vaccines should be avoided.

Special Monitoring of Rheumatoid Arthritis Patients: Before initiating treatment, a careful physical examination, including blood pressure measurements (on at least two occasions) and two creatinine levels to estimate baseline should be performed. Blood pressure and serum creatinine should be evaluated every 2 weeks during the initial 3 months and then monthly if the patient is stable. It is advisable to monitor serum creatinine and blood pressure always after an increase of the dose of nonsteroidal anti-inflammatory drugs and after initiation of new nonsteroidal anti-inflammatory drug therapy during Gengraf™ (cyclosporine capsules, USP **[MODIFIED]**) treatment. If co-administered with methotrexate, CBC and liver function tests are recommended to be monitored monthly (*see also PRECAUTIONS, General, Hypertension*).

In patients who are receiving cyclosporine, the dose of Gengraf™ should be decreased by 25%–50% if hypertension occurs. If hypertension persists, the dose of Gengraf™ should be further reduced or blood pressure should be controlled with antihypertensive agents. In most cases, blood pressure has returned to baseline when cyclosporine was discontinued.

In placebo-controlled trials of rheumatoid arthritis patients, systolic hypertension (defined as an occurrence of two systolic blood pressure readings >140 mmHg) and diastolic hypertension (defined as two diastolic blood pressure readings >90 mmHg) occurred in 33% and 19% of patients treated with cyclosporine, respectively. The corresponding placebo rates were 22% and 8%.

Special Monitoring for Psoriasis Patients: Before initiating treatment, a careful dermatological and physical examination, including blood pressure measurements (on at least two occasions) should be performed. Since Gengraf™ (cyclosporine capsules, USP **[MODIFIED]**) is an immunosuppressive agent, patients should be evaluated for the presence of occult infection on their first physical examination and for the presence of tumors initially, and throughout treatment with Gengraf™. Skin lesions not typical for psoriasis should be biopsied before starting Gengraf™. Patients with malignant or premalignant changes of the skin should be treated with Gengraf™ only after appropriate treatment of such lesions and if no other treatment option exists.

Baseline laboratories should include serum creatinine (on two occasions), BUN, CBC, serum magnesium, potassium, uric acid, and lipids.

The risk of cyclosporine nephropathy is reduced when the starting dose is low (2.5 mg/kg/day), the maximum dose does not exceed 4.0 mg/kg/day, serum creatinine is monitored regularly while cyclosporine is administered, and the dose of Gengraf™ is decreased when the rise in creatinine is greater than or equal to 25% above the patients pretreatment level. The increase in creatinine is generally reversible upon timely decrease of the dose of Gengraf™ or its discontinuation.

Serum creatinine and BUN should be evaluated every 2 weeks during the initial 3 months of therapy and then monthly if the patient is stable. If the serum creatinine is greater than or equal to 25% above the patient's pretreatment level, serum creatinine should be repeated within two weeks. If the change in serum creatinine remains greater than or equal to 25% above baseline, Gengraf™ should be reduced by 25%–50%. If at **any time** the serum creatinine increases by greater than or equal to 50% above pretreatment level, Gengraf™ should be reduced by 25%–50%. Gengraf™ should be discontinued if reversibility (within 25% of baseline) of serum creatinine is not achievable after two dosage modifications. It is advisable to monitor serum creatinine after an increase of the dose of nonsteroidal anti-inflammatory drug and after initiation of new nonsteroidal anti-inflammatory therapy during Gengraf™ treatment.

Blood pressure should be evaluated every 2 weeks during the initial 3 months of therapy and then monthly if the patient is stable, or more frequently when dosage adjustments are made. Patients without a history of previous hypertension before initiation of treatment with Gengraf™, should have the drug reduced by 25%-50% if found to have sustained hypertension. If the patient continues to be hypertensive despite multiple reductions of Gengraf™, then Gengraf™ should be discontinued. For patients with treated hypertension, before the initiation of Gengraf™ therapy, their medication should be adjusted to control hypertension while on Gengraf™. Gengraf™ should be discontinued if a change in hypertension management is not effective or tolerable.

CBC, uric acid, potassium, lipids, and magnesium should also be monitored every 2 weeks for the first 3 months of therapy, and then monthly if the patient is stable or more frequently when dosage adjustments are made. Gengraf™ dosage should be reduced by 25%–50% for any abnormality of clinical concern.

In controlled trials of cyclosporine in psoriasis patients, cyclosporine blood concentrations did not correlate well with either improvement or with side effects such as renal dysfunction.

Information for Patients: Patients should be advised that any change of cyclosporine formulation should be made cautiously and only under physician supervision because it may result in the need for a change in dosage.

Patients should be informed of the necessity of repeated laboratory tests while they are receiving cyclosporine. Patients should be advised of the potential risks during pregnancy and informed of the increased risk of neoplasia. Patients should also be informed of the risk of hypertension and renal dysfunction.

Patients should be advised that during treatment with cyclosporine, vaccination may be less effective and the use of live attenuated vaccines should be avoided.

Patients should be advised to take Gengraf™ on a consistent schedule with regard to time of day and relation to meals. Grapefruit and grapefruit juice affect metabolism, increasing blood concentration of cyclosporine, thus should be avoided.

Laboratory Tests: In all patients treated with cyclosporine, renal and liver functions should be assessed repeatedly by measurement of serum creatinine, BUN, serum bilirubin, and liver enzymes. Serum lipids, magnesium, and potassium should also be monitored. Cyclosporine blood concentrations should be routinely monitored in transplant patients (*see DOSAGE AND ADMINISTRATION, Blood Concentration Monitoring in Transplant Patients*), and periodically monitored in rheumatoid arthritis patients.

Drug Interactions: All of the individual drugs cited below are well substantiated to interact with cyclosporine. In addition, concomitant non-steroidal anti-inflammatory drugs, particularly in the setting of dehydration, may potentiate renal dysfunction.

Drugs That May Potentiate Renal Dysfunction

[See table above]

Drugs That Alter Cyclosporine Concentrations: Cyclosporine is extensively metabolized. Cyclosporine concentrations may be influenced by drugs that affect microsomal enzymes, particularly cytochrome P-450 III-A. Substances that inhibit this enzyme could decrease metabolism and increase cyclosporine concentrations. Substances that are inducers of cytochrome P-450 activity could increase metabolism and decrease cyclosporine concentrations. Monitoring of circulating cyclosporine concentrations and appropriate Gengraf™ (cyclosporine capsules, USP **[MODIFIED]**) dosage adjustment are essential when these drugs are used concomitantly (*see DOSAGE AND ADMINISTRATION, Blood Concentration Monitoring*).

Drugs That Increase Cyclosporine Concentrations

Calcium Channel Blockers	*Antibiotics*	*Other Drugs*
diltiazem	clarithromycin	allopurinol
nicardipine	erythromycin	bromocriptine
verapamil		danazol
		metoclopramide
Antifungals	*Glucocorticoids*	
fluconazole	methylprednisolone	
itraconazole		
ketoconazole		

The HIV protease inhibitors (e.g., indinavir, nelfinavir, ritonavir, and saquinavir) are known to inhibit cytochrome P-450 III-A and increase the concentrations of drugs metabolized by the cytochrome P-450 system. The interaction between HIV protease inhibitors and cyclosporine has not been studied. Care should be exercised when these drugs are administered concomitantly.

Grapefruit and grapefruit juice affect metabolism, increasing blood concentrations of cyclosporine, thus should be avoided.

Continued on next page

Gengraf—Cont.

Drugs That Decrease Cyclosporine Concentrations

Antibiotics	*Anticonvulsants*	*Other Drugs*
nafcillin	carbamazepine	octreotide
rifampin	phenobarbital	ticlopidine
	phenytoin	

Rifabutin is known to increase the metabolism of other drugs metabolized by the cytochrome P-450 system. The interaction between rifabutin and cyclosporine has not been studied. Care should be exercised when these two drugs are administered concomitantly.

Nonsteroidal Anti-inflammatory Drug (NSAID) Interactions: Clinical status and serum creatinine should be closely monitored when cyclosporine is used with nonsteroidal anti-inflammatory agents in rheumatoid arthritis patients (*see WARNINGS*).

Pharmacodynamic interactions have been reported to occur between cyclosporine and both naproxen and sulindac, in that concomitant use is associated with additive decreases in renal function, as determined by ^{99m}Tc-diethylenetriaminepentaacetic acid (DTPA) and (*p*-aminohippuric acid) PAH clearances. Although concomitant administration of diclofenac does not affect blood levels of cyclosporine, it has been associated with approximate doubling of diclofenac blood levels and occasional reports of reversible decreases in renal function. Consequently, the dose of diclofenac should be in the lower end of the therapeutic range.

Methotrexate Interaction: Preliminary data indicate that when methotrexate and cyclosporine were co-administered to rheumatoid arthritis patients (N=20), methotrexate concentrations (AUCs) were increased approximately 30% and the concentrations (AUCs) of its metabolite, 7-hydroxy methotrexate, were decreased by approximately 80%. The clinical significance of this interaction is not known. Cyclosporine concentrations do not appear to have been altered (N=6).

Other Drug Interactions: Reduced clearance of prednisolone, digoxin, and lovastatin has been observed when these drugs are administered with cyclosporine. In addition, a decrease in the apparent volume of distribution of digoxin has been reported after cyclosporine administration. Severe digitalis toxicity has been seen within days of starting cyclosporine in several patients taking digoxin. Cyclosporine should not be used with potassium-sparing diuretics because hyperkalemia can occur.

During treatment with cyclosporine, vaccination may be less effective. The use of live vaccines should be avoided. Myositis has occurred with concomitant lovastatin, frequent gingival hyperplasia with nifedipine, and convulsions with high dose methylprednisolone.

Psoriasis patients receiving other immunosuppressive agents or radiation therapy (including PUVA and UVB) should not receive concurrent cyclosporine because of the possibility of excessive immunosuppression.

Carcinogenesis, Mutagenesis, and Impairment of Fertility: Carcinogenicity studies were carried out in male and female rats and mice. In the 78-week mouse study, evidence of a statistically significant trend was found for lymphocytic lymphomas in females, and the incidence of hepatocellular carcinomas in mid-dose males significantly exceeded the control value. In the 24-month rat study, pancreatic islet cell adenomas significantly exceeded the control rate in the low dose level. Doses used in the mouse and rat studies were 0.01 to 0.16 times the clinical maintenance dose (6 mg/kg). The hepatocellular carcinomas and pancreatic islet cell adenomas were not dose related. Published reports indicate the co-treatment of hairless mice with UV irradiation and cyclosporine or other immunosuppressive agents shorten the time to skin tumor formation compared to UV irradiation alone.

Cyclosporine was not mutagenic in appropriate test systems. Cyclosporine has not been found to be mutagenic/genotoxic in the Ames Test, the V79-HGPRT Test, the micronucleus test in mice and Chinese hamsters, the chromosome-aberration tests in Chinese hamster bone-marrow, the mouse dominant lethal assay, and the DNA-repair test in sperm from treated mice. A recent study analyzing sister chromatid exchange (SCE) induction by cyclosporine using human lymphocytes *in vitro* gave indication of a positive effect (i.e., induction of SCE), at high concentrations in this system.

No impairment in fertility was demonstrated in studies in male and female rats.

Widely distributed papillomatosis of the skin was observed after chronic treatment of dogs with cyclosporine at 9 times the human initial psoriasis treatment dose of 2.5 mg/kg, where doses are expressed on a body surface area basis. This papillomatosis showed a spontaneous regression upon discontinuation of cyclosporine.

An increased incidence of malignancy is a recognized complication of immunosuppression in recipients of organ transplants and patients with rheumatoid arthritis and psoriasis. The most common forms of neoplasms are non-Hodgkin's lymphoma and carcinomas of the skin. The risk of malignancies in cyclosporine recipients is higher than in the normal, healthy population but similar to that in patients receiving other immunosuppressive therapies. Reduction or discontinuance of immunosuppression may cause the lesions to regress.

In psoriasis patients on cyclosporine, development of malignancies, especially those of the skin has been reported (*see*

Body System	Adverse Reactions	Randomized Kidney Patients: Cyclosporine (NON-MODIFIED) (N=227) %	Randomized Kidney Patients: Azathioprine (N=228) %	Cyclosporine Patients Cyclosporine, (NON-MODIFIED): Kidney (N=705) %	Heart (N=112) %	Liver (N=75) %
Genitourinary	Renal Dysfunction	32	6	25	38	37
Cardiovascular	Hypertension	26	18	13	53	27
	Cramps	4	<1	2	<1	0
Skin	Hirsutism	21	<1	21	28	45
	Acne	6	8	2	2	1
Central Nervous System	Tremor	12	0	21	31	55
	Convulsions	3	1	1	4	5
	Headache	2	<1	2	15	4
Gastrointestinal	Gum Hyperplasia	4	0	9	5	16
	Diarrhea	3	<1	3	4	8
	Nausea/Vomiting	2	<1	4	10	4
	Hepatotoxicity	<1	<1	4	7	4
	Abdominal Discomfort	<1	0	<1	7	0
Autonomic Nervous	Paresthesia	3	0	1	2	1
System	Flushing	<1	0	4	0	4
Hematopoietic	Leukopenia	2	19	<1	6	0
	Lymphoma	<1	0	1	6	1
Respiratory	Sinusitis	<1	0	4	3	7
Miscellaneous	Gynecomastia	<1	0	<1	4	3

Infectious Complications in Historical Randomized Studies in Renal Transplant Patients Using Cyclosporine (NON-MODIFIED)

Complication	Cyclosporine Treatment (N=227) % of Complications	Azathioprine with Steroids* (N=228) % of Complications
Septicemia	5.3	4.8
Abscesses	4.4	5.3
Systemic Fungal Infection	2.2	3.9
Local Fungal Infection	7.5	9.6
Cytomegalovirus	4.8	12.3
Other Viral Infections	15.9	18.4
Urinary Tract Infections	21.1	20.2
Wound and Skin Infections	7.0	10.1
Pneumonia	6.2	9.2

*Some patients also received ALG.

WARNINGS). Skin lesions not typical for psoriasis should be biopsied before starting cyclosporine treatment. Patients with malignant or premalignant changes of the skin should be treated with cyclosporine only after appropriate treatment of such lesions and if no other treatment option exists.

Pregnancy: ***Pregnancy Category C.*** Cyclosporine was not teratogenic in appropriate test systems. Only at dose levels toxic to dams, were adverse effects seen in reproduction studies in rats. Cyclosporine has been shown to be embryo- and fetotoxic in rats and rabbits following oral administration at maternally toxic doses. Fetal toxicity was noted in rats at 0.8 and rabbits at 5.4 times the transplant doses in humans of 6.0 mg/kg, where dose corrections are based on body surface area. Cyclosporine was embryo- and fetotoxic as indicated by increased pre- and postnatal mortality and reduced fetal weight together with related skeletal retardation.

There are no adequate and well-controlled studies in pregnant women. Gengraf™ (cyclosporine capsules, USP **[MODIFIED]**) should be used during pregnancy only if the potential benefit justifies the potential risk to the fetus.

The following data represent the reported outcomes of 116 pregnancies in women receiving cyclosporine during pregnancy, 90% of whom were transplant patients, and most of whom received cyclosporine throughout the entire gestational period. The only consistent patterns of abnormality were premature birth (gestational period of 28 to 36 weeks) and low birth weight for gestational age. Sixteen fetal losses occurred. Most of the pregnancies (85 of 100) were complicated by disorders; including, pre-eclampsia, eclampsia, premature labor, abruptio placentae, oligohydramnios, Rh incompatibility and fetoplacental dysfunction. Pre-term delivery occurred in 47%. Seven malformations were reported in 5 viable infants and in 2 cases of fetal loss. Twenty-eight percent of the infants were small for gestational age. Neonatal complications occurred in 27%. Therefore, the risks and benefits of using Gengraf™ during pregnancy should be carefully weighed.

Because of the possible disruption of maternal-fetal interaction, the risk/benefit ratio of using Gengraf™ in psoriasis patients during pregnancy should carefully be weighed with serious consideration for discontinuation of Gengraf™.

Nursing Mothers: Since cyclosporine is excreted in human milk, breast-feeding should be avoided.

Pediatric Use: Although no adequate and well-controlled studies have been completed in children, transplant recipients as young as one year of age have received cyclosporine **(MODIFIED)** with no unusual adverse effects. The safety and efficacy of cyclosporine **(MODIFIED)** treatment in pediatric patients with juvenile rheumatoid arthritis or psoriasis below the age of 18 have not been established.

Geriatric Use: In rheumatoid arthritis clinical trials with cyclosporine, 17.5% of patients were age 65 or older. These patients were more likely to develop systolic hypertension on therapy, and more likely to show serum creatinine rises ≥50% above the baseline after 3–4 months of therapy.

ADVERSE REACTIONS

Kidney, Liver, and Heart Transplantation: The principal adverse reactions of cyclosporine therapy are renal dysfunction, tremor, hirsutism, hypertension, and gum hyperplasia.

Hypertension, which is usually mild to moderate, may occur in approximately 50% of patients following renal transplantation and in most cardiac transplant patients.

Glomerular capillary thrombosis has been found in patients treated with cyclosporine and may progress to graft failure. The pathologic changes resembled those seen in the hemolytic-uremic syndrome and include thrombosis of the renal microvasculature, with platelet-fibrin thrombi occluding glomerular capillaries and afferent arterioles, microangiopathic hemolytic anemia, thrombocytopenia, and decreased renal function. Similar findings have been observed when other immunosuppressives have been employed post-transplantation.

Hypomagnesemia has been reported in some, but not all, patients exhibiting convulsions while on cyclosporine therapy. Although magnesium-depletion studies in normal subjects suggest that hypomagnesemia is associated with neurologic disorders, multiple factors, including hypertension, high dose methylprednisolone, hypocholesterolemia, and nephrotoxicity associated with high plasma concentrations of cyclosporine appear to be related to the neurological manifestations of cyclosporine toxicity.

In controlled studies, the nature, severity and incidence of the adverse events that were observed in 493 transplanted patients treated with cyclosporine **(MODIFIED)** were comparable with those observed in 208 transplanted patients who received cyclosporine **(NON-MODIFIED)** in these same studies when the dosage of the two drugs was adjusted to achieve the same cyclosporine blood trough concentrations.

Based on the historical experience with cyclosporine **(NON-MODIFIED)**, the following reactions occurred in 3% or greater of 892 patients involved in clinical trials of kidney, heart, and liver transplants.

[See first table above]

Among 705 kidney transplant patients treated with cyclosporine oral solution **(NON-MODIFIED)** in clinical trials, the reason for treatment discontinuation was renal toxicity in 5.4%, infection in 0.9%, lack of efficacy in 1.4%, acute tubular necrosis in 1.0%, lymphoproliferative disorders in 0.3%, hypertension in 0.3%, and other reasons in 0.7% of the patients.

The following reactions occurred in 2% or less of cyclosporine **(NON-MODIFIED)**-treated patients: allergic reactions, anemia, anorexia, confusion, conjunctivitis, edema, fever, brittle fingernails, gastritis, hearing loss, hiccups, hyperglycemia, muscle pain, peptic ulcer, thrombocytopenia, tinnitus.

The following reactions occurred rarely: anxiety, chest pain, constipation, depression, hair breaking, hematuria, joint pain, lethargy, mouth sores, myocardial infarction, night sweats, pancreatitis, pruritus, swallowing difficulty, tingling, upper GI bleeding, visual disturbance, weakness, weight loss.

[See second table above]

Rheumatoid Arthritis: The principal adverse reactions associated with the use of cyclosporine in rheumatoid arthritis are renal dysfunction (see *WARNINGS*), hypertension (see *PRECAUTIONS*), headache, gastrointestinal disturbances and hirsutism/hypertrichosis.

Cyclosporine (MODIFIED)/Cyclosporine (NON-MODIFIED) Rheumatoid Arthritis
Percentage of Patients with Adverse Events ≥3% in any Cyclosporine Treated Group

		Studies 651 + 652 + 2008	Study 302	Study 654	Study 654	Study 302	Studies 651 + 652 + 2008
Body System	**Preferred Term**	**Cyclosporine (NON-MODIFIED)† (N=269)**	**Cyclosporine (NON-MODIFIED) (N=155)**	**Methotrexate & Cyclosporine (NON-MODIFIED) (N=74)**	**Methotrexate & Placebo (N=73)**	**Cyclosporine (MODIFIED) (N=143)**	**Placebo (N=201)**
Autonomic Nervous System Disorders	Flushing	2%	2%	3%	0%	5%	2%
Body As A Whole - General Disorders	Accidental Trauma	0%	1%	10%	4%	4%	0%
	Edema NOS*	5%	14%	12%	4%	10%	<1%
	Fatigue	6%	3%	8%	12%	3%	7%
	Fever	2%	3%	0%	0%	2%	4%
	Influenza-like symptoms	<1%	6%	1%	0%	3%	2%
	Pain	6%	9%	10%	15%	13%	4%
	Rigors	1%	1%	4%	0%	3%	1%
Cardiovascular Disorders	Arrhythmia	2%	5%	5%	6%	2%	1%
	Chest Pain	4%	5%	1%	1%	6%	1%
	Hypertension	8%	26%	16%	12%	25%	2%
Central and Peripheral Nervous System Disorders	Dizziness	8%	6%	7%	3%	8%	3%
	Headache	17%	23%	22%	11%	25%	9%
	Migraine	2%	3%	0%	0%	3%	1%
	Parethesia	8%	7%	8%	4%	11%	1%
	Tremor	8%	7%	7%	3%	13%	4%
Gastrointestinal System Disorders	Abdominal Pain	15%	15%	15%	7%	15%	10%
	Anorexia	3%	3%	1%	0%	3%	3%
	Diarrhea	12%	12%	18%	15%	13%	8%
	Dyspepsia	12%	12%	10%	8%	8%	4%
	Flatulence	5%	5%	5%	4%	4%	1%
	Gastrointestinal Disorder NOS*	0%	2%	1%	4%	4%	0%
	Gingivitis	4%	3%	0%	0%	0%	1%
	Gum Hyperplasia	2%	4%	1%	3%	4%	1%
	Nausea	23%	14%	24%	15%	18%	14%
	Rectal Hemorrhage	0%	3%	0%	0%	1%	1%
	Stomatitis	7%	5%	16%	12%	6%	8%
	Vomiting	9%	8%	14%	7%	6%	5%
Hearing and Vestibular Disorders	Eat Disorders NOS*	0%	5%	0%	0%	1%	0%
Metabolic and Nutritional Disorders	Hypomagnesemia	0%	4%	0%	0%	6%	0%
Musculoskeletal System Disorders	Arthropathy	0%	5%	0%	1%	4%	0%
	Leg Cramps/Involuntary Muscle Contractions	2%	11%	11%	3%	12%	1%
Psychiatric Disorders	Depression	3%	6%	3%	1%	1%	2%
	Insomnia	4%	1%	1%	0%	3%	2%
Renal	Creatinine elevations ≥30%	43%	39%	55%	19%	48%	13%
	Creatinine elevations ≥50%	24%	18%	26%	8%	18%	3%
Reproductive Disorders, Female	Leukorrhea	1%	0%	4%	0%	1%	0%
	Menstrual Disorder	3%	2%	1%	0%	1%	1%
Respiratory System Disorders	Bronchitis	1%	3%	1%	0%	1%	3%
	Coughing	5%	3%	5%	7%	4%	4%
	Dyspnea	5%	1%	3%	3%	1%	2%
	Infection NOS*	9%	5%	0%	7%	3%	10%
	Pharyngitis	3%	5%	5%	6%	4%	4%
	Pneumonia	1%	0%	4%	0%	1%	1%
	Rhinitis	0%	3%	11%	10%	1%	0%
	Sinusitis	4%	4%	8%	4%	3%	3%
	Upper Respiratory Tract	0%	14%	23%	15%	13%	0%
Skin and Appendages Disorders	Alopecia	3%	0%	1%	1%	4%	4%
	Bullous Eruption	1%	0%	4%	1%	1%	1%
	Hypertrichosis	19%	17%	12%	0%	15%	3%
	Rash	7%	12%	10%	7%	8%	10%
	Skin Ulceration	1%	1%	3%	4%	0%	2%
Urinary System Disorders	Dysuria	0%	0%	11%	3%	1%	2%
	Micturition Frequency	2%	4%	3%	1%	2%	2%
	NPN, Increased	0%	19%	12%	0%	18%	0%
	Urinary Tract Infection	0%	3%	5%	4%	3%	0%
Vascular (Extracardiac) Disorders	Pupura	3%	4%	1%	1%	2%	0%

†Includes patients in 2.5 mg/kg/day dose group only. *NOS = Not Otherwise Specified.

In rheumatoid arthritis patients treated in clinical trials within the recommended dose range, cyclosporine therapy was discontinued in 5.3% of the patients because of hypertension and in 7% of the patients because of increased creatinine. These changes are usually reversible with timely dose decrease or drug discontinuation. The frequency and severity of serum creatinine elevations increase with dose and duration of cyclosporine therapy. These elevations are likely to become more pronounced without dose reduction or discontinuation.

The following adverse events occurred in controlled clinical trials:

[See table above]

In addition, the following adverse events have been reported in 1% to <3% of the rheumatoid arthritis patients in the cyclosporine treatment group in controlled clinical trials.

Autonomic Nervous System: dry mouth, increased sweating;

Body as a Whole: allergy, asthenia, hot flushes, malaise, overdose, procedure NOS*, tumor NOS*, weight decrease, weight increase;

Cardiovascular: abnormal heart sounds, cardiac failure, myocardial infarction, peripheral ischemia;

Central and Peripheral Nervous System: hypoesthesia, neuropathy, vertigo;

Endocrine: goiter;

Gastrointestinal: constipation, dysphagia, enanthema, eructation, esophagitis, gastric ulcer, gastritis, gastroenteritus, gingival bleeding, glossitis, peptic ulcer, salivary gland enlargement, tongue disorder, tooth disorder;

Infection: abscess, bacterial infection, cellulitis, folliculitis, fungal infection, herpes simplex, herpes zoster, renal abscess, moniliasis, tonsillitis, viral infection;

Hematologic: anemia, epistaxis, leukopenia, lymphadenopathy;

Liver and Biliary System: bilirubinemia;

Metabolic and Nutritional: diabetes mellitus, hyperkalemia, hyperuricemia, hypoglycemia;

Musculoskeletal System: arthralgia, bone fracture, bursitis, joint dislocation, myalgia, stiffness, synovial cyst, tendon disorder;

Neoplasms: breast fibroadenosis, carcinoma;

Psychiatric: anxiety, confusion, decreased libido, emotional lability, impaired concentration, increased libido, nervousness, paroniria, somnolence;

Reproductive (Female): breast pain, uterine hemorrhage;

Respiratory System: abnormal chest sounds, bronchospasm;

Skin and Appendages: abnormal pigmentation, angioedema, dermatitis, dry skin, eczema, nail disorder, pruritus, skin disorder, urticaria;

Special Senses: abnormal vision, cataract, conjunctivitis, deafness, eye pain, taste perversion, tinnitus, vestibular disorder;

Urinary System: abnormal urine, hematuria, increased BUN, micturition urgency, nocturia, polyuria, pyelonephritis, urinary incontinence.

*NOS = Not Otherwise Specified.

Psoriasis: The principal adverse reactions associated with the use of cyclosporine in patients with psoriasis are renal dysfunction, headache, hypertension, hypertriglyceridemia, hirsutism/hypertrichosis, paresthesia or hyperesthesia, influenza-like symptoms, nausea/vomiting, diarrhea, abdominal discomfort, lethargy, and musculoskeletal or joint pain. In psoriasis patients treated in U.S. controlled clinical studies within the recommended dose range, cyclosporine therapy was discontinued in 1.0% of the patients because of hypertension and in 5.4% of the patients because of increased creatinine. In the majority of cases, these changes were reversible after dose reduction or discontinuation of cyclosporine.

There has been one reported death associated with the use of cyclosporine in psoriasis. A 27 year old male developed renal deterioration and was continued on cyclosporine. He had progressive renal failure leading to death.

Frequency and severity of serum creatinine increases with dose and duration of cyclosporine therapy. These elevations are likely to become more pronounced and may result in irreversible renal damage without dose reduction or discontinuation.

Continued on next page

Gengraf—Cont.

[See table below]

The following events occurred in 1% to less than 3% of psoriasis patients treated with cyclosporine:

Body as a Whole: fever, flushes, hot flushes; ***Cardiovascular:*** chest pain; ***Central and Peripheral Nervous System:*** appetite increased, insomnia, dizziness, nervousness, vertigo; ***Gastrointestinal:*** abdominal distention, constipation, gingival bleeding; ***Liver and Biliary System:*** hyperbilirubinemia; ***Neoplasms:*** skin malignancies [squamous cell (0.9%) and basal cell (0.4%) carcinomas]; ***Reticuloendothelial:*** platelet, bleeding, and clotting disorders, red blood cell disorder; ***Respiratory:*** infection, viral and other infection; ***Skin and Appendages***: acne, folliculitis, keratosis, pruritus, rash, dry skin; ***Urinary System:*** micturition frequency; ***Vision:*** abnormal vision.

Mild hypomagnesemia and hyperkalemia may occur but are asymptomatic. Increases in uric acid may occur and attacks of gout have been rarely reported. A minor and dose related hyperbilirubinemia has been observed in the absence of hepatocellular damage. Cyclosporine therapy may be associated with a modest increase of serum triglycerides or cholesterol. Elevations of triglycerides (>750 mg/dL) occur in about 15% of psoriasis patients; elevations of cholesterol (>300 mg/dL) are observed in less than 3% of psoriasis patients. Generally these laboratory abnormalities are reversible upon dose reduction or discontinuation of cyclosporine.

OVERDOSAGE

There is a minimal experience with cyclosporine overdosage. Forced emesis can be of value up to 2 hours after administration of Gengraf™ (cyclosporine capsules, USP **[MODIFIED]**). Transient hepatotoxicity and nephrotoxicity may occur which should resolve following drug withdrawal. General supportive measures and symptomatic treatment should be followed in all cases of overdosage. Cyclosporine is not dialyzable to any great extent, nor is it cleared well by charcoal hemoperfusion. The oral dosage at which half of experimental animals are estimated to die is 31 times, 39 times and >54 times the human maintenance dose for transplant patients (6 mg/kg; corrections based on body surface area) in mice, rats, and rabbits.

DOSAGE AND ADMINISTRATION

Gengraf™ (cyclosporine capsules, USP [MODIFIED]) has increased bioavailability in comparison to Sandimmune®* (cyclosporine [NON-MODIFIED]). Gengraf™ and Sandimmune®* (cyclosporine [NON-MODIFIED]) are not bioequivalent and cannot be used interchangeably without physician supervision.

The daily dose of Gengraf™ (cyclosporine capsules, USP **[MODIFIED]**) should always be given in two divided doses (BID). It is recommended that Gengraf™ be administered on a consistent schedule with regard to time of day and relation to meals. Grapefruit and grapefruit juice affect metabolism, increasing blood concentration of cyclosporine, thus should be avoided.

Newly Transplanted Patients: The initial oral dose of Gengraf™ (cyclosporine capsules, USP **[MODIFIED]**) can be given 4–12 hours prior to transplantation or be given postoperatively. The initial dose of Gengraf™ varies depending on the transplanted organ and the other immunosuppressive agents included in the immunosuppressive protocol. In newly transplanted patients, the initial oral dose of Gengraf™ is the same as the initial oral dose of cyclosporine (**NON-MODIFIED**). Suggested initial doses are available from the results of a 1994 survey of the use of cyclosporine (**NON-MODIFIED**) in U.S. transplant centers. The mean $\pm$ SD initial doses were 9$\pm$3 mg/kg/day for renal transplant patients (75 centers), 8$\pm$4 mg/kg/day for liver transplant patients (30 centers), and 7$\pm$3 mg/kg/day for heart transplant patients (24 centers). Total daily doses were divided into two equal daily doses. The Gengraf™ dose is subsequently adjusted to achieve a pre-defined cyclosporine blood concentration (*see DOSAGE AND ADMINISTRATION, Blood Concentration Monitoring in Transplant Patients, below*). If cyclosporine trough blood concentrations are used, the target range is the same for Gengraf™ as for cyclosporine (**NON-MODIFIED**). Using the same trough concentration target range for Gengraf™ as for cyclosporine (**NON-MODIFIED**) results in greater cyclosporine exposure when Gengraf™ is administered (*see CLINICAL PHARMACOLOGY, Pharmacokinetics, Absorption*). Dosing should be titrated based on clinical assessments of rejection and tolerability. Lower Gengraf™ doses may be sufficient as maintenance therapy. Adjunct therapy with adrenal corticosteroids is recommended initially. Different tapering dosage schedules of prednisone appear to achieve similar results. A representative dosage schedule based on the patient's weight started with 2.0 mg/kg/day for the first 4 days tapered to 1.0 mg/kg/day by 1 week, 0.6 mg/kg/day by 2 weeks, 0.3 mg/kg/day by 1 month, and 0.15 mg/kg/day by 2 months and thereafter as a maintenance dose. Steroid doses may be further tapered on an individualized basis depending on status of patient and function of graft. Adjustments in dosage of prednisone must be made according to the clinical situation.

Conversion from Sandimmune®* (cyclosporine [NON-MODIFIED]) to Gengraf™ (cyclosporine capsules, USP [MODIFIED]) in Transplant Patients: In transplanted patients who are considered for conversion to Gengraf™ from Sandimmune®* (cyclosporine [**NON-MODIFIED**]), Gengraf™ should be started with the same daily dose as was previously used with Sandimmune®* (cyclosporine [**NON-MODIFIED**]) (1:1 dose conversion). The Gengraf™ dose should subsequently be adjusted to attain the pre-conversion cyclosporine blood trough concentration. Using the same trough concentration target range for Gengraf™ as for Sandimmune®* (cyclosporine [**NON-MODIFIED**]) results in greater cyclosporine exposure when Gengraf™ is administered (*see CLINICAL PHARMACOLOGY, Pharmacokinetics, Absorption*). Patients with suspected poor absorption of Sandimmune®* (cyclosporine [**NON-MODIFIED**]) require different dosing strategies (*see DOSAGE AND ADMINISTRATION, Transplant Patients with Poor Absorption of Sandimmune®* (cyclosporine [NON-MODIFIED]), below*). In some patients, the increase in blood trough concentration is more pronounced and may be of clinical significance.

Until the blood trough concentration attains the pre-conversion value, it is strongly recommended that the cyclosporine blood trough concentration be monitored every 4 to 7 days after conversion to Gengraf™. In addition, clinical safety parameters such as serum creatinine and blood pressure should be monitored every two weeks during the first two months after conversion. If the blood trough concentrations are outside the desired range and/or if the clinical safety parameters worsen, the dosage of Gengraf™ must be adjusted accordingly.

Transplant Patients with Poor Absorption of Sandimmune®* (cyclosporine [NON-MODIFIED]): Patients with lower than expected cyclosporine blood trough concentrations in relation to the oral dose of Sandimmune®* (cyclosporine [**NON-MODIFIED**]) may have poor or inconsistent absorption of cyclosporine from Sandimmune®* (cyclosporine [**NON-MODIFIED**]). After conversion to Gengraf™ (cyclosporine capsules, USP [**MODIFIED**]), patients tend to have higher cyclosporine concentrations. **Due to the increase in bioavailability of cyclosporine following conversion to Gengraf™, the cyclosporine blood trough concentration may exceed the target range. Particular caution should be exercised when converting patients to Gengraf™ at doses greater than 10 mg/kg/day.** The dose of Gengraf™ should be titrated individually based on cyclosporine trough concentrations, tolerability, and clinical response. In this population the cyclosporine blood trough concentration should be measured more frequently, at least twice a week (daily, if initial dose exceeds 10 mg/kg/day) until the concentration stabilizes within the desired range.

Rheumatoid Arthritis: The initial dose of Gengraf™ (cyclosporine capsules, USP **[MODIFIED]**) is 2.5 mg/kg/day, taken twice daily as a divided (BID) oral dose. Salicylates, nonsteroidal anti-inflammatory agents, and oral corticosteroids may be continued (*see WARNINGS and PRECAUTIONS: Drug Interactions*). Onset of action generally occurs between 4 and 8 weeks. If insufficient clinical benefit is seen and tolerability is good (including serum creatinine less than 30% above baseline), the dose may be increased by 0.5–0.75 mg/kg/day after 8 weeks and again after 12 weeks to a maximum of 4 mg/kg/day. If no benefit is seen by 16 weeks of therapy, Gengraf™ therapy should be discontinued.

Dose decreases by 25%-50% should be made at any time to control adverse events, e.g., hypertension elevations in serum creatinine (30% above patient's pretreatment level) or clinically significant laboratory abnormalities (*see WARNINGS and PRECAUTIONS*). If dose reduction is not effective in controlling abnormalities or if the adverse event or abnormality is severe, Gengraf™ should be discontinued. The same initial dose and dosage range should be used if Gengraf™ is combined with the recommended dose of methotrexate. Most patients can be treated with Gengraf™ doses of 3 mg/kg/day or below when combined with methotrexate doses of up to 15 mg/week (*see CLINICAL PHARMACOLOGY, Clinical Trials*).

There is limited long-term treatment data. Recurrence of rheumatoid arthritis disease activity is generally apparent within four weeks after stopping cyclosporine.

Psoriasis: The initial dose of Gengraf™ (cyclosporine capsules, USP **[MODIFIED]**) should be 2.5 mg/kg/day. Gengraf™ should be taken twice daily, as a divided (1.25 mg/kg BID) oral dose. Patients should be kept at that dose for at least 4 weeks, barring adverse events. If significant clinical improvement has not occurred in patients by that time, the patient's dosage should be increased at 2 week intervals. Based on patient response, dose increases of approximately 0.5 mg/kg/day should be made to a maximum of 4.0 mg/kg/day.

Dose decreases by 25%-50% should be made at any time to control adverse events, e.g., hypertension, elevations in serum creatinine ($\geq$25% above the patient's pretreatment level), or clinically significant laboratory abnormalities. If dose reduction is not effective in controlling abnormalities, or if the adverse event or abnormality is severe, Gengraf™ should be discontinued (*see PRECAUTIONS, Special Monitoring of Psoriasis Patients*).

Patients generally show some improvement in the clinical manifestations of psoriasis in 2 weeks. Satisfactory control and stabilization of the disease may take 12–16 weeks to achieve. Results of a dose-titration clinical trial with Gengraf™ indicate that an improvement of psoriasis by 75% or more (based on PASI) was achieved in 51% of the patients after 8 weeks and in 79% of the patients after 12 weeks. Treatment should be discontinued if satisfactory response cannot be achieved after 6 weeks at 4 mg/kg/day or the patient's maximum tolerated dose. Once a patient is adequately controlled and appears stable the dose of Gengraf™ should be lowered, and the patient treated with the lowest dose that maintains an adequate response (this should not necessarily be total clearing of the patient). In clinical trials, cyclosporine doses at the lower end of the recommended dosage range were effective in maintaining a satisfactory response in 60% of the patients. Doses below 2.5 mg/kg/day may also be equally effective.

Upon stopping treatment with cyclosporine, relapse will occur in approximately six weeks (50% of the patients) to 16

Adverse Events Occurring in 3% or More of Psoriasis Patients in Controlled Clinical Trials

Body System*	Preferred Term	Cyclosporine (MODIFIED) (N=182)	Cyclosporine (NON-MODIFIED) (N=185)
Infection or Partial Infection		24.7%	24.3%
	Influenza-like Symptoms	9.9%	8.1%
	Upper Respiratory Tract Infections	7.7%	11.3%
Cardiovascular System		28.0%	25.4%
	Hypertension**	27.5%	25.4%
Urinary System		24.2%	16.2%
	Increased Creatinine	19.8%	15.7%
Central and Peripheral Nervous System		26.4%	20.5%
	Headache	15.9%	14.0%
	Paresthesia	7.1%	4.8%
Musculoskeletal System		13.2%	8.7%
	Arthralgia	6.0%	1.1%
Body As a Whole - General		29.1%	22.2%
	Pain	4.4%	3.2%
Metabolic and Nutritional		9.3%	9.7%
Reproductive, Female		8.5% (4 of 47 females)	11.5% (6 of 52 females)
Resistance Mechanism		18.7%	21.1%
Skin and Appendages		17.6%	15.1%
	Hypertrichosis	6.6%	5.4%
Respiratory System		5.0%	6.5%
	Bronchospasm, Coughing, Dyspnea, Rhinitis	5.0%	4.9%
Psychiatric		5.0%	3.8%
Gastrointestinal System		19.8%	28.7%
	Abdominal Pain	2.7%	6.0%
	Diarrhea	5.0%	5.9%
	Dyspepsia	2.2%	3.2%
	Gum Hyperplasia	3.8%	6.0%
	Nausea	5.5%	5.9%
White cell and RES		4.4%	2.7%

* Total percentage of events within the system.
** Newly occurring hypertension = SBP $\geq$160 mm Hg and/or DBP $\geq$90 mm Hg.

weeks (75% of the patients). In the majority of patients rebound does not occur after cessation of treatment with cyclosporine. Thirteen cases of transformation of chronic plaque psoriasis to more severe forms of psoriasis have been reported. There were 9 cases of pustular and 4 cases of erythrodermic psoriasis. Long term experience with Gengraf™ in psoriasis patients is limited and continuous treatment for extended periods greater than one year is not recommended. Alternation with other forms of treatment should be considered in the long term management of patients with this life long disease.

Blood Concentration Monitoring in Transplant Patients: Transplant centers have found blood concentration monitoring of cyclosporine to be an essential component of patient management. Of importance to blood concentration analysis are the type of assay used, the transplanted organ, and other immunosuppressant agents being administered. While no fixed relationship has been established, blood concentration monitoring may assist in the clinical evaluation of rejection and toxicity, dose adjustments, and the assessment of compliance.

Various assays have been used to measure blood concentrations of cyclosporine. Older studies using a non-specific assay often cited concentrations that were roughly twice those of the specific assays. Therefore, comparison between concentrations in the published literature and an individual patient concentration using current assays must be made with detailed knowledge of the assay methods employed. Current assay results are also not interchangeable and their use should be guided by their approved labeling. A discussion of the different assay methods is contained in *Annals of Clinical Biochemistry* 1994;31:420-446. While several assays and assay matrices are available, there is a consensus that parent-compound-specific assays correlate best with clinical events. Of these, HPLC is the standard reference, but the monoclonal antibody RIAs and the monoclonal antibody FPIA offer sensitivity, reproducibility, and convenience. Most clinicians base their monitoring on trough cyclosporine concentrations. *Applied Pharmacokinetics, Principles of Therapeutic Drug Monitoring* (1992) contains a broad discussion of cyclosporine pharmacokinetics and drug monitoring techniques. Blood concentration monitoring is not a replacement for renal function monitoring or tissue biopsies.

HOW SUPPLIED

Gengraf™ Capsules (cyclosporine capsules, USP [MODIFIED])

25 mg

Oval, white imprinted in blue, the corporate logo, 25 mg, and the Abbo-Code OR.

Packages of 30 unit-dose blisters. (**NDC** 0074-6463-32).

100 mg

Oval, white, with two blue stripes, imprinted in blue, the corporate logo, 100 mg, and Abbo-Code OT.

Packages of 30 unit-dose blisters. (**NDC** 0074-6479-32).

Store and Dispense: In the original unit-dose container at controlled room temperature 15°–30°C (59°–86°F). (See USP).

*Sandimmune® is a registered trademark of Novartis Pharmaceuticals Corporation.

TM-Trademark ©Abbott

Manufactured by: Abbott Laboratories North Chicago, IL 60064, U.S.A.

Distributed by: SangStat Medical Corporation Fremont, CA 94555, U.S.A.

Revised: January, 2000

Ref. 03-4999-R1

Shown in Product Identification Guide, page 303

HYTRIN® ℞

(terazosin hydrochloride)

Capsules

DESCRIPTION

HYTRIN (terazosin hydrochloride), an alpha-1-selective adrenoceptor blocking agent, is a quinazoline derivative represented by the following chemical name and structural formula:

(RS)-Piperazine, 1-(4-amino-6,7-dimethoxy-2-quinazolinyl)-4-[(tetra-hydro-2-furanyl)carbonyl]-, monohydrochloride, dihydrate.

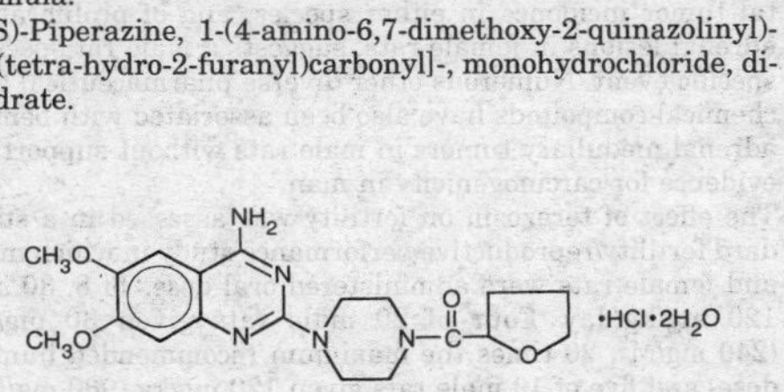

Terazosin hydrochloride is a white, crystalline substance, freely soluble in water and isotonic saline and has a molecular weight of 459.93. HYTRIN capsules (terazosin hydrochloride capsules) for oral ingestion are supplied in four dosage strengths containing terazosin hydrochloride equivalent to 1 mg, 2 mg, 5 mg, or 10 mg of terazosin.

Inactive Ingredients:

1 mg capsules: gelatin, glycerin, iron oxide, methylparaben, mineral oil, polyethylene glycol, povidone, propylparaben, titanium dioxide, and vanillin.

2 mg capsules: D&C yellow No. 10, gelatin, glycerin, methylparaben, mineral oil, polyethylene glycol, povidone, propylparaben, titanium dioxide, and vanillin.

5 mg capsules: D&C red No. 28, FD&C red No. 40, gelatin, glycerin, methylparaben, mineral oil, polyethylene glycol, povidone, propylparaben, titanium dioxide, and vanillin.

10 mg capsules: FD&C blue No. 1, gelatin, glycerin, methylparaben, mineral oil, polyethylene glycol, povidone, propylparaben, titanium dioxide, and vanillin.

CLINICAL PHARMACOLOGY

Pharmacodynamics:

A. Benign Prostatic Hyperplasia (BPH)

The symptoms associated with BPH are related to bladder outlet obstruction, which is comprised of two underlying components: a static component and a dynamic component. The static component is a consequence of an increase in prostate size. Over time, the prostate will continue to enlarge. However, clinical studies have demonstrated that the size of the prostate does not correlate with the severity of BPH symptoms or the degree of urinary obstruction. The dynamic component is a function of an increase in smooth muscle tone in the prostate and bladder neck, leading to constriction of the bladder outlet. Smooth muscle tone is mediated by sympathetic nervous stimulation of alpha-l adrenoceptors, which are abundant in the prostate, prostatic capsule and bladder neck. The reduction in symptoms and improvement in urine flow rates following administration of terazosin is related to relaxation of smooth muscle produced by blockade of alpha-l adrenoceptors in the bladder neck and prostate. Because there are relatively few alpha-l adrenoceptors in the bladder body, terazosin is able to reduce the bladder outlet obstruction without affecting bladder contractility.

Terazosin has been studied in 1222 men with symptomatic BPH. In three placebo-controlled studies, symptom evaluation and uroflowmetric measurements were performed approximately 24 hours following dosing. Symptoms were quantified using the Boyarsky Index. The questionnaire evaluated both obstructive (hesitancy, intermittency, terminal dribbling, impairment of size and force of stream, sensation of incomplete bladder emptying) and irritative (nocturia, daytime frequency, urgency, dysuria) symptoms by rating each of the 9 symptoms from 0–3, for a total score of 27 points. Results from these studies indicated that terazosin statistically significantly improved symptoms and peak urine flow rates over placebo as follows:

	Symptom Score (Range 0-27)			Peak Flow Rate (mL/sec)		
	N	Mean Baseline	Mean Change (%)	N	Mean Baseline	Mean Change (%)
Study 1 (10 mg)[a] **Titration to fixed dose (12 wks)**						
Placebo	55	9.7	−2.3 (24)	54	10.1	+1.0 (10)
Terazosin	54	10.1	−4.5 (45)*	52	8.8	+3.0 (34)*
Study 2 (2, 5, 10, 20 mg)[b] **Titration to response (24 wks)**						
Placebo	89	12.5	−3.8 (30)	88	8.8	+1.4 (16)
Terazosin	85	12.2	−5.3 (43)*	84	8.4	+2.9 (35)*
Study 3 (1, 2, 5, 10 mg)[c] **Titration to response (24 wks)**						
Placebo	74	10.4	−1.1 (11)	74	8.8	+1.2 (14)
Terazosin	73	10.9	−4.6 (42)*	73	8.6	+2.6 (30)*

[a] Highest dose 10 mg shown.
[b] 23% of patients on 10 mg, 41% of patients on 20 mg.
[c] 67% of patients on 10 mg.
* Significantly (p ≤ 0.05) more improvement than placebo.

In all three studies, both symptom scores and peak urine flow rates showed statistically significant improvement from baseline in patients treated with terazosin from week 2 (or the first clinic visit) and throughout the study duration.

Analysis of the effect of terazosin on individual urinary symptoms demonstrated that compared to placebo, terazosin significantly improved the symptoms of hesitancy, intermittency, impairment in size and force of urinary stream, sensation of incomplete emptying, terminal dribbling, daytime frequency and nocturia.

Global assessments of overall urinary function and symptoms were also performed by investigators who were blinded to patient treatment assignment. In studies 1 and 3, patients treated with terazosin had a significantly (p ≤ 0.001) greater overall improvement compared to placebo treated patients.

In a short term study (Study 1), patients were randomized to either 2, 5 or 10 mg of terazosin or placebo. Patients randomized to the 10 mg group achieved a statistically significant response in both symptoms and peak flow rate compared to placebo (Figure 1).

[See figure 1 at top of next column]

In a long-term, open-label, non-placebo controlled clinical trial, 181 men were followed for 2 years and 58 of these men were followed for 30 months. The effect of terazosin on urinary symptom scores and peak flow rates was maintained throughout the study duration (Figures 2 and 3):

Figure 1
Study 1

Mean Change in Total Symptom Score from Baseline+ **Mean Increase in Peak Flow Rate (mL/sec) from Baseline+**

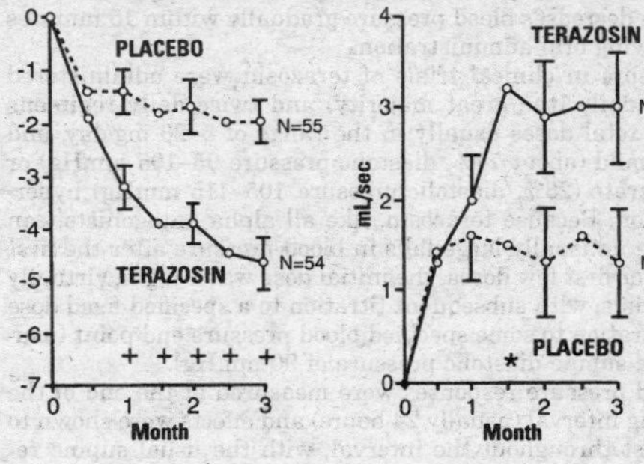

+ for baseline values see above table
* p ≤ 0.05, compared to placebo group

Figure 2
Mean Change in Total Symptom Score from Baseline Long-Term, Open-Label, Non-Placebo Controlled Study (N=494)

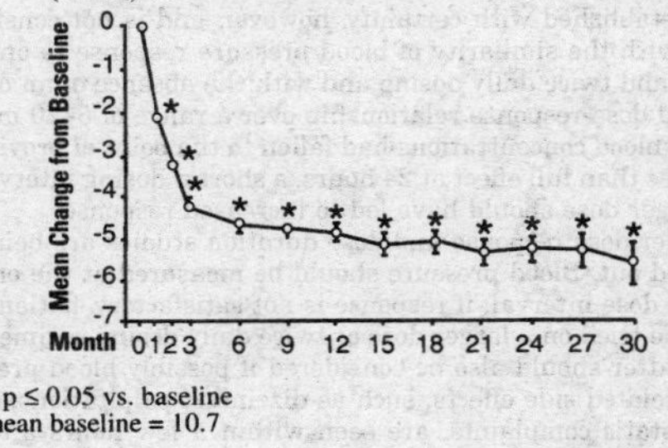

* p ≤ 0.05 vs. baseline
mean baseline = 10.7

Figure 3
Mean Change in Peak Flow Rate from Baseline Long-Term, Open-Label, Non-Placebo Controlled Study (N=494)

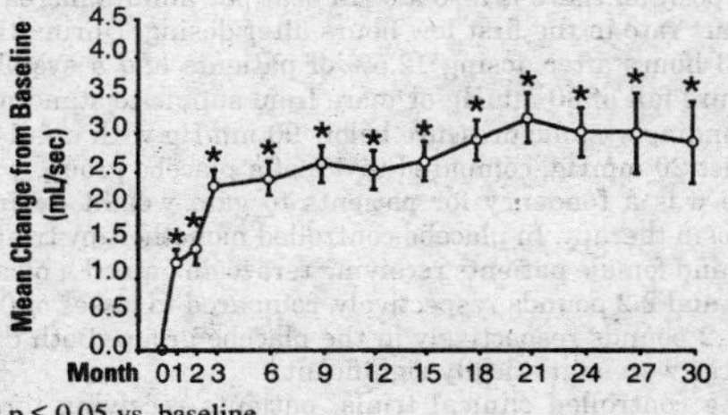

* p ≤ 0.05 vs. baseline
mean baseline = 9.9

In this long-term trial, both symptom scores and peak urinary flow rates showed statistically significant improvement suggesting a relaxation of smooth muscle cells.

Although blockade of alpha-1 adrenoceptors also lowers blood pressure in hypertensive patients with increased peripheral vascular resistance, terazosin treatment of normotensive men with BPH did not result in a clinically significant blood pressure lowering effect:

Mean Changes in Blood Pressure from Baseline to Final Visit in all Double-Blind, Placebo-Controlled Studies

	Group	Normotensive Patients DBP ≤90 mm Hg N	Mean Change	Hypertensive Patients DBP >90 mm Hg N	Mean Change
SBP (mm Hg)	**Placebo**	293	−0.1	45	−5.8
	Terazosin	519	−3.3*	65	−14.4*
DBP (mm Hg)	**Placebo**	293	+0.4	45	−7.1
	Terazosin	519	−2.2*	65	−15.1*

*p ≤ 0.05 vs. placebo

B. Hypertension

In animals, terazosin causes a decrease in blood pressure by decreasing total peripheral vascular resistance. The vasodilatory hypotensive action of terazosin appears to be pro-

Continued on next page

Hytrin—Cont.

duced mainly by blockade of alpha-1 adrenoceptors. Terazosin decreases blood pressure gradually within 15 minutes following oral administration.

Patients in clinical trials of terazosin were administered once daily (the great majority) and twice daily regimens with total doses usually in the range of 5–20 mg/day, and had mild (about 77%, diastolic pressure 95–105 mmHg) or moderate (23%, diastolic pressure 105–115 mmHg) hypertension. Because terazosin, like all alpha antagonists, can cause unusually large falls in blood pressure after the first dose or first few doses, the initial dose was 1 mg in virtually all trials, with subsequent titration to a specified fixed dose or titration to some specified blood pressure end point (usually a supine diastolic pressure of 90 mmHg).

Blood pressure responses were measured at the end of the dosing interval (usually 24 hours) and effects were shown to persist throughout the interval, with the usual supine responses 5–10 mmHg systolic and 3.5–8 mmHg diastolic greater than placebo. The responses in the standing position tended to be somewhat larger, by 1–3 mmHg, although this was not true in all studies. The magnitude of the blood pressure responses was similar to prazosin and less than hydrochlorothiazide (in a single study of hypertensive patients). In measurements 24 hours after dosing, heart rate was unchanged.

Limited measurements of peak response (2–3 hours after dosing) during chronic terazosin administration indicate that it is greater than about twice the trough (24 hour) response, suggesting some attenuation of response at 24 hours, presumably due to a fall in blood terazosin concentrations at the end of the dose interval. This explanation is not established with certainty, however, and is not consistent with the similarity of blood pressure response to once daily and twice daily dosing and with the absence of an observed dose-response relationship over a range of 5–20 mg, i.e., if blood concentrations had fallen to the point of providing less than full effect at 24 hours, a shorter dosing interval or larger dose should have led to increased response.

Further dose response and dose duration studies are being carried out. Blood pressure should be measured at the end of the dose interval; if response is not satisfactory, patients may be tried on a larger dose or twice daily dosing regimen. The latter should also be considered if possibly blood pressure-related side effects, such as dizziness, palpitations, or orthostatic complaints, are seen within a few hours after dosing.

The greater blood pressure effect associated with peak plasma concentrations (first few hours after dosing) appears somewhat more position-dependent (greater in the erect position) than the effect of terazosin at 24 hours and in the erect position there is also a 6–10 beat per minute increase in heart rate in the first few hours after dosing. During the first 3 hours after dosing 12.5% of patients had a systolic pressure fall of 30 mmHg or more from supine to standing, or standing systolic pressure below 90 mmHg with a fall of at least 20 mmHg, compared to 4% of a placebo group.

There was a tendency for patients to gain weight during terazosin therapy. In placebo-controlled monotherapy trials, male and female patients receiving terazosin gained a mean of 1.7 and 2.2 pounds respectively, compared to losses of 0.2 and 1.2 pounds respectively in the placebo group. Both differences were statistically significant.

During controlled clinical trials, patients receiving terazosin monotherapy had a small but statistically significant decrease (a 3% fall) compared to placebo in total cholesterol and the combined low-density and very-low-density lipoprotein fractions. No significant changes were observed in high-density lipoprotein fraction and triglycerides compared to placebo.

Analysis of clinical laboratory data following administration of terazosin suggested the possibility of hemodilution based on decreases in hematocrit, hemoglobin, white blood cells, total protein and albumin. Decreases in hematocrit and total protein have been observed with alpha-blockade and are attributed to hemodilution.

Pharmacokinetics:

Terazosin hydrochloride administered as HYTRIN capsules is essentially completely absorbed in man. Administration of capsules immediately after meals had a minimal effect on the extent of absorption. The time to reach peak plasma concentration however, was delayed by about 40 minutes. Terazosin has been shown to undergo minimal hepatic first-pass metabolism and nearly all of the circulating dose is in the form of parent drug. The plasma levels peak about one hour after dosing, and then decline with a half-life of approximately 12 hours. In a study that evaluated the effect of age on terazosin pharmacokinetics, the mean plasma half-lives were 14.0 and 11.4 hours for the age group ≥ 70 years and the age group of 20–39 years, respectively. After oral administration the plasma clearance was decreased by 31.7% in patients 70 years of age or older compared to that in patients 20–39 years of age.

The drug is 90–94% bound to plasma proteins and binding is constant over the clinically observed concentration range. Approximately 10% of an orally administered dose is excreted as parent drug in the urine and approximately 20% is excreted in the feces. The remainder is eliminated as metabolites. Impaired renal function had no significant effect on the elimination of terazosin, and dosage adjustment of terazosin to compensate for the drug removal during hemodialysis (approximately 10%) does not appear to be necessary. Overall, approximately 40% of the administered dose is excreted in the urine and approximately 60% in the feces. The disposition of the compound in animals is qualitatively similar to that in man.

INDICATIONS AND USAGE

HYTRIN (terazosin hydrochloride) is indicated for the treatment of symptomatic benign prostatic hyperplasia (BPH). There is a rapid response, with approximately 70% of patients experiencing an increase in urinary flow and improvement in symptoms of BPH when treated with HYTRIN. The long-term effects of HYTRIN on the incidence of surgery, acute urinary obstruction or other complications of BPH are yet to be determined.

HYTRIN is also indicated for the treatment of hypertension. It can be used alone or in combination with other antihypertensive agents such as diuretics or beta-adrenergic blocking agents.

CONTRAINDICATIONS

HYTRIN capsules are contraindicated in patients known to be hypersensitive to terazosin hydrochloride.

WARNINGS

Syncope and "First-dose" Effect:

HYTRIN capsules, like other alpha-adrenergic blocking agents, can cause marked lowering of blood pressure, especially postural hypotension, and syncope in association with the first dose or first few days of therapy. A similar effect can be anticipated if therapy is interrupted for several days and then restarted. Syncope has also been reported with other alpha-adrenergic blocking agents in association with rapid dosage increases or the introduction of another antihypertensive drug. Syncope is believed to be due to an excessive postural hypotensive effect, although occasionally the syncopal episode has been preceded by a bout of severe supraventricular tachycardia with heart rates of 120–160 beats per minute. Additionally, the possibility of the contribution of hemodilution to the symptoms of postural hypotension should be considered. To decrease the likelihood of syncope or excessive hypotension, treatment should always be initiated with a 1 mg dose of terazosin, given at bedtime. The 2 mg, 5 mg and 10 mg capsules are not indicated as initial therapy. Dosage should then be increased slowly, according to recommendations in the Dosage and Administration section and additional antihypertensive agents should be added with caution. The patient should be cautioned to avoid situations, such as driving or hazardous tasks, where injury could result should syncope occur during initiation of therapy.

In early investigational studies, where increasing single doses up to 7.5 mg were given at 3 day intervals, tolerance to the first dose phenomenon did not necessarily develop and the "first-dose" effect could be observed at all doses. Syncopal episodes occurred in 3 of the 14 subjects given terazosin at doses of 2.5, 5 and 7.5 mg, which are higher than the recommended initial dose; in addition, severe orthostatic hypotension (blood pressure falling to 50/0 mmHg) was seen in two others and dizziness, tachycardia, and lightheadedness occurred in most subjects. These adverse effects all occurred within 90 minutes of dosing.

In three placebo-controlled BPH studies 1, 2, and 3 (see CLINICAL PHARMACOLOGY), the incidence of postural hypotension in the terazosin treated patients was 5.1%, 5.2%, and 3.7% respectively.

In multiple dose clinical trials involving nearly 2000 hypertensive patients treated with terazosin, syncope was reported in about 1% of patients. Syncope was not necessarily associated only with the first dose.

If syncope occurs, the patient should be placed in a recumbent position and treated supportively as necessary. There is evidence that the orthostatic effect of terazosin is greater, even in chronic use, shortly after dosing. The risk of the events is greatest during the initial seven days of treatment, but continues at all time intervals.

Priapism:

Rarely, (probably less than once in every several thousand patients) terazosin and other α_1-antagonists have been associated with priapism (painful penile erection, sustained for hours and unrelieved by sexual intercourse or masturbation). Two or three dozen cases have been reported. Because this condition can lead to permanent impotence if not promptly treated, patients must be advised about the seriousness of the condition (see **PRECAUTIONS: Information for Patients**).

PRECAUTIONS

General:

Prostatic Cancer

Carcinoma of the prostate and BPH cause many of the same symptoms. These two diseases frequently co-exist. Therefore, patients thought to have BPH should be examined prior to starting HYTRIN therapy to rule out the presence of carcinoma of the prostate.

Orthostatic Hypotension

While syncope is the most severe orthostatic effect of terazosin (see Warnings), other symptoms of lowered blood pressure, such as dizziness, lightheadedness and palpitations, were more common and occurred in some 28% of patients in clinical trials of hypertension. In BPH clinical trials, 21% of the patients experienced one or more of the following: dizziness, hypotension, postural hypotension, syncope, and vertigo. Patients with occupations in which such events represent potential problems should be treated with particular caution.

Information for Patients (see Patient Package Insert):

Patients should be made aware of the possibility of syncopal and orthostatic symptoms, especially at the initiation of therapy, and to avoid driving or hazardous tasks for 12 hours after the first dose, after a dosage increase and after interruption of therapy when treatment is resumed. They should be cautioned to avoid situations where injury could result should syncope occur during initiation of terazosin therapy. They should also be advised of the need to sit or lie down when symptoms of lowered blood pressure occur, although these symptoms are not always orthostatic, and to be careful when rising from a sitting or lying position. If dizziness, lightheadedness, or palpitations are bothersome they should be reported to the physician, so that dose adjustment can be considered.

Patients should also be told that drowsiness or somnolence can occur with terazosin, requiring caution in people who must drive or operate heavy machinery.

Patients should be advised about the possibility of priapism as a result of treatment with HYTRIN and other similar medications. Patients should know that this reaction to HYTRIN is extremely rare, but that if it is not brought to immediate medical attention, it can lead to permanent erectile dysfunction (impotence).

Laboratory Tests:

Small but statistically significant decreases in hematocrit, hemoglobin, white blood cells, total protein and albumin were observed in controlled clinical trials. These laboratory findings suggested the possibility of hemodilution. Treatment with terazosin for up to 24 months had no significant effect on prostate specific antigen (PSA) levels.

Drug Interactions:

In controlled trials, terazosin has been added to diuretics, and several beta-adrenergic blockers; no unexpected interactions were observed. Terazosin has also been used in patients on a variety of concomitant therapies; while these were not formal interaction studies, no interactions were observed. Terazosin has been used concomitantly in at least 50 patients on the following drugs or drug classes: 1) analgesic/anti-inflammatory (e.g., acetaminophen, aspirin, codeine, ibuprofen, indomethacin); 2) antibiotics (e.g., erythromycin, trimethoprim and sulfamethoxazole); 3) anti cholinergic/sympathomimetics (e.g., phenylephrine hydrochloride, phenylpropanolamine hydrochloride, pseudoephedrine hydrochloride); 4) antigout (e.g., allopurinol); 5) antihistamines (e.g., chlorpheniramine); 6) cardiovascular agents (e.g., atenolol, hydrochlorothiazide, methyclothiazide, propranolol); 7) corticosteroids; 8) gastrointestinal agents (e.g., antacids); 9) hypoglycemics; 10) sedatives and tranquilizers (e.g., diazepam).

Use with Other Drugs:

In a study (n=24) where terazosin and verapamil were administered concomitantly, terazosin's mean AUC_{0-24} increased 11% after the first verapamil dose and after 3 weeks of verapamil treatment it increased by 24% with associated increases in C_{max}(25%) and C_{min} (32%) means. Terazosin mean T_{max} decreased from 1.3 hours to 0.8 hours after 3 weeks of verapamil treatment. Statistically significant differences were not found in the verapamil level with and without terazosin. In a study (n=6) where terazosin and captopril were administered concomitantly, plasma disposition of captopril was not influenced by concomitant administration of terazosin and terazosin maximum plasma concentrations increased linearly with dose at steady-state after administration of terazosin plus captopril (see Dosage and Administration).

Carcinogenesis, Mutagenesis, Impairment of Fertility:

Terazosin was devoid of mutagenic potential when evaluated *in vivo* and *in vitro* (the Ames test, *in vivo* cytogenetics, the dominant lethal test in mice, *in vivo* Chinese hamster chromosome aberration test and V79 forward mutation assay).

Terazosin, administered in the feed to rats at doses of 8, 40, and 250 mg/kg/day (70, 350, and 2100 mg/M^2/day), for two years, was associated with a statistically significant increase in benign adrenal medullary tumors of male rats exposed to the 250 mg/kg dose. This dose is 175 times the maximum recommended human dose of 20 mg (12 mg/M^2). Female rats were unaffected. Terazosin was not oncogenic in mice when administered in feed for 2 years at a maximum tolerated dose of 32 mg/kg/day (110 mg/M^2; 9 times the maximum recommended human dose). The absence of mutagenicity in a battery of tests, of tumorigenicity of any cell type in the mouse carcinogenicity assay, of increased total tumor incidence in either species, and of proliferative adrenal lesions in female rats, suggests a male rat species-specific event. Numerous other diverse pharmaceutical and chemical compounds have also been associated with benign adrenal medullary tumors in male rats without supporting evidence for carcinogenicity in man.

The effect of terazosin on fertility was assessed in a standard fertility/reproductive performance study in which male and female rats were administered oral doses of 8, 30 and 120 mg/kg/day. Four of 20 male rats given 30 mg/kg (240 mg/M^2; 20 times the maximum recommended human dose) and five of 19 male rats given 120 mg/kg (960 mg/M^2; 80 times the maximum recommended human dose) failed to sire a litter. Testicular weights and morphology were unaffected by treatment. Vaginal smears at 30 and 120 mg/kg/day, however, appeared to contain less sperm than smears from control matings and good correlation was reported between sperm count and subsequent pregnancy.

Oral administration of terazosin for one or two years elicited a statistically significant increase in the incidence of testicular atrophy in rats exposed to 40 and 250 mg/kg/day (29 and 175 times the maximum recommended human dose), but not in rats exposed to 8 mg/kg/day (> 6 times the maximum recommended human dose). Testicular atrophy was also observed in dogs dosed with 300 mg/kg/day (> 500 times the maximum recommended human dose) for three months but not after one year when dosed with 20 mg/kg/day (38 times the maximum recommended human dose). This lesion has also been seen with Minipress®, another (marketed) selective-alpha-1 blocking agent.

Pregnancy:

Teratogenic effects: Pregnancy Category C. Terazosin was not teratogenic in either rats or rabbits when administered at oral doses up to 280 and 60 times, respectively, the maximum recommended human dose. Fetal resorptions occurred in rats dosed with 480 mg/kg/day, approximately 280 times the maximum recommended human dose. Increased fetal resorptions, decreased fetal weight and an increased number of supernumerary ribs were observed in offspring of rabbits dosed with 60 times the maximum recommended human dose. These findings (in both species) were most likely secondary to maternal toxicity. There are no adequate and well-controlled studies in pregnant women and the safety of terazosin in pregnancy has not been established. HYTRIN is not recommended during pregnancy unless the potential benefit justifies the potential risk to the mother and fetus.

Nonteratogenic effects: In a peri- and post-natal development study in rats, significantly more pups died in the group dosed with 120 mg/kg/day (> 75 times the maximum recommended human dose) than in the control group during the three-week postpartum period.

Nursing Mothers:

It is not known whether terazosin is excreted in breast milk. Because many drugs are excreted in breast milk, caution should be exercised when terazosin is administered to a nursing woman.

Pediatric Use:

Safety and effectiveness in children have not been determined.

ADVERSE REACTIONS

Benign Prostatic Hyperplasia

The incidence of treatment-emergent adverse events has been ascertained from clinical trials conducted worldwide. All adverse events reported during these trials were recorded as adverse reactions. The incidence rates presented below are based on combined data from six placebo-controlled trials involving once-a-day administration of terazosin at doses ranging from 1 to 20 mg. Table 1 summarizes those adverse events reported for patients in these trials when the incidence rate in the terazosin group was at least 1% and was greater than that for the placebo group, or where the reaction is of clinical interest. Asthenia, postural hypotension, dizziness, somnolence, nasal congestion/rhinitis, and impotence were the only events that were significantly ($p \leq 0.05$) more common in patients receiving terazosin than in patients receiving placebo. The incidence of urinary tract infection was significantly lower in the patients receiving terazosin than in patients receiving placebo. An analysis of the incidence rate of hypotensive adverse events (see PRECAUTIONS) adjusted for the length of drug treatment has shown that the risk of the events is greatest during the initial seven days of treatment, but continues at all time intervals.

TABLE 1
ADVERSE REACTIONS DURING PLACEBO-CONTROLLED TRIALS BENIGN PROSTATIC HYPERPLASIA

Body System	Terazosin (N=636)	Placebo (N=360)
BODY AS A WHOLE		
† Asthenia	7.4%*	3.3%
Flu Syndrome	2.4%	1.7%
Headache	4.9%	5.8%
CARDIOVASCULAR SYSTEM		
Hypotension	0.6%	0.6%
Palpitations	0.9%	1.1%
Postural Hypotension	3.9%*	0.8%
Syncope	0.6%	0.0%
DIGESTIVE SYSTEM		
Nausea	1.7%	1.1%
METABOLIC AND NUTRITIONAL DISORDERS		
Peripheral Edema	0.9%	0.3%
Weight Gain	0.5%	0.0%
NERVOUS SYSTEM		
Dizziness	9.1%*	4.2%
Somnolence	3.6%*	1.9%
Vertigo	1.4%	0.3%
RESPIRATORY SYSTEM		
Dyspnea	1.7%	0.8%
Nasal Congestion/Rhinitis	1.9%*	0.0%
SPECIAL SENSES		
Blurred Vision/Amblyopia	1.3%	0.6%
UROGENITAL SYSTEM		
Impotence	1.6%*	0.6%
Urinary Tract Infection	1.3%	3.9%*

† Includes weakness, tiredness, lassitude and fatigue.
* $p \leq 0.05$ comparison between groups.

Additional adverse events have been reported, but these are, in general, not distinguishable from symptoms that might have occurred in the absence of exposure to terazosin. The safety profile of patients treated in the long-term open-label study was similar to that observed in the controlled studies.

The adverse events were usually transient and mild or moderate in intensity, but sometimes were serious enough to interrupt treatment. In the placebo-controlled clinical trials, the rates of premature termination due to adverse events were not statistically different between the placebo and terazosin groups. The adverse events that were bothersome, as judged by their being reported as reasons for discontinuation of therapy by at least 0.5% of the terazosin group and being reported more often than in the placebo group, are shown in Table 2.

TABLE 2
DISCONTINUATION DURING PLACEBO-CONTROLLED TRIALS BENIGN PROSTATIC HYPERPLASIA

Body System	Terazosin (N=636)	Placebo (N=360)
BODY AS A WHOLE		
Fever	0.5%	0.0%
Headache	1.1%	0.8%
CARDIOVASCULAR SYSTEM		
Postural Hypotension	0.5%	0.0%
Syncope	0.5%	0.0%
DIGESTIVE SYSTEM		
Nausea	0.5%	0.3%
NERVOUS SYSTEM		
Dizziness	2.0%	1.1%
Vertigo	0.5%	0.0%
RESPIRATORY SYSTEM		
Dyspnea	0.5%	0.3%
SPECIAL SENSES		
Blurred Vision/Amblyopia	0.6%	0.0%
UROGENITAL SYSTEM		
Urinary Tract Infection	0.5%	0.3%

Hypertension

The prevalence of adverse reactions has been ascertained from clinical trials conducted primarily in the United States. All adverse experiences (events) reported during these trials were recorded as adverse reactions. The prevalence rates presented below are based on combined data from fourteen placebo-controlled trials involving once-a-day administration of terazosin, as monotherapy or in combination with other antihypertensive agents, at doses ranging from 1 to 40 mg. Table 3 summarizes those adverse experiences reported for patients in these trials where the prevalence rate in the terazosin group was at least 5%, where the prevalence rate for the terazosin group was at least 2% and was greater than the prevalence rate for the placebo group, or where the reaction is of particular interest. Asthenia, blurred vision, dizziness, nasal congestion, nausea, peripheral edema, palpitations and somnolence were the only symptoms that were significantly ($p < 0.05$) more common in patients receiving terazosin than in patients receiving placebo. Similar adverse reaction rates were observed in placebo-controlled monotherapy trials.

TABLE 3
ADVERSE REACTIONS DURING PLACEBO-CONTROLLED TRIALS HYPERTENSION

Body System	Terazosin (N=859)	Placebo (N=506)
BODY AS A WHOLE		
† Asthenia	11.3%*	4.3%
Back Pain	2.4%	1.2%
Headache	16.2%	15.8%
CARDIOVASCULAR SYSTEM		
Palpitations	4.3%*	1.2%
Postural Hypotension	1.3%	0.4%
Tachycardia	1.9%	1.2%
DIGESTIVE SYSTEM		
Nausea	4.4%*	1.4%
METABOLIC AND NUTRITIONAL DISORDERS		
Edema	0.9%	0.6%
Peripheral Edema	5.5%*	2.4%
Weight Gain	0.5%	0.2%
MUSCULOSKELETAL SYSTEM		
Pain-Extremities	3.5%	3.0%
NERVOUS SYSTEM		
Depression	0.3%	0.2%
Dizziness	19.3%*	7.5%
Libido Decreased	0.6%	0.2%
Nervousness	2.3%	1.8%
Paresthesia	2.9%	1.4%
Somnolence	5.4%*	2.6%
RESPIRATORY SYSTEM		
Dyspnea	3.1%	2.4%
Nasal Congestion	5.9%*	3.4%
Sinusitis	2.6%	1.4%
SPECIAL SENSES		
Blurred Vision	1.6%*	0.0%
UROGENITAL SYSTEM		
Impotence	1.2%	1.4%

† Includes weakness, tiredness, lassitude and fatigue.
* Statistically significant at p=0.05 level.

Additional adverse reactions have been reported, but these are, in general, not distinguishable from symptoms that might have occurred in the absence of exposure to terazosin. The following additional adverse reactions were reported by at least 1% of 1987 patients who received terazosin in controlled or open, short- or long-term clinical trials or have been reported during marketing experience: *Body as a Whole:* chest pain, facial edema, fever, abdominal pain, neck pain, shoulder pain; *Cardiovascular System:* arrhythmia, vasodilation; *Digestive System:* constipation, diarrhea, dry mouth, dyspepsia, flatulence, vomiting; *Metabolic/Nutritional Disorders:* gout; *Musculoskeletal System:* arthralgia, arthritis, joint disorder, myalgia; *Nervous System:* anxiety, insomnia; *Respiratory System:* bronchitis, cold symptoms, epistaxis, flu symptoms, increased cough, pharyngitis, rhinitis; *Skin and Appendages:* pruritus, rash, sweating; *Special Senses:* abnormal vision, conjunctivitis, tinnitus; *Urogenital System:* urinary frequency, urinary incontinence primarily reported in postmenopausal women, urinary tract infection.

Post-marketing experience indicates that in rare instances patients may develop allergic reactions, including anaphylaxis, following administration of terazosin hydrochloride. There have been reports of priapism during post-marketing surveillance.

The adverse reactions were usually mild or moderate in intensity but sometimes were serious enough to interrupt treatment. The adverse reactions that were most bothersome, as judged by their being reported as reasons for discontinuation of therapy by at least 0.5% of the terazosin group and being reported more often than in the placebo group, are shown in Table 4.

TABLE 4
DISCONTINUATIONS DURING PLACEBO-CONTROLLED TRIALS HYPERTENSION

Body System	Terazosin (N=859)	Placebo (N=506)
BODY AS A WHOLE		
Asthenia	1.6%	0.0%
Headache	1.3%	1.0%
CARDIOVASCULAR SYSTEM		
Palpitations	1.4%	0.2%
Postural Hypotension	0.5%	0.0%
Syncope	0.5%	0.2%
Tachycardia	0.6%	0.0%
DIGESTIVE SYSTEM		
Nausea	0.8%	0.0%
METABOLIC AND NUTRITIONAL DISORDERS		
Peripheral Edema	0.6%	0.0%
NERVOUS SYSTEM		
Dizziness	3.1%	0.4%
Paresthesia	0.8%	0.2%
Somnolence	0.6%	0.2%
RESPIRATORY SYSTEM		
Dyspnea	0.9%	0.6%
Nasal Congestion	0.6%	0.0%
SPECIAL SENSES		
Blurred Vision	0.6%	0.0%

OVERDOSAGE

Should overdosage of HYTRIN lead to hypotension, support of the cardiovascular system is of first importance. Restoration of blood pressure and normalization of heart rate may be accomplished by keeping the patient in the supine position. If this measure is inadequate, shock should first be treated with volume expanders. If necessary, vasopressors

Continued on next page

Hytrin—Cont.

should then be used and renal function should be monitored and supported as needed. Laboratory data indicate that terazosin is 90–94% protein bound; therefore, dialysis may not be of benefit.

DOSAGE AND ADMINISTRATION

If HYTRIN administration is discontinued for several days, therapy should be reinstituted using the initial dosing regimen.

Benign Prostatic Hyperplasia:

Initial Dose:

1 mg at bedtime is the starting dose for all patients, and this dose should not be exceeded as an initial dose. Patients should be closely followed during initial administration in order to minimize the risk of severe hypotensive response.

Subsequent Doses:

The dose should be increased in a stepwise fashion to 2 mg, 5 mg, or 10 mg once daily to achieve the desired improvement of symptoms and/or flow rates. Doses of 10 mg once daily are generally required for the clinical response. Therefore, treatment with 10 mg for a minimum of 4–6 weeks may be required to assess whether a beneficial response has been achieved. Some patients may not achieve a clinical response despite appropriate titration. Although some additional patients responded at a 20 mg daily dose, there was an insufficient number of patients studied to draw definitive conclusions about this dose. There are insufficient data to support the use of higher doses for those patients who show inadequate or no response to 20 mg daily. **If terazosin administration is discontinued for several days or longer, therapy should be reinstituted using the initial dosing regimen.**

Use with Other Drugs:

Caution should be observed when HYTRIN is administered concomitantly with other antihypertensive agents, especially the calcium channel blocker verapamil, to avoid the possibility of developing significant hypotension. When using HYTRIN and other antihypertensive agents concomitantly, dosage reduction and retitration of either agent may be necessary (see Precautions).

Hypertension:

The dose of HYTRIN and the dose interval (12 or 24 hours) should be adjusted according to the patient's individual blood pressure response. The following is a guide to its administration:

Initial Dose:

1 mg at bedtime is the starting dose for all patients, and this dose should not be exceeded. This initial dosing regimen should be strictly observed to minimize the potential for severe hypotensive effects.

Subsequent Doses:

The dose may be slowly increased to achieve the desired blood pressure response. The usual recommended dose range is 1 mg to 5 mg administered once a day; however, some patients may benefit from doses as high as 20 mg per day. Doses over 20 mg do not appear to provide further blood pressure effect and doses over 40 mg have not been studied. Blood pressure should be monitored at the end of the dosing interval to be sure control is maintained throughout the interval. It may also be helpful to measure blood pressure 2–3 hours after dosing to see if the maximum and minimum responses are similar, and to evaluate symptoms such as dizziness or palpitations which can result from excessive hypotensive response. If response is substantially diminished at 24 hours an increased dose or use of a twice daily regimen can be considered. **If terazosin administration is discontinued for several days or longer, therapy should be reinstituted using the initial dosing regimen.** In clinical trials, except for the initial dose, the dose was given in the morning.

Use With Other Drugs: (see above)

HOW SUPPLIED

HYTRIN capsules (terazosin hydrochloride capsules) are available in four dosage strengths:

1 mg grey capsules (imprinted with ⊟ and the Abbo-Code HH):

Bottles of 100 .... (**NDC** 0074-3805-13),
Abbo-Pac® unit dose strip packages
of 100 capsules .... (**NDC** 0074-3805-11).

2 mg yellow capsules (imprinted with ⊟ and the Abbo-Code HY):

Bottles of 100 .... (**NDC** 0074-3806-13),
Abbo-Pac® unit dose strip packages
of 100 capsules .... (**NDC** 0074-3806-11).

5 mg red capsules (imprinted with ⊟ and the Abbo-Code HK):

Bottles of 100 .... (**NDC** 0074-3807-13),
Abbo-Pac® unit dose strip packages
of 100 capsules .... (**NDC** 0074-3807-11).

10 mg blue capsules (imprinted with ⊟ and the Abbo-Code HN):

Bottles of 100 .... (**NDC** 0074-3808-13),
Abbo-Pac® unit dose strip packages
of 100 capsules .... (**NDC** 0074-3808-11).

Recommended storage: Store at controlled room temperature between 20–25°C (68–77°F). See USP. Protect from light and moisture.

Revised: October, 1996
Ref. 03-4655-R3-Rev. Oct., 1996
ABBOTT LABORATORIES
NORTH CHICAGO, IL 60064, U.S.A

PATIENT INFORMATION ABOUT HYTRIN® (HI-TRIN)

Generic Name: terazosin (ter-A-zo-sin) hydrochloride
When used to treat
HYPERTENSION or BENIGN PROSTATIC HYPERPLASIA (BPH)

Please read this leaflet before you start taking HYTRIN. Also, read it each time you get a new prescription. This is a summary and should NOT take the place of a full discussion with your doctor who has additional information about HYTRIN. You and your doctor should discuss HYTRIN and your condition before you start taking it and at your regular check-ups.

HYTRIN is used to treat high blood pressure (hypertension). HYTRIN is also used to treat benign prostatic hyperplasia (BPH) in men. This leaflet describes HYTRIN as a treatment for hypertension or BPH.

What is hypertension (high blood pressure)?

Blood pressure is the tension of the blood within the blood vessels. If blood is pumped too forcefully, or if the blood vessels are too narrow, the pressure of the blood against the walls of the vessels rises.

If high blood pressure is not treated, over time, the increased pressure can damage blood vessels or it can cause the heart to work too hard and may decrease the flow of blood to the heart, brain, and kidneys. As a result, these organs may become damaged and not function correctly. If high blood pressure is controlled, this damage is less likely to happen.

Treatment options for hypertension

Non-drug treatments are sometimes effective in controlling mild hypertension. The most important lifestyle changes to lower blood pressure are to lose weight, reduce salt, fat, and alcohol in the diet, quit smoking, and exercise regularly. However, many hypertensive patients require one or more ongoing medications to control their blood pressure. There are different kinds of medication used to treat hypertension. Your doctor has prescribed HYTRIN for you.

What HYTRIN does to treat hypertension

HYTRIN works by relaxing blood vessels so that blood passes through them more easily. This helps to lower blood pressure.

What is BPH?

The prostate is a gland located below the bladder of men. It surrounds the urethra (you-REETH-rah), which is a tube that drains urine from the bladder. BPH is an enlargement of the prostate gland. The symptoms of BPH, however, can be caused by an increase in the tightness of muscles in the prostate. If the muscles inside the prostate tighten, they can squeeze the urethra and slow the flow of urine. This can lead to symptoms such as:

- a weak or interrupted stream when urinating
- a feeling that you cannot empty your bladder completely
- a feeling of delay when you start to urinate
- a need to urinate often, especially at night, or
- a feeling that you must urinate right away.

Treatment options for BPH:

There are three main treatment options for BPH:

- Program of monitoring or "Watchful Waiting". Some men have an enlarged prostate gland, but no symptoms, or symptoms that are not bothersome. If this applies, you and your doctor may decide on a program of monitoring including regular checkups, instead of medication or surgery.
- Medication. There are different kinds of medication used to treat BPH. Your doctor has prescribed HYTRIN for you. See "What HYTRIN does to treat BPH" below.
- Surgery. Some patients may need surgery. Your doctor can describe several different surgical procedures to treat BPH. Which procedure is best depends on your symptoms and medical condition.

What HYTRIN does to treat BPH

HYTRIN relaxes the tightness of a certain type of muscle in the prostate and at the opening of the bladder. This may increase the rate of urine flow and/or decrease the symptoms you are having.

- HYTRIN helps relieve the symptoms of BPH. It does NOT change the size of the prostate, which may continue to grow. However, a larger prostate does not necessarily cause more or worse symptoms.
- If HYTRIN is helping you, you should notice an effect on your particular symptoms in 2 to 4 weeks of starting to take the medication.
- Even though you take HYTRIN and it may help you, HYTRIN may not prevent the need for surgery in the future.

Other important facts about HYTRIN for BPH

- You should see an effect on your symptoms in 2 to 4 weeks. So, you will need to continue seeing your doctor to check your progress regarding your blood pressure in addition to your other regular check-ups.
- Your doctor has prescribed HYTRIN for your BPH and not for prostate cancer. However, a man can have BPH and prostate cancer at the same time. Doctors usually recommend that men be checked for prostate cancer once a year when they turn 50 (or 40 if a family member has had prostate cancer). These checks should continue even if you are taking HYTRIN. HYTRIN is not a treatment for prostate cancer.
- About Prostate Specific Antigen (PSA). Your doctor may have done a blood test called PSA. Your doctor is aware that HYTRIN does not affect PSA levels. You may want to ask your doctor more about this if you have had a PSA test done.

What you should know while taking HYTRIN for hypertension or BPH

WARNINGS

HYTRIN Can Cause A Sudden Drop in Blood Pressure After the VERY FIRST DOSE. You may feel dizzy, faint, or "lightheaded" particularly after you get up from bed or from a chair. This is more likely to occur after you've taken the first few doses, but can occur at any time while you are taking the drug. It can also occur if you stop taking the drug and then re-start treatment.

Because of this effect, your doctor may have told you to take HYTRIN at bedtime. If you take HYTRIN at bedtime but need to get up from bed to go to the bathroom, get up slowly and cautiously until you are sure how the medicine affects you. It is also important to get up slowly from a chair or bed at any time until you learn how you react to HYTRIN. You should not drive or do any hazardous tasks until you are used to the effects of the medication. If you begin to feel dizzy, sit or lie down until you feel better.

- You will start with a 1 mg dose of HYTRIN. Then the dose will be increased as your body gets used to the effect of the medication.
- Other side effects you could have while taking HYTRIN include drowsiness, blurred or hazy vision, nausea, or "puffiness" of the feet or hands. Discuss any unexpected effects you notice with your doctor.

Extremely rarely, HYTRIN and similar medications have caused painful erection of the penis, sustained for hours and unrelieved by sexual intercourse or masturbation. This condition is serious, and if untreated it can be followed by permanent inability to have an erection. If you have a prolonged abnormal erection, call your doctor or go to an emergency room as soon as possible.

How to take HYTRIN

Follow your doctor's instructions about how to take HYTRIN. You must take it every day at the dose prescribed. Talk with your doctor if you don't take if for a few days, you may have to restart it at a 1 mg dose and be cautious about possible dizziness. Do not share HYTRIN with anyone else; it was prescribed only for you.

Keep HYTRIN and all medicines out of the reach of children.

Store capsules between 68-77°F (20-25°C).

Protect from light and moisture.

FOR MORE INFORMATION ABOUT HYTRIN AND HYPERTENSION OR BPH, TALK WITH YOUR DOCTOR, NURSE, PHARMACIST OR HEALTH CARE PROVIDER.

Revised Oct., 1999
Ref. 03-4995-R2-Rev. Oct., 1999
ABBOTT LABORATORIES
NORTH CHICAGO, IL 60064, U.S.A
PRINTED IN U.S.A.

Shown in Product Identification Guide, page 303

IBERET–FOLIC–500® Filmtab® Tablets ℞

Controlled-Release Iron with Vitamin C, and B-Complex including Folic Acid

See combined listing under FERO-FOLIC-500.

K–LOR™ 20 mEq. ℞

[k 'lor]

(Potassium Chloride for Oral Solution, USP)

DESCRIPTION

Natural fruit-flavored K-LOR (potassium chloride for oral solution, USP) is an oral potassium supplement offered in individual packets as a powder for reconstitution. Each packet of K-LOR 20 mEq powder contains potassium 20 mEq and chloride 20 mEq provided by potassium chloride 1.5 g.

K-LOR powder is an electrolyte replenisher. The chemical name is potassium chloride, and the structural formula is KCl. Potassium chloride, USP, occurs as a white, granular powder or as colorless crystals. It is odorless and has a saline taste. Its solutions are neutral to litmus. It is freely soluble in water and insoluble in alcohol.

Inactive Ingredients: FD&C Yellow No. 6, maltodextrin (contains corn derivative), malic acid, saccharin, silica gel and natural flavoring.

CLINICAL PHARMACOLOGY

Potassium ion is the principal intracellular cation of most body tissues. Potassium ions participate in a number of essential physiological processes including the maintenance of intracellular tonicity, the transmission of nerve impulses, the contraction of cardiac, skeletal and smooth muscle, and the maintenance of normal renal function.

The intracellular concentration of potassium is approximately 150 to 160 mEq per liter. The normal adult plasma concentration is 3.5 to 5 mEq per liter. An active ion transport system maintains this gradient across the plasma membrane.

Potassium is a normal dietary constituent and under steady state conditions the amount of potassium absorbed from the gastrointestinal tract is equal to the amount excreted in the urine. The usual dietary intake of potassium is 50 to 100 mEq per day.

Potassium depletion will occur whenever the rate of potassium loss through renal excretion and/or loss from the gastrointestinal tract exceeds the rate of potassium intake. Such depletion usually develops as a consequence of therapy with diuretics, primary or secondary hyperaldosteronism, diabetic ketoacidosis, or inadequate replacement of potassium in patients on prolonged parenteral nutrition. Depletion can develop rapidly with severe diarrhea, especially if associated with vomiting. Potassium depletion due to these causes is usually accompanied by a concomitant loss of chloride and is manifested by hypokalemia and metabolic alkalosis. Potassium depletion may produce weakness, fatigue, disturbances of cardiac rhythm (primarily ectopic beats), prominent U-waves in the electrocardiogram, and, in advanced cases, flaccid paralysis and/or impaired ability to concentrate urine.

If potassium depletion associated with metabolic alkalosis cannot be managed by correcting the fundamental cause of the deficiency, e.g., where the patient requires long term diuretic therapy, supplemental potassium in the form of high potassium food or potassium chloride may restore normal potassium levels.

In rare circumstances, (e.g., patients with renal tubular acidosis), potassium depletion may be associated with metabolic acidosis and hyperchloremia. In such patients potassium replacement should be accomplished with potassium salts other than the chloride, such as potassium bicarbonate, potassium citrate, potassium acetate, or potassium gluconate.

INDICATIONS AND USAGE

1. For the treatment of patients with hypokalemia with or without metabolic alkalosis, in digitalis intoxication, and in patients with hypokalemic familial periodic paralysis. If hypokalemia is the result of diuretic therapy, consideration should be given to the use of a lower dose of diuretic, which may be sufficient without leading to hypokalemia.
2. For the prevention of hypokalemia in patients who would be at particular risk if hypokalemia were to develop, e.g., digitalized patients or patients with significant cardiac arrhythmias.

The use of potassium salts in patients receiving diuretics for uncomplicated essential hypertension is often unnecessary when such patients have a normal dietary pattern, and when low doses of the diuretic are used. Serum potassium should be checked periodically, however, and, if hypokalemia occurs, dietary supplementation with potassium-containing foods may be adequate to control milder cases. In more severe cases, and if dose adjustment of the diuretic is ineffective or unwarranted, supplementation with potassium salts may be indicated.

CONTRAINDICATIONS

Potassium supplements are contraindicated in patients with hyperkalemia since a further increase in serum potassium concentration in such patients can produce cardiac arrest. Hyperkalemia may complicate any of the following conditions: chronic renal failure, systemic acidosis such as diabetic acidosis, acute dehydration, extensive tissue breakdown as in severe burns, adrenal insufficiency, or the administration of a potassium-sparing diuretic, e.g., spironolactone, triamterene, or amiloride (see OVERDOSAGE).

K-LOR (potassium chloride for oral solution) is contraindicated in patients with known hypersensitivity to any ingredient in this product.

WARNINGS

Hyperkalemia (See OVERDOSAGE)

In patients with impaired mechanisms for excreting potassium, the administration of potassium salts can produce hyperkalemia and cardiac arrest. This occurs most commonly in patients given potassium intravenously, but may also occur in patients given potassium orally. Potentially fatal hyperkalemia can develop rapidly and can be asymptomatic. The use of potassium salts in patients with chronic renal disease, or any other condition which impairs potassium excretion, requires particularly careful monitoring of the serum potassium concentration and appropriate dosage adjustment.

Interaction with Potassium-Sparing Diuretics

Hypokalemia should not be treated by the concomitant administration of potassium salts and a potassium-sparing diuretic, e.g., spironolactone, triamterene, or amiloride, since the simultaneous administration of these agents can produce severe hyperkalemia.

Interaction with Angiotensin Converting Enzyme Inhibitors

Angiotensin converting enzyme (ACE) inhibitors (e.g., captopril, enalapril) will produce some potassium retention by inhibiting aldosterone production. Potassium supplements should be given to patients receiving ACE inhibitors only with close monitoring.

Metabolic Acidosis

Hypokalemia in patients with metabolic acidosis should be treated with an alkalinizing potassium salt such as potassium bicarbonate, potassium citrate, potassium acetate or potassium gluconate.

PRECAUTIONS

General: The diagnosis of potassium depletion is ordinarily made by demonstrating hypokalemia in a patient with a clinical history suggesting some cause for potassium depletion. In interpreting the serum potassium level, the physician should bear in mind that acute alkalosis *per se* can produce hypokalemia in the absence of a deficit in total body potassium, while acute acidosis *per se* can increase the serum potassium concentration to within the normal range even in the presence of a reduced total body potassium. The treatment of potassium depletion, particularly in the presence of cardiac disease, renal disease, or acidosis, requires careful attention to acid-base balance and appropriate monitoring of serum electrolytes, the electrocardiogram, and the clinical status of the patient.

Information for Patients: Physicians should consider reminding the patient of the following:

To dilute each packet of powder in 1/2 glassful of water or other liquid and take each dose after a meal.

To take this medicine following the frequency and amount prescribed by the physician. This is especially important if the patient is also taking diuretics and/or digitalis preparations.

Laboratory Tests: When blood is drawn for analysis of plasma potassium it is important to recognize that artifactual elevations can occur after improper venipuncture technique or as a result of *in vitro* hemolysis of the sample.

Drug Interactions: Potassium-sparing diuretics, angiotensin converting enzyme inhibitors (see WARNINGS).

Carcinogenesis, Mutagenesis, Impairment of Fertility: Carcinogenicity, mutagenicity and fertility studies in animals have not been performed. Potassium is a normal dietary constituent.

Pregnancy Category C: Animal reproduction studies have not been conducted with K-LOR powder. It is unlikely that potassium supplementation that does not lead to hyperkalemia would have an adverse effect on the fetus or would affect reproductive capacity.

Nursing Mothers: The normal potassium ion content of human milk is about 13 mEq per liter. Since oral potassium becomes part of the body potassium pool, as long as body potassium is not excessive, the contribution of potassium chloride supplementation should have little or no effect on the level in human milk.

Pediatric Use: Safety and effectiveness in children have not been established.

ADVERSE REACTIONS

One of the most severe adverse effects is hyperkalemia (see CONTRAINDICATIONS, WARNINGS and OVERDOSAGE).

The most common adverse reactions to oral potassium salts are nausea, vomiting, flatulence, abdominal pain/discomfort, and diarrhea. These symptoms are due to irritation of the gastrointestinal tract and are best managed by diluting the preparation further, taking the dose with meals, or reducing the amount taken at one time.

Skin rash has been reported rarely.

OVERDOSAGE

The administration of oral potassium salts to persons with normal excretory mechanisms for potassium rarely causes serious hyperkalemia. However, if excretory mechanisms are impaired or if intravenous administration is too rapid, potentially fatal hyperkalemia can result (see CONTRAINDICATIONS and WARNINGS). It is important to recognize that hyperkalemia is usually asymptomatic and may be manifested only by an increased serum potassium concentration (6.5–8.0 mEq/L) and characteristic electrocardiographic changes (peaking of T-waves, loss of P-waves, depression of S-T segments, and prolongation of the QT intervals). Late manifestations include muscle paralysis and cardiovascular collapse from cardiac arrest (9–12 mEq/L).

Treatment measures for hyperkalemia include the following:

1. Elimination of foods and medications containing potassium and of any agents with potassium-sparing properties;
2. Intravenous administration of 300 to 500 ml/hr of 10% dextrose solution containing 10–20 units of crystalline insulin per 1,000 ml;
3. Correction of acidosis, if present, with intravenous sodium bicarbonate;
4. Use of exchange resins, hemodialysis, or peritoneal dialysis.

In treating hyperkalemia, it should be recalled that in patients who have been stabilized on digitalis, lowering the serum potassium concentration too rapidly can produce digitalis toxicity.

DOSAGE AND ADMINISTRATION

The usual dietary potassium intake by the average adult is 50 to 100 mEq per day. Potassium depletion sufficient to cause hypokalemia usually requires the loss of 200 or more mEq of potassium from the total body store.

Dosage must be adjusted to the individual needs of each patient. The dose for the prevention of hypokalemia is typically in the range of 20 mEq per day. Doses of 40–100 mEq per day or more are used for the treatment of potassium depletion. Dosage should be divided if more than 20 mEq per day is given such that no more than 20 mEq is given in a single dose. The dose should be taken after a meal.

K-LOR 20 mEq powder provides 20 mEq of potassium chloride.

Each 20 mEq (one K-LOR mEq packet) of potassium should be dissolved in at least 4 oz (approximately 1/2 glassful) cold water or juice. This preparation, like other potassium supplements, must be properly diluted to avoid the possibility of gastrointestinal irritation.

HOW SUPPLIED

K-LOR 20 mEq (Potassium Chloride for Oral Solution, USP) is supplied in cartons of 30 packets (**NDC** 0074-3611-01), and in cartons of 100 packets (**NDC** 0074-3611-02). Each packet contains potassium, 20 mEq, and chloride, 20 mEq, provided by potassium chloride, 1.5 g.

Recommended storage: Store below 86°F (30°C)

Caution: Federal (U.S.A.) law prohibits dispensing without prescription.

Revised: June, 1994

Ref. 13-1379-5/R2

K-Tab® ℞

[*k 'tâb*]

(Potassium Chloride Extended-Release Tablets, USP)

DESCRIPTION

K-TAB (potassium chloride extended-release tablets) is a solid oral dosage form of potassium chloride containing 750 mg of potassium chloride, USP, equivalent to 10 mEq of potassium in a film-coated (not enteric-coated), wax matrix tablet. This formulation is intended to slow the release of potassium so that the likelihood of a high localized concentration of potassium chloride within the gastrointestinal tract is reduced. The expended inert, porous, wax/polymer matrix is not absorbed and may be excreted intact in the stool.

K-TAB tablets are an electrolyte replenisher. The chemical name is potassium chloride, and the structural formula is KCl. Potassium chloride, USP, occurs as a white, granular powder or as colorless crystals. It is odorless and has a saline taste. Its solutions are neutral to litmus. It is freely soluble in water and insoluble in alcohol.

Inactive Ingredients

Castor oil, cellulosic polymers, colloidal silicon dioxide, D&C Yellow No. 10, magnesium stearate, paraffin, polyvinyl acetate, titanium dioxide, vanillin and vitamin E.

CLINICAL PHARMACOLOGY

Potassium ion is the principal intracellular cation of most body tissues. Potassium ions participate in a number of essential physiological processes including the maintenance of intracellular tonicity, the transmission of nerve impulses, the contraction of cardiac, skeletal, and smooth muscle, and the maintenance of normal renal function.

The intracellular concentration of potassium is approximately 150 to 160 mEq per liter. The normal adult plasma concentration is 3.5 to 5 mEq per liter. An active ion transport system maintains this gradient across the plasma membrane.

Potassium is a normal dietary constituent and under steady state conditions the amount of potassium absorbed from the gastrointestinal tract is equal to the amount excreted in the urine. The usual dietary intake of potassium is 50 to 100 mEq per day.

Potassium depletion will occur whenever the rate of potassium loss through renal excretion and/or loss from the gastrointestinal tract exceeds the rate of potassium intake. Such depletion usually develops as a consequence of therapy with diuretics, primary or secondary hyperaldosteronism, diabetic ketoacidosis, or inadequate replacement of potassium in patients on prolonged parenteral nutrition. Depletion can develop rapidly with severe diarrhea, especially if associated with vomiting. Potassium depletion due to these causes is usually accompanied by a concomitant loss of chloride and is manifested by hypokalemia and metabolic alkalosis. Potassium depletion may produce weakness, fatigue, disturbances of cardiac rhythm (primarily ectopic beats), prominent U-waves in the electrocardiogram, and, in advanced cases, flaccid paralysis and/or impaired ability to concentrate urine.

If potassium depletion associated with metabolic alkalosis cannot be managed by correcting the fundamental cause of the deficiency, e.g., where the patient requires long term diuretic therapy, supplemental potassium in the form of high potassium food or potassium chloride may restore normal potassium levels.

In rare circumstances, (e.g., patients with renal tubular acidosis) potassium depletion may be associated with metabolic acidosis and hyperchloremia. In such patients potassium replacement should be accomplished with potassium salts other than the chloride, such as potassium bicarbonate, potassium citrate, potassium acetate, or potassium gluconate.

INDICATIONS AND USAGE

BECAUSE OF REPORTS OF INTESTINAL AND GASTRIC ULCERATION AND BLEEDING WITH CONTROLLED-RELEASE POTASSIUM CHLORIDE PREPARATIONS, THESE DRUGS SHOULD BE RESERVED FOR THOSE PATIENTS WHO CANNOT TOLERATE OR REFUSE TO TAKE LIQUID OR EFFERVESCENT POTASSIUM PREPARATIONS, OR FOR PATIENTS WITH WHOM THERE IS A PROBLEM OF COMPLIANCE WITH THESE PREPARATIONS.

1. For the treatment of patients with hypokalemia with or without metabolic alkalosis, in digitalis intoxication, and in patients with hypokalemic familial periodic paralysis. If hypokalemia is the result of diuretic therapy, consideration should be given to the use of a lower dose of diuretic, which may be sufficient without leading to hypokalemia.

Continued on next page

K-Tab—Cont.

2. For the prevention of hypokalemia in patients who would be at particular risk if hypokalemia were to develop, e.g., digitalized patients or patients with significant cardiac arrhythmias.

The use of potassium salts in patients receiving diuretics for uncomplicated essential hypertension is often unnecessary when such patients have a normal dietary pattern, and when low doses of the diuretic are used. Serum potassium should be checked periodically, however, and, if hypokalemia occurs, dietary supplementation with potassium-containing foods may be adequate to control milder cases. In more severe cases and if dose adjustment of the diuretic is ineffective or unwarranted supplementation with potassium salts may be indicated.

CONTRAINDICATIONS

Potassium supplements are contraindicated in patients with hyperkalemia since a further increase in serum potassium concentration in such patients can produce cardiac arrest. Hyperkalemia may complicate any of the following conditions: chronic renal failure, systemic acidosis such as diabetic acidosis, acute dehydration, extensive tissue breakdown as in severe burns, adrenal insufficiency, or the administration of potassium-sparing diuretic, e.g., spironolactone, triamterene, or amiloride (see OVERDOSAGE).
K-TAB tablets are contraindicated in patients with known hypersensitivity to any ingredient in this product.
Controlled-release formulations of potassium chloride have produced esophageal ulceration in certain cardiac patients with esophageal compression due to an enlarged left atrium. Potassium supplementation, when indicated in such patients, should be given as a liquid preparation.
All solid oral dosage forms of potassium chloride are contraindicated in any patient in whom there is structural, pathological, e.g., diabetic gastroparesis, or pharmacologic (use of anticholinergic agents or other agents with anticholinergic properties at sufficient doses to exert anticholinergic effects) cause for arrest or delay in tablet passage through the gastrointestinal tract.

WARNINGS

Hyperkalemia (see OVERDOSAGE)
In patients with impaired mechanisms for excreting potassium, the administration of potassium salts can produce hyperkalemia and cardiac arrest. This occurs most commonly in patients given potassium intravenously, but may also occur in patients given potassium orally. Potentially fatal hyperkalemia can develop rapidly and can be asymptomatic. The use of potassium salts in patients with chronic renal disease, or any other condition which impairs potassium excretion, requires particularly careful monitoring of the serum potassium concentration and appropriate dosage adjustment.
Interaction with Potassium-Sparing Diuretics
Hypokalemia should not be treated by the concomitant administration of potassium salts and a potassium-sparing diuretic, e.g., spironolactone, triamterene, or amiloride, since the simultaneous administration of these agents can produce severe hyperkalemia.
Interaction with Angiotensin Converting Enzyme Inhibitors
Angiotensin converting enzyme (ACE) inhibitors (e.g., captopril, enalapril) will produce some potassium retention by inhibiting aldosterone production. Potassium supplements should be given to patients receiving ACE inhibitors only with close monitoring.
Gastrointestinal Lesions
Solid oral dosage forms of potassium chloride can produce ulcerative and/or stenotic lesions of the gastrointestinal tract. Based on spontaneous adverse reaction reports, enteric-coated preparations of potassium chloride are associated with an increased frequency of small bowel lesions (40-50 per 100,000 patient years) compared to sustained-release wax matrix formulations (less than one per 100,000 patient years). Because of the lack of extensive marketing experience with microencapsulated products, a comparison between such products and wax matrix or enteric-coated products is not available. K-TAB tablets consist of a wax matrix formulated to provide a controlled rate of release potassium chloride and thus to minimize the possibility of a high local concentration of potassium near the gastrointestinal wall.
Prospective trials have been conducted in normal human volunteers in which the upper gastrointestinal tract was evaluated by endoscopic inspection before and after one week of solid oral potassium chloride therapy. The ability of this model to predict events occuring in usual clinical practice is unknown. Trials which approximated usual clinical practice did not reveal any clear differences between the wax matrix and microencapsulated dosage forms. In contrast, there was a higher incidence of gastric and duodenal lesions in subjects receiving a high dose of a wax matrix controlled-release formulation under conditions which did not resemble usual or recommended clinical practice, i.e., 96 mEq per day in divided doses of potassium chloride administered, to fasted patients in the presence of an anticholinergic drug to delay gastric emptying. The upper gastrointestinal lesions observed by endoscopy were asymptomatic and were not accompanied by evidence of bleeding (hemoccult testing). The relevance of these findings to the usual conditions, i.e., nonfasting, no anticholinergic agent, and smaller doses, under which controlled-release potassium chloride products are used is uncertain. Epidemiologic studies have not identified an elevated risk, compared to microencapsulated products, for upper gastrointestinal lesions in patients receiving wax matrix formulations. K-TAB tablets should be discontinued immediately and the possibility of ulceration, obstruction or perforation considered if severe vomiting, abdominal pain, distention, or gastrointestinal bleeding occurs.
Metabolic Acidosis
Hypokalemia in patients with metabolic acidosis should be treated with an alkalinizing potassium salt such as potassium bicarbonate, potassium citrate, potassium acetate, or potassium gluconate.

PRECAUTIONS

General: The diagnosis of potassium depletion is ordinarily made by demonstrating hypokalemia in a patient with a clinical history suggesting some cause for potassium depletion. In interpreting the serum potassium level, the physician should bear in mind that acute alkalosis *per se* can produce hypokalemia in the absence of a deficit in total body potassium, while acute acidosis *per se* can increase the serum potassium concentration to within the normal range even in the presence of a reduced total body potassium. The treatment of potassium depletion, particularly in the presence of cardiac disease, renal disease, or acidosis, requires careful attention to acid-base balance and appropriate monitoring of serum electrolytes, the electrocardiogram, and the clinical status of the patient.
Information for Patients: Physicians should consider reminding the patient of the following:
To take each dose with meals and with a full glass of water or other liquid.
To take this medicine following the frequency and amount prescribed by the physician. This is especially important if the patient is also taking diuretics and/or digitalis preparations.
To check with the physician if there is trouble swallowing tablets or if the tablets seem to stick in the throat.
To check with the physician at once if tarry stools or other evidence of gastrointestinal bleeding is noticed.
To take each dose without crushing, chewing or sucking the tablets.
Laboratory Tests: When blood is drawn for analysis of plasma potassium it is important to recognize that artifactual elevations can occur after improper venipuncture technique or as a result of *in vitro* hemolysis of the sample.
Drug Interactions: Potassium-sparing diuretics, angiotensin converting enzyme inhibitors (see WARNINGS).
Carcinogenesis, Mutagenesis, Impairment of Fertility: Carcinogenicity, mutagenicity and fertility studies in animals have not been performed. Potassium is a normal dietary constituent.
Pregnancy Category C: Animal reproduction studies have not been conducted with K-TAB tablets. It is unlikely that potassium supplementation that does not lead to hyperkalemia would have an adverse effect on the fetus or would affect reproductive capacity.
Nursing Mothers: The normal potassium ion content of human milk is about 13 mEq per liter. Since oral potassium becomes part of the body potassium pool, as long as body potassium is not excessive, the contribution of potassium chloride supplementation should have little or no effect on the level in human milk.
Pediatric Use: Safety and effectiveness in children have not been established.

ADVERSE REACTIONS

One of the most severe adverse effects is hyperkalemia (see CONTRAINDICATIONS, WARNINGS, and OVERDOSAGE). There also have been reports of upper and lower gastrointestinal conditions including obstruction, bleeding, ulceration, and perforation (see CONTRAINDICATIONS and WARNINGS).
The most common adverse reactions to oral potassium salts are nausea, vomiting, flatulence, abdominal pain/discomfort, and diarrhea. These symptoms are due to irritation of the gastrointestinal tract and are best managed by taking the dose with meals, or reducing the amount taken at one time.
Skin rash has been reported rarely.

OVERDOSAGE

The administration of oral potassium salts to persons with normal excretory mechanisms for potassium rarely causes serious hyperkalemia. However, if excretory mechanisms are impaired or if intravenous administration is too rapid, potentially fatal hyperkalemia can result (see CONTRAINDICATIONS and WARNINGS). It is important to recognize that hyperkalemia is usually asymptomatic and may be manifested only by an increased serum potassium concentration (6.5-8.0 mEq/L) and characteristic electrocardiographic changes (peaking of T-waves, loss P-waves, depression of S-T segments, and prolongation of QT intervals). Late manifestations include muscle paralysis and cardiovascular collapse from cardiac arrest (9-12 mEq/L).
Treatment measures for hyperkalemia include the following:

1. Elimination of foods and medications containing potassium and of any agents with potassium-sparing properties;
2. Intravenous administration of 300 to 500 mL/hr of 10% dextrose solution containing 10-20 units of crystalline insulin per 1,000 mL;
3. Correction of acidosis, if present, with intravenous sodium bicarbonate;
4. Use of exchange resins, hemodialysis, or peritoneal dialysis.

In treating hyperkalemia, it should be recalled that in patients who have been stabilized on digitalis, lowering the serum potassium concentration too rapidly can produce digitalis toxicity.

DOSAGE AND ADMINISTRATION

The usual dietary potassium intake by the average adult is 50 to 100 mEq per day. Potassium depletion sufficient to cause hypokalemia usually requires the loss of 200 or more mEq of potassium from the total body store.
Dosage must be adjusted to the individual needs of each patient. The dose for the prevention of hypokalemia is typically in the range of 20 mEq per day. Doses of 40-100 mEq per day or more are used for the treatment of potassium depletion. Dosage should be divided if more than 20 mEq per day is given such that no more than 20 mEq is given in a single dose.
K-TAB tablets provide 10 mEq of potassium chloride.
K-TAB tablets should be taken with meals and with a glass of water or other liquid. This product should not be taken on an empty stomach because of its potential for gastric irritation (see WARNINGS).
NOTE: K-TAB tablets are to be swallowed whole without crushing, chewing or sucking the tablets.

HOW SUPPLIED

K-TAB (potassium chloride extended-release tablets, USP) contains 750 mg of potassium chloride (equivalent to 10 mEq). K-TAB tablets are provided as yellow, ovaloid, extended-release Filmtab® tablets in bottles of 100 (**NDC** 0074-7804-13), 1000 (**NDC** 0074-7804-19) and 5000 (**NDC** 0074-7804-59) and in ABBO-PAC® unit dose packages of 100 (**NDC** 0074-7804-11).
Recommended storage: Store below 86°F (30°C).
Revised: October, 1998

Filmtab—Film-sealed tablets, Abbott
Ref. 03-4915-R15-Rev. October, 1998
Shown in Product Identification Guide, page 303

NEMBUTAL® SODIUM CAPSULES ℂ ℞

[*nĕm-bū-tal sō-dī-um*]
(pentobarbital sodium capsules, USP)

WARNING—MAY BE HABIT FORMING

DESCRIPTION

The barbiturates are nonselective central nervous system depressants which are primarily used as sedative hypnotics. The barbiturates and their sodium salts are subject to control under the Federal Controlled Substances Act (See "Drug Abuse and Dependence" section).
Barbiturates are substituted pyrimidine derivatives in which the basic structure common to these drugs is barbituric acid, a substance which has no central nervous system (CNS) activity. CNS activity is obtained by substituting alkyl, alkenyl, or aryl groups on the pyrimidine ring. Nembutal (pentobarbital sodium) is chemically represented by sodium 5-ethyl-5-(1-methylbutyl) barbiturate.
The structural formula for pentobarbitol sodium is:

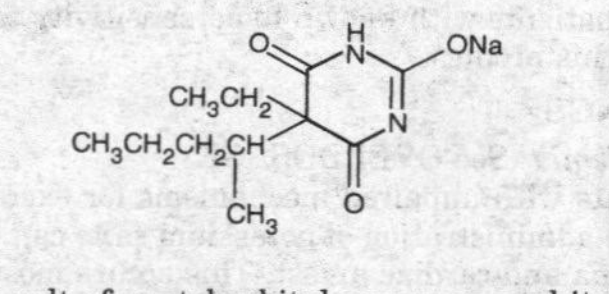

The sodium salt of pentobarbital occurs as a white, slightly bitter powder which is freely soluble in water and alcohol but practically insoluble in benzene and ether. Nembutal Sodium capsules for oral administration contain either 50 mg or 100 mg of pentobarbital sodium.
Inactive Ingredients: 50 mg Capsule: FD&C Blue No. 1, FD&C Red No. 3, FD&C Yellow No. 6, gelatin, lactose, magnesium stearate, polacrilin potassium and potassium chloride.
100 mg Capsule: colloidal silicon dioxide, corn starch, FD&C Blue No. 1, FD&C Red No. 3, FD&C Yellow No. 5 (tartrazine), FD&C Yellow No. 6, gelatin, magnesium stearate and potassium chloride.

CLINICAL PHARMACOLOGY

Barbiturates are capable of producing all levels of CNS mood alteration from excitation to mild sedation, to hypnosis, and deep coma. Overdosage can produce death. In high enough therapeutic doses, barbiturates induce anesthesia.
Barbiturates depress the sensory cortex, decrease motor activity, alter cerebellar function, and produce drowsiness, sedation, and hypnosis.
Barbiturate-induced sleep differs from physiological sleep. Sleep laboratory studies have demonstrated that barbiturates reduce the amount of time spent in the rapid eye movement (REM) phase of sleep or dreaming stage. Also, Stages III and IV sleep are decreased. Following abrupt cessation of barbiturates used regularly, patients may experience markedly increased dreaming, nightmares, and/or insomnia. Therefore, withdrawal of a single therapeutic dose over 5 or 6 days has been recommended to lessen the REM rebound and disturbed sleep which contribute to drug withdrawal syndrome (for example, decrease the dose from 3 to 2 doses a day for 1 week).

In studies, secobarbital sodium and pentobarbital sodium have been found to lose most of their effectiveness for both inducing and maintaining sleep by the end of 2 weeks of continued drug administration at fixed doses. The short-, intermediate-, and, to a lesser degree, long-acting barbiturates have been widely prescribed for treating insomnia. Although the clinical literature abounds with claims that the short-acting barbiturates are superior for producing sleep while the intermediate-acting compounds are more effective in maintaining sleep, controlled studies have failed to demonstrate these differential effects. Therefore, as sleep medications, the barbiturates are of limited value beyond short-term use.

Barbiturates have little analgesic action at subanesthetic doses. Rather, in subanesthetic doses these drugs may increase the reaction to painful stimuli. All barbiturates exhibit anticonvulsant activity in anesthetic doses. However, of the drugs in this class, only phenobarbital, mephobarbital, and metharbital have been clinically demonstrated to be effective as oral anticonvulsants in subhypnotic doses.

Barbiturates are respiratory depressants. The degree of respiratory depression is dependent upon dose. With hypnotic doses, respiratory depression produced by barbiturates is similar to that which occurs during physiologic sleep with slight decrease in blood pressure and heart rate.

Studies in laboratory animals have shown that barbiturates cause reduction in the tone and contractility of the uterus, ureters, and urinary bladder. However, concentrations of the drugs required to produce this effect in humans are not reached with sedative-hypnotic doses.

Barbiturates do not impair normal hepatic function, but have been shown to induce liver microsomal enzymes, thus increasing and/or altering the metabolism of barbiturates and other drugs. (See "Precautions—*Drug Interactions*" section).

Pharmacokinetics: Barbiturates are absorbed in varying degrees following oral, rectal, or parenteral administration. The salts are more rapidly absorbed than are the acids. The rate of absorption is increased if the sodium salt is ingested as a dilute solution or taken on an empty stomach.

The onset of action for oral or rectal administration varies from 20 to 60 minutes.

Duration of action, which is related to the rate at which the barbiturates are redistributed throughout the body, varies among persons and in the same person from time to time. In Table 1, the barbiturates are classified according to their duration of action. This classification should not be used to predict the exact duration of effect, but the grouping of drugs should be used as a guide in the selection of barbiturates.

No studies have demonstrated that the different routes of administration are equivalent with respect to bioavailability.

[See Table 1 above.]

Table 1.—*Classification, Onset, and Duration of Action of Commonly used Barbiturates Taken Orally*

Classification	Onset of action	Duration of action
Long-acting Phenobarbital.	1 hour or longer	10 to 12 hours
Intermediate Amobarbital Butabarbital.	$^3/_4$ to 1 hour	6 to 8 hours
Short-acting Pentobarbital Secobarbital.	10 to 15 minutes	3 to 4 hours

Barbiturates are weak acids that are absorbed and rapidly distributed to all tissues and fluids with high concentrations in the brain, liver, and kidneys. Lipid solubility of the barbiturates is the dominant factor in their distribution within the body. The more lipid soluble the barbiturate, the more rapidly it penetrates all tissues of the body. Barbiturates are bound to plasma and tissue proteins to a varying degree with the degree of binding increasing directly as a function of lipid solubility.

Phenobarbital has the lowest lipid solubility, lowest plasma binding, lowest brain protein binding, the longest delay in onset of activity, and the longest duration of action. At the opposite extreme is secobarbital which has the highest lipid solubility, plasma protein binding, brain protein binding, the shortest delay in onset of activity, and the shortest duration of action. Butabarbital is classified as an intermediate barbiturate.

The plasma half-life for pentobarbital in adults is 15 to 50 hours and appears to be dose dependent.

Barbiturates are metabolized primarily by the hepatic microsomal enzyme system, and the metabolic products are excreted in the urine, and less commonly, in the feces. Approximately 25 to 50 percent of a dose of aprobarbital or phenobarbital is eliminated unchanged in the urine, whereas the amount of other barbiturates excreted unchanged in the urine is negligible. The excretion of unmetabolized barbiturate is one feature that distinguishes the long-acting category from those belonging to other categories which are almost entirely metabolized. The inactive metabolites of the barbiturates are excreted as conjugates of glucuronic acid.

INDICATIONS AND USAGE

Oral:

a. Sedatives.
b. Hypnotics, for the short-term treatment of insomnia, since they appear to lose their effectiveness for sleep induction and sleep maintenance after 2 weeks (See "Clinical Pharmacology" section).
c. Preanesthetics.

CONTRAINDICATIONS

Barbiturates are contraindicated in patients with known barbiturate sensitivity. Barbiturates are also contraindicated in patients with a history of manifest or latent porphyria.

WARNINGS

1. *Habit forming:* Barbiturates may be habit forming. Tolerance, psychological and physical dependence may occur with continued use. (See "Drug Abuse and Dependence" and "Pharmacokinetics" sections). Patients who have psychological dependence on barbiturates may increase the dosage or decrease the dosage interval without consulting a physician and may subsequently develop a physical dependence on barbiturates. To minimize the possibility of overdosage or the development of dependence, the prescribing and dispensing of sedative-hypnotic barbiturates should be limited to the amount required for the interval until the next appointment. Abrupt cessation after prolonged use in the dependent person may result in withdrawal symptoms, including delirium, convulsions, and possibly death. Barbiturates should be withdrawn gradually from any patient known to be taking excessive dosage over long periods of time. (See "Drug Abuse and Dependence" section).
2. *Acute or chronic pain:* Caution should be exercised when barbiturates are administered to patients with acute or chronic pain, because paradoxical excitement could be induced or important symptoms could be masked. However, the use of barbiturates as sedatives in the postoperative surgical period and as adjuncts to cancer chemotherapy is well established.
3. *Use in pregnancy:* Barbiturates can cause fetal damage when administered to a pregnant woman. Retrospective, case-controlled studies have suggested a connection between the maternal consumption of barbiturates and a higher than expected incidence of fetal abnormalities. Following oral or parenteral administration, barbiturates readily cross the placental barrier and are distributed throughout fetal tissues with highest concentrations found in the placenta, fetal liver, and brain.
   Withdrawal symptoms occur in infants born to mothers who receive barbiturates throughout the last trimester of pregnancy. (See "Drug Abuse and Dependence" section). If this drug is used during pregnancy, or if the patient becomes pregnant while taking this drug, the patient should be apprised of the potential hazard to the fetus.
4. *Synergistic effects:* The concomitant use of alcohol or other CNS depressants may produce additive CNS depressant effects.

PRECAUTIONS

General: Barbiturates may be habit forming. Tolerance and psychological and physical dependence may occur with continuing use. (See "Drug Abuse and Dependence" section). Barbiturates should be administered with caution, if at all, to patients who are mentally depressed, have suicidal tendencies, or a history of drug abuse.

Elderly or debilitated patients may react to barbiturates with marked excitement, depression, and confusion. In some persons, barbiturates repeatedly produce excitement rather than depression.

In patients with hepatic damage, barbiturates should be administered with caution and initially in reduced doses. Barbiturates should not be administered to patients showing the premonitory signs of hepatic coma.

The 100 mg dosage strength of Nembutal Sodium capsules contains FD&C Yellow No. 5 (tartrazine) which may cause allergic-type reactions (including bronchial asthma) in certain susceptible individuals. Although the overall incidence of FD&C Yellow No. 5 (tartrazine) sensitivity in the general population is low, it is frequently seen in patients who also have aspirin hypersensitivity.

Information for the patient: Practitioners should give the following information and instructions to patients receiving barbiturates.

1. The use of barbiturates carries with it an associated risk of psychological and/or physical dependence. The patient should be warned against increasing the dose of the drug without consulting a physician.
2. Barbiturates may impair mental and/or physical abilities required for the performance of potentially hazardous tasks (e.g., driving, operating machinery, etc.).
3. Alcohol should not be consumed while taking barbiturates. Concurrent use of the barbiturates with other CNS depressants (e.g., alcohol, narcotics, tranquilizers, and antihistamines) may result in additional CNS depressant effects.

Laboratory tests: Prolonged therapy with barbiturates should be accompanied by periodic laboratory evaluation of organ systems, including hematopoietic, renal, and hepatic systems. (See "Precautions—General" and "Adverse Reactions" sections).

Drug interactions: Most reports of clinically significant drug interactions occurring with the barbiturates have involved phenobarbital. However, the application of these data to other barbiturates appears valid and warrants serial blood level determinations of the relevant drugs when there are multiple therapies.

1. *Anticoagulants:* Phenobarbital lowers the plasma levels of dicumarol (name previously used: bishydroxycoumarin) and causes a decrease in anticoagulant activity as measured by the prothrombin time. Barbiturates can induce hepatic microsomal enzymes resulting in increased metabolism and decreased anticoagulant response of oral anticoagulants (e.g., warfarin, acenocoumarol, dicumarol and phenprocoumon). Patients stabilized on anticoagulant therapy may require dosage adjustments if barbiturates are added to or withdrawn from their dosage regimen.
2. *Corticosteroids:* Barbiturates appear to enhance the metabolism of exogenous corticosteroids probably through the induction of hepatic microsomal enzymes. Patients stabilized on corticosteroid therapy may require dosage adjustments if barbiturates are added to or withdrawn from their dosage regimen.
3. *Griseofulvin:* Phenobarbital appears to interfere with the absorption of orally administered griseofulvin, thus decreasing its blood level. The effect of the resultant decreased blood levels of griseofulvin on therapeutic response has not been established. However, it would be preferable to avoid concomitant administration of these drugs.
4. *Doxycycline:* Phenobarbital has been shown to shorten the half-life of doxycycline for as long as 2 weeks after barbiturate therapy is discontinued.
   This mechanism is probably through the induction of hepatic microsomal enzymes that metabolize the antibiotic. If phenobarbital and doxycycline are administered concurrently, the clinical response to doxycycline should be monitored closely.
5. *Phenytoin, sodium valproate, valproic acid:* The effect of barbiturates on the metabolism of phenytoin appears to be variable. Some investigators report an accelerating effect, while others report no effect. Because the effect of barbiturates on the metabolism of phenytoin is not predictable, phenytoin and barbiturate blood levels should be monitored more frequently if these drugs are given concurrently. Sodium valproate and valproic acid appear to decrease barbiturate metabolism; therefore, barbiturate blood levels should be monitored and appropriate dosage adjustments made as indicated.
6. *Central nervous system depressants:* The concomitant use of other central nervous system depressants, including other sedatives or hypnotics, antihistamines, tranquilizers, or alcohol, may produce additive depressant effects.
7. *Monoamine oxidase inhibitors (MAOI):* MAOI prolong the effects of barbiturates probably because metabolism of the barbiturate is inhibited.
8. *Estradiol, estrone, progesterone and other steroidal hormones:* Pretreatment with or concurrent administration of phenobarbital may decrease the effect of estradiol by increasing its metabolism. There have been reports of patients treated with antiepileptic drugs (e.g., phenobarbital) who became pregnant while taking oral contraceptives. An alternate contraceptive method might be suggested to women taking phenobarbital.

Carcinogenesis: 1. Animal data. Phenobarbital sodium is carcinogenic in mice and rats after lifetime administration. In mice, it produced benign and malignant liver cell tumors. In rats, benign liver cell tumors were observed very late in life.

2. Human data. In a 29-year epidemiological study of 9,136 patients who were treated on an anticonvulsant protocol that included phenobarbital, results indicated a higher than normal incidence of hepatic carcinoma. Previously, some of these patients were treated with thorotrast, a drug that is known to produce hepatic carcinomas. Thus, this study did not provide sufficient evidence that phenobarbital sodium is carcinogenic in humans.

Data from one retrospective study of 235 children in which the types of barbiturates are not identified suggested an association between exposure to barbiturates prenatally and an increased incidence of brain tumor. (Gold, E., et al., "Increased Risk of Brain Tumors in Children Exposed to Barbiturates," Journal of National Cancer Institute, 61:1031–1034, 1978).

Pregnancy: 1. Teratogenic effects. Pregnancy Category D—See "Warnings—Use in Pregnancy" section.

2. *Nonteratogenic effects.* Reports of infants suffering from long-term barbiturate exposure in utero included the acute withdrawal syndrome of seizures and hyperirritability from birth to a delayed onset of up to 14 days. (See "Drug Abuse and Dependence" section).

Labor and delivery: Hypnotic doses of these barbiturates do not appear to significantly impair uterine activity during labor. Full anesthetic doses of barbiturates decrease the

Continued on next page

Nembutal Capsules—Cont.

force and frequency of uterine contractions. Administration of sedative-hypnotic barbiturates to the mother during labor may result in respiratory depression in the newborn. Premature infants are particularly susceptible to the depressant effects of barbiturates. If barbiturates are used during labor and delivery, resuscitation equipment should be available.

Data are currently not available to evaluate the effect of these barbiturates when forceps delivery or other intervention is necessary. Also, data are not available to determine the effect of these barbiturates on the later growth, development, and functional maturation of the child.

Nursing mothers: Caution should be exercised when a barbiturate is administered to a nursing woman since small amounts of barbiturates are excreted in the milk.

ADVERSE REACTIONS

The following adverse reactions and their incidence were compiled from surveillance of thousands of hospitalized patients. Because such patients may be less aware of certain of the milder adverse effects of barbiturates, the incidence of these reactions may be somewhat higher in fully ambulatory patients.

More than 1 in 100 patients. The most common adverse reaction estimated to occur at a rate of 1 to 3 patients per 100 is: *Nervous System:* Somnolence.

Less than 1 in 100 patients. Adverse reactions estimated to occur at a rate of less than 1 in 100 patients listed below, grouped by organ system, and by decreasing order of occurrence are:

Nervous system: Agitation, confusion, hyperkinesia, ataxia, CNS depression, nightmares, nervousness, psychiatric disturbance, hallucinations, insomnia, anxiety, dizziness, thinking abnormality.

Respiratory system: Hypoventilation, apnea.

Cardiovascular system: Bradycardia, hypotension, syncope.

Digestive system: Nausea, vomiting, constipation.

Other reported reactions: Headache, injection site reactions, hypersensitivity reactions (angioedema, skin rashes, exfoliative dermatitis), fever, liver damage, megaloblastic anemia following chronic phenobarbital use.

DRUG ABUSE AND DEPENDENCE

Pentobarbital sodium capsules are subject to control by the Federal Controlled Substances Act under DEA schedule II. Barbiturates may be habit forming. Tolerance, psychological dependence, and physical dependence may occur especially following prolonged use of high doses of barbiturates. Daily administration in excess of 400 milligrams (mg) of pentobarbital or secobarbital for approximately 90 days is likely to produce some degree of physical dependence. A dosage of from 600 to 800 mg taken for at least 35 days is sufficient to produce withdrawal seizures. The average daily dose for the barbiturate addict is usually about 1.5 grams. As tolerance to barbiturates develops, the amount needed to maintain the same level of intoxication increases; tolerance to a fatal dosage, however, does not increase more than two-fold. As this occurs, the margin between an intoxicating dosage and fatal dosage becomes smaller.

Symptoms of acute intoxication with barbiturates include unsteady gait, slurred speech, and sustained nystagmus. Mental signs of chronic intoxication include confusion, poor judgment, irritability, insomnia, and somatic complaints.

Symptoms of barbiturate dependence are similar to those of chronic alcoholism. If an individual appears to be intoxicated with alcohol to a degree that is radically disproportionate to the amount of alcohol in his or her blood the use of barbiturates should be suspected. The lethal dose of a barbiturate is far less if alcohol is also ingested.

The symptoms of barbiturate withdrawal can be severe and may cause death. Minor withdrawal symptoms may appear 8 to 12 hours after the last dose of a barbiturate. These symptoms usually appear in the following order: anxiety, muscle twitching, tremor of hands and fingers, progressive weakness, dizziness, distortion in visual perception, nausea, vomiting, insomnia, and orthostatic hypotension. Major withdrawal symptoms (convulsions and delirium) may occur within 16 hours and last up to 5 days after abrupt cessation of these drugs. Intensity of withdrawal symptoms gradually declines over a period of approximately 15 days. Individuals susceptible to barbiturate abuse and dependence include alcoholics and opiate abusers, as well as other sedative-hypnotic and amphetamine abusers.

Drug dependence to barbiturates arises from repeated administration of a barbiturate or agent with barbiturate-like effect on a continuous basis, generally in amounts exceeding therapeutic dose levels. The characteristics of drug dependence to barbiturates include: (a) a strong desire or need to continue taking the drug; (b) a tendency to increase the dose; (c) a psychic dependence on the effects of the drug related to subjective and individual appreciation of those effects; and (d) a physical dependence on the effects of the drug requiring its presence for maintenance of homeostasis and resulting in a definite, characteristic, and self-limited abstinence syndrome when the drug is withdrawn.

Treatment of barbiturate dependence consists of cautious and gradual withdrawal of the drug. Barbiturate-dependent patients can be withdrawn by using a number of different withdrawal regimens. In all cases withdrawal takes an extended period of time. One method involves substituting a 30 mg dose of phenobarbital for each 100 to 200 mg dose of barbiturate that the patient has been taking. The total daily amount of phenobarbital is then administered in 3 to 4 divided doses, not to exceed 600 mg daily. Should signs of withdrawal occur on the first day of treatment, a loading dose of 100 to 200 mg of phenobarbital may be administered IM in addition to the oral dose. After stabilization on phenobarbital, the total daily dose is decreased by 30 mg a day as long as withdrawal is proceeding smoothly. A modification of this regimen involves initiating treatment at the patient's regular dosage level and decreasing the daily dosage by 10 percent if tolerated by the patient.

Infants physically dependent on barbiturates may be given phenobarbital 3 to 10 mg/kg/day. After withdrawal symptoms (hyperactivity, disturbed sleep, tremors, hyperreflexia) are relieved, the dosage of phenobarbital should be gradually decreased and completely withdrawn over a 2 week period.

OVERDOSAGE

The toxic dose of barbiturates varies considerably. In general, an oral dose of 1 gram of most barbiturates produces serious poisoning in an adult. Death commonly occurs after 2 to 10 grams of ingested barbiturate. Barbiturate intoxication may be confused with alcoholism, bromide intoxication, and with various neurological disorders.

Acute overdosage with barbiturates is manifested by CNS and respiratory depression which may progress to Cheyne-Stokes respiration, areflexia, constriction of the pupils to a slight degree (though in severe poisoning they may show paralytic dilation), oliguria, tachycardia, hypotension, lowered body temperature, and coma. Typical shock syndrome (apnea, circulatory collapse, respiratory arrest, and death) may occur.

In extreme overdose, all electrical activity in the brain may cease, in which case a "flat" EEG normally equated with clinical death cannot be accepted. This effect is fully reversible unless hypoxic damage occurs. Consideration should be given to the possibility of barbiturate intoxication even in situations that appear to involve trauma.

Complications such as pneumonia, pulmonary edema, cardiac arrhythmias, congestive heart failure, and renal failure may occur. Uremia may increase CNS sensitivity to barbiturates. Differential diagnosis should include hypoglycemia, head trauma, cerebrovascular accidents, convulsive states, and diabetic coma. Blood levels from acute overdosage for some barbiturates are listed in Table 2.

[See table 2 below]

Treatment of overdosage is mainly supportive and consists of the following:

1. Maintenance of an adequate airway, with assisted respiration and oxygen administration as necessary.
2. Monitoring of vital signs and fluid balance.
3. If the patient is conscious and has not lost the gag reflex, emesis may be induced with ipecac. Care should be taken to prevent pulmonary aspiration of vomitus. After completion of vomiting, 30 grams activated charcoal in a glass of water may be administered.
4. If emesis is contraindicated, gastric lavage may be performed with a cuffed endotracheal tube in place with the patient in the face down position. Activated charcoal may be left in the emptied stomach and a saline cathartic administered.
5. Fluid therapy and other standard treatment for shock, if needed.
6. If renal function is normal, forced diuresis may aid in the elimination of the barbiturate. Alkalinization of the urine increases renal excretion of some barbiturates, especially phenobarbital, also aprobarbital, and mephobarbital (which is metabolized to phenobarbital).
7. Although not recommended as a routine procedure, hemodialysis may be used in severe barbiturate intoxications or if the patient is anuric or in shock.
8. Patient should be rolled from side to side every 30 minutes.
9. Antibiotics should be given if pneumonia is suspected.
10. Appropriate nursing care to prevent hypostatic pneumonia, decubiti, aspiration, and other complications of patients with altered states of consciousness.

DOSAGE AND ADMINISTRATION

Adults: The usual hypnotic dose consists of 100 mg at bedtime.

Children: The preoperative dose is 2 to 6 mg/kg/24 hours (maximum 100 mg), depending on age, weight, and the desired degree of sedation.

The proper hypnotic dose for children must be judged on the basis of individual age and weight.

Dosages of barbiturates must be individualized with full knowledge of their particular characteristics and recommended rate of administration. Factors of consideration are the patient's age, weight, and condition.

Special patient population: Dosage should be reduced in the elderly or debilitated because these patients may be more sensitive to barbiturates. Dosage should be reduced for patients with impaired renal function or hepatic disease.

HOW SUPPLIED

NEMBUTAL Sodium Capsules (pentobarbital sodium capsules, USP) are supplied as follows:

50 mg transparent and orange-colored capsules (imprinted with a and the Abbo-Code CF) in bottles of 100 (**NDC** 0074-3150-11)

100 mg yellow capsules (imprinted with a and the Abbo-Code CH) in bottles of 100 (**NDC** 0074-3114-01), and in the Abbo-Pac® unit dose packages of 100 (**NDC** 0074-3114-21).

Recommended Storage: Store below 86°F (30°C).

Revised: September, 1997

Ref. 03-4785-R11

Shown in Product Identification Guide, page 303

NEMBUTAL® SODIUM SOLUTION C-II ℞

PENTOBARBITAL SODIUM INJECTION, USP

WARNING—MAY BE HABIT FORMING

Ampuls—Vials

DO NOT USE IF MATERIAL HAS PRECIPITATED

DESCRIPTION

The barbiturates are nonselective central nervous system depressants which are primarily used as sedative hypnotics and also anticonvulsants in subhypnotic doses. The barbiturates and their sodium salts are subject to control under the Federal Controlled Substances Act (See "Drug Abuse and Dependence" section).

The sodium salts of amobarbital, pentobarbital, phenobarbital, and secobarbital are available as sterile parenteral solutions.

Barbiturates are substituted pyrimidine derivatives in which the basic structure common to these drugs is barbituric acid, a substance which has no central nervous system (CNS) activity. CNS activity is obtained by substituting alkyl, alkenyl, or aryl groups on the pyrimidine ring.

NEMBUTAL Sodium Solution (pentobarbital sodium injection) is a sterile solution for intravenous or intramuscular injection. Each ml contains pentobarbital sodium 50 mg, in a vehicle of propylene glycol, 40%, alcohol, 10% and water for injection, to volume. The pH is adjusted to approximately 9.5 with hydrochloric acid and/or sodium hydroxide.

NEMBUTAL Sodium is a short-acting barbiturate, chemically designated as sodium 5-ethyl-5-(1-methylbutyl) barbiturate. The structural formula for pentobarbital sodium is:

O H ONa
CH_3CH_2
$CH_3CH_2CH_2CH$
CH_3 O

The sodium salt occurs as a white, slightly bitter powder which is freely soluble in water and alcohol but practically insoluble in benzene and ether.

CLINICAL PHARMACOLOGY

Barbiturates are capable of producing all levels of CNS mood alteration from excitation to mild sedation, to hypno-

Table 2.—*Concentration of Barbiturate in the Blood Versus Degree of CNS Depression*

Blood barbiturate level in ppm (µg/ml)

Barbiturate	Onset/duration	Degree of depression in nontolerant persons* 1	2	3	4	5
Pentobarbital	Fast/short	≤2	0.5 to 3	10 to 15	12 to 25	15 to 40
Secobarbital	Fast/short	≤2	0.5 to 5	10 to 15	15 to 25	15 to 40
Amobarbital	Intermediate/ intermediate	≤3	2 to 10	30 to 40	30 to 60	40 to 80
Butabarbital	Intermediate/ intermediate	≤5	3 to 25	40 to 60	50 to 80	60 to 100
Phenobarbital	Slow/long	≤10	5 to 40	50 to 80	70 to 120	100 to 200

* Categories of degree of depression in nontolerant persons:
1. Under the influence and appreciably impaired for purposes of driving a motor vehicle or performing tasks requiring alertness and unimpaired judgment and reaction time.
2. Sedated, therapeutic range, calm, relaxed, and easily aroused.
3. Comatose, difficult to arouse, significant depression of respiration.
4. Compatible with death in aged or ill persons or in presence of obstructed airway, other toxic agents, or exposure to cold.
5. Usual lethal level, the upper end of the range includes those who received some supportive treatment.

sis, and deep coma. Overdosage can produce death. In high enough therapeutic doses, barbiturates induce anesthesia.
Barbiturates depress the sensory cortex, decrease motor activity, alter cerebellar function, and produce drowsiness, sedation, and hypnosis.
Barbiturate-induced sleep differs from physiological sleep. Sleep laboratory studies have demonstrated that barbiturates reduce the amount of time spent in the rapid eye movement (REM) phase of sleep or dreaming stage. Also, Stages III and IV sleep are decreased. Following abrupt cessation of barbiturates used regularly, patients may experience markedly increased dreaming, nightmares, and/or insomnia. Therefore, withdrawal of a single therapeutic dose over 5 or 6 days has been recommended to lessen the REM rebound and disturbed sleep which contribute to drug withdrawal syndrome (for example, decrease the dose from 3 to 2 doses a day for 1 week).
In studies, secobarbital sodium and pentobarbital sodium have been found to lose most of their effectiveness for both inducing and maintaining sleep by the end of 2 weeks of continued drug administration at fixed doses. The short-, intermediate-, and, to a lesser degree, long-acting barbiturates have been widely prescribed for treating insomnia. Although the clinical literature abounds with claims that the short-acting barbiturates are superior for producing sleep while the intermediate-acting compounds are more effective in maintaining sleep, controlled studies have failed to demonstrate these differential effects. Therefore, as sleep medications, the barbiturates are of limited value beyond short-term use.
Barbiturates have little analgesic action at subanesthetic doses. Rather, in subanesthetic doses these drugs may increase the reaction to painful stimuli. All barbiturates exhibit anticonvulsant activity in anesthetic doses. However, of the drugs in this class, only phenobarbital, mephobarbital, and metharbital have been clinically demonstrated to be effective as oral anticonvulsants in subhypnotic doses.
Barbiturates are respiratory depressants. The degree of respiratory depression is dependent upon dose. With hypnotic doses, respiratory depression produced by barbiturates is similar to that which occurs during physiologic sleep with slight decrease in blood pressure and heart rate.
Studies in laboratory animals have shown that barbiturates cause reduction in the tone and contractility of the uterus, ureters, and urinary bladder. However, concentrations of the drugs required to produce this effect in humans are not reached with sedative-hypnotic doses.
Barbiturates do not impair normal hepatic function, but have been shown to induce liver microsomal enzymes, thus increasing and/or altering the metabolism of barbiturates and other drugs. (See "Precautions—*Drug Interactions*" section).

Pharmacokinetics:
Barbiturates are absorbed in varying degrees following oral, rectal, or parenteral administration. The salts are more rapidly absorbed than are the acids.
The onset of action for oral or rectal administration varies from 20 to 60 minutes. For IM administration, the onset of action is slightly faster. Following IV administration, the onset of action ranges from almost immediately for pentobarbital sodium to 5 minutes for phenobarbital sodium. Maximal CNS depression may not occur until 15 minutes or more after IV administration for phenobarbital sodium.
Duration of action, which is related to the rate at which the barbiturates are redistributed throughout the body, varies among persons and in the same person from time to time.
No studies have demonstrated that the different routes of administration are equivalent with respect to bioavailability.
Barbiturates are weak acids that are absorbed and rapidly distributed to all tissues and fluids with high concentrations in the brain, liver, and kidneys. Lipid solubility of the barbiturates is the dominant factor in their distribution within the body. The more lipid soluble the barbiturate, the more rapidly it penetrates all tissues of the body. Barbiturates are bound to plasma and tissue proteins to a varying degree with the degree of binding increasing directly as a function of lipid solubility.
Phenobarbital has the lowest lipid solubility, lowest plasma binding, lowest brain protein binding, the longest delay in onset of activity, and the longest duration of action. At the opposite extreme is secobarbital which has the highest lipid solubility, plasma protein binding, brain protein binding, the shortest delay in onset of activity, and the shortest duration of action. Butabarbital is classified as an intermediate barbiturate.
The plasma half-life for pentobarbital in adults is 15 to 50 hours and appears to be dose dependent.
Barbiturates are metabolized primarily by the hepatic microsomal enzyme system, and the metabolic products are excreted in the urine, and less commonly, in the feces. Approximately 25 to 50 percent of a dose of aprobarbital or phenobarbital is eliminated unchanged in the urine, whereas the amount of other barbiturates excreted unchanged in the urine is negligible. The excretion of unmetabolized barbiturate is one feature that distinguishes the long-acting category from those belonging to other categories which are almost entirely metabolized. The inactive metabolites of the barbiturates are excreted as conjugates of glucuronic acid.

INDICATIONS AND USAGE

Parenteral:
a. Sedatives.
b. Hypnotics, for the short-term treatment of insomnia, since they appear to lose their effectiveness for sleep induction and sleep maintenance after 2 weeks (See "Clinical Pharmacology" section).
c. Preanesthetics.
d. Anticonvulsant, in anesthetic doses, in the emergency control of certain acute convulsive episodes, e.g., those associated with status epilepticus, cholera, eclampsia, meningitis, tetanus, and toxic reactions to strychnine or local anesthetics.

CONTRAINDICATIONS

Barbiturates are contraindicated in patients with known barbiturate sensitivity. Barbiturates are also contraindicated in patients with a history of manifest or latent porphyria.

WARNINGS

1. *Habit forming:* Barbiturates may be habit forming. Tolerance, psychological and physical dependence may occur with continued use. (See "Drug Abuse and Dependence" and "Pharmacokinetics" sections). Patients who have psychological dependence on barbiturates may increase the dosage or decrease the dosage interval without consulting a physician and may subsequently develop a physical dependence on barbiturates. To minimize the possibility of overdosage or the development of dependence, the prescribing and dispensing of sedative-hypnotic barbiturates should be limited to the amount required for the interval until the next appointment. Abrupt cessation after prolonged use in the dependent person may result in withdrawal symptoms, including delirium, convulsions, and possibly death. Barbiturates should be withdrawn gradually from any patient known to be taking excessive dosage over long periods of time. (See "Drug Abuse and Dependence" section).
2. *IV administration:* Too rapid administration may cause respiratory depression, apnea, laryngospasm, or vasodilation with fall in blood pressure.
3. *Acute or chronic pain:* Caution should be exercised when barbiturates are administered to patients with acute or chronic pain, because paradoxical excitement could be induced or important symptoms could be masked. However, the use of barbiturates as sedatives in the postoperative surgical period and as adjuncts to cancer chemotherapy is well established.
4. *Use in pregnancy:* Barbiturates can cause fetal damage when administered to a pregnant woman. Retrospective, case-controlled studies have suggested a connection between the maternal consumption of barbiturates and a higher than expected incidence of fetal abnormalities. Following oral or parenteral administration, barbiturates readily cross the placental barrier and are distributed throughout fetal tissues with highest concentrations found in the placenta, fetal liver, and brain. Fetal blood levels approach maternal blood levels following parenteral administration.
   Withdrawal symptoms occur in infants born to mothers who receive barbiturates throughout the last trimester of pregnancy. (See "Drug Abuse and Dependence" section). If this drug is used during pregnancy, or if the patient becomes pregnant while taking this drug, the patient should be apprised of the potential hazard to the fetus.
5. *Synergistic effects:* The concomitant use of alcohol or other CNS depressants may produce additive CNS depressant effects.

PRECAUTIONS

General:
Barbiturates may be habit forming. Tolerance and psychological and physical dependence may occur with continuing use. (See "Drug Abuse and Dependence" section). Barbiturates should be administered with caution, if at all, to patients who are mentally depressed, have suicidal tendencies, or a history of drug abuse.
Elderly or debilitated patients may react to barbiturates with marked excitement, depression, and confusion. In some persons, barbiturates repeatedly produce excitement rather than depression.
In patients with hepatic damage, barbiturates should be administered with caution and initially in reduced doses. Barbiturates should not be administered to patients showing the premonitory signs of hepatic coma.
Parenteral solutions of barbiturates are highly alkaline. Therefore, extreme care should be taken to avoid perivascular extravasation or intra-arterial injection. Extravascular injection may cause local tissue damage with subsequent necrosis; consequences of intra-arterial injection may vary from transient pain to gangrene of the limb. Any complaint of pain in the limb warrants stopping the injection.

Information for the patient:
Practitioners should give the following information and instructions to patients receiving barbiturates.
1. The use of barbiturates carries with it an associated risk of psychological and/or physical dependence. The patient should be warned against increasing the dose of the drug without consulting a physician.
2. Barbiturates may impair mental and/or physical abilities required for the performance of potentially hazardous tasks (e.g., driving, operating machinery, etc.).
3. Alcohol should not be consumed while taking barbiturates. Concurrent use of the barbiturates with other CNS depressants (e.g., alcohol, narcotics, tranquilizers, and antihistamines) may result in additional CNS depressant effects.

Laboratory tests:
Prolonged therapy with barbiturates should be accompanied by periodic laboratory evaluation of organ systems, including hematopoietic, renal, and hepatic systems. (See "Precautions-*General*" and "Adverse Reactions" sections).

Drug interactions:
Most reports of clinically significant drug interactions occurring with the barbiturates have involved phenobarbital. However, the application of these data to other barbiturates appears valid and warrants serial blood level determinations of the relevant drugs when there are multiple therapies.
1. *Anticoagulants:* Phenobarbital lowers the plasma levels of dicumarol (name previously used: bishydroxycoumarin) and causes a decrease in anticoagulant activity as measured by the prothrombin time. Barbiturates can induce hepatic microsomal enzymes resulting in increased metabolism and decreased anticoagulant response of oral anticoagulants (e.g., warfarin, acenocoumarol, dicumarol, and phenprocoumon). Patients stabilized on anticoagulant therapy may require dosage adjustments if barbiturates are added to or withdrawn from their dosage regimen.
2. *Corticosteroids:* Barbiturates appear to enhance the metabolism of exogenous corticosteroids probably through the induction of hepatic microsomal enzymes. Patients stabilized on corticosteroid therapy may require dosage adjustments if barbiturates are added to or withdrawn from their dosage regimen.
3. *Griseofulvin:* Phenobarbital appears to interfere with the absorption of orally administered griseofulvin, thus decreasing its blood level. The effect of the resultant decreased blood levels of griseofulvin on therapeutic response has not been established. However, it would be preferable to avoid concomitant administration of these drugs.
4. *Doxycycline:* Phenobarbital has been shown to shorten the half-life of doxycycline for as long as 2 weeks after barbiturate therapy is discontinued.

This mechanism is probably through the induction of hepatic microsomal enzymes that metabolize the antibiotic. If phenobarbital and doxycycline are administered concurrently, the clinical response to doxycycline should be monitored closely.

5. *Phenytoin, sodium valproate, valproic acid:* The effect of barbiturates on the metabolism of phenytoin appears to be variable. Some investigators report an accelerating effect, while others report no effect. Because the effect of barbiturates on the metabolism of phenytoin is not predictable, phenytoin and barbiturate blood levels should be monitored more frequently if these drugs are given concurrently. Sodium valproate and valproic acid appear to decrease barbiturate metabolism; therefore, barbiturate blood levels should be monitored and appropriate dosage adjustments made as indicated.
6. *Central nervous system depressants:* The concomitant use of other central nervous system depressants, including other sedatives or hypnotics, antihistamines, tranquilizers, or alcohol, may produce additive depressant effects.
7. *Monoamine oxidase inhibitors (MAOI):* MAOI prolong the effects of barbiturates probably because metabolism of the barbiturate is inhibited.
8. *Estradiol, estrone, progesterone and other steroidal hormones:* Pretreatment with or concurrent administration of phenobarbital may decrease the effect of estradiol by increasing its metabolism. There have been reports of patients treated with antiepileptic drugs (e.g., phenobarbital) who became pregnant while taking oral contraceptives. An alternate contraceptive method might be suggested to women taking phenobarbital.

Carcinogenesis:
1. *Animal data.* Phenobarbital sodium is carcinogenic in mice and rats after lifetime administration. In mice, it produced benign and malignant liver cell tumors. In rats, benign liver cell tumors were observed very late in life.
2. *Human data.* In a 29-year epidemiological study of 9,136 patients who were treated on an anticonvulsant protocol that included phenobarbital, results indicated a higher than normal incidence of hepatic carcinoma. Previously, some of these patients were treated with thorotrast, a drug that is known to produce hepatic carcinomas. Thus, this study did not provide sufficient evidence that phenobarbital sodium is carcinogenic in humans.

Data from one retrospective study of 235 children in which the types of barbiturates are not identified suggested an association between exposure to barbiturates prenatally and an increased incidence of brain tumor. (Gold, E., et al., "Increased Risk of Brain Tumors in Children Exposed to Barbiturates," Journal of National Cancer Institute, 61:1031-1034, 1978).

Pregnancy:
1. *Teratogenic effects.* Pregnancy Category D—See "Warnings—Use in Pregnancy" section.
2. *Nonteratogenic effects.* Reports of infants suffering from long-term barbiturate exposure *in utero* included the acute withdrawal syndrome of seizures and hyperirritability from birth to a delayed onset of up to 14 days. (See "Drug Abuse and Dependence" section).

Labor and delivery:
Hypnotic doses of these barbiturates do not appear to significantly impair uterine activity during labor. Full anes-

Continued on next page

Nembutal Solution—Cont.

thetic doses of barbiturates decrease the force and frequency of uterine contractions. Administration of sedative-hypnotic barbiturates to the mother during labor may result in respiratory depression in the newborn. Premature infants are particularly susceptible to the depressant effects of barbiturates. If barbiturates are used during labor and delivery, resuscitation equipment should be available.
Data are currently not available to evaluate the effect of these barbiturates when forceps delivery or other intervention is necessary. Also, data are not available to determine the effect of these barbiturates on the later growth, development, and functional maturation of the child.
Nursing mothers:
Caution should be exercised when a barbiturate is administered to a nursing woman since small amounts of barbiturates are excreted in the milk.

ADVERSE REACTIONS

The following adverse reactions and their incidence were compiled from surveillance of thousands of hospitalized patients. Because such patients may be less aware of certain of the milder adverse effects of barbiturates, the incidence of these reactions may be somewhat higher in fully ambulatory patients.
More than 1 in 100 patients. The most common adverse reaction estimated to occur at a rate of 1 to 3 patients per 100 is: *Nervous System:* Somnolence.
Less than 1 in 100 patients. Adverse reactions estimated to occur at a rate of less than 1 in 100 patients listed below, grouped by organ system, and by decreasing order of occurrence are:
Nervous system: Agitation, confusion, hyperkinesia, ataxia, CNS depression, nightmares, nervousness, psychiatric disturbance, hallucinations, insomnia, anxiety, dizziness, thinking abnormality.
Respiratory system: Hypoventilation, apnea.
Cardiovascular system: Bradycardia, hypotension, syncope.
Digestive system: Nausea, vomiting, constipation.
Other reported reactions: Headache, injection site reactions, hypersensitivity reactions (angioedema, skin rashes, exfoliative dermatitis), fever, liver damage, megaloblastic anemia following chronic phenobarbital use.

DRUG ABUSE AND DEPENDENCE

Pentobarbital sodium injection is subject to control by the Federal Controlled Substances Act under DEA schedule II.
Barbiturates may be habit forming. Tolerance, psychological dependence, and physical dependence may occur especially following prolonged use of high doses of barbiturates. Daily administration in excess of 400 milligrams (mg) of pentobarbital or secobarbital for approximately 90 days is likely to produce some degree of physical dependence. A dosage of from 600 to 800 mg taken for at least 35 days is sufficient to produce withdrawal seizures. The average daily dose for the barbiturate addict is usually about 1.5 grams. As tolerance to barbiturates develops, the amount needed to maintain the same level of intoxication increases; tolerance to a fatal dosage, however, does not increase more than two-fold. As this occurs, the margin between an intoxicating dosage and fatal dosage becomes smaller.
Symptoms of acute intoxication with barbiturates include unsteady gait, slurred speech, and sustained nystagmus. Mental signs of chronic intoxication include confusion, poor judgment, irritability, insomnia, and somatic complaints.
Symptoms of barbiturate dependence are similar to those of chronic alcoholism. If an individual appears to be intoxicated with alcohol to a degree that is radically disproportionate to the amount of alcohol in his or her blood the use of barbiturates should be suspected. The lethal dose of a barbiturate is far less if alcohol is also ingested.
The symptoms of barbiturate withdrawal can be severe and may cause death. Minor withdrawal symptoms may appear 8 to 12 hours after the last dose of a barbiturate. These symptoms usually appear in the following order: anxiety, muscle twitching, tremor of hands and fingers, progressive weakness, dizziness, distortion in visual perception, nausea, vomiting, insomnia, and orthostatic hypotension. Major withdrawal symptoms (convulsions and delirium) may occur within 16 hours and last up to 5 days after abrupt cessation of these drugs. Intensity of withdrawal symptoms gradually declines over a period of approximately 15 days. Individuals susceptible to barbiturate abuse and dependence include alcoholics and opiate abusers, as well as other sedative-hypnotic and amphetamine abusers.
Drug dependence to barbiturates arises from repeated administration of a barbiturate or agent with barbiturate-like effect on a continuous basis, generally in amounts exceeding therapeutic dose levels. The characteristics of drug dependence to barbiturates include: (a) a strong desire or need to continue taking the drug; (b) a tendency to increase the dose; (c) a psychic dependence on the effects of the drug related to subjective and individual appreciation of those effects; and (d) a physical dependence on the effects of the drug requiring its presence for maintenance of homeostasis and resulting in a definite, characteristic, and self-limited abstinence syndrome when the drug is withdrawn.
Treatment of barbiturate dependence consists of cautious and gradual withdrawal of the drug. Barbiturate-dependent patients can be withdrawn by using a number of different withdrawal regimens. In all cases withdrawal takes an extended period of time. One method involves substituting a 30 mg dose of phenobarbital for each 100 to 200 mg dose of barbiturate that the patient has been taking. The total daily amount of phenobarbital is then administered in 3 to 4 divided doses, not to exceed 600 mg daily. Should signs of withdrawal occur on the first day of treatment, a loading dose of 100 to 200 mg of phenobarbital may be administered IM in addition to the oral dose. After stabilization on phenobarbital, the total daily dose is decreased by 30 mg a day as long as withdrawal is proceeding smoothly. A modification of this regimen involves initiating treatment at the patient's regular dosage level and decreasing the daily dosage by 10 percent if tolerated by the patient.
Infants physically dependent on barbiturates may be given phenobarbital 3 to 10 mg/kg/day. After withdrawal symptoms (hyperactivity, disturbed sleep, tremors, hyperreflexia) are relieved, the dosage of phenobarbital should be gradually decreased and completely withdrawn over a 2-week period.

OVERDOSAGE

The toxic dose of barbiturates varies considerably. In general, an oral dose of 1 gram of most barbiturates produces serious poisoning in an adult. Death commonly occurs after 2 to 10 grams of ingested barbiturate. Barbiturate intoxication may be confused with alcoholism, bromide intoxication, and with various neurological disorders.
Acute overdosage with barbiturates is manifested by CNS and respiratory depression which may progress to Cheyne-Stokes respiration, areflexia, constriction of the pupils to a slight degree (though in severe poisoning they may show paralytic dilation), oliguria, tachycardia, hypotension, lowered body temperature, and coma. Typical shock syndrome (apnea, circulatory collapse, respiratory arrest, and death) may occur.
In extreme overdose, all electrical activity in the brain may cease, in which case a "flat" EEG normally equated with clinical death cannot be accepted. This effect is fully reversible unless hypoxic damage occurs. Consideration should be given to the possibility of barbiturate intoxication even in situations that appear to involve trauma.
Complications such as pneumonia, pulmonary edema, cardiac arrhythmias, congestive heart failure, and renal failure may occur. Uremia may increase CNS sensitivity to barbiturates. Differential diagnosis should include hypoglycemia, head trauma, cerebrovascular accidents, convulsive states, and diabetic coma. Blood levels from acute overdosage for some barbiturates are listed in Table 1.
[See table 1 below]
Treatment of overdosage is mainly supportive and consists of the following:

1. Maintenance of an adequate airway, with assisted respiration and oxygen administration as necessary.
2. Monitoring of vital signs and fluid balance.
3. Fluid therapy and other standard treatment for shock, if needed.
4. If renal function is normal, forced diuresis may aid in the elimination of the barbiturate. Alkalinization of the urine increases renal excretion of some barbiturates, especially phenobarbital, also aprobarbital and mephobarbital (which is metabolized to phenobarbital).
5. Although not recommended as a routine procedure, hemodialysis may be used in severe barbiturate intoxications or if the patient is anuric or in shock.
6. Patient should be rolled from side to side every 30 minutes.
7. Antibiotics should be given if pneumonia is suspected.
8. Appropriate nursing care to prevent hypostatic pneumonia, decubiti, aspiration, and other complications of patients with altered states of consciousness.

DOSAGE AND ADMINISTRATION

Dosages of barbiturates must be individualized with full knowledge of their particular characteristics and recommended rate of administration. Factors of consideration are the patient's age, weight, and condition. Parenteral routes should be used only when oral administration is impossible or impractical.
Intramuscular Administration: IM injection of the sodium salts of barbiturates should be made deeply into a large muscle, and a volume of 5 ml should not be exceeded at any one site because of possible tissue irritation. After IM injection of a hypnotic dose, the patient's vital signs should be monitored. The usual adult dosage of NEMBUTAL Sodium Solution is 150 to 200 mg as a single IM injection; the recommended pediatric dosage ranges from 2 to 6 mg/kg as a single IM injection not to exceed 100 mg.
Intravenous Administration: NEMBUTAL Sodium Solution should not be admixed with any other medication or solution. IV injection is restricted to conditions in which other routes are not feasible, either because the patient is unconscious (as in cerebral hemorrhage, eclampsia, or status epilepticus), or because the patient resists (as in delirium), or because prompt action is imperative. Slow IV injection is essential, and patients should be carefully observed during administration. This requires that blood pressure, respiration, and cardiac function be maintained, vital signs be recorded, and equipment for resuscitation and artificial ventilation be available. The rate of IV injection should not exceed 50 mg/min for pentobarbital sodium.
There is no average intravenous dose of NEMBUTAL Sodium Solution (pentobarbital sodium injection) that can be relied on to produce similar effects in different patients. The possibility of overdose and respiratory depression is remote when the drug is injected slowly in fractional doses.
A commonly used initial dose for the 70 kg adult is 100 mg. Proportional reduction in dosage should be made for pediatric or debilitated patients. At least one minute is necessary to determine the full effect of intravenous pentobarbital. If necessary, additional small increments of the drug may be given up to a total of from 200 to 500 mg for normal adults.
Anticonvulsant use: In convulsive states, dosage of NEMBUTAL Sodium Solution should be kept to a minimum to avoid compounding the depression which may follow convulsions. The injection must be made slowly with due regard to the time required for the drug to penetrate the blood-brain barrier.
Special patient population: Dosage should be reduced in the elderly or debilitated because these patients may be more sensitive to barbiturates. Dosage should be reduced for patients with impaired renal function or hepatic disease.
Inspection: Parenteral drug products should be inspected visually for particulate matter and discoloration prior to administration, whenever solution containers permit. Solutions for injection showing evidence of precipitation should not be used.

HOW SUPPLIED

NEMBUTAL Sodium Solution (pentobarbital sodium injection, USP) is available in the following sizes: 20-ml multiple-dose vial, 1 g per vial (**NDC** 0074-3778-04); and 50-ml multiple-dose vial, 2.5 g per vial (**NDC** 0074-3778-05).
Each ml contains:
Pentobarbital Sodium, derivative of
barbituric acid .... 50 mg
Warning - May be habit forming.
Propylene glycol .... 40% v/v
Alcohol 10%
Water for Injection .... qs
(pH adjusted to approximately 9.5 with hydrochloric acid and/or sodium hydroxide.)
Exposure of pharmaceutical products to heat should be minimized. Avoid excessive heat. Protect from freezing. It is recommended that the product be stored at room temperature-86°F (30°C); however, brief exposure up to 104° F (40°C) does not adversely affect the product.
Revised: February, 1998
Ref. 03-4715-R7
ABBOTT LABORATORIES
NORTH CHICAGO, IL 60064, U.S.A.

Table 1.— *Concentration of Barbiturate in the Blood Versus Degree of CNS Depression*

		Blood barbiturate level in ppm (μg/ml)				
		Degree of depression in nontolerant persons*				
Barbiturate	Onset/duration	1	2	3	4	5
Pentobarbital	Fast/short	≤2	0.5 to 3	10 to 15	12 to 25	15 to 40
Secobarbital	Fast/short	≤2	0.5 to 5	10 to 15	15 to 25	15 to 40
Amobarbital	Intermediate/intermediate	≤3	2 to 10	30 to 40	30 to 60	40 to 80
Butabarbital	Intermediate/intermediate	≤5	3 to 25	40 to 60	50 to 80	60 to 100
Phenobarbital	Slow/long	≤10	5 to 40	50 to 80	70 to 120	100 to 200

* Categories of degree of depression in nontolerant persons:
1. Under the influence and appreciably impaired for purposes of driving a motor vehicle or performing tasks requiring alertness and unimpaired judgment and reaction time.
2. Sedated, therapeutic range, calm, relaxed, and easily aroused.
3. Comatose, difficult to arouse, significant depression of respiration.
4. Compatible with death in aged or ill persons or in presence of obstructed airway, other toxic agents, or exposure to cold.
5. Usual lethal level, the upper end of the range includes those who received some supportive treatment.

NEMBUTAL® SODIUM SUPPOSITORIES

Ⓒ Ⅲ ℞

[*nĕm-bū 'tal*]
(PENTOBARBITAL SODIUM SUPPOSITORIES)

WARNING: MAY BE HABIT FORMING

DESCRIPTION

The barbiturates are nonselective central nervous system depressants which are primarily used as sedative hypnotics. The barbiturates and their sodium salts are subject to control under the Federal Controlled Substances Act (See "Drug Abuse and Dependence" section).

Barbiturates are substituted pyrimidine derivatives in which the basic structure common to these drugs is barbituric acid, a substance which has no central nervous system (CNS) activity. CNS activity is obtained by substituting alkyl, alkenyl, or aryl groups on the pyrimidine ring. Nembutal (pentobarbital sodium) is chemically represented by sodium 5-ethyl-5-(1-methylbutyl) barbiturate.

The structural formula for pentobarbital sodium is:

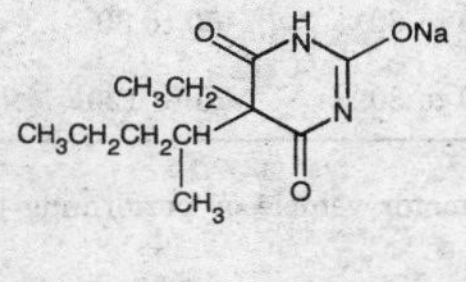

The sodium salt of pentobarbital occurs as a white, slightly bitter powder which is freely soluble in water and alcohol but practically insoluble in benzene and ether. Each rectal suppository contains either 30 mg, 60 mg, 120 mg, or 200 mg of pentobarbital sodium.

Inactive Ingredients: Semi-synthetic glycerides.

CLINICAL PHARMACOLOGY

Barbiturates are capable of producing all levels of CNS mood alteration from excitation to mild sedation, to hypnosis, and deep coma. Overdosage can produce death. In high enough therapeutic doses, barbiturates induce anesthesia. Barbiturates depress the sensory cortex, decrease motor activity, alter cerebellar function, and produce drowsiness, sedation, and hypnosis.

Barbiturate-induced sleep differs from physiological sleep. Sleep laboratory studies have demonstrated that barbiturates reduce the amount of time spent in the rapid eye movement (REM) phase of sleep or dreaming stage. Also, Stages III and IV sleep are decreased. Following abrupt cessation of barbiturates used regularly, patients may experience markedly increased dreaming, nightmares, and/or insomnia. Therefore, withdrawal of a single therapeutic dose over 5 or 6 days has been recommended to lessen the REM rebound and disturbed sleep which contribute to drug withdrawal syndrome (for example, decrease the dose from 3 to 2 doses a day for 1 week).

In studies, secobarbital sodium and pentobarbital sodium have been found to lose most of their effectiveness for both inducing and maintaining sleep by the end of 2 weeks of continued drug administration at fixed doses. The short-, intermediate-, and, to a lesser degree, long-acting barbiturates have been widely prescribed for treating insomnia. Although the clinical literature abounds with claims that the short-acting barbiturates are superior for producing sleep while the intermediate-acting compounds are more effective in maintaining sleep, controlled studies have failed to demonstrate these differential effects. Therefore, as sleep medications, the barbiturates are of limited value beyond short-term use.

Barbiturates have little analgesic action at subanesthetic doses. Rather, in subanesthetic doses these drugs may increase the reaction to painful stimuli. All barbiturates exhibit anticonvulsant activity in anesthetic doses. However, of the drugs in this class, only phenobarbital, mephobarbital, and metharbital have been clinically demonstrated to be effective as oral anticonvulsants in subhypnotic doses.

Barbiturates are respiratory depressants. The degree of respiratory depression is dependent upon dose. With hypnotic doses, respiratory depression produced by barbiturates is similar to that which occurs during physiologic sleep with slight decrease in blood pressure and heart rate.

Studies in laboratory animals have shown that barbiturates cause reduction in the tone and contractility of the uterus, ureters, and urinary bladder. However, concentrations of the drugs required to produce this effect in humans are not reached with sedative-hypnotic doses.

Barbiturates do not impair normal hepatic function, but have been shown to induce liver microsomal enzymes, thus increasing and/or altering the metabolism of barbiturates and other drugs. (See "Precautions—*Drug Interactions*" section).

Pharmacokinetics: Barbiturates are absorbed in varying degrees following oral, rectal, or parenteral administration. The onset of action for oral or rectal administration varies from 20 to 60 minutes.

Duration of action, which is related to the rate at which the barbiturates are redistributed throughout the body, varies among persons and in the same person from time to time. No studies have demonstrated that the different routes of administration are equivalent with respect to bioavailability.

Barbiturates are weak acids that are absorbed and rapidly distributed to all tissues and fluids with high concentrations in the brain, liver, and kidneys. Lipid solubility of the barbiturates is the dominant factor in their distribution within the body. The more lipid soluble the barbiturate, the more rapidly it penetrates all tissues of the body. Barbiturates are bound to plasma and tissue proteins to a varying degree with the degree of binding increasing directly as a function of lipid solubility.

Phenobarbital has the lowest lipid solubility, lowest plasma binding, lowest brain protein binding, the longest delay in onset of activity, and the longest duration of action. At the opposite extreme is secobarbital which has the highest lipid solubility, plasma protein binding, brain protein binding, the shortest delay in onset of activity, and the shortest duration of action. Butabarbital is classified as an intermediate barbiturate.

The plasma half-life for phentobarbital in adults is 15 to 50 hours and appears to be dose dependent.

Barbiturates are metabolized primarily by the hepatic microsomal enzyme system, and the metabolic products are excreted in the urine, and less commonly, in the feces. Approximately 25 to 50 percent of a dose of aprobarbital or phenobarbital is eliminated unchanged in the urine, whereas the amount of other barbiturates excreted unchanged in the urine is negligible. The excretion of unmetabolized barbiturate is one feature that distinguishes the long-acting category from those belonging to other categories which are almost entirely metabolized. The inactive metabolites of the barbiturates are excreted as conjugates of glucuronic acid.

INDICATIONS AND USAGE

Rectal: Barbiturates administered rectally are absorbed from the colon and are used when oral or parenteral administration may be undesirable.

1. Sedative.
2. Hypnotic, for the short-term treatment of insomnia, since they appear to lose their effectiveness for sleep induction and sleep maintenance after 2 weeks (See "Clinical Pharmacology" section).

CONTRAINDICATIONS

Barbiturates are contraindicated in patients with known barbiturate sensitivity. Barbiturates are also contraindicated in patients with a history of manifest or latent porphyria.

WARNINGS

1. *Habit forming:* Barbiturates may be habit forming. Tolerance, psychological and physical dependence may occur with continued use. (See "Drug Abuse and Dependence" and "Pharmacokinetics" sections). Patients who have psychological dependence on barbiturates may increase the dosage or decrease the dosage interval without consulting a physician and may subsequently develop a physical dependence on barbiturates. To minimize the possibility of overdosage or the development of dependence, the prescribing and dispensing of sedative-hypnotic barbiturates should be limited to the amount required for the interval until the next appointment. Abrupt cessation after prolonged use in the dependent person may result in withdrawal symptoms, including delirium, convulsions, and possibly death. Barbiturates should be withdrawn gradually from any patient known to be taking excessive dosage over long periods of time. (See "Drug Abuse and Dependence" section).

2. *Acute or chronic pain:* Caution should be exercised when barbiturates are administered to patients with acute or chronic pain, because paradoxical excitement could be induced or important symptoms could be masked. However, the use of barbiturates as sedatives in the postoperative surgical period and as adjuncts to cancer chemotherapy is well established.

3. *Use in pregnancy:* Barbiturates can cause fetal damage when administered to a pregnant woman. Retrospective, case-controlled studies have suggested a connection between the maternal consumption of barbiturates and a higher than expected incidence of fetal abnormalities. Following oral or parenteral administration, barbiturates readily cross the placental barrier and are distributed throughout fetal tissues with highest concentrations found in the placenta, fetal liver, and brain. It is presumed that this effect will also be seen following rectal administration. Withdrawal symptoms occur in infants born to mothers who receive barbiturates throughout the last trimester of pregnancy. (See "Drug Abuse and Dependence" section). If this drug is used during pregnancy, or if the patient becomes pregnant while taking this drug, the patient should be apprised of the potential hazard to the fetus.

4. *Synergistic effects:* The concomitant use of alcohol or other CNS depressants may produce additive CNS depressant effects.

PRECAUTIONS

General: Barbiturates may be habit forming. Tolerance and psychological and physical dependence may occur with continuing use. (See "Drug Abuse and Dependence" section). Barbiturates should be administered with caution, if at all, to patients who are mentally depressed, have suicidal tendencies, or a history of drug abuse.

Elderly or debilitated patients may react to barbiturates with marked excitement, depression, and confusion. In some persons, barbiturates repeatedly produce excitement rather than depression.

In patients with hepatic damage, barbiturates should be administered with caution and initially in reduced doses. Barbiturates should not be administered to patients showing the premonitory signs of hepatic coma.

Information for the patient: Practitioners should give the following information and instructions to patients receiving barbiturates.

1. The use of barbiturates carries with it an associated risk of psychological and/or physical dependence. The patient should be warned against increasing the dose of the drug without consulting a physician.
2. Barbiturates may impair mental and/or physical abilities required for the performance of potentially hazardous tasks (e.g., driving, operating machinery, etc.)
3. Alcohol should not be consumed while taking barbiturates. Concurrent use of the barbiturates with other CNS depressants (e.g., alcohol, narcotics, tranquilizers, and antihistamines) may result in additional CNS depressant effects.

Laboratory tests: Prolonged therapy with barbiturates should be accompanied by periodic laboratory evaluation of organ systems, including hematopoietic, renal, and hepatic systems. (See "Precautions — *General*" and "Adverse Reactions" sections).

Drug interactions: Most reports of clinically significant drug interactions occurring with the barbiturates have involved phenobarbital. However, the application of these data to other barbiturates appears valid and warrants serial blood level determinations of the relevant drugs when there are multiple therapies.

1. *Anticoagulants:* Phenobarbital lowers the plasma levels of dicumarol (name previously used: bishydroxycoumarin) and causes a decrease in anticoagulant activity as measured by the prothrombin time. Barbiturates can induce hepatic microsomal enzymes resulting in increased metabolism and decreased anticoagulant response of oral anticoagulants (e.g., warfarin, acenocoumarol, dicumarol, and phenprocoumon). Patients stabilized on anticoagulant therapy may require dosage adjustments if barbiturates are added to or withdrawn from their dosage regimen.
2. *Corticosteroids:* Barbiturates appear to enhance the metabolism of exogenous corticosteroids probably through the induction of hepatic microsomal enzymes. Patients stabilized on corticosteroid therapy may require dosage adjustments if barbiturates are added to or withdrawn from their dosage regimen.
3. *Griseofulvin:* Phenobarbital appears to interfere with the absorption of orally administered griseofulvin, thus decreasing its blood level. The effect of the resultant decreased blood levels of griseofulvin on therapeutic response has not been established. However, it would be preferable to avoid concomitant administration of these drugs.
4. *Doxycycline:* Phenobarbital has been shown to shorten the half-life of doxycycline for as long as 2 weeks after barbiturate therapy is discontinued.
   This mechanism is probably through the induction of hepatic microsomal enzymes that metabolize the antibiotic. If phenobarbital and doxycycline are administered concurrently, the clinical response to doxycycline should be monitored closely.
5. *Phenytoin, sodium valproate, valproic acid:* The effect of barbiturates on the metabolism of phenytoin appears to be variable. Some investigators report an accelerating effect, while others report no effect. Because the effect of barbiturates on the metabolism of phenytoin is not predictable, phenytoin and barbiturate blood levels should be monitored more frequently if these drugs are given concurrently. Sodium valproate and valproic acid appear to decrease barbiturate metabolism; therefore, barbiturate blood levels should be monitored and appropriate dosage adjustments made as indicated.
6. *Central nervous system depressants:* The concomitant use of other central nervous system depressants, including other sedatives or hypnotics, antihistamines, tranquilizers, or alcohol, may produce additive depressant effects.
7. *Monoamine oxidase inhibitors (MAOI):* MAOI prolong the effects of barbiturates probably because metabolism of the barbiturate is inhibited.
8. *Estradiol, estrone, progesterone and other steroidal hormones:* Pretreatment with or concurrent administration of phenobarbital may decrease the effect of estradiol by increasing its metabolism. There have been reports of patients treated with antiepileptic drugs (e.g., phenobarbital) who became pregnant while taking oral contraceptives. An alternate contraceptive method might be suggested to women taking phenobarbital.

Carcinogenesis:

1. Animal data. Phenobarbital sodium is carcinogenic in mice and rats after lifetime administration. In mice, it produced benign and malignant liver cell tumors. In rats, benign liver cell tumors were observed very late in life.
2. Human data. In a 29-year epidemiological study of 9,136 patients who were treated on an anticonvulsant protocol that included phenobarbital, results indicated a higher than normal incidence of hepatic carcinoma. Previously, some of these patients were treated with thorotrast, a drug that is known to produce hepatic carcinomas. Thus, this study did not provide sufficient evidence that phenobarbital sodium is carcinogenic in humans.

Data from one retrospective study of 235 children in which the types of barbiturates are not identified suggested an association between exposure to barbiturates prenatally and an increased incidence of brain tumor. (Gold, E., et al., "Increased Risk of Brain Tumors in Children Exposed to Barbiturates," Journal of National Cancer Institute, 61:1031–1034, 1978).

Pregnancy: *1. Teratogenic effects.* Pregnancy Category D — See "Warnings — Use in Pregnancy" section.

2. *Nonteratogenic effects.* Reports of infants suffering from long-term barbiturate exposure in utero included the acute

Continued on next page

Nembutal Suppositories—Cont.

withdrawal syndrome of seizures and hyperirritability from birth to a delayed onset of up to 14 days. (See "Drug Abuse and Dependence" section).

Labor and delivery: Hypnotic doses of these barbiturates do not appear to significantly impair uterine activity during labor. Full anesthetic doses of barbiturates decrease the force and frequency of uterine contractions. Administration of sedative-hypnotic barbiturates to the mother during labor may result in respiratory depression in the newborn. Premature infants are particularly susceptible to the depressant effects of barbiturates. If barbiturates are used during labor and delivery, resuscitation equipment should be available.

Data are currently not available to evaluate the effect of these barbiturates when forceps delivery or other intervention is necessary. Also, data are not available to determine the effect of these barbiturates on the later growth, development, and functional maturation of the child.

Nursing mothers: Caution should be exercised when a barbiturate is administered to a nursing woman since small amounts of barbiturates are excreted in the milk.

ADVERSE REACTIONS

The following adverse reactions and their incidence were compiled from surveillance of thousands of hospitalized patients. Because such patients may be less aware of certain of the milder adverse effects of barbiturates, the incidence of these reactions may be somewhat higher in fully ambulatory patients.

More than 1 in 100 patients. The most common adverse reaction estimated to occur at a rate of 1 to 3 patients per 100 is: *Nervous System:* Somnolence.

Less than 1 in 100 patients. Adverse reactions estimated to occur at a rate of less than 1 in 100 patients listed below, grouped by organ system, and by decreasing order of occurrence are:

Nervous system: Agitation, confusion, hyperkinesia, ataxia, CNS depression, nightmares, nervousness, psychiatric disturbance, hallucinations, insomnia, anxiety, dizziness, thinking abnormality.

Respiratory system: Hypoventilation, apnea.

Cardiovascular system: Bradycardia, hypotension, syncope.

Digestive system: Nausea, vomiting, constipation.

Other reported reactions: Headache, injection site reactions, hypersensitivity reactions (angioedema, skin rashes, exfoliative dermatitis), fever, liver damage, megaloblastic anemia following chronic phenobarbital use.

DRUG ABUSE AND DEPENDENCE

Pentobarbital sodium suppositories are subject to control by the Federal Controlled Substances Act under DEA schedule III.

Barbiturates may be habit forming. Tolerance, psychological dependence, and physical dependence may occur especially following prolonged use of high doses of barbiturates. Daily administration in excess of 400 milligrams (mg) of pentobarbital or secobarbital for approximately 90 days is likely to produce some degree of physical dependence. A dosage of from 600 to 800 mg taken for at least 35 days is sufficient to produce withdrawal seizures. The average daily dose for the barbiturate addict is usually about 1.5 grams. As tolerance to barbiturates develops, the amount needed to maintain the same level of intoxication increases; tolerance to a fatal dosage, however, does not increase more than two-fold. As this occurs, the margin between an intoxicating dosage and fatal dosage becomes smaller.

Symptoms of acute intoxication with barbiturates include unsteady gait, slurred speech, and sustained nystagmus. Mental signs of chronic intoxication include confusion, poor judgment, irritability, insomnia, and somatic complaints.

Symptoms of barbiturate dependence are similar to those of chronic alcoholism. If an individual appears to be intoxicated with alcohol to a degree that is radically disproportionate to the amount of alcohol in his or her blood the use of barbiturates should be suspected. The lethal dose of a barbiturate is far less if alcohol is also ingested.

The symptoms of barbiturate withdrawal can be severe and may cause death. Minor withdrawal symptoms may appear 8 to 12 hours after the last dose of a barbiturate. These symptoms usually appear in the following order: anxiety, muscle twitching, tremor of hands and fingers, progressive weakness, dizziness, distortion in visual perception, nausea, vomiting, insomnia, and orthostatic hypotension. Major withdrawal symptoms (convulsions and delirium) may occur within 16 hours and last up to 5 days after abrupt cessation of these drugs. Intensity of withdrawal symptoms gradually declines over a period of approximately 15 days. Individuals susceptible to barbiturate abuse and dependence include alcoholics and opiate abusers, as well as other sedative-hypnotic and amphetamine abusers.

Drug dependence to barbiturates arises from repeated administration of a barbiturate or agent with barbiturate-like effect on a continuous basis, generally in amounts exceeding therapeutic dose levels. The characteristics of drug dependence to barbiturates include: (a) a strong desire or need to continue taking the drug; (b) a tendency to increase the dose; (c) a psychic dependence on the effects of the drug related to subjective and individual appreciation of those effects; and (d) a physical dependence on the effects of the drug requiring its presence for maintenance of homeostasis and resulting in a definite, characteristic, and self-limited abstinence syndrome when the drug is withdrawn.

Table 1.—*Concentration of Barbiturate in the Blood Versus Degree of CNS Depression*

Barbiturate	Onset/ duration	Blood barbiturate level in ppm (μg/ml)				
		Degree of depression in nontolerant persons*				
		1	2	3	4	5
Pentobarbital	Fast/short	≤2	0.5 to 3	10 to 15	12 to 25	15 to 40
Secobarbital	Fast/short	≤2	0.5 to 5	10 to 15	15 to 25	15 to 40
Amobarbital	Intermediate/ intermediate	≤3	2 to 10	30 to 40	30 to 60	40 to 80
Butabarbital	Intermediate/ intermediate	≤5	3 to 25	40 to 60	50 to 80	60 to 100
Phenobarbital	Slow/long	≤10	5 to 40	50 to 80	70 to 120	100 to 200

* Categories of degree of depression in nontolerant persons:
1. Under the influence and appreciably impaired for purposes of driving a motor vehicle or performing tasks requiring alertness and unimpaired judgment and reaction time.
2. Sedated, therapeutic range, calm, relaxed, and easily aroused.
3. Comatose, difficult to arouse, significant depression of respiration.
4. Compatible with death in aged or ill persons or in presence of obstructed airway, other toxic agents, or exposure to cold.
5. Usual lethal level, the upper end of the range includes those who received some supportive treatment.

Treatment of barbiturate dependence consists of cautious and gradual withdrawal of the drug. Barbiturate-dependent patients can be withdrawn by using a number of different withdrawal regimens. In all cases withdrawal takes an extended period of time. One method involves substituting a 30 mg dose of phenobarbital for each 100 to 200 mg dose of barbiturate that the patient has been taking. The total daily amount of phenobarbital is then administered in 3 to 4 divided doses, not to exceed 600 mg daily. Should signs of withdrawal occur on the first day of treatment, a loading dose of 100 to 200 mg of phenobarbital may be administered IM in addition to the oral dose. After stabilization on phenobarbital, the total daily dose is decreased by 30 mg a day as long as withdrawal is proceeding smoothly. A modification of this regimen involves initiating treatment at the patient's regular dosage level and decreasing the daily dosage by 10 percent if tolerated by the patient.

Infants physically dependent on barbiturates may be given phenobarbital 3 to 10 mg/kg/day. After withdrawal symptoms (hyperactivity, disturbed sleep, tremors, hyperreflexia) are relieved, the dosage of phenobarbital should be gradually decreased and completely withdrawn over a 2 week period.

OVERDOSAGE

The toxic dose of barbiturates varies considerably. In general, an oral dose of 1 gram of most barbiturates produces serious poisoning in an adult. Death commonly occurs after 2 to 10 grams of ingested barbiturate. Barbiturate intoxication may be confused with alcoholism, bromide intoxication, and with various neurological disorders.

Acute overdosage with barbiturates is manifested by CNS and respiratory depression which may progress to Cheyne-Stokes respiration, areflexia, constriction of the pupils to a slight degree (though in severe poisoning they may show paralytic dilation), oliguria, tachycardia, hypotension, lowered body temperature, and coma. Typical shock syndrome (apnea, circulatory collapse, respiratory arrest, and death) may occur.

In extreme overdose, all electrical activity in the brain may cease, in which case a "flat" EEG normally equated with clinical death cannot be accepted. This effect is fully reversible unless hypoxic damage occurs. Consideration should be given to the possibility of barbiturate intoxication even in situations that appear to involve trauma.

Complications such as pneumonia, pulmonary edema, cardiac arrhythmias, congestive heart failure, and renal failure may occur. Uremia may increase CNS sensitivity to barbiturates. Differential diagnosis should include hypoglycemia, head trauma, cerebrovascular accidents, convulsive states, and diabetic coma. Blood levels from acute overdosage for some barbiturates are listed in Table 1.

[See table 1 above]

Treatment of overdosage is mainly supportive and consists of the following:

1. Maintenance of an adequate airway, with assisted respiration and oxygen administration as necessary.
2. Monitoring of vital signs and fluid balance.
3. Fluid therapy and other standard treatment for shock, if needed.
4. If renal function is normal, forced diuresis may aid in the elimination of the barbiturate. Alkalinization of the urine increases renal excretion of some barbiturates, especially phenobarbital, also aprobarbital, and mephobarbital (which is metabolized to phenobarbital).
5. Although not recommended as a routine procedure, hemodialysis may be used in severe barbiturate intoxications or if the patient is anuric or in shock.
6. Patient should be rolled from side to side every 30 minutes.
7. Antibiotics should be given if pneumonia is suspected.
8. Appropriate nursing care to prevent hypostatic pneumonia, decubiti, aspiration, and other complications of patients with altered states of consciousness.

DOSAGE AND ADMINISTRATION

Typical hypnotic doses for adults and children are given below. These are intended only as a guide, and administration should be adjusted to the individual needs of each patient. For sedation, in children 5–14 years and in adults, reduce dose appropriately.

Adults (average to above average weight)— one 120 mg or one 200 mg suppository.

Children —

12–14 years (80–110 lbs)	one 60 mg or one 120 mg suppository
5–12 years (40–80 lbs)	one 60 mg suppository
1–4 years (20–40 lbs)	one 30 mg or one 60 mg suppository
2 months–1 year (10–20 lbs)	one 30 mg suppository

Suppositories should not be divided.

Dosages of barbiturates must be individualized with full knowledge of their particular characteristics and recommended rate of administration. Factors of consideration are the patient's age, weight, and condition.

Special patient population: Dosage should be reduced in the elderly or debilitated because these patients may be more sensitive to barbiturates. Dosage should be reduced for patients with impaired renal function or hepatic disease.

HOW SUPPLIED

NEMBUTAL Sodium Suppositories (pentobarbital sodium suppositories) are available as suppositories containing pentobarbital sodium in the amount of 30 mg (**NDC** 0074-3272-01); 60 mg (**NDC** 0074-3148-01); 120 mg (**NDC** 0074-3145-01) and 200 mg (**NDC** 0074-3164-01). Supplied in boxes of 12 suppositories.

Store in a refrigerator (36°–46°F).

Revised: June, 1994

Ref. 03-4514-R13

NORVIR® ℞

[*nŏr-vĭr*]

(ritonavir capsules) Soft Gelatin

(ritonavir oral solution)

> **WARNING**
> CO-ADMINISTRATION OF NORVIR WITH CERTAIN NONSEDATING ANTIHISTAMINES, SEDATIVE HYPNOTICS, ANTIARRHYTHMICS, OR ERGOT ALKALOID PREPARATIONS MAY RESULT IN POTENTIALLY SERIOUS AND/OR LIFE-THREATENING ADVERSE EVENTS DUE TO POSSIBLE EFFECTS OF NORVIR ON THE HEPATIC METABOLISM OF CERTAIN DRUGS. SEE **CONTRAINDICATIONS** AND **PRECAUTIONS** SECTIONS.

DESCRIPTION

NORVIR (ritonavir) is an inhibitor of HIV protease with activity against the Human Immunodeficiency Virus (HIV).

Ritonavir is chemically designated as 10-Hydroxy-2-methyl-5-(1-methylethyl)-1-[2-(1-methylethyl)-4-thiazolyl]-3,6-dioxo-8,11-bis(phenylmethyl)-2,4,7,12-tetraazatridecan-13-oic acid, 5-thiazolylmethyl ester, [5S-(5R*,8R*,10R*,11R*)]. Its molecular formula is $C_{37}H_{48}N_6O_5S_2$, and its molecular weight is 720.95. Ritonavir has the following structural formula:

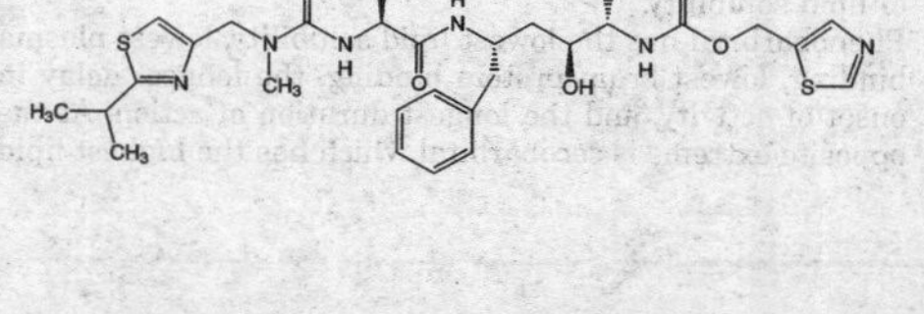

Ritonavir is a white-to-light-tan powder. Ritonavir has a bitter metallic taste. It is freely soluble in methanol and ethanol, soluble in isopropanol and practically insoluble in water.

NORVIR soft gelatin capsules are available for oral administration in a strength of 100 mg ritonavir with the following inactive ingredients: Butylated hydroxytoluene, ethanol, gelatin, iron oxide, oleic acid, polyoxyl 35 castor oil, and titanium dioxide.

NORVIR oral solution is available for oral administration as 80 mg/mL of ritonavir in a peppermint and caramel flavored vehicle. Each 8-ounce bottle contains 19.2 grams of ritonavir. NORVIR oral solution also contains ethanol, water, polyoxyl 35 castor oil, propylene glycol, anhydrous citric acid to adjust pH, saccharin sodium, peppermint oil, creamy caramel flavoring, and FD&C Yellow No. 6.

CLINICAL PHARMACOLOGY

Microbiology

Mechanism of action: Ritonavir is a peptidomimetic inhibitor of both the HIV-1 and HIV-2 proteases. Inhibition of HIV protease renders the enzyme incapable of processing the *gag-pol* polyprotein precursor which leads to production of non-infectious immature HIV particles.

Antiviral activity *in vitro*: The activity of ritonavir was assessed *in vitro* in acutely infected lymphoblastoid cell lines and in peripheral blood lymphocytes. The concentration of drug that inhibits 50% (EC_{50}) of viral replication ranged from 3.8 to 153 nM depending upon the HIV-1 isolate and the cells employed. The average EC_{50} for low passage clinical isolates was 22 nM (n=13). In MT_4 cells, ritonavir demonstrated additive effects against HIV-1 in combination with either zidovudine (ZDV) or didanosine (ddI). Studies which measured cytotoxicity of ritonavir on several cell lines showed that >20 μM was required to inhibit cellular growth by 50% resulting in an *in vitro* therapeutic index of at least 1000.

Resistance: HIV-1 isolates with reduced susceptibility to ritonavir have been selected *in vitro*. Genotypic analysis of these isolates showed mutations in the HIV protease gene at amino acid positions 84 (Ile to Val), 82 (Val to Phe), 71 (Ala to Val), and 46 (Met to Ile). Phenotypic (n=18) and genotypic (n=44) changes in HIV isolates from selected patients treated with ritonavir were monitored in phase I/II trials over a period of 3 to 32 weeks. Mutations associated with the HIV viral protease in isolates obtained from 41 patients appeared to occur in a stepwise and ordered fashion; in sequence, these mutations were position 82 (Val to Ala/Phe), 54 (Ile to Val), 71 (Ala to Val/Thr), and 36 (Ile to Leu), followed by combinations of mutations at an additional 5 specific amino acid positions. Of 18 patients for which both phenotypic and genotypic analysis were performed on free virus isolated from plasma, 12 showed reduced susceptibility to ritonavir *in vitro*. All 18 patients possessed one or more mutations in the viral protease gene. The 82 mutation appeared to be necessary but not sufficient to confer phenotypic resistance. Phenotypic resistance was defined as a ≥5-fold decrease in viral sensitivity *in vitro* from baseline. The clinical relevance of phenotypic and genotypic changes associated with ritonavir therapy has not been established.

Cross-resistance to other antiretrovirals: Among protease inhibitors variable cross-resistance has been recognized. Serial HIV isolates obtained from six patients during ritonavir therapy showed a decrease in ritonavir susceptibility *in vitro* but did not demonstrate a concordant decrease in susceptibility to saquinavir *in vitro* when compared to matched baseline isolates. However, isolates from two of these patients demonstrated decreased susceptibility to indinavir *in vitro* (8-fold). Isolates from 5 patients were also tested for cross-resistance to amprenavir and nelfinavir; isolates from 2 patients had a decrease in susceptibility to nelfinavir (12- to 14-fold), and none to amprenavir. Cross-resistance between ritonavir and reverse transcriptase inhibitors is unlikely because of the different enzyme targets involved. One ZDV-resistant HIV isolate tested *in vitro* retained full susceptibility to ritonavir.

Pharmacokinetics

The pharmacokinetics of ritonavir have been studied in healthy volunteers and HIV-infected patients (CD_4 ≥ 50 cells/μL). See Table 1 for ritonavir pharmacokinetic characteristics.

The absolute bioavailability of ritonavir has not been determined. After a 600 mg dose of oral solution, peak concentrations of ritonavir were achieved approximately 2 hours and 4 hours after dosing under fasting and non-fasting (514 KCal; 9% fat, 12% protein, and 79% carbohydrate) conditions, respectively. When the oral solution was given under non-fasting conditions, peak ritonavir concentrations decreased 23% and the extent of absorption decreased 7% relative to fasting conditions. Dilution of the oral solution, within one hour of administration, with 240 mL of chocolate milk, Advera® or Ensure® did not significantly affect the extent and rate of ritonavir absorption. After a single 600 mg dose under non-fasting conditions, in two separate studies, the soft gelatin capsule (n=57) and oral solution (n=18) formulations yielded mean ± SD areas under the plasma concentration-time curve (AUCs) of 121.7 ± 53.8 and 129.0 ± 39.3 μg•h/mL, respectively. Relative to fasting conditions, the extent of absorption of ritonavir from the soft gelatin capsule formulation was 13% higher when administered with a meal (615 KCal; 14.5% fat, 9% protein, and 76% carbohydrate).

Table 1
Ritonavir Pharmacokinetic Characteristics

Parameter	n	Values (Mean ± SD)
C_{max} SS†	10	11.2 ± 3.6 μg/mL
C_{trough} SS†	10	3.7 ± 2.6 μg/mL
V_{β}/F‡	91	0.41 ± 0.25 L/kg
$t_{1/2}$		3 – 5 h
CL/F SS†	10	8.8 ± 3.2 L/h
CL/F‡	91	4.6 ± 1.6 L/h
CL_R	62	<0.1 L/h
RBC/Plasma Ratio		0.14
Percent Bound*		98 to 99%

† SS = steady state; patients taking ritonavir 600 mg q12h.
‡ Single ritonavir 600 mg dose.
* Primarily bound to human serum albumin and alpha-1 acid glycoprotein over the ritonavir concentration range of 0.01 to 30 μg/mL.

Nearly all of the plasma radioactivity after a single oral 600 mg dose of ^{14}C-ritonavir oral solution (n=5) was attributed to unchanged ritonavir. Five ritonavir metabolites have been identified in human urine and feces. The isopropylthiazole oxidation metabolite (M-2) is the major metabolite and has antiviral activity similar to that of parent drug; however, the concentrations of this metabolite in plasma are low. *In vitro* studies utilizing human liver microsomes have demonstrated that cytochrome P450 3A (CYP3A) is the major isoform involved in ritonavir metabolism, although CYP2D6 also contributes to the formation of M-2.

In a study of five subjects receiving a 600 mg dose of ^{14}C-ritonavir oral solution, 11.3 ± 2.8% of the dose was excreted into the urine, with 3.5 ± 1.8% of the dose excreted as unchanged parent drug. In that study, 86.4 ± 2.9% of the dose was excreted in the feces with 33.8 ± 10.8% of the dose excreted as unchanged parent drug. Upon multiple dosing, ritonavir accumulation is less than predicted from a single dose possibly due to a time and dose-related increase in clearance.

[See table 1 above]

The pharmacokinetic profile of ritonavir in pediatric patients below the age of 2 years has not been established. Steady-state pharmacokinetics were evaluated in 37 HIV-infected patients ages 2 to 14 years receiving doses ranging from 250 mg/m^2 b.i.d. to 400 mg/m^2 b.i.d. Across dose groups, ritonavir steady-state oral clearance (CL/F/m^2) was approximately 1.5 times faster in pediatric patients than in adult subjects. Ritonavir concentrations obtained after 350 to 400 mg/m^2 twice daily in pediatric patients were comparable to those obtained in adults receiving 600 mg (approximately 330 mg/m^2) twice daily.

Special Populations:

Gender, Race and Age: No age-related pharmacokinetic differences have been observed in adult patients (18 to 63 years). Ritonavir pharmacokinetics have not been studied in older patients. A study of ritonavir pharmacokinetics in healthy males and females showed no statistically significant differences in the pharmacokinetics of ritonavir. Pharmacokinetic differences due to race have not been identified.

Renal Insufficiency: Ritonavir pharmacokinetics have not been studied in patients with renal insufficiency; however, since renal clearance is negligible, a decrease in total body clearance is not expected in patients with renal insufficiency.

Hepatic Insufficiency: Ritonavir pharmacokinetics have not been studied in subjects with hepatic insufficiency (see **PRECAUTIONS**).

Drug-Drug Interactions: Table 2 summarizes the effects on AUC and C_{max}, with 95% confidence intervals (95% CI), of co-administration of ritonavir with a variety of drugs. For information about clinical recommendations see **PRECAUTIONS—Drug Interactions.**

[See table 2 at top of next page]

INDICATIONS AND USAGE

NORVIR is indicated in combination with other antiretroviral agents for the treatment of HIV-infection. This indication is based on the results from a study in patients with advanced HIV disease that showed a reduction in both mortality and AIDS-defining clinical events for patients who received NORVIR either alone or in combination with nucleoside analogues. Median duration of follow-up in this study was 13.5 months.

Description of Clinical Studies

The activity of NORVIR as monotherapy or in combination with nucleoside analogues has been evaluated in 1446 patients enrolled in two double-blind, randomized trials.

Advanced Patients with Prior Antiretroviral Therapy

Study 247 was a randomized, double-blind trial (with open-label follow-up) conducted in HIV-infected patients with at least nine months of prior antiretroviral therapy and baseline CD_4 cell counts ≤ 100 cells/μL. NORVIR 600 mg b.i.d. or placebo was added to each patient's baseline antiretroviral therapy regimen, which could have consisted of up to two approved antiretroviral agents. The study accrued 1090 patients, with mean baseline CD_4 cell count at study entry of 32 cells/μL. After the clinical benefit of NORVIR therapy was demonstrated, all patients were eligible to switch to open-label NORVIR for the duration of the follow-up period. Median duration of double-blind therapy with NORVIR and placebo was 6 months. The median duration of follow-up through the end of the open-label phase was 13.5 months for patients randomized to NORVIR and 14 months for patients randomized to placebo.

The cumulative incidence of clinical disease progression or death during the double-blind phase of Study 247 was 26% for patients initially randomized to NORVIR compared to 42% for patients initially randomized to placebo. This difference in rates was statistically significant (see Figure 1).

Figure 1
Time to Disease Progression or Death During the Double-Blind Phase of Study 247

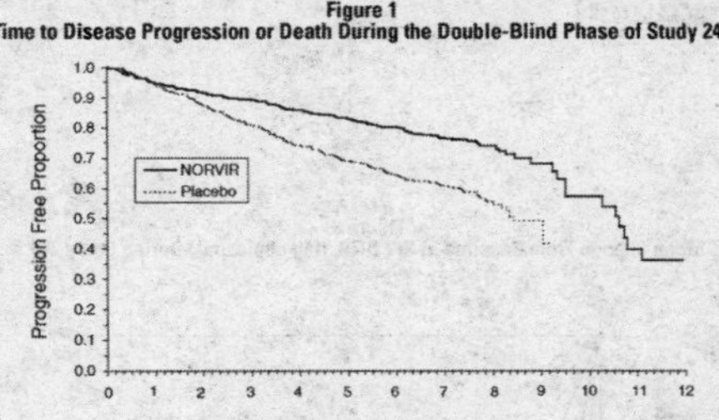

The cumulative mortality through the end of the open-label follow-up phase for patients enrolled in Study 247 was 18% for patients initially randomized to NORVIR compared to 26% for patients initially randomized to placebo. This difference in rates was statistically significant (see Figure 2). Since the analysis at the end of the open-label phase includes patients in the placebo arm who were switched from placebo to NORVIR therapy, the survival benefit of NORVIR cannot be precisely estimated.

Figure 2
Survival of Patients by Randomized Treatment Regimen in Study 247

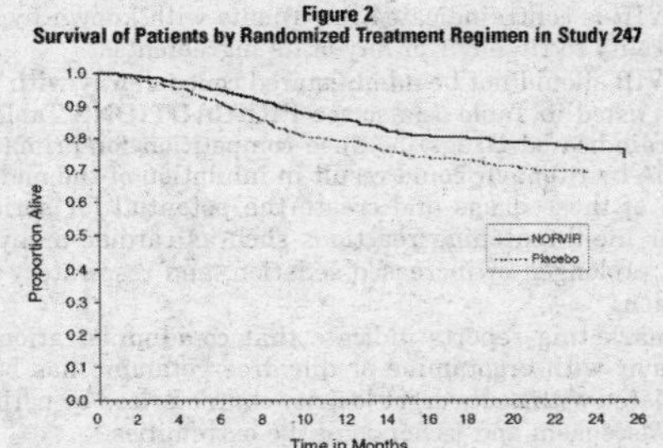

Figures 3 and 4 summarize the mean change from baseline for CD_4 cell count and plasma HIV RNA (copies/mL), respectively, during the first 24 weeks for the double-blind phase of Study 247.

Figure 3
Mean Change From Baseline in CD_4 Cell Count (cells/μL) During the Double-Blind Phase of Study 247

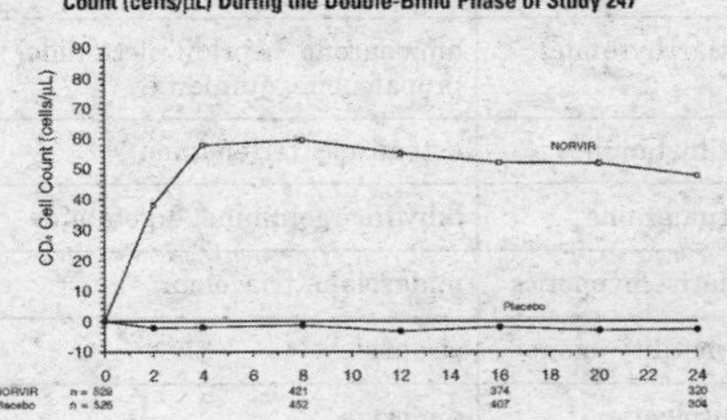

Figure 4
Mean Change From Baseline in HIV RNA (log copies/mL) During the Double-Blind Phase of Study 247

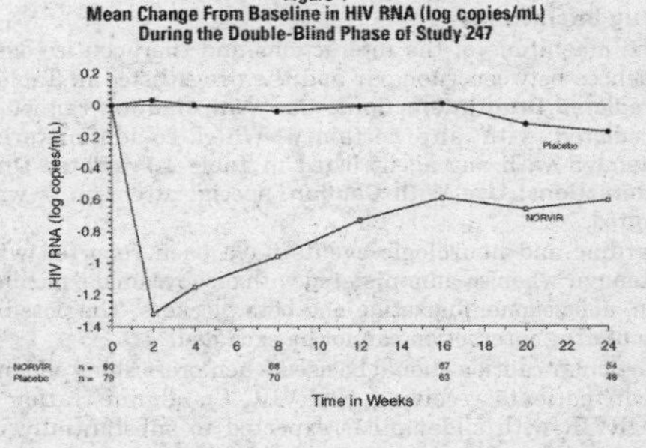

Continued on next page

Norvir—Cont.

Patients Without Prior Antiretroviral Therapy

In Study 245, 356 antiretroviral-naive HIV-infected patients (mean baseline CD_4 = 364 cells/μL) were randomized to receive either NORVIR 600 mg b.i.d., zidovudine 200 mg t.i.d., or a combination of these drugs. Figures 5 and 6 summarize the mean change from baseline for CD_4 cell count and plasma HIV RNA (copies/mL), respectively, during the first 24 weeks for the double-blind phase of Study 245.

Figure 5
Mean Change From Baseline in CD_4 Cell Count (cells/μL) During Study 245

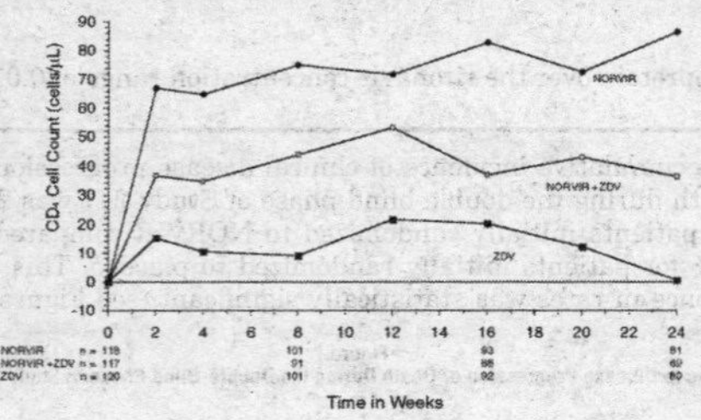

Figure 6
Mean Change From Baseline in HIV RNA (log copies/mL) During Study 245

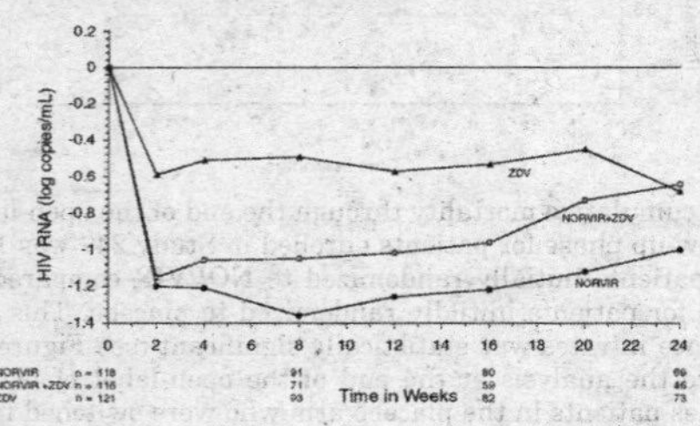

CONTRAINDICATIONS

NORVIR is contraindicated in patients with known hypersensitivity to ritonavir or any of its ingredients.

NORVIR should not be administered concurrently with the drugs listed in Table 3 (also see **PRECAUTIONS** Table 4: Contraindicated Drugs) because competition for primarily CYP3A by ritonavir could result in inhibition of the metabolism of these drugs and create the potential for serious and/or life-threatening reactions such as cardiac arrhythmias, prolonged or increased sedation, and respiratory depression.

Postmarketing reports indicate that co-administration of ritonavir with ergotamine or dihydroergotamine has been associated with acute ergot toxicity characterized by peripheral vasospasm and ischemia of the extremities.

Table 3
DRUGS THAT ARE CONTRAINDICATED WITH NORVIR USE

Drug Class	Drugs Within Class That Are CONTRAINDICATED With NORVIR
Antiarrhythmics	amiodarone, bepridil, flecainide, propafenone, quinidine
Antihistamines	astemizole, terfenadine
Antimigraine	dihydroergotamine, ergotamine
Sedative/hypnotics	midazolam, triazolam
GI motility agent	cisapride
Neuroleptic	pimozide

WARNINGS

Drug Interactions

The magnitude of the interactions and therapeutic consequences between ritonavir and the drugs listed in Table 4 **Predicted Drug Interactions: Use With Caution** cannot be predicted with any certainty. When co-administering ritonavir with any agent listed in Table 4 **Predicted Drug Interactions: Use With Caution**, special attention is warranted.

Cardiac and neurologic events have been reported with ritonavir when co-administered with disopyramide, mexiletine, nefazodone, fluoxetine and beta blockers. The possibility of drug interaction cannot be excluded.

Particular caution should be used when prescribing sildenafil in patients receiving NORVIR. Co-administration of NORVIR with sildenafil is expected to substantially increase sildenafil concentrations (11-fold increase in AUC) and may result in an increase in sildenafil-associated adverse events, including hypotension, syncope, visual changes, and prolonged erection (see **PRECAUTIONS: Drug Interactions**, Table 4 **Established Drug Interactions: Alteration in Dose or Regimen Recommended Based on Drug Interaction Studies** and the complete prescribing information for sildenafil).

Concomitant use of NORVIR with lovastatin or simvastatin is not recommended. Caution should be exercised if HIV protease inhibitors, including NORVIR, are used concurrently with other HMG-CoA reductase inhibitors that are also metabolized by the CYP3A4 pathway (e.g., atorvastatin or cerivastatin). The risk of myopathy including rhabdomyolysis may be increased when HIV protease inhibitors, including NORVIR, are used in combination with these drugs.

Concomitant use of NORVIR, and St. John's wort (hypericum perforatum) or products containing St. John's wort is not recommended. Coadministration of protease inhibitors, including NORVIR, with St. John's wort is expected to substantially decrease protease inhibitor concentrations and may result in sub-optimal levels of NORVIR and lead to loss of virologic response and possible resistance to NORVIR or to the class of protease inhibitors.

Table 2
Effects of Co-administered Drug on Ritonavir Plasma AUC and C_{max}

Drug	Ritonavir Dosage	n	AUC % (95% CI)	C_{max} % (95% CI)
		Effect on Ritonavir		
Clarithromycin 500 mg q12h 4 days	200 mg q8h 4 days	22	↑ 12% (2, 23%)	↑ 15% (2, 28%)
Didanosine 200 mg q12h 4 days	600 mg q12h 4 days	12	↔	↔
Fluconazole 400 mg day 1, 200 mg daily 4 days	200 mg q6h 4 days	8	↑ 12% (5, 20%)	↑ 15% (7, 22%)
Fluoxetine 30 mg q12h 8 days	600 mg single dose	16	↑ 19% (7, 34%)	↔
Ketoconazole 200 mg daily 7 days	500 mg q12h 10 days	12	↑ 18% (-3, 52%)	↑ 10% (-11, 36%)
Rifampin 600 mg or 300 mg daily 10 days	500 mg q12h 20 days	7,9*	↓ 35% (7, 55%)	↓ 25% (-5, 46%)
Zidovudine 200 mg q8h 4 days	300 mg q6h 4 days	10	↔	↔

Effects of Ritonavir on Co-administered Drug Plasma AUC and C_{max}

Drug	Ritonavir Dosage	n	AUC % (95% CI)	C_{max} % (95% CI)
Alprazolam 1 mg single dose	500 mg q12h 10 days	12	↓ 12% (-5, 30%)	↓ 16% (5, 27%)
Clarithromycin 500 mg q12h 4 days	200 mg q8h 4 days	22	↑ 77% (56, 103%)	↑ 31% (15, 51%)
14-OH clarithromycin metabolite			↓ 100%	↓ 99%
Desipramine 100 mg single dose	500 mg q12h 12 days	14	↑ 145% (103, 211%)	↑ 22% (12, 35%)
2-OH desipramine metabolite			↓ 15% (3, 26%)	↓ 67% (62, 72%)
Didanosine 200 mg q12h 4 days	600 mg q12h 4 days	12	↓ 13% (0, 23%)	↓ 16% (5, 26%)
Ethinyl estradiol 50 μg single dose	500 mg q12h 16 days	23	↓ 40% (31, 49%)	↓ 32% (24, 39%)
Indinavir 400 mg q12h Day 14[1]	400 mg q12h 15 days	10	↑ 6% (-14, 29%)	↓ 51% (40, 61%)
Indinavir 400 mg q12h Day 15[1]	400 mg q12h 15 days	10	↓ 7% (-25, 16%)	↓ 62% (52, 70%)
Ketoconazole 200 mg daily 7 days	500 mg q12h 10 days	12	↑ 3.4-fold (2.8, 4.3X)	↑ 55% (40, 72%)
Meperidine 50 mg oral single dose	500 mg q12h 10 days	8	↓ 62% (59, 65%)	↓ 59% (42, 72%)
Normeperidine metabolite		6	↑ 47% (-24, 345%)	↑ 87% (42, 147%)
Methadone 5 mg single dose[2]	500 mg q12h 15 days	11	↓ 36% (16, 52%)	↓ 38% (28, 46%)
Rifabutin 150 mg daily 16 days	500 mg q12h 10 days	5,11*	↑ 4-fold (2.8, 6.1X)	↑ 2.5-fold (1.9, 3.4X)
25-O-desacetyl rifabutin metabolite			↑ 35-fold (25, 78X)	↑ 16-fold (14, 20X)
Saquinavir 400 mg bid steady-state[3]	400 mg bid steady-state	7	↑ 17-fold (9, 31X)	↑ 14-fold (7, 28X)
Sildenafil 100 mg single dose	500 mg bid 8 days	28	↑ 11-fold	↑ 4-fold
Sulfamethoxazole 800 mg single dose[4]	500 mg q12h 12 days	15	↓ 20% (16, 23%)	↔
Theophylline 3 mg/kg q8h 15 days	500 mg q12h 10 days	13,11*	↓ 43% (42, 45%)	↓ 32% (29, 34%)
Trimethoprim 160 mg single dose[4]	500 mg q12h 12 days	15	↑ 20% (3, 43%)	↔
Zidovudine 200 mg q8h 4 days	300 mg q6h 4 days	9	↓ 25% (15, 34%)	↓ 27% (4, 45%)

[1] Ritonavir and indinavir were coadministered for 15 days; Day 14 doses were administered after a 15%-fat breakfast (757 Kcal) and 9%-fat evening snack (236 Kcal), and Day 15 doses were administered after a 15%-fat breakfast (757 Kcal) and 32%-fat dinner (815 Kcal). Indinavir C_{min} was also increased 4-fold. Effects were assessed relative to an indinavir 800 mg q8h regimen under fasting conditions.

[2] Effects were assessed on a dose-normalized comparison to a methadone 20 mg single dose.

[3] Comparison to a standard saquinavir HGC 600 mg t.i.d. regimen (n=114).

[4] Sulfamethoxazole and trimethoprim taken as single combination tablet.

↑ Indicates increase.
↓ Indicates decrease.
↔ Indicates no change.
* Parallel group design; entries are subjects receiving combination and control regimens, respectively.

Allergic Reactions

Allergic reactions including urticaria, mild skin eruptions, bronchospasm, and angioedema have been reported. Rare cases of anaphylaxis and Stevens-Johnson syndrome have also been reported.

Hepatic Reactions

Hepatic transaminase elevations exceeding 5 times the upper limit of normal, clinical hepatitis, and jaundice have occurred in patients receiving NORVIR alone or in combination with other antiretroviral drugs (see Table 6). There may be an increased risk for transaminase elevations in patients with underlying hepatitis B or C. Therefore, caution should be exercised when administering NORVIR to patients with pre-existing liver diseases, liver enzyme abnormalities, or hepatitis. Increased AST/ALT monitoring should be considered in these patients, especially during the first three months of NORVIR treatment.

There have been postmarketing reports of hepatic dysfunction, including some fatalities. These have generally occurred in patients taking multiple concomitant medications and/or with advanced AIDS.

Pancreatitis

Pancreatitis has been observed in patients receiving NORVIR therapy, including those who developed hypertriglyceridemia. In some cases fatalities have been observed. Patients with advanced HIV disease may be at increased risk of elevated triglycerides and pancreatitis.

Pancreatitis should be considered if clinical symptoms (nausea, vomiting, abdominal pain) or abnormalities in laboratory values (such as increased serum lipase or amylase values) suggestive of pancreatitis should occur. Patients who exhibit these signs or symptoms should be evaluated and NORVIR therapy should be discontinued if a diagnosis of pancreatitis is made.

Diabetes Mellitus/Hyperglycemia

New onset diabetes mellitus, exacerbation of pre-existing diabetes mellitus, and hyperglycemia have been reported during postmarketing surveillance in HIV-infected patients receiving protease inhibitor therapy. Some patients required either initiation or dose adjustments of insulin or oral hypoglycemic agents for treatment of these events. In some cases, diabetic ketoacidosis has occurred. In those patients who discontinued protease inhibitor therapy, hyperglycemia persisted in some cases. Because these events have been reported voluntarily during clinical practice, estimates of frequency cannot be made and a causal relationship between protease inhibitor therapy and these events has not been established.

PRECAUTIONS

General

Ritonavir is principally metabolized by the liver. Therefore, caution should be exercised when administering this drug to patients with impaired hepatic function (see **WARNINGS**).

Resistance/Cross-resistance

Varying degrees of cross-resistance among protease inhibitors have been observed. Continued administration of ritonavir therapy following loss of viral suppression may increase the likelihood of cross-resistance to other protease inhibitors (see **MICROBIOLOGY**).

Hemophilia

There have been reports of increased bleeding, including spontaneous skin hematomas and hemarthrosis, in patients with hemophilia type A and B treated with protease inhibitors. In some patients additional factor VIII was given. In more than half of the reported cases, treatment with protease inhibitors was continued or reintroduced. A causal relationship has not been established.

Fat Redistribution

Redistribution/accumulation of body fat including central obesity, dorsocervical fat enlargement (buffalo hump), peripheral wasting, breast enlargement, and "cushingoid appearance" have been observed in patients receiving protease inhibitors. The mechanism and long-term consequences of these events are currently unknown. A causal relationship has not been established.

Lipid Disorders

Treatment with NORVIR therapy alone or in combination with saquinavir has resulted in substantial increases in the concentration of total triglycerides and cholesterol. Triglyceride and cholesterol testing should be performed prior to initiating NORVIR therapy and at periodic intervals during therapy. Lipid disorders should be managed as clinically appropriate. See **PRECAUTIONS** Table 4 for additional information on potential drug interactions with NORVIR and HMG CoA reductase inhibitors.

Information For Patients

Patients should be informed that NORVIR is not a cure for HIV infection and that they may continue to acquire illnesses associated with advanced HIV infection, including opportunistic infections.

Patients should be told that the long-term effects of NORVIR are unknown at this time. They should be informed that NORVIR therapy has not been shown to reduce the risk of transmitting HIV to others through sexual contact or blood contamination.

Patients should be advised to take NORVIR with food, if possible.

Patients should be informed to take NORVIR every day as prescribed. Patients should not alter the dose or discontinue NORVIR without consulting their doctor. If a dose is missed, patients should take the next dose as soon as possible. However, if a dose is skipped, the patient should not double the next dose.

Patients should be informed that redistribution or accumulation of body fat may occur in patients receiving protease inhibitors and that the cause and long-term health effects of these conditions are not known at this time.

NORVIR may interact with some drugs; therefore, patients should be advised to report to their doctor the use of any other prescription, non-prescription medication or herbal products, particularly St. John's wort.

Laboratory Tests

Ritonavir has been shown to increase triglycerides, cholesterol, SGOT (AST), SGPT (ALT), GGT, CPK, and uric acid. Appropriate laboratory testing should be performed prior to initiating NORVIR therapy and at periodic intervals or if any clinical signs or symptoms occur during therapy. For comprehensive information concerning laboratory test alterations associated with nucleoside analogues, physicians should refer to the complete product information for each of these drugs.

Drug Interactions

Ritonavir has been found to be an inhibitor of cytochrome P450 3A (CYP3A) both *in vitro* and *in vivo* (Table 2). Agents that are extensively metabolized by CYP3A and have high first pass metabolism appear to be the most susceptible to large increases in AUC (>3-fold) when co-administered with ritonavir. Ritonavir also inhibits CYP2D6 to a lesser extent. Co-administration of substrates of CYP2D6 with ritonavir could result in increases (up to 2-fold) in the AUC of the other agent, possibly requiring a proportional dosage reduction. Ritonavir also appears to induce CYP3A as well as other enzymes, including glucuronosyl transferase, CYP1A2, and possibly CYP2C9.

Drugs that are contraindicated specifically due to the expected magnitude of interaction and potential for serious adverse events are listed both in **CONTRAINDICATIONS** Table 3 and under **Contraindicated Drugs** in Table 4.

Those drug interactions that have been established based on drug interaction studies are listed with the pharmacokinetic results in **CLINICAL PHARMACOLOGY**, Table 2. The clinical recommendations based on the results of these studies are listed in Table 4 **Established Drug Interactions: Alteration in Dose or Regimen Recommended Based on Drug Interaction Studies.**

A systematic review of over 200 medications prescribed to HIV-infected patients was performed to identify potential drug interactions with ritonavir.[2] There are a number of agents in which CYP3A or CYP2D6 partially contribute to the metabolism of the agent. In these cases, the magnitude of the interaction and therapeutic consequences cannot be predicted with any certainty.

When co-administering ritonavir with calcium channel blockers, immunosuppressants, some HMG-CoA reductase inhibitors (see **WARNINGS**, **Drug Interactions**), some steroids, or other substrates of CYP3A, or most antidepressants, certain antiarrhythmics, and some narcotic analgesics which are partially mediated by CYP2D6 metabolism, it is possible that substantial increases in concentrations of these other agents may occur, possibly requiring a dosage reduction (>50%); examples are listed in Table 4 **Predicted Drug Interactions: Use With Caution, Dose Decrease May be Needed.**

When co-administering ritonavir with any agent having a narrow therapeutic margin, such as anticoagulants, anticonvulsants, and antiarrhythmics, special attention is warranted. With some agents, the metabolism may be induced, resulting in decreased concentrations (see Table 4 **Predicted Drug Interactions: Use With Caution, Dose Increase May be Needed**).

Table 4
Drug Interactions With NORVIR
CONTRAINDICATED DRUGS
(Same as Table 3)

DRUGS THAT ARE CONTRAINDICATED WITH NORVIR USE

Drug Class	Drugs Within Class That Are CONTRAINDICATED With NORVIR
Antiarrhythmics	amiodarone, bepridil, flecainide, propafenone, quinidine
Antihistamines	astemizole, terfenadine
Antimigraine	dihydroergotamine, ergotamine
Sedative/hypnotics	midazolam, triazolam
GI motility agent	cisapride
Neuroleptic	pimozide

[See table at top of page]

Established Drug Interactions: Alteration in Dose or Regimen Recommended Based on Drug Interaction Studies
(see CLINICAL PHARMACOLOGY, Table 2 for Magnitude or Interaction)

Drug Name	Effect	Clinical Comment
Clarithromycin	↑ clarithromycin concentration	For patients with renal impairment the following dosage adjustments should be considered: • For patients with CL_{CR} 30 to 60 mL/min the dose of clarithromycin should be reduced by 50%. • For patients with CL_{CR} < 30 mL/min the dose of clarithromycin should be decreased by 75%. No dose adjustment for patients with normal renal function is necessary.
Desipramine	↑ desipramine concentration	Dosage reduction and concentration monitoring of desipramine is recommended
Didanosine		Dosing of didanosine and ritonavir should be separated by 2.5 hours to avoid formulation incompatibility
Disulfiram/Metronidazole		Ritonavir formulations contain alcohol, which can produce disulfiram-like reactions when co-administered with disulfiram or other drugs that produce this reaction (e.g., metronidazole)
Indinavir	↑ indinavir concentration	Appropriate doses for this combination, with respect to efficacy and safety, have not been established
Ketoconazole	↑ ketoconazole concentration	High doses of ketoconazole (>200 mg/day) are not recommended
Meperidine	↓ meperidine concentration/ ↑ normeperidine concentration (metabolite)	Dosage increase and long-term use of meperidine with ritonavir are not recommended due to the increased concentrations of the metabolite normeperidine which has both analgesic activity and CNS stimulant activity (e.g., seizures)
Methadone	↓ methadone concentration	Dosage increase of methadone may be considered
Oral Contraceptives	↓ ethinyl estradiol concentration	Dosage increase or alternate contraceptive measures should be considered
Rifabutin	↑ rifabutin and rifabutin metabolite concentration	Dosage reduction of rifabutin by at least three-quarters of the usual dose of 300 mg/day is recommended (e.g., 150 mg every other day or three times a week). Further dosage reduction may be necessary
Rifampin	↓ ritonavir concentration	Alternate antimycobacterial agents such as rifabutin should be considered (see Rifabutin, for dose reduction recommendations)
Saquinavir	↑ saquinavir concentration	When used in combination therapy for up to 24 weeks, doses of 400 mg b.i.d. of ritonavir and saquinavir were better tolerated than the higher doses of the combination. Saquinavir plasma concentrations achieved with Invirase® (saquinavir mesylate) (400 mg b.i.d.) and ritonavir (400 mg b.i.d.) are similar to those achieved with Fortovase™ (saquinavir) (400 mg b.i.d.) and ritonavir (400 mg b.i.d.)
Sildenafil	↑ sildenafil concentration	Sildenafil should not exceed a maximum single dose of 25 mg in a 48-hour period in patients receiving concomitant ritonavir therapy (see **WARNINGS**)
Theophylline	↓ theophylline concentration	Increased dosage of theophylline may be required; therapeutic monitoring should be considered

Continued on next page

Norvir—Cont.

Predicted Drug Interactions: Use With Caution, Dose Decrease of Coadministered Drug May Be Needed (see WARNINGS)

Examples of Drugs in Which Plasma Concentrations May Be Increased By Co-Administration With NORVIR

Drug Class	Examples of Drugs
Analgesics, narcotic	tramadol, propoxyphene
Antiarrhythmics	disopyramide, lidocaine, mexilitine
Anticonvulsants	carbamazepine, clonazepam, ethosuximide
Antidepressants	bupropion, nefazodone, selective serotonin reuptake inhibitors (SSRIs), tricyclics
Antiemetics	dronabinol
Antiparasitics	quinine
β-blockers	metoprolol, timolol
Calcium channel blockers	diltiazem, nifedipine, verapamil
Hypolipidemics, HMG CoA reductase inhibitors[1]	atorvastatin, cerivastatin, lovastatin, simvastatin
Immunosuppressants	cyclosporine, tacrolimus
Neuroleptics	perphenazine, risperidone, thioridazine
Sedative/hypnotics	clorazepate, diazepam, estazolam, flurazepam, zolpidem
Steroids	dexamethasone, prednisone
Stimulants	methamphetamine

[1] Coadministration with lovastatin and simvastatin is not recommended (see **WARNINGS, Drug Interactions**).

Predicted Drug Interactions: Use With Caution, Dose Increase of Coadministered Drug May Be Needed (see WARNINGS)

Examples of Drugs in Which Plasma Concentrations May Be Decreased By Co-Administration With NORVIR

Drug Class	Examples of Drugs
Anticoagulants	warfarin
Anticonvulsants	phenytoin, divalproex, lamotrigine
Antiparasitics	atovaquone

Post-Marketing Experience with Drugs Listed in Table 4

Cardiac and neurologic events have been reported when ritonavir has been co-administered with disopyramide, mexiletine, nefazodone, fluoxetine, and beta blockers. The possibility of drug interaction cannot be excluded.

Carcinogenesis and Mutagenesis

Long-term carcinogenicity studies of ritonavir in animal systems have not been completed. However, ritonavir was not mutagenic or clastogenic in a battery of *in vitro* and *in vivo* assays including bacterial reverse mutation (Ames) using *S. typhimurium* and *E. coli*, mouse lymphoma, mouse micronucleus, and chromosome aberrations in human lymphocytes.

Pregnancy, Fertility, and Reproduction

Pregnancy Category B: Ritonavir produced no effects on fertility in rats at drug exposures approximately 40% (male) and 60% (female) of that achieved with the proposed therapeutic dose. Higher dosages were not feasible due to hepatic toxicity.

No treatment-related malformations were observed when ritonavir was administered to pregnant rats or rabbits. Developmental toxicity observed in rats (early resorptions, decreased fetal body weight and ossification delays and developmental variations) occurred at a maternally toxic dosage at an exposure equivalent to approximately 30% of that achieved with the proposed therapeutic dose. A slight increase in the incidence of cryptorchidism was also noted in rats at an exposure approximately 22% of that achieved with the proposed therapeutic dose.

Developmental toxicity observed in rabbits (resorptions, decreased litter size and decreased fetal weights) also occurred at a maternally toxic dosage equivalent to 1.8 times the proposed therapeutic dose based on a body surface area conversion factor.

There are, however, no adequate and well-controlled studies in pregnant women. Because animal reproduction studies are not always predictive of human response, this drug should be used during pregnancy only if clearly needed.

Nursing Mothers: It is not known whether this drug is excreted in human milk. Because many drugs are excreted in human milk, caution should be exercised when ritonavir is administered to a nursing woman. However, the U.S. Public Health Service Centers for Disease Control and Prevention advises HIV-infected women not to breast-feed to avoid postnatal transmission of HIV to a child who may not be infected.

Pediatric Use

The safety and pharmacokinetic profile of ritonavir in pediatric patients below the age of 2 years have not been established. In HIV-infected patients age 2 to 16 years, the adverse event profile seen during a clinical trial and postmarketing experience was similar to that for adult patients. The evaluation of the antiviral activity of ritonavir in pediatric patients in clinical trials is ongoing.

ADVERSE REACTIONS

The safety of NORVIR alone and in combination with nucleoside analogues was studied in 1270 patients. Table 5 lists treatment-emergent adverse events (at least possibly related and of at least moderate intensity) that occurred in 2% or greater of patients receiving NORVIR alone or in combination with nucleosides in Study 245 or Study 247 and in combination with saquinavir in ongoing Study 462. In that study, 141 protease inhibitor-naive, HIV-infected patients with mean baseline CD_4 of 300 cells/μL were randomized to one of four regimens of NORVIR + saquinavir, including NORVIR 400 mg b.i.d. + saquinavir 400 mg b.i.d. Overall the most frequently reported clinical adverse events, other than asthenia, among patients receiving NORVIR were gastrointestinal and neurological disturbances including nausea, diarrhea, vomiting, anorexia, abdominal pain, taste perversion, and circumoral and peripheral paresthesias. Similar adverse event profiles were reported in patients receiving ritonavir in other trials.

[See table 5 above]

Table 5
Percentage of Patients with Treatment-Emergent Adverse Events[1] of Moderate or Severe Intensity Occurring in ≥2% of Patients Receiving NORVIR

Adverse Events	Study 245 Naive Patients[2]			Study 247 Advanced Patients[3]		Study 462 PI-Naive Patients[4]
	NORVIR + ZDV n=116	NORVIR n=117	ZDV n=119	NORVIR n=541	Placebo n=545	NORVIR + Saquinavir n=141
Body as a Whole						
Abdominal Pain	5.2	6.0	5.9	8.3	5.1	2.1
Asthenia	28.4	10.3	11.8	15.3	6.4	16.3
Fever	1.7	0.9	1.7	5.0	2.4	0.7
Headache	7.8	6.0	6.7	6.5	5.7	4.3
Malaise	5.2	1.7	3.4	0.7	0.2	2.8
Pain (unspecified)	0.9	1.7	0.8	2.2	1.8	4.3
Cardiovascular						
Syncope	0.9	1.7	0.8	0.6	0.0	2.1
Vasodilation	3.4	1.7	0.8	1.7	0.0	3.5
Digestive						
Anorexia	8.6	1.7	4.2	7.8	4.2	4.3
Constipation	3.4	0.0	0.8	0.2	0.4	1.4
Diarrhea	25.0	15.4	2.5	23.3	7.9	22.7
Dyspepsia	2.6	0.0	1.7	5.9	1.5	0.7
Fecal Incontinence	0.0	0.0	0.0	0.0	0.0	2.8
Flatulence	2.6	0.9	1.7	1.7	0.7	3.5
Local Throat Irritation	0.9	1.7	0.8	2.8	0.4	1.4
Nausea	46.6	25.6	26.1	29.8	8.4	18.4
Vomiting	23.3	13.7	12.6	17.4	4.4	7.1
Metabolic and Nutritional						
Weight Loss	0.0	0.0	0.0	2.4	1.7	0.0
Musculoskeletal						
Arthralgia	0.0	0.0	0.0	1.7	0.7	2.1
Myalgia	1.7	1.7	0.8	2.4	1.1	2.1
Nervous						
Anxiety	0.9	0.0	0.8	1.7	0.9	2.1
Circumoral Paresthesia	5.2	3.4	0.0	6.7	0.4	6.4
Confusion	0.0	0.9	0.0	0.6	0.6	2.1
Depression	1.7	1.7	2.5	1.7	0.7	7.1
Dizziness	5.2	2.6	3.4	3.9	1.1	8.5
Insomnia	3.4	2.6	0.8	2.0	1.8	2.8
Paresthesia	5.2	2.6	0.0	3.0	0.4	2.1
Peripheral Paresthesia	0.0	6.0	0.8	5.0	1.1	5.7
Somnolence	2.6	2.6	0.0	2.4	0.2	0.0
Thinking Abnormal	2.6	0.0	0.8	0.9	0.4	0.7
Respiratory						
Pharyngitis	0.9	2.6	0.0	0.4	0.4	1.4
Skin and Appendages						
Rash	0.9	0.0	0.8	3.5	1.5	0.7
Sweating	3.4	2.6	1.7	1.7	1.1	2.8
Special Senses						
Taste Perversion	17.2	11.1	8.4	7.0	2.2	5.0
Urogenital						
Nocturia	0.0	0.0	0.0	0.2	0.0	2.8

[1] Includes those adverse events at least possibly related to study drug or of unknown relationship and excludes concurrent HIV conditions.
[2] The median duration of treatment for patients randomized to regimens containing NORVIR in Study 245 was 9.1 months.
[3] The median duration of treatment for patients randomized to regimens containing NORVIR in Study 247 was 9.4 months.
[4] The median duration of treatment for patients in ongoing Study 462 was 48 weeks.

Adverse events occurring in less than 2% of patients receiving NORVIR in all phase II/phase III studies and considered at least possibly related or of unknown relationship to treatment and of at least moderate intensity are listed below by body system.

Body as a Whole: Abdomen enlarged, accidental injury, allergic reaction, back pain, cachexia, chest pain, chills, facial edema, facial pain, flu syndrome, hormone level altered, hypothermia, kidney pain, neck pain, neck rigidity, pelvic pain, photosensitivity reaction, and substernal chest pain.

Cardiovascular System: Cardiovascular disorder, cerebral ischemia, cerebral venous thrombosis, hypertension, hypotension, migraine, myocardial infarct, palpitation, peripheral vascular disorder, phlebitis, postural hypotension, tachycardia and vasospasm.

Digestive System: Abnormal stools, bloody diarrhea, cheilitis, cholestatic jaundice, colitis, dry mouth, dysphagia, eructation, esophageal ulcer, esophagitis, gastritis, gastroenteritis, gastrointestinal disorder, gastrointestinal hemorrhage, gingivitis, hepatic coma, hepatitis, hepatomegaly, hepatosplenomegaly, ileus, liver damage, melena, mouth ulcer, pancreatitis, pseudomembranous colitis, rectal disorder, rectal hemorrhage, sialadenitis, stomatitis, tenesmus, thirst, tongue edema, and ulcerative colitis.

Endocrine System: Adrenal cortex insufficiency and diabetes mellitus.

Hemic and Lymphatic System: Acute myeloblastic leukemia, anemia, ecchymosis, leukopenia, lymphadenopathy, lymphocytosis, myeloproliferative disorder, and thrombocytopenia.

Metabolic and Nutritional Disorders: Albuminuria, alcohol intolerance, avitaminosis, BUN increased, dehydration, edema, enzymatic abnormality, glycosuria, gout, hypercholesteremia, peripheral edema, and xanthomatosis.

Musculoskeletal System: Arthritis, arthrosis, bone disorder, bone pain, extraocular palsy, joint disorder, leg cramps, muscle cramps, muscle weakness, myositis, and twitching.

Nervous System: Abnormal dreams, abnormal gait, agitation, amnesia, aphasia, ataxia, coma, convulsion, dementia,

Table 6
Percentage of Patients, by Study and Treatment Group, with Chemistry and Hematology Abnormalities Occurring in > 3% of Patients Receiving NORVIR

		Study 245 Naive Patients			Study 247 Advanced Patients		Study 462 PI-Naive Patients
Variable	Limit	NORVIR + ZDV	NORVIR	ZDV	NORVIR	Placebo	NORVIR + Saquinavir
Chemistry	High						
Cholesterol	>240 mg/dL	30.7	44.8	9.3	36.5	8.0	65.2
CPK	>1000 IU/L	9.6	12.1	11.0	9.1	6.3	9.9
GGT	>300 IU/L	1.8	5.2	1.7	19.6	11.3	9.2
SGOT (AST)	>180 IU/L	5.3	9.5	2.5	6.4	7.0	7.8
SGPT (ALT)	>215 IU/L	5.3	7.8	3.4	8.5	4.4	9.2
Triglycerides	>800 mg/dL	9.6	17.2	3.4	33.6	9.4	23.4
Triglycerides	>1500 mg/dL	1.8	2.6	-	12.6	0.4	11.3
Triglycerides Fasting	>1500 mg/dL	1.5	1.3	-	9.9	0.3	-
Uric Acid	>12 mg/dL	-	-	-	3.8	0.2	1.4
Hematology	Low						
Hematocrit	<30%	2.6	-	0.8	17.3	22.0	0.7
Hemoglobin	<8.0 g/dL	0.9	-	-	3.8	3.9	-
Neutrophils	≤0.5 × 10^9/L	-	-	-	6.0	8.3	-
RBC	<3.0 × 10^{12}/L	1.8	-	5.9	18.6	24.4	-
WBC	<2.5 × 10^9/L	-	0.9	6.8	36.9	59.4	3.5

[1] ULN = upper limit of the normal range.
- Indicates no events reported.

Pediatric Dosage Guidelines[1]

Body Surface Area* (m^2)	Twice Daily Dose 250 mg/m^2	Twice Daily Dose 300 mg/m^2	Twice Daily Dose 350 mg/m^2	Twice Daily Dose 400 mg/m^2
0.25	0.8 mL (62.5 mg)	0.9 mL (75 mg)	1.1 mL (87.5 mg)	1.25 mL (100 mg)
0.50	1.6 mL (125 mg)	1.9 mL (150 mg)	2.2 mL (175 mg)	2.5 mL (200 mg)
1.00	3.1 mL (250 mg)	3.75 mL (300 mg)	4.4 mL (350 mg)	5 mL (400 mg)
1.25	3.9 mL (312.5 mg)	4.7 mL (375 mg)	5.5 mL (437.5 mg)	6.25 mL (500 mg)
1.50	4.7 mL (375 mg)	5.6 mL (450 mg)	6.6 mL (525 mg)	7.5 mL (600 mg)

* Body surface area can be calculated with the following equation: $BSA\ (m^2) = \sqrt{\frac{Ht\ (cm) \times Wt\ (kg)}{3600}}$

depersonalization, diplopia, emotional lability, euphoria, grand mal convulsion, hallucinations, hyperesthesia, hyperkinesia, hypesthesia, incoordination, libido decreased, manic reaction, nervousness, neuralgia, neuropathy, paralysis, peripheral neuropathic pain, peripheral neuropathy, peripheral sensory neuropathy, personality disorder, sleep disorder, speech disorder, stupor, subdural hematoma, tremor, urinary retention, vertigo, and vestibular disorder.

Respiratory System: Asthma, bronchitis, dyspnea, epistaxis, hiccup, hypoventilation, increased cough, interstitial pneumonia, larynx edema, lung disorder, rhinitis, and sinusitis.

Skin and Appendages: Acne, contact dermatitis, dry skin, eczema, erythema multiforme, exfoliative dermatitis, folliculitis, fungal dermatitis, furunculosis, maculopapular rash, molluscum contagiosum, onychomycosis, pruritus, psoriasis, pustular rash, seborrhea, skin discoloration, skin disorder, skin hypertrophy, skin melanoma, urticaria, and vesiculobullous rash.

Special Senses: Abnormal electro-oculogram, abnormal electroretinogram, abnormal vision, amblyopia/blurred vision, blepharitis, conjunctivitis, ear pain, eye disorder, eye pain, hearing impairment, increased cerumen, iritis, parosmia, photophobia, taste loss, tinnitus, uveitis, visual field defect, and vitreous disorder.

Urogenital System: Acute kidney failure, breast pain, cystitis, dysuria, hematuria, impotence, kidney calculus, kidney failure, kidney function abnormal, kidney pain, menorrhagia, penis disorder, polyuria, urethritis, urinary frequency, urinary tract infection, and vaginitis.

Post-Marketing Experience:

There have been postmarketing reports of seizure. Cause and effect relationship has not been established.

Dehydration, usually associated with gastrointestinal symptoms, and sometimes resulting in hypotension, syncope, or renal insufficiency has been reported. Syncope, orthostatic hypotension, and renal insufficiency have also been reported without known dehydration.

Redistribution/accumulation of body fat has been reported (see **PRECAUTIONS, Fat Redistribution**). There have been reports of increased bleeding in patients with hemophilia A or B (see **PRECAUTIONS, Hemophilia**).

Laboratory Abnormalities

Table 6 shows the percentage of patients who developed marked laboratory abnormalities.

[See table 6 above]

OVERDOSAGE

Acute Overdosage

Human Overdose Experience: Human experience of acute overdose with NORVIR is limited. One patient in clinical trials took NORVIR 1500 mg/day for two days. The patient reported paresthesias which resolved after the dose was decreased. A post-marketing case of renal failure with eosinophilia has been reported with ritonavir overdose.

The approximate lethal dose was found to be greater than 20 times the related human dose in rats and 10 times the related human dose in mice.

Management of Overdosage

Treatment of overdose with NORVIR consists of general supportive measures including monitoring of vital signs and observation of the clinical status of the patient. There is no specific antidote for overdose with NORVIR. If indicated, elimination of unabsorbed drug should be achieved by emesis or gastric lavage; usual precautions should be observed to maintain the airway. Administration of activated charcoal may also be used to aid in removal of unabsorbed drug. Since ritonavir is extensively metabolized by the liver and is highly protein bound, dialysis is unlikely to be beneficial in significant removal of the drug. A Certified Poison Control Center should be consulted for up-to-date information on the management of overdose with NORVIR.

DOSAGE AND ADMINISTRATION

NORVIR is administered orally. It is recommended that NORVIR be taken with meals if possible. Patients may improve the taste of NORVIR oral solution by mixing with chocolate milk, Ensure®, or Advera® within one hour of dosing. The effects of antacids on the absorption of ritonavir have not been studied.

Adults

The recommended dosage of ritonavir is 600 mg twice daily by mouth. Use of a dose titration schedule may help to reduce treatment-emergent adverse events while maintaining appropriate ritonavir plasma levels. Ritonavir should be started at no less than 300 mg twice daily and increased at 2 to 3 day intervals by 100 mg twice daily. If saquinavir and ritonavir are used in combination, the dosage of saquinavir should be reduced to 400 mg twice daily. The optimum dosage of NORVIR (400 mg or 600 mg twice daily), in combination with saquinavir, has not been determined; however, the combination regimen was better tolerated in patients who received NORVIR 400 mg twice daily.

Pediatric Patients

Ritonavir should be used in combination with other antiretroviral agents (see **General Dosing Guidelines**). The recommended dosage of ritonavir is 400 mg/m^2 twice daily by mouth and should not exceed 600 mg twice daily. Ritonavir should be started at 250 mg/m^2 and increased at 2 to 3 day intervals by 50 mg/m^2 twice daily. If patients do not tolerate 400 mg/m^2 twice daily due to adverse events, the highest tolerated dose may be used for maintenance therapy in combination with other antiretroviral agents; however, alternative therapy should be considered. When possible, dose should be administered using a calibrated dosing syringe.

[See second table above]

General Dosing Guidelines

Patients should be aware that frequently observed adverse events, such as mild to moderate gastrointestinal disturbances and paraesthesias, may diminish as therapy is continued. In addition, patients initiating combination regimens with NORVIR and nucleosides may improve gastrointestinal tolerance by initiating NORVIR alone and subsequently adding nucleosides before completing two weeks of NORVIR monotherapy.

HOW SUPPLIED

NORVIR (ritonavir capsules) soft gelatin are white capsules imprinted with the corporate logo, 100 and the Abbo-Code DS, available in the following package size:

Bottles of 120 capsules each .... (**NDC** 0074-6633-22).

Recommended storage: Store soft gelatin capsules in the refrigerator between 36-46°F (2-8°C) until dispensed. Refrigeration of NORVIR soft gelatin capsules by the patient is recommended, but not required if used within 30 days and stored below 77°F (25°C). Protect from light. Avoid exposure to excessive heat.

NORVIR (ritonavir oral solution) is an orange-colored liquid, supplied in amber-colored, multi-dose bottles containing 600 mg ritonavir per 7.5 mL marked dosage cup (80 mg/mL) in the following size:

240 mL bottles .... (**NDC** 0074-1940-63).

Recommended storage: Store NORVIR oral solution at room temperature 68°F to 77°F (20°C to 25°C). Do not refrigerate. Shake well before each use. Use by product expiration date. Product should be stored and dispensed in the original container.

Avoid exposure to excessive heat. Keep cap tightly closed.

NORVIR oral solution is manufactured by Abbott Laboratories, North Chicago, IL 60064, U.S.A. or Abbott Laboratories LTD, Queenborough, Kent, England. Distributed by Abbott Laboratories, North Chicago, IL 60064, U.S.A.

REFERENCES

1. Sewester CS. Calculations. In: Drug Facts and Comparisons. St. Louis, MO: J.B. Lippincott Co; January 1997: xix.
2. Bertz RJ and Granneman GR. Use of *in vitro* and *in vivo* data to estimate the likelihood of metabolic pharmacokinetic interactions. *Clin Pharmacokinet* 1997; 32(3):210–258.

Revised: March, 2000

ABBOTT LABORATORIES

NORTH CHICAGO, IL 60064, U.S.A.

NORVIR®

(ritonavir capsules) Soft Gelatin
(ritonavir oral solution)

Patient Information

NORVIR®
(Nor-veer)
Generic Name: ritonavir
(rit-ON-uh-veer)

Please read this leaflet carefully before you start taking NORVIR. Also, read it each time you get your NORVIR prescription refilled, just in case something has changed. Remember that this information does not take the place of careful discussions with your doctor when you start this medication and at check ups.

You should remain under a doctor's care when taking NORVIR and you should not change or stop treatment without first talking with your doctor.

You should tell your doctor about any drug you are taking or planning to take because taking NORVIR with some medications can result in serious or life-threatening problems.

Talk to your doctor if you have any questions about NORVIR. Your doctor or pharmacist can also give you more information about NORVIR.

What is NORVIR and how does it work?

NORVIR is in a class of drugs called the HIV protease (PRO-tee-ase) inhibitors. NORVIR is used in combination with other anti-HIV drugs to treat people with human immunodeficiency virus (HIV) infection. HIV infection leads to the destruction of CD_4 (T) cells, which are important to the immune system. After a large number of CD_4 (T) cells have been destroyed, acquired immune deficiency syndrome (AIDS) develops.

NORVIR works by blocking HIV protease (a protein-cutting enzyme), which is required for HIV to multiply. NORVIR has been shown to significantly reduce the amount of HIV in the blood and increase the number of CD_4 (T) cells. Patients who took NORVIR in clinical studies had significant reductions in both death and AIDS defining diseases; however NORVIR may not have these effects in all patients.

Does NORVIR cure HIV or AIDS?

NORVIR is not a cure for HIV infection or AIDS. The long-term effects of NORVIR are not known at this time. People taking NORVIR may still develop opportunistic infections or other conditions associated with HIV infection. Some of these conditions are pneumonia, herpes virus infections, and *Mycobacterium avium* complex (MAC) infections.

Does NORVIR reduce the risk of passing HIV to others?

NORVIR does not reduce the risk of passing HIV to others through sexual contact or blood contamination. Continue to practice safe sex and do not use or share dirty needles.

How should I take NORVIR?

- NORVIR is available only with a doctor's prescription.
- It is very important that you take NORVIR every day exactly as your doctor prescribed it.
- The usual dose for adults is six 100 mg capsules or 7.5 mL of the oral solution twice a day (morning and night), in combination with other anti-HIV drugs.

Continued on next page

Norvir—Cont.

- The dosing of NORVIR may be different for you than for other patients. Follow the directions from your doctor, exactly as written on the label.
- Children from 2 to 16 years of age can also take NORVIR. The child's doctor will decide the right dose based on the child's height and weight.
- Take NORVIR with food if possible.
- NORVIR Oral Solution is peppermint/caramel flavored. You can take it alone, or improve the taste by mixing it with 8 ounces of chocolate milk, Ensure®, or Advera®. NORVIR Oral Solution should be taken within 1 hour if mixed with these items. Ask your doctor, nurse or pharmacist about other ways to improve the taste of NORVIR Oral Solution.
- Do not alter or discontinue the daily dose of NORVIR without first consulting with your health care provider.
- Be sure to set up a schedule and follow it carefully.
- Only take medicine that has been prescribed specifically for you. Do not give NORVIR to others or take medicine prescribed for someone else.

What should I do if I miss a dose of NORVIR?

It is important that you do not miss any doses. If you miss a dose of NORVIR, take it as soon as possible and then take your next scheduled dose at its regularly scheduled time. If it is almost time for your next dose, wait and take the next dose at the regularly scheduled time. Do not double the next dose.

Who should not take NORVIR?

Together with your doctor, you need to decide whether NORVIR is appropriate for you.

- Do not take NORVIR if you have had a serious allergic reaction to NORVIR or any of its ingredients.
- Do not take NORVIR if you are taking certain medications. Taking certain drugs with NORVIR could create the potential for serious side effects that could be life threatening. You must tell your doctor about all the drugs you are taking or are planning to take before you take NORVIR. More information about drugs that interact with NORVIR can be found in the section **"Can I take NORVIR with other medicines?"**

Can I take NORVIR with other medications?*

NORVIR may interact with other drugs, including those you take without a prescription. You must tell your doctor about all the drugs you are taking or are planning to take before you take NORVIR.

- *You should not take the following drugs with NORVIR because serious or life-threatening problems such as irregular heartbeat, breathing difficulties or excessive sleepiness could occur:*
  - Cordarone® (amiodarone)
  - Ergotamine and dihydroergotamine such as Cafergot®, Migranal®, D.H.E 45®, and others
  - Halcion® (triazolam)
  - Hismanal® (astemizole)
  - Orap® (pimozide)
  - Propulsid® (cisapride)
  - Quinidine, also known as Quinaglute®, Cardioquin®, Quinidex®, and others
  - Rythmol® (propafenone)
  - Seldane® (terfenadine)
  - Tambocor® (flecainide)
  - Vascor® (bepridil)
  - Versed® (midazolam)
- Taking NORVIR with St. John's wort (hypericum perforatum), an herbal product sold as a dietary supplement or products containing St. John's wort is not recommended. Talk with your doctor if you are taking or are planning to take St. John's wort. Taking St. John's wort may decrease NORVIR levels and lead to increased viral load and possible resistance to NORVIR or cross-resistance to other antiretroviral drugs.

Drugs that require dosage adjustments:

It is possible that your doctor may need to increase or decrease the dose of other drugs when you are also taking NORVIR. Remember to tell your doctor all drugs you are taking or plan to take.

- The following drugs require dose reduction if taken with NORVIR:
  - Mycobutin® (rifabutin) Your doctor will lower your dose of Mycobutin
  - Viagra® (sildenafil)

Before you take Viagra with NORVIR, talk to your doctor about possible drug interactions and side effects. If you take Viagra and NORVIR together, you may be at risk of side effects of Viagra such as low blood pressure, visual changes, and penile erection lasting more than 4 hours. If an erection lasts longer than 4 hours, you should get medical help immediately to avoid permanent damage to your penis. Your doctor can explain these symptoms to you.

- If you are taking Oral contraceptives ("the pill") to prevent pregnancy, your doctor should increase the dose or you should use a different type of contraception since NORVIR may reduce the effectiveness of oral contraceptives.

The following drug reduces blood levels of NORVIR:

Rifampin, also known as Rimactane®, Rifadin®, Rifater®, or Rifamate®

Be sure to tell your doctor if you are taking rifampin.

What side effects might I have while taking NORVIR?

- This list of side effects is **not** complete. Your doctor or pharmacist can discuss with you a more complete list of possible side effects with NORVIR. Talk to your doctor promptly about any side effects you have.
- The most commonly reported side effects are: feeling weak/tired, nausea, vomiting, diarrhea, loss of appetite, abdominal pain, changes in taste, tingling feeling or numbness in hands or feet or around the lips, headache, and dizziness.
- Abnormal liver function tests have been reported in patients taking NORVIR. Liver problems including rare cases of death have occurred in patients taking NORVIR. People with pre-existing liver disease may have worsening of liver disease. Some patients had other illnesses or were taking other drugs. It is uncertain if NORVIR caused these liver problems.
- Diabetes and high blood sugar (hyperglycemia) have occurred in patients taking protease inhibitors. Some patients had diabetes before starting protease inhibitors, others did not. Some patients required adjustments to their diabetes medication. Others needed new diabetes medication.
- Changes in body fat have been seen in some patients taking protease inhibitors. These changes may include increased amount of fat in the upper back and neck ("buffalo hump"), breast and abdomen. Loss of fat from the face, legs, and arms may also happen. The cause and long-term health effects of these conditions are not known at this time.
- Inflammation of their pancreas (pancreatitis), including some deaths, have occurred in some patients taking NORVIR.
- Some patients have had large increases in triglycerides and cholesterol. The long-term risks for complications such as heart attacks or stroke due to increases in triglycerides and cholesterol are not known at this time.
- Increased bleeding has been reported in some patients with hemophilia.
- Allergic reactions ranging from mild to severe have occurred in patients taking NORVIR.

There have been other side effects noted in patients receiving NORVIR; however, these side effects may have been due to other drugs that patients were taking or to the illness itself. If you have questions about side effects, ask your doctor, nurse, or pharmacist. You should report any new or persistent symptoms to your doctor immediately.

What should I tell my doctor before taking NORVIR?

- *If you are pregnant:* The effects of NORVIR on pregnant women or their unborn babies are not known. If you are pregnant or plan to become pregnant, you should tell your doctor before taking NORVIR.
- *If you are breast-feeding:* You should not breast-feed if you have HIV. If you are a woman who has or will have a baby, talk with your doctor about the best way to feed your baby. You should be aware that if your baby does not already have HIV, there is a chance that HIV can be transmitted through breast-feeding.
- *If you have liver disease:* If you have liver disease, you should tell your doctor before taking NORVIR.
- *Other medical problems:* Certain medical problems may affect the use of NORVIR. Some people taking protease inhibitors have developed new or more serious diabetes or high blood sugar. Some people with hemophilia have had increased bleeding. It is not known whether the protease inhibitors caused these problems. Be sure to tell your doctor if you have hemophilia types A and B, diabetes mellitus, or an increase in thirst and/or frequent urination.

How do I store NORVIR?

- Keep NORVIR and all other medicines out of the reach of children.
- Store NORVIR Oral Solution at room temperature. Do not refrigerate NORVIR Oral Solution. Avoid exposing NORVIR Oral Solution to excessive heat or cold.
- Refrigeration of NORVIR soft gelatin capsules by the patient is recommended, but not required if used within 30 days and stored below 77°F (25°C). Avoid exposing NORVIR soft gelatin capsules to excessive heat or cold.
- Store NORVIR soft gelatin capsules and NORVIR Oral Solution in the original container.
- Shake NORVIR Oral Solution well before each use.
- Use NORVIR Oral Solution by the expiration date on the bottle.

Do not keep medicine that is out of date or that you no longer need. Be sure that if you throw any medicine away, it is out of the reach of children.

Whom should I call if I have questions about NORVIR?

If you would like more information about NORVIR, ask your doctor or pharmacist. If you have any questions or concerns about taking NORVIR, talk with your doctor.

If you suspect that you took more than the prescribed dose of this medicine, contact your local poison control center or emergency room immediately.

* The brands listed are trademarks of their respective owners and are not trademarks of Abbott Laboratories. The makers of these brands are not affiliated with and do not endorse Abbott Laboratories or its products.

Ref. 03-5026-R14

Revised: March, 2000

ABBOTT LABORATORIES

NORTH CHICAGO, IL 60064, U.S.A.

Shown in Product Identification Guide, page 303

OMNICEF® ℞

(cefdinir) capsules

[omnē-sĕf]

OMNICEF®

(cefdinir) for oral suspension

DESCRIPTION

OMNICEF® (cefdinir) capsules and OMNICEF® (cefdinir) for oral suspension contain the active ingredient cefdinir, an extended-spectrum, semisynthetic cephalosporin, for oral administration. Chemically, cefdinir is [6R-[6α,7β (Z)]]-7-[[(2-amino-4-thiazolyl)(hydroxyimino)acetyl]amino]-3-ethenyl-8-oxo-5-thia-1-azabicyclo[4.2.0]oct-2-ene-2-carboxylic acid. Cefdinir is a white to slightly brownish-yellow solid. It is slightly soluble in dilute hydrochloric acid and sparingly soluble in 0.1 M pH 7.0 phosphate buffer. The empirical formula is $C_{14}H_{13}N_5O_5S_2$ and the molecular weight is 395.42. Cefdinir has the structural formula shown below:

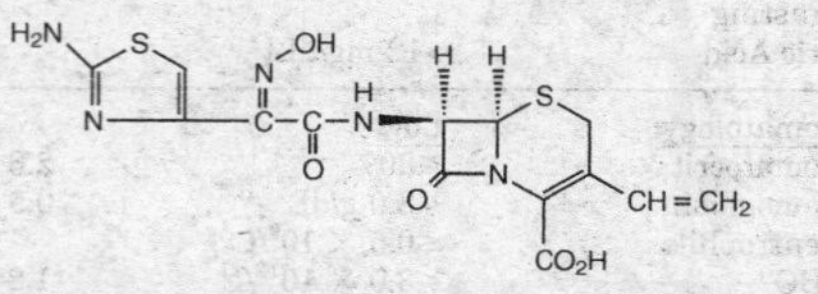

OMNICEF Capsules contain 300 mg cefdinir and the following inactive ingredients: carboxymethylcellulose calcium, NF; polyoxyl 40 stearate, NF; magnesium stearate, NF; and silicon dioxide, NF. The capsule shells contain FD&C Blue #1; FD&C Red #40; D&C Red #28; titanium dioxide, NF; gelatin, NF; and sodium lauryl sulfate, NF.

OMNICEF for Oral Suspension, after reconstitution, contains 125 mg cefdinir per 5 mL and the following inactive ingredients: sucrose, NF; citric acid, USP; sodium citrate, USP; sodium benzoate, NF; xanthan gum, NF; guar gum, NF; artificial strawberry and cream flavors; silicon dioxide, NF; and magnesium stearate, NF.

CLINICAL PHARMACOLOGY

Pharmacokinetics and Drug Metabolism

Absorption:

Oral Bioavailability: Maximal plasma cefdinir concentrations occur 2 to 4 hours postdose following capsule or suspension administration. Plasma cefdinir concentrations increase with dose, but the increases are less than dose-proportional from 300 mg (7 mg/kg) to 600 mg (14 mg/kg). Following administration of suspension to healthy adults, cefdinir bioavailability is 120% relative to capsules. Estimated bioavailability of cefdinir capsules is 21% following administration of a 300 mg capsule dose, and 16% following administration of a 600 mg capsule dose. Estimated absolute bioavailability of cefdinir suspension is 25%.

Effect of Food: Although the rate (C_{max}) and extent (AUC) of cefdinir absorption from the capsules are reduced by 16% and 10%, respectively, when given with a high-fat meal, the magnitude of these reductions is not likely to be clinically significant. Therefore, cefdinir may be taken without regard to food.

Cefdinir Capsules: Cefdinir plasma concentrations and pharmacokinetic parameter values following administration of single 300- and 600-mg oral doses of cefdinir to adult subjects are presented in the following table:

[See first table at top of next page]

Cefdinir Suspension: Cefdinir plasma concentrations and pharmacokinetic parameter values following administration of single 7- and 14-mg/kg oral doses of cefdinir to pediatric subjects (age 6 months–12 years) are presented in the following table:

[See second table at top of next page]

Multiple Dosing: Cefdinir does not accumulate in plasma following once- or twice-daily administration to subjects with normal renal function.

Distribution: The mean volume of distribution (Vd_{area}) of cefdinir in adult subjects is 0.35 L/kg (±0.29); in pediatric subjects (age 6 months–12 years), cefdinir Vd_{area} is 0.67 L/kg (±0.38).Cefdinir is 60% to 70% bound to plasma proteins in both adult and pediatric subjects; binding is independent of concentration.

Skin Blister: In adult subjects, median (range) maximal blister fluid cefdinir concentrations of 0.65 (0.33–1.1) and 1.1 (0.49–1.9) µg/mL were observed 4 to 5 hours following administration of 300- and 600-mg doses, respectively. Mean (±SD) blister C_{max} and AUC (0-∞) values were 48% (±13) and 91% (±18) of corresponding plasma values.

Tonsil Tissue: In adult patients undergoing elective tonsillectomy, respective median tonsil tissue cefdinir concentrations 4 hours after administration of single 300- and 600-mg doses were 0.25 (0.22–0.46) and 0.36 (0.22–0.80) µg/g. Mean tonsil tissue concentrations were 24% (±8) of corresponding plasma concentrations.

Sinus Tissue: In adult patients undergoing elective maxillary and ethmoid sinus surgery, respective median sinus tissue cefdinir concentrations 4 hours after administration of single 300- and 600-mg doses were <0.12 (<0.12–0.46) and 0.21 (<0.12–2.0) µg/g. Mean sinus tissue concentrations were 16% (±20) of corresponding plasma concentrations.

Lung Tissue: In adult patients undergoing bronchoscopy, respective median bronchial mucosa cefdinir concentrations 4 hours after administration of single 300- and 600-mg doses were 0.78 (<0.06–1.33) and 1.14 (<0.06–1.92) µg/mL, and were 31% (±18) of corresponding plasma concentrations. Respective median epithelial lining fluid concentra-

tions were 0.29 (<0.3–4.73) and 0.49 (<0.3–0.59) μg/mL, and were 35% (±83) of corresponding plasma concentrations.
Middle Ear Fluid: In 14 pediatric patients with acute bacterial otitis media, respective median middle ear fluid cefdinir concentrations 3 hours after administration of single 7- and 14-mg/kg doses were 0.21 (<0.09–0.94) and 0.72 (0.14–1.42) μg/mL. Mean middle ear fluid concentrations were 15% (±15) of corresponding plasma concentrations.
CSF: Data on cefdinir penetration into human cerebrospinal fluid are not available.
Metabolism and Excretion: Cefdinir is not appreciably metabolized. Activity is primarily due to parent drug. Cefdinir is eliminated principally via renal excretion with a mean plasma elimination half-life ($t_{1/2}$) of 1.7 (±0.6) hours. In healthy subjects with normal renal function, renal clearance is 2.0 (±1.0) mL/min/kg, and apparent oral clearance is 11.6 (±6.0) and 15.5 (±5.4) mL/min/kg following doses of 300- and 600-mg, respectively. Mean percent of dose recovered unchanged in the urine following 300- and 600-mg doses is 18.4% (±6.4) and 11.6% (±4.6), respectively. Cefdinir clearance is reduced in patients with renal dysfunction (see **Special Populations:** *Patients with Renal Insufficiency*). Because renal excretion is the predominant pathway of elimination, dosage should be adjusted in patients with markedly compromised renal function or who are undergoing hemodialysis (see **DOSAGE AND ADMINISTRATION**).
Special Populations:
Patients with Renal Insufficiency: Cefdinir pharmacokinetics were investigated in 21 adult subjects with varying degrees of renal function. Decreases in cefdinir elimination rate, apparent oral clearance (CL/F), and renal clearance were approximately proportional to the reduction in creatinine clearance (CL_{cr}). As a result, plasma cefdinir concentrations were higher and persisted longer in subjects with renal impairment than in those without renal impairment. In subjects with CL_{cr} between 30 and 60 mL/min, C_{max} and $t_{1/2}$ increased by approximately 2-fold and AUC by approximately 3-fold. In subjects with CL_{cr} <30 mL/min, C_{max} increased by approximately 2-fold, $t_{1/2}$ by approximately 5-fold, and AUC by approximately 6-fold. Dosage adjustment is recommended in patients with markedly compromised renal function (creatinine clearance <30 mL/min; see **DOSAGE AND ADMINISTRATION**).
Hemodialysis: Cefdinir pharmacokinetics were studied in 8 adult subjects undergoing hemodialysis. Dialysis (4 hours duration) removed 63% of cefdinir from the body and reduced apparent elimination $t_{1/2}$ from 16 (±3.5) to 3.2 (±1.2) hours. Dosage adjustment is recommended in this patient population (see **DOSAGE AND ADMINISTRATION**).
Hepatic Disease: Because cefdinir is predominantly renally eliminated and not appreciably metabolized, studies in patients with hepatic impairment were not conducted. It is not expected that dosage adjustment will be required in this population.
Geriatric Patients: The effect of age on cefdinir pharmacokinetics after a single 300-mg dose was evaluated in 32 subjects 19 to 91 years of age. Systemic exposure to cefdinir was substantially increased in older subjects (N=16), C_{max} by 44% and AUC by 86%. This increase was due to a reduction in cefdinir clearance. The apparent volume of distribution was also reduced, thus no appreciable alterations in apparent elimination $t_{1/2}$ were observed (elderly: 2.2 ± 0.6 hours vs young: 1.8 ± 0.4 hours). Since cefdinir clearance has been shown to be primarily related to changes in renal function rather than age, elderly patients do not require dosage adjustment unless they have markedly compromised renal function (creatinine clearance <30 mL/min, see *Patients with Renal Insufficiency*, above).
Gender and Race: The results of a meta-analysis of clinical pharmacokinetics (N=217) indicated no significant impact of either gender or race on cefdinir pharmacokinetics.
Microbiology
As with other cephalosporins, bactericidal activity of cefdinir results from inhibition of cell wall synthesis. Cefdinir is stable in the presence of some, but not all, β-lactamase enzymes. As a result, many organisms resistant to penicillins and some cephalosporins are susceptible to cefdinir.
Cefdinir has been shown to be active against most strains of the following microorganisms, both *in vitro* and in clinical infections as described in **INDICATIONS AND USAGE**.
Aerobic Gram-Positive Microorganisms:
Staphylococcus aureus (including β-lactamase producing strains)
NOTE: Cefdinir is inactive against methicillin-resistant staphylococci.
Streptococcus pneumoniae (penicillin-susceptible strains only)
Streptococcus pyogenes
Aerobic Gram-Negative Microorganisms:
Haemophilus influenzae (including β-lactamase producing strains)
Haemophilus parainfluenzae (including β-lactamase producing strains)
Moraxella catarrhalis (including β-lactamase producing strains)
The following *in vitro* data are available, **but their clinical significance is unknown.**
Cefdinir exhibits *in vitro* minimum inhibitory concentrations (MICs) of 1 μg/mL or less against (≥90%) strains of the following microorganisms; however, the safety and efficacy of cefdinir in treating clinical infections due to these microorganisms have not been established in adequate and well-controlled clinical trials.
Aerobic Gram-Positive Microorganisms:
Staphylococcus epidermidis (methicillin-susceptible strains only)
Streptococcus agalactiae
Viridans group streptococci
NOTE: Cefdinir is inactive against Enterococcus and methicillin-resistant *Staphylococcus* species.
Aerobic Gram-Negative Microorganisms:
Citrobacter diversus
Escherichia coli
Klebsiella pneumoniae
Proteus mirabilis
NOTE: Cefdinir is inactive against *Pseudomonas* and *Enterobacter* species.
Susceptibility Tests:
Dilution Techniques: Quantitative methods are used to determine antimicrobial minimum inhibitory concentrations (MICs). These MICs provide estimates of the susceptibility of bacteria to antimicrobial compounds. The MICs should be determined using a standardized procedure. Standardized procedures are based on a dilution method[(1)] (broth or agar) or equivalent with standardized inoculum concentrations and standardized concentrations of cefdinir powder. The MIC values should be interpreted according to the following criteria:

For organisms other than *Haemophilus* spp. and *Streptococcus* spp:

MIC (μg/mL)	Interpretation
≤1	Susceptible (S)
2	Intermediate (I)
≥4	Resistant (R)

For *Haemophilus* spp:[a]

MIC (μg/mL)	Interpretation[b]
≤1	Susceptible (S)

[a] These interpretive standards are applicable only to broth microdilution susceptibility tests with *Haemophilus* spp. using *Haemophilus* Test Medium (HTM).[(1)]
[b] The current absence of data on resistant strains precludes defining any results other than "Susceptible." Strains yielding MIC results suggestive of a "nonsusceptible" category should be submitted to a reference laboratory for further testing.

For *Streptococcus* spp:
Streptococcus pneumoniae that are susceptible to penicillin (MIC ≤0.06 μg/mL), or streptococci other than S. pneumoniae that are susceptible to penicillin (MIC ≤0.12 μg/mL), can be considered susceptible to cefdinir. Testing of cefdinir against penicillin-intermediate or penicillin-resistant isolates is not recommended. Reliable interpretive criteria for cefdinir are not available.
A report of "Susceptible" indicates that the pathogen is likely to be inhibited if the antimicrobial compound in the blood reaches the concentration usually achievable. A report of "Intermediate" indicates that the result should be considered equivocal, and, if the microorganism is not fully susceptible to alternative, clinically feasible drugs, the test should be repeated. This category implies possible clinical applicability in body sites where the drug is physiologically concentrated or in situations where high dosage of drug can be used. This category also provides a buffer zone which prevents small uncontrolled technical factors from causing major discrepancies in interpretation. A report of "Resistant" indicates that the pathogen is not likely to be inhibited if the antimicrobial compound in the blood reaches the concentrations usually achievable; other therapy should be selected.
Standardized susceptibility test procedures require the use of laboratory control microorganisms to control the technical aspects of laboratory procedures. Standard cefdinir powder should provide the following MIC values:

Microorganism	MIC Range (μg/mL)
Escherichia coli ATCC 25922	0.12–0.5
Haemophilus influenzae ATCC 49766[c]	0.12–0.5
Staphylococcus aureus ATCC 29213	0.12–0.5

[c] This quality control range is applicable only to *H. influenzae* ATCC 49766 tested by a broth microdilution procedure using HTM.

Diffusion Techniques: Quantitative methods that require measurement of zone diameters also provide reproducible estimates of the susceptibility of bacteria to antimicrobial compounds. One such standardized procedure[(2)] requires the use of standardized inoculum concentrations. This procedure uses paper disks impregnated with 5-μg cefdinir to test the susceptibility of microorganisms to cefdinir.
Reports from the laboratory providing results of the standard single-disk susceptibility test with a 5-μg cefdinir disk should be interpreted according to the following criteria:

For organisms other than *Haemophilus* spp. and *Streptococcus* spp:[d]

Zone Diameter (mm)	Interpretation
≥20	Susceptible (S)
17–19	Intermediate (I)
≤16	Resistant (R)

[d] Because certain strains of *Citrobacter, Providencia,* and *Enterobacter* spp. have been reported to give false susceptible results with the cefdinir disk, strains of these genera should not be tested and reported with this disk.

For *Haemophilus* spp:[e]

Zone Diameter (mm)	Interpretation[f]
≥20	Susceptible (S)

[e] These zone diameter standards are applicable only to tests with *Haemophilus* spp. using HTM.[(2)]
[f] The current absence of data on resistant strains precludes defining any results other than "Susceptible." Strains yielding MIC results suggestive of a "nonsusceptible" category should be submitted to a reference laboratory for further testing.

For *Streptococcus* spp:
Isolates of *Streptococcus pneumoniae* should be tested against a 1-μg oxacillin disk. Isolates with oxacillin zone sizes ≥20 mm are susceptible to penicillin and can be considered susceptible to cefdinir. Streptococci other than *S. pneumoniae* should be tested with a 10-unit penicillin disk. Isolates with penicillin zone sizes ≥28 mm are susceptible to penicillin and can be considered susceptible to cefdinir.
As with standardized dilution techniques, diffusion methods require the use of laboratory control microorganisms to control the technical aspects of laboratory procedures. For the diffusion technique, the 5-μg cefdinir disk should provide the following zone diameters in these laboratory quality control strains:

Organism	Zone Diameter (mm)
Escherichia coli ATCC 25922	24–28
Haemophilus influenzae ATCC 49766[g]	24–31
Staphylococcus aureus ATCC 25923	25–32

[g] This quality control range is applicable only to *H. influenzae* ATCC 49766 using HTM.

Mean (±SD) Plasma Cefdinir Pharmacokinetic Parameter Values Following Administration of Capsules to Adult Subjects

Dose	C_{max} (μg/mL)	t_{max} (hr)	AUC (μg•hr/mL)
300 mg	1.60 (0.55)	2.9 (0.89)	7.05 (2.17)
600 mg	2.87 (1.01)	3.0 (0.66)	11.1 (3.87)

Mean (±SD) Plasma Cefdinir Pharmacokinetic Parameter Values Following Administration of Suspension to Pediatric Subjects

Dose	C_{max} (μg/mL)	t_{max} (hr)	AUC (μg•hr/mL)
7 mg/kg	2.30 (0.65)	2.2 (0.6)	8.31 (2.50)
14 mg/kg	3.86 (0.62)	1.8 (0.4)	13.4 (2.64)

Continued on next page

Omnicef—Cont.

INDICATIONS AND USAGE

OMNICEF (cefdinir) capsules and OMNICEF (cefdinir) for oral suspension are indicated for the treatment of patients with mild to moderate infections caused by susceptible strains of the designated microorganisms in the conditions listed below.

Adults and Adolescents

Community-Acquired Pneumonia caused by *Haemophilus influenzae* (including β-lactamase producing strains), *Haemophilus parainfluenzae* (including β-lactamase producing strains), *Streptococcus pneumoniae* (penicillin-susceptible strains only), and *Moraxella catarrhalis* (including β-lactamase producing strains) (see **CLINICAL STUDIES**).

Acute Exacerbations of Chronic Bronchitis caused by *Haemophilus influenzae* (including β-lactamase producing strains), *Haemophilus parainfluenzae* (including β-lactamase producing strains), *Streptococcus pneumoniae* (penicillin-susceptible strains only), and *Moraxella catarrhalis* (including β-lactamase producing strains).

Acute Maxillary Sinusitis caused by *Haemophilus influenzae* (including β-lactamase producing strains), *Streptococcus pneumoniae* (penicillin-susceptible strains only), and *Moraxella catarrhalis* (including β-lactamase producing strains).

NOTE: For information on use in pediatric patients, See **Pediatric Use** and **DOSAGE AND ADMINISTRATION.**

Pharyngitis/Tonsillitis caused by *Streptococcus pyogenes* (see **CLINICAL STUDIES**).

NOTE: Cefdinir is effective in the eradication of *S. pyogenes* from the oropharynx. Cefdinir has not, however, been studied for the prevention of rheumatic fever following *S. pyogenes* pharyngitis/tonsillitis. Only intramuscular penicillin has been demonstrated to be effective for the prevention of rheumatic fever.

Uncomplicated Skin and Skin Structure Infections caused by *Staphylococcus aureus* (including β-lactamase producing strains) and *Streptococcus pyogenes*.

Pediatric Patients

Acute Bacterial Otitis Media caused by *Haemophilus influenzae* (including β-lactamase producing strains), *Streptococcus pneumoniae* (penicillin-susceptible strains only) and *Moraxella catarrhalis* (including β-lactamase producing strains).

Pharyngitis/Tonsillitis caused by Streptococcus pyogenes (see **CLINICAL STUDIES**).

NOTE: Cefdinir is effective in the eradication of *S. pyogenes* from the oropharynx. Cefdinir has not, however, been studied for the prevention of rheumatic fever following *S. pyogenes* pharyngitis/tonsillitis. Only intramuscular penicillin has been demonstrated to be effective for the prevention of rheumatic fever.

Uncomplicated Skin and Skin Structure Infections caused by *Staphylococcus aureus* (including β-lactamase producing strains) and *Streptococcus pyogenes*.

CONTRAINDICATIONS

OMNICEF (cefdinir) is contraindicated in patients with known allergy to the cephalosporin class of antibiotics.

WARNINGS

BEFORE THERAPY WITH OMNICEF (CEFDINIR) IS INSTITUTED, CAREFUL INQUIRY SHOULD BE MADE TO DETERMINE WHETHER THE PATIENT HAS HAD PREVIOUS HYPERSENSITIVITY REACTIONS TO CEFDINIR, OTHER CEPHALOSPORINS, PENICILLINS, OR OTHER DRUGS. IF CEFDINIR IS TO BE GIVEN TO PENICILLIN-SENSITIVE PATIENTS, CAUTION SHOULD BE EXERCISED BECAUSE CROSS-HYPERSENSITIVITY AMONG β-LACTAM ANTIBIOTICS HAS BEEN CLEARLY DOCUMENTED AND MAY OCCUR IN UP TO 10% OF PATIENTS WITH A HISTORY OF PENICILLIN ALLERGY. IF AN ALLERGIC REACTION TO CEFDINIR OCCURS, THE DRUG SHOULD BE DISCONTINUED. SERIOUS ACUTE HYPERSENSITIVITY REACTIONS MAY REQUIRE TREATMENT WITH EPINEPHRINE AND OTHER EMERGENCY MEASURES, INCLUDING OXYGEN, INTRAVENOUS FLUIDS, INTRAVENOUS ANTIHISTAMINES, CORTICOSTEROIDS, PRESSOR AMINES, AND AIRWAY MANAGEMENT, AS CLINICALLY INDICATED.

Pseudomembranous colitis has been reported with nearly all antibacterial agents, including cefdinir, and may range from mild- to life-threatening. Therefore, it is important to consider this diagnosis in patients who present with diarrhea subsequent to the administration of antibacterial agents.

Treatment with antibacterial agents alters the normal flora of the colon and may permit overgrowth of clostridia. Studies indicate that a toxin produced by *Clostridium difficile* is a primary cause of "antibiotic-associated colitis."

After the diagnosis of pseudomembranous colitis has been established, appropriate therapeutic measures should be initiated. Mild cases of pseudomembranous colitis usually respond to drug discontinuation alone. In moderate to severe cases, consideration should be given to management with fluids and electrolytes, protein supplementation, and treatment with an antibacterial drug clinically effective against *Clostridium difficile*.

PRECAUTIONS

General

As with other broad-spectrum antibiotics, prolonged treatment may result in the possible emergence and overgrowth of resistant organisms. Careful observation of the patient is essential. If superinfection occurs during therapy, appropriate alternative therapy should be administered.

Cefdinir, as with other broad-spectrum antimicrobials (antibiotics), should be prescribed with caution in individuals with a history of colitis.

In patients with transient or persistent renal insufficiency (creatinine clearance <30 mL/min), the total daily dose of OMNICEF should be reduced because high and prolonged plasma concentrations of cefdinir can result following recommended doses (see **DOSAGE AND ADMINISTRATION**).

Information for Patients

Antacids containing magnesium or aluminum interfere with the absorption of cefdinir. If this type of antacid is required during OMNICEF therapy, OMNICEF should be taken at least 2 hours before or after the antacid.

Iron supplements, including multivitamins that contain iron, interfere with the absorption of cefdinir. If iron supplements are required during OMNICEF therapy, OMNICEF should be taken at least 2 hours before or after the supplement.

Iron-fortified infant formula does not significantly interfere with the absorption of cefdinir. Therefore, OMNICEF for Oral Suspension can be administered with iron-fortified infant formula.

Diabetic patients and caregivers should be aware that the oral suspension contains 2.86 g of sucrose per teaspoon.

Drug Interactions

Antacids: (aluminum- or magnesium-containing): Concomitant administration of 300-mg cefdinir capsules with 30 mL Maalox® TC suspension reduces rate (C_{max}) and extent (AUC) of absorption by approximately 40%. Time to reach C_{max} is also prolonged by 1 hour. There are no significant effects on cefdinir pharmacokinetics if the antacid is administered 2 hours before or 2 hours after cefdinir. If antacids are required during OMNICEF therapy, OMNICEF should be taken at least 2 hours before or after the antacid.

Probenecid: As with other β-lactam antibiotics, probenecid inhibits the renal excretion of cefdinir, resulting in an approximate doubling in AUC, a 54% increase in peak cefdinir plasma levels, and a 50% prolongation in the apparent elimination $t_{1/2}$.

Iron Supplements and Foods Fortified With Iron: Concomitant administration of cefdinir with a therapeutic iron

ADVERSE EVENTS ASSOCIATED WITH CEFDINIR CAPSULES US TRIALS IN ADULT AND ADOLESCENT PATIENTS (N=3841)[a]

Incidence ≥1%	Diarrhea	15%
	Vaginal moniliasis	4% of women
	Nausea	3%
	Headache	2%
	Abdominal pain	1%
	Vaginitis	1% of women
Incidence <1% but >0.1%	Rash	0.9%
	Dyspepsia	0.7%
	Flatulence	0.7%
	Vomiting	0.7%
	Abnormal stools	0.3%
	Anorexia	0.3%
	Constipation	0.3%
	Dizziness	0.3%
	Dry Mouth	0.3%
	Asthenia	0.2%
	Insomnia	0.2%
	Leukorrhea	0.2% of women
	Moniliasis	0.2%
	Pruritus	0.2%
	Somnolence	0.2%

[a]1733 males, 2108 females

LABORATORY VALUE CHANGES OBSERVED WITH CEFDINIR CAPSULES US TRIALS IN ADULT AND ADOLESCENT PATIENTS (N=3841)

Incidence ≥ 1%	↑ Urine leukocytes	2%
	↑ Urine protein	2%
	↑ Gamma-glutamyltransferase[a]	1%
	↓ Lymphocytes, ↑ Lymphocytes	1%, 0.2%
	↑ Microhematuria	1%
Incidence <1% but >0.1%	↑ Glucose[a]	0.9%
	↑ Urine glucose	0.9%
	↑ White blood cells, ↓ White blood cells	0.9%, 0.7%
	↑ Alanine aminotransferase (ALT)	0.7%
	↑ Eosinophils	0.7%
	↑ Urine specific gravity, ↓ Urine specific gravity[a]	0.6%, 0.2%
	↓ Bicarbonate[a]	0.6%
	↑ Phosphorus, ↓ Phosphorus[a]	0.6, 0.3%
	↑ Aspartate aminotransferase (AST)	0.4%
	↑ Alkaline phosphatase	0.3%
	↑ Blood urea nitrogen (BUN)	0.3%
	↓ Hemoglobin	0.3%
	↑ Polymorphonuclear neutrophils (PMNs), ↓ PMNs	0.3%, 0.2%
	↑ Bilirubin	0.2%
	↑ Lactate dehydrogenase[a]	0.2%
	↑ Platelets	0.2%
	↑ Potassium[a]	0.2%
	↑ Urine pH[a]	0.2%

[a]N<3841 for these parameters

ADVERSE EVENTS ASSOCIATED WITH CEFDINIR SUSPENSION US TRIALS IN PEDIATRIC PATIENTS (N = 1783)[a]

Incidence ≥ 1%	Diarrhea	8%
	Rash	3%
	Vomiting	1%
Incidence <1% but >0.1%	Cutaneous moniliasis	0.9%
	Abdominal pain	0.8%
	Leukopenia[b]	0.3%
	Vaginal moniliasis	0.3% of girls
	Vaginitis	0.3% of girls
	Abnormal stools	0.2%
	Dyspepsia	0.2%
	Hyperkinesia	0.2%
	Increased AST[b]	0.2%
	Maculopapular rash	0.2%
	Nausea	0.2%

[a] 977 males, 806 females

[b] Laboratory changes were occasionally reported as adverse events.

supplement containing 60 mg of elemental iron (as $FeSO_4$) or vitamins supplemented with 10 mg of elemental iron reduced extent of absorption by 80% and 31%, respectively. If iron supplements are required during OMNICEF therapy, OMNICEF should be taken at least 2 hours before or after the supplement.
The effect of foods highly fortified with elemental iron (primarily iron-fortified breakfast cereals) on cefdinir absorption has not been studied.
Concomitantly administered iron-fortified infant formula (2.2 mg elemental iron/6 oz) has no significant effect on cefdinir pharmacokinetics. Therefore, OMNICEF for Oral Suspension can be administered with iron-fortified infant formula.
There have been rare reports of reddish stools in patients who have received cefdinir in Japan. The reddish color is due to the formation of a nonabsorbable complex between cefdinir or its breakdown products and iron in the gastrointestinal tract.

Drug/Laboratory Test Interactions
A false-positive reaction for ketones in the urine may occur with tests using nitroprusside, but not with those using nitroferricyanide. The administration of cefdinir may result in a false-positive reaction for glucose in urine using Clinitest®, Benedict's solution, or Fehling's solution. It is recommended that glucose tests based on enzymatic glucose oxidase reactions (such as Clinistix® or Tes-Tape®) be used. Cephalosporins are known to occasionally induce a positive direct Coombs' test.

Carcinogenesis, Mutagenesis, Impairment of Fertility
The carcinogenic potential of cefdinir has not been evaluated. No mutagenic effects were seen in the bacterial reverse mutation assay (Ames) or point mutation assay at the hypoxanthineguanine phosphoribosyltransferase locus (HGPRT) in V79 Chinese hamster lung cells. No clastogenic effects were observed *in vitro* in the structural chromosome aberration assay in V79 Chinese hamster lung cells or *in vivo* in the micronucleus assay in mouse bone marrow. In rats, fertility and reproductive performance were not affected by cefdinir at oral doses up to 1000 mg/kg/day (70 times the human dose on mg/kg/day, 11 times based on mg/m^2/day).

Pregnancy—Teratogenic Effects
Pregnancy Category B: Cefdinir was not teratogenic in rats at oral doses up to 1000 mg/kg/day (70 times the human dose on mg/kg/day, 11 times based on mg/m^2/day) or in rabbits at oral doses up to 10 mg/kg/day (0.7 times the human dose based on mg/kg/day, 0.23 times based on mg/m^2/day). Maternal toxicity (decreased body weight gain) was observed in rabbits at the maximum tolerated dose of 10 mg/kg/day without adverse effects on offspring. Decreased body weight occurred in rat fetuses at ≥100 mg/kg/day, and in rat offspring at ≥32 mg/kg/day. No effects were observed on maternal reproductive parameters or offspring survival, development, behavior, or reproductive function.
There are, however, no adequate and well-controlled studies in pregnant women. Because animal reproduction studies are not always predictive of human response, this drug should be used during pregnancy only if clearly needed.

Labor and Delivery
Cefdinir has not been studied for use during labor and delivery.

Nursing Mothers
Following administration of single 600-mg doses, cefdinir was not detected in human breast milk.

Pediatric Use
Safety and efficacy in neonates and infants less than 6 months of age have not been established. Use of cefdinir for the treatment of acute maxillary sinusitis in pediatric patients (age 6 months through 12 years) is supported by evidence from adequate and well-controlled studies in adults and adolescents, the similar pathophysiology of acute sinusitis in adult and pediatric patients, and comparative pharmacokinetic data in the pediatric population.

Geriatric Use
Efficacy is comparable in geriatric patients and younger adults. While cefdinir has been well-tolerated in all age groups, in clinical trials geriatric patients experienced a lower rate of adverse events, including diarrhea, than younger adults. Dose adjustment in elderly patients is not necessary unless renal function is markedly compromised (see **DOSAGE AND ADMINISTRATION**).

ADVERSE EVENTS

Clinical Trials—OMNICEF Capsules (Adult and Adolescent Patients):
In clinical trials, 5093 adult and adolescent patients (3841 US and 1252 non-US) were treated with the recommended dose of cefdinir capsules (600 mg/day). Most adverse events were mild and self-limiting. No deaths or permanent disabilities were attributed to cefdinir. One hundred forty-seven of 5093 (3%) patients discontinued medication due to adverse events thought by the investigators to be possibly, probably, or definitely associated with cefdinir therapy. The discontinuations were primarily for gastrointestinal disturbances, usually diarrhea or nausea. Nineteen of 5093 (0.4%) patients were discontinued due to rash thought related to cefdinir administration.
In the US, the following adverse events were thought by the investigators to be possibly, probably, or definitely related to cefdinir capsules in the mulitple-dose clinical trials (N = 3841 cefdinir-treated patients):
[See first table at top of previous page]

LABORATORY VALUE CHANGES OF POSSIBLE CLINICAL SIGNIFICANCE OBSERVED WITH CEFDINIR SUSPENSION US TRIALS IN PEDIATRIC PATIENTS (N = 1783)

Incidence ≥1%	↑ Lymphocytes, ↓ Lymphocytes	2, 0.8%
	↑ Alkaline phosphatase	1%
	↓ Bicarbonate[a]	1%
	↑ Eosinophils	1%
	↑ Lactate dehydrogenase	1%
	↑ Platelets	1%
	↑ PMNs, ↓ PMNs	1, 1%
	↑ Urine protein	1%
Incidence <1% but >0.1%	↑ Phosphorus, ↓ Phosphorus	0.9, 0.4%
	↑ Urine pH	0.8%
	↓ White blood cells, ↑ White blood cells	0.7, 0.3%
	↓ Calcium[a]	0.5%
	↓ Hemoglobin	0.5%
	↑ Urine leukocytes	0.5%
	↑ Monocytes	0.4%
	↑ AST	0.3%
	↑ Potassium[a]	0.3%
	↑ Urine specific gravity, ↓ Urine specific gravity	0.3, 0.1%
	↓ Hematocrit[a]	0.2%

[a] N = 1387 for these parameters.

Adults and Adolescents (Age 13 Years and Older)

Type of Infection	Dosage	Duration
Community-Acquired Pneumonia	300 mg q12h	10 days
Acute Exacerbations of Chronic Bronchitis	300 mg q12h	5 to 10 days
	or	
	600 mg q24h	10 days
Acute Maxillary Sinusitis	300 mg q12h	10 days
	or	
	600 mg q24h	10 days
Pharyngitis/Tonsillitis	300 mg q12h	5 to 10 days
	or	
	600 mg q24h	10 days
Uncomplicated Skin and Skin Structure Infections	300 mg q12h	10 days

Pediatric Patients (Age 6 Months Through 12 Years)

Type of Infection	Dosage	Duration
Acute Bacterial Otitis Media	7 mg/kg q12h	5 to 10 days
	or	
	14 mg/kg q24h	10 days
Acute Maxillary Sinusitis	7 mg/kg q12h	10 days
	or	
	14 mg/kg q24h	10 days
Pharyngitis/Tonsillitis	7 mg/kg q12h	5 to 10 days
	or	
	14 mg/kg q24h	10 days
Uncomplicated Skin and Skin Structure Infections	7 mg/kg q12h	10 days

OMNICEF FOR ORAL SUSPENSION PEDIATRIC DOSAGE CHART

Weight	125 mg/5 mL
9 kg/20 lbs	2.5 mL (½ tsp) q12h or 5 mL (1 tsp) q24h
18 kg/40 lbs	5 mL (1 tsp) q12h or 10 mL (2 tsp) q24h
27 kg/60 lbs	7.5 mL (1½ tsp) q12h or 15 mL (3 tsp) q24h
36 kg/80 lbs	10 mL (2 tsp) q12h or 20 mL (4 tsp) q24h
≥ 43 kg[a]/95 lbs	12 mL (2½ tsp) q12h or 24 mL (5 tsp) q24h

[a] Pediatric patients who weigh ≥43 kg should receive the maximum daily dose of 600 mg.

Directions for Mixing Omnicef for Oral Suspension

Final Concentration	Final Volume (mL)	Amount of Water	Directions
125 mg/5 mL	60	38 mL	Tap bottle to loosen powder, then add water in 2 portions. Shake well after each aliquot.
	100	63 mL	

The following laboratory value changes of possible clinical significance, irrespective of relationship to therapy with cefdinir, were seen during clinical trials conducted in the US:
[See second table on previous page]

Clinical Trials—OMNICEF for Oral Suspension (Pediatric Patients):
In clinical trials, 2289 pediatric patients (1783 US and 506 non-US) were treated with the recommended dose of cefdinir suspension (14 mg/kg/day). Most adverse events were mild and self-limiting. No deaths or permanent disabilities were attributed to cefdinir. Forty of 2289 (2%) patients discontinued medication due to adverse events considered by the investigators to be possibly, probably, or definitely associated with cefdinir therapy. Discontinuation were primarily for gastrointestinal disturbances, usually diarrhea. Five of 2289 (0.2%) patients were discontinued due to rash thought related to cefdinir administration.
In the US, the following adverse events were thought by investigators to be possibly, probably, or definitely related to cefdinir suspension in multiple-dose clinical trials (N=1783 cefdinir-treated patients):
[See third table on previous page]
NOTE: In both cefdinir- and control-treated patients, rates of diarrhea and rash were higher in the youngest pediatric patients. The incidence of cefdinir-treated patients ≤2 years of age was 17% (95/557) compared with 4% (51/1226) in those >2 years old. The incidence of rash (primarily diaper rash in the younger patients) was 8% (43/557) in patients ≤2 years of age compared with 1% (8/1226) in those >2 years old.
The following laboratory value changes of possible clinical significance, irrespective of relationship to therapy with cefdinir, were seen during clinical trials conducted in the US:
[See first table above]

Continued on next page

Omnicef—Cont.

Postmarketing Experience

The following adverse experiences and altered laboratory tests, regardless of their relationship to cefdinir, have been reported during extensive postmarketing experience, beginning with approval in Japan in 1991: Stevens-Johnson syndrome, toxic epidermal necrolysis, exfoliative dermatitis, erythema multiforme, erythema nodosum, conjunctivitis, stomatitis, acute hepatitis, cholestasis, fulminant hepatitis, hepatic failure, jaundice, increased amylase, shock, anaphylaxis, facial and laryngeal edema, feeling of suffocation, acute enterocolitis, bloody diarrhea, hemorrhagic colitis, melena, pseudomembranous colitis, pancytopenia, granulocytopenia, leukopenia, thrombocytopenia, idiopathic thrombocytopenic purpura, hemolytic anemia, acute respiratory failure, asthmatic attack, drug-induced pneumonia, eosinophilic pneumonia, idiopathic interstitial pneumonia, fever, acute renal failure, nephropathy, bleeding tendency, coagulation disorder, disseminated intravascular coagulation, upper GI bleed, peptic ulcer, ileus, loss of consciousness, allergic vasculitis, possible cefdinir-diclofenac interaction, cardiac failure, chest pain, myocardial infarction, hypertension, involuntary movements, and rhabdomyolysis.

Cephalosporin Class Adverse Events

The following adverse events and altered laboratory tests have been reported for cephalosporin-class antibiotics in general:

Allergic reactions, anaphylaxis, Stevens-Johnson syndrome, erythema multiforme, toxic epidermal necrolysis, renal dysfunction, toxic nephropathy, hepatic dysfunction including cholestasis, aplastic anemia, hemolytic anemia, hemorrhage, false-positive test for urinary glucose, neutropenia, pancytopenia, and agranulocytosis.

Pseudomembranous colitis symptoms may begin during or after antibiotic treatment (see **WARNINGS**).

Several cephalosporins have been implicated in triggering seizures, particularly in patients with renal impairment when the dosage was not reduced (see **DOSAGE AND ADMINISTRATION** and **OVERDOSAGE**). If seizures associated with drug therapy occur, the drug should be discontinued. Anticonvulsant therapy can be given if clinically indicated.

OVERDOSAGE

Information on cefdinir overdosage in humans is not available. In acute rodent toxicity studies, a single oral 5600-mg/kg dose produced no adverse effects. Toxic signs and symptoms following overdosage with other β-lactam antibiotics have included nausea, vomiting, epigastric distress, diarrhea, and convulsions. Hemodialysis removes cefdinir from the body. This may be useful in the event of a serious toxic reaction from overdosage, particularly if renal function is compromised.

DOSAGE AND ADMINISTRATION

(see **INDICATIONS AND USAGE** for Indicated Pathogens)

Capsules

The recommended dosage and duration of treatment for infections in adults and adolescents are described in the following chart; the total daily dose for all infections is 600 mg. Once-daily dosing for 10 days is as effective as BID dosing. Once-daily dosing has not been studied in pneumonia or skin infections; therefore, OMNICEF Capsules should be administered twice daily in these infections. OMNICEF Capsules may be taken without regard to meals.

[See second table on previous page]

Powder for Oral Suspension

The recommended dosage and duration of treatment for infections in pediatric patients are described in the following chart; the total daily dose for all infections is 14 mg/kg, up to a maximum dose of 600 mg per day. Once-daily dosing for 10 days is as effective as BID dosing. Once-daily dosing has not been studied in skin infections; therefore, OMNICEF for Oral Suspension should be administered twice daily in this infection. OMNICEF for Oral Suspension may be administered without regard to meals.

[See third table on previous page]
[See fourth table on previous page]

Patients With Renal Insufficiency

For adult patients with creatinine clearance <30 mL/min, the dose of cefdinir should be 300 mg given once daily.

Creatinine clearance is difficult to measure in outpatients. However, the following formula may be used to estimate creatinine clearance (CL_{cr}) in adult patients. For estimates to be valid, serum creatinine levels should reflect steady-state levels of renal function.

$$\text{Males:}\quad CL_{cr} = \frac{(\text{weight})\,(140 - \text{age})}{(72)\,(\text{serum creatinine})}$$

$$\text{Females:}\quad CL_{cr} = 0.85 \times \text{above value}$$

where creatinine clearance is in mL/min, age is in years, weight is in kilograms, and serum creatinine is in mg/dL.[3]

The following formula may be used to estimate creatinine clearance in pediatric patients:

$$CL_{cr} = K \times \frac{\text{body length or height}}{\text{serum creatinine}}$$

where K=0.55 for pediatric patients older than 1 years[4] and 0.45 for infants (up to 1 year)[5].

US Community-Acquired Pneumonia Study
Cefdinir vs Cefaclor

	Cefdinir BID	Cefaclor TID	Outcome
Clinical Cure Rates	150/187 (80%)	147/186 (79%)	Cefdinir equivalent to control
Eradication Rates			
Overall	177/195 (91%)	184/200 (92%)	Cefdinir equivalent to control
S. pneumoniae	31/31 (100%)	35/35 (100%)	
H. influenzae	55/65 (85%)	60/72 (83%)	
M. catarrhalis	10/10 (100%)	11/11 (100%)	
H. parainfluenzae	81/89 (91%)	78/82 (95%)	

European Community-Acquired Pneumonia Study
Cefdinir vs Amoxicillin/Clavulanate

	Cefdinir BID	Amoxicillin/ Clavulanate TID	Outcome
Clinical Cure Rates	83/104 (80%)	86/97 (89%)	Cefdinir not equivalent to control
Eradication Rates			
Overall	85/96 (89%)	84/90 (93%)	Cefdinir equivalent to control
S. pneumoniae	42/44 (95%)	43/44 (98%)	
H. influenzae	26/35 (74%)	21/26 (81%)	
M. catarrhalis	6/6 (100%)	8/8 (100%)	
H. parainfluenzae	11/11 (100%)	12/12 (100%)	

Pharyngitis/Tonsillitis Studies
Cefdinir (10 days) vs Penicillin (10 days)

Study	Efficacy Parameter	Cefdinir QD	Cefdinir BID	Penicillin QID	Outcome
Adults/ Adolescents	Eradication of *S. pyogenes*	192/210 (91%)	199/217 (92%)	181/217 (83%)	Cefdinir superior to control
	Clinical Cure Rates	199/210 (95%)	209/217 (96%)	193/217 (89%)	Cefdinir superior to control
Pediatric Patients	Eradication of *S. pyogenes*	215/228 (94%)	214/227 (94%)	159/227 (70%)	Cefdinir superior to control
	Clinical Cure Rates	222/228 (97%)	218/227 (96%)	196/227 (86%)	Cefdinir superior to control

Pharyngitis/Tonsillitis Studies
Cefdinir (5 days) vs Penicillin (10 days)

Study	Efficacy Parameter	Cefdinir BID	Penicillin QID	Outcome
Adults/ Adolescents	Eradication of *S. pyogenes*	193/218 (89%)	176/214 (82%)	Cefdinir equivalent to control
	Clinical Cure Rates	194/218 (89%)	181/214 (85%)	Cefdinir equivalent to control
Pediatric Patients	Eradication of *S. pyogenes*	176/196 (90%)	135/193 (70%)	Cefdinir superior to control
	Clinical Cure Rates	179/196 (91%)	173/193 (90%)	Cefdinir equivalent to control

In the above equation, creatinine clearance is in mL/min/1.73 m^2, body length or height is in centimeters, and serum creatinine is in mg/dL.

For pediatric patients with a creatinine clearance of <30 mL/min/1.73 m^2, the dose of cefdinir should be 7 mg/kg (up to 300 mg) given once daily.

Patients on Hemodialysis

Hemodialysis removes cefdinir from the body. In patients maintained on chronic hemodialysis, the recommended initial dosage regimen is 300-mg or 7-mg/kg dose every other day. At the conclusion of each hemodialysis session, 300 mg (or 7 mg/kg) should be given. Subsequent doses (300 mg or 7 mg/kg) are then administered every other day.

[See fifth table on previous page]

After mixing, the suspension can be stored at room temperature (25°C/77°F). The container should be kept tightly closed, and the suspension should be shaken well before each administration. The suspension may be used for 10 days, after which any unused portion must be discarded.

HOW SUPPLIED

OMNICEF Capsules, containing 300 mg cefdinir, as lavender and turquoise capsules imprinted with the product name, are available as follows:

60 Capsules/Bottle **NDC** 0074-3769-60

OMNICEF for Oral Suspension is a cream-colored powder formulation that, when reconstituted as directed, contains 125 mg cefdinir/5 mL. The reconstituted suspension has a cream color and strawberry flavor. The powder is available as follows:

60-mL bottles **NDC** 0074-3771-60
100-mL bottles **NDC** 0074-3771-13

Store the capsules and unsuspended powder at 25°C (77°F); excursions permitted to 15°–30°C (59°–86°F) [see USP Controlled Room Temperature]. Once reconstituted, the oral suspension can be stored at controlled room temperature for 10 days.

CLINICAL STUDIES

Community-Acquired Bacterial Pneumonia

In a controlled, double-blind study in adults and adolescents conducted in the US, cefdinir BID was compared with cefaclor 500 mg TID. Using strict evaluability and microbiological/clinical response criteria 6 to 14 days posttherapy, the following clinical cure rates, presumptive microbiologic eradication rates, and statistical outcomes were obtained:

[See first table above]

In a second controlled, investigator-blind study in adults and adolescents conducted primarily in Europe, cefdinir BID was compared with amoxicillin/clavulanate 500/125 mg TID. Using strict evaluability and clinical response criteria 6 to 14 days posttherapy, the following clinical cure rates, presumptive microbiologic eradication rates, and statistical outcomes were obtained:

[See second table above]

Streptococcal Pharyngitis/Tonsillitis

In four controlled studies conducted in the US, cefdinir was compared with 10 days of penicillin in adult, adolescent, and pediatric patients. Two studies (one in adults and adolescents, the other in pediatric patients) compared 10 days of cefdinir QD or BID to penicillin 250 mg or 10 mg/kg QID. Using strict evaluability and microbiologic/clinical response criteria 5 to 10 days posttherapy, the following clinical cure rates, microbiologic eradication rates, and statistical outcomes were obtained:

[See third table above]

Two studies (one in adults and adolescents, the other in pediatric patients) compared 5 days of cefdinir BID to 10 days of penicillin 250 mg or 10 mg/kg QID. Using strict evaluability and microbiologic/clinical response criteria 4 to 10 days posttherapy, the following clinical cure rates, microbiologic eradication rates, and statistical outcomes were obtained:

[See fourth table above]

REFERENCES

1. National Committee for Clinical Laboratory Standards. Methods for Dilution Antimicrobial Susceptibility Tests for Bacteria That Grow Aerobically, 4th ed. Approved Standard, NCCLS Document M7-A4, Vol 17(2). NCCLS, Villanova, PA, Jan 1997.
2. National Committee for Clinical Laboratory Standards. Performance Standards for Antimicrobial Disk Susceptibility Tests, 6th ed. Approved Standard, NCCLS Document M2-A6, Vol 17(1). NCCLS, Villanova, PA, Jan 1997.
3. Cockcroft DW, Gault MH. Prediction of creatinine clearance from serum creatinine. Nephron, 1976;16:31–41.
4. Schwartz GJ, Haycock GB, Edelmann CM, Spitzer A. A simple estimate of glomerular filtration rate in children derived from body length and plasma creatinine. Pediatrics 1976;58:259–63.
5. Schwartz GJ, Feld LG, Langford DJ. A simple estimate of glomerular filtration rate in full-term infants during the first year of life. J Pediatrics 1984;104:849–54.

℞ only

Ref. 03-5005-R1
Revised January, 2000
Manufactured by:
Lilly del Caribe, Inc.
Carolina, Puerto Rico 00986
For:
Abbott Laboratories
North Chicago, IL 60064
Under License of:
Fujisawa Pharmaceutical Co., Ltd.
Osaka, Japan

Shown in Product Identification Guide, page 303

PANHEMATIN® ℞

[*pan-hē 'ma-tin*]
HEMIN FOR INJECTION
For I.V. Use Only

PANHEMATIN (hemin for injection) should only be used by physicians experienced in the management of porphyrias in hospitals where the recommended clinical and laboratory diagnostic and monitoring techniques are available.
PANHEMATIN therapy should be considered after an appropriate period of alternate therapy (i.e., 400 g glucose/day for 1 to 2 days). (See "WARNINGS", "PRECAUTIONS" and "DOSAGE AND ADMINISTRATION" sections.)

DESCRIPTION

PANHEMATIN (hemin for injection) is an enzyme inhibitor derived from processed red blood cells. Hemin for injection was known previously as hematin. The term hematin has been used to describe the chemical reaction product of hemin and sodium carbonate solution. Hemin is an iron containing metalloporphyrin. Chemically hemin is represented as chloro [7,12-diethenyl-3,8,13,17-tetramethyl-21H,23H-porphine-2,18-dipropanoato (2-)-N^{21},N^{22}, N^{23}, N^{24}] iron. The structural formula for hemin is:

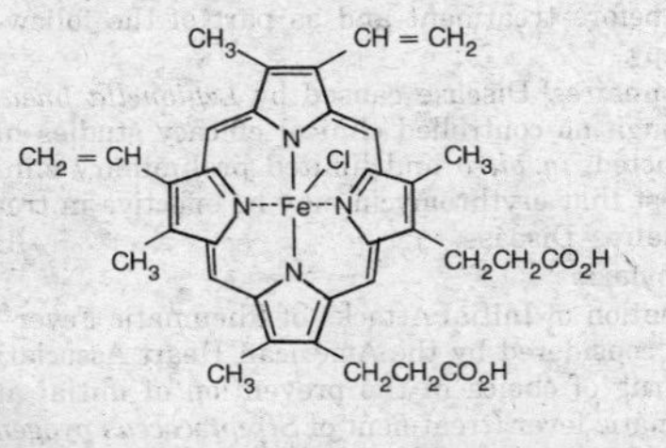

PANHEMATIN is a sterile, lyophilized powder suitable for intravenous administration after reconstitution. Each dispensing vial of PANHEMATIN contains the equivalent of 313 mg hemin, 215 mg sodium carbonate and 300 mg of sorbitol. The pH may have been adjusted with hydrochloric acid; the product contains no preservatives. When mixed as directed with Sterile Water for Injection, USP, each 43 mL provides the equivalent of approximately 301 mg hematin (7 mg/mL).

CLINICAL PHARMACOLOGY

Heme acts to limit the hepatic and/or marrow synthesis of porphyrin. This action is likely due to the inhibition of δ-aminolevulinic acid synthetase, the enzyme which limits the rate of the porphyrin/heme biosynthetic pathway. The exact mechanism by which hematin produces symptomatic improvement in patients with acute episodes of the hepatic porphyrias has not been elucidated.[1,9]
Following intravenous administration of hematin in non-jaundiced human patients, an increase in fecal urobilinogen can be observed which is roughly proportional to the amount of hematin administered. This suggests an enterohepatic pathway as at least one route of elimination. Bilirubin metabolites are also excreted in the urine following hematin injections.[2]
PANHEMATIN (hemin for injection) therapy for the acute porphyrias is not curative. After discontinuation of PANHEMATIN treatment, symptoms generally return although in some cases remission is prolonged. Some neurological symptoms have improved weeks to months after therapy although little or no response was noted at the time of treatment.
Other aspects of human pharmacokinetics have not been defined.

INDICATIONS AND USAGE

PANHEMATIN (hemin for injection) is indicated for the amelioration of recurrent attacks of acute intermittent porphyria temporally related to the menstrual cycle in susceptible women.
Manifestations such as pain, hypertension, tachycardia, abnormal mental status and mild to progressive neurologic signs may be controlled in selected patients with this disorder.
Similar findings have been reported in other patients with acute intermittent porphyria, porphyria variegata and hereditary coproporphyria. PANHEMATIN is not indicated in porphyria cutanea tarda.

CONTRAINDICATIONS

Hemin for injection is contraindicated in patients with known hypersensitivity to this drug.

WARNINGS

PANHEMATIN (hemin for injection) is made from human blood. Products made from human blood may contain infectious agents, such as viruses, that can cause disease. The risk that such products will transmit an infectious agent has been reduced by screening blood donors for prior exposure to certain viruses, by testing for the presence of certain current virus infections, and by inactivating certain viruses. Despite these measures, such products can still potentially transmit disease. There is also the possibility that unknown infectious agents may be present in such products. ALL infections thought by a physician possibly to have been transmitted by this product should be reported by the physician or other healthcare provider to Abbott Laboratories, (800) 633-9110. The physician should discuss the risks and benefits of this product with the patient.
PANHEMATIN therapy is intended to limit the rate of porphyria/heme biosynthesis possibly by inhibiting the enzyme δ-aminolevulinic acid synthetase. For this reason, drugs such as estrogens, barbituric acid derivatives and steroid metabolites which increase the activity of δ-aminolevulinic acid synthetase should be avoided.
Also, because PANHEMATIN has exhibited transient, mild anticoagulant effects during clinical studies, concurrent anticoagulant therapy should be avoided.[9] The extent and duration of the hypocoagulable state induced by PANHEMATIN has not been established.

PRECAUTIONS

General: Clinical benefit from PANHEMATIN depends on prompt administration. Attacks of porphyria may progress to a point where irreversible neuronal damage has occurred. PANHEMATIN therapy is intended to prevent an attack from reaching the critical stage of neuronal degeneration. PANHEMATIN is not effective in repairing neuronal damage.[9]
Recommended dosage guidelines should be strictly followed. Reversible renal shutdown has been observed in a case where an excessive hematin dose (12.2 mg/kg) was administered in a single infusion. Oliguria and increased nitrogen retention occurred although the patient remained asymptomatic.[4] No worsening of renal function has been seen with administration of recommended dosages of hematin.[9]
A large arm vein or a central venous catheter should be utilized for the administration of hemin for injection to avoid the possibility of phlebitis.
Since reconstituted PANHEMATIN is not transparent, any undissolved particulate matter is difficult to see when inspected visually. Therefore, terminal filtration through a sterile 0.45 micron or smaller filter is recommended.
Tests for Diagnosis and Monitoring of Therapy: Before PANHEMATIN therapy is begun, the presence of acute porphyria must be diagnosed using the following criteria:[9]
a. Presence of clinical symptoms.
b. Positive Watson-Schwartz or Hoesch test. (A negative Watson-Schwartz or Hoesch test indicates a porphyric attack is highly unlikely. When in doubt quantitative measures of δ-aminolevulinic acid and porphobilinogen in serum or urine may aid in diagnosis.)

Urinary concentrations of the following compounds may be *monitored* during PANHEMATIN therapy. Drug effect will be demonstrated by a decrease in one or more of the following compounds:[3–6]

ALA-δ-aminolevulinic acid
UPG-uroporphyrinogen
PBG-porphobilinogen
coproporphyrin

Carcinogenesis, Mutagenesis, Impairment of Fertility: No data are available on potential for carcinogenicity, mutagenicity or impairment of fertility in animals or humans.
Pregnancy: Teratogenic effects: Pregnancy Category C. Animal reproduction studies have not been conducted with hematin. It is also not known whether hematin can cause fetal harm when administered to a pregnant woman or can affect reproduction capacity. For this reason hemin for injection should not be given to a pregnant woman unless the expected benefits are sufficiently important to the health and welfare of the patient to outweigh the unknown hazard to the fetus.
Nursing Mothers: It is not known whether this drug is excreted in human milk. Because many drugs are excreted in human milk, caution should be exercised when hemin for injection is administered to a nursing woman.
Pediatric Use: Safety and effectiveness in pediatric patients under 16 years of age have not been established.

ADVERSE REACTIONS

Reversible renal shutdown has occurred with administration of excessive doses (See "PRECAUTIONS" section).
Phlebitis with or without leucocytosis and with or without mild pyrexia has occurred after administration of hematin through small arm veins.
There has been one report in the literature[8] of coagulopathy occurring in a patient receiving hematin therapy. This patient exhibited prolonged prothrombin time and partial thromboplastin time, thrombocytopenia, mild hypofibrinogenemia, mild elevation of fibrin split products and a 10% fall in hematocrit.

OVERDOSAGE

Reversible renal shutdown has been observed in a case where an excessive hematin dose (12.2 mg/kg) was administered in a single infusion. Treatment of this case consisted of ethacrynic acid and mannitol.[7]

DOSAGE AND ADMINISTRATION

Before administering hemin for injection, an appropriate period of alternate therapy (i.e., 400 g glucose/day for 1 to 2 days) must be considered. If improvement is unsatisfactory for the treatment of acute attacks of porphyria, an intravenous infusion of PANHEMATIN containing a dose of 1 to 4 mg/kg/day of hematin should be given over a period of 10 to 15 minutes for 3 to 14 days based on the clinical signs. In more severe cases this dose may be repeated no earlier than every 12 hours. No more than 6 mg/kg of hematin should be given in any 24-hour period.
After reconstitution each mL of PANHEMATIN contains the equivalent of approximately 7 mg of hematin. The drug may be administered directly from the vial.

Dosage Calculation Table

1 mg hematin equivalent = 0.14 mL PANHEMATIN
2 mg hematin equivalent = 0.28 mL PANHEMATIN
3 mg hematin equivalent = 0.42 mL PANHEMATIN
4 mg hematin equivalent = 0.56 mL PANHEMATIN

Since reconstituted PANHEMATIN is not transparent, any undissolved particulate matter is difficult to see when inspected visually. Therefore, terminal filtration through a sterile 0.45 micron or smaller filter is recommended.
Preparation of Solution: Reconstitute PANHEMATIN by aseptically adding 43 mL of Sterile Water for Injection, USP, to the dispensing vial. Immediately after adding diluent, the product should be shaken well for a period of 2 to 3 minutes to aid dissolution. **NOTE: Because PANHEMATIN contains no preservative and because PANHEMATIN undergoes rapid chemical decomposition in solution, it should not be reconstituted until immediately before use. After the first withdrawal from the vial, any solution remaining must be discarded.**
No drug or chemical agent should be added to a PANHEMATIN fluid admixture unless its effect on the chemical and physical stability has first been determined.

HOW SUPPLIED

PANHEMATIN (hemin for injection) is supplied as a sterile, lyophilized black powder in single dose dispensing vials (**NDC** 0074-2000-43). When mixed as directed with Sterile Water for Injection, USP, each 43 mL provides the equivalent of approximately 301 mg hematin (7 mg/mL). Store lyophilized powder in refrigerator (2–8°C) until time of use.

REFERENCES

1. Bickers, D., Treatment of the Porphyrias: Mechanisms of Action, *J Invest Dermatol* 77(1):107–113, 1981.
2. Watson, C. J., Hematin and Porphyria, editorial, *N Engl J Med* 293(12):605–607, September 18, 1975.
3. Lamon, J. M., Hematin Therapy for Acute Porphyria, *Medicine* 58(3):252–269, 1979.
4. Dhar, G. J., et al., Effects of Hematin in Hepatic Porphyria, *Ann Intern Med* 83:20–30, 1975.
5. Watson, C. J., et al., Use of Hematin in the Acute Attack of the "Inducible" Hepatic Porphyrias, *Adv Intern Med* 23:265–286, 1978.
6. McColl, K. E., et al., Treatment with Haematin in Acute Hepatic Porphyria, *Q J Med,* New Series L (198):161–174, Spring, 1981.
7. Dhar, G. J., et al., Transitory Renal Failure Following Rapid Administration of a Relatively Large Amount of Hematin in a Patient with Acute Intermittent Porphyria in Clinical Remission, *Acta Med Scand* 203:437–443, 1978.
8. Morris, D. L., et al., Coagulopathy Associated with Hematin Treatment for Acute Intermittent Porphyria, *Ann Intern Med* 95:700–701, 1981.
9. Pierach, C. A., Hematin Therapy for the Porphyric Attack, *Semin Liver Dis* 2(2):125–131, May, 1982.

Revised: August, 1998
Ref. 58-0458-R6

Continued on next page

PCE® ℞

[*p-c-ē*]
(erythromycin particles in tablets)
Dispertab® Tablets
Rx only

DESCRIPTION

PCE (erythromycin particles in tablets) is an antibacterial product containing specially coated erythromycin base particles for oral administration. The coating protects the antibiotic from the inactivating effects of gastric acidity and permits efficient absorption of the antibiotic in the small intestine. PCE is available in two strengths containing either 333 mg or 500 mg of erythromycin base. PCE 500 mg tablets contain no synthetic dyes or artificial colors.
Erythromycin is produced by a strain of *Saccharopolyspora erythraea* (formerly *Streptomyces erythraeus*) and belongs to the macrolide group of antibiotics. It is basic and readily forms salts with acids. Erythromycin is a white to off-white powder, slightly soluble in water, and soluble in alcohol, chloroform, and ether. Erythromycin is known chemically as (3R*, 4S*, 5S*, 6R*, 7R*, 9R*, 11R*, 12R*, 13S*, 14R*)-4-[(2,6-dideoxy-3-C-methyl-3-O-methyl-α-L-*ribo*-hexopyranosyl)oxy]-14-ethyl-7,12,13-trihydroxy-3,5,7,9,11,13-hexamethyl-6-[[3,4,6-trideoxy-3-(dimethylamino)-β-D-*xylo*-hexopyranosyl]oxy]oxacyclotetradecane-2,10-dione. The molecular formula is $C_{37}H_{67}NO_{13}$, and the molecular weight is 733.94. The structural formula is:

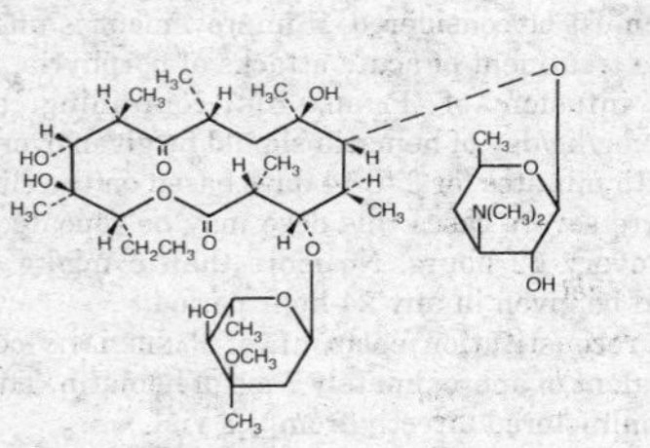

Inactive Ingredients:
PCE 333 mg tablets: Cellulosic polymers, citrate ester, colloidal silicon dioxide, D&C Red No. 30, hydrogenated vegetable oil wax, lactose, magnesium stearate, microcrystalline cellulose, povidone, propylene glycol, sodium starch glycolate, stearic acid and vanillin.
PCE 500 mg tablets: Cellulosic polymers, citrate ester, colloidal silicon dioxide, crospovidone, hydrogenated vegetable oil wax, iron oxide, microcrystalline cellulose, polyethylene glycol, povidone, propylene glycol, stearic acid, talc, titanium dioxide and vanillin.

CLINICAL PHARMACOLOGY

Orally administered erythromycin base and its salts are readily absorbed in the microbiologically active form. Interindividual variations in the absorption of erythromycin are, however, observed, and some patients do not achieve optimal serum levels. Erythromycin is largely bound to plasma proteins. After absorption, erythromycin diffuses readily into most body fluids. In the absence of meningeal inflammation, low concentrations are normally achieved in the spinal fluid but the passage of the drug across the blood-brain barrier increases in meningitis. Erythromycin crosses the placental barrier, but fetal plasma levels are low. The drug is excreted in human milk. Erythromycin is not removed by peritoneal dialysis or hemodialysis.
In the presence of normal hepatic function, erythromycin is concentrated in the liver and is excreted in the bile; the effect of hepatic dysfunction on biliary excretion of erythromycin is not known. After oral administration, less than 5% of the administered dose can be recovered in the active form in the urine.
The erythromycin particles in PCE tablets are coated with a polymer whose dissolution is pH dependent. This coating allows for minimal release of erythromycin in acidic environments, e.g. stomach. This delivery system is designed for optimal drug release and absorption in the small intestine. In multiple-dose, steady-state studies, PCE tablets have demonstrated rapid and generally adequate drug delivery in both fasting and nonfasting conditions. However, the presence of food results in lower blood levels, and optimal blood levels are obtained when PCE tablets are given in the fasting state (at least 1/2 hour and preferably 2 hours before meals). Bioavailability data are available from Abbott Laboratories, Dept. 42W.

Microbiology:
Erythromycin acts by inhibition of protein synthesis by binding 50 S ribosomal subunits of susceptible organisms. It does not affect nucleic acid synthesis. Antagonism has been demonstrated *in vitro* between erythromycin and clindamycin, lincomycin, and chloramphenicol.
Many strains of *Haemophilus influenzae* are resistant to erythromycin alone, but are susceptible to erythromycin and sulfonamides used concomitantly.
Staphylococci resistant to erythromycin may emerge during a course of erythromycin therapy.
Erythromycin has been shown to be active against most strains of the following microorganisms, both *in vitro* and in clinical infections as described in the **INDICATIONS AND USAGE** section.

Gram-positive organisms:
Corynebacterium diphtheriae
Corynebacterium minutissimum
Listeria monocytogenes
Staphylococcus aureus (resistant organisms may emerge during treatment)
Streptococcus pneumoniae
Streptococcus pyogenes
Gram-negative organisms:
Bordetella pertussis
Legionella pneumophila
Neisseria gonorrhoeae
Other microorganisms:
Chlamydia trachomatis
Entamoeba histolytica
Mycoplasma pneumoniae
Treponema pallidum
Ureaplasma urealyticum

The following *in vitro* data are available, **but their clinical significance is unknown**.
Erythromycin exhibits *in vitro* minimal inhibitory concentrations (MIC's) of 0.5 µg/mL or less against most (≥ 90%) strains of the following microorganisms; however, the safety and effectiveness of erythromycin in treating clinical infections due to these microorganisms have not been established in adequate and well-controlled clinical trials.
Gram-positive organisms:
Viridans group streptococci
Gram-negative organisms:
Moraxella catarrhalis

Susceptibility Tests:
Dilution Techniques:
Quantitative methods are used to determine antimicrobial minimum inhibitory concentrations (MIC's). These MIC's provide estimates of the susceptibility of bacteria to antimicrobial compounds. The MIC's should be determined using a standardized procedure. Standardized procedures are based on a dilution method[1] (broth or agar) or equivalent with standardized inoculum concentrations and standardized concentrations of erythromycin powder. The MIC values should be interpreted according to the following criteria:

MIC (µg/mL)	Interpretation
≤0.5	Susceptible (S)
1–4	Intermediate (I)
≥8	Resistant (R)

A report of "Susceptible" indicates that the pathogen is likely to be inhibited if the antimicrobial compound in the blood reaches the concentrations usually achievable. A report of "Intermediate" indicates that the result should be considered equivocal, and, if the microorganism is not fully susceptible to alternative, clinically feasible drugs, the test should be repeated. This category implies possible clinical applicability in body sites where the drug is physiologically concentrated or in situations where high dosage of drug can be used. This category also provides a buffer zone which prevents small uncontrolled technical factors from causing major discrepancies in interpretation. A report of "Resistant" indicates that the pathogen is not likely to be inhibited if the antimicrobial compound in the blood reaches the concentrations usually achievable; other therapy should be selected.
Standardized susceptibility test procedures require the use of laboratory control microorganisms to control the technical aspects of the laboratory procedures. Standard erythromycin powder should provide the following MIC values:

Microorganism	MIC (µg/mL)
S. aureus ATCC 29213	0.12–0.5
E. faecalis ATCC 29212	1–4

Diffusion Techniques:
Quantitative methods that require measurement of zone diameters also provide reproducible estimates of the susceptibility of bacteria to antimicrobial compounds. One such standardized procedure[2] requires the use of standardized inoculum concentrations. This procedure uses paper disks impregnated with 15-µg erythromycin to test the susceptibility of microorganisms to erythromycin.
Reports from the laboratory providing results of the standard single-disk susceptibility test with a 15-µg erythromycin disk should be interpreted according to the following criteria:

Zone Diameter (mm)	Interpretation
≥23	Susceptible (S)
14–22	Intermediate (I)
≤13	Resistant (R)

Interpretation should be as stated above for results using dilution techniques. Interpretation involves correlation of the diameter obtained in the disk test with the MIC for erythromycin.
As with standardized dilution techniques, diffusion methods require the use of laboratory control microorganisms that are used to control the technical aspects of the laboratory procedures. For the diffusion technique, the 15-µg erythromycin disk should provide the following zone diameters in these laboratory test quality control strains:

Microorganism	Zone Diameter (mm)
S. aureus ATCC 25923	22–30

INDICATIONS AND USAGE

PCE tablets are indicated in the treatment of infections caused by susceptible strains of the designated microorganisms in the diseases listed below:
Upper respiratory tract infections of mild to moderate degree caused by *Streptococcus pyogenes; Streptococcus pneumoniae; Haemophilus influenzae* (when used concomitantly with adequate doses of sulfonamides, since many strains of *H. influenzae* are not susceptible to the erythromycin concentrations ordinarily achieved). (See appropriate sulfonamide labeling for prescribing information.)
Lower respiratory tract infections of mild to moderate severity caused by *Streptococcus pyogenes* or *Streptococcus pneumoniae*.
Listeriosis caused by *Listeria monocytogenes*.
Respiratory tract infections due to *Mycoplasma pneumoniae*.
Skin and skin structure infections of mild to moderate severity caused by *Streptococcus pyogenes* or *Staphylococcus aureus* (resistant staphylococci may emerge during treatment).
Pertussis (whooping cough) caused by *Bordetella pertussis*. Erythromycin is effective in eliminating the organism from the nasopharynx of infected individuals, rendering them noninfectious. Some clinical studies suggest that erythromycin may be helpful in the prophylaxis of pertussis in exposed susceptible individuals.
Diphtheria: Infections due to *Corynebacterium diphtheriae*, as an adjunct to antitoxin, to prevent establishment of carriers and to eradicate the organism in carriers.
Erythrasma—In the treatment of infections due to *Corynebacterium minutissimum*.
Intestinal amebiasis caused by *Entamoeba histolytica* (oral erythromycins only). Extraenteric amebiasis requires treatment with other agents.
Acute pelvic inflammatory disease caused by *Neisseria gonorrhoeae*: Erythrocin® Lactobionate-I.V. (erythromycin lactobionate for injection, USP) followed by erythromycin base orally, as an alternative drug in treatment of acute pelvic inflammatory disease caused by *N. gonorrhoeae* in female patients with a history of sensitivity to penicillin. Patients should have a serologic test for syphilis before receiving erythromycin as treatment of gonorrhea and a follow-up serologic test for syphilis after 3 months.
Erythromycins are indicated for treatment of the following infections caused by *Chlamydia trachomatis*: conjunctivitis of the newborn, pneumonia of infancy, and urogenital infections during pregnancy. When tetracyclines are contraindicated or not tolerated, erythromycin is indicated for the treatment of uncomplicated urethral, endocervical, or rectal infections in adults due to *Chlamydia trachomatis*.
When tetracyclines are contraindicated or not tolerated, erythromycin is indicated for the treatment of nongonococcal urethritis caused by *Ureaplasma urealyticum*.
Primary syphilis caused by *Treponema pallidum*. Erythromycin (oral forms only) is an alternative choice of treatment for primary syphilis in patients allergic to the penicillins. In treatment of primary syphilis, spinal fluid should be examined before treatment and as part of the follow-up after therapy.
Legionnaires' Disease caused by *Legionella pneumophila*. Although no controlled clinical efficacy studies have been conducted, *in vitro* and limited preliminary clinical data suggest that erythromycin may be effective in treating Legionnaires' Disease.

Prophylaxis
Prevention of Initial Attacks of Rheumatic Fever—Penicillin is considered by the American Heart Association to be the drug of choice in the prevention of initial attacks of rheumatic fever (treatment of *Streptococcus pyogenes* infections of the upper respiratory tract e.g., tonsillitis, or pharyngitis).[3] Erythromycin is indicated for the treatment of penicillin-allergic patients. The therapeutic dose should be administered for ten days.
Prevention of Recurrent Attacks of Rheumatic Fever—Penicillin or sulfonamides are considered by the American Heart Association to be the drugs of choice in the prevention of recurrent attacks of rheumatic fever. In patients who are allergic to penicillin and sulfonamides, oral erythromycin is recommended by the American Heart Association in the long-term prophylaxis of streptococcal pharyngitis (for the prevention of recurrent attacks of rheumatic fever).[3]

CONTRAINDICATIONS

Erythromycin is contraindicated in patients with known hypersensitivity to this antibiotic.
Erythromycin is contraindicated in patients taking terfenadine, astemizole, or cisapride. (See **PRECAUTIONS**-*Drug Interactions*.)

WARNINGS

There have been reports of hepatic dysfunction, including increased liver enzymes, and hepatocellular and/or cholestatic hepatitis, with or without jaundice, occurring in patients receiving oral erythromycin products.
There have been reports suggesting that erythromycin does not reach the fetus in adequate concentration to prevent

congenital syphilis. Infants born to women treated during pregnancy with oral erythromycin for early syphilis should be treated with an appropriate penicillin regimen.

Rhabdomyolysis with or without renal impairment has been reported in seriously ill patients receiving erythromycin concomitantly with lovastatin. Therefore, patients receiving concomitant lovastatin and erythromycin should be carefully monitored for creatine kinase (CK) and serum transaminase levels. (See package insert for lovastatin.)

Pseudomembranous colitis has been reported with nearly all antibacterial agents, including erythromycin, and may range in severity from mild to life threatening. Therefore, it is important to consider this diagnosis in patients who present with diarrhea subsequent to the administration of antibacterial agents.

Treatment with antibacterial agents alters the normal flora of the colon and may permit overgrowth of clostridia. Studies indicate that a toxin produced by *Clostridium difficile* is a primary cause of "antibiotic-associated colitis".

After the diagnosis of pseudomembranous colitis has been established, therapeutic measures should be initiated. Mild cases of pseudomembranous colitis usually respond to discontinuation of the drug alone. In moderate to severe cases, consideration should be given to management with fluids and electrolytes, protein supplementation, and treatment with an antibacterial drug clinically effective against *Clostridium difficile* colitis.

PRECAUTIONS

General: Since erythromycin is principally excreted by the liver, caution should be exercised when erythromycin is administered to patients with impaired hepatic function. (See **CLINICAL PHARMACOLOGY** and **WARNINGS**.)

There have been reports that erythromycin may aggravate the weakness of patients with myasthenia gravis.

Prolonged or repeated use of erythromycin may result in an overgrowth of nonsusceptible bacteria or fungi. If superinfection occurs, erythromycin should be discontinued and appropriate therapy instituted.

When indicated, incision and drainage or other surgical procedures should be performed in conjunction with antibiotic therapy.

Drug Interactions: Erythromycin use in patients who are receiving high doses of theophylline may be associated with an increase in serum theophylline levels and potential theophylline toxicity. In case of theophylline toxicity and/or elevated serum theophylline levels, the dose of theophylline should be reduced while the patient is receiving concomitant erythromycin therapy.

Concomitant administration of erythromycin and digoxin has been reported to result in elevated digoxin serum levels.

There have been reports of increased anticoagulant effects when erythromycin and oral anticoagulants were used concomitantly. Increased anticoagulation effects due to interactions of erythromycin with oral anticoagulants may be more pronounced in the elderly.

Concurrent use of erythromycin and ergotamine or dihydroergotamine has been associated in some patients with acute ergot toxicity characterized by severe peripheral vasospasm and dysesthesia.

Erythromycin has been reported to decrease the clearance of triazolam and midazolam and, thus, may increase the pharmacologic effect of these benzodiazepines.

The use of erythromycin in patients concurrently taking drugs metabolized by the cytochrome P450 system may be associated with elevations in serum levels of these other drugs. There have been reports of interactions of erythromycin with carbamazepine, cyclosporine, tacrolimus, hexobarbital, phenytoin, alfentanil, cisapride, disopyramide, lovastatin, bromocriptine, valproate, terfenadine, and astemizole. Serum concentrations of drugs metabolized by the cytochrome P450 system should be monitored closely in patients concurrently receiving erythromycin.

Erythromycin has been reported to significantly alter the metabolism of the nonsedating antihistamines terfenadine and astemizole when taken concomitantly. Rare cases of serious cardiovascular adverse events, including electrocardiographic QT/QT_c interval prolongation, cardiac arrest, torsades de pointes, and other ventricular arrhythmias, have been observed. (See **CONTRAINDICATIONS**.) In addition, deaths have been reported rarely with concomitant administration of terfenadine and erythromycin.

There have been post-marketing reports of drug interactions when erythromycin was coadministered with cisapride, resulting in QT prolongation, cardiac arrhythmias, ventricular tachycardia, ventricular fibrillation, and torsades de pointes, most likely due to the inhibition of hepatic metabolism of cisapride by erythromycin. Fatalities have been reported. (See **CONTRAINDICATIONS**).

Drug/Laboratory Test interactions: Erythromycin interferes with the fluorometric determination of urinary catecholamines.

Carcinogenesis, Mutagenesis, Impairment of Fertility: Long-term (2-year) oral studies conducted in rats with erythromycin base did not provide evidence of tumorigenicity. Mutagenicity studies have not been conducted. There was no apparent effect on male or female fertility in rats fed erythromycin (base) at levels up to 0.25 percent of diet.

Pregnancy: Teratogenic effects. Pregnancy Category B: There is no evidence of teratogenicity or any other adverse effect on reproduction in female rats fed erythromycin base (up to 0.25 percent of diet) prior to and during mating, during gestation, and through weaning of two successive litters. There are, however, no adequate and well-controlled studies in pregnant women. Because animal reproduction studies are not always predictive of human response, this drug should be used during pregnancy only if clearly needed.

Labor and Delivery: The effect of erythromycin on labor and delivery is unknown.

Nursing Mothers: Erythromycin is excreted in human milk. Caution should be exercised when erythromycin is administered to a nursing woman.

Pediatric Use: See **INDICATIONS AND USAGE** and **DOSAGE AND ADMINISTRATION**.

ADVERSE REACTIONS

The most frequent side effects of oral erythromycin preparations are gastrointestinal and are dose-related. They include nausea, vomiting, abdominal pain, diarrhea and anorexia. Symptoms of hepatitis, hepatic dysfunction and/or abnormal liver function test results may occur. (See **WARNINGS**.)

Onset of pseudomembranous colitis symptoms may occur during or after antibacterial treatment. (See **WARNINGS**.)

Rarely, erythromycin has been associated with the production of ventricular arrhythmias, including ventricular tachycardia and torsades de pointes, in individuals with prolonged QT interval.

Allergic reactions ranging from urticaria to anaphylaxis have occurred. Skin reactions ranging from mild eruptions to erythema multiforme, Stevens-Johnson syndrome, and toxic epidermal necrolysis have been reported rarely.

There have been isolated reports of reversible hearing loss occurring chiefly in patients with renal insufficiency and in patients receiving high doses of erythromycin.

OVERDOSAGE

In case of overdosage, erythromycin should be discontinued. Overdosage should be handled with the prompt elimination of unabsorbed drug and all other appropriate measures should be instituted.

Erythromycin is not removed by peritoneal dialysis or hemodialysis.

DOSAGE AND ADMINISTRATION

In most patients, PCE tablets are well absorbed and may be dosed orally without regard to meals. However, optimal blood levels are obtained when either PCE 333 mg or PCE 500 mg tablets are given in the fasting state (at least 1/2 hour and preferably 2 hours before meals).

Adults: The usual dosage of PCE is one 333 mg tablet every 8 hours or one 500 mg tablet every 12 hours. Dosage may be increased up to 4 g per day according to the severity of the infection. However, twice-a-day dosing is not recommended when doses larger than 1 g daily are administered.

Children: Age, weight, and severity of the infection are important factors in determining the proper dosage. The usual dosage is 30 to 50 mg/kg/day, in equally divided doses. For more severe infections this dosage may be doubled but should not exceed 4 g per day.

In the treatment of streptococcal infections of the upper respiratory tract (e.g., tonsillitis or pharyngitis), the therapeutic dosage of erythromycin should be administered for at least ten days.

The American Heart Association suggests a dosage of 250 mg of erythromycin orally, twice a day in long-term prophylaxis of streptococcal upper respiratory tract infections for the prevention of recurring attacks of rheumatic fever in patients allergic to penicillin and sulfonamides.[3]

Conjunctivitis of the newborn caused by *Chlamydia trachomatis*: Oral erythromycin suspension 50 mg/kg/day in 4 divided doses for at least 2 weeks.[3]

Pneumonia of infancy caused by *Chlamydia trachomatis*: Although the optimal duration of therapy has not been established, the recommended therapy is oral erythromycin suspension 50 mg/kg/day in 4 divided doses for at least 3 weeks.

Urogenital infections during pregnancy due to *Chlamydia trachomatis*: Although the optimal dose and duration of therapy have not been established, the suggested treatment is 500 mg of erythromycin by mouth four times a day or two erythromycin 333 mg tablets orally every 8 hours on an empty stomach for at least 7 days. For women who cannot tolerate this regimen, a decreased dose of one erythromycin 500 mg tablet orally every 12 hours, one 333 mg tablet orally every 8 hours or 250 mg by mouth four times a day should be used for at least 14 days.[4]

For adults with uncomplicated urethral, endocervical, or rectal infections caused by *Chlamydia trachomatis*, when tetracycline is contraindicated or not tolerated: 500 mg of erythromycin by mouth four times a day or two 333 mg tablets orally every 8 hours for at least 7 days.[4]

For patients with nongonococcal urethritis caused by *Ureaplasma urealyticum* when tetracycline is contraindicated or not tolerated: 500 mg of erythromycin by mouth four times a day or two 333 mg tablets orally every 8 hours for at least seven days.[4]

Primary syphilis: 30 to 40 g given in divided doses over a period of 10 to 15 days.

Acute pelvic inflammatory disease caused by *N. gonorrhoeae*: 500 mg Erythrocin Lactobionate-I.V. (erythromycin lactobionate for injection, USP) every 6 hours for 3 days, followed by 500 mg of erythromycin base orally every 12 hours, or 333 mg of erythromycin base orally every 8 hours for 7 days.

Intestinal amebiasis: Adults: 500 mg every 12 hours, 333 mg every 8 hours or 250 mg every 6 hours for 10 to 14 days. Children: 30 to 50 mg/kg/day in divided doses for 10 to 14 days.

Pertussis: Although optimal dosage and duration have not been established, doses of erythromycin utilized in reported clinical studies were 40 to 50 mg/kg/day, given in divided doses for 5 to 14 days.

Legionnaires' Disease: Although optimal dosage has not been established, doses utilized in reported clinical data were 1 to 4 g daily in divided doses.

HOW SUPPLIED

PCE (erythromycin particles in tablets) is supplied as unscored, ovaloid, Dispertab® tablets in the following strengths and packages.

333 mg, pink-speckled white (imprinted with and PCE):
Bottles of 60 .... (**NDC** 0074-6290-60).
500 mg, white (imprinted with and EK):
Bottles of 100 .... (**NDC** 0074-3389-13).
Recommended Storage: Store below 86°F (30°C).

REFERENCES

1. National Committee for Clinical Laboratory Standards. *Methods for Dilution Antimicrobial Susceptibility Tests for Bacteria that Grow Aerobically*, Third Edition. Approved Standard NCCLS Document M7-A3, Vol. 13, No. 25 NCCLS, Villanova, PA, December 1993.
2. National Committee for Clinical Laboratory Standards, *Performance Standards for Antimicrobial Disk Susceptibility Tests*, Fifth Edition. Approved Standard NCCLS Document M2-A5, Vol. 13, No. 24 NCCLS, Villanova, PA, December 1993.
3. Committee on Rheumatic Fever, Endocarditis, and Kawasaki Disease of the Council on Cardiovascular Disease in the Young, the American Heart Association: Prevention of Rheumatic Fever. *Circulation*. 78(4):1082-1086, October 1988.
4. Data on file, Abbott Laboratories.

Ref. 03-5015-R7
Revised: February, 2000
PCE 333 mg: U.S. Pat. No. 4,874,614.
PCE 500 mg: U.S. Pat. No. 4,874,614 and 5,009,897.
ABBOTT LABORATORIES
NORTH CHICAGO, IL 60064, U.S.A.

Shown in Product Identification Guide, page 303

PROSOM™ Ⓒ ℞

[*prō-som*]
(estazolam tablets)

DESCRIPTION

ProSom (estazolam), a triazolobenzodiazepine derivative, is an oral hypnotic agent. Estazolam occurs as a fine, white, odorless powder that is soluble in alcohol and practically insoluble in water. The chemical name for estazolam is 8-chloro-6-phenyl-4H-s-triazolo[4,3-α] [1,4]benzodiazepine. The empirical formula is $C_{16}H_{11}ClN_4$. The structural formula is represented as follows:

ProSom tablets are scored and contain either 1 mg or 2 mg of estazolam.

Inactive Ingredients: colloidal silicon dioxide, lactose, povidone, stearic acid, and sodium starch glycolate.

In addition, the 2 mg tablets contain FD&C Red No. 40.

CLINICAL PHARMACOLOGY

Pharmacokinetics: ProSom tablets have been found to be equivalent in absorption to an orally administered solution of estazolam. Independent of concentration, estazolam in plasma is 93% protein bound.

In healthy subjects who received up to three times the recommended dose of ProSom, peak estazolam plasma concentrations occurred within two hours after dosing (range 0.5 to 6.0 hours) and were proportional to the administered dose, suggesting linear pharmacokinetics over the dosage range tested.

The range of estimates for the mean elimination half-life of estazolam varied from 10 to 24 hours. The clearance of benzodiazepines is accelerated in smokers compared to nonsmokers, and there is evidence that this occurs with estazolam. This decrease in half-life, presumably due to enzyme induction by smoking, is consistent with other drugs with similar hepatic clearance characteristics. In all subjects and at all doses, the mean elimination half-life appeared to be independent of the dose.

In a small study (N=8) using various doses in older subjects (59 to 68 years), peak estazolam concentrations were found to be similar to those observed in younger subjects with a mean elimination half-life of 18.4 hours (range 13.5 to 34.6 hours).

Estazolam is extensively metabolized, and the metabolites are excreted primarily in the urine. Less than 5% of a 2 mg dose of estazolam is excreted unchanged in the urine, with

Continued on next page

Prosom—Cont.

only 4% of the dose appearing in the feces. 4′-hydroxy estazolam is the major metabolite in plasma, with concentrations approaching 12% of those of the parent eight hours after administration. While it and the lesser metabolite, 1-oxo-estazolam, have some pharmacologic activity, their low potencies and low concentrations preclude any significant contribution to the hypnotic effect of ProSom.

Postulated relationship between elimination rate of benzodiazepine hypnotics and their profile of common untoward effects: The type and duration of hypnotic effects and the profile of unwanted effects during administration of benzodiazepine drugs may be influenced by the biologic half-life of administered drug and any active metabolites formed. If half-lives are long, drug or metabolites may accumulate during periods of nightly administration and may be associated with impairments of cognitive and/or motor performance during waking hours; the possibility of interaction with other psychoactive drugs or alcohol will be increased. In contrast, if half-lives are short, drug and metabolites will be cleared before the next dose is ingested, and carry-over effects related to excessive sedation or CNS depression should be minimal or absent. However, during nightly use for an extended period, pharmacodynamic tolerance or adaptation to some effects of benzodiazepine hypnotics may develop. If the drug has a short elimination half-life, it is possible that a relative deficiency of the drug or its active metabolites (ie, in relationship to the receptor site) may occur at some point in the interval between each night's use. This sequence of events may account for two clinical findings reported to occur after several weeks of nightly use of rapidly eliminated benzodiazepine hypnotics, namely, increased wakefulness during the last third of the night and increased daytime anxiety in selected patients.

Controlled Trials Supporting Efficacy: In three 7-night, double-blind, parallel-group trials comparing estazolam 1 mg and/or 2 mg with placebo in adult outpatients with chronic insomnia, estazolam 2 mg was consistently superior to placebo in subjective measures of sleep induction (latency) and sleep maintenance (duration, number of awakenings, depth and quality of sleep); estazolam 1 mg was similarly superior to placebo on all measures of sleep maintenance, however, it significantly improved sleep induction in only one of two studies. In a similarly designed trial comparing estazolam 0.5 mg and 1 mg with placebo in geriatric outpatients with chronic insomnia, only the 1 mg estazolam dose was consistently superior to placebo in sleep induction (latency) and in only one measure of sleep maintenance (ie, duration of sleep).

In a single-night, double-blind, parallel-group trial comparing estazolam 2 mg and placebo in patients admitted for elective surgery and requiring sleep medications, estazolam was superior to placebo in subjective measures of sleep induction and maintenance.

In a 12-week, double-blind, parallel-group trial including a comparison of estazolam 2 mg and placebo in adult outpatients with chronic insomnia, estazolam was superior to placebo in subjective measures of sleep induction (latency) and maintenance (duration, number of awakenings, total wake time during sleep) at week 2, but produced consistent improvement over 12 weeks only for sleep duration and total wake time during sleep. Following withdrawal at week 12, rebound insomnia was seen at the first withdrawal week, but there was no difference between drug and placebo by the second withdrawal week in all parameters except latency, for which normalization did not occur until the fourth withdrawal week.

Adult outpatients with chronic insomnia were evaluated in a sleep laboratory trial comparing four doses of estazolam (0.25, 0.50, 1.0 and 2.0 mg) and placebo, each administered for 2 nights in a crossover design. The higher estazolam doses were superior to placebo in most EEG measures of sleep induction and maintenance, especially at the 2 mg dose, but only for sleep duration in subjective measures of sleep.

INDICATIONS AND USAGE

ProSom (estazolam) is indicated for the short-term management of insomnia characterized by difficulty in falling asleep, frequent nocturnal awakenings, and/or early morning awakenings. Both outpatient studies and a sleep laboratory study have shown that ProSom administered at bedtime improved sleep induction and sleep maintenance (see CLINICAL PHARMACOLOGY).

Because insomnia is often transient and intermittent, the prolonged administration of ProSom is generally neither necessary nor recommended. Since insomnia may be a symptom of several other disorders, the possibility that the complaint may be related to a condition for which there is a more specific treatment should be considered.

There is evidence to support the ability of ProSom to enhance the duration and quality of sleep for intervals up to 12 weeks (see CLINICAL PHARMACOLOGY).

CONTRAINDICATIONS

Benzodiazepines may cause fetal damage when administered during pregnancy. An increased risk of congenital malformations associated with the use of diazepam and chlordiazepoxide during the first trimester of pregnancy has been suggested in several studies. Transplacental distribution has resulted in neonatal CNS depression and also withdrawal phenomena following the ingestion of therapeutic doses of a benzodiazepine hypnotic during the last weeks of pregnancy.

ProSom is contraindicated in pregnant women. If there is a likelihood of the patient becoming pregnant while receiving ProSom she should be warned of the potential risk to the fetus and instructed to discontinue the drug prior to becoming pregnant. The possibility that a woman of childbearing potential is pregnant at the time of institution of therapy should be considered.

WARNINGS

ProSom, like other benzodiazepines, has CNS depressant effects. For this reason, patients should be cautioned against engaging in hazardous occupations requiring complete mental alertness, such as operating machinery or driving a motor vehicle, after ingesting the drug, including potential impairment of the performance of such activities that may occur the day following ingestion of ProSom. Patients should also be cautioned about possible combined effects with alcohol and other CNS depressant drugs.

As with all benzodiazepines, amnesia, paradoxical reactions (eg, excitement, agitation, etc.), and other adverse behavioral effects may occur unpredictably.

There have been reports of withdrawal signs and symptoms of the type associated with withdrawal from CNS depressant drugs following the rapid decrease or the abrupt discontinuation of benzodiazepines (see DRUG ABUSE AND DEPENDENCE).

PRECAUTIONS

General: Impaired motor and/or cognitive performance attributable to the accumulation of benzodiazepines and their active metabolites following several days of repeated use at their recommended doses is a concern in certain vulnerable patients (eg, those especially sensitive to the effects of benzodiazepines or those with a reduced capacity to metabolize and eliminate them) (see DOSAGE AND ADMINISTRATION).

Elderly or debilitated patients and those with impaired renal or hepatic function should be cautioned about these risks and advised to monitor themselves for signs of excessive sedation or impaired conditions.

ProSom appears to cause dose-related respiratory depression that is ordinarily not clinically relevant at recommended doses in patients with normal respiratory function. However, patients with compromised respiratory function may be at risk and should be monitored appropriately. As a class, benzodiazepines have the capacity to depress respiratory drive; there are insufficient data available, however, to characterize their relative potency in depressing respiratory drive at clinically recommended doses.

As with other benzodiazepines, ProSom should be administered with caution to patients exhibiting signs or symptoms of depression. Suicidal tendencies may be present in such patients and protective measures may be required. Intentional overdosage is more common in this group of patients; therefore, the least amount of drug that is feasible should be prescribed for the patient at any one time.

Information for Patients: To assure the safe and effective use of ProSom, the following information and instructions should be given to patients:

1. Inform your physician about any alcohol consumption and medicine you are taking now, including drugs you may buy without a prescription. Alcohol should not be used during treatment with hypnotics.
2. Inform your physician if you are planning to become pregnant, if you are pregnant, or if you become pregnant while you are taking this medicine.
3. You should not take this medicine if you are nursing, as the drug may be excreted in breast milk.
4. Until you experience the way this medicine affects you, do not drive a car, operate potentially dangerous machinery, or engage in hazardous occupations requiring complete mental alertness after taking this medicine.
5. Since benzodiazepines may produce psychological and physical dependence, you should not increase the dose before consulting your physician. In addition, since the abrupt discontinuation of ProSom may be associated with temporary sleep disturbances, you should consult your physician before abruptly discontinuing doses of 2 mg per night or more.

Laboratory Tests: Laboratory tests are not ordinarily required in otherwise healthy patients. When treatment with ProSom is protracted, periodic blood counts, urinalyses, and blood chemistry analyses are advisable.

Drug Interactions: If ProSom is given concomitantly with other drugs acting on the central nervous system, careful consideration should be given to the pharmacology of all agents. The action of the benzodiazepines may be potentiated by anticonvulsants, antihistamines, alcohol, barbiturates, monoamine oxidase inhibitors, narcotics, phenothiazines, psychotropic medications, or other drugs that produce CNS depression. Smokers have an increased clearance of benzodiazepines as compared to nonsmokers; this was seen in studies with estazolam (see CLINICAL PHARMACOLOGY).

Carcinogenesis, Mutagenesis, Impairment of Fertility: Two-year carcinogenicity studies were conducted in mice and rats at dietary doses of 0.8, 3, and 10 mg/kg/day and 0.5, 2, and 10 mg/kg/day, respectively. Evidence of tumorigenicity was not observed in either study. Incidence of hyperplastic liver nodules increased in female mice given the mid- and high-dose levels. The significance of such nodules in mice is not known at this time.

In vitro and *in vivo* mutagenicity tests including the Ames test, DNA repair in *B. subtilis, in vivo* cytogenetics in mice and rats, and the dominant lethal test in mice did not show a mutagenic potential for estazolam.

Fertility in male and female rats was not affected by doses up to 30 times the usual recommended human dose.

Pregnancy:

1. Teratogenic Effects: Pregnancy Category X (see CONTRAINDICATIONS).
2. Nonteratogenic Effects: The child born of a mother taking benzodiazepines may be at some risk for withdrawal symptoms during the postnatal period. Neonatal flaccidity has been reported in an infant born of a mother who received benzodiazepines during pregnancy.

Labor and Delivery: ProSom has no established use in labor or delivery.

Nursing Mothers: Human studies have not been conducted; however, studies in lactating rats indicate that estazolam and/or its metabolites are secreted in the milk. The use of ProSom in nursing mothers is not recommended.

Pediatric Use: Safety and effectiveness in pediatric patients below the age of 18 have not been established.

Geriatric Use: Approximately 18% of individuals participating in the premarketing clinical trials of ProSom were 60 years of age or older. Overall, the adverse event profile did not differ substantively from that observed in younger individuals. Care should be exercised when prescribing benzodiazepines to small or debilitated elderly patients (see DOSAGE AND ADMINISTRATION).

ADVERSE REACTIONS

Commonly Observed: The most commonly observed adverse events associated with the use of ProSom, not seen at an equivalent incidence among placebo-treated patients were somnolence, hypokinesia, dizziness, and abnormal coordination.

Associated with Discontinuation of Treatment: Approximately 3% of 1277 patients who received ProSom in US premarketing clinical trials discontinued treatment because of an adverse clinical event. The only event commonly associated with discontinuation, accounting for 1.3% of the total, was somnolence.

Incidence in Controlled Clinical Trials: The table below enumerates adverse events that occurred at an incidence of 1% or greater among patients with insomnia who received ProSom in 7-night, placebo-controlled trials. Events reported by investigators were classified into standard dictionary (COSTART) terms to establish event frequencies. Event frequencies reported were not corrected for the occurrence of these events at baseline. The frequencies were obtained from data pooled across six studies: ProSom, N=685; placebo, N=433. The prescriber should be aware that these figures cannot be used to predict the incidence of side effects in the course of usual medical practice in which patient characteristics and other factors differ from those that prevailed in these six clinical trials. Similarly, the cited frequencies cannot be compared with figures obtained from other clinical investigators involving related drug products and uses, since each group of drug trials was conducted under a different set of conditions. However, the cited figures provide the physician with a basis of estimating the relative contribution of drug and nondrug factors to the incidence of side effects in the population studied.

[See table at top of next page]

Other Adverse Events:

During clinical trials conducted by Abbott, some of which were not placebo-controlled, ProSom was administered to approximately 1300 patients. Untoward events associated with this exposure were recorded by clinical investigators using terminology of their own choosing. To provide a meaningful estimate of the proportion of individuals experiencing adverse events, similar types of untoward events must be grouped into a smaller number of standardized event categories. In the tabulations that follow, a standard COSTART dictionary terminology has been used to classify reported adverse events. The frequencies presented, therefore, represent the proportion of the 1277 individuals exposed to ProSom who experienced an event of the type cited on at least one occasion while receiving ProSom. All reported events are included except those already listed in the previous table, those COSTART terms too general to be informative, and those events where a drug cause was remote. Events are further classified within body system categories and enumerated in order of decreasing frequency using the following definitions: frequent adverse events are defined as those occurring on one or more occasions in at least 1/100 patients; infrequent adverse events are those occurring in 1/100 to 1/1000 patients; rare events are those occurring in less than 1/1000 patients. It is important to emphasize that, although the events reported did occur during treatment with ProSom, they were not necessarily caused by it.

Body as a Whole—Infrequent: allergic reaction, chills, fever, neck pain, upper extremity pain; Rare: edema, jaw pain, swollen breast.

INCIDENCE OF ADVERSE EXPERIENCES IN PLACEBO-CONTROLLED CLINICAL TRIALS
(Percentage of Patients Reporting)

Body System/ Adverse Event*	ProSom (N=685)	Placebo (N=433)
Body as a Whole		
Headache	16	27
Asthenia	11	8
Malaise	5	5
Lower extremity pain	3	2
Back pain	2	2
Body pain	2	2
Abdominal pain	1	2
Chest pain	1	1
Digestive System		
Nausea	4	5
Dyspepsia	2	2
Musculoskeletal System		
Stiffness	1	—
Nervous System		
Somnolence	42	27
Hypokinesia	8	4
Nervousness	8	11
Dizziness	7	3
Coordination abnormal	4	1
Hangover	3	2
Confusion	2	—
Depression	2	3
Dream abnormal	2	2
Thinking abnormal	2	1
Respiratory System		
Cold symptoms	3	5
Pharyngitis	1	2
Skin and Appendages		
Pruritus	1	—

*Events reported by at least 1% of ProSom patients.

Cardiovascular System—Infrequent: flushing, palpitation; Rare: arrhythmia, syncope.
Digestive System—Frequent: constipation, dry mouth; Infrequent: decreased appetite, flatulence, gastritis, increased appetite, vomiting; Rare: enterocolitis, melena, ulceration of the mouth.
Endocrine System—Rare: thyroid nodule.
Hematologic and Lymphatic System—Rare: leukopenia, purpura, swollen lymph nodes.
Metabolic/Nutritional Disorders—Infrequent: thirst; Rare: increased SGOT, weight gain, weight loss.
Musculoskeletal System—Infrequent: arthritis, muscle spasm, myalgia; Rare: arthralgia.
Nervous System—Frequent: anxiety; Infrequent: agitation, amnesia, apathy, emotional lability, euphoria, hostility, paresthesia, seizure, sleep disorder, stupor, twitch; Rare: ataxia, circumoral paresthesia, decreased libido, decreased reflexes, hallucinations, neuritis, nystagmus, tremor.
Minor changes in EEG patterns, usually low-voltage fast activity, have been observed in patients during ProSom therapy or withdrawal and are of no known clinical significance.
Respiratory System—Infrequent: asthma, cough, dyspnea, rhinitis, sinusitis; Rare: epistaxis, hyperventilation, laryngitis.
Skin and Appendages—Infrequent: rash, sweating, urticaria; Rare: acne, dry skin.
Special Senses—Infrequent: abnormal vision, ear pain, eye irritation, eye pain, eye swelling, perverse taste, photophobia, tinnitus; Rare: decreased hearing, diplopia, scotomata.
Urogenital System—Infrequent: frequent urination, menstrual cramps, urinary hesitancy, urinary urgency, vaginal discharge/itching; Rare: hematuria, nocturia, oliguria, penile discharge, urinary incontinence.
Postintroduction Reports—Voluntary reports of non-US postmarketing experience with estazolam have included rare occurrences of photosensitivity, Stevens-Johnson syndrome, and agranulocytosis. Because of the uncontrolled nature of these spontaneous reports, a causal relationship to estazolam treatment has not been determined.

DRUG ABUSE AND DEPENDENCE

Controlled Substance: ProSom tablets are a controlled substance in Schedule IV.
Abuse and Dependence: Withdrawal symptoms similar to those noted with sedatives/hypnotics and alcohol have occurred following the abrupt discontinuation of drugs in the benzodiazepine class. The symptoms can range from mild dysphoria and insomnia to a major syndrome that may include abdominal and muscle cramps, vomiting, sweating, tremors, and convulsions.
Although withdrawal symptoms are more commonly noted after the discontinuation of higher than therapeutic doses of benzodiazepines, a proportion of patients taking benzodiazepines chronically at therapeutic doses may become physically dependent on them. Available data, however, cannot provide a reliable estimate of the incidence of dependency or the relationship of the dependency to dose and duration of treatment. There is some evidence to suggest that gradual reduction of dosage will attenuate or eliminate some withdrawal phenomena. In most instances, withdrawal phenomena are relatively mild and transient; however, life-threatening events (eg, seizures, delirium, etc.) have been reported.
Gradual withdrawal is the preferred course for any patient taking benzodiazepines for a prolonged period. Patients with a history of seizures, regardless of their concomitant antiseizure drug therapy, should not be withdrawn abruptly from benzodiazepines.
Individuals with a history of addiction to or abuse of drugs or alcohol should be under careful surveillance when receiving benzodiazepines because of the risk of habituation and dependence to such patients.

OVERDOSAGE

As with other benzodiazepines, experience with ProSom indicates that manifestations of overdosage include somnolence, respiratory depression, confusion, impaired coordination, slurred speech, and ultimately, coma. Patients have recovered from overdosage as high as 40 mg. As in the management of intentional overdose with any drug, the possibility should be considered that multiple agents may have been taken.
Gastric evacuation, either by the induction of emesis, lavage, or both, should be performed immediately. Maintenance of adequate ventilation is essential. General supportive care, including frequent monitoring of the vital signs and close observation of the patient, is indicated. Fluids should be administered intravenously to maintain blood pressure and encourage diuresis. The value of dialysis in treatment of benzodiazepine overdose has not been determined. The physician may wish to consider contacting a Poison Control Center for up-to-date information on the management of hypnotic drug product overdose.
Flumazenil, a specific benzodiazepine receptor antagonist, is indicated for the complete or partial reversal of the sedative effects of benzodiazepines and may be used in situations when an overdose with a benzodiazepine is known or suspected. Prior to the administration of flumazenil, necessary measures should be instituted to secure airway, ventilation, and intravenous access. Flumazenil is intended as an adjunct to, not as a substitute for, proper management of benzodiazepine overdose. Patients treated with flumazenil should be monitored for resedation, respiratory depression, and other residual benzodiazepine effects for an appropriate period after treatment. **The prescriber should be aware of a risk of seizure in association with flumazenil treatment, particularly in long-term benzodiazepine users and in cyclic antidepressant overdose.** The complete flumazenil package insert including CONTRAINDICATIONS, WARNINGS, and PRECAUTIONS should be consulted prior to use.

DOSAGE AND ADMINISTRATION

The recommended initial dose for adults is 1 mg at bedtime; however, some patients may need a 2 mg dose. In healthy elderly patients, 1 mg is also the appropriate starting dose, but increases should be initiated with particular care. In small or debilitated older patients, a starting dose of 0.5 mg, while only marginally effective in the overall elderly population, should be considered.

HOW SUPPLIED

ProSom tablets are scored tablets supplied as:
ProSom Tablets 1 mg white tablets bearing the Abbott logo and UC (Abbo-Code).
Bottles of 100 .... (**NDC** 0074-3735-13)
ProSom Tablets 2 mg pink tablets bearing the Abbott logo and UD (Abbo-Code).
Bottles of 100 .... (**NDC** 0074-3736-13)
Recommended storage: Store below 86°F (30°C).
Revised: June, 1998
Ref. 03-4889-R7
ABBOTT LABORATORIES
NORTH CHICAGO, IL 60064, U.S.A.

TRANXENE® Ⓒ℞

[*tran' zēen*]
T-Tab® Tablets
CLORAZEPATE DIPOTASSIUM
TRANXENE®-SD™
& TRANXENE®-SD™ HALF STRENGTH
CLORAZEPATE DIPOTASSIUM SINGLE DOSE TABLETS

DESCRIPTION

Chemically, TRANXENE is a benzodiazepine. The empirical formula is $C_{16}H_{11}ClK_2N_2O_4$; the molecular weight is 408.92; and the structural formula may be represented as follows:

The compound occurs as a fine, light yellow, practically odorless powder. It is insoluble in the common organic solvents, but very soluble in water. Aqueous solutions are unstable, clear, light yellow, and alkaline.
TRANXENE T-TAB tablets contain either 3.75 mg, 7.5 mg or 15 mg of clorazepate dipotassium for oral administration. TRANXENE-SD and TRANXENE-SD HALF STRENGTH tablets contain 22.5 mg and 11.25 mg of clorazepate dipotassium respectively. TRANXENE-SD and TRANXENE-SD HALF STRENGTH tablets gradually release clorazepate and are designed for once-a-day administration in patients already stabilized on TRANXENE T-TAB tablets.
Inactive ingredients for TRANXENE T-TAB® Tablets: Colloidal silicon dioxide, FD&C Blue No. 2 (3.75 mg only), FD&C Yellow No. 6 (7.5 mg only), FD&C Red No. 3 (15 mg only), magnesium oxide, magnesium stearate, microcrystalline cellulose, potassium carbonate, potassium chloride, and talc. Inactive ingredients for TRANXENE-SD and TRANXENE-SD HALF STRENGTH Tablets: Castor oil wax, FD&C Blue No. 2 (SD Half Strength, 11.25 mg only), iron oxide (SD, 22.5 mg only), lactose, magnesium oxide, magnesium stearate, potassium carbonate, potassium chloride, and talc.

CLINICAL PHARMACOLOGY

Pharmacologically, clorazepate dipotassium has the characteristics of the benzodiazepines. It has depressant effects on the central nervous system. The primary metabolite, nordiazepam, quickly appears in the blood stream. The serum half-life is about 2 days. The drug is metabolized in the liver and excreted primarily in the urine.
Studies in healthy men have shown that clorazepate dipotassium has depressant effects on the central nervous system. Prolonged administration of single daily doses as high as 120 mg was without toxic effects. Abrupt cessation of high doses was followed in some patients by nervousness, insomnia, irritability, diarrhea, muscle aches, or memory impairment.
Since orally administered clorazepate dipotassium is rapidly decarboxylated to form nordiazepam, there is essentially no circulating parent drug. Nordiazepam, the primary metabolite, quickly appears in the blood and is eliminated from the plasma with an apparent half-life of about 40 to 50 hours. Plasma levels of nordiazepam increase proportionally with TRANXENE dose and show moderate accumulation with repeated administration. The protein binding of nordiazepam in plasma is high (97-98%).
Within 10 days after oral administration of a 15 mg (50µCi) dose of ^{14}C-TRANXENE to two volunteers, 62–67% of the radioactivity was excreted in the urine and 15–19% was eliminated in the feces. Both subjects were still excreting measurable amounts of radioactivity in the urine (about 1% of the ^{14}C-dose) on day ten.
Nordiazepam is further metabolized by hydroxylation. The major urinary metabolite is conjugated oxazepam (3-hydroxynordiazepam), and smaller amounts of conjugated p-hydroxynordiazepam and nordiazepam are also found in the urine.

INDICATIONS AND USAGE

TRANXENE is indicated for the management of anxiety disorders or for the short-term relief of the symptoms of anxiety. Anxiety or tension associated with the stress of everyday life usually does not require treatment with an anxiolytic.
TRANXENE tablets are indicated as adjunctive therapy in the management of partial seizures.
The effectiveness of TRANXENE tablets in long-term management of anxiety, that is, more than 4 months, has not been assessed by systematic clinical studies. Long-term studies in epileptic patients, however, have shown continued therapeutic activity. The physician should reassess periodically the usefulness of the drug for the individual patient.
TRANXENE tablets are indicated for the symptomatic relief of acute alcohol withdrawal.

CONTRAINDICATIONS

TRANXENE tablets are contraindicated in patients with a known hypersensitivity to the drug and in those with acute narrow angle glaucoma.

Continued on next page

Tranxene—Cont.

WARNINGS

TRANXENE tablets are not recommended for use in depressive neuroses or in psychotic reactions.

Patients taking TRANXENE tablets should be cautioned against engaging in hazardous occupations requiring mental alertness, such as operating dangerous machinery including motor vehicles.

Since TRANXENE has a central nervous system depressant effect, patients should be advised against the simultaneous use of other CNS-depressant drugs, and cautioned that the effects of alcohol may be increased.

Because of the lack of sufficient clinical experience, TRANXENE tablets are not recommended for use in patients less than 9 years of age.

Physical and Psychological Dependence:

Withdrawal symptoms (similar in character to those noted with barbiturates and alcohol) have occurred following abrupt discontinuance of clorazepate. Withdrawal symptoms associated with the abrupt discontinuation of benzodiazepines have included convulsions, delirium, tremor, abdominal and muscle cramps, vomiting, sweating, nervousness, insomnia, irritability, diarrhea, and memory impairment. The more severe withdrawal symptoms have usually been limited to those patients who had received excessive doses over an extended period of time. Generally milder withdrawal symptoms have been reported following abrupt discontinuance of benzodiazepines taken continuously at therapeutic levels for several months. Consequently, after extended therapy, abrupt discontinuation of clorazepate should generally be avoided and a gradual dosage tapering schedule followed.

Caution should be observed in patients who are considered to have a psychological potential for drug dependence.

Evidence of drug dependence has been observed in dogs and rabbits which was characterized by convulsive seizures when the drug was abruptly withdrawn or the dose was reduced; the syndrome in dogs could be abolished by administration of clorazepate.

Usage in Pregnancy: **An increased risk of congenital malformations associated with the use of minor tranquilizers (chlordiazepoxide, diazepam, and meprobamate) during the first trimester of pregnancy has been suggested in several studies. Clorazepate dipotassium, a benzodiazepine derivative, has not been studied adequately to determine whether it, too, may be associated with an increased risk of fetal abnormality. Because use of these drugs is rarely a matter of urgency, their use during this period should almost always be avoided. The possibility that a woman of childbearing potential may be pregnant at the time of institution of therapy should be considered. Patients should be advised that if they become pregnant during therapy or intend to become pregnant they should communicate with their physician about the desirability of discontinuing the drug.**

Usage during Lactation:

TRANXENE tablets should not be given to nursing mothers since it has been reported that nordiazepam is excreted in human breast milk.

PRECAUTIONS

In those patients in which a degree of depression accompanies the anxiety, suicidal tendencies may be present and protective measures may be required. The least amount of drug that is feasible should be available to the patient.

Patients taking TRANXENE tablets for prolonged periods should have blood counts and liver function tests periodically. The usual precautions in treating patients with impaired renal or hepatic function should also be observed.

In elderly or debilitated patients, the initial dose should be small, and increments should be made gradually, in accordance with the response of the patient, to preclude ataxia or excessive sedation.

Information for Patients:

To assure the safe and effective use of benzodiazepines, patients should be informed that, since benzodiazepines may produce psychological and physical dependence, it is essential that they consult with their physician before either increasing the dose or abruptly discontinuing this drug.

Pediatric Use: See **WARNINGS**.

ADVERSE REACTIONS

The side effect most frequently reported was drowsiness. Less commonly reported (in descending order of occurrence) were: dizziness, various gastrointestinal complaints, nervousness, blurred vision, dry mouth, headache, and mental confusion. Other side effects included insomnia, transient skin rashes, fatigue, ataxia, genitourinary complaints, irritability, diplopia, depression, tremor, and slurred speech.

There have been reports of abnormal liver and kidney function tests and of decrease in hematocrit.

Decrease in systolic blood pressure has been observed.

DOSAGE AND ADMINISTRATION

For the symptomatic relief of anxiety:

TRANXENE T-TAB® tablets are administered orally in divided doses. The usual daily dose is 30 mg. The dose should be adjusted gradually within the range of 15 to 60 mg daily in accordance with the response of the patient. In elderly or debilitated patients it is advisable to initiate treatment at a daily dose of 7.5 to 15 mg.

TRANXENE tablets may also be administered in a single dose daily at bedtime; the recommended initial dose is 15 mg. After the initial dose, the response of the patient may require adjustment of subsequent dosage. Lower doses may be indicated in the elderly patient. Drowsiness may occur at the initiation of treatment and with dosage increment.

TRANXENE-SD (22.5 mg) tablets may be administered as a single dose every 24 hours. This tablet is intended as an alternate dosage form for the convenience of patients stabilized on a dose of 7.5 mg tablets three times a day. TRANXENE-SD tablets should not be used to initiate therapy.

TRANXENE-SD HALF STRENGTH (11.25 mg) tablets may be administered as a single dose every 24 hours. This tablet is intended as an alternate dosage form for the convenience of patients stabilized on a dose of 3.75 mg tablets three times a day. TRANXENE-SD HALF STRENGTH should not be used to initiate therapy.

For the symptomatic relief of acute alcohol withdrawal:

The following dosage schedule is recommended:

1st 24 hours (Day 1)	30 mg initially; followed by 30 to 60 mg in divided doses
2nd 24 hours (Day 2)	45 to 90 mg in divided doses
3rd 24 hours (Day 3)	22.5 to 45 mg in divided doses
Day 4	15 to 30 mg in divided doses

Thereafter, gradually reduce the daily dose to 7.5 to 15 mg. Discontinue drug therapy as soon as patient's condition is stable.

The maximum recommended total daily dose is 90 mg. Avoid excessive reductions in the total amount of drug administered on successive days.

As an Adjunct to Antiepileptic Drugs:

In order to minimize drowsiness, the recommended initial dosages and dosage increments should not be exceeded.

Adults: The maximum recommended initial dose in patients over 12 years old is 7.5 mg three times a day. Dosage should be increased by no more than 7.5 mg every week and should not exceed 90 mg/day.

Children (9-12 years): The maximum recommended initial dose is 7.5 mg two times a day. Dosage should be increased by no more than 7.5 mg every week and should not exceed 60 mg/day.

DRUG INTERACTIONS

If TRANXENE is to be combined with other drugs acting on the central nervous system, careful consideration should be given to the pharmacology of the agents to be employed. Animal experience indicates that clorazepate dipotassium prolongs the sleeping time after hexobarbital or after ethyl alcohol, increases the inhibitory effects of chlorpromazine, but does not exhibit monoamine oxidase inhibition. Clinical studies have shown increased sedation with concurrent hypnotic medications. The actions of the benzodiazepines may be potentiated by barbiturates, narcotics, phenothiazines, monoamine oxidase inhibitors or other antidepressants.

If TRANXENE tablets are used to treat anxiety associated with somatic disease states, careful attention must be paid to possible drug interaction with concomitant medication.

In bioavailability studies with normal subjects, the concurrent administration of antacids at therapeutic levels did not significantly influence the bioavailability of TRANXENE tablets.

OVERDOSAGE

Overdosage is usually manifested by varying degrees of CNS depression ranging from slight sedation to coma. As in the management of overdosage with any drug, it should be borne in mind that multiple agents may have been taken.

The treatment of overdosage should consist of the general measures employed in the management of overdosage of any CNS depressant. Gastric evacuation either by the induction of emesis, lavage, or both, should be performed immediately. General supportive care, including frequent monitoring of the vital signs and close observation of the patient, is indicated. Hypotension, though rarely reported, may occur with large overdoses. In such cases the use of agents such as Levophed® Bitartrate (norepinephrine bitartrate injection, USP) or Aramine® Injection (metaraminol bitartrate injection, USP) should be considered.

While reports indicate that individuals have survived overdoses of clorazepate dipotassium as high as 450 to 675 mg, these doses are not necessarily an accurate indication of the amount of drug absorbed since the time interval between ingestion and the institution of treatment was not always known. Sedation in varying degrees was the most common physiological manifestation of clorazepate dipotassium overdosage. Deep coma when it occurred was usually associated with the ingestion of other drugs in addition to clorazepate dipotassium.

Flumazenil, a specific benzodiazepine receptor antagonist, is indicated for the complete or partial reversal of the sedative effects of benzodiazepines and may be used in situations when an overdose with a benzodiazepine is known or suspected. Prior to the administration of flumazenil, necessary measures should be instituted to secure airway, ventilation, and intravenous access. Flumazenil is intended as an adjunct to, not as a substitute for, proper management of benzodiazepine overdose. Patients treated with flumazenil should be monitored for resedation, respiratory depression, and other residual benzodiazepine effects for an appropriate period after treatment. **The prescriber should be aware of a risk of seizure in association with flumazenil treatment, particularly in long-term benzodiazepine users and in cyclic antidepressant overdose.** The complete flumazenil package insert including CONTRAINDICATIONS, WARNINGS, and PRECAUTIONS should be consulted prior to use.

ANIMAL PHARMACOLOGY AND TOXICOLOGY

Studies in rats and monkeys have shown a substantial difference between doses producing tranquilizing, sedative and toxic effects. In rats, conditioned avoidance response was inhibited at an oral dose of 10 mg/kg; sedation was induced at 32 mg/kg; the LD_{50} was 1320 mg/kg. In monkeys aggressive behavior was reduced at an oral dose of 0.25 mg/kg; sedation (ataxia) was induced at 7.5 mg/kg; the LD_{50} could not be determined because of the emetic effect of large doses, but the LD_{50} exceeds 1600 mg/kg.

Twenty-four dogs were given clorazepate dipotassium orally in a 22-month toxicity study; doses up to 75 mg/kg were given. Drug-related changes occurred in the liver; weight was increased and cholestasis with minimal hepatocellular damage was found, but lobular architecture remained well preserved.

Eighteen rhesus monkeys were given oral doses of clorazepate dipotassium from 3 to 36 mg/kg daily for 52 weeks. All treated animals remained similar to control animals. Although total leucocyte count remained within normal limits it tended to fall in the female animals on the highest doses. Examination of all organs revealed no alterations attributable to clorazepate dipotassium. There was no damage to liver function or structure.

Reproduction Studies: Standard fertility, reproduction, and teratology studies were conducted in rats and rabbits. Oral doses in rats up to 150 mg/kg and in rabbits up to 15 mg/kg produced no abnormalities in the fetuses. TRANXENE did not alter the fertility indices or reproductive capacity of adult animals. As expected, the sedative effect of high doses interfered with care of the young by their mothers (*see Usage in Pregnancy*).

HOW SUPPLIED

TRANXENE® 3.75 mg, scored T-TAB® tablets are supplied as blue-colored tablets bearing the Abbott logo, the distinctive T shape and a two-letter Abbo-Code designation, TL:

Bottles of 100 .... (**NDC** 0074-4389-13).
Bottles of 500 .... (**NDC** 0074-4389-53).
ABBO-PAC® unit dose packages:
100 .... (**NDC** 0074-4389-11).

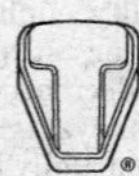
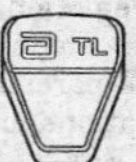

7.5 mg scored T-TAB® tablets are supplied as peach-colored tablets bearing the Abbott logo, the distinctive T shape and a two-letter Abbo-Code designation, TM:

Bottles of 100 .... (**NDC** 0074-4390-13).
Bottles of 500 .... (**NDC** 0074-4390-53).
ABBO-PAC® unit dose packages:
100 .... (**NDC** 0074-4390-11).

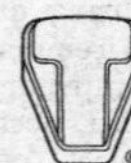
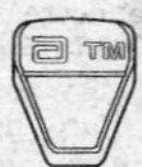

15 mg scored T-TAB® tablets are supplied as lavender-colored tablets bearing the Abbott logo, the distinctive T shape and a two-letter Abbo-Code designation, TN:

Bottles of 100 .... (**NDC** 0074-4391-13).
Bottles of 500 .... (**NDC** 0074-4391-53).
ABBO-PAC® unit dose packages:
100 .... (**NDC** 0074-4391-11).

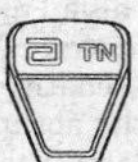

TRANXENE®-SD™ 22.5 mg single dose tablets are supplied as tan-colored tablets bearing the Abbott logo and a two-letter Abbo-Code designation, TY:

Bottles of 100 .... (**NDC** 0074-2997-13).

TRANXENE®-SD™ HALF STRENGTH 11.25 mg single dose tablets are supplied as blue-colored tablets bearing the Abbott logo and a two-letter Abbo-Code designation, TX:

Bottles of 100 .... (**NDC** 0074-2699-13).

T-TAB, tablet appearance and shape are trademarks of Abbott Laboratories.

Recommended storage: Store below 77°F (25°C)

U.S. Design Pat. No. D–300,879

Ref. 03-4833-R14

Abbott Laboratories

North Chicago, IL 60064, U.S.A.

Revised: December, 1997

Shown in Product Identification Guide, page 303

TRICOR® ℞
[*trī cōr*]
(fenofibrate capsules), micronized
Rx only

DESCRIPTION

TRICOR® (fenofibrate capsules), micronized, is a lipid regulating agent available as capsules for oral administration. Each capsule contains 67 mg, 134 mg or 200 mg of micronized fenofibrate. The chemical name for fenofibrate is 2-[4-(4-chlorobenzoyl) phenoxy]-2-methyl-propanoic acid, 1-methylethyl ester with the following structural formula:

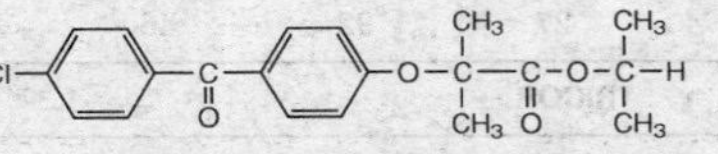

The empirical formula is $C_{20}H_{21}O_4Cl$ and the molecular weight is 360.83; fenofibrate is insoluble in water. The melting point is 79–82°C. Fenofibrate is a white solid which is stable under ordinary conditions.

Inactive Ingredients: Each capsule also contains crospovidone, iron oxide, lactose, magnesium stearate, pregelatinized starch, sodium lauryl sulfate, and titanium dioxide.

CLINICAL PHARMACOLOGY

A variety of clinical studies have demonstrated that elevated levels of total cholesterol (total-C), low density lipoprotein cholesterol (LDL-C), and apolipoprotein B (apo B), an LDL membrane complex, are associated with human atherosclerosis. Similarly, decreased levels of high density lipoprotein cholesterol (HDL-C) and its transport complex, apolipoprotein A (apo AI and apo AII) are associated with the development of atherosclerosis. Epidemiologic investigations have established that cardiovascular morbidity and mortality vary directly with the level of total-C, LDL-C, and triglycerides, and inversely with the level of HDL-C. The independent effect of raising HDL-C or lowering triglycerides (TG) on the risk of cardiovascular morbidity and mortality has not been determined.

Fenofibric acid, the active metabolite of fenofibrate, produces reductions in total cholesterol, LDL cholesterol, apolipoprotein B, total triglycerides and triglyceride rich lipoprotein (VLDL) in treated patients. In addition, treatment with fenofibrate results in increases in high density lipoprotein (HDL) and apoproteins apoAI and apoAII.

The effects of fenofibric acid seen in clinical practice have been explained *in vivo* in transgenic mice and *in vitro* in human hepatocyte cultures by the activation of peroxisome proliferator activated receptor α (PPARα). Through this mechanism, fenofibrate increases lipolysis and elimination of triglyceride-rich particles from plasma by activating lipoprotein lipase and reducing production of apoprotein C-III (an inhibitor of lipoprotein lipase activity). The resulting fall in triglycerides produces an alteration in the size and composition of LDL from small, dense particles (which are thought to be atherogenic due to their susceptibility to oxidation), to large buoyant particles. These larger particles have a greater affinity for cholesterol receptors and are catabolized rapidly. Activation of PPARα also induces an increase in the synthesis of apoproteins A-I, A-II and HDL-cholesterol.

Fenofibrate also reduces serum uric acid levels in hyperuricemic and normal individuals by increasing the urinary excretion of uric acid.

Pharmacokinetics/Metabolism

Clinical experience has been obtained with two different formulations of fenofibrate: a "micronized" and "non-micronized" formulation, which have been demonstrated to be bioequivalent. Comparisons of blood levels following oral administration of both formulations in healthy volunteers demonstrate that a single capsule containing 67 mg of the "micronized" formulation is bioequivalent to 100 mg of the "non-micronized" formulation. Three capsules containing 67 mg TRICOR are bioequivalent to a single 200 mg TRICOR capsule.

Absorption

The absolute bioavailability of fenofibrate cannot be determined as the compound is virtually insoluble in aqueous media suitable for injection. However, fenofibrate is well absorbed from the gastrointestinal tract. Following oral administration in healthy volunteers, approximately 60% of a single dose of radiolabelled fenofibrate appeared in urine, primarily as fenofibric acid and its glucuronate conjugate, and 25% was excreted in the feces. Peak plasma levels of fenofibric acid occur within 6 to 8 hours after administration.

The absorption of fenofibrate is increased when administered with food. With micronized fenofibrate, the absorption is increased by approximately 35% under fed as compared to fasting conditions.

Distribution

In healthy volunteers, steady-state plasma levels of fenofibric acid were shown to be achieved within 5 days of dosing with single oral doses equivalent to 67 mg TRICOR and did not demonstrate accumulation across time following multiple dose administration. Serum protein binding was approximately 99% in normal and hyperlipidemic subjects.

Metabolism

Following oral administration, fenofibrate is rapidly hydrolyzed by esterases to the active metabolite, fenofibric acid; no unchanged fenofibrate is detected in plasma.

Table 1
Mean Percent Change in Lipid Parameters at End of Treatment†

Treatment Group	Total-C	LDL-C	HDL-C	TG
Pooled Cohort				
Mean baseline lipid values (n=646)	306.9 mg/dL	213.8 mg/dL	52.3 mg/dL	191.0 mg/dL
All FEN (n=361)	−18.7%*	−20.6%*	+11.0%*	−28.9*
Placebo (n=285)	−0.4%	−2.2%	+0.7%	+7.7%
Baseline LDL-C > 160 mg/dL and TG < 150 mg/dL (Type IIa)				
Mean baseline lipid values (n=334)	307.7 mg/dL	227.7 mg/dL	58.1 mg/dL	101.7 mg/dL
All FEN (n=193)	−22.4%*	−31.4%*	+9.8%*	−23.5%*
Placebo (n=141)	+0.2%	−2.2%	+2.6%	+11.7%
Baseline LDL-C > 160 mg/dL and TG ≥ 150 mg/dL (Type IIb)				
Mean baseline lipid values (n=242)	312.8 mg/dL	219.8 mg/dL	46.7 mg/dL	231.9 mg/dL
All (FEN (n=126)	−16.8%*	−20.1%*	+14.6%*	+35.9%*
Placebo (n=116)	−3.0%	−6.6%	+2.3%	+0.9%

†Duration of study treatment was 3 to 6 months.
*p= <0.05 vs. Placebo

Fenofibric acid is primarily conjugated with glucuronic acid and then excreted in urine. A small amount of fenofibric acid is reduced at the carbonyl moiety to a benzhydrol metabolite which is, in turn, conjugated with glucuronic acid and excreted in urine.

In vivo metabolism data indicate that neither fenofibrate nor fenofibric acid undergo oxidative metabolism (e.g., cytochrome P450) to a significant extent.

Excretion

After absorption, fenofibrate is mainly excreted in the urine in the form of metabolites, primarily fenofibric acid and fenofibric acid glucuronide. After administration of radiolabelled fenofibrate, approximately 60% of the dose appeared in the urine and 25% was excreted in the feces.

Fenofibric acid is eliminated with a half-life of 20 hours, allowing once daily administration in a clinical setting.

Special Populations

Geriatrics

In elderly volunteers 77–87 years of age, the oral clearance of fenofibric acid following a single oral dose of fenofibrate was 1.2 L/h, which compares to 1.1 L/h in young adults. This indicates that a similar dosage regimen can be used in the elderly, without increasing accumulation of the drug or metabolites.

Pediatrics

TRICOR has not been investigated in adequate and well-controlled trials in pediatric patients.

Gender

No pharmacokinetic difference between males and females has been observed for fenofibrate.

Race

The influence of race on the pharmacokinetics of fenofibrate has not been studied, however fenofibrate is not metabolized by enzymes known for exhibiting inter-ethnic variability. Therefore, inter-ethnic pharmacokinetic differences are very unlikely.

Renal insufficiency

In a study in patients with severe renal impairment (creatinine clearance < 50 mL/min), the rate of clearance of fenofibric acid was greatly reduced, and the compound accumulated during chronic dosage. However, in patients having moderate renal impairment (creatinine clearance of 50 to 90 mL/min), the oral clearance and the oral volume of distribution of fenofibric acid are increased compared to healthy adults (2.1 L/h and 95 L versus 1.1 L/h and 30 L, respectively). Therefore, the dosage of TRICOR should be minimized in patients who have severe renal impairment, while no modification of dosage is required in patients having moderate renal impairment.

Hepatic insufficiency

No pharmacokinetic studies have been conducted in patients having hepatic insufficiency.

Drug-drug interactions

In vitro studies using human liver microsomes indicate that fenofibrate and fenofibric acid are not inhibitors of cytochrome (CYP) P450 isoforms CYP3A4, CYP2D6, CYP2E1, or CYP1A2. They are weak inhibitors of CYP2C19 and CYP2A6, and mild-to-moderate inhibitors of CYP2C9 at therapeutic concentrations.

Potentiation of coumarin-type anticoagulants has been observed with prolongation of the prothrombin time/INR.

Bile acid sequestrants have been shown to bind other drugs given concurrently. Therefore, fenofibrate should be taken at least 1 hour before or 4–6 hours after a bile acid binding resin to avoid impeding its absorption. (See WARNINGS and PRECAUTIONS).

Clinical Trials

Hypercholesterolemia (Heterozygous Familial and Nonfamilial) and Mixed Dyslipidemia (Fredrickson Types IIa and IIb)

The effects of fenofibrate at a dose equivalent to 200 mg TRICOR per day were assessed from four randomized, placebo-controlled, double-blind, parallel-group studies including patients with the following mean baseline lipid values: total-C 306.9 mg/dL; LDL-C 213.8 mg/dL; HDL-C 52.3 mg/dL; and triglycerides 191.0 mg/dL. TRICOR therapy lowered LDL-C, Total-C, and the LDL-C/HDL-C ratio. TRICOR therapy also lowered triglycerides and raised HDL-C (see Table 1).

[See table 1 above]

In a subset of the subjects, measurements of apo B were conducted. TRICOR treatment significantly reduced apo B from baseline to endpoint as compared with placebo (−25.1% vs. 2.4%, p<0.0001, n=213 and 143 respectively).

Hypertriglyceridemia (Fredrickson Type IV and V)

The effects of fenofibrate on serum triglycerides were studied in two randomized, double-blind, placebo-controlled clinical trials[1] of 147 hypertriglyceridemic patients (Fredrickson Types IV and V). Patients were treated for eight weeks under protocols that differed only in that one entered patients with baseline triglyceride (TG) levels of 500 to 1500 mg/dL, and the other TG levels of 350 to 500 mg/dL. In patients with hypertriglyceridemia and normal cholesterolemia with or without hyperchylomicronemia (Type IV/V hyperlipidemia), treatment with fenofibrate at dosages equivalent to 200 mg TRICOR per day decreased primarily very low density lipoprotein (VLDL) triglycerides and VLDL cholesterol. Treatment of patients with Type IV hyperlipoproteinemia and elevated triglycerides often results in an increase of low density lipoprotein (LDL) cholesterol (see Table 2).

[See table 2 at top of next page]

The effect of TRICOR on cardiovascular morbidity and mortality has not been determined.

INDICATIONS AND USAGE

Treatment of Hypercholesterolemia

TRICOR (fenofibrate capsules), micronized, is indicated as adjunctive therapy to diet for the reduction of LDL-C, Total-C, Triglycerides and Apo B in adult patients with primary hypercholesterolemia or mixed dyslipidemia (Fredrickson Types IIa and IIb). Lipid-altering agents should be used in addition to a diet restricted in saturated fat and cholesterol when response to diet and non-pharmacological interventions alone has been inadequate (see National Cholesterol Education Program [NCEP] Treatment Guidelines, below).

Treatment of Hypertriglyceridemia

TRICOR is also indicated as adjunctive therapy to diet for treatment of adult patients with hypertriglyceridemia (Fredrickson Types IV and V hyperlipidemia). Improving glycemic control in diabetic patients showing fasting chylomicronemia will usually reduce fasting triglycerides and eliminate chylomicronemia thereby obviating the need for pharmacologic intervention.

Markedly elevated levels of serum triglycerides (e.g. > 2,000 mg/dL) may increase the risk of developing pancreatitis. The effect of TRICOR therapy on reducing this risk has not been adequately studied.

Drug therapy is not indicated for patients with Type I hyperlipoproteinemia, who have elevations of chylomicrons and plasma triglycerides, but who have normal levels of very low density lipoprotein (VLDL). Inspection of plasma refrigerated for 14 hours is helpful in distinguishing Types I, IV and V hyperlipoproteinemia[2].

The initial treatment for dyslipidemia is dietary therapy specific for the type of lipoprotein abnormality. Excess body weight and excess alcoholic intake may be important factors in hypertriglyceridemia and should be addressed prior to any drug therapy. Physical exercise can be an important ancillary measure. Diseases contributory to hyperlipidemia, such as hypothyroidism or diabetes mellitus should be looked for and adequately treated. Estrogen therapy, like thiazide diuretics and beta-blockers, is sometimes associated with massive rises in plasma triglycerides, especially in subjects with familial hypertriglyceridemia. In such cases, discontinuation of the specific etiologic agent may obviate the need for specific drug therapy of hypertriglyceridemia.

Continued on next page

Tricor—Cont.

The use of drugs should be considered only when reasonable attempts have been made to obtain satisfactory results with non-drug methods. If the decision is made to use drugs, the patient should be instructed that this does not reduce the importance of adhering to diet. (See WARNINGS and PRECAUTIONS).
[See second table at right]

The NCEP Treatment Guidelines

Definite Athero-sclerotic Disease[a]	Two or More Other Risk Factors[b]	LDL-Cholesterol mg/dL (mmol/L) Initiation Level	Goal
No	No	≥ 190 (≥4.9)	<160 (< 4.1)
No	Yes	≥ 160 (≥4.1)	<130 (< 3.4)
Yes	Yes or No	≥ 130[c] (≥3.4)	<100 (< 2.6)

(a) Coronary heart disease or peripheral vascular disease (including symptomatic carotid artery disease).
(b) Other risk factors for coronary heart disease (CHD) include: age (males: ≥45 years; females: ≥55 years or premature menopause without estrogen replacement therapy); family history of premature CHD; current cigarette smoking; hypertension; confirmed HDL-C <35 mg/dL (<0.91 mmol/L); and diabetes mellitus. Subtract 1 risk factor if HDL-C is ≥60 mg/dL (≥1.6 mmol/L).
(c) In CHD patients with LDL-C levels 100 to 129 mg/dL, the physician should exercise clinical judgment in deciding whether to initiate drug treatment.

CONTRAINDICATIONS

TRICOR is contraindicated in patients who exhibit hypersensitivity to fenofibrate.
TRICOR is contraindicated in patients with hepatic or severe renal dysfunction, including primary biliary cirrhosis, and patients with unexplained persistent liver function abnormality.
TRICOR is contraindicated in patients with preexisting gallbladder disease (see WARNINGS).

WARNINGS

Liver Function: Fenofibrate at doses equivalent to 134 mg to 200 mg TRICOR per day has been associated with increases in serum transaminases [AST (SGOT) or ALT (SGPT)]. In a pooled analysis of 10 placebo-controlled trials, increases to > 3 times the upper limit of normal occurred in 5.3% of patients taking fenofibrate versus 1.1% of patients treated with placebo.
When transaminases determinations were followed either after discontinuation of treatment or during continued treatment, a return to normal limits was usually observed. The incidence of increases in transaminase related to fenofibrate therapy appear to be dose related. In an 8-week dose-ranging study, the incidence of ALT or AST elevations to at least three times the upper limit of normal was 13% in patients receiving dosages equivalent to 134 mg to 200 mg TRICOR per day and was 0% in those receiving dosages equivalent to 34 mg or 67 mg TRICOR per day, or placebo. Hepatocellular, chronic active and cholestatic hepatitis associated with fenofibrate therapy have been reported after exposures of weeks to several years. In extremely rare cases, cirrhosis has been reported in association with chronic active hepatitis.
Regular periodic monitoring of liver function, including serum ALT (SGPT) should be performed for the duration of therapy with TRICOR, and therapy discontinued if enzyme levels persist above three times the normal limit.
Cholelithiasis: Fenofibrate, like clofibrate and gemfibrozil, may increase cholesterol excretion into the bile, leading to cholelithiasis. If cholelithiasis is suspected, gallbladder studies are indicated. TRICOR therapy should be discontinued if gallstones are found.
Concomitant Oral Anticoagulants: Caution should be exercised when anticoagulants are given in conjunction with TRICOR because of the potentiation of coumarin-type anticoagulants in prolonging the prothrombin time/INR. The dosage of the anticoagulant should be reduced to maintain the prothrombin time/INR at the desired level to prevent bleeding complications. Frequent prothrombin time/INR determinations are advisable until it has been definitely determined that the prothrombin time/INR has stabilized.
Concomitant HMG-CoA reductase inhibitors: The combined use of TRICOR and HMG-CoA reductase inhibitors should be avoided unless the benefit of further alterations in lipid levels is likely to outweigh the increased risk of this drug combination.
In a single-dose drug interaction study in 23 healthy adults the concomitant administration of TRICOR and pravastatin resulted in no clinically important difference in the pharmacokinetics of fenofibric acid, pravastatin or its active metabolite 3a-hydroxy iso-pravastatin when compared to either drug given alone.
The combined use of fibric acid derivatives and HMG-CoA reductase inhibitors has been associated, in the absence of a marked pharmacokinetic interaction, in numerous case reports, with rhabdomyolysis, markedly elevated creatine kinase (CK) levels and myoglobinuria, leading in a high proportion of cases to acute renal failure.

Table 2
Effects of TRICOR in Patients With Fredrickson Type IV/V Hyperlipidemia

Study 1	Placebo				TRICOR			
Baseline TG levels 350 to 499 mg/dL	N	Baseline (Mean)	Endpoint (Mean)	% Change (Mean)	N	Baseline (Mean)	Endpoint (Mean)	% Change (Mean)
Triglycerides	28	449	450	−0.5	27	432	223	−46.2*
VLDL Triglycerides	19	367	350	2.7	19	350	178	−44.1*
Total Cholesterol	28	255	261	2.8	27	252	227	−9.1*
HDL Cholesterol	28	35	36	4	27	34	40	19.6*
LDL Cholesterol	28	120	129	12	27	128	137	14.5
VLDL Cholesterol	27	99	99	5.8	27	92	46	−44.7*
Study 2	**Placebo**				**TRICOR**			
Baseline TG levels 500 to 1500 mg/dL	**N**	**Baseline (Mean)**	**Endpoint (Mean)**	**% Change (Mean)**	**N**	**Baseline (Mean)**	**Endpoint (Mean)**	**% Change (Mean)**
Triglycerides	44	710	750	7.2	48	726	308	−54.5*
VLDL Triglycerides	29	537	571	18.7	33	543	205	−50.6*
Total Cholesterol	44	272	271	0.4	48	261	223	−13.8*
HDL Cholesterol	44	27	28	5.0	48	30	36	22.9*
LDL Cholesterol	42	100	90	−4.2	45	103	131	45.0*
VLDL Cholesterol	42	137	142	11.0	45	126	54	−49.4*

* = p<0.05 vs. Placebo

Fredrickson Classification of Hyperlipoproteinemias

Type	Lipoprotein Elevated	Lipid Elevation Major	Minor
I (rare)	chylomicrons	TG	↑↔C
IIa	LDL	C	–
IIb	LDL, VLDL	C	TG
III (rare)	IDL	C, TG	–
IV	VLDL	TG	↑↔C
V (rare)	chylomicrons, VLDL	TG	↑↔

C=cholesterol
TG=triglycerides
LDL=low density lipoprotein
VLDL=very low density lipoprotein
IDL=intermediate density lipoprotein

The use of fibrates alone, including TRICOR (fenofibrate capsules), micronized, may occasionally be associated with myositis, myopathy, or rhabdomyolysis. Patients receiving TRICOR and complaining of muscle pain, tenderness, or weakness should have prompt medical evaluation for myopathy, including serum creatine kinase level determination. If myopathy/myositis is suspected or diagnosed, TRICOR therapy should be stopped.
Mortality: The effect of TRICOR on coronary heart disease morbidity and mortality and non-cardiovascular mortality has not been established.
Other Considerations: In the Coronary Drug Project, a large study of post myocardial infarction of patients treated for 5 years with clofibrate, there was no difference in mortality seen between the clofibrate group and the placebo group. There was however, a difference in the rate of cholelithiasis and cholecystitis requiring surgery between the two groups (3.0% vs. 1.8%).
Because of chemical, pharmacological, and clinical similarities between TRICOR (fenofibrate capsules), micronized, Atromid-S (clofibrate), and Lopid (gemfibrozil), the adverse findings in 4 large randomized, placebo-controlled clinical studies with these other fibrate drugs may also apply to TRICOR.
In a study conducted by the World Health Organization (WHO), 5000 subjects without known coronary artery disease were treated with placebo or clofibrate for 5 years and followed for an additional one year. There was a statistically significant, higher age-adjusted all-cause mortality in the clofibrate group compared with the placebo group (5.70% vs. 3.96%, p=<0.01). Excess mortality was due to a 33% increase in non-cardiovascular causes, including malignancy, post-cholecystectomy complications, and pancreatitis. This appeared to confirm the higher risk of gallbladder disease seen in clofibrate-treated patients studied in the Coronary Drug Project.
The Helsinki Heart Study was a large (n=4081) study of middle-aged men without a history of coronary artery disease. Subjects received either placebo or gemfibrozil for 5 years, with a 3.5 year open extension afterward. Total mortality was numerically higher in the gemfibrozil randomization group but did not achieve statistical significance (p=0.19, 95% confidence interval for relative risk G:P=.91–1.64). Although cancer deaths trended higher in the gemfibrozil group (p=0.11), cancers (excluding basal cell carcinoma) were diagnosed with equal frequency in both study groups. Due to the limited size of the study, the relative risk of death from any cause was not shown to be different than that seen in the 9 year follow-up data from World Health Organization study (RR=1.29). Similarly, the numerical excess of gallbladder surgeries in the gemfibrozil group did not differ statistically from that observed in the WHO study.
A secondary prevention component of the Helsinki Heart Study enrolled middle-aged men excluded from the primary prevention study because of known or suspected coronary heart disease. Subjects received gemfibrozil or placebo for 5 years. Although cardiac deaths trended higher in the gemfibrozil group, this was not statistically significant (hazard ratio 2.2, 95% confidence interval: 0.94-5.05). The rate of gallbladder surgery was not statistically significant between study groups, but did trend higher in the gemfibrozil group, (1.9% vs. 0.3%, p=0.07). There was a statistically significant difference in the number of appendectomies in the gemfibrozil group (6/311 vs. 0/317, p=0.029).

PRECAUTIONS

Initial therapy: Laboratory studies should be done to ascertain that the lipid levels are consistently abnormal before instituting TRICOR therapy. Every attempt should be made to control serum lipids with appropriate diet, exercise, weight loss in obese patients, and control of any medical problems such as diabetes mellitus and hypothyroidism that are contributing to the lipid abnormalities. Medications known to exacerbate hypertriglyceridemia (beta-blockers, thiazides, estrogens) should be discontinued or changed if possible prior to consideration of triglyceride-lowering drug therapy.
Continued therapy: Periodic determination of serum lipids should be obtained during initial therapy in order to establish the lowest effective dose of TRICOR. Therapy should be withdrawn in patients who do not have an adequate response after two months of treatment with the maximum recommended dose of 200 mg per day.
Pancreatitis: Pancreatitis has been reported in patients taking fenofibrate, gemfibrozil, and clofibrate. This occurrence may represent a failure of efficacy in patients with severe hypertriglyceridemia, a direct drug effect, or a secondary phenomenon mediated through biliary tract stone or sludge formation with obstruction of the common bile duct.
Hypersensitivity Reactions: Acute hypersensitivity reactions including severe skin rashes requiring patient hospitalization and treatment with steroids have occurred very rarely during treatment with fenofibrate, including rare spontaneous reports of Stevens-Johnson syndrome, and toxic epidermal necrolysis. Urticaria was seen in 1.1 vs. 0%, and rash in 1.4 vs. 0.8% of fenofibrate and placebo patients respectively in controlled trials.
Hematologic Changes: Mild to moderate hemoglobin, hematocrit, and white blood cell decreases have been observed in patients following initiation of fenofibrate therapy. However, these levels stabilize during long-term administration. Extremely rare spontaneous reports of thrombocytopenia and agranulocytosis have been received during post-marketing surveillance outside of the U.S. Periodic blood counts are recommended during the first 12 months of TRICOR administration.
Skeletal muscle: The use of fibrates alone, including TRICOR, may occasionally be associated with myopathy. Treatment with drugs of the fibrate class has been associated on rare occasions with rhabdomyolysis, usually in patients with impaired renal function. Myopathy should be

considered in any patient with diffuse myalgias, muscle tenderness or weakness, and/or marked elevations of creatine phosphokinase levels.

Patients should be advised to report promptly unexplained muscle pain, tenderness or weakness, particularly if accompanied by malaise or fever. CPK levels should be assessed in patients reporting these symptoms, and fenofibrate therapy should be discontinued if markedly elevated CPK levels occur or myopathy is diagnosed.

Drug Interactions

Oral Anticoagulants: CAUTION SHOULD BE EXERCISED WHEN COUMARIN ANTICOAGULANTS ARE GIVEN IN CONJUNCTION WITH TRICOR. THE DOSAGE OF THE ANTICOAGULANTS SHOULD BE REDUCED TO MAINTAIN THE PROTHROMBIN TIME/INR AT THE DESIRED LEVEL TO PREVENT BLEEDING COMPLICATIONS. FREQUENT PROTHROMBIN TIME/INR DETERMINATIONS ARE ADVISABLE UNTIL IT HAS BEEN DEFINITELY DETERMINED THAT THE PROTHROMBIN TIME/INR HAS STABILIZED.

HMG-CoA reductase inhibitors: The combined use of TRICOR and HMG-CoA reductase inhibitors should be avoided unless the benefit of further alterations in lipid levels is likely to outweigh the increased risk of this drug combination (see WARNINGS).

Resins: Since bile acid sequestrants may bind other drugs given concurrently, patients should take TRICOR (fenofibrate capsules), micronized, at least 1 hour before or 4–6 hours after a bile acid binding resin to avoid impeding its absorption.

Cyclosporine: Because cyclosporine can produce nephrotoxicity with decreases in creatinine clearance and rises in serum creatinine, and because renal excretion is the primary elimination route of fibrate drugs including TRICOR, there is a risk that an interaction will lead to deterioration. The benefits and risks of using TRICOR with immunosuppressants and other potentially nephrotoxic agents should be carefully considered, and the lowest effective dose employed.

Carcinogenesis, Mutagenesis, Impairment of Fertility: In a 24-month study in rats (10, 45, and 200 mg/kg; 0.3, 1, and 6 times the maximum recommended human dose on the basis of mg/meter^2 of surface area), the incidence of liver carcinoma was significantly increased at 6 times the maximum recommended human dose in males and females. A statistically significant increase in pancreatic carcinomas occurred in males at 1 and 6 times the maximum recommended human dose; there were also increases in pancreatic adenomas and benign testicular interstitial cell tumors at 6 times the maximum recommended human dose in males. In a second 24-month study in a different strain of rats (doses of 10 and 60 mg/kg; 0.3 and 2 times the maximum recommended human dose based on mg/meter^2 surface area), there were significant increases in the incidence of pancreatic acinar adenomas in both sexes and increases in interstitial cell tumors of the testes at 2 times the maximum recommended human dose.

A comparative carcinogenicity study was done in rats comparing three drugs: fenofibrate (10 and 70 mg/kg; 0.3 and 1.6 times the maximum recommended human dose), clofibrate (400 mg/kg; 1.6 times the human dose), and gemfibrozil (250 mg/kg; 1.7 times the human dose) (multiples based on mg/meter^2 surface area). Pancreatic acinar adenomas were increased in males and females on fenofibrate; hepatocellular carcinoma and pancreatic acinar adenomas were increased in males and hepatic neoplastic nodules in females treated with clofibrate; hepatic neoplastic nodules were increased in males and females treated with gemfibrozil while testicular interstitial cell tumors were increased in males on all three drugs.

In a 21-month study in mice at doses of 10, 45, and 200 mg/kg (approximately 0.2, 0.7 and 3 times the maximum recommended human dose on the basis of mg/meter^2 surface area), there were statistically significant increases in liver carcinoma at 3 times the maximum recommended human dose in both males and females. In a second 18-month study at the same doses, there was a significant increase in liver carcinoma in male mice and liver adenoma in female mice at 3 times the maximum recommended human dose.

Electron microscopy studies have demonstrated peroxisomal proliferation following fenofibrate administration to the rat. An adequate study to test for peroxisome proliferation in humans has not been done, but changes in peroxisome morphology and numbers have been observed in humans after treatment with other members of the fibrate class when liver biopsies were compared before and after treatment in the same individual.

Fenofibrate has been demonstrated to be devoid of mutagenic potential in the following tests: Ames, mouse lymphoma, chromosomal aberration and unscheduled DNA synthesis.

Pregnancy Category C: Fenofibrate has been shown to be embryocidal and teratogenic in rats when given in doses 7 to 10 times the maximum recommended human dose and embryocidal in rabbits when given at 9 times the maximum recommended human dose (on the basis of mg/meter^2 surface area). There are no adequate and well-controlled studies in pregnant women. Fenofibrate should be used during pregnancy only if the potential benefit justifies the potential risk to the fetus.

Administration of 9 times the maximum recommended human dose of fenofibrate to female rats before and throughout gestation caused 100% of dams to delay delivery and resulted in a 60% increase in post-implantation loss, a decrease in litter size, a decrease in birth weight, a 40% survival of pups at birth, a 4% survival of pups as neonates, and a 0% survival of pups to weaning, and an increase in spina bifida.

BODY SYSTEM Adverse Event	Fenofibrate* (N=439)	Placebo (N=365)
BODY AS A WHOLE		
Abdominal Pain	4.6%	4.4%
Back Pain	3.4%	2.5%
Headache	3.2%	2.7%
Asthenia	2.1%	3.0%
Flu Syndrome	2.1%	2.7%
DIGESTIVE		
Liver Function Tests Abnormal	7.5%**	1.4%
Diarrhea	2.3%	4.1%
Nausea	2.3%	1.9%
Constipation	2.1%	1.4%
METABOLIC AND NUTRITIONAL DISORDERS		
SGPT Increased	3.0%	1.6%
Creatine Phosphokinase Increased	3.0%	1.4%
SGOT Increased	3.4%**	0.5%
RESPIRATORY		
Respiratory Disorder	6.2%	5.5%
Rhinitis	2.3%	1.1%

* Dosage equivalent to 200 mg TRICOR (fenofibrate capsules), micronized

** Significantly different from Placebo

Administration of 10 times the maximum recommended human dose to female rats on days 6–15 of gestation caused an increase in gross, visceral and skeletal findings in fetuses (domed head/hunched shoulders/rounded body/abnormal chest, kyphosis, stunted fetuses, elongated sternal ribs, malformed sternebrae, extra foramen in palatine, misshapen vertebrae, supernumerary ribs).

Administration of 7 times the maximum recommended human dose to female rats from day 15 of gestation through weaning caused a delay in delivery, a 40% decrease in live births, a 75% decrease in neonatal survival, and decreases in pup weight, at birth as well as on days 4 and 21 postpartum.

Administration of 9 and 18 times the maximum recommended human dose to female rabbits caused abortions in 10% of dams at 9 times and 25% of dams at 18 times the maximum recommended human dose and death of 7% of fetuses at 18 times the maximum recommended human dose.

Nursing mothers: Fenofibrate should not be used in nursing mothers. Because of the potential for tumorigenicity seen in animal studies, a decision should be made whether to discontinue nursing or to discontinue the drug.

Pediatric Use: Safety and efficacy in pediatric patients have not been established.

Geriatric Use: Fenofibric acid is known to be substantially excreted by the kidney, and the risk of adverse reactions to this drug may be greater in patients with impaired renal function. Because elderly patients are more likely to have decreased renal function, care should be taken in dose selection.

ADVERSE REACTIONS

CLINICAL: Adverse events reported by 2% or more of patients treated with fenofibrate during the double-blind, placebo-controlled trials, regardless of causality, are listed in the table below. Adverse events led to discontinuation of treatment in 5.0% of patients treated with fenofibrate and in 3.0% treated with placebo. Increases in liver function tests were the most frequent events, causing discontinuation of fenofibrate treatment in 1.6% of patients in double-blind trials.

[See table above]

Additional adverse events reported by three or more patients in placebo- controlled trials or reported in other controlled or open trials, regardless of causality are listed below.

BODY AS A WHOLE: Chest pain, pain (unspecified), infection, malaise, allergic reaction, cyst, hernia, fever, photosensitivity reaction, and accidental injury.

CARDIOVASCULAR SYSTEM: Angina pectoris, hypertension, vasodilatation, coronary artery disorder, electrocardiogram abnormal, ventricular extrasystoles, myocardial infarct, peripheral vascular disorder, migraine, varicose vein, cardiovascular disorder, hypotension, palpitation, vascular disorder, arrhythmia, phlebitis, tachycardia, extrasystoles, and atrial fibrillation.

DIGESTIVE SYSTEM: Dyspepsia, flatulence, nausea, increased appetite, gastroenteritis, cholelithiasis, rectal disorder, esophagitis, gastritis, colitis, tooth disorder, vomiting, anorexia, gastrointestinal disorder, duodenal ulcer, nausea and vomiting, peptic ulcer, rectal hemorrhage, liver fatty deposit, cholecystitis, eructation, gamma glutamyl transpeptidase, and diarrhea.

ENDOCRINE SYSTEM: Diabetes mellitus

HEMIC AND LYMPHATIC SYSTEM: Anemia, leukopenia, ecchymosis, eosinophilia, lymphadenopathy, and thrombocytopenia.

METABOLIC AND NUTRITIONAL DISORDERS: Creatinine increased, weight gain, hypoglycemia, gout, weight loss, edema, hyperuricemia, and peripheral edema.

MUSCULOSKELETAL SYSTEM: Myositis, myalgia, arthralgia, arthritis, tenosynovitis, joint disorder, arthrosis, leg cramps, bursitis, and myasthenia.

NERVOUS SYSTEM: Dizziness, insomnia, depression, vertigo, libido decreased, anxiety, paresthesia, dry mouth, hypertonia, nervousness, neuralgia, and somnolence.

RESPIRATORY SYSTEM: Pharyngitis, bronchitis, cough increased, dyspnea, asthma, pneumonia, laryngitis, and sinusitis.

SKIN AND APPENDAGES: Rash, pruritus, eczema, herpes zoster, urticaria, acne, sweating, fungal dermatitis, skin disorder, alopecia, contact dermatitis, herpes simplex, maculopapular rash, nail disorder, and skin ulcer.

SPECIAL SENSES: Conjunctivitis, eye disorder, amblyopia, ear pain, otitis media, abnormal vision, cataract specified, and refraction disorder.

UROGENITAL SYSTEM: Urinary frequency, prostatic disorder, dysuria, kidney function abnormal, urolithiasis, gynecomastia, unintended pregnancy, vaginal moniliasis, and cystitis.

OVERDOSAGE

There is no specific treatment for overdose with TRICOR. General supportive care of the patient is indicated, including monitoring of vital signs and observation of clinical status, should an overdose occur. If indicated, elimination of unabsorbed drug should be achieved by emesis or gastric lavage; usual precautions should be observed to maintain the airway. Because fenofibrate is highly bound to plasma proteins, hemodialysis should not be considered.

DOSAGE AND ADMINISTRATION

Patients should be placed on an appropriate lipid-lowering diet before receiving TRICOR, and should continue this diet during treatment with TRICOR. TRICOR should be given with meals, thereby optimizing the bioavailability of the medication.

For the treatment of adult patients with primary hypercholesterolemia or mixed hyperlipidemia, the initial dose of TRICOR is 200 mg per day.

For adult patients with hypertriglyceridemia, the initial dose is 67 to 200 mg per day. Dosage should be individualized according to patient response, and should be adjusted if necessary following repeat lipid determinations at 4 to 8 week intervals. The maximum dose is 200 mg per day.

Treatment with TRICOR should be initiated at a dose of 67 mg/day in patients having impaired renal function, and increased only after evaluation of the effects on renal function and lipid levels at this dose. In the elderly, the initial dose should likewise be limited to 67 mg/day.

Lipid levels should be monitored periodically and consideration should be given to reducing the dosage of TRICOR if lipid levels fall significantly below the targeted range.

HOW SUPPLIED

TRICOR® (fenofibrate capsules), micronized, is available as hard gelatin capsules in three strengths:

67 mg yellow capsules, imprinted with ▭ on cap and Abbo-Code identification letters FR on body, available in bottles of 90 (**NDC** 0074-4342-90).

134 mg white capsules, imprinted with ▭ on cap and Abbo-Code identification letters AR on body, available in bottles of 90 (**NDC** 0074-6447-90).

200 mg orange capsules, imprinted with ▭ on cap and Abbo-Code identification letters SR on body, available in bottles of 90 (**NDC** 0074-6415-90).

Storage

Store at controlled room temperature, 15-30°C (59–86°F). Keep out of the reach of children. Protect from moisture.

Manufactured for Abbott Laboratories, North Chicago, IL 60064, U.S.A. by Laboratoires Fournier, S.A., 21300 Chenôve, France

Made in France

REFERENCES

1. GOLDBERG AC, *et al*. Fenofibrate for the Treatment of Type IV and V Hyperlipoproteinemias: A Double-Blind, Placebo-Controlled Multicenter US Study. *Clinical Therapeutics*, 11, pp. 69–83, 1989.
2. NIKKILA EA. Familial Lipoprotein Lipase Deficiency and Related Disorders of Chylomicron Metabolism. In Stanbury J.B., *et al.* (eds.): *The Metabolic Basis of Inherited Disease*, 5th edition, McGraw-Hill, 1983, Chap. 30, pp. 622–642.

Continued on next page

Tricor—Cont.

3. BROWN WV, et al. Effects of Fenofibrate on Plasma Lipids: Double-Blind, Multicenter Study In Patients with Type IIA or IIB Hyperlipidemia. *Arteriosclerosis.* 6, pp. 670–678, 1986.

Revised: April, 2000
Ref. 03-5037-R4-Rev. April 2000
ABBOTT LABORATORIES
NORTH CHICAGO, IL 60064, U.S.A.

Shown in Product Identification Guide, page 303

ZEMPLAR™ ℞

[*zĕm 'plär*]
(paricalcitol injection)
Fliptop Vial

DESCRIPTION

Zemplar™ (paricalcitol injection) is a synthetically manufactured vitamin D analog. It is available as a sterile, clear, colorless, aqueous solution for intravenous injection. Each mL contains paricalcitol, 5 mcg; propylene glycol, 30% (v/v); and alcohol, 20% (v/v).

Paricalcitol is a white powder chemically designated as 19-nor-1α,3β,25-trihydroxy-9,10-secoergosta-5(Z),7(E),22(E)-triene and has the following structural formula:

Molecular formula is $C_{27}H_{44}O_3$.
Molecular weight is 416.65.

CLINICAL PHARMACOLOGY

Mechanism of Action

Paricalcitol is a synthetic vitamin D analog. Vitamin D and paricalcitol have been shown to reduce parathyroid hormone (PTH) levels.

Pharmacokinetics

Distribution

The pharmacokinetics of paricalcitol have been studied in patients with chronic renal failure (CRF) requiring hemodialysis. Zemplar™ is administered as an intravenous bolus injection. Within two hours after administering doses ranging from 0.04 to 0.24 mcg/kg, concentrations of paricalcitol decreased rapidly; thereafter, concentrations of paricalcitol declined log-linearly with a mean half-life of about 15 hours. No accumulation of paricalcitol was observed with multiple dosing.

Elimination

In healthy subjects, plasma radioactivity after a single 0.16 mcg/kg intravenous bolus dose of ^{3}H-paricalcitol (n=4) was attributed to parent drug. Paricalcitol was eliminated primarily by hepatobiliary excretion, as 74% of the radioactive dose was recovered in feces and only 16% was found in urine.

Metabolism

Several unknown metabolites were detected in both the urine and feces, with no detectable paricalcitol in the urine. These metabolites have not been characterized and have not been identified. Together, these metabolites contributed 51% of the urinary radioactivity and 59% of the fecal radioactivity. *In vitro* plasma protein binding of paricalcitol was extensive (>99.9%) and nonsaturable over the concentration range of 1 to 100 ng/mL.

Paricalcitol Pharmacokinetic Characteristics in CRF Patients (0.24 mcg/kg dose)

Parameter	n	Values (Mean ± SD)
C_{max} (5 min. after bolus)	6	1850 ± 664 (pg/mL)
$AUC_{0-\infty}$	5	27382 ± 8230 (pg•hr/mL)
CL	5	0.72 ± 0.24 (L/hr)
V_{SS}	5	6 ± 2 (L)

Laboratory Tests

In placebo-controlled studies, paricalcitol reduced serum total alkaline phosphatase levels.

Special Populations

Paricalcitol pharmacokinetics have not been investigated in special populations (geriatric, pediatric, hepatic insufficiency), or for drug-drug interactions. Pharmacokinetics were not gender-dependent.

Clinical Studies

In three 12-week, placebo-controlled, phase 3 studies in chronic renal failure patients on dialysis, the dose of Zemplar™ was started at 0.04 mcg/kg 3 times per week. The dose was increased by 0.04 mcg/kg every 2 weeks until intact parathyroid hormone (iPTH) levels were decreased at least 30% from baseline or a fifth escalation brought the dose to 0.24 mcg/kg, or iPTH fell to less than 100 pg/mL, or the Ca × P product was greater than 75 within any 2 week period, or serum calcium became greater than 11.5 mg/dL at any time.

	Group (No. of Pts.)	Baseline Mean (Range)	Mean (SE) Change From Baseline to Final Evaluation
PTH (pg/mL)	Zemplar™ (n=40)	783 (291–2076)	-379 (43.7)
	placebo (n=38)	745 (320–1671)	-69.6 (44.8)
Alkaline Phosphatase (U/L)	Zemplar™ (n=31)	150 (40–600)	-41.5 (10.6)
	placebo (n=34)	169 (56–911)	+2.6 (10.1)
Calcium (mg/dL)	Zemplar™ (n=40)	9.3 (7.2–10.4)	+0.47 (0.1)
	placebo (n=38)	9.1 (7.8–10.7)	+0.02 (0.1)
Phosphorus (mg/dL)	Zemplar™ (n=40)	5.8 (3.7–10.2)	+0.47 (0.3)
	placebo (n=38)	6.0 (2.8–8.8)	-0.47 (0.3)
Calcium x	Zemplar™ (n=40)	54 (32–106)	+7.9 (2.2)
Phosphorus Product	placebo (n=38)	54 (26–77)	-3.9 (2.3)

Adverse Event Incidence Rates for All Treated Patients In All Placebo-Controlled Studies

Adverse Event	Zemplar™ (n=62)%	Placebo (n=51)%
Overall	71	78
Body as a Whole		
Chills	5	0
Feeling unwell	3	0
Fever	5	2
Flu	5	4
Sepsis	5	2
Cardiovascular System		
Palpitation	3	0
Digestive System		
Dry mouth	3	2
Gastrointestinal bleeding	5	2
Nausea	13	8
Vomiting	8	4
Metabolic and Nutritional Disorders		
Edema	7	0
Nervous System		
Light-headedness	5	2
Respiratory System		
Pneumonia	5	0

Patients treated with Zemplar™ achieved a mean iPTH reduction of 30% within 6 weeks. In these studies, there was no significant difference in the incidence of hypercalcemia or hyperphosphatemia between Zemplar™ and placebo-treated patients. The results from these studies are as follows:

[See first table above]

A long-term, open-label safety study of 164 CRF patients (mean dose of 7.5 mcg three times per week), demonstrated that mean serum Ca, P, and Ca × P remained within clinically appropriate ranges with PTH reduction (mean decrease of 319 pg/mL at 13 months).

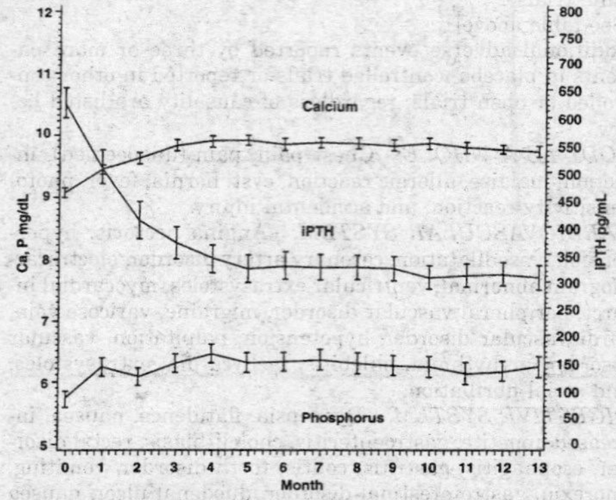

INDICATIONS AND USAGE

Zemplar™ is indicated for the prevention and treatment of secondary hyperparathyroidism associated with chronic renal failure. Studies in patients with chronic renal failure show that Zemplar™ suppresses PTH levels with no significant difference in the incidence of hypercalcemia or hyperphosphatemia when compared to placebo. However, the serum phosphorus, calcium and calcium × phosphorus product (Ca × P) may increase when Zemplar™ is administered.

CONTRAINDICATIONS

Zemplar™ should not be given to patients with evidence of vitamin D toxicity, hypercalcemia, or hypersensitivity to any ingredient in this product (see **PRECAUTIONS, General**).

WARNINGS

Acute overdose of Zemplar™ may cause hypercalcemia, and require emergency attention. During dose adjustment, serum calcium and phosphorus levels should be monitored closely (e.g., twice weekly). If clinically significant hypercalcemia develops, the dose should be reduced or interrupted. Chronic administration of Zemplar™ may place patients at risk of hypercalcemia, elevated Ca × P product, and metastatic calcification. Signs and symptoms of vitamin D intoxication associated with hypercalcemia include:

Early

Weakness, headache, somnolence, nausea, vomiting, dry mouth, constipation, muscle pain, bone pain, and metallic taste.

Late

Anorexia, weight loss, conjunctivitis (calcific), pancreatitis, photophobia, rhinorrhea, pruritus, hyperthermia, decreased libido, elevated BUN, hypercholesterolemia, elevated AST and ALT, ectopic calcification, hypertension, cardiac arrhythmias, somnolence, death, and rarely, overt psychosis.

Treatment of patients with clinically significant hypercalcemia consists of immediate dose reduction or interruption of Zemplar™ therapy and includes a low calcium diet, withdrawal of calcium supplements, patient mobilization, attention to fluid and electrolyte imbalances, assessment of electrocardiographic abnormalities (critical in patients receiving digitalis), and hemodialysis or peritoneal dialysis against a calcium-free dialysate, as warranted. Serum calcium levels should be monitored frequently until normocalcemia ensues.

Phosphate or vitamin D-related compounds should not be taken concomitantly with Zemplar™.

PRECAUTIONS

General: Digitalis toxicity is potentiated by hypercalcemia of any cause, so caution should be applied when digitalis compounds are prescribed concomitantly with Zemplar™. Adynamic bone lesions may develop if PTH levels are suppressed to abnormal levels.

Information for the Patient: The patient should be instructed that, to ensure effectiveness of Zemplar™ therapy, it is important to adhere to a dietary regimen of calcium supplementation and phosphorus restriction. Appropriate types of phosphate-binding compounds may be needed to control serum phosphorus levels in patients with chronic renal failure (CRF), but excessive use of aluminum containing compounds should be avoided. Patients should also be carefully informed about the symptoms of elevated calcium.

Essential Laboratory Tests: During the initial phase of medication, serum calcium and phosphorus should be determined frequently (e.g., twice weekly). Once dosage has been established, serum calcium and phosphorus should be measured at least monthly. Measurements of serum or plasma PTH are recommended every 3 months. An intact PTH (iPTH) assay is recommended for reliable detection of biologically active PTH in patients with CRF. During dose adjustment of Zemplar™, laboratory tests may be required more frequently.

Drug Interactions: Specific interaction studies were not performed. Digitalis toxicity is potentiated by hypercalcemia of any cause, so caution should be applied when digitalis compounds are prescribed concomitantly with Zemplar™.

Carcinogenesis, Mutagenesis, Impairment of Fertility:
Long-term studies in animals to evaluate the carcinogenic potential of paricalcitol have not been completed. Paricalcitol did not exhibit genetic toxicity *in vitro* with or without metabolic activation in the microbial mutagenesis assay (Ames Assay), mouse lymphoma mutagenesis assay (L5178Y), or a human lymphocyte cell chromosomal aberration assay. There was also no evidence of genetic toxicity in an *in vivo* mouse micronucleus assay. Zemplar™ had no effect on fertility (male or female) in rats at intravenous doses up to 20 mcg/kg/dose [equivalent to 13 times the highest recommended human dose (0.24 mcg/kg) based on surface area, mg/m^2].

Pregnancy: *Pregnancy Category C.* Paricalcitol has been shown to cause minimal decreases in fetal viability (5%) when administered daily to rabbits at a dose 0.5 times the 0.24 mcg/kg human dose (based on surface area, mg/m^2) and when administered to rats at a dose 2 times the 0.24 mcg/kg human dose (based on plasma levels of exposure). At the highest dose tested (20 mcg/kg 3 times per week in rats, 13 times the 0.24 mcg/kg human dose based on surface area), there was a significant increase of the mortality of newborn rats at doses that were maternally toxic (hypercalcemia). No other effects on offspring development were observed. Paricalcitol was not teratogenic at the doses tested.
There are no adequate and well-controlled studies in pregnant women. Zemplar™ should be used during pregnancy only if the potential benefit justifies the potential risk to the fetus.

Nursing Mothers: It is not known whether paricalcitol is excreted in human milk. Because many drugs are excreted in human milk, caution should be exercised when Zemplar™ is administered to a nursing woman.

Pediatric Use: Safety and efficacy of Zemplar™ in pediatric patients have not been established.

Geriatric Use: Of the 40 patients receiving Zemplar™ in the three phase 3 placebo-controlled CRF studies, 10 patients were 65 years or over. In these studies, no overall differences in efficacy or safety were observed between patients 65 years or older and younger patients.

ADVERSE REACTIONS

Zemplar™ has been evaluated for safety in clinical studies in 454 CRF patients. In four, placebo-controlled, double-blind, multicenter studies, discontinuation of therapy due to any adverse event occurred in 6.5% of 62 patients treated with Zemplar™ (dosage titrated as tolerated, see **CLINICAL PHARMACOLOGY, Clinical Studies**) and 2.0% of 51 patients treated with placebo for one to three months. Adverse events occurring with greater frequency in the Zemplar™ group at a frequency of 2% or greater, regardless of causality, are presented in the following table:

[See second table on previous page]

A patient who reported the same medical term more than once was counted only once for that medical term.
Safety parameters (changes in mean Ca, P, Ca × P) in an open-label safety study up to 13 months in duration support the long-term safety of Zemplar™ in this patient population.

OVERDOSAGE

Overdosage of Zemplar™ may lead to hypercalcemia (see **WARNINGS**).

DOSAGE AND ADMINISTRATION

The currently accepted target range for iPTH levels in CRF patients is no more than 1.5 to 3 times the non-uremic upper limit of normal.
The recommended initial dose of Zemplar™ is 0.04 mcg/kg to 0.1 mcg/kg (2.8–7 mcg) administered as a bolus dose no more frequently than every other day at any time during dialysis. Doses as high as 0.24 mcg/kg (16.8 mcg) have been safely administered.
If a satisfactory response is not observed, the dose may be increased by 2 to 4 mcg at 2- to 4-week intervals. During any dose adjustment period, serum calcium and phosphorus levels should be monitored more frequently, and if an elevated calcium level or a Ca × P product greater than 75 is noted, the drug dosage should be immediately reduced or interrupted until these parameters are normalized. Then, Zemplar™ should be reinitiated at a lower dose. Doses may need to be decreased as the PTH levels decrease in response to therapy. Thus, incremental dosing must be individualized.
The following table is a suggested approach in dose titration:

Suggested Dosing Guidelines

PTH Level	Zemplar™ Dose
the same or increasing	increase
decreasing by <30%	increase
decreasing by >30%, <60%	maintain
decreasing by >60%	decrease
one and one-half to three times upper limit of normal	maintain

Parenteral drug products should be inspected visually for particulate matter and discoloration prior to administration whenever solution and container permit.
Discard unused portion.

HOW SUPPLIED

Zemplar™ (paricalcitol injection) 5 mcg/mL is supplied as 1 and 2 mL single-dose Fliptop Vials.

List No.	Volume/ Container	Concentration	Total Content
1658	1 mL/Fliptop Vial	5 mcg/mL	5 mcg
1658	2 mL/Fliptop Vial	5 mcg/mL	10 mcg

Store at 25°C (77°F). Excursions permitted to 15°–30°C (59°–86°F).
U.S. patents: 5,246,925; 5,587,497
Reference 58-6026

ABBOTT LABORATORIES, NORTH CHICAGO, IL 60064, USA

ZYFLO™ FILMTAB® ℞

[zī-flo]
(zileuton tablets)

DESCRIPTION

Zileuton is an orally active inhibitor of 5-lipoxygenase, the enzyme that catalyzes the formation of leukotrienes from arachidonic acid. Zileuton has the chemical name (±)-1-(1-Benzo[b]thien-2-ylethyl)-1-hydroxyurea and the following chemical structure:

Zileuton has the molecular formula $C_{11}H_{12}N_2O_2S$ and a molecular weight of 236.29. It is a racemic mixture (50:50) of R(+) and S(-) enantiomers. Zileuton is a practically odorless, white, crystalline powder that is soluble in methanol and ethanol, slightly soluble in acetonitrile, and practically insoluble in water and hexane. The melting point ranges from 144.2°C to 145.2°C. ZYFLO tablets for oral administration is supplied in one dosage strength containing 600 mg of zileuton.

Inactive Ingredients: crospovidone, hydroxypropyl cellulose, hydroxypropyl methylcellulose, magnesium stearate, microcrystalline cellulose, pregelatinized starch, propylene glycol, sodium starch glycolate, talc, and titanium dioxide.

CLINICAL PHARMACOLOGY

Mechanism of Action:
Zileuton is a specific inhibitor of 5-lipoxygenase and thus inhibits leukotriene (LTB_4, LTC_4, LTD_4, and LTE_4) formation. Both the R(+) and S(-) enantiomers are pharmacologically active as 5-lipoxygenase inhibitors in *in vitro* systems. Leukotrienes are substances that induce numerous biological effects including augmentation of neutrophil and eosinophil migration, neutrophil and monocyte aggregation, leukocyte adhesion, increased capillary permeability, and smooth muscle contraction. These effects contribute to inflammation, edema, mucus secretion, and bronchoconstriction in the airways of asthmatic patients. Sulfido-peptide leukotrienes (LTC_4, LTD_4, LTE_4, also known as the slow-releasing substances of anaphylaxis) and LTB_4, a chemoattractant for neutrophils and eosinophils, can be measured in a number of biological fluids including bronchoalveolar lavage fluid (BALF) from asthmatic patients.
Zileuton is an orally active inhibitor of *ex vivo* LTB_4 formation in several species, including dogs, monkeys, rats, sheep, and rabbits. Zileuton inhibits arachidonic acid-induced ear edema in mice, neutrophil migration in mice in response to polyacrylamide gel, and eosinophil migration into the lungs of antigen-challenged sheep.
Zileuton inhibits leukotriene-dependent smooth muscle contractions *in vitro* in guinea pig and human airways. The compound inhibits leukotriene-dependent bronchospasm in antigen and arachidonic acid-challenged guinea pigs. In antigen-challenged sheep, zileuton inhibits late-phase bronchoconstriction and airway hyperreactivity. In humans, pretreatment with zileuton attenuated bronchoconstriction caused by cold air challenge in patients with asthma.

PHARMACOKINETICS

Zileuton is rapidly absorbed upon oral administration with a mean time to peak plasma concentration (T_{max}) of 1.7 hours and a mean peak level (C_{max}) of 4.98 µg/mL. The absolute bioavailability of ZYFLO is unknown. Systemic exposure (mean AUC) following 600 mg ZYFLO administration is 19.2 µg.hr/mL. Plasma concentrations of zileuton are proportional to dose, and steady-state levels are predictable from single-dose pharmacokinetic data. Administration of ZYFLO with food resulted in a small but statistically significant increase (27%) in zileuton C_{max} without significant changes in the extent of absorption (AUC) or T_{max}. Therefore, ZYFLO can be administered with or without food (see **DOSAGE AND ADMINISTRATION**).
The apparent volume of distribution (V/F) of zileuton is approximately 1.2 L/kg. Zileuton is 93% bound to plasma proteins, primarily to albumin, with minor binding to α1-acid glycoprotein.
Elimination of zileuton is predominantly via metabolism with a mean terminal half-life of 2.5 hours. Apparent oral clearance of zileuton is 7.0 mL/min/kg. ZYFLO activity is primarily due to the parent drug. Studies with radiolabeled drug demonstrated that orally administered zileuton is well absorbed into the systemic circulation with 94.5% and 2.2% of the radiolabeled dose recovered in urine and feces, respectively. Several zileuton metabolites have been identified in human plasma and urine. These include two diastereomeric O-glucuronide conjugates (major metabolites) and an N-dehydroxylated metabolite of zileuton. The urinary excretion of the inactive N-dehydroxylated metabolite and unchanged zileuton each accounted for less than 0.5% of the dose. *In vitro* studies utilizing human liver microsomes have shown that zileuton and its N-dehydroxylated metabolite can be oxidatively metabolized by the cytochrome P450 isoenzymes 1A2, 2C9 and 3A4 (CYP1A2, CYP2C9 and CYP3A4).

Special populations:
Effect of age: Zileuton pharmacokinetics were similar in healthy elderly subjects (>65 years) compared to healthy younger adults (18 to 40 years).
Effect of gender: Across several studies, no significant gender effects were observed on the pharmacokinetics of zileuton.
Renal insufficiency: The pharmacokinetics of zileuton were similar in healthy subjects and in subjects with mild, moderate, and severe renal insufficiency. In subjects with renal failure requiring hemodialysis, zileuton pharmacokinetics were not altered by hemodialysis and a very small percentage of the administered zileuton dose (<0.5%) was removed by hemodialysis. Hence, dosing adjustment in patients with renal dysfunction or undergoing hemodialysis is not necessary.
Hepatic insufficiency: ZYFLO is contraindicated in patients with active liver disease (see **CONTRAINDICATIONS** and **PRECAUTIONS, Hepatic**).

CLINICAL STUDIES

Two double-blind, parallel, placebo-controlled, multi-center studies have established the efficacy of ZYFLO in the treatment of asthma. Three hundred seventy-three (373) patients were enrolled in the 6-month, double-blind phase of Study 1, and 401 patients were enrolled in the 3-month double-blind phase of Study 2. In these studies, the patients were mild-to-moderate asthmatics who had a mean baseline FEV_1 of approximately 2.3 liters and who used inhaled beta-agonists as needed, the mean being approximately 6 puffs of albuterol per day from a metered-dose inhaler. In each study, patients were randomized to receive either ZYFLO 400 mg four times daily, ZYFLO 600 mg four times daily, or placebo. Only the ZYFLO 600 mg four times daily dosage regimen was shown to be efficacious by demonstrating statistically significant improvement across several parameters.
Efficacy endpoints measured in Study 1 are shown in Table 1 below as mean change from baseline to the end of the study (six months). Statistically significant differences from placebo at the $p<0.05$ level are indicated by an asterisk(*). Similar results were observed after three months in Study 2.

Table 1
MEAN CHANGE FROM BASELINE TO END OF STUDY (Six-Month Study)

Efficacy Endpoint	ZYFLO 600 mg 4 times/ day	Placebo
Trough FEV_1(L)	0.27	0.14
AM PEFR (L/min)	30.60*	5.04
PM PEFR (L/min)	24.59*	7.98
β-Agonist Use (puffs/day)	-1.77*	-0.22
Daily Symptom Score (0–3 Scale)	-0.49*	-0.28
Nocturnal Symptom Score (0–3 Scale)	-0.29*	-0.04

Continued on next page

Zyflo—Cont.

Figure 1 shows the mean effect of ZYFLO versus placebo for the primary efficacy variable, trough FEV_1, over the course of Study 1.

Figure 1
Mean Change From Baseline in Trough FEV_1 (L)

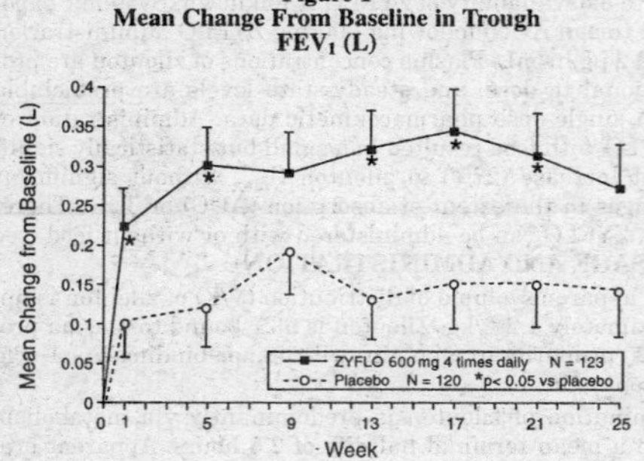

Of all the patients in Study 1 and Study 2, 7.0% of those administered ZYFLO 600 mg four times daily required systemic corticosteroid therapy for exacerbation of asthma, whereas 18.7% of the placebo group required corticosteroid treatment. This difference was statistically significant.

In these trials, there was a statistically significant improvement from baseline in FEV_1, which occurred 2 hours after initial administration of ZYFLO. This mean increase was approximately 0.10 L greater than that in placebo-treated patients.

These studies evaluated patients receiving as-needed inhaled beta-agonist as their only asthma therapy. In this patient population, post-hoc analyses suggested that individuals with lower FEV_1 values at baseline showed a greater improvement.

The role of ZYFLO in the management of patients with more severe asthma, patients receiving anti-asthma therapy other than as-needed, inhaled beta-agonists, or patients receiving it as an oral or inhaled corticosteroid-sparing agent remains to be fully characterized.

INDICATIONS AND USAGE

ZYFLO is indicated for the prophylaxis and chronic treatment of asthma in adults and children 12 years of age and older.

CONTRAINDICATIONS

ZYFLO tablets are contraindicated in patients with:

- Active liver disease or transaminase elevations greater than or equal to three times the upper limit of normal (≥3×ULN) (see **PRECAUTIONS, Hepatic**).
- Hypersensitivity to zileuton or any of its inactive ingredients.

WARNINGS

ZYFLO is not indicated for use in the reversal of bronchospasm in acute asthma attacks, including status asthmaticus. Therapy with ZYFLO can be continued during acute exacerbations of asthma.

Co-administration of ZYFLO and theophylline results in, on average, an approximate doubling of serum theophylline concentrations. Theophylline dosage in these patients should be reduced and serum theophylline concentrations monitored closely (see **PRECAUTIONS, Drug Interactions**).

Co-administration of ZYFLO and warfarin results in a clinically significant increase in prothrombin time (PT). Patients on oral warfarin therapy and ZYFLO should have their prothrombin times monitored closely and anticoagulant dose adjusted accordingly (see **PRECAUTIONS, Drug Interactions**).

Co-administration of ZYFLO and propranolol results in doubling of propranolol AUC and consequent increased beta-blocker activity. Patients on ZYFLO and propranolol should be closely monitored and the dose of the propranolol reduced as necessary (see **PRECAUTIONS, Drug Interactions**).

PRECAUTIONS

Hepatic: Elevations of one or more liver function tests may occur during ZYFLO therapy. These laboratory abnormalities may progress, remain unchanged, or resolve with continued therapy. In a few cases, initial transaminase elevations were first noted after discontinuing treatment, usually within 2 weeks. The ALT (SGPT) test is considered the most sensitive indicator of liver injury. In placebo-controlled clinical trials, the frequency of ALT elevations greater than or equal to three times the upper limit of normal (3×ULN) was 1.9% for ZYFLO-treated patients, compared with 0.2% for placebo-treated patients.

In a long-term safety surveillance study, 2458 patients received ZYFLO in addition to their usual asthma care and 489 received their usual asthma care. In patients treated for up to 12 months with ZYFLO in addition to their usual asthma care, 4.6% developed an ALT of at least 3×ULN, compared with 1.1% of patients receiving only their usual asthma care. Sixty-one percent of these elevations occurred during the first two months of ZYFLO therapy. After two months of treatment, the rate of new ALT elevations ≥3×ULN stabilized at a mean of 0.30% per month for patients receiving ZYFLO-plus-usual-asthma care compared with 0.11% per month for patients receiving usual asthma care alone. Of the 61 ZYFLO-plus-usual-asthma-care patients with ALT elevations between 3 to 5×ULN, 32 patients (52%) had ALT values decrease to below 2×ULN while continuing ZYFLO therapy. Twenty-one of the 61 patients (34%) had further increases in ALT levels to ≥ 5×ULN and were withdrawn from the study in accordance with the study protocol. In patients who discontinued ZYFLO, elevated ALT levels returned to < 2×ULN in an average of 32 days (range 1–111 days).

In controlled and uncontrolled clinical trials involving more than 5000 patients treated with ZYFLO, the overall rate of ALT elevation ≥ 3×ULN was 3.2%. In these trials, one patient developed symptomatic hepatitis with jaundice, which resolved upon discontinuation of therapy. An additional 3 patients with transaminase elevations developed mild hyperbilirubinemia that was less than three times the upper limit of normal. There was no evidence of hypersensitivity or other alternative etiologies for these findings. In subset analyses, females over the age of 65 appeared to be at an increased risk for ALT elevations. Patients with pre-existing transaminase elevations may also be at an increased risk for ALT elevations (see **CONTRAINDICATIONS**).

It is recommended that hepatic transaminases be evaluated at initiation of, and during therapy with, ZYFLO. Serum ALT should be monitored before treatment begins, once-a-month for the first 3 months, every two to three months for the remainder of the first year, and periodically thereafter for patients receiving long-term ZYFLO therapy. If clinical signs and/or symptoms of liver dysfunction (e.g., right upper quadrant pain, nausea, fatigue, lethargy, pruritus, jaundice, or "flu-like" symptoms) develop or transaminase elevations greater than 5 times the ULN occur, ZYFLO should be discontinued and transaminase levels followed until normal.

Since treatment with ZYFLO may result in increased hepatic transaminases, ZYFLO should be used with caution in patients who consume substantial quantities of alcohol and/or have a past history of liver disease.

Information for Patients: Patients should be told that:

- ZYFLO is indicated for the chronic treatment of asthma and should be taken regularly as prescribed, even during symptom-free periods.
- ZYFLO is not a bronchodilator and should not be used to treat acute episodes of asthma.
- When taking ZYFLO, they should not decrease the dose or stop taking any other antiasthma medications unless instructed by a physician.
- While using ZYFLO, medical attention should be sought if short-acting bronchodilators are needed more often than usual, or if more than the maximum number of inhalations of short-acting bronchodilator treatment prescribed for a 24-hour period are needed.
- The most serious side effect of ZYFLO is elevation of liver enzyme tests and that, while taking ZYFLO, they must return for liver enzyme test monitoring on a regular basis.
- If they experience signs and/or symptoms of liver dysfunction (e.g., right upper quadrant pain, nausea, fatigue, lethargy, pruritus, jaundice, or "flu-like" symptoms), they should contact their physician immediately.
- ZYFLO can interact with other drugs and that, while taking ZYFLO, they should consult their doctor before starting or stopping any prescription or non-prescription medicines.

A patient leaflet is included with the tablets.

Drug Interactions: In a drug-interaction study in 16 healthy volunteers, co-administration of multiple doses of zileuton (800 mg every 12 hours) and theophylline (200 mg every 6 hours) for 5 days resulted in a significant decrease (approximately 50%) in steady-state clearance of theophylline, an approximate doubling of theophylline AUC, and an increase in theophylline C_{max} (by 73%). The elimination half-life of theophylline was increased by 24%. Also, during co-administration, theophylline-related adverse events were observed more frequently than after theophylline alone. Upon initiation of ZYFLO in patients receiving theophylline, the theophylline dosage should be reduced by approximately one-half and plasma theophylline concentrations monitored. Similarly, when initiating therapy with theophylline in a patient receiving ZYFLO, the maintenance dose and/or dosing interval of theophylline should be adjusted accordingly and guided by serum theophylline determinations (see **WARNINGS**).

Concomitant administration of multiple doses of ZYFLO (600 mg every 6 hours) and warfarin (fixed daily dose obtained by titration in each subject) to 30 healthy male volunteers resulted in a 15% decrease in R-warfarin clearance and an increase in AUC of 22%. The pharmacokinetics of S-warfarin were not affected. These pharmacokinetic changes were accompanied by a clinically significant increase in prothrombin times. Monitoring of prothrombin time, or other suitable coagulation tests, with the appropriate dose titration of warfarin is recommended in patients receiving concomitant ZYFLO and warfarin therapy (see **WARNINGS**).

Co-administration of ZYFLO and propranolol results in a significant increase in propranolol concentrations. Administration of a single 80-mg dose of propranolol in 16 healthy male volunteers who received ZYFLO 600 mg every 6 hours for 5 days resulted in a 42% decrease in propranolol clearance. This resulted in an increase in propranolol C_{max}, AUC, and elimination half-life by 52%, 104%, and 25%, respectively. There was an increase in β-blockade and decrease in heart rate associated with the co-administration of these drugs. Patients on ZYFLO and propranolol should be closely monitored and the dose of propranolol reduced as necessary (see **WARNINGS**). No formal drug-drug interaction studies between ZYFLO and other beta-adrenergic blocking agents (i.e., β-blockers) have been conducted. It is reasonable to employ appropriate clinical monitoring when these drugs are co-administered with ZYFLO.

In a drug interaction study in 16 healthy volunteers, co-administration of multiple doses of terfenadine (60 mg every 12 hours) and ZYFLO (600 mg every 6 hours) for 7 days resulted in a decrease in clearance of terfenadine by 22% leading to a statistically significant increase in mean AUC and C_{max} of terfenadine of approximately 35%. This increase in terfenadine plasma concentration in the presence of ZYFLO was not associated with a significant prolongation of the QTc interval. Although there was no cardiac effect in this small number of healthy volunteers, given the high inter-individual pharmacokinetic variability of terfenadine, co-administration of ZYFLO and terfenadine is not recommended.

Drug-drug interaction studies conducted in healthy volunteers between ZYFLO and prednisone and ethinyl estradiol (oral contraceptive), drugs known to be metabolized by the P450 3A4 (CYP3A4) isoenzyme, have shown no significant interaction. However, no formal drug-drug interaction studies between ZYFLO and dihydropyridine, calcium channel blockers, cyclosporine, cisapride, and astemizole, also metabolized by CYP3A4, have been conducted. It is reasonable to employ appropriate clinical monitoring when these drugs are co-administered with ZYFLO.

Drug-drug interaction studies in healthy volunteers have been conducted with ZYFLO and digoxin, phenytoin, sulfasalazine, and naproxen. There was no significant interaction between ZYFLO and any of these drugs.

Carcinogenesis, Mutagenesis, Impairment of Fertility: In 2-year carcinogenicity studies, increases in the incidence of liver, kidney, and vascular tumors in female mice and a trend towards an increase in the incidence of liver tumors in male mice were observed at 450 mg/kg/day (providing approximately 4 times [females] or 7 times [males] the systemic exposure [AUC] achieved at the maximum recommended human daily oral dose). No increase in the incidence of tumors was observed at 150 mg/kg/day (providing approximately 2 times the systemic exposure [AUC] achieved at the maximum recommended human daily oral dose). In rats, an increase in the incidence of kidney tumors was observed in both sexes at 170 mg/kg/day (providing approximately 6 times [males] or 14 times [females] the systemic exposure [AUC] achieved at the maximum recommended human daily oral dose). No increased incidence of kidney tumors was seen at 80 mg/kg/day (providing approximately 4 times [males] or 6 times [females] the systemic exposure [AUC] achieved at the maximum recommended human daily oral dose). Although a dose-related increased incidence of benign Leydig cell tumors was observed, Leydig cell tumorigenesis was prevented by supplementing male rats with testosterone.

Zileuton was negative in genotoxicity studies including bacterial reverse mutation (Ames) using *S. typhimurium* and *E. coli*, chromosome aberration in human lymphocytes, *in vitro* unscheduled DNA synthesis (UDS), in rat hepatocytes with or without zileuton pretreatment and in mouse and rat kidney cells with zileuton pretreatment, and mouse micronucleus assays. However, a dose-related increase in DNA adduct formation was reported in kidneys and livers of female mice treated with zileuton. Although some evidence of DNA damage was observed in a UDS assay in hepatocytes isolated from Aroclor-1254 treated rats, no such finding was noticed in hepatocytes isolated from monkeys, where the metabolic profile of zileuton is more similar to that of humans.

In reproductive performance/fertility studies, zileuton produced no effects on fertility in rats at oral doses up to 300 mg/kg/day (providing approximately 8 times [male rats] and 18 times [female rats] the systemic exposure [AUC] achieved at the maximum recommended human daily oral dose). Comparative systemic exposure (AUC) is based on measurements in male rats or nonpregnant female rats at similar dosages. However, reduction in fetal implants was observed at oral doses of 150 mg/kg/day and higher (providing approximately 9 times the systemic exposure [AUC] achieved at the maximum recommended human daily oral dose). Increases in gestation length, prolongation of estrous cycle, and increases in stillbirths were observed at oral doses of 70 mg/kg/day and higher (providing approximately 4 times the systemic exposure (AUC) achieved at the maximum recommended human daily oral dose). In a perinatal/postnatal study in rats, reduced pup survival and growth were noted at an oral dose of 300 mg/kg/day (providing approximately 18 times the systemic exposure [AUC] achieved at the maximum recommended human daily oral dose).

Pregnancy: Pregnancy Category C: Developmental studies indicated adverse effects (reduced body weight and increased skeletal variations) in rats at an oral dose of 300 mg/kg/day (providing approximately 18 times the systemic exposure [AUC] achieved at the maximum recommended human daily oral dose). Comparative systemic exposure [AUC] is based on measurements in nonpregnant female rats at a similar dosage. Zileuton and/or its metabolites cross the placental barrier of rats. Three of 118 (2.5%) rabbit fetuses had cleft palates at an oral dose of 150 mg/kg/day (equivalent to the maximum recommended human daily oral dose on a mg/m^2 basis). There are no adequate and well-controlled studies in pregnant women.

ZYFLO should be used during pregnancy only if the potential benefit justifies the potential risk to the fetus.

Nursing Mothers: Zileuton and/or its metabolites are excreted in rat milk. It is not known if zileuton is excreted in human milk. Because many drugs are excreted in human milk, and because of the potential for tumorigenicity shown for ZYFLO in animal studies, a decision should be made whether to discontinue nursing or to discontinue the drug, taking into account the importance of the drug to the mother.

Pediatric Use: The safety and effectiveness of ZYFLO in pediatric patients under 12 years of age have not been established.

ADVERSE REACTIONS

Clinical Studies: A total of 5542 patients have been exposed to zileuton in clinical trials, 2252 of them for greater than 6 months and 742 for greater than 1 year.

Adverse events most frequently occurring (frequency ≥3%) in ZYFLO-treated patients and at a frequency greater than placebo-treated patients are summarized in Table 2.

TABLE 2
Proportion of Patients Experiencing Adverse Events in Placebo-Controlled Studies in Asthma

BODY SYSTEM/Event	ZYFLO 600 mg 4 times daily % Occurrence (N = 475)	Placebo % Occurrence (N = 491)
BODY AS A WHOLE		
Headache	24.6	24.0
Pain (unspecified)	7.8	5.3
Abdominal Pain	4.6	2.4
Asthenia	3.8	2.4
Accidental Injury	3.4	2.0
DIGESTIVE SYSTEM		
Dyspepsia	8.2*	2.9
Nausea	5.5	3.7
MUSCULOSKELETAL		
Myalgia	3.2	2.9

* p≤0.05 vs placebo

Less common adverse events occurring at a frequency of greater than 1% and more commonly in ZYFLO-treated patients included: arthralgia, chest pain, conjunctivitis, constipation, dizziness, fever, flatulence, hypertonia, insomnia, lymphadenopathy, malaise, neck pain/rigidity, nervousness, pruritus, somnolence, urinary tract infection, vaginitis, and vomiting.

The frequency of discontinuation from the asthma clinical studies due to any adverse event was comparable between ZYFLO (9.7%) and placebo-treated (8.4%) groups.

In placebo-controlled clinical trials, the frequency of ALT elevations ≥3×ULN was 1.9% for ZYFLO-treated patients, compared with 0.2% for placebo-treated patients. In controlled and uncontrolled trials, one patient developed symptomatic hepatitis with jaundice, which resolved upon discontinuation of therapy. An additional 3 patients with transaminase elevations developed mild hyperbilirubinemia that was less than three times the upper limit of normal. There was no evidence of hypersensitivity or other alternative etiologies for these findings. ZYFLO is contraindicated in patients with active liver disease or transaminase elevations greater than or equal to 3×ULN (see **CONTRAINDICATIONS**). It is recommended that hepatic transaminases be evaluated at initiation of and during therapy with ZYFLO (see **PRECAUTIONS, Hepatic**).

Occurrences of low white blood cell count (≤ 2.8×10^9/L) were observed in 1.0% of 1,678 patients taking ZYFLO and 0.6% of 1,056 patients taking placebo in placebo-controlled studies. These findings were transient and the majority of cases returned toward normal or baseline with continued ZYFLO dosing. All remaining cases returned toward normal or baseline after discontinuation of ZYFLO. Similar findings were also noted in a long-term safety surveillance study of 2458 patients treated with ZYFLO plus usual asthma care versus 489 patients treated only with usual asthma care for up to one year. The clinical significance of these observations is not known.

In the long-term safety surveillance trial of ZYFLO plus usual asthma care versus usual asthma care alone, a similar adverse event profile was seen as in other clinical trials.

Post-Marketing Experience: Rash and urticaria have been reported with ZYFLO.

OVERDOSAGE

Human experience of acute overdose with zileuton is limited. A patient in a clinical trial took between 6.6 and 9.0 grams of zileuton in a single dose. Vomiting was induced and the patient recovered without sequelae. Zileuton is not removed by dialysis. Should an overdose occur, the patient should be treated symptomatically and supportive measures instituted as required. If indicated, elimination of unabsorbed drug should be achieved by emesis or gastric lavage; usual precautions should be observed to maintain the airway. A Certified Poison Control Center should be consulted for up-to-date information on management of overdose with ZYFLO.

The oral minimum lethal doses in mice and rats were 500–4000 and 300–1000 mg/kg in various preparations, respectively (providing greater than 3 and 9 times the systemic exposure [AUC] achieved at the maximum recommended human daily oral dose, respectively). No deaths occurred, but nephritis was reported in dogs at an oral dose of 1000 mg/kg (providing in excess of 12 times the systemic exposure [AUC] achieved at the maximum recommended human daily oral dose).

DOSAGE AND ADMINISTRATION

The recommended dosage of ZYFLO for the symptomatic treatment of patients with asthma is one 600-mg tablet four times a day for a total daily dose of 2400 mg. For ease of administration, ZYFLO may be taken with meals and at bedtime. Hepatic transaminases should be evaluated prior to initiation of ZYFLO and periodically during treatment (see **PRECAUTIONS, Hepatic**).

HOW SUPPLIED

ZYFLO Filmtab Tablets are available as 1 dosage strength: 600-mg white ovaloid tablets with single bisect, debossed on bisect side with Abbott logo and ZL (Abbo-Code), and 600 on the opposite side:

High-density polyethylene
bottles of 120 .... (**NDC** 0074-8036-22)

Recommended storage: Store tablets at controlled room temperature between 20°–25°C, (68°–77°F). See USP. Protect from light.

TM – Trademark
Filmtab - Film-sealed tablets, Abbott
Revised March 1998
Ref. 03-4854-R2
ABBOTT LABORATORIES
NORTH CHICAGO, IL 60064, U.S.A.

ZYFLO™ FILMTAB®
(zileuton tablets)

Patient Information
Medication Guide
Zyflo™ Filmtab® Tablets
Generic Name: zileuton

Please read this leaflet carefully before you start taking Zyflo™ Filmtab® tablets. Also, read it each time you get your Zyflo prescription refilled.

This leaflet provides important information about taking Zyflo. It is not meant to take the place of your doctor's specific instructions. Talk to your doctor if you have any questions about Zyflo. Your doctor or pharmacist can also provide you with additional information about Zyflo.

What is the most important information I should know about Zyflo?

The most important things to remember are to take all your doses of Zyflo every day and to make sure that you return to your doctor's office for scheduled liver enzyme tests.

You should also know that you should seek medical help immediately if you need more "puffs" of your bronchodilator inhaler than normal or if you use the maximum number of "puffs" prescribed for one 24-hour period. These could be a sign of worsening asthma which means that your asthma therapy may need to be changed.

What is Zyflo?

Zyflo, which contains the active ingredient zileuton, blocks the formation of certain chemicals (leukotrienes) that may contribute to your asthma symptoms.

Who should not take Zyflo?

You should not take Zyflo if you:

- have active liver disease or have liver enzymes that are elevated.
- have ever had an allergic reaction to this medicine.

Your doctor will determine if it is safe for you to take Zyflo.

What should I tell my doctor before I take the first dose of Zyflo?

You should tell your doctor if you:

- have ever had liver disease, hepatitis, jaundice (yellow eyes or skin), or dark urine.
- drink alcohol.
- are taking any prescription or nonprescription medicines. Your doctor may adjust the doses of some of your other medicines while you are taking Zyflo.
- if you are taking theophylline for your asthma, the blood-thinning medication warfarin, or the blood-pressure medication propranolol. Your doctor may need to change the doses of these drugs.
- are pregnant, planning to become pregnant, or are breast-feeding.

How should I take Zyflo?

- Zyflo is taken four times a day with or without food. It may be easier to remember to take Zyflo if you make it part of your daily routine such as with meals and at bedtime.
- For Zyflo to help control your asthma symptoms, it must be taken every day as prescribed by your doctor. Zyflo WILL NOT relieve an asthma attack that has already started. While taking Zyflo, it is important to keep taking your other asthma medicines as directed and to follow all of your doctor's instructions.
- Even if you have no asthma symptoms, do not decrease the dose of Zyflo or stop taking the medicine without talking to your doctor first. Feeling good is a sign that the medicine is working.
- When you take your dose of Zyflo, the tablets may be swallowed whole or split in half to make them easier to swallow.

What should I avoid while taking Zyflo?

- Because Zyflo may affect how other medications work, always talk to your doctor before you start or stop taking any medicines while taking Zyflo. This includes all prescription and nonprescription medicines.
- Never take a larger dose of Zyflo or take it more often than your doctor has prescribed.
- It is also important for you to know that it may take several days or a few weeks to get the full benefit from Zyflo and that you should not stop taking it if you do not feel better right away.

What are the possible side effects of Zyflo?

All medicines, including Zyflo, cause side effects in some people. Some of the most common side effects are abdominal pain, upset stomach, and nausea. You should tell your doctor if you experience any new or unusual symptoms while taking Zyflo.

One side effect that occurs in a small number of patients is an increased release of substances from the liver called "enzymes." Liver enzymes can be measured by a simple blood test. It is important that your doctor makes sure that your liver enzymes do not become too high and that it is safe for you to continue taking Zyflo. To insure your safety, your doctor will do this blood test before you first start taking Zyflo and repeat it on a regular basis while you are taking the medicine.

Usually, even if your liver enzymes are increased, you will not notice any symptoms. However, some symptoms of increased liver enzymes are feeling more tired than normal, "flu-like" symptoms, itching, yellow skin and/or yellow color in the whites of the eyes, or urine that is darker than normal.

If you notice these or any other symptoms that you think may be caused by Zyflo, call your doctor immediately. Once the medicine is stopped, these symptoms usually go away. Even if you do not have any of these symptoms, you should continue to see your doctor for regular check-ups and liver enzyme tests.

Where should I keep my supply of Zyflo?

Keep Zyflo and all medicines out of the reach of children. In case of an accidental overdose, call your doctor or a Poison Control Center immediately.

Protect Zyflo from light and replace the child-resistant cap each time after use. Store Zyflo between 68°–77°F (20°–25°C).

If you would like more information about Zyflo, ask your doctor or pharmacist. If you have any questions or concerns about taking Zyflo, discuss them with your doctor.

Filmtab - Film-sealed tablets, Abbott
TM - Trademark
Revised March, 1998
Ref. 03-4854-R2
ABBOTT LABORATORIES
NORTH CHICAGO, IL 60064, U.S.A.

Shown in Product Identification Guide, page 303

Advanced Nutritional Technology®, Inc.

6988 SIERRA CT.
DUBLIN, CA 94568

Direct Inquiries to:
(925) 828–2128
FAX: (925) 828–6848

NUTR-E-SOL® OTC
(Water Soluble Natural Vitamin E (TPGS) For Maximum Absorption)

FORMULATION

400 I.U. Water Soluble Natural Vitamin E (TPGS) per tablespoon

PHYSIOLOGICAL CONSIDERATIONS

Advanced Nutritional Technology's Nutr-E-Sol is a high potency water soluble natural vitamin E designed for fast absorption.

Nutr-E-Sol contains a unique form of vitamin E (d-α-tocopheryl polyethylene glycol 1000 succinate or TPGS) that is absorbed directly through the intestinal wall without the use of bile for emulsification. Nutr-E-Sol is useful in raising vitamin E blood levels in diseases such as Cystic Fibrosis, Crohn's Disease, Short Bowel Syndrome, Biliary Cirrhosis and Cholestatis, where vitamin E blood levels are low.

Nutr-E-Sol may be taken alone or mixed with drinks. This product is tasteless and sugar-free for better compliance with the young and diabetic.

Studies indicate that Nutr-E-Sol's form of Vitamin E is absorbed better than other water-soluble vitamin E supplements, dry vitamin E supplements and emulsified forms of vitamin E.

DOSAGE

Liquid—One to three tablespoon per day

Continued on next page

Nutr-E-Sol—Cont.

HOW SUPPLIED

	SIZE	NDC #
Nutr-E-Sol	8 oz	62617-515-10
Nutr-E-Sol	16 oz	62617-515-20

SUPEREPA 2000® OTC
(Eicosapentaenoic Acid and Docosahexaenoic Acid)

FORMULATION

Each softgel contains 1000 mg omega-3 (EPA 500 mg, DHA 310 mg, Other Omega-3 Fatty Acid 190 mg)
All strengths are cholesterol free! No vitamin A & D or sodium are added and each product is free of toxic metals.

PHYSIOLOGICAL CONSIDERATIONS

SuperEPA 2000® softgels are highly concentrated, cholesterol free fish oils providing up to three times the strength of other omega-3 fatty acid nutritional supplements. SuperEPA 2000® is recommended as part of a dietary intervention plan for people at early risk of coronary heart disease. Such a plan should include reduction of cholesterol and total dietary fat intake and an increase in the ratio of polyunsaturated to saturated fats. SuperEPA 2000® is being studied around the world in areas such as blood lipid control, inflammation, diabetes, arthritis schizoaffective disorder and cognitive functioning in patients with schizophrenia.

DOSAGE

One to three softgels daily, taken with meals.

HOW SUPPLIED

	SIZE	NDC #
SuperEPA 2000®	90's	62617-050-03

ULTRA ZN
Prostate Formula **OTC**

PHYSIOLOGICAL CONSIDERATIONS

Ultra Zn has been proven a significant difference reduce in frequency urine flow measurement; dysuria residuile urine; perineal heaviness, nocturia, interval between two diurnal voilings, sensation of incomplete voiding

DOSAGE

One or two tablets daily, taken with meals.

HOW SUPPLIED

	SIZE	NDC #
Ultra Zn	60's	62617-460-02

Agouron Pharmaceuticals, Inc.

**10350 NORTH TORREY PINES ROAD
LA JOLLA, CA 92037-1020**

Direct Inquiries to:
Customer Communications
(888) VIRACEPT
FAX: (858) 678–8266
Medical Emergency Contact:
Medical Affairs
(888) VIRACEPT
FAX: (858) 678–8245

RESCRIPTOR® ℞
[rē 'scrĭp-tor]
(delavirdine mesylate) tablets

> **WARNING:** RESCRIPTOR Tablets are indicated for the treatment of HIV-1 infection in combination with appropriate antiretroviral agents when therapy is warranted. This indication is based on surrogate marker changes in clinical studies. Clinical benefit was not demonstrated for RESCRIPTOR based on survival or incidence of AIDS-defining clinical events in a completed trial comparing RESCRIPTOR plus didanosine with didanosine monotherapy (see DESCRIPTION OF CLINICAL STUDIES).
> Resistant virus emerges rapidly when RESCRIPTOR is administered as monotherapy. Therefore, RESCRIPTOR should always be administered in combination with appropriate antiretroviral therapy.

DESCRIPTION

RESCRIPTOR Tablets contain delavirdine mesylate, a synthetic non-nucleoside reverse transcriptase inhibitor of the human immunodeficiency virus type 1 (HIV-1). The chemical name of delavirdine mesylate is piperazine, 1-[3-[(1-methyl-ethyl)amino]-2-pyridinyl]-4-[[5-[(methylsulfonyl)-amino]-1*H*-indol-2-yl]carbonyl]-, monomethanesulfonate. Its molecular formula is $C_{22}H_{28}N_6O_3S \cdot CH_4O_3S$, and its molecular weight is 552.68. The structural formula is:

Delavirdine mesylate is an odorless white-to-tan crystalline powder. The aqueous solubility of delavirdine free base at 23°C is 2,942 µg/mL at pH 1.0, 295 µg/mL at pH 2.0, and 0.81 µg/mL at pH 7.4.
Each RESCRIPTOR Tablet, for oral administration, contains 100 or 200 mg of delavirdine mesylate (henceforth referred to as delavirdine). Inactive ingredients consist of lactose, microcrystalline cellulose, croscarmellose sodium magnesium stearate, colloidal silicon dioxide, and carnauba wax. In addition, the 100-mg tablet contains Opadry White YS-1-7000-E and the 200-mg tablet contains hydroxypropyl methylcellulose, Opadry White YS-1-18202-A, and Pharmaceutical Ink Black.

MICROBIOLOGY

Mechanism of action: Delavirdine is a non-nucleoside reverse transcriptase inhibitor (NNRTI) of HIV-1. Delavirdine binds directly to reverse transcriptase (RT) and blocks RNA-dependent and DNA-dependent polymerase activities. Delavirdine does not compete with template: primer or deoxynucleoside triphosphates. HIV-2 RT and human cellular DNA polymerases α, γ, or δ are not inhibited by delavirdine. In addition, HIV-1 group O, a group of highly divergent strains that are uncommon in North America, may not be inhibited by delavirdine.
In vitro HIV-1 susceptibility: In vitro anti–HIV-1 activity of delavirdine was assessed by infecting cell lines of lymphoblastic and monocytic origin and peripheral blood lymphocytes with laboratory and clinical isolates of HIV-1. IC_{50} and IC_{90} values (50% and 90% inhibitory concentrations) for laboratory isolates (N=5) ranged from 0.005 to 0.030 µM and 0.04 to 0.10 µM, respectively. Mean IC_{50} of clinical isolates (N=74) was 0.038 µM (range 0.001 to 0.69 µM); 73 of 74 clinical isolates had an $IC_{50} \leq 0.18$ µM. The IC_{90} of 24 of these clinical isolates ranged from 0.05 to 0.10 µM. In drug combination studies of delavirdine with zidovudine, didanosine, zalcitabine, lamivudine, interferon-α, and protease inhibitors, additive to synergistic anti–HIV-1 activity was observed in cell culture. The relationship between the in vitro susceptibility of HIV-1 RT inhibitors and the inhibition of HIV replication in humans has not been established.
Drug resistance: Phenotypic analyses of isolates from patients treated with delavirdine as monotherapy showed a 50-fold to 500-fold reduction in sensitivity in 14 of 15 patients by week 8 of therapy. Genotypic analyses of HIV-1 isolates from patients receiving delavirdine plus zidovudine combination therapy (N=19) showed mutations in 16 of 19 isolates by week 24 of therapy. Mutations occurred predominantly at position 103 and less frequently at positions 181 and 236. In a separate study, an average 86-fold increase in the zidovudine sensitivity of patient isolates (N=24) was observed after 24 weeks on delavirdine and zidovudine combination therapy. The clinical relevance of the phenotypic and the genotypic changes associated with delavirdine therapy has not been determined.
Cross-resistance: Rapid emergence of HIV strains that are cross-resistant to certain NNRTIs has been observed in vitro. Mutations at positions 103 and 181 have been associated with resistance to other NNRTIs. RESCRIPTOR may confer cross-resistance to other non-nucleoside reverse transcriptase inhibitors when used alone or in combination.
The potential for cross-resistance between delavirdine and protease inhibitors is low because of the different enzyme targets involved. The potential for cross-resistance between NNRTIs and nucleoside analogue RT inhibitors is low because of different sites of binding on the viral RT and distinct mechanisms of action.

CLINICAL PHARMACOLOGY

Pharmacokinetics

Absorption and Bioavailability: Delavirdine is rapidly absorbed following oral administration, with peak plasma concentrations occurring at approximately one hour. Following administration of delavirdine 400 mg tid (n=67, HIV-1–infected patients), the mean ± SD steady-state peak plasma concentration (C_{max}) was 35 ± 20 µM (range 2 to 100 µM), systemic exposure (AUC) was 180 ± 100 µM • hr (range 5 to 515 µM • hr) and trough concentration (C_{min}) was 15 ± 10 µM (range 0.1 to 45 µM). The single-dose bioavailability of delavirdine tablets relative to an oral solution was 85 ± 25% (n=16, non-HIV–infected subjects). The single-dose bioavailability of delavirdine tablets (100-mg strength) was increased by approximately 20% when a slurry of drug was prepared by allowing delavirdine tablets to disintegrate in water before administration (n=16, non-HIV–infected subjects). The bioavailability of the 200-mg strength delavirdine tablets has not been evaluated when administered as a slurry, because they are not readily dispersed in water (see DOSAGE AND ADMINISTRATION).
Delavirdine may be administered with or without food. Following single-dose administration of delavirdine tablets with a high-fat meal (874 kcal, 57 g fat), mean C_{max} was decreased by 60% and mean AUC was decreased by 26%, relative to fasted administration (n=12, non-HIV–infected subjects). In a multiple-dose study, delavirdine was administered every eight hours with food or every eight hours, one hour before or two hours after a meal (n=13, HIV-1–infected patients). Patients remained on their typical diet throughout the study; meal content was not standardized. When multiple doses of delavirdine were administered with food, mean C_{max} was reduced by 22% but AUC and C_{min} were not altered.
Distribution: Delavirdine is extensively bound (approximately 98%) to plasma proteins, primarily albumin. The percentage of delavirdine that is protein bound is constant over a delavirdine concentration range of 0.5 to 196 µM. In five HIV-1–infected patients whose total daily dose of delavirdine ranged from 600 to 1200 mg, cerebrospinal fluid concentrations of delavirdine averaged 0.4% ± 0.07% of the corresponding plasma delavirdine concentrations; this represents about 20% of the fraction not bound to plasma proteins. Steady-state delavirdine concentrations in saliva (n=5, HIV-1–infected patients who received delavirdine 400 mg tid) and semen (n=5 healthy volunteers who received delavirdine 300 mg tid) were about 6% and 2%, respectively, of the corresponding plasma delavirdine concentrations collected at the end of a dosing interval.
Metabolism and Elimination: Delavirdine is extensively converted to several inactive metabolites. Delavirdine is primarily metabolized by cytochrome P450 3A (CYP3A), but in vitro data suggest that delavirdine may also be metabolized by CYP2D6. The major metabolic pathways for delavirdine are N-desalkylation and pyridine hydroxylation. Delavirdine exhibits nonlinear steady-state elimination pharmacokinetics, with apparent oral clearance decreasing by about 22-fold as the total daily dose of delavirdine increases from 60 to 1200 mg/day. In a study of ^{14}C-delavirdine in six healthy volunteers who received multiple doses of delavirdine tablets 300 mg tid, approximately 44% of the radiolabeled dose was recovered in feces, and approximately 51% of the dose was excreted in urine. Less than 5% of the dose was recovered unchanged in urine. The apparent plasma half-life of delavirdine increases with dose; mean half-life following 400 mg tid is 5.8 hours, with a range of 2 to 11 hours.
In vitro and in vivo studies have shown that delavirdine reduces CYP3A activity and inhibits its own metabolism. In vitro studies have also shown that delavirdine reduces CYP2C9 and CYP2C19 activity. Inhibition of CYP3A by delavirdine is reversible within 1 week after discontinuation of drug.

Special Populations

Hepatic or Renal Impairment: The pharmacokinetics of delavirdine in patients with hepatic or renal impairment have not been investigated (see PRECAUTIONS).
Age: The pharmacokinetics of delavirdine have not been studied in patients <16 years or >65 years of age.
Gender: Following administration of delavirdine (400 mg every eight hours), median delavirdine AUC was 31% higher in female patients (n=12) than in male patients (n=55).
Race: No significant differences in the mean trough delavirdine concentrations were observed between different racial or ethnic groups.

Drug Interactions (see also PRECAUTIONS-Drug Interactions)

Antacids: In a single-dose study in twelve healthy volunteers, simultaneous administration of 300 mg delavirdine with alumina and magnesia oral suspension resulted in a 41 ± 19% reduction in delavirdine AUC (see PRECAUTIONS-Drug Interactions).
Clarithromycin: In a study in six HIV-1–infected patients, coadministration of clarithromycin (500 mg bid) with delavirdine (300 mg tid) resulted in a 44 ± 50% increase in delavirdine AUC. Compared to historical data, clarithromycin AUC was increased by approximately 100% and 14-hydroxyclarithromycin AUC was decreased by 75%.
Didanosine: In a study of nine HIV-1–infected patients, simultaneous administration of didanosine (125 mg or 250 mg bid) with delavirdine (400 mg tid) for two weeks resulted in an approximately 20% decrease in both didanosine AUC and delavirdine AUC, relative to when administration of delavirdine and didanosine was separated by at least one hour (see PRECAUTIONS-Drug Interactions).
Fluconazole: In a study in eight HIV-1–infected patients, coadministration of fluconazole (400 mg once daily) with delavirdine (300 mg tid) did not significantly alter the pharmacokinetics of delavirdine. Compared to historical data, fluconazole pharmacokinetics were not altered by delavirdine.
Fluoxetine: Population pharmacokinetic data available for 36 patients suggest that fluoxetine increases trough plasma delavirdine concentrations by about 50%.
Indinavir: Preliminary data (n=14) indicate that delavirdine inhibits the metabolism of indinavir such that coadministration of a 400 mg single dose of indinavir with delavirdine (400 mg tid) resulted in indinavir AUC values slightly less than those observed following administration of an 800 mg dose of indinavir alone. Also, coadministration of a 600 mg dose of indinavir with delavirdine (400 mg tid) resulted in indinavir AUC values approximately 40% greater than those observed following administration of an 800 mg dose of indinavir alone. Indinavir had no effect on delavirdine pharmacokinetics (see PRECAUTIONS-Drug Interactions).
Ketoconazole: Population pharmacokinetic data available for 26 patients suggest that ketoconazole increases trough plasma delavirdine concentrations by about 50%.
Phenytoin, Phenobarbital, and Carbamazepine: Population pharmacokinetic data available for eight patients sug-

gest that coadministration of phenytoin, phenobarbital, or carbamazepine with delavirdine results in a substantial reduction in trough plasma delavirdine concentrations (see PRECAUTIONS-Drug Interactions).

Rifabutin: In a study in seven HIV-1–infected patients, coadministration of rifabutin (300 mg once daily) with delavirdine (400 mg tid) resulted in an 80 ± 10% decrease in delavirdine AUC. Compared to historical data, rifabutin AUC was increased by at least 100% (see PRECAUTIONS-Drug Interactions).

Rifampin: In a study in seven HIV-1–infected patients, coadministration of rifampin (600 mg once daily) with delavirdine (400 mg tid) resulted in a 96 ± 4% decrease in delavirdine AUC (see PRECAUTIONS-Drug Interactions).

Ritonavir: Preliminary data (n=13) indicate that coadministration of delavirdine (400 mg or 600 mg bid) with ritonavir (300 mg bid) did not alter ritonavir pharmacokinetics. Coadministration of ritonavir (300 mg bid) with delavirdine (400 mg bid) did not significantly alter delavirdine pharmacokinetics (n=9). The pharmacokinetic interaction between delavirdine and ritonavir at their recommended doses has not been studied (see PRECAUTIONS-Drug Interactions).

Saquinavir: In 13 healthy volunteers, coadministration of saquinavir (600 mg tid) with delavirdine (400 mg tid) resulted in a five-fold increase in saquinavir AUC. In seven healthy volunteers, coadministration of saquinavir (600 mg tid) with delavirdine (400 mg tid) resulted in a 15 ± 16% decrease in delavirdine AUC (see PRECAUTIONS-Drug Interactions).

Sulfamethoxazole and Trimethoprim/Sulfamethoxazole (TMP/SMX): Population pharmacokinetic data available for 311 patients suggest that the pharmacokinetics of delavirdine are not affected by sulfamethoxazole or TMP/SMX.

Zidovudine: Zidovudine and delavirdine do not alter one another's pharmacokinetics.

INDICATIONS AND USAGE

RESCRIPTOR Tablets are indicated for the treatment of HIV-1 infection in combination with appropriate antiretroviral agents when therapy is warranted. This indication is based on surrogate marker changes in clinical studies. Clinical benefit was not demonstrated for RESCRIPTOR based on survival or incidence of AIDS-defining clinical events in a completed trial comparing RESCRIPTOR plus didanosine with didanosine monotherapy (see DESCRIPTION OF CLINICAL STUDIES).

Resistant virus emerges rapidly when RESCRIPTOR is administered as monotherapy. Therefore, RESCRIPTOR should always be administered in combination with appropriate antiretroviral therapy.

DESCRIPTION OF CLINICAL STUDIES

In two of the clinical studies described below (Study 0021, Part 1 and Study 0017), an experimental HIV nucleic acid amplification assay was used to estimate the level of circulating HIV RNA in plasma. In the clinical study ACTG 261, also described below, an approved HIV nucleic acid amplification assay was used.

Figures 1–3 below present results for all patients with data available at the time points shown. The decrease in sample size reflects patients leaving the study, missed visits, and those who had not reached specified time points at data cutoff. In general, patients who left the study had lower CD4 cell counts and higher plasma HIV RNA values than patients remaining on study. Therefore, absolute changes from baseline are overstated in all treatment arms, increasingly so at later time points. However, the added effect of delavirdine treatment relative to the control arms does not appear to be significantly affected by patient dropout.

Study 0021, Part 1: RESCRIPTOR-Zidovudine Dual Therapy Trial

Study 0021, Part 1 was a randomized, double-blind trial comparing treatment with RESCRIPTOR plus zidovudine and zidovudine monotherapy in 718 HIV-1–infected patients (median age 34.3 years [range 17 to 70 years], 19% female, 32% non-Caucasian). Patients were treatment naive or had received less than 6 months of prior zidovudine therapy. Mean baseline CD4 cell count was 334 cells/mm^3 (range 75 to 696 cells/mm^3) and mean baseline plasma HIV-1 RNA was 5.25 $\log_{10}$ copies/mL. Treatment doses were RESCRIPTOR 200 mg, 300 mg, or 400 mg tid plus zidovudine 200 mg tid or zidovudine monotherapy 200 mg tid. No statistically significant difference in CD4 cell count for the combination of RESCRIPTOR plus zidovudine compared with zidovudine monotherapy was observed in a planned analysis at 24 weeks. The mean change from baseline in $\log_{10}$ copies/mL plasma HIV-1 RNA is summarized in Fig 1 for RESCRIPTOR 400 mg tid plus zidovudine and zidovudine monotherapy. All patients had not completed 52 weeks at the time of this analysis.

[See figure 1 at top of next column]

Study 0017 RESCRIPTOR-Didanosine Dual Therapy Trial

Study 0017 was a randomized, double-blind trial comparing treatment with RESCRIPTOR plus didanosine versus didanosine monotherapy in 1,190 HIV-1–infected patients (median age 37.4 years [range 19 to 78 years], 13% female, 32% non-Caucasian). Patients had received up to 4 months prior didanosine therapy; there were no restrictions on prior zidovudine use. Mean baseline CD4 cell count was 142 cells/mm^3 (range 0 to 541 cells/mm^3) and mean baseline plasma HIV-1 RNA was 5.77 $\log_{10}$ copies/mL. Treatment doses were RESCRIPTOR 400 mg tid plus didanosine or didanosine

Fig 1: Mean Change From Baseline in Plasma HIV-1 RNA* Study 0021

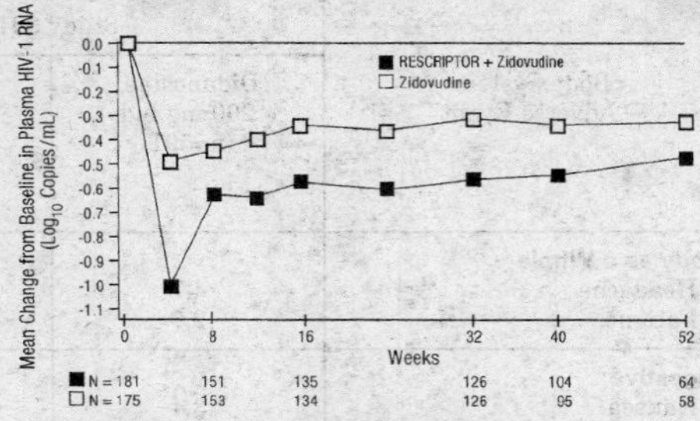

* Clinical significance of changes in plasma HIV-1 RNA levels has not been established.

monotherapy. The dose of didanosine was adjusted by body weight (<60 kg, 125 mg bid; >60 kg, 200 mg bid). Mean changes from baseline in CD4 cell count and $\log_{10}$ copies/mL plasma HIV-1 RNA are summarized in Figs 2 and 3, respectively. All patients had not completed 52 weeks at the time of this analysis.

Fig 2: Mean Change From Baseline in CD4 Cell Counts Study 0017

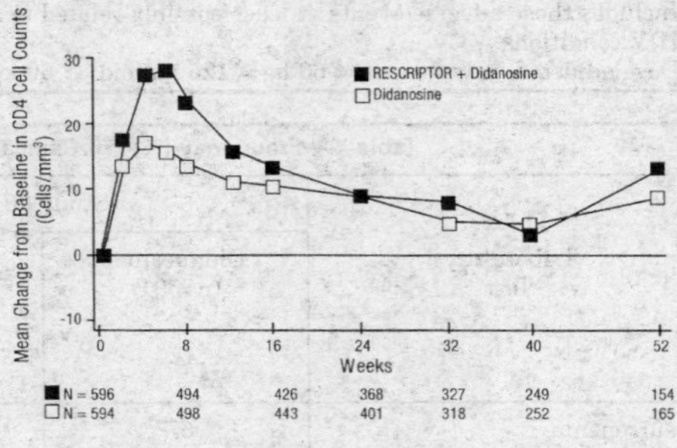

Fig 3: Mean Change From Baseline in Plasma HIV-1 RNA* Study 0017

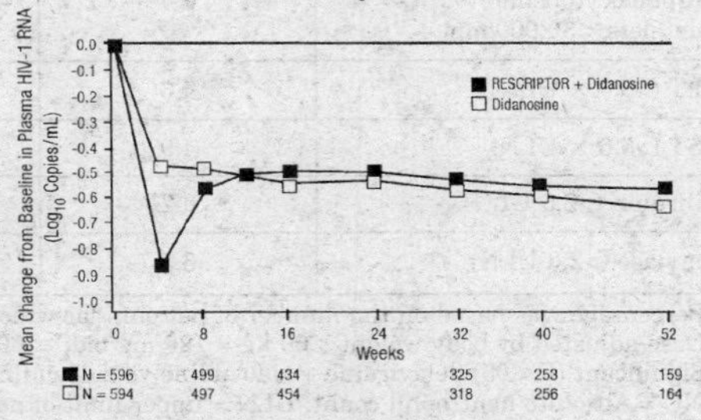

* Clinical significance of changes in plasma HIV-1 RNA levels has not been established.

An analysis of clinical efficacy end points (death, clinical progression defined as time to AIDS or death) was performed when all patients had completed at least 6 months in the trial. Comparable rates of deaths and AIDS progression between the didanosine monotherapy arm and the combination of RESCRIPTOR plus didanosine arm were observed. Refer to Fig 4.

Fig 4: Time to Clinical Progression or Death Study 0017

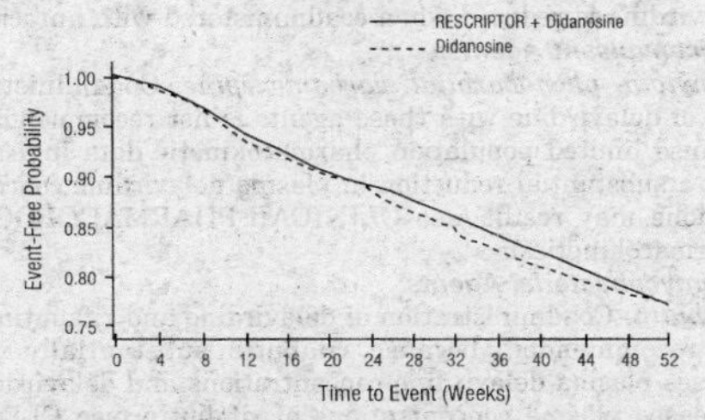

ACTG 261: RESCRIPTOR-Zidovudine-Didanosine Triple Therapy Trial

AIDS Clinical Trials Group (ACTG) Protocol 261 was a randomized trial comparing the following four treatment regimens: RESCRIPTOR plus didanosine, RESCRIPTOR plus zidovudine, RESCRIPTOR plus didanosine and zidovudine, and zidovudine plus didanosine. The study enrolled 544 HIV-1–infected patients (median age 35 years, 18% female and 44% non-Caucasian patients) who were either nucleoside treatment naive or had prior treatment with zidovudine or didanosine (not both) for less than 6 months. Thirty-seven percent reported previous antiretroviral therapy (194 patients with zidovudine and 6 with didanosine). Mean baseline CD4 cell count was 296 cells/mm^3 (range 55 to 640 cells/mm^3). Median baseline plasma HIV-1 RNA level (available for 229 patients) was 4.45 $\log_{10}$ copies/mL (28,260 copies/mL). Treatment doses were RESCRIPTOR 400 mg tid, zidovudine 200 mg tid, and didanosine dose adjusted by body weight (<60 kg, 125 mg bid; >60 kg, 200 mg bid). Preliminary results showed no statistically significant difference in CD4 cell count for the three drug combination of RESCRIPTOR, zidovudine, and didanosine compared with the combination of zidovudine plus didanosine. No statistically significant difference in plasma HIV-1 RNA for three-drug combination of RESCRIPTOR, zidovudine, and didanosine compared with the combination of zidovudine plus didanosine was observed. The mean change from baseline in CD4 cell count is shown in Fig 5. The mean change from baseline in plasma HIV-1 RNA is displayed through week 32 due to the small number of subjects having HIV-1 RNA determinations at week 48 and is shown in Fig 6.

Fig 5: Mean Change From Baseline in CD4 Cell Counts ACTG 261

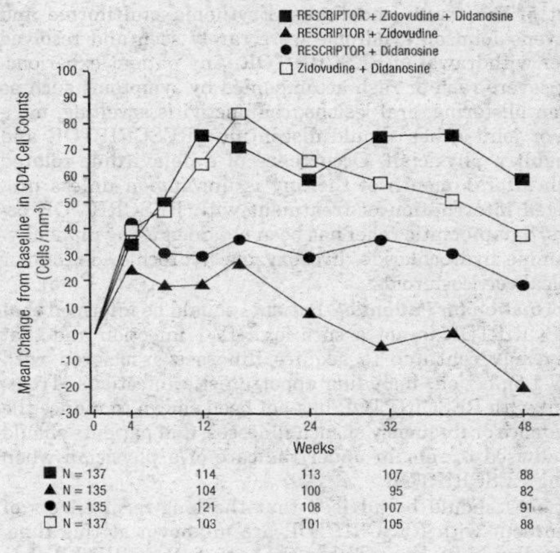

Fig 6: Mean Change From Baseline in Plasma HIV-1 RNA*, ACTG 261

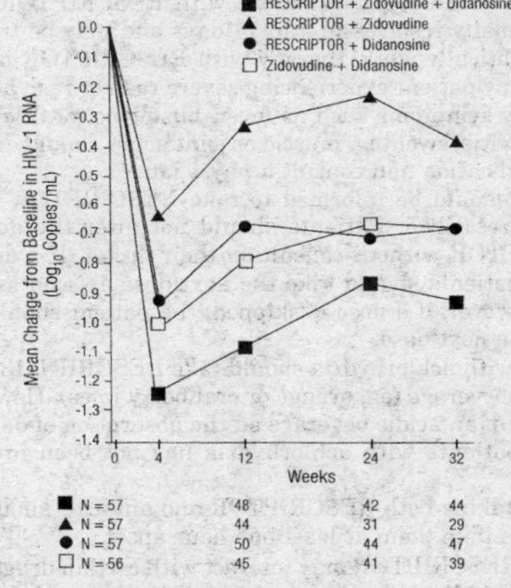

* Clinical significance of changes in plasma HIV-1 RNA levels has not been established.

CONTRAINDICATIONS

RESCRIPTOR Tablets are contraindicated in patients with previously demonstrated clinically significant hypersensitivity to any of the components of the formulation.

WARNINGS

Coadministration of RESCRIPTOR Tablets with certain nonsedating antihistamines, sedative hypnotics, antiarrhythmics, calcium channel blockers, ergot alkaloid preparations, amphetamines, cisapride, and sildenafil, may result in potentially serious and/or life-threatening adverse events due to possible effects of RESCRIPTOR on the hepatic metabolism of certain drugs (see PRECAUTIONS section).

PRECAUTIONS

General: Delavirdine is metabolized primarily by the liver. Therefore, caution should be exercised when administering RESCRIPTOR Tablets to patients with impaired hepatic function.

Resistance/Cross-Resistance: Non-nucleoside reverse transcriptase inhibitors, when used alone or in combination, may confer cross-resistance to other non-nucleoside reverse transcriptase inhibitors.

Skin Rash: Skin rash attributable to RESCRIPTOR has occurred in 18% of all patients in combination regimens in phase II and III controlled trials who received RESCRIPTOR 400 mg tid. Forty-two percent to 50% of patients treated with RESCRIPTOR 400 mg tid in Studies 0021 and 0017 experienced rash compared with 24% to 32% of patients receiving monotherapy with zidovudine or didanosine, respectively. In Studies 0021 and 0017, 4.3% of

Continued on next page

Rescriptor—Cont.

patients treated with RESCRIPTOR 400 mg tid discontinued treatment due to rash.

Dose titration did not significantly reduce the incidence of rash. Rash was typically diffuse, maculopapular, erythematous, and often pruritic. Skin rash was more common in patients with lower CD4 cell counts and usually occurred within 1 to 3 weeks (median = 11 days) of treatment. Rash classified as severe was observed in 3.6% of patients in Studies 0021 and 0017. In most cases, the duration of the rash was less than 2 weeks and did not require dose reduction or discontinuation of RESCRIPTOR. Most patients were able to resume therapy after rechallenge with RESCRIPTOR following a treatment interruption due to rash. The distribution of the rash was mainly on the upper body and proximal arms, with decreasing intensity of the lesions on the neck and face, and progressively less on the rest of the trunk and limbs. Erythema multiforme and Stevens-Johnson syndrome were rarely seen and resolved after withdrawal of RESCRIPTOR. Any patient experiencing severe rash or rash accompanied by symptoms such as fever, blistering, oral lesions, conjunctivitis, swelling, muscle or joint aches should discontinue RESCRIPTOR and consult a physician. Occurrence of a delavirdine-related rash after 1 month of therapy is uncommon unless prolonged interruption of treatment with RESCRIPTOR occurs. Symptomatic relief has been obtained using diphenhydramine hydrochloride, hydroxyzine hydrochloride, and/or topical corticosteroids.

Information for Patients: Patients should be informed that RESCRIPTOR is not a cure for HIV-1 infection and that they may continue to acquire illnesses associated with HIV-1 infection, including opportunistic infections. Treatment with RESCRIPTOR has not been shown to reduce the incidence or frequency of such illnesses, and patients should be advised to remain under the care of a physician when using RESCRIPTOR.

Patients should be advised that the long-term effects of treatment with RESCRIPTOR are unknown at this time. They should be advised that the use of RESCRIPTOR has not been shown to reduce the risk of transmission of HIV-1.

Patients should be instructed that the major toxicity of RESCRIPTOR is rash and should be advised to promptly notify their physician should rash occur. The majority of rashes associated with RESCRIPTOR occur within 1 to 3 weeks after initiating treatment with RESCRIPTOR. The rash normally resolves in 3 to 14 days and may be treated symptomatically while therapy with RESCRIPTOR is continued. Any patient experiencing severe rash or rash accompanied by symptoms such as fever, blistering, oral lesions, conjunctivitis, swelling, muscle or joint aches should discontinue medication and consult a physician.

Patients should be informed to take RESCRIPTOR every day as prescribed. Patients should not alter the dose of RESCRIPTOR without consulting their doctor. If a dose is missed, patients should take the next dose as soon as possible. However, if a dose is skipped, the patient should not double the next dose.

Patients with achlorhydria should take RESCRIPTOR with an acidic beverage (eg, orange or cranberry juice). However, the effect of an acidic beverage on the absorption of delavirdine in patients with achlorhydria has not been investigated.

Patients taking both RESCRIPTOR and antacids should be advised to take them at least one hour apart.

Because RESCRIPTOR may interact with certain drugs, patients should be advised to report to their doctor the use of any prescription or over-the-counter medications.

Drug Interactions (see also CLINICAL PHARMACOLOGY-Pharmacokinetics-Drug Interactions)

General: Coadministration of RESCRIPTOR with certain nonsedating antihistamines, sedative hypnotics, antiarrhythmics, calcium channel blockers, ergot alkaloid preparations, amphetamines, cisapride, and sildenafil, may result in potentially serious and/or life-threatening adverse events. Due to the inhibitory effect of delavirdine on CYP3A and CYP2C9, coadministration of RESCRIPTOR with drugs primarily metabolized by these liver enzymes may result in increased plasma concentrations. Higher plasma concentrations of these drugs could increase or prolong both therapeutic and adverse effects (Table 1). Therefore, appropriate dose adjustments may be necessary for these drugs. Drugs that induce CYP3A may also reduce plasma delavirdine concentrations (Table 2). Physicians should consider using alternatives to drugs that induce CYP3A while a patient is taking RESCRIPTOR.

Table 1. Selected Drugs that are Predicted to Have Plasma Concentrations Increased by Delavirdine*

HIV protease inhibitors: indinavir, saquinavir
Antihistamines: terfenadine,† astemizole†
Antimicrobial agents: clarithromycin, dapsone, rifabutin
Anti-migraine agents: ergot derivatives
Benzodiazepines: alprazolam,† midazolam,† triazolam†
Calcium channel blockers: dihydropyridines, eg, nifedipine
GI motility agents: cisapride†
Other: sildenafil, quinidine, warfarin

*This table is not all inclusive.
† See WARNINGS.

Table 3.—Adverse Events of Moderate or Severe Intensity in ≥2% of Patients Receiving RESCRIPTOR*

Body System/ Adverse Event	Study 0017		Study 0021	
	Didanosine† 200 mg bid (n=591)	Delavirdine 400 mg tid + Didanosine† 200 mg bid (n=594)	Zidovudine 200 mg tid (n=271)	Delavirdine 400 mg tid + Zidovudine 200 mg tid (n=287)
Body as a Whole				
Headache	4.7	5.6	4.8	5.6
Fatigue	2.7	2.9	4.8	5.2
Digestive				
Nausea	3.4	4.9	6.6	10.8
Diarrhea	4.4	4.5	2.2	3.5
Vomiting	1.2	2.4	1.1	2.8
Metabolic and Nutritional				
Increased ALT (SGPT)	3.6	5.2	0.7	2.4
Increased AST (SGOT)	3.0	4.5	0.7	1.7
Skin				
Rash	3.0	9.8	1.5	12.5
Maculopapular rash	2.0	6.6	1.1	4.5
Pruritus	1.7	2.2	1.5	3.1

*Includes those adverse events at least possibly related to study drug or of unknown relationship and excludes concurrent HIV conditions.
† Dose adjusted body weight < 60 kg = 125 mg bid; ≥ 60 kg = 200 mg bid.

Table 4.—Frequency (%)* of Clinically Important Laboratory Abnormalities

Laboratory Test	Study 0017		Study 0021	
	Didanosine† (n=591)	Delavirdine 400 mg tid + Didanosine† (n=594)	Zidovudine 200 mg tid (n=271)	Delavirdine 400 mg tid + Zidovudine 200 mg tid (n=287)
Neutropenia (ANC<750mm^3)	6.7	5.7	7.7‡	3.5
Anemia (Hgb <7.0 g/dL)	0.2	0.7	1.1	1.0
Thrombocytopenia (platelets <50,000/mm^3)	1.4	1.5	0.0	0.0
ALT (>5.0 × ULN)	4.6	6.7	3.7	3.8
AST (>5.0 × ULN)	4.9	5.6	3.0	2.1
Bilirubin (>2.5 ULN)	0.7	0.5	0.4	1.0
Amylase (>2.0 ULN)	6.5	5.2	1.1	0.0

*Percentage was based on the number of patients for which data on that laboratory test was available.
† Dose adjusted by body weight <60 kg = 125 mg bid; ≥ 60 kg = 200 mg bid.
‡ Significant (P<.05) delavirdine + zidovudine vs zidovudine.
ANC = Absolute neutrophil count; ULN = upper limit of normal.

Table 2. Selected Drugs that are Predicted to Decrease Plasma Delavirdine Concentrations‡§

Anticonvulsants: carbamazepine, phenobarbital, phenytoin
Antimycobacterial agents: rifabutin, rifampin

‡ This table is not all inclusive.
§ RESCRIPTOR may not be effective when administered concomitantly with these drugs.

Antacids: Doses of an antacid and RESCRIPTOR should be separated by at least one hour, because the absorption of delavirdine is reduced when coadministered with antacids.

Anticonvulsant Agents:

Phenytoin, phenobarbital, carbamazepine: Coadministration of delavirdine with these agents is not recommended, because limited population pharmacokinetic data indicate that a substantial reduction in plasma delavirdine concentrations may result (see CLINICAL PHARMACOLOGY-Pharmacokinetics).

Antimycobacterial Agents:

Rifabutin: Coadministration of delavirdine and rifabutin is not recommended, because rifabutin substantially decreases plasma delavirdine concentrations and delavirdine increases plasma concentrations of rifabutin (see CLINICAL PHARMACOLOGY-Pharmacokinetics).

Rifampin: Delavirdine should not be coadministered with rifampin, because rifampin reduces delavirdine systemic exposure (AUC) by almost 100% (see CLINICAL PHARMACOLOGY-Pharmacokinetics).

Erectile Dysfunction Agents:

Sildenafil: Caution should be used when prescribing sildenafil in patients receiving delavirdine, because delavirdine inhibits CYP3A4 which may result in an increase of sildenafil concentrations. Patients receiving delavirdine and sildenafil should be advised that they may be at an increased risk for sildenafil-associated adverse events, including hypotension visual changes, and prolonged erection, and should report these symptoms promptly to their physician. Currently, there are no safety and efficacy data available from the use of this combination. If delavirdine and sildenafil are used concomitantly, a single sildenafil dose of 25 mg in a 48-hour period should not be exceeded. This recommendation is based on data from a ritonavir/sildenafil drug-interaction study.

H_2Receptor Antagonists:

Cimetidine, famotidine, nizatidine, and ranitidine: These agents increase gastric pH and may reduce the absorption of delavirdine. Although the effect of these drugs on delavirdine absorption has not been evaluated, chronic use of these drugs with delavirdine is not recommended.

Nucleoside Analogue Reverse Transcriptase Inhibitors:

Didanosine: Administration of didanosine and delavirdine should be separated by at least one hour, because coadministration if didanosine and delavirdine resulted in reduced systemic exposure to both drugs by approximately 20% (see CLINICAL PHARMACOLOGY-Pharmacokinetics).

Protease Inhibitors (see CLINICAL PHARMACOLOGY-Pharmacokinetics):

Amprenavir: Delavirdine has the potential to increase serum concentrations of amprenavir.

Indinavir: Due to an increase in indinavir plasma concentrations (preliminary results), a dose reduction of indinavir to 600 mg tid should be considered when delavirdine and indinavir are coadministered. Currently, there are no safety and efficacy data available from the use of this combination.

Ritonavir: No studies have been conducted with combination therapy of delavirdine and ritonavir at their recommended doses. Preliminary results indicate there is no evidence of an interaction at doses of delavirdine 400 mg to 600 mg bid and ritonavir 300 mg bid. Currently, there are no safety and efficacy data available from the use of this combination.

Saquinavir: Saquinavir AUC increased 5-fold when delavirdine (400 mg tid) and saquinavir (600 mg tid) were administered in combination. Currently, there are limited safety and no efficacy data available from the use of this combination. In a small, preliminary study, hepatocellular enzyme elevations occurred in 13% of subjects during the first several weeks of the delavirdine and saquinavir combination (6% grade 3 or 4). Hepatocellular enzymes (ALT/AST) should be monitored frequently if this combination is prescribed.

Carcinogenesis, Mutagenesis and Impairment of Fertility: Long-term carcinogenicity studies with delavirdine in animals have not been completed. A battery of genetic toxicology tests was conducted with delavirdine, including the Ames assay, in vitro unscheduled DNA synthesis (UDS) assay, an in vitro cytogenetics (chromosome aberration) assay in human peripheral lymphocytes, a mammalian mutation assay in Chinese hamster ovary cells, and the micronucleus test in mice. The results were negative indicating delavirdine is not mutagenic.

Delavirdine at doses of 20, 100, and 200 mg/kg/day did not cause impairment of fertility in rats when males were treated for 70 days and females were treated for 14 days prior to mating.

Pregnancy: Pregnancy Category C: Delavirdine has been shown to be teratogenic in rats. Delavirdine caused ventricular septal defects in rats at doses of 50, 100, and 200 mg/kg/day when administered during the period of organogenesis. The lowest dose of delavirdine that caused malformations produced systemic exposures in pregnant rats equal to or lower than the expected human exposure to RESCRIPTOR ($C_{min} \approx 15\ \mu M$) at the recommended dose. Exposure in rats approximately 5-fold higher than the expected human exposure resulted in marked maternal toxicity, embryotoxicity, fetal developmental delay, and reduced pup survival. Additionally, reduced pup survival on postpartum day 0 occurred at an exposure (mean C_{min}) approximately equal to the expected human exposure. Delavirdine was excreted in the milk of lactating rats at a concentration three to five times that of rat plasma.

Delavirdine at doses of 200 and 400 mg/kg/day administered during the period of organogenesis caused maternal toxicity, embryotoxicity and abortions in rabbits. The lowest dose of delavirdine that resulted in these toxic effects produced systemic exposures in pregnant rabbits approximately 6-fold higher than the expected human exposure to RESCRIPTOR ($C_{min} \approx 15\ \mu M$) at the recommended dose. The no-observed-adverse-effect dose in the pregnant rabbit was 100 mg/kg/day. Various malformations were observed at this dose, but the incidence of such malformations was not statistically significantly different from those observed in the control group. Systemic exposures in pregnant rabbits at a dose of 100 mg/kg/day were lower than those expected in humans at the recommended clinical dose. Malformations were not apparent at 200 and 400 mg/kg/day; however, only a limited number of fetuses were available for examination as a result of maternal and embryo death.

No adequate and well-controlled studies in pregnant women have been conducted. RESCRIPTOR should be used during pregnancy only if the potential benefit justifies the potential risk to the fetus. Of 7 unplanned pregnancies reported in premarketing clinical studies, 3 were ectopic pregnancies and 3 pregnancies resulted in healthy live births. One infant was born prematurely with a small muscular ventricular septal defect to a patient who received approximately six weeks of treatment with delavirdine and zidovudine early in the course of the pregnancy.

Nursing Mothers: The U.S. Public Health Services Centers for Disease Control and Prevention advises HIV-infected women not to breast-feed to avoid postnatal transmission of HIV to a child who may not yet be infected.

Pediatric Use: Safety and effectiveness of delavirdine in combination with other antiretroviral agents have not been established in HIV-1–infected individuals younger than 16 years of age.

ADVERSE REACTIONS

The safety of RESCRIPTOR Tablets alone and in combination with other therapies has been studied in 1,969 patients receiving RESCRIPTOR.

Adverse events of moderate or severe intensity reported in ≥2% of patients receiving RESCRIPTOR in combination with didanosine or zidovudine in Studies 0017 and 0021 are summarized in Table 3. The median duration of treatment in Studies 0017 and 0021 was 34 and 42 weeks (up to 107 weeks for both studies), respectively, at the time of the safety assessment. The most frequently reported drug-related medical event was rash (see PRECAUTIONS-Skin Rash).

[See table 3 at top of previous page]

Medical events occurring in less than 2% of patients receiving RESCRIPTOR (in combination treatment) in all phase II and III studies, considered possibly related to treatment, and of at least ACTG grade 2 in intensity are listed below by body system.

Body as a Whole: Abdominal cramps, abdominal distention, abdominal pain (generalized or localized), allergic reaction, asthenia, back pain, chest pain, chills, edema (generalized or localized), epidermal cyst, fever, flank pain, flu syndrome, lethargy, lip edema, malaise, neck rigidity, pain (generalized or localized), sebaceous cyst, trauma, and upper respiratory infection.

Cardiovascular System: Bradycardia, migraine, pallor, palpitation, postural hypotension, syncope, tachycardia, and vasodilation.

Digestive System: Anorexia, aphthous stomatitis, bloody stool, colitis, constipation, decreased appetite, diarrhea (*Clostridium difficile*), diverticulitis, duodenitis, dry mouth, dyspepsia, dysphagia, enteritis, esophagitis, fecal incontinence, flatulence, gagging, gastritis, gastroesophageal reflux, gastrointestinal bleeding, gastrointestinal disorder, gingivitis, gum hemorrhage, increased appetite, increased saliva, increased thirst, mouth ulcer, nonspecific hepatitis, pancreatitis, rectal disorder, sialadenitis, stomatitis, and tongue edema or ulceration.

Hemic and Lymphatic System: Anemia, bruise, ecchymosis, eosinophilia, granulocytosis, neutropenia, pancytopenia, petechia, prolonged partial thromboplastin time, purpura, spleen disorder, and thrombocytopenia.

Metabolic and Nutritional Disorders: Alcohol intolerance, bilirubinemia, hyperkalemia, hyperuricemia, hypocalcemia, hyponatremia, hypophosphatemia, increased gamma glutamyl transpeptidase, increased lipase, increased serum alkaline phosphatase, increased serum amylase, increased serum creatine phosphokinase, increased serum creatinine, peripheral edema, and weight increase or decrease.

Musculoskeletal System: Arthralgia or arthritis of single and multiple joints, bone disorder, bone pain, leg cramps, muscular weakness, myalgia, tendon disorder, tenosynovitis, and tetany.

Nervous System: Abnormal coordination, agitation, amnesia, anxiety, change in dreams, cognitive impairment, confusion, decreased libido, depressive symptoms, disorientation, dizziness, emotional lability, hallucination, hyperesthesia, hyperreflexia, hypesthesia, impaired concentration, insomnia, manic symptoms, muscle cramp, nervousness, neuropathy, nightmares, nystagmus, paralysis, paranoid symptoms, paresthesia, restlessness, somnolence, tingling, tremor, vertigo, and weakness.

Respiratory System: Bronchitis, chest congestion, cough, dyspnea, epistaxis, laryngismus, pharyngitis, rhinitis, and sinusitis.

Skin and Appendages: Angioedema, dermal leukocytoclastic vasculitis, dermatitis, desquamation, diaphoresis, dry skin, erythema, erythema multiforme, folliculitis, fungal dermatitis, hair loss, nail disorder, petechial rash, seborrhea, skin disorder, skin nodule, Stevens-Johnson syndrome, urticaria, and vesiculobullous rash.

Special Senses: Blepharitis, conjunctivitis, diplopia, dry eyes, ear pain, photophobia, taste perversion, and tinnitus.

Urogenital System: Breast enlargement, calculi of the kidney, epididymitis, hematuria, hemospermia, impotence, kidney pain, metrorrhagia, nocturia, polyuria, proteinuria, and vaginal moniliasis.

Laboratory Abnormalities: The frequency of clinically important laboratory abnormalities observed during therapy in Studies 0017 and 0021 is summarized in Table 4. There was no significant difference in ACTG grades 3 and 4 laboratory abnormalities between treatment groups except a two-fold reduction in neutropenia in the delavirdine plus zidovudine combination group compared with the zidovudine monotherapy group in Study 0021.

[See table 4 on previous page]

OVERDOSAGE

No reports of overdose with RESCRIPTOR Tablets are available in humans. Several patients have received up to 850 mg tid for up to 6 months with no serious drug-related medical events.

Management of Overdosage: Treatment of overdosage with RESCRIPTOR should consist of general supportive measures, including monitoring of vital signs and observation of the patient's clinical status. There is no specific antidote for overdosage with RESCRIPTOR. If indicated, elimination of unabsorbed drug should be achieved by emesis or gastric lavage. Since delavirdine is extensively metabolized by the liver and is highly protein bound, dialysis is unlikely to result in significant removal of the drug.

DOSAGE AND ADMINISTRATION

The recommended dosage for RESCRIPTOR Tablets is 400 mg (four 100-mg or two 200-mg tablets) three times daily. RESCRIPTOR should be used in combination with other appropriate antiretroviral therapy. The complete prescribing information for other antiretroviral agents should be consulted for information on dosage and administration.

The 100-mg RESCRIPTOR Tablets may be dispersed in water prior to consumption. To prepare a dispersion, add four 100-mg RESCRIPTOR Tablets to at least 3 ounces of water, allow to stand for a few minutes, and then stir until a uniform dispersion occurs (see CLINICAL PHARMACOLOGY-Pharmacokinetics-Absorption and Bioavailability). The dispersion should be consumed promptly. The glass should be rinsed with water and the rinse swallowed to insure the entire dose is consumed. **The 200-mg tablets should be taken as intact tablets, because they are not readily dispersed in water.** Note: The 200-mg tablets are approximately one third smaller in size than the 100-mg tablets.

RESCRIPTOR Tablets may be administered with or without food (see CLINICAL PHARMACOLOGY-Pharmacokinetics-Absorption and Bioavailability). Patients with achlorhydria should take RESCRIPTOR with an acidic beverage (eg, orange or cranberry juice). However, the effect of an acidic beverage on the absorption of delavirdine in patients with achlorhydria has not been investigated.

Patients taking both RESCRIPTOR and antacids should be advised to take them at least one hour apart.

HOW SUPPLIED

RESCRIPTOR Tablets are available as follows:

100 mg: white, capsule-shaped tablets marked with "U 3761".

Bottles of 360 tablets NDC 0009-3761-03

200 mg: white, capsule-shaped tablets marked with "RESCRIPTOR 200 mg".

Bottles of 180 tablets NDC 0009-7576-01

Store at controlled room temperature 20° to 25°C (68° to 77°F) [see USP]. Keep container tightly closed. Protect from high humidity.

℞ only

ANIMAL TOXICOLOGY

Toxicities among various organs and organ systems in rats, mice, rabbits, dogs, and monkeys were observed following the administration of delavirdine. Necrotizing vasculitis was the most significant toxicity that occurred in dogs when mean nadir serum concentrations of delavirdine were at least 7-fold higher than the expected human exposure to RESCRIPTOR ($C_{min} \approx 15\ \mu M$) at the recommended dose. Vasculitis in dogs was not reversible during a 2.5-month recovery period; however, partial resolution of the vascular lesion characterized by reduced inflammation, diminished necrosis, and intimal thickening occurred during this period. Other major target organs included the gastrointestinal tract, endocrine organs, liver, kidneys, bone marrow, lymphoid tissue, lung, and reproductive organs.

US Patent No. 5,563,142

Pharmacia & Upjohn Company
Kalamazoo, Michigan 49001, USA
Revised July 1999

Shown in Product Identification Guide, page 303

VIRACEPT® ℞

[*vī 'ră-cĕpt*]

(nelfinavir mesylate)

TABLETS and ORAL POWDER

DESCRIPTION

VIRACEPT® (nelfinavir mesylate) is an inhibitor of the human immunodeficiency virus (HIV) protease. VIRACEPT Tablets are available for oral administration as a light blue, capsule-shaped tablet with a clear film coating in a 250 mg strength (as nelfinavir free base). Each tablet also contains the following inactive ingredients: calcium silicate, crospovidone, magnesium stearate, FD&C blue #2 powder, hydroxypropyl methylcellulose and triacetin. VIRACEPT Oral Powder is available for oral administration in a 50 mg/g strength (as nelfinavir free base) in bottles. The oral powder also contains the following inactive ingredients: microcrystalline cellulose, maltodextrin, dibasic potassium phosphate, crospovidone, hydroxypropyl methylcellulose, aspartame, sucrose palmitate, and natural and artificial flavor. The chemical name for nelfinavir mesylate is [3*S*-[2(2*S**, 3*S**), 3α,4aβ,8aβ]]-*N*-(1,1-dimethylethyl)decahydro-2-[2-hydroxy-3-[(3-hydroxy-2-methylbenzoyl)amino]-4-(phenylthio)butyl]-3-isoquinolinecarboxamide mono-methanesulfonate (salt) and the molecular weight is 663.90 (567.79 as the free base). Nelfinavir mesylate has the following structural formula:

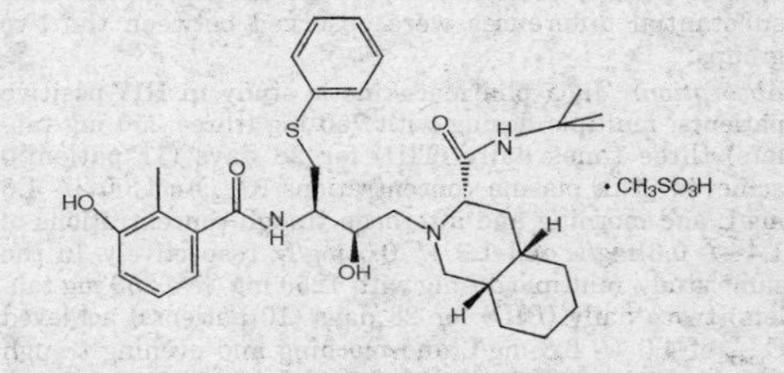

Nelfinavir mesylate is a white to off-white amorphous powder, slightly soluble in water at pH ≤4 and freely soluble in methanol, ethanol, isopropanol and propylene glycol.

Microbiology

Mechanism of Action: Nelfinavir is an inhibitor of the HIV-1 protease. Inhibition of the viral protease prevents cleavage of the gag-pol polyprotein resulting in the production of immature, non-infectious virus.

Antiviral Activity In Vitro: The antiviral activity of nelfinavir *in vitro* has been demonstrated in both acute and/or chronic HIV infections in lymphoblastoid cell lines, peripheral blood lymphocytes and monocytes/macrophages. Nelfinavir was found to be active against several laboratory strains of HIV-1 and several clinical isolates of HIV-1 and the HIV-2 strain ROD. The EC_{95} (95% effective concentration) of nelfinavir ranged from 7 to 196 nM. In combination with reverse transcriptase inhibitors, nelfinavir demonstrated additive (didanosine or stavudine) to synergistic (zidovudine, lamivudine or zalcitabine) antiviral activity *in vitro* without enhanced cytotoxicity. Drug combination studies with protease inhibitors (ritonavir, saquinavir or indinavir) showed variable results ranging from antagonistic to synergistic.

Drug Resistance: HIV-1 isolates with reduced susceptibility to nelfinavir have been selected *in vitro*. HIV isolates from selected patients treated with nelfinavir alone or in combination with reverse transcriptase inhibitors were monitored for phenotypic (n=19) and genotypic (n=195, 157 of which were evaluable) changes in clinical trials over a period of 2 to 82 weeks. One or more virus protease mutations at amino acid positions 30, 35, 36, 46, 71, 77 and 88 were detected in >10% of patients with evaluable isolates. Of 19 patients for which both phenotypic and genotypic analyses were performed on clinical isolates, 9 showed reduced sus-

Continued on next page

Viracept—Cont.

ceptibility (5- to 93-fold) to nelfinavir *in vitro*. All 9 patients possessed one or more mutations in the virus protease gene. Amino acid position 30 appeared to be the most frequent mutation site.

The overall incidence of the D30N mutation in the virus protease of evaluable patients (n=157) receiving nelfinavir monotherapy or nelfinavir in combination with zidovudine and lamivudine or stavudine was 54.8%. The overall incidence of other mutations associated with primary protease inhibitor resistance was 9.6% for the L90M substitution whereas substitutions at 48, 82, or 84 were not observed.

Cross-resistance: Preclinical Studies-HIV isolates obtained from 5 patients during nelfinavir therapy showed a 5- to 93-fold decrease in nelfinavir susceptibility *in vitro* when compared to matched baseline isolates, but did not demonstrate a concordant decrease in susceptibility to indinavir, ritonavir, saquinavir or amprenavir, *in vitro*. Conversely, following ritonavir therapy 6 of 7 clinical isolates with decreased ritonavir susceptibility (8- to 113-fold) *in vitro* compared to baseline also exhibited decreased susceptibility to nelfinavir *in vitro* (5- to 40-fold). An HIV isolate obtained from a patient receiving saquinavir therapy showed decreased susceptibility to saquinavir (7-fold), but did not demonstrate a concordant decrease in susceptibility to nelfinavir. Cross-resistance between nelfinavir and reverse transcriptase inhibitors is unlikely because different enzyme targets are involved. Clinical isolates (n=5) with decreased susceptibility to zidovudine, lamivudine, or nevirapine remain fully susceptible to nelfinavir *in vitro*.

Clinical Studies-There have been no controlled or comparative studies evaluating the virologic response to subsequent protease inhibitor-containing regimens in patients who have demonstrated loss of virologic response to a nelfinavir-containing regimen. However, virologic response was evaluated in a single-arm prospective study of 26 patients with extensive prior antiretroviral experience with reverse transcriptase inhibitors (mean 2.9) who had received VIRACEPT for a mean duration of 59.7 weeks and were switched to a ritonavir (400 mg BID)/saquinavir hard-gel (400 mg BID) containing regimen after a prolonged period of VIRACEPT failure (median 48 weeks). Sequence analysis of HIV-1 isolates prior to switch demonstrated a D30N or an L90M substitution in 18 and 6 patients, respectively. Subjects remained on therapy for a mean of 48 weeks (range 40 to 56 weeks) where 17 of 26 (65%) subjects and 13 of 26 (50%) subjects were treatment responders with HIV RNA below the assay limit of detection (Chiron bDNA) at 24 and 48 weeks, respectively.

CLINICAL PHARMACOLOGY

Pharmacokinetics

The pharmacokinetic properties of nelfinavir were evaluated in healthy volunteers and HIV-infected patients; no substantial differences were observed between the two groups.

Absorption: In a pharmacokinetic study in HIV-positive patients, multiple dosing with 750 mg (three 250 mg tablets) three times daily (TID) for 28 days (11 patients) achieved peak plasma concentrations (C_{max}) of 3.0 +/- 1.6 mg/L and morning and afternoon trough concentrations of 1.4 +/- 0.6 mg/L and 1.0 +/- 0.5 mg/L, respectively. In the same study, multiple dosing with 1250 mg (five 250 mg tablets) twice daily (BID) for 28 days (10 patients) achieved C_{max} of 4.0 +/- 0.8 mg/L and morning and evening trough concentrations of 2.2 +/- 1.3 mg/L and 0.7 +/- 0.4 mg/L, respectively. The difference between morning and afternoon or evening trough concentrations for the TID and BID regimens was also observed in healthy volunteers who were dosed at precise 8- or 12-hour intervals.

Effect of Food on Oral Absorption: Maximum plasma concentrations and area under the plasma concentration-time curve (AUC) were 2 to 3-fold higher under fed conditions compared to fasting. The effect of food on nelfinavir absorption was evaluated in two studies (n=14, total). The meals evaluated contained 517 to 759 Kcal, with 153 to 313 Kcal derived from fat.

Distribution: The apparent volume of distribution following oral administration of nelfinavir was 2-7 L/kg. Nelfinavir in serum is extensively protein-bound (>98%).

Metabolism: Unchanged nelfinavir comprised 82–86% of the total plasma radioactivity after a single oral 750 mg dose of ^{14}C-nelfinavir. *In vitro*, multiple cytochrome P-450 isoforms including CYP3A are responsible for metabolism of nelfinavir. One major and several minor oxidative metabolites were found in plasma. The major oxidative metabolite has *in vitro* antiviral activity comparable to the parent drug.

Elimination: The terminal half-life in plasma was typically 3.5 to 5 hours. The majority (87%) of an oral 750 mg dose containing ^{14}C-nelfinavir was recovered in the feces; fecal radioactivity consisted of numerous oxidative metabolites (78%) and unchanged nelfinavir (22%). Only 1-2% of the dose was recovered in urine, of which unchanged nelfinavir was the major component.

Special Populations

Hepatic or Renal Insufficiency: The pharmacokinetics of nelfinavir have not been studied in patients with hepatic or renal insufficiency; however, less than 2% of nelfinavir is excreted in the urine, so the impact of renal impairment on nelfinavir elimination should be minimal.

Table 1: Drug Interactions
Effect of Nelfinavir on Coadministered Drug Plasma AUC and C_{max}

		Coadministered Drug		
Coadministered Drug	Nelfinavir Dose	N	AUC (95% CI)	C_{max} (95% CI)
Lamivudine 150 mg Single Dose	750 mg q8h × 7-10 days	11	↑10% (1–20%)	↑31% (5–62%)
Stavudine 30–40 mg bid × 56 days	750 mg tid × 56 days	8	↔	↔
Zidovudine 200 mg Single Dose	750 mg q8h × 7-10 days	11	↓35% (28–41%)	↓31% (8–49%)
Indinavir 800 mg Single Dose	750 mg q8h × 7 days	6	↑51% (25–83%)	↔
Ritonavir 500 mg Single Dose	750 mg q8h × 5 doses	10	↔	↔
Saquinavir 1200 mg Single Dose[1]	750 mg tid × 4 days	14	↑392% (271–553%)	↑179% (105–280%)
Efavirenz 600 mg qd × 7 days	750 mg q8h × 7 days	10	↔	↔
Ethinyl estradiol 35 μg qd × 15 days	750 mg q8h × 7 days	12	↓47% (41–63%)	↓28% (14–39%)
Norethindrone 0.4 mg qd × 15 days	750 mg q8h × 7 days	12	↓18% (12–27%)	↔
Rifabutin 150 mg qd × 8 days[2]	750 mg q8h × 7-8 days[3]	12	↑83% (69–99%)	↑19% (9–30%)
Rifabutin 300 mg qd × 8 days	750 mg q8h × 7-8 days	10	↑207% (151–276%)	↑146% (112–186%)

↑ Indicates increase
↓ Indicates decrease
↔Indicates no change (p value > 0.05)
[1] Using the soft gelatin capsule_formulation of saquinavir 1200mg
[2] Rifabutin 150mg qd changes in Table 1 are relative to Rifabutin 300mg qd × 8 days without coadministration with nelfinavir
[3] Comparable changes in rifabutin concentrations were observed with VIRACEPT 1250mg q12h × 7 days

Table 2: Drug Interactions
Effect of Coadministered Drug on Nelfinavir Plasma AUC and C_{max}

		Nelfinavir		
Coadministered Drug	Nelfinavir Dose	N	AUC (95% CI)	C_{max} (95% CI)
Didanosine 200 mg Single Dose	750 mg Single Dose	9	↔	↔
Zidovudine 200 mg + Lamivudine 150 mg Single Dose	750 mg q8h × 7–10 days	11	↔	↔
Indinavir 800 mg q8h × 7 days	750 mg Single Dose	6	↑83% (34–150%)	↑31% (13–52%)
Ritonavir 500 mg q12h × 3 doses	750 mg Single Dose	10	↑152% (86–242%)	↑44% (25–67%)
Saquinavir 1200 mg tid × 4 days[1]	750 mg Single Dose	14	↑18% (5–33%)	↔
Efavirenz 600 mg qd × 7 days	750 mg q8h × 7 days	10	↑20% (5–38%)	↑21% (8–36%)
Ketoconazole 400 mg qd × 7 days	500 mg q8h × 5–6 days	12	↑35% (21–49%)	↑25% (8–44%)
Nevirapine 200 mg qd × 14 days Followed by 200 mg bid × 14 days	750 mg tid × 36 days	23	↔	↔
Rifabutin 150 mg qd × 8 days	750 mg q8h × 7–8 days 1250 mg q12h × 7–8 days	11 11	↓23% (12–33%) ↔	↓18% (6–29%) ↔
Rifabutin 300 mg qd × 8 days	750 mg q8h × 7–8 days	10	↓32% (10–48%)	↓25% (6–38%)
Rifampin 600 mg qd × 7 days	750 mg q8h × 5–6 days	12	↓82% (77–86%)	↓76% (67–83%)

↑ Indicates increase
↓ Indicates decrease
↔Indicates no change (p value > 0.05)
[1] Using the soft gelatin capsule_formulation of saquinavir 1200mg
[2] Rifabutin 150mg qd changes in Table 1 are relative to Rifabutin 300mg qd × 8 days without coadministration with nelfinavir
[3] Comparable changes in rifabutin concentrations were observed with VIRACEPT 1250mg q12h × 7 days

Gender and Race: No significant pharmacokinetic differences have been detected between males and females. Pharmacokinetic differences due to race have not been evaluated.

Pediatrics: see PRECAUTIONS: Pediatric Use

Geriatric Patients: The pharmacokinetics of nelfinavir have not been studied in patients over 65 years of age.

Drug Interactions (also see CONTRAINDICATIONS, WARNINGS, PRECAUTIONS: Drug Interactions)

The potential ability of nelfinavir to inhibit the major human cytochrome P450 isoforms (CYP3A, CYP2C19, CYP2D6, CYP2C9, CYP1A2 and CYP2E1) has been investigated *in vitro*. Only CYP3A was inhibited at concentrations in the therapeutic range.

Specific drug interaction studies were performed with nelfinavir and a number of drugs. Tables 1 summarizes the effects of nelfinavir on the geometric mean AUC and C_{max} of coadministered drugs. Table 2 shows the effects of coadministered drugs on the geometric mean AUC and C_{max} of nelfinavir.

[See table 1 above]
[See table 2 above]

For information regarding clinical recommendations, see CONTRAINDICATIONS, WARNINGS, PRECAUTIONS: Drug Interactions.

INDICATIONS AND USAGE

VIRACEPT in combination with other antiretroviral agents is indicated for the treatment of HIV infection.

Description of Studies

In the clinical studies described below, efficacy was evaluated by the percent of patients with plasma HIV RNA < 400 copies/mL (Studies 511 and 542) or < 500 copies/mL (Study ACTG 364), using the Roche RT-PCR (Amplicor) HIV-1 Monitor or < 50 copies/mL, using the Roche HIV-1 Ultrasensitive assay (Study Avanti 3). In the analysis presented in each figure, patients who terminated the study early for any reason, switched therapy due to inadequate efficacy or who had a missing HIV-RNA measurement that was either preceded or followed by a measurement above the limit of assay quantification were considered to have HIV-RNA above 400 copies/mL, above 500 copies/mL, or above 50 copies/mL at subsequent time points, depending on the assay that was used.

a. Studies in Antiretroviral Treatment Naïve Patients

Study 511: VIRACEPT + zidovudine + lamivudine versus zidovudine + lamivudine

Study 511 was a double-blind, randomized, placebo controlled trial comparing treatment with zidovudine (ZDV; 200mg TID) and lamivudine (3TC; 150mg BID) plus 2 doses of VIRACEPT (750mg and 500mg TID) to zidovudine (200mg TID) and lamivudine (150mg BID) alone in 297 antiretroviral naive HIV-1 infected patients (median age 35 years [range 21 to 63], 89% male and 78% Caucasian). Mean baseline CD4 cell count was 288 cells/mm^3 and mean baseline plasma HIV RNA was 5.21 $\log_{10}$ copies/mL (160,394 copies/mL). The percent of patients with plasma HIV RNA < 400 copies/mL and mean changes in CD4 cell count are summarized in Figures 1 and 2, respectively.

Figure 1
Study 511: Percentage of Patients With HIV RNA Below 400 Copies/mL

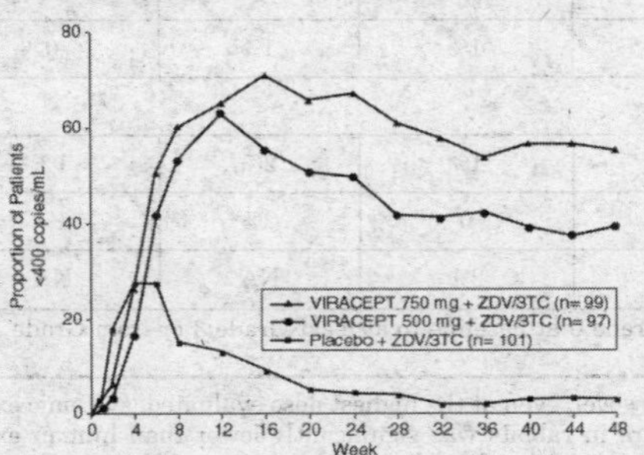

Figure 2
Study 511: Mean Change From Baseline in CD4 Cell Counts

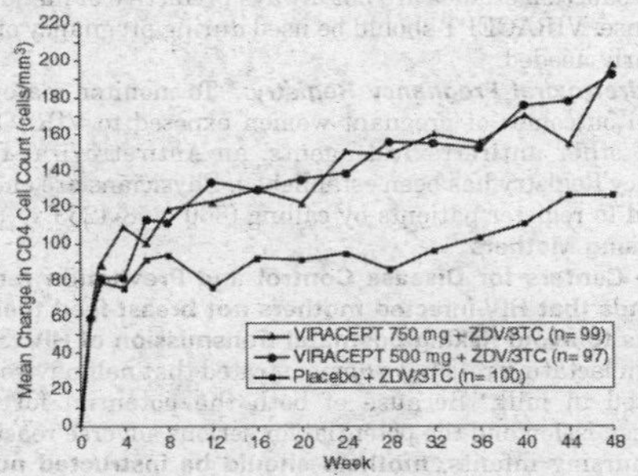

Study 542: VIRACEPT BID + stavudine + lamivudine compared to VIRACEPT TID + stavudine + lamivudine

Study 542 is an ongoing, randomized, open-label trial comparing the HIV RNA suppression achieved by VIRACEPT 1250 mg BID versus VIRACEPT 750 mg TID in patients also receiving stavudine (d4T; 30–40mg BID) and lamivudine (3TC; 150mg BID). Patients had a median age of 36 years (range 18 to 83), were 84% male, and were 91% Caucasian. Patients had received less than 6 months of therapy with nucleoside transcriptase inhibitors and were naïve to protease inhibitors. Mean baseline CD4 cell count was 296 cells/mm^3 and mean baseline plasma HIV RNA was 5.0 $\log_{10}$ copies/mL (100,706 copies/mL).

Results showed that there was no significant difference in mean CD4 count among treatment groups; the mean increases from baseline for the BID and TID arms were 150 cells/mm^3 at 24 weeks and approximately 200 cells/mm^3 at 48 weeks.

The percent of patients with HIV RNA <400 copies/mL is summarized in Figure 3. The outcomes of patients through 48 weeks of treatment are summarized in Table 3.

[See figure at top of next column]

Figure 3
Study 542: Percentage of Patients With HIV RNA Below 400 Copies/mL

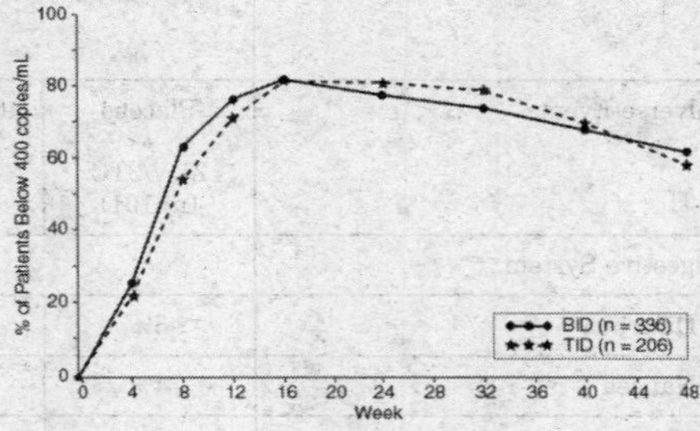

Table 3
Outcomes of Randomized Treatment Through 48 Weeks

Outcome	Viracept 1250 mg BID Regimen	Viracept 750 mg TID Regimen
Number of patients evaluable*	323	192
HIV RNA < 400 copies/ml	198 (61%)	111 (58%)
HIV RNA ≥ 400 copies/ml	46 (14%)	22 (11%)
Discontinued due to VIRACEPT toxicity**	9 (3%)	2 (1%)
Discontinued due to other antiretroviral agents' toxicity**	3 (1%)	3 (2%)
Others***	67 (21%)	54 (28%)

*Twelve patients in the BID arm and fourteen patients in the TID arm have not yet reached 48 weeks of therapy

**These rates only reflect dose-limiting toxicities that were counted as the initial reason for treatment failure in the analysis (See ADVERSE REACTIONS for a description of the safety profile of these regimens).

***Consent withdrawn, lost to follow-up, intercurrent illness, noncompliance or missing data; all assumed as failures

Study Avanti 3: VIRACEPT TID + zidovudine + lamivudine compared to zidovudine + lamivudine.

Study Avanti 3 was a placebo-controlled, randomized, double-blind study designed to evaluate the safety and efficacy of VIRACEPT (750 mg TID) in combination with zidovudine (ZDV; 300 mg BID) and lamivudine (3TC; 150 mg BID) versus placebo in combination with ZDV and 3TC administered to antiretroviral-naive patients with HIV infection and a CD4 lymphocyte count between 150 and 500 cells/µL. Patients had a mean age of 35 (range 22–59) were 89% male and 88% Caucasian. Mean baseline CD4 cell count was 304 cells/mm^3 and mean baseline plasma HIV RNA was 4.8 $\log_{10}$ copies/mL (57,887 copies/mL). The percent of patients with plasma HIV RNA <50 copies/mL at 52 weeks was 54% for the VIRACEPT + ZDV + 3TC treatment group and 13% for the ZDV + 3TC treatment group.

b. Studies in Antiretroviral Treatment Experienced Patients

Study ACTG 364: VIRACEPT TID + 2NRTIs compared to efavirenz + 2NRTIs compared to VIRACEPT + efavirenz + 2NRTIs

Study ACTG 364 was a randomized, double-blind study that evaluated the combination of VIRACEPT 750 mg TID and/or efavirenz 600 mg QD with 2 NRTIs (either didanosine [ddI]+ d4T, ddI + 3TC, or d4T + 3TC) in patients with prolonged prior nucleoside exposure who had completed 2 previous ACTG studies. Patients had a mean age of 41 years (range 18 to 75), were 88% male, and were 74% Caucasian. Mean baseline CD4 cell count was 389 cells/mm^3 and mean baseline plasma HIV RNA was 3.9 $\log_{10}$ copies/mL (7,954 copies/mL).

The percent of patients with plasma HIV RNA < 500 copies/mL at 48 weeks was 42%, 62%, and 72% for the VIRACEPT, EFV, and VIRACEPT+EFV treatment groups, respectively. The 4-drug combination of VIRACEPT + EFV + 2 NRTIs was more effective in suppressing plasma HIV RNA in these patients than either 3-drug regimen.

CONTRAINDICATIONS

VIRACEPT is contraindicated in patients with clinically significant hypersensitivity to any of its components.

VIRACEPT should not be administered concurrently with cisapride, triazolam, midazolam, ergot derivatives, amiodarone or quinidine because VIRACEPT may affect the hepatic metabolism of these drugs and create the potential for serious and/or life-threatening adverse events.

WARNINGS

Patients with Phenylketonuria: VIRACEPT Oral Powder contains 11.2 mg phenylalanine per gram of powder.

New onset diabetes mellitus, exacerbation of pre-existing diabetes mellitus and hyperglycemia have been reported during post-marketing surveillance in HIV-infected patients receiving protease inhibitor therapy. Some patients required either initiation or dose adjustments of insulin or oral hypoglycemic agents for treatment of these events. In some cases diabetic ketoacidosis has occurred. In those patients who discontinued protease inhibitor therapy, hyperglycemia persisted in some cases. Because these events have been reported voluntarily during clinical practice, estimates of frequency cannot be made and a causal relationship between protease inhibitor therapy and these events has not been established.

Concomitant use of VIRACEPT with lovastatin or simvastatin is not recommended. Caution should be exercised if HIV protease inhibitors, including VIRACEPT, are used concurrently with other HMG-CoA reductase inhibitors that are also metabolized by the CYP3A4 pathway (e.g., atorvastatin or cerivastatin). The risk of myopathy including rhabdomyolysis may be increased when protease inhibitors, including VIRACEPT, are used in combination with these drugs.

Particular caution should be used when prescribing sildenafil in patients receiving protease inhibitors, including VIRACEPT. Coadministration of a protease inhibitor with sildenafil is expected to substantially increase sildenafil concentrations and may result in an increase in sildenafil-associated adverse events, including hypotension, visual changes, and priapism. (see PRECAUTIONS, Drug Interactions and Information for Patients, and the complete prescribing information for sildenafil)

Concomitant use of St. John's wort (hypericum perforatum) or St. John's wort containing products and VIRACEPT is not recommended. Coadministration of St. John's wort with protease inhibitors, including VIRACEPT, is expected to substantially decrease protease inhibitor concentrations and may result in sub-optimal levels of VIRACEPT and lead to loss of virologic response and possible resistance to VIRACEPT or to the class of protease inhibitors.

PRECAUTIONS

General

Nelfinavir is principally metabolized by the liver. Therefore, caution should be exercised when administering this drug to patients with hepatic impairment.

Resistance/Cross Resistance

HIV cross-resistance between protease inhibitors has been observed. (see Microbiology)

Hemophilia

There have been reports of increased bleeding, including spontaneous skin hematomas and hemarthrosis, in patients with hemophilia type A and B treated with protease inhibitors. In some patients, additional factor VIII was given. In more than half of the reported cases, treatment with protease inhibitors was continued or reintroduced. A causal relationship has not been established.

Redistribution/Accumulation of Body Fat

Redistribution/accumulation of body fat including central obesity, dorsocervical fat enlargement (buffalo hump), peripheral wasting, breast enlargement, and "cushingoid appearance" have been observed in patients receiving antiretroviral therapy. The mechanism and long-term consequences of these events are currently unknown. A causal relationship has not been established.

Information For Patients

For optimal absorption, patients should be advised to take VIRACEPT with food (See CLINICAL PHARMACOLOGY: Pharmacokinetics and DOSAGE AND ADMINISTRATION).

Patients should be informed that VIRACEPT is not a cure for HIV infection and that they may continue to acquire illnesses associated with advanced HIV infection, including opportunistic infections.

Patients should be told that there is currently no data demonstrating that VIRACEPT therapy can reduce the risk of transmitting HIV to others through sexual contact or blood contamination.

Patients should be told that sustained decreases in plasma HIV RNA have been associated with a reduced risk of progression to AIDS and death. Patients should be advised to take VIRACEPT and other concomitant antiretroviral therapy every day as prescribed. Patients should not alter the dose or discontinue therapy without consulting with their doctor. If a dose of VIRACEPT is missed, patients should take the dose as soon as possible and then return to their normal schedule. However, if a dose is skipped, the patient should not double the next dose.

Patients should be informed that VIRACEPT Tablets are film-coated and that this film-coating is intended to make the tablets easier to swallow.

The most frequent adverse event associated with VIRACEPT is diarrhea, which can usually be controlled with non-prescription drugs, such as loperamide, which slow gastrointestinal motility.

Patients should be informed that redistribution or accumulation of body fat may occur in patients receiving antiretroviral therapy including protease inhibitors and that the cause and long term health effects of these conditions are not known at this time.

VIRACEPT may interact with some drugs, therefore, patients should be advised to report to their doctor the use of any other prescription, non-prescription medication or herbal products, particularly St. John's wort.

Patients receiving oral contraceptives should be instructed that alternate or additional contraceptive measures should be used during therapy with VIRACEPT.

Patients receiving sildenafil and nelfinavir should be advised that they may be at an increased risk of sildenafil-

Continued on next page

Viracept—Cont.

associated adverse events including hypotension, visual changes, and prolonged penile erection, and should promptly report any symptoms to their doctor.

Drug Interactions (Also see CONTRAINDICATIONS, WARNINGS, CLINICAL PHARMACOLOGY: Drug Interactions)

Nelfinavir is an inhibitor of CYP3A (cytochrome P450 3A). Coadministration of VIRACEPT and drugs primarily metabolized by CYP3A (e.g., dihydropyridine calcium channel blockers, HMG-CoA reductase inhibitors, immunosuppressants and sildenafil) may result in increased plasma concentrations of the other drug that could increase or prolong both its therapeutic and adverse effects, see Tables 4, 5 and 6. Nelfinavir is metabolized in part by CYP3A. Coadministration of VIRACEPT and drugs that induce CYP3A, such as rifampin, may decrease nelfinavir plasma concentrations and reduce its therapeutic effect. Coadministration of VIRACEPT and drugs that inhibit CYP3A may increase nelfinavir plasma concentrations.

Drug interaction studies reveal no clinically significant drug interactions between nelfinavir and didanosine, lamivudine, stavudine, zidovudine, efavirenz or ketoconazole and no dose adjustments are needed. In the case of didanosine, it is recommended that didanosine be administered on an empty stomach; therefore, nelfinavir should be administered with food one hour after or more than 2 hours before didanosine.

Based on known metabolic profiles, clinically significant drug interactions are not expected between VIRACEPT and dapsone, trimethoprim/sulfamethoxazole, clarithromycin, azithromycin, erythromycin, itraconazole or fluconazole.

Table 4
Drugs That Should Not Be Coadministered With VIRACEPT

Drug Class	Drugs Within Class Not to be Coadministered With VIRACEPT
Antiarrhythmics	amiodarone, quinidine
Antimigraine	ergot derivatives
Antimycobacterial agents	rifampin
Benzodiazepines	midazolam, triazolam
GI motility agents	cisapride
HMG-CoA reductase inhibitors	lovastatin, simvastatin

Table 5
Established Drug Interactions: Alteration in Dose or Regimen Recommended Based on Drug Interaction Studies (see CLINICAL PHARMACOLOGY, for Magnitude of Interaction, Tables 1 and 2)

Drug Name	Effect on Concentration	Clinical Comment
Rifabutin	↑ rifabutin ↓ nelfinavir (750 mg TID) ↔ nelfinavir (1250 mg BID)	It is recommended that the dose of rifabutin be reduced to one-half the usual dose when administered with VIRACEPT; 1250 mg BID is the preferred dose of VIRACEPT when coadministered with rifabutin.
Indinavir	↑ nelfinavir ↑ indinavir	Appropriate doses for this combination with respect to safety and efficacy have not been established.
Ritonavir	↑ nelfinavir	Appropriate doses for this combination, with respect to safety and efficacy, have not been established.
Saquinavir	↑ saquinavir	Appropriate doses for this combination with respect to safety and efficacy have not been established.
Oral contraceptives	↓ ethinyl estradiol	Alternative or additional contraceptive measures should be used when oral contraceptives and VIRACEPT are coadministered.

Table 6
Other Potentially Significant Clinical Drug Interactions With VIRACEPT*

Anticonvulsants: carbamazepine, phenobarbital, phenytoin	May decrease nelfinavir plasma concentrations**
HMG-CoA reductase inhibitors: atorvastatin, cerivastatin,	Plasma concentrations may be increased by VIRACEPT.
Immunosuppressants: cyclosporine tacrolimus	Plasma concentrations may be increased by VIRACEPT.
Erectile dysfunction agents: sildenafil	Expected to substantially increase sildenafil concentrations (sildenafil should not exceed a maximum single dose of 25 mg in a 48 hour period when administered in patients receiving protease inhibitors; consult sildenafil prescribing information).

* This table is not all inclusive.
** VIRACEPT may not be effective due to decreased nelfinavir plasma concentrations in patients taking these agents concomitantly.

Table 7
Percentage of Patients with Treatment-Emergent[1] Adverse Events of Moderate or Severe Intensity Reported in ≥2% of Patients

	Study 511 24 weeks			Study 542 48 weeks	
Adverse Events	Placebo + ZDV/3TC (n=101)	500 mg TID VIRACEPT + ZDV/3TC (n=97)	750 mg TID VIRACEPT + ZDV/3TC (n=100)	1250 mg BID VIRACEPT + d4T/3TC (n=344)	750 mg TID VIRACEPT + d4T/3TC (n=210)
Digestive System					
Diarrhea	3%	14%	20%	20%	15%
Nausea	4%	3%	7%	3%	3%
Flatulence	0	5%	2%	1%	1%
Skin/Appendages					
Rash	1%	1%	3%	2%	1%

[1] Includes those adverse events at least possibly related to study drug or of unknown relationship and excludes concurrent HIV conditions

Table 8
Percentage of Patients by Treatment Group With Marked Laboratory Abnormalities[1] in >2% of Patients

	Study 511			Study 542	
	Placebo + ZDV/3TC (n=101)	500 mg TID VIRACEPT + ZDV/3TC (n=97)	750 mg TID VIRACEPT + ZDV/3TC (n=100)	1250 mg BID VIRACEPT + d4T/3TC (n=344)	750 mg TID VIRACEPT + d4T/3TC (n=210)
Hematology					
Hemoglobin	6%	3%	2%	0	0
Neutrophils	4%	3%	5%	2%	1%
Lymphocytes	1%	6%	1%	1%	0
Chemistry					
ALT (SGPT)	6%	1%	1%	2%	1%
AST (SGOT)	4%	1%	0	2%	1%
Creatine Kinase	7%	2%	2%	NA	NA

[1] Marked laboratory abnormalities are defined as a shift from Grade 0 at baseline to at least Grade 3 or from Grade 1 to Grade 4

Carcinogenesis and Mutagenesis

Carcinogenicity studies in animals have not yet been completed. Nelfinavir was not, however, mutagenic or clastogenic in a battery of *in vitro* and *in vivo* tests including microbial mutagenesis (Ames), mouse lymphoma, chromosome aberrations in human lymphocytes, and an *in vivo* rat micronucleus assay.

Pregnancy, Fertility and Reproduction - Pregnancy Category B

Comparisons of systemic exposure are based on the steady-state area under the plasma concentration time curve (AUC) observed in humans receiving the recommended therapeutic dose. Nelfinavir produced no effects on either male or female mating and fertility or embryo survival in rat studies at exposures comparable to human therapeutic exposure. There were also no effects on fetal development or maternal toxicity when nelfinavir was administered to pregnant rats at systemic exposures comparable to human exposure. Administration of nelfinavir to pregnant rabbits resulted in no fetal development effects up to a dose at which a slight decrease in maternal body weight was observed; however, even at the highest dose evaluated, systemic exposure in rabbits was significantly lower than human exposure. Additional studies in rats indicated that exposure to nelfinavir in females from mid-pregnancy through lactation had no effect on the survival, growth, and development of the offspring to weaning. Subsequent reproductive performance of these offspring was also not affected by maternal exposure to nelfinavir. However, there are no adequate and well-controlled studies in pregnant women. Because animal reproduction studies are not always predictive of human response, VIRACEPT should be used during pregnancy only if clearly needed.

Antiretroviral Pregnancy Registry: To monitor maternal-fetal outcomes of pregnant women exposed to VIRACEPT and other antiretroviral agents, an Antiretroviral Pregnancy Registry has been established. Physicians are encouraged to register patients by calling (800) 258-4263.

Nursing Mothers

The Centers for Disease Control and Prevention recommends that HIV-infected mothers not breast-feed their infants to avoid risking postnatal transmission of HIV. Studies in lactating rats have demonstrated that nelfinavir is excreted in milk. Because of both the potential for HIV transmission and the potential for serious adverse reactions in nursing infants, **mothers should be instructed not to breast-feed if they are receiving VIRACEPT.**

Pediatric Use

Nelfinavir was studied in one open-label, uncontrolled trial in 38 pediatric patients ranging in age from 2 to 13 years. In order to achieve plasma concentrations in pediatric patients which approximate those observed in adults, the recommended pediatric dose is 20–30 mg/kg given three times daily with a meal or light snack, not to exceed 750 mg three times a day. (see DOSAGE AND ADMINISTRATION).

A similar adverse event profile was seen during the pediatric clinical trial as in adult patients. The evaluation of the antiviral activity of nelfinavir in pediatric patients is ongoing. The evaluation of the safety, effectiveness and pharmacokinetics of nelfinavir in pediatric patients below the age of 2 years is ongoing.

Geriatric Use

Clinical studies of VIRACEPT did not include sufficient numbers of subjects aged 65 and over to determine whether they respond differently from younger subjects.

ADVERSE REACTIONS

The safety of VIRACEPT was studied in over 5000 patients who received drug either alone or in combination with nucleoside analogues. The majority of adverse events were of

Table 9
Pediatric Dose to be Administered Three Times Daily

Body Weight Kg.	lbs.	Number of Level 1 gm Scoops	Number of Level Teaspoons	Number of Tablets
7 to < 8.5	15.5 to < 18.5	4	1	—
8.5 to < 10.5	18.5 to < 23	5	1 1/4	—
10.5 to < 12	23 to < 26.5	6	1 1/2	—
12 to < 14	26.5 to < 31	7	1 3/4	—
14 to < 16	31 to < 35	8	2	—
16 to < 18	35 to < 39.5	9	2 1/4	—
18 to < 23	39.5 to < 50.5	10	2 1/2	2
≥ 23	≥ 50.5	15	3 3/4	3

mild intensity. The most frequently reported adverse event among patients receiving VIRACEPT was diarrhea, which was generally of mild to moderate intensity.

Drug-related clinical adverse experiences of moderate or severe intensity in ≥2% of patients treated with VIRACEPT coadministered with d4T and 3TC (Study 542) for up to 48 weeks or with ZDV plus 3TC (Study 511) for up to 24 weeks are presented in Table 7.

[See table 7 at top of previous page]

Adverse events occurring in less than 2% of patients receiving VIRACEPT in all phase II/III clinical trials and considered at least possibly related or of unknown relationship to treatment and of at least moderate severity are listed below.

Body as a Whole: abdominal pain, accidental injury, allergic reaction, asthenia, back pain, fever, headache, malaise, pain and redistribution/accumulation of body fat (see PRECAUTIONS, Fat Redistribution.)

Digestive System: anorexia, dyspepsia, epigastric pain, gastrointestinal bleeding, hepatitis, mouth ulceration, pancreatitis and vomiting.

Hemic/Lymphatic System: anemia, leukopenia and thrombocytopenia.

Metabolic/Nutritional System: increases in alkaline phosphate, amylase, creatine phosphokinase, lactic dehydrogenase, SGOT, SGPT and gamma glutamyl transpeptidase; hyperlipemia, hyperuricemia, hyperglycemia, hypoglycemia, dehydration, and liver function tests abnormal.

Musculoskeletal System: arthralgia, arthritis, cramps, myalgia, myasthenia and myopathy.

Nervous System: anxiety, depression, dizziness, emotional lability, hyperkinesia, insomnia, migraine, paresthesia, seizures, sleep disorder, somnolence and suicide ideation.

Respiratory System: dyspnea, pharyngitis, rhinitis, and sinusitis.

Skin/Appendages: dermatitis, folliculitis, fungal dermatitis, maculopapular rash, pruritus, sweating, and urticaria.

Special Senses: acute iritis and eye disorder.

Urogenital System: kidney calculus, sexual dysfunction and urine abnormality.

Post-Marketing Experience

The following additional adverse experiences have been reported from postmarketing surveillance as at least possibly related or of unknown relationship to VIRACEPT:

Body as a Whole: Hypersensitivity reactions (including bronchospasm, moderate to severe rash, fever and edema).

Digestive System: jaundice

Metabolic/Nutritional System: bilirubinemia, metabolic acidosis

Laboratory Abnormalities

The percentage of patients with marked laboratory abnormalities in Studies 542 and 511 are presented in Table 8. Marked laboratory abnormalities are defined as a Grade 3 or 4 abnormality in a patient with a normal baseline value or a Grade 4 abnormality in a patient with a Grade 1 abnormality at baseline.

[See table 8 on previous page]

OVERDOSAGE

Human experience of acute overdose with VIRACEPT is limited. There is no specific antidote for overdose with VIRACEPT. If indicated, elimination of unabsorbed drug should be achieved by emesis or gastric lavage. Administration of activated charcoal may also be used to aid removal of unabsorbed drug. Since nelfinavir is highly protein bound, dialysis is unlikely to significantly remove drug from blood.

DOSAGE AND ADMINISTRATION

Adults: The recommended dose is 1250 mg (five 250 mg tablets) twice daily or 750 mg (three 250 mg tablets) three times daily. VIRACEPT should be taken with a meal or light snack. It is recommended that VIRACEPT be used in combination with nucleoside analogues. Patients unable to swallow tablets may place whole tablets or crushed tablets in a small amount of water to dissolve before ingestion or they may mix crushed tablets in a small amount food. Once mixed with food or dissolved in water, the entire contents must be consumed within 6 hours in order to obtain the full dose.

Pediatric Patients (2–13 years): The recommended oral dose of VIRACEPT for pediatric patients 2 to 13 years of age is 20–30 mg/kg per dose, three times daily with a meal or a light snack. The pharmacokinetics of twice daily dosing of VIRACEPT in pediatric patients has not been established. For children unable to take tablets, VIRACEPT Oral Powder may be administered. The oral powder may be mixed with a small amount of water, milk, formula, soy formula, soy milk or dietary supplements; once mixed, the entire contents must be consumed in order to obtain the full dose. The recommended use period for storage of the product in these media is 6 hours. Acidic food or juice (e.g., orange juice, apple juice or apple sauce) are not recommended to be used in combination with VIRACEPT, because the combination may result in a bitter taste. VIRACEPT Oral Powder should not be reconstituted with water in its original container. The recommended pediatric dose of VIRACEPT to be administered three times daily is described in Table 9.

[See table 9 above]

HOW SUPPLIED

VIRACEPT (nelfinavir mesylate) Tablets, 250 mg, are light blue, capsule-shaped tablets with a clear film coating engraved with "VIRACEPT" on one side and "250 mg" on the other.

Available as:
NDC 63010-010-27, bottle containing 270 tablets
NDC 63010-010-30, bottle containing 300 tablets

VIRACEPT (nelfinavir mesylate) Oral Powder, 50 mg/g is an off-white powder containing 50 mg (as nelfinavir free base) in each level scoopful (1 gram).

Available as:
NDC 63010-011-90, multiple use bottle containing 144 grams of powder with scoop.

VIRACEPT Tablets and Oral Powder should be stored at 15 to 30 °C (59° to 86 °F).

Keep container tightly closed. Dispense in original container.

VIRACEPT is a registered trademark of Agouron Pharmaceuticals, Inc.

Issued 5/18/2000

Shown in Product Identification Guide, page 303

Alcon Laboratories, Inc.

and its affiliates
CORPORATE HEADQUARTERS
6201 SOUTH FREEWAY
FORT WORTH, TX 76134

Direct Inquiries to:
Pharmaceutical/Consumer: (800) 451-3937
(Therapeutic Drugs/Lens Care)
Surgical: (800) 862-5266
(Instrumentation/Surgical Meds)
6201 South Freeway
Fort Worth, TX 76134
(817) 293-0450 (Main Switchboard)

OPHTHALMIC PRODUCTS

For information on Alcon ophthalmic products, consult the PDR For Ophthalmology. See a complete listing of products in the Manufacturers' Index section of this book. For information, literature, samples or service items contact Alcon at the phone numbers listed above.

AZOPT® ℞
(brinzolamide ophthalmic suspension) 1%

DESCRIPTION

AZOPT® (brinzolamide ophthalmic suspension) 1% contains a carbonic anhydrase inhibitor formulated for multi-dose topical ophthalmic use. Brinzolamide is described chemically as: (R)-(+)-4-Ethylamino-2-(3-methoxypropyl)-3,4-dihydro-2H-thieno [3,2-e]-1,2-thiazine-6-sulfonamide-1,1-doxide. Its empirical formula is $C_{12}H_{21}N_3O_5S_3$.

Brinzolamide has a molecular weight of 383.5 and a melting point of about 131°C. It is a white powder, which is insoluble in water, very soluble in methanol and soluble in ethanol.

AZOPT 1% is supplied as a sterile, aqueous suspension of brinzolamide which has been formulated to be readily suspended and slow settling, following shaking. It has a pH of approximately 7.5 and an osmolality of 300 mOsm/kg. Each mL of AZOPT 1% contains 10 mg brinzolamide. Inactive ingredients are mannitol, carbomer 974P, tyloxapol, edetate disodium, sodium chloride, hydrochloric acid and/or sodium hydroxide (to adjust pH), and purified water. Benzalkonium chloride 0.01% is added as a preservative.

CLINICAL PHARMACOLOGY

Carbonic anhydrase (CA) is an enzyme found in many tissues of the body including the eye. It catalyzes the reversible reaction involving the hydration of carbon dioxide and the dehydration of carbonic acid. In humans, carbonic anhydrase exists as a number of isoenzymes, the most active being carbonic anhydrase II (CA-II), found primarily in red blood cells (RBCs), but also in other tissues. Inhibition of carbonic anhydrase in the ciliary processes of the eye decreases aqueous humor secretion, presumably by slowing the formation of bicarbonate ions with subsequent reduction in sodium and fluid transport.

The result is a reduction in intraocular pressure (IOP).

AZOPT 1% contains brinzolamide, an inhibitor of carbonic anhydrase II (CA-II). Following topical ocular administration, brinzolamide inhibits aqueous humor formation and reduces elevated intraocular pressure. Elevated intraocular pressure is a major risk factor in the pathogenesis of optic nerve damage and glaucomatous visual field loss.

Following topical ocular administration, brinzolamide is absorbed into the systemic circulation. Due to its affinity for CA-II, brinzolamide distributes extensively into the RBCs and exhibits a long half-life in whole blood (approximately 111 days). In humans, the metabolite N-desethyl brinzolamide is formed, which also binds to CA and accumulates in RBCs. This metabolite binds mainly to CA-I in the presence of brinzolamide. In plasma, both parent brinzolamide and N-desethyl brinzolamide concentrations are low and generally below assay quantitation limits (<10 ng/mL). Binding to plasma proteins is approximately 60%. Brinzolamide is eliminated predominantly in the urine as unchanged drug. N-Desethyl brinzolamide is also found in the urine along with lower concentrations of the N-desmethoxypropyl and O-desmethyl metabolites.

An oral pharmacokinetic study was conducted in which healthy volunteers received 1 mg capsules of brinzolamide twice per day for up to 32 weeks. This regimen approximates the amount of drug delivered by topical ocular administration of AZOPT® (brinzolamide ophthalmic suspension) 1% dosed to both eyes three times per day and simulates systemic drug and metabolite concentrations similar to those achieved with long-term topical dosing. RBC CA activity was measured to assess the degree to systemic CA inhibition. Brinzolamide saturation of RBC CA-II was achieved within 4 weeks (RBC concentrations of approximately 20 μM). N-Desethyl brinzolamide accumulated in RBCs to steady-state within 20–28 weeks reaching concentrations ranging from 6–30 μM. The inhibition of CA-II activity at steady-state was approximately 70–75%, which is below the degree of inhibition expected to have a pharmacological effect on renal function or respiration in healthy subjects.

In two, three-month clinical studies, AZOPT (brinzolamide ophthalmic suspension) 1% dosed three times per day (TID) in patients with elevated intraocular pressure (IOP), produced significant reductions in IOPs (4–5 mmHg). These IOP reductions are equivalent to the reductions observed with TRUSOPT* (dorzolamide hydrochloride ophthalmic solution) 2% dosed TID in the same studies.

In two clinical studies in patients with elevated intraocular pressure, AZOPT 1% was associated with less stinging and burning upon instillation than TRUSOPT* 2%.

INDICATIONS AND USAGE

AZOPT® Ophthalmic Suspension 1% is indicated in the treatment of elevated intraocular pressure in patients with ocular hypertension or open-angle glaucoma.

CONTRAINDICATIONS

AZOPT® is contraindicated in patients who are hypersensitive to any component of this product.

WARNINGS

AZOPT® is a sulfonamide and although administered topically it is absorbed systemically. Therefore, the same types of adverse reactions that are attributable to sulfonamides may occur with topical administration of AZOPT. Fatalities have occurred, although rarely, due to severe reactions to sulfonamides including Stevens-Johnson syndrome, toxic epidermal necrolysis, fulminant hepatic necrosis, agranulocytosis, aplastic anemia, and other blood dyscrasias. Sensitization may recur when a sulfonamide is re-administered irrespective of the route of administration. If signs of serious reactions or hypersensitivity occur, discontinue the use of this preparation.

PRECAUTIONS

General:

Carbonic anhydrase activity has been observed in both the cytoplasm and around the plasma membranes of the corneal endothelium. The effect of continued administration of AZOPT on the corneal endothelium has not been fully evaluated. The management of patients with acute angle-clo-

Continued on next page

Azopt—Cont.

sure glaucoma requires therapeutic interventions in addition to ocular hypotensive agents. AZOPT has not been studied in patients with acute angle-closure glaucoma.

AZOPT has not been studied in patients with severe renal impairment (CrCl <30 mL/min). Because AZOPT and its metabolite are excreted predominantly by the kidney, AZOPT is not recommended in such patients.

AZOPT® has not been studied in patients with hepatic impairment and should be used with caution in such patients. There is a potential for an additive effect on the known systemic effects of carbonic anhydrase inhibition in patients receiving an oral carbonic anhydrase inhibitor and AZOPT. The concomitant administration of AZOPT and oral carbonic anhydrase inhibitors is not recommended.

Information For Patients:

AZOPT® is a sulfonamide and although administered topically, it is absorbed systemically; therefore, the same type of adverse reactions attributable to sulfonamides may occur with topical administration. Patients should be advised that if serious or unusual ocular or systemic reactions or signs of hypersensitivity occur, they should discontinue the use of the product and consult their physician (see **Warnings**).

Vision may be temporarily blurred following dosing with AZOPT. Care should be exercised in operating machinery or driving a motor vehicle.

Patients should be instructed to avoid allowing the tip of the dispensing container to contact the eye or surrounding structures or other surfaces, since the product can become contaminated by common bacteria known to cause ocular infections. Serious damage to the eye and subsequent loss of vision may result from using contaminated solutions.

Patients should also be advised that if they have ocular surgery or develop an intercurrent ocular condition (e.g., trauma or infection), they should immediately seek their physician's advice concerning the continued use of the present multidose container.

If more than one topical ophthalmic drug is being used, the drugs should be administered at least ten minutes apart.

The preservative in AZOPT® Ophthalmic Suspension, benzalkonium chloride, may be absorbed by soft contact lenses. Contact lenses should be removed during instillation of AZOPT, but may be reinserted 15 minutes after instillation.

Drug Interactions:

AZOPT® Ophthalmic Suspension 1% contains a carbonic anhydrase inhibitor. Acid-base and electrolyte alterations were not reported in the clinical trials with brinzolamide. However, in patients treated with oral carbonic anhydrase inhibitors, rare instances of drug interactions have occurred with high-dose salicylate therapy. Therefore, the potential for such drug interaction should be considered in patients receiving AZOPT.

Carcinogenesis, Mutagenesis, Impairment of Fertility:

Carcinogenicity data on brinzolamide are not available. The following tests for mutagenic potential were negative: (1) *in vivo* mouse micronucleus assay; (2) *in vivo* sister chromatid exchange assay; and (3) Ames *E. coli* test. The *in vitro* mouse lymphoma forward mutation assay was negative in the absence of activation, but positive in the presence of microsomal activation.

In reproduction studies of brinzolamide in rats, there were no adverse effects on the fertility or reproductive capacity of males or females at doses up to 18 mg/kg/day (375 times the recommended human ophthalmic dose).

Pregnancy:

Teratogenic Effects: Pregnancy Category C. Developmental toxicity studies with brinzolamide in rabbits at oral doses of 1, 3, and 6 mg/kg/day (20, 62, and 125 times the recommended human ophthalmic dose) produced maternal toxicity at 6 mg/kg/day and a significant increase in the number of fetal variations, such as accessory skull bones, which was only slightly higher than the historic value at 1 and 6 mg/kg. In rats, statistically decreased body weights of fetuses from dams receiving oral doses of 18 mg/kg/day (375 times the recommended human ophthalmic dose) during gestation were proportional to the reduced maternal weight gain, with no statistically significant effects on organ or tissue development. Increases in unossified sternebrae, reduced ossification of the skull, and unossified hyoid that occurred at 6 and 18 mg/kg were not statistically significant. No treatment-related malformations were seen. Following oral administration of ^{14}C-brinzolamide to pregnant rats, radioactivity was found to cross the placenta and was present in the fetal tissues and blood.

There are no adequate and well-controlled studies in pregnant women. AZOPT® should be used during pregnancy only if the potential benefit justifies the potential risk to the fetus.

Nursing Mothers:

In a study of brinzolamide in lactating rats, decreases in body weight gain in offspring at an oral dose of 15 mg/kg/day (312 times the recommended human ophthalmic dose) were seen during lactation. No other effects were observed. However, following oral administration of ^{14}C-brinzolamide to lactating rats, radioactivity was found in milk at concentrations below those in the blood and plasma.

It is not known whether this drug is excreted in human milk. Because many drugs are excreted in human milk and because of the potential for serious adverse reactions in nursing infants from AZOPT, a decision should be made whether to discontinue nursing or to discontinue the drug, taking into account the importance of the drug to the mother.

Pediatric Use:

Safety and effectiveness in pediatric patients have not been established.

ADVERSE REACTIONS

In clinical studies of AZOPT (brinzolamide ophthalmic suspension) 1%, the most frequently reported adverse events associated with AZOPT 1% were blurred vision and bitter, sour or unusual taste. These events occurred in approximately 5–10% of patients. Blepharitis, dermatitis, dry eye, foreign body sensation, headache, hyperemia, ocular discharge, ocular discomfort, ocular keratitis, ocular pain, ocular pruritus and rhinitis were reported at an incidence of 1–5%.

The following adverse reactions were reported at an incidence below 1%: allergic reactions, alopecia, chest pain, conjunctivitis, diarrhea, diplopia, dizziness, dry mouth, dyspnea, dyspepsia, eye fatigue, hypertonia, keratoconjunctivitis, keratopathy, kidney pain, lid margin crusting or sticky sensation, nausea, pharyngitis, tearing and urticaria.

OVERDOSAGE

Although no human data are available, electrolyte imbalance, development of an acidotic state, and possible nervous system effects may occur following oral administration of an overdose. Serum electrolyte levels (particularly potassium) and blood pH levels should be monitored.

DOSAGE AND ADMINISTRATION

Shake well before use. The recommended dose is 1 drop of AZOPT® Ophthalmic Suspension in the affected eye(s) three times daily.

AZOPT may be used concomitantly with other topical ophthalmic drug products to lower intraocular pressure.

If more than one topical ophthalmic drug is being used, the drugs should be administered at least ten minutes apart.

HOW SUPPLIED

AZOPT® Ophthalmic Suspension 1% is supplied in plastic DROP-TAINER® dispensers with a controlled dispensing-tip as follows:

NDC 0065-0275-24	2.5 mL
NDC 0065-0275-05	5 mL
NDC 0065-0275-10	10 mL
NDC 0065-0275-15	15 mL

Storage: Store AZOPT Ophthalmic Suspension 1% at 4–30°C (39–86°F).

Rx Only

U.S. Patent Numbers: 5,240,923; 5,378,703; 5,461,081; patents pending.

*TRUSOPT is a registered trademark of Merck & Co., Inc.

BETAXON™ ℞

(levobetaxolol hydrochloride ophthalmic suspension) 0.5% as base

DESCRIPTION

BETAXON™ (levobetaxolol hydrochloride ophthalmic suspension) 0.5% contains levobetaxolol hydrochloride, a cardioselective beta-adrenergic receptor blocking agent, in a sterile resin suspension formulation. Levobetaxolol hydrochloride is a white, crystalline powder with a molecular weight of 343.89.

Empirical Formula: $C_{18}H_{29}NO_3{\bullet}HCl$

Chemical Name:

(S)-1-[p-[2-(cyclopropylmethoxy)ethyl]phenoxy]-3-(isopropylamino)-2-propanol hydrochloride.

Each mL of BETAXON™ (levobetaxolol hydrochloride ophthalmic suspension) 0.5% contains:

Active: levobetaxolol HCl 5.6 mg equivalent to 5.0 mg of levobetaxolol free base.

Preservative: benzalkonium chloride 0.01%. **Inactives:** mannitol, poly(styrene-divinyl benzene) sulfonic acid, Carbomer 974P, boric acid, N-lauroylsarcosine, edetate disodium, hydrochloric acid or tromethamine (to adjust pH) and purified water. It has a pH of 5.5 to 7.5 and an osmolality of 260 to 340 mOsm per kg.

CLINICAL PHARMACOLOGY

Levobetaxolol is a cardioselective (beta-1-adrenergic) receptor blocking agent that does not have significant membrane-stabilizing (local anesthetic) activity and is devoid of intrinsic sympathomimetic action. Animal studies suggest levobetaxolol (S-isomer) is the more active enantiomer of betaxolol (racemate).

When instilled in the eye, BETAXON™ Ophthalmic Suspension has the action of reducing elevated intraocular pressure. Elevated IOP presents a major risk factor in glaucomatous field loss. The higher the level of IOP, the greater the likelihood of optic nerve damage and visual field loss. In two well-controlled clinical studies in which a total of 356 patients were dosed for three months, BETAXON™ Ophthalmic Suspension produced clinically relevant reductions in IOP at all follow-up visits. At 8 AM after nighttime dosing (trough), IOP was reduced from baseline approximately 4 to 5 mmHg (16% to 21%). At 10 AM, two hours after dosing (peak), IOP was reduced from baseline approximately 5 to 6 mmHg (20% to 23%).

Since racemic betaxolol and other beta-adrenergic antagonists have been shown to reduce intraocular pressure by a reduction of aqueous production as demonstrated by tonography and aqueous fluorophotometry, it is assumed that the mechanism of action of levobetaxolol is similar. The intraocular pressure lowering effect of racemic betaxolol can generally be noted within 30 minutes and the maximal effect can usually be detected two hours after topical administration. It is assumed that the intraocular pressure lowering time profile of levobetaxolol is similar. A single dose provides approximately a 12-hour reduction of intraocular pressure.

BETAXON™ Ophthalmic Suspension 0.5% (levobetaxolol hydrochloride ophthalmic suspension) was dosed topically for 7 days to steady-state in 20 normal volunteers. An average maximal levobetaxolol plasma concentration (Cmax) of 0.5 ± 0.14 ng/mL was reached about three hours after the last dose: The mean half-life of levobetaxolol was approximately 20 hours.

In comparisons between BETAXON™ Ophthalmic Suspension and non-cardioselective beta blockers in reactive airway subjects, BETAXON™ Ophthalmic Suspension is expected to demonstrate less effect on pulmonary function [FEV_1 and Forced Vital Capacity (FVC)].

The cardiovascular effects of BETAXON™ Ophthalmic Suspension 0.5% and betaxolol ophthalmic solution 1% were compared in double-masked, crossover studies to timolol maleate ophthalmic solution 0.5%. Levobetaxolol and betaxolol were shown during exercise to have significantly less effect on heart rate and systolic blood pressure than timolol maleate.

INDICATIONS AND USAGE

BETAXON™ (levobetaxolol hydrochloride ophthalmic suspension) 0.5% is indicated for lowering intraocular pressure in patients with chronic open-angle glaucoma or ocular hypertension.

CONTRAINDICATIONS

Hypersensitivity to any component of this product. BETAXON™ Ophthalmic Suspension is contraindicated in patients with sinus bradycardia, greater than a first degree atrioventricular block, cardiogenic shock, or patients with overt cardiac failure.

WARNING

Topically applied beta-adrenergic blocking agents may be absorbed systemically. The same adverse reactions found with systemic administration of beta-adrenergic blocking agents may occur with topical administration. For example, severe respiratory reactions and cardiac reactions, including death due to bronchospasm in patients with asthma, and rarely death in association with cardiac failure, have been reported with topical application of beta-adrenergic blocking agents.

BETAXON™ Ophthalmic Suspension has been shown to have a minor effect on heart rate and blood pressure in clinical studies. Caution should be used in treating patients with a history of cardiac failure or heart block. Treatment with BETAXON™ Ophthalmic Suspension should be discontinued at the first signs of cardiac failure.

PRECAUTIONS

General:

Diabetes Mellitus. Beta-adrenergic blocking agents should be administered with caution in patients subject to spontaneous hypoglycemia or to diabetic patients (especially those with labile diabetes) who are receiving insulin or oral hypoglycemic agents. Beta-adrenergic receptor blocking agents may mask the signs and symptoms of acute hypoglycemia.

Thyrotoxicosis. Beta-adrenergic blocking agents may mask certain clinical signs (e.g., tachycardia) of hyperthyroidism. Patients suspected of developing thyrotoxicosis should be managed carefully to avoid abrupt withdrawal of beta-adrenergic blocking agents, which might precipitate a thyroid storm.

Muscle Weakness. Beta-adrenergic blockade has been reported to potentiate muscle weakness consistent with certain myasthenic symptoms (e.g., diplopia, ptosis and generalized weakness).

Major Surgery. Consideration should be given to the gradual withdrawal of beta-adrenergic blocking agents prior to general anesthesia because of the reduced ability of the heart to respond to beta-adrenergically mediated sympathetic reflex stimuli.

Pulmonary. Caution should be exercised in the treatment of glaucoma patients with excessive restriction of pulmonary function. There have been reports of asthmatic attacks and pulmonary distress during betaxolol treatment. Although rechallenges of some such patients with ophthalmic betaxolol has not adversely affected pulmonary function test results, the possibility of adverse pulmonary effects in patients sensitive to beta blockers cannot be ruled out.

Information for Patients: Do not touch dropper tip to any surface, as this may contaminate the contents. Do not use with contact lenses in eyes.

Drug Interactions: Patients who are receiving a beta-adrenergic blocking agent orally and BETAXON™ Ophthalmic Suspension should be observed for a potential additive effect either on the intraocular pressure or on the known systemic effects of beta blockade. Close observation of the patient is recommended when a beta blocker is administered to patients receiving catecholamine-depleting drugs such as reserpine, because of possible additive effects and the production of hypotension and/or bradycardia. Levobetaxolol is an adrenergic blocking agent; therefore, caution should be exercised in patients using concomitant adrenergic psychotropic drugs.

Risk from anaphylactic reaction: While taking beta-blockers, patients with a history of atopy or a history of severe anaphylactic reaction to a variety of allergens may be more reactive to repeated accidental, diagnostic, or therapeutic challenge with such allergens. Such patients may be unresponsive to the usual doses of epinephrine used to treat anaphylactic reactions.

Ocular: In patients with angle-closure glaucoma, the immediate treatment objective is to reopen the angle by constriction of the pupil with a miotic agent. Racemic betaxolol has little or no effect on the pupil. It is expected that levobetaxolol will also have little or no effect on the pupil. When BETAXON™ Ophthalmic Suspension is used to reduce elevated intraocular pressure in angle-closure glaucoma, it should be used with a miotic and not alone.

Carcinogenesis, Mutagenesis, Impairment of Fertility: In lifetime studies in mice at oral doses of 6, 20 and 60 mg/kg/day and in rats at oral doses of 3, 12 and 48 mg/kg/day, betaxolol HCl demonstrated no carcinogenic effect. Higher dose levels were not tested. Levobetaxolol was not mutagenic in the Ames assay, chromosomal aberration, mouse lymphoma, and cell transformation assays *in vitro.* Levobetaxolol demonstrated potential mutagenicity in the sister chromatid exchange assay in Chinese Hamster Ovarian cell *in vitro* in the presence of metabolic activation systems.

Pregnancy: Pregnancy Category C. Reproduction, teratology, and peri- and postnatal studies have been conducted with orally administered betaxolol HCl and levobetaxlol HCl in rats and rabbits. There was evidence of drug related postimplantation loss in rabbits with levobetaxolol HCl at 12 mg/kg/day and sternebrae malformations at 4 mg/kg/day. No other adverse effects on reproduction were noted at subtoxic dose levels. There are no adequate and well-controlled studies in pregnant women.

BETAXON™ Ophthalmic Suspension should be used during pregnancy only if the potential benefit justifies the potential risk to the fetus.

Nursing Mothers: It is not known whether BETAXON™ Ophthalmic Suspension is excreted in human milk. Because many drugs are excreted in human milk, caution should be exercised when BETAXON™ Ophthalmic Suspension is administered to nursing women.

Pediatric Use: Safety and effectiveness in pediatric patients have not been established.

Geriatric Use: No overall differences in safety or effectiveness have been observed between elderly and other adult patients.

ADVERSE REACTIONS

Ocular: In clinical trials, the most frequent event associated with the use of BETAXON™ Ophthalmic Suspension 0.5% has been transient ocular discomfort upon instillation (11%). Transient blurred vision has been reported in approximately 2% of patients. Other ocular events have been reported in less than 2% of patients and include: cataracts, and vitreous disorders. All other ocular events occurred one time at an incidence of less than 0.2%.

Systemic: Systemic reactions following administration of BETAXON™ Ophthalmic Suspension 0.5% and other topical ocular formulations of betaxolol have been at an incidence of less than 2%.

These include:

Cardiovascular: Bradycardia, heart block, hypertension, hypotension, tachycardia, and vascular anomaly.

Central Nervous System: Anxiety, dizziness, hypertonia, and vertigo.

Digestive: Constipation and dyspepsia.

Endocrine: Diabetes and hypothyroidism.

Metabolic and Nutritional Disorders: Gout, hypercholesteremia, and hyperlipidemia.

Musculoskelatal: Arthritis and tendonitis.

Pulmonary: Pulmonary distress characterized by bronchitis, dyspnea, pharyngitis, pneumonia, rhinitis, and sinusitis.

Skin and Appendages: Alopecia, dermatitis, and psoriasis.

Special Senses: Ear pain, otitis media, taste perversion, and tinnitus.

Urogenital: Breast abscess and cystitis.

Other: Accidental injury, headache, and infection.

OVERDOSAGE

No information is available on overdosage in humans. The oral maximum tolerated dose (MTD) of levobetaxolol in rats was 1250 mg/kg. The symptoms which might be expected with an overdose of a systemically administered beta-1-adrenergic receptor blocking agent are bradycardia, hypotension and acute cardiac failure.

DOSAGE AND ADMINISTRATION

The recommended dose is one drop of BETAXON™ (levobetaxolol hydrochloride ophthalmic suspension) 0.5% in the affected eye(s) twice daily. In some patients, the intraocular pressure lowering responses to BETAXON™ Ophthalmic Suspension may require a few weeks to stabilize. As with any new medication, careful monitoring of patients is advised. The concomitant use of two topical beta-adrenergic agents is not recommended.

HOW SUPPLIED

BETAXON™ (levobetaxolol hydrochloride ophthalmic suspension) 0.5% is supplied as follows: 5, 10 and 15 mL in a clear LDPE plastic ophthalmic DROP-TAINER® dispenser and a yellow polypropylene screw cap.

5 mL: NDC 0065-0239-05
10 mL: NDC 0065-0239-10
15 mL: NDC 0065-0239-15

STORAGE: Store upright 39° to 77°F (4° to 25°C).

Protect from Light.

Shake well before using.

Rx Only

U.S. Patent Nos. 4,911,920; 5,520,920; 5,540,918; 4,342,783; 4,252,984 and Pat. Pending. Revised May, 2000

BETOPTIC S® ℞

(betaxolol HCl)
0.25% as base
Sterile Ophthalmic Suspension

DESCRIPTION

BETOPTIC S® Ophthalmic Suspension 0.25% contains betaxolol hydrochloride, a cardioselective beta-adrenergic receptor blocking agent, in a sterile resin suspension formulation. Betaxolol hydrochloride is a white, crystalline powder, with a molecular weight of 343.89.

Chemical Name:

(±)-1-[p-[2-(cyclopropylmethoxy)ethyl] phenoxy]-3-(isopropylamino)-2-propanol hydrochloride.

Each mL of BETOPTIC S Ophthalmic Suspension contains: **Active:** betaxolol HCl 2.8 mg equivalent to 2.5 mg of betaxolol base. **Preservative:** benzalkonium chloride 0.01%. **Inactive:** Mannitol, Poly(Styrene-Divinyl Benzene) sulfonic acid, Carbomer 934P, edetate disodium, hydrochloric acid or sodium hydroxide (to adjust pH) and purified water.

CLINICAL PHARMACOLOGY

Betaxolol HCl, a cardioselective (beta-1-adrenergic) receptor blocking agent, does not have significant membrane-stabilizing (local anesthetic) activity and is devoid of intrinsic sympathomimetic action. Orally administered beta-adrenergic blocking agents reduce cardiac output in healthy subjects and patients with heart disease. In patients with severe impairment of myocardial function, beta-adrenergic receptor antagonists may inhibit the sympathetic stimulatory effect necessary to maintain adequate cardiac function.

When instilled in the eye, BETOPTIC S Ophthalmic Suspension 0.25% has the action of reducing elevated intraocular pressure, whether or not accompanied by glaucoma. Ophthalmic betaxolol has minimal effect on pulmonary and cardiovascular parameters.

Elevated IOP presents a major risk factor in glaucomatous field loss. The higher the level of IOP, the greater the likelihood of optic nerve damage and visual field loss. Betaxolol has the action of reducing elevated as well as normal intraocular pressure and the mechanism of ocular hypotensive action appears to be a reduction of aqueous production as demonstrated by tonography and aqueous fluorophotometry. The onset of action with betaxolol can generally be noted within 30 minutes and the maximal effect can usually be detected 2 hours after topical administration. A single dose provides a 12-hour reduction in intraocular pressure.

In controlled, double-masked studies, the magnitude and duration of the ocular hypotensive effect of BETOPTIC S Ophthalmic Suspension 0.25% and BETOPTIC Ophthalmic Solution 0.5% were clinically equivalent. BETOPTIC S Suspension was significantly more comfortable than BETOPTIC Solution.

Ophthalmic betaxolol solution at 1% (one drop in each eye) was compared to placebo in a crossover study challenging nine patients with reactive airway disease. Betaxolol HCl had no significant effect on pulmonary function as measured by FEV_1, Forced Vital Capacity (FVC), FEV_1/FVC and was not significantly different from placebo. The action of isoproterenol, a beta stimulant, administered at the end of the study was not inhibited by ophthalmic betaxolol.

No evidence of cardiovascular beta adrenergic-blockade during exercise was observed with betaxolol in a double-masked, crossover study in 24 normal subjects comparing ophthalmic betaxolol and placebo for effects on blood pressure and heart rate.

INDICATIONS AND USAGE

BETOPTIC S Ophthalmic Suspension 0.25% has been shown to be effective in lowering intraocular pressure and may be used in patients with chronic open-angle glaucoma and ocular hypertension. It may be used alone or in combination with other intraocular pressure lowering medications.

CONTRAINDICATIONS

Hypersensitivity to any component of this product. BETOPTIC S Ophthalmic Suspension 0.25% is contraindicated in patients with sinus bradycardia, greater than a first degree atrioventricular block, cardiogenic shock, or patients with overt cardiac failure.

WARNING

Topically applied beta-adrenergic blocking agents may be absorbed systemically. The same adverse reactions found with systemic administration of beta-adrenergic blocking agents may occur with topical administration. For example, severe respiratory reactions and cardiac reactions, including death due to bronchospasm in patients with asthma, and rarely death in association with cardiac failure, have been reported with topical application of beta-adrenergic blocking agents.

BETOPTIC S Ophthalmic Suspension 0.25% has been shown to have a minor effect on heart rate and blood pressure in clinical studies. Caution should be used in treating patients with a history of cardiac failure or heart block. Treatment with BETOPTIC S Ophthalmic Suspension 0.25% should be discontinued at the first signs of cardiac failure.

PRECAUTIONS

General:

Diabetes Mellitus. Beta-adrenergic blocking agents should be administered with caution in patients subject to spontaneous hypoglycemia or to diabetic patients (especially those with labile diabetes) who are receiving insulin or oral hypoglycemic agents. Beta-adrenergic receptor blocking agents may mask the signs and symptoms of acute hypoglycemia.

Thyrotoxicosis. Beta-adrenergic blocking agents may mask certain clinical signs (e.g., tachycardia) of hyperthyroidism. Patients suspected of developing thyrotoxicosis should be managed carefully to avoid abrupt withdrawal of beta-adrenergic blocking agents, which might precipitate a thyroid storm.

Muscle Weakness. Beta-adrenergic blockade has been reported to potentiate muscle weakness consistent with certain myasthenic symptoms (e.g., diplopia, ptosis and generalized weakness).

Major Surgery. Consideration should be given to the gradual withdrawal of beta-adrenergic blocking agents prior to general anesthesia because of the reduced ability of the heart to respond to beta-adrenergically mediated sympathetic reflex stimuli.

Pulmonary. Caution should be exercised in the treatment of glaucoma patients with excessive restriction of pulmonary function. There have been reports of asthmatic attacks and pulmonary distress during betaxolol treatment. Although rechallenges of some such patients with ophthalmic betaxolol has not adversely affected pulmonary function test results, the possibility of adverse pulmonary effects in patients sensitive to beta blockers cannot be ruled out.

Information for Patients: Do not touch dropper tip to any surface, as this may contaminate the contents. Do not use with contact lenses in eyes.

Drug Interactions: Patients who are receiving a beta-adrenergic blocking agent orally and BETOPTIC S Ophthalmic Suspension 0.25% should be observed for a potential additive effect either on the intraocular pressure or on the known systemic effects of beta blockade.

Close observation of the patient is recommended when a beta blocker is administered to patients receiving catecholamine-depleting drugs such as reserpine, because of possible additive effects and the production of hypotension and/or bradycardia.

Betaxolol is an adrenergic blocking agent; therefore, caution should be exercised in patients using concomitant adrenergic psychotropic drugs.

Risk from anaphylactic reaction: While taking beta-blockers, patients with a history of atopy or a history of severe anaphylactic reaction to a variety of allergens may be more reactive to repeated accidental, diagnostic, or therapeutic challenge with such allergens. Such patients may be unresponsive to the usual doses of epinephrine used to treat anaphylactic reactions.

Ocular: In patients with angle-closure glaucoma, the immediate treatment objective is to reopen the angle by constriction of the pupil with a miotic agent. Betaxolol has little or no effect on the pupil. When BETOPTIC S Ophthalmic Suspension 0.25% is used to reduce elevated intraocular pressure in angle-closure glaucoma, it should be used with a miotic and not alone.

Carcinogenesis, Mutagenesis, Impairment of Fertility: Lifetime studies with betaxolol HCl have been completed in mice at oral doses of 6, 20 or 60 mg/kg/day and in rats at 3, 12 or 48 mg/kg/day; betaxolol HCl demonstrated no carcinogenic effect. Higher dose levels were not tested.

In a variety of *in vitro* and *in vivo* bacterial and mammalian cell assays, betaxolol HCl was nonmutagenic.

Pregnancy: Pregnancy Category C. Reproduction, teratology, and peri- and postnatal studies have been conducted with orally administered betaxolol HCl in rats and rabbits. There was evidence of drug related postimplantation loss in rabbits and rats at dose levels above 12 mg/kg and 128 mg/kg, respectively. Betaxolol HCl was not shown to be teratogenic, however, and there were no other adverse effects on reproduction at subtoxic dose levels. There are no adequate and well-controlled studies in pregnant women. BETOPTIC S should be used during pregnancy only if the potential benefit justifies the potential risk to the fetus.

Nursing Mothers: It is not known whether betaxolol HCl is excreted in human milk. Because many drugs are excreted in human milk, caution should be exercised when BETOPTIC S Ophthalmic Suspension 0.25% is administered to nursing women.

Pediatric Use: Safety and effectiveness in pediatric patients have not been established.

ADVERSE REACTIONS

Ocular: In clinical trials, the most frequent event associated with the use of BETOPTIC S Ophthalmic Suspension 0.25% has been transient ocular discomfort. The following other conditions have been reported in small numbers of patients: blurred vision, corneal punctate keratitis, foreign

Continued on next page

Betoptic S—Cont.

body sensation, photophobia, tearing, itching, dryness of eyes, erythema, inflammation, discharge, ocular pain, decreased visual acuity and crusty lashes.
Additional medical events reported with other formulations of betaxolol include allergic reactions, decreased corneal sensitivity, corneal punctate staining which may appear in dendritic formations, edema and anisocoria.
Systemic: Systemic reactions following administration of BETOPTIC S Ophthalmic Suspension 0.25% or BETOPTIC Ophthalmic Solution 0.5% have been rarely reported. These include:
Cardiovascular: Bradycardia, heart block and congestive failure.
Pulmonary: Pulmonary distress characterized by dyspnea, bronchospasm, thickened bronchial secretions, asthma and respiratory failure.
Central Nervous System: Insomnia, dizziness, vertigo, headaches, depression, lethargy, and increase in signs and symptoms of myasthenia gravis.
Other: Hives, toxic epidermal necrolysis, hair loss, and glossitis. Perversions of taste and smell have been reported.

OVERDOSAGE

No information is available on overdosage of humans. The oral LD50 of the drug ranged from 350–920 mg/kg in mice and 860–1050 mg/kg in rats. The symptoms which might be expected with an overdose of a systemically administered beta-1-adrenergic receptor blocking agent are bradycardia, hypotension and acute cardiac failure.
A topical overdose of BETOPTIC S Ophthalmic Suspension 0.25% may be flushed from the eye(s) with warm tap water.

DOSAGE AND ADMINISTRATION

The recommended dose is one to two drops of BETOPTIC S Ophthalmic Suspension 0.25% in the affected eye(s) twice daily. In some patients, the intraocular pressure lowering responses to BETOPTIC S may require a few weeks to stabilize. As with any new medication, careful monitoring of patients is advised.
If the intraocular pressure of the patient is not adequately controlled on this regimen, concomitant therapy with pilocarpine and other miotics, and/or epinephrine and/or carbonic anhydrase inhibitors can be instituted.

HOW SUPPLIED

BETOPTIC S Ophthalmic Suspension 0.25% is supplied as follows: 2.5, 5, 10 and 15 mL in plastic ophthalmic DROP-TAINER® dispensers.

2.5 mL: **NDC** 0065-0246-20
5 mL: **NDC** 0065-0246-05
10 mL: **NDC** 0065-0246-10
15 mL: **NDC** 0065-0246-15

STORAGE

Store upright at room temperature. Shake well before using.
Rx Only.
U.S. Patents Nos. 4,252,984; 4,311,708; 4,342,783; 4,911,920.

BION® TEARS OTC
Lubricant Eye Drops

DESCRIPTION

BION® TEARS are specially designed to be physiologically compatible with the surface of the eye and to treat dry eye symptoms by replacing needed tear components. BION® TEARS advanced formula contains:
The unique DUASORB® polymeric system which combines with natural tears to soothe sensitive dry spots.
A special lubricating vehicle designed to match the electrolyte balance of sodium, potassium, calcium, magnesium, zinc and bicarbonate found in natural tears.
No preservatives or decongestants that may cause irritation or limit use. BION® TEARS may be used as often as necessary to provide relief.
BION® TEARS special formula requires special packaging. Airtight foil pouches are used to maintain the delicate balance of ingredients until the product is ready for use in the eye. **To ensure optimal effectiveness once the pouch is opened, the containers inside the pouch must be used within four days (96 hours).**
PLEASE READ THESE WARNINGS PRIOR TO USING BION® TEARS LUBRICANT EYE DROPS AND KEEP THIS INSERT FOR FUTURE REFERENCE.

WARNINGS

If you experience eye pain, changes in vision, continued redness or irritation of the eye, or if the condition worsens or persists for more than 72 hours, discontinue use and consult a doctor.
If solution changes color or becomes cloudy, do not use. To avoid contamination, do not touch tip of container to any surface. Do not reuse. Once opened, discard. Keep this and all drugs out of the reach of children. In case of accidental ingestion, seek professional assistance or contact a Poison Control Center immediately.

HOW SUPPLIED

BION® TEARS Lubricant Eye Drops are supplied in boxes of 28 0.015 fl. oz. single-use containers.
Product Code 0065-0419-18

CILOXAN® ℞
(Ciprofloxacin HCl)
0.3% as base
Sterile Ophthalmic Solution and Ointment

DESCRIPTION

CILOXAN® (Ciprofloxacin HCl) Ophthalmic Solution and Ointment are synthetic, sterile, multiple dose, antimicrobial for topical ophthalmic use. Ciprofloxacin is a fluoroquinolone antibacterial active against a broad spectrum of gram-positive and gram-negative ocular pathogens. It is available as the monohydrochloride monohydrate salt of 1-cyclopropyl-6-fluoro-1,4-dihydro-4-oxo-7-(1-piperazinyl)-3-quinoline-carboxylic acid. It is a faint to light yellow crystalline powder with a molecular weight of 385.8. Its empirical formula is $C_{17}H_{18}FN_3O_3 \cdot HCl \cdot H_2O$.
Ciprofloxacin differs from other quinolones in that it has a fluorine atom at the 6-position, a piperazine moiety at the 7-position, and a cyclopropyl ring at the 1-position.
Each mL of CILOXAN Ophthalmic Solution contains: **Active:** Ciprofloxacin HCl 3.5 mg equivalent to 3 mg base. **Preservative:** Benzalkonium Chloride 0.006%. **Inactive:** Sodium Acetate, Acetic Acid, Mannitol 4.6%, Edetate Disodium 0.05%, Hydrochloric Acid and/or Sodium Hydroxide (to adjust pH) and Purified Water. The pH is approximately 4.5 and the osmolality is approximately 300 mOsm.
Each gram of CILOXAN Ophthalmic Ointment contains: **Active:** Ciprofloxacin HCl 3.33 mg equivalent to 3 mg base. **Inactives:** Mineral Oil, White Petrolatum.

CLINICAL PHARMACOLOGY

Systemic Absorption: A systemic absorption study was performed in which CILOXAN Ophthalmic Solution was administerd in each eye every two hours while awake for two days followed by every four hours while awake for an additional 5 days. The maximum reported plasma concentration of ciprofloxacin was less than 5 ng/mL. The mean concentration was usually less than 2.5 ng/mL. Ointment mean concentration levels have not been determined but are expected to be similar.
Microbiology: Ciprofloxacin has *in vitro* activity against a wide range of gram-negative and gram-positive organisms. The bactericidal action of ciprofloxacin results from interference with the enzyme DNA gyrase which is needed for the synthesis of bacterial DNA.
Ciprofloxacin has been shown to be active against most strains of the following organisms both *in vitro* and in clinical infections. (See INDICATIONS AND USAGE section).

Gram-Positive:
Staphylococcus aureus (including methicillin-susceptible and methicillin-resistant strains)
Staphylococcus epidermidis
Streptococcus pneumoniae
Streptococcus (Viridans Group)

Gram-Negative:
Haemophilus influenzae
Pseudomonas aeruginosa
Serratia marcescens

Ciprofloxacin has been shown to be active *in vitro* against most strains of the following organisms, however, the clinical significance of these data is unknown:

Gram-Positive:
Bacillus species
Corynobacterium species
Enterococcus faecalis (Many strains are only moderately susceptible)
Staphylococcus haemolyticus
Staphylococcus hominis
Staphylococcus saprophyticus
Streptococcus pyogenes

Gram-Negative:
Acinetobacter caloacetius subsp anitratus
Aeromonas caviae
Aeromonas hydrophilia
Brucella melitensis
Campylobacter coli
Campylobacter jejuni
Citrobacter diversus
Citrobacter freundii
Edwardsiella tarda
Enterobacter aerogenes
Enterobacter cloacae
Eschricia coli
Haemophilius ducreyl
Haemophilius parainfluenzae
Klebsiella pneumoniae
Klebsiella oxytoca
Legionella pneumophilia
Moraxella (Branhamella) catarrhalis
Morganella morganii
Neisseria gonorrhoeae
Neisseria meningitidis
Pasteurella multocida
Proteus mirabilis
Proteus vulgaris
Providencia rettgeri
Providencia stuartii
Salmonella enteritidis
Salmonella typhi
Shigella sonneii
Shigella flexneri
Vibrio cholerae
Vibrio parahaemolyticus
Vibrio vulnificus
Yersinia enterocolitica

Other Organisms:
Chlamydia trachomatis (only moderately susceptible) and Mycobacterium tuberculosis (only moderately susceptible).
Most strains of Pseudomonas cepacia and Burkholderia cepacia and some strains of Pseudomonas maltophilia and Stenotrophomonas maltophilia are resistant to ciprofloxacin as are most anaerobic bacteria, including Bacteroides fragilis and Clostridium difficile.
The minimal bactericidal concentration (MBC) generally does not exceed the minimal inhibitory concentration (MIC) by more than a factor of 2. Resistance to ciprofloxacin *in vitro* usually develops slowly (multiple-step mutation).
Ciprofloxacin does not cross-react with other antimicrobial agents such as beta-lactams or aminoglycosides; therefore, organisms resistant to these drugs may be susceptible to ciprofloxacin. Organisms resistant to ciprofloxacin may be susceptible to beta-lactams or aminoglycosides.
Clinical Studies:
Following therapy with CILOXAN® Ophthalmic Solution, 76% of the patients with corneal ulcers and positive bacterial cultures were clinically cured and complete re-epithelialization occurred in about 92% of the ulcers.
In 3 and 7 day multicenter clinical trials, 52% of the patients with conjunctivitis and positive conjunctival cultures were clinically cured and 70–80% had all causative pathogens eradicated by the end of treatment. In multicenter clinical trials, approximately 75% of the patients with signs and symptoms of bacterial conjunctivitis and positive conjunctival cultures were clinically cured and approximately 80% had presumed pathogens eradicated by the end of treatment (day 7).

INDICATIONS AND USAGE

CILOXAN Ophthalmic Solution and CILOXAN Ophthalmic Ointment are indicated for the treatment of infections caused by susceptible strains of the designated microorganisms in the conditions listed below:
Conjunctivitis — Solution and Ointment:
Haemophilus influenzae
Staphylococcus aureus
Staphylococcus epidermidis
Streptococcus pneumoniae
Streptococcus (Viridans Group)
Corneal Ulcers — Solution only:
Pseudomonas aeruginosa
Serratia marcescens*
Staphylococcus aureus
Staphylococcus epidermidis
Streptococcus pneumoniae
Streptococcus (Viridans Group)*
*Efficacy for these organisms was studied in fewer than 10 infections.

CONTRAINDICATIONS

A history of hypersensitivity to ciprofloxacin or any other component of the medication is a contraindication to its use. A history of hypersensitivity to other quinolones may also contraindicate the use of ciprofloxacin.

WARNINGS

NOT FOR INJECTION INTO THE EYE.
Serious and occasionally fatal hypersensitivity (anaphylactic) reactions, some following the first dose, have been reported in patients receiving systemic quinolone therapy. Some reactions were accompanied by cardiovascular collapse, loss of consciousness, tingling, pharyngeal or facial edema, dyspnea, urticaria, and itching. Only a few patients had a history of hypersensitivity reactions. Serious anaphylactic reactions require immediate emergency treatment with epinephrine and other resuscitation measures, including oxygen, intravenous fluids, intravenous antihistamines, corticosteroids, pressor amines and airway management, as clinically indicated. Remove contact lenses before using.

PRECAUTIONS

General: As with other antibacterial preparations, prolonged use of ciprofloxacin may result in overgrowth of nonsusceptible organisms, including fungi. If superinfection occurs, appropriate therapy should be initiated. Whenever clinical judgment dictates, the patient should be examined with the aid of magnification, such as slit lamp biomicroscopy and, where appropriate, fluorescein staining.
Ciprofloxacin should be discontinued at the first appearance of a skin rash or any other sign of hypersensitivity reaction.
Ophthalmic ointments may retard corneal healing and cause visual blurring. Patients should be advised not to wear contact lenses if they have signs and symptoms of bacterial conjunctivitis.
In clinical studies of patients with bacterial corneal ulcer, a white crystalline precipitate located in the superficial portion of the corneal defect was observed in 35 (16.6%) of 210 patients. The onset of the precipitate was within 24 hours to 7 days after starting therapy. In one patient, the precipitate was immediately irrigated out upon its appearance. In 17 patients, resolution of the precipitate was seen in 1 to 8 days (seven within the first 24–72 hours), in five patients, resolution was noted in 10–13 days. In nine patients, exact resolution days were unavailable; however, at follow-up examinations, 18–44 days after onset of the event, complete resolution of the precipitate was noted. In three patients,

outcome information was unavailable. The precipitate did not preclude continued use of ciprofloxacin, nor did it adversely affect the clinical course of the ulcer or visual outcome. (SEE ADVERSE REACTIONS).

Information for patients: Do not touch tip of any surface, as this may contaminate the product.

Drug Interactions: Specific drug interaction studies have not been conducted with ophthalmic ciprofloxacin. However, the systemic administration of some quinolones has been shown to elevate plasma concentrations of theophylline, interfere with the metabolism of caffeine, enhance the effects of the oral anticoagulant, warfarin, and its derivatives and has been associated with transient elevations in serum creatinine in patients receiving cyclosporine concomitantly.

Carcinogenesis, Mutagenesis, Impairment of Fertility: Eight *in vitro* mutagenicity tests have been conducted with ciprofloxacin and the test results are listed below:

Salmonella/Microsome Test (Negative)
E. coli DNA Repair Assay (Negative)
Mouse Lymphoma Cell Forward Mutation Assay (Positive)
Chinese Hamster V_{79} Cell HGPRT Test (Negative)
Syrian Hamster Embryo Cell Transformation Assay (Negative)
Saccharomyces cerevisiae Point Mutation Assay (Negative)
Saccharomyces cerevisiae Mitotic Crossover and Gene Conversion Assay (Negative)
Rat Hepatocyte DNA Repair Assay (Positive)

Thus, two of the eight tests were positive, but the results of the following three *in vivo* test systems gave negative results:

Rat Hepatocyte DNA Repair Assay
Micronucleus Test (Mice)
Dominant Lethal Test (Mice)

Long term carcinogenicity studies in mice and rats have been completed. After daily oral dosing for up to two years, there is no evidence that ciprofloxacin had any carcinogenic or tumorigenic effects in these species.

Pregnancy—Pregnancy Category C: Reproduction studies have been performed in rats and mice at doses up to six times the usual daily human oral dose and have revealed no evidence of impaired fertility or harm to the fetus due to ciprofloxacin. In rabbits, as with most antimicrobial agents, ciprofloxacin (30 and 100 mg/kg orally) produced gastrointestinal disturbances resulting in maternal weight loss and an increased incidence of abortion. No teratogenicity was observed at either dose. After intravenous administration, at doses up to 20 mg/kg, no maternal toxicity was produced and no embryotoxicity or teratogenicity was observed. There are no adequate and well controlled studies in pregnant women. CILOXAN® should be used during pregnancy only if the potential benefit justifies the potential risk to the fetus.

Nursing Mothers: It is not known whether topically applied ciprofloxacin is excreted in human milk; however, it is known that orally administered ciprofloxacin is excreted in the milk of lactating rats and oral ciprofloxacin has been reported in human breast milk after a single 500 mg dose. Caution should be exercised when CILOXAN is administered to a nursing mother.

Pediatric Use: Safety and effectiveness in pediatric patients below the age of 1 year (solution) and 2 years (ointment) have not been established.

Although ciprofloxacin and other quinolones cause arthropathy in immature Beagle dogs/animals after oral administration, topical ocular administration of ciprofloxacin to immature animals did not cause any arthropathy and there is no evidence that the ophthalmic dosage form has any effect on the weight bearing joints.

ADVERSE REACTIONS

The most frequently reported drug related adverse reaction was local burning or discomfort. In corneal ulcer studies with frequent administration of the drug, white crystalline precipitates were seen in approximately 17% (solution) and 13% (ointment) of patients (SEE PRECAUTIONS). Other reactions occurring in less than 10% of patients included lid margin crusting, crystals/scales, foreign body sensation, itching, conjunctival hyperemia and a bad taste following instillation. Additional events occurring in less than 1% of patients included corneal staining, keratopathy/keratitis, allergic reactions, lid edema, tearing, photophobia, corneal infiltrates, nausea and decreased vision, blurred vision, dry eye, epitheliopathy, eye pain, irritation and dermatitis.

OVERDOSAGE

A topical overdose of CILOXAN Opththalmic Solution may be flushed from the (eye(s) with warm tap water.

DOSAGE AND ADMINISTRATION

Corneal Ulcers: The recommended dosage regimen for the treatment of corneal ulcers is two drops of the Solution into the affected eye every 15 minutes for the first six hours and then two drops into the affected eye every 30 minutes for the remainder of the first day. On the second day, instill two drops in the affected eye hourly. On the third through the fourteenth day, place two drops in the affected eye every four hours. Treatment may be continued after 14 days if corneal re-epithelialization has not occurred.

Bacterial Conjunctivitis: Solution: The recommended dosage regimen for the treatment of bacterial conjunctivitis is one or two drops of CILOXAN Ophthalmic Solution instilled into the conjunctival sac(s) every two hours while awake for two days and one or two drops every four hours while awake for the next five days. Ointment: Apply a ½" ribbon into the conjunctival sac three times a day on the first two days, then apply a ½" ribbon two times a day for the next five days.

HOW SUPPLIED

As a sterile ophthalmic solution in 2.5 mL (NDC 0065-0656-25), 5 mL (NDC 0065-0656-05) and 10 mL (NDC 0065-0656-10) in plastic DROP-TAINER® dispensers. Sterile ophthalmic ointment in 3.5 g ophthalmic tube (NDC 0065-0654-35).

STORAGE

Solution: Store at 2° to 25°C (36° to 77°F). Protect from light.

Ointment: Store at 36°F to 77°F (2°C to 25°C)

ANIMAL PHARMACOLOGY

Ciprofloxacin and related drugs have been shown to cause arthropathy in immature animals of most species tested following oral administration. However, a one-month topical ocular study using immature Beagle dogs did not demonstrate any articular lesions.

Rx Only

U.S. Patent No. 4,670,444

CIPRO® HC OTIC ℞

(ciprofloxacin hydrochloride and hydrocortisone otic suspension)

DESCRIPTION

CIPRO® HC OTIC (ciprofloxacin hydrochloride and hydrocortisone otic suspension) contains the synthetic broad spectrum antibacterial agent, ciprofloxacin hydrochloride, combined with the anti-inflammatory corticosteroid, hydrocortisone, in a preserved, nonsterile suspension for otic use. Each mL of CIPRO HC OTIC contains ciprofloxacin hydrochloride (equivalent to 2 mg ciprofloxacin), 10 mg hydrocortisone, and 9 mg benzyl alcohol as a preservative. The inactive ingredients are polyvinyl alcohol, sodium chloride, sodium acetate, glacial acetic acid, phospholipon 90HB (modified lecithin), polysorbate, and purified water. Sodium hydroxide or hydrochloric acid may be added for adjustment of pH.

Ciprofloxacin, a fluoroquinolone, is available as the monohydrochloride monohydrate salt of 1-cyclopropyl-6-fluoro-1,4-dihydro-4-oxo-7-(1-piperazinyl)-3-quinolinecarboxylic acid. Its empirical formula is $C_{17}H_{18}FN_3O_3 \bullet HCl \bullet H_2O$.

Hydrocortisone, pregn-4-ene-3, 20-dione, 11, 17, 21-trihydroxy-(11β)-, is an anti-inflammatory corticosteroid. Its empirical formula is $C_{21}H_{30}O_5$.

CLINICAL PHARMACOLOGY

The plasma concentrations of ciprofloxacin were not measured following three drops of otic suspension administration because the systemic exposure to ciprofloxacin is expected to be below the limit of quantitation of the assay (0.05 µg/mL).

Similarly, the predicted C_{max} of hydrocortisone is within the range of endogenous hydrocortisone concentration (0–150 ng/mL), and therefore can not be differentiated from the endogenous cortisol.

Preclinical studies have shown that CIPRO HC OTIC was not toxic to the guinea pig cochlea when administered intratympanically twice daily for 30 days and was only weakly irritating to rabbit skin upon repeated exposure.

Hydrocortisone has been added to aid in the resolution of the inflammatory response accompanying bacterial infection.

Microbiology

Ciprofloxacin has *in vitro* activity against a wide range of gram-positive and gram-negative microorganisms. The bactericidal action of ciprofloxacin results from interference with the enzyme, DNA gyrase, which is needed for the synthesis of bacterial DNA. Cross-resistance has been observed between ciprofloxacin and other fluoroquinolones. There is generally no cross-resistance between ciprofloxacin and other classes of antibacterial agents such as beta-lactams or aminoglycosides.

Ciprofloxacin has been shown to be active against most strains of the following microorganisms, both *in vitro* and in clinical infections of acute otitis externa as described in the **INDICATIONS AND USAGE** section:

Aerobic gram-positive microorganism
Staphylococcus aureus
Aerobic gram-negative microorganisms
Proteus mirabilis
Pseudomonas aeruginosa

INDICATIONS AND USAGE

CIPRO® HC OTIC is indicated for the treatment of acute otitis externa in adult and pediatric patients, one year and older, due to susceptible strains of *Pseudomonas aeruginosa, Staphylococcus aureus,* and *Proteus mirabilis.*

CONTRAINDICATIONS

CIPRO HC OTIC is contraindicated in persons with a history of hypersensitivity to hydrocortisone, ciprofloxacin or any member of the quinolone class of antimicrobial agents. This nonsterile product should not be used in the tympanic membrane is perforated. Use of this product is contraindicated in viral infections of the external canal including varicella and herpes simplex infections.

WARNINGS

NOT FOR OPHTHALMIC USE. NOT FOR INJECTION.

CIPRO HC OTIC should be discontinued at the first appearance of a skin rash or any other sign of hypersensitivity. Serious and occasionally fatal hypersensitivity (anaphylactic) reactions, some following the first dose, have been reported in patients receiving systemic quinolones. Serious acute hypersensitivity reactions may require immediate emergency treatment.

PRECAUTIONS

GENERAL: As with other antibiotic preparations, use of this product may result in overgrowth of nonsusceptible organisms, including fungi. If the infection is not improved after one week of therapy, cultures should be obtained to guide further treatment.

Information for Patients:

If rash or allergic reaction occurs, discontinue use immediately and contact your physician.
Do not use in the eyes.
Avoid contaminating the dropper with material from the ear, fingers, or other sources.
Protect from light.
Shake well immediately before using.
Discard unused portion after therapy is completed.

Carcinogenesis, Mutagenesis, Impairment of Fertility: Eight *in vitro* mutagenicity tests have been conducted with ciprofloxacin, and the test results are listed below:

Salmonella/Microsome Test (Negative)
E. coli DNA Repair Assay (Negative)
Mouse Lymphoma Cell Forward Mutation Assay (Positive)
Chinese Hamster V_{79} Cell HGPRT Test (Negative)
Syrian Hamster Embryo Cell Transformation Assay (Negative)
Saccharomyces cerevisiae Point Mutation Assay (Negative)
Saccharomyces cerevisiae Mitotic Crossover and Gene Conversion Assay (Negative)
Rat Hepatocyte DNA Repair Assay (Positive)

Thus, 2 of the 8 tests were positive, but results of the following 3 *in vivo* test systems gave negative results:

Rat Hepatocyte DNA Repair Assay
Micronucleus Test (Mice)
Dominant Lethal Test (Mice)

Long-term carcinogenicity studies in mice and rats have been completed for ciprofloxacin. After daily oral doses of 750 mg/kg (mice) and 250 mg/kg (rats) were administered for up to 2 years, there was no evidence that ciprofloxacin had any carcinogenic or tumorigenic effects in these species. No long term studies of CIPRO® HC OTIC suspension have been performed to evaluate carcinogenic potential.

Fertility studies performed in rats at oral doses of ciprofloxacin up to 100 mg/kg/day revealed no evidence of impairment. This would be over 1000 times the maximum recommended clinical dose of ototopical ciprofloxacin based upon body surface area, assuming total absorption of ciprofloxacin from the ear of a patient treated with CIPRO® HC OTIC twice per day.

Long term studies have not been performed to evaluate the carcinogenic potential or the effect on fertility of topical hydrocortisone. Mutagenicity studies with hydrocortisone were negative.

Pregnancy: Teratogenic Effects. Pregnancy Category C: Reproduction studies have been performed in rats and mice using oral doses of up to 100 mg/kg and IV doses up to 30 mg/kg and have revealed no evidence of harm to the fetus as a result of ciprofloxacin. In rabbits, ciprofloxacin (30 and 100 mg/kg orally) produced gastrointestinal disturbances resulting in maternal weight loss and an increased incidence of abortion, but no teratogenicity was observed at either dose. After intravenous administration of doses up to 20 mg/kg, no maternal toxicity was produced in the rabbit, and no embryotoxicity or teratogenicity was observed.

Corticosteroids are generally teratogenic in laboratory animals when administered systemically at relatively low dosage levels. The more potent corticosteroids have been shown to be teratogenic after dermal application in laboratory animals.

Animal reproduction studies have not been conducted with CIPRO HC OTIC. No adequate and well controlled studies have been performed in pregnant women. Caution should be exercised when CIPRO HC OTIC is used by a pregnant woman.

Nursing Mothers: Ciprofloxacin is excreted in human milk with systemic use. It is not known whether ciprofloxacin is excreted in human milk following topical otic administration. Because of the potential for serious adverse reactions in nursing infants, a decision should be made whether to discontinue nursing or to discontinue the drug, taking into account the importance of the drug to the mother.

Pediatric use: The safety and efficacy of CIPRO HC OTIC have been established in pediatric patients 2 years and older (131 patients) in adequate and well-controlled clinical trials. Although no data are available on patients less than age 2 years, there are no known safety concerns or differences in the disease process in this population which would preclude use of this product in patients one year and older. **See DOSAGE AND ADMINISTRATION.**

ADVERSE REACTIONS

In Phase 3 clinical trials, a total of 564 patients were treated with CIPRO® HC OTIC. Adverse events with at least remote relationship to treatment included headache (1.2%) and pruritus (0.4%). The following treatment-related

Continued on next page

Cipro HC—Cont.

adverse events were each reported in a single patient: migraine, hypesthesia, paresthesia, fungal dermatitis, cough, rash, urticaria, and alopecia.

DOSAGE AND ADMINISTRATION

SHAKE WELL IMMEDIATELY BEFORE USING.

For children (age 1 year and older) and adults, 3 drops of the suspension should be instilled into the affected ear twice daily for seven days. The suspension should be warmed by holding the bottle in the hand for 1–2 minutes to avoid the dizziness which may result from the instillation of a cold solution into the ear canal. The patient should lie with the affected ear upward and then the drops should be instilled. This position should be maintained for 30–60 seconds to facilitate penetration of the drops into the ear. Repeat, if necessary, for the opposite ear. Discard unused portion after therapy is completed.

HOW SUPPLIED

CIPRO HC OTIC is supplied as a white to off-white opaque suspension in a 10 mL bottle with a dropper dispenser.

NDC 0065-8531-10

Store below 77° F (25° C). Avoid freezing. Protect from light.

U.S. Patent Nos. 4,670,444; 4,844,902; 5,843,930; and Pat. Pending.

CIPRO® is a registered trademark of Bayer AG.

Licensed by **Bayer AG**

Manufactured by **Bayer Corporation**.

Rx Only

Shown in Product Identification Guide, page 303

NAPHCON® A — OTC

Eye Drops
Relieves Itching & Redness
EYE ALLERGY RELIEF

Temporary relief of the minor eye symptoms of itching and redness caused by ragweed, pollen, grass, animal hair, and dander.

DESCRIPTION

Active: Pheniramine Maleate 0.3%, Naphazoline Hydrochloride 0.025%. **Preservative:** Benzalkonium Chloride 0.01%. **Inactive:** Sodium Chloride, Boric Acid, Sodium Borate, Edetate Disodium 0.01%, Sodium Hydroxide and/or Hydrochloric Acid (to adjust pH), Purified Water. The sterile ophthalmic solution has a pH of about 6 and a tonicity of about 270 mOsm/Kg.

DIRECTIONS

Instill 1 or 2 drops in the affected eye(s) up to 4 times daily.

WARNINGS

To avoid contamination, do not touch tip of container to any surface. Replace cap after using. If solution changes color or becomes cloudy, do not use.

If you experience eye pain, changes in vision, continued redness or irritation of the eye, or if the condition worsens, or persists for more than 72 hours, discontinue use and consult a physician. Overuse of this product may produce increased redness of the eye.

If you are sensitive to any ingredient in this product, do not use. Do not use use this product if you have heart disease, high blood pressure, difficulty in urination due to enlargement of the prostate gland or narrow angle glaucoma unless directed by a physician.

Accidental oral ingestion in infants and children may lead to coma and marked reduction in body temperature. Before using in children under 6 years of age, consult your physician. Keep this and all drugs out of reach of children. In case of accidental ingestion, seek professional assistance or contact a Poison Control Center immediately.

Remove contact lenses before using.

Store at 36°–80°F (2°–27°C).

Protect from light.

Use before the expiration date marked on the carton or bottle.

PATANOL® — ℞

(olopatadine hydrochloride ophthalmic solution) 0.1%

DESCRIPTION

PATANOL® (olopatadine hydrochloride ophthalmic solution) 0.1% is a sterile ophthalmic solution containing olopatadine, a relatively selective H_1-receptor antagonist and inhibitor of histamine release from the mast cell for topical administration to the eyes. Olopatadine hydrochloride is a white, crystalline, water-soluble powder with a molecular weight of 373.88.

Chemical Name: 11-[(Z)-3-(Dimethylamino)propylidene]-6-11-dihydrodibenz[b,e] oxepin-2-acetic acid hydrochloride

Each mL of PATANOL contains: **Active:** 1.11 mg olopatadine hydrochloride equivalent to 1 mg olopatadine. **Preservative:** benzalkonium chloride 0.01%. **Inactives:** dibasic sodium phosphate; sodium chloride; hydrochloric acid/sodium hydroxide (adjust pH); and purified water.

It has a pH of approximately 7 and an osmolality of approximately 300 mOsm/kg.

CLINICAL PHARMACOLOGY

Olopatadine is an inhibitor of the release of histamine from the mast cell and a relatively selective histamine H_1-antagonist that inhibits the *in vivo* and *in vitro* type 1 immediate hypersensitivity reaction including inhibition of histamine induced effects on human conjunctival epithelial cells. Olopatadine is devoid of effects on alpha-adrenergic, dopamine, muscarinic type 1 and 2, and serotonin receptors. Following topical ocular administration in man, olopatadine was shown to have low systemic exposure. Two studies in normal volunteers (totaling 24 subjects) dosed bilaterally with olopatadine 0.15% ophthalmic solution once every 12 hours for 2 weeks demonstrated plasma concentrations to be generally below the quantitation limit of the assay (<0.5 ng/mL). Samples in which olopatadine was quantifiable were typically found within 2 hours of dosing and ranged from 0.5 to 1.3 ng/mL. The half-life in plasma was approximately 3 hours, and elimination was predominantly through renal excretion. Approximately 60–70% of the dose was recovered in the urine as parent drug. Two metabolites, the monodesmethyl and the N-oxide, were detected at low concentrations in the urine.

INDICATIONS AND USAGE

PATANOL (olopatadine hydrochloride ophthalmic solution) 0.1% is indicated for the treatment of the signs and symptoms of allergic conjunctivitis.

CONTRAINDICATIONS

PATANOL is contraindicated in persons with a known hypersensitivity to olopatadine hydrochloride or any components of PATANOL.

WARNINGS

PATANOL® is for topical use only and not for injection or oral use.

PRECAUTIONS: Information for Patients: To prevent contaminating the dropper tip and solution, care should be taken not to touch the eyelids or surrounding areas with the dropper tip of the bottle. Keep bottle tightly closed when not in use.

Carcinogenesis, Mutagenesis, Impairment of Fertility: Olopatadine administered orally was not carcinogenic in mice and rats in doses up to 500 mg/kg/day and 200 mg/kg/day, respectively. Based on a 40 µl drop size, these doses were 78,125 and 31,250 times higher than the maximum recommended ocular human dose (MROHD). No mutagenic potential was observed when olopatadine was tested in an *in vitro* bacterial reverse mutation (Ames) test, an *in vitro* mammalian chromosome aberration assay or an *in vivo* mouse micronucleus test. Olopatadine administered to male and female rats at oral doses of 62,500 times MROHD level resulted in a slight decrease in the fertility index and reduced implantation rate; no effects on reproductive function were observed at doses of 7,800 times the maximum recommended ocular human use level.

Pregnancy: Pregnancy Category C. Olopatadine was found not to be teratogenic in rats and rabbits. However, rats treated at 600 mg/kg/day, or 93,750 times the MROHD and rabbits treated at 400 mg/kg/day, or 62,500 times the MROHD, during organogenesis showed a decrease in live fetuses. There are, however, no adequate and well controlled studies in pregnant women. Because animal studies are not always predictive of human responses, this drug should be used in pregnant women only if the potential benefit to the mother justifies the potential risk to the embryo or fetus.

Nursing Mothers: Olopatadine has been identified in the milk of nursing rats following oral administration. It is not known whether topical ocular administration could result in sufficient systemic absorption to produce detectable quantities in the human breast milk. Nevertheless, caution should be exercised when PATANOL® is administered to a nursing mother.

Pediatric Use: Safety and effectiveness in pediatric patients below the age of 3 years have not been established.

ADVERSE REACTIONS

Headaches have been reported at an incidence of 7%. The following adverse experiences have been reported in less than 5% of patients: Asthenia, blurred vision, burning or stinging, cold syndrome, dry eye, foreign body sensation, hyperemia, hypersensitivity, keratitis, lid edema, nausea, pharyngitis, pruritus, rhinitis, sinusitis, and taste perversion. Some of these events were similar to the underlying disease being studied.

DOSAGE AND ADMINISTRATION

The recommended dose is one drop in each affected eye two times per day at an interval of 6 to 8 hours.

HOW SUPPLIED

PATANOL® (olopatadine hydrochloride ophthalmic solution) 0.1% is supplied as follows: 5 mL in plastic DROP-TAINER® dispenser.

5 mL: NDC 0065-0271-05

Storage: Store at 39°F to 77°F (4°C to 25°C).

U.S. Patents Nos. 4,871,865; 4,923,892; 5,116,863; 5,641,805.

Rx Only.

TEARS NATURALE® II — OTC

Lubricant Eye Drops

TEARS NATURALE FREE®

Lubricant Eye Drops

DESCRIPTION

TEARS NATURALE® II is the only lubricant eye drop preserved with safe, nonsensitizing POLYQUAD® 0.001%. *In vitro* studies have shown that POLYQUAD substantially avoids the damaging effects of epithelial cell toxicity possible with other tear substitute preservatives and allows epithelial cell growth. POLYQUAD has been shown to be 99% reaction-free in normal subjects and 97% reaction-free in subjects known to be preservative sensitive.

TEARS NATURALE® FREE is a preservative-free version of TEARS NATURALE II.

With their unique mucin like polymeric formulation, and with their natural pH, low viscosity, and isotonicity, TEARS NATURALE II and TEARS NATURALE FREE provide dry eye patients with comfort and prompt relief of dry eye symptoms.

Sterile-For Topical Eye Use Only

INGREDIENTS

TEARS NATURALE II: Each mL contains: **Active:** DUASORB®, a water soluble polymeric system containing Dextran 70 0.1% and Hydroxypropyl Methylcellulose 2910 0.3%.

Preservative: POLYQUAD® (Polyquaternium-1) 0.001%. **Inactive:** Sodium Borate, Potassium Chloride, Sodium Chloride, Purified Water. May contain Hydrochloric Acid and/or Sodium Hydroxide to adjust pH.

TEARS NATURALE FREE: Each mL contains: **Active:** DUASORB®, a water soluble polymeric system containing Dextran 70 0.1% and Hydroxypropyl Methylcellulose 2910 0.3%.

Inactives: Sodium Borate, Potassium Chloride, Sodium Chloride, Purified Water. May contain Hydrochloric Acid and/or Sodium Hydroxide to adjust pH.

INDICATIONS

For the temporary relief of burning and irritation due to dryness of the eye and for use as a protectant against further irritation. For the temporary relief of discomfort due to minor irritations of the eye or to exposure to wind or sun.

WARNINGS

If you experience eye pain, changes in vision, continued redness or irritation of the eye, or if the condition worsens or persists for more than 72 hours, discontinue use and consult a doctor.

If solution changes color or becomes cloudy, do not use.

To avoid contamination, do not touch tip of container to any surface. Replace cap after using. Keep this and all drugs out of the reach of children. In case of accidental ingestion, seek professional assistance or contact a Poison Control Center immediately.

DIRECTIONS

TEARS NATURALE® II: Instill 1 or 2 drops in the affected eye(s) as needed. TEARS NATURALE® FREE: Make sure container is intact before use. To open, completely TWIST off tab. DO NOT pull off. Instill 1 or 2 drops in the affected eye(s) as needed. To close, press tab down over container tip and twist. Reclosed vial may leak under pressure.

DISCARD CONTAINER 12 HOURS AFTER OPENING.

HOW SUPPLIED

TEARS NATURALE II Lubricant Eye Drops are supplied in 15 mL and 30 mL plastic DROP-TAINER® bottles.

15 mL NDC 0065-0418-15
30 mL NDC 0065-0418-30

TEARS NATURALE FREE Lubricant Eye Drops are supplied in boxes of 36 0.03 fl. oz. re-closable vials.

NDC 0065-0416-32

STORAGE: Store at room temperature.

TOBRADEX® — ℞

(tobramycin and dexamethasone ophthalmic suspension)
Sterile

DESCRIPTION

TOBRADEX® (tobramycin and dexamethasone ophthalmic suspension) is a sterile, multiple dose antibiotic and steroid combination for topical ophthalmic use.

Each mL of TOBRADEX® Suspension contains: Actives: Tobramycin 0.3% (3 mg) and Dexamethasone 0.1% (1 mg). **Preservative:** Benzalkonium Chloride 0.01%. **Inactives:** Tyloxapol, Edetate Disodium, Sodium Chloride, Hydroxyethyl Cellulose, Sodium Sulfate, Sulfuric Acid and/or Sodium Hydroxide (to adjust pH) and Purified Water.

CLINICAL PHARMACOLOGY

Corticoids suppress the inflammatory response to a variety of agents and they probably delay or slow healing. Since corticoids may inhibit the body's defense mechanism against infection, a concomitant antimicrobial drug may be used when this inhibition is considered to be clinically significant. Dexamethasone is a potent corticoid.

The antibiotic component in the combination (tobramycin) is included to provide action against susceptible organisms.

In vitro studies have demonstrated that tobramycin is active against susceptible strains of the following microorganisms:
Staphylococci, including *S. aureus* and *S. epidermidis* (coagulase-positive and coagulase-negative), including penicillin-resistant strains.
Streptococci, including some of the Group A-beta-hemolytic species, some nonhemolytic species, and some *Streptococcus pneumoniae*.
Pseudomonas aeruginosa, Escherichia coli, Klebsiella pneumoniae, Enterobacter aerogenes, Proteus mirabilis, Morganella morganii, most *Proteus vulgaris* strains, *Haemophilus influenzae* and *H. aegyptius, Moraxella lacunata, Acinetobacter calcoaceticus* and some *Neisseria* species.
Bacterial susceptibility studies demonstrate that in some cases microorganisms resistant to gentamicin remain susceptible to tobramycin.
No data are available on the extent of systemic absorption from TOBRADEX Ophthalmic Suspension; however, it is known that some systemic absorption can occur with ocularly applied drugs. If the maximum dose of TOBRADEX Ophthalmic Suspension is given for the first 48 hours (two drops in each eye every 2 hours) and complete systemic absorption occurs, which is highly unlikely, the daily dose of dexamethasone would be 2.4 mg. The usual physiologic replacement dose is 0.75 mg daily. If TOBRADEX Ophthalmic Suspension is given after the first 48 hours as two drops in each eye every 4 hours, the administered dose of dexamethasone would be 1.2 mg daily.

INDICATIONS AND USAGE

TOBRADEX Ophthalmic Suspension is indicated for steroid-responsive inflammatory ocular conditions for which a corticosteroid is indicated and where superficial bacterial ocular infection or a risk of bacterial ocular infection exists.
Ocular steroids are indicated in inflammatory conditions of the palpebral and bulbar conjunctiva, cornea and anterior segment of the globe where the inherent risk of steroid use in certain infective conjunctivitides is accepted to obtain a diminution in edema and inflammation. They are also indicated in chronic anterior uveitis and corneal injury from chemical, radiation or thermal burns, or penetration of foreign bodies.
The use of a combination drug with an anti-infective component is indicated where the risk of superficial ocular infection is high or where there is an expectation that potentially dangerous numbers of bacteria will be present in the eye.
The particular anti-infective drug in this product is active against the following common bacterial eye pathogens:
Staphylococci, including *S. aureus* and *S. epidermidis* (coagulase-positive and coagulase-negative), including penicillin-resistant strains.
Streptococci, including some of the Group A-beta-hemolytic species, some nonhemolytic species, and some *Streptococcus pneumoniae*.
Pseudomonas aeruginosa, Escherichia coli, Klebsiella pneumoniae, Enterobacter aerogenes, Proteus mirabilis, Morganella morganii, most *Proteus vulgaris* strains, *Haemophilus influenzae* and *H. aegyptius, Moraxella lacunata, Acinetobacter calcoaceticus* and some *Neisseria* species.

CONTRAINDICATIONS

Epithelial herpes simplex keratitis (dendritic keratitis), vaccinia, varicella, and many other viral diseases of the cornea and conjunctiva. Mycobacterial infection of the eye. Fungal diseases of ocular structures. Hypersensitivity to a component of the medication.

WARNINGS

NOT FOR INJECTION INTO THE EYE. Sensitivity to topically applied aminoglycosides may occur in some patients. If a sensitivity reaction does occur, discontinue use.
Prolonged use of steroids may result in glaucoma, with damage to the optic nerve, defects in visual acuity and fields of vision, and posterior subcapsular cataract formation. Intraocular pressure should be routinely monitored even though it may be difficult in pediatric patients and uncooperative patients. Prolonged use may suppress the host response and thus increase the hazard of secondary ocular infections. In those diseases causing thinning of the cornea or sclera, perforations have been known to occur with the use of topical steroids. In acute purulent conditions of the eye, steroids may mask infection or enhance existing infection.

PRECAUTIONS

General. The possibility of fungal infections of the cornea should be considered after long-term steroid dosing. As with other antibiotic preparations, prolonged use may result in overgrowth of nonsusceptible organisms, including fungi. If superinfection occurs, appropriate therapy should be initiated. When multiple prescriptions are required, or whenever clinical judgement dictates, the patient should be examined with the aid of magnification, such as slit lamp biomicroscopy and, where appropriate, fluorescein staining.
Cross-sensitivity to other aminoglycoside antibiotics may occur; if hypersensitivity develops with this product, discontinue use and institute appropriate therapy.
Information for Patients: Do not touch dropper tip to any surface, as this may contaminate the contents. Contact lenses should not be worn during the use of this product.
Carcinogenesis, Mutagenesis, Impairment of Fertility: No studies have been conducted to evaluate the carcinogenic or mutagenic potential. No impairment of fertility was noted in studies of subcutaneous tobramycin in rats at doses of 50 and 100 mg/kg/day.
Pregnancy Category C. Corticosteroids have been found to be teratogenic in animal studies. Ocular administration of 0.1% dexamethasone resulted in 15.6% and 32.3% incidence of fetal anomalies in two groups of pregnant rabbits. Fetal growth retardation and increased mortality rates have been observed in rats with chronic dexamethasone therapy. Reproduction studies have been performed in rats and rabbits with tobramycin at doses up to 100 mg/kg/day parenterally and have revealed no evidence of impaired fertility or harm to the fetus. There are no adequate and well controlled studies in pregnant women. TOBRADEX® Ophthalmic Suspension should be used during pregnancy only if the potential benefit justifies the potential risk to the fetus.
Nursing Mothers. Systemically administered corticosteroids appear in human milk and could suppress growth, interfere with endogenous corticosteroid production, or cause other untoward effects. It is not known whether topical administration of corticosteroids could result in sufficient systemic absorption to produce detectable quantities in human milk. Because many drugs are excreted in human milk, caution should be exercised when TOBRADEX® Ophthalmic Suspension is administered to a nursing woman.
Pediatric Use. Safety and effectiveness in pediatric patients below the age of 2 years have not been established.

ADVERSE REACTIONS

Adverse reactions have occurred with steroid/anti-infective combination drugs which can be attributed to the steroid component, the anti-infective component, or the combination. Exact incidence figures are not available. The most frequent adverse reactions to topical ocular tobramycin (TOBREX®) are hypersensitivity and localized ocular toxicity, including lid itching and swelling, and conjunctival erythema. These reactions occur in less than 4% of patients. Similar reactions may occur with the topical use of other aminoglycoside antibiotics. Other adverse reactions have not been reported; however, if topical ocular tobramycin is administered concomitantly with systemic aminoglycoside antibiotics, care should be taken to monitor the total serum concentration. The reactions due to the steroid component are: elevation of intraocular pressure (IOP) with possible development of glaucoma, and infrequent optic nerve damage; posterior subcapsular cataract formation; and delayed wound healing.
Secondary Infection. The development of secondary infection has occurred after use of combinations containing steroids and antimicrobials. Fungal infections of the cornea are particularly prone to develop coincidentally with long-term applications of steroids. The possibility of fungal invasion must be considered in any persistent corneal ulceration where steroid treatment has been used. Secondary bacterial ocular infection following suppression of host responses also occurs.

OVERDOSAGE

Clinically apparent signs and symptoms of an overdosage of TOBRADEX® Ophthalmic Suspension (punctate keratitis, erythema, increased lacrimation, edema and lid itching) may be similar to adverse reaction effects seen in some patients.

DOSAGE AND ADMINISTRATION

One or two drops instilled into the conjuctival sac(s) every four to six hours. During the initial 24 to 48 hours, the dosage may be increased to one or two drops every two (2) hours. Frequency should be decreased gradually as warranted by improvement in clinical signs. Care should be taken not to discontinue therapy prematurely.
Not more than 20 mL should be prescribed initially and the prescription should not be refilled without further evaluation as outlined in PRECAUTIONS above.

HOW SUPPLIED

Sterile ophthalmic suspension in 2.5 mL (**NDC** 0065-0647-25), 5 mL (**NDC** 0065-0647-05) and 10 mL (**NDC** 0065-0647-10) DROP-TAINER® dispensers.
STORAGE: Store at 8° to 27°C (46° to 80°F).
Store suspension upright and shake well before using.
Rx Only
U.S. Patent No. 5,149,694

TOBRADEX® ℞
(tobramycin and dexamethasone ophthalmic ointment)
Sterile

DESCRIPTION

TOBRADEX® (tobramycin and dexamethasone ophthalmic ointment) is a sterile, multiple dose antibiotic and steroid combination for topical ophthalmic use.
Each gram of TOBRADEX® Ointment contains: Actives: Tobramycin 0.3% (3mg) and Dexamethasone 0.1% (1mg). **Preservative:** Chlorobutanol 0.5%. **Inactives:** Mineral Oil and White Petrolatum.

CLINICAL PHARMACOLOGY

Corticoids suppress the inflammatory response to a variety of agents and they probably delay or slow healing. Since corticoids may inhibit the body's defense mechanism against infection, a concomitant antimicrobial drug may be used when this inhibition is considered to be clinically signficant. Dexamethasone is a potent corticoid.
The antibiotic component in the combination (tobramycin) is included to provide action against susceptible organisms.
In vitro studies have demonstrated that tobramycin is active against susceptible strains of the following microorganisms:
Staphylococci, including *S. aureus* and *S. epidermidis* (coagulase-positive and coagulase-negative), including penicillin-resistant strains.
Streptococci, including some of the Group A-beta-hemolytic species, some nonhemolytic species, and some *Streptococcus pneumoniae*.
Pseudomonas aeruginosa, Escherichia coli, Klebsiella pneumoniae, Enterobacter aerogenes, Proteus mirabilis, Morganella morganii, most *Proteus vulgaris* strains, *Haemophilus influenzae* and *H. aegyptius, Moraxella lacunata, Acinetobacter calcoaceticus* and some *Neisseria* species.
Bacterial susceptibility studies demonstrate that in some cases microorganisms resistant to gentamicin remain susceptible to tobramycin.
No data are available on the extent of systemic absorption from TOBRADEX Ophthalmic Ointment; however, it is known that some systemic absorption can occur with ocularly applied drugs. The usual physiologic replacement dose is 0.75 mg daily. The administered dose for TOBRADEX Ophthalmic Ointment in both eyes four times daily would be 0.4 mg of dexamethasone daily.

INDICATIONS AND USAGE

TOBRADEX Ophthalmic Ointment is indicated for steroid-responsive inflammatory ocular conditions for which a corticosteroid is indicated and where superficial bacterial ocular infection or a risk of bacterial ocular infection exists.
Ocular steroids are indicated in inflammatory conditions of the palpebral and bulbar conjunctiva, cornea and anterior segment of the globe where the inherent risk of steroid use in certain infective conjunctivitides is accepted to obtain a diminution in edema and inflammation. They are also indicated in chronic anterior uveitis and corneal injury from chemical, radiation or thermal burns, or penetration of foreign bodies.
The use of a combination drug with an anti-infective component is indicated where the risk of superficial ocular infection is high or where there is an expectation that potentially dangerous numbers of bacteria will be present in the eye.
The particular anti-infective drug in this product is active against the following common bacterial eye pathogens:
Staphylococci, including *S. aureus* and *S. epidermidis* (coagulase-positive and coagulase-negative), including penicillin-resistant strains.
Streptococci, including some of the Group A-beta-hemolytic species, some nonhemolytic species, and some *Streptococcus pneumoniae*.
Pseudomonas aeruginosa, Escherichia coli, Klebsiella pneumoniae, Enterobacter aerogenes, Proteus mirabilis, Morganella morganii, most *Proteus vulgaris* strains, *Haemophilus influenzae* and *H. aegyptius, Moraxella lacunata, Acinetobacter calcoaceticus* and some *Neisseria* species.

CONTRAINDICATIONS

Epithelial herpes simplex keratitis (dendritic keratitis), vaccinia, varicella, and many other viral diseases of the cornea and conjunctiva. Mycobacterial infection of the eye. Fungal diseases of ocular structures. Hypersensitivity to a component of the medication.

WARNINGS

NOT FOR INJECTION INTO THE EYE. Sensitivity to topically applied aminoglycosides may occur in some patients. If a sensitivity reaction does occur, discontinue use.
Prolonged use of steroids may result in glaucoma, with damage to the optic nerve, defects in visual acuity and fields of vision, and posterior subcapsular cataract formation. Intraocular pressure should be routinely monitored even though it may be difficult in pediatric patients and uncooperative patients. Prolonged use may suppress the host response and thus increase the hazard of secondary ocular infections. In those diseases causing thinning of the cornea or sclera, perforations have been known to occur with the use of topical steroids. In acute purulent conditions of the eye, steroids may mask infection or enhance existing infection.

PRECAUTIONS

General. The possibility of fungal infections of the cornea should be considered after long-term steroid dosing. As with other antibiotic preparations, prolonged use may result in overgrowth of nonsusceptible organisms, including fungi. If superinfection occurs, appropriate therapy should be initiated. When multiple prescriptions are required, or whenever clinical judgement dictates, the patient should be examined with the aid of magnification, such as slit lamp biomicroscopy and, where appropriate, fluorescein staining.
Cross-sensitivity to other aminoglycoside antibiotics may occur; if hypersensitivity develops with this product, discontinue use and institute appropriate therapy.
Ophthalmic ointment may retard corneal wound healing.
Information for Patients: Do not touch tube tip to any surface, as this may contaminate the contents. Contact lenses should not be worn during the use of this product.
Carcinogenesis, Mutagenesis, Impairment of Fertility. No studies have been conducted to evaluate the carcinogenic or mutagenic potential. No impairment of fertility was noted in studies of subcutaneous tobramycin in rats at doses of 50 and 100 mg/kg/day.
Pregnancy Category C. Corticosteroids have been found to be teratogenic in animal studies. Ocular administration of

Continued on next page

TobraDex—Cont.

0.1% dexamethasone resulted in 15.6% and 32.3% incidence of fetal anomalies in two groups of pregnant rabbits. Fetal growth retardation and increased mortality rates have been observed in rats with chronic dexamethasone therapy. Reproduction studies have been performed in rats and rabbits with tobramycin at doses up to 100 mg/kg/day parenterally and have revealed no evidence of impaired fertility or harm to the fetus. There are no adequate and well controlled studies in pregnant women. TOBRADEX® Ophthalmic Ointment should be used during pregnancy only if the potential benefit justifies the potential risk to the fetus.

Nursing Mothers. Systemically administered corticosteroids appear in human milk and could suppress growth, interfere with endogenous corticosteroid production, or cause other untoward effects. It is not known whether topical administration of corticosteroids could result in sufficient systemic absorption to produce detectable quantities in human milk. Because many drugs are excreted in human milk, caution should be exercised when TOBRADEX® Ophthalmic Ointment is administered to a nursing woman.

Pediatric Use. Safety and effectiveness in pediatric patients below the age of 2 years have not been established.

ADVERSE REACTIONS

Adverse reactions have occurred with steroid/anti-infective combination drugs which can be attributed to the steroid component, the anti-infective component, or the combination. Exact incidence figures are not available. The most frequent adverse reactions to topical ocular tobramycin (TOBREX®) are hypersensitivity and localized ocular toxicity, including lid itching and swelling, and conjunctival erythema. These reactions occur in less than 4% of patients. Similar reactions may occur with the topical use of other aminoglycoside antibiotics. Other adverse reactions have not been reported; however, if topical ocular tobramycin is administered concomitantly with systemic aminoglycoside antibiotics, care should be taken to monitor the total serum concentration. The reactions due to the steroid component are: elevation of intraocular pressure (IOP) with possible development of glaucoma, and infrequent optic nerve damage; posterior subcapsular cataract formation; and delayed wound healing.

Secondary Infection. The development of secondary infection has occurred after use of combinations containing steroids and antimicrobials. Fungal infections of the cornea are particularly prone to develop coincidentally with long-term applications of steroids. The possibility of fungal invasion must be considered in any persistent corneal ulceration where steroid treatment has been used. Secondary bacterial ocular infection following suppression of host responses also occurs.

OVERDOSAGE

Clinically apparent signs and symptoms of an overdose of TOBRADEX® Ophthalmic Ointment (punctate keratitis, erythema, increased lacrimation, edema and lid itching) may be similar to adverse reaction effects seen in some patients.

DOSAGE AND ADMINISTRATION

Apply a small amount (approximately 1/2 inch ribbon) into the conjunctival sac(s) up to three or four times daily.

How to apply TOBRADEX Ophthalmic Ointment:

1. Tilt your head back.
2. Place a finger on your cheek just under your eye and gently pull down until a "V" pocket is formed between your eyeball and your lower lid.
3. Place a small amount (about 1/2 inch) of TOBRADEX Ophthalmic Ointment in the "V" pocket. Do not let the tip of the tube touch your eye.
4. Look downward before closing your eye.

Not more than 8 g should be prescribed initially and the prescription should not be refilled without further evaluations as outlined in the PRECAUTIONS above.

HOW SUPPLIED

Sterile ophthalmic ointment in 3.5 g ophthalmic tube (NDC 0065-0648-35).

STORAGE: Store at 8° to 27°C (46° to 80°F).

Rx Only

U.S. Patent No. 5,149,694

Allergan, Inc.

2525 DUPONT DRIVE
P.O. BOX 19534
IRVINE, CA 92623-9534

Direct Inquiries to:
(714) 246-4500

OPHTHALMIC PRODUCTS

For information on Allergan, Inc., prescription, OTC, and ophthalmic products, consult the Physicians' Desk Reference for Ophthalmology. For literature, service items, or sample material, contact Allergan directly. See a complete listing of products in the Manufacturers' Index section of this book.

ACULAR® ℞

(ketorolac tromethamine ophthalmic solution) 0.5%
Sterile

PRODUCT OVERVIEW

ACULAR® (ketorolac tromethamine ophthalmic solution) 0.5% is the only topical NSAID indicated for the temporary relief of ocular itching due to seasonal allergic conjunctivitis. ACULAR® is also indicated for the treatment of postoperative inflammation in patients who have undergone cataract extraction.

ACULAR® relieves the ocular itch associated with seasonal allergic conjunctivitis and inflammation following cataract surgery due in part to its ability to inhibit prostaglandin biosynthesis.

In two double-masked, paired studies (N=241), ACULAR® Solution was found to be significantly more effective than its vehicle in relieving the ocular itch of seasonal allergic conjunctivitis.

Two controlled clinical studies showed that patients treated for two weeks with ACULAR® ophthalmic solution were less likely to have measurable signs of inflammation (cell and flare) than patients treated with its vehicle.

ACULAR® Solution is also proven safe in clinical trials, and avoids steroid-like side effects (e.g., no significant effect upon IOP).[1] There is no significant ocular toxicity reported in clinical studies to date with ACULAR®.

The most frequently reported adverse events have been transient stinging and burning on instillation (approximately 40%). Caution should be used in patients with sensitivities to other NSAIDs.

ACULAR® Solution is available in 3 mL, 5 mL and 10 mL plastic bottles with a controlled-dropper tip.

Please see full prescribing information included.

ACULAR®, a registered trademark of Syntex (U.S.A.) Inc., is manufactured and distributed by Allergan, Inc. under license from its developer, Syntex (U.S.A.) Inc., Palo Alto, CA.

ACULAR® is marketed by Allergan, Inc.

PRESCRIBING INFORMATION

ACULAR® ℞

(ketorolac tromethamine ophthalmic solution) 0.5%
Sterile

DESCRIPTION

ACULAR® (ketorolac tromethamine ophthalmic solution) is a member of the pyrrolo-pyrrole group of nonsteroidal anti-inflammatory drugs (NSAIDs) for ophthalmic use. Its chemical name is (±)-5-benzoyl-2,3-dihydro-1*H*-pyrrolizine-1-carboxylic acid compound with 2-amino-2-(hydroxymethyl)-1,3-propanediol (1:1).

ACULAR® is supplied as a sterile isotonic aqueous 0.5% solution, with a pH of 7.4. ACULAR® is a racemic mixture of R-(+)- and S-(-)- ketorolac tromethamine. Ketorolac tromethamine may exist in three crystal forms. All forms are equally soluble in water. The pKa of ketorolac is 3.5. This white to off-white crystalline substance discolors on prolonged exposure to light. The molecular weight of ketorolac tromethamine is 376.41. Each mL of ACULAR® ophthalmic solution contains: Active: ketorolac tromethamine 0.5%. Preservative: benzalkonium chloride 0.01%. Inactives: edetate disodium 0.1%; octoxynol 40; sodium chloride; hydrochloric acid and/or sodium hydroxide to adjust the pH; and purified water. The osmolality of ACULAR® is 290 mOsmol/kg.

ANIMAL PHARMACOLOGY

Ketorolac tromethamine prevented the development of increased intraocular pressure induced in rabbits with topically applied arachidonic acid. Ketorolac did not inhibit rabbit lens aldose reductase *in vitro.*

Ketorolac tromethamine ophthalmic solution did not enhance the spread of ocular infections induced in rabbits with *Candida albicans, Herpes simplex* virus type one, or *Pseudomonas aeruginosa.*

CLINICAL PHARMACOLOGY

Ketorolac tromethamine is nonsteroidal anti-inflammatory drug which, when administered systemically, has demonstrated analgesic, anti-inflammatory, and anti-pyretic activity. The mechanism of its action is thought to be due, in part, to its ability to inhibit prostaglandin biosynthesis. Ketorolac tromethamine given systemically does not cause pupil constriction.

Prostaglandins have been shown in many animal models to be mediators of certain kinds of intraocular inflammation. In studies performed in animal eyes, prostaglandins have been shown to produce disruption of the blood-aqueous humor barrier, vasodilation, increased vascular permeability, leukocytosis, and increased intraocular pressure. Prostaglandins also appear to play a role in the miotic response produced during ocular surgery by constricting the iris sphincter independently of cholinergic mechanisms.

Two drops (0.1 mL) of 0.5% ACULAR® ophthalmic solution instilled into the eyes of patients 12 hours and 1 hour prior to cataract extraction achieved measurable levels in 8 of 9 patients' eyes (mean ketorolac concentration 95 ng/mL aqueous humor, range 40 to 170 ng/mL). Ocular administration of ketorolac tromethamine reduces prostaglandin E_2 (PGE_2) levels in aqueous humor. The mean concentration of PGE_2 was 80 pg/mL in the aqueous humor of eyes receiving vehicle and 28 pg/mL in the eyes receiving ACULAR® 0.5% ophthalmic solution.

One drop (0.05 mL) of 0.5% ACULAR® ophthalmic solution was instilled into one eye and one drop of vehicle into the other eye TID in 26 normal subjects. Only 5 of 26 subjects had a detectable amount of ketorolac in their plasma (range 10.7 to 22.5 ng/mL) at Day 10 during topical ocular treatment. When ketorolac tromethamine 10 mg is administered systemically every 6 hours, peak plasma levels at steady state are around 960 ng/mL.

Two controlled clinical studies showed that ACULAR® ophthalmic solution was significantly more effective than its vehicle in relieving ocular itching caused by seasonal allergic conjunctivitis.

Two controlled clinical studies showed that patients treated for two weeks with ACULAR® ophthalmic solution were less likely to have measurable signs of inflammation (cell and flare) than patients treated with its vehicle.

Results from clinical studies indicate that ACULAR® has no significant effect upon intraocular pressure; however, changes in intraocular pressure may occur following cataract surgery.

ACULAR® ophthalmic solution has been safely administered in conjunction with other ophthalmic medications such as antibiotics, beta blockers, carbonic anhydrase inhibitors, cycloplegics, and mydriatics.

INDICATIONS AND USAGE

ACULAR® ophthalmic solution is indicated for the temporary relief of ocular itching due to seasonal allergic conjunctivitis. ACULAR® is also indicated for the treatment of postoperative inflammation in patients who have undergone cataract extraction.

CONTRAINDICATIONS

ACULAR® ophthalmic solution is contraindicated in patients with previously demonstrated hypersensitivity to any of the ingredients in the formulation.

WARNINGS

There is the potential for cross-sensitivity to acetylsalicylic acid, phenylacetic acid derivatives, and other nonsteroidal anti-inflammatory agents. Therefore, caution should be used when treating individuals who have previously exhibited sensitivities to these drugs.

With some nonsteroidal anti-inflammatory drugs, there exists the potential for increased bleeding time due to interference with thrombocyte aggregation. There have been reports that ocularly applied nonsteroidal anti-inflammatory drugs may cause increased bleeding of ocular tissues (including hyphemas) in conjunction with ocular surgery.

PRECAUTIONS

General: It is recommended that ACULAR® ophthalmic solution be used with caution in patients with known bleeding tendencies or who are receiving other medications which may prolong bleeding time.

Information for Patients: ACULAR® should not be administered while wearing contact lenses.

Carcinogenesis, Mutagenesis, and Impairment of Fertility: An 18-month study in mice at oral doses of ketorolac tromethamine equal to the parenteral MRHD (Maximum Recommended Human Dose) and a 24-month study in rats at oral doses 2.5 times the parenteral MRHD, showed no evidence of tumorigenicity.

Ketorolac tromethamine was not mutagenic in Ames test, unscheduled DNA synthesis and repair, and in forward mutation assays. Ketorolac did not cause chromosome breakage in the *in vivo* mouse micronucleus assay. At 1590 ug/mL (approximately 1000 times the average human plasma levels) and at higher concentrations, ketorolac tromethamine increased the incidence of chromosomal aberrations in Chinese hamster ovarian cells.

Impairment of fertility did not occur in male or female rats at oral doses of 9 mg/kg and 16 mg/kg respectively.

Pregnancy:

Pregnancy Category C. Reproduction studies have been performed in rabbits, using daily oral doses at 3.6 mg/kg and in rats at 10 mg/kg during organogenesis. Results of these studies did not reveal evidence of teratogenicity to the fetus. Oral doses of ketorolac tromethamine at 1.5 mg/kg, which was half of the human oral exposure, administered after gestation day 17 caused dystocia and higher pup mortality in rats. There are no adequate and well-controlled studies in pregnant women. Ketorolac tromethamine should be used during pregnancy only if the potential benefit justifies the potential risk to the fetus.

Nonteratogenic Effects: Because of the known effects of prostaglandin-inhibiting drugs on the fetal cardiovascular system (closure of the ductus arteriosus), the use of ACULAR® ophthalmic solution during late pregnancy should be avoided.

Nursing Mothers: Caution should be exercised when ACULAR® is administered to a nursing woman.

Pediatric Use: Safety and efficacy in pediatric patients below the age of 12 have not been established.

ADVERSE REACTIONS

In controlled clinical studies, the most frequent adverse events reported with the use of ACULAR® ophthalmic solution have been transient stinging and burning on instillation. These events were reported by up to 40% of patients treated with ACULAR® ophthalmic solution. In all development studies conducted, other adverse events occurring less than 5% of the time during treatment with ACULAR® included ocular irritation, allergic reactions, superficial ocular infections, and superficial keratitis.

Other adverse events reported rarely with the use of ACULAR® ophthalmic solution include: eye dryness, corneal infiltrates, corneal ulcer, and visual disturbance (blurry vision).

DOSAGE AND ADMINISTRATION

The recommended dose of ACULAR® ophthalmic solution is one drop (0.25 mg) four times a day for relief of ocular itching due to seasonal allergic conjunctivitis.

For the treatment of postoperative inflammation in patients who have undergone cataract extraction, one drop of ACULAR® ophthalmic solution should be applied to the affected eye(s) four times daily beginning 24 hours after cataract surgery and continuing through the first 2 weeks of the postoperative period.

HOW SUPPLIED

ACULAR® (ketorolac tromethamine ophthalmic solution) is available for topical ophthalmic administration as a 0.5% sterile solution, and is supplied in white opaque plastic bottles with a controlled dropper tip in the following sizes:

3 mL —NDC 0023-2181-03
5 mL —NDC 0023-2181-05
10 mL—NDC 0023-2181-10

Store at controlled room temperature 15–30°C (59–86°F) with protection from light.

Rx only

U.S. Patent Nos. 4,089,969; 4,454,151; 5,110,493

ACULAR®, a registered trademark of Syntex (U.S.A.) Inc., is manufactured and distributed by Allergan, Inc. under license from its developer, Syntex (U.S.A.) Inc., Palo Alto, California, U.S.A.

ALLERGAN

Irvine, CA 92612

Shown in Product Identification Guide, page 303

ACULAR® PF ℞

(ketorolac tromethamine ophthalmic solution) 0.5% Preservative-Free

DESCRIPTION

ACULAR® PF (ketorolac tromethamine ophthalmic solution) Preservative-Free is a member of the pyrrolo-pyrrole group of nonsteroidal anti-inflammatory drugs (NSAIDs) for ophthalmic use. Ketorolac tromethamine's chemical name is (±)-5-benzoyl-2,3-dihydro-1*H* pyrrolizine-1-carboxylic acid compound with 2-amino-2-(hydroxymethyl)-1,3-propanediol (1:1).

ACULAR® PF is a racemic mixture of R-(+) and S-(-)-ketorolac tromethamine. Ketorolac tromethamine may exist in three crystal forms. All forms are equally soluble in water. The pKa of ketorolac is 3.5. This white to off-white crystalline substance discolors on prolonged exposure to light. The molecular weight of ketorolac tromethamine is 376.41. The osmolality of ACULAR® PF is 290 mOsmol/kg. Each ml of ACULAR® PF contains: Active ingredient: ketorolac tromethamine 0.5%. Inactives: sodium chloride; hydrochloric acid and/or sodium hydroxide to adjust the pH to 7.4; and purified water.

CLINICAL PHARMACOLOGY

Ketorolac tromethamine is a nonsteroidal anti-inflammatory drug which, when administered systemically, has demonstrated analgesic, anti-inflammatory, and anti-pyretic activity. The mechanism of its action is thought to be due to its ability to inhibit prostaglandin biosynthesis. Ketorolac tromethamine given systemically does not cause pupil constriction.

One drop (0.05 mL) of ketorolac tromethamine (preserved) was instilled into one eye and one drop of vehicle into the other eye TID in 26 normal subjects. Only 5 of 26 subjects had a detectable amount of ketorolac in their plasma (range 10.7 to 22.5 ng/mL) at day 10 during topical ocular treatment. When ketorolac tromethamine 10 mg is administered systemically every 6 hours, peak plasma levels at steady state are around 960 ng/mL.

In two double-masked, multi-centered, parallel-group studies, 340 patients who had undergone incisional refractive surgery received ACULAR® PF or its vehicle QID for up to 3 days. Significant differences favored ACULAR® PF for the treatment of ocular pain and photophobia.

Results from clinical studies indicate that ketorolac tromethamine has no significant effect upon intraocular pressure.

INDICATIONS AND USAGE

ACULAR® PF ophthalmic solution is indicated for the reduction of ocular pain and photophobia following incisional refractive surgery.

CONTRAINDICATIONS

ACULAR® PF is contraindicated in patients with previously demonstrated hypersensitivity to any of the ingredients in the formulation.

WARNINGS

There is the potential for cross-sensitivity to acetylsalicylic acid, phenylacetic acid derivatives, and other nonsteroidal anti-inflammatory agents. Therefore, caution should be used when treating individuals who have previously exhibited sensitivities to these drugs.

With some nonsteroidal anti-inflammatory drugs, there exists the potential for increased bleeding time due to interference with thrombocyte aggregation. There have been reports that ocularly applied nonsteroidal anti-inflammatory drugs may cause increased bleeding of ocular tissues (including hyphemas) in conjunction with ocular surgery.

PRECAUTIONS

General: It is recommended that ACULAR® PF be used with caution in surgical patients with known bleeding tendencies or who are receiving other medications which may prolong bleeding time.

Wound healing may be delayed with the use of ACULAR® PF.

Information for Patients: ACULAR® PF should not be administered while wearing contact lenses.

The solution from one individual single-use vial is to be used immediately after opening for administration to one or both eyes, and the remaining contents should be discarded immediately after administration. To avoid contamination, do not touch tip of unit-dose vial to eye or any other surface.

Carcinogenesis, Mutagenesis, and Impairment of Fertility: An 18-month study in mice at oral doses of ketorolac tromethamine equal to the parenteral MRHD (Maximum Recommended Human Dose) and a 24-month study in rats at oral doses 2.5 times the parenteral MRHD, showed no evidence of tumorigenicity.

Ketorolac tromethamine was not mutagenic in the Ames test, unscheduled DNA synthesis and repair, and forward mutation assays. Ketorolac did not cause chromosome breakage in the *in vivo* mouse micronucleus assay. At 1590 μg/mL (approximately 1000 times the average human plasma levels) and at higher concentrations, ketorolac tromethamine increased the incidence of chromosomal aberrations in Chinese hamster ovarian cells.

Impairment of fertility did not occur in male or female rats at oral doses of 9 mg/kg and 16 mg/kg, respectively.

Pregnancy: Teratogenic Effects: Pregnancy Category C: Reproduction studies have been performed in rabbits, using daily oral doses at 3.6 mg/kg and in rats at 10 mg/kg during organogenesis. Results of these studies did not reveal evidence of teratogenicity to the fetus. Oral doses of ketorolac tromethamine at 1.5 mg/kg, which was half of the human oral exposure, administered after gestation day 17 caused dystocia and higher pup mortality in rats. There are no adequate and well-controlled studies in pregnant women. Ketorolac tromethamine should be used during pregnancy only if the potential benefit justifies the potential risk to the fetus.

Nonteratogenic Effects: Because of the known effects of prostaglandin-inhibiting drugs on the fetal cardiovascular system (closure of the ductus arteriosus), the use of ACULAR® PF during late pregnancy should be avoided.

Nursing Mothers: Caution should be exercised when ACULAR® PF is administered to a nursing woman.

Pediatric Use: Safety and efficacy in pediatric patients below the age of 12 years have not been established.

ADVERSE REACTIONS

The most frequent adverse events reported with the use of ketorolac tromethamine ophthalmic solutions have been transient stinging and burning on instillation. These events were reported by approximately 20% of patients participating in clinical trials.

Other adverse events occurring 1%–10% of the time during treatment with ketorolac tromethamine ophthalmic solutions included ocular irritation, allergic reactions, superficial ocular infections, superficial keratitis, ocular inflammation, corneal edema, and iritis.

Other adverse events reported rarely with the use of ketorolac tromethamine ophthalmic solutions include: eye dryness, corneal infiltrates, corneal ulcer, visual disturbance (blurry vision), and headaches.

DOSAGE AND ADMINISTRATION

The recommended dose of ACULAR® PF Preservative-Free is one drop (0.25 mg) four times a day in the operated eye as needed for pain and photophobia for up to 3 days after incisional refractive surgery.

HOW SUPPLIED

ACULAR® PF (ketorolac tromethamine ophthalmic solution) 0.5% Preservative-Free is available as a sterile solution supplied in single-use vials as follows: ACULAR® PF 12 Single-Use Vials 0.4 mL each - NDC 0023-9055-04. Store ACULAR® PF between 15°C–30°C (59°F–86°F) with protection from light.

Rx only

U.S. Patent Nos. 4,089,969; 4,454,151; 5,110,493

ALLERGAN Irvine, CA 92612, U.S.A.

ACULAR® is a registered trademark of SYNTEX (U.S.A.) Inc. ACULAR® PF is manufactured and distributed by ALLERGAN under license from its developer, SYNTEX (U.S.A.) Inc., Palo Alto, California, U.S.A. November 1997

Shown in Product Identification Guide, page 303

ALOCRIL™ ℞

(nedocromil sodium ophthalmic solution) 2% Sterile

DESCRIPTION

ALOCRIL™ (nedocromil sodium ophthalmic solution) 2% is a clear, yellow, sterile solution for topical ophthalmic use. Nedocromil sodium is represented by the following structural formula:

NaO_2C ... CO_2Na

$C_{19}H_{15}NNa_2O_7$ Mol. Wt. 415.30 CAS: 69049-74-7

Chemical Name: 4H-Pyrano[3,2-g] quinoline-2, 8-dicarboxylic acid, 9-ethyl-6, 9-dihydro-4, 6-dioxo-10-propyl-, disodium salt.

Each mL contains: Active: Nedocromil sodium 20 mg (2%); **Preservative:** Benzalkonium chloride 0.01%; **Inactives:** Sodium chloride 0.5%, edetate disodium 0.05% and purified water. It has a pH of 4.0 to 5.5.

CLINICAL PHARMACOLOGY

Nedocromil sodium is a mast cell stabilizer. Nedocromil sodium inhibits the release of mediators from cells involved in hypersensitivity reactions. Decreased chemotaxis and decreased activation of eosinophils have also been demonstrated.

In vitro studies with adult human bronchoalveolar cells showed that nedocromil sodium inhibits histamine release from a population of mast cells having been defined as belonging to the mucosal sub type and beta-glucuronidase release from macrophages.

Pharmacokinetics and Bioavailability

Nedocromil sodium exhibits low systemic absorption. When administered as a 2% ophthalmic solution in adult human volunteers, less than 4% of the total dose was systemically absorbed following multiple dosing. Absorption is mainly through the nasolacrimal duct rather than through the conjunctiva. It is not metabolized and is eliminated primarily unchanged in urine (70%) and feces (30%).

INDICATIONS AND USAGE

ALOCRIL™ is indicated for the treatment of itching associated with allergic conjunctivitis.

CONTRAINDICATIONS

ALOCRIL™ is contraindicated in those patients who have shown hypersensitivity to nedocromil sodium or to any of the other ingredients.

PRECAUTIONS

Information for Patients

Patients should be advised to follow the patient instructions listed on the Information for Patients sheet.

Users of contact lenses should refrain from wearing lenses while exhibiting the signs and symptoms of allergic conjunctivitis.

Carcinogenesis, Mutagenesis, and Impairment of Fertility

A two-year inhalation carcinogenicity study of nedocromil sodium at a dose of 24 mg/kg/day (approximately 400 times the maximum recommended human daily ocular dose on a mg/kg basis) in Wistar rats showed no carcinogenic potential.

Nedocromil sodium showed no mutagenic potential in the Ames Salmonella/microsome plate assay, mitotic gene conversion in Saccharomyces cerevisiae, mouse lymphoma forward mutation and mouse micronucleus assays.

Reproduction and fertility studies in mice and rats showed no effects on male and female fertility at a subcutaneous dose of 100 mg/kg/day (more than 1600 times the maximum recommended human daily ocular dose).

Pregnancy: Teratogenic Effects: Pregnancy Category B

Reproduction studies performed in mice, rats and rabbits using a subcutaneous dose of 100 mg/kg/day (more than 1600 times the maximum human daily ocular dose on a mg/kg basis) revealed no evidence of teratogenicity or harm to the fetus due to nedocromil sodium. There are, however, no adequate and well-controlled studies in pregnant women. Because animal reproduction studies are not always predictive of human response, ALOCRIL™ should be used during pregnancy only if clearly needed.

Nursing Mothers

After intravenous administration to lactating rats, nedocromil was excreted in milk. It is not known whether this drug

Continued on next page

Alocril—Cont.

is excreted in human milk. Because many drugs are excreted in human milk, caution should be exercised when ALOCRIL™ is administered to a nursing woman.

Pediatric Use

Safety and effectiveness in children below the age of 3 years have not been established.

Geriatric Use

No overall differences in safety or effectiveness have been observed between elderly and younger patients.

ADVERSE REACTIONS

The most frequently reported adverse experience was headache (~40%).

Ocular burning, irritation and stinging, unpleasant taste, and nasal congestion have been reported to occur in 10-30% of patients. Other events occurring between 1-10% included asthma, conjunctivitis, eye redness, photophobia, and rhinitis.

Some of these events were similar to the underlying ocular disease being studied.

DOSAGE AND ADMINISTRATION

The recommended dosage is one or two drops in each eye twice a day. ALOCRIL™ should be used at regular intervals.

Treatment should be continued throughout the period of exposure (i.e., until the pollen season is over or until exposure to the offending allergen is terminated), even when symptoms are absent.

HOW SUPPLIED

ALOCRIL™ (nedocromil sodium ophthalmic solution) 2% is supplied as 5 mL of solution in a natural, low-density polyethylene round eye drop bottle with a controlled dropper tip, and a natural polypropylene cap.

5 mL NDC 0023-8842-05

Storage

Store between 2°-25°C (36°-77°F). Keep tightly closed and out of the reach of children.

Rx Only

Manufactured by
Laboratoires FISONS SA
Le Trait, France

Distributed by
Allergan
Irvine, CA 92612, USA

 71338US11 H 8729X

Shown in Product Identification Guide, page 303

ALPHAGAN® ℞
(brimonidine tartrate ophthalmic solution) 0.2%

DESCRIPTION

ALPHAGAN® (brimonidine tartrate ophthalmic solution) 0.2% is a relatively selective alpha-2 adrenergic agonist for ophthalmic use. The chemical name of brimonidine tartrate is 5-bromo-6-(2-imidazolidinylideneamino) quinoxaline L-tartrate. It is an off-white, pale yellow to pale pink powder. In solution, ALPHAGAN® has a clear, greenish-yellow color. It has a molecular weight of 442.24 as the tartrate salt and is water soluble (34 mg/mL). The molecular formula is $C_{11}H_{10}BrN_5 \cdot C_4H_6O_6$.

ALPHAGAN® (brimonidine tartrate ophthalmic solution) 0.2% is a sterile ophthalmic solution. Each mL of ALPHAGAN® Solution contains:

ACTIVE: brimonidine tartrate 2 mg (equivalent to 1.32 mg as brimonidine free base).

PRESERVATIVE: benzalkonium chloride (0.05 mg)

INACTIVES: polyvinyl alcohol; sodium chloride; sodium citrate; citric acid; and purified water. Hydrochloric acid and/or sodium hydroxide may be added to adjust pH (6.3–6.5).

CLINICAL PHARMACOLOGY

Mechanism of Action

ALPHAGAN® is an alpha adrenergic receptor agonist. It has a peak ocular hypotensive effect occurring at two hours post-dosing. Fluorophotometric studies in animals and humans suggest that brimonidine tartrate has a dual mechanism of action by reducing aqueous humor production and increasing uveoscleral outflow.

Pharmacokinetics

After ocular administration of a 0.2% solution, plasma concentrations peaked within 1 to 4 hours and declined with a systemic half-life of approximately 3 hours.

In humans, systemic metabolism of brimonidine is extensive. It is metabolized primarily by the liver. Urinary excretion is the major route of elimination of the drug and its metabolites. Approximately 87% of an orally-administered radioactive dose was eliminated within 120 hours, with 74% found in the urine.

Clinical Studies

Elevated IOP presents a major risk factor in glaucomatous field loss. The higher the level of IOP, the greater the likelihood of optic nerve damage and visual field loss. ALPHAGAN® has the action of lowering intraocular pressure with minimal effect on cardiovascular and pulmonary parameters. In comparative clinical studies with timolol 0.5%, lasting up to one year, the IOP lowering effect of ALPHAGAN® was approximately 4–6 mm Hg compared with approximately 6 mm Hg for timolol. In these studies, both patient groups were dosed BID, however, due to the duration of action of ALPHAGAN®, it is recommended that ALPHAGAN® be dosed TID. Eight percent of the subjects were discontinued from studies due to inadequately controlled intraocular pressure, which in 30% of these patients occurred during the first month of therapy. Approximately 20% were discontinued due to adverse experiences.

INDICATIONS AND USAGE

ALPHAGAN® is indicated for lowering intraocular pressure in patients with open-angle glaucoma or ocular hypertension. The IOP lowering efficacy of ALPHAGAN® Ophthalmic Solution diminishes over time in some patients. This loss of effect appears with a variable time of onset in each patient and should be closely monitored.

CONTRAINDICATIONS

ALPHAGAN® is contraindicated in patients with hypersensitivity to brimonidine tartrate or any component of this medication. It is also contraindicated in patients receiving monoamine oxidase (MAO) inhibitor therapy.

PRECAUTIONS

General: Although ALPHAGAN® had minimal effect on blood pressure of patients in clinical studies, caution should be exercised in treating patients with severe cardiovascular disease. ALPHAGAN® has not been studied in patients with hepatic or renal impairment; caution should be used in treating such patients. ALPHAGAN® should be used with caution in patients with depression, cerebral or coronary insufficiency, Raynaud's phenomenon, orthostatic hypotension or thromboangiitis obliterans. During the studies there was a loss of effect in some patients. The IOP-lowering efficacy observed with ALPHAGAN® Ophthalmic Solution during the first month of therapy may not always reflect the long-term level of IOP reduction. Patients prescribed IOP-lowering medication should be routinely monitored for IOP.

Information for Patients: The preservative in ALPHAGAN®, benzalkonium chloride, may be absorbed by soft contact lenses. Patients wearing soft contact lenses should be instructed to wait at least 15 minutes after instilling ALPHAGAN® to insert soft contact lenses. As with other drugs in this class, ALPHAGAN® may cause fatigue and/or drowsiness in some patients. Patients who engage in hazardous activities should be cautioned of the potential for a decrease in mental alertness.

Drug Interactions: Although specific drug interaction studies have not been conducted with ALPHAGAN®, the possibility of an additive or potentiating effect with CNS depressants (alcohol, barbiturates, opiates, sedatives, or anesthetics) should be considered. ALPHAGAN® did not have significant effects on pulse and blood pressure in clinical studies. However, since alpha-agonists, as a class, may reduce pulse and blood pressure, caution in using concomitant drugs such as beta-blockers (ophthalmic and systemic), antihypertensives and/or cardiac glycosides is advised. Tricyclic antidepressants have been reported to blunt the hypotensive effect of systemic clonidine. It is not known whether the concurrent use of these agents with ALPHAGAN® can lead to an interference in IOP lowering effect. No data on the level of circulating catecholamines after ALPHAGAN® is instilled are available. Caution, however, is advised in patients taking tricyclic antidepressants which can affect the metabolism and uptake of circulating amines.

Carcinogenesis, Mutagenesis, Impairment of Fertility: No compound-related carcinogenic effects were observed in 21 month and 2 year studies in mice and rats given oral doses of 2.5 mg/kg/day (as the free base) and 1.0 mg/kg/day, respectively (~77 and 118 times, respectively, the human plasma drug concentration following the recommended ophthalmic dose). ALPHAGAN® was not mutagenic or cytogenic in a series of *in vitro* and *in vivo* studies including the Ames test, host-mediated assay, chromosomal aberration assay in Chinese Hamster Ovary (CHO) cells, cytogenic studies in mice and dominant lethal assay.

Pregnancy: Teratogenic Effects: Pregnancy Category B. Reproduction studies performed in rats with oral doses of 0.66 mg base/kg revealed no evidence of impaired fertility or harm to the fetus due to ALPHAGAN®. Dosing at this level produced 100 times the plasma drug concentration level seen in humans following multiple ophthalmic doses. There are no studies of ALPHAGAN® in pregnant women, however in animal studies, brimonidine crossed the placenta and entered into the fetal circulation to a limited extent. ALPHAGAN® should be used during pregnancy only if the potential benefit to the mother justifies the potential risk to the fetus.

Nursing Mothers: It is not known whether ALPHAGAN® is excreted in human milk, although in animal studies, brimonidine tartrate has been shown to be excreted in breast milk. A decision should be made whether to discontinue nursing or to discontinue the drug, taking into account the importance of the drug to the mother.

Pediatric Use: Safety and effectiveness in pediatric patients have not been established. Agitation, apnea, bradycardia, convulsions, cyanosis, depression, dyspnea, emotional instability, hypotension, hypothermia, hypotonia, hypoventilation, irritability, lethargy, somnolence, and stupor have been reported in pediatric patients.

Geriatric Use: No overall differences in safety or effectiveness have been observed between elderly and other adult patients.

ADVERSE REACTIONS

Adverse events occurring in approximately 10–30% of the subjects, in descending order of incidence, included oral dryness, ocular hyperemia, burning and stinging, headache, blurring, foreign body sensation, fatigue/drowsiness, conjunctival follicles, ocular allergic reactions, and ocular pruritus. Events occurring in approximately 3–9% of the subjects, in descending order included corneal staining/erosion, photophobia, eyelid erythema, ocular ache/pain, ocular dryness, tearing, upper respiratory symptoms, eyelid edema, conjunctival edema, dizziness, blepharitis, ocular irritation, gastrointestinal symptoms, asthenia, conjunctival blanching, abnormal vision and muscular pain. The following adverse reactions were reported in less than 3% of the patients: lid crusting, conjunctival hemorrhage, abnormal taste, insomnia, conjunctival discharge, depression, hypertension, anxiety, palpitations/arrhythmias, nasal dryness and syncope.

OVERDOSAGE

No information is available on overdosage in humans. Treatment of an oral overdose includes supportive and symptomatic therapy; a patent airway should be maintained.

DOSAGE AND ADMINISTRATION

The recommended dose is one drop of ALPHAGAN® in the affected eye(s) three times daily, approximately 8 hours apart.

HOW SUPPLIED

ALPHAGAN® (brimonidine tartrate ophthalmic solution) 0.2% is supplied sterile in white opaque plastic dropper bottles as follows:

5 mL NDC 0023-8665-05
10 mL NDC 0023-8665-10
15 mL NDC 0023-8665-15

NOTE: Store at or below 25° C (77° F).

Rx only

ALLERGAN

Shown in Product Identification Guide, page 304

AZELEX® ℞
(azelaic acid cream) 20%
For Dermatologic Use Only
Not for Ophthalmic Use

DESCRIPTION

AZELEX® (azelaic acid cream) 20% contains azelaic acid, a naturally occurring saturated dicarboxylic acid.

Structural Formula: HOOC-$(CH_2)_7$-COOH. Chemical Name: 1,7-heptanedicarboxylic acid. Empirical Formula: $C_9H_{16}O_4$. Molecular Weight: 188.22.

Active Ingredient: Each gram of AZELEX® contains azelaic acid .... 0.2 gm (20% w/w).

Inactive Ingredients: cetearyl octanoate, glycerin, glyceryl stearate and cetearyl alcohol and cetyl palmitate and cocoglycerides, PEG-5 glyceryl stearate, propylene glycol and purified water. Benzoic acid is present as a preservative.

CLINICAL PHARMACOLOGY

The exact mechanism of action of azelaic acid is not known. The following *in vitro* data are available, but their clinical significance is unknown. Azelaic acid has been shown to possess antimicrobial activity against *Propionibacterium acnes* and *Staphylococcus epidermidis*. The antimicrobial action may be attributable to inhibition of microbial cellular protein synthesis.

A normalization of keratinization leading to an anticomedonal effect of azelaic acid may also contribute to its clinical activity. Electron microscopic and immunohistochemical evaluation of skin biopsies from human subjects treated with AZELEX® demonstrated a reduction in the thickness of the stratum corneum, a reduction in number and size of keratohyalin granules, and a reduction in the amount and distribution of filaggrin (a protein component of keratohyalin) in epidermal layers. This is suggestive of the ability to decrease microcomedo formation.

Pharmacokinetics: Following a single application of AZELEX® to human skin *in vitro,* azelaic acid penetrates into the stratum corneum (approximately 3 to 5% of the applied dose) and other viable skin layers (up to 10% of the dose is found in the epidermis and dermis). Negligible cutaneous metabolism occurs after topical application. Approximately 4% of the topically applied azelaic acid is systemically absorbed. Azelaic acid is mainly excreted unchanged in the urine but undergoes some β-oxidation to shorter chain dicarboxylic acids. The observed half-lives in healthy subjects are approximately 45 minutes after oral dosing and 12 hours after topical dosing, indicating percutaneous absorption rate-limited kinetics.

Azelaic acid is a dietary constituent (whole grain cereals and animal products), and can be formed endogenously from longer-chain dicarboxylic acids, metabolism of oleic acid, and ω-oxidation of monocarboxylic acids. Endogenous plasma concentration (20 to 80 ng/mL) and daily urinary excretion (4 to 28 mg) of azelaic acid are highly dependent on dietary intake. After topical treatment with AZELEX® in humans, plasma concentration and urinary excretion of azelaic acid are not significantly different from baseline levels.

INDICATIONS AND USAGE

AZELEX® is indicated for the topical treatment of mild-to-moderate inflammatory acne vulgaris.

CONTRAINDICATIONS

AZELEX® is contraindicated in individuals who have shown hypersensitivity to any of its components.

WARNINGS

AZELEX® is for dermatologic use only and not for ophthalmic use.

There have been isolated reports of hypopigmentation after use of azelaic acid. Since azelaic acid has not been well studied in patients with dark complexions, these patients should be monitored for early signs of hypopigmentation.

PRECAUTIONS

General: If sensitivity or severe irritation develop with the use of AZELEX®, treatment should be discontinued and appropriate therapy instituted.

Information for patients: Patients should be told: 1. To use AZELEX® for the full prescribed treatment period. 2. To avoid the use of occlusive dressings or wrappings. 3. To keep AZELEX® away from the mouth, eyes and other mucous membranes. If it does come in contact with the eyes, they should wash their eyes with large amounts of water and consult a physician if eye irritation persists. 4. If they have dark complexions, to report abnormal changes in skin color to their physician. 5. Due in part to the low pH of azelaic acid, temporary skin irritation (pruritus, burning, or stinging) may occur when AZELEX® is applied to broken or inflamed skin, usually at the start of treatment. However, this irritation commonly subsides if treatment is continued. If it continues, AZELEX® should be applied only once-a-day, or the treatment should be stopped until these effects have subsided. If troublesome irritation persists, use should be discontinued, and patients should consult their physician. (See **ADVERSE REACTIONS**.)

Carcinogenesis, mutagenesis, impairment of fertility: Azelaic acid is a human dietary component of a simple molecular structure that does not suggest carcinogenic potential, and it does not belong to a class of drugs for which there is a concern about carcinogenicity. Therefore, animal studies to evaluate carcinogenic potential with AZELEX® Cream were not deemed necessary. In a battery of tests (Ames assay, HGPRT test in Chinese hamster ovary cells, human lymphocyte test, dominant lethal assay in mice), azelaic acid was found to be nonmutagenic. Animal studies have shown no adverse effects on fertility.

Pregnancy: Teratogenic Effects: Pregnancy Category B. Embryotoxic effects were observed in Segment I and Segment II oral studies with rats receiving 2500 mg/kg/day of azelaic acid. Similar effects were observed in Segment II studies in rabbits given 150 to 500 mg/kg/day and in monkeys given 500 mg/kg/day. The doses at which these effects were noted were all within toxic dose ranges for the dams. No teratogenic effects were observed. There are, however, no adequate and well-controlled studies in pregnant women. Because animal reproduction studies are not always predictive of human response, this drug should be used during pregnancy only if clearly needed.

Nursing Mothers: Equilibrium dialysis was used to assess human milk partitioning *in vitro*. At an azelaic acid concentration of 25 µg/mL, the milk/plasma distribution coefficient was 0.7 and the milk/buffer distribution was 1.0, indicating that passage of drug into maternal milk may occur. Since less than 4% of a topically applied dose is systemically absorbed, the uptake of azelaic acid into maternal milk is not expected to cause a significant change from baseline azelaic acid levels in the milk. However, caution should be exercised when AZELEX® is administered to a nursing mother.

Pediatric Use: Safety and effectiveness in pediatric patients under 12 years of age have not been established.

ADVERSE REACTIONS

During U.S. clinical trials with AZELEX®, adverse reactions were generally mild and transient in nature. The most common adverse reactions occurring in approximately 1–5% of patients were pruritus, burning, stinging and tingling. Other adverse reactions such as erythema, dryness, rash, peeling, irritation, dermatitis, and contact dermatitis were reported in less than 1% of subjects. There is the potential for experiencing allergic reactions with use of AZELEX®.

In patients using azelaic acid formulations, the following additional adverse experiences have been reported rarely: worsening of asthma, vitiligo depigmentation, small depigmented spots, hypertrichosis, reddening (signs of keratosis pilaris), and exacerbation of recurrent herpes labialis.

DOSAGE AND ADMINISTRATION

After the skin is thoroughly washed and patted dry, a thin film of AZELEX® should be gently but thoroughly massaged into the affected areas twice daily, in the morning and evening. The hands should be washed following application. The duration of use of AZELEX® can vary from person to person and depends on the severity of the acne. Improvement of the condition occurs in the majority of patients with inflammatory lesions within four weeks.

HOW SUPPLIED

AZELEX® is supplied in collapsible tubes in the following sizes:

30 g—NDC 0023-8694-30.
50 g—NDC 0023-8694-50.

Note: Protect from freezing. Store between 15°–30°C (59°–86°F).

Rx only

Distributed under license; U.S. Patent No. 4,386,104.
April 1997
Distributed by
ALLERGAN
Irvine, California 92612, U.S.A.

Made in Germany

BLEPHAMIDE® ℞

(sulfacetamide sodium and prednisolone acetate ophthalmic ointment USP)
10%/0.2% sterile

DESCRIPTION

BLEPHAMIDE® (sulfacetamide sodium and prednisolone acetate ophthalmic ointment USP) is a sterile topical ophthalmic ointment combining an antibacterial and a corticosteroid.

Contains: Actives: sulfacetamide sodium 10% and prednisolone acetate 0.2%. Inactives: phenylmercuric acetate (0.0008%); mineral oil; white petrolatum; and petrolatum (and) lanolin alcohol.

Chemical Names: Sulfacetamide sodium: N-sulfanilylacetamide monosodium salt monohydrate.

Prednisolone acetate: 11β, 17, 21-trihydroxypregna-1,4-diene-3, 20-dione, 21-acetate.

CLINICAL PHARMACOLOGY

Corticosteroids suppress the inflammatory response to a variety of agents and they probably delay or slow healing. Since corticosteroids may inhibit the body's defense mechanism against infection, a concomitant antibacterial drug may be used when this inhibition is considered to be clinically significant in a particular case.

When a decision to administer both a corticosteroid and an antibacterial is made, the administration of such drugs in combination has the advantage of greater patient compliance and convenience, with the added assurance that the appropriate dosage of both drugs is administered, plus assured compatibility of ingredients when both types of drugs are in the same formulation and, particularly, that the correct volume of drug is delivered and retained.

The relative potency of corticosteroids depends on the molecular structure, concentration and release from the vehicle.

Microbiology: Sulfacetamide exerts a bacteriostatic effect against susceptible bacteria by restricting the synthesis of folic acid required for growth through competition with p-amino benzoic acid.

Some strains of these bacteria may be resistant to sulfacetamide or resistant strains may emerge *in vivo*.

The anti-infective component in BLEPHAMIDE® ointment is included to provide action against specific organisms susceptible to it. Sulfacetamide sodium is active *in vitro* against susceptible strains of the following microorganisms: *Escherichia coli, Staphylococcus aureus, Streptococcus pneumoniae, Streptococcus* (viridans group), *Haemophilus influenzae, Klebsiella* species, and *Enterobacter* species. This product does not provide adequate coverage against: *Neisseria* species, *Pseudomonas* species, and *Serratia marcescens* (see **INDICATIONS AND USAGE**).

INDICATIONS AND USAGE

BLEPHAMIDE® ophthalmic ointment is indicated for steroid-responsive inflammatory ocular conditions for which a corticosteroid is indicated and where superficial bacterial ocular infection or a risk of bacterial ocular infection exists. Ocular corticosteroids are indicated in inflammatory conditions of the palpebral and bulbar conjunctiva, cornea, and anterior segment of the globe where the inherent risk of corticosteroid use in certain infective conjunctivitides is accepted to obtain diminution in edema and inflammation. They are also indicated in chronic anterior uveitis and corneal injury from chemical, radiation or thermal burns or penetration of foreign bodies.

The use of a combination drug with an anti-infective component is indicated where the risk of superficial ocular infection is high or where there is an expectation that potentially dangerous numbers of bacteria will be present in the eye.

The particular antibacterial drug in this product is active against the following common bacterial eye pathogens: *Escherichia coli, Staphylococcus aureus, Streptococcus pneumoniae, Streptococcus* (viridans group), *Haemophilus influenzae, Klebsiella* species, and *Enterobacter* species.

The product does not provide adequate coverage against: *Neisseria* species, *Pseudomonas* species, and *Serratia marcescens.*

A significant percentage of staphylococcal isolates are completely resistant to sulfa drugs.

CONTRAINDICATIONS

BLEPHAMIDE® ophthalmic ointment is contraindicated in most viral diseases of the cornea and conjunctiva including epithelial herpes simplex keratitis (dendritic keratitis), vaccinia, and varicella, and also in mycobacterial infection of the eye and fungal diseases of ocular structures.

This product is also contraindicated in individuals with known or suspected hypersensitivity to any of the ingredients of this preparation, to other sulfonamides and to other corticosteroids. See **WARNINGS**. (Hypersensitivity to the antimicrobial component occurs at a higher rate than for other components).

WARNINGS

NOT FOR INJECTION INTO THE EYE.

Prolonged use of corticosteroids may result in ocular hypertension/glaucoma with damage to the optic nerve, defects in visual acuity and fields of vision, and in posterior subcapsular cataract formation.

Acute anterior uveitis may occur in susceptible individuals, primarily Blacks.

Prolonged use of BLEPHAMIDE® ophthalmic ointment may suppress the host response and thus increase the hazard of secondary ocular infections. In those diseases causing thinning of the cornea or sclera, perforation has been known to occur with the use of topical corticosteroids. In acute purulent conditions of the eye, corticosteroids may mask infection or enhance existing infection.

If the product is used for 10 days or longer, intraocular pressure should be routinely monitored even though it may be difficult in children and uncooperative patients. Corticosteroids should be used with caution in the presence of glaucoma. Intraocular pressure should be checked frequently.

A significant percentage of staphylococcal isolates are completely resistant to sulfonamides.

The use of steroids after cataract surgery may delay healing and increase the incidence of filtering blebs.

The use of ocular corticosteroids may prolong the course and may exacerbate the severity of many viral infections of the eye (including herpes simplex). Employment of corticosteroid medication in the treatment of herpes simplex requires great caution.

Topical steroids are not effective in mustard gas keratitis and Sjogren's keratoconjunctivitis.

Fatalities have occurred, although rarely, due to severe reactions to sulfonamides including Stevens-Johnson syndrome, toxic epidermal necrolysis, fulminant hepatic necrosis, agranulocytosis, aplastic anemia and other blood dyscrasias. Sensitization may recur when a sulfonamide is readministered, irrespective of the route of administration. If signs of hypersensitivity or other serious reactions occur, discontinue use of this preparation. Cross-sensitivity among corticosteroids has been demonstrated (see **ADVERSE REACTIONS**).

PRECAUTIONS

General: The initial prescription and renewal of the medication order beyond 8 g of ointment should be made by a physician only after examination of the patient with the aid of magnification, such as slit lamp biomicroscopy and, where appropriate, fluorescein staining. If signs and symptoms fail to improve after two days, the patient should be re-evaluated. The possibility of fungal infections of the cornea should be considered after prolonged corticosteroid dosing. Use with caution in patients with severe dry eye. Fungal cultures should be taken when appropriate.

The p-amino benzoic acid present in purulent exudates competes with sulfonamides and can reduce their effectiveness. Ophthalmic ointments may retard corneal healing.

Information for Patients: If inflammation or pain persists longer than 48 hours or becomes aggravated, the patient should be advised to discontinue use of the medication and consult a physician (see **WARNINGS**).

This product is sterile when packaged. To prevent contamination, care should be taken to avoid touching the tube tip to eyelids or to any other surface. The use of this tube by more than one person may spread infection. Keep tube tightly closed when not in use. Keep out of the reach of children.

Laboratory Tests: Eyelid cultures and tests to determine the susceptibility of organisms to sulfacetamide may be indicated if signs and symptoms persist or recur in spite of the recommended course of treatment with BLEPHAMIDE® ophthalmic ointment.

Drug Interactions: BLEPHAMIDE® ophthalmic ointment is incompatible with silver preparations. Local anesthetics related to p-amino benzoic acid may antagonize the action of the sulfonamides.

Carcinogenesis, Mutagenesis, Impairment of Fertility: Prednisolone has been reported to be noncarcinogenic. Long-term animal studies for carcinogenic potential have not been performed with sulfacetamide.

One author detected chromosomal nondisjunction in the yeast *Saccharomyces cerevisiae* following application of sulfacetamide sodium. The significance of this finding to topical ophthalmic use of sulfacetamide sodium in the human is unknown.

Mutagenic studies with prednisolone have been negative. Studies on reproduction and fertility have not been performed with sulfacetamide. A long-term chronic toxicity study in dogs showed that high oral doses of prednisolone prevented estrus. A decrease in fertility was seen in male and female rats that were mated following oral dosing with another glucocorticosteroid.

Pregnancy: Teratogenic Effects: Pregnancy Category C. Animal reproduction studies have not been conducted with sulfacetamide sodium. Prednisolone has been shown to be teratogenic in rabbits, hamsters, and mice. In mice, pred-

Continued on next page

Blephamide Ointment—Cont.

nisolone has been shown to be teratogenic when given in doses 1 to 10 times the human ocular dose. Dexamethasone, hydrocortisone and prednisolone were ocularly applied to both eyes of pregnant mice five times per day on days 10 through 13 of gestation. A significant increase in the incidence of cleft palate was observed in the fetuses of the treated mice. There are no adequate well-controlled studies in pregnant women dosed with corticosteroids.
Kernicterus may be precipitated in infants by sulfonamides being given systemically during the third trimester of pregnancy. It is not known whether sulfacetamide sodium can cause fetal harm when administered to a pregnant woman or whether it can affect reproductive capacity.
BLEPHAMIDE® ophthalmic ointment should be used during pregnancy only if the potential benefit justifies the potential risk to the fetus.
Nursing Mothers: It is not known whether topical administration of corticosteroids could result in sufficient systemic absorption to produce detectable quantities in human milk. Systemically administered corticosteroids appear in human milk and could suppress growth, interfere with endogenous corticosteroid production, or cause other untoward effects. Systemically administered sulfonamides are capable of producing kernicterus in infants of lactating women. Because of the potential for serious adverse reactions in nursing infants from sulfacetamide sodium and prednisolone acetate ophthalmic ointments, a decision should be made whether to discontinue nursing or to discontinue the medication.
Pediatric Use: Safety and effectiveness in children below the age of six have not been established.

ADVERSE REACTIONS

Adverse reactions have occurred with corticosteroid/antibacterial combination drugs which can be attributed to the corticosteroid component, the antibacterial component, or the combination. Exact incidence figures are not available since no denominator of treated patients is available.
Reactions occurring most often from the presence of the antibacterial ingredient are allergic sensitizations. Fatalities have occurred, although rarely, due to severe reactions to sulfonamides including Stevens-Johnson syndrome, toxic epidermal necrolysis, fulminant hepatic necrosis, agranulocytosis, aplastic anemia, and other blood dyscrasias (See **WARNINGS**).
Sulfacetamide sodium may cause local irritation.
The reactions due to the corticosteroid component in decreasing order of frequency are: elevation of intraocular pressure (IOP) with possible development of glaucoma and infrequent optic nerve damage, posterior subcapsular cataract formation, and delayed wound healing.
Although systemic effects are extremely uncommon, there have been rare occurrences of systemic hypercorticoidism after use of topical steroids.
Corticosteroid-containing preparations can also cause acute anterior uveitis or perforation of the globe. Mydriasis, loss of accommodation and ptosis have occasionally been reported following local use of corticosteroids.
Secondary Infection: The development of secondary infection has occurred after use of combinations containing corticosteroids and antibacterials. Fungal and viral infections of the cornea are particularly prone to develop coincidentally with long-term applications of corticosteroid. The possibility of fungal invasion must be considered in any persistent corneal ulceration where corticosteroid treatment has been used.
Secondary bacterial ocular infection following suppression of host responses also occurs.

DOSAGE AND ADMINISTRATION

A small amount, approximately $^1/_2$ inch ribbon of ointment, should be applied in the conjunctival sac three or four times daily and once or twice at night.
Not more than 8 g should be prescribed initially.
The dosing of BLEPHAMIDE® ophthalmic ointment may be reduced, but care should be taken not to discontinue therapy prematurely. In chronic conditions, withdrawal of treatment should be carried out by gradually decreasing the frequency of application.
If signs and symptoms fail to improve after two days, the patient should be re-evaluated (see **PRECAUTIONS**).

HOW SUPPLIED

BLEPHAMIDE® (sulfacetamide sodium and prednisolone acetate ophthalmic ointment USP) 10%/0.2% is supplied sterile in 3.5 gram ointment tubes:
NDC 0023-0313-04.
Note: Store away from heat.
Rx only

Shown in Product Identification Guide, page 304

BLEPHAMIDE® ℞
(sulfacetamide sodium-prednisolone acetate ophthalmic suspension)

DESCRIPTION

BLEPHAMIDE® ophthalmic suspension is a topical anti-inflammatory/anti-infective combination product for ophthalmic use.
Chemical Names:
Sulfacetamide sodium: N-Sulfanilylacetamide monosodium salt monohydrate.
Prednisolone acetate: 11β, 17, 21-Trihydroxypregna-1, 4-diene-3, 20-dione 21-acetate.
Contains:
Actives: sulfacetamide sodium 10.0%, prednisolone acetate (microfine suspension) 0.2%: Preservative: benzalkonium chloride (0.004%): Inactives: polyvinyl alcohol 1.4%; polysorbate 80; edetate disodium; sodium phosphate, dibasic; potassium phosphate, monobasic; sodium thiosulfate; hydrochloric acid and/or sodium hydroxide to adjust the pH; and purified water.

CLINICAL PHARMACOLOGY

Corticosteroids suppress the inflammatory response to a variety of agents and they probably delay or slow healing. Since corticosteroids may inhibit the body's defense mechanism against infection, a concomitant antibacterial drug may be used when this inhibition is considered to be clinically significant in a particular case.
When a decision to administer both a corticosteroid and an antibacterial is made, the administration of such drugs in combination has the advantage of greater patient compliance and convenience, with the added assurance that the appropriate dosage of both drugs is administered. When both types of drugs are in the same formulation, compatibility of ingredients is assured and the correct volume of drug is delivered and retained. The relative potency of corticosteroids depends on the molecular structure, concentration, and release from the vehicle.
Microbiology: Sulfacetamide sodium exerts a bacteriostatic effect against susceptible bacteria by restricting the synthesis of folic acid required for growth through competition with p-aminobenzoic acid.
Some strains of these bacteria may be resistant to sulfacetamide or resistant strains may emerge *in vivo*.
The anti-infective component in these products is included to provide action against specific organisms susceptible to it. Sulfacetamide sodium is active *in vitro* against susceptible strains of the following microorganisms: *Escherichia coli, Staphylococcus aureus, Streptococcus pneumoniae, Streptococcus (viridans* group), *Haemophilus influenzae, Klebsiella* species, and *Enterobacter* species. This product does not provide adequate coverage against: *Neisseria* species, *Pseudomonas* species, and *Serratia marcescens* (see **INDICATIONS AND USAGE**).

INDICATIONS AND USAGE

A steroid/anti-infective combination is indicated for steroid-responsive inflammatory ocular conditions for which a corticosteroid is indicated and where superficial bacterial infection or a risk of bacterial ocular infection exists.
Ocular corticosteroids are indicated in inflammatory conditions of the palpebral and bulbar conjunctiva, cornea, and anterior segment of the globe where the inherent risk of corticosteroid use in certain infective conjunctivitides is accepted to obtain a diminution in edema and inflammation. They are also indicated in chronic anterior uveitis and corneal injury from chemical, radiation, or thermal burns or penetration of foreign bodies.
The use of a combination drug with an anti-infective component is indicated where the risk of superficial ocular infection is high or where there is an expectation that potentially dangerous numbers of bacteria will be present in the eye.
The particular antibacterial drug in this product is active against the following common bacterial eye pathogens: *Escherichia coli, Staphylococcus aureus, Streptococcus pneumoniae, Streptococcus* (viridans group), *Haemophilus influenzae, Klebsiella* species, and *Enterobacter* species.
This product does not provide adequate coverage against *Neisseria* species, *Pseudomonas* species, and *Serratia marcescens*.
A significant percentage of staphlococcal isolates are completely resistant to sulfa drugs.

CONTRAINDICATIONS

BLEPHAMIDE® ophthalmic suspension is contraindicated in most viral diseases of the cornea and conjunctiva including epithelial herpes simplex keratitis (dendritic keratitis), vaccinia, and varicella, and also in mycobacterial infection of the eye and fungal diseases of ocular structures.
This product is also contraindicated in individuals with known or suspected hypersensitivity to any of the ingredients of this preparation, to other sulfonamides and to other corticosteroids. See **WARNINGS.** (Hypersensitivity to the antimicrobial component occurs at a higher rate than for other components.)

WARNINGS

NOT FOR INJECTION INTO THE EYE.
Prolonged use of corticosteroids may result in ocular hypertension/glaucoma with damage to the optic nerve, defects in visual acuity and fields of vision, and in posterior subcapsular cataract formation.
Acute anterior uveitis may occur in susceptible individuals, primarily Blacks.
Prolonged use of BLEPHAMIDE® ophthalmic suspension may suppress the host response and thus increase the hazard of secondary ocular infections. In those diseases causing thinning of the cornea or sclera, perforation has been known to occur with the use of topical corticosteroids. In acute purulent conditions of the eye, corticosteroids may mask infection or enhance existing infection.
If the product is used for 10 days or longer, intraocular pressure should be routinely monitored even though it may be difficult in children and uncooperative patients. Corticosteroids should be used with caution in the presence of glaucoma. Intraocular pressure should be checked frequently.
A significant percentage of staphylococcal isolates are completely resistant to sulfonamides.
The use of steroids after cataract surgery may delay healing and increase the incidence of filtering blebs.
The use of ocular corticosteroids may prolong the course and may exacerbate the severity of many viral infections of the eye (including herpes simplex). Employment of corticosteroid medication in the treatment of herpes simplex requires great caution.
Topical steroids are not effective in mustard gas keratitis and Sjogren's keratoconjunctivitis.
Fatalities have occurred, although rarely, due to severe reactions to sulfonamides including Stevens-Johnson syndrome, toxic epidermal necrolysis, fulminant hepatic necrosis, agranulocytosis, aplastic anemia and other blood dyscrasias. Sensitization may recur when a sulfonamide is readministered, irrespective of the route of administration. If signs of hypersensitivity or other serious reactions occur, discontinue use of this preparation. Cross-sensitivity among corticosteroids has been demonstrated (see **ADVERSE REACTIONS**).

PRECAUTIONS

General: The initial prescription and renewal of the medication order beyond 20 milliliters of the suspension should be made by a physician only after examination of the patient with the aid of magnification, such as slit lamp biomicroscopy and, where appropriate, fluorescein staining. If signs and symptoms fail to improve after two days, the patient should be re-evaluated.
The possibility of fungal infections of the cornea should be considered after prolonged corticosteroid dosing. Use with caution in patients with severe dry eye. Fungal cultures should be taken when appropriate.
The p-amino benzoic acid present in purulent exudates competes with sulfonamides and can reduce their effectiveness.
Information for Patients: If inflammation or pain persists longer than 48 hours or becomes aggravated, the patient should be advised to discontinue use of the medication and consult a physician (see **WARNINGS**). Contact lenses should not be worn during the use of this product.
This product is sterile when packaged. To prevent contamination, care should be taken to avoid touching the applicator tip to eyelids or to any other surface. The use of this bottle by more than one person may spread infection. Keep bottle tightly closed when not in use. Protect from light. Sulfonamide solutions darken on prolonged standing and exposure to heat and light. Do not use if solution has darkened. Yellowing does not affect activity. Keep out of the reach of children.
Laboratory Tests: Eyelid cultures and tests to determine the susceptibility of organisms to sulfacetamide may be indicated if signs and symptoms persist or recur in spite of the recommended course of treatment with BLEPHAMIDE® ophthalmic suspension.
Drug Interactions: BLEPHAMIDE® ophthalmic suspension is incompatible with silver preparations. Local anesthetics related to p-amino benzoic acid may antagonize the action of the sulfonamides.
Carcinogenesis, Mutagenesis, Impairment of Fertility: Prednisolone has been reported to be noncarcinogenic. Long-term animal studies for carcinogenic potential have not been performed with sulfacetamide.
One author detected chromosomal nondisjunction in the yeast *Saccharomyces cerevisiae* following application of sulfacetamide sodium. The significance of this finding to topical ophthalmic use of sulfacetamide sodium in the human is unknown.
Mutagenic studies with prednisolone have been negative. Studies on reproduction and fertility have not been performed with sulfacetamide. A long-term chronic toxicity study in dogs showed that high oral doses of prednisolone prevented estrus. A decrease in fertility was seen in male and female rats that were mated following oral dosing with another glucocorticosteroid.
Pregnancy: Teratogenic Effects: Pregnancy Category C. Animal reproduction studies have not been conducted with sulfacetamide sodium. Prednisolone has been shown to be teratogenic in rabbits, hamsters, and mice. In mice, prednisolone has been shown to be teratogenic when given in doses 1 to 10 times the human ocular dose. Dexamethasone, hydrocortisone and prednisolone were ocularly applied to both eyes of pregnant mice five times per day on days 10 through 13 of gestation. A significant increase in the incidence of cleft palate was observed in the fetuses of the treated mice. There are no adequate well-controlled studies in pregnant women dosed with corticosteroids.
Kernicterus may be precipitated in infants by sulfonamides being given systemically during the third trimester of pregnancy. It is not known whether sulfacetamide sodium can cause fetal harm when administered to a pregnant woman or whether it can affect reproductive capacity.
BLEPHAMIDE® ophthalmic suspension should be used during pregnancy only if the potential benefit justifies the potential risk to the fetus.
Nursing Mothers: It is not known whether topical administration of corticosteroids could result in sufficient systemic absorption to produce detectable quantities in human milk. Systemically administered corticosteroids appear in human

milk and could suppress growth, interfere with endogenous corticosteroid production, or cause other untoward effects. Systemically administered sulfonamides are capable of producing kernicterus in infants of lactating women. Because of the potential for serious adverse reactions in nursing infants from sulfacetamide sodium and prednisolone acetate ophthalmic suspensions, a decision should be made whether to discontinue nursing or to discontinue the medication.

Pediatric Use: Safety and effectiveness in pediatric patients below the age of six have not been established.

ADVERSE REACTIONS

Adverse reactions have occurred with corticosteroid/antibacterial combination drugs which can be attributed to the corticosteroid component, the antibacterial component, or the combination. Exact incidence figures are not available since no denominator of treated patients is available.

Reactions occurring most often from the presence of the anti-bacterial ingredient are allergic sensitizations. Fatalities have occurred, although rarely, due to severe reactions to sulfonamides including Stevens-Johnson syndrome, toxic epidermal necrolysis, fulminant hepatic necrosis, agranulocytosis, aplastic anemia, and other blood dyscrasias (See **WARNINGS**).

Sulfacetamide sodium may cause local irritation.

The reactions due to the corticosteroid component in decreasing order of frequency are: elevation of intraocular pressure (IOP) with possible development of glaucoma and infrequent optic nerve damage, posterior subcapsular cataract formation, and delayed wound healing.

Although systemic effects are extremely uncommon, there have been rare occurrences of systemic hypercorticoidism after use of topical corticosteroids.

Corticosteroid-containing preparations can also cause acute anterior uveitis or perforation of the globe. Mydriasis, loss of accommodation and ptosis have occasionally been reported following local use of corticosteroids.

Secondary Infection: The development of secondary infection has occurred after use of combinations containing corticosteroids and antibacterials. Fungal and viral infections of the cornea are particularly prone to develop coincidentally with long-term applications of corticosteroid. The possibility of fungal invasion must be considered in any persistent corneal ulceration where corticosteroid treatment has been used.

Secondary bacterial ocular infection following suppression of host responses also occurs.

DOSAGE AND ADMINISTRATION

SHAKE WELL BEFORE USING. Two drops should be instilled into the conjunctival sac every four hours during the day and at bedtime.

Not more than 20 milliliters should be prescribed initially, and the prescription should not be refilled without further evaluation as outlined in **PRECAUTIONS** above.

BLEPHAMIDE® dosage may be reduced, but care should be taken not to discontinue therapy prematurely. In chronic conditions, withdrawal of treatment should be carried out by gradually decreasing the frequency of application.

If signs and symptoms fail to improve after two days, the patient should be re-evaluated (see **PRECAUTIONS**).

HOW SUPPLIED

BLEPHAMIDE® ophthalmic suspension is supplied in plastic dropper bottles in the following sizes:

5 mL—NDC 11980-022-05 10 mL—NDC 11980-022-10

Note: Protect from freezing. **Shake well before using.**

Storage: Store BLEPHAMIDE® at 8°–24°C (46°–75°F) in an upright position.

PROTECT FROM LIGHT

Sulfonamide solutions darken on prolonged standing and exposure to heat and light. Do not use if solution has darkened. Yellowing does not affect activity.

KEEP OUT OF REACH OF CHILDREN

Rx only.

Shown in Product Identification Guide, page 304

BOTOX® ℞

(Botulinum Toxin Type A) Purified Neurotoxin Complex

DESCRIPTION

BOTOX® (Botulinum Toxin Type A) Purified Neurotoxin Complex is a sterile, vacuum-dried form of purified botulinum toxin type A, produced from a culture of the Hall strain of *Clostridium botulinum* grown in a medium containing N-Z amine and yeast extract. It is purified from the culture solution by a series of acid precipitations to a crystalline complex consisting of the active high molecular weight toxin protein and an associated hemagglutinin protein. The crystalline complex is re-dissolved in a solution containing saline and albumin and sterile filtered (0.2 microns) prior to vacuum-drying. **BOTOX®** is to be reconstituted with sterile non-preserved saline prior to intramuscular injection.

Each vial of **BOTOX®** Purified Neurotoxin Complex contains 100 units (U) of *Clostridium botulinum* toxin type A, 0.5 milligrams of albumin (human), and 0.9 milligrams of sodium chloride in a sterile, vacuum-dried form without a preservative. One unit (U) corresponds to the calculated median lethal intraperitoneal dose (LD/50) in mice of the reconstituted **BOTOX®** injected.

CLINICAL PHARMACOLOGY

BOTOX® (Botulinum Toxin Type A) Purified Neurotoxin Complex blocks neuromuscular conduction by binding to receptor sites on motor nerve terminals, entering the nerve terminals, and inhibiting the release of acetylcholine. When injected intramuscularly at therapeutic doses, **BOTOX®** produces a localized chemical denervation muscle paralysis. When the muscle is chemically denervated, it atrophies and may develop extrajunctional acetylcholine receptors. There is evidence that the nerve can sprout and reinnervate the muscle, with the weakness thus being reversible.

The paralytic effect on muscles injected with **BOTOX®** Purified Neurotoxin Complex is useful in reducing the excessive, abnormal contractions associated with blepharospasm. When used for the treatment of strabismus, it is postulated that the administration of **BOTOX®** affects muscle pairs by inducing an atrophic lengthening of the injected muscle and a corresponding shortening of the muscle's antagonist. Following peri-ocular injection of **BOTOX®**, distant muscles show electrophysiologic changes but no clinical weakness or other clinical change for a period of several weeks or months, parallel to the duration of local clinical paralysis.

In one study, botulinum toxin was evaluated in 27 patients with essential blepharospasm. Twenty-six of the patients had previously undergone drug treatment utilizing benztropine mesylate, clonazepam and/or baclofen without adequate clinical results. Three of these patients then underwent muscle stripping surgery still without an adequate outcome. One patient of the 27 was previously untreated. Upon using botulinum toxin, 25 of the 27 patients reported improvement within 48 hours. One of the other patients was later controlled with a higher dosage. The remaining patient reported only mild improvement but remained functionally impaired.

In another study, 12 patients with blepharospasm were evaluated in a double-blind, placebo-controlled study. All patients receiving botulinum toxin (n=8) were improved compared with no improvements in the placebo group (n=4). The mean dystonia score improved by 72%, the self-assessment score rating improved by 61%, and a videotape evaluation rating improved by 39%. The effects of the treatment lasted a mean of 12.5 weeks.

One thousand six hundred eighty-four patients with blepharospasm evaluated in an open trial showed clinical improvement lasting an average of 12.5 weeks prior to the need for re-treatment.

Six hundred seventy-seven patients with strabismus treated with one or more injections of **BOTOX®** Purified Neurotoxin Complex were evaluated in an open trial. Fifty-five percent of these patients were improved to an alignment of 10 prism diopters or less when evaluated six months or more following injection. These results are consistent with results from additional open label trials which were conducted for this indication.

INDICATIONS AND USAGE

BOTOX® (Botulinum Toxin Type A) Purified Neurotoxin Complex is indicated for the treatment of strabismus and blepharospasm associated with dystonia, including benign essential blepharospasm or VII nerve disorders in patients 12 years of age and above.

The efficacy of **BOTOX®** Purified Neurotoxin Complex in deviations over 50 prism diopters, in restrictive strabismus, in Duane's syndrome with lateral rectus weakness, and in secondary strabismus caused by prior surgical over-recession of the antagonist is doubtful, or multiple injections over time may be required. **BOTOX®** is ineffective in chronic paralytic strabismus except to reduce antagonist contracture in conjunction with surgical repair.

Presence of antibodies to botulinum toxin type A may reduce the effectiveness of **BOTOX®** Purified Neurotoxin Complex therapy. In clinical studies, reduction in effectiveness due to antibody production has occurred in one patient with blepharospasm receiving three doses of **BOTOX®** over a six week period totalling 92 U, and in several patients with torticollis who received multiple doses experimentally, totalling over 300 U in a one-month period. For this reason, the dose of **BOTOX®** for strabismus and blepharospasm should be kept below 200 U in a one month period.

CONTRAINDICATIONS

BOTOX® (Botulinum Toxin Type A) Purified Neurotoxin Complex is contraindicated in individuals with known hypersensitivity to any ingredient in the formulation.

WARNINGS

The recommended dosages and frequencies of administration for **BOTOX®** Purified Neurotoxin Complex should not be exceeded. There have not been any reported instances of systemic toxicity resulting from accidental injection or oral ingestion of **BOTOX®**. Should accidental injection or oral ingestion occur, the person should be medically supervised for several days on an office or outpatient basis for signs or symptoms of systemic weakness or muscle paralysis. The entire contents of a vial is below the estimated dose for systemic toxicity in humans weighing 6 kg. or greater.

In the event of overdosage or injection into the wrong muscle, additional information may be obtained by contacting Allergan, Inc. at (800) 433-8871 from 8:00 a.m. to 4:00 p.m. Pacific Time, or at (714) 246-5954 for a recorded message at other times.

The effect of botulinum toxin may be potentiated by aminoglycoside antibiotics or any other drugs that interfere with neuromuscular transmission. Caution should be exercised when **BOTOX®** Purified Neurotoxin Complex is used in patients taking any of these drugs. This product contains albumin, a derivative of human blood. Based on effective donor screening and product manufacturing processes, it carries an extremely remote risk for transmission of viral diseases. A theoretical risk for transmission of Creutzfeldt-Jakob disease (CJD) also is considered extremely remote. No cases of transmission of viral diseases or CJD have ever been identified for albumin.

PRECAUTIONS

General: The safe and effective use of **BOTOX®** (Botulinum Toxin Type A) Purified Neurotoxin Complex depends upon proper storage of the product, selection of the correct dose, and proper reconstitution and administration techniques. Physicians administering **BOTOX®** must understand the relevant neuromuscular and orbital anatomy and any alterations to the anatomy due to prior surgical procedures, and standard electromyographic techniques.

As with all biologic products, epinephrine and other precautions as necessary should be available should an anaphylactic reaction occur.

During the administration of **BOTOX®** Purified Neurotoxin Complex for the treatment of strabismus, retrobulbar hemorrhages sufficient to compromise retinal circulation have occurred from needle penetrations into the orbit. It is recommended that appropriate instruments to decompress the orbit be accessible. Ocular (globe) penetrations by needles have also occurred. An ophthalmoscope to diagnose this condition should be available.

Reduced blinking from **BOTOX®** Purified Neurotoxin Complex injection of the orbicularis muscle can lead to corneal exposure, persistent epithelial defect and corneal ulceration, especially in patients with VII nerve disorders. One case of corneal perforation in an aphakic eye requiring corneal grafting has occurred because of this effect. Careful testing of corneal sensation in eyes previously operated upon, avoidance of injection into the lower lid area to avoid ectropion, and vigorous treatment of any epithelial defect should be employed. This may require protective drops, ointment, therapeutic soft contact lenses, or closure of the eye by patching or other means.

Information for Patients: Patients with blepharospasm may have been extremely sedentary for a long time. Sedentary patients should be cautioned to resume activity slowly and carefully following the administration of **BOTOX®** Purified Neurotoxin Complex.

Drug Interactions: The effect of botulinum toxin may be potentiated by aminoglycoside antibiotics or any other drugs that interfere with neuromuscular transmission. Caution should be exercised when **BOTOX®** Purified Neurotoxin Complex is used in patients taking any of these drugs. (See **Warnings**).

Pregnancy: ***Pregnancy Category C:*** Animal reproduction studies have not been conducted with **BOTOX®** Purified Neurotoxin Complex. It is also not known whether **BOTOX®** can cause fetal harm when administered to a pregnant woman or can affect reproduction capacity. **BOTOX®** should be administered to pregnant women only if clearly needed.

Carcinogenesis, Mutagenesis, Impairment of Fertility: Long term studies in animals have not been performed to evaluate carcinogenic potential of **BOTOX®** Purified Neurotoxin Complex.

Nursing Mothers: It is not known whether this drug is excreted in human milk. Because many drugs are excreted in human milk, caution should be exercised when **BOTOX®** Purified Neurotoxin Complex is administered to a nursing woman.

Pediatric Use: Safety and effectiveness in children below the age of 12 have not been established.

ADVERSE REACTIONS

There have been reports of seven cases of diffuse skin rash and two cases of local swelling of the eyelid skin lasting for several days following eyelid injection.

Strabismus: Inducing paralysis in one or more extraocular muscles may produce spatial disorientation, double vision, or past-pointing. Covering the affected eye may alleviate these symptoms. Extraocular muscles adjacent to the injection site are often affected, causing ptosis or vertical deviation, especially with higher doses of **BOTOX®** (Botulinum Toxin Type A) Purified Neurotoxin Complex. The incidence rates of these side effects in 2058 adults who received 3650 injections for horizontal strabismus are listed below:

Ptosis	15.7%
Vertical deviation	16.9%

The incidence of ptosis was much less after inferior rectus injection (0.9%) and much greater after superior rectus injection (37.7%).

The incidence rates of these side effects persisting for over six months in an enlarged series of 5587 injections of horizontal muscles in 3104 patients are listed below:

Ptosis lasting over 180 days	0.3%
Vertical deviation greater than 2 prism diopters lasting over 180 days	2.1%

In these patients, the injection procedure itself caused nine scleral perforations. A vitreous hemorrhage occurred and later cleared in one case. No retinal detachment or visual loss occurred in any case. Sixteen retrobulbar hemorrhages occurred. Decompression of the orbit after five minutes was done to restore retinal circulation in one case. No eye lost

Continued on next page

Botox—Cont.

vision from retrobulbar hemorrhage. Five eyes had pupillary change consistent with ciliary ganglion damage (Adies pupil).

Blepharospasm: In 1684 patients who received 4258 treatments (involving multiple injections) for blepharospasm, the incidence rates of adverse reactions per treated eye are listed below:

Ptosis	11.0%
Irritation/Tearing	10.0%

(includes dry eye, lagophthalmos, and photophobia)

Ectropion, keratitis, diplopia and entropion were reported rarely (incidence less than 1%)

Ecchymosis occurs easily in the soft eyelid tissues. This can be prevented by applying pressure at the injection site immediately after the injection.

In two cases of VII nerve disorder (one case of an aphakic eye) reduced blinking from **BOTOX®** Purified Neurotoxin Complex injection of the orbicularis muscle led to serious corneal exposure, persistent epithelial defect and corneal ulceration. Perforation requiring corneal grafting occurred in one case, an aphakic eye. Avoidance of injection into the lower lid area to avoid ectropion may reduce this hazard. Vigorous treatment of any corneal epithelial defect should be employed. This may require protective drops, ointment, therapeutic soft contact lenses, or closure of the eye by patching or other means.

Two patients previously incapacitated by blepharospasm experienced cardiac collapse attributed to over-exertion within three weeks following **BOTOX®** Purified Neurotoxin Complex therapy. Sedentary patients should be cautioned to resume activity slowly and carefully following the administration of **BOTOX®**.

OVERDOSAGE

In the event of overdosage or injection into the wrong muscle, additional information may be obtained by contacting Allergan, Inc. at (800) 433-8871 from 8:00 a.m. to 4:00 p.m. Pacific Time, or at (714) 246-5954 for a recorded message at other times.

DOSAGE AND ADMINISTRATION

Strabismus: **BOTOX®** (Botulinum Toxin Type A) Purified Neurotoxin Complex is intended for injection into extraocular muscles utilizing the electrical activity recorded from the tip of the injection needle as a guide to placement within the target muscle. Injection without surgical exposure or electromyographic guidance should not be attempted. Physicians should be familiar with electromyographic technique.

An injection of **BOTOX®** Purified Neurotoxin Complex is prepared by drawing into a sterile 1.0 mL tuberculin syringe an amount of the properly diluted toxin (see Dilution Table) slightly greater than the intended dose. Air bubbles in the syringe barrel are expelled and the syringe is attached to the electromyographic injection needle, preferably a 1.5 inch, 27 gauge needle. Injection volume in excess of the intended dose is expelled through the needle into an appropriate waste container to assure patency of the needle and to confirm that there is no syringe-needle leakage. A new, sterile needle and syringe should be used to enter the vial on each occasion for dilution or removal of **BOTOX®**.

To prepare the eye for **BOTOX®** Purified Neurotoxin Complex injection, it is recommended that several drops of a local anesthetic and an ocular decongestant be given several minutes prior to injection.

Note: The volume of **BOTOX®** Purified Neurotoxin Complex injected for treatment of strabismus should be between 0.05 mL to 0.15 mL per muscle.

Strabismus dosage: The initial listed doses of the diluted **BOTOX®** Purified Neurotoxin Complex (see Dilution Table below) typically create paralysis of injected muscles beginning one to two days after injection and increasing in intensity during the first week. The paralysis lasts for 2–6 weeks and gradually resolves over a similar time period. Overcorrections lasting over 6 months have been rare. About one half of patients will require subsequent doses because of inadequate paralytic response of the muscle to the initial dose, or because of mechanical factors such as large deviations or restrictions, or because of the lack of binocular motor fusion to stabilize the alignment.

I. Initial doses in units (abbreviated as U). Use the lower listed doses for treatment of small deviations. Use the larger doses only for large deviations.
   A. For vertical muscles, and for horizontal strabismus of less than 20 prism diopters: 1.25 U to 2.5 U in any one muscle.
   B. For horizontal strabismus of 20 prism diopters to 50 prism diopters: 2.5 U to 5.0 U in any one muscle.
   C. For persistent VI nerve palsy of one month or longer duration: 1.25 U to 2.5 U in the medial rectus muscle.

II. Subsequent doses for residual or recurrent strabismus.
   A. It is recommended that patients be re-examined 7–14 days after each injection to assess the effect of that dose.
   B. Patients experiencing adequate paralysis of the target muscle that require subsequent injections should receive a dose comparable to the initial dose.
   C. Subsequent doses for patients experiencing incomplete paralysis of the target muscle may be increased up to twice the size of the previously administered dose.
   D. Subsequent injections should not be administered until the effects of the previous dose have dissipated as evidenced by substantial function in the injected and adjacent muscles.
   E. The maximum recommended dose as a single injection for any one muscle is 25 U.

Blepharospasm: For blepharospasm, diluted **BOTOX®** Purified Neurotoxin Complex (see Dilution Table) is injected using a sterile, 27–30 gauge needle without electromyographic guidance. 1.25 U to 2.5 U (0.05 mL to 0.1 mL volume at each site) injected into the medial and lateral pre-tarsal orbicularis oculi of the upper lid and into the lateral pre-tarsal orbicularis oculi of the lower lid is the initial recommended dose. In general, the initial effect of the injections is seen within three days and reaches a peak at one to two weeks post-treatment. Each treatment lasts approximately three months, following which the procedure can be repeated indefinitely. At repeat treatment sessions, the dose may be increased up to two-fold if the response from the initial treatment is considered insufficient—usually defined as an effect that does not last longer than two months. However there appears to be little benefit obtainable from injecting more than 5.0 U per site. Some tolerance may be found when **BOTOX®** is used in treating blepharospasm if treatments are given any more frequently than every three months, and it is rare to have the effect be permanent.

The cumulative dose of **BOTOX®** Purified Neurotoxin Complex in a 30-day period should not exceed 200 U.

DILUTION TECHNIQUE

To reconstitute vacuum-dried **BOTOX®** (Botulinum Toxin Type A) Purified Neurotoxin Complex, use sterile normal saline **without** a preservative; 0.9% Sodium Chloride Injection is the recommended diluent. Draw up the proper amount of diluent in the appropriate size syringe. Since **BOTOX®** is denatured by bubbling or similar violent agitation, inject the diluent into the vial gently. Discard the vial if a vacuum does not pull the diluent into the vial. Record the date and time of reconstitution on the space on the label. **BOTOX®** should be administered within 4 hours after reconstitution.

During this time period, reconstituted **BOTOX®** Purified Neurotoxin Complex should be stored in a refrigerator (2° to 8°C). Reconstituted **BOTOX®** should be clear, colorless and free of particulate matter. Parenteral drug products should be inspected visually for particulate matter and discoloration prior to administration and whenever the solution and the container permit. The use of one vial for more than one patient is not recommended because the product and diluent do not contain a preservative.

Dilution Table

Diluent Added (0.9% Sodium Chloride Injection)	Resulting dose in Units per 0.1 mL
1.0 mL	10.0 U
2.0 mL	5.0 U
4.0 mL	2.5 U
8.0 mL	1.25 U

Note: These dilutions are calculated for an injection volume of 0.1 mL. A decrease or increase in the **BOTOX®** Purified Neurotoxin Complex dose is also possible by administering a smaller or larger injection volume—from 0.05 mL (50% decrease in dose) to 0.15 mL (50% increase in dose).

HOW SUPPLIED

Each vial contains 100 U of vacuum-dried *Clostridium botulinum* toxin type A. NDC 0023-1145-01.

Rx only

STORAGE

Store the vacuum-dried product in a freezer at or below −5°C. Administer **BOTOX®** (Botulinum Toxin Type A) Purified Neurotoxin Complex within four hours after the vial is removed from the freezer and reconstituted. During these four hours, reconstituted **BOTOX®** should be stored in a refrigerator (2° to 8°C). Reconstituted **BOTOX®** should be clear, colorless and free of particulate matter.

All vials, including expired vials, or equipment used with the drug should be disposed of carefully as is done with all medical waste.

September 1999

ELIMITE® Cream (permethrin) 5% * ℞

DESCRIPTION

ELIMITE® (permethrin) 5% Cream is a topical scabicidal agent for the treatment of infestation with *Sarcoptes scabiei* (scabies). It is available in an off-white, vanishing cream base. ELIMITE® Cream is for topical use only.

Chemical Name: The permethrin used is an approximate 1:3 mixture of the cis and trans isomers of the pyrethroid 3-(2,2-dichloroethenyl)-2,2-dimethylcyclopropanecarboxylic acid, (3-phenoxyphenyl) methyl ester. Permethrin has a molecular formula of $C_{21}H_{20}Cl_2O_3$ and a molecular weight of 391.29. It is a yellow to light orange-brown, low melting solid or viscous liquid.

Active Ingredient: Each gram contains permethrin 50 mg (5%).

Inactive Ingredients: Butylated hydroxytoluene, carbomer 934P, fractionated coconut oil, glycerin, glyceryl monostearate, isopropyl myristate, lanolin alcohols, mineral oil, polyoxyethylene cetyl ethers, purified water, and sodium hydroxide. Formaldehyde 1 mg (0.1%) is added as a preservative.

CLINICAL PHARMACOLOGY

Permethrin, a pyrethroid, is active against a broad range of pests including lice, ticks, fleas, mites, and other arthropods. It acts on the nerve cell membrane to disrupt the sodium channel current by which the polarization of the membrane is regulated. Delayed repolarization and paralysis of the pests are the consequences of this disturbance.

Permethrin is rapidly metabolized by ester hydrolysis to inactive metabolites which are excreted primarily in the urine. Although the amount of permethrin absorbed after a single application of the 5% cream has not been determined precisely, data from studies with ^{14}C-labeled permethrin and absorption studies of the cream applied to patients with moderate to severe scabies indicate it is 2% or less of the amount applied.

INDICATIONS AND USAGE

ELIMITE® (permethrin) 5% Cream is indicated for the treatment of infestation with *Sarcoptes scabiei* (scabies).

CONTRAINDICATIONS

ELIMITE® is contraindicated in patients with known hypersensitivity to any of its components, to any synthetic pyrethroid or pyrethrin.

WARNINGS

If hypersensitivity to ELIMITE® occurs, discontinue use.

PRECAUTIONS

General: Scabies infestation is often accompanied by pruritus, edema and erythema. Treatment with ELIMITE® may temporarily exacerbate these conditions.

Information for patients: Patients with scabies should be advised that itching, mild burning and/or stinging may occur after application of ELIMITE®. In clinical trials approximately 75% of patients treated with ELIMITE® who continued to manifest pruritus at 2 weeks had cessation by 4 weeks. If irritation persists, they should consult their physician. ELIMITE® may be very mildly irritating to the eyes. Patients should be advised to avoid contact with eyes during application and to flush with water immediately if ELIMITE® gets in the eyes.

Carcinogenesis, mutagenesis, impairment of fertility: Six carcinogenicity bioassays were evaluated with permethrin, three each in rats and mice. No tumorigenicity was seen in the rat studies. However, species-specific increases in pulmonary adenomas, a common benign tumor of mice of high spontaneous background incidence, were seen in the three mouse studies. In one of these studies there was an increased incidence of pulmonary alveolar-cell carcinomas and benign liver adenomas only in female mice when permethrin was given in their food at a concentration of 5000 ppm. Mutagenicity assays, which give useful correlative data for interpreting results from carcinogenicity bioassays in rodents, were negative. Permethrin showed no evidence of mutagenic potential in a battery of *in vitro* and *in vivo* genetic toxicity studies.

Permethrin did not have any adverse effect on reproductive function at a dose of 180 mg/kg/day orally in a three-generation rat study.

Pregnancy: *teratogenic effects:* Pregnancy Category B: Reproduction studies have been performed in mice, rats, and rabbits (200 to 400 mg/kg/day orally) and have revealed no evidence of impaired fertility or harm to the fetus due to permethrin. There are, however, no adequate and well-controlled studies in pregnant women. Because animal reproduction studies are not always predictive of human response, this drug should be used during pregnancy only if clearly needed.

Nursing mothers: It is not known whether this drug is excreted in human milk. Because many drugs are excreted in human milk and because of the evidence for tumorigenic potential of permethrin in animal studies, consideration should be given to discontinuing nursing temporarily or withholding the drug while the mother is nursing.

Pediatric use: ELIMITE® is safe and effective in pediatric patients two months of age and older. Safety and effectiveness in infants less than two months of age have not been established.

ADVERSE REACTIONS

In clinical trials, generally mild and transient burning and stinging followed application with ELIMITE® in 10% of patients and was associated with the severity of infestation. Pruritus was reported in 7% of patients at various times post-application. Erythema, numbness, tingling, and rash were reported in 1 to 2% or less of patients (see PRECAUTIONS: General).

OVERDOSAGE

No instance of accidental ingestion of ELIMITE® has been reported. If ingested, gastric lavage and general supportive measures should be employed.

DOSAGE AND ADMINISTRATION

Adults and children: Thoroughly massage ELIMITE® into the skin from the head to the soles of the feet. Scabies rarely infests the scalp of adults, although the hairline, neck, temple, and forehead may be infested in infants and geriatric patients. Usually 30 grams is sufficient for an average adult. The cream should be removed by washing (shower or

bath) after 8 to 14 hours. Infants should be treated on the scalp, temple and forehead. ONE APPLICATION IS GENERALLY CURATIVE.
Patients may experience persistent pruritus after treatment. This is rarely a sign of treatment failure and is not an indication for retreatment. Demonstrable living mites after 14 days indicate that retreatment is necessary.

HOW SUPPLIED

ELIMITE® (permethrin) 5% (wt./wt.) Cream is supplied in tubes in the following size: 60 g NDC 0023-7915-60.
Note: Store at 15° to 25°C (59° to 77°F).
Rx only
Manufactured for:
Allergan, Inc.
Irvine, CA 92612, U.S.A.
by Catalytica Pharmaceuticals, Inc.
Research Triangle Park, NC 27709

EXSEL® Lotion/Shampoo ℞
(Selenium Sulfide Lotion, USP) 2.5%

Active Ingredient: selenium sulfide .... 2.5% (w/v) in aqueous suspension.
Inactive Ingredients: edetate disodium; bentonite; sodium dodecylbenzene sulfonate; sodium C14-16 olefin sulfonate; glyceryl ricinoleate; dimethicone copolyol; titanium dioxide; citric acid monohydrate; sodium phosphate monobasic, monohydrate; fragrance; and purified water.

HOW SUPPLIED

EXSEL® is available in a 4 fl oz plastic bottle—NDC 0023-0817-99

FLUOROPLEX® ℞
(fluorouracil)
1% Topical Cream
and
1% Topical Solution

PRODUCT OVERVIEW

KEY FACTS

Effective treatment for multiple Actinic Keratoses sites.
Provides effective treatment for both clinical and subclinical lesions.
FLUOROPLEX® Cream does not contain irritating parabens or propylene glycol.

MAJOR USES

Multiple actinic keratoses.

SAFETY INFORMATION

Contraindicated in persons hypersensitive to fluorouracil or its listed ingredients.
Contraindicated in pregnancy.
Prolonged exposure to sunlight or other forms of ultraviolet irradiation may increase intensity of reaction.
Adequate long-term studies in animals to evaluate carcinogenic potential have not been conducted with fluorouracil.

PRESCRIBING INFORMATION

FLUOROPLEX® ℞
(fluorouracil)
1% Topical Cream
and
1% Topical Solution

DESCRIPTION

FLUOROPLEX® (fluorouracil) 1% Topical Cream and 1% Topical Solution are antineoplastic/antimetabolite products for dermatological use. Fluorouracil has the empirical formula $C_4H_3FN_2O_2$ and a molecular weight of 130.08. It is sparingly soluble in water and slightly soluble in alcohol. The pH is approximately 8.5 for FLUOROPLEX® Topical Cream and 9.2 for FLUOROPLEX® Topical Solution.
Chemical Name:
2,4(*1H, 3H*)-Pyrimidinedione, 5-fluoro-.
FLUOROPLEX 1% Topical Cream contains:
Active Ingredient: fluorouracil .... 1.0%.
Inactive Ingredients: benzyl alcohol, emulsifying wax, mineral oil, isopropyl myristate, sodium hydroxide and purified water.
FLUOROPLEX® 1% Topical Solution contains:
Active Ingredient: fluorouracil 1.0%
Inactive Ingredients: propylene glycol, sodium hydroxide and/or hydrochloric acid to adjust the pH, and purified water.

CLINICAL PHARMACOLOGY

There is evidence that fluorouracil (or its metabolites) blocks the methylation reaction of deoxyuridylic acid to thymidylic acid. In this fashion, fluorouracil interferes with the synthesis of deoxyribonucleic acid (DNA) and to a lesser extent inhibits the formation of ribonucleic acid (RNA).

INDICATIONS AND USAGE

FLUOROPLEX® is indicated for the topical treatment of multiple actinic (solar) keratoses.

CONTRAINDICATIONS

Fluorouracil is contraindicated in women who are or may become pregnant. These products should not be used by patients who are allergic to any of their components.

WARNINGS

There exists the potential for a delayed hypersensitivity reaction to fluorouracil. Patch testing to prove hypersensitivity may be inconclusive.[1]
If an occlusive dressing is used, there may be an increase in the incidence of inflammatory reactions in the adjacent normal skin.
The patient should avoid prolonged exposure to sunlight or other forms of ultraviolet irradiation during treatment with FLUOROPLEX®, as the intensity of the reaction may be increased.

PRECAUTIONS

General: There is a possibility of increased absorption through ulcerated or inflamed skin.
Information for patients: The medication should be applied with care near the eyes, nose and mouth. Excessive reaction in these areas may occur due to irritation from accumulation of drug. If FLUOROPLEX® is applied with the fingers, the hands should be washed immediately afterward.
The reaction to FLUOROPLEX® in treated areas may be unsightly during therapy, and, in some cases, for several weeks following cessation of therapy.
Laboratory Tests: To rule out the presence of a frank neoplasm, a biopsy should be made of those areas failing to respond to treatment or recurring after treatment.
Carcinogenesis, mutagenesis, impairment of fertility: Adequate long-term studies in animals to evaluate carcinogenic potential have not been conducted with fluorouracil. In three *in vitro* cell transformation assays, fluorouracil produced morphological transformation of cells. Morphological transformation was also produced in one of these *in vitro* assays by a metabolite of fluorouracil and the transformed cells produced malignant tumors when injected into immunosuppressed syngeneic mice. Fluorouracil has been shown to exert mutagenic activity in the yeast cells, **Bacillus subtilis,** and **Drosophila** assays. In addition, fluorouracil has produced chromosome damage at concentrations of 1.0 and 2.0 mcg/mL in an *in vitro* hamster fibroblast assay and increases in micronuclei formation in the bone marrow of mice at intraperitoneal doses within the human therapeutic dose range of 12–15 mg/kg/day. Patients receiving cumulative doses of 0.24–1.0 g of fluorouracil parenterally have shown an increase in numerical and structural chromosome aberrations in peripheral blood lymphocytes. Fluorouracil has been shown to impair fertility after parenteral administration in rats. In mice, single-dose intravenous and intraperitoneal injections of fluorouracil have been reported to kill differentiated spermatogonia and spermatocytes at a dose of 500 mg/kg and produce abnormalities in spermatids at 50 mg/kg.
Fluorouracil was negative in the dominant lethal mutation assay performed in mice.
Pregnancy: Teratogenic effects: Pregnancy Category X: Fluorouracil may cause fetal harm when administered to a pregnant woman. Fluorouracil administered parenterally has been shown to be teratogenic in mice, rats and hamsters, and embryolethal in monkeys. Fluorouracil is contraindicated in women who are or may become pregnant. If this drug is used during pregnancy, or if the patient becomes pregnant while taking this drug, the patient should be apprised of the potential hazard to the fetus.
Nursing mothers: It is not known whether this drug is excreted in human milk. Because many drugs are excreted in human milk, and because there is some systemic absorption of fluorouracil after topical administration (see **PRECAUTIONS: General**), mothers should not nurse their infants while receiving this drug.
Pediatric use: Safety and effectiveness in pediatric patients have not been established.

ADVERSE REACTIONS

Pain, pruritus, burning, irritation, inflammation, allergic contact dermatitis and telangiectasia have been reported. Occasionally, hyperpigmentation and scarring have also been reported.

OVERDOSAGE

Ordinarily, overdosage will not cause acute problems. If FLUOROPLEX® accidentally comes in contact with the eye(s), flush the eye(s) with water or normal saline. If FLUOROPLEX® is accidentally ingested, induce emesis and gastric lavage. Administer symptomatic and supportive care as needed.

DOSAGE AND ADMINISTRATION

The patient should be instructed to apply sufficient medication to cover the entire face or other affected areas.
Apply medication twice daily with non-metallic applicator or fingertips and wash hands afterwards. A treatment period of 2–6 weeks is usually required.
Increasing the frequency of application and a longer period of administration with FLUOROPLEX® may be required on areas other than the head and neck.
When FLUOROPLEX® is applied to keratotic skin, a response occurs with the following sequence: erythema, usually followed by scaling, tenderness, erosion, ulceration, necrosis and re-epithelization. When the inflammatory reaction reaches the erosion, ulceration and necrosis stages, the use of the drug should be terminated. Responses may sometimes occur in areas which appear clinically normal. These may be sites of subclinical actinic (solar) keratosis which the medication is affecting.

HOW SUPPLIED

FLUOROPLEX® (fluorouracil) 1% Topical Cream is available in 30 g tubes (NDC 0023-0812-30).
FLUOROPLEX® (fluorouracil) 1% Topical Solution is available in 30 mL plastic dropper bottles (NDC 0023-0810-30).
Note: Avoid freezing. Store at 15°–30°C (59°–86 °F) in tight containers.
Rx only

REFERENCE

1. Epstein E. Testing for 5-fluorouracil allergy: patch and intradermal tests. *Contact Dermatitis* 1984; 10:311.

MAXIFLOR® ℞
(diflorasone diacetate)
Cream, USP, 0.05%
Ointment, USP, 0.05%

DESCRIPTION

MAXIFLOR® Cream Contains:
Active Ingredient: 0.5 mg diflorasone diacetate, USP, in an emulsified and hydrophilic cream base.
Inactive Ingredients: Propylene glycol, stearic acid, polysorbate 60, sorbitan monostearate and monooleate, sorbic acid, citric acid and water. The corticosteroid is formulated as a solution in the vehicle using 15 percent propylene glycol to optimize drug delivery.
MAXIFLOR® Ointment Contains:
Active Ingredient: 0.5 mg diflorasone diacetate, USP, in an emollient, occlusive base. *Inactive Ingredients:* Polyoxypropylene 15-stearyl ether, stearic acid, lanolin alcohol and white petrolatum.

HOW SUPPLIED

MAXIFLOR® (diflorasone diacetate) Cream, USP, 0.05% is available in collapsible tubes in the following sizes:
30 gram NDC 0023-0766-30
60 gram NDC 0023-0766-60
MAXIFLOR® (diflorasone diacetate) Ointment, USP, 0.05% is available in collapsible tubes in the following sizes:
30 gram NDC 0023-0770-30
60 gram NDC 0023-0770-60
Manufactured for ALLERGAN
Irvine, California 92612, USA
by Pharmacia & Upjohn Company
Kalamazoo, Michigan 49001

OCUFLOX® ℞
(ofloxacin ophthalmic solution)
0.3% sterile

DESCRIPTION

OCUFLOX® (ofloxacin ophthalmic solution) 0.3% is a sterile ophthalmic solution. It is a fluorinated carboxyquinolone anti-infective for topical ophthalmic use.
Structural Formula:

ofloxacin

$C_{18}H_{20}FN_3O_4$ Mol Wt 361.37

Chemical Name: (±)-9-Fluoro-2,3-dihydro-3-methyl-10-(4-methyl-1-piperazinyl)-7-oxo-7H-pyrido[1,2,3-de]-1,4 benzoxazine-6-carboxylic acid.
Contains:

Active:	ofloxacin 0.3% (3 mg/mL);
Preservative:	benzalkonium chloride (0.005%);
Inactives:	sodium chloride and purified water. May also contain hydrochloric acid and/or sodium hydroxide to adjust pH.

OCUFLOX® solution is unbuffered and formulated with a pH of 6.4 (range—6.0 to 6.8). It has an osmolality of 300 mOsm/kg. Ofloxacin is a fluorinated 4-quinolone which differs from other fluorinated 4-quinolones in that there is a six member (pyridobenzoxazine) ring from positions 1 to 8 of the basic ring structure.

CLINICAL PHARMACOLOGY

Pharmacokinetics: Serum, urine and tear concentrations of ofloxacin were measured in 30 healthy women at various

Continued on next page

Ocuflox—Cont.

time points during a ten-day course of treatment with OCUFLOX® solution. The mean serum ofloxacin concentration ranged from 0.4 ng/mL to 1.9 ng/mL. Maximum ofloxacin concentration increased from 1.1 ng/mL on day one to 1.9 ng/mL on day 11 after QID dosing for 10½ days. Maximum serum ofloxacin concentrations after ten days of topical ophthalmic dosing were more than 1000 times lower than those reported after standard oral doses of ofloxacin.

Tear ofloxacin concentrations ranged from 5.7 to 31 μg/g during the 40 minute period following the last dose on day 11. Mean tear concentration measured four hours after topical ophthalmic dosing was 9.2 μg/g.

Corneal tissue concentrations of 4.4 μg/mL were observed four hours after beginning topical ocular application of two drops of OCUFLOX® ophthalmic solution every 30 minutes. Ofloxacin was excreted in the urine primarily unmodified.

Microbiology: Ofloxacin has in vitro activity against a broad range of gram-positive and gram-negative aerobic and anaerobic bacteria. Ofloxacin is bactericidal at concentrations equal to or slightly greater than inhibitory concentrations. Ofloxacin is thought to exert a bactericidal effect on susceptible bacterial cells by inhibiting DNA gyrase, an essential bacterial enzyme which is a critical catalyst in the duplication, transcription, and repair of bacterial DNA.

Cross-resistance has been observed between ofloxacin and other fluoroquinolones. There is generally no cross-resistance between ofloxacin and other classes of antibacterial agents such as beta-lactams or aminoglycosides.

Ofloxacin has been shown to be active against most strains of the following organisms both in vitro and clinically, in conjunctival and/or corneal ulcer infections as described in the **INDICATIONS AND USAGE** section.

AEROBES, GRAM-POSITIVE:

Staphylococcus aureus
Staphylococcus epidermidis
Streptococcus pneumoniae

AEROBES, GRAM-NEGATIVE:

Enterobacter cloacae
Haemophilus influenzae
Proteus mirabilis
Pseudomonas aeruginosa
*Serratia marcescens**

ANAEROBIC SPECIES:

Propionibacterium acnes

*Efficacy for this organism was studied in fewer than 10 infections.

The safety and effectiveness of OCUFLOX® ophthalmic solution in treating ophthalmologic infections due to the following organisms have not been established in adequate and well-controlled clinical trials. OCUFLOX® ophthalmic solution has been shown to be active in vitro against most strains of these organisms but the clinical significance in ophthalmologic infections is unknown.

AEROBES, GRAM-POSITIVE:

Enterococcus faecalis
Listeria monocytogenes
Staphylococcus capitis
Staphylococcus hominus
Staphylococcus simulans
Streptococcus pyogenes

AEROBES, GRAM-NEGATIVE:

Acinetobacter calcoaceticus var. *anitratus*
Acinetobacter calcoaceticus var. *Iwoffii*
Citrobacter diversus
Citrobacter freundii
Enterobacter aerogenes
Enterobacter agglomerans
Escherichia coli
Haemophilus parainfluenzae
Klebsiella oxytoca
Klebsiella pneumoniae
Moraxella (Branhamella) catarrhalis
Moraxella lacunata
Morganella morganii
Neisseria gonorrhoeae
Pseudomonas acidovorans
Pseudomonas fluorescens
Shigella sonnei

OTHER:

Chlamydia trachomatis

Clinical Studies:

Conjunctivitis: In a randomized, double-masked, multicenter clinical trial, OCUFLOX® ophthalmic solution was superior to its vehicle after 2 days of treatment in patients with conjunctivitis and positive conjunctival cultures. Clinical outcomes for the trial demonstrated a clinical improvement rate of 86% (54/63) for the ofloxacin treated group versus 72% (48/67) for the placebo treated group after 2 days of therapy. Microbiological outcomes for the same clinical trial demonstrated an eradication rate for causative pathogens of 65% (41/63) for the ofloxacin treated group versus 25% (17/67) for the vehicle treated group after 2 days of therapy. Please note that microbiologic eradication does not always correlate with clinical outcome in anti-infective trials.

Corneal Ulcers: In a randomized, double-masked, multicenter trial of 140 subjects with positive cultures, OCUFLOX® ophthalmic solution treated subjects had an overall clinical success rate (complete re-epithelialization and no progression of the infiltrate for two consecutive visits) of 82% (61/74) compared to 80% (53/66) for the fortified antibiotic group, consisting of 1.5% tobramycin and 10% cefazolin solutions. The median time to clinical success was 11 days for the ofloxacin treated group and 10 days for the fortified treatment group.

INDICATIONS AND USAGE

OCUFLOX® ophthalmic solution is indicated for the treatment of infections caused by susceptible strains of the following bacteria in the conditions listed below:

CONJUNCTIVITIS:

Gram-positive bacteria:

Staphylococcus aureus
Staphylococcus epidermidis
Streptococcus pneumoniae

Gram-negative bacteria:

Enterobacter cloacae
Haemophilus influenzae
Proteus mirabilis
Pseudomonas aeruginosa

CORNEAL ULCERS:

Gram-positive bacteria:

Staphylococcus aureus
Staphylococcus epidermidis
Streptococcus pneumoniae

Gram-negative bacteria:

Pseudomonas aeruginosa
*Serratia marcescens**

Anaerobic species:

Propionibacterium acnes

*Efficacy for this organism was studied in fewer than 10 infections.

CONTRAINDICATIONS

OCUFLOX® solution is contraindicated in patients with a history of hypersensitivity to ofloxacin, to other quinolones, or to any of the components in this medication.

WARNINGS

NOT FOR INJECTION.

OCUFLOX® solution should not be injected subconjunctivally, nor should it be introduced directly into the anterior chamber of the eye.

Serious and occasionally fatal hypersensitivity (anaphylactic) reactions, some following the first dose, have been reported in patients receiving systemic quinolones, including ofloxacin. Some reactions were accompanied by cardiovascular collapse, loss of consciousness, angioedema (including laryngeal, pharyngeal or facial edema), airway obstruction, dyspnea, urticaria, and itching. A rare occurrence of Stevens-Johnson syndrome, which progressed to toxic epidermal necrolysis, has been reported in a patient who was receiving topical ophthalmic ofloxacin. If an allergic reaction to ofloxacin occurs, discontinue the drug. Serious acute hypersensitivity reactions may require immediate emergency treatment. Oxygen and airway management, including intubation should be administered as clinically indicated.

PRECAUTIONS

General: As with other anti-infectives, prolonged use may result in overgrowth of nonsusceptible organisms, including fungi. If superinfection occurs, discontinue use and institute alternative therapy. Whenever clinical judgment dictates, the patient should be examined with the aid of magnification, such as slit lamp biomicroscopy and, where appropriate, fluorescein staining. Ofloxacin should be discontinued at the first appearance of a skin rash or any other sign of hypersensitivity reaction.

The systemic administration of quinolones, including ofloxacin, has led to lesions or erosions of the cartilage in weight-bearing joints and other signs of arthropathy in immature animals of various species. Ofloxacin, administered systemically at 10 mg/kg/day in young dogs (equivalent to 110 times the maximum recommended daily *adult ophthalmic* dose) has been associated with these types of effects.

Information for Patients: Avoid contaminating the applicator tip with material from the eye, fingers, or other source. Systemic quinolones, including ofloxacin, have been associated with hypersensitivity reactions, even following a single dose. Discontinue use immediately and contact your physician at the first sign of a rash or allergic reaction.

Drug Interactions: Specific drug interaction studies have not been conducted with OCUFLOX® ophthalmic solution. However, the systemic administration of some quinolones has been shown to elevate plasma concentrations of theophylline, interfere with the metabolism of caffeine, and enhance the effects of the oral anticoagulant warfarin and its derivatives, and has been associated with transient elevations in serum creatinine in patients receiving cyclosporine concomitantly.

Carcinogenesis, Mutagenesis, Impairment of Fertility: Long term studies to determine the carcinogenic potential of ofloxacin have not been conducted.

Ofloxacin was not mutagenic in the Ames test, in vitro and in vivo cytogenic assay, sister chromatid exchange assay (Chinese hamster and human cell lines), unscheduled DNA synthesis (UDS) assay using human fibroblasts, the dominant lethal assay, or mouse micronucleus assay. Ofloxacin was positive in the UDS test using rat hepatocyte, and in the mouse lymphoma assay.

In fertility studies in rats, ofloxacin did not affect male or female fertility or morphological or reproductive performance at oral dosing up to 360 mg/kg/day (equivalent to 4000 times the maximum recommended daily ophthalmic dose).

Pregnancy: Teratogenic Effects. Pregnancy Category C: Ofloxacin has been shown to have embryocidal effect in rats and in rabbits when given in doses of 810 mg/kg/day (equivalent to 9000 times the maximum recommended daily ophthalmic dose) and 160 mg/kg/day (equivalent to 1800 times the maximum recommended daily ophthalmic dose). These dosages resulted in decreased fetal body weight and increased fetal mortality in rats and rabbits, respectively. Minor fetal skeletal variations were reported in rats receiving doses of 810 mg/kg/day. Ofloxacin has not been shown to be teratogenic at doses as high as 810 mg/kg/day and 160 mg/kg/day when administered to pregnant rats and rabbits, respectively.

Nonteratogenic Effects: Additional studies in rats with doses up to 360 mg/kg/day during late gestation showed no adverse effect on late fetal development, labor, delivery, lactation, neonatal viability, or growth of the newborn.

There are, however, no adequate and well-controlled studies in pregnant women. OCUFLOX® solution should be used during pregnancy only if the potential benefit justifies the potential risk to the fetus.

Nursing Mothers: In nursing women a single 200 mg oral dose resulted in concentrations of ofloxacin in milk which were similar to those found in plasma. It is not known whether ofloxacin is excreted in human milk following topical ophthalmic administration. Because of the potential for serious adverse reactions from ofloxacin in nursing infants, a decision should be made whether to discontinue nursing or to discontinue the drug, taking into account the importance of the drug to the mother.

Pediatric Use: Safety and effectiveness in infants below the age of one year have not been established.

Quinolones, including ofloxacin, have been shown to cause arthropathy in immature animals after oral administration; however, topical ocular administration of ofloxacin to immature animals has not shown any arthropathy. There is no evidence that the ophthalmic dosage form of ofloxacin has any effect on weight bearing joints.

Geriatric Use: No overall differences in safety or effectiveness have been observed between elderly and younger patients.

ADVERSE REACTIONS

Ophthalmic Use: The most frequently reported drug-related adverse reaction was transient ocular burning or discomfort. Other reported reactions include stinging, redness, itching, chemical conjunctivitis/keratitis, ocular/periocular/facial edema, foreign body sensation, photophobia, blurred vision, tearing, dryness, and eye pain. Rare reports of dizziness and nausea have been received.

DOSAGE AND ADMINISTRATION

The recommended dosage regimen for the treatment of **bacterial conjunctivitis** is:

Days 1 and 2
Instill one to two drops every two to four hours in the affected eye(s).
Days 3 through 7
Instill one to two drops four times daily.

The recommended dosage regimen for the treatment of **bacterial corneal ulcer** is:

Days 1 and 2
Instill one to two drops into the affected eye every 30 minutes, while awake. Awaken at approximately four and six hours after retiring and instill one to two drops.
Days 3 through 7 to 9
Instill one to two drops hourly, while awake.
Days 7 to 9 through treatment completion
Instill one to two drops, four times daily.

HOW SUPPLIED

OCUFLOX® (ofloxacin ophthalmic solution) 0.3% is supplied sterile in plastic dropper bottles of the following sizes:

1 mL—NDC 11980-779-01
5 mL—NDC 11980-779-05
10 mL—NDC 11980-779-10

Note: Store at 15–25°C (59–77°F)

Rx only

Revised March 2000

Allergan America, Hormigueros, Puerto Rico 00660

Licensed from: Daiichi Pharmaceutical Co., Ltd., Tokyo, Japan and Santen Pharmaceutical Co., Ltd., Osaka, Japan

U.S. PAT. NOS. 4,382,892; 4,551,456

 7651X 70829US11H

Shown in Product Identification Guide, page 304

OPTICROM® ℞

(cromolyn sodium ophthalmic solution, USP) 4%
Sterile

Prescribing Information

DESCRIPTION

OPTICROM® (cromolyn sodium ophthalmic solution, USP) 4% is a clear, colorless, sterile solution intended for topical ophthalmic use.

Cromolyn sodium is represented by the following structural formula:

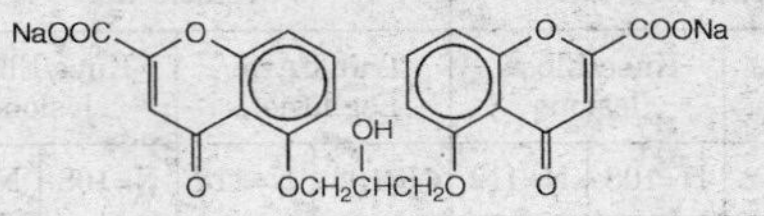

$C_{23}H_{14}Na_2O_{11}$ Mol. Wt 512.34

Chemical Name: Disodium 5-5′ - [(2-hydroxy-trimethylene) dioxy] bis [4-oxo-4*H*-1-benzopyran-2-carboxylate].
Pharmacologic Category: Mast cell stabilizer
Each mL contains: **Active**: Cromolyn sodium 40 mg (4%); **Preservative**: Benzalkonium chloride 0.01%; **Inactives**: Edetate disodium 0.1% and purified water. It has a pH of 4.0 to 7.0.

CLINICAL PHARMACOLOGY

In vitro and *in vivo* animal studies have shown that cromolyn sodium inhibits the degranulation of sensitized mast cells which occurs after exposure to specific antigens. Cromolyn sodium acts by inhibiting the release of histamine and SRS-A (slow-reacting substance of anaphylaxis) from the mast cell.
Another activity demonstrated *in vitro* is the capacity of cromolyn sodium to inhibit the degranulation of non-sensitized rat mast cells by phospholipase A and the subsequent release of chemical mediators. Another study showed that cromolyn sodium did not inhibit the enzymatic activity of released phospholipase A on its specific substrate.
Cromolyn sodium has no intrinsic vasoconstrictor, antihistamine, or anti-inflammatory activity.
Cromolyn sodium is poorly absorbed. When multiple doses of cromolyn sodium ophthalmic solution are instilled into normal rabbit eyes, less than 0.07% of the administered dose of cromolyn sodium is absorbed into the systemic circulation (presumably by way of the eye, nasal passages, buccal cavity, and gastrointestinal tract). Trace amounts (less than 0.01%) of the cromolyn sodium dose penetrate into the aqueous humor and clearance from this chamber is virtually complete within 24 hours after treatment is stopped.
In normal volunteers, analysis of drug excretion indicates that approximately 0.03% of cromolyn sodium is absorbed following administration to the eye.

INDICATIONS AND USAGE

OPTICROM® is indicated in the treatment of vernal keratoconjunctivitis, vernal conjunctivitis, and vernal keratitis.

CONTRAINDICATIONS

OPTICROM® is contraindicated in those patients who have shown hypersensitivity to cromolyn sodium or to any of the other ingredients.

PRECAUTIONS

General: Patients may experience a transient stinging or burning sensation following application of OPTICROM®. The recommended frequency of administration should not be exceeded (see **DOSAGE AND ADMINISTRATION**).
Information for Patients: Patients should be advised to follow the patient instructions listed on the Information for Patients sheet.
Users of contact lenses should refrain from wearing lenses while exhibiting the signs and symptoms of vernal keratoconjunctivitis, vernal conjunctivitis, or vernal keratitis. Do not wear contact lenses during treatment with OPTICROM®.
Carcinogenesis, Mutagenesis, and Impairment of Fertility: Long term studies of cromolyn sodium in mice (12 months intraperitoneal administration at doses up to 150 mg/kg three days per week), hamsters (intraperitoneal administration at doses up to 52.6 mg/kg three days per week for 15 weeks followed by 17.5 mg/kg three days per week for 37 weeks), and rats (18 months subcutaneous administration at doses up to 75 mg/kg six days per week) showed no neoplastic effects. The average daily maximum dose levels administered in these studies were 192.9 mg/m^2 for mice, 47.2 mg/m^2 for hamsters and 385.8 mg/m^2 for rats. These doses correspond to approximately 6.8, 1.7, and 14 times the maximum daily human dose of 28 mg/m^2.
Cromolyn sodium showed no mutagenic potential in the Ames *Salmonella*/microsome plate assays, mitotic gene conversion in *Saccharomyces cerevisiae* and in an *in vitro* cytogenetic study in human peripheral lymphocytes.
No evidence of impaired fertility was shown in laboratory reproduction studies conducted subcutaneously in rats at the highest doses tested, 175 mg/kg/day (1050 mg/m^2) in males and 100 mg/kg/day (600 mg/m^2) in females. These doses are approximately 37 and 21 times the maximum daily human dose, respectively, based on mg/m^2.
Pregnancy
Teratogenic Effects: Pregnancy Category B. Reproduction studies with cromolyn sodium administered subcutaneously to pregnant mice and rats at maximum daily doses of 540 mg/kg (1620 mg/m^2) and 164 mg/kg (984 mg/m^2), respectively, and intravenously to rabbits at a maximum daily dose of 485 mg/kg (5820 mg/m^2) produced no evidence of fetal malformation. These doses represent approximately 57, 35, and 205 times the maximum daily human dose, respectively, on a mg/m^2 basis. Adverse fetal effects (increased resorption and decreased fetal weight) were noted only at the very high parenteral doses that produced maternal toxicity. There are, however, no adequate and well-controlled studies in pregnant women. Because animal reproduction studies are not always predictive of human response, this drug should be used during pregnancy only if clearly needed.
Nursing Mothers: It is not known whether this drug is excreted in human milk. Because many drugs are excreted in human milk, caution should be exercised when OPTICROM® is administered to a nursing woman.
Pediatric Use: Safety and effectiveness in children below the age of 4 years have not been established.

ADVERSE REACTIONS

The most frequently reported adverse reaction attributed to the use of OPTICROM®, on the basis of reoccurrence following readministration, is transient ocular stinging or burning upon instillation.
The following adverse reactions have been reported as infrequent events. It is unclear whether they are attributed to the drug:
Conjunctival injection; watery eyes; itchy eyes; dryness around the eye; puffy eyes; eye irritation; and styes.
Immediate hypersensitivity reactions have been reported rarely and include dyspnea, edema, and rash.

DOSAGE AND ADMINISTRATION

The dose is 1–2 drops in each eye 4–6 times a day at regular intervals. One drop contains approximately 1.6 mg cromolyn sodium.
Patients should be advised that the effect of OPTICROM® therapy is dependent upon its administration at regular intervals, as directed.
Symptomatic response to therapy (decreased itching, tearing, redness, and discharge) is usually evident within a few days, but longer treatment for up to six weeks is sometimes required. Once symptomatic improvement has been established, therapy should be continued for as long as needed to sustain improvement. If required, corticosteroids may be used concomitantly with OPTICROM®.

HOW SUPPLIED

OPTICROM® (cromolyn sodium ophthalmic solution, USP) 4% is supplied as 10 mL of solution in an opaque polyethylene eye drop bottle.
10 mL **NDC** 0023-6422-10
Store at Controlled Room Temperature 20–25°C (68–77°F). Protect from light - store in original carton. Keep tightly closed and out of the reach of children.
Rx only
ALLERGAN

Revised February 1998
IN-F9541
70568 US 10D RX9419

POLYTRIM® ℞
(TRIMETHOPRIM SULFATE AND POLYMYXIN B SULFATE OPHTHALMIC SOLUTION) Sterile

DESCRIPTION

POLYTRIM® (trimethoprim sulfate and polymyxin B sulfate ophthalmic solution) is a sterile antimicrobial solution for topical ophthalmic use. It has pH of 4.0 to 6.2 and osmolality of 270 to 310 mOsm/kg.
Chemical Names: Trimethoprim sulfate, 2,4-Diamino-5-(3,4,5-trimethoxybenzyl)pyrimidine sulfate is a white, odorless, crystalline powder with a molecular weight of 678.72.
Polymyxin B sulfate is the sulfate salt of polymyxin B_1 and B_2 which are produced by the growth of *Bacillus polymyxa* (Prazmowski) Migula (Fam. Bacillaceae). It has a potency of not less than 6,000 polymyxin B units per mg, calculated on an anhydrous basis.
Contains: Actives: trimethoprim sulfate equivalent to 1 mg/mL; polymyxin B sulfate 10,000 units/mL. Preservative: benzalkonium chloride 0.04 mg/mL. Inactives: sodium chloride; sulfuric acid and purified water. May also contain sodium hydroxide for pH adjustment.

CLINICAL PHARMACOLOGY

Trimethoprim is a synthetic antibacterial drug active against a wide variety of aerobic gram-positive and gram-negative ophthalmic pathogens. Trimethoprim blocks the production of tetrahydrofolic acid from dihydrofolic acid by binding to and reversibly inhibiting the enzyme dihydrofolate reductase. This binding is stronger for the bacterial enzyme than for the corresponding mammalian enzyme and therefore selectively interferes with bacterial biosynthesis of nucleic acids and proteins.
Polymyxin B, a cyclic lipopeptide antibiotic, is bactericidal for a variety of gram-negative organisms, especially *Pseudomonas aeruginosa*. It increases the permeability of the bacterial cell membrane by interacting with the phospholipid components of the membrane.
Blood samples were obtained from 11 human volunteers at 20 minutes, 1 hour and 3 hours following instillation in the eye of 2 drops of ophthalmic solution containing 1 mg trimethoprim and 10,000 units polymyxin B per mL. Peak serum concentrations were approximately 0.03 µg/mL trimethoprim and 1 unit/mL polymyxin B.
Microbiology: *In vitro* studies have demonstrated that the anti-infective components of POLYTRIM® are active against the following bacterial pathogens that are capable of causing external infections of the eye:
Trimethoprim: *Staphylococcus aureus* and *Staphylococcus epidermidis, Streptococcus pyogenes, Streptococcus faecalis, Streptococcus pneumoniae, Haemophilus influenzae, Haemophilus aegyptius, Escherichia coli, Klebsiella pneumoniae, Proteus mirabilis* (indole-negative), *Proteus vulgaris* (indole-positive), *Enterobacter aerogenes,* and *Serratia marcescens.*
Polymyxin B: *Pseudomonas aeruginosa, Escherichia coli, Klebsiella pneumoniae, Enterobacter aerogenes* and *Haemophilus influenzae.*

INDICATIONS AND USAGE

POLYTRIM® Ophthalmic Solution is indicated in the treatment of surface ocular bacterial infections, including acute bacterial conjunctivitis, and blepharoconjunctivitis, caused by susceptible strains of the following microorganisms: *Staphylococcus aureus, Staphylococcus epidermidis, Streptococcus pneumoniae, Streptococcus viridans, Haemophilus influenzae* and *Pseudomonas aeruginosa.**

*Efficacy for this organism in this organ system was studied in fewer than 10 infections.

CONTRAINDICATIONS

POLYTRIM® Ophthalmic Solution is contraindicated in patients with known hypersensitivity to any of its components.

WARNINGS

NOT FOR INJECTION INTO THE EYE. If a sensitivity reaction to POLYTRIM® occurs, discontinue use. POLYTRIM® Ophthalmic Solution is not indicated for the prophylaxis or treatment of ophthalmia neonatorum.

PRECAUTIONS

General: As with other antimicrobial preparations, prolonged use may result in overgrowth of nonsusceptible organisms, including fungi. If superinfection occurs, appropriate therapy should be initiated.
Information for Patients: Avoid contaminating the applicator tip with material from the eye, fingers, or other source. This precaution is necessary if the sterility of the drops is to be maintained.
If redness, irritation, swelling or pain persists or increases, discontinue use immediately and contact your physician. Patients should be advised not to wear contact lenses if they have signs and symptoms of ocular bacterial infections.
Carcinogenesis, Mutagenesis, Impairment of Fertility:
Carcinogenesis: Long-term studies in animals to evaluate carcinogenic potential have not been conducted with polymyxin B sulfate or trimethoprim.
Mutagenesis: Trimethoprim was demonstrated to be non-mutagenic in the Ames assay. In studies at two laboratories no chromosomal damage was detected in cultured Chinese hamster ovary cells at concentrations approximately 500 times human plasma levels after oral administration; at concentrations approximately 1000 times human plasma levels after oral administration in these same cells, a low level of chromosomal damage was induced at one of the laboratories. Studies to evaluate mutagenic potential have not been conducted with polymyxin B sulfate.
Impairment of Fertility: Polymyxin B sulfate has been reported to impair the motility of equine sperm, but its effects on male or female fertility are unknown.
No adverse effects on fertility or general reproductive performance were observed in rats given trimethoprim in oral dosages as high as 70 mg/kg/day for males and 14 mg/kg/day for females.
Pregnancy: ***Teratogenic Effects:*** Pregnancy Category C. Animal reproduction studies have not been conducted with polymyxin B sulfate. It is not known whether polymyxin B sulfate can cause fetal harm when administered to a pregnant woman or can affect reproduction capacity.
Trimethoprim has been shown to be teratogenic in the rat when given in oral doses 40 times the human dose. In some rabbit studies, the overall increase in fetal loss (dead and resorbed and malformed conceptuses) was associated with oral doses 6 times the human therapeutic dose.
While there are no large well-controlled studies on the use of trimethoprim in pregnant women, Brumfitt and Pursell, in a retrospective study, reported the outcome of 186 pregnancies during which the mother received either placebo or oral trimethoprim in combination with sulfamethoxazole. The incidence of congenital abnormalities was 4.5% (3 of 66) in those who received placebo and 3.3% (4 of 120) in those receiving trimethoprim and sulfamethoxazole. There were no abnormalities in the 10 children whose mothers received the drug during the first trimester. In a separate survey, Brumfitt and Pursell also found no congenital abnormalities in 35 children whose mothers had received oral trimethoprim and sulfamethoxazole at the time of conception or shortly thereafter.
Because trimethoprim may interfere with folic acid metabolism, trimethoprim should be used during pregnancy only if the potential benefit justifies the potential risk to the fetus.
Nonteratogenic Effects: The oral administration of trimethoprim to rats at a dose of 70 mg/kg/day commencing with the last third of gestation and continuing through parturition and lactation caused no deleterious effects on gestation or pup growth and survival.
Nursing mothers: It is not known whether this drug is excreted in human milk. Because many drugs are excreted

Continued on next page

Polytrim—Cont.

in human milk, caution should be exercised when POLYTRIM® Ophthalmic Solution is administered to a nursing woman.

Pediatric Use: Safety and effectiveness in children below the age of 2 months have not been established (see WARNINGS).

ADVERSE REACTIONS

The most frequent adverse reaction to POLYTRIM® Ophthalmic Solution is local irritation consisting of increased redness, burning, stinging, and/or itching. This may occur on instillation, within 48 hours, or at any time with extended use. There are also multiple reports of hypersensitivity reactions consisting of lid edema, itching, increased redness, tearing, and/or circumocular rash. Photosensitivity has been reported in patients taking oral trimethoprim.

DOSAGE AND ADMINISTRATION

In mild to moderate infections, instill one drop in the affected eye(s) every three hours (maximum of 6 doses per day) for a period of 7 to 10 days.

HOW SUPPLIED

A sterile ophthalmic solution, each mL contains trimethoprim sulfate equivalent to 1 mg trimethoprim and polymyxin B sulfate 10,000 units in a plastic dropper bottle of 10 mL (NDC 0023-7824-10). 5 mL (NDC 0023-7824-05).

Note: Store at 15°–25°C (59°–77°F) and protect from light.

Rx only

TAZORAC® ℞

[tăz ō răc]

(tazarotene topical gel) 0.05%
(tazarotene topical gel) 0.1%

FOR DERMATOLOGIC USE ONLY
NOT FOR OPHTHALMIC USE

DESCRIPTION

TAZORAC® is a translucent, aqueous gel and contains the compound tazarotene, a member of the acetylenic class of retinoids. It is for topical dermatologic use only. The active ingredient is represented by the following structural formula:

OCH$_2$CH$_3$

TAZAROTENE

$C_{21}H_{21}NO_2S$

Molecular Weight: **351.46**

Chemical Name: ethyl 6-[2-(4,4-dimethylthiochroman-6-yl)-ethynyl] nicotinate

Contains:

Active: Tazarotene .... 0.05% or 0.1% (w/w)

Preservative: Benzyl alcohol .... 1.0% (w/w)

Inactives: Ascorbic acid, butylated hydroxyanisole, butylated hydroxytoluene, carbomer 934P, edetate disodium, hexylene glycol, purified water, poloxamer 407, polyethylene glycol 400, polysorbate 40, and tromethamine.

CLINICAL PHARMACOLOGY

Tazarotene is a retinoid prodrug which is converted to its active form, the cognate carboxylic acid of tazarotene (AGN 190299), by rapid deesterification in most biological systems. AGN 190299 binds to all three members of the retinoic acid receptor (RAR) family: RARα, RARβ, and RARγ, but shows relative selectivity for RARβ, and RARγ and may modify gene expression. The clinical significance of these findings is unknown.

Psoriasis: The mechanism of tazarotene action in psoriasis is not defined. Topical tazarotene blocks induction of mouse epidermal ornithine decarboxylase (ODC) activity, which is associated with cell proliferation and hyperplasia. In cell culture and *in vitro* models of skin, tazarotene suppresses expression of MRP8, a marker of inflammation present in the epidermis of psoriasis subjects at high levels. In human keratinocyte cultures, it inhibits cornified envelope formation, whose build-up is an element of the psoriatic scale. The clinical significance of these findings is unknown.

Acne: The mechanism of tazarotene action in acne is not defined. Tazarotene inhibited corneocyte accumulation in rhino mouse skin and cross-linked envelope formation in cultured human keratinocytes. The clinical significance of these findings is unknown.

Pharmacokinetics:

Following topical application, tazarotene undergoes esterase hydrolysis to form its active metabolite, AGN 190299. Little parent compound could be detected in the plasma. AGN 190299 was highly bound to plasma proteins (>99%). Tazarotene and AGN 190299 were metabolized to sulfoxides, sulfones and other polar metabolites which were eliminated through urinary and fecal pathways. The half-life of AGN 190299 following topical application of tazarotene was similar in normal and psoriatic subjects, approximately 18 hours.

Plaque Elevation, Scaling and Erythema in Two Controlled Clinical Trials for Psoriasis

		TAZORAC® 0.05% Gel				TAZORAC® 0.1% Gel				Vehicle Gel			
		Trunk/Arm/ Leg lesions		Knee/Elbow lesions		Trunk/Arm/ Leg lesions		Knee/Elbow lesions		Trunk/Arm/ Leg lesions		Knee/Elbow lesions	
		N=108	N=111	N=108	N=111	N=108	N=112	N=108	N=112	N=108	N=113	N=108	N=113
Plaque elevation	B* C-12* C-24*	2.5 -1.4 -1.2	2.6 -1.3	2.6 -1.3 -1.1	2.6 -1.1	2.5 -1.4 -1.1	2.6 -1.4	2.6 -1.5 -1.0	2.6 -1.3	2.4 -0.8 -0.9	2.6 -0.7	2.6 -0.7 -0.7	2.6 -0.6
Scaling	B* C-12* C-24*	2.4 -1.1 -0.9	2.5 -1.1	2.5 -1.1 -0.8	2.6 -0.9	2.4 -1.3 -1.0	2.6 -1.3	2.5 -1.2 -0.8	2.7 -1.2	2.4 -0.7 -0.8	2.6 -0.7	2.5 -0.6 -0.7	2.7 -0.6
Erythema	B* C-12* C-24*	2.4 -1.0 -1.1	2.7 -0.8	2.2 -0.9 -0.7	2.5 -0.8	2.4 -1.0 -0.9	2.8 -1.1	2.3 -1.0 -0.8	2.5 -0.8	2.3 -0.6 -0.7	2.7 -0.5	2.2 -0.5 -0.6	2.5 -0.5

Plaque elevation, scaling and erythema scored on a 0-4 scale with 0=none, 1=mild, 2=moderate, 3=severe and 4=very severe.

*B=Mean Baseline Severity: C-12=Mean Change from Baseline at end of 12 weeks of therapy: C-24=Mean Change from Baseline at week 24 (12 weeks after the end of therapy).

Global improvement over baseline at the end of 12 weeks of treatment in these two studies is shown in the following table:

	TAZORAC® 0.05% Gel		TAZORAC® 0.1% Gel		Vehicle Gel	
	N=81	N=93	N=79	N=69	N=84	N=91
100% improvement	2 (2%)	1 (1%)	0	0	1 (1%)	0
≥75% improvement	23 (28%)	17 (18%)	30 (38%)	17 (25%)	10 (12%)	9 (10%)
≥50% improvement	42 (52%)	39 (42%)	51 (65%)	36 (52%)	28 (33%)	21 (23%)
1-49% improvement	21 (26%)	32 (34%)	18 (23%)	23 (33%)	27 (32%)	32 (35%)
No change or worse	18 (22%)	22 (24%)	10 (13%)	10 (14%)	29 (35%)	38 (42%)

Reduction in Lesion Counts after 12 Weeks of Treatment in Two Controlled Clinical Trials for Acne

	TAZORAC® 0.1% Gel		Vehicle Gel	
	N=150	N=149	N=148	N=149
Noninflammatory lesions	55%	43%	35%	27%
Inflammatory lesions	42%	47%	30%	28%
Total lesions	52%	45%	33%	27%

The human *in vivo* studies described below were conducted with tazarotene gel applied topically at approximately 2 mg/cm^2 and left on the skin for 10 to 12 hours. Both the peak plasma concentration (Cmax) and area under the plasma concentration time curve (AUC) refer to the active metabolite only.

Two single, topical dose studies were conducted using ^{14}C-tazarotene gel. Systemic absorption, as determined from radioactivity in the excreta, was less than 1% of the applied dose (without occlusion) in six psoriatic patients and approximately 5% of the applied dose (under occlusion) in six healthy subjects. One non-radiolabeled single-dose study comparing the 0.05% gel to the 0.1% gel in healthy subjects indicated that the Cmax and AUC were 40% higher for the 0.1% gel.

After 7 days of topical dosing with measured doses of tazarotene 0.1% gel on 20% of the total body surface without occlusion in 24 healthy subjects, the Cmax was 0.72 ± 0.58 ng/mL (mean ± SD) occurring 9 hours after the last dose, and the AUC_{0-24hr} was 10.1 ± 7.2 ng·hr/mL. Systemic absorption was 0.91 ± 0.67% of the applied dose.

In a 14-day study in five psoriatic patients, measured doses of tazarotene 0.1% gel were applied daily by nursing staff to involved skin without occlusion (8 to 18% of total body surface area; mean ± SD: 13 ± 5%). The Cmax was 12.0 ± 7.6 ng/mL occurring 6 hours after the final dose, and the AUC_{0-24hr} was 105 ± 55 ng·hr/mL. Systemic absorption was 14.8 ± 7.6% of the applied dose. Extrapolation of these results to represent dosing on 20% of total body surface yielded estimates of Cmax of 18.9 ± 10.6 ng/mL and AUC_{0-24hr} of 172 ± 88 ng·hr/mL.

An *in vitro* percutaneous absorption study, using radiolabeled drug and freshly excised human skin or human cadaver skin, indicated that approximately 4 to 5% of the applied dose was in the stratum corneum (tazarotene: AGN 190299 = 5:1) and 2 to 4% was in the viable epidermis-dermis layer (tazarotene: AGN 190299 = 2:1) 24 hours after topical application of the gel.

Clinical Studies:

Psoriasis:

In two large vehicle-controlled clinical studies, tazarotene 0.05% and 0.1% gels applied once daily for 12 weeks were significantly more effective than vehicle in reducing the severity of the clinical signs of stable plaque psoriasis covering up to 20% of body surface area. In one of the studies, patients were followed up for an additional 12 weeks following cessation of therapy with TAZORAC®. Mean baseline scores and changes from baseline (reductions) after treatment in these two studies are shown in the following table:

[See first table above]
[See second table above]

The 0.1% gel was more effective than the 0.05% gel, but the 0.05% gel was associated with less local irritation than the 0.1% gel (see ADVERSE REACTIONS section).

Acne:

In two large vehicle-controlled studies, tazarotene 0.1% gel applied once daily was significantly more effective than vehicle in the treatment of facial acne vulgaris of mild to moderate severity. Percent reductions in lesion counts after treatment for 12 weeks in these two studies are shown in the following table:

[See third table above]
[See table at top of next page]

INDICATIONS AND USAGE

TAZORAC® (tazarotene topical gel) 0.05% and 0.1% are indicated for the topical treatment of patients with stable plaque psoriasis of up to 20% body surface area involvement.

TAZORAC® (tazarotene topical gel) 0.1% is also indicated for the topical treatment of patients with facial acne vulgaris of mild to moderate severity.

The efficacy of TAZORAC® in the treatment of acne previously treated with other retinoids or resistant to oral antibiotics has not been established.

CONTRAINDICATIONS

Retinoids may cause fetal harm when administered to a pregnant woman.

In rats, tazarotene 0.05%, administered **topically** during gestation days 6 through 17 at 0.25 mg/kg/day (1.5 mg/m^2/day) resulted in reduced fetal body weights and reduced skeletal ossification. Rabbits dosed **topically** with 0.25 mg/kg/day (2.75 mg/m^2 total body surface area/day) tazarotene during gestation days 6 through 18 were noted with single incidences of known retinoid malformations, including spina bifida, hydrocephaly, and heart anomalies. As with other retinoids, when tazarotene was given **orally** to experimental animals, developmental delays were seen in rats, and teratogenic effects and post-implantation fetal loss were seen in rats and rabbits at doses producing 0.7 and 13

Global improvement over baseline at the end of 12 weeks of treatment in these two studies is shown in the following table:

	TAZORAC® 0.1% Gel		Vehicle Gel	
	N=105	N=117	N=117	N=110
100% improvement	1 (1%)	0	0	0
≥75% improvement	40 (38%)	21 (18%)	23 (20%)	11 (10%)
≥50% improvement	71 (68%)	56 (48%)	47 (40%)	32 (29%)
1-49% improvement	23 (22%)	49 (42%)	48 (41%)	46 (42%)
No change or worse	11 (10%)	12 (10%)	22 (19%)	32 (29%)

times, respectively, the systemic exposure (AUC_{0-24hr}) in human psoriasis patients, when extrapolated for **topical** treatment of 20% of body surface area. THUS, SYSTEMIC EXPOSURE IN TOPICALLY TREATED PSORIASIS PATIENTS (FOR USE ON UP TO 20% OF BODY SURFACE AREA) COULD BE IN THE SAME ORDER OF MAGNITUDE AS IN THESE ORALLY TREATED ANIMALS.

Systemic exposure anticipated in the treatment of facial acne may be less, due to a more limited area of application.

Six women inadvertently exposed to TAZORAC® during pregnancy in clinical trials have subsequently delivered healthy babies. As the exact timing and extent of exposure in relation to the gestation time are not certain, the significance of these findings is not known.

TAZORAC® is contraindicated in women who are or may become pregnant. If this drug is used during pregnancy, or if the patient becomes pregnant while taking this drug, treatment should be discontinued and the patient apprised of the potential hazard to the fetus. Women of childbearing potential should be warned of the potential risk and use adequate birth-control measures when TAZORAC® is used. The possibility that a woman of childbearing potential is pregnant at the time of institution of therapy should be considered. A negative result for pregnancy test having a sensitivity down to at least 50 mIU/mL for human chorionic gonadotropin (hCG) should be obtained within 2 weeks prior to TAZORAC® therapy, which should begin during a normal menstrual period.

TAZORAC® is contraindicated in individuals who have shown hypersensitivity to any of its components.

WARNINGS

Pregnancy Category X: See CONTRAINDICATIONS section. Women of childbearing potential should be warned of the potential risk and use adequate birth-control measures when TAZORAC® is used. The possibility that a woman of childbearing potential is pregnant at the time of institution of therapy should be considered. A negative result for pregnancy test having a sensitivity down to at least 50 mIU/mL for hCG should be obtained within 2 weeks prior to TAZORAC® therapy, which should begin during a normal menstrual period.

PRECAUTIONS

General: TAZORAC® should only be applied to the affected areas. For external use only. Avoid contact with eyes, eyelids, and mouth. If contact with eyes occurs, rinse thoroughly with water. The safety of use over more than 20% of body surface area has not been established in psoriasis or acne.

Retinoids should not be used on eczematous skin, as they may cause severe irritation.

Because of heightened burning susceptibility, exposure to sunlight (including sunlamps) should be avoided unless deemed medically necessary, and in such cases, exposure should be minimized during the use of TAZORAC®. Patients must be warned to use sunscreens (minimum SPF of 15) and protective clothing when using TAZORAC®. Patients with sunburn should be advised not to use TAZORAC® until fully recovered. Patients who may have considerable sun exposure due to their occupation and those patients with inherent sensitivity to sunlight should exercise particular caution when using TAZORAC® and ensure that the precautions outlined in the Information for Patients subsection are observed.

TAZORAC® should be administered with caution if the patient is also taking drugs known to be photosensitizers (e.g., thiazides, tetracyclines, fluoroquinolones, phenothiazines, sulfonamides) because of the increased possibility of augmented photosensitivity.

If pruritus, burning, skin redness or peeling is excessive, the medication should be discontinued until the integrity of the skin is restored.

Weather extremes, such as wind or cold, may be more irritating to patients using TAZORAC®.

Information for Patients: See attached Patient Package Insert.

Drug Interactions: Concomitant dermatologic medications and cosmetics that have a strong drying effect should be avoided. It is also advisable to "rest" a patient's skin until the effects of such preparations subside before use of TAZORAC® is begun.

Carcinogenesis, mutagenesis, impairment of fertility: Long-term studies of tazarotene following oral administration of 0.025, 0.050, and 0.125 mg/kg/day to rats showed no indications of increased carcinogenic risks. However, in other rat studies, oral doses twice that of the highest dose in the rat carcinogenicity study produced an AUC_{0-24hr} that was less (0.7 times) than that in topically treated psoriatic patients extrapolated for treatment of 20% of body surface area. In evaluation of photocarcinogenicity, median time to onset of tumors was decreased and the number of tumors increased in hairless mice following chronic topical dosing with intercurrent exposure to ultraviolet radiation at tazarotene concentrations of 0.001%, 0.005%, and 0.01% for up to 40 weeks.

A long-term topical application study in mice terminated at 88 weeks showed that dose levels of 0.05, 0.125, 0.25 and 1.0 mg/kg/day (reduced to 0.5 mg/kg/day for males after 41 weeks due to severe dermal irritation) revealed no apparent carcinogenic effects when compared to vehicle control animals; untreated control animals were not completely evaluated. The AUC_{0-12hr}'s for these doses were 82.7, 137, 183, 136 (males at 1.0/0.5 mg/kg) and 344 ng·hr/mL (females at 1.0 mg/kg), respectively. The mean AUC_{0-24hr} for psoriatic patients was 172 ng·hr/mL, extrapolated for 20% total body surface area.

Tazarotene was found to be non-mutagenic in the Ames assay and did not produce structural chromosomal aberrations in a human lymphocyte assay. Tazarotene was also non-mutagenic in the CHO/HPRT mammalian cell forward gene mutation assay and was non-clastogenic in the *in vivo* mouse micronucleus test.

No impairment of fertility occurred in rats when male animals were treated for 70 days prior to mating and female animals were treated for 14 days prior to mating and continuing through gestation and lactation with topical doses of TAZORAC® gel of up to 0.125 mg/kg/day (0.738 mg/m^2/day).

Reproductive capabilities of F1 animals, including F2 survival and development, were not affected by topical administration of TAZORAC® gel to female F0 parental rats from gestation day 16 through lactation day 20 at the maximum tolerated dose of 0.125 mg/kg/day (0.738 mg/m^2/day).

Pregnancy: Teratogenic Effects: Pregnancy Category X: See CONTRAINDICATIONS section. Women of childbearing potential should use adequate birth-control measures when TAZORAC® is used. The possibility that a woman of childbearing potential is pregnant at the time of institution of therapy should be considered. A negative result for pregnancy test having a sensitivity down to at least 50 mIU/mL for hCG should be obtained within 2 weeks prior to TAZORAC® therapy, which should begin during a normal menstrual period.

Nursing Mothers: After single topical doses of ^{14}C-tazarotene to the skin of lactating rats, secretion of radioactivity was detected in milk, suggesting that there would be transfer of drug-related material to the offspring via milk. It is not known whether this drug is excreted in human milk. Caution should be exercised when tazarotene is administered to a nursing woman.

Pediatric Use: The safety and efficacy of tazarotene have not been established in pediatric patients under the age of 12 years.

ADVERSE REACTIONS

Psoriasis:

The most frequent adverse events reported with TAZORAC® 0.05% and 0.1% gels were limited to the skin. Those occurring in 10 to 30% of patients, in descending order, included pruritus, burning/stinging, erythema, worsening of psoriasis, irritation, and skin pain. Events occurring in 1 to 10% of patients included rash, desquamation, irritant contact dermatitis, skin inflammation, fissuring, bleeding and dry skin. Increases in "psoriasis worsening" and "sun-induced erythema" were noted in some patients over the 4th to 12th months as compared to the first three months of a 1 year study. In general, the incidence of adverse events with TAZORAC® 0.05% gel was 2 to 5% lower than that seen with TAZORAC® 0.1% gel.

Acne:

The most frequent adverse events reported with TAZORAC® 0.1% gel were limited to the skin. Those events occurring in 10 to 30% of patients, in descending order, included desquamation, burning/stinging, dry skin, erythema and pruritus. Events occurring in 1 to 10% of patients included irritation, skin pain, fissuring, localized edema and skin discoloration.

In human dermal safety studies, tazarotene 0.05% and 0.1% gels did not induce contact sensitization, phototoxicity or photoallergy.

OVERDOSAGE

Excessive topical use of TAZORAC® may lead to marked redness, peeling, or discomfort (see PRECAUTIONS).

TAZORAC® is not for oral use. Oral ingestion of the drug may lead to the same adverse effects as those associated with excessive oral intake of Vitamin A (hypervitaminosis A) or other retinoids. If oral ingestion occurs, the patient should be monitored, and appropriate supportive measures should be administered as necessary.

DOSAGE AND ADMINISTRATION

General: Application may cause a transitory feeling of burning or stinging. If irritation is excessive, application should be discontinued.

For psoriasis: Apply TAZORAC® once a day, in the evening, to psoriatic lesions, using enough (2 mg/cm^2) to cover only the lesion with a thin film to no more than 20% of body surface area. If a bath or shower is taken prior to application, the skin should be dry before applying the gel. Because unaffected skin may be more susceptible to irritation, application of tazarotene to these areas should be carefully avoided. TAZORAC® was investigated for up to 12 months during clinical trials for psoriasis.

For acne: Cleanse the face gently. After the skin is dry, apply a thin film of TAZORAC® (2 mg/cm^2) once a day, in the evening, to the skin where acne lesions appear. Use enough to cover the entire affected area. TAZORAC® was investigated for up to 12 weeks during clinical trials for acne.

HOW SUPPLIED

TAZORAC® (tazarotene topical gel) is available in concentrations of 0.05% and 0.1%. It comes in collapsible aluminum tubes, in 30 gm and 100 gm sizes.

	TAZORAC® Gel 0.05%	TAZORAC® Gel 0.1%
30 mg	NDC 0023-8335-03	NDC 0023-0042-03
100 mg	NDC 0023-8335-10	NDC 0023-0042-10

NOTE: TAZORAC® gel should be stored at 25°C (77°F): excursion permitted to 15–30°C (59–86°F).

Rx only

ALLERGAN
Irvine, California 92612, USA December 1998

70967 US 12 D

Alpha Therapeutic Corporation

5555 VALLEY BLVD.
LOS ANGELES, CA 90032

Direct Inquiries to:
CONTACTS:
Medical Director: (323) 227-7077
Professional Services: (800) 292-6118
After Hours Emergency Orders: (800) 421-0008
Direct Inquiries: (323) 225-2221
Customer Service: (800) 421-0008
Fax: (323) 227-7027

ALBUTEIN® 5% ℞
Albumin (Human), USP, 5% Solution

10 bottles per case.
250mL bottle & IV set NDC 49669-5211-1
500mL bottle & IV set NDC 49669-5211-2

ALBUTEIN® 25% ℞
Albumin (Human), USP, 25% Solution

10 bottles per case.
50mL bottle & IV set NDC 49669-5213-2
100mL bottle & IV set NDC 49669-5213-3

ALPHANATE® ℞
Antihemophilic Factor, (Human)
Solvent Detergent/Heat Treated

DESCRIPTION

Alphanate® Antihemophilic Factor (Human) Solvent Detergent/Heat Treated is a highly purified Factor VIII product for the treatment of Hemophilia A and acquired Factor VIII deficiency. It is intended for intravenous administration. The product is purified by column chromatography and utilizes a solvent detergent treatment and heat treatment for viral inactivation.

HOW SUPPLIED

The product is available in the following potencies:

Factor VIII Activity	Diluent	NDC Number
250 i.u.	5 mL	49669-4600-01
500 i.u.	5 mL	49669-4600-01
1000 i.u.	10 mL	49669-4600-02
1500 i.u.	10 mL	49669-4600-02

Each carton contains a single dose vial of concentrate, sterile water for injection, a double ended transfer needle and microaggragate filter, and a package insert with full prescribing information. 12 vials per case.

Continued on next page

ALPHANINE® SD ℞
Coagulation Factor IX (Human)
Solvent Detergent Treated/Virus Filtered

DESCRIPTION
AlphaNine® SD, Coagulation Factor IX (Human) is a highly purified Factor IX product for the treatment of Hemophilia B. It is intended for intravenous administration. The product is purified by a dual affinity column process and includes both solvent detergent treatment and virus filtration for added safeguards.

HOW SUPPLIED
The product is available in the following potencies:

Factor IX Activity	Diluent	NDC Number
500 IU	10 mL	49669-3600-02
1000 IU	10 mL	49669-3600-02
1500 IU	10 mL	49669-3600-02

Each carton contains a single dose vial of concentrate, sterile water for injection, a double-ended transfer needle, microaggregate filter, and a package insert with full prescribing information. 12 vials per case.

PROFILNINE® SD ℞
Factor IX Complex
Solvent Detergent Treated

DESCRIPTION
Profilnine® SD, Factor IX Complex, Solvent Detergent Treated is a lyophilized concentrate containing factors II, IX, and X plus low levels of factor VII. The product is available in single dose vials of Factor IX for the treatment of Hemophilia B (Factor IX deficiency).

HOW SUPPLIED
The product is available in the following potencies:

Factor IX Activity	Diluent	NDC Number
500 i.u.	5 mL	49669-3200-02
1000 i.u.	10 mL	49669-3200-03
1500 i.u.	10 mL	49669-3200-03

Each individual carton contains a single dose vial of Factor IX, sterile water for injection, transfer needle, microaggregate filter, and a package insert with full prescribing information. 12 vials per case.

VENOGLOBULIN®–S 5% Solution ℞
Immune Globulin Intravenous (Human)
SOLVENT DETERGENT TREATED

Venoglobulin®-S 5% Solution, Solvent Detergent Treated is a sterile, highly purified solution of intact, unmodified human immunoglobulin G intended for intravenous use. IgG is isolated from large pools of human plasma using the Cohn-Oncley cold alcohol fractionation process, followed by polyethylene glycol fractionation and ion exchange chromatography. The manufacturing process includes treatment with a mixture of tri-n-butyl phosphate (TNBP) and polysorbate 80.
The process used to produce Venoglobulin®-S inactivates and/or partitions up to 13 cumulative logs of Human Immunodeficiency Virus Type 1 (HIV-1) based on *in vitro* studies. Additional solvent-detergent treatment further removes greater than 10 logs of HIV-1 and greater than 6 logs of HIV-2 as demonstrated *in vitro,* thereby providing an extra measure of safety.
Venoglobulin®-S contains all IgG antibody activities present in the donor population. The distribution of IgG subclasses corresponds to that of normal human plasma. Gamma globulin is isolated without additional chemical or enzymatic modification and the Fc portion of the molecule is maintained functionally intact. Typically IgG purity exceeds 99%.
The composition of Venoglobulin®-S is as follows:

Component	Quantity/mL
Human immunoglobulin G	50 mg
D-sorbitol	50 mg
Albumin (Human)	<1.3 mg
Polyethylene glycol	<100 mcg
Polysorbate 80	<100 mcg
Tri-n-butyl phosphate	< 10 mcg

This formulation contains no preservatives. The pH of the solution ranges from 5.2 to 5.8. The osmolarity is approximately 300 mOsm/L.

HOW SUPPLIED

Vial size	Grams of IgG	NDC Number
50 mL	2.5 g	49669-1612-1
100 mL	5.0 g	49669-1613-1
200 mL	10.0 g	49669-1614-1

All sizes are packaged with a sterile I.V. administration set. 10 vials per case. Store at or below 25°C or 77°F. Do not freeze.

VENOGLOBULIN®-S 10% Solution ℞
Immune Globulin Intravenous (Human)
SOLVENT DETERGENT TREATED

DESCRIPTION
Venoglobulin®-S 10% Solution, Solvent Detergent Treated is a sterile, highly purified solution of intact, unmodified human immunoglobulin G intended for intravenous use. IgG is isolated from large pools of human plasma using the Cohn-Oncley cold alcohol fractionation process, followed by polyethylene glycol fractionation and ion exchange chromatography. The manufacturing process also includes a solvent detergent viral inactivation step.
The composition of Venoglobulin-S 10% is as follows:

Component	Quantity/mL
Human immunoglobulin G	100 mg
D-sorbitol	50 mg
Albumin (Human)	≤2.6 mg
Polyethylene glycol	≤200 mcg
Polysorbate 80	≤200 mcg
Tri-n-butyl phosphate	≤20 mcg

This formulation contains no preservatives. The pH of the solution ranges from 5.2 to 5.8. The osmolarity is approximately 330 mOsm/L.

HOW SUPPLIED

Vial size	Grams of IgG	NDC Number
50 mL	5.0 g	49669-1622-1
100 mL	10.0 g	49669-1623-1
200 mL	20.0 g	49669-1624-1

All sizes are packaged with a sterile IV administration set. 10 vials per case. Store at 2–8°C (36–46°F). Do not freeze. Warm to room temperature before infusion.

EDUCATIONAL MATERIAL

Scientific publications, monographs, product literature, brochures and formulary kits available upon request.

Alpharma®
U.S. Pharmaceuticals Division
7205 WINDSOR BLVD.
BALTIMORE, MD 21244

For General Inquiries Contact:
Customer Service
(800) 638–9096

LINDANE LOTION USP 1% ℞

DESCRIPTION
Lindane Lotion USP, 1% is an ectoparasiticide and ovicide effective against *Sarcoptes scabiei* (scabies). In addition to the active ingredient, lindane, it contains glycerol monostearate, cetyl alcohol, stearic acid, trolamine, carrageenan, 2-amino-2-methyl-1-propanol, methylparaben, butylparaben, perfume and water to form a non-greasy lotion. Lindane, which is the highly purified gamma isomer of 1, 2, 3, 4, 5, 6, hexachlorocyclohexane, has the following structural formula:

$C_6H_6Cl_6$ 290.83

CLINICAL PHARMACOLOGY
Lindane exerts its parasiticidal action by being directly absorbed into the parasites and their ova. Feldmann and Maibach[1] reported approximately 10% absorption of a lindane acetone solution applied to the forearm and left in place for 24 hours. Dale, et al[2], reported a blood level of 290 ng/mL associated with convulsions following the accidental ingestion of a lindane-containing product. Ginsburg[3] found a mean peak blood level of 28 ng/mL 6 hours after total body application of lindane lotion to scabietic infants and children. The half-life was determined to be 18 hours.

INDICATIONS AND USAGE
Because post-treatment pruritus is common and may lead to misuse, lindane lotion is indicated only for the treatment of patients infested with *Sarcoptes scabiei* (scabies) who have either failed to respond to adequate doses, or are intolerant of, other approved therapies. Reinfestation should be considered carefully before attributing the posttreatment presence of ectoparasites to a failure of response to adequate doses of other approved therapies.

CONTRAINDICATIONS
Lindane lotion is contraindicated for premature neonates because their skin may be more permeable than full term infants and their liver enzymes may not be sufficiently developed. It is also contraindicated for patients with Norwegian (crusted) scabies due to possible increased absorption. It is also contraindicated for patients with known seizure disorders and for individuals with a known sensitivity to the product or any of its components.

WARNINGS
LINDANE PENETRATES HUMAN SKIN AND HAS THE POTENTIAL FOR CNS TOXICITY (SEE CLINICAL PHARMACOLOGY SECTION). LINDANE LOTION SHOULD BE USED ACCORDING TO RECOMMENDED DOSAGE (SEE DIRECTIONS FOR USE) ESPECIALLY ON INFANTS, PREGNANT WOMEN AND NURSING MOTHERS. ANIMAL STUDIES INDICATE THAT POTENTIAL TOXIC EFFECTS OF TOPICALLY APPLIED LINDANE ARE GREATER IN THE YOUNG. SEIZURES AND, IN RARE INSTANCES, DEATHS HAVE BEEN REPORTED AFTER EXCESS DOSAGE, OVER-EXPOSURE, FREQUENT REAPPLICATIONS, AND ACCIDENTAL AND INTENTIONAL INGESTION OF LINDANE. THESE INSTANCES OF PATIENT MISUSE HAVE BEEN ASSOCIATED WITH LACK OF PATIENT UNDERSTANDING OF DIRECTIONS OF USE, PRESCRIBING OR DISPENSING EXCESSIVE QUANTITIES, AND IMPROPER REAPPLICATIONS. IN EXCEEDINGLY RARE CASES SEIZURES HAVE BEEN REPORTED WHEN USED ACCORDING TO DIRECTIONS. NO RESIDUAL EFFECTS OF LINDANE TREATMENT HAS BEEN DEMONSTRATED; THEREFORE, THIS PRODUCT SHOULD NOT BE USED TO WARD OFF A POSSIBLE INFESTATION. If accidental ingestion occurs, prompt gastric lavage is indicated. Because oils may enhance absorption, saline rather than oily cathartics should be used. Central nervous excitation can be controlled by the administration of pentobarbital, phenobarbital or diazepam.

PRECAUTIONS
General: Care should be taken to avoid contact with the eyes. If such contact occurs, eyes should be immediately flushed with water. If irritation or sensitization occurs, the patient should be advised to consult a physician.
Geriatric: Dosage may have to be reduced due to the possibility of increased absorption through elderly skin.
Information for Patients: Patients must be instructed on the proper use of the medication, especially as to amount applied and duration of use. Patient's Directions for Use must accompany the product.
Laboratory Tests: No laboratory tests are needed for the proper use of this medication.
Drug Interactions: Oils may enhance absorption; therefore, simultaneous use of creams, ointments or oils should be avoided.
Carcinogenesis: Although no studies have been conducted with lindane lotion, numerous long-term feeding studies have been conducted in mice and rats to evaluate the carcinogenic potential of the technical grade of hexachlorocyclohexane (BHC) as well as the alpha, beta, gamma (lindane) and delta isomers. Both oral and topical applications have been evaluated. Nagasaki[4], Goto[5] and Hanada[6] found varying amounts of benign and malignant hepatomas associated with BHC and the alpha, delta and epsilon isomers. None reported a carcinogenic potential for lindane. Tumors were found only in the animals which had received the alpha isomer. Weisse and Herbst[7] also evaluated the carcinogenic potential of lindane in mice but could find no evidence of lindane carcinogenicity. The National Cancer Institute[8] also found no evidence of carcinogenicity.
Thorpe and Walker[9] compared beta BHC with lindane, dieldrin, DDT and hexabarbital in mice. Despite the unusually high incidence of tumors in the control group, they concluded that 600 ppm of lindane was associated with a significant increase in the incidence of hepatoma and thus, considered it a tumorigen.
Orr[10] and Kashyap, et al[11], evaluated the carcinogenic potential in mice of topically applied BHC. In neither study was there any evidence of a tumorigenic or carcinogenic potential associated with topical application of BHC.
Mutagenicity tests have been used as predictive information about the carcinogenicity of various chemical compounds. Numerous types of mutagenicity tests have been performed with lindane. The results of these tests do not indicate that lindane is mutagenic.
Pregnancy: *Teratogenic Effects*-Pregnancy Category B. Reproduction, including multigeneration studies have been

performed in mice, rats, rabbits, pigs, and dogs at doses up to 10 times the human dose and have revealed no evidence of impaired fertility or harm to the fetus due to orally administered lindane. There are, however, no adequate and well-controlled studies in pregnant women. Because animal reproduction studies are not always predictive of human response, the recommended dosage should not be exceeded on pregnant women. They should be treated no more than twice during a pregnancy.

Nursing Mothers: Lindane is secreted in human milk in low concentrations. Studies conducted in the United States as well as in Europe and South America found levels of lindane in human milk ranging from 0 to 113 ppb, as the result of ingestion of foods which had been treated with lindane. There appeared to be no difference in concentrations between country and urban dwellers. Although the levels of lindane found in blood after topical application with lindane lotion make it unlikely that amounts of lindane sufficient to cause serious adverse reactions will be excreted in the milk of nursing mothers who have used lindane lotion, if there is any concern, an alternate method of feeding may be used for 4 days.

Pediatric Use: Refer to the CONTRAINDICATIONS and WARNINGS sections.

ADVERSE REACTIONS

Lindane has been reported to cause central nervous stimulation ranging from dizziness to convulsions. Cases of convulsions have been reported in connection with lindane lotion therapy. However, these incidents were almost always associated with accidental oral ingestion or misuse of the product. In exceedingly rare cases, seizures have been reported when used according to directions. Eczematous eruptions due to irritation from this product have also been reported. Incidence of these adverse reactions is relatively infrequent, occurring in less than 1 in 100,000 patients.

DRUG ABUSE AND DEPENDENCE

Lindane lotion is not subject to abuse, nor is there any dependence on the drug.

OVERDOSAGE

Overdosage or oral ingestion of lindane lotion can cause central nervous system excitation and if taken in sufficient quantities, convulsions may occur. If accidental ingestion occurs, prompt gastric lavage should be instituted. However, since oils favor absorption, saline cathartics for intestinal evacuation should be given rather than oil laxatives. If central nervous system manifestations occur, they can be antagonized by the administration of pentobarbital, phenobarbital or diazepam.

DOSAGE AND ADMINISTRATION

CAUTION: USE ONLY AS DIRECTED. DO NOT EXCEED RECOMMENDED DOSAGE.

No residual effects have been demonstrated, therefore, this product should not be used to ward off a possible infestation. However, sexual contacts should be treated simultaneously.

NOTE: PLEASE READ CAREFULLY.

DIRECTIONS FOR USE:

WARNING:

THIS PRODUCT CAN BE POISONOUS IF MISUSED. CHILDREN MUST NOT BE ALLOWED TO APPLY THIS DRUG WITHOUT DIRECT ADULT SUPERVISION. USE LOTION FOR SCABIES ONLY. APPLY ONLY ONCE. USE ONLY ENOUGH TO COVER THE BODY IN A THIN LAYER. 1 OUNCE (HALF OF A 2 OUNCE CONTAINER) SHOULD BE ALL THAT IS NEEDED FOR CHILDREN UNDER 6 YEARS OF AGE; 1 TO 2 OUNCES FOR OLDER CHILDREN AND ADULTS. DO NOT LEAVE ON FOR MORE THAN 12 HOURS. DO NOT INGEST. KEEP AWAY FROM MOUTH AND EYES. COVER INFANTS' HANDS AND FEET DURING TREATMENT TO PREVENT SUCKING AND LICKING OF LOTION. DO NOT USE IF OPEN WOUNDS, CUTS OR SORES ARE PRESENT, UNLESS DIRECTED BY YOUR PHYSICIAN.

(LOTION: SHAKE WELL)

1. APPLY THIS PREPARATION TO DRY SKIN IN A THIN LAYER AND RUB IN THOROUGHLY.
2. TRIM NAILS AND APPLY UNDER NAILS WITH TOOTHBRUSH (THROW AWAY TOOTHBRUSH AFTER USE).
3. IF A WARM BATH IS TAKEN BEFORE APPLICATION, ALLOW THE SKIN TO DRY AND COOL COMPLETELY BEFORE APPLYING THE MEDICATION.
4. A TOTAL BODY APPLICATION SHOULD BE MADE FROM THE NECK DOWN, INCLUDING SOLES OF FEET, UNLESS OTHERWISE DIRECTED BY YOUR PHYSICIAN.
5. THE LOTION SHOULD BE LEFT ON FOR 8 TO 12 HOURS (USUALLY OVERNIGHT) AND THEN REMOVED BY THOROUGH WASHING (BATH OR SHOWER).
6. AVOID UNNECESSARY CONTACT WITH YOUR SKIN IF YOU ARE APPLYING TO ANOTHER PERSON. IF TREATING MORE THAN ONE PERSON, PERSON APPLYING LOTION (ESPECIALLY PREGNANT OR NURSING WOMEN) SHOULD WEAR RUBBER GLOVES.
7. ALL RECENTLY WORN CLOTHING, UNDERWEAR AND PAJAMAS, AND USED SHEETS, PILLOW CASES, AND TOWELS SHOULD BE WASHED IN VERY HOT WATER OR DRY-CLEANED.

AFTER ONE APPLICATION, ITCHING WILL CONTINUE FOR SEVERAL WEEKS. THIS IS NORMAL AND DOES NOT REQUIRE REAPPLICATION.

IF YOU HAVE ANY QUESTIONS OR CONCERNS ABOUT YOUR CONDITION OR USE OF THE LOTION, CONTACT YOUR PHYSICIAN.

HOW SUPPLIED

Lindane Lotion USP, 1% in patient-size 2 fl oz (59 mL) and pharmacy-size only pint (473 mL) bottles.

SHAKE WELL BEFORE USING.

Store at controlled room temperature 15°–30°C (59°–86°F). Dispense in a tight, light-resistant container as defined in the USP, with a child-resistant closure.

REFERENCES

1. Feldmann, R.J. and Maibach, H.I., *Toxicol. Applied. Pharmacol.*, 28:126, 1974.
2. Dale, W.E., Curly, A. and Cueto, C. *Life Sci* 5:47, 1966.
3. Ginsburg, C.M., et al., *J. Pediatr.* 91:6, 998–1000, 1977.
4. Nagasaki, T., Tomii, S., Mega, T., Marugami, M. and Ito. N. *Gann* (Cancer) 63(3):393, 1972.
5. Goto, M., Hattori, M., Miyagawa, T. and Enomoto, M., *Chemosphere* 6:279, 1972.
6. Hanada, M., Yatani, C., Miyaji, T., *Gann* 64:511, 1973.
7. Weisse, I., and Herbst, M., *Toxicol.* 7:233, 1977.
8. Technical Report Series, NCI-CG-TR-14, *HEW PUBLICATIONS,* No. (NIH) 77–814.
9. Thorpe, E., and Walker, A.I.T., *Food Cosmetic Toxicol.* 11:433, 1973.
10. Orr, J.W., *Nature* 162:189, 1948.
11. Kashyap, S.K. et. al., *J. Environ, Sci. Health* 14:305–318, 1979.

Manufactured by
Alpharma USPD Inc.
Baltimore, MD 21244

FORM NO. 0570-02 Rev. 3/00
VC 1661

PHARMACIST—DETACH AND GIVE TO PATIENT

LINDANE LOTION USP 1%
DIRECTIONS FOR USE

WARNING:

THIS PRODUCT CAN BE POISONOUS IF MISUSED. CHILDREN MUST NOT BE ALLOWED TO APPLY THIS DRUG WITHOUT DIRECT ADULT SUPERVISION. USE LOTION FOR SCABIES ONLY. APPLY ONLY ONCE. USE ONLY ENOUGH TO COVER THE BODY IN A THIN LAYER. 1 OUNCE (HALF OF A 2 OUNCE CONTAINER) SHOULD BE ALL THAT IS NEEDED FOR CHILDREN UNDER 6 YEARS OF AGE; 1 TO 2 OUNCES FOR OLDER CHILDREN AND ADULTS. DO NOT LEAVE ON FOR MORE THAN 12 HOURS. DO NOT INGEST. KEEP AWAY FROM MOUTH AND EYES. COVER INFANTS' HANDS AND FEET DURING TREATMENT TO PREVENT SUCKING AND LICKING OF LOTION. DO NOT USE IF OPEN WOUNDS, CUTS OR SORES ARE PRESENT, UNLESS DIRECTED BY YOUR PHYSICIAN.

(Lotion: Shake Well)

1. Apply this preparation to dry skin in a thin layer and rub in thoroughly.
2. Trim nails and apply under nails with toothbrush (throw away toothbrush after use).
3. If a warm bath is taken before application, allow the skin to dry and cool completely before applying the medication.
4. A total body application should be made from the neck down, including soles of feet, unless otherwise directed by your physician.
5. The lotion should be left on for 8 to 12 hours (usually overnight) and then removed by thorough washing (bath or shower).
6. If applying lotion to another person, wear rubber gloves, especially if you are pregnant or a nursing mother.
7. All recently worn clothing, underwear and pajamas, and used sheets, pillow cases, and towels should be washed in very hot water or dry-cleaned.

After one application, itching will continue for several weeks. This is normal and does not require reapplication.

If you have any questions or concerns about your condition or use of the lotion, contact your physician.

VC 1661

LINDANE SHAMPOO, USP 1% ℞

DESCRIPTION

Lindane Shampoo, USP 1% is an ectoparasiticide and ovicide effective against *Pediculosis capitis* (head lice), *Pediculosis pubis* (crab lice) and their ova. In addition to the active ingredient, lindane, it contains trolamine lauryl sulfate, polysorbate 60, acetone and water to form a cosmetically pleasant shampoo. The pH may be adjusted with Citric Acid and/or Trolamine. Lindane, which is the highly purified gamma isomer of 1, 2, 3, 4, 5, 6, hexachlorocyclohexane, has the following structural formula:

Cl Cl Cl Cl Cl Cl

$C_6H_6Cl_6$ 290.83

CLINICAL PHARMACOLOGY

Lindane exerts its parasiticidal action by being directly absorbed into the parasites and their ova. Dale, et al[1], reported a blood level of 290 ng/mL associated with convulsions following the accidental ingestion of a lindane containing product. Analysis of blood taken from subjects before and after the use of lindane shampoo showed a mean peak blood level of only 3 ng/mL which appeared at six hours and disappeared at eight hours after the shampoo was applied.

INDICATIONS AND USAGE

Because post-treatment pruritus is common and may lead to misuse, lindane shampoo is indicated only for the treatment of patients with pediculosis capitis (head lice) and pediculosis pubis (crab lice) who have either failed to respond to adequate doses, or are intolerant of, other approved therapies. Reinfestation should be considered carefully before attributing the posttreatment presence of ectoparasites to a failure of response to adequate doses of other approved therapies.

CONTRAINDICATIONS

Lindane shampoo is contraindicated for premature neonates because their skin may be more permeable than full term infants and their liver enzymes may not be sufficiently developed. It is also contraindicated for patients with known seizure disorders and for individuals with a known sensitivity to the product or any of its components.

WARNINGS

LINDANE PENETRATES HUMAN SKIN AND HAS THE POTENTIAL FOR CNS TOXICITY (SEE CLINICAL PHARMACOLOGY SECTION). LINDANE SHAMPOO SHOULD BE USED ACCORDING TO RECOMMENDED DOSAGE (SEE DIRECTIONS FOR USE) ESPECIALLY ON INFANTS, PREGNANT WOMEN AND NURSING MOTHERS. ANIMAL STUDIES INDICATE THAT POTENTIAL TOXIC EFFECTS OF TOPICALLY APPLIED LINDANE ARE GREATER IN THE YOUNG. SEIZURES AND, IN RARE INSTANCES, DEATHS HAVE BEEN REPORTED AFTER EXCESS DOSAGE, OVER-EXPOSURE, FREQUENT REAPPLICATIONS, AND ACCIDENTAL AND INTENTIONAL INGESTION OF LINDANE. THESE INSTANCES OF PATIENT MISUSE HAVE BEEN ASSOCIATED WITH LACK OF PATIENT UNDERSTANDING OF DIRECTIONS FOR USE, PRESCRIBING OR DISPENSING EXCESSIVE QUANTITIES, AND IMPROPER REAPPLICATIONS. IN EXCEEDINGLY RARE CASES SEIZURES HAVE BEEN REPORTED WHEN USED ACCORDING TO DIRECTIONS. NO RESIDUAL EFFECTS OF LINDANE TREATMENT HAVE BEEN DEMONSTRATED, THEREFORE, THIS PRODUCT SHOULD NOT BE USED TO WARD OFF A POSSIBLE INFESTATION.

If accidental ingestion occurs, prompt gastric lavage is indicated. Because oils may enhance absorption, saline rather than oily cathartics should be used. Central nervous excitation can be controlled by the administration of pentobarbital, phenobarbital or diazepam.

PRECAUTIONS

General: Care should be taken to avoid contact with the eyes. If such contact occurs, eyes should be immediately flushed with water. If irritation or sensitization occurs, the patient should be advised to consult a physician.

Information for Patients: Patients must be instructed on the proper use of the medication, especially as to amount applied and duration of use. Patient's Directions for Use must accompany the product.

Laboratory Tests: No laboratory tests are needed for the proper use of this medication.

Drug Interactions: Oils may enhance absorption, therefore, avoid using oil treatments, or oil based hair dressings or conditioners immediately before and after applying lindane shampoo.

Carcinogenesis: Although no studies have been conducted with lindane shampoo, numerous long-term feeding studies have been conducted in mice and rats to evaluate the carcinogenic potential of the technical grade of hexachlorocyclohexane (BHC) as well as the alpha, beta, gamma (lindane) and delta isomers. Both oral and topical applications have been evaluated. Nagasaki[2], Goto[3] and Hanada[4] found varying amounts of benign and malignant hepatomas associated with BHC and the alpha, delta and epsilon isomers. None reported a carcinogenic potential for lindane. Tumors were found only in the animals which had received the alpha isomer. Weisse and Herbst[5] also evaluated the carcinogenic potential of lindane in mice but could find no evidence of lindane carcinogenicity. The National Cancer Institute[6] had also found no evidence of carcinogenicity.

Thorpe and Walker[7] compared beta BHC with lindane, dieldrin, DDT and hexabarbital in mice. Despite the unusually high incidence of tumors in the control group, they concluded that 600 ppm of lindane was associated with a significant increase in the incidence of hepatoma and thus, considered it a tumorigen.

Orr[8] and Kashyap, et al[9] evaluated the carcinogenic potential in mice of topically applied BHC. In neither study was there any evidence of a tumorigenic or carcinogenic potential associated with topical application of BHC.

Mutagenicity tests have been used as predictive information about the carcinogenicity of various chemical com-

Continued on next page

Lindane Shampoo—Cont.

pounds. Numerous types of mutagenicity tests have been performed with lindane. The results of these tests do not indicate that lindane is mutagenic.

Pregnancy: *Teratogenic Effects*—Pregnancy Category B. Reproduction, including multigeneration, studies have been performed in mice, rats, rabbits, pigs, and dogs at doses up to 10 times the human dose and have revealed no evidence of impaired fertility or harm to the fetus due to orally administered lindane. There are, however, no adequate and well-controlled studies in pregnant women. Because animal reproduction studies are not always predictive of human response, the recommended dosage should not be exceeded on pregnant women. They should be treated no more than twice during a pregnancy.

Nursing Mothers: Lindane is secreted in human milk in low concentrations. Studies conducted in the United States as well as in Europe and South America found levels of lindane in human milk ranging from 0 to 113 ppb, as the result of ingestion of foods which had been treated with lindane. There appeared to be no difference in concentrations between country and urban dwellers. Although the levels of lindane found in blood after topical application with lindane shampoo make it unlikely that amounts of lindane sufficient to cause serious adverse reactions will be excreted in the milk of nursing mothers who have used lindane shampoo, if there is any concern, an alternate method of feeding may be used for 4 days.

Pediatric Use: Refer to the CONTRAINDICATIONS and WARNINGS sections.

ADVERSE REACTIONS

Lindane has been reported to cause central nervous stimulation ranging from dizziness to convulsions. Cases of convulsions have been reported in connection with lindane shampoo therapy. However, these incidents were almost always associated with accidental oral ingestion or misuse of the product. In exceedingly rare cases, seizures have been reported when used according to directions. Eczematous eruptions due to irritation from this product have also been reported. Incidence of these adverse reactions is relatively infrequent, occurring in less than 1 in 100,000 patients.

DRUG ABUSE AND DEPENDENCE

Lindane shampoo is not subject to abuse, nor is there any dependence on the drug.

OVERDOSAGE

Overdosage or oral ingestion of lindane shampoo can cause central nervous system excitation and, if taken in sufficient quantities, convulsions may occur.

If accidental ingestion occurs, prompt gastric lavage should be instituted. However, since oils favor absorption, saline cathartics for intestinal evacuation should be given rather than oil laxatives. If central nervous system manifestations occur, they can be antagonized by the administration of pentobarbital, phenobarbital or diazepam.

DOSAGE AND ADMINISTRATION

CAUTION: USE ONLY AS DIRECTED. DO NOT EXCEED RECOMMENDED DOSAGE.

No residual effects of lindane shampoo treatment have been demonstrated, therefore, this product should not be used to ward off a possible infestation. However, sexual contacts should be treated simultaneously.

NOTE: PLEASE READ CAREFULLY.
DIRECTIONS FOR USE:
WARNING:
THIS PRODUCT CAN BE POISONOUS IF MISUSED. CHILDREN MUST NOT BE ALLOWED TO APPLY THIS DRUG WITHOUT DIRECT ADULT SUPERVISION. USE SHAMPOO FOR HEAD AND PUBIC LICE ONLY. DO NOT USE FOR SCABIES. USE ONLY IN AMOUNTS DIRECTED BELOW. IN NO CASE SHOULD MORE THAN 2 OUNCES BE USED BY ONE PERSON IN ONE APPLICATION. DO NOT INGEST. KEEP AWAY FROM MOUTH AND EYES. DO NOT USE IF OPEN WOUNDS, CUTS OR SORES ARE PRESENT ON SCALP OR GROIN, UNLESS DIRECTED BY YOUR PHYSICIAN.
AVOID USING OIL TREATMENTS, OIL BASED HAIR DRESSINGS OR CONDITIONERS IMMEDIATELY BEFORE AND AFTER APPLYING LINDANE SHAMPOO.
(SHAKE WELL)

1. BEFORE APPLYING LINDANE SHAMPOO, USE REGULAR SHAMPOO (WITHOUT CONDITIONERS), RINSE AND COMPLETELY DRY HAIR.
2. USE 1 OUNCE (HALF OF A 2 OUNCE BOTTLE) FOR SHORT HAIR; 1.5 OUNCES (THREE-QUARTERS OF A 2 OUNCE BOTTLE) FOR MEDIUM LENGTH HAIR; AND FULL 2 OUNCE BOTTLE FOR LONG HAIR.
3. APPLY SHAMPOO DIRECTLY TO DRY HAIR WITHOUT ADDING WATER. WORK THOROUGHLY INTO THE HAIR AND ALLOW TO REMAIN IN PLACE FOR 4 MINUTES ONLY.
4. AFTER 4 MINUTES, ADD SMALL QUANTITIES OF WATER TO HAIR UNTIL A GOOD LATHER FORMS.
5. IMMEDIATELY RINSE ALL LATHER AWAY. AVOID UNNECESSARY CONTACT OF LATHER WITH OTHER BODY SURFACES.
6. TOWEL BRISKLY AND REMOVE NITS WITH NIT COMB OR TWEEZERS.
7. AVOID UNNECESSARY CONTACT WITH YOUR SKIN IF YOU ARE APPLYING SHAMPOO TO ANOTHER PERSON. IF TREATING MORE THAN ONE PERSON, PERSON APPLYING SHAMPOO (ESPECIALLY PREGNANT AND/OR NURSING WOMEN) SHOULD WEAR RUBBER GLOVES.

RE-TREATMENT IS USUALLY NOT NECESSARY, BUT PRESENCE OF LIVING LICE IN HAIR 7 DAYS AFTER TREATMENT INDICATES THAT RE-TREATMENT MAY BE NECESSARY. DO NOT RETREAT WITHOUT THE ADVICE OF A PHYSICIAN.

HOW SUPPLIED

Lindane Shampoo, USP 1% in patient-size 2 fl oz (59 mL) and pharmacy-size only pint (473 mL) bottles.
SHAKE WELL BEFORE USING.
Store at controlled room temperature 15°–30°C (59°–86°F).
Dispense in a tight, light-resistant container as defined in the USP, with a child-resistant closure.

REFERENCES

1. Dale, W.E., Curly, A. and Cueto, C. *Life Sci* 5:47, 1966.
2. Nagasaki, T., Tomii, S., Mega, T., Marugami, M. and Ito, N. *Gann* (Cancer) 63(3):373, 1972.
3. Goto, M., Hattori, M., Miyagawa, T. and Enomoto, M., *Chemosphere* 6:279, 1972.
4. Hanada, M., Yatani, C., Miyaji, T., *Gann* 64:511, 1973.
5. Weisse, I., and Herbst, M., *Toxicol.* 7:233, 1977.
6. Technical Report Series, NCl-CG-TR-14, *HEW PUBLICATIONS*, No. (NIH) 77–814.
7. Thorpe, E., and Walker, A.I.T., *Food Cosmetic Toxicol. 11: 433, 1973.*
8. Orr, J.W., *Nature* 162:189, 1948.
9. Kashyap, S.K. et al, *J. Environ. Sci. Health* 14:305–318, 1979.

Manufactured by
Alpharma USPD Inc.
Baltimore, MD 21244

FORM NO. 0572-02 Rev. 3/00
VC 1664

PHARMACIST — DETACH AND GIVE TO PATIENT

LINDANE SHAMPOO, USP 1%
A SHAMPOO
FOR THE TREATMENT OF HEAD OR PUBIC LICE

CAUTION: USE ONLY AS DIRECTED. DO NOT EXCEED RECOMMENDED DOSE.
NOTE: PLEASE READ CAREFULLY.
DIRECTIONS FOR USE:
WARNING:
THIS PRODUCT CAN BE POISONOUS IF MISUSED. CHILDREN MUST NOT BE ALLOWED TO APPLY THIS DRUG WITHOUT DIRECT ADULT SUPERVISION. USE SHAMPOO FOR HEAD AND PUBIC LICE ONLY. DO NOT USE FOR SCABIES. USE ONLY IN AMOUNTS DIRECTED BELOW. IN NO CASE SHOULD MORE THAN 2 OUNCES BE USED BY ONE PERSON IN ONE APPLICATION. DO NOT INGEST. KEEP AWAY FROM MOUTH AND EYES. DO NOT USE IF OPEN WOUNDS, CUTS OR SORES ARE PRESENT ON SCALP OR GROIN, UNLESS DIRECTED BY YOUR PHYSICIAN.
AVOID USING OIL TREATMENTS, OIL BASED HAIR DRESSINGS OR CONDITIONERS IMMEDIATELY BEFORE AND AFTER APPLYING LINDANE SHAMPOO.
(SHAKE WELL)

1. BEFORE APPLYING LINDANE SHAMPOO, USE REGULAR SHAMPOO (WITHOUT CONDITIONERS), RINSE AND COMPLETELY DRY HAIR.
2. USE 1 OUNCE (HALF OF A 2 OUNCE BOTTLE) FOR SHORT HAIR; 1.5 OUNCES (THREE-QUARTERS OF A 2 OUNCE BOTTLE) FOR MEDIUM LENGTH HAIR; AND FULL 2 OUNCE BOTTLE FOR LONG HAIR.
3. APPLY SHAMPOO DIRECTLY TO DRY HAIR WITHOUT ADDING WATER. WORK THOROUGHLY INTO THE HAIR AND ALLOW TO REMAIN IN PLACE FOR 4 MINUTES ONLY.
4. AFTER 4 MINUTES, ADD SMALL QUANTITIES OF WATER TO HAIR UNTIL A GOOD LATHER FORMS.
5. IMMEDIATELY RINSE ALL LATHER AWAY. AVOID UNNECESSARY CONTACT OF LATHER WITH OTHER BODY SURFACES.
6. TOWEL BRISKLY AND REMOVE NITS WITH NIT COMB OR TWEEZERS.
7. AVOID UNNECESSARY CONTACT WITH YOUR SKIN IF YOU ARE APPLYING SHAMPOO TO ANOTHER PERSON. IF TREATING MORE THAN ONE PERSON, PERSON APPLYING SHAMPOO (ESPECIALLY PREGNANT AND/OR NURSING WOMEN) SHOULD WEAR RUBBER GLOVES.

RE-TREATMENT IS USUALLY NOT NECESSARY, BUT PRESENCE OF LIVING LICE IN HAIR 7 DAYS AFTER TREATMENT INDICATES THAT RE-TREATMENT MAY BE NECESSARY. DO NOT RE-TREAT WITHOUT THE ADVICE OF A PHYSICIAN.

VC 1664

For information on over-the-counter drugs, consult **PDR For Nonprescription Drugs**.

ALZA Pharmaceuticals,

A division of ALZA Corporation
1900 CHARLESTON ROAD
MOUNTAIN VIEW, CA 94043

Direct Inquiries to:
Customer Service
(800) 227-9953
FAX: (888) 261-8045

For Medical Information or Medical Emergencies Contact:
Medical Communications
(800) 634-8977 or (800) 506-4959
FAX: (650) 962-2488

BICITRA® ℞

[bye"si-trah]
Brand of sodium citrate and citric acid oral solution, USP

DESCRIPTION

BICITRA® is a stable and pleasant-tasting oral systemic alkalizer solution containing sodium citrate and citric acid in a sugar-free base. It is a nonparticulate neutralizing buffer.
BICITRA® contains in each teaspoonful (5 mL):
SODIUM CITRATE Dihydrate 500 mg (0.34 Molar)
CITRIC ACID Monohydrate 334 mg (0.32 Molar)
Each mL contains 1 mEq sodium ion and is equivalent to 1 mEq bicarbonate (HCO_3). BICITRA® also contains butylparaben, flavoring, maltitol, and sodium saccharin.

HOW SUPPLIED

BICITRA® is a grape flavored citrate solution supplied as:
16 fl. oz. (473 mL)
(NDC 17314-9330-1);
30 mL Unit Dose
(NDC 17314-9330-5);
15 mL Unit Dose
(NDC 17314-9330-4).

Keep tightly closed and protect from excessive heat or freezing.

Rx only

under license to
ALZA Corporation
Distributed by:
ALZA Corporation
Mountain View, CA 94043
Mfd. by:
Draxis Pharma Inc.
Kirkland, Quebec H9H 4J4
Canada
ALZA Pharmaceuticals
A division of ALZA Corp.
Mountain View, CA 94043
1001721 Rev 9804
REV9804 (212001)

DITROPAN® ℞

(oxybutynin chloride)
Tablets and Syrup

DESCRIPTION

Each scored biconvex, engraved blue DITROPAN® Tablet contains 5 mg of oxybutynin chloride. Each 5 mL of DITROPAN® Syrup contains 5 mg of oxybutynin chloride. Chemically, oxybutynin chloride is d,l (racemic) 4-diethylamino-2-butynyl phenylcyclohexylglycolate hydrochloride. The empirical formula of oxybutynin chloride is $C_{22}H_{31}NO_3 \cdot HCl$. The structural formula appears below:

Oxybutynin chloride is a white crystalline solid with a molecular weight of 393.9. It is readily soluble in water and acids, but relatively insoluble in alkalis.
DITROPAN® Tablets
Also contains: calcium stearate, FD&C Blue #1 Lake, lactose, and microcrystalline cellulose.
DITROPAN® Syrup
Also contains: citric acid, FD&C Green #3, glycerin, methylparaben, flavor, sodium citrate, sorbitol, sucrose, and water.
DITROPAN® Tablets and Syrup are for oral administration.
Therapeutic Category: Antispasmodic, anticholinergic.

HOW SUPPLIED

DITROPAN® (oxybutynin chloride) Tablets are supplied in bottles of 100 tablets (NDC 17314-9200-1) and 1000 tablets (NDC 17314-9200-2) and in Unit Dose Identification Paks of 100 tablets (NDC 17314-9200-3).

Blue scored tablets (5 mg) are engraved with DITROPAN on one side with 92 and 00, separated by a horizontal score, on the other side.
DITROPAN® Syrup (5 mg/5 mL) is supplied in bottles of 16 fluid ounces (473 mL) (NDC 17314-9201-4).
Pharmacist: Dispense in tight, light-resistant container as defined in the USP.
Store at controlled room temperature (59–86°F).
Rx ONLY

Manufactured by Hoechst Marion Roussel, Inc., Kansas City, MO 64137

Distributed by ALZA Corporation, Mountain View, CA 94043 50016519
Edition: 01/98

DITROPAN XL® ℞
(oxybutynin chloride)
Extended Release Tablets

DESCRIPTION

DITROPAN XL® (oxybutynin chloride) is an antispasmodic, anticholinergic agent. Each DITROPAN XL® Extended Release Tablet contains 5 mg, 10 mg or 15 mg of oxybutynin chloride USP, formulated as a once-a-day controlled-release tablet for oral administration. Oxybutynin chloride is administered as a racemate of R- and S- enantiomers.
Chemically, oxybutynin chloride is d,l (racemic) 4-diethylamino-2-butynyl phenylcyclohexyl-glycolate hydrochloride. The empirical formula of oxybutynin chloride is $C_{22}H_{31}NO_3 \bullet HCl$.
Its structural formula is:

Oxybutynin chloride is a white crystalline solid with a molecular weight of 393.9. It is readily soluble in water and acids, but relatively insoluble in alkalis.
DITROPAN XL® also contains the following inert ingredients: cellulose acetate, hydroxypropyl methylcellulose, lactose, magnesium stearate, polyethylene glycol, polyethylene oxide, synthetic iron oxides, titanium dioxide, polysorbate 80, sodium chloride, and butylated hydroxytoluene.

System Components and Performance

DITROPAN XL® uses osmotic pressure to deliver oxybutynin chloride at a controlled rate over approximately 24 hours. The system, which resembles a conventional tablet in appearance, comprises an osmotically active bilayer core surrounded by a semipermeable membrane. The bilayer core is composed of a drug layer containing the drug and excipients, and a push layer containing osmotically active components. There is a precision-laser drilled orifice in the semipermeable membrane on the drug-layer side of the tablet. In an aqueous environment, such as the gastrointestinal tract, water permeates through the membrane into the tablet core, causing the drug to go into suspension and the push layer to expand. This expansion pushes the suspended drug out through the orifice. The semipermeable membrane controls the rate at which water permeates into the tablet core, which in turn controls the rate of drug delivery. The controlled rate of drug delivery into the gastrointestinal lumen is thus independent of pH or gastrointestinal motility. The function of DITROPAN XL® depends on the existence of an osmotic gradient between the contents of the bilayer core and the fluid in the gastrointestinal tract. Since the osmotic gradient remains constant, drug delivery remains essentially constant. The biologically inert components of the tablet remain intact during gastrointestinal transit and are eliminated in the feces as an insoluble shell.

CLINICAL PHARMACOLOGY

Oxybutynin chloride exerts a direct antispasmodic effect on smooth muscle and inhibits the muscarinic action of acetylcholine on smooth muscle. Oxybutynin chloride exhibits only one-fifth of the anticholinergic activity of atropine on the rabbit detrusor muscle, but four to ten times the antispasmodic activity. No blocking effects occur at skeletal neuromuscular junctions or autonomic ganglia (antinicotinic effects).
Oxybutynin chloride relaxes bladder smooth muscle. In patients with conditions characterized by involuntary bladder contractions, cystometric studies have demonstrated that oxybutynin increases bladder (vesical) capacity, diminishes the frequency of uninhibited contractions of the detrusor muscle, and delays the initial desire to void. Oxybutynin thus decreases urgency and the frequency of both incontinent episodes and voluntary urination.
Antimuscarinic activity resides predominantly in the R-isomer. A metabolite, desethyloxybutynin, has pharmacological activity similar to that of oxybutynin in in vitro studies.

Pharmacokinetics

Absorption

Following the first dose of DITROPAN XL®, oxybutynin plasma concentrations rise for 4 to 6 hours; thereafter steady concentrations are maintained for up to 24 hours, minimizing fluctuations between peak and trough concentrations associated with oxybutynin.

Number of Urge Urinary Incontinence Episodes Per Week

Study 1	N	DITROPAN XL®	N	Placebo
Mean Baseline	34	15.9	16	20.9
Mean (SD) Change from Baseline†	34	-15.8 (8.9)	16	-7.6 (8.6)
95% Confidence Interval for Difference (DITROPAN XL® - Placebo)			(-13.6, -2.8)*	

* The difference between DITROPAN XL® and placebo was statistically significant.
† Covariate adjusted mean with missing observations set to baseline values

Study 2	N	DITROPAN XL®	N	oxybutynin
Mean Baseline	53	27.6	52	23.0
Mean (SD) Change from Baseline†	53	-17.6 (11.9)	52	-19.4 (11.9)
95% Confidence Interval for Difference (DITROPAN XL® - oxybutynin)			(-2.8, 6.5)	

† Covariate adjusted mean with missing observations set to baseline values

Study 3	N	DITROPAN XL®	N	oxybutynin
Mean Baseline	111	18.9	115	19.5
Mean (SD) Change from Baseline†	111	-14.5 (8.7)	115	-13.8 (8.6)
95% Confidence Interval for Difference (DITROPAN XL® - oxybutynin)			(-3.0, 1.6)**	

** The difference between DITROPAN XL® and oxybutynin fulfilled the criteria for comparable efficacy.
† Covariate adjusted mean with missing observations set to baseline values

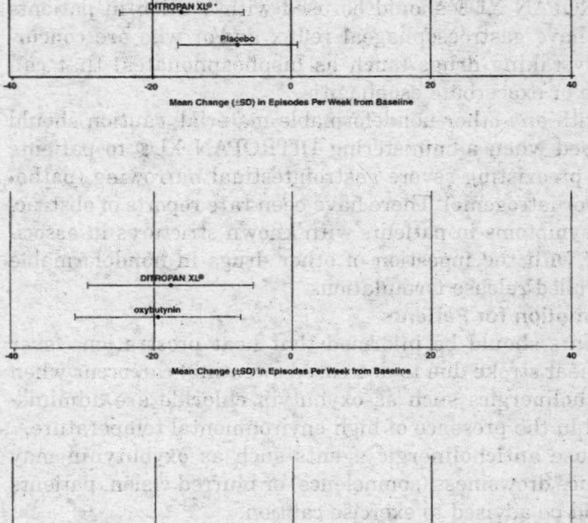

The relative bioavailabilities of R- and S-oxybutynin from DITROPAN XL® are 156% and 187%, respectively, compared with oxybutynin. The mean pharmacokinetic parameters for R- and S-oxybutynin are summarized in Table 1. The plasma concentration-time profiles for R- and S-oxybutynin are similar in shape; Figure 1 shows the profile for R-oxybutynin.

Table 1
Mean (SD) R- and S-Oxybutynin Pharmacokinetic Parameters Following a Single Dose of DITROPAN XL® 10 mg (n=43)

Parameters (units)	R-Oxybutynin		S-Oxybutynin	
C_{max} (ng/mL)	1.0	(0.6)	1.8	(1.0)
T_{max} (h)	12.7	(5.4)	11.8	(5.3)
$t_{½}$ (h)	13.2	(6.2)	12.4	(6.1)
$AUC_{(0-48)}$ (ng•h/mL)	18.4	(10.3)	34.2	(16.9)
AUC_{inf} (ng•h/mL)	21.3	(12.2)	39.5	(21.2)

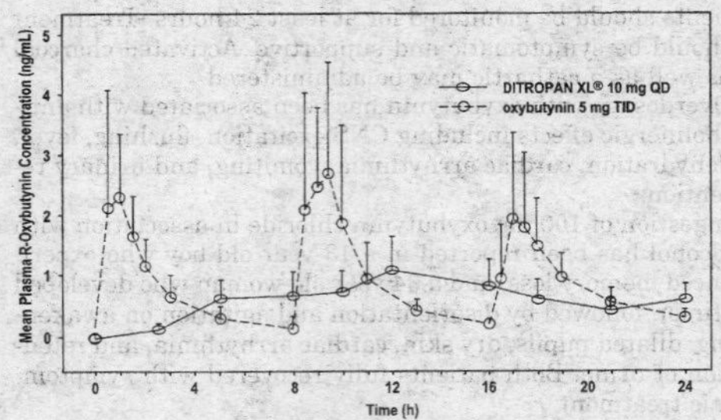

Figure 1. Mean R-oxybutynin plasma concentrations following a single dose of DITROPAN XL® 10 mg and oxybutynin 5 mg administered every 8 hours (n=23 for each treatment).

Steady-state oxybutynin plasma concentrations are achieved by Day 3 of repeated DITROPAN XL® dosing, with no observed drug accumulation or change in oxybutynin and desethyloxybutynin pharmacokinetic parameters.

Food Effects

The rate and extent of absorption and metabolism of oxybutynin are similar under fed and fasted conditions.

Distribution

Plasma concentrations of oxybutynin decline biexponentially following intravenous or oral administration. The volume of distribution is 193 L after intravenous administration of 5 mg oxybutynin chloride.

Metabolism

Oxybutynin is metabolized primarily by the cytochrome P450 enzyme systems, particularly CYP3A4 found mostly in the liver and gut wall. Its metabolic products include phenylcyclohexylglycolic acid, which is pharmacologically inactive, and desethyloxybutynin, which is pharmacologically active. Following DITROPAN XL® administration, plasma concentrations of R- and S-desethyloxybutynin are 73% and 92%, respectively, of concentrations observed with oxybutynin.

Excretion

Oxybutynin is extensively metabolized by the liver, with less than 0.1% of the administered dose excreted unchanged in the urine. Also, less than 0.1% of the administered dose is excreted as the metabolite desethyloxybutynin.

Dose Proportionality

Pharmacokinetic parameters of oxybutynin and desethyloxybutynin (C_{max} and AUC) following administration of 5–20 mg of DITROPAN XL® are dose proportional.

Special Populations

Geriatric: The pharmacokinetics of DITROPAN XL® were similar in all patients studied (up to 78 years of age).
Pediatric: The pharmacokinetics of DITROPAN XL® were not evaluated in individuals younger than 18 years of age. See **PRECAUTIONS**: Pediatric Use.
Gender: There are no significant differences in the pharmacokinetics of oxybutynin in healthy male and female volunteers following administration of DITROPAN XL®.
Race: Available data suggest that there are no significant differences in the pharmacokinetics of oxybutynin based on race in healthy volunteers following administration of DITROPAN XL®.
Renal Insufficiency: There is no experience with the use of DITROPAN XL® in patients with renal insufficiency.
Hepatic Insufficiency: There is no experience with the use of DITROPAN XL® in patients with hepatic insufficiency.
Drug-Drug Interactions: See **PRECAUTIONS:** Drug Interactions.

Clinical Studies

DITROPAN XL® was evaluated for the treatment of patients with overactive bladder with symptoms of urge urinary incontinence, urgency, and frequency in three controlled studies and one open label study. The majority of patients were Caucasian (89.0%) and female (91.9%) with a mean age of 59 years (range, 18 to 98 years). Entry criteria required that patients have urge or mixed incontinence (with a predominance of urge) as evidenced by ≥ 6 urge incontinence episodes per week and ≥ 10 micturitions per day. Study 1 was a forced dose escalation design, whereas the other studies used a dose adjustment design in which each patient's final dose was adjusted to a balance between improvement of incontinence symptoms and tolerability of side effects. Controlled studies included patients known to be responsive to oxybutynin or other anticholinergic medications, and these patients were maintained on a final dose for up to 2 weeks.
The efficacy results for the three controlled trials are presented in the following tables and figures.
[See tables & figures at top of page]

INDICATIONS AND USAGE

DITROPAN XL® is a once-daily controlled-release tablet indicated for the treatment of overactive bladder with symptoms of urge urinary incontinence, urgency, and frequency.

CONTRAINDICATIONS

DITROPAN XL® is contraindicated in patients with urinary retention, gastric retention, or uncontrolled narrow-angle glaucoma and in patients who are at risk for these conditions.
DITROPAN XL® is also contraindicated in patients who have demonstrated hypersensitivity to the drug substance or other components of the product.

PRECAUTIONS

General

DITROPAN XL® should be used with caution in patients with hepatic or renal impairment.
Urinary Retention:
DITROPAN XL® should be administered with caution to patients with clinically significant bladder outflow obstruction because of the risk of urinary retention (see **CONTRAINDICATIONS**).
Gastrointestinal Disorders:
DITROPAN XL® should be administered with caution to patients with gastrointestinal obstructive disorders because of the risk of gastric retention (see **CONTRAINDICATIONS**).

Continued on next page

Ditropan XL—Cont.

DITROPAN XL®, like other anticholinergic drugs, may decrease gastrointestinal motility and should be used with caution in patients with conditions such as ulcerative colitis, intestinal atony, and myasthenia gravis.

DITROPAN XL® should be used with caution in patients who have gastroesophageal reflux and/or who are concurrently taking drugs (such as bisphosphonates) that can cause or exacerbate esophagitis.

As with any other nondeformable material, caution should be used when administering DITROPAN XL® to patients with preexisting severe gastrointestinal narrowing (pathologic or iatrogenic). There have been rare reports of obstructive symptoms in patients with known strictures in association with the ingestion of other drugs in nondeformable controlled-release formulations.

Information for Patients

Patients should be informed that heat prostration (fever and heat stroke due to decreased sweating) can occur when anticholinergics such as oxybutyin chloride are administered in the presence of high environmental temperature.

Because anticholinergic agents such as oxybutynin may produce drowsiness (somnolence) or blurred vision, patients should be advised to exercise caution.

Patients should be informed that alcohol may enhance the drowsiness caused by anticholinergic agents such as oxybutynin.

Patients should be informed that DITROPAN XL® should be swallowed whole with the aid of liquids. Patients should not chew, divide, or crush tablets. The medication is contained within a nonabsorbable shell designed to release the drug at a controlled rate. The tablet shell is eliminated from the body; patients should not be concerned if they occasionally notice in their stool something that looks like a tablet.

Drug Interactions

The concomitant use of oxybutynin with other anticholinergic drugs or with other agents which produce dry mouth, constipation, somnolence (drowsiness), and/or other anticholinergic-like effects may increase the frequency and/or severity of such effects.

Anticholinergic agents may potentially alter the absorption of some concomitantly administered drugs due to anticholinergic effects on gastrointestinal motility.

Pharmacokinetic studies with patients concomitantly receiving cytochrome P450 enzyme inhibitors, such as antimycotic agents (e.g. ketoconazole, itraconazole, and miconazole) or macrolide antibiotics (e.g. erythromycin and clarithromycin), have not been performed.

No specific drug-drug interaction studies have been performed with DITROPAN XL®.

Carcinogenesis, Mutagenesis, Impairment of Fertility

A 24-month study in rats at dosages of oxybutynin chloride of 20, 80 and 160 mg/kg/day showed no evidence of carcinogenicity. These doses are approximately 6, 25 and 50 times the maximum human exposure, based on surface area.

Oxybutynin chloride showed on increase of mutagenic activity when tested in *Schizosaccharomyces pompholiciformis, Saccharomyces cerevisiae,* and *Salmonella typhimurium* test systems.

Reproduction studies with oxybutynin chloride in the mouse, rat, hamster, and rabbit showed no definite evidence of impaired fertility.

Pregnancy: Teratogenic Effects

Pregnancy Category B

Reproduction studies with oxybutynin chloride in the mouse, rat, hamster, and rabbit showed no definite evidence of impaired fertility or harm to the animal fetus. The safety of DITROPAN XL® administration to women who are or who may become pregnant has not been established. Therefore, DITROPAN XL® should not be given to pregnant women unless, in the judgment of the physician, the probable clinical benefits outweigh the possible hazards.

Nursing Mothers

It is not known whether oxybutynin is excreted in human milk. Because many drugs are excreted in human milk, caution should be exercised when DITROPAN XL® is administered to a nursing woman.

Pediatric Use

The safety and efficacy of DITROPAN XL® in pediatric patients have not been established.

Geriatric Use

The rate and severity of anticholinergic effects reported by patients less than 65 years old and those 65 years and older were similar (See **CLINICAL PHARMACOLOGY, Pharmacokinetics,** ***Special Populations:*** *Gender*).

ADVERSE REACTIONS

Adverse Events with DITROPAN XL®

The safety and efficacy of DITROPAN XL® was evaluated in a total of 580 participants who received DITROPAN XL® in clinical trials (429 patients, 151 healthy volunteers). These participants were treated with 5–30 mg/day for up to 4.5 months. Safety information is provided for 429 patients from three controlled clinical studies and one open label study (Table 2). The adverse events are reported regardless of causality.

Table 2
Incidence (%) of Adverse Events Reported by ≥5% of Patients Using DITROPAN XL® (5–30 mg/day)

Body System	Adverse Event	DITROPAN XL® 5–30 mg/day (n=429)
General	headache	9.8
	asthenia	6.8
	pain	6.8
Digestive	dry mouth	60.8
	constipation	13.1
	diarrhea	9.1
	nausea	8.9
	dyspepsia	6.8
Nervous	somnolence	11.9
	dizziness	6.3
Respiratory	rhinitis	5.6
Special senses	blurred vision	7.7
	dry eyes	6.1
Urogenital	urinary tract infection	5.1

The most common adverse events reported by patients receiving 5–30 mg/day DITROPAN XL® were the expected side effects of anticholinergic agents. The incidence of dry mouth was dose-related.

The discontinuation rate for all adverse events was 6.8%. The most frequent adverse event causing early discontinuation of study medication was nausea (1.9%), while discontinuation due to dry mouth was 1.2%.

In addition, the following adverse events were reported by 2 to <5% of patients using DITROPAN XL® (5–30 mg/day) in all studies. *General:* abdominal pain, dry nasal and sinus mucous membranes, accidental injury, back pain, flu syndrome; *Cardiovascular:* hypertension, palpitation, vasodilatation; *Digestive:* flatulence, gastroesophageal reflux; *Musculoskeletal:* arthritis; *Nervous:* insomnia, nervousness, confusion; *Respiratory:* upper respiratory tract infection, cough, sinusitis, bronchitis, pharyngitis; *Skin:* dry skin, rash; *Urogenital:* impaired urination (hesitancy), increased post void residual volume, urinary retention, cystitis.

Adverse Events with Oxybutynin Chloride

Other adverse events have been reported with oxybutynin chloride: tachycardia, hallucinations, cycloplegia, mydriasis, impotence, and suppression of lactation.

OVERDOSAGE

The continuous release of oxybutynin from DITROPAN XL® should be considered in the treatment of overdosage. Patients should be monitored for at least 24 hours. Treatment should be symptomatic and supportive. Activated charcoal as well as a cathartic may be administered.

Overdosage with oxybutynin has been associated with anticholinergic effects including CNS excitation, flushing, fever, dehydration, cardiac arrhythmia, vomiting, and urinary retention.

Ingestion of 100 mg oxybutynin chloride in association with alcohol has been reported in a 13 year old boy who experienced memory loss, and a 34 year old woman who developed stupor, followed by disorientation and agitation on awakening, dilated pupils, dry skin, cardiac arrhythmia, and retention of urine. Both patients fully recovered with symptomatic treatment.

DOSAGE AND ADMINISTRATION

DITROPAN XL® must be swallowed whole with the aid of liquids, and must not be chewed, divided, or crushed.

DITROPAN XL® may be administered with or without food.

The recommended starting dose of DITROPAN XL® is 5 mg once daily. Dosage may be adjusted in 5-mg increments to achieve a balance of efficacy and tolerability (up to a maximum of 30 mg/day). In general dosage adjustment may proceed at approximately weekly intervals.

HOW SUPPLIED

DITROPAN XL® (oxybutynin chloride) Extended Release Tablets are available in three dosage strengths, 5 mg (pale yellow), 10 mg (pink) and 15 mg (gray) and are imprinted with "5 XL", "10 XL" or "15 XL". DITROPAN XL® (oxybutynin chloride) Extended Release Tablets are supplied in bottles of 100 tablets.

5 mg	100 count bottle	NDC 17314-8500-1
10 mg	100 count bottle	NDC 17314-8501-1
15 mg	100 count bottle	NDC 17314-8502-1

Storage

Store at 25°C (77°F); excursions permitted to 15–30°C (59–86°F) [see USP Controlled Room Temperature]. Protect from moisture and humidity.

Rx only

For more information call 1-888-395-1232 or visit www.DitropanXL.com

Manufactured, distributed, and marketed by
ALZA Corporation, Mountain View, CA 94043.
Marketed by
UCB Pharma, Inc., Smyrna, GA 30080.
00096531 Edition: 7/99

Shown in Product Identification Guide, page 304

DOXIL® ℞

[dŏk'sĭl]

(doxorubicin HCl liposome injection)
FOR INTRAVENOUS INFUSION ONLY
A product of ALZA Pharmaceuticals
A division of ALZA Corporation
Mountain View, CA 94043 USA

WARNINGS

1. Experience with Doxil® (doxorubicin HCl liposome injection) at high cumulative doses is too limited to have established its effects on the myocardium. It should therefore be assumed that Doxil® will have myocardial toxicity similar to conventional formulations of doxorubicin HCl. Irreversible myocardial toxicity leading to congestive heart failure often unresponsive to cardiac supportive therapy may be encountered as the total dosage of doxorubicin HCl approaches 550 mg/m^2. Prior use of other anthracyclines or anthracenediones will reduce the total dose of doxorubicin HCl that can be given without cardiac toxicity. Cardiac toxicity also may occur at lower cumulative doses in patients with prior mediastinal irradiation or who are receiving concurrent cyclophosphamide therapy.
   Doxil® should be administered to patients with a history of cardiovascular disease only when the benefit outweighs the risk to the patient.
2. Acute infusion-associated reactions (flushing, shortness of breath, facial swelling, headache, chills, back pain, tightness in the chest or throat, and/or hypotension) have occurred in about 5% to 10% of patients treated with Doxil®. In most patients, these reactions resolve over the course of several hours to a day once the infusion is terminated. In some patients, the reaction has resolved with slowing of the infusion rate. Doxil® should be administered at an initial rate of 1 mg/min to minimize the risk of infusion reactions. (See **WARNINGS—Infusion Reactions.**)
3. Severe myelosuppression may occur. (See **WARNINGS—Myelosuppression.**)
4. Dosage should be reduced in patients with impaired hepatic function. (See **DOSAGE AND ADMINISTRATION.**)
5. Accidental substitution of Doxil® for doxorubicin HCl has resulted in severe side effects. Doxil® should not be substituted for doxorubicin HCl on a mg per mg basis. (See **DESCRIPTION** and **DOSAGE AND ADMINISTRATION.**)
6. Doxil® should be administered only under the supervision of a physician who is experienced in the use of cancer chemotherapeutic agents.

DESCRIPTION

Doxil® (doxorubicin HCl liposome injection) is doxorubicin hydrochloride (HCl) encapsulated in STEALTH® liposomes for intravenous administration.

Note: Liposomal encapsulation can substantially affect a drug's functional properties relative to those of the unencapsulated drug. In addition, different liposomal drug products may vary from one another in the chemical composition and physical form of the liposomes. Such differences can substantially affect the functional properties of liposomal drug products. DO NOT SUBSTITUTE.

Doxorubicin is a cytotoxic anthracycline antibiotic isolated from *Streptomyces peucetius* var. *caesius.*

Doxorubicin HCl, which is the established name for (8*S*,10*S*)-10-[(3-amino-2,3,6-trideoxy-α-L-*lyxo*-hexopyranosyl)oxy]-8-glycolyl-7,8,9,10-tetrahydro-6,8,11-trihydroxy-1-methoxy-5,12-naphthacenedione hydrochloride, has the following structure:

The molecular formula of the drug is $C_{27}H_{29}NO_{11}$•HCl; its molecular weight is 579.99.

Doxil® is provided as a sterile, translucent, red liposomal dispersion in 10-mL or 30-mL glass, single use vials. Each vial contains 20 mg or 50 mg doxorubicin HCl at a concentration of 2 mg/mL and a pH of 6.5. The STEALTH® liposome carriers are composed of N-(carbonyl-methoxypolyethylene glycol 2000)-1,2-distearoyl-*sn*-glycero-3-phosphoethanolamine sodium salt (MPEG-DSPE), 3.19 mg/mL; fully hydrogenated soy phosphatidylcholine (HSPC), 9.58 mg/mL; and cholesterol, 3.19 mg/mL. Each mL also contains ammonium sulfate, approximately 2 mg; histidine as a buffer; hydrochloric acid and/or sodium hydroxide for pH control; and sucrose to maintain isotonicity. Greater than 90% of the drug is encapsulated in the STEALTH® liposomes.

MPEG-DSPE has the following structural formula:

$CH_3[OCH_2CH_2]_nOC(=O)NHCH_2CH_2O-P(=O)(O^- Na^+)-OCH_2-CH(OC(=O)(CH_2)_{16}CH_3)-CH_2OC(=O)(CH_2)_{16}CH_3$

n = ca. 45

HSPC has the following structural formula:

$(CH_3)_3N^+-CH_2CH_2O-P(=O)(O^-)-OCH_2-CH(OC(=O)(CH_2)_mCH_3)-CH_2OC(=O)(CH_2)_nCH_3$

m, n = 14 or 16

CLINICAL PHARMACOLOGY

Mechanism of Action

The active ingredient of Doxil® is doxorubicin HCl. The mechanism of action of doxorubicin HCl is thought to be related to its ability to bind DNA and inhibit nucleic acid synthesis. Cell structure studies have demonstrated rapid cell penetration and perinuclear chromatin binding, rapid inhibition of mitotic activity and nucleic acid synthesis, and induction of mutagenesis and chromosomal aberrations.

Doxil® is doxorubicin HCl encapsulated in long-circulating STEALTH® liposomes. Liposomes are microscopic vesicles composed of a phospholipid bilayer that are capable of encapsulating active drugs. The STEALTH® liposomes of Doxil® are formulated with surface-bound methoxypolyethylene glycol (MPEG), a process often referred to as pegylation, to protect liposomes from detection by the mononuclear phagocyte system (MPS) and to increase blood circulation time.

Representation of a STEALTH® liposome:

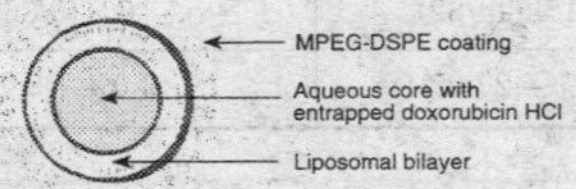

STEALTH® liposomes have a half-life of approximately 55 hours in humans. They are stable in blood, and direct measurement of liposomal doxorubicin shows that at least 90% of the drug (the assay used cannot quantify less than 5–10% free doxorubicin) remains liposome-encapsulated during circulation.

It is hypothesized that because of their small size (ca. 100 nm) and persistence in the circulation, the pegylated Doxil® liposomes are able to penetrate the altered and often compromised vasculature of tumors. This hypothesis is supported by studies using colloidal gold-containing STEALTH® liposomes, which can be visualized microscopically. Evidence of penetration of STEALTH® liposomes from blood vessels and their entry and accumulation in tumors has been seen in mice with C-26 colon carcinoma tumors and in transgenic mice with Kaposi's sarcoma-like lesions. Once the STEALTH® liposomes distribute to the tissue compartment, the encapsulated doxorubicin HCl becomes available. The exact mechanism of release is not understood.

Pharmacokinetics

The plasma pharmacokinetics of Doxil® were evaluated in 42 patients with AIDS-related Kaposi's sarcoma (KS) who received single doses of 10 or 20 mg/m² administered by a 30-minute infusion. Twenty-three of these patients received single doses of both 10 and 20 mg/m² with a 3-week washout period between doses. The pharmacokinetic parameter values of Doxil®, given for total doxorubicin (mostly liposomally bound), are presented in the following table.

[See table at top of page]

Doxil® displayed linear pharmacokinetics over the range of 10 to 20 mg/m². Disposition occurred in two phases after Doxil® administration, with a relatively short first phase (≈ 5 hours) and a prolonged second phase (≈ 55 hours) that accounted for the majority of the area under the curve (AUC).

The pharmacokinetics of Doxil® at a 50 mg/m² dose is reported to be non-linear. At this dose, the elimination half-life of Doxil® is expected to be longer and the clearance lower compared to a 20 mg/m² dose. The exposure (AUC) is thus expected to be more than proportional at a 50 mg/m² dose when compared with the lower doses.

Distribution: In contrast to the pharmacokinetics of doxorubicin, which displays a large volume of distribution, ranging from 700 to 1100 L/m², the small steady state volume of distribution of Doxil® shows that Doxil® is confined mostly to the vascular fluid volume. Plasma protein binding of Doxil® has not been determined; the plasma protein binding of doxorubicin is approximately 70%.

Metabolism: Doxorubicinol, the major metabolite of doxorubicin, was detected at very low levels (range: of 0.8 to 26.2 ng/mL) in the plasma of patients who received 10 or 20 mg/m² Doxil®.

Excretion: The plasma clearance of Doxil® was slow, with a mean clearance value of 0.041 L/h/m² at a dose of 20 mg/m². This is in contrast to doxorubicin, which displays a plasma clearance value ranging from 24 to 35 L/h/m².

Pharmacokinetic Parameters of Doxil® in AIDS Patients with Kaposi's Sarcoma

Parameter (units)	Dose 10 mg/m²	Dose 20 mg/m²
Peak Plasma Concentration (µg/mL)	4.12 ± 0.215	8.34 ± 0.49
Plasma Clearance (L/h/m²)	0.056 ± 0.01	0.041 ± 0.004
Steady State Volume of Distribution (L/m²)	2.83 ± 0.145	2.72 ± 0.120
AUC (µg/mL•h)	277 ± 32.9	590 ± 58.7
First Phase (λ 1) Half-Life (h)	4.7 ± 1.1	5.2 ± 1.4
Second Phase (λ 2) Half-Life (h)	52.3 ± 5.6	55.0 ± 4.8

N = 23
Mean ± Standard Error

Because of its slower clearance, the AUC of Doxil®, primarily representing the circulation of liposome-encapsulated doxorubicin, is approximately two to three orders of magnitude larger than the AUC for a similar dose of conventional doxorubicin HCl as reported in the literature.

Special Populations: The pharmacokinetics of Doxil® have not been separately evaluated in women, in members of different ethnic groups, or in individuals with renal or hepatic insufficiency.

Drug-Drug Interactions: Although the patient populations for the current indications are on various medications, drug-drug interactions between Doxil® and other drugs, including antiviral agents, have not been evaluated.

Tissue Distribution

Kaposi's sarcoma lesions and normal skin biopsies were obtained at 48 and 96 hours postinfusion of 20 mg/m² Doxil® in 11 patients. The concentration of Doxil® in KS lesions was a median of 19 (range, 3–53) times higher than in normal skin at 48 hours posttreatment; however, this was not corrected for likely differences in blood content between KS lesions and normal skin. The corrected ratio may lie between 1 and 22 times. Thus, higher concentrations of Doxil® are delivered to KS lesions than to normal skin.

Clinical Studies

Ovarian Carcinoma

Doxil® (doxorubicin HCl liposome injection) was studied in three open-label, single-arm, clinical trials of 176 patients with metastatic ovarian carcinoma. One hundred forty-five (145) of these patients were refractory to both paclitaxel- and platinum-based chemotherapy regimens. Refractory patients are defined as those having progressive disease while on treatment, or within 6 months of completing treatment. Patients in these studies received Doxil® at 50 mg/m² infused over one hour every 3 or 4 weeks for 3–6 cycles or longer in the absence of dose-limiting toxicity or progression of disease.

The baseline demographics and clinical characteristics of the refractory patients are shown in the following table.

[See first table at top of next page]

The primary efficacy parameter was response rate for the population of patients refractory to both paclitaxel and a platinum-containing regimen. Assessment of response was based on Southwest Oncology Group (SWOG) criteria, and required confirmation four weeks after the initial observation. Secondary efficacy parameters were time to response, duration of response, and time to progression.

The response rates for the individual phase 2 trials are given in the following table:

[See second table at top of next page]

When the data from the single arm trials are combined, the response rate for all patients refractory to paclitaxel and platinum agents was 13.8% (20/145) (95% CI 8.1% to 19.3%). The median time to progression was 15.9 weeks, the median time to response was 17.6 weeks, and the duration of response was 39.4 weeks.

Preliminary Results of Ovarian Cancer Randomized Trial

Data were also provided from an interim analysis of a randomized comparative study of Doxil®. Of the 44 patients in the Doxil® arm with tumors refractory to paclitaxel and platinum compounds, 6 had objective responses, a response rate of 13.6% (95% CI 5.2% to 27.4%).

AIDS-Related Kaposi's Sarcoma

Doxil® was studied in an open-label, single-arm, multicenter study utilizing Doxil® at 20 mg/m² by intravenous infusion every three weeks, generally until progression or intolerance occurred. In an interim analysis, the treatment history of 383 patients was reviewed, and a cohort of 77 patients was retrospectively identified as having disease progression on prior systemic combination chemotherapy (at least 2 cycles of a regimen containing at least two of three treatments: bleomycin, vincristine or vinblastine, or doxorubicin) or as being intolerant to such therapy. Forty-nine of the 77 (64%) patients had received prior doxorubicin HCl.

These 77 patients were predominantly white, homosexual males with a median CD4 count of 10 cells/mm³. Their age ranged from 24 to 54 years, with a mean age of 38 years. Using the ACTG staging criteria,[1] 78% of the patients were at poor risk for tumor burden, 96% at poor risk for immune system, and 58% at poor risk for systemic illness at baseline. Their mean Karnofsky status score was 74%. All 77 patients had cutaneous or subcutaneous lesions, 40% also had oral lesions, 26% pulmonary lesions, and 14% of patients had lesions of the stomach/intestine. The majority of these patients had disease progression on prior systemic combination chemotherapy.

The median time on study for these 77 patients was 155 days and ranged from 1 to 456 days. The median cumulative dose was 154 mg/m² and ranged from 20 to 620 mg/m².

Two analyses of tumor response were used to evaluate the effectiveness of Doxil®: one analysis based on investigator assessment of changes in lesions over the entire body, and one analysis based on changes in indicator lesions.

Investigator Assessment

Investigator response was based on modified ACTG criteria.[1] Partial response was defined as no new lesions, sites of disease, or worsening edema; flattening of ≥ 50% of previously raised lesions or area of indicator lesions decreasing by ≥ 50%; and response lasting at least 21 days with no prior progression.

Indicator Lesion Assessment

A retrospectively defined analysis was conducted based on assessment of the response of up to five prospectively identified representative indicator lesions. A partial response was defined as flattening of ≥ 50% of previously raised indicator lesions, or > 50% decrease in the area of indicator lesions and lasting at least 21 days with no prior progression.

Only patients with adequate documentation of baseline status and follow-up assessments were considered evaluable for response. Patients who received concomitant KS treatment during study, who completed local radiotherapy to sites encompassing one or more of the indicator lesions within two months of study entry, who had less than four indicator lesions, or who had less than three raised indicator lesions at baseline (the latter applies solely to indicator lesion assessment) were considered nonevaluable for response. Of the 77 patients who had disease progression on prior systemic combination chemotherapy or who were intolerant to such therapy, 34 were evaluable for investigator assessment and 42 were evaluable for indicator lesion assessment.

Responses are summarized in the tables below.

Response in Refractory[a] AIDS-KS

Investigator Assessment	All Evaluable Patients (n = 34)	Evaluable Patients Who Received Prior Doxorubicin (n = 20)
Response[b]		
Partial (PR)	27%	30%
Stable	29%	40%
Progression	44%	30%
Duration of PR (days)		
Median	73	89
Range	43+ – 210+	42+ – 210+
Time to PR (days)		
Median	43	53
Range	15 – 133	15 – 109

Indicator Lesion Assessment	All Evaluable Patients (n = 42)	Evaluable Patients Who Received Prior Doxorubicin (n = 23)
Response[b]		
Partial (PR)	48%	52%
Stable	26%	30%
Progression	26%	17%
Duration of PR (days)		
Median	71	79
Range	22+ – 210+	35 – 210+
Time to PR (days)		
Median	22	48
Range	15 – 109	15 – 109

[a] Patients with disease that progressed on prior combination chemotherapy or who were intolerant to such therapy.
[b] There were no complete responses in this population.

INDICATIONS AND USAGE

Doxil® (doxorubicin HCl liposome injection) is indicated for:

1. The treatment of metastatic carcinoma of the ovary in patients with disease that is refractory to both paclitaxel- and platinum-based chemotherapy regimens. Refractory disease is defined as disease that has progressed while on treatment, or within 6 months of completing treatment.

Continued on next page

Doxil—Cont.

2. The treatment of AIDS-related Kaposi's sarcoma in patients with disease that has progressed on prior combination chemotherapy or in patients who are intolerant to such therapy.

These indications are based on objective tumor response rates. No results are available from controlled trials that demonstrate a clinical benefit resulting from this treatment, such as improvement in disease-related symptoms or increased survival.

CONTRAINDICATIONS

Doxil® (doxorubicin HCl liposome injection) is contraindicated in patients who have a history of hypersensitivity reactions to a conventional formulation of doxorubicin HCl or the components of Doxil®.
Doxil® is contraindicated in nursing mothers.

WARNINGS

Cardiac Toxicity

Experience with large cumulative doses of Doxil® (doxorubicin HCl liposome injection) is limited. Doxil's cardiac risk and its risk compared to conventional doxorubicin formulations have not been adequately evaluated. At present, therefore, warnings related to the use of conventional formulation doxorubicin HCl should be observed.

Special attention must be given to the cardiac toxicity exhibited by doxorubicin HCl. Acute left ventricular failure can occur with doxorubicin, particularly in patients who have received total doxorubicin dosage exceeding the currently recommended limit of 550 mg/m^2. Lower (400 mg/m^2) doses appear to cause heart failure in patients who have received radiotherapy to the mediastinal area or concomitant therapy with other potentially cardiotoxic agents such as cyclophosphamide.

Caution should be observed in patients who have received other anthracyclines, and the total dose of doxorubicin HCl given should take into account any previous or concomitant therapy with other anthracyclines or related compounds.

Congestive heart failure and/or cardiomyopathy may be encountered after discontinuation of therapy. Patients with a history of cardiovascular disease should be administered Doxil® only when the potential benefit of treatment outweighs the risk.

Cardiac function should be carefully monitored in patients treated with Doxil®. The most definitive test for anthracycline myocardial injury is endomyocardial biopsy. Other methods, such as echocardiography or gated radionuclide scans, have been used to monitor cardiac function during anthracycline therapy. Any of these methods should be employed to monitor potential cardiac toxicity during Doxil® therapy. If these test results indicate possible cardiac injury associated with Doxil® therapy, the benefit of continued therapy must be carefully weighed against the risk of myocardial injury.

In the AIDS-KS studies, 68 (9.6%) patients experienced cardiac-related adverse events. In 30 patients (4.3%), the event was thought to be possibly or probably related to Doxil®. Nine cases of possibly or probably related cardiomyopathy and/or congestive heart failure were reported. Seven (1.0%) of the possibly or probably related cardiac events were severe. These severe events included arrhythmia (nonspecific), cardiomyopathy, heart failure, pericardial effusion, and tachycardia. Three patients discontinued study due to cardiac events.

Myelosuppression

In ovarian cancer patients, myelosuppression was generally moderate and reversible. Anemia was the most common hematologic adverse event (52.6%), followed by neutropenia (51.7%), leukopenia (42.2%) and thrombocytopenia (24.2%). In ovarian cancer patients, 3.3% received G-CSF (or GM-CSF) to support their blood counts. (See **DOSAGE AND ADMINISTRATION, Dose Modification Guidelines.**)

In AIDS-KS patients, who often present with baseline myelosuppression due to such factors as their HIV disease or concomitant medications, myelosuppression appears to be the dose-limiting adverse event, at the recommended dose of 20 mg/m^2 (see Hematology Data table in **ADVERSE REACTIONS, AIDS-KS Patients**). Leukopenia is the most common adverse event experienced in this population; anemia and thrombocytopenia can also be expected. Sepsis occurred in 5% of patients; for 0.7% of patients the event was considered possibly or probably related to Doxil®. Eleven patients (1.6%) discontinued study because of bone marrow suppression or neutropenia.

In all patients, because of the potential for bone marrow suppression, careful hematologic monitoring is required during use of Doxil®, including white blood cell, neutrophil, platelet counts, and Hgb/Hct. With the recommended dosage schedule, leukopenia is usually transient. Hematologic toxicity may require dose reduction or delay or suspension of Doxil® therapy. Persistent severe myelosuppression may result in superinfection, neutropenic fever, or hemorrhage. Development of sepsis in the setting of neutropenia has resulted in discontinuation of treatment and in rare cases, death.

Doxil® may potentiate the toxicity of other anticancer therapies. In particular, hematologic toxicity may be more severe when Doxil® is administered in combination with other agents that cause bone marrow suppression.

Infusion Reactions

Acute infusion-related reactions, characterized by flushing, shortness of breath, facial swelling, headache, chills, back pain, tightness in the chest and throat, and/or hypotension have occurred in 5% to 10% of patients treated with Doxil®. In most patients, these reactions resolve over the course of several hours to a day once the infusion is terminated. In some patients, the reaction resolves when the rate of infusion is slowed. The majority of infusion-related events occurred during the first infusion. Six AIDS-KS patients (0.9%) and 13 (1.7%) solid tumor patients discontinued Doxil® therapy because of infusion-related reactions. Similar reactions have not been reported with conventional doxorubicin and they presumably represent a reaction to the Doxil® liposomes or one of its surface components.

The initial rate of infusion should be 1 mg/min to help minimize the risk of infusion reactions. (See **DOSAGE AND ADMINISTRATION.**)

Patient Demographics for Refractory Patients from Phase 2 Ovarian Cancer Studies

	Study 1 (U.S.) (n = 27)	Study 2 (U.S.) (n = 82)	Study 3 (non-U.S.) (n = 36)
Age at diagnosis (years)			
Median	64	61.5	51.5
Range	46 – 75	34 – 85	22 – 80
Drug-Free Interval (months)			
Median	1.8	1.7	2.6
Range	0.5 – 15.6	0.6 – 7.0	0.7 – 15.2
Sum of Lesions at Baseline (cm^2)			
Median	25	18.3	32.4
Range	1.2 – 230.0	1.3 – 285.0	0.3 – 114.0
FIGO Staging			
I	1 (3.7%)	3 (3.7%)	4 (11.1%)
II	3 (11.1%)	3 (3.7%)	1 (2.8%)
III	15 (55.6%)	60 (73.2%)	24 (66.7%)
IV	8 (29.6%)	16 (19.5%)	6 (16.7%)
Not Specified	—	—	1 (2.8%)
CA-125 at Baseline			
Median	123.5	199.0	1004.5
Range	20 – 14,012	7 – 46,594	20 – 12,089
Number of Prior Chemotherapy Regimens			
1	7 (25.9%)	13 (15.9%)	9 (25.0%)
2	11 (40.7%)	44 (53.7%)	19 (52.8%)
3	6 (22.2%)	25 (30.5%)	8 (22.8%)
4	3 (11.1%)	—	—

Response Rates in Refractory Patients from single arm Ovarian Cancer Studies

	Study 1 (U.S.)	Study 2 (U.S.)	Study 3 (non-U.S.)
Response Rate	22.2% (6/27)	17.1% (14/82)	0% (0/36)
95% Confidence Interval	8.6% – 42.3%	9.7% – 27.0%	0.0% – 9.7%

Palmar-Plantar Erythrodysesthesia

In ovarian cancer patients, 37.4% of patients experienced PPE (developed palmar-plantar skin eruptions characterized by swelling, pain, erythema and, for some patients, desquamation of the skin on the hands and the feet), with 16.4% of the patients reporting Grade 3 or 4 events. Thirteen (3.5%) of the ovarian cancer patients discontinued treatment due to PPE or other skin toxicity. (See definitions of PPE grades in **DOSAGE AND ADMINISTRATION, Dose Modification Guidelines.**)

Among 705 patients with AIDS-related Kaposi's sarcoma treated with Doxil® at 20 mg/m^2, 24 (3.4%) developed PPE, with 3 (0.9%) discontinuing.

PPE was generally seen after 2 or 3 cycles of treatment but may occur earlier. In most patients the reaction is mild and resolves in one to two weeks so that prolonged delay of therapy need not occur. However, dose modification may be required to manage PPE. (See **DOSAGE AND ADMINISTRATION, Dose Modification Guidelines.**) The reaction can be severe and debilitating in some patients and may require discontinuation of treatment.

Pregnancy Category D

Doxil® can cause fetal harm when administered to a pregnant woman. Doxil® is embryotoxic at doses of 1 mg/kg/day in rats and is embryotoxic and abortifacient at 0.5 mg/kg/day in rabbits (both doses are about one-eighth the 50 mg/m^2 human dose on a mg/m^2 basis). Embryotoxicity was characterized by increased embryo-fetal deaths and reduced live litter sizes.

There are no adequate and well-controlled studies in pregnant women. If Doxil® is to be used during pregnancy, or if the patient becomes pregnant during therapy, the patient should be apprised of the potential hazard to the fetus. If pregnancy occurs in the first few months following treatment with Doxil, the prolonged half-life of the drug must be considered. Women of childbearing potential should be advised to avoid pregnancy.

Toxicity Potentiation

The doxorubicin in Doxil® may potentiate the toxicity of other anti-cancer therapies. Exacerbation of cyclophosphamide-induced hemorrhagic cystitis and enhancement of the hepatotoxicity of 6-mercaptopurine have been reported with the conventional formulation of doxorubicin HCl. Radiation-induced toxicity to the myocardium, mucosae, skin, and liver have been reported to be increased by the administration of doxorubicin HCl.

Injection Site Effects

Doxil® is not a vesicant, but should be considered an irritant and precautions should be taken to avoid extravasation. With intravenous administration of Doxil®, extravasation may occur with or without an accompanying stinging or burning sensation, even if blood returns well on aspiration of the infusion needle. (See **DOSAGE AND ADMINISTRATION.**) If any signs or symptoms of extravasation have occurred, the infusion should be immediately terminated and restarted in another vein. The application of ice over the site of extravasation for approximately 30 minutes may be helpful in alleviating the local reaction. **Doxil® must not be given by the intramuscular or subcutaneous route.**

In studies with rabbits, lesions that were induced by subcutaneous injection of Doxil® were minor and reversible compared to more severe and irreversible lesions and tissue necrosis that were induced after subcutaneous injection of conventional doxorubicin HCl.

Hepatic Impairment

The pharmacokinetics of Doxil® has not been adequately evaluated in patients with hepatic impairment. Doxorubicin is eliminated in large part by the liver. Thus, Doxil® dosage should be reduced in patients with impaired hepatic function. (See **DOSAGE AND ADMINISTRATION.**)

Prior to Doxil® administration, evaluation of hepatic function is recommended using conventional clinical laboratory tests such as SGOT, SGPT, alkaline phosphatase and bilirubin. (See **DOSAGE AND ADMINISTRATION.**)

Carcinogenesis, Mutagenesis, Impairment of Fertility

Secondary acute myelogenous leukemia has been reported in patients treated with topoisomerase II inhibitors, including anthracyclines.

Although no studies have been conducted with Doxil®, doxorubicin HCl and related compounds have been shown to have mutagenic and carcinogenic properties when tested in experimental models.

STEALTH® liposomes without drug were negative when tested in Ames, mouse lymphoma and chromosomal aberration assays in vitro, and mammalian micronucleus assay in vivo.

The possible adverse effects on fertility in males and females in humans or experimental animals have not been adequately evaluated. However, Doxil® resulted in mild to moderate ovarian and testicular atrophy in mice after a single dose of 36 mg/kg (about twice the 50 mg/m^2 human dose on a mg/m^2 basis). Decreased testicular weights and hypospermia were present in rats after repeat doses $\geq$ 0.25 mg/kg/day (about on thirtieth the 50 mg/m^2 human dose on a mg/m^2 basis), and diffuse degeneration of the seminiferous tubules and a marked decrease in spermatogenesis were observed in dogs after repeat doses of 1 mg/kg/day (about one half the 50 mg/m^2 human dose on a mg/m^2 basis).

PRECAUTIONS

General

Patients receiving therapy with Doxil® should be monitored by a physician experienced in the use of cancer chemotherapeutic agents. Most adverse events are manageable with dose reductions or delays. (See **DOSAGE AND ADMINISTRATION, Dose Modification Guidelines.**)

Laboratory Tests

Complete blood counts, including platelet counts, should be obtained frequently and at a minimum prior to each dose of Doxil®.

Drug Interactions

No formal drug interaction studies have been conducted with Doxil®. Until specific compatibility data are available, it is not recommended that Doxil® be mixed with other drugs. Doxil® may interact with drugs known to interact with the conventional formulation of doxorubicin HCl.

Pregnancy

Pregnancy Category D: (See **WARNINGS.**)

Nursing Mothers

It is not known whether this drug is excreted in human milk. Because many drugs, including anthracyclines, are excreted in human milk and because of the potential for serious adverse reactions in nursing infants from Doxil®, mothers should discontinue nursing prior to taking this drug.

Pediatric Use

The safety and effectiveness of Doxil® in pediatric patients have not been established.

Geriatric Use

Of the 373 ovarian cancer patients, 29% were 60 to 69 years old, while 22.8% were 70 years and over. No overall differences were observed between these subjects and younger subjects, but greater sensitivity of some older individuals cannot be ruled out. There are insufficient data for a comparative evaluation of efficacy according to age.

Radiation Therapy

Recall of skin reaction due to prior radiotherapy has occurred with Doxil® administration.

Information for the Patient

Patients and patients' caregivers should be informed of the expected adverse effects of Doxil®, particularly hand-foot syndrome, stomatitis, and neutropenia and its complications of neutropenic fever, infection, and sepsis.

Hand-Foot Syndrome (Palmar-Plantar Erythrodysesthesia): Patients who experience tingling or burning, redness, flaking, bothersome swelling, small blisters, or small sores on the palms of their hands or soles of their feet (symptoms of Hand-Foot Syndrome) should notify their physician.

Stomatitis: Patients who experience painful redness, swelling, or sores in the mouth (symptoms of stomatitis) should notify their physician.

Fever and Neutropenia: Patients who develop a fever of 100.5°F or higher should notify their physician.

Nausea, vomiting, tiredness, weakness, rash, or mild hair loss: Patients who develop any of these symptoms should notify their physician.

ADVERSE REACTIONS

Ovarian Cancer Patients

Safety data are available from 373 ovarian cancer patients treated with Doxil® in 4 clinical studies. The patient population was predominantly white (93.6%) with a median age of 60 years. Patients received a median cycle dose of 50 mg/m^2 administered with a median cycle length of 29.5 days. They remained on study drug for a median of 56 days and received a median cumulative dose of 137.5 mg/m^2. Patients received a median of 3 cycles of Doxil®, although some patients remained on study drug for a prolonged period, with 46 patients (12.3%) receiving more than 10 cycles of treatment.

Adverse events (AEs) were reported in all but 2 of the 361 patients who had at least one AE form collected. A total of 3,124 AEs were reported, an average of 8.6 AEs per patient. Most (91.7%) patients had AEs that were considered related to study drug.

Hematology Data Reported in Ovarian Cancer Patients

	% Ovarian Patients (n=373)
Leukopenia	
< 4,000/mm^3	42.2
< 1,000/mm^3	8.3
G-CSF or GM-CSF support*	3.3
Neutropenia	
< 2000/mm^3	51.7
< 500/mm^3	8.3
Febrile neutropenia	0.3
Anemia	
< 10 g/dL	52.6
< 8 g/dL	25.0
RBC transfusions	12.9
Epoetin alpha support*	2.1
Thrombocytopenia	
< 150,000/mm^3	24.2
< 25,000/mm^3	1.1
Platelet transfusions*	1.4

Drug-Related Non-Hematologic Adverse Events Reported in ≥ 5% of Ovarian Cancer Patients

Non-Hematologic Adverse Event	% Ovarian Patients (n=361)
Palmar-plantar erythrodysesthesia	
All Grades	37.4
Grade 3 & 4	16.4
Stomatitis	
All Grades	37.4
Grade 3 & 4	7.7
Nausea	
All Grades	37.7
Grade 3 & 4	4.2
Asthenia	33.0
Vomiting	22.4
Rash	21.6
Alopecia	15.2
Constipation	12.7
Anorexia	11.9
Mucous Membrane Disorder	11.6
Diarrhea	10.0
Abdominal Pain	8.0
Paresthesia	7.8
Pain	7.2
Fever	6.9
Pharyngitis	5.5
Dry Skin	5.5
Headache	5.3

*From concomitant medication or transfusion logs, not reported as AEs.

The following additional (not in table) adverse events were observed in ovarian cancer patients with doses administered every four weeks; only events considered at least possibly drug-related by investigators are included.

Incidence 1% to 5%

Body as a Whole: allergic reaction, chills, infection, chest pain, back pain, abdomen enlarged, malaise.
Digestive System: dyspepsia, oral moniliasis, mouth ulceration, esophagitis, dysphagia.
Metabolic and Nutritional System: peripheral edema, dehydration.
Musculoskeletal System: myalgia.
Nervous System: somnolence, dizziness, depression, insomnia, anxiety.
Respiratory System: dyspnea, cough increased, rhinitis.
Cutaneous: pruritus, skin discoloration, skin disorder, vesiculobullous rash, maculopapular rash, exfoliative dermatitis, herpes zoster, sweating.
Special Senses: conjunctivitis, taste perversion.

Incidence Less Than 1%

Body As A Whole: cellulitis, anaphylactoid reaction, ascites, flu syndrome, neck pain, moniliasis, injection site pain, face edema, chills and fever, pelvic pain, chest pain substernal, injection site inflammation.
Cardiovascular System: hypertension, angina pectoris, pericardial effusion, postural hypotension, hypotension, palpitation, syncope, shock, bradycardia, arrhythmia, phlebitis, tachycardia, cardiomegaly, heart failure, hemorrhage.
Digestive System: gingivitis, eructation, increased salivation, melena, gastrointestinal hemorrhage, proctitis, jaundice, ileus, periodontal abscess, flatulence, aphthous stomatitis, gastritis, glossitis, gum hemorrhage.
Hemic and Lymphatic System: hypochromic anemia, lymphadenopathy, eccymosis, petechia.
Metabolic/Nutritional Disorders: SGOT increase, creatinine increase, hypocalcemia, hyperglycemia, hypokalemia, hypermagnesemia, hyponatremia, weight gain, bilirubinemia, generalized edema, cachexia, hypochloremia.
Musculoskeletal System: arthralgia, bone pain, myasthenia.
Nervous System: peripheral neuritis, incoordination, thinking abnormal, confusion, hypertonia, nervousness, hyperesthesia, hypesthesia, neuropathy, ataxia.
Respiratory System: pleural effusion, asthma, hiccup, pneumothorax, laryngitis, sinusitis, voice alteration, epistaxis, pneumonia.
Skin and Appendages: skin ulcer, herpes simplex, contact dermatitis, fungal dermatitis, furunculosis, skin nodule, urticaria, acne.
Special Senses: amblyopia, blepheritis, parosmia, taste loss.
Urogenital System: urinary tract infection, leukorrhea, cystitis, nocturia, dysuria, breast pain, mastitis, oliguria, vaginitis, kidney function abnormal, vaginal hemorrhage, hydronephrosis, vaginal moniliasis.

AIDS-KS Patients

Information on adverse events is based on the experience reported in 753 patients with AIDS-related KS enrolled in four studies. The majority of patients were treated with 20 mg/m^2 of Doxil® (doxorubicin HCl liposome injection) every two to three weeks. The median time on study was 127 days and ranged from 1 to 811 days. The median cumulative dose was 120 mg/m^2 and ranged from 3.3 to 798.6 mg/m^2. Twenty-six patients (3.0%) received cumulative doses of greater than 450 mg/m^2.

Of these 753 patients, 61.2% were considered poor risk for KS tumor burden, 91.5% poor for immune system, and 46.9% for systemic illness; 36.2% were poor risk for all three categories. Patients' median CD4 count was 21.0 cells/mm^3, with 50.8% of patients having less than 50 cells/mm^3. The mean absolute neutrophil count at study entry was approximately 3000 cells/mm^3.

Patients received a variety of potentially myelotoxic drugs in combination with Doxil®. Of the 693 patients with concomitant medication information, 58.7% were on one or more antiretroviral medications; 34.9% patients were on zidovudine (AZT), 20.8% on didanosine (ddI), 16.5% on zalcitabine (ddC), and 9.5% on stavudine (D4T). A total of 85.1% patients were on PCP prophylaxis, most (54.4%) on sulfamethoxazole/trimethoprim. Eighty-five percent of patients were receiving antifungal medications, primarily fluconazole (75.8%). Seventy-two percent of patients were receiving antivirals, 56.3% acyclovir, 29% ganciclovir, and 16% foscarnet. In addition, 47.8% patients received colony stimulating factors (sargramostim/filgrastim) sometime during their course of treatment.

Of the 753 patients enrolled in the Doxil® clinical trials, adverse event information was available for 705 patients. In many instances it was difficult to determine whether adverse events resulted from Doxil®, from concomitant therapy, or from the patients' underlying disease(s).

Eighty-three percent of the patients reported adverse events that were considered to be possibly or probably related to the treatment with Doxil®.

Adverse reactions only infrequently (5%) led to discontinuation of treatment. Those that did so included bone marrow suppression, cardiac adverse events, infusion-related reactions, toxoplasmosis, palmar-plantar erythrodysesthesia, pneumonia, cough/dyspnea, fatigue, optic neuritis, progression of a non-KS tumor, allergy to penicillin, and unspecified reasons.

Hematology Data Reported in AIDS-KS Patients

	Refractory or Intolerant AIDS-KS Patients (n=74)	Total AIDS-KS Patients (n=720)
Leukopenia		
< 4,000/mm^3	65 (87.8%)	658 (91.4%)
< 1,000/mm^3	7 (9.5%)	83 (11.5%)
Neutropenia		
< 2000/mm^3	57 (77.0%)	612 (85.0%)
< 500/mm^3	8 (10.8%)	96 (13.3%)
Anemia		
< 10 g/dL	43 (58.1%)	399 (55.4%)
< 8 g/dL	12 (16.2%)	131 (18.2%)
Thrombocytopenia		
< 150,000/mm^3	45 (60.8%)	439 (60.9%)
< 25,000/mm^3	1 (1.4%)	30 (4.2%)

Probably and Possibly Drug-Related Non-Hematologic *Adverse Events Reported in ≥ 5% of AIDS-KS Patients*

Adverse Event	Refractory or Intolerant AIDS-KS Patients (n=77)	Total AIDS-KS Patients (n=705)
Nausea	14 (18.2%)	119 (16.9%)
Asthenia	5 (6.5%)	70 (9.9%)
Fever	6 (7.8%)	64 (9.1%)
Alopecia	7 (9.1%)	63 (8.9%)
Alkaline Phosphatase Increase	1 (1.3%)	55 (7.8%)
Vomiting	6 (7.8%)	55 (7.8%)
Hypochromic Anemia	4 (5.2%)	69 (9.8%)
Diarrhea	4 (5.2%)	55 (7.8%)
Stomatitis	4 (5.2%)	48 (6.8%)
Oral Moniliasis	1 (1.3%)	39 (5.5%)

The following additional (not in table) adverse events were observed in AIDS-KS patients; only events considered at least possibly drug-related by investigators are included.

Incidence 1% to 5%

Body as a Whole: headache, back pain, infection, allergic reaction, chills.
Cardiovascular: chest pain, hypotension, tachycardia.
Cutaneous: Herpes simplex, rash, itching.
Digestive System: mouth ulceration, glossitis, constipation, aphthous stomatitis, anorexia, dysphagia, abdominal pain.
Hematologic: hemolysis, increased prothrombin time.
Metabolic/Nutritional: SGPT increase, weight loss, hypocalcemia, hyperbilirubinemia, hyperglycemia.
Other: dyspnea, albuminuria, pneumonia, retinitis, emotional lability, dizziness, somnolence.

Incidence Less Than 1%

Body As A Whole: face edema, cellulitis, sepsis, abscess, radiation injury, flu syndrome, moniliasis, hypothermia, injection site hemorrhage, injection site pain, cryptococcosis, ascites.
Cardiovascular System: thrombophlebitis, cardiomyopathy, pericardial effusion, hemorrhage, palpitation, syncope, bundle branch block, congestive heart failure, cardiomegaly, heart arrest, migraine, thrombosis, ventricular arrhythmia.

Continued on next page

Doxil—Cont.

Digestive System: dyspepsia, cholestatic jaundice, gastritis, gingivitis, ulcerative proctitis, colitis, esophageal ulcer, esophagitis, gastrointestinal hemorrhage, hepatic failure, leukoplakia of mouth, pancreatitis, ulcerative stomatitis, hepatitis, hepatosplenomegaly, increased appetite, jaundice, sclerosing cholangitis, tenesmus, fecal impaction.
Endocrine System: diabetes mellitus.
Hemic and Lymphatic System: eosinophilia, lymphadenopathy, lymphangitis, lymphedema, petechia, thromboplastin decrease.
Metabolic/Nutritional Disorders: lactic dehydrogenase increase, hypernatremia, creatinine increase, BUN increase, dehydration, edema, hypercalcemia, hyperkalemia, hyperlipemia, hyperuricemia, hypoglycemia, hypokalemia, hypolipemia, hypomagnesemia, hyponatremia, hypophosphatemia, hypoproteinemia, ketosis, weight gain.
Musculoskeletal System: myalgia, arthralgia, bone pain, myositis.
Nervous System: paresthesia, insomnia, peripheral neuritis, depression, neuropathy, anxiety, convulsion, hypotonia, acute brain syndrome, confusion, hemiplegia, hypertonia, hypokinesia, vertigo.
Respiratory System: pleural effusion, asthma, bronchitis, cough increase, hyperventilation, pharyngitis, pneumothorax, rhinitis, sinusitis.
Skin and Appendages: maculopapular rash, skin ulcer, skin discoloration, herpes zoster, exfoliative dermatitis, cutaneous moniliasis, erythema multiforme, erythema nodosum, furunculosis, psoriasis, pustular rash, skin necrosis, urticaria, vesiculbullous rash.
Special Senses: otitis media, taste perversion, abnormal vision, blindness, conjunctivitis, eye pain, optic neuritis, tinnitus, visual field defect.
Urogenital System: hematuria, balanitis, cystitis, dysuria, genital edema, glycosuria, kidney failure.

OVERDOSAGE

Acute overdosage with doxorubicin HCl causes increases in mucositis, leukopenia and thrombocytopenia.
Treatment of acute overdosage consists of treatment of the severely myelosuppressed patient with hospitalization, antibiotics, platelet and granulocyte transfusions and symptomatic treatment of mucositis.

DOSAGE AND ADMINISTRATION

Ovarian Cancer Patients

Doxil® (doxorubicin HCl liposome injection) should be administered intravenously at a dose of 50 mg/m^2 (doxorubicin HCl equivalent) at an initial rate of 1 mg/min to minimize the risk of infusion reactions. If no infusion-related AEs are observed, the rate of infusion can be increased to complete administration of the drug over one hour. The patient should be dosed once every 4 weeks, for as long as the patient does not progress, shows no evidence of cardiotoxicity (see **WARNINGS**), and continues to tolerate treatment. A minimum of 4 courses is recommended because median time to response in clinical trials was 4 months. To manage adverse events such as PPE, stomatitis, or hematologic toxicity the doses may be delayed or reduced (see Dose Modification Guidelines below). Pretreatment with or concomitant use of antiemetics should be considered.

AIDS-KS Patients

Doxil® (doxorubicin HCl liposome injection) should be administered intravenously at a dose of 20 mg/m^2 (doxorubicin HCl equivalent) over 30 minutes, once every three weeks, for as long as patients respond satisfactorily and tolerate treatment.

General

Do not administer as a bolus injection or an undiluted solution. Rapid infusion may increase the risk of infusion-related reactions. (See **WARNINGS—Infusion Reactions.**)
Each 10-mL vial contains 20 mg doxorubicin HCl at a concentration of 2 mg/mL. Each 30-mL vial contains 50 mg doxorubicin HCl at a concentration of 2 mg/mL.
Until specific compatibility data are available, it is not recommended that Doxil® be mixed with other drugs.
Doxil® should be considered an irritant and precautions should be taken to avoid extravasation. With intravenous administration of Doxil®, extravasation may occur with or without an accompanying stinging or burning sensation, even if blood returns well on aspiration of the infusion needle. If any signs or symptoms of extravasation have occurred the infusion should be immediately terminated and restarted in another vein. The application of ice over the site of extravasation for approximately 30 minutes may be helpful in alleviating the local reaction. **Doxil® must not be given by the intramuscular or subcutaneous route.**

Dose Modification Guidelines

Doxil® exhibits nonlinear pharmacokinetics as 50 mg/m^2; therefore, dose adjustments may result in a non-proportional greater change in plasma concentration and exposure to the drug. (see **CLINICAL PHARMACOLOGY, Pharmacokinetics**.)
Patients should be carefully monitored for toxicity. Adverse events, such as PPE, hematologic toxicities, and stomatitis may be managed by dose delays and adjustments. Following the first appearance of a Grade 2 or higher adverse event, the dosing should be adjusted or delayed as described in the following tables. Once the dose has been reduced, it should not be increased at a later time.

Recommended Dose Modification Guidelines

PALMAR-PLANTAR ERYTHRODYSESTHESIA

Toxicity Grade	Dose Adjustment
1 (mild erythema, swelling, or desquamation not interfering with daily activities)	**Redose unless patient has experienced previous Grade 3 or 4 toxicity.** If so, delay up to 2 weeks and decrease dose by 25%. Return to original dose interval.
2 (erythema, desquamation, or swelling interfering with, but not precluding normal physical activities; small blisters or ulcerations less than 2 cm in diameter.)	**Delay dosing up to 2 weeks or until resolved to Grade 0-1.** If after 2 weeks there is no resolution, Doxil® should be discontinued.
3 (blistering, ulceration, or swelling interfering with walking or normal daily activities; cannot wear regular clothing)	**Delay dosing up to 2 weeks or until resolved to Grade 0-1.** Decrease dose by 25% and return to original dose interval. If after 2 weeks there is no resolution, Doxil® should be discontinued.
4 (diffuse or local process causing infectious complications, or a bed ridden state or hospitalization)	**Delay dosing up to 2 weeks or until resolved to Grade 0-1.** Decrease dose by 25% and return to original dose interval. If after 2 weeks there is no resolution, Doxil® should be discontinued.

[See table at top of page]

HEMATOLOGICAL TOXICITY

GRADE	ANC	PLATELETS	MODIFICATION
1	1500 – 1900	75,000 – 150,000	Resume treatment with no dose reduction
2	1000 – <1500	50,000 – <75,000	Wait until ANC ≥1,500 and platelets ≥ 75,000; redose with no dose reduction
3	500 – 999	25,000 – <50,000	Wait until ANC ≥ 1,500 and platelets ≥ 75,000; redose with no dose reduction
4	<500	<25,000	Wait until ANC ≥ 1,500 and platelets ≥ 75,000; redose at 25% dose reduction or continue full dose with cytokine support.

STOMATITIS

Toxicity Grade	Dose Adjustment
1 (painless ulcers, erythema, or mild soreness)	**Redose unless patient has experienced previous Grade 3 or 4 toxicity.** If so, delay up to 2 weeks and decrease dose by 25%. Return to original dose interval.
2 (painful erythema, edema, or ulcers, but can eat)	**Delay dosing up to 2 weeks or until resolved to Grade 0-1.** If after 2 weeks there is no resolution, Doxil® should be discontinued.
3 (painful erythema, edema, or ulcers, and cannot eat)	**Delay dosing up to 2 weeks or until resolved to Grade 0-1.** Decrease dose by 25% and return to original dose interval. If after 2 weeks there is no resolution, Doxil® should be discontinued.
4 (requires parenteral or enteral support)	**Delay dosing up to 2 weeks or until resolved to Grade 0-1.** Decrease dose by 25% and return to original dose interval. If after 2 weeks there is no resolution, Doxil® should be discontinued.

Patients with Impaired Hepatic Function

Limited clinical experience exists in treating hepatically impaired patients with Doxil®. Based on experience with doxorubicin HCl, it is recommended that Doxil® dosage be reduced if the bilirubin is elevated as follows: Serum bilirubin 1.2 to 3.0 mg/dL give ½ normal dose, >3 mg/dL give ¼ normal dose.

Preparation for Intravenous Administration

The appropriate dose of Doxil®, up to a maximum of 90 mg, must be diluted in 250 mL of 5% Dextrose Injection, USP prior to administration. Aseptic technique must be strictly observed since no preservative or bacteriostatic agent is present in Doxil®. Diluted Doxil® should be refrigerated at 2°C to 8°C (36°F to 46°F) and administered within 24 hours.
Do not use with in-line filters.
Do not mix with other drugs.
Do not mix with any diluent other than 5% Dextrose Injection.
Do not use any bacteriostatic agent, such as benzyl alcohol.
Doxil® is not a clear solution but a translucent, red liposomal dispersion.
Parenteral drug products should be inspected visually for particulate matter and discoloration prior to administration, whenever solution and container permit. Do not use if a precipitate or foreign matter is present.

Storage and Stability

Refrigerate unopened vials of Doxil® at 2°C to 8°C (36°F to 46°F). Avoid freezing. Prolonged freezing may adversely affect liposomal drug products; however, short-term freezing (less than 1 month) does not appear to have a deleterious effect on Doxil®.

Procedure for Proper Handling and Disposal

Caution should be exercised in the handling and preparation of Doxil®.
The use of gloves is required.
If Doxil® comes into contact wth skin or mucosa, immediately wash thoroughly with soap and water.
Doxil® should be considered an irritant and precautions should be taken to avoid extravasation. With intravenous administration of Doxil®, extravasation may occur with or without an accompanying stinging or burning sensation, even if blood returns well on aspiration of the infusion needle. If any signs or symptoms of extravasation have occurred, the infusion should be immediately terminated and restarted in another vein. Doxil® must not be given by the intramuscular or subcutaneous route.
Doxil® should be handled and disposed of in a manner consistent with other anticancer drugs. Several guidelines on this subject exist.[2–8]

HOW SUPPLIED

Doxil® (doxorubicin HCl liposome injection) is supplied as a sterile, translucent, red liposomal dispersion in 10-mL or 30-mL glass, single use vials.
Each 10-mL vial contains 20 mg doxorubicin HCl at a concentration of 2 mg/mL.
Each 30-mL vial contains 50 mg doxorubicin HCl at a concentration of 2 mg/mL.
Refrigerate at 2°–8°C. Avoid freezing. Prolonged freezing may adversely affect liposomal drug products; however, short-term freezing (less than 1 month) does not appear to have a deleterious effect on Doxil®.
The following packages of six individually cartoned vials are available:

mg in vial	fill volume	vial size	NDC #'s
20 mg vial	10-mL	10-mL	17314-9600-1
50 mg vial	25-mL	30-mL	17314-9600-2

REFERENCES

1. Krown et al. Kaposi's sarcoma in the acquired immune deficiency syndrome: A proposal for uniform evaluation, response, and staging criteria. J Clin Oncol. 1989; 7(9): 1201–1207.
2. Recommendations for the safe handling of cytotoxic drugs. NIH Publication No. 92-2621. US Government Printing Office, Washington, DC 20402.
3. OSHA Work-Practice guidelines for personnel dealing with cytotoxic (antineoplastic) drugs. Am J Hosp Pharm. 1986; 43:1193–1204.
4. American Society of Hospital Pharmacists Technical Assistance Bulletin on Handling Cytotoxic and Hazardous Drugs. Am J Hosp Pharm. 1985; 42:131–137.
5. National Study Commission on Cytotoxic Exposure—Recommendations for Handling Cytotoxic Agents. Available from Louis P. Jeffrey, Sc.D., Chairman, National Study Commission on Cytotoxic Exposure, Massachusetts College of Pharmacy and Allied Health Sciences, 179 Longwood Avenue, Boston, Massachusetts 02115.
6. AMA Council Report. Guidelines for handling parenteral antineoplastics. JAMA 1985; 253(11):1590–1592.
7. Clinical Oncologic Society of Australia: Guidelines and recommendation for safe handling of antineoplastic agents. Med. J. Australia 1983; 1:426–428.
8. Jones RB, et al. Safe handling of chemotherapeutic agents: a report from the Mount Sinai Medical Center. Ca–A Cancer Journal for Clinicians. 1983; Sept/Oct:258–263.

Rx only
Manufactured by:
Ben Venue Laboratories, Inc., Bedford, Ohio 44146
Distributed by:
ALZA Pharmaceuticals, Inc.,
A division of ALZA Corporation
Mountain View, CA 94043 USA
Last revised: July 2000
00091913

Shown in Product Identification Guide, page 304

ELMIRON®-100 mg ℞
(pentosan polysulfate sodium)
Capsules

DESCRIPTION

Pentosan polysulfate sodium is a semi-synthetically produced heparin-like macromolecular carbohydrate derivative which chemically and structurally resembles glycosaminoglycans. It is a white odorless powder, slightly hygroscopic and soluble in water to 50% at pH 6. It has a molecular weight of 4000 to 6000 Dalton with the following structural formula:

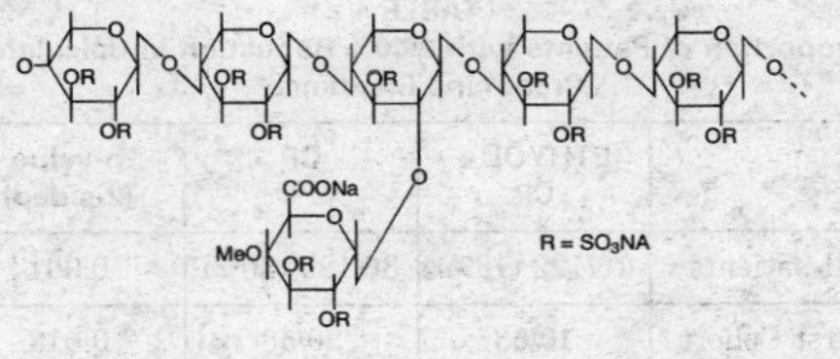

ELMIRON® is supplied in white opaque hard gelatin capsules containing 100 mg pentosan polysulfate sodium, microcrystalline cellulose, and magnesium stearate. It is formulated for oral use.

CLINICAL PHARMACOLOGY

GENERAL: Pentosan polysulfate sodium is a low molecular weight heparin-like compound. It has anticoagulant and fibrinolytic effects. The mechanism of action of pentosan polysulfate sodium in interstitial cystitis is not known.

PHARMACOKINETICS:

Absorption: In preliminary clinical studies with different doses of radio labeled pentosan polysulfate sodium, absorption was approximately 3% of the administered dose (n=3).

Distribution: Preclinical studies with parenterally administered radio labeled pentosan polysulfate sodium showed distribution to the uroepithelium of the genitourinary tract with lesser amounts found in the liver, spleen, lung, skin, periosteum, and bone marrow. Erythrocyte penetration is low in animals.

Metabolism: Preliminary literature studies of metabolism in 5 healthy volunteers with radio labeled drug suggest that 68% of the dose, at about 1 hour after IV administration, undergoes partial desulfation in the liver and spleen. In another study of 3 healthy volunteers, partial depolymerization occurs in the kidney. Both the desulfation and depolymerization can be saturated with continued dosing.

Excretion: In preliminary clinical studies in 8 healthy male volunteers, the elimination half-life of pentosan polysulfate sodium had a mean value at 24 hours after IV injection of 40 mg.

The elimination half-life in urine following orally administered radio labeled pentosan polysulfate sodium was determined to be 4.8 hours for the unchanged drug.

In preliminary human studies in 3 healthy male volunteers, after single doses of radio labeled drug, urinary excretion averaged 3.5% of the administered dose. After multiple doses of pentosan polysulfate sodium, urine excretion of radioactivity averaged 11% of the administered dose.

Further analyses of the urinary fraction obtained after repeated dosing showed that about 3% of the dose may be unchanged pentosan polysulfate sodium.

Special Populations: Dose adjustments in geriatric patients and in patients with hepatic or renal impairment were not studied.

PHARMACODYNAMICS:

The mechanism by which pentosan polysulfate sodium achieves its effects in patients is unknown. In preliminary clinical models, pentosan polysulfate sodium adhered to the bladder wall mucosal membrane. The drug may act as a buffer to control cell permeability preventing irritating solutes in the urine from reaching the cells.

Food effects: The effect of food on absorption of pentosan polysulfate sodium is now known. In clinical trials, ELMIRON® was administered with water 1 hour before or 2 hours after meals.

Drug-Drug Interactions:
Not studied.

CLINICAL TRIALS

ELMIRON® was evaluated in two clinical trials for the relief of pain in patients with chronic interstitial cystitis (IC). All patients met the NIH definition of IC based upon the results of cystoscopy, cytology, and biopsy. One blinded, randomized, placebo controlled study evaluated 151 patients (145 women, 5 men, 1 unknown) with a mean age of 44 years (range 18 to 81). Approximately equal numbers of patients received either placebo or ELMIRON® 100 mg three times a day for 3 months. Clinical improvement in bladder pain was based upon the patient's own assessment. In this study, 28/74 (38%) of patients who received ELMIRON® and 13/74 (18%) of patients who received placebo, showed greater than 50% improvement in bladder pain (p=0.005).

A second clinical trial, the physician's usage study, was a prospectively designed retrospective analysis of 2499 patients who received ELMIRON® 300 mg a day without blinding. Of the 2499 patients, 2220 were women, 254 were men, and 25 were of unknown sex. The patients had a mean age of 47 years and 23% were over 60 years of age. By 3 months, 1307 (52%) of the patients had dropped out or were ineligible for analysis, overall, 1192 (48%) received ELMIRON® for 3 months; 892 (36%) received ELMIRON® for 6 months; and 598 (24%) received ELMIRON® for one year. Patients had unblinded evaluations every 3 months for the patient's rating of overall change in pain in comparison to baseline and for the difference calculated in "pain/discomfort" scores. At baseline, pain/discomfort scores for the original 2499 patients were severe or unbearable in 60%, moderate in 33% and mild or none in 7% of patients. The extent of the patients' pain improvement is shown in Table 1.

At 3 months, 722/2499 (29%) of the patients originally in the study had pain scores that improved by one or two categories. By 6 months, in the 892 patients who continued taking ELMIRON®, an additional 116/2499 (5%) of patients had improved pain scores. After 6 months, the percent of patients who reported the first onset of pain relief was less than 1.5% of patients who originally entered in the study (see Table 2).

Table 1:
Pain Scores in Reference to Baseline in Open Label Physician's Usage Study (N=2499)[1]

Efficacy Parameter	3 months[2]	6 months[2]
Patient Rating of Overall Change in Pain (Recollection of difference between current pain and baseline pain)[2]	N=1161 Median=3 Mean=3.44 Cl: (3.37, 3.51)	N=724 Median=4 Mean=3.91 Cl: (3.83, 3.99)
Change in Pain/ Discomfort Score (Calculated difference in scores at the time point and baseline)[4]	N=1440 Median=1 Mean=0.51 Cl: (0.45, 0.57)	N=904 Median=1 Mean=0.66 Cl: (0.61, 0.71)

[1] Trial not designed to detect onset of pain relief.
[2] Cl=95% confidence interval.
[3] 6-point-scale: 1 = worse, 2 = no better, 3 = slightly improved, 4 = moderately improved, 5 = greatly improved, 6=symptom gone.
[4] 3-point scale: 1=none or mild, 2=moderate, 3=severe or unbearable.

Table 2:
Number (%) of Patients with New Relief of Pain/Discomfort' in the Open-Label Physician's Usage Study (N=2499)

	at 3 months[2] (n=1192)	at 6 months[3] (n=892)
Considering only the patients who continued treatment	722/1192 (61%)	116/892 (13%)
Considering all the patients originally enrolled in the study	722/2499 (29%)	116/2499 (5%)

[1]First-time improvement in pain/discomfort score by 1 or 2 categories.
[2]Number (%) of patients with improvement of pain/discomfort score at 3 months when compared to baseline.
[2]Number (%) of patients without pain/ discomfort improvement at 3 months who had improvement at 6 months.

INDICATIONS AND USAGE

ELMIRON® (pentosan polysulfate sodium) is indicated for the relief of bladder pain or discomfort associated with interstitial cystitis.

CONTRAINDICATIONS

ELMIRON® (pentosan polysulfate sodium) is contraindicated in patients with known hypersensitivity to the drug, structurally related compounds, or excipients.

WARNINGS

None.

PRECAUTIONS

GENERAL:

ELMIRON® (pentosan polysulfate sodium) is a weak anticoagulant (1/15 the activity of heparin). Bleeding complications of ecchymosis, epistaxis, and gum hemorrhage have been reported (see **ADVERSE REACTIONS**). Patients undergoing invasive procedures or having signs/symptoms of underlying coagulopathy or other increased risk of bleeding (due to other therapies such as coumarin anticoagulants, heparin, t-PA streptokinase, or high dose aspirin) should be evaluated for hemorrhage. Patients with diseases such as aneurysms, thrombocytopenia, hemophilia, gastrointestinal ulcerations, polyps, or diverticula should be carefully evaluated before starting ELMIRON®.

A similar product that was given subcutaneously, sublingually, or intramuscularly (and not initially metabolized by the liver) is associated with delayed immunoallergic thrombocytopenia with symptoms of thrombosis and hemorrhage. Caution should be exercised when using ELMIRON® in patients who have a history of heparin induced thrombocytopenia.

Hepatic Insufficiency: Pentosan polysulfate sodium is desulfated by both the liver and the spleen. The extent to which hepatic insufficiency or splenic disorders may increase the bioavailability of the parent or active metabolites of pentosan polysulfate sodium is not known. Caution should be exercised when using ELMIRON® in these patients.

Mildly (<2.5 × normal) elevated transaminase, alkaline phosphatase, γ-glutamyl transpeptidase, and lactic dehydrogenase occurred in 1.2% of patients. The increases usually appeared 3 to 12 months after the start of ELMIRON® therapy, and were not associated with jaundice or other clinical signs or symptoms. These abnormalities are usually transient, may remain essentially unchanged, or may rarely progress with continued use. Increases in PTT and PT (<1% for both) or thrombocytopenia (0.2%) were noted.

Alopecia is associated with pentosan polysulfate and with heparin products. In clinical trials of ELMIRON®, alopecia could begin within the first 4 weeks of treatment. Ninety-seven percent (97%) of the cases of alopecia reported were alopecia areata, limited to a single area on the scalp.

INFORMATION FOR PATIENTS:

Patients should take the drug as prescribed, in the dosage prescribed, and no more frequently than prescribed. Patients should be reminded that ELMIRON® has a weak anticoagulant effect. This effect may increase bleeding times.

LABORATORY TEST FINDINGS:

Pentosan polysulfate sodium did not affect prothrombin time (PT) or partial thromboplastin time (PTT) up to 1200 mg per day in 24 healthy male subjects treated for 8 days. Pentosan polysulfate sodium also inhibits the generation of factor Xa in plasma and inhibits thrombin-induced platelet aggregation in human platelet rich plasma ex vivo. (See **PRECAUTIONS**-Hepatic Insufficiency Section for additional information).

CARCINOGENICITY, MUTAGENESIS, IMPAIRMENT OF FERTILITY:

Long term studies in animals have not been performed to evaluate the carcinogenic potential of ELMIRON®. Pentosan polysulfate sodium was not clastogenic or mutagenic when tested in the mouse micronucleus test or the Ames test (*S. typhimurium*). The effect of pentosan polysulfate sodium on spermatogenesis has not been investigated.

PREGNANCY CATEGORY B:

Reproduction studies have been performed in mice and rats with intravenous daily doses of 15 mg/kg, and in rabbits with 7.5 mg/kg. These doses are 0.42 and 0.14 times the daily oral human doses of ELMIRON® when normalized to body surface area. These studies did not reveal evidence of impaired fertility or harm to the fetus from ELMIRON®. Direct in vitro bathing of cultured mouse embryos with pentosan polysulfate sodium (PPS) at a concentration of 1 mg/mL may cause reversible limb bud abnormalities. Adequate and well controlled studies have not been performed in pregnant women. Because animal studies are not always predictive of human response, this drug should be used in pregnancy only if clearly needed.

NURSING MOTHERS:

It is not known whether this drug is excreted in human milk. Because many drugs are excreted in human milk, caution should be exercised when ELMIRON® is administered to a nursing woman.

PEDIATRIC USE:

Safety and effectiveness in pediatric patients below the age of 16 years have not been established.

ADVERSE REACTIONS

ELMIRON® was evaluated in clinical trials in a total of 2627 patients (2343 women, 262 men, 22 unknown) with a mean age of 47 [range 18 to 88 with 581 (22%) over 60 years of age]. Of the 2627 patients, 128 patients were in a 3 month trial and the remaining 2499 patients were in a long term, unblinded trial.

Continued on next page

Elmiron—Cont.

Deaths occurred in 6/2627 (0.2%) patients who received the drug over a period of 3 to 75 months. The deaths appear to be related to other concurrent illnesses or procedures, except in one patient for whom the cause was not known. Serious adverse events occurred in 33/2627 (1.3%) patients. Two patients had severe abdominal pain or diarrhea and dehydration that required hospitalization. Because there was not a control group of patients with interstitial cystitis who were concurrently evaluated, it is difficult to determine which events are associated with ELMIRON® and which events are associated with concurrent illness, medicine, or other factors.

Adverse Experience in Placebo-Controlled Clinical Trials of ELMIRON® 100 mg Three Times a Day for 3 Months

Body System/ Adverse Experience		Elmiron® n=128	Placebo n=130
CNS	Overall Number of Patients*	3	5
	Insomnia	1	0
	Headache	1	3
	Severe Emotional Lability/Depression	2	1
	Nystagmus/Dizziness	1	1
	Hyperkinesia		1
GI	Overall Number of Patients*	7	7
	Nausea	3	3
	Diarrhea	3	6
	Dyspepsia	1	0
	Jaundice	0	1
	Vomiting	0	2
Skin/Allergic	Overall Number of Patients*	2	4
	Rash	0	2
	Pruritus	0	2
	Lacrimation	1	1
	Rhinitis	1	1
	Increased Sweating	1	0
Other	Overall Number of Patients*	1	3
	Amenorrhea	0	1
	Arthralgia	0	1
	Vaginitis	1	1
Total Events		17	27
Total Number of Patients Reporting Adverse Events		13	19

* Within a body system, the individual events do not sum to equal overall number of patients because a patient may have more than one event.

The adverse events described below were reported in an unblinded clinical trial of 2499 interstitial cystitis patients treated with ELMIRON®. Of the original 2499 patients, 1192 (48%) received ELMIRON® for 3 months; 892 (36%) received ELMIRON® for 6 months; and 598 (24%) received ELMIRON® for one year, 355 (14%) received ELMIRON ® for 2 years, and 145 (6%) for 4 years.

FREQUENCY (1 to 4%): Alopecia (4%), diarrhea (4%), nausea (4%), headache (3%), rash (3%), dyspepsia (2%), abdominal pain (2%), liver function abnormalities (1%), dizziness (1%).

FREQUENCY (≤1%):

Digestive: Vomiting, mouth ulcer, colitis, esophagitis, gastritis, flatulence, constipation, anorexia, gum hemorrhage.

Hematologic: Anemia, ecchymosis, increased prothrombin time, increased partial thromboplastin time, leukopenia, thrombocytopenia.

Hypersensitive Reactions: Allergic reaction, photosensitivity.

Respiratory System: Pharyngitis, rhinitis, epistaxis, dyspnea.

Skin and Appendages: Pruritus, urticaria.

Special Senses: Conjunctivitis, tinnitus, optic neuritis, amblyopia, retinal hemorrhage.

OVERDOSAGE

Overdose has not been reported. Based upon the pharmacodynamics of the drug, toxicity is likely to be reflected as anticoagulation, bleeding, thrombocytopenia, liver function abnormalities, and gastric distress. (See **CLINICAL PHARMACOLOGY** and **PRECAUTIONS** sections). In the event of acute overdosage, the patient should be given gastric lavage if possible, carefully observed and given symptomatic and supportive treatment.

DOSAGE AND ADMINISTRATION

The recommended dose of ELMIRON® is 300 mg/day taken as one 100 mg capsule orally three times daily. The capsules should be taken with water at least 1 hour before meals or 2 hours after meals.

Patients receiving ELMIRON® should be reassessed after 3 months. If improvement has not occurred and if limiting adverse events are not present, ELMIRON® may be continued for another 3 months.

The clinical value and risks of continued treatment in patients whose pain has not improved by 6 months is not known.

HOW SUPPLIED

ELMIRON® is supplied in white opaque hard gelatin capsules imprinted "BNP7600" containing 100 mg pentosan polysulfate sodium. Supplied in bottles of 100 capsules. NDC NUMBER 17314-9300-1

STORAGE

Store at controlled room temperature
15°–30°C (59°–86°F).

Rx only

ELMIRON® is a Registered Trademark of Baker Norton Pharmaceuticals, Inc. under license to ALZA Corporation.

ALZA Pharmaceuticals
A division of ALZA Corp.
Mountain View, CA 94043
Manufactured by:
Zenith Coldline Pharmaceuticals, Inc.
Miami, FL 33137
Distributed by
ALZA Corporation
Mountain View, CA 94043
1001719 REV 9810
Patent #5, 180, 715

Shown in Product Identification Guide, page 304

ETHYOL® ℞
[a-thī-ol]
(amifostine)
for Injection
Rx only

DESCRIPTION

ETHYOL (amifostine) is an organic thiophosphate cytoprotective agent known chemically as 2-[(3-aminopropyl)amino]ethanethiol dihydrogen phosphate (ester) and has the following structural formula:

$$H_2N(CH_2)_3NH(CH_2)_2S\text{-}PO_3H_2$$

Amifostine is a white crystalline powder which is freely soluble in water. Its empirical formula is $C_5H_{15}N_2O_3PS$ and it has a molecular weight of 214.22.

ETHYOL is the trihydrate form of amifostine and is supplied as a sterile lyophilized powder requiring reconstitution for intravenous infusion. Each single-use 10 mL vial contains 500 mg of amifostine on the anhydrous basis.

CLINICAL PHARMACOLOGY

ETHYOL is a prodrug that is dephosphorylated by alkaline phosphatase in tissues to a pharmacologically active free thiol metabolite. This metabolite is believed to be responsible for the reduction of the cumulative renal toxicity of cisplatin and for the reduction of the toxic effects of radiation on normal oral tissues. The ability of ETHYOL to differentially protect normal tissues is attributed to the higher capillary alkaline phosphatase activity, higher pH and better vascularity of normal tissues relative to tumor tissue, which results in a more rapid generation of the active thiol metabolite as well as a higher rate constant for uptake into cells. The higher concentration of the thiol metabolite in normal tissues is available to bind to, and thereby detoxify, reactive metabolites of cisplatin. This thiol metabolite can also scavenge reactive oxygen species generated by exposure to either cisplatin or radiation.

Pharmacokinetics: Clinical pharmacokinetic studies show that ETHYOL is rapidly cleared from the plasma with a distribution half-life of <1 minute and an elimination half-life of approximately 8 minutes. Less than 10% of ETHYOL remains in the plasma 6 minutes after drug administration. ETHYOL is rapidly metabolized to an active free thiol metabolite. A disulfide metabolite is produced subsequently and is less active than the free thiol. After a 10-second bolus dose of 150 mg/m² of ETHYOL, renal excretion of the parent drug and its two metabolites was low during the hour following drug administration, averaging 0.69%, 2.64% and 2.22% of the administered dose for the parent, thiol and disulfide, respectively. Measurable levels of the free thiol metabolite have been found in bone marrow cells 5–8 minutes after intravenous infusion of ETHYOL. Pretreatment with dexamethasone or metoclopramide has no effect on ETHYOL pharmacokinetics.

Clinical Studies

Chemotherapy for Ovarian Cancer and Non-Small Cell Lung Cancer. A randomized controlled trial compared six cycles of cylophosphamide 1000 mg/m², and cisplatin 100 mg/m² with or without ETHYOL pretreatment at 910 mg/m², in two successive cohorts of 121 patients with advanced ovarian cancer. In both cohorts, after multiple cycles of chemotherapy, pretreatment with ETHYOL significantly reduced the cumulative renal toxicity associated with cisplatin as assessed by the proportion of patients who had ≥40% decrease in creatinine clearance from pretreatment values, protracted elevations in serum creatinine (>1.5 mg/dL), or severe hypomagnesemia. Subgroup analyses suggested that the effect of ETHYOL was present in patients who had received nephrotoxic antibiotics, or who had preexisting diabetes or hypertension (and thus may have been at increased risk for significant nephrotoxicity), as well as in patients who lacked these risks. Selected analyses of the effects of ETHYOL in reducing the cumulative renal toxicity of cisplatin in the randomized ovarian cancer study are provided in TABLES 1 and 2, below.

TABLE 1
Proportion of Patients with ≥40% Reduction in Calculated Creatinine Clearance*

	ETHYOL + CP	CP	p-value (2-sided)
All patients	16/122 (13%)	36/120 (30%)	0.001
First Cohort	10/63	20/58	0.018
Second Cohort	6/59	16/62	0.026

*Creatinine clearance values were calculated using the Cockcroft-Gault formula, *Nephron* 1976;16:31–41.

[See table 2 below]

In the randomized ovarian cancer study, ETHYOL had no detectable effect on the antitumor efficacy of cisplatin-cyclophosphamide chemotherapy. Objective response rates (including pathologically confirmed complete remission rates), time to progression, and survival duration were all similar in the ETHYOL and control study groups. The table below summarizes the principal efficacy findings of the randomized ovarian cancer study.

[See table 3 at top of next page]

A Phase II trial of ETHYOL, 740–910 mg/m², and cisplatin, 120 mg/m², administered on day 1 and vinblastine, 5mg/m², administered on days 1, 8, 15 and 22 of each monthly cycle was conducted in 25 patients with Stage IV non-small cell lung cancer. This regimen was repeated until disease progression or unacceptable toxicity occurred, or a maximum of six cycles had been administered. Among 13 patients who received 4 or more cycles of this intensive cisplatin regimen, 1 had a ≥40% reduction in creatinine clearance. These results are consistent with the randomized ovarian cancer trial.

Sixteen of the 25 patients treated demonstrated a partial response to chemotherapy. With a median follow-up of 19 months, the median survival was 17 months. At one year, 64% of the patients were alive. These results indicate that ETHYOL may not adversely affect the efficacy of this chemotherapy for non-small cell lung cancer.

Radiotherapy for Head and Neck Cancer. A randomized controlled trial of standard fractionated radiation (1.8 Gy—2.0 Gy/day for 5 days/week for 5–7 weeks) with or without ETHYOL, administered at 200 mg/m² as a 3 minute i.v. infusion 15–30 minutes prior to each fraction of radiation, was conducted in 315 patients with head and neck cancer. Patients were required to have at least 75% of both parotid glands in the radiation field. The incidence of Grade 2 or higher acute (90 days or less from start of radiation) and late xerostomia (9–12 months following radiation) as assessed by RTOG Acute and Late Morbidity Scoring Criteria,

TABLE 2
NCI Toxicity Grades of Serum Magnesium Levels for Each Patient's Last Cycle of Therapy

NCI-CTC Grade: (mEq/L)	0 >1.4	1 ≤1.4->1.1	2 ≤1.1->0.8	3 ≤0.8->0.5	4 ≤0.5	p-value*
All Patients						0.001
ETHYOL + CP	92	13	3	0	0	
CP	73	18	7	5	1	
First Cohort						0.017
ETHYOL + CP	49	10	3	0	0	
CP	35	8	6	3	1	
Second Cohort						0.012
ETHYOL + CP	43	3	0	0	0	
CP	38	10	1	2	0	

*Based on 2-sided Mantel-Haenszel Chi-Square statistic.

TABLE 3
Comparison of Principal Efficacy Findings

	ETHYOL + CP	CP
Complete pathologic tumor response rate	21.3%	15.8%
Time to progression (months)		
Median (± 95% CI)	15.8 (13.2, 25.1)	18.1 (12.5, 20.4)
Mean (± Std error)	19.8 (±1.04)	19.1 (±1.58)
Hazard ratio (95% Confidence Interval)	.98 (.64, 1.4)	
Survival (months)		
Median (± 95% CI)	31.3 (28.3, 38.2)	31.8 (26.3, 39.8)
Mean (± Std error)	33.7 (±2.03)	34.3 (±2.04)
Hazard ratio (95% Confidence Interval)	.97 (.69, 1.32)	

was significantly reduced in patients receiving ETHYOL (TABLE 4).

TABLE 4
Incidence of Grade 2 or Higher Xerostomia (RTOG criteria)

	ETHYOL + RT	RT	p-value
Acute (≤90 days from start of radiation	51% (75/148)	78% (120/153)	p<0.0001
Late[a] (9–12 months post radiation)	35% (36/103)	57% (63/111)	p=0.0016

[a]Based on the number of patients for whom actual data were available.

At one year following radiation, whole saliva collection following radiation showed that more patients given ETHYOL produced >0.1 gm of saliva (72% vs. 49%). In addition, the median saliva production at one year was higher in those patients who received ETHYOL (0.26 gm vs. 0.1 gm). Stimulated saliva collections did not show a difference between treatment arms. These improvements in saliva production were supported by the patients' subjective responses to a questionnaire regarding oral dryness.

In the randomized head and neck cancer study, locoregional control, disease-free survival and overall survival were all comparable in the two treatment groups after one year of follow-up (see TABLE 5).

[See table 5 below]

INDICATIONS AND USAGE

ETHYOL (amifostine) is indicated to reduce the cumulative renal toxicity associated with repeated administration of cisplatin in patients with advanced ovarian cancer or non-small cell lung cancer.

ETHYOL is indicated to reduce the incidence of moderate to severe xerostomia in patients undergoing post-operative radiation treatment for head and neck cancer, where the radiation port includes a substantial portion of the parotid glands (see Clinical Studies).

For the approved indications, the clinical data do not suggest that the effectiveness of cisplatin based chemotherapy regimens or radiation therapy is altered by ETHYOL. There are at present only limited data on the effects of ETHYOL on the efficacy of chemotherapy or radiotherapy in other settings. ETHYOL should not be administered to patients in other settings where chemotherapy can produce a significant survival benefit or cure, or in patients receiving definitive radiotherapy, except in the context of a clinical study (see WARNINGS).

CONTRAINDICATIONS

ETHYOL is contraindicated in patients with known sensitivity to aminothiol compounds.

WARNINGS

1. Effectiveness of the Cytotoxic Regimen

Limited data are currently available regarding the preservation of antitumor efficacy when ETHYOL is administered prior to cisplatin therapy in settings other than advanced ovarian cancer or non-small cell lung cancer. Although some animal data suggest interference is possible, in most tumor models the antitumor effects of chemotherapy are not altered by amifostine. ETHYOL should not be used in patients receiving chemotherapy for other malignancies in which chemotherapy can produce a significant survival benefit or cure (e.g., certain malignancies of germ cell origin), except in the context of a clinical study.

2. Effectiveness of Radiotherapy

ETHYOL should not be administered in patients receiving definitive radiotherapy, except in the context of a clinical trial, since there are at present insufficient data to exclude a tumor-protective effect in this setting. ETHYOL was studied only with standard fractionated radiotherapy and only when ≥75% of both parotid glands were exposed to radiation. The effects of ETHYOL on the incidence of xerostomia and on toxicity in the setting of combined chemotherapy and radiotherapy and in the setting of accelerated and hyperfractionated therapy have not been systematically studied.

3. Hypotension

Patients who are hypotensive or in a state of dehydration should not receive ETHYOL. Patients receiving ETHYOL at doses recommended for chemotherapy who are taking antihypertensive therapy that cannot be stopped for 24 hours preceding ETHYOL treatment, should not receive ETHYOL. Patients should be adequately hydrated prior to ETHYOL infusion and kept in a supine position during the infusion. Blood pressure should be monitored every 5 minutes during the infusion, and thereafter as clinically indicated. It is important that the duration of the 910 mg/m^2 infusion not exceed 15 minutes, as administration of ETHYOL as a longer infusion is associated with a higher incidence of side effects. For infusion durations less than 5 minutes, blood pressure should be monitored at least before and immediately after the infusion, and thereafter as clinically indicated. If hypotension occurs, patients should be placed in the Trendelenburg position and be given an infusion of normal saline using a separate i.v. line. Guidelines for interrupting and restarting ETHYOL infusion if a decrease in systolic blood pressure should occur are provided in the DOSAGE AND ADMINISTRATION section. Hypotension may occur during or shortly after ETHYOL infusion, despite adequate hydration and positioning of the patient (see ADVERSE REACTIONS and GENERAL PRECAUTIONS). Hypotension has been reported to be associated with dyspnea, apnea, hypoxia, and in rare cases seizures, unconsciousness, respiratory arrest and renal failure.

4. Nausea and Vomiting

Antiemetic medication should be administered prior to and in conjunction with ETHYOL (see DOSAGE AND ADMINISTRATION). When ETHYOL is administered with highly emetogenic chemotherapy, the fluid balance of the patient should be carefully monitored.

5. Hypocalcemia

Serum calcium levels should be monitored in patients at risk of hypocalcemia, such as those with nephrotic syndrome or patients receiving multiple doses of ETHYOL (see ADVERSE REACTIONS). If necessary, calcium supplements can be administered.

PRECAUTIONS

General

Patients should be adequately hydrated prior to the ETHYOL infusion and blood pressure should be monitored (see DOSAGE AND ADMINISTRATION).

The safety of ETHYOL administration has not been established in elderly patients, or in patients with preexisting cardiovascular or cerebrovascular conditions such as ischemic heart disease, arrhythmias, congestive heart failure, or history of stroke or transient ischemic attacks. ETHYOL should be used with particular care in these and other patients in whom the common ETHYOL adverse effects of nausea/vomiting and hypotension may be more likely to have serious consequences.

Prior to chemotherapy, ETHYOL should be administered as a 15-minute infusion (see DOSAGE AND ADMINISTRATION). Blood pressure should be monitored every 5 minutes during the infusion, and thereafter as clinically indicated.

Prior to radiation therapy, ETHYOL should be administered as a 3-minute infusion (see DOSAGE AND ADMINISTRATION). Blood pressure should be monitored at least before and immediately after the infusion, and thereafter as clinically indicated.

Drug Interactions

Special consideration should be given to the administration of ETHYOL in patients receiving antihypertensive medications or other drugs that could cause or potentiate hypotension.

Carcinogenesis, Mutagenesis, Impairment of Fertility

No long term animal studies have been performed to evaluate the carcinogenic potential of ETHYOL. ETHYOL was negative in the Ames test and in the mouse micronucleus test. The free thiol metabolite was positive in the Ames test with S9 microsomal fraction in the TA1535 *Salmonella typhimurium* strain and at the TK locus in the mouse L5178Y cell assay. The metabolite was negative in the mouse micronucleus test and negative for clastogenicity in human lymphocytes.

Pregnancy

Pregnancy Category C. ETHYOL has been shown to be embryotoxic in rabbits at doses of 50 mg/kg, approximately sixty percent of the recommended dose in humans on a body surface area basis. There are no adequate and well-controlled studies in pregnant women. ETHYOL should be used during pregnancy only if the potential benefit justifies the potential risk to the fetus.

Nursing Mothers

No information is available on the excretion of ETHYOL or its metabolites into human milk. Because many drugs are excreted in human milk and because of the potential for adverse reactions in nursing infants, it is recommended that breast feeding be discontinued if the mother is treated with ETHYOL.

Pediatric Use

The safety and effectiveness in pediatric patients have not been established.

ADVERSE REACTONS

In the randomized study of patients with ovarian cancer given ETHYOL at a dose of 910 mg/m^2 prior to chemotherapy, transient hypotension was observed in 62% of patients treated. The mean time of onset was 14 minutes into the 15-minute period of ETHYOL infusion, and the mean duration was 6 minutes. In some cases, the infusion had to be prematurely terminated due to a more pronounced drop in systolic blood pressure. In general, the blood pressure returned to normal within 5–15 minutes. Fewer than 3% of patients discontinued ETHYOL due to blood pressure reductions. In the randomized study of patients with head and neck cancer given ETHYOL at a dose of 200 mg/m^2 prior to

Continued on next page

TABLE 5
Comparison of Principal Efficacy Findings at 1 Year

	ETHYOL + RT	RT
Locoregional Control Rate[a]	76.1%	75.0%
Hazard Ratio[b]	1.013	
95% Confidence Interval	(0.671, 1.530)	
Disease-Free Survival Rate[a]	74.6%	70.4%
Hazard Ratio[b]	1.035	
95% Confidence Interval	(0.702, 1.528)	
Overall Survival Rate[a]	89.4%	82.4%
Hazard Ratio[b]	1.585	
95% Confidence Interval	(0.961, 2.613)	

[a]1 year rates estimated using Kaplan-Meier method
[b]Hazard ratio >1.0 is in favor of the ETHYOL + RT arm

TABLE 6
Incidence of Common Adverse Events in Patients Receiving ETHYOL

	Phase III Ovarian Cancer Trial (WR-1) 910 mg/m^2		Phase III Head and Neck Cancer Trial (WR-38) 200 mg/m^2	
	Per Patient	Per Infusion	Per Patient	Per Infusion
Nausea/Vomiting				
≥Grade 3	36/122 (30%)	53/592 (9%)	12/150 (8%)	13/4314 (<1%)
All Grades	117/122 (96%)	520/592 (88%)	80/150 (53%)	233/4314 (5%)
Hypotension				
≥Grade 3[a]	10/122 (8%)		4/150 (3%)	
All Grades	75/122 (61%)	159/592 (27%)	22/150 (15%)	46/4314 (1%)

[a]According to protocol-defined criteria. WR-1: requiring interruption of infusion; WR-38: drop of >20mm Hg.

Ethyol—Cont.

radiotherapy, hypotension was observed in 15% of patients treated.
Hypotension that requires interruption of the ETHYOL infusion should be treated with fluid infusion and postural management of the patient (supine or Trendelenburg position). If the blood pressure returns to normal within 5 minutes and the patient is asymptomatic, the infusion may be restarted, so that the full dose of ETHYOL can be administered.
Short term, reversible loss of consciousness has been reported rarely. Blood pressure reductions during ETHYOL administration have not been reported to cause long term CNS, cardiovascular or renal sequelae, but clinical studies performed to date have not evaluated the safety of ETHYOL in elderly patients or in patients with preexisting cardiovascular or cerebrovascular conditions.
Nausea and/or vomiting occur frequently after ETHYOL infusion and may be severe. In the ovarian cancer randomized study, the incidence of severe nausea/vomiting on day 1 of cyclophosphamide-cisplatin chemotherapy was 10% in patients who did not receive ETHYOL, and 19% in patients who did receive ETHYOL. In the randomized study of patients with head and neck cancer, the incidence of severe nausea/vomiting was 8% in patients who received ETHYOL and 1% in patients who did not receive ETHYOL.
Other effects which have been described during or following ETHYOL infusion are flushing/feeling of warmth, chills/feeling of coldness, fever, dizziness, somnolence, hiccups and sneezing. These effects have not generally precluded the completion of therapy.
Decrease in serum calcium concentrations is a known pharmacological effect of ETHYOL. At the recommended doses, clinically significant hypocalcemia has occurred rarely (<1%) (see WARNINGS).
Allergic reactions have been reported with the use of ETHYOL. The majority of cases presented with the following symptoms: hypotension, fever, chills/rigors, dyspnea, skin rashes and urticaria. Other skin reactions including erythema multiforme, and in rare cases Stevens-Johnson Syndrome and toxic epidermal necrolysis, have been reported.
There have been rare reports of anaphylactoid reactions including hypoxia, laryngeal edema, chest tightness, and possible cardiac arrest.
There have been rare reports of seizures in patients receiving ETHYOL.
TABLE 6 contains a summary of the more common adverse events from the two approved doses of ETHYOL:
[See table 6 at bottom of previous page]
In the randomized study of patients with head and neck cancer, 17% (26/150) discontinued ETHYOL due to adverse events. All but one of these patients continued to receive radiation treatment until completion.

OVERDOSAGE

In clinical trials, the maximum single dose of ETHYOL was 1300 mg/m^2. No information is available on single doses higher than this in adults. In the setting of a clinical trial, pediatric patients have received single ETHYOL doses of up to 2700 mg/m^2. At the higher doses, anxiety and reversible urinary retention occurred.
Administration of ETHYOL at 2 and 4 hours after the initial dose has not led to increased nausea and vomiting or hypotension. The most likely symptom of overdosage is hypotension, which should be managed by infusion of normal saline and other supportive measures, as clinically indicated.

DOSAGE AND ADMINISTRATION

For Reduction of Cumulative Renal Toxicity with Chemotherapy: The recommended starting dose of ETHYOL is 910 mg/m^2 administered once daily as a 15-minute i.v. infusion, starting 30 minutes prior to chemotherapy.
The 15-minute infusion is better tolerated than more extended infusions. Further reductions in infusion times for chemotherapy regimens have not been systematically investigated.
Patients should be adequately hydrated prior to ETHYOL infusion and kept in a supine position during the infusion. Blood pressure should be monitored every 5 minutes during the infusion, and thereafter as clinically indicated.
The infusion of ETHYOL should be interrupted if the systolic blood pressure decreases significantly from the baseline value as listed in the guideline below:

Guideline for Interrupting ETHYOL Infusion Due to Decrease in Systolic Blood Pressure

	Baseline Systolic Blood Pressure (mm Hg)				
	<100	100–119	120–139	140–179	≥180
Decrease in systolic blood pressure during infusion of ETHYOL (mm Hg)	20	25	30	40	50

If the blood pressure returns to normal within 5 minutes and the patient is asymptomatic, the infusion may be restarted so that the full dose of ETHYOL may be administered. If the full dose of ETHYOL cannot be administered, the dose of ETHYOL for subsequent chemotherapy cycles should be 740 mg/m^2.
It is recommended that antiemetic medication, including dexamethasone 20 mg i.v. and a serotonin 5HT$_3$ receptor antagonist, be administered prior to and in conjunction with ETHYOL. Additional antiemetics may be required based on the chemotherapy drugs administered.
For Reduction of Moderate to Severe Xerostomia from Radiation of the Head and Neck: The recommended dose of ETHYOL is 200 mg/m^2 administered once daily as a 3-minute i.v. infusion, starting 15–30 minutes prior to standard fraction radiation therapy (1.8–2.0 Gy).
Patients should be adequately hydrated prior to ETHYOL infusion. Blood pressure should be monitored at least before and immediately after the infusion, and thereafter as clinically indicated.
It is recommended that antiemetic medication be administered prior to and in conjunction with ETHYOL. Oral 5HT$_3$ receptor antagonists, alone or in combination with other antiemetics, have been used effectively in the radiotherapy setting.

Reconstitution
ETHYOL (amifostine) for Injection is supplied as a sterile lyophilized powder requiring reconstitution for intravenous infusion. Each single-use vial contains 500 mg of amifostine on the anhydrous basis.
Prior to intravenous injection, ETHYOL is reconstituted with 9.7 mL of sterile 0.9% Sodium Chloride Injection, USP. The reconstituted solution (500 mg amifostine/10 mL) is chemically stable for up to 5 hours at room temperature (approximately 25°C) or up to 24 hours under refrigeration (2°C to 8°C).
ETHYOL prepared in polyvinylchloride (PVC) bags at concentrations ranging from 5 mg/mL to 40 mg/mL is chemically stable for up to 5 hours when stored at room temperature (approximately 25°C) or up to 24 hours when stored under refrigeration (2°C to 8°C).
CAUTION: Parenteral products should be inspected visually for particulate matter and discoloration prior to administration whenever solution and container permit. Do not use if cloudiness or precipitate is observed.

Incompatibilities
The compatibility of ETHYOL with solutions other than 0.9% Sodium Chloride for Injection, or Sodium Chloride solutions with other additives, has not been examined. The use of other solutions is not recommended.

HOW SUPPLIED

ETHYOL (amifostine) for Injection is supplied as a sterile lyophilized powder in 10 mL single-use vials (NDC 17314-7253-1). Each single-use vial contains 500 mg of amifostine on the anhydrous basis. The vials are available packaged as follows:
3 pack—3 vials per carton (NDC 17314-7253-3)
Store the lyophilized dosage form at Controlled Room Temperature 20°–25°C (68°–77°F) [See USP].
U.S. Patents 5,424,471; 5,591,731
Manufactured by:
USB Pharma B.V.
6545 CG Nijmegen
The Netherlands
Or:
Ben Venue, Inc.
Bedford, Ohio 44146
Marketed by:
ALZA Pharmaceuticals
A division of ALZA Corporation
Palo Alto,
California 94303
And:
U.S. Bioscience, Inc.
West Conshohocken,
Pennsylvania 19428
1-800-506-4959

Revision Date 6/99 N-LB2022 PE
Shown in Product Identification Guide, page 304

MYCELEX® ℞
(clotrimazole) TROCHE
FOR TOPICAL ORAL ADMINISTRATION

DESCRIPTION

Each Mycelex® Troche contains 10mg clotrimazole [1-(o-chloro-α,α-diphenylbenzyl) imidazole], a synthetic antifungal agent, for topical use in the mouth.
Structural Formula:

Chemical Formula: $C_{22}H_{17}ClN_2$

The troche dosage from is a large, slowly dissolving tablet (lozenge) containing 10 mg of clotrimazole dispersed in dextrose, microcrystalline cellulose, povidone, and magnesium stearate.

CLINICAL PHARMACOLOGY

Clotrimazole is a broad-spectrum antifungal agent that inhibits the growth of pathogenic yeasts by altering the permeability of cell membranes. The action of clotrimazole is fungistatic at concentrations of drug up to 20 mcg/mL and may be fungicidal *in vitro* against *Candida albicans* and other species of the genus *Candida* at higher concentrations. No single-step or multiple-step resistance to clotrimazole has developed during successive passages of *Candida albicans* in the laboratory; however, individual organism tolerance has been observed during successive passages in the laboratory. Such *in vitro* tolerance has resolved once the organism has been removed from the antifungal environment.
After oral administration of a 10 mg clotrimazole troche to healthy volunteers, concentrations sufficient to inhibit most species of *Candida* persist in saliva for up to three hours following the approximately 30 minutes needed for a troche to dissolve. The long term persistence of drug in saliva appears to be related to the slow release of clotrimazole from the oral mucosa to which the drug is apparently bound. Repetitive dosing at three hour intervals maintains salivary levels above the minimum inhibitory concentrations of most strains of *Candida;* however, the relationship between *in vitro* susceptibility of pathogenic fungi to clotrimazole and prophylaxis or cure of infections in humans has not been established.
In another study, the mean serum concentrations were 4.98 ± 3.7 and 3.23 ± 1.4 nanograms/mL of clotrimazole at 30 and 60 minutes, respectively, after administration as a troche.

INDICATIONS AND USAGE

Mycelex® Troches are indicated for the local treatment of oropharyngeal candidiasis. The diagnosis should be confirmed by a KOH smear and/or culture prior to treatment.
Mycelex® Troches are also indicated prophylactically to reduce the incidence of oropharyngeal candidiasis in patients immunocompromised by conditions that include chemotherapy, radiotherapy, or steroid therapy utilized in the treatment of leukemia, solid tumors, or renal transplantation. There are no data from adequate and well-controlled trials to establish the safety and efficacy of this product for prophylactic use in patients immunocompromised by etiologies other than those listed in the previous sentence (See DOSAGE AND ADMINISTRATION.)

CONTRAINDICATIONS

Mycelex® Troches are contra-indicated in patients who are hypersensitive to any of its components.

WARNING

Mycelex® Troches are not indicated for the treatment of systemic mycoses including systemic candidiasis.

PRECAUTIONS

Abnormal liver function tests have been reported in patients treated with clotrimazole troches; elevated SGOT levels were reported in about 15% of patients in the clinical trials. In most cases the elevations were minimal and it was often impossible to distinguish effects of clotrimazole from those of other therapy and the underlying disease (malignancy in most cases). Periodic assessment of hepatic function is advisable particularly in patients with pre-existing hepatic impairment.
Since patients must be instructed to allow each troche to dissolve slowly in the mouth in order to achieve maximum effect of the medication, they must be of such an age and physical and/or mental condition to comprehend such instructions.
Carcinogenesis: An 18 month dosing study with clotrimazole in rats has not revealed any carcinogenic effect.
Usage in Pregnancy: Pregnancy Category C: Clotrimazole has been shown to be embryotoxic in rats and mice when given in doses 100 times the adult human dose (in mg/kg), possibly secondary to maternal toxicity. The drug was not teratogenic in mice, rabbits, and rats when given in doses up to 200, 180, and 100 times the human dose.
Clotrimazole given orally to mice from nine weeks before mating through weaning at a dose 120 times the human dose was associated with impairment of mating, decreased number of viable young, and decreased survival to weaning. No effects were observed at 60 times the human dose. When the drug was given to rats during a similar time period at 50 times the human dose, there was a slight decrease in the number of pups per litter and decreased pup viability.
There are no adequate and well controlled studies in pregnant women. Clotrimazole troches should be used during pregnancy only if the potential benefit justifies the potential risk to the fetus.
PEDIATRIC USE Safety and effectiveness of clotrimazole in children below the age of 3 years have not been established; therefore, its use in such patients is not recommended.
The safety and efficacy of the prophylactic use of clotrimazole troches in children have not been established.

	Strength	NDC Code	Tablet Identification
Bottles of 70:	10 mg	NDC 17314-9400-1	MYCELEX 10
Bottles of 140:	10 mg	NDC 17314-9400-3	MYCELEX 10
Unit Dose Package of 70:	10 mg	NDC 17314-9400-2	MYCELEX 10

ADVERSE REACTIONS

Abnormal liver function tests have been reported in patients treated with clotrimazole troches; elevated SGOT levels were reported in about 15% of patients in the clinical trials (See Precautions section).

Nausea, vomiting, unpleasant mouth sensations and pruritus have also been reported with the use of the troche.

OVERDOSAGE

No data available.

DRUG ABUSE AND DEPENDENCE

No data available.

DOSAGE AND ADMINISTRATION

Mycelex® Troches are administered only as a lozenge that must be slowly dissolved in the mouth. The recommended dose is one troche five times a day for fourteen consecutive days. Only limited data are available on the safety and effectiveness of the clotrimazole troche after prolonged administration; therefore, therapy should be limited to short term use, if possible.

For prophylaxis to reduce the incidence of oropharyngeal candidiasis in patients immunocompromised by conditions that include chemotherapy, radiotherapy, or steroid therapy utilized in the treatment of leukemia, solid tumors, or renal transplantation, the recommended dose is one troche three times daily for the duration of chemotherapy or until steroids are reduced to maintenance levels.

HOW SUPPLIED

Mycelex® Troches, white discoid, uncoated tablets are supplied in bottles of 70 and 140. Mycelex® Troches are also available for institutional use in foil packages of 70 tablets. Each tablet will be identified with the following: Mycelex 10.

[See table above]

Store below 86°F (30°C).

Avoid freezing.

Rx only

Manufactured by Bayer Corporation
West Haven, CT 06516

Distributed by ALZA Pharmaceuticals
A Division of ALZA Corporation
Mountain View, CA 94043

PD100799 6/98 BAY 5097

©1998 Bayer Corporation 8349

Shown in Product Identification Guide, page 304

POLYCITRA® SYRUP ℞
POLYCITRA®-LC ℞

[*polly "si-trah*]

(tricitrates oral solution)

DESCRIPTION

Syrup POLYCITRA® and POLYCITRA®-LC are stable and pleasant-tasting oral systemic alkalizers containing potassium citrate, sodium citrate, and citric acid. Syrup POLYCITRA® is a sugar-base preparation. POLYCITRA®-LC is a sugar-free solution, to be used by patients who desire a low-carbohydrate diet. Both products are non-alcoholic and contain identical amounts of active ingredients.

HOW SUPPLIED

POLYCITRA®-Syrup
16 fl. oz. (473 mL)
(NDC 17314-9322-1)

POLYCITRA®-LC
16 fl. oz. (473 mL)
(NDC 17314-9323-1)

Keep tightly closed and protect from excessive heat and freezing.

Rx only

©1998Baker Norton Pharmaceuticals, Inc.

POLYCITRA® and POLYCITRA®-LC are Registered Trademarks of Baker Norton Pharmaceuticals, Inc. under license to ALZA Corporation.

Distributed by:
ALZA Corporation
Mountain View, CA 94043

Manufactured by:
Draxis Pharma Inc.
Kirkland, Quebec H9H 4J4
Canada
MADE IN CANADA

ALZA Pharmaceuticals
A division of ALZA Corp.
Mountain View, CA 94043

1001739 REV9804
(212011)

POLYCITRA–K CRYSTALS® ℞

[*polly "si-trah- kāy*]

(Potassium Citrate and Citric Acid for Oral Solution)

DESCRIPTION

POLYCITRA–K CRYSTALS® is a pleasant-tasting oral systemic alkalizer containing potassium citrate and citric acid in a sugar-free base.

HOW SUPPLIED

POLYCITRA-K CRYSTALS®

—Unit Dose Packets, 100/box (NDC 17314–9320–1).

Protect from excessive heat or freezing.

Rx only

©1998 Baker Norton Pharmaceuticals, Inc.

POLYCITRA-K Crystals® is a registered Trademark of Baker Norton Pharmaceuticals, Inc. under license to ALZA Corporation

POLYCITRA-K Crystals® is Distributed by
ALZA Corporation
Mountain view, CA 94043

Manufactured by
Zenith Goldline Pharmaceuticals, Inc.
Miami, FL 33137

ALZA Pharmaceuticals
A division of
ALZA Corp.
Mountain View, CA 94043

1001734 REV9802

POLYCITRA®–K ORAL SOLUTION ℞

[*polly" si-trah-kāy*]

Potassium Citrate and Citric Acid Oral Solution, USP

DESCRIPTION

POLYCITRA®-K is a stable and pleasant-tasting oral systemic alkalizer containing potassium citrate and citric acid in a sugar-free non-alcoholic base.

HOW SUPPLIED

POLYCITRA®-K ORAL SOLUTION

—16 fl. oz. (473 mL)
(NDC 17314-9321-1).

Keep tightly closed and protect from excessive heat or freezing.

Rx only

©1998 Baker Norton Pharmaceuticals, Inc.

POLYCITRA®-K is a Registered Trademark of Baker Norton Pharmaceuticals, Inc. under license to ALZA Corporation.

Distributed by:
ALZA Corporation
Mountain View, CA 94043

Manufactured by:
Draxis Pharma Inc.
Kirkland, Quebec H9H 4J4
Canada
MADE IN CANADA

ALZA Pharmaceuticals
A division of ALZA Corp.
Mountain View, CA 94043

1001729 REV 9804
(212021)

TESTODERM® TTS Ⓒⅲ

[*tes-tō-derm*]

Testosterone Transdermal System
5 mg/day

TESTODERM®

Testosterone Transdermal System
4 or 6 mg/day

TESTODERM® WITH ADHESIVE

Testosterone Transdermal System
6 mg/day

CONTROLLED DELIVERY
FOR ONCE-DAILY APPLICATION

DESCRIPTION

TESTODERM® TTS, TESTODERM®, and TESTODERM® WITH ADHESIVE Testosterone Transdermal Systems (referred to collectively as the TESTODERM® products) are designed to release controlled amounts of testosterone, the primary circulating endogenous androgen, continuously upon application to the arm, back or upper buttocks (TESTODERM® TTS) or scrotal skin (TESTODERM® and TESTODERM® WITH ADHESIVE). The TESTODERM® products are described below.

[See table at top of next page]

The active component of each of the systems is testosterone. Testosterone USP is a white or creamy-white crystalline powder or crystals chemically described as 17-beta hydroxyandrost-4-en-3-one. The remaining components of the systems are pharmacologically inactive.

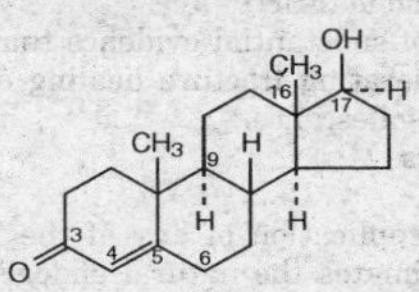

Testosterone
$C_{19}H_{28}O_2$ **MW 288.43**

TESTODERM® TTS is composed of the following layers: a flexible backing of transparent polyester/ethylene-vinyl acetate copolymer film, a drug reservoir of testosterone USP and 1.2 mL alcohol USP gelled with hydroxypropyl cellulose, and an ethylene-vinyl acetate copolymer membrane coated with a layer of polyisobutylene adhesive formulation that controls the rate of release of testosterone from the system. A protective liner of silicone-coated polyester covers the adhesive surface. The liner must be removed before application.

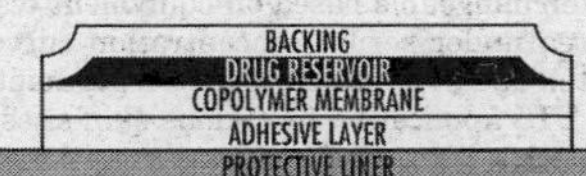

TESTODERM® is composed of two layers: a soft flexible backing of polyester and a testosterone-containing film of ethylene-vinyl acetate copolymer that contacts the skin surface and modulates the availability of the steroid. A protective liner of fluorocarbon diacrylate or silicone-coated polyester covers the drug film. The liner must be removed before application.

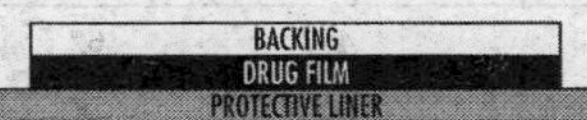

TESTODERM® WITH ADHESIVE is composed of three layers: a soft flexible backing of polyester and a testosterone-containing film of ethylene-vinyl acetate copolymer. The surface of the drug film is partially covered by the third layer: thin and narrow adhesive stripes composed of polyisobutylene and colloidal silicon dioxide. A protective liner of fluorocarbon diacrylate-coated polyester covers the adhesive stripes and the adhesive-free area of the drug film. The liner must be removed before application.

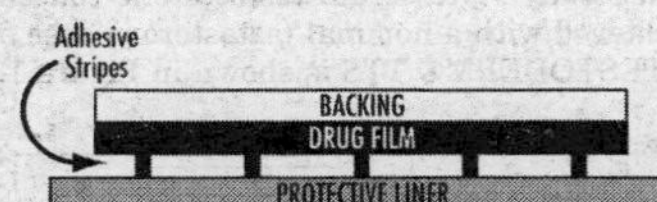

CLINICAL PHARMACOLOGY

Testosterone

The TESTOSDERM® products deliver physiologic amounts of testosterone, the primary endogenous androgenic hormone. Endogenous testosterone serum concentrations in normal males follow a circadian pattern. Daily morning application of any of the TESTODERM® products results in a serum testosterone profile that approximates the natural endogenous pattern of normal men.

General Androgen Effects

Endogenous androgens, including testosterone and dihydrotestosterone (DHT), are responsible for the normal growth and development of the male sex organs and for maintenance of secondary sex characteristics. These effects include the growth and maturation of prostate, seminal vesicles, penis, and scrotum; the development of male hair distribution, such as facial, pubic, chest, and axillary hair; laryngeal enlargement, vocal chord thickening, alterations in body musculature, and fat distribution. DHT is necessary for the normal development of secondary sex characteristics.

Male hypogonadism results from insufficient secretion of testosterone and is characterized by low serum testosterone concentrations. Symptoms associated with male hypogonadism include impotence and decreased sexual desire, fatigue and loss of energy, mood depression, and regression of secondary sexual characteristics.

Drugs in the androgen class also cause retention of nitrogen, sodium, potassium, phosphorus, and decreased urinary excretion of calcium. Androgens have been reported to increase protein anabolism and decrease protein catabolism. Nitrogen balance is improved only when there is sufficient intake of calories and protein.

Androgens are responsible for the growth spurt of adolescence and for the eventual termination of linear growth brought about by fusion of the epiphyseal growth centers. In children, exogenous androgens accelerate linear growth rates but may cause a disproportionate advancement in bone maturation. Use over long periods may result in fusion of the epiphyseal growth centers and termination of the growth process. Androgens have been reported to stimulate the production of red blood cells by enhancing the production of erythropoietin.

During exogenous administration of androgens, endogenous testosterone release may be inhibited through feedback inhibition of pituitary luteinizing hormone (LH). At large

Continued on next page

Testoderm—Cont.

doses of exogenous androgens, spermatogenesis may also be suppressed through feedback inhibition of pituitary follicle-stimulating hormone (FSH).
There is a lack of substantial evidence that androgens are effective in accelerating fracture healing or in shortening post-surgical convalescence.

Pharmacokinetics

Absorption

Daily morning application of any of the TESTODERM® products approximates the natural endogenous pattern of serum testosterone of normal males. Following application, testosterone is continuously absorbed during the 24-hour dosing period. The serum testosterone concentrations rise to a maximum at 2 to 4 hours and return toward baseline within approximately 2 hours after system removal. The testosterone levels achieved with the TESTODERM® products generally are within the range for normal men. Patients vary in their ability to absorb testosterone transdermally (see **Clinical Studies**).

TESTODERM® TTS

For TESTODERM® TTS three skin sites (arm, back, and upper buttocks), representing recommended application sites, are interchangeable based on equivalent testosterone $AUC_{(0-27)}$ (area under serum concentration curve) values. The estimated mean pharmacokinetic parameters after Testoderm® TTS application to various skin sites are presented in Table 1.

Table 1
Mean Serum Testosterone Pharmacokinetic Parameters after Application of Testoderm® TTS to Three Different Skin Sites (n=13)

PARAMETERS	TREATMENTS Upper Buttocks	Arm	Back
C_{max} (ng/dL)	482	462	499
*T_{max} (h)	3.9	4.0	3.9
AUC (ng•h/dL)	9,560	8,651	8,988

*Median value

In clinical trials, 94% of patients on TESTODERM® TTS treatment achieved maximum and average serum testosterone concentrations (C_{max} and C_{avg}, respectively) within the normal range; the average C_{max} and C_{avg} serum testosterone concentrations were 531 ng/dL and 366 ng/dL, respectively. Within-subject coefficient of variation in testosterone C_{avg} for subjects on TESTODERM® TTS therapy was 17%. The typical steady state serum testosterone concentration pattern achieved with a nominal testosterone dose of 5 mg/day from TESTODERM® TTS is shown in Figure 1.

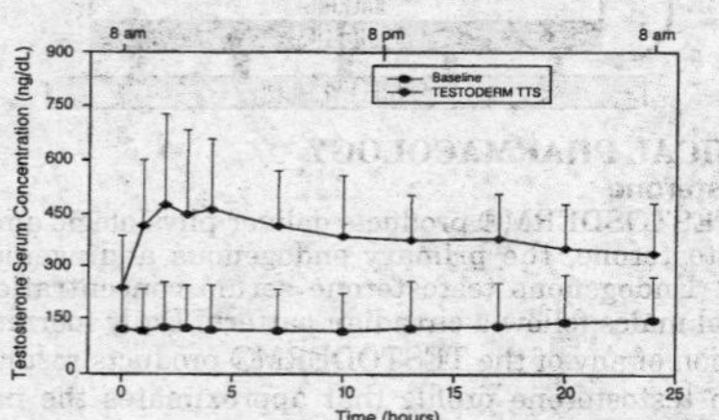

Figure 1. *Serum concentrations of testosterone (mean ± SD) during pretreatment baseline or while wearing a TESTODERM® TTS system on the upper buttocks (n=32). Systems were applied at 0 hours (8 AM) and removed 24 hours later.*

Normal range serum testosterone concentrations are reached during the first day of dosing.
There is no accumulation of testosterone following repeated application of TESTODERM® TTS.
Two TESTODERM® TTS systems deliver a testosterone dose which is twice that delivered by a single system.
There is no first-pass skin metabolism of testosterone to DHT when applied to arm, back or upper buttocks skin sites as recommended.

TESTODERM®

Scrotal skin is at least five times more permeable to testosterone than other skin sites. TESTODERM® or TESTODERM® WITH ADHESIVE will not produce adequate serum testosterone concentrations if applied to non-scrotal skin.
Hypogonadal men using TESTODERM® therapy have trough serum testosterone concentrations that are about 15% of peak levels. Serum levels reach a plateau at 3 to 4 weeks.

TESTODERM® WITH ADHESIVE

Data from a pharmacokinetic trial in 50 normal male subjects show that TESTODERM® WITH ADHESIVE applied to scrotal skin is equivalent to TESTODERM® with respect to rate (C_{max}) and extent (AUC) of testosterone delivery.

Distribution

Circulating testosterone is chiefly bound in the serum to sex hormone-binding globulin (SHBG) and albumin. The albumin-bound fraction of testosterone easily dissociates from albumin and is presumed to be bioactive. The portion of testosterone bound to SHBG is not considered biologically active. The amount of SHBG in the serum and the total testosterone level will determine the distribution of bioactive and nonbioactive androgen. SHBG-binding capacity is high in prepubertal children, declines during puberty and adulthood, and increases again during the later decades of life.

	Dose (mg/day)	Size (cm^2)	Application Site
Testoderm® TTS	5	60	Arm, Back, Upper Buttocks
Testoderm®*	6	60	Scrotum
Testoderm®*	4	40	Scrotum
Testoderm® with Adhesive	6	60	Scrotum

* The composition of the two sizes per unit area is identical.

Metabolism

There is considerable variation in the half-life of testosterone as reported in the literature, ranging from 10 to 100 minutes. Testosterone is a substrate for conversion to an active metabolite, dihydrotestosterone (DHT). Testosterone is metabolized to various 17-keto steroids through two different pathways, and the major active metabolites are estradiol and DHT. Concentrations of estradiol in normal men are 1.0 to 5.0 ng/dL. DHT concentrations in normal male serum are 30 to 85 ng/dL. DHT binds with greater affinity to SHBG than does testosterone. In many tissues the activity of testosterone appears to depend on reduction to DHT, which binds to cytosol receptor proteins. The steroid-receptor complex is transported to the nucleus where it initiates transcription and cellular changes related to androgen action. In reproductive tissues, DHT is further metabolized to 3-alpha and 3-beta androstanediol.
Composite results of all studies with TESTODERM® show elevated DHT concentrations and a change in the ratio of testosterone to DHT (T/DHT) during treatment. The range in this ratio ws 0.7–12.5, as compared with a ratio of 3.6–15.2 in normal untreated men. The long-term effects of the change in this ratio are not known.
The T/DHT ratio during TESTODERM® TTS treatment was not statistically significantly different from placebo treatment.

Excretion

About 90% of a dose of testosterone given intramuscularly is excreted in the urine as glucuronic and sulfuric acid conjugates of testosterone and its metabolites; about 6% of a dose is excreted in the feces, mostly in the unconjugated form. Inactivation of testosterone occurs primarily in the liver.

Special Populations

Geriatric

In clinical trials with TESTODERM® TTS, C_{avg} testosterone concentrations were not different between men aged 65 and older and younger adult males.

Race

There is insufficient information available from trials with the TESTODERM® products to compare testosterone pharmacokinetics in different racial groups.

Renal Insufficiency

There is no experience with the use of the TESTODERM® products in patients with renal insufficiency.

Hepatic Insufficiency

There is no experience with the use of the TESTODERM® products in patients with hepatic insufficiency.

Drug-Drug Interactions

See PRECAUTIONS: Drug Interactions.

Clinical Studies

TESTODERM® TTS

Of 32 hypogonadal men receiving daily application of a single TESTODERM® TTS system, 94% achieved normal serum concentrations of testosterone as determined by C_{max} and C_{avg} (200-1000 ng/dL). Mean free testosterone, estradiol, and dihydrotestosterone concentrations were also in the normal range after application of TESTODERM® TTS.

TESTODERM® and TESTODERM® WITH ADHESIVE

After at least 3 weeks of TESTODERM® therapy when steady-state is obtained, 30 hypogonadal men treated with 6 mg/day systems for 22 hours daily achieved mean maximum serum testosterone concentrations of 593 ng/dL at 2 to 4 hours post application. Sixty percent of the patients achieved individual maximal testosterone concentrations >500 ng/dL. The mean 24 hour steady-state AUC (area under the curve) value was 9132 ng/dL. The mean DHT serum concentrations ranged from 134 to 162 ng/dL. Normal levels of testosterone have been maintained in patients who have worn the systems for up to six years. DHT levels also remain stable. The increase in serum testosterone concentration is proportional to the size of the system.
The variability of total testosterone concentrations among patients receiving TESTODERM® treatment was 35% to 49%. The coefficient of variation of total testosterone concentrations within individual patients was 30% to 41%. This variability is comparable to the values reported in the literature for both normal and hypogonadal men.
In two 12-week clinical studies in 72 hypogonadal men, TESTODERM® therapy produced positive effects on mood and sexual behavior. By five weeks, 45 patients not previously treated with TESTODERM® showed statistically significant increases in sexual activity. Compared to baseline, mean sexual events per week increased for sexual intercourse (0.3 to 0.8), orgasm (0.4 to 1.2), waking erections (1.0 to 3.5), and spontaneous erections (0.4 to 2.8).
Changes in nonfasting serum lipid concentrations were observed during TESTODERM® therapy. By three months total cholesterol and high-density lipoprotein cholesterol decreased an average of 8% and 13%, respectively. High-density lipoprotein cholesterol remained stable thereafter. Total cholesterol continued to decrease through two years. At the end of two years, the total cholesterol/high-density lipoprotein cholesterol ratio was not different from pretreatment values.
Estradiol levels increased to the normal range with treatment. Sporadic elevations of estradiol above the normal range for men were observed in 3 of 72 patients and these were not associated with feminizing side effects.

INDICATIONS AND USAGE

The TESTODERM® products are indicated for replacement therapy in males for conditions associated with a deficiency or absence of endogenous testosterone:

1. Primary hypogonadism (congenital or acquired) – testicular failure due to cryptorchidism, bilateral torsion, orchitis, vanishing testis syndrome, orchidectomy, Klinefelter's syndrome, chemotherapy, or toxic damage from alcohol or heavy metals. These men usually have low serum testosterone levels and gonadotropins (FSH, LH) above the normal range.
2. Hypogonadotropic hypogonadism (congenital or acquired)—idiopathic gonadotropin or LHRH deficiency or pituitary-hypothalamic injury from tumors, trauma, or radiation. These men have low testosterone serum levels but have gonadotropins in the normal or low range.
   The TESTODERM® products have not been evaluated clinically in males under 18 years of age.

CONTRAINDICATIONS

Androgens are contraindicated in men with carcinoma of the breast or known or suspected carcinoma of the prostate.
The TESTODERM® products are not indicated for use in women, have not been evaluated in women, and must not be used in women. Testosterone may cause fetal harm.
The TESTODERM® products should not be used in patients with known hypersensitivity to any components of the respective systems, e.g., ethanol (alcohol USP is a component of TESTODERM® TTS).

WARNINGS

1. Prolonged use of high doses of orally active 17-alpha-alkyl androgens (e.g., methyltestosterone) has been associated with serious hepatic adverse effects (peliosis hepatis, hepatic neoplasms, cholestatic hepatitis, and jaundice). Peliosis hepatis can be a life-threatening or fatal complication. Long-term therapy with testosterone enanthate, which elevates blood levels for prolonged periods, has produced multiple hepatic adenomas. Testosterone is not known to produce these adverse effects.
2. Geriatric patients treated with androgens may be at an increased risk for the development of prostatic hyperplasia and prostatic carcinoma.
3. Geriatric patients and other patients with clinical or demographic characteristics that are recognized to be associated with an increased risk of prostate cancer should be evaluated for the presence of prostate cancer prior to initiation of testosterone replacement therapy. In men receiving testosterone replacement therapy, surveillance for prostate cancer should be consistent with current practices for eugonadal men (see **PRECAUTIONS:** Carcinogenesis, Mutagenesis, Impairment of Fertility and Laboratory Tests).
4. Edema with or without congestive heart failure may be a serious complication in patients with preexisting cardiac, renal, or hepatic disease. In addition to discontinuation of the drug, diuretic therapy may be required.
5. Gynecomastia frequently develops and occasionally persists in patients being treated for hypogonadism.
6. There are literature reports that the treatment of hypogonadal men with testosterone esters may potentiate sleep apnea in some patients,[1,2] especially those with risk factors such as obesity or chronic lung diseases.[3,4,5]

PRECAUTIONS

General

The physician should instruct patients to report any of the following:

- Too frequent or persistent erections of the penis.
- Any nausea, vomiting, changes in skin color, or ankle swelling.
- Breathing disturbances, including those associated with sleep.

Virilization of female partners has been reported with use of a topical testosterone solution. Percutaneous creams leave as much as 90 mg residual testosterone on the skin. The results from one study indicated that, after removal of a TESTODERM® system, the potential for transfer of testosterone to a sexual partner was 6 µg, 1/45th the daily endogenous testosterone production by the female body. TESTODERM® TTS, unlike TESTODERM® or TESTODERM® WITH ADHESIVE, has an occlusive backing that prevents the partner from coming in contact with the active material in the system. If a TESTODERM® TTS system is inadvertently transferred to a female partner, it should be removed immediately and the contacted skin washed. Changes in body hair distribution or significant increase in acne of the female partner should be brought to the attention of a physician.

Information for Patients

An information brochure containing instructions for the use of TESTODERM® TTS is available. A separate instruction booklet is available for TESTODERM® and TESTODERM® WITH ADHESIVE. These booklets contain important information and instructions on how to properly use and dispose of the TESTODERM® products. Patients should be encouraged to ask questions of the physician and pharmacist.

Advise patients of the following:

- TESTODERM® TTS should not be applied to the scrotum.
- TESTODERM® and TESTODERM® WITH ADHESIVE are designed for application to scrotal skin only.
- The TESTODERM® products should be applied once daily to dry, clean skin. If the TESTODERM® product has come off after it has been worn for more than 12 hours and it cannot be reapplied, the patient may wait until the next routine application time to apply a new system.

Laboratory Tests

1. Hemoglobin and hematocrit levels should be checked periodically (to detect polycythemia) in patients on long-term androgen therapy.
2. Liver function, prostatic specific antigen, cholesterol, and high-density lipoprotein should be checked periodically.
3. To ensure proper dosing, serum testosterone concentrations may be measured (see **DOSAGE AND ADMINISTRATION**).

Drug Interactions

Anticoagulants: C-17 substituted derivatives of testosterone, such as methandrostenolone, have been reported to decrease the anticoagulant requirements of patients receiving oral anticoagulants. Patients receiving oral anticoagulant therapy require close monitoring, especially when androgens are started or stopped.

Oxyphenbutazone: Concurrent administration of oxyphenbutazone and androgens may result in elevated serum levels of oxyphenbutazone.

Insulin: In diebetic patients, the metabolic effects of androgens may decrease blood glucose and, therefore, insulin requirements.

Propranolol: In a published pharmacokinetic study of an injectable testosterone product, administration of testosterone cypionate led to an increased clearance of propranolol in the majority of men tested.[6]

Corticosteroids: The concurrent administration of testosterone with ACTH or corticosteroids may enhance edema formation; thus these drugs should be administered cautiously, particularly in patients with cardiac or hepatic disease.[7]

Drug/Laboratory Test Interactions

Androgens may decrease levels of thyroxin-binding globulin, resulting in decreased total T_4 serum levels and increased resin uptake of T_3 and T_4. Free thyroid hormone levels remain unchanged, however, and there is no clinical evidence of thyroid dysfunction.

Carcinogenesis, Mutagenesis, Impairment of Fertility Animal Data: Testosterone has been tested by subcutaneous injection and implantation in mice and rats. In mice, the implant induced cervical-uterine tumors, which metastasized in some cases. There is suggestive evidence that injection of testosterone into some strains of female mice increases their susceptibility to hepatoma. Testosterone is also known to increase the number of tumors and decrease the degree of differentiation of chemically induced carcinomas of the liver in rats.

Human Data: There are rare reports of hepatocellular carcinoma in patients receiving long-term therapy with androgens in high doses. Withdrawal of the drugs did not lead to regression of the tumors in all cases.

Geriatric patients treated with androgens may be at an increased risk for the development of prostatic hyperplasia and prostatic carcinoma.

Geriatric patients and other patients with clinical or demographic characteristics that are recognized to be associated with an increased risk of prostate cancer should be evaluated for the presence of prostate cancer prior to initiation of testosterone replacement therapy.

In men receiving testosterone replacement therapy, surveillance for prostate cancer should be consistent with current practices for eugonadal men.

Pregnancy Category X (see Contraindications). Teratogenic Effects: The TESTODERM® products are not indicated for women and must not be used in women.

Nursing Mothers: The TESTODERM® products are not indicated for women and must not be used in women.

Pediatric Use: Safety and efficacy of the TESTODERM® products in pediatric patients has not been established.

ADVERSE REACTIONS

Adverse events are reported in this section by product. Adverse events reported during use of a given product may occur in patients who are treated with any TESTODERM® product.

Adverse Events with TESTODERM® TTS

In clinical studies of 457 participants (116 hypogonadal males and 341 healthy adult males) treated for up to 6 weeks with TESTODERM® TTS, the most commonly reported adverse events were application site reactions of transient itching (12%) and moderate or severe erythema (3%).

Table 2
Adverse events reported in clinical trials in males (n=457) receiving TESTODERM® TTS by 1% or more of users.

Event	Percent of Patients
Itching (ASR)*	12
Headache	5
Erythema† (ASR)*	3
Myalgia	2
Accidental injury	2
Pruritus	2
Pain	2
Asthenia	1
Flu syndrome	1
Libido increased	1
Burning sensation (ASR)*	1
Rash	1

* ASR = Application Site Reaction
† Moderate or severe

Adverse events reported by less than 1% of TESTODERM® TTS users in clinical trials that were of probable or unknown relationship to drug were: *Body as a Whole:* abdominal pain, back pain, infection; *Cardiovascular System:* congestive heart failure, hypertension, tachycardia; *Digestive System:* diarrhea, nausea; *Metabolic and Nutritional System:* hyperglycemia, hyperlipemia, hyponatremia; *Musculoskeletal System:* arthralgia; *Nervous System:* nervousness, depression, dizziness, dry mouth, insomnia, decreased libido, personality disorder, CNS stimulation; *Respiratory System:* bronchitis; *Skin System:* application site reactions – papules/pustules, edema, vesicles, pain, other—, acne, alopecia, hirsutism; *Urogenital System:* abnormal ejaculation, breast pain, dysuria, urinary tract infection, and impaired urination.

Topical Reactions

Of 457 study participants, 3 men (1%) discontinued prematurely because of application site reactions.

There were no clinically significant differences in skin tolerability in younger (<65 years old) and older (≥ 65 years old) subjects.

A contact sensitization rate of 0.5% for TESTODERM® TTS was observed in a 6-week study of 233 normal male volunteers.

In one study with 14 days of daily use, 42% of patients reported 3 or more detachments of their TESTODERM® TTS; of these detachments, 33% occurred during exercise.

Adverse Events with TESTODERM®

In clinical studies of 104 patients treated with TESTODERM®, the most common adverse effects reported were local effects. In US clinical trials, most of the 72 patients filling out a daily questionnaire reported scrotal itching, discomfort, or irritation at some time during therapy. Of all the daily questionnaire responses, 7% reported itching, 4% discomfort, and 2% irritation. All topical reactions decreased with duration of use.

The following adverse effects (greater than 1%) were reported in association with TESTODERM® therapy in 104 patients using the product for up to three years. These effects are listed in decreasing frequency of occurrence with the percentages of patients reporting the effect in parentheses: Gynecomastia (5%), acne (4%), prostatitis/urinary tract infection (4%), breast tenderness (3%), stroke (2%). For this same patient population, the following adverse effects were reported by 1% of users: memory loss, pupillary dilation, abnormal liver enzymes, scrotal cellulitis, deep vein phlebitis, benign prostatic hyperplasia, rectal mucosal lesion over prostate, hematuria/bladder cancer, papilloma on scrotum, and congestive heart failure.

See **CLINICAL PHARMACOLOCY**, Clinical Studies, regarding effects on serum lipids.

Adverse Events with TESTODERM® WITH ADHESIVE

In a pharmacokinetic study in 50 normal men, skin assessment scores following a single 24-hour application of TESTODERM® WITH ADHESIVE to scrotal skin were similar to those for TESTODERM®. Other adverse events reported during the study were headache (6%), dizziness (6%), back pain, pain, nausea, and pustular rash (1% each).

General Adverse Events with Androgen Replacement Therapy

Skin and Appendages: Hirsutism, male pattern baldness, seborrhea, and acne.

Endocrine and Urogenital: Gynecomastia and excessive frequency and duration of penile erections. Oligospermia may occur at high doses (see **CLINICAL PHARMACOLOGY**).

Fluid and Electrolyte Disturbances: Retention of sodium, chloride, water, potassium, calcium, and inorganic phosphates.

Gastrointestinal: Nausea, cholestatic jaundice, alterations in liver function tests. Rare instances of hepatocellular neoplasms and peliosis hepatis have occurred (see **WARNINGS**).

Hematologic: Suppression of clotting factors II, V, VII, and X, bleeding in patients on concomitant anticoagulant therapy, and polycythemia.

Nervous System: Increased or decreased libido, headache, anxiety, depression, and generalized paresthesia.

Metabolic: Increased serum cholesterol.

Miscellaneous: Rarely, anaphylactoid reactions.

DRUG ABUSE AND DEPENDENCE

The TESTODERM® products contain a Schedule III controlled substance as defined by the Anabolic Steroids Control Act.

TESTODERM® TTS is designed for application to arm, back or upper buttocks skin.

TESTODERM® and TESTODERM® WITH ADHESIVE are designed for application to scrotal skin only. Because scrotal skin is at least five times more permeable to testosterone than other skin sites, TESTODERM® or TESTODERM® WITH ADHESIVE will not produce adequate serum testosterone concentrations if applied to non-scrotal skin.

Ingestion of testosterone, or the contents of any of the TESTODERM® products will not result in clinically significant serum testosterone concentrations due to extensive first-pass metabolism. In addition, an intramuscular injection of testosterone from any of the TESTODERM® products will not produce adequate serum testosterone levels due to its short half-life (about 10 minutes).

OVERDOSAGE

There is one report of acute overdosage by injection of testosterone enanthate: testosterone levels of up to 11,400 ng/dL were implicated in a cerebrovascular accident.

DOSAGE AND ADMINISTRATION

TESTODERM® TTS

One system is applied at about the same time each day. The adhesive side of the TESTODERM® TTS system should be placed on a clean, dry area of skin on the arm, back or upper buttocks immediately upon removal from the protective pouch. DO NOT APPLY TO THE SCROTUM. The area selected should not be oily, damaged, or irritated. The system should be pressed firmly in place with the palm of the hand for about 10 seconds, making sure there is good contact, especially around the edges. In the event that a system should fall off, the same system may be reapplied. If the system comes off after it has been worn for more than 12 hours and it cannot be reapplied, a new system may be applied at the next routine application time. In either case, the daily treatment schedule should be continued. The TESTODERM® TTS system should be worn approximately 24 hours and then replaced. To ensure proper dosing, serum testosterone concentration may be measured 2–4 hours after an application of TESTODERM® TTS. If the serum testosterone concentrations are low, the dosing regimen may be increased to 2 systems. Because of variability in analytical values among diagnostic laboratories, all testosterone measurements should be performed at the same laboratory.

TESTODERM® and TESTODERM® WITH ADHESIVE

Patients should start therapy with a 6 mg/day system of either TESTODERM® or TESTODERM® WITH ADHESIVE applied daily; if the scrotal area cannot accommodate a 6 mg/day system, a 4 mg/day TESTODERM® system should be used. One TESTODERM® or TESTODERM® WITH ADHESIVE system should be placed on clean, dry, scrotal skin. Scrotal hair should be dry-shaved for optimal skin contact. Chemical depilatories should not be used (see Patient Information). TESTODERM® or TESTODERM® WITH ADHESIVE should be worn 22–24 hours.

After 3–4 weeks of daily system use, blood should be drawn 2–4 hours after system application for determination of serum total testosterone. Because of variability in analytical values among diagnostic laboratories, this laboratory work and later analyses for assessing the effect of the TESTODERM® and TESTODERM® WITH ADHESIVE therapy should be performed at the same laboratory.

If patients have not achieved desired results by the end of 6–8 weeks of treatment with any of the TESTODERM® products, another form of testosterone replacement therapy should be considered.

HOW SUPPLIED

TESTODERM® TTS, TESTODERM®, and TESTODERM® WITH ADHESIVE testosterone transdermal systems contain a Schedule III controlled substance as defined by the Anabolic Steroids Control Act.

TESTODERM® TTS

TESTODERM® TTS systems are supplied as individually pouched systems, 30 per carton. TESTODERM® TTS 5 mg/day (Testosterone Transdermal System) – each 60 cm^2 system contains 328 mg testosterone USP for nominal dose of 5 mg/day

Carton of 30 TESTODERM® TTS 5 mg/day systems .... NDC 17314-4717-3

TESTODERM® and TESTODERM® WITH ADHESIVE

TESTODERM® and TESTODERM® WITH ADHESIVE systems are supplied as individually pouched systems, 30 per carton.

TESTODERM® 4 mg/day (Testosterone Transdermal System) – each 40 cm^2 system contains 10 mg testosterone USP for nominal delivery of 4 mg for one day.

Carton of 30 TESTODERM® 4 mg/day systems .... NDC 17314-4608-3

TESTODERM® and TESTODERM® WITH ADHESIVE

6 mg/day (Testosterone Transdermal System) – each 60 cm^2 system contains 15 mg testosterone USP for nominal delivery of 6 mg for one day.

Carton of 30 TESTODERM® 6 mg/day systems .... NDC 17314-4609-3

Carton of 30 TESTODERM® WITH ADHESIVE 6 mg/day systems .... NDC 17314-2836-3

Storage

TESTODERM® TTS

Store at controlled room temperature below 25°C (77°F).

TESTODERM® and TESTODERM® WITH ADHESIVE

Store at room temperature 15°–30°C (59°–86°F).

Continued on next page

Testoderm—Cont.

Disposal
TESTODERM® products should be discarded in household trash in a manner that prevents accidental application or ingestion by children or pets.

REFERENCES

1. Matsumoto AM, Sandblom RE, Schoene RB et al. *Testosterone replacement in hypogonadal men: Effects on obstructive sleep apnoea, respiratory drives, and sleep.* Clin Endocrinol (1985) 22: 713–721.
2. Schneider BK, Pickett CK, Zwillich CW et al. *Influence of testosterone on breathing during sleep.* J Appl Physiol (1986) 61: 618–623.
3. Matsumoto AM. *Hormonal therapy of male hypogonadism.* Endocrinol Metab Clin North Am. (1994) 23: 857–875.
4. Bardin CW, Swerdloff RS, Santen RJ. *Androgens: Risks and benefits.* J Clin Endocinol Metab (1991) 73: 4–7.
5. Nieschlag E, Wang CCL. *Guidelines for the use of androgens in men.* Geneva: World Health Organization (1992); 1–16.
6. Walle T, Walle UK, Mathur RS et al. *Propranolol metabolism in normal subjects: Association with sex steroid hormones.* Curr Pharmacol Ther (1994) 56:127–132.
7. Physicians' Generic Rx: The Complete Drug Reference. (1996); II-1972

Rx only
Manufactured by ALZA Corporation, Palo Alto, CA 94304, USA.

ALZA PHARMACEUTICALS
A DIVISION OF ALZA CORPORATION
Edition: 01/98

00071212
Shown in Product Identification Guide, page 304

URISPAS® ℞
[*yore 'eh-spaz*]
brand of
flavoxate HCl
100 mg tablets

DESCRIPTION
Urispas (flavoxate HCl) tablets contain flavoxate hydrochloride, a synthetic urinary tract spasmolytic.
Chemically, flavoxate hydrochloride is 2-piperidinoethyl 3-methyl-4-oxo-2-phenyl-4H-1-benzopyran-8-carboxylate hydrochloride. The empirical formula of flavoxate hydrochloride is $C_{24}H_{25}NO_4 \bullet HCl$. The molecular weight is 427.94. The structural formula appears below.

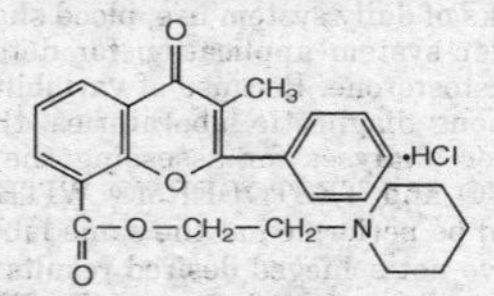

Urispas is supplied in tablets for oral administration. Each round, white, film-coated *Urispas* tablet is debossed URISPAS SKF and contains flavoxate hydrochloride, 100 mg. Inactive ingredients consist of calcium phosphate, castor oil, cellulose acetate phthalate, magnesium stearate, polyethylene glycol, starch and talc.

HOW SUPPLIED
Urispas (flavoxate HCl), 100 mg, is supplied as round, white, film-coated tablets debossed with the product name URISPAS and SKF, in bottles of 100 and in Single Unit Packages of 100 (intended for institutional use only).
100 mg 100's: NDC 17314-9220-1
100 mg SUP 100's: NDC 17314-9220-2
Store between 15° and 30°C (59° and 86°F).
Revision of Date: June 2000
Manufactured by
SmithKline Beecham Pharmaceuticals
Philadelphia, PA 19101
Distributed by
ALZA Corporation
Mountain View, CA 94043
UR:L19 675762

For EMERGENCY telephone numbers,
consult the **Manufacturers' Index.**

Amarin Pharmaceuticals Inc.
25 INDEPENDENCE BLVD.
WARREN NJ 07059

Direct Inquiries to:
For Medical Information Contact:
1-888-952-7462

To Report Adverse Events Contact:
1-888-952-7462

BONTRIL® PDM Ⓒ III
[*bŏn 'tril*]
(phendimetrazine tartrate tablets, USP 35 mg)

HOW SUPPLIED
Three-layered green, white and yellow tablet with 8648 on the scored side and the letter "C" on the other. Bontril® PDM tablets containing 35 mg of phendimetrazine tartrate are available in bottles of 100 (NDC 0086-0048-10) and 1,000 (NDC 0086-0048-90).

CAUTION
Rx only
See product insert for complete information.
Manufactured for Amarin Pharmaceuticals Inc.

BONTRIL® SLOW-RELEASE Ⓒ III
[*bŏn 'tril*]
(brand of phendimetrazine tartrate slow-release capsules 105 mg)

DESCRIPTION
Phendimetrazine tartrate, as the dextro isomer, has the chemical name of (+)-3,4-Dimethyl-2-phenylmorpholine Tartrate.
The structural formula is as follows:

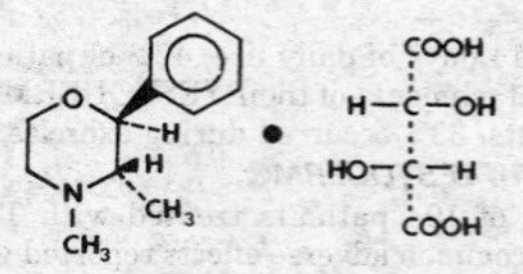

M.W. 341

Phendimetrazine tartrate is a white, odorless powder with a bitter taste. It is soluble in water, methanol and ethanol. Bontril Slow-Release capsules contain FD&C Yellow No. 6 as a color additive.

ACTIONS
Phendimetrazine tartrate is a sympathomimetic amine with pharmacological activity similar to the prototype drugs of this class used in obesity, the amphetamines. Actions include central nervous system stimulation and elevation of blood pressure. Tachyphylaxis and tolerance have been demonstrated with all drugs of this class in which these phenomena have been looked for.
Drugs of this class used in obesity are commonly known as "anorectics" or "anorexigenics". It has not been established, however, that the action of such drugs in treating obesity is primarily one of appetite suppression. Other central nervous system actions or metabolic effects may be involved.
Adult obese subjects instructed in dietary management and treated with anorectic drugs lose more weight on the average than those treated with placebo and diet, as determined in relatively short term clinical trials.
The magnitude of increased weight loss of drug-treated patients over placebo-treated patients is only a fraction of a pound a week. The rate of weight loss is greatest in the first weeks of therapy for both drug and placebo subjects and tends to decrease in succeeding weeks. The possible origin of the increased weight loss due to the various drug effects is not established. The amount of weight loss associated with the use of an anorectic drug varies from trial to trial, and the increased weight loss appears to be related in part to variables other than the drug prescribed, such as the physician investigator, the population treated, and the diet prescribed. Studies do not permit conclusions as to the relative importance of the drug and non-drug factors on weight loss.
The natural history of obesity is measured in years, whereas the studies cited are restricted to a few weeks duration; thus, the total impact of drug-induced weight loss over that of diet alone must be considered clinically limited.
The active drug 105 mg of phendimetrazine tartrate in each capsule of this special slow-release dosage form approximates the action of three 35 mg non-time release doses taken at 4 hours intervals.
The major route of elimination is via the kidneys where most of the drug and metabolites are excreted. Some of the drug is metabolized to phenmetrazine and also phendimetrazine-N-oxide.
The average half-life of elimination when studied under controlled conditions is about 1.9 hours for the non-time and 9.8 hours for the slow-release dosage form. The absorption half-life of the drug from conventional non-time 35 mg phendimetrazine tartrate tablets is approximately the same. These data indicate that the slow-release product has a similar onset of action to the conventional non-time-release product and, in addition, has a prolonged therapeutic effect.

INDICATIONS
Phendimetrazine tartrate is indicated in the management of exogenous obesity as a short term adjunct (a few weeks) in a regimen of weight reduction based on caloric restriction. The limited usefulness of agents of this class (see ACTIONS) should be measured against possible risk factors inherent in their use such as those described below.

CONTRAINDICATIONS
Advanced arteriosclerosis, symptomatic cardiovascular disease, moderate and severe hypertension, hyperthyroidism, known hypersensitivity, or idiosyncrasy to the sympathomimetic amines, glaucoma. Agitated states. Patients with a history of drug abuse. Use in patients taking other CNS stimulants including monoamine oxidase inhibitors.

WARNINGS
Tolerance to the anorectic effect usually develops within a few weeks. When this occurs, the recommended dose should not be exceeded in an attempt to increase the effect; rather, the drug should be discontinued.
Use of phendimetrazine tartrate within 14 days following the administration of monoamine oxidase inhibitors may result in a hypertensive crisis.
Abrupt cessation of administration following prolonged high dosage results in extreme fatigue and depression. Because of the effect on the central nervous system phendimetrazine tartrate may impair the ability of the patient to engage in potentially hazardous activities such as operating machinery or driving a motor vehicle; the patient should therefore be cautioned accordingly.

PRECAUTIONS
Caution is to be exercised in prescribing phendimetrazine tartrate for patients with even mild hypertension.
Insulin requirements in diabetes mellitus may be altered in association with the use of phendimetrazine tartrate and the concomitant dietary regimen.
Phendimetrazine tartrate may decrease the hypotensive effect of guanethidine.
The least amount feasible should be prescribed or dispensed at one time in order to minimize the possibility of overdosage.
Usage in Pregnancy: Safe use in pregnancy has not been established. Until more information is available, phendimetrazine tartrate should not be taken by women who are or may become pregnant unless, in the opinion of the physician, the potential benefits outweigh the possible hazards.
Usage in Children: Phendimetrazine tartrate is not recommended for use in children under 12 years of age.

ADVERSE REACTIONS
Cardiovascular: Palpitation, tachycardia, elevation of blood pressure.
Central Nervous System: Overstimulation, restlessness, dizziness, insomnia, tremor, headache; rarely psychotic episodes at recommended doses, agitation, flushing, sweating, blurring of vision.
Gastrointestinal: Dryness of the mouth, diarrhea, constipation, nausea, stomach pain.
Genitourinary: Changes in libido, urinary frequency, dysuria.

DRUG ABUSE AND DEPENDENCE
Controlled Substance: Phendimetrazine tartrate is a Schedule III controlled substance.
Dependence: Phendimetrazine Tartrate is related chemically and pharmacologically to the amphetamines. Amphetamines and related stimulant drugs have been extensively abused, and the possibility of abuse of phendimetrazine should be kept in mind when evaluating the desirability of including a drug as part of a weight reduction program. Abuse of amphetamines and related drugs may be associated with intense psychological dependence and severe social dysfunction. There are reports of patients who have increased the dosage to many times that recommended. Abrupt cessation following prolonged high dosage administration results in extreme fatigue and mental depression; changes are also noted on the sleep EEG. Manifestations of chronic intoxication with anorectic drugs include severe dermatoses, marked insomnia, irritability, hyperactivity and personality changes. The most severe manifestation of chronic intoxications is psychosis, often clinically indistinguishable from schizophrenia.

OVERDOSAGE
Manifestations of acute overdosage may include restlessness, tremor, hyperreflexia, rapid respiration, confusion, assaultiveness, hallucinations, panic states.
Fatigue and depression usually follow the central stimulation.
Cardiovascular effects include arrhythmias, hypertension, or hypotension and circulatory collapse. Gastrointestinal symptoms include nausea, vomiting, diarrhea, and abdominal cramps. Poisoning may result in convulsions, coma, and death.

Management of acute intoxication is largely symptomatic and includes lavage and sedation with a barbiturate. Experience with hemodialysis or peritoneal dialysis is inadequate to permit recommendation in this regard.
Acidification of the urine increases phendimetrazine tartrate excretion.
Intravenous phentolamine (Regitine) has been suggested for possible acute, severe hypertension, if this complicates overdosage.

DOSAGE AND ADMINISTRATION

One Slow-Release Capsule (105 mg) in the morning, taken 30-60 minutes before the morning meal.
Phendimetrazine Tartrate is not recommended for use in children under twelve years of age.

HOW SUPPLIED

Phendimetrazine Tartrate Slow-Release Capsules, 105 mg is supplied in bottles of 100 opaque green and clear yellow capsules, imprinted with the letter "A" and 047. NDC # 65234-047-10.
Store at controlled room temperature, 15°– 30°C(59°–86°F).

CAUTION

Rx only
Manufactured for Amarin Pharmaceuticals Inc.

CAPITAL® AND CODEINE ORAL SUSPENSION Ⓒ
(acetaminophen and codeine phosphate oral suspension USP)

HOW SUPPLIED

CAPITAL® AND CODEINE ORAL SUSPENSION contains 120 mg of acetaminophen and 12 mg of codeine phosphate/5 mL and is given orally. CAPITAL® AND CODEINE ORAL SUSPENSION is a fruit punch-flavored pink suspension available in 16 fluid oz. (473 mL) bottles, NDC 0086-0046-16.
SHAKE WELL BEFORE USING
Store at controlled room temperature 15°–30°C (59°–86°F).
Dispense in tight, light-resistant glass container and label "Shake Well Before Using."

CAUTION

Rx only
See product insert for complete information.
Manufactured for Amarin Pharmaceuticals Inc.

EXGEST® LA ℞
(phenylpropanolamine hydrochloride/guaifenesin)

HOW SUPPLIED

EXGEST® LA is available as a white, lightly blue-speckled, oval, scored, long-acting tablet for oral administration. It is inscribed with "8673" on the scored side and "C" on the other. Each long-acting tablet contains phenylpropanolamine hydrochloride 75 mg and guaifenesin 400 mg. Supplied in bottles of 100 tablets (NDC 0086-0063-10) and in bottles of 500 tablets (NDC 0086-0063-50).
Store at controlled room temperature, 15°–30°C (59°–86°F.)

CAUTION

Rx only
Manufactured for Amarin Pharmaceuticals Inc.

HYDROCET® CAPSULES Ⓒ III
(HYDROCODONE BITARTRATE AND ACETAMINOPHEN CAPSULES)

HOW SUPPLIED

Blue and white, opaque capsules imprinted with the letter "C" and 8657.
Each capsule contains Hydrocodone Bitartrate*, USP 5 mg and Acetaminophen, USP 500 mg. Keep in tight, light resistant containers.
Supplied in bottles of 100 capsules NDC 0086-0057-10.
Store at controlled room temperature, 15°–30°C (59°–86°F).
Manufactured for:
Amarin Pharmaceuticals Inc.

MOTOFEN® Ⓒ IV
Tablets
(difenoxin hydrochloride with atropine sulfate)
antidiarrheal

DESCRIPTION

Each five-sided dye free MOTOFEN® tablet contains:
Difenoxin (as the hydrochloride) .... 1.0 mg
Atropine sulfate .... 0.025 mg
Difenoxin hydrochloride, 1-(3-cyano-3,3-diphenylpropyl)-4-phenyl-4-piperidinecarboxylic acid monohydrochloride, is an orally administered antidiarrheal agent which is chemically related to the narcotic meperidine.
The structural formula is:

HOOC — N—CH_2CH_2—C(CN) — • HCl

Difenoxin Hydrochloride

Atropine sulfate is present to discourage deliberate overdosage.
Atropine sulfate, an anticholinergic, is endo (±)-α-(hydroxymethyl) benzeneacetic acid 8-methyl-8-azabicyclo[3.2.1] oct-3-yl ester sulfate (2:1) (salt) monohydrate and has the following structural formula:

[N—CH_3 ; CH_2OH ; OOCCH ; C_6H_5]$_2$ • H_2SO_4 • H_2O

Atropine Sulfate

Inactive ingredients: calcium stearate, cellulose, lactose, corn starch.

CLINICAL PHARMACOLOGY

Animal studies have shown that difenoxin hydrochloride manifests its antidiarrheal effect by slowing intestinal motility. The mechanism of action is by a local effect on the gastrointestinal wall.
Difenoxin is the principal active metabolite of diphenoxylate.
Following oral administration of MOTOFEN®, difenoxin is rapidly and extensively absorbed. Mean peak plasma levels of approximately 160 ng/mL occurred within 40 to 60 minutes in most patients following an oral dose of 2mg. Plasma levels decline to less than 10% of their peak values within 24 hours and to less than 1% of their peak values within 72 hours. This decline parallels the appearance of difenoxin and its metabolites in the urine. Difenoxin is metabolized to an inactive hydroxylated metabolite. Both the drug and its metabolites are excreted, mainly as conjugates, in urine and feces.

INDICATIONS AND USAGE

MOTOFEN® (difenoxin hydrochloride with atropine sulfate) is indicated as adjunctive therapy in the management of acute nonspecific diarrhea and acute exacerbations of chronic functional diarrhea.

CONTRAINDICATIONS

MOTOFEN® is contraindicated in patients with diarrhea associated with organisms that penetrate the intestinal mucosa (toxigenic *E. coli, Salmonella* species, *Shigella*) and pseudomembranous colitis associated with broad spectrum antibiotics. Antiperistaltic agents should not be used in these conditions because they may prolong and/or worsen diarrhea.
MOTOFEN® is *contraindicated in children under 2 years of age* because of the decreased margin of safety of drugs in this class in younger age groups.
MOTOFEN® is contraindicated in patients with a known hypersensitivity to difenoxin, atropine, or any of the inactive ingredients, and in patients who are jaundiced.

WARNINGS

MOTOFEN® IS *NOT* AN INNOCUOUS DRUG AND DOSAGE RECOMMENDATIONS SHOULD BE STRICTLY ADHERED TO. MOTOFEN IS NOT RECOMMENDED FOR CHILDREN UNDER 2 YEARS OF AGE. OVERDOSAGE MAY RESULT IN SEVERE RESPIRATORY DEPRESSION AND COMA, POSSIBLY LEADING TO PERMANENT BRAIN DAMAGE OR DEATH (SEE *OVERDOSAGE*). THEREFORE, KEEP THIS MEDICATION OUT OF THE REACH OF CHILDREN.
FLUID AND ELECTROLYTE BALANCE—THE USE OF MOTOFEN® DOES NOT PRECLUDE THE ADMINISTRATION OF APPROPRIATE FLUID AND ELECTROLYTE THERAPY. DEHYDRATION, PARTICULARLY IN CHILDREN, MAY FURTHER INFLUENCE THE VARIABILITY OF RESPONSE TO MOTOFEN AND MAY PREDISPOSE TO DELAYED DIFENOXIN INTOXICATION. DRUG-INDUCED INHIBITION OF PERISTALSIS MAY RESULT IN FLUID RETENTION IN THE COLON, AND THIS MAY FURTHER AGGRAVATE DEHYDRATION AND ELECTROLYTE IMBALANCE.
IF SEVERE DEHYDRATION OR ELECTROLYTE IMBALANCE IS MANIFESTED, MOTOFEN® SHOULD BE WITHHELD UNTIL APPROPRIATE CORRECTIVE THERAPY HAS BEEN INITIATED.
Ulcerative Colitis —In some patients with acute ulcerative colitis, agents which inhibit intestinal motility or delay intestinal transit time have been reported to induce toxic megacolon. Consequently, patients with acute ulcerative colitis should be carefully observed and MOTOFEN® therapy should be discontinued promptly if abdominal distention occurs or if other untoward symptoms develop.
Liver and Kidney Disease —MOTOFEN® (difenoxin hydrochloride with atropine sulfate) should be used with extreme caution in patients with advanced hepatorenal disease and in all patients with abnormal liver function tests since hepatic coma may be precipitated.
Atropine —A subtherapeutic dose of atropine has been added to difenoxin hydrochloride to discourage deliberate overdosage. Usage of MOTOFEN® in recommended doses is not likely to cause prominent anticholinergic side effects, but MOTOFEN® should be avoided in patients in whom anticholinergic drugs are contraindicated. The warnings and precautions for use of anticholinergic agents should be observed. In children, signs of atropinism may occur even with recommended doses of MOTOFEN®, particularly in patients with Down's Syndrome.

PRECAUTIONS

Information for Patients
CAUTION PATIENTS TO ADHERE STRICTLY TO RECOMMENDED DOSAGE SCHEDULES. THE MEDICATION SHOULD BE KEPT OUT OF REACH OF CHILDREN SINCE ACCIDENTAL OVERDOSAGE MAY RESULT IN SEVERE, EVEN FATAL, RESPIRATORY DEPRESSION.
MOTOFEN® may produce drowsiness or dizziness. The patient should be cautioned regarding activities requiring mental alertness, such as driving or operating dangerous machinery.
Drug Interactions
Since the chemical structure of difenoxin hydrochloride is similar to meperidine hydrochloride, the concurrent use of MOTOFEN® with monoamine oxidase inhibitors may, in theory, precipitate a hypertensive crisis.
MOTOFEN® may potentiate the action of barbiturates, tranquilizers, narcotics, and alcohol. When these medications are used concomitantly with MOTOFEN®, the patient should be closely monitored.
Diphenoxylate hydrochloride, from which the principal active metabolite difenoxin is derived, was found to inhibit the hepatic microsomal enzyme system at a dose of 2 mg/kg/day in studies conducted with male rats. Therefore, difenoxin has the potential to prolong the biological half-lives of drugs for which the rate of elimination is dependent on the microsomal drug metabolizing enzyme system.
Carcinogenesis, Mutagenesis, Impairment of Fertility
No evidence of carcinogenesis was found in a long-term study of difenoxin hydrochloride/atropine in the rat. In this 104 week study, rats received dietary doses of 0, 1.25, 2.5, or 5 mg/kg/day difenoxin/atropine (20:1 ratio).
No experiments have been conducted to determine the mutagenic potential of MOTOFEN®. MOTOFEN® did not significantly impair fertility in rats.
Pregnancy/Teratogenic Effects
Pregnancy Category C. Reproduction studies in rats and rabbits with doses at 31 and 61 times the human therapeutic dose respectively, on a mg/kg basis, demonstrated no evidence of teratogenesis due to MOTOFEN® (difenoxin hydrochloride with atropine sulfate).
Pregnant rats receiving oral doses of difenoxin hydrochloride/atropine 20 times the maximum human dose had an increase in delivery time as well as a significant increase in the percent of stillbirths.
Neonatal survival in rats was also reduced with most deaths occurring within four days of delivery.
There are no well controlled studies in pregnant women. MOTOFEN® should be used during pregnancy only if the potential benefit justifies the potential risk to the fetus.
Nursing Mothers
Because of the potential for serious adverse reactions in nursing infants from MOTOFEN®, a decision should be made whether to discontinue nursing or to discontinue the drug, taking into account the importance of the drug to the mother.
Pediatric Use
SAFETY AND EFFECTIVENESS IN CHILDREN BELOW THE AGE OF 12 HAVE NOT BEEN ESTABLISHED. MOTOFEN® IS CONTRAINDICATED IN CHILDREN UNDER 2 YEARS OF AGE. See OVERDOSAGE section for information on hazards from accidental poisoning in children.

ADVERSE REACTIONS

In view of the small amount of atropine present (0.025 mg/tablet), effects such as dryness of the skin and mucous membranes, flushing, hyperthermia, tachycardia and urinary retention are very unlikely to occur, except perhaps in children.
Many of the adverse effects reported during clinical investigation of MOTOFEN® are difficult to distinguish from symptoms associated with the diarrheal syndrome. However, the following events were reported at the stated frequencies:
Gastrointestinal: Nausea, 1 in 15 patients; vomiting, 1 in 30 patients; dry mouth, 1 in 30 patients; epigastric distress, 1 in 100 patients; and constipation, 1 in 300 patients.
Central Nervous System: Dizziness and light-headedness, 1 in 20 patients; drowsiness, 1 in 25 patients; and headache, 1 in 40 patients; tiredness, nervousness, insomnia and confusion ranged from 1 in 200 to 1 in 600 patients.
Other less frequent reactions: Burning eyes and blurred vision occurred in a few cases.
The following adverse reactions have been reported in patients receiving chemically-related drugs: numbness of extremities, euphoria, depression, sedation, anaphylaxis, an-

Continued on next page

Motofen—Cont.

gioneurotic edema, urticaria, swelling of the gums, pruritus, toxic megacolon, paralytic ileus, pancreatitis, and anorexia.

THIS MEDICATION SHOULD BE KEPT IN A CHILD-RESISTANT CONTAINER AND OUT OF THE REACH OF CHILDREN SINCE AN OVERDOSAGE MAY RESULT IN SEVERE RESPIRATORY DEPRESSION AND COMA, POSSIBLY LEADING TO PERMANENT BRAIN DAMAGE OR DEATH.

DRUG ABUSE AND DEPENDENCE

MOTOFEN® (difenoxin hydrochloride with atropine sulfate) tablets are a Schedule IV controlled substance.

Addiction to (dependence on) difenoxin hydrochloride is theoretically possible at high dosage. Therefore, the recommended dosage should not be exceeded. Because of the structural and pharmacological similarities of difenoxin hydrochloride to drugs with a definite addiction potential, MOTOFEN® should be administered with considerable caution to patients who are receiving addicting drugs, to individuals known to be addiction prone, or to those in whom histories suggest may increase the dosage on their own initiative.

OVERDOSAGE

Diagnosis and Treatment

In the event of overdosage (initial signs may include dryness of the skin and mucous membranes, flushing, hyperthermia and tachycardia followed by lethargy or coma, hypotonic reflexes, nystagmus, pinpoint pupils and respiratory depression) gastric lavage, establishment of a patent airway and possibly mechanically assisted respiration are advised.

The narcotic antagonist naloxone may be used in the treatment of respiratory depression caused by narcotic analgesics or pharmacologically related compounds such as MOTOFEN® tablets. When naloxone is administered intravenously, the onset of action is generally apparent within two minutes. Naloxone may also be administered subcutaneously or intramuscularly providing a slightly less rapid onset of action but a more prolonged effect.

To counteract respiratory depression caused by MOTOFEN® overdosage, the following dosage schedule for naloxone should be followed:

Adult Dosage: The usual initial adult dose of naloxone is 0.4 mg (one mL) administered intravenously. If respiratory function does not adequately improve after the initial dose, the same IV dose may be repeated at two-to-three minute intervals.

Children: The usual adult dose of naloxone for children is 0.01 mg/kg of body weight administered intravenously and repeated at two-to-three minute intervals if necessary.

Since the duration of action of difenoxin hydrochloride is longer than that of naloxone, improvement of respiration following administration may be followed by recurrent respiratory depression. Consequently, continuous observation is necessary until the effect of difenoxin hydrochloride on respiration (which effect may persist for many hours) has passed. Supplemental intramuscular doses of naloxone may be utilized to produce a longer lasting effect. TREAT ALL POSSIBLE MOTOFEN® OVERDOSAGES AS SERIOUS AND MAINTAIN MEDICAL OBSERVATION FOR AT LEAST 48 HOURS, PREFERABLY UNDER CONTINUOUS HOSPITAL CARE.

Although signs of overdosage and respiratory depression may not be evident soon after ingestion of difenoxin hydrochloride, respiratory depression may occur from 12 to 30 hours later.

DOSAGE AND ADMINISTRATION

The recommended starting dose of MOTOFEN® tablets in adults is 2 tablets (2 mg), then 1 tablet (1 mg) after each loose stool or 1 tablet (1 mg) every 3 to 4 hours as needed, but the total dosage during any 24-hour treatment period should not exceed 8 tablets (8 mg). In the treatment of diarrhea, if clinical improvement is not observed in 48 hours, continued administration of this type medication is not recommended. For acute diarrheas and acute exacerbations of functional diarrhea, treatment beyond 48 hours is usually not necessary.

Studies in children below the age of 12 have been inadequate to evaluate the safety and effectiveness of MOTOFEN® in this age group. MOTOFEN® is contraindicated in children under 2 years of age.

HOW SUPPLIED

MOTOFEN® is available as a white, dye-free, five-sided, scored tablet with "8674" on the scored side and "C" on the other. Each tablet contains 1.0 mg difenoxin (as the hydrochloride salt) and 0.025 mg atropine sulfate. Supplied in bottles of 100 tablets (NDC 0086-0074-10) and in bottles of 50 tablets (NDC 0086-0074-05).

Store at controlled room temperature, 15°–30°C (59°–86°F).

Rx only

Manufactured for: Amarin Pharmaceuticals Inc.

NOLAMINE® ℞

[*nō 'lă-mēn '*]

DESCRIPTION

Each timed-release tablet contains:

Phenindamine tartrate .... 24 mg

Chlorpheniramine maleate .... 4 mg

Phenylpropanolamine hydrochloride .... 50 mg

HOW SUPPLIED

Pink, timed release tablets coded C 86204 in bottles of 100 (NDC 0086-0204-10) and 250 (NDC 0086-0204-25). Store at controlled room temperature, 15°–30°C (59°–86°F) and keep away from light.

Manufactured for Amarin Pharmaceuticals Inc.

PHRENILIN® ℞

[*fren 'ĭ-lin*]

(Butalbital 50 mg and Acetaminophen 325 mg Tablet)

and

PHRENILIN® FORTE ℞

(Butalbital 50 mg and Acetaminophen 650 mg Capsule)

DESCRIPTION

PHRENILIN®: Each PHRENILIN® tablet, for oral administration, contains Butalbital, USP 50 mg, Acetaminophen, USP 325 mg.

In addition each PHRENILIN® Tablet contains the following inactive ingredients: alginic acid, cornstarch, D&C Red No. 27—Aluminum Lake, FD&C Blue No. 1—Aluminum Lake, gelatin, magnesium stearate, microcrystalline cellulose and pregelatinized starch.

PHRENILIN® FORTE: Each PHRENILIN® FORTE capsule, for oral administration, contains Butalbital, USP 50 mg, Acetaminophen, USP 650 mg.

In addition each PHRENILIN® FORTE capsule may also contain the following inactive ingredients: benzyl alcohol, butylparaben, D&C Red No. 28, D&C Red No. 33, edetate calcium disodium, FD&C Blue No. 1, FD&C Red No. 40, gelatin, methylparaben, propylparaben, silicon dioxide, sodium lauryl sulfate, sodium propionate and titanium dioxide.

Butalbital (5-allyl-5-isobutylbarbituric acid), a slightly bitter, white, odorless, crystalline powder, is a short to intermediate-acting barbiturate. It has the following structural formula:

$C_{11}H_{16}N_2O_3$ MW = 224.26

Acetaminophen, (4'-hydroxyacetanilide), a slightly bitter, white, odorless, crystalline powder, is a non-opiate, non-salicylate analgesic and antipyretic. It has the following structural formula:

$C_8H_9NO_2$ MW = 151.16

CLINICAL PHARMACOLOGY

This combination drug product is intended as a treatment for tension headache.

It consists of a fixed combination of butalbital and acetaminophen. The role each component plays in the relief of the complex of symptoms known as tension headache is incompletely understood.

Pharmacokinetics: The behavior of the individual components is described below.

Butalbital: Butalbital is well absorbed from the gastrointestinal tract and is expected to distribute to most tissues in the body. Barbiturates in general may appear in breast milk and readily cross the placental barrier. They are bound to plasma and tissue proteins to a varying degree and binding increases directly as a function of lipid solubility.

Elimination of butalbital is primarily via the kidney (59% to 88% of the dose) as unchanged drug or metabolites. The plasma half-life is about 35 hours. Urinary excretion products include parent drug (about 3.6% of the dose), 5-isobutyl-5-(2,3-dihydroxypropyl) barbituric acid (about 24% of the dose), 5-allyl-5(3-hydroxy-2- methyl-1-propyl) barbituric acid (about 4.8% of the dose), products with the barbituric acid ring hydrolyzed with excretion of urea (about 14% of the dose), as well as unidentified materials. Of the material excreted in the urine, 32% is conjugated.

See OVERDOSAGE for toxicity information.

Acetaminophen: Acetaminophen is rapidly absorbed from the gastrointestinal tract and is distributed throughout most body tissues. The plasma half-life is 1.25 to 3 hours, but may be increased by liver damage and following overdosage. Elimination of acetaminophen is principally by liver metabolism (conjugation) and subsequent renal excretion of metabolites. Approximately 85% of an oral dose appears in the urine within 24 hours of administration, most as the glucuronide conjugate, with small amounts of other conjugates and unchanged drug.

See OVERDOSAGE for toxicity information.

INDICATIONS AND USAGE

PHRENILIN® tablets & PHRENILIN® FORTE capsules are indicated for the relief of the symptom complex of tension (or muscle contraction) headache.

Evidence supporting the efficacy and safety of this combination product in the treatment of multiple recurrent headaches is unavailable. Caution in this regard is required because butalbital is habit-forming and potentially abusable.

CONTRAINDICATIONS

This product is contraindicated under the following conditions:

- Hypersensitivity or intolerance to any component of this product.
- Patients with porphyria.

WARNINGS

Butalbital is habit-forming and potentially abusable. Consequently, the extended use of this product is not recommended.

PRECAUTIONS

General: PHRENILIN® tablets & PHRENILIN® FORTE capsules (Butalbital and Acetaminophen) should be prescribed with caution in certain special-risk patients, such as the elderly or debilitated, and those with severe impairment of renal or hepatic function, or acute abdominal conditions.

Information for Patients: This product may impair mental and/or physical abilities required for the performance of potentially hazardous tasks such as driving a car or operating machinery. Such tasks should be avoided while taking this product.

Alcohol and other CNS depressants may produce an additive CNS depression, when taken with this combination product, and should be avoided.

Butalbital may be habit-forming. Patients should take the drug only for as long as it is prescribed, in the amounts prescribed, and no more frequently than prescribed.

Laboratory Tests: In patients with severe hepatic or renal disease, effects of therapy should be monitored with serial liver and/or renal function tests.

Drug Interactions: The CNS effects of butalbital may be enhanced by monoamine oxidase (MAO) inhibitors.

Butalbital and acetaminophen may enhance the effects of: other narcotic analgesics, alcohol, general anesthetics, tranquilizers such as chlordiazepoxide, sedative-hypnotics, or other CNS depressants, causing increased CNS depression.

Drug/Laboratory Test Interactions: Acetaminophen may produce false-positive test results for urinary 5-hydroxyindoleacetic acid.

Carcinogenesis, Mutagenesis, Impairment of Fertility: No adequate studies have been conducted in animals to determine whether acetaminophen or butalbital have a potential for carcinogenesis, mutagenesis or impairment of fertility.

Pregnancy: ***Teratogenic Effects:*** Pregnancy Category C: Animal reproduction studies have not been conducted with this combination product. It is also not known whether butalbital and acetaminophen can cause fetal harm when administered to a pregnant woman or can affect reproduction capacity. These products should be given to a pregnant woman only when clearly needed.

Nonteratogenic Effects: Withdrawal seizures were reported in a two-day-old male infant whose mother had taken a butalbital-containing drug during the last two months of pregnancy. Butalbital was found in the infant's serum. The infant was given phenobarbital 5 mg/kg, which was tapered without further seizure or other withdrawal symptoms.

Nursing Mothers: Barbiturates and acetaminophen are excreted in breast milk in small amounts, but the significance of their effects on nursing infants is not known. Because of potential for serious adverse reactions in nursing infants from butalbital and acetaminophen, a decision should be made whether to discontinue nursing or to discontinue the drug, taking into account the importance of the drug to the mother.

Pediatric Use: Safety and effectiveness in children below the age of 12 have not been established.

ADVERSE REACTIONS

Frequently Observed: The most frequently reported adverse reactions are drowsiness, lightheadedness, dizziness, sedation, shortness of breath, nausea, vomiting, abdominal pain, and intoxicated feeling.

Infrequently Observed: All adverse events tabulated below are classified as infrequent.

Central Nervous: headache, shaky feeling, tingling, agitation, fainting, fatigue, heavy eyelids, high energy, hot spells, numbness, sluggishness, seizure. Mental confusion, excitement or depression can also occur due to intolerance, particularly in elderly or debilitated patients, or due to overdosage of butalbital.

Autonomic Nervous: dry mouth, hyperhidrosis.

Gastrointestinal: difficulty swallowing, heartburn, flatulence, constipation.

Cardiovascular: tachycardia.

Musculoskeletal: leg pain, muscle fatigue.

Genitourinary: diuresis.

Miscellaneous: pruritus, fever, earache, nasal congestion, tinnitus, euphoria, allergic reactions.

Several cases of dermatological reactions, including toxic epidermal necrolysis and erythema multiforme, have been reported.

The following adverse drug events may be borne in mind as potential effects of the components of this product. Potential effects of high dosage are listed in the OVERDOSAGE section.

Acetaminophen: allergic reactions, rash, thrombocytopenia, agranulocytosis.

DRUG ABUSE AND DEPENDENCE

Abuse and Dependence:

Butalbital: *Barbiturates may be habit-forming:* Tolerance, psychological dependence, and physical dependence may occur especially following prolonged use of high doses of barbiturates. The average daily dose for the barbiturate addict is usually about 1500 mg. As tolerance to barbiturates develops, the amount needed to maintain the same level of intoxication increases; tolerance to a fatal dosage, however, does not increase more than two-fold. As this occurs, the margin between an intoxication dosage and fatal dosage becomes smaller. The lethal dose of a barbiturate is far less if alcohol is also ingested. Major withdrawal symptoms (convulsions and delirium) may occur within 16 hours and last up to 5 days after abrupt cessation of these drugs. Intensity of withdrawal symptoms gradually declines over a period of approximately 15 days. Treatment of barbiturate dependence consists of cautious and gradual withdrawal of the drug. Barbiturate-dependent patients can be withdrawn by using a number of different withdrawal regimens. One method involves initiating treatment at the patient's regular dosage level and gradually decreasing the daily dosage as tolerated by the patient.

OVERDOSAGE

Following an acute overdosage of butalbital and acetaminophen, toxicity may result from the barbiturate or acetaminophen.

Signs and Symptoms: Toxicity from barbiturate poisoning include drowsiness, confusion, and coma; respiratory depression; hypotension; and hypovolemic shock.

In acetaminophen overdosage: dose-dependent, potentially fatal hepatic necrosis is the most serious adverse effect. Renal tubular necroses, hypoglycemic coma and thrombocytopenia may also occur. Early symptoms following a potentially hepatotoxic overdose may include: nausea, vomiting, diaphoresis and general malaise. Clinical and laboratory evidence of hepatic toxicity may not be apparent until 48 to 72 hours post-ingestion. In adults hepatic toxicity has rarely been reported with acute overdoses of less than 10 grams, or fatalities with less than 15 grams.

Treatment: A single or multiple overdose with these combination products is a potentially lethal polydrug overdose, and consultation with a regional poison control center is recommended.

Immediate treatment includes support of cardiorespiratory function and measures to reduce drug absorption. Vomiting should be induced mechanically, or with syrup of ipecac, if the patient is alert (adequate pharyngeal and laryngeal reflexes). Oral activated charcoal (1 g/kg) should follow gastric emptying. The first dose should be accompanied by an appropriate cathartic. If repeated doses are used, the cathartic might be included with alternate doses as required. Hypotension is usually hypovolemic and should respond to fluids. Pressors should be avoided. A cuffed endotracheal tube should be inserted before gastric lavage of the unconscious patient and, when necessary, to provide assisted respiration. If renal function is normal, forced diuresis may aid in the elimination of the barbiturate. Alkalinization of the urine increases renal excretion of some barbiturates, especially phenobarbital.

Meticulous attention should be given to maintaining adequate pulmonary ventilation. In severe cases of intoxication, peritoneal dialysis, or preferably hemodialysis may be considered. If hypoprothrombinemia occurs due to acetaminophen overdose, vitamin K should be administered intravenously.

If the dose of acetaminophen may have exceeded 140 mg/kg, acetylcysteine should be administered as early as possible. Serum acetaminophen levels should be obtained, since levels four or more hours following ingestion help predict acetaminophen toxicity. Do not await acetaminophen assay results before initiating treatment. Hepatic enzymes should be obtained initially, and repeated at 24-hour intervals.

Methemoglobinemia over 30% should be treated with methylene blue by slow intravenous administration.

Toxic Doses (for adults):

PHRENILIN® tablets (Butalbital 50 mg and Acetaminophen 325 mg tablets)

Butalbital: toxic dose 1 g (20 tablets)

Acetaminophen: toxic dose 10 g (30 tablets)

PHRENILIN® FORTE capsules (Butalbital 50 mg and Acetaminophen 650 mg capsules)

Butalbital: toxic dose 1 g (20 capsules)

Acetaminophen: toxic dose 10 g (15 capsules)

DOSAGE AND ADMINISTRATION

PHRENILIN®: One or two tablets every four hours. Total daily dosage should not exceed 6 tablets.

PHRENILIN® FORTE: One capsule every four hours. Total daily dosage should not exceed 6 capsules.

Extended and repeated use of these products is not recommended because of the potential for physical dependence.

HOW SUPPLIED

PHRENILIN®: Pale violet scored tablets with the letter C on one side and 8650 on the other, in bottles of 100 (NDC 0086-0050-10) in bottles of 500 (NDC 0086-0050-50). Each tablet contains butalbital, USP 50 mg and acetaminophen, USP 325 mg.

PHRENILIN® FORTE: Amethyst, opaque capsules imprinted with the letter C and 8656, in bottles of 100 (NDC 0086-0056-10) in bottles of 500 (NDC 0086-0056-50). Each capsule contains butalbital, USP 50 mg and acetaminophen USP 650 mg.

Store PHRENILIN® and PHRENILIN® FORTE (Butalbital and Acetaminophen) at controlled room temperature, 15°–30°C (59°–86°F). Dispense in a tight container as defined in the USP.

Rx only

Manufactured for Amarin Pharmaceuticals Inc.

SALFLEX® ℞
(salsalate tablets USP)

HOW SUPPLIED

SALFLEX® 500 mg tablets:

Each round, white, dye-free, film-coated SALFLEX® tablet is inscribed with 8671 on one side and "C" on the other. Each tablet contains 500 mg salsalate and is available in bottles of 100 tablets (NDC 0086-0071-10).

SALFLEX® 750 mg tablets:

Each oval, white, dye-free, film-coated SALFLEX® tablet is inscribed with 8672 on the scored side and "C" on the other. Each tablet contains 750 mg salsalate and is available in bottles of 100 tablets (NDC 0086-0072-10) and 500 tablets (NDC 0086-0072-50).

Store at controlled room temperature, 15°–30°C (59°–86°F). Dispense in a tight container as defined in the USP.

CAUTION: Rx only

Manufactured for Amarin Pharmaceuticals Inc.

American Lecithin Company
115 HURLEY ROAD, UNIT 2B
OXFORD, CT 06478

Direct Inquiries to:
Randall E. Zigmont
(203) 262-7100
Fax: (203) 262-7101

For Medical Emergencies Contact:
In Emergencies:
Randall E. Zigmont
(203) 262-7100
Fax: (203) 262-7101

PHOSCHOL® OTC
[fos 'kol]
Phosphatidylcholine (highly purified lecithin)
Softgels and Concentrate

DESCRIPTION

PhosChol 900 contains 900 mg of pure phosphatidylcholine in each softgel.

PhosChol Concentrate contains 3000 mg of pure phosphatidylcholine in each teaspoonful.

ACTION & USES

Choline circulating in the blood after PC ingestion is taken up into all cells of the body. The brain has a unique way of ensuring that its nerve cells will receive adequate supplies of circulating choline.

A special protein molecule within the brain's capillaries traps the circulating choline, and then transports it across the blood-brain barrier, into the brain. Once in the brain, choline is incorporated into the brain's own PC, which is an essential and major part of neuronal membranes. Circulating choline transported into the brain has an additional very important function for a special group of nerve cells that make a biochemical, acetylcholine, which is released into synapses as a neurotransmitter. It provides the essential precursor used to synthesize acetylcholine. Moreover, when nerve cells are active, firing frequently and releasing large quantities of acetylcholine, their ability to make adequate amounts of the neurotransmitter requires that they receive adequate amounts of choline from the blood stream. In the absence of adequate choline, the ability of nerve cells to transmit messages to other cells across synapses is impaired and neuronal cell membranes can be depleted of PC causing cell damage. In contrast, when supplemental choline is provided, these messages can be amplified and membrane structure maintained.

PhosChol® brand of highly purified lecithin has been carefully developed to contain the highest concentration of phosphatidylcholine commercially available and can provide for the highest blood choline levels.

[See figure 1 at top of next column]

ADMINISTRATION

PhosChol® nutritional supplements may be recommended for two purposes:

To guard against low blood choline levels, and to restore blood choline levels in patients suffering from selected brain disorders. Amounts of PC sufficient to increase blood choline levels would help support normal cellular membrane composition and repair; they would also provide sufficient precursor choline for the maintenance of acetylcholine biosynthesis. Taken according to these schedules, dietary supplements of PC are an aid to good health, and protect against low choline stores.

Figure 1.
LEVELS OF CHOLINE IN HUMAN PLASMA AFTER THE ADMINISTRATION OF 3, 6, 9, AND 18 GRAM DOSES OF PHOSCHOL

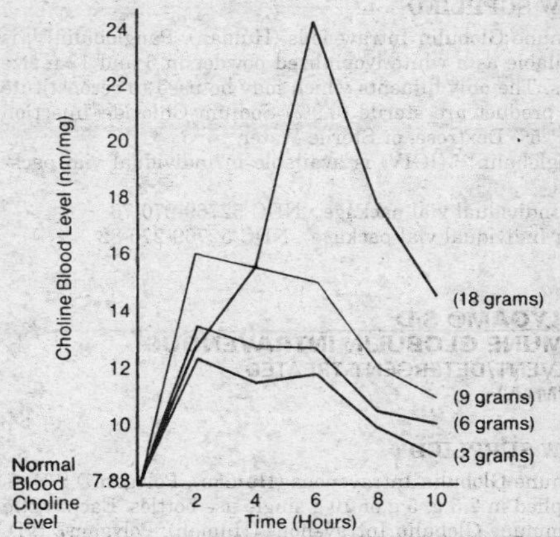

(One 9-gram dose at baseline, one 9-gram dose at 4 hours)

To increase blood choline by 50%, patients should take 3 grams of PhosChol before meals by noon. To double blood choline levels, patients should take 9 grams of PhosChol before meals by noon. If ingestion before meals causes intestinal distress, it is recommended that PhosChol be taken either with meals or immediately thereafter.

ADVERSE REACTIONS

No major side effects have been reported in connection with consumption of large quantities of phosphatidylcholine or commercially available (less pure) lecithin.

Minor side effects may be seen such as increased salivation, nausea and upset stomach.

HOW SUPPLIED

Two strengths as clear, amber colored, one-piece sealed softgels.

PhosChol 900 contains 900 mg of pure phosphatidylcholine in each softgel and is available in bottles of 30, 100 and 300 softgels. Ten softgels a day provide 9 grams of phosphatidylcholine.

One strength as a liquid concentrate.

PhosChol Concentrate contains 3000 mg of pure phosphatidylcholine in each teaspoonful and is available in 8 oz., and 16 oz. bottles. Three teaspoonsful a day provide 9 grams of phosphatidylcholine.

American Red Cross
NATIONAL HEADQUARTERS
BIOMEDICAL SERVICES
1616 FORT MYER DRIVE, 17th FLOOR
ARLINGTON, VA 22209-3100

Direct Inquiries to:
Professional Services Department
800-293-5023
FAX: 703-312-8742
Customer Service Department
800-446-8883
FAX: 703-312-8746

ALBUMARC® 5% ℞
ALBUMIN (HUMAN), USP, 5% SOLUTION

6 bottles per case	NDC #
250mL bottle	52769-450-25
500mL bottle	52769-450-50

ALBUMARC® 25% ℞
ALBUMIN (HUMAN), USP, 25% SOLUTION

10 bottles per case	NDC #
50mL bottle	52769-451-05
100mL bottle	52769-451-10

MONARC-M™ ℞
ANTIHEMOPHILIC FACTOR (HUMAN)
Method M
Monoclonal Purified

HOW SUPPLIED

MONARC–M™, is available as single dose bottles. Each bottle is labeled with the potency in International Units, and is packaged together with 10 mL of Sterile Water for Injection, USP, a double-ended needle, and a filter needle. NDC 52769-460-01

Continued on next page

PANGLOBULIN™ ℞
IMMUNE GLOBULIN INTRAVENOUS (HUMAN)

CAUTION: US Federal law prohibits dispensing wihtout prescription.

HOW SUPPLIED

Immune Globulin Intravenous (Human), Panglobulin™, is available as a white lyophilized powder in 6 and 12 g size vials. The only diluents which may be used to reconstitute the product are sterile (0.9%) Sodium Chloride Injection USP, 5% Dextrose, or Sterile Water.
Panglobulin™ (IGIV) is available in individual vial packages.
6 g Individual vial package NDC 52769-270-76
12 g Individual vial package NDC 52769-270-82

POLYGAM® S/D
IMMUNE GLOBULIN INTRAVENOUS ℞
SOLVENT/DETERGENT TREATED
(HUMAN)

HOW SUPPLIED

Immune Globulin Intravenous (Human), Polygam® S/D, is supplied in 2.5 g, 5 g or 10 g single use bottles. Each bottle of Immune Globulin Intravenous (Human), Polygam® S/D, is furnished with a suitable volume of Sterile Water for Injection, USP, a transfer device and an administration set which contains an integral airway and a 15 micron filter.
5g NDC 52769-471-75
10g NDC 52769-471-80

Amgen
AMGEN INC.
ONE AMGEN CENTER DRIVE
THOUSAND OAKS, CA 91320-1789

Direct Inquiries to:
Customer Service Department
(800) 282-6436
FAX: (800) 292-6436

For Medical Information Contact:
Professional Services Department
(800) 772-6436
FAX: 805-376-8550
In Emergencies:
(800) 772-6436
After Hours and Weekends:
(800) 772-6436

Sales and Ordering:
Customer Service Department
(800) 282-6436
FAX: (800) 292-6436

EPOGEN® ℞
EPOETIN ALFA
RECOMBINANT
For Injection

DESCRIPTION

Erythropoietin is a glycoprotein which stimulates red blood cell production. It is produced in the kidney and stimulates the division and differentiation of committed erythroid progenitors in the bone marrow. EPOGEN® (Epoetin alfa), a 165 amino acid glycoprotein manufactured by recombinant DNA technology, has the same biological effects as endogenous erythropoietin.[1] It has a molecular weight of 30,400 daltons and is produced by mammalian cells into which the human erythropoietin gene has been introduced. The product contains the identical amino acid sequence of isolated natural erythropoietin.
EPOGEN® is formulated as a sterile, colorless liquid in an isotonic sodium chloride/sodium citrate buffered solution or a sodium chloride/sodium phosphate buffered solution for intravenous (IV) or subcutaneous (SC) administration.
Single-dose, Preservative-free Vial: Each 1 mL of solution contains 2000, 3000, 4000 or 10,000 Units of Epoetin alfa, 2.5 mg Albumin (Human), 5.8 mg sodium citrate, 5.8 mg sodium chloride, and 0.06 mg citric acid in Water for Injection, USP (pH 6.9 ± 0.3). This formulation contains no preservative.
Single-dose, Preservative-free Vial: 1 mL (40,000 Units/mL). Each 1 mL of solution contains 40,000 Units of Epoetin alfa, 2.5 mg Albumin (Human), 1.2 mg sodium phosphate monobasic monohydrate, 1.8 mg sodium phosphate dibasic anhydrate, 0.7 mg sodium citrate, 5.8 mg sodium chloride, and 6.8 mg citric acid in Water for Injection, USP (pH 6.9 ± 0.3). This formulation contains no preservative.
Multidose, Preserved Vial: 2 mL (20,000 Units, 10,000 Units/mL). Each 1 mL of solution contains 10,000 Units of Epoetin alfa, 2.5 mg Albumin (Human), 1.3 mg sodium citrate, 8.2 mg sodium chloride, 0.11 mg citric acid, and 1% benzyl alcohol as preservative in Water for Injection, USP (pH 6.1 ± 0.3).
Multidose, Preserved Vial: 1 mL (20,000 Units/mL). Each 1 mL of solution contains 20,000 Units of Epoetin alfa, 2.5 mg Albumin (Human), 1.3 mg sodium citrate, 8.2 mg sodium chloride, 0.11 mg citric acid, and 1% benzyl alcohol as preservative in Water for Injection, USP (pH 6.1 ± 0.3).

CLINICAL PHARMACOLOGY

Chronic Renal Failure Patients

Endogenous production of erythropoietin is normally regulated by the level of tissue oxygenation. Hypoxia and anemia generally increase the production of erythropoietin, which in turn stimulates erythropoiesis.[2] In normal subjects, plasma erythropoietin levels range from 0.01 to 0.03 Units/mL and increase up to 100- to 1000-fold during hypoxia or anemia.[2] In contrast, in patients with chronic renal failure (CRF), production of erythropoietin is impaired, and this erythropoietin deficiency is the primary cause of their anemia.[3,4]
Chronic renal failure is the clinical situation in which there is a progressive and usually irreversible decline in kidney function. Such patients may manifest the sequelae of renal dysfunction, including anemia, but do not necessarily require regular dialysis. Patients with end-stage renal disease (ESRD) are those patients with CRF who require regular dialysis or kidney transplantation for survival.
EPOGEN® has been shown to stimulate erythropoiesis in anemic patients with CRF, including both patients on dialysis and those who do not require regular dialysis.[4–13] The first evidence of a response to the three times weekly (TIW) administration of EPOGEN® is an increase in the reticulocyte count within 10 days, followed by increases in the red cell count, hemoglobin, and hematocrit, usually within 2 to 6 weeks.[4,5] Because of the length of time required for erythropoiesis—several days for erythroid progenitors to mature and be released into the circulation—a clinically significant increase in hematocrit is usually not observed in less than 2 weeks and may require up to 6 weeks in some patients. Once the hematocrit reaches the suggested target range (30% to 36%), that level can be sustained by EPOGEN® therapy in the absence of iron deficiency and concurrent illnesses.
The rate of hematocrit increase varies between patients and is dependent upon the dose of EPOGEN®, within a therapeutic range of approximately 50 to 300 Units/kg TIW.[4] A greater biologic response is not observed at doses exceeding 300 Units/kg TIW.[6] Other factors affecting the rate and extent of response include availability of iron stores, the baseline hematocrit, and the presence of concurrent medical problems.

Zidovudine-treated HIV-infected Patients

Responsiveness to EPOGEN® in HIV-infected patients is dependent upon the endogenous serum erythropoietin level prior to treatment. Patients with endogenous serum erythropoietin levels ≤ 500 mUnits/mL, and who are receiving a dose of zidovudine ≤ 4200 mg/week, may respond to EPOGEN® therapy. Patients with endogenous serum erythropoietin levels > 500 mUnits/mL do not appear to respond to EPOGEN® therapy. In a series of four clinical trials involving 255 patients, 60% to 80% of HIV-infected patients treated with zidovudine had endogenous serum erythropoietin levels ≤ 500 mUnits/mL.
Response to EPOGEN® in zidovudine-treated HIV-infected patients is manifested by reduced transfusion requirements and increased hematocrit.

Cancer Patients on Chemotherapy

Anemia in cancer patients may be related to the disease itself or the effect of concomitantly administered chemotherapeutic agents. EPOGEN® has been shown to increase hematocrit and decrease transfusion requirements after the first month of therapy (months 2 and 3), in anemic cancer patients undergoing chemotherapy.
A series of clinical trials enrolled 131 anemic cancer patients who were receiving cyclic cisplatin- or non cisplatin-containing chemotherapy. Endogenous baseline serum erythropoietin levels varied among patients in these trials with approximately 75% (n = 83/110) having endogenous serum erythropoietin levels ≤ 132 mUnits/mL, and approximately 4% (n = 4/110) of patients having endogenous serum erythropoietin levels > 500 mUnits/mL. In general, patients with lower baseline serum erythropoietin levels responded more vigorously to EPOGEN® than patients with higher baseline erythropoietin levels. Although no specific serum erythropoietin level can be stipulated above which patients would be unlikely to respond to EPOGEN® therapy, treatment of patients with grossly elevated serum erythropoietin levels (eg, > 200 mUnits/mL) is not recommended.

Pharmacokinetics

Intravenously administered EPOGEN® is eliminated at a rate consistent with first order kinetics with a circulating half-life ranging from approximately 4 to 13 hours in adult and pediatric patients with CRF.[14–16] Within the therapeutic dose range, detectable levels of plasma erythropoietin are maintained for at least 24 hours.[7] After SC administration of EPOGEN® to patients with CRF, peak serum levels are achieved within 5 to 24 hours after administration and decline slowly thereafter. There is no apparent difference in half-life between adult patients not on dialysis whose serum creatinine levels were greater than 3, and adult patients maintained on dialysis.
In normal volunteers, the half-life of IV administered EPOGEN® is approximately 20% shorter than the half-life in CRF patients. The pharmacokinetics of EPOGEN® have not been studied in HIV-infected patients.
The pharmacokinetic profile of EPOGEN® in children and adolescents appears to be similar to that of adults. Limited data are available in neonates.[17]
It has been demonstrated in normal volunteers that the 10,000 Units/mL citrate-buffered Epoetin alfa formulation and the 40,000 Units/mL phosphate-buffered Epoetin alfa formulation are bioequivalent after SC administration of single 750 Units/kg doses. The C_{max} and $t_{1/2}$ after administration of the phosphate buffered Epoetin alfa formulation were 1.8 ± 0.7 Units/mL and 19.0 ± 5.9 hours (mean ± SD), respectively. The corresponding mean ± SD values for the citrate-buffered Epoetin alfa formulation were 2 ± 0.9 Units/mL and 16.3 ± 3.0 hours. There was no notable accumulation in serum after two weekly 750 Units/kg SC doses of Epoetin alfa.

INDICATIONS AND USAGE

Treatment of Anemia of Chronic Renal Failure Patients

EPOGEN® is indicated for the treatment of anemia associated with CRF, including patients on dialysis (ESRD) and patients not on dialysis. EPOGEN® is indicated to elevate or maintain the red blood cell level (as manifested by the hematocrit or hemoglobin determinations) and to decrease the need for transfusions in these patients.
Non-dialysis patients with symptomatic anemia considered for therapy should have a hematocrit less than 30%.
EPOGEN® is not intended for patients who require immediate correction of severe anemia. EPOGEN® may obviate the need for maintenance transfusions but is not a substitute for emergency transfusion.
Prior to initiation of therapy, the patient's iron stores should be evaluated. Transferrin saturation should be at least 20% and ferritin at least 100 ng/mL. Blood pressure should be adequately controlled prior to initiation of EPOGEN® therapy, and must be closely monitored and controlled during therapy.
EPOGEN® should be administered under the guidance of a qualified physician (see DOSAGE AND ADMINISTRATION).

Treatment of Anemia in Zidovudine-treated HIV-infected Patients

EPOGEN® is indicated for the treatment of anemia related to therapy with zidovudine in HIV-infected patients. EPOGEN® is indicated to elevate or maintain the red blood cell level (as manifested by the hematocrit or hemoglobin determinations) and to decrease the need for transfusions in these patients. EPOGEN® is not indicated for the treatment of anemia in HIV-infected patients due to other factors such as iron or folate deficiencies, hemolysis or gastrointestinal bleeding, which should be managed appropriately.
EPOGEN®, at a dose of 100 Units/kg TIW, is effective in decreasing the transfusion requirement and increasing the red blood cell level of anemic, HIV-infected patients treated with zidovudine, when the endogenous serum erythropoietin level is ≤ 500 mUnits/mL and when patients are receiving a dose of zidovudine ≤ 4200 mg/week.

Treatment of Anemia in Cancer Patients on Chemotherapy

EPOGEN® is indicated for the treatment of anemia in patients with non-myeloid malignancies where anemia is due to the effect of concomitantly administered chemotherapy. EPOGEN® is indicated to decrease the need for transfusions in patients who will be receiving concomitant chemotherapy for a minimum of 2 months. EPOGEN® is not indicated for the treatment of anemia in cancer patients due to other factors such as iron or folate deficiencies, hemolysis or gastrointestinal bleeding, which should be managed appropriately.

Reduction of Allogeneic Blood Transfusion in Surgery Patients

EPOGEN® is indicated for the treatment of anemic patients (hemoglobin > 10 to ≤ 13 g/dL) scheduled to undergo elective, noncardiac, nonvascular surgery to reduce the need for allogeneic blood transfusions.[18–20] EPOGEN® is indicated for patients at high risk for perioperative transfusions with significant, anticipated blood loss. EPOGEN® is not indicated for anemic patients who are willing to donate autologous blood. The safety of the perioperative use of EPOGEN® has been studied only in patients who are receiving anticoagulant prophylaxis.

CLINICAL EXPERIENCE: RESPONSE TO EPOGEN®

Chronic Renal Failure Patients

Response to EPOGEN® was consistent across all studies. In the presence of adequate iron stores (see IRON EVALUATION), the time to reach the target hematocrit is a function of the baseline hematocrit and the rate of hematocrit rise. The rate of increase in hematocrit is dependent upon the dose of EPOGEN® administered and individual patient variation. In clinical trials at starting doses of 50 to 150 Units/kg TIW, adult patients responded with an average rate of hematocrit rise of:

STARTING DOSE (TIW IV)	HEMATOCRIT INCREASE POINTS/DAY	POINTS/2 WEEKS
50 Units/kg	0.11	1.5
100 Units/kg	0.18	2.5
150 Units/kg	0.25	3.5

Over this dose range, approximately 95% of all patients responded with a clinically significant increase in hematocrit, and by the end of approximately 2 months of therapy virtually all patients were transfusion-independent. Changes in the quality of life of adult patients treated with EPOGEN® were assessed as part of a phase 3 clinical trial.[5,8] Once the target hematocrit (32% to 38%) was achieved, statistically significant improvements were demonstrated for most quality of life parameters measured, including energy and activity level, functional ability, sleep and eating behavior, health status, satisfaction with health, sex life, well-being, psychological effect, life satisfaction, and happiness. Patients also reported improvement in their disease symptoms. They showed a statistically significant increase in exercise capacity (VO_2 max), energy, and strength with a significant reduction in aching, dizziness, anxiety, shortness of breath, muscle weakness, and leg cramps.[8,21]

Adult Patients on Dialysis: Thirteen clinical studies were conducted, involving IV administration to a total of 1010 anemic patients on dialysis for 986 patient-years of EPOGEN® therapy. In the three largest of these clinical trials, the median maintenance dose necessary to maintain the hematocrit between 30% to 36% was approximately 75 Units/kg TIW. In the US multicenter Phase 3 study, approximately 65% of the patients required doses of 100 Units/kg TIW, or less, to maintain their hematocrit at approximately 35%. Almost 10% of patients required a dose of 25 Units/kg, or less, and approximately 10% required a dose of more than 200 Units/kg TIW to maintain their hematocrit at this level. A multicenter unit dose study was also conducted in 119 patients receiving peritoneal dialysis who self-administered EPOGEN® subcutaneously for approximately 109 patient-years of experience. Patients responded to EPOGEN® administered SC in a manner similar to patients receiving IV administration.[22]

Pediatric Patients on Dialysis: One hundred twenty-eight children from 2 months to 19 years of age with CRF requiring dialysis were enrolled in 4 clinical studies of EPOGEN®. The largest study was a placebo-controlled, randomized trial in 113 children with anemia (hematocrit ≤ 27%) undergoing peritoneal dialysis or hemodialysis. The initial dose of EPOGEN® was 50 Units/kg IV or SC TIW. The dose of study drug was titrated to achieve either a hematocrit of 30% to 36% or an absolute increase in hematocrit of 6 percentage points over baseline.

At the end of the initial 12 weeks, a statistically significant rise in mean hematocrit (9.4% vs 0.9%) was observed only in the EPOGEN® arm. The proportion of children achieving a hematocrit of 30%, or an increase in hematocrit of 6 percentage points over baseline, at any time during the first 12 weeks was higher in the EPOGEN® arm (96% vs 58%). Within 12 weeks of initiating EPOGEN® therapy, 92.3% of the pediatric patients were transfusion-independent as compared to 65.4% who received placebo. Among patients who received 36 weeks of EPOGEN®, hemodialysis patients required a higher median maintenance dose (167 Units/kg/week [n = 28] vs 76 Units/kg/week [n = 36]) and took longer to achieve a hematocrit of 30% to 36% (median time to response 69 days vs 32 days) than patients undergoing peritoneal dialysis.

Patients With CRF Not Requiring Dialysis

Four clinical trials were conducted in patients with CRF not on dialysis involving 181 patients treated with EPOGEN® for approximately 67 patient-years of experience. These patients responded to EPOGEN® therapy in a manner similar to that observed in patients on dialysis. Patients with CRF not on dialysis demonstrated a dose-dependent and sustained increase in hematocrit when EPOGEN® was administered by either an IV or SC route, with similar rates of rise of hematocrit when EPOGEN® was administered by either route. Moreover, EPOGEN® doses of 75 to 150 Units/kg per week have been shown to maintain hematocrits of 36% to 38% for up to 6 months. Correcting the anemia of progressive renal failure will allow patients to remain active even though their renal function continues to decrease.[23-24]

Zidovudine-treated HIV-infected Patients

EPOGEN® has been studied in four placebo-controlled trials enrolling 297 anemic (hematocrit < 30%) HIV-infected (AIDS) patients receiving concomitant therapy with zidovudine (all patients were treated with Epoetin alfa manufactured by Amgen Inc.). In the subgroup of patients (89/125 EPOGEN® and 88/130 placebo) with prestudy endogenous serum erythropoietin levels ≤ 500 mUnits/mL EPOGEN® reduced the mean cumulative number of units of blood transfused per patient by approximately 40% as compared to the placebo group.[25] Among those patients who required transfusions at baseline, 43% of patients treated with EPOGEN® versus 18% of placebo-treated patients were transfusion-independent during the second and third months of therapy. EPOGEN® therapy also resulted in significant increases in hematocrit in comparison to placebo. When examining the results according to the weekly dose of zidovudine received during month 3 of therapy, there was a statistically significant ($p < 0.003$) reduction in transfusion requirements in patients treated with EPOGEN® (n = 51) compared to placebo treated patients (n = 54) whose mean weekly zidovudine dose was ≤ 4200 mg/week.[25]

Approximately 17% of the patients with endogenous serum erythropoietin levels ≤ 500 mUnits/mL receiving EPOGEN® in doses from 100 to 200 Units/kg TIW achieved a hematocrit of 38% without administration of transfusions or significant reduction in zidovudine dose. In the subgroup of patients whose prestudy endogenous serum erythropoietin levels were > 500 mUnits/mL, EPOGEN® therapy did not reduce transfusion requirements or increase hematocrit, compared to the corresponding responses in placebo-treated patients.

In a six month open-label EPOGEN® study, patients responded with decreased transfusion requirements and sustained increases in hematocrit and hemoglobin with doses of EPOGEN® up to 300 Units/kg TIW.[25-27]

Responsiveness to EPOGEN® therapy may be blunted by intercurrent infectious/inflammatory episodes and by an increase in zidovudine dosage. Consequently, the dose of EPOGEN® must be titrated based on these factors to maintain the desired erythropoietic response.

Cancer Patients on Chemotherapy

EPOGEN® has been studied in a series of placebo-controlled, double-blind trials in a total of 131 anemic cancer patients. Within this group, 72 patients were treated with concomitant non cisplatin-containing chemotherapy regimens and 59 patients were treated with concomitant cisplatin-containing chemotherapy regimens. Patients were randomized to EPOGEN® 150 Units/kg or placebo subcutaneously TIW for 12 weeks.

EPOGEN® therapy was associated with a significantly ($p < 0.008$) greater hematocrit response than in the corresponding placebo-treated patients (see table).[25]

HEMATOCRIT (%):
MEAN CHANGE FROM BASELINE TO FINAL VALUE*

STUDY	*EPOGEN®*	*PLACEBO*
Chemotherapy	7.6	1.3
Cisplatin	6.9	0.6

*Significantly higher in EPOGEN® patients than in placebo patients ($p < 0.008$)

In the two types of chemotherapy studies (utilizing an EPOGEN® dose of 150 Units/kg TIW), the mean number of units of blood transfused per patient after the first month of therapy was significantly ($p < 0.02$) lower in patients treated with EPOGEN® (0.71 units in months 2, 3) than in corresponding placebo-treated patients (1.84 units in months 2, 3). Moreover, the proportion of patients transfused during months 2 and 3 of therapy combined was significantly ($p < 0.03$) lower in the patients treated with EPOGEN® than in the corresponding placebo-treated patients (22% vs 43%).[25]

Comparable intensity of chemotherapy in the EPOGEN® and placebo groups in the chemotherapy trials was suggested by a similar area under the neutrophil time curve in patients treated with EPOGEN® and placebo-treated patients as well as by a similar proportion of patients in groups treated with EPOGEN® and placebo-treated groups whose absolute neutrophil counts fell below 1000 cells/μL. Available evidence suggests that patients with lymphoid and solid cancers respond equivalently to EPOGEN® therapy, and that patients with or without tumor infiltration of the bone marrow respond equivalently to EPOGEN® therapy.

Surgery Patients

EPOGEN® has been studied in a placebo-controlled, double-blind trial enrolling 316 patients scheduled for major, elective orthopedic hip or knee surgery who were expected to require ≥ 2 units of blood and who were not able or willing to participate in an autologous blood donation program. Based on previous studies which demonstrated that pretreatment hemoglobin is a predictor of risk of receiving transfusion,[20,28] patients were stratified into one of three groups based on their pretreatment hemoglobin [≤ 10 (n = 2), > 10 to ≤ 13 (n = 96), and > 13 to ≤ 15 g/dL (n = 218)] and then randomly assigned to receive 300 IU/kg EPOGEN®, 100 IU/kg EPOGEN®, or placebo by SC injection for 10 days before surgery, on the day of surgery, and for four days after surgery.[18] All patients received oral iron and a low-dose post-operative warfarin regimen.[18]

Treatment with EPOGEN® 300 IU/kg significantly ($p = 0.024$) reduced the risk of allogeneic transfusion in patients with a pretreatment hemoglobin of > 10 to ≤ 13 g/dL; 5/31 (16%) of EPOGEN® 300 IU/kg, 6/26 (23%) of EPOGEN® 100 IU/kg, and 13/29 (45%) of placebo-treated patients were transfused.[18] There was no significant difference in the number of patients transfused between EPOGEN® (9% 300 IU/kg, 6% 100 IU/kg) and placebo (13%) in the > 13 to ≤ 15 g/dL hemoglobin stratum. There were too few patients in the ≤ 10 g/dL group to determine if EPOGEN® is useful in this hemoglobin strata. In the > 10 to ≤ 13 g/dL pretreatment stratum, the mean number of units transfused per EPOGEN® treated patient (0.45 units blood for 300 IU/kg, 0.42 units blood for 100 IU/kg) was less than the mean transfused per placebo-treated patient (1.14 units) (overall $p = 0.028$). In addition, mean hemoglobin, hematocrit and reticulocyte counts increased significantly during the presurgery period in patients treated with EPOGEN®.[18]

EPOGEN® was also studied in an open-label, parallel-group trial enrolling 145 subjects with a pretreatment hemoglobin level of ≥ 10 to ≤ 13 g/dL who were scheduled for major orthopedic hip or knee surgery and who were not participating in an autologous program.[19] Subjects were randomly assigned to receive one of two SC dosing regimens of EPOGEN® (600 IU/kg once weekly for 3 weeks prior to surgery and on the day of surgery, or 300 IU/kg once daily for 10 days prior to surgery, on the day of surgery and for 4 days after surgery). All subjects received oral iron and appropriate pharmacologic anticoagulation therapy.

From pretreatment to presurgery, the mean increase in hemoglobin in the 600 IU/kg weekly group (1.44 g/dL) was greater than observed in the 300 IU/kg daily group.[19] The mean increase in absolute reticulocyte count was smaller in the weekly group ($0.11 \times 10^6/mm^3$) compared to the daily group ($0.17 \times 10^6/mm^3$). Mean hemoglobin levels were similar for the two treatment groups throughout the postsurgical period.

The erythropoietic response observed in both treatment groups resulted in similar transfusion rates [11/69 (16%) in the 600 IU/kg weekly group and 14/71 (20%) in the 300 IU/kg daily group].[19] The mean number of units transfused per subject was approximately 0.3 units in both treatment groups.

CONTRAINDICATIONS

EPOGEN® is contraindicated in patients with:

1. Uncontrolled hypertension.
2. Known hypersensitivity to mammalian cell-derived products.
3. Known hypersensitivity to Albumin (Human).

WARNINGS

Pediatric Use

The multidose preserved formulation contains benzyl alcohol. Benzyl alcohol has been reported to be associated with an increased incidence of neurological and other complications in premature infants which are sometimes fatal.

Thrombotic Events and Increased Mortality

A randomized, prospective trial of 1265 hemodialysis patients with clinically evident cardiac disease (ischemic heart disease or congestive heart failure) was conducted in which patients were assigned to EPOGEN® treatment targeted to a maintenance hematocrit of either 42 ± 3% or 30 ± 3%. Increased mortality was observed in 634 patients randomized to a target hematocrit of 42% [221 deaths (35% mortality)] compared to 631 patients targeted to remain at a hematocrit of 30% [185 deaths (29% mortality)]. The reason for the increased mortality observed in these studies is unknown, however, the incidence of non-fatal myocardial infarctions (3.1% vs 2.3%), vascular access thromboses (39% vs 29%), and all other thrombotic events (22% vs 18%) were also higher in the group randomized to achieve a hematocrit of 42%.

Increased mortality was also observed in a randomized placebo-controlled study of EPOGEN® in adult patients who did not have CRF who were undergoing coronary artery bypass surgery (7 deaths in 126 patients randomized to EPOGEN® versus no deaths among 56 patients receiving placebo). Four of these deaths occurred during the period of study drug administration and all 4 deaths were associated with thrombotic events. While the extent of the population affected is unknown, in patients at risk for thrombosis, the anticipated benefits of EPOGEN® treatment should be weighed against the potential for increased risks associated with therapy.

Chronic Renal Failure Patients

Hypertension: Patients with uncontrolled hypertension should not be treated with EPOGEN®; blood pressure should be controlled adequately before initiation of therapy. Up to 80% of patients with CRF have a history of hypertension.[29] Although there does not appear to be any direct pressor effects of EPOGEN®, blood pressure may rise during EPOGEN® therapy. During the early phase of treatment when the hematocrit is increasing, approximately 25% of patients on dialysis may require initiation of, or increases in, antihypertensive therapy. Hypertensive encephalopathy and seizures have been observed in patients with CRF treated with EPOGEN®.

Special care should be taken to closely monitor and aggressively control blood pressure in patients treated with EPOGEN®. Patients should be advised as to the importance of compliance with antihypertensive therapy and dietary restrictions. If blood pressure is difficult to control by initiation of appropriate measures, the hematocrit may be reduced by decreasing or withholding the dose of EPOGEN®. A clinically significant decrease in hematocrit may not be observed for several weeks.

It is recommended that the dose of EPOGEN® be decreased if the hematocrit increase exceeds 4 points in any 2-week period, because of the possible association of excessive rate of rise of hematocrit with an exacerbation of hypertension. In CRF patients on hemodialysis with clinically evident ischemic heart disease or congestive heart failure, the hematocrit should be managed carefully, not to exceed 36% (SEE THROMBOTIC EVENTS).

Seizures: Seizures have occurred in patients with CRF participating in EPOGEN® clinical trials.

In adult patients on dialysis, there was a higher incidence of seizures during the first 90 days of therapy (occurring in approximately 2.5% of patients) as compared with later timepoints.

Given the potential for an increased risk of seizures during the first 90 days of therapy, blood pressure and the presence of premonitory neurologic symptoms should be monitored closely. Patients should be cautioned to avoid potentially hazardous activities such as driving or operating heavy machinery during this period.

While the relationship between seizures and the rate of rise of hematocrit is uncertain, it is recommended that the dose of EPOGEN® be decreased if the hematocrit increase exceeds 4 points in any 2-week period.

Thrombotic Events: During hemodialysis, patients treated with EPOGEN® may require increased anticoagulation with heparin to prevent clotting of the artificial kidney (see ADVERSE REACTIONS for more information about thrombotic events).

Other thrombotic events (eg, myocardial infarction, cerebrovascular accident, transient ischemic attack) have occurred in clinical trials at an annualized rate of less than 0.04 events per patient year of EPOGEN® therapy. These trials

Continued on next page

Epogen—Cont.

were conducted in adult patients with CRF (whether on dialysis or not) in whom the target hematocrit was 32% to 40%. However, the risk of thrombotic events, including vascular access thrombosis, was significantly increased in adult patients with ischemic heart disease or congestive heart failure receiving EPOGEN® therapy with the goal of reaching a normal hematocrit (42%) as compared to a target hematocrit of 30%. Patients with pre-existing cardiovascular disease should be monitored closely.

Zidovudine-treated HIV-infected Patients

In contrast to CRF patients, EPOGEN® therapy has not been linked to exacerbation of hypertension, seizures, and thrombotic events in HIV-infected patients.

PRECAUTIONS

The parenteral administration of any biologic product should be attended by appropriate precautions in case allergic or other untoward reactions occur (see CONTRAINDICATIONS). In clinical trials, while transient rashes were occasionally observed concurrently with EPOGEN® therapy, no serious allergic or anaphylactic reactions were reported (see ADVERSE REACTIONS for more information regarding allergic reactions).

The safety and efficacy of EPOGEN® therapy have not been established in patients with a known history of a seizure disorder or underlying hematologic disease (eg, sickle cell anemia, myelodysplastic syndromes, or hypercoagulable disorders).

In some female patients, menses have resumed following EPOGEN® therapy; the possibility of pregnancy should be discussed and the need for contraception evaluated.

Hematology

Exacerbation of porphyria has been observed rarely in patients with CRF treated with EPOGEN®. However, EPOGEN® has not caused increased urinary excretion of porphyrin metabolites in normal volunteers, even in the presence of a rapid erythropoietic response. Nevertheless, EPOGEN® should be used with caution in patients with known porphyria.

In preclinical studies in dogs and rats, but not in monkeys, EPOGEN® therapy was associated with subclinical bone marrow fibrosis. Bone marrow fibrosis is a known complication of CRF in humans and may be related to secondary hyperparathyroidism or unknown factors. The incidence of bone marrow fibrosis was not increased in a study of adult patients on dialysis who were treated with EPOGEN® for 12 to 19 months, compared to the incidence of bone marrow fibrosis in a matched group of patients who had not been treated with EPOGEN®.

Hematocrit in CRF patients should be measured twice a week; zidovudine-treated HIV-infected and cancer patients should have hematocrit measured once a week until hematocrit has been stabilized, and measured periodically thereafter.

Delayed or Diminished Response

If the patient fails to respond or to maintain a response to doses within the recommended dosing range, the following etiologies should be considered and evaluated:

1. Iron deficiency: Virtually all patients will eventually require supplemental iron therapy (see IRON EVALUATION).
2. Underlying infectious, inflammatory, or malignant processes.
3. Occult blood loss.
4. Underlying hematologic diseases (ie, thalassemia, refractory anemia, or other myelodysplastic disorders).
5. Vitamin deficiencies: Folic acid or vitamin B12.
6. Hemolysis.
7. Aluminum intoxication.
8. Osteitis fibrosa cystica.

Iron Evaluation

During EPOGEN® therapy, absolute or functional iron deficiency may develop. Functional iron deficiency, with normal ferritin levels but low transferrin saturation, is presumably due to the inability to mobilize iron stores rapidly enough to support increased erythropoiesis. Transferrin saturation should be at least 20% and ferritin should be at least 100 ng/mL.

Prior to and during EPOGEN® therapy, the patient's iron status, including transferrin saturation (serum iron divided by iron binding capacity) and serum ferritin, should be evaluated. Virtually all patients will eventually require supplemental iron to increase or maintain transferrin saturation to levels which will adequately support erythropoiesis stimulated by EPOGEN®. All surgery patients being treated with EPOGEN® should receive adequate iron supplementation throughout the course of therapy in order to support erythropoiesis and avoid depletion of iron stores.

Drug Interaction

No evidence of interaction of EPOGEN® with other drugs was observed in the course of clinical trials.

Carcinogenesis, Mutagenesis, and Impairment of Fertility

Carcinogenic potential of EPOGEN® has not been evaluated. EPOGEN® does not induce bacterial gene mutation (Ames Test), chromosomal aberrations in mammalian cells, micronuclei in mice, or gene mutation at the HGPRT locus. In female rats treated IV with EPOGEN®, there was a trend for slightly increased fetal wastage at doses of 100 and 500 Units/kg.

Pregnancy Category C

EPOGEN® has been shown to have adverse effects in rats when given in doses 5 times the human dose. There are no adequate and well-controlled studies in pregnant women. EPOGEN® should be used during pregnancy only if potential benefit justifies the potential risk to the fetus.

In studies in female rats, there were decreases in body weight gain, delays in appearance of abdominal hair, delayed eyelid opening, delayed ossification, and decreases in the number of caudal vertebrae in the F1 fetuses of the 500 Units/kg group. In female rats treated IV, there was a trend for slightly increased fetal wastage at doses of 100 and 500 Units/kg. EPOGEN® has not shown any adverse effect at doses as high as 500 Units/kg in pregnant rabbits (from day 6 to 18 of gestation).

Nursing Mothers

Postnatal observations of the live offspring (F1 generation) of female rats treated with EPOGEN® during gestation and lactation revealed no effect of EPOGEN® at doses of up to 500 Units/kg. There were, however, decreases in body weight gain, delays in appearance of abdominal hair, eyelid opening, and decreases in the number of caudal vertebrae in the F1 fetuses of the 500 Units/kg group. There were no EPOGEN®-related effects on the F2 generation fetuses.

It is not known whether EPOGEN® is excreted in human milk. Because many drugs are excreted in human milk, caution should be exercised when EPOGEN® is administered to a nursing woman.

Pediatric Use

See WARNINGS, Pediatric Use.

Pediatric Patients on Dialysis: EPOGEN® is indicated in infants (1 month to 2 years), children (2 years to 12 years), and adolescents (12 years to 16 years) for the treatment of anemia associated with CRF requiring dialysis. Safety and effectiveness in pediatric patients less than 1 month old have not been established (see CLINICAL EXPERIENCE, Chronic Renal Failure, *Pediatric Patients on Dialysis*). The safety data from these studies show that there is no increased risk to pediatric CRF patients on dialysis when compared to the safety profile of EPOGEN® in adult CRF patients (see ADVERSE REACTIONS and WARNINGS). Published literature [31–33] provides supportive evidence of the safety and effectiveness of EPOGEN® in pediatric CRF patients on dialysis.

Pediatric Patients Not Requiring Dialysis: Published literature[33,34] has reported the use of EPOGEN® in 133 pediatric patients with anemia associated with CRF not requiring dialysis, ages 3 months to 20 years, treated with 50 to 250 Units/kg SC or IV, QW to TIW. Dose-dependent increases in hemoglobin and hematocrit were observed with reductions in transfusion requirements.

Pediatric HIV-infected Patients: Published literature [35,36] has reported the use of EPOGEN® in 20 zidovudine-treated anemic HIV-infected pediatric patients ages 8 months to 17 years, treated with 50 to 400 Units/kg SC or IV, 2 to 3 times per week. Increases in hemoglobin levels and in reticulocyte counts, and decreases in or elimination of blood transfusions were observed.

Pediatric Cancer Patients on Chemotherapy: Published literature[37,38] has reported the use of EPOGEN® in approximately 64 anemic pediatric cancer patients ages 6 months to 18 years, treated with 25 to 300 Units/kg SC or IV, 3 to 7 times per week. Increases in hemoglobin and decreases in transfusion requirements were noted.

Chronic Renal Failure Patients

Patients with CRF Not Requiring Dialysis

Blood pressure and hematocrit should be monitored no less frequently than for patients maintained on dialysis. Renal function and fluid and electrolyte balance should be closely monitored, as an improved sense of well-being may obscure the need to initiate dialysis in some patients.

Hematology: Sufficient time should be allowed to determine a patient's responsiveness to a dosage of EPOGEN® before adjusting the dose. Because of the time required for erythropoiesis and the red cell half-life, an interval of 2 to 6 weeks may occur between the time of a dose adjustment (initiation, increase, decrease, or discontinuation) and a significant change in hematocrit.

In order to avoid reaching the suggested target hematocrit too rapidly, or exceeding the suggested target range (hematocrit of 30% to 36%), the guidelines for dose and frequency of dose adjustments (see DOSAGE AND ADMINISTRATION) should be followed.

For patients who respond to EPOGEN® with a rapid increase in hematocrit (eg, more than 4 points in any 2-week period), the dose of EPOGEN® should be reduced because of the possible association of excessive rate of rise of hematocrit with an exacerbation of hypertension.

The elevated bleeding time characteristic of CRF decreases toward normal after correction of anemia in adult patients treated with EPOGEN®. Reduction of bleeding time also occurs after correction of anemia by transfusion.

Laboratory Monitoring: The hematocrit should be determined twice a week until it has stabilized in the suggested target range and the maintenance dose has been established. After any dose adjustment, the hematocrit should also be determined twice weekly for at least 2 to 6 weeks until it has been determined that the hematocrit has stabilized in response to the dose change. The hematocrit should then be monitored at regular intervals.

A complete blood count with differential and platelet count should be performed regularly. During clinical trials, modest increases were seen in platelets and white blood cell counts. While these changes were statistically significant, they were not clinically significant and the values remained within normal ranges.

In patients with CRF, serum chemistry values [including blood urea nitrogen (BUN), uric acid, creatinine, phosphorus, and potassium] should be monitored regularly. During clinical trials in adult patients on dialysis, modest increases were seen in BUN, creatinine, phosphorus, and potassium. In some adult patients with CRF not on dialysis treated with EPOGEN®, modest increases in serum uric acid and phosphorus were observed. While changes were statistically significant, the values remained within the ranges normally seen in patients with CRF.

Diet: As the hematocrit increases and patients experience an improved sense of well-being and quality of life, the importance of compliance with dietary and dialysis prescriptions should be reinforced. In particular, hyperkalemia is not uncommon in patients with CRF. In US studies in patients on dialysis, hyperkalemia has occurred at an annualized rate of approximately 0.11 episodes per patient-year of EPOGEN® therapy, often in association with poor compliance to medication, diet, and/or dialysis.

Dialysis Management: Therapy with EPOGEN® results in an increase in hematocrit and a decrease in plasma volume which could affect dialysis efficiency. In studies to date, the resulting increase in hematocrit did not appear to adversely affect dialyzer function[9,10] or the efficiency of high flux hemodialysis.[11] During hemodialysis, patients treated with EPOGEN® may require increased anticoagulation with heparin to prevent clotting of the artificial kidney.

Patients who are marginally dialyzed may require adjustments in their dialysis prescription. As with all patients on dialysis, the serum chemistry values (including BUN, creatinine, phosphorus, and potassium) in patients treated with EPOGEN® should be monitored regularly to assure the adequacy of the dialysis prescription.

Information for Patients: In those situations in which the physician determines that a home dialysis patient can safely and effectively self-administer EPOGEN®, the patient should be instructed as to the proper dosage and administration. Home dialysis patients should be referred to the full "Information for Home Dialysis Patients" insert; it is not a disclosure of all possible effects. Patients should be informed of the signs and symptoms of allergic drug reaction and advised of appropriate actions. If home use is prescribed for a home dialysis patient, the patient should be thoroughly instructed in the importance of proper disposal and cautioned against the reuse of needles, syringes, or drug product. A puncture-resistant container for the disposal of used syringes and needles should be available to the patient. The full container should be disposed of according to the directions provided by the physician.

Renal Function: In adult patients with CRF not on dialysis, renal function and fluid and electrolyte balance should be closely monitored, as an improved sense of well-being may obscure the need to initiate dialysis in some patients. In patients with CRF not on dialysis, placebo-controlled studies of progression of renal dysfunction over periods of greater than 1 year have not been completed. In shorter term trials in adult patients with CRF not on dialysis, changes in creatinine and creatinine clearance were not significantly different in patients treated with EPOGEN®, compared with placebo-treated patients. Analysis of the slope of 1/serum creatinine versus time plots in these patients indicates no significant change in the slope after the initiation of EPOGEN® therapy.

Zidovudine-treated HIV-infected Patients

Hypertension: Exacerbation of hypertension has not been observed in zidovudine-treated HIV-infected patients treated with EPOGEN®. However, EPOGEN® should be withheld in these patients if pre-existing hypertension is uncontrolled, and should not be started until blood pressure is controlled. In double-blind studies, a single seizure has been experienced by a patient treated with EPOGEN®.[25]

Cancer Patients on Chemotherapy

Hypertension: Hypertension, associated with a significant increase in hematocrit, has been noted rarely in patients treated with EPOGEN®. Nevertheless, blood pressure in patients treated with EPOGEN® should be monitored carefully, particularly in patients with an underlying history of hypertension or cardiovascular disease.

Seizures: In double-blind, placebo-controlled trials, 3.2% (n = 2/63) of patients treated with EPOGEN® and 2.9% (n = 2/68) of placebo-treated patients had seizures. Seizures in 1.6% (n = 1/63) of patients treated with EPOGEN® occurred in the context of a significant increase in blood pressure and hematocrit from baseline values. However, both patients treated with EPOGEN® also had underlying CNS pathology which may have been related to seizure activity.

Thrombotic Events: In double-blind, placebo-controlled trials, 3.2% (n = 2/63) of patients treated with EPOGEN® and 11.8% (n = 8/68) of placebo-treated patients had thrombotic events (eg, pulmonary embolism, cerebrovascular accident).

Growth Factor Potential: EPOGEN® is a growth factor that primarily stimulates red cell production. However, the possibility that EPOGEN® can act as a growth factor for any tumor type, particularly myeloid malignancies, cannot be excluded.

Surgery Patients

Thrombotic/Vascular Events: In perioperative clinical trials with orthopedic patients, the overall incidence of thrombotic/vascular events was similar in Epoetin alfa and placebo-treated patients who had a pretreatment hemoglobin of

> 10 to ≤ 13 g/dL. In patients with a hemoglobin of > 13 g/dL treated with 300 IU/kg of Epoetin alfa, the possibility that EPOGEN® treatment may be associated with an increased risk of postoperative thrombotic/vascular events cannot be excluded.[14–16,24]

In one study in which Epoetin alfa was administered in the perioperative period to patients undergoing coronary artery bypass graft surgery, there were seven deaths in the group treated with Epoetin alfa (n = 126) and no deaths in the placebo-treated group (n = 56). Among the seven deaths in the patients treated with Epoetin alfa, four were at the time of therapy (between study day 2 and 8). The four deaths at the time of therapy (3%) were associated with thrombotic/vascular events. A causative role of Epoetin alfa cannot be excluded (see WARNINGS).

Hypertension: Blood pressure may rise in the perioperative period in patients being treated with EPOGEN®. Therefore, blood pressure should be monitored carefully.

ADVERSE REACTIONS

Chronic Renal Failure Patients

EPOGEN® is generally well-tolerated. The adverse events reported are frequent sequelae of CRF and are not necessarily attributable to EPOGEN® therapy. In double-blind, placebo-controlled studies involving over 300 patients with CRF, the events reported in greater than 5% of patients treated with EPOGEN® during the blinded phase were:

[See first table at right]

Significant adverse events of concern in patients with CRF treated in double-blind, placebo-controlled trials occurred in the following percent of patients during the blinded phase of the studies:

Seizure	1.1%	1.1%
CVA/TIA	0.4%	0.6%
MI	0.4%	1.1%
Death	0%	1.7%

In the US EPOGEN® studies in adult patients on dialysis (over 567 patients), the incidence (number of events per patient-year) of the most frequently reported adverse events were: hypertension (0.75), headache (0.40), tachycardia (0.31), nausea/vomiting (0.26), clotted vascular access (0.25), shortness of breath (0.14), hyperkalemia (0.11), and diarrhea (0.11). Other reported events occurred at a rate of less than 0.10 events per patient per year.

Events reported to have occurred within several hours of administration of EPOGEN® were rare, mild, and transient, and included injection site stinging in dialysis patients and flu-like symptoms such as arthralgias and myalgias. In all studies analyzed to date, EPOGEN® administration was generally well-tolerated, irrespective of the route of administration.

Pediatric CRF Patients: In pediatric patients with CRF on dialysis, the pattern of most adverse events was similar to that found in adults. Additional adverse events reported during the double-blind phase in > 10% of pediatric patients in either treatment group were: abdominal pain, dialysis access complications including access infections and peritonitis in those receiving peritoneal dialysis, fever, upper respiratory infection, cough, pharyngitis, and constipation. The rates are similar between the treatment groups for each event.

Hypertension: Increases in blood pressure have been reported in clinical trials, often during the first 90 days of therapy. On occasion, hypertensive encephalopathy and seizures have been observed in patients with CRF treated with EPOGEN®. When data from all patients in the US Phase 3 multicenter trial were analyzed, there was an apparent trend of more reports of hypertensive adverse events in patients on dialysis with a faster rate of rise of hematocrit (greater than 4 hematocrit points in any 2-week period). However, in a double-blind, placebo-controlled trial, hypertensive adverse events were not reported at an increased rate in the group treated with EPOGEN® (150 Units/kg TIW) relative to the placebo group.

Seizures: There have been 47 seizures in 1010 patients on dialysis treated with EPOGEN® in clinical trials, with an exposure of 986 patient-years for a rate of approximately 0.048 events per patient-year. However, there appeared to be a higher rate of seizures during the first 90 days of therapy (occurring in approximately 2.5% of patients) when compared to subsequent 90-day periods. The baseline incidence of seizures in the untreated dialysis population is difficult to determine; it appears to be in the range of 5% to 10% per patient-year.[39,40,41]

Thrombotic Events: In clinical trials where the maintenance hematocrit was 35 ± 3% on EPOGEN®, clotting of the vascular access (A-V shunt) has occurred at an annualized rate of about 0.25 events per patient-year, and other thrombotic events (eg, myocardial infarction, cerebral vascular accident, transient ischemic attack, and pulmonary embolism) occurred at a rate of 0.04 events per patient-year. In a separate study of 1111 untreated dialysis patients, clotting of the vascular access occurred at a rate of 0.50 events per patient-year. However, in CRF patients on hemodialysis who also had clinically evident ischemic heart disease or congestive heart failure, the risk of A-V shunt thrombosis was higher (39% vs 29%, $p < 0.001$), and myocardial infarctions, vascular ischemic events, and venous thrombosis were increased, in patients targeted to a hematocrit of 42 ± 3% compared to those maintained at 30 ± 3% (see WARNINGS).

In patients treated with commercial EPOGEN®, there have been rare reports of serious or unusual thrombo-embolic events including migratory thrombophlebitis, microvascular thrombosis, pulmonary embolus, and thrombosis of the retinal artery, and temporal and renal veins. A causal relationship has not been established.

Allergic Reactions: There have been no reports of serious allergic reactions or anaphylaxis associated with EPOGEN® administration during clinical trials. Skin rashes and urticaria have been observed rarely and when reported have generally been mild and transient in nature. There have been rare reports of potentially serious allergic reactions including urticaria with associated respiratory symptoms or circumoral edema, or urticaria alone. Most reactions occurred in situations where a causal relationship could not be established. Symptoms recurred with rechallenge in a few instances, suggesting that allergic reactivity may occasionally be associated with EPOGEN® therapy.

There has been no evidence for development of antibodies to erythropoietin in patients tested to date, including those receiving EPOGEN® for over 4 years. Nevertheless, if an anaphylactoid reaction occurs, EPOGEN® should be immediately discontinued and appropriate therapy initiated.

Zidovudine-treated HIV-infected Patients

Adverse events reported in clinical trials with EPOGEN® in zidovudine-treated HIV-infected patients were consistent with the progression of HIV infection. In double-blind, placebo-controlled studies of three-months duration involving approximately 300 zidovudine-treated HIV-infected patients, adverse events with an incidence of ≥ 10% in either patients treated with EPOGEN® or placebo-treated patients were:

[See second table above]

There were no statistically significant differences between treatment groups in the incidence of the above events.

In the 297 patients studied, EPOGEN® was not associated with significant increases in opportunistic infections or mortality.[25] In 71 patients from this group treated with EPOGEN® at 150 Units/kg TIW, serum p24 antigen levels did not appear to increase.[27] Preliminary data showed no enhancement of HIV replication in infected cell lines *in vitro*.[25]

Peripheral white blood cell and platelet counts are unchanged following EPOGEN® therapy.

Allergic Reactions: Two zidovudine-treated HIV-infected patients had urticarial reactions within 48 hours of their first exposure to study medication. One patient was treated with EPOGEN® and one was treated with placebo (EPOGEN® vehicle alone). Both patients had positive immediate skin tests against their study medication with a negative saline control. The basis for this apparent preexisting hypersensitivity to components of the EPOGEN® formulation is unknown, but may be related to HIV-induced immunosuppression or prior exposure to blood products.

Seizures: In double-blind and open-label trials of EPOGEN® in zidovudine-treated HIV-infected patients, 10 patients have experienced seizures.[25] In general, these seizures appear to be related to underlying pathology such as meningitis or cerebral neoplasms, not EPOGEN® therapy.

Cancer Patients on Chemotherapy

Adverse experiences reported in clinical trials with EPOGEN® in cancer patients were consistent with the underlying disease state. In double-blind, placebo-controlled studies of up to 3 months duration involving 131 cancer patients, adverse events with an incidence > 10% in either patients treated with EPOGEN® or placebo-treated patients were as indicated below:

[See first table at top of next page]

Although some statistically significant differences between patients being treated with EPOGEN®-and placebo-treated patients were noted, the overall safety profile of EPOGEN® appeared to be consistent with the disease process of advanced cancer. During double-blind and subsequent open-label therapy in which patients (n = 72 for total exposure to EPOGEN®) were treated for up to 32 weeks with doses as

Continued on next page

PERCENT OF PATIENTS REPORTING EVENT

Event	Patients Treated with EPOGEN® (n = 200)	Placebo-Treated Patients (n = 135)
Hypertension	24%	19%
Headache	16%	12%
Arthralgias	11%	6%
Nausea	11%	9%
Edema	9%	10%
Fatigue	9%	14%
Diarrhea	9%	6%
Vomiting	8%	5%
Chest Pain	7%	9%
Skin Reaction, Administration Site	7%	12%
Asthenia	7%	12%
Dizziness	7%	13%
Clotted Access	7%	2%

PERCENT OF PATIENTS REPORTING EVENT

Event	Patients Treated with EPOGEN® (n = 144)	Placebo-Treated Patients (n = 153)
Pyrexia	38%	29%
Fatigue	25%	31%
Headache	19%	14%
Cough	18%	14%
Diarrhea	16%	18%
Rash	16%	8%
Congestion, Respiratory	15%	10%
Nausea	15%	12%
Shortness of Breath	14%	13%
Asthenia	11%	14%
Skin Reaction, Medication Site	10%	7%
Dizziness	9%	10%

Epogen—Cont.

high as 927 Units/kg, the adverse experience profile of EPOGEN® was consistent with the progression of advanced cancer.

Based on comparable survival data and on the percentage of patients treated with EPOGEN® and placebo-treated patients who discontinued therapy due to death, disease progression, or adverse experiences (22% and 13%, respectively; p = 0.25), the clinical outcome in patients treated with EPOGEN® and placebo-treated patients appeared to be similar. Available data from animal tumor models and measurement of proliferation of solid tumor cells from clinical biopsy specimens in response to EPOGEN® suggest that EPOGEN® does not potentiate tumor growth. Nevertheless, as a growth factor, the possibility that EPOGEN® may potentiate growth of some tumors, particularly myeloid tumors, cannot be excluded. A randomized controlled Phase 4 study is currently ongoing to further evaluate this issue. The mean peripheral white blood cell count was unchanged following EPOGEN® therapy compared to the corresponding value in the placebo-treated group.

Surgery Patients

Adverse events with an incidence of ≥ 10% are shown in the following table:

[See second table at right]

Thrombotic/Vascular Events: In three double-blind, placebo-controlled orthopedic surgery studies, the rate of deep venous thrombosis (DVT) was similar among Epoetin alfa and placebo-treated patients in the recommended population of patients with a pretreatment hemoglobin of > 10 to ≤ 13 g/dL.[18,20,28] However, in 2 of 3 orthopedic surgery studies the overall rate (all pretreatment hemoglobin groups combined) of DVTs detected by postoperative ultrasonography and/or surveillance venography was higher in the group treated with Epoetin alfa than in the placebo-treated group (11% vs 6%). This finding was attributable to the difference in DVT rates observed in the subgroup of patients with pretreatment hemoglobin > 13 g/dL. However, the incidence of DVTs was within the range of that reported in the literature for orthopedic surgery patients.

In the orthopedic surgery study of patients with pretreatment hemoglobin of > 10 to ≤ 13 g/dL which compared two dosing regimens (600 IU/kg weekly × 4 and 300 IU/kg daily × 15), 4 subjects in the 600 IU/kg weekly EPOGEN® group (5%) and no subjects in the 300 IU/kg daily group had a thrombotic vascular event during the study period.[19]

In a study examining the use of Epoetin alfa in 182 patients scheduled for coronary artery bypass graft surgery, 23% of patients treated with Epoetin alfa and 29% treated with placebo experienced thrombotic/vascular events. There were 4 deaths among the Epoetin alfa-treated patients that were associated with a thrombotic/vascular event. A causative role of Epoetin alfa cannot be excluded (see WARNINGS).

OVERDOSAGE

The maximum amount of EPOGEN® that can be safely administered in single or multiple doses has not been determined. Doses of up to 1500 Units/kg TIW for 3 to 4 weeks have been administered to adults without any direct toxic effects of EPOGEN® itself.[6] Therapy with EPOGEN® can result in polycythemia if the hematocrit is not carefully monitored and the dose appropriately adjusted. If the suggested target range is exceeded, EPOGEN® may be temporarily withheld until the hematocrit returns to the suggested target range; EPOGEN® therapy may then be resumed using a lower dose (see DOSAGE AND ADMINISTRATION). If polycythemia is of concern, phlebotomy may be indicated to decrease the hematocrit.

DOSAGE AND ADMINISTRATION

Chronic Renal Failure Patients

The recommended range for the starting dose of EPOGEN® is 50 to 100 Units/kg TIW for adult patients. The recommended starting dose for pediatric CRF patients on dialysis is 50 Units/kg TIW. The dose of EPOGEN® should be reduced as the hematocrit approaches 36% or increases by more than 4 points in any 2-week period. The dosage of EPOGEN® must be individualized to maintain the hematocrit within the suggested target range. At the physician's discretion, the suggested target hematocrit range may be expanded to achieve maximal patient benefit.

EPOGEN® may be given either as an IV or SC injection. In patients on hemodialysis, EPOGEN® usually has been administered as an IV bolus TIW. While the administration of EPOGEN® is independent of the dialysis procedure, EPOGEN® may be administered into the venous line at the end of the dialysis procedure to obviate the need for additional venous access. In adult patients with CRF not on dialysis, EPOGEN® may be given either as an IV or SC injection.

Patients who have been judged competent by their physicians to self-administer EPOGEN® without medical or other supervision may give themselves either an IV or SC injection. The table below provides general therapeutic guidelines for patients with CRF:

[See table at top of next page]

During therapy, hematological parameters should be monitored regularly (see LABORATORY MONITORING).

Pre-therapy Iron Evaluation: Prior to and during EPOGEN® therapy, the patient's iron stores, including transferrin saturation (serum iron divided by iron binding capacity) and serum ferritin, should be evaluated. Transferrin saturation should be at least 20%, and ferritin should be at least 100 ng/mL. Virtually all patients will eventually require supplemental iron to increase or maintain transferrin saturation to levels that will adequately support erythropoiesis stimulated by EPOGEN®.

Dose Adjustment: Following EPOGEN® therapy, a period of time is required for erythroid progenitors to mature and be released into circulation resulting in an eventual increase in hematocrit. Additionally, red blood cell survival time affects hematocrit and may vary due to uremia. As a result, the time required to elicit a clinically significant change in hematocrit (increase or decrease) following any dose adjustment may be 2 to 6 weeks.

Dose adjustment should not be made more frequently than once a month, unless clinically indicated. After any dose adjustment, the hematocrit should be determined twice weekly for at least 2 to 6 weeks (see LABORATORY MONITORING).

- If the hematocrit is increasing and approaching 36%, the dose should be reduced to maintain the suggested target hematocrit range. If the reduced dose does not stop the rise in hematocrit, and it exceeds 36%, doses should be temporarily withheld until the hematocrit begins to decrease, at which point therapy should be reinitiated at a lower dose.
- At any time, if the hematocrit increases by more than 4 points in a 2-week period, the dose should be immediately decreased. After the dose reduction, the hematocrit should be monitored twice weekly for 2 to 6 weeks, and further dose adjustments should be made as outlined in MAINTENANCE DOSE.
- If a hematocrit increase of 5 to 6 points is not achieved after an 8-week period and iron stores are adequate (see DELAYED OR DIMINISHED RESPONSE), the dose of EPOGEN® may be incrementally increased. Further increases may be made at 4 to 6 week intervals until the desired response is attained.

Maintenance Dose: The maintenance dose must be individualized for each patient on dialysis. In the US Phase 3

PERCENT OF PATIENTS REPORTING EVENT

Event	Patients Treated with EPOGEN® (n = 63)	Placebo-Treated Patients (n = 48)
Pyrexia	29%	19%
Diarrhea	21%[a]	7%
Nausea	17%[b]	32%
Vomiting	17%	15%
Edema	17%[c]	1%
Asthenia	13%	16%
Fatigue	13%	15%
Shortness of Breath	13%	9%
Parasthesia	11%	6%
Upper Respiratory Infection	11%	4%
Dizziness	5%	12%
Trunk Pain	3%[d]	16%

[a]p = 0.041,
[b]p = 0.069,
[c]p = 0.0016,
[d]p = 0.017

PERCENT OF PATIENTS REPORTING EVENT

Event	Patients Treated with EPOGEN® 300 IU/kg (n = 112)[a]	Patients Treated with EPOGEN® 100 IU/kg (n = 101)[a]	Placebo-treated Patients (n = 103)[a]	Patients Treated with EPOGEN® 600 IU/kg (n = 73)[b]	Patients Treated with EPOGEN® 300 IU/kg (n = 72)[b]
Pyrexia	51%	50%	60%	47%	42%
Nausea	48%	43%	45%	45%	58%
Constipation	43%	42%	43%	51%	53%
Skin reaction, Medication site	25%	19%	22%	26%	29%
Vomiting	22%	12%	14%	21%	29%
Skin Pain	18%	18%	17%	5%	4%
Pruritus	16%	16%	14%	14%	22%
Insomnia	13%	16%	13%	21%	18%
Headache	13%	11%	9%	10%	19%
Dizziness	12%	9%	12%	11%	21%
Urinary Tract Infection	12%	3%	11%	11%	8%
Hypertension	10%	11%	10%	5%	10%
Diarrhea	10%	7%	12%	10%	6%
Deep Venous Thrombosis	10%	3%	5%	0%[c]	0%[c]
Dyspepsia	9%	11%	6%	7%	8%
Anxiety	7%	2%	11%	11%	4%
Edema	6%	11%	8%	11%	7%

[a] Study including patients undergoing orthopedic surgery treated with EPOGEN® or placebo for 15 days
[b] Study including patients undergoing orthopedic surgery treated with EPOGEN® 600 IU/kg weekly × 4 or 300 IU/kg daily × 15
[c] Determined by clinical symptoms

Starting Dose:	
Adults	50 to 100 Units/kg TIW; IV or SC
Pediatric Patients	50 Units/kg TIW; IV or SC
Reduce Dose When:	1. Hct. approaches 36% or, 2. Hct. increases > 4 points in any 2-week period
Increase Dose If:	Hct. does not increase by 5 to 6 points after 8 weeks of therapy, and hct. is below suggested target range
Maintenance Dose:	Individually titrate
Suggested Target Hct. Range:	30% to 36%

multicenter trial in patients on hemodialysis, the median maintenance dose was 75 Units/kg TIW, with a range from 12.5 to 525 Units/kg TIW. Almost 10% of the patients required a dose of 25 Units/kg, or less, and approximately 10% of the patients required more than 200 Units/kg TIW to maintain their hematocrit in the suggested target range. In pediatric hemodialysis and peritoneal dialysis patients, the median maintenance dose was 167 Units/kg/week (49 to 447 Units/kg per week) and 76 Units/kg/week (24 to 323 Units/kg per week) administered in divided doses (TIW or BIW), respectively to achieve the target range of 30% to 36%.

If the hematocrit remains below, or falls below, the suggested target range, iron stores should be re-evaluated. If the transferrin saturation is less than 20%, supplemental iron should be administered. If the transferrin saturation is greater than 20%, the dose of EPOGEN® may be increased. Such dose increases should not be made more frequently than once a month, unless clinically indicated, as the response time of the hematocrit to a dose increase can be 2 to 6 weeks. Hematocrit should be measured twice weekly for 2 to 6 weeks following dose increases. In adult patients with CRF not on dialysis, the maintenance dose must also be individualized. EPOGEN® doses of 75 to 150 Units/kg/week have been shown to maintain hematocrits of 36% to 38% for up to 6 months.

Delayed or Diminished Response: Over 95% of patients with CRF responded with clinically significant increases in hematocrit, and virtually all patients were transfusion-independent within approximately 2 months of initiation of EPOGEN® therapy.

If a patient fails to respond or maintain a response, other etiologies should be considered and evaluated as clinically indicated (see PRECAUTIONS for discussion of delayed or diminished response).

Zidovudine-treated HIV-infected Patients

Prior to beginning EPOGEN®, it is recommended that the endogenous serum erythropoietin level be determined (prior to transfusion). Available evidence suggests that patients receiving zidovudine with endogenous serum erythropoietin levels > 500 mUnits/mL are unlikely to respond to therapy with EPOGEN®.

Starting Dose: For adult patients with serum erythropoietin levels ≤ 500 mUnits/mL who are receiving a dose of zidovudine ≤ 4200 mg/week, the recommended starting dose of EPOGEN® is 100 Units/kg as an IV or SC injection TIW for 8 weeks. For pediatric patients, see PRECAUTIONS, Pediatric Use.

Increase Dose: During the dose adjustment phase of therapy, the hematocrit should be monitored weekly. If the response is not satisfactory in terms of reducing transfusion requirements or increasing hematocrit after 8 weeks of therapy, the dose of EPOGEN® can be increased by 50 to 100 Units/kg TIW. Response should be evaluated every 4 to 8 weeks thereafter and the dose adjusted accordingly by 50 to 100 Units/kg increments TIW. If patients have not responded satisfactorily to an EPOGEN® dose of 300 Units/kg TIW, it is unlikely that they will respond to higher doses of EPOGEN®.

Maintenance Dose: After attainment of the desired response (ie, reduced transfusion requirements or increased hematocrit), the dose of EPOGEN® should be titrated to maintain the response based on factors such as variations in zidovudine dose and the presence of intercurrent infectious or inflammatory episodes. If the hematocrit exceeds 40%, the dose should be discontinued until the hematocrit drops to 36%. The dose should be reduced by 25% when treatment is resumed and then titrated to maintain the desired hematocrit.

Cancer Patients on Chemotherapy

Baseline endogenous serum erythropoietin levels varied among patients in these trials with approximately 75% (n = 83/110) having endogenous serum erythropoietin levels < 132 mUnits/mL, and approximately 4% (n = 4/110) of patients having endogenous serum erythropoietin levels > 500 mUnits/mL. In general, patients with lower baseline serum erythropoietin levels responded more vigorously to EPOGEN® than patients with higher erythropoietin levels. Although no specific serum erythropoietin level can be stipulated above which patients would be unlikely to respond to EPOGEN® therapy, treatment of patients with grossly elevated serum erythropoietin levels (eg, > 200 mUnits/mL) is not recommended. The hematocrit should be monitored on a weekly basis in patients receiving EPOGEN® therapy until hematocrit becomes stable.

Starting Dose: The recommended starting dose of EPOGEN® for adults is 150 Units/kg SC TIW. For pediatric patients, see PRECAUTIONS, Pediatric Use.

Dose Adjustment: If the response is not satisfactory in terms of reducing transfusion requirements or increasing hematocrit after 8 weeks of therapy, the dose of EPOGEN® can be increased up to 300 Units/kg TIW. If patients have not responded satisfactorily to an EPOGEN® dose of 300 Units/kg TIW, it is unlikely that they will respond to higher doses of EPOGEN®. If the hematocrit exceeds 40%, the dose of EPOGEN® should be withheld until the hematocrit falls to 36%. The dose of EPOGEN® should be reduced by 25% when treatment is resumed and titrated to maintain the desired hematocrit. If the initial dose of EPOGEN® includes a very rapid hematocrit response (eg, an increase of more than 4 percentage points in any 2-week period), the dose of EPOGEN® should be reduced.

Surgery Patients

Prior to initiating treatment with EPOGEN® a hemoglobin should be obtained to establish that it is > 10 to ≤ 13 g/dL.[18] The recommended dose of EPOGEN® is 300 IU/kg/day subcutaneously for 10 days before surgery, on the day of surgery, and for 4 days after surgery.

An alternate dose schedule is 600 IU/kg EPOGEN® subcutaneously in once weekly doses (21, 14, and 7 days before surgery) plus a fourth dose on the day of surgery.[19]

All patients should receive adequate iron supplementation. Iron supplementation should be initiated no later than the beginning of treatment with EPOGEN® and should continue throughout the course of therapy.

PREPARATION AND ADMINISTRATION OF EPOGEN®

1. Do not shake. It is not necessary to shake EPOGEN®. Prolonged vigorous shaking may denature any glycoprotein, rendering it biologically inactive.
2. Parenteral drug products should be inspected visually for particulate matter and discoloration prior to administration. Do not use any vials exhibiting particulate matter or discoloration.
3. Using aseptic techniques, attach a sterile needle to a sterile syringe. Remove the flip top from the vial containing EPOGEN®, and wipe the septum with a disinfectant. Insert the needle into the vial, and withdraw into the syringe an appropriate volume of solution.
4. **Single-dose** 1 mL vial contains no preservative. Use one dose per vial; do not re-enter the vial. Discard unused portions.
   Multidose 1 mL and 2 mL vials contain preservative. Store at 2° to 8°C after initial entry and between doses. Discard 21 days after initial entry.
5. Do not dilute or administer in conjunction with other drug solutions. However, at the time of SC administration, preservative-free EPOGEN® from single-use vials may be admixed in a syringe with bacteriostatic 0.9% sodium chloride injection, USP, with benzyl alcohol 0.9% (bacteriostatic saline) at a 1:1 ratio using aseptic technique. The benzyl alcohol in the bacteriostatic saline acts as a local anesthetic which may ameliorate SC injection site discomfort. Admixing is not necessary when using the multidose vials of EPOGEN® containing benzyl alcohol.

HOW SUPPLIED

EPOGEN®, containing Epoetin alfa, is available in the following packages:

1 mL **Single-dose, Preservative-free** Solution
- 2000 Units/mL (NDC 55513-126-10)
- 3000 Units/mL (NDC 55513-267-10)
- 4000 Units/mL (NDC 55513-148-10)
- 10,000 Units/mL (NDC 55513-144-10)
- 40,000 Units/mL (NDC 55513-823-10)

Supplied in cartons containing 10 single-dose vials.

2 mL **Multidose, Preserved** Solution
- 10,000 Units/mL (NDC 55513-283-10)

1 mL **Multidose, Preserved** Solution
- 20,000 Units/mL (NDC 55513-478-10)

Supplied in cartons containing 10 multidose vials.

STORAGE

Store at 2° to 8°C (36° to 46°F). Do not freeze or shake.

REFERENCES

1. Egrie JC, Strickland TW, Lane J, et al. Characterization and Biological Effects of Recombinant Human Erythropoietin. *Immunobiol.* 1986;72:213–224.
2. Graber SE, Krantz SB. Erythropoietin and the Control of Red Cell Production. *Ann Rev Med.* 1978;29:51–66.
3. Eschbach JW, Adamson JW. Anemia of End-Stage Renal Disease (ESRD). *Kidney Intl.* 1985;28:1–5.
4. Eschbach JW, Egrie JC, Downing MR, et al. Correction of the Anemia of End-Stage Renal Disease with Recombinant Human Erythropoietin. *NEJM.* 1987;316:73–78.
5. Eschbach JW, Abdulhadi MH, Browne JK, et al. Recombinant Human Erythropoietin in Anemic Patients with End-Stage Renal Disease. *Ann Intern Med.* 1989;111:992–1000.
6. Eschbach JW, Egrie JC, Downing MR, et al. The Use of Recombinant Human Erythropoietin (r-HuEPO): Effect in End-Stage Renal Disease (ESRD). In: Friedman, Beyer, DeSanto, Giordano, eds. *Prevention of Chronic Uremia*. Philadelphia, PA: Field and Wood Inc; 1989:148–155.
7. Egrie JC, Eschbach JW, McGuire T, Adamson JW. Pharmacokinetics of Recombinant Human Erythropoietin (r-HuEPO) Administered to Hemodialysis (HD) Patients. *Kidney Intl.* 1988;33:262.
8. Evans RW, Rader B, Manninen DL, et al. The Quality of Life of Hemodialysis Recipients Treated with Recombinant Human Erythropoietin. *JAMA.* 1990;263:825–830.
9. Paganini E, Garcia J, Ellis P, et al. Clinical Sequelae of Correction of Anemia with Recombinant Human Erythropoietin (r-HuEPO); Urea Kinetics, Dialyzer Function and Reuse. *Am J Kid Dis.* 1988;11:16.
10. Delano BG, Lundin AP, Golansky R, et al. Dialyzer Urea and Creatinine Clearances Not Significantly Changed in r-HuEPO Treated Maintenance Hemodialysis (MD) Patients. *Kidney Intl.* 1988;33:219.
11. Stivelman J, Van Wyck D, Ogden D. Use of Recombinant Erythropoietin (r-HuEPO) with High Flux Dialysis (HFD) Does Not Worsen Azotemia or Shorten Access Survival. *Kidney Intl.* 1988;33:239.
12. Lim VS, DeGowin RL, Zavala D, et al. Recombinant Human Erythropoietin Treatment in Pre-Dialysis Patients: A Double-Blind Placebo Controlled Trial. *Ann Int Med.* 1989;110:108–114.
13. Stone WJ, Graber SE, Krantz SB, et al. Treatment of the Anemia of Pre-Dialysis Patients with Recombinant Human Erythropoietin: A Randomized, Placebo-Controlled Trial. *Am J Med Sci.* 1988;296:171–179.
14. Braun A, Ding R, Seidel C, Fies T, Kurtz A, Scharer K. Pharmacokinetics of recombinant human erythropoietin applied subcutaneously to children with chronic renal failure. *Pediatr Nephrol.* 1993;7:61–64.
15. Geva P, Sherwood JB. Pharmacokinetics of recombinant human erythropoietin (rHuEPO) in pediatric patients on chronic cycling peritoneal dialysis (CCPD). *Blood.* 1991;78 (Suppl 1):91a.
16. Jabs K, Grant JR, Harmon W, et al. Pharmacokinetics of Epoetin alfa (rHuEPO) in pediatric hemodialysis (HD) patients. *J Am Soc Nephrol.* 1991;2:380.
17. Kling PJ, Widness JA, Guillery EN, Veng-Pedersen P, Peters C, DeAlarcon PA. Pharmacokinetics and pharmacodynamics of erythropoietin during therapy in an infant with renal failure. *J Pediatr.* 1992;121:822–825.
18. deAndrade JR and Jove M. Baseline Hemoglobin as a Predictor of Risk of Transfusion and Response to Epoetin alfa in Orthopedic Surgery Patients. *Am. J. of Orthoped.* 1996;25 (8):533–542.
19. Goldberg MA and McCutchen JW. A Safety and Efficacy Comparison Study of Two Dosing Regimens of Epoetin alfa in Patients Undergoing Major Orthopedic Surgery. *Am. J. of Orthoped.* 1996;25 (8):544–552.
20. Faris PM and Ritter MA. The Effects of Recombinant Human Erythropoietin on Perioperative Transfusion Requirements in Patients Having a Major Orthopedic Operation. *J. Bone and Joint Surgery.* 1996;78-A:62–72.
21. Lundin AP, Akerman MJH, Chesler RM, et al. Exercise in Hemodialysis Patients after Treatment with Recombinant Human Erythropoietin. *Nephron.* 1991;58:315–319.
22. Amgen Inc., data on file.
23. Eschbach JW, Kelly MR, Haley NR, et al. Treatment of the Anemia of Progressive Renal Failure with Recombinant Human Erythropoietin. *NEJM.* 1989;321:158–163.
24. The US Recombinant Human Erythropoietin Predialysis Study Group. Double-Blind, Placebo-Controlled Study of the Therapeutic Use of Recombinant Human Erythropoietin for Anemia Associated with Chronic Renal Failure in Predialysis Patients. *Am J Kid Dis.* 1991;18:50–59.
25. Ortho Biologics, Inc., data on file.
26. Danna RP, Rudnick SA, Abels RI. Erythropoietin Therapy for the Anemia Associated with AIDS and AIDS Therapy and Cancer. In: MB Garnick, ed. *Erythropoietin in Clinical Applications—An International Perspective.* New York, NY: Marcel Dekker; 1990:301–324.
27. Fischl M, Galpin JE, Levine JD, et al. Recombinant Human Erythropoietin for Patients with AIDS Treated with Zidovudine. *NEJM.* 1990;322:1488–1493.
28. Laupacis A. Effectiveness of Perioperative Recombinant Human Eyrthropoietin in Elective Hip Replacement. *Lancet.* 1993;341:1228–1232.

Continued on next page

Epogen—Cont.

29. Kerr DN. Chronic Renal Failure. In: Beeson PB, McDermott W, Wyngaarden JB, eds. *Cecil Textbook of Medicine*. Philadelphia, PA: W.B. Saunders; 1979:1351–1367.
30. Campos A, Garin EH. Therapy of renal anemia in children and adolescents with recombinant human erythropoietin (rHuEPO). *Clin Pediatr* (Phila). 1992;31:94–99.
31. Montini G, Zacchello G, Baraldi E, et al. Benefits and risks of anemia correction with recombinant human erythropoietin in children maintained by hemodialysis. *J Pediatr*. 1990;117:556–560.
32. Offner G, Hoyer PF, Latta K, Winkler L, Brodehl J, Scigalla P. One year's experience with recombinant erythropoietin in children undergoing continuous ambulatory or cycling peritoneal dialysis. *Pediatr Nephrol*. 1990;4:498–500.
33. Muller-Wiefel DE, Scigalla P. Specific problems of renal anemia in childhood. *Contrib Nephrol*. 1988;66: 71–84.
34. Scharer K, Klare B, Dressel P, Gretz N. Treatment of renal anemia by subcutaneous erythropoietin in children with preterminal chronic renal failure. *Acta Paediatr*. 1993;82:953–958.
35. Mueller BU, Jacobsen RN, Jarosinski P, et al. Erythropoietin for zidovudine-associated anemia in children with HIV infection. *Pediatr AIDS and HIV Infect: Fetus to Adolesc*. 1994;5:169–173.
36. Zuccotti GV, Plebani A, Biasucci G, et al. Granulocyte-colony stimulating factor and erythropoietin therapy in children with human immunodeficiency virus infection. *J Int Med Res*. 1996;24:115–121.
37. Beck MN, Beck D. Recombinant erythropoietin in acute chemotherapy-induced anemia of children with cancer. *Med Pediatr Oncol*. 1995;25:17–21.
38. Bennetts G, Bertolone S, Bray G, Dinndorf P, Feusner J, Cairo M. Erythropoietin reduces volumes of red cell transfusions required in some subsets of children with acute lymphocytic leukemia. *Blood*. 1995;86:853a.
39. Raskin NH, Fishman RA. Neurologic Disorders in Renal Failure (First of Two Parts). *NEJM*. 1976;294:143–148.
40. Raskin NH and Fishman RA. Neurologic Disorders in Renal Failure (Second of Two Parts). *NEJM*. 1976;294:204–210.
41. Messing RO, Simon RP. Seizures as a Manifestation of Systemic Disease. *Neurologic Clinics*. 1986;4:563–584.

Manufactured by:
Amgen Inc.
One Amgen Center Drive
Thousand Oaks, CA
91320-1799
Issue Date: 07/26/99

MC 10547
50M/9-99 P30490
Shown in Product Identification Guide, page 304

INFERGEN® ℞
(Interferon alfacon-1)

DESCRIPTION

Interferon alfacon-1 is a recombinant non-naturally occurring type-I interferon. The 166-amino acid sequence of Interferon alfacon-1 was derived by scanning the sequences of several natural interferon alpha subtypes and assigning the most frequently observed amino acid in each corresponding position.[1] Four additional amino acid changes were made to facilitate the molecular construction, and a corresponding synthetic DNA sequence was constructed using chemical synthesis methodology. Interferon alfacon-1 differs from interferon alfa-2 at 20/166 amino acids (88% homology), and comparison with interferon-beta shows identity at over 30% of the amino acid positions. Interferon alfacon-1 is produced in *Escherichia coli* (*E coli*) cells that have been genetically altered by insertion of a synthetically constructed sequence that codes for Interferon alfacon-1. Prior to final purification, Interferon alfacon-1 is allowed to oxidize to its native state, and its final purity is achieved by sequential passage over a series of chromatography columns. This protein has a molecular weight of 19,434 daltons. Infergen® is the Amgen Inc. trademark for Interferon alfacon-1.

Infergen is a sterile, clear, colorless, preservative-free liquid formulated with 100 mM sodium chloride and 25 mM sodium phosphate at pH 7.0 ± 0.2. The product is available in single-use vials and prefilled syringes containing 9 mcg and 15 mcg Interferon alfacon-1 at a fill volume of 0.3 mL and 0.5 mL, respectively. Infergen vials and prefilled syringes contain 0.03 mg/mL of Interferon alfacon-1, 5.9 mg/mL sodium chloride, and 3.8 mg/mL sodium phosphate in Water for Injection, USP. The Infergen SingleJect™ prefilled syringe has a glass barrel and a 26 gauge, 5/8 inch needle. Infergen is to be administered undiluted by subcutaneous (SC) injection.

Formulation, filling, and packaging operations for Infergen are performed by Amgen Puerto Rico, a wholly-owned subsidiary of Amgen Inc.

CLINICAL PHARMACOLOGY

General

Interferons are a family of naturally occurring, small protein molecules with molecular weights of 15,000 to 21,000 daltons that are produced and secreted by cells in response to viral infections or to various synthetic and biological inducers. Two major classes of interferons have been identified (ie, type-I and type-II). Type-I interferons include a family of more than 25 interferon alphas as well as interferon beta and interferon omega. While all alpha interferons have similar biological effects, not all the activities are shared by each alpha interferon and, in many cases, the extent of activity varies substantially for each interferon subtype.

All type-I interferons share common biological activities generated by binding of interferon to the cell-surface receptor, leading to the production of several interferon-stimulated gene products. Type-I interferons induce pleiotropic biologic responses which include antiviral, antiproliferative and immunomodulatory effects, regulation of cell surface major histocompatibility antigen (HLA class I and class II) expression and regulation of cytokine expression. Examples of interferon-stimulated gene products include 2′5′ oligoadenylate synthetase (2′5′ OAS) and β-2 microglobulin.

The antiviral, antiproliferative, NK cell activation, and gene-induction activities of Infergen have been compared with other recombinant alfa interferons in *in vitro* assays and have demonstrated similar ranges of activity. Infergen exhibited at least five times higher specific activity *in vitro* than Interferon alfa-2a and Interferon alfa-2b.[2] Comparison of Infergen with a WHO international potency standard for recombinant interferon alfa (83/514) revealed that the specific activity of Infergen in both an *in vitro* antiviral cytopathic effect assay and an antiproliferative assay was 1×10^9 U/mg. However, correlation between *in vitro* activity and clinical activity of any interferon is unknown.

Pharmacokinetics and Pharmacodynamics

The pharmacokinetic properties of Infergen have not been evaluated in patients with chronic hepatitis C. Pharmacokinetic profiles were evaluated in normal, healthy volunteer subjects after SC injection of 1, 3, or 9 mcg Interferon alfacon-1. Plasma levels of Infergen after SC administration of any dose were too low to be detected by either ELISA or by inhibition of viral cytopathic effect. However, analysis of Infergen-induced cellular products (induction of 2′5′ OAS and β-2 microglobulin) after treatment in these subjects revealed a statistically significant, dose-related increase in the area under the curve (AUC) for the levels of 2′5′ OAS or β-2 microglobulin induced over time ($p < 0.001$ for all comparisons). Concentrations of 2′5′ OAS were maximal at 24 hours after dosing, while serum levels of β-2 microglobulin appeared to reach a maximum 24 to 36 hours after dosing. The dose-response relationships observed for 2′5′ OAS and β-2 microglobulin were indicative of biological activity after SC administration of 1 to 9 mcg Infergen.

Preclinical Experience

All interferons have been shown to be highly species specific. Antiviral activity of Infergen was observed in the rhesus monkey LLC cell line and golden Syrian hamster BHK cell line. Antiviral activity of Infergen in the golden Syrian hamster was confirmed further *in vivo*.[3] Pharmacokinetic studies of Infergen in golden Syrian hamsters and rhesus monkeys demonstrated rapid absorption following SC injection. Peak serum concentrations of Infergen were observed at 1 hour and 4 hours in golden Syrian hamsters and in rhesus monkeys, respectively. Subcutaneous bioavailability was high in both species, averaging 99% in golden Syrian hamsters and 83% to 104% in rhesus monkeys. Clearance of Infergen, averaging 1.99 mL/minute/kg in golden Syrian hamsters and 0.71 to 0.92 mL/minute/kg in rhesus monkeys, was due predominantly to catabolism and excretion by the kidneys. The terminal half-life of Infergen following SC dosing was 1.3 hours in golden Syrian hamsters and 3.4 in rhesus monkeys. Upon 7-day multiple SC dosing, no accumulation of serum levels was observed in golden Syrian hamsters.

In preclinical toxicology studies in golden Syrian hamsters and rhesus monkeys, administration of Infergen at doses of up to 100 mcg/kg/day was associated with decreased body weight, decreased food consumption, and bone marrow suppression. High-dose chronic exposure at doses of 10 to 100 mcg/kg/day (50- to 500-fold higher than the maximum clinical dose given daily) in rhesus monkeys was not tolerated for greater than 1 month, due to the development of vascular leak syndrome.

Reproductive toxicity studies in pregnant rhesus monkeys and golden Syrian hamsters demonstrated an increase in fetal loss in hamsters treated with Infergen at doses of greater than 150 mcg/kg/day, and in rhesus monkeys at doses of 3 and 10 mcg/kg/day. The Infergen toxicity profile described is consistent with the known toxicity profile of other alfa interferons.[4]

CLINICAL EXPERIENCE: RESPONSE TO INFERGEN

Infergen was studied in an open label dose escalation study using 3, 6, 9, 12, or 15 mcg administered three times per week (TIW) to patients with compensated liver disease secondary to chronic hepatitis C virus (HCV) infection. The 15 mcg dose was the maximal tolerated dose. All doses demonstrated an acceptable safety profile and preliminary evidence of efficacy.

The efficacy of 3 and 9 mcg doses of Infergen in the treatment of chronic HCV infection was examined in a randomized, double-blind clinical trial involving 704 patients previously untreated with alfa interferon. Patients were 18 years or older, had compensated liver disease, tested positive for HCV RNA, and had elevated serum alanine aminotransferase (ALT) concentrations averaging > 1.5 times the upper limit of normal. Staging of chronic liver disease was confirmed by a liver biopsy taken within 1 year prior to enrollment. Other causes of chronic liver disease were ruled out prior to randomization. Notable exclusion criteria were decompensated liver disease, thyroid abnormality, or history of depression.

Efficacy of Infergen therapy was assessed on an intent to treat basis and was determined by measurement of serum ALT concentrations at the end of therapy (24 weeks) and following 24 weeks of observation after the end of treatment. Serum HCV RNA was also assessed using a quantitative reverse transcriptase polymerase chain reaction (RT-PCR) assay with a lower limit of sensitivity of 100 copies/mL. Liver histology was assessed by comparing the histology activity index (HAI) score[5] of a pretreatment biopsy specimen with the HAI score from a specimen obtained 24 weeks after cessation of interferon therapy.

Patients enrolled in the study were randomized to one of three treatment groups: Infergen at a dose of 3 mcg (n = 232), Infergen at a dose of 9 mcg (n = 232), or Interferon alfa-2b recombinant [IFN α-2b, Intron® A (Intron® is a registered trademark of the Schering Corporation)] at a dose of 3 million international units (IU) (approximately 15 mcg) (n = 240). All patients were scheduled to receive their respective interferons SC TIW for 24 weeks (end of treatment). Following treatment, patients were observed for an additional 24 weeks to assess durability of ALT normalization (end of post-treatment observation). In all patients, a complete response was defined as a decrease in serum ALT concentration to at or below the upper limit of normal (48 U/L) at the end of the post-treatment observation period, even if ALT normalization had not been observed at the end of treatment. Complete response was dependent on two consecutive normal serum ALT values determined 4 weeks apart. Reduction of HCV RNA to < 100 copies/mL was measured as a secondary efficacy endpoint (two consecutive measurements).

Sustained response rates by ALT normalization and HCV RNA reductions to below detectable limits are included in Table 1. Among the Infergen treatment groups in this study, the 9 mcg dosage arm demonstrated a similar efficacy profile when compared to the IFN α-2b dosage arm. The 3 mcg Infergen dosage arm had lesser efficacy; 3% of patients receiving 3 mcg Infergen had sustained reduction in their ALT concentrations to within the normal range and 3% had sustained reduction in HCV RNA to below detectable limits.

[See table 1 below]

In this study, liver biopsies were taken at baseline and at the end of post-treatment observation. Similar improvement in liver histology, assessed by HAI score,[5] was observed in the 9 mcg Infergen (68%), 3 mcg Infergen (63%), and IFN α-2b (65%) dosage arms.

Subsequent treatment with 15 mcg of Infergen was evaluated in an open-label clinical trial in 107 patients who had failed initial therapy with either 9 mcg Infergen or 3 million IU (approximately 15 mcg) IFN α-2b. Of these patients, 74/107 had failed to normalize ALT concentrations during either the initial treatment period or the post-treatment observation period, while 33/107 achieved a normal ALT concentration during initial treatment, but experienced relapse (return of abnormal ALT concentration) during post-treatment observation. Patients were assessed for normalization of ALT (ALT response rate) and HCV RNA reduction to < 100 copies/mL (HCV response rate) at the end of 24 weeks of observation. Response rates (expressed as fraction of patients, percentage of patients, and 95% confidence interval of percentage) are presented for all patients and two subsets of: patients who had relapsed following initial therapy and patients who had never normalized following initial therapy.

Overall 16/107 [15% (9–23% CI)] patients had a sustained ALT response. Of patients who had relapsed following initial therapy 10/33 [30% (16–49% CI)] had a sustained ALT response and 6/74 [8% (3–17% CI)] who never normalized their ALT concentration had a sustained ALT response. Overall 10/107 [9% (5–17% CI)] patients had a sustained HCV response (< 100 copies/mL). Of patients who had re-

Table 1. Rates (95% CI[a]) of ALT Normalization and HCV RNA Reductions to Below Detectable Limits

	End of 24-week Treatment		End of Observation (Sustained Response Rate)	
	Infergen 9 mcg	IFN α-2b 3 Million IU[b]	Infergen 9 mcg	IFN α-2b 3 Million IU[b]
Normalized ALT	39% (33%, 46%)	35% (29%, 41%)	17% (12%, 22%)	17% (13%, 22%)
HCV RNA Negative	33% (27%, 39%)	25% (19%, 31%)	9% (6%, 14%)	8% (5%, 13%)

[a]CI = Confidence Interval.
[b]3 million IU IFN α-2b is equivalent to approximately 15 mcg IFN α-2b.

lapsed following initial therapy 8/32 [25% (11–43% CI)] had a sustained HCV response and 2/75 [3% (0–9% CI)] who never had a reduction in HCV RNA to < 100 copies/mL had a sustained HCV response.

Serum antibody levels were measured in all patients using both an Infergen-binding radioimmunoassay and an IFN α-2b-binding ELISA. A patient was considered to have developed binding antibodies if, using serum samples from two consecutive time points, a positive response was detected in either assay. The number of patients developing positive binding antibody responses in either assay was similar in the 9 mcg Infergen (11%) and 3 million IU IFN α-2b groups (15%). The titer of neutralizing antibodies to interferon was not measured. Sustained ALT response rates in patients treated with Infergen who developed binding antibodies (4/25) were similar to sustained ALT response rates in patients who did not develop detectable antibody titers (40/195). The most frequently observed time to first antibody response was week 16 of interferon treatment. Following cessation of interferon therapy, the number of patients with a positive antibody response declined during post-treatment observation.

INDICATIONS AND USAGE

Infergen is indicated for the treatment of chronic HCV infection in patients 18 years of age or older with compensated liver disease who have anti-HCV serum antibodies and/or the presence of HCV RNA. Other causes of hepatitis, such as viral hepatitis B or autoimmune hepatitis should be ruled out prior to initiation of therapy with Infergen. In some patients with chronic HCV infection, Infergen normalizes serum ALT concentrations, reduces serum HCV RNA concentrations to undetectable quantities (< 100 copies/mL), and improves liver histology.

CONTRAINDICATIONS

Infergen is contraindicated in patients with known hypersensitivity to alpha interferons, to *E coli*-derived products, or to any component of the product.

WARNINGS

Treatment with Infergen should be administered under the guidance of a qualified physician, and may lead to moderate-to-severe adverse experiences requiring dose reduction, temporary dose cessation, or discontinuation of further therapy.

Withdrawal from study for adverse events occurred in 7% of patients treated with 9 mcg Infergen (including 4% due to psychiatric events).

SEVERE PSYCHIATRIC ADVERSE EVENTS MAY MANIFEST IN PATIENTS RECEIVING THERAPY WITH INTERFERON, INCLUDING INFERGEN. DEPRESSION, SUICIDAL IDEATION, AND SUICIDE ATTEMPT MAY OCCUR. The incidence of pyschiatric events of suicidal ideation was small (1%) for patients treated with 9 mcg Infergen compared to the overall incidence (55%) of psychiatric events. Infergen should be used with caution in patients who report a history of depression and physicians should monitor all patients for evidence of depression. Physicians should inform patients of the possible development of depression prior to initiation of Infergen therapy, and patients should report any sign or symptom of depression immediately. Other prominent psychiatric adverse events may also occur, including nervousness, anxiety, emotional lability, abnormal thinking, agitation, or apathy (see PRECAUTIONS).

INFERGEN SHOULD BE ADMINISTERED WITH CAUTION TO PATIENTS WITH PRE-EXISTING CARDIAC DISEASE. Hypertension and supraventricular arrhythmias, chest pain and myocardial infarction have been associated with interferon therapies.[6]

No studies with Infergen have been conducted in patients with decompensated hepatic disease. Patients with decompensated hepatic disease should not be treated with Infergen, and patients who develop symptoms of hepatic decompensation, such as jaundice, ascites, coagulopathy, or decreased serum albumin, should halt further interferon therapy.

PRECAUTIONS

General

Since the use of type-I interferons has been associated with depression, Infergen therapy should not be used in patients with a history of severe psychiatric disorders and should be discontinued in patients developing severe depression, suicidal ideation, or other severe psychiatric disorders (see WARNINGS).

Infergen should be used with caution in patients with a history of cardiac disease. Hypertension (5%), tachycardia (4%), and palpitation (3%) were the most common cardiovascular adverse events reported for 9 mcg Infergen therapy, with 1% of patients reporting tachyarrhythmias which were dose-limiting (see WARNINGS).

Infergen should be used cautiously in patients with abnormally low peripheral blood cell counts or who are receiving agents that are known to cause myelosuppression. Leukopenia, particularly granulocytopenia, may be severe in patients treated with alpha interferons, including Infergen, and may necessitate dose reduction or temporary dose cessation. Thrombocytopenia is a common, but less severe, event often associated with alpha interferon therapy. Therapy should be withheld if the absolute neutrophil count (ANC) is $< 500 \times 10^6$/L or if the platelet count is $< 50 \times 10^9$/L. Transplantation patients, or other chronically immunosuppressed patients, should receive Infergen therapy with caution.

Table 2. Patient Incidence of Adverse Events in Phase 3 Clinical Trials Regardless of Attribution[a]

Body System	Preferred Term	Initial Treatment[b]		Subsequent Treatment[b]
		Infergen 9 mcg (n = 231)	IFN α-2b 3 Million IU (n = 236)	Infergen 15 mcg (n = 165)
		% of Patients		% of Patients
APPLICATION SITE				
	Injection Site Erythema	23	15	17
	Injection Site Pain	9	3	8
	Injection Site Ecchymosis	6	7	5
BODY AS A WHOLE				
	Body Pain	54	45	39
	Influenza-like Symptoms[c]	15	11	8
	Hot Flushes	13	7	7
	Pain Chest–Non-cardiac	13	14	5
	Malaise	11	10	2
	Asthenia	9	11	10
	Edema Peripheral	9	8	4
	Access Pain	8	9	1
	Allergic Reaction	7	5	3
	Weight Decrease	5	7	5
CARDIOVASCULAR				
	Hypertension	5	3	2
	Palpitation	3	6	5
CNS/PNS	Insomnia	39	30	24
	Dizziness	22	25	18
	Paresthesia	13	10	9
	Amnesia	10	6	2
	Hypoesthesia	10	8	8
	Hypertonia	7	10	6
	Confusion	4	6	4
	Somnolence	4	8	5
ENDOCRINE DISORDERS				
	Thyroid Test Abnormal	9	5	4
FLU-LIKE SYMPTOMS				
	Headache	82	83	78
	Fatigue	69	67	65
	Fever	61	45	58
	Myalgia	58	56	51
	Rigors	57	45	62
	Arthralgia	51	45	43
	Sweating Increased	12	11	13
GASTRO-INTESTINAL				
	Abdominal Pain	41	40	24
	Nausea	40	36	30
	Diarrhea	29	24	24
	Anorexia	24	17	21
	Dyspepsia	21	18	12
	Vomiting	12	11	13
	Constipation	9	6	5
	Flatulence	8	9	6
	Tooth Ache	7	7	3
	Hemorrhoids	6	3	1
	Saliva Decreased	6	7	4
HEARING—VESTIBULAR				
	Tinnitus	6	4	4
	Earache	5	7	5
	Otitis	2	5	1
HEMATOLOGIC	Granulocytopenia	23	25	42
	Thrombocytopenia	19	16	18
	Leukopenia	15	13	19
	Ecchymosis	6	4	4
	Lymphadenopathy	6	8	4
	Lymphocytosis	5	7	11
	PT Increased	3	5	1

Serious acute hypersensitivity reactions have been reported in rare instances following treatment with alpha interferons. If hypersensitivity reactions occur (eg, urticaria, angioedema, bronchoconstriction, anaphylaxis), the drug should be discontinued immediately and appropriate medical treatment instituted.

Infergen should be administered with caution to patients with a history of endocrine disorders. Abnormal thyroid stimulating hormone (TSH) and free thyroxine (T_4) level with hypothyroidism occurred in 4% of patients administered 9 mcg Infergen, and thyroid supplements were required in approximately two thirds of those patients.

Ophthalmologic disorders have been reported with treatment with alpha interferons. Investigators using alpha interferons have reported the occurrence of retinal hemorrhages, cotton wool spots, and retinal artery or vein obstruction in rare instances. Any patient complaining of loss of visual acuity or visual field should have an eye examination. Because these ocular events may occur in conjunction with other disease states, a visual exam prior to initiation of interferon therapy is recommended in patients with diabetes mellitus or hypertension.

Exacerbation of autoimmune disease has been reported in patients receiving type-I interferon therapy. Infergen should not be used in patients with autoimmune hepatitis and be used with caution in patients with other autoimmune disorders.

While fever may be related to the flu-like symptoms reported in patients treated with Infergen, when fever occurs, other possible causes of persistent fever should be ruled out.

Information for Patients

If home use is determined to be desirable by the physician, instruction on appropriate use should be given by a health care professional. The patient must be instructed as to the proper dosage and administration. Information included in the full "Information for Patients" leaflet (provided separately) should be fully reviewed with the patient; it is not a disclosure of all, or possible, adverse effects. The most common adverse reactions occurring with Infergen therapy are flu-like symptoms including fatigue, fever, rigors, headache, arthralgia, myalgia, and increased sweating. Non-narcotic analgesics and bedtime administration of Infergen may be used to prevent or lessen some of these symptoms. Additionally, patients must be thoroughly instructed in the importance of proper disposal procedures and cautioned against the reuse of needles, syringes, or re-entry of the drug product. A puncture-resistant container for the disposal of used syringes and needles should be used by the patient and should be disposed of according to the directions provided by the health care provider.

Laboratory Tests

Laboratory tests are recommended for all patients on Infergen therapy, prior to beginning treatment (baseline), 2 weeks after initiation of therapy, and periodically thereafter during the 24 weeks of therapy at the discretion of the phy-

Continued on next page

Infergen—Cont.

sician. Following completion of Infergen therapy, any abnormal test values should be monitored periodically. The entrance criteria that were used for the clinical study of Infergen may be considered as a guideline to acceptable baseline values for initiation of treatment:

- Platelet count $\geq 75 \times 10^9$/L
- Hemoglobin concentration $\geq$ 100 g/L
- ANC $\geq 1500 \times 10^6$/L
- Serum creatinine concentration < 180 µmol/L (< 2.0 mg/dL) or creatinine clearance > 0.83 mL/second (> 50 mL/minute)
- Serum albumin concentration $\geq$ 25 g/L
- Bilirubin within normal limits
- TSH and T_4 within normal limits

Neutropenia, thrombocytopenia, hypertriglyceridemia, and thyroid disorders have been reported with administration of Infergen (see ADVERSE REACTIONS). Therefore, these laboratory parameters should be monitored closely.

Drug Interactions

No formal drug interaction studies have been conducted with Infergen. Infergen should be used cautiously in patients who are receiving agents that are known to cause myelosuppression or with agents known to be metabolized via the cytochrome P-450 pathway.[7] Patients taking drugs that are metabolized by this pathway should be monitored closely for changes in the therapeutic and/or toxic levels of concomitant drugs.

Carcinogenesis, Mutagenesis, Impairment of Fertility

Carcinogenesis: No carcinogenicity data for Infergen are available in animals or humans.

Mutagenesis: Infergen was not mutagenic when tested in several *in vitro* assays, including the Ames bacterial mutagenicity assay and an *in vitro* cytogenetic assay in human lymphocytes, either in the presence or absence of metabolic activation.

Impairment of Fertility: Infergen at doses as high as 100 mcg/kg did not selectively affect reproductive performance or the development of the offspring when administered SC to male and female golden Syrian hamsters for 70 and 14 days before mating, respectively, and then through mating and to day 7 of pregnancy.

Pregnancy Category C

Infergen has been shown to have embryolethal or abortifacient effects in golden Syrian hamsters when given at 135 times the human dose and in cynomolgus and rhesus monkeys when given at 9 to 81 times (based on body surface area) the human dose. There are no adequate and well-controlled studies in pregnant women. Infergen should not be used during pregnancy. If a woman becomes pregnant or plans to become pregnant while taking Infergen, she should be informed of the potential hazards to the fetus. Males and females treated with Infergen should be advised to use effective contraception.

Nursing Mothers

It is not known whether Infergen is excreted in human milk. Because many drugs are excreted in human milk, caution should be exercised if Infergen is administered to a nursing woman. The effect on the nursing neonate of orally ingested Infergen in breast milk has not been evaluated.

Pediatric Use

The safety and effectiveness of Infergen have not been established in patients below the age of 18 years. Infergen therapy is not recommended in pediatric patients.

ADVERSE REACTIONS

Adverse experiences that were reported, regardless of attribution to treatment, in at least 5% of the patients in the 9 mcg Infergen or 3 million IU IFN α-2b groups of the pivotal study are presented in Table 2, listed in decreasing order by the 9 mcg Infergen group. The incidence of adverse events is expressed based on the number of patients experiencing each event at least once during treatment or post-treatment of the study.

Most adverse events were mild-to-moderate in severity and abated with cessation of therapy. Flu-like symptoms (ie, headache, fatigue, fever, rigors, myalgia, sweating increased, and arthralgia) were the most frequently reported treatment-related adverse reactions. Most were short-lived and could be treated symptomatically.

Depression, usually mild-to-moderate in severity, was reported in 26% of patients who received 9 mcg Infergen and was the most common adverse event resulting in study drug discontinuation.

In patients who had tolerated previous interferon therapy and failed to normalize ALT concentration or who had achieved normalization of ALT concentration during the treatment period but who relapsed during the post-treatment observation period, further treatment with 15 mcg TIW of Infergen for 24 weeks was generally tolerated (see Table 2). The higher dose of Infergen used in these patients was associated with a greater incidence of leukopenia and granulocytopenia, and one or more dose reduction for all causes were required in 33% of patients. Patients who do not tolerate initial standard interferon therapy should not receive therapy with 15 mcg TIW of Infergen.

[See table 2 at top of previous page and above]

Laboratory Values

The following laboratory variables were found to be affected by therapy with Infergen in the 231 patients who received treatment with 9 mcg Infergen.

Table 2. Patient Incidence of Adverse Events in Phase 3 Clinical Trials Regardless of Attribution[a]

		Initial Treatment[b]		Subsequent Treatment[b]
		Infergen 9 mcg (n = 231)	IFN α-2b 3 Million IU (n = 236)	Infergen 15 mcg (n = 165)
Body System	Preferred Term	% of Patients		% of Patients
LIVER AND BILIARY				
	Liver Tender	5	3	5
	Hepatomegaly	3	5	5
METABOLIC—NUTRITION				
	Hypertriglyceridemia	6	7	5
MUSCULO-SKELETAL				
	Back Pain	42	37	29
	Limb Pain	26	25	13
	Neck Pain	14	13	8
	Skeletal Pain	14	14	10
	Musculo-Skeletal Disorder	4	4	7
PSYCHIATRIC DISORDER				
	Nervousness	31	29	16
	Depression	26	25	18
	Anxiety	19	18	10
	Emotional Lability	12	11	6
	Thinking Abnormal	8	12	10
	Agitation	6	6	4
	Libido Decreased	5	5	5
REPRODUCTIVE—FEMALE				
	Dysmenorrhea	9	9	2
	Vaginitis	8	2	5
	Menstrual Disorder	6	5	2
	Moniliasis Genital	2	6	2
	Pain Breast	0	5	2
RESISTANCE MECHANISM				
	Infection	3	5	2
RESPIRATORY	Pharyngitis	34	31	17
	Infection Upper Respiratory	31	34	16
	Cough	22	17	12
	Sinusitis	17	22	12
	Rhinitis	13	16	7
	Respiratory Tract Congestion	12	7	5
	Upper Respiratory Tract Congestion	10	14	7
	Epistaxis	8	12	6
	Dyspnea	7	12	8
	Bronchitis	6	6	2
SKIN AND APPENDAGES				
	Alopecia	14	25	10
	Pruritus	14	14	11
	Rash	13	15	13
	Erythema	6	6	6
	Skin Dry	6	5	2
	Wound	4	7	3
SPECIAL SENSES				
	Taste Perversion	3	6	3
VISION DISORDERS				
	Conjunctivitis	8	8	4
	Eye Pain	5	6	4
	Vision Abnormal	3	5	5

[a] Only events that occurred at a frequency of ≥5% in any treatment group are included. Patients can appear more than once in Table 2. Because the two studies were conducted at different times with nonidentical patient groups, the adverse events profile for the subsequent treatment study is not directly comparable to the initial treatment study.

[b] Adverse events reported in patients during treatment or post-treatment observation in the pivotal initial treatment and subsequent treatment studies are listed regardless of attribution to treatment.

[c] Influenza-like Symptoms: presumed viral etiology.

Hemoglobin and Hematocrit: Treatment with Infergen was associated with gradual decreases in mean values for hemoglobin and hematocrit, which were 4% and 5% below baseline at the end of treatment. Decreases from baseline of 20% or more in hemoglobin or hematocrit were seen in 1% of patients or less.

White Blood Cells: Infergen treatment was associated with decreases in mean values for both total white blood cell (WBC) count and ANC within the first 2 weeks of treatment. By the end of treatment, mean decreases from baseline of 19% for WBCs and 23% for ANC were observed. These effects reversed during the post-treatment observation period. In two Infergen-treated patients in the phase 3 trial, decreases in ANC to levels below 500×10^6 cells/L were seen. In both cases, the ANC returned to clinically acceptable levels with reduction of the dose of Infergen, and these transient decreases in neutrophils were not associated with infections.

Platelets: Infergen treatment was associated with alterations in platelet count. Decreases in mean platelet count of 16% compared to baseline were seen by the end of treatment. These decreases were reversed during the post-treatment observation period. Values below normal were common during treatment with 3% of patients developing values less than 50×10^9 cells/L, usually necessitating dose reduction.

Triglycerides: Mean values for serum triglyceride increased shortly after the start of administration of Infergen, with increases of 41%, compared with baseline, at the end of the treatment period. Seven percent of the patients developed values which were at least three times above pretreatment levels during treatment. This effect was promptly reversed after discontinuation of treatment.

Thyroid Function: Infergen treatment was associated with biochemical changes consistent with hypothyroidism including increases in TSH and decreases in T_4 mean values. Increases in TSH to greater than 7 mU/L were seen in 10% of 9 mcg Infergen-treated patients either during the treatment period or the 24-week post-treatment observation period. Thyroid supplements were instituted in approximately one third of these patients.

Laboratory Values for Subsequent Treatment: From a database of 165 patients receiving treatment with 15 mcg of Infergen after failing initial interferon therapy, similar changes in the laboratory variables as outlined above were observed. However, mean decreases from baseline of 23% for WBCs and 27% for ANC were observed, which was greater than during initial treatment. Reductions in WBCs and ANC resulted in alteration of doses in 11 patients (7%). Two patients experienced reversible reduction in ANC to < 500 $\times 10^6$ cells/L, which were not associated with infectious complications. No patients discontinued as a result of hematologic toxicity.

OVERDOSAGE

In Infergen trials, the maximum overdose reported was a dose of 150 mcg Infergen administered SC in a patient enrolled in a phase 1 advanced malignancy trial. The patient received 10 times the prescribed dosage for 3 days. The patient experienced a mild increase in anorexia, chills, fever, and myalgia. Increases in ALT (15 to 127 IU/L), aspartate transaminase (AST) (15 to 164 IU/L), and lactic dehydrogenase (LDH) (183 to 281 IU/L) were reported. These laboratory values returned to normal or to the patient's baseline values within 30 days.

DOSAGE AND ADMINISTRATION

The recommended dose of Infergen for treatment of chronic HCV infection is 9 mcg TIW administered SC as a single injection for 24 weeks. At least 48 hours should elapse between doses of Infergen. Should a patient miss a scheduled dose, the missed dose should be taken as soon as possible, and the administration schedule revised at the physician's discretion.

Patients who tolerated previous interferon therapy and did not respond or relapsed following its discontinuation may be subsequently treated with 15 mcg of Infergen TIW for 6 months. Patients should not be treated with 15 mcg of Infergen TIW if they have not received, or have not tolerated, an initial course of interferon therapy.

There are significant differences in specific activities among interferons. Health care providers should be aware that changes in interferon brand may require adjustments of dosage and/or change in route of administration. Patients should be warned not to change brands of interferon without medical consultation. Patients should also be instructed by their physician not to reduce the dosage of Infergen prior to medical consultation.

Dose Reduction

For patients who experience a severe adverse reaction on Infergen, dosage should be withheld temporarily. If the adverse reaction dose not become tolerable, therapy should be discontinued. Dose reduction to 7.5 mcg may be necessary following an intolerable adverse event. In the pivotal study, 11% of patients (26/231) who initially received Infergen at a dose of 9 mcg (0.3 mL) were dose-reduced to 7.5 mcg (0.25 mL).

If adverse reactions continue to occur at the reduced dosage, the physician may discontinue treatment or reduce dosage further. However, decreased efficacy may result from continued treatment at dosages below 7.5 mcg.

During subsequent treatment with 15 mcg of Infergen, 33% of patients required dose reduction in 3 mcg increments.

Administration of Infergen

If home use is determined to be desirable by the physician, instruction on appropriate use should be given by a health care professional. After administration of Infergen, it is essential to follow the procedure for proper disposal of syringes and needles. See "Information For Patients" leaflet for detailed instructions provided separately.

Storage

Infergen should be stored in the refrigerator at 2° to 8°C (36° to 46°F). Do not freeze. Avoid vigorous shaking and exposure to direct sunlight. Just prior to injection, Infergen may be allowed to reach room temperature.

Parenteral drug products should be inspected visually for particulate matter and discoloration prior to administration; if particulates or discoloration are observed, the container should not be used.

HOW SUPPLIED

Use only one dose per vial; do not re-enter the vial. Discard unused portions. Do not save unused drug for later administration.

Use only on dose per prefilled syringe. Discard unused portions. Do not save unused drug for later administration.

Vials

Single-dose, preservative-free vials containing 9 mcg (0.3 mL) of Interferon alfacon-1 are available in dispensing packs of six vials (NDC 55513-554-06).

Single-dose, preservative-free vials containing 15 mcg (0.5 mL) of Interferon alfacon-1 are available in dispensing packs of six vials (NDC 55513-562-06).

Prefilled Syringes (SingleJect™)

Single-dose, preservative-free prefilled syringes containing 9 mcg (0.3 mL) of Interferon alfacon-1 are available in dispensing packs of six prefilled syringes (NDC 55513-926-06).

Single-dose, preservative-free prefilled syringes containing 15 mcg (0.5 mL) of Interferon alfacon-1 are available in dispensing packs of six prefilled syringes (NDC 55513-927-06).

Infergen should be stored at 2° to 8°C (36° to 46°F). Do not freeze. Avoid vigorous shaking.

REFERENCES

1. Alton K, Stabinsky Y, Richards R, et al. Production, characterization and biological effects of recombinant DNA derived human IFN-α and IFN-γ analogs. In: De Maeyer E, Schellekens H, eds. *The Biology of the Interferon System 1983*. Elsevier Science Publishers: Amsterdam. 1983;119–128.
2. Blatt LM, Davis J, Klein SB, Taylor MW. The biologic activity and molecular characterization of a novel synthetic interferon-alpha species, consensus interferon. *J Interferon Cytokine Res.* 1996;16:489–499.
3. Fish EN, Banerjee K, Levin HL, Stebbing N. Antiherpetic effects of a human alpha interferon analog, IFN-alpha Con_1, in hamsters. *Antimicrob Agents Chemother.* 1986;30:52–56.
4. Trown PW, Willis RJ, Kamm JJ. The preclinical development of Roferon®-A. *Cancer.* 1986;57:1648–1656.
5. Knodell RG, Ishak KG, Black WC, et al. Formulation and application of a numerical scoring system for assessing histological activity in asymptomatic chronic active hepatitis. *Hepatology.* 1981;1:431–435.
6. Vial T, Descotes J. Clinical toxicity of interferons. *Drug Safety.* 1994;10:115–150.
7. Horsmans Y, Brenard R, Geubel AP. Short report: interferon-α decreases ^{14}C-aminopyrine breath test values in patients with chronic hepatitis C. *Aliment Pharmacol Ther.* 1994;8:353–355.

This product and its use are covered by the following US Patent Nos.: 4,695,623; 5,372,808; 5,541,293.

Manufactured by:
Amgen Inc.
One Amgen Center Drive
Thousand Oaks
California 91320-1799

Issue Date: 11/30/98

MC10557
7500/1-99 P80080A

Shown in Product Identification Guide, page 304

NEUPOGEN® ℞
(Filgrastim)

DESCRIPTION

Filgrastim is a human granulocyte colony-stimulating factor (G-CSF), produced by recombinant DNA technology. NEUPOGEN® is the Amgen Inc. trademark for Filgrastim, which has been selected as the name for recombinant methionyl human granulocyte colony-stimulating factor (r-metHuG-CSF).

NEUPOGEN® is a 175 amino acid protein manufactured by recombinant DNA technology.[1] NEUPOGEN® is produced by *Escherichia coli* (*E coli*) bacteria into which has been inserted the human granulocyte colony-stimulating factor gene. NEUPOGEN® has a molecular weight of 18,800 daltons. The protein has an amino acid sequence that is identical to the natural sequence predicted from human DNA sequence analysis, except for the addition of an N-terminal methionine necessary for expression in *E coli*. Because NEUPOGEN® is produced in *E coli*, the product is nonglycosylated and thus differs from G-CSF isolated from a human cell.

NEUPOGEN® is a sterile, clear, colorless, preservative-free liquid for parenteral administration containing Filgrastim at a specific activity of $1.0 \pm 0.6 \times 10^8$ U/mg, (as measured by a cell mitogenesis assay). The product is available in single use vials and prefilled syringes. The single use vials contain either 300 mcg or 480 mcg Filgrastim at a fill volume of 1.0 mL or 1.6 mL, respectively. The single use prefilled syringes contain either 300 mcg or 480 mcg Filgrastim at a fill volume of 0.5 mL or 0.8 mL, respectively. See table below for product composition of each single use vial or prefilled syringe.

[See first table at top of next page]

CLINICAL PHARMACOLOGY

Colony-stimulating Factors

Colony-stimulating factors are glycoproteins which act on hematopoietic cells by binding to specific cell surface receptors and stimulating proliferation, differentiation commitment, and some end-cell functional activation.

Endogenous G-CSF is a lineage specific colony-stimulating factor which is produced by monocytes, fibroblasts, and endothelial cells. G-CSF regulates the production of neutrophils within the bone marrow and affects neutrophil progenitor proliferation,[2,3] differentiation,[2,4] and selected end-cell functional activation (including enhanced phagocytic ability,[5] priming of the cellular metabolism associated with respiratory burst,[6] antibody dependent killing,[7] and the increased expression of some functions associated with cell surface antigens[8]). G-CSF is not species specific and has been shown to have minimal direct in vivo or in vitro effects on the production of hematopoietic cell types other than the neutrophil lineage.

Preclinical Experience

Filgrastim was administered to monkeys, dogs, hamsters, rats, and mice as part of a preclinical toxicology program which included single-dose acute, repeated-dose subacute, subchronic, and chronic studies. Single-dose administration of Filgrastim by the oral, intravenous (IV), subcutaneous (SC), or intraperitoneal (IP) routes resulted in no significant toxicity in mice, rats, hamsters, or monkeys. Although no deaths were observed in mice, rats, or monkeys at dose levels up to 3450 mcg/kg or in hamsters using single doses up to approximately 860 mcg/kg, deaths were observed in a subchronic (13-week) study in monkeys. In this study, evidence of neurological symptoms was seen in monkeys treated with doses of Filgrastim greater than 1150 mcg/kg/day for up to 18 days. Deaths were seen in five of the eight treated animals and were associated with 15- to 28-fold increases in peripheral leukocyte counts, and neutrophil-infiltrated hemorrhagic foci were seen in both the cerebrum and cerebellum. In contrast, no monkeys died following 13 weeks of daily IV administration of Filgrastim at a dose level of 115 mcg/kg. In an ensuing 52-week study, one 115 mcg/kg dose female monkey died after 18 weeks of daily IV administration of Filgrastim. Death was attributed to cardiopulmonary insufficiency.

In subacute, repeated-dose studies, changes observed were attributable to the expected pharmacological actions of Filgrastim (ie, dose-dependent increases in white cell counts, increased circulating segmented neutrophils, and increased myeloid:erythroid ratio in bone marrow). In all species, histopathologic examination of the liver and spleen revealed evidence of ongoing extramedullary granulopoiesis; increased spleen weights were seen in all species and appeared to be dose-related. A dose-dependent increase in serum alkaline phosphatase was observed in rats, and may reflect increased activity of osteoblasts and osteoclasts. Changes in serum chemistry values were reversible following discontinuation of treatment.

In rats treated at doses of 1150 mcg/kg/day for 4 weeks (5 of 32 animals) and for 13 weeks at doses of 100 mcg/kg/day (4 of 32 animals) and 500 mcg/kg/day (6 of 32 animals), articular swelling of the hind legs was observed. Some degree of hind leg dysfunction was also observed; however, symptoms reversed following cessation of dosing. In rats, osteoclasis and osteoanagenesis were found in the femur, humerus, coccyx, and hind legs (where they were accompanied by synovitis) after IV treatment for 4 weeks (115 to 1150 mcg/kg/day), and in the sternum after IV treatment for 13 weeks (115 to 575 mcg/kg/day). These effects reversed to normal within 4 to 5 weeks following cessation of treatment.

In the 52-week chronic, repeated-dose studies performed in rats (IP injection up to 57.5 mcg/kg/day), and cynomolgus monkeys (IV injection of up to 115 mcg/kg/day), changes observed were similar to those noted in the subacute studies. Expected pharmacological actions of Filgrastim included dose-dependent increases in white cell counts, increased circulating segmented neutrophils and alkaline phosphatase levels, and increased myeloid:erythroid ratios in the bone marrow. Decreases in platelet counts were also noted in primates. In no animals tested were hemorrhagic complications observed. Rats displayed dose-related swelling of the hind limb, accompanied by some degree of hind limb dysfunction; osteopathy was noted microscopically. Enlarged spleens (both species) and livers (monkeys), reflective of ongoing extramedullary granulopoiesis, as well as myeloid hyperplasia of the bone marrow, were observed in a dose-dependent manner.

Pharmacologic Effects of NEUPOGEN®

In phase 1 studies involving 96 patients with various nonmyeloid malignancies, NEUPOGEN® administration resulted in a dose-dependent increase in circulating neutrophil counts over the dose range of 1 to 70 mcg/kg/day.[9–11] This increase in neutrophil counts was observed whether NEUPOGEN® was administered IV (1 to 70 mcg/kg twice daily),[9] SC (1 to 3 mcg/kg once daily),[11] or by continuous SC infusion (3 to 11 mcg/kg/day).[10] With discontinuation of NEUPOGEN® therapy, neutrophil counts returned to baseline, in most cases within 4 days. Isolated neutrophils displayed normal phagocytic (measured by zymosan-stimulated chemoluminescence) and chemotactic [measured by migration under agarose using N-formyl-methionyl-leucyl-phenylalanine (fMLP) as the chemotaxin] activity in vitro.

The absolute monocyte count was reported to increase in a dose-dependent manner in most patients receiving NEUPOGEN®, however, the percentage of monocytes in the differential count remained within the normal range. In all studies to date, absolute counts of both eosinophils and basophils did not change and were within the normal range following administration of NEUPOGEN®. Increases in lymphocyte counts following NEUPOGEN® administration have been reported in some normal subjects and cancer patients.

White blood cell (WBC) differentials obtained during clinical trials have demonstrated a shift towards earlier granulocyte progenitor cells (left shift), including the appearance of promyelocytes and myeloblasts, usually during neutrophil recovery following the chemotherapy-induced nadir. In addition, Dohle bodies, increased granulocyte granulation, as well as hypersegmented neutrophils have been observed. Such changes were transient, and were not associated with clinical sequelae nor were they necessarily associated with infection.

Pharmacokinetics

Absorption and clearance of NEUPOGEN® follows first-order pharmacokinetic modeling without apparent concentration dependence. A positive linear correlation occurred between the parenteral dose and both the serum concentration and area under the concentration-time curves. Continuous IV infusion of 20 mcg/kg of NEUPOGEN® over 24 hours resulted in mean and median serum concentrations of approximately 48 and 56 ng/mL, respectively. Subcutaneous administration of 3.45 mcg/kg and 11.5 mcg/kg resulted in maximum serum concentrations of 4 and 49 ng/mL, respectively, within 2 to 8 hours. The volume of distribution averaged 150 mL/kg in both normal subjects and cancer patients. The elimination half-life, in both normal subjects and cancer patients, was approximately 3.5 hours. Clearance rates of NEUPOGEN® were approximately 0.5 to 0.7 mL/minute/kg. Single parenteral doses or daily IV doses, over a 14-day period, resulted in comparable half-lives. The half-lives were similar for IV administration (231 minutes, following doses of 34.5 mcg/kg) and for SC administration (210 minutes, following NEUPOGEN® doses of 3.45 mcg/kg). Continuous 24-hour IV infusions of 20 mcg/kg over an 11- to 20-day period produced steady-state serum concentrations of NEUPOGEN® with no evidence of drug accumulation over the time period investigated.

CLINICAL EXPERIENCE

Cancer Patients Receiving Myelosuppressive Chemotherapy

NEUPOGEN® has been shown to be safe and effective in accelerating the recovery of neutrophil counts following a variety of chemotherapy regimens. In a phase 3 clinical trial in small cell lung cancer, patients received SC administration of NEUPOGEN® (4 to 8 mcg/kg/day, days 4 to 17) or placebo. In this study, the benefits of NEUPOGEN® therapy were shown to be prevention of infection as manifested by febrile neutropenia, decreased hospitalization, and decreased IV antibiotic usage. No difference in survival or disease progression was demonstrated.

In the phase 3, randomized, double-blind, placebo-controlled trial conducted in patients with small cell lung cancer, patients were randomized to receive NEUPOGEN® (n =

Continued on next page

Neupogen—Cont.

99) or placebo (n = 111) starting on day 4, after receiving standard dose chemotherapy with cyclophosphamide, doxorubicin, and etoposide. A total of 210 patients were evaluated for efficacy and 207 evaluated for safety. Treatment with NEUPOGEN® resulted in a clinically and statistically significant reduction in the incidence of infection, as manifested by febrile neutropenia; the incidence of at least one infection over all cycles of chemotherapy was 76% (84/111) for placebo-treated patients, versus 40% (40/99) for NEUPOGEN®-treated patients ($p < 0.001$). The following secondary analyses were also performed. The requirements for in-patient hospitalization and antibiotic use were also significantly decreased during the first cycle of chemotherapy; incidence of hospitalization was 69% (77/111) for placebo-treated patients in cycle 1, versus 52% (51/99) for NEUPOGEN®-treated patients (p = 0.032). The incidence of IV antibiotic usage was 60% (67/111) for placebo-treated patients in cycle 1, versus 38% (38/99) for NEUPOGEN®-treated patients (p = 0.003). The incidence, severity, and duration of severe neutropenia [absolute neutrophil count (ANC) < 500/mm^3] following chemotherapy were all significantly reduced. The incidence of severe neutropenia in cycle 1 was 84% (83/99) for patients receiving NEUPOGEN® versus 96% (106/110) for patients receiving placebo (p = 0.004). Over all cycles, patients randomized to NEUPOGEN® had a 57% (286/500 cycles) rate of severe neutropenia versus 77% (416/543 cycles) for patients randomized to placebo. The median duration of severe neutropenia in cycle 1 was reduced from 6 days (range 0 to 10 days) for patients receiving placebo to 2 days (range 0 to 9 days) for patients receiving NEUPOGEN® ($p < 0.001$). The mean duration of neutropenia in cycle 1 was 5.64 ± 2.27 days for patients receiving placebo versus 2.44 ± 1.90 days for patients receiving NEUPOGEN®. Over all cycles, the median duration of neutropenia was 3 days for patients randomized to placebo versus 1 day for patients randomized to NEUPOGEN®. The median severity of neutropenia (as measured by ANC nadir) was 72/mm^3 (range 0/mm^3 to 7912/mm^3) in cycle 1 for patients receiving NEUPOGEN® versus 38/mm^3 (range 0/mm^3 to 9520/mm^3) for patients receiving placebo (p = 0.012). The mean severity of neutropenia in cycle 1 was 496/mm^3 ± 1382/mm^3 for patients receiving NEUPOGEN® versus 204/mm^3 ± 953/mm^3 for patients receiving placebo. Over all cycles, the ANC nadir for patients randomized to NEUPOGEN® was 403/mm^3, versus 161/mm^3 for patients randomized to placebo. Administration of NEUPOGEN® resulted in an earlier ANC nadir following chemotherapy than was experienced by patients receiving placebo (day 10 vs day 12). NEUPOGEN® was well-tolerated when given SC daily at doses of 4 to 8 mcg/kg for up to 14 consecutive days following each cycle of chemotherapy (see ADVERSE REACTIONS).

Several other phase 1/2 studies, which did not directly measure the incidence of infection, but which did measure increases in neutrophils, support the efficacy of NEUPOGEN®. The regimens are presented to provide some background on the clinical experience with NEUPOGEN®. No claim regarding the safety or efficacy of the chemotherapy regimens is made. The effects of NEUPOGEN® on tumor growth or on the anti-tumor activity of the chemotherapy were not assessed. The doses of NEUPOGEN® used in these studies are considerably greater than those found to be effective in the phase 3 study described above. Such phase 1/2 studies are summarized in the following table.

[See second table above]

Patients With Acute Myeloid Leukemia Receiving Induction or Consolidation Chemotherapy

In a randomized, double-blind, placebo-controlled, multicenter, phase 3 clinical trial, 521 patients (median age 54, range 16 to 89 years) were treated for de novo acute myeloid leukemia (AML). Following a standard induction chemotherapy regimen comprising daunorubicin, cytosine arabinoside, and etoposide[15] (DAV 3+7+5), patients received either NEUPOGEN® at 5 mcg/kg/day or placebo, SC, from 24 hours after the last dose of chemotherapy until neutrophil recovery (ANC 1000/mm^3 for 3 consecutive days or 10,000/mm^3 for 1 day) or for a maximum of 35 days.

Treatment with NEUPOGEN® significantly reduced the median time to ANC recovery and the median duration of fever, antibiotic use, and hospitalization following induction chemotherapy. In the NEUPOGEN®-treated group, the median time from initiation of chemotherapy to ANC recovery (ANC ≥ 500/mm^3) was 20 days (vs 25 days in the control group, p = 0.0001), the median duration of fever was reduced by 1.5 days (p = 0.009), and there were statistically significant reductions in the durations of IV antibiotic use and hospitalization. During consolidation therapy (DAV 2+5+5), patients treated with NEUPOGEN® also experienced significant reductions in the incidence of severe neutropenia, time to neutrophil recovery, the incidence and duration of fever, and in the durations of IV antibiotic use and hospitalization. Patients treated with a further course of standard (DAV 2+5+5) or high-dose cytosine arabinoside consolidation also experienced significant reductions in the duration of neutropenia.

There were no statistically significant differences between NEUPOGEN® and placebo groups in complete remission rate (69% NEUPOGEN® vs 68% placebo, p = 0.77), disease-free survival [median 342 days NEUPOGEN® (n = 178), 322 days placebo (n = 177), p = 0.99], time to progression of all randomized patients (median 165 days NEUPOGEN®, 186 days placebo, p = 0.87), or overall survival (median 380 days NEUPOGEN®, 425 days placebo, p = 0.83).

	300 mcg/ 1.0 mL Vial	480 mcg/ 1.6 mL Vial	300 mcg/ 0.5 mL Syringe	480 mcg/ 0.8 mL Syringe
Filgrastim	300 mcg	480 mcg	300 mcg	480 mcg
Acetate	0.59 mg	0.94 mg	0.295 mg	0.472 mg
Sorbitol	50.0 mg	80.0 mg	25.0 mg	40.0 mg
Tween® 80	0.004%	0.004%	0.004%	0.004%
Sodium	0.035 mg	0.056 mg	0.0175 mg	0.028 mg
Water for Injection				
USP q.s. ad	1.0 mL	1.6 mL	0.5 mL	0.8 mL

Type of Malignancy	Regimen	Chemotherapy Dose	No. Pts.	Trial Phase	NEUPOGEN® Daily Dosage[a]
Small Cell					
Lung Cancer	Cyclophosphamide	1 g/m^2/day	210	3	4–8 mcg/kg SC
	Doxorubicin	50 mg/m^2/day			days 4–17
	Etoposide	120 mg/m^2/day × 3			
		q 21 days			
Small Cell					
Lung Cancer[11]	Ifosfamide	5 g/m^2/day	12	1/2	5.75–46 mcg/kg IV
	Doxorubicin	50 mg/m^2/day			days 4–17
	Etoposide	120 mg/m^2/day × 3			
	Mesna	8 g/m^2/day			
		q 21 days			
Urothelial					
Cancer[12]	Methotrexate	30 mg/m^2/day × 2	40	1/2	3.45–69 mcg/kg IV
	Vinblastine	3 mg/m^2/day × 2			days 4–11
	Doxorubicin	30 mg/m^2/day			
	Cisplatin	70 mg/m^2/day			
		q 28 days			
Various					
Nonmyeloid					
Malignancies[13]	Cyclophosphamide	2.5 g/m^2/day × 2	18	1/2	23–69 mcg/kg[b] IV
	Etoposide	500 mg/m^2/day × 3			days 8–28
	Cisplatin	50 mg/m^2/day × 3			
		q 28 days			
Breast/Ovarian					
Cancer[14]	Doxorubicin[c]	75 mg/m^2	21	2	11.5 mcg/kg IV
		100 mg/m^2			days 2–9
		125 mg/m^2			5.75 mcg/kg IV
		150 mg/m^2			days 10–12
		q 14 days			
Neuroblastoma	Cyclophosphamide	150 mg/m^2 × 7	12	2	5.45–17.25 mcg/kg SC
	Doxorubicin	35 mg/m^2			days 6–19
	Cisplatin	90 mg/m^2			
		q 28 days			
		(cycles 1,3,5)[d]			

[a] NEUPOGEN® doses were those that accelerated neutrophil production. Doses which provided no additional acceleration beyond that achieved at the next lower dose are not reported.

[b] Lowest dose(s) tested in the study.

[c] Patients received doxorubicin at either 75, 100, 125, or 150 mg/m^2.

[d] Cycles 2,6 = cyclophosphamide 150 mg/m^2 × 7 and etoposide 280 mg/m^2 × 3. Cycle 4 = cisplatin 90 mg/m^2 × 1 and etoposide 280 mg/m^2 × 3.

Cancer Patients Receiving Bone Marrow Transplant

In two separate randomized, controlled trials, patients with Hodgkin's disease (HD) and non-Hodgkin's lymphoma (NHL) were treated with myeloablative chemotherapy and autologous bone marrow transplantation (ABMT). In one study (n = 54), NEUPOGEN® was administered at doses of 10 or 30 mcg/kg/day; a third treatment group in this study received no NEUPOGEN®. A statistically significant reduction in the median number of days of severe neutropenia (ANC < 500/mm^3) occurred in the NEUPOGEN®-treated group versus the control group (23 days in the control group, 11 days in the 10 mcg/kg/day group, and 14 days in the 30 mcg/kg/day group, [11 days in the combined treatment groups, p = 0.004]). In the second study (n = 44, 43 patients evaluable), NEUPOGEN® was administered at doses of 10 or 20 mcg/kg/day; a third treatment group in this study received no NEUPOGEN®. A statistically significant reduction in the median number of days of severe neutropenia occurred in the NEUPOGEN®-treated group versus the control group (21.5 days in the control group and 10 days in both treatment groups, $p < 0.001$). The number of days of febrile neutropenia was also reduced significantly in this study [13.5 days in the control group, 5 days in the 10 mcg/kg/day group, and 5.5 days in the 20 mcg/kg/day group, (5 days in the combined treatment groups, $p < 0.0001$)]. Reductions in the number of days of hospitalization and antibiotic use were also seen, although these reductions were not statistically significant. There were no effects on red blood cell or platelet levels.

In a randomized, placebo-controlled trial, 70 patients with myeloid and nonmyeloid malignancies were treated with myeloablative therapy and allogeneic bone marrow transplant followed by 300 mcg/m^2/day of a Filgrastim product. A statistically significant reduction in the median number of days of severe neutropenia occurred in the treated group versus the control group (19 days in the control group and 15 days in the treatment group, $p < 0.001$) and time to recovery of ANC to ≥ 500/mm^3 (21 days in the control group and 16 days in the treatment group, $p < 0.001$).

In three nonrandomized studies (n = 119), patients received ABMT and treatment with NEUPOGEN®. One study (n = 45) involved patients with breast cancer and malignant melanoma. A second study (n = 39) involved patients with HD. The third study (n = 35) involved patients with NHL, acute lymphoblastic leukemia (ALL), and germ cell tumor. In these studies, the recovery of the ANC to ≥ 500/mm^3 ranged from a median of 11.5 to 13 days.

None of the conditioning regimens used in the ABMT studies included radiation therapy.

While these studies were not designed to compare survival, this information was collected and evaluated. The overall survival and disease progression of patients receiving NEUPOGEN® in these studies were similar to those observed in the respective control groups and to historical data.

Peripheral Blood Progenitor Cell Collection and Therapy in Cancer Patients

All patients in the Amgen-sponsored trials received a similar mobilization/collection regimen: NEUPOGEN® was administered for 6 to 7 days, with an apheresis procedure on days 5, 6, and 7 (except for a limited number of patients receiving apheresis on days 4, 6, and 8). In a non-Amgen-sponsored study, patients underwent mobilization to a target number of mononuclear cells (MNC), with apheresis starting on day 5. There are no data on the mobilization of peripheral blood progenitor cells (PBPC) after days 4 to 5 that are not confounded by leukapheresis.

Mobilization: Mobilization of PBPC was studied in 50 heavily pretreated patients (median number of prior cycles = 9.5) with NHL, HD, or ALL (Amgen study 1). CFU-GM was used as the marker for engraftable PBPC. The median CFU-GM level on each day of mobilization was determined from the data available (CFU-GM assays were not obtained on all patients on each day of mobilization). These data are presented below.

The data from Amgen study 1 were supported by data from Amgen study 2 in which 22 pretreated breast cancer patients (median number of prior cycles = 3) were studied. Both the CFU-GM and $CD34^+$ cells reached a maximum on day 5 at > 10-fold over baseline and then remained elevated with leukapheresis.

[See first table at top of next page]

In three studies of patients with prior exposure to chemotherapy, the median CFU-GM yield in the leukapheresis product ranged from 20.9 to 32.7 × 10^4/kg body weight (n = 105). In two of these studies where $CD34^+$ yields in the leukapheresis product were also determined, the median $CD34^+$ yields were 3.11 and 2.80 × 10^6/kg, respectively (n = 56). In an additional study of 18 chemotherapy-naive patients, the median CFU-GM yield was 123.4 × 10^4/kg.

Engraftment: Engraftment following NEUPOGEN®-mobilized PBPC is summarized for 101 patients in the table below. In all studies a Cox regression model showed that the total number of CFU-GM and/or CD34+ cells collected was a significant predictor of time to platelet recovery.

In a randomized unblinded study of patients with HD or NHL undergoing myeloablative chemotherapy (Amgen study 3), 27 patients received NEUPOGEN®-mobilized PBPC followed by NEUPOGEN® and 31 patients received ABMT followed by NEUPOGEN®. Patients randomized to the NEUPOGEN®-mobilized PBPC group compared to the ABMT group had significantly fewer days of platelet transfusions (median 6 vs 10 days), a significantly shorter time to a sustained platelet count > 20,000/mm^3 (median 16 vs 23 days), a significantly shorter time to recovery of a sustained ANC ≥ 500/mm^3 (median 11 vs 14 days), significantly fewer days of red blood cell transfusions (median 2 vs 3 days) and a significantly shorter duration of posttransplant hospitalization.

[See second table at right]

Three of the 101 patients (3%) did not achieve the criteria for engraftment as defined by a platelet count ≥ 20,000/mm^3 by day 28. In clinical trials of NEUPOGEN® for the mobilization of PBPC, NEUPOGEN® was administered to patients at 5 to 24 mcg/kg/day after reinfusion of the collected cells until a sustainable ANC (≥ 500/mm^3) was reached. The rate of engraftment of these cells in the absence of NEUPOGEN® posttransplantation has not been studied.

Patients With Severe Chronic Neutropenia

Severe chronic neutropenia (SCN) (idiopathic, cyclic, and congenital) is characterized by a selective decrease in the number of circulating neutrophils and an enhanced susceptibility to bacterial infections.

The daily administration of NEUPOGEN® has been shown to be safe and effective in causing a sustained increase in the neutrophil count and a decrease in infectious morbidity in children and adults with the clinical syndrome of SCN.[16]

In the phase 3 trial, summarized in the following table, daily treatment with NEUPOGEN® resulted in significant beneficial changes in the incidence and duration of infection, fever, antibiotic use, and oropharyngeal ulcers. In this trial, 120 patients with a median age of 12 years (range 1 to 76 years) were treated.

[See third table at right]

The incidence for each of these five clinical parameters was lower in the NEUPOGEN® arm compared to the control arm for cohorts in each of the three major diagnostic categories. All three diagnostic groups showed favorable trends in favor of treatment. An analysis of variance showed no significant interaction between treatment and diagnosis, suggesting that efficacy did not differ substantially in the different diseases. Although NEUPOGEN® substantially reduced neutropenia in all patient groups, in patients with cyclic neutropenia, cycling persisted but the period of neutropenia was shortened to 1 day.

As a result of the lower incidence and duration of infections, there was also a lower number of episodes of hospitalization (28 hospitalizations in 62 patients in the treated group vs 44 hospitalizations in 60 patients in the control group over a 4-month period [p = 0.0034]). Patients treated with NEUPOGEN® also reported a lower number of episodes of diarrhea, nausea, fatigue, and sore throat.

In the phase 3 trial, untreated patients had a median ANC of 210/mm^3 (range 0 to 1550/mm^3). NEUPOGEN® therapy was adjusted to maintain the median ANC between 1500 and 10,000/mm^3. Overall, the response to NEUPOGEN® was observed in 1 to 2 weeks. The median ANC after 5 months of NEUPOGEN® therapy for all patients was 7460/mm^3 (range 30 to 30,880/mm^3). NEUPOGEN® dosing requirements were generally higher for patients with congenital neutropenia (2.3 to 40 mcg/kg/day) than for patients with idiopathic (0.6 to 11.5 mcg/kg/day) or cyclic (0.5 to 6 mcg/kg/day) neutropenia.

Progenitor Cell Levels in Peripheral Blood by Mobilization Day

	Overall Study 1 CFU-GM/mL		Study 2 CFU-GM/mL		Study 2 CD34+ (×10^4/mL)	
	No. Samples	Median (25%–75%)	No. Samples	Median (25%–75%)	No. Samples	Median (25%–75%)
Day 1	11	18 (13–62)	20	42 (15–151)	20	0.13 (0.02–0.66)
Day 2	7	22 (3–61)	n/a	n/a	n/a	n/a
Day 3	10	138 (39–364)	n/a	n/a	n/a	n/a
Day 4	18	365 (158–864)	18	576 (108–1819)	17	2.11 (0.58–3.93)
Day 5	36	781 (391–1608)	21	960 (72–1677)	22	3.16 (1.08–6.11)
Day 6	46	505 (199–1397)	22	756 (70–3486)	22	2.67 (1.09–4.40)
Day 7	37	333 (111–938)	22	597 (118–2009)	21	2.64 (0.78–4.22)
Day 8	15	383 (94–815)	12	51 (10–746)	12	1.61 (0.38–4.31)

n/a = not available

	Amgen-sponsored Study 1 N = 13	Amgen-sponsored Study 2 N = 22	Amgen-sponsored Study 3 N = 27	Non-Amgen-sponsored Study N = 39
Median PBPC/kg Collected				
MNC	9.5 × 10^8	9.5 × 10^8	8.1 × 10^8	10.3 × 10^8
CD34+	n/a	3.1 × 10^6	2.8 × 10^6	6.2 × 10^6
CFU-GM	63.9 × 10^4	25.3 × 10^4	32.6 × 10^4	n/a
Days to ANC ≥ 500/mm^3				
Median	9	10	11	10
Range	8–10	8–15	9–38	7–40
Days to Plt. ≥ 20,000/mm^3				
Median	10	12.5	16	15.5
Range	7–16	10–30	8–52	7–63

n/a = not available

Overall Significant Changes in Clinical Endpoints Median Incidence[a] (Events) or Duration (Days) per 28-day Period

	Control Patients[b]	NEUPOGEN®-treated Patients	p-value
Incidence of Infection	0.50	0.20	<0.001
Incidence of Fever	0.25	0.20	<0.001
Duration of Fever	0.63	0.20	0.005
Incidence of Oropharyngeal Ulcers	0.26	0.00	<0.001
Incidence of Antibiotic Use	0.49	0.20	<0.001

[a] Incidence values were calculated for each patient, and are defined as the total number of events experienced divided by the number of 28-day periods of exposure (on-study). Median incidence values were then reported for each patient group.
[b] Control patients were observed for a 4-month period.

INDICATIONS AND USAGE

Cancer Patients Receiving Myelosuppressive Chemotherapy

NEUPOGEN® is indicated to decrease the incidence of infection, as manifested by febrile neutropenia, in patients with nonmyeloid malignancies receiving myelosuppressive anti-cancer drugs associated with a significant incidence of severe neutropenia with fever (see CLINICAL EXPERIENCE). A complete blood count (CBC) and platelet count should be obtained prior to chemotherapy, and twice per week (see LABORATORY MONITORING) during NEUPOGEN® therapy to avoid leukocytosis and to monitor the neutrophil count. In phase 3 clinical studies, NEUPOGEN® therapy was discontinued when the ANC was ≥ 10,000/mm^3 after the expected chemotherapy-induced nadir.

Patients With Acute Myeloid Leukemia Receiving Induction or Consolidation Chemotherapy

NEUPOGEN® is indicated for reducing the time to neutrophil recovery and the duration of fever, following induction or consolidation chemotherapy treatment of adults with AML.

Cancer Patients Receiving Bone Marrow Transplant

NEUPOGEN® is indicated to reduce the duration of neutropenia and neutropenia-related clinical sequelae, eg, febrile neutropenia, in patients with nonmyeloid malignancies undergoing myeloablative chemotherapy followed by marrow transplantation (see CLINICAL EXPERIENCE). It is recommended that CBCs and platelet counts be obtained at a minimum of three times per week (see LABORATORY MONITORING) following marrow infusion to monitor the recovery of marrow reconstitution.

Patients Undergoing Peripheral Blood Progenitor Cell Collection and Therapy

NEUPOGEN® is indicated for the mobilization of hematopoietic progenitor cells into the peripheral blood for collection by leukapheresis. Mobilization allows for the collection of increased numbers of progenitor cells capable of engraftment compared with collection by leukapheresis without mobilization or bone marrow harvest. After myeloablative chemotherapy, the transplantation of an increased number of progenitor cells can lead to more rapid engraftment, which may result in a decreased need for supportive care (see CLINICAL EXPERIENCE).

Patients With Severe Chronic Neutropenia

NEUPOGEN® is indicated for chronic administration to reduce the incidence and duration of sequelae of neutropenia (eg, fever, infections, oropharyngeal ulcers) in symptomatic patients with congenital neutropenia, cyclic neutropenia, or idiopathic neutropenia (see CLINICAL EXPERIENCE). It is essential that serial CBCs with differential and platelet counts, and an evaluation of bone marrow morphology and karyotype be performed prior to initiation of NEUPOGEN® therapy (see WARNINGS). The use of NEUPOGEN® prior to confirmation of SCN may impair diagnostic efforts and may thus impair or delay evaluation and treatment of an underlying condition, other than SCN, causing the neutropenia.

CONTRAINDICATIONS

NEUPOGEN® is contraindicated in patients with known hypersensitivity to *E coli*-derived proteins, Filgrastim, or any component of the product.

WARNINGS

Allergic-type reactions occurring on initial or subsequent treatment have been reported in < 1 in 4000 patients treated with NEUPOGEN®. These have generally been characterized by systemic symptoms involving at least two body systems, most often skin (rash, urticaria, facial edema), respiratory (wheezing, dyspnea), and cardiovascular (hypotension, tachycardia). Some reactions occurred on initial exposure. Reactions tended to occur within the first 30 minutes after administration and appeared to occur more frequently in patients receiving NEUPOGEN® IV. Rapid resolution of symptoms occurred in most cases after administration of antihistamines, steroids, bronchodilators, and/or epinephrine. Symptoms recurred in more than half the patients who were rechallenged.

Patients With Severe Chronic Neutropenia

The safety and efficacy of NEUPOGEN® in the treatment of neutropenia due to other hematopoietic disorders (eg, myelodysplastic syndrome [MDS]) have not been established. Care should be taken to confirm the diagnosis of SCN before initiating NEUPOGEN® therapy.

MDS and AML have been reported to occur in the natural history of congenital neutropenia without cytokine therapy.[17] Cytogenetic abnormalities, transformation to MDS, and AML have also been observed in patients treated with NEUPOGEN® for SCN. Based on available data including a postmarketing surveillance study, the risk of developing MDS and AML appears to be confined to the subset of patients with congenital neutropenia (see ADVERSE REACTIONS). Abnormal cytogenetics and MDS have been associated with the eventual development of myeloid leukemia. The effect of NEUPOGEN® on the development of abnormal cytogenetics and the effect of continued NEUPOGEN® administration in patients with abnormal cytogenetics or MDS are unknown. If a patient with SCN develops abnormal cytogenetics or myelodysplasia, the risks and benefits of continuing NEUPOGEN® should be carefully considered.

PRECAUTIONS

General

Simultaneous Use With Chemotherapy and Radiation Therapy

The safety and efficacy of NEUPOGEN® given simultaneously with cytotoxic chemotherapy have not been estab-

Continued on next page

Neupogen—Cont.

lished. Because of the potential sensitivity of rapidly dividing myeloid cells to cytotoxic chemotherapy, do not use NEUPOGEN® in the period 24 hours before through 24 hours after the administration of cytotoxic chemotherapy (see DOSAGE AND ADMINISTRATION).
The efficacy of NEUPOGEN® has not been evaluated in patients receiving chemotherapy associated with delayed myelosuppression (eg, nitrosoureas) or with mitomycin C or with myelosuppressive doses of antimetabolites such as 5-fluorouracil.
The safety and efficacy of NEUPOGEN® have not been evaluated in patients receiving concurrent radiation therapy. Simultaneous use of NEUPOGEN® with chemotherapy and radiation therapy should be avoided.

Potential Effect on Malignant Cells

NEUPOGEN® is a growth factor that primarily stimulates neutrophils. However, the possibility that NEUPOGEN® can act as a growth factor for any tumor type cannot be excluded. In a randomized study evaluating the effects of NEUPOGEN® versus placebo in patients undergoing remission induction for AML, there was no significant difference in remission rate, disease-free or overall survival (see CLINICAL EXPERIENCE).
The safety of NEUPOGEN® in chronic myeloid leukemia (CML) and myelodysplasia has not been established.
When NEUPOGEN® is used to mobilize PBPC, tumor cells may be released from the marrow and subsequently collected in the leukapheresis product. The effect of reinfusion of tumor cells has not been well-studied, and the limited data available are inconclusive.

Leukocytosis

Cancer Patients Receiving Myelosuppressive Chemotherapy

White blood cell counts of 100,000/mm^3 or greater were observed in approximately 2% of patients receiving NEUPOGEN® at doses above 5 mcg/kg/day. There were no reports of adverse events associated with this degree of leukocytosis. In order to avoid the potential complications of excessive leukocytosis, a CBC is recommended twice per week during NEUPOGEN® therapy (see LABORATORY MONITORING).

Premature Discontinuation of NEUPOGEN® Therapy

Cancer Patients Receiving Myelosuppressive Chemotherapy

A transient increase in neutrophil counts is typically seen 1 to 2 days after initiation of NEUPOGEN® therapy. However, for a sustained therapeutic response, NEUPOGEN® therapy should be continued following chemotherapy until the post nadir ANC reaches 10,000/mm^3. Therefore, the premature discontinuation of NEUPOGEN® therapy, prior to the time of recovery from the expected neutrophil nadir, is generally not recommended (see DOSAGE AND ADMINISTRATION).

Other

In studies of NEUPOGEN® administration following chemotherapy, most reported side effects were consistent with those usually seen as a result of cytotoxic chemotherapy (see ADVERSE REACTIONS). Because of the potential of receiving higher doses of chemotherapy (ie, full doses on the prescribed schedule), the patient may be at greater risk of thrombocytopenia, anemia, and nonhematologic consequences of increased chemotherapy doses (please refer to the prescribing information of the specific chemotherapy agents used). Regular monitoring of the hematocrit and platelet count is recommended. Furthermore, care should be exercised in the administration of NEUPOGEN® in conjunction with other drugs known to lower the platelet count.
In septic patients receiving NEUPOGEN®, the physician should be alert to the theoretical possibility of adult respiratory distress syndrome, due to the possible influx of neutrophils at the site of inflammation.
There have been rare reports (< 1 in 7000 patients) of cutaneous vasculitis in patients treated with NEUPOGEN®. In most cases, the severity of cutaneous vasculitis was moderate or severe. Most of the reports involved patients with SCN receiving long-term NEUPOGEN® therapy. Symptoms of vasculitis generally developed simultaneously with an increase in the ANC and abated when the ANC decreased. Many patients were able to continue NEUPOGEN® at a reduced dose.

Information for Patients

In those situations in which the physician determines that the patient can safely and effectively self-administer NEUPOGEN®, the patient should be instructed as to the proper dosage and administration. Patients should be referred to the "Information for Patients" labeling included with the package insert in each dispensing carton of NEUPOGEN®. This patient information, however, is not intended to be a disclosure of all known or possible effects. If home use is prescribed, patients should be thoroughly instructed in the importance of proper disposal and cautioned against the reuse of needles, syringes, or drug product. A puncture-resistant container for the disposal of used syringes and needles should be available to the patient. The full container should be disposed of according to the directions provided by the physician.

Laboratory Monitoring

Cancer Patients Receiving Myelosuppressive Chemotherapy

A CBC and platelet count should be obtained prior to chemotherapy, and at regular intervals (twice per week) during NEUPOGEN® therapy. Following cytotoxic chemotherapy, the neutrophil nadir occurred earlier during cycles when NEUPOGEN® was administered, and WBC differentials demonstrated a left shift, including the appearance of promyelocytes and myeloblasts. In addition, the duration of severe neutropenia was reduced, and was followed by an accelerated recovery in the neutrophil counts. Therefore, regular monitoring of WBC counts, particularly at the time of the recovery from the postchemotherapy nadir, is recommended in order to avoid excessive leukocytosis.

Cancer Patients Receiving Bone Marrow Transplant

Frequent CBCs and platelet counts are recommended (at least three times per week) following marrow transplantation.

Patients With Severe Chronic Neutropenia

During the initial 4 weeks of NEUPOGEN® therapy and during the 2 weeks following any dose adjustment, a CBC with differential and platelet count should be performed twice weekly. Once a patient is clinically stable, a CBC with differential and platelet count should be performed monthly during the first year of treatment. Thereafter, if clinically stable, routine monitoring with regular CBCs (ie, as clinically indicated but at least quarterly) is recommended. Additionally, for those patients with congenital neutropenia, annual bone marrow and cytogenetic evaluations should be performed throughout the duration of treatment (see WARNINGS, ADVERSE REACTIONS).
In clinical trials, the following laboratory results were observed:

- Cyclic fluctuations in the neutrophil counts were frequently observed in patients with congenital or idiopathic neutropenia after initiation of NEUPOGEN® therapy.
- Platelet counts were generally at the upper limits of normal prior to NEUPOGEN® therapy. With NEUPOGEN® therapy, platelet counts decreased but usually remained within normal limits (see ADVERSE REACTIONS).
- Early myeloid forms were noted in peripheral blood in most patients, including the appearance of metamyelocytes and myelocytes. Promyelocytes and myeloblasts were noted in some patients.
- Relative increases were occasionally noted in the number of circulating eosinophils and basophils. No consistent increases were observed with NEUPOGEN® therapy.
- As in other trials, increases were observed in serum uric acid, lactic dehydrogenase, and serum alkaline phosphatase.

Drug Interaction

Drug interactions between NEUPOGEN® and other drugs have not been fully evaluated. Drugs which may potentiate the release of neutrophils, such as lithium, should be used with caution.

Carcinogenesis, Mutagenesis, Impairment of Fertility

The carcinogenic potential of NEUPOGEN® has not been studied. NEUPOGEN® failed to induce bacterial gene mutations in either the presence or absence of a drug metabolizing enzyme system. NEUPOGEN® had no observed effect on the fertility of male or female rats, or on gestation at doses up to 500 mcg/kg.

Pregnancy Category C

NEUPOGEN® has been shown to have adverse effects in pregnant rabbits when given in doses 2 to 10 times the human dose. Since there are no adequate and well-controlled studies in pregnant women, the effect, if any, of NEUPOGEN® on the developing fetus or the reproductive capacity of the mother is unknown. However, the scientific literature describes transplacental passage of NEUPOGEN® when administered to pregnant rats during the latter part of gestation[18] and apparent transplacental passage of NEUPOGEN® when administered to pregnant humans by ≤ 30 hours prior to preterm delivery (≤ 30 weeks gestation).[19] NEUPOGEN® should be used during pregnancy only if the potential benefit justifies the potential risk to the fetus.
In rabbits, increased abortion and embryolethality were observed in animals treated with NEUPOGEN® at 80 mcg/kg/day. NEUPOGEN® administered to pregnant rabbits at doses of 80 mcg/kg/day during the period of organogenesis was associated with increased fetal resorption, genitourinary bleeding, developmental abnormalities, decreased body weight, live births, and food consumption. External abnormalities were not observed in the fetuses of dams treated at 80 mcg/kg/day. Reproductive studies in pregnant rats have shown that NEUPOGEN® was not associated with lethal, teratogenic, or behavioral effects on fetuses when administered by daily IV injection during the period of organogenesis at dose levels up to 575 mcg/kg/day.
In Segment III studies in rats, offspring of dams treated at > 20 mcg/kg/day exhibited a delay in external differentiation (detachment of auricles and descent of testes) and slight growth retardation, possibly due to lower body weight of females during rearing and nursing. Offspring of dams treated at 100 mcg/kg/day exhibited decreased body weights at birth, and a slightly reduced 4-day survival rate.

Nursing Mothers

It is not known whether NEUPOGEN® is excreted in human milk. Because many drugs are excreted in human milk, caution should be exercised if NEUPOGEN® is administered to a nursing woman.

Pediatric Use

In a phase 3 study to assess the safety and efficacy of NEUPOGEN® in the treatment of SCN, 120 patients with a median age of 12 years were studied. Of the 120 patients, 12 were infants (1 month to 2 years of age), 47 were children (2 to 12 years of age), and 9 were adolescents (12 to 16 years of age). Additional information is available from a SCN postmarketing surveillance study, which includes long-term follow-up of patients in the clinical studies and information from additional patients who entered directly into the postmarketing surveillance study. Of the 531 patients in the surveillance study as of December 31, 1997, 32 were infants, 200 were children, and 68 were adolescents (see CLINICAL EXPERIENCE, INDICATIONS AND USAGE, LABORATORY MONITORING, DOSAGE AND ADMINISTRATION).
Pediatric patients with congenital types of neutropenia (Kostmann's syndrome, congenital agranulocytosis, or Schwachman-Diamond syndrome) have developed cytogenetic abnormalities and have undergone transformation to MDS and AML while receiving chronic NEUPOGEN® treatment. The relationship of these events to NEUPOGEN® administration is unknown (see WARNINGS, ADVERSE REACTIONS).
Long-term follow-up data from the postmarketing surveillance study suggest that height and weight are not adversely affected in patients who received up to 5 years of NEUPOGEN® treatment. Limited data from patients who were followed in the phase 3 study for 1.5 years did not suggest alterations in sexual maturation or endocrine function.
The safety and efficacy in neonates and patients with autoimmune neutropenia of infancy have not been established.
In the cancer setting, 12 pediatric patients with neuroblastoma have received up to 6 cycles of cyclophosphamide, cisplatin, doxorubicin, and etoposide chemotherapy concurrently with NEUPOGEN®; in this population, NEUPOGEN® was well-tolerated. There was one report of palpable splenomegaly associated with NEUPOGEN® therapy, however, the only consistently reported adverse event was musculoskeletal pain, which is no different from the experience in the adult population.

ADVERSE REACTIONS

Cancer Patients Receiving Myelosuppressive Chemotherapy

In clinical trials involving over 350 patients receiving NEUPOGEN® following nonmyeloablative cytotoxic chemotherapy, most adverse experiences were the sequelae of the underlying malignancy or cytotoxic chemotherapy. In all phase 2 and 3 trials, medullary bone pain, reported in 24% of patients, was the only consistently observed adverse reaction attributed to NEUPOGEN® therapy. This bone pain was generally reported to be of mild-to-moderate severity, and could be controlled in most patients with non-narcotic analgesics; infrequently, bone pain was severe enough to require narcotic analgesics. Bone pain was reported more frequently in patients treated with higher doses (20 to 100 mcg/kg/day) administered IV, and less frequently in patients treated with lower SC doses of NEUPOGEN® (3 to 10 mcg/kg/day).
In the randomized, double-blind, placebo-controlled trial of NEUPOGEN® therapy following combination chemotherapy in patients (n = 207) with small cell lung cancer, the following adverse events were reported during blinded cycles of study medication (placebo or NEUPOGEN® at 4 to 8 mcg/kg/day). Events are reported as exposure-adjusted since patients remained on double-blind NEUPOGEN® a median of 3 cycles versus 1 cycle for placebo.
[See first table at top of next page]
In this study, there were no serious, life-threatening, or fatal adverse reactions attributed to NEUPOGEN® therapy. Specifically, there were no reports of flu-like symptoms, pleuritis, pericarditis, or other major systemic reactions to NEUPOGEN®.
Spontaneously reversible elevations in uric acid, lactate dehydrogenase, and alkaline phosphatase occurred in 27% to 58% of 98 patients receiving blinded NEUPOGEN® therapy following cytotoxic chemotherapy; increases were generally mild-to-moderate. Transient decreases in blood pressure (< 90/60 mmHg), which did not require clinical treatment, were reported in 7 of 176 patients in phase 3 clinical studies following administration of NEUPOGEN®. Cardiac events (myocardial infarctions, arrhythmias) have been reported in 11 of 375 cancer patients receiving NEUPOGEN® in clinical studies; the relationship to NEUPOGEN® therapy is unknown. No evidence of interaction of NEUPOGEN® with other drugs was observed in the course of clinical trials (see PRECAUTIONS).
There has been no evidence for the development of antibodies or of a blunted or diminished response to NEUPOGEN® in treated patients, including those receiving NEUPOGEN® daily for almost 2 years.

Patients With Acute Myeloid Leukemia

In a randomized phase 3 clinical trial, 259 patients received NEUPOGEN® and 262 patients received placebo postchemotherapy. Overall, the frequency of all reported adverse events was similar in both the NEUPOGEN® and placebo groups (83% vs 82% in Induction 1, 61% vs 64% in Consolidation 1). Adverse events reported more frequently in the NEUPOGEN®-treated group included: petechiae (17% vs 14%), epistaxis (9% vs 5%), and transfusion reactions (10% vs 5%). There were no significant differences in the frequency of these events.
There were a similar number of deaths in each treatment group during induction (25 NEUPOGEN® vs 27 placebo). The primary causes of death included infection (9 vs 18), persistent leukemia (7 vs 5), and hemorrhage (6 vs 3). Of the hemorrhagic deaths, five cerebral hemorrhages were reported in the NEUPOGEN® group and one in the placebo group. Other serious nonfatal hemorrhagic events were reported in the respiratory tract (4 vs 1), skin (4 vs 4), gastrointestinal tract (2 vs 2), urinary tract (1 vs 1), ocular (1 vs 0), and other nonspecific sites (2 vs 1). While 19 (7%) patients in the NEUPOGEN® group and five (2%) patients in the placebo group experienced severe or fatal hemorrhagic events, overall, hemorrhagic adverse events were reported

at a similar frequency in both groups (40% vs 38%). The time to transfusion-independent platelet recovery and the number of days of platelet transfusions were similar in both groups.

Cancer Patients Receiving Bone Marrow Transplant

In clinical trials, the reported adverse effects were those typically seen in patients receiving intensive chemotherapy followed by bone marrow transplant (BMT). The most common events reported in both control and treatment groups included stomatitis, nausea, and vomiting, generally of mild-to-moderate severity and were considered unrelated to NEUPOGEN®. In the randomized studies of BMT involving 167 patients who received study drug, the following events occurred more frequently in patients treated with Filgrastim than in controls: nausea (10% vs 4%), vomiting (7% vs 3%), hypertension (4% vs 0%), rash (12% vs 10%), and peritonitis (2% vs 0%). None of these events were reported by the Investigator to be related to NEUPOGEN®. One event of erythema nodosum was reported moderate in severity and possibly related to NEUPOGEN®.

Generally, adverse events observed in nonrandomized studies were similar to those seen in randomized studies, occurred in a minority of patients, and were of mild-to-moderate severity. In one study (n = 45), three serious adverse events reported by the Investigator were considered possibly related to NEUPOGEN®. These included two events of renal insufficiency and one event of capillary leak syndrome. The relationship of these events to NEUPOGEN® remains unclear since they occurred in patients with culture-proven infection with clinical sepsis who were receiving potentially nephrotoxic antibacterial and antifungal therapy.

Cancer Patients Undergoing Peripheral Blood Progenitor Cell Collection and Therapy

In clinical trials, 126 patients received NEUPOGEN® for PBPC mobilization. In this setting, NEUPOGEN® was generally well-tolerated. Adverse events related to NEUPOGEN® consisted primarily of mild-to-moderate musculoskeletal symptoms, reported in 44% of patients. These symptoms were predominantly events of medullary bone pain (33%). Headache was reported related to NEUPOGEN® in 7% of patients. Transient increases in alkaline phosphatase related to NEUPOGEN® were reported in 21% of the patients who had serum chemistries measured; most were mild-to-moderate.

All patients had increases in neutrophil counts during mobilization, consistent with the biological effects of NEUPOGEN®. Two patients had a WBC count > 100,000/mm^3. No sequelae were associated with any grade of leukocytosis.

Sixty-five percent of patients had mild-to-moderate anemia and 97% of patients had decreases in platelet counts; five patients (out of 126) had decreased platelet counts to < 50,000/mm^3. Anemia and thrombocytopenia have been reported to be related to leukapheresis; however, the possibility that NEUPOGEN® mobilization may contribute to anemia or thrombocytopenia has not been ruled out.

Patients With Severe Chronic Neutropenia

Mild-to-moderate bone pain was reported in approximately 33% of patients in clinical trials. This symptom was readily controlled with non-narcotic analgesics. Generalized musculoskeletal pain was also noted in higher frequency in patients treated with NEUPOGEN®. Palpable splenomegaly was observed in approximately 30% of patients. Abdominal or flank pain was seen infrequently, and thrombocytopenia (< 50,000/mm^3) was noted in 12% of patients with palpable spleens. Fewer than 3% of all patients underwent splenectomy, and most of these had a prestudy history of splenomegaly. Fewer than 6% of patients had thrombocytopenia (< 50,000/mm^3) during NEUPOGEN® therapy, most of whom had a pre-existing history of thrombocytopenia. In most cases, thrombocytopenia was managed by NEUPOGEN® dose reduction or interruption. An additional 5% of patients had platelet counts between 50,000 to 100,000/mm^3. There were no associated serious hemorrhagic sequelae in these patients. Epistaxis was noted in 15% of patients treated with NEUPOGEN®, but was associated with thrombocytopenia in 2% of patients. Anemia was reported in approximately 10% of patients, but in most cases appeared to be related to frequent diagnostic phlebotomy, chronic illness, or concomitant medications. Other adverse events infrequently observed and possibly related to NEUPOGEN® therapy were: injection site reaction, rash, hepatomegaly, arthralgia, osteoporosis, cutaneous vasculitis, hematuria/proteinuria, alopecia, and exacerbation of some pre-existing skin disorders (eg, psoriasis).

Cytogenetic abnormalities, transformation to MDS, and AML have been observed in patients treated with NEUPOGEN® for SCN (see WARNINGS, PRECAUTIONS: Pediatric Use). As of December 31, 1997, data were available from a postmarketing surveillance study of 531 SCN patients with an average follow-up of 4.0 years. Based on analysis of these data, the risk of developing MDS and AML appears to be confined to the subset of patients with congenital neutropenia. A life-table analysis of these data revealed that the cumulative risk of developing leukemia or MDS by the end of the 8th year of NEUPOGEN® treatment in a patient with congenital neutropenia was 16.5 % (95% C.I. = 9.8%, 23.3%); this represents an annual rate of approximately 2%. Cytogenetic abnormalities, most commonly involving chromosome 7, have been reported in patients treated with NEUPOGEN® who had previously documented normal cytogenetics. It is unknown whether the development of cytogenetic abnormalities, MDS, or AML is related to chronic daily NEUPOGEN® administration or to the natural history of congenital neutropenia. It is also unknown if the rate of conversion in patients who have not received NEUPOGEN® is different from that of patients who have received NEUPOGEN®. Routine monitoring through regular CBCs is recommended for all SCN patients. Additionally, annual bone marrow and cytogenetic evaluations are recommended in all patients with congenital neutropenia (see LABORATORY MONITORING).

% of Blinded Cycles with Events

Event	NEUPOGEN® N = 384 Patient Cycles	Placebo N = 257 Patient Cycles
Nausea/Vomiting	57	64
Skeletal Pain	22	11
Alopecia	18	27
Diarrhea	14	23
Neutropenic Fever	13	35
Mucositis	12	20
Fever	12	11
Fatigue	11	16
Anorexia	9	11
Dyspnea	9	11
Headache	7	9
Cough	6	8
Skin Rash	6	9
Chest Pain	5	6
Generalized Weakness	4	7
Sore Throat	4	9
Stomatitis	5	10
Constipation	5	10
Pain (Unspecified)	2	7

Absolute Neutrophil Count	NEUPOGEN® Dose Adjustment
When ANC > 1000/mm^3 for 3 consecutive days then:	Reduce to 5 mcg/kg/day[a]
If ANC remains > 1000/mm^3 for 3 more consecutive days then:	Discontinue NEUPOGEN®
If ANC decreases to < 1000/mm^3	Resume at 5 mcg/kg/day

[a] If ANC decreases to < 1000/mm^3 at any time during the 5 mcg/kg/day administration, NEUPOGEN® should be increased to 10 mcg/kg/day, and the above steps should then be followed.

OVERDOSAGE

In cancer patients receiving NEUPOGEN® as an adjunct to myelosuppressive chemotherapy, it is recommended, to avoid the potential risks of excessive leukocytosis, that NEUPOGEN® therapy be discontinued if the ANC surpasses 10,000/mm^3 after the chemotherapy-induced ANC nadir has occurred. Doses of NEUPOGEN® that increase the ANC beyond 10,000/mm^3 may not result in any additional clinical benefit.

The maximum tolerated dose of NEUPOGEN® has not been determined. Efficacy was demonstrated at doses of 4 to 8 mcg/kg/day in the phase 3 study of nonmyeloablative chemotherapy. Patients in the BMT studies received up to 138 mcg/kg/day without toxic effects, although there was a flattening of the dose response curve above daily doses of greater than 10 mcg/kg/day.

In NEUPOGEN® clinical trials of cancer patients receiving myelosuppressive chemotherapy, WBC counts > 100,000/mm^3 have been reported in less than 5% of patients, but were not associated with any reported adverse clinical effects.

In cancer patients receiving myelosuppressive chemotherapy, discontinuation of NEUPOGEN® therapy usually results in a 50% decrease in circulating neutrophils within 1 to 2 days, with a return to pretreatment levels in 1 to 7 days.

DOSAGE AND ADMINISTRATION

Cancer Patients Receiving Myelosuppressive Chemotherapy

The recommended starting dose of NEUPOGEN® is 5 mcg/kg/day, administered as a single daily injection by SC bolus injection, by short IV infusion (15 to 30 minutes), or by continuous SC or continuous IV infusion. A CBC and platelet count should be obtained before instituting NEUPOGEN® therapy, and monitored twice weekly during therapy. Doses may be increased in increments of 5 mcg/kg for each chemotherapy cycle, according to the duration and severity of the ANC nadir.

NEUPOGEN® should be administered no earlier than 24 hours after the administration of cytotoxic chemotherapy. NEUPOGEN® should not be administered in the period 24 hours before the administration of chemotherapy (see PRECAUTIONS). NEUPOGEN® should be administered daily for up to 2 weeks, until the ANC has reached 10,000/mm^3 following the expected chemotherapy-induced neutrophil nadir. The duration of NEUPOGEN® therapy needed to attenuate chemotherapy-induced neutropenia may be dependent on the myelosuppressive potential of the chemotherapy regimen employed. NEUPOGEN® therapy should be discontinued if the ANC surpasses 10,000/mm^3 after the expected chemotherapy-induced neutrophil nadir (see PRECAUTIONS). In phase 3 trials, efficacy was observed at doses of 4 to 8 mcg/kg/day.

Cancer Patients Receiving Bone Marrow Transplant

The recommended dose of NEUPOGEN® following BMT is 10 mcg/kg/day given as an IV infusion of 4 or 24 hours, or as a continuous 24-hour SC infusion. For patients receiving BMT, the first dose of NEUPOGEN® should be administered at least 24 hours after cytotoxic chemotherapy and at least 24 hours after bone marrow infusion.

During the period of neutrophil recovery, the daily dose of NEUPOGEN® should be titrated against the neutrophil response as follows:

[See second table above]

Peripheral Blood Progenitor Cell Collection and Therapy in Cancer Patients

The recommended dose of NEUPOGEN® for the mobilization of PBPC is 10 mcg/kg/day SC, either as a bolus or a continuous infusion. It is recommended that NEUPOGEN® be given for at least 4 days before the first leukapheresis procedure and continued until the last leukapheresis. Although the optimal duration of NEUPOGEN® administration and leukapheresis schedule have not been established, administration of NEUPOGEN® for 6 to 7 days with leukaphereses on days 5, 6, and 7 was found to be safe and effective (see CLINICAL EXPERIENCE for schedules used in clinical trials). Neutrophil counts should be monitored after 4 days of NEUPOGEN®, and NEUPOGEN® dose modification should be considered for those patients who develop a WBC count > 100,000/mm^3.

In all clinical trials of NEUPOGEN® for the mobilization of PBPC, NEUPOGEN® was also administered after reinfusion of the collected cells (see CLINICAL EXPERIENCE).

Patients With Severe Chronic Neutropenia

NEUPOGEN® should be administered to those patients in whom a diagnosis of congenital, cyclic, or idiopathic neutropenia has been definitively confirmed. Other diseases associated with neutropenia should be ruled out.

Starting Dose:

Congenital Neutropenia: The recommended daily starting dose is 6 mcg/kg BID SC every day.

Idiopathic or Cyclic Neutropenia: The recommended daily starting dose is 5 mcg/kg as a single injection SC every day.

Dose Adjustments:

Chronic daily administration is required to maintain clinical benefit. Absolute neutrophil count should not be used as the sole indication of efficacy. The dose should be individually adjusted based on the patients' clinical course as well as ANC. In the SCN postmarketing surveillance study, the reported median daily doses of NEUPOGEN® were: 6.0 mcg/kg (congenital neutropenia), 2.1 mcg/kg (cyclic neutropenia), and 1.2 mcg/kg (idiopathic neutropenia). In rare instances, patients with congenital neutropenia have required doses of NEUPOGEN® ≥ 100 mcg/kg/day.

Dilution

If required, NEUPOGEN® may be diluted in 5% dextrose. NEUPOGEN® diluted to concentrations between 5 and 15 mcg/mL should be protected from adsorption to plastic materials by the addition of Albumin (Human) to a final concentration of 2 mg/mL. When diluted in 5% dextrose or 5% dextrose plus Albumin (Human), NEUPOGEN® is compatible with glass bottles, PVC and polyolefin IV bags, and polypropylene syringes.

Dilution of NEUPOGEN® to a final concentration of less than 5 mcg/mL is not recommended at any time. **Do not dilute with saline at any time; product may precipitate.**

Storage

NEUPOGEN® should be stored in the refrigerator at 2° to 8°C (36° to 46°F). Avoid shaking. Prior to injection, NEUPOGEN® may be allowed to reach room temperature for a

Continued on next page

Neupogen—Cont.

maximum of 24 hours. Any vial or prefilled syringe left at room temperature for greater than 24 hours should be discarded. Parenteral drug products should be inspected visually for particulate matter and discoloration prior to administration, whenever solution and container permit; if particulates or discoloration are observed, the container should not be used.

HOW SUPPLIED

NEUPOGEN®: Use only one dose per vial; do not re-enter the vial. Discard unused portions. Do not save unused drug for later administration.

Use only one dose per prefilled syringe. Discard unused portions. Do not save unused drug for later administration.

Vials

Single-dose, preservative-free vials containing 300 mcg (1 mL) of Filgrastim (300 mcg/mL). Dispensing packs of 10 (NDC 55513-530-10).

Single-dose, preservative-free vials containing 480 mcg (1.6 mL) of Filgrastim (300 mcg/mL). Dispensing packs of 10 (NDC 55513-546-10).

Prefilled Syringes (Singleject™)

Single-dose, preservative-free, prefilled syringes with 26 gauge, 5/8 inch needles containing 300 mcg (0.5 mL) of Filgrastim (600 mcg/mL). Dispensing packs of 10 (NDC 55513-924-10).

Single-dose, preservative-free, prefilled syringes with 26 gauge, 5/8 inch needles containing 480 mcg (0.8 mL) of Filgrastim (600 mcg/mL). Dispensing packs of 10 (NDC 55513-209-10).

NEUPOGEN® should be stored at 2° to 8°C (36° to 46°F). Avoid shaking.

REFERENCES

1. Zsebo KM, Cohen AM, Murdock DC, et al. Recombinant human granulocyte colony-stimulating factor: Molecular and biological characterization. *Immunobiol.* 1986;172: 175–184.
2. Welte K, Bonilla MA, Gillio AP, et al. Recombinant human G-CSF: Effects on hematopoiesis in normal and cyclophosphamide treated primates. *J Exp Med.* 1987;165: 941–948.
3. Duhrsen U, Villeval JL, Boyd J, et al. Effects of recombinant human granulocyte colony-stimulating factor on hematopoietic progenitor cells in cancer patients. *Blood.* 1988;72:2074–2081.
4. Souza LM, Boone TC, Gabrilove J, et al. Recombinant human granulocyte colony-stimulating factor: Effects on normal and leukemic myeloid cells. *Science.* 1986;232: 61–65.
5. Weisbart RH, Kacena A, Schuh A, Golde DW. GM-CSF induces human neutrophil IgA-mediated phagocytosis by an IgA Fc receptor activation mechanism. *Nature.* 1988;332:647–648.
6. Kitagawa S, Yuo A, Souza LM, Saito M, Miura Y, Takaku F. Recombinant human granulocyte colony-stimulating factor enhances superoxide release in human granulocytes stimulated by chemotactic peptide. *Biochem Biophys Res Commun.* 1987;1443:1146.
7. Glaspy JA, Baldwin GC, Robertson PA, et al. Therapy for neutropenia in hairy cell leukemia with recombinant human granulocyte colony-stimulating factor. *Ann Int Med.* 1988;109:789–795.
8. Yuo A, Kitagawa S, Ohsaka A, et al. Recombinant human granulocyte colony-stimulating factor as an activator of human granulocytes: Potentiation of responses triggered by receptor-mediated agonists and stimulation of C3bi receptor expression and adherance. *Blood.* 1989;74:2144–2149.
9. Gabrilove JL, Jakubowski A, Fain K, et al. Phase I study of granulocyte colony-stimulating factor in patients with transitional cell carcinoma of the urothelium. *J Clin Invest.* 1988;82:1454–1461.
10. Morstyn G, Souza L, Keech J, et al. Effect of granulocyte colony-stimulating factor on neutropenia induced by cytotoxic chemotherapy. *Lancet.* 1988;1:667–672.
11. Bronchud MH, Scarffe JH, Thatcher N, et al. Phase I/II study of recombinant human granulocyte colony-stimulating factor in patients receiving intensive chemotherapy for small cell lung cancer. *Br J Cancer.* 1987;56:809–813.
12. Gabrilove JL, Jakubowski A, Scher H, et al. Effect of granulocyte colony-stimulating factor on neutropenia and associated morbidity due to chemotherapy for transitional cell carcinoma of the urothelium. *N Engl J Med.* 1988;318:1414–1422.
13. Neidhart J, Mangalik A, Kohler W, et al. Granulocyte colony-stimulating factor stimulates recovery of granulocytes in patients receiving dose-intensive chemotherapy without bone-marrow transplantation. *J Clin Oncol.* 1989;7:1685–1691.
14. Bronchud MH, Howell A, Crowther D, et al. The use of granulocyte colony-stimulating factor to increase the intensity of treatment with doxorubicin in patients with advanced breast and ovarian cancer. *Br J Cancer.* 1989;60:121–128.
15. Heil G, Hoelzer D, Sanz MA, et al. A randomized, double-blind, placebo-controlled, phase III study of Filgrastim in remission induction and consolidation therapy for adults with de novo Acute Myeloid Leukemia. *Blood.* 1997;90:4710–4718.
16. Dale DC, Bonilla MA, Davis MW, et al. A randomized controlled phase III trial of recombinant human granulocyte colony-stimulating factor (Filgrastim) for treatment of severe chronic neutropenia. *Blood.* 1993;81: 2496–2502.
17. Schroeder TM and Kurth R. Spontaneous chromosomal breakage and high incidence of leukemia in inherited disease. *Blood.* 1971;37:96–112.
18. Medlock, ES, et al. G-CSF crosses the placenta and stimulates fetal rat granulopoiesis. *Blood.* 1993;81:916–922.
19. Calhoun, DA, et al. Transplacental passage of recombinant huG-CSF in women with an imminent preterm delivery. *Am J Obstet Gynecol.* 1996;174:1306–1311.

This product and its use are covered by the following US Patent Nos.: 4,810,643; 4,999,291; 5,528,823; 5,580,755.

Manufactured by:
Amgen Inc.
One Amgen Center Drive
Thousand Oaks, California 91320-1799

Issue Date: 06/30/00

Shown in Product Identification Guide, page 304

Anesta Corp.

4745 WILEY POST WAY
SALT LAKE CITY, UT 84116

Direct Inquiries to:
(801) 595-1405
FAX: (801) 595-1406
www.anesta.com

ACTIQ® Ⓒ℞
[act' ic]
(oral transmucosal fentanyl citrate)

PHYSICIANS AND OTHER HEALTHCARE PROVIDERS MUST BECOME FAMILIAR WITH THE IMPORTANT WARNINGS IN THIS LABEL.
***Actiq* is indicated only for the management of breakthrough cancer pain in patients with malignancies who are already receiving and who are tolerant to opioid therapy for their underlying persistent cancer pain.** Patients considered opioid tolerant are those who are taking at least 60 mg morphine/day, 50 mcg transdermal fentanyl/hour, or an equianalgesic dose of another opioid for a week or longer.
Because life-threatening hypoventilation could occur at any dose in patients not taking chronic opiates, *Actiq* is contraindicated in the management of acute or postoperative pain. This product **must not** be used in opioid non-tolerant patients.
Actiq is intended to be used only in the care of cancer patients and only by oncologists and pain specialists who are knowledgeable of and skilled in the use of Schedule II opioids to treat cancer pain.
Patients and their caregivers must be instructed that *Actiq* contains a medicine in an amount which can be fatal to a child. Patients and their caregivers must be instructed to keep all units out of the reach of children and to discard open units properly. (See Information for Patients and Their Caregivers for disposal instructions.)

WARNING: May be habit forming

DESCRIPTION

Actiq (oral transmucosal fentanyl citrate) is a solid formulation of fentanyl citrate, a potent opioid analgesic, intended for oral transmucosal administration. *Actiq* is formulated as a white to off-white solid drug matrix on a handle that is radiopaque and is fracture resistant (ABS plastic) under normal conditions when used as directed.

Actiq is designed to be dissolved slowly in the mouth in a manner to facilitate transmucosal absorption. The handle allows the *Actiq* unit to be removed from the mouth if signs of excessive opioid effects appear during administration.

Active Ingredient: Fentanyl citrate, USP is *N*-(1-Phenethyl-4-piperidyl) propionanilide citrate (1:1). Fentanyl is a highly lipophilic compound (octanol-water partition coefficient at pH 7.4 is 816:1) that is freely soluble in organic solvents and sparingly soluble in water (1:40). The molecular weight of the free base is 336.5 (the citrate salt is 528.6). The pKa of the tertiary nitrogens are 7.3 and 8.4. The compound has the following structural formula:

CH_3CH_2CON–(piperidyl)–N–CH_2CH_2–(phenyl) · HO–$C(CH_2COOH)_2$–$COOH$

Actiq is available in six strengths equivalent to 200, 400, 600, 800, 1200, or 1600 mcg fentanyl base that is identified by the text on the foil pouch, the shelf carton, and the dosage unit handle.

Inactive Ingredients: Sucrose, liquid glucose, artificial raspberry flavor, and white dispersion G.B. dye.

CLINICAL PHARMACOLOGY AND PHARMACOKINETICS

Pharmacology:

Fentanyl, a pure opioid agonist, acts primarily through interaction with opioid mu-receptors located in the brain, spinal cord and smooth muscle. The primary site of therapeutic action is the central nervous system (CNS). The most clinically useful pharmacologic effects of the interaction of fentanyl with mu-receptors are analgesia and sedation.

Other opioid effects may include somnolence, hypoventilation, bradycardia, postural hypotension, pruritus, dizziness, nausea, diaphoresis, flushing, euphoria and confusion or difficulty in concentrating at clinically relevant doses.

Clinical Pharmacology

Analgesia:

The analgesic effects of fentanyl are related to the blood level of the drug, if proper allowance is made for the delay into and out of the CNS (a process with a 3-to-5-minute half-life). In opioid non-tolerant individuals, fentanyl provides effects ranging from analgesia at blood levels of 1 to 2 ng/mL, all the way to surgical anesthesia and profound respiratory depression at levels of 10–20 ng/mL.

In general, the minimum effective concentration and the concentration at which toxicity occurs rise with increasing tolerance to any and all opioids. The rate of development of tolerance varies widely among individuals. As a result, the dose of *Actiq* should be individually titrated to achieve the desired effect (see **DOSAGE AND ADMINISTRATION**).

Gastrointestinal (GI) Tract and Other Smooth Muscle:

Opioids increase the tone and decrease contractions of the smooth muscle of the gastrointestinal (GI) tract. This results in prolongation in GI transit time and may be responsible for the constipating effect of opioids. Because opioids may increase biliary tract pressure, some patients with biliary colic may experience worsening of pain.

While opioids generally increase the tone of urinary tract smooth muscle, the overall effect tends to vary, in some cases producing urinary urgency, in others, difficulty in urination.

Respiratory System:

All opioid mu-receptor agonists, including fentanyl, produce dose dependent respiratory depression. The risk of respiratory depression is less in patients receiving chronic opioid therapy who develop tolerance to respiratory depression and other opioid effects. During the titration phase of the clinical trials, somnolence, which may be a precursor to respiratory depression, did increase in patients who were treated with higher doses of *Actiq*. In studies of opioid non-tolerant subjects, respiratory rate and oxygen saturation typically decrease as fentanyl blood concentration increases. Typically, peak respiratory depressive effects (decrease in respiratory rate) are seen 15 to 30 minutes from the start of oral transmucosal fentanyl citrate (OTFC®) administration and may persist for several hours.

Serious or fatal respiratory depression can occur, even at recommended doses, in vulnerable individuals. As with other potent opioids, fentanyl has been associated with cases of serious and fatal respiratory depression in opioid non-tolerant individuals.

Fentanyl depresses the cough reflex as a result of its CNS activity. Although not observed with *Actiq* in clinical trials, fentanyl given rapidly by intravenous injection in large doses may interfere with respiration by causing rigidity in the muscles of respiration. Therefore, physicians and other healthcare providers should be aware of this potential complication.

(See BOX WARNING, CONTRAINDICATIONS, WARNINGS, PRECAUTIONS, ADVERSE REACTIONS, and OVERDOSAGE for additional information on hypoventilation.)

Pharmacokinetics

Absorption:

The absorption pharmacokinetics of fentanyl from the oral transmucosal dosage form is a combination of an initial rapid absorption from the buccal mucosa and a more prolonged absorption of swallowed fentanyl from the GI tract. Both the blood fentanyl profile and the bioavailability of fentanyl will vary depending on the fraction of the dose that is absorbed through the oral mucosa and the fraction swallowed.

Absolute bioavailability, as determined by area under the concentration-time curve, of 15 mcg/kg in 12-adult males was 50% compared to intravenous fentanyl.

Normally, approximately 25% of the total dose of *Actiq* is rapidly absorbed from the buccal mucosa and becomes systemically available. The remaining 75% of the total dose is swallowed with the saliva and then is slowly absorbed from the GI tract. About 1/3 of this amount (25% of the total dose) escapes hepatic and intestinal first-pass elimination and becomes systemically available. Thus, the generally observed 50% bioavailability of *Actiq* is divided equally between rapid transmucosal and slower GI absorption. Therefore, a unit dose of *Actiq*, if chewed and swallowed, might result in lower peak concentrations and lower bioavailability than when consumed as directed.

Dose proportionality among four of the available strengths of *Actiq* (200, 400, 800, and 1600 mcg) has been demonstrated in a balanced crossover design in adult subjects. Mean serum fentanyl levels following these four doses of *Actiq* are shown in Figure 1. The curves for each dose level are similar in shape with increasing dose levels producing increasing serum fentanyl levels. C_{max} and $AUC_{0\to\infty}$ increased in a dose-dependent manner that is approximately proportional to the *Actiq* administered.

Figure 1.
Mean Serum Fentanyl Concentration (ng/mL) in Adult Subjects Comparing 4 Doses of *Actiq*

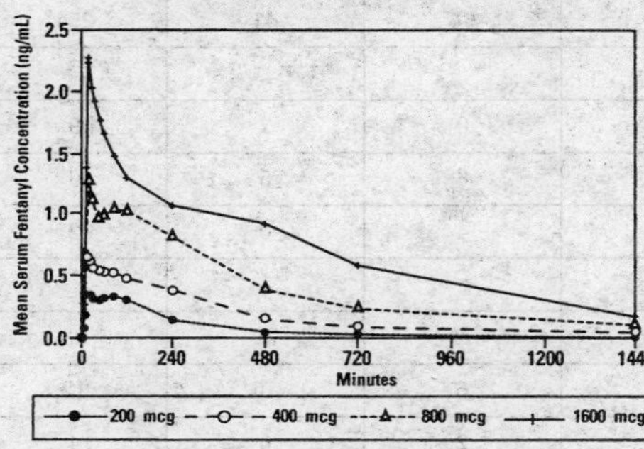

The pharmacokinetic parameters of the four strengths of *Actiq* tested in the dose-proportionality study are shown in Table 1. The mean C_{max} ranged from 0.39 – 2.51 ng/mL. The median time of maximum plasma concentration (T_{max}) across these four doses of *Actiq* varied from 20 – 40 minutes (range of 20-480 minutes) after a standardized consumption time of 15 minutes.

[See table 1 above]

Distribution:

Fentanyl is highly lipophilic. Animal data showed that following absorption, fentanyl is rapidly distributed to the brain, heart, lungs, kidneys and spleen followed by a slower redistribution to muscles and fat. The plasma protein binding of fentanyl is 80–85%. The main binding protein is alpha-1-acid glycoprotein, but both albumin and lipoproteins contribute to some extent. The free fraction of fentanyl increases with acidosis. The mean volume of distribution at steady state (V_{ss}) was 4 L/kg.

Metabolism:

Fentanyl is metabolized in the liver and in the intestinal mucosa to norfentanyl by cytochrome P450 3A4 isoform. Norfentanyl was not found to be pharmacologically active in animal studies (see **PRECAUTIONS: Drug Interactions** for additional information).

Elimination:

Fentanyl is primarily (more than 90%) eliminated by biotransformation to N-dealkylated and hydroxylated inactive metabolites. Less than 7% of the dose is excreted unchanged in the urine, and only about 1% is excreted unchanged in the feces. The metabolites are mainly excreted in the urine, while fecal excretion is less important. The total plasma clearance of fentanyl was 0.5 L/hr/kg (range 0.3 – 0.7 L/hr/kg). The terminal elimination half-life after *OTFC* administration is about 7 hours.

Special Populations:

Elderly Patients:

Elderly patients have been shown to be twice as sensitive to the effects of fentanyl when administered intravenously, compared with the younger population. While a formal study evaluating the safety profile of *Actiq* in the elderly population has not been performed, in the 257 opioid tolerant cancer patients studied with *Actiq*, approximately 20% were over age 65 years. No difference was noted in the safety profile in this group compared to those aged less than 65 years, though they did titrate to lower doses than younger patients (see **PRECAUTIONS**).

Patients with Renal or Hepatic Impairment:

Actiq should be administered with caution to patients with liver or kidney dysfunction because of the importance of these organs in the metabolism and excretion of drugs and effects on plasma-binding proteins (see **PRECAUTIONS**). Although fentanyl kinetics are known to be altered in both hepatic and renal disease due to alterations in metabolic clearance and plasma proteins, individualized doses of *Actiq* have been used successfully for breakthrough cancer pain in patients with hepatic and renal disorders. The duration of effect for the initial dose of fentanyl is determined by redistribution of the drug, such that diminished metabolic clearance may only become significant with repeated dosing or with excessively large single doses. For these reasons, while doses titrated to clinical effect are recommended for all patients, special care should be taken in patients with severe hepatic or renal disease.

Gender

Both male and female opioid-tolerant cancer patients were studied for the treatment of breakthrough cancer pain. No clinically relevant gender differences were noted either in dosage requirement or in observed adverse events.

CLINICAL TRIALS

Breakthrough Cancer Pain:

Actiq was investigated in clinical trials involving 257 opioid tolerant adult cancer patients experiencing breakthrough cancer pain. Breakthrough cancer pain was defined as a transient flare of moderate-to-severe pain occurring in cancer patients experiencing persistent cancer pain otherwise controlled with maintenance doses of opioid medications including at least 60 mg morphine/day, 50 mcg transdermal fentanyl/hour, or an equianalgesic dose of another opioid for a week or longer.

Table 1.
Pharmacokinetic Parameters in Adult Subjects Receiving 200, 400, 800, and 1600 mcg Units of Actiq

Pharmacokinetic Parameter	200 mcg	400 mcg	800 mcg	1600 mcg
T_{max}, minute median (range)	40 (20–120)	25 (20–240)	25 (20–120)	20 (20–480)
C_{max}, ng/mL mean (% CV)	0.39 (23)	0.75 (33)	1.55 (30)	2.51 (23)
AUC_{0-1440}, ng/mL minute mean (% CV)	102 (65)	243 (67)	573 (64)	1026 (67)
$t_{1/2}$, minute mean (% CV)	193 (48)	386 (115)	381 (55)	358 (45)

In two dose titration studies 95 of 127 patients (75%) who were on stable doses of either long-acting oral opioids or transdermal fentanyl for their persistent cancer pain titrated to a successful dose of *Actiq* to treat their breakthrough cancer pain within the dose range offered (200, 400, 600, 800, 1200 and 1600 mcg). In these studies 11% of patients withdrew due to adverse events and 14% withdrew due to other reasons. A "successful" dose was defined as a dose where one unit of *Actiq* could be used consistently for at least two consecutive days to treat breakthrough cancer pain without unacceptable side effects.

The successful dose of *Actiq* for breakthrough cancer pain was not predicted from the daily maintenance dose of opioid used to manage the persistent cancer pain and is thus best determined by dose titration.

A double-blind placebo controlled crossover study was performed in cancer patients to evaluate the effectiveness of *Actiq* for the treatment of breakthrough cancer pain. Of 130 patients who entered the study 92 patients (71%) achieved a successful dose during the titration phase. The distribution of successful doses is shown in Table 2.

Table 2.
Successful Dose of *Actiq* Following Initial Titration

Actiq Dose	Total No (%) (N=92)
200 mcg	13 (14)
400 mcg	19 (21)
600 mcg	14 (15)
800 mcg	18 (20)
1200 mcg	13 (14)
1600 mcg	15 (16)
Mean ±SD	789±468 mcg

On average, patients over 65 years of age titrated to a mean dose that was about 200 mcg less than the mean dose to which younger adult patients were titrated.

Actiq produced statistically significantly more pain relief compared with placebo at 15, 30, 45 and 60 minutes following administration (see Figure 2).

Figure 2
Pain Relief (PR) Scores (Mean±SD) During the Double-Blind Phase-All Patients with Evaluable Episodes on Both *Actiq* and Placebo (N=86)

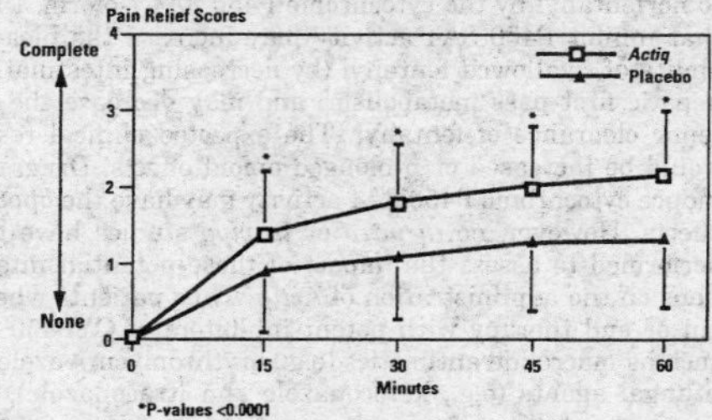

In this same study patients also rated the performance of medication to treat their breakthrough cancer pain using a different scale ranging from "poor" to "excellent." On average, placebo was rated "fair" and *Actiq* was rated "good."

INDICATIONS AND USAGE

(See BOX WARNING and CONTRAINDICATIONS)

Actiq is indicated only for the management of breakthrough cancer pain in patients with malignancies who are **already receiving and who are tolerant to opioid therapy for their underlying persistent cancer pain**. Patients considered opioid tolerant are those who are taking at least 60 mg morphine/day, 50 mcg transdermal fentanyl/hour, or an equianalgesic dose of another opioid for a week or longer.

Because life-threatening hypoventilation could occur at any dose in patients not taking chronic opiates, *Actiq* is contraindicated in the management of acute or postoperative pain. This product **must not** be used in opioid non-tolerant patients.

Actiq is intended to be used only in the care of cancer patients only by oncologists and pain specialists who are knowledgeable of and skilled in the use of Schedule II opioids to treat cancer pain.

Actiq should be individually titrated to a dose that provides adequate analgesia and minimizes side effects. If signs of excessive opioid effects appear before the unit is consumed, the dosage unit should be removed from the patient's mouth immediately, disposed of properly, and subsequent doses should be decreased (see **DOSAGE AND ADMINISTRATION**).

Patients and their caregivers must be instructed that *Actiq* contains a medicine in an amount that can be fatal to a child. Patients and their caregivers must be instructed to keep all units out of the reach of children and to discard opened units properly in a secured container.

CONTRAINDICATIONS

Because life-threatening hypoventilation could occur at any dose in patients not taking chronic opiates, *Actiq* is contraindicated in the management of acute or postoperative pain. The risk of respiratory depression begins to increase with fentanyl plasma levels of 2.0 ng/mL in opioid non-tolerant individuals (see **Pharmacokinetics**). This product **must not** be used in opioid non-tolerant patients.

Patients considered opioid tolerant are those who are taking at least 60 mg morphine/day, 50 mcg transdermal fentanyl/hour, or an equianalgesic dose of another opioid for a week or longer.

Actiq is contraindicated in patients with known intolerance or hypersensitivity to any of its components or the drug fentanyl.

WARNINGS

See BOX WARNING

The concomitant use of other CNS depressants, including other opioids, sedatives or hypnotics, general anesthetics, phenothiazines, tranquilizers, skeletal muscle relaxants, sedating antihistamines, potent inhibitors of cytochrome P450 3A4 isoform (e.g., erythromycin, ketoconazole, and certain protease inhibitors), and alcoholic beverages may produce increased depressant effects. Hypoventilation, hypotension, and profound sedation may occur.

Actiq is not recommended for use in patients who have received MAO inhibitors within 14 days, because severe and unpredictable potentiation by MAO inhibitors has been reported with opioid analgesics.

Pediatric Use: The appropriate dosing and safety of *Actiq* in opioid tolerant children with breakthrough cancer pain have not been established below the age of 16 years.

Patients and their caregivers must be instructed that *Actiq* contains a medicine in an amount which can be fatal to a child. Patients and their caregivers must be instructed to keep both used and unused dosage units out of the reach of children. While all units should be disposed of immediately after use, partially consumed units represent a special risk to children. In the event that a unit is not completely consumed it must be properly disposed as soon as possible. (See **SAFETY AND HANDLING, PRECAUTIONS,** and **PATIENT LEAFLET** for specific patient instructions.)

Physicians and dispensing pharmacists must specifically question patients or caregivers about the presence of children in the home on a full time or visiting basis and counsel them regarding the dangers to children from inadvertent exposure.

PRECAUTIONS

General

The initial dose of *Actiq* to treat episodes of breakthrough cancer pain should be 200 mcg. Each patient should be individually titrated to provide adequate analgesia while minimizing side effects.

Opioid analgesics impair the mental and/or physical ability required for the performance of potentially dangerous tasks (e.g., driving a car or operating machinery). Patients taking *Actiq* should be warned of these dangers and should be counseled accordingly.

The use of concomitant CNS active drugs requires special patient care and observation. (See **WARNINGS**.)

Hypoventilation (Respiratory Depression)

As with all opioids, there is a risk of clinically significant hypoventilation in patients using *Actiq*. Accordingly, all patients should be followed for symptoms of respiratory depression. Hypoventilation may occur more readily when opioids are given in conjunction with other agents that depress respiration.

Continued on next page

Actiq—Cont.

Chronic Pulmonary Disease
Because potent opioids can cause hypoventilation, *Actiq* should be titrated with caution in patients with chronic obstructive pulmonary disease or pre-existing medical conditions predisposing them to hypoventilation. In such patients, even normal therapeutic doses of *Actiq* may further decrease respiratory drive to the point of respiratory failure.

Head Injuries and Increased Intracranial Pressure
Actiq should only be administered with extreme caution in patients who may be particularly susceptible to the intracranial effects of CO_2 retention such as those with evidence of increased intracranial pressure or impaired consciousness. Opioids may obscure the clinical course of a patient with a head injury and should be used only if clinically warranted.

Cardiac Disease
Intravenous fentanyl may produce bradycardia. Therefore, *Actiq* should be used with caution in patients with bradyarrhythmias.

Hepatic or Renal Disease
Actiq should be administered with caution to patients with liver or kidney dysfunction because of the importance of these organs in the metabolism and excretion of drugs and effects on plasma binding proteins (see **PHARMACOKINETICS**).

Information for Patients and Their Caregivers
Patients and their caregivers must be instructed that *Actiq* contains medicine in an amount that could be fatal to a child. Patients and their caregivers must be instructed to keep both used and unused dosage units out of the reach of children. Partially consumed units represent a special risk to children. In the event that a unit is not completely consumed it must be properly disposed as soon as possible. (See **SAFETY AND HANDLING, WARNINGS,** and **PATIENT LEAFLET** for specific patient instructions.)
Patients and their caregivers should be provided with an *Actiq* Welcome Kit, which contains educational materials and safe storage containers to help patients store *Actiq* and other medicines out of the reach of children. Patients and their caregivers should also have an opportunity to watch the patient safety video, which provides proper product use, storage, handling and disposal directions. Patients should also have an opportunity to discuss the video with their health care providers. Health care professionals should call 1-888-818-4113 to obtain a supply of welcome kits or videos for patient viewing.

Disposal of Used *Actiq* Units
Patients must be instructed to dispose of completely used and partially used *Actiq* units.
1) After consumption of the unit is complete and the matrix is totally dissolved, throw away the handle in a trash container that is out of the reach of children.
2) If any of the drug matrix remains on the handle, place the handle under hot running tap water until all of the drug matrix is dissolved, and then dispose of the handle in a place that is out of the reach of children.
3) Handles in the child-resistant container should be disposed of (as described in steps 1 and 2) at least once a day.

If the patient does not entirely consume the unit and the remaining drug cannot be immediately dissolved under hot running water, the patient or caregiver must temporarily store the *Actiq* unit in the specially provided child-resistant container out of the reach of children until proper disposal is possible.

Disposal of Unopened *Actiq* Units When No Longer Needed
Patients and members of their household must be advised to dispose of any unopened units remaining from a prescription as soon as they are no longer needed.
To dispose of the unused *Actiq* units:
1) Remove the *Actiq* unit from its pouch using scissors, and hold the *Actiq* by its handle over the toilet bowl.
2) Using wire-cutting pliers cut off the drug matrix end so that it falls into the toilet.
3) Dispose of the handle in a place that is out of the reach of children.
4) Repeat steps 1, 2, and 3 for each *Actiq* unit. Flush the toilet twice after 5 units have been cut and deposited into the toilet.

Do not flush the entire *Actiq* units, *Actiq* handles, foil pouches, or cartons down the toilet. The handle should be disposed of where children cannot reach it (see **SAFETY AND HANDLING**).
Detailed instructions for the proper storage, administration, disposal, and important instructions for managing an overdose of *Actiq* are provided in the *Actiq* Patient Leaflet. Patients should be encouraged to read this information in its entirety and be given an opportunity to have their questions answered.
In the event that a caregiver requires additional assistance in disposing of excess unusable units that remain in the home after a patient has expired, they should be instructed to call the toll-free number (1-888-453-1041) or seek assistance from their local DEA office.

Laboratory Tests
The effects of *Actiq* on laboratory tests have not been evaluated.

Drug Interactions
See **WARNINGS**.

Table 3.
Percent of Patients with Specific Adverse Events Commonly Associated with Opioid Administration or of Particular Clinical Interest Which Occurred During Titration (Events in 1% or More of Patients)

Dose Group	200 600 mcg	800–1400 mcg	1600 mcg	>1600 mcg	Any
Number of Patients	230	138	54	41	254
Body As A Whole					
Asthenia	6	4	0	7	9
Headache	3	4	6	5	6
Accidental Injury	1	1	4	0	2
Digestive					
Nausea	14	15	11	22	23
Vomiting	7	6	6	15	12
Constipation	1	4	2	0	4
Nervous					
Dizziness	10	16	6	15	17
Somnolence	9	9	11	20	17
Confusion	1	6	2	0	4
Anxiety	3	0	2	0	3
Abnormal Gait	0	1	4	0	2
Dry Mouth	1	1	2	0	2
Nervousness	1	1	0	0	2
Vasodilatation	2	0	2	0	2
Hallucinations	0	1	2	2	1
Insomnia	0	1	2	0	1
Thinking Abnormal	0	1	2	0	1
Vertigo	1	0	0	0	1
Respiratory					
Dyspnea	2	3	6	5	4
Skin					
Pruritus	1	0	0	5	2
Rash	1	1	0	2	2
Sweating	1	1	2	2	2
Special Senses					
Abnormal Vision	1	0	2	0	2

Fentanyl is metabolized in the liver and intestinal mucosa to norfentanyl by the cytochrome P450 3A4 isoform. Drugs that inhibit P450 3A4 activity may increase the bioavailability of swallowed fentanyl (by decreasing intestinal and hepatic first pass metabolism) and may decrease the systemic clearance of fentanyl. The expected clinical results would be increased or prolonged opioid effects. Drugs that induce cytochrome P450 3A4 activity may have the opposite effects. However, no *in vitro* or *in vivo* studies have been performed to assess the impact of those potential interactions on the administration of *Actiq*. Thus patients who begin or end therapy with potent inhibitors of CYP450 3A4 such as macrolide antibiotics (e.g., erythromycin), azole antifungal agents (e.g., ketoconazole and itraconazole), and protease inhibitors (e.g., ritanovir) while receiving *Actiq* should be monitored for a change in opioid effects and, if warranted, the dose of *Actiq* should be adjusted.

Carcinogenesis, Mutagenesis, and Impairment of Fertility
Because animal carcinogenicity studies have not been conducted with fentanyl citrate, the potential carcinogenic effect of *Actiq* is unknown.
Standard mutagenicity testing of fentanyl citrate has been conducted. There was no evidence of mutagenicity in the Ames *Salmonella* or *Escherichia* mutagenicity assay, the *in-vitro* mouse lymphoma mutagenesis assay, and the *in-vivo* micronucleus cytogenetic assay in the mouse.
Reproduction studies in rats revealed a significant decrease in the pregnancy rate of all experimental groups. This decrease was most pronounced in the high dose group (1.25 mg/kg subcutaneously) in which one of twenty animals became pregnant.

Pregnancy - Category C
Fentanyl has been shown to impair fertility and to have an embryocidal effect with an increase in resorptions in rats when given for a period of 12 to 21 days in doses of 30 mcg/kg IV or 160 mcg/kg subcutaneously.
No evidence of teratogenic effects has been observed after administration of fentanyl citrate to rats. There are no adequate and well-controlled studies in pregnant women. *Actiq* should be used during pregnancy only if the potential benefit justifies the potential risk to the fetus.

Labor and Delivery
Actiq is not indicated for use in labor and delivery.

Nursing Mothers
Fentanyl is excreted in human milk; therefore *Actiq* should not be used in nursing women because of the possibility of sedation and/or respiratory depression in their infants.

Pediatric Use
See **WARNINGS**.

Geriatric Use
Of the 257 patients in clinical studies of *Actiq* in breakthrough cancer pain, 61 (24%) were 65 and over, while 15 (6%) were 75 and over.
Those patients over the age of 65 titrated to a mean dose that was about 200 mcg less than the mean dose titrated to by younger patients. Previous studies with intravenous fentanyl showed that elderly patients are twice as sensitive to the effects of fentanyl as the younger population.
No difference was noted in the safety profile of the group over 65 as compared to younger patients in *Actiq* clinical trials. However, greater sensitivity in older individuals cannot be ruled out. Therefore, caution should be exercised in individually titrating *Actiq* in elderly patients to provide adequate efficacy while minimizing risk.

ADVERSE REACTIONS

Pre-Marketing Clinical Trial Experience
The safety of *Actiq* has been evaluated in 257 opioid tolerant chronic cancer pain patients. The duration of *Actiq* use varied during the open-label study. Some patients were followed for over 21 months. The average duration of therapy in the open-label study was 129 days.
The adverse events seen with *Actiq* are typical opioid side effects. Frequently, these adverse events will cease or decrease in intensity with continued use of *Actiq*, as the patient is titrated to the proper dose. Opioid side effects should be expected and managed accordingly.

The most serious adverse effects associated with all opioids are respiratory depression (potentially leading to apnea or respiratory arrest), circulatory depression, hypotension, and shock. All patients should be followed for symptoms of respiratory depression.

Because the clinical trials of *Actiq* were designed to evaluate safety and efficacy in treating breakthrough cancer pain, all patients were also taking concomitant opioids, such as sustained-release morphine or transdermal fentanyl, for their persistent cancer pain. The adverse event data presented here reflect the actual percentage of patients experiencing each adverse effect among patients who received *Actiq* for breakthrough cancer pain along with a concomitant opioid for persistent cancer pain. There has been no attempt to correct for concomitant use of other opioids, duration of *Actiq* therapy, or cancer-related symptoms. Adverse events are included regardless of causality or severity.

Three short-term clinical trials with similar titration schemes were conducted in 257 patients with malignancy and breakthrough cancer pain. Data are available for 254 of these patients. The goal of titration in these trials was to find the dose of *Actiq* that provided adequate analgesia with acceptable side effects (successful dose). Patients were titrated from a low dose to a successful dose in a manner similar to current titration dosing guidelines. Table 3 lists by dose groups, adverse events with an overall frequency of 1% or greater that occurred during titration and are commonly associated with opioid administration or are of particular clinical interest. The ability to assign a dose-response relationship to these adverse events is limited by the titration schemes used in these studies. Adverse events are listed in descending order of frequency within each body system.

[See table 3 at top of previous page]

The following adverse events not reflected in Table 3 occurred during titration with an overall frequency of 1% or greater and are listed in descending order of frequency within each body system.

Body as a Whole: Pain, fever, abdominal pain, chills, back pain, chest pain, infection
Cardiovascular: Migraine
Digestive: Diarrhea, dyspepsia, flatulence
Metabolic and Nutritional: Peripheral edema, dehydration
Nervous: Hypesthesia
Respiratory: Pharyngitis, cough increased

The following events occurred during titration with an overall frequency of less than 1% and are listed in descending order of frequency within each body system.

Body as a Whole: Flu syndrome, abscess, bone pain
Cardiovascular: Deep thrombophlebitis, hypertension, hypotension
Digestive: Anorexia, eructation, esophageal stenosis, fecal impaction, gum hemorrhage, mouth ulceration, oral moniliasis
Hemic and Lymphatic: Anemia, leukopenia
Metabolic and Nutritional: Edema, hypercalcemia, weight loss
Musculoskeletal: Myalgia, pathological fracture, myasthenia
Nervous: Abnormal dreams, urinary retention, agitation, amnesia, emotional lability, euphoria, incoordination, libido decreased, neuropathy, paresthesia, speech disorder
Respiratory: Hemoptysis, pleural effusion, rhinitis, asthma, hiccup, pneumonia, respiratory insufficiency, sputum increased
Skin and Appendages: Alopecia, exfoliative dermatitis
Special Senses: Taste perversion
Urogenital: Vaginal hemorrhage, dysuria, hematuria, urinary incontinence, urinary tract infection

A long-term extension study was conducted in 156 patients with malignancy and breakthrough cancer pain who were treated for an average of 129 days. Data are available for 152 of these patients. Table 4 lists by dose groups, adverse events with an overall frequency of 1% or greater that occurred during the long-term extension study and are commonly associated with opioid administration or are of particular clinical interest. Adverse events are listed in descending order of frequency within each body system.

[See table 4 above]

Table 4.
Percent of Patients with Adverse Events Commonly Associated with Opioid Administration or of Particular Clinical Interest Which Occurred During Long Term Treatment (Events in 1% or More of Patients)

Dose Group	200–600 mcg	800–1400 mcg	1600 mcg	>1600 mcg	Any
Number of Patients	**98**	**83**	**53**	**27**	**152**
Body As A Whole					
Asthenia	25	30	17	15	38
Headache	12	17	13	4	20
Accidental Injury	4	6	4	7	9
Hypertonia	2	2	2	0	3
Digestive					
Nausea	31	36	25	26	45
Vomiting	21	28	15	7	31
Constipation	14	11	13	4	20
Intestinal Obstruction	0	2	4	0	3
Cardiovascular					
Hypertension	1	1	0	0	1
Nervous					
Dizziness	12	10	9	0	16
Anxiety	9	8	8	7	15
Somnolence	8	13	8	7	15
Confusion	2	5	13	7	10
Depression	9	4	2	7	9
Insomnia	5	1	8	4	7
Abnormal Gait	5	1	0	0	4
Dry Mouth	3	1	2	4	4
Nervousness	2	2	0	4	3
Stupor	4	1	0	0	3
Vasodilatation	1	1	4	0	3
Thinking Abnormal	2	1	0	0	2
Abnormal Dreams	1	1	0	0	1
Convulsion	0	1	2	0	1
Myoclonus	0	0	4	0	1
Tremor	0	1	2	0	1
Vertigo	0	0	4	0	1
Respiratory					
Dyspnea	15	16	8	7	22
Skin					
Rash	3	5	8	4	8
Sweating	3	2	2	0	4
Pruritus	2	0	2	0	2
Special Senses					
Abnormal Vision	2	2	0	0	3
Urogenital					
Urinary Retention	1	2	0	0	2

The following events not reflected in Table 4 occurred with an overall frequency of 1% or greater in the long-term extension study and are listed in descending order of frequency within each body system.

Body as a Whole: Pain, fever, back pain, abdominal pain, chest pain, flu syndrome, chills, infection, abdomen enlarged, bone pain, ascites, sepsis, neck pain, viral infection, fungal infection, cachexia, cellulitis, malaise, pelvic pain
Cardiovascular: Deep thrombophlebitis, migraine, palpitation, vascular disorder
Digestive: Diarrhea, anorexia, dyspepsia, dysphagia, oral moniliasis, mouth ulceration, rectal disorder, stomatitis, flatulence, gastrointestinal hemorrhage, gingivitis, jaundice, periodontal abscess, eructation, glossitis, rectal hemorrhage
Hemic and Lymphatic: Anemia, leukopenia, thrombocytopenia, ecchymosis, lymphadenopathy, lymphedema, pancytopenia
Metabolic and Nutritional: Peripheral edema, edema, dehydration, weight loss, hyperglycemia, hypokalemia, hypercalcemia, hypomagnesemia
Musculoskeletal: Myalgia, pathological fracture, joint disorder, leg cramps, arthralgia, bone disorder
Nervous: Hypesthesia, paresthesia, hypokinesia, neuropathy, speech disorder
Respiratory: Cough increased, pharyngitis, pneumonia, rhinitis, sinusitis, bronchitis, epistaxis, asthma, hemoptysis, sputum increased
Skin and Appendages: Skin ulcer, alopecia
Special Senses: Tinnitus, conjunctivitis, ear disorder, taste perversion
Urogenital: Urinary tract infection, urinary incontinence, breast pain, dysuria, hematuria, scrotal edema, hydronephrosis, kidney failure, urinary urgency, urination impaired, breast neoplasm, vaginal hemorrhage, vaginitis

The following events occurred with a frequency of less than 1% in the long-term extension study and are listed in descending order of frequency within each body system.

Body as a Whole: Allergic reaction, cyst, face edema, flank pain, granuloma, bacterial infection, injection site pain, mucous membrane disorder, neck rigidity
Cardiovascular: Angina pectoris, hemorrhage, hypotension, peripheral vascular disorder, postural hypotension, tachycardia
Digestive: Cheilitis, esophagitis, fecal incontinence, gastroenteritis, gastrointestinal disorder, gum hemorrhage, hemorrhage of colon, hepatorenal syndrome, liver tenderness, tooth caries, tooth disorder
Hemic and Lymphatic: Bleeding time increased
Metabolic and Nutritional: Acidosis, generalized edema, hypocalcemia, hypoglycemia, hyponatremia, hypoproteinemia, thirst
Musculoskeletal: Arthritis, muscle atrophy, myopathy, synovitis, tendon disorder

Continued on next page

Actiq—Cont.

Nervous: Acute brain syndrome, agitation, cerebral ischemia, facial paralysis, foot drop, hallucinations, hemiplegia, miosis, subdural hematoma
Respiratory: Hiccup, hyperventilation, lung disorder, pneumothorax, respiratory failure, voice alteration
Skin and Appendages: Herpes zoster, maculopapular rash, skin discoloration, urticaria, vesiculobullous rash
Special Senses: Ear pain, eye hemorrhage, lacrimation disorder, partial permanent deafness, partial transitory deafness
Urogenital: Kidney pain, nocturia, oliguria, polyuria, pyelonephritis

DRUG ABUSE AND DEPENDENCE

Fentanyl is a mu-opioid agonist and a Schedule II controlled substance that can produce drug dependence of the morphine type. *Actiq* may be subject to misuse, abuse and addiction.
The administration of *Actiq* should be guided by the response of the patient. Physical dependence, per se, is not ordinarily a concern when one is treating a patient with chronic cancer pain, and fear of tolerance and physical dependence should not deter using doses that adequately relieve the pain.
Opioid analgesics may cause physical dependence. Physical dependence results in withdrawal symptoms in patients who abruptly discontinue the drug. Withdrawal also may be precipitated through the administration of drugs with opioid antagonist activity, e.g., naloxone, nalmefene, or mixed agonist/antagonist analgesics (pentazocine, butorphanol, buprenorphine, nalbuphine).
Physical dependence usually does not occur to a clinically significant degree until after several weeks of continued opioid usage. Tolerance, in which increasingly larger doses are required in order to produce the same degree of analgesia, is initially manifested by a shortened duration of analgesic effect, and subsequently, by decreases in the intensity of analgesia.
The handling of *Actiq* should be managed to minimize the risk of diversion, including restriction of access and accounting procedures as appropriate to the clinical setting and as required by law (see **SAFETY AND HANDLING**).

OVERDOSAGE

Clinical Presentation
The manifestations of *Actiq* overdosage are expected to be similar in nature to intravenous fentanyl and other opioids, and are an extension of its pharmacological actions with the most serious significant effect being hypoventilation (see **CLINICAL PHARMACOLOGY**).
General
Immediate management of opioid overdose includes removal of the *Actiq* unit, if still in the mouth, ensuring a patent airway, physical and verbal stimulation of the patient, and assessment of level of consciousness, ventilatory and circulatory status.
Treatment of Overdosage (Accidental Ingestion) in the Opioid NON-Tolerant Person
Ventilatory support should be provided, intravenous access obtained, and naloxone or other opioid antagonists should be employed as clinically indicated. The duration of respiratory depression following overdose may be longer than the effects of the opioid antagonist's action (e.g., the half-life of naloxone ranges from 30 to 81 minutes) and repeated administration may be necessary. Consult the package insert of the individual opioid antagonist for details about such use.
Treatment of Overdose in Opioid-Tolerant Patients
Ventilatory support should be provided and intravenous access obtained as clinically indicated. Judicious use of naloxone or another opioid antagonist may be warranted in some instances, but it is associated with the risk of precipitating an acute withdrawal syndrome.
General Considerations for Overdose
Management of severe *Actiq* overdose includes: securing a patent airway, assisting or controlling ventilation, establishing intravenous access, and GI decontamination by lavage and/or activated charcoal, once the patient's airway is secure. In the presence of hypoventilation or apnea, ventilation should be assisted or controlled and oxygen administered as indicated.
Patients with overdose should be carefully observed and appropriately managed until their clinical condition is well controlled.
Although muscle rigidity interfering with respiration has not been seen following the use of *Actiq*, this is possible with fentanyl and other opioids. If it occurs, it should be managed by the use of assisted or controlled ventilation, by an opioid antagonist, and as a final alternative, by a neuromuscular blocking agent.

DOSAGE AND ADMINISTRATION

***Actiq* is contraindicated in non-opioid tolerant individuals.**
Actiq should be individually titrated to a dose that provides adequate analgesia and minimizes side effects (see **Dose Titration**).
As with all opioids, the safety of patients using such products is dependent on health care professionals prescribing them in strict conformity with their approved labeling with respect to patient selection, dosing, and proper conditions for use.
Physicians and dispensing pharmacists must specifically question patients and caregivers about the presence of children in the home on a full time or visiting basis and counsel accordingly regarding the dangers to children of inadvertent exposure to *Actiq*.
Administration of *Actiq*
The foil package should be opened with scissors immediately prior to product use. The patient should place the *Actiq* unit in his or her mouth between the cheek and lower gum, occasionally moving the drug matrix from one side to the other using the handle. The *Actiq* unit should be sucked, not chewed. A unit dose of *Actiq*, if chewed and swallowed, might result in lower peak concentrations and lower bioavailability than when consumed as directed.
The *Actiq* unit should be consumed over a 15-minute period. Longer or shorter consumption times may produce less efficacy than reported in *Actiq* clinical trials. If signs of excessive opioid effects appear before the unit is consumed, the drug matrix should be removed from the patient's mouth immediately and future doses should be decreased.
Patients and caregivers must be instructed that Actiq contains medicine in an amount that could be fatal to a child. While all units should be disposed of immediately after use, partially used units represent a special risk and must be disposed of as soon as they are consumed and/or no longer needed. Patients and caregivers should be advised to dispose of any units remaining from a prescription as soon as they are no longer needed (see **Disposal Instructions**).
Dose Titration
Starting Dose: *The initial dose of Actiq to treat episodes of breakthrough cancer pain should be 200 mcg.* Patients should be prescribed an initial titration supply of six 200 mcg *Actiq* units, thus limiting the number of units in the home during titration. Patients should use up all units before increasing to a higher dose.
From this initial dose, patients should be closely followed and the dosage level changed until the patient reaches a dose that provides adequate analgesia using a single *Actiq* dosage unit per breakthrough cancer pain episode.
Patients should record their use of *Actiq* over several episodes of breakthrough cancer pain and review their experience with their physicians to determine if a dosage adjustment is warranted.
Redosing Within a Single Episode: Until the appropriate dose is reached, patients may find it necessary to use an additional *Actiq* unit during a single episode. Redosing may start 15 minutes after the previous unit has been completed (30 minutes after the start of the previous unit). While patients are in the titration phase and consuming units which individually may be subtherapeutic, no more than two units should be taken for each individual breakthrough cancer pain episode.
Increasing the Dose: If treatment of several consecutive breakthrough cancer pain episodes requires more than one *Actiq* per episode, an increase in dose to the next higher available strength should be considered. At each new dose of *Actiq* during titration, it is recommended that six units of the titration dose be prescribed. Each new dose of *Actiq* used in the titration period should be evaluated over several episodes of breakthrough cancer pain (generally 1–2 days) to determine whether it provides adequate efficacy with acceptable side effects. The incidence of side effects is likely to be greater during this initial titration period compared to later, after the effective dose is determined.
Daily Limit: Once a successful dose has been found (i.e., an average episode is treated with a single unit), patients should limit consumption to four or fewer units per day. If consumption increases above four units/day, the dose of the long-acting opioid used for persistent cancer pain should be re-evaluated.

***Actiq* Titration Process**
See BOX WARNING

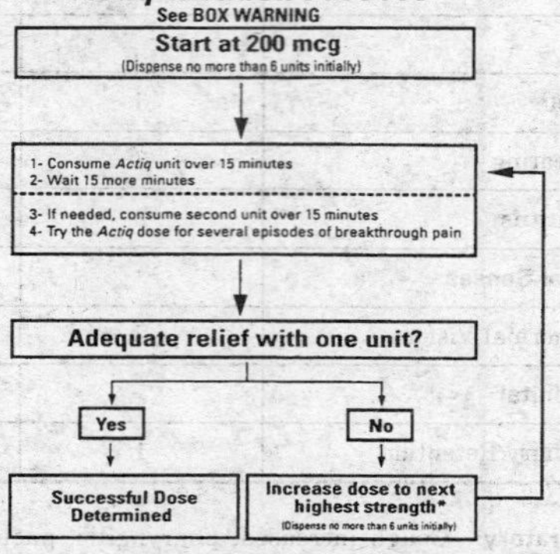

Start at 200 mcg
(Dispense no more than 6 units initially)

1- Consume *Actiq* unit over 15 minutes
2- Wait 15 more minutes
3- If needed, consume second unit over 15 minutes
4- Try the *Actiq* dose for several episodes of breakthrough pain

Adequate relief with one unit?

Yes → Successful Dose Determined

No → Increase dose to next highest strength* (Dispense no more than 6 units initially)

*Available dosage strengths include: 200, 400, 600, 800, 1200, and 1600 mcg.

Dosage Adjustment
Experience in a long-term study of *Actiq* used in the treatment of breakthrough cancer pain suggests that dosage adjustment of both *Actiq* and the maintenance (around-the-clock) opioid analgesic may be required in some patients to continue to provide adequate relief of breakthrough cancer pain.
Generally, the *Actiq* dose should be increased when patients require more than one dosage unit per breakthrough cancer pain episode for several consecutive episodes. When titrating to an appropriate dose, small quantities (six units) should be prescribed at each titration step. Physicians should consider increasing the around-the-clock opioid dose used for persistent cancer pain in patients experiencing more than four breakthrough cancer pain episodes daily.
Discontinuation of *Actiq*
For patients requiring discontinuation of opioids, a gradual downward titration is recommended because it is not known at what dose level the opioid may be discontinued without producing the signs and symptoms of abrupt withdrawal.

SAFETY AND HANDLING

Actiq is supplied in individually sealed child-resistant foil pouches. The amount of fentanyl contained in *Actiq* can be fatal to a child. Patients and their caregivers must be instructed to keep *Actiq* out of the reach of children (see **BOX WARNING, WARNINGS, PRECAUTIONS** and **PATIENT LEAFLET**).
Store at 25°C (77°F) with excursions permitted between 15° and 30°C (59° to 86°F) until ready to use. (See USP Controlled Room Temperature.)
Actiq should be protected from freezing and moisture. Do not store above 25°C. Do not use if the foil pouch has been opened.

DISPOSAL OF ACTIQ

Patients must be advised to dispose of any units remaining from a prescription as soon as they are no longer needed. While all units should be disposed of immediately after use, partially consumed units represent a special risk because they are no longer protected by the child resistant pouch, yet may contain enough medicine to be fatal to a child (see **Information for Patients**).
A temporary storage bottle is provided as part of the *Actiq* Welcome Kit (see **Information for Patients and Their Caregivers**). This container is to be used by patients or their caregivers in the event that a partially consumed unit cannot be disposed of promptly. Instructions for usage of this container are included in the patient leaflet.
Patients and members of their household must be advised to dispose of any units remaining from a prescription as soon as they are no longer needed. Instructions are included in **Information for Patients and Their Caregivers** and in the patient leaflet. If additional assistance is required, referral to the *Actiq* 800# (1-888-453-1041) should be made.

HOW SUPPLIED

Actiq is supplied in six dosage strengths. Each unit is individually wrapped in a child-resistant, protective foil pouch. These foil pouches are packed 24 per shelf carton for use when patients have been titrated to the appropriate dose.
Patients should be prescribed an initial titration supply of six 200 mcg *Actiq* units. At each new dose of *Actiq* during titration, it is recommended that only six units of the next higher dose be prescribed.
Each dosage unit has a white to off-white color. The dosage strength of each unit is marked on the handle, the foil pouch and the carton. See foil pouch and carton for product information.

Dosage Strength (fentanyl base)	Carton/Foil Pouch Color	NDC Number
200 mcg	Gray	NDC 0074-2460-24
400 mcg	Blue	NDC 0074-2461-24
600 mcg	Orange	NDC 0074-2462-24
800 mcg	Purple	NDC 0074-2463-24
1200 mcg	Green	NDC 0074-2464-24
1600 mcg	Burgundy	NDC 0074-2465-24

Note: Colors are a secondary aid in product identification. Please be sure to confirm the printed dosage before dispensing.
℞ only.
DEA order form required. A Schedule CII narcotic.
Manufactured by ABBOTT LABORATORIES, NORTH CHICAGO, IL 60064, USA
Distributed by ABBOTT LABORATORIES, INC., NORTH CHICAGO, IL 60064, USA
Under license from ANESTA CORP., Salt Lake City, UT 84116, USA
U. S. Patent No. 4,671,953
Reference 58-0645-R2-Rev. Feb., 1999

ABBOTT LABORATORIES, NORTH CHICAGO, IL 60064, USA
Shown in Product Identification Guide, page 304

Apothecon

A Bristol-Myers Squibb Company
P.O. BOX 4500
PRINCETON, NJ 08543-4500

For Medical Information Contact:
Generally:
Bristol-Myers Squibb Drug Information Department
P.O. Box 4500
Princeton, NJ 08543-4500
(800) 321-1335
Adverse Drug Experiences
and Product Defects Reporting call
between 8:30 am-4:30 pm EST:
(609) 818-3737

Sales and Ordering:
Orders for Apothecon Products may be placed by:
1. Calling toll-free between 8:30 am-6:00 pm EST:
   (800) 631-5244
2. Mailing your purchase orders to:
   Apothecon
   Attn: Customer Service Department
   P.O. Box 5250
   Princeton, NJ 08543-5250
3. Faxing your purchase orders to:
   Customer Service Department
   (800) 523-2965

UNILOG®
(Tablet and Capsule Identification Code)
ALPHABETICAL INDEX

Unilog Number	Product
AP 4168	**Acyclovir Capsules,** 200 mg
AP 4165	**Acyclovir Tablets,** 400 mg
AP 4166	**Acyclovir Tablets,** 800 mg
INV 211	**Amantadine Hydrochloride Capsules, USP** 100 mg
INV 259	**Atenolol Tablets** 25 mg
INV 256	**Atenolol Tablets** 50 mg
INV 257	**Atenolol Tablets** 100 mg
AP 2593	**Atenolol and Chlorthalidone Tablets, USP** 100 mg/25mg
AP 2592	**Atenolol and Chlorthalidone Tablets, USP** 50 mg/25mg
INV 208	**Benztropine Mesylate Tablets, USP** 0.5 mg
INV 209	**Benztropine Mesylate Tablets, USP** 1 mg
INV 210	**Benztropine Mesylate Tablets, USP** 2 mg
AP 8818	**Buspirone HCl Tablets** 5 mg
AP 8819	**Buspirone HCl Tablets** 10 mg
AP 7045	**Captopril Tablets, USP** 12.5 mg
AP 7046	**Captopril Tablets, USP** 25 mg
AP 7047	**Captopril Tablets, USP** 50 mg
AP 7048	**Captopril Tablets, USP** 100 mg
AP 5160	**Captopril and Hydrochlorothiazide Tablets, USP** 25mg/15mg
AP 5161	**Captopril and Hydrochlorothiazide Tablets, USP** 25mg/25mg
AP 5162	**Captopril and Hydrochlorothiazide Tablets, USP** 50mg/15mg
AP 5163	**Captopril and Hydrochlorothiazide Tablets, USP** 50mg/25mg
AP 7491	**Cefaclor Capsules** 250 mg
AP 7494	**Cefaclor Capsules** 500 mg
Bristol 7271	**Cefadroxil Capsules, USP** 500 mg
7375 Bristol	**Cephalexin Capsules USP** 250 mg
7376 Bristol	**Cephalexin Capsules USP** 500 mg
Squibb 181	**Cephalexin Capsules USP** 250 mg
Squibb 239	**Cephalexin Capsules USP** 500 mg
INV 321	**Clomipramine HCl Capsules** 25 mg
INV 322	**Clomipramine HCl Capsules** 50 mg
INV 323	**Clomipramine HCl Capsules** 75 mg
INV 353	**Clonazepam Tablets** .5 mg
INV 354	**Clonazepam Tablets** 1 mg
INV 355	**Clonazepam Tablets** 2 mg
INV 252	**Cyclobenzaprine Hydrochloride Tablets, USP** 10 mg
MJ 775	**Desyrel Tablets** (Trazodone Hydrochloride Tablets) 50 mg
MJ 776	**Desyrel Tablets** (Trazodone Hydrochloride Tablets) 100 mg
MJ 778	**Desyrel Dividose Tablets** (Trazodone Hydrochloride Tablets) 150 mg
MJ 796	**Desyrel Dividose Tablets** (Trazodone Hydrochloride Tablets) 300 mg
INV 383	**Diclofenac Potassium Tablets, USP** 50 mg
Squibb W048	**Dicloxacillin Sodium Capsules USP** 250 mg
Squibb W058	**Dicloxacillin Sodium Capsules USP** 500 mg
7892	**Dynapen Capsules** (Dicloxacillin Sodium Capsules USP) 125 mg
W048	**Dynapen Capsules** (Dicloxacillin Sodium Capsules USP) 250 mg
W058	**Dynapen Capsules** (Dicloxacillin Sodium Capsules USP) 500 mg
AP 025	**Estradiol Tablets** .5 mg
AP 026	**Estradiol Tablets** 1.0 mg
AP 027	**Estradiol Tablets** 2.0 mg
INV 359	**Etodolac Capsules** 200 mg
INV 360	**Etodolac Capsules** 300 mg
INV 350	**Etodolac Capsules** 400 mg
Squibb 429	**Florinef Tablets** Fludrocortisone Acetate Tablets USP) 0.1 mg
INV 250	**Hydroxychloroquine Sulfate Tablets, USP** 200 mg
INV 246	**Indapamide Tablets, USP** 1.25 mg
INV 247	**Indapamide Tablets, USP** 2.5 mg
Bristol 3506	**Kantrex Capsules** (Kanamycin Sulfate Capsules) 500 mg
BL 770	**Klotrix Tablets** (Potassium Chloride Tablets) 10 mEq
531 MD	**Methylphenidate HCl Tablets,** 5 mg
530 MD	**Methylphenidate HCl Tablets,** 10 mg
562 MD	**Methylphenidate HCl Tablets,** 20 mg ER
532 MD	**Methylphenidate HCl Tablets** 20 mg
INV 351	**Methylprednisolone Tablets** 4 mg
INV 263	**Metoclopramide Tablets, USP** 5 mg
INV 264	**Metoclopramide Tablets, USP** 10 mg
BMS W921	**Metoprolol Tartrate Tablets, USP** 50 mg
BMS W933	**Metoprolol Tartrate Tablets, USP** 100 mg
Squibb 580	**Mycostatin Oral Tablets** (Nystatin Tablets USP) 500,000 u.
AP 2461	**Nadolol Tablets, USP** 20 mg
AP 2462	**Nadolol Tablets, USP** 40 mg
AP 2463	**Nadolol Tablets, USP** 80 mg
AP 2464	**Nadolol Tablets, USP** 120 mg
AP 2465	**Nadolol Tablets, USP** 160 mg
BL N1	**Naldecon Tablets**
INV 289	**Naproxen Sodium Delayed Release Tablets, USP** 375 mg
INV 290	**Naproxen Sodium Delayed Release Tablets, USP** 500 mg
PPP 606	**Naturetin Tablets** (Bendroflumethiazide Tablets USP) 5 mg
PPP 618	**Naturetin Tablets** (Bendroflumethazide Tablets USP) 10 mg
Squibb 611	**Niacin Tablets USP** 50 mg
Squibb 612	**Niacin Tablets USP** 100 mg
Squibb 537	**Niacin Tablets USP** 500 mg
INV 265	**Orphenadrine Citrate 25 mg,** Aspirin 385 mg, Caffeine 30 mg Tablets
INV 266	**Orphenadrine Citrate 50 mg,** Aspirin 770 mg, Caffeine 60 mg Tablets
INV 336	**Orphenadrine Citrate** Extended Release Tablets, 100mg
AP 6910	**Potassium Chloride Extended Release Tablets** 10 meq
Bristol 7992	**Principen Capsules** (Ampicillin Capsules USP) 250 mg
Bristol 7993	**Principen Capsules** (Ampicillin Capsules USP) 500 mg
INV 275	**Prochlorperazine Maleate Tablets, USP** 5 mg
INV 276	**Prochlorperazine Maleate Tablets, USP** 10 mg
PPP 863	**Prolixin Tablets** (Fluphenazine Hydrochloride Tablets USP) 1 mg
PPP 864	**Prolixin Tablets** (Fluphenazine Hydrochloride Tablets USP) 2.5 mg
PPP 877	**Prolixin Tablets** (Fluphenazine Hydrochloride Tablets USP) 5 mg
PPP 956	**Prolixin Tablets** (Fluphenazine Hydrochloride Tablets USP) 10 mg
PPP 758	**Pronestyl Capsules** (Procainamide Hydrochloride Capsules USP) 250 mg
PPP 756	**Pronestyl Capsules** (Procainamide Hydrochloride Capsules USP) 375 mg
PPP 757	**Pronestyl Capsules** (Procainamide Hydrochloride Capsules USP) 500 mg
PPP 431	**Pronestyl Tablets** (Procainamide Hydrochloride Tablets USP) 250 mg
PPP 434	**Pronestyl Tablets** (Procainamide Hydrochloride Tablets USP) 375 mg
PPP 438	**Pronestyl Tablets** (Procainamide Hydrochloride Tablets USP) 500 mg
PPP 775	**Pronestyl-SR Tablets** (Procainamide Hydrochloride Tablets) 500 mg
PPP 769	**Rauzide Tablets** (Rauwolfia Serpentina with Bendroflumethiazide Tablets) 50 mg - 4 mg
Squibb 655	**Sumycin Capsules** (Tetracycline Hydrochloride Capsules USP) 250 mg
Squibb 763	**Sumycin Capsules** (Tetracycline Hydrochloride Capsules USP) 500 mg
Squibb 663	**Sumycin Tablets** (Tetracycline Hydrochloride Tablets USP) 250 mg
Squibb 603	**Sumycin Tablets** (Tetracycline Hydrochloride Tablets USP) 500 mg
Squibb 535	**Theragran Hematinic Tablets**
AP 3171	**Trazodone Hydrochloride Tablets,** 150 mg
BMS 37	**Trimox Tablets, USP (Chewable)** 125 mg
BMS 38	**Trimox Tablets, USP (Chewable)** 250 mg
Bristol 7278	**Trimox Capsules** (Amoxicillin Capsules USP) 250 mg
Bristol 7279	**Trimox Capsules** (Amoxicillin Capsules USP) 500 mg
MJ 543	**Vasodilan Tablets** (Isoxsuprine Hydrochloride) 10 mg
MJ 544	**Vasodilan Tablets** (Isoxsuprine Hydrochloride) 20 mg
BL V1	**Veetids Tablets** (Penicillin V Potassium Tablets, USP) 250 mg
BL V2	**Veetids Tablets** (Penicillin V Potassium Tablets, USP) 500 mg
Squibb 113	**Velosef '250' Capsules** (Cephradine Capsules USP) 250 mg
Squibb 114	**Velosef '500' Capsules** (Cephradine Capsules USP) 500 mg

Arco Pharmaceuticals, Inc.

105 ORVILLE DRIVE
BOHEMIA, NY 11716

Direct Inquiries to:
Professional Service Department
(631) 567-9500

ARCO-LASE® OTC
(broad pH spectrum digestant)

COMPOSITION
Each soft, mint flavored tablet contains Trizyme*, 38 mg., and Lipase, 25 mg.
*Contains the following standardized enzymes: amylolytic 30 mg.; proteolytic 6 mg.; cellulolytic 2 mg.

ACTION AND USES
Indicated for most gastrointestinal disorders due to poor digestion. Flatulence, gas and bloating, dyspepsia, distention, fullness, heartburn, or in any condition where normal digestion is impaired by digestive insufficiencies. Arcolase provides the highest standardized enzymatic activity, plus the protective action of the widest pH range. Thus it is effective throughout the entire G.I. tract. Requiring no enteric coating, there is assurance of a positive breakdown of its factors. This is advantageous, because quite often patients with digestive disorders cannot digest their food properly, let alone hard, or enteric coated capsules or tablets.

SIDE EFFECTS
None.

ADMINISTRATION AND DOSAGE
One tablet with or immediately following meals. Tablet may be swallowed or chewed.

SUPPLIED
Bottles of 50's. NDC 275-4040.

ARCO–LASE® PLUS ℞

COMPOSITION
Same as Arco-Lase, plus the addition of Hyoscyamine sulfate 0.10 mg., atropine sulfate 0.02 mg. and phenobarbital $^{1}/_{8}$ gr. (Warning: may be habit forming.)

ACTION AND USES
Gastrointestinal disturbances, such as cramps, bloating, spasms, diarrhea, nausea, vomiting and peptic ulcer. The enzymes correct the digestive insufficiencies.
The antispasmodic and phenobarbital contribute to the symptomatic relief of hypermotility and nervous tension, which usually accompanies functional disturbances of the bowel.

ADMINISTRATION AND DOSAGE
One tablet following meals.

SIDE EFFECTS
May cause rapid pulse, dryness of mouth and blurred vision.

Continued on next page

Arco-Lase Plus—Cont.

CONTRAINDICATIONS
This product is contraindicated in the presence of glaucoma or prostatic hypertrophy.

SUPPLIED
Bottles of 50's. NDC 275-45-45.

LITERATURE AVAILABLE
Yes.

MEGA-B® OTC
(super potency vitamin B complex, sugar & starch free)

COMPOSITION
Each Mega-B Tablet contains the following Mega Vitamins:

B_1 (Thiamine Mononitrate)	100 mg.
B_2 (Riboflavin)	100 mg.
B_6 (Pyridoxine Hydrochloride)	100 mg.
B_{12} (Cyanocobalamin)	100 mcg.
Choline Bitartrate	100 mg.
Inositol	100 mg.
Niacinamide	100 mg.
Folic Acid	100 mcg.
Pantothenic Acid	100 mg.
d-Biotin	100 mcg.
Para-Aminobenzoic Acid (PABA)	100 mg.

In a base of yeast to provide the identified and unidentified B-Complex Factors.

ADVANTAGES
Each Mega-B capsule-shaped tablet provides the highest vitamin B complex available in a single dose.
Mega-B was designed for those patients who require truly Mega vitamin potencies with the convenience of minimum dosage.

INDICATIONS
Mega-B is indicated in conditions characterized by depletions or increased demand of the water-soluble B-complex vitamins. It may be useful in the nutritional management of patients during prolonged convalescence associated with major surgery. It is also indicated for stress conditions, as an adjunct to antibiotics and diuretic therapy, pre and post operative cases, liver conditions, gastrointestinal disorders interfering with intake or absorption of water-soluble vitamins, prolonged or wasting diseases, diabetes, burns, fractures, severe infections, and some psychological disorders.

WARNING
NOT INTENDED FOR TREATMENT OF PERNICIOUS ANEMIA, OR OTHER PRIMARY OR SECONDARY ANEMIAS.

DOSAGE
Usual dosage is one Mega-B tablet daily, or varied, depending on clinical needs.

SUPPLIED
Yellow capsule shaped tablets in bottles of 30, 100 and 500.

MEGADOSE™ OTC
(multiple mega-vitamin formula with minerals, sugar and starch free)

COMPOSITION

Vitamin A	25,000	USP Units
Vitamin D	1,000	USP Units
Vitamin C w/Rose Hips	250	mg.
Vitamin E	100	IU
Folic Acid	400	mcg.
Vitamin B_1	80	mg.
Vitamin B_2	80	mg.
Niacinamide	80	mg.
Vitamin B_6	80	mg.
Vitamin B_{12}	80	mcg.
Biotin	80	mcg.
Pantothenic Acid	80	mg.
Choline Bitartrate	80	mg.
Inositol	80	mg.
Para-Aminobenzoic Acid	80	mg.
Rutin	30	mg.
Citrus Bioflavonoids	30	mg.
Betaine Hydrochloride	30	mg.
Glutamic Acid	30	mg.
Hesperidin Complex	5	mg.
Iodine (from Kelp)	0.15	mg.
Calcium Gluconate*	50	mg.
Zinc Gluconate*	25	mg.
Potassium Gluconate*	10	mg.
Ferrous Gluconate*	10	mg.
Magnesium Gluconate*	7	mg.
Manganese Gluconate*	6	mg.
Copper Gluconate*	0.5	mg.

*Natural mineral chelates in a base containing natural ingredients.

DOSAGE
One tablet daily.

SUPPLIED
Capsule shaped tablets in bottles of 30, 100 and 250.

Astra Merck Inc.
See AstraZeneca LP

Astra Pharmaceuticals, L.P.
See AstraZeneca LP

AstraZeneca LP
WILMINGTON, DE 19850-5437

For Medical Information, Adverse Drug Experiences, and Customer Service Contact: (800) 236-9933

AQUASOL A® ℞
Parenteral
water-miscible vitamin A Palmitate

50,000 USP Units
(15 mg retinol)/mL

with 0.5% chlorobutanol as preservative; 12% polysorbate 80, 0.1% citric acid, 0.03% butylated hydroxyanisole, 0.03% butylated hydroxytoluene; and sodium hydroxide to adjust pH.

THIS IS A STERILE PRODUCT FOR INTRAMUSCULAR INJECTION

DESCRIPTION
AQUASOL A PARENTERAL (water-miscible vitamin A Palmitate) provides 50,000 USP Units of vitamin A per mL as retinol ($C_{20}H_{30}O$) in the form of vitamin A palmitate, a light yellow to amber oil. The structural formula of retinol is:

CH3 CH3 / C / H2C C–CH=CH–C(CH3)=CH–CH=CH–C(CH3)=CHCH2OH / H2C C–CH3 / CH2

Ordinarily oil-soluble, the vitamin A in this product has been water solubilized by special processing* and is available in a water solution for intramuscular injection.
One USP Unit is equivalent to one international unit (IU) and to 0.3 mcg of retinol or 0.6 mcg of beta-carotene.

CLINICAL PHARMACOLOGY
Beta-carotene, retinol, and retinal have effective and reliable vitamin A activity. Retinal and retinol are in chemical equilibrium in the body and have equivalent antixerophthalmic activity. Retinal combines with the rod pigment, opsin, in the retina to form rhodopsin, necessary for visual dark adaptation. Vitamin A prevents retardation of growth and preserves the epithelial cells' integrity. Normal adult liver storage is sufficient to satisfy two years' requirements of vitamin A.
Vitamin A is readily absorbed from the gastrointestinal tract, where the biosynthesis of vitamin A from beta-carotene takes place. Vitamin A absorption requires bile salts, pancreatic lipase, and dietary fat. It is transported in the blood to the liver by the chylomicron fraction of the lymph. Vitamin A is stored in Kupffer cells of the liver mainly as the palmitate. Normal serum vitamin A is 80–300 Units per 100 mL (plasma range is 30–70 μg per dl) and for carotenoids 270–753 Units per 100 mL. The normal adult liver contains approximately 100 to 300 micrograms per gram, mostly as retinol palmitate.

*Oil-soluble vitamin A water solubilized with polysorbate 80.

INDICATIONS
Vitamin A injection is effective for the treatment of vitamin A deficiency.
The parenteral administration is indicated when the oral administration is not feasible as in anorexia, nausea, vomiting, pre- and post- operative conditions, or it is not available as in the "Malabsorption Syndrome" with accompanying steatorrhea.

CONTRAINDICATIONS
The intravenous administration. Hypervitaminosis A. Sensitivity to any of the ingredients in this preparation.
Use in Pregnancy: Safety of amounts exceeding 6,000 Units of vitamin A daily during pregnancy has not been established at this time. The use of vitamin A in excess of the recommended dietary allowance may cause fetal harm when administered to a pregnant woman. Animal reproduction studies have shown fetal abnormalities associated with overdosage in several species. Malformations of the central nervous system, the eye, the palate, and the urogenital tract are recorded. Vitamin A in excess of the recommended dietary allowance is contraindicated in women who are or may become pregnant. If vitamin A is used during pregnancy, or if the patient becomes pregnant while taking vitamin A, the patient should be apprised of the potential hazard to the fetus.

WARNINGS
Avoid overdosage. Keep out of the reach of children.

PRECAUTIONS
General: Protect from light. Prolonged daily dose administration over 25,000 Units vitamin A should be under close supervision. Blood level assays are not a direct measure of liver storage. Liver storage should be adequate before discontinuing therapy. Single vitamin A deficiency is rare. Multiple vitamin deficiency is expected in any dietary deficiency.
Drug Interactions: Women on oral contraceptives have shown a significant increase in plasma vitamin A levels.
Carcinogenesis: There are no studies that show that administration of vitamin A will cause or prevent cancer.
Pregnancy Category X:
See CONTRAINDICATIONS section.
Nursing Mothers: The U.S. Recommended Daily Allowance (RDA) of vitamin A (5,000 Units) is recommended for nursing mothers.

ADVERSE REACTIONS
See OVERDOSAGE section. Anaphylactic shock and death have been reported using the intravenous route. Allergic reactions have been reported rarely with administration of Aquasol A Parenteral including one case of an anaphylactoid type reaction.

OVERDOSAGE
The following amounts have been found to be toxic orally. Toxicity manifestations depend on the age, dosage, size, and duration of administration.
Acute toxicity—single dose (25,000 Units/kg body weight)
Infant: 350,000 Units
Adult: Over 2 million Units
Chronic toxicity (4,000 Units/kg body weight for 6 to 15 months)
Infants 3 to 6 months old: 18,500 Units (water dispersed)/day for one to three months.
Adult: 1 million Units daily for three days; 50,000 Units daily for longer than 18 months; 500,000 Units daily for two months.

Hypervitaminosis A Syndrome:
1. *General manifestations:*
Fatigue, malaise, lethargy, abdominal discomfort, anorexia, and vomiting.
2. *Specific manifestations:*
a. Skeletal: slow growth, hard tender cortical thickening over the radius and tibia, migratory arthralgia and premature closure of the epiphysis.
b. Central Nervous System: irritability, headache, and increased intracranial pressure as manifested by bulging fontanels, papilledema, and exophthalmos.
c. Dermatologic: fissures of the lips, drying and cracking of the skin, alopecia, scaling, massive desquamation, and increased pigmentation.
d. Systemic: hypomenorrhea, hepatosplenomegaly, jaundice, leukopenia, vitamin A plasma level over 1,200 Units/100 mL.

The treatment of hypervitaminosis A consists of immediate withdrawal of the vitamin along with symptomatic and supportive treatment.

DOSAGE AND ADMINISTRATION
For intramuscular use.
I. Adults
100,000 Units daily for three days followed by 50,000 daily for two weeks.
II. Children 1 to 8 years old
17,500 to 35,000 Units daily for 10 days.
III. Infants
7,500 to 15,000 Units daily for 10 days.

Follow-up therapy with an oral therapeutic multi-vitamin preparation, containing 10,000 to 20,000 Units vitamin A for persons over 8 years old and 5,000 to 10,000 Units for infants and children, is recommended daily for two months. In malabsorption, the parenteral route must be used for an equivalent preparation.
Poor dietary habits should be corrected and an abundant and well-balanced dietary intake should be prescribed.

HOW SUPPLIED
Aquasol A Parenteral (water-miscible vitamin A Palmitate) is available as: NDC 0186-4239-62; 50,000 USP Units (15 mg retinol/mL); 2 mL single-dose vial, box of 10.
Store at 2°–8°C (36°–46°F). Do not freeze.
Caution: Federal law prohibits dispensing without prescription.

Manufactured by:
Centeon L.L.C., Kankakee, IL 60901

Manufactured for:
Astra USA, Inc., Westborough, MA 01581
021646R01 Rev. 6/96

ASTRAMORPH/PF™ Ⓒ

[ăs ′-trâ-mŏrf ″]

(morphine sulfate Injection, USP) Preservative-Free

DESCRIPTION

Morphine is the most important alkaloid of opium and is a phenanthrene derivative. It is available as the sulfate, having the following structural formula:

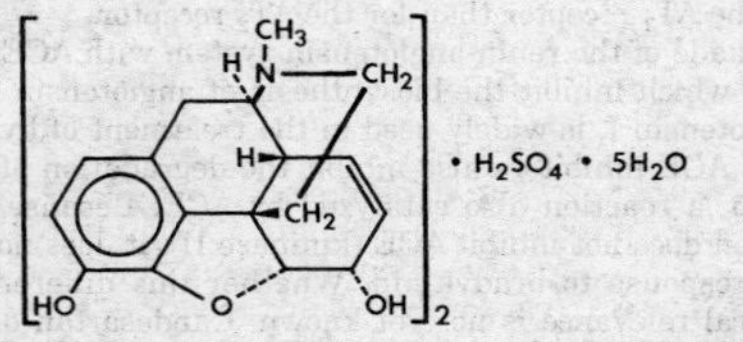

• H_2SO_4 • $5H_2O$

7,8-Didehydro-4,5-epoxy-17-methyl-(5α,6α)-morphinan-3,6-diol sulfate (2:1) (salt), pentahydrate

Preservative-free Astramorph/PF (morphine sulfate Injection, USP) is a sterile, pyrogen-free, isobaric solution free of antioxidants, preservatives or other potentially neurotoxic additives, and is intended for intravenous, epidural or intrathecal administration as a narcotic analgesic. Each milliliter contains morphine sulfate 0.5 mg or 1 mg (Warning: May Be Habit Forming) and sodium chloride 9 mg in Water for Injection. pH may be adjusted with hydrochloric acid to 2.5–6.5. Containers are sealed under nitrogen. Each container is intended for SINGLE USE ONLY. Discard any unused portion. DO NOT AUTOCLAVE.

CLINICAL PHARMACOLOGY

Morphine exerts its primary effects on the central nervous system and organs containing smooth muscle. Pharmacologic effects include analgesia, drowsiness, alteration in mood (euphoria), reduction in body temperature (at low doses), dose-related depression of respiration, interference with adrenocortical response to stress (at high doses), reduction in peripheral resistance with little or no effect on cardiac index and miosis.

Morphine, as other opioids, acts as an agonist interacting with stereo-specific and saturable binding sites/receptors in the brain, spinal cord and other tissues. These sites have been classified as μ receptors and are widely distributed throughout the central nervous system being present in highest concentration in the limbic system (frontal and temporal cortex, amygdala and hippocampus), thalamus, striatum, hypothalamus, midbrain and laminae I, II, IV and V of the dorsal horn in the spinal cord. It has been postulated that exogenously administered morphine exerts its analgesic effect, in part, by altering the central release of neurotransmitter from afferent nerves sensitive to noxious stimuli. Peripheral threshold or responsiveness to noxious stimuli is unaffected leaving monosynaptic reflexes such as the patellar or the Achilles tendon reflex intact.

Autonomic reflexes are not affected by epidural or intrathecal morphine, however morphine exerts spasmogenic effects on the gastrointestinal tract that result in decreased peristaltic activity.

Central nervous system effects of intravenously administered morphine sulfate are influenced by ability to cross the blood-brain barrier.

The delay in the onset of analgesia following epidural or intrathecal injection may be attributed to its relatively poor lipid solubility (i.e., an oil/water partition coefficient of 1.42), and its slow access to the receptor sites. The hydrophilic character of morphine may also explain its retention in the CNS and its slow release into the systemic circulation, resulting in a prolonged effect.

Nausea and vomiting may be prominent and are thought to be the result of central stimulation of the chemoreceptor trigger zone. Histamine release is common; allergic manifestations of urticaria and, rarely, anaphylaxis may occur. Bronchoconstriction may occur either as an idiosyncratic reaction or from large dosages.

Approximately one-third of intravenous morphine is bound to plasma proteins. Free morphine is rapidly redistributed in parenchymatous tissues. The major metabolic pathway is through conjugation with glucuronic acid in the liver. Elimination half-life is approximately 1.5 to 2 hours in healthy volunteers. For intravenously administered morphine, 90% is excreted in the urine within 24 hours and traces are detectable in urine up to 48 hours. About 7–10% of administered morphine eventually appears in the feces as conjugated morphine.

Peak serum levels following epidural or intrathecal administration of Astramorph/PF are reached within 30 minutes in most subjects and decline to very low levels during the next 2 to 4 hours. The onset of action occurs in 15 to 60 minutes following epidural administration or intrathecal administration; analgesia may last up to 24 hours. Due to this extended duration of action, sustained pain relief can be provided with lower daily doses (by these two routes) than are usually required with intravenous or intramuscular morphine administration.

INDICATIONS AND USAGE

Preservative-free Astramorph/PF is a systemic narcotic analgesic for administration by the intravenous, epidural or intrathecal routes. It is used for the management of pain not responsive to non-narcotic analgesics. Morphine sulfate, administered epidurally or intrathecally, provides pain relief for extended periods without attendant loss of motor, sensory or sympathetic function.

CONTRAINDICATIONS

Astramorph/PF is contraindicated in those medical conditions which would preclude the administration of opioids by the intravenous route—allergy to morphine or other opiates, acute bronchial asthma, upper airway obstruction.

Administration of morphine by the epidural or intrathecal route is contraindicated in the presence of infection at the injection site, anticoagulant therapy, bleeding diathesis, parenterally administered corticosteroids within a two week period or other concomitant drug therapy or medical condition which would contraindicate the technique of epidural or intrathecal analgesia.

WARNINGS

Astramorph/PF administration should be limited to use by those familiar with the management of respiratory depression, and in the case of epidural or intrathecal administration, familiar with the techniques and patient management problems associated with epidural or intrathecal drug administration. Because epidural administration has been associated with lessened potential for immediate or late adverse effects than intrathecal administration, the epidural route should be used whenever possible. Rapid intravenous administration may result in chest wall rigidity.

FACILITIES WHERE ASTRAMORPH/PF IS ADMINISTERED MUST BE EQUIPPED WITH RESUSCITATIVE EQUIPMENT, OXYGEN, NALOXONE INJECTION, AND OTHER RESUSCITATIVE DRUGS. WHEN THE EPIDURAL OR INTRATHECAL ROUTE OF ADMINISTRATION IS EMPLOYED, PATIENTS MUST BE OBSERVED IN A FULLY EQUIPPED AND STAFFED ENVIRONMENT FOR AT LEAST 24 HOURS.

SEVERE RESPIRATORY DEPRESSION UP TO 24 HOURS FOLLOWING EPIDURAL OR INTRATHECAL ADMINISTRATION HAS BEEN REPORTED.

Morphine sulfate may be habit forming. (See DRUG ABUSE AND DEPENDENCE section.)

PRECAUTIONS

General: Preservative-free Astramorph/PF (morphine sulfate Injection, USP) should be administered with extreme caution in aged or debilitated patients, in the presence of increased intracranial/intraocular pressure and in patients with head injury. Pupillary changes (miosis) may obscure the course of intracranial pathology. Care is urged in patients who have a decreased respiratory reserve (e.g., emphysema, severe obesity, kyphoscoliosis).

Seizures may result from high doses. Patients with known seizure disorders should be carefully observed for evidence of morphine-induced seizure activity.

It is recommended that administration of Astramorph/PF by the epidural or intrathecal routes be limited to the lumbar area. Intrathecal use has been associated with a higher incidence of respiratory depression than epidural use.

Smooth muscle hypertonicity may result in biliary colic, difficulty in urination and possible urinary retention requiring catheterization. Consideration should be given to risks inherent in urethral catheterization, e.g., sepsis, when epidural or intrathecal administration is considered, especially in the perioperative period.

Elimination half-life may be prolonged in patients with reduced metabolic rates and with hepatic or renal dysfunction. Hence, care should be exercised in administering morphine in these conditions, particularly with repeated dosing.

Patients with reduced circulating blood volume, impaired myocardial function or on sympatholytic drugs should be observed carefully for orthostatic hypotension, particularly in transport.

Patients with chronic obstructive pulmonary disease and patients with acute asthmatic attack may develop acute respiratory failure with administration of morphine. Use in these patients should be reserved for those whose conditions require endotracheal intubation and respiratory support or control of ventilation.

Drug Interactions: Depressant effects of morphine are potentiated by either concomitant administration or in the presence of other CNS depressants such as alcohol, sedatives, antihistaminics or psychotropic drugs (e.g., MAO inhibitors, phenothiazines, butyrophenones and tricyclic antidepressants). Premedication or intra-anesthetic use of neuroleptics with morphine may increase the risk of respiratory depression.

Carcinogenesis, Mutagenesis, Impairment of Fertility: Studies of morphine sulfate in animals to evaluate the carcinogenic and mutagenic potential or the effect on fertility have not been conducted.

Pregnancy: *Teratogenic Effects—Pregnancy Category C*
Animal reproduction studies have not been conducted with morphine sulfate. It is also not known whether morphine sulfate can cause fetal harm when administered to a pregnant woman or can affect reproductive capacity. Morphine sulfate should be given to a pregnant woman only if clearly needed.

Nonteratogenic effects—Infants born from mothers who have been taking morphine chronically may exhibit withdrawal symptoms.

Labor and Delivery: *Intravenous* morphine readily passes into the fetal circulation and may result in respiratory depression in the neonate. Naloxone and resuscitative equipment should be available for reversal of narcotic-induced respiratory depression in the neonate. In addition, intravenous morphine may reduce the strength, duration and frequency of uterine contraction resulting in prolonged labor. *Epidurally and intrathecally* administered morphine readily passes into the fetal circulation and may result in respiratory depression of the neonate. Controlled clinical studies have shown that *epidural* administration has little or no effect on the relief of labor pain.

However, studies have suggested that in most cases 0.2 to 1 mg of morphine *intrathecally* provides adequate pain relief with little effect on the duration of first stage labor. The second stage labor, though, may be prolonged if the parturient is not encouraged to bear down. A continuous intravenous infusion of naloxone, 0.6 mg/hr, for 24 hours after intrathecal injection may be employed to reduce the incidence of potential side effects.

Nursing Mothers: Morphine is excreted in maternal milk. Effect on the nursing infant is not known.

Pediatric Use: Safety and effectiveness in children have not been established.

ADVERSE REACTIONS

The most serious side effect is respiratory depression. Because of delay in maximum CNS effect with intravenously administered drug (30 min), rapid administration may result in overdosing. Bolus administration by the epidural or intrathecal route may result in early respiratory depression due to direct venous redistribution of morphine to the respiratory centers in the brain. Late (up to 24 hours) onset of acute respiratory depression has been reported with administration by the epidural or intrathecal route and is believed to be the result of rostral spread. Reports of respiratory depression following intrathecal administration have been more frequent, but the dosage used in most of these cases has been considerably higher than that recommended. This depression may be severe and could require intervention (see WARNINGS and OVERDOSAGE sections). Even without clinical evidence of ventilatory inadequacy, a diminished CO_2 ventilation response may be noted for up to 22 hours following epidural or intrathecal administration.

While low doses of intravenously administered morphine have little effect on cardiovascular stability, high doses are excitatory, resulting from sympathetic hyperactivity and increase in circulating catecholamines. Excitation of the central nervous system resulting in convulsions may accompany high doses of morphine given intravenously. Dysphoric reactions may occur and toxic psychoses have been reported.

Epidural or intrathecal administration is accompanied by a high incidence of pruritus which is dose related but not confined to site of administration. Nausea and vomiting are frequently seen in patients following morphine administration. Urinary retention which may persist for 10–20 hours following single epidural or intrathecal administration has been reported in approximately 90% of males. Incidence is somewhat lower in females. Patients may require catheterization (see PRECAUTIONS). Pruritus, nausea/vomiting and urinary retention frequently can be alleviated by the intravenous administration of low doses of naloxone (0.2 mg).

Tolerance and dependence to chronically administered morphine, by whatever route, is known to occur (see DRUG ABUSE AND DEPENDENCE section).

Miscellaneous side effects include constipation, headache, anxiety, depression of cough reflex, interference with thermal regulation and oliguria. Evidence of histamine release such as urticaria, wheals and/or local tissue irritation may occur.

In general, side effects are amenable to reversal by narcotic antagonists. **NALOXONE HYDROCHLORIDE INJECTION AND RESUSCITATIVE EQUIPMENT SHOULD BE IMMEDIATELY AVAILABLE FOR ADMINISTRATION IN CASE OF LIFE THREATENING OR INTOLERABLE SIDE EFFECTS.**

DRUG ABUSE AND DEPENDENCE

Controlled Substance: Morphine sulfate Injection is a Schedule II substance under the Drug Enforcement Administration classification.

Abuse: Morphine has recognized abuse and dependence potential.

Dependence: Cerebral and spinal receptors may develop tolerance/dependence independently, as a function of local dosage. Care must be taken to avert withdrawal in those patients who have been maintained on parenteral/oral narcotics when epidural or intrathecal administration is considered. Withdrawal may occur following chronic epidural or intrathecal administration, as well as the development of tolerance to morphine by these routes. (See NONTERATOGENIC EFFECTS under Pregnancy).

OVERDOSAGE

Overdosage is characterized by respiratory depression with or without concomitant CNS depression. Since respiratory arrest may result either through direct depression of the respiratory center or as the result of hypoxia, primary attention should be given to the establishment of adequate respiratory exchange through provision of a patent airway and institution of assisted or controlled ventilation. The narcotic antagonist, naloxone hydrochloride, is a specific an-

Continued on next page

Astramorph/PF—Cont.

tidote. Naloxone hydrochloride (see package insert for full prescribing information) should be administered intravenously, simultaneously with respiratory resuscitation. *As the duration of effect of naloxone is considerably shorter than that of epidural or intrathecal morphine, repeated administration may be necessary.* Patients should be closely observed for evidence of renarcotization. *Note: Respiratory depression may be delayed in onset up to 24 hours* following epidural or intrathecal administration. In painful conditions, reversal of narcotic effect may result in acute onset of pain and release of catecholamines. Careful administration of naloxone may permit reversal of side effects without affecting analgesia. Parenteral administration of narcotics in patients receiving epidural or intrathecal morphine may result in overdosage.

DOSAGE AND ADMINISTRATION

Preservative-free Astramorph/PF (morphine sulfate Injection, USP) is intended for intravenous, epidural or intrathecal administration.

Intravenous Administration

Dosage—The initial dose of morphine sulfate should be 2 mg to 10 mg/70 kg of body weight. Patients under the age of 18; no information available.

Epidural Administration

ASTRAMORPH/PF SHOULD BE ADMINISTERED EPIDURALLY ONLY BY PHYSICIANS EXPERIENCED IN THE TECHNIQUES OF EPIDURAL ADMINISTRATION AND WHO ARE THOROUGHLY FAMILIAR WITH THE LABELING. IT SHOULD BE ADMINISTERED ONLY IN SETTINGS WHERE ADEQUATE PATIENT MONITORING IS POSSIBLE. RESUSCITATIVE EQUIPMENT AND A SPECIFIC ANTAGONIST (NALOXONE HYDROCHLORIDE INJECTION) SHOULD BE IMMEDIATELY AVAILABLE FOR THE MANAGEMENT OF RESPIRATORY DEPRESSION AS WELL AS COMPLICATIONS WHICH MIGHT RESULT FROM INADVERTENT INTRATHECAL OR INTRAVASCULAR INJECTION. (NOTE: INTRATHECAL DOSAGE IS USUALLY 1/10 THAT OF EPIDURAL DOSAGE.) PATIENT MONITORING SHOULD BE CONTINUED FOR AT LEAST 24 HOURS AFTER EACH DOSE, SINCE DELAYED RESPIRATORY DEPRESSION MAY OCCUR.

Proper placement of a needle or catheter in the epidural space should be verified before Astramorph/PF is injected. Acceptable techniques for verifying proper placement include: a) aspiration to check for absence of blood or cerebrospinal fluid, or b) administration of 5 mL (3 mL in obstetric patients) of UNPRESERVED 1.5% Lidocaine and Epinephrine (1:200,000) Injection and then observe the patient for lack of tachycardia (this indicates that vascular injection has *not* been made) and lack of sudden onset of segmental anesthesia (this indicates that intrathecal injection has *not* been made).

Epidural Adult Dosage—Initial injection of 5 mg in the lumbar region may provide satisfactory pain relief for up to 24 hours. If adequate pain relief is not achieved within one hour, careful administration of incremental doses of 1 to 2 mg at intervals sufficient to assess effectiveness may be given. No more than 10 mg/24 hr should be administered.

Thoracic administration has been shown to dramatically increase the incidence of early and late respiratory depression even at doses of 1 to 2 mg.

For continuous infusion an initial dose of 2 to 4 mg/24 hours is recommended. Further doses of 1 to 2 mg may be given if pain relief is not achieved initially.

Aged or debilitated patients–Administer with extreme caution (see PRECAUTIONS section). Doses of less than 5 mg may provide satisfactory pain relief for up to 24 hours.

Epidural Pediatric Use—No information on use in pediatric patients is available.

Intrathecal Administration

NOTE: INTRATHECAL DOSAGE IS USUALLY 1/10 THAT OF EPIDURAL DOSAGE.

ASTRAMORPH/PF SHOULD BE ADMINISTERED INTRATHECALLY ONLY BY PHYSICIANS EXPERIENCED IN THE TECHNIQUES OF INTRATHECAL ADMINISTRATION AND WHO ARE THOROUGHLY FAMILIAR WITH THE LABELING. IT SHOULD BE ADMINISTERED ONLY IN SETTINGS WHERE ADEQUATE PATIENT MONITORING IS POSSIBLE. RESUSCITATIVE EQUIPMENT AND A SPECIFIC ANTAGONIST (NALOXONE HYDROCHLORIDE INJECTION) SHOULD BE IMMEDIATELY AVAILABLE FOR THE MANAGEMENT OF RESPIRATORY DEPRESSION AS WELL AS COMPLICATIONS WHICH MIGHT RESULT FROM INADVERTENT INTRAVASCULAR INJECTION. **PATIENT MONITORING SHOULD BE CONTINUED FOR AT LEAST 24 HOURS AFTER EACH DOSE, SINCE DELAYED RESPIRATORY DEPRESSION MAY OCCUR. RESPIRATORY DEPRESSION (BOTH EARLY AND LATE ONSET) HAS OCCURRED MORE FREQUENTLY FOLLOWING INTRATHECAL ADMINISTRATION.**

Intrathecal Adult Dosage—A single injection of 0.2 to 1 mg may provide satisfactory pain relief for up to 24 hours. **(CAUTION: THIS IS ONLY 0.4 TO 2 ML OF THE 0.5 MG/ML POTENCY OR 0.2 to 1 ML OF THE 1 MG/ML POTENCY OF ASTRAMORPH/PF.) DO NOT INJECT INTRATHECALLY MORE THAN 2 ML OF THE 0.5 MG/ML POTENCY OR 1 ML OF THE 1 MG/ML POTENCY. USE IN THE LUMBAR AREA ONLY IS RECOMMENDED.** Repeated intrathecal injections of Astramorph/PF are not recommended. A constant intravenous infusion of naloxone hydrochloride, 0.6 mg/hr, for 24 hours after intrathecal injection may be used to reduce the incidence of potential side effects.

Aged or debilitated patients–Administer with extreme caution (see PRECAUTIONS section). A lower dosage is usually satisfactory.

Repeat Dosage—If pain recurs, alternative routes of administration should be considered, since experience with repeated doses of morphine by the intrathecal route is limited.

Intrathecal Pediatric Use—No information on use in pediatric patients is available.

Parenteral drug products should be inspected for particulate matter and discoloration prior to administration, whenever solution and container permit.

HOW SUPPLIED

The following strengths and container types of Astramorph/PF are available:

0.5 mg/mL

NDC 0186-1159-03	2 mL (1 mg) Ampule, Boxes of 10
NDC 0186-1150-02	10 mL (5 mg) Ampule, Boxes of 5
NDC 0186-1152-12	10 mL (5 mg) Single Dose Vial, Boxes of 5 Astra E-Z OFF® vial closure

1 mg/mL

NDC 0186-1160-03	2 mL (2 mg) Ampule, Boxes of 10
NDC 0186-1151-02	10 mL (10 mg) Ampule, Boxes of 5
NDC 0186-1153-12	10 mL (10 mg) Single Dose Vial, Boxes of 5 Astra E-Z OFF® vial closure

Storage

Protect from light. Store in carton at controlled room temperature, 15° to 30°C (59° to 86°F) until ready to use. Astramorph/PF contains no preservative. DISCARD ANY UNUSED PORTION. DO NOT AUTOCLAVE. Do not use the injection if darker than pale yellow or if discolored in any other way, or if it contains a precipitate.

Caution: Federal law prohibits dispensing without prescription.

021865R04 Rev. 5/97

ATACAND® ℞

(candesartan cilexetil)
TABLETS

USE IN PREGNANCY
When used in pregnancy during the second and third trimesters, drugs that act directly on the renin-angiotensin system can cause injury and even death to the developing fetus. When pregnancy is detected, ATACAND should be discontinued as soon as possible. See WARNINGS, Fetal/Neonatal Morbidity and Mortality.

DESCRIPTION

ATACAND* (candesartan cilexetil), a prodrug, is hydrolyzed to candesartan during absorption from the gastrointestinal tract. Candesartan is a selective AT_1 subtype angiotensin II receptor antagonist.

Candesartan cilexetil, a nonpeptide, is chemically described as (±)-1-[[(cyclohexyloxy)carbonyl]oxy]ethyl 2-ethoxy-1-[[2'-(1H-tetrazol-5-yl) [1,1'-biphenyl] -4-yl] methyl] -1H-benzimidazole-7-carboxylate.

Its empirical formula is $C_{33}H_{34}N_6O_6$, and its structural formula is

CH3CH2O— N=N HN COO—C—OCOO— H CH3

↓ site of ester hydrolysis.

Candesartan cilexetil is a white to off-white powder with a molecular weight of 610.67. It is practically insoluble in water and sparingly soluble in methanol. Candesartan cilexetil is a racemic mixture containing one chiral center at the cyclohexyloxycarbonyloxy ethyl ester group. Following oral administration, candesartan cilexetil undergoes hydrolysis at the ester link to form the active drug, candesartan, which is achiral.

ATACAND is available for oral use as tablets containing either 4 mg, 8 mg, 16 mg, or 32 mg of candesartan cilexetil and the following inactive ingredients: hydroxypropyl cellulose, polyethylene glycol, lactose, corn starch, carboxymethylcellulose calcium, and magnesium stearate. Ferric oxide (reddish brown) is added to the 8-mg, 16-mg, and 32-mg tablets as a colorant.

*Registered trademark of the AstraZeneca group of companies

CLINICAL PHARMACOLOGY

Mechanism of Action

Angiotensin II is formed from angiotensin I in a reaction catalyzed by angiotensin-converting enzyme (ACE, kininase II). Angiotensin II is the principal pressor agent of the renin-angiotensin system, with effects that include vasoconstriction, stimulation of synthesis and release of aldosterone, cardiac stimulation, and renal reabsorption of sodium. Candesartan blocks the vasoconstrictor and aldosterone-secreting effects of angiotensin II by selectively blocking the binding of angiotensin II to the AT_1 receptor in many tissues, such as vascular smooth muscle and the adrenal gland. Its action is, therefore, independent of the pathways for angiotensin II synthesis.

There is also an AT_2 receptor found in many tissues, but AT_2 is not known to be associated with cardiovascular homeostasis. Candesartan has much greater affinity (>10,000-fold) for the AT_1 receptor than for the AT_2 receptor.

Blockade of the renin-angiotensin system with ACE inhibitors, which inhibit the biosynthesis of angiotensin II from angiotensin I, is widely used in the treatment of hypertension. ACE inhibitors also inhibit the degradation of bradykinin, a reaction also catalyzed by ACE. Because candesartan does not inhibit ACE (kininase II), it does not affect the response to bradykinin. Whether this difference has clinical relevance is not yet known. Candesartan does not bind to or block other hormone receptors or ion channels known to be important in cardiovascular regulation.

Blockade of the angiotensin II receptor inhibits the negative regulatory feedback of angiotensin II on renin secretion, but the resulting increased plasma renin activity and angiotensin II circulating levels do not overcome the effect of candesartan on blood pressure.

Pharmacokinetics

General

Candesartan cilexetil is rapidly and completely bioactivated by ester hydrolysis during absorption from the gastrointestinal tract to candesartan, a selective AT_1 subtype angiotensin II receptor antagonist. Candesartan is mainly excreted unchanged in urine and feces (via bile). It undergoes minor hepatic metabolism by O-deethylation to an inactive metabolite. The elimination half-life of candesartan is approximately 9 hours. After single and repeated administration, the pharmacokinetics of candesartan are linear for oral doses up to 32 mg of candesartan cilexetil. Candesartan and its inactive metabolite do not accumulate in serum upon repeated once-daily dosing.

Following administration of candesartan cilexetil, the absolute bioavailability of candesartan was estimated to be 15%. After tablet ingestion, the peak serum concentration (C_{max}) is reached after 3 to 4 hours. Food with a high fat content does not affect the bioavailability of candesartan after candesartan cilexetil administration.

Metabolism and Excretion

Total plasma clearance of candesartan is 0.37 mL/min/kg, with a renal clearance of 0.19 mL/min/kg. When candesartan is administered orally, about 26% of the dose is excreted unchanged in urine. Following an oral dose of ^{14}C-labeled candesartan cilexetil, approximately 33% of radioactivity is recovered in urine and approximately 67% in feces. Following an intravenous dose of ^{14}C-labeled candesartan, approximately 59% of radioactivity is recovered in urine and approximately 36% in feces. Biliary excretion contributes to the elimination of candesartan.

Distribution

The volume of distribution of candesartan is 0.13 L/kg. Candesartan is highly bound to plasma proteins (>99%) and does not penetrate red blood cells. The protein binding is constant at candesartan plasma concentrations well above the range achieved with recommended doses. In rats, it has been demonstrated that candesartan crosses the blood-brain barrier poorly, if at all. It has also been demonstrated in rats that candesartan passes across the placental barrier and is distributed in the fetus.

Special Populations

Pediatric—The pharmacokinetics of candesartan cilexetil have not been investigated in patients <18 years of age.

Geriatric and Gender—The pharmacokinetics of candesartan have been studied in the elderly (≥65 years) and in both sexes. The plasma concentration of candesartan was higher in the elderly (C_{max} was approximately 50% higher, and AUC was approximately 80% higher) compared to younger subjects administered the same dose. The pharmacokinetics of candesartan were linear in the elderly, and candesartan and its inactive metabolite did not accumulate in the serum of these subjects upon repeated, once-daily administration. No initial dosage adjustment is necessary. (See DOSAGE AND ADMINISTRATION.) There is no difference in the pharmacokinetics of candesartan between male and female subjects.

Renal Insufficiency—In hypertensive patients with renal insufficiency, serum concentrations of candesartan were elevated. After repeated dosing, the AUC and C_{max} were approximately doubled in patients with severe renal impairment (creatinine clearance <30 mL/min/1.73m²) compared to patients with normal kidney function. The pharmacokinetics of candesartan in hypertensive patients undergoing hemodialysis are similar to those in hypertensive patients with severe renal impairment. Candesartan cannot be removed by hemodialysis. No initial dosage adjustment is necessary in patients with renal insufficiency. (See DOSAGE AND ADMINISTRATION.)

Hepatic Insufficiency—No differences in the pharmacokinetics of candesartan were observed in patients with mild to moderate chronic liver disease. The pharmacokinetics after candesartan cilexetil administration have not been investigated in patients with severe hepatic insufficiency. No initial dosage adjustment is necessary in patients with mild hepatic disease. (See DOSAGE AND ADMINISTRATION.)

Drug Interactions

See PRECAUTIONS, Drug Interactions.

Pharmacodynamics

Candesartan inhibits the pressor effects of angiotensin II infusion in a dose-dependent manner. After 1 week of once-daily dosing with 8 mg of candesartan cilexetil, the pressor effect was inhibited by approximately 90% at peak with approximately 50% inhibition persisting for 24 hours.

Plasma concentrations of angiotensin I and angiotensin II, and plasma renin activity (PRA), increased in a dose-dependent manner after single and repeated administration of candesartan cilexetil to healthy subjects and hypertensive patients. ACE activity was not altered in healthy subjects after repeated candesartan cilexetil administration. The once-daily administration of up to 16 mg of candesartan cilexetil to healthy subjects did not influence plasma aldosterone concentrations, but a decrease in the plasma concentration of aldosterone was observed when 32 mg of candesartan cilexetil was administered to hypertensive patients. In spite of the effect of candesartan cilexetil on aldosterone secretion, very little effect on serum potassium was observed.

In multiple-dose studies with hypertensive patients, there were no clinically significant changes in metabolic function including serum levels of total cholesterol, triglycerides, glucose, or uric acid. In a 12-week study of 161 patients with noninsulin-dependent (type 2) diabetes mellitus and hypertension, there was no change in the level of HbA_{1c}.

Clinical Trials

The antihypertensive effects of ATACAND were examined in 14 placebo-controlled trials of 4- to 12-weeks duration, primarily at daily doses of 2 to 32 mg per day in patients with baseline diastolic blood pressures of 95 to 114 mmHg. Most of the trials were of candesartan cilexetil as a single agent, but it was also studied as add-on to hydrochlorothiazide and amlodipine. These studies included a total of 2350 patients randomized to one of several doses of candesartan cilexetil and 1027 to placebo. Except for a study in diabetics, all studies showed significant effects, generally dose related, of 2 to 32 mg on trough (24 hour) systolic and diastolic pressures compared to placebo, with doses of 8 to 32 mg giving effects of about 8–12/4–8 mmHg. There were no exaggerated first-dose effects in these patients. Most of the antihypertensive effect was seen within 2 weeks of initial dosing, and the full effect in 4 weeks. With once-daily dosing, blood pressure effect was maintained over 24 hours, with trough to peak ratios of blood pressure effect generally over 80%. Candesartan cilexetil had an additional blood pressure lowering effect when added to hydrochlorothiazide.

The antihypertensive effect was similar in men and women and in patients older and younger than 65. Candesartan was effective in reducing blood pressure regardless of race, although the effect was somewhat less in blacks (usually a low-renin population). This has been generally true for angiotensin II antagonists and ACE inhibitors.

In long-term studies of up to 1 year, the antihypertensive effectiveness of candesartan cilexetil was maintained, and there was no rebound after abrupt withdrawal.

There were no changes in the heart rate of patients treated with candesartan cilexetil in controlled trials.

INDICATIONS AND USAGE

ATACAND is indicated for the treatment of hypertension. It may be used alone or in combination with other antihypertensive agents.

CONTRAINDICATIONS

ATACAND is contraindicated in patients who are hypersensitive to any component of this product.

WARNINGS

Fetal/Neonatal Morbidity and Mortality

Drugs that act directly on the renin-angiotensin system can cause fetal and neonatal morbidity and death when administered to pregnant women. Several dozen cases have been reported in the world literature in patients who were taking angiotensin-converting enzyme inhibitors. When pregnancy is detected, ATACAND should be discontinued as soon as possible.

The use of drugs that act directly on the renin-angiotensin system during the second and third trimesters of pregnancy has been associated with fetal and neonatal injury, including hypotension, neonatal skull hypoplasia, anuria, reversible or irreversible renal failure, and death. Oligohydramnios has also been reported, presumably resulting from decreased fetal renal function; oligohydramnios in this setting has been associated with fetal limb contractures, craniofacial deformation, and hypoplastic lung development. Prematurity, intrauterine growth retardation, and patent ductus arteriosus have also been reported, although it is not clear whether these occurrences were due to exposure to the drug.

These adverse effects do not appear to have resulted from intrauterine drug exposure that has been limited to the first trimester. Mothers whose embryos and fetuses are exposed to an angiotensin II receptor antagonist only during the first trimester should be so informed. Nonetheless, when patients become pregnant, physicians should have the patient discontinue the use of ATACAND as soon as possible.

Rarely (probably less often than once in every thousand pregnancies), no alternative to a drug acting on the renin-angiotensin system will be found. In these rare cases, the mothers should be apprised of the potential hazards to their fetuses, and serial ultrasound examinations should be performed to assess the intra-amniotic environment.

If oligohydramnios is observed, ATACAND should be discontinued unless it is considered life saving for the mother. Contraction stress testing (CST), a nonstress test (NST), or biophysical profiling (BPP) may be appropriate, depending upon the week of pregnancy. Patients and physicians should be aware, however, that oligohydramnios may not appear until after the fetus has sustained irreversible injury.

Infants with histories of *in utero* exposure to an angiotensin II receptor antagonist should be closely observed for hypotension, oliguria, and hyperkalemia. If oliguria occurs, attention should be directed toward support of blood pressure and renal perfusion. Exchange transfusion or dialysis may be required as means of reversing hypotension and/or substituting for disordered renal function.

There is no clinical experience with the use of ATACAND in pregnant women. Oral doses ≥ 10 mg of candesartan cilexetil/kg/day administered to pregnant rats during late gestation and continued through lactation were associated with reduced survival and an increased incidence of hydronephrosis in the offspring. The 10-mg/kg/day dose in rats is approximately 2.8 times the maximum recommended daily human dose (MRHD) of 32 mg on a mg/m^2 basis (comparison assumes human body weight of 50 kg). Candesartan cilexetil given to pregnant rabbits at an oral dose of 3 mg/kg/day (approximately 1.7 times the MRHD on a mg/m^2 basis) caused maternal toxicity (decreased body weight and death) but, in surviving dams had no adverse effects on fetal survival, fetal weight, or external, visceral or skeletal development. No maternal toxicity or adverse effects on fetal development were observed when oral doses up to 1000 mg of candesartan cilexetil/kg/day (approximately 138 times the MRHD on a mg/m^2 basis) were administered to pregnant mice.

Hypotension in Volume- and Salt-Depleted Patients

In patients with an activated renin-angiotensin system, such as volume- and/or salt-depleted patients (eg, those being treated with diuretics), symptomatic hypotension may occur. These conditions should be corrected prior to administration of ATACAND, or the treatment should start under close medical supervision (see DOSAGE AND ADMINISTRATION).

If hypotension occurs, the patients should be placed in the supine position and, if necessary, given an intravenous infusion of normal saline. A transient hypotensive response is not a contraindication to further treatment which usually can be continued without difficulty once the blood pressure has stabilized.

PRECAUTIONS

General

Impaired Renal Function—As a consequence of inhibiting the renin-angiotensin-aldosterone system, changes in renal function may be anticipated in susceptible individuals treated with ATACAND. In patients whose renal function may depend upon the activity of the renin-angiotensin-aldosterone system (eg, patients with severe congestive heart failure), treatment with angiotensin-converting enzyme inhibitors and angiotensin receptor antagonists has been associated with oliguria and/or progressive azotemia and (rarely) with acute renal failure and/or death. Similar results may be anticipated in patients treated with ATACAND. (See CLINICAL PHARMACOLOGY, Special Populations.)

In studies of ACE inhibitors in patients with unilateral or bilateral renal artery stenosis, increases in serum creatinine or blood urea nitrogen (BUN) have been reported. There has been no long-term use of ATACAND in patients with unilateral or bilateral renal artery stenosis, but similar results may be expected.

Information for Patients

Pregnancy—Female patients of childbearing age should be told about the consequences of second- and third-trimester exposure to drugs that act on the renin-angiotensin system, and they should also be told that these consequences do not appear to have resulted from intrauterine drug exposure that has been limited to the first trimester. These patients should be asked to report pregnancies to their physicians as soon as possible.

Drug Interactions

No significant drug interactions have been reported in studies of candesartan cilexetil given with other drugs such as glyburide, nifedipine, digoxin, warfarin, hydrochlorothiazide and oral contraceptives in healthy volunteers. Because candesartan is not significantly metabolized by the cytochrome P450 system and at therapeutic concentrations has no effects on P450 enzymes, interactions with drugs that inhibit or are metabolized by those enzymes would not be expected.

Carcinogenesis, Mutagenesis, Impairment of Fertility

There was no evidence of carcinogenicity when candesartan cilexetil was orally administered to mice and rats for up to 104 weeks at doses up to 100 and 1000 mg/kg/day, respectively. Rats received the drug by gavage; whereas, mice received the drug by dietary administration. These (maximally-tolerated) doses of candesartan cilexetil provided systemic exposures to candesartan (AUCs) that were, in mice, approximately 7 times and, in rats, more than 70 times the exposure in man at the maximum recommended daily human dose (32 mg).

Candesartan cilexetil was not genotoxic in the microbial mutagenesis and mammalian cell mutagenesis assays and in the *in vivo* chromosomal aberration and rat unscheduled DNA synthesis assays. In addition, candesartan was not genotoxic in the microbial mutagenesis, mammalian cell mutagenesis, and *in vitro* and *in vivo* chromosome aberration assays.

Fertility and reproductive performance were not affected in studies with male and female rats given oral doses of up to 300 mg/kg/day (83-times the maximum daily human dose of 32 mg on a body surface area basis).

Pregnancy

Pregnancy Categories C (first trimester) *and D* (second and third trimesters). See WARNINGS, Fetal/Neonatal Morbidity and Mortality.

Nursing Mothers

It is not known whether candesartan is excreted in human milk, but candesartan has been shown to be present in rat milk. Because of the potential for adverse effects on the nursing infant, a decision should be made whether to discontinue nursing or discontinue the drug, taking into account the importance of the drug to the mother.

Pediatric Use

Safety and effectiveness in pediatric patients have not been established.

Geriatric Use

Of the total number of subjects in clinical studies of ATACAND, 21% were 65 and over, while 3% were 75 and over. No overall differences in safety or effectiveness were observed between these subjects and younger subjects, and other reported clinical experience has not identified differences in responses between the elderly and younger patients, but greater sensitivity of some older individuals cannot be ruled out. In a placebo-controlled trial of about 200 elderly hypertensive patients (ages 65 to 87 years), administration of candesartan cilexetil was well tolerated and lowered blood pressure by about 12/6 mmHg more than placebo.

ADVERSE REACTIONS

ATACAND has been evaluated for safety in more than 3600 patients/subjects, including more than 3200 patients treated for hypertension. About 600 of these patients were studied for at least 6 months and about 200 for at least 1 year. In general, treatment with ATACAND was well tolerated. The overall incidence of adverse events reported with ATACAND was similar to placebo.

The rate of withdrawals due to adverse events in all trials in patients (7510 total) was 3.3% (ie, 108 of 3260) of patients treated with candesartan cilexetil as monotherapy and 3.5% (ie, 39 of 1106) of patients treated with placebo. In placebo-controlled trials, discontinuation of therapy due to clinical adverse events occurred in 2.4% (ie, 57 of 2350) of patients treated with ATACAND and 3.4% (ie, 35 of 1027) of patients treated with placebo.

The most common reasons for discontinuation of therapy with ATACAND were headache (0.6%) and dizziness (0.3%).

The adverse events that occurred in placebo-controlled clinical trials in at least 1% of patients treated with ATACAND and at a higher incidence in candesartan cilexetil (n=2350) than placebo (n=1027) patients included back pain (3% vs. 2%), dizziness (4% vs. 3%), upper respiratory tract infection (6% vs. 4%), pharyngitis (2% vs. 1%), and rhinitis (2% vs. 1%).

The following adverse events occurred in placebo-controlled clinical trials at a more than 1% rate but at about the same or greater incidence in patients receiving placebo compared to candesartan cilexetil: fatigue, peripheral edema, chest pain, headache, bronchitis, coughing, sinusitis, nausea, abdominal pain, diarrhea, vomiting, arthralgia, albuminuria.

Other potentially important adverse events that have been reported, whether or not attributed to treatment, with an incidence of 0.5% or greater from the more than 3200 patients worldwide treated with ATACAND are listed below. It cannot be determined whether these events were causally related to ATACAND. **Body as a Whole:** asthenia, fever; **Central and Peripheral Nervous System:** paresthesia, vertigo; **Gastrointestinal System Disorder:** dyspepsia, gastroenteritis; **Heart Rate and Rhythm Disorders:** tachycardia, palpitation; **Metabolic and Nutritional Disorders:** creatine phosphokinase increased, hyperglycemia, hypertriglyceridemia, hyperuricemia; **Musculoskeletal System Disorders:** myalgia; **Platelet/Bleeding-Clotting Disorders:** epistaxis; **Psychiatric Disorders:** anxiety, depression, somnolence; **Respiratory System Disorders:** dyspnea; **Skin and Appendages Disorders:** rash, sweating increased; **Urinary System Disorders:** hematuria.

Other reported events seen less frequently included angina pectoris, myocardial infarction, and angioedema.

Adverse events occurred at about the same rates in men and women, older and younger patients, and black and nonblack patients.

Post-Marketing Experience

Other adverse events reported for candesartan cilexetil where a causal relationship could not be established include very rare cases of neutropenia, leukopenia and agranulocytosis.

Laboratory Test Findings

In controlled clinical trials, clinically important changes in standard laboratory parameters were rarely associated with the administration of ATACAND.

Continued on next page

Atacand—Cont.

Creatinine, Blood Urea Nitrogen—Minor increases in blood urea nitrogen (BUN) and serum creatinine were observed infrequently.
Hyperuricemia—Hyperuricemia was rarely found (19 or 0.6% of 3260 patients treated with candesartan cilexetil and 5 or 0.5% of 1106 patients treated with placebo).
Hemoglobin and Hematocrit—Small decreases in hemoglobin and hematocrit (mean decreases of approximately 0.2 grams/dL and 0.5 volume percent, respectively) were observed in patients treated with ATACAND alone but were rarely of clinical importance. Anemia, leukopenia, and thrombocytopenia were associated with withdrawal of one patient each from clinical trials.
Potassium—A small increase (mean increase of 0.1 mEq/L) was observed in patients treated with ATACAND alone but was rarely of clinical importance. One patient from a congestive heart failure trial was withdrawn for hyperkalemia (serum potassium = 7.5 mEq/L). This patient was also receiving spironolactone.
Liver Function Tests—Elevations of liver enzymes and/or serum bilirubin were observed infrequently. Five patients assigned to candesartan cilexetil in clinical trials were withdrawn because of abnormal liver chemistries. All had elevated transaminases. Two had mildly elevated total bilirubin, but one of these patients was diagnosed with Hepatitis A.

OVERDOSAGE

No lethality was observed in acute toxicity studies in mice, rats, and dogs given single oral doses of up to 2000 mg/kg of candesartan cilexetil. In mice given single oral doses of the primary metabolite, candesartan, the minimum lethal dose was greater than 1000 mg/kg but less than 2000 mg/kg.
Limited data are available in regard to overdosage in humans. In one recorded case of an intentional overdose, a 43-year-old female patient (Body Mass Index of 31 kg/m^2) ingested an estimated 160 mg of candesartan cilexetil in conjunction with multiple other pharmaceutical agents (ibuprofen, naproxen sodium, diphenhydramine hydrochloride, and ketoprofen). Gastric lavage was performed; the patient was monitored in hospital for several days and was discharged without sequelae.
Candesartan cannot be removed by hemodialysis.
Treatment—To obtain up-to-date information about the treatment of overdose, consult your Regional Poison Control Center. Telephone numbers of certified poison control centers are listed in the *Physicians' Desk Reference (PDR)*. In managing overdose, consider the possibilities of multiple-drug overdoses, drug-drug interactions, and altered pharmacokinetics in your patient.
The most likely manifestation of overdosage with ATACAND would be hypotension, dizziness, and tachycardia; bradycardia could occur from parasympathetic (vagal) stimulation. If symptomatic hypotension should occur, supportive treatment should be instituted.

DOSAGE AND ADMINISTRATION

Dosage must be individualized. Blood pressure response is dose related over the range of 2 to 32 mg. The usual recommended starting dose of ATACAND is 16 mg once daily when it is used as monotherapy in patients who are not volume depleted. ATACAND can be administered once or twice daily with total daily doses ranging from 8 mg to 32 mg. Larger doses do not appear to have a greater effect, and there is relatively little experience with such doses. Most of the antihypertensive effect is present within 2 weeks, and maximal blood pressure reduction is generally obtained within 4 to 6 weeks of treatment with ATACAND.
No initial dosage adjustment is necessary for elderly patients, for patients with mildly impaired renal function, or for patients with mildly impaired hepatic function (see CLINICAL PHARMACOLOGY, Special Populations). For patients with possible depletion of intravascular volume (eg, patients treated with diuretics, particularly those with impaired renal function), ATACAND should be initiated under close medical supervision and consideration should be given to administration of a lower dose (see WARNINGS, Hypotension in Volume- and Salt-Depleted Patients).
ATACAND may be administered with or without food.
If blood pressure is not controlled by ATACAND alone, a diuretic may be added. ATACAND may be administered with other antihypertensive agents.

HOW SUPPLIED

No. 3782—Tablets ATACAND, 4 mg, are white to off-white, circular/biconvex-shaped, non-film-coated tablets, coded ACF on one side and 004 on the other. They are supplied as follows:
NDC 0186-0004-31 unit of use bottles of 30.
No. 3780—Tablets ATACAND, 8 mg, are light pink, circular/biconvex-shaped, non-film-coated tablets, coded ACG on one side and 008 on the other. They are supplied as follows:
NDC 0186-0008-31 unit of use bottles of 30.
No. 3781—Tablets ATACAND, 16 mg, are pink, circular/biconvex-shaped, non-film-coated tablets, coded ACH on one side and 016 on the other. They are supplied as follows:
NDC 0186-0016-31 unit of use bottles of 30
NDC 0186-0016-54 unit of use bottles of 90
NDC 0186-0016-28 unit dose packages of 100.
No. 3791—Tablets ATACAND, 32 mg, are pink, circular/biconvex-shaped, non-film-coated tablets, coded ACL on one side and 032 on the other. They are supplied as follows:
NDC 0186-0032-31 unit of use bottles of 30
NDC 0186-0032-54 unit of use bottles of 90
NDC 0186-0032-28 unit dose packages of 100.

Storage
Store at 25°C (77°F); excursions permitted to 15–30°C (59–86°F) [see USP Controlled Room Temperature]. Keep container tightly closed.
Manufactured under the license
from Takeda Chemical Industries, Ltd.
by: Astra AB, S-151 85 Södertälje, Sweden.
Packaged by:
Merck & Co., Inc., West Point, PA 19486
Distributed by:
Astra Pharmaceuticals, L.P., Wayne, PA 19087
610002-04 Revised February 2000
Shown in Product Identification Guide, page 304

CALCITONIN-SALMON INJECTION, SYNTHETIC ℞

DESCRIPTION

Calcitonin is a polypeptide hormone secreted by the parafollicular cells of the thyroid gland in mammals and by the ultimobranchial gland of birds and fish.
Calcitonin-salmon injection, synthetic is a synthetic polypeptide of 32 amino acids in the same linear sequence that is found in calcitonin of salmon origin. This is shown by the following graphic formula:

H—Cys—Ser—Asn—Leu—Ser—Thr—Cys—Val—Leu—Gly—Lys—Leu—Ser—Gln—Glu—Leu—
1 2 3 4 5 6 7 8 9 10 11 12 13 14 15 16

His—Lys—Leu—Gln—Thr—Tyr—Pro—Arg—Thr—Asn—Thr—Gly—Ser—Gly—Thr—Pro—NH_2
17 18 19 20 21 22 23 24 25 26 27 28 29 30 31 32

It is provided in sterile solution for subcutaneous or intramuscular injection. Each milliliter contains 200 I.U. calcitonin-salmon; 5 mg phenol (as preservative); with sodium chloride, sodium acetate, glacial acetic acid, and sodium hydroxide to adjust tonicity and pH between 3.9 and 4.5. Filled under nitrogen.
The activity of calcitonin-salmon is stated in International Units based on bioassay in comparison with the International Reference Preparation of calcitonin-salmon for Bioassay, distributed by the National Institute for Biological Standards and Control, Holly Hill, London.

HOW SUPPLIED

Calcitonin-salmon injection, synthetic is available as:
NDC 0186-1608-13; 2 mL multiple dose vial containing 200 I.U. per mL Box of 1
Store in refrigerator, between 2°-8°C (36°-46°F).
Caution: Federal law prohibits dispensing without prescription.
021713R02 Rev. 2/97

DURANEST® ℞

[*dur 'a-nest*]
(etidocaine hydrochloride)
Injections for infiltration and nerve block

DESCRIPTION

Duranest (etidocaine HCl) Injections are sterile aqueous solutions that contain a local anesthetic agent and are administered parenterally by injection. See INDICATIONS AND USAGE for specific uses. The specific quantitative composition of each available solution is shown in Table 1.
Duranest Injections contain etidocaine HCl, which is chemically designated as butanamide, N-(2,6-dimethylphenyl)-2-(ethylpropylamine)-, monohydrochloride and has the following structural formula:

Epinephrine is (-)-3, 4-Dihydroxy-α-[(methylamino) methyl] benzyl alcohol and has the following structural formula:

The pK_a of etidocaine (7.74) is similar to that of lidocaine (7.86). However, etidocaine possesses a greater degree of lipid solubility and protein binding capacity than does lidocaine. Duranest Injections are sterile and, except for the 1.5% concentration, are available with or without epinephrine 1:200,000. Single dose containers of Duranest Injection without epinephrine may be reautoclaved if necessary.
See Table 1 for composition of available injections.
[See table 1 at top of next page]

CLINICAL PHARMACOLOGY

Mechanism of Action: Etidocaine stabilizes the neuronal membrane by inhibiting the ionic fluxes required for the initiation and conduction of impulses, thereby effecting local anesthetic action.
Onset and Duration of Action: *In vivo* animal studies have shown that etidocaine has a rapid onset (3–5 minutes) and a prolonged duration of action (5–10 hours). Based on comparative clinical studies of lidocaine and etidocaine, the anesthetic properties of etidocaine in man may be characterized as follows: Initial onset of sensory analgesia and motor blockade is rapid (usually 3–5 minutes) and similar to that produced by lidocaine. Duration of sensory analgesia is 1.5 to 2 times longer than that of lidocaine by the peridural route. The difference in analgesic duration between etidocaine and lidocaine may be even greater following peripheral nerve blockade than following central neural block. Duration of analgesia in excess of 9 hours is not infrequent when etidocaine is used for peripheral nerve blocks such as brachial plexus blockade. Etidocaine produces a profound degree of motor blockade and abdominal muscle relaxation when used for peridural analgesia.
Hemodynamics: Excessive blood levels may cause changes in cardiac output, total peripheral resistance, and mean arterial pressure. With central neural blockade these changes may be attributable to block of autonomic fibers, a direct depressant effect of the local anesthetic agent on various components of the cardiovascular system, and/or the beta-adrenergic receptor stimulating action of epinephrine when present. The net effect is normally a modest hypotension when the recommended dosages are not exceeded.
Pharmacokinetics and Metabolism: Information derived from diverse formulations, concentrations and usages reveals that etidocaine is completely absorbed following parenteral administration, its rate of absorption depending, for example, upon such factors as the site of administration and the presence or absence of a vasconstrictor agent. Except for intravenous administration, the highest blood levels are obtained following intercostal nerve block and the lowest after subcutaneous administration.
The plasma binding of etidocaine is dependent on drug concentration, and the fraction bound decreases with increasing concentration. At 0.5–1.0 μg/mL, 95% is bound to plasma protein.
Etidocaine crosses the blood-brain and placental barriers, presumably by passive diffusion.
Etidocaine is metabolized rapidly by the liver, and metabolites and unchanged drug are excreted by the kidney. Biotransformation includes oxidative N-dealkylation, ring hydroxylation, cleavage of the amide linkage, and conjugation. To date, approximately 20 metabolites of etidocaine have been found in the urine. The percent of dose excreted as unchanged drug is less than 10%.
The mean elimination half-life of etidocaine following a bolus intravenous injection is about 2.5 hours. Because of the rapid rate at which etidocaine is metabolized, any condition that affects liver function may alter etidocaine kinetics. Renal dysfunction may not affect etidocaine kinetics but may increase the accumulation of metabolites.
Factors such as acidosis and the concomitant use of CNS stimulants and depressants affect the CNS levels of etidocaine required to produce overt systemic effects. In the rhesus monkey, arterial blood levels of 4.5 μg/mL have been shown to be threshold for convulsive activity.

INDICATIONS AND USAGE

Duranest (etidocaine HCl) Injections are indicated for infiltration anesthesia, peripheral nerve blocks (e.g., brachial plexus, intercostal, retrobulbar, ulnar, inferior alveolar), and central neural block (i.e., lumbar or caudal epidural blocks).

CONTRAINDICATIONS

Etidocaine is contraindicated in patients with a known history of hypersensitivity to local anesthetics of the amide type.

WARNINGS

DURANEST INJECTIONS FOR INFILTRATION AND NERVE BLOCK SHOULD BE EMPLOYED ONLY BY CLINICIANS WHO ARE WELL VERSED IN DIAGNOSIS AND MANAGEMENT OF DOSE-RELATED TOXICITY AND OTHER ACUTE EMERGENCIES THAT MIGHT ARISE FROM THE BLOCK TO BE EMPLOYED AND THEN ONLY AFTER ENSURING THE *IMMEDIATE* AVAILABILITY OF OXYGEN, OTHER RESUSCITATIVE DRUGS, CARDIOPULMONARY EQUIPMENT, AND THE PERSONNEL NEEDED FOR PROPER MANAGEMENT OF TOXIC REACTIONS AND RELATED EMERGENCIES (see also ADVERSE REACTIONS and PRECAUTIONS). DELAY IN PROPER MANAGEMENT OF DOSE-RELATED TOXICITY, UNDERVENTILATION FROM ANY CAUSE AND/OR ALTERED SENSITIVITY MAY LEAD TO THE DEVELOPMENT OF ACIDOSIS, CARDIAC ARREST, AND POSSIBLY DEATH.
To avoid intravascular injection, aspiration should be performed before the local anesthetic solution is injected. The needle must be repositioned until no return of blood can be elicited by aspiration. Note, however, that the absence of blood in the syringe does not guarantee that intravascular injection has been avoided.
Local anesthetic solutions containing antimicrobial preservatives (e.g., methylparaben) should not be used for epidu-

ral anesthesia because the safety of these agents has not been established with regard to intrathecal injection, either intentional or accidental.

Vasopressor agents administered for the treatment of hypotension related to caudal or other epidural blocks should not be used in the presence of ergot-type oxytocic drugs, since severe persistent hypertension and even rupture of cerebral blood vessels may occur.

Duranest with epinephrine solutions contain sodium metabisulfite, a sulfite that may cause allergic-type reactions including anaphylactic symptoms and life-threatening or less severe asthmatic episodes in certain susceptible people. The overall prevalence of sulfite sensitivity in the general population is unknown and probably low. Sulfite sensitivity is seen more frequently in asthmatic than in nonasthmatic people.

PRECAUTIONS

General: The safety and effectiveness of etidocaine depend on proper dosage, correct technique, adequate precautions, and readiness for emergencies. Standard textbooks should be consulted for specific techniques and precautions for various regional anesthetic procedures. Resuscitative equipment, oxygen, and other resuscitative drugs should be available for immediate use. (See WARNINGS and ADVERSE REACTIONS.) The lowest dosage that results in effective anesthesia should be used to avoid high plasma levels and serious adverse effects. Syringe aspirations should also be performed before and during each supplemental injection when using indwelling catheter techniques. During the administration of epidural anesthesia, it is recommended that a test dose be administered initially and that the patient be monitored for central nervous system toxicity and cardiovascular toxicity, as well as for signs of unintended intrathecal administration, before proceeding. When clinical conditions permit, consideration should be given to employing local anesthetic solutions that contain epinephrine for the test dose because circulatory changes compatible with epinephrine may also serve as a warning sign of unintended intravascular injection. An intravascular injection is still possible even if aspirations for blood are negative. Repeated doses of etidocaine may cause significant increases in blood levels with each repeated dose because of slow accumulation of the drug or its metabolites. Tolerance to elevated blood levels varies with the status of the patient. Debilitated, elderly patients, acutely ill patients, and children should be given reduced doses commensurate with their age and physical condition.

Etidocaine should also be used with caution in patients with severe shock or heart block.

Lumbar and caudal epidural anesthesia should be used with extreme caution in persons with the following conditions: existing neurological disease, spinal deformities, septicemia, and severe hypertension.

Local anesthetic solutions containing a vasoconstrictor should be used cautiously and in carefully circumscribed quantities in areas of the body supplied by end arteries or having otherwise compromised blood supply. Patients with peripheral vascular disease and those with hypertensive vascular disease may exhibit exaggerated vasoconstrictor response. Ischemic injury or necrosis may result. Preparations containing a vasoconstrictor should be used with caution in patients during or following the administration of potent general anesthetic agents, since cardiac arrhythmias may occur under such conditions.

Careful and constant monitoring of cardiovascular and respiratory (adequacy of ventilation) vital signs and the patient's state of consciousness should be accomplished after each local anesthetic injection. It should be kept in mind at such times that restlessness, anxiety, tinnitus, dizziness, blurred vision, tremors, depression or drowsiness may be early warning signs of central nervous system toxicity.

Since amide-type local anesthetics are metabolized by the liver, Duranest Injections should be used with caution in patients with hepatic disease.

Patients with severe hepatic disease, because of their inability to metabolize local anesthetics normally, are at greater risk of developing toxic plasma concentrations. Duranest Injection should also be used with caution in patients with impaired cardiovascular function since they may be less able to compensate for functional changes associated with the prolongation of A-V conduction produced by these drugs.

Many drugs used during the conduct of anesthesia are considered potential triggering agents for familial malignant hyperthermia. Since it is not known whether amide-type local anesthetics may trigger this reaction and since the need for supplemental general anesthesia cannot be predicted in advance, it is suggested that a standard protocol for the management of malignant hyperthermia should be available. Early unexplained signs of tachycardia, tachypnea, labile blood pressure and metabolic acidosis may precede temperature elevation. Successful outcome is dependent on early diagnosis, prompt discontinuance of the suspect triggering agent(s) and institution of treatment, including oxygen therapy, indicated supportive measures and dantrolene (consult dantrolene sodium intravenous package insert before using).

Etidocaine should be used with caution in persons with known drug sensitivities. Patients allergic to para-aminobenzoic acid derivatives (procaine, tetracaine, benzocaine, etc.) have not shown cross sensitivity to etidocaine.

Use in the Head and Neck Area: Small doses of local anesthetics injected into the head and neck area, including retrobulbar, dental and stellate ganglion blocks, may produce adverse reactions similar to systemic toxicity seen with unintentional intravascular injections of larger doses. The injection procedures require the utmost care. Confusion, convulsions, respiratory depression and/or respiratory arrest, and cardiovascular stimulation or depression have been reported. These reactions may be due to intra-arterial injection of the local anesthetic with retrograde flow to the cerebral circulation. They may also be due to puncture of the dural sheath of the optic nerve during retrobulbar block with diffusion of any local anesthetic along the subdural space to the midbrain. Patients receiving these blocks should have their circulation and respiration monitored and be constantly observed. Resuscitative equipment and personnel for treating adverse reactions should be immediately available. Dosage recommendations should not be exceeded. (See DOSAGE AND ADMINISTRATION.)

Table 1. Composition of Available Injections

Product Identification				Formula		
Duranest (etidocaine HCl) Concentration % (mg/mL)		Epinephrine Dilution (as the bitartrate) (mg/mL)	pH	Sodium chloride (mg/mL)	Single Dose Vials/ Dental Cartridge Sodium metabisulfite (mg/mL)	Citric acid (mg/mL)
1.0	(10)	None	4.0–5.0	7.1	None	—
1.0	(10)	1:200,000 (0.005 mg/mL)	3.0–4.5	7.1	0.5	0.2
1.5	(15)	1:200,000 (0.005 mg/mL)	3.0–4.5	6.2	0.5	0.2

NOTE: pH of all solutions adjusted with sodium hydroxide and/or hydrochloric acid. Duranest dental cartridges are only available as 1.5% solution with epinephrine 1:200,000. Filled under nitrogen.

Use in Ophthalmic Surgery: When local anesthetic injections are employed for retrobulbar block, lack of corneal sensation should not be relied upon to determine whether or not the patient is ready for surgery. This is because complete lack of corneal sensation usually precedes clinically acceptable external ocular muscle akinesia.

Use in Dentistry: Because of the long duration of anesthesia, when Duranest 1.5% with epinephrine is used for dental injections, patients should be cautioned about the possibility of inadvertent trauma to tongue, lips and buccal mucosa and advised not to chew solid foods or test the anesthetized area by biting or probing.

Information for Patients: When appropriate, patients should be informed in advance that they may experience temporary loss of sensation and motor activity, usually in the lower half of the body, following proper administration of epidural anesthesia.

Clinically Significant Drug Interactions: The administration of local anesthetic solutions containing epinephrine or norepinephrine to patients receiving monoamine oxidase inhibitors, tricyclic antidepressants or phenothiazines may produce severe, prolonged hypotension or hypertension. Concurrent use of these agents should generally be avoided. In situations when concurrent therapy is necessary, careful patient monitoring is essential.

Concurrent administration of vasopressor drugs (for the treatment of hypotension related to epidural blocks) and ergot-type oxytocic drugs may cause severe, persistent hypertension or cerebrovascular accidents.

Drug Laboratory Test Interactions: The intramuscular injection of etidocaine may result in an increase in creatine phosphokinase levels. Thus, the use of this enzyme determination, without isoenzyme separation, as a diagnostic test for the presence of acute myocardial infarction may be compromised by the intramuscular injection of etidocaine.

Carcinogenesis, Mutagenesis, Impairment of Fertility: Studies of etidocaine in animals to evaluate the carcinogenic and mutagenic potential have not been conducted. Studies in rats at 1.7 times the maximum recommended human dose have revealed no impairment of fertility.

Use in Pregnancy: Teratogenic Effects. Pregnancy Category B. Reproduction studies have been performed in rats and rabbits at doses up to 1.7 times the human dose and have revealed no evidence of harm to the fetus caused by etidocaine. There are, however, no adequate and well-controlled studies in pregnant women. Animal reproduction studies are not always predictive of human response. General consideration should be given to this fact before administering etidocaine to women of childbearing potential, especially during early pregnancy when maximum organogenesis takes place.

Labor and Delivery: Local anesthetics rapidly cross the placenta and when used for epidural, paracervical, pudendal or caudal block anesthesia, can cause varying degrees of maternal, fetal and neonatal toxicity. (See CLINICAL PHARMACOLOGY—Pharmacokinetics.) The incidence and degree of toxicity depend upon the procedure performed, the type and amount of drug used, and the technique of drug administration. Adverse reactions in the parturient, fetus and neonate involve alterations of the central nervous system, peripheral vascular tone and cardiac function.

Maternal hypotension has resulted from regional anesthesia. Local anesthetics produce vasodilation by blocking sympathetic nerves. Elevating the patient's legs and positioning her on her left side will help prevent decreases in blood pressure. The fetal heart rate also should be monitored continuously and electronic fetal monitoring is highly advisable.

Epidural anesthesia may alter the forces of parturition through changes in uterine contractility or maternal expulsive efforts. Because Duranest Injection may produce profound motor block, it is not recommended for epidural anesthesia in normal delivery. Duranest Injection is, however, recommended for epidural anesthesia when caesarean section is to be performed.

The use of some local anesthetic drug products during labor and delivery may be followed by diminished muscle strength and tone for the first day or two of life. The long-term significance of these observations is unknown.

Fetal bradycardia may occur in 20 to 30 percent of patients receiving paracervical nerve block anesthesia with the amide-type local anesthetics and may be associated with fetal acidosis. Fetal heart rate should always be monitored during paracervical anesthesia. The physician should weigh the possible advantages against risks when considering paracervical block in prematurity, toxemia of pregnancy, and fetal distress. Careful adherence to recommended dosage is of the utmost importance in obstetrical paracervical block. Failure to achieve adequate analgesia with recommended doses should arouse suspicion of intravascular or fetal intracranial injection. Cases compatible with unintended fetal intracranial injection of local anesthetic solution have been reported following intended paracervical or pudendal block or both. Babies so affected present with unexplained neonatal depression at birth, which correlates with high local anesthetic serum levels, and often manifest seizures within six hours. Prompt use of supportive measures combined with forced urinary excretion of the local anesthetic has been used successfully to manage this complication. Case reports of maternal convulsions and cardiovascular collapse following use of some local anesthetics for paracervical block in early pregnancy (as anesthesia for elective abortion) suggest that systemic absorption under these circumstances may be rapid. There are inadequate data in support of safe and effective use of etidocaine for obstetrical or non-obstetrical paracervical block, therefore, such use is not recommended.

Nursing Mothers: It is not known whether this drug is excreted in human milk. Because many drugs are excreted in human milk, caution should be exercised when etidocaine is administered to a nursing woman.

Pediatric Use: No information is currently available on appropriate pediatric doses.

ADVERSE REACTIONS

Systemic: Adverse experiences following the administration of etidocaine are similar in nature to those observed with other amide local anesthetic agents. These adverse experiences are, in general, dose-related and may result from high plasma levels caused by excessive dosage, rapid absorption or unintended intravascular injection, or may result from a hypersensitivity, idiosyncrasy or diminished tolerance on the part of the patient. Serious adverse experiences are generally systemic in nature. The following types are those most commonly reported:

Central Nervous System: CNS manifestations are excitatory and/or depressant and may be characterized by lightheadedness, nervousness, apprehension, euphoria, confusion, dizziness, drowsiness, tinnitus, blurred or double vision, vomiting, sensations of heat, cold or numbness, twitching, tremors, convulsions, unconsciousness, respiratory depression and arrest. The excitatory manifestations may be very brief or may not occur at all, in which case the first manifestation of toxicity may be drowsiness merging into unconsciousness and respiratory arrest.

Drowsiness following the administration of etidocaine is usually an early sign of a high blood level of the drug and may occur as a consequence of rapid absorption.

Cardiovascular System: Cardiovascular manifestations are usually depressant and are characterized by bradycardia, hypotension, and cardiovascular collapse, which may lead to cardiac arrest.

Allergic: Allergic reactions are characterized by cutaneous lesions, urticaria, edema or anaphylactoid reactions. Allergic reactions may occur as a result of sensitivity either to local anesthetic agents or to the methylparaben used as a preservative in multiple dose vials. The detection of sensitivity by skin testing is of doubtful value.

Neurologic: The incidences of adverse reactions associated with the use of local anesthetics may be related to the total dose of local anesthetic administered and are also dependent upon the particular drug used, the route of administration and the physical status of the patient.

In the practice of caudal or lumbar epidural block, occasional unintentional penetration of the subarachnoid space by the catheter may occur. Subsequent adverse effects may depend partially on the amount of drug administered subdurally. These may include spinal block of varying magnitude (including total spinal block), hypotension secondary to

Continued on next page

Duranest—Cont.

spinal block, loss of bladder and bowel control, and loss of perineal sensation and sexual function. Persistent motor, sensory and/or autonomic (sphincter control) deficit of some lower spinal segments with slow recovery (several months) or incomplete recovery have been reported in rare instances when caudal or lumbar epidural block has been attempted. Backache and headache have also been noted following use of these anesthetic procedures.
There have been reported cases of permanent injury to extraocular muscles requiring surgical repair following retrobulbar administration.
Other: There have been rare reports of TRISMUS in patients who have received Duranest (etidocaine HCl) for dental anesthesia. Onset of symptoms occurs within hours or days upon resolution of blockade. No correlation has been demonstrated with dosage, administration technique or dental procedure. In most patients, symptoms resolved within days to weeks, although some reports have suggested that symptoms were present for many months. Symptomatic treatment with analgesics, moist heat and physiotherapy was helpful in some cases.

OVERDOSAGE

Acute emergencies from local anesthetics are generally related to high plasma levels encountered during therapeutic use of local anesthetics or to unintended subarachnoid injection of local anesthetic solution (see ADVERSE REACTIONS, WARNINGS, and PRECAUTIONS).
Management of Local Anesthetic Emergencies: The first consideration is prevention, best accomplished by careful and constant monitoring of cardiovascular and respiratory vital signs and the patient's state of consciousness after each local anesthetic injection. At the first sign of change, oxygen should be administered.
The first step in the management of convulsions, as well as underventilation or apnea due to unintentional subarachnoid injection of drug solution, consists of immediate attention to the maintenance of a patent airway and assisted or controlled ventilation with oxygen and a delivery system capable of permitting immediate positive airway pressure by mask. Immediately after the institution of these ventilatory measures, the adequacy of the circulation should be evaluated, keeping in mind that drugs used to treat convulsions sometimes depress the circulation when administered intravenously. Should convulsions persist despite adequate respiratory support, and if the status of the circulation permits, small increments of an ultra-short acting barbiturate (such as thiopental or thiamylal) or a benzodiazepine (such as diazepam) may be administered intravenously. The clinician should be familiar, prior to use of local anesthetics, with these anticonvulsant drugs. Supportive treatment of circulatory depression may require administration of intravenous fluids and, when appropriate, a vasopressor as directed by the clinical situation (e.g., ephedrine).
If not treated immediately, both convulsions and cardiovascular depression can result in hypoxia, acidosis, bradycardia, arrhythmias and cardiac arrest. Underventilation or apnea due to unintentional subarachnoid injection of local anesthetic solution may produce these same signs and also lead to cardiac arrest if ventilatory support is not instituted. If cardiac arrest should occur, standard cardiopulmonary resuscitative measures should be instituted.
Endotracheal intubation, employing drugs and techniques familiar to the clinician, may be indicated, after initial administration of oxygen by mask, if difficulty is encountered in the maintenance of a patent airway or if prolonged ventilatory support (assisted or controlled) is indicated.
Dialysis is of negligible value in the treatment of acute overdosage with etidocaine.
The intravenous LD_{50} of etidocaine HCl in female mice is 7.6 (6.6–8.5) mg/kg and the subcutaneous LD_{50} is 112 (96–166) mg/kg.

DOSAGE AND ADMINISTRATION

As with all local anesthetic agents, the dose of Duranest (etidocaine HCl) Injection to be employed will depend upon the area to be anesthetized, the vascularity of the tissues, the number of neuronal segments to be blocked, the type of regional anesthetic technique, and the physical condition and tolerance of the individual patient.
The maximum dose to be employed as a single injection should be determined on the basis of the status of the patient and the type of regional anesthetic technique to be performed. Although single injections of 450 mg have been employed for regional anesthesia without adverse effects, at present it is strongly recommended that the maximal dose as a single injection should not exceed 400 mg (approximately 8.0 mg/kg or 3.6 mg/lb based on a 50 kg person) with epinephrine 1:200,000 and 300 mg (approximately 6 mg/kg or 2.7 mg/lb based on a 50 kg person) without epinephrine. Because etidocaine has been shown to disappear quite rapidly from blood, toxicity is influenced by rapidity of administration, and therefore, slow injection in vascular areas is highly recommended. Incremental doses of Duranest Injection may be repeated at 2–3 hour intervals.
Caudal and Lumbar Epidural Block: As a precaution against the adverse experiences sometimes observed following unintentional penetration of the subarachnoid space, a test dose of 2–5 mL should be administered at least 5 minutes prior to injecting the total volume required for a lumbar or caudal epidural block. The test dose should be repeated if the patient is moved in a manner that may have displaced the catheter. Epinephrine, if contained in the test dose (10–15 μg have been suggested), may serve as a warning of unintentional intravascular injection. If injected into a blood vessel, this amount of epinephrine is likely to produce a transient "epinephrine response" within 45 seconds, consisting of an increase in heart rate and systolic blood pressure, circumoral pallor, palpitations and nervousness in the unsedated patient. The sedated patient may exhibit only a pulse rate increase of 20 or more beats per minute for 15 or more seconds. Patients on beta-blockers may not manifest changes in heart rate, but blood pressure monitoring can detect an evanescent rise in systolic blood pressure. Adequate time should be allowed for onset of anesthesia after administration of each test dose. The rapid injection of a large volume of Duranest Injection through the catheter should be avoided, and when feasible, fractional doses should be administered.
In the event of the known injection of a large volume of local anesthetic solution into the subarachnoid space, after suitable resuscitation, and if the catheter is in place, consider attempting the recovery of drug by draining a moderate amount of cerebrospinal fluid (such as 10 mL) through the epidural catheter.
Use in Dentistry: When used for local anesthesia in dental procedures the dosage of Duranest (etidocaine HCl) Injection depends on the physical status of the patient, the area of the oral cavity to be anesthetized, the vascularity of the oral tissues, and the technique of anesthesia. The least volume of solution that results in effective local anesthesia should be administered. For specific techniques and procedures of local anesthesia in the oral cavity, refer to standard textbooks.
Dosage requirements should be determined on an individual basis. In maxillary infiltration and/or inferior alveolar nerve block, initial dosages of 1.0–5.0 mL (1/2–2 1/2 cartridges) of Duranest Injection 1.5% with epinephrine 1:200,000 are usually effective.
Aspiration is recommended since it reduces the possibility of intravascular injection, thereby keeping the incidence of side effects and anesthetic failures to a minimum.
The following dosage recommendations are intended as guides for the use of Duranest Injection in the average adult patient. As indicated previously, the dosage should be reduced for elderly or debilitated patients or patients with severe renal disease.

Table 2. Dosage Recommendations

PROCEDURE	Duranest HCl with epinephrine 1:200,000 Conc. (%)	Vol. (mL)	Total Dose (mg)	PROCEDURE	Duranest HCl with epinephrine 1:200,000 Conc. (%)	Vol. (mL)	Total Dose (mg)
Peripheral Nerve Block	1.0	5–40	50–400	Caudal	1.0	10–30	100–300
Central Neural Block Lumbar Peridural				Retrobulbar	1.0 or 1.5	2–4	20–60
Intra-abdominal or Pelvic Surgery Lower Limb Surgery Caesarean Section	1.0 or 1.5	10–30 10–20	100–300 150–300	Maxillary Infiltration and/or inferior Alveolar Nerve Block	1.5	1–5	15–75

Dosage Form and Volume	Duranest Injection Concentration	Epinephrine Dilution (as the bitartrate)	pH	NDC Number
Single Dose Vials* 30 mL	1.0%	None	4.0–5.0	0186-0820-01
	1.0%	1:200,000	3.0–4.5	0186-0825-01
20 mL	1.5%	1:200,000	3.0–4.5	0186-0836-03
Dental Cartridge** 1.8 mL	1.5%	1:200,000	3.0–4.5	0186-0840-14

Solutions containing epinephrine should be protected from light.
*Store at controlled room temperature 15°–30°C (59°–86°F).
**Store at room temperature, approx. 25°C (77°F).

NOTE:
Parenteral drug products should be inspected visually for particulate matter and discoloration prior to administration whenever the solution and container permit. The Injection is not to be used if its color is pinkish or darker than slightly yellow or if it contains a precipitate.
[See table 2 above]

HOW SUPPLIED

[See second table above]
021842R31 Rev. 3/97

EMLA® Anesthetic Disc ℞
(lidocaine 2.5% and prilocaine 2.5% cream)
Topical Adhesive System
EMLA® CREAM
(lidocaine 2.5% and prilocaine 2.5%)

DESCRIPTION

EMLA Cream (lidocaine 2.5% and prilocaine 2.5%) is an emulsion in which the oil phase is a eutectic mixture of lidocaine and prilocaine in a ratio of 1:1 by weight. This eutectic mixture has a melting point below room temperature and therefore both local anesthetics exist as a liquid oil rather than as crystals. It is packaged in 5 gram and 30 gram tubes. It is also packaged in the Anesthetic Disc, which is a single-dose unit of EMLA contained within an occlusive dressing. The Anesthetic Disc is composed of a laminate backing, an absorbent cellulose disc, and an adhesive tape ring. The disc contains 1 gram of EMLA emulsion, the active contact surface being approximately 10 cm^2. The surface area of the entire anesthetic disc is approximately 40 cm^2.
Lidocaine is chemically designated as acetamide, 2-(diethylamino)-N-(2,6-dimethylphenyl), has an octanol:water partition ratio of 43 at pH 7.4, and has the following structure:

CH_3 / $-NH-CO-CH_2-N(C_2H_5)_2$ / CH_3

$C_{14}H_{22}N_2O$ M.W. 234.3

Prilocaine is chemically designated as propanamide, N-(2-methylphenyl)-2-(propylamino), has an octanol:water partition ratio of 25 at pH 7.4, and has the following structure:

CH_3 / $-NH-CO-CH(CH_3)-NH-CH_2-CH_2-CH_3$

$C_{13}H_{20}N_2O$ M.W. 220.3

Each gram of EMLA contains lidocaine 25 mg, prilocaine 25 mg, polyoxyethylene fatty acid esters (as emulsifiers), carboxypolymethylene (as a thickening agent), sodium hydroxide to adjust to a pH approximating 9, and purified water to 1 gram. EMLA contains no preservative, however it passes the USP antimicrobial effectiveness test due to the pH. The specific gravity of EMLA Cream is 1.00.

CLINICAL PHARMACOLOGY

Mechanism of Action: EMLA (lidocaine 2.5% and prilocaine 2.5%), applied to intact skin under occlusive dressing, provides dermal analgesia by the release of lidocaine and prilocaine from the cream into the epidermal and dermal layers of the skin and by the accumulation of lidocaine and prilocaine in the vicinity of dermal pain receptors and nerve endings. Lidocaine and prilocaine are amide-type local anesthetic agents. Both lidocaine and prilocaine stabilize neuronal membranes by inhibiting the ionic fluxes required for the initiation and conduction of impulses, thereby effecting local anesthetic action.

The onset, depth and duration of dermal analgesia provided by EMLA depends primarily on the duration of application. To provide sufficient analgesia for clinical procedures such as intravenous catheter placement and venipuncture, EMLA should be applied under an occlusive dressing for at least 1 hour. To provide dermal analgesia for clinical procedures such as split skin graft harvesting, EMLA should be applied under occlusive dressing for at least 2 hours. Satisfactory dermal analgesia is achieved 1 hour after application, reaches maximum at 2 to 3 hours, and persists for 1 to 2 hours after removal.

Dermal application of EMLA may cause a transient, local blanching followed by a transient, local redness or erythema.

Pharmacokinetics: EMLA is a eutectic mixture of lidocaine 2.5% and prilocaine 2.5% formulated as an oil in water emulsion. In this eutectic mixture, both anesthetics are liquid at room temperature (see DESCRIPTION) and the penetration and subsequent systemic absorption of both prilocaine and lidocaine are enhanced over that which would be seen if each component in crystalline form was applied separately as a 2.5% topical cream.

Absorption—The amount of lidocaine and prilocaine systemically absorbed from EMLA is directly related to both the duration of application and to the area over which it is applied. In two pharmacokinetic studies, 60 g of EMLA Cream (1.5 g lidocaine and 1.5 g prilocaine) was applied to 400 cm^2 of intact skin on the lateral thigh and then covered by an occlusive dressing. The subjects were then randomized such that one-half of the subjects had the occlusive dressing and residual cream removed after 3 hours, while the remainder left the dressing in place for 24 hours. The results from these studies are summarized below.

[See table 1 above]

TABLE 1
Absorption of Lidocaine and Prilocaine from EMLA Cream: Normal Volunteers (N=16)

EMLA (g)	Area (cm^2)	Time on (hrs)	Drug Content (mg)	Absorbed (mg)	Cmax (μg/mL)	Tmax (hr)
60	400	3	lidocaine 1500	54	0.12	4
			prilocaine 1500	92	0.07	4
60	400	24*	lidocaine 1500	243	0.28	10
			prilocaine 1500	503	0.14	10

*Maximum recommended duration of exposure is 4 hours.

When 60 g of EMLA Cream was applied over 400 cm^2 for 24 hours, peak blood levels of lidocaine are approximately 1/20 the systemic toxic level. Likewise, the maximum prilocaine level is about 1/36 the toxic level. In a pharmacokinetic study, EMLA Cream was applied to penile skin in 20 adult male patients in doses ranging from 0.5 g to 3.3 g for 15 minutes. Plasma concentrations of lidocaine and prilocaine following EMLA Cream application in this study were consistently low (2.5–16 ng/mL for lidocaine and 2.5–7 ng/mL for prilocaine). The application of EMLA to broken or inflamed skin, or to 2,000 cm^2 or more of skin where more of both anesthetics are absorbed, could result in higher plasma levels that could, in susceptible individuals, produce a systemic pharmacologic response.

Distribution—When each drug is administered intravenously, the steady-state volume of distribution is 1.1 to 2.1 L/kg (mean 1.5, ±0.3 SD, n=13) for lidocaine and is 0.7 to 4.4 L/kg (mean 2.6, ±1.3 SD, n=13) for prilocaine. The larger distribution volume for prilocaine produces the lower plasma concentrations of prilocaine observed when equal amounts of prilocaine and lidocaine are administered. At concentrations produced by application of EMLA, lidocaine is approximately 70% bound to plasma proteins, primarily alpha-1-acid glycoprotein. At much higher plasma concentrations (1 to 4 μg/mL of free base) the plasma protein binding of lidocaine is concentration dependent. Prilocaine is 55% bound to plasma proteins. Both lidocaine and prilocaine cross the placental and blood brain barrier, presumably by passive diffusion.

Metabolism—It is not known if lidocaine or prilocaine are metabolized in the skin. Lidocaine is metabolized rapidly by the liver to a number of metabolites including monoethylglycinexylidide (MEGX) and glycinexylidide (GX), both of which have pharmacologic activity similar to, but less potent than that of lidocaine. The metabolite, 2,6-xylidine, has unknown pharmacologic activity but is carcinogenic in rats (see Carcinogenesis subsection of PRECAUTIONS). Following intravenous administration, MEGX and GX concentrations in serum range from 11 to 36% and from 5 to 11% of lidocaine concentrations, respectively. Prilocaine is metabolized in both the liver and kidneys by amidases to various metabolites including *ortho*-toluidine and N-n-propylalanine. It is not metabolized by plasma esterases. The *ortho*-toluidine metabolite has been shown to be carcinogenic in several animal models (see Carcinogenesis subsection of PRECAUTIONS). In addition, *ortho*-toluidine can produce methemoglobinemia following systemic doses of prilocaine approximating 8 mg/kg (see ADVERSE REACTIONS). Very young patients, patients with glucose-6-phosphate deficiencies and patients taking oxidizing drugs such as antimalarials and sulfonamides are more susceptible to methemoglobinemia (see Methemoglobinemia subsection of PRECAUTIONS).

Elimination—The half-life of lidocaine elimination from the plasma following IV administration is approximately 65 to 150 minutes (mean 110, ±24 SD, n=13). More than 98% of an absorbed dose of lidocaine can be recovered in the urine as metabolites or parent drug. The systemic clearance is 10 to 20 mL/min/kg (mean 13, ± 3 SD, n=13). The elimination half-life of prilocaine is approximately 10 to 150 minutes (mean 70, ±48 SD, n=13). The systemic clearance is 18 to 64 mL/min/kg (mean 38, ±15 SD, n=13).

Pediatrics: Some pharmacokinetic (PK) data are available in infants (1 month to <2 years old) and children (2 to <12 years old). One PK study was conducted in 9 full-term neonates (mean age: 7 days and mean gestational age: 38.8 weeks). The study results show that neonates had comparable plasma lidocaine and prilocaine concentrations and blood methemoglobin concentrations as those found in previous pediatric PK studies and clinical trials. There was a tendency towards an increase in methemoglobin formation. However, due to assay limitations and very little amount of blood that could be collected from neonates, large variations in the above reported concentrations were found.

Special Populations: No specific PK studies were conducted. The half-life may be increased in cardiac or hepatic dysfunction. Prilocaine's half-life also may be increased in hepatic or renal dysfunction since both of these organs are involved in prilocaine formation.

CLINICAL STUDIES

EMLA Cream application in adults prior to IV cannulation or venipuncture was studied in 200 patients in four clinical studies in Europe. Application for at least 1 hour provided significantly more dermal analgesia than placebo cream or ethyl chloride. EMLA Cream was comparable to subcutaneous lidocaine, but was less efficacious than intradermal lidocaine. Most patients found EMLA Cream treatment preferable to lidocaine infiltration or ethyl chloride spray.

EMLA Cream was compared with 0.5% lidocaine infiltration prior to skin graft harvesting in one open label study in 80 adult patients in England. Application of EMLA Cream for 2 to 5 hours provided dermal analgesia comparable to lidocaine infiltration.

EMLA Cream application in children was studied in seven non-US studies (320 patients) and one US study (100 patients). In controlled studies, application of EMLA Cream for at least 1 hour with or without presurgical medication prior to needle insertion provided significantly more pain reduction than placebo. In children under the age of seven years, EMLA Cream was less effective than in older children or adults.

EMLA Cream was compared with placebo in the laser treatment of facial port-wine stains in 72 pediatric patients (ages 5–16). EMLA Cream was effective in providing pain relief during laser treatment.

EMLA Cream alone was compared to EMLA Cream followed by lidocaine infiltration and lidocaine infiltration alone prior to cryotherapy for the removal of male genital warts. The data from 121 patients demonstrated that EMLA Cream was not effective as a sole anesthetic agent in managing the pain from the surgical procedure. The administration of EMLA Cream prior to lidocaine infiltration provided significant relief of discomfort associated with local anesthetic infiltration and thus was effective in the overall reduction of pain from the procedure only when used in conjunction with local anesthetic infiltration of lidocaine.

EMLA Cream was studied in 105 full term neonates (gestational age: 37 weeks) for blood drawing and circumcision procedures. When considering the use of EMLA in neonates, the primary concerns are the systemic absorption of the active ingredients and the subsequent formation of methemoglobin. In clinical studies performed in neonates, the plasma levels of lidocaine, prilocaine, and methemoglobin were not reported in a range expected to cause clinical symptoms.

Local dermal effects associated with EMLA Cream application in these studies on intact skin included paleness, redness and edema and were transient in nature (see ADVERSE REACTIONS).

Individualization of Dose: The dose of EMLA which provides effective analgesia depends on the duration of the application over the treated area.

All pharmacokinetic and clinical studies employed a thick layer of EMLA Cream (1–2 g/10 cm^2). The duration of application prior to venipuncture was 1 hour. The duration of application prior to taking split thickness skin grafts was 2 hours. Although a thinner application may be efficacious, such has not been studied and may result in less complete analgesia or a shorter duration of adequate analgesia.

The systemic absorption of lidocaine and prilocaine is a side effect of the desired local effect. The amount of drug absorbed depends on surface area and duration of application. The systemic blood levels depend on the amount absorbed and patient size (weight) and rate of systemic drug elimination. Long duration of application, large treatment area, small patients, or impaired elimination may result in high blood levels. The systemic blood levels are typically a small fraction (1/20 to 1/36) of the blood levels which produce toxicity. Table 2 which follows gives maximum recommended doses, application areas and application times for infants and children.

[See table 2 at top of next page]

An IV antiarrhythmic dose of lidocaine is 1 mg/kg (70 mg/70 kg) and gives a blood level of about 1 μg/mL. Toxicity would be expected at blood levels above 5 μg/mL. Smaller areas of treatment are recommended in a debilitated patient, a small child or a patient with impaired elimination. Decreasing the duration of application is likely to decrease the analgesic effect.

INDICATIONS AND USAGE

EMLA (a eutectic mixture of lidocaine 2.5% and prilocaine 2.5%) is indicated as a topical anesthetic for use on **normal intact skin** for local analgesia.

EMLA is not recommended for use on mucous membranes because limited studies show much greater absorption of lidocaine and prilocaine than through intact skin. Safe dosing recommendations for use on mucous membranes cannot be made because it has not been studied adequately.

EMLA is not recommended in any clinical situation in which penetration or migration beyond the tympanic membrane into the middle ear is possible because of the ototoxic effects observed in animal studies (see WARNINGS).

CONTRAINDICATIONS

EMLA (lidocaine 2.5% and prilocaine 2.5%) is contraindicated in patients with a known history of sensitivity to local anesthetics of the amide type or to any other component of the product.

WARNINGS

Application of EMLA to larger areas or for longer times than those recommended could result in sufficient absorption of lidocaine and prilocaine resulting in serious adverse effects (see Individualization of Dose).

Studies in laboratory animals (guinea pigs) have shown that EMLA has an ototoxic effect when instilled into the middle ear. In these same studies, animals exposed to EMLA Cream in the external auditory canal only, showed no abnormality. EMLA should not be used in any clinical situation in which its penetration or migration beyond the tympanic membrane into the middle ear is possible.

Methemoglobinemia: EMLA should not be used in those rare patients with congenital or idiopathic methemoglobinemia and in infants under the age of twelve months who are receiving treatment with methemoglobin-inducing agents. Very young patients or patients with glucose-6-phosphate deficiencies are more susceptible to methemoglobinemia.

Patients taking drugs associated with drug-induced methemoglobinemia such as sulfonamides, acetaminophen, acetanilid, aniline dyes, benzocaine, chloroquine, dapsone, naphthalene, nitrates and nitrites, nitrofurantoin, nitroglycerin, nitroprusside, pamaquine, para-aminosalicylic acid, phenacetin, phenobarbital, phenytoin, primaquine, quinine, are also at greater risk for developing methemoglobinemia.

There have been reports of significant methemoglobinemia (20–30%) in infants and children following excessive applications of EMLA Cream. These cases involved the use of large doses, larger than recommended areas of application, or infants under the age of 3 months who did not have fully mature enzyme systems. In addition, a few of these cases involved the concomitant administration of methemoglobin-inducing agents. Most patients recovered spontaneously after removal of the cream. Treatment with IV methylene blue may be effective if required.

Physicians are cautioned to make sure that parents or other caregivers understand the need for careful application of EMLA, to ensure that the doses and areas of application recommended in Table 2 are not exceeded (especially in children under the age of 3 months) and to limit the period of application to the minimum required to achieve the desired anesthesia.

PRECAUTIONS

General: Repeated doses of EMLA may increase blood levels of lidocaine and prilocaine. EMLA should be used with caution in patients who may be more sensitive to the systemic effects of lidocaine and prilocaine including acutely ill, debilitated, or elderly patients.

EMLA coming in contact with the eye should be avoided because animal studies have demonstrated severe eye irritation. Also the loss of protective reflexes can permit corneal irritation and potential abrasion. Absorption of EMLA in conjunctival tissues has not been determined. If eye contact occurs, immediately wash out the eye with water or saline and protect the eye until sensation returns.

Patients allergic to para-aminobenzoic acid derivatives (procaine, tetracaine, benzocaine, etc.) have not shown cross sensitivity to lidocaine and/or prilocaine, however, EMLA should be used with caution in patients with a history of drug sensitivities, especially if the etiologic agent is uncertain.

Continued on next page

Emla—Cont.

Patients with severe hepatic disease, because of their inability to metabolize local anesthetics normally, are at greater risk of developing toxic plasma concentrations of lidocaine and prilocaine.
Lidocaine and prilocaine have been shown to inhibit viral and bacterial growth. The effect of EMLA on **intradermal** injections of **live** vaccines has not been determined.
Information for Patients: When EMLA is used, the patient should be aware that the production of dermal analgesia may be accompanied by the block of all sensations in the treated skin. For this reason, the patient should avoid inadvertent trauma to the treated area by scratching, rubbing, or exposure to extreme hot or cold temperatures until complete sensation has returned.
Drug Interactions: EMLA should be used with caution in patients receiving Class I antiarrhythmic drugs (such as tocainide and mexiletine) since the toxic effects are additive and potentially synergistic.
Prilocaine may contribute to the formation of methemoglobin in patients treated with other drugs known to cause this condition (see Methemoglobinemia subsection of WARNINGS).
Carcinogenesis, Mutagenesis, Impairment of Fertility:
Carcinogenesis—Metabolites of both lidocaine and prilocaine have been shown to be carcinogenic in laboratory animals. In the animal studies reported below, doses or blood levels are compared to the Single Dermal Administration (SDA) of 60 g of EMLA Cream to 400 cm^2 for 3 hours to a small person (50 kg). The typical application of EMLA Cream for one or two treatments for venipuncture sites (2.5 or 5 g) would be 1/24 or 1/12 of that dose in an adult or about the same mg/kg dose in an infant. The typical application of EMLA Anesthetic Disc for one or two treatments for venipuncture sites (1 or 2 g) would be 1/60 or 1/30 of that dose in an adult or about half the mg/kg dose in an infant.
A two-year oral toxicity study of 2,6-xylidine, a metabolite of lidocaine, has shown that in both male and female rats 2,6-xylidine in daily doses of 900 mg/m^2 (60 times SDA) resulted in carcinomas and adenomas of the nasal cavity. With daily doses of 300 mg/m^2 (20 times SDA), the increase in incidence of nasal carcinomas and/or adenomas in each sex of the rat were not statistically greater than the control group. In the low dose (90 mg/m^2; 6 times SDA) and control groups, no nasal tumors were observed. A rhabdomyosarcoma, a rare tumor, was observed in the nasal cavity of both male and female rats at the high dose of 900 mg/m^2. In addition, the compound caused subcutaneous fibromas and/or fibrosarcomas in both male and female rats and neoplastic nodules of the liver in the female rats with a significantly positive trend test; pairwise comparisons using Fisher's Exact Test showed significance only at the high dose of 900 mg/m^2. The animal study was conducted at oral doses of 15, 50, and 150 mg/kg/day. The dosages have been converted to mg/m^2 for the SDA calculations above.
Chronic oral toxicity studies of *ortho*-toluidine, a metabolite of prilocaine, in mice (900 to 14,400 mg/m^2; 60 to 960 times SDA) and rats (900 to 4,800 mg/m^2; 60 to 320 times SDA) have shown that *ortho*-toluidine is a carcinogen in both species. The tumors included hepatocarcinomas/adenomas in female mice, multiple occurrences of hemangiosarcomas/hemangiomas in both sexes of mice, sarcomas of multiple organs, transitional-cell carcinomas/papillomas of urinary bladder in both sexes of rats, subcutaneous fibromas/fibrosarcomas and mesotheliomas in male rats, and mammary gland fibroadenomas/adenomas in female rats. The lowest dose tested (900 mg/m^2; 60 times SDA) was carcinogenic in both species. Thus the no-effect dose must be less than 60 times SDA. The animal studies were conducted at 150 to 2,400 mg/kg in mice and at 150 to 800 mg/kg in rats. The dosages have been converted to mg/m^2 for the SDA calculations above.
Mutagenesis—The mutagenic potential of lidocaine HCl has been tested in the Ames Salmonella/mammalian microsome test and by analysis of structural chromosome aberrations in human lymphocytes *in vitro*, and by the mouse micronucleus test *in vivo*. There was no indication in these three tests of any mutagenic effects.
The mutagenicity of 2,6-xylidine, a metabolite of lidocaine, has been studied in different tests with mixed results. The compound was found to be weakly mutagenic in the Ames test only under metabolic activation conditions. In addition, 2,6-xylidine was observed to be mutagenic at the thymidine kinase locus, with or without activation, and induced chromosome aberrations and sister chromatid exchanges at concentrations at which the drug precipitated out of the solution (1.2 mg/mL). No evidence of genotoxicity was found in the *in vivo* assays measuring unscheduled DNA synthesis in rat hepatocytes, chromosome damage in polychromatic erythrocytes or preferential killing of DNA repair-deficient bacteria in liver, lung, kidney, testes and blood extracts from mice. However, covalent binding studies of DNA from liver and ethmoid turbinates in rats indicate that 2,6-xylidine may be genotoxic under certain conditions *in vivo*.
Ortho-toluidine, a metabolite of prilocaine, (0.5 μg/mL) showed positive results in *Escherichia coli* DNA repair and phage-induction assays. Urine concentrates from rats treated with *ortho*-toluidine (300 mg/kg orally; 300 times SDA) were mutagenic for *Salmonella typhimurium* with metabolic activation. Several other tests on *ortho*-toluidine, including reverse mutations in five different *Salmonella typhimurium* strains with or without metabolic activation and with single strand breaks in DNA of V79 Chinese hamster cells, were negative.
Impairment of Fertility—See Use in Pregnancy.

TABLE 2
EMLA MAXIMUM RECOMMENDED DOSE, APPLICATION AREA, AND APPLICATION TIME BY AGE AND WEIGHT*
For Infants and Children Based on Application to Intact Skin

Age and Body Weight Requirements	Maximum Total Dose of EMLA	Maximum Application Area**	Maximum Applicaton Time
0 up to 3 months or <5 kg	1 g	10 cm^2	1 hour
3 up to 12 months and >5 kg	2 g	20 cm^2	4 hours
1 to 6 years and >10 kg	10 g	100 cm^2	4 hours
7 to 12 years and >20 kg	20 g	200 cm^2	4 hours

Please note: If a patient greater than 3 months old does not meet the minimum weight requirement, the maximum total dose of EMLA should be restricted to that which corresponds to the patient's **weight.**
* These are broad guidelines for avoiding systemic toxicity in applying EMLA to patients with normal intact skin and with normal renal and hepatic function.
** For more individualized calculation of how much lidocaine and prilocaine may be absorbed, physicians can use the following estimates of lidocaine and prilocaine absorption for children and adults:
The estimated mean (±SD) absorption of lidocaine is 0.045 (±0.016) mg/cm^2/hr.
The estimated mean (±SD) absorption of prilocaine is 0.077 (±0.036) mg/cm^2/hr.

Age and Body Weight Requirements	Maximum Total Dose of EMLA	Maximum Application Area	Maximum Application Time
0 up to 3 months or < 5 kg	1 g	10 cm^2	1 hour
3 up to 12 months and > 5 kg	2 g	20 cm^2	4 hours
1 to 6 years and > 10 kg	10 g	100 cm^2	4 hours
7 to 12 years and > 20 kg	20 g	200 cm^2	4 hours

Use in Pregnancy: Teratogenic Effects: Pregnancy Category B.
Reproduction studies with lidocaine have been performed in rats and have revealed no evidence of harm to the fetus (30 mg/kg subcutaneously; 22 times SDA). Reproduction studies with prilocaine have been performed in rats and have revealed no evidence of impaired fertility or harm to the fetus (300 mg/kg intramuscularly; 188 times SDA). There are, however, no adequate and well-controlled studies in pregnant women. Because animal reproduction studies are not always predictive of human response, EMLA should be used during pregnancy only if clearly needed.
Reproduction studies have been performed in rats receiving subcutaneous administration of an aqueous mixture containing lidocaine HCl and prilocaine HCl at 1:1 (w/w). At 40 mg/kg each, a dose equivalent to 29 times SDA lidocaine and 25 times SDA prilocaine, no teratogenic, embryotoxic or fetotoxic effects were observed.
Labor and Delivery: Neither lidocaine nor prilocaine are contraindicated in labor and delivery. Should EMLA be used concomitantly with other products containing lidocaine and/or prilocaine, total doses contributed by all formulations must be considered.
Nursing Mothers: Lidocaine, and probably prilocaine, are excreted in human milk. Therefore, caution should be exercised when EMLA is administered to a nursing mother since the milk:plasma ratio of lidocaine is 0.4 and is not determined for prilocaine.
Pediatric Use: Controlled studies of EMLA Cream in children under the age of seven years have shown less overall benefit than in older children or adults. These results illustrate the importance of emotional and psychological support of younger children undergoing medical or surgical procedures.
EMLA should be used with care in patients with conditions or therapy associated with methemoglobinemia (see Methemoglobinemia subsection of WARNINGS).
When using EMLA in young children, especially infants under the age of 3 months, care must be taken to insure that the caregiver understands the need to limit the dose and area of application, and to prevent accidental ingestion (see DOSAGE AND ADMINISTRATION and Methemoglobinemia).
In neonates (minimum gestation age: 37 weeks) and children weighing less than 20 kg, the area and duration of application should be limited (see TABLE 2 in Individualization of Dose).

ADVERSE REACTIONS

Localized Reactions: During or immediately after treatment with EMLA, the skin at the site of treatment may develop erythema or edema or may be the locus of abnormal sensation. Rare cases of discrete purpuric or petechial reactions at the application site have been reported. Rare cases of hyperpigmentation following the use of EMLA Cream have been reported. The relationship to EMLA Cream or the underlying procedure has not been established. In clinical studies involving over 1,300 EMLA Cream-treated subjects, one or more such local reactions were noted in 56% of patients, and were generally mild and transient, resolving spontaneously within 1 or 2 hours. There were no serious reactions which were ascribed to EMLA Cream.
In patients treated with EMLA Cream, local effects observed in the trials included: paleness (pallor or blanching) 37%, redness (erythema) 30%, alterations in temperature sensations 7%, edema 6%, itching 2% and rash, less than 1%.
Allergic Reactions: Allergic and anaphylactoid reactions associated with lidocaine or prilocaine can occur. They are characterized by urticaria, angioedema, bronchospasm, and shock. If they occur they should be managed by conventional means. The detection of sensitivity by skin testing is of doubtful value.
Systemic (Dose Related) Reactions: Systemic adverse reactions following appropriate use of EMLA are unlikely due to the small dose absorbed (see Pharmacokinetics subsection of CLINICAL PHARMACOLOGY). Systemic adverse effects of lidocaine and/or prilocaine are similar in nature to those observed with other amide local anesthetic agents including CNS excitation and/or depression (light-headedness, nervousness, apprehension, euphoria, confusion, dizziness, drowsiness, tinnitus, blurred or double vision, vomiting, sensations of heat, cold or numbness, twitching, tremors, convulsions, unconsciousness, respiratory depression and arrest). Excitatory CNS reactions may be brief or not occur at all, in which case the first manifestation may be drowsiness merging into unconsciousness. Cardiovascular manifestations may include bradycardia, hypotension and cardiovascular collapse leading to arrest.

OVERDOSAGE

Peak blood levels following a 60 g application to 400 cm^2 for 3 hours are 0.05 to 0.16 μg/mL for lidocaine and 0.02 to 0.10μg/mL for prilocaine. Toxic levels of lidocaine (>5 μg/mL) and/or prilocaine (>6 μg/mL) cause decreases in cardiac output, total peripheral resistance and mean arterial pressure. These changes may be attributable to direct depressant effects of these local anesthetic agents on the cardiovascular system. In the absence of massive topical overdose or oral ingestion, evaluation should include evaluation of other etiologies for the clinical effects or overdosage from other sources of lidocaine, prilocaine or other local anesthetics. Consult the package inserts for parenteral Xylocaine (lidocaine HCl) or Citanest (prilocaine HCl) for further information for the management of overdose.

DOSAGE AND ADMINISTRATION

Adult Patients
EMLA Cream and Anesthetic Disc
A thick layer of EMLA Cream is applied to intact skin and covered with an occlusive dressing, or alternatively, an EMLA Anesthetic Disc is applied to intact skin:
Minor Dermal Procedures: For minor procedures such as intravenous cannulation and venipuncture, apply 2.5 grams of EMLA Cream (1/2 the 5 g tube) over 20 to 25 cm^2 of skin surface, or 1 EMLA Anesthetic Disc (1g over 10 cm^2) for at least 1 hour. In controlled clinical trials using EMLA Cream, two sites were usually prepared in case there was a technical problem with cannulation or venipuncture at the first site.
EMLA Cream
A thick layer of EMLA Cream is applied to intact skin and covered with an occlusive dressing:
Major Dermal Procedures: For more painful dermatological procedures involving a larger skin area such as split thickness skin graft harvesting, apply 2 grams of EMLA Cream per 10 cm^2 of skin and allow to remain in contact with the skin for at least 2 hours.
Adult Male Genital Skin: As an adjunct prior to local anesthetic infiltration, apply a thick layer of EMLA Cream (1 g/10 cm^2) to the skin surface for 15 minutes. Local anesthetic infiltration should be performed immediately after removal of EMLA Cream.
Dermal analgesia can be expected to increase for up to 3 hours under occlusive dressing and persist for 1 to 2 hours after removal of the cream. The amount of lidocaine and prilocaine absorbed during the period of application can be estimated from the information in Table 2, ** footnote, in Individualization of Dose.
Pediatric Patients
The following are the maximum recommended doses, application areas and application times for EMLA based on a child's age and weight:
[See second table above]

Please note: If a patient greater than 3 months old does not meet the minimum weight requirement, the maximum total dose of EMLA should be restricted to that which corresponds to the patient's **weight**.
Practitioners should carefully instruct caregivers to avoid application of excessive amounts of EMLA (see PRECAUTIONS).
When applying EMLA to the skin of young children, care must be taken to maintain careful observation of the child to prevent accidental ingestion of EMLA, the occlusive dressing, or the anesthetic disc. A secondary protective covering to prevent inadvertent disruption of the application site may be useful.
EMLA should not be used in neonates with a gestational age less than 37 weeks nor in infants under the age of twelve months who are receiving treatment with methemoglobin-inducing agents (see Methemoglobinemia subsection of WARNINGS).
When EMLA (lidocaine 2.5% and prilocaine 2.5%) is used concomitantly with other products containing local anesthetic agents, the amount absorbed from all formulations must be considered (see Individualization of Dose). The amount absorbed in the case of EMLA is determined by the area over which it is applied and the duration of application under occlusion (see Table 2, ** footnote, in Individualization of Dose).
Although the incidence of systemic adverse reactions with EMLA is very low, caution should be exercised, particularly when applying it over large areas and leaving it on for longer than 2 hours. The incidence of systemic adverse reactions can be expected to be directly proportional to the area and time of exposure (see Individualization of Dose).

HOW SUPPLIED

EMLA Cream is available as the following:
NDC 0186-1515-01 5 gram tube, box of 1, contains 2 Tegaderm® dressings (6 cm × 7 cm)
NDC 0186-1515-01
Product No. 0186-1515-03 5 gram tube, box of 5, contains 12 Tegaderm® dressings (6 cm × 7 cm)
NDC 0186-1516-01 30 gram tube, box of 1
EMLA Anesthetic Disc is available in the following:
NDC 0186-1512-70 1 gram Anesthetic Disc, box of 2
NDC 0186-1512-70
Product No. 0186-1512-71 1 gram Anesthetic Disc, box of 10
NOT FOR OPHTHALMIC USE.
KEEP CONTAINER TIGHTLY CLOSED AT ALL TIMES WHEN NOT IN USE.
Store at controlled room temperature 15–30°C (59–86°F).
EMLA Anesthetic Disc manufactured by:
Astra Pharmaceutical Production, AB
Södertälje, Sweden
EMLA Cream manufactured by:
Astra Pharmaceuticals, L.P., Wayne, PA 19087

INSTRUCTIONS FOR APPLICATION

EMLA®
Anesthetic Disc
(lidocaine 2.5% and prilocaine 2.5% cream)
Topical Adhesive System

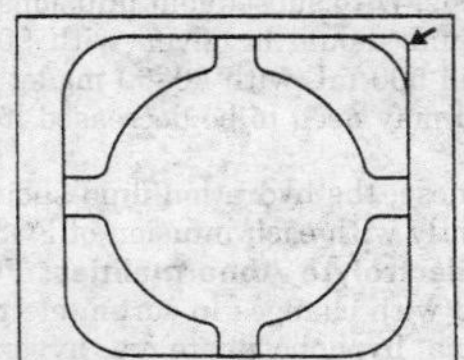

1. Make sure that the area to be anesthetized is clean and dry. Take hold of the aluminum flap at the corner of the Anesthetic Disc and bend it backwards. Next, take hold of the corner of the beige-colored Anesthetic Disc layer.

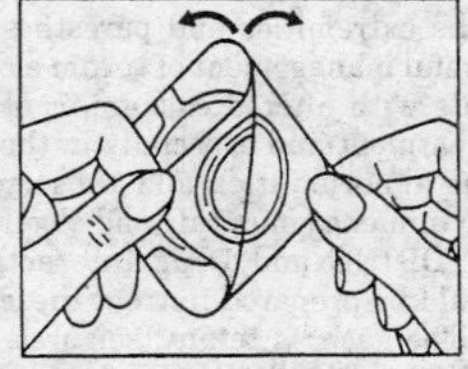

2. Pull the two layers apart, separating the adhesive surface from the protective liner, as shown. Make sure that you do not touch the white, round disc, which contains EMLA.

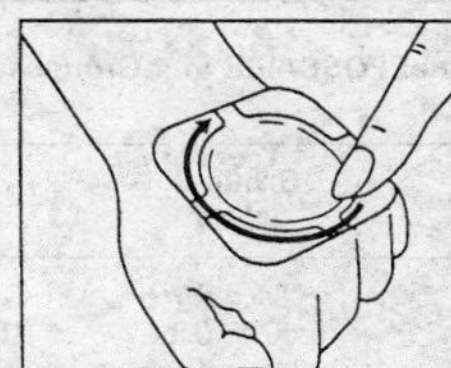

3. Press firmly around the *edges* of the Anesthetic Disc to ensure good adhesion to the skin. **Do not press on the center of the Anesthetic Disc.** This may cause EMLA to spread under the adhesive.

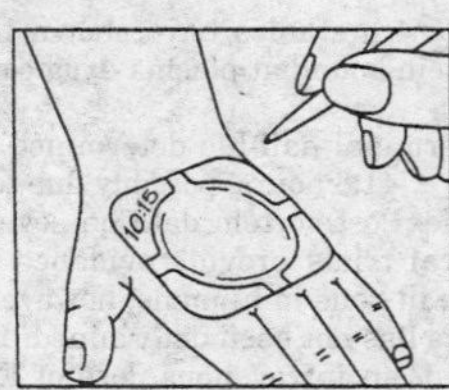

4. The time of application may be easily marked along the border of the Anesthetic Disc. (A ballpoint pen may be used for this purpose.)
EMLA Anesthetic Disc must be applied at least **one hour** before the start of a procedure.
PRECAUTIONS
1. Do not apply near eyes or on open wounds.
2. Keep out of reach of children.

Manufactured by: Astra Pharmaceutical Production, AB
Södertälje, Sweden
Manufactured for:
Astra Pharmaceuticals, L.P., Wayne, PA 19087
021792R03 Rev. 4/99

INSTRUCTIONS FOR APPLICATION

EMLA®
CREAM (lidocaine 2.5% and prilocaine 2.5%)

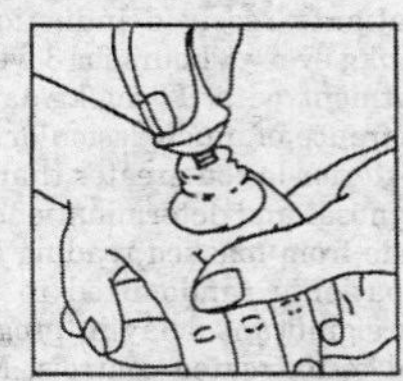

1. In adults, apply 2.5 g of cream (1/2 the 5 g tube) per 20 to 25 cm^2 (approx. 2 in. by 2 in.) of skin in a thick layer at the site of the procedure. For pediatric patients, apply ONLY as prescribed by your physician. If your child is below the age of 3 months or small for their age, please inform your doctor before applying EMLA, which can be harmful, if applied over too much skin at one time in young children.
If your child becomes very dizzy, excessively sleepy, or develops duskiness of the face or lips after applying EMLA, remove the cream and contact your physician at once.

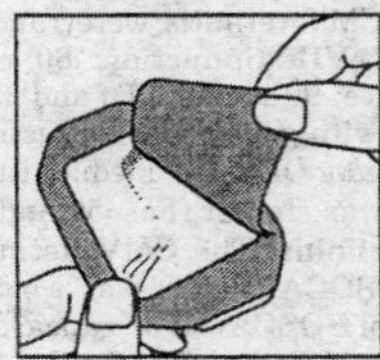

2. Take an occlusive dressing (provided with the 5 g tubes only) and remove the center cut-out piece.

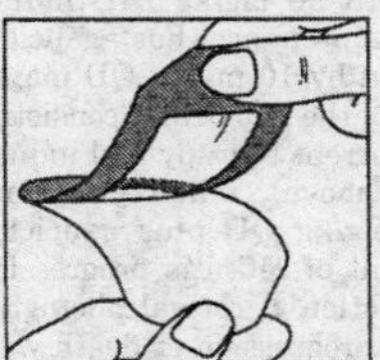

3. Peel the paper liner from the paper framed dressing.

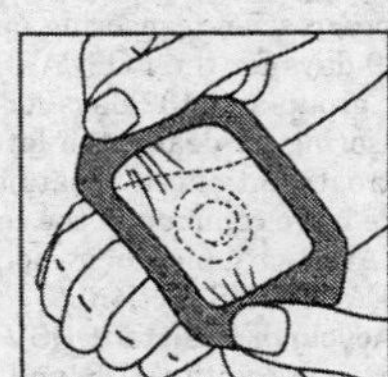

4. Cover the EMLA® Cream so that you get a thick layer underneath. Do not spread out the cream. Smooth down the dressing edges carefully and ensure it is secure to avoid leakage. (This is especially important when the patient is a child.)

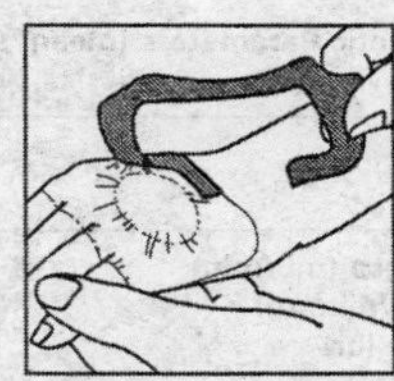

5. Remove the paper frame. The time of application can easily be marked directly on the occlusive dressing. EMLA® must be applied at least 1 hour before the start of a routine procedure and for 2 hours before the start of a painful procedure.

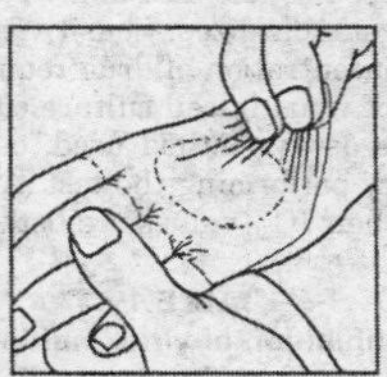

6. Remove the occlusive dressing, wipe off the EMLA® Cream, clean the entire area with an antiseptic solution and prepare the patient for the procedure. The duration of effective skin anesthesia will be at least 1 hour after removal of the occlusive dressing.
PRECAUTIONS
1. Do not apply near eyes or on open wounds.
2. Keep out of reach of children.

Astra Pharmaceuticals, L.P., Wayne, PA 19087
021700R04 Rev. 7/99
Shown in Product Identification Guide, page 304

FOSCAVIR® (foscarnet sodium) Injection ℞

WARNING
RENAL IMPAIRMENT IS THE MAJOR TOXICITY OF FOSCAVIR. FREQUENT MONITORING OF SERUM CREATININE, WITH DOSE ADJUSTMENT FOR CHANGES IN RENAL FUNCTION, AND ADEQUATE HYDRATION WITH ADMINISTRATION OF FOSCAVIR, IS IMPERATIVE. (See ADMINISTRATION section; Hydration.)
SEIZURES, RELATED TO ALTERATIONS IN PLASMA MINERALS AND ELECTROLYTES, HAVE BEEN ASSOCIATED WITH FOSCAVIR TREATMENT. THEREFORE, PATIENTS MUST BE CAREFULLY MONITORED FOR SUCH CHANGES AND THEIR POTENTIAL SEQUELAE. MINERAL AND ELECTROLYTE SUPPLEMENTATION MAY BE REQUIRED.
FOSCAVIR IS INDICATED FOR USE ONLY IN IMMUNOCOMPROMISED PATIENTS WITH CMV RETINITIS AND MUCOCUTANEOUS ACYCLOVIR-RESISTANT HSV INFECTIONS. (See INDICATIONS section.)

DESCRIPTION

FOSCAVIR is the brand name for foscarnet sodium. The chemical name of foscarnet sodium is phosphonoformic acid, trisodium salt. Foscarnet sodium is a white, crystalline powder containing 6 equivalents of water of hydration with an empirical formula of $Na_3CO_5P \bullet 6\ H_20$ and a molecular weight of 300.1. The structural formula is:

$$3\ Na^+ \left[{}^{-}O-\overset{\displaystyle O}{\overset{\|}{P}}-\overset{\displaystyle O}{\overset{\|}{C}} \atop \quad\;\; O^- \qquad O^- \right] \bullet 6\ H_2O$$

FOSCAVIR has the potential to chelate divalent metal ions, such as calcium and magnesium, to form stable coordination compounds. FOSCAVIR INJECTION is a sterile, isotonic aqueous solution for intravenous administration only. The solution is clear and colorless. Each milliliter of FOSCAVIR contains 24 mg of foscarnet sodium hexahydrate in Water for Injection, USP. Hydrochloric acid and/or sodium hydroxide may have been added to adjust the pH of the solution to 7.4. FOSCAVIR INJECTION contains no preservatives.

VIROLOGY

Mechanism of Action: FOSCAVIR is an organic analogue of inorganic pyrophosphate that inhibits replication of herpesviruses *in vitro* including cytomegalovirus (CMV) and herpes simplex virus types 1 and 2 (HSV-1 and HSV-2).
FOSCAVIR exerts its antiviral activity by a selective inhibition at the pyrophosphate binding site on virus-specific DNA polymerases at concentrations that do not affect cellular DNA polymerases. FOSCAVIR does not require activation (phosphorylation) by thymidine kinase or other kinases and therefore is active *in vitro* against HSV TK deficient mutants and CMV UL97 mutants. Thus, HSV strains resistant to acyclovir or CMV strains resistant to ganciclovir may be sensitive to FOSCAVIR. However, acyclovir or ganciclovir resistant mutants with alterations in the viral DNA polymerase may be resistant to FOSCAVIR and may not respond to therapy with FOSCAVIR. The combination of FOSCAVIR and ganciclovir has been shown to have enhanced activity *in vitro*.
Antiviral Activity *in vitro* and *in vivo*: The quantitative relationship between the *in vitro* susceptibility of human cytomegalovirus (CMV) or herpes simplex virus 1 and 2 (HSV-1 and HSV-2) to FOSCAVIR and clinical response to

Continued on next page

Foscavir—Cont.

therapy has not been established and virus sensitivity testing has not been standardized. Sensitivity test results, expressed as the concentration of drug required to inhibit by 50% the growth of virus in cell culture (IC_{50}), vary greatly depending on the assay method used, cell type employed and the laboratory performing the test. A number of sensitive viruses and their IC_{50} values are listed below (Table 1).

TABLE 1
FOSCARNET Inhibition of virus multiplication in cell culture

Virus	IC_{50} (μM)
CMV	50–800*
HSV-1, HSV-2	10–130
Ganciclovir resistant CMV	190
HSV-TK negative mutant	67
HSV-DNA polymerase mutants	5–443

* Mean = 269 μM

Statistically significant decreases in positive CMV cultures from blood and urine have been demonstrated in two studies (FOS-03 and ACTG-015/915) of patients treated with FOSCAVIR. Although median time to progression of CMV retinitis was increased in patients treated with FOSCAVIR, reductions in positive blood or urine cultures have not been shown to correlate with clinical efficacy in individual patients.

TABLE 2
BLOOD AND URINE CULTURE RESULTS FROM CMV RETINITIS PATIENTS*

Blood	+CMV	−CMV
Baseline	27	34
End of Induction**	1	60
Urine	**+CMV**	**−CMV**
Baseline	52	6
End of Induction**	21	37

* A total of 77 patients was treated with FOSCAVIR in two clinical trials (FOS-03 and ACTG-015/915). Not all patients had blood or urine cultures done and some patients had results from both cultures.
** (60 mg/kg FOSCAVIR TID for 2–3 weeks).

Resistance: Strains of both HSV and CMV that are resistant to FOSCAVIR can be readily selected *in vitro* by passage of wild type virus in the presence of increasing concentrations of the drug. All FOSCAVIR resistant mutants are known to be generated through mutation in the viral DNA polymerase gene. CMV strains with double mutations conferring resistance to both FOSCAVIR and ganciclovir have been isolated from patients with AIDS. The possibility of viral resistance should be considered in patients who show poor clinical response or experience persistent viral excretion during therapy.

CLINICAL PHARMACOLOGY

Pharmacokinetics: The pharmacokinetics of foscarnet have been determined after administration as an intermittent intravenous infusion during induction therapy in AIDS patients with CMV retinitis. Observed plasma foscarnet concentrations in four studies (FOS-01, ACTG-015, FP48PK, FP49PK) are summarized in Table 3:

TABLE 3
Foscarnet Pharmacokinetic Characteristics*

Parameter	60 mg/kg Q8h	90 mg/kg Q12h
C_{max} at steady-state (μM)	589 ± 192 (24)	623 ± 132 (19)
C_{trough} at steady-state (μM)	114 ± 91 (24)	63 ± 57 (17)
Volume of distribution (L/kg)	0.41 ± 0.13 (12)	0.52 ± 0.20 (18)
Plasma half-life (hr)	4.0 ± 2.0 (24)	3.3 ± 1.4 (18)
Systemic clearance (L/hr)	6.2 ± 2.1 (24)	7.1 ± 2.7 (18)
Renal clearance (L/hr)	5.6 ± 1.9 (5)	6.4 ± 2.5 (13)
CSF:plasma ratio	0.69 ± 0.19 (9)†	0.66 ± 0.11 (5)‡

* Values expressed as mean ± S.D. (number of subjects studied) for each parameter
† 50 mg/kg Q8h for 28 days, samples taken 3 hrs after end of 1 hr infusion (Astra Report 815-04 AC025-1)
‡ 90 mg/kg Q12h for 28 days, samples taken 1 hr after end of 2 hr infusion (Hengge et al., 1993)

Distribution: *In vitro* studies have shown that 14–17% of foscarnet is protein bound at plasma drug concentrations of 1–1000 μM.

The foscarnet terminal half-life determined by urinary excretion was 87.5 ± 41.8 hours, possibly due to release of foscarnet from bone. Postmortem data on several patients in European clinical trials provide evidence that foscarnet does accumulate in bone in humans; however, the extent to which this occurs has not been determined. In animal studies (mice), 40% of an intravenous dose of FOSCAVIR was deposited in bone in young animals and 7% was deposited in adult animals.

Special Populations:

Adults with Impaired Renal Function—The pharmacokinetic properties of foscarnet have been determined in a small group of adult subjects with normal and impaired renal function, as summarized in Table 4:

[See table 4 below]

Total systemic clearance (CL) of foscarnet decreased and half-life increased with diminishing renal function (as expressed by creatinine clearance). Based on these observations, it is necessary to modify the dosage of foscarnet in patients with renal impairment (see DOSAGE AND ADMINISTRATION).

CLINICAL TRIALS

CMV Retinitis: A prospective, randomized, controlled clinical trial (FOS-03) was conducted in 24 patients with AIDS and CMV retinitis comparing treatment with FOSCAVIR to no treatment. Patients received induction treatment of FOSCAVIR, 60 mg/kg every 8 hours for 3 weeks, followed by maintenance treatment with 90 mg/kg/day until retinitis progression (appearance of a new lesion or advancement of the border of a posterior lesion greater than 750 microns in diameter). All diagnoses and determinations of retinitis progression were made from masked reading of retinal photographs. The 13 patients randomized to treatment with FOSCAVIR had a significant delay in progression of CMV retinitis compared to untreated controls. Median times to retinitis progression from study entry were 93 days (range 21– >364) and 22 days (range 7–42), respectively.

In another prospective clinical trial of CMV retinitis in patients with AIDS (ACTG-915), 33 patients were treated with two to three weeks of FOSCAVIR induction (60 mg/kg TID) and then randomized to either 90 mg/kg/day or 120 mg/kg/day maintenance therapy. The median times from study entry to retinitis progression were not significantly different between the treatment groups, 96 (range 14– >176) days and 140 (range 16– >233) days, respectively. In study ACTG 129/FGCRT SOCA study 107 patients with newly diagnosed CMV retinitis were randomized to treatment with FOSCAVIR (induction: 60 mg/kg TID for 2 weeks; maintenance: 90 mg/kg QD) and 127 were randomized to treatment with ganciclovir (induction: 5 mg/kg BID; maintenance: 5 mg/kg QD). The median time to progression on the two drugs was similar (Fos=59 and Gcv=56 days).

Relapsed CMV Retinitis: The CMV Retinitis Retreatment Trial (ACTG 228/SOCA CRRT) was a randomized, open-label comparison of FOSCAVIR or ganciclovir monotherapy to the combination of both drugs for the treatment of persistently active or relapsed CMV retinitis in patients with AIDS. Subjects were randomized to one of the three treatments: FOSCAVIR 90 mg/kg BID induction followed by 120 mg/kg QD maintenance (Fos); ganciclovir 5 mg/kg BID induction followed by 10 mg/kg QD maintenance (Gcv); or the combination of the two drugs, consisting of continuation of the subject's current therapy and induction dosing of the other drug (as above), followed by maintenance with FOSCAVIR 90 mg/kg QD plus ganciclovir 5 mg/kg QD (Cmb). Assessment of retinitis progression was performed by masked evaluation of retinal photographs. The median times to retinitis progression or death were 39 days for the FOSCAVIR group, 61 days for the ganciclovir group and 105 days for the combination group. For the alternative endpoint of retinitis progression (censoring on death), the median times were 39 days for the FOSCAVIR group, 61 days for the ganciclovir group and 132 days for the combination group. Due to censoring on death, the latter analysis may overestimate the treatment effect. Treatment modifications due to toxicity were more common in the combination group than in the FOSCAVIR or ganciclovir monotherapy groups (see ADVERSE REACTIONS section).

Mucocutaneous Acyclovir-Resistant HSV Infections: In a controlled trial, patients with AIDS and mucocutaneous, acyclovir-resistant HSV infection were randomized to either FOSCAVIR (N=8) at a dose of 40 mg/kg TID or vidarabine (N=6) at a dose of 15 mg/kg per day. Eleven patients were non-randomly assigned to receive treatment with FOSCAVIR because of prior intolerance to vidarabine. Lesions in the eight patients randomized to FOSCAVIR healed after 11 to 25 days; seven of the 11 patients non-randomly treated with FOSCAVIR healed their lesions in 10 to 30 days. Vidarabine was discontinued because of intolerance (N=4) or poor therapeutic response (N=2). In a second trial, forty AIDS patients and three bone marrow transplant recipients with mucocutaneous, acyclovir-resistant HSV infections were randomized to receive FOSCAVIR at a dose of either 40 mg/kg BID or 40 mg/kg TID. Fifteen of the 43 patients had healing of their lesions in 11 to 72 days with no difference in response between the two treatment groups.

INDICATIONS

CMV Retinitis: FOSCAVIR is indicated for the treatment of CMV retinitis in patients with acquired immunodeficiency syndrome (AIDS). Combination therapy with FOSCAVIR and ganciclovir is indicated for patients who have relapsed after monotherapy with either drug. SAFETY AND EFFICACY OF FOSCAVIR HAVE NOT BEEN ESTABLISHED FOR TREATMENT OF OTHER CMV INFECTIONS (e.g., PNEUMONITIS, GASTROENTERITIS); CONGENITAL OR NEONATAL CMV DISEASE; OR NON-IMMUNOCOMPROMISED INDIVIDUALS.

Mucocutaneous Acyclovir-Resistant HSV Infections: FOSCAVIR is indicated for the treatment of acyclovir-resistant mucocutaneous HSV infections in immunocompromised patients. SAFETY AND EFFICACY OF FOSCAVIR HAVE NOT BEEN ESTABLISHED FOR TREATMENT OF OTHER HSV INFECTIONS (e.g., RETINITIS, ENCEPHALITIS); CONGENITAL OR NEONATAL HSV DISEASE; OR HSV IN NON-IMMUNOCOMPROMISED INDIVIDUALS.

CONTRAINDICATIONS

FOSCAVIR is contraindicated in patients with clinically significant hypersensitivity to foscarnet sodium.

WARNINGS

Renal Impairment: THE MAJOR TOXICITY OF FOSCAVIR IS RENAL IMPAIRMENT (see ADVERSE REACTIONS section). Renal impairment is most likely to become clinically evident during the second week of induction therapy, but may occur at any time during FOSCAVIR treatment. Renal function should be monitored carefully during both induction and maintenance therapy (see PATIENT MONITORING section). Elevations in serum creatinine are usually, but not always, reversible following discontinuation or dose adjustment of FOSCAVIR. Safety and efficacy data for patients with baseline serum creatinine levels greater than 2.8 mg/dL or measured 24-hour creatinine clearances <50 mL/min are limited.

BECAUSE OF FOSCAVIR'S POTENTIAL TO CAUSE RENAL IMPAIRMENT, DOSE ADJUSTMENT BASED ON SERUM CREATININE IS NECESSARY. Hydration may reduce the risk of nephrotoxicity. It is recommended that 750–1000 mL of normal saline or 5% dextrose solution should be given prior to the first infusion of FOSCAVIR to establish diuresis. With subsequent infusions, 750–1000 mL of hydration fluid should be given with 90-120 mg/kg of FOSCAVIR, and 500 mL with 40–60 mg/kg of FOSCAVIR. Hydration fluid may need to be decreased if clinically warranted.

After the first dose, the hydration fluid should be administered concurrently with each infusion of FOSCAVIR.

Mineral and Electrolyte Abnormalities: FOSCAVIR has been associated with changes in serum electrolytes including hypocalcemia, hypophosphatemia, hyperphosphatemia, hypomagnesemia, and hypokalemia (see ADVERSE REACTIONS section). FOSCAVIR may also be associated with a dose-related decrease in ionized serum calcium which may not be reflected in total serum calcium. This effect is likely to be related to chelation of divalent metal ions such as calcium by foscarnet. Patients should be advised to report symptoms of low ionized calcium such as perioral tingling, numbness in the extremities and paresthesias. Particular caution and careful management of serum electrolytes is advised in patients with altered calcium or other electrolyte levels before treatment and especially in those with neurologic or cardiac abnormalities and those receiving other drugs known to influence minerals and electrolytes (see PATIENT MONITORING and Drug Interactions sections). Physicians should be prepared to treat these abnormalities and their sequelae such as tetany, seizures or cardiac disturbances. The rate of FOSCAVIR infusion may also affect the decrease in ionized calcium. **Therefore, an infusion pump must be used for administration to prevent rapid intravenous infusion (see DOSAGE AND ADMINISTRA-**

TABLE 4
Pharmacokinetic Parameters (mean ± S.D.) After a Single 60 mg/kg Dose of FOSCAVIR in 4 Groups* of Adults with Varying Degrees of Renal Function

Parameter	Group 1 (N=6)	Group 2 (N=6)	Group 3 (N=6)	Group 4 (N=4)
Creatinine clearance (mL/min)	108 ± 16	68 ± 8	34 ± 9	20 ± 4
Foscarnet CL (mL/min/kg)	2.13 ± 0.71	1.33 ± 0.43	0.46 ± 0.14	0.43 ± 0.26
Foscarnet half-life (hr)	1.93 ± 0.12	3.35 ± 0.87	13.0 ± 4.05	25.3 ± 18.7

* Group 1 patients had normal renal function defined as a creatinine clearance (CrCl) of >80 mL/min, Group 2 CrCl was 50–80 mL/min, Group 3 CrCl was 25–49 mL/min and Group 4 CrCl was 10–24 mL/min.

TION section). Slowing the infusion rate may decrease or prevent symptoms.

Seizures: Seizures related to mineral and electrolyte abnormalities have been associated with FOSCAVIR treatment (see WARNING section; Mineral and Electrolyte Abnormalities). Several cases of seizures were associated with death. Risk factors associated with seizures included impaired baseline renal function, low total serum calcium, and underlying CNS conditions.

PRECAUTIONS

General: Care must be taken to infuse solutions containing FOSCAVIR only into veins with adequate blood flow to permit rapid dilution and distribution to avoid local irritation (see DOSAGE AND ADMINISTRATION). Local irritation and ulcerations of penile epithelium have been reported in male patients receiving FOSCAVIR, possibly related to the presence of drug in the urine. One case of vulvovaginal ulcerations in a female receiving FOSCAVIR has been reported. Adequate hydration with close attention to personal hygiene may minimize the occurrence of such events.

Hemopoietic System: Anemia has been reported in 33% of patients receiving FOSCAVIR in controlled studies. Granulocytopenia has been reported in 17% of patients receiving FOSCAVIR in controlled studies; however, only 1% (2/189) were terminated from these studies because of neutropenia.

Information for Patients

CMV Retinitis—Patients should be advised that FOSCAVIR is not a cure for CMV retinitis, and that they may continue to experience progression of retinitis during or following treatment. They should be advised to have regular ophthalmologic examinations.

Mucocutaneous Acyclovir-Resistant HSV Infections—Patients should be advised that FOSCAVIR is not a cure for HSV infections. While complete healing is possible, relapse occurs in most patients. Because relapse may be due to acyclovir-sensitive HSV, sensitivity testing of the viral isolate is advised. In addition, repeated treatment with FOSCAVIR has led to the development of resistance associated with poorer response. In the case of poor therapeutic response, sensitivity testing of the viral isolate also is advised.

General—Patients should be informed that the major toxicities of foscarnet are renal impairment, electrolyte disturbances, and seizures, and that dose modifications and possibly discontinuation may be required. The importance of close monitoring while on therapy must be emphasized. Patients should be advised of the importance of reporting to their physicians symptoms of perioral tingling, numbness in the extremities or paresthesias during or after infusion as possible symptoms of electrolyte abnormalities. Should such symptoms occur, the infusion of FOSCAVIR should be stopped, appropriate laboratory samples for assessment of electrolyte concentrations obtained, and a physician consulted before resuming treatment. The rate of infusion must be no more than 1 mg/kg/minute. The potential for renal impairment may be minimized by accompanying FOSCAVIR administration with hydration adequate to establish and maintain a diuresis during dosing.

Drug Interactions: A possible drug interaction of FOSCAVIR and intravenous pentamidine has been described. Concomitant treatment of four patients in the United Kingdom with FOSCAVIR and intravenous pentamidine may have caused hypocalcemia; one patient died with severe hypocalcemia. Toxicity associated with concomitant use of aerosolized pentamidine has not been reported.

Because of foscarnet's tendency to cause renal impairment, the use of FOSCAVIR should be avoided in combination with potentially nephrotoxic drugs such as aminoglycosides, amphotericin B and intravenous pentamidine (see above) unless the potential benefits outweigh the risks to the patient.

Abnormal renal function in connection with the use of FOSCAVIR in combination with ritonavir and/or saquinavir has been observed in clinical practice.

Since FOSCAVIR decreases serum concentrations of ionized calcium, concurrent treatment with other drugs known to influence serum calcium concentrations should be used with particular caution.

Ganciclovir—The pharmacokinetics of foscarnet and ganciclovir were not altered in 13 patients receiving either concomitant therapy or daily alternating therapy for maintenance of CMV disease.

Carcinogenesis, Mutagenesis, Impairment of Fertility: Carcinogenicity studies were conducted in rats and mice at oral doses of 500 mg/kg/day and 250 mg/kg/day. Oral bioavailability in unfasted rodents is < 20%. No evidence of oncogenicity was reported at plasma drug levels equal to 1/3 and 1/5, respectively, of those in humans (at the maximum recommended human daily dose) as measured by the area-under-the-time/concentration curve (AUC).

FOSCAVIR showed genotoxic effects in the BALB/3T3 *in vitro* transformation assay at concentrations greater than 0.5 mcg/mL and an increased frequency of chromosome aberrations in the sister chromatid exchange assay at 1000 mcg/mL. A high dose of foscarnet (350 mg/kg) caused an increase in micronucleated polychromatic erythrocytes *in vivo* in mice at doses that produced exposures (area under curve) comparable to that anticipated clinically.

Pregnancy: Teratogenic Effect:

Pregnancy, Category C: FOSCAVIR did not adversely affect fertility and general reproductive performance in rats. The results of peri- and post-natal studies in rats were also negative. However, these studies used exposures that are inadequate to define the potential for impairment of fertility at human drug exposure levels.

Daily subcutaneous doses up to 75 mg/kg administered to female rats prior to and during mating, during gestation, and 21 days post-partum caused a slight increase (< 5%) in the number of skeletal anomalies compared with the control group. Daily subcutaneous doses up to 75 mg/kg administered to rabbits and 150 mg/kg administered to rats during gestation caused an increase in the frequency of skeletal anomalies/variations. On the basis of estimated drug exposure (as measured by AUC), the 150 mg/kg dose in rats and 75 mg/kg dose in rabbits were approximately one-eighth (rat) and one-third (rabbit) the estimated maximal daily human exposure. These studies are inadequate to define the potential teratogenicity at levels to which women will be exposed.

There are no adequate and well controlled studies in pregnant women. Because animal reproductive studies are not always predictive of human response, FOSCAVIR should be used during pregnancy only if clearly needed.

Nursing Mothers: It is not known whether FOSCAVIR is excreted in human milk; however, in lactating rats administered 75 mg/kg, FOSCAVIR was excreted in maternal milk at concentrations three times higher than peak maternal blood concentrations.

Pediatric Use: The safety and effectiveness of FOSCAVIR in pediatric patients have not been established. FOSCAVIR is deposited in teeth and bone and deposition is greater in young and growing animals. FOSCAVIR has been demonstrated to adversely affect development of tooth enamel in mice and rats. The effects of this deposition on skeletal development have not been studied. Since deposition in human bone has also been shown to occur, it is likely that it does so to a greater degree in developing bone in pediatric patients. Administration to pediatric patients should be undertaken only after careful evaluation and only if the potential benefits for treatment outweigh the risks.

Use in the Elderly: No studies of the efficacy or safety of FOSCAVIR in persons over age 65 have been conducted. Since these individuals frequently have reduced glomerular filtration, particular attention should be paid to assessing renal function before and during FOSCAVIR administration (see DOSAGE AND ADMINISTRATION).

ADVERSE REACTIONS

THE MAJOR TOXICITY OF FOSCAVIR IS RENAL IMPAIRMENT (see WARNINGS section). Approximately 33% of 189 patients with AIDS and CMV retinitis who received FOSCAVIR (60 mg/kg TID), without adequate hydration, developed significant impairment of renal function (serum creatinine ≥ 2.0 mg/dL). The incidence of renal impairment in subsequent clinical trials in which 1000 mL of normal saline or 5% dextrose solution was given with each infusion of FOSCAVIR was 12% (34/280).

FOSCAVIR has been associated with changes in serum electrolytes including hypocalcemia (15–30%), hypophosphatemia (8–26%) and hyperphosphatemia (6%), hypomagnesemia (15–30%), and hypokalemia (16–48%) (see WARNINGS section). The higher percentages were derived from those patients receiving hydration.

FOSCAVIR treatment was associated with seizures in 18/189 (10%) AIDS patients in the initial five controlled studies (see WARNINGS section). Risk factors associated with seizures included impaired baseline renal function, low total serum calcium, and underlying CNS conditions predisposing the patient to seizures. The rate of seizures did not increase with duration of treatment. Three cases were associated with overdoses of FOSCAVIR (see OVERDOSAGE section).

In five controlled U.S. clinical trials the most frequently reported adverse events in patients with AIDS and CMV retinitis are shown in Table 5. These figures were calculated without reference to drug relationship or severity.

TABLE 5—Adverse Events Reported in Five Controlled US Clinical Trials

	n = 189		n = 189
Fever	65%	**Abnormal Renal Function**	27%
Nausea	47%	**Vomiting**	26%
Anemia	33%	**Headache**	26%
Diarrhea	30%	**Seizures**	10%

From the same controlled studies, adverse events categorized by investigator as "severe" are shown in Table 6. Although death was specifically attributed to FOSCAVIR in only one case, other complications of FOSCAVIR (i.e., renal impairment, electrolyte abnormalities, and seizures) may have contributed to patient deaths (see WARNINGS section).

TABLE 6—Severe Adverse Events

	n = 189
Death	14%
Abnormal Renal Function	14%
Marrow Suppression	10%
Anemia	9%
Seizures	7%

From the five initial U.S. controlled trials of FOSCAVIR, the following list of adverse events has been compiled regardless of causal relationship to FOSCAVIR. Evaluation of these reports was difficult because of the diverse manifestations of the underlying disease and because most patients received numerous concomitant medications.

Incidence 5% or Greater

Body as a Whole: fever, fatigue, rigors, asthenia, malaise, pain, infection, sepsis, death

Central and Peripheral Nervous System: headache, paresthesia, dizziness, involuntary muscle contractions, hypoesthesia, neuropathy, seizures including grand mal seizures (see WARNINGS)

Gastrointestinal System: anorexia, nausea, diarrhea, vomiting, abdominal pain

Hematologic: anemia, granulocytopenia, leukopenia (see PRECAUTIONS)

Metabolic and Nutritional: mineral and electrolyte imbalances (see WARNINGS) including hypokalemia, hypocalcemia, hypomagnesemia, hypophosphatemia, hyperphosphatemia

Psychiatric: depression, confusion, anxiety

Respiratory System: coughing, dyspnea

Skin and Appendages: rash, increased sweating

Urinary: alterations in renal function including increased serum creatinine, decreased creatinine clearance, and abnormal renal function (see WARNINGS)

Special Senses: vision abnormalities

Incidence between 1% and 5%

Application Site: injection site pain, injection site inflammation

Body as a Whole: back pain, chest pain, edema, influenza-like symptoms, bacterial infections, moniliasis, fungal infections, abscess

Cardiovascular: hypertension, palpitations, ECG abnormalities including sinus tachycardia, first degree AV block and non-specific ST-T segment changes, hypotension, flushing, cerebrovascular disorder (see WARNINGS)

Central and Peripheral Nervous System: tremor, ataxia, dementia, stupor, generalized spasms, sensory disturbances, meningitis, aphasia, abnormal coordination, leg cramps, EEG abnormalities (see WARNINGS)

Gastrointestinal: constipation, dysphagia, dyspepsia, rectal hemorrhage, dry mouth, melena, flatulence, ulcerative stomatitis, pancreatitis

Hematologic: thrombocytopenia, platelet abnormalities, thrombosis, white blood cell abnormalities, lymphadenopathy

Liver and Biliary: abnormal A-G ratio, abnormal hepatic function, increased SGPT, increased SGOT

Metabolic and Nutritional: hyponatremia, decreased weight, increased alkaline phosphatase, increased LDH, increased BUN, acidosis, cachexia, thirst, hypercalcemia (see WARNINGS)

Musculo-Skeletal: arthralgia, myalgia

Neoplasms: lymphoma-like disorder, sarcoma

Psychiatric: insomnia, somnolence, nervousness, amnesia, agitation, aggressive reaction, hallucination

Respiratory System: pneumonia, sinusitis, pharyngitis, rhinitis, respiratory disorders, respiratory insufficiency, pulmonary infiltration, stridor, pneumothorax, hemoptysis, bronchospasm

Skin and Appendages: pruritus, skin ulceration, seborrhea, erythematous rash, maculo-papular rash, skin discoloration

Special Senses: taste perversions, eye abnormalities, eye pain, conjunctivitis

Urinary System: albuminuria, dysuria, polyuria, urethral disorder, urinary retention, urinary tract infections, acute renal failure, nocturia, facial edema

Selected adverse events occurring at a rate of less than 1% in the five initial U.S. controlled clinical trials of FOSCAVIR include: syndrome of inappropriate antidiuretic hormone secretion, pancytopenia, hematuria, dehydration, hypoproteinemia, increases in amylase and creatinine phosphokinase, cardiac arrest, coma, and other cardiovascular and neurologic complications.

Selected adverse event data from the Foscarnet vs. Ganciclovir CMV Retinitis Trial (FGCRT), performed by the Studies of the Ocular Complications of AIDS (SOCA) Research Group, are shown in Table 7 (see CLINICAL TRIALS section).

[See table 7 at top of next page]

Selected adverse events from ACTG Study 228 (CRRT) comparing combination therapy with FOSCAVIR or ganciclovir monotherapy are shown in Table 8. The most common reason for a treatment change in patients assigned to either FOSCAVIR or ganciclovir was retinitis progression. The most frequent reason for a treatment change in the combination treatment group was toxicity.

[See table 8 on next page]

Adverse events that have been reported in post-marketing surveillance include: ventricular arrhythmia, prolongation of QT interval, diabetes insipidus (usually nephrogenic), renal calculus, and muscle disorders including myopathy, myositis, muscle weakness and rare cases of rhabdomyolysis. Cases of vesiculobullous eruptions including erythema multiforme, toxic epidermal necrolysis, and Stevens-Johnson Syndrome have been reported. In most cases, patients were taking other medications that have been associated with toxic epidermal necrolysis or Stevens-Johnson Syndrome.

OVERDOSAGE

In controlled clinical trials performed in the United States, overdosage with FOSCAVIR was reported in 10 out of 189 patients. All 10 patients experienced adverse events and all except one made a complete recovery. One patient died after receiving a total daily dose of 12.5 g for three days instead of the intended 10.9 g. The patient suffered a grand mal sei-

Continued on next page

Foscavir—Cont.

zure and became comatose. Three days later the patient expired with the cause of death listed as respiratory/cardiac arrest. The other nine patients received doses ranging from 1.14 times to 8 times their recommended doses with an average of 4 times their recommended doses. Overall, three patients had seizures, three patients had renal function impairment, four patients had paresthesias either in limbs or periorally, and five patients had documented electrolyte disturbances primarily involving calcium and phosphate.
The pattern of adverse events associated with overdose in post-marketing surveillance is consistent with the symptoms previously observed during foscarnet therapy.
There is no specific antidote for FOSCAVIR overdose. Hemodialysis and hydration may be of benefit in reducing drug plasma levels in patients who receive an overdosage of FOSCAVIR, but the effectiveness of these interventions has not been evaluated. The patient should be observed for signs and symptoms of renal impairment and electrolyte imbalance. Medical treatment should be instituted if clinically warranted.

DOSAGE AND ADMINISTRATION

CAUTION—DO NOT ADMINISTER FOSCAVIR BY RAPID OR BOLUS INTRAVENOUS INJECTION. THE TOXICITY OF FOSCAVIR MAY BE INCREASED AS A RESULT OF EXCESSIVE PLASMA LEVELS. CARE SHOULD BE TAKEN TO AVOID UNINTENTIONAL OVERDOSE BY CAREFULLY CONTROLLING THE RATE OF INFUSION. THEREFORE, AN INFUSION PUMP MUST BE USED. IN SPITE OF THE USE OF AN INFUSION PUMP, OVERDOSES HAVE OCCURRED.

ADMINISTRATION

FOSCAVIR is administered by controlled intravenous infusion, either by using a central venous line or by using a peripheral vein. The standard 24 mg/mL solution may be used with or without dilution when using a central venous catheter for infusion. When a peripheral vein catheter is used, the 24 mg/mL solution <u>must</u> be diluted to 12 mg/mL with 5% dextrose in water or with a normal saline solution prior to administration to avoid local irritation of peripheral veins. Since the dose of FOSCAVIR is calculated on the basis of body weight, it may be desirable to remove and discard any unneeded quantity from the bottle before starting with the infusion to avoid overdosage. Dilutions and/or removals of excess quantities should be accomplished under aseptic conditions. Solutions thus prepared should be used within 24 hours of first entry into a sealed bottle. *To reduce the risk of nephrotoxicity, creatinine clearance (mL/min/kg) should be calculated even if serum creatinine is within the normal range, and doses should be adjusted accordingly.*

Hydration: Hydration may reduce the risk of nephrotoxicity. It is recommended that 750–1000 mL of normal saline or 5% dextrose solution should be given prior to the first infusion of FOSCAVIR to establish diuresis. With subsequent infusions, 750–1000 mL of hydration fluid should be given with 90–120 mg/kg of FOSCAVIR, and 500 mL with 40–60 mg/kg of FOSCAVIR. Hydration fluid may need to be decreased if clinically warranted.
After the first dose, the hydration fluid should be administered concurrently with each infusion of FOSCAVIR.

Compatibility With Other Solutions/Drugs: Other drugs and supplements can be administered to a patient receiving FOSCAVIR. However, care must be taken to ensure that FOSCAVIR is only administered with normal saline or 5% dextrose solution and that no other drug or supplement is administered concurrently via the same catheter. Foscarnet has been reported to be chemically incompatible with 30% dextrose, amphotericin B, and solutions containing calcium such as Ringer's lactate and TPN. Physical incompatibility with other IV drugs has also been reported including acyclovir sodium, ganciclovir, trimetrexate glucuronate, pentamidine isethionate, vancomycin, trimethoprim/sulfamethoxazole, diazepam, midazolam, digoxin, phenytoin, leucovorin, and prochlorperazine. Because of foscarnet's chelating properties, a precipitate can potentially occur when divalent cations are administered concurrently in the same catheter.
Parenteral drug products must be inspected visually for particulate matter and discoloration prior to administration whenever the solution and container permit. Solutions that are discolored or contain particulate matter should not be used.

Accidental Exposure: Accidental skin and eye contact with foscarnet sodium solution may cause local irritation and burning sensation. If accidental contact occurs, the exposed area should be flushed with water.

DOSAGE

THE RECOMMENDED DOSAGE, FREQUENCY, OR INFUSION RATES SHOULD NOT BE EXCEEDED. ALL DOSES MUST BE INDIVIDUALIZED FOR PATIENTS' RENAL FUNCTION.

Induction Treatment: The recommended initial dose of FOSCAVIR for patients with normal renal function is:

- For CMV retinitis patients, either 90 mg/kg (1-1/2 to 2 hour infusion) every twelve hours or 60 mg/kg (minimum one hour infusion) every eight hours over 2-3 weeks depending on clinical response.
- For acyclovir-resistant HSV patients, 40 mg/kg (minimum one hour infusion) either every 8 or 12 hours for 2-3 weeks or until healed.

TABLE 7—FGCRT: SELECTED ADVERSE EVENTS*

EVENT	GANCICLOVIR			FOSCARNET		
	No. of Events	No. of Patients	Rates§	No. of Events	No. of Patients	Rates§
Absolute neutrophil count decreasing to $<0.50 \times 10^9$ per liter	63	41	1.30	31	17	0.72
Serum creatinine increasing to >260 μmol per liter (>2.9 mg/dL)	6	4	0.12	13	9	0.30
Seizure‡	21	13	0.37	19	13	0.37
Catheterization-related infection	49	27	1.26	51	28	1.46
Hospitalization	209	91	4.74	202	75	5.03

* Values for the treatment groups refer only to patients who completed at least one follow-up visit—i.e., 113 to 119 patients in the ganciclovir group and 93 to 100 in the foscarnet group. "Events" denotes all events observed and "patients" the number of patients with one or more of the indicated events.
‡ Final frozen SOCA I database dated October 1991.
§ Per person-year at risk

TABLE 8
CRRT: Selected Adverse Events

	Foscavir N=88			Ganciclovir N=93			Combination N=93		
	No. Events	No. Pts.†	Rate‡	No. Events	No. Pts.†	Rate‡	No. Events	No. Pts.†	Rate‡
Anemia (Hgb <70 g/L)	11	7	0.20	9	7	0.14	19	15	0.33
Neutropenia§									
ANC $<0.75 \times 10^9$ cells/L	86	32	1.53	95	41	1.51	107	51	1.91
ANC $<0.50 \times 10^9$ cells/L	50	25	0.91	49	28	0.80	50	28	0.85
Thrombocytopenia									
Platelets $<50 \times 10^9$/L	28	14	0.50	19	8	0.43	40	15	0.56
Platelets $<20 \times 10^9$/L	1	1	0.01	6	2	0.05	7	6	0.18
Nephrotoxicity Creatinine >260 μmol/L (>2.9 mg/dL)	9	7	0.15	10	7	0.17	11	10	0.20
Seizures	6	6	0.17	7	6	0.15	10	5	0.18
Hospitalizations	86	53	1.86	111	59	2.36	118	64	2.36

† Pts. = patients with event;
‡ Rate = events/person/year;
§ ANC = absolute neutrophil count

TABLE 9
FOSCAVIR DOSING GUIDE
INDUCTION

CrCl (mL/min/kg)	HSV: Equivalent to 80 mg/kg/day total (40 mg/kg Q12h)	HSV: Equivalent to 120 mg/kg/day total (40 mg/kg Q8h)	CMV: Equivalent to 180 mg/kg/day total (60 mg/kg Q8h)	CMV: Equivalent to 180 mg/kg/day total (90 mg/kg Q12h)
>1.4	40 Q12h	40 Q8h	60 Q8h	90 Q12h
>1.0–1.4	30 Q12h	30 Q8h	45 Q8h	70 Q12h
>0.8–1.0	20 Q12h	**35 Q12h**	**50 Q12h**	50 Q12h
>0.6–0.8	**35 Q24h**	**25 Q12h**	**40 Q12h**	**80 Q24h**
>0.5–0.6	**25 Q24h**	40 Q24h	60 Q24h	**60 Q24h**
≥0.4–0.5	**20 Q24h**	35 Q24h	50 Q24h	**50 Q24h**
<0.4	Not Recommended	Not Recommended	Not Recommended	Not Recommended

MAINTENANCE

CrCl (mL/min/kg)	CMV: Equivalent to 90 mg/kg/day (once daily)	CMV: Equivalent to 120 mg/kg/day (once daily)
>1.4	90 Q24h	120 Q24h
>1.0–1.4	70 Q24h	90 Q24h
>0.8–1.0	50 Q24h	65 Q24h
>0.6–0.8	**80 Q48h**	**105 Q48h**
>0.5–0.6	**60 Q48h**	**80 Q48h**
≥0.4–0.5	**50 Q48h**	**65 Q48h**
<0.4	Not Recommended	Not Recommended

> means "greater than"; ≥ means "greater than or equal to"; < means "less than"

An infusion pump must be used to control the rate of infusion. Adequate hydration is recommended to establish a diuresis (see Hydration for recommendation), both prior to and during treatment to minimize renal toxicity (see WARNINGS), provided there are no clinical contraindications.

Maintenance Treatment: Following induction treatment the recommended maintenance dose of FOSCAVIR for CMV retinitis is 90 mg/kg/day to 120 mg/kg/day (individualized for renal function) given as an intravenous infusion over 2 hours. Because the superiority of the 120 mg/kg/day has not been established in controlled trials, and given the likely relationship of higher plasma foscarnet levels to toxicity, it is recommended that most patients be started on maintenance treatment with a dose of 90 mg/kg/day. Escalation to 120 mg/kg/day may be considered should early reinduction be required because of retinitis progression. Some patients who show excellent tolerance to FOSCAVIR may benefit from initiation of maintenance treatment at 120 mg/kg/day earlier in their treatment.
An infusion pump must be used to control the rate of infusion with all doses. Again, hydration to establish diuresis both prior to and during treatment is recommended to minimize renal toxicity, provided there are no clinical contraindications (see WARNINGS).
Patients who experience progression of retinitis while receiving FOSCAVIR maintenance therapy may be retreated with the induction and maintenance regimens given above or with a combination of FOSCAVIR and ganciclovir (see CLINICAL TRIALS section). **Because of physical incompatibility, FOSCAVIR and ganciclovir must NOT be mixed.**

Use in Patients with Abnormal Renal Function: FOSCAVIR should be used with caution in patients with abnormal renal function because reduced plasma clearance of foscarnet will result in elevated plasma levels (see CLINICAL PHARMACOLOGY). In addition, FOSCAVIR has the potential to further impair renal function (see WARNINGS). Safety and efficacy data for patients with baseline serum creatinine levels greater than 2.8 mg/dL or measured 24-hour creatinine clearances < 50 mL/min are limited.

Renal function must be monitored carefully at baseline and during induction and maintenance therapy with appropriate dose adjustments for FOSCAVIR as outlined below (see Dose Adjustment and PATIENT MONITORING). During FOSCAVIR therapy if creatinine clearance falls below the limits of the dosing nomograms (0.4 mL/min/kg), FOSCAVIR should be discontinued, the patient hydrated, and monitored daily until resolution of renal impairment is ensured.

Dose Adjustment: FOSCAVIR dosing must be individualized according to the patient's renal function status. Refer to Table 9 below for recommended doses and adjust the dose as indicated. Even patients with serum creatinine in the normal range may require dose adjustment; therefore, the dose should be calculated at baseline and frequently thereafter. To use this dosing guide, actual 24-hour creatinine clearance (mL/min) must be divided by body weight (kg), or the estimated creatinine clearance in mL/min/kg can be calculated from serum creatinine (mg/dL) using the following formula (modified Cockcroft and Gault equation):

For males:

$$\frac{140 - \text{age}}{\text{serum creatinine} \times 72} \quad (\times\ 0.85 \text{ for females}) = \text{mL/min/kg}$$

[See table 9 at top of previous page]

PATIENT MONITORING

The majority of patients will experience some decrease in renal function due to FOSCAVIR administration. Therefore it is recommended that creatinine clearance, either measured or estimated using the modified Cockcroft and Gault equation based on serum creatinine, be determined at baseline, 2–3 times per week during induction therapy and at least every one to two weeks during maintenance therapy, with FOSCAVIR dose adjusted accordingly (see Dose Adjustment). More frequent monitoring may be required for some patients. It is also recommended that a 24-hour creatinine clearance be determined at baseline and periodically thereafter to ensure correct dosing (assuming verification of an adequate collection using creatinine index). FOSCAVIR should be discontinued if creatinine clearance drops below 0.4 mL/min/kg.

Due to FOSCAVIR's propensity to chelate divalent metal ions and alter levels of serum electrolytes, patients must be monitored closely for such changes. It is recommended that a schedule similar to that recommended for serum creatinine (see above) be used to monitor serum calcium, magnesium, potassium and phosphorus. Particular caution is advised in patients with decreased total serum calcium or other electrolyte levels before treatment, as well as in patients with neurologic or cardiac abnormalities, and in patients receiving other drugs known to influence serum calcium levels. Any clinically significant metabolic changes should be corrected. Also, patients who experience mild (e.g., perioral numbness or paresthesias) or severe (e.g., seizures) symptoms of electrolyte abnormalities should have serum electrolyte and mineral levels assessed as close in time to the event as possible.

Careful monitoring and appropriate management of electrolytes, calcium, magnesium and creatinine are of particular importance in patients with conditions that may predispose them to seizures (see WARNINGS).

HOW SUPPLIED

FOSCAVIR (foscarnet sodium) INJECTION, 24 mg/mL for intravenous infusion, is supplied in glass bottles as follows:

NDC 0186-1906-01 500 mL bottles, cases of 12
NDC 0186-1905-01 250 mL bottles, cases of 12

FOSCAVIR INJECTION should be stored at controlled room temperature, 15°–30°C (59°– 86°F), and should be protected from excessive heat (above 40°C) and from freezing. FOSCAVIR INJECTION should be used only if the bottle and seal are intact, a vacuum is present, and the solution is clear and colorless.

Rx only

Manufactured by:
Abbott Laboratories, North Chicago, IL 60064
Manufactured for:
Astra Pharmaceuticals, L.P., Wayne, PA 19087
000571R09 Rev. 2/99

LEXXEL® ℞
(enalapril maleate-felodipine ER)
TABLETS

USE IN PREGNANCY

When used in pregnancy during the second and third trimesters, ACE inhibitors can cause injury and even death to the developing fetus. When pregnancy is detected, LEXXEL should be discontinued as soon as possible. See WARNINGS, Fetal/Neonatal Morbidity and Mortality.

DESCRIPTION

LEXXEL* (enalapril maleate-felodipine ER) is a combination product, consisting of an outer layer of enalapril maleate surrounding a core tablet of an extended-release felodipine formulation.

Enalapril maleate is the maleate salt of enalapril, the ethyl ester of a long-acting angiotensin converting enzyme inhibitor, enalaprilat. Enalapril maleate is chemically described as (*S*)-1-[*N*-[1-(ethoxycarbonyl)-3-phenylpropyl]-L-alanyl]-L-proline, (*Z*)-2-butenedioate salt (1:1). Its empirical formula is $C_{20}H_{28}N_2O_5 \bullet C_4H_4O_4$, and its structural formula is: [See chemical structure at top of next column]

Enalapril maleate is a white to off-white, crystalline powder with a molecular weight of 492.53. It is sparingly soluble in water, soluble in ethanol, and freely soluble in methanol.

Felodipine, a calcium channel blocker, is a dihydropyridine derivative that is chemically described as ± ethyl methyl 4-(2,3-dichlorophenyl)-1,4-dihydro-2,6-dimethyl-3,5-pyridinedicarboxylate. Its empirical formula is $C_{18}H_{19}Cl_2NO_4$ and its structural formula is:

Felodipine is a slightly yellowish, crystalline powder with a molecular weight of 384.26. It is insoluble in water and is freely soluble in dichloromethane and ethanol. Felodipine is a racemic mixture; however, *S*-felodipine is the more biologically active enantiomer.

LEXXEL is available for oral use in two tablet combinations of enalapril maleate with felodipine as an extended-release formulation: LEXXEL 5-2.5, containing 5 mg of enalapril maleate and 2.5 mg of felodipine ER and LEXXEL 5-5, containing 5 mg of enalapril maleate and 5 mg of felodipine ER. Inactive ingredients include: propyl gallate, polyoxyl 40 hydrogenated castor oil, cellulose compounds, lactose, aluminum silicate, sodium stearyl fumarate, carnauba wax, and iron oxides. The tablets are imprinted with an ink of synthetic red iron oxide (LEXXEL 5-2.5) or synthetic black iron oxide (LEXXEL 5-5) which contains pharmaceutical glaze in SD-45, n-butyl alcohol, propylene glycol, isopropyl alcohol, ammonium hydroxide, and simethicone (LEXXEL 5-2.5) and methyl alcohol (LEXXEL 5-5).

*LEXXEL is a trademark of the AstraZeneca group of companies

CLINICAL PHARMACOLOGY

Mechanism of Action: The two components of LEXXEL have complementary antihypertensive actions. **Enalapril** is a prodrug; following oral administration, it is bioactivated by hydrolysis of the ethyl ester to enalaprilat, which is the active angiotensin converting enzyme (ACE) inhibitor. Enalaprilat inhibits angiotensin-converting enzyme in humans and animals. ACE is a peptidyl dipeptidase that catalyzes the conversion of angiotensin I to the vasoconstrictor substance, angiotensin II. Angiotensin II also stimulates aldosterone secretion by the adrenal cortex. The beneficial effects of enalapril in hypertension appear to result primarily from suppression of the renin-angiotensin-aldosterone system.

Inhibition of ACE results in decreased plasma angiotensin II, which leads to decreased vasopressor activity and to decreased aldosterone secretion. Although the latter decrease is small, it results in small increases of serum potassium. In hypertensive patients treated with enalapril maleate alone for up to 48 weeks, mean increases in serum potassium of approximately 0.2 mEq/L were observed. In patients treated with enalapril maleate plus a thiazide diuretic, there was essentially no change in serum potassium. (See PRECAUTIONS.) Removal of angiotensin II negative feedback on renin secretion leads to increased plasma renin activity.

ACE is identical to kininase, an enzyme that degrades bradykinin. Whether increased levels of bradykinin, a potent vasodepressor peptide, play a role in the therapeutic effects of enalapril maleate remains to be elucidated.

While the mechanism through which enalapril lowers blood pressure is believed to be primarily suppression of the renin-angiotensin-aldosterone system, enalapril is antihypertensive even in patients with low-renin hypertension. Although enalapril was antihypertensive in all races studied, black hypertensive patients (usually a low-renin hypertensive population) had a smaller average response to enalapril monotherapy than non-black patients.

Felodipine is a dihydropyridine calcium channel blocker that reduces the influx of Ca^{++} by an effect on the voltage dependent L-channels in vascular smooth muscle and cultured rabbit atrial cells, and blocks potassium-induced contracture of the rat portal vein.

Pharmacologic studies show that the effects of felodipine on contractile processes are selective, with greater effects on vascular smooth muscle than cardiac muscle. Negative inotropic effects can be detected *in vitro*, but such effects have not been seen in intact animals.

The consequences of vasodilation produced by felodipine include a modest, short-lived reflex increase in heart rate. A mild diuretic effect is seen in several animal species and man, but most of the effects of felodipine are accounted for by its effects on peripheral vascular resistance.

Pharmacokinetics and Metabolism: Concomitant administration of enalapril and felodipine as an extended-release formulation has little effect on the bioavailability of either compound. The rate and extent of absorption of enalapril from LEXXEL is not significantly different from that of enalapril in VASOTEC** (enalapril maleate). The rate and extent of absorption of felodipine from LEXXEL has not been directly compared to the extended-release formulation of felodipine in PLENDIL*** (felodipine).

Following oral administration of LEXXEL, peak concentrations of enalapril occur within about one hour. Enalapril is hydrolyzed to enalaprilat, which is a more potent angiotensin converting enzyme inhibitor than enalapril. Peak serum concentrations of enalaprilat occur about three hours after an oral dose of LEXXEL. Based on urinary recovery, the extent of absorption of enalapril is approximately 60%.

**Registered trademark of Merck & Co., Inc.
***Trademark of the AstraZeneca group of companies

Peak concentrations of the isomers of felodipine are generally seen at 3–6 hours after administration of LEXXEL. Following oral administration, felodipine is almost completely absorbed and undergoes extensive first-pass metabolism; the systemic bioavailability of felodipine ER is approximately 20%.

When LEXXEL is taken with food (a substantial meal of 650 kcal or greater), some of the pharmacokinetics of its components are changed. Although the $AUC_{(0\text{–}48\ hr)}$ of felodipine is not changed, the peak concentration of its isomers is almost doubled, and the trough concentration is approximately halved. The bioavailability of enalapril, as measured by total urinary recovery of enalaprilat, is slightly reduced. As with other dihydropyridine calcium channel blockers, the bioavailability of felodipine was increased when taken with grapefruit juice, compared to when taken with water or orange juice.

The systemic plasma clearance of felodipine in young healthy subjects is about 0.8 L/min, and the apparent volume of distribution is 10 L/kg. Approximately 99% of felodipine is bound to plasma proteins.

Following administration of ^{14}C-labeled intravenous or immediate-release oral felodipine in man, about 70% of the dose of radioactivity was recovered in urine and 10% in the feces. A negligible amount of intact felodipine was recovered in the urine and feces (<0.5%). Six metabolites, which account for 23% of the oral dose, have been identified; none has significant vasodilating activity. Following oral administration of the immediate-release formulation, the plasma levels of felodipine declined polyexponentially with a mean terminal half-life of 11 to 16 hours.

Excretion of enalaprilat and enalapril is primarily renal. Approximately 94% of the dose is recovered in the urine and feces as enalaprilat or enalapril. The principal components in urine are enalaprilat, accounting for about 40% of the dose, and intact enalapril. There is no evidence of metabolites of enalapril, other than enalaprilat. The serum concentration profile of enalaprilat exhibits a prolonged terminal phase, apparently representing a small fraction of the administered dose that has been bound to ACE. The amount bound does not increase with dose, indicating a saturable site of binding. The effective half-life for accumulation of enalaprilat following multiple doses of enalapril maleate is 11 hours.

The disposition of enalapril and enalaprilat in patients with renal insufficiency is similar to that in patients with normal renal function until the glomerular filtration rate is reduced to 30 mL/min or less. With glomerular filtration rate ≤30 mL/min, peak and trough enalaprilat levels increase, time to peak concentration increases, and time to steady state may be delayed. The effective half-life of enalaprilat following multiple doses of enalapril maleate is prolonged at this level of renal insufficiency. Enalaprilat is dialyzable at a rate of 62 mL/min.

Plasma concentrations of felodipine, after a single dose and at steady state, increase with age. Mean clearance of felodipine in elderly hypertensives (mean age 74) was only 45% of that for young volunteers (mean age 26). At steady state, the mean AUC for young patients was 39% of that for the elderly. Data for intermediate age ranges suggest that the AUCs fall between the extremes of the young and the elderly.

In patients with hepatic disease, the clearance of felodipine was reduced to about 60% of that seen in normal young volunteers.

Blood Brain Barrier and Blood Placental Barrier—Animal studies have shown that felodipine crosses the blood brain

Continued on next page

Lexxel—Cont.

barrier. The plasma to brain concentration ratio of felodipine is about 20:1. Felodipine crosses the placenta. Fetal plasma levels of felodipine are similar to maternal plasma levels. Studies in dogs indicate that enalapril crosses the blood brain barrier poorly, if at all; enalaprilat does not enter the brain. Multiple doses of enalapril maleate in rats do not result in accumulation in any tissues. Milk of lactating rats contains radioactivity following administration of ^{14}C enalapril maleate. Radioactivity was found to cross the placenta following administration of labeled drug to pregnant hamsters.

Pharmacodynamics: Administration of **enalapril** maleate to patients with hypertension of severity ranging from mild to severe results in a reduction of both supine and standing blood pressure, usually with no orthostatic component. Symptomatic postural hypotension is infrequent with enalapril alone, although it might be anticipated in volume-depleted patients. (See WARNINGS.) In most patients studied, after oral administration of a single dose of enalapril, onset of antihypertensive activity was seen at one hour, with peak reduction of blood pressure achieved by 4 to 6 hours. At recommended doses, antihypertensive effects have been maintained for at least 24 hours. In some patients the effects may diminish toward the end of the dosing interval. In most patients, achievement of optimal blood pressure reduction may require several weeks of therapy. The antihypertensive effects of enalapril have continued during long-term therapy. Abrupt withdrawal of enalapril has not been associated with a rapid increase in blood pressure. In hemodynamic studies in patients with essential hypertension, blood pressure reduction was accompanied by a reduction in peripheral arterial resistance with an increase in cardiac output and little or no change in heart rate. Following administration of enalapril maleate, there is an increase in renal blood flow; glomerular filtration rate is usually unchanged. The effects appear to be similar in patients with renovascular hypertension.

In a clinical pharmacology study, indomethacin or sulindac was administered to hypertensive patients receiving enalapril. In this study there was no evidence of a blunting of the antihypertensive action of enalapril.

The effect of **felodipine** on blood pressure is principally a consequence of a dose-related decrease in peripheral vascular resistance. Blood pressure response following administration of felodipine ER to hypertensive patients is correlated with dose and plasma concentrations of felodipine. A reduction in blood pressure generally occurs within 2 to 5 hours. During chronic administration, substantial blood pressure control lasts for 24 hours, with trough reductions in diastolic blood pressure approximately 40–50% of peak reductions. A reflex increase in heart rate frequently occurs during the first week of therapy; this increase attenuates over time. Heart rate increases of 5–10 beats per minute may be seen during chronic dosing. The increase is inhibited by beta-blocking agents.

Felodipine has no significant effect on cardiac conduction (P-R, P-Q, and H-V intervals). In clinical trials in hypertensive patients without clinical evidence of left ventricular dysfunction, no symptoms suggestive of a negative inotropic effect were noted; however, none would be expected in this population.

In an 8-week, fixed-dose, parallel-group, double-blind study, 707 hypertensive patients were randomized among all possible combinations of enalapril (0, 5, or 20 mg), and extended-release felodipine (0, 2.5, 5, or 10 mg), both taken once daily. Each of the non-placebo combinations was significantly more effective than placebo in reducing seated systolic and diastolic blood pressure at peak (3 to 5 hours after dosing) and trough (24 hours after dosing). Enalapril and felodipine contributed additively to the effect, so that each active-active combination was significantly more effective than either of its component monotherapies. Most of the drug effect seen at peak was still present at trough. The efficacy of combination therapy relative to monotherapy was not significantly affected by race, sex, or age.

During chronic dosing with LEXXEL, the maximum reduction in blood pressure is generally achieved after one to two weeks. The antihypertensive effects of LEXXEL have continued during chronic therapy for at least one year.

INDICATIONS AND USAGE

LEXXEL is indicated for the treatment of hypertension.

This fixed combination drug is not indicated for the initial therapy of hypertension. (See DOSAGE AND ADMINISTRATION.)

In using LEXXEL, consideration should be given to the fact that another angiotensin converting enzyme inhibitor, captopril, has caused agranulocytosis, particularly in patients with renal impairment or collagen vascular disease, and that available data are insufficient to show that enalapril (a component of LEXXEL) does not have a similar risk. (See WARNINGS, Neutropenia/Agranulocytosis.)

In considering use of LEXXEL, it should be noted that black patients receiving ACE inhibitors have been reported to have a higher incidence of angioedema compared to non-blacks. (See WARNINGS, Angioedema.)

CONTRAINDICATIONS

LEXXEL is contraindicated in patients who are hypersensitive to any component of this product. Because of the enalapril component, LEXXEL is contraindicated in patients with a history of angioedema related to previous treatment with an angiotensin converting enzyme inhibitor and in patients with hereditary or idiopathic angioedema.

WARNINGS

Anaphylactoid and Possibly Related Reactions: Presumably because angiotensin-converting enzyme inhibitors affect the metabolism of eicosanoids and polypeptides, including endogenous bradykinin, patients receiving ACE inhibitors (including LEXXEL) may be subject to a variety of adverse reactions, some of them serious.

Angioedema: Angioedema of the face, extremities, lips, tongue, glottis and/or larynx has been reported in patients treated with angiotensin converting enzyme inhibitors, including enalapril. This may occur at any time during treatment. In such cases LEXXEL should be promptly discontinued, and appropriate therapy and monitoring should be provided until complete and sustained resolution of signs and symptoms has occurred. In instances where swelling has been confined to the face and lips the condition has generally resolved without treatment, although antihistamines have been useful in relieving symptoms. Angioedema associated with laryngeal edema may be fatal. **Where there is involvement of the tongue, glottis or larynx, likely to cause airway obstruction, appropriate therapy, e.g., subcutaneous epinephrine solution 1:1000 (0.3 mL to 0.5 mL) and/or measures necessary to ensure a patent airway, should be promptly provided.** (See ADVERSE REACTIONS.)

Patients with a history of angioedema unrelated to ACE inhibitor therapy may be at increased risk of angioedema while receiving an ACE inhibitor (see also INDICATIONS AND USAGE and CONTRAINDICATIONS.)

Anaphylactoid Reactions During Desensitization: Two patients undergoing desensitizing treatment with hymenoptera venom while receiving ACE inhibitors sustained life-threatening anaphylactoid reactions. In the same patients, these reactions were avoided when ACE inhibitors were temporarily withheld, but they reappeared upon inadvertent rechallenge.

Anaphylactoid Reactions During Membrane Exposure: Anaphylactoid reactions have been reported in patients dialyzed with high-flux membranes and treated concomitantly with an ACE inhibitor. Anaphylactoid reactions have also been reported in patients undergoing low-density lipoprotein apheresis with dextran sulfate absorption.

Hypotension: LEXXEL can occasionally cause symptomatic hypotension.

Excessive hypotension is rare in uncomplicated hypertensive patients treated with enalapril alone. Patients at risk for excessive hypotension, sometimes associated with oliguria and/or progressive azotemia, and rarely with acute renal failure and/or death, include those with the following conditions or characteristics: heart failure, hyponatremia, high dose diuretic therapy, recent intensive diuresis or increase in diuretic dose, renal dialysis, or severe volume and/or salt depletion of any etiology. It may be advisable to eliminate the diuretic (except in patients with heart failure), reduce the diuretic dose or increase salt intake cautiously before initiating therapy with enalapril maleate in patients at risk for excessive hypotension who are able to tolerate such adjustments. (See PRECAUTIONS, Drug Interactions and ADVERSE REACTIONS.) In patients at risk for excessive hypotension, therapy should be started under very close medical supervision and such patients should be followed closely for the first 2 weeks of treatment and whenever the dose of enalapril and/or diuretic is increased. Similar considerations may apply to patients with ischemic heart or cerebrovascular disease, in whom an excessive fall in blood pressure could result in a myocardial infarction or cerebrovascular accident.

If excessive hypotension occurs, the patient should be placed in the supine position and, if necessary, receive an intravenous infusion of normal saline. A transient hypotensive response is not a contraindication to further doses of enalapril maleate, which usually can be given without difficulty once the blood pressure has stabilized. If symptomatic hypotension develops, a dose reduction or discontinuation of enalapril or diuretic may be necessary.

Felodipine, like other calcium channel blockers, may occasionally precipitate significant hypotension and rarely syncope. It may lead to reflex tachycardia which in susceptible individuals may precipitate angina pectoris. (See ADVERSE REACTIONS.)

Neutropenia/Agranulocytosis: Another angiotensin converting enzyme inhibitor, captopril, has been shown to cause agranulocytosis and bone marrow depression, rarely in uncomplicated patients but more frequently in patients with renal impairment, especially if they also have a collagen vascular disease. Available data from clinical trials of enalapril are insufficient to show that enalapril does not cause agranulocytosis at similar rates. Marketing experience has revealed cases of neutropenia or agranulocytosis in which a causal relationship to enalapril cannot be excluded. Periodic monitoring of white blood cell counts in patients with collagen vascular disease and renal disease should be considered.

Hepatic Failure: Rarely, ACE inhibitors have been associated with a syndrome that starts with cholestatic jaundice and progresses to fulminant hepatic necrosis and (sometimes) death. The mechanism of this syndrome is not understood. Patients receiving ACE inhibitors who develop jaundice or marked elevations of hepatic enzymes should discontinue the ACE inhibitor and receive appropriate medical follow-up.

Fetal/Neonatal Morbidity and Mortality: ACE inhibitors can cause fetal and neonatal morbidity and death when administered to pregnant women. Several dozen cases have been reported in the world literature. When pregnancy is detected, LEXXEL should be discontinued as soon as possible.

The use of ACE inhibitors during the second and third trimesters of pregnancy has been associated with fetal and neonatal injury, including hypotension, neonatal skull hypoplasia, anuria, reversible or irreversible renal failure, and death. Oligohydramnios has also been reported, presumably resulting from decreased fetal renal function; oligohydramnios in this setting has been associated with fetal limb contractures, craniofacial deformation, and hypoplastic lung development. Prematurity, intrauterine growth retardation, and patent ductus arteriosus have also been reported, although it is not clear whether these occurrences were due to the ACE-inhibitor exposure.

These adverse effects do not appear to have resulted from intrauterine ACE-inhibitor exposure that has been limited to the first trimester. Mothers whose embryos and fetuses are exposed to ACE inhibitors only during the first trimester should be so informed. Nonetheless, when patients become pregnant, physicians should make every effort to discontinue the use of LEXXEL as soon as possible.

Rarely (probably less often than once in every thousand pregnancies), no alternative to ACE inhibitors will be found. In these rare cases, the mothers should be apprised of the potential hazards to their fetuses, and serial ultrasound examinations should be performed to assess the intra-amniotic environment.

If oligohydramnios is observed, LEXXEL should be discontinued unless it is considered lifesaving for the mother. Contraction stress testing (CST), a non-stress test (NST), or biophysical profiling (BPP) may be appropriate, depending upon the week of pregnancy. Patients and physicians should be aware, however, that oligohydramnios may not appear until after the fetus has sustained irreversible injury.

Infants with histories of *in utero* exposure to ACE inhibitors should be closely observed for hypotension, oliguria, and hyperkalemia. If oliguria occurs, attention should be directed toward support of blood pressure and renal perfusion. Exchange transfusion or dialysis may be required as means of reversing hypotension and/or substituting for disordered renal function. Enalapril, which crosses the placenta, has been removed from neonatal circulation by peritoneal dialysis with some clinical benefit, and theoretically may be removed by exchange transfusion, although there is no experience with the latter procedure.

No teratogenic effects of enalapril were seen in studies of pregnant rats and rabbits. On a body surface area basis, the doses used were 57 times and 12 times, respectively, the maximum recommended human daily dose (MRHDD).

In rats administered the combination of enalapril and felodipine (enalapril [E]=1.9-felodipine [F]=2.5 mg/kg/day), an increased incidence of fetuses with dilated renal pelvis/ureter was observed. However, there was no evidence of this effect in the offspring postweaning. In mice, with doses of E=23, F=30 mg/kg/day or greater, there was an increased incidence of both early and late *in utero* deaths. Other than a transient and slight decrease in body weight gain in the first generation offspring, there were no adverse effects in offspring with regard to sexual maturation, behavioral development, fertility or fecundity.

Enalapril-felodipine given to pregnant mice (enalapril 20.8, felodipine 27 mg/kg/day) and rats (enalapril =17.3, felodipine =22.5 mg/kg/day) produced plasma levels (C_{max} and AUC values) of enalapril/enalaprilat that were 76 to 418-fold greater and plasma levels of felodipine that were 151 to 433–fold greater than those expected in humans (non-pregnant) at the dose to be used in humans.

PRECAUTIONS

General

Aortic Stenosis/Hypertrophic Cardiomyopathy—As with all vasodilators, enalapril should be given with caution to patients with obstruction in the outflow tract of the left ventricle.

Impaired Renal Function—As a consequence of inhibiting the renin-angiotensin-aldosterone system, changes in renal function may be anticipated in susceptible individuals treated with enalapril. In patients with severe heart failure whose renal function may depend on the activity of the renin-angiotensin-aldosterone system, treatment with angiotensin converting enzyme inhibitors, including enalapril, may be associated with oliguria and/or progressive azotemia and rarely with acute renal failure and/or death.

In clinical studies in hypertensive patients with unilateral or bilateral renal artery stenosis, increases in blood urea nitrogen and serum creatinine were observed in 20% of patients treated with enalapril. These increases were almost always reversible upon discontinuation of enalapril and/or diuretic therapy. In such patients, renal function should be monitored during the first few weeks of therapy.

Some enalapril-treated patients with hypertension or heart failure, with no apparent pre-existing renal vascular disease, have developed increases in blood urea and serum creatinine, usually minor and transient, especially when enalapril has been given concomitantly with a diuretic. This is more likely to occur in patients with pre-existing renal impairment. Dosage reduction of enalapril or discontinuation of the diuretic may be required.

Evaluation of the hypertensive patient should always include assessment of renal function.

Hyperkalemia—Elevated serum potassium (greater than 5.7 mEq/L) was observed in approximately 1% of hypertensive patients in clinical trials treated with enalapril alone. In most cases these were isolated values which resolved despite continued therapy. Hyperkalemia was a cause of discontinuation of therapy in 0.28% of hypertensive patients. In clinical trials in heart failure, hyperkalemia was observed in 3.8% of patients but was not a cause for discontinuation.

Risk factors for the development of hyperkalemia include renal insufficiency, diabetes mellitus, and the concomitant use of potassium-sparing diuretics, potassium supplements and/or potassium-containing salt substitutes, which should be used cautiously, if at all, with enalapril. (See Drug Interactions.)

Elderly Patients or Patients with Impaired Liver Function—Patients over 65 years of age or patients with impaired liver function may have elevated plasma concentrations of felodipine. (See DOSAGE AND ADMINISTRATION.)

Cough—Presumably due to the inhibition of the degradation of endogenous bradykinin, persistent nonproductive cough has been reported with all ACE inhibitors, always resolving after discontinuation of therapy. ACE inhibitor-induced cough should be considered in the diagnosis of cough.

Surgery/Anesthesia—In patients undergoing major surgery or during anesthesia with agents that produce hypotension, enalapril may block angiotensin II formation secondary to compensatory renin release. If hypotension occurs and is considered to be due to this mechanism, it can be corrected by volume expansion.

Peripheral Edema—Peripheral edema, generally mild and not associated with generalized fluid retention, was the most common adverse event in the felodipine clinical trials. The incidence of peripheral edema was both dose and age dependent. This adverse event generally occurs within 2–3 weeks of the initiation of treatment.

Information for Patients: Patients should be instructed to take LEXXEL whole and not to divide, crush or chew the tablet.

All patients should be advised to consult their physician if they experience any of the following conditions:

Angioedema—Angioedema, including laryngeal edema, may occur at any time during treatment with angiotensin converting enzyme inhibitors, including enalapril. Patients should be so advised and told to report immediately any signs or symptoms suggesting angioedema (swelling of face, extremities, eyes, lips, tongue, difficulty in swallowing or breathing) and to take no more drug until they have consulted with the prescribing physician.

Hypotension—Patients should be cautioned to report light headedness especially during the first few days of therapy. If actual syncope occurs, the patients should be told to discontinue LEXXEL until they have consulted with the prescribing physician. All patients should be cautioned that excessive perspiration and dehydration may lead to an excessive fall in blood pressure because of reduction in fluid volume. Other causes of volume depletion, such as vomiting or diarrhea, may also lead to a fall in blood pressure; patients should be advised to consult with the physician.

Hyperkalemia—Patients should be told not to use salt substitutes containing potassium without consulting their physician.

Neutropenia—Patients should be told to report promptly any indication of infection (e.g., sore throat, fever) which may be a sign of neutropenia.

Pregnancy—Female patients of childbearing age should be told about the consequences of second- and third-trimester exposure to ACE inhibitors, and they should also be told that these consequences do not appear to have resulted from intrauterine ACE-inhibitor exposure that has been limited to the first trimester. These patients should be asked to report pregnancies to their physicians as soon as possible.

Gingival Hyperplasia—Patients should be told that mild gingival hyperplasia (gum swelling) has been reported. Good dental hygiene decreases its incidence and severity.

Note: As with many other drugs, certain advice to patients being treated with LEXXEL is warranted. This information is intended to aid in the safe and effective use of this medication. It is not disclosure of all possible adverse or intended effects.

Drug Interactions: *Hypotension—Patients on Diuretic Therapy:* Patients on diuretics, and especially those in whom diuretic therapy was recently instituted, may occasionally experience an excessive reduction of blood pressure after initiation of therapy with enalapril. The possibility of hypotensive effects with enalapril can be minimized by either discontinuing the diuretic or increasing the salt intake prior to initiation of treatment with enalapril. If it is necessary to continue the diuretic, provide close medical supervision after the initial dose for at least two hours and until blood pressure has stabilized for at least an additional hour. (See WARNINGS and DOSAGE AND ADMINISTRATION.)

Agents Causing Renin Release—The antihypertensive effect of enalapril is augmented by antihypertensive agents that cause renin release (e.g., diuretics).

Non-steroidal Anti-inflammatory Agents—In some patients with compromised renal function who are being treated with non-steroidal anti-inflammatory drugs, the coadministration of enalapril may result in a further deterioration of renal function. These effects are usually reversible.

Agents Increasing Serum Potassium—Enalapril attenuates potassium loss caused by thiazide-type diuretics. Potassium-sparing diuretics (e.g., spironolactone, triamterene, or amiloride), potassium supplements, or potassium-containing salt substitutes may lead to significant increases in serum potassium. Therefore, if concomitant use of these agents is indicated because of demonstrated hypokalemia, they should be used with caution and with frequent monitoring of serum potassium.

Lithium—Lithium toxicity has been reported in patients receiving lithium concomitantly with drugs which cause elimination of sodium, including ACE inhibitors. A few cases of lithium toxicity have been reported in patients receiving concomitant enalapril and lithium and were reversible upon discontinuation of both drugs. It is recommended that serum lithium levels be monitored frequently if enalapril is administered concomitantly with lithium.

Beta-Blocking Agents—Enalapril has been used concomitantly with beta adrenergic-blocking agents without evidence of clinically significant adverse interactions.

A pharmacokinetic study of felodipine in conjunction with metoprolol demonstrated no significant effects on the pharmacokinetics of felodipine. The AUC and C_{max} of metoprolol, however, were increased approximately 31% and 38%, respectively. In controlled clinical trials, however, beta blockers including metoprolol were concurrently administered with felodipine and were well tolerated.

Cimetidine—In healthy subjects, pharmacokinetic studies showed an approximately 50% increase in the area under the plasma concentration time curve (AUC) as well as the C_{max} of felodipine when given concomitantly with cimetidine. It is anticipated that a clinically significant interaction may occur in some hypertensive patients.

Digoxin—Enalapril has been used concomitantly with digoxin without evidence of clinically significant adverse interactions.

When given concomitantly with felodipine ER, the pharmacokinetics of digoxin in patients with heart failure were not significantly altered.

Anticonvulsants—In a pharmacokinetic study, maximum plasma concentrations of felodipine were considerably lower in epileptic patients on long-term anticonvulsant therapy (e.g., phenytoin, carbamazepine, or phenobarbital) than in healthy volunteers. In such patients, the mean area under the felodipine plasma concentration-time curve was also reduced to approximately 6% of that observed in healthy volunteers. Since a clinically significant interaction may be anticipated, alternative antihypertensive therapy should be considered in these patients.

Other Concomitant Therapy—In healthy subjects, there were no clinically significant interactions when felodipine was given concomitantly with indomethacin or spironolactone.

Enalapril has been used concomitantly with methyldopa, nitrates, hydralazine, and prazosin without evidence of clinically significant adverse interactions.

Carcinogenesis, Mutagenesis, Impairment of Fertility: No long-term carcinogenicity tests have been performed with the combination. Enalapril-felodipine was not mutagenic with or without metabolic activation *in vitro* in the Ames microbial mutation assay, the V-79 mammalian cell forward mutation assay, the alkaline elution assay with rat hepatocytes or the CHO mammalian cell cytogenetics assay. An *in vivo* mouse bone marrow cytogenetics assay was also negative.

In rats given enalapril-felodipine, there was no effect on fertility in males at doses up to 6.9/9 mg/kg/day, and in females at doses up to 17.3/22.5 mg/kg/day.

There was no evidence of a tumorigenic effect when enalapril was administered for 106 weeks to male and female rats at doses up to 90 mg/kg/day or for 94 weeks to male and female mice at doses up to 90 and 180 mg/kg/day, respectively. These doses are 26 times (in rats and female mice) and 13 times (in male mice) the maximum recommended human daily dose (MRHDD) when compared on a body surface area basis.

Neither enalapril maleate nor the active diacid was mutagenic in the Ames microbial mutagen test with or without metabolic activation. Enalapril was also negative in the following genotoxicity studies: rec-assay, reverse mutation assay with *E. coli*, sister chromatid exchange with cultured mammalian cells, and the micronucleus test with mice, as well as in an *in vivo* cytogenic study using mouse bone marrow.

There were no adverse effects on reproductive performance of male and female rats treated with up to 90 mg/kg/day of enalapril (26 times the MRHDD when compared on a body surface area basis).

In a 2-year carcinogenicity study in rats fed felodipine at doses of 7.7, 23.1 or 69.3 mg/kg/day (up to 61 times[†] the maximum recommended human dose on a mg/m^2 basis), a dose-related increase in the incidence of benign interstitial cell tumors of the testes (Leydig cell tumors) was observed in treated male rats. These tumors were not observed in a similar study in mice at doses up to 138.6 mg/kg/day (61 times[†] the maximum recommended human dose on a mg/m^2 basis). Felodipine, at the doses employed in the 2-year rat study, has been shown to lower testicular testosterone and to produce a corresponding increase in serum luteinizing hormone in rats. The Leydig cell tumor development is possibly secondary to these hormonal effects which have not been observed in man.

[†]Based on patient weight of 50 kg

In this same rat study, a dose-related increase in the incidence of focal squamous cell hyperplasia, compared to control, was observed in the esophageal groove of male and female rats in all dose groups. No other drug-related esophageal or gastric pathology was observed in the rats or with chronic administration in mice and dogs. The latter species, like man, has no anatomical structure comparable to the esophageal groove.

Felodipine was not carcinogenic when fed to mice at doses of up to 138.6 mg/kg/day (61 times[†] the maximum recommended human dose on a mg/m^2 basis) for periods of up to 80 weeks in males and 99 weeks in females.

Felodipine did not display any mutagenic activity *in vitro* in the Ames microbial mutagenicity test or in the mouse lymphoma forward mutation assay. No clastogenic potential was seen *in vivo* in the mouse micronucleus test at oral doses up to 2500 mg/kg (1100 times[†] the maximum recommended human dose on a mg/m^2 basis) or *in vitro* in a human lymphocyte chromosome aberration assay.

A fertility study in which male and female rats were administered doses of 3.8, 9.6, or 26.9 mg/kg/day showed no significant effect of felodipine on reproductive performance.

Pregnancy: *Pregnancy Categories C* (first trimester) *and D* (second and third trimesters). See WARNINGS, Fetal/Neonatal Morbidity and Mortality.

Teratogenic Effects—Studies in pregnant rabbits administered doses of felodipine 0.46, 1.2, 2.3, and 4.6 mg/kg/day (from 0.5 to 5 times[†] the maximum recommended human dose on a mg/m^2 basis) showed digital anomalies consisting of reduction in size and degree of ossification of the terminal phalanges in the fetuses. The frequency and severity of the changes appeared dose-related and were noted even at the lowest dose. These changes have been shown to occur with other members of the dihydropyridine class and are possibly a result of compromised uterine blood flow. Similar fetal anomalies were not observed in rats given felodipine.

In a teratology study in cynomolgus monkeys, no reduction in the size of the terminal phalanges was observed, but an abnormal position of the distal phalanges was noted in about 40% of the fetuses.

Nonteratogenic Effects—A prolongation of parturition with difficult labor and an increased frequency of fetal and early postnatal deaths were observed in rats administered felodipine doses of 9.6 mg/kg/day (8 times[†] the maximum human dose on a mg/m^2 basis) and above.

Significant enlargement of the mammary glands, in excess of the normal enlargement for pregnant rabbits, was found with doses greater than or equal to 1.2 mg/kg/day (1.4 times the maximum human dose on a mg/m^2 basis). This effect occurred only in pregnant rabbits and regressed during lactation. Similar changes in the mammary glands were not observed in rats or monkeys.

There are no adequate and well-controlled studies with felodipine in pregnant women. If felodipine is used during pregnancy, or if the patient becomes pregnant while taking this drug, she should be apprised of the potential hazard to the fetus, possible digital anomalies of the infant, and the potential effects of felodipine on labor and delivery, and on the mammary glands of pregnant females.

[†] Based on patient weight of 50 kg

Nursing Mothers: Enalapril and enalaprilat are detected in human breast milk. It is not known whether felodipine administered as monotherapy is secreted in human milk; studies of the combination of enalapril and felodipine in rats indicate that felodipine concentrates in milk to a level almost ten-fold that found in plasma. Because of the potential for serious adverse reactions from enalapril and felodipine in the infant, a decision should be made either to discontinue nursing or to discontinue the drug, taking into account the importance of the drug to the mother. Therefore, caution should be exercised when LEXXEL is given to a nursing mother.

Pediatric Use: Safety and effectiveness in pediatric patients have not been established.

ADVERSE REACTIONS

In a factorial study, combinations of enalapril at doses of 0, 5, and 20 mg and felodipine ER at doses of 0, 2.5, 5, and 10 mg were evaluated for safety in more than 700 patients with hypertension. In addition more than 500 patients received various combinations of enalapril (5 or 10 mg) and felodipine ER (2.5, 5, or 10 mg) with or without hydrochlorothiazide (12.5 mg) in an open-labeled study up to 52 weeks (mean 33 weeks). Adverse events were similar to those described with the individual components.

In general, treatment with enalapril maleate-felodipine ER was well tolerated and adverse events were mild and transient in nature. In the placebo-controlled, double-blind trial, discontinuation of therapy due to adverse events considered related (possibly, probably or definitely) occurred in 2.8% vs 1.3% of patients treated with the combination or placebo, respectively. The most frequently observed clinical adverse events considered related to treatment with the combination were headache, edema or swelling, and dizziness.

Continued on next page

Lexxel—Cont.

Clinical adverse events considered related (possibly, probably, or definitely) to treatment with enalapril-felodipine ER that occurred with an incidence of 1% or greater with the combination during the placebo-controlled, double-blind trial are compared to individual components and placebo in the table below:

[See table below]

Other clinical adverse events considered related (possibly, probably, or definitely) to treatment with enalapril-felodipine ER that occurred with an incidence of less than 1% in the placebo-controlled, double-blind trial are listed below. These events are listed in order of decreasing frequency within each category. ***Body as a Whole:*** Syncope, facial edema, orthostatic effects, chest pain; ***Cardiovascular:*** Palpitation, hypotension, bradycardia, premature ventricular contraction, increased blood pressure; ***Digestive:*** Dry mouth, constipation, dyspepsia, flatulence, acid regurgitation, vomiting, diarrhea, nausea, anal/rectal pain; ***Metabolic:*** Gout; ***Musculoskeletal:*** Neck pain, joint swelling; ***Nervous/Psychiatric:*** Insomnia, nervousness, somnolence, ataxia, agitation, paresthesia, tremor; ***Respiratory:*** Dyspnea, respiratory congestion, pharyngeal discomfort, dry throat; ***Skin:*** Rash, angioedema, pruritus, alopecia, dry skin; ***Special Senses:*** Increased intraocular pressure; ***Urogenital:*** Impotence, hot flashes.

Other infrequently reported adverse events were seen in clinical trials with enalapril-felodipine ER (causal relationship unknown). These included: ***Body as a Whole:*** Abdominal pain, fever; ***Digestive:*** Dental pain; ***Metabolic:*** Increased ALT and AST, hyperglycemia; ***Musculoskeletal:*** Back pain, myalgia, foot pain, knee pain, shoulder pain, tendinitis; ***Respiratory:*** Upper respiratory infection, sinusitis, pharyngitis, bronchitis, nasal congestion, influenza, sinus disorder; ***Special Senses:*** Conjunctivitis; ***Urogenital:*** Proteinuria, pyuria, urinary tract infection.

Enalapril Maleate: Other adverse events that have been reported with enalapril, without regard to causality, are listed (in decreasing severity) below:

Angioedema—Angioedema has been reported in patients receiving enalapril maleate, with an incidence higher in black than in non-black patients. Angioedema associated with laryngeal edema may be fatal. If angioedema of the face, extremities, lips, tongue, glottis and/or larynx occurs, treatment with LEXXEL should be discontinued and appropriate therapy instituted immediately. (See WARNINGS.)

Body as a Whole: Anaphylactoid reactions (see WARNINGS, Anaphylactoid and Possibly Related Reactions); ***Cardiovascular:*** Cardiac arrest, myocardial infarction or cerebrovascular accident, possibly secondary to excessive hypotension in high risk patients (see WARNINGS, Hypotension), orthostatic hypotension, pulmonary embolism and infarction, pulmonary edema, rhythm disturbances including atrial tachycardia and bradycardia, atrial fibrillation, angina pectoris; ***Digestive:*** Ileus, pancreatitis, hepatic failure, hepatitis (hepatocellular [proven on rechallenge] or cholestatic jaundice) (see WARNINGS, Hepatic Failure), melena, anorexia, glossitis, stomatitis; ***Hematologic:*** Rare cases of neutropenia, thrombocytopenia and bone marrow depression; ***Musculoskeletal:*** Muscle cramps; ***Nervous/Psychiatric:*** Depression, confusion, peripheral neuropathy (e.g. paresthesia, dysesthesia), vertigo; ***Respiratory:*** Bronchospasm, rhinorrhea, sore throat and hoarseness, asthma, pneumonia, pulmonary infiltrates, eosinophilic pneumonitis; ***Skin:*** Exfoliative dermatitis, toxic epidermal necrolysis, Stevens-Johnson syndrome, pemphigus, herpes zoster, erythema multiforme, urticaria, diaphoresis, photosensitivity; ***Special Senses:*** Blurred vision, taste alteration, anosmia, tinnitus, dry eyes, tearing; ***Urogenital:*** Renal failure, oliguria, renal dysfunction (see PRECAUTIONS), flank pain, gynecomastia; ***Miscellaneous:*** A symptom complex has been reported which may include a positive ANA, an elevated erythrocyte sedimentation rate, arthralgia/arthritis, myalgia/myositis, fever, serositis, vasculitis, leukocytosis, eosinophilia, photosensitivity rash and other dermatologic manifestations; ***Fetal/Neonatal Morbidity and Mortality:*** See WARNINGS, Fetal/Neonatal Morbidity and Mortality.

Felodipine as an Extended-Release Formulation: Other adverse events that have been reported with felodipine ER, without regard to causality, are listed (in decreasing severity) below:

Body as a Whole: Flu-like illness; ***Cardiovascular:*** Myocardial infarction, angina pectoris, arrhythmia, tachycardia, premature beats; ***Digestive:*** Gingival hyperplasia; ***Endocrine:*** Gynecomastia; ***Hematologic:*** Anemia; ***Musculoskeletal:*** Arthralgia, leg pain, muscle cramps, arm pain, hip pain; ***Nervous/Psychiatric:*** Depression, anxiety disorders, irritability, decreased libido; ***Respiratory:*** Upper respiratory infection, rhinorrhea, sneezing, pharyngitis, influenza, epistaxis, respiratory infection; ***Skin:*** Contusion, erythema, urticaria; ***Special Senses:*** Visual disturbances; ***Urogenital:*** Urinary frequency, urinary urgency, dysuria, polyuria.

Laboratory Test Findings: In controlled clinical trials with enalapril-felodipine ER, clinically important changes in standard laboratory parameters associated with administration of LEXXEL were rare. No changes peculiar to the combination treatment were observed.

Serum Electrolytes—See PRECAUTIONS.

Creatinine—Minor reversible increases in serum creatinine were observed in patients treated with LEXXEL. Increases in creatinine are more likely to occur in patients with renal insufficiency or those pretreated with a diuretic and based on experience with other ACE inhibitors, would be expected to be especially likely in patients with renal artery stenosis (see PRECAUTIONS).

Other—Minor reversible increases or decreases in serum potassium were infrequently observed in patients treated with LEXXEL; rarely were these measurements outside the normal range.

OVERDOSAGE

Limited data are available in regard to enalapril overdosage in humans. In a suicide attempt, one patient took 150 mg felodipine together with 15 tablets each of atenolol and spironolactone and 20 tablets of nitrazepam. The patient's blood pressure and heart rate were normal on admission to hospital; he subsequently recovered without significant sequelae.

Human overdoses with any combination of enalapril and felodipine ER have not been reported.

Single oral doses of enalapril above 1000 mg/kg and ≥1775 mg/kg were associated with lethality in mice and rats, respectively. Oral doses of felodipine at 240 mg/kg and 264 mg/kg in male and female mice, respectively, and 2390 mg/kg and 2250 mg/kg in male and female rats, respectively, caused significant lethality.

In interaction studies on the acute oral toxicity of the combination in mice, pretreatment with felodipine (50 mg/kg) for one hour led to an increase in mortality at doses of enalapril maleate that exceeded 1000 mg/kg. Significant lethality with felodipine was not increased by pretreatment of mice for one hour with 100 mg/kg of enalapril maleate.

Treatment: To obtain up-to-date information about the treatment of overdose, consult your Regional Poison-Control Center. Telephone numbers of certified poison-control centers are listed in the *Physicians' Desk Reference (PDR)*. In managing overdose, consider the possibilities of multiple-drug overdoses, drug-drug interactions, and unusual drug kinetics in your patient.

The most likely effect of overdose with LEXXEL is vasodilation, with consequent hypotension and tachycardia. Repletion of central fluid volume (Trendelenburg positioning, infusion of crystalloids) may be sufficient therapy, but pressor agents (norepinephrine or high-dose dopamine) may be required.

Enalaprilat may be removed from general circulation by hemodialysis at a rate of 62 mL/min and has been removed from neonatal circulation by peritoneal dialysis. (See Warnings, Anaphylactoid reactions during membrane exposure.) It has not been established whether felodipine can be removed from the circulation by hemodialysis.

DOSAGE AND ADMINSTRATION

LEXXEL is an effective treatment for hypertension. This fixed combination drug is not indicated for initial therapy of hypertension.

The recommended initial dose of enalapril maleate for hypertension in patients not receiving diuretics is 5 mg once a day. The usual dosage range of enalapril maleate for hypertension is 10–40 mg per day administered in a single dose or two divided doses. In some patients treated once daily with enalapril, the antihypertensive effect may diminish toward the end of the dosing interval. In such patients, an increase in dosage or twice daily administration should be considered. The recommended initial dose of felodipine ER is 5 mg once a day with a usual dosage range of 2.5 mg-10 mg once a day. In elderly or hepatically impaired patients, the recommended initial dose of felodipine is 2.5 mg. When LEXXEL is taken with food, the peak concentration of felodipine is almost doubled, and the trough (24-hour) concentration is approximately halved (see CLINICAL PHARMACOLOGY, Pharmacokinetics and Metabolism).

In clinical trials of enalapril-felodipine ER combination therapy using enalapril doses of 5–20 mg and felodipine ER doses of 2.5–10 mg once daily, the antihypertensive effects increased with increasing doses of each component in all patient groups.

The hazards (see WARNINGS and ADVERSE REACTIONS) of enalapril are generally independent of dose; those of felodipine are a mixture of dose-dependent phenomena (primarily peripheral edema) and dose-independent phenomena, the former much more common than the latter. Therapy with any combination of enalapril and felodipine will thus be associated with both sets of dose-independent hazards.

Rarely, the dose-independent hazards associated with enalapril or felodipine are serious. To minimize dose-independent hazards, it is usually appropriate to begin therapy with LEXXEL only after a patient has failed to achieve the desired antihypertensive effect with one or the other monotherapy.

Replacement Therapy: Although the felodipine component of LEXXEL has not been shown to be bioequivalent to the available extended-release felodipine (PLENDIL), patients receiving enalapril and felodipine from separate tablets once a day may instead wish to receive the tablets of LEXXEL containing the same component doses.

Therapy Guided By Clinical Effect: A patient whose blood pressure is not adequately controlled with felodipine (or another dihydropyridine) or enalapril (or another ACE inhibitor) alone may be switched to combination therapy with LEXXEL, initially one tablet daily, usually LEXXEL 5-5. If blood pressure control is inadequate after a week or two, the dose may be increased to 2 tablets LEXXEL 5-5 administered once daily. The next incremental effect can be achieved with 4 tablets LEXXEL 5-2.5 administered once daily. If control remains unsatisfactory, consider addition of a thiazide diuretic.

Use in Patients with Metabolic Impairments: Regimens of therapy with LEXXEL need not be adjusted for renal function as long as the patient's creatinine clearance is >30 mL/min/1.73m^2 (serum creatinine roughly ≤3 mg/dL or 265 μmol/L). In patients with more severe renal impairment, the recommended initial dose of enalapril is 2.5 mg. LEXXEL should regularly be taken either without food or with a light meal (see CLINICAL PHARMACOLOGY, Pharmacokinetics and Metabolism). LEXXEL should be swallowed whole and not divided, crushed or chewed.

HOW SUPPLIED

No. 3771—Tablets LEXXEL, 5-2.5 are white, round/biconvex-shaped, film-coated tablets, coded LEXXEL 2, 5-2.5 on one side and no markings on the other. Each tablet contains 5 mg of enalapril maleate and 2.5 mg of felodipine as an extended-release formulation. They are supplied as follows:

NDC 0186-0002-31 unit of use bottles of 30 (with desiccants)

No. 3661—Tablets LEXXEL, 5-5 are white, round/biconvex-shaped, film-coated tablets, coded LEXXEL 1, 5-5 on one side and no markings on the other. Each tablet contains 5 mg of enalapril maleate and 5 mg of felodipine as an extended-release formulation. They are supplied as follows:

NDC 0186-0001-31 unit of use bottles of 30 (with desiccants)

NDC 0186-0001-68 bottles of 100 (with desiccants)

Storage: Store at 25°C (77°F); excursions permitted between 15°C and 30°C (59°F and 86°F) [See USP Controlled Room Temperature]. Keep container tightly closed. Protect from moisture and light. Dispense in a tight container, if product package is subdivided.

Manufactured by: Merck & Co., Inc.,
West Point, PA 19486,
Distributed by:
Astra Pharmaceuticals, L.P.
Wayne, PA 19087,
620008-04 Revised January 2000

Shown in Product Identification Guide, page 304

Percent of Patients with Adverse Events in the Double-Blind Trial
(Percent discontinuation shown in parentheses)

Body System Adverse Event	Enalapril[a] Felodipine ER[b] N=319	Enalapril[a] N=133	Felodipine ER[b] N=176	Placebo N=79
Body as a Whole				
Edema/Swelling	4.1(0.3)	2.3(0.0)	10.8(1.7)	1.3(0.0)
Asthenia/Fatigue	1.9(0.0)	2.3(0.8)	0.6(0.6)	3.8(0.0)
Nervous/Psychiatric				
Headache	10.3(0.6)	3.8(0.0)	10.2(1.1)	7.6(1.3)
Dizziness	4.4(0.3)	1.5(0.0)	2.8(0.6)	0.0(0.0)
Respiratory				
Cough	2.2(0.6)	2.3(0.0)	0.6(0.0)	0.0(0.0)
Skin				
Flushing	1.6(0.3)	0.0(0.0)	2.3(1.1)	0.0(0.0)

[a]Combination of dose of 5 and 20 mg daily
[b]Combination of dose 2.5, 5 and 10 mg daily

M.V.I.®-12 ℞

Multi-Vitamin Infusion

For dilution in intravenous infusions only.

(For details of indications, dosage and administration, precautions, and adverse reactions, see circular in package.)

After M.V.I.-12 is diluted in an intravenous infusion, the resulting solution is ready for immediate use. Some of the vitamins in this product, particularly A and D and riboflavin, are light sensitive, and exposure to light should be minimized.

Store at 2°–8°C (36°–46°F).

HOW SUPPLIED

M.V.I.-12—NDC 0186-1199-38 Boxes of 10 and cartons of 100. Each box contains two vials—Vial 1 (5 mL) and Vial 2 (5 mL), both vials to be used for a single dose.

M.V.I.-12 Multi-Dose (PHARMACY BULK PACKAGE)–NDC 0186-1199-71 Boxes of 20 vials, 50 mL each (10 Vial 1 and 10 Vial 2). Mix contents of Vial 1 with Vial 2 to provide ten single doses.

Astra USA, Inc., Westborough, MA 01581

021901R01 Rev. 7/99

HOW SUPPLIED

M.V.I.-12 UNIT VIAL—NDC 0186-1199-41 Boxes of 10 two-chambered 10 mL vials.

Made by:
Astra USA, Inc., Westborough, MA 01581
Sterilized and Filled by:
The Liposome Manufacturing Company, Inc.
Indianapolis, IN 46268
004352R00 Iss. 4/98

M.V.I.® PEDIATRIC ℞

Multi-Vitamins for Infusion

For dilution in intravenous infusions only.

(For details of indications, dosage and administration, precautions, and adverse reactions, see circular in package.)

DISCARD ANY UNUSED PORTION.

Parenteral drug products should be inspected visually for particulate matter and discoloration prior to administration, whenever solution and container permit.

After M.V.I. Pediatric is reconstituted it should be immediately diluted into the intravenous solution. The resulting solution should be administered immediately. Some of the vitamins in this product, particularly vitamins A and D and riboflavin, are light-sensitive and exposure to light should be minimized.

HOW SUPPLIED

M.V.I Pediatric is available as:
NDC 0186-1839-31, Single Dose Vial, Boxes of 10.
Store under refrigeration, 2–8°C (36–46°F).
Manufactured by: Catalytica Pharmaceuticals, Inc
Greenville, NC 27834
Manufactured for: Astra Pharmaceuticals, L.P.
Wayne, PA 19087
704101-01 Rev. 1/00

NALBUPHINE HCl INJECTION ℞

(For details of indications, dosage and administration, precautions, and adverse reactions, see circular in package.)

HOW SUPPLIED

Nalbuphine HCl Injection for intramuscular, subcutaneous or intravenous use is available in the following dosage forms:

Vials
10 mg/mL, 10 mL vial (box of 1), NDC 0186-1262-12
20 mg/mL, 10 mL vial (box of 1), NDC 0186-1266-12
Store at controlled room temperature 15°–30°C (59°–86°F). Protect from light.
021886R05 Rev. 6/97

NAROPIN™ ℞

[nă-rōpin]
(ropivacaine HCl Injection)

DESCRIPTION

Naropin™ (ropivacaine HCl Injection) is a member of the amino amide class of local anesthetics. Naropin injections are sterile, isotonic solutions that contain the enantiomerically pure drug substance, sodium chloride for isotonicity and Water for Injection. Sodium hydroxide and/or hydrochloric acid may be used for pH adjustment. These solutions are administered parenterally.

Naropin contains ropivacaine HCl which is chemically described as S-(-)-1-propyl-2′,6′-pipecoloxylidide hydrochloride monohydrate. The drug substance is a white crystalline powder, with a chemical formula of $C_{17}H_{26}N_2O{\cdot}HCl{\cdot}H_2O$, molecular weight of 328.89 and the following structural formula:

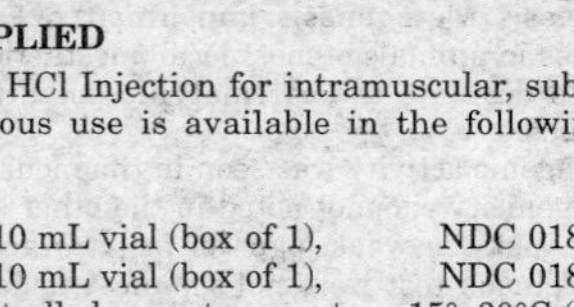

At 25°C ropivacaine HCl has a solubility of 53.8 mg/mL in water, a distribution ratio between n-octanol and phosphate buffer at pH 7.4 of 141 and a pKa of 8.07 in 0.1 M KCl solution. The pKa of ropivacaine is approximately the same as bupivacaine (8.1) and is similar to that of mepivacaine (7.7). However, ropivacaine has an intermediate degree of lipid solubility compared to bupivacaine and mepivacaine.

Naropin is preservative free and is available in single dose containers in 2.0, 5.0, 7.5 and 10.0 mg/mL concentrations. The specific gravity of Naropin solutions range from 1.002 to 1.005 at 25°C.

CLINICAL PHARMACOLOGY

Mechanism of Action: Ropivacaine is a member of the amino amide class of local anesthetics and is supplied as the pure S-(-)-enantiomer. Local anesthetics block the generation and the conduction of nerve impulses, presumably by increasing the threshold for electrical excitation in the nerve, by slowing the propagation of the nerve impulse, and by reducing the rate of rise of the action potential. In general, the progression of anesthesia is related to the diameter, myelination and conduction velocity of affected nerve fibers. Clinically, the order of loss of nerve function is as follows: (1) pain, (2) temperature, (3) touch, (4) proprioception, and (5) skeletal muscle tone.

PHARMACOKINETICS

Absorption: The systemic concentration of ropivacaine is dependent on the total dose and concentration of drug administered, the route of administration, the patient's hemodynamic/circulatory condition and the vascularity of the administration site.

From the epidural space, ropivacaine shows complete and biphasic absorption. The half-lives of the two phases, (mean ± SD) are 14 ± 7 minutes and 4.2 ± 0.9 h, respectively. The slow absorption is the rate limiting factor in the elimination of ropivacaine which explains why the terminal half-life is longer after epidural than after intravenous administration. Ropivacaine shows dose-proportionality up to the highest intravenous dose studied, 80 mg, corresponding to a mean ± SD peak plasma concentration of 1.9 ±0.3 μg/mL.

Distribution: After intravascular infusion, ropivacaine has a steady state volume of distribution of 41 ± 7 liters. Ropivacaine is 94% protein bound, mainly to α_1-acid glycoprotein. An increase in total plasma concentrations during continuous epidural infusion has been observed, related to a postoperative increase of α_1-acid glycoprotein. Variations in unbound, i.e. pharmacologically active, concentrations have been less than in total plasma concentration. Ropivacaine readily crosses the placenta and equilibrium in regard to unbound concentration will be rapidly reached (see PRECAUTIONS, Labor and Delivery).

Metabolism: Ropivacaine is extensively metabolized in the liver, predominantly by aromatic hydroxylation mediated by cytochrome P4501A to 3-hydroxy ropivacaine. Approximately 37% of the total dose is excreted in the urine as both free and conjugated 3-hydroxy ropivacaine. Low concentrations of 3-hydroxy ropivacaine have been found in the plasma. Urinary excretion of the 4-hydroxy and both the 3-hydroxy and 4-hydroxy N-dealkylated metabolites accounts for less than 3% of dose. An additional metabolite, 2-hydroxy-methyl-ropivacaine, has been identified but not quantified in the urine. Both 3-hydroxy and 4-hydroxy ropivacaine have a local anesthetic activity in animal models less than that of ropivacaine. There is no evidence of *in vivo* racemization in urine of S-(-)-ropivacaine to R-(+)-ropivacaine.

Elimination: The kidney is the main excretory organ for most local anesthetic metabolites. In total, 86% of the ropivacaine dose is excreted in the urine after intravenous administration of which only 1% relates to unchanged drug. Ropivacaine has a mean ± SD total plasma clearance of 387 ± 107 mL/min, an unbound plasma clearance of 7.2 ± 1.6 L/min, and a renal clearance of 1 mL/min. The mean ± SD terminal half-life is 1.8 ± 0.7 h after intravascular administration and 4.2 ± 1.0 h after epidural administration (see Absorption).

Pharmacodynamics: Studies in humans have demonstrated that, unlike most other local anesthetics, the presence of epinephrine has no major effect on either the time of onset or the duration of action of ropivacaine. Likewise, addition of epinephrine to ropivacaine has no effect on limiting systemic absorption of ropivacaine.

Systemic absorption of local anesthetics can produce effects on the central nervous and cardiovascular systems. At blood concentrations achieved with therapeutic doses, changes in cardiac conduction, excitability, refractoriness, contractility, and peripheral vascular resistance are minimal. However, toxic blood concentrations depress cardiac conduction and excitability, which may lead to atrioventricular block, ventricular arrhythmias and to cardiac arrest, sometimes resulting in fatalities. In addition, myocardial contractility is depressed and peripheral vasodilation occurs, leading to decreased cardiac output and arterial blood pressure.

Following systemic absorption, local anesthetics can produce central nervous system stimulation, depression or both. Apparent central stimulation is usually manifested as restlessness, tremors and shivering, progressing to convulsions, followed by depression and coma, progressing ultimately to respiratory arrest. However, the local anesthetics have a primary depressant effect on the medulla and on higher centers. The depressed stage may occur without a prior excited stage.

In two clinical pharmacology studies (total n=24) ropivacaine and bupivacaine were infused (10 mg/min) in human volunteers until the appearance of CNS symptoms, e.g., visual or hearing disturbances, perioral numbness, tingling and others. Similar symptoms were seen with both drugs. In one study, the mean ± SD maximum tolerated intravenous dose of ropivacaine infused (124 ± 38 mg) was significantly higher than that of bupivacaine (99 ± 30 mg) while in the other study the doses were not different (115 ± 29 mg of ropivacaine and 103 ± 30 mg of bupivacaine). In the latter study, the number of subjects reporting each symptom was similar for both drugs with the exception of muscle twitching which was reported by more subjects with bupivacaine than ropivacaine at comparable intravenous doses. At the end of the infusion, ropivacaine in both studies caused significantly less depression of cardiac conductivity (less QRS widening) than bupivacaine. Ropivacaine and bupivacaine caused evidence of depression of cardiac contractility, but there were no changes in cardiac output.

In nonclinical pharmacology studies comparing ropivacaine and bupivacaine in several animal species, the cardiac toxicity of ropivacaine was less than that of bupivacaine, although both were considerably more toxic than lidocaine. Arrhythmogenic and cardiodepressant effects were seen in animals at significantly higher doses of ropivacaine than bupivacaine. The incidence of successful resuscitation was not significantly different between the ropivacaine and bupivacaine groups.

Clinical Trials: Ropivacaine was studied as a local anesthetic both for surgical anesthesia and for acute pain management. (See DOSAGE AND ADMINISTRATION.)

The onset, depth and duration of sensory block are, in general, similar to bupivacaine. However, the depth and duration of motor block, in general, are less than that with bupivacaine.

Epidural Administration In Surgery—There were 25 clinical studies performed in 900 patients to evaluate Naropin epidural injection for general surgery. Naropin was used in doses ranging from 75 to 250 mg. In doses of 100-200 mg, the median (1st-3rd quartile) onset time to achieve a T10 sensory block was 10 (5-13) minutes and the median (1st-3rd quartile) duration at the T10 level was 4 (3-5) hours. (See DOSAGE AND ADMINISTRATION.)

Higher doses produced a more profound block with a greater duration of effect.

Epidural Administration In Cesarean Section—There were 8 studies performed in 218 patients to evaluate Naropin for cesarean section. 5 mg/mL (0.5%) Naropin was used in doses up to 150 mg. Median onset measured at T6 ranged from 11 to 26 minutes. Median duration of sensory block at T6 ranged from 1.7 to 3.2 h, and duration of motor block ranged from 1.4 to 2.9 h. Naropin provided adequate muscle relaxation for surgery in all cases.

Epidural Administration In Labor And Delivery—There were 10 double-blind clinical studies performed to evaluate Naropin versus bupivacaine for epidural block for management of labor pain (Naropin, n=258; bupivacaine, n=231). When administered in doses up to 278 mg as intermittent injections or as a continuous infusion, Naropin produced adequate pain relief.

A prospective meta-analysis on 6 of these studies provided detailed evaluation of the delivered newborns and showed no difference in clinical outcomes compared to bupivacaine. There were significantly fewer instrumental deliveries in mothers receiving ropivacaine as compared to bupivacaine.

LABOR AND DELIVERY META-ANALYSIS: MODE OF DELIVERY

Delivery Mode	Naropin n=199		Bupivacaine n=188	
	n	%	n	%
Spontaneous Vertex	116	58	92	49
Vacuum Extractor	26	27* (Vacuum Extractor + Forceps)	33	40 (Vacuum Extractor + Forceps)
Forceps	28		42	
Cesarean Section	29	15	21	11

* p=0.004 versus bupivacaine

Epidural Administration In Postoperative Pain Management—There were 8 clinical studies performed in 382 patients to evaluate Naropin for postoperative pain management after upper and lower abdominal surgery and after orthopedic surgery. The studies utilized intravascular morphine via PCA as a rescue medication and as an efficacy variable. Epidural anesthesia with Naropin was used intraoperatively for each of these procedures prior to initiation of postoperative Naropin. The incidence and intensity of the motor block were dependent on the dose rate of Naropin and the site of injection. Cumulative doses of up to 770 mg of ropivacaine were administered over 24 hours (intraoperative block plus postoperative continuous infusion). The overall quality of pain relief, as judged by the patients, in the ropivacaine groups was rated as good or excellent (73% to 100%). The frequency of motor block was greatest at 4 hours and decreased during the infusion period in all groups. At least 80% of patients in the upper and lower abdominal studies and 42% in the orthopedic studies had no motor block at the end of the 21-hour infusion period. Sensory block was also dose rate-dependent and a decrease in spread was observed during the infusion period. Clinical studies with 2 mg/mL (0.2%) Naropin have demonstrated that infusion rates of 6–10 mL (12–20 mg) per hour provide adequate analgesia with only slight and non-progressive motor block in cases of moderate to severe postoperative pain. In these studies, this technique resulted in a signifi-

Continued on next page

Naropin—Cont.

cant reduction in patients' morphine rescue dose-requirement. Clinical experience supports the use of Naropin epidural infusions for up to 24 hours.
Epidural infusion of Naropin has, in some cases, been associated with transient increases in temperature to > 38.5°C. This occurred more frequently at doses >16 mg/h.
Peripheral Nerve Block—Naropin, 5 mg/mL, (0.5%), was evaluated for its ability to provide anesthesia for surgery using the techniques of Peripheral Nerve Block. There were 13 studies performed including a series of 4 pharmacodynamic and pharmacokinetic studies performed on minor nerve blocks. From these, 235 Naropin treated patients were evaluable for efficacy. Naropin was used in doses up to 275 mg. When used for brachial plexus block, onset depended on technique used. Supraclavicular blocks were consistently more successful than axillary blocks. The median onset of sensory block (anesthesia) produced by ropivacaine 0.5% via axillary block ranged from 10 minutes (medial brachial cutaneous nerve) to 45 minutes (musculocutaneous nerve). Median duration ranged from 3.7 hours (medial brachial cutaneous nerve) to 8.7 hours (ulnar nerve). The 5 mg/mL (0.5%) Naropin solution gave success rates from 56% to 86% for axillary blocks, compared with 92% for supraclavicular blocks.
Local Infiltration—There were 7 clinical studies performed to evaluate the local infiltration of Naropin to produce anesthesia for surgery and analgesia in postoperative pain management. In these studies, 297 patients who received Naropin in doses up to 200 mg were evaluable for efficacy. With infiltration of 100–200 mg Naropin, the time to first request for analgesic was 2–6 hours. When compared to placebo, Naropin produced lower pain scores and a reduction of analgesic consumption.

INDICATIONS AND USAGE

Naropin is indicated for the production of local or regional anesthesia for surgery, for postoperative pain management and for obstetrical procedures.

Surgical Anesthesia:	epidural block for surgery including cesarean section; major nerve block; local infiltration
Acute Pain Management:	epidural continuous infusion or intermittent bolus e.g., postoperative or labor; local infiltration

Standard current textbooks should be consulted to determine the accepted procedures and techniques for the administration of local anesthetic agents.

CONTRAINDICATIONS

Naropin is contraindicated in patients with a known hypersensitivity to Naropin or to any local anesthetic agent of the amide type.

WARNINGS

FOR CESAREAN SECTION, THE 5 MG/ML (0.5%) NAROPIN SOLUTION IN DOSES UP TO 150 MG IS RECOMMENDED. AS WITH ALL LOCAL ANESTHETICS, NAROPIN SHOULD BE ADMINISTERED IN INCREMENTAL DOSES. SINCE NAROPIN SHOULD NOT BE INJECTED RAPIDLY IN LARGE DOSES, IT IS NOT RECOMMENDED FOR EMERGENCY SITUATIONS, WHERE A FAST ONSET OF SURGICAL ANESTHESIA IS NECESSARY. HISTORICALLY, PREGNANT PATIENTS WERE REPORTED TO HAVE A HIGH RISK FOR CARDIAC ARRHYTHMIAS, CARDIAC/ CIRCULATORY ARREST AND DEATH WHEN BUPIVACAINE WAS INADVERTENTLY RAPIDLY INJECTED INTRAVENOUSLY.
LOCAL ANESTHETICS SHOULD ONLY BE EMPLOYED BY CLINICIANS WHO ARE WELL VERSED IN THE DIAGNOSIS AND MANAGEMENT OF DOSE RELATED TOXICITY AND OTHER ACUTE EMERGENCIES WHICH MIGHT ARISE FROM THE BLOCK TO BE EMPLOYED, AND THEN ONLY AFTER INSURING THE **IMMEDIATE (WITHOUT DELAY)** AVAILABILITY OF OXYGEN, OTHER RESUSCITATIVE DRUGS, CARDIOPULMONARY RESUSCITATIVE EQUIPMENT, AND THE PERSONNEL RESOURCES NEEDED FOR PROPER MANAGEMENT OF TOXIC REACTIONS AND RELATED EMERGENCIES (See also ADVERSE REACTIONS and PRECAUTIONS). DELAY IN PROPER MANAGEMENT OF DOSE RELATED TOXICITY, UNDERVENTILATION FROM ANY CAUSE AND/OR ALTERED SENSITIVITY MAY LEAD TO THE DEVELOPMENT OF ACIDOSIS, CARDIAC ARREST AND, POSSIBLY, DEATH.
SOLUTIONS OF NAROPIN SHOULD NOT BE USED FOR THE PRODUCTION OF OBSTETRICAL PARACERVICAL BLOCK ANESTHESIA, RETROBULBAR BLOCK OR SPINAL ANESTHESIA (SUBARACHNOID BLOCK) DUE TO INSUFFICIENT DATA TO SUPPORT SUCH USE. INTRAVENOUS REGIONAL ANESTHESIA (BIER BLOCK) SHOULD NOT BE PERFORMED DUE TO A LACK OF CLINICAL EXPERIENCE AND THE RISK OF ATTAINING TOXIC BLOOD LEVELS OF NAROPIN.
It is essential that aspiration for blood, or cerebrospinal fluid (where applicable), be done prior to injecting any local anesthetic, both the original dose and all subsequent doses, to avoid intravascular or subarachnoid injection. However, a negative aspiration does *not* ensure against an intravascular or subarachnoid injection.
A well-known risk of epidural anesthesia may be an unintentional subarachnoid injection of local anesthetic. Two clinical studies have been performed to verify the safety of Naropin at a volume of 3 mL injected into the subarachnoid space since this dose represents an incremental epidural volume that could be unintentionally injected. The 15 and 22.5 mg doses injected resulted in sensory levels as high as T5 and T4, respectively. Sensory analgesia started in the sacral dermatomes in 2-3 minutes, extended to the T10 level in 10–13 minutes and lasted for approximately 2 hours. The results of these two clinical studies showed that a 3 mL dose did not produce any serious adverse events when spinal anesthesia blockade was achieved.
Naropin should be used with caution in patients receiving other local anesthetics or agents structurally related to amide-type local anesthetics, since the toxic effects of these drugs are additive.

PRECAUTIONS

General: The safe and effective use of local anesthetics depends on proper dosage, correct technique, adequate precautions and readiness for emergencies.
Resuscitative equipment, oxygen and other resuscitative drugs should be available for immediate use (see WARNINGS and ADVERSE REACTIONS). The lowest dosage that results in effective anesthesia should be used to avoid high plasma levels and serious adverse effects. Injections should be made slowly and incrementally, with frequent aspirations before and during the injection to avoid intravascular injection. When a continuous catheter technique is used, syringe aspirations should also be performed before and during each supplemental injection. During the administration of epidural anesthesia, it is recommended that a test dose of a local anesthetic with a fast onset be administered initially and that the patient be monitored for central nervous system and cardiovascular toxicity, as well as for signs of unintended intrathecal administration before proceeding. When clinical conditions permit, consideration should be given to employing local anesthetic solutions which contain epinephrine for the test dose because circulatory changes compatible with epinephrine may also serve as a warning sign of unintended intravascular injection. An intravascular injection is still possible even if aspirations for blood are negative. Administration of higher than recommended doses of Naropin to achieve greater motor blockade or increased duration of sensory blockade may negate the advantages of Naropin's favorable cardiovascular depression profile in the event that an inadvertent intravascular injection occurs.
Injection of repeated doses of local anesthetics may cause significant increases in plasma levels with each repeated dose due to slow accumulation of the drug or its metabolites or to slow metabolic degradation. Tolerance to elevated blood levels varies with the physical condition of the patient. Debilitated, elderly patients, and acutely ill patients and children should be given reduced doses commensurate with their age and physical condition. Local anesthetics should also be used with caution in patients with hypotension, hypovolemia or heart block.
Careful and constant monitoring of cardiovascular and respiratory vital signs (adequacy of ventilation) and the patient's state of consciousness should be performed after each local anesthetic injection. It should be kept in mind at such times that restlessness, anxiety, incoherent speech, lightheadedness, numbness and tingling of the mouth and lips, metallic taste, tinnitus, dizziness, blurred vision, tremors, twitching, depression, or drowsiness may be early warning signs of central nervous system toxicity.
Because amide-type local anesthetics such as Naropin are metabolized by the liver, these drugs, especially repeat doses, should be used cautiously in patients with hepatic disease. Patients with severe hepatic disease, because of their inability to metabolize local anesthetics normally, are at a greater risk of developing toxic plasma concentrations. Local anesthetics should also be used with caution in patients with impaired cardiovascular function because they may be less able to compensate for functional changes associated with the prolongation of A-V conduction produced by these drugs.
Many drugs used during the conduct of anesthesia are considered potential triggering agents for malignant hyperthermia. Amide-type local anesthetics are not known to trigger this reaction. However, since the need for supplemental general anesthesia cannot be predicted in advance, it is suggested that a standard protocol for management should be available.
Epidural Anesthesia: During epidural administration, Naropin should be administered in incremental doses of 3 to 5 mL with sufficient time between doses to detect toxic manifestations of unintentional intravascular or intrathecal injection. Syringe aspirations should also be performed before and during each supplemental injection in continuous (intermittent) catheter techniques. An intravascular injection is still possible even if aspirations for blood are negative. During the administration of epidural anesthesia, it is recommended that a test dose be administered initially and the effects monitored before the full dose is given. When clinical conditions permit, the test dose should contain epinephrine (10 to 15 μg have been suggested) to serve as a warning of unintentional intravascular injection. If injected into a blood vessel, this amount of epinephrine is likely to produce a transient "epinephrine response" within 45 seconds, consisting of an increase in heart rate and systolic blood pressure, circumoral pallor, palpitations and nervousness in the unsedated patient. The sedated patient may exhibit only a pulse rate increase of 20 or more beats per minute for 15 or more seconds. Therefore, following the test dose, the heart should be continuously monitored for a heart rate increase. Patients on beta-blockers may not manifest changes in heart rate, but blood pressure monitoring can detect a rise in systolic blood pressure. A test dose of a short-acting amide anesthetic such as 30 to 40 mg of lidocaine is recommended to detect an unintentional intrathecal administration. This will be manifested within a few minutes by signs of spinal block (e.g., decreased sensation of the buttocks, paresis of the legs, or, in the sedated patient, absent knee jerk). An intravascular or subarachnoid injection is still possible even if results of the test dose are negative. The test dose itself may produce a systemic toxic reaction, high spinal or epinephrine-induced cardiovascular effects.
Use in Head and Neck Area: Small doses of local anesthetics injected into the head and neck area may produce adverse reactions similar to systemic toxicity seen with unintentional intravascular injections of larger doses. The injection procedures require the utmost care. Confusion, convulsions, respiratory depression, and/or respiratory arrest, and cardiovascular stimulation or depression have been reported. These reactions may be due to intra-arterial injection of the local anesthetic with retrograde flow to the cerebral circulation. Patients receiving these blocks should have their circulation and respiration monitored and be constantly observed. Resuscitative equipment and personnel for treating adverse reactions should be immediately available. Dosage recommendations should not be exceeded (see DOSAGE AND ADMINISTRATION).
Use in Ophthalmic Surgery: The use of Naropin in retrobulbar blocks for ophthalmic surgery has not been studied. Until appropriate experience is gained, the use of Naropin for such surgery is not recommended.
Information for Patients: When appropriate, patients should be informed in advance that they may experience temporary loss of sensation and motor activity in the anesthetized part of the body following proper administration of lumbar epidural anesthesia. Also, when appropriate, the physician should discuss other information including adverse reactions in the Naropin package insert.
Clinically Significant Drug-Drug Interactions: Naropin should be used with caution in patients receiving other local anesthetics or agents structurally related to amide-type local anesthetics, since the toxic effects of these drugs are additive.
In vitro studies indicate that cytochrome P4501A is involved in the formation of 3-hydroxy ropivacaine, the major metabolite. Thus agents likely to be administered concomitantly with Naropin, which are metabolized by this isozyme family may potentially interact with Naropin. Such interaction might be a possibility with drugs known to be metabolized by P4501A2 via competitive inhibition such as theophylline, imipramine and with potent inhibitors such as fluvoxamine and verapamil.
Carcinogenesis, Mutagenesis, Impairment of Fertility: Long term studies in animals of most local anesthetics, including Naropin, to evaluate the carcinogenic potential have not been conducted.
Weak mutagenic activity was seen in the mouse lymphoma test. Mutagenicity was not noted in the other assays, demonstrating that the weak signs of *in vitro* activity in the mouse lymphoma test were not manifest under diverse *in vivo* conditions.
Studies performed with ropivacaine in rats did not demonstrate an effect on fertility or general reproductive performance over two generations.
Pregnancy Category B: Teratogenicity studies in rats and rabbits did not show evidence of any adverse effects on organogenesis or early fetal development in rats or rabbits. The doses used were approximately equal to 5 and 2.5 times, respectively, the maximum recommended human dose (250 mg) based on body weight. There were no treatment related effects on late fetal development, parturition, lactation, neonatal viability or growth of the offspring in 2 perinatal and postnatal studies in rats, at dose levels up to approximately 5 times the maximum recommended human dose based on body weight. In another study with a higher dose, 23 mg/kg, an increased pup loss was seen during the first 3 days postpartum, which was considered secondary to impaired maternal care due to maternal toxicity.
There are no adequate and well-controlled studies in pregnant women of the effects of Naropin on the developing fetus. Naropin should be used during pregnancy only if clearly needed. This does not preclude the use of Naropin after fetal organogenesis is completed or for obstetrical anesthesia or analgesia. (See Labor and Delivery).
Labor and Delivery: Local anesthetics, including Naropin, rapidly cross the placenta, and when used for epidural block can cause varying degrees of maternal, fetal and neonatal toxicity (see CLINICAL PHARMACOLOGY, PHARMACOKINETICS). The incidence and degree of toxicity depend upon the procedure performed, the type and amount of drug used, and the technique of drug administration. Adverse reactions in the parturient, fetus and neonate involve alterations of the central nervous system, peripheral vascular tone and cardiac function.
Maternal hypotension has resulted from regional anesthesia with Naropin for obstetrical pain relief. Local anesthetics produce vasodilation by blocking sympathetic nerves. Elevating the patient's legs and positioning her on her left side will help prevent decreases in blood pressure. The fetal heart rate also should be monitored continuously, and electronic fetal monitoring is highly advisable.

Epidural anesthesia has been reported to prolong the second stage of labor by removing the parturient's reflex urge to bear down or by interfering with motor function. Spontaneous vertex delivery occurred more frequently in patients receiving Naropin than in those receiving bupivacaine.

Nursing Mothers: Some local anesthetic drugs are excreted in human milk and caution should be exercised when they are administered to a nursing woman. The excretion of ropivacaine or its metabolites in human milk has not been studied. Based on the milk/plasma concentration ratio in rats, the estimated daily dose to a pup will be about 4% of the dose given to the mother. Assuming that the milk/plasma concentration in humans is of the same order, the total Naropin dose to which the baby is exposed by breast feeding is far lower than by exposure *in utero* in pregnant women at term (see PRECAUTIONS).

Pediatric Use: No special studies were conducted in pediatrics. Until further experience is gained in children younger than 12 years, administration of Naropin in this age group is not recommended.

ADVERSE REACTIONS

Reactions to Naropin are characteristic of those associated with other amide-type local anesthetics. A major cause of adverse reactions to this group of drugs may be associated with excessive plasma levels, which may be due to overdosage, unintentional intravascular injection or slow metabolic degradation.

The reported adverse events are derived from controlled clinical trials in the U.S. and other countries. The reference drug was usually bupivacaine. The studies were conducted using a variety of premedications, sedatives, and surgical procedures of varying length. Most adverse events reported were mild and transient, and may reflect the surgical procedures, patient characteristics (including disease) and/or medications administered.

Of the 3558 patients enrolled in the clinical trials, 2404 were exposed to Naropin. Each patient was counted once for each type of adverse event.

Incidence >5%: hypotension, fetal bradycardia, nausea, bradycardia, vomiting, paresthesia, back pain

Incidence 1-5%: fever, headache, pain, postoperative complications, urinary retention, dizziness, pruritus, rigors, anemia, hypertension, tachycardia, anxiety, oliguria, hypoesthesia, chest pain, fetal disorders including tachycardia and fetal distress, and neonatal disorders including jaundice, tachypnea, fever, respiratory disorder and vomiting

A comparison has been made between Naropin and bupivacaine for events with a frequency of 1% or greater. Tables 1a and 1b show adverse events (number and percentage) in patients exposed to *similar doses* in double-blind controlled clinical trials. In the trials, Naropin was administered as an epidural anesthetic/analgesic for surgery, labor, or cesarean section. In addition, patients that received Naropin for peripheral nerve block or local infiltration are included.

Table 1a.
Adverse Events Reported in ≥1% of Adult Patients Receiving Regional Or Local Anesthesia (Surgery, Labor, Cesarean Section, Peripheral Nerve Block and Local Infiltration)

Adverse Reaction	Naropin total N = 742		Bupivacaine total N = 737	
	N	(%)	N	(%)
hypotension	237	(31.9)	225	(30.5)
nausea	92	(12.4)	96	(13.0)
paresthesia	51	(6.9)	44	(6.0)
vomiting	48	(6.5)	38	(5.2)
back pain	36	(4.9)	47	(6.4)
pain	39	(5.3)	40	(5.4)
bradycardia	32	(4.3)	38	(5.2)
headache	23	(3.1)	26	(3.5)
fever	25	(3.4)	20	(2.7)
chills	16	(2.2)	14	(1.9)
dizziness	18	(2.4)	10	(1.4)
pruritus	16	(2.2)	11	(1.5)
urinary retention	10	(1.3)	12	(1.6)
hypoesthesia	8	(1.1)	10	(1.4)

Table 1b.
Adverse Events Reported in ≥1% of Fetuses or Neonates of Mothers Who Received Regional Anesthesia (Cesarean Section and Labor Studies)

Adverse Reaction	Naropin total N = 337		Bupivacaine total N = 317	
	N	(%)	N	(%)
fetal bradycardia	58	(17.2)	53	(16.7)
neonatal jaundice	12	(3.6)	12	(3.8)
neonatal tachypnea	8	(2.4)	11	(3.5)
fetal tachycardia	7	(2.1)	8	(2.5)
neonatal fever	6	(1.8)	8	(2.5)
fetal distress	4	(1.2)	8	(2.5)
neonatal respiratory distress	5	(1.5)	4	(1.3)
neonatal vomiting	5	(1.5)	1	(0.3)

Incidence <1%: The following list includes all adverse and intercurrent events which were recorded in more than one patient, but occurred at an overall rate of less than one percent, and were considered clinically relevant.

Table 2. Common Events (Epidural Administration)

Adverse Reaction	Naropin 5 mg/mL total N=256		Naropin 7.5 mg/mL total N=297		Naropin 10 mg/mL total N=207		Bupivacaine 5 mg/mL total N=236		Bupivacaine 7.5 mg/mL total N=174	
	N	(%)	N	(%)	N	(%)	N	(%)	N	(%)
hypotension	99	(38.7)	146	(49.2)	113	(54.6)	91	(38.6)	89	(51.1)
nausea	34	(13.3)	68	(22.9)			41	(17.4)	36	(20.7)
bradycardia	29	(11.3)	58	(19.5)	40	(19.3)	32	(13.6)	25	(14.4)
back pain	18	(7.0)	23	(7.7)	34	(16.4)	21	(8.9)	23	(13.2)
vomiting	18	(7.0)	33	(11.1)	23	(11.1)	19	(8.1)	14	(8.0)
headache	12	(4.7)	20	(6.7)	16	(7.7)	13	(5.5)	9	(5.2)
fever	8	(3.1)	5	(1.7)	18	(8.7)	11	(4.7)		
chills	6	(2.3)	7	(2.4)	6	(2.9)	4	(1.7)	3	(1.7)
urinary retention	5	(2.0)	8	(2.7)	10	(4.8)	10	(4.2)		
paresthesia	5	(2.0)	10	(3.4)	5	(2.4)	7	(3.0)		
pruritus			14	(4.7)	3	(1.4)			7	(4.0)

Application Site Reactions - injection site pain
Cardiovascular System- vasovagal reaction, syncope, postural hypotension, non-specific ECG abnormalities
Female Reproductive - poor progression of labor, uterine atony
Gastrointestinal System - fecal incontinence, tenesmus
General and Other Disorders - hypothermia, malaise, asthenia, accident and/or injury
Hearing and Vestibular - tinnitus, hearing abnormalities
Heart Rate and Rhythm - extrasystoles, non-specific arrhythmias, atrial fibrillation
Liver and Biliary System - jaundice
Metabolic Disorders - hypokalemia, hypomagnesemia
Musculoskeletal System - myalgia, cramps
Myo/Endo/Pericardium - ST segment changes, myocardial infarction
Nervous System - tremor, Horner's syndrome, paresis, dyskinesia, neuropathy, vertigo, coma, convulsion, hypokinesia, hypotonia, ptosis, stupor
Psychiatric Disorders - agitation, confusion, somnolence, nervousness, amnesia, hallucination, emotional lability, insomnia, nightmares
Respiratory System - dyspnea, bronchospasm, coughing
Skin Disorders - rash, urticaria
Urinary System Disorders - urinary incontinence, urinary tract infection, micturition disorder
Vascular - deep vein thrombosis, phlebitis, pulmonary embolism
Vision - vision abnormalities

For the indication epidural anesthesia for surgery, the 15 most common adverse events were compared between different concentrations of Naropin and bupivacaine. Table 2 is based on data from trials in the U.S. and other countries where Naropin was administered as an epidural anesthetic for surgery.

[See table 2 above]

Using data from the same studies, the number (%) of patients experiencing hypotension is displayed by patient age, drug and concentration in Table 4. In Table 3, the adverse events for Naropin are broken down by gender.

Table 3.
Most Common Adverse Events by Gender (Epidural Administration)
Total N: Females = 405, Males = 355

Adverse Reaction	Female		Male	
	N	(%)	N	(%)
hypotension	220	(54.3)	138	(38.9)
nausea	119	(29.4)	23	(6.5)
bradycardia	65	(16.0)	56	(15.8)
vomiting	59	(14.6)	8	(2.3)
back pain	41	(10.1)	23	(6.5)
headache	33	(8.1)	17	(4.8)
chills	18	(4.4)	5	(1.4)
fever	16	(4.0)	3	(0.8)
pruritus	16	(4.0)	1	(0.3)
pain	12	(3.0)	4	(1.1)
urinary retention	11	(2.7)	7	(2.0)
dizziness	9	(2.2)	4	(1.1)
hypoesthesia	8	(2.0)	2	(0.6)
paresthesia	8	(2.0)	10	(2.8)

[See table 4 at top of next page]

Systemic Reactions: The most commonly encountered acute adverse experiences that demand immediate countermeasures are related to the central nervous system and the cardiovascular system. These adverse experiences are generally dose-related and due to high plasma levels which may result from overdosage, rapid absorption from the injection site, diminished tolerance or from unintentional intravascular injection of the local anesthetic solution. In addition to systemic dose-related toxicity, unintentional subarachnoid injection of drug during the intended performance of lumbar epidural block or nerve blocks near the vertebral column (especially in the head and neck region) may result in underventilation or apnea ("Total or High Spinal"). Also, hypotension due to loss of sympathetic tone and respiratory paralysis or underventilation due to cephalad extension of the motor level of anesthesia may occur. This may lead to secondary cardiac arrest if untreated. Factors influencing plasma protein binding, such as acidosis, systemic diseases that alter protein production or competition with other drugs for protein binding sites, may diminish individual tolerance.

Central Nervous System Reactions: These are characterized by excitation and/or depression. Restlessness, anxiety, dizziness, tinnitus, blurred vision or tremors may occur, possibly proceeding to convulsions. However, excitement may be transient or absent, with depression being the first manifestation of an adverse reaction. This may quickly be followed by drowsiness merging into unconsciousness and respiratory arrest. Other central nervous system effects may be nausea, vomiting, chills, and constriction of the pupils.

The incidence of convulsions associated with the use of local anesthetics varies with the route of administration and the total dose administered. In a survey of studies of epidural anesthesia, overt toxicity progressing to convulsions occurred in approximately 0.1% of local anesthetic administrations.

Cardiovascular System Reactions: High doses or unintentional intravascular injection may lead to high plasma levels and related depression of the myocardium, decreased cardiac output, heart block, hypotension, bradycardia, ventricular arrhythmias, including ventricular tachycardia and ventricular fibrillation, and possibly cardiac arrest. (See WARNINGS, PRECAUTIONS, and OVERDOSAGE sections.)

Allergic Reactions: Allergic type reactions are rare and may occur as a result of sensitivity to the local anesthetic (see WARNINGS). These reactions are characterized by signs such as urticaria, pruritus, erythema, angioneurotic edema (including laryngeal edema), tachycardia, sneezing, nausea, vomiting, dizziness, syncope, excessive sweating, elevated temperature, and possibly, anaphylactoid symptomatology (including severe hypotension). Cross sensitivity among members of the amide-type local anesthetic group has been reported. The usefulness of screening for sensitivity has not been definitively established.

Neurologic Reactions: The incidence of adverse neurologic reactions associated with the use of local anesthetics may be related to the total dose and concentration of local anesthetic administered and are also dependent upon the particular drug used, the route of administration and the physical status of the patient. Many of these observations may be related to local anesthetic techniques, with or without a contribution from the drug.

During lumbar epidural block, occasional unintentional penetration of the subarachnoid space by the catheter or needle may occur. Subsequent adverse effects may depend partially on the amount of drug administered intrathecally and the physiological and physical effects of a dural puncture. These observations may include spinal block of varying magnitude (including high or total spinal block), hypotension secondary to spinal block, urinary retention, loss of bladder and bowel control (fecal and urinary incontinence), and loss of perineal sensation and sexual function. Signs and symptoms of subarachnoid block typically start within 2-3 minutes of injection. Doses of 15 and 22.5 mg of Naropin resulted in sensory levels as high as T5 and T4, respectively. Sensory analgesia started in the sacral dermatomes in 2-3 minutes and extended to the T10 level in 10-13 minutes and lasted for approximately 2 hours. Other neurological effects following unintentional subarachnoid administration during epidural anesthesia may include persistent anesthesia, paresthesia, weakness, paralysis of the lower extremities and loss of sphincter control, all of which may have slow, incomplete or no recovery. Headache, septic meningitis, meningismus, slowing of labor, increased incidence of forceps delivery, or cranial nerve palsies due to traction on nerves from loss of cerebrospinal fluid have been reported (see DOSAGE AND ADMINISTRATION discussion of Lumbar Epidural Block). A high spinal is characterized by paralysis of the arms, loss of consciousness, respiratory paralysis and bradycardia.

OVERDOSAGE

Acute emergencies from local anesthetics are generally related to high plasma levels encountered during therapeutic use of local anesthetics or to unintended subarachnoid or intravascular injection of local anesthetic solution. (See ADVERSE REACTIONS, WARNINGS, and PRECAUTIONS.)

Continued on next page

Naropin—Cont.

Management of Local Anesthetic Emergencies: The practitioner should be familiar with standard contemporary textbooks that address the management of local anesthetic emergencies. No specific information is available on the treatment of overdosage with Naropin; treatment should be symptomatic and supportive. Therapy with Naropin should be discontinued.

The first consideration is prevention, best accomplished by incremental injection of Naropin, careful and constant monitoring of cardiovascular and respiratory vital signs and the patient's state of consciousness after each local anesthetic injection and during continuous infusion. At the first sign of change, oxygen should be administered.

The first step in the management of systemic toxic reactions, as well as underventilation or apnea due to unintentional subarachnoid injection of drug solution, consists of immediate attention to the establishment and maintenance of a patent airway and effective assisted or controlled ventilation with 100% oxygen with a delivery system capable of permitting immediate positive airway pressure by mask. This may prevent convulsions if they have not already occurred.

If necessary, use drugs to control convulsions. Intravenous barbiturates, anticonvulsant agents, or muscle relaxants should only be administered by those familiar with their use. Immediately after the institution of these ventilatory measures, the adequacy of the circulation should be evaluated. Supportive treatment of circulatory depression may require administration of intravenous fluids, and, when appropriate, a vasopressor dictated by the clinical situation (such as ephedrine or epinephrine to enhance myocardial contractile force).

The mean dosages of ropivacaine producing seizures, after intravenous infusion in dogs, nonpregnant and pregnant sheep were 4.9, 6.1 and 5.9 mg/kg, respectively. These doses were associated with peak arterial total plasma concentrations of 11.4, 4.3 and 5.0 μg/mL, respectively. In rats, the LD_{50} is 9.9 and 12 mg/kg by the intravenous route for males and females respectively.

In human volunteers given intravenous Naropin, the mean maximum tolerated total and free arterial plasma concentrations were 4.3 and 0.6 μg/mL respectively, at which time moderate CNS symptoms (muscle twitching) were noted.

Clinical data from patients experiencing local anesthetic induced convulsions demonstrated rapid development of hypoxia, hypercarbia and acidosis within a minute of the onset of convulsions. These observations suggest that oxygen consumption and carbon dioxide production are greatly increased during local anesthetic convulsions and emphasize the importance of immediate and effective ventilation with oxygen which may avoid cardiac arrest.

If difficulty is encountered in the maintenance of a patent airway or if prolonged ventilatory support (assisted or controlled) is indicated, endotracheal intubation, employing drugs and techniques familiar to the clinician, may be indicated after initial administration of oxygen by mask.

The supine position is dangerous in pregnant women at term because of aorta-caval compression by the gravid uterus. Therefore, during treatment of systemic toxicity, maternal hypotension or fetal bradycardia following regional block, the parturient should be maintained in the left lateral decubitus position if possible, or manual displacement of the uterus off the great vessels should be accomplished. Resuscitation of obstetrical patients may take longer than resuscitation of non-pregnant patients and closed-chest cardiac compression may be ineffective. Rapid delivery of the fetus may improve the response to resuscitative efforts.

DOSAGE AND ADMINISTRATION

The rapid injection of a large volume of local anesthetic solution should be avoided and fractional (incremental) doses should always be used. The smallest dose and concentration required to produce the desired result should be administered.

The dose of any local anesthetic administered varies with the anesthetic procedure, the area to be anesthetized, the vascularity of the tissues, the number of neuronal segments to be blocked, the depth of anesthesia and degree of muscle relaxation required, the duration of anesthesia desired, individual tolerance, and the physical condition of the patient. Patients in poor general condition due to aging or other compromising factors such as partial or complete heart conduction block, advanced liver disease or severe renal dysfunction require special attention although regional anesthesia is frequently indicated in these patients. To reduce the risk of potentially serious adverse reactions, attempts should be made to optimize the patient's condition before major blocks are performed, and the dosage should be adjusted accordingly.

Use an adequate test dose (3-5 mL of a short acting local anesthetic solution containing epinephrine) prior to induction of complete block. This test dose should be repeated if the patient is moved in such a fashion as to have displaced the epidural catheter. Allow adequate time for onset of anesthesia following administration of each test dose.

Parenteral drug products should be inspected visually for particulate matter and discoloration prior to administration, whenever solution and container permit. Solutions which are discolored or which contain particulate matter should not be administered. For specific techniques and procedures, refer to standard contemporary textbooks.

[See second table above]

Table 4.
Effects of Age on Hypotension (Epidural Administration)
Total N: Naropin = 760, bupivacaine = 410

	Naropin						Bupivacaine			
AGE	**5 mg/mL**		**7.5 mg/mL**		**10 mg/mL**		**5 mg/mL**		**7.5 mg/mL**	
	N	**(%)**	**N**	**(%)**	**N**	**(%)**	**N**	**(%)**	**N**	**(%)**
<65	68	(32.2)	99	(43.2)	87	(51.5)	64	(33.5)	73	(48.3)
≥65	31	(68.9)	47	(69.1)	26	(68.4)	27	(60.0)	16	(69.6)

Dosage Recommendations

	Conc. mg/mL	(%)	Volume mL	Dose mg	Onset min	Duration hours
SURGICAL ANESTHESIA						
Lumbar Epidural Administration	5.0	(0.5%)	15–30	75–150	15–30	2–4
	7.5	(0.75%)	15–25	113–188	10–20	3–5
Surgery	10.0	(1.0%)	15–20	150–200	10–20	4–6
Lumbar Epidural Administration Cesarean Section	5.0	(0.5%)	20–30	100–150	15–25	2–4
Thoracic Epidural Administration To establish block for postoperative pain relief	5.0	(0.5%)	5–15	25–75	10–20	n/a[1]
Major Nerve Block (e.g., brachial plexus block)	5.0	(0.5%)	35–50	175–250	15–30	5–8
Field Block (e.g., minor nerve blocks and infiltration)	5.0	(0.5%)	1–40	5–200	1–15	2–6
LABOR PAIN MANAGEMENT						
Lumbar Epidural Administration						
Initial Dose	2.0	(0.2%)	10–20	20–40	10–15	0.5–1.5
Continuous infusion[2]	2.0	(0.2%)	6–14 mL/h	12–28 mg/h	n/a[1]	n/a[1]
Incremental injections (top-up)[2]	2.0	(0.2%)	10–15 mL/h	20–30 mg/h	n/a[1]	n/a[1]
POSTOPERATIVE PAIN MANAGEMENT						
Lumbar Epidural Administration						
Continuous infusion[3]	2.0	(0.2%)	6–10 mL/h	12–20 mg/h	n/a[1]	n/a[1]
Thoracic Epidural Administration Continuous infusion[3]	2.0	(0.2%)	4–8 mL/h	8–16 mg/h	n/a[1]	n/a[1]
Infiltration	2.0	(0.2%)	1–100	2–200	1–5	2–6
(e.g., minor nerve block)	5.0	(0.5%)	1–40	5–200	1–5	2–6

1 = Not Applicable
2 = Median dose of 21 mg per hour was administered by continuous infusion or by incremental injections (top-ups) over a median delivery time of 5.5 hours.
3 = Cumulative doses up to 770 mg of Naropin over 24 hours for postoperative pain management have been well tolerated in adults.

The doses in the table are those considered to be necessary to produce a successful block and should be regarded as guidelines for use in adults. Individual variations in onset and duration occur. The figures reflect the expected average dose range needed. For other local anesthetic techniques standard current textbooks should be consulted.

When prolonged blocks are used, either through continuous infusion or through repeated bolus administration, the risks of reaching a toxic plasma concentration or inducing local neural injury must be considered. Experience to date indicates that a cumulative dose of up to 770 mg Naropin administered over 24 hours is well tolerated in adults when used for postoperative pain management.

For treatment of postoperative pain, the following technique can be recommended: If regional anesthesia was not used intraoperatively, then an epidural block with Naropin is induced via an epidural catheter. Analgesia is maintained with an infusion of Naropin, 2 mg/mL (0.2%). Clinical studies have demonstrated that infusion rates of 6-10 mL (12-20 mg), per hour provide adequate analgesia with only slight and nonprogressive motor block in cases of moderate to severe postoperative pain. If patients require additional pain relief, higher infusion rates of up to 14 mL (28 mg) per hour may be used. With this technique a significant reduction in the need for opioids was demonstrated. Clinical experience supports the use of Naropin epidural infusions for up to 24 hours.

HOW SUPPLIED

Naropin™ Astra E-Z Off® Single Dose Vials:

7.5 mg/mL	10 mL	NDC 0186-0867-41
10.0 mg/mL	10 mL	NDC 0186-0868-41

Naropin™ Single Dose Vials:

2.0 mg/mL	20 mL	NDC 0186-0859-51
5.0 mg/mL	30 mL	NDC 0186-0863-61
7.5 mg/mL	20 mL	NDC 0186-0867-51
10.0 mg/mL	20 mL	NDC 0186-0868-51

Naropin™ Single Dose Ampules:

2.0 mg/mL	20 mL	NDC 0186-0859-52
5.0 mg/mL	30 mL	NDC 0186-0863-62
7.5 mg/mL	20 mL	NDC 0186-0867-52
10.0 mg/mL	20 mL	NDC 0186-0868-52

Naropin™ Single Dose Infusion Bottles:

2.0 mg/mL	100 mL	NDC 0186-0859-81
2.0 mg/mL	200 mL	NDC 0186-0859-91

Naropin™ Sterile-Pak® Single Dose Vials:

2.0 mg/mL	20 mL	Product Code 0859-59
5.0 mg/mL	30 mL	Product Code 0863-69
7.5 mg/mL	20 mL	Product Code 0867-59
10.0 mg/mL	20 mL	Product Code 0868-59

Naropin™ Polyamp DuoFit™ Sterile Pak®:

2.0 mg/mL	10 mL	NDC 0186-0859-47
2.0 mg/mL	20 mL	NDC 0186-0859-57
5.0 mg/mL	10 mL	NDC 0186-0863-47
5.0 mg/mL	20 mL	NDC 0186-0863-57
7.5 mg/mL	10 mL	NDC 0186-0867-47
7.5 mg/mL	20 mL	NDC 0186-0867-57
10.0 mg/mL	10 mL	NDC 0186-0868-47
10.0 mg/mL	20 mL	NDC 0186-0868-57

The solubility of ropivacaine is limited at pH above 6. Thus care must be taken as precipitation may occur if Naropin is mixed with alkaline solutions.

Disinfecting agents containing heavy metals, which cause release of respective ions (mercury, zinc, copper, etc.) should not be used for skin or mucous membrane disinfection since they have been related to incidents of swelling and edema. When chemical disinfection of the container surface is desired, either isopropyl alcohol (91%) or ethyl alcohol (70%) is recommended. It is recommended that chemical disinfection be accomplished by wiping the ampule or vial stopper thoroughly with cotton or gauze that has been moistened with the recommended alcohol just prior to use. When a container is required to have a sterile outside, a Sterile-Pak should be chosen. Glass containers may, as an alternative, be autoclaved once. Stability has been demonstrated using a targeted F_0 of 7 minutes at 121°C .

Solutions should be stored at controlled room temperature 20° - 25°C (68° - 77°F) [see USP].

These products are intended for single use and are free from preservatives. Any solution remaining from an opened container should be discarded promptly. In addition, continuous infusion bottles should not be left in place for more than 24 hours.

Rx only

021683R01 Rev. 1/99

Shown in Product Identification Guide, page 304

NESACAINE® ℞
(chloroprocaine HCl Injection, USP)
[nes' a-caine]
NESACAINE®-MPF
(chloroprocaine HCl Injection, USP)
For Infiltration and Nerve Block.

DESCRIPTION

Nesacaine and Nesacaine-MPF Injections are sterile non pyrogenic local anesthetics. The active ingredient in Nesacaine and Nesacaine-MPF Injections is chloroprocaine HCl (benzoic acid, 4-amino-2-chloro-2-(diethylamino) ethyl ester, monohydrochloride), which is represented by the following structural formula:

$$NH_2-C_6H_3(Cl)-COOCH_2CH_2N(C_2H_5)_2 \cdot HCl$$

[See table 1 above]

The solutions are adjusted to pH 2.7–4.0 by means of sodium hydroxide and/or hydrochloric acid. Filled under nitrogen.

Nesacaine and Nesacaine-MPF Injections should not be resterilized by autoclaving.

Table 1: Composition of Available Injections

Product Identification	Chloroprocaine HCl	Sodium Chloride	Disodium EDTA dihydrate	Methylparaben
	Formula (mg/mL)			
Nesacaine 1%	10	6.7	0.111	1
Nesacaine 2%	20	4.7	0.111	1
Nesacaine-MPF 2%	20	4.7	—	—
Nesacaine-MPF 3%	30	3.3	—	—

CLINICAL PHARMACOLOGY

Chloroprocaine, like other local anesthetics, blocks the generation and the conduction of nerve impulses, presumably by increasing the threshold for electrical excitation in the nerve, by slowing the propagation of the nerve impulse and by reducing the rate of rise of the action potential. In general, the progression of anesthesia is related to the diameter, myelination and conduction velocity of affected nerve fibers. Clinically, the order of loss of nerve function is as follows: (1) pain, (2) temperature, (3) touch, (4) proprioception, and (5) skeletal muscle tone.

Systemic absorption of local anesthetics produces effects on the cardiovascular and central nervous systems. At blood concentrations achieved with normal therapeutic doses, changes in cardiac conduction, excitability, refractoriness, contractility, and peripheral vascular resistance are minimal. However, toxic blood concentrations depress cardiac conduction and excitability, which may lead to atrioventricular block and ultimately to cardiac arrest. In addition, with toxic blood concentrations myocardial contractility may be depressed and peripheral vasodilation may occur, leading to decreased cardiac output and arterial blood pressure.

Following systemic absorption, toxic blood concentrations of local anesthetics can produce central nervous system stimulation, depression, or both. Apparent central stimulation may be manifested as restlessness, tremors and shivering, which may progress to convulsions. Depression and coma may occur, possibly progressing ultimately to respiratory arrest.

However, the local anesthetics have a primary depressant effect on the medulla and on higher centers. The depressed stage may occur without a prior stage of central nervous system stimulation.

PHARMACOKINETICS

The rate of systemic absorption of local anesthetic drugs is dependent upon the total dose and concentration of drug administered, the route of administration, the vascularity of the administration site, and the presence or absence of epinephrine in the anesthetic injection. Epinephrine usually reduces the rate of absorption and plasma concentration of local anesthetics and is sometimes added to local anesthetic injections in order to prolong the duration of action. The onset of action with chloroprocaine is rapid (usually within 6 to 12 minutes), and the duration of anesthesia, depending upon the amount used and the route of administration, may be up to 60 minutes.

Local anesthetics appear to cross the placenta by passive diffusion. However, the rate and degree of diffusion varies considerably among the different drugs as governed by: (1) the degree of plasma protein binding, (2) the degree of ionization, and (3) the degree of lipid solubility. Fetal/maternal ratios of local anesthetics appear to be inversely related to the degree of plasma protein binding, since only the free, unbound drug is available for placental transfer. Thus, drugs with the highest protein binding capacity may have the lowest fetal/maternal ratios. The extent of placental transfer is also determined by the degree of ionization and lipid solubility of the drug. Lipid soluble, nonionized drugs readily enter the fetal blood from the maternal circulation. Depending upon the route of administration, local anesthetics are distributed to some extent to all body tissues, with high concentrations found in highly perfused organs such as the liver, lungs, heart, and brain.

Various pharmacokinetic parameters of the local anesthetics can be significantly altered by the presence of hepatic or renal disease, addition of epinephrine, factors affecting urinary pH, renal blood flow, the route of administration, and the age of the patient. The *in vitro* plasma half-life of chloroprocaine in adults is 21 ± 2 seconds for males and 25 ± 1 seconds for females. The *in vitro* plasma half-life in neonates is 43 ± 2 seconds.

Chloroprocaine is rapidly metabolized in plasma by hydrolysis of the ester linkage by pseudocholinesterase. The hydrolysis of chloroprocaine results in the production of β-diethylaminoethanol and 2-chloro-4-aminobenzoic acid, which inhibits the action of the sulfonamides (see PRECAUTIONS).

The kidney is the main excretory organ for most local anesthetics and their metabolites. Urinary excretion is affected by urinary perfusion and factors affecting urinary pH.

INDICATIONS AND USAGE

Nesacaine 1% and 2% Injections, in multidose vials with methylparaben as preservative, are indicated for the production of local anesthesia by infiltration and peripheral nerve block. They are not to be used for lumbar or caudal epidural anesthesia.

Nesacaine-MPF 2% and 3% Injections, in single dose vials without preservative and without EDTA, are indicated for the production of local anesthesia by infiltration, peripheral and central nerve block, including lumbar and caudal epidural blocks.

Nesacaine and Nesacaine-MPF Injections are not to be used for subarachnoid administration.

CONTRAINDICATIONS

Nesacaine and Nesacaine-MPF Injections are contraindicated in patients hypersensitive (allergic) to drugs of the PABA ester group.

Lumbar and caudal epidural anesthesia should be used with extreme caution in persons with the following conditions: existing neurological disease, spinal deformities, septicemia, and severe hypertension.

WARNINGS

LOCAL ANESTHETICS SHOULD ONLY BE EMPLOYED BY CLINICIANS WHO ARE WELL VERSED IN DIAGNOSIS AND MANAGEMENT OF DOSE RELATED TOXICITY AND OTHER ACUTE EMERGENCIES WHICH MIGHT ARISE FROM THE BLOCK TO BE EMPLOYED, AND THEN ONLY AFTER ENSURING THE *IMMEDIATE* AVAILABILITY OF OXYGEN, OTHER RESUSCITATIVE DRUGS, CARDIOPULMONARY RESUSCITATIVE EQUIPMENT, AND THE PERSONNEL RESOURCES NEEDED FOR PROPER MANAGEMENT OF TOXIC REACTIONS AND RELATED EMERGENCIES (see also ADVERSE REACTIONS and PRECAUTIONS). DELAY IN PROPER MANAGEMENT OF DOSE RELATED TOXICITY, UNDERVENTILATION FROM ANY CAUSE AND/OR ALTERED SENSITIVITY MAY LEAD TO THE DEVELOPMENT OF ACIDOSIS, CARDIAC ARREST AND, POSSIBLY, DEATH. NESACAINE (chloroprocaine HCl Injection, USP) contains methylparaben and should not be used for lumbar or caudal epidural anesthesia because safety of this antimicrobial preservative has not been established with regard to intrathecal injection, either intentional or unintentional. NESACAINE-MPF Injection contains no preservative; discard unused injection remaining in vial after initial use.

Vasopressors should not be used in the presence of ergot type oxytocic drugs, since a severe persistent hypertension may occur.

To avoid intravascular injection, aspiration should be performed before the anesthetic solution is injected. The needle must be repositioned until no blood return can be elicited. However, the absence of blood in the syringe does not guarantee that intravascular injection has been avoided.

Mixtures of local anesthetics are sometimes employed to compensate for the slower onset of one drug and the shorter duration of action of the second drug. Experiments in primates suggest that toxicity is probably additive when mixtures of local anesthetics are employed, but some experiments in rodents suggest synergism. Caution regarding toxic equivalence should be exercised when mixtures of local anesthetics are employed.

PRECAUTIONS

General: The safety and effective use of chloroprocaine depend on proper dosage, correct technique, adequate precautions and readiness for emergencies. Resuscitative equipment, oxygen and other resuscitative drugs should be available for immediate use. (See WARNINGS and ADVERSE REACTIONS.) The lowest dosage that results in effective anesthesia should be used to avoid high plasma levels and serious adverse effects. Injections should be made slowly, with frequent aspirations before and during the injection to avoid intravascular injection. Syringe aspirations should also be performed before and during each supplemental injection in continuous (intermittent) catheter techniques. During the administration of epidural anesthesia, it is recommended that a test dose be administered (3 mL of 3% or 5 mL of 2% Nesacaine-MPF Injection) initially and that the patient be monitored for central nervous system toxicity and cardiovascular toxicity, as well as for signs of unintended intrathecal administration, before proceeding. When clinical conditions permit, consideration should be given to employing a chloroprocaine solution that contains epinephrine for the test dose because circulatory changes characteristic of epinephrine may also serve as a warning sign of unintended intravascular injection. An intravascular injection is still possible even if aspirations for blood are negative. With the use of continuous catheter techniques, it is recommended that a fraction of each supplemental dose be administered as a test dose in order to verify proper location of the catheter.

Injection of repeated doses of local anesthetics may cause significant increases in plasma levels with each repeated dose due to slow accumulation of the drug or its metabolites. Tolerance to elevated blood levels varies with the physical condition of the patient. Debilitated, elderly patients, acutely ill patients, and children should be given reduced doses commensurate with their age and physical status. Local anesthetics should also be used with caution in patients with hypotension or heart block.

Careful and constant monitoring of cardiovascular and respiratory (adequacy of ventilation) vital signs and the patient's state of consciousness should be accomplished after each local anesthetic injection. It should be kept in mind at such times that restlessness, anxiety, tinnitus, dizziness, blurred vision, tremors, depression or drowsiness may be early warning signs of central nervous system toxicity.

Local anesthetic injections containing a vasoconstrictor should be used cautiously and in carefully circumscribed quantities in areas of the body supplied by end arteries or having otherwise compromised blood supply. Patients with peripheral vascular disease and those with hypertensive vascular disease may exhibit exaggerated vasoconstrictor response. Ischemic injury or necrosis may result.

Since ester-type local anesthetics are hydrolyzed by plasma cholinesterase produced by the liver, chloroprocaine should be used cautiously in patients with hepatic disease.

Local anesthetics should also be used with caution in patients with impaired cardiovascular function since they may be less able to compensate for functional changes associated with the prolongation of A-V conduction produced by these drugs.

Use in Ophthalmic Surgery—When local anesthetic injections are employed for retrobulbar block, lack of corneal sensation should not be relied upon to determine whether or not the patient is ready for surgery. This is because complete lack of corneal sensation usually precedes clinically acceptable external ocular muscle akinesia.

Information for Patients: When appropriate, patients should be informed in advance that they may experience temporary loss of sensation and motor activity, usually in the lower half of the body, following proper administration of epidural anesthesia.

Clinically Significant Drug Interactions: The administration of local anesthetic solutions containing epinephrine or norepinephrine to patients receiving monoamine oxidase inhibitors, tricyclic antidepressants or phenothiazines may produce severe, prolonged hypotension or hypertension. Concurrent use of these agents should generally be avoided. In situations when concurrent therapy is necessary, careful patient monitoring is essential.

Concurrent administration of vasopressor drugs (for the treatment of hypotension related to obstetric blocks) and ergot-type oxytocic drugs may cause severe, persistent hypertension or cerebrovascular accidents.

The para-aminobenzoic acid metabolite of chloroprocaine inhibits the action of sulfonamides. Therefore, chloroprocaine should not be used in any condition in which a sulfonamide drug is being employed.

Carcinogenesis, Mutagenesis, and Impairment of Fertility: Long-term studies in animals to evaluate carcinogenic potential and reproduction studies to evaluate mutagenesis or impairment of fertility have not been conducted with chloroprocaine.

Pregnancy: Category C: Animal reproduction studies have not been conducted with chloroprocaine. It is also not known whether chloroprocaine can cause fetal harm when administered to a pregnant woman or can affect reproduction capacity. Chloroprocaine should be given to a pregnant woman only if clearly needed. This does not preclude the use of chloroprocaine at term for the production of obstetrical anesthesia.

Labor and Delivery: Local anesthetics rapidly cross the placenta, and when used for epidural, paracervical, pudendal or caudal block anesthesia, can cause varying degrees of maternal, fetal and neonatal toxicity. (See CLINICAL PHARMACOLOGY and PHARMACOKINETICS.)

The incidence and degree of toxicity depend upon the procedure performed, the type and amount of drug used, and the technique of drug administration. Adverse reactions in the parturient, fetus and neonate involve alterations of the central nervous system, peripheral vascular tone and cardiac function.

Continued on next page

Nesacaine/Nesacaine-MPF—Cont.

Maternal hypotension has resulted from regional anesthesia. Local anesthetics produce vasodilation by blocking sympathetic nerves. Elevating the patient's legs and positioning her on her left side will help prevent decreases in blood pressure. The fetal heart rate also should be monitored continuously, and electronic fetal monitoring is highly advisable.

Epidural, paracervical, or pudendal anesthesia may alter the forces of parturition through changes in uterine contractility or maternal expulsive efforts. In one study, paracervical block anesthesia was associated with a decrease in the mean duration of first stage labor and facilitation of cervical dilation. However, epidural anesthesia has also been reported to prolong the second stage of labor by removing the parturient's reflex urge to bear down or by interfering with motor function. The use of obstetrical anesthesia may increase the need for forceps assistance.

The use of some local anesthetic drug products during labor and delivery may be followed by diminished muscle strength and tone for the first day or two of life. The long-term significance of these observations is unknown.

Careful adherence to recommended dosage is of the utmost importance in obstetrical paracervical block. Failure to achieve adequate analgesia with recommended doses should arouse suspicion of intravascular or fetal intracranial injection. Cases compatible with unintended fetal intracranial injection of local anesthetic injection have been reported following intended paracervical or pudendal block or both. Babies so affected present with unexplained neonatal depression at birth which correlates with high local anesthetic serum levels and usually manifest seizures within six hours. Prompt use of supportive measures combined with forced urinary excretion of the local anesthetic has been used successfully to manage this complication.

Case reports of maternal convulsions and cardiovascular collapse following use of some local anesthetics for paracervical block in early pregnancy (as anesthesia for elective abortion) suggest that systemic absorption under these circumstances may be rapid. The recommended maximum dose of each drug should not be exceeded. Injection should be made slowly and with frequent aspiration. Allow a 5-minute interval between sides.

There are no data concerning use of chloroprocaine for obstetrical paracervical block when toxemia of pregnancy is present or when fetal distress or prematurity is anticipated in advance of the block; such use is, therefore, not recommended.

The following information should be considered by clinicians who select chloroprocaine for obstetrical paracervical block anesthesia:

1. Fetal bradycardia (generally a heart rate of less than 120 per minute for more than 2 minutes) has been noted by electronic monitoring in about 5 to 10 percent of the cases (various studies) where initial total doses of 120 mg to 400 mg of chloroprocaine were employed. The incidence of bradycardia, within this dose range, might not be dose related.
2. Fetal acidosis has not been demonstrated by blood gas monitoring around the time of bradycardia or afterwards. These data are limited and generally restricted to nontoxemic cases where fetal distress or prematurity was not anticipated in advance of the block.
3. No intact chloroprocaine and only trace quantities of a hydrolysis product, 2-chloro-4-aminobenzoic acid, have been demonstrated in umbilical cord arterial or venous plasma following properly administered paracervical block with chloroprocaine.
4. The role of drug factors and non-drug factors associated with fetal bradycardia following paracervical block are unexplained at this time.

Nursing Mothers: It is not known whether this drug is excreted in human milk. Because many drugs are excreted in human milk, caution should be exercised when chloroprocaine is administered to a nursing woman.

Pediatric Use: Guidelines for the administration of Nesacaine and Nesacaine-MPF Injections to children are presented in DOSAGE AND ADMINISTRATION.

ADVERSE REACTIONS

Systemic: The most commonly encountered acute adverse experiences that demand immediate countermeasures are related to the central nervous system and the cardiovascular system. These adverse experiences are generally dose related and may result from rapid absorption from the injection site, diminished tolerance, or from unintentional intravascular injection of the local anesthetic solution. In addition to systemic dose-related toxicity, unintentional subarachnoid injection of drug during the intended performance of caudal or lumbar epidural block or nerve blocks near the vertebral column (especially in the head and neck region) may result in underventilation or apnea ("Total Spinal"). Factors influencing plasma protein binding, such as acidosis, systemic diseases that alter protein production, or competition of other drugs for protein binding sites, may diminish individual tolerance. Plasma cholinesterase deficiency may also account for diminished tolerance to ester type local anesthetics.

Central Nervous System Reactions: These are characterized by excitation and/or depression. Restlessness, anxiety, dizziness, tinnitus, blurred vision or tremors may occur, possibly proceeding to convulsions. However, excitement may be transient or absent, with depression being the first manifestation of an adverse reaction. This may quickly be followed by drowsiness merging into unconsciousness and respiratory arrest.

The incidence of convulsions associated with the use of local anesthetics varies with the procedure used and the total dose administered. In a survey of studies of epidural anesthesia, overt toxicity progressing to convulsions occurred in approximately 0.1 percent of local anesthetic administrations.

Cardiovascular System Reactions: High doses, or unintended intravascular injection, may lead to high plasma levels and related depression of the myocardium, hypotension, bradycardia, ventricular arrhythmias, and, possibly, cardiac arrest.

Allergic: Allergic type reactions are rare and may occur as a result of sensitivity to the local anesthetic or to other formulation ingredients, such as the antimicrobial preservative methylparaben, contained in multiple dose vials. These reactions are characterized by signs such as urticaria, pruritis, erythema, angioneurotic edema (including laryngeal edema), tachycardia, sneezing, nausea, vomiting, dizziness, syncope, excessive sweating, elevated temperature, and possibly, anaphylactoid type symptomatology (including severe hypotension). Cross sensitivity among members of the ester-type local anesthetic group has been reported. The usefulness of screening for sensitivity has not been definitely established.

Neurologic: In the practice of caudal or lumbar epidural block, occasional unintentional penetration of the subarachnoid space by the catheter may occur (see PRECAUTIONS). Subsequent adverse observations may depend partially on the amount of drug administered intrathecally. These observations may include spinal block of varying magnitude (including total spinal block), hypotension secondary to spinal block, loss of bladder and bowel control, and loss of perineal sensation and sexual function. Arachnoiditis, persistent motor, sensory and/or autonomic (sphincter control) deficit of some lower spinal segments with slow recovery (several months) or incomplete recovery have been reported in rare instances. (See DOSAGE AND ADMINISTRATION discussion of Caudal and Lumbar Epidural Block.) Backache and headache have also been noted following lumbar epidural or caudal block.

OVERDOSAGE

Acute emergencies from local anesthetics are generally related to high plasma levels encountered during therapeutic use of local anesthetics or to unintended subarachnoid injection of local anesthetic solution (see ADVERSE REACTIONS, WARNINGS and PRECAUTIONS).

In mice, the intravenous LD_{50} of chloroprocaine HCl is 97 mg/kg and the subcutaneous LD_{50} of chloroprocaine HCl is 950 mg/kg.

Management of Local Anesthetic Emergencies: The first consideration is prevention, best accomplished by careful and constant monitoring of cardiovascular and respiratory vital signs and the patient's state of consciousness after each local anesthetic injection. At the first sign of change, oxygen should be administered.

The first step in the management of convulsions, as well as underventilation or apnea due to unintentional subarachnoid injection of drug solution, consists of immediate attention to the maintenance of a patent airway and assisted or controlled ventilation with oxygen and a delivery system capable of permitting immediate positive airway pressure by mask. Immediately after the institution of these ventilatory measures, the adequacy of the circulation should be evaluated, keeping in mind that drugs used to treat convulsions sometimes depress the circulation when administered intravenously. Should convulsions persist despite adequate respiratory support, and if the status of the circulation permits, small increments of an ultra-short acting barbiturate (such as thiopental or thiamylal) or a benzodiazepine (such as diazepam) may be administered intravenously; the clinician should be familiar, prior to the use of anesthetics, with these anticonvulsant drugs. Supportive treatment of circulatory depression may require administration of intravenous fluids and, when appropriate, a vasopressor dictated by the clinical situation (such as ephedrine to enhance myocardial contractile force).

If not treated immediately, both convulsions and cardiovascular depression can result in hypoxia, acidosis, bradycardia, arrhythmias and cardiac arrest. Underventilation or apnea due to unintentional subarachnoid injection of local anesthetic solution may produce these same signs and also lead to cardiac arrest if ventilatory support is not instituted. If cardiac arrest should occur, standard cardiopulmonary resuscitative measures should be instituted. Recovery has been reported after prolonged resuscitative efforts.

Endotracheal intubation, employing drugs and techniques familiar to the clinician, may be indicated, after initial administration of oxygen by mask, if difficulty is encountered in the maintenance of a patent airway or if prolonged ventilatory support (assisted or controlled) is indicated.

DOSAGE AND ADMINISTRATION

Chloroprocaine may be administered as a single injection or continuously through an indwelling catheter. As with all local anesthetics, the dose administered varies with the anesthetic procedure, the vascularity of the tissues, the depth of anesthesia and degree of muscle relaxation required, the duration of anesthesia desired, and the physical condition of the patient. The smallest dose and concentration required to produce the desired result should be used. Dosage should be reduced for children, elderly and debilitated patients and patients with cardiac and/or liver disease. The maximum single recommended doses of chloroprocaine in adults are: without epinephrine, 11 mg/kg, not to exceed a maximum total dose of 800 mg; with epinephrine (1:200,000), 14 mg/kg, not to exceed a maximum total dose of 1000 mg. For specific techniques and procedures, refer to standard textbooks.

Caudal and Lumbar Epidural Block: In order to guard against adverse experiences sometimes noted following unintended penetration of the subarachnoid space, the following procedure modifications are recommended:

1. Use an adequate test dose (3 mL of Nesacaine-MPF 3% Injection or 5 mL of Nesacaine-MPF 2% Injection) prior to induction of complete block. This test dose should be repeated if the patient is moved in such a fashion as to have displaced the epidural catheter. Allow adequate time for onset of anesthesia following administration of each test dose.
2. Avoid the rapid injection of a large volume of local anesthetic injection through the catheter. Consider fractional doses, when feasible.
3. In the event of the known injection of a large volume of local anesthetic injection into the subarachnoid space, after suitable resuscitation and if the catheter is in place, consider attempting the recovery of drug by draining a moderate amount of cerebrospinal fluid (such as 10 mL) through the epidural catheter.

As a guide for some routine procedures, suggested doses are given below:

1. Infiltration and Peripheral Nerve Block: NESACAINE or NESACAINE-MPF (chloroprocaine HCl Injection, USP)
[See table below]
2. Caudal and Lumbar Epidural Block: NESACAINE-MPF INJECTION. For caudal anesthesia, the initial dose is 15 to 25 mL of a 2% or 3% solution. Repeated doses may be given at 40 to 60 minute intervals.
For lumbar epidural anesthesia, 2 to 2.5 mL per segment of a 2% or 3% solution can be used. The usual total volume of Nesacaine-MPF Injection is from 15 to 25 mL. Repeated doses 2 to 6 mL less than the original dose may be given at 40 to 50 minute intervals.

The above dosages are recommended as a guide for use in the average adult. Maximum dosages of all local anesthetics must be individualized after evaluating the size and physical condition of the patient and the rate of systemic absorption from a particular injection site.

Pediatric Dosage: It is difficult to recommend a maximum dose of any drug for children, since this varies as a function of age and weight. For children over 3 years of age who have a normal lean body mass and normal body development, the maximum dose is determined by the child's age and weight and should not exceed 11 mg/kg (5 mg/lb). For example, in a child of 5 years weighing 50 lbs (23 kg), the dose of chloroprocaine HCl without epinephrine would be 250 mg. Concentrations of 0.5–1.0% are suggested for infiltration and 1.0–1.5% for nerve block. In order to guard against systemic toxicity, the lowest effective concentration and lowest effective dose should be used at all times. Some of the lower concentrations for use in infants and smaller children are not available in pre-packaged containers; it will be necessary to dilute available concentrations with the amount of 0.9% sodium chloride injection necessary to obtain the required final concentration of chloroprocaine injection.

Preparation of Epinephrine Injections—To prepare a 1:200,000 epinephrine-chloroprocaine HCl injection, add 0.1 mL of a 1 to 1000 Epinephrine Injection USP to 20 mL of Nesacaine-MPF Injection.

Chloroprocaine is incompatible with caustic alkalis and their carbonates, soaps, silver salts, iodine and iodides.

Parenteral drug products should be inspected visually for particulate matter and discoloration prior to administration, whenever injection and container permit. As with other anesthetics having a free aromatic amino group, Nesacaine and Nesacaine-MPF Injections are slightly photosensitive and may become discolored after prolonged exposure to light. It is recommended that these vials be stored in the original outer containers, protected from direct sunlight. Discolored injection should not be administered. If exposed to low temperatures, Nesacaine and Nesacaine-MPF Injec-

Anesthetic Procedure	Solution Concentration %	Volume (mL)	Total Dose (mg)
Mandibular	2	2–3	40–60
Infraorbital	2	0.5–1	10–20
Brachial plexus	2	30–40	600–800
Digital (without epinephrine)	1	3–4	30–40
Pudendal	2	10 each side	400
Paracervical (see also PRECAUTIONS)	1	3 per each of 4 sites	up to 120

tions may deposit crystals of chloroprocaine HCl which will redissolve with shaking when returned to room temperature. The product should not be used if it contains undissolved (e.g., particulate) material.

HOW SUPPLIED

NESACAINE (chloroprocaine HCl Injection, USP) with preservatives is supplied as follows:

1% solution (NDC 0186-0971-66) in 30 mL multiple dose vials

2% solution (NDC 0186-0972-66) in 30 mL multiple dose vials

NESACAINE-MPF (chloroprocaine HCl Injection, USP) without preservatives and without EDTA is supplied as follows:

2% solution (NDC 0186-0991-66) in 20 mL single dose vials

3% solution (NDC 0186-0992-66) in 20 mL single dose vials

Keep from freezing. Protect from light. Store at controlled room temperature 15°–30°C (59°–86°F).

021849R11 Rev. 2/97

TABLETS
PLENDIL® ℞
(Felodipine)
EXTENDED-RELEASE TABLETS

DESCRIPTION

PLENDIL* (felodipine) is a calcium antagonist (calcium channel blocker). Felodipine is a dihydropyridine derivative that is chemically described as ± ethyl methyl 4-(2,3-dichlorophenyl)-1,4-dihydro-2,6-dimethyl-3,5-pyridinedicarboxylate. Its empirical formula is $C_{18}H_{19}Cl_2NO_4$ and its structural formula is:

Felodipine is a slightly yellowish, crystalline powder with a molecular weight of 384.26. It is insoluble in water and is freely soluble in dichloromethane and ethanol. Felodipine is a racemic mixture.

Tablets PLENDIL provide extended release of felodipine. They are available as tablets containing 2.5 mg, 5 mg, or 10 mg of felodipine for oral administration. In addition to the active ingredient felodipine, the tablets contain the following inactive ingredients: Tablets PLENDIL 2.5 mg — hydroxypropyl cellulose, lactose, FD&C Blue 2, sodium stearyl fumarate, titanium dioxide, yellow iron oxide, and other ingredients. Tablets PLENDIL 5 mg and 10 mg — cellulose, red and yellow oxide, lactose, polyethylene glycol, sodium stearyl fumarate, titanium dioxide and other ingredients.

*Registered trademark of Astra AB

CLINICAL PHARMACOLOGY

Mechanism of Action: Felodipine is a member of the dihydropyridine class of calcium channel antagonists (calcium channel blockers). It reversibly competes with nitrendipine and/or other calcium channel blockers for dihydropyridine binding sites, blocks voltage-dependent Ca^{++} currents in vascular smooth muscle and cultured rabbit atrial cells, and blocks potassium-induced contracture of the rat portal vein.

In vitro studies show that the effects of felodipine on contractile processes are selective, with greater effects on vascular smooth muscle than cardiac muscle. Negative inotropic effects can be detected *in vitro,* but such effects have not been seen in intact animals.

The effect of felodipine on blood pressure is principally a consequence of a dose-related decrease of peripheral vascular resistance in man, with a modest reflex increase in heart rate (see Cardiovascular Effects). With the exception of a mild diuretic effect seen in several animal species and man, the effects of felodipine are accounted for by its effects on peripheral vascular resistance.

Pharmacokinetics and Metabolism: Following oral administration, felodipine is almost completely absorbed and undergoes extensive first-pass metabolism. The systemic bioavailability of PLENDIL is approximately 20%. Mean peak concentrations following the administration of PLENDIL are reached in 2.5 to 5 hours. Both peak plasma concentration and the area under the plasma concentration time curve (AUC) increase linearly with doses up to 20 mg. Felodipine is greater than 99% bound to plasma proteins.

Following intravenous administration, the plasma concentration of felodipine declined triexponentially with mean disposition half-lives of 4.8 minutes, 1.5 hours, and 9.1 hours. The mean contributions of the three individual phases to the overall AUC were 15, 40, and 45%, respectively, in the order of increasing $t_{1/2}$.

Following oral administration of the immediate-release formulation, the plasma level of felodipine also declined polyexponentially with a mean terminal $t_{1/2}$ of 11 to 16 hours. The mean peak and trough steady-state plasma concentrations achieved after 10 mg of the immediate-release formulation given once a day to normal volunteers, were 20 and 0.5 nmol/L, respectively. The trough plasma concentration of felodipine in most individuals was substantially below the concentration needed to effect a half-maximal decline in blood pressure (EC_{50}) [4–6 nmol/L for felodipine], thus precluding once-a-day dosing with the immediate-release formulation.

Following administration of a 10-mg dose of PLENDIL, the extended-release formulation, to young, healthy volunteers, mean peak and trough steady-state plasma concentrations of felodipine were 7 and 2 nmol/L, respectively. Corresponding values in hypertensive patients (mean age 64) after a 20-mg dose of PLENDIL were 23 and 7 nmol/L. Since the EC_{50} for felodipine is 4 to 6 nmol/L, a 5- to 10-mg dose of PLENDIL in some patients, and a 20-mg dose in others, would be expected to provide an antihypertensive effect that persists for 24 hours (see Cardiovascular Effects below and DOSAGE AND ADMINISTRATION).

The systemic plasma clearance of felodipine in young healthy subjects is about 0.8 L/min, and the apparent volume of distribution is about 10 L/kg.

Following an oral or intravenous dose of ^{14}C-labeled felodipine in man, about 70% of the dose of radioactivity was recovered in urine and 10% in the feces. A negligible amount of intact felodipine is recovered in the urine and feces (< 0.5%). Six metabolites, which account for 23% of the oral dose, have been identified; none has significant vasodilating activity.

Following administration of PLENDIL to hypertensive patients, mean peak plasma concentrations at steady state are about 20% higher than after a single dose. Blood pressure response is correlated with plasma concentrations of felodipine.

The bioavailability of PLENDIL is influenced by the presence of food. When administered either with a high fat or carbohydrate diet, C_{max} is increased by approximately 60%; AUC is unchanged. When PLENDIL was administered after a light meal (orange juice, toast, and cereal), however, there is no effect on felodipine's pharmacokinetics. The bioavailability of felodipine was increased approximately two-fold when taken with grapefruit juice. Orange juice does not appear to modify the kinetics of PLENDIL. A similar finding has been seen with other dihydropyridine calcium antagonists, but to a lesser extent than that seen with felodipine.

Age Effects—Plasma concentrations of felodipine, after a single dose and at steady state, increase with age. Mean clearance of felodipine in elderly hypertensives (mean age 74) was only 45% of that of young volunteers (mean age 26). At steady state mean AUC for young patients was 39% of that for the elderly. Data for intermediate age ranges suggest that the AUCs fall between the extremes of the young and the elderly.

Hepatic Dysfunction—In patients with hepatic disease, the clearance of felodipine was reduced to about 60% of that seen in normal young volunteers.

Renal impairment does not alter the plasma concentration profile of felodipine; although higher concentrations of the metabolites are present in the plasma due to decreased urinary excretion, these are inactive.

Animal studies have demonstrated that felodipine crosses the blood-brain barrier and the placenta.

Cardiovascular Effects: Following administration of PLENDIL, a reduction in blood pressure generally occurs within 2 to 5 hours. During chronic administration, substantial blood pressure control lasts for 24 hours, with trough reductions in diastolic blood pressure approximately 40–50% of peak reductions. The antihypertensive effect is dose dependent and correlates with the plasma concentration of felodipine.

A reflex increase in heart rate frequently occurs during the first week of therapy; this increase attenuates over time. Heart rate increases of 5–10 beats per minute may be seen during chronic dosing. The increase is inhibited by beta-blocking agents.

The P-R interval of the ECG is not affected by felodipine when administered alone or in combination with a beta-blocking agent. Felodipine alone or in combination with a beta-blocking agent has been shown, in clinical and electrophysiologic studies, to have no significant effect on cardiac conduction (P-R, P-Q, and H-V intervals).

In clinical trials in hypertensive patients without clinical evidence of left ventricular dysfunction, no symptoms suggestive of a negative inotropic effect were noted; however, none would be expected in this population (see PRECAUTIONS).

Renal/Endocrine Effects: Renal vascular resistance is decreased by felodipine while glomerular filtration rate remains unchanged. Mild diuresis, natriuresis, and kaliuresis have been observed during the first week of therapy. No significant effects on serum electrolytes were observed during short- and long-term therapy.

In clinical trials in patients with hypertension, increases in plasma noradrenaline levels have been observed.

Clinical Studies: Felodipine produces dose-related decreases in systolic and diastolic blood pressure as demonstrated in six placebo-controlled, dose response studies using either immediate-release or extended-release dosage forms. These studies enrolled over 800 patients on active treatment, at total daily doses ranging from 2.5 to 20 mg. In those studies felodipine was administered either as monotherapy or was added to beta blockers. The results of the 2 studies with PLENDIL given once daily as monotherapy are shown in the table below:

MEAN REDUCTIONS IN BLOOD PRESSURE (mmHg)*
Systolic/Diastolic

Dose	N	Mean Peak Response	Mean Trough Response	Trough/ Peak Ratios (%s)
Study 1 (8 weeks)				
2.5 mg	68	9.4/4.7	2.7/2.5	29/53
5 mg	69	9.5/6.3	2.4/3.7	25/59
10 mg	67	18.0/10.8	10.0/6.0	56/56
Study 2 (4 weeks)				
10 mg	50	5.3/7.2	1.5/3.2	33/40**
20 mg	50	11.3/10.2	4.5/3.2	43/34**

*Placebo response subtracted
**Different number of patients available for peak and trough measurements

INDICATIONS AND USAGE

PLENDIL is indicated for the treatment of hypertension. PLENDIL may be used alone or concomitantly with other antihypertensive agents.

CONTRAINDICATIONS

PLENDIL is contraindicated in patients who are hypersensitive to this product.

PRECAUTIONS

General: *Hypotension*—Felodipine, like other calcium antagonists, may occasionally precipitate significant hypotension and, rarely, syncope. It may lead to reflex tachycardia which in susceptible individuals may precipitate angina pectoris. (See ADVERSE REACTIONS.)

Heart Failure—Although acute hemodynamic studies in a small number of patients with NYHA Class II or III heart failure treated with felodipine have not demonstrated negative inotropic effects, safety in patients with heart failure has not been established. Caution, therefore, should be exercised when using PLENDIL in patients with heart failure or compromised ventricular function, particularly in combination with a beta blocker.

Elderly Patients or Patients with Impaired Liver Function—Patients over 65 years of age or patients with impaired liver function may have elevated plasma concentrations of felodipine and may respond to lower doses of PLENDIL; therefore, a starting dose of 2.5 mg once a day is recommended. These patients should have their blood pressure monitored closely during dosage adjustment of PLENDIL. (See CLINICAL PHARMACOLOGY and DOSAGE AND ADMINISTRATION.)

Peripheral Edema—Peripheral edema, generally mild and not associated with generalized fluid retention, was the most common adverse event in the clinical trials. The incidence of peripheral edema was both dose and age dependent. Frequency of peripheral edema ranged from about 10% in patients under 50 years of age taking 5 mg daily to about 30% in those over 60 years of age taking 20 mg daily. This adverse effect generally occurs within 2–3 weeks of the initiation of treatment.

Information for Patients: Patients should be instructed to take PLENDIL whole and not to crush or chew the tablets. They should be told that mild gingival hyperplasia (gum swelling) has been reported. Good dental hygiene decreases its incidence and severity.

NOTE: As with many other drugs, certain advice to patients being treated with PLENDIL is warranted. This information is intended to aid in the safe and effective use of this medication. It is not a disclosure of all possible adverse or intended effects.

Drug Interactions: *CYP3A4 Inhibitors*—Felodipine is metabolized by CYP3A4. Co-administration of CYP3A4 inhibitors (e.g., ketoconazole, itraconazole, erythromycin, grapefruit juice, cimetidine) with felodipine may lead to several-fold increases in the plasma levels of felodipine, either due to an increase in bioavailability or due to a decrease in metabolism. These increases in concentration may lead to increased effects, (lower blood pressure and increased heart rate). These effects have been observed with co-administration of itraconazole (a potent CYP3A4 inhibitor). Caution should be used when CYP3A4 inhibitors are co-administered with felodipine. A conservative approach to dosing felodipine should be taken. The following specific interactions have been reported:

Itraconazole—Co-administration of another extended release formulation of felodipine with itraconazole resulted in approximately 8-fold increase in the AUC, more than 6-fold increase in the C_{max}, and 2-fold prolongation in the half-life of felodipine.

Erythromycin—Co-administration of felodipine (PLENDIL) with erythromycin resulted in approximately 2.5-fold increase in the AUC and C_{max}, and about 2-fold prolongation in the half-life of felodipine.

Continued on next page

Plendil—Cont.

Grapefruit juice—Co-administration of felodipine with grapefruit juice resulted in more than 2-fold increase in the AUC and C_{max}, but no prolongation in the half-life of felodipine.

Cimetidine—Co-administration of felodipine with cimetidine (a non-specific CYP-450 inhibitor) resulted in an increase of approximately 50% in the AUC and the C_{max}, of felodipine.

Beta-Blocking Agents—A pharmacokinetic study of felodipine in conjunction with metoprolol demonstrated no significant effects on the pharmacokinetics of felodipine. The AUC and C_{max} of metoprolol, however, were increased approximately 31 and 38%, respectively. In controlled clinical trials, however, beta blockers including metoprolol were concurrently administered with felodipine and were well tolerated.

Digoxin—When given concomitantly with PLENDIL the pharmacokinetics of digoxin in patients with heart failure were not significantly altered.

Anticonvulsants—In a pharmacokinetic study, maximum plasma concentrations of felodipine were considerably lower in epileptic patients on long-term anticonvulsant therapy (e.g., phenytoin, carbamazepine, or phenobarbital) than in healthy volunteers. In such patients, the mean area under the felodipine plasma concentration-time curve was also reduced to approximately 6% of that observed in healthy volunteers. Since a clinically significant interaction may be anticipated, alternative antihypertensive therapy should be considered in these patients.

Other Concomitant Therapy—In healthy subjects there were no clinically significant interactions when felodipine was given concomitantly with indomethacin or spironolactone.

Interaction with Food—See CLINICAL PHARMACOLOGY, Pharmacokinetics and Metabolism.

Carcinogenesis, Mutagenesis, Impairment of Fertility: In a 2-year carcinogenicity study in rats fed felodipine at doses of 7.7, 23.1 or 69.3 mg/kg/day (up to 28 times** the maximum recommended human dose on a mg/m^2 basis), a dose-related increase in the incidence of benign interstitial cell tumors of the testes (Leydig cell tumors) was observed in treated male rats. These tumors were not observed in a similar study in mice at doses up to 138.6 mg/kg/day (28 times** the maximum recommended human dose on a mg/m^2 basis). Felodipine, at the doses employed in the 2-year rat study, has been shown to lower testicular testosterone and to produce a corresponding increase in serum luteinizing hormone in rats. The Leydig cell tumor development is possibly secondary to these hormonal effects which have not been observed in man.

In this same rat study a dose-related increase in the incidence of focal squamous cell hyperplasia compared to control was observed in the esophageal groove of male and female rats in all dose groups. No other drug-related esophageal or gastric pathology was observed in the rats or with chronic administration in mice and dogs. The latter species, like man, has no anatomical structure comparable to the esophageal groove.

Felodipine was not carcinogenic when fed to mice at doses up to 138.6 mg/kg/day (28 times** the maximum recommended human dose on a mg/m^2 basis) for periods of up to 80 weeks in males and 99 weeks in females.

Felodipine did not display any mutagenic activity *in vitro* in the Ames microbial mutagenicity test or in the mouse lymphoma forward mutation assay. No clastogenic potential was seen *in vivo* in the mouse micronucleus test at oral doses up to 2500 mg/kg (506 times** the maximum recommended human dose on a mg/m^2 basis) or *in vitro* in a human lymphocyte chromosome aberration assay.

A fertility study in which male and female rats were administered doses of 3.8, 9.6 or 26.9 mg/kg/day showed no significant effect of felodipine on reproductive performance.

PREGNANCY

Pregnancy Category C.

Teratogenic Effects—Studies in pregnant rabbits administered doses of 0.46, 1.2, 2.3, and 4.6 mg/kg/day (from 0.4 to 4 times** the maximum recommended human dose on a mg/m^2 basis) showed digital anomalies consisting of reduction in size and degree of ossification of the terminal phalanges in the fetuses. The frequency and severity of the changes appeared dose related and were noted even at the lowest dose. These changes have been shown to occur with other members of the dihydropyridine class and are possibly a result of compromised uterine blood flow. Similar fetal anomalies were not observed in rats given felodipine.

In a teratology study in cynomolgus monkeys, no reduction in the size of the terminal phalanges was observed, but an abnormal position of the distal phalanges was noted in about 40% of the fetuses.

Nonteratogenic Effects—A prolongation of parturition with difficult labor and an increased frequency of fetal and early postnatal deaths were observed in rats administered doses of 9.6 mg/kg/day (4 times** the maximum human dose on a mg/m^2 basis) and above.

Significant enlargement of the mammary glands, in excess of the normal enlargement for pregnant rabbits, was found with doses greater than or equal to 1.2 mg/kg/day (equal to the maximum human dose on a mg/m^2 basis). This effect occurred only in pregnant rabbits and regressed during lactation. Similar changes in the mammary glands were not observed in rats or monkeys.

There are no adequate and well-controlled studies in pregnant women. If felodipine is used during pregnancy, or if the patient becomes pregnant while taking this drug, she should be apprised of the potential hazard to the fetus, possible digital anomalies of the infant, and the potential effects of felodipine on labor and delivery, and on the mammary glands of pregnant females.

Nursing Mothers: It is not known whether this drug is secreted in human milk and because of the potential for serious adverse reactions from felodipine in the infant, a decision should be made whether to discontinue nursing or to discontinue the drug, taking into account the importance of the drug to the mother.

Pediatric Use: Safety and effectiveness in pediatric patients have not been established.

**Based on patient weight of 50 kg

ADVERSE REACTIONS

In controlled studies in the United States and overseas, approximately 3000 patients were treated with felodipine as either the extended-release or the immediate-release formulation.

The most common clinical adverse events reported with PLENDIL administered as monotherapy at the recommended dosage range of 2.5 mg to 10 mg once a day were peripheral edema and headache. Peripheral edema was generally mild, but it was age and dose related and resulted in discontinuation of therapy in about 3% of the enrolled patients. Discontinuation of therapy due to any clinical adverse event occurred in about 6% of the patients receiving PLENDIL, principally for peripheral edema, headache, or flushing.

Adverse events that occurred with an incidence of 1.5% or greater at any of the recommended doses of 2.5 mg to 10 mg once a day (PLENDIL, N = 861; Placebo, N = 334), without regard to causality, are compared to placebo and are listed by dose in the table below. These events are reported from controlled clinical trials with patients who were randomized to a fixed dose of PLENDIL or titrated from an initial dose of 2.5 mg or 5 mg once a day. A dose of 20 mg once a day has been evaluated in some clinical studies. Although the antihypertensive effect of PLENDIL is increased at 20 mg once a day, there is a disproportionate increase in adverse events, especially those associated with vasodilatory effects (see DOSAGE and ADMINISTRATION).

[See table below]

Adverse events that occurred in 0.5 up to 1.5% of patients who received PLENDIL in all controlled clinical trials at the recommended dosage range of 2.5 mg to 10 mg once a day, and serious adverse events that occurred at a lower rate, or events reported during marketing experience (those lower rate events are in italics) are listed below. These events are listed in order of decreasing severity within each category, and the relationship of these events to administration of PLENDIL is uncertain: ***Body as a Whole:*** Chest pain, facial edema, flu-like illness; ***Cardiovascular:*** *Myocardial infarction, hypotension, syncope, angina pectoris, arrhythmia,* tachycardia, premature beats; ***Digestive:*** Abdominal pain, diarrhea, vomiting, dry mouth, flatulence, acid regurgitation; ***Endocrine:*** Gynecomastia; ***Hematologic:*** *Anemia;* ***Metabolic:*** ALT (SGPT) increased; ***Musculoskeletal:*** Arthralgia, back pain, leg pain, foot pain, muscle cramps, myalgia, arm pain, knee pain, hip pain; ***Nervous/Psychiatric:*** Insomnia, depression, anxiety disorders, irritability, nervousness, somnolence, decreased libido; ***Respiratory:*** Dyspnea, pharyngitis, bronchitis, influenza, sinusitis, epistaxis, respiratory infection; ***Skin:*** Contusion, erythema, urticaria; ***Special Senses:*** Visual disturbances; ***Urogenital:*** Impotence, urinary frequency, urinary urgency, dysuria, polyuria.

Gingival Hyperplasia—Gingival hyperplasia, usually mild, occurred in <0.5% of patients in controlled studies. This condition may be avoided or may regress with improved dental hygiene. (See PRECAUTIONS, Information for Patients.)

Clinical Laboratory Test Findings: *Serum Electrolytes*—No significant effects on serum electrolytes were observed during short- and long-term therapy (see CLINICAL PHARMACOLOGY, Renal/Endocrine Effects).

Serum Glucose—No significant effects on fasting serum glucose were observed in patients treated with PLENDIL in the U.S. controlled study.

Liver Enzymes—1 of 2 episodes of elevated serum transaminases decreased once drug was discontinued in clinical studies; no follow-up was available for the other patient.

OVERDOSAGE

Oral doses of 240 mg/kg and 264 mg/kg in male and female mice, respectively, and 2390 mg/kg and 2250 mg/kg in male and female rats, respectively, caused significant lethality.

In a suicide attempt, one patient took 150 mg felodipine together with 15 tablets each of atenolol and spironolactone and 20 tablets of nitrazepam. The patient's blood pressure and heart rate were normal on admission to hospital; he subsequently recovered without significant sequelae.

Overdosage might be expected to cause excessive peripheral vasodilation with marked hypotension and possibly bradycardia.

If severe hypotension occurs, symptomatic treatment should be instituted. The patient should be placed supine with the legs elevated. The administration of intravenous fluids may be useful to treat hypotension due to overdosage with calcium antagonists. In case of accompanying bradycardia, atropine (0.5–1 mg) should be administered intravenously. Sympathomimetic drugs may also be given if the physician feels they are warranted.

It has not been established whether felodipine can be removed from the circulation by hemodialysis.

To obtain up-to-date information about the treatment of overdose, consult your Regional Poison-Control Center. Telephone numbers of certified poison-control centers are listed in the *Physicians' Desk Reference (PDR)*. In managing overdose, consider the possibilities of multiple-drug overdoses, drug-drug interactions, and unusual drug kinetics in your patient.

DOSAGE AND ADMINISTRATION

The recommended starting dose is 5 mg once a day. Depending on the patient's response, the dosage can be decreased to 2.5 mg or increased to 10 mg once a day. These adjustments should occur generally at intervals of not less than 2 weeks. The recommended dosage range is 2.5–10 mg once daily. In clinical trials, doses above 10 mg daily showed an increased blood pressure response but a large increase in the rate of peripheral edema and other vasodilatory adverse events (see ADVERSE REACTIONS). Modification of the recommended dosage is usually not required in patients with renal impairment.

PLENDIL should regularly be taken either without food or with a light meal (see CLINICAL PHARMACOLOGY, Pharmacokinetics and Metabolism). PLENDIL should be swallowed whole and not crushed or chewed.

Use in the Elderly or Patients with Impaired Liver Function—Patients over 65 years of age, or patients with impaired liver function, may develop higher plasma concentra-

Percent of Patients with Adverse Events in Controlled Trials* of PLENDIL (N=861) as Monotherapy without Regard to Causality (Incidence of discontinuations shown in parentheses)

Body System Adverse Events	Placebo N=334	2.5 mg N=255	5 mg N=581	10 mg N=408
Body as a Whole				
Peripheral Edema	3.3 (0.0)	2.0 (0.0)	8.8 (2.2)	17.4 (2.5)
Asthenia	3.3 (0.0)	3.9 (0.0)	3.3 (0.0)	2.2 (0.0)
Warm Sensation	0.0 (0.0)	0.0 (0.0)	0.9 (0.2)	1.5 (0.0)
Cardiovascular				
Palpitation	2.4 (0.0)	0.4 (0.0)	1.4 (0.3)	2.5 (0.5)
Digestive				
Nausea	1.5 (0.9)	1.2 (0.0)	1.7 (0.3)	1.0 (0.7)
Dyspepsia	1.2 (0.0)	3.9 (0.0)	0.7 (0.0)	0.5 (0.0)
Constipation	0.9 (0.0)	1.2 (0.0)	0.3 (0.0)	1.5 (0.2)
Nervous				
Headache	10.2 (0.9)	10.6 (0.4)	11.0 (1.7)	14.7 (2.0)
Dizziness	2.7 (0.3)	2.7 (0.0)	3.6 (0.5)	3.7 (0.5)
Paresthesia	1.5 (0.3)	1.6 (0.0)	1.2 (0.0)	1.2 (0.2)
Respiratory				
Upper Respiratory Infection	1.8 (0.0)	3.9 (0.0)	1.9 (0.0)	0.7 (0.0)
Cough	0.3 (0.0)	0.8 (0.0)	1.2 (0.0)	1.7 (0.0)
Rhinorrhea	0.0 (0.0)	1.6 (0.0)	0.2 (0.0)	0.2 (0.0)
Sneezing	0.0 (0.0)	1.6 (0.0)	0.0 (0.0)	0.0 (0.0)
Skin				
Rash	0.9 (0.0)	2.0 (0.0)	0.2 (0.0)	0.2 (0.0)
Flushing	0.9 (0.3)	3.9 (0.0)	5.3 (0.7)	6.9 (1.2)

* Patients in titration studies may have been exposed to more than one dose level of PLENDIL.

tions of felodipine; therefore, a starting dose of 2.5 mg once a day is recommended. Dosage may be adjusted as described above. (See PRECAUTIONS.)

HOW SUPPLIED

No. 3584—Tablets PLENDIL, 2.5 mg, are sage green, round convex tablets, with code 450 on one side and PLENDIL on the other. They are supplied as follows:
NDC 0186-0450-28 unit dose packages of 100
NDC 0186-0450-58 unit of use bottles of 100
NDC 0186-0450-31 unit of use bottles of 30.
No. 3585—Tablets PLENDIL, 5 mg, are light red-brown, round convex tablets, with code 451 on one side and PLENDIL on the other. They are supplied as follows:
NDC 0186-0451-28 unit dose packages of 100
NDC 0186-0451-58 unit of use bottles of 100
NDC 0186-0451-31 unit of use bottles of 30
No. 3586—Tablets PLENDIL, 10 mg, are red-brown, round convex tablets, with code 452 on one side and PLENDIL on the other. They are supplied as follows:
NDC 0186-0452-28 unit dose packages of 100
NDC 0186-0452-58 unit of use bottles of 100
NDC 0186-0452-31 unit of use bottles of 30

Storage
Store below 30°C (86°F). Keep container tightly closed. Protect from light.
Manufactured by:
Merck & Co., Inc., West Point, PA 19486
Distributed by:
Astra Pharmaceuticals, L.P., Wayne, PA 19087
63000212 Revised October 1999
Shown in Product Identification Guide, page 304

POLOCAINE® ℞
[pō ′-lō-caine ″]
(Mepivacaine Hydrochloride Injection, USP)

POLOCAINE®-MPF
(Mepivacaine Hydrochloride Injection, USP)
THESE SOLUTIONS ARE NOT INTENDED FOR SPINAL ANESTHESIA OR DENTAL USE

(For details of indications, dosage and administration, precautions, and adverse reactions, see circular in package.)

HOW SUPPLIED

POLOCAINE-MPF (Mepivacaine HCl Injection, USP) without preservatives is available as follows:
1% Single-dose vials of 30 mL (NDC 0186-0412-01)
1.5% Single-dose vials of 30 mL (NDC 0186-0418-01)
2% Single-dose vials of 20 mL (NDC 0186-0422-01)
POLOCAINE (Mepivacaine HCl Injection, USP) with preservatives is available as follows:
1% Multiple-dose vials of 50 mL (NDC 0186-0410-01)
2% Multiple-dose vials of 50 mL (NDC 0186-0420-01)
Unused portions of solutions not containing preservatives should be discarded.
Store at controlled room temperature 15°–30°C (59°–86°F).
021668R00 Iss. 1/92

PRILOSEC® ℞
(omeprazole)
DELAYED-RELEASE CAPSULES

DESCRIPTION

The active ingredient in PRILOSEC* (omeprazole) Delayed-Release Capsules is a substituted benzimidazole, 5-methoxy-2-[[(4-methoxy-3, 5-dimethyl-2-pyridinyl) methyl] sulfinyl]-1*H*-benzimidazole, a compound that inhibits gastric acid secretion. Its empirical formula is $C_{17}H_{19}N_3O_3S$, with a molecular weight of 345.42. The structural formula is:

[structural formula: H, O, N, S, CH_2, N, H_3CO, H_3C, CH_3, OCH_3]

,

Omeprazole is a white to off-white crystalline powder which melts with decomposition at about 155°C. It is a weak base, freely soluble in ethanol and methanol, and slightly soluble in acetone and isopropanol and very slightly soluble in water. The stability of omeprazole is a function of pH; it is rapidly degraded in acid media, but has acceptable stability under alkaline conditions.

PRILOSEC is supplied as delayed-release capsules for oral administration. Each delayed-release capsule contains either 10 mg, 20 mg or 40 mg of omeprazole in the form of enteric-coated granules with the following inactive ingredients: cellulose, disodium hydrogen phosphate, hydroxypropyl cellulose, hydroxypropyl methylcellulose, lactose, mannitol, sodium lauryl sulfate and other ingredients. The capsule shells have the following inactive ingredients: gelatin-NF, FD&C Blue #1, FD&C Red #40, D&C Red #28, titanium dioxide, synthetic black iron oxide, isopropanol, butyl alcohol, FD&C Blue #2, D&C Red #7 Calcium Lake, and, in addition, the 10 mg and 40 mg capsule shells also contain D&C Yellow #10.

*Registered trademark of the AstraZeneca Group

CLINICAL PHARMACOLOGY

Pharmacokinetics and Metabolism: Omeprazole

PRILOSEC Delayed-Release Capsules contain an enteric-coated granule formulation of omeprazole (because omeprazole is acid-labile), so that absorption of omeprazole begins only after the granules leave the stomach. Absorption is rapid, with peak plasma levels of omeprazole occurring within 0.5 to 3.5 hours. Peak plasma concentrations of omeprazole and AUC are approximately proportional to doses up to 40 mg, but because of a saturable first-pass effect, a greater than linear response in peak plasma concentration and AUC occurs with doses greater than 40 mg. Absolute bioavailability (compared to intravenous administration) is about 30–40% at doses of 20–40 mg, due in large part to presystemic metabolism. In healthy subjects the plasma half-life is 0.5 to 1 hour, and the total body clearance is 500–600 mL/min. Protein binding is approximately 95%.

The bioavailability of omeprazole increases slightly upon repeated administration of PRILOSEC Delayed-Release Capsules.

Following single dose oral administration of a buffered solution of omeprazole, little if any unchanged drug was excreted in urine. The majority of the dose (about 77%) was eliminated in urine as at least six metabolites. Two were identified as hydroxyomeprazole and the corresponding carboxylic acid. The remainder of the dose was recoverable in feces. This implies a significant biliary excretion of the metabolites of omeprazole. Three metabolites have been identified in plasma—the sulfide and sulfone derivatives of omeprazole, and hydroxyomeprazole. These metabolites have very little or no antisecretory activity.

In patients with chronic hepatic disease, the bioavailability increased to approximately 100% compared to an I.V. dose, reflecting decreased first-pass effect, and the plasma half-life of the drug increased to nearly 3 hours compared to the half-life in normals of 0.5–1 hour. Plasma clearance averaged 70 mL/min, compared to a value of 500–600 mL/min in normal subjects.

In patients with chronic renal impairment, whose creatinine clearance ranged between 10 and 62 mL/min/1.73 m^2, the disposition of omeprazole was very similar to that in healthy volunteers, although there was a slight increase in bioavailability. Because urinary excretion is a primary route of excretion of omeprazole metabolites, their elimination slowed in proportion to the decreased creatinine clearance.

The elimination rate of omeprazole was somewhat decreased in the elderly, and bioavailability was increased. Omeprazole was 76% bioavailable when a single 40 mg oral dose of omeprazole (buffered solution) was administered to healthy elderly volunteers, versus 58% in young volunteers given the same dose. Nearly 70% of the dose was recovered in urine as metabolites of omeprazole and no unchanged drug was detected. The plasma clearance of omeprazole was 250 mL/min (about half that of young volunteers) and its plasma half-life averaged one hour, about twice that of young healthy volunteers.

In pharmacokinetic studies of single 20 mg omeprazole doses, an increase in AUC of approximately four-fold was noted in Asian subjects compared to Caucasians.

Dose adjustment, particularly where maintenance of healing of erosive esophagitis is indicated, for the hepatically impaired and Asian subjects should be considered.

Pharmacokinetics: Combination Therapy with Antimicrobials

Omeprazole 40 mg daily was given in combination with clarithromycin 500 mg every 8 hours to healthy adult male subjects. The steady state plasma concentrations of omeprazole were increased (C_{max}, AUC_{0-24}, and $T_{½}$ increases of 30%, 89% and 34% respectively) by the concomitant administration of clarithromycin. The observed increases in omeprazole plasma concentration were associated with the following pharmacological effects. The mean 24-hour gastric pH value was 5.2 when omeprazole was administered alone and 5.7 when co-administered with clarithromycin.

The plasma levels of clarithromycin and 14-hydroxy-clarithromycin were increased by the concomitant administration of omeprazole. For clarithromycin, the mean C_{max} was 10% greater, the mean C_{min} was 27% greater, and the mean AUC_{0-8} was 15% greater when clarithromycin was administered with omeprazole than when clarithromycin was administered alone. Similar results were seen for 14-hydroxy-clarithromycin, the mean C_{max} was 45% greater, the mean C_{min} was 57% greater, and the mean AUC_{0-8} was 45% greater. Clarithromycin concentrations in the gastric tissue and mucus were also increased by concomitant administration of omeprazole.

Clarithromycin Tissue Concentrations 2 hours after Dose[1]

Tissue	Clarithromycin	Clarithromycin + Omeprazole
Antrum	10.48 ± 2.01 (n = 5)	19.96 ± 4.71 (n = 5)
Fundus	20.81 ± 7.64 (n = 5)	24.25 ± 6.37 (n = 5)
Mucus	4.15 ± 7.74 (n = 4)	39.29 ± 32.79 (n = 4)

[1] Mean ± SD (μg/g)

For information on clarithromycin pharmacokinetics and microbiology, consult the clarithromycin package insert, CLINICAL PHARMACOLOGY section.
The pharmacokinetics of omeprazole, clarithromycin, and amoxicillin have not been adequately studied when all three drugs are administered concomitantly.
For information on amoxicillin pharmacokinetics and microbiology, see the amoxicillin package insert, ACTIONS, PHARMACOLOGY and MICROBIOLOGY sections.

Pharmacodynamics

Mechanism of Action

Omeprazole belongs to a new class of antisecretory compounds, the substituted benzimidazoles, that do not exhibit anticholinergic or H_2 histamine antagonistic properties, but that suppress gastric acid secretion by specific inhibition of the H^+/K^+ ATPase enzyme system at the secretory surface of the gastric parietal cell. Because this enzyme system is regarded as the acid (proton) pump within the gastric mucosa, omeprazole has been characterized as a gastric acid-pump inhibitor, in that it blocks the final step of acid production. This effect is dose-related and leads to inhibition of both basal and stimulated acid secretion irrespective of the stimulus. Animal studies indicate that after rapid disappearance from plasma, omeprazole can be found within the gastric mucosa for a day or more.

Antisecretory Activity

After oral administration, the onset of the antisecretory effect of omeprazole occurs within one hour, with the maximum effect occurring within two hours. Inhibition of secretion is about 50% of maximum at 24 hours and the duration of inhibition lasts up to 72 hours. The antisecretory effect thus lasts far longer than would be expected from the very short (less than one hour) plasma half-life, apparently due to prolonged binding to the parietal H^+/K^+ ATPase enzyme. When the drug is discontinued, secretory activity returns gradually, over 3 to 5 days. The inhibitory effect of omeprazole on acid secretion increases with repeated once-daily dosing, reaching a plateau after four days.

Results from numerous studies of the antisecretory effect of multiple doses of 20 mg and 40 mg of omeprazole in normal volunteers and patients are shown below. The "max" value represents determinations at a time of maximum effect (2–6 hours after dosing), while "min" values are those 24 hours after the last dose of omeprazole.

Range of Mean Values from Multiple Studies of the Mean Antisecretory Effects of Omeprazole After Multiple Daily Dosing

Parameter	Omeprazole 20 mg		Omeprazole 40 mg	
	Max	Min	Max	Min
% Decrease in Basal Acid Output	78*	58–80	94*	80–93
% Decrease in Peak Acid Output	79*	50–59	88*	62–68
% Decrease in 24-hr. Intragastric Acidity		80–97		92–94

*Single Studies

Single daily oral doses of omeprazole ranging from a dose of 10 mg to 40 mg have produced 100% inhibition of 24-hour intragastric acidity in some patients.

Enterochromaffin-like (ECL) Cell Effects

In 24-month carcinogenicity studies in rats, a dose-related significant increase in gastric carcinoid tumors and ECL cell hyperplasia was observed in both male and female animals (see PRECAUTIONS, Carcinogenesis, Mutagenesis, Impairment of Fertility). Carcinoid tumors have also been observed in rats subjected to fundectomy or long-term treatment with other proton pump inhibitors or high doses of H_2-receptor antagonists.

Human gastric biopsy specimens have been obtained from more than 3000 patients treated with omeprazole in long-term clinical trials. The incidence of ECL cell hyperplasia in these studies increased with time; however, no case of ECL cell carcinoids, dysplasia, or neoplasia has been found in these patients. (See also CLINICAL PHARMACOLOGY, Pathological Hypersecretory Conditions.)

Serum Gastrin Effects

In studies involving more than 200 patients, serum gastrin levels increased during the first 1 to 2 weeks of once-daily administration of therapeutic doses of omeprazole in parallel with inhibition of acid secretion. No further increase in serum gastrin occurred with continued treatment. In comparison with histamine H_2-receptor antagonists, the median increases produced by 20 mg doses of omeprazole were higher (1.3 to 3.6 fold vs. 1.1 to 1.8 fold increase). Gastrin values returned to pretreatment levels, usually within 1 to 2 weeks after discontinuation of therapy.

Other Effects

Systemic effects of omeprazole in the CNS, cardiovascular and respiratory systems have not been found to date. Omeprazole, given in oral doses of 30 or 40 mg for 2 to 4 weeks, had no effect on thyroid function, carbohydrate metabolism, or circulating levels of parathyroid hormone, cortisol, estradiol, testosterone, prolactin, cholecystokinin or secretin.

No effect on gastric emptying of the solid and liquid components of a test meal was demonstrated after a single dose of omeprazole 90 mg. In healthy subjects, a single I.V. dose of omeprazole (0.35 mg/kg) had no effect on intrinsic factor se-

Continued on next page

Prilosec—Cont.

cretion. No systematic dose-dependent effect has been observed on basal or stimulated pepsin output in humans. However, when intragastric pH is maintained at 4.0 or above, basal pepsin output is low, and pepsin activity is decreased.

As do other agents that elevate intragastric pH, omeprazole administered for 14 days in healthy subjects produced a significant increase in the intragastric concentrations of viable bacteria. The pattern of the bacterial species was unchanged from that commonly found in saliva. All changes resolved within three days of stopping treatment.

Clinical Studies

Duodenal Ulcer Disease

Active Duodenal Ulcer—In a multicenter, double-blind, placebo-controlled study of 147 patients with endoscopically documented duodenal ulcer, the percentage of patients healed (per protocol) at 2 and 4 weeks was significantly higher with PRILOSEC 20 mg once a day than with placebo ($p \leq 0.01$).

Treatment of Active Duodenal Ulcer
% of Patients Healed

	PRILOSEC 20 mg a.m. (n = 99)	Placebo a.m. (n = 48)
Week 2	*41	13
Week 4	*75	27

*(p≤0.01)

Complete daytime and nighttime pain relief occurred significantly faster ($p \leq 0.01$) in patients treated with PRILOSEC 20 mg than in patients treated with placebo. At the end of the study, significantly more patients who had received PRILOSEC had complete relief of daytime pain ($p \leq 0.05$) and nighttime pain ($p \leq 0.01$).

In a multicenter, double-blind study of 293 patients with endoscopically documented duodenal ulcer, the percentage of patients healed (per protocol) at 4 weeks was significantly higher with PRILOSEC 20 mg once a day than with ranitidine 150 mg b.i.d. ($p < 0.01$).

Treatment of Active Duodenal Ulcer
% of Patients Healed

	PRILOSEC 20 mg a.m. (n = 145)	Ranitidine 150 mg b.i.d (n = 148)
Week 2	42	34
Week 4	*82	63

*(p<0.01)

Healing occurred significantly faster in patients treated with PRILOSEC than in those treated with ranitidine 150 mg b.i.d. ($p < 0.01$).

In a foreign multinational randomized, double-blind study of 105 patients with endoscopically documented duodenal ulcer, 20 mg and 40 mg of PRILOSEC were compared to 150 mg b.i.d. of ranitidine at 2, 4 and 8 weeks. At 2 and 4 weeks both doses of PRILOSEC were statistically superior (per protocol) to ranitidine, but 40 mg was not superior to 20 mg of PRILOSEC, and at 8 weeks there was no significant difference between any of the active drugs.

Treatment of Active Duodenal Ulcer
% of Patients Healed

	PRILOSEC 20 mg (n = 34)	PRILOSEC 40 mg (n = 36)	Ranitidine 150 mg b.i.d. (n = 35)
Week 2	*83	*83	53
Week 4	*97	*100	82
Week 8	100	100	94

*(p≤0.01)

H. pylori Eradication in Patients with Duodenal Ulcer Disease

Triple Therapy (PRILOSEC/clarithromycin/amoxicillin)—Three U.S., randomized, double-blind clinical studies in patients with *H. pylori* infection and duodenal ulcer disease (n = 558) compared PRILOSEC plus clarithromycin plus amoxicillin to clarithromycin plus amoxicillin. Two studies (126 and 127) were conducted in patients with an active duodenal ulcer, and the other study (M96–446) was conducted in patients with a history of a duodenal ulcer in the past 5 years but without an ulcer present at the time of enrollment. The dose regimen in the studies was PRILOSEC 20 mg b.i.d. plus clarithromycin 500 mg b.i.d. plus amoxicillin 1 g b.i.d. for 10 days; or clarithromycin 500 mg b.i.d. plus amoxicillin 1 g b.i.d. for 10 days. In studies 126 and 127, patients who took the omeprazole regimen also received an additional 18 days of PRILOSEC 20 mg q.d. Endpoints studied were eradication of *H. pylori* and duodenal ulcer healing (studies 126 and 127 only). *H. pylori* status was determined by CLOtest®, histology and culture in all three studies. For a given patient, *H. pylori* was considered eradicated if at least two of these tests were negative, and none was positive.

The combination of omeprazole plus clarithromycin plus amoxicillin was effective in eradicating *H. pylori*.

[See first table above]

Per-Protocol and Intent-to-Treat *H. pylori* Eradication Rates
% of Patients Cured [95% Confidence Interval]

	PRILOSEC +clarithromycin +amoxicillin		Clarithromycin +amoxicillin	
	Per-Protocol†	Intent-to-Treat‡	Per-Protocol†	Intent-to-Treat‡
Study 126	*77 [64, 86] (n = 64)	*69 [57, 79] (n = 80)	43 [31, 56] (n = 67)	37 [27, 48] (n = 84)
Study 127	*78 [67, 88] (n = 65)	*73 [61, 82] (n = 77)	41 [29, 54] (n = 68)	36 [26, 47] (n = 83)
Study M96-446	*90 [80, 96] (n = 69)	*83 [74, 91] (n = 84)	33 [24, 44] (n = 93)	32 [23, 42] (n = 99)

†Patients were included in the analysis if they had confirmed duodenal ulcer disease (active ulcer, studies 126 and 127; history of ulcer within 5 years, study M96-446) and *H. pylori* infection at baseline defined as at least two of three positive endoscopic tests from CLOtest®, histology, and/or culture. Patients were included in the analysis if they completed the study. Additionally, if patients dropped out of the study due to an adverse event related to the study drug, they were included in the analysis as failures of therapy. The impact of eradication on ulcer recurrence has not been assessed in patients with a past history of ulcer.
‡Patients were included in the analysis if they had documented *H. pylori* infection at baseline and had confirmed duodenal ulcer disease. All dropouts were included as failures of therapy.
*($p<0.05$) versus clarithromycin plus amoxicillin.

H. pylori Eradication Rates (Per-Protocol Analysis at 4 to 6 Weeks)
% of Patients Cured [95% Confidence Interval]

	PRILOSEC + Clarithromycin	PRILOSEC	Clarithromycin
U.S. Studies			
Study M93-067	74 [60, 85]†‡ (n = 53)	0 [0, 7] (n = 54)	31 [18, 47] (n = 42)
Study M93-100	64 [51, 76]†‡ (n = 61)	0 [0, 6] (n = 59)	39 [24, 55] (n = 44)
Non U.S. Studies			
Study M92-812b	83 [71, 92]‡ (n = 60)	1 [0, 7] (n = 74)	N/A
Study M93-058	74 [64, 83]‡ (n = 86)	1 [0, 6] (n = 90)	N/A

†Statistically significantly higher than clarithromycin monotherapy ($p < 0.05$)
‡Statistically significantly higher than omeprazole monotherapy ($p < 0.05$)

Dual Therapy (PRILOSEC/clarithromycin)—Four randomized, double-blind, multi-center studies (M93–067, M93–100, M92–812b, and M93–058) evaluated PRILOSEC 40 mg q.d. plus clarithromycin 500 mg t.i.d. for 14 days, followed by PRILOSEC 20 mg q.d. (M93–067, M93–100, M93–058) or by PRILOSEC 40 mg q.d. (M92–812b) for an additional 14 days in patients with active duodenal ulcer associated with *H. pylori*. Studies M93–067 and M93–100 were conducted in the U.S. and Canada and enrolled 242 and 256 patients, respectively. *H. pylori* infection and duodenal ulcer were confirmed in 219 patients in Study M93–067 and 228 patients in Study M93–100. These studies compared the combination regimen to PRILOSEC and clarithromycin monotherapies. Studies M92–812b and M93–058 were conducted in Europe and enrolled 154 and 215 patients, respectively. *H. pylori* infection and duodenal ulcer were confirmed in 148 patients in study M92–812b and 208 patients in Study M93–058. These studies compared the combination regimen to omeprazole monotherapy. The results for the efficacy analyses for these studies are described below. *H. pylori* eradication was defined as no positive test (culture or histology) at 4 weeks following the end of treatment, and two negative tests were required to be considered eradicated of *H. pylori*. In the per-protocol analysis, the following patients were excluded: dropouts, patients with missing *H. pylori* tests post-treatment, and patients that were not assessed for *H. pylori* eradication because they were found to have an ulcer at the end of treatment.

The combination of omeprazole and clarithromycin was effective in eradicating *H. pylori*.

[See second table above]

Ulcer healing was not significantly different when clarithromycin was added to omeprazole therapy compared to omeprazole therapy alone.

The combination of omeprazole and clarithromycin was effective in eradicating *H. pylori* and reduced duodenal ulcer recurrence.

Duodenal Ulcer Recurrence Rates by *H. pylori* Eradication Status, % of Patients with Ulcer Recurrence

	H. pylori eradicated#	*H. pylori* not eradicated#
U.S. Studies†		
6 months post-treatment		
Study M93-067	*35 (n = 49)	60 (n = 88)
Study M93-100	*8 (n = 53)	60 (n = 106)
Non U.S. Studies‡		
6 months post-treatment		
Study M92-812b	*5 (n = 43)	46 (n = 78)
Study M93-058	*6 (n = 53)	43 (n = 107)
12 months post-treatment		
Study M92-812b	*5 (n = 39)	68 (n = 71)

#*H. pylori* eradication status assessed at same timepoint as ulcer recurrence
†Combined results for PRILOSEC + clarithromycin, PRILOSEC, and clarithromycin treatment arms
‡Combined results for PRILOSEC + clarithromycin and PRILOSEC treatment arms
*($p \leq 0.01$) versus proportion with duodenal ulcer recurrence who were not *H. pylori* eradicated

Gastric Ulcer

In a U.S. multicenter, double-blind, study of omeprazole 40 mg once a day, 20 mg once a day, and placebo in 520 patients with endoscopically diagnosed gastric ulcer, the following results were obtained.

Treatment of Gastric Ulcer
% of Patients Healed
(All Patients Treated)

	PRILOSEC 20 mg q.d. (n = 202)	PRILOSEC 40 mg q.d. (n = 214)	Placebo (n = 104)
Week 4	47.5**	55.6**	30.8
Week 8	74.8**	82.7**,+	48.1

**($p < 0.01$) PRILOSEC 40 mg or 20 mg versus placebo
+($p < 0.05$) PRILOSEC 40 mg versus 20 mg

For the stratified groups of patients with ulcer size less than or equal to 1 cm, no difference in healing rates between 40 mg and 20 mg was detected at either 4 or 8 weeks. For patients with ulcer size greater than 1 cm, 40 mg was significantly more effective than 20 mg at 8 weeks.

In a foreign, multinational, double-blind study of 602 patients with endoscopically diagnosed gastric ulcer, omeprazole 40 mg once a day, 20 mg once a day, and ranitidine 150 mg twice a day were evaluated.

Treatment of Gastric Ulcer
% of Patients Healed
(All Patients Treated)

	PRILOSEC 20 mg q.d. (n = 200)	PRILOSEC 40 mg q.d. (n = 187)	Ranitidine 150 mg b.i.d. (n = 199)
Week 4	63.5	78.1**,++	56.3
Week 8	81.5	91.4**,++	78.4

**($p < 0.01$) PRILOSEC 40 mg versus ranitidine
++($p < 0.01$) PRILOSEC 40 mg versus 20 mg

Gastroesophageal Reflux Disease (GERD)

Symptomatic GERD

A placebo controlled study was conducted in Scandinavia to compare the efficacy of omeprazole 20 mg or 10 mg once daily for up to 4 weeks in the treatment of heartburn and other symptoms in GERD patients without erosive esophagitis. Results are shown below.

% Successful Symptomatic Outcome[a]

	PRILOSEC 20 mg a.m.	PRILOSEC 10 mg a.m.	Placebo a.m.
All patients	46*† (n = 205)	31† (n = 199)	13 (n = 105)
Patients with confirmed GERD	56*† (n = 115)	36† (n = 109)	14 (n = 59)

[a]Defined as complete resolution of heartburn
*($p < 0.005$) versus 10 mg
†($p < 0.005$) versus placebo

Erosive Esophagitis

In a U.S. multicenter double-blind placebo controlled study of 20 mg or 40 mg of PRILOSEC Delayed-Release Capsules in patients with symptoms of GERD and endoscopically diagnosed erosive esophagitis of grade 2 or above, the percentage healing rates (per protocol) were as follows:

Week	20 mg PRILOSEC (n = 83)	40 mg PRILOSEC (n = 87)	Placebo (n = 43)
4	39**	45**	7
8	74**	75**	14

**($p < 0.01$) PRILOSEC versus placebo.

In this study, the 40 mg dose was not superior to the 20 mg dose of PRILOSEC in the percentage healing rate. Other controlled clinical trials have also shown that PRILOSEC is effective in severe GERD. In comparisons with histamine H_2-receptor antagonists in patients with erosive esophagitis, grade 2 or above, PRILOSEC in a dose of 20 mg was significantly more effective than the active controls. Complete daytime and nighttime heartburn relief occurred significantly faster ($p < 0.01$) in patients treated with PRILOSEC than in those taking placebo or histamine H_2-receptor antagonists.

In this and five other controlled GERD studies, significantly more patients taking 20 mg omeprazole (84%) reported complete relief of GERD symptoms than patients receiving placebo (12%).

Long Term Maintenance Treatment of Erosive Esophagitis

In a U.S. double-blind, randomized, multicenter, placebo controlled study, two dose regimens of PRILOSEC were studied in patients with endoscopically confirmed healed esophagitis. Results to determine maintenance of healing of erosive esophagitis are shown below.

Life Table Analysis

	PRILOSEC 20 mg q.d. (n = 138)	PRILOSEC 20 mg 3 days per week. (n = 137)	Placebo (n = 131)
Percent in endoscopic remission at 6 months	*70	34	11

*($p < 0.01$) PRILOSEC 20 mg q.d. versus PRILOSEC 20 mg 3 consecutive days per week or placebo.

In an international multicenter double-blind study, PRILOSEC 20 mg daily and 10 mg daily were compared to ranitidine 150 mg twice daily in patients with endoscopically confirmed healed esophagitis. The table below provides the results of this study for maintenance of healing of erosive esophagitis.

Life Table Analysis

	PRILOSEC 20 mg q.d. (n = 131)	PRILOSEC 10 mg q.d. (n = 133)	Ranitidine 150 mg b.i.d. (n = 128)
Percent in endoscopic remission at 12 months	*77	‡58	46

*($p = 0.01$) PRILOSEC 20 mg q.d. versus PRILOSEC 10 mg q.d. or Ranitidine.

‡($p = 0.03$) PRILOSEC 10 mg q.d. versus Ranitidine.

In patients who initially had grades 3 or 4 erosive esophagitis, for maintenance after healing 20 mg daily of PRILOSEC was effective, while 10 mg did not demonstrate effectiveness.

Pathological Hypersecretory Conditions

In open studies of 136 patients with pathological hypersecretory conditions, such as Zollinger-Ellison (ZE) syndrome with or without multiple endocrine adenomas, PRILOSEC Delayed-Release Capsules significantly inhibited gastric acid secretion and controlled associated symptoms of diarrhea, anorexia, and pain. Doses ranging from 20 mg every other day to 360 mg per day maintained basal acid secretion below 10 mEq/hr in patients without prior gastric surgery, and below 5 mEq/hr in patients with prior gastric surgery. Initial doses were titrated to the individual patient need, and adjustments were necessary with time in some patients (see DOSAGE AND ADMINISTRATION). PRILOSEC was well tolerated at these high dose levels for prolonged periods (> 5 years in some patients). In most ZE patients, serum gastrin levels were not modified by PRILOSEC. However, in some patients serum gastrin increased to levels greater than those present prior to initiation of omeprazole therapy. At least 11 patients with ZE syndrome on long-term treatment with PRILOSEC developed gastric carcinoids. These findings are believed to be a manifestation of the underlying condition, which is known to be associated with such tumors, rather than the result of the administration of PRILOSEC. (See ADVERSE REACTIONS.)

Microbiology

Omeprazole and clarithromycin dual therapy and omeprazole, clarithromycin and amoxicillin triple therapy have been shown to be active against most strains of *Helicobacter pylori in vitro* and in clinical infections as described in the INDICATIONS AND USAGE section.

Helicobacter

Helicobacter pylori

Pretreatment Resistance

Clarithromycin pretreatment resistance rates were 3.5% (4/113) in the omeprazole/clarithromycin dual therapy studies (M93-067, M93-100) and 9.3% (41/439) in omeprazole/clarithromycin/amoxicillin triple therapy studies (126, 127, M96-446).

Clarithromycin Susceptibility Test Results and Clinical/Bacteriological Outcomes[a]

Clarithromycin Pretreatment Results		Clarithromycin Post-treatment Results: *H. pylori* negative-eradicated	*H. pylori* positive-not eradicated — Post-treatment susceptibility results: S[b]	I[b]	R[b]	No MIC
Dual Therapy - (omeprazole 40 mg q.d./clarithromycin 500 mg t.i.d. for 14 days followed by omeprazole 20 mg q.d. for another 14 days) (Studies M93-067, M93-100)						
Susceptible[b]	108	72	1		26	9
Intermediate[b]	1				1	
Resistant[b]	4				4	
Triple Therapy - (omeprazole 20 mg b.i.d./clarithromycin 500 mg b.i.d./amoxicillin 1 g b.i.d. for 10 days - Studies 126, 127, M96-446; followed by omeprazole 20 mg q.d. for another 18 days - Studies 126, 127)						
Susceptible[b]	171	153	7		3	8
Intermediate[b]						
Resistant[b]	14	4	1		6	3

[a] Includes only patients with pretreatment clarithromycin susceptibility test results

[b] Susceptible (S) MIC ≤ 0.25 μg/mL, Intermediate (I) MIC 0.5-1.0 μg/mL, Resistant (R) MIC ≥ 2 μg/mL

Amoxicillin pretreatment susceptible isolates (≤ 0.25 μg/mL) were found in 99.3% (436/439) of the patients in the omeprazole/clarithromycin/amoxicillin triple therapy studies (126, 127, M96-446). Amoxicillin pretreatment minimum inhibitory concentrations (MICs) > 0.25 μg/mL occurred in 0.7% (3/439) of the patients, all of whom were in the clarithromycin and amoxicillin study arm. One patient had an unconfirmed pretreatment amoxicillin minimum inhibitory concentration (MIC) of > 256 μg/mL by Etest®.

Clarithromycin Susceptibility Test Results and Clinical/Bacteriological Outcomes

[See table above]

Patients not eradicated of *H. pylori* following omeprazole/clarithromycin/amoxicillin triple therapy or omeprazole/clarithromycin dual therapy will likely have clarithromycin resistant *H. pylori* isolates. Therefore, clarithromycin susceptibility testing should be done, if possible. Patients with clarithromycin resistant *H. pylori* should not be treated with any of the following: omeprazole/clarithromycin dual therapy, omeprazole/clarithromycin/amoxicillin triple therapy, or other regimens which include clarithromycin as the sole antimicrobial agent.

Amoxicillin Susceptibility Test Results and Clinical/Bacteriological Outcomes

In the triple therapy clinical trials, 84.9% (157/185) of the patients in the omeprazole/clarithromycin/amoxicillin treatment group who had pretreatment amoxicillin susceptible MICs (≤ 0.25 μg/mL) were eradicated of *H. pylori* and 15.1% (28/185) failed therapy. Of the 28 patients who failed triple therapy, 11 had no post-treatment susceptibility test results and 17 had post-treatment *H. pylori* isolates with amoxicillin susceptible MICs. Eleven of the patients who failed triple therapy also had post-treatment *H. pylori* isolates with clarithromycin resistant MICs.

Susceptibility Test for *Helicobacter pylori*

The reference methodology for susceptibility testing of *H. pylori* is agar dilution MICs[1]. One to three microliters of an inoculum equivalent to a No. 2 McFarland standard ($1 \times 10^7 - 1 \times 10^8$ CFU/mL for *H. pylori*) are inoculated directly onto freshly prepared antimicrobial containing Mueller-Hinton agar plates with 5% aged defibrinated sheep blood (≥ 2 weeks old). The agar dilution plates are incubated at 35°C in a microaerobic environment produced by a gas generating system suitable for campylobacters. After 3 days of incubation, the MICs are recorded as the lowest concentration of antimicrobial agent required to inhibit growth of the organism. The clarithromycin and amoxicillin MIC values should be interpreted according to the following criteria:

Clarithromycin MIC (μg/mL)[a]	Interpretation	
≤0.25	Susceptible	(S)
0.5–1.0	Intermediate	(I)
≥2.0	Resistant	(R)

Amoxicillin MIC (μg/mL)[a,b]	Interpretation	
≤0.25	Susceptible	(S)

[a] These are tentative breakpoints for the agar dilution methodology and they should not be used to interpret results obtained using alternative methods.

[b] There were not enough organisms with MICs > 0.25 μg/mL to determine a resistance breakpoint.

Standardized susceptibility test procedures require the use of laboratory control microorganisms to control the technical aspects of the laboratory procedures. Standard clarithromycin and amoxicillin powders should provide the following MIC values:

Microorganism	Antimicrobial Agent	MIC (μg/mL)[a]
H. pylori ATCC 43504	Clarithromycin	0.015-0.12 (μg/mL)
H. pylori ATCC 43504	Amoxicillin	0.015-0.12 (μg/mL)

[a] These are quality control ranges for the agar dilution methodology and they should not be used to control test results obtained using alternative methods.

[1] National Committee for Clinical Laboratory Standards. Summary Minutes, Subcommittee on Antimicrobial Susceptibility Testing, Tampa FL, January 11-13, 1998.

INDICATIONS AND USAGE

Duodenal Ulcer

PRILOSEC Delayed-Release Capsules are indicated for short-term treatment of active duodenal ulcer. Most patients heal within four weeks. Some patients may require an additional four weeks of therapy.

PRILOSEC Delayed-Release Capsules, in combination with clarithromycin and amoxicillin, are indicated for treatment of patients with *H. pylori* infection and duodenal ulcer disease (active or up to 1-year history) to eradicate *H. pylori*.

PRILOSEC Delayed-Release Capsules, in combination with clarithromycin, are indicated for treatment of patients with *H. pylori* infection and duodenal ulcer disease to eradicate *H. pylori*.

Eradication of *H. pylori* has been shown to reduce the risk of duodenal ulcer recurrence (see CLINICAL PHARMACOLOGY, Clinical Studies and DOSAGE AND ADMINISTRATION).

Among patients who fail therapy, PRILOSEC with clarithromycin is more likely to be associated with the development of clarithromycin resistance as compared with triple therapy. In patients who fail therapy, susceptibility testing should be done. If resistance to clarithromycin is demonstrated or susceptibility testing is not possible, alternative antimicrobial therapy should be instituted. (See Microbiology section, and the clarithromycin package insert, MICROBIOLOGY section.)

Gastric Ulcer

PRILOSEC Delayed-Release Capsules are indicated for short-term treatment (4–8 weeks) of active benign gastric ulcer. (See CLINICAL PHARMACOLOGY, Clinical Studies, Gastric Ulcer.)

Treatment of Gastroesophageal Reflux Disease (GERD)

Symptomatic GERD

PRILOSEC Delayed-Release Capsules are indicated for the treatment of heartburn and other symptoms associated with GERD.

Erosive Esophagitis

PRILOSEC Delayed-Release Capsules are indicated for the short-term treatment (4–8 weeks) of erosive esophagitis which has been diagnosed by endoscopy.

(See CLINICAL PHARMACOLOGY, Clinical Studies.)

The efficacy of PRILOSEC used for longer than 8 weeks in these patients has not been established. In the rare instance of a patient not responding to 8 weeks of treatment, it may be helpful to give up to an additional 4 weeks of treatment. If there is recurrence of erosive esophagitis or GERD symptoms (e.g. heartburn), additional 4-8 week courses of omeprazole may be considered.

Maintenance of Healing of Erosive Esophagitis

PRILOSEC Delayed-Release Capsules are indicated to maintain healing of erosive esophagitis.

Controlled studies do not extend beyond 12 months.

Continued on next page

Prilosec—Cont.

Pathological Hypersecretory Conditions
PRILOSEC Delayed-Release Capsules are indicated for the long-term treatment of pathological hypersecretory conditions (e.g., Zollinger-Ellison syndrome, multiple endocrine adenomas and systemic mastocytosis).

CONTRAINDICATIONS

Omeprazole
PRILOSEC Delayed-Release Capsules are contraindicated in patients with known hypersensitivity to any component of the formulation.

Clarithromycin
Clarithromycin is contraindicated in patients with a known hypersensitivity to any macrolide antibiotic.
Concomitant administration of clarithromycin with cisapride, pimozide, or terfenadine is contraindicated. There have been post-marketing reports of drug interactions when clarithromycin and/or erythromycin are co-administered with cisapride, pimozide, or terfenadine resulting in cardiac arrhythmias (QT prolongation, ventricular tachycardia, ventricular fibrillation, and torsades de pointes) most likely due to inhibition of hepatic metabolism of these drugs by erythromycin and clarithromycin. Fatalities have been reported. (Please refer to full prescribing information for clarithromycin before prescribing.)

Amoxicillin
Amoxicillin is contraindicated in patients with a history of allergic reaction to any of the penicillins. (Please refer to full prescribing information for amoxicillin before prescribing.)

WARNINGS

Clarithromycin
CLARITHROMYCIN SHOULD NOT BE USED IN PREGNANT WOMEN EXCEPT IN CLINICAL CIRCUMSTANCES WHERE NO ALTERNATIVE THERAPY IS APPROPRIATE. IF PREGNANCY OCCURS WHILE TAKING CLARITHROMYCIN, THE PATIENT SHOULD BE APPRISED OF THE POTENTIAL HAZARD TO THE FETUS. (See WARNINGS in prescribing information for clarithromycin.)

Amoxicillin
SERIOUS AND OCCASIONALLY FATAL HYPERSENSITIVITY (anaphylactic) REACTIONS HAVE BEEN REPORTED IN PATIENTS ON PENICILLIN THERAPY. THESE REACTIONS ARE MORE LIKELY TO OCCUR IN INDIVIDUALS WITH A HISTORY OF PENICILLIN HYPERSENSITIVITY AND/OR A HISTORY OF SENSITIVITY TO MULTIPLE ALLERGENS. BEFORE INITIATING THERAPY WITH AMOXICILLIN, CAREFUL INQUIRY SHOULD BE MADE CONCERNING PREVIOUS HYPERSENSITIVITY REACTIONS TO PENICILLINS, CEPHALOSPORINS OR OTHER ALLERGENS. IF AN ALLERGIC REACTION OCCURS, AMOXICILLIN SHOULD BE DISCONTINUED AND APPROPRIATE THERAPY INSTITUTED. **SERIOUS ANAPHYLACTIC REACTIONS REQUIRE IMMEDIATE EMERGENCY TREATMENT WITH EPINEPHRINE. OXYGEN, INTRAVENOUS STEROIDS AND AIRWAY MANAGEMENT, INCLUDING INTUBATION, SHOULD ALSO BE ADMINISTERED AS INDICATED.** (See WARNINGS in prescribing information for amoxicillin.)

Antimicrobials
Pseudomembranous colitis has been reported with nearly all antibacterial agents and may range in severity from mild to life-threatening. Therefore, it is important to consider this diagnosis in patients who present with diarrhea subsequent to the administration of antibacterial agents. (See WARNINGS in prescribing information for clarithromycin and amoxicillin.)

PRECAUTIONS

General
Symptomatic response to therapy with omeprazole does not preclude the presence of gastric malignancy.
Atrophic gastritis has been noted occasionally in gastric corpus biopsies from patients treated long-term with omeprazole.

Information for Patients
PRILOSEC Delayed-Release Capsules should be taken before eating. Patients should be cautioned that the PRILOSEC Delayed-Release Capsule should not be opened, chewed or crushed, and should be swallowed whole.

Drug Interactions
Other
Omeprazole can prolong the elimination of diazepam, warfarin and phenytoin, drugs that are metabolized by oxidation in the liver. Although in normal subjects no interaction with theophylline or propranolol was found, there have been clinical reports of interaction with other drugs metabolized via the cytochrome P-450 system (e.g., cyclosporine, disulfiram, benzodiazepines). Patients should be monitored to determine if it is necessary to adjust the dosage of these drugs when taken concomitantly with PRILOSEC.
Because of its profound and long lasting inhibition of gastric acid secretion, it is theoretically possible that omeprazole may interfere with absorption of drugs where gastric pH is an important determinant of their bioavailability (e.g., ketoconazole, ampicillin esters, and iron salts). In the clinical trials, antacids were used concomitantly with the administration of PRILOSEC.
Combination Therapy with Clarithromycin
Co-administration of omeprazole and clarithromycin have resulted in increases in plasma levels of omeprazole, clarithromycin, and 14-hydroxy-clarithromycin. (See also CLINICAL PHARMACOLOGY, Pharmacokinetics: Combination Therapy with Antimicrobials.)
Concomitant administration of clarithromycin with cisapride, pimozide, or terfenadine is contraindicated.
There have been reports of an interaction between erythromycin and astemizole resulting in QT prolongation and torsades de pointes. Concomitant administration of erythromycin and astemizole is contraindicated. Because clarithromycin is also metabolized by cytochrome P450, concomitant administration of clarithromycin with astemizole is not recommended. (See also CONTRAINDICATIONS, Clarithromycin, above. Please refer to full prescribing information for clarithromycin before prescribing.)

Carcinogenesis, Mutagenesis, Impairment of Fertility
In two 24-month carcinogenicity studies in rats, omeprazole at daily doses of 1.7, 3.4, 13.8, 44.0 and 140.8 mg/kg/day (approximately 4 to 352 times the human dose, based on a patient weight of 50 kg and a human dose of 20 mg) produced gastric ECL cell carcinoids in a dose-related manner in both male and female rats; the incidence of this effect was markedly higher in female rats, which had higher blood levels of omeprazole. Gastric carcinoids seldom occur in the untreated rat. In addition, ECL cell hyperplasia was present in all treated groups of both sexes. In one of these studies, female rats were treated with 13.8 mg omeprazole/kg/day (approximately 35 times the human dose) for one year, then followed for an additional year without the drug. No carcinoids were seen in these rats. An increased incidence of treatment-related ECL cell hyperplasia was observed at the end of one year (94% treated vs 10% controls). By the second year the difference between treated and control rats was much smaller (46% vs 26%) but still showed more hyperplasia in the treated group. An unusual primary malignant tumor in the stomach was seen in one rat (2%). No similar tumor was seen in male or female rats treated for two years. For this strain of rat no similar tumor has been noted historically, but a finding involving only one tumor is difficult to interpret. A 78-week mouse carcinogenicity study of omeprazole did not show increased tumor occurrence, but the study was not conclusive.
Omeprazole was not mutagenic in an *in vitro* Ames *Salmonella typhimurium* assay, an *in vitro* mouse lymphoma cell assay and an *in vivo* rat liver DNA damage assay. A mouse micronucleus test at 625 and 6250 times the human dose gave a borderline result, as did an *in vivo* bone marrow chromosome aberration test. A second mouse micronucleus study at 2000 times the human dose, but with different (suboptimal) sampling times, was negative.
In a rat fertility and general reproductive performance test, omeprazole in a dose range of 13.8 to 138.0 mg/kg/day (approximately 35 to 345 times the human dose) was not toxic or deleterious to the reproductive performance of parental animals.

Pregnancy
Omeprazole
Pregnancy Category C
Teratology studies conducted in pregnant rats at doses up to 138 mg/kg/day (approximately 345 times the human dose) and in pregnant rabbits at doses up to 69 mg/kg/day (approximately 172 times the human dose) did not disclose any evidence for a teratogenic potential of omeprazole.
In rabbits, omeprazole in a dose range of 6.9 to 69.1 mg/kg/day (approximately 17 to 172 times the human dose) produced dose-related increases in embryo-lethality, fetal resorptions and pregnancy disruptions. In rats, dose-related embryo/fetal toxicity and postnatal developmental toxicity were observed in offspring resulting from parents treated with omeprazole 13.8 to 138.0 mg/kg/day (approximately 35 to 345 times the human dose). There are no adequate or well-controlled studies in pregnant women. Sporadic reports have been received of congenital abnormalities occurring in infants born to women who have received omeprazole during pregnancy. Omeprazole should be used during pregnancy only if the potential benefit justifies the potential risk to the fetus.

Clarithromycin
Pregnancy Category C. See WARNINGS (above) and full prescribing information for clarithromycin before using in pregnant women.

Nursing Mothers
It is not known whether omeprazole is excreted in human milk. In rats, omeprazole administration during late gestation and lactation at doses of 13.8 to 138 mg/kg/day (35 to 345 times the human dose) resulted in decreased weight gain in pups. Because many drugs are excreted in human milk, because of the potential for serious adverse reactions in nursing infants from omeprazole, and because of the potential for tumorigenicity shown for omeprazole in rat carcinogenicity studies, a decision should be made whether to discontinue nursing or to discontinue the drug, taking into account the importance of the drug to the mother.

Pediatric Use
Safety and effectiveness in pediatric patients have not been established.

Geriatric Use
Omeprazole was administered to over 2000 elderly individuals (≥ 65 years of age) in clinical trials in the US and Europe. There were no differences in safety and effectiveness between the elderly and younger subjects. Other reported clinical experience has not identified differences in response between the elderly and younger subjects, but greater sensitivity of some older individuals cannot be ruled out.
Pharmacokinetic studies have shown the elimination rate was somewhat decreased in the elderly and bioavailability was increased. The plasma clearance of omeprazole was 250 mL/min (about half that of young volunteers) and its plasma half-life averaged one hour, about twice that of young healthy volunteers. However, no dosage adjustment is necessary in the elderly. (See CLINICAL PHARMACOLOGY.)

ADVERSE REACTIONS

PRILOSEC Delayed-Release Capsules were generally well tolerated during domestic and international clinical trials in 3096 patients.
In the U.S. clinical trial population of 465 patients (including duodenal ulcer, Zollinger-Ellison syndrome and resistant ulcer patients), the following adverse experiences were reported to occur in 1% or more of patients on therapy with PRILOSEC. Numbers in parentheses indicate percentages of the adverse experiences considered by investigators as possibly, probably or definitely related to the drug:

	Omeprazole (n = 465)	Placebo (n = 64)	Ranitidine (n = 195)
Headache	6.9 (2.4)	6.3	7.7 (2.6)
Diarrhea	3.0 (1.9)	3.1 (1.6)	2.1 (0.5)
Abdominal Pain	2.4 (0.4)	3.1	2.1
Nausea	2.2 (0.9)	3.1	4.1 (0.5)
URI	1.9	1.6	2.6
Dizziness	1.5 (0.6)	0.0	2.6 (1.0)
Vomiting	1.5 (0.4)	4.7	1.5 (0.5)
Rash	1.5 (1.1)	0.0	0.0
Constipation	1.1 (0.9)	0.0	0.0
Cough	1.1	0.0	1.5
Asthenia	1.1 (0.2)	1.6 (1.6)	1.5 (1.0)
Back Pain	1.1	0.0	0.5

The following adverse reactions which occurred in 1% or more of omeprazole-treated patients have been reported in international double-blind, and open-label, clinical trials in which 2,631 patients and subjects received omeprazole.

Incidence of Adverse Experiences ≥ 1%
Causal Relationship not Assessed

	Omeprazole (n = 2631)	Placebo (n = 120)
Body as a Whole, site unspecified		
Abdominal pain	5.2	3.3
Asthenia	1.3	0.8
Digestive System		
Constipation	1.5	0.8
Diarrhea	3.7	2.5
Flatulence	2.7	5.8
Nausea	4.0	6.7
Vomiting	3.2	10.0
Acid regurgitation	1.9	3.3
Nervous System/Psychiatric		
Headache	2.9	2.5

Additional adverse experiences occurring in < 1% of patients or subjects in domestic and/or international trials, or occurring since the drug was marketed, are shown below within each body system. In many instances, the relationship to PRILOSEC was unclear.
Body As a Whole: Allergic reactions, including, rarely, anaphylaxis (see also *Skin* below), fever, pain, fatigue, malaise, abdominal swelling
Cardiovascular: Chest pain or angina, tachycardia, bradycardia, palpitation, elevated blood pressure, peripheral edema
Gastrointestinal: Pancreatitis (some fatal), anorexia, irritable colon, flatulence, fecal discoloration, esophageal candidiasis, mucosal atrophy of the tongue, dry mouth. During treatment with omeprazole, gastric fundic gland polyps have been noted rarely. These polyps are benign and appear to be reversible when treatment is discontinued.
Gastro-duodenal carcinoids have been reported in patients with ZE syndrome on long-term treatment with PRILOSEC. This finding is believed to be a manifestation of the underlying condition, which is known to be associated with such tumors.
Hepatic: Mild and, rarely, marked elevations of liver function tests [ALT (SGPT), AST (SGOT), γ-glutamyl transpeptidase, alkaline phosphatase, and bilirubin (jaundice)]. In rare instances, overt liver disease has occurred, including hepatocellular, cholestatic, or mixed hepatitis, liver necrosis (some fatal), hepatic failure (some fatal), and hepatic encephalopathy.
Metabolic/Nutritional: Hyponatremia, hypoglycemia, weight gain
Musculoskeletal: Muscle cramps, myalgia, muscle weakness, joint pain, leg pain
Nervous System/Psychiatric: Psychic disturbances including depression, aggression, hallucinations, confusion, insomnia, nervousness, tremors, apathy, somnolence, anxiety, dream abnormalities; vertigo; paresthesia; hemifacial dysesthesia
Respiratory: Epistaxis, pharyngeal pain
Skin: Rash and, rarely, cases of severe generalized skin reactions including toxic epidermal necrolysis (TEN; some fatal), Stevens-Johnson syndrome, and erythema multiforme (some severe); purpura and/or petechiae (some with rechallenge); skin inflammation, urticaria, angioedema, pruritus, alopecia, dry skin, hyperhidrosis
Special Senses: Tinnitus, taste perversion

Urogenital: Interstitial nephritis (some with positive rechallenge), urinary tract infection, microscopic pyuria, urinary frequency, elevated serum creatinine, proteinuria, hematuria, glycosuria, testicular pain, gynecomastia
Hematologic: Rare instances of pancytopenia, agranulocytosis (some fatal), thrombocytopenia, neutropenia, anemia, leucocytosis, and hemolytic anemia have been reported.
The incidence of clinical adverse experiences in patients greater than 65 years of age was similar to that in patients 65 years of age or less.

Combination Therapy for *H. pylori* Eradication
In clinical trials using either dual therapy with PRILOSEC and clarithromycin, or triple therapy with PRILOSEC, clarithromycin, and amoxicillin, no adverse experiences peculiar to these drug combinations have been observed. Adverse experiences that have occurred have been limited to those that have been previously reported with omeprazole, clarithromycin, or amoxicillin.
Triple Therapy (PRILOSEC/clarithromycin/amoxicillin)—The most frequent adverse experiences observed in clinical trials using combination therapy with PRILOSEC, clarithromycin, and amoxicillin (n = 274) were diarrhea (14%), taste perversion (10%), and headache (7%). None of these occurred at a higher frequency than that reported by patients taking the antimicrobial drugs alone.
For more information on clarithromycin or amoxicillin, refer to the respective package inserts, ADVERSE REACTIONS sections.
Dual Therapy (PRILOSEC/clarithromycin)—Adverse experiences observed in controlled clinical trials using combination therapy with PRILOSEC and clarithromycin (n=346) which differed from those previously described for omeprazole alone were: Taste perversion (15%), tongue discoloration (2%), rhinitis (2%), pharyngitis (1%) and flu syndrome (1%).
For more information on clarithromycin, refer to the clarithromycin package insert, ADVERSE REACTIONS section.

OVERDOSAGE

Rare reports have been received of overdosage with omeprazole. Doses ranged from 320 mg to 900 mg (16–45 times the usual recommended clinical dose). Manifestations were variable, but included confusion, drowsiness, blurred vision, tachycardia, nausea, diaphoresis, flushing, headache, and dry mouth. Symptoms were transient, and no serious clinical outcome has been reported. No specific antidote for omeprazole overdosage is known. Omeprazole is extensively protein bound and is, therefore, not readily dialyzable. In the event of overdosage, treatment should be symptomatic and supportive.
Lethal doses of omeprazole after single oral administration are about 1500 mg/kg in mice and greater than 4000 mg/kg in rats, and about 100 mg/kg in mice and greater than 40 mg/kg in rats given single intravenous injections. Animals given these doses showed sedation, ptosis, convulsions, and decreased activity, body temperature, and respiratory rate and increased depth of respiration.

DOSAGE AND ADMINISTRATION

Short-Term Treatment of Active Duodenal Ulcer
The recommended adult oral dose of PRILOSEC is 20 mg once daily. Most patients heal within four weeks. Some patients may require an additional four weeks of therapy. (See INDICATIONS AND USAGE.)

***H. pylori* Eradication for the Reduction of the Risk of Duodenal Ulcer Recurrence**
Triple Therapy (PRILOSEC/clarithromycin/amoxicillin)—The recommended adult oral regimen is PRILOSEC 20 mg plus clarithromycin 500 mg plus amoxicillin 1000 mg each given twice daily for 10 days. In patients with an ulcer present at the time of initiation of therapy, an additional 18 days of PRILOSEC 20 mg once daily is recommended for ulcer healing and symptom relief.
Dual Therapy (PRILOSEC/clarithromycin)—The recommended adult oral regimen is PRILOSEC 40 mg once daily plus clarithromycin 500 mg t.i.d. for 14 days. In patients with an ulcer present at the time of initiation of therapy, an additional 14 days of PRILOSEC 20 mg once daily is recommended for ulcer healing and symptom relief.
Please refer to clarithromycin full prescribing information for CONTRAINDICATIONS and WARNING, and for information regarding dosing in elderly and renally impaired patients (PRECAUTIONS: General, PRECAUTIONS: Geriatric Use and PRECAUTIONS: Drug Interactions).
Please refer to amoxicillin full prescribing information for CONTRAINDICATIONS and WARNINGS.

Gastric Ulcer
The recommended adult oral dose is 40 mg once a day for 4-8 weeks. (See CLINICAL PHARMACOLOGY, Clinical Studies, Gastric Ulcer, and INDICATIONS AND USAGE, Gastric Ulcer.)

Gastroesophageal Reflux Disease (GERD)
The recommended adult oral dose for the treatment of patients with symptomatic GERD and no esophageal lesions is 20 mg daily for up to 4 weeks. The recommended adult oral dose for the treatment of patients with erosive esophagitis and accompanying symptoms due to GERD is 20 mg daily for 4 to 8 weeks. (See INDICATIONS AND USAGE.)

Maintenance of Healing of Erosive Esophagitis
The recommended adult oral dose is 20 mg daily. (See CLINICAL PHARMACOLOGY, Clinical Studies.)

Pathological Hypersecretory Conditions
The dosage of PRILOSEC in patients with pathological hypersecretory conditions varies with the individual patient. The recommended adult oral starting dose is 60 mg once a day. Doses should be adjusted to individual patient needs and should continue for as long as clinically indicated. Doses up to 120 mg t.i.d. have been administered. Daily dosages of greater than 80 mg should be administered in divided doses. Some patients with Zollinger-Ellison syndrome have been treated continuously with PRILOSEC for more than 5 years.
No dosage adjustment is necessary for patients with renal impairment, hepatic dysfunction or for the elderly.
PRILOSEC Delayed-Release Capsules should be taken before eating. In the clinical trials, antacids were used concomitantly with PRILOSEC.
Patients should be cautioned that the PRILOSEC Delayed-Release Capsule should not be opened, chewed or crushed, and should be swallowed whole.

HOW SUPPLIED

No. 3426—PRILOSEC Delayed-Release Capsules, 10 mg, are opaque, hard gelatin, apricot and amethyst colored capsules, coded 606 on cap and PRILOSEC 10 on the body. They are supplied as follows:
NDC 0186-0606-31 unit of use bottles of 30
NDC 0186-0606-68 bottles of 100
NDC 0186-0606-28 unit dose packages of 100
NDC 0186-0606-82 bottles of 1000.
No. 3440—PRILOSEC Delayed-Release Capsules, 20 mg, are opaque, hard gelatin, amethyst colored capsules, coded 742 on cap and PRILOSEC 20 on body. They are supplied as follows:
NDC 0186-0742-31 unit of use bottles of 30
NDC 0186-0742-28 unit dose package of 100
NDC 0186-0742-82 bottles of 1000.
No. 3428—PRILOSEC Delayed-Release Capsules, 40 mg, are opaque, hard gelatin, apricot and amethyst colored capsules, coded 743 on cap and PRILOSEC 40 on the body. They are supplied as follows:
NDC 0186-0743-31 unit of use bottles of 30
NDC 0186-0743-68 bottles of 100
NDC 0186-0743-28 unit dose packages of 100
NDC 0186-0743-82 bottles of 1000.

Storage
Store PRILOSEC Delayed-Release Capsules in a tight container protected from light and moisture. Store between 15°C and 30°C (59°F and 86°F).
Trademarks herein are the property of the AstraZeneca Group

Manufactured for: AstraZeneca LP, Wilmington, DE 19850
By: Merck & Co., Inc., Whitehouse Station, NJ 08889, USA
640004-32 Revised April 2000
Shown in Product Identification Guide, page 305

PULMICORT TURBUHALER® 200 mcg ℞
[*pull'mĭ-cŏrt*]
(budesonide inhalation powder)
For Oral Inhalation Only.

DESCRIPTION

Budesonide, the active component of PULMICORT TURBUHALER 200 mcg, is a corticosteroid designated chemically as (RS)-11β,16α,17,21-Tetrahydroxypregna-1,4-diene-3,20-dione cyclic 16,17-acetal with butyraldehyde. Budesonide is provided as a mixture of two epimers (22R and 22S). The empirical formula of budesonide is $C_{25}H_{34}O_6$ and its molecular weight is 430.5. Its structural formula is:

Budesonide is a white to off-white, tasteless, odorless powder that is practically insoluble in water and in heptane, sparingly soluble in ethanol, and freely soluble in chloroform. Its partition coefficient between octanol and water at pH 7.4 is 1.6×10^3.
PULMICORT TURBUHALER is an inhalation-driven multi-dose dry powder inhaler which contains only micronized budesonide. Each actuation of PULMICORT TURBUHALER provides 200 mcg budesonide per metered dose, which delivers approximately 160 mcg budesonide from the mouthpiece (based on *in vitro* testing at 60 L/min for 2 sec). The amount of drug delivered to the lung will depend on patient factors such as inspiratory flow (see Patient's Instructions for Use). In adult patients with asthma (mean FEV_1 2.9 L [0.8–5.1 L]) mean peak inspiratory flow (PIF) through PULMICORT TURBUHALER was 78 (40–111) L/min. Similar results (mean PIF 82 [43–125] L/min) were obtained in asthmatic children (6 to 15 years, mean FEV_1 2.1 L [0.9–5.4 L]).

CLINICAL PHARMACOLOGY

Budesonide is an anti-inflammatory corticosteroid that exhibits potent glucocorticoid activity and weak mineralocorticoid activity. In standard *in vitro* and animal models, budesonide has approximately a 200-fold higher affinity for the glucocorticoid receptor and a 1000-fold higher topical anti-inflammatory potency than cortisol (rat croton oil ear edema assay). As a measure of systemic activity, budesonide is 40 times more potent than cortisol when administered subcutaneously and 25 times more potent when administered orally in the rat thymus involution assay.
The precise mechanism of corticosteroid actions on inflammation in asthma is not known. Corticosteroids have been shown to have a wide range of inhibitory activities against multiple cell types (e.g., mast cells, eosinophils, neutrophils, macrophages, and lymphocytes) and mediators (e.g., histamine, eicosanoids, leukotrienes, and cytokines) involved in allergic and non-allergic-mediated inflammation. These anti-inflammatory actions of corticosteroids may contribute to their efficacy in asthma.
Studies in asthmatic patients have shown a favorable ratio between topical anti-inflammatory activity and sytemic corticosteroid effects over a wide range of doses from PULMICORT TURBUHALER. This is explained by a combination of a relatively high local anti-inflammatory effect, extensive first pass hepatic degradation of orally absorbed drug (85–95%), and the low potency of formed metabolites (see below).

Pharmacokinetics
The activity of PULMICORT TURBUHALER is due to the parent drug, budesonide. In glucocorticoid receptor affinity studies, the 22R form was two times as active as the 22S epimer. *In vitro* studies indicated that the two forms of budesonide do not interconvert. The 22R form was preferentially cleared by the liver with systemic clearance of 1.4 L/min vs. 1.0 L/min for the 22S form. The terminal half-life, 2 to 3 hours, was the same for both epimers and was independent of dose. In asthmatic patients, budesonide showed a linear increase in AUC and C_{max} with increasing dose after both a single dose and repeated dosing from PULMICORT TURBUHALER.
Absorption: After oral administration of budesonide, peak plasma concentration was achieved in about 1 to 2 hours and the absolute systemic availability was 6–13%. In contrast, most of budesonide delivered to the lungs is systemically absorbed. In healthy subjects, 34% of the metered dose was deposited in the lungs (as assessed by plasma concentration method) with an absolute systemic availability of 39% of the metered dose. Pharmacokinetics of budesonide do not differ significantly in healthy volunteers and asthmatic patients. Peak plasma concentrations of budesonide occurred within 30 minutes of inhalation from PULMICORT TURBUHALER.
Distribution: The volume of distribution of budesonide was approximately 3 L/kg. It was 85–90% bound to plasma proteins. Protein binding was constant over the concentration range (1–100 nmol/L) achieved with, and exceeding, recommended doses of PULMICORT TURBUHALER. Budesonide showed little or no binding to corticosteroid binding globulin. Budesonide rapidly equilibrated with red blood cells in a concentration independent manner with a blood/plasma ratio of about 0.8.
Metabolism: *In vitro* studies with human liver homogenates have shown that budesonide is rapidly and extensively metabolized. Two major metabolites formed via cytochrome P450 3A catalyzed biotransformation have been isolated and identified as 16α-hydroxyprednisolone and 6β-hydroxybudesonide. The corticosteroid activity of each of these two metabolites is less than 1% of that of the parent compound. No qualitative difference between the *in vitro* and *in vivo* metabolic patterns have been detected. Negligible metabolic inactivation was observed in human lung and serum preparations.
Excretion: Budesonide was excreted in urine and feces in the form of metabolites. Approximately 60% of an intravenous radiolabelled dose was recovered in the urine. No unchanged budesonide was detected in the urine.
Special Populations: No pharmacokinetic differences have been identified due to race, gender or advanced age.
Pediatric: Following intravenous dosing in pediatric patients age 10–14 years, plasma half-life was shorter than in adults (1.5 hrs vs 2.0 hrs in adults). In the same population following inhalation of budesonide via a pressurized metered-dose inhaler, absolute systemic availability was similar to that in adults.
Hepatic Insufficiency: Reduced liver function may affect the elimination of corticosteroids. The pharmacokinetics of budesonide were affected by compromised liver function as evidenced by a doubled systemic availability after oral ingestion. The intravenous pharmacokinetics of budesonide were, however, similar in cirrhotic patients and in healthy subjects.
Drug-drug Interactions: Ketoconazole, a potent inhibitor of cytochrome P450 3A, the main metabolic enzyme for corticosteroids, increased plasma levels of orally ingested budesonide. At recommended doses, cimetidine had a slight but clinically insignificant effect on the pharmacokinetics of oral budesonide.

Pharmacodynamics
To confirm that systemic absorption is not a significant factor in the clinical efficacy of inhaled budesonide, a clinical study in patients with asthma was performed comparing 400 mcg budesonide administered via a pressurized metered dose inhaler with a tube spacer to 1400 mcg of oral budesonide and placebo. The study demonstrated the efficacy of inhaled budesonide but not orally ingested budesonide despite comparable systemic levels. Thus, the therapeutic effect of conventional doses of orally inhaled budesonide are largely explained by its direct action on the respiratory tract.

Continued on next page

Pulmicort Turbuhaler—Cont.

Generally, PULMICORT TURBUHALER has a relatively rapid onset of action for an inhaled corticosteroid. Improvement in asthma control following inhalation of PULMICORT TURBUHALER can occur within 24 hours of beginning treatment although maximum benefit may not be achieved for 1 to 2 weeks, or longer.

PULMICORT TURBUHALER has been shown to decrease airway reactivity to various challenge models, including histamine, methacholine, sodium metabisulfite, and adenosine monophosphate in hyperreactive patients. The clinical relevance of these models is not certain.

Pretreatment with PULMICORT TURBUHALER 1600 mcg daily (800 mcg twice daily) for 2 weeks reduced the acute (early-phase reaction) and delayed (late-phase reaction) decrease in FEV_1 following inhaled allergen challenge.

The effects of PULMICORT TURBUHALER on the hypothalamic-pituitary-adrenal (HPA) axis were studied in 905 adults and 404 pediatric patients with asthma. For most patients, the ability to increase cortisol production in response to stress, as assessed by cosyntropin (ACTH) stimulation test, remained intact with PULMICORT TURBUHALER treatment at recommended doses. For adult patients treated with 100, 200, 400, or 800 mcg twice daily for 12 weeks, 4%, 2%, 6%, and 13% respectively, had an abnormal stimulated cortisol response (peak cortisol <14.5 mcg/dL assessed by liquid chromatography following short-cosyntropin test) as compared to 8% of patients treated with placebo. Similar results were obtained in pediatric patients. In another study in adults, doses of 400, 800 and 1600 mcg budesonide twice daily via PULMICORT TURBUHALER for 6 weeks were examined; 1600 mcg twice daily (twice the maximum recommended dose) resulted in a 27% reduction in stimulated cortisol (6-hour ACTH infusion) while 10 mg prednisone resulted in a 35% reduction. In this study, no patient on PULMICORT TURBUHALER at doses of 400 and 800 mcg twice daily met the criterion for an abnormal stimulated cortisol response (peak cortisol <14.5 mcg/dL assessed by liquid chromatography) following ACTH infusion. An open-label, long-term follow-up of 1133 patients for up to 52 weeks confirmed the minimal effect on the HPA axis (both basal and stimulated plasma cortisol) of PULMICORT TURBUHALER when administered at recommended doses.

In patients who had previously been oral steroid-dependent, use of PULMICORT TURBUHALER in recommended doses was associated with higher stimulated cortisol response compared to baseline following 1 year of therapy.

The administration of budesonide via PULMICORT TURBUHALER in doses up to 800 mcg/day (mean daily dose 445 mcg/day) or via a pressurized metered-dose inhaler in doses up to 1200 mcg/day (mean daily dose 620 mcg/day) to 216 pediatric patients (age 3 to 11 years) for 2 to 6 years had no significant effect on statural growth compared with non-corticosteroid therapy in 62 matched control patients. However, the long-term effect of PULMICORT TURBUHALER on growth is not fully known.

CLINICAL TRIALS

The therapeutic efficacy of PULMICORT TURBUHALER has been evaluated in controlled clinical trials involving more than 1300 patients (6 years and older) with asthma of varying disease duration (<1 year to >20 years) and severity.

Double-blind, parallel, placebo-controlled clinical trials of 12 weeks duration and longer have shown that, compared with placebo, PULMICORT TURBUHALER significantly improved lung function (measured by PEF and FEV_1), significantly decreased morning and evening symptoms of asthma, and significantly reduced the need for as needed inhaled β_2-agonist use at doses of 400 mcg to 1600 mcg per day (200 mcg to 800 mcg twice daily) in adults and 400 mcg to 800 mcg per day (200 mcg to 400 mcg twice daily) in pediatric patients 6 years of age and older.

Improved lung function (morning PEF) was observed within 24 hours of initiating treatment in both adult and pediatric patients 6 years of age and older, although maximum benefit was not achieved for 1 to 2 weeks, or longer, after starting treatment. Improved lung function was maintained throughout the 12 weeks of the double-blind portion of the trials.

Patients Not Receiving Corticosteroid Therapy

In a 12-week clinical trial in 273 patients with mild to moderate asthma (mean baseline FEV_1 2.27 L) who were not well controlled by bronchodilators alone, PULMICORT TURBUHALER was evaluated at doses of 200 mcg twice daily and 400 mcg twice daily versus placebo. The FEV_1 results from this trial are shown in the figure below. Pulmonary function improved significantly on both doses of PULMICORT TURBUHALER compared with placebo.

[See figure at top of next column]

In a 12-month controlled trial in 75 patients not previously receiving corticosteroids, PULMICORT TURBUHALER at 200 mcg twice daily resulted in improved lung function (measured by PEF) and reduced bronchial hyperreactivity compared to placebo.

Patients Previously Maintained on Inhaled Corticosteroids

The safety and efficacy of PULMICORT TURBUHALER was also evaluated in adult and pediatric patients (age 6 to 18 years) previously maintained on inhaled corticosteroids (adults: N=473, mean baseline FEV_1 2.04 L, baseline doses of beclomethasone dipropionate 126-1008 mcg/day; pediatrics: N=404, mean baseline FEV_1 2.09 L, baseline doses of

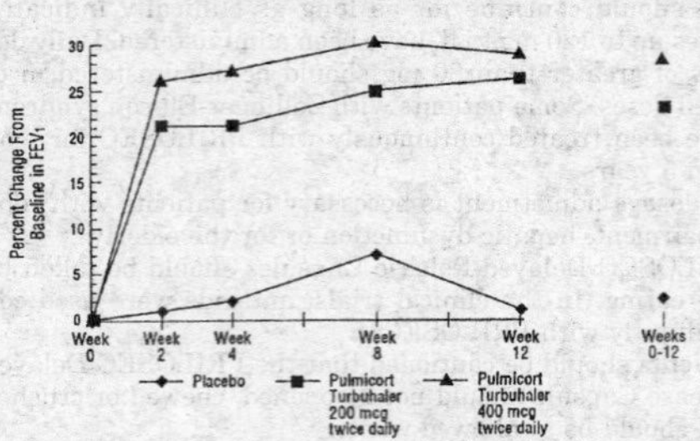

beclomethasone dipropionate 126-672 mcg/day or triamcinolone acetonide 300-1800 mcg/day). The FEV_1 results of these two trials, both 12 weeks in duration, are presented in the following figures. Pulmonary function improved significantly with all doses of PULMICORT TURBUHALER compared to placebo in both trials.

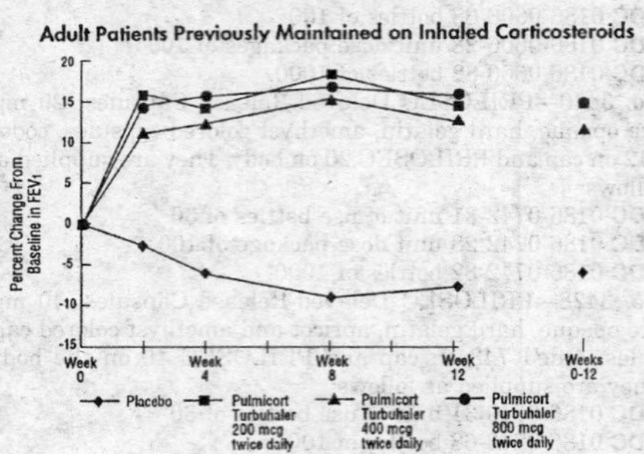

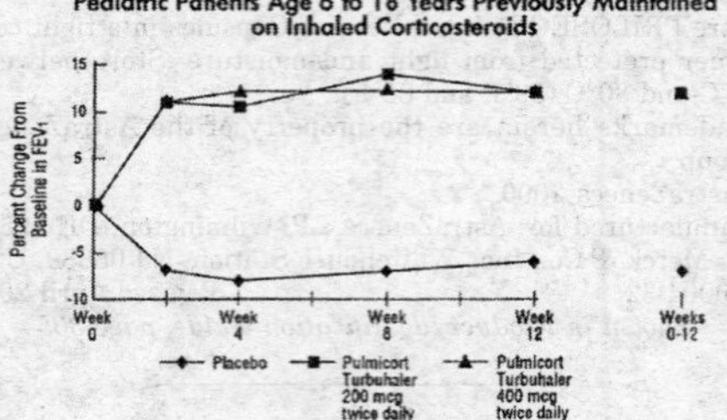

Patients Receiving PULMICORT TURBUHALER Once Daily

The efficacy and safety of once-daily administration of PULMICORT TURBUHALER 200 mcg and 400 mcg and placebo were also evaluated in 309 adult asthmatic patients (mean baseline FEV_1 2.7 L) in an 18-week study. Compared with placebo, patients receiving Pulmicort 200 or 400 mcg once daily showed significantly better asthma stability as assessed by PEF and FEV_1 over an initial 6-week treatment period, which was maintained with a 200 mcg daily dose over the subsequent 12 weeks. Although the study population included both patients previously treated with inhaled corticosteroids, as well as patients not previously receiving corticosteroid therapy, the results showed that once-daily dosing was most clearly effective for those patients previously maintained on orally inhaled corticosteroids (see DOSAGE AND ADMINISTRATION).

Patients Previously Maintained on Oral Corticosteroids

In a clinical trial in 159 severe asthmatic patients requiring chronic oral prednisone therapy (mean baseline prednisone dose 19.3 mg/day) PULMICORT TURBUHALER at doses of 400 mcg twice daily and 800 mcg twice daily was compared to placebo over a 20-week period. Approximately two-thirds (68% on 400 mcg twice daily and 64% on 800 mcg twice daily) of PULMICORT TURBUHALER-treated patients were able to achieve sustained (at least 2 weeks) oral corticosteroid cessation (compared with 8% of placebo-treated patients) and improved asthma control. The average oral corticosteroid dose was reduced by 83% on 400 mcg twice daily and 79% on 800 mcg twice daily for PULMICORT TURBUHALER-treated patients vs. 27% for placebo. Additionally, 58 out of 64 patients (91%) who completely eliminated oral corticosteroids during the double-blind phase of the trial remained off oral corticosteroids for an additional 12 months while receiving PULMICORT TURBUHALER.

INDICATIONS AND USAGE

PULMICORT TURBUHALER is indicated for the maintenance treatment of asthma as prophylactic therapy in adult and pediatric patients six years of age or older. It is also indicated for patients requiring oral corticosteroid therapy for asthma. Many of those patients may be able to reduce or eliminate their requirement for oral corticosteroids over time.

PULMICORT TURBUHALER is NOT indicated for the relief of acute bronchospasm.

CONTRAINDICATIONS

PULMICORT TURBUHALER is contraindicated in the primary treatment of status asthmaticus or other acute episodes of asthma where intensive measures are required.

Hypersensitivity to budesonide contraindicates the use of PULMICORT TURBUHALER.

WARNINGS

Particular care is needed for patients who are transferred from systemically active corticosteroids to PULMICORT TURBUHALER because deaths due to adrenal insufficiency have occurred in asthmatic patients during and after transfer from systemic corticosteroids to less systemically available inhaled corticosteroids. After withdrawal from systemic corticosteroids, a number of months are required for recovery of HPA function.

Patients who have been previously maintained on 20 mg or more per day of prednisone (or its equivalent) may be most susceptible, particularly when their systemic corticosteroids have been almost completely withdrawn. During this period of HPA suppression, patients may exhibit signs and symptoms of adrenal insufficiency when exposed to trauma, surgery, or infection (particularly gastroenteritis) or other conditions associated with severe electrolyte loss. Although PULMICORT TURBUHALER may provide control of asthma symptoms during these episodes, in recommended doses it supplies less than normal physiological amounts of glucocorticoid systemically and does NOT provide the mineralocorticoid activity that is necessary for coping with these emergencies.

During periods of stress or a severe asthma attack, patients who have been withdrawn from systemic corticosteroids should be instructed to resume oral corticosteroids (in large doses) immediately and to contact their physicians for further instruction. These patients should also be instructed to carry a medical identification card indicating that they may need supplementary systemic corticosteroids during periods of stress or a severe asthma attack.

Transfer of patients from systemic corticosteroid therapy to PULMICORT TURBUHALER may unmask allergic conditions previously suppressed by the systemic corticosteroid therapy, e.g., rhinitis, conjunctivitis, and eczema (see Dosage and Administration).

Patients who are on drugs which suppress the immune system are more susceptible to infection than healthy individuals. Chicken pox and measles, for example, can have a more serious or even fatal course in susceptible pediatric patients or adults on immunosuppressant doses of corticosteroids. In pediatric or adult patients who have not had these diseases, particular care should be taken to avoid exposure. How the dose, route and duration of corticosteroid administration affects the risk of developing a disseminated infection is not known. The contribution of the underlying disease and/or prior corticosteroid treatment to the risk is also not known. If exposed, therapy with varicella zoster immune globulin (VZIG) or pooled intravenous immunoglobulin (IVIG), as appropriate, may be indicated. If exposed to measles, prophylaxis with pooled intramuscular immunoglobulin (IG) may be indicated. (See the respective package insert for complete VZIG and IG prescribing information.) If chicken pox develops, treatment with antiviral agents may be considered.

PULMICORT TURBUHALER is not a bronchodilator and is not indicated for rapid relief of bronchospasm or other acute episodes of asthma.

As with other inhaled asthma medications, bronchospasm, with an immediate increase in wheezing, may occur after dosing. If bronchospasm occurs following dosing with PULMICORT TURBUHALER, it should be treated immediately with a fast-acting inhaled bronchodilator. Treatment with PULMICORT TURBUHALER should be discontinued and alternate therapy instituted.

Patients should be instructed to contact their physician immediately when episodes of asthma not responsive to their usual doses of bronchodilators occur during treatment with PULMICORT TURBUHALER. During such episodes, patients may require therapy with oral corticosteroids.

PRECAUTIONS

General: During withdrawal from oral corticosteroids, some patients may experience symptoms of systemically active corticosteroid withdrawal, e.g., joint and/or muscular pain, lassitude, and depression, despite maintenance or even improvement of respiratory function.

PULMICORT TURBUHALER will often permit control of asthma symptoms with less suppression of HPA function than therapeutically equivalent oral doses of prednisone. Since budesonide is absorbed into the circulation and can be systemically active at higher doses, the full beneficial effects of PULMICORT TURBUHALER in minimizing HPA dysfunction may be expected only when recommended dosages are not exceeded and individual patients are titrated to the lowest effective dose. Since individual sensitivity to effects on cortisol production exists, physicians should consider this information when prescribing PULMICORT TURBUHALER.

Because of the possibility of systemic absorption of inhaled corticosteroids, patients treated with these drugs should be observed carefully for any evidence of systemic corticosteroid effects. Particular care should be taken in observing patients postoperatively or during periods of stress for evidence of inadequate adrenal response.

It is possible that systemic corticosteroid effects such as hypercorticism and adrenal suppression may appear in a small number of patients, particularly at higher doses. If

such changes occur, PULMICORT TURBUHALER should be reduced slowly, consistent with accepted procedures for management of asthma symptoms and for tapering of systemic steroids.
A reduction of growth velocity in children or teenagers may occur as a result of inadequate control of chronic diseases such as asthma or from use of corticosteroids for treatment. Physicians should closely follow the growth of all pediatric patients taking corticosteroids by any route and weigh the benefits of corticosteroid therapy and asthma control against the possibility of growth suppression (see PRECAUTIONS, Pediatric Use section).
Although patients in clinical trials have received PULMICORT TURBUHALER on a continuous basis for periods of 1 to 2 years, the long-term local and systemic effects of PULMICORT TURBUHALER in human subjects are not completely known. In particular, the effects resulting from chronic use of PULMICORT TURBUHALER on developmental or immunological processes in the mouth, pharynx, trachea, and lung are unknown.
In clinical trials with PULMICORT TURBUHALER, localized infections with Candida albicans occurred in the mouth and pharynx in some patients. If oropharyngeal candidiasis develops, it should be treated with appropriate local or systemic (i.e., oral) antifungal therapy while still continuing with PULMICORT TURBUHALER therapy, but at times therapy with PULMICORT TURBUHALER may need to be temporarily interrupted under close medical supervision.
Inhaled corticosteroids should be used with caution, if at all, in patients with active or quiescent tuberculosis infection of the respiratory tract, untreated systemic fungal, bacterial, viral or parasitic infections; or ocular herpes simplex.
Rare instances of glaucoma, increased intraocular pressure, and cataracts have been reported following the inhaled administration of corticosteroids.

Information for Patients: For proper use of PULMICORT TURBUHALER and to attain maximum improvement, the patient should read and follow the accompanying Patient's Instructions for Use carefully. In addition, patients being treated with PULMICORT TURBUHALER should receive the following information and instructions. This information is intended to aid the patient in the safe and effective use of the medication. It is not a disclosure of all possible adverse or intended effects.

- Patients should use PULMICORT TURBUHALER at regular intervals as directed since its effectiveness depends on regular use. The patient should not alter the prescribed dosage unless advised to do so by the physician.
- PULMICORT TURBUHALER is not a bronchodilator and is not intended to treat acute or life-threatening episodes of asthma.
- PULMICORT TURBUHALER must be in the upright position (mouthpiece on top) during loading in order to provide the correct dose. PULMICORT TURBUHALER must be primed when the unit is used for the very first time. To prime the unit, hold the unit in an upright position and turn the brown grip fully to the right, then fully to the left until it clicks. Repeat. The unit is now primed and ready to load the first dose by turning the grip fully to the right and fully to the left until it clicks.
  On subsequent uses, it is not necessary to prime the unit. However, it must be loaded in the upright position immediately prior to use. Turn the brown grip fully to the right, then fully to the left until it clicks. During inhalation, PULMICORT TURBUHALER must be held in the upright (mouthpiece up) or horizontal position. Do not shake the inhaler. Place the mouthpiece between lips and inhale forcefully and deeply. The powder is then delivered to the lungs.
- Patients should not exhale through PULMICORT TURBUHALER.
- Due to the small volume of powder, the patient may not taste or sense the presence of any medication entering the lungs when inhaling from TURBUHALER. This lack of "sensation" does not indicate that the patient is not receiving benefit from PULMICORT TURBUHALER.
- Rinsing the mouth with water without swallowing after each dosing may decrease the risk of the development of oral candidiasis.
- When there are 20 doses remaining in PULMICORT TURBUHALER, a red mark will appear in the indicator window.
- PULMICORT TURBUHALER should not be used with a spacer.
- The mouthpiece should not be bitten or chewed.
- The cover should be replaced securely after each opening.
- Keep PULMICORT TURBUHALER clean and dry at all times.
- Improvement in asthma control following inhalation of PULMICORT TURBUHALER can occur within 24 hours of beginning treatment although maximum benefit may not be achieved for 1 to 2 weeks, or longer. If symptoms do not improve in that time frame, or if the condition worsens, the patient should be instructed to contact the physician.
- Patients should be warned to avoid exposure to chicken pox or measles and if they are exposed, to consult their physicians without delay.
- For proper use of PULMICORT TURBUHALER and to attain maximum improvement, the patient should read and follow the accompanying Patient's Instructions for Use.

Drug Interactions: In clinical studies, concurrent administration of budesonide and other drugs commonly used in the treatment of asthma has not resulted in an increased frequency of adverse events. Ketoconazole, a potent inhibitor of cytochrome P450 3A, may increase plasma levels of budesonide during concomitant dosing. The clinical significance of concomitant administration of ketoconazole with PULMICORT TURBUHALER is not known, but caution may be warranted.

Carcinogenesis, Mutagenesis, Impairment of Fertility: Long-term studies were conducted in mice and rats using oral administration to evaluate the carcinogenic potential of budesonide.
There was no evidence of a carcinogenic effect when budesonide was administered orally for 91 weeks to mice at doses up to 200 mcg/kg/day (approximately ½ the maximum recommended daily inhalation dose in adults and children on a mcg/m^2 basis).
In a 104-week oral study in Sprague-Dawley rats, a statistically significant increase in the incidence of gliomas was observed in male rats receiving an oral dose of 50 mcg/kg/day (approximately ¼ the maximum recommended daily inhalation dose on a mcg/m^2 basis); no such changes were seen in male rats receiving oral doses of 10 and 25 mcg/kg/day (approximately $^1/_{20}$ and $^1/_8$ the maximum recommended daily inhalation dose on a mcg/m^2 basis) or in female rats at oral doses up to 50 mcg/kg/day (approximately $^1/_4$ the maximum recommended human daily inhalation dose on a mcg/m^2 basis).
Two additional 104-week carcinogenicity studies have been performed with oral budesonide at doses of 50 mcg/kg/day (approximately $^1/_3$ the maximum recommended daily inhalation dose in adults and children on a mcg/m^2 basis) in male Sprague-Dawley and Fischer rats. These studies did not demonstrate an increased glioma incidence in budesonide-treated animals as compared with concurrent controls or reference corticosteroid-treated groups (prednisolone and triamcinolone acetonide). Compared with concurrent controls, a statistically significant increase in the incidence of hepatocellular tumors was observed in all three steroid groups (budesonide, prednisolone, triamcinolone acetonide) in these studies.
The mutagenic potential of budesonide was evaluated in six different test systems; Ames Salmonella/microsome plate test, mouse micronucleus test, mouse lymphoma test, chromosome aberration test in human lymphocytes, sex-linked recessive lethal test in Drosophila melanogaster, and DNA repair analysis in rat hepatocyte culture. Budesonide was not mutagenic or clastogenic in any of these tests.
The effect of subcutaneous budesonide on fertility and general reproductive performance was studied in rats. At 20 mcg/kg/day (approximately $^1/_8$ the maximum recommended daily inhalation dose in adults on a mcg/m^2 basis), decreases in maternal body weight gain, prenatal viability, and viability of the young at birth and during lactation were observed. No such effects were noted at 5 mcg/kg (approximately $^1/_{32}$ the maximum recommended daily inhalation dose in adults on a mcg/m^2 basis).

Pregnancy: Teratogenic Effects: Pregnancy Category C: As with other glucocorticoids, budesonide produced fetal loss, decreased pup weight and skeletal abnormalities at subcutaneous doses of 25 mcg/kg/day in rabbits (approximately $^1/_3$ the maximum recommended daily inhalation dose in adults on a mcg/m^2 basis) and 500 mcg/kg/day in rats (approximately 3 times the maximum recommended daily inhalation dose in adults on a mcg/m^2 basis).
No teratogenic or embryocidal effects were observed in rats when budesonide was administered by inhalation at doses up to 250 mcg/kg/day (approximately 2 times the maximum recommended daily inhalation dose in adults on a mcg/m^2 basis).
There are no adequate and well-controlled studies in pregnant women. Budesonide should be used during pregnancy only if the potential benefit justifies the potential risk to the fetus.
Experience with oral corticosteroids since their introduction in pharmacologic as opposed to physiologic doses suggests that rodents are more prone to teratogenic effects from corticosteroids than humans.

Nonteratogenic Effects: Hypoadrenalism may occur in infants born of mothers receiving corticosteroids during pregnancy. Such infants should be carefully observed.

Nursing Mothers: Corticosteroids are secreted in human milk. Because of the potential for adverse reactions in nursing infants from any corticosteroid, a decision should be made whether to discontinue nursing or discontinue the drug, taking into account the importance of the drug to the mother. Actual data for budesonide are lacking.

Pediatric Use: Safety and effectiveness of PULMICORT TURBUHALER in pediatric patients below 6 years of age have not been established.
In pediatric asthma patients the frequency of adverse events observed with PULMICORT TURBUHALER was similar between the 6- to 12-year age group (N=172) compared with the 13- to 17-year age group (N=124).
Oral corticosteroids have been shown to cause growth suppression in pediatric and adolescent patients, particularly with higher doses over extended periods. If a pediatric or adolescent patient on any corticosteroid appears to have growth suppression, the possibility that they are particularly sensitive to this effect of corticosteroids should be considered (see PRECAUTIONS).

Geriatric Use: One hundred patients 65 years or older were included in the US and non-US controlled clinical trials of PULMICORT TURBUHALER. There were no differences in the safety and efficacy of the drug compared to those seen in younger patients.

ADVERSE REACTIONS

The following adverse reactions were reported in patients treated with PULMICORT TURBUHALER.
The incidence of common adverse events is based upon double-blind, placebo-controlled US clinical trials in which 1,116 adult and pediatric patients age 6–70 years (472 females and 644 males) were treated with PULMICORT TURBUHALER (200 to 800 mcg twice daily for 12 to 20 weeks) or placebo.
The following table shows the incidence of adverse events in patients previously receiving bronchodilators and/or inhaled corticosteroids in US controlled clinical trials. This population included 232 male and 62 female pediatric patients (age 6 to 17 years) and 332 male and 331 female adult patients (age 18 years and greater).
[See table above]

Adverse Events with ≥3% Incidence reported by Patients on PULMICORT TURBUHALER

Adverse Event	Placebo N=284 %	PULMICORT TURBUHALER 200 mcg twice daily N=286 %	400 mcg twice daily N=289 %	800 mcg twice daily N=98 %
Respiratory System				
Respiratory infection	17	20	24	19
Pharyngitis	9	10	9	5
Sinusitis	7	11	7	2
Voice alteration	0	1	2	6
Body As A Whole				
Headache	7	14	13	14
Flu syndrome	6	6	6	14
Pain	2	5	5	5
Back pain	1	2	3	6
Fever	2	2	4	0
Digestive System				
Oral candidiasis	2	2	4	4
Dyspepsia	2	1	2	4
Gastroenteritis	1	1	2	3
Nausea	2	2	1	3
Average Duration of Exposure (days)	59	79	80	80

The table above includes all events (whether considered drug-related or non drug-related by the investigators) that occurred at a rate of ≥3% in any one PULMICORT TURBUHALER group and were more common than in the placebo group. In considering these data, the increased average duration of exposure for PULMICORT TURBUHALER patients should be taken into account.
The following other adverse events occurred in these clinical trials using PULMICORT TURBUHALER with an incidence of 1 to 3% and were more common on PULMICORT TURBUHALER than on placebo.
Body As A Whole: neck pain
Cardiovascular: syncope
Digestive: abdominal pain, dry mouth, vomiting
Metabolic and Nutritional: weight gain
Musculoskeletal: fracture, myalgia
Nervous: hypertonia, migraine
Platelet, Bleeding and Clotting: ecchymosis
Psychiatric: insomnia
Resistance Mechanisms: infection
Special Senses: taste perversion

Continued on next page

Pulmicort Turbuhaler—Cont.

In a 20-week trial in adult asthmatics who previously required oral corticosteroids, the effects of PULMICORT TURBUHALER 400 mcg twice daily (N=53) and 800 mcg twice daily (N=53) were compared with placebo (N=53) on the frequency of reported adverse events. Adverse events, whether considered drug-related or non drug-related by the investigators, reported in more than five patients in the PULMICORT TURBUHALER group and which occurred more frequently with PULMICORT TURBUHALER than placebo are shown below (% PULMICORT TURBUHALER and % placebo). In considering these data, the increased average duration of exposure for PULMICORT TURBUHALER patients (78 days for PULMICORT TURBUHALER vs. 41 days for placebo) should be taken into account.

Body As A Whole:	asthenia (9% and 2%)
	headache (12% and 2%)
	pain (10% and 2%)
Digestive:	dyspepsia (8% and 0%)
	nausea (6% and 0%)
	oral candidiasis (10% and 0%)
Musculoskeletal:	arthralgia (6% and 0%)
Respiratory:	cough increased (6% and 2%)
	respiratory infection (32% and 13%)
	rhinitis (6% and 2%)
	sinusitis (16% and 11%)

Patient Receiving PULMICORT TURBUHALER Once Daily
The adverse event profile of once-daily administration of PULMICORT TURBUHALER 200 mcg and 400 mcg, and placebo, was evaluated in 309 adult asthmatic patients in an 18-week study. The study population included both patients previously treated with inhaled corticosteroids, and patients not previously receiving corticosteroid therapy. There was no clinically relevant difference in the pattern of adverse events following once-daily administration of PULMICORT TURBUHALER when compared to twice-daily dosing.

Pediatric Studies: In a 12-week placebo-controlled trial in 404 pediatric patients 6 to 18 years of age previously maintained on inhaled corticosteroids, the frequency of adverse events for each age category (6 to 12 years, 13 to 18 years) was comparable for PULMICORT TURBUHALER (at 100, 200 and 400 mcg twice daily) and placebo. There were no clinically relevant differences in the pattern or severity of adverse events in children compared with those reported in adults.

Adverse Event Reports From Other Sources: Rare adverse events reported in the published literature or from marketing experience include: immediate and delayed hypersensitivity reactions including rash, contact dermatitis, urticaria, angioedema and bronchospasm; symptoms of hypocorticism and hypercorticism; psychiatric symptoms including depression, aggressive reactions, irritability, anxiety and psychosis.

OVERDOSAGE

The potential for acute toxic effects following overdose of PULMICORT TURBUHALER is low. If used at excessive doses for prolonged periods, systemic corticosteroid effects such as hypercorticism may occur (see PRECAUTIONS). PULMICORT TURBUHALER at twice the highest recommended dose (3200 mcg daily) administered for 6 weeks caused a significant reduction (27%) in the plasma cortisol response to a 6-hour infusion of ACTH compared with placebo (+1%). The corresponding effect of 10 mg prednisone daily was a 35% reduction in the plasma cortisol response to ACTH.

The minimal inhalation lethal dose in mice was 100 mg/kg (approximately 320 times the maximum recommended daily inhalation dose in adults and approximately 380 times the maximum recommended daily inhalation dose in children on a mcg/m^2 basis). There were no deaths following the administration of an inhalation dose of 68 mg/kg in rats (approximately 430 times the maximum recommended daily inhalation dose in adults and approximately 510 times the maximum recommended daily inhalation dose in children on a mcg/m^2 basis). The minimal oral lethal dose was 200 mg/kg in mice (approximately 630 times the maximum recommended daily inhalation dose in adults and approximately 750 times the maximum recommended daily inhalation dose in children on a mcg/m^2 basis) and less than 100 mg/kg in rats (approximately 630 times the maximum recommended daily inhalation dose in adults and approximately 750 times the maximum recommended daily inhalation dose in children based on a mcg/m^2 basis).

DOSAGE AND ADMINISTRATION

PULMICORT TURBUHALER should be administered by the orally inhaled route in asthmatic patients age 6 years and older. Individual patients will experience a variable onset and degree of symptom relief. Generally, PULMICORT TURBUHALER has a relatively rapid onset of action for an inhaled corticosteroid. Improvement in asthma control following inhaled administration of PULMICORT TURBUHALER can occur within 24 hours of initiation of treatment, although maximum benefit may not be achieved for 1 to 2 weeks, or longer. The safety and efficacy of PULMICORT TURBUHALER when administered in excess of recommended doses have not been established.

The recommended starting dose and the highest recommended dose of PULMICORT TURBUHALER, based on prior asthma therapy, are listed in the following table.

	Previous Therapy	Recommended Starting Dose	Highest Recommended Dose
Adults:	Bronchodilators alone	200 to 400 mcg twice daily	400 mcg twice daily
	Inhaled Corticosteroids*	200 to 400 mcg twice daily	800 mcg twice daily
	Oral Corticosteroids	400 to 800 mcg twice daily	800 mcg twice daily
Children:	Bronchodilators alone	200 mcg twice daily	400 mcg twice daily
	Inhaled Corticosteroids*	200 mcg twice daily	400 mcg twice daily
	Oral Corticosteroids	The highest recommended dose in children is 400 mcg twice daily	

*In patients with mild to moderate asthma who are well controlled on inhaled corticosteroids, dosing with PULMICORT TURBUHALER 200 mcg or 400 mcg once daily may be considered. PULMICORT TURBUHALER can be administered once daily either in the morning or in the evening.

[See table above]
If the once-daily treatment with PULMICORT TURBUHALER does not provide adequate control of asthma symptoms, the total daily dose should be increased and/or administered as a divided dose.

Patients Maintained on Chronic Oral Corticosteroids
Initially, PULMICORT TURBUHALER should be used concurrently with the patient's usual maintenance dose of systemic corticosteroid. After approximately one week, gradual withdrawal of the systemic corticosteroid is started by reducing the daily or alternate daily dose. The next reduction is made after an interval of one or two weeks, depending on the response of the patient. Generally, these decrements should not exceed 2.5 mg of prednisone or its equivalent. A slow rate of withdrawal is strongly recommended. During reduction of oral corticosteroids, patients should be carefully monitored for asthma instability, including objective measures of airway function, and for adrenal insufficiency (see WARNINGS). During withdrawal, some patients may experience symptoms of systemic corticosteroid withdrawal, e.g., joint and/or muscular pain, lassitude and depression, despite maintenance or even improvement in pulmonary function. Such patients should be encouraged to continue with PULMICORT TURBUHALER but should be monitored for objective signs of adrenal insufficiency. If evidence of adrenal insufficiency occurs, the systemic corticosteroid doses should be increased temporarily and thereafter withdrawal should continue more slowly. During periods of stress or a severe asthma attack, transfer patients may require supplementary treatment with systemic corticosteroids.

NOTE: In all patients it is desirable to titrate to the lowest effective dose once asthma stability is achieved. Patients should be instructed to prime PULMICORT TURBUHALER prior to its initial use, and instructed to inhale deeply and forcefully each time the unit is used. Rinsing the mouth after inhalation is also recommended.

Directions for Use: Illustrated Patient's Instructions for Use accompany each package of PULMICORT TURBUHALER.

HOW SUPPLIED

PULMICORT TURBUHALER consists of a number of assembled plastic details, the main parts being the dosing mechanism, the storage unit for drug substance and the mouthpiece. The inhaler is protected by a white outer tubular cover screwed onto the inhaler. The body of the inhaler is white and the turning grip is brown. The following wording is printed on the grip in raised lettering, "Pulmicort™ 200 mcg." TURBUHALER cannot be refilled and should be discarded when empty.

PULMICORT TURBUHALER is available as 200 mcg/dose, 200 doses.

Store at controlled room temperature 20°C to 25°C (68°F to 77°F) [see USP].

PATIENT'S INSTRUCTIONS FOR USE

PULMICORT TURBUHALER® 200 mcg
(budesonide inhalation powder)

Please read this leaflet carefully before you start to take your medicine. It provides a summary of information on your medicine.

FOR FURTHER INFORMATION ASK YOUR DOCTOR OR PHARMACIST.

WHAT YOU SHOULD KNOW ABOUT PULMICORT TURBUHALER
Your doctor has prescribed Pulmicort Turbuhaler 200 mcg. It contains a medication called budesonide, which is a synthetic corticosteroid.

Corticosteroids are natural substances found in the body that help fight inflammation. They are used to treat asthma because they reduce the swelling and irritation in the walls of the small air passages in the lungs and ease breathing problems. When inhaled regularly, corticosteroids also help to prevent attacks of asthma.

Pulmicort Turbuhaler treats the inflammation—the "quiet part" of asthma that you cannot hear, see, or feel.

When inflammation is left untreated, your asthma symptoms and attacks can increase. Pulmicort Turbuhaler works to prevent and reduce your asthma symptoms and attacks.

IMPORTANT POINTS TO REMEMBER ABOUT PULMICORT TURBUHALER
1. **MAKE SURE** that this medicine is suitable for you (see "BEFORE USING YOUR PULMICORT TURBUHALER" below).
2. It is important that you inhale each dose as your doctor has advised.
3. Use your Turbuhaler as directed by your doctor. **DO NOT STOP TREATMENT OR REDUCE YOUR DOSE EVEN IF YOU FEEL BETTER,** unless told to do so by your doctor.
4. **DO NOT** inhale more doses or use your Turbuhaler more often than instructed by your doctor.
5. This medicine is **NOT** intended to provide rapid relief of your breathing difficulties during an asthma attack. It must be taken at regular intervals as recommended by your doctor, and not as an emergency measure.
6. Your doctor may prescribe additional medication (such as bronchodilators) for emergency relief if an acute asthma attack occurs. Please contact your doctor if:
→ an asthma attack does not respond to the additional medication,
→ you require more of the additional medication than usual.
7. If you also use another medicine by inhalation, you should consult your doctor for instructions on when to use it in relation to using your Pulmicort Turbuhaler.

BEFORE USING YOUR PULMICORT TURBUHALER
TELL YOUR DOCTOR BEFORE STARTING TO TAKE THIS MEDICINE:
→ if you are pregnant (or intending to become pregnant),
→ if you are breast-feeding a baby,
→ if you are allergic to budesonide or any other orally inhaled corticosteroid.

In some circumstances, this medicine may not be suitable and your doctor may wish to give you a different medicine. Make sure that your doctor knows what other medicines you are taking.

USING YOUR PULMICORT TURBUHALER
→ Follow the instructions shown on the other side. If you have any problems, tell your doctor or pharmacist.
→ It is important that you inhale each dose as directed by your doctor. The pharmacy label will usually tell you what dose to take and how often. If it doesn't, or you are not sure, ask your doctor or pharmacist.

DOSAGE
→ Use as directed by your doctor.
→ It is **VERY IMPORTANT** that you follow your doctor's instructions as to how many inhalations to take and how often to use your Pulmicort Turbuhaler.
→ **DO NOT** inhale more doses or use your Pulmicort Turbuhaler more often than your doctor advises.
→ It may take 1 to 2 weeks or longer before you feel maximum improvement, so **IT IS VERY IMPORTANT THAT YOU USE PULMICORT TURBUHALER REGULARLY. DO NOT STOP TREATMENT OR REDUCE YOUR DOSE EVEN IF YOU ARE FEELING BETTER,** unless told to do so by your doctor.
→ If you miss a dose, just take your regularly scheduled next dose when it is due. **DO NOT DOUBLE** the dose.

HOW TO USE YOUR PULMICORT TURBUHALER
Read the complete instructions carefully and use only as directed.

BEFORE YOU USE A NEW PULMICORT TURBUHALER
Before you use a new Pulmicort Turbuhaler for the first time, you should prime it. To do this, turn the cover and lift off. Hold Pulmicort Turbuhaler upright (with mouthpiece up), then twist the brown grip fully to the right and back again to the left. Repeat. Now you are ready to use it. **You do not have to prime it any other time after this, even if you put it aside for a prolonged period of time.**

FOLLOW THE INSTRUCTIONS BELOW:

1 LOADING A DOSE
→ Twist the cover and lift off.
→ In order to provide the correct dose, **Pulmicort Turbuhaler must be held in the upright position (mouthpiece up) whenever a dose of medication is being loaded.**
→ Twist the brown grip fully to the right as far as it will go. Twist it back again fully to the left.
→ You will hear a click.

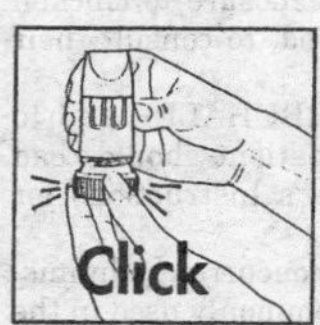

→ Turn your head away from the inhaler and breathe out. **Do not blow or exhale into the inhaler. Do not shake the inhaler after loading it.**

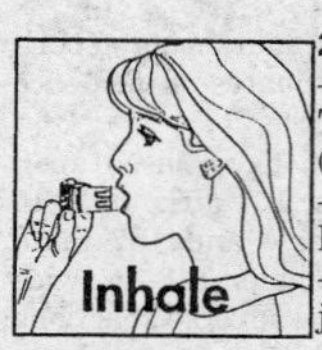

2 INHALING THE DOSE
→ When you are inhaling, Pulmicort Turbuhaler must be held in the upright (mouthpiece up) or horizontal position.
→ Place the mouthpiece between your lips and inhale deeply and forcefully.
→ If more than one dose is required, just repeat the steps above.
→ **When you are finished, place the cover back on** the inhaler and twist shut. **Rinse your mouth with water. Do not swallow.**
→ **Keep your Pulmicort Turbuhaler clean and dry at all times.**

STORING YOUR PULMICORT TURBUHALER
→ After each use, place the white cover back on and twist it firmly into place.
→ Keep Pulmicort Turbuhaler in a dry place at controlled room temperature, 68° to 77°F (20° to 25°C).
→ Keep your Pulmicort Turbuhaler out of the **reach of young children.**
→ **DO NOT** use after the date shown on the body of your Turbuhaler.

HOW TO KNOW WHEN YOUR PULMICORT TURBUHALER IS EMPTY

THERE ARE 200 DOSES IN EACH PULMICORT TURBUHALER.
Your Pulmicort Turbuhaler has a convenient dose indicator window just below the mouthpiece.

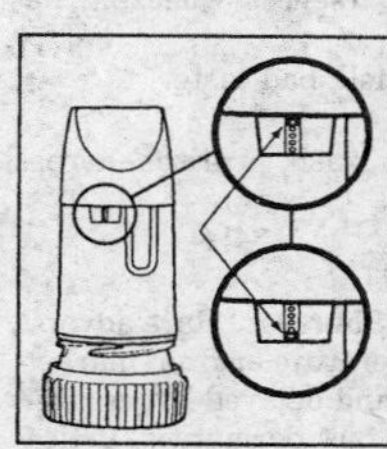

→ **When a red mark appears at the top of the window, there are 20 doses of medicine remaining.** Now is the time to get your next Pulmicort Turbuhaler.
→ **When the red mark reaches the bottom of the window, your inhaler is empty. Discard it.** (You may still hear a sound if you shake it—this sound is not the medicine. This sound is produced by the drying agent inside Turbuhaler.)
→ **Do not immerse it in water to find out if it is empty. Simply check your dose indicator window.**

FURTHER INFORMATION ABOUT PULMICORT TURBUHALER
→ Pulmicort Turbuhaler delivers your medicine as a very fine powder **that you may not taste, smell, or feel.** By following the instructions for use in this leaflet, you can be confident that you have received the correct dose.
→ Pulmicort Turbuhaler should not be used with a spacer.
→ Pulmicort Turbuhaler contains only budesonide and does not contain any inactive ingredients.
→ Pulmicort Turbuhaler is specially designed to deliver only one dose at a time, no matter how often you click the brown grip. If you accidentally blow into your inhaler after loading a dose, simply follow the instructions for loading a new dose.

This leaflet does not contain the complete information about your medicine. If you have any questions, or are not sure about something, then you should ask your doctor or pharmacist.
You may want to read this leaflet again. Please DO NOT THROW IT AWAY until you have finished your medicine.
REMEMBER: This medicine has been prescribed for you by your doctor. DO NOT give this medicine to anyone else.
USE THIS PRODUCT AS DIRECTED, UNLESS INSTRUCTED TO DO OTHERWISE BY YOUR DOCTOR.
If you have further questions about the use of Pulmicort Turbuhaler, call:
1-800-343-4777

000641R02 Rev. 10/98

Shown in Product Identification Guide, page 305

RHINOCORT® Nasal Inhaler ℞
(budesonide)
For Intranasal Use Only. Shake Well Before Use.

DESCRIPTION
Budesonide, the active component of Rhinocort® Nasal Inhaler, is an anti-inflammatory glucocorticosteroid. It is designated chemically as (RS)-11β,16α,17,21-Tetrahydroxypregna-1,4-diene-3,20-dione cyclic 16,17-acetal with butyraldehyde. Budesonide is provided as a mixture of two epimers (22R and 22S). The empirical formula of budesonide is $C_{25}H_{34}O_6$ and its molecular weight is 430.5. Its structural formula is:

Budesonide is a white to off-white odorless powder that is practically insoluble in water and in heptane, sparingly soluble in ethanol, and freely soluble in chloroform. Its partition coefficient between octanol and water at pH 7.4 is 1.6×10^3.
Rhinocort Nasal Inhaler is a metered-dose pressurized aerosol unit containing a suspension of micronized budesonide in a mixture of propellants, (dichlorodifluoromethane, trichloromonofluoromethane, and dichlorotetrafluoroethane) and sorbitan trioleate.
Each actuation releases 50 μg budesonide from the valve and delivers approximately 32 μg budesonide from the nasal adapter (dose to patient). Throughout the package insert 32 μg per actuation is used to calculate the dose administered. One canister provides at least 200 metered doses.

CLINICAL PHARMACOLOGY
Budesonide is a glucocorticosteroid having a potent glucocorticoid and weak mineralocorticoid activity. In standard *in vitro* and animal models, budesonide has an approximately 200 fold higher affinity for the glucocorticoid receptor and a 1000 fold higher topical anti-inflammatory potency than cortisol (rat croton oil ear edema assay). As a measure of systemic activity, budesonide is 40 times more potent than cortisol when administered subcutaneously and 25 times more potent when administered orally in the rat thymus involution assay.
The precise mechanism of glucocorticosteroid actions on allergic and nonallergic rhinitis is not known. Glucocorticosteroids have been shown to have a wide range of inhibitory activities against multiple cell types (e.g., mast cells, eosinophils, neutrophils, macrophages and lymphocytes) and mediators (e.g., histamine, eicosanoids, leukotrienes and cytokines) involved in allergic and nonallergic/irritant-mediated inflammation.
Corticoids affect the delayed (6 hour) response to an allergen challenge more than the histamine-associated immediate response (20 minute). The clinical significance of these findings is unknown.

Pharmacokinetics: The pharmacokinetics of budesonide have been studied following nasal, oral and intravenous administration. Pharmacokinetic studies were performed with doses higher than those used clinically because at clinical doses the resulting plasma levels are below the limits of detection.
The results are as follows:
[See table above]

Route of Administration		Mean* [range] T_{max} (hr)	C_{max}** (nmol/L)	Systemic Availability***	V_D (L)	Clearance (L/min)
Nasal Inhaler	(N=9)	0.6 [0.3–2]	0.52 [0.24–0.88]	21 [16–27]	—	—
Oral Capsule	(N=11)	1.0 [0.5–2]	0.33 [0.19–0.50]	12 [8–20]	—	—
I.V.	(N=11)	—	—	100	201 [102–275]	1.2 [0.8–1.5]

* mean of the two epimers
** dose normalized to a 256 μg dose
*** % of delivered dose

Only about 20% of an intranasal dose from the Rhinocort Nasal Inhaler reaches the systemic circulation.
While budesonide is well absorbed from the GI tract, the oral bioavailability of budesonide is low (~10%) primarily due to extensive first pass metabolism in the liver. After reaching the systemic circulation, plasma levels decline in a log linear manner with an apparent elimination half-life of approximately 2 hours.
Budesonide has a volume of distribution of approximately 200 L and is 88% protein bound in the plasma. Budesonide is a mixture of two epimers, 22R and 22S. In glucocorticoid receptor affinity studies, the 22R form is two times as active as the 22S epimer. It is also preferentially cleared by the liver with an apparent systemic clearance of 1.4 +/− 0.3 L/min., vs. 1.0 +/− 0.2 L/min. for the 22S form. *In vitro* studies indicate that the two forms of budesonide do not interconvert.
Budesonide is rapidly and extensively metabolized in man by the liver. *In vitro* studies looking at sites of metabolism showed negligible metabolism in skin, lung, and serum. After intranasal administration of a radiolabeled dose, $^2/_3$ of the radioactivity was found in the urine and the remainder in the feces by 96 hours. The primary metabolites of budesonide in the urine following IV administration are 16α-hydroxyprednisolone (24%) and 6β-hydroxybudesonide (5%). An additional 34% of the radioactivity recovered in the urine were conjugates. No unchanged budesonide was found in the urine. These results regarding the metabolic fate of budesonide parallel results obtained in *in vitro* metabolic studies using human liver homogenates.
In vitro studies of the binding of the two primary metabolites to the glucocorticoid receptor indicate that they have less than 1% of the affinity for the receptor as the parent compound budesonide.

Pharmacodynamics: The effect of Rhinocort Nasal Inhaler at a dosage of two sprays in each nostril morning and evening (total daily dose of 256 μg) on hypothalamic-pituitary-adrenal (HPA) axis function has been evaluated in 275 adults and 61 children following short-term use (<2 months) and in 113 adults and 116 children following longer use (6–48 months). Early morning plasma cortisol and the short cosyntropin stimulation test (30–60 minutes) were the most commonly performed assessments of HPA function.
Twenty-four hour urinary cortisol levels were determined in 50 adults (short term) and 96 children (long term). There were no statistically significant changes from baseline measurements in early morning plasma cortisol or 24-hour urinary cortisol excretion or in response to cosyntropin.
In a crossover trial using single doses of 200, 400 and 800 μg of an aqueous formulation of budesonide administered intranasally at 10 P.M., a dose-dependent decrease in urinary cortisol excretion was found between 10 P.M. and 8 A.M. the following morning. The same study has not been performed with Rhinocort Nasal Inhaler. However, in a study using the Rhinocort Nasal Inhaler administered at 10 P.M., doses four (1024 μg) and eight (2048 μg) times higher than the recommended daily dose (256 μg) were followed by a significant decrease in plasma cortisol levels at 8 A.M. the following morning (17% and 22%, respectively).
A 3 week clinical study in seasonal rhinitis, comparing Rhinocort Nasal Inhaler and orally ingested budesonide with placebo in 98 patients with allergic rhinitis due to birch pollen, demonstrated that the therapeutic effect of budesonide can be attributed to the topical effects of budesonide. Intranasally, 128 μg of budesonide applied twice daily (55 μg systemically absorbed/day) provided clinically and statistically significant evidence of efficacy, whereas 250 μg of budesonide ingested twice a day as a capsule (65 μg systemically absorbed/day) was no different from placebo in reducing nasal symptoms.

Clinical Trials: The prophylactic and therapeutic efficacy of Rhinocort Nasal Inhaler has been evaluated in 20 controlled clinical trials of seasonal or perennial rhinitis. The number of patients treated with budesonide in these studies was 50 male and 33 female patients ages 6 to 12 years old, 77 males and 62 females ages 13 to 18 years old, 185 males and 246 females ages 19 to 64 and 1 male and 2 females over 64. The patients were predominantly caucasian.
Double-blind clinical trials of two to four weeks duration have shown that, compared with placebo, Rhinocort Nasal Inhaler 128 μg b.i.d. (two sprays in each nostril morning and evening) or 256 μg q.d. (four sprays in each nostril in the morning) provides statistically significant relief of nasal symptoms such as blockage, rhinorrhea, itching, and sneezing in adults and children with seasonal allergic rhinitis or perennial allergic rhinitis. Similar improvement has also been demonstrated in adults with nonallergic perennial rhinitis.
The therapeutic effect of Rhinocort Nasal Inhaler compared with placebo has been demonstrated by rhinoscopic examinations in children and adults with seasonal or perennial allergic rhinitis and adults with nonallergic perennial rhinitis. Biopsies of the nasal mucosa of 50 adult patients after 12 months of treatment and of 10 patients after 3–5 years of therapy showed no histopathological evidence of adverse effects. The clinical significance of either of these findings is unknown.

Individualization of Dosage: It is recommended that the starting dose for all adults be 256 μg daily, as either two sprays in each nostril twice per day, morning and evening, or as four sprays in each nostril once a day in the morning. The effect should be assessed 3–7 days after initiating treatment and then periodically until the patient's symptoms are stable.
If adequate relief of symptoms is not achieved after 3 weeks of treatment, then Rhinocort Nasal Inhaler should be discontinued.
In patients who do achieve a good result it is desirable, once the maximum benefit seems to have been achieved, to titrate an individual patient to the minimum effective dose. Because of the generally short duration of therapy for seasonal allergic rhinitis, it is usually not necessary to do this. In patients with perennial allergic rhinitis, once adequate relief has been obtained the dose should be gradually decreased every 2–4 weeks as long as the desired clinical effect is maintained. If symptoms return, the dose may briefly be increased to the patient's starting dose and then returned to the dose the patient was on before symptoms reoccurred.
As with other aerosolized nasal glucocorticosteroids, the vehicle used to deliver the glucocorticosteroid may cause symptoms that are difficult to distinguish from the patient's rhinitis symptoms. The corticoid may suppress symptoms caused by the vehicle at higher doses but as the dose is decreased symptoms from the vehicle may emerge. If a patient needs chronic treatment and the daily dose cannot be decreased from the starting dose, it may be advisable to try alternative therapy.

INDICATIONS AND USAGE
Rhinocort Nasal Inhaler is indicated for the management of symptoms of seasonal or perennial allergic rhinitis in adults and children and nonallergic perennial rhinitis in adults.
Rhinocort Nasal Inhaler is not recommended for treatment of nonallergic rhinitis in children because adequate numbers of such children have not been studied.

Continued on next page

Rhinocort—Cont.

CONTRAINDICATIONS

Hypersensitivity to any of the ingredients of this preparation contraindicates its use.

WARNINGS

The replacement of a systemic glucocorticosteroid with a topical glucocorticosteroid can be accompanied by signs of adrenal insufficiency, and in addition some patients may experience symptoms of withdrawal, e.g., joint and/or muscular pain, lassitude and depression. Patients previously treated for prolonged periods with systemic glucocorticosteroids and transferred to topical glucocorticosteroids should be carefully monitored for acute adrenal insufficiency in response to stress. In those patients who have asthma or other clinical conditions requiring long-term systemic glucocorticosteroid treatment, too rapid a decrease in systemic glucocorticosteroids may cause a severe exacerbation of their symptoms.

The use of Rhinocort Nasal Inhaler with alternate-day systemic prednisone could increase the likelihood of hypothalamic-pituitary-adrenal (HPA) suppression compared with a therapeutic dose of either one alone. Therefore, Rhinocort Nasal Inhaler should be used with caution in patients already receiving alternate-day prednisone treatment for any disease. In addition, the concomitant use of Rhinocort Nasal Inhaler with other inhaled glucocorticosteroids could increase the risk of signs or symptoms of hypercorticism and/or suppression of the HPA-axis.

Patients who are on drugs which suppress the immune system are more susceptible to infections than healthy individuals. Chicken pox and measles, for example, can have a more serious or even fatal course in non-immune children or adults on immunosuppressant doses of corticosteroids. In such children or adults, who have not had these diseases, particular care should be taken to avoid exposure. How the dose, route and duration of corticosteroid administration affects the risk of developing a disseminated infection is not known. The contribution of the underlying disease and/or prior corticosteroid treatment to the risk is also not known. If exposed to chicken pox, prophylaxis with varicella zoster immune globulin (VZIG) may be indicated. If exposed to measles, prophylaxis with pooled intramuscular immunoglobulin (IG) may be indicated. (See the respective package insert for complete VZIG and IG prescribing information). If chicken pox develops, treatment with antiviral agents may be considered.

PRECAUTIONS

General: Rarely, immediate hypersensitivity reactions or contact dermatitis may occur after the intranasal administration of budesonide. Rare instances of wheezing, nasal septum perforation and increased intraocular pressure have been reported following the intranasal application of aerosolized glucocorticosteroids.

Like other glucocorticosteroids, budesonide is absorbed into the circulation. Use of excessive doses of glucocorticosteroids may lead to signs or symptoms of hypercorticism, suppression of HPA function and/or suppression of growth in children or teenagers. In short term studies of the acute effect of inhaled budesonide 256 μg/day on lower leg growth (knemometry), it like other inhaled and intramuscular corticoids which have been studied showed a decrease in the rate of lower leg growth. The clinical significance of this finding is not known. In two one-year studies in 92 children taking recommended doses of Rhinocort Nasal Inhaler, height and skeletal stature were consistent with chronological age. Physicians should closely follow the growth of children taking corticoids, by any route, and weigh the benefits of corticoid therapy against the possibility of growth suppression if a child's growth appears slowed.

Although systemic effects have been minimal with recommended doses of Rhinocort Nasal Inhaler, this potential risk increases with larger doses. Therefore, larger than recommended doses of Rhinocort Nasal Inhaler should be avoided.

When used at larger doses, systemic glucocorticosteroid effects such as hypercorticism and adrenal suppression may appear. If such changes occur, the dosage of Rhinocort Nasal Inhaler should be discontinued slowly, consistent with accepted procedures for discontinuing oral glucocorticosteroid therapy.

In clinical studies with budesonide administered intranasally, the development of localized infections of the nose and pharynx with Candida albicans has occurred only rarely. When such an infection develops, it may require treatment with appropriate local therapy and discontinuation of treatment with Rhinocort Nasal Inhaler. Patients using Rhinocort Nasal Inhaler over several months or longer should be examined periodically for evidence of Candida infection or other signs of adverse effects on the nasal mucosa.

Rhinocort Nasal Inhaler should be used with caution, if at all, in patients with active or quiescent tuberculous infections, untreated fungal, bacterial, or systemic viral infections, or ocular herpes simplex.

Because of the inhibitory effect of glucocorticosteroids on wound healing, patients who have experienced recent nasal septal ulcers, nasal surgery, or nasal trauma should not use a nasal glucocorticosteroid until healing has occurred.

Information for Patients: Patients being treated with Rhinocort Nasal Inhaler should receive the following information and instructions.

Patients should use Rhinocort Nasal Inhaler as prescribed. A decrease in symptoms may occur as soon as 24 hours after starting glucocorticosteroid therapy and generally can be expected to occur within a few days of initiating therapy in allergic rhinitis. The patient should contact the physician if symptoms do not improve by three weeks, or if the condition worsens. Nasal irritation and/or burning after use of the spray occur only rarely with this product. The patient should contact the physician if they occur repeatedly.

Patients who are on corticosteroids should be warned to avoid exposure to chicken pox or measles. Patients should also be advised that if they are exposed, they should consult their physician without delay.

For the proper use of this unit and to attain maximum improvement, the patient should read and follow the accompanying patient instructions carefully.

Carcinogenesis, Mutagenesis, Impairment of Fertility: Long-term studies were conducted in mice and rats using oral administration to evaluate the carcinogenic potential of budesonide.

There was no evidence of a carcinogenic effect when budesonide was administered orally for 91 weeks to mice at doses up to 200 μg/kg/day (600 μg/m^2/day).

In a 104-week carcinogenicity study in Sprague-Dawley rats (41), a statistically significant increase in the incidence of gliomas was observed in male rats receiving 50 μg/kg/day (300 μg/m^2/day) orally; no such changes were seen in male rats receiving doses of 10 and 25 μg/kg/day (60 and 150 μg/m^2/day) or in female rats at any dose. Two additional 104-week carcinogenicity studies have been performed with oral budesonide at doses of 50 μg/kg/day (300 μg/m^2/day) in male Sprague-Dawley and Fischer rats. These studies did not demonstrate an increased glioma incidence in budesonide treated animals as compared with concurrent controls or reference glucocorticosteroid treated groups (prednisolone and triamcinolone acetonide).

Compared with concurrent control male Sprague-Dawley rats there was a statistically significant increase in the incidence of hepatocellular tumors. This finding was confirmed in all three steroid groups (budesonide, prednisolone, triamcinolone acetonide) in the second study in male Sprague-Dawley rats.

The mutagenic potential of budesonide was evaluated in six different test systems; Ames Salmonella/microsome plate test, mouse micronucleus test, mouse lymphoma test, chromosome aberration test in human lymphocytes, sex-linked recessive lethal test in Drosophila melanogaster, and DNA repair analysis in rat hepatocyte culture. No mutagenic or clastogenic properties of budesonide were found in any of the tests.

The effect upon fertility and general reproductive performance was studied in rats given budesonide subcutaneously. At 20 μg/kg/day (120 μg/m^2/day) and higher dose levels, a decrease in maternal body-weight gain was observed along with a decrease in prenatal viability and viability of the young at birth and during lactation. No such effects were noted at the dose level 5 μg/kg/day (30 μg/m^2/day).

Pregnancy: Teratogenic Effects: Pregnancy Category C: As with other glucocorticoids budesonide has been shown to be teratogenic and embryocidal in rabbits and rats when given subcutaneously in doses exceeding 5 and 100 μg/kg/day (59 and 600 μg/m^2/day), respectively. In these studies budesonide at 25 μg/kg/day (295 μg/m^2/day) given to rabbits and 500 μg/kg/day (3000 μg/m^2/day) given to rats was found to produce fetal loss, decreased pup weights and skeletal abnormalities. No teratogenic or embryocidal effects have been seen in rats when budesonide was administered by inhalation at doses of 100–250 μg/kg/day (600–1500 μg/m^2/day, approximately 27–68 times the human recommended starting dose based on μg/kg/day or 4–10 times the human dose based on μg/m^2/day).

There are no adequate and well-controlled studies in pregnant women. Budesonide should be used during pregnancy only if the potential benefit justifies the potential risk to the fetus. Experience with oral glucocorticosteroids since their introduction in pharmacologic, as opposed to physiologic, doses suggests that rodents are more prone to teratogenic effects from glucocorticosteroids than humans. In addition, because there is a natural increase in glucocorticosteroid production during pregnancy, most women will require a lower exogenous glucocorticosteroid dose and many will not need glucocorticosteroid treatment during pregnancy.

Nonteratogenic Effects: Hypoadrenalism may occur in infants born of mothers receiving glucocorticosteroids during pregnancy. Such infants should be carefully observed.

Nursing Mothers: It is not known whether budesonide is excreted in human milk. Because other glucocorticosteroids are excreted in human milk, caution should be exercised when Rhinocort Nasal Inhaler is administered to nursing women.

Pediatric Use: Safety and effectiveness in children below 6 years of age have not been established. Oral glucocorticosteroids have been shown to cause growth suppression in children and teenagers with extended use. If a child or teenager on any glucocorticosteroid appears to have growth suppression, the possibility that they are particularly sensitive to this effect of glucocorticosteroids should be considered (see PRECAUTIONS).

ADVERSE REACTIONS

Adverse reaction information is derived from blinded-controlled clinical trials (see Clinical Trials), open label studies and marketing experience. In the description below, rates of rare events are derived principally from marketing experience and publications, and accurate estimates of incidence are not possible.

The incidence of common adverse reactions is based upon controlled clinical trials in 606 patients [101 girls and 145 boys (<19 years of age) and 203 female and 157 male adults] treated with Rhinocort Nasal Inhaler 128 μg twice daily over 2–4 weeks. The most common adverse reactions were symptoms of irritation of the nasal mucous membranes. All common adverse reactions were reported with approximately the same frequency by placebo patients suggesting the possibility that the vehicle or the rhinitis itself was responsible for the symptoms. Sneezing after use of the inhaler occurred in 2% of Rhinocort treated patients and in 11% of patients using the placebo.

Systemic glucocorticosteroid side-effects were not reported during controlled clinical studies with Rhinocort Nasal Inhaler. If recommended doses are exceeded, however, or if individuals are particularly sensitive, symptoms of hypercorticism, i.e., Cushing's syndrome, could occur.

Incidence Greater than 1% (Based on controlled clinical trials):

Respiratory: nasal irritation*, pharyngitis*, cough increased*, epistaxis*.

Digestive: dry mouth, dyspepsia.

*incidence 3 to 9%; incidence of unmarked reactions 1 to 3%.

Incidence Less than 1% (Based on controlled clinical trials):

Respiratory: dyspnea, moniliasis, hoarseness, wheezing, nasal pain.

Special Senses: reduced sense of smell, bad taste.

Digestive: nausea.

Skin and Appendages: facial edema, rash, pruritus, herpes simplex.

Nervous System: nervousness.

Musculoskeletal: myalgia, arthralgia.

Adverse Event Reports from Other Sources: Rare adverse events reported in the published literature or from marketing experience include: immediate and delayed hypersensitivity reactions including rash, contact dermatitis, urticaria, angioedema, and bronchospasm; nasal septal disorders including atrophy, necrosis and/or perforation; symptoms of hypocorticism and hypercorticism; alopecia; psychiatric symptoms including depression, aggressive reactions, irritability, anxiety and psychosis.

OVERDOSAGE

Acute overdosage with this dosage form is unlikely since one canister of Rhinocort Nasal Inhaler only contains approximately 12.7 mg of budesonide. Chronic overdosage may result in signs/symptoms of hypercorticism (see WARNINGS and PRECAUTIONS).

DOSAGE AND ADMINISTRATION

Adults and children 6 years of age and older: The recommended starting dose is 256 μg daily, given as either two sprays in each nostril morning and evening or as four sprays in each nostril in the morning.

A decrease in symptoms may occur as soon as 24 hours after onset of treatment with Rhinocort Nasal Inhaler but generally it takes 3–7 days to reach maximum benefit.

If no improvement has been obtained by the third week of treatment with Rhinocort Nasal Inhaler, treatment should be discontinued.

After the desired clinical effect has been obtained, the maintenance dose should be reduced to the smallest amount necessary for control of symptoms (see Individualization of Dosage, CLINICAL PHARMACOLOGY section).

If glucocorticosteroids are discontinued when they still are needed, symptoms may not recur for several days.

At recommended doses, Rhinocort's therapeutic effects are localized to the nose, therefore, concomitant treatment may be necessary to counteract allergic eye symptoms. Doses exceeding 256 μg daily (4 sprays/nostril) are not recommended. Rhinocort Nasal Inhaler is not recommended for children below 6 years of age or for children with nonallergic perennial rhinitis because adequate numbers of these children have not been studied.

Directions for Use: Illustrated Patient's Instructions for Use accompany each package of Rhinocort Nasal Inhaler.

HOW SUPPLIED

Rhinocort Nasal Inhaler is supplied in a 7.0 g canister containing 200 metered doses provided with a metering valve and nasal adapter together with Patient's Instructions for Use. Each actuation delivers approximately 32 μg of micronized budesonide from the nasal adapter to the patient.

Rx only. Rhinocort Nasal Inhaler should be stored between 15°C (59°F) and 30°C (86°F) with the valve up. Shake well before use.

Each inhaler with actuator is packaged in an aluminum foil pouch to protect the product from moisture. After opening the aluminum pouch, the product should be used within 6 months and storage in an area of high humidity should be avoided.

Contents under pressure. Do not puncture. Do not use or store near heat or open flame. Exposure to temperatures above 50°C (120°F) may cause the canister to explode. Never throw the container into fire or an incinerator. Keep out of reach of children.

Note: The indented statement below is required by the Federal government's Clean Air Act for all products containing or manufactured with chlorofluorocarbons (CFCs).

WARNING: Contains trichloromonofluoromethane, dichlorotetrafluoroethane, and dichlorodifluoromethane, substances which harm public health and environment by destroying ozone in the upper atmosphere.

A notice similar to the above WARNING has been placed in the patient information leaflet of this product pursuant to EPA regulations.

Patient's Instructions For Use

Use a pair of scissors to cut the pouch open. Read the information before using Rhinocort Nasal Inhaler.

Follow the directions carefully.

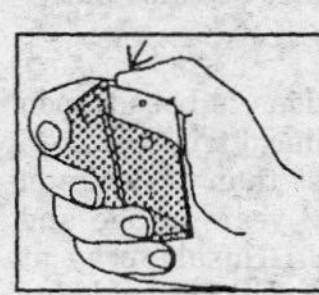

1. Blow your nose. Open the nasal inhaler by pressing on the arrow and rotating until it clicks into the locked position. Shake the canister thoroughly before using.

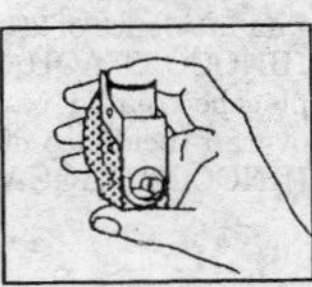

2. Place your thumb on the bottom of the unit (on the grid) while placing your index finger on the top of the canister. Wrap your fingers securely around the back. Press straight down on the canister to deliver a dose. Spray into the air 4 times before using for the first time.

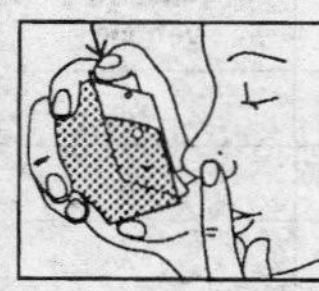

3. Close one nostril and insert the end of the inhaler tube into the other nostril. Hold your breath and deliver a dose. For optimum results, shake the canister between sprays.

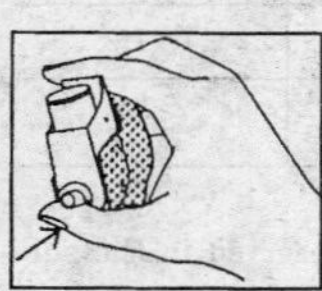

4. Rotate the unit closed for storage.

5. If Rhinocort is unused for 8 weeks, spray into the air 4 times before reuse.

WARNING: Contains trichloromonofluoromethane, dichlorotetrafluoroethane, and dichlorodifluoromethane, substances which harm the environment by destroying ozone in the upper atmosphere. Your physician has determined that this product is likely to help your personal health. USE THIS PRODUCT AS DIRECTED, UNLESS INSTRUCTED TO DO OTHERWISE BY YOUR PHYSICIAN. If you have any questions about alternatives, consult with your physician.

N.B.

Follow your doctor's directions and do not use Rhinocort Nasal Inhaler more often than prescribed. Contact your doctor if you find the effect strongly reduced.

Rhinocort Nasal Inhaler does not give immediate relief. Generally it will take a few days to achieve full effect. It is therefore very important that Rhinocort is used regularly.

Rhinocort Nasal Inhaler should be used within 6 months after the aluminum pouch has been opened. After opening the pouch, avoid storage in areas of high humidity.

Cleaning: Remove the aerosol container and wash the plastic parts regularly in warm-not hot-water with addition of mild detergent if necessary. Allow the plastic parts to dry completely and then replace the container.

Contents under pressure. Do not puncture or throw container into incinerator. Using or storing near open flame or heating above 120°F (50°C) may cause container to burst.

Manufactured for: Astra USA, Inc., Westborough, MA 01581

001053R03 Rev. 5/98

Shown in Product Identification Guide, page 305

RHINOCORT® AQUA™ ℞

[rhīnō-cōrt aquă]

(budesonide)

NASAL SPRAY 32 mcg

For Intranasal Inhalation Only.

℞ Only

DESCRIPTION

Budesonide, the active ingredient of RHINOCORT AQUA Nasal Spray, is an anti-inflammatory synthetic corticosteroid.

It is designated chemically as [(RS)-11-beta, 16-alpha, 17, 21-Tetrahydroxypregna-1,4,-diene-3,20-dione cyclic 16, 17-acetal with butyraldehyde].

Budesonide is provided as the mixture of two epimers (22R and 22S).

The empirical formula of budesonide is $C_{25}H_{34}O_6$ and its molecular weight is 430.5.

Its structural formula is:

Budesonide is a white to off-white, odorless powder that is practically insoluble in water and in heptane, sparingly soluble in ethanol, and freely soluble in chloroform.

Its partition coefficient between octanol and water at pH 5 is 1.6×10^3.

RHINOCORT AQUA is an unscented, metered-dose, manual-pump spray formulation containing a micronized suspension of budesonide in an aqueous medium. Microcrystalline cellulose and carboxymethyl cellulose sodium, dextrose anhydrous, polysorbate 80, disodium edetate, potassium sorbate and purified water are contained in this medium; hydrochloric acid is added to adjust the pH to a target of 4.5.

RHINOCORT AQUA Nasal Spray delivers 32 mcg of budesonide per spray.

Each bottle of RHINOCORT AQUA Nasal Spray 32 mcg contains 60 metered sprays after initial priming.

Prior to initial use, the container must be shaken gently and the pump must be primed by actuating eight times. If used daily, the pump does not need to be reprimed. If not used for two consecutive days, reprime with one spray or until a fine spray appears. If not used for more than 14 days, rinse the applicator and reprime with two sprays or until a fine spray appears.

CLINICAL PHARMACOLOGY

Budesonide is a synthetic corticosteroid having potent glucocorticoid activity and weak mineralocorticoid activity. In standard *in-vitro* and animal models, budesonide has approximately a 200-fold higher affinity for the glucocorticoid receptor and a 1000-fold higher topical anti-inflammatory potency than cortisol (rat croton oil ear edema assay). As a measure of systemic activity, budesonide is 40 times more potent than cortisol when administered subcutaneously and 25 times more potent when administered orally in the rat thymus involution assay. In glucocorticoid receptor affinity studies, the 22R form was twice as active as the 22S epimer. The precise mechanism of corticosteroid actions in seasonal and perennial allergic rhinitis is not known. Corticosteroids have been shown to have a wide range of inhibitory activities against multiple cell types (*e.g.* mast cells, eosinophils, neutrophils, macrophages, and lymphocytes) and mediators (*e.g.* histamine eicosanoids, leukotrienes, and cytokines) involved in allergic mediated inflammation.

Corticosteroids affect the delayed (6 hour) response to an allergen challenge more than the histamine-associated immediate response (20 minute). The clinical significance of these findings is unknown.

Pharmacokinetics: The pharmacokinetics of budesonide have been studied following nasal, oral and intravenous administration. Budesonide is relatively well absorbed after both inhalation and oral administration, and is rapidly metabolized into metabolites with low corticosteroid potency. The clinical activity of RHINOCORT AQUA Nasal Spray is therefore believed to be due to the parent drug, budesonide. *In-vitro* studies indicate that the two epimeric forms of budesonide do not interconvert.

Absorption: Following intranasal administration of RHINOCORT AQUA, the mean peak plasma concentration occurs at approximately 0.7 hours. Compared to an intravenous dose, approximately 34% of the delivered intranasal dose reaches the systemic circulation, most of which is absorbed through the nasal mucosa. While budesonide is well absorbed from the GI tract, the oral bioavailability of budesonide is low (~10%) primarily due to extensive first pass metabolism in the liver.

Distribution: Budesonide has a volume of distribution of approximately 2–3 L/kg. The volume of distribution for the 22R epimer is almost twice that of the 22S epimer. Protein binding of budesonide *in-vitro* is constant (85–90%) over a concentration range (1–100 nmol/L) which exceeded that achieved after administration of recommended doses. Budesonide shows little to no binding to glucocorticosteroid binding globulin. It rapidly equilibrates with red blood cells in a concentration independent manner with a blood/plasma ratio of about 0.8.

Metabolism: Budesonide is rapidly and extensively metabolized in humans by the liver. Two major metabolites (16α-hydroxyprednisolone and 6β-hydroxybudesonide) are formed via cytochrome P450 3A isoenzyme-catalyzed biotransformation. Known metabolic inhibitors of cytochrome P450 3A (*e.g.,* ketoconazole), or significant hepatic impairment, may increase the systemic exposure of unmetabolized budesonide (see WARNINGS and PRECAUTIONS). *In-vitro* studies on the binding of the two primary metabolites to the glucocorticoid receptor indicate that they have less than 1% of the affinity for the receptor as the parent compound budesonide. *In-vitro* studies have evaluated sites of metabolism and showed negligible metabolism in skin, lung, and serum. No qualitative difference between the *in-vitro* and *in-vivo* metabolic patterns could be detected.

Elimination: Budesonide is excreted in the urine and feces in the form of metabolites. After intranasal administration of a radio labeled dose, 2/3 of the radioactivity was found in the urine and the remainder in the feces. The main metabolites of budesonide in the 0-24 hour urine sample following IV administration are 16α-hydroxyprednisolone (24%) and 6β-hydroxybudesonide (5%). An additional 34% of the radioactivity recovered in the urine was identified as conjugates. The 22R form was preferentially cleared with clearance value of 1.4 L/min vs. 1.0 L/min for the 22S form. The terminal half-life, 2 to 3 hours, was similar for both epimers and it appeared to be independent of dose.

Special Populations

Geriatric: No specific pharmacokinetic study has been undertaken in subjects >65 years of age.

Pediatric: After administration of RHINOCORT AQUA Nasal Spray, the time to reach peak drug concentrations and plasma half-life were similar in children and in adults. Children had plasma concentrations approximately twice those observed in adults due primarily to differences in weight between children and adults.

Gender: No specific pharmacokinetic study has been conducted to evaluate the effect of gender on budesonide pharmacokinetics. However, following administration of 400 mcg RHINOCORT AQUA Nasal Spray to 7 male and 8 female volunteers in a pharmacokinetic study, no major gender differences in the pharmacokinetic parameters were found.

Race: No specific study has been undertaken to evaluate the effect of race on budesonide pharmacokinetics.

Renal Insufficiency: The pharmacokinetics of budesonide have not been investigated in patients with renal insufficiency.

Hepatic Insufficiency: Reduced liver function may affect the elimination of corticosteroids. The pharmacokinetics of orally administered budesonide were affected by compromised liver function as evidenced by a doubled systemic availability. The relevance of this finding to intranasally administered budesonide has not been established.

Pharmacodynamics: A 3-week clinical study in seasonal rhinitis, comparing RHINOCORT Nasal Inhaler, orally ingested budesonide, and placebo in 98 patients with allergic rhinitis due to birch pollen, demonstrated that the therapeutic effect of RHINOCORT Nasal Inhaler can be attributed to the topical effects of budesonide.

The effects of RHINOCORT AQUA Nasal Spray on adrenal function have been evaluated in several clinical trials. In a four-week clinical trial, 61 adult patients who received 256 mcg daily of RHINOCORT AQUA Nasal Spray demonstrated no significant differences from patients receiving placebo in plasma cortisol levels measured before and 60 minutes after 0.25 mg intramuscular cosyntropin. There were no consistent differences in 24-hour urinary cortisol measurements in patients receiving up to 400 mcg daily. Similar results were seen in a study of 150 children and adolescents aged 6 to 17 with perennial rhinitis who were treated with 256 mcg daily for up to 12 months.

After treatment with the recommended maximal daily dose of RHINOCORT AQUA (256 mcg) for seven days, there was a small, but statistically significant decrease in the area under the plasma cortisol-time curve over 24 hours (AUC_{0-24h}) in healthy adult volunteers.

A dose-related suppression of 24-hour urinary cortisol excretion was observed after administration of RHINOCORT AQUA doses ranging from 100–800 mcg daily for up to four days in 78 healthy adult volunteers. The clinical relevance of these results is unknown.

Clinical Trials: The therapeutic efficacy of RHINOCORT AQUA Nasal Spray has been evaluated in placebo-controlled clinical trials of seasonal and perennial allergic rhinitis of 3–6 weeks duration.

The number of patients treated with budesonide in these studies was 90 males and 51 females aged 6–12 years and 691 males and 694 females 12 years and above. The patients were predominantly Caucasian.

Overall, the results of these clinical trials showed that RHINOCORT AQUA Nasal Spray administered once daily provides statistically significant reduction in the severity of nasal symptoms of seasonal and perennial allergic rhinitis including runny nose, sneezing, and nasal congestion.

In some studies, improvement versus placebo has been shown to occur within 24 hours of initiating treatment with RHINOCORT AQUA Nasal Spray. Maximum benefit is generally not achieved until 2 weeks after initiation of treatment.

INDICATIONS AND USAGE

RHINOCORT AQUA Nasal Spray is indicated for the management of nasal symptoms of seasonal or perennial allergic rhinitis in adults and children six years of age and older.

CONTRAINDICATIONS

Hypersensitivity to any of the ingredients in this preparation contraindicates the use of RHINOCORT AQUA Nasal Spray.

WARNINGS

The replacement of a systemic corticosteroid with a topical corticosteroid can be accompanied by signs of adrenal insufficiency, and in addition some patients may experience symptoms of corticosteroid withdrawal, *e.g.* joint and/or muscular pain, lassitude and depression. Patients previously treated for prolonged periods with systemic corticosteroids and transferred to topical corticosteroids should be carefully monitored for acute adrenal insufficiency in response to stress. In those patients who have asthma or

Continued on next page

Rhinocort Aqua—Cont.

other clinical conditions requiring long-term systemic corticosteroid treatment, too rapid a decrease in systemic corticosteroids may cause a severe exacerbation of their symptoms.

Patients who are on drugs which suppress the immune system are more susceptible to infections than healthy individuals. Chicken pox and measles, for example, can have a more serious or even fatal course in non-immune children or adults on immunosuppressant doses of corticosteroids. In such children or adults, who have not had these diseases, particular care should be taken to avoid exposure. How the dose, route and duration of corticosteroid administration affects the risk of developing a disseminated infection is not known. The contribution of the underlying disease and/or prior corticosteroid treatment to the risk is also not known. If exposed to chicken pox, prophylaxis with varicella zoster immune globulin (VZIG) may be indicated. If exposed to measles, prophylaxis with pooled intramuscular immunoglobulin (IG) may be indicated. (See the respective package inserts for complete VZIG and IG prescribing information). If chicken pox develops, treatment with antiviral agents may be considered.

PRECAUTIONS

General: Intranasal corticosteroids may cause a reduction in growth velocity when administered to pediatric patients (see PRECAUTIONS, Pediatric Use).

Rarely, immediate and/or delayed hypersensitivity reactions may occur after the intranasal administration of budesonide. Rare instances of wheezing, nasal septum perforation, and increased intraocular pressure have been reported following the intranasal application of corticosteroids, including budesonide.

Although systemic effects have been minimal with recommended doses of RHINOCORT AQUA Nasal Spray, any such effect is dose dependent. Therefore, larger than recommended doses of RHINOCORT AQUA Nasal Spray should be avoided and the minimal effective dose for the patient should be used (see DOSAGE AND ADMINISTRATION).

When used at larger doses, systemic corticosteroid effects such as hypercorticism and adrenal suppression may appear. If such changes occur, the dosage of RHINOCORT AQUA Nasal Spray should be discontinued slowly consistent with accepted procedures for discontinuing oral corticosteroid therapy.

In clinical studies with budesonide administered intranasally, the development of localized infections of the nose and pharynx with *Candida albicans* has occurred only rarely. When such an infection develops, it may require treatment with appropriate local or systemic therapy and discontinuation of treatment with RHINOCORT AQUA Nasal Spray. Patients using RHINOCORT AQUA Nasal Spray over several months or longer should be examined periodically for evidence of *Candida* infection or other signs of adverse effects on the nasal mucosa.

RHINOCORT AQUA Nasal Spray should be used with caution, if at all, in patients with active or quiescent tuberculous infection, untreated fungal, bacterial, or systemic viral infections, or ocular herpes simplex.

Because of the inhibitory effect of corticosteroids on wound healing, patients who have experienced recent nasal septal ulcers, nasal surgery, or nasal trauma should not use a nasal corticosteroid until healing has occurred.

Hepatic dysfunction influences the pharmacokinetics of budesonide, similar to the effect on other corticosteroids, with a reduced elimination rate and increased systemic availability (see CLINICAL PHARMACOLOGY, Special Populations).

Information for Patients: Patients being treated with RHINOCORT AQUA Nasal Spray should receive the following information and instructions. Patients who are on immunosuppressant doses of corticosteroids should be warned to avoid exposure to chicken pox or measles and, if exposed, to obtain medical advice.

Patients should use RHINOCORT AQUA Nasal Spray at regular intervals since its effectiveness depends on its regular use (see DOSAGE and ADMINISTRATION).

An improvement in nasal symptoms may be seen within the first 24 hours after initiation of treatment. Maximum benefit is generally not achieved until 2 weeks after initiation of treatment. Initial assessment for response should be made during this time frame and periodically until the patient's symptoms are stabilized.

The patient should take the medication as directed and should not exceed the prescribed dosage. The patient should contact the physician if symptoms do not improve after two weeks, or if the condition worsens. Patients who experience recurrent episodes of epistaxis (nosebleeds) or nasal septum discomfort while taking this medication should contact their physician. For proper use of this unit and to attain maximum improvement, the patient should read and follow the accompanying patient instructions carefully.

It is important to shake the bottle well before each use. The RHINOCORT AQUA Nasal Spray 32 mcg bottle should be discarded after 60 sprays after initial priming, since the amount of budesonide delivered per spray thereafter may be substantially less than the labeled dose. Do not transfer any remaining suspension to another bottle.

Drug Interactions: The main route of metabolism of budesonide, as well as other corticosteroids, is via cytochrome P450 3A (CYP3A). After oral administration of ketoconazole, a potent inhibitor of cytochrome P450 3A, the mean plasma concentration of orally administered budesonide increased by more than seven fold. Concomitant administration of other known inhibitors of CYP3A (*e.g.* itraconazole, clarithromycin, erythromycin, etc.) may inhibit the metabolism of, and increase the systemic exposure to, budesonide (see WARNINGS, PRECAUTIONS, General).

Omeprazole, an inhibitor of cytochrome P450 2C19, did not have effects on the pharmacokinetics of oral budesonide, while cimetidine, primarily an inhibitor of cytochrome P450 1A2, caused a slight decrease in budesonide clearance and corresponding increase in its oral bioavailability.

Carcinogenesis, Mutagenesis, Impairment of Fertility: In a two-year study in Sprague-Dawley rats, budesonide caused a statistically significant increase in the incidence of gliomas in the male rats receiving an oral dose of 50 mcg/kg (approximately twice the maximum recommended daily intranasal dose in adults and children on a mcg/m^2 basis). No tumorigenicity was seen in male and female rats at respective oral doses up to 25 and 50 mcg/kg (approximately equal to and two times the maximum recommended daily intranasal dose in adults and children on a mcg/m^2 basis, respectively). In two additional two-year studies in male Fischer and Sprague-Dawley rats, budesonide caused no gliomas at an oral dose of 50 mcg/kg (approximately twice the maximum recommended daily intranasal dose in adults and children on a mcg/m^2 basis). However, in male Sprague-Dawley rats, budesonide caused a statistically significant increase in the incidence of hepatocellular tumors at an oral dose of 50 mcg/kg (approximately twice the maximum recommended daily intranasal dose in adults and children on a mcg/m^2 basis). The concurrent reference corticosteroids (prednisolone and triamcinolone acetonide) in these two studies showed similar findings.

In a 91-week study in mice, budesonide caused no treatment-related carcinogenicity at oral doses up to 200 mcg/kg (approximately 3 times the maximum recommended daily intranasal dose in adults and children on a mcg/m^2 basis).

Budesonide was not mutagenic or clastogenic in six different test systems: Ames, *salmonella*/microsome plate test, mouse micronucleus test, mouse lymphoma test, chromosome aberration test in human lymphocytes, sex-linked recessive lethal test in *Drosophila melanogaster*, and DNA repair analysis in rat hematocyte culture.

In rats, budesonide caused a decrease in prenatal viability and viability of the pups at birth and during lactation, along with a decrease in maternal body-weight gain, at subcutaneous doses of 20 mcg/kg and above (less than the maximum recommended daily intranasal dose in adults on a mcg/m^2 basis). No such effects were noted at 5 mcg/kg (less than the maximum recommended daily intranasal dose in adults on a mcg/m^2 basis).

Pregnancy: Teratogenic Effects: Pregnancy Category C: Budesonide was teratogenic and embryocidal in rabbits and rats. Budesonide produced fetal loss, decreased pup weights, and skeletal abnormalities at subcutaneous doses of 25 mcg/kg in rabbits and 500 mcg/kg in rats (approximately 2 and 16 times the maximum recommended daily intranasal dose in adults on a mcg/m^2 basis). In another study in rats, no teratogenic or embryocidal effects were seen at inhalation doses up to 250 mcg/kg (approximately 8 times the maximum recommended daily intranasal dose in adults on a mcg/m^2 basis).

There are no adequate and well-controlled studies in pregnant women. RHINOCORT AQUA Nasal Spray should be used during pregnancy only if the potential benefit justifies the potential risk to the fetus.

Experience with oral corticosteroids since their introduction in pharmacologic, as opposed to physiologic, doses suggests that rodents are more prone to teratogenic effects from corticosteroids than humans. In addition, because there is a natural increase in corticosteroid production during pregnancy, most women will require a lower exogenous corticosteroid dose and many will not need corticosteroid treatment during pregnancy.

Nonteratogenic Effects: Hypoadrenalism may occur in infants born of mothers receiving corticosteroids during pregnancy. Such infants should be carefully observed.

Nursing Mothers: It is not known whether budesonide is excreted in human milk. Because other corticosteroids are excreted in human milk, caution should be exercised when RHINOCORT AQUA Nasal Spray is administered to nursing women.

Pediatric Use: Safety and effectiveness in pediatric patients below 6 years of age have not been established.

Controlled clinical studies have shown that intranasal corticosteroids may cause a reduction in growth velocity in pediatric patients. This effect has been observed in the absence of laboratory evidence of hypothalamic-pituitary-adrenal (HPA) axis suppression, suggesting that growth velocity is a more sensitive indicator of systemic corticosteroid exposure in pediatric patients than some commonly used tests of HPA axis function. The long-term effects of this reduction in growth velocity associated with intranasal corticosteroids, including the impact on final adult height, are unknown. The potential for "catch up" growth following discontinuation of treatment with intranasal corticosteroids has not been adequately studied. The growth of pediatric patients receiving intranasal corticosteroids, including RHINOCORT AQUA Nasal Spray, should be monitored routinely (*e.g.*, via stadiometry). The potential growth effects of prolonged treatment should be weighed against clinical benefits obtained and the availability of safe and effective non-corticosteroid treatment alternatives. To minimize the systemic effects of intranasal corticosteroids, including RHINOCORT AQUA Nasal Spray, each patient should be titrated to the lowest dose that effectively controls his/her symptoms.

Geriatic Use: Of the 2,461 patients in clinical studies of RHINOCORT AQUA Nasal Spray, 5% were 60 years of age and over. No overall differences in safety or effectiveness were observed between these subjects and younger subjects, except for an adverse event reporting frequency of epistaxis which increased with age. Further, other reported clinical experience has not identified any other differences in responses between elderly and younger patients, but greater sensitivity of some older individuals cannot be ruled out.

ADVERSE REACTIONS

The incidence of common adverse reactions is based upon two U.S. and five non-U.S. controlled clinical trials in 1526 patients [110 females and 239 males less than 18 years of age, and 635 females and 542 males 18 years of age and older] treated with RHINOCORT AQUA Nasal Spray at doses up to 400 mcg once daily for 3–6 weeks. The table below describes adverse events occurring at an incidence of 2% or greater and more common among RHINOCORT AQUA Nasal Spray-treated patients than in placebo-treated patients in controlled clinical trials. The overall incidence of adverse events was similar between RHINOCORT AQUA and Placebo.

Adverse Event	RHINOCORT AQUA	Placebo Vehicle
Epistaxis	8%	5%
Pharyngitis	4%	3%
Bronchospasm	2%	1%
Coughing	2%	<1%
Nasal Irritation	2%	<1%

A similar adverse event profile was observed in the subgroup of pediatric patients 6 to 12 years of age.

Two to three percent (2–3%) of patients in clinical trials discontinued because of adverse events. Systemic corticosteroid side-effects were not reported during controlled clinical studies with RHINOCORT AQUA Nasal Spray.

If recommended doses are exceeded, however, or if individuals are particularly sensitive, symptoms of hypercorticism, *i.e.*, Cushing's Syndrome, could occur.

Rare adverse events reported from post-marketing experience include: nasal septum perforation, pharynx disorders (throat irritation, throat pain, swollen throat, burning throat, and itchy throat), angioedema, anosmia, and palpitations.

Cases of growth suppression have been reported for intranasal corticosteroids including RHINOCORT AQUA Nasal Spray (see PRECAUTIONS, Pediatric Use).

OVERDOSAGE

Acute overdosage with this dosage form is unlikely since one 60 spray bottle of RHINOCORT AQUA Nasal Spray 32 mcg only contains approximately 3.2 mg of budesonide. Chronic overdosage may result in signs/symptoms of hypercorticism (see WARNINGS and PRECAUTIONS).

DOSAGE AND ADMINISTRATION

The recommended starting dose for adults and children 6 years of age and older is 64 mcg per day administered as one spray per nostril of RHINOCORT AQUA 32 mcg Nasal Spray once daily. The maximum recommended dose for adults (12 years of age and older) is 256 mcg per day administered as four sprays per nostril once daily of RHINOCORT AQUA 32 mcg Nasal Spray and the maximum recommended dose for pediatrics (<12 years of age) is 128 mcg per day administered as two sprays per nostril once daily of RHINOCORT AQUA 32 mcg Nasal Spray (see HOW SUPPLIED).

Prior to initial use, the container must be shaken gently and the pump must be primed by actuating eight times. If used daily, the pump does not need to be reprimed. If not used for two consecutive days, reprime with one spray or until a fine spray appears. If not used for more than 14 days, rinse the applicator and reprime with two sprays or until a fine spray appears.

Individualization of Dosage: It is always desirable to titrate an individual patient to the minimum effective dose to reduce the possibility of side effects. In adults and children 6 years of age and older, the recommended starting dose is 64 mcg daily administered as one spray per nostril of RHINOCORT AQUA Nasal Spray 32 mcg, once-daily. Some patients who do not achieve symptom control at the recommended starting dose may benefit from an increased dose. The maximum daily dose is 256 mcg for adults and 128 mcg for pediatric patients (<12 years of age). When the maximum benefit has been achieved and symptoms have been controlled, reducing the dose may be effective in maintaining control of the allergic rhinitis symptoms in patients who were initially controlled on higher doses.

An improvement in symptoms may be seen in some patients within the first 24 hours after initiating treatment. Maximum benefit is generally not achieved until 2 weeks after initiation of treatment. Initial assessment for response should be made during this time frame and periodically until the patient's symptoms are stabilized.

Directions for Use: Illustrated Patient's Instructions for Use accompany each package of RHINOCORT AQUA 32 mcg Nasal Spray.

HOW SUPPLIED

RHINOCORT AQUA Nasal Spray is available as 32 mcg per spray, in a 10 mL green coated glass bottle with a metered-dose pump spray with a green protection cap and patient instructions for use. Each spray delivers 32 mcg of budesonide to the patient. RHINOCORT AQUA Nasal Spray 32 mcg dose is available in bottles containing 60 metered sprays, after initial priming.

NDC 0186-1070-06
RHINOCORT AQUA Nasal Spray
32 mcg, 60 metered sprays.

RHINOCORT AQUA Nasal Spray should be stored at controlled room temperature, 20 to 25°C (68 to 77°F) with the valve up. Do not freeze. Protect from light. **Shake gently before use.** Do not spray in eyes.

Manufactured by:
Astra Pharmaceutical Production, AB, Södertälje, Sweden
Manufactured for:
Astra Pharmaceuticals, L.P., Wayne, PA 19087
72179100 Iss. 10/99

Shown in Product Identification Guide, page 305

SENSORCAINE® ℞
[*sén-sor-caine*]
(bupivacaine HCl Injection, USP)
SENSORCAINE®–MPF
(bupivacaine HCl Injection, USP)
SENSORCAINE® with Epinephrine
(bupivacaine HCl and epinephrine Injection, USP)
1:200,000 (as bitartrate)
SENSORCAINE®–MPF with Epinephrine
(bupivacaine HCl and epinephrine Injection, USP)
1:200,000 (as bitartrate)

DESCRIPTION

Sensorcaine® (bupivacaine HCl) injections are sterile isotonic solutions that contain a local anesthetic agent with and without epinephrine (as bitartrate) 1:200,000 and are administered parenterally by injection. See INDICATIONS AND USAGE for specific uses. Solutions of bupivacaine HCl may be autoclaved if they do not contain epinephrine.

Sensorcaine® injections contain bupivacaine HCl which is chemically designated as 2-piperidinecarboxamide, 1-butyl-N-(2,6-dimethylphenyl)-, monohydrochloride, monohydrate and has the following structure:

$CH_2(CH_2)_2CH_3$ CH_3 N CONH • HCl • H_2O CH_3

Epinephrine is (-)-3,4-Dihydroxy-α [(methylamino)methyl] benzyl alcohol. It has the following structural formula:

OH HO C CH_2NHCH_3 H HO

The pK_a of bupivacaine (8.1) is similar to that of lidocaine (7.86). However, bupivacaine possesses a greater degree of lipid solubility and is protein bound to a greater extent than lidocaine.

Bupivacaine is related chemically and pharmacologically to the aminoacyl local anesthetics. It is a homologue of mepivacaine and is chemically related to lidocaine. All three of these anesthetics contain an amide linkage between the aromatic nucleus and the amino or piperidine group. They differ in this respect from the procaine-type local anesthetics, which have an ester linkage.

Dosage forms listed as Sensorcaine-MPF indicates single dose solutions that are Methyl Paraben Free (MPF).

Sensorcaine-MPF is a sterile isotonic solution containing sodium chloride. Sensorcaine in multiple dose vials, each mL also contains 1 mg methylparaben as antiseptic preservative. The pH of these solutions is adjusted to between 4.0 and 6.5 with sodium hydroxide and/or hydrochloric acid.

Sensorcaine-MPF with Epinephrine 1:200,000 (as bitartrate) is a sterile isotonic solution containing sodium chloride. Each mL contains bupivacaine hydrochloride and 0.005 mg epinephrine, with 0.5 mg sodium metabisulfite as an antioxidant and 0.2 mg citric acid (anhydrous) as stabilizer. Sensorcaine with Epinephrine 1:200,000 (as bitartrate) in multiple dose vials, each mL also contains 1 mg methylparaben as antiseptic preservative. The pH of these solutions is adjusted to between 3.3 to 5.5 with sodium hydroxide and/or hydrochloric acid. Filled under nitrogen.

Note: The user should have an appreciation and awareness of the formulations and their intended uses. (See DOSAGE AND ADMINISTRATION.)

CLINICAL PHARMACOLOGY

Local anesthetics block the generation and the conduction of nerve impulses, presumably by increasing the threshold for electrical excitation in the nerve, by slowing the propagation of the nerve impulse, and by reducing the rate of rise of the action potential. In general, the progression of anesthesia is related to the diameter, myelination and conduction velocity of affected nerve fibers. Clinically, the order of loss of nerve function is as follows: (1) pain, (2) temperature, (3) touch, (4) proprioception, and (5) skeletal muscle tone.

Systemic absorption of local anesthetics produces effects on the cardiovascular and central nervous systems. At blood concentrations achieved with therapeutic doses, changes in cardiac conduction, excitability, refractoriness, contractility, and peripheral vascular resistance are minimal. However, toxic blood concentrations depress cardiac conduction and excitability, which may lead to atrioventricular block, ventricular arrhythmias and to cardiac arrest, sometimes resulting in fatalities. In addition, myocardial contractility is depressed and peripheral vasodilation occurs, leading to decreased cardiac output and arterial blood pressure. Recent clinical reports and animal research suggest that these cardiovascular changes are more likely to occur after unintended intravascular injection of bupivacaine. Therefore, incremental dosing is necessary.

Following systemic absorption, local anesthetics can produce central nervous system stimulation, depression or both. Apparent central stimulation is usually manifested as restlessness, tremors and shivering, progressing to convulsions, followed by depression and coma, progressing ultimately to respiratory arrest. However, the local anesthetics have a primary depressant effect on the medulla and on higher centers. The depressed stage may occur without a prior excited stage.

Pharmacokinetics: The rate of systemic absorption of local anesthetics is dependent upon the total dose and concentration of drug administered, the route of administration, the vascularity of the administration site, and the presence or absence of epinephrine in the anesthetic solution. A dilute concentration of epinephrine (1:200,000 or 5 μg/mL) usually reduces the rate of absorption and peak plasma concentration of bupivacaine, permitting the use of moderately larger total doses and sometimes prolonging the duration of action.

The onset of action with bupivacaine is rapid and anesthesia is long-lasting. The duration of anesthesia is significantly longer with bupivacaine than with any other commonly used local anesthetic. It has also been noted that there is a period of analgesia that persists after the return of sensation, during which time the need for potent analgesics is reduced.

Local anesthetics are bound to plasma proteins in varying degrees. Generally, the lower the plasma concentration of drug, the higher the percentage of drug bound to plasma proteins.

Local anesthetics appear to cross the placenta by passive diffusion. The rate and degree of diffusion is governed by: (1) the degree of plasma protein binding, (2) the degree of ionization, and (3) the degree of lipid solubility. Fetal/maternal ratios of local anesthetics appear to be inversely related to the degree of plasma protein binding, because only the free, unbound drug is available for placental transfer. Bupivacaine, with a high protein binding capacity (95%), has a low fetal/maternal ratio (0.2–0.4). The extent of placental transfer is also determined by the degree of ionization and lipid solubility of the drug. Lipid soluble, nonionized drugs readily enter the fetal blood from the maternal circulation.

Depending upon the route of administration, local anesthetics are distributed to some extent to all body tissues, with high concentrations found in highly perfused organs such as the liver, lungs, heart, and brain.

Pharmacokinetic studies on the plasma profile of bupivacaine after direct intravenous injection suggest a three-compartment open model. The first compartment is represented by the rapid intravascular distribution of the drug. The second compartment represents the equilibration of the drug throughout the highly perfused organs such as the brain, myocardium, lungs, kidneys, and liver. The third compartment represents an equilibration of the drug with poorly perfused tissues, such as muscle and fat. The elimination of drug from tissue depends largely upon the ability of binding sites in the circulation to carry it to the liver where it is metabolized.

After injection of Sensorcaine for caudal, epidural or peripheral nerve block in man, peak levels of bupivacaine in the blood are reached in 30 to 45 minutes, followed by a decline to insignificant levels during the next 3 to 6 hours.

Various pharmacokinetic parameters of the local anesthetics can be significantly altered by the presence of hepatic or renal disease, addition of epinephrine, factors affecting urinary pH, renal blood flow, the route of drug administration, and the age of the patient. The half-life of bupivacaine in adults is 3.5 ± 2.0 hours and in neonates 8.1 hours.

Amide-type local anesthetics such as bupivacaine are metabolized primarily in the liver via conjugation with glucuronic acid.

Patients with hepatic disease, especially those with severe hepatic disease, may be more susceptible to the potential toxicities of the amide-type local anesthetics. The major metabolite of bupivacaine is 2,6-pipecoloxylidine.

The kidney is the main excretory organ for most local anesthetics and their metabolites. Urinary excretion is affected by renal perfusion and factors affecting urinary pH. Only 5% of bupivacaine is excreted unchanged in the urine.

When administered in recommended doses and concentrations, Sensorcaine does not ordinarily produce irritation or tissue damage and does not cause methemoglobinemia.

INDICATIONS AND USAGE

Sensorcaine is indicated for the production of local or regional anesthesia or analgesia for surgery, for oral surgery procedures, for diagnostic and therapeutic procedures, and for obstetrical procedures. Only the 0.25% and 0.5% concentrations are indicated for obstetrical anesthesia. (See WARNINGS.)

Experience with non-obstetrical surgical procedures in pregnant patients is not sufficient to recommend use of the 0.75% concentration in these patients. Sensorcaine is not recommended for intravenous regional anesthesia (Bier Block). (See WARNINGS.)

The routes of administration and indicated Sensorcaine concentrations are:

local infiltration	0.25%
peripheral nerve block	0.25%, 0.5%
retrobulbar block	0.75%
sympathetic block	0.25%
lumbar epidural	0.25%, 0.5% and 0.75% (non-obstetrical)
caudal	0.25%, 0.5%
epidural test dose (see PRECAUTIONS)	

(See DOSAGE AND ADMINISTRATION for additional information.) Standard textbooks should be consulted to determine the accepted procedures and techniques for the administration of Sensorcaine.

Use only the single dose ampules and single dose vials for caudal or epidural anesthesia; the multiple dose vials contain a preservative and, therefore, should not be used for these procedures.

CONTRAINDICATIONS

Sensorcaine is contraindicated in obstetrical paracervical block anesthesia. Its use by this technique has resulted in fetal bradycardia and death.

Sensorcaine is contraindicated in patients with a known hypersensitivity to it or to any local anesthetic agent of the amide type or to other components of bupivacaine solutions.

WARNINGS

THE 0.75% CONCENTRATION OF SENSORCAINE INJECTION IS NOT RECOMMENDED FOR OBSTETRICAL ANESTHESIA. THERE HAVE BEEN REPORTS OF CARDIAC ARREST WITH DIFFICULT RESUSCITATION OR DEATH DURING USE OF BUPIVACAINE FOR EPIDURAL ANESTHESIA IN OBSTETRICAL PATIENTS. IN MOST CASES, THIS HAS FOLLOWED USE OF THE 0.75% CONCENTRATION. RESUSCITATION HAS BEEN DIFFICULT OR IMPOSSIBLE DESPITE APPARENTLY ADEQUATE PREPARATION AND APPROPRIATE MANAGEMENT. CARDIAC ARREST HAS OCCURRED AFTER CONVULSIONS RESULTING FROM SYSTEMIC TOXICITY, PRESUMABLY FOLLOWING UNINTENTIONAL INTRAVASCULAR INJECTION. THE 0.75% CONCENTRATION SHOULD BE RESERVED FOR SURGICAL PROCEDURES WHERE A HIGH DEGREE OF MUSCLE RELAXATION AND PROLONGED EFFECT ARE NECESSARY.

LOCAL ANESTHETICS SHOULD ONLY BE EMPLOYED BY CLINICIANS WHO ARE WELL VERSED IN DIAGNOSIS AND MANAGEMENT OF DOSE-RELATED TOXICITY AND OTHER ACUTE EMERGENCIES WHICH MIGHT ARISE FROM THE BLOCK TO BE EMPLOYED, AND THEN ONLY AFTER INSURING THE *IMMEDIATE* AVAILABILITY OF OXYGEN, OTHER RESUSCITATIVE DRUGS, CARDIOPULMONARY RESUSCITATIVE EQUIPMENT, AND THE PERSONNEL RESOURCES NEEDED FOR PROPER MANAGEMENT OF TOXIC REACTIONS AND RELATED EMERGENCIES. (See also ADVERSE REACTIONS, PRECAUTIONS, and OVERDOSAGE.) DELAY IN PROPER MANAGEMENT OF DOSE-RELATED TOXICITY, UNDERVENTILATION FROM ANY CAUSE AND/OR ALTERED SENSITIVITY MAY LEAD TO THE DEVELOPMENT OF ACIDOSIS, CARDIAC ARREST AND, POSSIBLY, DEATH.

Local anesthetic solutions containing antimicrobial preservatives, i.e., those supplied in multiple dose vials, should not be used for epidural or caudal anesthesia because safety has not been established with regard to intrathecal injection, either intentional or unintentional, of such preservatives.

It is essential that aspiration for blood or cerebrospinal fluid (where applicable) be done prior to injecting any local anesthetic, both the original dose and all subsequent doses, to avoid intravascular or subarachnoid injection. However, a negative aspiration does *not* ensure against an intravascular or subarachnoid injection.

Bupivacaine and Epinephrine Injection or other vasopressors should not be used concomitantly with ergot-type oxytocic drugs, because a severe persistent hypertension may occur. Likewise, solutions of bupivacaine containing a vasoconstrictor, such as epinephrine, should be used with extreme caution in patients receiving monoamine oxidase

Continued on next page

Sensorcaine/Sensorcaine-MPF—Cont

(MAO) inhibitors or antidepressants of the triptyline or imipramine types, because severe prolonged hypertension may result.
Until further experience is gained in children younger than 12 years, administration of bupivacaine in this age group is not recommended.
Reports of cardiac arrest and death have occurred with the use of bupivacaine for intravenous regional anesthesia (Bier Block). Information on safe dosages or techniques of administration of this product are lacking; therefore, bupivacaine is not recommended for use by this technique.
Prior use of chloroprocaine may interfere with subsequent use of bupivacaine. Because of this, and because safety of intercurrent use of bupivacaine and chloroprocaine has not been established, such use is not recommended.
Sensorcaine with epinephrine solutions contain sodium metabisulfite, a sulfite that may cause allergic-type reactions including anaphylactic symptoms and life-threatening or less severe asthmatic episodes in certain susceptible people. The overall prevalence of sulfite sensitivity in the general population is unknown and probably low. Sulfite sensitivity is seen more frequently in asthmatic than in nonasthmatic people.

PRECAUTIONS

General: The safety and effectiveness of local anesthetics depend on proper dosage, correct technique, adequate precautions and readiness for emergencies. Resuscitative equipment, oxygen, and other resuscitative drugs should be available for immediate use. (See WARNINGS, ADVERSE REACTIONS, and OVERDOSAGE.) During major regional nerve blocks, the patient should have I.V. fluids running via an indwelling catheter to assure a functioning intravenous pathway. The lowest dosage of local anesthetic that results in effective anesthesia should be used to avoid high plasma levels and serious adverse effects. The rapid injection of a large volume of local anesthetic solution should be avoided and fractional (incremental) doses should be used when feasible.
Epidural Anesthesia: During epidural administration of bupivacaine, concentrated solutions (0.5–0.75%) should be administered in incremental doses of 3 to 5 mL with sufficient time between doses to detect toxic manifestations of unintentional intravascular or intrathecal injection. Syringe aspirations should also be performed before and during each supplemental injection in continuous (intermittent) catheter techniques. An intravascular injection is still possible even if aspirations for blood are negative.
During the administration of epidural anesthesia, it is recommended that a test dose be administered initially and the effects monitored before the full dose is given. When using a "continuous" catheter technique, test doses should be given prior to both the original and all reinforcing doses, because plastic tubing in the epidural space can migrate into a blood vessel or through the dura. When clinical conditions permit, the test dose should contain epinephrine (10 to 15 μg have been suggested) to serve as a warning of unintentional intravascular injection. If injected into a blood vessel, this amount of epinephrine is likely to produce a transient "epinephrine response" within 45 seconds, consisting of an increase in heart rate and systolic blood pressure, circumoral pallor, palpitations and nervousness in the unsedated patient. The sedated patient may exhibit only a pulse rate increase of 20 or more beats per minute for 15 or more seconds. Therefore, following the test dose, the heart rate should be monitored for a heart rate increase. Patients on beta-blockers may not manifest changes in heart rate, but blood pressure monitoring can detect an evanescent rise in systolic blood pressure. The test dose should also contain 10 to 15 mg of Sensorcaine or an equivalent dose of a short-acting amide anesthetic such as 30 to 40 mg of lidocaine, to detect an unintentional intrathecal administration. This will be manifested within a few minutes by signs of spinal block (e.g., decreased sensation of the buttocks, paresis of the legs, or, in the sedated patient, absent knee jerk). An intravascular or subarachnoid injection is still possible even if results of the test dose are negative. The test dose itself may produce a systemic toxic reaction, high spinal or epinephrine-induced cardiovascular effects.
Injection of repeated doses of local anesthetics may cause significant increases in plasma levels with each repeated dose due to slow accumulation of the drug or its metabolites or to slow metabolic degradation. Tolerance to elevated blood levels varies with the physical condition of the patient. Debilitated, elderly patients, acutely ill patients and children should be given reduced doses commensurate with their age and physical condition. Local anesthetics should also be used with caution in patients with hypotension or heart block.
Careful and constant monitoring of cardiovascular and respiratory vital signs (adequacy of ventilation) and the patient's state of consciousness should be performed after each local anesthetic injection. It should be kept in mind at such times that restlessness, anxiety, incoherent speech, lightheadedness, numbness and tingling of the mouth and lips, metallic taste, tinnitus, dizziness, blurred vision, tremors, twitching, depression, or drowsiness may be early warning signs of central nervous system toxicity.
Local anesthetic solutions containing a vasoconstrictor should be used cautiously and in carefully restricted quantities in areas of the body supplied by end arteries or having otherwise compromised blood supply such as digits, nose, external ear, penis, etc. Patients with hypertensive vascular disease may exhibit exaggerated vasoconstrictor response. Ischemic injury or necrosis may result.
Because amide-type local anesthetics such as bupivacaine are metabolized by the liver, these drugs, especially repeat doses, should be used cautiously in patients with hepatic disease. Patients with severe hepatic disease, because of their inability to metabolize local anesthetics normally, are at a greater risk of developing toxic plasma concentrations.
Local anesthetics should also be used with caution in patients with impaired cardiovascular function because they may be less able to compensate for functional changes associated with the prolongation of A-V conduction produced by these drugs.
Serious dose-related cardiac arrhythmias may occur if preparations containing a vasoconstrictor such as epinephrine are employed in patients during or following the administration of potent inhalation anesthetics. In deciding whether to use these products concurrently in the same patient, the combined action of both agents upon the myocardium, the concentration and volume of vasoconstrictor used, and the time since injection, when applicable, should be taken into account.
Many drugs used during the conduct of anesthesia are considered potential triggering agents for familial malignant hyperthermia. Because it is not known whether amide-type local anesthetics may trigger this reaction and because the need for supplemental general anesthesia cannot be predicted in advance, it is suggested that a standard protocol for management should be available. Early unexplained signs of tachycardia, tachypnea, labile blood pressure and metabolic acidosis may precede temperature elevation. Successful outcome is dependent on early diagnosis, prompt discontinuance of the suspect triggering agent(s) and prompt treatment, including oxygen therapy, dantrolene (consult dantrolene sodium intravenous package insert before using) and other supportive measures.
Use in Head and Neck Area: Small doses of local anesthetics injected into the head and neck area, including retrobulbar, dental and stellate ganglion blocks, may produce adverse reactions similar to systemic toxicity seen with unintentional intravascular injections of larger doses. The injection procedures require the utmost care. Confusion, convulsions, respiratory depression and/or respiratory arrest, and cardiovascular stimulation or depression have been reported. These reactions may be due to intraarterial injection of the local anesthetic with retrograde flow to the cerebral circulation. They may also be due to puncture of the dural sheath of the optic nerve during retrobulbar block with diffusion of any local anesthetic along the subdural space to the midbrain. Patients receiving these blocks should have their circulation and respiration monitored and be constantly observed. Resuscitative equipment and personnel for treating adverse reactions should be immediately available. Dosage recommendations should not be exceeded (see DOSAGE AND ADMINISTRATION).
Use in Ophthalmic Surgery: Clinicians who perform retrobulbar blocks should be aware that there have been reports of respiratory arrest following local anesthetic injection. Prior to retrobulbar block, as with all other regional procedures, the immediate availability of equipment, drugs, and personnel to manage respiratory arrest or depression, convulsions, and cardiac stimulation or depression should be assured (see also WARNINGS and *Use in Head and Neck Area*, above). As with other anesthetic procedures, patients should be constantly monitored following ophthalmic blocks for signs of these adverse reactions, which may occur following relatively low total doses. A concentration of 0.75% bupivacaine is indicated for retrobulbar block; however, this concentration is not indicated for any other peripheral nerve block, including the facial nerve and not indicated for local infiltration, including the conjunctiva (see INDICATIONS and PRECAUTIONS, *General*). Mixing Sensorcaine (bupivacaine HCl) with other local anesthetics is not recommended because of insufficient data on the clinical use of such mixtures.
When Sensorcaine 0.75% is used for retrobulbar block, complete corneal anesthesia usually precedes onset of clinically acceptable external ocular muscle akinesia. Therefore, presence of akinesia rather than anesthesia alone should determine readiness of the patient for surgery.
Information for Patients: When appropriate, patients should be informed in advance that they may experience temporary loss of sensation and motor activity, usually in the lower half of the body following proper administration of caudal or lumbar epidural anesthesia. Also, when appropriate, the physician should discuss other information including adverse reactions in the Sensorcaine package insert.
Clinically Significant Drug Interactions: The administration of local anesthetic solutions containing epinephrine or norepinephrine to patients receiving monoamine oxidase inhibitors or tricyclic antidepressants may produce severe, prolonged hypertension. Concurrent use of these agents should generally be avoided. In situations in which concurrent therapy is necessary, careful patient monitoring is essential.
Concurrent administration of vasopressor drugs and of ergot-type oxytocic drugs may cause severe, persistent hypertension or cerebrovascular accidents.
Phenothiazines and butyrophenones may reduce or reverse the pressor effect of epinephrine.
Carcinogenesis, Mutagenesis, and Impairment of Fertility: Long-term studies in animals of most local anesthetics, including bupivacaine, to evaluate the carcinogenic potential have not been conducted. Mutagenic potential or the effect on fertility has not been determined. There is no evidence from human data that bupivacaine may be carcinogenic or mutagenic or that it impairs fertility.
Pregnancy Category C: Decreased pup survival in rats and embryocidal effect in rabbits have been observed when bupivacaine HCl was administered to these species in doses comparable to nine and five times, respectively, the maximum recommended daily human dose (400 mg). There are no adequate and well-controlled studies in pregnant women of the effect of bupivacaine on the developing fetus. Sensorcaine should be used during pregnancy only if the potential benefit justifies the potential risk to the fetus. This does not exclude the use of Sensorcaine (0.25% and 0.5% concentrations) at term for obstetrical anesthesia or analgesia. (See *Labor and Delivery*.)
Labor and Delivery: See Box WARNINGS regarding obstetrical use in 0.75% concentration.
Sensorcaine is contraindicated in obstetrical paracervical block anesthesia.
Local anesthetics rapidly cross the placenta, and when used for epidural, caudal or pudendal block anesthesia, can cause varying degrees of maternal, fetal and neonatal toxicity. (See *Pharmacokinetics* in CLINICAL PHARMACOLOGY.) The incidence and degree of toxicity depend upon the procedure performed, the type and amount of drug used, and the technique of drug administration. Adverse reactions in the parturient, fetus and neonate involve alterations of the central nervous system, peripheral vascular tone and cardiac function.
Maternal hypotension has resulted from regional anesthesia. Local anesthetics produce vasodilation by blocking sympathetic nerves. Elevating the patient's legs and positioning her on her left side will help prevent decreases in blood pressure. The fetal heart rate also should be monitored continuously, and electronic fetal monitoring is highly advisable.
Epidural, caudal, or pudendal anesthesia may alter the forces of parturition through changes in uterine contractility or maternal expulsive efforts. Epidural anesthesia has been reported to prolong the second stage of labor by removing the parturient's reflex urge to bear down or by interfering with motor function. The use of obstetrical anesthesia may increase the need for forceps assistance.
The use of some local anesthetic drug products during labor and delivery may be followed by diminished muscle strength and tone for the first day or two of life. This has not been reported with Sensorcaine.
It is extremely important to avoid aortocaval compression by the gravid uterus during administration of regional block to parturients. To do this, the patient must be maintained in the left lateral decubitus position or a blanket roll or sandbag may be placed beneath the right hip and the gravid uterus displaced to the left.
Nursing Mothers: It is not known whether local anesthetic drugs are excreted in human milk. Because many drugs are excreted in human milk, caution should be exercised when local anesthetics are administered to a nursing mother.
Pediatric Use: Until further experience is gained in children younger than 12 years, administration of Sensorcaine (bupivacaine HCl) Injection in this age group is not recommended.

ADVERSE REACTIONS

Reactions to bupivacaine are characteristic of those associated with other amide-type local anesthetics. A major cause of adverse reactions to this group of drugs may be associated with its excessive plasma levels, which may be due to overdosage, unintentional intravascular injection or slow metabolic degradation.
Systemic: The most commonly encountered acute adverse experiences that demand immediate countermeasures are related to the central nervous system and the cardiovascular system. These adverse experiences are generally dose related and due to high plasma levels which may result from overdosage, rapid absorption from the injection site, diminished tolerance or from unintentional intravascular injection of the local anesthetic solution. In addition to systemic dose-related toxicity, unintentional subarachnoid injection of drug during the intended performance of caudal or lumbar epidural block or nerve blocks near the vertebral column (especially in the head and neck region) may result in underventilation or apnea ("Total or High Spinal"). Also, hypotension due to loss of sympathetic tone and respiratory paralysis or underventilation due to cephalad extension of the motor level of anesthesia may occur. This may lead to secondary cardiac arrest if untreated. Factors influencing plasma protein binding, such as acidosis, systemic diseases that alter protein production or competition with other drugs for protein binding sites, may diminish individual tolerance.
Central Nervous System Reactions: These are characterized by excitation and/or depression. Restlessness, anxiety, dizziness, tinnitus, blurred vision or tremors may occur, possibly proceeding to convulsions. However, excitement may be transient or absent, with depression being the first manifestation of an adverse reaction. This may quickly be followed by drowsiness merging into unconsciousness and respiratory arrest. Other central nervous system effects may be nausea, vomiting, chills, and constriction of the pupils.
The incidence of convulsions associated with the use of local anesthetics varies with the procedure used and the total

dose administered. In a survey of studies of epidural anesthesia, overt toxicity progressing to convulsions occurred in approximately 0.1 percent of local anesthetic administrations.

Cardiovascular System Reactions: High doses or unintentional intravascular injection may lead to high plasma levels and related depression of the myocardium, decreased cardiac output, heart block, hypotension, bradycardia, ventricular arrhythmias, including ventricular tachycardia and ventricular fibrillation, and cardiac arrest. (See WARNINGS, PRECAUTIONS, and OVERDOSAGE sections.)

Allergic: Allergic type reactions are rare and may occur as a result of sensitivity to the local anesthetic or to other formulation ingredients, such as the antimicrobial preservative methylparaben contained in multiple dose vials or sulfites in epinephrine-containing solutions (see WARNINGS). These reactions are characterized by signs such as urticaria, pruritus, erythema, angioneurotic edema (including laryngeal edema), tachycardia, sneezing, nausea, vomiting, dizziness, syncope, excessive sweating, elevated temperature, and possibly, anaphylactoid symptomatology (including severe hypotension). Cross sensitivity among members of the amide-type local anesthetic group has been reported. The usefulness of screening for sensitivity has not been definitely established.

Neurologic: The incidence of adverse neurologic reactions associated with the use of local anesthetics may be related to the total dose of local anesthetic administered and are also dependent upon the particular drug used, the route of administration and the physical status of the patient. Many of these effects may be related to local anesthetic techniques, with or without a contribution from the drug.

In the practice of caudal or lumbar epidural block, occasional unintentional penetration of the subarachnoid space by the catheter or needle may occur. Subsequent adverse effects may depend partially on the amount of drug administered intrathecally and the physiological and physical effects of a dural puncture. A high spinal is characterized by paralysis of the legs, loss of consciousness, respiratory paralysis and bradycardia.

Neurologic effects following unintentional subarachnoid administration during epidural or caudal anesthesia may include spinal block by varying magnitude (including high or total spinal block); hypotension secondary to spinal block; urinary retention; fecal and urinary incontinence; loss of perineal sensation and sexual function; persistent anesthesia, paresthesia, weakness, paralysis of the lower extremities and loss of sphincter control, all of which may have slow, incomplete or no recovery; headache; backache; septic meningitis; meningismus; slowing of labor; increased incidence of forceps delivery; or cranial nerve palsies due to traction on nerves from loss of cerebrospinal fluid.

OVERDOSAGE

Acute emergencies from local anesthetics are generally related to high plasma levels encountered during therapeutic use of local anesthetics or to unintended subarachnoid injection of local anesthetic solution. (See ADVERSE REACTIONS, WARNINGS, and PRECAUTIONS.)

Management of Local Anesthetic Emergencies: The first consideration is prevention, best accomplished by careful and constant monitoring of cardiovascular and respiratory vital signs and the patient's state of consciousness after each local anesthetic injection. At the first sign of change, oxygen should be administered.

The first step in the management of systemic toxic reactions, as well as underventilation or apnea due to unintentional subarachnoid injection of drug solution, consists of ***immediate*** *attention to the establishment and maintenance of a patent airway and effective assisted or controlled ventilation with 100% oxygen with a delivery system capable of permitting immediate positive airway pressure by mask.* This may prevent convulsions if they have not already occurred.

If necessary, use drugs to control the convulsions. A 50 to 100 mg bolus I.V. injection of succinylcholine will paralyze the patient without depressing the central nervous or cardiovascular systems and facilitate ventilation. A bolus I.V. dose of 5 to 10 mg of diazepam or 50 to 100 mg of thiopental will permit ventilation and counteract central nervous system stimulation, but these drugs also depress the central nervous system, respiratory and cardiac function, add to postictal depression, and may result in apnea. Intravenous barbiturates, anticonvulsant agents, or muscle relaxants should only be administered by those familiar with their use. Immediately after the institution of these ventilatory measures, the adequacy of the circulation should be evaluated. Supportive treatment of circulatory depression may require administration of intravenous fluids, and, when appropriate, a vasopressor dictated by the clinical situation (such as ephedrine or epinephrine to enhance myocardial contractile force).

If difficulty is encountered in the maintenance of a patent airway or if prolonged ventilatory support (assisted or controlled) is indicated, endotracheal intubation, employing drugs and techniques familiar to the clinician, may be indicated after initial administration of oxygen by mask.

Recent clinical data from patients experiencing local anesthetic induced convulsions demonstrated rapid development of hypoxia, hypercarbia, and acidosis with bupivacaine within a minute of the onset of convulsions. These observations suggest that oxygen consumption and carbon dioxide production are greatly increased during local anesthetic convulsions and emphasize the importance of immediate and effective ventilation with oxygen which may avoid cardiac arrest.

TABLE 1. DOSAGE RECOMMENDATIONS—SENSORCAINE (bupivacaine HCl) INJECTIONS

Type of Block	Conc.	Each Dose (mL)	Each Dose (mg)	Motor Block[1]
Local Infiltration	0.25%[4]	up to max.	up to max.	—
Epidural	0.75%[2,4]	10–20	75–150	complete
	0.5%[4]	10–20	50–100	moderate to complete
	0.25%[4]	10–20	25–50	partial to moderate
Caudal	0.5%[4]	15–30	75–150	moderate to complete
	0.25%[4]	15–30	37.5–75	moderate
Peripheral Nerves	0.5%[4]	5 to max.	25 to max.	moderate to complete
	0.25%[4]	5 to max.	12.5 to max.	moderate to complete
Retrobulbar[3]	0.75%[4]	2–4	15–30	complete
Sympathetic	0.25%	20–50	50–125	—
Epidural[3]	0.5%	2–3	10–15	—
Test Dose	w/epi		(See PRECAUTIONS)	

[1]With continuous (intermittent) techniques, repeat doses increase the degree of motor block. The first repeat dose of 0.5% may produce complete motor block. Intercostal nerve block with 0.25% may also produce complete motor block for intra-abdominal surgery.
[2]For single dose use, not for intermittent (catheter) epidural technique. Not for obstetric anesthesia.
[3]See PRECAUTIONS.
[4]Solutions with or without epinephrine.

Sensorcaine-MPF (methylparaben free) is available in the following forms:	
Single Dose Ampules:	
5 mL	0.5% with epinephrine 1:200,000
30 mL	0.25%, 0.5% and 0.75% without epinephrine
	0.5% and 0.75% with epinephrine 1:200,000
Single Dose Vials:	
10 mL with Astra E-Z Off® vial closure;	0.25%, 0.5% and 0.75% without epinephrine
	0.25%, 0.5% and 0.75% with epinephrine 1:200,000
30 mL	0.25%, 0.5% and 0.75% without epinephrine
	0.25%, 0.5% and 0.75% with epinephrine 1:200,000
Sensorcaine is available in the following forms:	
Multiple Dose Vials:	
50 mL	0.25% and 0.5% without epinephrine
	0.25% and 0.5% with epinephrine 1:200,000

If not treated immediately, convulsions with simultaneous hypoxia, hypercarbia and acidosis, plus myocardial depression from the direct effects of the local anesthetic may result in cardiac arrhythmias, bradycardia, asystole, ventricular fibrillation, or cardiac arrest. Respiratory abnormalities, including apnea, may occur. Underventilation or apnea due to unintentional subarachnoid injection of local anesthetic solution may produce these same signs and also lead to cardiac arrest if ventilatory support is not instituted. *If cardiac arrest should occur, a successful outcome may require prolonged resuscitative efforts.*

The supine position is dangerous in pregnant women at term because of aortocaval compression by the gravid uterus. Therefore, during treatment of systemic toxicity, maternal hypotension or fetal bradycardia following regional block, the parturient should be maintained in the left lateral decubitus position if possible, or manual displacement of the uterus off the great vessels be accomplished.

The mean seizure dosage of bupivacaine in rhesus monkeys was found to be 4.4 mg/kg with mean arterial plasma concentration of 4.5 mcg/mL. The intravenous and subcutaneous LD_{50} in mice is 6 to 8 mg/kg and 38 to 54 mg/kg respectively.

DOSAGE AND ADMINISTRATION

The dose of any local anesthetic administered varies with the anesthetic procedure, the area to be anesthetized, the vascularity of the tissues, the number of neuronal segments to be blocked, the depth of anesthesia and degree of muscle relaxation required, the duration of anesthesia desired, individual tolerance, and the physical condition of the patient. The smallest dose and concentration required to produce the desired result should be administered. Dosages of Sensorcaine should be reduced for young, elderly and debilitated patients and patients with cardiac and/or liver disease. The rapid injection of a large volume of local anesthetic solution should be avoided and fractional (incremental) doses should be used when feasible.

For specific techniques and procedures, refer to standard textbooks.

In recommended doses, Sensorcaine produces complete sensory block, but the effect on motor function differs among the three concentrations.

0.25%—when used for caudal, epidural, or peripheral nerve block, produces incomplete motor block. Should be used for operations in which muscle relaxation is not important, or when another means of providing muscle relaxation is used concurrently. Onset of action may be slower than with the 0.5% or 0.75% solutions.

0.5%—provides motor blockade for caudal, epidural, or nerve block, but muscle relaxation may be inadequate for operations in which complete muscle relaxation is essential.

0.75%—produces complete motor block. Most useful for epidural block in abdominal operations requiring complete muscle relaxation, and for retrobulbar anesthesia. Not for obstetrical anesthesia.

The duration of anesthesia with Sensorcaine is such that for most indications, a single dose is sufficient.

Maximum dosage limit must be individualized in each case after evaluating the size and physical status of the patient, as well as the usual rate of systemic absorption from a particular injection site. Most experience to date is with single doses of Sensorcaine up to 225 mg with epinephrine 1:200,000 and 175 mg without epinephrine; more or less drug may be used depending on individualization of each case.

These doses may be repeated up to once every three hours. In clinical studies to date, total daily doses up to 400 mg have been reported. Until further experience is gained, this dose should not be exceeded in 24 hours. The duration of anesthetic effect may be prolonged by the addition of epinephrine.

The dosages in Table 1 have generally proved satisfactory and are recommended as a guide for use in the average adult. These dosages should be reduced for young, elderly or debilitated patients. Until further experience is gained Sensorcaine is not recommended for children younger than 12 years. Sensorcaine is contraindicated for obstetrical paracervical blocks, and is not recommended for intravenous regional anesthesia (Bier Block).

Use in Epidural Anesthesia: During epidural administration of Sensorcaine, 0.5% and 0.75% solutions should be administered in incremental doses of 3 mL to 5 mL with sufficient time between doses to detect toxic manifestations of unintentional intravascular or intrathecal injection. In obstetrics, only the 0.5% and 0.25% concentrations should be used; incremental doses of 3 mL to 5 mL of the 0.5% solution not exceeding 50 mg to 100 mg at any dosing interval are recommended. Repeat doses should be preceded by a test dose containing epinephrine if not contraindicated. Use only the single dose ampules and single dose vials for caudal or epidural anesthesia; the multiple dose vials contain a preservative and therefore should not be used for these procedures.

Test dose for Caudal and Lumbar Epidural Blocks: See PRECAUTIONS.

Unused portions of solutions in single dose containers should be discarded, since this product form contains no preservatives.

[See table 1 above]

NOTE: Parenteral drug products should be inspected visually for particulate matter and discoloration prior to administration whenever the solution and container permit. The Injection is not to be used if its color is pinkish or darker than slightly yellow or if it contains a precipitate.

HOW SUPPLIED

SOLUTIONS OF SENSORCAINE (BUPIVACAINE HYDROCHLORIDE) SHOULD NOT BE USED FOR THE PRODUCTION OF SPINAL ANESTHESIA (SUBARACHNOID BLOCK) BECAUSE OF INSUFFICIENT DATA TO SUPPORT SUCH USE.

[See second table above]

Disinfecting agents containing heavy metals, which cause release of respective ions (mercury, zinc, copper, etc.), should not be used for skin or mucous membrane disinfection since they have been related to incidents of swelling and edema. When chemical disinfection of the container surface is desired, either isopropyl alcohol (91%) or ethyl alcohol (70%) is recommended. It is recommended that chem-

Continued on next page

Sensorcaine/Sensorcaine-MPF—Cont

ical disinfection be accomplished by wiping the ampule or vial stopper thoroughly with cotton or gauze that has been moistened with the recommended alcohol just prior to use. Solutions should be stored at controlled room temperature 15° to 30°C (59°–86°F).
Solutions containing epinephrine should be protected from light.
Caution: Federal law prohibits dispensing without prescription.
021680R03 Rev. 3/97
Shown in Product Identification Guide, page 305

SENSORCAINE®-MPF SPINAL INJECTION ℞

[*sén-sor-caine*]
(bupivacaine HCl in dextrose Injection, USP)
bupivacaine HCl 0.75% in dextrose 8.25% Injection
Sterile Hyperbaric Solution for Spinal Anesthesia

(For details of indications, dosage and administration, precautions, and adverse reactions, see circular in package.)

HOW SUPPLIED

NDC 0186-1026-03 2 mL ampule (15 mg bupivacaine HCl with 165 mg dextrose), boxes of 10.
Store at controlled room temperature, between 15°C and 30°C (59°F and 86°F).
021868R04 Rev. 5/97

STREPTASE® ℞

(Streptokinase)

DESCRIPTION

Streptase®, Streptokinase, is a sterile, purified preparation of a bacterial protein elaborated by group C β-hemolytic streptococci. It is supplied as a lyophilized white powder containing 25 mg cross-linked gelatin polypeptides, 25 mg sodium L-glutamate, sodium hydroxide to adjust pH, and 100 mg Albumin (Human) per vial or infusion bottle as stabilizers. The preparation contains no preservatives and is intended for intravenous and intracoronary administration.

CLINICAL PHARMACOLOGY

Streptase, Streptokinase, acts with plasminogen to produce an "activator complex" that converts plasminogen to the proteolytic enzyme plasmin. The $t_{1/2}$ of the activator complex is about 23 minutes; the complex is inactivated, in part, by antistreptococcal antibodies. The mechanism by which dissociated streptokinase is eliminated is clearance by sites in the liver; however, no metabolites of streptokinase have been identified. Plasmin degrades fibrin clots as well as fibrinogen and other plasma proteins. Plasmin is inactivated by circulating inhibitors, such as α-2-plasmin inhibitor or α-2-macroglobulin. These inhibitors are rapidly consumed at high doses of streptokinase.
Intravenous infusion of Streptokinase is followed by increased fibrinolytic activity, which decreases plasma fibrinogen levels for 24 to 36 hours. The decrease in plasma fibrinogen is associated with decreases in plasma and blood viscosity and red blood cell aggregation. The hyperfibrinolytic effect disappears within a few hours after discontinuation, but a prolonged thrombin time may persist for up to 24 hours due to the decrease in plasma levels of fibrinogen and an increase in the amount of circulating fibrin(ogen) degradation products (FDP). Depending upon the dosage and duration of infusion of Streptokinase, the thrombin time will decrease to less than two times the normal control value within 4 hours, and return to normal by 24 hours.
Intravenous administration has been shown to reduce blood pressure and total peripheral resistance with a corresponding reduction in cardiac afterload. These expected responses were not studied with the intracoronary administration of Streptase, Streptokinase. The quantitative benefit has not been evaluated.
Variable amounts of circulating antistreptokinase antibody are present in individuals as a result of recent streptococcal infections. The recommended dosage schedule usually obviates the need for antibody titration.
Two very large, randomized, placebo-controlled studies[1,2] involving almost 30,000 patients have demonstrated that a 60-minute intravenous infusion of 1,500,000 IU of Streptokinase significantly reduces mortality following a myocardial infarction. One of these studies also evaluated concomitant oral administration of low dose aspirin (160 mg/d over one month).
In the GISSI study the reduction in mortality was time dependent. There was a 47% reduction in mortality among patients treated within one hour of the onset of chest pain, a 23% reduction among patients treated within three hours, and a 17% reduction among patients treated between three and six hours. There was also a reduction in mortality in patients treated between six and twelve hours from the onset of symptoms, but the reduction was not statistically significant.
In the ISIS-2 study the reduction in mortality was also time dependent. If Streptokinase and aspirin were administered within the first hour after symptom onset, the reduction in mortality was 44%. The reduction in the odds of death in patients treated within four hours was 53% for the combination of Streptokinase and aspirin, and 35% for Streptokinase alone. However, the reduction was still significant when treatment was started 5–24 hours after symptom onset: 33% for the combined therapy and 17% for Streptokinase alone. Overall, in the 0–24 hour time period there was a 42% reduction in the odds of death with combined treatment (Streptokinase and aspirin) versus placebo ($2p<0.00001$) and a 25% reduction in the odds of death with Streptokinase alone versus placebo ($2p<0.00001$).
One of eight smaller studies using a similar dosing schedule showed a statistically significant reduction in mortality. When all of these studies were pooled, the overall decrease in mortality was approximately 23%. Results from pooling several studies using different dosages with long term infusion corroborate these observations.
In addition, studies measuring left ventricular ejection fraction (LVEF) at discharge showed the mean LVEFs were 3–6 percentage points higher in the Streptokinase group than in the control group. This difference was statistically significant in some of the studies[3,4]. Furthermore, some studies reported greater improvement in LVEF among patients treated within three hours than in patients treated later.
Results from a randomized controlled trial in over 11,000 patients show that, following treatment with IV Streptokinase, there is a reduction in the number of patients with clinical congestive heart failure during the 14–21 day in-hospital period. Clinical congestive heart failure occurred in 12.8% of Streptokinase-treated patients compared with 15% of the control patients ($p=0.001$)[1].
The rate of reocclusion of the infarct-related vessel has been reported to be approximately 15–20%. The rate of reocclusion depends on dosage, additional anticoagulant therapy and residual stenosis. When the reinfarctions were evaluated in studies involving 8800 Streptokinase-treated patients, the overall rate was 3.8% (range 2–15%). In over 8500 control patients, the rate of reinfarction was 2.4%. However, the ISIS-2 study showed that an increase in reinfarction was avoided when Streptokinase was combined with low dose aspirin. The rate of reinfarction in the combination group was 1.8% vs. 1.9% in the group given aspirin alone.
Streptase, Streptokinase, administered by the intracoronary route has resulted in thrombolysis usually within one hour, and ensuing reperfusion results in improvement of cardiac function and reduction of mortality[5,6]. LVEF was increased in patients treated with Streptokinase when compared to patients treated with conventional therapy. When the initial LVEF was low, the Streptokinase-treated patients showed greater improvement than did the controls.
Spontaneous reperfusion is known to occur and has been observed with angiography at various time points after infarction. Data from one study show that 73% of Streptokinase-treated patients and 47% of the placebo-allocated patients reperfused during hospitalization. The relationship between coronary artery patency and clinical efficacy has not been established.
Studies with thrombolytic therapy for pulmonary embolism show no significant difference in lung perfusion scan between the thrombolysis group and the heparin group at one-year follow-up. However, measurements of pulmonary capillary blood volumes and diffusing capacities at two weeks and one year after therapy indicate that a more complete resolution of thrombotic obstruction and normalization of pulmonary physiology was achieved with thrombolytic therapy, thus preventing the long term sequelae of pulmonary hypertension and pulmonary failure[7].
The long term benefit of Streptase, Streptokinase, therapy for deep vein thrombosis (DVT) has been evaluated venographically[8]. The combined results of five randomized studies show no residual thrombotic material in 60-75% of patients treated with Streptokinase versus only 10% of those treated with heparin. Thrombolytic therapy also preserves venous valve function in a majority of cases, thus avoiding the pathologic venous changes that produce the clinical post-phlebitic syndrome which occurs in 90% of the DVT patients treated with heparin.
There is a time-related decrease in effectiveness when Streptase, Streptokinase, is used in the management of peripheral arterial thromboembolism. When administered three to ten days after onset of obstruction, rates of clearance of 50–75% were reported.

INDICATIONS AND USAGE

Acute Evolving Transmural Myocardial Infarction: Streptase, Streptokinase, is indicated for use in the management of acute myocardial infarction (AMI) in adults, for the lysis of intracoronary thrombi, the improvement of ventricular function, and the reduction of mortality associated with AMI, when administered by either the intravenous or the intracoronary route, as well as for the reduction of infarct size and congestive heart failure associated with AMI when administered by the intravenous route. Earlier administration of Streptokinase is correlated with greater clinical benefit. (See CLINICAL PHARMACOLOGY.)
Pulmonary Embolism: Streptase, Streptokinase, is indicated for the lysis of objectively diagnosed (angiography or lung scan) pulmonary emboli, involving obstruction of blood flow to a lobe or multiple segments, with or without unstable hemodynamics.
Deep Vein Thrombosis: Streptase, Streptokinase, is indicated for the lysis of objectively diagnosed (preferably ascending venography), acute, extensive thrombi of the deep veins such as those involving the popliteal and more proximal vessels.
Arterial Thrombosis or Embolism: Streptase, Streptokinase, is indicated for the lysis of acute arterial thrombi and emboli. Streptokinase is not indicated for arterial emboli originating from the left side of the heart due to the risk of new embolic phenomena such as cerebral embolism.
Occlusion of Arteriovenous Cannulae: Streptase, Streptokinase, is indicated as an alternative to surgical revision for clearing totally or partially occluded arteriovenous cannulae when acceptable flow cannot be achieved.

CONTRAINDICATIONS

Because thrombolytic therapy increases the risk of bleeding, Streptase, Streptokinase, is contraindicated in the following situations:

- active internal bleeding
- recent (within 2 months) cerebrovascular accident, intracranial or intraspinal surgery (see WARNINGS)
- intracranial neoplasm
- severe uncontrolled hypertension

Streptokinase should not be administered to patients having experienced severe allergic reaction to the product.

WARNINGS

Bleeding: Following intravenous high-dose brief-duration Streptokinase therapy in acute myocardial infarction, severe bleeding complications requiring transfusion are extremely rare (0.3–0.5%), and combined therapy with low dose aspirin does not appear to increase the risk of major bleeding. The addition of aspirin to Streptokinase may cause a slight increase in the risk of minor bleeding (3.1% without aspirin vs. 3.9% with)[2].
Streptokinase will cause lysis of hemostatic fibrin deposits such as those occurring at sites of needle punctures, particularly when infused over several hours, and bleeding may occur from such sites. In order to minimize the risk of bleeding during treatment with Streptokinase, venipunctures and physical handling of the patient should be performed carefully and as infrequently as possible, and intramuscular injections must be avoided.
Should an arterial puncture be necessary during intravenous therapy, upper extremity vessels are preferable. Pressure should be applied for at least 30 minutes, a pressure dressing applied, and the puncture site checked frequently for evidence of bleeding.
In the following conditions the risks of therapy may be increased and should be weighed against the anticipated benefits.

- Recent (within 10 days) major surgery, obstetrical delivery, organ biopsy, previous puncture of noncompressible vessels
- Recent (within 10 days) serious gastrointestinal bleeding
- Recent (within 10 days) trauma including cardiopulmonary resuscitation
- Hypertension: systolic BP >180 mm Hg and/or diastolic BP >110 mm Hg
- High likelihood of left heart thrombus, e.g., mitral stenosis with atrial fibrillation
- Subacute bacterial endocarditis
- Hemostatic defects including those secondary to severe hepatic or renal disease
- Pregnancy
- Age >75 years
- Cerebrovascular disease
- Diabetic hemorrhagic retinopathy
- Septic thrombophlebitis or occluded AV cannula at seriously infected site
- Any other condition in which bleeding constitutes a significant hazard or would be particularly difficult to manage because of its location.

Should serious spontaneous bleeding (not controllable by local pressure) occur, the infusion of Streptase, Streptokinase, should be terminated immediately and treatment instituted as described under ADVERSE REACTIONS.
Bleeding into the pericardium, sometimes associated with myocardial rupture, has been seen in individual cases and has resulted in fatalities.
Arrhythmias: Rapid lysis of coronary thrombi has been shown to cause reperfusion atrial or ventricular dysrhythmias requiring immediate treatment. Careful monitoring for arrhythmia is recommended during and immediately following administration of Streptase, Streptokinase, for acute myocardial infarction. Occasionally, tachycardia and bradycardia have been observed.
Hypotension: Hypotension, sometimes severe, not secondary to bleeding or anaphylaxis has been observed during intravenous Streptase, Streptokinase, infusion in 1% to 10% of patients. Patients should be monitored closely and, should symptomatic or alarming hypotension occur, appropriate treatment should be administered. This treatment may include a decrease in the intravenous Streptokinase infusion rate. Smaller hypotensive effects are common and have not required treatment.
Cholesterol Embolism: Cholesterol embolism has been reported rarely in patients treated with all types of thrombolytic agents; the true incidence is unknown. This serious condition, which can be lethal, is also associated with invasive vascular procedures (e.g., cardiac catheterization, angiography, vascular surgery) and/or anticoagulant therapy. Clinical features of cholesterol embolism may include livedo reticularis, "purple toe" syndrome, acute renal failure, gangrenous digits, hypertension, pancreatitis, myocardial infarction, cerebral infarction, spinal cord infarction, retinal artery occlusion, bowel infarction, and rhabdomyolysis.

Other: Non-cardiogenic pulmonary edema has been reported rarely in patients treated with Streptase, Streptokinase. The risk of this appears greatest in patients who have large myocardial infarctions and are undergoing thrombolytic therapy by the intracoronary route.
Rarely, polyneuropathy has been temporally related to the use of Streptase, Streptokinase, with some cases described as Guillain Barré Syndrome.
Should pulmonary embolism or recurrent pulmonary embolism occur during Streptase, Streptokinase, therapy, the originally planned course of treatment should be completed in an attempt to lyse the embolus. While pulmonary embolism may occasionally occur during Streptokinase treatment, the incidence is no greater than when patients are treated with heparin alone. In addition to pulmonary embolism, embolization to other sites during Streptase treatment, has been observed.

PRECAUTIONS

General: There have been rare cases where Streptase, Streptokinase, has been administered for suspected AMI subsequently diagnosed as pancreatitis. Fatalities have occurred under these circumstances.
Repeated Administration — Because of the increased likelihood of resistance due to antistreptokinase antibody, Streptase, Streptokinase, may not be effective if administered between five days and twelve months of prior Streptokinase or Anistreplase administration, or streptococcal infections, such as streptococcal pharyngitis, acute rheumatic fever, or acute glomerulonephritis secondary to a streptococcal infection.

Laboratory Tests

Intravenous or Intracoronary Infusion for Myocardial Infarction — Intravenous administration of Streptase, Streptokinase, will cause marked decreases in plasminogen and fibrinogen and increases in thrombin time (TT), activated partial thromboplastin time (APTT), and prothrombin time (PT), which usually normalize within 12–24 hours. These changes may also occur in some patients with intracoronary administration of Streptokinase.
Intravenous Infusion for Other Indications — Before commencing thrombolytic therapy, it is desirable to obtain an activated partial thromboplastin time (APTT), a prothrombin time (PT), a thrombin time (TT), or fibrinogen levels, and a hematocrit and platelet count. If heparin has been given, it should be discontinued and the TT or APTT should be less than twice the normal control value before thrombolytic therapy is started.
During the infusion, decreases in plasminogen and fibrinogen levels and an increase in the level of FDP (the latter two causing a prolongation in the clotting times of coagulation tests) will generally confirm the existence of a lytic state. Therefore, lytic therapy can be confirmed by performing the TT, APTT, PT, or fibrinogen levels approximately 4 hours after initiation of therapy. If heparin is to be (re)instituted following the Streptase, Streptokinase, infusion, the TT or APTT should be less than twice the normal control value (see manufacturer's prescribing information for proper use of heparin).

Drug Interactions: The interaction of Streptase, Streptokinase, with other drugs has not been well studied.
Use of Anticoagulants and Antiplatelet Agents — Streptase, Streptokinase, alone or in combination with antiplatelet agents and anticoagulants, may cause bleeding complications. Therefore, careful monitoring is advised. In the treatment of acute MI, aspirin, when not otherwise contraindicated, should be administered with Streptokinase (*see below*).
Anticoagulation and Antiplatelets After Treatment for Myocardial Infarction — In the treatment of acute myocardial infarction, the use of aspirin has been shown to reduce the incidence of reinfarction and stroke. The addition of aspirin to Streptokinase causes a minimal increase in the risk of minor bleeding (3.9% vs. 3.1%), but does not appear to increase the incidence of major bleeding (see ADVERSE REACTIONS)[2]. The use of anticoagulants following administration of Streptokinase increases the risk of bleeding, but has not yet been shown to be of unequivocal clinical benefit. Therefore, whereas the use of aspirin is recommended unless otherwise contraindicated, the use of anticoagulants should be decided by the treating physician.
Anticoagulation After IV Treatment for Other Indications — Continuous intravenous infusion of heparin, without a loading dose, has been recommended following termination of Streptase, Streptokinase, infusion for treatment of pulmonary embolism or deep vein thrombosis to prevent rethrombosis. The effect of Streptokinase on thrombin time (TT) and activated partial thromboplastin time (APTT) will usually diminish within 3 to 4 hours after Streptokinase therapy, and heparin therapy without a loading dose can be initiated when the TT or the APTT is less than twice the normal control value.

Pregnancy

Pregnancy Category C — Animal reproduction studies have not been conducted with Streptase, Streptokinase. It is also not known whether Streptokinase can cause fetal harm when administered to a pregnant woman or can affect reproduction capacity. Streptokinase should be given to a pregnant woman only if clearly needed.

Pediatric Use: Controlled clinical studies have not been conducted in children to determine safety and efficacy in the pediatric population. The evidence of clinical benefits and risks is solely based on anecdotal reports in patients ranging in age from <1 month to 16 years. The largest number of patient reports have pertained to the use of streptokinase in arterial occlusions. For arterial occlusions the most frequently used loading dose was 1000 IU/kg; fewer numbers of patients received 3000 IU/kg. Loading dose durations have typically ranged from 5 minutes to 30 minutes. Continuous infusion doses were frequently 1000 IU/kg/hr; fewer were at 1500 IU/kg/hr. Infusions were maintained for ≤ 12 hours in approximately half of the published cases; a smaller proportion were between 12 hours and 24 hours. Reported adverse events associated with the use of streptokinase in the pediatric population are similar in nature to those associated with its use in adults. Rates of all bleeding complications have been variable, and as high as 50% at catheter sites in some studies. Occasionally bleeding has required transfusion. Careful monitoring of patient status is necessary.

TABLE 1
SUGGESTED DILUTIONS AND INFUSION RATES

Dosage	Vial Size (IU)	Total Solution Volume	Infusion Rate
1. Acute Myocardial Infarction			
A. Intravenous Infusion	1,500,000	45 mL	Infuse 45 mL within 60 min.
B. Intracoronary Infusion	250,000	125 mL	
1. 20,000 IU bolus			1. Loading Dose of 10 mL
2. 2,000 IU/minute for 60 minutes			2. Then 60 mL/hour
II. Pulmonary Embolism, Deep Vein Thrombosis, Arterial Thrombosis or Embolism			
Intravenous Infusion			
A. 1. 250,000 IU loading dose over 30 minutes	1,500,000	90 mL	1. Infuse 30 mL/hour for 30 minutes
2. 100,000 IU/hour maintenance dose			2. Infuse 6 mL per hour
B. SAME	1,500,000 infusion bottle	45 mL	1. 15 mL/hour for 30 minutes 2. Infuse 3 mL per hour

ADVERSE REACTIONS

The following adverse reactions have been associated with intravenous therapy and may also occur with intracoronary artery infusion:

Bleeding: The reported incidence of bleeding (major or minor) has varied widely depending on the indication, dose, route and duration of administration, and concomitant therapy.
Minor bleeding can be anticipated mainly at invaded or disturbed sites. If such bleeding occurs, local measures should be taken to control the bleeding.
Severe internal bleeding involving gastrointestinal (including hepatic bleeding), genitourinary, retroperitoneal, or intracerebral sites has occurred and has resulted in fatalities. In the treatment of acute myocardial infarction with intravenous Streptokinase, the GISSI and ISIS-2 studies reported a rate of major bleeding (requiring transfusion) of 0.3–0.5%. However, rates as high as 16% have been reported in studies which required administration of anticoagulants and invasive procedures.
Major bleed rates are difficult to determine for other dosages and patient populations because of the different dosing and intervals of infusions. The rates reported appear to be within the ranges reported for intravenous administration in acute myocardial infarction.
Should uncontrollable bleeding occur, Streptokinase infusion should be terminated immediately, rather than slowing the rate of administration of or reducing the dose of Streptokinase. If necessary, bleeding can be reversed and blood loss effectively managed with appropriate replacement therapy. Although the use of aminocaproic acid in humans as an antidote for Streptokinase has not been documented, it may be considered in an emergency situation.

Allergic Reactions: Fever and shivering, occurring in 1–4% of patients[1,2], are the most commonly reported allergic reactions with intravenous use of Streptase, Streptokinase, in acute myocardial infarction. Anaphylactic and anaphylactoid reactions ranging in severity from minor breathing difficulty to bronchospasm, periorbital swelling or angioneurotic edema have been observed rarely. Other milder allergic effects such as urticaria, itching, flushing, nausea, headache and musculoskeletal pain have also been observed, as have delayed hypersensitivity reactions such as vasculitis and interstitial nephritis. Anaphylactic shock is very rare, having been reported in 0–0.1% of patients[1,2,4].
Mild or moderate allergic reactions may be managed with concomitant antihistamine and/or corticosteroid therapy. Severe allergic reactions require immediate discontinuation of Streptase, Streptokinase, with adrenergic, antihistamine, and/or corticosteroid agents administered intravenously as required.

Respiratory: There have been reports of respiratory depression in patients receiving Streptokinase. In some cases, it was not possible to determine whether the respiratory depression was associated with Streptokinase or was a symptom of the underlying process. If respiratory depression is associated with Streptokinase, the occurrence is believed to be rare.

Other Adverse Reactions: Transient elevations of serum transaminases have been observed. The source of these enzyme rises and their clinical significance is not fully understood.
There have been reports in the literature of cases of back pain associated with the use of Streptokinase. In most cases the pain developed during Streptokinase intravenous infusion and ceased within minutes of discontinuation of the infusion.

DOSAGE AND ADMINISTRATION

Acute Evolving Transmural Myocardial Infarction: Administer Streptokinase as soon as possible after onset of symptoms. The greatest benefit in mortality reduction was observed when Streptokinase was administered within four hours, but statistically significant benefit has been reported up to 24 hours (see CLINICAL PHARMACOLOGY).

Route	Total Dose	Dosage/Duration
Intravenous infusion	1,500,000 IU	1,500,000 IU within 60 min.
Intracoronary infusion	140,000 IU	20,000 IU by bolus followed by 2,000 IU/min. for 60 min.

Pulmonary Embolism, Deep Vein Thrombosis, Arterial Thrombosis or Embolism: Streptase, Streptokinase, treatment should be instituted as soon as possible after onset of the thrombotic event, preferably within 7 days. Any delay in instituting lytic therapy to evaluate the effect of heparin therapy decreases the potential for optimal efficacy. Since human exposure to streptococci is common, antibodies to Streptokinase are prevalent. Thus, a loading dose of Streptokinase sufficient to neutralize these antibodies is required. A dose of 250,000 IU of Streptokinase infused into a peripheral vein over 30 minutes has been found appropriate in over 90% of patients. Furthermore, if the thrombin time or any other parameter of lysis after 4 hours of therapy is not significantly different from the normal control level, discontinue Streptokinase because excessive resistance is present.

Indication	Loading Dose	IV Infusion Dosage/Duration
Pulmonary Embolism	250,000 IU/30 min.	100,000 IU/hr for 24 hr (72 hrs if concurrent DVT is suspected).
Deep Vein Thrombosis	250,000 IU/30 min.	100,000 IU/hr for 72 hr
Arterial Thrombosis or Embolism	250,000 IU/30 min.	100,000 IU/hr for 24–72 hr

Arteriovenous Cannulae Occlusion: Before using Streptase, Streptokinase, an attempt should be made to clear the cannula by careful syringe technique, using heparinized saline solution. If adequate flow is not re-established, Streptokinase may be employed. Allow the effect of any pretreatment anticoagulants to diminish. Instill 250,000 IU Streptokinase in 2 mL of solution into each occluded limb of the cannula slowly. Clamp off cannula limb(s) for 2 hours. Observe the patient closely for possible adverse effects. After treatment, aspirate contents of infused cannula limb(s), flush with saline, reconnect cannula.

Pediatric Patients: Specific dosage and administration recommendations cannot be made based on the limited data available. However, published experience generally used loading and continuous infusion doses administered on a weight-adjusted basis. See Precautions, Pediatric Use.

Reconstitution and Dilution: The protein nature and lyophilized form of Streptase, Streptokinase, require careful reconstitution and dilution. Slight flocculation (described as thin translucent fibers) of reconstituted Streptokinase occurred occasionally during clinical trials but did not interfere with the safe use of the solution. The following reconstitution and dilution procedures are recommended:

Vials and Infusion Bottles

1. Slowly add 5 mL Sodium Chloride Injection, USP or 5% Dextrose Injection, USP to the Streptase, Streptokinase, vial, directing the diluent at the side of the vacuum-packed vial rather than into the drug powder.
2. Roll and tilt the vial gently to reconstitute. Avoid shaking. (Shaking may cause foaming.) (If necessary, total volume may be increased to a maximum of 500 mL in glass or 50 mL in plastic containers, and the infusion pump rate in Table 1 should be adjusted accordingly.) To facilitate setting the infusion pump rate, a total volume of 45 mL, or a multiple thereof, is recommended.
3. Withdraw the entire reconstituted contents of the vial; slowly and carefully dilute further to a total volume as recommended in Table 1. Avoid shaking and agitation on dilution.
4. When diluting the 1,500,000 IU infusion bottle (50 mL), slowly add 5 mL Sodium Chloride Injection,

Continued on next page

Streptase—Cont.

USP, or 5% Dextrose Injection, USP, directing it at the side of the bottle rather than into the drug powder. Roll and tilt the bottle gently to reconstitute. Avoid shaking as it may cause foaming. Add an additional 40 mL of diluent to the bottle, avoiding shaking and agitation. (Total volume = 45 mL). Administer by infusion pump at the rate indicated in Table 1.

5. Parenteral drug products should be inspected visually for particulate matter and discoloration prior to administration. (The Albumin (Human) may impart a slightly yellow color to the solution.)
6. The reconstituted solution can be filtered through a 0.8 μm or larger pore size filter.
7. Because Streptase, Streptokinase, contains no preservatives, it should be reconstituted immediately before use. The solution may be used for direct intravenous administration within eight hours following reconstitution if stored at 2–8°C (36–46°F).
8. Do not add other medication to the container of Streptase, Streptokinase.
9. Unused reconstituted drug should be discarded.

[See table 1 at top of previous page]

For Use In Arteriovenous Cannulae: Slowly reconstitute the contents of 250,000 IU Streptase, Streptokinase, vacuum-packed vial with 2 mL Sodium Chloride Injection, USP or 5% Dextrose Injection, USP.

HOW SUPPLIED

Streptase, Streptokinase, is supplied as a lyophilized white powder in 50 mL infusion bottles (1,500,000 IU) or in 6.5 mL vials with a color-coded label corresponding to the amount of purified Streptokinase in each vial as follows:

green	250,000 IU	NDC 0186-1770-01	box of 1
blue	750,000 IU	NDC 0186-1771-01	box of 1
red	1,500,000 IU	NDC 0186-1773-01	box of 1 (vials)
red	1,500,000 IU	NDC 0186-1774-01	box of 1 (infusion bottles)

Store unopened vials at controlled room temperature (15–30°C or 59–86°F).

REFERENCES

1. GISSI: Effectiveness of intravenous thrombolytic treatment in acute myocardial infarction. Lancet I: 397-402, 1986.
2. ISIS-2 Collaborative Group: Randomized trial of streptokinase, oral aspirin, both, or neither among 17,187 cases of suspected acute myocardial infarction: ISIS-2. Lancet II:349-360, 1988.
3. White, H., Norris, R., Brown, M., et al: Effect of intravenous streptokinase on left ventricular function and early survival after acute myocardial infarction. N Engl J Med 317: 850-5, 1987.
4. The I.S.A.M. Study Group: A prospective trial of intravenous streptokinase in acute myocardial infarction (I.S.A.M.). N Engl J Med 314: 1465-1471, 1986.
5. Anderson, J., Marshall, H., Bray, B., et al: A randomized trial of intracoronary streptokinase in the treatment of acute myocardial infarction. N Engl J Med 308: 1312-8, 1983.
6. Kennedy, J., Ritchie, J., Davis, K., Fritz, J.: Western Washington randomized trial of intracoronary streptokinase in acute myocardial infarction. N Engl J Med 309: 1477-82, 1983.
7. Sharma, G., Burleson, V., Sasahara, A.: Effect of thrombolytic therapy on pulmonary-capillary blood volume in patients with pulmonary embolism. N Engl J Med 303: 842-5, 1980.
8. Arnesen, H., Heilo, A., Jakobsen, E., et al: A prospective study of streptokinase and heparin in the treatment of venous thrombosis. Acta Med Scand 203: 457-463, 1978.

Manufactured by Hoechst Marion Roussel Deutschland GmbH in Marburg/Lahn, Germany US License No. 1232
Distributed by Astra USA, Inc., Westborough, MA 01581
021596R11 (Revised 9/98)

TABLETS
TONOCARD® ℞
(tocainide HCl)

WARNINGS

Blood Dyscrasias: Agranulocytosis, bone marrow depression, leukopenia, neutropenia, aplastic/hypoplastic anemia, thrombocytopenia and sequelae such as septicemia and septic shock have been reported in patients receiving TONOCARD. Most of these patients received TONOCARD within the recommended dosage range. Fatalities have occurred (with approximately 25% mortality in reported agranulocytosis cases). Since most of these events have been noted during the first 12 weeks of therapy, it is recommended that complete blood counts, including white cell, differential and platelet counts be performed, optimally, at weekly intervals for the first 3 months of therapy; and frequently thereafter. Complete blood counts should be performed promptly if the patient develops any signs of infection (such as fever, chills, sore throat, or stomatitis), bruising, or bleeding. If any of these hematologic disorders is identified, TONOCARD should be discontinued and appropriate treatment should be instituted if necessary. Blood counts usually return to normal within 1 month of discontinuation. Caution should be used in patients with pre-existing marrow failure or cytopenia of any type. (See ADVERSE REACTIONS.)

Pulmonary Fibrosis: Pulmonary fibrosis, interstitial pneumonitis, fibrosing alveolitis, pulmonary edema, and pneumonia have been reported in patients receiving TONOCARD. Many of these events occurred in patients who were seriously ill. Fatalities have been reported. The experiences are usually characterized by bilateral infiltrates on x-ray and are frequently associated with dyspnea and cough. Fever may or may not be present. Patients should be instructed to promptly report the development of any pulmonary symptoms such as exertional dyspnea, cough or wheezing. Chest x-rays are advisable at that time. If these pulmonary disorders develop, TONOCARD should be discontinued. (See ADVERSE REACTIONS.)

DESCRIPTION

TONOCARD* (tocainide HCl) is a primary amine analog of lidocaine with antiarrhythmic properties useful in the treatment of ventricular arrhythmias. The chemical name for tocainide hydrochloride is 2-amino-*N*-(2,6-dimethylphenyl) propanamide hydrochloride. Its empirical formula is $C_{11}H_{16}N_2O \bullet HCl$, with a molecular weight of 228.72. The structural formula is:

CH_3
—$NHCOCHCH_3 \cdot HCl$
NH_2
CH_3

Tocainide hydrochloride is a white crystalline powder with a bitter taste and is freely soluble in water. It is supplied as 400 mg and 600 mg tablets for oral administration. Each tablet contains the following inactive ingredients: hydroxypropyl methylcellulose, iron oxide, magnesium stearate, methylcellulose, polyethylene glycol, and titanium dioxide.

*Registered trademark of Astra Pharmaceuticals, L.P.

CLINICAL PHARMACOLOGY

Action: Tocainide, like lidocaine, produces dose dependent decreases in sodium and potassium conductance, thereby decreasing the excitability of myocardial cells. In experimental animal models, the dose-related depression of sodium current is more pronounced in ischemic tissue than in normal tissue.

Electrophysiology: Tocainide is a Class I antiarrhythmic compound with electrophysiologic properties in man similar to those of lidocaine, but dissimilar from quinidine, procainamide, and disopyramide.

In studies of isolated dog Purkinje fibers, tocainide in concentrations of 1–50 mcg/mL had no significant effect on resting membrane potential, but reduced the amplitude and rate of depolarization (dv/dt) of the action potential. Tocainide decreased the effective refractory period (ERP) to a lesser extent than the action potential duration (APD) resulting in an increase in the ERP/APD ratio.

In patients with cardiac disease, TONOCARD produced no clinically significant changes in sinus nodal function, effective refractory periods, or intracardiac conduction times when studied under electrophysiologic testing procedures.

Tocainide, like lidocaine, characteristically does not prolong ventricular depolarization (QRS duration) or repolarization (QT intervals) as measured by electrocardiography. Theoretically, therefore, TONOCARD may be useful in the treatment of ventricular arrhythmias associated with a prolonged QT interval.

Patients who respond to lidocaine also respond to TONOCARD in a majority of cases. Failure to respond to lidocaine usually predicts failure to respond to TONOCARD, but there are exceptions to this.

In a controlled comparison with quinidine, 600 mg b.i.d. of TONOCARD produced a mean reduction of 42% in PVC count, compared to a 54% reduction by quinidine 300 mg every 6 hours. Among all patients entered into the study, about one-fifth of tocainide recipients and one-third of quinidine recipients had 75% or greater reductions in PVC count or had elimination of ventricular tachycardia.

Pharmacokinetics: Following oral administration of tocainide, peak plasma concentrations occur within 0.5 to 2 hours. The average plasma half-life in patients is approximately 15 hours. Although the effective plasma concentration may vary from patient to patient, the usual therapeutic plasma range (as defined by 50–80% PVC suppression) is 4–10 mcg/mL (18–45 micromole/L), expressed as tocainide hydrochloride. Tocainide is approximately 10% bound to plasma protein.

In contrast to lidocaine, tocainide undergoes negligible first pass hepatic degradation. Following oral administration, the bioavailability of TONOCARD approaches 100%. The extent of its bioavailability is unaffected by food. Tocainide has no cardioactive metabolites. Approximately 40% of the administered dose of tocainide is excreted unchanged in the urine. Acidification of the urine has not been shown to significantly alter tocainide excretion in the urine, but alkalinization of the urine results in a significant decrease in the percent of tocainide excreted unchanged in the urine. Animal data indicate that tocainide crosses the blood-brain barrier; however, it has less lipid solubility than lidocaine.

Hemodynamics: Cardiac catheterization studies in man utilizing intravenous tocainide infusions (0.5–0.75 mg/kg/min over 15 min) have shown that tocainide usually produces a small degree of depression of parameters of left ventricular function, such as left ventricular dP/dt, and left ventricular end diastolic pressure. There were usually no changes in cardiac output or clinical evidence of increasing congestive heart failure in the well-compensated patients studied. Small but statistically significant increases in aortic and pulmonary arterial pressures have been consistently observed and are probably related to small increases in vascular resistance. When used concomitantly with a beta-blocking drug, tocainide further reduced cardiac index and left ventricular dP/dt and further increased pulmonary wedge pressure.

No clinically significant changes in heart rate, blood pressure, or signs of myocardial depression were observed in a study of 72 post-myocardial infarction patients receiving long-term therapy with oral TONOCARD at usual doses (400 mg q8h). When tocainide was administered orally at a dose of 120 mg/kg to anesthetized dogs (14 times the initial maximum dose recommended for humans), a negative inotropic effect was observed: the rate of change of left ventricular pressure decreased by up to 29% of control at 3 hours after administration. This effect was not observed at lower doses (60 mg/kg). Tocainide has been used safely in patients with acute myocardial infarction and various degrees of congestive heart failure. It has, however, a small negative inotropic effect and can increase peripheral resistance slightly. It therefore should be used cautiously in patients with known heart failure, particularly if a beta blocker is given as well. (See PRECAUTIONS.)

INDICATIONS AND USAGE

TONOCARD is indicated for the treatment of documented ventricular arrhythmias, such as sustained ventricular tachycardia, that, in the judgment of the physician, are life-threatening. Because of the proarrhythmic effects of TONOCARD, as well as its potential for other serious adverse effects, (see WARNINGS), its use to treat lesser arrhythmias is not recommended. Treatment of patients with asymptomatic ventricular premature contractions should be avoided.

Initiation of treatment with TONOCARD, as with other antiarrhythmic agents used to treat life-threatening arrhythmias, should be carried out in the hospital. It is essential that each patient given TONOCARD be evaluated electrocardiographically and clinically prior to, and during, therapy with TONOCARD to determine whether the response to TONOCARD supports continued treatment.

Antiarrhythmic drugs have not been shown to enhance survival in patients with ventricular arrhythmias.

CONTRAINDICATIONS

Patients who are hypersensitive to this product or to local anesthetics of the amide type.

Patients with second or third degree atrioventricular block in the absence of an artificial ventricular pacemaker.

WARNINGS

Mortality: **In the National Heart, Lung and Blood Institute's Cardiac Arrhythmia Suppression Trial (CAST), a long-term, multi-center, randomized, double-blind study in patients with asymptomatic non-life-threatening ventricular arrhythmias who had a myocardial infarction more than 6 days but less than 2 years previously, an excessive mortality or non-fatal cardiac arrest rate (7.7%) was seen in patients treated with encainide or flecainide compared with that seen in patients assigned to carefully matched placebo-treated groups (3.0%). The average duration of treatment with encainide or flecainide in this study was 10 months.**

The applicability of the CAST results to other populations (e.g., those without recent myocardial infarction) is uncertain. Considering the known proarrhythmic properties of TONOCARD (tocainide HCl) and the lack of evidence of improved survival for any antiarrhythmic drug in patients without life-threatening arrhythmias, the use of TONOCARD as well as other antiarrhythmic agents should be reserved for patients with life-threatening ventricular arrhythmias.

Acceleration of Ventricular Rate: Acceleration of ventricular rate occurs infrequently when antiarrhythmics are administered to patients with atrial flutter or fibrillation (see ADVERSE REACTIONS).

PRECAUTIONS

General: In patients with known heart failure or minimal cardiac reserve, TONOCARD should be used with caution because of the potential for aggravating the degree of heart failure.

Caution should be used in the institution or continuation of antiarrhythmic therapy in the presence of signs of increasing depression of cardiac conductivity.

In patients with severe liver or kidney disease, the rate of drug elimination may be significantly decreased (see DOSAGE AND ADMINISTRATION).

Since antiarrhythmic drugs may be ineffective in patients with hypokalemia, the possibility of a potassium deficit should be explored and, if present, the deficit should be corrected.

Like all other oral antiarrhythmics, TONOCARD has been reported to increase arrhythmias in some patients (see ADVERSE REACTIONS).

Information for Patients: Patients should be instructed to promptly report the development of bruising or bleeding; any signs of infections such as fever, chills, sore throat, or soreness and ulcers in the mouth; any pulmonary symptoms, such as exertional dyspnea, cough, or wheezing; rash.

Laboratory Tests: As with other antiarrhythmics, abnormal liver function tests, particularly in the early stages of therapy, have been reported. Periodic monitoring of liver function should be considered. Hepatitis and jaundice have been reported in some patients.

Drug Interactions: Tocainide and lidocaine are pharmacodynamically similar. The concomitant use of these 2 agents may cause an increased incidence of adverse reactions, including central nervous system adverse reactions such as seizure.

Specific interaction studies with cimetidine, digoxin, metoprolol and warfarin have been conducted, no clinically significant interaction was seen with cimetidine, digoxin or warfarin; but tocainide and metoprolol had additive effects on wedge pressure and cardiac index. TONOCARD has also been used in open studies with digitalis, beta-blocking agents, other antiarrhythmic agents, anticoagulants, and diuretics, without evidence of clinically significant interactions. Nevertheless, caution should be exercised in the use of multiple drug therapy.

TONOCARD is equally effective in digitalized and non-digitalized patients. In 17 patients with refractory ventricular arrhythmias on concomitant therapy, serum digoxin levels (1.1 ± 0.4 ng/mL) remained in the expected normal range (0.5–2.5 ng/mL) during tocainide administration.

Carcinogenesis, Mutagenesis, Impairment of Fertility: The carcinogenic potential of tocainide was studied in mice using oral doses up to 300 mg/kg/day (about 6 times the maximum recommended human dose) for up to 94 weeks in males and 102 weeks in females and in rats at doses up to 200 mg/kg/day for 24 months. Tocainide did not affect the type or incidence of neoplasia in the 2 studies.

Tocainide did not show any mutagenic potential when evaluated *in vivo* in the micronucleus test using mice at oral doses up to 187.5 mg/kg/day (about 7 times the usual human dose). Also, no mutagenic activity was seen *in vitro* in the Ames microbial mutagen test or in the mouse lymphoma forward mutation assay.

Reproduction and fertility studies in rats showed no adverse effects on male or female fertility at oral doses up to 200 mg/kg/day (about 8 times the usual human dose).

Pregnancy: *Pregnancy Category C.* In a teratogenicity study in rabbits, tocainide was administered orally at doses of 25, 50, and 100 mg/kg/day (about 1 to 4 times the usual human dose). No evidence of a drug-related teratogenic effect was noted; however, these doses were maternotoxic and produced a dose-related increase in abortions and stillbirths. In a teratogenicity study in rats, an oral dose of 300 mg/kg/day (about 12 times the usual human dose) showed no evidence of treatment-related fetal malformations, but maternotoxicity and an increase in fetal resorptions were noted. An oral dose of 30 mg/kg/day (about twice the usual human dose) did not produce any adverse effects.

In reproduction studies in rats at maternotoxic oral doses of 200 and 300 mg/kg/day (about 8 and 12 times the usual human dose, respectively), dystocia, and delayed parturition occurred which was accompanied by an increase in stillbirths and decreased survival in offspring during the first week postpartum. Growth and viability of surviving offspring were not affected for the remainder of the lactation period.

There are no adequate and well-controlled studies in pregnant women. TONOCARD should be used during pregnancy only if the potential benefit justifies the potential risk to the fetus.

Nursing Mothers: It is not known whether tocainide is secreted in human milk. Because many drugs are secreted in human milk and because of the potential for serious adverse reactions in nursing infants from TONOCARD, a decision should be made whether to discontinue nursing or to discontinue the drug, taking into account the importance of the drug to the mother.

Pediatric Use: Safety and effectiveness in pediatric patients have not been established.

Geriatric Use: Clinical studies of TONOCARD did not include sufficient numbers of subjects aged 65 and over to determine whether they respond differently from younger subjects. Other reported clinical experience has not identified differences in responses between the elderly and younger patients. In general, dose selection for an elderly patient should be cautious, usually starting at the low end of the dosing range, reflecting the greater frequency of decreased hepatic, renal, or cardiac function, and of concomitant disease or other drug therapy.

ADVERSE REACTIONS

TONOCARD commonly produces minor, transient, nervous system and gastrointestinal adverse reactions, but is otherwise generally well tolerated. TONOCARD has been evaluated in both short-term (n = 1,358) and long-term (n = 262) controlled studies as well as a compassionate use program. Dosages were lower in most of the controlled studies (1200 mg/day) and higher in the compassionate use program (1800 mg and more). In long-term (2–6 months) controlled studies, the most frequent adverse reactions were dizziness/vertigo (15.3%), nausea (14.5%), paresthesia (9.2%), and tremor (8.4%). These reactions were generally mild, transient, dose-related and reversible with a reduction in dosage, by taking the drug with food, or by therapy discontinuation. Tremor, when present, may be useful as a clinical indicator that the maximum dose is being approached. Adverse reactions leading to therapy discontinuation occurred in 21% of patients in long-term controlled trials and were usually related to the nervous system or digestive system.

Adverse reactions occurring in greater than 1% of patients from the short-term and long-term controlled studies appear in the following table:

	Percent of Patients Controlled Studies	
	Short-term (n = 1,358)	Long-term (n = 262)
BODY AS A WHOLE		
Tiredness/drowsiness/fatigue/lethargy/lassitude/sleepiness	1.6	0.8
Hot/cold feelings	0.5	1.5
CARDIOVASCULAR		
Hypotension	3.4	2.7
Bradycardia	1.8	0.4
Palpitations	1.8	0.4
Chest pain	1.6	0.4
Conduction disorders	1.5	0.0
Left ventricular failure	1.4	0.0
DIGESTIVE		
Nausea	15.2	14.5
Vomiting	8.3	4.6
Anorexia	1.2	1.9
Diarrhea/loose stools	0.0	3.8
NERVOUS SYSTEM/PSYCHIATRIC		
Dizziness/vertigo	8.0	15.3
Paresthesia	3.5	9.2
Tremor	2.9	8.4
Confusion/disorientation/hallucinations	2.1	2.7
Headache	2.1	4.6
Nervousness	1.5	0.4
Altered mood/awareness	1.5	3.4
Incoordination/unsteadiness/walking disturbances	1.2	0.0
Anxiety	1.1	1.5
Ataxia	0.2	3.0
SKIN		
Diaphoresis	5.1	2.3
Rash/skin lesion	0.4	8.4
SPECIAL SENSES		
Blurred vision/visual disturbances	1.3	1.5
Tinnitus/hearing loss	0.4	1.5
Nystagmus	0.0	1.1

An additional group of about 2,000 patients has been treated in a program allowing for the use of TONOCARD under compassionate use circumstances. These patients were seriously ill with the large majority on multiple drug therapy, and comparatively high doses of TONOCARD were used. Fifty-four percent of the patients continued in the program for 1 year or longer, and 12% were treated for longer than 3 years, with the longest duration of therapy being 9 years. Adverse reactions leading to therapy discontinuation occurred in 12% of patients (usually central nervous system effects or rash). A tabulation of adverse reactions occurring in 1% or more of patients follows:

	Percent of Patients Compassionate Use (n = 1,927)
CARDIOVASCULAR	
Increased ventricular arrhythmias/PVCs	10.9
CHF/progression of CHF	4.0
Tachycardia	3.2
Hypotension	1.8
Conduction disorders	1.3
Bradycardia	1.0
DIGESTIVE	
Nausea	24.6
Anorexia	11.3
Vomiting	9.0
Diarrhea/loose stools	6.8
MUSCULOSKELETAL	
Arthritis/arthralgia	4.7
Myalgia	1.7
NERVOUS SYSTEM/PSYCHIATRIC	
Dizziness/vertigo	25.3
Tremor	21.6
Nervousness	11.5
Confusion/disorientation/hallucinations	11.2
Altered mood/awareness	11.0
Ataxia	10.8
Paresthesia	9.2
SKIN	
Rash/skin lesion	12.2
Diaphoresis	8.3
Lupus	1.6
SPECIAL SENSES	
Blurred vision/vision disturbances	10.0
Nystagmus	1.1

Adverse reactions occurring in less than 1% of patients in either the controlled studies or the compassionate use program or since the drug was marketed are as follows:

Body as a Whole: Septicemia; septic shock; syncope; vasovagal episodes; edema; fever; chills; cinchonism; asthenia; malaise.

Cardiovascular: Ventricular fibrillation; extension of acute myocardial infarction; cardiogenic shock; pulmonary embolism; angina; AV block; hypertension; claudication; increased QRS duration; pleurisy/pericarditis; prolonged QT interval; right bundle branch block; cardiomegaly; sinus arrest; vasculitis; orthostatic hypotension; cold extremities.

Digestive: Hepatitis, jaundice (see PRECAUTIONS), abnormal liver function tests; pancreatitis; abdominal pain/discomfort; constipation; dysphagia; gastrointestinal symptoms (including dyspepsia); stomatitis; dry mouth; thirst.

Hematologic: Agranulocytosis; bone marrow depression; aplastic/hypoplastic anemia; hemolytic anemia; anemia; leukopenia; neutropenia; thrombocytopenia; eosinophilia.

Metabolic and Immune: Hypersensitivity Reaction (including some of the following symptoms or signs: rash, fever, joint pains, abnormal liver function tests, eosinophilia); increased ANA.

Musculoskeletal: Muscle cramps; muscle twitching/spasm; neck pain; pain radiating from neck; pressure on shoulder.

Nervous System/Psychiatric: Coma; convulsions/seizures; myasthenia gravis; depression; psychosis; psychic disturbances; agitation; decreased mental acuity; dysarthria; impaired memory; increased stuttering/slurred speech; insomnia/sleeping disturbances; local anesthesia; dream abnormalities.

Respiratory: Respiratory arrest; pulmonary edema; pulmonary fibrosis; fibrosing alveolitis; pneumonia; interstitial pneumonitis; dyspnea; hiccough; yawning.

Skin: Stevens-Johnson syndrome; exfoliative dermatitis; erythema multiforme; urticaria; alopecia; pruritus; pallor/flushed face.

Special Senses: Diplopia; earache; taste perversion/smell perversion.

Urogenital: Urinary retention; polyuria/increased diuresis.

Agranulocytosis, bone marrow depression, leukopenia, neutropenia, aplastic/hypoplastic anemia, and thrombocytopenia have been reported (0.18%) in patients receiving TONOCARD in controlled trials and the compassionate use program. Most of these events have been noted during the first 12 weeks of therapy. (See Box WARNINGS.)

Pulmonary fibrosis, interstitial pneumonitis, fibrosing alveolitis, pulmonary edema, and pneumonia, have been reported in patients receiving TONOCARD. The incidence of pulmonary fibrosis (including interstitial pneumonitis and fibrosing alveolitis) was 0.11% in controlled trials and the compassionate use program. These events usually occurred in seriously ill patients. Symptoms of these pulmonary disorders and/or x-ray changes usually occurred following 3–18 weeks of therapy. Fatalities have been reported. (See Box WARNINGS.)

A number of disorders, in which a causal relationship with TONOCARD has not been established, have been reported in seriously ill patients. These include: renal failure, renal dysfunction, myocardial infarction, cerebrovascular accidents and transient ischemic attacks. These disorders may be related to the patient's underlying condition.

DRUG ABUSE AND DEPENDENCE

Drug withdrawal after chronic treatment has not shown any indication of psychological or physical dependence.

OVERDOSAGE

The initial and most important signs and symptoms of overdosage would be expected to be related to the central nervous system. Other adverse reactions, such as gastrointestinal disturbances, may follow. (See ADVERSE REACTIONS.)

Should convulsions or cardiopulmonary depression or arrest develop, the patency of the airway and adequacy of ventilation must be assured immediately. Should convulsions persist despite ventilatory therapy with oxygen, small increments of anticonvulsive agents may be given intravenously. Examples of such agents include a benzodiazepine (e.g., diazepam), an ultrashort-acting barbiturate (e.g., thiopental or thiamylal), or a short-acting barbiturate (e.g., pentobarbital or secobarbital).

The oral LD_{50} of tocainide was calculated to be about 800 mg/kg in mice, 1000 mg/kg in rats, and 230 mg/kg in guinea pigs; deaths were usually preceded by convulsions. Studies in normal individuals to date indicate that tocainide has a hemodialysis clearance approximately equivalent to its renal clearance.

DOSAGE AND ADMINISTRATION

The dosage of TONOCARD must be individualized on the basis of antiarrhythmic response and tolerance, both of which are dose-related. Clinical and electrocardiographic

Continued on next page

Tonocard—Cont.

evaluation (including Holter monitoring if necessary for evaluation) are needed to determine whether the desired antiarrhythmic response has been obtained and to guide titration and dose adjustment. Adverse effects appearing shortly after dosing, for example, suggest a need for dividing the dose further with a shorter dose-interval. Loss of arrhythmia control prior to the next dose suggests use of a shorter dose interval and/or a dose increase. Absence of a clear response suggests reconsideration of therapy.

The recommended initial dosage is 400 mg every 8 hours. The usual adult dosage is between 1200 and 1800 mg/day in a three dose daily divided regimen. Doses beyond 2400 mg per day have been administered infrequently. Patients who tolerate the t.i.d. regimen may be tried on a twice daily regimen with careful monitoring.

Some patients, particularly those with renal or hepatic impairment, may be adequately treated with less than 1200 mg/day.

HOW SUPPLIED

No. 3409—Tablets TONOCARD, 400 mg, are oval, yellow, scored, film-coated tablets, coded 707 on one side and TONOCARD on the other side. They are supplied as follows:

NDC 0186-0707-68 bottles of 100

No. 3410—Tablets TONOCARD, 600 mg, are oblong, yellow, scored, film-coated tablets, coded 709 on one side and TONOCARD on the other side. They are supplied as follows:

NDC 0186-0709-68 bottles of 100

Storage

Store at 25°C (77°F), excursions permitted to 15–30°C (59–86°F) [see USP Controlled Room Temperature]. Keep container tightly closed.

Manufactured by: Merck & Co., Inc.
West Point, PA 19486
Distributed by:
Astra Pharmaceuticals, L.P., Wayne, PA 19087
65000216 Revised October 1999

Shown in Product Identification Guide, page 305

TOPROL-XL® TABLETS ℞

(metoprolol succinate)
Extended Release Tablets
Tablets: 50 mg, 100 mg, and 200 mg

DESCRIPTION

Toprol-XL, metoprolol succinate, is a beta$_1$-selective (cardioselective) adrenoceptor blocking agent, for oral administration, available as extended release tablets. Toprol-XL has been formulated to provide a controlled and predictable release of metoprolol for once daily administration. The tablets comprise a multiple unit system containing metoprolol succinate in a multitude of controlled release pellets. Each pellet acts as a separate drug delivery unit and is designed to deliver metoprolol continuously over the dosage interval. The tablets contain 47.5 mg, 95 mg and 190 mg of metoprolol succinate equivalent to 50, 100 and 200 mg of metoprolol tartrate, USP, respectively. Its chemical name is (±)1-(isopropylamino)-3-[p-(2-methoxyethyl)phenoxy]-2-propanol succinate (2:1) (salt). Its structural formula is:

[OH; $OCH_2CHCH_2NHCH(CH_3)_2$; $CH_2CH_2OCH_3$]$_2$ · COOH–CH_2–CH_2–COOH

Metoprolol succinate is a white crystalline powder with a molecular weight of 652.8. It is freely soluble in water; soluble in methanol; sparingly soluble in ethanol; slightly soluble in dichloromethane and 2-propanol; practically insoluble in ethyl-acetate, acetone, diethylether and heptane. Inactive ingredients: silicon dioxide, cellulose compounds, sodium stearyl fumarate, polyethylene glycol, titanium dioxide, paraffin.

CLINICAL PHARMACOLOGY

Metoprolol is a beta$_1$-selective (cardioselective) adrenergic receptor blocking agent. This preferential effect is not absolute, however, and at higher plasma concentrations, metoprolol also inhibits beta$_2$-adrenoreceptors, chiefly located in the bronchial and vascular musculature. Metoprolol has no intrinsic sympathomimetic activity, and membrane-stabilizing activity is detectable only at plasma concentrations much greater than required for beta-blockade. Animal and human experiments indicate that metoprolol slows the sinus rate and decreases AV nodal conduction.

Clinical pharmacology studies have confirmed the beta-blocking activity of metoprolol in man, as shown by (1) reduction in heart rate and cardiac output at rest and upon exercise, (2) reduction of systolic blood pressure upon exercise, (3) inhibition of isoproterenol-induced tachycardia, and (4) reduction of reflex orthostatic tachycardia.

The relative beta$_1$-selectivity of metoprolol has been confirmed by the following: (1) In normal subjects, metoprolol is unable to reverse the beta$_2$-mediated vasodilating effects of epinephrine. This contrasts with the effect of nonselective beta-blockers, which completely reverse the vasodilating effects of epinephrine. (2) In asthmatic patients, metoprolol reduces FEV_1 and FVC significantly less than a nonselective beta-blocker, propranolol, at equivalent beta$_1$-receptor blocking doses.

In five controlled studies in normal healthy subjects, the same daily doses of Toprol-XL and immediate release metoprolol were compared in terms of the extent and duration of beta$_1$-blockade produced. Both formulations were given in a dose range equivalent to 100–400 mg of immediate release metoprolol per day. In these studies, Toprol-XL was administered once a day and immediate release metoprolol was administered once to four times a day. A sixth controlled study compared the beta$_1$-blocking effects of a 50 mg daily dose of the two formulations. In each study, beta$_1$-blockade was expressed as the percent change from baseline, in exercise heart rate following standardized submaximal exercise tolerance tests at steady state. Toprol-XL administered once a day, and immediate release metoprolol administered once to four times a day, provided comparable total beta$_1$-blockade over 24 hours (area under the beta$_1$-blockade versus time curve) in the dose range 100–400 mg. At a dosage of 50 mg once daily, Toprol-XL produced significantly higher total beta$_1$-blockade over 24 hours than immediate release metoprolol. For Toprol-XL, the percent reduction in exercise heart rate was relatively stable throughout the entire dosage interval and the level of beta$_1$-blockade increased with increasing doses from 50 to 300 mg daily. The effects at peak/ trough (i.e. at 24 hours post dosing) were; 14/9, 16/10, 24/14, 27/22 and 27/20% reduction in exercise heart rate for doses of 50, 100, 200, 300 and 400 mg Toprol-XL once a day, respectively. In contrast to Toprol-XL immediate release metoprolol given at a dose of 50–100 mg once a day, produced a significantly larger peak effect on exercise tachycardia, but the effect was not evident at 24 hours. To match the peak to trough ratio obtained with Toprol-XL over the dosing range of 200 to 400 mg, a t.i.d. to q.i.d. divided dosing regimen was required for immediate release metoprolol.

The relationship between plasma metoprolol levels and reduction in exercise heart rate is independent of the pharmaceutical formulation. Using the E_{max} model, the maximal beta$_1$-blocking effect has been estimated to produce a 28.3% reduction in exercise heart rate. Beta$_1$-blocking effects in the range of 30–80% of the maximal effect (corresponding to approximately 8–23% reduction in exercise heart rate) are expected to occur at metoprolol plasma concentrations ranging from 30–540 nmol/L. The concentration-effect curve begins reaching a plateau between 200–300 nmol/L, and higher plasma levels produce little additional beta$_1$-blocking effect. The relative beta$_1$-selectivity of metoprolol diminishes and blockade of beta$_2$-adrenoceptors increases at higher plasma concentrations.

Although beta-adrenergic receptor blockade is useful in the treatment of angina and hypertension, there are situations in which sympathetic stimulation is vital. In patients with severely damaged hearts, adequate ventricular function may depend on sympathetic drive. In the presence of AV block, beta-blockade may prevent the necessary facilitating effect of sympathetic activity on conduction. Beta$_2$-adrenergic blockade results in passive bronchial constriction by interfering with endogenous adrenergic bronchodilator activity in patients subject to bronchospasm and may also interfere with exogenous bronchodilators in such patients.

Hypertension: The mechanism of the antihypertensive effects of beta-blocking agents has not been elucidated. However, several possible mechanisms have been proposed: (1) competitive antagonism of catecholamines at peripheral (especially cardiac) adrenergic neuron sites, leading to decreased cardiac output; (2) a central effect leading to reduced sympathetic outflow to the periphery; and (3) suppression of renin activity.

In controlled clinical studies, an immediate release dosage form of metoprolol has been shown to be an effective antihypertensive agent when used alone or as concomitant therapy with thiazide-type diuretics at dosages of 100–450 mg daily. Toprol-XL, in dosages of 100 to 400 mg once daily, has been shown to possess comparable β_1-blockade as conventional metoprolol tablets administered two to four times daily. In addition, Toprol-XL administered at a dose of 50 mg once daily has been shown to lower blood pressure 24-hours post-dosing in placebo controlled studies. In controlled, comparative, clinical studies, immediate release metoprolol appeared comparable as an antihypertensive agent to propranolol, methyldopa, and thiazide-type diuretics, and affected both supine and standing blood pressure. Because of variable plasma levels attained with a given dose and lack of a consistent relationship of antihypertensive activity to drug plasma concentration, selection of proper dosage requires individual titration.

Angina Pectoris: By blocking catecholamine-induced increases in heart rate, in velocity and extent of myocardial contraction, and in blood pressure, metoprolol reduces the oxygen requirements of the heart at any given level of effort, thus making it useful in the long-term management of angina pectoris. However, in patients with heart failure, beta-adrenergic blockade may increase oxygen requirements by increasing left ventricular fiber length and end-diastolic pressure.

In controlled clinical trials, an immediate release formulation of metoprolol has been shown to be an effective antianginal agent, reducing the number of angina attacks and increasing exercise tolerance. The dosage used in these studies ranged from 100 to 400 mg daily. Toprol-XL, in dosages of 100 to 400 mg once daily, has been shown to possess comparable β_1-blockade as conventional metoprolol tablets administered two to four times daily.

Pharmacokinetics: In man, absorption of metoprolol is rapid and complete. Plasma levels following oral administration of conventional metoprolol tablets, however, approximate 50% of levels following intravenous administration, indicating about 50% first-pass metabolism. Metoprolol crosses the blood-brain barrier and has been reported in the CSF in a concentration 78% of the simultaneous plasma concentration.

Plasma levels achieved are highly variable after oral administration. Only a small fraction of the drug (about 12%) is bound to human serum albumin. Elimination is mainly by biotransformation in the liver, and the plasma half-life ranges from approximately 3 to 7 hours. Less than 5% of an oral dose of metoprolol is recovered unchanged in the urine; the rest is excreted by the kidneys as metabolites that appear to have no clinical significance. Following intravenous administration of metoprolol, the urinary recovery of unchanged drug is approximately 10%. The systemic availability and half-life of metoprolol in patients with renal failure do not differ to a clinically significant degree from those in normal subjects. Consequently, no reduction in dosage is usually needed in patients with chronic renal failure.

In comparison to conventional metoprolol, the plasma metoprolol levels following administration of Toprol-XL are characterized by lower peaks, longer time to peak and significantly lower peak to trough variation. The peak plasma levels following once daily administration of Toprol-XL average one-fourth to one-half the peak plasma levels obtained following a corresponding dose of conventional metoprolol, administered once daily or in divided doses. At steady state the average bioavailability of metoprolol following administration of Toprol- XL, across the dosage range of 50 to 400 mg once daily, was 77% relative to the corresponding single or divided doses of conventional metoprolol. Nevertheless, over the 24 hour dosing interval, β_1-blockade is comparable and dose-related (see CLINICAL PHARMACOLOGY). The bioavailability of metoprolol shows a dose-related, although not directly proportional increase with dose and is not significantly affected by food following Toprol-XL administration.

INDICATIONS AND USAGE

Hypertension: Toprol-XL tablets are indicated for the treatment of hypertension. They may be used alone or in combination with other antihypertensive agents.

Angina Pectoris: Toprol-XL tablets are indicated in the long-term treatment of angina pectoris.

CONTRAINDICATIONS

Hypertension and Angina: Toprol-XL is contraindicated in sinus bradycardia, heart block greater than first degree, cardiogenic shock, and overt cardiac failure (see WARNINGS).

WARNINGS

Hypertension and Angina

Cardiac Failure—Sympathetic stimulation is a vital component supporting circulatory function in congestive heart failure, and beta-blockade carries the potential hazard of further depressing myocardial contractility and precipitating more severe failure. In hypertensive and angina patients who have congestive heart failure controlled by digitalis and diuretics, Toprol-XL should be administered cautiously. Both digitalis and Toprol-XL slow AV conduction.

In Patients Without a History of Cardiac Failure—Continued depression of the myocardium with beta-blocking agents over a period of time can, in some cases, lead to cardiac failure. At the first sign or symptom of impending cardiac failure, patients should be fully digitalized and/or given a diuretic. The response should be observed closely. If cardiac failure continues, despite adequate digitalization and diuretic therapy, Toprol-XL should be withdrawn.

Ischemic Heart Disease: Following abrupt cessation of therapy with certain beta-blocking agents, exacerbations of angina pectoris and, in some cases, myocardial infarction have occurred. When discontinuing chronically administered Toprol-XL, particularly in patients with ischemic heart disease, the dosage should be gradually reduced over a period of 1–2 weeks and the patient should be carefully monitored. If angina markedly worsens or acute coronary insufficiency develops, Toprol-XL administration should be reinstated promptly, at least temporarily, and other measures appropriate for the management of unstable angina should be taken. Patients should be warned against interruption or discontinuation of therapy without the physician's advice. Because coronary artery disease is common and may be unrecognized, it may be prudent not to discontinue Toprol-XL therapy abruptly even in patients treated only for hypertension.

Bronchospastic Diseases—PATIENTS WITH BRONCHOSPASTIC DISEASES SHOULD, IN GENERAL, NOT RECEIVE BETA-BLOCKERS. Because of its relative beta$_1$-selectivity, however, Toprol-XL may be used with caution in patients with bronchospastic disease who do not respond to, or cannot tolerate, other antihypertensive treatment. Since beta$_1$-selectivity is not absolute, a beta$_2$-stimulating agent should be administered concomitantly, and the lowest possible dose of Toprol-XL should be used (see DOSAGE AND ADMINISTRATION).

Major Surgery—The necessity or desirability of withdrawing beta-blocking therapy prior to major surgery is controversial; the impaired ability of the heart to respond to reflex adrenergic stimuli may augment the risks of general anesthesia and surgical procedures.

Toprol-XL like other beta-blockers, is a competitive inhibitor of beta-receptor agonists, and its effects can be reversed by administration of such agents, e.g., dobutamine or isoproterenol. However, such patients may be subject to protracted severe hypotension. Difficulty in restarting and maintaining the heart beat has also been reported with beta-blockers.

Diabetes and Hypoglycemia—Toprol-XL should be used with caution in diabetic patients if a beta-blocking agent is required. Beta-blockers may mask tachycardia occurring with hypoglycemia, but other manifestations such as dizziness and sweating may not be significantly affected.

Thyrotoxicosis—Beta-adrenergic blockade may mask certain clinical signs (e.g., tachycardia) of hyperthyroidism. Patients suspected of developing thyrotoxicosis should be managed carefully to avoid abrupt withdrawal of beta-blockade, which might precipitate a thyroid storm.

PRECAUTIONS

General: Toprol-XL should be used with caution in patients with impaired hepatic function.

Information for Patients: Patients should be advised to take Toprol-XL regularly and continuously, as directed, preferably with or immediately following meals. If a dose should be missed, the patient should take only the next scheduled dose (without doubling it). Patients should not discontinue Toprol-XL without consulting the physician.

Patients should be advised (1) to avoid operating automobiles and machinery or engaging in other tasks requiring alertness until the patient's response to therapy with Toprol- XL has been determined; (2) to contact the physician if any difficulty in breathing occurs; (3) to inform the physician or dentist before any type of surgery that he or she is taking Toprol-XL.

Laboratory Tests: Clinical laboratory findings may include elevated levels of serum transaminase, alkaline phosphatase, and lactate dehydrogenase.

Drug Interactions: Catecholamine-depleting drugs (e.g., reserpine) may have an additive effect when given with beta-blocking agents. Patients treated with Toprol-XL plus a catecholamine depletor should therefore be closely observed for evidence of hypotension or marked bradycardia, which may produce vertigo, syncope, or postural hypotension.

Carcinogenesis, Mutagenesis, Impairment of Fertility: Long-term studies in animals have been conducted to evaluate the carcinogenic potential of metoprolol tartrate. In 2-year studies in rats at three oral dosage levels of up to 800 mg/kg/day, there was no increase in the development of spontaneously occurring benign or malignant neoplasms of any type. The only histologic changes that appeared to be drug related were an increased incidence of generally mild focal accumulation of foamy macrophages in pulmonary alveoli and a slight increase in biliary hyperplasia. In a 21-month study in Swiss albino mice at three oral dosage levels of up to 750 mg/kg/day, benign lung tumors (small adenomas) occurred more frequently in female mice receiving the highest dose than in untreated control animals. There was no increase in malignant or total (benign plus malignant) lung tumors, nor in the overall incidence of tumors or malignant tumors. This 21-month study was repeated in CD-1 mice, and no statistically or biologically significant differences were observed between treated and control mice of either sex for any type of tumor.

All mutagenicity tests performed on metoprolol tartrate (a dominant lethal study in mice, chromosome studies in somatic cells, a Salmonella/mammalian-microsome mutagenicity test, and a nucleus anomaly test in somatic interphase nuclei) and metoprolol succinate (a Salmonella/mammalian-microsome mutagenicity test) were negative.

No evidence of impaired fertility due to metoprolol tartrate was observed in a study performed in rats at doses up to 55.5 times the maximum daily human dose of 450 mg.

Pregnancy Category C: Metoprolol tartrate has been shown to increase post-implantation loss and decrease neonatal survival in rats at doses up to 55.5 times the maximum daily human dose of 450 mg. Distribution studies in mice confirm exposure of the fetus when metoprolol tartrate is administered to the pregnant animal. These studies have revealed no evidence of impaired fertility or teratogenicity. There are no adequate and well-controlled studies in pregnant women. Because animal reproduction studies are not always predictive of human response, this drug should be used during pregnancy only if clearly needed.

Nursing Mothers: Metoprolol is excreted in breast milk in very small quantities. An infant consuming 1 liter of breast milk daily would receive a dose of less than 1 mg of the drug. Caution should be exercised when Toprol-XL is administered to a nursing woman.

Pediatric Use: Safety and effectiveness in pediatric patients have not been established.

Risk of Anaphylactic Reactions: While taking beta-blockers, patients with a history of severe anaphylactic reactions to a variety of allergens may be more reactive to repeated challenge, either accidental, diagnostic or therapeutic. Such patients may be unresponsive to the usual doses of epinephrine used to treat allergic reaction.

ADVERSE REACTIONS

Hypertension and Angina: Most adverse effects have been mild and transient. The following adverse reactions have been reported for metoprolol tartrate.

Central Nervous System—Tiredness and dizziness have occurred in about 10 of 100 patients. Depression has been reported in about 5 of 100 patients. Mental confusion and short-term memory loss have been reported. Headache, somnolence, nightmares, and insomnia have also been reported.

Cardiovascular—Shortness of breath and bradycardia have occurred in approximately 3 of 100 patients. Cold extremities; arterial insufficiency, usually of the Raynaud type; palpitations; congestive heart failure; peripheral edema; syncope; chest pain; and hypotension have been reported in about 1 of 100 patients (see CONTRAINDICATIONS, WARNINGS and PRECAUTIONS).

Respiratory—Wheezing (bronchospasm) and dyspnea have been reported in about 1 of 100 patients (see WARNINGS).

Gastrointestinal—Diarrhea has occurred in about 5 of 100 patients. Nausea, dry mouth, gastric pain, constipation, flatulence, digestive tract disorders and heartburn have been reported in about 1 of 100 patients.

Hypersensitive Reactions—Pruritus or rash have occurred in about 5 of 100 patients. Worsening of psoriasis has also been reported.

Miscellaneous—Peyronie's disease has been reported in fewer than 1 of 100,000 patients. Musculoskeletal pain, blurred vision, decreased libido and tinnitus have also been reported.

There have been rare reports of reversible alopecia, agranulocytosis, and dry eyes. Discontinuation of the drug should be considered if any such reaction is not otherwise explicable. The oculomucocutaneous syndrome associated with the beta-blocker practolol has not been reported with metoprolol.

Potential Adverse Reactions: A variety of adverse reactions not listed above have been reported with other beta-adrenergic blocking agents and should be considered potential adverse reactions to Toprol-XL.

Central Nervous System—Reversible mental depression progressing to catatonia; an acute reversible syndrome characterized by disorientation for time and place, short-term memory loss, emotional lability, slightly clouded sensorium, and decreased performance on neuropsychometrics.

Cardiovascular—Intensification of AV block (see CONTRAINDICATIONS).

Hematologic—Agranulocytosis, nonthrombocytopenic purpura, thrombocytopenic purpura.

Hypersensitive Reactions—Fever combined with aching and sore throat, laryngospasm, and respiratory distress.

OVERDOSAGE

Acute Toxicity: There have been a few reports of overdosage with Toprol-XL and no specific overdosage information was obtained with this drug, with the exception of animal toxicology data. However, since Toprol-XL (metoprolol succinate salt) contains the same active moiety, metoprolol, as conventional metoprolol tablets (metoprolol tartrate salt), the recommendations on overdosage for metoprolol conventional tablets are applicable to Toprol-XL.

Signs and Symptoms: Potential signs and symptoms associated with overdosage with metoprolol are bradycardia, hypotension, bronchospasm, and cardiac failure.

Treatment: There is no specific antidote.

In general, patients with acute or recent myocardial infarction may be more hemodynamically unstable than other patients and should be treated accordingly. On the basis of the pharmacologic actions of metoprolol tartrate, the following general measures should be employed.

Elimination of the Drug—Gastric lavage should be performed.

Bradycardia—Atropine should be administered. If there is no response to vagal blockade, isoproterenol should be administered cautiously.

Hypotension—A vasopressor should be administered, e.g., levarterenol or dopamine.

Bronchospasm—A $beta_2$-stimulating agent and/or a theophylline derivative should be administered.

Cardiac Failure—A digitalis glycoside and diuretics should be administered. In shock resulting from inadequate cardiac contractility, administration of dobutamine, isoproterenol or glucagon may be considered.

DOSAGE AND ADMINISTRATION

Toprol-XL is an extended release tablet intended for once-a-day administration. When switching from immediate release metoprolol tablet to Toprol-XL, the same total daily dose of Toprol-XL should be used.

As with immediate release metoprolol, dosages of Toprol-XL should be individualized and titration may be needed in some patients.

Toprol-XL tablets are scored and can be divided; however, the whole or half tablet should be swallowed whole and not chewed or crushed.

Hypertension: The usual initial dosage is 50 to 100 mg daily in a single dose, whether used alone or added to a diuretic. The dosage may be increased at weekly (or longer) intervals until optimum blood pressure reduction is achieved. In general, the maximum effect of any given dosage level will be apparent after 1 week of therapy. Dosages above 400 mg per day have not been studied.

Angina Pectoris: The dosage of Toprol-XL should be individualized. The usual initial dosage is 100 mg daily, given in a single dose. The dosage may be gradually increased at weekly intervals until optimum clinical response has been obtained or there is a pronounced slowing of the heart rate. Dosages above 400 mg per day have not been studied. If treatment is to be discontinued, the dosage should be reduced gradually over a period of 1–2 weeks (see WARNINGS).

HOW SUPPLIED

Tablets 50 mg:
Contain 47.5 mg of metoprolol succinate equivalent to 50 mg of metoprolol tartrate, USP
Are white, biconvex, round, film-coated
Engraved A/mo on one side and scored on the other
Bottles of 100 NDC 0186-1090-05

Tablets 100 mg:
Contain 95 mg of metoprolol succinate equivalent to 100 mg of metoprolol tartrate, USP
Are white, biconvex, round, film-coated
Engraved A/ms on one side and scored on the other
Bottles of 100 NDC 0186-1092-05

Tablets 200 mg:
Contain 190 mg of metoprolol succinate equivalent to 200 mg of metoprolol tartrate, USP
Are white, biconvex, oval, film-coated
Engraved A/my and scored on one side
Bottles of 100 NDC 0186-1094-05

Store at controlled room temperature 15–30°C (59–86°F).

All trademarks are the property of the AstraZeneca Group.

64133-39 Rev. 5/00

Manufactured for: AstraZeneca LP
Wilmington, DE 19850
By: AstraZeneca AB
S-151 85 Södertälje, Sweden

Shown in Product Identification Guide, page 305

XYLOCAINE® (lidocaine HCl Injection, USP) ℞

[*zī 'lo-caine*]

XYLOCAINE®

(lidocaine HCl and epinephrine Injection, USP)

For Infiltration and Nerve Block

DESCRIPTION

Xylocaine (lidocaine HCl) Injections are sterile, non pyrogenic, aqueous solutions that contain a local anesthetic agent with or without epinephrine and are administered parenterally by injection. See INDICATIONS for specific uses.

Xylocaine solutions contain lidocaine HCl, which is chemically designated as acetamide, 2-(diethylamino)-N-(2,6-dimethylphenyl)-, monohydrochloride and has the molecular wt. 270.8. Lidocaine HCl ($C_{14}H_{22}N_2O \bullet HCl$) has the following structural formula:

CH_3 / NH—CO—CH_2—N(C_2H_5)(C_2H_5) · HCl / CH_3

Epinephrine is (-) -3, 4-Dihydroxy-α-[(methylamino) methyl] benzyl alcohol and has the molecular wt. 183.21. Epinephrine ($C_9H_{13}NO_3$) has the following structural formula:

HO / HO — C(OH)(H) — CH_2NHCH_3

Dosage forms listed as Xylocaine-MPF indicate single dose solutions that are Methyl Paraben Free (MPF).

Xylocaine MPF is a sterile, non pyrogenic, isotonic solution containing sodium chloride. Xylocaine in multiple dose vials, each mL also contains 1 mg methylparaben as antiseptic preservative. The pH of these solutions is adjusted to approximately 6.5 (5.0–7.0) with sodium hydroxide and/or hydrochloric acid.

Xylocaine MPF with Epinephrine is a sterile, non pyrogenic, isotonic solution containing sodium chloride. Each mL contains lidocaine hydrochloride and epinephrine, with 0.5 mg sodium metabisulfite as an antioxidant and 0.2 mg citric acid as a stabilizer. Xylocaine with Epinephrine in multiple dose vials, each mL also contains 1 mg methylparaben as antiseptic preservative. The pH of these solutions is adjusted to approximately 4.5 (3.3–5.5) with sodium hydroxide and/or hydrochloric acid. Filled under nitrogen.

CLINICAL PHARMACOLOGY

Mechanism of Action: Lidocaine stabilizes the neuronal membrane by inhibiting the ionic fluxes required for the initiation and conduction of impulses thereby effecting local anesthetic action.

Hemodynamics: Excessive blood levels may cause changes in cardiac output, total peripheral resistance, and mean arterial pressure. With central neural blockade these changes may be attributable to block of autonomic fibers, a direct depressant effect of the local anesthetic agent on various components of the cardiovascular system, and/or the beta-adrenergic receptor stimulating action of epinephrine when

Continued on next page

Xylocaine/Xylocaine w/Epi.—Cont.

present. The net effect is normally a modest hypotension when the recommended dosages are not exceeded.

Pharmacokinetics and Metabolism: Information derived from diverse formulations, concentrations and usages reveals that lidocaine is completely absorbed following parenteral administration, its rate of absorption depending, for example, upon various factors such as the site of administration and the presence or absence of a vasoconstrictor agent. Except for intravascular administration, the highest blood levels are obtained following intercostal nerve block and the lowest after subcutaneous administration.

The plasma binding of lidocaine is dependent on drug concentration, and the fraction bound decreases with increasing concentration. At concentrations of 1 to 4 µg of free base per mL 60 to 80 percent of lidocaine is protein bound. Binding is also dependent on the plasma concentration of the alpha-1-acid glycoprotein.

Lidocaine crosses the blood-brain and placental barriers, presumably by passive diffusion.

Lidocaine is metabolized rapidly by the liver, and metabolites and unchanged drug are excreted by the kidneys. Biotransformation includes oxidative N-dealkylation, ring hydroxylation, cleavage of the amide linkage, and conjugation. N-dealkylation, a major pathway of biotransformation, yields the metabolites monoethylglycinexylidide and glycinexylidide. The pharmacological/toxicological actions of these metabolites are similar to, but less potent than, those of lidocaine. Approximately 90% of lidocaine administered is excreted in the form of various metabolites, and less than 10% is excreted unchanged. The primary metabolite in urine is a conjugate of 4-hydroxy-2,6-dimethylaniline.

The elimination half-life of lidocaine following an intravenous bolus injection is typically 1.5 to 2.0 hours. Because of the rapid rate at which lidocaine is metabolized, any condition that affects liver function may alter lidocaine kinetics. The half-life may be prolonged two-fold or more in patients with liver dysfunction. Renal dysfunction does not affect lidocaine kinetics but may increase the accumulation of metabolites.

Factors such as acidosis and the use of CNS stimulants and depressants affect the CNS levels of lidocaine required to produce overt systemic effects. Objective adverse manifestations become increasingly apparent with increasing venous plasma levels above 6.0 µg free base per mL. In the rhesus monkey arterial blood levels of 18–21 µg/mL have been shown to be threshold for convulsive activity.

INDICATIONS AND USAGE

Xylocaine (lidocaine HCl) Injections are indicated for production of local or regional anesthesia by infiltration techniques such as percutaneous injection and intravenous regional anesthesia by peripheral nerve block techniques such as brachial plexus and intercostal and by central neural techniques such as lumbar and caudal epidural blocks, when the accepted procedures for these techniques as described in standard textbooks are observed.

CONTRAINDICATIONS

Lidocaine is contraindicated in patients with a known history of hypersensitivity to local anesthetics of the amide type.

WARNINGS

XYLOCAINE INJECTIONS FOR INFILTRATION AND NERVE BLOCK SHOULD BE EMPLOYED ONLY BY CLINICIANS WHO ARE WELL VERSED IN DIAGNOSIS AND MANAGEMENT OF DOSE-RELATED TOXICITY AND OTHER ACUTE EMERGENCIES THAT MIGHT ARISE FROM THE BLOCK TO BE EMPLOYED AND THEN ONLY AFTER ENSURING THE *IMMEDIATE* AVAILABILITY OF OXYGEN, OTHER RESUSCITATIVE DRUGS, CARDIOPULMONARY EQUIPMENT AND THE PERSONNEL NEEDED FOR PROPER MANAGEMENT OF TOXIC REACTIONS AND RELATED EMERGENCIES. (See also ADVERSE REACTIONS and PRECAUTIONS.) DELAY IN PROPER MANAGEMENT OF DOSE-RELATED TOXICITY, UNDERVENTILATION FROM ANY CAUSE AND/OR ALTERED SENSITIVITY MAY LEAD TO THE DEVELOPMENT OF ACIDOSIS, CARDIAC ARREST AND, POSSIBLY, DEATH.

To avoid intravascular injection, aspiration should be performed before the local anesthetic solution is injected. The needle must be repositioned until no return of blood can be elicited by aspiration. Note, however, that the absence of blood in the syringe does not guarantee that intravascular injection has been avoided.

Local anesthetic solutions containing antimicrobial preservatives, (e.g., methylparaben) should not be used for epidural or spinal anesthesia because the safety of these agents has not been established with regard to intrathecal injection, either intentional or accidental.

Xylocaine with epinephrine solutions contain sodium metabisulfite, a sulfite that may cause allergic-type reactions including anaphylactic symptoms and life-threatening or less severe asthmatic episodes in certain susceptible people. The overall prevalence of sulfite sensitivity in the general population is unknown and probably low. Sulfite sensitivity is seen more frequently in asthmatic than in non-asthmatic people.

PRECAUTIONS

General: The safety and effectiveness of lidocaine depend on proper dosage, correct technique, adequate precautions, and readiness for emergencies. Standard textbooks should be consulted for specific techniques and precautions for various regional anesthetic procedures.

Resuscitative equipment, oxygen, and other resuscitative drugs should be available for immediate use. (See WARNINGS and ADVERSE REACTIONS.) The lowest dosage that results in effective anesthesia should be used to avoid high plasma levels and serious adverse effects. Syringe aspirations should also be performed before and during each supplemental injection when using indwelling catheter techniques. During the administration of epidural anesthesia, it is recommended that a test dose be administered initially and that the patient be monitored for central nervous system toxicity and cardiovascular toxicity, as well as for signs of unintended intrathecal administration, before proceeding. When clinical conditions permit, consideration should be given to employing local anesthetic solutions that contain epinephrine for the test dose because circulatory changes compatible with epinephrine may also serve as a warning sign of unintended intravascular injection. An intravascular injection is still possible even if aspirations for blood are negative. Repeated doses of lidocaine may cause significant increases in blood levels with each repeated dose because of slow accumulation of the drug or its metabolites. Tolerance to elevated blood levels varies with the status of the patient. Debilitated, elderly patients, acutely ill patients, and children should be given reduced doses commensurate with their age and physical condition. Lidocaine should also be used with caution in patients with severe shock or heart block.

Lumbar and caudal epidural anesthesia should be used with extreme caution in persons with the following conditions: existing neurological disease, spinal deformities, septicemia and severe hypertension.

Local anesthetic solutions containing a vasoconstrictor should be used cautiously and in carefully circumscribed quantities in areas of the body supplied by end arteries or having otherwise compromised blood supply. Patients with peripheral vascular disease and those with hypertensive vascular disease may exhibit exaggerated vasoconstrictor response. Ischemic injury or necrosis may result. Preparations containing a vasoconstrictor should be used with caution in patients during or following the administration of potent general anesthetic agents, since cardiac arrhythmias may occur under such conditions.

Careful and constant monitoring of cardiovascular and respiratory (adequacy of ventilation) vital signs and the patient's state of consciousness should be accomplished after each local anesthetic injection. It should be kept in mind at such times that restlessness, anxiety, tinnitus, dizziness, blurred vision, tremors, depression or drowsiness may be early warning signs of central nervous system toxicity.

Since amide-type local anesthetics are metabolized by the liver, Xylocaine Injection should be used with caution in patients with hepatic disease. Patients with severe hepatic disease, because of their inability to metabolize local anesthetics normally, are at greater risk of developing toxic plasma concentrations. Xylocaine Injection should also be used with caution in patients with impaired cardiovascular function since they may be less able to compensate for functional changes associated with the prolongation of A-V conduction produced by these drugs.

Many drugs used during the conduct of anesthesia are considered potential triggering agents for familial malignant hyperthermia. Since it is not known whether amide-type local anesthetics may trigger this reaction and since the need for supplemental general anesthesia cannot be predicted in advance, it is suggested that a standard protocol for the management of malignant hyperthermia should be available. Early unexplained signs of tachycardia, tachypnea, labile blood pressure and metabolic acidosis may precede temperature elevation. Successful outcome is dependent on early diagnosis, prompt discontinuance of the suspect triggering agent(s) and institution of treatment, including oxygen therapy, indicated supportive measures and dantrolene (consult dantrolene sodium intravenous package insert before using).

Proper tourniquet technique, as described in publications and standard textbooks, is essential in the performance of intravenous regional anesthesia. Solutions containing epinephrine or other vasoconstrictors should not be used for this technique.

Lidocaine should be used with caution in persons with known drug sensitivities. Patients allergic to para-aminobenzoic acid derivatives (procaine, tetracaine, benzocaine, etc.) have not shown cross sensitivity to lidocaine.

Use in the Head and Neck Area: Small doses of local anesthetics injected into the head and neck area, including retrobulbar, dental and stellate ganglion blocks, may produce adverse reactions similar to systemic toxicity seen with unintentional intravascular injections of larger doses. Confusion, convulsions, respiratory depression and/or respiratory arrest, and cardiovascular stimulation or depression have been reported. These reactions may be due to intra-arterial injection of the local anesthetic with retrograde flow to the cerebral circulation. Patients receiving these blocks should have their circulation and respiration monitored and be constantly observed. Resuscitative equipment and personnel for treating adverse reactions should be immediately available. Dosage recommendations should not be exceeded. (See DOSAGE and ADMINISTRATION.)

Information for Patients: When appropriate, patients should be informed in advance that they may experience temporary loss of sensation and motor activity, usually in the lower half of the body, following proper administration of epidural anesthesia.

Clinically Significant Drug Interactions: The administration of local anesthetic solutions containing epinephrine or norepinephrine to patients receiving monoamine oxidase inhibitors or tricyclic antidepressants may produce severe, prolonged hypertension.

Phenothiazines and butyrophenones may reduce or reverse the pressor effect of epinephrine.

Concurrent use of these agents should generally be avoided. In situations when concurrent therapy is necessary, careful patient monitoring is essential.

Concurrent administration of vasopressor drugs (for the treatment of hypotension related to obstetric blocks) and ergot-type oxytocic drugs may cause severe, persistent hypertension or cerebrovascular accidents.

Drug/Laboratory Test Interactions: The intramuscular injection of lidocaine may result in an increase in creatine phosphokinase levels. Thus, the use of this enzyme determination, without isoenzyme separation, as a diagnostic test for the presence of acute myocardial infarction may be compromised by the intramuscular injection of lidocaine.

Carcinogenesis, Mutagenesis, Impairment of Fertility: Studies of lidocaine in animals to evaluate the carcinogenic and mutagenic potential or the effect on fertility have not been conducted.

Pregnancy: *Teratogenic Effects:* Pregnancy Category B. Reproduction studies have been performed in rats at doses up to 6.6 times the human dose and have revealed no evidence of harm to the fetus caused by lidocaine. There are, however, no adequate and well-controlled studies in pregnant women. Animal reproduction studies are not always predictive of human response. General consideration should be given to this fact before administering lidocaine to women of childbearing potential, especially during early pregnancy when maximum organogenesis takes place.

Labor and Delivery: Local anesthetics rapidly cross the placenta and when used for epidural, paracervical, pudendal or caudal block anesthesia, can cause varying degrees of maternal, fetal and neonatal toxicity. (see CLINICAL PHARMACOLOGY, Pharmacokinetics.) The potential for toxicity depends upon the procedure performed, the type and amount of drug used, and the technique of drug administration. Adverse reactions in the parturient, fetus and neonate involve alterations of the central nervous system, peripheral vascular tone and cardiac function.

Maternal hypotension has resulted from regional anesthesia. Local anesthetics produce vasodilation by blocking sympathetic nerves. Elevating the patient's legs and positioning her on her left side will help prevent decreases in blood pressure.

The fetal heart rate also should be monitored continuously, and electronic fetal monitoring is highly advisable.

Epidural, spinal, paracervical, or pudendal anesthesia may alter the forces of parturition through changes in uterine contractility or maternal expulsive efforts. In one study, paracervical block anesthesia was associated with a decrease in the mean duration of first stage labor and facilitation of cervical dilation. However, spinal and epidural anesthesia have also been reported to prolong the second stage of labor by removing the parturient's reflex urge to bear down or by interfering with motor function. The use of obstetrical anesthesia may increase the need for forceps assistance.

The use of some local anesthetic drug products during labor and delivery may be followed by diminished muscle strength and tone for the first day or two of life. The long-term significance of these observations is unknown. Fetal bradycardia may occur in 20 to 30 percent of patients receiving paracervical nerve block anesthesia with the amide-type local anesthetics and may be associated with fetal acidosis. Fetal heart rate should always be monitored during paracervical anesthesia. The physician should weigh the possible advantages against risks when considering a paracervical block in prematurity, toxemia of pregnancy, and fetal distress. Careful adherence to recommended dosage is of the utmost importance in obstetrical paracervical block. Failure to achieve adequate analgesia with recommended doses should arouse suspicion of intravascular or fetal intracranial injection. Cases compatible with unintended fetal intracranial injection of local anesthetic solution have been reported following intended paracervical or pudendal block or both. Babies so affected present with unexplained neonatal depression at birth, which correlates with high local anesthetic serum levels, and often manifest seizures within six hours. Prompt use of supportive measures combined with forced urinary excretion of the local anesthetic has been used successfully to manage this complication.

Case reports of maternal convulsions and cardiovascular collapse following use of some local anesthetics for paracervical block in early pregnancy (as anesthesia for elective abortion) suggest that systemic absorption under these circumstances may be rapid. The recommended maximum dose of each drug should not be exceeded. Injection should be made slowly and with frequent aspiration. Allow a 5-minute interval between sides.

Nursing Mothers: It is not known whether this drug is excreted in human milk. Because many drugs are excreted in human milk, caution should be exercised when lidocaine is administered to a nursing woman.

Pediatric Use: Dosages in children should be reduced, commensurate with age, body weight and physical condition. See DOSAGE AND ADMINISTRATION.

HOW SUPPLIED

Xylocaine (lidocaine HCl) Concentration	Epinephrine Dilution (if present)	Xylocaine-MPF: Ampules (mL) 2	5	10	20	30	Polyamp DuoFit™ (mL) 10	20	Single Dose Vial (mL) 2	5	10	20	30	50	Xylocaine: Multiple Dose Vial (mL) 10	20	50
0.5%														X			X
0.5%	1:200,000																X
1%		X	X			X	X	X	X	X	X		X		X	X	X
1%	1:100,000														X	X	X
1%	1:200,000					X				X	X		X				
1.5%					X		X	X			X	X					
1.5%	1:200,000		X			X				X	X		X				
2%		X		X			X		X	X	X				X	X	X
2%	1:100,000														X	X	X
2%	1:200,000				X					X	X	X					

ADVERSE REACTIONS

Systemic: Adverse experiences following the administration of lidocaine are similar in nature to those observed with other amide local anesthetic agents. These adverse experiences are, in general, dose-related and may result from high plasma levels caused by excessive dosage, rapid absorption or inadvertent intravascular injection, or may result from a hypersensitivity, idiosyncrasy or diminished tolerance on the part of the patient. Serious adverse experiences are generally systemic in nature. The following types are those most commonly reported:

Central Nervous System: CNS manifestations are excitatory and/or depressant and may be characterized by lightheadedness, nervousness, apprehension, euphoria, confusion, dizziness, drowsiness, tinnitus, blurred or double vision, vomiting, sensations of heat, cold or numbness, twitching, tremors, convulsions, unconsciousness, respiratory depression and arrest. The excitatory manifestations may be very brief or may not occur at all, in which case the first manifestation of toxicity may be drowsiness merging into unconsciousness and respiratory arrest.

Drowsiness following the administration of lidocaine is usually an early sign of a high blood level of the drug and may occur as a consequence of rapid absorption.

Cardiovascular System: Cardiovascular manifestations are usually depressant and are characterized by bradycardia, hypotension, and cardiovascular collapse, which may lead to cardiac arrest.

Allergic: Allergic reactions are characterized by cutaneous lesions, urticaria, edema or anaphylactoid reactions. Allergic reactions may occur as a result of sensitivity either to local anesthetic agents or to the methylparaben used as a preservative in the multiple dose vials. Allergic reactions as a result of sensitivity to lidocaine are extremely rare and, if they occur, should be managed by conventional means. The detection of sensitivity by skin testing is of doubtful value.

Neurologic: The incidences of adverse reactions associated with the use of local anesthetics may be related to the total dose of local anesthetic administered and are also dependent upon the particular drug used, the route of administration and the physical status of the patient. In a prospective review of 10,440 patients who received lidocaine for spinal anesthesia, the incidences of adverse reactions were reported to be about 3 percent each for positional headaches, hypotension and backache; 2 percent for shivering; and less than 1 percent each for peripheral nerve symptoms, nausea, respiratory inadequacy and double vision. Many of these observations may be related to local anesthetic techniques, with or without a contribution from the local anesthetic.

In the practice of caudal or lumbar epidural block, occasional unintentional penetration of the subarachnoid space by the catheter may occur. Subsequent adverse effects may depend partially on the amount of drug administered subdurally. These may include spinal block of varying magnitude (including total spinal block), hypotension secondary to spinal block, loss of bladder and bowel control, and loss of perineal sensation and sexual function. Persistent motor, sensory and/or autonomic (sphincter control) deficit of some lower spinal segments with slow recovery (several months) or incomplete recovery have been reported in rare instances when caudal or lumbar epidural block has been attempted. Backache and headache have also been noted following use of these anesthetic procedures.

There have been reported cases of permanent injury to extraocular muscles requiring surgical repair following retrobulbar administration.

OVERDOSAGE

Acute emergencies from local anesthetics are generally related to high plasma levels encountered during therapeutic use of local anesthetics or to unintended subarachnoid injection of local anesthetic solution (see ADVERSE REACTIONS, WARNINGS, and PRECAUTIONS).

Management of Local Anesthetic Emergencies: The first consideration is prevention, best accomplished by careful and constant monitoring of cardiovascular and respiratory vital signs and the patient's state of consciousness after each local anesthetic injection. At the first sign of change, oxygen should be administered.

The first step in the management of convulsions, as well as underventilation or apnea due to unintended subarachnoid injection of drug solution, consists of immediate attention to the maintenance of a patent airway and assisted or controlled ventilation with oxygen and a delivery system capable of permitting immediate positive airway pressure by mask. Immediately after the institution of these ventilatory measures, the adequacy of the circulation should be evaluated, keeping in mind that drugs used to treat convulsions sometimes depress the circulation when administered intravenously. Should convulsions persist despite adequate respiratory support, and if the status of the circulation permits, small increments of an ultra-short acting barbiturate (such as thiopental or thiamylal) or a benzodiazepine (such as diazepam) may be administered intravenously. The clinician should be familiar, prior to the use of local anesthetics, with these anticonvulsant drugs. Supportive treatment of circulatory depression may require administration of intravenous fluids and, when appropriate, a vasopressor as directed by the clinical situation (e.g., ephedrine).

If not treated immediately, both convulsions and cardiovascular depression can result in hypoxia, acidosis, bradycardia, arrhythmias and cardiac arrest. Underventilation or apnea due to unintentional subarachnoid injection of local anesthetic solution may produce these same signs and also lead to cardiac arrest if ventilatory support is not instituted. If cardiac arrest should occur, standard cardiopulmonary resuscitative measures should be instituted.

Endotracheal intubation, employing drugs and techniques familiar to the clinician, may be indicated, after initial administration of oxygen by mask, if difficulty is encountered in the maintenance of a patent airway or if prolonged ventilatory support (assisted or controlled) is indicated.

Dialysis is of negligible value in the treatment of acute overdosage with lidocaine.

The oral LD_{50} of lidocaine HCl in non-fasted female rats is 459 (346–773) mg/kg (as the salt) and 214 (159–324) mg/kg (as the salt) in fasted female rats.

DOSAGE AND ADMINISTRATION

Table 1 (Recommended Dosages) summarizes the recommended volumes and concentrations of Xylocaine Injection for various types of anesthetic procedures. The dosages suggested in this table are for normal healthy adults and refer to the use of epinephrine-free solutions. When larger volumes are required, only solutions containing epinephrine should be used except in those cases where vasopressor drugs may be contraindicated.

These recommended doses serve only as a guide to the amount of anesthetic required for most routine procedures. The actual volumes and concentrations to be used depend on a number of factors such as type and extent of surgical procedure, depth of anesthesia and degree of muscular relaxation required, duration of anesthesia required, and the physical condition of the patient. In all cases the lowest concentration and smallest dose that will produce the desired result should be given. Dosages should be reduced for children and for the elderly and debilitated patients and patients with cardiac and/or liver disease.

The onset of anesthesia, the duration of anesthesia and the degree of muscular relaxation are proportional to the volume and concentration (i.e., total dose) of local anesthetic used. Thus, an increase in volume and concentration of Xylocaine Injection will decrease the onset of anesthesia, prolong the duration of anesthesia, provide a greater degree of muscular relaxation and increase the segmental spread of anesthesia. However, increasing the volume and concentration of Xylocaine Injection may result in a more profound fall in blood pressure when used in epidural anesthesia. Although the incidence of side effects with lidocaine is quite low, caution should be exercised when employing large volumes and concentrations, since the incidence of side effects is directly proportional to the total dose of local anesthetic agent injected.

For intravenous regional anesthesia, only the 50 mL single dose vial containing Xylocaine (lidocaine HCl) 0.5% Injection should be used.

Epidural Anesthesia: For epidural anesthesia, only the following dosage forms of Xylocaine Injection are recommended:

1% without epinephrine	10 mL Polyamp DuoFit™
1% without epinephrine	20 mL Polyamp DuoFit™
1% without epinephrine	30 mL single dose solutions
1% with epinephrine 1:200,000	30 mL single dose solutions
1.5% without epinephrine	10 mL Polyamp DuoFit™
1.5% without epinephrine	20 mL Polyamp DuoFit™
1.5% without epinephrine	20 mL ampules, 20 mL single dose solutions
1.5% with epinephrine 1:200,000	30 mL ampules, 30 mL single dose solutions
2% without epinephrine	10 mL Polyamp DuoFit™
2% without epinephrine	10 mL ampules, 10 mL single dose solutions
2% with epinephrine 1:200,000	20 mL ampules, 20 mL single dose solutions

Although these solutions are intended specifically for epidural anesthesia, they may also be used for infiltration and peripheral nerve block, provided they are employed as single dose units. These solutions contain no bacteriostatic agent.

In epidural anesthesia, the dosage varies with the number of dermatomes to be anesthetized (generally 2–3 mL of the indicated concentration per dermatome).

Caudal and Lumbar Epidural Block: As a precaution against the adverse experience sometimes observed following unintentional penetration of the subarachnoid space, a test dose such as 2–3 mL of 1.5% lidocaine should be administered at least 5 minutes prior to injecting the total volume required for a lumbar or caudal epidural block. The test dose should be repeated if the patient is moved in a manner that may have displaced the catheter. Epinephrine, if contained in the test dose, (10–15 µg have been suggested), may serve as a warning of unintentional intravascular injection. If injected into a blood vessel, this amount of epinephrine is likely to produce a transient "epinephrine response" within 45 seconds, consisting of an increase in heart rate and systolic blood pressure, circumoral pallor, palpitations and nervousness in the unsedated patient. The sedated patient may exhibit only a pulse rate increase of 20 or more beats per minute for 15 or more seconds. Patients on beta blockers may not manifest changes in heart rate, but blood pressure monitoring can detect an evanescent rise in systolic blood pressure. Adequate time should be allowed for onset of anesthesia after administration of each test dose. The rapid injection of a large volume of Xylocaine Injection through the catheter should be avoided, and, when feasible, fractional doses should be administered.

In the event of the known injection of a large volume of local anesthetic solution into the subarachnoid space, after suitable resuscitation and if the catheter is in place, consider attempting the recovery of drug by draining a moderate amount of cerebrospinal fluid (such as 10 mL) through the epidural catheter.

MAXIMUM RECOMMENDED DOSAGES

Adults: For normal healthy adults, the individual maximum recommended dose of lidocaine HCl with epinephrine should not exceed 7 mg/kg (3.5 mg/lb) of body weight, and in general it is recommended that the maximum total dose not exceed 500 mg. When used without epinephrine the maximum individual dose should not exceed 4.5 mg/kg (2 mg/lb) of body weight, and in general it is recommended that the maximum total dose does not exceed 300 mg. For continuous epidural or caudal anesthesia, the maximum recommended dosage should not be administered at intervals of less than 90 minutes. When continuous lumbar or caudal epidural anesthesia is used for non-obstetrical procedures, more drug may be administered if required to produce adequate anesthesia.

The maximum recommended dose per 90 minute period of lidocaine hydrochloride for paracervical block in obstetrical patients and non-obstetrical patients is 200 mg total. One half of the total dose is usually administered to each side. Inject slowly, five minutes between sides. (See also discussion of paracervical block in PRECAUTIONS.)

For intravenous regional anesthesia, the dose administered should not exceed 4 mg/kg in adults.

Continued on next page

Xylocaine/Xylocaine w/Epi.—Cont.

Children: It is difficult to recommend a maximum dose of any drug for children, since this varies as a function of age and weight. For children over 3 years of age who have a normal lean body mass and normal body development, the maximum dose is determined by the child's age and weight. For example, in a child of 5 years weighing 50 lbs the dose of lidocaine HCl should not exceed 75–100 mg (1.5–2 mg/lb). The use of even more dilute solutions (i.e., 0.25–0.5%) and total dosages not to exceed 3 mg/kg (1.4 mg/lb) are recommended for induction of intravenous regional anesthesia in children.
In order to guard against systemic toxicity, the lowest effective concentration and lowest effective dose should be used at all times. In some cases it will be necessary to dilute available concentrations with 0.9% sodium chloride injection in order to obtain the required final concentration.
NOTE: Parenteral drug products should be inspected visually for particulate matter and discoloration prior to administration whenever the solution and container permit. The injection is not to be used if its color is pinkish or darker than slightly yellow or if it contains a precipitate.

Table 1. Recommended Dosages

Procedure	Xylocaine (lidocaine hydrochloride) Injection (without epinephrine) Conc (%)	Vol (mL)	Total Dose (mg)
Infiltration			
Percutaneous	0.5 or 1	1–60	5–300
Intravenous regional	0.5	10–60	50–300
Peripheral Nerve Blocks, e.g.			
Brachial	1.5	15–20	225–300
Dental	2	1–5	20–100
Intercostal	1	3	30
Paravertebral	1	3–5	30–50
Pudendal (each side)	1	10	100
Paracervical			
Obstetrical analgesia (each side)	1	10	100
Sympathetic Nerve Blocks, e.g.			
Cervical (stellate ganglion)	1	5	50
Lumbar	1	5–10	50–100
Central Neural Blocks			
Epidural*			
Thoracic	1	20–30	200–300
Lumbar			
Analgesia	1	25–30	250–300
Anesthesia	1.5	15–20	225–300
	2	10–15	200–300
Caudal			
Obstetrical analgesia	1	20–30	200–300
Surgical anesthesia	1.5	15–20	225–300

* Dose determined by number of dermatomes to be anesthetized (2–3 mL/dermatome).

THE ABOVE SUGGESTED CONCENTRATIONS AND VOLUMES SERVE ONLY AS A GUIDE. OTHER VOLUMES AND CONCENTRATIONS MAY BE USED PROVIDED THE TOTAL MAXIMUM RECOMMENDED DOSE IS NOT EXCEEDED.

STERILIZATION, STORAGE AND TECHNICAL PROCEDURES
Disinfecting agents containing heavy metals, which cause release of respective ions (mercury, zinc, copper, etc.) should not be used for skin or mucous membrane disinfection as they have been related to incidents of swelling and edema. When chemical disinfection of multi-dose vials is desired, either isopropyl alcohol (91%) or ethyl alcohol (70%) is recommended. Many commercially available brands of rubbing alcohol, as well as solutions of ethyl alcohol not of U.S.P. grade, contain denaturants which are injurious to rubber and therefore are not to be used.
Dosage forms listed as Xylocaine-MPF indicate single dose solutions that are Methyl Paraben Free (MPF).
[See table at top of previous page]
All solutions should be stored at room temperature, approximately 25°C (77°F).
Protect from light.
Trademarks herein are the property of the AstraZeneca Group

702201-03 Rev. 4/00
Shown in Product Identification Guide, page 305

XYLOCAINE® ℞
[zī 'lo-caine]
(lidocaine HCl Injection, USP)
For Ventricular Arrhythmias

(For details of indications, dosage and administration, precautions, and adverse reactions, see circular in package.)

DESCRIPTION
Xylocaine (lidocaine HCl Injection, USP) is a sterile non pyrogenic solution of an antiarrhythmic agent administered intravenously by either direct injection or continuous infusion.
Xylocaine Injections are composed of aqueous solutions of lidocaine hydrochloride. Lidocaine HCl ($C_{14}H_{22}N_2O{\cdot}HCl$) is chemically designated acetamide, 2-(diethylamino)-N-(2,6 dimethylphenyl)-, monohydrochloride.

HOW SUPPLIED
For direct intravenous injection, Xylocaine (lidocaine HCl Injection, USP) without preservatives is supplied in the following dosage forms:

NDC 0186-0615-01	50 mg	5 mL Prefilled Syringe with a 21 G 15/16″ Needle
NDC 0186-0611-01	100 mg	5 mL Prefilled Syringe with a 21 G 15/16″ Needle
NDC 0186-0232-03	100 mg	5 mL Ampule

For preparing solutions for intravenous infusions, Xylocaine (lidocaine HCl Injection, USP) without sodium chloride or preservatives is supplied in the following dosage forms:

NDC 0186-0166-01	1 gram	25 mL Single Use Vial without transfer unit
NDC 0186-0169-01	2 grams	50 mL Single Use Vial without transfer unit
NDC 0186-0167-01	1 gram	25 mL Single Use Vial with presterilized transfer unit
NDC 0186-0168-01	2 grams	50 mL Single Use Vial with presterilized transfer unit

Solutions should be stored at controlled room temperature 15°–30°C (59°–86°F).
021679R03 Rev. 6/97

4% XYLOCAINE®-MPF (lidocaine HCl) ℞
[zī 'lo-caine]
Sterile Solution

(For details of indications, dosage and administration, precautions, and adverse reactions, see circular in package.)

DESCRIPTION
4% Xylocaine-MPF (lidocaine HCl) Sterile Solution (Methylparaben Free) contains a local anesthetic agent and is administered topically or by injection. See INDICATIONS for specific uses.
4% Xylocaine-MPF Sterile Solution contains lidocaine HCl, which is chemically designated as acetamide, 2-(diethylamino)-N-(2,6-dimethylphenyl)-mono-hydrochloride.
4% Xylocaine-MPF Sterile Solution in 5 mL ampules may be autoclaved repeatedly if necessary.
Composition of 4% Xylocaine-MPF Sterile Solution
Each mL contains lidocaine HCl, 40.0 mg, and sodium hydroxide and/or hydrochloric acid to adjust pH to 5.0–7.0. A sterile, aqueous solution.

HOW SUPPLIED
4% Xylocaine-MPF (lidocaine HCl) Sterile Solution, 5 mL ampule (NDC 0186-0235-03) and 5 mL prefilled sterile disposable syringe packaged in a presterilized kit containing a laryngotracheal cannula (NDC 0186-0235-72).
Store at controlled room temperature: 15°–30°C (59°–86°F).
021562R09 Rev. 2/97

4% XYLOCAINE® (lidocaine HCl) ℞
[zī 'lo-caine]
TOPICAL SOLUTION

(For details of indications, dosage and administration, precautions, and adverse reactions, see circular in package.)

DESCRIPTION
Xylocaine (lidocaine HCl) 4% Topical Solution contains a local anesthetic agent and is administered topically. See INDICATIONS for specific uses.
Xylocaine 4% Topical Solution contains lidocaine HCl, which is chemically designated as acetamide, 2-(diethylamino)-N-(2, 6-dimethylphenyl)-, monohydrochloride.
The 50 mL screw-cap bottle should not be autoclaved, because the closure employed cannot withstand autoclaving temperatures and pressures. Composition of Xylocaine (lidocaine HCl) 4% Topical Solution: Each mL contains lidocaine HCl, 40 mg, methylparaben, and sodium hydroxide and/or hydrochloric acid to adjust pH to 6.0 – 7.0.
An aqueous solution. NOT FOR INJECTION.

HOW SUPPLIED
Xylocaine (lidocaine HCl) 4% Topical Solution 50 mL screw-cap bottle, cartoned (NDC 0186-0320-01). NOT FOR INJECTION.
Store at controlled room temperature 15°-30°C (59°-86°F).
021708R00 Rev. 4/97

1.5% XYLOCAINE®-MPF with Dextrose 7.5% Injection ℞
(lidocaine HCl and dextrose anhydrous Injection)
For Spinal Anesthesia in Obstetrics.

(For details of indications, dosage and administration, precautions, and adverse reactions, see circular in package.)

HOW SUPPLIED
Xylocaine-MPF 1.5% with Dextrose 7.5% Injection (lidocaine HCl and dextrose anhydrous Injection), NDC 0186-0212-03, is supplied in 2 mL ampules in packages of 10.
Store at controlled room temperature 15°–30°C (59°-86°F).
021836R09 Rev. 9/97

5% XYLOCAINE®-MPF With Glucose 7.5% Injection ℞
[zī 'lo-cain]
(lidocaine HCl and dextrose anhydrous Injection)

(For details of indications, dosage and administration, precautions, and adverse reactions, see circular in package.)

HOW SUPPLIED
Xylocaine-MPF 5% with Glucose 7.5% Injection (lidocaine HCl and dextrose anhydrous Injection), NDC 0186-0225-03, is supplied in 2 mL ampules in packages of 10.
Store at controlled room temperature 15°–30°C (59°–86°F).
021564R14 Rev. 9/97

XYLOCAINE® 2% Jelly (lidocaine hydrochloride) ℞
[zī 'lo-caine]

(For details of indications, dosage and administration, precautions, and adverse reactions, see circular in package.)

DESCRIPTION
Xylocaine (lidocaine HCl) 2% Jelly is a sterile aqueous product that contains a local anesthetic agent and is administered topically. (See INDICATIONS for specific uses.)
Xylocaine 2% Jelly contains lidocaine HCl which is chemically designated as acetamide, 2-(diethylamino)-N-(2,6-dimethylphenyl)-, monohydrochloride.
Xylocaine 2% Jelly also contains hydroxypropylmethylcellulose, and the resulting mixture maximizes contact with mucosa and provides lubrication for instrumentation. The unused portion should be discarded after initial use.
Composition of Xylocaine 2% Jelly (30 mL and 5 mL tubes): Each mL contains 20 mg of lidocaine HCl. The formulation also contains methylparaben, propylparaben, hydroxypropylmethylcellulose, and sodium hydroxide and/or hydrochloric acid to adjust pH to 6.0–7.0.
Composition of Xylocaine 2% Jelly (10 mL and 20 mL syringes): Each mL contains 20 mg of lidocaine HCl. The formulation also contains hydroxypropylmethylcellulose, and sodium hydroxide and/or hydrochloric acid to adjust pH to 6.2–6.8.

HOW SUPPLIED
Xylocaine (lidocaine HCl) 2% Jelly is supplied in the listed dosage forms.
NDC 0186-0330-01 30 mL aluminum tube, Box of 1
A detachable applicator cone and a key for expressing the contents are included.
NDC 0186-0330-36 5 mL plastic tube, Box of 10
NDC 0186-0336-43 10 mL polypropylene syringe, Box of 10
NDC 0186-0336-53 20 mL polypropylene syringe, Box of 10
Store at controlled room temperature 20–25°C (68–77°F) [see USP].
Trademarks herein are the property of the AstraZeneca Group

Xylocaine Jelly Syringes are manufactured by AstraZeneca AB, Karlskoga, Sweden.
AstraZeneca LP, Wilmington, DE 19850
700831-00 Rev. 4/00
Shown in Product Identification Guide, page 305

5% XYLOCAINE® OINTMENT (lidocaine) ℞
[zī 'lo-caine]

(For details of indications, dosage and administration, precautions, and adverse reactions, see circular in package.)

DESCRIPTION
Xylocaine (lidocaine) 5% Ointment contains a local anesthetic agent and is administered topically. See INDICATIONS for specific uses.
Xylocaine 5% Ointment contains lidocaine, which is chemically designated as acetamide, 2-(diethylamino)-N-(2,6-dimethylphenyl)-.
Composition of Xylocaine 5% Ointment:
Each gram of the plain and flavored ointments contains lidocaine, 50 mg, polyethylene glycol 540 blend, polyethylene glycol 3350 and propylene glycol. The flavored ointment contains sodium saccharin, peppermint oil and spearmint oil.

HOW SUPPLIED
Xylocaine (lidocaine) 5% Ointment (NDC 0186-0315-21) is available in 35 gm tubes.

Xylocaine (lidocaine) 5% Ointment Flavored for application within the oral cavity, is dispensed in 3.5 gram tubes, 10 tubes per carton (NDC 0186-0350-03), and in 35-gram jars (NDC 0186-0350-01).
KEEP CONTAINER TIGHTLY CLOSED AT ALL TIMES WHEN NOT IN USE.
Store at controlled room temperature 15°–30°C (59°–86°F).
021563R00 Rev. 5/97

XYLOCAINE ® 2.5% OINTMENT (lidocaine) OTC
[zī 'lo-cain]

(See PDR For Nonprescription Drugs.)

2% XYLOCAINE® Viscous ℞
(lidocaine HCl) Solution
[zī 'lo-caine]
A Topical Anesthetic for the Mucous Membranes of the Mouth and Pharynx

(For details of indications, dosage and administration, precautions, and adverse reactions, see circular in package.)

DESCRIPTION

Xylocaine (lidocaine HCl) 2% Viscous Solution contains a local anesthetic agent and is administered topically. Xylocaine 2% Viscous Solution contains lidocaine HCl, which is chemically designated as acetamide, 2-(diethylamino)-N-(2,6-dimethylphenyl)-, monohydrochloride.
The molecular formula of lidocaine is $C_{14}H_{22}N_2O$. The molecular weight is 234.34.

HOW SUPPLIED

Xylocaine 2% (lidocaine HCl) Viscous Solution is available in 100 mL (NDC 0186-0360-01) and 450 mL (NDC 0186-0360-11) polyethylene squeeze bottles and in unit of use (adult dose) packages of 25 (20 mL) polyethylene bottles (NDC 0186-0361-78).
The solutions should be stored at controlled room temperature 15–30°C (59–86°F).
808165-00 3/00

AstraZeneca Pharmaceuticals LP

1800 CONCORD PIKE
WILMINGTON, DE 19850-5437 USA

For Product and Business Information, and Adverse Drug Experiences:
Information Center
1-800-236-9933

For Product Ordering:
Trade Customer Service
1-800-842-9920

Internet: www.astrazeneca-us.com

ACCOLATE® Tablets ℞
[acc'late]
(zafirlukast)

DESCRIPTION

Zafirlukast is a synthetic, selective peptide leukotriene receptor antagonist (LTRA), with the chemical name 4-(5-cyclopentyloxy-carbonylamino-1-methyl-indol-3-ylmethyl)-3-methoxy-N-o-tolylsulfonylbenzamide. The molecular weight of zafirlukast is 575.7 and the structure formula is:

The empirical formula is: $C_{31}H_{33}N_3O_6S$
Zafirlukast, a fine white to pale yellow amorphous powder, is practically insoluble in water. It is slightly soluble in methanol and freely soluble in tetrahydrofuran, dimethylsulfoxide, and acetone.
ACCOLATE is supplied as 10 and 20 mg tablets for oral administration.
Inactive Ingredients: Film-coated tablets containing croscarmellose sodium, lactose, magnesium stearate, microcrystalline cellulose, povidone, hydroxypropylmethylcellulose and titanium dioxide.

CLINICAL PHARMACOLOGY

Mechanism of Action: Zafirlukast is a selective and competitive receptor antagonist of leukotriene D_4 and E_4 (LTD_4 and LTE_4), components of slow-reacting substance of anaphylaxis (SRSA). Cysteinyl leukotriene production and receptor occupation have been correlated with the pathophysiology of asthma, including airway edema, smooth muscle constriction, and altered cellular activity associated with the inflammatory process, which contribute to the signs and symptoms of asthma. Patients with asthma were found in one study to be 25–100 times more sensitive to the bronchoconstricting activity of inhaled LTD_4 than nonasthmatic subjects.
In vitro studies demonstrated that zafirlukast antagonized the contractile activity of three leukotrienes (LTC_4, LTD_4 and LTE_4) in conducting airway smooth muscle from laboratory animals and humans. Zafirlukast prevented intradermal LTD_4-induced increases in cutaneous vascular permeability and inhibited inhaled LTD_4-induced influx of eosinophils into animal lungs. Inhalational challenge studies in sensitized sheep showed that zafirlukast suppressed the airway responses to antigen; this included both the early- and late-phase response and the nonspecific hyperresponsiveness.
In humans, zafirlukast inhibited bronchoconstriction caused by several kinds of inhalational challenges. Pretreatment with single oral doses of zafirlukast inhibited the bronchoconstriction caused by sulfur dioxide and cold air in patients with asthma. Pretreatment with single doses of zafirlukast attenuated the early- and late-phase reaction caused by inhalation of various antigens such as grass, cat dander, ragweed, and mixed antigens in patients with asthma. Zafirlukast also attenuated the increase in bronchial hyperresponsiveness to inhaled histamine that followed inhaled allergen challenge.

Clinical Pharmacokinetics and Bioavailability:

Absorption

Zafirlukast is rapidly absorbed following oral administration. Peak plasma concentrations are generally achieved 3 hours after oral administration. The absolute bioavailability of zafirlukast is unknown. In two separate studies, one using a high fat and the other a high protein meal, administration of zafirlukast with food reduced the mean bioavailability by approximately 40%.

Distribution

Zafirlukast is more than 99% bound to plasma proteins, predominantly albumin. The degree of binding was independent of concentration in the clinically relevant range. The apparent steady-state volume of distribution (V_{ss}/F) is approximately 70 L, suggesting moderate distribution into tissues. Studies in rats using radiolabeled zafirlukast indicate minimal distribution across the blood-brain barrier.

Metabolism

Zafirlukast is extensively metabolized. The most common metabolic products are hydroxylated metabolites which are excreted in the feces. The metabolites of zafirlukast identified in plasma are at least 90 times less potent as LTD_4 receptor antagonists than zafirlukast in a standard *in vitro* test of activity. *In vitro* studies using human liver microsomes showed that the hydroxylated metabolites of zafirlukast excreted in the feces are formed through the cytochrome P450 2C9 (CYP2C9) pathway. Additional *in vitro* studies utilizing human liver microsomes show that zafirlukast inhibits the cytochrome P450 CYP3A4 and CYP2C9 isoenzymes at concentrations close to the clinically achieved total plasma concentrations. (see Drug Interactions)

Excretion

The apparent oral clearance (CL/f) of zafirlukast is approximately 20 L/h. Studies in the rat and dog suggest that biliary excretion is the primary route of excretion. Following oral administration of radiolabeled zafirlukast to volunteers, urinary excretion accounts for approximately 10% of the dose and the remainder is excreted in feces. Zafirlukast is not detected in urine.
In the pivotal bioequivalence study, the mean terminal half-life of zafirlukast is approximately 10 hours in both normal adult subjects and patients with asthma. In other studies, the mean plasma half-life of zafirlukast ranged from approximately 8 to 16 hours in both normal subjects and patients with asthma. The pharmacokinetics of zafirlukast are approximately linear over the range from 5 mg to 80 mg. Steady-state plasma concentrations of zafirlukast are proportional to the dose and predictable from single-dose pharmacokinetic data. Accumulation of zafirlukast in the plasma following twice daily dosing is approximately 45%.
The pharmacokinetic parameters of zafirlukast 20 mg administered as a single dose to 36 male volunteers are shown with the table below.

Mean (%Coefficient of Variation) pharmacokinetic parameters of zafirlukast following single 20 mg oral dose administration to male volunteers (n=36)

Cmax ng/ml	tmax[1] h	AUC ng.h/mL	t1/2 h	CL/f L/h
326 (31.0)	2 (0.5-5.0)	1137 (34)	13.3 (75.6)	19.4 (32)

[1]Median and range

Special Populations

Gender: The pharmacokinetics of zafirlukast are similar in males and females. Weight-adjusted apparent oral clearance does not differ due to gender.
Race: No differences in the pharmacokinetics of zafirlukast due to race have been observed.
Elderly: The apparent oral clearance of zafirlukast decreases with age. In patients above 65 years of age, there is an approximately 2–3 fold greater C_{max} and AUC compared to young adult patients.
Children: Following administration of a 20 mg dose of zafirlukast to 20 boys and girls between 7 and 11 years of age, a mean (% coefficient of variation) peak drug concentration of 601 ng/mL (45%) was obtained at about 2.5 hrs. Zafirlukast systemic exposure as determined by mean AUC was 2027 ng.h/mL (38%). Weight unadjusted apparent clearance was 11.4 L/h (42%) which resulted in greater systemic drug exposure than that obtained in adults for an identical dose. Zafirlukast disposition was unchanged after multiple dosing (20 mg twice daily) in children and the degree of accumulation in plasma was similar to that observed in adults.
Hepatic Insufficiency: In a study of patients with hepatic impairment (biopsy-proven cirrhosis), there was a reduced clearance of zafirlukast resulting in a 50–60% greater C_{max} and AUC compared to normal subjects.
Renal Insufficiency: Based on a cross-study comparison, there are no apparent differences in the pharmacokinetics of zafirlukast between renally-impaired patients and normal subjects.
Drug Interactions: The following drug interaction studies have been conducted with zafirlukast. (see **PRECAUTIONS: Drug Interactions**)

- Co-administration of multiple doses of zafirlukast (160 mg/day) to steady state with a single 25 mg dose of warfarin (a substrate of CYP2C9) resulted in a significant increase in the mean AUC (+63%) and half-life (+36%) of S-warfarin. The mean prothrombin time increased by approximately 35%. The pharmacokinetics of zafirlukast were unaffected by coadministration with warfarin.
- Co-administration of zafirlukast (80 mg/day) at steady state with a single dose of a liquid theophylline preparation (6 mg/kg) in 13 asthmatic patients, 18 to 44 years of age, resulted in decreased mean plasma concentrations of zafirlukast by approximately 30%, but no effect on plasma theophylline concentrations was observed.
- Co-administration of zafirlukast (20 mg/day) or placebo at steady state with a single dose of sustained release theophylline preparation (16 mg/kg) in 16 healthy boys and girls (6 through 11 years of age) resulted in no significant differences in the pharmacokinetic parameters of theophylline.
- Co-administration of zafirlukast dosed at 40 mg twice daily in a single-blind, parallel-group, 3-week study in 39 healthy female subjects taking oral contraceptives, resulted in no significant effect on ethinyl estradiol plasma concentrations or contraceptive efficacy.
- Co-administration of zafirlukast (40 mg/day) with aspirin (650 mg four times daily) resulted in mean increased plasma concentrations of zafirlukast by approximately 45%.
- Co-administration of a single dose of zafirlukast (40 mg) with erythromycin (500 mg three times daily for 5 days) to steady state in 11 asthmatic patients, resulted in decreased mean plasma concentrations of zafirlukast by approximately 40% due to a decrease in zafirlukast bioavailability.

Clinical Studies:

Three U.S. double-blind, randomized, placebo-controlled, 13-week clinical trials in 1,380 adults and children 12 years of age and older with mild-to-moderate asthma demonstrated that ACCOLATE improved daytime asthma symptoms, nighttime awakenings, mornings with asthma symptoms, rescue beta$_2$-agonist use, FEV_1, and morning peak expiratory flow rate. In these studies, the patients had a mean baseline FEV_1 of approximately 75% of predicted normal and a mean baseline beta-agonist requirement of approximately 4–5 puffs of albuterol per day. The results of the largest of the trials are shown in the table below.
[See table at top of next page]
In a second and smaller study, the effect of ACCOLATE on most efficacy parameters was comparable to the active control (inhaled cromolyn sodium 1600 µg four times per day) and superior to placebo at endpoint for decreasing rescue beta-agonist use (figure below).

Mean ß$_2$-agonist use (puffs/day)

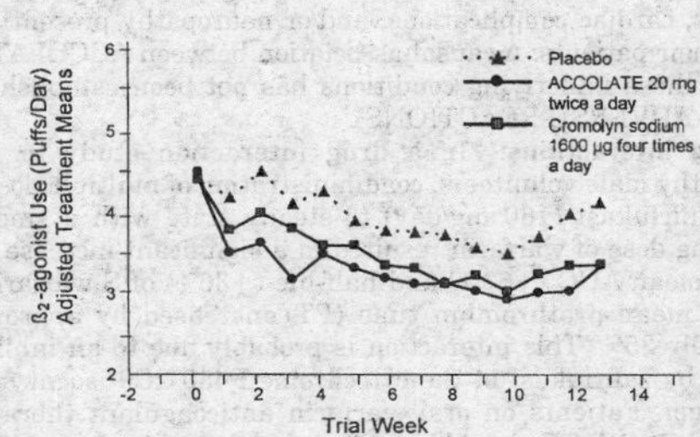

In these trials, improvement in asthma symptoms occurred within one week of initiating treatment with ACCOLATE. The role of ACCOLATE in the management of patients with more severe asthma, patients receiving antiasthma therapy

Continued on next page

Accolate—Cont.

other than as-needed, inhaled beta$_2$-agonists, or as an oral or inhaled corticosteroid-sparing agent remains to be fully characterized.

INDICATIONS AND USAGE

ACCOLATE is indicated for the prophylaxis and chronic treatment of asthma in adults and children 7 years of age and older.

CONTRAINDICATIONS

ACCOLATE is contraindicated in patients who are hypersensitive to zafirlukast or any of its inactive ingredients.

WARNINGS

ACCOLATE is not indicated for use in the reversal of bronchospasm in acute asthma attacks, including status asthmaticus. Therapy with ACCOLATE can be continued during acute exacerbations of asthma.

Coadministration of zafirlukast with warfarin results in a clinically significant increase in prothrombin time (PT). Patients on oral warfarin anticoagulant therapy and ACCOLATE should have their prothrombin times monitored closely and anticoagulant dose adjusted accordingly. (See PRECAUTIONS, Drug Interactions.)

PRECAUTIONS

Information for Patients: ACCOLATE is indicated for the chronic treatment of asthma and should be taken regularly as prescribed, even during symptom-free periods. ACCOLATE is not a bronchodilator and should not be used to treat acute episodes of asthma. Patients receiving ACCOLATE should be instructed not to decrease the dose or stop taking any other antiasthma medications unless instructed by a physician. Women who are breast-feeding should be instructed not to take ACCOLATE (see PRECAUTIONS, Nursing Mothers). Alternative antiasthma medication should be considered in such patients.

The bioavailability of ACCOLATE may be decreased when taken with food. Patients should be instructed to take ACCOLATE at least 1 hour before or 2 hours after meals.

Patients should be told that a rare side effect of ACCOLATE is hepatic dysfunction, and to contact their physician immediately if they experience symptoms of hepatic dysfunction (e.g., right upper quadrant abdominal pain, nausea, fatigue, lethargy, pruritus, jaundice, flu-like symptoms, and anorexia).

Hepatic: Rarely, elevations of one or more liver enzymes have occurred in patients receiving ACCOLATE in controlled clinical trials. In clinical trials, most of these have been observed at doses four times higher than the recommended dose. The following hepatic events (which have occurred predominantly in females) have been reported from postmarketing adverse event surveillance of patients who have received the recommended dose of ACCOLATE (40 mg/day): cases of symptomatic hepatitis (with or without hyperbilirubinemia) without other attributable cause; and rarely, hyperbilirubinemia without other elevated liver function tests. In most, but not all, postmarketing reports, the patient's symptoms abated and the liver enzymes returned to normal or near normal after stopping ACCOLATE. In rare cases, patients have progressed to hepatic failure.

If liver dysfunction is suspected based upon clinical signs or symptoms (e.g., right upper quadrant abdominal pain, nausea, fatigue, lethargy, pruritus, jaundice, flu-like symptoms, anorexia, and enlarged liver) ACCOLATE should be discontinued. Liver function tests, in particular serum ALT, should be measured immediately and the patient managed accordingly. If liver function tests are consistent with hepatic dysfunction, ACCOLATE therapy should not be resumed. Patients in whom ACCOLATE was withdrawn because of hepatic dysfunction where no other attributable cause is identified should not be re-exposed to ACCOLATE. (See PRECAUTIONS, Information for Patients and ADVERSE REACTIONS sections.)

Eosinophilic Conditions: In rare cases, patients on ACCOLATE therapy may present with systemic eosinophilia, sometimes presenting with clinical features of vasculitis consistent with Churg-Strauss syndrome, a condition which is often treated with systemic steroid therapy. These events usually, but not always, have been associated with the reduction of oral steroid therapy. Physicians should be alert to eosinophilia, vasculitic rash, worsening pulmonary symptoms, cardiac complications, and/or neuropathy presenting in their patients. A causal association between ACCOLATE and these underlying conditions has not been established (See ADVERSE REACTIONS).

Drug Interactions: In a drug interaction study in 16 healthy male volunteers, coadministration of multiple doses of zafirlukast (160 mg/day) to steady state with a single 25-mg dose of warfarin resulted in a significant increase in the mean AUC (+63%) and half-life (+36%) of S-warfarin. The mean prothrombin time (PT) increased by approximately 35%. This interaction is probably due to an inhibition by zafirlukast of the cytochrome P450 2C9 isoenzyme system. Patients on oral warfarin anticoagulant therapy and ACCOLATE should have their prothrombin times monitored closely and anticoagulant dose adjusted accordingly (see WARNINGS). No formal drug-drug interaction studies with ACCOLATE and other drugs known to be metabolized by the cytochrome P450 2C9 isoenzyme (e.g., tolbutamide, phenytoin, carbamazepine) have been conducted; however, care should be exercised when ACCOLATE is co-administered with these drugs.

Table 1. Mean Change from Baseline at Study Endpoint

	ACCOLATE 20 mg twice daily N=514	Placebo N=248
Daytime Asthma symptom score (0-3 scale)	−0.44*	−0.25
Nightime Awakenings (number per week)	−1.27*	−0.43
Mornings with Asthma Symptoms (days per week)	−1.32*	−0.75
Rescue β2-agonist use (puffs per day)	−1.15*	−0.24
FEV1 (L)	+0.15*	+0.05
Morning PEFR (L/min)	+22.06*	+7.63
Evening PEFR (L/min)	+13.12	+10.14

*$p<0.05$, compared to placebo

In a drug interaction study in 11 asthmatic patients, coadministration of a single dose of zafirlukast (40 mg) with erythromycin (500 mg three times daily for 5 days) to steady state resulted in decreased mean plasma levels of zafirlukast by approximately 40% due to a decrease in zafirlukast bioavailability.

Co-administration of zafirlukast (20 mg/day) or placebo at steady state with a single dose of sustained release theophylline preparation (16 mg/kg) in 16 healthy boys and girls (6 through 11 years of age) resulted in no significant differences in the pharmacokinetic parameters of theophylline.

Co-administration of zafirlukast (80 mg/day) at steady state with a single dose of a liquid theophylline preparation (6 mg/kg) in 13 asthmatic patients, 18 to 44 years of age, resulted in decreased mean plasma levels of zafirlukast by approximately 30%, but no effect on plasma theophylline levels was observed.

Rare cases of patients experiencing increased theophylline levels with or without clinical signs or symptoms of theophylline toxicity after the addition of ACCOLATE to an existing theophylline regimen have been reported. The mechanism of the interaction between ACCOLATE and theophylline in these patients in unknown (see ADVERSE REACTIONS).

Co-administration of zafirlukast (40 mg/day) with aspirin (650 mg four times daily) resulted in mean increased plasma levels of zafirlukast by approximately 45%.

In a single-blind, parallel-group, 3-week study in 39 healthy female subjects taking oral contraceptives, 40 mg twice daily of zafirlukast had no significant effect on ethinyl estradiol plasma concentrations or contraceptive efficacy.

No formal drug-drug interaction studies between ACCOLATE and marketed drugs known to be metabolized by the P450 3A4 (CYP 3A4) isoenzyme (e.g dihydropyridine calcium-channel blockers, cyclosporin, cisapride) have been conducted. As ACCOLATE is known to be an inhibitor of CYP 3A4 in vitro, it is reasonable to employ appropriate clinical monitoring when these drugs are coadministered with ACCOLATE.

Carcinogenesis, Mutagenesis, Impairment of Fertility: In two-year carcinogenicity studies, zafirlukast was administered at dietary doses of 10, 100, and 300 mg/kg to mice and 40, 400, and 2000 mg/kg to rats. Male mice given 300 mg/kg/day (approximately 75 times the maximum recommended daily oral dose in adults and in children based on a comparison of the plasma area-under the curves [AUCs] values of total drug exposure) showed an increased incidence of hepatocellular adenomas; female mice at this dose showed a greater incidence of whole body histocytic sarcomas. Male and female rats given a dietary dose of 2000 mg/kg/day (approximately 630 times the maximum recommended daily oral dose in adults and in children based on a comparison of the AUCs of total drug exposure) of zafirlukast showed an increased incidence of urinary bladder transitional cell papillomas. Zafirlukast was not tumorigenic at dietary doses up to 100 mg/kg (approximately 40 times the maximum recommended daily oral dose in adults and in children based on comparison of the AUC of total drug exposure) in mice and at dietary doses up to 400 mg/kg (approximately 550 times the maximum recommended daily oral dose in adults and in children based on a comparison of the AUCs of total drug exposure) in rats. The clinical significance of these findings for the long-term use of ACCOLATE is unknown.

Zafirlukast showed no evidence of mutagenic potential in the reverse microbial assay, in 2 forward point mutation (CHO-HGPRT and mouse lymphoma) assays or in two assays for chromosomal aberrations (an in vitro human peripheral blood lymphocyte clastogenic assay and a rat bone marrow micronucleus assay).

No evidence of impairment of fertility and reproduction was seen in male and female rats treated with zafirlukast at oral doses up to 2000 mg/kg (approximately 410 times the maximum recommended daily oral dose in adults on a mg/m^2 basis).

Pregnancy Category B: No teratogenicity was observed at oral doses up to 1600 mg/kg/day in mice (approximately 160 times the maximum recommended daily oral dose in adults on a mg/m^2 basis), 2000 mg/kg/day in rats (approximately 410 times the maximum recommended daily oral dose in adults on a mg/m^2 basis) and 2000 mg/kg/day in cynomolgus monkeys (approximately 120 times the maximum recommended daily oral dose in adults based on comparison of the AUCs of total drug exposure). At an oral dose of 2000 mg/kg/day (approximately 410 times the maximum recommended daily oral dose in adults on a mg/m^2 basis) in rats, maternal toxicity and deaths were seen with increased incidence of early fetal resorption. Spontaneous abortions occurred in cynomolgus monkeys at a maternally toxic dose of 2000 mg/kg/day. There are no adequate and well-controlled trials in pregnant women. Because animal reproduction studies are not always predictive of human response, ACCOLATE should be used during pregnancy only if clearly needed.

Nursing Mothers: Zafirlukast is excreted in breast milk. Following repeated 40-mg twice-a-day dosing in healthy women, average steady-state concentrations of zafirlukast in breast milk were 50 ng/mL compared to 255 ng/mL in plasma. Because of the potential for tumorigenicity shown for zafirlukast in mouse and rat studies and the enhanced sensitivity of neonatal rats and dogs to the adverse effects of zafirlukast, ACCOLATE should not be administered to mothers who are breast-feeding.

Pediatric Use: The safety of ACCOLATE at doses of 10 mg twice daily has been demonstrated in 205 pediatric patients aged 5 through 11 years in placebo-controlled trials lasting up to six weeks and with 179 patients in this age range participating in 52 weeks of treatment in an open label extension.

The effectiveness of ACCOLATE for the prophylaxis and chronic treatment of asthma in pediatric patients aged 7 to 11 years is based on an extrapolation of the demonstrated efficacy of ACCOLATE in adults with asthma and the likelihood that the disease course, and pathophysiology and the drug's effect are substantially similar between the two populations. The recommended dose for the patients 7–11 years of age is based upon a cross-study comparison of the pharmacokinetics of zafirlukast in adults and pediatric subjects, and on the safety profile of zafirlukast in both adult and pediatric patients at doses equal to or higher than the recommended dose.

The effective dose of zafirlukast in pediatric patients 5 and 6 years of age has not been established. The safety and effectiveness of zafirlukast for pediatric patients less than 5 years of age has not been established.

Geriatric Use: Based on cross study comparison, the clearance of zafirlukast is reduced in patients 65 years of age and older such that C_{max} and AUC are approximately 2- to 3-fold greater than those of younger patients (see DOSAGE AND ADMINISTRATION, and CLINICAL PHARMACOLOGY sections).

A total of 8,094 patients were exposed to zafirlukast in North American and European short-term placebo-controlled clinical trials. Of these, 243 patients were elderly (age 65 years and older). No overall difference in adverse events was seen in the elderly patients, except for an increase in the frequency of infection among zafirlukast-treated elderly patients compared to placebo treated elderly patients (7.0% vs. 2.9%). The infections were not severe, occurred mostly in the lower respiratory tract, and did not necessitate withdrawal of therapy.

An open-label, uncontrolled, 4-week trial of 3759 asthma patients compared the safety and efficacy of ACCOLATE 20 mg given twice daily in three patient age groups, adolescents (12–17 years), adults (18–65 years), and elderly (greater than 65 years). A higher percentage of elderly patients (n=384) reported adverse events when compared to adults and adolescents. These elderly patients showed less improvement in efficacy measures. In the elderly patients, adverse events occurring in greater than 1% of the population included headache (4.7%), diarrhea and nausea (1.8%), and pharyngitis (1.3%). The elderly reported the lowest percentage of infections of all three age groups in this study.

ADVERSE REACTIONS

Adults and Children 12 years of age and older

The safety database for ACCOLATE consists of more than 4,000 healthy volunteers and patients who received ACCOLATE, of which 1723 were asthmatics enrolled in trials of 13 weeks duration or longer. A total of 671 patients received ACCOLATE for 1 year or longer. The majority of the patients were 18 years of age or older; however, 222 patients between the age of 12 and 18 years received ACCOLATE.

A comparison of adverse events reported by ≥ 1% of zafirlukast-treated patients, and at rates numerically greater than in placebo-treated patients, is shown for all trials in the table below.

Table 2

Adverse Event	ACCOLATE N=4058	PLACEBO N=2032
Headache	12.9%	11.7%
Infection	3.5%	3.4%
Nausea	3.1%	2.0%
Diarrhea	2.8%	2.1%
Pain (generalized)	1.9%	1.7%
Asthenia	1.8%	1.6%
Abdominal Pain	1.8%	1.1%
Accidental Injury	1.6%	1.5%
Dizziness	1.6%	1.5%
Myalgia	1.6%	1.5%
Fever	1.6%	1.1%
Back Pain	1.5%	1.2%
Vomiting	1.5%	1.1%
SGPT Elevation	1.5%	1.1%
Dyspepsia	1.3%	1.2%

The frequency of less common adverse events was comparable between ACCOLATE and placebo.

Rarely, elevations of one or more liver enzymes have occurred in patients receiving ACCOLATE in controlled clinical trials. In clinical trials, most of these have been observed at doses four times higher than the recommended dose. The following hepatic events (which have occurred predominantly in females) have been reported from postmarketing adverse event surveillance of patients who have received the recommended dose of ACCOLATE (40 mg/day): cases of symptomatic hepatitis (with or without hyperbilirubinemia) without other attributable cause; and rarely, hyperbilirubinemia without other elevated liver function tests. In most, but not all, postmarketing reports, the patient's symptoms abated and the liver enzymes returned to normal or near normal after stopping ACCOLATE. In rare cases, patients have progressed to hepatic failure.

In clinical trials, an increased proportion of zafirlukast patients over the age of 55 years reported infections as compared to placebo-treated patients. A similar finding was not observed in other age groups studied. These infections were mostly mild or moderate in intensity and predominantly affected the respiratory tract. Infections occurred equally in both sexes, were dose-proportional to total milligrams of zafirlukast exposure, and were associated with coadministration of inhaled corticosteroids. The clinical significance of this finding is unknown.

In rare cases, patients on ACCOLATE therapy may present with systemic eosinophilia, sometimes presenting with clinical features of vasculitis consistent with Churg-Strauss syndrome, a condition which is often treated with systemic steroid therapy. These events usually, but not always, have been associated with the reduction of oral steroid therapy. Physicians should be alert to eosinophilia, vasculitic rash, worsening pulmonary symptoms, cardiac complications, and/or neuropathy presenting in their patients. A causal association between ACCOLATE and these underlying conditions has not been established. (see PRECAUTIONS—Eosinophilic Conditions).

Hypersensitivity reactions, including urticaria, angioedema and rashes, with or without blistering, have been reported in association with ACCOLATE therapy. Additionally, there have been reports of patients experiencing agranulocytosis, bleeding, bruising, or edema, arthralgia and myalgia in association with ACCOLATE therapy.

Rare cases of patients experiencing increased theophylline levels with or without clinical signs or symptoms of theophylline toxicity after the addition of ACCOLATE to an existing theophylline regimen have been reported. The mechanism of the interaction between ACCOLATE and theophylline in these patients is unknown and not predicted by available *in vitro* metabolism data and the results of two clinical drug interaction studies (see CLINICAL PHARMACOLOGY and PRECAUTIONS—Drug Interactions sections).

Pediatric Patients 5 through 11 years of Age

ACCOLATE has been evaluated for safety in 788 pediatric patients 5 through 11 years of age. Cumulatively, 313 pediatric patients were treated with ACCOLATE 10 mg bid or higher for at least 6 months, and 113 of them were treated for one year or longer in clinical trials. The safety profile of ACCOLATE 10 mg twice daily-versus placebo in the 4 and 6-week double-blind trials was generally similar to that observed in the adult clinical trials with ACCOLATE 20 mg twice daily.

In pediatric patients receiving ACCOLATE in multi-dose clinical trials, the following events occurred with a frequency of ≥2% and more frequently than in pediatric patients who received placebo, regardless of causality assessment: headache (4.5 vs. 4.2%) and abdominal pain (2.8 vs. 2.3%).

OVERDOSAGE

No deaths occurred at oral zafirlukast doses of 2000 mg/kg in mice (approximately 200 times the maximum recommended daily oral dose in adults on a mg/m^2 basis and approximately 300 times the maximum recommended daily oral dose in children on a mg/m^2 basis), 2000 mg/kg in rats (approximately 410 times the maximum recommended daily oral dose in adults on a mg/m^2 basis and approximately 600 times the maximum recommended daily oral dose in children on a mg/m^2 basis), and 500 mg/kg in dogs (approximately 340 times the maximum recommended daily oral dose in adults on a mg/m^2 basis and approximately 500 times the maximum recommended daily oral dose in children on a mg/m^2 basis).

Overdosage with ACCOLATE has been reported in four patients surviving reported doses as high as 200 mg. The predominant symptoms reported following ACCOLATE overdose were rash and upset stomach. There were no acute toxic effects in humans that could be consistently ascribed to the administration of ACCOLATE. It is reasonable to employ the usual supportive measures in the event of an overdose; e.g., remove unabsorbed material from the gastrointestinal tract, employ clinical monitoring, and institute supportive therapy, if required.

DOSAGE AND ADMINISTRATION

Adults and Children 12 years of age and older

The recommended dose of ACCOLATE is 20 mg twice daily in adults and children 12 years and older.

Pediatric Patients 7 through 11 years of Age

The recommended dose of ACCOLATE in children 7 through 11 years of age is 10 mg twice daily.

Since food reduces the bioavailability of zafirlukast, ACCOLATE should be taken at least 1 hour before or 2 hours after meals.

Elderly Patients: Based on cross-study comparisons, the clearance of zafirlukast is reduced in elderly patients (65 years of age and older), such that C_{max} and AUC are approximately twice those of younger adults. In clinical trials, a dose of 20 mg twice daily was not associated with an increase in the overall incidence of adverse events or withdrawals because of adverse events in elderly patients.

Patients with Hepatic Impairment: The clearance of zafirlukast is reduced in patients with stable alcoholic cirrhosis such that the C_{max} and AUC are approximately 50–60% greater than those of normal adults. ACCOLATE has not been evaluated in patients with hepatitis or in long-term studies of patients with cirrhosis.

Patients with Renal Impairment: Dosage adjustment is not required for patients with renal impairment.

HOW SUPPLIED

ACCOLATE 10 mg Tablets, (NDC 0310-0401) white, unflavored, round, biconvex, film-coated, mini-tablets identified with "ZENECA" debossed on one side and "ACCOLATE 10" debossed on the other side are supplied in opaque HDPE bottles of 60 tablets and Hospital Unit Dose blister packages of 100 tablets.

ACCOLATE 20 mg Tablets, (NDC 0310-0402) white, round, biconvex, coated tablets identified with "ZENECA" debossed on one side and "ACCOLATE 20" debossed on the other side are supplied in opaque HDPE bottles of 60 tablets and hospital Unit Dose blister packages of 100 tablets.

Store at controlled room temperature, (20°–25° C) (68°–77°F) [see USP]. Protect from light and moisture. Dispense in the original air-tight container.

ZENECA
Manufactured for:
Zeneca Pharmaceuticals
A Business Unit of Zeneca Inc.
Wilmington, Delaware 19850-5437
By: IPR Pharmaceuticals Inc.
Carolina, Puerto Rico 00984-1967
Rev N 06/00 PCC 64160-01
SIC 670201

Shown in Product Identification Guide, page 305

ARIMIDEX® ℞
anastrozole
TABLETS

DESCRIPTION

ARIMIDEX® (anastrozole) tablets for oral administration contain 1 mg of anastrozole, a non-steroidal aromatase inhibitor. It is chemically described as 1,3-Benzenediacetonitrile, α, α, α', α'-tetramethyl-5-(1H-1,2,4-triazol-1-ylmethyl). Its molecular formula is $C_{17}H_{19}N_5$ and its structural formula is:

H₃C CH₃ H₃C CH₃ CN CN N N N

Anastrozole is an off-white powder with a molecular weight of 293.4. Anastrozole has moderate aqueous solubility (0.5 mg/mL at 25°C); solubility is independent of pH in the physiological range. Anastrozole is freely soluble in methanol, acetone, ethanol, and tetrahydrofuran, and very soluble in acetonitrile.

Each tablet contains as inactive ingredients: lactose, magnesium stearate, hydroxypropylmethylcellulose, polyethylene glycol, povidone, sodium starch glycolate, and titanium dioxide.

CLINICAL PHARMACOLOGY

Mechanism of Action

Many breast cancers have estrogen receptors and growth of these tumors can be stimulated by estrogens. In post-menopausal women, the principal source of circulating estrogen (primarily estradiol) is conversion of adrenally-generated androstenedione to estrone by aromatase in peripheral tissues, such as adipose tissue, with further conversion of estrone to estradiol. Many breast cancers also contain aromatase; the importance of tumor-generated estrogens is uncertain.

Treatment of breast cancer has included efforts to decrease estrogen levels by ovariectomy premenopausally and by use of anti-estrogens and progestational agents both pre- and post-menopausally, and these interventions lead to decreased tumor mass or delayed progression of tumor growth in some women.

Anastrozole is a potent and selective non-steroidal aromatase inhibitor. It significantly lowers serum estradiol concentrations and has no detectable effect on formation of adrenal corticosteroids or aldosterone.

Pharmacokinetics

Inhibition of aromatase activity is primarily due to anastrozole, the parent drug. Studies with radiolabeled drug have demonstrated that orally administered anastrozole is well absorbed into the systemic circulation with 83 to 85% of the radiolabel recovered in urine and feces. Food does not affect the extent of absorption. Elimination of anastrozole is primarily via hepatic metabolism (approximately 85%) and to a lesser extent, renal excretion (approximately 11%), and anastrozole has a mean terminal elimination half-life of approximately 50 hours in postmenopausal women. The major circulating metabolite of anastrozole, triazole, lacks pharmacologic activity. The pharmacokinetic parameters are similar in patients and in healthy postmenopausal volunteers. The pharmacokinetics of anastrozole are linear over the dose range of 1 to 20 mg and do not change with repeated dosing. Consistent with the approximately 2-day terminal elimination half-life, plasma concentrations approach steady-state levels at about 7 days of once daily dosing and steady-state levels are approximately three- to four-fold higher than levels observed after a single dose of ARIMIDEX. Anastrozole is 40% bound to plasma proteins in the therapeutic range.

Metabolism and Excretion: Studies of postmenopausal women demonstrated that anastrozole is extensively metabolized with about 10% of the dose excreted in the urine as unchanged drug within 72 hours of dosing, and the remainder (about 60% of the dose) excreted in the urine as metabolites. Metabolism of anastrozole occurs by N-dealkylation, hydroxylation and glucoronidation. Three metabolites of anastrozole have been identified in human plasma and urine. The known metabolites are triazole, a glucuronide conjugate of hydroxy-anastrozole, and a glucuronide of anastrozole itself. Several minor (less than 5% of the radioactive dose) metabolites have not been identified.

Because renal elimination is not a significant pathway of elimination, total body clearance of anastrozole is unchanged even in severe (creatinine clearance less than 30 mL/min/1.73m^2) renal impairment; dosing adjustment in patients with renal dysfunction is not necessary (see Special Populations and DOSAGE AND ADMINISTRATION sections). Dosage adjustment is also unnecessary in patients with stable hepatic cirrhosis (see Special Populations and DOSAGE AND ADMINISTRATION sections).

Special Populations

Geriatric: Anastrozole pharmacokinetics have been investigated in postmenopausal female volunteers and patients with breast cancer. No age related effects were seen over the range <50 to >80 years.

Race: Anastrozole pharmacokinetic differences due to race have not been studied.

Renal Insufficiency: Anastrozole pharmacokinetics have been investigated in subjects with renal insufficiency. Anastrozole renal clearance decreased proportionally with creatinine clearance and was approximately 50% lower in volunteers with severe renal impairment (creatinine clearance less than 30 mL/min/1.73m^2) compared to controls. Since only about 10% of anastrozole is excreted unchanged in the urine, the reduction in renal clearance did not influence the total body clearance (see DOSAGE AND ADMINISTRATION).

Hepatic Insufficiency: Hepatic metabolism accounts for approximately 85% of anastrozole elimination. Anastrozole pharmacokinetics have been investigated in subjects with hepatic cirrhosis related to alcohol abuse. The apparent oral clearance (CL/F) of anastrozole was approximately 30% lower in subjects with stable hepatic cirrhosis than in control subjects with normal liver function. However, plasma anastrozole concentrations in the subjects with hepatic cirrhosis were within the range of concentrations seen in normal subjects across all clinical trials (see DOSAGE AND ADMINISTRATION), so that no dosage adjustment is needed.

Drug-Drug Interactions: Anastrozole inhibited reactions catalyzed by cytochrome P450 1A2, 2C8/9, and 3A4 *in vitro* with Ki values which were approximately 30 times higher than the mean steady-state C_{max} values observed following a 1-mg daily dose. Anastrozole had no inhibitory effect on reactions catalyzed by cytochrome P450 2A6 or 2D6 *in vitro*. Administration of a single 30 mg/kg or multiple 10 mg/kg doses of anastrozole to subjects had no effect on the clearance of antipyrine or urinary recovery of antipyrine metab-

Continued on next page

Arimidex—Cont.

olites. Based on these *in vitro* and *in vivo* results, it is unlikely that co-administration of ARIMIDEX 1 mg with other drugs will result in clinically significant inhibition of cytochrome P450 mediated metabolism.

Pharmacodynamics

Effect on Estradiol: Mean serum concentrations of estradiol were evaluated in multiple daily dosing trials with 0.5, 1, 3, 5, and 10 mg of ARIMIDEX in postmenopausal women with advanced breast cancer. Clinically significant suppression of serum estradiol was seen with all doses. Doses of 1 mg and higher resulted in suppression of mean serum concentrations of estradiol to the lower limit of detection (3.7 pmol/L). The recommended daily dose, ARIMIDEX 1 mg, reduced estradiol by approximately 70% within 24 hours and by approximately 80% after 14 days of daily dosing. Suppression of serum estradiol was maintained for up to 6 days after cessation of daily dosing with ARIMIDEX 1 mg.

Effect on Corticosteroids: In multiple daily dosing trials with 3, 5, and 10 mg, the selectivity of anastrozole was assessed by examining effects on corticosteroid synthesis. For all doses, anastrozole did not effect cortisol or aldosterone secretion at baseline or in response to ACTH. No glucocorticoid or mineralocorticoid replacement therapy is necessary with anastrozole.

Other Endocrine Effects: In multiple daily dosing trials with 5 and 10 mg, thyroid stimulation hormone (TSH) was measured; there was no increase in TSH during the administration of ARIMIDEX. ARIMIDEX does not possess direct progestogenic, androgenic, or estrogenic activity in animals, but does perturb the circulating levels of progesterone, androgens, and estrogens.

Clinical Studies

Anastrozole was studied in two well-controlled clinical trials (0004, a North American study; 0005, a predominately European study) in postmenopausal women with advanced breast cancer who had disease progression following tamoxifen therapy for either advanced or early breast cancer. Some of the patients had also received previous cytotoxic treatment. Most patients were ER-positive; a smaller fraction were ER-unknown or ER-negative (the ER-negative patients were eligible only if they had had a positive response to tamoxifen). Eligible patients with measurable and non-measurable disease were randomized to receive either a single daily dose of 1 mg or 10 mg of ARIMIDEX or megestrol acetate 40 mg four times a day. The studies were double-blinded with respect to ARIMIDEX. Time to progression and objective response (only patients with measurable disease could be considered partial responders) rates were the primary efficacy variables. Objective response rates were calculated based on the Union Internationale Contre le Cancer (UICC) criteria. The rate of prolonged (more than 24 weeks) stable disease, the rate of progression, and survival were also calculated.

Both trials included over 375 patients; demographics and other baseline characteristics were similar for the three treatment groups in each trial. Patients in the 0005 trial had responded better to prior tamoxifen treatment. Of the patients entered who had prior tamoxifen therapy for advanced disease (58% in Trial 0004; 57% in Trial 0005), 18% of these patients in Trial 0004 and 42% in Trial 0005 were reported by the primary investigator to have responded. In Trial 0004, 81% of patients were ER-positive, 13% were ER-unknown, and 6% were ER-negative. In Trial 0005, 58% of patients were ER-positive, 37% were ER-unknown, and 5% were ER-negative. In Trial 0004, 62% of patients had measurable disease compared to 79% in Trial 0005. The sites of metastatic disease were similar among treatment groups for each trial. On average, 40% of the patients had soft tissue metastases, 60% had bone metastases, and 40% had visceral (15% liver) metastases.

As shown in the table below, similar results were observed among treatment groups and between the two trials. None of the within-trial differences were statistically significant.

	ARIMIDEX 1 mg	ARIMIDEX 10 mg	Megestrol Acetate 160 mg
Trial 0004 (N. America)	(n=128)	(n=130)	(n=128)
Median Follow-up (months)*	31.3	30.9	32.9
Median Time to Death (months)	29.6	25.7	26.7
2 Year Survival Probability (%)	62.0	58.0	53.1
Median Time to Progression (months)	5.7	5.3	5.1
Objective Response (all patients) (%)	12.5	10.0	10.2
Stable Disease for >24 weeks (%)	35.2	29.2	32.8
Progression (%)	86.7	85.4	90.6
Trial 0005 (Europe, Australia, S.Africa)	(n=135)	(n=118)	(n=125)
Median Follow-up (months)*	31.0	30.9	31.5
Median Time to Death (months)	24.3	24.8	19.8
2 Year Survival Probability (%)	50.5	50.9	39.1
Median Time to Progression (months)	4.4	5.3	3.9
Objective Response (all patients) (%)	12.6	15.3	14.4
Stable Disease for >24 weeks (%)	24.4	25.4	23.2
Progression (%)	91.9	89.8	92.0

* Surviving Patients

More than 1/3 of the patients in each treatment group in both studies had either an objective response or stabilization of their disease for greater than 24 weeks. Among the 263 patients who received ARIMIDEX 1 mg, there were 11 complete responders and 22 partial responders. In patients who had an objective response, more than 80% were still responding at 6 months from randomization and more than 45% were still responding at 12 months from randomization.

When data from the two controlled trials are pooled, the objective response rates and median times to progression and death were similar for patients randomized to ARIMIDEX 1 mg and megestrol acetate. There is, in this data, no indication that ARIMIDEX 10 mg is superior to ARIMIDEX 1 mg.

	ARIMIDEX 1 mg	ARIMIDEX 10 mg	Megestrol Acetate 160 mg
Trials 0004 & 0005 (Pooled Data)	(n=263)	(n=248)	(n=253)
Median Time to Death (months)	26.7	25.5	22.5
2 Year Survival Probability (%)	56.1	54.6	46.3
Median Time to Progression (months)	4.8	5.3	4.6
Objective Response (all patients) (%)	12.5	12.5	12.3

Objective response rates and median times to progression and death for ARIMIDEX 1 mg were similar to megestrol acetate for women over or under 65. There were too few non-white patients studied to draw conclusions about racial differences in response.

INDICATIONS AND USAGE

ARIMIDEX is indicated for the treatment of advanced breast cancer in postmenopausal women with disease progression following tamoxifen therapy.

Patients with ER-negative disease and patients who did not respond to previous tamoxifen therapy rarely responded to ARIMIDEX.

CONTRAINDICATIONS

None known.

WARNINGS

ARIMIDEX can cause fetal harm when administered to a pregnant woman. Anastrozole has been found to cross the placenta following oral administration of 0.1 mg/kg in rats and rabbits (about $^3/_4$ and 1.5 times the recommended human dose, respectively, on a mg/m^2 basis. Studies in both rats and rabbits at doses equal to or greater than 0.1 and 0.02 mg/kg/day, respectively (about $^3/_4$ and $^1/_3$, respectively, the recommended human dose on a mg/m^2 basis), administered during the period of organogenesis showed that anastrozole increased pregnancy loss (increased pre- and/or post-implantation loss, increased resorption, and decreased numbers of live fetuses); effects were dose-related in rats. Placental weights were significantly increased in rats at doses of 0.1 mg/kg/day or more.

Evidence of fetotoxicity, including delayed fetal development (i.e., incomplete ossification and depressed fetal body weights), was observed in rats administered doses of 1 mg/kg/day (which produced plasma anastrozole C_{ssmax} and $AUC_{0-24\ hr}$ that were 19 times and 9 times higher than the respective values found in healthy post-menopausal humans at the recommended dose). There was no evidence of teratogenicity in rats administered doses up to 1.0 mg/kg/day. In rabbits, anastrozole caused pregnancy failure at doses equal to or greater than 1.0 mg/kg/day (about 16 times the recommended human dose on a mg/m^2 basis); there was no evidence of teratogenicity in rabbits administered 0.2 mg/kg/day (about 3 times the recommended human dose on a mg/m^2 basis).

There are no adequate and well-controlled studies in pregnant women using ARIMIDEX. If ARIMIDEX is used during pregnancy or if the patient becomes pregnant while receiving this drug, the patient should be apprised of the potential hazard to the fetus or potential risk for loss of the pregnancy.

PRECAUTIONS

General: Before starting treatment with ARIMIDEX, pregnancy must be excluded (see WARNINGS).

ARIMIDEX should be administered under the supervision of a qualified physician experienced in the use of anticancer agents.

Laboratory Tests: Three-fold elevations of mean serum gamma glutamyl transferase (GT) levels have been observed among patients with liver metastases receiving ARIMIDEX or megestrol acetate. These changes were likely related to the progression of liver metastases in these patients, although other contributing factors could not be ruled out.

Drug Interactions: (See CLINICAL PHARMACOLOGY)

Anastrozole inhibited *in vitro* metabolic reactions catalyzed by cytochromes P450 1A2, 2C8/9, and 3A4 but only at relatively high concentrations. Anastrozole did not inhibit P450 2A6 or the polymorphic P450 2D6 in human liver microsomes. Anastrozole did not alter the pharmacokinetics of antipyrine. Although there have been no formal interaction studies other than with antipyrine, based on these *in vivo* and *in vitro* studies, it is unlikely that co-administration of a 1-mg dose of ARIMIDEX with other drugs will result in clinically significant drug inhibition of cytochrome P450-mediated metabolism of the other drugs.

Drug/Laboratory Test Interactions: No clinically significant changes in the results of clinical laboratory tests have been observed.

Carcinogenesis: No long-term animal studies have been conducted to assess the carcinogenic potential of ARIMIDEX.

Mutagenesis: ARIMIDEX has not been shown to be mutagenic in *in vitro* tests (Ames and E. coli bacterial tests, CHO-K1 gene mutation assay) or clastogenic either *in vitro* (chromosome aberrations in human lymphocytes) or *in vivo* (micronucleus test in rats).

Impairment of Fertility: Studies to investigate the effect of ARIMIDEX on fertility have not been conducted; however, chronic studies indicated hypertrophy of the ovaries and the presence of follicular cysts in rats administered doses equal to or greater than 1 mg/kg/day (which produced plasma anastrozole C_{ssmax} and $AUC_{0-24\ hr}$ that were 19 and 9 times higher than the respective values found in healthy post-menopausal humans at the recommended dose). In addition, hyperplastic uteri were observed in chronic studies of female dogs administered doses equal to or greater than 1 mg/kg/day (which produced plasma anastrozole C_{ssmax} and $AUC_{0-24\ hr}$ that were 22 times and 16 times higher than the respective values found in post-menopausal humans at the recommended dose). It is not known whether these effects on the reproductive organs of animals are associated with impaired fertility in humans.

Pregnancy: Pregnancy Category D: (See WARNINGS).

Nursing Mothers: It is not known if anastrozole is excreted in human milk. Because many drugs are excreted in human milk, caution should be exercised when ARIMIDEX is administered to a nursing woman (see WARNINGS and PRECAUTIONS).

Pediatric Use: The safety and efficacy of ARIMIDEX in pediatric patients have not been established.

Geriatric Use: Fifty percent of patients in studies 0004 and 0005 were 65 or older. Response rates and time to progression were similar for the over 65 and younger patients.

ADVERSE REACTIONS

ARIMIDEX was generally well tolerated in two well-controlled clinical trials (i.e., Trials 0004 and 0005), with less than 3.3% of the ARIMIDEX-treated patients and 4.0% of the megestrol acetate-treated patients withdrawing due to an adverse event.

The principal adverse event more common with ARIMIDEX than megestrol acetate was diarrhea. Adverse events reported in greater than 5% of the patients in any of the treatment groups in these two well-controlled clinical trials, regardless of causality, are presented below:

Number (n) and Percentage of Patients with Adverse Event †

	ARIMIDEX 1 mg (n=262)		ARIMIDEX 10 mg (n=246)		Megestrol Acetate 160 mg (n=253)	
Adverse Event	n	%	n	%	n	%
Asthenia	42	(16.0)	33	(13.4)	47	(18.6)
Nausea	41	(15.6)	48	(19.5)	28	(11.1)
Headache	34	(13.0)	44	(17.9)	24	(9.5)
Hot Flushes	32	(12.2)	29	(10.6)	21	(8.3)
Pain	28	(10.7)	38	(15.4)	29	(11.5)
Back Pain	28	(10.7)	26	(10.6)	19	(7.5)
Dyspnea	24	(9.2)	27	(11.0)	53	(20.9)
Vomiting	24	(9.2)	26	(10.6)	16	(6.3)
Cough Increased	22	(8.4)	18	(7.3)	19	(7.5)
Diarrhea	22	(8.4)	18	(7.3)	7	(2.8)
Constipation	18	(6.9)	18	(7.3)	21	(8.3)
Abdominal Pain	18	(6.9)	14	(5.7)	18	(7.1)
Anorexia	18	(6.9)	19	(7.7)	11	(4.3)
Bone Pain	17	(6.5)	26	(11.8)	19	(7.5)
Pharyngitis	16	(6.1)	23	(9.3)	15	(5.9)
Dizziness	16	(6.1)	12	(4.9)	15	(5.9)
Rash	15	(5.7)	15	(6.1)	19	(7.5)
Dry Mouth	15	(5.7)	11	(4.5)	13	(5.1)
Peripheral Edema	14	(5.3)	21	(8.5)	28	(11.1)
Pelvic Pain	14	(5.3)	17	(6.9)	13	(5.1)
Depression	14	(5.3)	6	(2.4)	5	(2.0)
Chest Pain	13	(5.0)	18	(7.3)	13	(5.1)
Paresthesia	12	(4.6)	15	(6.1)	9	(3.6)
Vaginal Hemorrhage	6	(2.3)	4	(1.6)	13	(5.1)

Weight Gain	4	(1.5)	9	(3.7)	30	(11.9)
Sweating	4	(1.5)	3	(1.2)	16	(6.3)
Increased Appetite	0	(0)	1	(0.4)	13	(5.1)

† A patient may have more than one adverse event.

Other less frequent (2% to 5%) adverse experiences reported in patients receiving ARIMIDEX 1 mg in either Trial 0004 or Trial 0005 are listed below. These adverse experiences are listed by body system and are in order of decreasing frequency within each body system regardless of assessed causality.
Body as a Whole: Flu syndrome; fever; neck pain; malaise; accidental injury; infection
Cardiovascular: Hypertension; thrombophlebitis
Hepatic: Gamma GT increased; SGOT increased; SGPT increased
Hematologic: Anemia; leukopenia
Metabolic and Nutritional: Alkaline phosphatase increased; weight loss
Mean serum total cholesterol levels increased by 0.5 mmol/L among patients receiving ARIMIDEX. Increases in LDL cholesterol have been shown to contribute to these changes.
Musculoskeletal: Myalgia; arthralgia; pathological fracture
Nervous: Somnolence; confusion; insomnia; anxiety; nervousness
Respiratory: Sinusitis; bronchitis; rhinitis
Skin and Appendages: Hair thinning; pruritus
Urogenital: Urinary tract infection; breast pain
Vaginal bleeding has been reported infrequently, mainly in patients during the first few weeks after changing from existing hormonal therapy to treatment with ARIMIDEX. If bleeding persists, further evaluation should be considered.
The incidences of the following adverse event groups, potentially causally related to one or both of the therapies because of their pharmacology, were statistically analyzed: weight gain, edema, thromboembolic disease, gastrointestinal disturbance, hot flushes, and vaginal dryness. These six groups, and the adverse events captured in the groups, were prospectively defined. The results are shown in the table below.

Number (n) and Percentage of Patients

	ARIMIDEX 1 mg (n=262)		ARIMIDEX 10 mg (n=246)		Megestrol Acetate 160 mg (n=253)	
Adverse Event Group	n	%	n	%	n	%
Gastrointestinal Disturbance	77	(29.4)	81	(32.9)	54	(21.3)
Hot Flushes	33	(12.6)	29	(11.8)	35	(13.8)
Edema	19	(7.3)	28	(11.4)	35	(13.8)
Thomboembolic Disease	9	(3.4)	4	(1.6)	12	(4.7)
Vaginal Dryness	5	(1.9)	3	(1.2)	2	(0.8)
Weight Gain	4	(1.5)	10	(4.1)	30	(11.9)

More patients treated with megestrol acetate reported weight gain as an adverse event compared to patients treated with ARIMIDEX 1 mg ($p<0.0001$). Other differences were not statistically significant.
An examination of the magnitude of change in weight in all patients was also conducted. Thirty-four percent (87/253) of the patients treated with megestrol acetate experienced weight gain of 5% or more and 11% (27/253) of the patients treated with megestrol acetate experienced weight gain of 10% or more. Among patients treated with ARIMIDEX 1 mg, 13 % (33/262) experienced weight gain of 5% or more and 3% (6/262) experienced weight gain of 10% or more. On average, this 5 to 10% weight gain represented between 6 and 12 pounds.
No patients receiving ARIMIDEX or megestrol acetate discontinued treatment due to drug-related weight gain.

OVERDOSAGE

Clinical trials have been conducted with ARIMIDEX, up to 60 mg in a single dose given to healthy male volunteers and up to 10 mg daily given to postmenopausal women with advanced breast cancer; these dosages were well tolerated. A single dose of ARIMIDEX that results in life-threatening symptoms has not been established. In rats, lethality was observed after single oral doses that were greater than 100 mg/kg (about 800 times the recommended human dose on a mg/m^2 basis) and was associated with severe irritation to the stomach (necrosis, gastritis, ulceration, and hemorrhage).
There is no specific antidote to overdosage and treatment must be symptomatic. In the management of an overdose, consider that multiple agents may have been taken. Vomiting may be induced if the patient is alert. Dialysis may be helpful because ARIMIDEX is not highly protein bound. General supportive care, including frequent monitoring of vital signs and close observation of the patient, is indicated.

DOSAGE AND ADMINISTRATION

The dose of ARIMIDEX is one 1-mg tablet taken once a day. Patients treated with ARIMIDEX do not require glucocorticoid or mineralocorticoid replacement therapy.
Patients with Hepatic Impairment: (See CLINICAL PHARMACOLOGY) Hepatic metabolism accounts for approximately 85% of anastrozole elimination. Although clearance of anastrozole was decreased in patients with cirrhosis due to alcohol abuse, plasma anastrozole concentrations stayed in the usual range seen in patients without liver disease. Therefore, no changes in dose are recommended for patients with mild-to-moderate hepatic impairment, although patients should be monitored for side effects. ARIMIDEX has not been studied in patients with severe hepatic impairment.
Patients with Renal Impairment: No changes in dose are necessary for patients with renal impairment.

HOW SUPPLIED

White, biconvex, film-coated tablets containing 1 mg of anastrozole. The tablets are impressed on one side with a logo consisting of a letter "A" (upper case) with an arrowhead attached to the foot of the extended right leg of the "A" and on the reverse with the tablet strength marking "Adx 1". These tablets are supplied in bottles of 30 tablets (NDC 0310-0201-30)
Store at controlled room temperature, 20°–25°C (68°–77°F) [see USP].
ZENECA Pharmaceuticals
A Business Unit of Zeneca Inc.
Wilmington, Delaware 19850-5437
64076-04 Rev F 07/98
Shown in Product Identification Guide, page 305

CASODEX® ℞
bicalutamide tablets

DESCRIPTION

CASODEX® (bicalutamide) Tablets for oral administration contain 50 mg of bicalutamide, a non-steroidal antiandrogen with no other known endocrine activity. The chemical name is propanamide, N-[4-cyano-3-(trifluoromethyl)phenyl]-3-[(4-fluorophenyl)sulfonyl]-2-hydroxy-2-methyl-,(+ −).
The structural and empirical formulas are:

$C_{18}H_{14}N_2O_4F_4S$

Bicalutamide has a molecular weight of 430.37. The pKa' is approximately 12. Bicalutamide is a fine white to off-white powder which is practically insoluble in water at 37°C (5 mg per 1000 mL), slightly soluble in chloroform and absolute ethanol, sparingly soluble in methanol, and soluble in acetone and tetrahydrofuran.
CASODEX is a racemate with its antiandrogenic activity being almost exclusively exhibited by the R-enantiomer of bicalutamide; the S-enantiomer is essentially inactive.
The inactive ingredients of CASODEX Tablets are lactose, magnesium stearate, methylhydroxypropylcellulose, polyethylene glycol, polyvidone, sodium starch glycollate, and titanium dioxide.

CLINICAL PHARMACOLOGY

Mechanism of Action: CASODEX is a non-steroidal antiandrogen. It competitively inhibits the action of androgens by binding to cytosol androgen receptors in the target tissue. Prostatic carcinoma is known to be androgen sensitive and responds to treatment that counteracts the effect of androgen and/or removes the source of androgen.
When CASODEX is combined with luteinizing hormone-releasing hormone (LHRH) analogue therapy, the suppression of serum testosterone induced by the LHRH analogue is not affected. However, in clinical trials with CASODEX as a single agent for prostate cancer, rises in serum testosterone and estradiol have been noted.
Pharmacokinetics
Absorption: Bicalutamide is well-absorbed following oral administration, although the absolute bioavailability is unknown. Co-administration of bicalutamide with food has no clinically significant effect on rate or extent of absorption.
Distribution: Bicalutamide is highly protein-bound (96%). See Drug-Drug Interactions below.
Metabolism/Elimination: Bicalutamide undergoes stereospecific metabolism. The S (inactive) isomer is metabolized primarily by glucuronidation. The R (active) isomer also undergoes glucuronidation but is predominantly oxidized to an inactive metabolite followed by glucuronidation. Both the parent and metabolite glucuronides are eliminated in the urine and feces. The S-enantiomer is rapidly cleared relative to the R-enantiomer, with the R-enantiomer accounting for about 99% of total steady-state plasma levels.
Special Populations
Geriatric: In two studies in patients given 50 or 150 mg daily, no significant relationship between age and steady-state levels of total bicalutamide or the active R-enantiomer has been shown.
Hepatic Insufficiency: No clinically significant difference in the pharmacokinetics of either enantiomer of bicalutamide was noted in patients with mild-to-moderate hepatic disease as compared to healthy controls. However, the half-life of the R-enantiomer was increased approximately 76% (5.9 and 10.4 days for normal and impaired patients, respectively) in patients with severe liver disease (n=4).
Renal Insufficiency: Renal impairment (as measured by creatinine clearance) had no significant effect on the elimination of total bicalutamide or the active R-enantiomer.
Women, Pediatrics: Bicalutamide has not been studied in women or pediatric subjects.
Drug-Drug Interactions: Clinical studies have not shown any drug interactions between bicalutamide and LHRH analogues (goserelin or leuprolide). There is no evidence that bicalutamide induces hepatic enzymes. *In vitro* protein-binding studies have shown that bicalutamide can displace coumarin anticoagulants from binding sites. Prothrombin times should be closely monitored in patients already receiving coumarin anticoagulants who are started on CASODEX.
Pharmacokinetics of the active enantiomer of CASODEX in normal males and patients with prostate cancer are presented in Table 1.

Table 1

Parameter	Mean	Standard Deviation
Normal Males (n=30)		
Apparent Oral Clearance (L/hr)	0.320	0.103
Single Dose Peak Concentration (μg/mL)	0.768	0.178
Single Dose Time to Peak Concentration (hours)	31.3	14.6
Half-Life (days)	5.8	2.29
Patients with Prostate Cancer (n=40)		
C_{SS} (μg/mL)	8.939	3.504

C_{SS} = Mean Steady-State Concentration

Clinical Studies
In a multicenter, double-blind, controlled clinical trial, 813 patients with previously untreated advanced prostate cancer were randomized to receive CASODEX 50 mg once daily (404 patients) or flutamide 250 mg (409 patients) three times a day, each in combination with LHRH analogues (either goserelin acetate implant or leuprolide acetate depot). In an analysis conducted after a median follow-up of 160 weeks was reached, 213 (52.7%) patients treated with CASODEX-LHRH analogue therapy and 235 (57.5%) patients treated with flutamide-LHRH analogue therapy had died. There was no significant difference in survival between treatment groups (see Figure 1). The hazard ratio for time to death (survival) was 0.87 (95% confidence interval 0.72 to 1.05).

Figure 1
The Kaplan-Meier Probability of Death For Both Antiandrogen Treatment Groups

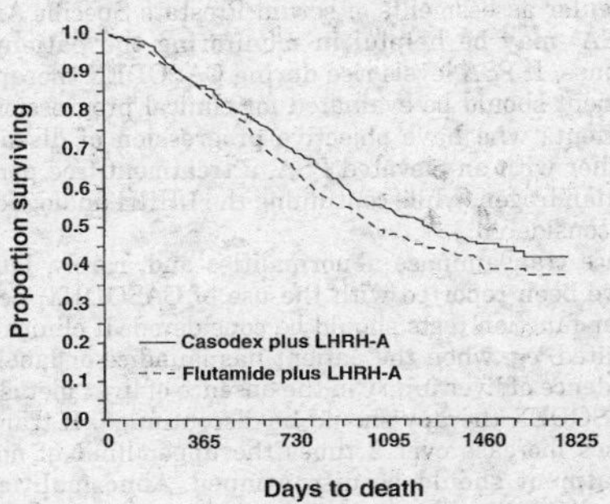

There was no significant difference in time to objective tumor progression between treatment groups (see Figure 2). Objective tumor progression was defined as the appearance of any bone metastases or the worsening of any existing bone metastases on bone scan attributable to metastatic disease, or an increase by 25% or more of any existing measurable extraskeletal metastases. The hazard ratio for time to progression of CASODEX plus LHRH analogue to that of flutamide plus LHRH analogue was 0.93 (95% confidence interval, 0.79 to 1.10).
[See figure 2 at top of next column]
Quality of life was assessed with self-administered patient questionnaires on pain, social functioning, emotional well-being, vitality, activity limitation, bed disability, overall health, physical capacity, general symptoms, and treatment related symptoms. Assessment of the Quality of Life questionnaires did not indicate consistent significant differences between the two treatment groups.

Continued on next page

Casodex—Cont.

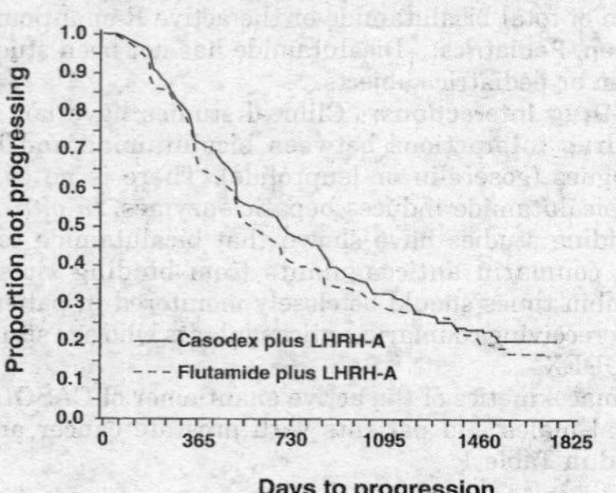

Figure 2
The Kaplan-Meier Curve For Time to Progression For Both Antiandrogen Treatment Groups

INDICATIONS AND USAGE

CASODEX is indicated for use in combination therapy with a luteinizing hormone-releasing hormone (LHRH) analogue for the treatment of Stage D_2 metastatic carcinoma of the prostate.

CONTRAINDICATIONS

CASODEX is contraindicated in any patient who has shown a hypersensitivity reaction to the drug or any of the tablet's components.

CASODEX is not indicated in women. Further, CASODEX is contraindicated in women who are or may become pregnant. If this drug is used during pregnancy, or if the patient becomes pregnant while taking this drug, the patient should be apprised of the potential hazard to the fetus. CASODEX may cause fetal harm when administered to pregnant women. The male offspring of rats receiving doses of 10 mg/kg/day (plasma drug concentrations in rats equal to approximately 2/3 human therapeutic concentrations*) and above were observed to have reduced anogenital distance and hypospadias in reproductive toxicology studies. These pharmacological effects have been observed with other antiandrogens. No other teratogenic effects were observed in rabbits receiving doses up to 200 mg/kg/day (approximately 1/3 human therapeutic concentrations*) or rats receiving doses up to 250 mg/kg/day (approximately 2 times human therapeutic concentrations*).

*Based on a maximum dose of 50 mg/day of bicalutamide for an average 70 kg patient.

PRECAUTIONS

General

1. CASODEX should be used with caution in patients with moderate-to-severe hepatic impairment. CASODEX is extensively metabolized by the liver. Limited data in subjects with severe hepatic impairment suggest that excretion of CASODEX may be delayed and could lead to further accumulation. Periodic liver function tests should be considered for patients on long-term therapy.
2. In clinical trials with CASODEX as a single agent for prostate cancer, gynecomastia and breast pain have been reported in up to 38% and 39% of patients, respectively.
3. Regular assessments of serum Prostate Specific Antigen (PSA) may be helpful in monitoring the patient's response. If PSA levels rise during CASODEX therapy, the patient should be evaluated for clinical progression. For patients who have objective progression of disease together with an elevated PSA, a treatment-free period of antiandrogen, while continuing the LHRH analogue, may be considered.
4. Since transaminase abnormalities and, rarely, jaundice have been reported with the use of CASODEX, periodic liver function tests should be considered. If clinically indicated, eg, when the patient has jaundice or laboratory evidence of liver injury in the absence of liver metastases, CASODEX therapy should be discontinued. If transaminases increase over 2 times the upper limit of normal, treatment should be discontinued. Abnormalities are usually reversible upon discontinuation.

Information for Patients: Patients should be informed that therapy with CASODEX and the LHRH analogue should be initiated concomitantly, and that they should not interrupt or stop taking these medications without consulting their physician. Treatment with CASODEX should be started at the same time as treatment with an LHRH analogue.

Drug Interactions: *In vitro* studies have shown CASODEX can displace coumarin anticoagulants, such as warfarin, from their protein-binding sites. It is recommended that if CASODEX is started in patients already receiving coumarin anticoagulants, prothrombin times should be closely monitored and adjustment of the anticoagulant dose may be necessary (see CLINICAL PHARMACOLOGY, Drug-Drug Interactions).

Carcinogenesis, Mutagenesis, Impairment of Fertility: Two-year oral carcinogenicity studies were conducted in both male and female rats and mice at doses of 5, 15 or 75 mg/kg/day of bicalutamide. A variety of tumor target organ effects were identified and were attributed to the antiandrogenicity of bicalutamide, namely, testicular benign interstitial (Leydig) cell tumors in male rats at all dose levels (the steady-state plasma concentration with the 5 mg/kg/day dose is approximately 2/3 human therapeutic concentrations*) and uterine adenocarcinoma in female rats at 75 mg/kg/day (approximately 1 1/2 times the human therapeutic concentrations*). There is no evidence of Leydig cell hyperplasia in patients; uterine tumors are not relevant to the indicated patient population.

A small increase in the incidence of hepatocellular carcinoma in male mice given 75 mg/kg/day of bicalutamide (approximately 4 times human therapeutic concentrations*) and an increased incidence of benign thyroid follicular cell adenomas in rats given 5 mg/kg/day (approximately 2/3 human therapeutic concentrations*) and above were recorded. These neoplastic changes were progressions of non-neoplastic changes related to hepatic enzyme induction observed in animal toxicity studies. Enzyme induction has not been observed following bicalutamide administration in man. There were no tumorigenic effects suggestive of genotoxic carcinogenesis.

A comprehensive battery of both *in vitro* and *in vivo* genotoxicity tests (yeast gene conversion, Ames, *E. coli*, CHO/HGPRT, human lymphocyte cytogenetic, mouse micronucleus, and rat bone marrow cytogenetic tests) has demonstrated that CASODEX does not have genotoxic activity.

Administration of CASODEX may lead to inhibition of spermatogenesis. The long-term effects of CASODEX on male fertility have not been studied.

In male rats dosed at 250 mg/kg/day (approximately 2 times human therapeutic concentrations*), the precoital interval and time to successful mating were increased in the first pairing but no effects on fertility following successful mating were seen. These effects were reversed by 7 weeks after the end of an 11-week period of dosing.

No effects on female rats dosed at 10, 50 and 250 mg/kg/day (approximately 2/3, 1 and 2 times human therapeutic concentrations, respectively*) or their female offspring were observed. Administration of bicalutamide to pregnant females resulted in feminization of the male offspring leading to hypospadias at all dose levels. Affected male offspring were also impotent.

*Based on a maximum dose of 50 mg/day of bicalutamide for an average 70 kg patient.

Pregnancy: Pregnancy Category X (see CONTRAINDICATIONS).

Nursing Mothers: CASODEX is not indicated for use in women. It is not known whether this drug is excreted in human milk. Because many drugs are excreted in human milk, caution should be exercised when CASODEX is administered to a nursing woman.

Pediatric Use: Safety and effectiveness of CASODEX in pediatric patients have not been established.

ADVERSE REACTIONS

In patients with advanced prostate cancer treated with CASODEX in combination with an LHRH analogue, the most frequent adverse experience was hot flashes (53%).

In the multicenter, double-blind, controlled clinical trial comparing CASODEX 50 mg once daily with flutamide 250 mg three times a day, each in combination with an LHRH analogue, the following adverse experiences with an incidence of 5% or greater, regardless of causality, have been reported.

Table 2
Incidence of Adverse Events (≥5% in Either Treatment Group) Regardless of Causality

Body System Adverse Event	Treatment Group Number of Patients (%)			
	CASODEX Plus LHRH Analogue (n = 401)		Flutamide Plus LHRH Analogue (n = 407)	
Body as a Whole				
Pain (General)	142	(35)	127	(31)
Back Pain	102	(25)	105	(26)
Asthenia	89	(22)	87	(21)
Pelvic Pain	85	(21)	70	(17)
Infection	71	(18)	57	(14)
Abdominal Pain	46	(11)	46	(11)
Chest Pain	34	(8)	34	(8)
Headache	29	(7)	27	(7)
Flu Syndrome	28	(7)	30	(7)
Cardiovascular				
Hot Flashes	211	(53)	217	(53)
Hypertension	34	(8)	29	(7)
Digestive				
Constipation	87	(22)	69	(17)
Nausea	62	(15)	58	(14)
Diarrhea	49	(12)	107	(26)
Increased Liver Enzyme Test†	30	(7)	46	(11)
Dyspepsia	30	(7)	23	(6)
Flatulence	26	(6)	22	(5)
Anorexia	25	(6)	29	(7)
Vomiting	24	(6)	32	(8)
Hemic and Lymphatic				
Anemia††	45	(11)	53	(13)
Metabolic and Nutritional				
Peripheral Edema	53	(13)	42	(10)
Weight Loss	30	(7)	39	(10)
Hyperglycemia	26	(6)	27	(7)
Alkaline Phosphatase Increased	22	(5)	24	(6)
Weight Gain	22	(5)	18	(4)
Musculoskeletal				
Bone Pain	37	(9)	43	(11)
Myasthenia	27	(7)	19	(5)
Arthritis	21	(5)	29	(7)
Pathological Fracture	17	(4)	32	(8)
Nervous System				
Dizziness	41	(10)	35	(9)
Paresthesia	31	(8)	40	(10)
Insomnia	27	(7)	39	(10)
Anxiety	20	(5)	9	(2)
Depression	16	(4)	33	(8)
Respiratory System				
Dyspnea	51	(13)	32	(8)
Cough Increased	33	(8)	24	(6)
Pharyngitis	32	(8)	23	(6)
Bronchitis	24	(6)	22	(3)
Pneumonia	18	(4)	19	(5)
Rhinitis	15	(4)	22	(5)
Skin and Appendages				
Rash	35	(9)	30	(7)
Sweating	25	(6)	20	(5)
Urogenital				
Nocturia	49	(12)	55	(14)
Hematuria	48	(12)	26	(6)
Urinary Tract Infection	35	(9)	36	(9)
Gynecomastia	36	(9)	30	(7)
Impotence	27	(7)	35	(9)
Breast Pain	23	(6)	15	(4)
Urinary Frequency	23	(6)	29	(7)
Urinary Retention	20	(5)	14	(3)
Urination Impaired	19	(5)	15	(4)
Urinary Incontinence	15	(4)	32	(8)

† Increased liver enzyme test includes increases in AST, ALT or both.

†† Anemia includes anemia, hypochromic- and iron deficiency anemia.

Other adverse experiences (greater than or equal to 2%, but less than 5%) reported in the CASODEX-LHRH analogue treatment group are listed below by body system and are in order of decreasing frequency within each body system regardless of causality.

Body as a Whole: Neoplasm; Neck pain; Fever; Chills; Sepsis; Hernia; Cyst

Cardiovascular: Angina pectoris; Congestive heart failure; Myocardial infarct; Heart arrest; Coronary artery disorder; Syncope

Digestive: Melena; Rectal hemorrhage; Dry mouth; Dysphagia; Gastrointestinal disorder; Periodontal abscess; Gastrointestinal carcinoma

Metabolic and Nutritional: Edema; BUN increased; Creatinine increased; Dehydration; Gout; Hypercholesteremia

Musculoskeletal: Myalgia; Leg cramps

Nervous: Hypertonia; Confusion; Somnolence; Libido decreased; Neuropathy; Nervousness

Respiratory: Lung disorder; Asthma; Epistaxis; Sinusitis

Skin and Appendages: Dry skin; Alopecia; Pruritus; Herpes zoster; Skin carcinoma; Skin disorder

Special Senses: Cataract specified

Urogenital: Dysuria; Urinary urgency; Hydronephrosis; Urinary tract disorder

Abnormal Laboratory Test Values: Laboratory abnormalities including elevated AST, ALT, bilirubin, BUN, and creatinine and decreased hemoglobin and white cell count have been reported in both CASODEX-LHRH analogue treated and flutamide-LHRH analogue treated patients.

OVERDOSAGE

Long-term clinical trials have been conducted with dosages up to 200 mg of CASODEX daily and these dosages have been well tolerated. A single dose of CASODEX that results in symptoms of an overdose considered to be life-threatening has not been established.

There is no specific antidote; treatment of an overdose should be symptomatic.

In the management of an overdose with CASODEX, vomiting may be induced if the patient is alert. It should be remembered that, in this patient population, multiple drugs may have been taken. Dialysis is not likely to be helpful since CASODEX is highly protein bound and is extensively metabolized. General supportive care, including frequent monitoring of vital signs and close observation of the patient, is indicated.

DOSAGE AND ADMINISTRATION

The recommended dose for CASODEX therapy in combination with an LHRH analogue is one 50 mg tablet once daily (morning or evening), with or without food. It is recommended that CASODEX be taken at the same time each day. Treatment with CASODEX should be started at the same time as treatment with an LHRH analogue.

Dosage Adjustment in Renal Impairment: No dosage adjustment is necessary for patients with renal impairment (see CLINICAL PHARMACOLOGY, Special Populations, Renal Insufficiency).

Dosage Adjustment in Hepatic Impairment: No dosage adjustment is necessary for patients with mild to moderate hepatic impairment. Although there is a 76% (5.9 and 10.4 days for normal and impaired patients, respectively) increase in the half-life of the active enantiomer of bicalutamide in patients with severe liver impairment (n=4), no dosage adjustment is necessary (see CLINICAL PHARMACOLOGY, Special Populations, Hepatic Impairment and PRECAUTIONS sections).

HOW SUPPLIED

50 mg Tablets. (NDC 0310-0705) White, film-coated tablets (identified on one side with "CDX50" and on the reverse with the "CASODEX logo") are supplied in unit dose blisters of 30 tablets per carton (0310-0705-39), bottles of 30 tablets (0310-0705-30) and bottles of 100 tablets (0310-0705-10).

Store at controlled room temperature, 20°-25°C (68°-77°F).

Made in Germany

Manufactured for

Zeneca
Pharmaceuticals
A Business Unit of Zeneca Inc.
Wilmington, Delaware 19850-5437 USA
by Zeneca GmbH, Plankstadt, Germany

64145-00 Rev J 03/98

Shown in Product Identification Guide, page 305

CEFOTAN® ℞

[cef 'o-tan]

cefotetan disodium for injection
For Intravenous or Intramuscular Use

CEFOTAN® ℞

cefotetan injection
In GALAXY® Plastic Container (PL 2040)
For Intravenous Use Only

DESCRIPTION

CEFOTAN (cefotetan disodium for injection) and CEFOTAN (cefotetan injection) in Galaxy®* plastic container (PL 2040) as cefotetan disodium are sterile, semisynthetic, broad-spectrum, beta-lactamase resistant, cephalosporin (cephamycin) antibiotics for parenteral administration. It is the disodium salt of [6R-(6*a*,7*a*)]-7-[[[4-(2-amino-1-carboxy-2-oxoethylidene)-1,3-dithietan-2-yl]carbonyl]amino]-7-methoxy-3-[[(1-methyl-1*H*-tetrazol-5-yl)thio]methyl]-8-oxo-5-thia-1-azabicyclo[4.2.0]oct-2-ene-2-carboxylic acid. Its molecular formula is $C_{17}H_{15}N_7Na_2O_8S_4$ with a molecular weight of 619.57.

Structural Formula

CEFOTAN (cefotetan disodium for injection) is supplied in vials containing 80 mg (3.5 mEq) of sodium per gram of cefotetan activity. It is a white to pale yellow powder which is very soluble in water. Reconstituted solutions of CEFOTAN (cefotetan disodium for injection) are intended for intravenous and intramuscular administration. The solution varies from colorless to yellow depending on the concentration. The pH of freshly reconstituted solutions is usually between 4.5 to 6.5.

CEFOTAN in the ADD-Vantage Vial† is intended for intravenous use only after dilution with the appropriate volume of ADD-Vantage diluent solution.

CEFOTAN is available in two vial strengths. Each CEFOTAN 1 g vial contains cefotetan disodium equivalent to 1 g cefotetan activity. Each CEFOTAN 2 g vial contains cefotetan disodium equivalent to 2 g cefotetan activity.

CEFOTAN (cefotetan injection) in the Galaxy® plastic container (PL 2040) is a frozen, iso-osmotic, sterile, nonpyrogenic premixed 50 mL solution containing 1 g or 2 g cefotetan as cefotetan disodium. Dextrose, USP has been added to adjust the osmolality to 300 mOsmol/kg (approximately 1.9 g and 1.1 g to the 1 g and 2 g dosages, respectively); sodium bicarbonate has been added to convert cefotetan free acid to the sodium salt. The pH has been adjusted between 4 and 6.5 with sodium bicarbonate and may have been adjusted with hydrochloric acid. CEFOTAN (cefotetan injection) in the Galaxy® plastic container (PL 2040) contains 80 mg (3.5 mEq) of sodium per gram of cefotetan activity. After thawing to room temperature, the solution is intended for intravenous use only.

This Galaxy® container is fabricated from a specially designed multilayer plastic (PL 2040). Solutions are in contact with the polyethylene layer of this container and can leach out certain chemical components of the plastic in very small amounts within the expiration dating period. The suitability of the plastic has been confirmed in tests in animals according to the USP biological tests for plastic containers as well as by tissue culture toxicity.

CLINICAL PHARMACOLOGY

High plasma levels of cefotetan are attained after intravenous and intramuscular administration of single doses to normal volunteers.

PLASMA CONCENTRATIONS AFTER 1 GRAM IV [a] OR IM DOSE
Mean Plasma Concentration (µg/mL)
Time After Injection

Route	15 min	30 min	1h	2h	4h	8h	12h
IV	92	158	103	72	42	18	9
IM	34	56	71	68	47	20	9

[a]30-minute infusion

PLASMA CONCENTRATIONS AFTER 2 GRAM IV [a] OR IM DOSE
Mean Plasma Concentration (µg/mL)
Time After Injection

Route	5 min	10 min	1h	3h	5h	9h	12h
IV	237	223	135	74	48	22	12[b]
IM	—	20	75	91	69	33	19

[a] Injected over 3 minutes
[b] Concentrations estimated from regression line

The plasma elimination half-life of cefotetan is 3 to 4.6 hours after either intravenous or intramuscular administration.

Repeated administration of CEFOTAN does not result in accumulation of the drug in normal subjects.

Cefotetan is 88% plasma protein bound.

No active metabolites of cefotetan have been detected; however, small amounts (less than 7%) of cefotetan in plasma and urine may be converted to its tautomer, which has antimicrobial activity similar to the parent drug.

In normal patients, from 51% to 81% of an administered dose of CEFOTAN is excreted unchanged by the kidneys over a 24 hour period, which results in high and prolonged urinary concentrations. Following intravenous doses of 1 gram and 2 grams, urinary concentrations are highest during the first hour and reach concentrations of approximately 1700 and 3500 µg/mL respectively.

In volunteers with reduced renal function, the plasma half-life of cefotetan is prolonged. The mean terminal half-life increases with declining renal function, from approximately 4 hours in volunteers with normal renal function to about 10 hours in those with moderate renal impairment. There is a linear correlation between the systemic clearance of cefotetan and creatinine clearance. When renal function is impaired, a reduced dosing schedule based on creatinine clearance must be used. (see DOSAGE AND ADMINISTRATION).

Therapeutic levels of cefotetan are achieved in many body tissues and fluids including:

skin	ureter
muscle	bladder
fat	maxillary sinus mucosa
myometrium	tonsil
endometrium	bile
cervix	peritoneal fluid
ovary	umbilical cord serum
kidney	amniotic fluid

Microbiology

The bactericidal action of cefotetan results from inhibition of cell wall synthesis. Cefotetan has *in vitro* activity against a wide range of aerobic and anaerobic gram-positive and gram-negative organisms. The methoxy group in the 7-alpha position provides cefotetan with a high degree of stability in the presence of beta-lactamases including both penicillinases and cephalosporinase of gram-negative bacteria. Cefotetan has been shown to be active against most strains of the following organisms **both *in vitro* and in clinical infections** (see **INDICATIONS AND USAGE**).

Gram-Negative Aerobes
Escherichia coli
Haemophilus influenzae (including ampicillin-resistant strains)
Klebsiella species (including *K. pneumoniae*)
Morganella morganii
Neisseria gonorrhoeae (nonpenicillinase-producing strains)
Proteus mirabilis
Proteus vulgaris
Providencia rettgeri
Serratia marcescens

NOTE: Approximately one-half of the usually clinically significant strains of *Enterobacter* species (e.g., *E. aerogenes* and *E. cloacae*) are resistant to cefotetan. Most strains of *Pseudomonas aeruginosa* and *Acinetobacter* species are resistant to cefotetan.

Gram-Positive Aerobes
Staphylococcus aureus (including penicillinase- and nonpenicillinase-producing strains)
Staphylococcus epidermidis
Streptococcus agalactiae (group B beta-hemolytic streptococcus)
Streptococcus pneumoniae
Streptococcus pyogenes

NOTE: Methicillin-resistant staphylococci are resistant to cephalosporins. Some strains of *Staphylococcus epidermidis* and most strains of enterococci, e.g., *Enterococcus faecalis* (formerly *Streptococcus faecalis*) are resistant to cefotetan.

Anaerobes
Prevotella bivia (formerly *Bacteroides bivius*)
Prevotella disiens (formerly *Bacteroides disiens*)
Bacteroides fragilis
Prevotella melaninogenica (formerly Bacteroides melaninogenicus)
Bacteroides vulgatus
Fusobacterium species
Gram-positive bacilli (including *Clostridium* species; see WARNINGS)

NOTE: Most strains of *C. difficile* are resistant (see WARNINGS).
Peptococcus niger
Peptostreptococcus species

NOTE: Many strains of *B. distasonis*, *B. ovatus* and *B. thetaiotaomicron* are resistant to cefotetan *in vitro*. However, the therapeutic utility of cefotetan against these organisms cannot be accurately predicted on the basis of *in vitro* susceptibility tests alone.

The following *in vitro* data are available but their clinical significance is unknown. Cefotetan has been shown to be active *in vitro* against most strains of the following organisms:

Gram-Negative Aerobes
Citrobacter species (including *C. diversus* and *C. freundii*)
Klebsiella oxytoca
Moraxella (Branhamella) catarrhalis
Neisseria gonorrhoeae (penicillinase-producing strains)
Salmonella species
Serratia species
Shigella species
Yersinia enterocolitica

Anaerobes
Porphyromonas asaccharolytica (formerly *Bacteroides asaccharolyticus*)
Prevotella oralis (formerly *Bacteroides oralis*)
Bacteroides splanchnicus
Clostridium difficile (see WARNINGS)
Propionibacterium species
Veillonella species

Susceptibility Tests

Dilution Techniques: Quantitative methods are used to determine antimicrobial minimal inhibitory concentrations (MIC's). These MIC's provide estimates of the susceptibility of bacteria to antimicrobial compounds. The MICs should be determined using a standardized procedure. Standardized procedures are based on a dilution method[1] (broth or agar) or equivalent with standardized inoculum concentrations and standardized concentrations or cefotetan powder. The MIC values should be interpreted according to the following criteria:

MIC (µg/mL)	Interpretation
≤16	Susceptible (S)
32	Intermediate (I)
≥64	Resistant (R)

A report of 'Susceptible' indicates that the pathogen is likely to be inhibited if the antimicrobial compound in the blood reaches the concentrations usually achievable. A report of 'Intermediate' indicates that the result should be considered equivocal, and if the microorganism is not fully susceptible to alternative, clinically feasible drugs, the test should be repeated. This category implies possible clinical applicability in body sites where the drug is physiologically concentrated or in situations where high dosage of drug can be used. This category also provides a buffer zone which prevents small uncontrolled technical factors from causing major discrepancies in interpretation. A report of 'Resistant' indicates that the pathogen is not likely to be inhibited if the antimicrobial compound in the blood reaches the concentrations usually achievable; other therapy should be selected.

Standardized susceptibility test procedures require the use of laboratory control microorganisms to control the technical aspects of the laboratory procedures. Standard cefotetan powder should provide the following MIC values:

Microorganism	MIC (µg/mL)
E. coli ATCC 25922	0.06–0.25
S. aureus ATCC 29213	4–16

Diffusion Techniques: Quantitative methods that require measurement of zone diameters also provide reproducible estimates of the susceptibility of bacteria to antimicrobial compounds. One such standardized procedure[2] requires the use of the standardized inoculum concentrations. This procedure uses paper disks impregnated with 30 µg cefotetan to test the susceptibility of microorganisms to cefotetan.

Reports from the laboratory providing results of the standard single-disk susceptibility test with a 30 µg cefotetan disk should be interpreted according to the following criteria:

Zone Diameter (mm)	Interpretation
≥16	Susceptible (S)
13–15	Intermediate (I)
≤12	Resistant (R)

Interpretation should be as stated above for results using dilution techniques. Interpretation involves correlation of the diameter obtained in the disk test with the MIC for cefotetan.

As with standardized dilution techniques, diffusion methods require the use of laboratory control microorganisms that

Continued on next page

Cefotan—Cont.

are used to control the technical aspects of the laboratory procedures. For the diffusion technique, the 30 µg cefotetan disk should provide the following zone diameters in these laboratory test quality control strains.

Microorganism	Zone Diameter (mm)
E. coli ATCC 25922	28–34
S. aureus ATCC 25923	17–23

Anaerobic Techniques: For anaerobic bacteria, the susceptibility to cefotetan as MIC's can be determined by standardized test methods[3]. The MIC values obtained should be interpreted according to the following criteria:

MIC (µg/mL)	Interpretation
≤16	Susceptible (S)
32	Intermediate (I)
≥64	Resistant (R)

Interpretation is identical to that stated above for results using dilution techniques.
As with other susceptibility techniques, the use of laboratory control microorganisms is required to control the technical aspects of the laboratory standardized procedures. Standardized cefotetan powder should provide the following MIC values:

Microorganism	MIC (µg/mL)
Bacteroides fragilis ATCC 25285	4–16
Bacteroides thetaiotaomicron ATCC 29741	32–128
Eubacterium lentum ATCC 43055	32–128

INDICATIONS AND USAGE

Treatment

CEFOTAN is indicated for the therapeutic treatment of the following infections when caused by susceptible strains of the designated organisms:

Urinary Tract Infections caused by *E. coli, Klebsiella* spp (including *K. pneumoniae*), *Proteus mirabilis* and *Proteus* spp (which may include the organisms now called *Proteus vulgaris, Providencia rettgeri*, and *Morganella morganii*).

Lower Respiratory Tract Infections caused by *Streptococcus pneumoniae, Staphylococcus aureus* (penicillinase- and nonpenicillinase-producing strains), *Haemophilus influenzae* (including ampicillin- resistant strains), *Klebsiella* species (including *K. pneumoniae*), *E. coli, Proteus mirabilis*, and *Serratia marcescens**.

Skin and Skin Structure Infections due to *Staphylococcus aureus* (penicillinase- and nonpenicillinase-producing strains), *Staphylococcus epidermidis, Streptococcus pyogenes, Streptococcus* species (excluding enterococci), *Escherichia coli, Klebsiella pneumoniae, Peptococcus niger**, *Peptostreptococcus species.*

Gynecologic Infections caused by *Staphylococcus aureus*, (including penicillinase- and nonpenicillinase-producing strains), *Staphylococcus epidermidis, Streptococcus* species (excluding enterococci), *Streptococcus agalactiae, E. coli, Proteus mirabilis, Neisseria gonorrhoeae*, Bacteroides species (excluding *B. distasonis, B. ovatus, B. thetaiotaomicron*), *Fusobacterium* species*, and gram-positive anaerobic cocci (including *Peptococcus niger* and *Peptostreptococcus* species).

Cefotetan, like other cephalosporins, has no activity against *Chlamydia trachomatis*. Therefore, when cephalosporins are used in the treatment of pelvic inflammatory disease, and *C. trachomatis* is one of the suspected pathogens, appropriate antichlamydial coverage should be added.

Intra-abdominal Infections caused by *E. coli, Klebsiella* species (including *K. pneumoniae*), *Streptococcus* species (excluding enterococci), *Bacteroides* species (excluding *B. distasonis, B. ovatus, B. thetaiotaomicron*) and *Clostridium* species*.

Bone and Joint Infections caused by *Staphylococcus aureus.**

*Efficacy for this organism in this organ system was studied in fewer than ten infections.

Specimens for bacteriological examination should be obtained in order to isolate and identify causative organisms and to determine their susceptibilities to cefotetan. Therapy may be instituted before results of susceptibility studies are known; however, once these results become available, the antibiotic treatment should be adjusted accordingly.

In cases of confirmed or suspected gram-positive or gram-negative sepsis or in patients with other serious infections in which the causative organism has not been identified, it is possible to use CEFOTAN concomitantly with an aminoglycoside. Cefotetan combinations with aminoglycosides have been shown to be synergistic *in vitro* against many Enterobacteriaceae and also some other gram-negative bacteria. The dosage recommended in the labeling of both antibiotics may be given and depends on the severity of the infection and the patient's condition.

NOTE: Increases in serum creatinine have occurred when CEFOTAN was given alone. If CEFOTAN and an aminoglycoside are used concomitantly, renal function should be carefully monitored, because nephrotoxicity may be potentiated.

Prophylaxis

The preoperative administration of CEFOTAN may reduce the incidence of certain postoperative infections in patients undergoing surgical procedures that are classified as clean contaminated or potentially contaminated (e.g., cesarean section, abdominal or vaginal hysterectomy, transurethral surgery, biliary tract surgery, and gastrointestinal surgery).
If there are signs and symptoms of infection, specimens for culture should be obtained for identification of the causative organism so that appropriate therapeutic measures may be initiated.

General Guidelines for Dosage of CEFOTAN

Type of Infection	Daily Dose	Frequency and Route
Urinary Tract	1–4 grams	500 mg every 12 hours IV or IM 1 or 2 g every 24 hours IV or IM 1 or 2 g every 12 hours IV or IM
Skin & Skin Structure Mild–Moderate[a]	2 grams	2 g every 24 hours IV 1 g every 12 hours IV or IM
Severe	4 grams	2 g every 12 hours IV
Other Sites	2–4 grams	1 or 2 g every 12 hours IV or IM
Severe	4 grams	2 g every 12 hours IV
Life-Threatening	6 grams[b]	3 g every 12 hours IV

[a] *Klebsiella pneumoniae* skin and skin structure infections should be treated with 1 or 2 grams every 12 hours IV or IM.
[b] Maximum daily dosage should not exceed 6 grams.

CONTRAINDICATIONS

CEFOTAN is contraindicated in patients with a known allergy to the cephalosporin group of antibiotics and in those individuals who have experienced a cephalosporin associated hemolytic anemia.

WARNINGS

BEFORE THERAPY WITH CEFOTAN IS INSTITUTED, CAREFUL INQUIRY SHOULD BE MADE TO DETERMINE WHETHER THE PATIENT HAS HAD PREVIOUS HYPERSENSITIVITY REACTIONS TO CEFOTETAN, CEPHALOSPORINS, PENICILLINS, OR OTHER DRUGS. IF THIS PRODUCT IS TO BE GIVEN TO PENICILLIN-SENSITIVE PATIENTS, CAUTION SHOULD BE EXERCISED BECAUSE CROSS-HYPERSENSITIVITY AMONG BETA-LACTAM ANTIBIOTICS HAS BEEN CLEARLY DOCUMENTED AND MAY OCCUR IN UP TO 10% OF PATIENTS WITH A HISTORY OF PENICILLIN ALLERGY. IF AN ALLERGIC REACTION TO CEFOTAN OCCURS, DISCONTINUE THE DRUG. SERIOUS ACUTE HYPERSENSITIVITY REACTIONS MAY REQUIRE TREATMENT WITH EPINEPHRINE AND OTHER EMERGENCY MEASURES, INCLUDING OXYGEN, INTRAVENOUS FLUIDS, INTRAVENOUS ANTIHISTAMINES, CORTICOSTEROIDS, PRESSOR AMINES, AND AIRWAY MANAGEMENT, AS CLINICALLY INDICATED.

AN IMMUNE MEDIATED HEMOLYTIC ANEMIA HAS BEEN OBSERVED IN PATIENTS RECEIVING CEPHALOSPORIN CLASS ANTIBIOTICS. SEVERE CASES OF HEMOLYTIC ANEMIA, INCLUDING FATALITIES, HAVE BEEN REPORTED IN ASSOCIATION WITH THE ADMINISTRATION OF CEFOTETAN. SUCH REPORTS ARE UNCOMMON. IF A PATIENT DEVELOPS ANEMIA ANYTIME WITHIN 2–3 WEEKS SUBSEQUENT TO THE ADMINISTRATION OF CEFOTETAN, THE DIAGNOSIS OF A CEPHALOSPORIN ASSOCIATED ANEMIA SHOULD BE CONSIDERED AND THE DRUG STOPPED UNTIL THE ETIOLOGY IS DETERMINED WITH CERTAINTY. BLOOD TRANSFUSIONS MAY BE CONSIDERED AS NEEDED (See **CONTRAINDICATIONS**).

PATIENTS WHO RECEIVE PROLONGED COURSES OF CEFOTETAN FOR TREATMENT OF INFECTIONS SHOULD HAVE PERIODIC MONITORING FOR SIGNS AND SYMPTOMS OF HEMOLYTIC ANEMIA INCLUDING A MEASUREMENT OF HEMATOLOGICAL PARAMETERS WHERE APPROPRIATE.

Pseudomembranous colitis has been reported with nearly all antibacterial agents, including cefotetan, and may range in severity from mild to life-threatening. Therefore, it is important to consider this diagnosis in patients who present with diarrhea subsequent to the administration of antibacterial agents.

Treatment with antibacterial agents alters the normal flora of the colon and may permit overgrowth of clostridia. Studies indicate that a toxin produced by *Clostridium difficile* is a primary cause of "antibiotic-associated colitis".

After the diagnosis of pseudomembranous colitis has been established, appropriate therapeutic measures should be initiated. Mild cases of pseudomembranous colitis usually respond to drug discontinuation alone. In moderate to severe cases, consideration should be given to management with fluids and electrolytes, protein supplementation, and treatment with an antibacterial drug clinically effective against *Clostridium difficile* colitis. (See ADVERSE REACTIONS.)

In common with many other broad-spectrum antibiotics, CEFOTAN may be associated with a fall in prothrombin activity and, possibly, subsequent bleeding. Those at increased risk include patients with renal or hepatobiliary impairment or poor nutritional state, the elderly, and patients with cancer. Prothrombin time should be monitored and exogenous vitamin K administered as indicated.

PRECAUTIONS

General: As with other broad-spectrum antibiotics, prolonged use of CEFOTAN may result in overgrowth of nonsusceptible organisms. Careful observation of the patient is essential. If superinfection does occur during therapy, appropriate measures should be taken.

CEFOTAN should be used with caution in individuals with a history of gastrointestinal disease, particularly colitis.

Information for Patients: As with some other cephalosporins, a disulfiram-like reaction characterized by flushing, sweating, headache, and tachycardia may occur when alcohol (beer, wine, etc.) is ingested within 72 hours after CEFOTAN administration. Patients should be cautioned about the ingestion of alcoholic beverages following the administration of CEFOTAN.

Drug Interactions: Increases in serum creatinine have occurred when CEFOTAN was given alone. If CEFOTAN and an aminoglycoside are used concomitantly, renal function should be carefully monitored, because nephrotoxicity may be potentiated.

Drug/Laboratory Test Interactions: The administration of CEFOTAN may result in a false positive reaction for glucose in the urine using Clinitest®‡, Benedict's solution, or Fehling's solution. It is recommended that glucose tests based on enzymatic glucose oxidase be used.

As with other cephalosporins, high concentrations of cefotetan may interfere with measurement of serum and urine creatinine levels by Jaffe' reaction and produce false increases in the levels of creatinine reported.

Carcinogenesis, Mutagenesis, Impairment of Fertility: Although long-term studies in animals have not been performed to evaluate carcinogenic potential, no mutagenic potential of cefotetan was found in standard laboratory tests. Cefotetan has adverse effects on the testes of prepubertal rats. Subcutaneous administration of 500 mg/kg/day (approximately 8-16 times the usual adult human dose) on days 6-35 of life (thought to be developmentally analogous to late childhood and prepuberty in humans) resulted in reduced testicular weight and seminiferous tubule degeneration in 10 of 10 animals. Affected cells included spermatogonia and spermatocytes; Sertoli and Leydig cells were unaffected. Incidence and severity of lesions were dose-dependent; at 120 mg/kg/day (approximately 2-4 times the usual human dose) only 1 of 10 treated animals was affected, and the degree of degeneration was mild.

Similar lesions have been observed in experiments of comparable design with other methylthiotetrazole-containing antibiotics and impaired fertility has been reported, particularly at high dose levels. No testicular effects were observed in 7-week-old rats treated with up to 1000 mg/kg/day SC for 5 weeks, or in infant dogs (3 weeks old) that received up to 300 mg/kg/day IV for 5 weeks. The relevance of these findings to humans is unknown.

Pregnancy: Teratogenic Effects. Pregnancy Category B: Reproduction studies have been performed in rats and monkeys at doses up to 20 times the human dose and have revealed no evidence of impaired fertility or harm to the fetus due to cefotetan. There are, however, no adequate and well-controlled studies in pregnant women. Because animal reproductive studies are not always predictive of human response, this drug should be used during pregnancy only if clearly needed.

Nursing Mothers: Cefotetan is excreted in human milk in very low concentrations. Caution should be exercised when cefotetan is administered to a nursing woman.

Pediatric Use: Safety and effectiveness in children have not been established.

ADVERSE REACTIONS

In clinical studies, the following adverse effects were considered related to CEFOTAN therapy. Those appearing in italics have been reported during postmarketing experience.

Gastrointestinal symptoms occurred in 1.5% of patients, the most frequent were diarrhea (1 in 80) and nausea (1 in 700); *pseudomembranous colitis*. Onset of pseudomembranous colitis symptoms may occur during or after antibiotic treatment or surgical prophylaxis. (See **WARNINGS**.)

Hematologic laboratory abnormalities occurred in 1.4% of patients and included eosinophilia (1 in 200), positive direct Coombs' test (1 in 250), and thrombocytosis (1 in 300); *agranulocytosis, hemolytic anemia, leukopenia, thrombocytopenia,* and *prolonged prothrombin time with or without bleeding.*

Hepatic enzyme elevations occurred in 1.2% of patients and included a rise in ALT (SGPT) (1 in 150), AST (SGOT) (1 in 300), alkaline phosphatase (1 in 700), and LDH (1 in 700).

Hypersensitivity reactions were reported in 1.2% of patients and included rash (1 in 150) and itching (1 in 700); *anaphylactic reactions and urticaria.*

Local: effects were reported in less than 1% of patients and included phlebitis at the site of injection (1 in 300), and discomfort (1 in 500).

Renal: *Elevations in BUN and serum creatinine have been reported.*
Urogenital: *Nephrotoxicity has rarely been reported.*
Miscellaneous: *Fever*
In addition to the adverse reactions listed above which have been observed in patients treated with cefotetan, the following adverse reactions and altered laboratory tests have been reported for cephalosporin-class antibiotics: pruritus, Stevens-Johnson syndrome, erythema multiforme, toxic epidermal necrolysis, vomiting, abdominal pain, colitis, superinfection, vaginitis including vaginal candidiasis, renal dysfunction, toxic nephropathy, hepatic dysfunction including cholestasis, aplastic anemia, hemorrhage, elevated bilirubin, pancytopenia, and neutropenia.
Several cephalosporins have been implicated in triggering seizures, particularly in patients with renal impairment, when the dosage was not reduced. (See DOSAGE AND ADMINISTRATION and OVERDOSAGE.) If seizures associated with drug therapy occur, the drug should be discontinued. Anticonvulsant therapy can be given if clinically indicated.

OVERDOSAGE

Information on overdosage with CEFOTAN in humans is not available. If overdosage should occur, it should be treated symptomatically and hemodialysis considered, particularly if renal function is compromised.

DOSAGE AND ADMINISTRATION

Treatment
Cefotetan injection in Galaxy® plastic container should not be used for intramuscular administration.
CEFOTAN in the ADD-Vantage Vial is intended for intravenous infusion only, after dilution with the appropriate volume of ADD-Vantage diluent solution.
The usual adult dosage is 1 or 2 grams of CEFOTAN (cefotetan disodium for injection) administered intravenously or intramuscularly or CEFOTAN (cefotetan injection) in the Galaxy® plastic container (PL 2040) administered intravenously every 12 hours for 5 to 10 days. Proper dosage and route of administration should be determined by the condition of the patient, severity of the infection, and susceptibility of the causative organism.
[See table at top of previous page]
If *Chlamydia trachomatis* is a suspected pathogen in gynecologic infections, appropriate antichlamydial coverage should be added, since cefotetan has no activity against this organism.
Prophylaxis:
To prevent postoperative infection in clean contaminated or potentially contaminated surgery in adults, the recommended dosage is 1 or 2 g of CEFOTAN administered once, intravenously, 30 to 60 minutes prior to surgery. In patients undergoing cesarean section, the dose should be administered as soon as the umbilical cord is clamped.
Impaired Renal Function:
When renal function is impaired, a reduced dosage schedule must be employed. The following dosage guidelines may be used.
[See table above]

DOSAGE GUIDELINES FOR PATIENTS WITH IMPAIRED RENAL FUNCTION

Creatinine Clearance mL/min	Dose	Frequency
>30	Usual Recommended Dosage*	Every 12 hours
10–30	Usual Recommended Dosage*	Every 24 hours
<10	Usual Recommended Dosage*	Every 48 hours

* Dose determined by the type and severity of infection, and susceptibility of the causative organism.

Alternatively, the dosing interval may remain constant at 12 hour intervals, but the dose reduced to one-half the usual recommended dose for patients with a creatinine clearance of 10-30 mL/min, and one-quarter the usual recommended dose for patients with a creatinine clearance of less than 10 mL/min.
When only serum creatinine levels are available, creatinine clearance may be calculated from the following formula. The serum creatinine level should represent a steady state of renal function.

Males: $\frac{\text{Weight (kg)} \times (140 - \text{age})}{72 \times \text{serum creatinine (mg/100 mL)}}$

Females: $0.9 \times$ value for males

Cefotetan is dialyzable and it is recommended that for patients undergoing intermittent hemodialysis, one-quarter of the usual recommended dose be given every 24 hours on days between dialysis and one-half the usual recommended dose on the day of dialysis.

CEFOTETAN DISODIUM FOR INJECTION

Preparation of Solution From Cefotetan Disodium For Injection
For Intravenous Use: Reconstitute with Sterile Water for Injection. Shake to dissolve and let stand until clear.

Vial Size	Amount of Diluent Added (mL)	Approximate Withdrawable Vol (mL)	Approximate Average Concentration (mg/mL)
1 gram	10	10.5	95
2 gram	10–20	11–21	182–95

Infusion bottles (100 mL) may be reconstituted with 50 to 100 mL of Dextrose Injection 5% or Sodium Chloride Injection 0.9%.
NOTE: ADD-VANTAGE VIALS ARE NOT TO BE USED IN THIS MANNER
For ADD-Vantage Vials: ADD-Vantage Vials of CEFOTAN are to be reconstituted only with Sodium Chloride Injection 0.9% or Dextrose Injection 5% in the 50 mL, 100 mL or 250 mL Flexible Diluent Containers. CEFOTAN supplied in single-use ADD-Vantage Vials should be prepared as directed.

Directions for Use of CEFOTAN (cefotetan disodium for injection) in ADD-Vantage Vials:
To Open Diluent Container: Peel overwrap from the corner and remove container. Some opacity of the plastic due to moisture absorption during the sterilization process may be observed. This is normal and does not affect the solution quality or safety. The opacity will diminish gradually.
To Assemble ADD-Vantage Vial and Flexible Diluent Container: (Use Aseptic Technique)
1. Remove the protective covers from the top of the vial and the vial port on the diluent container as follows:
   a. To remove the breakaway vial cap, swing the pull ring over the top of the vial and pull down far enough to start the opening (See Figure 1), then pull straight up to remove the cap. (See Figure 2.) **NOTE:** Once the breakaway cap has been removed, do not access vial with syringe.

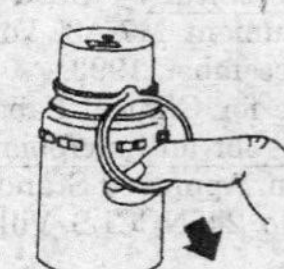
Figure 1

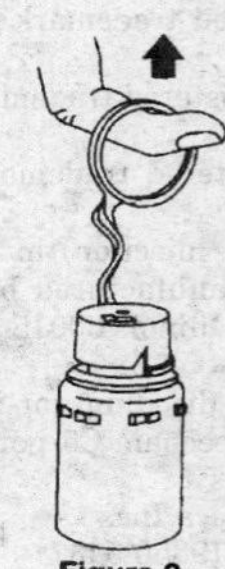
Figure 2

   b. To remove the vial port cover, grasp the tab on the pull ring, pull up to break the three tie strings, then pull back to remove the cover. (See Figure 3.)

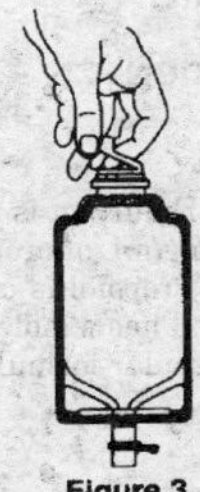
Figure 3

2. Screw the vial into the vial port until it will go no further. THE VIAL MUST BE SCREWED IN TIGHTLY TO ASSURE A SEAL. This occurs approximately 1/2 turn (180°) after the first audible click. (See Figure 4.) The clicking sound does not assure a seal; the vial must be turned as far as it will go. **NOTE:** ONCE VIAL IS SEATED, DO NOT ATTEMPT TO REMOVE. (See Figure 4.)

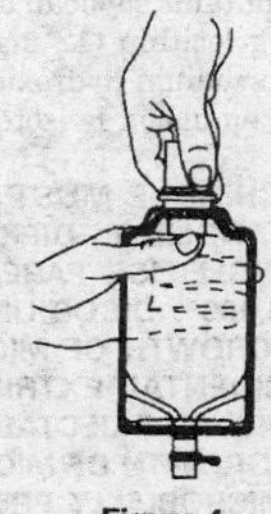
Figure 4

3. Recheck the vial to assure that it is tight by trying to turn it further in the direction of assembly.
4. Label appropriately.

To Prepare Admixture:
1. Squeeze the bottom of the diluent container gently to inflate the portion of the container surrounding the end of the drug vial.
2. With the other hand, push the drug vial down into the container telescoping the walls of the container. Grasp the inner cap of the vial through the walls of the container. (See Figure 5.)

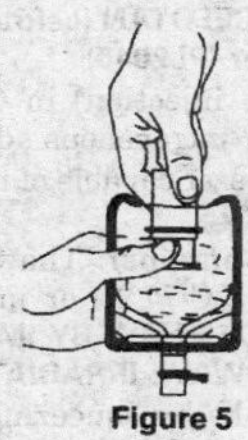
Figure 5

3. Pull the inner cap from the drug vial. (See Figure 6.) Verify that the rubber stopper has been pulled out and invert the system several times, allowing the drug and diluent to mix.

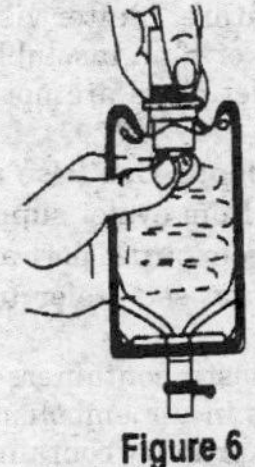
Figure 6

4. Mix contents thoroughly and use within the specified time.

Preparation For Administration: (Use Aseptic Technique)
1. Confirm the activation and admixture of vial contents.
2. Check for leaks by squeezing container firmly. If leaks are found, discard unit as sterility may be impaired.
3. Close flow control clamp of administration set.
4. Remove cover from outlet port at bottom of container.
5. Insert piercing pin of administration set into port with a twisting motion until the pin is firmly seated. **NOTE:** See full directions on administration set carton.
6. Lift the free end of the hanger loop on the bottom of the vial, breaking the two tie strings. Bend the loop outward to lock it in the upright position, then suspend container from hanger.
7. Squeeze and release drip chamber to establish proper fluid level in chamber.
8. Open flow control clamp and clear air from set. Close clamp.
9. Attach set to venipuncture device. If device is not indwelling, prime and make venipuncture.
10. Regulate rate of administration with flow control clamp.

WARNING: Do not use flexible container in series connections.
For Intramuscular Use: Reconstitute with Sterile Water for Injection; Bacteriostatic Water for Injection; Sodium Chloride Injection 0.9%, USP; 0.5% Lidocaine HCl; or 1% Lidocaine HCl. Shake to dissolve and let stand until clear.

Vial Size	Amount of Diluent Added (mL)	Approximate Withdrawable Vol (mL)	Average Concentration (mg/mL)
1 gram	2	2.5	400
2 gram	3	4	500

Intravenous Administration:
The intravenous route is preferable for patients with bacteremia, bacterial septicemia, or other severe or life-threatening infections, or for patients who may be poor risks because of lowered resistance resulting from such debilitating conditions as malnutrition, trauma, surgery, diabetes, heart failure, or malignancy, particularly if shock is present or impending.
For intermittent intravenous administration, a solution containing 1 gram or 2 grams of CEFOTAN (cefotetan disodium for injection) in Sterile Water for Injection can be injected over a period of three to five minutes. Using an infusion system, the solution may also be given over a longer period of time through the tubing system by which the patient may be receiving other intravenous solutions. Butterfly® or scalp vein- type needles are preferred for this type of

Continued on next page

Cefotan—Cont.

infusion. However, during infusion of the solution containing CEFOTAN (cefotetan disodium for injection), it is advisable to discontinue temporarily the administration of other solutions at the same site.

NOTE: Solutions of CEFOTAN must not be admixed with solutions containing aminoglycosides. If CEFOTAN and aminoglycosides are to be administered to the same patient, they must be administered separately and not as a mixed injection.

Intramuscular Administration:

As with all intramuscular preparations, (cefotetan disodium for injection) should be injected well within the body of a relatively large muscle such as the upper outer quadrant of the buttock (i.e., gluteus maximus); aspiration is necessary to avoid inadvertent injection into a blood vessel.

CEFOTETAN INJECTION

Directions for Use of CEFOTAN (cefotetan injection) in Galaxy® Plastic Container (PL2040)

CEFOTAN (cefotetan injection) in Galaxy® plastic container (PL 2040) is for intravenous administration only.

Storage: Store in a freezer capable of maintaining a temperature of -20°C/-4°F.

Thawing of Plastic Container: Thaw frozen container at room temperature (25°C/77°F) or in a refrigerator (5°C/41°F). **[DO NOT FORCE THAW BY IMMERSION IN WATER BATHS OR BY MICROWAVE IRRADIATION.]**

Check for minute leaks by squeezing container firmly. If leaks are detected, discard solution as sterility may be impaired.

The container should be visually inspected. Components of the solution may precipitate in the frozen state and will dissolve upon reaching room temperature with little or no agitation. Potency is not affected. Agitate after solution has reached room temperature. If after visual inspection the solution remains cloudy or if an insoluble precipitate is noted or if any seals or outlet ports are not intact, the container should be discarded.

Preparation of Intravenous Use (Use aseptic technique):

1. Suspend container from eyelet support.
2. Remove protector from outlet port at bottom of container.
3. Attach administration set. Refer to complete directions accompanying set.

Caution: Do not use plastic containers in series connections. Such use could result in air embolism due to residual air being drawn from the primary container before administration of the fluid from the secondary container is complete.

Intravenous Administration:

The intravenous route is preferable for patients with bacteremia, bacterial septicemia, or other severe or life threatening infections, or for patients who may be poor risks because of lowered resistance resulting from such debilitating conditions as malnutrition, trauma, surgery, diabetes, heart failure, or malignancy, particularly if shock is present or impending.

Using an infusion system, CEFOTAN (cefotetan injection) in Galaxy® plastic container (PL 2040) should be given over 20 to 60 minutes through the tubing system by which the patient may be receiving other intravenous solutions. Butterfly® or scalp vein-type needles are preferred for this type of infusion. However, during infusion of the solution containing CEFOTAN (cefotetan injection) in Galaxy® plastic container (PL 2040), it is advisable to discontinue temporarily the administration of other solutions at the same site.

Compatibility and Stability of CEFOTAN Products:

Frozen samples should be thawed at room temperature before use. After the periods mentioned below, any unused solutions or frozen material should be discarded. **DO NOT REFREEZE.**

NOTE: Solutions of CEFOTAN must not be admixed-with solutions containing aminoglycosides. If CEFOTAN and aminoglycosides are to be administered to the same patient, they must be administered separately and not as a mixed injection. **DO NOT ADD SUPPLEMENTARY MEDICATION.**

CEFOTETAN DISODIUM FOR INJECTION

CEFOTAN (cefotetan disodium for injection) reconstituted as described above (PREPARATION OF SOLUTION) maintains satisfactory potency for 24 hours at room temperature (25°C/77°F), for 96 hours under refrigeration (5°C/41°F), and for at least 1 week in the frozen state (-20°C/-4°F). After reconstitution and subsequent storage in disposable glass or plastic syringes, CEFOTAN (cefotetan disodium for injection) is stable for 24 hours at room temperature and 96 hours under refrigeration.

ADD-Vantage Vials:

Ordinarily, ADD-Vantage Vials should be reconstituted only when it is certain that the patient is ready to receive the drug. However, ADD-Vantage Vials of CEFOTAN reconstituted as described in Preparation of Solution, for ADD-Vantage Vials, maintains satisfactory potency for 24 hours at room temperature (25°C/77°F).

(DO NOT REFRIGERATE OR FREEZE CEFOTAN IN ADD-VANTAGE VIALS.)

CEFOTETAN INJECTION

The thawed solution in Galaxy® plastic container (PL 2040) remains chemically stable for 48 hours at room temperature (25°C/77°F) or for 21 days under refrigeration (5°C/41°F).

NOTE: Parenteral drug products should be inspected visually for particulate matter and discoloration prior to administration whenever solution and container permit.

HOW SUPPLIED

CEFOTAN (cefotetan disodium for injection) is a dry, white to pale yellow powder supplied in vials containing cefotetan disodium equivalent to 1 g and 2 g cefotetan activity for intravenous and intramuscular administration. The vials should not be stored at temperatures above 22° C (72° F) and should be protected from light.

1 g ADD-Vantage Vial (NDC 0310-0376-31)
2 g ADD-Vantage Vial (NDC 0310-0377-32)
1 g Vial (NDC 0310-0376-10)
2 g Vial (NDC 0310-0377-20)
1 g Piggyback Vial (NDC 0310-0376-11)
2 g Piggyback Vial (NDC 0310-0377-21)

CEFOTAN is also available as a 10 g pharmacy bulk package.

10g in 100 mL Vial (NDC 0310-0375-10)

CEFOTAN (cefotetan injection) is supplied as a frozen, iso-osmotic, premixed solution in single dose Galaxy® plastic containers (PL 2040) as follows:

1 g in 50 mL plastic container (NDC 0310-0378-51)
2 g in 50 mL plastic container (NDC 0310-0379-51)

Store containers at or below -20°C/-4°F. **[See DIRECTIONS FOR USE OF CEFOTAN (cefotetan injection) IN GALAXY® PLASTIC CONTAINER (PL 2040)].**

REFERENCES

1. National Committee for Clinical Laboratory Standards. Methods for Dilution Antimicrobial Susceptibility Tests for Bacteria that Grow Aerobically—Third Edition. Approved Standard NCCLS Document M7-A3, Vol. 13, No. 25, NCCLS, Villanova, PA, December, 1993.
2. National Committee for Clinical Laboratory Standards. Performance Standards for antimicrobial Disk Susceptibility Tests—Fifth Edition. Approved Standard NCCLS Document M2-A5, Vol. 13, No. 24, NCCLS, Villanova, PA, December 1993.
3. National Committee for Clinical Laboratory Standards. Methods for Antimicrobial Susceptibility Testing of Anaerobic Bacteria—Third Edition. Approved Standard NCCLS Document M11-A3, Vol 13, No. 26, NCCLS, Villanova, PA, December 1993.

*Galaxy® is a registered trademark of Baxter Healthcare Corporation.

†ADD-Vantage is a registered trademark of Abbott Laboratories Inc.

‡ Clinitest® is a registered trademark of Ames Division, Miles Laboratories, Inc.

CEFOTAN® (cefotetan injection) in Galaxy® plastic container (PL 2040) is manufactured by Baxter Healthcare Corporation, Deerfield, Illinois 60015 USA for Zeneca Pharmaceuticals.

CEFOTAN® (cefotetan disodium for injection) is manufactured by SmithKline Beecham Corporation for:
Zeneca Pharmaceuticals
A Business Unit of Zeneca Inc.
Wilmington, Delaware 19850-5437
Rev J 03/99 SIC 64065-04

Shown in Product Identification Guide, page 305

DIPRIVAN® 1% ℞
INJECTABLE EMULSION
10 mg/mL propofol
FOR I.V. ADMINISTRATION

DESCRIPTION

DIPRIVAN® Injectable Emulsion is a sterile, nonpyrogenic emulsion containing 10mg/mL of propofol suitable for intravenous administration. Propofol is chemically described as 2,6-diisopropylphenol and has a molecular weight of 178.27. The structural and molecular formulas are:

$(CH_3)_2CH$–[benzene ring with OH]–$CH(CH_3)_2$

$C_{12}H_{18}O$

Propofol is very slightly soluble in water and, thus, is formulated in a white, oil-in-water emulsion. The pKa is 11. The octanol/water partition coefficient for propofol 6761:1 at a pH of 6–8.5. In addition to the active component, propofol, the formulation also contains soybean oil (100 mg/mL), glycerol (22.5 mg/mL), egg lecithin (12 mg/mL), and disodium edetate (0.005%); with sodium hydroxide to adjust pH. The DIPRIVAN Injectable emulsion is isotonic and has a pH of 7–8.5.

STRICT ASEPTIC TECHNIQUE MUST ALWAYS BE MAINTAINED DURING HANDLING. DIPRIVAN INJECTABLE EMULSION IS A SINGLE-USE PARENTERAL PRODUCT WHICH CONTAINS 0.005% DISODIUM EDETATE TO RETARD THE RATE OF GROWTH OF MICROORGANISMS IN THE EVENT OF ACCIDENTAL EXTRINSIC CONTAMINATION. HOWEVER, DIPRIVAN INJECTABLE EMULSION CAN STILL SUPPORT THE GROWTH OF MICROORGANISMS AS IT IS NOT AN ANTIMICROBIALLY PRESERVED PRODUCT UNDER USP STANDARDS. ACCORDINGLY, STRICT ASEPTIC TECHNIQUE MUST STILL BE ADHERED TO. DO NOT USE IF CONTAMINATION IS SUSPECTED. DISCARD UNUSED PORTIONS AS DIRECTED WITHIN THE REQUIRED TIME LIMITS (SEE DOSAGE AND ADMINISTRATION, HANDLING PROCEDURES). THERE HAVE BEEN REPORTS IN WHICH FAILURE TO USE ASEPTIC TECHNIQUE WHEN HANDLING DIPRIVAN INJECTABLE EMULSION WAS ASSOCIATED WITH MICROBIAL CONTAMINATION OF THE PRODUCT AND WITH FEVER, INFECTION/SEPSIS, OTHER LIFE-THREATENING ILLNESS, AND/OR DEATH.

CLINICAL PHARMACOLOGY

General

DIPRIVAN Injectable Emulsion is an intravenous sedative-hypnotic agent for use in the induction and maintenance of anesthesia or sedation. Intravenous injection of a therapeutic dose of propofol produces hypnosis rapidly with minimal excitation, usually within 40 seconds from the start of an injection (the time for one arm-brain circulation). As with other rapidly acting intravenous anesthetic agents, the half-time of the blood-brain equilibration is approximately 1 to 3 minutes, and this accounts for the rapid induction of anesthesia.

Pharmacodynamics

Pharmacodynamic properties of propofol are dependent upon the therapeutic blood propofol concentrations. Steady state propofol blood concentrations are generally proportional to infusion rates, especially within an individual patient. Undesirable side effects such as cardiorespiratory depression are likely to occur at higher blood concentrations which result from bolus dosing or rapid increase in infusion rate. An adequate interval (3 to 5 minutes) must be allowed between clinical dosage adjustments in order to assess drug effects.

The hemodynamic effects of DIPRIVAN Injectable Emulsion during induction of anesthesia vary. If spontaneous ventilation is maintained, the major cardiovascular effects are arterial hypotension (sometimes greater than a 30% decrease) with little or no change in heart rate and no appreciable decrease in cardiac output. If ventilation is assisted or controlled (positive pressure ventilation), the degree and incidence of decrease in cardiac output are accentuated. Addition of a potent opioid (e.g., fentanyl) when used as a premedicant further decreases cardiac output and respiratory drive.

If anesthesia is continued by infusion of DIPRIVAN Injectable Emulsion, the stimulation of endotracheal intubation and surgery may return arterial pressure towards normal. However, cardiac output may remain depressed. Comparative clinical studies have shown that the hemodynamic effects of DIPRIVAN Injectable Emulsion during induction of anesthesia are generally more pronounced than with other IV induction agents traditionally used for this purpose.

Clinical and preclinical studies suggest that DIPRIVAN Injectable Emulsion is rarely associated with elevation of plasma histamine levels.

Induction of anesthesia with DIPRIVAN Injectable Emulsion is frequently associated with apnea in both adults and children. In 1573 adult patients who received DIPRIVAN Injectable Emulsion (2 to 2.5 mg/kg), apnea lasted less than 30 seconds in 7% of patients, 30-60 seconds in 24% of patients, and more than 60 seconds in 12% of patients. In the 213 pediatric patients between the ages of 3 and 12 years assessable for apnea who received DIPRIVAN Injectable Emulsion (1 to 3.6 mg/kg), apnea lasted less than 30 seconds in 12% of patients, 30-60 seconds in 10% of patients, and more than 60 seconds in 5% of patients.

During maintenance, DIPRIVAN Injectable Emulsion causes a decrease in ventilation usually associated with an increase in carbon dioxide tension which may be marked depending upon the rate of administration and other concurrent medications (e.g., opioids, sedatives, etc.).

During monitored anesthesia care (MAC) sedation, attention must be given to the cardiorespiratory effects of DIPRIVAN Injectable Emulsion. Hypotension, oxyhemoglobin desaturation, apnea, airway obstruction, and/or oxygen desaturation can occur, especially following a rapid bolus of DIPRIVAN Injectable Emulsion. During initiation of MAC sedation, slow infusion or slow injection techniques are preferable over rapid bolus administration, and during maintenance of MAC sedation, a variable rate infusion is preferable over intermittent bolus administration in order to minimize undesirable cardiorespiratory effects. In the elderly, debilitated, or ASA III/IV patients, rapid (single or repeated) bolus dose administration should not be used for MAC sedation. (See WARNINGS.) DIPRIVAN Injectable Emulsion is not recommended for MAC Sedation in children because safety and effectiveness have not been established.

Clinical studies in humans and studies in animals show that DIPRIVAN Injectable Emulsion does not suppress the adrenal response to ACTH. Preliminary findings in patients with normal intraocular pressure indicate that DIPRIVAN Injectable Emulsion anesthesia produces a decrease in intraocular pressure which may be associated with a concomitant decrease in systemic vascular resistance.

Animal studies and limited experience in susceptible patients have not indicated any propensity of DIPRIVAN Injectable Emulsion to induce malignant hyperthermia.

Studies to date indicate that DIPRIVAN Injectable Emulsion when used in combination with hypocarbia increases cerebrovascular resistance and decreases cerebral blood flow, cerebral metabolic oxygen consumption, and intracranial pressure. DIPRIVAN Injectable Emulsion does not affect cerebrovascular reactivity to changes in arterial carbon dioxide tension. (see Clinical Trials-Neuroanesthesia).

Hemosiderin deposits have been observed in the liver of dogs receiving DIPRIVAN Injectable Emulsion containing 0.005% disodium edetate over a four week period; the clinical significance is unknown.

Pharmacokinetics

The proper use of DIPRIVAN Injectable Emulsion requires an understanding of the disposition and elimination characteristics of propofol.

The pharmacokinetics of propofol are well described by a three compartment linear model with compartments representing the plasma, rapidly equilibrating tissues, and slowly equilibrating tissues.

Following an IV bolus dose, there is rapid equilibration between the plasma and the highly perfused tissue of the brain, thus accounting for the rapid onset of anesthesia. Plasma levels initially decline rapidly as a result of both rapid distribution and high metabolic clearance. Distribution accounts for about half of this decline following a bolus of propofol.

However, distribution is not constant over time, but decreases as body tissues equilibrate with plasma and become saturated. The rate at which equilibration occurs is a function of the rate and duration of the infusion. When equilibration occurs there is no longer a net transfer of propofol between tissues and plasma.

Discontinuation of the recommended doses of DIPRIVAN Injectable Emulsion after the maintenance of anesthesia for approximately one-hour, or for sedation in the ICU for one-day, results in a prompt decrease in blood propofol concentrations and rapid awakening. Longer infusions (10 days of ICU sedation) result in accumulation of significant tissue stores of propofol, such that the reduction in circulating propofol is slowed and the time to awakening is increased.

By daily titration of DIPRIVAN Injectable Emulsion dosage to achieve only the minimum effective therapeutic concentration, rapid awakening within 10 to 15 minutes will occur even after long term administration. If, however, higher than necessary infusion levels have been maintained for a long time, propofol will be redistributed from fat and muscle to the plasma, and this return of propofol from peripheral tissues will slow recovery.

The figure below illustrates the fall of plasma propofol levels following ICU sedation infusions of various durations.

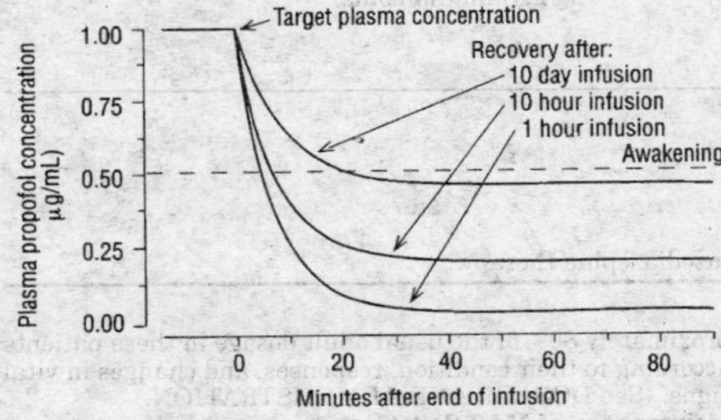

The large contribution of distribution (about 50%) to the fall of propofol plasma levels following brief infusions means that after very long infusions (at steady state), about half the initial rate will maintain the same plasma levels. Failure to reduce the infusion rate in patients receiving DIPRIVAN Injectable Emulsion for extended periods may result in excessively high blood concentrations of the drug. Thus, titration to clinical response and daily evaluation of sedation levels are important during use of DIPRIVAN Injectable Emulsion infusion for ICU sedation, especially of long duration.

Adults:

Propofol clearance ranges from 23–50mL/kg/min (1.6 to 3.4 L/min in 70 kg adults). It is chiefly eliminated by hepatic conjugation to inactive metabolites which are excreted by the kidney. A glucuronide conjugate accounts for about 50% of the administered dose. Propofol has a steady state volume of distribution (10-day infusion) approaching 60 L/kg in healthy adults. A difference in pharmacokinetics due to gender has not been observed. The terminal half-life of propofol after a 10-day infusion is 1 to 3 days.

Geriatrics:

With increasing patient age, the dose of propofol needed to achieve a defined anesthetic endpoint (dose-requirement) decreases. This does not appear to be an age-related change of pharmacodynamics or brain sensitivity, as measured by EEG burst suppression. With increasing patient age pharmacokinetic changes are such that for a given IV bolus dose, higher peak plasma concentrations occur, which can explain the decreased dose requirement. These higher peak plasma concentrations in the elderly can predispose patients to cardiorespiratory effects including hypotension, apnea, airway obstruction and/or oxygen desaturation. The higher plasma levels reflect an age-related decrease in volume of distribution and reduced intercompartmental clearance. Lower doses are thus recommended for initiation and maintenance of sedation/anesthesia in elderly patients. (See CLINICAL PHARMACOLOGY - Individualization of Dosage.)

Pediatrics:

The pharmacokinetics of propofol were studied in 53 children between the ages of 3 and 12 years who received DIPRIVAN Injectable Emulsion for periods of approximately 1-2 hours. The observed distribution and clearance of propofol in these children was similar to adults.

Organ Failure:

The pharmacokinetics of propofol do not appear to be different in people with chronic hepatic cirrhosis or chronic renal impairment compared to adults with normal hepatic and renal function. The effects of acute hepatic or renal failure on the pharmacokinetics of propofol have not been studied.

Clinical Trials

Anesthesia and Monitored Anesthesia Care (MAC) Sedation

DIPRIVAN Injectable Emulsion was compared to intravenous and inhalational anesthetic or sedative agents in 91 trials involving a total of 5,135 patients. Of these 3,354 received DIPRIVAN Injectable Emulsion and comprised the overall safety database for anesthesia and MAC sedation. Fifty-five of these trials, 20 for anesthesia induction and 35 for induction and maintenance of anesthesia or MAC sedation, were carried out in the US or Canada and provided the basis for dosage recommendations and the adverse event profile during anesthesia or MAC sedation.

Pediatric Anesthesia

DIPRIVAN Injectable Emulsion was compared to standard anesthetic agents in 12 clinical trials involving 534 patients receiving DIPRIVAN Injectable Emulsion. Of these, 349 were from US/Canadian clinical trials and comprised the overall safety database for Pediatric Anesthesia.

TABLE 1. PEDIATRIC ANESTHESIA CLINICAL TRIALS
Patients Receiving DIPRIVAN Injectable Emulsion Median and (Range)

	Induction Only	Induction and Maintenance
Number of Patients*	243	105
Induction Bolus Dosages	2.5 mg/kg (1–3.5)	3 mg/kg (2–3.6)
Injection Duration	20 sec (6–45)	
Maintenance Dosage	—	181 µg/kg/min (107–418)
Maintenance Duration	—	78 min (29–268)

*Body weight not recorded for one patient.

Neuroanesthesia

DIPRIVAN Injectable Emulsion was studied in 50 patients undergoing craniotomy for supratentorial tumors in two clinical trials. The mean lesion size (anterior/posterior and lateral) was 31 mm and 32 mm in one trial and 55 mm and 42 mm in the other trial respectively.

[See table 2 above]

TABLE 2. NEUROANESTHESIA CLINICAL TRIALS
Patients Receiving DIPRIVAN Injectable Emulsion Median and (Range)

Patient Type	No. of Patients	Induction Bolus Dosages (mg/kg)	Maintenance Dosage (µg/kg/min)	Maintenance Duration (min)
Craniotomy patients	50	136 (0.9–6.9)	146 (68–425)	285 (48–622)

In ten of these patients, DIPRIVAN Injectable Emulsion was administered by infusion in a controlled clinical trial to evaluate the effect of DIPRIVAN Injectable Emulsion on cerebrospinal fluid pressure (CSFP). The mean arterial pressure was maintained relatively constant over 25 minutes with a change from baseline of −4% ± 17% (mean ± SD), whereas the percent change in cerebrospinal fluid pressure (CSFP) was −46% ± 14%. As CSFP is an indirect measure of intracranial pressure (ICP), when given by infusion or slow bolus, DIPRIVAN Injectable Emulsion, in combination with hypocarbia, is capable of decreasing ICP independent of changes in arterial pressure.

Intensive Care Unit (ICU) Sedation

DIPRIVAN Injectable Emulsion was compared to benzodiazepines and/or opioids in 14 clinical trials involving a total of 550 ICU patients. Of these, 302 received DIPRIVAN Injectable Emulsion and comprise the overall safety database for ICU sedation. Six of these studies were carried out in the US or Canada and provide the basis for dosage recommendations and the adverse event profile.

Information from 193 literature reports of DIPRIVAN Injectable Emulsion used for ICU sedation in over 950 patients and information from the clinical trials are summarized below:

[See table 3 at top of next page]

Cardiac Anesthesia

DIPRIVAN Injectable Emulsion was evaluated in 5 clinical trials conducted in the US and Canada, involving a total of 569 patients undergoing coronary artery bypass graft (CABG). Of these, 301 patients received DIPRIVAN Injectable Emulsion. They comprise the safety database for cardiac anesthesia and provide the basis for dosage recommendations in this patient population, in conjunction with reports in the published literature.

Individualization of Dosage

General:

STRICT ASEPTIC TECHNIQUE MUST ALWAYS BE MAINTAINED DURING HANDLING. DIPRIVAN INJECTABLE EMULSION IS A SINGLE-USE PARENTERAL PRODUCT WHICH CONTAINS 0.005% DISODIUM EDETATE TO RETARD THE RATE OF GROWTH OF MICROORGANISMS IN THE EVENT OF ACCIDENTAL EXTRINSIC CONTAMINATION. HOWEVER, DIPRIVAN INJECTABLE EMULSION CAN STILL SUPPORT THE GROWTH OF MICROORGANISMS AS IT IS NOT AN ANTIMICROBIALLY PRESERVED PRODUCT UNDER USP STANDARDS. ACCORDINGLY, STRICT ASEPTIC TECHNIQUE MUST STILL BE ADHERED TO. DO NOT USE IF CONTAMINATION IS SUSPECTED. DISCARD UNUSED PORTIONS AS DIRECTED WITHIN THE REQUIRED TIME LIMITS (SEE DOSAGE AND ADMINISTRATION, HANDLING PROCEDURES). THERE HAVE BEEN REPORTS IN WHICH FAILURE TO USE ASEPTIC TECHNIQUE WHEN HANDLING DIPRIVAN INJECTABLE EMULSION WAS ASSOCIATED WITH MICROBIAL CONTAMINATION OF THE PRODUCT AND WITH FEVER, INFECTION/SEPSIS, OTHER LIFE-THREATENING ILLNESS, AND/OR DEATH.

Propofol blood concentrations at steady state are generally proportional to infusion rates, especially in individual patients. Undesirable effects such as cardiorespiratory depression are likely to occur at higher blood concentrations which result from bolus dosing or rapid increases in the infusion rate. An adequate interval (3 to 5 minutes) must be allowed between clinical dosage adjustments in order to assess drug effects.

When administering DIPRIVAN Injectable Emulsion by infusion, syringe pumps or volumetric pumps are recommended to provide controlled infusion rates. When infusing DIPRIVAN Injectable Emulsion to patients undergoing magnetic resonance imaging, metered control devices may be utilized if mechanical pumps are impractical.

Changes in vital signs (increases in pulse rate, blood pressure, sweating and/or tearing) that indicate a response to surgical stimulation or lightening of anesthesia may be controlled by the administration of DIPRIVAN Injectable Emulsion 25 mg (2.5 mL) to 50 mg (5 mL) incremental boluses and/or by increasing the infusion rate.

For minor surgical procedures (e.g. body surface) nitrous oxide (60%-70%) can be combined with a variable rate DIPRIVAN Injectable Emulsion infusion to provide satisfactory anesthesia. With more stimulating surgical procedures (e.g. intra-abdominal), or if supplementation with nitrous oxide is not provided, administration rate(s) of DIPRIVAN Injectable Emulsion and/or opioids should be increased in order to provide adequate anesthesia.

Infusion rates should always be titrated downward in the absence of clinical signs of light anesthesia until a mild response to surgical stimulation is obtained in order to avoid administration of DIPRIVAN Injectable Emulsion at rates higher than are clinically necessary. Generally, rates of 50 to 100 µg/kg/min in adults, should be achieved during maintenance in order to optimize recovery times.

Other drugs that cause CNS depression (hypnotics/sedatives, inhalational anesthetics and opioids) can increase CNS depression induced by propofol. Morphine premedication (0.15 mg/kg) with nitrous oxide 67% in oxygen has been shown to decrease the necessary propofol injection maintenance infusion rate and therapeutic blood concentrations when compared to non-narcotic (lorazepam) premedication.

Induction of General Anesthesia

Adult Patients:

Most adult patients under 55 years of age and classified ASA I/II require 2 to 2.5 mg/kg of DIPRIVAN Injectable Emulsion for induction when unpremedicated or when premedicated with oral benzodiazepines or intramuscular opioids. For induction, DIPRIVAN Injectable Emulsion should be titrated (approximately 40 mg every 10 seconds) against the response of the patient until the clinical signs show the onset of anesthesia. As with other sedative-hypnotic agents, the amount of intravenous opioid and/or benzodiazepine premedication will influence the response of the patient to an induction dose of DIPRIVAN Injectable Emulsion.

Elderly, Debilitated, or ASA III/IV Patients:

It is important to be familiar and experienced with the intravenous use of DIPRIVAN Injectable Emulsion before treating elderly, debilitated or ASA III/IV patients. Due to the reduced clearance and higher blood concentrations, most of these patients require approximately 1 to 1.5 mg/kg (approximately 20 mg every 10 seconds) of DIPRIVAN Injectable Emulsion for induction of anesthesia according to their condition and responses. A rapid bolus should not be used as this will increase the likelihood of undesirable cardiorespiratory depression including hypotension, apnea, airway obstruction and/or oxygen desaturation. (See DOSAGE AND ADMINISTRATION.)

Neurosurgical Patients:

Slower induction is recommended using boluses of 20 mg every 10 seconds. Slower boluses or infusions of DIPRIVAN Injectable Emulsion for induction of anesthesia, titrated to clinical responses, will generally result in reduced induction dosage requirements (1 to 2 mg/kg). (See PRECAUTIONS and DOSAGE AND ADMINISTRATION.)

Cardiac Anesthesia:

DIPRIVAN Injectable Emulsion has been well-studied in patients with coronary artery disease, but experience in patients with hemodynamically significant valvular or congenital heart disease is limited. As with other anesthetic and sedative-hypnotic agents, DIPRIVAN Injectable Emulsion

Continued on next page

Diprivan—Cont.

in healthy patients causes a decrease in blood pressure that is secondary to decreases in preload (ventricular filling volume at the end of the diastole) and afterload (arterial resistance at the beginning of the systole). The magnitude of these changes is proportional to the blood and effect site concentrations achieved. These concentrations depend upon the dose and speed of the induction and maintenance infusion rates.

In addition, lower heart rates are observed during maintenance with DIPRIVAN Injectable Emulsion, possibly due to reduction of the sympathetic activity and/or resetting of the baroreceptor reflexes. Therefore, anticholinergic agents should be administered when increases in vagal tone are anticipated.

As with other anesthetic agents, DIPRIVAN Injectable Emulsion reduces myocardial oxygen consumption. Further studies are needed to confirm and delineate the extent of these effects on the myocardium and the coronary vascular system.

Morphine premedication (0.15 mg/kg) with nitrous oxide 67% in oxygen has been shown to decrease the necessary DIPRIVAN Injectable Emulsion maintenance infusion rates and therapeutic blood concentrations when compared to non narcotic (lorazepam) premedication. The rate of DIPRIVAN Injectable Emulsion administration should be determined based on the patient's premedication and adjusted according to clinical responses.

A rapid bolus induction should be avoided. A slow rate of approximately 20 mg every 10 seconds until induction onset (0.5 to 1.5 mg/kg) should be used. In order to assure adequate anesthesia, when DIPRIVAN Injectable Emulsion is used as the primary agent, maintenance infusion rates should not be less than 100 µg/kg/min and should be supplemented with analgesic levels of continuous opioid administration. When an opioid is used as the primary agent, DIPRIVAN Injectable Emulsion maintenance rates should not be less than 50 µg/kg/min and care should be taken to insure amnesia with concomitant benzodiazepines. Higher doses of DIPRIVAN Injectable Emulsion will reduce the opioid requirements (see Table 4). When DIPRIVAN Injectable Emulsion is used as the primary anesthetic, it should not be administered with the high-dose opioid technique as this may increase the likelihood of hypotension (see PRECAUTIONS - Cardiac Anesthesia).

[See table 4 above]

Maintenance of General Anesthesia

In adults, anesthesia can be maintained by administering DIPRIVAN Injectable Emulsion by infusion or intermittent IV bolus injection. The patient's clinical response will determine the infusion rate or the amount and frequency of incremental injections.

Continuous Infusion:

DIPRIVAN Injectable Emulsion 100 to 200 µg/kg/min administered in a variable rate infusion with 60%–70% nitrous oxide and oxygen provides anesthesia for patients undergoing general surgery. Maintenance by infusion of DIPRIVAN Injectable Emulsion should immediately follow the induction dose in order to provide satisfactory or continuous anesthesia during the induction phase. During this initial period following the induction dose higher rates of infusion are generally required (150 to 200 µg/kg/min) for the first 10 to 15 minutes. Infusion rates should subsequently be decreased 30%–50% during the first half-hour of maintenance.

Other drugs that cause CNS depression (hypnotics/sedatives, inhalational anesthetics and opioids) can increase the CNS depression induced by propofol.

Intermittent Bolus:

Increments of DIPRIVAN Injectable Emulsion 25 mg (2.5 mL) to 50mg (5mL) may be administered with nitrous oxide in adult patients undergoing general surgery. The incremental boluses should be administered when changes in vital signs indicate a response to surgical stimulation or light anesthesia.

DIPRIVAN Injectable Emulsion has been used with a variety of agents commonly used in anesthesia such as atropine, scopolamine, glycopyrrolate, diazepam, depolarizing and nondepolarizing muscle relaxants, and opioid analgesics, as well as with inhalational and regional anesthetic agents.

In the elderly, debilitated or ASA III/IV patients, rapid bolus doses should not be used as this will increase cardiorespiratory effects including hypotension, apnea, airway obstruction and/or oxygen desaturation.

Pediatric Anesthesia

Induction of General Anesthesia:

Most pediatric patients 3 years of age or older and classified ASA I or II require 2.5 to 3.5 mg/kg of DIPRIVAN Injectable Emulsion for induction when unpremedicated or when lightly premedicated with oral benzodiazepines or intramuscular opioids. Within this dosage range, younger children may require larger induction doses than older children. As with other sedative-hypnotic agents, the amount of intravenous opioid and/or benzodiazepine premedication will influence the response of the patient to an induction dose of DIPRIVAN Injectable Emulsion. In addition, a lower dosage is recommended for children classified ASA III or IV. Attention should be paid to minimize pain on injection when administering DIPRIVAN Injectable Emulsion to pediatric patients. Rapid boluses of DIPRIVAN Injectable Emulsion

TABLE 3. ICU SEDATION CLINICAL TRIALS AND LITERATURE

Patients receiving DIPRIVAN Injectable Emulsion Median and (Range)

ICU Patient Type	Number of Patients: Trials	Number of Patients: Literature	Sedation Dose: µg/kg/min	Sedation Dose: mg/kg/h	Sedation Duration: Hours
Post-CABG	41	—	11	.66	10
			(0.1–30)	(0.006–1.8)	(2–14)
	—	334	(5–100)	(0.3–6)	(4–24)
Post-Surgical	60	—	20	1.2	18
			(6–53)	(0.4–3.2)	(0.3–187)
	—	142	(23–82)	(1.4–4.9)	(6–96)
Neuro/Head Trauma	7	—	25	1.5	168
			(13–37)	(0.8–2.2)	(112–282)
	—	184	(8.3–87)	(0.5–5.2)	(8 hr–5 days)
Medical	49	—	41	2.5	72
			(9–131)	(0.5–7.9)	(0.4–337)
	—	76	(3.3–62)	(0.2–3.7)	(4–96)
Special Patients					
ARDS/Resp. Failure	—	56	(10–142)	(0.6–8.5)	(1 hr–8 days)
COPD/Asthma	—	49	(17–75)	(1.4–5)	(1–8 days)
Status Epilepticus	—	15	(25–167)	(1.5–10)	(1–21 days)
Tetanus	—	11	(5–100)	(0.3–6)	(1–25 days)

Trials (Individual patients from clinical studies)
Literature (Individual patients from published reports)
CABG (Coronary Artery Bypass Graft)
ARDS (Adult Respiratory Distress Syndrome)

Table 4. Cardiac Anesthesia Techniques

Primary Agent	Rate	Secondary Agent/Rate (Following Induction with Primary Agent)
DIPRIVAN Injectable Emulsion		OPIOID[a]/0.05–0.075 µg/kg/min (no bolus)
Preinduction anxiolysis	25 µg/kg/min	
Induction	0.5–1.5 mg/kg over 60 sec	
Maintenance (Titrated to Clinical Response)	100–150 µg/kg/min	
OPIOID[b]		DIPRIVAN Injectable Emulsion/50–100 µg/kg/min (no bolus)
Induction	25–50 µg/kg	
Maintenance	0.2–0.3 µg/kg/min	

[a] OPIOID is defined in terms of fentanyl equivalents, i.e.
1 µg of fentanyl =5 µg of alfentanil (for bolus)
=10 µg of alfentanil (for maintenance)
or
=0.1 µg of sufentanil

[b] Care should be taken to ensure amnesia with concomitant benzodiazepine therapy

may be administered if small veins are pretreated with lidocaine or when antecubital or larger veins are utilized (See PRECAUTIONS - General).

DIPRIVAN Injectable Emulsion administered in a variable rate infusion with nitrous oxide 60-70% provides satisfactory anesthesia for most pediatric patients 3 years of age or older, ASA I or II, undergoing general anesthesia.

Maintenance of General Anesthesia:

Maintenance by infusion of DIPRIVAN Injectable Emulsion at a rate of 200–300 µg/kg/min should immediately follow the induction dose. Following the first half hour of maintenance, if clinical signs of light anesthesia are not present, the infusion rate should be decreased; during this period, infusion rates of 125–150 µg/kg/min are typically needed. However, younger children (5 years of age or less) may require larger maintenance infusion rates than older children.

Monitored Anesthesia Care (MAC) Sedation in Adults

When DIPRIVAN Injectable Emulsion is administered for MAC sedation, rates of administration should be individualized and titrated to clinical response. In most patients the rates of DIPRIVAN Injectable Emulsion administration will be in the range of 25–75 µg/kg/min.

During initiation of MAC sedation, slow infusion or slow injection techniques are preferable over rapid bolus administration. During maintenance of MAC sedation, a variable rate infusion is preferable over intermittent bolus dose administration. In the elderly, debilitated, or ASA III/IV patients, rapid (single or repeated) bolus dose administration should not be used for MAC sedation. (See WARNINGS.) **A rapid bolus injection can result in undesirable cardiorespiratory depression including hypotension, apnea, airway obstruction, and/or oxygen desaturation.**

Initiation of MAC Sedation:

For initiation of MAC sedation, either an infusion or a slow injection method may be utilized while closely monitoring cardiorespiratory function. With the infusion method, sedation may be initiated by infusing DIPRIVAN Injectable Emulsion at 100 to 150 µg/kg/min (6 to 9 mg/kg/h) for a period of 3 to 5 minutes and titrating to the desired level of sedation while closely monitoring respiratory function. With the slow injection method for initiation, patients will require approximately 0.5 mg/kg administered over 3 to 5 minutes and titrated to clinical responses. When DIPRIVAN Injectable Emulsion is administered slowly over 3 to 5 minutes, most patients will be adequately sedated and the peak drug effect can be achieved while minimizing undesirable cardiorespiratory effects occurring at high plasma levels.

In the elderly, debilitated, or ASA III/IV patients, rapid (single or repeated) bolus dose administration should not be used for MAC sedation. (See WARNINGS.) The rate of administration should be over 3-5 minutes and the dosage of DIPRIVAN Injectable Emulsion should be reduced to approximately 80% of the usual adult dosage in these patients according to their condition, responses, and changes in vital signs. (See DOSAGE AND ADMINISTRATION.)

Maintenance of MAC Sedation:

For maintenance of sedation, a variable rate infusion method is preferable over an intermittent bolus dose method. With the variable rate infusion method, patients will generally require maintenance rates of 25 to 75 µg/kg/min (1.5 to 4.5 mg/kg/h) during the first 10 to 15 minutes of sedation maintenance. Infusion rates should subsequently be decreased over time to 25 to 50 µg/kg/min and adjusted to clinical responses. In titrating to clinical effect, allow approximately 2 minutes for onset of peak drug effect.

Infusion rates should always be titrated downward in the absence of clinical signs of light sedation until mild responses to stimulation are obtained in order to avoid sedative administration of DIPRIVAN Injectable Emulsion at rates higher than are clinically necessary.

If the intermittent bolus dose method is used, increments of DIPRIVAN Injectable Emulsion 10 mg (1 mL) or 20 mg (2 mL) can be administered and titrated to desired level of sedation. With the intermittent bolus method of sedation maintenance there is the potential for respiratory depression, transient increases in sedation depth, and/or prolongation of recovery.

In the elderly, debilitated, or ASA III/IV patients, rapid (single or repeated) bolus dose administration should not be used for MAC sedation. (See WARNINGS.) The rate of administration and the dosage of DIPRIVAN Injectable Emulsion should be reduced to approximately 80% of the usual adult dosage in these patients according to their condition, responses, and changes in vital signs. (See DOSAGE AND ADMINISTRATION.)

DIPRIVAN Injectable Emulsion can be administered as the sole agent for maintenance of MAC sedation during surgical/diagnostic procedures. When DIPRIVAN Injectable Emulsion sedation is supplemented with opioid and/or benzodiazepine medications, these agents increase the sedative and respiratory effects of DIPRIVAN Injectable Emulsion and may also result in a slower recovery profile. (See PRECAUTIONS, Drug Interactions.)

ICU Sedation:

(**See WARNINGS and DOSAGE AND ADMINISTRATION, Handling Procedures.**) For intubated, mechanically ventilated adult patients, Intensive Care Unit (ICU) sedation should be initiated slowly with a continuous infusion in order to titrate to desired clinical effect and minimize hypotension. (See DOSAGE AND ADMINISTRATION.)

Across all 6 US/Canadian clinical studies, the mean infusion maintenance rate for all DIPRIVAN Injectable Emulsion patients was 27± 21 µg/kg/min. The maintenance infusion rates required to maintain adequate sedation ranged from 2.8 µg/kg/min to 130 µg/kg/min. The infusion rate was lower in patients over 55 years of age (approximately 20 µg/

kg/min) compared to patients under 55 years of age (approximately 38 µg/kg/min). In these studies, morphine or fentanyl was used as needed for analgesia.

Most adult ICU patients recovering from the effects of general anesthesia or deep sedation will require maintenance rates of 5 to 50 µg/kg/min (0.3 to 3 mg/kg/h) individualized and titrated to clinical response. (See DOSAGE AND ADMINISTRATION.) With medical ICU patients or patients who have recovered from the effects of general anesthesia or deep sedation, the rate of administration of 50 µg/kg/min or higher may be required to achieve adequate sedation. These higher rates of administration may increase the likelihood of patients developing hypotension.

Although there are reports of reduced analgesic requirements, most patients received opioids for analgesia during maintenance of ICU sedation. Some patients also received benzodiazepines and/or neuromuscular blocking agents. During long term maintenance of sedation, some ICU patients were awakened once or twice every 24 hours for assessment of neurologic or respiratory function. (See Clinical Trials, Table 3.)

In post-CABG (coronary artery bypass graft) patients, the maintenance rate of propofol administration was usually low (median 11 µg/kg/min) due to the intraoperative administration of high opioid doses. Patients receiving DIPRIVAN Injectable Emulsion required 35% less nitroprusside than midazolam patients; this difference was statistically significant ($P<0.05$). During initiation of sedation in Post-CABG patients, a 15% to 20% decrease in blood pressure was seen in the first 60 minutes. It was not possible to determine cardiovascular effects in patients with severely compromised ventricular function (See Clinical Trials, Table 3).

In Medical or Postsurgical ICU studies comparing DIPRIVAN Injectable Emulsion to benzodiazepine infusion or bolus, there were no apparent differences in maintenance of adequate sedation, mean arterial pressure, or laboratory findings. Like the comparators, DIPRIVAN Injectable Emulsion reduced blood cortisol during sedation while maintaining responsivity to challenges with adrenocorticotropic hormone (ACTH). Case reports from the published literature generally reflect that DIPRIVAN Injectable Emulsion has been used safely in patients with a history of porphyria or malignant hyperthermia.

In hemodynamically stable head trauma patients ranging in age from 19–43 years, adequate sedation was maintained with DIPRIVAN Injectable Emulsion or morphine (N=7 in each group). There were no apparent differences in adequacy of sedation, intracranial pressure, cerebral perfusion pressure, or neurologic recovery between the treatment groups. In literature reports from Neurosurgical ICU and severely head-injured patients DIPRIVAN Injectable Emulsion infusion with or without diuretics and hyperventilation controlled intracranial pressure while maintaining cerebral perfusion pressure. In some patients bolus doses resulted in decreased blood pressure and compromised cerebral perfusion pressure. (See Clinical Trials, Table 3.)

DIPRIVAN Injectable Emulsion was found to be effective in status epilepticus which was refractory to the standard anticonvulsant therapies. For these patients as well as for ARDS/respiratory failure and tetanus patients sedation maintenance dosages were generally higher than those for other critically ill patient populations. (See Clinical Trials, Table 3.)

Abrupt discontinuation of DIPRIVAN Injectable Emulsion prior to weaning or for daily evaluation of sedation levels should be avoided. This may result in rapid awakening with associated anxiety, agitation and resistance to mechanical ventilation. Infusions of DIPRIVAN Injectable Emulsion should be adjusted to maintain a light level of sedation through the weaning process or evaluation of sedation level. (See PRECAUTIONS.)

INDICATIONS AND USAGE

DIPRIVAN Injectable Emulsion is an IV sedative-hypnotic agent that can be used for both induction and/or maintenance of anesthesia as part of a balanced anesthetic technique for inpatient and outpatient surgery in adults and in children 3 years of age or older.

DIPRIVAN Injectable Emulsion, when administered intravenously as directed, can be used to initiate and maintain monitored anesthesia care (MAC) sedation during diagnostic procedures in adults. DIPRIVAN Injectable Emulsion may also be used for MAC sedation in conjunction with local/regional anesthesia in patients undergoing surgical procedures. (See PRECAUTIONS.)

DIPRIVAN Injectable Emulsion should only be administered to intubated, mechanically ventilated adult patients in the Intensive Care Unit (ICU) to provide continuous sedation and control of stress responses. In this setting, DIPRIVAN Injectable Emulsion should be administered only by persons skilled in the medical management of critically ill patients and trained in cardiovascular resuscitation and airway management.

DIPRIVAN Injectable Emulsion is not recommended for obstetrics, including cesarean section deliveries. DIPRIVAN Injectable Emulsion crosses the placenta, and as with other general anesthetic agents, the administration of DIPRIVAN Injectable Emulsion may be associated with neonatal depression. (See PRECAUTIONS.)

DIPRIVAN Injectable Emulsion is not recommended for use in nursing mothers because DIPRIVAN Injectable Emulsion has been reported to be excreted in human milk and the effects of oral absorption of small amounts of propofol are not known. (See PRECAUTIONS.)

DIPRIVAN Injectable Emulsion is not recommended for anesthesia in children below the age of 3 years because safety and effectiveness have not been established. DIPRIVAN Injectable Emulsion is not recommended for MAC sedation in children because safety and effectiveness have not been established. DIPRIVAN Injectable Emulsion is not recommended for pediatric ICU sedation because safety and effectiveness have not been established.

CONTRAINDICATIONS

DIPRIVAN Injectable Emulsion is contraindicated in patients with a known hypersensitivity to DIPRIVAN Injectable Emulsion or its components, or when general anesthesia or sedation are contraindicated.

WARNINGS

For general anesthesia or monitored anesthesia care (MAC) sedation, DIPRIVAN Injectable Emulsion should be administered only by persons trained in the administration of general anesthesia and not involved in the conduct of the surgical/diagnostic procedure. Patients should be continuously monitored, and facilities for maintenance of a patent airway, artificial ventilation, and oxygen enrichment and circulatory resuscitation must be immediately available.

For sedation of intubated, mechanically ventilated adult patients in the Intensive Care Unit (ICU), DIPRIVAN Injectable Emulsion should be administered only by persons skilled in the management of critically ill patients and trained in cardiovascular resuscitation and airway management.

In the elderly, debilitated or ASA III/IV patients, rapid (single or repeated) bolus administration should not be used during general anesthesia or MAC sedation in order to minimize undesirable cardiorespiratory depression including hypotension, apnea, airway obstruction and/or oxygen desaturation.

MAC sedation patients should be continuously monitored by persons not involved in the conduct of the surgical or diagnostic procedure; oxygen supplementation should be immediately available and provided where clinically indicated; and oxygen saturation should be monitored in all patients. Patients should be continuously monitored for early signs of hypotension, apnea, airway obstruction and/or oxygen desaturation. These cardiorespiratory effects are more likely to occur following rapid initiation (loading) boluses or during supplemental maintenance boluses, especially in the elderly, debilitated, or ASA III/IV patients.

DIPRIVAN Injectable Emulsion should not be coadministered through the same IV catheter with blood or plasma because compatibility has not been established. *In vitro* tests have shown that aggregates of the globular component of the emulsion vehicle have occurred with blood/plasma/serum from humans and animals. The clinical significance is not known.

STRICT ASEPTIC TECHNIQUE MUST ALWAYS BE MAINTAINED DURING HANDLING. DIPRIVAN INJECTABLE EMULSION IS A SINGLE-USE PARENTERAL PRODUCT WHICH CONTAINS 0.005% DISODIUM EDETATE TO RETARD THE RATE OF GROWTH OF MICROORGANISMS IN THE EVENT OF ACCIDENTAL EXTRINSIC CONTAMINATION. HOWEVER, DIPRIVAN INJECTABLE EMULSION CAN STILL SUPPORT THE GROWTH OF MICROORGANISMS AS IT IS NOT AN ANTIMICROBIALLY PRESERVED PRODUCT UNDER USP STANDARDS. ACCORDINGLY, STRICT ASEPTIC TECHNIQUE MUST STILL BE ADHERED TO. DO NOT USE IF CONTAMINATION IS SUSPECTED. DISCARD UNUSED PORTIONS AS DIRECTED WITHIN THE REQUIRED TIME LIMITS (SEE DOSAGE AND ADMINISTRATION, HANDLING PROCEDURES). THERE HAVE BEEN REPORTS IN WHICH FAILURE TO USE ASEPTIC TECHNIQUE WHEN HANDLING DIPRIVAN INJECTABLE EMULSION WAS ASSOCIATED WITH MICROBIAL CONTAMINATION OF THE PRODUCT AND WITH FEVER, INFECTION/SEPSIS, OTHER LIFE-THREATENING ILLNESS, AND/OR DEATH.

PRECAUTIONS

General:

A lower induction dose and a slower maintenance rate of administration should be used in elderly, debilitated, or ASA III/IV patients. (See CLINICAL PHARMACOLOGY - Individualization of Dosage.) Patients should be continuously monitored for early signs of significant hypotension and/or bradycardia. Treatment may include increasing the rate of intravenous fluid, elevation of lower extremities, use of pressor agents, or administration of atropine. Apnea often occurs during induction and may persist for more than 60 seconds. Ventilatory support may be required. Because DIPRIVAN Injectable Emulsion is an emulsion, caution should be exercised in patients with disorders of lipid metabolism such as primary hyperlipoproteinemia, diabetic hyperlipemia, and pancreatitis.

Very rarely the use of DIPRIVAN Injectable Emulsion may be associated with the development of a period of postoperative unconsciousness which may be accompanied by an increase in muscle tone. This may or may not be preceded by a brief period of wakefulness. Recovery is spontaneous. The clinical criteria for discharge from the recovery/day surgery area established for each institution should be satisfied before discharge of the patient from the care of the anesthesiologist.

When DIPRIVAN Injectable Emulsion is administered to an epileptic patient, there may be a risk of seizure during the recovery phase.

In adults and children, attention should be paid to minimize pain on administration of DIPRIVAN Injectable Emulsion. Transient local pain can be minimized if the larger veins of the forearm or antecubital fossa are used. Pain during intravenous injection may also be reduced by prior injection of IV lidocaine (1 mL of a 1% solution). Pain on injection occurred frequently in pediatric patients (45%) when a small vein of the hand was utilized without lidocaine pretreatment. With lidocaine pretreatment or when antecubital veins were utilized, pain was minimal (incidence less than 10%) and well tolerated.

Venous sequelae (phlebitis or thrombosis) have been reported rarely (<1%). In two well-controlled clinical studies using dedicated intravenous catheters, no instances of venous sequelae were observed up to 14 days following induction.

Intra-arterial injection in animals did not induce local tissue effects. Accidental intra-arterial injection has been reported in patients, and, other than pain, there were no major sequelae.

Intentional injection into subcutaneous or perivascular tissues of animals caused minimal tissue reaction. During the post-marketing period there have been rare reports of local pain, swelling, blisters, and/or tissue necrosis following accidental extravasation of DIPRIVAN Injectable Emulsion.

Perioperative myoclonia, rarely including convulsions and opisthotonos, has occurred in temporal relationship in cases in which DIPRIVAN Injectable Emulsion has been administered.

Clinical features of anaphylaxis, which may include angioedema, bronchospasm, erythema and hypotension, occur rarely following DIPRIVAN Injectable Emulsion administration, although use of other drugs in most instances makes the relationship to DIPRIVAN Injectable Emulsion unclear.

There have been rare reports of pulmonary edema in temporal relationship to the administration of DIPRIVAN Injectable Emulsion, although a causal relationship is unknown.

Very rarely, cases of unexplained postoperative pancreatitis (requiring hospital admission) have been reported after anesthesia in which DIPRIVAN Injectable Emulsion was one of the induction agents used. Due to a variety of confounding factors in these cases, including concomitant medications, a causal relationship to DIPRIVAN Injectable Emulsion is unclear.

DIPRIVAN Injectable Emulsion has no vagolytic activity. Reports of bradycardia, asystole, and rarely, cardiac arrest have been associated with DIPRIVAN Injectable Emulsion. The intravenous administration of anticholinergic agents (e.g., atropine or glycopyrrolate) should be considered to modify potential increases in vagal tone due to concomitant agents (e.g., succinylcholine) or surgical stimuli.

Intensive Care Unit Sedation:

(See WARNINGS and DOSAGE AND ADMINISTRATION, Handling Procedures.) The administration of DIPRIVAN Injectable Emulsion should be initiated as a continuous infusion and changes in the rate of administration made slowly (>5 min) in order to minimize hypotension and avoid acute overdosage. (See CLINICAL PHARMACOLOGY- Individualization of Dosage.)

Patients should be monitored for early signs of significant hypotension and/or cardiovascular depression, which may be profound. These effects are responsive to discontinuation of DIPRIVAN Injectable Emulsion, IV fluid administration, and/or vasopressor therapy.

As with other sedative medications, there is wide interpatient variability in DIPRIVAN Injectable Emulsion dosage requirements, and these requirements may change with time.

Failure to reduce the infusion rate in patients receiving DIPRIVAN Injectable Emulsion for extended periods may result in excessively high blood concentrations of the drug. Thus, titration to clinical response and daily evaluation of sedation levels are important during use of DIPRIVAN Injectable Emulsion infusion for ICU sedation, especially of long duration.

Opioids and paralytic agents should be discontinued and respiratory function optimized prior to weaning patients from mechanical ventilation. Infusions of DIPRIVAN Injectable Emulsion should be adjusted to maintain a light level of sedation prior to weaning patients from mechanical ventilatory support. Throughout the weaning process this level of sedation may be maintained in the absence of respiratory depression. Because of the rapid clearance of DIPRIVAN Injectable Emulsion, abrupt discontinuation of a patient's infusion may result in rapid awakening of the patient with associated anxiety, agitation, and resistance to mechanical ventilation, making weaning from mechanical ventilation difficult. It is therefore recommended that administration of DIPRIVAN Injectable Emulsion be continued in order to maintain a light level of sedation throughout the weaning process until 10-15 minutes prior to extubation at which time the infusion can be discontinued.

There have been very rare reports of rhabdomyolysis associated with the administration of DIPRIVAN Injectable Emulsion for ICU sedation.

Since DIPRIVAN Injectable Emulsion is formulated in an oil-in-water emulsion, elevations in serum triglycerides may occur when DIPRIVAN Injectable Emulsion is administered for extended periods of time. Patients at risk of hyperlipidemia should be monitored for increases in serum triglycerides or serum turbidity. Administration of DIPRIVAN In-

Continued on next page

Diprivan—Cont.

jectable Emulsion should be adjusted if fat is being inadequately cleared from the body. A reduction in the quantity of concurrently administered lipids is indicated to compensate for the amount of lipid infused as part of the DIPRIVAN Injectable Emulsion formulation; 1 mL of DIPRIVAN Injectable Emulsion contains approximately 0.1 g of fat (1.1 kcal). In patients who are predisposed to zinc deficiency, such as those with burns, diarrhea, and/or major sepsis, the need for supplemental zinc should be considered during prolonged therapy with DIPRIVAN Injectable Emulsion.

EDTA is a strong chelator of trace metals—including zinc. Calcium disodium edetate has been used in gram quantities to treat heavy metal toxicity. When used in this manner it is possible that as much as 10 mg of elemental zinc can be lost per day via this mechanism. Although with DIPRIVAN Injectable Emulsion there are no reports of decreased zinc levels or zinc deficiency-related adverse events, DIPRIVAN Injectable Emulsion should not be infused for longer than 5 days without providing a drug holiday to safely replace estimated or measured urine zinc losses.

At high doses (2–3 grams per day), EDTA has been reported, on rare occasions, to be toxic to the renal tubules. Studies to-date, in patients with normal or impaired renal function have not shown any alteration in renal function with DIPRIVAN Injectable Emulsion containing 0.005% disodium edetate. In patients at risk for renal impairment, urinalysis and urine sediment should be checked before initiation of sedation and then be monitored on alternate days during sedation.

The long-term administration of DIPRIVAN Injectable Emulsion to patients with renal failure and/or hepatic insufficiency has not been evaluated.

Neurosurgical Anesthesia:

When DIPRIVAN Injectable Emulsion is used in patients with increased intracranial pressure or impaired cerebral circulation, significant decreases in mean arterial pressure should be avoided because of the resultant decreases in cerebral perfusion pressure. To avoid significant hypotension and decreases in cerebral perfusion pressure, an infusion or slow bolus of approximately 20 mg every 10 seconds should be utilized instead of rapid, more frequent, and/or larger boluses of DIPRIVAN Injectable Emulsion. Slower induction titrated to clinical responses, will generally result in reduced induction dosage requirements (1 to 2 mg/kg). When increased ICP is suspected, hyperventilation and hypocarbia should accompany the administration of DIPRIVAN Injectable Emulsion. (See DOSAGE AND ADMINISTRATION.)

Cardiac Anesthesia:

Slower rates of administration should be utilized in premedicated patients, geriatric patients, patients with recent fluid shifts, or patients who are hemodynamically unstable. Any fluid deficits should be corrected prior to administration of DIPRIVAN Injectable Emulsion. In those patients where additional fluid therapy may be contraindicated, other measures, e.g., elevation of lower extremities, or use of pressor agents, may be useful to offset the hypotension which is associated with the induction of anesthesia with DIPRIVAN Injectable Emulsion.

Information for Patients:

Patients should be advised that performance of activities requiring mental alertness, such as operating a motor vehicle, or hazardous machinery or signing legal documents may be impaired for some time after general anesthesia or sedation.

Drug Interactions:

The induction dose requirements of DIPRIVAN Injectable Emulsion may be reduced in patients with intramuscular or intravenous premedication, particularly with narcotics (e.g., morphine, meperidine, and fentanyl, etc.) and combinations of opioids and sedatives (e.g., benzodiazepines, barbiturates, chloral hydrate, droperidol, etc.). These agents may increase the anesthetic or sedative effects of DIPRIVAN Injectable Emulsion and may also result in more pronounced decreases in systolic, diastolic, and mean arterial pressures and cardiac output.

During maintenance of anesthesia or sedation, the rate of DIPRIVAN Injectable Emulsion administration should be adjusted according to the desired level of anesthesia or sedation and may be reduced in the presence of supplemental analgesic agents (e.g., nitrous oxide or opioids). The concurrent administration of potent inhalational agents (e.g., isoflurane, enflurane, and halothane) during maintenance with DIPRIVAN Injectable Emulsion has not been extensively evaluated. These inhalational agents can also be expected to increase the anesthetic or sedative and cardiorespiratory effects of DIPRIVAN Injectable Emulsion.

DIPRIVAN Injectable Emulsion does not cause a clinically significant change in onset, intensity or duration of action of the commonly used neuromuscular blocking agents (e.g., succinylcholine and nondepolarizing muscle relaxants).

No significant adverse interactions with commonly used premedications or drugs used during anesthesia or sedation (including a range of muscle relaxants, inhalational agents, analgesic agents, and local anesthetic agents) have been observed.

Carcinogenesis, Mutagenesis, Impairment of Fertility:

Animal carcinogenicity studies have not been performed with propofol.

In vitro and *in vivo* animal tests failed to show any potential for mutagenicity by propofol. Tests for mutagenicity included the Ames (using *Salmonella* sp) mutation test, gene

Incidence greater than 1%—Probably Causally Related

	Anesthesia/MAC Sedation	ICU Sedation
Cardiovascular:	Bradycardia Hypotension* [Peds: 17%] [Hypertension Peds: 8%] (see also CLINICAL PHARMACOLOGY)	Bradycardia, Decreased Cardiac Output, Hypotension 26%
Central Nervous System:	Movement* [Peds: 17%]	
Injection Site:	Burning/Stinging or Pain, 17.6% [Peds: 10%]	
Metabolic/Nutritional:		Hyperlipemia*
Respiratory:	Apnea (see also CLINICAL PHARMACOLOGY)	Respiratory Acidosis
Skin and Appendages:	Rash [Peds: 5%]	

Events without an * or % had an incidence of 1%–3%
* Incidence of events 3% to 10%

Incidence less than 1%—Probably Causally Related

	Anesthesia/MAC Sedation	ICU Sedation
Body as a Whole:	Anaphylaxis/Anaphylactoid Reaction, Perinatal Disorder	
Cardiovascular:	Premature Atrial Contractions, Syncope	
Central Nervous System:	Hypertonia/Dystonia, Paresthesia	Agitation
Digestive:	Hypersalivation	
Musculoskeletal:	Myalgia	
Respiratory:	Wheezing	Decreased Lung Function
Skin and Appendages:	Flushing, Pruritus	
Special Senses:	Amblyopia	
Urogenital:	Cloudy Urine	Green Urine

Incidence less than 1%—Causal Relationship Unknown

	Anesthesia/MAC Sedation	ICU Sedation
Body as a Whole:	Asthenia, Awareness, Chest Pain Extremities Pain, Fever, Increased Drug Effect, Neck Rigidity/Stiffness, Trunk Pain	Fever, Sepsis, Trunk Pain, Whole Body Weakness
Cardiovascular:	Arrhythmia, Atrial Fibrillation, Atrioventricular Heart Block, Bigeminy, Bleeding, Bundle Branch Block, Cardiac Arrest, ECG Abnormal, Edema, Extrasystole, Heart Block, Hypertension, Myocardial Infarction, Myocardial Ischemia, Premature Ventricular Contractions, ST Segment Depression, Supraventricular Tachycardia, Tachycardia, Ventricular Fibrillation	Arrhythmia, Atrial Fibrillation, Bigeminy, Cardiac Arrest Extrasystole, Right Heart Failure, Ventricular Tachycardia
Central Nervous System:	Abnormal Dreams, Agitation, Amorous Behavior, Anxiety, Bucking/Jerking/Thrashing, Chills/Shivering, Clonic Myoclonic Movement, Combativeness, Confusion, Delirium, Depression, Dizziness, Emotional Lability, Euphoria, Fatigue, Hallucinations, Headache, Hypotonia, Hysteria, Insomnia, Moaning, Neuropathy, Opisthotonos, Rigidity, Seizures, Somnolence, Tremor, Twitching	Chills/Shivering, Intracranial Hypertension, Seizures, Somnolence, Thinking Abnormal
Digestive:	Cramping, Diarrhea, Dry Mouth, Enlarged Parotid, Nausea, Swallowing, Vomiting	Ileus, Liver Function Abnormal
Hematologic/Lymphatic:	Coagulation Disorder, Leukocytosis	
Injection Site:	Hives/Itching, Phlebitis, Redness/Discoloration	
Metabolic/Nutritional:	Hyperkalemia, Hyperlipemia	BUN Increased, Creatinine Increased, Dehydration, Hyperglycemia, Metabolic Acidosis, Osmolality Increased
Respiratory:	Bronchospasm, Burning in Throat, Cough, Dyspnea, Hiccough, Hyperventilation, Hypoventilation, Hypoxia, Laryngospasm, Pharyngitis, Sneezing, Tachypnea, Upper Airway Obstruction	Hypoxia
Skin and Appendages:	Conjunctival Hyperemia, Diaphoresis, Urticaria	Rash
Special Senses:	Diplopia, Ear Pain, Eye Pain, Nystagmus, Taste Perversion, Tinnitus	
Urogenital:	Oliguria, Urine Retention	Kidney Failure

mutation/gene conversion using Saccharomyces cerevisiae, invitro cytogenetic studies in Chinese hamsters and a mouse micronucleus test.

Studies in female rats at intravenous doses up to 15 mg/kg/day (6 times the maximum recommended human induction dose) for 2 weeks before pregnancy to day 7 of gestation did not show impaired fertility. Male fertility in rats was not affected in a dominant lethal study at intravenous doses up to 15 mg/kg/day for 5 days.

Pregnancy Category B:

Reproduction studies have been performed in rats and rabbits at intravenous doses of 15 mg/kg/day (6 times the recommended human induction dose) and have revealed no evidence of impaired fertility or harm to the fetus due to propofol. Propofol, however, has been shown to cause maternal deaths in rats and rabbits and decreased pup survival during the lactating period in dams treated with 15 mg/kg/day (or 6 times the recommended human induction dose). The pharmacological activity (anesthesia) of the drug on the mother is probably responsible for the adverse effects seen in the offspring. There are, however, no adequate and well-controlled studies in pregnant women. Because animal reproduction studies are not always predictive of human responses, this drug should be used during pregnancy only if clearly needed.

Labor and Delivery:

DIPRIVAN Injectable Emulsion is not recommended for obstetrics, including cesarean section deliveries. DIPRIVAN Injectable Emulsion crosses the placenta, and as with other general anesthetic agents, the administration of DIPRIVAN Injectable Emulsion may be associated with neonatal depression.

Nursing Mothers:

DIPRIVAN Injectable Emulsion is not recommended for use in nursing mothers because DIPRIVAN Injectable Emulsion has been reported to be excreted in human milk and the effects of oral absorption of small amounts of propofol are not known.

Pediatrics:

DIPRIVAN Injectable Emulsion is not recommended for use in pediatric patients for ICU or MAC sedation. In addition, DIPRIVAN Injectable Emulsion is not recommended for general anesthesia for children below the age of 3 years because safety and effectiveness have not been established. Although no causal relationship has been established, serious adverse events (including fatalities) have been reported in children given DIPRIVAN Injectable Emulsion for ICU sedation. These events were seen most often in children with respiratory tract infections given doses in excess of those recommended for adults.

Geriatric use
The effect of age on induction dose requirements for propofol was assessed in an open study involving 211 unpremedicated patients with approximately 30 patients in each decade between the ages of 16 and 80. The average dose to induce anesthesia was calculated for patients up to 54 years of age and for patients 55 years of age or older. The average dose to induce anesthesia in patients up to 54 years of age was 1.99 mg/kg and in patients above 54 it was 1.66 mg/kg. Subsequent clinical studies have demonstrated lower dosing requirements for subjects greater than 60 years of age.

ADVERSE REACTIONS

General
Adverse event information is derived from controlled clinical trials and worldwide marketing experience. In the description below, rates of the more common events represent US/Canadian clinical study results. Less frequent events are also derived from publications and marketing experience in over 8 million patients; there are insufficient data to support an accurate estimate of their incidence rates. These studies were conducted using a variety of premedicants, varying lengths of surgical/diagnostic procedures and various other anesthetic/sedative agents. Most adverse events were mild and transient.

Anesthesia and MAC Sedation in Adults
The following estimates of adverse events for DIPRIVAN Injectable Emulsion include data from clinical trials in general anesthesia/MAC sedation (N=2889 adult patients). The adverse events listed below as probably causally related are those events in which the actual incidence rate in patients treated with DIPRIVAN Injectable Emulsion was greater than the comparator incidence rate in these trials. Therefore, incidence rates for anesthesia and MAC sedation in adults generally represent estimates of the percentage of clinical trial patients which appeared to have probable causal relationship.
The adverse experience profile from reports of 150 patients in the MAC sedation clinical trials is similar to the profile established with DIPRIVAN Injectable Emulsion during anesthesia (see below). During MAC sedation clinical trials, significant respiratory events included cough, upper airway obstruction, apnea, hypoventilation, and dyspnea.

Anesthesia in Children
Generally the adverse experience profile from reports of 349 DIPRIVAN Injectable Emulsion pediatric patients between the ages of 3 and 12 years in the US/Canadian anesthesia clinical trials is similar to the profile established with DIPRIVAN Injectable Emulsion during anesthesia in adults (see Pediatric percentages [Peds %] below). Although not reported as an adverse event in clinical trials, apnea is frequently observed in pediatric patients.

ICU Sedation in Adults
The following estimates of adverse events include data from clinical trials in ICU sedation (N=159) patients. Probably related incidence rates for ICU sedation were determined by individual case report form review. Probable causality was based upon an apparent dose response relationship and/or positive responses to rechallenge. In many instances the presence of concomitant disease and concomitant therapy made the causal relationship unknown. Therefore, incidence rates for ICU sedation generally represent estimates of the percentage of clinical trial patients which appeared to have a probable causal relationship.
[See table at top of previous page]

DRUG ABUSE AND DEPENDENCE

Rare cases of self administration of DIPRIVAN Injectable Emulsion by health care professionals have been reported, including some fatalities. DIPRIVAN Injectable Emulsion should be managed to prevent the risk of diversion, including restriction of access and accounting procedures as appropriate to the clinical setting.

OVERDOSAGE

If overdosage occurs, DIPRIVAN Injectable Emulsion administration should be discontinued immediately. Overdosage is likely to cause cardiorespiratory depression. Respiratory depression should be treated by artificial ventilation with oxygen. Cardiovascular depression may require repositioning of the patient by raising the patient's legs, increasing the flow rate of intravenous fluids and administering pressor agents and/or anticholinergic agents.

DOSAGE AND ADMINISTRATION

Dosage and rate of administration should be individualized and titrated to the desired effect, according to clinically relevant factors, including preinduction and concomitant medications, age, ASA physical classification, and level of debilitation of the patient.
The following is abbreviated dosage and administration information which is only intended as a general guide in the use of DIPRIVAN Injectable Emulsion. Prior to administering DIPRIVAN Injectable Emulsion, it is imperative that the physician review and be completely familiar with the specific dosage and administration information detailed in the CLINICAL PHARMACOLOGY - Individualization of Dosage section. In the elderly, debilitated , or ASA III/IV patients, rapid bolus doses should not be the method of administration. (See WARNINGS.)

Intensive Care Unit Sedation:
STRICT ASEPTIC TECHNIQUE MUST ALWAYS BE MAINTAINED DURING HANDLING. DIPRIVAN INJECTABLE EMULSION IS A SINGLE-USE PARENTERAL PRODUCT WHICH CONTAINS 0.005% DISODIUM EDETATE TO RETARD THE RATE OF GROWTH OF MICROORGANISMS IN THE EVENT OF ACCIDENTAL EXTRINSIC CONTAMINATION. HOWEVER, DIPRIVAN INJECTABLE EMULSION CAN STILL SUPPORT THE GROWTH OF MICROORGANISMS AS IT IS NOT AN ANTIMICROBIALLY PRESERVED PRODUCT UNDER USP STANDARDS. ACCORDINGLY, STRICT ASEPTIC TECHNIQUE MUST STILL BE ADHERED TO. DO NOT USE IF CONTAMINATION IS SUSPECTED. (See DOSAGE AND ADMINISTRATION, Handling Procedures.)
DIPRIVAN Injectable Emulsion should be individualized according to the patient's condition and response, blood lipid profile, and vital signs. (See PRECAUTIONS- ICU sedation.) For intubated, mechanically ventilated adult patients, Intensive Care Unit (ICU) sedation should be initiated slowly with a continuous infusion in order to titrate to desired clinical effect and minimize hypotension. When indicated, initiation of sedation should begin at 5 µg/kg/min (0.3 mg/kg/h). The infusion rate should be increased by increments of 5 to 10 µg/kg/min (0.3 to 0.6 mg/kg/h) until the desired level of sedation is achieved. A minimum period of 5 minutes between adjustments should be allowed for onset of peak drug effect. Most adult patients require maintenance rates of 5 to 50 µg/kg/min (0.3 to 3 mg/kg/h) or higher. Dosages of DIPRIVAN Injectable Emulsion should be reduced in patients who have received large dosages of narcotics. Conversely, the DIPRIVAN Injectable Emulsion dosage requirement may be reduced by adequate management of pain with analgesic agents. As with other sedative medications, there is interpatient variability in dosage requirements, and these requirements may change with time. (see dosage guide.) EVALUATION OF LEVEL OF SEDATION AND ASSESSMENT OF CNS FUNCTION SHOULD BE CARRIED OUT DAILY THROUGHOUT MAINTENANCE TO DETERMINE THE MINIMUM DOSE OF DIPRIVAN INJECTABLE EMULSION REQUIRED FOR SEDATION (SEE **CLINICAL TRIALS**, **ICU SEDATION**). Bolus administration of 10 or 20 mg should only be used to rapidly increase depth of sedation in patients where hypotension is not likely to occur. Patients with compromised myocardial function, intravascular volume depletion, or abnormally low vascular tone (e.g., sepsis) may be more susceptible to hypotension. (See PRECAUTIONS.)
EDTA is a strong chelator of trace metals — including zinc. Calcium disodium edetate has been used in gram quantities to treat heavy metal toxicity. When used in this manner it is possible that as much as 10 mg of elemental zinc can be lost per day via this mechanism. Although with DIPRIVAN Injectable Emulsion there are no reports of decreased zinc levels or zinc deficiency-related adverse events, DIPRIVAN Injectable Emulsion should not be infused for longer than 5 days without providing a drug holiday to safely replace estimated or measured urine zinc losses.
At high doses (2–3 grams per day), EDTA has been reported, on rare occasions, to be toxic to the renal tubules. Studies to-date, in patients with normal or impaired renal function have not shown any alteration in renal function with DIPRIVAN Injectable Emulsion containing 0.005% disodium edetate. In patients at risk for renal impairment, urinalysis and urine sediment should be checked before initiation of sedation and then be monitored on alternate days during sedation.
SUMMARY OF DOSAGE GUIDELINES - Dosages and rates of administration in the following table should be individualized and titrated to clinical response. Safety and dosage requirements in pediatric patients have only been established for induction and maintenance of anesthesia. For complete dosage information, see CLINICAL PHARMACOLOGY - Individualization of Dosage.
[See table above]
Compatibility and Stability: DIPRIVAN Injectable Emulsion should not be mixed with other therapeutic agents prior to administration.

INDICATION	DOSAGE AND ADMINISTRATION
Induction of General Anesthesia	**Healthy Adults Less Than 55 Years of Age:** 40 mg every 10 seconds until induction onset (2 to 2.5 mg/kg). **Elderly, Debilitated, or ASA III/IV Patients:** 20 mg every 10 seconds until induction onset (1 to 1.5 mg/kg). **Cardiac Anesthesia:** 20 mg every 10 seconds until induction onset (0.5 to 1.5 mg/kg). **Neurosurgical Patients:** 20 mg every 10 seconds until induction onset (1 to 2 mg/kg). **Pediatric —healthy, 3 years of age or older:** 2.5 to 3.5 mg/kg administered over 20–30 seconds.
Maintenance of General Anesthesia:	**Infusion** **Healthy Adults Less Than 55 Years of Age:** 100 to 200 µg/kg/min (6 to 12 mg/kg/h). **Elderly, Debilitated, ASA III/IV Patients:** 50 to 100 µg/kg/min (3 to 6 mg/kg/h). **Cardiac Anesthesia:** Most patients require: Primary DIPRIVAN Injectable Emulsion with Secondary Opioid—100–150 µg/kg/min Low Dose DIPRIVAN Injectable Emulsion with Primary Opioid—50–100 µg/kg/min (See CLINICAL PHARMACOLOGY—Table 4) **Neurosurgical Patients:** 100 to 200 µg/kg/min (6 to 12 mg/kg/h). **Pediatric—healthy, 3 years of age or older:** 125 to 300 µg/kg/min (7.5 to 18 mg/kg/h)
Maintenance of General Anesthesia:	**Intermittent Bolus** **Healthy Adults Less Than 55 Years of Age:** Increments of 20 to 50 mg as needed.
Initiation of MAC Sedation	**Healthy Adults Less Than 55 Years of Age:** Slow infusion or slow injection techniques are recommended to avoid apnea or hypotension. Most patients require an infusion of 100 to 150 µg/kg/min (6 to 9 mg/kg/h) for 3 to 5 minutes or a slow injection of 0.5 mg/kg over 3 to 5 minutes followed immediately by a maintenance infusion. **Elderly, Debilitated, Neurological, or ASA III/IV Patients:** Most patients require dosages similar to healthy adults. Rapic boluses are to be avoided. (See WARNINGS.)
Maintenance of MAC Sedation	**Healthy Adults Less Than 55 Years of Age:** A variable rate infusion technique is preferable over an intermittent bolus technique. Most patients require an infusion of 25 to 75 µg/kg/min (1.5 to 4.5 mg/kg/h) or incremental bolus doses of 10 mg or 20 mg. **In Elderly, Debilitated, Neurological, or ASA III/IV Patients:** Most patients require 80% of the usual adult dose. A rapid (single or repeated) bolus dose should not be used. (See WARNINGS.)
Initiation and Maintenance of ICU Sedation in Intubated, Mechanically Ventilated	Adult Patients—Because of the lingering effects of previous anesthetic or sedative agents, in most patients the initial infusion should be 5 µg/kg/min (0.3 mg/kg/h) for at least 5 minutes. Subsequent increments of 5 to 10 µg/kg/min (0.3 to 0.6 mg/kg/h) over 5 to 10 minutes may be used until desired level of sedation is achieved. Maintenance rates of 5 to 50 µg/kg/min (0.3 to 3 mg/kg/h) or higher may be required. **Evaluation of level of sedation and assessment of CNS function should be carried out daily throughout maintenance to determine the minimum dose of DIPRIVAN Injectable Emulsion required for sedation.** **The tubing and any unused portions of DIPRIVAN Injectable Emulsion should be discarded after 12 hours because DIPRIVAN Injectable Emulsion contains no preservatives and is capable of supporting growth of microorganisms. (See WARNINGS, and DOSAGE AND ADMINISTRATION.)**

Continued on next page

Diprivan—Cont.

Dilution Prior to Administration: DIPRIVAN Injectable Emulsion is provided as a ready to use formulation. However, should dilution be necessary, it should only be diluted with 5% Dextrose Injection, USP, and it should not be diluted to a concentration less than 2 mg/mL because it is an emulsion. In diluted form it has been shown to be more stable when in contact with glass than with plastic (95% potency after 2 hours of running infusion in plastic).

Administration with Other Fluids: Compatibility of DIPRIVAN Injectable Emulsion with the coadministration of blood/serum/plasma has not been established. (See WARNINGS.) DIPRIVAN Injectable Emulsion has been shown to be compatible when administered with the following intravenous fluids.

— 5% Dextrose Injection, USP
— Lactated Ringers Injection, USP
— Lactated Ringers and 5% Dextrose Injection
— 5% Dextrose and 0.45% Sodium Chloride Injection, USP
— 5% Dextrose and 0.2% Sodium Chloride Injection, USP

Assembly Instructions for Pre-Filled Syringe

1. Remove the Luer connector from packaging.
2. Remove glass syringe barrel from tray and check for cracks or leaks. Shake. Remove the plastic cover. Applying moderate pressure, disinfect the surface of the rubber stopper using the alcohol swab provided in the package prior to attachment of the Luer connector.
3. Pull off needle cover from Luer connector. The bevel of the needle spike is slightly bent (c-tip) to prevent potential coring.
4. Stand the syringe barrel vertically on a hard surface and push Luer connector on to syringe barrel so needle penetrates rubber seal and connector slides over the aluminum seal until firmly seated. (Fig. 1)

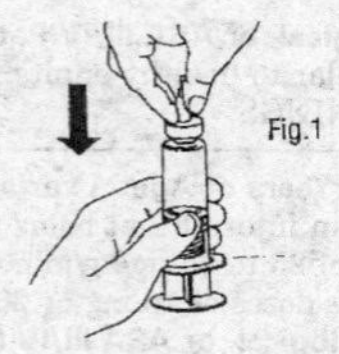

5. Add plunger rod by screwing clockwise. CAUTION: the rod must be fully screwed on, otherwise it may detach which could result in siphoning of the syringe contents. (Fig. 2)

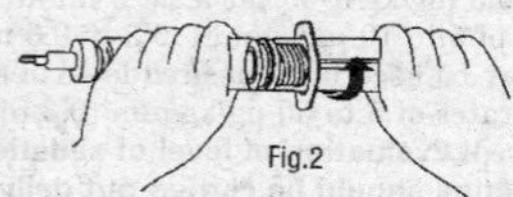

6. Unscrew Luer cover remove excess nitrogen gas from the syringe (a small nitrogen gas bubble may remain). Assemble administration line and connect syringe.

Handling Procedures

General

Parenteral drug products should be inspected visually for particulate matter and discoloration prior to administration whenever solution and container permit.

Clinical experience with the use of in-line filters and DIPRIVAN Injectable Emulsion during anesthesia or ICU/MAC sedation is limited. DIPRIVAN Injectable Emulsion should only be administered through a filter with a pore size of 5 µm or greater unless it has been demonstrated that the filter does not restrict the flow of DIPRIVAN Injectable Emulsion and/or cause the breakdown of the emulsion. Filters should be used with caution and where clinically appropriate. Continuous monitoring is necessary due to the potential for restricted flow and/or breakdown of the emulsion. Do not use if there is evidence of separation of the phases of the emulsion.

Rare cases of self administration of DIPRIVAN Injectable Emulsion, by health care professionals have been reported, including some fatalities (See DRUG ABUSE AND DEPENDENCE).

STRICT ASEPTIC TECHNIQUE MUST ALWAYS BE MAINTAINED DURING HANDLING. DIPRIVAN INJECTABLE EMULSION IS A SINGLE-USE PARENTERAL PRODUCT; WHICH CONTAINS 0.005% DISODIUM EDETATE TO RETARD THE RATE OF GROWTH OF MICROORGANISMS IN THE EVENT OF ACCIDENTAL EXTRINSIC CONTAMINATION. HOWEVER, DIPRIVAN INJECTABLE EMULSION CAN STILL SUPPORT THE GROWTH OF MICROORGANISMS AS IT IS NOT AN ANTIMICROBIALLY PRESERVED PRODUCT UNDER USP STANDARDS. ACCORDINGLY, STRICT ASEPTIC TECHNIQUE MUST STILL BE ADHERED TO. DO NOT USE IF CONTAMINATION IS SUSPECTED. DISCARD UNUSED PORTIONS AS DIRECTED WITHIN THE REQUIRED TIME LIMITS (SEE DOSAGE AND ADMINISTRATION, HANDLING PROCEDURES). THERE HAVE BEEN REPORTS IN WHICH FAILURE TO USE ASEPTIC TECHNIQUE WHEN HANDLING DIPRIVAN INJECTABLE EMULSION WAS ASSOCIATED WITH MICROBIAL CONTAMINATION OF THE PRODUCT AND WITH FEVER, INFECTION/SEPSIS, OTHER LIFE-THREATENING ILLNESS, AND/OR DEATH.

Guideline for Aseptic Technique for General Anesthesia/MAC Sedation

DIPRIVAN Injectable Emulsion should be prepared for use just prior to initiation of each individual anesthetic/sedative procedure. The ampoule neck surface, or vial/pre-filled syringe rubber stopper should be disinfected using 70% isopropyl alcohol. DIPRIVAN Injectable Emulsion should be drawn into sterile syringes immediately after ampoules or vials are opened. When withdrawing DIPRIVAN Injectable Emulsion from vials, a sterile vent spike should be used. The syringe(s) should be labeled with appropriate information including the date and time the ampoule or vial was opened. Administration should commence promptly and be completed within 6 hours after the ampoules, vials, pre-filled syringes have been opened.

DIPRIVAN Injectable Emulsion should be prepared for single patient use only. Any unused portions of DIPRIVAN Injectable Emulsion, reservoirs, dedicated administration tubing and/or solutions containing DIPRIVAN Injectable Emulsion must be discarded at the end of the anesthetic procedure or at 6 hours, whichever occurs sooner. The IV line should be flushed every 6 hours and at the end of the anesthetic procedure to remove residual DIPRIVAN Injectable Emulsion.

Guidelines for Aseptic Technique for ICU Sedation

DIPRIVAN Injectable Emulsion should be prepared for single-patient use only. When DIPRIVAN Injectable Emulsion is administered directly from the vial/pre-filled syringe, strict aseptic techniques must be followed. The vial/pre-filled syringe rubber stopper should be disinfected using 70% isopropyl alcohol. A sterile vent spike and sterile tubing must be used for administration of DIPRIVAN Injectable Emulsion. As with other lipid emulsions, the number of IV line manipulations should be minimized. Administration should commence promptly and must be completed within 12 hours after the vial has been spiked. The tubing and any unused portions of DIPRIVAN Injectable Emulsion must be discarded after 12 hours.

If DIPRIVAN Injectable Emulsion is transferred to a syringe or other container prior to administration, the handling procedures for General anesthesia/MAC sedation should be followed, and the product should be discarded and administration lines changed after 6 hours.

HOW SUPPLIED

DIPRIVAN Injectable Emulsion is available in ready to use 20 mL ampoules, 20 mL infusion vials, 50 mL infusion vials, 100 mL infusion vials, and 50 mL pre-filled syringes containing 10 mg/mL of propofol.

20 mL ampoules (NDC 0310-0300-20)
20 mL infusion vials (NDC 0310-0300-22)
50 mL infusion vials (NDC 0310-0300-50)
100 mL infusion vials (NDC 0310-0300-11)
50 mL pre-filled syringes (NDC 0310-0300-54)

Propofol undergoes oxidative degradation, in the presence of oxygen, and is therefore packaged under nitrogen to eliminate this degradation path.

Store between 4–22°C (40–72°F). Do not freeze. Shake well before use.

Manufactured for:
ZENECA
Pharmaceuticals
A Business Unit of Zeneca Inc.
Wilmington, Delaware 19850-5437
By: Zeneca S.p.A., Caponago, Italy
Made in Italy
SIC 64168-01 Rev M 02/00

Shown in Product Identification Guide, page 305

ELAVIL® ℞
(AMITRIPTYLINE HCl)
Tablets and Injection

DESCRIPTION

Amitriptyline HCl is 3-(10,11-dihydro-5*H*-dibenzo [*a,d*] cycloheptene-5-ylidene)-*N,N*-dimethyl-1-propanamine hydrochloride. Its empirical formula is $C_{20}H_{23}N \cdot HCl$ and its structural formula is:

• HCl
$CHCH_2CH_2N(CH_3)_2$

Amitriptyline HCl, a dibenzocycloheptadiene derivative, has a molecular weight of 313.87. It is a white, odorless, crystalline compound which is freely soluble in water.

ELAVIL* (Amitriptyline HCl) is supplied as 10 mg, 25 mg, 50 mg, 75 mg, 100 mg, and 150 mg tablets and as a sterile solution for intramuscular use. Inactive ingredients of the tablets are calcium phosphate, cellulose, colloidal silicon dioxide, hydroxypropyl cellulose, hydroxypropyl methylcellulose, lactose, magnesium stearate, starch, stearic acid, talc, and titanium dioxide. Tablets ELAVIL 10 mg also contain FD&C Blue 1. Tablets ELAVIL 25 mg also contain D&C Yellow 10, FD&C Blue 1, and FD&C Yellow 6. Tablets ELAVIL 50 mg also contain D&C Yellow 10, FD&C Yellow 6 and iron oxide. Tablets ELAVIL 75 mg also contain FD&C Yellow 6. Tablets ELAVIL 100 mg also contain FD&C Blue 2 and FD&C Red 40. Tablets ELAVIL 150 mg also contain FD&C Blue 2 and FD&C Yellow 6. Each milliliter of the sterile solution contains:

Amitriptyline hydrochloride	10 mg
Dextrose	44 mg
Water for Injection, q.s.	1 mL
Added as preservatives:	
Methylparaben	1.5 mg
Propylparaben	0.2 mg

ACTIONS

ELAVIL is an antidepressant with sedative effects. Its mechanism of action in man is not known. It is not a monoamine oxidase inhibitor and it does not act primarily by stimulation of the central nervous system.

Amitriptyline inhibits the membrane pump mechanism responsible for uptake of norepinephrine and serotonin in adrenergic and serotonergic neurons. Pharmacologically this action may potentiate or prolong neuronal activity since reuptake of these biogenic amines is important physiologically in terminating transmitting activity. This interference with the reuptake of norepinephrine and/or serotonin is believed by some to underlie the antidepressant activity of amitriptyline.

INDICATIONS

For the relief of symptoms of depression. Endogenous depression is more likely to be alleviated than are other depressive states.

CONTRAINDICATIONS

ELAVIL is contraindicated in patients who have shown prior hypersensitivity to it.

It should not be given concomitantly with monoamine oxidase inhibitors. Hyperpyretic crises, severe convulsions, and deaths have occurred in patients receiving tricyclic antidepressant and monoamine oxidase inhibiting drugs simultaneously. When it is desired to replace a monoamine oxidase inhibitor with ELAVIL, a minimum of 14 days should be allowed to elapse after the former is discontinued. ELAVIL should then be initiated cautiously with gradual increase in dosage until optimum response is achieved.

This drug is not recommended for use during the acute recovery phase following myocardial infarction.

WARNINGS

ELAVIL may block the antihypertensive action of guanethidine or similarly acting compounds.

It should be used with caution in patients with a history of seizures and, because of its atropine-like action, in patients with a history of urinary retention, angle-closure glaucoma or increased intraocular pressure. In patients with angle-closure glaucoma, even average doses may precipitate an attack.

Patients with cardiovascular disorders should be watched closely. Tricyclic antidepressant drugs, including ELAVIL, particularly when given in high doses, have been reported to produce arrhythmias, sinus tachycardia, and prolongation of the conduction time. Myocardial infarction and stroke have been reported with drugs of this class.

Close supervision is required when ELAVIL is given to hyperthyroid patients or those receiving thyroid medication.

ELAVIL may enhance the response to alcohol and the effects of barbiturates and other CNS depressants. In patients who may use alcohol excessively, it should be borne in mind that the potentiation may increase the danger inherent in any suicide attempt or overdosage. Delirium has been reported with concurrent administration of amitriptyline and disulfiram.

Usage in Pregnancy: Pregnancy Category C: Teratogenic effects were not observed in mice, rats, or rabbits when amitriptyline was given orally at doses of 2 to 40 mg/kg/day (up to 13 times the maximum recommended human dose**). Studies in literature have shown amitriptyline to be teratogenic in mice and hamsters when given by various routes of administration at doses of 28 to 100 mg/kg/day (9 to 33 times the maximum recommended human dose), producing multiple malformations. Another study in the rat reported that an oral dose of 25 mg/kg/day (8 times the maximum recommended human dose) produced delays in ossification of fetal vertebral bodies without other signs of embryotoxicity. In rabbits, an oral dose of 60 mg/kg/day (20 times the maximum recommended human dose) was reported to cause incomplete ossification of the cranial bones.

Amitriptyline has been shown to cross the placenta. Although a causal relationship has not been established, there have been a few reports of adverse events, including CNS effects, limb deformities, or developmental delay, in infants whose mothers had taken amitriptyline during pregnancy. There are no adequate and well-controlled studies in pregnant women. ELAVIL should be used during pregnancy only if the potential benefit to the mother justifies the potential risk to the fetus.

Nursing Mothers: Amitriptyline is excreted into breast milk. In one report in which a patient received amitriptyline 100 mg/day while nursing her infant, levels of 83–141 ng/mL were detected in the mother's serum. Levels of 135–151 ng/mL were found in the breast milk, but no trace of the drug could be detected in the infant's serum.

Because of the potential for serious adverse reactions in nursing infants from amitriptyline, a decision should be made whether to discontinue nursing or to discontinue the drug, taking into account the importance of the drug to the mother.

Usage in Pediatric Patients: In view of the lack of experience with the use of this drug in pediatric patients, it is not recommended at the present time for patients under 12 years of age.

PRECAUTIONS

Schizophrenic patients may develop increased symptoms of psychosis; patients with paranoid symptomatology may have an exaggeration of such symptoms. Depressed patients, particularly those with known manic-depressive illness, may experience a shift to mania or hypomania. In these circumstances the dose of amitriptyline may be reduced or a major tranquilizer such as perphenazine may be administered concurrently.

The possibility of suicide in depressed patients remains until significant remission occurs. Potentially suicidal patients should not have access to large quantities of this drug. Prescriptions should be written for the smallest amount feasible.

Concurrent administration of ELAVIL and electroshock therapy may increase the hazards associated with such therapy. Such treatment should be limited to patients for whom it is essential.

When possible, the drug should be discontinued several days before elective surgery.

Both elevation and lowering of blood sugar levels have been reported.

ELAVIL should be used with caution in patients with impaired liver function.

Drug Interactions: Drugs Metabolized by P450 2D6—The biochemical activity of the drug metabolizing isozyme cytochrome P450 2D6 (debrisoquin hydroxylase) is reduced in a subset of the Caucasian population (about 7–10% of Caucasians are so called "poor metabolizers"); reliable estimates of the prevalence of reduced P450 2D6 isozyme activity among Asian, African and other populations are not yet available. Poor metabolizers have higher than expected plasma concentrations of tricyclic antidepressants (TCAs) when given usual doses. Depending on the fraction of drug metabolized by P450 2D6, the increase in plasma concentration may be small, or quite large (8-fold increase in plasma AUC of the TCA).

In addition, certain drugs inhibit the activity of this isozyme and make normal metabolizers resemble poor metabolizers. An individual who is stable on a given dose of TCA may become abruptly toxic when given one of these inhibiting drugs as concomitant therapy. The drugs that inhibit cytochrome P450 2D6 include some that are not metabolized by the enzyme (quinidine; cimetidine) and many that are substrates for P450 2D6 (many other antidepressants, phenothiazines, and the Type 1C antiarrhythmics propafenone and flecainide). While all the selective serotonin reuptake inhibitors (SSRIs), e.g., fluoxetine, sertraline, and paroxetine, inhibit P450 2D6, they may vary in the extent of inhibition. The extent to which SSRI-TCA interactions may pose clinical problems will depend on the degree of inhibition and the pharmacokinetics of the SSRI involved. Nevertheless, caution is indicated in the coadministration of TCAs with any of the SSRIs and also in switching from one class to the other. Of particular importance, sufficient time must elapse before initiating TCA treatment in a patient being withdrawn from fluoxetine, given the long half-life of the parent and active metabolite (at least 5 weeks may be necessary).

Concomitant use of tricyclic antidepressants with drugs that can inhibit cytochrome P450 2D6 may require lower doses than usually prescribed for either the tricyclic antidepressant or the other drug. Furthermore, whenever one of these other drugs is withdrawn from co-therapy, an increased dose of tricyclic antidepressant may be required. It is desirable to monitor TCA plasma levels whenever a TCA is going to be coadministered with another drug known to be an inhibitor of P450 2D6.

Monoamine oxidase inhibitors—see CONTRAINDICATIONS section. Guanethidine or similarly acting compounds; thyroid medication; alcohol, barbiturates and other CNS depressants; and disulfiram— see WARNINGS section.

When ELAVIL is given with anticholinergic agents or sympathomimetic drugs, including epinephrine combined with local anesthetics, close supervision and careful adjustment of dosages are required.

Hyperpyrexia has been reported when ELAVIL is administered with anticholinergic agents or with neuroleptic drugs, particularly during hot weather.

Paralytic ileus may occur in patients taking tricyclic antidepressants in combination with anticholinergic-type drugs.

Cimetidine is reported to reduce hepatic metabolism of certain tricyclic antidepressants, thereby delaying elimination and increasing steady-state concentrations of these drugs. Clinically significant effects have been reported with the tricyclic antidepressants when used concomitantly with cimetidine. Increases in plasma levels of tricyclic antidepressants, and in the frequency and severity of side effects, particularly anticholinergic, have been reported when cimetidine was added to the drug regimen. Discontinuation of cimetidine in well-controlled patients receiving tricyclic antidepressants and cimetidine may decrease the plasma levels and efficacy of the antidepressants.

Caution is advised if patients receive large doses of ethchlorvynol concurrently. Transient delirium has been reported in patients who were treated with one gram of ethchlorvynol and 75–150 mg of ELAVIL.

Information for Patients: While on therapy with ELAVIL, patients should be advised as to the possible impairment of mental and/or physical abilities required for performance of hazardous tasks, such as operating machinery or driving a motor vehicle.

Geriatric Use: Clinical experience has not identified differences in responses between elderly and younger patients. In general, dose selection for an elderly patient should be cautious, usually starting at the low end of the dosing range, reflecting the greater frequency of decreased hepatic function, concomitant disease and other drug therapy in elderly patients.

Geriatric patients are particularly sensitive to the anticholinergic side effects of tricyclic antidepressants including ELAVIL. Peripheral anticholinergic effects include tachycardia, urinary retention, constipation, dry mouth, blurred vision, and exacerbation of narrow-angle glaucoma. Central nervous system anticholinergic effects include cognitive impairment, psychomotor slowing, confusion, sedation, and delirium. Elderly patients taking ELAVIL may be at increased risk for falls. Elderly patients should be started on low doses of ELAVIL and observed closely (see DOSAGE AND ADMINISTRATION).

ADVERSE REACTIONS

Within each category the following adverse reactions are listed in order of decreasing severity. Included in the listing are a few adverse reactions which have not been reported with this specific drug. However, pharmacological similarities among the tricyclic antidepressant drugs require that each of the reactions be considered when amitriptyline is administered.

Cardiovascular: Myocardial infarction; stroke; nonspecific ECG changes and changes in AV conduction; heart block; arrhythmias; hypotension, particularly orthostatic hypotension; syncope; hypertension; tachycardia; palpitation.

CNS and Neuromuscular: Coma; seizures; hallucinations; delusions; confusional states; disorientation; incoordination; ataxia; tremors; peripheral neuropathy; numbness, tingling, and paresthesias of the extremities; extrapyramidal symptoms including abnormal involuntary movements and tardive dyskinesia; dysarthria; disturbed concentration; excitement; anxiety; insomnia; restlessness; nightmares; drowsiness; dizziness; weakness; fatigue; headache; syndrome of inappropriate ADH (antidiuretic hormone) secretion; tinnitus; alteration in EEG patterns.

Anticholinergic: Paralytic ileus; hyperpyrexia; urinary retention; dilatation of the urinary tract; constipation; blurred vision, disturbance of accommodation, increased ocular pressure, mydriasis; dry mouth.

Allergic: Skin rash; urticaria; photosensitization; edema of face and tongue.

Hematologic: Bone marrow depression including agranulocytosis, leukopenia, thrombocytopenia; purpura; eosinophilia.

Gastrointestinal: Rarely hepatitis (including altered liver function and jaundice); nausea; epigastric distress; vomiting; anorexia; stomatitis; peculiar taste; diarrhea; parotid swelling; black tongue.

Endocrine: Testicular swelling and gynecomastia in the male; breast enlargement and galactorrhea in the female; increased or decreased libido; impotence; elevation and lowering of blood sugar levels.

Other: Alopecia; edema; weight gain or loss; urinary frequency; increased perspiration.

Withdrawal Symptoms: After prolonged administration, abrupt cessation of treatment may produce nausea, headache, and malaise. Gradual dosage reduction has been reported to produce, within two weeks, transient symptoms including irritability, restlessness, and dream and sleep disturbance.

These symptoms are not indicative of addiction. Rare instances have been reported of mania or hypomania occurring within 2–7 days following cessation of chronic therapy with tricyclic antidepressants.

Causal Relationship Unknown: Other reactions, reported under circumstances where a causal relationship could not be established, are listed to serve as alerting information to physicians:

Body as a Whole: Lupus-like syndrome (migratory arthritis, positive ANA and rheumatoid factor).

Digestive: Hepatic failure, ageusia.

Postmarketing Adverse Events

A syndrome resembling neuroleptic malignant syndrome (NMS) has been very rarely reported after starting or increasing the dose of ELAVIL, with and without concomitant medications known to cause NMS. Symptoms have included muscle rigidity, fever, mental status changes, diaphoresis, tachycardia, and tremor.

Very rare cases of serotonin syndrome (SS) have been reported with ELAVIL in combination with other drugs that have a recognized association with SS.

DOSAGE AND ADMINISTRATION

Oral Dosage

Dosage should be initiated at a low level and increased gradually, noting carefully the clinical response and any evidence of intolerance.

Initial Dosage for Adults: For outpatients 75 mg of amitriptyline HCl a day in divided doses is usually satisfactory. If necessary, this may be increased to a total of 150 mg per day. Increases are made preferably in the late afternoon and/or bedtime doses. A sedative effect may be apparent before the antidepressant effect is noted, but an adequate therapeutic effect may take as long as 30 days to develop.

An alternate method of initiating therapy in outpatients is to begin with 50 to 100 mg amitriptyline HCl at bedtime. This may be increased by 25 or 50 mg as necessary in the bedtime dose to a total of 150 mg per day.

Hospitalized patients may require 100 mg a day initially. This can be increased gradually to 200 mg a day if necessary. A small number of hospitalized patients may need as much as 300 mg a day.

Adolescent and Elderly Patients: In general, lower dosages are recommended for these patients. Ten milligrams 3 times a day with 20 mg at bedtime may be satisfactory in adolescent and elderly patients who do not tolerate higher dosages.

Maintenance: The usual maintenance dosage of amitriptyline HCl is 50 to 100 mg per day. In some patients 40 mg per day is sufficient. For maintenance therapy the total daily dosage may be given in a single dose preferably at bedtime. When satisfactory improvement has been reached, dosage should be reduced to the lowest amount that will maintain relief of symptoms. It is appropriate to continue maintenance therapy 3 months or longer to lessen the possibility of relapse.

Intramuscular Dosage

Initially, 20 to 30 mg (2 to 3 mL) four times a day.

When ELAVIL Injection is administered intramuscularly, the effects may appear more rapidly than with oral administration.

When ELAVIL Injection is used for initial therapy in patients unable or unwilling to take ELAVIL Tablets, the tablets should replace the injection as soon as possible.

Usage in Pediatric Patients

In view of the lack of experience with the use of this drug in pediatric patients, it is not recommended at the present time for patients under 12 years of age.

Plasma Levels

Because of the wide variation in the absorption and distribution of tricyclic antidepressants in body fluids, it is difficult to directly correlate plasma levels and therapeutic effect. However, determination of plasma levels may be useful in identifying patients who appear to have toxic effects and may have excessively high levels, or those in whom lack of absorption or noncompliance is suspected. Because of increased intestinal transit time and decreased hepatic metabolism in elderly patients, plasma levels are generally higher for a given oral dose of ELAVIL than in younger patients. Elderly patients should be monitored carefully and quantitative serum levels obtained as clinically appropriate. Adjustments in dosage should be made according to the patient's clinical response and not on the basis of plasma levels.***

OVERDOSAGE

Deaths may occur from overdosage with this class of drugs. Multiple drug ingestion (including alcohol) is common in deliberate tricyclic antidepressant overdose. As the management is complex and changing, it is recommended that the physician contact a poison control center for current information on treatment. Signs and symptoms of toxicity develop rapidly after tricyclic antidepressant overdose, therefore, hospital monitoring is required as soon as possible.

Manifestations: Critical manifestations of overdose include: cardiac dysrhythmias, severe hypotension, convulsions, and CNS depression, including coma. Changes in the electrocardiogram, particularly in QRS axis or width, are clinically significant indicators of tricyclic antidepressant toxicity.

Other signs of overdose may include: impaired myocardial contractility, confusion, disturbed concentration, transient visual hallucinations, dilated pupils, disorders of ocular motility, agitation, hyperactive reflexes, polyradiculoneuropathy, stupor, drowsiness, muscle rigidity, vomiting, hypothermia, hyperpyrexia, or any of the symptoms listed under ADVERSE REACTIONS.

Management:

General: Obtain an ECG and immediately initiate cardiac monitoring. Protect the patient's airway, establish an intravenous line and initiate gastric decontamination. A minimum of six hours of observation with cardiac monitoring and observation for signs of CNS or respiratory depression, hypotension, cardiac dysrhythmias and/or conduction blocks, and seizures is necessary. If signs of toxicity occur at any time during the period, extended monitoring is required. There are case reports of patients succumbing to fatal dysrhythmias late after overdose; these patients had clinical evidence of significant poisoning prior to death and most received inadequate gastrointestinal decontamination. Monitoring of plasma drug levels should not guide management of the patient.

Gastrointestinal Decontamination: All patients suspected of tricyclic antidepressant overdose should receive gastrointestinal decontamination. This should include large volume gastric lavage followed by activated charcoal. If consciousness is impaired, the airway should be secured prior to lavage. EMESIS IS CONTRAINDICATED.

Cardiovascular: A maximal limb-lead QRS duration of ≥0.10 seconds may be the best indication of the severity of the overdose. Intravenous sodium bicarbonate should be used to maintain the serum pH in the range of 7.45 to 7.55. If the pH response is inadequate, hyperventilation may also be used. Concomitant use of hyperventilation and sodium bicarbonate should be done with extreme caution, with frequent pH monitoring. A pH > 7.60 or a pCO_2 < 20mm Hg is

Continued on next page

Elavil—Cont.

undesirable. Dysrhythmias unresponsive to sodium bicarbonate therapy/hyperventilation may respond to lidocaine, bretylium or phenytoin. Type 1A and 1C antiarrhythmics are generally contraindicated (e.g., quinidine, disopyramide, and procainamide).

In rare instances, hemoperfusion may be beneficial in acute refractory cardiovascular instability in patients with acute toxicity. However, hemodialysis, peritoneal dialysis, exchange transfusions, and forced diuresis generally have been reported as ineffective in tricyclic antidepressant poisoning.

CNS: In patients with CNS depression, early intubation is advised because of the potential for abrupt deterioration. Seizures should be controlled with benzodiazepines, or if these are ineffective, other anticonvulsants (e.g., phenobarbital, phenytoin). Physostigmine is not recommended except to treat life-threatening symptoms that have been unresponsive to other therapies, and then only in consultation with a poison control center.

Psychiatric Follow-up: Since overdosage is often deliberate, patients may attempt suicide by other means during the recovery phase. Psychiatric referral may be appropriate.

Pediatric Management: The principles of management of pediatric and adult overdosages are similar. It is strongly recommended that the physician contact the local poison control center for specific pediatric treatment.

HOW SUPPLIED

Tablets ELAVIL, 10 mg, are blue, round, film coated tablets, identified with "40" debossed on one side and "ELAVIL" on the other side. They are supplied as follows:
NDC 0310-0040-10 bottles of 100
Tablets ELAVIL, 25 mg, are yellow, round, film coated tablets, identified with "45" debossed on one side and "ELAVIL" on the other side. They are supplied as follows:
NDC 0310-0045-10 bottles of 100
NDC 0310-0045-50 bottles of 5000
Tablets ELAVIL, 50 mg, are beige, round, film coated tablets, identified with "41" debossed on one side and "ELAVIL" on the other side. They are supplied as follows:
NDC 0310-0041-10 bottles of 100
Tablets ELAVIL, 75 mg, are orange, round, film coated tablets, identified with "42" debossed on one side and "ELAVIL" on the other side. They are supplied as follows:
NDC 0310-0042-10 bottles of 100
Tablets ELAVIL, 100 mg, are mauve, round, film coated tablets, identified with "43" debossed on one side and "ELAVIL" on the other side. They are supplied as follows:
NDC 0310-0043-10 bottles of 100
Tablets ELAVIL, 150 mg, are blue, capsule shaped, film coated tablets, identified with "47" debossed on one side and "ELAVIL" on the other side. They are supplied as follows:
NDC 0310-0047-30 bottles of 30
NDC 0310-0047-10 bottles of 100
Injection ELAVIL, 10 mg/mL, is a clear, colorless solution, and is supplied as follows:
NDC 0310-0049-10 in 10 mL vials

Storage: Store Tablets ELAVIL in a well-closed container. Avoid storage at temperatures above 30°C (86°F). In addition, Tablets ELAVIL 10 mg must be protected from light and stored in a well-closed, light-resistant container.

Protect ELAVIL Injection from freezing and avoid storage above 30°C (86°F).

METABOLISM

Studies in man following oral administration of ^{14}C-labeled drug indicated that amitriptyline is rapidly absorbed and metabolized. Radioactivity of the plasma was practically negligible, although significant amounts of radioactivity appeared in the urine by 4 to 6 hours and one-half to one-third of the drug was excreted within 24 hours.

Amitriptyline is metabolized by N-demethylation and bridge hydroxylation in man, rabbit, and rat. Virtually the entire dose is excreted as glucuronide or sulfate conjugate of metabolites, with little unchanged drug appearing in the urine. Other metabolic pathways may be involved.

REFERENCES

Ayd FJ Jr: Amitriptyline (ELAVIL) therapy for depressive reactions. Psychosomatics 1960;1:320-325.

Diamond S: Human metabolizer of amitriptyline tagged with carbon 14. Curr Ther Res, Mar 1965, pp 170-175.

Dorfman W: Clinical experiences with amitriptyline (ELAVIL): A preliminary report. Psychosomatics 1960;1: 153-155.

Fallette JM, Stasney CR, Mintz AA: Amitriptyline poisoning treated with physostigmine. South Med J 1970;63:1492-1493.

Hollister LE, Overall JE, Johnson M, et al: Controlled comparison of amitriptyline, imipramine and placebo in hospitalized depressed patients. J Nerv Ment Dis 1964;139:370-375.

Hordern A, Burt CG, Holt NF: Depressive states: A pharmacotherapeutic study, Springfield study. Springfield, Ill, Charles C. Thomas, 1965.

Jenike MA: Treatment of Affective Illness in the Elderly with Drugs and Electroconvulsive Therapy. J Geriatr Psychiatry 1989; 22(1): 77–112.

Klerman GL, Cole JO: Clinical pharmacology of imipramine and related antidepressant compounds. Int J Psychiatry 1976:3:267-304.

Liu B, Anderson G, Mittman N, et al: Use of selective serotonin-reuptake inhibitors or tricyclic antidepressants and risk of hip fractures in elderly people. Lancet 1998; 351(9112): 1303–1307.

McConaghy N, Joffe AD, Kingston WR, et al: Correlation of clinical features of depressed out-patients with response to amitriptyline and protriptyline. Br J Psychiatry 1968;114: 103-106.

McDonald IM, Perkins M, Marjerrison G, et al: A controlled comparison of amitriptyline and electroconvulsive therapy in the treatment of depression. Am J Psychiatry 1966;122: 1427-1431.

Slovis T, Ott J, Teitelbaum D, et al: Physostigmine therapy in acute tricyclic antidepressant poisoning. Clin Toxicol 1971;4:451-459.

Symposium on depression with special studies of a new antidepressant, amitriptyline. Dis Nerv Syst, (Sect 2) May 1961, pp 5-56.

* Registered trademark of ZENECA Inc.
** Based on a maximum recommended amitriptyline dose of 150 mg/day or 3mg/kg/day for a 50 kg patient.
*** Hollister LE: Monitoring Tricyclic Antidepressant Plasma Concentrations. JAMA 1979; 241(23): 2530–2533.

Manufactured for:
Zeneca Pharmaceuticals
A Business Unit of Zeneca Inc.
Wilmington, Delaware 19850-5437
by MERCK & Co., Inc. West Point, PA 19486 USA
64134-02 Rev H 08/98
90883-16*
*Elavil Injection

Shown in Product Identification Guide, page 305

HIBICLENS® Antiseptic/Antimicrobial Skin Cleanser (chlorhexidine gluconate) OTC

[hi 'bi-klenz]

DESCRIPTION

HIBICLENS is an antiseptic antimicrobial skin cleanser possessing bactericidal activities. HIBICLENS contains 4% w/v HIBITANE® (chlorhexidine gluconate), a chemically unique hexamethylenebis biguanide with inactive ingredients: Fragrance, isopropyl alcohol 4%, purified water, Red 40, and other ingredients, in a mild, sudsing base adjusted to pH 5.0–6.5 for optimal activity and stability as well as compatibility with the normal pH of the skin.

ACTION

HIBICLENS is bactericidal on contact. It has antiseptic activity and a persistent antimicrobial effect with rapid bactericidal activity against a wide range of microorganisms, including gram-positive bacteria, and gram-negative bacteria such as *Pseudomonas aeruginosa*. The effectiveness of HIBICLENS is not signficantly reduced by the presence of organic matter, such as blood.[1]

In a study[2] simulating surgical use, the immediate bactericidal effect of HIBICLENS after a single six-minute scrub resulted in a 99.9% reduction in resident bacterial flora, with a reduction of 99.98% after the eleventh scrub. Reductions on surgically gloved hands were maintained over the six-hour test period.

HIBICLENS displays persistent antimicrobial action. In one study[2], 93% of a radiolabeled formulation of HIBICLENS remained present on uncovered skin after five hours.

HIBICLENS prevents skin infection thereby reducing the risk of cross-infection.

INDICATIONS

HIBICLENS is indicated for use as a surgical scrub, as a health-care personnel handwash, for patient preoperative showering and bathing, as a patient preoperative skin preparation, and as a skin wound cleanser and general skin cleanser.

SAFETY

The extensive use of chlorhexidine gluconate for over 20 years outside the United States has produced no evidence of absorption of the compound through intact skin. The potential for producing skin reactions is extremely low. HIBICLENS can be used many times a day without causing irritation, dryness, or discomfort. Experimental studies indicate that when used for cleaning superficial wounds, HIBICLENS will neither cause additional tissue injury nor delay healing.

WARNINGS

FOR EXTERNAL USE ONLY. KEEP OUT OF EYES, EARS AND MOUTH. HIBICLENS SHOULD NOT BE USED AS A PREOPERATIVE SKIN PREPARATION OF THE FACE OR HEAD. MISUSE OF HIBICLENS HAS BEEN REPORTED TO CAUSE SERIOUS AND PERMANENT EYE INJURY WHEN IT HAS BEEN PERMITTED TO ENTER AND REMAIN IN THE EYE DURING SURGICAL PROCEDURES. IF HIBICLENS SHOULD CONTACT THESE AREAS, RINSE OUT PROMPTLY AND THOROUGHLY WITH WATER. Avoid contact with meninges. HIBICLENS should not be used by persons who have a sensitivity to it or its components. Chlorhexidine gluconate has been reported to cause deafness when instilled in the middle ear through perforated ear drums. Irritation, sensitization and generalized allergic reactions have been reported with chlorhexidine-containing products, especially in the genital areas. If adverse reactions occur, discontinue use immediately and if severe, contact a physician. Keep this and all drugs out of the reach of children. In case of accidental ingestion, seek professional assistance or contact a Poison Control Center immediately.

Accidental ingestion: Chlorhexidine gluconate taken orally is poorly absorbed. Treat with gastric lavage using milk, egg white, gelatin or mild soap. Employ supportive measures as appropriate.

Avoid excessive heat (above 104°F).

DIRECTIONS FOR USE

Skin Wound and General Skin Cleansing

Wounds which involve more than the superficial layers of the skin should not be routinely treated with HIBICLENS. HIBICLENS should not be used for repeated general skin cleansing of large body areas except in those patients whose underlying condition makes it necessary to reduce the bacterial population of the skin. To use, thoroughly rinse the area to be cleansed with water. Apply the minimum amount of HIBICLENS necessary to cover the skin or wound area and wash gently. Rinse again thoroughly.

Preoperative Skin Preparation

Apply HIBICLENS liberally to surgical site and swab for at least two minutes. Dry with a sterile towel. Repeat procedure for an additional two minutes and dry with a sterile towel.

Preoperative Showering and Whole-Body bathing

The patient should be instructed to wash the entire body, including the scalp, on two consecutive occasions immediately prior to surgery. Each procedure should consist of two consecutive thorough applications of HIBICLENS followed by thorough rinsing. If the patient's condition allows, showering is recommended for whole-body bathing. The recommended procedure is: Wet the body, including hair. Wash the hair using 25 mL of HIBICLENS and the body with another 25 mL of HIBICLENS. Rinse. Repeat. Rinse thoroughly after second application.

HEALTH-CARE PERSONNEL USE

SURGICAL HAND SCRUB

Directions for use of HIBICLENS Liquid: Wet hands and forearms with water. Scrub for 3 minutes with about 5 mL of HIBICLENS and a wet brush, paying particular attention to the nails, cuticles, and interdigital spaces. A separate nail cleaner may be used. Rinse thoroughly. Wash for an additional 3 minutes with 5 mL of HIBICLENS and rinse under running water. Dry thoroughly.

Personnel Hand Wash

Wet hands with warm water. (Avoid using very cold or very hot water.) Dispense about 5 mL of HIBICLENS into cupped hands. Wash for 15 seconds. (Do not use excessive pressure to produce additional lather.) Rinse thoroughly with warm water. Dry thoroughly.

Directions for use of HIBICLENS® Sponge/Brush: Open package and remove nail cleaner. Wet hands. Use nail cleaner under fingernails and to clean cuticles. Wet hands and forearms to the elbow with warm water. (Avoid using very cold or very hot water.) Wet sponge side of sponge/brush. Squeeze and pump immediately to work up adequate lather. Apply lather to hands and forearms using *sponge* side of the product. *Start 3 minute scrub* by using the brush side of the product to scrub *only* nails, cuticles, and interdigital areas. Use sponge side for scrubbing hands and forearms. (Avoid using brush on these more sensitive areas.) Rinse thoroughly with warm water. Scrub for an additional 3 minutes *using sponge side* only. To produce additional lather, add a small amount of water and pump the sponge. (While scrubbing, do not use excessive pressure to produce lather—a small amount of lather is all that is required to adequately cleanse skin with HIBICLENS.) Rinse and dry thoroughly, blotting hands and forearms with a soft sterile towel.

IMPORTANT LAUNDERING ADVICE FOR HOSPITAL STAFF AND OTHER USERS OF ANTISEPTIC PATIENT SKIN PREPARATIONS CONTAINING CHLORHEXIDINE GLUCONATE

Chlorhexidine gluconate is a unique agent that most closely fits the definition of an ideal antimicrobial agent, having (among others) one of the most important characteristics of persistent activity. This persistence is due to chlorhexidine gluconate binding to the protein of the skin and, thus, being available for residual activity over a relatively long period of time.

Chlorhexidine gluconate, however, binds not only to protein of the skin, but also to many fabrics, particularly cotton. Thus, special laundering procedures should be considered when such products contact these fabrics. As a result of such contact, chlorhexidine gluconate may become adsorbed onto the fabric and not be removed by washing. If sufficient available chlorine is present during the washing procedure, a fast brown stain may develop due to a chemical reaction between chlorhexidine gluconate and chlorine.

SUGGESTED LAUNDERING PROCEDURES TO LIMIT STAINING

1. **Not Aging.** Avoid allowing the product to age (set) on unwashed linens.
2. **Flushing and Washing.** A flush operation as the initial step in the wash process is helpful in the laundering of linen exposed to chlorhexidine gluconate. Such flushing is also important in the laundering of linen which contains organic materials such as blood or pus. For best results, warm water flushes (90°–100°F) are recommended. After

Operation	Water Level	Temperature	Time (Min)	Supplies/ 100 lb
Break	Low	180°F	20	1.5 lb oxalic acid
Flush	High	Cold	1	—
Emulsify	Low	160°F	5	18 oz emulsifier
Flush	High	Cold	1	—
Bleach	Low	180°F	20	2 lb alkali builder and 1 lb organic bleach
Rinse	High	Cold	1	—
Antichlor	High	Cold	2	4 oz antichlor
Rinse	High	Cold	1	—
Rinse	High	Cold	1	—
Sour	Low	Cold	4	2 oz rust removing sour

a number of initial flushings followed by a washing with a low alkaline/nonchlorine detergent, most articles which come in contact with chlorhexidine gluconate should have an acceptable level of whiteness. If a rewash process using bleach is necessary to achieve a greater degree of whiteness, the bleach used should be a nonchlorine bleach.

3. **Not Using Chlorine Bleach.** Modern laundering methods often make the use of chlorine bleach unnecessary. It is worthwhile trying to wash without chlorine to ascertain if the resulting degree of whiteness is acceptable. Omission of chlorine from the laundering process can extend the useful life of cotton articles since oxidizing bleaches such as chlorine may cause some damage to cellulose even when used in low concentration.
4. **Changing to a Peroxide-Type Bleach, Such as Sodium Perborate, Sodium Percarbonate or Hydrogen Peroxide.** This should eliminate the reaction which could occur with the use of chlorine bleaches. If a chlorine bleach must be used, a concentration of less than 7 ppm available chlorine ($^1/_{10}$ the normal bleach level) is suggested to minimize possible staining.

A NOTE ON LAUNDERING OF PERSONAL CLOTHING

The laundering procedures set forth above using low alkaline, nonchlorinated laundry detergents are also applicable to laundering of uniforms and lab coats. Commercially available laundry detergents which do not contain chlorine include Borax, Borateem, Dreft, Oxydol, and Ivory Snow. These products, however, will not remove stains previously set into the fabric.

RECLAMATION OF STAINED LINENS

For those linens which previously have been stained due to the chemical reaction between chlorhexidine gluconate and chlorine, the following laundering procedure may be helpful in reducing the visible stain:

[See table above]

HOW SUPPLIED

For general handwashing locations: pocket-size, 15 mL foil Packettes; plastic disposable bottles of 4 oz and 8 oz with dispenser caps; and 16 oz filled globes. *For surgical scrub areas:* disposable, unit-of-use 22 mL impregnated Sponge/Brushes with nail cleaner; plastic disposable bottles of 32 oz and 1 gal. The 32-oz bottle is designed for a special foot-operated wall dispenser. A hand-operated wall dispenser is available for the 16-oz globe. Hand pumps are available for 16 oz, 32 oz, and 1 gal sizes. Liquid: NDC 0310-0575. Sponge/Brush: NDC 0310-0577.

Store at controlled room temperature, 20–25°C (68–77°F) [see USP].

REFERENCES

1. Lowbury, EJL and Lilly, HA: The effect of blood on disinfection of surgeons' hands, Brit. J. Surg. 61:19–21 (Jan.) 1974.
2. Peterson AF, Rosenberg A, Alatary SD: Comparative evaluation of surgical scrub preparations, Surg. Gynecol. Obstet. 146:63–65 (Jan.) 1978.

Zeneca Pharmaceuticals
A Business Unit of Zeneca Inc.
Wilmington, DE 19850-5437 USA

Shown in Product Identification Guide, page 305

HIBISTAT® Germicidal Hand Rinse OTC
HIBISTAT® TOWELETTE
Germicidal Handwipe
[*hi 'bi-stat*]
(chlorhexidine gluconate)

DESCRIPTION

HIBISTAT is a germicidal hand rinse which provides rapid bactericidal action and has a persistent antimicrobial effect against a wide range of microorganisms. HIBISTAT is a clear, colorless liquid containing 0.5% w/w HIBITANE® (chlorhexidine gluconate) with inactive ingredients: emollients, isopropyl alcohol 70%, purified water.

INDICATIONS

HIBISTAT is indicated for health-care personnel use as a germicidal hand rinse. HIBISTAT is indicated for hand hygiene on physically clean hands. It is used in those situations where hands are physically clean, but in need of degerming, when routine handwashing is not convenient or desirable.

HIBISTAT provides rapid germicidal action and has a persistent effect.

HIBISTAT should be used in-between patients and procedures where there are no sinks available or continued return to the sink area is inconvenient. HIBISTAT can be used as an alternative to detergent-based products when hands are physically clean. Also, HIBISTAT is an effective germicidal hand rinse following a soap and water handwash.

WARNINGS

Flammable. This product is alcohol based. Alcohol is extremely flammable. It should be kept away from flame or devices which may generate an electrical spark.

FOR EXTERNAL USE ONLY. KEEP OUT OF EYES, EARS AND MOUTH. HIBISTAT SHOULD NOT BE USED AS A PREOPERATIVE SKIN PREPARATION OF THE FACE OR HEAD. MISUSE OF CHLORHEXIDINE-CONTAINING PRODUCTS HAS BEEN REPORTED TO CAUSE SERIOUS AND PERMANENT EYE INJURY WHEN IT HAS BEEN PERMITTED TO ENTER AND REMAIN IN THE EYE DURING SURGICAL PROCEDURES. IF HIBISTAT SHOULD CONTACT THESE AREAS, RINSE OUT PROMPTLY AND THOROUGHLY WITH WATER.

Avoid contact with meninges. HIBISTAT should not be used by persons who have a sensitivity to it or its components. Chlorhexidine gluconate has been reported to cause deafness when instilled in the middle ear through perforated ear drums. Irritation, sensitization, and generalized allergic reactions have been reported with chlorhexidine-containing products, especially in the genital areas. If adverse reactions occur, discontinue use immediately and if severe, contact a physician. Keep this and all drugs out of the reach of children. In case of accidental ingestion, seek professional assistance or contact a Poison Control Center immediately. Avoid excessive heat (above 104°F).

Accidental ingestion: Chlorhexidine gluconate taken orally is poorly absorbed. Treat with gastric lavage using milk, egg white, gelatin or mild soap avoiding pulmonary aspiration. Do not use apomorphine. Assist respiration if necessary and keep patient warm. Intravenous levulose can accelerate alcohol metabolism. In severe cases, hemodialysis or peritoneal dialysis may be appropriate.

DIRECTIONS FOR USE

HIBISTAT Towelette: Rub hands vigorously with HIBISTAT Towelette for approximately 15 seconds, paying particular attention to nails and interdigital spaces. HIBISTAT dries rapidly in use. No water or towel drying are necessary. The emollients contained in the HIBISTAT Towelette protect the hands from the potential drying effect of alcohol.

HIBISTAT Liquid: Dispense about 5 mL of HIBISTAT into cupped hands and rub vigorously until dry (about 15 seconds), paying particular attention to nails and interdigital spaces. HIBISTAT dries rapidly in use. No water or toweling are necessary. The emollients contained in HIBISTAT protect the hands from the potential drying effect of alcohol.

LAUNDERING

Chlorhexidine gluconate chemically reacts with chlorine to form a brown stain on fabric. Fabric which has come in contact with chlorhexidine gluconate should be rinsed well and washed without the addition of chlorine products. If bleach is desired, only nonchlorine bleach should be used. Full laundering instructions are packed with each case of HIBISTAT. (Please see HIBICLENS® for full laundering instructions.)

HOW SUPPLIED

In disposable towelettes containing 5 mL, packaged 50 towelettes to a carton.
NDC 0310-0587 (towelettes)
Manufactured For:
Zeneca Pharmaceuticals
A Business Unit of Zeneca Inc.
Wilmington, DE 19850-5437 USA
by ACCUPAC, Inc

Shown in Product Identification Guide, page 305

MERREM® I.V. ℞
(meropenem for injection)
For Intravenous Use Only

DESCRIPTION

MERREM® I.V. (meropenem for injection) is a sterile, pyrogen-free, synthetic, broad-spectrum, carbapenem antibiotic for intravenous administration. It is (4R,5S,6S)-3-[[(3S,5S)-5-(Dimethylcarbamoyl)- 3-pyrrolidinyl]thio]-6-[(1R)-1-hydroxyethyl]-4-methyl-7-oxo-1-azabicyclo[3.2.0]hept-2-ene-2-carboxylic acid trihydrate. Its empirical formula is $C_{17}H_{25}N_3O_5S \bullet 3H_2O$ with a molecular weight of 437.52. Its structural formula is:

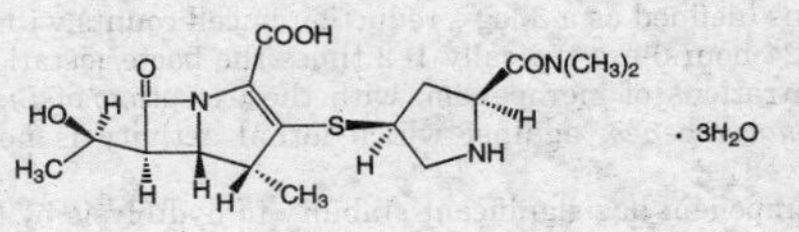

MERREM I.V. is a white to pale yellow crystalline powder. The solution varies from colorless to yellow depending on the concentration. The pH of freshly constituted solutions is between 7.3 and 8.3. Meropenem is soluble in 5% monobasic potassium phosphate solution, sparingly soluble in water, very slightly soluble in hydrated ethanol, and practically insoluble in acetone or ether.

When constituted as instructed (see **DOSAGE AND ADMINISTRATION; PREPARATION OF SOLUTION**), each 1 g MERREM I.V. vial will deliver 1 g of meropenem and 90.2 mg of sodium as sodium carbonate (3.92 mEq). Each 500 mg MERREM I.V. vial will deliver 500 mg meropenem and 45.1 mg of sodium as sodium carbonate (1.96 mEq).

MERREM I.V. in the ADD-Vantage† vial is intended for intravenous use only after dilution with the appropriate volume of diluent solution in the Abbott ADD-Vantage® diluent container. (See **DOSAGE AND ADMINISTRATION-PREPARATION OF SOLUTION.**) MERREM I.V. in the ADD-Vantage vial is available in two strengths. Each 1 g ADD-Vantage vial of MERREM I.V. will deliver 90.2 mg of sodium as sodium carbonate (3.92 mEq), and each 500 mg ADD-Vantage vial will deliver 45.1 mg of sodium as sodium carbonate (1.96 mEq).

CLINICAL PHARMACOLOGY

At the end of a 30-minute intravenous infusion of a single dose of MERREM I.V. in normal volunteers, mean peak plasma concentrations are approximately 23 μg/mL (range 14–26) for the 500 mg dose and 49 μg/mL (range 39–58) for the 1 g dose. A 5-minute intravenous bolus injection of MERREM I.V. in normal volunteers results in mean peak plasma concentrations of approximately 45 μg/mL (range 18–65) for the 500 mg dose and 112 μg/mL (range 83–140) for the 1 g dose.

Following intravenous doses of 500 mg, mean plasma concentrations of meropenem usually decline to approximately 1 μg/mL at 6 hours after administration.

In subjects with normal renal function, the elimination half-life of MERREM I.V. is approximately 1 hour. Approximately 70% of the intravenously administered dose is recovered as unchanged meropenem in the urine over 12 hours, after which little further urinary excretion is detectable. Urinary concentrations of meropenem in excess of 10 μg/mL are maintained for up to 5 hours after a 500 mg dose. No accumulation of meropenem in plasma or urine was observed with regimens using 500 mg administered every 8 hours or 1 g administered every 6 hours in volunteers with normal renal function.

Plasma protein binding of meropenem is approximately 2%. There is one metabolite which is microbiologically inactive. Meropenem penetrates well into most body fluids and tissues including cerebrospinal fluid, achieving concentrations matching or exceeding those required to inhibit most susceptible bacteria. After a single intravenous dose of MERREM I.V., the highest mean concentrations of meropenem were found in tissues and fluids at 1 hour (0.5 to 1.5 hours) after the start of infusion, except where indicated in the tissues and fluids listed in the table below.

[See table at top of next page]

The pharmacokinetics of MERREM I.V. in pediatric patients 2 years of age or older are essentially similar to those in adults. The elimination half-life for meropenem was approximately 1.5 hours in pediatric patients of age 3 months to 2 years. The pharmacokinetics are linear over the dose range from 10 to 40 mg/kg.

Pharmacokinetic studies with MERREM I.V. in patients with renal insufficiency have shown that the plasma clearance of meropenem correlates with creatinine clearance. Dosage adjustments are necessary in subjects with renal impairment. (See **DOSAGE AND ADMINISTRATION-Use in Adults with Renal Impairment.**) A pharmacokinetic study with MERREM I.V. in elderly patients with renal insufficiency has shown a reduction in plasma clearance of meropenem that correlates with age-associated reduction in creatinine clearance.

Meropenem I.V. is hemodialyzable. However, there is no information on the usefulness of hemodialysis to treat overdosage. (See **OVERDOSAGE.**)

A pharmacokinetic study with MERREM I.V. in patients with hepatic impairment has shown no effects of liver disease on the pharmacokinetics of meropenem.

Microbiology

The bactericidal activity of meropenem results from the inhibition of cell wall synthesis. Meropenem readily penetrates the cell wall of most gram-positive and gram-negative bacteria to reach penicillin-binding-protein (PBP) tar-

Continued on next page

Merrem—Cont.

gets. Its strongest affinities are toward PBPs 2, 3 and 4 of *Escherichia coli* and *Pseudomonas aeruginosa*; and PBPs 1, 2 and 4 of *Staphylococcus aureus*. Bactericidal concentrations (defined as a 3 $\log_{10}$ reduction in cell counts within 12 to 24 hours) are typically 1–2 times the bacteriostatic concentrations of meropenem, with the exception of *Listeria monocytogenes*, against which lethal activity is not observed.

Meropenem has significant stability to hydrolysis by β-lactamases of most categories, both penicillinases and cephalosporinases produced by gram-positive and gram-negative bacteria, with the exception of metallo-β-lactamases. Meropenem should not be used to treat methicillin-resistant staphylococci. Cross-resistance is sometimes observed with strains resistant to other carbapenems.

In vitro tests show meropenem to act synergistically with aminoglycoside antibiotics against some isolates of *Pseudomonas aeruginosa*.

Meropenem has been shown to be active against most strains of the following microorganisms, both *in vitro* and in clinical infections as described in the **INDICATIONS AND USAGE** section.

Gram-Positive Aerobes
Streptococcus pneumoniae (excluding penicillin-resistant strains)
Viridans group streptococci

NOTE: Penicillin-resistant strains had meropenem MIC_{90} values of 1 or 2 μg/mL, which is above the 0.25 μg/mL susceptible breakpoint for this species.

Gram-Negative Aerobes
Escherichia coli
Haemophilus influenzae (β-lactamase and non-β-lactamase-producing)
Klebsiella pneumoniae
Neisseria meningitidis
Pseudomonas aeruginosa

Anaerobes
Bacteroides fragilis
Bacteroides thetaiotaomicron
Peptostreptococcus species

The following *in vitro* data are available, **but their clinical significance is unknown.**

Meropenem exhibits *in vitro* minimum inhibitory concentrations (MICs) of 0.25 μg/mL against most (≥ 90%) strains of *Streptococcus pneumoniae*, 0.5 μg/mL or less against most (≥ 90%) strains of *Haemophilus influenzae*, and 4 μg/mL or less against most (≥ 90%) strains of the other microorganisms in the following list; however, the safety and effectiveness of meropenem in treating clinical infections due to these microorganisms have not been established in adequate and well-controlled clinical trials.

Gram-Positive Aerobes
Staphylococcus aureus (β-lactamase and non β-lactamase producing)
Staphylococcus epidermidis (β-lactamase and non β-lactamase-producing)

NOTE: Staphylococci which are resistant to methicillin/oxacillin must be considered resistant to meropenem.

Gram-Negative Aerobes
Acinetobacter species
Aeromonas hydrophila
Campylobacter jejuni
Citrobacter diversus
Citrobacter freundii
Enterobacter cloacae
Haemophilus influenzae (ampicillin-resistant, non-β-lactamase producing strains [BLNAR strains])
Hafnia alvei
Klebsiella oxytoca
Moraxella catarrhalis (β-lactamase and non-β-lactamase-producing strains)
Morganella morganii
Pasteurella multocida
Proteus mirabilis
Proteus vulgaris
Salmonella species
Serratia marcescens
Shigella species
Yersinia enterocolitica

Anaerobes
Bacteroides distasonis
Bacteroides ovatus
Bacteroides uniformis
Bacteroides ureolyticus
Bacteroides vulgatus
Clostridium difficile
Clostridium perfringens
Eubacterium lentum
Fusobacterium species
Prevotella bivia
Prevotella intermedia
Prevotella melaninogenica
Porphyromonas asaccharolytica
Propionibacterium acnes

Susceptibility Tests

Dilution Techniques:
Quantitative methods are used to determine antimicrobial minimum inhibitory concentrations (MIC's). These MIC's provide estimates of the susceptibility of bacteria to antimicrobial compounds. The MIC's should be determined using a standardized procedure. Standardized procedures are based on a dilution method[1] (broth or agar) or equivalent with standardized inoculum concentrations and standardized concentrations of meropenem powder. The MIC values should be interpreted according to the following criteria for indicated aerobic organisms other than *Haemophilus* species and streptococci:

MIC (μg/mL)	Interpretation
≤ 4	(S) Susceptible
8	(I) Intermediate
≥ 16	(R) Resistant

Haemophilus Test Media (HTM) and the following interpretive criteria should be used when testing *Haemophilus* species:

MIC (μg/mL)	Interpretation
≤ 0.5	(S) Susceptible

The current absence of resistant strains precludes defining any categories other than "Susceptible". Strains yielding results suggestive of a "Nonsusceptible" category should be submitted to a reference laboratory for further testing.

The following criteria should be used when testing streptococci including *Streptococcus pneumoniae*.

When testing *S. pneumoniae*:

MIC (μg/mL)	Interpretation
≤ 0.12	(S) Susceptible
0.5	(I) Intermediate
≥ 1	(R) Resistant

When testing viridans group streptococci:

MIC (μg/mL)	Interpretation
≤ 0.5	(S) Susceptible

The current absence of resistant strains precludes defining any categories other than "Susceptible". Strains yielding results suggestive of a "Nonsusceptible" category should be submitted to a reference laboratory for further testing.

A report of 'Susceptible' indicates that the pathogen is likely to be inhibited if the antimicrobial compound in the blood reaches the concentrations usually achievable. A report of 'Intermediate' indicates that the result should be considered equivocal, and, if the microorganism is not fully susceptible to alternative, clinically feasible drugs, the test should be repeated. This category implies possible clinical applicability in body sites where the drug is physiologically concentrated or in situations where high dosage of drug can be used. This category also provides a buffer zone which prevents small uncontrolled technical factors from causing major discrepancies in interpretation. A report of 'Resistant' indicates that the pathogen is not likely to be inhibited if the antimicrobial compound in the blood reaches the concentrations usually achievable; other therapy should be selected.

Standardized susceptibility test procedures require the use of laboratory control microorganisms to control the technical aspects of the laboratory procedures. Standard meropenem powder should provide the following MIC values:

Microorganism	ATCC	MIC (μg/mL)
Enterococcus faecalis	29212	2.0–8.0
Escherichia coli	25922	0.008–0.06
Haemophilus influenzae	49766	0.03–0.12
Pseudomonas aeruginosa	27853	0.25–1.0
Streptococcus pneumoniae	49619	0.06–0.25

Diffusion Techniques:
Quantitative methods that require measurement of zone diameters also provide reproducible estimates of the susceptibility of bacteria to antimicrobial compounds. One such standardized procedure[2] requires the use of standardized inoculum concentrations. This procedure uses paper disks impregnated with 10–μg of meropenem to test the susceptibility of microorganisms to meropenem.

Reports from the laboratory providing results of the standard single-disk susceptibility test with a 10-μg disk should be interpreted according to the following criteria for indicated aerobic organisms other than *Haemophilus* species and streptococci:

Zone Diameter (mm)	Interpretation
≥ 16	(S) Susceptible
14–15	(I) Intermediate
≤ 13	(R) Resistant

Haemophilus Test Media and the following criteria should be used when testing *Haemophilus* species:

Zone Diameter (mm)	Interpretation
≥ 20	(S) Susceptible

The current absence of resistant strains precludes defining any categories other than "Susceptible". Strains yielding results suggestive of a "Nonsusceptible" category should be submitted to a reference laboratory for further testing.

Streptococcus pneumoniae isolates should be tested using 1-μg/mL oxacillin disk. Isolates with oxacillin zone sizes of ≥ 20 mm are susceptible (MIC ≤ 0.06 μg/mL) to penicillin and can be considered susceptible to meropenem for approved indications, and meropenem need not be tested. A meropenem MIC should be determined on isolates of *S. pneumoniae* with oxacillin zone sizes of ≤ 19 mm. The disk test does not distinguish penicillin intermediate strains (i.e., MIC's = 0.25–1.0 μg/mL) from strains that are penicillin resistant (i.e., MIC's ≥ 2 μg/mL). Viridans group streptococci should be tested for meropenem susceptibility using an MIC method. Reliable disk diffusion tests for meropenem do not yet exist for testing streptococci.

Interpretation should be as stated above for results using dilution techniques. Interpretation involves correlation of the diameter obtained in the disk test with the MIC for meropenem.

As with standardized dilution techniques, diffusion methods require the use of laboratory control microorganisms that are used to control the technical aspects of the laboratory procedures. For the diffusion technique, the 10-μg meropenem disk should provide the following zone diameters in these laboratory test quality control strains:

Microorganism	ATCC	Zone Diameter (mm)
Escherichia coli	25922	28–34
Haemophilus influenzae	49247	20–28
Pseudomonas aeruginosa	27853	27–33

Anaerobic Techniques:
For anaerobic bacteria, susceptibility to meropenem as MICs can be determined by standardized test methods.[3] The MIC values obtained should be interpreted according to the following criteria:

MIC (μg/mL)	Interpretation
≤ 4	(S) Susceptible
8	(I) Intermediate
≥ 16	(R) Resistant

Interpretation is identical to that stated above for results using dilution techniques.

As with other susceptibility techniques, the use of laboratory control microorganisms is required to control the technical aspects of the laboratory standardized procedures. Standardized meropenem powder should provide the following MIC values:

Microorganism	ATCC	MIC (μg/mL)
Bacteroides fragilis	25285	0.06–0.25
Bacteroides thetaiotaomicron	29741	0.125–0.5

INDICATIONS AND USAGE

MERREM I.V. is indicated as single agent therapy for the treatment of the following infections when caused by susceptible strains of the designated microorganisms:

Meropenem Concentrations in Selected Tissues (Highest Concentrations Reported)

Tissue	I.V. Dose (g)	Number of Samples	Mean [μg/mL or μg/(g)]***	Range [μg/mL or μg/(g)]
Endometrium	0.5	7	4.2	1.7–10.2
Myometrium	0.5	15	3.8	0.4–8.1
Ovary	0.5	8	2.8	0.8–4.8
Cervix	0.5	2	7.0	5.4–8.5
Fallopian tube	0.5	9	1.7	0.3–3.4
Skin	0.5	22	3.3	0.5–12.6
Skin	1.0	10	5.3	1.3–16.7
Colon	1.0	2	2.6	2.5–2.7
Bile	1.0	7	14.6 (3 h)	4.0–25.7
Gallbladder	1.0	1	—	3.9
Interstitial fluid	1.0	5	26.3	20.9–37.4
Peritoneal fluid	1.0	9	30.2	7.4–54.6
Lung	1.0	2	4.8 (2 h)	1.4–8.2
Bronchial mucosa	1.0	7	4.5	1.3–11.1
Muscle	1.0	2	6.1 (2 h)	5.3–6.9
Fascia	1.0	9	8.8	1.5–20
Heart valves	1.0	7	9.7	6.4–12.1
Myocardium	1.0	10	15.5	5.2–25.5
CSF (inflamed)	20 mg/kg*	8	1.1 (2 h)	0.2–2.8
	40 mg/kg**	5	3.3 (3 h)	0.9–6.5
CSF (uninflamed)	1.0	4	0.2 (2 h)	0.1–0.3

*in pediatric patients of age 5 months to 8 years
**in pediatric patients of age 1 month to 15 years
***at 1 hour unless otherwise noted

Intra-abdominal Infections
Complicated appendicitis and peritonitis caused by viridans group streptococci, *Escherichia coli, Klebsiella pneumoniae, Pseudomonas aeruginosa, Bacteroides fragilis, B. thetaiotaomicron,* and *Peptostreptococcus* species.

Bacterial Meningitis (Pediatric patients ≥ 3 months only)
Bacterial meningitis caused by *Streptococcus pneumoniae*‡, *Haemophilus influenzae* (β-lactamase and non-β-lactamase-producing strains), and *Neisseria meningitidis.*

‡The efficacy of meropenem as monotherapy in the treatment of meningitis caused by penicillin nonsusceptible strains of *Streptococcus pneumoniae* has not been established.

MERREM I.V. has been found to be effective in eliminating concurrent bacteremia in association with bacterial meningitis.

For information regarding use in pediatric patients (3 months of age and older) see **PRECAUTIONS - Pediatrics, ADVERSE REACTIONS,** and **DOSAGE AND ADMINISTRATION** sections.

Appropriate cultures should usually be performed before initiating antimicrobial treatment in order to isolate and identify the organisms causing infection and determine their susceptibility to MERREM I.V.

MERREM I.V. is useful as presumptive therapy in the indicated condition (i.e., intra-abdominal infections) prior to the identification of the causative organisms because of its broad spectrum of bactericidal activity.

Antimicrobial therapy should be adjusted, if appropriate, once the results of culture(s) and antimicrobial susceptibility testing are known.

CONTRAINDICATIONS

MERREM I.V. is contraindicated in patients with known hypersensitivity to any component of this product or to other drugs in the same class or in patients who have demonstrated anaphylactic reactions to β-lactams.

WARNINGS

SERIOUS AND OCCASIONALLY FATAL HYPERSENSITIVITY (ANAPHYLACTIC) REACTIONS HAVE BEEN REPORTED IN PATIENTS RECEIVING THERAPY WITH β-LACTAMS. THESE REACTIONS ARE MORE LIKELY TO OCCUR IN INDIVIDUALS WITH A HISTORY OF SENSITIVITY TO MULTIPLE ALLERGENS.

THERE HAVE BEEN REPORTS OF INDIVIDUALS WITH A HISTORY OF PENICILLIN HYPERSENSITIVITY WHO HAVE EXPERIENCED SEVERE HYPERSENSITIVITY REACTIONS WHEN TREATED WITH ANOTHER β-LACTAM. BEFORE INITIATING THERAPY WITH MERREM I.V., CAREFUL INQUIRY SHOULD BE MADE CONCERNING PREVIOUS HYPERSENSITIVITY REACTIONS TO PENICILLINS, CEPHALOSPORINS, OTHER β-LACTAMS, AND OTHER ALLERGENS. IF AN ALLERGIC REACTION TO MERREM I.V. OCCURS, DISCONTINUE THE DRUG IMMEDIATELY. **SERIOUS ANAPHYLACTIC REACTIONS REQUIRE IMMEDIATE EMERGENCY TREATMENT WITH EPINEPHRINE, OXYGEN, INTRAVENOUS STEROIDS, AND AIRWAY MANAGEMENT, INCLUDING INTUBATION. OTHER THERAPY MAY ALSO BE ADMINISTERED AS INDICATED.**

Seizures and other CNS adverse experiences have been reported during treatment with MERREM I.V. (See **PRECAUTIONS** and **ADVERSE REACTIONS**.)

Pseudomembranous colitis has been reported with nearly all antibacterial agents, including meropenem, and may range in severity from mild to life-threatening. Therefore, it is important to consider this diagnosis in patients who present with diarrhea subsequent to the administration of antibacterial agents.

Treatment with antibacterial agents alters the normal flora of the colon and may permit overgrowth of clostridia. Studies indicate that a toxin produced by *Clostridium difficile* is a primary cause of "antibiotic-associated colitis".

After the diagnosis of pseudomembranous colitis has been established, therapeutic measures should be initiated. Mild cases of pseudomembranous colitis usually respond to drug discontinuation alone. In moderate-to-severe cases, consideration should be given to management with fluids and electrolytes, protein supplementation, and treatment with an antibacterial drug clinically effective against *Clostridium difficile* colitis.

PRECAUTIONS

General: Seizures and other CNS adverse experiences have been reported during treatment with MERREM I.V. These experiences have occurred most commonly in patients with CNS disorders (e.g., brain lesions or history of seizures) or with bacterial meningitis and/or compromised renal function.

During the initial clinical investigations, 2038 immunocompetent adult patients were treated for infections outside the CNS with MERREM I.V. (500 mg or 1000 mg q 8 hours). Overall seizures, whether drug related or not, occurred in 0.5% of the meropenem-treated patients. All meropenem-treated patients with seizures had pre-existing contributing factors. Among these are included prior history of seizures or CNS abnormality and concomitant medications with seizure potential. Dosage adjustment is recommended in patients with advanced age and/or reduced renal function. (See **DOSAGE AND ADMINISTRATION - Use in Adults with Renal Impairment.**)

Close adherence to the recommended dosage regimens is urged, especially in patients with known factors that predispose to convulsive activity. Anticonvulsant therapy should be continued in patients with known seizure disorders. If focal tremors, myoclonus, or seizures occur, patients should be evaluated neurologically, placed on anticonvulsant therapy if not already instituted, and the dosage of MERREM I.V. re-examined to determine whether it should be decreased or the antibiotic discontinued.

In patients with renal dysfunction, thrombocytopenia has been observed but no clinical bleeding reported. (See **DOSAGE AND ADMINISTRATION - Use in Adults with Renal Impairment.**)

There is inadequate information regarding the use of MERREM I.V. in patients on hemodialysis.

As with other broad-spectrum antibiotics, prolonged use of meropenem may result in overgrowth of nonsusceptible organisms. Repeated evaluation of the patient is essential. If superinfection does occur during therapy, appropriate measures should be taken.

Laboratory Tests: While MERREM I.V. possesses the characteristic low toxicity of the beta-lactam group of antibiotics, periodic assessment of organ system functions, including renal, hepatic, and hematopoietic, is advisable during prolonged therapy.

Drug Interactions: Probenecid competes with meropenem for active tubular secretion and thus inhibits the renal excretion of meropenem. This led to statistically significant increases in the elimination half-life (38%) and in the extent of systemic exposure (56%). Therefore, the coadministration of probenecid with meropenem is not recommended.

Other than probenecid, no specific drug interaction studies were conducted.

Carcinogenesis, Mutagenesis, Impairment of Fertility:
Carcinogenesis: Carcinogenesis studies have not been performed.

Mutagenesis: Genetic toxicity studies were performed with meropenem using the bacterial reverse mutation test, the Chinese hamster ovary HGPRT assay, cultured human lymphocytes cytogenic assay, and the mouse micronucleus test. There was no evidence of mutagenic potential found in any of these tests.

Impairment of fertility: Reproductive studies were performed with meropenem in rats at doses up to 1000 mg/kg/day, and cynomolgus monkeys at doses up to 360 mg/kg/day (on the basis of AUC comparisons, approximately 1.8 times and 3.7 times, respectively, to the human exposure at the usual dose of 1 g every 8 hours). There was no reproductive toxicity seen.

Pregnancy Category B: Reproductive studies have been performed with meropenem in rats at doses of up to 1000 mg/kg/day, and cynomolgus monkeys at doses of up to 360 mg/kg/day (on the basis of AUC comparisons, approximately 1.8 times and 3.7 times respectively, to the human exposure at the usual dose of 1 g every 8 hours). These studies revealed no evidence of impaired fertility or harm to the fetus due to meropenem, although there were slight changes in fetal body weight at doses of 250 mg/kg/day (on the basis of AUC comparisons, 0.4 times the human exposure at a dose of 1 g every 8 hours) and above in rats. There are, however, no adequate and well-controlled studies in pregnant women. Because animal reproduction studies are not always predictive of human response, this drug should be used during pregnancy only if clearly needed.

Pediatrics: The safety and effectiveness of MERREM I.V. have been established for pediatric patients ≥ 3 months of age. Use of MERREM I.V. in pediatric patients with bacterial meningitis is supported by evidence from adequate and well-controlled studies in the pediatric population. Use of MERREM I.V. in pediatric patients with intra-abdominal infections is supported by evidence from adequate and well-controlled studies with adults with additional data from pediatric pharmacokinetics studies and controlled clinical trials in pediatric patients. (See **CLINICAL PHARMACOLOGY, INDICATIONS AND USAGE, ADVERSE REACTIONS, DOSAGE AND ADMINISTRATION,** and **CLINICAL STUDIES** sections.)

Nursing Mothers: It is not known whether this drug is excreted in human milk. Because many drugs are excreted in human milk, caution should be exercised when MERREM I.V. is administered to a nursing woman.

Geriatric Use: Of the total number of subjects in clinical studies of MERREM I.V., approximately 1100 (30%) were 65 years of age and older, while 400 (11%) were 75 years and older. No overall differences in safety or effectiveness were observed between these subjects and younger subjects; spontaneous reports and other reported clinical experience have not identified differences in responses between the elderly and younger patients, but greater sensitivity of some older individuals cannot be ruled out.

A pharmacokinetic study with MERREM I.V. in elderly patients with renal insufficiency has shown a reduction in plasma clearance of meropenem that correlates with age-associated reduction in creatinine clearance. (See **DOSAGE AND ADMINISTRATION; Use in Adults with Renal Impairment:**).

MERREM I.V. is known to be substantially excreted by the kidney, and the risk of toxic reactions to this drug may be greater in patients with impaired renal function. Because elderly patients are more likely to have decreased renal function, care should be taken in dose selection, and it may be useful to monitor renal function.

ADVERSE REACTIONS

Adult Patients:
During the initial clinical investigations, 2038 immunocompetent adult patients were treated for infections outside the CNS with MERREM I.V. (500 mg or 1000 mg q 8 hours). Deaths in 3 patients were assessed as possibly related to meropenem; 28 (1.4%) patients had meropenem discontinued because of adverse events. Many patients in these trials were severely ill and had multiple background diseases, physiological impairments and were receiving multiple other drug therapies. In the seriously ill population, it was not possible to determine the relationship between observed adverse events and therapy with MERREM I.V.

The following adverse reaction frequencies were derived from the clinical trials in the 2038 patients treated with MERREM I.V.

Local Adverse Reactions
Local adverse reactions that were reported irrespective of the relationship to therapy with MERREM I.V. were as follows:

Inflammation at the injection site	3.0%
Phlebitis/thrombophlebitis	1.2%
Injection site reaction	1.1%
Pain at the injection site	0.4%
Edema at the injection site	0.2%

Systemic Adverse Reactions
Systemic adverse clinical reactions that were reported irrespective of the relationship to MERREM I.V. occurring in greater than 1.0% of the patients were diarrhea (5.0%), nausea/vomiting (3.9%), headache (2.8%), rash (1.7%), pruritus (1.6%), apnea (1.2%), and constipation (1.2%).

Additional adverse systemic clinical reactions that were reported irrespective of relationship to therapy with MERREM I.V. and occurring in less than 1.0% but greater than 0.1% of the patients are listed below within each body system in order of decreasing frequency:

Bleeding events [gastrointestinal hemorrhage, melena, epistaxis, and hemoperitoneum] occurred in 0.7% of meropenem patients.

Body as a Whole: pain, abdominal pain, chest pain, sepsis, shock, fever, abdominal enlargement, back pain, hepatic failure

Cardiovascular: heart failure, heart arrest, tachycardia, hypertension, myocardial infarction, pulmonary embolus, bradycardia, hypotension, syncope

Digestive System: oral moniliasis, anorexia, cholestatic jaundice/jaundice, flatulence, ileus

Hemic/Lymphatic: anemia

Metabolic/Nutritional: peripheral edema, hypoxia

Nervous System: insomnia, agitation/delirium, confusion, dizziness, seizure (see **PRECAUTIONS**), nervousness, paresthesia, hallucinations, somnolence, anxiety, depression

Respiratory: respiratory disorder, dyspnea

Skin and Appendages: urticaria, sweating

Urogenital System: dysuria, kidney failure

Adverse Laboratory Changes
Adverse laboratory changes that were reported irrespective of relationship to MERREM I.V. and occurring in greater than 0.2% of the patients were as follows:

Hepatic: increased SGPT (ALT), SGOT (AST), alkaline phosphatase, LDH, and bilirubin

Hematologic: increased platelets, increased eosinophils, prolonged prothrombin time, prolonged partial thromboplastin time, decreased platelets, positive direct or indirect Coombs test, decreased hemoglobin, decreased hematocrit, decreased WBC, shortened prothrombin time and shortened partial thromboplastin time.

Renal: increased creatinine and increased BUN

NOTE: It is not known if the safety profile of MERREM I.V. is changed in patients with varying degrees of renal impairment.

Urinalysis: presence of urine red blood cells

Pediatric Patients:

Clinical Adverse Reactions
MERREM I.V. was studied in 417 pediatric patients (≥ 3 months to <13 years of age) with serious bacterial infections at dosages of 10 to 20 mg/kg every 8 hours. The types of clinical adverse events seen in these patients are similar to the adults, with the most common adverse events reported as possibly, probably or definitely related to MERREM I.V. and their rates of occurrence as follows:

Diarrhea	4.3%
Rash	1.4%
Vomiting	1.0%

MERREM I.V. was studied in 198 pediatric patients (≥ 3 months to <17 years of age) with meningitis at a dosage of 40 mg/kg every 8 hours. The types of clinical adverse events seen in these patients are similar to the adults, with the most common adverse events reported as possibly, probably, or definitely related to MERREM I.V. and their rates of occurrence as follows:

Rash (mostly diaper area moniliasis)	3.5%
Diarrhea	3.5%
Oral Moniliasis	2.0%
Glossitis	1.0%

In the meningitis studies the rates of seizure activity during therapy were comparable between patients with no CNS abnormalities who received meropenem and those who received comparator agents (either cefotaxime or ceftriaxone). In the MERREM I.V. treated group, 12/15 patients with seizures had late onset seizures (defined as occurring on day 3 or later) versus 7/20 in the comparator arm.

Adverse Laboratory Changes:
Laboratory abnormalities seen in the pediatric-aged patients in both the pediatric and the meningitis studies are similar to those reported in adult patients.

There is no experience in pediatric patients with renal impairment.

Post-marketing Experience:
No post-marketing experience is available.

Continued on next page

Merrem—Cont.

OVERDOSAGE

In mice and rats, large intravenous doses of meropenem (2200-4000 mg/kg) have been associated with ataxia, dyspnea, convulsions, and mortalities.

Intentional overdosing of MERREM I.V. is unlikely, although accidental overdosing might occur if large doses are given to patients with reduced renal function. The largest dose of meropenem administered in clinical trials has been 2 g given intravenously every 8 hours. At this dosage, no adverse pharmacological effects or increased safety risks have been observed.

No specific information is available for the treatment of MERREM I.V. overdosage. In the event of an overdose, MERREM I.V. should be discontinued and general supportive treatment given until renal elimination takes place. Meropenem and its metabolite are readily dialyzable and effectively removed by hemodialysis; however, no information is available on the use of hemodialysis to treat overdosage.

CLINICAL STUDIES

Intra-abdominal:

One controlled clinical study of complicated intra-abdominal infection was performed in the United States where meropenem was compared to clindamycin/tobramycin. Three controlled clinical studies of complicated intra-abdominal infections were performed in Europe; meropenem was compared to imipenem (two trials) and cefotaxime/metronidazole (one trial).

Using strict evaluability criteria and microbiologic eradication and clinical cures at follow-up which occurred 7 or more days after completion of therapy, the following presumptive microbiologic eradication/clinical cure rates and statistical findings were obtained:

[See table above]

Treatment Arm	No. evaluable/ No. enrolled (%)	Microbiologic Eradication Rate	Clinical Cure Rate	Outcome
meropenem	146/516 (28%)	98/146 (67%)	101/146 (69%)	
imipenem	65/220 (30%)	40/65 (62%)	42/65 (65%)	Meropenem equivalent to control
cefotaxime/ metronidazole	26/85 (30%)	22/26 (85%)	22/26 (85%)	Meropenem not equivalent to control
clindamycin/ tobramycin	50/212 (24%)	38/50 (76%)	38/50 (76%)	Meropenem equivalent to control

The finding that meropenem was not statistically equivalent to cefotaxime/metronidazole may have been due to uneven assignment of more seriously ill patients to the meropenem arm. Currently there is no additional information available to further interpret this observation.

Bacterial Meningitis:

Four hundred forty-six patients (397 pediatric patients ≥ 3 months to < 17 years of age) were enrolled in 4 separate clinical trials and randomized to treatment with meropenem (n=225) at a dose of 40 mg/kg q 8 hours or a comparator drug, i.e., cefotaxime (n=187) or ceftriaxone (n=34), at the approved dosing regimens. A comparable number of patients were found to be clinically evaluable (ranging from 61–68%) and with a similar distribution of pathogens isolated on initial CSF culture.

Patients were defined as clinically not cured if any one of the following three criteria were met:

1. At the 5–7 week post-completion of therapy visit, the patient had any one of the following: moderate to severe motor, behavior or development deficits, hearing loss of >60 decibels in one or both ears, or blindness.
2. During therapy the patient's clinical status necessitated the addition of other antibiotics.
3. Either during or post-therapy, the patient developed a large subdural effusion needing surgical drainage, or a cerebral abscess, or a bacteriologic relapse.

Using the definition, the following efficacy rates were obtained, per organism. The values represent the number of patients clinically cured/number of clinically evaluable patients, with the percent cure in parentheses.

MICROORGANISM	MERREM I.V.	COMPARATOR
S. pneumoniae	17/24 (71)	19/30 (63)
H. influenzae (+)	8/10 (80)	6/6 (100)
H. influenzae (-/NT)	44/59 (75)	44/60 (73)
N. meningitidis	30/35 (86)	35/39 (90)
TOTAL (including others)	102/131 (78)	108/140 (77)

(+) β-lactamase-producing; (-/NT) non-β-lactamase-producing or not tested

Sequelae were the most common reason patients were assessed as clinically not cured.

Five patients were found to be bacteriologically not cured, 3 in the comparator group (1 relapse and 2 patients with cerebral abscesses) and 2 in the meropenem group (1 relapse and 1 with continued growth of *Pseudomonas aeruginosa).*

The adverse events seen were comparable between the two treatment groups both in type and frequency. The meropenem group did have a statistically higher number of patients with transient elevation of liver enzymes. (See **ADVERSE REACTIONS**.) Rates of seizure activity during therapy were comparable between patients with no CNS abnormalities who received meropenem and those who received comparator agents. In the MERREM I.V. treated group, 12/15 patients with seizures had late onset seizures (defined as occurring on day 3 or later) versus 7/20 in the comparator arm.

With respect to hearing loss, 263 of the 271 evaluable patients had at least one hearing test performed post-therapy. The following table shows the degree of hearing loss between the meropenem-treated patients and the comparator-treated patients.

Degree of Hearing Loss (in one or both ears)	Meropenem n=128	Comparator n=135
No loss	61%	56%
20–40 decibels	20%	24%
>40–60 decibels	8%	7%
>60 decibels	9%	10%

DOSAGE AND ADMINISTRATION

Adults: One gram (1 g) by intravenous administration every 8 hours. MERREM I.V. should be given by intravenous infusion, over approximately 15 to 30 minutes or as an intravenous bolus injection (5 to 20 mL) over approximately 3–5 minutes.

Use in Adults with Renal Impairment: Dosage should be reduced in patients with creatinine clearance less than 51 mL/min. (see dosing table below).

Recommended MERREM I.V. Dosage Schedule for Adults With Impaired Renal Function

Creatinine Clearance (mL/min)	Dose (dependent on type of infection)	Dosing Interval
26–50	recommended dose (1000 mg)	every 12 hours
10–25	one-half recommended dose	every 12 hours
<10	one-half recommended dose	every 24 hours

When only serum creatinine is available, the following formula (Cockcroft and Gault equation)[4] may be used to estimate creatinine clearance.

Males: Creatinine Clearance (mL/min) =

$$\frac{\text{Weight (kg)} \times (140 - \text{age})}{72 \times \text{serum creatinine (mg/dL)}}$$

Females: 0.85 × above value

There is inadequate information regarding the use of MERREM I.V. in patients on hemodialysis.

There is no experience with peritoneal dialysis.

Use in Adults With Hepatic Insufficiency: No dosage adjustment is necessary in patients with impaired hepatic function.

Use in Elderly Patients: No dosage adjustment is required for elderly patients with creatinine clearance values above 50 mL/min.

Use in Pediatric Patients: For pediatric patients from 3 months of age and older, the MERREM I.V. dose is 20 or 40 mg/kg every 8 hours (maximum dose is 2 g every 8 hours), depending on the type of infection (intra-abdominal or meningitis). (See Dosing Table Below.) Pediatric patients weighing over 50 kg should be administered MERREM I.V. at a dose of 1 g every 8 hours for intra-abdominal infections and 2 g every 8 hours for meningitis. MERREM I.V. should be given as intravenous infusion over approximately 15 to 30 minutes or as an intravenous bolus injection (5 to 20 mL) over approximately 3–5 minutes.

Recommended MERREM I.V. Dosage Schedule for Pediatrics With Normal Renal Function

Type of Infection	Dose (mg/kg)	Dosing Interval
Intra-abdominal	20	every 8 hours
Meningitis	40	every 8 hours

There is no experience in pediatric patients with renal impairment.

PREPARATION OF SOLUTION

For Intravenous Bolus Administration

Constitute injection vials (500 mg and 1 g) with sterile Water for Injection. (See table below.) Shake to dissolve and let stand until clear.

Vial Size	Amount of Diluent Added (mL)	Approximate Withdrawable Volume (mL)	Approximate Average Concentration (mg/mL)
500 mg	10	10	50
1 g	20	20	50

For Infusion

Infusion vials (500 mg and 1 g) may be directly constituted with a compatible infusion fluid. (See **COMPATIBILITY AND STABILITY**.) Alternatively, an injection vial may be constituted, then the resulting solution added to an I.V. container and further diluted with an appropriate infusion fluid. (See **COMPATIBILITY AND STABILITY**.)

NOTE: ADD-VANTAGE VIALS ARE NOT TO BE USED IN THIS MANNER.

For ADD-Vantage Vials

ADD-Vantage vials of MERREM I.V. are to be constituted only with Sodium Chloride Injection 0.45%, Sodium Chloride Injection 0.9% or Dextrose Injection 5% in the 50, 100, and 250 mL Abbott ADD-Vantage® flexible diluent containers. MERREM I.V. supplied in single-use ADD-Vantage vials should be prepared as directed.

DIRECTIONS FOR USE OF MERREM I.V. (meropenem for injection) IN ADD-VANTAGE VIALS:

To Open Diluent Container: Peel overwrap from the corner and remove from container. Some opacity of the plastic due to moisture absorption during the sterilization process may be observed. This is normal and does not affect the solution quality or safety. The opacity will diminish gradually.

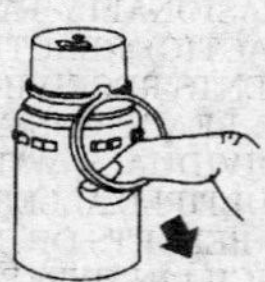

Figure 1

To Assemble ADD-Vantage Vial and Flexible Diluent Container: (Use Aseptic Technique)

1. Remove the protective covers from the top of the vial and the vial port on the diluent container as follows:
   a. To remove the breakaway vial cap, swing the pull ring over the top of the vial and pull down far enough to start the opening (See Figure 1), then pull straight up to remove the cap. (See Figure 2.)
   NOTE: Once the breakaway cap has been removed, do not access vial with syringe.

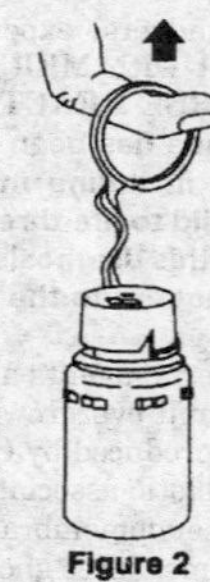

Figure 2

   b. To remove the vial port cover, grasp the tab on the pull ring, pull up to break the three tie strings, then pull back to remove the cover. (See Figure 3.)

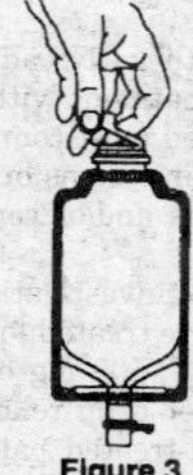

Figure 3

2. Screw the vial into the vial port until it will go no further. THE VIAL MUST BE SCREWED IN TIGHTLY TO ASSURE A SEAL. This occurs approximately ½ turn (180°) after the first audible click. (See Figure 4.) The clicking sound does not assure a seal; the vial must be turned as far as it will go.
   NOTE: ONCE VIAL IS SEATED, DO NOT ATTEMPT TO REMOVE.

3. Recheck the vial to assure that it is tight by trying to turn it further in the direction of assembly.
4. Label appropriately.

To Prepare Admixture:

1. Squeeze the bottom of the diluent container gently to inflate the portion of the container surrounding the end of the drug vial.

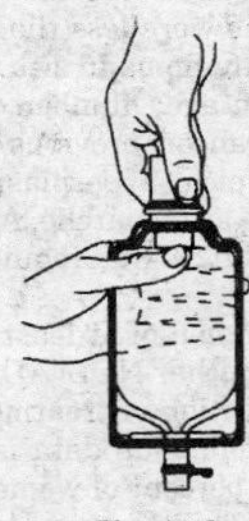

Figure 4

2. With the other hand, push the drug vial down into the container telescoping the walls of the container. Grasp the inner cap of the vial through the walls of the container. (See Figure 5.)

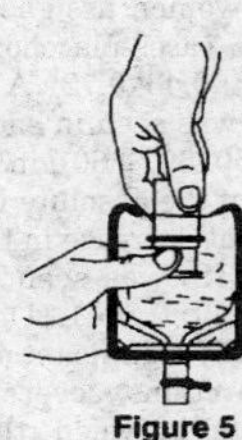

Figure 5

3. Pull the inner cap from the drug vial. (See Figure 6.) Verify that the rubber stopper has been pulled out and invert the system several times, allowing the drug and diluent to mix.

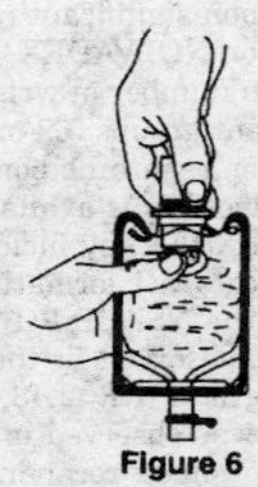

Figure 6

4. Mix contents thoroughly and use within the specified time.

Preparation For Administration: (Use Aseptic Technique)

1. Confirm the activation and admixture of vial contents.
2. Check for leaks by squeezing container firmly. If leaks are found, discard unit as sterility may be impaired.
3. Close flow control clamp of administration set.
4. Remove cover from outlet port at bottom of container.
5. Insert piercing pin of administration set into port with a twisting motion until the pin is firmly seated. **NOTE:** See full directions on administration set carton.
6. Lift the free end of the hanger loop on the bottom of the vial, breaking the two tie strings. Bend the loop outward to lock it in the upright position, then suspend container from hanger.
7. Squeeze and release drip chamber to establish proper fluid level in chamber.
8. Open flow control clamp and clear air from set. Close clamp.
9. Attach set to venipuncture device. If device is not indwelling, prime and make venipuncture.
10. Regulate rate of administration with flow control clamp.

WARNING: Do not use flexible container in series connections.

COMPATIBILITY AND STABILITY

Compatibility of MERREM I.V. with other drugs has not been established. MERREM I.V. should not be mixed with or physically added to solutions containing other drugs.

Freshly prepared solutions of MERREM I.V. should be used whenever possible. However, constituted solutions of MERREM I.V. maintain satisfactory potency at controlled room temperature 15–25°C (59–77°F) or under refrigeration at 4°C (39°F) as described below. Solutions of intravenous MERREM I.V. should not be frozen.

Intravenous Bolus Administration

MERREM I.V. injection vials constituted with sterile Water for Injection for bolus administration (up to 50 mg/mL of MERREM I.V.) may be stored for up to 2 hours at controlled room temperature 15–25°C (59–77°F) or for up to 12 hours at 4°C (39°F).

Intravenous Infusion Administration

Stability in Infusion Vials: MERREM I.V. infusion vials constituted with Sodium Chloride Injection 0.9% (MERREM I.V. concentrations ranging from 2.5 to 50 mg/mL) are stable for up to 2 hours at controlled room temperature 15–25°C (59–77°F) or for up to 18 hours at 4°C (39°F). Infusion vials of MERREM I.V. constituted with Dextrose Injection 5% (MERREM I.V. concentrations ranging from 2.5 to 50 mg/mL) are stable for up to 1 hour at controlled room temperature 15–25°C (59–77°F) or for up to 8 hours at 4°C (39°F).

Stability in Plastic I.V. Bags: Solutions prepared for infusion (MERREM I.V. concentrations ranging from 1 to 20 mg/mL) may be stored in plastic intravenous bags with diluents as shown below:

	Number of Hours Stable at Controlled Room Temperature 15–25°C (59–77°F)	Number of Hours Stable at 4°C (39°F)
Sodium Chloride Injection 0.9%	4	24
Dextrose Injection 5.0%	1	4
Dextrose Injection 10.0%	1	2
Dextrose and Sodium Chloride Injection 5.0%/0.9%	1	2
Dextrose and Sodium Chloride Injection 5.0%/0.2%	1	4
Potassium Chloride in Dextrose Injection 0.15%/5.0%	1	6
Sodium Bicarbonate in Dextrose Injection 0.02%/5.0%	1	6
Dextrose Injection 5.0% in Normosol®-M	1	8
Dextrose Injection 5.0% in Ringers Lactate Injection	1	4
Dextrose and Sodium Chloride Injection 2.5%/0.45%	3	12
Mannitol Injection 2.5%	2	16
Ringers Injection	4	24
Ringers Lactate Injection	4	12
Sodium Lactate Injection 1/6 N	2	24
Sodium Bicarbonate Injection 5.0%	1	4

Stability in Baxter Minibag Plus: Solutions of MERREM I.V. (MERREM I.V. concentrations ranging from 2.5 to 20 mg/mL) in Baxter Minibag Plus bags with Sodium Chloride Injection 0.9% may be stored for up to 4 hours at controlled room temperatures 15–25°C (59–77°F) or for up to 24 hours at 4°C (39°F). Solutions of MERREM I.V. (MERREM I.V. concentrations ranging from 2.5 to 20 mg/mL) in Baxter Minibag Plus bags with Dextrose Injection 5.0% may be stored up to 1 hour at controlled room temperatures 15–25°C (59–77°F) or for up to 6 hours at 4°C (39°F).

Stability in Plastic Syringes, Tubing and Intravenous Infusion Sets: Solutions of MERREM I.V. (MERREM I.V. concentrations ranging from 1 to 20 mg/mL) in Water for Injection or Sodium Chloride Injection 0.9% (for up to 4 hours) or in Dextrose Injection 5.0% (for up to 2 hours) at controlled room temperatures 15–25°C (59–77°F) are stable in plastic tubing and volume control devices of common intravenous infusion sets. Solutions of MERREM I.V. (MERREM I.V. concentrations ranging from 1 to 20mg/mL) in Water for Injection or Sodium Chloride Injection 0.9% (for up to 48 hours) or in Dextrose Injection 5% (for up to 6 hours) are stable at 4°C (39°F) in plastic syringes.

ADD-Vantage Vials: ADD-Vantage vials diluted in Sodium Chloride Injection 0.45% (MERREM I.V. concentrations ranging from 5 to 20 mg/mL) may be stored for up to 6 hours at controlled room temperature 15–25°C (59–77°F) or for 24 hours at 4°C (39°F). ADD-Vantage vials diluted in Sodium Chloride Injection 0.9% (MERREM I.V. concentrations ranging from 1–20 mg/mL) may be stored for up to 4 hours at controlled room temperature 15–25°C (59–77°F) or for 24 hours at 4°C (39°F). ADD-Vantage vials diluted with Dextrose Injection 5.0% (MERREM I.V. concentrations ranging from 1–20 mg/mL) may be stored for up to 1 hour at controlled room temperature 15–25°C (59–77°F) or for 8 hours at 4°C (39°F).

NOTE: Parenteral drug products should be inspected visually for particulate matter and discoloration prior to administration, whenever solution and container permit.

HOW SUPPLIED

MERREM I.V. is supplied in 20 mL and 30 mL injection vials containing sufficient meropenem to deliver 500 mg or 1 g for intravenous administration, respectively. MERREM I.V. is supplied in 100 mL infusion vials containing sufficient meropenem to deliver 500 mg or 1 g for intravenous administration. The dry powder should be stored at controlled room temperature 20–25°C (68–77°F) [see USP].

MERREM I.V. is also supplied as ADD-Vantage Vials containing sufficient meropenem to deliver 500 mg or 1 g for intravenous administration.

500 mg Injection Vial (NDC 0310-0325-20)
500 mg Infusion Vial (NDC 0310-0325-11)
1 g Injection Vial (NDC 0310-0321-30)
1 g Infusion Vial (NDC 0310-0321-11)
500 mg ADD-Vantage (NDC 0310-0325-15)
1 g ADD-Vantage (NDC 0310-0321-15)

REFERENCES

1. National Committee for Clinical Laboratory Standards. Methods for Dilution Antimicrobial Susceptibility Tests for Bacteria that Grow Aerobically — Third Edition. Approved Standard NCCLS Document M7-A3, Vol. 13, No. 25, NCCLS, Villanova, PA, December, 1993.
2. National Committee for Clinical Laboratory Standards. Performance Standards for Antimicrobial Disk Susceptibility Tests — Fifth Edition. Approved Standard NCCLS Document M2-A5, Vol. 13, No. 24, NCCLS, Villanova, PA. December 1993.
3. National Committee for Clinical Laboratory Standards. Methods for Antimicrobial Susceptibility Testing of Anaerobic Bacteria – Third Edition. Approved Standard NCCLS Document M11-A3, Vol. 13, No. 26, NCCLS, Villanova, PA. December 1993.
4. Cockcroft DW, Gault MH. Prediction of creatinine clearance from serum creatinine. Nephron. 1976; 16:31-41.

†ADD-Vantage is a registered trademark of Abbott Laboratories Inc.

ZENECA

Manufactured for:
Zeneca Pharmaceuticals
A Business Unit of Zeneca Inc.
Wilmington, Delaware 19850-5437
By: Sumitomo Pharmaceuticals Co., Ltd.
Ibaraki-shi, Osaka 567, Japan
Made in Japan
SIC 64155-02 Rev G 8/99

Shown in Product Identification Guide, page 305

NOLVADEX® ℞

[*nol 'va-dex*]
tamoxifen citrate

DESCRIPTION

NOLVADEX® (tamoxifen citrate) Tablets, a nonsteroidal antiestrogen, are for oral administration. NOLVADEX Tablets are available as:

10 mg Tablets. Each tablet contains 15.2 mg of tamoxifen citrate which is equivalent to 10 mg of tamoxifen.

20 mg Tablets. Each tablet contains 30.4 mg of tamoxifen citrate which is equivalent to 20 mg of tamoxifen.

Inactive Ingredients: carboxymethylcellulose calcium, magnesium stearate, mannitol and starch.

Chemically, NOLVADEX is the trans-isomer of a triphenylethylene derivative. The chemical name is (Z)2-[4-(1,2-diphenyl-1-butenyl) phenoxy]-N, N-dimethylethanamine 2-hydroxy-1,2,3- propanetricarboxylate (1:1). The structural and empirical formulas are:

$(CH_3)_2N(CH_2)_2O$— C = C — C_2H_5 • $C_6H_8O_7$
$(C_{32}H_{37}NO_8)$

Tamoxifen citrate has a molecular weight of 563.62, the pKa' is 8.85, the equilibrium solubility in water at 37°C is 0.5 mg/mL and in 0.02 N HCl at 37°C, it is 0.2 mg/mL.

CLINICAL PHARMACOLOGY

NOLVADEX is a nonsteroidal agent that has demonstrated potent antiestrogenic properties in animal test systems. The antiestrogenic effects may be related to its ability to compete with estrogen for binding sites in target tissues such as breast. Tamoxifen inhibits the induction of rat mammary carcinoma induced by dimethylbenzanthracene (DMBA) and causes the regression of already established DMBA-induced tumors. In this rat model, tamoxifen appears to exert its antitumor effects by binding the estrogen receptors. In cytosols derived from human breast adenocarcinomas, tamoxifen competes with estradiol for estrogen receptor protein.

Tamoxifen is extensively metabolized after oral administration. Studies in women receiving 20 mg of ^{14}C tamoxifen have shown that approximately 65% of the administered dose is excreted from the body over a period of 2 weeks with fecal excretion the primary route of elimination. The drug is excreted mainly as polar conjugates, with unchanged drug and unconjugated metabolites accounting for less than 30% of the total fecal radioactivity.

N-desmethyl tamoxifen is the major metabolite found in patients' plasma. The biological activity of N-desmethyl tamoxifen appears to be similar to that of tamoxifen. 4-Hydroxytamoxifen and a side chain primary alcohol derivative of tamoxifen have been identified as minor metabolites in plasma.

Following a single oral dose of 20 mg tamoxifen, an average peak plasma concentration of 40 ng/mL (range 35 to 45 ng/mL) occurred approximately 5 hours after dosing. The decline in plasma concentrations of tamoxifen is biphasic with a terminal elimination half-life of about 5 to 7 days. The average peak plasma concentration of N-desmethyl tamoxifen is 15 ng/mL (range 10 to 20 ng/mL). Chronic administration of 10 mg tamoxifen given twice daily for 3

Continued on next page

Nolvadex—Cont.

months to patients results in average steady-state plasma concentrations of 120 ng/mL (range 67–183 ng/mL) for tamoxifen and 336 ng/mL (range 148–654 ng/mL) for N-desmethyl tamoxifen. The average steady-state plasma concentrations of tamoxifen and N-desmethyl tamoxifen after administration of 20 mg tamoxifen once daily for 3 months are 122 ng/mL (range 71–183 ng/mL) and 353 ng/mL (range 152–706 ng/mL), respectively. After initiation of therapy, steady state concentrations for tamoxifen are achieved in about 4 weeks and steady state concentrations for N-desmethyl tamoxifen are achieved in about 8 weeks, suggesting a half-life of approximately 14 days for this metabolite.

In a 3-month crossover steady-state bioavailability study with NOLVADEX 10 mg twice a day vs. NOLVADEX 20 mg given once daily, NOLVADEX 20 mg taken once daily had similar bioavailability to NOLVADEX 10 mg taken twice a day.

Clinical Studies—Metastatic Breast Cancer

Premenopausal Women (NOLVADEX vs. Ablation)—Three prospective, randomized studies (Ingle, Pritchard, Buchanan) compared NOLVADEX to ovarian ablation (oophorectomy or ovarian irradiation) in premenopausal women with advanced breast cancer. Although the objective response rate, time to treatment failure, and survival were similar with both treatments, the limited patient accrual prevented a demonstration of equivalence. In an overview analysis of survival data from the 3 studies, the hazard ratio for death (NOLVADEX/ovarian ablation) was 1.00 with two-sided 95% confidence intervals of 0.73 to 1.37. Elevated serum and plasma estrogens have been observed in premenopausal women receiving NOLVADEX, but the data from the randomized studies do not suggest an adverse effect of this increase. A limited number of premenopausal patients with disease progression during NOLVADEX therapy responded to subsequent ovarian ablation.

Male Breast Cancer—Published results from 122 patients (119 evaluable) and case reports in 16 patients (13 evaluable) treated with NOLVADEX have shown that NOLVADEX is effective for the palliative treatment of male breast cancer. Sixty-six of these 132 evaluable patients responded to NOLVADEX which constitutes a 50% objective response rate.

Clinical Studies—Adjuvant Breast Cancer

Overview—The Early Breast Cancer Trialists' Collaborative Group (EBCTCG) conducted worldwide overviews of systemic adjuvant therapy for early breast cancer in 1985, 1990, and again in 1995. In 1998, 10-year outcome data were reported for 36,689 women in 55 randomized trials of adjuvant NOLVADEX using doses of 20–40 mg/day for 1–5+ years. Twenty-five percent of patients received 1 year or less of trial treatment, 52% received 2 years, and 23% received about 5 years. Forty-eight percent of tumors were estrogen receptor (ER) positive (>10 fmol/mg), 21% were ER poor (<10 fmol/l), and 31% were ER unknown. Among 29,441 patients with ER positive or unknown breast cancer, 58% were entered into trials comparing NOLVADEX to no adjuvant therapy and 42% were entered into trials comparing NOLVADEX in combination with chemotherapy vs. the same chemotherapy alone. Among these patients, 54% had node positive disease and 46% had node negative disease.

Among women with ER positive or unknown breast cancer and positive nodes who received about 5 years of treatment, overall survival at 10 years was 61.4% for NOLVADEX vs. 50.5% for control (logrank 2p < 0.00001). The recurrence free rate at 10 years was 59.7% for NOLVADEX vs. 44.5% for control (logrank 2p < 0.00001). Among women with ER positive or unknown breast cancer and negative nodes who received about 5 years of treatment, overall survival at 10 years was 78.9% for NOLVADEX vs. 73.3% for control (logrank 2p < 0.00001). The recurrence free rate at 10 years was 79.2% for NOLVADEX versus 64.3% for control (logrank 2p < 0.00001).

The effect of the scheduled duration of tamoxifen may be described as follows. In women with ER positive or unknown breast cancer receiving 1 year or less, 2 years or about 5 years of NOLVADEX, the proportional reductions in mortality were 12%, 17% and 26%, respectively (trend significant at 2p < 0.003). The corresponding reductions in breast cancer recurrence were 21%, 29% and 47% (trend significant at 2p < 0.00001).

Benefit is less clear for women with ER poor breast cancer in whom the proportional reduction in recurrence was 10% (2p = 0.007) for all durations taken together, or 9% (2p = 0.02) if contralateral breast cancers are excluded. The corresponding reduction in mortality was 6% (NS). The effects of about 5 years of NOLVADEX on recurrence and mortality were similar regardless of age and concurrent chemotherapy. There was no indication that doses greater than 20 mg per day were more effective.

Node Positive—Individual Studies—Two studies (Hubay and NSABP B-09) demonstrated an improved disease-free survival following radical or modified radical mastectomy in postmenopausal women or women 50 years of age or older with surgically curable breast cancer with positive axillary nodes when NOLVADEX was added to adjuvant cytotoxic chemotherapy. In the Hubay study, NOLVADEX was added to "low-dose" CMF (cyclophosphamide, methotrexate and fluorouracil). In the NSABP B-09 study, NOLVADEX was added to melphalan [L-phenylalanine mustard (P)] and fluorouracil (F).

In the Hubay study, patients with a positive (more than 3 fmol) estrogen receptor were more likely to benefit. In the NSABP B-09 study in women age 50–59 years, only women with both estrogen and progesterone receptor levels 10 fmol or greater clearly benefited, while there was a nonstatistically significant trend toward adverse effect in women with both estrogen and progesterone receptor levels less than 10 fmol. In women age 60–70 years, there was a trend toward a beneficial effect of NOLVADEX without any clear relationship to estrogen or progesterone receptor status.

Three prospective studies (ECOG-1178, Toronto, NATO) using NOLVADEX adjuvantly as a single agent demonstrated an improved disease-free survival following total mastectomy and axillary dissection for postmenopausal women with positive axillary nodes compared to placebo/no treatment controls. The NATO study also demonstrated an overall survival benefit.

Node Negative—Individual Studies—NSABP B-14, a prospective, double-blind, randomized study, compared NOLVADEX to placebo in women with axillary node-negative, estrogen-receptor positive (≥ 10 fmol/mg cytosol protein) breast cancer (as adjuvant therapy, following total mastectomy and axillary dissection, or segmental resection, axillary dissection, and breast radiation). After five years of treatment, there was a significant improvement in disease-free survival in women receiving NOLVADEX. This benefit was apparent both in women under age 50 and in women at or beyond age 50.

One additional randomized study (NATO) demonstrated improved disease-free survival for NOLVADEX compared to no adjuvant therapy following total mastectomy and axillary dissection in postmenopausal women with axillary node-negative breast cancer. In this study, the benefits of NOLVADEX appeared to be independent of estrogen receptor status.

Duration of Therapy—In the EBCTCG 1995 overview, the reduction in recurrence and mortality was greater in those studies that used tamoxifen for about 5 years than in those that used tamoxifen for a shorter period of therapy.

In the NSABP B-14 trial, in which patients were randomized to NOLVADEX 20 mg/day for 5 years vs. placebo and were disease-free at the end of this 5-year period were offered rerandomization to an additional 5 years of NOLVADEX or placebo. With 4 years of follow-up after this rerandomization, 92% of the women that received 5 years of NOLVADEX were alive and disease-free, compared to 86% of the women scheduled to receive 10 years of NOLVADEX (p=0.003). Overall survivals were 96% and 94%, respectively (p=0.08). Results of the B-14 study suggest that continuation of therapy beyond 5 years does not provide additional benefit.

A Scottish trial of 5 years of tamoxifen versus indefinite treatment found a disease-free survival of 70% in the five-year group and 61% in the indefinite group, with 6.2 years median follow-up (HR=1.27, 95% CI 0.87–1.85).

In a large randomized trial conducted by the Swedish Breast Cancer Cooperative Group of adjuvant NOLVADEX 40 mg/day for 2 or 5 years, overall survival at 10 years was estimated to be 80% in the patients in the 5-year tamoxifen group, compared with 74% among corresponding patients in the 2-year treatment group (p=0.03). Disease-free survival at 10 years was 73% in the 5-year group and 67% in the 2-year group (p=0.009). Compared with 2 years of tamoxifen treatment, 5 years of treatment resulted in a slightly greater reduction in the incidence of contralateral breast cancer at ten years, but this difference was not statistically significant.

Contralateral Breast Cancer—The incidence of contralateral breast cancer is reduced in breast cancer patients (premenopausal and postmenopausal) receiving NOLVADEX compared to placebo. Data on contralateral breast cancer are available from 32,422 out of 36,689 patients in the 1995 overview analysis of the Early Breast Cancer Trialists Collaborative Group (EBCTCG). In clinical trials with NOLVADEX of 1 year or less, 2 years, and about 5 years duration, the proportional reductions in the incidence rate of contralateral breast cancer among women receiving NOLVADEX were 13% (NS), 26% (2p = 0.004) and 47% (2p < 0.00001), with a significant trend favoring longer tamoxifen duration (2p = 0.008). The proportional reduction in the incidence of contralateral breast cancer were independent of age and ER status of the primary tumor. Treatment with about 5 years of NOLVADEX reduced the annual incidence rate of contralateral breast cancer from 7.6 per 1000 patients in the control group compared with 3.9 per 1000 patients in the tamoxifen group.

In a large randomized trial in Sweden (the Stockholm Trial) of adjuvant NOLVADEX 40 mg/day for 2–5 years, the incidence of second primary breast tumors was reduced 40% (p < 0.008) on tamoxifen compared to control. In the NSABP B-14 trial in which patients were randomized to NOLVADEX 20 mg/day for 5 years vs. placebo, the incidence of second primary breast cancers was also significantly reduced (p < 0.01). In NSABP B-14, the annual rate of contralateral breast cancer was 8.0 per 1,000 patients in the placebo group compared with 5.0 per 1,000 patients in the tamoxifen group, at 10 years after first randomization.

Clinical Studies—Reduction in Breast Cancer Incidence in High Risk Women

The Breast Cancer Prevention Trial (BCPT, NSABP P-1) was a double-blind, randomized, placebo controlled trial with a primary objective to determine whether five years of NOLVADEX therapy (20 mg/day) would reduce the incidence of invasive breast cancer in women at high risk for the disease (See **INDICATIONS AND USAGE**). Secondary objectives included an evaluation of the incidence of ischemic heart disease; the effects on the incidence of bone fractures; and other events that might be associated with the use of NOLVADEX, including: endometrial cancer, pulmonary embolus, deep vein thrombosis, stroke, and cataract formation and surgery (See **WARNINGS**).

The Gail Model was used to calculate predicted breast cancer risk for women who were less than 60 years of age and did not have lobular carcinoma in situ (LCIS). The following risk factors were used: age; number of first-degree female relatives with breast cancer; previous breast biopsies; presence or absence of atypical hyperplasia; nulliparity; age at first live birth; and age at menarche. A 5-year predicted risk of breast cancer of ≥ 1.67% was required for entry into the trial.

In this trial, 13,388 women of at least 35 years of age were randomized to receive either NOLVADEX or placebo for five years. The median duration of treatment was 3.5 years. As of January 31, 1998, follow-up data is available for 13,114 women. Twenty-seven percent of women randomized to placebo (1,782) and 24% of women randomized to NOLVADEX (1,596) completed 5 years of therapy. The demographic characteristics of women on the trial with follow-up data are shown in Table 1.

[See table 1 at bottom of next page]

Results are shown in Table 2. After a median follow-up of 4.2 years, the incidence of invasive breast cancer was reduced by 44% among women assigned to NOLVADEX (86 cases-NOLVADEX, 156 cases-placebo; p<0.00001; relative risk (RR)=0.56, 95% CI: 0.43–0.72). A reduction in the incidence of breast cancer was seen in each prospectively specified age group (≤49, 50–59, ≥60), in women with or without LCIS, and in each of the absolute risk levels specified in Table 2. A non-significant decrease in the incidence of ductal carcinoma in situ (DCIS) was seen (23-NOLVADEX, 35-placebo; RR=0.66; 95% CI: 0.39–1.11).

There was no statistically significant difference in the number of myocardial infarctions, severe angina, or acute ischemic cardiac events between the two groups (61-NOLVADEX, 59-placebo; RR=1.04, 95% CI: 0.73–1.49).

No overall difference in mortality (53 deaths in NOLVADEX group vs. 65 deaths in placebo group) was present. No difference in breast cancer-related mortality was observed (4 deaths in NOLVADEX group versus 5 deaths in placebo group).

Although there was a non-significant reduction in the number of hip fractures (9 on NOLVADEX, 20 on placebo) in the NOLVADEX group, the number of wrist fractures was similar in the two treatment groups (69 on NOLVADEX, 74 on placebo). No information regarding bone mineral density or other markers of osteoporosis is available.

The risks of NOLVADEX therapy include endometrial cancer, DVT, PE, stroke, cataract formation and cataract surgery (See Table 2). In the NSABP P-1 trial, 33 cases of endometrial cancer were observed in the NOLVADEX group vs. 14 in the placebo group (RR=2.48, 95% CI: 1.27–4.92). Deep vein thrombosis was observed in 30 women receiving NOLVADEX vs. 19 in women receiving placebo (RR=1.59, 95% CI: 0.86-2.98). Eighteen cases of pulmonary embolism were observed in the NOLVADEX group vs. 6 in the placebo group (RR=3.01, 95% CI: 1.15–9.27). There were 34 strokes on the NOLVADEX arm and 24 on the placebo arm (RR=1.42; 95% CI: 0.82–2.51). Cataract formation in women without cataracts at baseline was observed in 540 women taking NOLVADEX vs. 483 women receiving placebo (RR=1.13, 95% CI: 1.00–1.28). Cataract surgery (with or without cataracts at baseline) was performed in 201 women taking NOLVADEX vs. 129 women receiving placebo (RR=1.51, 95% CI 1.21–1.89) (See **WARNINGS**).

Table 2 summarizes the major outcomes of the NSABP P-1 trial. For each endpoint, the following results are presented: the number of events and rate per 1,000 women per year for the placebo and NOLVADEX groups; and the relative risk (RR) and its associated 95% confidence interval (CI) between NOLVADEX and placebo. Relative risks less than 1.0 indicate a benefit of NOLVADEX therapy. The limits of the confidence intervals can be used to assess the statistical significance of the benefits or risks of NOLVADEX therapy. If the upper limit of the CI is less than 1.0, then a statistically significant benefit exists.

For most participants, multiple risk factors would have been required for eligibility. This table considers risk factors individually, regardless of other co-existing risk factors, for women who developed breast cancer. The 5-year predicted absolute breast cancer risk accounts for multiple risk factors in an individual and should provide the best estimate of individual benefit (See **INDICATIONS AND USAGE**).

[See table 2 on page 636]

Table 3 describes the characteristics of the breast cancers in the NSABP P-1 trial and includes tumor size, nodal status, ER status. NOLVADEX decreased the incidence of small estrogen receptor positive tumors, but did not alter the incidence of estrogen receptor negative tumors or larger tumors.

[See table 3 on page 636]

Interim results from 2 trials in addition to the NSABP P-1 trial examining the effects of tamoxifen in reducing breast cancer incidence have been reported.

The first was the Italian Tamoxifen Prevention trial. In this trial women between the ages of 35 and 70, who had had a total hysterectomy, were randomized to receive 20 mg tamoxifen or matching placebo for 5 years. The primary endpoints were occurrence of, and death from, invasive breast cancer. Women without any specific risk factors for breast cancer were to be entered. Between 1992 and 1997, 5,408 women were randomized. Hormone Replacement Therapy (HRT) was used in 14% of participants. The trial closed in 1997 due to the large number of dropouts during the first year of treatment (26%). After 46 months of follow-up there were 22 breast cancers in women on placebo and 19 in women on tamoxifen. Although no decrease in breast cancer incidence was observed, there was a trend for a reduction in breast cancer among women receiving protocol therapy for at least 1 year (19-placebo, 11-tamoxifen). The small numbers of participants along with the low level of risk in this otherwise healthy group precluded an adequate assessment of the effect of tamoxifen in reducing the incidence of breast cancer.

The second trial, the Royal Marsden Trial (RMT) was reported as an interim analysis. The RMT was begun in 1986 as a feasibility study of whether larger scale trials could be mounted. The trial was subsequently extended to a pilot trial to accrue additional participants to further assess the safety of tamoxifen. Twenty-four hundred and seventy-one women were entered between 1986 and 1996; they were selected on the basis of a family history of breast cancer. HRT was used in 40% of participants. In this trial, with a 70-month median follow-up, 34 and 36 breast cancers (8 noninvasive, 4 on each arm) were observed among women on tamoxifen and placebo, respectively. Patients in this trial were younger than those in the NSABP P-1 trial and may have been more likely to develop ER (-) tumors, which are unlikely to be reduced in number by tamoxifen therapy. Although women were selected on the basis of family history and were thought to have a high risk of breast cancer, few events occurred, reducing the statistical power of the study. These factors are potential reasons why the RMT may not have provided an adequate assessment of the effectiveness of tamoxifen in reducing the incidence of breast cancer.

In these trials, an increased number of cases of deep vein thrombosis, pulmonary embolus, stroke, and endometrial cancer were observed on the tamoxifen arm compared to the placebo arm. The frequency of events was consistent with the safety data observed in the NSABP P-1 trial.

INDICATIONS AND USAGE

Metastatic Breast Cancer: NOLVADEX is effective in the treatment of metastatic breast cancer in women and men. In premenopausal women with metastatic breast cancer, NOLVADEX is an alternative to oophorectomy or ovarian irradiation. Available evidence indicates that patients whose tumors are estrogen receptor positive are more likely to benefit from NOLVADEX therapy.

Adjuvant Treatment of Breast Cancer: NOLVADEX is indicated for the treatment of node-positive breast cancer in postmenopausal women following total mastectomy or segmental mastectomy, axillary dissection, and breast irradiation. In some NOLVADEX adjuvant studies, most of the benefit to date has been in the subgroup with 4 or more positive axillary nodes.

NOLVADEX is indicated for the treatment of axillary node-negative breast cancer in women following total mastectomy or segmental mastectomy, axillary dissection, and breast irradiation. Data are insufficient to predict which women are most likely to benefit and to determine if NOLVADEX provides any benefit in women with tumors less than 1 cm.

NOLVADEX reduces the occurrence of contralateral breast cancer in patients receiving adjuvant NOLVADEX therapy for breast cancer.

Current data from clinical trials support five years of adjuvant NOLVADEX therapy for patients with breast cancer.

The estrogen and progesterone receptor values may help to predict whether adjuvant NOLVADEX therapy is likely to be beneficial.

Reduction in Breast Cancer Incidence in High Risk Women: NOLVADEX is indicated to reduce the incidence of breast cancer in women at high risk for breast cancer. This effect was shown in a study of 5 years planned duration with a median follow-up of 4.2 years. Twenty-five percent of the participants received drug for 5 years. The longer term effects are not known. In this study, there was no impact of tamoxifen on overall or breast cancer-related mortality.

NOLVADEX is indicated only for high-risk women. "High risk" is defined as women at least 35 years of age with a 5-year predicted risk of breast cancer ≥ 1.67%, as calculated by the Gail Model.

Examples of combinations of factors predicting a 5-year risk ≥ 1.67% are:

Age 35 or older and any of the following combination of factors:

- One first degree relative with a history of breast cancer, 2 or more benign biopsies, and a history of a breast biopsy showing atypical hyperplasia; or
- At least 2 first degree relatives with a history of breast cancer, and a personal history of at least 1 breast biopsy; or
- LCIS

Age 40 or older and any of the following combination of factors:

- One first degree relative with a history of breast cancer, 2 or more benign biopsies, age at first live birth 25 or older, and age at menarche 11 or younger; or
- At least 2 first degree relatives with a history of breast cancer, and age at first live birth 19 or younger; or
- One first degree relative with a history of breast cancer, and a personal history of a breast biopsy showing atypical hyperplasia.

Age 45 or older and any of the following combination of factors:

- At least 2 first degree relatives with history a of breast cancer and age at first live birth 24 or younger; or
- One first degree relative with a history of breast cancer with a personal history of a benign breast biopsy, age at menarche 11 or less and age at first live birth 20 or more.

Age 50 or older and any of the following combination of factors:

- At least 2 first degree relatives with a history of breast cancer; or
- History of 1 breast biopsy showing atypical hyperplasia, and age at first live birth 30 or older and age at menarche 11 or less; or
- History of at least 2 breast biopsies with a history of atypical hyperplasia, and age at first live birth 30 or more.

Age 55 and any of the following combination of factors:

- One first degree relative with a history of breast cancer with a personal history of a benign breast biopsy, and age at menarche 11 or less; or
- History of at least 2 breast biopsies with a history of atypical hyperplasia, and age at first live birth 20 or older.

Age 60 or older and:

- 5 year predicted risk of breast cancer ≥ 1.67%, as calculated by the Gail Model.

For women whose risk factors are not described in the above examples, the Gail Model is necessary to estimate absolute breast cancer risk. Health Care Professionals can obtain a Gail Model Risk Assessment Tool by dialing 1-800-544-2007.

There are no data available regarding the effect of NOLVADEX on breast cancer incidence in women with inherited mutations (BRCA1, BRCA2).

After an assessment of the risk of developing breast cancer, the decision regarding therapy with NOLVADEX for the reduction in breast cancer incidence should be based upon an individual assessment of the benefits and risks of NOLVADEX therapy. In the NSABP P-1 trial, NOLVADEX treatment lowered the risk of developing breast cancer during the follow-up period of the trial, but did not eliminate breast cancer risk (See Table 2 in **CLINICAL PHARMACOLOGY**).

CONTRAINDICATIONS

NOLVADEX is contraindicated in patients with known hypersensitivity to the drug or any of its ingredients.

Reduction in Breast Cancer Incidence in High Risk Women: NOLVADEX is contraindicated in women who require concomitant coumarin-type anticoagulant therapy or in women with a history of deep vein thrombosis or pulmonary embolus.

WARNINGS

Effects in Metastatic Breast Cancer Patients: As with other additive hormonal therapy (estrogens and androgens), hypercalcemia has been reported in some breast cancer patients with bone metastases within a few weeks of starting treatment with NOLVADEX. If hypercalcemia does occur, appropriate measures should be taken and, if severe, NOLVADEX should be discontinued.

Effects on the Uterus-Endometrial Cancer: As with other additive hormonal therapy (estrogens), an increased incidence of endometrial cancer has been reported in association with NOLVADEX treatment. The underlying mechanism is unknown, but may be related to the estrogen-like effect of NOLVADEX. Any patients receiving or having previously received NOLVADEX, who report abnormal vaginal bleeding should be promptly evaluated. Patients receiving or having previously received NOLVADEX should have routine gynecological care and they should promptly inform their physician if they experience any abnormal gynecological symptoms, eg, menstrual irregularities, abnormal vaginal bleeding, changes in vaginal discharge, or pelvic pain or pressure.

In a large randomized trial in Sweden of adjuvant NOLVADEX 40 mg/day for 2–5 years, an increased incidence of uterine cancer was noted. Twenty three of 1,372 patients randomized to receive NOLVADEX versus 4 of 1,357 patients randomized to the observation group developed cancer of the uterus [RR = 5.6 (1.9–16.2), p<.001]. One of the patients with cancer of the uterus who was randomized to receive NOLVADEX never took the drug. After approximately 6.8 years of follow-up in the NSABP B-14 trial, 15 of 1,419 women randomized to receive NOLVADEX 20 mg/day for 5 years developed uterine cancer and 2 of the 1,424 women randomized to receive placebo, who subsequently were treated with NOLVADEX, also developed uterine cancer. Most of the uterine cancers were diagnosed at an early stage, but deaths from uterine cancer have been reported.

In the NSABP P-1 trial, among participants randomized to NOLVADEX there was a statistically significant increase in the incidence of endometrial cancer (33 cases of invasive endometrial cancer, compared to 14 cases among participants randomized to placebo (RR=2.48, 95% CI: 1.27–4.92). This increase was primarily observed among women at least 50 years of age at the time of randomization (26 cases of invasive endometrial cancer, compared to 6 cases among participants randomized to placebo (RR=4.50, 95% CI: 1.78–13.16). Among women ≤ 49 years of age at the time of randomization there were 7 cases of invasive endometrial cancer, compared to 8 cases among participants randomized to placebo (RR=0.94, 95% CI: 0.28–2.89). If age at the time of diagnosis is considered, there were 4 cases of endometrial cancer among participants ≤ 49 randomized to NOLVADEX compared to 2 among participants randomized to placebo (RR=2.21, 95% CI: 0.4–12.0). For women ≥ 50 at the time of diagnosis, there were 29 cases among participants random-

Continued on next page

Table 1. Demographic Characteristics of Women in the NSABP P-1 Trial

Characteristic	Placebo #	Placebo %	Tamoxifen #	Tamoxifen %
Age (yrs.)				
35–39	184	3	158	2
40–49	2,394	36	2,411	37
50–59	2,011	31	2.019	31
60–69	1,588	24	1,563	24
≥70	393	6	393	6
Age at first live birth (yrs.)				
Nulliparous	1,202	18	1,205	18
12–19	915	14	946	15
20–24	2,448	37	2,449	37
25–29	1,399	21	1,367	21
≥30	606	9	577	9
Race				
White	6,333	96	6,323	96
Black	109	2	103	2
Other	128	2	118	2
Age at menarche				
≥14	1,243	19	1,170	18
12–13	3,610	55	3,610	55
≤11	1,717	26	1,764	27
# of first degree relatives with breast cancer				
0	1,584	24	1,525	23
1	3,714	57	3,744	57
2+	1,272	19	1,275	20
Prior Hysterectomy				
No	4,173	63.5	4,018	62.4
Yes	2,397	36.5	2,464	37.7
# of previous breast biopsies				
0	2,935	45	2,923	45
1	1,833	28	1,850	28
≥2	1,802	27	1,771	27
History of atypical hyperplasia in the breast				
No	5,958	91	5,969	91
Yes	612	9	575	9
History of LCIS at entry				
No	6,165	94	6,135	94
Yes	405	6	409	6
5-year predicted breast cancer risk (%)				
≤2.00	1,646	25	1,626	25
2.01–3.00	2,028	31	2,057	31
3.01–5.00	1,787	27	1,707	26
≥5.01	1,109	17	1,162	18
TOTAL	6,570	100.0	6,544	100.0

Nolvadex—Cont.

ized to NOLVADEX compared to 12 among women on placebo (RR=2.5, 95% CI: 1.3–4.9). The risk ratios were similar in the two groups, although fewer events occurred in younger women. Most (29 of 33 cases in the NOLVADEX group) endometrial cancers were diagnosed in symptomatic women; although 5 of 33 cases in the NOLVADEX group occurred in asymptomatic women. Among women receiving NOLVADEX the events appeared between 1 and 61 months (average = 32 months) from the start of treatment.

Among participants receiving NOLVADEX, there were 33 cases of FIGO stage I [20 IA, 12 IB, and 1 IC] endometrial cancer. Among participants receiving placebo, there were 13 FIGO stage I cases [8 IA and 5 IB]. There was a single FIGO Stage IV endometrial cancer in a participant receiving placebo (See Table 2 in **CLINICAL PHARMACOLOGY**). The distribution of FIGO stage was similar between participants receiving NOLVADEX and placebo. Five women receiving NOLVADEX and 1 receiving placebo with FIGO Stage IB disease received postoperative radiation therapy in addition to surgery.

Endometrial sampling did not alter the endometrial cancer detection rate compared to women who did not undergo endometrial sampling (0.6% with sampling, 0.5% without sampling) for women with an intact uterus. There are no data to suggest that routine endometrial sampling in asymptomatic women taking NOLVADEX to reduce the incidence of breast cancer would be beneficial.

Non-Malignant Effects on the Uterus: An increased incidence of endometrial changes including hyperplasia and polyps have been reported in association with NOLVADEX treatment. The incidence and pattern of this increase suggest that the underlying mechanism is related to the estrogenic properties of NOLVADEX.

There have been a few reports of endometriosis and uterine fibroids in women receiving NOLVADEX. The underlying mechanism may be due to the partial estrogenic effect of NOLVADEX. Ovarian cysts have also been observed in a small number of premenopausal patients with advanced breast cancer who have been treated with NOLVADEX.

Thromboembolic Effects of NOLVADEX: As with other additive hormonal therapy (estrogen), there is evidence of an increased incidence of thromboembolic events, including deep vein thrombosis and pulmonary embolism, during NOLVADEX therapy. When NOLVADEX is coadminstered with chemotherapy, there may be a further increase in the incidence of thromboembolic effects. For treatment of breast cancer, the risks and benefits of NOLVADEX should be carefully considered in women with a history of thromboembolic events.

Data from the NSABP P-1 trial show that participants receiving NOLVADEX without a history of pulmonary emboli (PE) had a statistically significant increase in pulmonary emboli (18-NOLVADEX, 6-placebo, RR=3.01, 95% CI: 1.15–9.27). Three of the pulmonary emboli, all in the NOLVADEX arm, were fatal. Eighty-seven percent of the cases of pulmonary embolism occurred in women at least 50 years of age at randomization. Among women receiving NOLVADEX, the events appeared between 2 and 60 months (average = 27 months) from the start of treatment.

In this same population, a non-statistically significant increase in deep vein thrombosis (DVT) was seen in the NOLVADEX group (30-NOLVADEX, 19-placebo; RR=1.59, 95% CI: 0.86–2.98). The same increase in relative risk was seen in women ≤ 49 and in women ≥ 50, although fewer events occurred in younger women. Women with thromboembolic events were at risk for a second related event (7 out of 25 women on placebo, 5 out of 48 women on NOLVADEX) and were at risk for complications of the event and its treatment (0/25 on placebo, 4/48 on NOLVADEX). Among women receiving NOLVADEX, deep vein thrombosis events occurred between 2 and 57 months (average = 19 months) from the start of treatment.

There was a non-statistically significant increase in stroke among patients randomized to NOLVADEX (24-Placebo; 34-NOLVADEX; RR=1.42; 95% CI: 0.82–2.51). Six of the 24 strokes in the placebo group were considered hemorrhagic in origin and 10 of the 34 strokes in the NOLVADEX group were categorized as hemorrhagic. Seventeen of the 34 strokes in the NOLVADEX group were considered occlusive and 7 were considered to be of unknown etiology. Fourteen of the 24 strokes on the placebo arm were reported to be occlusive and 4 of unknown etiology. Among these strokes 3 strokes in the placebo group and 4 strokes in the NOLVADEX group were fatal. Eighty-eight percent of the strokes occurred in women at least 50 years of age at the time of randomization. Among women receiving NOLVADEX, the events occurred between 1 and 63 months (average = 30 months) from the start of treatment.

Effects on the liver: Liver cancer: In the Swedish trial using adjuvant NOLVADEX 40 mg/day for 2–5 years, 3 cases of liver cancer have been reported in the NOLVADEX-treated group vs. 1 case in the observation group (See **PRECAUTIONS—Carcinogenesis**). In other clinical trials evaluating NOLVADEX, no cases of liver cancer have been reported to date.

No cases of liver cancer were reported in the NSABP P-1 trial with a median follow-up of 4.2 years.

Effects on the liver: Non-malignant effects: NOLVADEX has been associated with changes in liver enzyme levels, and on rare occasions, a spectrum of more severe liver abnormalities including fatty liver, cholestasis, hepatitis and

Table 2: Major Outcomes of the NSABP P-1 Trial

Type of Event	# Of Events Placebo	# Of Events Nolvadex	Rate/1000 Women/Year Placebo	Rate/1000 Women/Year Nolvadex	RR	95% CI LIMITS
Invasive Breast Cancer	156	86	6.49	3.58	0.56	0.43–0.72
Age ≤49	59	38	6.34	4.11	0.65	0.43–0.98
Age 50–59	46	25	6.31	3.53	0.56	0.35–0.91
Age ≥60	51	23	7.17	3.22	0.45	0.27–0.74
Risk Factors for Breast Cancer History, LCIS						
No	140	78	6.23	3.51	0.56	0.43–0.74
Yes	16	8	12.73	6.33	0.50	0.21–1.17
History, Atypical Hyperplasia						
No	138	84	6.37	3.89	0.61	0.47–0.80
Yes	18	2	8.69	1.05	0.12	0.03–0.52
# First Degree Relatives						
0	32	17	5.97	3.26	0.55	0.30–0.98
1	80	45	5.81	3.31	0.57	0.40–0.82
2	35	18	8.92	4.67	0.52	0.30–0.92
≥3	9	6	13.33	7.58	0.57	0.20–1.59
5-Year Predicted Breast Cancer Risk (as calculated by the Gail Model)						
≤2.00%	31	13	5.36	2.26	0.42	0.22–0.81
2.01–3.00%	39	28	5.25	3.83	0.73	0.45–1.18
3.01–5.00%	36	26	5.37	4.06	0.76	0.46–1.26
≥5.00%	50	19	13.15	4.71	0.36	0.21–0.61
DCIS	35	23	1.47	0.97	0.66	0.39–1.11
Fractures (protocol-specified sites)	92[1]	76[1]	3.87	3.20	0.61	0.83–1.12
Hip	20	9	0.84	0.38	0.45	0.18–1.04
Wrist[2]	74	69	3.11	2.91	0.93	0.67–1.29
Total Ischemic Events	59	61	2.47	2.57	1.04	0.71–1.51
Myocardial Infarction	27	27	1.13	1.13	1.00	0.57–1.78
Fatal	8	7	0.33	0.29	0.88	0.27–2.77
Nonfatal	19	20	0.79	0.84	1.06	0.54–2.09
Angina[3]	12	12	0.50	0.50	1.00	0.41–2.44
Acute Ischemic Syndrome[4]	20	22	0.84	0.92	1.11	0.58–2.13
Invasive Endometrial Cancer (among women without a hysterectomy)	14	33	0.92	2.29	2.48	1.27–4.92
Stroke[5]	24	34	1.00	1.43	1.42	0.82–2.51
Transient Ischemic Attack	21	18	0.88	0.75	0.86	0.43–1.70
Pulmonary Emboli[6]	6	18	0.25	0.75	3.01	1.15–9.27
Deep-Vein Thrombosis[7]	19	30	0.79	1.26	1.59	0.86–2.98
Cataracts Developing on Study[8]	483	540	22.51	25.41	1.13	1.00–1.28
Underwent Cataract Surgery[8]	63	101	31.43	46.62	1.48	1.08–2.03
Underwent Cataract Surgery[9]	129	201	37.58	56.81	1.51	1.21–1.89

1 Two women had hip and wrist fractures
2 Includes Colles' and other lower radius fractures
3 Requiring angioplasty or CABG
4 New Q-wave on ECG; no angina or elevation of serum enzymes; or angina requiring hospitalization without surgery
5 Seven cases were fatal; three in the placebo group and four in the NOLVADEX group
6 Three cases in the NOLVADEX group were fatal
7 All but three cases in each group required hospitalization
8 Based on women without cataracts at baseline (6,230-Placebo, 6,199-NOLVADEX)
9 All women (6,707-Placebo, 6,681-NOLVADEX)

Table 3: Characteristics of Breast Cancer in NSABP P-1 Trial

Staging Parameter	Placebo N=156	Tamoxifen N=86	Total N=242	Staging Parameter	Placebo N=156	Tamoxifen N=86	Total N=242
Tumor Size:				**Stage:**			
T1	117	60	177	I	88	47	135
T2	28	20	48	II: node negative	15	9	24
T3	7	3	10	II: node positive	33	22	55
T4	1	2	3	III	6	4	10
Unknown	3	1	4	IV	2[1]	1	3
				Unknown	12	3	15
Nodal Status:							
Negative	103	56	159	**Estrogen receptor:**			
1–3 positive nodes	29	14	43	Positive	115	38	153
≥ 4 positive nodes	10	12	22	Negative	27	36	63
Unknown	14	4	18	Unknown	14	12	26

1 One participant presented with a suspicious bone scan but did not have documented metastases. She subsequently died of metastatic breast cancer.

hepatic necrosis. A few of these serious cases included fatalities. In most reported cases the relationship to NOLVADEX is uncertain. However, some positive rechallenges and dechallenges have been reported.

In the NSABP P-1 trial, few grade 3–4 changes in liver function (SGOT, SGPT, bilirubin, alkaline phosphatase) were observed (10 on placebo and 6 on NOLVADEX). Serum lipids were not systematically collected.

Other cancers: A number of second primary tumors, occurring at sites other than the endometrium, have been reported following the treatment of breast cancer with NOLVADEX in clinical trials. Data from the NSABP B-14 and P-1 studies show no increase in other (non-uterine) cancers among patients receiving NOLVADEX. Whether an increased risk for other (non-uterine) cancers is associated with NOLVADEX is still uncertain and continues to be evaluated.

Effects on the Eye: Ocular disturbances, including corneal changes, decrement in color vision perception, retinal vein thrombosis, and retinopathy have been reported in patients receiving NOLVADEX. An increased incidence of cataracts and the need for cataract surgery have been reported in patients receiving NOLVADEX.

In the NSABP P-1 trial, an increased risk of borderline significance of developing cataracts among those women without cataracts at baseline (540-NOLVADEX; 483-placebo; RR=1.13, 95% CI: 1.00–1.28) was observed. Among these same women, NOLVADEX was associated with an increased risk of having cataract surgery (101-NOLVADEX; 63-placebo; RR=1.62, 95% CI: 1.17–2.25) (See Table 2 in **CLINICAL PHARMACOLOGY**). Among all women on the trial (with or without cataracts at baseline), NOLVADEX was associated with an increased risk of having cataract surgery (201-NOLVADEX; 129-placebo; RR=1.51, 95% CI: 1.21–1.89). Eye examinations were not required during the study. No other conclusions regarding non-cataract ophthalmic events can be made.

Pregnancy Category D: NOLVADEX may cause fetal harm when administered to a pregnant woman. Women should be advised not to become pregnant while taking NOLVADEX and should use barrier or nonhormonal contraceptive measures if sexually active. Effects on reproductive functions are expected from the antiestrogenic properties of the drug. In reproductive studies in rats at dose levels equal to or below the human dose, nonteratogenic developmental skeletal changes were seen and were found reversible. In addition, in fertility studies in rats and in teratology studies in rabbits using doses at or below those used in humans, a lower incidence of embryo implantation and a higher incidence of fetal death or retarded in utero growth were observed, with slower learning behavior in some rat pups when compared to historical controls. Several pregnant marmosets were dosed during organogenesis or in the last half of pregnancy. No deformations were seen and, although the dose was high enough to terminate pregnancy in some animals, those that did maintain pregnancy showed no evidence of teratogenic malformations.

In rodent models of fetal reproductive tract development, tamoxifen (at doses 0.3 to 2.4-fold the human maximum recommended dose on a mg/m^2 basis) caused changes in both sexes that are similar to those caused by estradiol, ethynylestradiol and diethylstilbestrol. Although the clinical relevance of these changes is unknown, some of these changes, especially vaginal adenosis, are similar to those seen in young women who were exposed to diethylstilbestrol in utero and who have a 1 in 1,000 risk of developing clear-cell adenocarcinoma of the vagina or cervix. To date, in utero exposure to tamoxifen has not been shown to cause vaginal adenosis, or clear-cell adenocarcinoma of the vagina or cervix, in young women. However, only a small number of young women have been exposed to tamoxifen in utero, and a smaller number have been followed long enough (to age 15–20) to determine whether vaginal or cervical neoplasia could occur as a result of this exposure.

There are no adequate and well controlled trials of tamoxifen in pregnant women. There have been a small number of reports of vaginal bleeding, spontaneous abortions, birth defects, and fetal deaths in pregnant women. If this drug is used during pregnancy, or the patient becomes pregnant while taking this drug, or within approximately two months after discontinuing therapy, the patient should be apprised of the potential risks to the fetus including the potential long term risk of a DES-like syndrome.

Reduction in Breast Cancer Incidence in High Risk Women—Pregnancy Category D: For sexually active women of child-bearing potential, NOLVADEX therapy should be initiated during menstruation. In women with menstrual irregularity, a negative B-HCG immediately prior to the initiation of therapy is sufficient (See **PRECAUTIONS—Information for Patients—Reduction in Breast Cancer Incidence in High Risk Women**).

PRECAUTIONS

General: Decreases in platelet counts, usually to 50,000–100,000/mm^3, infrequently lower, have been occasionally reported in patients taking NOLVADEX for breast cancer. In patients with significant thrombocytopenia, rare hemorrhagic episodes have occurred, but it is uncertain if these episodes are due to NOLVADEX therapy. Leukopenia has been observed, sometimes in association with anemia and/or thrombocytopenia. There have been rare reports of neutropenia and pancytopenia in patients receiving NOLVADEX; this can sometimes be severe.

In the NSABP P-1 trial, 6 women on NOLVADEX and 2 on placebo experienced grade 3–4 drops in platelet counts ($\leq$50,000/mm^3).

Information for Patients:

Reduction in Breast Cancer Incidence in High Risk Women: Women who are at high risk for breast cancer can consider taking NOLVADEX therapy to reduce the incidence of breast cancer. Whether the benefits of treatment are considered to outweigh the risks depends on a woman's personal health history and on how she weighs the benefits and risks. NOLVADEX therapy to reduce the incidence of breast cancer may therefore not be appropriate for all women at high risk for breast cancer. Women who are considering NOLVADEX therapy should consult their health care professional for an assessment of the potential benefits and risks prior to starting therapy for reduction in breast cancer incidence (See Table 2 in **CLINICAL PHARMACOLOGY**).

Women should understand that NOLVADEX reduces the incidence of breast cancer, but may not eliminate risk. NOLVADEX decreased the incidence of small estrogen receptor positive tumors, but did not alter the incidence of estrogen receptor negative tumors or larger tumors. In women with breast cancer who are at high risk of developing a second breast cancer, treatment with about 5 years of NOLVADEX reduced the annual incidence rate of a second breast cancer by approximately 50%.

Women who are pregnant or who plan to become pregnant should not take NOLVADEX to reduce her risk of breast cancer. Effective nonhormonal contraception must be used by all premenopausal women taking NOLVADEX if they are sexually active. For sexually active women of child-bearing potential, NOLVADEX therapy should be initiated during menstruation. In women with menstrual irregularity, a negative B-HCG immediately prior to the initiation of therapy is sufficient (See **WARNINGS—Pregnancy Category D**).

Two European trials of tamoxifen to reduce the risk of breast cancer were conducted and showed no difference in the number of breast cancer cases between the tamoxifen and placebo arms. These studies had trial designs that differed from that of NSABP P-1, were smaller than NSABP P-1, and enrolled women at a lower risk for breast cancer than those in P-1.

Monitoring During NOLVADEX Therapy: Women taking or having previously taken NOLVADEX should be instructed to seek prompt medical attention for new breast lumps, vaginal bleeding, gynecologic symptoms (menstrual irregularities, changes in vaginal discharge, or pelvic pain or pressure), symptoms of leg swelling or tenderness, unexplained shortness of breath, or changes in vision. Women should inform all care providers, regardless of the reason for evaluation, that they take NOLVADEX.

Women taking NOLVADEX to reduce the incidence of breast cancer should have a breast examination, a mammogram, and a gynecologic examination prior to the initiation of therapy. These studies should be repeated at regular intervals while on therapy, in keeping with good medical practice. Women taking NOLVADEX as adjuvant breast cancer therapy should follow the same monitoring procedures as for

Adverse Reactions*	NOLVADEX All Effects % of Women n=104	OVARIAN ABLATION All Effects % of Women n=100
Flush	33	46
Amenorrhea	16	69
Altered Menses	13	5
Oligomenorrhea	9	1
Bone Pain	6	6
Menstrual Disorder	6	4
Nausea	5	4
Cough/Coughing	4	1
Edema	4	1
Fatigue	4	1
Musculoskeletal Pain	3	0
Pain	3	4
Ovarian Cyst(s)	3	2
Depression	2	2
Abdominal Cramps	1	2
Anorexia	1	2

* Some women had more than one adverse reaction.

women taking NOLVADEX for the reduction in the incidence of breast cancer. Women taking NOLVADEX as treatment for metastatic breast cancer should review this monitoring plan with their care provider and select the appropriate modalities and schedule of evaluation.

Laboratory Tests: Periodic complete blood counts, including platelet counts, and periodic liver function tests should be obtained.

Drug Interactions: When NOLVADEX is used in combination with coumarin-type anticoagulants, a significant increase in anticoagulant effect may occur. Where such coadministration exists, careful monitoring of the patient's prothrombin time is recommended.

In the NSABP P-1 trial, women who required coumarin-type anticoagulants for any reason were ineligible for participation in the trial (See **CONTRAINDICATIONS**).

There is an increased risk of thromboembolic events occurring when cytotoxic agents are used in combination with NOLVADEX.

Tamoxifen, N-desmethyl tamoxifen and 4-hydroxytamoxifen have been found to be potent inhibitors of hepatic cytochrome p-450 mixed function oxidases. The effect of tamoxifen on metabolism and excretion of other antineoplastic drugs, such as cyclophosphamide and other drugs that require mixed function oxidases for activation, is not known. One patient receiving NOLVADEX with concomitant phenobarbital exhibited a steady state serum level of tamoxifen lower than that observed for other patients (ie, 26 ng/mL vs. mean value of 122 ng/mL). However, the clinical significance of this finding is not known.

Concomitant bromocriptine therapy has been shown to elevate serum tamoxifen and N-desmethyl tamoxifen.

Drug/Laboratory Testing Interactions: During postmarketing surveillance, T_4 elevations were reported for a few postmenopausal patients which may be explained by increases in thyroid-binding globulin. These elevations were not accompanied by clinical hyperthyroidism.

Variations in the karyopyknotic index on vaginal smears and various degrees of estrogen effect on Pap smears have been infrequently seen in postmenopausal patients given NOLVADEX.

In the postmarketing experience with NOLVADEX, infrequent cases of hyperlipidemias have been reported. Periodic monitoring of plasma triglycerides and cholesterol may be indicated in patients with pre-existing hyperlipidemias (See **ADVERSE REACTIONS—Postmarketing experience** section).

Carcinogenesis: A conventional carcinogenesis study in rats (doses of 5, 20, and 35 mg/kg/day for up to 2 years) revealed hepatocellular carcinoma at all doses, and the incidence of these tumors was significantly greater among rats given 20 or 35 mg/kg/day (69%) than those given 5 mg/kg/day (14%). The incidence of these tumors in rats given 5 mg/kg/day (29.5 mg/m^2) was significantly greater than in controls.

In addition, preliminary data from 2 independent reports of 6-month studies in rats reveal liver tumors which in one study are classified as malignant (See **WARNINGS**).

Endocrine changes in immature and mature mice were investigated in a 13-month study. Granulosa cell ovarian tumors and interstitial cell testicular tumors were found in mice receiving NOLVADEX, but not in the controls.

Mutagenesis: Although no genotoxic potential was found in a conventional battery of in vivo and in vitro tests with pro- and eukaryotic test systems with drug metabolizing systems present, increased levels of DNA adducts have been found in the livers of rats exposed to tamoxifen. Tamoxifen also has been found to increase levels of micronucleus formation in vitro in human lymphoblastoid cell line (MCL-5). Based on these findings, tamoxifen is genotoxic in rodent and human MCL-5 cells.

Impairment of Fertility: Fertility in female rats was decreased following administration of 0.04 mg/kg for two weeks prior to mating through day 7 of pregnancy. There was a decreased number of implantations, and all fetuses were found dead.

Following administration to rats of 0.16 mg/kg from days 7–17 of pregnancy, there were increased numbers of fetal deaths. Administration of 0.125 mg/kg to rabbits during days 6–18 of pregnancy resulted in abortion or premature delivery. Fetal deaths occurred at higher doses. There were no teratogenic changes in either rat or rabbit segment II studies. Several pregnant marmosets were dosed with 10 mg/kg/day either during organogenesis or in the last half of pregnancy. No deformations were seen, and although the dose was high enough to terminate pregnancy in some animals, those that did maintain pregnancy showed no evidence of teratogenic malformations. Rats given 0.16 mg/kg from day 17 of pregnancy to 1 day before weaning demonstrated increased numbers of dead pups at parturition. It was reported that some rat pups showed slower learning behavior, but this did not achieve statistical significance in one study, and in another study where significance was reported, this was obtained by comparing dosed animals with controls of another study.

The recommended daily human dose of 20–40 mg corresponds to 0.4–0.8 mg/kg for an average 50 kg woman.

Pregnancy Category D: See **WARNINGS**.

Nursing Mothers: It is not known whether this drug is excreted in human milk. Because many drugs are excreted in human milk and because of the potential for serious adverse reactions in nursing infants from NOLVADEX, a decision should be made whether to discontinue nursing or to discontinue the drug, taking into account the importance of the drug to the mother.

Pediatric Use: The safety and efficacy of NOLVADEX in pediatric patients have not been established.

Geriatric Use: In the NSABP P-1 trial, the percentage of women at least 65 years of age was 16%. Women at least 70 years of age accounted for 6% of the participants. A reduction in breast cancer incidence was seen among participants in each of the subsets: A total of 28 and 10 invasive breast cancers were seen among participants 65 and older in the placebo and NOLVADEX groups, respectively. Across all other outcomes, the results in this subset reflect the results observed in the subset of women at least 50 years of age. No overall differences in tolerability were observed between older and younger patients (See **CLINICAL PHARMACOLOGY—Clinical Studies—Reduction in Breast Cancer Incidence in High Risk Women** section).

ADVERSE REACTIONS

Adverse reactions to NOLVADEX are relatively mild and rarely severe enough to require discontinuation of treatment in breast cancer patients.

Continued clinical studies have resulted in further information which better indicates the incidence of adverse reactions with NOLVADEX as compared to placebo.

Metastatic Breast Cancer: Increased bone and tumor pain and, also, local disease flare have occurred, which are sometimes associated with a good tumor response. Patients with increased bone pain may require additional analgesics. Patients with soft tissue disease may have sudden increases in the size of preexisting lesions, sometimes associated with marked erythema within and surrounding the lesions and/or the development of new lesions. When they occur, the bone pain or disease flare are seen shortly after starting NOLVADEX and generally subside rapidly.

In patients treated with NOLVADEX for metastatic breast cancer, the most frequent adverse reaction to NOLVADEX is hot flashes.

Other adverse reactions which are seen infrequently are hypercalcemia, peripheral edema, distaste for food, pruritus vulvae, depression, dizziness, light-headedness, headache, hair thinning and/or partial hair loss, and vaginal dryness.

Premenopausal Women: The following table summarizes the incidence of adverse reactions reported at a frequency of 2% or greater from clinical trials (Ingle, Pritchard, Buchanan) which compared NOLVADEX therapy to ovarian ablation in premenopausal patients with metastatic breast cancer.

[See table above]

Male Breast Cancer: NOLVADEX is well tolerated in males with breast cancer. Reports from the literature and case reports suggest that the safety profile of NOLVADEX in males is similar to that seen in women. Loss of libido and impotence have resulted in discontinuation of tamoxifen therapy in male patients. Also, in oligospermic males treated with tamoxifen, LH, FSH, testosterone and estrogen levels were elevated. No significant clinical changes were reported.

Adjuvant Breast Cancer: In the NSABP B-14 study, women with axillary node-negative breast cancer were randomized to 5 years of NOLVADEX 20 mg/day or placebo following primary surgery. The reported adverse effects are tabulated below (mean follow-up of approximately 6.8 years) showing adverse events more common on NOLVADEX than on placebo. The incidence of hot flashes (64% vs. 48%), vaginal discharge (30% vs. 15%), and irregular menses (25% vs. 19%) were higher with NOLVADEX compared with placebo. All other adverse effects occurred with similar frequency in the 2 treatment groups, with the

Continued on next page

Nolvadex—Cont.

exception of thrombotic events, a higher incidence was seen in NOLVADEX-treated patients (through 5 years, 1.7% vs. 0.4%). Two of the patients treated with NOLVADEX who had thrombotic events died.

[See table above]

In the Eastern Cooperative Oncology Group (ECOG) adjuvant breast cancer trial, NOLVADEX or placebo was administered for 2 years to women following mastectomy. When compared to placebo, NOLVADEX showed a significantly higher incidence of hot flashes (19% vs. 8% for placebo). The incidence of all other adverse reactions was similar in the 2 treatment groups with the exception of thrombocytopenia where the incidence for NOLVADEX was 10% vs. 3% for placebo, an observation of borderline statistical significance.

In other adjuvant studies, Toronto and NOLVADEX Adjuvant Trial Organization (NATO), women received either NOLVADEX or no therapy. In the Toronto study, hot flashes were observed in 29% of patients, for NOLVADEX vs. 1% in the untreated group. In the NATO trial, hot flashes and vaginal bleeding were reported in 2.8%, and 2.0% of women, respectively, for NOLVADEX vs. 0.2% for each in the untreated group.

Reduction in Breast Cancer Incidence in High Risk Women: In the NSABP P-1 Trial, there was an increase in five serious adverse effects in the NOLVADEX group: endometrial cancer (33 cases in the NOLVADEX group vs. 14 in the placebo group); pulmonary embolism (18 cases in the NOLVADEX group vs. 6 in the placebo group); deep vein thrombosis (30 cases in the NOLVADEX group vs. 19 in the placebo group); stroke (34 cases in the NOLVADEX group vs. 24 in the placebo group); cataract formation (540 cases in the NOLVADEX group vs. 483 in the placebo group) and cataract surgery (101 cases in the NOLVADEX group vs. 63 in the placebo group) (See **WARNINGS** and Table 2 in **CLINICAL PHARMACOLOGY**).

The following table presents the adverse events observed in NSABP P-1 by treatment arm. Only adverse events more common on NOLVADEX than placebo are shown.

[See table above]

In the NSABP P-1 trial, 15.0% and 9.7% of participants receiving NOLVADEX and placebo therapy, respectively withdrew from the trial for medical reasons. The following are the medical reasons for withdrawing from NOLVADEX and placebo therapy, respectively: Hot flashes (3.1% vs. 1.5%) and Vaginal Discharge (0.5% vs. 0.1%).

In the NSABP P-1 Trial, 8.7% and 9.6% of participants receiving NOLVADEX and placebo therapy, respectively withdrew for non-medical reasons.

On the NSABP P-1 Trial, hot flashes of any severity occurred in 68% of women on placebo and in 80% of women on NOLVADEX. Severe hot flashes occurred in 28% of women on placebo and 45% of women on NOLVADEX. Vaginal discharge occurred in 35% and 55% of women on placebo and NOLVADEX respectively; and was severe in 4.5% and 12.3% respectively. There was no difference in the incidence of vaginal bleeding between treatment arms.

Postmarketing experience: Less frequently reported adverse reactions are vaginal bleeding, vaginal discharge, menstrual irregularities, skin rash and headaches. Usually these have not been of sufficient severity to require dosage reduction or discontinuation of treatment. Very rare reports of erythema multiforme, Stevens-Johnson syndrome, bullous pemphigoid and rare reports of hypersensitivity reactions including angioedema have been reported with NOLVADEX therapy. Rarely, elevation of serum triglyceride levels, in some cases with pancreatitis, may be associated with the use of NOLVADEX (see **PRECAUTIONS—Drug/Laboratory Testing Interactions** section).

OVERDOSAGE

Signs observed at the highest doses following studies to determine LD_{50} in animals were respiratory difficulties and convulsions.

Acute overdosage in humans has not been reported. In a study of advanced metastatic cancer patients which specifically determined the maximum tolerated dose of NOLVADEX in evaluating the use of very high doses to reverse multidrug resistance, acute neurotoxicity manifested by tremor, hyperreflexia, unsteady gait and dizziness were noted. These symptoms occurred within 3–5 days of beginning NOLVADEX and cleared within 2–5 days after stopping therapy. No permanent neurologic toxicity was noted. One patient experienced a seizure several days after NOLVADEX was discontinued and neurotoxic symptoms had resolved. The causal relationship of the seizure to NOLVADEX therapy is unknown. Doses given in these patients were all greater than 400 mg/m^2 loading dose, followed by maintenance doses of 150 mg/m^2 of NOLVADEX given twice a day.

In the same study, prolongation of the QT interval on the electrocardiogram was noted when patients were given doses higher than 250 mg/m^2 loading dose, followed by maintenance doses of 80 mg/m^2 of NOLVADEX given twice a day. For a woman with a body surface area of 1.5 m^2 the minimal loading dose and maintenance doses given at which neurological symptoms and QT changes occurred were at least 6 fold higher in respect to the maximum recommended dose.

No specific treatment for overdosage is known; treatment must be symptomatic.

NSABP B-14 Study

Adverse Effect	% of Women NOLVADEX (n=1422)	PLACEBO (n=1437)	Adverse Effect	% of Women NOLVADEX (n=1422)	PLACEBO (n=1437)
Hot Flashes	64	48	Increased Bilirubin	2	1
Fluid Retention	32	30	Increased Creatinine	2	1
Vaginal Discharge	30	15	Thrombocytopenia*	2	1
Nausea	26	24	Thrombotic Events		
Irregular Menses	25	19	Deep Vein Thrombosis	0.8	0.2
Weight Loss (>5%)	23	18	Pulmonary Embolism	0.5	0.2
Skin Changes	19	15	Superficial Phlebitis	0.4	0.0
Increased SGOT	5	3			

* Defined as a platelet count of $<100{,}000/\text{mm}^3$

NSABP P-1 Trial: All Adverse Events

	% of Women NOLVADEX N=6681	PLACEBO N=6707		% of Women NOLVADEX N=6681	PLACEBO N=6707
Self Reported Symptoms	N=6441[1]	N=6469[1]	**Adverse Effects**	N=6492[3]	N=6484[3]
Hot Flashes	80	68	**Other Toxicities**		
Vaginal Discharges	55	35	Mood	11.6	10.8
Vaginal Bleeding	23	22	Infection/Sepsis	6.0	5.1
			Constipation	4.4	3.2
Laboratory Abnormalities	N=6520[2]	N=6535[2]	Alopecia	5.2	4.4
Platelets decreased	0.7	0.3	Skin	5.6	4.7
			Allergy	2.5	2.1

[1] Number with Quality of Life Questionnaires
[2] Number with Treatment Follow-up Forms
[3] Number with Adverse Drug Reaction Forms

DOSAGE AND ADMINISTRATION

For patients with breast cancer, the recommended daily dose is 20–40 mg. Dosages greater than 20 mg per day should be given in divided doses (morning and evening).

In three single agent adjuvant studies in women, one 10 mg NOLVADEX tablet was administered two (ECOG and NATO) or three (Toronto) times a day for two years. In the NSABP B-14 adjuvant study in women with node-negative breast cancer, one 10 mg NOLVADEX tablet was given twice a day for at least five years. Results of the B-14 study suggest that continuation of therapy beyond five years does not provide additional benefit (see **CLINICAL PHARMACOLOGY**). In the EBCTCG 1995 overview, the reduction in recurrence and mortality was greater in those studies that used tamoxifen for about 5 years than in those that used tamoxifen for a shorter period of therapy. There was no indication that doses greater than 20 mg per day were more effective. Current data from clinical trials support five years of adjuvant NOLVADEX therapy for patients with breast cancer.

Reduction in Breast Cancer Incidence in High Risk Women: The recommended dose is NOLVADEX 20 mg daily for 5 years. There are no data to support the use of NOLVADEX other than for 5 years (See **CLINICAL PHARMACOLOGY—Clinical Studies—Reduction in Breast Cancer Incidence in High Risk Women**).

HOW SUPPLIED

10 mg Tablets containing tamoxifen as the citrate in an amount equivalent to 10 mg of tamoxifen (round, biconvex, uncoated, white tablet identified with NOLVADEX 600 debossed on one side and a cameo debossed on the other side) are supplied in bottles of 60 tablets, 180 tablets and 2500 tablets. NDC 0310-0600.

20 mg Tablets containing tamoxifen as the citrate in an amount equivalent to 20 mg of tamoxifen (round, biconvex, uncoated, white tablet identified with NOLVADEX 604 debossed on one side and a cameo debossed on the other side) are supplied in bottles of 30 tablets, 90 tablets and 1250 tablets. NDC 0310-0604.

Store at controlled room temperature, 20–25°C (68–77°F) [see USP]. Dispense in a well-closed, light-resistant container.

Patient Information about
NOLVADEX® (tamoxifen citrate) Tablets

for Breast Cancer Treatment and Reduction in the Incidence of Breast Cancer

Brand Name: **NOLVADEX®** (Nol 'va dex) Generic Name: Tamoxifen (ta-MOX-i-fen)

Please read this information carefully before you begin taking NOLVADEX. It is important to read this information each time your prescription is filled or refilled in case new information is available. This summary does not tell you everything about NOLVADEX. Your health care professional is the best source of information about this medicine. You should talk with him or her before you begin taking NOLVADEX and at regular checkups. In addition, the professional package insert contains more detailed information on NOLVADEX.

What are the most important things I should know about NOLVADEX?

NOLVADEX has been shown to help women with advanced breast cancer and in clinical trials of over 30,000 women with early breast cancer it has been shown to reduce the risk of recurrence. Also in a trial of 13,000 women at high risk of breast cancer, NOLVADEX reduced the risk of developing the disease.

Like all medicines, NOLVADEX has some side effects. Most are mild and relate to its hormonal mode of action. NOLVADEX can, however, also increase the risk of some serious and potentially life-threatening conditions, including, uterine cancer, blood clots, and stroke. It can also increase the risk of getting cataracts or of needing cataract surgery. If you experience symptoms of any of these, tell your doctor **immediately** (see **"What should I avoid or do while taking NOLVADEX?"**). You and your doctor must carefully discuss your personal medical conditions, history, and preferences to decide whether the good NOLVADEX may do for you outweighs its potential risks. If you and your doctor decide that NOLVADEX therapy is right for you, you should look for symptoms indicating you might be experiencing one of NOLVADEX's known risks.

What is NOLVADEX?

- NOLVADEX is a prescription medicine used to reduce the risk of getting breast cancer in women who have a high risk of getting breast cancer.

This effect was shown in the Breast Cancer Prevention Trial (BCPT, NSABP P-1), a large study where over 13,000 women at high risk for breast cancer were to take NOLVADEX or placebo (a pill without tamoxifen) for 5 years. High risk women were those who were at least 35 years old and had a combination of risks that made their chances of developing breast cancer greater than 1.67% in the next five years. The risk factors included early age at first menstrual period, late age at first pregnancy, no pregnancies, close family members with breast cancer (mother, sister, or daughter), history of previous breast biopsies, or high-risk changes in the breast seen on a biopsy. Twenty-five percent of the women in the study completed 5 years of treatment, and most women in this study have been followed for about 4 years. The study showed that NOLVADEX reduced the chance of getting breast cancer by 44%. The longer term effects of NOLVADEX on reducing the chance of getting breast cancer are not known.

We do not know whether taking NOLVADEX for 5 years only delays the appearance of cancer, or actually decreases the number of tumors that will ever develop since long-term studies have not been completed. Some women in this study also experienced serious side effects of NOLVADEX. They are described in detail in the section, **What are the possible side effects of NOLVADEX?**. Some of these women experienced complications related to the treatment of these side effects.

The following table of the major results from the study is intended to be an aid in weighing the potential benefit of a reduction in risk of breast cancer against the potential risk of serious side effects of NOLVADEX.

[See table at bottom of next page]

Two European trials of NOLVADEX in women with a high risk of breast cancer were also conducted. They showed no difference in the number of breast cancer cases between the women who took tamoxifen and those who got placebo. These studies had trial designs that differed from that of NSABP P-1, were smaller than P-1, and enrolled women at a lower risk for breast cancer than those in the P-1 trial.

- NOLVADEX is used to treat advanced breast cancer in women and men.

  Three studies compared NOLVADEX to surgery or radiation to the ovaries in premenopausal women with advanced breast cancer and found that NOLVADEX was similar to surgery or radiation in causing tumor shrinkage.

  Published studies have demonstrated that NOLVADEX is effective for the treatment of advanced breast cancer in men.

- NOLVADEX is used to reduce the recurrence of breast cancer in women who have had surgery and/or radiation therapy to treat early breast cancer. NOLVADEX is also used in women with breast cancer who are at risk of developing a second breast cancer in the opposite breast. The Early Breast Cancer Trialists Collaborative Group reviewed the 10-year results of studies of NOLVADEX for early breast cancer. Treatment with NOLVADEX for about 5 years reduced the risk of recurrence of breast cancer and improved overall survival. Treatment with about 5 years of NOLVADEX also reduced the chance of getting a second breast cancer in the opposite breast by approximately 50%, a result similar to that seen in the NSABP P-1 study.

- NOLVADEX is a tablet available in two dosage strengths: 10 mg tablets and 20 mg tablets. The active ingredient in each tablet is tamoxifen citrate.

How does NOLVADEX work?

NOLVADEX belongs to a group of medicines called anti-estrogens. Anti-estrogens work by blocking the effects of the hormone estrogen in the body. Estrogen may cause the growth of some types of breast tumors. NOLVADEX may block the growth of tumors that respond to estrogen.

Who should not take NOLVADEX?

- You should not take NOLVADEX to reduce the risk of getting breast cancer if you have ever had blood clots or if you develop blood clots that require medical treatment. However, if you are taking NOLVADEX for treatment of early or advanced breast cancer, the benefits of NOLVADEX may outweigh the risks associated with developing new blood clots. Your health care professional can assist you in deciding whether NOLVADEX is right for you.
- You should not take NOLVADEX if you are taking medicines to thin your blood (anticoagulants) like warfarin (Coumadin®*).
- You should not take NOLVADEX if you plan to become pregnant while taking NOLVADEX or during the two months after you stop taking it because NOLVADEX may harm your unborn child. You should see your doctor immediately and stop taking NOLVADEX if you become pregnant while taking the drug. Please talk with your doctor about birth control recommendations. If you are capable of becoming pregnant, you should start NOLVADEX during a menstrual period or if you have irregular periods have a negative pregnancy test before beginning to take NOLVADEX.
- You should not take NOLVADEX if you are breast feeding.
- You should not take NOLVADEX if you have ever had an allergic reaction to NOLVADEX or tamoxifen citrate (the chemical name) or any of its ingredients.
- NOLVADEX is not known to reduce the risk of breast cancer in women with changes in breast cancer genes (BRCA1 or BRCA2).
- You should not take NOLVADEX to decrease the chance of getting breast cancer if you are less than age 35 because NOLVADEX has not been tested in younger women.
- You should not take NOLVADEX to reduce the risk of breast cancer unless you are at high risk of getting breast cancer. Certain conditions put women at high risk and it is possible to calculate this risk for any woman. Breast cancer risk assessment tools to help calculate your risk of breast cancer have been developed and are available to your health care professional. You should discuss your risks with your health care professional.
- Children should not take NOLVADEX because treatment for them has not been sufficiently studied.

How should I take NOLVADEX?

- Follow your doctor's instructions about when and how to take NOLVADEX. Read the label on the container. If you are unsure or have questions, ask your doctor or pharmacist.
- You will take NOLVADEX differently, depending on your diagnosis.
- For treatment of breast cancer in adult women and men, the usual dose is 20–40 mg a day. Take the tablets once or twice a day depending on the tablet strength prescribed. If your doctor has prescribed a different dose, do not change it unless he or she tells you to do so. For women with early breast cancer, NOLVADEX should be taken for 5 years. For women with advanced cancer, NOLVADEX should be taken until your doctor feels it is no longer indicated.
- For reduction of the risk of breast cancer, the usual dose is 20 mg a day, for five years.
- Take your medicine each day. You may find it easier to remember to take your medicine if you take it at the same time each day. If you forget to take a dose, take it as soon as you remember and then take the next dose as usual.
- Swallow the tablets whole with a drink of water.
- You can take NOLVADEX with or without food.
- Do not stop taking your tablets unless your doctor tells you to do so.

Are there other important factors to consider before taking NOLVADEX?

- Tell your doctor if you have ever had blood clots that required medical treatment.
- Because NOLVADEX may affect how other medicines work, always tell your doctor if you are taking any other prescription or non-prescription (over-the-counter) medications, particularly if you are taking warfarin to thin your blood.
- You should not become pregnant when taking NOLVADEX or during the two months after you stop taking it as NOLVADEX may harm your unborn child. Please contact your doctor for birth control recommendations. You should see your doctor immediately if you think you may have become pregnant after starting to take NOLVADEX.

What should I avoid/or do while taking NOLVADEX?

- You should contact your doctor immediately if you notice any of the following symptoms. Some of these symptoms may suggest that you are experiencing a rare but serious side effect associated with NOLVADEX (see **"What are the possible side effects of NOLVADEX?"**).
  - — new breast lumps
  - — vaginal bleeding
  - — changes in your menstrual cycle
  - — changes in vaginal discharge
  - — pelvic pain or pressure
  - — swelling or tenderness in your calf
  - — unexplained breathlessness (shortness of breath)
  - — sudden chest pain
  - — coughing up blood
  - — changes in your vision

  If you see a health care professional who is new to you (an emergency room doctor, another doctor in the practice), tell him or her that you take NOLVADEX.
- Because NOLVADEX may affect how other medicines work, always tell your doctor if you are taking any other prescription or non-prescription (over-the-counter) medicines. Be sure to tell your doctor if you are taking warfarin (coumadin) to thin your blood.
- You should not become pregnant when taking NOLVADEX or during the two months after you stop taking it because NOLVADEX may harm your unborn child. You should see your doctor immediately if you think you may have become pregnant after starting to take NOLVADEX. Please talk with your doctor about birth control recommendations. If you are taking NOLVADEX to reduce your risk of getting breast cancer, and you are sexually active, NOLVADEX should be started during your menstrual period. If you have irregular periods, you should have a negative pregnancy test before you start NOLVADEX.
- If you are taking NOLVADEX to reduce your risk of getting breast cancer, you should know that NOLVADEX does not prevent all breast cancers. While you are taking NOLVADEX and in keeping with your doctor's recommendation, you should have annual gynecological check-ups which should include breast exams and mammograms. If breast cancer occurs, there is no guarantee that it will be detected at an early stage. This is why it is important to continue with regular check-ups.

What are the possible side effects of NOLVADEX?

Like many medicines, NOLVADEX causes side effects in most patients. The majority of the side effects seen with NOLVADEX have been mild and do not usually cause breast cancer patients to stop taking the medication. In women with breast cancer, withdrawal from NOLVADEX therapy is about 5%. Approximately 15% of women who took NOLVADEX to reduce the chance of getting breast cancer stopped treatment because of side effects.

The most common side effects reported with NOLVADEX are: hot flashes; vaginal discharge or bleeding; and menstrual irregularities (these side effects may be mild or may be a sign of a more serious side effect). Women may experience hair loss, skin rashes (itching or peeling skin) or headaches; however, hair loss is uncommon and is usually mild.

A rare but serious side effect of NOLVADEX is a blood clot in the veins. Blood clots stop the flow of blood and can cause serious medical problems, disability or death. Women who take NOLVADEX are at increased risk for developing blood clots in the lungs and legs. Some women may develop more than one blood clot, even if NOLVADEX is stopped. Women may also have complications from treating the clot, such as bleeding from thinning the blood too much. Symptoms of a blood clot in the lungs may include sudden chest pain, shortness of breath or coughing up blood. Symptoms of a blood clot in the legs are pain or swelling in the calves. A blood clot in the legs may move to the lungs. If you experience any of these symptoms of a blood clot, contact your doctor immediately.

	Cases per year out of 1000 Women taking NOLVADEX	Cases per year out of 1000 Women taking Placebo
Breast Cancer	3.6	6.5
Endometrial Cancer*	2.3	0.9
Blood clot in the lungs	0.8	0.3
Blood clot in the veins	1.3	0.8
Stroke	1.4	1.0
Cataracts	25.4	22.5
Cataract surgery	46.6	31.4

* In women with a uterus.

NOLVADEX increases the chance of having a stroke, which can cause serious medical problems, disability, or death. If you experience any symptoms of stroke, such as weakness, difficulty walking or talking, or numbness, contact your doctor immediately.

NOLVADEX increases the chance of changes occurring in the lining of your uterus (endometrium), which can be serious and could include cancer of the uterus. If you have not had a hysterectomy (removal of the uterus), it is important for you to contact your doctor immediately if you experience any unusual vaginal discharge, vaginal bleeding, or menstrual irregularities; or pain or pressure in the pelvis (lower stomach). These may be caused by changes to the lining of your uterus (endometrium). It is important to bring them to your doctor's attention without delay as they can occasionally indicate the start of something more serious, and could include cancer of the uterus or other changes to the uterus.

NOLVADEX may cause cataracts or changes to parts of the eye known as the cornea or retina. NOLVADEX can increase the chance of needing cataract surgery, and can cause blood clots in the veins of the eye. NOLVADEX can result in difficulty in distinguishing different colors. If you experience any changes in your vision, tell your doctor immediately.

Rare side effects, which may be serious, include certain liver problems such as jaundice (which may be seen as yellowing of the whites of the eyes) or hypertriglyceridemia (increased levels of fats in the blood) sometimes with pancreatitis (pain or tenderness in the upper abdomen). Stop taking NOLVADEX and contact your doctor immediately if you develop angioedema (swelling of the face, lips, tongue and/or throat).

If you are a woman receiving NOLVADEX for treatment of advanced breast cancer, and you experience excessive nausea, vomiting or thirst, tell your doctor immediately. This may mean that there are changes in the amount of calcium in your blood (hypercalcemia). Your doctor will evaluate this.

In patients with breast cancer, a temporary increase in the size of the tumor may occur and sometimes results in muscle aches/bone pain and skin redness. This condition may occur shortly after starting NOLVADEX and may be associated with a good response to treatment.

Many of these side effects happen only rarely. However, you should contact your doctor if you think you have any of these or any other problems with your NOLVADEX. Some side effects of NOLVADEX may become apparent soon after starting the drug, but others may first appear at any time during therapy.

This summary does not include all possible side effects with NOLVADEX. It is important to talk to your health care professional about possible side effects. If you want to read more, ask your doctor or pharmacist to give you the professional labeling.

How should I store NOLVADEX?

NOLVADEX Tablets should be stored at room temperature (68–77°F). Keep in a well-closed, light-resistant container. Keep out of the reach of children.

Do not take your tablets after the expiration date on the container. Be sure that any discarded tablets are out of the reach of children.

This leaflet provides you with a summary of information about NOLVADEX. Medicines are sometimes prescribed for uses other than those listed. NOLVADEX has been prescribed specifically for you by your doctor. Do not give your medicine to anyone else, even if they have a similar condition, because it may harm them.

If you have any questions or concerns, contact your doctor or pharmacist. Your pharmacist also has a longer leaflet about NOLVADEX written for health care professionals that you can ask to read. For more information about NOLVADEX or breast cancer, call 1-800-34 LIFE 4.

*Coumadin® is a registered trademark of DuPont Pharmaceuticals.

ZENECA Pharmaceuticals
A Business Unit of Zeneca Inc.
Wilmington, Delaware 19850-5437
64156-00 Rev W 9/99

Shown in Product Identification Guide, page 306

SEROQUEL® ℞
[*serō-quĕl*]
(quetiapine fumarate)
tablets

DESCRIPTION

SEROQUEL (quetiapine fumarate) is an antipsychotic drug belonging to a new chemical class, the dibenzothiazepine derivatives. The chemical designation is 2-[2-(4-dibenzo *[b,f]* [1,4]thiazepin-11-yl-1-piperazinyl)ethoxy]-ethanol fumarate (2:1) (salt). It is present in tablets as the fumarate salt. All doses and tablet strengths are expressed as milligrams of base, not as fumarate salt. Its molecular formula is

Continued on next page

Seroquel—Cont.

$C_{42}H_{50}N_6O_4S_2 \cdot C_4H_4O_4$ and it has a molecular weight of 883.11 (fumarate salt). The structural formula is:

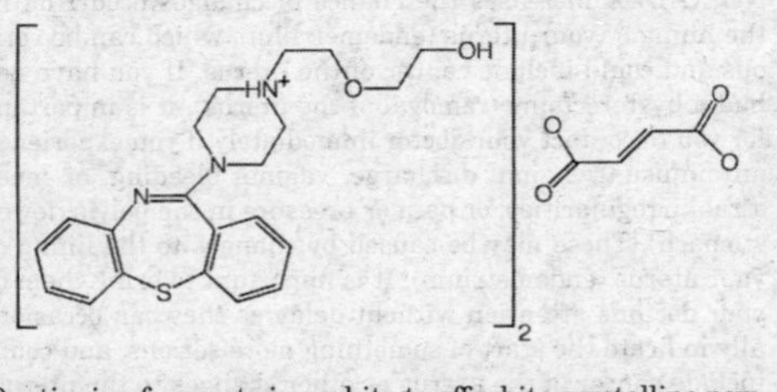

Quetiapine fumarate is a white to off-white crystalline powder which is moderately soluble in water.

SEROQUEL is supplied for oral administration as 25 mg (peach), 100 mg (yellow) and 200 mg (white) tablets.

Inactive ingredients are povidone, dibasic dicalcium phosphate dihydrate, microcrystalline cellulose, sodium starch glycolate, lactose monohydrate, magnesium stearate, hydroxypropyl methylcellulose, polyethylene glycol, and titanium dioxide.

The 25 mg tablets contain red ferric oxide and yellow ferric oxide and the 100 mg tablets contain only yellow ferric oxide.

CLINICAL PHARMACOLOGY

Pharmacodynamics

SEROQUEL is an antagonist at multiple neurotransmitter receptors in the brain; serotonin $5HT_{1A}$ and $5HT_2$ (IC_{50s}=717 & 148nM respectively), dopamine D_1 and D_2 (IC_{50s}= 1268 & 329nM respectively), histamine H_1 (IC_{50}=30nM), and adrenergic α_1 and α_2 receptors (IC_{50s}=94 & 271nM, respectively). SEROQUEL has no appreciable affinity at cholinergic muscarinic and benzodiazepine receptors (IC_{50s}>5000 nM).

The mechanism of action of SEROQUEL, as with other antipsychotic drugs, is unknown. However, it has been proposed that this drug's antipsychotic activity is mediated through a combination of dopamine type 2 (D_2) and serotonin type 2 ($5\text{-}HT_2$) antagonism. Antagonism at receptors other than dopamine and $5HT_2$ with similar receptor affinities may explain some of the other effects of SEROQUEL.

SEROQUEL'S antagonism of histamine H_1 receptors may explain the somnolence observed with this drug.

SEROQUEL'S antagonism of adrenergic α_1 receptors may explain the orthostatic hypotension observed with this drug.

Pharmacokinetics

Quetiapine fumarate activity is primarily due to the parent drug. The multiple-dose pharmacokinetics of quetiapine are dose-proportional within the proposed clinical dose range, and quetiapine accumulation is predictable upon multiple dosing. Elimination of quetiapine is mainly via hepatic metabolism with a mean terminal half-life of about 6 hours within the proposed clinical dose range. Steady state concentrations are expected to be achieved within two days of dosing. Quetiapine is unlikely to interfere with the metabolism of drugs metabolized by cytochrome P450 enzymes.

Absorption: Quetiapine fumarate is rapidly absorbed after oral administration, reaching peak plasma concentrations in 1.5 hours. The tablet formulation is 100% bioavailable relative to solution. The bioavailability of quetiapine is marginally affected by administration with food, with C_{max} and AUC values increased by 25% and 15%, respectively.

Distribution: Quetiapine is widely distributed throughout the body with an apparent volume of distribution of 10±4 L/kg. It is 83% bound to plasma proteins at therapeutic concentrations. *In vitro*, quetiapine did not affect the binding of warfarin or diazepam to human serum albumin. In turn, neither warfarin nor diazepam altered the binding of quetiapine.

Metabolism and Elimination: Following a single oral dose of ^{14}C-quetiapine, less than 1% of the administered dose was excreted as unchanged drug, indicating that quetiapine is highly metabolized. Approximately 73% and 20% of the dose was recovered in the urine and feces, respectively.

Quetiapine is extensively metabolized by the liver. The major metabolic pathways are sulfoxidation to the sulfoxide metabolite and oxidation to the parent acid metabolite; both metabolites are pharmacologically inactive. *In vitro* studies using human liver microsomes revealed that the cytochrome P450 3A4 isoenzyme is involved in the metabolism of quetiapine to its major, but inactive, sulfoxide metabolite.

Population Subgroups

Age: Oral clearance of quetiapine was reduced by 40% in elderly patients (≥ 65 years, n=9) compared to young patients (n=12), and dosing adjustment may be necessary (See **DOSAGE AND ADMINISTRATION**).

Gender: There is no gender effect on the pharmacokinetics of quetiapine.

Race: There is no race effect on the pharmacokinetics of quetiapine.

Smoking: Smoking has no effect on the oral clearance of quetiapine.

Renal Insufficiency: Patients with severe renal impairment (Clcr=10–30 mL/min/1.73 m^2, n=8) had a 25% lower mean oral clearance than normal subjects (Clcr > 80 mL/min/1.73 m^2, n=8), but plasma quetiapine concentrations in the subjects with renal insufficiency were within the range of concentrations seen in normal subjects receiving the same dose. Dosage adjustment is therefore not needed in these patients.

Hepatic Insufficiency: Hepatically impaired patients (n=8) had a 30% lower mean oral clearance of quetiapine than normal subjects. In two of the 8 hepatically impaired patients, AUC and C_{max} were 3-times higher than those observed typically in healthy subjects. Since quetiapine is extensively metabolized by the liver, higher plasma levels are expected in the hepatically impaired population, and dosage adjustment may be needed. (See **DOSAGE AND ADMINISTRATION**).

Drug-Drug Interactions: *In vitro* enzyme inhibition data suggest that quetiapine and 9 of its metabolites would have little inhibitory effect on *in vivo* metabolism mediated by cytochromes P450 1A2, 2C9, 2C19, 2D6, and 3A4.

Quetiapine oral clearance is increased by the prototype cytochrome P450 3A4 inducer, phenytoin, and decreased by the prototype cytochrome P450 3A4 inhibitor, ketoconazole. Dose adjustment of quetiapine will be necessary if it is coadministered with phenytoin or ketoconazole. (See **DRUG INTERACTIONS** under **PRECAUTIONS** and **DOSAGE AND ADMINISTRATION**).

Quetiapine oral clearance is not inhibited by the non-specific enzyme inhibitor, cimetidine.

Quetiapine at doses of 750 mg/day did not affect the single dose pharmacokinetics of antipyrine, lithium, or lorazepam. (See **DRUG INTERACTIONS** under **PRECAUTIONS**).

Clinical Efficacy Data

The efficacy of SEROQUEL in the management of the manifestations of psychotic disorders was established in 3 short-term (6-week) controlled trials of psychotic inpatients who met DSM III-R criteria for schizophrenia. Although a single fixed dose haloperidol arm was included as a comparative treatment in one of the three trials, this single haloperidol dose group was inadequate to provide a reliable and valid comparison of SEROQUEL and haloperidol.

Several instruments were used for assessing psychiatric signs and symptoms in these studies, among them the Brief Psychiatric Rating Scale (BPRS), a multi-item inventory of general psychopathology traditionally used to evaluate the effects of drug treatment in psychosis. The BPRS psychosis cluster (conceptual disorganization, hallucinatory behavior, suspiciousness, and unusual thought content) is considered a particularly useful subset for assessing actively psychotic schizophrenic patients. A second traditional assessment, the Clinical Global Impression (CGI), reflects the impression of a skilled observer, fully familiar with the manifestations of schizophrenia, about the overall clinical state of the patient. In addition, the Scale for Assessing Negative Symptoms (SANS), a more recently developed but less well evaluated scale, was employed for assessing negative symptoms.

The results of the trials follow:

(1) In a 6-week, placebo-controlled trial (n=361) involving 5 fixed doses of SEROQUEL (75, 150, 300, 600, and 750 mg/day on a tid schedule), the 4 highest doses of SEROQUEL were generally superior to placebo on the BPRS total score, the BPRS psychosis cluster, and the CGI severity score, with the maximum effect seen at 300 mg/day, and the effects of doses of 150 to 750 were generally indistinguishable. SEROQUEL, at a dose of 300 mg/day, was superior to placebo on the SANS.

(2) In a 6-week, placebo-controlled trial (n=286) involving titration of SEROQUEL in high (up to 750 mg/day on a tid schedule) and low (up to 250 mg/day on a tid schedule) doses, only the high dose of SEROQUEL group (mean dose, 500 mg/day) was generally superior to placebo on the BPRS total score, the BPRS psychosis cluster, the CGI severity score, and the SANS.

(3) In a 6-week dose and dose regimen comparison trial (n=618) involving two fixed doses of SEROQUEL (450 mg/day on both bid and tid schedules and 50 mg/day on a bid schedule), only the 450 mg/day (225 mg bid schedule) dose group was generally superior to the 50 mg/day (25 mg bid) SEROQUEL dose group on the BPRS total score, the BPRS psychosis cluster, the CGI severity score, and on the SANS.

Examination of population subsets (race, gender, and age) did not reveal any differential responsiveness on the basis of race or gender, with an apparently greater effect in patients under the age of 40 compared to those older than 40. The clinical significance of this finding is unknown.

INDICATIONS AND USAGE

SEROQUEL is indicated for the management of the manifestations of psychotic disorders.

The antipsychotic efficacy of SEROQUEL was established in short-term (6-week) controlled trials of schizophrenic inpatients (See **CLINICAL PHARMACOLOGY**).

The effectiveness of SEROQUEL in long-term use, that is, for more than 6 weeks, has not been systematically evaluated in controlled trials. Therefore, the physician who elects to use SEROQUEL for extended periods should periodically reevaluate the long-term usefulness of the drug for the individual patient (See **DOSAGE AND ADMINISTRATION**).

CONTRAINDICATIONS

SEROQUEL is contraindicated in individuals with a known hypersensitivity to this medication or any of its ingredients.

WARNINGS

Neuroleptic Malignant Syndrome (NMS)

A potentially fatal symptom complex sometimes referred to as Neuroleptic Malignant Syndrome (NMS) has been reported in association with administration of antipsychotic drugs. Two possible cases of NMS [2/2387 (0.1%)] have been reported in clinical trials with SEROQUEL. Clinical manifestations of NMS are hyperpyrexia, muscle rigidity, altered mental status, and evidence of autonomic instability (irregular pulse or blood pressure, tachycardia, diaphoresis, and cardiac dysrhythmia). Additional signs may include elevated creatinine phosphokinase, myoglobinuria (rhabdomyolysis), and acute renal failure.

The diagnostic evaluation of patients with this syndrome is complicated. In arriving at a diagnosis, it is important to exclude cases where the clinical presentation includes both serious medical illness (e.g., pneumonia, systemic infection, etc.) and untreated or inadequately treated extrapyramidal signs and symptoms (EPS). Other important considerations in the differential diagnosis include central anticholinergic toxicity, heat stroke, drug fever, and primary central nervous system (CNS) pathology.

The management of NMS should include: 1) immediate discontinuation of antipsychotic drugs and other drugs not essential to concurrent therapy; 2) intensive symptomatic treatment and medical monitoring; and 3) treatment of any concomitant serious medical problems for which specific treatments are available. There is no general agreement about specific pharmacological treatment regimens for NMS.

If a patient requires antipsychotic drug treatment after recovery from NMS, the potential reintroduction of drug therapy should be carefully considered. The patient should be carefully monitored since recurrences of NMS have been reported.

Tardive Dyskinesia

A syndrome of potentially irreversible, involuntary, dyskinetic movements may develop in patients treated with antipsychotic drugs. Although the prevalence of the syndrome appears to be highest among the elderly, especially elderly women, it is impossible to rely upon prevalence estimates to predict, at the inception of antipsychotic treatment, which patients are likely to develop the syndrome. Whether antipsychotic drug products differ in their potential to cause tardive dyskinesia is unknown.

The risk of developing tradive dyskinesia and the likelihood that it will become irreversible are believed to increase as the duration of treatment and the total cumulative dose of antipsychotic drugs administered to the patient increase. However, the syndrome can develop, although much less commonly, after relatively brief treatment periods at low doses.

There is no known treatment for established cases of tardive dyskinesia, although the syndrome may remit, partially or completely, if antipsychotic treatment is withdrawn. Antipsychotic treatment, itself, however, may suppress (or partially suppress) the signs and symptoms of the syndrome and thereby may possibly mask the underlying process. The effect that symptomatic suppression has upon the long-term course of the syndrome is unknown.

Given these considerations, SEROQUEL should be prescribed in a manner that is most likely to minimize the occurrence of tardive dyskinesia. Chronic antipsychotic treatment should generally be reserved for patients who appear to suffer from a chronic illness that (1) is known to respond to antipsychotic drugs, and (2) for whom alternative, equally effective, but potentially less harmful treatments are not available or appropriate. In patients who do require chronic treatment, the smallest dose and the shortest duration of treatment producing a satisfactory clinical response should be sought. The need for continued treatment should be reassessed periodically.

If signs and symptoms of tardive dyskinesia appear in a patient on SEROQUEL, drug discontinuation should be considered. However, some patients may require treatment with SEROQUEL despite the presence of the syndrome.

PRECAUTIONS

General

Orthostatic Hypotension: SEROQUEL may induce orthostatic hypotension associated with dizziness, tachycardia and, in some patients, syncope, especially during the initial dose-titration period, probably reflecting its "1-adrenergic antagonist properties. Syncope was reported in 1% (22/2162) of the patients treated with SEROQUEL, compared with 0% (0/206) on placebo and about 0.5% (2/420) on active control drugs. The risk of orthostatic hypotension and syncope may be minimized by limiting the initial dose to 25 mg bid (See **DOSAGE AND ADMINISTRATION**). If hypotension occurs during titration to the target dose, a return to the previous dose in the titration schedule is appropriate.

SEROQUEL should be used with particular caution in patients with known cardiovascular disease (history of myocardial infarction or ischemic heart disease, heart failure or conduction abnormalities), cerebrovascular disease or conditions which would predispose patients to hypotension (dehydration, hypovolemia, and treatment with antihypertensive medications).

Cataracts: The development of cataracts was observed in association with quetiapine treatment in chronic dog studies (see Animal Toxicology). Lens changes have also been observed in patients during long-term SEROQUEL treatment, but a causal relationship to SEROQUEL use has not been established. Nevertheless, the possibility of lenticular changes cannot be excluded at this time. Therefore, examination of the lens by methods adequate to detect cataract formation, such as slit lamp exam or other appropriately sensitive methods, is recommended at initiation of treatment or shortly thereafter, and at 6 month intervals during chronic treatment.

Seizures: During clinical trials, seizures occurred in 0.8% (18/2387) of patients treated with SEROQUEL compared to 0.5% (1/206) on placebo and 1% (4/420) on active control drugs. As with other antipsychotics, SEROQUEL should be used cautiously in patients with a history of seizures or with conditions that potentially lower the seizure threshold, e.g., Alzheimer's dementia. Conditions that lower the seizure threshold may be more prevalent in a population of 65 years or older.

Hypothyroidism: Clinical trials with SEROQUEL demonstrated a dose-related decrease in total and free thyroxine (T4) of approximately 20% at the higher end of the therapeutic dose range was maximal in the first two to four weeks of treatment and maintained without adaptation or progression during more chronic therapy. Generally, these changes were of no clinical significance and TSH was unchanged in most patients, and levels of TBG were unchanged. In nearly all cases, cessation of SEROQUEL treatment was associated with a reversal of the effects on total and free T4, irrespective of the duration of treatment. About 0.4% (10/2386) of SEROQUEL patients did experience TSH increases. Six of the patients with TSH increases needed replacement thyroid treatment.

Cholesterol and Triglyceride Elevations: In a pool of 3- to 6-week placebo-controlled trials, SEROQUEL-treated patients had increases from baseline in cholesterol and triglyceride of 11% and 17%, respectively, compared to slight decreases for placebo patients. These changes were only weakly related to the increases in weight observed in SEROQUEL-treated patients.

Hyperprolactinemia: Although an elevation of prolactin levels was not demonstrated in clinical trials with SEROQUEL, increased prolactin levels were observed in rat studies with this compound and were associated with an increase in mammary gland neoplasia in rats (see Carcinogenesis). Tissue culture experiments indicate that approximately one-third of human breast cancers are prolactin dependent *in vitro*, a factor of potential importance if the prescription of these drugs is contemplated in a patient with previously detected breast cancer. Although disturbances such as galactorrhea, amenorrhea, gynecomastia, and impotence have been reported with prolactin-elevating compounds, the clinical significance of elevated serum prolactin levels is unknown for most patients. Neither clinical studies nor epidemiologic studies conducted to date have shown as association between chronic administration of this class of drugs and tumorigenesis in humans; the available evidence is considered too limited to be conclusive at this time.

Transaminase Elevations: Asymptomatic, transient, and reversible elevations in serum transaminases (primarily ALT) have been reported. The proportions of patients with transaminase elevations of > 3 times the upper limits of the normal reference range in a pool of 3- to 6-week placebo-controlled trials were approximately 6% for SEROQUEL compared to 1% for placebo. These hepatic enzyme elevations usually occurred within the first 3 weeks of drug treatment and promptly returned to prestudy levels with ongoing treatment with SEROQUEL.

Potential for Cognitive and Motor Impairment: Somnolence was a commonly reported adverse event reported in patients treated with SEROQUEL especially during the 3-5 day period of initial dose-titration. In the 3- to 6-week placebo-controlled trials, somnolence was reported in 18% of patients on SEROQUEL compared to 11% of placebo patients. Since SEROQUEL has the potential to impair judgment, thinking, or motor skills, patients should be cautioned about performing activities requiring mental altertness, such as operating a motor vehicle (including automobiles) or operating hazardous machinery until they are reasonably certain that SEROQUEL therapy does not affect them adversely.

Priapism: One case of priapism in a patient receiving SEROQUEL has been reported prior to market introduction. While a causal relationship to use of SEROQUEL has not been established, other drugs with alpha-adrenergic blocking effects have been reported to induce priapism, and it is possible that SEROQUEL may share this capacity. Severe priapism may require surgical intervention.

Body Temperature Regulation: Although not reported with SEROQUEL, disruption of the body's ability to reduce core body temperature has been attributed to antipsychotic agents. Appropriate care is advised when prescribing SEROQUEL for patients who will be experiencing conditions which may contribute to an elevation in core body temperature, e.g., exercising strenuously, exposure to extreme heat, receiving concomitant medication with anticholinergic activity, or being subject to dehydration.

Dysphagia: Esophageal dysmotility and aspiration have been associated with antipsychotic drug use. Aspiration pneumonia is a common cause of morbidity and mortality in elderly patients, in particular those with advanced Alzheimer's dementia. SEROQUEL and other antipsychotic drugs should be used cautiously in patients at risk for aspiration pneumonia.

Suicide: The possibility of a suicide attempt is inherent in schizophrenia, and close supervision of high-risk patients should accompany drug therapy. Prescriptions for SEROQUEL should be written for the smallest quantity of tablets consistent with good patient management in order to reduce the risk of overdose.

Use in Patients with Concomitant Illness: Clinical experience with SEROQUEL in patients with certain concomitant systemic illnesses (see Renal and Impairment and Hepatic Impairment under **CLINICAL PHARMACOLOGY**, Special Populations) is limited.

SEROQUEL has not been evaluated or used to any appreciable extent in patients with a recent history of myocardial infarction or unstable heart disease. Patients with these diagnoses were excluded from premarketing clinical studies. Because of the risk of orthostatic hypotension with SEROQUEL, caution should be observed in cardiac patients (see Orthostatic Hypotension).

Information for Patients

Physicians are advised to discuss the following issues with patients for whom they prescribe SEROQUEL.

Orthostatic Hypotension: Patients should be advised of the risk of orthostatic hypotension, especially during the 3–5 day period of initial dose titration, and also at times of re-initiating treatment or increases in dose.

Interference with Cognitive and Motor Performance: Since somnolence was a commonly reported adverse event associated with SEROQUEL treatment, patients should be advised of the risk of somnolence, especially during the 3–5 day period of initial dose titration. Patients should be cautioned about performing any activity requiring mental altertness, such as operating a motor vehicle (including automobiles) or operating hazardous machinery, until they are reasonably certain that SEROQUEL therapy does not affect them adversely.

Pregnancy: Patients should be advised to notify their physician if they become pregnant or intend to become pregnant during therapy.

Nursing: Patients should be advised not to breast feed if they are taking SEROQUEL.

Concomitant Medication: As with other medications, patients should be advised to notify their physicians if they are taking, or plan to take, any prescription or over-the-counter drugs.

Alcohol: Patients should be advised to avoid consuming alcoholic beverages while taking SEROQUEL.

Heat Exposure and Dehydration: Patients should be advised regarding appropriate care in avoiding overheating and dehydration.

Laboratory Tests

No specific laboratory tests are recommended.

Drug Interactions

The risks of using SEROQUEL in combination with other drugs have not been extensively evaluated in systematic studies. Given the primary CNS effects of SEROQUEL, caution should be used when it is taken in combination with other centrally acting drugs. SEROQUEL potentiated the cognitive and motor effects of alcohol in a clinical trial in subjects with selected psychotic disorders, and alcoholic beverages should be avoided while taking SEROQUEL.

Because of its potential for inducing hypotension, SEROQUEL may enhance the effects of certain antihypertensive agents.

SEROQUEL may antagonize the effects of levodopa and dopamine agonists.

The Effect of Other Drugs on SEROQUEL

Phenytoin: Coadministration of quetiapine (250 mg tid) and phenytoin (100 mg tid) increased the mean oral clearance of quetiapine by 5-fold. Increased doses of SEROQUEL may be required to maintain control of psychotic symptoms in patients receiving quetiapine and phenytoin, or other hepatic enzyme inducers (e.g., carbamazepine, barbiturates, rifampin, glucocorticoids). Caution should be taken if phenytoin is withdrawn and replaced with a noninducer (e.g., valproate) (see **DOSAGE AND ADMINISTRATION**).

Thioridazine: Thioridazine (200 mg bid) increased the oral clearance of quetiapine (300 mg bid) by 65%.

Cimetidine: Administration of multiple daily doses of cimetidine (400 mg tid for 4 days) resulted in a 20% decrease in the mean oral clearance of quetiapine (150 mg tid). Dosage adjustment for quetiapine is not required when it is given with cimetidine.

P450 3A Inhibitors: Coadministration of ketoconazole (200 mg once daily for 4 days), a potent inhibitor of cytochrome P450 3A, reduced oral clearance of quetiapine by 84%, resulting in a 335% increase in maximum plasma concentration of quetiapine. Caution is indicated when SEROQUEL is administered with ketoconazole and other inhibitors of cytochrome P450 3A (e.g., itraconazole, fluconazole, and erythromycin).

Fluoxetine, Imipramine, Haloperidol, and Risperidone: Coadministration of fluoxetine (60 mg once daily); imipramine (75 mg bid), haloperidol (7.5 mg bid), or risperidone (3 mg bid) with quetiapine (300 mg bid) did not alter the steady state pharmacokinetics of quetiapine.

Effect of Quetiapine on Other Drugs:

Lorazepam: The mean oral clearance of lorazepam (2 mg, single dose) was reduced by 20% in the presence of quetiapine administered as 250 mg tid dosing.

Lithium: Concomitant administration of quetiapine (250 mg tid) with lithium had no effect on any of the steady state pharmacokinetic parameters of lithium.

Antipyrine: Administration of multiple daily doses up to 750 mg/day (one a tid schedule) of quetiapine to subjects with selected psychotic disorders had no clinically relevant effect on the clearance of antipyrine or urinary recovery of antipyrine metabolites. These results indicate that quetiapine does not significantly induce hepatic enzymes responsible for cytochrome P450 mediated metabolism of antipyrine.

Carcinogenesis, Mutagenesis, Impairment of Fertility

Carcinogenesis: Carcinogenicity studies were conducted in C57BL mice and Wistar rats. Quetiapine was administered in the diet to mice at doses of 20, 75, 250, and 750 mg/kg and to rats by gavage at doses of 25, 75, and 250 mg/kg for two years. These doses are equivalent to 0.1, 0.5, 1.5, and 4.5 times the maximum human dose (800 mg/day) on a mg/m^2 basis (mice) or 0.3, 0.9, and 3.0 times the maximum human dose on a mg/m^2 basis (rats). There were statistically significant increases in thyroid gland follicular adenomas in male mice at doses of 250 and 750 mg/kg or 1.5 and 4.5 times the maximum human dose on a mg/m^2 basis and in male rats at a dose of 250 mg/kg or 3.0 times the maximum human dose on a mg/m^2 basis. Mammary gland adenocarcinomas were statistically significantly increased in female rats at all doses tested (25, 75, and 250 mg/kg or 0.3, 0.9, and 3.0 times the maximum recommended human dose on a mg/m^2 basis).

Thyroid follicular cell adenomas may have resulted from chronic stimulation of the thyroid gland by thyroid stimulating hormone (TSH) resulting from enhanced metabolism and clearance of thyroxine by rodent liver. Changes in TSH, thyroxine, and thyroxine clearance consistent with this mechanism were observed in subchronic toxicity studies in rat and mouse and in a 1-year toxicity study in rat; however, the result of these studies were not definitive. The relevance of the increases in thyroid follicular cell adenomas to human risk, through whatever mechanism, is unknown.

Antipsychotic drugs have been shown to chronically elevate prolactin levels in rodents. Serum measurements in a 1-yr toxicity study showed that quetiapine increased median serum prolactin levels a maximum of 32- and 13-fold in male and female rats, respectively. Increases in mammary neoplasms have been found in rodents after chronic administration of other antipsychotic drugs and are considered to be prolactin-mediated. The relevance of this increased incidence of prolactin-mediated mammary gland tumors in rats to human risk is unknown (see Hyperprolactinemia in **PRECAUTIONS, General**).

Mutagenesis: The mutagenic potential of quetiapine was tested in six *in vitro* bacterial gene mutation assays and in an *in vitro* mammalian gene mutation assay in Chinese Hamster Ovary cells. However, sufficiently high concentrations of quetiapine may not have been used for all tester strains. Quetiapine did produce a reproducible increase in mutations in one *Salmonella typhimurium* tester strain in the presence of metabolic activation. No evidence of clastogenic potential was obtained in an *in vitro* chromosomal aberration assay in cultured human lymphocytes or in the *in vivo* micronucleus assay in rats.

Impairment of Fertility: Quetiapine decreased mating and fertility in male Sprague-Dawley rats at oral doses of 50 and 150 mg/kg or 0.6 and 1.8 times the maximum human dose on a mg/m^2 basis. Drug-related effects included increases in interval to mate and in the number of matings required for successful impregnation. These effects continued to be observed at 150 mg/kg even after a two-week period without treatment. The no-effect dose for impaired mating and fertility in male rats was 25 mg/kg, or 0.3 times the maximum human dose on a mg/m^2 basis. Quetiapine adversely affected mating and fertility in female Sprague-Dawley rats at an oral dose of 50 mg/kg, or 0.6 times the maximum human dose on a mg/m^2 basis. Drug-related effects included decreases in matings and in matings resulting in pregnancy, and an increase in the interval to mate. An increase in irregular estrus cycles was observed at doses of 10 and 50 mg/kg, or 0.1 and 0.6 times the maximum human dose on a mg/m^2 basis. The no-effect dose in female rats was 1 mg/kg, or 0.01 times the maximum human dose on a mg/m^2 basis.

Pregnancy

Pregnancy Category C

The teratogenic potential of quetiapine was studied in Wistar rats and Dutch Belted rabbits dosed during the period of organogenesis. No evidence of a teratogenic effect was detected in rats at doses of 25 to 200 mg/kg or 0.3 to 2.4 times the maximum human dose on a mg/m^2 basis or in rabbits at 25 to 100 mg/kg or 0.6 to 2.4 times the maximum human dose on a mg/m^2 basis. There was, however, evidence of embryo/fetal toxicity. Delays in skeletal ossification were detected in rat fetuses at doses of 50 and 200 mg/kg (0.6 and 2.4 times the maximum human dose on a mg/m^2 basis) and in rabbits at 50 and 100 mg/kg (1.2 and 2.4 times the maximum human dose on a mg/m^2 basis). Fetal body weight was reduced in rat fetuses at 200 mg/kg and rabbit fetuses at 100 mg/kg (2.4 times the maximum human dose on a mg/m^2 basis for both species). There was an increased incidence of a minor soft tissue anomaly (carpal/tarsal flexure) in rabbit fetuses at a dose of 100 mg/kg (2.4 times the maximum human dose on a mg/m^2 basis). Evidence of maternal toxicity (i.e., decreases in body weight gain and/or death) was observed at the high dose in the rat study and at all doses in the rabbit study. In a peri/postnatal reproductive study in rats, no drug-related effects were observed at doses of 1, 10, and 20 mg/kg or 0.01, 0.12, and 0.24 times the maximum human dose on a mg/m^2 basis. However, in a preliminary peri/postnatal study, there were increases in fetal and pup death, and decreases in mean litter weight at 150 mg/kg, or 3.0 times the maximum human dose on a mg/m^2 basis.

There are no adequate and well-controlled studies in pregnant women, and quetiapine should be used during pregnancy only if the potential benefit justifies the potential risk to the fetus.

Labor and Delivery: The effect of SEROQUEL on labor and delivery in humans is unknown.

Nursing Mothers: SEROQUEL was excreted in milk of treated animals during lactation. It is not known if SEROQUEL is excreted in human milk. It is recommended that women receiving SEROQUEL should not breast feed.

Pediatric Use: The safety and effectiveness of SEROQUEL in pediatric patients have not been established.

Continued on next page

Seroquel—Cont.

Geriatric Use: Of the approximately 2400 patients in clinical studies with SEROQUEL, 8% (190) were 65 years of age or over. In general, there was no indication of any different tolerability of SEROQUEL in the elderly compared to younger adults. Nevertheless, the presence of factors that might decrease pharmacokinetic clearance, increase the pharmacodynamic response to SEROQUEL, or cause poorer tolerance or orthostasis, should lead to consideration of a lower starting dose, slower titration, and careful monitoring during the initial dosing period in the elderly. The mean plasma clearance of SEROQUEL was reduced by 30% to 50% in elderly patients when compared to younger patients. (see Pharmacokinetics under **CLINICAL PHARMACOLOGY** and **DOSAGE AND ADMINISTRATION**).

ADVERSE REACTIONS

The premarketing development program for SEROQUEL included over 2600 patients and/or normal subjects exposed to 1 or more doses of SEROQUEL. Of these 2600 subjects, approximately 2300 were patients who participated in multiple dose effectiveness trials, and their experience corresponded to approximately 865 patient-years. The conditions and duration of treatment with SEROQUEL varied greatly and included (in overlapping categories) open-label and double-blind phases of studies, inpatients and outpatients, fixed-dose and dose-titration studies, and short-term or longer-term exposure. Adverse reactions were assessed by collecting adverse events, results of physical examinations, vital signs, weights, laboratory analyses, ECGs, and results of ophthalmologic examinations.

Adverse events during exposure were obtained by general inquiry and recorded by clinical investigators using terminology of their own choosing. Consequently, it is not possible to provide a meaningful estimate of the proportion of individuals experiencing adverse events without first grouping similar types of events into a smaller number of standardized event categories. In the tables and tabulations that follow, standard COSTART terminology has been used to classify reported adverse events.

The stated frequencies of adverse events represent the proportion of individuals who experienced, at least once, a treatment-emergent adverse event of the type listed. An event was considered treatment emergent if it occurred for the first time or worsened while receiving therapy following baseline evaluation.

Adverse Findings Observed in Short-Term, Controlled Trials

Adverse Events Associated with Discontinuation of Treatment in Short-Term, Placebo-Controlled Trials

Overall, there was little difference in the incidence of discontinuation due to adverse events (4% of SEROQUEL vs. 3% for placebo) in a pool of controlled trials. However, discontinuations due to somnolence and hypotension were considered to be drug related (see **PRECAUTIONS**):

Adverse Event	SEROQUEL	Placebo
Somnolence	0.8%	0%
Hypotension	0.4%	0%

Adverse Events Occurring at an Incidence of 1% or More Among SEROQUEL Treated Patients in Short-Term, Placebo-Controlled Trials: Table 1 enumerates the incidence, rounded in the nearest percent, of treatment-emergent adverse events that occurred during acute therapy (up to 6 weeks) of schizophrenia in 1% or more of patients treated with SEROQUEL (doses ranging from 75 to 750 mg/day) where the incidence in patients treated with SEROQUEL was greater than the incidence in placebo-treated patients.

The prescriber should be aware that the figures in the tables and tabulations cannot be used to predict the incidence of side effects in the course of usual medical practice where patient characteristics and other factors differ from those that prevailed in the clinical trials. Similarly, the cited frequencies cannot be compared with figures obtained from other clinical investigations involving different treatments, uses, and investigators. The cited figures, however, do provide the prescribing physician with some basis for estimating the relative contribution of drug and nondrug factors to the side effect incidence in the population studied.

In these studies, the most commonly observed adverse events associated with the use of SEROQUEL (incidence of 5% or greater) and observed at a rate on SEROQUEL at least twice that of placebo were dizziness (10%), postural hypotension (7%), dry mouth (7%), and dyspepsia (6%).

[See first table above]

Table 1. Treatment-Emergent Adverse Experience Incidence in 3- to 6-Week Placebo-Controlled Clinical Trials[1]

Body System/ Preferred Term	SEROQUEL (n=510)	Placebo (n=206)
Body as a Whole		
Headache	19%	18%
Asthenia	4%	3%
Abdominal pain	3%	1%
Back pain	2%	1%
Fever	2%	1%
Nervous System		
Somnolence	18%	11%
Dizziness	10%	4%
Digestive System		
Constipation	9%	5%
Dry Mouth	7%	3%
Dyspepsia	6%	2%
Cardiovascular System		
Postural hypotension	7%	2%
Tachycardia	7%	5%
Metabolic and Nutritional Disorders		
Weight gain	2%	0%
Skin and Appendages		
Rash	4%	3%
Respiratory System		
Rhinitis	3%	1%
Special Senses		
Ear pain	1%	0%

[1] Events for which the SEROQUEL incidence was equal to or less than placebo are not listed in the table, but included the following: pain, infection, chest pain, hostility, accidental injury, hypertension, hypotension, nausea, vomiting, diarrhea, myalgia, agitation, insomnia, anxiety, nervousness, akathisia, hypertonia, tremor, depression, paresthesia, pharyngitis, dry skin, amblyopia, and urinary tract infection.

Explorations for interactions on the basis of gender, age, and race did not reveal any clinically meaningful differences in the adverse event occurrence on the basis of these demographic factors.

Dose Dependency of Adverse Events in Short-Term, Placebo-Controlled Trials

Dose-related Adverse Events: Spontaneously elicited adverse event data from a study comparing five fixed doses of SEROQUEL (75 mg, 150 mg, 300 mg, 600 mg, and 750 mg/day) to placebo were explored for dose-relatedness of adverse events. Logistic regression analyses revealed a positive dose response ($p<0.05$) for the following adverse events: dyspepsia, abdominal pain, and weight gain.

Extrapyramidal Symptoms: Data from one 6-week clinical trial comparing five fixed doses of SEROQUEL (75, 150, 300, 600, 750 mg/day) provided evidence for the lack of treatment-emergent extrapyramidal symptoms (EPS) and dose-relatedness of EPS associated with SEROQUEL treatment. Three methods were used to measure EPS (1) Simpson-Angus total score (mean change from baseline) which evaluates parkinsonism and akathisia, (2) incidence of spontaneous complaints of EPS (akathisia, akinesia, cogwheel rigidity, extrapyramidal syndrome, hypertonia, hypokinesia, neck rigidity, and tremor), and (3) use of anticholinergic medications to treat emergent EPS.

[See second table above]

Dose Groups	Placebo	SEROQUEL 75 mg	150 mg	300 mg	600 mg	750 mg
Parkinsonism	-0.6	-1.0	-1.2	-1.6	-1.8	-1.8
EPS incidence	16%	6%	6%	4%	8%	6%
Anticholinergic Medications	14%	11%	10%	8%	12%	11%

In three additional placebo-controlled clinical trials using variable doses of SEROQUEL, there were no differences between the SEROQUEL and placebo treatment groups in the incidence of EPS, as assessed by Simpson-Angus total scores, spontaneous complaints of EPS, and the use of concomitant anticholinergic medications to treat EPS.

Vital Sign Changes: SEROQUEL is associated with orthostatic hypotension (see **PRECAUTIONS**).

Weight Gain: The proportions of patients meeting a weight gain criterion of ≥7% of body weight were compared in a pool of four 3- to 6-week placebo-controlled clinical trials, revealing a statistically significantly greater incidence of weight gain for SEROQUEL (23%) compared to placebo (6%).

Laboratory Changes: An assessment of the premarketing experience for SEROQUEL suggested that it is associated with asymptomatic increases in SGPT and increases in both total cholesterol and triglycerides (see **PRECAUTIONS**).

An assessment of hematological parameters in short-term, placebo-controlled trials revealed no clinical important differences between SEROQUEL and placebo.

ECG Changes: Between group comparisons for pooled placebo-controlled trials revealed no statistically significant SEROQUEL/placebo differences in the proportions of patients experiencing potentially important changes in ECG parameters, including QT, QTc, and PR intervals. However, the proportions of patients meeting the criteria for tachycardia were compared in four 3-6-week-placebo-controlled clinical trials revealing a 1% (4/399) incidence for SEROQUEL compared to 0.6% (1/156) incidence for placebo. SEROQUEL use was associated with a mean increase in heart rate, assessed by ECG, of 7 beats per minute compared to a mean increase of 1 beat per minute among placebo patients. This slight tendency to tachycardia may be related to SEROQUEL's potential for inducing orthostatic changes (see **PRECAUTIONS**).

Other Adverse Events Observed During the Premarketing Evaluation of SEROQUEL

Following is a list of COSTART terms that reflect treatment-emergent adverse events as defined in the introduction to the ADVERSE REACTIONS section reported by patients treated with SEROQUEL at multiple doses ≥ 75 mg/day during any phase of a trial within the premarketing database of approximately 2200 patients. All reported events are included except those already listed in Table 1 or elsewhere in labeling, those events for which a drug cause was remote, and those event terms which were so general as to be uninformative. It is important to emphasize that, although the events reported occurred during treatment with SEROQUEL, they were not necessarily caused by it.

Events are further categorized by body system and listed in order of decreasing frequency according to the following definitions: frequent adverse events are those occurring in at least 1/100 patients (only those not already listed in the tabulated results from placebo-controlled trials appear in this listing); infrequent adverse events are those occurring in 1/100 to 1/1000 patients; rare events are those occurring in fewer than 1/1000 patients.

Nervous System: ***Frequent:*** hypertonia, dysarthria; ***Infrequent:*** abnormal dreams, dyskinesia, thinking abnormal, tardive dyskinesia, vertigo, involuntary movements, confusion, amnesia, psychosis, hallucinations, hyperkinesia, libido increased*, urinary retention, incoordination, paranoid reaction, abnormal gait, myoclonus, delusions, manic reaction, apathy, ataxia, depersonalization, stupor, bruxism, catatonic reaction, hemiplegia; ***Rare:*** aphasia, buccoglossal syndrome, choreoathetosis, delirium, emotional lability, euphoria, libido decreased*, neuralgia, stuttering, subdural hematoma.

Body as a Whole: ***Frequent:*** flu syndrome; ***Infrequent:*** neck pain, pelvic pain*, suicide attempt, malaise, photosensitivity reaction, chills, face edema, moniliasis; ***Rare:*** abdomen enlarged.

Digestive System: ***Frequent:*** anorexia; ***Infrequent:*** increased salivation, increased appetite, gamma glutamyl transpeptidase increased, gingivitis, dysphagia, flatulence, gastroenteritis, gastritis, hemorrhoids, stomatitis, thirst, tooth caries, fecal incontinence, gastroesophageal reflux, gum hemorrhage, mouth ulceration, rectal hemorrhage, tongue edema; ***Rare:*** glossitis, hematemesis, intestinal obstruction, melena, pancreatitis.

Cardiovascular System: ***Frequent:*** palpitation; ***Infrequent:*** vasodilatation, QT interval prolonged, migraine, bradycardia, cerebral ischemia, irregular pulse, T wave abnormality, bundle branch block, cerebrovascular accidenct, deep thrombophlebitis, T wave inversion; ***Rare:*** angina pectoris, atrial fibrillation, AV block first degree, congestive heart failure, ST elevated, thrombophlebitis, T wave flattening, ST abnormality, increased QRS duration.

Respiratory System: ***Frequent:*** pharyngitis, rhinitis, cough increased, dyspnea; ***Infrequent:*** pneumonia, epistaxis, asthma; ***Rare:*** hiccup, hyperventilation.

Metabolic and Nutritional System: ***Frequent:*** peripheral edema; ***Infrequent:*** weight loss, alkaline phosphatase increased, hyperlipemia, alcohol intolerance, dehydration, hyperglycemia, creatinine increased, hypoglycemia; ***Rare:*** glycosuria, gout, hand edema, hypokalemia, water intoxication.

Skin and Appendages System: ***Frequent:*** sweating; ***Infrequent:*** pruritis, acne, eczema, contact dermatitis, maculopapular rash, seborrhea, skin ulcer; ***Rare:*** exfoliative dermatitis, psoriasis, skin discoloration.

Urogenital System: ***Infrequent:*** dysmenorrhea*, vaginitis*, urinary incontinence, metrorrhagia*, impotence*, dysuria, vaginal moniliasis*, abnormal ejaculation*, cystitis,

urinary frequency, amenorrhea*, female lactation*, leukorrhea*, vaginal hemorrhage*, vulvovaginitis* orchitis*; ***Rare:*** gynecomastia*, nocturia, polyuria, acute kidney failure.
Special Senses: ***Infrequent:*** conjunctivitis, abnormal vision, dry eyes, tinnitus, taste perversion, blepharitis, eye pain; ***Rare:*** abnormality of accommodation, deafness, glaucoma.
Musculoskeletal System: ***Infrequent:*** pathological fracture, myasthenia, twitching, arthralgia, arthritis, leg cramps, bone pain.
Hemic and Lymphatic System: ***Frequent:*** leukopenia; ***Infrequent:*** leukocytosis, anemia, ecchymosis, eosinophilia, hypochromic anemia; lymphadenopathy, cyanosis; ***Rare:*** hemolysis, thrombocytopenia.
Endorcine System: ***Infrequent:*** hypothyroidism, diabetes mellitus; ***Rare:*** hyperthyroidism.
*adjusted for gender
Post Marketing Experience: Adverse events reported since market introduction which were temporally related to SEROQUEL therapy include the following: rarely leukopenia/neutropenia. If a patient develops a low white cell count consider discontinuation of therapy. Possible risk factors for leukopenia/neutropenia include pre-existing low white cell count and history of drug induced leukopenia/neutropenia.

DRUG ABUSE AND DEPENDENCE

Controlled Substance Class: SEROQUEL is not a controlled substance.
Physical and Psychologic dependence: SEROQUEL has not been systematically studied, in animals or humans, for its potential for abuse, tolerance, or physical dependence. While the clinical trials did not reveal any tendency for any drug-seeking behavior, these observations were not systematic, and it is not possible to predict on the basis of this limited experience the extent to which a CNS-active drug will be misused, diverted, and/or abused once marketed. Consequently, patients should be evaluated carefully for a history of drug abuse, and such patients should be observed closely for signs of misuse or abuse of SEROQUEL, e.g., development of tolerance, increases in dose, drug-seeking behavior.

OVERDOSAGE

Human experience: Experience with SEROQUEL® (quetiapine fumarate) in acute overdosage was limited in the clinical trial database (6 reports) with estimated doses ranging from 1200 mg to 9600 mg and no fatalities. In general, reported signs and symptoms were those resulting from an exaggeration of the drug's known pharmacological effects, i.e., drowsiness and sedation, tachycardia and hypotension. One case, involving an estimated overdose of 9600 mg, was associated with hypokalemia and first degree heart block.
Management of Overdosage: In case of acute overdosage, establish and maintain an airway and ensure adequate oxygenation and ventilation. Gastric lavage (after intubation, if patient is unconscious) and administration of activated charcoal together with a laxative should be considered. The possibility of obtundation, seizure or dystonic reaction of the head and neck following overdose may create a risk of aspiration with induced emesis. Cardiovascular monitoring should commence immediately and should include continuous electrocardiographic monitoring to detect possible arrhythmias. If antiarrhythmic therapy is administered, disopyramide, procainamide and quinidine carry a theoretical hazard of additive QT-prolonging effects when administered in patients with acute overdosage of SEROQUEL. Similarly it is reasonable to expect that the alpha-adrenergic-blocking properties of bretylium might be additive to those of quetiapine, resulting in problematic hypotension.
There is no specific antidote to SEROQUEL. Therefore appropriate supportive measures should be instituted. The possibility of multiple drug involvement should be considered. Hypotension and circulatory collapse should be treated with appropriate measures such as intravenous fluids and/or sympathomimetic agents (epinephrine and dopamine should not be used, since beta stimulation may worsen hypotension in the setting of quetiapine-induced alpha blockade). In case of severe extrapyramidal symptoms, anticholinergic medication should be administered. Close medical supervision and monitoring should continue until the patient recovers.

DOSAGE AND ADMINISTRATION

Usual Dose: SEROQUEL should generally be administered with an initial dose of 25 mg bid, with increases in increments of 25–50 mg bid or tid on the second and third day, as tolerated, to a target dose range of 300 to 400 mg daily by the fourth day, given bid or tid. Further dosage adjustments, if indicated, should generally occur at intervals of not less than 2 days, as steady state for SEROQUEL would not be achieved for approximately 1–2 days in the typical patient. When dosage adjustments are necessary, dose increments/decrements of 25–50 mg bid are recommended. Most efficacy data with SEROQUEL were obtained using tid regimens, but in one controlled trial 225 mg bid was also effective.
Antipsychotic efficacy was demonstrated in a dose range of 150 to 750 mg/day in the clinical trials supporting the effectiveness of SEROQUEL. In a dose response study, doses above 300 mg/day were not demonstrated to be more efficacious than the 300 mg/day dose. In other studies, however, doses in the range of 400–500 mg/day appeared to be needed. The safety of doses above 800 mg/day has not been evaluated in clinical trials.
Dosing in Special Populations
Consideration should be given to a slower rate of dose titration and a lower target dose in the elderly, and in patients who are debilitated or who had a predisposition to hypotensive reactions (see **CLINICAL PHARMACOLOGY**). When indicated, dose escalation should be performed with caution in these patients.
Patients with hepatic impairment should be started on 25 mg/day. The dose should be increased daily in increments of 25–50 mg/day to an effective dose, depending on the clinical response and tolerability of the patient.
The elimination of quetiapine was enhanced in the presence of phenytoin. Higher maintenance doses of quetiapine may be required when it is coadministered with phenytoin and other enzyme inducers such as carbamazepine and phenobarbital. (See Drug Interactions under **PRECAUTIONS**)
Maintenance Treatment: While there is no body of evidence available to answer the question of how long the patient treated with SEROQUEL should remain on it, the effectiveness of maintenance treatment is well established for many other antipsychotic drugs. It is recommended that responding patients be continued on SEROQUEL, but at the lowest dose needed to maintain remission. Patients should be periodically reassessed to determine the need for maintenance treatment.
Reinitiation of Treatment in Patients Previously Discontinued: Although there are no data to specifically address reinitiation of treatment, it is recommended that when restarting patients who have had an interval of less than one week off SEROQUEL, titration of SEROQUEL is not required, and the maintenance dose may be reinitiated. When restarting therapy of patients who have been off SEROQUEL for more than one week, the initial titration schedule should be followed.
Switching from Other Antipsychotics: There are no systematically collected data to specifically address switching from other antipsychotics to SEROQUEL.

HOW SUPPLIED

25 mg Tablets (NDC 0310-0275) peach, round, biconvex, film coated tablets, identified with 'SEROQUEL' and '25' on one side and plain on the other side, are supplied in bottles of 100 tablets and hospital unit dose packages of 100 tablets.
100 mg Tablets (NDC 0310-0271) yellow, round, biconvex film coated tablets, identified with 'SEROQUEL' and '100' on one side and plain on the other side, are supplied in bottles of 100 tablets and hospital unit dose packages of 100 tablets.
200 mg Tablets (NDC 0310-0272) white, round, biconvex, film coated tablets, identified with 'SEROQUEL' and '200' on one side and plain on the other side, are supplied in bottles of 100 tablets and hospital unit dose packages of 100 tablets.
Store at 25°C (77°F); excursions permitted to 15–30°C (59–86°F) [See USP].

ANIMAL TOXICOLOGY

Quetiapine caused a dose-related increase in pigment deposition in thyroid gland in rat toxicity studies which were 4 weeks in duration or longer and in a mouse 2-year carcinogenicity study. Doses were 10–250 mg/kg in rats, 75–750 mg/kg in mice; these doses are 0.1–3.0, and 0.1–4.5 times the maximum recommended human dose (on a mg/m^2 basis), respectively. Pigment deposition was shown to be irreversible in rats. The identity of the pigment could not be determined, but was found to be co-localized with quetiapine in thyroid gland follicular epithelial cells. The functional effects and the relevance of this finding to human risk are unknown.
In dogs receiving quetiapine for 6 or 12 months, but not for 1 month, focal triangular cataracts occurred at the junction of posterior sutures in the outer cortex of the lens at a dose of 100 mg/kg, or 4 times the maximum recommended human dose on a mg/m^2 basis. This finding may be due to inhibition of cholesterol biosynthesis by quetiapine. Quetiapine caused a dose related reduction in plasma cholesterol levels in repeat-dose dog and monkey studies; however, there was no correlation between plasma cholesterol and the presence of cataracts in individual dogs. The appearance of delta-8-cholestanol in plasma is consistent with inhibition of a late stage in cholesterol biosynthesis in these species. There also was a 25% reduction in cholesterol content of the outer cortex of the lens observed in a special study in quetiapine treated female dogs. Drug-related cataracts have not been seen in any other species; however, in a 1-year study in monkeys, a striated appearance of the anterior lens surface was detected in 2/7 females at a dose of 225 mg/kg or 5.5 times the maximum recommended human dose on a mg/m^2 basis.
Manufactured by:
ZENECA
Pharmaceuticals
A Business Unit of Zeneca Inc.
Wilmington, Delaware 19850-5437
64149-00 Rev I 5/99
Shown in Product Identification Guide, page 306

SORBITRATE® ℞

[sorb 'i-trate]
(Isosorbide Dinitrate)

DESCRIPTION

Isosorbide dinitrate (ISDN) is 1,4:3,6-dianhydro-D-glucitol 2,5-dinitrate, an organic nitrate whose structural formula is:
[See chemical structure at top of next column]

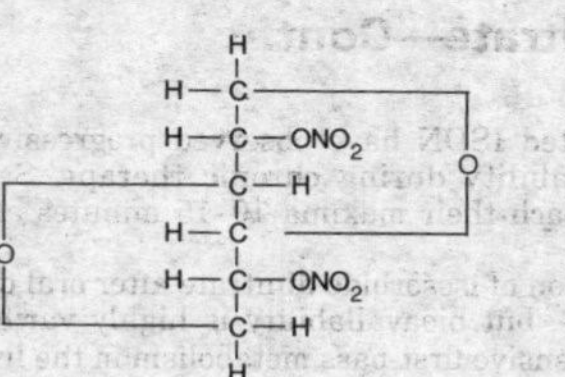

and whose molecular weight is 236.14. The organic nitrates are vasodilators, active on both arteries and veins.
Isosorbide dinitrate is a white, crystalline, odorless compound which is stable in air and in solution, has a melting point of 70°C and has an optical rotation of +134° (c = 1.0, alcohol, 20°C). Isosorbide dinitrate is freely soluble in organic solvents such as acetone, alcohol, and ether; but is only sparingly soluble in water.
SORBITRATE is available as:
SORBITRATE® CHEWABLE TABLETS USP
5 mg Chewable Tablet. Each tablet contains 5 mg of isosorbide dinitrate. Inactive Ingredients: Blue 1, confectioner's sugar, corn starch, flavor, hydrogenated vegetable oil, magnesium stearate, mannitol, povidone, Yellow 10.
SORBITRATE® ORAL TABLETS USP
5 mg Oral Tablet. Each tablet contains 5 mg of isosorbide dinitrate. Inactive Ingredients: Blue 1, corn starch, lactose (hydrous), magnesium stearate, pregelatinized starch, Yellow 10.
10 mg Oral Tablet. Each tablet contains 10 mg of isosorbide dinitrate. Inactive Ingredients: corn starch, lactose (hydrous), magnesium stearate, pregelatinized starch, Yellow 10.
20 mg Oral Tablet. Each tablet contains 20 mg of isosorbide dinitrate. Inactive Ingredients: Blue 1, corn starch, lactose (hydrous), magnesium stearate, pregelatinized starch.
40 mg Oral Tablet. Each tablet contains 40 mg of isosorbide dinitrate. Inactive Ingredients: Blue 1, corn starch, lactose (hydrous), magnesium stearate, pregelatinized starch.

CLINICAL PHARMACOLOGY

The principal pharmacological action of isosorbide dinitrate is relaxation of vascular smooth muscle and consequent dilatation of peripheral arteries and veins, especially the latter. Dilatation of the veins promotes peripheral pooling of blood and decreases venous return to the heart, thereby reducing left ventricular end-diastolic pressure and pulmonary capillary wedge pressure (preload). Arteriolar relaxation reduces systemic vascular resistance, systolic arterial pressure, and mean arterial pressure (afterload). Dilatation of the coronary arteries also occurs. The relative importance of preload reduction, afterload reduction, and coronary dilatation remains undefined.
Dosing regimens for most chronically used drugs are designed to provide plasma concentrations that are continuously greater than a minimally effective concentration. This strategy is inappropriate for organic nitrates. Several well-controlled clinical trials have used exercise testing to assess the anti-anginal efficacy of continuously-delivered nitrates. In the large majority of these trials, active agents were no more effective than placebo after 24 hours (or less) of continuous therapy. Attempts to overcome nitrate tolerance by dose escalation, even to doses far in excess of those used acutely, have consistently failed. Only after nitrates have been absent from the body for several hours has their anti-anginal efficacy been restored.
Pharmacokinetics: Once absorbed, the distribution volume of isosorbide dinitrate is 2–4 L/kg, and this volume is cleared at the rate of 2–4 L/min, so ISDN's half-life in serum is about an hour. Since the clearance exceeds hepatic blood flow, considerable extrahepatic metabolism must also occur. Clearance is effected primarily by denitration to the 2-mononitrate (15%–25%) and the 5-mononitrate (75%–85%).
Both metabolites have biological activity, especially the 5-mononitrate. With an overall half-life of about 5 hours, the 5-mononitrate is cleared from the serum by denitration to isosorbide; glucuronidation to the 5-mononitrate glucuronide; and denitration/hydration to sorbitol. The 2-mononitrate has been less well studied, but it appears to participate in the same metabolic pathways, with a half-life of about 2 hours.
The daily dose-free interval sufficient to avoid tolerance to organic nitrates has not been well defined. Studies of nitroglycerin (an organic nitrate with a very short half-life) have shown that daily dose-free intervals of 10–12 hours are usually sufficient to minimize tolerance. Daily dose-free intervals that have succeeded in avoiding tolerance during trials of moderate doses (eg, 30 mg) of immediate-release ISDN have generally been somewhat longer (at least 14 hours), but this is consistent with the longer half-lives of ISDN and its active metabolites.
Few well-controlled clinical trials of organic nitrates have been designed to detect rebound or withdrawal effects. In one such trial, however, subjects receiving nitrogylcerin had *less* exercise tolerance at the end of the daily dose-free interval than the parallel group receiving placebo. The incidence, magnitude, and clinical significance of similar phenomena in patients receiving ISDN have not been studied.
Bioavailability of ISDN after single sublingual doses is 40%–50%. Multiple-dose studies of sublingual ISDN pharmacokinetics have not been reported; multiple-dose studies

Continued on next page

Sorbitrate—Cont.

of ingested ISDN have observed progressive increases in bioavailability during chronic therapy. Serum levels of ISDN reach their maxima 10–15 minutes after sublingual dosing.

Absorption of isosorbide dinitrate after oral dosing is nearly complete, but bioavailability is highly varible (10%–90%), with extensive first-pass metabolism in the liver. Serum levels reach their maxima about an hour after ingestion. The average bioavailability of ISDN is about 25%; most studies have observed progressive increases in bioavailability during chronic therapy.

The absorption kinetics of chewable isosorbide dinitrate tablets have not been studied. Absorption of ingested ISDN is known to be nearly complete, although bioavailability is highly variable. Ingested ISDN undergoes extensive first-pass metabolism in the liver; it is not known what portion of this first-pass effect is avoided by buccal absorption of the chewable formulation.

Kinetic studies of absorption of immediate-release formulations of ISDN have found highly variable bioavailability with extensive first-pass metabolism in the liver. Most such studies have observed progressive increases in bioavailability during chronic therapy.

Clinical Trials: In a controlled trial in which 0.4 mg of sublingual nitroglycerin took 1.9 minutes to begin to produce an anti-anginal effect, 5 mg of sublingual ISDN took 3.4 minutes to begin to produce a similar effect. In the same trial, the anti-anginal effect of the sublingual nitrogylcerin was evident for about an hour, while that of the sublingual ISDN lasted about 2 hours.

In other controlled trials, the anti-anginal efficacy of sublingual ISDN has persisted for periods ranging from 30 minutes up to 4 hours.

Multiple-dose trials of sublingual ISDN have not been reported. Multiple-dose trials of ingested formulations of ISDN have shown that ISDN's anti-anginal efficacy is substantially attenuated by tolerance unless the daily regimen does not include at least one interdosing interval of at least 14 hours. The daily interdosing interval necessary in any chronic regimen using sublingual ISDN is not known.

In clinical trials, immediate-release oral isosorbide dinitrate has been administered in a variety of regimens, with total daily doses ranging from 30 mg to 480 mg.

Controlled trials of single oral doses of isosorbide dinitrate have demonstrated effective reductions in exercise-related angina for up to 8 hours. Anti-anginal activity is present about 1 hour after dosing.

Most controlled trials of multiple-dose oral ISDN taken every 12 hours (or more frequently) for several weeks have shown statistically significant anti-anginal efficacy for only 2 hours after dosing. Once-daily regimens, and regimens with at least one daily interval of at least 14 hours (eg, a regimen providing doses at 0800, 1400 and 1800) have shown efficacy after the first dose of each day that was similar to that shown in the single-dose studies cited above.

In controlled trials in which sublingual nitroglycerin took $1^1/_2$–2 minutes to begin to produce an anti-anginal effect, chewable ISDN tablets took $2^1/_2$–3 minutes to begin to produce a similar effect. In these same trials, the anti-anginal effect of sublingual nitroglycerin was evident for about 1–$1^1/_2$ hours, while that of chewable ISDN lasted about an hour longer.

Clinical trials of chewable ISDN have used doses of 5 and 10 mg. It is not known whether lower doses would be equally effective.

Multiple-dose trials of chewable ISDN have not been reported. Multiple-dose trials of ingested formulations of ISDN have shown that ISDN's anti-anginal efficacy is substantially attenuated by tolerance unless the daily regimen does not include at least one interdosing interval of at least 14 hours. The daily interdosing interval necessary in any chronic regimen using chewable ISDN is, because of the rapid onset of action of this formulation, probably somewhat longer.

From large, well-controlled studies of other nitrates, it is reasonable to believe that the maximal achievable daily duration of anti-anginal effect from isosorbide dinitrate is about 12 hours. No dosing regimen for isosorbide dinitrate has, however, ever actually been shown to achieve this duration of effect. In the absence of data from multiple-dose trials, and considering the capacity of organic nitrates to induce tolerance, it is not reasonable to assume that multiple sublingual ISDN tablets taken during the course of a day will all have similar effects.

INDICATIONS AND USAGE

SORBITRATE sublingual and chewable tablets are indicated for the prevention and treatment of angina pectoris due to coronary artery disease. However, because the onset of action of these tablets is significantly slower than that of sublingual nitroglycerin, they are not the drugs of first choice for abortion of an acute anginal episode.

SORBITRATE oral tablets are indicated for the prevention of angina pectoris due to coronary artery disease. The onset of action of immediate release oral isosorbide dinitrate is not sufficiently rapid for this product to be useful in aborting an acute anginal episode.

CONTRAINDICATIONS

Allergic reactions to organic nitrates are extremely rare, but they do occur. Isosorbide dinitrate is contraindicated in patients who are allergic to it or other nitrates.

WARNINGS

Amplification of the vasodilatory effects of SORBITRATE by sildenafil can result in severe hypotension. The time course and dose dependence of this interaction have not been studied. Appropriate supportive care has not been studied, but it seems reasonable to treat this as a nitrate overdose, with elevation of the extremities and with central volume expansion.

The benefits of isosorbide dinitrate in patients with acute myocardial infarction or congestive heart failure have not been established. If one elects to use isosorbide dinitrate in these conditions, careful clinical or hemodynamic monitoring must be used to avoid the hazards of hypotension and tachycardia. Because the effects of oral and chewable ISDN tablets are so difficult to terminate rapidly, this formulation is not recommended in these settings.

PRECAUTIONS

General: Severe hypotension, particularly with upright posture, may occur with even small doses of isosorbide dinitrate. This drug should therefore be used with caution in patients who may be volume depleted or who, for whatever reason (eg, diuretics), are already hypotensive. Hypotension induced by isosorbide dinitrate may be accompanied by paradoxical bradycardia and increased angina pectoris.

Nitrate therapy may aggravate the angina caused by hypertrophic cardiomyopathy.

As tolerance to isosorbide dinitrate develops, the effect of sublingual nitroglycerin on exercise tolerance, allthough still observable, is somewhat blunted.

In industrial workers who have had long-term exposure to unknown (presumably high) doses of organic nitrates, tolerance clearly occurs. Chest pain, acute myocardial infarction, and even sudden death have occurred during temporary withdrawal of nitrates from these workers, demonstrating the existence of true physical dependence.

Some clinical trials in angina patients have provided nitroglycerin for about 12 continuous hours of every 24-hour day. During the daily dose-free intervals in some of these trials, anginal attacks have been more easily provoked than before treatment, and patients have demonstrated hemodynamic rebound and decreased exercise tolerance. The importance of these observations to the routine, clinical use of isosorbide dinitrate is not known. It may be prudent to gradually withdraw patients from ISDN when the therapy is being terminated, rather than stopping the drug abruptly.

Information for Patients: Patients should be told that the anti-anginal efficacy of isosorbide dinitrate is strongly related to its dosing regimen, so the prescribed schedule of dosing should be followed carefully. In particular, daily headaches sometimes accompany treatment with isosorbide dinitrate. In patients who get these headaches, the headaches are a marker of the activity of the drug. Patients should resist the temptation to avoid headaches by altering the schedule of their treatment with isosorbide dinitrate, since loss of headache may be associated with simultaneous loss of anti-anginal efficacy. Aspirin and/or acetaminophen, on the other hand, often successfully relieve isosorbide dinitrate-induced headaches with no deleterious effect on isosorbide dinitrate's anti-anginal efficacy.

Treatment with isosorbide dinitrate may be associated with lightheadedness on standing, especially just after rising from a recumbent or seated position. This effect may be more frequent in patients who have also consumed alcohol.

DRUG INTERACTIONS:

The vasodilating effects of isosorbide dinitrate may be additive with those of other vasodilators. Alcohol, in particular, has been found to exhibit additive effects of this variety.

ISDN acts directly on vascular smooth muscle; therefore, any other agent that acts on vascular smooth muscle can be expected to have decreased or increased effect depending on the agents.

Marked symptomatic, orthostatic hypotension has been reported when calcium channel blockers and organic nitrates were used in combination. Dose adjustment of either class of agents may be necessary.

Carcinogenesis, Mutagenesis, and Impairment of Fertility: No long-term studies in animals have been performed to evaluate the carcinogenic potential of isosorbide dinitrate. In a modified two-litter reproduction study, there was no remarkable gross pathology and no altered fertility or gestation among rats fed isosorbide dinitrate at 25 or 100 mg/kg/day.

Pregnancy: Pregnancy Category C: At oral doses 35 and 150 times the maximum recommended human daily dose, isosorbide dinitrate has been shown to cause a dose-related increase in embryotoxicity (increase in mummified pups) in rabbits. There are no adequate, well-controlled studies in pregnant women. Isosorbide dinitrate should be used during pregnancy only if the potential benefit justifies the potential risk to the fetus.

Nursing Mothers: It is not known whether isosorbide dinitrate is excreted in human milk. Because many drugs are excreted in human milk, caution should be exercised when isosorbide dinitrate is administered to a nursing woman.

Pediatric Use: Safety and effectiveness in pediatric patients have not been established.

ADVERSE REACTIONS

Adverse reactions to isosorbide dinitrate are generally dose-related, and almost all of these reactions are the result of isosorbide dinitrate's activity as a vasodilator. Headache, which may be severe and persistent, is the most commonly reported side effect. Headache may be recurrent with each daily dose, especially at higher doses. Cutaneous vasodilation with flushing may occur. Transient episodes of lightheadedness, dizziness, and weakness, as well as other signs of cerebral ischemia associated with postural hypotension, may also occur. Hypotension occurs infrequently, but in some patients it may be severe enough to warrant discontinuation of therapy. (See OVERDOSAGE.)

Syncope, crescendo angina, and rebound hypertension have been reported but are uncommon.

Extremely rarely, ordinary doses of organic nitrates have caused methemoglobinemia in normal seeming patients. Methemoglobinemia is so infrequent at these doses that further discussion of its diagnosis and treatment is deferred. (See OVERDOSAGE.)

Data are not available to allow estimation of the frequency of adverse reactions during treatment with SORBITRATE tablets.

OVERDOSAGE

Hemodynamic Effects: The ill effects of isosorbide dinitrate overdose are generally the results of isosorbide dinitrate's capacity to induce vasodilatation, venous pooling, reduced cardiac output, and hypotension. These hemodynamic changes may have protean manifestations, including increased intracranial pressure, with any or all of the following: persistent throbbing headache, confusion, and moderate fever; vertigo; palpitations; visual disturbances; nausea and vomiting (possibly with colic and even bloody diarrhea); syncope (especially in the upright posture); initial hyperpnea; air hunger; and dyspnea, later followed by slow breathing and/or reduced ventilatory effort; diaphoresis, with the skin either flushed or cold and clammy; heart block and bradycardia; paralysis; coma; seizures; and death.

Laboratory determinations of serum levels of isosorbide dinitrate and its metabolites are not widely available, and such determinations have, in any event, no established role in the management of isosorbide dinitrate overdose.

There are no data suggesting what dose of isosorbide dinitrate is likely to be life-threatening in humans. In rats, the median acute lethal dose (LD_{50}) was found to be 1100 mg/kg (approximately 500 times the recommended therapeutic dose in humans).

No data are available to suggest physiological maneuvers (eg, maneuvers to change the pH of the urine) that might accelerate elimination of isosorbide dinitrate and its active metabolites. Similarly, it is not known which—if any—of these substances can usefully be removed from the body by hemodialysis.

No specific antagonist to the vasodilator effects of isosorbide dinitrate is known, and no intervention has been subject to controlled study as a therapy of isosorbide dinitrate overdose. Because the hypotension associated with isosorbide dinitrate overdose is the result of venodilatation and arterial hypovolemia, prudent therapy in this situation should be directed toward increase in central fluid volume. Passive elevation of the patient's legs and passive movement of extremities may be sufficient, but intravenous infusion of normal saline or similar fluid may also be necessary.

The use epinephrine or other arterial vasoconstrictors in this setting is likely to do more harm than good.

In patients with renal disease or congestive heart failure, therapy resulting in central volume expansion is not without hazard. Treatment of isosorbide dinitrate overdose in these patients may be subtle and difficult, and invasive monitoring may be required.

Methemoglobinemia: Nitrate ions liberated during metabolism of isosorbide dinitrate can oxidize hemoglobin into methemoglobin. Even in patients totally without cytochrome b_5 reductase activity, however, and even assuming that the nitrate moieties of isosorbide dinitrate are quantitatively applied to oxidation of hemoglobin, about 1 mg/kg of isosorbide dinitrate should be required before any of these patients manifests clinically significant ($\geq$10%) methemoglobinemia. In patients with normal reductase function, significant production of methemoglobin should require even larger doses of isosorbide dinitrate. In one study in which 36 patients received 2–4 weeks of continuous nitroglycerin therapy at 3.1 to 4.4 mg/hr (equivalent, in total administered dose of nitrate ions, to 4.8–6.9 mg of bioavailable isosorbide dinitrate per hour), the average methemoglobin level measured was 0.2%; this was comparable to that observed in parallel patients who received placebo.

Notwithstanding these observations, there are case reports of significant methemoglobinemia in association with moderate overdoses of organic nitrates. None of the affected patients had been thought to be unusually susceptible.

Methemoglobin levels are available from most clinical laboratories. The diagnosis should be suspected in patients who exhibit signs of impaired oxygen delivery despite adequate cardiac output and adequate arterial pO_2. Classically, methemoglobinemic blood is described as chocolate brown, without color change on exposure to air.

When methemoglobinemia is diagnosed, the treatment of choice is methylene blue, 1–2 mg/kg intravenously.

DOSAGE AND ADMINISTRATION

As noted above (**CLINICAL PHARMACOLOGY**), multiple studies with ISDN and other nitrates have shown that maintenance of continuous 24-hour plasma levels results in refractory tolerance. Every dosing regimen for ISDN must provide a daily dose-free interval to minimize the development of this tolerance. To achieve the necessary nitrate-free interval with immediate-release oral ISDN, it appears that at least one of the daily dose-free intervals must be at least

14 hours long. In the case of sublingual and chewable tablets, it is probably true that one of the daily dose-free intervals must be somewhat longer than 14 hours.

As also noted above (**CLINICAL PHARMACOLOGY**), the effects of the second and later doses have been smaller and shorter-lasting than the effects of the first.

Large controlled studies with other nitrates suggest that no dosing regimen with SORBITRATE Tablets should be expected to provide more than about 12 hours of continuous anti-anginal efficacy per day.

A patient anticipating activity likely to cause angina should take one SORBITRATE Chewable Tablet, 5 mg, about 15 minutes before the activity is expected to begin. SORBITRATE Sublingual Tablet, 2.5 mg to 5 mg, may be used to abort an acute anginal episode, but this use is recommended only in patients who fail to respond to sublingual nitroglycerin.

In clinical trials, immediate-release oral isosorbide dinitrate has been administered in a variety of regimens, with total daily doses ranging from 30 mg to 480 mg.

As with all titratable drugs, it is important to administer the minimum dose that produces the desired effect. The usual starting dose of SORBITRATE Oral Tablets is 5 mg to 20 mg, two or three times daily. For maintenance therapy, 10 mg to 40 mg, two to three times daily is recommended. Some patients may require higher doses. A daily dose-free interval of at least 14 hours is advisable to minimize tolerance. The optimal interval will vary with the individual patient, dose and regimen.

HOW SUPPLIED

SORBITRATE®Chewable Tablets USP

5 mg Chewable Tablets. (NDC-0310-0810) Green, round, scored tablets (identified front "S", reverse "810") are supplied in bottles of 100 and 500.

SORBITRATE Oral Tablets USP

5 mg Oral Tablets. (NDC-0310-0770) Green, oval-shaped, scored tablets (identified front "S", reverse "770") are supplied in bottles of 100 and 500.

10 mg Oral Tablets. (NDC-0310-0780) Yellow, oval-shaped, scored tablets (identified front "S", reverse "780") are supplied in bottles of 100, 500.

20 mg Oral Tablets. (NDC-0310-0820) Blue, oval-shaped, scored tablets (identified front "S", reverse "820") are supplied in bottles of 100.

40 mg Oral Tablets. (NDC-0310-0774) Light Blue, oval-shaped, scored tablets (identified front "S", reverse "774") are supplied in bottles of 100.

Avoid storage at temperatures above 25°C (77°F).

Zeneca Pharmaceuticals
A Business Unit of Zeneca Inc.
Wilmington, DE 19850-5437
Rev R 11/98 SIC 64119-01

Shown in Product Identification Guide, page 306

SULAR® ℞
(Nisoldipine)
Extended Release Tablets
For Oral Use

DESCRIPTION

SULAR® (nisoldipine) is an extended release tablet dosage form of the dihydropyridine calcium channel blocker nisoldipine. Nisoldipine is 3,5-pyridinedicarboxylic acid, 1,4-dihydro-2,6-dimethyl-4-(2-nitrophenyl)-, methyl 2-methylpropyl ester, $C_{20}H_{24}N_2O_6$, and has the structural formula:

NO_2 H_3COOC $COOCH_2CH(CH_3)_2$ H_3C N H CH_3

Nisoldipine is a yellow crystalline substance, practically insoluble in water but soluble in ethanol. It has a molecular weight of 388.4. SULAR tablets consist of an external coat and an internal core. Both coat and core contain nisoldipine, the coat as a slow release formulation and the core as a fast release formulation. SULAR tablets contain either 10, 20, 30 or 40 mg of nisoldipine for once-a-day oral administration.

Inert ingredients in the formulation are: hydroxypropylcellulose, lactose, corn starch, crospovidone, microcrystalline cellulose, sodium lauryl sulfate, povidone and magnesium stearate. The inert ingredients in the film coating are: hydroxypropylmethylcellulose, polyethylene glycol, ferric oxide, and titanium dioxide.

CLINICAL PHARMACOLOGY

Mechanism of Action

Nisoldipine is a member of the dihydropyridine class of calcium channel antagonists (calcium ion antagonists or slow channel blockers) that inhibit the transmembrane influx of calcium into vascular smooth muscle and cardiac muscle. It reversibly competes with other dihydropyridines for binding to the calcium channel. Because the contractile process of vascular smooth muscle is dependent upon the movement of extracellular calcium into the muscle through specific ion channels, inhibition of the calcium channel results in dilation of the arterioles. *In vitro* studies show that the effects of nisoldipine on contractile processes are selective, with greater potency on vascular smooth muscle than on cardiac muscle. Although, like other dihydropyridine calcium channel blockers, nisoldipine has negative inotropic effects *in vitro*, studies conducted in intact anesthetized animals have shown that the vasodilating effect occurs at doses lower than those that affect cardiac contractility.

The effect of nisoldipine on blood pressure is principally a consequence of a dose-related decrease of peripheral vascular resistance. While nisoldipine, like other dihydropyridines, exhibits a mild diuretic effect, most of the antihypertensive activity is attributed to its effect on peripheral vascular resistance.

Pharmacokinetics and Metabolism

Nisoldipine pharmacokinetics are independent of the dose in the range of 20 to 60 mg, with plasma concentrations proportional to dose. Nisoldipine accumulation, during multiple dosing, is predictable from a single dose.

Nisoldipine is relatively well absorbed into the systemic circulation with 87% of the radiolabeled drug recovered in urine and feces. The absolute bioavailability of nisoldipine is about 5%. Nisoldipine's low bioavailability is due, in part, to pre-systemic metabolism in the gut wall, and this metabolism decreases from the proximal to the distal parts of the intestine. Food with a high fat content has a pronounced effect on the release of nisoldipine from the coat-core formulation and results in a significant increase in peak concentration (C_{max}) by up to 300%. Total exposure, however, is decreased about 25%, presumably because more of the drug is released proximally. This effect appears to be specific for nisoldipine in the controlled release formulation, as a less pronounced food effect was seen with the immediate release tablet. Concomitant intake of a high fat meal with SULAR should be avoided.

Maximal plasma concentrations of nisoldipine are reached 6 to 12 hours after dosing. The terminal elimination half-life (reflecting post absorption clearance of nisoldipine) ranges from 7 to 12 hours. C_{max} and AUC increase by factors of approximately 1.3 and 1.5, respectively, from first dose to steady state. After oral administration, the concentration of (+) nisoldipine, the active enantiomer, is about 6 times higher than the (−) inactive enantiomer. The plasma protein binding of nisoldipine is very high, with less than 1% unbound over the plasma concentration range of 100 ng/mL to 10 mcg/mL.

Nisoldipine is highly metabolized; 5 major urinary metabolites have been identified. Although 60–80% of an oral dose undergoes urinary excretion, only traces of unchanged nisoldipine are found in urine. The major biotransformation pathway appears to be the hydroxylation of the isobutyl ester. A hydroxylated derivative of the side chain, present in plasma at concentrations approximately equal to the parent compound, appears to be the only active metabolite, and has about 10% of the activity of the parent compound. Cytochrome P_{450} enzymes are believed to play a major role in the metabolism of nisoldipine. The particular isoenzyme system responsible for its metabolism has not been identified, but other dihydropyridines are metabolized by cytochrome P_{450} IIIA4. Nisoldipine should not be administered with grapefruit juice as this has been shown, in a study of 12 subjects, to interfere with nisoldipine metabolism, resulting in a mean increase in C_{max} of about 3-fold (ranging up to about 7-fold) and AUC of almost 2-fold (ranging up to about 5-fold). A similar phenomenon has been seen with several other dihydropyridine calcium channel blockers.

Special Populations

Renal dysfunction: Because renal elimination is not an important pathway, bioavailability and pharmacokinetics of SULAR were not significantly different in patients with various degrees of renal impairment. Dosing adjustments in patients with mild to moderate renal impairment are not necessary.

Geriatric: Elderly patients have been found to have 2 to 3 fold higher plasma concentrations (C_{max} and AUC) than young subjects. This should be reflected in more cautious dosing (See DOSAGE AND ADMINISTRATION).

Hepatic Insufficiency: In patients with liver cirrhosis given 10 mg SULAR, plasma concentrations of the parent compound were 4 to 5 times higher than those in healthy young subjects. Lower starting and maintenance doses should be used in cirrhotic patients (See DOSAGE AND ADMINISTRATION).

Gender and Race: The effect of gender or race on the pharmacokinetics of nisoldipine has not been investigated.

Disease States: Hypertension does not significantly alter the pharmacokinetics of nisoldipine.

Pharmacodynamics

Hemodynamic Effects

Administration of a single dose of nisoldipine leads to decreased systemic vascular resistance and blood pressure with a transient increase in heart rate. The change in heart rate is greater with immediate release nisoldipine preparations. The effect on blood pressure is directly related to the initial degree of elevation above normal. Chronic administration of nisoldipine results in a sustained decrease in vascular resistance and small increases in stroke index and left ventricular ejection fraction. A study of the immediate release formulation showed no effect of nisoldipine on the renin-angiotensin-aldosterone system or on plasma norepinephrine concentration in normals. Changes in blood pressure in hypertensive patients given SULAR were dose related over the range of 10–60 mg/day.

Nisoldipine does not appear to have significant negative inotropic activity in intact animals or humans, and did not lead to worsening of clinical heart failure in three small studies of patients with asymptomatic and symptomatic left ventricular dysfunction. There is little information, however, in patients with severe congestive heart failure, and all calcium channel blockers should be used with caution in any patient with heart failure.

Electropyhysiologic Effects

Nisoldipine has no clinically important chronotropic effects. Except for mild shortening of sinus cycle, SA conduction time and AH intervals, single oral doses up to 20 mg of immediate release nisoldipine did not significantly change other conduction parameters. Similar electrophysiologic effects were seen with single iv doses, which could be blunted in patients pre-treated with beta-blockers. Dose and plasma level related flattening or inversion of T-waves have been observed in a few small studies. Such reports were concentrated in patients receiving rapidly increased high doses in one study; the phenomenon has not been a cause of safety concern in large clinical trials.

Clinical Studies In Hypertension

The antihypertensive efficacy of SULAR was studied in 5 double-blind, placebo-controlled, randomized studies, in which over 600 patients were treated with SULAR as monotherapy and about 300 with placebo; 4 of the five studies compared 2 or 3 fixed doses while the fifth allowed titration from 10–40 mg. Once daily administration of SULAR produced sustained reductions in systolic and diastolic blood pressures over the 24 hour dosing interval in both supine and standing positions. The mean placebo-subtracted reductions in supine systolic and diastolic blood pressure at trough, 24 hours post-dose, in these studies, are shown below. Changes in standing blood pressure were similar:

MEAN SUPINE TROUGH SYSTOLIC AND DIASTOLIC BLOOD PRESSURE CHANGES (mm Hg)

SULAR Dose (mg/day)	10 mg	20 mg	30 mg	40 mg	60 mg	10–40 mg titrated
Systolic	8	11	11	14	15	15
Diastolic	3	5	7	7	10	8

In patients receiving atenolol, supine blood pressure reductions with SULAR at 20, 40 and 60 mg once daily were $^{12}/_{6}$, $^{19}/_{8}$ and $^{22}/_{10}$ mm Hg, respectively. The sustained antihypertensive effect of SULAR was demonstrated by 24 hour blood pressure monitoring and examination of peak and trough effects. The trough/peak ratios ranged from 70 to 100% for diastolic and systolic blood pressure. The mean change in heart rate in these studies was less than one beat per minute. In 4 of the 5 studies, patients received initial doses of 20–30 mg SULAR without incident (excessive effects on blood pressure or heart rate). The fifth study started patients on lower doses of SULAR.

Patient race and gender did not influence the blood pressure lowering effect of SULAR. Despite the higher plasma concentration of nisoldipine in the elderly, there was no consistent difference in their blood pressure response except that the 10 mg dose was somewhat more effective than in non-elderly patients. No postural effect on blood pressure was apparent and there was no evidence of tolerance to the antihypertensive effect of SULAR in patients treated for up to one year.

INDICATIONS AND USAGE

SULAR is indicated for the treatment of hypertension. It may be used alone or in combination with other antihypertensive agents.

CONTRAINDICATIONS

SULAR is contraindicated in patients with known hypersensitivity to dihydropyridine calcium channel blockers.

WARNINGS

Increased angina and/or myocardial infarction in patients with coronary artery disease: Rarely, patients, particularly those with severe obstructive coronary artery disease, have developed increased frequency, duration and/or severity of angina, or acute myocardial infarction on starting calcium channel blocker therapy or at the time of dosage increase. The mechanism of this effect has not been established. In controlled studies of SULAR in patients with angina this was seen about 1.5% of the time in patients given nisoldipine, compared with 0.9% in patients given placebo.

PRECAUTIONS

General

Hypotension: Because nisoldipine, like other vasodilators, decreases peripheral vascular resistance, careful monitoring of blood pressure during the initial administration and titration of SULAR is recommended. Close observation is especially important for patients already taking medications that are known to lower blood pressure. Although in most patients the hypotensive effect of SULAR is modest and well tolerated, occasional patients have had excessive

Continued on next page

Sular—Cont.

and poorly tolerated hypotension. These responses have usually occurred during initial titration or at the time of subsequent upward dosage adjustment.

Congestive Heart Failure: Although acute hemodynamic studies of nisoldipine in patients with NYHA Class II–IV heart failure have not demonstrated negative inotropic effects, safety of SULAR in patients with heart failure has not been established. Caution therefore should be exercised when using SULAR in patients with heart failure or compromised ventricular function, particularly in combination with a beta-blocker.

Patients with Hepatic Impairment: Because nisoldipine is extensively metabolized by the liver and, in patients with cirrhosis, it reaches blood concentrations about 5 times those in normals, SULAR should be administered cautiously in patients with severe hepatic dysfunction (See DOSAGE AND ADMINISTRATION).

Information for Patients: SULAR is an extended release tablet and should be swallowed whole. Tablets should not be chewed, divided or crushed. SULAR should not be administered with a high fat meal. Grapefruit juice, which has been shown to increase significantly the bioavailability of nisoldipine and other dihydropyridine type calcium channel blockers, should not be taken with SULAR.

Laboratory Tests: SULAR is not known to interfere with the interpretation of laboratory tests.

Drug Interactions: A 30 to 45% increase in AUC and C_{max} of nisoldipine was observed with concomitant administration of cimetidine 400 mg twice daily. Ranitidine 150 mg twice daily did not interact significantly with nisoldipine (AUC was decreased by 15–20%). No pharmacodynamic effects of either histamine H_2 receptor antagonist were observed.

Coadministration of phenytoin with 40 mg SULAR tablets in epileptic patients lowered the nisoldipine plasma concentrations to undetectable levels. Coadministration of SULAR with phenytoin or any known CYP3A4 inducer should be avoided and alternative antihypertensive therapy should be considered.

Pharmacokinetic interactions between nisoldipine and beta-blockers (atenolol, propranolol) were variable and not significant. Propranolol attenuated the heart rate increase following administration of immediate release nisoldipine. The blood pressure effect of SULAR tended to be greater in patients on atenolol than in patients on no other anithypertensive therapy.

Quinidine at 648 mg bid decreased the bioavailability (AUC) of nisoldipine by 26%, but not the peak concentration. The immediate release, but not the coat-core formulation of nisoldipine increased plasma quinidine concentrations by about 20%. This interaction was not accompanied by ECG changes and its clinical significance is not known. No significant interactions were found between nisoldipine and warfarin or digoxin.

Carcinogenesis, Mutagenesis, Impairment of Fertility: Dietary administration of nisoldipine to male and female rats for up to 24 months (mean doses up to 82 and 111 mg/kg/day, 16 and 19 times the maximum recommended human dose (MRHD) on a mg/m^2 basis, respectively) and female mice for up to 21 months (mean doses of up to 217 mg/kg/day, 20 times the MRHD on a mg/m^2 basis) revealed no evidence of tumorigenic effect of nisoldipine. In male mice receiving a mean dose of 163 mg nisolipine/kg/day (16 times the MRHD of 60 mg/day on a mg/m^2 basis), an increased frequency of stomach papilloma, but still within the historical range, was observed. No evidence of stomach neoplasia was observed at lower doses (up to 58 mg/kg/day). Nisoldipine was negative when tested in a battery of genotoxicity assays including the Ames test and the CHO/HGRPT assay for mutagenicity and the *in vivo* mouse micronucleus test and *in vitro* CHO cell test for clastogenicity.

When administered to male and female rats at doses of up to 30 mg/kg/day (about 5 times the MRHD on a mg/m^2 basis) nisoldipine had no effect on fertility.

Pregnancy Category C: Nisoldipine was neither teratogenic nor fetotoxic at doses that were not maternally toxic. Nisoldipine was fetotoxic but not teratogenic in rats and rabbits at doses resulting in maternal toxicity (reduced maternal body weight gain). In pregnant rats, increased fetal resporption (post-implantation loss) was observed at 100 mg/kg/day and decreased fetal weight was observed at both 30 and 100 mg/kg/day. These doses are, respectively, about 5 and 16 times the MRHD when compared on a mg/m^2 basis. In pregnant rabbits, decreased fetal and placental weights were observed at a dose of 30 mg/kg/day, about 10 times the MRHD when compared on a mg/m^2 basis. In a study in which pregnant monkeys (both treated and control) had high rates of abortion and mortality, the only surviving fetus from a group exposed to a maternal dose of 100 mg nisoldipine/kg/day (about 30 times the MRHD when compared on a mg/m^2 basis) presented with forelimb and vertebral abnormalities not previously seen in control monkeys of the same strain. There are no adequate and well controlled studies in pregnant women. SULAR should be used in pregnancy only if the potential benefit justifies the potential risk to the fetus.

Nursing Mothers: It is not known whether nisoldipine is excreted in human milk. Because many drugs are excreted in human milk, a decision should be made to discontinue nursing, or to discontinue SULAR, taking into account the importance of the drug to the mother.

Pediatric Use: Safety and effectiveness in pediatric patients have not been established.

Geriatric Use: Of the total number of subjects in the placebo-controlled clinical studies of nisoldipine for hypertension 12% were over 65 years of age.

Elderly patients have been found to have 2 to 3 fold higher plasma concentrations (Cmax and AUC) than younger subjects. No overall differences in safety of effectiveness were observed between these subjects and younger subjects (See CLINICAL PHARMACOLOGY—Special Population—Geriatrics).

Patients over 65 are expected to develop higher plasma concentrations of nisoldipine. In general, dose selection for an elderly patient should be cautious. A starting dose not exceeding 10 mg daily is recommended in this patient group. Blood pressure should be monitored closely during dose adjustment (See DOSAGE AND ADMINISTRATION).

ADVERSE EXPERIENCES

More than 6000 patients world-wide have received nisoldipine in clinical trials for the treatment of hypertension, either as the immediate release or the SULAR extended release formulation. Of about 1,500 patients who received SULAR in hypertension studies, about 55% were exposed for at least 2 months and about one third were exposed for over 6 months, the great majority at doses of 20 to 60 mg daily.

SULAR is generally well-tolerated. In the U.S. clinical trials of SULAR in hypertension, 10.9% of the 921 SULAR patients discontinued treatment due to adverse events compared with 2.9% of 280 placebo patients. The frequency of discontinuations due to adverse experiences was related to dose, with a 5.4% discontinuation rate at 10 mg daily and a 10.9% discontinuation rate at 60 mg daily.

The most frequently occurring adverse experiences with SULAR are those related to its vasodilator properties; these are generally mild and only occasionally lead to patient withdrawal from treatment. The table below, from U.S. placebo-controlled parallel dose response trials of SULAR using doses from 10–60 mg once daily in patients with hypertension, lists all of the adverse events, regardless of the causal relationship to SULAR, for which the overall incidence on SULAR was both >1% and greater with SULAR than with placebo.

Adverse Event	Nisoldipine (%) (n=663)	Placebo (%) (n=280)
Peripheral Edema	22	10
Headache	22	15
Dizziness	5	4
Pharyngitis	5	4
Vasodilation	4	2
Sinusitis	3	2
Palpitation	3	1
Chest Pain	2	1
Nausea	2	1
Rash	2	1

Only peripheral edema and possibly dizziness appear to be dose related.

Adverse Event	Placebo	SULAR 10 mg	20 mg	30 mg	40 mg	60 mg
(Rates in %)	N=280	N=30	N=170	N=105	N=139	N=137
Peripheral Edema	10	7	15	20	27	29
Dizziness	4	7	3	3	4	10

The common adverse events occurred at about the same rate in men as in women, and at a similar rate in patients over age 65 as in those under that age, except that headache was much less common in older patients. Except for peripheral edema and vasodilation, which were more common in whites, adverse event rates were similar in blacks and whites.

The following adverse events occurred in ≤1% of all patients treated for hypertension in U.S. and foreign clinical trials, or with unspecified incidence in other studies. Although a causal relationship of SULAR to these events cannot be established, they are listed to alert the physician to a possible relationship with SULAR treatment.

Body As A Whole: cellulitis, chills, facial edema, fever, flu syndrome, malaise

Cardiovascular: atrial fibrillation, cerebrovascular accident, congestive heart failure, first degree AV block, hypertension, hypotension, jugular venous distension, migraine, myocardial infarction, postural hypotension, ventricular extrasystoles, supraventricular tachycardia, syncope, systolic ejection murmur, T wave abnormalities on ECG (flattening, inversion, nonspecific changes), venous insufficiency

Digestive: abnormal liver function tests, anorexia, colitis, diarrhea, dry mouth, dyspepsia, dysphagia, flatulence, gastritis, gastrointestinal hemorrhage, gingival hyperplasia, glossitis, hepatomegaly, increased appetite, melena, mouth ulceration

Endocrine: diabetes mellitus, thyroiditis

Hemic and Lymphatic: anemia, ecchymoses, leukopenia, petechiae

Metabolic and Nutritional: gout, hypokalemia, increased serum creatine kinase, increased nonprotein nitrogen, weight gain, weight loss

Musculoskeletal: arthralgia, arthritis, leg cramps, myalgia, myasthenia, myositis, tenosynovitis

Nervous: abnormal dreams, abnormal thinking and confusion, amnesia, anxiety, ataxia, cerebral ischemia, decreased libido, depression, hypesthesia, hypertonia, insomnia, nervousness, paresthesia, somnolence, tremor, vertigo

Respiratory: asthma, dyspnea, end inspiratory wheeze and fine rales, epistaxis, increased cough, laryngitis, pharyngitis, pleural effusion, rhinitis, sinusitis

Skin and Appendages: acne, alopecia, dry skin, exfoliative dermatitis, fungal dermatitis, herpes simplex, herpes zoster, maculopapular rash, pruritus, pustular rash, skin discoloration, skin ulcer, sweating, urticaria

Special senses: abnormal vision, amblyopia, blepharitis, conjunctivitis, ear pain, glaucoma, itchy eyes, keratoconjunctivitis, otitis media, retinal detachment, tinnitus, watery eyes, taste disturbance, temporary unilateral loss of vision, vitreous floater, watery eyes

Urogenital: dysuria, hematuria, impotence, nocturia, urinary frequency, increased BUN and serum creatinine, vaginal hemorrhage, vaginitis.

The following postmarketing event has been reported very rarely in patients receiving SULAR: systemic hypersensitivity reaction which may include one or more of the following: angioedema, shortness of breath, tachycardia, chest tightness, hypotension, and rash. A definite causal relationship with SULAR has not been established. An unusual event observed with immediate release nisoldipine but not observed with SULAR was one case of photosensitivity. Gynecomastia has been associated with the use of calcium channel blockers.

OVERDOSAGE

There is no experience with nisoldipine overdosage. Generally, overdosage with other dihydropyridines leading to pronounced hypotension calls for active cardiovascular support including monitoring of cardiovascular and respiratory function, elevation of extremities, judicious use of calcium infusion, pressor agents and fluids. Clearance of nisoldipine would be expected to be slowed in patients with impaired liver function. Since nisoldipine is highly protein bound, dialysis is not likely to be of any benefit; however, plasmapheresis may be beneficial.

DOSAGE AND ADMINISTRATION

The dosage of SULAR must be adjusted to each patient's needs. Therapy usually should be initiated with 20 mg orally once daily, then increased by 10 mg per week or longer intervals, to attain adequate control of blood pressure. Usual maintenance dosage is 20 to 40 mg once daily. Blood pressure response increases over the 10–60 mg daily dose range but adverse event rates also increase. Doses beyond 60 mg once daily are not recommended. SULAR has been used safely with diuretics, ACE inhibitors, and beta-blocking agents.

Patients over age 65, or patients with impaired liver function are expected to develop higher plasma concentrations of nisoldipine. Their blood pressure should be monitored closely during any dosage adjustment. A starting dose not exceeding 10 mg daily is recommended in these patient groups.

SULAR tablets should be administered orally once daily. Administration with a high fat meal can lead to excessive peak drug concentration and should be avoided. Grapefruit products should be avoided before and after dosing. SULAR is an extended release dosage form and tablets should be swallowed whole, not bitten, divided or crushed.

HOW SUPPLIED

SULAR extended release tablets are supplied as 10 mg, 20 mg, 30 mg, and 40 mg round film coated tablets. The different strengths can be identified as follows:

Strength	Color	Markings
10 mg	Oyster	891 on one side and ZENECA 10 on the other side.
20 mg	Yellow Cream	892 on one side and ZENECA 20 on the other side.
30 mg	Mustard	893 on one side and ZENECA 30 on the other side.
40 mg	Burnt Orange	894 on one side and ZENECA 40 on the other side.

SULAR Tablets are supplied in:

	Strength	NDC Code
Bottles of 100	10 mg	0310-0891-10
	20 mg	0310-0892-10
	30 mg	0310-0893-10
	40 mg	0310-0894-10
Unit Dose Packages of 100	10 mg	0310-0891-39
	20 mg	0310-0892-39
	30 mg	0310-0893-39

Protect from light and moisture. Store at controlled room temperature, 20–25°C (68–77°F) [see USP]. Dispense in tight, light-resistant containers.

SULAR® is a trademark of Bayer AG, used under license by Zeneca Inc.

ZENECA
Manufactured for:
Zeneca Pharmaceuticals
A Business Unit of Zeneca Inc.
Wilmington, DE 19850-5437 USA
By: Bayer Ag, Leverkusen, Germany
Made in Germany
Rev M 03/99 SIC 64131-00
Shown in Product Identification Guide, page 306

TENORETIC® ℞

[ten "o-ret 'ic]
(atenolol and chlorthalidone)

DESCRIPTION

TENORETIC® (atenolol and chlorthalidone) is for the treatment of hypertension. It combines the antihypertensive activity of two agents: a $beta_1$-selective (cardioselective) hydrophilic blocking agent (atenolol, TENORMIN®) and a monosulfonamyl diuretic (chlorthalidone). Atenolol is Benzeneacetamide, 4-[2'-hydroxy-3'-[(1-methylethyl) amino] propoxy]-.

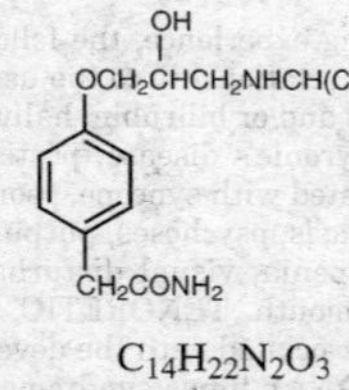

$C_{14}H_{22}N_2O_3$

Atenolol (free base) is a relatively polar hydrophilic compound with a water solubility of 26.5 mg/mL at 37° C. It is freely soluble in 1N HCl (300 mg/mL at 25°C) and less soluble in chloroform (3 mg/mL at 25°C).

Chlorthalidone is 2-Chloro-5-(1-hydroxy-3-oxo-1-isoindolinyl) benzene sulfonamide:

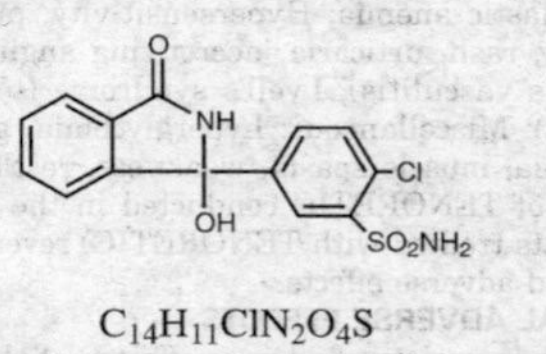

$C_{14}H_{11}ClN_2O_4S$

Chlorthalidone has a water solubility of 12 mg/100 mL at 20°C.

Each TENORETIC 100 Tablet contains:

Atenolol (TENORMIN®)	100 mg
Chlorthalidone	25 mg

Each TENORETIC 50 Tablet contains:

Atenolol (TENORMIN®)	50 mg
Chlorthalidone	25 mg

Inactive ingredients: magnesium stearate, microcrystalline cellulose, povidone, sodium starch glycolate.

CLINICAL PHARMACOLOGY

TENORETIC

Atenolol and chlorthalidone have been used singly and concomitantly for the treatment of hypertension. The antihypertensive effects of these agents are additive, and studies have shown that there is no interference with bioavailability when these agents are given together in the single combination tablet. Therefore, this combination provides a convenient formulation for the concomitant administration of these two entities. In patients with more severe hypertension, TENORETIC may be administered with other antihypertensives such as vasodilators.

Atenolol

Atenolol is a $beta_1$-selective (cardioselective) beta-adrenergic receptor blocking agent without membrane stabilizing or intrinsic sympathomimetic (partial agonist) activities. This preferential effect is not absolute, however, and at higher doses, atenolol inhibits $beta_2$-adrenoreceptors, chiefly located in the bronchial and vascular musculature.

Pharmacodynamics: In standard animal or human pharmacological tests, beta-adrenoreceptor blocking activity of atenolol has been demonstrated by: (1) reduction in resting and exercise heart rates and cardiac output, (2) reduction of systolic and diastolic blood pressure at rest and on exercise, (3) inhibition of isoproterenol induced tachycardia and (4) reduction in reflex orthostatic tachycardia.

A significant beta-blocking effect of atenolol, as measured by reduction of exercise tachycardia, is apparent within one hour following administration of a single dose. This effect is maximal at about 2 to 4 hours and persists for at least 24 hours. The effect at 24 hours is dose related and also bears a linear relationship to the logarithm of plasma atenolol concentration. However, as has been shown for all beta blocking agents, the antihypertensive effect does not appear to be related to plasma level.

In normal subjects, the $beta_1$-selectivity of atenolol has been shown by its reduced ability to reverse the $beta_2$-mediated vasodilating effect of isoproterenol as compared to equivalent beta-blocking doses of propranolol. In asthmatic patients, a dose of atenolol producing a greater effect on resting heart rate than propranolol resulted in much less increase in airway resistance. In a placebo controlled comparison of approximately equipotent oral doses of several beta-blockers, atenolol produced a significantly smaller decrease of FEV_1 than nonselective beta-blockers, such as propranolol and unlike those agents did not inhibit bronchodilation in response to isoproterenol.

Consistent with its negative chronotropic effect due to beta blockade of the SA node, atenolol increases sinus cycle length and sinus node recovery time. Conduction in the AV node is also prolonged. Atenolol is devoid of membrane stabilizing activity, and increasing the dose well beyond that producing beta blockade does not further depress myocardial contractility. Several studies have demonstrated a moderate (approximately 10%) increase in stroke volume at rest and exercise.

In controlled clinical trials, atenolol given as a single daily dose, was an effective antihypertensive agent providing 24-hour reduction of blood pressure. Atenolol has been studied in combination with thiazide-type diuretics and the blood pressure effects of the combination are approximately additive. Atenolol is also compatible with methyldopa, hydralazine and prazosin, the combination resulting in a larger fall in blood pressure than with the single agents. The dose range of atenolol is narrow, and increasing the dose beyond 100 mg once daily is not associated with increased antihypertensive effect. The mechanisms of the antihypertensive effects of beta-blocking agents have not been established. Several mechanisms have been proposed and include: (1) competitive antagonism of catecholamines at peripheral (especially cardiac) adrenergic neuron sites, leading to decreased cardiac output, (2) a central effect leading to reduced sympathetic outflow to the periphery and (3) suppression of renin activity. The results from long-term studies have not shown any diminution of the antihypertensive efficacy of atenolol with prolonged use.

Pharmacokinetics and Metabolism: In man, absorption of an oral dose is rapid and consistent but incomplete. Approximately 50% of an oral dose is absorbed from the gastrointestinal tract, the remainder being excreted unchanged in the feces. Peak blood levels are reached between 2 and 4 hours after ingestion. Unlike propranolol or metoprolol, but like nadolol, hydrophilic atenolol undergoes little or no metabolism by the liver, and the absorbed portion is eliminated primarily by renal excretion. Atenolol also differs from propranolol in that only a small amount (6–16%) is bound to proteins in the plasma. This kinetic profile results in relatively consistent plasma drug levels with about a fourfold interpatient variation. There is no information as to the pharmacokinetic effect of atenolol on chlorthalidone.

The elimination half-life of atenolol is approximately 6 to 7 hours and there is no alteration of the kinetic profile of the drug by chronic administration. Following doses of 50 mg or 100 mg, both beta-blocking and antihypertensive effects persist for at least 24 hours. When renal function is impaired, elimination of atenolol is closely related to the glomerular filtration rate; but significant accumulation does not occur until the creatinine clearance falls below 35 mL/ min/1.73m^2 (see circular for atenolol [TENORMIN®]).

Chlorthalidone

Chlorthalidone is a monosulfonamyl diuretic which differs chemically from thiazide diuretics in that a double ring system is incorporated in its structure. It is an oral diuretic with prolonged action and low toxicity. The diuretic effect of the drug occurs within 2 hours of an oral dose. It produces diuresis with greatly increased excretion of sodium and chloride. At maximal therapeutic dosage, chlorthalidone is approximately equal in its diuretic effect to comparable maximal therapeutic doses of benzothiadiazine diuretics. The site of action appears to be the cortical diluting segment of the ascending limb of Henle's loop of the nephron.

INDICATIONS AND USAGE

TENORETIC is indicated in the treatment of hypertension. This fixed dose combination drug is not indicated for initial therapy of hypertension. If the fixed dose combination represents the dose appropriate to the individual patient's needs, it may be more convenient than the separate components.

CONTRAINDICATIONS

TENORETIC is contraindicated in patients with: sinus bradycardia; heart block greater than first degree; cardiogenic shock; overt cardiac failure (see WARNINGS); anuria; hypersensitivity to this product or to sulfonamide-derived drugs.

WARNINGS

Cardiac Failure: Sympathetic stimulation is necessary in supporting circulatory function in congestive heart failure, and beta blockade carries the potential hazard of further depressing myocardial contractility and precipitating more severe failure. In patients who have congestive heart failure controlled by digitalis and/or diuretics, TENORETIC should be administered cautiously. Both digitalis and atenolol slow AV conduction.

IN PATIENTS WITHOUT A HISTORY OF CARDIAC FAILURE, continued depression of the myocardium with beta-blocking agents over a period of time can, in some cases, lead to cardiac failure. At the first sign or symptom of impending cardiac failure, patients should be treated appropriately according to currently recommended guidelines, and the response observed closely. If cardiac failure continues despite adequate treatment, TENORETIC should be withdrawn. (see DOSAGE AND ADMINISTRATION)

Renal and Hepatic Disease and Electrolyte Disturbances: Since atenolol is excreted via the kidneys, TENORETIC should be used with caution in patients with impaired renal function.

In patients with renal disease, thiazides may precipitate azotemia. Since cumulative effects may develop in the presence of impaired renal function, if progressive renal impairment becomes evident, TENORETIC should be discontinued.

In patients with impaired hepatic function or progressive liver disease, minor alterations in fluid and electrolyte balance may precipitate hepatic coma. TENORETIC should be used with caution in these patients.

Ischemic Heart Disease: Following abrupt cessation of therapy with certain beta-blocking agents in patients with coronary artery disease, exacerbations of angina pectoris and, in some cases, myocardial infarction have been reported. Therefore, such patients should be cautioned against interruption of therapy without the physician's advice. Even in the absence of overt angina pectoris, when discontinuation of TENORETIC is planned, the patient should be carefully observed and should be advised to limit physical activity to a minimum. TENORETIC should be reinstated if withdrawal symptoms occur. Because coronary artery disease is common and may be unrecognized, it may be prudent not to discontinue TENORETIC therapy abruptly even in patients treated only for hypertension.

Concomitant Use of Calcium Channel Blockers: Bradycardia and heart block can occur and the left ventricular end diastolic pressure can rise when beta-blockers are administered with verapamil or diltiazem. Patients with pre-existing conduction abnormalities or left ventricular dysfunction are particularly susceptible. (See **PRECAUTIONS**.)

Bronchospastic Diseases: PATIENTS WITH BRONCHOSPASTIC DISEASE SHOULD, IN GENERAL, NOT RECEIVE BETA BLOCKERS. Because of its relative $beta_1$-selectivity, however, TENORETIC may be used with caution in patients with bronchospastic disease who do not respond to or cannot tolerate, other antihypertensive treatment. Since $beta_1$-selectivity is not absolute, the lowest possible dose of TENORETIC should be used and a $beta_2$-stimulating agent (bronchodilator) should be made available. If dosage must be increased, dividing the dose should be considered in order to achieve lower peak blood levels.

Anesthesia and Major Surgery: It is not advisable to withdraw beta-adrenoreceptor blocking drugs prior to surgery in the majority of patients. However, care should be taken when using anesthetic agents such as those which may depress the myocardium. Vagal dominance, if it occurs, may be corrected with atropine (1–2 mg IV).

Beta blockers are competitive inhibitors of beta-receptor agonists and their effects on the heart can be reversed by administration of such agents; eg, dobutamine or isoproterenol with caution (see section on Overdosage).

Metabolic and Endocrine Effects: TENORETIC may be used with caution in diabetic patients. Beta blockers may mask tachycardia occurring with hypoglycemia, but other manifestations such as dizziness and sweating may not be significantly affected. At recommended doses atenolol does not potentiate insulin-induced hypoglycemia and, unlike nonselective beta blockers, does not delay recovery of blood glucose to normal levels.

Insulin requirements in diabetic patients may be increased, decreased or unchanged; latent diabetes mellitus may become manifest during chlorthalidone administration.

Beta-adrenergic blockade may mask certain clinical signs (eg, tachycardia) of hyperthyroidism. Abrupt withdrawal of beta blockade might precipitate a thyroid storm; therefore, patients suspected of developing thyrotoxicosis from whom TENORETIC therapy is to be withdrawn should be monitored closely.

Because calcium excretion is decreased by thiazides, TENORETIC should be discontinued before carrying out tests for parathyroid function. Pathologic changes in the parathyroid glands, with hypercalcemia and hypophosphatemia, have been observed in a few patients on prolonged thiazide therapy; however, the common complications of hyperparathyroidism such as renal lithiasis, bone resorption, and peptic ulceration have not been seen.

Hyperuricemia may occur, or acute gout may be precipitated in certain patients receiving thiazide therapy.

Untreated Pheochromocytoma: TENORETIC should not be given to patients with untreated pheochromocytoma.

Pregnancy and Fetal Injury: Atenolol can cause fetal harm when administered to a pregnant woman. Atenolol crosses the placental barrier and appears in cord blood. Administration of atenolol, starting in the second trimester of pregnancy, has been associated with the birth of infants that are small for gestational age. No studies have been performed on the use of atenolol in the first trimester and the possibility of fetal injury cannot be excluded. If this drug is used during pregnancy, or if the patient becomes pregnant while taking this drug, the patient should be apprised of the potential hazard to the fetus.

TENORETIC was studied for teratogenic potential in the rat and rabbit. Doses of atenolol/chlorthalidone of 8/2, 80/20, and 240/60 mg/kg/day were administered orally to pregnant rats with no evidence of embryofetotoxicity observed. Two studies were conducted in rabbits. In the first study, pregnant rabbits were dosed with 8/2, 80/20, and 160/40 mg/kg/day of atenolol/chlorthalidone. No teratogenic effects were noted, but embryonic resorptions were observed at all dose levels (ranging from approximately 5 times to 100

Continued on next page

Tenoretic—Cont.

times the maximum recommended human dose*). In the second rabbit study, doses of atenolol/chlorthalidone were 4/1, 8/2, and 20/5 mg/kg/day. No teratogenic or embryotoxic effects were demonstrated.

Atenolol—Atenolol has been shown to produce a dose-related increase in embryo-fetal resorptions in rats at doses equal to or greater than 50 mg/kg/day or 25 or more times the maximum recommended human antihypertensive dose.* Although similar effects were not seen in rabbits, the compound was not evaluated in rabbits at doses above 25 mg/kg/day or 12.5 times the maximum recommended human antihypertensive dose.*

*Based on the maximum dose of 100 mg/day in a 50 kg patient.

Chlorthalidone—Thiazides cross the placental barrier and appear in cord blood. The use of chlorthalidone and related drugs in pregnant women requires that the anticipated benefits of the drug be weighed against possible hazards to the fetus. These hazards include fetal or neonatal jaundice, thrombocytopenia and possibly other adverse reactions which have occurred in the adult.

PRECAUTIONS

General: TENORETIC may aggravate peripheral arterial circulatory disorders.

Electrolyte and Fluid Balance Status: Periodic determination of serum electrolytes to detect possible electrolyte imbalance should be performed at appropriate intervals.

Patients should be observed for clinical signs of fluid or electrolyte imbalance; ie, hyponatremia, hypochloremic alkalosis, and hypokalemia. Serum and urine electrolyte determinations are particularly important when the patient is vomiting excessively or receiving parenteral fluids. Warning signs or symptoms of fluid and electrolyte imbalance include dryness of the mouth, thirst, weakness, lethargy, drowsiness, restlessness, muscle pains or cramps, muscular fatigue, hypotension, oliguria, tachycardia, and gastrointestinal disturbances such as nausea and vomiting.

Measurement of potassium levels is appropriate especially in elderly patients, those receiving digitalis preparations for cardiac failure, patients whose dietary intake of potassium is abnormally low, or those suffering from gastrointestinal complaints.

Hypokalemia may develop especially with brisk diuresis, when severe cirrhosis is present, or during concomitant use of corticosteroids or ACTH.

Interference with adequate oral electrolyte intake will also contribute to hypokalemia. Hypokalemia can sensitize or exaggerate the response of the heart to the toxic effects of digitalis (eg, increased ventricular irritability). Hypokalemia may be avoided or treated by use of potassium supplements or foods with a high potassium content.

Any chloride deficit during thiazide therapy is generally mild and usually does not require specific treatment except under extraordinary circumstances (as in liver disease or renal disease). Dilutional hyponatremia may occur in edematous patients in hot weather; appropriate therapy is water restriction rather than administration of salt except in rare instances when the hyponatremia is life-threatening. In actual salt depletion, appropriate replacement is the therapy of choice.

Drug Interactions: TENORETIC may potentiate the action of other antihypertensive agents used concomitantly. Patients treated with TENORETIC plus a catecholamine depletor (eg, reserpine) should be closely observed for evidence of hypotension and/or marked bradycardia which may produce vertigo, syncope or postural hypotension.

Calcium channel blockers may also have an additive effect when given with TENORETIC. (See WARNINGS.)

Thiazides may decrease arterial responsiveness to norepinephrine. This diminution is not sufficient to preclude the therapeutic effectiveness of norepinephrine. Thiazides may increase the responsiveness to tubocurarine.

Concomitant use of prostaglandin synthase inhibiting drugs, e.g., indomethacin, may decrease the hypotensive effects of beta-blockers.

Lithium generally should not be given with diuretics because they reduce its renal clearance and add a high risk of lithium toxicity. Read circulars for lithium preparations before use of such preparations with TENORETIC.

Beta blockers may exacerbate the rebound hypertension which can follow the withdrawal of clonidine. If the two drugs are coadministered, the beta-blocker should be withdrawn several days before the gradual withdrawal of clonidine. If replacing clonidine by beta-blocker therapy, the introduction of beta-blockers should be delayed for several days after clonidine administration has stopped.

While taking beta blockers, patients with a history of anaphylactic reaction to a variety of allergens may have a more severe reaction on repeated challenge, either accidental, diagnostic or therapeutic. Such patients may be unresponsive to the usual doses of epinephrine used to treat the allergic reaction.

Other Precautions: In patients receiving thiazides, sensitivity reactions may occur with or without a history of allergy or bronchial asthma. The possible exacerbation or activation of systemic lupus erythematosus has been reported. The antihypertensive effects of thiazides may be enhanced in the postsympathectomy patient.

Carcinogenesis, Mutagenesis, Impairment of Fertility: Two long-term (maximum dosing duration of 18 or 24 months) rat studies and one long-term (maximum dosing duration of 18 months) mouse study, each employing dose levels as high as 300 mg/kg/day or 150 times the maximum recommended human antihypertensive dose,* did not indicate a carcinogenic potential of atenolol. A third (24 month) rat study, employing doses of 500 and 1,500 mg/kg/day (250 and 750 times the maximum recommended human antihypertensive dose*) resulted in increased incidences of benign adrenal medullary tumors in males and females, mammary fibroadenomas in females, and anterior pituitary adenomas and thyroid parafollicular cell carcinomas in males. No evidence of a mutagenic potential of atenolol was uncovered in the dominant lethal test (mouse), in vivo cytogenetics test (Chinese hamster) or Ames test (*S typhimurium*).

Fertility of male or female rats (evaluated at dose levels as high as 200 mg/kg/day or 100 times the maximum recommended human dose*) was unaffected by atenolol administration.

Animal Toxicology: Six month oral administration studies were conducted in rats and dogs using TENORETIC doses up to 12.5 mg/kg/day (atenolol/chlorthalidone 10/2.5 mg/kg/day—approximately five times the maximum recommended human antihypertensive dose*). There were no functional or morphological abnormalities resulting from dosing either compound alone or together other than minor changes in heart rate, blood pressure and urine chemistry which were attributed to the known pharmacologic properties of atenolol and/or chlorthalidone.

Chronic studies of atenolol performed in animals have revealed the occurrence of vacuolation of epithelial cells of Brunner's glands in the duodenum of both male and female dogs at all tested dose levels (starting at 15 mg/kg/day or 7.5 times the maximum recommended human antihypertensive dose*) and increased incidence of artrial degeneration of hearts of male rats at 300 but not 150 mg atenolol/kg/day (150 and 75 times the maximum recommended human antihypertensive dose*, respectively).

*Based on the maximum dose of 100 mg/day in a 50 kg patient.

Use in Pregnancy: Pregnancy Category D: See WARNINGS—Pregnancy and Fetal Injury.

Nursing Mothers: Atenolol is excreted in human breast milk at a ratio of 1.5 to 6.8 when compared to the concentration in plasma. Caution should be exercised when atenolol is administered to a nursing woman. Clinically significant bradycardia has been reported in breast fed infants. Premature infants, or infants with impaired renal function, may be more likely to develop adverse effects.

Pediatric Use: Safety and effectiveness in pediatric patients have not been established.

ADVERSE REACTIONS

TENORETIC is usually well tolerated in properly selected patients. Most adverse effects have been mild and transient. The adverse effects observed for TENORETIC are essentially the same as those seen with the individual components.

Atenolol: The frequency estimates in the following table were derived from controlled studies in which adverse reactions were either volunteered by the patient (US studies) or elicited, eg, by checklist (foreign studies). The reported frequency of elicited adverse effects was higher for both atenolol and placebo-treated patients than when these reactions were volunteered. Where frequency of adverse effects for atenolol and placebo is similar, causal relationship to atenolol is uncertain.

[See table below]

	Volunteered (US Studies)		Total-Volunteered and Elicited (Foreign + US Studies)	
	Atenolol (n = 164) %	Placebo (n = 206) %	Atenolol (n = 399) %	Placebo (n = 407) %
CARDIOVASCULAR				
Bradycardia	3	0	3	0
Cold Extremities	0	0.5	12	5
Postural Hypotension	2	1	4	5
Leg Pain	0	0.5	3	1
CENTRAL NERVOUS SYSTEM/ NEUROMUSCULAR				
Dizziness	4	1	13	6
Vertigo	2	0.5	2	0.2
Light-Headedness	1	0	3	0.7
Tiredness	0.6	0.5	26	13
Fatigue	3	1	6	5
Lethargy	1	0	3	0.7
Drowsiness	0.6	0	2	0.5
Depression	0.6	0.5	12	9
Dreaming	0	0	3	1
GASTROINTESTINAL				
Diarrhea	2	0	3	2
Nausea	4	1	3	1
RESPIRATORY (see Warnings)				
Wheezing	0	0	3	3
Dyspnea	0.6	1	6	4

During postmarketing experience, the following have been reported in temporal relationship to the use of the drug: elevated liver enzymes and/or bilirubin, hallucinations, headache, impotence, Peyronie's disease, postural hypotension which may be associated with syncope, psoriasiform rash or exacerbation of psoriasis, psychoses, purpura, reversible alopecia, thrombocytopenia, visual disturbance, sick sinus syndrome, and dry mouth. TENORETIC, like other beta-blockers, has been associated with the development of antinuclear antibodies (ANA), lupus syndrome, and Raynaud's phenomenon.

Chlorthalidone: Cardiovascular: orthostatic hypotension; Gastrointestinal: anorexia, gastric irritation, vomiting, cramping, constipation, jaundice (intrahepatic cholestatic jaundice), pancreatitis; CNS: vertigo, paresthesia, xanthopsia; Hematologic: leukopenia, agranulocytosis, thrombocytopenia, aplastic anemia; Hypersensitivity: purpura, photosensitivity, rash, urticaria, necrotizing angiitis (vasculitis) (cutaneous vasculitis), Lyell's syndrome (toxic epidermal necrolysis); Miscellaneous: hyperglycemia, glycosuria, hyperuricemia, muscle spasm, weakness, restlessness. Clinical trials of TENORETIC conducted in the United States (89 patients treated with TENORETIC) revealed no new or unexpected adverse effects.

POTENTIAL ADVERSE EFFECTS

In addition, a variety of adverse effects not observed in clinical trials with atenolol but reported with other beta-adrenergic blocking agents should be considered potential adverse effects of atenolol. Nervous System: Reversible mental depression progressing to catatonia; an acute reversible syndrome characterized by disorientation for time and place, short-term memory loss, emotional lability, slightly clouded sensorium, decreased performance on neuropsychometrics; Cardiovascular: Intensification of AV block (see CONTRAINDICATIONS); Gastrointestinal: Mesenteric arterial thrombosis, ischemic colitis; Hematologic: Agranulocytosis; Allergic: Erythematous rash, fever combined with aching and sore throat, laryngospasm and respiratory distress.

Miscellaneous: There have been reports of skin rashes and/or dry eyes associated with the use of beta-adrenergic blocking drugs. The reported incidence is small, and, in most cases, the symptoms have cleared when treatment was withdrawn. Discontinuance of the drug should be considered if any such reaction is not otherwise explicable. Patients should be closely monitored following cessation of therapy. (See DOSAGE AND ADMINISTRATION.)

The oculomucocutaneous syndrome associated with the beta blocker practolol has not been reported with atenolol (TENORMIN). Furthermore, a number of patients who had previously demonstrated established practolol reactions were transferred to atenolol (TENORMIN) therapy with subsequent resolution or quiescence of the reaction.

Clinical Laboratory Test Findings: Clinically important changes in standard laboratory parameters were rarely associated with the administration of TENORETIC. The changes in laboratory parameters were not progressive and usually were not associated with clinical manifestations. The most common changes were increases in uric acid and decreases in serum potassium.

OVERDOSAGE

No specific information is available with regard to overdosage and TENORETIC in humans. Treatment should be symptomatic and supportive and directed to the removal of any unabsorbed drug by induced emesis, or administration of activated charcoal. Atenolol can be removed from the general circulation by hemodialysis. Further consideration should be given to dehydration, electrolyte imbalance and hypotension by established procedures.

Atenolol: Overdosage with atenolol has been reported with patients surviving acute doses as high as 5 g. One death was reported in a man who may have taken as much as 10 g acutely.

The predominant symptoms reported following atenolol overdose are lethargy, disorder of respiratory drive, wheezing, sinus pause, and bradycardia. Additionally, common effects associated with overdosage of any beta-adrenergic blocking agent are congestive heart failure, hypotension, bronchospasm, and/or hypoglycemia. Other treatment modalities should be employed at the physician's discretion and may include:

BRADYCARDIA: Atropine 1–2 mg intravenously. If there is no response to vagal blockade, give isoproterenol cautiously. In refractory cases, a transvenous cardiac pacemaker may be indicated. Glucagon in a 10 mg intravenous bolus has been reported to be useful. If required, this may be repeated or followed by an intravenous infusion of glucagon 1–10 mg/h depending on response.

HEART BLOCK (SECOND OR THIRD DEGREE): Isoproterenol or transvenous pacemaker.

CONGESTIVE HEART FAILURE: Digitalize the patient and administer a diuretic. Glucagon has been reported to be useful.

HYPOTENSION: Vasopressors such as dopamine or norepinephrine (levarterenol). Monitor blood pressure continuously.

BRONCHOSPASM: A $beta_2$-stimulant such as isoproterenol or terbutaline and/or aminophylline.

HYPOGLYCEMIA: Intravenous glucose.

ELECTROLYTE DISTURBANCE: Monitor electrolyte levels and renal function. Institute measures to maintain hydration and electrolytes.

Based on the severity of symptoms, management may require intensive support care and facilities for applying cardiac and respiratory support.

Chlorthalidone: Symptoms of chlorthalidone overdose include nausea, weakness, dizziness and disturbances of electrolyte balance.

DOSAGE AND ADMINISTRATION

DOSAGE MUST BE INDIVIDUALIZED (See INDICATIONS AND USAGE)

Chlorthalidone is usually given at a dose of 25 mg daily; the usual initial dose of atenolol is 50 mg daily. Therefore, the initial dose should be one TENORETIC 50 tablet given once a day. If an optimal response is not achieved, the dosage should be increased to one TENORETIC 100 tablet given once a day.

When necessary, another antihypertensive agent may be added gradually beginning with 50 percent of the usual recommended starting dose to avoid an excessive fall in blood pressure.

Since atenolol is excreted via the kidneys, dosage should be adjusted in cases of severe impairment of renal function. No significant accumulation of atenolol occurs until creatinine clearance falls below 35 mL/min/1.73m^2 (normal range is 100–150 mL/min/1.73m^2); therefore, the following maximum dosages are recommended for patients with renal impairment.

Creatinine Clearance (mL/min/1.73m^2)	Atenolol Elimination Half-life (hrs)	Maximum Dosage
15–35	16–27	50 mg daily
<15	>27	50 mg every other day

HOW SUPPLIED

TENORETIC 50 Tablets (atenolol 50 mg and chlorthalidone 25 mg), NDC 0310-0115, (white, round, biconvex, uncoated tablets with TENORETIC on one side and 115 on the other side, bisected) are supplied in bottles of 100 tablets.

TENORETIC 100 Tablets (atenolol 100 mg and chlorthalidone 25 mg), NDC 0310-0117, (white, round, biconvex, uncoated tablets with TENORETIC on one side and 117 on the other side) are supplied in bottles of 100 tablets.

Store at controlled room temperature, 20–25°C (68–77°F) [see USP]. Dispense in well-closed, light-resistant containers.

ZENECA

Manufactured for:

Zeneca Pharmaceuticals

A Business Unit of Zeneca Inc.

Wilmington, Delaware 19850-5437

By: IPR Pharmaceuticals, Inc.

Carolina, Puerto Rico 00984-1967

Rev F 07/99 SIC 64112-02

PCC 620017

Shown in Product Identification Guide, page 306

TENORMIN® Tablets ℞
TENORMIN® I.V. Injection

[ten-or 'min]

(atenolol)

DESCRIPTION

TENORMIN (atenolol), a synthetic, $beta_1$-selective (cardioselective) adrenoreceptor blocking agent, may be chemically described as benzeneacetamide, 4-[2'-hydroxy-3'-[(1-methylethyl)amino]propoxy]-. The molecular and structural formulas are:

OH
|
$OCH_2CHCH_2NHCH(CH_3)_2$

$C_{14}H_{22}N_2O_3$

CH_2CONH_2

Atenolol (free base) has a molecular weight of 266. It is a relatively polar hydrophilic compound with a water solubility of 26.5 mg/mL at 37°C and a log partition coefficient (octanol/ water) of 0.23. It is freely soluble in 1N HCl (300 mg/mL at 25°C) and less soluble in chloroform (3 mg/mL at 25°C).

TENORMIN is available as 25, 50 and 100 mg tablets for oral administration. TENORMIN for parenteral administration is available as TENORMIN I.V. Injection containing 5 mg atenolol in 10 mL sterile, isotonic, citrate-buffered, aqueous solution. The pH of the solution is 5.5–6.5.

Inactive Ingredients: TENORMIN Tablets: Magnesium stearate, microcrystalline cellulose, povidone, sodium starch glycolate. TENORMIN I.V. Injection: Sodium chloride for isotonicity and citric acid and sodium hydroxide to adjust pH.

CLINICAL PHARMACOLOGY

TENORMIN is a $beta_1$-selective (cardioselective) beta-adrenergic receptor blocking agent without membrane stabilizing or intrinsic sympathomimetic (partial agonist) activities. This preferential effect is not absolute, however, and at higher doses, TENORMIN inhibits $beta_2$-adrenoreceptors, chiefly located in the bronchial and vascular musculature.

Pharmacokinetics and Metabolism: In man, absorption of an oral dose is rapid and consistent but incomplete. Approximately 50% of an oral dose is absorbed from the gastrointestinal tract, the remainder being excreted unchanged in the feces. Peak blood levels are reached between two (2) and four (4) hours after ingestion. Unlike propranolol or metoprolol, but like nadolol, TENORMIN undergoes little or no metabolism by the liver, and the absorbed portion is eliminated primarily by renal excretion. Over 85% of an intravenous dose is excreted in urine within 24 hours compared with approximately 50% for an oral dose. TENORMIN also differs from propranolol in that only a small amount (6%–16%) is bound to proteins in the plasma. This kinetic profile results in relatively consistent plasma drug levels with about a fourfold interpatient variation.

The elimination half-life of oral TENORMIN is approximately 6 to 7 hours, and there is no alteration of the kinetic profile of the drug by chronic administration. Following intravenous administration, peak plasma levels are reached within 5 minutes. Declines from peak levels are rapid (5- to 10-fold) during the first 7 hours; thereafter, plasma levels decay with a half-life similar to that of orally administered drug. Following oral doses of 50 mg or 100 mg, both beta-blocking and antihypertensive effects persist for at least 24 hours. When renal function is impaired, elimination of TENORMIN is closely related to the glomerular filtration rate; significant accumulation occurs when the creatinine clearance falls below 35 mL/min/1.73m^2. (See DOSAGE AND ADMINISTRATION).

Pharmacodynamics: In standard animal or human pharmacological tests, beta-adrenoreceptor blocking activity of TENORMIN has been demonstrated by: (1) reduction in resting and exercise heart rate and cardiac output, (2) reduction of systolic and diastolic blood pressure at rest and on exercise, (3) inhibition of isoproterenol induced tachycardia, and (4) reduction in reflex orthostatic tachycardia.

A significant beta-blocking effect of TENORMIN, as measured by reduction of exercise tachycardia, is apparent within one hour following oral administration of a single dose. This effect is maximal at about 2 to 4 hours, and persists for at least 24 hours. Maximum reduction in exercise tachycardia occurs within 5 minutes of an intravenous dose. For both orally and intravenously administered drug, the duration of action is dose related and also bears a linear relationship to the logarithm of plasma TENORMIN concentration. The effect on exercise tachycardia of a single 10 mg intravenous dose is largely dissipated by 12 hours, whereas beta-blocking activity of single oral doses of 50 mg and 100 mg is still evident beyond 24 hours following administration. However, as has been shown for all beta-blocking agents, the antihypertensive effect does not appear to be related to plasma level.

In normal subjects, the $beta_1$-selectivity of TENORMIN has been shown by its reduced ability to reverse the $beta_2$-mediated vasodilating effect of isoproterenol as compared to equivalent beta-blocking doses of propranolol. In asthmatic patients, a dose of TENORMIN producing a greater effect on resting heart rate than propranolol resulted in much less increase in airway resistance. In a placebo controlled comparison of approximately equipotent oral doses of several beta blockers, TENORMIN produced a significantly smaller decrease of FEV_1 than nonselective beta blockers such as propranolol and, unlike those agents, did not inhibit bronchodilation in response to isoproterenol.

Consistent with its negative chronotropic effect due to beta blockade of the SA node, TENORMIN increases sinus cycle length and sinus node recovery time. Conduction in the AV node is also prolonged. TENORMIN is devoid of membrane stabilizing activity, and increasing the dose well beyond that producing beta blockade does not further depress myocardial contractility. Several studies have demonstrated a moderate (approximately 10%) increase in stroke volume at rest and during exercise.

In controlled clinical trials, TENORMIN, given as a single daily oral dose, was an effective antihypertensive agent providing 24-hour reduction of blood pressure. TENORMIN has been studied in combination with thiazide-type diuretics, and the blood pressure effects of the combination are approximately additive. TENORMIN is also compatible with methyldopa, hydralazine, and prazosin, each combination resulting in a larger fall in blood pressure than with the single agents. The dose range of TENORMIN is narrow and increasing the dose beyond 100 mg once daily is not associated with increased antihypertensive effect. The mechanisms of the antihypertensive effects of beta-blocking agents have not been established. Several possible mechanisms have been proposed and include: (1) competitive antagonism of catecholamines at peripheral (especially cardiac) adrenergic neuron sites, leading to decreased cardiac output, (2) a central effect leading to reduced sympathetic outflow to the periphery, and (3) suppression of renin activity. The results from long-term studies have not shown any diminution of the antihypertensive efficacy of TENORMIN with prolonged use.

By blocking the positive chronotropic and inotropic effects of catecholamines and by decreasing blood pressure, atenolol generally reduces the oxygen requirements of the heart at any given level of effort, making it useful for many patients in the long-term management of angina pectoris. On the other hand, atenolol can increase oxygen requirements by increasing left ventricular fiber length and end diastolic pressure, particularly in patients with heart failure.

In a multicenter clinical trial (ISIS-1) conducted in 16,027 patients with suspected myocardial infarction, patients presenting within 12 hours (mean = 5 hours) after the onset of pain were randomized to either conventional therapy plus TENORMIN (n = 8,037), or conventional therapy alone (n = 7,990). Patients with a heart rate of <50 bpm or systolic blood pressure <100 mm Hg, or with other contraindications to beta blockade, were excluded. Thirty-eight percent of each group were treated within 4 hours of onset of pain. The mean time from onset of pain to entry was 5.0 ± 2.7 hours in both groups. Patients in the TENORMIN group were to receive TENORMIN I.V. Injection 5–10 mg given over 5 minutes plus TENORMIN Tablets 50 mg every 12 hours orally on the first study day (the first oral dose administered about 15 minutes after the IV dose) followed by either TENORMIN Tablets 100 mg once daily or TENORMIN Tablets 50 mg twice daily on days 2–7. The groups were similar in demographic and medical history characteristics and in electrocardiographic evidence of myocardial infarction, bundle branch block, and first degree atrioventricular block at entry.

During the treatment period (days 0–7), the vascular mortality rates were 3.89% in the TENORMIN group (313 deaths) and 4.57% in the control group (365 deaths). This absolute difference in rates, 0.68%, is statistically significant at the P <0.05 level. The absolute difference translates into a proportional reduction of 15% (3.89-4.57/4.57 = −0.15). The 95% confidence limits are 1%–27%. Most of the difference was attributed to mortality in days 0-1 (TENORMIN—121 deaths; control—171 deaths).

Despite the large size of the ISIS-1 trial, it is not possible to identify clearly subgroups of patients most likely or least likely to benefit from early treatment with atenolol. Good clinical judgment suggests, however, that patients who are dependent on sympathetic stimulation for maintenance of adequate cardiac output and blood pressure are not good candidates for beta blockade. Indeed, the trial protocol reflected that judgment by excluding patients with blood pressure consistently below 100 mm Hg systolic. The overall results of the study are compatible with the possibility that patients with borderline blood pressure (less than 120 mm Hg systolic), especially if over 60 years of age, are less likely to benefit.

The mechanism through which atenolol improves survival in patients with definite or suspected acute myocardial infarction is unknown, as is the case for other beta blockers in the postinfarction setting. Atenolol, in addition to its effects on survival, has shown other clinical benefits including reduced frequency of ventricular premature beats, reduced chest pain, and reduced enzyme elevation.

INDICATIONS AND USAGE

Hypertension: TENORMIN is indicated in the management of hypertension. It may be used alone or concomitantly with other antihypertensive agents, particularly with a thiazide-type diuretic.

Angina Pectoris Due to Coronary Atherosclerosis: TENORMIN is indicated for the long-term management of patients with angina pectoris.

Acute Myocardial Infarction: TENORMIN is indicated in the management of hemodynamically stable patients with definite or suspected acute myocardial infarction to reduce cardiovascular mortality. Treatment can be initiated as soon as the patient's clinical condition allows. (See DOSAGE AND ADMINISTRATION, CONTRAINDICATIONS, AND WARNINGS.) In general, there is no basis for treating patients like those who were excluded from the ISIS-1 trial (blood pressure less than 100 mm Hg systolic, heart rate less than 50 bpm) or have other reasons to avoid beta blockade. As noted above, some subgroups (eg, elderly patients with systolic blood pressure below 120 mm Hg) seemed less likely to benefit.

CONTRAINDICATIONS

TENORMIN is contraindicated in sinus bradycardia, heart block greater than first degree, cardiogenic shock, and overt cardiac failure. (See WARNINGS.)

TENORMIN is contraindicated in those patients with a history of hypersensitivity to the atenolol or any of the drug product's components.

Continued on next page

Tenormin—Cont.

WARNINGS

Cardiac Failure: Sympathetic stimulation is necessary in supporting circulatory function in congestive heart failure, and beta blockade carries the potential hazard of further depressing myocardial contractility and precipitating more severe failure. In patients who have congestive heart failure controlled by digitalis and/or diuretics, TENORMIN should be administered cautiously. Both digitalis and atenolol slow AV conduction.

In patients with acute myocardial infarction, cardiac failure which is not promptly and effectively controlled by 80 mg of intravenous furosemide or equivalent therapy is a contraindication to beta-blocker treatment.

In Patients Without a History of Cardiac Failure: Continued depression of the myocardium with beta-blocking agents over a period of time can, in some cases, lead to cardiac failure. At the first sign or symptom of impending cardiac failure, patients should be treated appropriately according to currently recommended guidelines, and the response observed closely. If cardiac failure continues despite adequate treatment, TENORMIN should be withdrawn. (See DOSAGE AND ADMINISTRATION.)

Cessation of Therapy with TENORMIN: Patients with coronary artery disease, who are being treated with TENORMIN, should be advised against abrupt discontinuation of therapy. Severe exacerbation of angina and the occurrence of myocardial infarction and ventricular arrhythmias have been reported in angina patients following the abrupt discontinuation of therapy with beta blockers. The last two complications may occur with or without preceding exacerbation of the angina pectoris. As with other beta blockers, when discontinuation of TENORMIN is planned, the patients should be carefully observed and advised to limit physical activity to a minimum. If the angina worsens or acute coronary insufficiency develops, it is recommenced that TENORMIN be promptly reinstituted, at least temporarily. Because coronary artery disease is common and may be unrecognized, it may be prudent not to discontinue TENORMIN therapy abruptly even in patients treated only for hypertension. (See DOSAGE AND ADMINISTRATION.)

Concomitant Use of Calcium Channel Blockers: Bradycardia and heart block can occur and the left ventricular end diastolic pressure can rise when beta blockers are administered with verapamil or diltiazem. Patients with pre-existing conduction abnormalities or left ventricular dysfunction are particularly susceptible. (See **PRECAUTIONS**.)

Bronchospastic Diseases: PATIENTS WITH BRONCHOSPASTIC DISEASE SHOULD, IN GENERAL, NOT RECEIVE BETA BLOCKERS. Because of its relative $beta_1$ selectivity, however, TENORMIN may be used with caution in patients with bronchospastic disease who do not respond to, or cannot tolerate, other antihypertensive treatment. Since $beta_1$ selectivity is not absolute, the lowest possible dose of TENORMIN should be used with therapy initiated at 50 mg and a $beta_2$-stimulating agent (bronchodilator) should be made available. If dosage must be increased, dividing the dose should be considered in order to achieve lower peak blood levels.

Anesthesia and Major Surgery: It is not advisable to withdraw beta-adrenoreceptor blocking drugs prior to surgery in the majority of patients. However, care should be taken when using anesthetic agents such as those which may depress the myocardium. Vagal dominance, if it occurs, may be corrected with atropine (1-2 mg IV).

Additionally, caution should be used when TENORMIN I.V. Injection is administered concomitantly with such agents.

TENORMIN, like other beta blockers, is a competitive inhibitor of beta-receptor agonists and its effects on the heart can be reversed by administration of such agents: eg, dobutamine or isoproterenol with caution (see section on OVERDOSAGE).

Diabetes and Hypoglycemia: TENORMIN should be used with caution in diabetic patients if a beta-blocking agent is required. Beta blockers may mask tachycardia occurring with hypoglycemia, but other manifestations such as dizziness and sweating may not be significantly affected. At recommended doses TENORMIN does not potentiate insulin-induced hypoglycemia and, unlike nonselective beta blockers, does not delay recovery of blood glucose to normal levels.

Thyrotoxicosis: Beta-adrenergic blockade may mask certain clinical signs (eg, tachycardia) of hyperthyroidism. Patients suspected of having thyroid disease should be monitored closely when adminstering TENORMIN I.V. Injection. Abrupt withdrawal of beta blockade might precipitate a thyroid storm; therefore, patients suspected of developing thyrotoxicosis from whom TENORMIN therapy is to be withdrawn should be monitored closely. (See DOSAGE AND ADMINISTRATION.)

Untreated Pheochromocytoma: TENORMIN and TENORMIN I.V. should not be given to patients with untreated pheochromocytoma.

Pregnancy and Fetal Injury: Atenolol can cause fetal harm when administered to a pregnant woman. Atenolol crosses the placental barrier and appears in cord blood. Administration of atenolol, starting in the second trimester of pregnancy, has been associated with the birth of infants that are small for gestational age. No studies have been performed on the use of atenolol in the first trimester and the possibility of fetal injury cannot be excluded. If this drug is used during pregnancy, or if the patient becomes pregnant while taking this drug, the patient should be apprised of the potential hazard to the fetus.

Atenolol has been shown to produce a dose-related increase in embryo/fetal resorptions in rats at doses equal to or greater than 50 mg/kg/day or 25 or more times the maximum recommended human antihypertensive dose*. Although similar effects were not seen in rabbits, the compound was not evaluated in rabbits at doses above 25 mg/kg/day or 12.5 times the maximum recommended human antihypertensive dose*.

*Based on the maximum dose of 100 mg/day in a 50 kg patient.

PRECAUTIONS

General: Patients already on a beta blocker must be evaluated carefully before TENORMIN is administered. Initial and subsequent TENORMIN dosages can be adjusted downward depending on clinical observations including pulse and blood pressure. TENORMIN may aggravate peripheral arterial circulatory disorders.

Impaired Renal Function: The drug should be used with caution in patients with impaired renal function. (See DOSAGE AND ADMINISTRATION.)

Drug Interactions: Catecholamine-depleting drugs (eg, reserpine) may have an additive effect when given with beta-blocking agents. Patients treated with TENORMIN plus a catecholamine depletor should therefore be closely observed for evidence of hypotension and/or marked bradycardia which may produce vertigo, syncope or postural hypotension.

Calcium channel blockers may also have an additive effect when given with TENORMIN (See WARNINGS.).

Beta blockers may exacerbate the rebound hypertension which can follow the withdrawal of clonidine. If the two drugs are coadministered, the beta blocker should be withdrawn several days before the gradual withdrawal of clonidine. If replacing clonidine by beta-blocker therapy, the introduction of beta blockers should be delayed for several days after clonidine administration has stopped.

Caution should be exercised with TENORMIN I.V. Injection when given in close proximity with drugs that may also have a depressant effect on myocardial contractility. On rare occasions, concomitant use of intravenous beta blockers and intravenous verapamil has resulted in serious adverse reactions, especially in patients with severe cardiomyopathy, congestive heart failure, or recent myocardial infarction.

Concomitant use of prostaglandin synthase inhibiting drugs, e.g., indomethacin, may decrease the hypotensive effects of beta-blockers.

Information on concurrent usage of atenolol and aspirin is limited. Data from several studies, ie, TIMI-II, ISIS-2, currently do not suggest any clinical interaction between aspirin and beta blockers in the acute myocardial infarction setting.

While taking beta blockers, patients with a history of anaphylactic reaction to a variety of allergens may have a more severe reaction on repeated challenge, either accidental, diagnostic or therapeutic. Such patients may be unresponsive to the usual doses of epinephrine used to treat the allergic reaction.

Carcinogenesis, Mutagenesis, Impairment of Fertility: Two long-term (maximum dosing duration of 18 or 24 months) rat studies and one long-term (maximum dosing duration of 18 months) mouse study, each employing dose levels as high as 300 mg/kg/day or 150 times the maximum recommended human antihypertensive dose,* did not indicate a carcinogenic potential of atenolol. A third (24 month) rat study, employing doses of 500 and 1,500 mg/kg/day (250 and 750 times the maximum recommended human antihypertensive dose*) resulted in increased incidences of benign adrenal medullary tumors in males and females, mammary fibroadenomas in females, and anterior pituitary adenomas and thyroid parafollicular cell carcinomas in males. No evidence of a mutagenic potential of atenolol was uncovered in the dominant lethal test (mouse), in vivo cytogenetics test (Chinese hamster) or Ames test (*S typhimurium*).

Fertility of male or female rats (evaluated at dose levels as high as 200 mg/kg/day or 100 times the maximum recommended human dose*) was unaffected by atenolol administration.

Animal Toxicology: Chronic studies employing oral atenolol performed in animals have revealed the occurrence of vacuolation of epithelial cells of Brunner's glands in the duodenum of both male and female dogs at all tested dose levels of atenolol (starting at 15 mg/kg/day or 7.5 times the maximum recommended human antihypertensive dose*) and increased incidence of atrial degeneration of hearts of male rats at 300 but not 150 mg atenolol/kg/day (150 and 75 times the maximum recommended human antihypertensive dose,* respectively).

*Based on the maximum dose of 100 mg/day in a 50 kg patient.

Usage in Pregnancy: Pregnancy Category D: See WARNINGS—Pregnancy and Fetal Injury.

Nursing Mothers: Atenolol is excreted in human breast milk at a ratio of 1.5 to 6.8 when compared to the concentration in plasma. Caution should be exercised when TENORMIN is administered to a nursing woman. Clinically significant bradycardia has been reported in breast fed infants. Premature infants, or infants with impaired renal function, may be more likely to develop adverse effects.

Pediatric Use: Safety and effectiveness in pediatric patients have not been established.

ADVERSE REACTIONS

Most adverse effects have been mild and transient.

The frequency estimates in the following table were derived from controlled studies in hypertensive patients in which adverse reactions were either volunteered by the patient (US studies) or elicited, eg, by checklist (foreign studies). The reported frequency of elicited adverse effects was higher for both TENORMIN and placebo-treated patients than when these reactions were volunteered. Where frequency of adverse effects of TENORMIN and placebo is similar, causal relationship to TENORMIN is uncertain.

[See table at left]

	Volunteered (US Studies)		Total—Volunteered and Elicited (Foreign + US Studies)	
	Atenolol (n = 164) %	Placebo (n = 206) %	Atenolol (n = 399) %	Placebo (n = 407) %
CARDIOVASCULAR				
Bradycardia	3	0	3	0
Cold Extremities	0	0.5	12	5
Postural Hypotension	2	1	4	5
Leg Pain	0	0.5	3	1
CENTRAL NERVOUS SYSTEM/NEUROMUSCULAR				
Dizziness	4	1	13	6
Vertigo	2	0.5	2	0.2
Light-headedness	1	0	3	0.7
Tiredness	0.6	0.5	26	13
Fatigue	3	1	6	5
Lethargy	1	0	3	0.7
Drowsiness	0.6	0	2	0.5
Depression	0.6	0.5	12	9
Dreaming	0	0	3	1
GASTROINTESTINAL				
Diarrhea	2	0	3	2
Nausea	4	1	3	1
RESPIRATORY (see WARNINGS)				
Wheeziness	0	0	3	3
Dyspnea	0.6	1	6	4

Acute Myocardial Infarction: In a series of investigations in the treatment of acute myocardial infarction, bradycardia and hypotension occurred more commonly, as expected for any beta blocker, in atenolol-treated patients than in control patients. However, these usually responded to atropine and/or to withholding further dosage of atenolol. The incidence of heart failure was not increased by atenolol. Inotropic agents were infrequently used. The reported frequency of these and other events occurring during these investigations is given in the following table.

In a study of 477 patients, the following adverse events were reported during either intravenous and/or oral atenolol administration:

[See first table at top of next page]

In the subsequent International Study of Infarct Survival (ISIS-1) including over 16,000 patients of whom 8,037 were randomized to receive TENORMIN treatment, the dosage of intravenous and subsequent oral TENORMIN was either discontinued or reduced for the following reasons:

[See second table at top of next page]

During postmarketing experience with TENORMIN, the following have been reported in temporal relationship to the use of the drug: elevated liver enzymes and/or bilirubin, hallucinations, headache, impotence, Peyronie's disease, postural hypotension which may be associated with syncope, psoriasiform rash or exacerbation of psoriasis, psychoses, purpura, reversible alopecia, thrombocytopenia, visual disturbances, sick sinus syndrome, and drymouth. TENORMIN, like other beta blockers, has been associated with the development of antinuclear antibodies (ANA), lupus syndrome, and Raynaud's phenomenon.

POTENTIAL ADVERSE EFFECTS

In addition, a variety of adverse effects have been reported with other beta-adrenergic blocking agents, and may be considered potential adverse effects of TENORMIN.

Hematologic: Agranulocytosis.

Allergic: Fever, combined with aching and sore throat, laryngospasm, and respiratory distress.

Central Nervous System: Reversible mental depression progressing to catatonia; an acute reversible syndrome characterized by disorientation of time and place; short-term memory loss; emotional lability with slightly clouded sensorium; and decreased performance on neuropsychometrics.

Gastrointestinal: Mesenteric arterial thrombosis, ischemic colitis.

Other: Erythematous rash.

Miscellaneous: There have been reports of skin rashes and/ or dry eyes associated with the use of beta-adrenergic blocking drugs. The reported incidence is small, and in most cases, the symptoms have cleared when treatment was withdrawn. Discontinuance of the drug should be considered if any such reaction is not otherwise explicable. Patients should be closely monitored following cessation of therapy. (SEE DOSAGE AND ADMINISTRATION.)

The oculomucocutaneous syndrome associated with the beta blocker practolol has not been reported with TENORMIN. Furthermore, a number of patients who had previously demonstrated established practolol reactions were transferred to TENORMIN therapy with subsequent resolution or quiescence of the reaction.

OVERDOSAGE

Overdosage with TENORMIN has been reported with patients surviving acute doses as high as 5 g. One death was reported in a man who may have taken as much as 10 g acutely.

The predominant symptoms reported following TENORMIN overdose are lethargy, disorder of respiratory drive, wheezing, sinus pause and bradycardia. Additionally, common effects associated with overdosage of any beta-adrenergic blocking agent and which might also be expected in TENORMIN overdose are congestive heart failure, hypotension, bronchospasm and/or hypoglycemia.

Treatment of overdose should be directed to the removal of any unabsorbed drug by induced emesis, gastric lavage, or administration of activated charcoal. TENORMIN can be removed from the general circulation by hemodialysis. Other treatment modalities should be employed at the physician's discretion and may include:

BRADYCARDIA: Atropine intravenously. If there is no response to vagal blockade, give isoproterenol cautiously. In refractory cases, a transvenous cardiac pacemaker may be indicated.

HEART BLOCK (SECOND OR THIRD DEGREE): Isoproterenol or transvenous cardiac pacemaker.

CARDIAC FAILURE: Digitalize the patient and administer a diuretic. Glucagon has been reported to be useful.

HYPOTENSION: Vasopressors such as dopamine or norepinephrine (levarterenol). Monitor blood pressure continuously.

BRONCHOSPASM: A beta$_2$ stimulant such as isoproterenol or terbutaline and/or aminophylline.

HYPOGLYCEMIA: Intravenous glucose.

Based on the severity of symptoms, management may require intensive support care and facilities for applying cardiac and respiratory support.

DOSAGE AND ADMINISTRATION

Hypertension: The initial dose of TENORMIN is 50 mg given as one tablet a day either alone or added to diuretic therapy. The full effect of this dose will usually be seen within one to two weeks. If an optimal response is not achieved, the dosage should be increased to TENORMIN 100 mg given as one tablet a day. Increasing the dosage beyond 100 mg a day is unlikely to produce any further benefit.

TENORMIN may be used alone or concomitantly with other antihypertensive agents including thiazide-type diuretics, hydralazine, prazosin, and alpha-methyldopa.

Angina Pectoris: The initial dose of TENORMIN is 50 mg given as one tablet a day. If an optimal response is not achieved within one week, the dosage should be increased to TENORMIN 100 mg given as one tablet a day. Some patients may require a dosage of 200 mg once a day for optimal effect.

Twenty-four hour control with once daily dosing is achieved by giving doses larger than necessary to achieve an immediate maximum effect. The maximum early effect on exercise tolerance occurs with doses of 50 to 100 mg, but at these doses the effect at 24 hours is attenuated, averaging about 50% to 75% of that observed with once a day oral doses of 200 mg.

Acute Myocardial Infarction: In patients with definite or suspected acute myocardial infarction, treatment with TENORMIN I.V. Injection should be initiated as soon as possible after the patient's arrival in the hospital and after eligibility is established. Such treatment should be initiated

	Conventional Therapy Plus Atenolol (n=244)		Conventional Therapy Alone (n=233)	
Bradycardia	43	(18%)	24	(10%)
Hypotension	60	(25%)	34	(15%)
Bronchospasm	3	(1.2%)	2	(0.9%)
Heart Failure	46	(19%)	56	(24%)
Heart Block	11	(4.5%)	10	(4.3%)
BBB + Major Axis Deviation	16	(6.6%)	28	(12%)
Supraventricular Tachycardia	28	(11.5%)	45	(19%)
Atrial Fibrillation	12	(5%)	29	(11%)
Atrial Flutter	4	(1.6%)	7	(3%)
Ventricular Tachycardia	39	(16%)	52	(22%)
Cardiac Reinfarction	0	(0%)	6	(2.6%)
Total Cardiac Arrests	4	(1.6%)	16	(6.9%)
Nonfatal Cardiac Arrests	4	(1.6%)	12	(5.1%)
Deaths	7	(2.9%)	16	(6.9%)
Cardiogenic Shock	1	(0.4%)	4	(1.7%)
Development of Ventricular Septal Defect	0	(0%)	2	(0.9%)
Development of Mitral Regurgitation	0	(0%)	2	(0.9%)
Renal Failure	1	(0.4%)	0	(0%)
Pulmonary Emboli	3	(1.2%)	0	(0%)

Reasons for Reduced Dosage	IV Atenolol Reduced Dose (<5 mg)*		Oral Partial Dose	
Hypotension/Bradycardia	105	(1.3%)	1168	(14.5%)
Cardiogenic Shock	4	(.04%)	35	(.44%)
Reinfarction	0	(0%)	5	(.06%)
Cardiac Arrest	5	(.06%)	28	(.34%)
Heart Block (> first degree)	5	(.06%)	143	(1.7%)
Cardiac Failure	1	(.01%)	233	(2.9%)
Arrhythmias	3	(.04%)	22	(.27%)
Bronchospasm	1	(.01%)	50	(.62%)

* Full dosage was 10 mg and some patients received less than 10 mg but more than 5 mg.

Creatinine Clearance (mL/min/1.73m^2)	Atenolol Elimination Half-Life (h)	Maximum Dosage (tablets)	Maximum Dosage (I.V.)
15–35	16–27	50 mg daily	50 mg daily
<15	>27	25 mg daily	50 mg daily

in a coronary care or similar unit immediately after the patient's hemodynamic condition has stabilized. Treatment should begin with the intravenous administration of 5 mg TENORMIN over 5 minutes followed by another 5 mg intravenous injection 10 minutes later. TENORMIN I.V. Injection should be administered under carefully controlled conditions including monitoring of blood pressure, heart rate, and electrocardiogram. Dilutions of TENORMIN I.V. Injection in Dextrose Injection USP, Sodium Chloride Injection USP, or Sodium Chloride and Dextrose Injection may be used. These admixtures are stable for 48 hours if they are not used immediately.

In patients who tolerate the full intravenous dose (10 mg), TENORMIN Tablets 50 mg should be initiated 10 minutes after the last intravenous dose followed by another 50 mg oral dose 12 hours later. Thereafter, TENORMIN can be given orally either 100 mg once daily or 50 mg twice a day for a further 6–9 days or until discharge from the hospital. If bradycardia or hypotension requiring treatment or any other untoward effects occur, TENORMIN should be discontinued. (See full prescribing information prior to initiating therapy with TENORMIN tablets.)

Data from other beta blocker trials suggest that if there is any question concerning the use of IV beta blocker or clinical estimate that there is a contraindication, the IV beta blocker may be eliminated and patients fulfilling the safety criteria may be given TENORMIN Tablets 50 mg twice daily or 100 mg once a day for at least seven days (if the IV dosing is excluded).

Although the demonstration of efficacy of TENORMIN is based entirely on data from the first seven postinfarction days, data from other beta blocker trials suggest that treatment with beta blockers that are effective in the postinfarction setting may be continued for one to three years if there are no contraindications.

TENORMIN is an additional treatment to standard coronary care unit therapy.

Elderly Patients or Patients with Renal Impairment: TENORMIN is excreted by the kidneys; consequently dosage should be adjusted in cases of severe impairment of renal function. Some reduction in dosage may also be appropriate for the elderly, since decreased kidney function is a physiologic consequence of aging. Atenolol excretion would be expected to decrease with advancing age.

No significant accumulation of TENORMIN occurs until creatinine clearance falls below 35 mL/min/1.73 m^2. Accumulation of atenolol and prolongation of its half-life were studied in subjects with creatinine clearance between 5 and 105 mL/min. Peak plasma levels were significantly increased in subjects with creatinine clearances below 30 mL/min.

The following maximum oral dosages are recommended for elderly, renally-impaired patients and for patients with renal impairment due to other causes:

[See third table above]

Some renally-impaired or elderly patients being treated for hypertension may require a lower starting dose of TENORMIN: 25 mg given as one tablet a day. If this 25 mg dose is used, assessment of efficacy must be made carefully. This should include measurement of blood pressure just prior to the next dose ("trough" blood pressure) to ensure that the treatment effect is present for a full 24 hours.

Although a similar dosage reduction may be considered for elderly and/or renally-impaired patients being treated for indications other than hypertension, data are not available for these patient populations.

Patients on hemodialysis should be given 25 mg or 50 mg after each dialysis; this should be done under hospital supervision as marked falls in blood pressure can occur.

Cessation of Therapy in Patients with Angina Pectoris: If withdrawal of TENORMIN therapy is planned, it should be achieved gradually and patients should be carefully observed and advised to limit physical activity to a minimum.

Parenteral drug products should be inspected visually for particulate matter and discoloration prior to administration, whenever solution and container permit.

HOW SUPPLIED

TENORMIN Tablets: Tablets of 25 mg atenolol, NDC 0310-0107 (round, flat, uncoated white tablets identified with "T" debossed on one side and 107 debossed on the other side) are supplied in bottles of 100 tablets.

Tablets of 50 mg atenolol, NDC 0310-0105 (round, flat, uncoated white tablets identified with "TENORMIN" debossed on one side and 105 debossed on the other side, bisected) are supplied in bottles of 100 tablets and 1000 tablets, and unit dose packages of 100 tablets.

Tablets of 100 mg atenolol, NDC 0310-0101 (round, flat, uncoated white tablets identified with "TENORMIN" debossed on one side and 101 debossed on the other side) are supplied in bottles of 100 tablets and unit dose packages of 100 tablets.

Store at controlled room temperature, 20–25°C (68–77°F) [see USP]. Dispense in well-closed, light resistant containers.

TENORMIN I.V. Injection:*

TENORMIN I.V. Injection, NDC 0310-0108, is supplied as 5 mg atenolol in 10 mL ampules of isotonic citrate-buffered aqueous solution.

Continued on next page

Tenormin—Cont.

Protect from light. Keep ampules in outer packaging until time of use. Store at controlled room temperature 20–25°C (68–77°F) [see USP].
ZENECA
Manufactured for:
Zeneca Pharmaceuticals
A Business Unit of Zeneca Inc.
Wilmington, Delaware 19850-5437
By: IPR Pharmaceuticals, Inc.
Carolina, Puerto Rico 00984-1967
TENORMIN I.V. Injection
is manufactured by:
Marsam Pharmaceuticals Inc.
Cherry Hill, NJ 08034
*64124-03/C0457b Rev N 07/99
610024 Rev M 07/99
Shown in Product Identification Guide, page 306

ZESTORETIC® ℞
[zes'tor-etic]
(Lisinopril and Hydrochlorothiazide)

USE IN PREGNANCY

When used in pregnancy during the second and third trimesters, ACE inhibitors can cause injury and even death to the developing fetus. When pregnancy is detected, ZESTORETIC should be discontinued as soon as possible. See WARNINGS, Pregnancy, Lisinopril, Fetal/Neonatal Morbidity and Mortality.

DESCRIPTION

ZESTORETIC® (Lisinopril and Hydrochlorothiazide) combines an angiotensin converting enzyme inhibitor, lisinopril, and a diuretic, hydrochlorothiazide.
Lisinopril, a synthetic peptide derivative, is an oral long-acting angiotensin converting enzyme inhibitor. It is chemically described as (S)-1-[N^2-(1-carboxy-3-phenylpropyl)-L-lysyl]-L-proline dihydrate. Its empirical formula is $C_{21}H_{31}N_3O_5 \bullet 2H_2O$ and its structural formula is:

Lisinopril is a white to off-white, crystalline powder, with a molecular weight of 441.53. It is soluble in water, sparingly soluble in methanol, and practically insoluble in ethanol.
Hydrochlorothiazide is 6-chloro-3,4-dihydro-2H-1,2,4-benzothiadiazine-7-sulfonamide 1,1-dioxide. Its empirical formula is $C_7H_8ClN_3O_4S_2$ and its structural formula is:

Hydrochlorothiazide is a white, or practically white, crystalline powder with a molecular weight of 297.72, which is slightly soluble in water, but freely soluble in sodium hydroxide solution.
ZESTORETIC is available for oral use in three tablet combinations of lisinopril with hydrochlorothiazide: ZESTORETIC 10–12.5 containing 10 mg lisinopril and 12.5 mg hydrochlorothiazide; ZESTORETIC 20–12.5 containing 20 mg lisinopril and 12.5 mg hydrochlorothiazide; and, ZESTORETIC 20–25 containing 20 mg lisinopril and 25 mg hydrochlorothiazide.

Inactive Ingredients:
10–12.5 Tablets—calcium phosphate, magnesium stearate, mannitol, red ferric oxide, starch, yellow ferric oxide.
20–12.5 Tablets—calcium phosphate, magnesium stearate, mannitol, starch.
20–25 Tablets—calcium phosphate, magnesium stearate, mannitol, red ferric oxide, starch, yellow ferric oxide.

CLINICAL PHARMACOLOGY

Lisinopril and Hydrochlorothiazide
As a result of its diuretic effects, hydrochlorothiazide increases plasma renin activity, increases aldosterone secretion, and decreases serum potassium. Administration of lisinopril blocks the renin-angiotensin aldosterone axis and tends to reverse the potassium loss associated with the diuretic.
In clinical studies, the extent of blood pressure reduction seen with the combination of lisinopril and hydrochlorothiazide was approximately additive. The ZESTORETIC 10–12.5 combination worked equally well in black and white patients. The ZESTORETIC 20–12.5 and ZESTORETIC 20–25 combinations appeared somewhat less effective in black patients, but relatively few black patients were studied. In most patients, the antihypertensive effect of ZESTORETIC was sustained for at least 24 hours.
In a randomized, controlled comparison, the mean antihypertensive effects of ZESTORETIC 20–12.5 and ZESTORETIC 20–25 were similar, suggesting that many patients who respond adequately to the latter combination may be controlled with ZESTORETIC 20–12.5. (See DOSAGE AND ADMINISTRATION.)
Concomitant administration of lisinopril and hydrochlorothiazide has little or no effect on the bioavailability of either drug. The combination tablet is bioequivalent to concomitant administration of the separate entities.

Lisinopril
Mechanism of Action: Lisinopril inhibits angiotensin-converting enzyme (ACE) in human subjects and animals. ACE is a peptidyl dipeptidase that catalyzes the conversion of angiotensin I to the vasoconstrictor substance, angiotensin II. Angiotensin II also stimulates aldosterone secretion by the adrenal cortex. Inhibition of ACE results in decreased plasma angiotensin II which leads to decreased vasopressor activity and to decreased aldosterone secretion. The latter decrease may result in a small increase of serum potassium. Removal of angiotensin II negative feedback on renin secretion leads to increased plasma renin activity. In hypertensive patients with normal renal function treated with lisinopril alone for up to 24 weeks, the mean increase in serum potassium was less than 0.1 mEq/L; however, approximately 15 percent of patients had increases greater than 0.5 mEq/L and approximately six percent had a decrease greater than 0.5 mEq/L. In the same study, patients treated with lisinopril plus a thiazide diuretic showed essentially no change in serum potassium. (See PRECAUTIONS.)
ACE is identical to kininase, an enzyme that degrades bradykinin. Whether increased levels of bradykinin, a potent vasodepressor peptide, play a role in the therapeutic effects of lisinopril remains to be elucidated.
While the mechanism through which lisinopril lowers blood pressure is believed to be primarily suppression of the renin-angiotensin-aldosterone system, lisinopril is antihypertensive even in patients with low-renin hypertension. Although lisinopril was antihypertensive in all races studied, black hypertensive patients (usually a low-renin hypertensive population) had a smaller average response to lisinopril monotherapy than nonblack patients.
Pharmacokinetics and Metabolism: Following oral administration of lisinopril, peak serum concentrations occur within about 7 hours. Declining serum concentrations exhibit a prolonged terminal phase which does not contribute to drug accumulation. This terminal phase probably represents saturable binding to ACE and is not proportional to dose. Lisinopril does not appear to be bound to other serum proteins.
Lisinopril does not undergo metabolism and is excreted unchanged entirely in the urine. Based on urinary recovery, the mean extent of absorption of lisinopril is approximately 25 percent, with large intersubject variability (6%–60%) at all doses tested (5–80 mg). Lisinopril absorption is not influenced by the presence of food in the gastrointestinal tract.
Upon multiple dosing, lisinopril exhibits an effective half-life of accumulation of 12 hours.
Impaired renal function decreases elimination of lisinopril, which is excreted principally through the kidneys, but this decrease becomes clinically important only when the glomerular filtration rate is below 30 mL/min. Above this glomerular filtration rate, the elimination half-life is little changed. With greater impairment, however, peak and trough lisinopril levels increase, time to peak concentration increases and time to attain steady state is prolonged. Older patients, on average, have (approximately doubled) higher blood levels and area under the plasma concentration time curve (AUC) than younger patients (See DOSAGE AND ADMINISTRATION.) Lisinopril can be removed by hemodialysis.
Studies in rats indicate that lisinopril crosses the blood-brain barrier poorly. Multiple doses of lisinopril in rats do not result in accumulation in any tissues. However, milk of lactating rats contains radioactivity following administration of ^{14}C lisinopril. By whole body autoradiography, radioactivity was found in the placenta following administration of labeled drug to pregnant rats, but none was found in the fetuses.
Pharmacodynamics: Administration of lisinopril to patients with hypertension results in a reduction of supine and standing blood pressure to about the same extent with no compensatory tachycardia. Symptomatic postural hypotension is usually not observed although it can occur and should be anticipated in volume and/or salt-depleted patients. (See WARNINGS.)
In most patients studied, onset of antihypertensive activity was seen at one hour after oral administration of an individual dose of lisinopril, with peak reduction of blood pressure achieved by six hours.
In some patients achievement of optimal blood pressure reduction may require two to four weeks of therapy.
At recommended single daily doses, antihypertensive effects have been maintained for at least 24 hours, after dosing, although the effect at 24 hours was substantially smaller than the effect six hours after dosing.
The antihypertensive effects of lisinopril have continued during long-term therapy. Abrupt withdrawal of lisinopril has not been associated with a rapid increase in blood pressure; nor with a significant overshoot of pretreatment blood pressure.
In hemodynamic studies in patients with essential hypertension, blood pressure reduction was accompanied by a reduction in peripheral arterial resistance with little or no change in cardiac output and in heart rate. In a study in nine hypertensive patients, following administration of lisinopril, there was an increase in mean renal blood flow that was not significant. Data from several small studies are inconsistent with respect to the effect of lisinopril on glomerular filtration rate in hypertensive patients with normal renal function, but suggest that changes, if any, are not large.
In patients with renovascular hypertension lisinopril has been shown to be well tolerated and effective in controlling blood pressure. (See PRECAUTIONS.)

Hydrochlorothiazide
The mechanism of the antihypertensive effect of thiazides is unknown. Thiazides do not usually affect normal blood pressure.
Hydrochlorothiazide is a diuretic and antihypertensive. It affects the distal renal tubular mechanism of electrolyte reabsorption. Hydrochlorothiazide increases excretion of sodium and chloride in approximately equivalent amounts. Natriuresis may be accompanied by some loss of potassium and bicarbonate.
After oral use diuresis begins within two hours, peaks in about four hours and lasts about 6 to 12 hours.
Hydrochlorothiazide is not metabolized but is eliminated rapidly by the kidney. When plasma levels have been followed for at least 24 hours, the plasma half-life has been observed to vary between 5.6 and 14.8 hours. At least 61 percent of the oral dose is eliminated unchanged within 24 hours. Hydrochlorothiazide crosses the placental but not the blood-brain barrier.

INDICATIONS AND USAGE

ZESTORETIC is indicated for the treatment of hypertension.
These fixed-dose combinations are not indicated for initial therapy (see DOSAGE AND ADMINISTRATION).
In using ZESTORETIC, consideration should be given to the fact that an angiotensin-converting enzyme inhibitor, captopril, has caused agranulocytosis, particularly in patients with renal impairment or collagen vascular disease, and that available data are insufficient to show that lisinopril does not have a similar risk. (See WARNINGS.)
In considering the use of ZESTORETIC, it should be noted that ACE inhibitors have been associated with a higher rate of angioedema in black than in nonblack patients (see WARNINGS, Lisinopril, Angioedema).

CONTRAINDICATIONS

ZESTORETIC is contraindicated in patients who are hypersensitive to any component of this product and in patients with a history of angioedema related to previous treatment with an angiotensin-converting enzyme inhibitor. Because of the hydrochlorothiazide component, this product is contraindicated in patients with anuria or hypersensitivity to other sulfonamide-derived drugs.

WARNINGS

Lisinopril
Anaphylactoid and Possibly Related Reactions: Presumably because angiotensin-converting enzyme inhibitors affect the metabolism of eicosanoids and polypeptides, including endogenous bradykinin, patients receiving ACE inhibitors (including ZESTORETIC) may be subject to a variety of adverse reactions, some of them serious.
Angioedema: Angioedema of the face, extremities, lips, tongue, glottis and/or larynx has been reported rarely in patients treated with angiotensin-converting enzyme inhibitors, including lisinopril. This may occur at any time during treatment. ACE inhibitors have been associated with a higher rate of angioedema in black than in nonblack patients. ZESTORETIC should be promptly discontinued and the appropriate therapy and monitoring should be provided until complete and sustained resolution of signs and symptoms has occurred. In instances where swelling has been confined to the face and lips the condition has generally resolved without treatment, although antihistamines have been useful in relieving symptoms. Angioedema associated with laryngeal edema may be fatal. **Where there is involvement of the tongue, glottis or larynx, likely to cause airway obstruction, subcutaneous epinephrine solution 1:1000 (0.3 mL to 0.5 mL) and/or measures necessary to ensure a patent airway should be promptly provided. (See ADVERSE REACTIONS.)**
Patients with a history of angioedema unrelated to ACE inhibitor therapy may be at increased risk of angioedema while receiving an ACE inhibitor (see also INDICATIONS AND USAGE and CONTRAINDICATIONS).
Anaphylactoid Reactions During Desensitization: Two patients undergoing desensitizing treatment with hymenoptera venom while receiving ACE inhibitors sustained life-threatening anaphylactoid reactions. In the same patients, these reactions were avoided when ACE inhibitors were temporarily withheld, but they reappeared upon inadvertent rechallenge.
Anaphylactoid Reactions During Membrane Exposure: Thiazide-containing combination products are not recommended in patients with severe renal dysfunction. Sudden and potentially life-threatening anaphylactoid reactions have been reported in some patients dialyzed with high-flux membranes (eg, AN69¶) and treated concomitantly with an ACE inhibitor. In such patients, dialysis must be stopped immediately, and aggressive therapy for anaphylactoid reactions be initiated. Symptoms have not been relieved by antihistamines in these situations. In these patients, consideration should be given to using a different type of dial-

ysis membrane or a different class of antihypertensive agent. Anaphylactoid reactions have also been reported in patients undergoing low-density lipoprotein apheresis with dextran sulfate absorption.

Hypotension and Related Effects: Excessive hypotension was rarely seen in uncomplicated hypertensive patients but is a possible consequence of lisinopril use in salt/volume-depleted persons such as those treated vigorously with diuretics or patients on dialysis. (See PRECAUTIONS, Drug Interactions and ADVERSE REACTIONS.)

Syncope has been reported in 0.8 percent of patients receiving ZESTORETIC. In patients with hypertension receiving lisinopril alone, the incidence of syncope was 0.1 percent. The overall incidence of syncope may be reduced by proper titration of the individual components. (See PRECAUTIONS, Drug Interactions, ADVERSE REACTIONS and DOSAGE AND ADMINISTRATION.)

In patients with severe congestive heart failure, with or without associated renal insufficiency, excessive hypotension has been observed and may be associated with oliguria and/or progressive azotemia, and rarely with acute renal failure and/or death. Because of the potential fall in blood pressure in these patients, therapy should be started under very close medical supervision. Such patients should be followed closely for the first two weeks of treatment and whenever the dose of lisinopril and/or diuretic is increased. Similar considerations apply to patients with ischemic heart or cerebrovascular disease in whom an excessive fall in blood pressure could result in a myocardial infarction or cerebrovascular accident.

If hypotension occurs, the patient should be placed in the supine position and, if necessary, receive an intravenous infusion of normal saline. A transient hypotensive response is not a contraindication to further doses which usually can be given without difficulty once the blood pressure has increased after volume expansion.

Leukopenia/Neutropenia/Agranulocytosis: Another angiotensin-converting enzyme inhibitor, captopril, has been shown to cause agranulocytosis and bone marrow depression, rarely in uncomplicated patients but more frequently in patients with renal impairment, especially if they also have a collagen vascular disease. Available data from clinical trials of lisinopril are insufficient to show that lisinopril does not cause agranulocytosis at similar rates. Marketing experience has revealed rare cases of leukopenia/neutropenia and bone marrow depression in which a causal relationship to lisinopril cannot be excluded. Periodic monitoring of white blood cell counts in patients with collagen vascular disease and renal disease should be considered.

Hepatic Failure: Rarely, ACE inhibitors have been associated with a syndrome that starts with cholestatic jaundice and progresses to fulminant hepatic necrosis and (sometimes) death. The mechanism of this syndrome is not understood. Patients receiving ACE inhibitors who develop jaundice or marked elevations of hepatic enzymes should discontinue the ACE inhibitor and receive appropriate medical follow-up.

Pregnancy

Lisinopril and Hydrochlorothiazide: Teratogenicity studies were conducted in mice and rats with up to 90 mg/kg/day of lisinopril (56 times the maximum recommended human dose) in combination with 10 mg/kg/day of hydrochlorothiazide (2.5 times the maximum recommended human dose). Maternal or fetotoxic effects were not seen in mice with the combination. In rats decreased maternal weight gain and decreased fetal weight occurred down to 3/10 mg/kg/day (the lowest dose tested). Associated with the decreased fetal weight was a delay in fetal ossification. The decreased fetal weight and delay in fetal ossification were not seen in saline-supplemented animals given 90/10 mg/kg/day.

When used in pregnancy during the second and third trimesters, ACE inhibitors can cause injury and even death to the developing fetus. When pregnancy is detected, ZESTORETIC should be discontinued as soon as possible. (See Lisinopril, Fetal/Neonatal Morbidity and Mortality below.)

Lisinopril

Fetal/Neonatal Morbidity and Mortality: ACE inhibitors can cause fetal and neonatal morbidity and death when administered to pregnant women. Several dozen cases have been reported in the world literature. When pregnancy is detected, ACE inhibitor therapy should be discontinued as soon as possible.

The use of ACE inhibitors during the second and third trimesters of pregnancy has been associated with fetal and neonatal injury, including hypotension, neonatal skull hypoplasia, anuria, reversible or irreversible renal failure, and death. Oligohydramnios has also been reported, presumably resulting from decreased fetal renal function; oligohydramnios in this setting has been associated with fetal limb contractures, craniofacial deformation, and hypoplastic lung development. Prematurity, intrauterine growth retardation, and patent ductus arteriosus have also been reported, although it is not clear whether these occurrences were due to the ACE-inhibitor exposure.

These adverse effects do not appear to have resulted from intrauterine ACE-inhibitor exposure that has been limited to the first trimester. Mothers whose embryos and fetuses are exposed to ACE inhibitors only during the first trimester should be so informed. Nonetheless, when patients become pregnant, physicians should make every effort to discontinue the use of ZESTORETIC as soon as possible.

Rarely (probably less often than once in every thousand pregnancies), no alternative to ACE inhibitors will be found. In these rare cases, the mothers should be apprised of the potential hazards to their fetuses, and serial ultrasound examinations should be performed to assess the intraamniotic environment.

If oligohydramnios is observed, ZESTORETIC should be discontinued unless it is considered lifesaving for the mother. Contraction stress testing (CST), a nonstress test (NST), or biophysical profiling (BPP) may be appropriate, depending upon the week of pregnancy. Patients and physicians should be aware, however, that oligohydramnios may not appear until after the fetus has sustained irreversible injury.

Infants with histories of in utero exposure to ACE inhibitors should be closely observed for hypotension, oliguria, and hyperkalemia. If oliguria occurs, attention should be directed toward support of blood pressure and renal perfusion. Exchange transfusion or dialysis may be required as means of reversing hypotension and/or substituting for disordered renal function. Lisinopril, which crosses the placenta, has been removed from neonatal circulation by peritoneal dialysis with some clinical benefit, and theoretically may be removed by exchange transfusion, although there is no experience with the latter procedure.

No teratogenic effects of lisinopril were seen in studies of pregnant rats, mice, and rabbits. On a mg/kg basis, the doses used were up to 625 times (in mice), 188 times (in rats), and 0.6 times (in rabbits) the maximum recommended human dose.

Hydrochlorothiazide

Teratogenic Effects: Reproduction studies in the rabbit, the mouse and the rat at doses up to 100 mg/kg/day (50 times the human dose) showed no evidence of external abnormalities of the fetus due to hydrochlorothiazide. Hydrochlorothiazide given in a two-litter study in rats at doses of 4–5.6 mg/kg/day (approximately 1–2 times the usual daily human dose) did not impair fertility or produce birth abnormalities in the offspring. Thiazides cross the placental barrier and appear in cord blood.

Nonteratogenic Effects: These may include fetal or neonatal jaundice, thrombocytopenia, and possibly other adverse reactions have occurred in the adult.

Hydrochlorothiazide

Thiazides should be used with caution in severe renal disease. In patients with renal disease, thiazides may precipitate azotemia. Cumulative effects of the drug may develop in patients with impaired renal function.

Thiazides should be used with caution in patients with impaired hepatic function or progressive liver disease, since minor alterations of fluid and electrolyte balance may precipitate hepatic coma.

Sensitivity reactions may occur in patients with or without a history of allergy or bronchial asthma.

The possibility of exacerbation or activation of systemic lupus erythematosus has been reported.

Lithium generally should not be given with thiazides. (See PRECAUTIONS, Drug Interactions, Lisinopril and Hydrochlorothiazide.)

PRECAUTIONS

General

Lisinopril

Impaired Renal Function: As a consequence of inhibiting the renin-angiotensin-aldosterone system, changes in renal function may be anticipated in susceptible individuals. In patients with severe congestive heart failure whose renal function may depend on activity of the renin-angiotensin-aldosterone system, treatment with angiotensin-converting enzyme inhibitors, including lisinopril, may be associated with oliguria and/or progressive azotemia and rarely with acute renal failure and/or death.

In hypertensive patients with unilateral or bilateral renal artery stenosis, increases in blood urea nitrogen and serum creatinine may occur. Experience with another angiotensin-converting enzyme inhibitor suggests that these increases are usually reversible upon discontinuation of lisinopril and/or diuretic therapy. In such patients renal function should be monitored during the first few weeks of therapy.

Some hypertensive patients with no apparent pre-existing renal vascular disease have devloped increases in blood urea and serum creatinine, usually minor and transient, especially when lisinopril has been given concomitantly with a diuretic. This is more likely to occur in patients with pre-existing renal impairment. Dosage reduction of lisinopril and/or discontinuation of the diuretic may be required.

Evaluation of the hypertensive patient should always include assessment of renal function (See DOSAGE AND ADMINISTRATION.)

Hyperkalemia: In clinical trials hyperkalemia (serum potassium greater than 5.7 mEq/L) occurred in approximately 1.4 percent of hypertensive patients treated with lisinopril plus hydrochlorothiazide. In most cases these were isolated values which resolved despite continued therapy. Hyperkalemia was not a cause of discontinuation of therapy. Risk factors for the development of hyperkalemia include renal insufficiency, diabetes mellitus, and the concomitant use of potassium-sparing diuretics, potassium supplements and/or potassium-containing salt substitutes, which should be used cautiously if at all with ZESTORETIC. (See Drug Interactions.)

Cough: Presumably due to the inhibition of the degradation of endogenous bradykinin, persistent nonproductive cough has been reported with all ACE inhibitors, almost always resolving after discontinuation of therapy. ACE inhibitor-induced cough should be considered in the differential diagnosis of cough.

Surgery/Anesthesia: In patients undergoing major surgery or during anesthesia with agents that produce hypotension, lisinopril may block angiotensin II formation secondary to compensatory renin release. If hypotension occurs and is considered to be due to this mechanism, it can be corrected by volume expansion.

Hydrochlorothiazide

Periodic determination of serum electrolytes to detect possible electrolyte imbalance should be performed at appropriate intervals.

All patients receiving thiazide therapy should be observed for clinical signs of fluid or electrolyte imbalance: namely, hyponatremia, hypochloremic alkalosis, and hypokalemia. Serum and urine electrolyte determinations are particularly important when the patient is vomiting excessively or receiving parenteral fluids. Warning signs or symptoms of fluid and electrolyte imbalance, irrespective of cause, include dryness of mouth, thirst, weakness, lethargy, drowsiness, restlessness, confusion, seizures, muscle pains or cramps, muscular fatigue, hypotension, oliguria, tachycardia, and gastrointestinal disturbances such as nausea and vomiting.

Hypokalemia may develop, especially with brisk diuresis, when severe cirrhosis is present, or after prolonged therapy. Interference with adequate oral electrolyte intake will also contribute to hypokalemia. Hypokalemia may cause cardiac arrhythmia and may also sensitize or exaggerate the response of the heart to the toxic effects of digitalis (eg, increased ventricular irritability). Because lisinopril reduces the production of aldosterone, concomitant therapy with lisinopril attenuates the diuretic-induced potassium loss. (See Drug Interactions, Agents Increasing Serum Potassium.)

Although any chloride deficit is generally mild and usually does not require specific treatment, except under extraordinary circumstances (as in liver disease or renal disease), chloride replacement may be required in the treatment of metabolic alkalosis.

Dilutional hyponatremia may occur in edematous patients in hot weather; appropriate therapy is water restriction, rather than administration of salt except in rare instances when the hyponatremia is life-threatening. In actual salt depletion, appropriate replacement is the therapy of choice.

Hyperuricemia may occur or frank gout may be precipitated in certain patients receiving thiazide therapy.

In diabetic patients dosage adjustments of insulin or oral hypoglycemic agents may be required. Hyperglycemia may occur with thiazide diuretics. Thus latent diabetes mellitus may become manifest during thiazide therapy.

The antihypertensive effects of the drug may be enhanced in the postsympathectomy patient.

If progressive renal impairment becomes evident consider withholding or discontinuing diuretic therapy.

Thiazides have been shown to increase the urinary excretion of magnesium; this may result in hypomagnesemia.

Thiazides may decrease urinary calcium excretion. Thiazides may cause intermittent and slight elevation of serum calcium in the absence of known disorders of calcium metabolism. Marked hypercalcemia may be evidence of hidden hyperparathyroidism. Thiazides should be discontinued before carrying out tests for parathyroid function.

Increases in cholesterol and triglyceride levels may be associated with thiazide diuretic therapy.

Information for Patients

Angioedema: Angioedema, including laryngeal edema, may occur at any time during treatment with angiotensin-converting enzyme inhibitors, including ZESTORETIC. Patients should be so advised and told to report immediately any signs or symptoms suggesting angioedema (swelling of face, extremities, eyes, lips, tongue, difficulty in swallowing or breathing) and to take no more drug until they have consulted with the prescribing physician.

Symptomatic Hypotension: Patients should be cautioned to report lightheadedness especially during the first few days of therapy. If actual syncope occurs, the patients should be told to discontinue the drug until they have consulted with the prescribing physician.

All patients should be cautioned that excessive perspiration and dehydration may lead to an excessive fall in blood pressure because of reduction in fluid volume. Other causes of volume depletion such as vomiting or diarrhea may also lead to a fall in blood pressure; patients should be advised to consult with their physician.

Hyperkalemia: Patients should be told not to use salt substitutes containing potassium without consulting their physician.

Leukopenia/Neutropenia: Patients should be told to report promptly any indication of infection (eg, sore throat, fever) which may be a sign of leukopenia/neutropenia.

Pregnancy: Female patients of childbearing age should be told about the consequences of second- and third-trimester exposure to ACE inhibitors, and they should also be told that these consequences do not appear to have resulted from intrauterine ACE-inhibitor exposure that has been limited to the first trimester. These patients should be asked to report pregnancies to their physicians as soon as possible.

NOTE: As with many other drugs, certain advice to patients being treated with ZESTORETIC is warranted. This

Continued on next page

Zestoretic—Cont.

information is intended to aid in the safe and effective use of this medication. It is not a disclosure of all possible adverse or intended effects.

Drug Interactions

Lisinopril

Hypotension—Patients on Diuretic Therapy: Patients on diuretics and especially those in whom diuretic therapy was recently instituted, may occasionally experience an excessive reduction of blood pressure after initiation of therapy with lisinopril. The possibility of hypotensive effects with lisinopril can be minimized by either discontinuing the diuretic or increasing the salt intake prior to initiation of treatment with lisinopril. If it is necessary to continue the diuretic, initiate therapy with lisinopril at a dose of 5 mg daily, and provide close medical supervision after the initial dose for at least two hours and until blood pressure has stabilized for at least an additional hour. (See WARNINGS, and DOSAGE AND ADMINISTRATION.) When a diuretic is added to the therapy of a patient receiving lisinopril, an additional antihypertensive effect is usually observed. (See DOSAGE AND ADMINISTRATION.)

Indomethacin: In a study in 36 patients with mild to moderate hypertension where the antihypertensive effects of lisinopril alone were compared to lisinopril given concomitantly with indomethacin, the use of indomethacin was associated with a reduced effect, although the difference between the two regimens was not significant.

Other Agents: Lisinopril has been used concomitantly with nitrates and/or digoxin without evidence of clinically significant adverse interactions. No meaningful clinically important pharmacokinetic interactions occurred when lisinopril was used concomitantly with propranolol, digoxin, or hydrochlorothiazide. The presence of food in the stomach does not alter the bioavailability of lisinopril.

Agents Increasing Serum Potassium: Lisinopril attenuates potassium loss caused by thiazide-type diuretics. Use of linisopril with potassium-sparing diuretics (eg, spironolactone, triameterene, or amiloride), potassium supplements, or potassium-containing salt substitutes may lead to significant increases in serum potassium. Therefore, if concomitant use of these agents is indicated, because of demonstrated hypokalemia, they should be used with caution and with frequent monitoring of serum potassium.

Lithium: Lithium toxicity has been reported in patients receiving lithium concomitantly with drugs which cause elimination of sodium, including ACE inhibitors. Lithium toxicity was usually reversible upon discontinuation of lithium and the ACE inhibitor. It is recommended that serum lithium levels be monitored frequently if lisinopril is administered concomitantly with lithium.

Hydrochlorothiazide

When administered concurrently the following drugs may interact with thiazide diuretics.

Alcohol, barbiturates, or narcotics—potentiation of orthostatic hypotension may occur.

Antidiabetic drugs (oral agents and insulin)—dosage adjustment of the antidiabetic drug may be required.

Other antihypertensive drugs—additive effect or potentiation.

Cholestyramine and colestipol resins—Absorption of hydrochlorothiazide is impaired in the presence of anionic exchange resins. Single doses of either cholestyramine or colestipol resins bind the hydrochlorothiazide and reduce its absorption from the gastrointestinal tract by up to 85 and 43 percent, respectively.

Corticosteroids, ACTH—intensified electrolyte depletion, particularly hypokalemia.

Pressor amines (eg, norepinephrine)—possible decreased response to pressor amines but not sufficient to preclude their use.

Skeletal muscle relaxants, nondepolarizing (eg, tubocurarine)—possible increased responsiveness to the muscle relaxant.

Lithium—should not generally be given with diuretics. Diuretic agents reduce the renal clearance of lithium and add a high risk of lithium toxicity. Refer to the package insert for lithium preparations before use of such preparations with ZESTORETIC.

Non-Steroidal Anti-inflammatory Drugs—In some patients, the administration of a non-steroidal anti-inflammatory agent can reduce the diuretic, natriuretic, and antihypertensive effects of loop, potassium-sparing and thiazide diuretics. Therefore, when ZESTORETIC and non-steroidal anti-inflammatory agents are used concomitantly, the patient should be observed closely to determine if the desired effect of ZESTORETIC is obtained.

Carcinogenesis, Mutagenesis, Impairment of Fertility

Lisinopril and Hydrochlorothiazide: Lisinopril in combination with hydrochlorothiazide was not mutagenic in a microbial mutagen test using *Salmonella typhimurium* (Ames test) or *Escherichia coli* with or without metabolic activation or in a forward mutation assay using Chinese hamster lung cells. Lisinopril and hydrochlorothiazide did not produce DNA single strand breaks in an *in vitro* alkaline elution rat hepatocyte assay. In addition, it did not produce increases in chromosomal aberrations in an *in vitro* test in Chinese hamster ovary cells or in an in vivo study in mouse bone marrow.

Lisinopril: There was no evidence of a tumorigenic effect when lisinopril was administered for 105 weeks to male and female rats at doses up to 90 mg/kg/day (about 56 or 9 times* the maximum daily human dose, based on body weight and body surface area, respectively). There was no evidence of carcinogenicity when lisinopril was administered for 92 weeks to (male and female) mice at doses up to 135 mg/kg/day (about 84 times* the maximum recommended daily human dose). This dose was 6.8 times the maximum human dose based on body surface area in mice.

*Calculations assume a human weight of 50 kg and human body surface area of $1.62m^2$.

Lisinopril was not mutagenic in the Ames microbial mutagen test with or without metabolic activation. It was also negative in a forward mutation assay using Chinese hamster lung cells. Lisinopril did not produce single strand DNA breaks in an *in vitro* alkaline elution rat hepatocyte assay. In addition, lisinopril did not produce increases in chromosomal aberrations in an *in vitro* test in Chinese hamster ovary cells or in an *in vivo* study in mouse bone marrow.

There were no adverse effects on reproductive performance in male and female rats treated with up to 300 mg/kg/day of lisinopril. This dose is 188 times and 30 times the maximum daily human dose based on mg/kg and mg/m^2, respectively.

Hydrochlorothiazide: Two-year feeding studies in mice and rats conducted under the auspices of the National Toxicology Program (NTP) uncovered no evidence of a carcinogenic potential of hydrochlorothiazide in female mice (at doses up to approximately 600 mk/kg/day) or in male and female rats (at doses of up to approximately 100 mg/kg/day). These doses are 150 times and 12 times for mice and 25 times and 4 times for rats the maximum human daily dose based on mg/kg and mg/m^2, respectively. The NTP, however, found equivocal evidence for hepatocarcinogenicity in male mice.

Hydrochlorothiazide was not genotoxic *in vitro* in the Ames mutagenicity assay of *Salmonella typhimurium* strains TA 98, TA 100, TA 1535, TA 1537, and TA 1538 and in the Chinese Hamster Ovary (CHO) test for chromosomal aberrations, or *in vivo* in assays using mouse germinal cell chromosomes, Chinese hamster bone marrow chromosomes, and the *Drosophila* sex-linked recessive lethal trait gene. Positive test results were obtained only in the *in vitro* CHO Sister Chromatid Exchange (clastogenicity) and in the Mouse Lymphoma Cell (mutagenicity) assays, using concentrations of hydrochlorothiazide from 43 to 1300 µg/mL, and in the *Aspergillus nidulans* nondisjunction assay at an unspecified concentration.

Hydrochlorothiazide had no adverse effects on the fertility of mice and rats of either sex in studies wherein these species were exposed, via their diet, to doses of up to 100 and 4 mg/kg, respectively, prior to conception and throughout gestation. In mice this dose is 25 times and 2 times the maximum daily human dose based on mg/kg and mg/m^2, respectively. In rats this dose is 1 times and 0.2 times the maximum daily human dose based on mg/kg and mg/m^2, respectively.

Pregnancy

Pregnancy Categories C (first trimester) and D (second and third trimesters). See WARNINGS, Pregnancy, Lisinopril, Fetal/Neonatal Morbidity and Mortality.

Nursing Mothers

It is not known whether lisinopril is excreted in human milk. However, milk of lactating rats contains radioactivity following administration of ^{14}C lisinopril. In another study, lisinopril was present in rat milk at levels similar to plasma levels in the dams. Thiazides do appear in human milk. Because of the potential for serious adverse reactions in nursing infants from ACE inhibitors and hydrochlorothiazide, a decision should be made whether to discontinue nursing and/or discontinue ZESTORETIC, taking into account the importance of the drug to the mother.

Pediatric Use

Safety and effectiveness in pediatric patients have not been established.

ADVERSE REACTIONS

ZESTORETIC has been evaluated for safety in 930 patients including 100 patients treated for 50 weeks or more.

In clinical trials with ZESTORETIC no adverse experiences peculiar to this combination drug have been observed. Adverse experiences that have occurred have been limited to those that have been previously reported with lisinopril or hydrochlorothiazide.

The most frequent clinical adverse experiences in controlled trials (including open label extension) with any combination of lisinopril and hydrochlorothiazide were: dizziness (7.5%), headache (5.2%), cough (3.9%), fatigue (3.7%) and orthostatic effects (3.2%) all of which were more common than in placebo-treated patients. Generally, adverse experiences were mild and transient in nature, but see WARNINGS regarding angioedema and excessive hypotension or syncope. Discontinuation of therapy due to adverse effects was required in 4.4% of patients principally because of dizziness, cough, fatigue and muscle cramps.

Adverse experiences occurring in greater than one percent of patients treated with lisinopril plus hydrochlorothiazide in controlled clinical trials are shown below.

Percent of Patients in Controlled Studies

	Lisinopril and Hydrochlorothiazide (n=930) Incidence	(discontinuation)	Placebo (n=207) Incidence
Dizziness	7.5	(0.8)	1.9
Headache	5.2	(0.3)	1.9
Cough	3.9	(0.6)	1.0
Fatigue	3.7	(0.4)	1.0
Orthostatic Effects	3.2	(0.1)	1.0
Diarrhea	2.5	(0.2)	2.4
Nausea	2.2	(0.1)	2.4
Upper Respiratory Infection	2.2	(0.0)	0.0
Muscle Cramps	2.0	(0.4)	0.5
Asthenia	1.8	(0.2)	1.0
Paresthesia	1.5	(0.1)	0.0
Hypotension	1.4	(0.3)	0.5
Vomiting	1.4	(0.1)	0.5
Dyspepsia	1.3	(0.0)	0.0
Rash	1.2	(0.1)	0.5
Impotence	1.2	(0.3)	0.0

Clinical adverse experiences occurring in 0.3% to 1.0% of patients in controlled trials included:

Body as a Whole: Chest pain, abdominal pain, syncope, chest discomfort, fever, trauma, virus infection. **Cardiovascular:** Palpitation, orthostatic hypotension. **Digestive:** Gastrointestinal cramps, dry mouth, constipation, heartburn. **Musculoskeletal:** Back pain, shoulder pain, knee pain, back strain, myalgia, foot pain. **Nervous/Psychiatric:** Decreased libido, vertigo, depression, somnolence. **Respiratory:** Common cold, nasal congestion, influenza, bronchitis, pharyngeal pain, dyspnea, pulmonary congestion, chronic sinusitis, allergic rhinitis, pharyngeal discomfort. **Skin:** Flushing, pruritus, skin inflammation, diaphoresis. **Special Senses:** Blurred vision, tinnitus, otalgia. **Urogenital:** Urinary tract infection.

Angioedema: Angioedema of the face, extremities, lips, tongue, glottis and/or larynx has been reported rarely. (See WARNINGS.)

Hypotension: In clinical trials, adverse effects relating to hypotension occurred as follows: hypotension (1.4%), orthostatic hypotension (0.5%), other orthostatic effects (3.2%). In addition syncope occurred in 0.8% of patients. (See WARNINGS.)

Cough: See PRECAUTIONS—Cough.

Clinical Laboratory Test Findings

Serum Electrolytes: (See PRECAUTIONS.)

Creatinine, Blood Urea Nitrogen: Minor reversible increases in blood urea nitrogen and serum creatinine were observed in patients with essential hypertension treated with ZESTORETIC. More marked increases have also been reported and were more likely to occur in patients with renal artery stenosis. (See PRECAUTIONS.)

Serum Uric Acid, Glucose, Magnesium, Cholesterol, Triglycerides and Calcium: (See PRECAUTIONS).

Hemoglobin and Hematocrit: Small decreases in hemoglobin and hematocrit (mean decreases of approximately 0.5 g% and 1.5 vol%, respectively) occurred frequently in hypertensive patients treated with ZESTORETIC but were rarely of clinical importance unless another cause of anemia coexisted. In clinical trials, 0.4% of patients discontinued therapy due to anemia.

Liver Function Tests: Rarely, elevations of liver enzymes and/or serum bilirubin have occurred. (See WARNINGS, Hepatic Failure.)

Other adverse reactions that have been reported with individual components are listed below:

Lisinopril—In clinical trials adverse reactions which occurred with lisinopril were also seen with ZESTORETIC. In addition, and since lisinopril has been marketed, the following adverse reactions have been reported with lisinopril and should be considered potential adverse reactions for ZESTORETIC: **Body as a Whole:** Anaphylactoid reactions (see WARNINGS, Anaphylactoid Reactions During Membrane Exposure), malaise, edema, facial edema, pain, pelvic pain, flank pain, chills; **Cardiovascular:** Cardiac arrest, myocardial infarction or cerebrovascular accident, possibly secondary to excessive hypotension in high risk patients (see WARNINGS, Hypotension), pulmonary embolism and infarction, worsening of heart failure, arrhythmias (including tachycardia, ventricular tachycardia, atrial tachycardia, atrial fibrillation, bradycardia, and premature ventricular contractions), angina pectoris, transient ischemic attacks, paroxysmal nocturnal dyspnea, decreased blood pressure, peripheral edema, vasculitis; **Digestive:** Pancreatitis, hepatitis (hepatocellular or cholestatic jaundice) (see WARNINGS, Hepatic Failure), gastritis, anorexia, flatulence, increased salivation; **Endocrine:** Diabetes mellitus; **Hematologic:** Rare cases of bone marrow depression, hemolytic anemia, leukopenia/Neutropenia, and thrombocytopenia have been reported in which a causal relationship to lisinopril can not be excluded; **Metabolic:** Gout, weight loss, dehydration, fluid overload, weight gain; **Musculoskeletal:** Arthritis, arthralgia, neck pain, hip pain, joint pain, leg pain, arm pain, lumbago; **Nervous System/Psychiatric:** Ataxia, memory impairment, tremor, insomnia, stroke, nervousness, confusion, peripheral neuropathy (eg, paresthesia, dysesthesia), spasm, hypersomnia, irritability; **Respiratory:** Malignant lung neoplasms, hemoptysis, pulmonary edema, pulmonary infiltrates, bronchospasm, asthma, pleural effusion, pneumonia, eosinophilic pneumonitis, wheezing, orthopnea, painful respiration, epistaxis, laryngitis, sinusitis, pharyngitis, rhinitis, rhinorrhea, chest sound abnormalities; **Skin:** Urticaria, alopecia, herpes zoster, photosensitivity, skin lesions, skin infections, pemphigus, erythema, rare cases of other severe skin reactions, including toxic epidermal necrolysis and Stevens-Johnson syndrome (causal relationship has not been established); **Special Senses:** Visual loss, diplopia, photophobia, taste alteration; **Urogenital:** Acute renal failure, oliguria, anuria, uremia, progressive azotemia, renal dysfunction (see PRECAUTIONS and DOSAGE AND ADMINISTRATION), pyelonephritis, dysuria, breast pain.

Miscellaneous: A symptom complex has been reported which may include a positive ANA, an elevated erythrocyte sedimentation rate, arthralgia/arthritis, myalgia, fever, vasculitis, eosinophilia and leukocytosis. Rash, photosensitivity or other dermatological manifestations may occur alone or in combination with these symptoms.

Fetal/Neonatal Morbidity and Mortality

See WARNINGS—Pregnancy, Lisinopril, Fetal/Neonatal Morbidity and Mortality.

Hydrochlorothiazide—Body as a Whole: Weakness; **Digestive:** Anorexia, gastric irritation, cramping, jaundice (intrahepatic cholestatic jaundice (See WARNINGS, Hepatic Failure), pancreatitis, sialoadenitis, constipation; **Hematologic:** Leukopenia, agranulocytosis, thrombocytopenia, aplastic anemia, hemolytic anemia; **Musculoskeletal:** Muscle spasm; **Nervous System/Psychiatric:** Restlessness; **Renal:** Renal failure, renal dysfunction, interstitial nephritis (see WARNINGS); **Skin:** Erythema multiforme including Stevens-Johnson syndrome, exfoliative dermatitis including toxic epidermal necrolysis, alopecia; **Special Senses:** Xanthopsia; **Hypersensitivity:** Purpura, photosensitivity, urticaria, necrotizing angiitis (vasculitis and cutaneous vasculitis), respiratory distress including pneumonitis and pulmonary edema, anaphylactic reactions.

OVERDOSAGE

No specific information is available on the treatment of overdosage with ZESTORETIC. Treatment is symptomatic and supportive. Therapy with ZESTORETIC should be discontinued and the patient observed closely. Suggested measures include induction of emesis and/or gastric lavage, and correction of dehydration, electrolyte imbalance and hypotension by established procedures.

Lisinopril: Following a single oral dose of 20 g/kg no lethality occurred in rats and death occurred in one of 20 mice receiving the same dose. The most likely manifestation of overdosage would be hypotension, for which the usual treatment would be intravenous infusion of normal saline solution.

Lisinopril can be removed by hemodialysis.

Hydrochlorothiazide: Oral administration of a single oral dose of 10 g/kg to mice and rats was not lethal. The most common signs and symptoms observed are those caused by electrolyte depletion (hypokalemia, hypochloremia, hyponatremia) and dehydration resulting from excessive diuresis. If digitalis has also been administered, hypokalemia may accentuate cardiac arrhythmias.

DOSAGE AND ADMINISTRATION

Lisinopril monotherapy is an effective treatment of hypertension in once-daily doses of 10–80 mg, while hydrochlorothiazide monotherapy is effective in doses of 12.5–50 mg per day. In clinical trials of lisinopril/hydrochlorothiazide combination therapy using lisinopril doses of 10–80 mg and hydrochlorothiazide doses of 6.25–50 mg, the antihypertensive response rates generally increased with increasing dosing of either component.

The side effects (see WARNINGS) of lisinopril are generally rare and apparently independent of dose; those of hydrochlorothiazide are a mixture of dose-dependent phenomena (primarily hypokalemia) and dose-independent phenomena (eg, pancreatitis), the former much more common than the latter. Therapy with any combination of lisinopril and hydrochlorothiazide may be associated with either or both dose-independent or dose-dependent side effects, but addition of lisinopril in clinical trials blunted the hypokalemia normally seen with diuretics.

To minimize dose-dependent side effects, it is usually appropriate to begin combination therapy only after a patient has failed to achieve the desired effect with monotherapy.

Dose Titration Guided by Clinical Effect: A patient whose blood pressure is not adequately controlled with either lisinopril or hydrochlorothiazide monotherapy may be switched to lisinopril/HCTZ 10/12.5 or lisinopril/HCTZ 20/12.5, depending on current monotherapy dose. Further increases of either or both components should depend on clinical response with blood pressure measured at the interdosing interval to ensure that there is an adequate antihypertensive effect at that time. The hydrochlorothiazide dose should generally not be increased until 2–3 weeks have elapsed. After addition of the diuretic it may be possible to reduce the dose of lisinopril. Patients whose blood pressures are adequately controlled with 25 mg of daily hydrochlorothiazide, but who experience significant potassium loss with this regimen may achieve similar or greater blood-pressure control without electrolyte disturbance if they are switched to lisinopril/HCTZ 10/12.5.

In patients who are currently being treated with a diuretic, symptomatic hypotension occasionally may occur following the initial dose of lisinopril. The diuretic should, if possible, be discontinued for two to three days before beginning therapy with lisinopril to reduce the likelihood of hypotension. (See WARNINGS.) If the patient's blood pressure is not controlled with lisinopril alone, diuretic therapy may be resumed.

If the diuretic cannot be discontinued, an initial dose of 5 mg of lisinopril should be used under medical supervision for at least two hours and until blood pressure has stabilized for at least an additional hour. (See WARNINGS and PRECAUTIONS, Drug Interactions.)

Concomitant administration of ZESTORETIC with potassium supplements, potassium salt substitutes or potassium-sparing diuretics may lead to increases of serum potassium. (See PRECAUTIONS.)

Replacement Therapy: The combination may be substituted for the titrated individual components.

Use in Elderly: In general, blood pressure response and adverse experiences were similar in younger and older patients given ZESTORETIC. However, in a multiple dose pharmacokinetic study in elderly versus young patients using the lisinopril/hydrochlorothiazide combination, area under the plasma concentration time curve (AUC) increased approximately 120% for lisinopril and approximately 80% for hydrochlorothiazide in older patients. Therefore, dosage adjustments in elderly patients should be made with particular caution.

Use in Renal Impairment: Regimens of therapy with lisinopril/HCTZ need not take account of renal function as long as the patient's creatinine clearance is >30 mL/min/1.7m^2 (serum creatinine roughly ≤3 mg/dL or 265 μmol/L). In patients with more severe renal impairment, loop diuretics are preferred to thiazides, so lisinopril/HCTZ is not recommended (see WARNINGS, Anaphylactoid Reactions During Membrane Exposure).

HOW SUPPLIED

ZESTORETIC 10–12.5 Tablets (NDC 0310-0141) Peach, round, biconvex, uncoated tablets identified with "141" debossed on one side and "ZESTORETIC" on the other side are supplied in bottles of 100 tablets.

ZESTORETIC 20–12.5 Tablets (NDC 0310-0142) White, round, biconvex, uncoated tablets identified with "142" debossed on one side and "ZESTORETIC" on the other side are supplied in bottles of 100 tablets.

ZESTORETIC 20–25 Tablets (NDC 0310-0145) Peach, round, biconvex, uncoated tablets identified with "145" debossed on one side and "ZESTORETIC" on the other side are supplied in bottles of 100 tablets.

Store at controlled room temperature, 20–25°C (68–77°F) [see USP]. Protect from excessive light and humidity.

¶Registered trademark of Hospal Ltd.

All other trademarks are the property of the AstraZeneca Group.

Manufactured for:
AstraZeneca Pharmaceuticals LP
Wilmington, DE 19850
By: IPR Pharmaceuticals, Inc.
Carolina, Puerto Rico 00984
Rev Q 03/00 PCC 660003
SIC 64157-00

Shown in Product Identification Guide, page 306

ONCE-DAILY ZESTRIL® (LISINOPRIL) ℞

USE IN PREGNANCY

When used in pregnancy during the second and third trimesters, ACE inhibitors can cause injury and even death to the developing fetus. When pregnancy is detected, ZESTRIL should be discontinued as soon as possible. See WARNINGS, Fetal/Neonatal Morbidity and Mortality.

DESCRIPTION

Lisinopril is an oral long-acting angiotensin converting enzyme inhibitor. Lisinopril, a synthetic peptide derivative, is chemically described as (S)-1-[N^2-(1-carboxy-3-phenylpropyl)-L-lysyl]-L-proline dihydrate. Its empirical formula is $C_{21}H_{31}N_3O_5 \bullet 2H_2O$ and its structural formula is:

Lisinopril is a white to off-white, crystalline powder, with a molecular weight of 441.53. It is soluble in water and sparingly soluble in methanol and practically insoluble in ethanol.

ZESTRIL is supplied as 2.5 mg, 5 mg, 10 mg, 20 mg, 30 mg and 40 mg tablets for oral administration.

Inactive Ingredients: 2.5 mg tablets—calcium phosphate, magnesium stearate, mannitol, starch.

5, 10, 20 and 30 mg tablets—calcium phosphate, magnesium stearate, mannitol, red ferric oxide, starch.

40 mg tablets—calcium phosphate, magnesium stearate, mannitol, starch, yellow ferric oxide.

CLINICAL PHARMACOLOGY

Mechanism of Action: Lisinopril inhibits angiotensin converting enzyme (ACE) in human subjects and animals. ACE is a peptidyl dipeptidase that catalyzes the conversion of angiotensin I to the vasoconstrictor substance, angiotensin II. Angiotensin II also stimulates aldosterone secretion by the adrenal cortex. The beneficial effects of lisinopril in hypertension and heart failure appear to result primarily from suppression of the renin-angiotensin-aldosterone system. Inhibition of ACE results in decreased plasma angiotensin II which leads to decreased vasopressor activity and to decreased aldosterone secretion. The latter decrease may result in a small increase of serum potassium. In hypertensive patients with normal renal function treated with ZESTRIL alone for up to 24 weeks, the mean increase in serum potassium was approximately 0.1 mEq/L; however, approximately 15% of patients had increases greater than 0.5 mEq/L and approximately 6% had a decrease greater than 0.5 mEq/L. In the same study, patients treated with ZESTRIL and hydrochlorothiazide for up to 24 weeks had a mean decrease in serum potassium of 0.1 mEq/L; approximately 4% of patients had increases greater than 0.5 mEq/L and approximately 12% had a decrease greater than 0.5 mEq/L. (See PRECAUTIONS.) Removal of angiotensin II negative feedback on renin secretion leads to increased plasma renin activity.

ACE is identical to kininase, an enzyme that degrades bradykinin. Whether increased levels of bradykinin, a potent vasodepressor peptide, play a role in the therapeutic effects of ZESTRIL remains to be elucidated.

While the mechanism through which ZESTRIL lowers blood pressure is believed to be primarily suppression of the renin-angiotensin-aldosterone system, ZESTRIL is antihypertensive even in patients with low-renin hypertension. Although ZESTRIL was antihypertensive in all races studied, black hypertensive patients (usually a low-renin hypertensive population) had a smaller average response to monotherapy than nonblack patients.

Concomitant administration of ZESTRIL and hydrochlorothiazide further reduced blood pressure in black and nonblack patients and any racial differences in blood pressure response were no longer evident.

Pharmacokinetics and Metabolism: Following oral administration of ZESTRIL, peak serum concentrations of lisinopril occur within about 7 hours, although there was a trend to a small delay in time taken to reach peak serum concentrations in acute myocardial infarction patients. Declining serum concentrations exhibit a prolonged terminal phase which does not contribute to drug accumulation. This terminal phase probably represents saturable binding to ACE and is not proportional to dose.

Lisinopril does not appear to be bound to other serum proteins. Lisinopril does not undergo metabolism and is excreted unchanged entirely in the urine. Based on urinary recovery, the mean extent of absorption of lisinopril is approximately 25%, with large intersubject variability (6%–60%) at all doses tested (5–80 mg). Lisinopril absorption is not influenced by the presence of food in the gastrointestinal tract. The absolute bioavailability of lisinopril is reduced to 16% in patients with stable NYHA Class II-IV congestive heart failure, and the volume of distribution appears to be slightly smaller than that in normal subjects. The oral bioavailability of lisinopril in patients with acute myocardial infarction is similar to that in healthy volunteers.

Upon multiple dosing, lisinopril exhibits an effective half-life of accumulation of 12 hours.

Impaired renal function decreases elimination of lisinopril, which is excreted principally through the kidneys, but this decrease becomes clinically important only when the glomerular filtration rate is below 30 mL/min. Above this glomerular filtration rate, the elimination half-life is little changed. With greater impairment, however, peak and trough lisinopril levels increase, time to peak concentration increases and time to attain steady state is prolonged. Older patients, on average, have (approximately doubled) higher blood levels and the area under the plasma concentration time curve (AUC) than younger patients. (See DOSAGE AND ADMINISTRATION.) Lisinopril can be removed by hemodialysis.

Studies in rats indicate that lisinopril crosses the blood-brain barrier poorly. Multiple doses of lisinopril in rats do not result in accumulation in any tissues. Milk of lactating rats contains radioactivity following administration of ^{14}C lisinopril. By whole body autoradiography, radioactivity was found in the placenta following administration of labeled drug to pregnant rats, but none was found in the fetuses.

Pharmacodynamics and Clinical Effects

Hypertension: Administration of ZESTRIL to patients with hypertension results in a reduction of both supine and standing blood pressure to about the same extent with no compensatory tachycardia. Symptomatic postural hypotension is usually not observed although it can occur and should be anticipated in volume and/or salt-depleted patients. (See WARNINGS.) When given together with thiazide-type diuretics, the blood pressure lowering effects of the two drugs are approximately additive.

In most patients studied, onset of antihypertensive activity was seen at one hour after oral administration of an individual dose of ZESTRIL, with peak reduction of blood pressure achieved by 6 hours. Although an antihypertensive effect was observed 24 hours after dosing with recommended

Continued on next page

Zestril—Cont.

single daily doses, the effect was more consistent and the mean effect was considerably larger in some studies with doses of 20 mg or more than with lower doses. However, at all doses studied, the mean antihypertensive effect was substantially smaller 24 hours after dosing than it was 6 hours after dosing.

In some patients achievement of optimal blood pressure reduction may require two to four weeks of therapy.

The antihypertensive effects of ZESTRIL are maintained during long-term therapy. Abrupt withdrawal of ZESTRIL has not been associated with a rapid increase in blood pressure, or a significant increase in blood pressure compared to pretreatment levels.

Two dose-response studies utilizing a once daily regimen were conducted in 438 mild to moderate hypertensive patients not on a diuretic. Blood pressure was measured 24 hours after dosing. An antihypertensive effect of ZESTRIL was seen with 5 mg in some patients. However, in both studies blood pressure reduction occurred sooner and was greater in patients treated with 10, 20 or 80 mg of ZESTRIL. In controlled clinical studies, ZESTRIL 20–80 mg has been compared in patients with mild to moderate hypertension to hydrochlorothiazide 12.5–50 mg and with atenolol 50–200 mg; and in patients with moderate to severe hypertension to metoprolol 100–200 mg. It was superior to hydrochlorothiazide in effects on systolic and diastolic pressure in a population that was 3/4 Caucasian. ZESTRIL was approximately equivalent to atenolol and metoprolol in effects on diastolic blood pressure, and had somewhat greater effects on systolic blood pressure.

ZESTRIL had similar effectiveness and adverse effects in younger and older (> 65 years) patients. It was less effective in blacks than in Caucasians.

In hemodynamic studies in patients with essential hypertension, blood pressure reduction was accompanied by a reduction in peripheral arterial resistance with little or no change in cardiac output and in heart rate. In a study in nine hypertensive patients, following administration of ZESTRIL, there was an increase in mean renal blood flow that was not significant. Data from several small studies are inconsistent with respect to the effect of lisinopril on glomerular filtration rate in hypertensive patients with normal renal function, but suggest that changes, if any, are not large.

In patients with renovascular hypertension ZESTRIL has been shown to be well tolerated and effective in controlling blood pressure. (See PRECAUTIONS.)

Heart Failure: During baseline-controlled clinical trials, in patients receiving digitalis and diuretics, single doses of ZESTRIL resulted in decreases in pulmonary capillary wedge pressure, systemic vascular resistance and blood pressure accompanied by an increase in cardiac output and no change in heart rate.

In two placebo controlled, 12-week clinical studies, using doses of ZESTRIL up to 20 mg, ZESTRIL as adjunctive therapy to digitalis and diuretics improved the following signs and symptoms due to congestive heart failure: edema, rales, paroxysmal nocturnal dyspnea and jugular venous distention. In one of the studies, beneficial response was also noted for: orthopnea, presence of third heart sound and the number of patients classified as NYHA Class III and IV. Exercise tolerance was also improved in this study. The once daily dosing for the treatment of congestive heart failure was the only dosage regimen used during clinical trial development and was determined by the measurement of hemodynamic response. A large (over 3000 patients) survival study, the ATLAS Trial, comparing 2.5 and 35 mg of lisinopril in patients with heart failure, showed that the higher dose of lisinopril had outcomes at least as favorable as the lower dose.

Acute Myocardial Infarction: The Gruppo Italiano per lo Studio della Sopravvienza nell'Infarto Miocardico (GISSI-3) study was a multicenter, controlled, randomized, unblinded clinical trial conducted in 19,394 patients with acute myocardial infarction admitted to a coronary care unit. It was designed to examine the effects of short-term (6 week) treatment with lisinopril, nitrates, their combination, or no therapy on short-term (6 week) mortality and on longer-term death and markedly impaired cardiac function. Patients presenting within 24 hours of the onset of symptoms who were hemodynamically stable were randomized, in a 2 × 2 factorial design, to six weeks of either 1) ZESTRIL alone (n=4841), 2) nitrates alone (n=4869), 3) ZESTRIL plus nitrates (n=4841), or 4) open control (n=4843). All patients received routine therapies, including thrombolytics (72%), aspirin (84%), and a beta-blocker (31%), as appropriate, normally utilized in acute myocardial infarction (MI) patients.

The protocol excluded patients with hypotension (systolic blood pressure ≤ 100 mmHg), severe heart failure, cardiogenic shock, and renal dysfunction (serum creatinine >2 mg/dL and/or proteinuria > 500 mg/24 h). Doses of ZESTRIL were adjusted as necessary according to protocol (see DOSAGE AND ADMINISTRATION).

Study treatment was withdrawn at six weeks except where clinical conditions indicated continuation of treatment.

The primary outcomes of the trial were the overall mortality at 6 weeks and a combined endpoint at 6 months after the myocardial infarction, consisting of the number of patients who died, had late (day 4) clinical congestive heart failure, or had extensive left ventricular damage defined as ejection fraction ≤ 35% or an akinetic-dyskinetic [A-D] score ≥ 45%.

Patients receiving ZESTRIL (n=9646), alone or with nitrates, had an 11% lower risk of death (2p [two-tailed] = 0.04) compared to patients receiving no ZESTRIL (n=9672) (6.4% vs. 7.2%, respectively) at six weeks. Although patients randomized to receive ZESTRIL for up to six weeks also fared numerically better on the combined end-point at 6 months, the open nature of the assessment of heart failure, substantial loss to follow-up echocardiography, and substantial excess use of lisinopril between 6 weeks and 6 months in the group randomized to 6 weeks of lisinopril, preclude any conclusion about this endpoint.

Patients with acute myocardial infarction, treated with ZESTRIL, had a higher (9.0% versus 3.7%) incidence of persistent hypotension (systolic blood pressure < 90 mmHg for more than 1 hour) and renal dysfunction (2.4% versus 1.1%) in-hospital and at six weeks (increasing creatinine concentration to over 3 mg/dL or a doubling or more of the baseline serum creatinine concentration). See ADVERSE REACTIONS—Acute Myocardial Infarction.

INDICATIONS AND USAGE

Hypertension: ZESTRIL is indicated for the treatment of hypertension. It may be used alone as initial therapy or concomitantly with other classes of antihypertensive agents.

Heart Failure: ZESTRIL is indicated as adjunctive therapy in the management of heart failure in patients who are not responding adequately to diuretics and digitalis.

Acute Myocardial Infarction: ZESTRIL is indicated for the treatment of hemodynamically stable patients within 24 hours of acute myocardial infarction, to improve survival. Patients should receive, as appropriate, the standard recommended treatments such as thrombolytics, aspirin and beta-blockers.

In using ZESTRIL, consideration should be given to the fact that another angiotensin converting enzyme inhibitor, captopril, has caused agranulocytosis, particularly in patients with renal impairment or collagen vascular disease, and that available data are insufficient to show that ZESTRIL does not have a similar risk. (See WARNINGS.)

In considering the use of ZESTRIL, it should be noted that in controlled trials ACE inhibitors have an effect on blood pressure that is less in black patients than in nonblacks. In addition, ACE inhibitors have been associated with a higher rate of angioedema in black than in nonblack patients (see WARNINGS, Angioedema).

CONTRAINDICATIONS

ZESTRIL is contraindicated in patients who are hypersensitive to this product and in patients with a history of angioedema related to previous treatment with an angiotensin converting enzyme inhibitor.

WARNINGS

Anaphylactoid and Possibly Related Reactions: Presumably because angiotensin-converting enzyme inhibitors affect the metabolism of eicosanoids and polypeptides, including endogenous bradykinin, patients receiving ACE inhibitors (including ZESTRIL) may be subject to a variety of adverse reactions, some of them serious.

Angioedema: Angioedema of the face, extremities, lips, tongue, glottis and/or larynx has been reported in patients treated with angiotensin converting enzyme inhibitors, including ZESTRIL. This may occur at any time during treatment. ACE inhibitors have been associated with a higher rate of angioedema in black than in nonblack patients. ZESTRIL should be promptly discontinued and appropriate therapy and monitoring should be provided until complete and sustained resolution of signs and symptoms has occurred. In instances where swelling has been confined to the face and lips the condition has generally resolved without treatment, although antihistamines have been useful in relieving symptoms. Angioedema associated with laryngeal edema may be fatal. **Where there is involvement of the tongue, glottis or larynx, likely to cause airway obstruction, appropriate therapy, e.g., subcutaneous epinephrine solution 1:1000 (0.3 mL to 0.5 mL) and/or measures necessary to ensure a patent airway should be promptly provided. (See ADVERSE REACTIONS.)**

Patients with a history of angioedema unrelated to ACE inhibitor therapy may be at increased risk of angioedema while receiving an ACE inhibitor. (See also INDICATIONS AND USAGE and CONTRAINDICATIONS).

Anaphylactoid Reactions During Desensitization: Two patients undergoing desensitizing treatment with hymenoptera venom while receiving ACE inhibitors sustained life-threatening anaphylactoid reactions. In the same patients, these reactions were avoided when ACE inhibitors were temporarily withheld, but they reappeared upon inadvertent rechallenge.

Anaphylactoid Reactions During Membrane Exposure: Sudden and potentially life-threatening anaphylactoid reactions have been reported in some patients dialyzed with high-flux membranes (e.g., AN69¶) and treated concomitantly with an ACE inhibitor. In such patients, dialysis must be stopped immediately, and aggressive therapy for anaphylactoid reactions be initiated. Symptoms have not been relieved by antihistamines in these situations. In these patients, consideration should be given to using a different type of dialysis membrane or a different class of antihypertensive agent. Anaphylactoid reactions have also been reported in patients undergoing low-density lipoprotein apheresis with dextran sulfate absorption.

Hypotension: Excessive hypotension is rare in patients with uncomplicated hypertension treated with ZESTRIL alone.

Patients with heart failure given ZESTRIL commonly have some reduction in blood pressure, with peak blood pressure reduction occurring 6 to 8 hours post dose. Evidence from the two-dose ATLAS trial suggested that incidence of hypotension may increase with dose of lisinopril in heart failure patients. Discontinuation of therapy because of continuing symptomatic hypotension usually is not necessary when dosing instructions are followed; caution should be observed when initiating therapy. (See DOSAGE AND ADMINISTRATION.)

Patients at risk of excessive hypotension, sometimes associated with oliguria and/or progressive azotemia, and rarely with acute renal failure and/or death, include those with the following conditions or characteristics: heart failure with systolic blood pressure below 100 mmHg, hyponatremia, high dose diuretic therapy, recent intensive diuresis or increase in diuretic dose, renal dialysis, or severe volume and/or salt depletion of any etiology. It may be advisable to eliminate the diuretic (except in patients with heart failure), reduce the diuretic dose or increase salt intake cautiously before initiating therapy with ZESTRIL in patients at risk for excessive hypotension who are able to tolerate such adjustments. (See PRECAUTIONS, Drug Interactions and ADVERSE REACTIONS.)

Patients with acute myocardial infarction in the GISSI-3 trial had a higher (9.0% versus 3.7%) incidence of persistent hypotension (systolic blood pressure < 90 mmHg for more than 1 hour) when treated with ZESTRIL. Treatment with ZESTRIL must not be initiated in acute myocardial infarction patients at risk of further serious hemodynamic deterioration after treatment with a vasodilator (e.g., systolic blood pressure at 100 mmHg or lower) or cardiogenic shock.

In patients at risk of excessive hypotension, therapy should be started under very close medical supervision and such patients should be followed closely for the first two weeks of treatment and whenever the dose of ZESTRIL and/or diuretic is increased. Similar considerations may apply to patients with ischemic heart or cerebrovascular disease, or in patients with acute myocardial infarction, in whom an excessive fall in blood pressure could result in a myocardial infarction or cerebrovascular accident.

If excessive hypotension occurs, the patient should be placed in the supine position and, if necessary, receive an intravenous infusion of normal saline. A transient hypotensive response is not a contraindication to further doses of ZESTRIL which usually can be given without difficulty once the blood pressure has stabilized. If symptomatic hypotension develops, a dose reduction or discontinuation of ZESTRIL or concomitant diuretic may be necessary.

Leukopenia/Neutropenia/Agranulocytosis: Another angiotensin converting enzyme inhibitor, captopril, has been shown to cause agranulocytosis and bone marrow depression, rarely in uncomplicated patients but more frequently in patients with renal impairment especially if they also have a collagen vascular disease. Available data from clinical trials of ZESTRIL are insufficient to show that ZESTRIL does not cause agranulocytosis at similar rates. Marketing experience has revealed rare cases of leukopenia/neutropenia and bone marrow depression in which a causal relationship to lisinopril cannot be excluded. Periodic monitoring of white blood cell counts in patients with collagen vascular disease and renal disease should be considered.

Hepatic Failure: Rarely, ACE inhibitors have been associated with a syndrome that starts with cholestatic jaundice and progresses to fulminant hepatic necrosis and (sometimes) death. The mechanism of this syndrome is not understood. Patients receiving ACE inhibitors who develop jaundice or marked elevations of hepatic enzymes should discontinue the ACE inhibitor and receive appropriate medical follow-up.

Fetal/Neonatal Morbidity and Mortality: ACE inhibitors can cause fetal and neonatal morbidity and death when administered to pregnant women. Several dozen cases have been reported in the world literature. When pregnancy is detected, ACE inhibitors should be discontinued as soon as possible.

The use of ACE inhibitors during the second and third trimesters of pregnancy has been associated with fetal and neonatal injury, including hypotension, neonatal skull hypoplasia, anuria, reversible or irreversible renal failure, and death. Oligohydramnios has also been reported, presumably resulting from decreased fetal renal function; oligohydramnios in this setting has been associated with fetal limb contractures, craniofacial deformation, and hypoplastic lung development. Prematurity, intrauterine growth retardation, and patent ductus arteriosus have also been reported, although it is not clear whether these occurrences were due to the ACE-inhibitor exposure.

These adverse effects do not appear to have resulted from intrauterine ACE-inhibitor exposure that has been limited to the first trimester. Mothers whose embryos and fetuses are exposed to ACE inhibitors only during the first trimester should be so informed. Nonetheless, when patients become pregnant, physicians should make every effort to discontinue the use of ZESTRIL as soon as possible.

Rarely (probably less often than once in every thousand pregnancies), no alternative to ACE inhibitors will be found. In these rare cases, the mothers should be apprised of the potential hazards to their fetuses, and serial ultrasound examinations should be performed to assess the intraamniotic environment.

If oligohydramnios is observed, ZESTRIL should be discontinued unless it is considered lifesaving for the mother. Contraction stress testing (CST), a nonstress test (NST), or biophysical profiling (BPP) may be appropriate, depending upon the week of pregnancy. Patients and physicians should be aware, however, that oligohydramnios may not appear until after the fetus has sustained irreversible injury.

Infants with histories of *in utero* exposure to ACE inhibitors should be closely observed for hypotension, oliguria, and hyperkalemia. If oliguria occurs, attention should be directed toward support of blood pressure and renal perfusion. Exchange transfusion or dialysis may be required as means of reversing hypotension and/or substituting for disordered renal function. Lisinopril, which crosses the placenta, has been removed from neonatal circulation by peritoneal dialysis with some clinical benefit, and theoretically may be removed by exchange transfusion, although there is no experience with the latter procedure.

No teratogenic effects of lisinopril were seen in studies of pregnant rats, mice, and rabbits. On a mg/kg basis, the doses used were up to 625 times (in mice), 188 times (in rats), and 0.6 times (in rabbits) the maximum recommended human dose.

PRECAUTIONS

General

Impaired Renal Function: As a consequence of inhibiting the renin-angiotensin-aldosterone system, changes in renal function may be anticipated in susceptible individuals. In patients with severe congestive heart failure whose renal function may depend on the activity of the renin-angiotensin-aldosterone system, treatment with angiotensin converting enzyme inhibitors, including ZESTRIL, may be associated with oliguria and/or progressive azotemia and rarely with acute renal failure and/or death.

In hypertensive patients with unilateral or bilateral renal artery stenosis, increases in blood urea nitrogen and serum creatinine may occur. Experience with another angiotensin converting enzyme inhibitor suggests that these increases are usually reversible upon discontinuation of ZESTRIL and/or diuretic therapy. In such patients, renal function should be monitored during the first few weeks of therapy. Some patients with hypertension or heart failure with no apparent pre-existing renal vascular disease have developed increases in blood urea nitrogen and serum creatinine, usually minor and transient, especially when ZESTRIL has been given concomitantly with a diuretic. This is more likely to occur in patients with pre-existing renal impairment. Dosage reduction and/or discontinuation of the diuretic and/or ZESTRIL may be required.

Patients with acute myocardial infarction in the GISSI-3 trial, treated with ZESTRIL had a higher (2.4% versus 1.1%) incidence of renal dysfunction in-hospital and at six weeks (increasing creatinine concentration to over 3 mg/dL or a doubling or more of the baseline serum creatinine concentration). In acute myocardial infarction, treatment with ZESTRIL should be initiated with caution in patients with evidence of renal dysfunction, defined as serum creatinine concentration exceeding 2 mg/dL. If renal dysfunction develops during treatment with ZESTRIL (serum creatinine concentration exceeding 3 mg/dL or a doubling from the pretreatment value) then the physician should consider withdrawal of ZESTRIL.

Evaluation of patients with hypertension, heart failure, or myocardial infarction should always include assessment of renal function. (See DOSAGE AND ADMINISTRATION.)

Hyperkalemia: In clinical trials hyperkalemia (serum potassium greater than 5.7 mEq/L) occurred in approximately 2.2% of hypertensive patients and 4.8% of patients with heart failure. In most cases these were isolated values which resolved despite continued therapy. Hyperkalemia was a cause of discontinuation of therapy in approximately 0.1% of hypertensive patients; 0.6% of patients with heart failure and 0.1% of patients with myocardial infarction. Risk factors for the development of hyperkalemia include renal insufficiency, diabetes mellitus, and the concomitant use of potassium-sparing diuretics, potassium supplements and/or potassium-containing salt substitutes, which should be used cautiously, if at all, with ZESTRIL. (See Drug Interactions.)

Cough: Presumably due to the inhibition of the degradation of endogenous bradykinin, persistent nonproductive cough has been reported with all ACE inhibitors, almost always resolving after discontinuation of therapy. ACE inhibitor-induced cough should be considered in the differential diagnosis of cough.

Surgery/Anesthesia: In patients undergoing major surgery or during anesthesia with agents that produce hypotension, ZESTRIL may block angiotensin II formation secondary to compensatory renin release. If hypotension occurs and is considered to be due to this mechanism, it can be corrected by volume expansion.

Information for Patients

Angioedema: Angioedema, including laryngeal edema, may occur at any time during treatment with angiotensin-converting enzyme inhibitors, including ZESTRIL. Patients should be so advised and told to report immediately any signs or symptoms suggesting angioedema (swelling of face, extremities, eyes, lips, tongue, difficulty in swallowing or breathing) and to take no more drug until they have consulted with the prescribing physician.

Symptomatic Hypotension: Patients should be cautioned to report lightheadedness especially during the first few days of therapy. If actual syncope occurs, the patient should be told to discontinue the drug until they have consulted with the prescribing physician.

PERCENT OF PATIENTS IN CONTROLLED STUDIES

	ZESTRIL (n=1349) Incidence (discontinuation)	ZESTRIL/ Hydrochlorothiazide (n=629) Incidence (discontinuation)	PLACEBO (n=207) Incidence (discontinuation)
Body as a Whole			
Fatigue	2.5 (0.3)	4.0 (0.5)	1.0 (0.0)
Asthenia	1.3 (0.5)	2.1 (0.2)	1.0 (0.0)
Orthostatic Effects	1.2 (0.0)	3.5 (0.2)	1.0 (0.0)
Cardiovascular			
Hypotension	1.2 (0.5)	1.6 (0.5)	0.5 (0.5)
Digestive			
Diarrhea	2.7 (0.2)	2.7 (0.3)	2.4 (0.0)
Nausea	2.0 (0.4)	2.5 (0.2)	2.4 (0.0)
Vomiting	1.1 (0.2)	1.4 (0.1)	0.5 (0.0)
Dyspepsia	0.9 (0.0)	1.9 (0.0)	0.0 (0.0)
Musculoskeletal			
Muscle Cramps	0.5 (0.0)	2.9 (0.8)	0.5 (0.0)
Nervous/Psychiatric			
Headache	5.7 (0.2)	4.5 (0.5)	1.9 (0.0)
Dizziness	5.4 (0.4)	9.2 (1.0)	1.9 (0.0)
Paresthesia	0.8 (0.1)	2.1 (0.2)	0.0 (0.0)
Decreased Libido	0.4 (0.1)	1.3 (0.1)	0.0 (0.0)
Vertigo	0.2 (0.1)	1.1 (0.2)	0.0 (0.0)
Respiratory			
Cough	3.5 (0.7)	4.6 (0.8)	1.0 (0.0)
Upper Respiratory Infection	2.1 (0.1)	2.7 (0.1)	0.0 (0.0)
Common Cold	1.1 (0.1)	1.3 (0.1)	0.0 (0.0)
Nasal Congestion	0.4 (0.1)	1.3 (0.1)	0.0 (0.0)
Influenza	0.3 (0.1)	1.1 (0.1)	0.0 (0.0)
Skin			
Rash	1.3 (0.4)	1.6 (0.2)	0.5 (0.5)
Urogenital			
Impotence	1.0 (0.4)	1.6 (0.5)	0.0 (0.0)

All patients should be cautioned that excessive perspiration and dehydration may lead to an excessive fall in blood pressure because of reduction in fluid volume. Other causes of volume depletion such as vomiting or diarrhea may also lead to a fall in blood pressure; patients should be advised to consult with their physician.

Hyperkalemia: Patients should be told not to use salt substitutes containing potassium without consulting their physician.

Leukopenia/Neutropenia: Patients should be told to report promptly any indication of infection (e.g., sore throat, fever) which may be a sign of leukopenia/neutropenia.

Pregnancy: Female patients of childbearing age should be told about the consequences of second- and third-trimester exposure to ACE inhibitors, and they should also be told that these consequences do not appear to have resulted from intrauterine ACE inhibitor exposure that has been limited to the first trimester. These patients should be asked to report pregnancies to their physicians as soon as possible.

NOTE: As with many other drugs, certain advice to patients being treated with ZESTRIL is warranted. This information is intended to aid in the safe and effective use of this medication. It is not a disclosure of all possible adverse or intended effects.

Drug Interactions

Hypotension—Patients on Diuretic Therapy: Patients on diuretics and especially those in whom diuretic therapy was recently instituted, may occasionally experience an excessive reduction of blood pressure after initiation of therapy with ZESTRIL. The possibility of hypotensive effects with ZESTRIL can be minimized by either discontinuing the diuretic or increasing the salt intake prior to initiation of treatment with ZESTRIL. If it is necessary to continue the diuretic, initiate therapy with ZESTRIL at a dose of 5 mg daily, and provide close medical supervision after the initial dose until blood pressure has stabilized. (See WARNINGS, and DOSAGE AND ADMINISTRATION.) When a diuretic is added to the therapy of a patient receiving ZESTRIL, an additional antihypertensive effect is usually observed. Studies with ACE inhibitors in combination with diuretics indicate that the dose of the ACE inhibitor can be reduced when it is given with a diuretic. (See DOSAGE AND ADMINISTRATION.)

Indomethacin: In a study in 36 patients with mild to moderate hypertension where the antihypertensive effects of ZESTRIL alone were compared to ZESTRIL given concomitantly with indomethacin, the use of indomethacin was associated with a reduced effect, although the difference between the two regimens was not significant.

Other Agents: ZESTRIL has been used concomitantly with nitrates and/or digoxin without evidence of clinically significant adverse interactions. This included post myocardial infarction patients who were receiving intravenous or transdermal nitroglycerin. No clinically important pharmacokinetic interactions occurred when ZESTRIL was used concomitantly with propranolol or hydrochlorothiazide. The presence of food in the stomach does not alter the bioavailability of ZESTRIL.

Agents Increasing Serum Potassium: ZESTRIL attenuates potassium loss caused by thiazide-type diuretics. Use of ZESTRIL with potassium-sparing diuretics (e.g., spironolactone, triamterene or amiloride), potassium supplements, or potassium-containing salt substitutes may lead to significant increases in serum potassium. Therefore, if concomitant use of these agents is indicated because of demonstrated hypokalemia, they should be used with caution and with frequent monitoring of serum potassium. Potassium-sparing agents should generally not be used in patients with heart failure who are receiving ZESTRIL.

Lithium: Lithium toxicity has been reported in patients receiving lithium concomitantly with drugs which cause elimination of sodium, including ACE inhibitors. Lithium toxicity was usually reversible upon discontinuation of lithium and the ACE inhibitor. It is recommended that serum lithium levels be monitored frequently if ZESTRIL is administered concomitantly with lithium.

Carcinogenesis, Mutagenesis, Impairment of Fertility: There was no evidence of a tumorigenic effect when lisinopril was administered for 105 weeks to male and female rats at doses up to 90 mg/kg/day (about 56 or 9 times* the maximum recommended daily human dose, based on body weight and body surface area, respectively). There was no evidence of carcinogenicity when lisinopril was administered for 92 weeks to (male and female) mice at doses up to 135 mg/kg/day (about 84 times* the maximum recommended daily human dose). This dose was 6.8 times the maximum human dose based on body surface area in mice.

*Calculations assume a human weight of 50 kg and human body surface area of 1.62 m^2.

Lisinopril was not mutagenic in the Ames microbial mutagen test with or without metabolic activation. It was also negative in a forward mutation assay using Chinese hamster lung cells. Lisinopril did not produce single strand DNA breaks in an *in vitro* alkaline elution rat hepatocyte assay. In addition, lisinopril did not produce increases in chromosomal aberrations in an *in vitro* test in Chinese hamster ovary cells or in an *in vivo* study in mouse bone marrow.

There were no adverse effects on reproductive performance in male and female rats treated with up to 300 mg/kg/day of lisinopril. This dose is 188 times and 30 times the maximum human dose when based on mg/kg and mg/m^2, respectively.

Pregnancy

Pregnancy Categories C (first trimester) and D (second and third trimesters): See WARNINGS, Fetal/Neonatal Morbidity and Mortality.

Nursing Mothers: Milk of lactating rats contains radioactivity following administration of ^{14}C lisinopril. It is not known whether this drug is excreted in human milk. Because many drugs are excreted in human milk and because of the potential for serious adverse reactions in nursing infants from ACE inhibitors, a decision should be made whether to discontinue nursing and/or discontinue ZESTRIL, taking into account the importance of the drug to the mother.

Pediatric Use: Safety and effectiveness in pediatric patients have not been established.

ADVERSE REACTIONS

ZESTRIL has been found to be generally well tolerated in controlled clinical trials involving 1969 patients with hypertension or heart failure. For the most part, adverse experiences were mild and transient.

Hypertension: In clinical trials in patients with hypertension treated with ZESTRIL, discontinuation of therapy due to clinical adverse experiences occurred in 5.7% of patients. The overall frequency of adverse experiences could not be related to total daily dosage within the recommended therapeutic dosage range.

Continued on next page

Zestril—Cont.

For adverse experiences occurring in greater than 1% of patients with hypertension treated with ZESTRIL or ZESTRIL plus hydrochlorothiazide in controlled clinical trials, and more frequently with ZESTRIL and/or ZESTRIL plus hydrochlorothiazide than placebo, comparative incidence data are listed in the table below:
[See table at top of previous page]
Chest pain and back pain were also seen, but were more common on placebo than ZESTRIL.

Heart Failure: In patients with heart failure treated with ZESTRIL for up to four years, discontinuation of therapy due to clinical adverse experiences occurred in 11.0% of patients. In controlled studies in patients with heart failure, therapy was discontinued in 8.1% of patients treated with ZESTRIL for 12 weeks, compared to 7.7% of patients treated with placebo for 12 weeks.

The following table lists those adverse experiences which occurred in greater than 1% of patients with heart failure treated with ZESTRIL or placebo for up to 12 weeks in controlled clinical trials, and more frequently on ZESTRIL than placebo.
[See table above]

	Controlled Trials	
	ZESTRIL (n=407) Incidence (discontinuation) 12 weeks	Placebo (n=155) Incidence (discontinuation) 12 weeks
Body as a Whole		
Chest Pain	3.4 (0.2)	1.3 (0.0)
Abdominal Pain	2.2 (0.7)	1.9 (0.0)
Cardiovascular		
Hypotension	4.4 (1.7)	0.6 (0.6)
Digestive		
Diarrhea	3.7 (0.5)	1.9 (0.0)
Nervous/Psychiatric		
Dizziness	11.8 (1.2)	4.5 (1.3)
Headache	4.4 (0.2)	3.9 (0.0)
Respiratory		
Upper Respiratory Infection	1.5 (0.0)	1.3 (0.0)
Skin		
Rash	1.7 (0.5)	0.6 (0.6)

Also observed at > 1% with ZESTRIL but more frequent or as frequent on placebo than ZESTRIL in controlled trials were asthenia, angina pectoris, nausea, dyspnea, cough, and pruritus.

Worsening of heart failure, anorexia, increased salivation, muscle cramps, back pain, myalgia, depression, chest sound abnormalities, and pulmonary edema were also seen in controlled clinical trials, but were more common on placebo than ZESTRIL.

In the two-dose ATLAS trial in heart failure patients, withdrawals due to adverse events were not different between the low and high groups, either in total number of discontinuation (17-18%) or in rare specific events (<1%). The following adverse events, mostly related to ACE inhibition, were reported more commonly in the high dose group:

% of patients Events	High Dose (N=1568)	Low Dose (N=1596)
Dizziness	18.9	12.1
Hypotension	10.8	6.7
Creatinine increased	9.9	7.0
Hyperkalemia	6.4	3.5
NPN* increased	9.2	6.5
Syncope	7.0	5.1

*NPN = Non-protein nitrogen

Acute Myocardial Infarction: In the GISSI-3 trial, in patients treated with ZESTRIL for six weeks following acute myocardial infarction, discontinuation of therapy occurred in 17.6% of patients.

Patients treated with ZESTRIL had a significantly higher incidence of hypotension and renal dysfunction compared with patients not taking ZESTRIL.

In the GISSI-3 trial, hypotension (9.7%), renal dysfunction (2.0%), cough (0.5%), post infarction angina (0.3%), skin rash and generalized edema (0.01%), and angioedema (0.01%) resulted in withdrawal of treatment. In elderly patients treated with ZESTRIL, discontinuation due to renal dysfunction was 4.2%.

Other clinical adverse experiences occurring in 0.3% to 1.0% of patients with hypertension or heart failure treated with ZESTRIL in controlled clinical trials and rarer, serious, possibly drug-related events reported in uncontrolled studies or marketing experience are listed below, and within each category are in order of decreasing severity:

Body as a Whole: Anaphylactoid reactions (see WARNINGS, Anaphylactoid Reactions During Membrane Exposure), syncope, orthostatic effects, chest discomfort, pain, pelvic pain, flank pain, edema, facial edema, virus infection, fever, chills, malaise.

Cardiovascular: Cardiac arrest; myocardial infarction or cerebrovascular accident possibly secondary to excessive hypotension in high risk patients (see WARNINGS, Hypotension); pulmonary embolism and infarction, arrhythmias (including ventricular tachycardia, atrial tachycardia, atrial fibrillation, bradycardia and premature ventricular contractions), palpitations, transient ischemic attacks, paroxysmal nocturnal dyspnea, orthostatic hypotension, decreased blood pressure, peripheral edema, vasculitis.

Digestive: Pancreatitis, hepatitis (hepatocellular or cholestatic jaundice) (see WARNINGS, Hepatic Failure), vomiting, gastritis, dyspepsia, heartburn, gastrointestinal cramps, constipation, flatulence, dry mouth.

Hematologic: Rare cases of bone marrow depression, hemolytic anemia, leukopenia/neutropenia and thrombocytopenia.

Endocrine: Diabetes mellitus.

Metabolic: Weight loss, dehydration, fluid overload, gout, weight gain.

Musculoskeletal: Arthritis, arthralgia, neck pain, hip pain, low back pain, joint pain, leg pain, knee pain, shoulder pain, arm pain, lumbago.

Nervous System/Psychiatric: Stroke, ataxia, memory impairment, tremor, peripheral neuropathy (e.g., dysesthesia), spasm, paresthesia, confusion, insomnia, somnolence, hypersomnia, irritability and nervousness.

Respiratory System: Malignant lung neoplasms, hemoptysis, pulmonary infiltrates, bronchospasm, asthma, pleural effusion, pneumonia, eosinophilic pneumonitis, bronchitis, wheezing, orthopnea, painful respiration, epistaxis, laryngitis, sinusitis, pharyngeal pain, pharyngitis, rhinitis, rhinorrhea.

Skin: Urticaria, alopecia, herpes zoster, photosensitivity, skin lesions, skin infections, pemphigus, erythema, flushing, diaphoresis. Other severe skin reactions have been reported rarely, including toxic epidermal necrolysis and Stevens-Johnson syndrome; causal relationship has not been established.

Special Senses: Visual loss, diplopia, blurred vision, tinnitus, photophobia, taste alteration.

Urogenital System: Acute renal failure, oliguria, anuria, uremia, progressive azotemia, renal dysfunction, (see PRECAUTIONS and DOSAGE AND ADMINISTRATION), pyelonephritis, dysuria, urinary tract infection, breast pain.

Miscellaneous: A symptom complex has been reported which may include a positive ANA, an elevated erythrocyte sedimentation rate, arthralgia/arthritis, myalgia, fever, vasculitis, eosinophilia and leukocytosis. Rash, photosensitivity or other dermatological manifestations may occur alone or in combination with these symptoms.

ANGIOEDEMA: Angioedema has been reported in patients receiving ZESTRIL (0.1%). Angioedema associated with laryngeal edema may be fatal. If angioedema of the face, extremities, lips, tongue, glottis and/or larynx occurs, treatment with ZESTRIL should be discontinued and appropriate therapy instituted immediately. (See WARNINGS.)

HYPOTENSION: In hypertensive patients, hypotension occurred in 1.2% and syncope occurred in 0.1% of patients. Hypotension or syncope was a cause of discontinuation of therapy in 0.5% of hypertensive patients. In patients with heart failure, hypotension occurred in 5.3% and syncope occurred in 1.8% of patients. These adverse experiences were possibly dose-related (see above data from ATLAS Trial) and caused discontinuation of therapy in 1.8% of these patients in the symptomatic trials. In patients treated with ZESTRIL for six weeks after acute myocardial infarction, hypotension (systolic blood pressure ≤100 mmHg) resulted in discontinuation of therapy in 9.7% of the patients. (See WARNINGS.)

Fetal/Neonatal Morbidity and Mortality: See WARNINGS, Fetal/Neonatal Morbidity and Mortality.

Cough: See PRECAUTIONS—Cough

Clinical Laboratory Test Findings

Serum Electrolytes: Hyperkalemia (See PRECAUTIONS), hyponatremia.

Creatinine, Blood Urea Nitrogen: Minor increases in blood urea nitrogen and serum creatinine, reversible upon discontinuation of therapy, were observed in about 2.0% of patients with essential hypertension treated with ZESTRIL alone. Increases were more common in patients receiving concomitant diuretics and in patients with renal artery stenosis. (See PRECAUTIONS.) Reversible minor increases in blood urea nitrogen and serum creatinine were observed in approximately 11.6% of patients with heart failure on concomitant diuretic therapy. Frequently, these abnormalities resolved when the dosage of the diuretic was decreased.

Hemoglobin and Hematocrit: Small decreases in hemoglobin and hematocrit (mean decreases of approximately 0.4 g% and 1.3 vol%, respectively) occurred frequently in patients treated with ZESTRIL but were rarely of clinical importance in patients without some other cause of anemia. In clinical trials, less than 0.1% of patients discontinued therapy due to anemia.

Liver Function Tests: Rarely, elevations of liver enzymes and/or serum bilirubin have occurred. (See WARNINGS, Hepatic Failure.)

In hypertensive patients, 2.0% discontinued therapy due to laboratory adverse experiences, principally elevations in blood urea nitrogen (0.6%), serum creatinine (0.5%) and serum potassium (0.4%).

In the heart failure trials, 3.4% of patients discontinued therapy due to laboratory adverse experiences; 1.8% due to elevations in blood urea nitrogen and/or creatinine and 0.6% due to elevations in serum potassium.

In the myocardial infarction trial, 2.0% of patients receiving ZESTRIL discontinued therapy due to renal dysfunction (increasing creatinine concentration to over 3 mg/dL or a doubling or more of the baseline serum creatinine concentration); less than 1.0% of patients discontinued therapy due to other laboratory adverse experiences: 0.1% with hyperkalemia and less than 0.1% with hepatic enzyme alterations.

OVERDOSAGE

Following a single oral dose of 20 g/kg no lethality occurred in rats, and death occurred in one of 20 mice receiving the same dose. The most likely manifestation of overdosage would be hypotension, for which the usual treatment would be intravenous infusion of normal saline solution.

Lisinopril can be removed by hemodialysis.

DOSAGE AND ADMINISTRATION

Hypertension

Initial Therapy: In patients with uncomplicated essential hypertension not on diuretic therapy, the recommended initial dose is 10 mg once a day. Dosage should be adjusted according to blood pressure response. The usual dosage range is 20 to 40 mg per day administered in a single daily dose. The antihypertensive effect may diminish toward the end of the dosing interval regardless of the administered dose, but most commonly with a dose of 10 mg daily. This can be evaluated by measuring blood pressure just prior to dosing to determine whether satisfactory control is being maintained for 24 hours. If it is not, an increase in dose should be considered. Doses up to 80 mg have been used but do not appear to give greater effect. If blood pressure is not controlled with ZESTRIL alone, a low dose of a diuretic may be added. Hydrochlorothiazide, 12.5 mg has been shown to provide an additive effect. After the addition of a diuretic, it may be possible to reduce the dose of ZESTRIL.

Diuretic Treated Patients: In hypertensive patients who are currently being treated with a diuretic, symptomatic hypotension may occur occasionally following the initial dose of ZESTRIL. The diuretic should be discontinued, if possible, for two to three days before beginning therapy with ZESTRIL to reduce the likelihood of hypotension. (See WARNINGS.) The dosage of ZESTRIL should be adjusted according to blood pressure response. If the patient's blood pressure is not controlled with ZESTRIL alone, diuretic therapy may be resumed as described above.

If the diuretic cannot be discontinued, an initial dose of 5 mg should be used under medical supervision for at least two hours and until blood pressure has stabilized for at least an additional hour. (See WARNINGS and PRECAUTIONS, Drug Interactions.)

Concomitant administration of ZESTRIL with potassium supplements, potassium salt substitutes, or potassium-sparing diuretics may lead to increases of serum potassium. (See PRECAUTIONS.)

Dosage Adjustment in Renal Impairment: The usual dose of ZESTRIL (10 mg) is recommended for patients with creatinine clearance > 30 mL/min (serum creatinine of up to approximately 3 mg/dL). For patients with creatinine clearance ≥ 10 mL/min ≤ 30 mL/min (serum creatinine ≥ 3 mg/dL), the first dose is 5 mg once daily. For patients with creatinine clearance < 10 mL/min (usually on hemodialysis) the recommended initial dose is 2.5 mg. The dosage may be titrated upward until blood pressure is controlled or to a maximum of 40 mg daily.

Renal Status	Creatinine Clearance mL/min	Initial Dose mg/day
Normal Renal Function to Mild Impairment	>30	10
Moderate to Severe Impairment	≥10≤30	5
Dialysis Patients*	<10	2.5**

* See WARNINGS, Anaphylactoid Reactions During Membrane Exposure.
**Dosage interval should be adjusted depending on the blood pressure response.

Heart Failure: ZESTRIL is indicated as adjunctive therapy with diuretics and (usually) digitalis. The recommended starting dose is 5 mg once a day. When initiating treatment with lisinopril in patients with heart failure, the initial dose should be administered under medical observation, especially in those patients with low blood pressure (systolic blood pressure below 100 mmHg). The mean peak blood pressure lowering occurs six to eight hours after dosing. Observation should continue until blood pressure is stable. The concomitant diuretic dose should be reduced, if possible, to help minimize hypovolemia which may contribute to hypotension. (See WARNINGS and PRECAUTIONS, Drug Interactions.) The appearance of hypotension after the initial dose of ZESTRIL does not preclude subsequent careful dose titration with the drug, following effective management of the hypotension.

The usual effective dosage range is 5 to 40 mg per day administered as a single dose. The dose of ZESTRIL can be increased by increments of no greater than 10 mg, at intervals of no less than 2 weeks to the highest tolerated dose, up to a maximum of 40 mg daily. Dose adjustment should be based on the clinical response of individual patients.

Dosage Adjustment in Patients with Heart Failure and Renal Impairment or Hyponatremia: In patients with heart failure who have hyponatremia (serum sodium < 130 mEq/L) or moderate to severe renal impairment (creatinine clearance ≤ 30 mL/min or serum creatinine > 3 mg/dL), therapy with ZESTRIL should be initiated at a dose of 2.5 mg once a day under close medical supervision. (See WARNINGS and PRECAUTIONS, Drug Interactions.)

Acute Myocardial Infarction: In hemodynamically stable patients within 24 hours of the onset of symptoms of acute myocardial infarction, the first dose of ZESTRIL is 5 mg given orally, followed by 5 mg after 24 hours, 10 mg after 48 hours and then 10 mg of ZESTRIL once daily. Dosing should continue for six weeks. Patients should receive, as appropriate, the standard recommended treatments such as thrombolytics, aspirin, and beta-blockers.

Patients with a low systolic blood pressure (≤ 120 mmHg) when treatment is started or during the first 3 days after the infarct should be given a lower 2.5 mg oral dose of ZESTRIL (see WARNINGS). If hypotension occurs (systolic blood pressure ≤ 100 mmHg) a daily maintenance dose of 5 mg may be given with temporary reductions to 2.5 mg if needed. If prolonged hypotension occurs (systolic blood pressure < 90 mmHg for more than 1 hour) ZESTRIL should be withdrawn. For patients who develop symptoms of heart failure, see DOSAGE AND ADMINISTRATION, Heart Failure.

Dosage Adjustment in Patients With Myocardial Infarction with Renal Impairment: In acute myocardial infarction, treatment with ZESTRIL should be initiated with caution in patients with evidence of renal dysfunction, defined as serum creatinine concentration exceeding 2 mg/dL. No evaluation of dosing adjustments in myocardial infarction patients with severe renal impairment has been performed.

Use in Elderly: In general, blood pressure response and adverse experiences were similar in younger and older patients given similar doses of ZESTRIL. Pharmacokinetic studies, however, indicate that maximum blood levels and area under the plasma concentration time curve (AUC) are doubled in older patients, so that dosage adjustments should be made with particular caution.

HOW SUPPLIED

2.5 mg Tablets (NDC 0310-0135) white, round, biconvex, uncoated tablets identified as "ZESTRIL 2 1/2" on one side and "135" on the other side are supplied in bottles of 100 tablets.

5 mg Tablets (NDC 0310-0130) pink, capsule-shaped, biconvex, bisected, uncoated tablets, identified "ZESTRIL" on one side and "130" on the other side are supplied in bottles of 100 tablets and 1000 tablets, and unit dose packages of 100 tablets.

10 mg Tablets (NDC 0310-0131) pink, round, biconvex, uncoated tablets identified "ZESTRIL 10" debossed on one side, and "131" debossed on the other side are supplied in bottles of 100 tablets, 1000 tablets, 3000 tablets, and unit dose packages of 100 tablets.

20 mg Tablets (NDC 0310-0132) red, round, biconvex, uncoated tablets identified "ZESTRIL 20" debossed on one side, and "132" debossed on the other side are supplied in bottles of 100 tablets, 1000 tablets, 3000 tablets, and unit dose packages of 100 tablets.

30 mg Tablets (NDC 0310-0133) red, round, biconvex, uncoated tablets identified "ZESTRIL 30" debossed on one side, and "133" debossed on the other side in bottles of 100 tablets.

40 mg Tablets (NDC 0310-0134) yellow, round, biconvex, uncoated tablets identified "ZESTRIL 40" debossed on one side, and "134" debossed on the other side are supplied in bottles of 100 tablets.

Store at controlled room temperature, 20–25°C (68–77°F)[see USP]. Protect from moisture, freezing and excessive heat. Dispense in a tight container.

¶Registered trademark of Hospal Ltd.

All other trademarks are the property of the AstraZeneca Group

Manufactured for:
AstraZeneca Pharmaceuticals LP
Wilmington, Delaware 19850
By: IPR Pharmaceuticals Inc.
Carolina, Puerto Rico 00984
Rev V 02/00 64150-00

Shown in Product Identification Guide, page 306

ZOLADEX® 3.6 mg ℞

[zōl'-ă-dĕx]

GOSERELIN ACETATE IMPLANT
Equivalent to 3.6 mg goserelin

DESCRIPTION

ZOLADEX® (goserelin acetate implant), contains a potent synthetic decapeptide analogue of luteinizing hormone-releasing hormone (LHRH), also known as a gonadotropin releasing hormone (GnRH) agonist analogue. Goserelin acetate is chemically described as an acetate salt of [D-Ser(Bu^t)^6,Azgly^{10}]LHRH. Its chemical structure is pyro-Glu-His-Trp-Ser-Tyr-D-Ser(Bu^t)-Leu-Arg-Pro-Azgly-NH$_2$ acetate [$C_{59}H_{84}N_{18}O_{14} \cdot (C_2H_4O_2)_x$ where x = 1 to 2.4].

Goserelin acetate is an off-white powder with a molecular weight of 1269 Daltons (free base). It is freely soluble in glacial acetic acid. It is soluble in water, 0.1M hydrochloric acid, 0.1M sodium hydroxide, dimethylformamide and dimethyl sulfoxide. Goserelin acetate is practically insoluble in acetone, chloroform and ether.

ZOLADEX is supplied as a sterile, biodegradable product containing goserelin acetate equivalent to 3.6 mg of goserelin. ZOLADEX is designed for subcutaneous injection with continuous release over a 28-day period. Goserelin acetate is dispersed in a matrix of D,L-lactic and glycolic acids copolymer (13.3-14.3 mg/dose) containing less than 2.5% acetic acid and up to 12% goserelin-related substances and presented as a sterile, white to cream colored 1-mm diameter cylinder, preloaded in a special single use syringe with a 16-gauge needle and overwrapped in a sealed, light and moisture proof, aluminum foil laminate pouch containing a desiccant capsule. Studies of the D,L-lactic and glycolic acids copolymer have indicated that it is completely biodegradable and has no demonstrable antigenic potential.

CLINICAL PHARMACOLOGY

Mechanism of Action: ZOLADEX is a synthetic decapeptide analogue of LHRH. ZOLADEX acts as a potent inhibitor of pituitary gonadotropin secretion when administered in the biodegradable formulation.

Following initial administration in males, ZOLADEX causes an initial increase in serum luteinizing hormone (LH) and follicle stimulating hormone (FSH) levels with subsequent increases in serum levels of testosterone. Chronic administration of ZOLADEX leads to sustained suppression of pituitary gonadotropins, and serum levels of testosterone consequently fall into the range normally seen in surgically castrated men approximately 2–4 weeks after initiation of therapy. This leads to accessory sex organ regression. In animal and in vitro studies, administration of goserelin resulted in the regression or inhibition of growth of the hormonally sensitive dimethylbenzanthracene (DMBA)-induced rat mammary tumor and Dunning R3327 prostate tumor. In clinical trials with follow-up of more than 2 years, suppression of serum testosterone to castrate levels has been maintained for the duration of therapy.

In females, a similar down-regulation of the pituitary gland by chronic exposure to ZOLADEX leads to suppression of gonadotropin secretion, a decrease in serum estradiol to levels consistent with the postmenopausal state, and would be expected to lead to a reduction of ovarian size and function, reduction in the size of the uterus and mammary gland, as well as a regression of sex hormone-responsive tumors, if present. Serum estradiol is suppressed to levels similar to those observed in postmenopausal women within 3 weeks following initial administration; however, after suppression was attained, isolated elevations of estradiol were seen in 10% of the patients enrolled in clinical trials. Serum LH and FSH are suppressed to follicular phase levels within four weeks after initial administration of drug and are usually maintained at that range with continued use of ZOLADEX. In 5% or less of women treated with ZOLADEX, FSH and LH levels may not be suppressed to follicular phase levels on day 28 post treatment with use of a single 3.6 mg depot injection. In certain individuals, suppression of any of these hormones to such levels may not be achieved with ZOLADEX. Estradiol, LH and FSH levels return to pretreatment values within 12 weeks following the last implant administration in all but rare cases.

Pharmacokinetics: The pharmacokinetics of ZOLADEX have been determined in both male and female healthy volunteers and patients. In these studies, ZOLADEX was administered as a single 250 µg (aqueous solution) dose and as a single or multiple 3.6 mg depot dose by subcutaneous route.

Absorption: The absorption of radiolabeled drug was rapid, and the peak blood radioactivity levels occurred between 0.5 and 1.0 hour after dosing. The mean (± standard deviation) pharmacokinetic parameter estimates of ZOLADEX after administration of 3.6 mg depot for 2 months in males and females are presented in the following table.

[See table at top of next page]

Pharmacokinetic data were obtained using a nonspecific RIA method.

Goserelin is released from the depot at a much slower rate initially for the first 8 days, and then there is more rapid and continuous release for the remainder of the 28-day dosing period. Despite the change in the releasing rate of goserelin, administration of ZOLADEX every 28 days resulted in testosterone levels that were suppressed to and maintained in the range normally seen in surgically castrated men.

When ZOLADEX 3.6 mg depot was used for treating male and female patients with normal renal and hepatic function, there was no significant evidence of drug accumulation. However, in clinical trials the minimum serum levels of a few patients were increased. These levels can be attributed to interpatient variation.

Distribution: The apparent volumes of distribution determined after subcutaneous administration of 250 µg aqueous solution of goserelin were 44.1 and 20.3 liters for males and females, respectively. The plasma protein binding of goserelin obtained from one sample was found to be 27.3%.

Metabolism: Metabolism of goserelin, by hydrolysis of the C-terminal amino acids, is the major clearance mechanism. The major circulating component in serum appeared to be 1–7 fragment, and the major component presented in urine of one healthy male volunteer was 5–10 fragment. The metabolism of goserelin in humans yields a similar but narrow profile of metabolites to that found in other species. All metabolites found in humans have also been found in toxicology species.

Excretion: Clearance of goserelin following subcutaneous administration of the solution formulation of goserelin is very rapid and occurs via a combination of hepatic metabolism and urinary excretion. More than 90% of a subcutaneous radiolabeled solution formulation dose of goserelin is excreted in urine. Approximately 20% of the dose in urine is accounted for by unchanged goserelin. The total body clearance of goserelin (administered subcutaneously as a 3.6 mg depot) was significantly ($p<0.05$) greater (163.9 versus 110.5 L/min) in females compared to males.

Special Populations

Renal Insufficiency: In clinical trials with the solution formulation of goserelin, male patients with impaired renal function (creatinine clearance < 20 mL/min) had a total body clearance and serum elimination half-life of 31.5 mL/min and 12.1 hours, respectively, compared to 133 mL/min and 4.2 hours for subjects with normal renal function (creatinine clearance > 70 mL/min). In females, the effects of reduced goserelin clearance due to impaired renal function on drug efficacy and toxicity are unknown. Pharmacokinetic studies using the aqueous formulation of goserelin in patients with renal impairment do not indicate a need for dose adjustment with the use of the depot formulation.

Hepatic Insufficiency: The total body clearances and serum elimination half-lives were similar between normal and hepatic impaired patients receiving 250 µg solution formulation of goserelin. Pharmacokinetic studies using the aqueous formulation of goserelin in patients with hepatic impairment do not indicate a need for dose adjustment with the use of the depot formulation.

Drug-Drug Interactions: No formal drug-drug interaction studies have been performed.

Clinical Studies - Prostatic Carcinoma: In controlled studies of patients with advanced prostatic cancer comparing ZOLADEX to orchiectomy, the long-term endocrine responses and objective responses were similar between the two treatment arms. Additionally, duration of survival was similar between the two treatment arms in a comparative trial.

Clinical Studies — Stage B2-C Prostatic Carcinoma: The effects of hormonal treatment combined with radiation were studied in 466 patients (231 ZOLADEX + flutamide + radiation, 235 radiation alone) with bulky primary tumors confined to the prostate (stage B2) or extending beyond the capsule (stage C), with or without pelvic node involvement.

In this multicentered, controlled trial, administration of ZOLADEX (3.6 mg depot) and flutamide capsules (250 mg t.i.d.) prior to and during radiation was associated with a significantly lower rate of local failure compared to radiation alone (16% vs 33% at 4 years, $P<0.001$). The combination therapy also resulted in a trend toward reduction in the incidence of distant metastases (27% vs 36% at 4 years, $P=0.058$). Median disease-free survival was significantly increased in patients who received complete hormonal therapy combined with radiation as compared to those patients who received radiation alone (4.4 vs 2.6 years, $P<0.001$). Inclusion of normal PSA level as a criterion for disease-free survival also resulted in significantly increased median disease-free survival in patients receiving the combination therapy (2.7 vs 1.5 years, $P<0.001$).

Clinical Studies — Endometriosis: In controlled clinical studies using the 3.6 mg formulation every 28 days for 6 months, ZOLADEX was shown to be as effective as danazol therapy in relieving clinical symptoms (dysmenorrhea, dyspareunia and pelvic pain) and signs (pelvic tenderness, pelvic induration) of endometriosis and decreasing the size of endometrial lesions as determined by laparoscopy. In one study comparing ZOLADEX with danazol (800 mg/day), 63% of ZOLADEX-treated patients and 42% of danazol-treated patients had a greater than or equal to 50% reduction in the extent of endometrial lesions. In the second study comparing ZOLADEX with danazol (600 mg/day), 62% of ZOLADEX-treated and 51% of danazol-treated patients had a greater than or equal to 50% reduction in the extent of endometrial lesions. The clinical significance of a decrease in endometriotic lesions is not known at this time; and in addition, laparoscopic staging of endometriosis does not necessarily correlate with severity of symptoms.

In these two studies, ZOLADEX led to amenorrhea in 92% and 80%, respectively, of all treated women within 8 weeks after initial administration. Menses usually resumed within 8 weeks following completion of therapy.

Continued on next page

Zoladex—Cont.

Within 4 weeks following initial administration, clinical symptoms were significantly reduced, and at the end of treatment were, on average, reduced by approximately 84%. During the first two months of ZOLADEX use, some women experience vaginal bleeding of variable duration and intensity. In all likelihood, this bleeding represents estrogen withdrawal bleeding, and is expected to stop spontaneously. There is insufficient evidence to determine whether pregnancy rates are enhanced or adversely affected by the use of ZOLADEX.

Clinical Studies — Breast Cancer: The Southwest Oncology Group conducted a prospective, randomized clinical trial (SWOG-8692 [INT-0075]) in premenopausal women with advanced estrogen receptor positive or progesterone receptor positive breast cancer which compared ZOLADEX with oophorectomy. On the basis of interim data from 124 women, the best objective response (CR+PR) for the ZOLADEX group is 22% versus 12% for the oophorectomy group. The median time to treatment failure is 6.7 months for patients treated with ZOLADEX and 5.5 months for patients treated with oophorectomy. The median survival time for the ZOLADEX arm is 33.2 months and for the oophorectomy arm is 33.6 months.

Subjective responses based on measures of pain control and performance status were observed with both treatments; 48% of the women in the ZOLADEX treatment group and 50% in the oophorectomy group had subjective responses. In the clinical trial (SWOG-8692 [INT 0075]), the mean post treatment estradiol level was reported as 17.8 pg/mL. (The mean estradiol level in post-menopausal women as reported in the literature is 13 pg/mL). During the conduct of the clinical trial, women whose estradiol levels were not reduced to the postmenopausal range, received two ZOLADEX depots, thus, increasing the dose of ZOLADEX from 3.6 mg to 7.2 mg.

Findings were similar in uncontrolled clinical trials involving patients with hormone receptor positive and negative breast cancer. Premenopausal women with estrogen receptor (ER) status of positive, negative, or unknown participated in the uncontrolled (Phase II and Trial 2302) clinical trials. Objective tumor responses were seen regardless of ER status, as shown in the following table.

OBJECTIVE RESPONSE BY ER STATUS

	CR + PR/Total No. (%)	
ER status	Phase II (N = 228)	Trial 2302 (N = 159)
Positive	43/119 (36)	31/86 (36)
Negative	6/33 (18)	3/26 (10)
Unknown	20/76 (26)	18/44 (41)

Clinical Studies-Endometrial Thinning: Two trials were conducted with ZOLADEX prior to endometrial ablation for dysfunctional uterine bleeding.

Trial 0022, was a double-blind, prospective, randomized, parallel-group multicenter trial conducted in 358 premenopausal women with dysfunctional uterine bleeding. Eligible patients were randomized to receive either two depots of ZOLADEX 3.6 mg (n=180) or two placebo injections (n=178) administered four weeks apart. 175 patients in each group underwent endometrial ablation using either diathermy loop alone or in combination with rollerball approximately 2 weeks after the second injection. Endometrial thickness was assessed immediately before surgery using a transvaginal ultrasonic probe. The incidence of amenorrhea was compared between the ZOLADEX and placebo groups at 24 weeks after endometrial ablation.

The median endometrial thickness before surgery was significantly less in the ZOLADEX treatment group (1.50 mm) compared to the placebo group (3.55 mm). Six months after surgery, 40% of patients (70/175) treated with ZOLADEX in Trial 0022 reported amenorrhea as compared with 26% who had received placebo injections (44/171), a difference that was statistically significant.

Trial 0003, was a single center, open-label, randomized trial in premenopausal women with dysfunctional uterine bleeding. The trial allowed for a comparison of 1 depot of ZOLADEX and 2 depots of ZOLADEX administered 4 weeks apart with ablation using Nd: YAG laser occurring 4 weeks after ZOLADEX administration. Forty patients were randomized into each of the ZOLADEX treatment groups.

The median endometrial thickness before surgery was significantly less in the group treated with two depots (0.5 mm) compared to the group treated with one depot (1 mm). No difference in the incidence of amenorrhea was found at 24 weeks (24% in both groups). Of the 74 patients that completed the trial, 53 % reported hypomenorrhea and 20% reported normal menses six months after surgery.

INDICATIONS AND USAGE

Prostatic Carcinoma: ZOLADEX is indicated in the palliative treatment of advanced carcinoma of the prostate.

Stage B2-C Prostatic Carcinoma: ZOLADEX is indicated for use in combination with flutamide for the management of locally confined Stage T2b-T4 (Stage B2-C) carcinoma of the prostate. Treatment with ZOLADEX and flutamide should start 8 weeks prior to initiating radiation therapy and continue during radiation therapy.

Endometriosis: ZOLADEX is indicated for the management of endometriosis, including pain relief and reduction of endometriotic lesions for the duration of therapy. Experience with ZOLADEX for the management of endometriosis has been limited to women 18 years of age and older treated for 6 months.

Parameters (Units)	Males n=7	Females n=9
Peak Plasma Concentration (ng/mL)	2.84 ± 1.81	1.46 ± 0.82
Time to Peak Concentration (days)	12–15	8–22
Area Under the Curve (0–28 days) (ng.h/mL)	27.8 ± 15.3	18.5 ± 10.3
Systemic Clearance (mL/min)	110.5 ± 47.5	163.9 ± 71.0
*Apparent Volume of Distribution (L)	44.1 ± 13.6	20.3 ± 4.1
*Elimination Half-life (h)	4.2 ± 1.1	2.3 ± 0.6

* The apparent volume of distribution and the elimination half-life were determined after subcutaneous administration of 250 μg aqueous solution of goserelin.

Advanced Breast Cancer: ZOLADEX is indicated for use in the palliative treatment of advanced breast cancer in pre- and perimenopausal women.

The estrogen and progesterone receptor values may help to predict whether ZOLADEX therapy is likely to be beneficial. (See CLINICAL PHARMACOLOGY.)

Endometrial Thinning: ZOLADEX is indicated for use as an endometrial-thinning agent prior to endometrial ablation for dysfunctional uterine bleeding.

CONTRAINDICATIONS

A report of an anaphylactic reaction to synthetic GnRH (Factrel) has been reported in the medical literature.

ZOLADEX is contraindicated in those patients who have a known hypersensitivity to LHRH, LHRH agonist analogues or any of the components in ZOLADEX.

ZOLADEX is contraindicated in women being treated for endometriosis or endometrial thinning who are or may become pregnant while receiving the drug. ZOLADEX can cause fetal harm when administered to a pregnant woman. Effects on reproductive function, as a result of antigonadotrophic properties of the drug, are expected to occur on chronic administration.

Effective nonhormonal contraception must be used by all premenopausal women during ZOLADEX therapy and for 12 weeks following discontinuation of therapy. There are no adequate and well-controlled studies in pregnant women using ZOLADEX. If this drug is used during pregnancy, or the patient being treated for endometriosis or endometrial thinning becomes pregnant while taking this drug, the patient should be apprised of the potential hazard to the fetus or potential risk for loss of the pregnancy. Women of childbearing potential should be advised to avoid becoming pregnant.

For a description of findings in animal reproductive toxicity studies, see **WARNINGS**.

ZOLADEX is contraindicated in women who are breast feeding (see Nursing Mothers Section).

WARNINGS

Before starting treatment with ZOLADEX, pregnancy must be excluded. Safe use of ZOLADEX in pregnancy has not been established. ZOLADEX can cause fetal harm when administered to a pregnant woman. ZOLADEX has been found to cross the placenta following subcutaneous administration of 50 and 1000 μg/kg in rats and rabbits, respectively. Studies in both rats and rabbits at doses equal to or greater than 2 and 20 μg/kg/day, respectively (about 1/10 and 2 times the daily maximum recommended human dose, respectively, on a mg/m^2 basis), administered during the period of organogenesis, have confirmed that ZOLADEX will increase pregnancy loss, and is embryotoxic/fetotoxic (characterized by increased preimplantation loss, increased resorption and an increase in umbilical hernia in rats at a dose of ≥ 10 μg/kg/day [about 1/2 the recommended human dose on a mg/m^2 basis]); effects were dose-related. In additional reproduction studies in rats, ZOLADEX was found to decrease fetus and pup survival.

There are no adequate and well-controlled studies in pregnant women using ZOLADEX. Women of childbearing potential should be advised to avoid becoming pregnant.

When used every 28 days, ZOLADEX usually inhibits ovulation and stops menstruation. Contraception is not ensured, however, by taking ZOLADEX. During treatment, pregnancy must be avoided by the use of nonhormonal methods of contraception. If ZOLADEX is used during pregnancy (in a patient with advanced breast cancer) or the patient becomes pregnant while receiving this drug, the patient must be apprised of the potential risk for loss of the pregnancy due to possible hormonal imbalance as a result of the expected pharmacologic action of ZOLADEX treatment. Following the last ZOLADEX injection, nonhormonal methods of contraception must be continued until the return of menses or for at least 12 weeks. (See **CONTRAINDICATIONS.**)

Prostate and Breast Cancer: Initially, ZOLADEX, like other LHRH agonists, causes transient increases in serum levels of testosterone in men with prostate cancer, and estrogen in women with breast cancer. Transient worsening of symptoms, or the occurrence of additional signs and symptoms of prostate or breast cancer, may occasionally develop during the first few weeks of ZOLADEX treatment. A small number of patients may experience a temporary increase in bone pain, which can be managed symptomatically. As with other LHRH agonists, isolated cases of ureteral obstruction and spinal cord compression have been observed in patients with prostate cancer. If spinal cord compression or renal impairment develops, standard treatment of these complications should be instituted. For extreme cases in prostate cancer patients, an immediate orchiectomy should be considered.

As with other LHRH agonists or hormonal therapies (antiestrogens, estrogens, etc.), hypercalcemia has been reported in some prostate and breast cancer patients with bone metastases after starting treatment with ZOLADEX. If hypercalcemia does occur, appropriate treatment measures should be initiated.

PRECAUTIONS

General: Hypersensitivity, antibody formation and acute anaphylactic reactions have been reported with LHRH agonist analogues.

Of 115 women worldwide treated with ZOLADEX and tested for development of binding to goserelin following treatment with ZOLADEX, one patient showed low-titer binding to goserelin. On further testing of this patient's plasma obtained following treatment, her goserelin binding component was found not to be precipitated with rabbit antihuman immunoglobulin polyvalent sera. These findings suggest the possibility of antibody formation.

The pharmacologic action of ZOLADEX on the uterus and cervix may cause an increase in cervical resistance. Therefore, care should be taken when dilating the cervix for endometrial ablation.

Information for Patients

Males: The use of ZOLADEX in patients at particular risk of developing ureteral obstruction or spinal cord compression should be considered carefully and the patients monitored closely during the first month of therapy. Patients with ureteral obstruction or spinal cord compression should have appropriate treatment prior to initiation of ZOLADEX therapy.

Females: Patients must be made aware of the following information:

1. Since menstruation should stop with effective doses of ZOLADEX the patient should notify her physician if regular menstruation persists. Patients missing one or more successive doses of ZOLADEX may experience breakthrough menstrual bleeding.
2. ZOLADEX should not be prescribed if the patient is pregnant, breast feeding, lactating, has nondiagnosed abnormal vaginal bleeding, or is allergic to any of the components of ZOLADEX.
3. Use of ZOLADEX in pregnancy is contraindicated in women being treated for endometriosis or endometrial thinning. Therefore, a nonhormonal method of contraception should be used during treatment. Patients should be advised that if they miss one or more successive doses of ZOLADEX, breakthrough menstrual bleeding or ovulation may occur with the potential for conception. If a patient becomes pregnant during treatment for endometriosis or endometrial thinning, ZOLADEX treatment should be discontinued and the patient should be advised of the possible risks to the pregnancy and fetus. (See CONTRAINDICATIONS.)
   For patients being treated for advanced breast cancer, see **WARNINGS**.
4. Those adverse events occurring most frequently in clinical studies with ZOLADEX are associated with hypoestrogenism; of these, the most frequently reported are hot flashes (flushes), headaches, vaginal dryness, emotional lability, change in libido, depression, sweating and change in breast size. Clinical studies in endometriosis suggest the addition of Hormone Replacement Therapy (estrogens and/or progestins) to ZOLADEX may decrease the occurrence of vasomotor symptoms and vaginal dryness associated with hypoestrogenism without compromising the efficacy of ZOLADEX in relieving pelvic symptoms. The optimal drugs, dose and duration of treatment has not been established.
5. As with other LHRH agonist analogues, treatment with ZOLADEX induces a hypoestrogenic state which results in a loss of bone mineral density (BMD) over the course of treatment, some of which may not be reversible. In patients with a history of prior treatment that may have resulted in bone mineral density loss and/or in patients with major risk factors for decreased bone mineral density such as chronic alcohol abuse and/or tobacco abuse, significant family history of osteoporosis, or chronic use of drugs that can reduce bone density such as anticonvulsants or corticosteroids, ZOLADEX therapy may pose an additional risk. In these patients the risks and benefits must be weighed carefully before therapy with ZOLADEX is instituted. Clinical studies suggest the addition of Hormone Replacement Therapy (estrogens and/or progestins) to ZOLADEX is effective in reducing the bone mineral loss which occurs with ZOLADEX alone. The optimal drugs, dose and duration of treatment has not been established.
6. Currently, there are no clinical data on the effects of retreatment or treatment of benign gynecological conditions with ZOLADEX for periods in excess of 6 months.

7. As with other hormonal interventions that disrupt the pituitary-gonadal axis, some patients may have delayed return to menses. The rare patient, however, may experience persistent amenorrhea.

Drug Interactions: No formal drug-drug interaction studies have been performed. No confirmed interactions have been reported between ZOLADEX and other drugs.

Drug/Laboratory Test Interactions: Administration of ZOLADEX in therapeutic doses results in suppression of the pituitary-gonadal system. Because of this suppression, diagnostic tests of pituitary-gonadotropic and gonadal functions conducted during treatment and until the resumption of menses may show results which are misleading. Normal function is usually restored within 12 weeks after treatment is discontinued.

Carcinogenesis, Mutagenesis, Impairment of Fertility: Subcutaneous implant of ZOLADEX in male and female rats once every 4 weeks for 1 year and recovery for 23 weeks at doses of about 80 and 150 µg/kg (males) and 50 and 100 µg/kg (females) daily (about 3 to 9 times the recommended human dose on a mg/m^2 basis) resulted in an increased incidence of pituitary adenomas. An increased incidence of pituitary adenomas was also observed following subcutaneous implant of ZOLADEX in rats at similar dose levels for a period of 72 weeks in males and 101 weeks in females. The relevance of the rat pituitary adenomas to humans has not been established. Subcutaneous implants of ZOLADEX every 3 weeks for 2 years delivered to mice at doses of up to 2400 µg/kg/day (about 70 times the recommended human dose on a mg/m^2 basis) resulted in an increased incidence of histiocytic sarcoma of the vertebral column and femur.

Mutagenicity tests using bacterial and mammalian systems for point mutations and cytogenetic effects have provided no evidence for mutagenic potential.

Administration of goserelin led to changes that were consistent with gonadal suppression in both male and female rats as a result of its endocrine action. In male rats administered 500–1000 µg/kg/day (about 30–60 times the recommended human dose on a mg/m^2 basis), a decrease in weight and atrophic histological changes were observed in the testes, epididymis, seminal vesicle and prostate gland with complete suppression of spermatogenesis. In female rats administered 50–1000 µg/kg/day (about 3–60 times the recommended daily human dose on a mg/m^2 basis), suppression of ovarian function led to decreased size and weight of ovaries and secondary sex organs; follicular development was arrested at the antral stage and the corpora lutea were reduced in size and number. Except for the testes, almost complete histologic reversal of these effects in males and females was observed several weeks after dosing was stopped; however, fertility and general reproductive performance were reduced in those that became pregnant after goserelin was discontinued. Fertile matings occurred within 2 weeks after cessation of dosing, even though total recovery of reproductive function may not have occurred before mating took place; and, the ovulation rate, the corresponding implantation rate, and number of live fetuses were reduced.

Based on histological examination, drug effects on reproductive organs were reversible in male and female dogs administered 107–214 µg/kg/day ZOLADEX (about 20–40 times the recommended daily human dose on a mg/m^2 basis) when drug treatment was stopped after continuous administration for 1 year.

Pregnancy: Pregnancy Category X for treatment of endometriosis and endometrial thinning. See **CONTRAINDICATIONS** and **WARNINGS** sections. **Pregnancy Category D** for treatment of advanced breast cancer in pre- and perimenopausal women. See WARNINGS section.

Nursing Mothers: ZOLADEX has been shown to be excreted in the milk of lactating rats. It is not known if this drug is excreted in human milk. Because many drugs are excreted in human milk, and because of the potential for serious adverse reactions from ZOLADEX in nursing infants, mothers should discontinue nursing prior to taking the drug.

Pediatric Use: The safety and efficacy of ZOLADEX in pediatric patients have not been established.

ADVERSE REACTIONS

General: Rarely, hypersensitivity reactions (including urticaria and anaphylaxis) have been reported in patients receiving ZOLADEX.

Changes in blood pressure, manifest as hypotension or hypertension, have been occasionally observed in patients administered ZOLADEX. The changes are usually transient, resolving either during continued therapy or after cessation of therapy with ZOLADEX. Rarely, such changes have been sufficient to require medical intervention including withdrawal of treatment from ZOLADEX.

Males - Prostatic Carcinoma: ZOLADEX has been found to be generally well tolerated in clinical trials. Adverse reactions reported in these trials were rarely severe enough to result in the patients' withdrawal from ZOLADEX treatment. As seen with other hormonal therapies, the most commonly observed adverse events during ZOLADEX therapy were due to the expected physiological effects from decreased testosterone levels. These included hot flashes, sexual dysfunction and decreased erections.

Initially, ZOLADEX, like other LHRH agonists, causes transient increases in serum levels of testosterone. A small percentage of patients experienced a temporary worsening of signs and symptoms (see WARNINGS section), usually manifested by an increase in cancer-related pain which was managed symptomatically. Isolated cases of exacerbation of disease symptoms, either ureteral obstruction or spinal cord

ADVERSE EVENTS DURING ACUTE RADIATION THERAPY
(within the first 90 days of radiation therapy)

	flutamide + ZOLADEX + Radiation (n=231) % All	Radiation Only (n=235) % All
Rectum/Large Bowel	80	76
Bladder	58	60
Skin	37	37

TREATMENT RECEIVED

ADVERSE EVENT	ZOLADEX (n=242) %	ORCHIECTOMY (n=254) %	ADVERSE EVENT	ZOLADEX (n=242) %	ORCHIECTOMY (n=254) %
Hot Flashes	62	53	Rash	6	1
Sexual Dysfunction	21	15	Sweating	6	4
Decreased Erections	18	16	Anorexia	5	2
Lower Urinary Tract Symptoms	13	8	Chronic Obstructive Pulmonary Disease	5	3
Lethargy	8	4	Congestive Heart Failure	5	1
Pain (worsened in the first 30 days)	8	3	Dizziness	5	4
Edema	7	8	Insomnia	5	1
Upper Respiratory Infection	7	2	Nausea	5	2
			Complications of Surgery	0	18†

† Complications related to surgery were reported in 18% of the orchiectomy patients, while only 3% of ZOLADEX patients reported adverse reactions at the injection site. The surgical complications included scrotal infection (5.9%), groin pain (4.7%), wound seepage (3.1%), scrotal hematoma (2.8%), incisional discomfort (1.6%) and skin necrosis (1.2%).

ADVERSE EVENTS DURING LATE RADIATION PHASE
(after 90 days of radiation therapy)

	flutamide + ZOLADEX + Radiation (n=231) % All	Radiation Only (n=235) % All
Diarrhea	36	40
Cystitis	16	16
Rectal Bleeding	14	20
Proctitis	8	8
Hematuria	7	12

TREATMENT RECEIVED

ADVERSE EVENT	ZOLADEX (n=411) %	DANAZOL (n=207) %	ADVERSE EVENT	ZOLADEX (n=411) %	DANAZOL (n=207) %
Hot Flashes	96	67	Hirsutism	7	15
Vaginitis	75	43	Insomnia	11	4
Headache	75	63	Breast Pain	7	4
Emotional Lability	60	56	Abdominal Pain	7	7
Libido Decreased	61	44	Back Pain	7	13
Sweating	45	30	Flu Syndrome	5	5
Depression	54	48	Dizziness	6	4
Acne	42	55	Application Site Reaction	6	—
Breast Atrophy	33	42	Voice Alterations	3	8
Seborrhea	26	52	Pharyngitis	5	2
Peripheral Edema	21	34	Hair Disorders	4	11
Breast Enlargement	18	15	Myalgia	3	11
Pelvic Symptoms	18	23	Nervousness	3	5
Pain	17	16	Weight Gain	3	23
Dyspareunia	14	5	Leg Cramps	2	6
Libido Increased	12	19	Increased Appetite	2	5
Infection	13	11	Pruritus	2	6
Asthenia	11	13	Hypertonia	1	10
Nausea	8	14			

compression, occurred at similar rates in controlled clinical trials with both ZOLADEX and orchiectomy. The relationship of these events to therapy is uncertain.

Changes in the hormonal environment following treatment with an LHRH analogue or orchiectomy may result in a loss in bone mineral density due to a marked reduction of testosterone concentrations.

In the controlled clinical trials of ZOLADEX versus orchiectomy, the following events were reported as adverse reactions in greater than 5% of the patients.

[See first table above]

The following additional adverse reactions were reported in greater than 1% but less than 5% of the patients treated with ZOLADEX: CARDIOVASCULAR — arrhythmia, cerebrovascular accident, hypertension, myocardial infarction, peripheral vascular disorder, chest pain; CENTRAL NERVOUS SYSTEM — anxiety, depression, headache; GASTROINTESTINAL — constipation, diarrhea, ulcer, vomiting; HEMATOLOGIC — anemia; METABOLIC/NUTRITIONAL — gout, hyperglycemia, weight increase; MISCELLANEOUS — chills, fever; UROGENITAL — renal insufficiency, urinary obstruction, urinary tract infection, breast swelling and tenderness.

Stage B2-C Prostatic Carcinoma: Treatment with ZOLADEX and flutamide did not add substantially to the toxicity of radiation treatment alone. The following adverse experiences were reported during a multicenter clinical trial comparing ZOLADEX + flutamide + radiation versus radiation alone. The most frequently reported (greater than 5%) adverse experiences are listed below:

[See second table above]

[See third table above]

Additional adverse event data was collected for the combination therapy with radiation group over both the hormonal treatment and hormonal treatment plus radiation phases of the study. Adverse experiences occurring in more than 5% of patients in this group, over both parts of the study, were hot flashes (46%), diarrhea (40%), nausea (9%), and skin rash (8%).

Females: As would be expected with a drug that results in hypoestrogenism, the most frequently reported adverse reactions were those related to this effect.

Endometriosis: In controlled clinical trials comparing ZOLADEX every 28 days and danazol daily for the treatment of endometriosis, the following events were reported at a frequency of 5% or greater:

[See fourth table above]

The following adverse events not already listed above were reported at a frequency of 1% or greater, regardless of causality, in ZOLADEX-treated women from all clinical trials: WHOLE BODY — allergic reaction, chest pain, fever, malaise; CARDIOVASCULAR — hemorrhage, hypertension, migraine, palpitations, tachycardia; DIGESTIVE — anorexia, constipation, diarrhea, dry mouth, dyspepsia, flatulence; HEMATOLOGIC — ecchymosis; METABOLIC AND NUTRITIONAL — edema; MUSCULOSKELETAL — arthralgia, joint disorder; CNS — anxiety, paresthesia, somnolence, thinking abnormal; RESPIRATORY — bronchitis, cough increased, epistaxis, rhinitis, sinusitis; SKIN — alopecia, dry skin, rash, skin discoloration; SPECIAL SENSES — amblyopia, dry eyes; UROGENITAL — dysmenorrhea, urinary frequency, urinary tract infection, vaginal hemorrhage.

Continued on next page

Zoladex—Cont.

Hormone Replacement Therapy: Clinical studies suggest the addition of Hormone Replacement Therapy (estrogens and/or progestins) to ZOLADEX may decrease the occurrence of vasomotor symptoms and vaginal dryness associated with hypoestrogenism without compromising the efficacy of ZOLADEX in relieving pelvic symptoms. The optimal drugs, dose and duration of treatment has not been established.
Changes in Bone Mineral Density: After 6 months of ZOLADEX treatment, 109 female patients treated with ZOLADEX showed an average 4.3% decrease of vertebral trabecular bone mineral density (BMD) as compared to pretreatment values. BMD was measured by dual-photon absorptiometry or dual energy x-ray absorptiometry. Sixty-six of these patients were assessed for BMD loss 6 months after the completion (posttherapy) of the 6-month therapy period. Data from these patients showed an average 2.4% BMD loss compared to pretreatment values. Twenty-eight of the 109 patients were assessed for BMD at 12 months posttherapy. Data from these patients showed an average decrease of 2.5% in BMD compared to pretreatment values. These data suggest a possibility of partial reversibility. Clinical studies suggest the addition of Hormone Replacement Therapy (estrogens and/or progestins) to ZOLADEX is effective in reducing the bone mineral loss which occurs with ZOLADEX alone without compromising the efficacy of ZOLADEX in relieving the symptoms of endometriosis. The optimal drugs, dose and duration of treatment has not been established.
Changes in Laboratory Values During Treatment
Plasma Enzymes. Elevation of liver enzymes (AST, ALT) have been reported in female patients exposed to ZOLADEX (representing less than 1% of all patients).
Lipids. In a controlled trial, ZOLADEX therapy resulted in a minor, but statistically significant effect on serum lipids. In patients treated for endometriosis at 6 months following initiation of therapy, danazol treatment resulted in a mean increase in LDL cholesterol of 33.3 mg/dL and a decrease in HDL cholesterol of 21.3 mg/dL compared to increases of 21.3 and 2.7 mg/dL in LDL cholesterol and HDL cholesterol, respectively, for ZOLADEX-treated patients. Triglycerides increased by 8.0 mg/dL in ZOLADEX-treated patients compared to a decrease of 8.9 mg/dL in danazol-treated patients.
In patients treated for endometriosis, ZOLADEX increased total cholesterol and LDL cholesterol during 6 months of treatment. However, ZOLADEX therapy resulted in HDL cholesterol levels which were significantly higher relative to danazol therapy. At the end of 6 months of treatment, HDL cholesterol fractions (HDL_2 and HDL_3) were decreased by 13.5 and 7.7 mg/dL, respectively, for danazol-treated patients compared to treatment increases of 1.9 and 0.8 mg/dL, respectively, for ZOLADEX treated patients.
Breast Cancer: The adverse event profile for women with advanced breast cancer treated with ZOLADEX is consistent with the profile described above for women treated with ZOLADEX for endometriosis. In a controlled clinical trial (SWOG-8692) comparing ZOLADEX with oophorectomy in premenopausal and perimenopausal women with advanced breast cancer, the following events were reported at a frequency of 5% or greater in either treatment group regardless of causality.

	TREATMENT RECEIVED	
ADVERSE EVENT	ZOLADEX (n=57) % of Pts.	OOPHORECTOMY (n=55) % of Pts.
Hot Flashes	70	47
Tumor Flare	23	4
Nausea	11	7
Edema	5	0
Malaise/Fatigue/ Lethargy	5	2
Vomiting	4	7

In the Phase II clinical trial program in 333 pre- and perimenopausal women with advanced breast cancer, hot flashes were reported in 75.9% of patients and decreased libido was noted in 47.7% of patients. These two adverse events reflect the pharmacological actions of ZOLADEX.

Injection site reactions were reported in less than 1% of patients.
Endometrial Thinning: The following adverse events were reported at a frequency of 5% or greater in premenopausal women presenting with dysfunctional uterine bleeding in Trial 0022 for endometrial thinning. These results indicate that headache, hot flushes and sweating, were more common in the ZOLADEX group than in the placebo group.
[See table at bottom of page]

OVERDOSAGE

The pharmacologic properties of ZOLADEX and its mode of administration make accidental or intentional overdosage unlikely. There is no experience of overdosage from clinical trials. Animal studies indicate that no increased pharmacologic effect occurred at higher doses or more frequent administration. Subcutaneous doses of the drug as high as 1 mg/kg/day in rats and dogs did not produce any nonendocrine related sequelae; this dose is greater than 400 times that proposed for human use. If overdosage occurs, it should be managed symptomatically.

DOSAGE AND ADMINISTRATION

ZOLADEX, at a dose of 3.6 mg, should be administered subcutaneously every 28 days into the upper abdominal wall using an aseptic technique under the supervision of a physician.
While a delay of a few days is permissible, every effort should be made to adhere to the 28-day schedule.
Prostate Cancer: For the management of advanced prostate cancer, ZOLADEX is intended for long-term administration unless clinically inappropriate.
Stage B2-C Prostatic Carcinoma: When ZOLADEX is given in combination with radiotherapy and flutamide for patients with Stage T2b-T4 (Stage B2-C) prostatic carcinoma, treatment should be started 8 weeks prior to initiating radiotherapy and should continue during radiation therapy. A treatment regimen using a ZOLADEX 3.6 mg depot 8 weeks before radiotherapy, followed in 28 days by the ZOLADEX 10.8 mg depot, can be administered. Alternatively, four injections of 3.6 mg depot can be administered at 28 day intervals, two depots preceding and two during radiotherapy.
Endometriosis: For the management of endometriosis, the recommended duration of administration is 6 months. Currently, there are no clinical data on the effect of treatment of benign gynecological conditions with ZOLADEX for periods in excess of 6 months.
Retreatment cannot be recommended for the management of endometriosis since safety data for retreatment are not available. If the symptoms of endometriosis recur after a course of therapy, and further treatment with ZOLADEX is contemplated, consideration should be given to monitoring bone mineral density. Clinical studies suggest the addition of Hormone Replacement Therapy (estrogens and/or progestins) to ZOLADEX is effective in reducing the bone mineral loss which occurs with ZOLADEX alone without compromising the efficacy of ZOLADEX in relieving the symptoms of endometriosis. The addition of Hormone Replacement Therapy may also reduce the occurrence of vasomotor symptoms and vaginal dryness associated with hypoestrogenism. The optimal drugs, dose and duration of treatment has not been established.
Breast Cancer: For the management of advanced breast cancer, ZOLADEX is intended for long-term administration unless clinically inappropriate.
Endometrial Thinning: For use as an endometrial-thinning agent prior to endometrial ablation, the dosing recommendation is one or two depots (with each depot given four weeks apart). When one depot is administered, surgery should be performed at four weeks. When two depots are administered, surgery should be performed within two to four weeks following administration of the second depot.
Renal or Hepatic Impairment: No dosage adjustment is necessary for patients with renal or hepatic impairment.
Administration Technique: The proper method of administration of ZOLADEX is described in the instructions that follow.

1. The package should be inspected for damage prior to opening. If the package is damaged, the syringe should not be used. Do not remove the sterile syringe from the package until immediately before use. Examine the syringe for damage, and check that ZOLADEX is visible in the translucent chamber.
2. Clean an area of the upper abdominal wall with an alcohol swab. (A local anesthetic may be used in the normal fashion at the option of the administrator or patient.)
3. Grasp red plastic safety clip tab, pull out and away from needle, and discard immediately. Then remove needle cover.
4. Using an aseptic technique, stretch or pinch the patient's skin with one hand, and grip syringe barrel. Insert the hypodermic needle into the subcutaneous tissue.

NOTE: The ZOLADEX syringe cannot be used for aspiration. If the hypodermic needle penetrates a large vessel, blood will be seen instantly in the syringe chamber. If a vessel is penetrated, withdraw the needle and inject with a new syringe elsewhere.

5. Change the direction of the needle so it parallels the abdominal wall. Push the needle in until the barrel hub touches the patient's skin. Withdraw the needle one centimeter to create a space to discharge ZOLADEX. Fully depress the plunger to discharge ZOLADEX.
6. Withdraw the needle. Then bandage the site. Confirm discharge of ZOLADEX by ensuring tip of the plunger is visible within the tip of the needle. Dispose of the used needle and syringe in a safe manner.

NOTE: In the unlikely event of the need to surgically remove ZOLADEX, it may be localized by ultrasound.

HOW SUPPLIED

ZOLADEX is supplied as a sterile and totally biodegradable D,L-lactic and glycolic acids copolymer (13.3-14.3 mg/dose) impregnated with goserelin acetate equivalent to 3.6 mg of goserelin in a disposable syringe device fitted with a 16 gauge hypodermic needle (NDC 0310-0960). The unit is sterile and comes in a sealed, light and moisture proof, aluminum foil laminate pouch containing a desiccant capsule. Store at room temperature (do not exceed 25°C).
Manufactured for:
Zeneca Pharmaceuticals
A business unit of Zeneca Inc.
Wilmington, Delaware 19850-5437
By: Zeneca Limited, Macclesfield, England
Made in the United Kingdom
64132-02 Rev G 02/99
Shown in Product Identification Guide, page 306

ZOLADEX® 3-MONTH ℞

[*zōl'-ă-dĕx*]
GOSERELIN ACETATE IMPLANT 10.8 mg
Equivalent to 10.8 mg goserelin
FOR USE IN MEN WITH PROSTATE CANCER

DESCRIPTION

ZOLADEX® (goserelin acetate implant), contains a potent synthetic decapeptide analogue of luteinizing hormone-releasing hormone (LHRH), also known as a gonadotropin releasing hormone (GnRH) agonist analogue. Goserelin acetate is chemically described as an acetate salt of [D-Ser(Bu^t)^6,Azgly^{10}]LHRH. Its chemical structure is pyro-Glu-His-Trp-Ser-Tyr-D-Ser(Bu^t)-Leu-Arg-Pro-Azgly-NH_2 acetate [$C_{59}H_{84}N_{18}O_{14} \cdot (C_2H_4O_2)_x$ where x = 1 to 2.4].
Goserelin acetate is an off-white powder with a molecular weight of 1269 Daltons (free base). It is freely soluble in glacial acetic acid. It is soluble in water, 0.1M hydrochloric acid, 0.1M sodium hydroxide, dimethylformamide and dimethyl sulfoxide. Goserelin acetate is practically insoluble in acetone, chloroform and ether.
ZOLADEX 10.8 mg implant is supplied as a sterile, biodegradable product containing goserelin acetate equivalent to 10.8 mg of goserelin. ZOLADEX is designed for subcutaneous implantation with continuous release over a 12-week period. Goserelin acetate is dispersed in a matrix of D,L-lactic and glycolic acids copolymer (12.82-14.76 mg/dose) containing less than 2% acetic acid and up to 10% goserelin-related substances and presented as a sterile, white to cream colored 1.5 mm diameter cylinder, preloaded in a special single-use syringe with a 14-gauge needle and overwrapped in a sealed, light- and moisture-proof, aluminum foil laminate pouch containing a desiccant capsule.
Studies of the D,L-lactic and glycolic acids copolymer have indicated that it is completely biodegradable and has no demonstrable antigenic potential.
ZOLADEX is also supplied as a sterile, biodegradable product containing goserelin acetate equivalent to 3.6 mg of goserelin designed for administration every 28 days.

CLINICAL PHARMACOLOGY

Mechanism of Action: ZOLADEX is a synthetic decapeptide analogue of LHRH. ZOLADEX acts as a potent inhibitor of pituitary gonadotropin secretion when administered in the biodegradable formulation.
Following initial administration, ZOLADEX causes an initial increase in serum-luteinizing hormone (LH) and follicle-stimulating hormone (FSH) levels with subsequent increases in serum levels of testosterone. Chronic administration of ZOLADEX leads to sustained suppression of pituitary gonadotropins, and serum levels of testosterone consequently fall into the range normally seen in surgically castrated men approximately 21 days after initiation of therapy. This leads to accessory sex organ regression.
In animal and in *in vitro* studies, administration of goserelin resulted in the regression or inhibition of growth of the

ADVERSE EVENTS REPORTED AT A FREQUENCY OF 5% OR GREATER IN ZOLADEX AND PLACEBO TREATMENT GROUPS OF TRIAL 0022

ADVERSE EVENT	ZOLADEX 3.6 mg (n=180) %	placebo (n=177) %	ADVERSE EVENT	ZOLADEX 3.6 mg (n=180) %	placebo (n=177) %
Whole body			**Respiratory**		
Headache	32	22	Pharyngitis	6	9
Abdominal Pain	11	10	Sinusitis	3	6
Pelvic Pain	9	6	**Skin and appendages**		
Back Pain	4	7	Sweating	16	5
Cardiovascular			**Urogenital**		
Vasodilatation	57	18	Dysmenorrhea	7	9
Migraine	7	4	Uterine Hemorrhage	6	4
Hypertension	6	2	Vulvovaginitis	5	1
Digestive			Menorrhagia	4	5
Nausea	5	6	Vaginitis	1	6
Nervous					
Nervousness	5	3			
Depression	3	7			

hormonally sensitive dimethylbenzanthracene (DMBA)-induced rat mammary tumor and Dunning R3327 prostate tumor.

In clinical trials using ZOLADEX 3.6 mg with follow-up of more than 2 years, suppression of serum testosterone to castrate levels has been maintained for the duration of therapy.

Pharmacokinetics:

Absorption: The pharmacokinetics of goserelin have been determined in healthy male volunteers and patients. In healthy males, radiolabeled goserelin was administered as a single 250 µg (aqueous solution) dose by the subcutaneous route. The absorption of radiolabeled drug was rapid, and the peak blood radioactivity levels occurred between 0.5 and 1.0 hour after dosing.

The overall pharmacokinetic profile of goserelin following administration of a ZOLADEX 10.8 mg depot to patients with prostate cancer was determined. The initial release of goserelin from the depot was relatively rapid resulting in a peak concentration at 2 hours after dosing. From Day 4 until the end of the 12-week dosing interval, the sustained release of goserelin from the depot produced reasonably stable systemic exposure. Mean (Standard Deviation) pharmacokinetic data are presented in Table 1. There is no clinically significant accumulation of goserelin following administration of four depots administered at 12-week intervals. Pharmacokinetic data were obtained using an RIA method, which has been shown to be specific for goserelin in the presence of its metabolites.

[See table 1 above]

Serum goserelin concentrations in prostate cancer patients administered three 3.6 mg depots followed by one 10.8 mg depot are displayed in Figure 1. The profiles for both formulations are primarily dependent upon the rate of drug release from the depots. For the 3.6 mg depot, mean concentrations gradually rise to reach a peak of about 3 ng/mL at around 15 days after administration and then decline to approximately 0.5 ng/mL by the end of the treatment period. For the 10.8 mg depot, mean concentrations increase to reach a peak of about 8 ng/mL within the first 24 hours and then decline rapidly up to Day 4. Thereafter, mean concentrations remain relatively stable in the range of about 0.3 to 1 ng/mL up to the end of the treatment period.

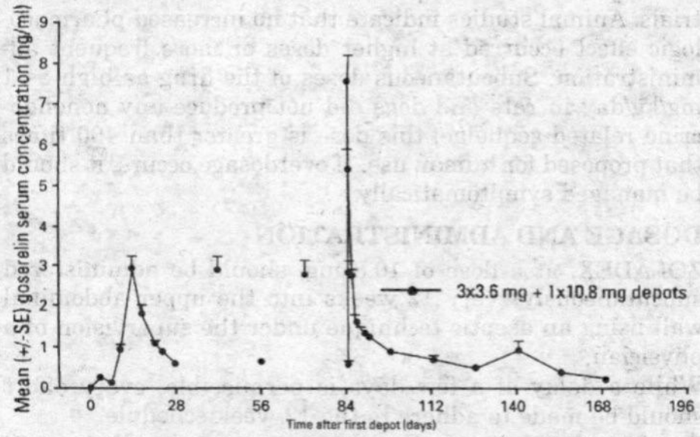

Figure 1: Goserelin serum concentrations during dosing three ZOLADEX 3.6 mg depots (0, 28, 56 days) then one ZOLADEX 10.8 mg depot (84 days) to prostate cancer patients.

Administration of four ZOLADEX 10.8 mg depots to patients with prostate cancer resulted in testosterone levels that were suppressed to and maintained within the range normally observed in surgically castrated men (0–1.73 nmol/L or 0–50 ng/dL), over the dosing interval in approximately 91% (145/160) of patients studied. In 6 of 15 patients that escaped from castrate range, serum testosterone levels were maintained below 2.0 nmol/L (58 ng/dL) and in only one of the 15 patients did the depot completely fail to maintain serum testosterone levels to within the castrate range over a 336-day period (4 depot injections). In the 8 additional patients, a transient escape was followed 14 days later by a level within the castrate range.

Distribution: The apparent volume of distribution determined after subcutaneous administration of 250 µg aqueous solution of goserelin was 44.1 ± 13.6 liters for healthy males. The plasma protein binding of goserelin was found to be 27%.

Metabolism: Metabolism of goserelin, by hydrolysis of the C-terminal amino acids, is the major clearance mechanism. The major circulating component in serum appeared to be 1–7 fragment, and the major component present in urine of one healthy male volunteer was 5–10 fragment. The metabolism of goserelin in humans yields a similar but narrow profile of metabolites to that found in other species. All metabolites found in humans have also been found in toxicology species.

Excretion: Clearance of goserelin following subcutaneous administration of a radiolabeled solution of goserelin was very rapid and occurred via a combination of hepatic and urinary excretion. More than 90% of a subcutaneous radiolabeled solution formulation dose of goserelin was excreted in urine. Approximately 20% of the dose recovered in urine was accounted for by unchanged goserelin.

Special Populations

Renal Insufficiency: In clinical trials with the solution formulation of goserelin, subjects with impaired renal function (creatinine clearance less than 20 mL/min) had a serum elimination half-life of 12.1 hours compared to 4.2 hours for subjects with normal renal function (creatinine clearance greater than 70 mL/min). However, there was no evidence for any accumulation of goserelin on multiple dosing of the ZOLADEX 10.8 mg depot to subjects with impaired renal function. There was no evidence for any increase in incidence of adverse events in renally impaired patients administered the 10.8 mg depot. These data indicate that there is no need for any dosage adjustment when administering ZOLADEX 10.8 mg to subjects with impaired renal function.

Table 1

Goserelin pharmacokinetic parameters for the 10.8 mg depot

Parameter	n	Mean	(SD)	95% CI Lower	95% CI Upper
Systemic clearance (mL/min)	41	121	(42.4)	108	134
C_{max} (ng/mL)	41	8.85	(2.83)	7.96	9.74
T_{max} (h)	41	1.80	(0.34)	1.70	1.92
C_{min} (ng/mL)	44	0.37	(0.21)	0.30	0.43
Elimination Half-life (h)¶	7	4.16	(1.12)	3.12	5.20

¶ = determined after subcutaneous administration of 250 µg aqueous solution of goserelin.
SD = standard deviation
95% CI = 95% confidence interval

Hepatic Insufficiency: The clearance and half-life of goserelin administered as an aqueous solution are not affected by hepatic impairment. These data indicate that there is no need for any dosage adjustment when administering ZOLADEX 10.8 mg to subjects with impaired hepatic function.

Geriatric: There is no need for any dosage adjustment when administering ZOLADEX 10.8 mg to geriatric patients.

Body Weight: A decline of approximately 1 to 2.5% in the AUC after administration of a 10.8 mg depot was observed with a kilogram increase in body weight. In obese patients who have not responded clinically, testosterone levels should be monitored closely.

Drug-Drug Interactions: No formal drug-drug interaction studies have been performed.

Clinical Studies - Prostatic Carcinoma: In two controlled clinical trials, 160 patients with advanced prostate cancer were randomized to receive either one 3.6 mg ZOLADEX implant every four weeks or a single 10.8 mg ZOLADEX implant every 12 weeks. Mean serum testosterone suppression was similar between the two arms. PSA falls at three months were 94% in patients who received the 10.8 mg implant and 92.5% in patients that received three 3.6 mg implants.

Periodic monitoring of serum testosterone levels should be considered if the anticipated clinical or biochemical response to treatment has not been achieved. A clinical outcome similar to that produced with the use of the 3.6 mg implant administered every 28 days is predicted with ZOLADEX 10.8 mg implant administered every 12 weeks (84 days). Total testosterone was measured by the DPC Coat-A-Count radioimmunoassay method which, as defined by the manufacturers, is highly specific and accurate. Acceptable variability of approximately 20% at low testosterone levels has been demonstrated in the clinical studies performed with the ZOLADEX 10.8 mg depot.

Clinical Studies - Stage B2-C Prostatic Carcinoma: The effects of hormonal treatment combined with radiation were studied in 466 patients (231 ZOLADEX + flutamide + radiation, 235 radiation alone) with bulky primary tumors confined to the prostate (stage B2) or extending beyond the capsule (stage C), with or without pelvic node involvement.

In this multicentered, controlled trial, administration of ZOLADEX (3.6 mg depot) and flutamide capsules (250 mg t.i.d.) prior to and during radiation was associated with a significantly lower rate of local failure compared to radiation alone (16% vs 33% at 4 years, P<0.001). The combination therapy also resulted in a trend toward reduction in the incidence of distant metastases (27% vs 36% at 4 years, P =0.058). Median disease-free survival was significantly increased in patients who received complete hormonal therapy combined with radiation as compared to those patients who received radiation alone (4.4 vs 2.6 years, P<0.001). Inclusion of normal PSA level as a criterion for disease-free survival also resulted in significantly increased median disease-free survival in patients receiving the combination therapy (2.7 vs 1.5 years, P<0.001).

INDICATIONS AND USAGE

Prostatic Carcinoma: ZOLADEX is indicated in the palliative treatment of advanced carcinoma of the prostate.

In controlled studies of patients with advanced prostatic cancer comparing ZOLADEX 3.6 mg to orchiectomy, the long-term endocrine responses and objective responses were similar between the two treatment arms. Additionally, duration of survival was similar between the two treatment arms in a major comparative trial.

In controlled studies of patients with advanced prostatic cancer, ZOLADEX 10.8 mg implant produced pharmacodynamically similar effect in terms of suppression of serum testosterone to that achieved with ZOLADEX 3.6 mg implant. Clinical outcome similar to that produced with the use of the ZOLADEX 3.6 mg implant administered every 28 days is predicted with the ZOLADEX 10.8 mg implant administered every 12 weeks.

Stage B2-C Prostatic Carcinoma: ZOLADEX is indicated for use in combination with flutamide for the management of locally confined Stage T2b-T4 (Stage B2-C) carcinoma of the prostate. Treatment with ZOLADEX and flutamide should start 8 weeks prior to initiating radiation therapy and continue during radiation therapy.

CONTRAINDICATIONS

A report of an anaphylactic reaction to synthetic GnRH (Factrel) has been reported in the medical literature. ZOLADEX is contraindicated in those patients who have a known hypersensitivity to LHRH, LHRH agonist analogues or any of the components in ZOLADEX.

ZOLADEX 10.8 mg implant is not indicated in women as the data are insufficient to support reliable suppression of serum estradiol. For female patients requiring treatment with goserelin, refer to the prescribing information for ZOLADEX 3.6 mg implant.

ZOLADEX is contraindicated in women who are or may become pregnant while receiving the drug. In studies in rats and rabbits, ZOLADEX increased preimplantation loss, resorptions, and abortions (see Pregnancy section). In rats and dogs, ZOLADEX suppressed ovarian function, decreased ovarian weight and size, and led to atrophic changes in secondary sex organs. Further evidence suggests that fertility was reduced in female rats that became pregnant after ZOLADEX was stopped. These effects are an expected consequence of the hormonal alterations produced by ZOLADEX in humans. If a patient becomes pregnant during treatment, the drug must be discontinued and the patient must be apprised of the potential risk for loss of the pregnancy due to possible hormonal imbalance as a result of the expected pharmacologic action of ZOLADEX treatment. In animal studies, there was no evidence that ZOLADEX possessed the potential to cause teratogenicity in rabbits; however, in rats the incidence of umbilical hernia was significantly increased with treatment. (See Pregnancy, Teratogenic Effects.)

WARNINGS

Initially, ZOLADEX, like other LHRH agonists, causes transient increases in serum levels of testosterone. Transient worsening of symptoms, or the occurrence of additional signs and symptoms of prostatic cancer, may occasionally develop during the first few weeks of ZOLADEX treatment. A small number of patients may experience a temporary increase in bone pain, which can be managed symptomatically. As with other LHRH agonists, isolated cases of ureteral obstruction and spinal cord compression have been observed. If spinal cord compression or renal impairment develops, standard treatment of these complications should be instituted, and in extreme cases an immediate orchiectomy considered.

PRECAUTIONS

General: Hypersensitivity, antibody formation and acute anaphylactic reactions have been reported with LHRH agonist analogues.

Of 115 women worldwide treated with ZOLADEX 3.6 mg and tested for development of binding to goserelin following treatment with ZOLADEX, one patient showed low-titer binding to goserelin. On further testing of this patient's plasma obtained following treatment, her goserelin binding component was found not to be precipitated with rabbit antihuman immunoglobulin polyvalent sera. These findings suggest the possibility of antibody formation.

Information for Patients: The use of ZOLADEX in patients at particular risk of developing ureteral obstruction or spinal cord compression should be considered carefully and the patients monitored closely during the first month of therapy. Patients with ureteral obstruction or spinal cord compression should have appropriate treatment prior to initiation of ZOLADEX therapy.

Drug Interactions: No drug interaction studies with other drugs have been conducted with ZOLADEX. No confirmed interactions have been reported between ZOLADEX and other drugs.

Drug/Laboratory Test Interactions: Administration of ZOLADEX in therapeutic doses results in suppression of the pituitary-gonadal system. Because of this suppression, diagnostic tests of pituitary-gonadotropic and gonadal functions conducted during treatment may show results which are misleading.

Carcinogenesis, Mutagenesis, Impairment of Fertility: Subcutaneous implant of ZOLADEX in male and female rats once every 4 weeks for 1 year and recovery for 23 weeks at doses of about 80 and 150 µg/kg (males) and 50 and 100 µg/kg (females) daily (about 3 to 9 times the recommended human dose on a mg/m^2 basis) resulted in an increased incidence of pituitary adenomas. An increased incidence of pituitary adenomas was also observed following subcutaneous implant of ZOLADEX in rats at similar dose levels for a period of 72 weeks in males and 101 weeks in females. The relevance of the rat pituitary adenomas to humans has not

Continued on next page

Zoladex 3 month—Cont.

been established. Subcutaneous implants of ZOLADEX every 3 weeks for 2 years delivered to mice at doses of up to 2400 μg/kg/day (about 70 times the recommended human dose on a mg/m² basis) resulted in an increased incidence of histiocytic sarcoma of the vertebral column and femur.

Mutagenicity tests using bacterial and mammalian systems for point mutations and cytogenetic effects have provided no evidence for mutagenic potential.

Administration of goserelin led to changes that were consistent with gonadal suppression in both male and female rats as a result of its endocrine action. In male rats administered 500-1000 μg/kg/day (about 30-60 times the recommended human dose on a mg/m² basis), a decrease in weight and atrophic histological changes were observed in the testes, epididymis, seminal vesicle and prostate gland with complete suppression of spermatogenesis. In female rats administered 50-1000 μg/kg/day (about 3-60 times the recommended daily human dose on a mg/m² basis), suppression of ovarian function led to decreased size and weight of ovaries and secondary sex organs; follicular development was arrested at the antral stage and the corpora lutea were reduced in size and number. Except for the testes, almost complete histologic reversal of these effects in males and females was observed several weeks after dosing was stopped; however, fertility and general reproductive performance were reduced in those that became pregnant after goserelin was discontinued. Fertile matings occurred within 2 weeks after cessation of dosing, even though total recovery of reproductive function may not have occurred before mating took place; and, the ovulation rate, the corresponding implantation rate, and number of live fetuses were reduced.

Based on histological examination, drug effects on reproductive organs seem to be completely reversible in male and female dogs when drug treatment was stopped after continuous administration for 1 year at 100 times the recommended monthly dose.

Pregnancy, Teratogenic Effects: Pregnancy Category X. See **CONTRAINDICATIONS** section. ZOLADEX 10.8 mg is not indicated in women as the data are insufficient to support reliable suppression of serum estradiol. Studies in both rats and rabbits at doses of 2, 10, 20, and 50 μg/kg/day and 20, 250, and 1,000 μg/kg/day, respectively (about 1/10 to 3 times and 2 to 100 times the daily maximum recommended human dose, respectively, on a mg/m² basis) administered during the period of organogenesis, have confirmed that ZOLADEX will increase pregnancy loss in a dose-related manner. While there was no evidence that ZOLADEX possessed the potential to cause teratogenicity in rabbits, in rats the incidence of umbilical hernia was significantly increased at doses greater than 10 mg/kg/day (about 1/2 the recommended dose on a mg/m² basis).

Nursing Mothers: It is not known if this drug is excreted in human milk. Many drugs are excreted in human milk and there is a potential for serious adverse reactions in nursing infants of mothers receiving ZOLADEX (See CONTRAINDICATIONS).

Pediatric Use: Safety and efficacy of ZOLADEX in pediatric patients have not been established.

ADVERSE REACTIONS

General: Rarely, hypersensitivity reactions (including urticaria and anaphylaxis) have been reported in patients receiving ZOLADEX.

As with other endocrine therapies, hypercalcemia (increased calcium) has rarely been reported in cancer patients with bone metastases following initiation of treatment with ZOLADEX or other LHRH agonists.

ZOLADEX has been found to be generally well tolerated in clinical trials. Adverse reactions reported in these trials were rarely severe enough to result in the patients' withdrawal from ZOLADEX treatment. As seen with other hormonal therapies, the most commonly observed adverse events during ZOLADEX therapy were due to the expected physiological effects from decreased testosterone levels. These included hot flashes, sexual dysfunction and decreased erections.

Initially, ZOLADEX, like other LHRH agonists, causes transient increases in serum levels of testosterone. A small percentage of patients experienced a temporary worsening of signs and symptoms (see WARNINGS section), usually manifested by an increase in cancer-related pain which was managed symptomatically. Isolated cases of exacerbation of disease symptoms, either ureteral obstruction or spinal cord compression, occurred at similar rates in controlled clinical trials with both ZOLADEX and orchiectomy. The relationship of these events to therapy is uncertain.

Changes in the hormonal environment following treatment with an LHRH analogue or orchiectomy may result in a loss in bone mineral density due to a marked reduction of testosterone concentrations.

Changes in blood pressure, manifest as hypotension or hypertension, have been occasionally observed in patients administered ZOLADEX. The changes are usually transient, resolving either during continued therapy or after cessation of therapy with ZOLADEX. Rarely, such changes have been sufficient to require medical intervention including withdrawal of treatment from ZOLADEX.

Two controlled clinical trials using ZOLADEX 10.8 mg versus ZOLADEX 3.6 mg were conducted. During a comparative phase, patients were randomized to receive either a single 10.8 mg implant or three consecutive 3.6 mg implants every 4 weeks over weeks 0-12. During this phase, the only adverse event reported in greater than 5% of patients was hot flashes, with an incidence of 47% in the ZOLADEX 10.8 mg group and 48% in the ZOLADEX 3.6 mg group.

From weeks 12-48 all patients were treated with a 10.8 mg implant every 12 weeks. During this noncomparative phase, the following adverse events were reported in greater than 5% of patients:

Adverse Event	ZOLADEX 10.8 mg (n = 157) %
Hot Flashes	64
Pain (General)	14
Gynecomastia	8
Pelvic Pain	6
Bone Pain	6
Asthenia	5

The following adverse events were reported in greater than 1%, but less than 5% of patients treated with ZOLADEX 10.8 mg implant every 12 weeks. Some of these are commonly reported in elderly patients.

WHOLE BODY - Abdominal pain, Back pain, Flu syndrome, Headache, Sepsis, Aggravation reaction
CARDIOVASCULAR - Angina pectoris, Cerebral ischemia, Cerebrovascular accident, Heart failure, Pulmonary embolus, Varicose veins
DIGESTIVE - Diarrhea, Hematemesis
ENDOCRINE - Diabetes mellitus
HEMATOLOGIC - Anemia
METABOLIC - Peripheral edema
NERVOUS SYSTEM - Dizziness, Paresthesia, Urinary retention
RESPIRATORY - Cough increased, Dyspnea, Pneumonia
SKIN - Herpes simplex, Pruritus
UROGENITAL - Bladder neoplasm, Breast pain, Hematuria, Impotence, Urinary frequency, Urinary incontinence, Urinary tract disorder, Urinary tract infection, Urination impaired.

The following adverse events not already listed above were reported in patients receiving ZOLADEX 3.6 mg in other clinical trials. Inclusion does not necessarily represent a causal relationship to ZOLADEX 10.8 mg.

WHOLE BODY: Allergic reaction, Chills, Fever, Infection, Injection site reaction, Lethargy, Malaise
CARDIOVASCULAR: Arrhythmia, Chest pain, Hemorrhage, Hypertension, Migraine, Myocardial infarction, Palpitations, Peripheral vascular disorder, Tachycardia
DIGESTIVE: Anorexia, Constipation, Dry mouth, Dyspepsia, Flatulence, Increased appetite, Nausea, Ulcer, Vomiting
HEMATOLOGIC: Ecchymosis
METABOLIC: Edema, Gout, Hyperglycemia, Weight increase
MUSCULOSKELETAL: Arthralgia, Hypertonia, Joint disorder, Leg cramps, Myalgia, Osteoporosis
NERVOUS SYSTEM: Anxiety, Depression, Emotional lability, Headache, Insomnia, Nervousness, Somnolence, Thinking abnormal
RESPIRATORY: Bronchitis, Chronic obstructive pulmonary disease, Epistaxis, Rhinitis, Sinusitis, Upper respiratory infection, Voice alterations
SKIN: Acne, Alopecia, Dry skin, Hair disorders, Rash, Seborrhea, Skin discoloration, Sweating
SPECIAL SENSES: Amblyopia, Dry eyes
UROGENITAL: Breast tenderness, Decreased erections, Renal insufficiency, Sexual dysfunction, Urinary obstruction

Stage B2-C Prostatic Carcinoma: Treatment with ZOLADEX and flutamide did not add substantially to the toxicity of radiation treatment alone. The following adverse experiences were reported during a multicenter clinical trial comparing ZOLADEX + flutamide + radiation versus radiation alone. The most frequently reported (greater than 5%) adverse experiences are listed below.

ADVERSE EVENTS DURING ACUTE RADIATION THERAPY
(within first 90 days of radiation therapy)

	(n=231) flutamide + ZOLADEX + Radiation % All	(n=235) Radiation Only % All
Rectum/Large Bowel	80	76
Bladder	58	60
Skin	37	37

ADVERSE EVENTS DURING LATE RADIATION PHASE
(after 90 days of radiation therapy)

	(n=231) flutamide + ZOLADEX + Radiation % All	(n=235) Radiation Only % All
Diarrhea	36	40
Cystitis	16	16
Rectal Bleeding	14	20
Proctitis	8	8
Hematuria	7	12

[See first table above]
[See second table above]

Additional adverse event data was collected for the combination therapy with radiation group over both the hormonal treatment and hormonal treatment plus radiation phases of the study. Adverse experiences occurring in more than 5% of patients in this group, over both parts of the study, were hot flashes (46%), diarrhea (40%), nausea (9%), and skin rash (8%).

Changes in Laboratory Values During Treatment

Plasma Enzymes: Elevation of liver enzymes (AST, ALT) have been reported in female patients exposed to ZOLADEX 3.6 mg (representing less than 1% of all patients). There was no other evidence of abnormal liver function. Causality between these changes and ZOLADEX have not been established.

Lipids: In a controlled trial in females, ZOLADEX 3.6 mg implant therapy resulted in a minor, but statistically significant effect on serum lipids (ie, increases in LDL cholesterol of 21.3 mg/dL; increases in HDL cholesterol of 2.7 mg/dL; and triglycerides increased by 8.0 mg/dL).

OVERDOSAGE

The pharmacologic properties of ZOLADEX and its mode of administration make accidental or intentional overdosage unlikely. There is no experience of overdosage from clinical trials. Animal studies indicate that no increased pharmacologic effect occurred at higher doses or more frequent administration. Subcutaneous doses of the drug as high as 1 mg/kg/day in rats and dogs did not produce any nonendocrine related sequelae; this dose is greater than 400 times that proposed for human use. If overdosage occurs, it should be managed symptomatically.

DOSAGE AND ADMINISTRATION

ZOLADEX, at a dose of 10.8 mg, should be administered subcutaneously every 12 weeks into the upper abdominal wall using an aseptic technique under the supervision of a physician.

While a delay of a few days is permissible, every effort should be made to adhere to the 12-week schedule.

Prostatic Carcinoma: For the management of advanced prostate cancer, ZOLADEX is intended for long-term administration unless clinically inappropriate.

Stage B2-C Prostatic Carcinoma: When ZOLADEX is given in combination with radiotherapy and flutamide for patients with Stage T2b-T4 (Stage B2-C) prostatic carcinoma, treatment should be started 8 weeks prior to initiating radiotherapy and should continue during radiation therapy. A treatment regimen using one ZOLADEX 3.6 mg depot, followed in 28 days by one ZOLADEX 10.8 mg depot, should be administered.

Renal or Hepatic Impairment: No dosage adjustment is necessary for patients with renal or hepatic impairment.

Females: ZOLADEX 10.8 mg implant is not indicated in women as the data are insufficient to support reliable suppression of serum estradiol. For female patients requiring treatment with goserelin, refer to the prescribing information for ZOLADEX 3.6 mg implant.

Administration Technique: The proper method of administration of ZOLADEX is described in the instructions that follow.

1. The package should be inspected for damage prior to opening. If the package is damaged, the syringe should not be used. Do not remove the sterile syringe from the package until immediately before use. Examine the syringe for damage, and check that ZOLADEX is visible in the translucent chamber.
2. Clean an area of the upper abdominal wall with an alcohol swab. (A local anesthetic may be used in the normal fashion at the option of the administrator or patient.)
3. Grasp blue plastic safety clip tab, pull out and away from needle, and discard immediately. Then remove needle cover.
4. Using an aseptic technique, stretch or pinch the patient's skin with one hand, and grip the syringe barrel. Insert the hypodermic needle into the subcutaneous tissue.
   NOTE: The ZOLADEX syringe cannot be used for aspiration. If the hypodermic needle penetrates a large vessel, blood will be seen instantly in the syringe chamber. If a vessel is penetrated, withdraw the needle and inject with a new syringe elsewhere.
5. Change the direction of the needle so it parallels the abdominal wall. Push the needle in until the barrel hub touches the patient's skin. Withdraw the needle one centimeter to create a space to discharge ZOLADEX. Fully depress the plunger to discharge ZOLADEX.

6. Withdraw the needle. Then bandage the site. Confirm discharge of ZOLADEX by ensuring tip of the plunger is visible within the tip of the needle. Dispose of the used needle and syringe in a safe manner.

NOTE: In the unlikely event of the need to surgically remove ZOLADEX, it may be localized by ultrasound.

HOW SUPPLIED

ZOLADEX 10.8 mg implant is supplied as a sterile and totally biodegradable D,L-lactic and glycolic acids copolymer (12.82-14.76 mg/dose) impregnated with goserelin acetate equivalent to 10.8 mg of goserelin in a disposable syringe device fitted with a 14-gauge hypodermic needle (NDC 0310-0961). The unit is sterile and comes in a sealed, light- and moisture-proof, aluminum foil laminate pouch containing a desiccant capsule. Store at room temperature (do not exceed 25°C).

Manufactured for:
Zeneca Pharmaceuticals
A Business Unit of Zeneca Inc.
Wilmington, Delaware 19850-5437
By: Zeneca Limited, Macclesfield, England
Made in the United Kingdom
64140-01 Rev G 02/99

ZOMIG® ℞

[*zō-mĭg*]
(zolmitriptan)
Tablets

DESCRIPTION

ZOMIG® (zolmitriptan) Tablets contain zolmitriptan, which is a selective 5-hydroxytryptamine $_{1B/1D}$ (5-$HT_{1B/1D}$) receptor agonist. Zolmitriptan is chemically designated as (S)-4-[[3-[2-(Dimethylamino)ethyl]-1H-indol-5-yl]methyl]-2-oxazolidinone and has the following chemical structure:

The empirical formula is $C_{16}H_{21}N_3O_2$, representing a molecular weight of 287.36. Zolmitriptan is a white to almost white powder that is readily soluble in water. ZOMIG is supplied as 2.5 mg (yellow) and 5 mg (pink) tablets for oral administration. The film-coated tablets contain anhydrous lactose NF, microcrystalline cellulose NF, sodium starch glycolate NF, magnesium stearate NF, hydroxypropyl methylcellulose USP, titanium dioxide USP, polyethylene glycol 400 NF, yellow iron oxide NF (2.5 mg tablet), red iron oxide NF (5 mg tablet), and polyethylene glycol 8000 NF.

CLINICAL PHARMACOLOGY

Mechanism of Action: Zolmitriptan binds with high affinity to human recombinant 5-HT_{1D} and 5-HT_{1B} receptors. Zolmitriptan exhibits modest affinity for 5-HT_{1A} receptors, but has no significant affinity (as measured by radioligand binding assays) or pharmacological activity at 5-HT_2, 5-HT_3, 5-HT_4, alpha$_{1-}$, alpha$_{2-}$, or beta$_{1-}$ adrenergic; H_1, H_2, histaminic; muscarinic; dopamine$_1$, or dopamine$_2$ receptors. The N-desmethyl metabolite also has high affinity for 5-$HT_{1B/1D}$ and modest affinity for 5-HT_{1A} receptors.

Current theories proposed to explain the etiology of migraine headache suggest that symptoms are due to local cranial vasodilatation and/or to the release of sensory neuropeptides (vasoactive intestinal peptide, substance P and calcitonin gene-related peptide) through nerve endings in the trigeminal system. The therapeutic activity of zolmitriptan for the treatment of migraine headache can most likely be attributed to the agonist effects at the 5-$HT_{1B/1D}$ receptors on intracranial blood vessels (including the arteriovenous anastomoses) and sensory nerves of the trigeminal system which result in cranial vessel constriction and inhibition of pro-inflammatory neuropeptide release.

Pharmacokinetics: Zolmitriptan is well absorbed after oral administration with peak plasma concentrations occurring in 2 hours. Mean absolute bioavailability is approximately 40%. Zolmitriptan displays linear kinetics over the dose range of 2.5 to 50 mg. The mean elimination half-life of zolmitriptan and of the active N-desmethyl metabolite is 3 hours. Zolmitriptan is converted to an active N-desmethyl metabolite such that the metabolite concentrations are about two thirds that of zolmitriptan. Because the 5-$HT_{1B/1D}$ potency of the metabolite is 2 to 6 times that of the parent, the metabolite may contribute a substantial portion of the overall effect after zolmitriptan administration. The T_{max} for this metabolite is approximately 2 to 3 hours. No accumulation occurred on multiple dosing. Food has no significant effect on the bioavailability of zolmitriptan.

The mean apparent volume of distribution is 7.0 L/kg. Plasma protein binding of zolmitriptan is 25% over the concentration range of 10–1000 ng/mL.

Total radioactivity recovered in urine and feces was 65% and 30% of the administered dose, respectively. About 8% of the dose was recovered in the urine as unchanged zolmitriptan. Indole acetic acid metabolite accounted for 31% of the dose, followed by N-oxide (7%) and N-desmethyl (4%) metabolites. The indole acetic acid and N-oxide metabolites are inactive.

Mean total plasma clearance is 31.5 mL/min/kg, of which one-sixth is renal clearance. The renal clearance is greater than the glomerular filtration rate suggesting renal tubular secretion.

During a moderate to severe migraine attack, mean AUC_{0-4} and C_{max} for zolmitriptan were decreased by 40% and 25%, respectively, and mean T_{max} was delayed by one-half hour compared to the same patients during a migraine-free period.

Special Populations

Age: Zolmitriptan pharmacokinetics in healthy elderly non-migraineur volunteers (age 65–76 yrs) were similar to those in younger non-migraineur volunteers (age 18–39 yrs).

Gender: Mean plasma concentrations of zolmitriptan were up to 1.5-fold higher in females than males.

Renal Impairment: Clearance of zolmitriptan was reduced by 25% in patients with severe renal impairment (Clcr $\geq$ 5 $\leq$ 25 mL/min) compared to the normal group (Clcr > = 70 mL/min); no significant change in clearance was observed in the moderately renally impaired group (Clcr $\geq$ 26 $\leq$ 50 mL/min).

Hepatic Impairment: In severely hepatically impaired patients, the mean C_{max}, T_{max}, and $AUC_{0-\infty}$ of zolmitriptan were increased 1.5, 2 (2 vs 4 hr), and 3-fold, respectively, compared to normals. Seven out of 27 patients experienced 20 to 80 mm Hg elevations in systolic and/or diastolic blood pressure after a 10 mg dose. Zolmitriptan should be administered with caution in subjects with liver disease, generally using doses less than 2.5 mg (see WARNINGS and PRECAUTIONS).

Hypertensive Patients: No differences in the pharmacokinetics of zolmitriptan or its effects on blood pressure were seen in mild to moderate hypertensive volunteers compared to normotensive controls.

Race: Retrospective analysis of pharmacokinetic data between Japanese and Caucasians revealed no significant differences.

Drug Interactions: All drug interaction studies were performed in healthy volunteers using a single 10 mg dose of zolmitriptan and a single dose of the other drug except where otherwise noted.

Fluoxetine: The pharmacokinetics of zolmitriptan, as well as its effect on blood pressure, were unaffected by 4 weeks of pretreatment with oral fluoxetine (20 mg/day).

MAO Inhibitors: Following one week of administration of 150 mg bid moclobemide, a specific MAO-A inhibitor, there was an increase of about 25% in both C_{max} and AUC for zolmitriptan and a 3-fold increase in the C_{max} and AUC of the active N-desmethyl metabolite of zolmitriptan (see CONTRAINDICATIONS and PRECAUTIONS).

Selegiline, a selective MAO-B inhibitor, at a dose of 10 mg/day for 1 week, had no effect on the pharmacokinetics of zolmitriptan and its metabolite.

Propranolol: C_{max} and AUC of zolmitriptan increased 1.5-fold after one week of dosing with propranolol (160 mg/day). C_{max} and AUC of the N-desmethyl metabolite were reduced by 30% and 15%, respectively. There were no interactive effects on blood pressure or pulse rate following administration of propranolol with zolmitriptan.

Acetaminophen: A single 1 g dose of acetaminophen does not alter the pharmacokinetics of zolmitriptan and its N-desmethyl metabolite. However, zolmitriptan delayed the T_{max} of acetaminophen by one hour.

Metoclopramide: A single 10 mg dose of metoclopramide had no effect on the pharmacokinetics of zolmitriptan or its metabolites.

Oral Contraceptives: Retrospective analysis of pharmacokinetic data across studies indicated that mean plasma concentrations of zolmitriptan were generally higher in females taking oral contraceptives compared to those not taking oral contraceptives. Mean C_{max} and AUC of zolmitriptan were found to be higher by 30% and 50%, respectively, and T_{max} was delayed by one-half hour in females taking oral contraceptives. The effect of zolmitriptan on the pharmacokinetics of oral contraceptives has not been studied.

Cimetidine: Following the administration of cimetidine, the half-life and AUC of a 5 mg dose of zolmitriptan and its active metabolite were approximately doubled (see PRECAUTIONS).

Clinical Studies: The efficacy of ZOMIG Tablets in the acute treatment of migraine headaches was demonstrated in five randomized, double blind, placebo controlled studies, of which 2 utilized the 1 mg dose, 2 utilized the 2.5 mg dose and 4 utilized the 5 mg dose; all studies used the marketed formulation. In study 1, patients treated their headaches in a clinic setting. In the other studies, patients treated their headaches as outpatients. In study 4, patients who had previously used sumatriptan were excluded, whereas in the other studies no such exclusion was applied. Patients enrolled in these 5 studies were predominantly female (82%) and Caucasian (97%) with a mean age of 40 yeas (range 12–65). Patients were instructed to treat a moderate to severe headache. Headache response, defined as a reduction in headache severity from moderate or severe pain to mild or no pain, was assessed at 1, 2, and, in most studies, 4 hours after dosing. Associated symptoms such as nausea, photophobia, and phonophobia were also assessed. Maintenance of response was assessed for up to 24 hours postdose. A second dose of ZOMIG Tablets or other medication was allowed 2 to 24 hours after the initial treatment for persistent and recurrent headache. The frequency and time to use of these additional treatments were also recorded. In all studies, the effect of zolmitriptan was compared to placebo in the treatment of a single migraine attack.

In all five studies, the percentage of patients achieving headache response 2 hours after treatment was significantly greater among patients receiving ZOMIG Tablets at all doses (except for the 1 mg dose in the smallest study) compared to those who received placebo. In the two studies that evaluated the 1 mg dose, there was a statistically significant greater percentage of patients with headache response at 2 hours in the higher dose groups (2.5 and/or 5 mg) compared to the 1 mg dose group. There were no statistically significant differences between the 2.5 and 5 mg dose groups (or of doses up to 20 mg) for the primary end point of headache response at 2 hours in any study. The results of these controlled clinical studies are summarized in Table 1.

Comparisons of drug performance based upon results obtained in different clinical trials are never reliable. Because studies are conducted at different times, with different samples of patients, by different investigators, employing different criteria and/or different interpretations of the same criteria, under different conditions (dose, dosing regimen, etc.), quantitative estimates of treatment response and the timing of response may be expected to vary considerably from study to study.

Table 1: Percentage of Patients with Headache Response (Mild or no Headache) 2 Hours Following Treatment (n = number of patients randomized).

	Placebo	ZOMIG 1.0 mg	ZOMIG 2.5 mg	ZOMIG 5 mg
Study 1[a]	16% (n=19)	27% (n=22)	NA	60%*# (n=20)
Study 2	19% (n=88)	NA	NA	66%* (n=179)
Study 3	34% (n=121)	50%* (n=140)	65%*# (n=260)	67%*# (n=245)
Study 4[b]	44% (n=55)	NA	NA	59%* (n=491)
Study 5	36% (n=92)	NA NA	62%* (n=178)	NA

* p<0.05 in comparison with placebo.
\# p<0.05 in comparison with 1 mg.
a This was the only study in which patients treated the headache in a clinic setting.
b This was the only study where patients were excluded who had previously used sumatriptan.
NA - not applicable

The estimated probability of achieving an initial headache response by 4 hours following treatment is depicted in Figure 1.

Figure 1: Estimated probability of Achieving initial headache response within 4 hours *

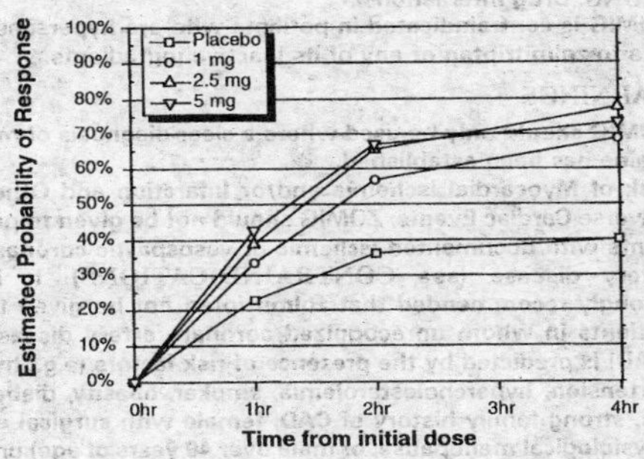

*Figure 1 shows the Kaplan Meier plot of the probability over time of obtaining headache response (no or mild pain) following treatment with zolmitriptan. The averages displayed are based on pooled data from 3 placebo controlled, outpatient, trials providing evidence of efficacy (Trials 2, 3 and 5). Patients not achieving headache response or taking additional treatment prior to 4 hours were censored at 4 hours.

For patients with migraine associated photophobia, phonophobia, and nausea at baseline, there was a decreased incidence of these symptoms following administration of ZOMIG as compared to placebo.

Two to 24 hours following the initial dose of study treatment, patients were allowed to use additional treatment for pain relief in the form of a second dose of study treatment or other medication. The estimated probability of patients taking a second dose or other medication for migraine over the 24 hours following the initial dose of study treatment is summarized in Figure 2.

[See figure 2 at top of next column]

The efficacy of ZOMIG was unaffected by presence of aura; duration of headache prior to treatment; relationship to menses; gender, age, or weight of the patient; pretreatment nausea, or concomitant use of common migraine prophylactic drugs.

INDICATIONS AND USAGE

ZOMIG is indicated for the acute treatment of migraine with or without aura in adults.

ZOMIG is not intended for the prophylactic therapy of migraine or for use in the management of hemiplegic or basi-

Continued on next page

Zomig—Cont.

Figure 2: The Estimated Probability Of Patients Taking A Second Dose Or Other Medication For Migraines Over The 24 Hours Following The Initial Dose Of Study Treatment *

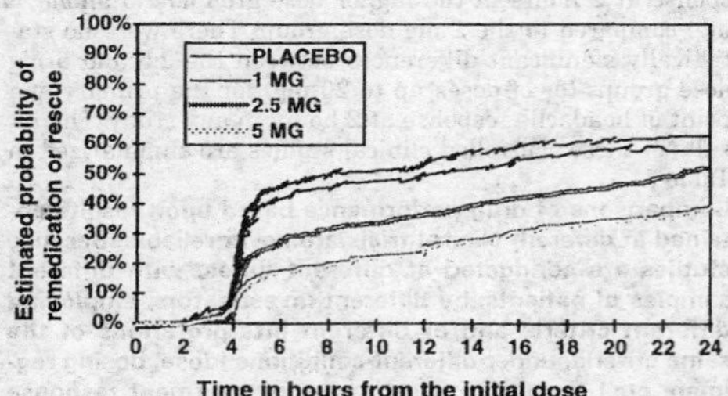

*This Kaplan-Meier plot is based on data obtained in 3 placebo controlled clinical trials (Study 2, 3 and 5). Patients not using additional treatments were censored at 24 hours. The plot includes both patients who had headache response at 2 hours and those who had no response to the initial dose. It should be noted that the protocols did not allow remedication within 2 hours post dose.

lar migraine (see CONTRAINDICATIONS). Safety and effectiveness of ZOMIG have not been established for cluster headache, which is present in an older, predominantly male population.

CONTRAINDICATIONS

ZOMIG should not be given to patients with ischemic heart disease (angina pectoris, history of myocardial infarction, or documented silent ischemia) or to patients who have symptoms or findings consistent with ischemic heart disease, coronary artery vasospasm, including Prinzmetal's variant angina, or other significant underlying cardiovascular disease (see WARNINGS).

Because ZOMIG may increase blood pressure, it should not be given to patients with uncontrolled hypertension (see WARNINGS).

ZOMIG should not be used within 24 hours of treatment with another 5-HT$_1$ agonist, or an ergotamine-containing or ergot-type medication like dihydroergotamine or methysergide.

ZOMIG should not be administered to patients with hemiplegic or basilar migraine.

Concurrent administration of MAO-A inhibitors or use of zolmitriptan within 2 weeks of discontinuation of MAO-A inhibitor therapy is contraindicated (see CLINICAL PHARMACOLOGY: Drug Interactions and PRECAUTIONS: Drug Interactions).

ZOMIG is contraindicated in patients who are hypersensitive to zolmitriptan or any of its inactive ingredients.

WARNINGS

ZOMIG should only be used where a clear diagnosis of migraine has been established.

Risk of Myocardial Ischemia and/or Infarction and Other Adverse Cardiac Events: ZOMIG should not be given to patients with documented ischemic or vasospastic coronary artery disease (see CONTRAINDICATIONS). It is strongly recommended that zolmitriptan not be given to patients in whom unrecognized coronary artery disease (CAD) is predicted by the presence of risk factors (e.g., hypertension, hypercholesterolemia, smoker, obesity, diabetes, strong family history of CAD, female with surgical or physiological menopause, or male over 40 years of age) unless a cardiovascular evaluation provides satisfactory clinical evidence that the patient is reasonably free of coronary artery and ischemic myocardial disease or other significant underlying cardiovascular disease. The sensitivity of cardiac diagnostic procedures to detect cardiovascular disease or predisposition to coronary artery vasospasm is modest, at best. If, during the cardiovascular evaluation, the patient's medical history, electrocardiographic or other investigations reveal findings indicative of, or consistent with, coronary artery vasospasm or myocardial ischemia, zolmitriptan should not be administered (see CONTRAINDICATIONS). For patients with risk factors predictive of CAD, who are determined to have a satisfactory cardiovascular evaluation, it is strongly recommended that administration of the first dose of zolmitriptan take place in the setting of a physician's office or similar medically staffed and equipped facility unless the patient has previously received zolmitriptan. Because cardiac ischemia can occur in the absence of clinical symptoms, consideration should be given to obtaining on the first occasion of use an electrocardiogram (ECG) during the interval immediately following ZOMIG, in these patients with risk factors.

It is recommended that patients who are intermittent long-term users of ZOMIG and who have or acquire risk factors predictive of CAD, as described above, undergo periodic interval cardiovascular evaluation as they continue to use ZOMIG.

The systematic approach described above is intended to reduce the likelihood that patients with unrecognized cardiovascular disease will be inadvertently exposed to zolmitriptan.

Cardiac Events and Fatalities: Serious adverse cardiac events, including acute myocardial infarction, have been reported within a few hours following administration of zolmitriptan. Life-threatening disturbances of cardiac rhythm, and death have been reported within a few hours following the administration of other 5-HT$_1$ agonists. Considering the extent of use of 5-HT$_1$ agonists in patients with migraine, the incidence of these events is extremely low.

ZOMIG can cause coronary vasospasm; at least one of these events occurred in a patient with no cardiac disease history and with documented absence of coronary artery disease. Because of the close proximity of the events to ZOMIG use, a causal relationship cannot be excluded. In the cases where there has been known underlying coronary artery disease, the relationship is uncertain.

Patients with symptomatic Wolff-Parkinson-White syndrome or arrhythmias associated with other cardiac accessory conduction pathway disorders should not receive ZOMIG.

Premarketing experience with zolmitriptan: Among the more than 2,500 patients with migraine who participated in premarketing controlled clinical trials of ZOMIG Tablets, no deaths or serious cardiac events were reported.

Postmarketing experience with zolmitriptan: Serious cardiovascular events have been reported in association with the use of ZOMIG. The uncontrolled nature of postmarketing surveillance, however, makes it impossible to determine definitively the proportion of the reported cases that were actually caused by zolmitriptan or to reliably assess causation in individual cases.

Cerebrovascular Events and Fatalities with 5-HT$_1$ agonists: Cerebral hemorrhage, subarachnoid hemorrhage, stroke, and other cerebrovascular events have been reported in patients treated with 5-HT$_1$ agonists; and some have resulted in fatalities. In a number of cases, it appears possible that the cerebrovascular events were primary, the agonist having been administered in the incorrect belief that the symptoms experienced were a consequence of migraine, when they were not. It should be noted that patients with migraine may be at increased risk of certain cerebrovascular events (eg, stroke, hemorrhage, transient ischemic attack).

Other Vasospasm-Related Events: 5-HT$_1$ agonists may cause vasospastic reactions other than coronary artery vasospasm. Both peripheral vascular ischemia and colonic ischemia with abdominal pain and bloody diarrhea have been reported with 5-HT$_1$ agonists.

Increase in Blood Pressure: Significant elevations in systemic blood pressure have been reported on rare occasions in patients with and without a history of hypertension treated with 5-HT$_1$ agonists. Zolmitriptan is contraindicated in patients with uncontrolled hypertension. In volunteers, an increase of 1 and 5 mm Hg in the systolic and diastolic blood pressure, respectively, was seen at 5 mg. In the headache trials, vital signs were measured only in the small inpatient study and no effect on blood pressure was seen. In a study of patients with moderate to severe liver disease, 7 of 27 experienced 20 to 80 mm Hg elevations in systolic and/or diastolic blood pressure after a dose of 10 mg of zolmitriptan (see CONTRAINDICATIONS).

An 18% increase in mean pulmonary artery pressure was seen following dosing with another 5-HT$_1$ agonist in a study evaluating subjects undergoing cardiac catheterization.

PRECAUTIONS

General: As with other 5-HT$_{1B/1D}$ agonists, sensations of tightness, pain, pressure, and heaviness have been reported after treatment with ZOMIG Tablets in the precordium, throat, neck, and jaw. Because zolmitriptan may cause coronary artery vasospasm, patients who experience signs or symptoms suggestive of angina following dosing should be evaluated for the presence of CAD or a predisposition to Prinzmetal's variant angina before receiving additional doses of medication, and should be monitored electrocardiographically if dosing is resumed and similar symptoms recur. Similarly, patients who experience other symptoms or signs suggestive of decreased arterial flow, such as ischemic bowel syndrome or Raynaud's syndrome following the use of any 5-HT agonist are candidates for further evaluation. (see WARNINGS).

Zolmitriptan should also be administered with caution to patients with diseases that may alter the absorption, metabolism, or excretion of drugs, such as impaired hepatic function (see CLINICAL PHARMACOLOGY).

For a given attack, if a patient does not respond to the first dose of zolmitriptan, the diagnosis of migraine headache should be reconsidered before administration of a second dose.

Binding to Melanin-Containing Tissues: When pigmented rats were given a single oral dose of 10 mg/kg of radiolabeled zolmitriptan, the radioactivity in the eye after 7 days, the latest time point examined, was still 75% of the value measured after 4 hours. This suggests that zolmitriptan and/or its metabolites may bind to the melanin of the eye. Because there could be accumulation in melanin rich tissues over time, this raises the possibility that zolmitriptan could cause toxicity in these tissues after extended use. However, no effects on the retina related to treatment with zolmitriptan were noted in any of the toxicity studies. Although no systematic monitoring of ophthalmologic function was undertaken in clinical trials, and no specific recommendations for ophthalmologic monitoring are offered, prescribers should be aware of the possibility of long-term ophthalmologic effects.

Information for Patients: See PATIENT INFORMATION at the end of this labeling for the text of the separate leaflet provided for patients.

Laboratory Tests: No monitoring of specific laboratory tests is recommended.

Drug Interactions: Ergot-containing drugs have been reported to cause prolonged vasospastic reactions. Because there is a theoretical basis that these effects may be additive, use of ergotamine-containing or ergot-type medications (like dihydroergotamine or methysergide) and zolmitriptan within 24 hours of each other should be avoided (see CONTRAINDICATIONS).

MAO-A inhibitors increase the systemic exposure of zolmitriptan. Therefore, the use of zolmitriptan in patients receiving MAO-A inhibitors is contraindicated (see CLINICAL PHARMACOLOGY and CONTRAINDICATIONS).

Concomitant use of other 5-HT$_{1B/1D}$ agonists within 24 hours of ZOMIG treatment is not recommended. (see CONTRAINDICATIONS).

Following administration of cimetidine, the half-life and AUC of zolmitriptan and its active metabolites were approximately doubled (see CLINICAL PHARMACOLOGY).

Selective serotonin reuptake inhibitors (SSRIs) (eg, fluoxetine, fluvoxamine, paroxetine, sertraline) have been reported, rarely, to cause weakness, hyperreflexia, and incoordination when coadministered with 5-HT$_1$ agonists. If concomitant treatment with zolmitriptan and an SSRI is clinically warranted, appropriate observation of the patient is advised.

Drug/Laboratory Test Interactions: Zolmitriptan is not known to interfere with commonly employed clinical laboratory tests.

Carcinogenesis, Mutagenesis, Impairment of Fertility: Carcinogenesis: Carcinogenicity studies by oral gavage were carried out in mice and rats at doses up to 400 mg/kg/day. Mice were dosed for 85 weeks (males) and 92 weeks (females). The exposure (plasma AUC of parent drug) at the highest dose level was approximately 800 times that seen in humans after a single 10 mg dose (the maximum recommended total daily dose). There was no effect of zolmitriptan on tumor incidence. Control, low dose, and middle dose rats were dosed for 104–105 weeks; the high dose group was sacrificed after 101 weeks (males) and 86 weeks (females) due to excess mortality. Aside from an increase in the incidence of thyroid follicular cell hyperplasia and thyroid follicular cell adenomas seen in male rats receiving 400 mg/kg/day, an exposure approximately 3000 times that seen in humans after dosing with 10 mg, no tumors were noted.

Mutagenesis: Zolmitriptan was mutagenic in an Ames test, in 2 of 5 strains of S. typhimurium tested, in the presence of, but not in the absence of, metabolic activation. It was not mutagenic in an *in vitro* mammalian gene cell mutation (CHO/HGPRT) assay. Zolmitriptan was clastogenic in an *in vitro* human lymphocyte assay both in the absence of and the presence of metabolic activation; it was not clastogenic in an *in vivo* mouse micronucleus assay. It was also not genotoxic in an unscheduled DNA synthesis study.

Impairment of Fertility: Studies of male and female rats administered zolmitriptan prior to and during mating and up to implantation have shown no impairment of fertility at doses up to 400 mg/kg/day. Exposure at this dose was approximately 3000 times exposure at the maximum recommended human dose of 10 mg/day.

Pregnancy: Pregnancy Category C: There are no adequate and well controlled studies in pregnant women; therefore, zolmitriptan should be used during pregnancy only if the potential benefit justifies the potential risk to the fetus.

In reproductive toxicity studies in rats and rabbits, oral administration of zolmitriptan to pregnant animals was associated with embryolethality and fetal abnormalities. When pregnant rats were administered oral zolmitriptan during the period of organogenesis at doses of 100, 400, and 1200 mg/kg/day, there was a dose-related increase in embryolethality which became statistically significant at the high dose. The maternal plasma exposures at these doses were approximately 280, 1100, and 5000 times the exposure in humans receiving the maximum recommended total daily dose of 10 mg. The high dose was maternally toxic, as evidenced by a decreased maternal body weight gain during gestation. In a similar study in rabbits, embryolethality was increased at the maternally toxic doses of 10 and 30 mg/kg/day (maternal plasma exposures equivalent to 11 and 42 times exposure in humans receiving the maximum recommended total daily dose of 10 mg), and increased incidences of fetal malformations (fused sternebrae, rib anomalies) and variations (major blood vessel variations, irregular ossification pattern of ribs) were observed at 30 mg/kg/day. Three mg/kg/day was a no effect dose (equivalent to human exposure at a dose of 10 mg). When female rats were given zolmitriptan during gestation, parturition, and lactation, an increased incidence of hydronephrosis was found in the offspring at the maternally toxic dose of 400 mg/kg/day (1100 times human exposure).

Nursing Mothers: It is not known whether zolmitriptan is excreted in human milk. Because many drugs are excreted in human milk, caution should be exercised when zolmitriptan is administered to a nursing woman. Lactating rats dosed with zolmitriptan had milk levels equivalent to maternal plasma levels at 1 hour and 4 times higher than plasma levels at 4 hours.

Pediatric Use: Safety and effectiveness of ZOMIG in pediatric patients have not been established.

Use in the Elderly: Although the pharmacokinetic disposition of the drug in the elderly is similar to that seen in younger adults, there is no information about the safety and effectiveness of zolmitriptan in this population because patients over age 65 were excluded from the controlled clinical trials. (see CLINICAL PHARMACOLOGY: Special Populations)

ADVERSE REACTIONS

Serious cardiac events, including myocardial infarction, have occurred following the use of ZOMIG Tablets. These events are extremely rare and most have been reported in patients with risk factors predictive of CAD. Events reported, in association with drugs of this class, have included coronary artery vasospasm, transient myocardial ischemia, myocardial infarction, ventricular tachycardia, and ventricular fibrillation (see CONTRAINDICATIONS, WARNINGS, and PRECAUTIONS).

Incidence in Controlled Clinical Trials: Among 2,633 patients treated with ZOMIG in the active and placebo controlled trials, no patients withdrew for reasons related to adverse events, but as patients treated a single headache in these trials, the opportunity for discontinuation was limited. In a long-term, open label study where patients were allowed to treat multiple migraine attacks for up to 1 year, 8% (167 out of 2,058) withdrew from the trial because of adverse experience. The most common events were paresthesia, asthenia, nausea, dizziness, pain, chest or neck tightness or heaviness, somnolence, and warm sensation.

Table 2 lists the adverse events that occurred in ≥ 2% of the 2,075 patients in any one of the ZOMIG 1 mg, ZOMIG 2.5 mg or ZOMIG 5 mg dose groups of the controlled clinical trials. Only events that were more frequent in a ZOMIG group compared to the placebo groups are included. The events cited reflect experience gained under closely monitored conditions of clinical trials in a highly selected patient population. In actual clinical practice or in other clinical trials, these frequency estimates may not apply, as the conditions of use, reporting behavior, and the kinds of patients treated may differ.

Several of the adverse events appear dose related, notably paresthesia, sensation of heaviness or tightness in chest, neck, jaw, and throat, dizziness, somnolence, and possibly asthenia and nausea.

[See table 2 above]

Table 2: Adverse Experience Incidence in Five Placebo-Controlled Migraine Clinical Trials: Events Reported By ≥2% Patients Treated With ZOMIG

Adverse Event Type	Placebo (n=401)	ZOMIG 1 mg (n=163)	ZOMIG 2.5 mg (n=498)	ZOMIG 5 mg (n=1012)
ATYPICAL SENSATIONS	**6%**	**12%**	**12%**	**18%**
Hypesthesia	1%	1%	1%	2%
Paresthesia (all types)	2%	5%	7%	9%
Sensation warm/cold	4%	6%	5%	7%
PAIN AND PRESSURE SENSATIONS	**7%**	**13%**	**14%**	**22%**
Chest - pain/tightness/pressure and/or heaviness	1%	2%	3%	4%
Neck/throat/jaw - pain/tightness/pressure	3%	4%	7%	10%
Heaviness other than chest or neck	1%	1%	2%	5%
Pain - location specified	1%	2%	2%	3%
Other - Pressure/tightness/heaviness	0%	2%	2%	2%
DIGESTIVE	**8%**	**11%**	**16%**	**14%**
Dry mouth	2%	5%	3%	3%
Dyspepsia	1%	3%	2%	1%
Dysphagia	0%	0%	0%	2%
Nausea	4%	4%	9%	6%
NEUROLOGICAL	**10%**	**11%**	**17%**	**21%**
Dizziness	4%	6%	8%	10%
Somnolence	3%	5%	6%	8%
Vertigo	0%	0%	0%	2%
OTHER				
Asthenia	3%	5%	3%	9%
Palpitations	1%	0%	<1%	2%
Myalgia	<1%	1%	1%	2%
Myasthenia	<1%	0%	1%	2%
Sweating	1%	0%	2%	3%

ZOMIG is generally well tolerated. Across all doses, most adverse reactions were mild and transient and did not lead to long-lasting effects. The incidence of adverse events in controlled clinical trials was not affected by gender, weight, or age of the patients; use of prophylactic medications; or presence of aura. There were insufficient data to assess the impact of race on the incidence of adverse events.

Other Events: In the paragraphs that follow, the frequencies of less commonly reported adverse clinical events are presented. Because the reports include events observed in open and uncontrolled studies, the role of ZOMIG in their causation cannot be reliably determined. Furthermore, variability associated with adverse event reporting, the terminology used to describe adverse events, etc., limit the value of the quantitative frequency estimates provided. Event frequencies are calculated as the number of patients who used ZOMIG (n=4,027) and reported an event divided by the total number of patients exposed to ZOMIG. All reported events are included except those already listed in the previous table, those too general to be informative, and those not reasonably associated with the use of the drug. Events are further classified within body system categories and enumerated in order of decreasing frequency using the following definitions: infrequent adverse events are those occurring in 1/100 to 1/1,000 patients and rare adverse events are those occurring in fewer than 1/1,000 patients.

Typical sensation: Infrequent was hyperesthesia

General: Infrequent were allergy reaction, chills, facial edema, fever, malaise, and photosensitivity.

Cardiovascular: Infrequent were arrhythmias, hypertension, and syncope. Rare were bradycardia, extrasystoles, postural hypotension, QT prolongation, tachycardia, and thrombophlebitis.

Digestive: Infrequent were increased appetite, tongue edema, esophagitis, gastroenteritis, liver function abnormality, and thirst. Rare were anorexia, constipation, gastritis, hematemesis, pancreatitis, melena, and ulcer.

Hemic: Infrequent was ecchymosis. Rare were cyanosis, thrombocytopenia, eosinophilia, and leukopenia.

Metabolic: Infrequent was edema. Rare were hyperglycemia and alkaline phosphatase increased.

Musculoskeletal: Infrequent were back pain, leg cramps, and tenosynovitis. Rare were arthritis, asthenia, tetany, and twitching.

Neurological: Infrequent were agitation, anxiety, depression, emotional lability, and insomnia; Rare were akathesia, amnesia, apathy, ataxia, dystonia, euphoria, hallucinations, cerebral ischemia, hyperkinesia, hypotonia, hypertonia, and irritability.

Respiratory: Infrequent were bronchitis, bronchospasm, epistaxis, hiccup, laryngitis, and yawn. Rare were apnea and voice alteration.

Skin: Infrequent were pruritus, rash, and urticaria.

Special Senses: Infrequent were dry eye, eye pain, hyperacusis, ear pain, parosmia, and tinnitus. Rare were diplopia and lacrimation.

Urogenital: Infrequent were hematuria, cystitis, polyuria, urinary frequency, and urinary urgency. Rare were miscarriage and dysmenorrhea.

Postmarketing Experience: The following section enumerates potentially important adverse events that have occurred in clinical practice and which have been reported spontaneously to various surveillance systems. The events enumerated represent reports arising from both domestic and non-domestic use of zolmitriptan. The events enumerated include all except those already listed in the ADVERSE REACTIONS section above or those too general to be informative. Because the reports cite events reported spontaneously from worldwide postmarketing experience, frequency of events and the role of zolmitriptan in their causation cannot be reliably determined.

Cardiovascular: Coronary artery vasospasm; transient myocardial ischemia, angina pectoris, and myocardial infarction.

DRUG ABUSE AND DEPENDENCE

The abuse potential of ZOMIG has not been assessed in clinical trials.

OVERDOSAGE

There is no experience with clinical overdose. Volunteers receiving single 50 mg oral doses of zolmitriptan commonly experienced sedation.

The elimination half-life of ZOMIG is 3 hours (see CLINICAL PHARMACOLOGY), and therefore monitoring of patients after overdose with ZOMIG should continue for at least 15 hours or while symptoms or signs persist.

There is no specific antidote to zolmitriptan. In cases of severe intoxication, intensive care procedures are recommended, including establishing and maintaining a patent airway, ensuring adequate oxygenation and ventilation, and monitoring and support of the cardiovascular system.

It is unknown what effect hemodialysis or peritoneal dialysis has on the plasma concentrations of zolmitriptan.

DOSAGE AND ADMINISTRATION

In controlled clinical trials, single doses of 1, 2.5 and 5 mg of zolmitriptan were effective for the acute treatment of migraines in adults. A greater proportion of patients had headache response following a 2.5 or 5 mg dose than following a 1 mg dose (see Table 1). In the only direct comparison of 2.5 and 5 mg, there was little added benefit from the larger dose, but side effects are generally increased at 5 mg (see Table 2). Patients should, therefore, be started on 2.5 mg or lower. A dose lower than 2.5 mg can be achieved by manually breaking a 2.5 mg tablet in half.

If the headache returns, the dose may be repeated after 2 hours, not to exceed 10 mg within a 24-hour period. Controlled trials have not adequately established the effectiveness of a second dose if the initial dose is ineffective.

The safety of treating an average of more than three headaches in a 30-day period has not been established.

Hepatic Impairment: Patients with moderate to severe hepatic impairment have decreased clearance of zolmitriptan and significant elevation in blood pressure was observed in some patients. Use of a low dose with blood pressure monitoring is recommended (see CLINICAL PHARMACOLOGY AND WARNINGS).

HOW SUPPLIED

2.5 mg Tablets—Yellow, biconvex, film-coated, scored tablets containing 2.5 mg of zolmitriptan identified with "ZOMIG" and "2.5" debossed on one side are supplied in cartons containing a blister pack of 6 tablets. (NDC 0310-0210-20).

5 mg Tablets—Pink, biconvex, film-coated tablets containing 5 mg of zolmitriptan identified with "ZOMIG" and "5" debossed on one side are supplied in cartons containing a blister pack of 3 tablets. (NDC 0310-0211-25).

Store at controlled room temperature, 20–25°C (68–77°F) [see USP]. Protect from light and moisture.

PATIENT INFORMATION

The following wording is contained in a separate leaflet provided for patients.

ZOMIG®
(zolmitriptan) Tablets
Patient Information about
ZOMIG (Zo-mig)
for Migraines

Generic Name: zolmitriptan (zol-mi-trip-tan)

Information for the Consumer on ZOMIG (zolmitriptan) Tablets: Please read this leaflet carefully before you administer ZOMIG Tablets. This provides a summary of the information available on your medicine. Please do not throw away this leaflet until you have finished your medicine. You may need to read this leaflet again. This leaflet does not contain all the information on ZOMIG Tablets. For further information or advice, ask your doctor or pharmacist.

Information About Your Medicine: The name of your medicine is ZOMIG Tablets. It can be obtained only by prescription from your doctor. The decision to use ZOMIG Tablets is one that you and your doctor should make jointly, taking into account your individual preferences and medical circumstances. If you have risk factors for heart disease (such as high blood pressure, high cholesterol, obesity, diabetes, smoking, strong family history of heart disease, or you are postmenopausal or a male over the age of 40), you should tell your doctor, who should evaluate you for heart disease in order to determine if ZOMIG Tablets are appropriate for you.

1. **The Purpose of Your Medicine:** ZOMIG Tablets are intended to relieve your migraine, but not to prevent or reduce the number of attacks you experience. Use ZOMIG Tablets only to treat an actual migraine attack.
2. **Important Questions to Consider Before Using ZOMIG Tablets:** If the answer to any of the following questions is **YES** or if you do not know the answer, then you must discuss it with your doctor before you use ZOMIG Tablets.
   - Do you have any chest pain, heart disease, shortness of breath, or irregular heartbeats? Have you had a heart attack?
   - Do you have risk factors for heart disease (such as high blood pressure, high cholesterol, obesity, diabetes, smoking, strong family history of heart disease, or you are postmenopausal or a male over the age of 40)?
   - Do you have high blood pressure?
   - Are you pregnant? Do you think you might be pregnant? Are you trying to become pregnant? Are you not using adequate contraception? Are you breast feeding an infant?
   - Have you ever had to stop taking this or any other medication because of an allergy or other problems?
   - Are you taking any other migraine medications, including 5-HT1 agonist or migraine medications containing ergotamine, dihydroergotamine, or methysergide?
   - Are you taking any medication for depression (monoamine oxidase inhibitors or selective serotonin reuptake inhibitors [SSRIs])?
   - Have you had, or do you have, any disease of the liver or kidney?
   - Have you had, or do you have, epilepsy or seizures?
   - Is this headache different from your usual migraine attacks?

   Remember, if you answered **YES** to any of the above questions, then you must discuss it with your doctor.
3. **The Use of ZOMIG Tablets During Pregnancy:** Do not use ZOMIG Tablets if you are pregnant, think you might

Continued on next page

Zomig—Cont.

be pregnant, are trying to become pregnant, or are not using adequate contraception, unless you have discussed this with your doctor.

4. **How to Use ZOMIG Tablets:** Adults should be started on a 2.5 mg dose or lower administered by mouth. A dose lower than 2.5 mg can be achieved by manually breaking a 2.5 mg tablet in half. If your headache comes back after your initial dose, a second dose may be administered anytime after 2 hours of administering the dose. For any attack where you have no response to the first dose, do not take a second dose without first consulting with your doctor. Do not administer more than a total of 10 mg of ZOMIG Tablets in any 24-hour period. Discard any unused tablets or its portion that have been removed from the blister packaging.
5. **Side Effects to Watch for:**
   - Some patients experience pain or tightness in the chest or throat when using ZOMIG Tablets. If this happens to you, then discuss it with your doctor before using any more ZOMIG Tablets. If the chest pain is severe or does not go away, call your doctor immediately.
   - Shortness of breath; wheeziness; heart throbbing; swelling of eyelids, face, or lips; or a skin rash, skin lumps, or hives happens rarely. If it happens to you, then tell your doctor immediately. Do not take any more ZOMIG Tablets unless your doctor tells you to do so.
   - Some people may have feelings of tingling, heat, heaviness, or pressure after treatment with ZOMIG Tablets. A few people may feel drowsy, dizzy, tired, or sick. Tell your doctor immediately if you have symptoms that you do not understand.
6. **What to Do if an Overdose Is Taken:** If you have taken more medication than you have been told, contact either your doctor, hospital emergency department, or nearest poison control center immediately. This medicine was prescribed for your particular condition and should not be used by others or for any other condition.
7. **Storing Your Medicine:** Keep your medicine in a safe place where children cannot reach it. It may be harmful to children. Store your medication away from heat, light, moisture, and at a controlled room temperature. If your medication has expired (the expiration date is printed on the treatment pack), throw it away as instructed. If your doctor decides to stop your treatment, do not keep any leftover medicine unless your doctor tells you to. Throw away your medicine as instructed. Be sure that discarded tablets are out of the reach of children.

Rev K 05/00 64161-00 680003

Manufactured for:
AstraZeneca Pharmaceuticals LP
Wilmington, DE 19850
By: IPR Pharmaceuticals, Inc.
Carolina, PR 00984
Shown in Product Identification Guide, page 306

Athena Neurosciences
800 GATEWAY BOULEVARD
SOUTH SAN FRANCISCO, CA 94080

For Medical Information Contact:
(888) NEURO-05
(888) 638-7605
To Report Adverse Events Contact:
(877) ELAN GSS
(877) 352-6477
The products below are distributed by Athena Neurosciences, a business unit of Elan Pharmaceuticals, Inc.

ATAMET® ℞
CARBIDOPA AND LEVODOPA TABLETS, USP

DESCRIPTION
When Carbidopa and Levodopa Tablets are to be given to patients who are being treated with levodopa, levodopa must be discontinued at least eight hours before therapy with this combination product is started. In order to reduce adverse reactions, it is necessary to individualize therapy. See the WARNINGS and DOSAGE AND ADMINISTRATION sections before initiating therapy.
Carbidopa, an inhibitor of aromatic amino acid decarboxylation, is a white, crystalline compound, slightly soluble in water. It is designated chemically as (–)-L-α-hydrazino-α-methyl-β-(3, 4-dihydroxybenzene) propanoic acid monohydrate, and has the following structural formula:

$C_{10}H_{14}N_2O_4 \cdot H_2O$ M.W. 244.25

Tablet content is expressed in terms of anhydrous carbidopa which has a molecular weight of 226.23.
Levodopa, an aromatic amino acid, is a white, crystalline compound, slightly soluble in water. It is designated chemically as (–)-L-α-amino-β-(3,4-dihydroxybenzene) propanoic acid, and has the following structural formula:

$C_9H_{11}NO_4$ M.W. 197.2

Carbidopa and Levodopa is supplied as tablets in two strengths:
Carbidopa and Levodopa Tablets 25 mg/100 mg, containing 25 mg of carbidopa and 100 mg of levodopa.
Carbidopa and Levodopa Tablets 25 mg/250 mg, containing 25 mg of carbidopa and 250 mg of levodopa.
Inactive ingredients are magnesium stearate, microcrystalline cellulose, pregelatinized starch, and corn starch. Carbidopa and Levodopa Tablets 25 mg/250 mg also contain FD&C Blue 2. Carbidopa and Levodopa Tablets 25 mg/100 mg contain D&C Yellow 10 and FD&C Yellow 6.

HOW SUPPLIED
Carbidopa and Levodopa Tablets 25 mg/100 mg NDC 59075-585-10 are available in the following form:
Mottled yellow, round, scored tablets, engraved A-"585" on the scored side, and packaged in bottles of 100.
Carbidopa and Levodopa Tablets 25 mg/250 mg NDC 59075-587-10 are available in the following form:
Mottled blue, round, scored tablets, engraved A-"587" on the scored side, and packaged in bottles of 100.
Store at controlled room temperature 15°–30°C (59°–86°F).
PROTECT FROM LIGHT.
Dispense in a tight, light-resistant container as defined in the USP, with a child-resistant closure (as required).
Rev. F 3/2000

Manufactured by:
TEVA PHARMACEUTICAL IND. LTD.
Jerusalem, 91010, Israel
Distributed by:
Elan Pharmaceuticals
South San Francisco, CA 94080
Atamet is a registered trademark of Elan Pharmaceuticals, Inc.

DIASTAT® Rectal Delivery System ℞
[dī'ă-stat]
(diazepam rectal gel)

(For full prescribing information please see Elan Pharma)

MYSOLINE® ℞
[mī'sō-lēn]
(primidone)
Anticonvulsant

(For full prescribing information please see Elan Pharma)

PERMAX® ℞
[pĕr 'măks]
(pergolide mesylate)

DESCRIPTION
Permax® (Pergolide Mesylate) is an ergot derivative dopamine receptor agonist at both D_1 and D_2 receptor sites. Pergolide mesylate is chemically designated as 8β-[(Methylthio)methyl]-6-propylergoline monomethanesulfonate; the structural formula is as follows:

The formula weight of the base is 314.5; 1 mg of base corresponds to 3.18 µmol.
Permax is provided for oral administration in tablets containing 0.05 mg (0.159 µmol), 0.25 mg (0.795 µmol), or 1 mg (3.18 µmol) pergolide as the base. The tablets also contain croscarmellose sodium, iron oxide, lactose, magnesium stearate, and povidone. The 0.05 mg tablet also contains methionine, and the 0.25 mg tablet also contains F D & C Blue No. 2.

CLINICAL PHARMACOLOGY
Pharmacodynamic Information —Pergolide mesylate is a potent dopamine receptor agonist. Pergolide is 10 to 1,000 times more potent than bromocriptine on a milligram per milligram basis in various in vitro and in vivo test systems. Pergolide mesylate inhibits the secretion of prolactin in humans; it causes a transient rise in serum concentrations of growth hormone and a decrease in serum concentrations of luteinizing hormone. In Parkinson's disease, pergolide mesylate is believed to exert its therapeutic effect by directly stimulating postsynaptic dopamine receptors in the nigrostriatal system.
Pharmacokinetic Information (Absorption, Distribution, Metabolism, and Elimination) —Information on oral systemic bioavailability of pergolide mesylate is unavailable because of the lack of a sufficiently sensitive assay to detect the drug after the administration of a single dose. However, following oral administration of ^{14}C radiolabeled pergolide mesylate, approximately 55% of the administered radioactivity can be recovered from the urine and 5% from expired CO_2, suggesting that a significant fraction is absorbed. Nothing can be concluded about the extent of presystemic clearance, if any. Data on postabsorption distribution of pergolide are unavailable.
At least 10 metabolites have been detected, including N-despropylpergolide, pergolide sulfoxide, and pergolide sulfone. Pergolide sulfoxide and pergolide sulfone are dopamine agonists in animals. The other detected metabolites have not been identified, and it is not known whether any other metabolites are active pharmacologically.
The major route of excretion is the kidney.
Pergolide is approximately 90% bound to plasma proteins. This extent of protein binding may be important to consider when pergolide mesylate is coadministered with other drugs known to affect protein binding.

INDICATIONS AND USAGE
Permax is indicated as adjunctive treatment to levodopa/carbidopa in the management of the signs and symptoms of Parkinson's disease.
Evidence to support the efficacy of pergolide mesylate as an antiparkinsonian adjunct was obtained in a multicenter study enrolling 376 patients with mild to moderate Parkinson's disease who were intolerant to *l* -dopa/carbidopa as manifested by moderate to severe dyskinesia and/or on-off phenomena. On average, the patients evaluated had been on *l* -dopa/carbidopa for 3.9 years (range, 2 days to 16.8 years). The administration of pergolide mesylate permitted a 5% to 30% reduction in the daily dose of *l* -dopa. On average these patients treated with pergolide mesylate maintained an equivalent or better clinical status than they exhibited at baseline.

CONTRAINDICATIONS
Pergolide mesylate is contraindicated in patients who are hypersensitive to this drug or other ergot derivatives.

WARNINGS
Symptomatic Hypotension —In clinical trials, approximately 10% of patients taking pergolide mesylate with *l* -dopa versus 7% taking placebo with *l* -dopa experienced symptomatic orthostatic and/or sustained hypotension, especially during initial treatment. With gradual dosage titration, tolerance to the hypotension usually develops. It is therefore important to warn patients of the risk, to begin therapy with low doses, and to increase the dosage in carefully adjusted increments over a period of 3 to 4 weeks (*see* Dosage and Administration).
Hallucinosis —In controlled trials, pergolide mesylate with *l* -dopa caused hallucinosis in about 14% of patients as opposed to 3% taking placebo with *l* -dopa. This was of sufficient severity to cause discontinuation of treatment in about 3% of those enrolled; tolerance to this untoward effect was not observed.
Fatalities —In the placebo-controlled trial, 2 of 187 patients treated with placebo died as compared with 1 of 189 patients treated with pergolide mesylate. Of the 2,299 patients treated with pergolide mesylate in premarketing studies evaluated as of October 1988, 143 died while on the drug or shortly after discontinuing it. Because the patient population under evaluation was elderly, ill, and at high risk for death, it seems unlikely that pergolide mesylate played any role in these deaths, but the possibility that pergolide shortens survival of patients cannot be excluded with absolute certainty.
In particular, a case-by-case review of the clinical course of the patients who died failed to disclose any unique set of signs, symptoms, or laboratory results that would suggest that treatment with pergolide caused their deaths. Sixty-eight percent (68%) of the patients who died were 65 years of age or older. No death (other than a suicide) occurred within the first month of treatment; most of the patients who died had been on pergolide for years. A relative frequency of the causes of death by organ system are: Pulmonary failure/Pneumonia, 35%; Cardiovascular, 30%; Cancer, 11%; Unknown, 8.4%; Infection, 3.5%; Extrapyramidal syndrome, 3.5%; Stroke, 2.1%; Dysphagia, 2.1%; Injury, 1.4%; Suicide, 1.4%; Dehydration, 0.7%; Glomerulonephritis, 0.7%.
Serous Inflammation and Fibrosis —There have been rare reports of pleuritis, pleural effusion, pleural fibrosis, pericarditis, pericardial effusion or retroperitoneal fibrosis in patients taking pergolide. Some patients had experienced similar events while taking the ergot derivative bromocriptine. Pergolide should be used with caution in patients with a history of these conditions, particularly those patients who experienced the events while taking ergot derivatives. Patients with a history of such events should be carefully monitored clinically and with appropriate radiographic and laboratory studies while taking pergolide.

PRECAUTIONS
General —Caution should be exercised when administering pergolide mesylate to patients prone to cardiac dysrhythmias.

In a study comparing pergolide mesylate and placebo, patients taking pergolide mesylate were found to have significantly more episodes of atrial premature contractions (APCs) and sinus tachycardia.

The use of pergolide mesylate in patients on *l*-dopa may cause and/or exacerbate preexisting states of confusion and hallucinations (*see* Warnings) and preexisting dyskinesia. Also, the abrupt discontinuation of pergolide mesylate in patients receiving it chronically as an adjunct to *l*-dopa may precipitate the onset of hallucinations and confusion; these may occur within a span of several days. Discontinuation of pergolide should be undertaken gradually whenever possible, even if the patient is to remain on *l*-dopa.

A symptom complex resembling the neuroleptic malignant syndrome (NMS) (characterized by elevated temperature, muscular rigidity, altered consciousness, and autonomic instability), with no other obvious etiology, has been reported in association with rapid dose reduction, withdrawal of, or changes in antiparkinsonian therapy, including pergolide.

Information for Patients—Patients and their families should be informed of the common adverse consequences of the use of pergolide mesylate (*see* Adverse Reactions) and the risk of hypotension (*see* Warnings).

Patients should be advised to notify their physician if they become pregnant or intend to become pregnant during therapy.

Patients should be advised to notify their physician if they are breast feeding an infant.

Laboratory Tests—No specific laboratory tests are deemed essential for the management of patients on Permax. Periodic routine evaluation of all patients, however, is appropriate.

Drug Interactions—Dopamine antagonists, such as the neuroleptics (phenothiazines, butyrophenones, thioxanthines) or metoclopramide, ordinarily should not be administered concurrently with Permax (a dopamine agonist); these agents may diminish the effectiveness of Permax.

Because pergolide mesylate is approximately 90% bound to plasma proteins, caution should be exercised if pergolide mesylate is coadministered with other drugs known to affect protein binding.

Carcinogenesis, Mutagenesis, and Impairment of Fertility—A 2-year carcinogenicity study was conducted in mice using dietary levels of pergolide mesylate equivalent to oral doses of 0.6, 3.7, and 36.4 mg/kg/day in males and 0.6, 4.4, and 40.8 mg/kg/day in females. A 2-year study in rats was conducted using dietary levels equivalent to oral doses of 0.04, 0.18, and 0.88 mg/kg/day in males and 0.05, 0.28, and 1.42 mg/kg/day in females. The highest doses tested in the mice and rats were approximately 340 and 12 times the maximum human oral dose administered in controlled clinical trials (6 mg/day equivalent to 0.12 mg/kg/day).

A low incidence of uterine neoplasms occurred in both rats and mice. Endometrial adenomas and carcinomas were observed in rats. Endometrial sarcomas were observed in mice. The occurrence of these neoplasms is probably attributable to the high estrogen/progesterone ratio that would occur in rodents as a result of the prolactin-inhibiting action of pergolide mesylate. The endocrine mechanisms believed to be involved in the rodents are not present in humans. However, even though there is no known correlation between uterine malignancies occurring in pergolide-treated rodents and human risk, there are no human data to substantiate this conclusion.

Pergolide mesylate was evaluated for mutagenic potential in a battery of tests that included an Ames bacterial mutation assay, a DNA repair assay in cultured rat hepatocytes, an in vitro mammalian cell-point-mutation assay in cultured L5178Y cells, and a determination of chromosome alteration in bone marrow cells of Chinese hamsters. A weak mutagenic response was noted in the mammalian cell-point-mutation assay only after metabolic activation with rat liver microsomes. No mutagenic effects were obtained in the 2 other in vitro assays and in the in vivo assay. The relevance of these findings in humans is unknown.

A fertility study in male and female mice showed that fertility was maintained at 0.6 and 1.7 mg/kg/day but decreased at 5.6 mg/kg/day. Prolactin has been reported to be involved in stimulating and maintaining progesterone levels required for implantation in mice, and, therefore, the impaired fertility at the high dose may have occurred because of depressed prolactin levels.

Usage in Pregnancy—Pregnancy Category B—Reproduction studies were conducted in mice at doses of 5, 16, and 45 mg/kg/day and in rabbits at doses of 2, 6, and 16 mg/kg/day. The highest doses tested in mice and rabbits were 375 and 133 times the 6 mg/day maximum human dose administered in controlled clinical trials. In these studies, there was no evidence of harm to the fetus due to pergolide mesylate. There are, however, no adequate and well-controlled studies in pregnant women. Among women who received pergolide mesylate for endocrine disorders in premarketing studies, there were 33 pregnancies that resulted in healthy babies and 6 pregnancies that resulted in congenital abnormalities (3 major, 3 minor); a causal relationship has not been established. Because human data are limited and because animal reproduction studies are not always predictive of human response, this drug should be used during pregnancy only if clearly needed.

Nursing Mothers—It is not known whether this drug is excreted in human milk. The pharmacologic action of pergolide mesylate suggests that it may interfere with lactation. Because many drugs are excreted in human milk and because of the potential for serious adverse reactions to pergolide mesylate in nursing infants, a decision should be made whether to discontinue nursing or to discontinue the drug, taking into account the importance of the drug to the mother.

Pediatric Use—Safety and effectiveness in pediatric patients have not been established.

Incidence of Treatment-Emergent Adverse Experiences in the Placebo-Controlled Clinical Trial

Body System/ Adverse Event*	Percentage of Patients Reporting Events	
	Pergolide Mesylate N = 189	Placebo N =187
Body as a Whole		
Pain	7.0	2.1
Abdominal pain	5.8	2.1
Injury, accident	5.8	7.0
Headache	5.3	6.4
Asthenia	4.2	4.8
Chest pain	3.7	2.1
Flu syndrome	3.2	2.1
Neck pain	2.7	1.6
Back pain	1.6	2.1
Surgical procedure	1.6	<1
Chills	1.1	0
Face edema	1.1	0
Infection	1.1	0
Cardiovascular		
Postural hypotension	9.0	7.0
Vasodilatation	3.2	<1
Palpitation	2.1	<1
Hypotension	2.1	<1
Syncope	2.1	1.1
Hypertension	1.6	1.1
Arrhythmia	1.1	<1
Myocardial infarction	1.1	<1
Digestive		
Nausea	24.3	12.8
Constipation	10.6	5.9
Diarrhea	6.4	2.7
Dyspepsia	6.4	2.1
Anorexia	4.8	2.7
Dry mouth	3.7	<1
Vomiting	2.7	1.6
Hemic and Lymphatic		
Anemia	1.1	<1
Metabolic and Nutritional		
Peripheral edema	7.4	4.3
Edema	1.6	0
Weight gain	1.6	0
Musculoskeletal		
Arthralgia	1.6	2.1
Bursitis	1.6	<1
Myalgia	1.1	<1
Twitching	1.1	0
Nervous System		
Dyskinesia	62.4	24.6
Dizziness	19.1	13.9
Hallucinations	13.8	3.2
Dystonia	11.6	8.0
Confusion	11.1	9.6
Somnolence	10.1	3.7
Insomnia	7.9	3.2
Anxiety	6.4	4.3
Tremor	4.2	7.5
Depression	3.2	5.4
Abnormal dreams	2.7	4.3
Personality disorder	2.1	<1
Psychosis	2.1	0
Abnormal gait	1.6	1.6
Akathisia	1.6	0
Extrapyramidal syndrome	1.6	1.1
Incoordination	1.6	<1
Paresthesia	1.6	3.2
Akinesia	1.1	1.1
Hypertonia	1.1	0
Neuralgia	1.1	<1
Speech disorder	1.1	1.6
Respiratory System		
Rhinitis	12.2	5.4
Dyspnea	4.8	1.1
Epistaxis	1.6	<1
Hiccup	1.1	0
Skin and Appendages		
Rash	3.2	2.1
Sweating	2.1	2.7
Special Senses		
Abnormal vision	5.8	5.4
Diplopia	2.1	0
Taste perversion	1.6	0
Eye disorder	1.1	0
Urogenital System		
Urinary frequency	2.7	6.4
Urinary tract infection	2.7	3.7
Hematuria	1.1	<1

* Events reported by at least 1% of patients receiving pergolide mesylate are included.

ADVERSE REACTIONS

Commonly Observed—In premarketing clinical trials, the most commonly observed adverse events associated with use of pergolide mesylate which were not seen at an equivalent incidence among placebo-treated patients were: nervous system complaints, including dyskinesia, hallucinations, somnolence, insomnia; digestive complaints, including nausea, constipation, diarrhea, dyspepsia; and respiratory system complaints, including rhinitis.

Associated With Discontinuation of Treatment—Twenty-seven percent (27%) of approximately 1,200 patients receiving pergolide mesylate for treatment of Parkinson's disease in premarketing clinical trials in the US and Canada dis-

Continued on next page

Permax—Cont.

continued treatment due to adverse reactions. The events most commonly causing discontinuation were related to the nervous system (15.5%), primarily hallucinations (7.8%) and confusion (1.8%).

Fatalities —*See* Warnings.

Incidence in Controlled Clinical Trials —The table that follows enumerates adverse events that occurred at a frequency of 1% or more among patients taking pergolide mesylate who participated in the premarketing controlled clinical trials comparing pergolide mesylate with placebo. In a double-blind, controlled study of 6 months' duration, patients with Parkinson's disease were continued on *l* -dopa/carbidopa and were randomly assigned to receive either pergolide mesylate or placebo as additional therapy.

The prescriber should be aware that these figures cannot be used to predict the incidence of side effects in the course of usual medical practice where patient characteristics and other factors differ from those which prevailed in the clinical trials. Similarly, the cited frequencies cannot be compared with figures obtained from other clinical investigations involving different treatments, uses, and investigators. The cited figures, however, do provide the prescribing physician with some basis for estimating the relative contribution of drug and nondrug factors to the side-effect incidence rate in the population studied.

[See table at top of previous page]

Events Observed During the Premarketing Evaluation of Permax— This section reports event frequencies evaluated as of October 1988 for adverse events occurring in a group of approximately 1,800 patients who took multiple doses of pergolide mesylate. The conditions and duration of exposure to pergolide mesylate varied greatly, involving well-controlled studies as well as experience in open and uncontrolled clinical settings. In the absence of appropriate controls in some of the studies, a causal relationship between these events and treatment with pergolide mesylate cannot be determined.

The following enumeration by organ system describes events in terms of their relative frequency of reporting in the data base. Events of major clinical importance are also described in the Warnings and Precautions sections.

The following definitions of frequency are used: frequent adverse events are defined as those occurring in at least 1/100 patients; infrequent adverse events are those occurring in 1/100 to 1/1,000 patients; rare events are those occurring in fewer than 1/1,000 patients.

Body as a Whole—*Frequent:* headache, asthenia, accidental injury, pain, abdominal pain, chest pain, back pain, flu syndrome, neck pain, fever; *Infrequent:* facial edema, chills, enlarged abdomen, malaise, neoplasm, hernia, pelvic pain, sepsis, cellulitis, moniliasis, abscess, jaw pain, hypothermia; *Rare:* acute abdominal syndrome, LE syndrome

Cardiovascular System—*Frequent:* postural hypotension, syncope, hypertension, palpitations, vasodilatations, congestive heart failure; *Infrequent:* myocardial infarction, tachycardia, heart arrest, abnormal electrocardiogram, angina pectoris, thrombophlebitis, bradycardia, ventricular extrasystoles, cerebrovascular accident, ventricular tachycardia, cerebral ischemia, atrial fibrillation, varicose vein, pulmonary embolus, AV block, shock; *Rare:* vasculitis, pulmonary hypertension, pericarditis, migraine, heart block, cerebral hemorrhage

Digestive System—*Frequent:* nausea, vomiting, dyspepsia, diarrhea, constipation, dry mouth, dysphagia; *Infrequent:* flatulence, abnormal liver function tests, increased appetite, salivary gland enlargement, thirst, gastroenteritis, gastritis, periodontal abscess, intestinal obstruction, nausea and vomiting, gingivitis, esophagitis, cholelithiasis, tooth caries, hepatitis, stomach ulcer, melena, hepatomegaly, hematemesis, eructation; *Rare:* sialadenitis, peptic ulcer, pancreatitis, jaundice, glossitis, fecal incontinence, duodenitis, colitis, cholecystitis, aphthous stomatitis, esophageal ulcer

Endocrine System—*Infrequent:* hypothyroidism, adenoma, diabetes mellitus, ADH inappropriate; *Rare:* endocrine disorder, thyroid adenoma

Hemic and Lymphatic System—*Frequent:* anemia; *Infrequent:* leukopenia, lymphadenopathy, leukocytosis, thrombocytopenia, petechia, megaloblastic anemia, cyanosis; *Rare:* purpura, lymphocytosis, eosinophilia, thrombocythemia, acute lymphoblastic leukemia, polycythemia, splenomegaly

Metabolic and Nutritional System—*Frequent:* peripheral edema, weight loss, weight gain; *Infrequent:* dehydration, hypokalemia, hypoglycemia, iron deficiency anemia, hyperglycemia, gout, hypercholesteremia; *Rare:* electrolyte imbalance, cachexia, acidosis, hyperuricemia

Musculoskeletal System—*Frequent:* twitching, myalgia, arthralgia; *Infrequent:* bone pain, tenosynovitis, myositis, bone sarcoma, arthritis; *Rare:* osteoporosis, muscle atrophy, osteomyelitis

Nervous System—*Frequent:* dyskinesia, dizziness, hallucinations, confusion, somnolence, insomnia, dystonia, paresthesia, depression, anxiety, tremor, akinesia, extrapyramidal syndrome, abnormal gait, abnormal dreams, incoordination, psychosis, personality disorder, nervousness, choreoathetosis, amnesia, paranoid reaction, abnormal thinking; *Infrequent:* akathisia, neuropathy, neuralgia, hypertonia, delusions, convulsion, libido increased, euphoria, emotional lability, libido decreased, vertigo, myoclonus, coma, apathy, paralysis, neurosis, hyperkinesia, ataxia, acute brain syndrome, torticollis, meningitis, manic reaction, hypokinesia, hostility, agitation, hypotonia; *Rare:* stupor, neuritis, intracranial hypertension, hemiplegia, facial paralysis, brain edema, myelitis, hallucinations and confusion after abrupt discontinuation

Respiratory System—*Frequent:* rhinitis, dyspnea, pneumonia, pharyngitis, cough increased; *Infrequent:* epistaxis, hiccup, sinusitis, bronchitis, voice alteration, hemoptysis, asthma, lung edema, pleural effusion, laryngitis, emphysema, apnea, hyperventilation; *Rare:* pneumothorax, lung fibrosis, larynx edema, hypoxia, hypoventilation, hemothorax, carcinoma of lung

Skin and Appendages System—*Frequent:* sweating, rash; *Infrequent:* skin discoloration, pruritus, acne, skin ulcer, alopecia, dry skin, skin carcinoma, seborrhea, hirsutism, herpes simplex, eczema, fungal dermatitis, herpes zoster; *Rare:* vesiculobullous rash, subcutaneous nodule, skin nodule, skin benign neoplasm, lichenoid dermatitis

Special Senses System—*Frequent:* abnormal vision, diplopia; *Infrequent:* otitis media, conjunctivitis, tinnitus, deafness, taste perversion, ear pain, eye pain, glaucoma, eye hemorrhage, photophobia, visual field defect; *Rare:* blindness, cataract, retinal detachment, retinal vascular disorder

Urogenital System—*Frequent:* urinary tract infection, urinary frequency, urinary incontinence, hematuria, dysmenorrhea; *Infrequent:* dysuria, breast pain, menorrhagia, impotence, cystitis, urinary retention, abortion, vaginal hemorrhage, vaginitis, priapism, kidney calculus, fibrocystic breast, lactation, uterine hemorrhage, urolithiasis, salpingitis, pyuria, metrorrhagia, menopause, kidney failure, breast carcinoma, cervical carcinoma; *Rare:* amenorrhea, bladder carcinoma, breast engorgement, epididymitis, hypogonadism, leukorrhea, nephrosis, pyelonephritis, urethral pain, uricaciduria, withdrawal bleeding

Postintroduction Reports—Voluntary reports of adverse events temporally associated with pergolide that have been received since market introduction and which may have no causal relationship with the drug, include the following: neuroleptic malignant syndrome.

OVERDOSAGE

There is no clinical experience with massive overdosage. The largest overdose involved a young hospitalized adult patient who was not being treated with pergolide mesylate but who intentionally took 60 mg of the drug. He experienced vomiting, hypotension, and agitation. Another patient receiving a daily dosage of 7 mg of pergolide mesylate unintentionally took 19 mg/day for 3 days, after which his vital signs were normal but he experienced severe hallucinations. Within 36 hours of resumption of the prescribed dosage level, the hallucinations stopped. One patient unintentionally took 14 mg/day for 23 days instead of her prescribed 1.4 mg/day dosage. She experienced severe involuntary movements and tingling in her arms and legs. Another patient who inadvertently received 7 mg instead of the prescribed 0.7 mg experienced palpitations, hypotension, and ventricular extrasystoles. The highest total daily dose (prescribed for several patients with refractory Parkinson's disease) has exceeded 30 mg.

Symptoms —Animal studies indicate that the manifestations of overdosage in man might include nausea, vomiting, convulsions, decreased blood pressure, and CNS stimulation. The oral median lethal doses in mice and rats were 54 and 15 mg/kg respectively.

Treatment —To obtain up-to-date information about the treatment of overdose, a good resource is your certified Regional Poison Control Center. Telephone numbers of certified poison control centers are listed in the *Physicians' Desk Reference (PDR).* In managing overdosage, consider the possibility of multiple drug overdoses, interaction among drugs, and unusual drug kinetics in your patient.

Management of overdosage may require supportive measures to maintain arterial blood pressure. Cardiac function should be monitored; an antiarrhythmic agent may be necessary. If signs of CNS stimulation are present, a phenothiazine or other butyrophenone neuroleptic agent may be indicated; the efficacy of such drugs in reversing the effects of overdose has not been assessed.

Protect the patient's airway and support ventilation and perfusion. Meticulously monitor and maintain, within acceptable limits, the patient's vital signs, blood gases, serum electrolytes, etc. Absorption of drugs from the gastrointestinal tract may be decreased by giving activated charcoal, which, in many cases, is more effective than emesis or lavage; consider charcoal instead of or in addition to gastric emptying. Repeated doses of charcoal over time may hasten elimination of some drugs that have been absorbed. Safeguard the patient's airway when employing gastric emptying or charcoal.

There is no experience with dialysis or hemoperfusion, and these procedures are unlikely to be of benefit.

DOSAGE AND ADMINISTRATION

Administration of Permax should be initiated with a daily dosage of 0.05 mg for the first 2 days. The dosage should then be gradually increased by 0.1 or 0.15 mg/day every third day over the next 12 days of therapy. The dosage may then be increased by 0.25 mg/day every third day until an optimal therapeutic dosage is achieved.

Permax is usually administered in divided doses 3 times per day. During dosage titration, the dosage of concurrent *l*-dopa/carbidopa may be cautiously decreased.

In clinical studies, the mean therapeutic daily dosage of Permax was 3 mg/day. The average concurrent daily dosage of *l*-dopa/carbidopa (expressed as *l*-dopa) was approximately 650 mg/day. The efficacy of Permax at doses above 5 mg/day has not been systematically evaluated.

HOW SUPPLIED

Tablets (scored):

0.05 mg, ivory, debossed with A615, in bottles of 30 (UC5336)—NDC 59075-615-30

0.25 mg, green, debossed with A625, in bottles of 100 (UC5337)—NDC 59075-625-10

1 mg, pink, debossed with A630, in bottles of 100 (UC5338)—NDC 59075-630-10

Store at controlled room temperature, 15° to 30°C (59° to 86°F).

PERMAX is a registered trademark of Eli Lilly and Company, and licensed exclusively in the U.S. to Elan Pharmaceuticals, Inc.

Literature revised March 20, 2000

Manufactured by:
Eli Lilly and Company
Indianapolis, IN 46285, USA

Distributed by:
Athena Neurosciences,
a business unit of
Elan Pharmacaeuticals, Inc.
South San Francisco, CA 94080
PV 2278 UCP

Shown in Product Identification Guide, page 306

ZANAFLEX® ℞

[*zañ-ă-flex*]
(tizanidine hydrochloride)
Tablets 2 and 4 mg

DESCRIPTION

ZANAFLEX* (tizanidine hydrochloride) is a centrally acting α_2-adrenergic agonist. Tizanidine HCl (tizanidine) is a white to off-white, fine crystalline powder, odorless or with a faint characteristic odor. Tizanidine is slightly soluble in water and methanol; solubility in water decreases as the pH increases. Its chemical name is 5-chloro-4-(2-imidazolin-2-ylamino)-2,1,3-benzothiodiazole hydrochloride. Tizanidine's molecular formula is $C_9H_8ClN_5S{\cdot}HCl$, its molecular weight is 290.2 and its structural formula is:

Zanaflex is supplied as 2 and 4 mg tablets for oral administration. Zanaflex tablets are composed of the active ingredient, tizanidine hydrochloride (2.288 mg equivalent to 2 mg tizanidine base and 4.576 mg equivalent to 4 mg tizanidine base), and the inactive ingredients, silicon dioxide colloidal, stearic acid, microcrystalline cellulose and anhydrous lactose.

* Registered trademark of Elan Pharmaceuticals, Inc.

CLINICAL PHARMACOLOGY

Mechanism of Action

Tizanidine is an agonist at α_2-adrenergic receptor sites and presumably reduces spasticity by increasing presynaptic inhibition of motor neurons. In animal models, tizanidine has no direct effect on skeletal muscle fibers or the neuromuscular junction, and no major effect on monosynaptic spinal reflexes. The effects of tizanidine are greatest on polysynaptic pathways. The overall effect of these actions is thought to reduce facilitation of spinal motor neurons.

The imidazoline chemical structure of tizanidine is related to that of the anti-hypertensive drug clonidine and other α_2-adrenergic agonists. Pharmacological studies in animals show similarities between the two compounds, but tizanidine was found to have one-tenth to one-fiftieth (1/50) of the potency of clonidine in lowering blood pressure.

Pharmacokinetics

Following oral administration, tizanidine is essentially completely absorbed and has a half-life of approximately 2.5 hours (coefficient of variation [CV] = 33%). Following administration of tizanidine, peak plasma concentrations occurred at 1.5 hours (CV = 40%) after dosing. Food increases C_{max} by approximately one-third and shortens time to peak concentration by approximately 40 minutes, but the extent of tizanidine absorption is not affected. Tizanidine has linear pharmacokinetics over a dose of 1 to 20 mg. The absolute oral bioavailability of tizanidine is approximately 40% (CV = 24%), due to extensive first-pass metabolism in the liver; approximately 95% of an administered dose is metabolized. Tizanidine metabolites are not known to be active; their half-lives range from 20 to 40 hours. Tizanidine is widely distributed throughout the body; mean steady state volume of distribution is 2.4 L/kg (CV = 21%) following intravenous administration in healthy adult volunteers.

Following single and multiple oral dosing of ^{14}C-tizanidine, an average of 60% and 20% of total radioactivity was recovered in the urine and feces, respectively.

Tizanidine is approximately 30% bound to plasma proteins, independent of concentration over the therapeutic range.

Special Populations

Age Effects: No specific pharmacokinetic study was conducted to investigate age effects. Cross study comparison of pharmacokinetic data following single dose administration of 6 mg tizanidine showed that younger subjects cleared the drug four times faster than the elderly subjects. Tizanidine has not been evaluated in children (see PRECAUTIONS).

Hepatic Impairment: Pharmacokinetic differences due to hepatic impairment have not been studied (see WARNINGS).

Renal Impairment: Tizanidine clearance is reduced by more than 50% in elderly patients with renal insufficiency (creatinine clearance < 25 mL/min) compared to healthy elderly subjects; this would be expected to lead to a longer duration of clinical effect. Tizanidine should be used with caution in renally impaired patients (see PRECAUTIONS).

Gender Effects: No specific pharmacokinetic study was conducted to investigate gender effects. Retrospective analysis of pharmacokinetic data, however, following single and multiple dose administration of 4 mg tizanidine showed that gender had no effect on the pharmacokinetics of tizanidine.

Race Effects: Pharmacokinetic differences due to race have not been studied.

Drug Interactions-Oral Contraceptives: No specific pharmacokinetic study was conducted to investigate interaction between oral contraceptives and tizanidine. Retrospective analysis of population pharmacokinetic data following single and multiple dose administration of 4 mg tizanidine, however, showed that women concurrently taking oral contraceptives had 50% lower clearance of tizanidine compared to women not on oral contraceptives (see PRECAUTIONS).

CLINICAL STUDIES

Tizanidine's capacity to reduce increased muscle tone associated with spasticity was demonstrated in two adequate and well controlled studies in patients with multiple sclerosis or spinal cord injury.

In one study, patients with multiple sclerosis were randomized to receive single oral doses of drug or placebo. Patients and assessors were blind to treatment assignment and efforts were made to reduce the likelihood that assessors would become aware indirectly of treatment assignment (e.g., they did not provide direct care to patients and were prohibited from asking questions about side effects). In all, 140 patients received either placebo, 8 mg or 16 mg of tizanidine.

Response was assessed by physical examination; muscle tone was rated on a 5 point scale (Ashworth score), with a score of 0 used to describe normal muscle tone. A score of 1 indicated a slight spastic catch while a score of 2 indicated more marked muscle resistance. A score of 3 was used to describe considerable increase in tone, making passive movement difficult. A muscle immobilized by spasticity was given a score of 4. Spasm counts were also collected.

Assessments were made at 1, 2, 3 and 6 hours after treatment. A statistically significant reduction of the Ashworth score for Zanaflex compared to placebo was detected at 1, 2 and 3 hours after treatment. Figure 1 below shows a comparison of the mean change in muscle tone from baseline as measured by the Ashworth scale. The greatest reduction in muscle tone was 1 to 2 hours after treatment. By 6 hours after treatment, muscle tone in the 8 and 16 mg tizanidine groups was indistinguishable from muscle tone in placebo treated patients. Within a given patient, improvement in muscle tone was correlated with plasma concentration. Plasma concentrations were variable from patient to patient at a given dose. Although 16 mg produced a larger effect, adverse events including hypotension were more common and more severe than in the 8 mg group. There were no differences in the number of spasms occurring in each group.

FIGURE 1: Single Dose Study - Mean Change in Muscle Tone from Baseline as Measured by the Ashworth Scale +/- 95% Confidence Interval
(A Negative Ashworth Score Signifies an Improvement in Muscle Tone from Baseline)

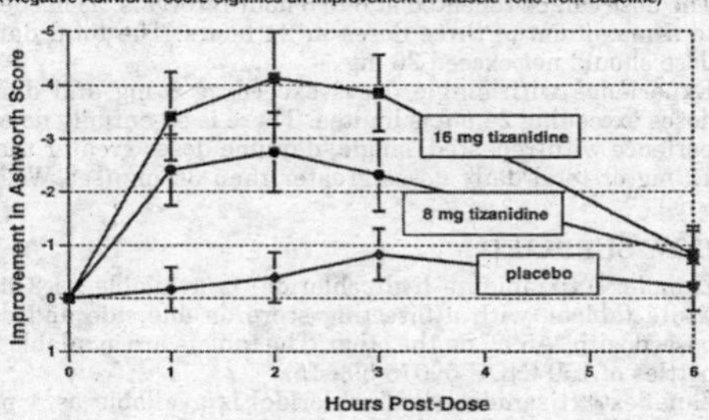

In a multiple dose study, 118 patients with spasticity secondary to spinal cord injury were randomized to either placebo or tizanidine. Steps similar to those taken in the first study were employed to ensure the integrity of blinding.

Patients were titrated over 3 weeks up to a maximum tolerated dose or 36 mg daily given in three unequal doses (e.g., 10 mg given in the morning and afternoon and 16 mg given at night). Patients were then maintained on their maximally tolerated dose for 4 additional weeks (i.e., maintenance phase). Throughout the maintenance phase, muscle tone was assessed on the Ashworth scale within a period of 2.5 hours following either the morning or afternoon dose. The number of daytime spasms was recorded daily by patients.

At endpoint (the protocol-specified time of outcome assessment), there was a statistically significant reduction in muscle tone and frequency of spasms in the tizanidine treated group compared to placebo. The reduction in muscle tone was not associated with a reduction in muscle strength (a desirable outcome) but also did not lead to any consistent advantage of tizanidine treated patients on measures of activities of daily living. Figure 2 below shows a comparison of the mean change in muscle tone from baseline as measured by the Ashworth scale.

FIGURE 2: Multiple Dose Study - Mean Change in Muscle Tone 0.5-2.5 Hours after Dosing as Measured by the Ashworth Scale +/- 95% Confidence Interval
(A Negative Ashworth Score Signifies an Improvement in Muscle Tone from Baseline)

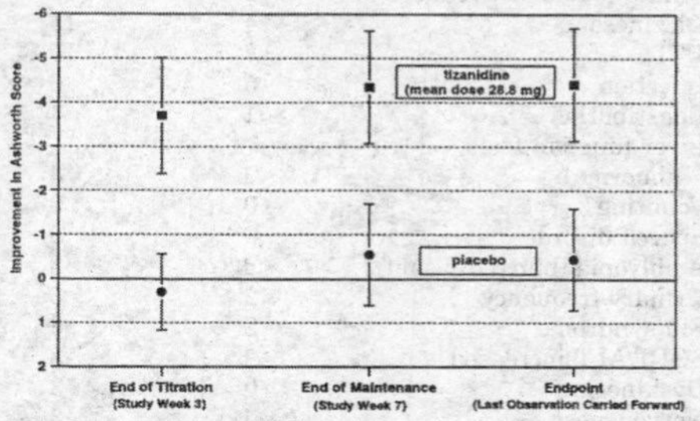

INDICATIONS AND USAGE

Tizanidine is a short-acting drug for the management of spasticity. Because of the short duration of effect, treatment with tizanidine should be reserved for those daily activities and times when relief of spasticity is most important (see DOSAGE AND ADMINISTRATION).

CONTRAINDICATIONS

Zanaflex is contraindicated in patients with known hypersensitivity to Zanaflex or its ingredients.

WARNINGS

Limited data base for chronic use of single doses above 8 mg and multiple doses above 24 mg per day

Clinical experience with long-term use of tizanidine at doses of 8 to 16 mg single doses or total daily doses of 24 to 36 mg (see DOSAGE AND ADMINISTRATION) is limited. Approximately 75 patients have been exposed to individual doses of 12 mg or more for at least one year or more and approximately 80 patients have been exposed to total daily doses of 30 to 36 mg/day for at least one year or more. There is essentially no long-term experience with single, daytime doses of 16 mg. Because long-term clinical study experience at high doses is limited, only those adverse events with a relatively high incidence are likely to have been identified (see WARNINGS, PRECAUTIONS and ADVERSE REACTIONS).

Hypotension

Tizanidine is an α_2-adrenergic agonist (like clonidine) and can produce hypotension. In a single dose study where blood pressure was monitored closely after dosing, two-thirds of patients treated with 8 mg of tizanidine had a 20% reduction in either the diastolic or systolic BP. The reduction was seen within 1 hour after dosing, peaked 2 to 3 hours after dosing and was associated, at times, with bradycardia, orthostatic hypotension, lightheadedness/dizziness and rarely syncope. The hypotensive effect is dose related and has been measured following single doses of ≥ 2 mg.

The chance of significant hypotension may possibly be minimized by titration of the dose and by focusing attention on signs and symptoms of hypotension prior to dose advancement. In addition, patients moving from a supine to a fixed upright position may be at increased risk for hypotension and orthostatic effects.

Caution is advised when tizanidine is to be used in patients receiving concurrent antihypertensive therapy and should not be used with other α_2-adrenergic agonists.

Risk of Liver Injury

Tizanidine occasionally causes liver injury, most often hepatocellular in type. In controlled clinical studies, approximately 5% of patients treated with tizanidine had elevations of liver function tests (ALT/SGPT, AST/SGOT) to greater than 3 times the upper limit of normal (or 2 times if baseline levels were elevated) compared to 0.4% in the control patients. Most cases resolved rapidly upon drug withdrawal with no reported residual problems. In occasional symptomatic cases, nausea, vomiting, anorexia and jaundice have been reported. In postmarketing experience, three deaths associated with liver failure have been reported in patients treated with tizanidine. In one case, a 49 year-old male developed jaundice and liver enlargement following 2 months of tizanidine treatment, primarily at 6 mg tid. A liver biopsy showed multilobular necrosis without eosinophilic infiltration. Treatment was discontinued and the patient died in hepatic coma 10 days later. There was no evidence of hepatitis B and C in this patient and other therapy included only oxezepam and ranitidine. There was thus no explanation, other than a reaction to tizanidine, to explain the liver injury. In the two other cases, patients were taking other drugs with known potential for liver toxicity. One patient, treated with tizanidine at a dose of 4 mg/day, was also on carbamazepine when he developed cholestatic jaundice after 2 months of treatment; this patient died with pneumonia about 20 days later. Another patient, treated with tizanidine for 11 days, was also treated with dantrolene for about 2 weeks prior to developing fatal fulminant hepatic failure.

Monitoring of aminotransferase levels is recommended during the first 6 months of treatment (e.g., baseline, 1, 3 and 6 months) and periodically thereafter, based on clinical status. Because of the potential toxic hepatic effect of tizanidine, the drug should be used only with extreme caution in patients with impaired hepatic function.

Sedation

In the multiple dose, controlled clinical studies, 48% of patients receiving any dose of tizanidine reported sedation as an adverse event. In 10% of these cases, the sedation was rated as severe compared to <1% in the placebo treated patients. Sedation may interfere with everyday activity.

The effect appears to be dose related. In a single dose study, 92% of the patients receiving 16 mg, when asked, reported that they were drowsy during the 6 hour study. This compares to 76% of the patients on 8 mg and 35% of the patients on placebo. Patients began noting this effect 30 minutes following dosing. The effect peaked 1.5 hours following dosing. Of the patients who received a single dose of 16 mg, 51% continued to report drowsiness 6 hours following dosing compared to 13% in the patients receiving placebo or 8 mg of tizanidine.

In the multiple dose studies, the prevalence of patients with sedation peaked following the first week of titration and then remained stable for the duration of the maintenance phase of the study.

Hallucinosis/Psychotic-Like Symptoms

Tizanidine use has been associated with hallucinations. Formed, visual hallucinations or delusions have been reported in 5 of 170 patients (3%) in two North American controlled clinical studies. These 5 cases occurred within the first 6 weeks. Most of the patients were aware that the events were unreal. One patient developed psychoses in association with the hallucinations. One patient among these 5 continued to have problems for at least 2 weeks following discontinuation of tizanidine.

PRECAUTIONS

Cardiovascular

Prolongation of the QT interval and bradycardia were noted in chronic toxicity studies in dogs at doses equal to the maximum human dose on a mg/m^2 basis. ECG evaluation was not performed in the controlled clinical studies. Reduction in pulse rate has been noted in association with decreases in blood pressure in the single dose controlled study (see WARNINGS).

Ophthalmic

Dose-related retinal degeneration and corneal opacities have been found in animal studies at doses equivalent to approximately the maximum recommended dose on a mg/m^2 basis. There have been no reports of corneal opacities or retinal degeneration in the clinical studies.

Use in Renally Impaired Patients

Tizanidine should be used with caution in patients with renal insufficiency (creatinine clearance < 25 mL/min), as clearance is reduced by more than 50%. In these patients, during titration, the individual doses should be reduced. If higher doses are required, individual doses rather than dosing frequency should be increased. These patients should be monitored closely for the onset or increase in severity of the common adverse events (dry mouth, somnolence, asthenia and dizziness) as indicators of potential overdose.

Use in Women Taking Oral Contraceptives

Tizanidine should be used with caution in women taking oral contraceptives, as clearance of tizanidine is reduced by approximately 50% in such patients. In these patients, during titration, the individual doses should be reduced.

Information for Patients

Patients should be advised of the limited clinical experience with tizanidine both in regard to duration of use and the higher doses required to reduce muscle tone (see WARNINGS).

Because of the possibility of tizanidine lowering blood pressure, patients should be warned about the risk of clinically significant orthostatic hypotension (see WARNINGS).

Because of the possibility of sedation, patients should be warned about performing activities requiring alertness, such as driving a vehicle or operating machinery (see WARNINGS). Patients should also be instructed that the sedation may be additive when Zanaflex is taken in conjunction with drugs (baclofen, benzodiazepines) or substances (e.g., alcohol) that act as CNS depressants.

Zanaflex should be used with caution where spasticity is utilized to sustain posture and balance in locomotion or whenever spasticity is utilized to obtain increased function.

Drug Interactions

In vitro studies of cytochrome P450 isoenzymes using human liver microsomes indicate that neither tizanidine nor the major metabolites are likely to affect the metabolism of other drugs metabolized by cytochrome P450 isoenzymes.

Acetaminophen: Tizanidine delayed the T_{max} of acetaminophen by 16 minutes. Acetaminophen did not affect the pharmacokinetics of tizanidine.

Alcohol: Alcohol increased the AUC of tizanidine by approximately 20% while also increasing its C_{max} by approximately 15%. This was associated with an increase in side effects of tizanidine. The CNS depressant effects of tizanidine and alcohol are additive.

Oral Contraceptives: No specific pharmacokinetic study was conducted to investigate interaction between oral contraceptives and tizanidine, but retrospective analysis of population pharmacokinetic data following single and multiple dose administration of 4 mg tizanidine showed that women concurrently taking oral contraceptives had 50% lower clearance of tizanidine than women not on oral contraceptives.

Carcinogenesis, Mutagenesis, Impairment of Fertility

No evidence for carcinogenicity was seen in two dietary studies in rodents. Tizanidine was administered to mice for

Continued on next page

Zanaflex—Cont.

78 weeks at doses up to 16 mg/kg, which is equivalent to 2 times the maximum recommended human dose on a mg/m^2 basis. Tizanidine was also administered to rats for 104 weeks at doses up to 9 mg/kg, which is equivalent to 2.5 times the maximum recommended human dose on a mg/m^2 basis. There was no statistically significant increase in tumors in either species.

Tizanidine was not mutagenic or clastogenic in the following *in vitro* assays: the bacterial Ames test and the mammalian gene mutation test and chromosomal aberration test in Chinese hamster cells. It was also negative in the following *in vivo* assays: the bone marrow micronucleus test in mice, the bone marrow micronucleus and cytogenicity test in Chinese hamsters, the dominant lethal mutagenicity test in mice, and the unscheduled DNA synthesis (UDS) test in mice.

Tizanidine did not affect fertility in male rats at doses of 10 mg/kg, approximately 2.7 times the maximum recommended human dose on a mg/m^2 basis, and in females at doses of 3 mg/kg, approximately equal to the maximum recommended human dose on a mg/m^2 basis; fertility was reduced in males receiving 30 mg/kg (8 times the maximum recommended human dose on a mg/m^2 basis) and in females receiving 10 mg/kg (2.7 times the maximum recommended human dose on a mg/m^2 basis). At these doses, maternal behavioral effects and clinical signs were observed including marked sedation, weight loss, and ataxia.

Pregnancy

Pregnancy Category C: Reproduction studies performed in rats at a dose of 3 mg/kg, equal to the maximum recommended human dose on a mg/m^2 basis, and in rabbits at 30 mg/kg, 16 times the maximum recommended human dose on a mg/m^2 basis, did not show evidence of teratogenicity. Tizanidine at doses that are equal to and up to 8 times the maximum recommended human dose on a mg/m^2 basis increased gestation duration in rats. Prenatal and postnatal pup loss was increased and developmental retardation occurred. Postimplantation loss was increased in rabbits at doses of 1 mg/kg or greater, equal to or greater than 0.5 times the maximum recommended human dose on a mg/m^2 basis. Tizanidine has not been studied in pregnant women. Tizanidine should be given to pregnant women only if clearly needed.

Labor and Delivery

The effect of tizanidine on labor and delivery in humans is unknown.

Nursing Mothers

It is not known whether tizanidine is excreted in human milk, although as a lipid soluble drug, it might be expected to pass into breast milk.

Geriatric Use

Tizanidine should be used with caution in elderly patients because clearance is decreased four-fold.

Pediatric Use

There are no adequate and well-controlled studies to document the safety and efficacy of tizanidine in children.

ADVERSE REACTIONS

In multiple dose, placebo-controlled clinical studies, 264 patients were treated with tizanidine and 261 with placebo. Adverse events, including severe adverse events, were more frequently reported with tizanidine than with placebo.

Common Adverse Events Leading to Discontinuation

Forty-five of 264 (17%) patients receiving tizanidine and 13 of 261 (5%) patients receiving placebo in three multiple dose, placebo-controlled clinical studies discontinued treatment for adverse events. When patients withdrew from the study, they frequently had more than one reason for discontinuing. The adverse events most frequently leading to withdrawal of tizanidine treated patients in the controlled clinical studies were asthenia (weakness, fatigue and/or tiredness) (3%), somnolence (3%), dry mouth (3%), increased spasm or tone (2%) and dizziness (2%).

Most Frequent Adverse Clinical Events Seen in Association With the Use of Tizanidine

In multiple dose, placebo-controlled clinical studies involving 264 patients with spasticity, the most frequent adverse events were dry mouth, somnolence/sedation, asthenia (weakness, fatigue and/or tiredness), and dizziness. Three-quarters of the patients rated the events as mild to moderate and one-quarter of the patients rated the events as being severe. These events appeared to be dose related.

Adverse Events Reported in Controlled Studies

The events cited reflect experience gained under closely monitored conditions of clinical studies in a highly selected patient population. In actual clinical practice or in other clinical studies, these frequency estimates may not apply, as the conditions of use, reporting behavior, and the kinds of patients treated may differ. Table 1 lists treatment emergent signs and symptoms that were reported in greater than 2% of patients in three multiple dose, placebo-controlled studies who received tizanidine where the frequency in the tizanidine group was at least as common as in the placebo group. These events are not necessarily related to tizanidine treatment. For comparison purposes, the corresponding frequency of the event (per 100 patients) among placebo treated patients is also provided.

TABLE 1: Multiple Dose, Placebo-Controlled Studies - Frequent (> 2%) Adverse Events Reported for Which Zanaflex Incidence is Greater Than Placebo

Event	Placebo N = 261 %	Zanaflex N = 264 %
Dry mouth	10	49
Somnolence	10	48
Asthenia (weakness, fatigue and/or tiredness)	16	41
Dizziness	4	16
UTI	7	10
Infection	5	6
Constipation	1	4
Liver function tests abnormal	<1	3
Vomiting	0	3
Speech disorder	0	3
Amblyopia (blurred vision)	<1	3
Urinary frequency	2	3
Flu syndrome	2	3
SGPT/ALT increased	<1	3
Dyskinesia	0	3
Nervousness	<1	3
Pharyngitis	1	3
Rhinitis	2	3

In the single dose, placebo-controlled study involving 142 patients with spasticity, the patients were specifically asked if they had experienced any of the four most common adverse events: dry mouth, somnolence (drowsiness), asthenia (weakness, fatigue and/or tiredness), and dizziness. In addition, hypotension and bradycardia were observed. The occurrence of these adverse events are summarized in Table 2. Other events were, in general, reported at a rate of 2% or less.

TABLE 2: Single Dose, Placebo-Controlled Study - Common Adverse Events Reported

Event	Placebo N = 48 %	Zanaflex 8 mg N = 45 %	Zanaflex 16 mg N = 49 %
Somnolence	31	78	92
Dry mouth	35	76	88
Asthenia (weakness, fatigue and/or tiredness)	40	67	78
Dizziness	4	22	45
Hypotension	0	16	33
Bradycardia	0	2	10

Other Adverse Events Observed During the Evaluation of Tizanidine

Tizanidine was administered to 1187 patients in additional clinical studies where adverse event information was available. The conditions and duration of exposure varied greatly, and included (in overlapping categories) double-blind and open-label studies, uncontrolled and controlled studies, inpatient and outpatient studies, and titration studies. Untoward events associated with this exposure were recorded by clinical investigators using terminology of their own choosing. Consequently, it is not possible to provide a meaningful estimate of the proportion of individuals experiencing adverse events without first grouping similar types of untoward events into a smaller number of standardized event categories.

In the tabulations that follow, reported adverse events were classified using a standard COSTART-based dictionary terminology. The frequencies presented, therefore, represent the proportion of the 1187 patients exposed to tizanidine who experienced an event of the type cited on at least one occasion while receiving tizanidine. All reported events are included except those already listed in Table 1. If the COSTART term for an event was so general as to be uninformative, it was replaced with a more informative term. It is important to emphasize that, although the events reported occurred during treatment with tizanidine, they were not necessarily caused by it.

Events are further categorized by body system and listed in order of decreasing frequency according to the following definitions: frequent adverse events are those occurring on one or more occasions in at least 1/100 patients (only those not already listed in the tabulated results from placebo-controlled studies appear in this listing); infrequent adverse events are those occurring in 1/100 to 1/1000 patients.

Body as a Whole: *Frequent:* fever; *Infrequent:* allergic reaction, moniliasis, malaise, abscess, neck pain, sepsis, cellulitis, death, overdose; *Rare:* carcinoma, congenital anomaly, suicide attempt.

Cardiovascular System: *Infrequent:* vasodilatation, postural hypotension, syncope, migraine, arrhythmia; *Rare:* angina pectoris, coronary artery disorder, heart failure, myocardial infarct, phlebitis, pulmonary embolus, ventricular extrasystoles, ventricular tachycardia.

Digestive System: *Frequent:* abdomen pain, diarrhea, dyspepsia; *Infrequent:* dysphagia, cholelithiasis, fecal impaction, flatulence, gastrointestinal hemorrhage, hepatitis, melena; *Rare:* gastroenteritis, hematemesis, hepatoma, intestinal obstruction, liver damage.

Hemic and Lymphatic System: *Infrequent:* ecchymosis, hypercholesteremia, anemia, hyperlipemia, leukopenia, leukocytosis, sepsis; *Rare:* petechia, purpura, thrombocythemia, thrombocytopenia.

Metabolic and Nutritional System: *Infrequent:* edema, hypothyroidism, weight loss; *Rare:* adrenal cortex insufficiency, hyperglycemia, hypokalemia, hyponatremia, hypoproteinemia, respiratory acidosis.

Musculoskeletal System: *Frequent:* myasthenia, back pain; *Infrequent:* pathological fracture, arthralgia, arthritis, bursitis.

Nervous System: *Frequent:* depression, anxiety, paresthesia; *Infrequent:* tremor, emotional lability, convulsion, paralysis, thinking abnormal, vertigo, abnormal dreams, agitation, depersonalization, euphoria, migraine, stupor, dysautonomia, neuralgia; *Rare:* dementia, hemiplegia, neuropathy.

Respiratory System: *Infrequent:* sinusitis, pneumonia, bronchitis; *Rare:* asthma.

Skin and Appendages: *Frequent:* rash, sweating, skin ulcer; *Infrequent:* pruritus, dry skin, acne, alopecia, urticaria; *Rare:* exfoliative dermatitis, herpes simplex, herpes zoster, skin carcinoma.

Special Senses: *Infrequent:* ear pain, tinnitus, deafness, glaucoma, conjunctivitis, eye pain, optic neuritis, otitis media, retinal hemorrhage, visual field defect; *Rare:* iritis, keratitis, optic atrophy.

Urogenital System: *Infrequent:* urinary urgency, cystitis, menorrhagia, pyelonephritis, urinary retention, kidney calculus, uterine fibroids enlarged, vaginal moniliasis, vaginitis; *Rare:* albuminuria, glycosuria, hematuria, metrorrhagia.

DRUG ABUSE AND DEPENDENCE

Abuse potential was not evaluated in human studies. Rats were able to distinguish tizanidine from saline in a standard discrimination paradigm, after training, but failed to generalize the effects of morphine, cocaine, diazepam or phenobarbital to tizanidine. Monkeys were shown to self-administer tizanidine in a dose-dependent manner, and abrupt cessation of tizanidine produced transient signs of withdrawal at doses > 35 times the maximum recommended human dose on a mg/m^2 basis. These transient withdrawal signs (increased locomotion, body twitching, and aversive behavior toward the observer) were not reversed by naloxone administration.

OVERDOSAGE

One significant overdosage of tizanidine has been reported. Attempted suicide by a 46 year-old male with multiple sclerosis resulted in coma very shortly after the ingestion of one-hundred 4 mg tizanidine tablets. Pupils were not dilated and nystagmus was not present. The patient had marked respiratory depression with Cheyne-Stokes respiration. Gastric lavage and forced diuresis with furosemide and mannitol were instituted. The patient recovered several hours later without sequelae. Laboratory findings were normal.

Should overdosage occur, basic steps to ensure the adequacy of an airway and the monitoring of cardiovascular and respiratory systems should be undertaken. For the most recent information concerning the management of overdose, contact a poison control center.

DOSAGE AND ADMINISTRATION

A single oral dose of 8 mg of tizanidine reduces muscle tone in patients with spasticity for a period of several hours. The effect peaks at approximately 1 to 2 hours and dissipates between 3 to 6 hours. Effects are dose-related.

Although single doses of less than 8 mg have not been demonstrated to be effective in controlled clinical studies, the dose-related nature of tizanidine's common adverse events make it prudent to begin treatment with single oral doses of 4 mg. Increase the dose gradually (2 to 4 mg steps) to optimum effect (satisfactory reduction of muscle tone at a tolerated dose).

The dose can be repeated at 6 to 8 hour intervals, as needed, to a maximum of three doses in 24 hours. The total daily dose should not exceed 36 mg.

Experience with single doses exceeding 8 mg and daily doses exceeding 24 mg is limited. There is essentially no experience with repeated, single, daytime doses greater than 12 mg or total daily doses greater than 36 mg (see WARNINGS).

HOW SUPPLIED

Zanaflex® (tizanidine hydrochloride) is available as 2 mg white tablets, with a bisecting score on one side and debossed with "A592" on the other. The tablets are available in bottles of 150 (NDC 59075-592-15).

Zanaflex® (tizanidine hydrochloride) is available as 4 mg white tablets, with a quadrisecting score on one side and debossed with "A594" on the other. The tablets are available in bottles of 150 (NDC 59075-594-15).

Store at 25°C (77°F); excursions permitted to 15–30°C (59–86°F) [see USP Controlled Room Temperature]. Dispense in containers with child resistant closure.

Rx Only

Manufactured by:
Novartis Pharma AG.
Basel, Switzerland
for

Athena Neurosciences
a business unit of Elan Pharmaceuticals
South San Francisco, California 94080

700045 Rev. 02-08-00

Shown in Product Identification Guide, page 306

Aventis Pharmaceuticals

399 INTERPACE PARKWAY
P.O. BOX 663
PARSIPPANY, NJ 07054

Direct Inquiries to:
Customer Service
399 Interpace Parkway
P.O. Box 663
Parsippany, NJ 07054
(800) 207-8049

For Medical Information Contact:
Generally:
Medical Informatics
399 Interpace Parkway
Parsippany, NJ 07054
(800) 633-1610

For information on the following products which are not described, contact the Customer Information Center at (800) 552-3656:
Bentyl® (dicyclomine hydrochloride USP) Capsules, Tablets, Injection, Syrup
Cantil® (mepenzolate bromide USP) Tablets
Cardizem® SR (diltiazem hydrochloride) Capsules
Cardizem® (diltiazem hydrochloride) Tablets
Cephulac® (lactulose solution)
Chronulac® (lactulose solution)
DDAVP® Rhinal Tube 2.5 mL (desmopressin acetate)
Hiprex® (methenamine hippurate)
Lasix® (furosemide) Tablets
Novafed® A (pseudoephedrine hydrochloride and chlorpheniramine maleate) Extended-Release Capsules
SLO-PHYLLIN® Tablets and Syrup (theophylline, anhydrous, USP)
SLO-PHYLLIN® GG Syrup (150 mg theophylline, anhydrous and 90 mg guaifenesin/15 mL)
Tenuate® (diethylpropion hydrochloride USP) Tablets/Dospan

PRODUCT IDENTIFICATION NUMERICAL SUMMARY SOLID ORAL DOSAGE FORMS

Aventis Pharmaceuticals
Parsippany, NJ 07054
To provide quick and positive identification of Aventis Pharmaceuticals prescription drug products, we have imprinted an identifying number and the name MARION on the following tablets.
1771 CARDIZEM® Tablets, 30 mg (diltiazem hydrochloride)
1772 CARDIZEM® Tablets, 60 mg (diltiazem hydrochloride)
ALLEGRA® 60-mg capsules are imprinted in black ink, with "allegra" on the cap and "60 mg" on the body.
ALLEGRA® 30-mg tablets have 03 on one side and 0088 on the other.
ALLEGRA® 60-mg tablets have 06 on one side and 0088 on the other.
ALLEGRA® 180-mg tablets have 018 on one side and 0088 on the other.
ALLEGRA-D® extended-release tablets are engraved with "Allegra-D".
AMARYL® (glimepiride) Tablets 1 mg, 2 mg, and 4 mg are imprinted with "AMARYL" on one side and the Hoechst logo on both sides of the bisect on the other side.
ANZEMET® 50 mg tablets are imprinted with "ANZEMET 50" on one side.
ANZEMET® 100 mg tablets are imprinted with "100" on one side and "ANZEMET" on the other.
ARAVA™ (leflunomide) Tablets, 10 mg, are embossed with "ZBN" on one side.
ARAVA™ Tablets, 20 mg, are embossed with "ZBO" on one side.
ARAVA™ Tablets, 100 mg, are embossed with "ZBP" on one side.
BENTYL® Capsules, 10 mg (dicyclomine hydrochloride USP) is imprinted BENTYL 10.
BENTYL® Tablets, 20 mg (dicyclomine hydrochloride USP) is debossed BENTYL 20.
CANTIL® Tablets, 25 mg (mepenzolate bromide USP) is debossed MERRELL 37.
CARAFATE® Tablets, 1 g (sucralfate) is identified by the brand name CARAFATE embossed on one side and 1712 on the reverse side.
CARDIZEM® Tablets, 90 mg (diltiazem hydrochloride) is imprinted with the brand name CARDIZEM on one side and 90 mg on the reverse side.
CARDIZEM® Tablets, 120 mg (diltiazem hydrochloride) is imprinted with the brand name CARDIZEM on one side and 120 mg on the reverse side.
CARDIZEM® SR Capsules, 60 mg (diltiazem hydrochloride) is imprinted with the Cardizem logo on one end and Cardizem SR 60 mg on the other.
CARDIZEM® SR Capsules, 90 mg (diltiazem hydrochloride) is imprinted with the Cardizem logo on one end and Cardizem SR 90 mg on the other.
CARDIZEM® SR Capsules, 120 mg (diltiazem hydrochloride) is imprinted with the Cardizem logo on one end and Cardizem SR 120 mg on the other.
CARDIZEM® CD Capsules, 120 mg (diltiazem hydrochloride) is imprinted with cardizem CD and 120 mg on one end.
CARDIZEM® CD Capsules, 180 mg (diltiazem hydrochloride) is imprinted with cardizem CD and 180 mg on one end.
CARDIZEM® CD Capsules, 240 mg (diltiazem hydrochloride) is imprinted with cardizem CD and 240 mg on one end.
CARDIZEM® CD Capsules, 300 mg (diltiazem hydrochloride) is imprinted with cardizem CD and 300 mg on one end.
CARDIZEM® CD Capsules, 360 mg (diltiazem hydrochloride) is imprinted with cardizem CD and 360 mg on one end.
CLOMID® Tablets, 50 mg (clomiphene citrate) is debossed CLOMID 50.
DDAVP® (desmopressin acetate) 0.1 mg Tablets are coded with "DDAVP" on one side of the bisect and "0.1" on the other side of the bisect. "RPR" is coded on the reverse.
DDAVP® (desmopressin acetate) 0.2 mg Tablets are coded with "DDAVP" on one side of the bisect and "0.2" on the other side of the bisect. "RPR" is coded on the reverse.
DIAβETA® (glyburide) Tablets 1.25 mg, 2.5 mg, and 5 mg are imprinted with "Hoechst" on one side and "Diaβ" on the other side.
HIPREX® Tablets, 1 g (methenamine hippurate) is debossed MERRELL 277.
LASIX® (furosemide) Tablets 20 mg are imprinted with "Lasix® " on one side and "HOECHST" on the other.
LASIX® (furosemide) Tablets 40 mg are imprinted with "Lasix® 40" on one side and the Hoechst logo on the other.
LASIX® (furosemide) Tablets 80 mg are imprinted with "Lasix® 80" on one side and the Hoechst logo on the other.
NILANDRON® Tablets have a triangular logo on one face and an internal reference number (168) on the other.
NORPRAMIN® Tablets, 10 mg (desipramine hydrochloride USP) is imprinted 68-7.
NORPRAMIN® Tablets, 25 mg (desipramine hydrochloride USP) is imprinted NORPRAMIN 25.
NORPRAMIN® Tablets, 50 mg (desipramine hydrochloride USP) is imprinted NORPRAMIN 50.
NORPRAMIN® Tablets, 75 mg (desipramine hydrochloride USP) is imprinted NORPRAMIN 75.
NORPRAMIN® Tablets, 100 mg (desipramine hydrochloride USP) is imprinted NORPRAMIN 100.
NORPRAMIN® Tablets, 150 mg (desipramine hydrochloride USP) is imprinted NORPRAMIN 150.
NOVAFED® A Capsules, 120 mg pseudoephedrine hydrochloride and 8 mg chlorpheniramine maleate is imprinted NOVAFED A.
Penetrex® (enoxacin) 200 mg Tablets are marked with "rPr" on one side and "5100" on the other.
Penetrex® (enoxacin) 400 mg Tablets are marked with "rPr" on one side and "5140" on the other.
RIFADIN® Capsules, 150 mg (rifampin) is imprinted RIFADIN 150.
RIFADIN® Capsules, 300 mg (rifampin) is imprinted RIFADIN 300.
RIFAMATE® Capsules, 300 mg rifampin and 150 mg isoniazid is imprinted RIFAMATE.
RIFATER® Tablets, 120 mg rifampin, 50 mg isoniazid, and 300 mg pyrazinamide is imprinted RIFATER.
Rilutek® (riluzole) 50 mg Tablets are engraved with "RPR 202" on one side.
Slo-Phyllin® (theophylline, anhydrous, USP) 100 mg Tablets are coded with "rPr" and "351" on one side.
Slo-Phyllin® (theophylline, anhydrous, USP) 200 mg Tablets are coded with "rPr" and "352" on one side.
TENUATE® Tablets, 25 mg (diethylpropion hydrochloride USP) is debossed TENUATE 25 or MERRELL 697.
TENUATE® DOSPAN® Controlled-Release Tablets, 75 mg (diethylpropion hydrochloride USP) is debossed TENUATE 75 or MERRELL 698.
TRENTAL® (pentoxifylline) Tablets are imprinted "TRENTAL".

ALLEGRA® ℞

[ə-ˈlĕgra]
(fexofenadine hydrochloride)
Capsules and Tablets

Prescribing Information as of February 2000

DESCRIPTION

Fexofenadine hydrochloride, the active ingredient of ALLEGRA, is a histamine H_1-receptor antagonist with the chemical name (±)-4-[1 hydroxy-4-[4-(hydroxydiphenylmethyl)-1-piperidinyl]-butyl]-α, α-dimethyl benzeneacetic acid hydrochloride. It has the following chemical structure

The molecular weight is 538.13 and the empirical formula is $C_{32}H_{39}NO_4 \cdot HCl$.

Fexofenadine hydrochloride is a white to off-white crystalline powder. It is freely soluble in methanol and ethanol, slightly soluble in chloroform and water, and insoluble in hexane. Fexofenadine hydrochloride is a racemate and exists as a zwitterion in aqueous media at physiological pH.

ALLEGRA is formulated as a capsule or tablet for oral administration. Each capsule contains 60 mg fexofenadine hydrochloride and the following excipients: croscarmellose sodium, gelatin, lactose, microcrystalline cellulose, and pregelatinized starch. The printed capsule shell is made from gelatin, iron oxide, silicon dioxide, sodium lauryl sulfate, titanium dioxide, and other ingredients.

Each tablet contains 30, 60, or 180 mg fexofenadine hydrochloride (depending on the dosage strength) and the following excipients: croscarmellose sodium, magnesium stearate, microcrystalline cellulose, and pregelatinized starch. The aqueous tablet film coating is made from hydroxypropyl methylcellulose, iron oxide blends, polyethylene glycol, povidone, silicone dioxide, and titanium dioxide.

CLINICAL PHARMACOLOGY

Mechanism of Action

Fexofenadine hydrochloride is an antihistamine with selective peripheral H_1-receptor antagonist activity. Both enantiomers of fexofenadine hydrochloride displayed approximately equipotent antihistaminic effects. Fexofenadine inhibited histamine release from peritoneal mast cells in rats. In laboratory animals, no anticholinergic, $alpha_1$-adrenergic or beta-adrenergic-receptor blocking effects were observed. No sedative or other central nervous system effects were observed. Radiolabeled tissue distribution studies in rats indicated that fexofenadine does not cross the blood-brain barrier.

Pharmacokinetics

Absorption:

Fexofenadine hydrochloride was rapidly absorbed following oral administration of a single dose of two 60 mg capsules to healthy male volunteers with a mean time to maximum plasma concentration occurring at 2.6 hours post-dose. After administration of a single 60 mg capsule to healthy subjects, the mean maximum plasma concentration was 131 ng/mL. Following single dose oral administrations of either the 60 and 180 mg tablet to healthy, adult male volunteers, mean maximum plasma concentrations were 142 and 494 ng/mL, respectively. The tablet formulations are bioequivalent to the capsule when administered at equal doses. Fexofenadine hydrochloride pharmacokinetics are linear for oral doses up to a total daily dose of 240 mg (120 mg twice daily).

Distribution:

Fexofenadine hydrochloride is 60% to 70% bound to plasma proteins, primarily albumin and α_1-acid glycoprotein.

Elimination:

The mean elimination half-life of fexofenadine was 14.4 hours following administration of 60 mg, twice daily, in normal volunteers.

Human mass balance studies documented a recovery of approximately 80% and 11% of the [^{14}C] fexofenadine hydrochloride dose in the feces and urine, respectively. Because the absolute bioavailability of fexofenadine hydrochloride has not been established, it is unknown if the fecal component represents unabsorbed drug or the result of biliary excretion.

Metabolism:

Approximately 5% of the total oral dose was metabolized.

Special Populations:

Special population pharmacokinetics (for geriatric subjects, renal and hepatic impairment), obtained after a single dose of 80 mg fexofenadine hydrochloride, were compared to those for normal subjects from a separate study of similar design. While subject weights were relatively uniform between studies, these adult special population patients were substantially older than the healthy, young volunteers. Thus, an age effect may be confounding the pharmacokinetic differences observed in some of the special populations.

Seasonal allergic rhinitis (SAR) and chronic idiopathic urticaria (CIU) patients. The pharmacokinetics of fexofenadine hydrochloride in seasonal allergic rhinitis and chronic idiopathic urticaria patients were similar to those in healthy subjects.

Geriatric Subjects. In older subjects (≥65 years old), peak plasma levels of fexofenadine were 99% greater than those observed in normal volunteers (<65 years old). Mean elimination half-lives were similar to those observed in normal volunteers.

Pediatric Patients. Cross study comparisons indicated that fexofenadine hydrochloride area under the curve (AUC) following oral administration of a 60 mg dose to 7–12 year old pediatric allergic rhinitis patients was 56% greater compared to healthy adult subjects given the same dose. Plasma exposure in pediatric patients given 30 mg fexofenadine hydrochloride is comparable to adults given 60 mg.

Renal Impairment. In patients with mild to moderate (creatinine clearance 41–80 mL/min) and severe (creatinine clearance 11–40 mL/min) renal impairment, peak plasma levels of fexofenadine were 87% and 111% greater, respectively, and mean elimination half-lives were 59% and 72% longer, respectively, than observed in normal volunteers. Peak plasma levels in patients on dialysis (creatinine clearance ≤10 mL/min) were 82% greater and half-life was 31% longer than observed in normal volunteers. Based on increases in bioavailability and half-life, a dose of 60 mg once daily is recommended as the starting dose in patients with decreased renal function. (See DOSAGE AND ADMINISTRATION).

Hepatic Impairment. The pharmacokinetics of fexofenadine hydrochloride in patients with hepatic disease did not differ substantially from that observed in healthy patients.

Continued on next page

Allegra—Cont.

Effect of Gender. Across several trials, no clinically significant gender-related differences were observed in the pharmacokinetics of fexofenadine hydrochloride.

Pharmacodynamics

Wheal and Flare. Human histamine skin wheal and flare studies following single and twice daily doses of 20 and 40 mg fexofenadine hydrochloride demonstrated that the drug exhibits an antihistamine effect by 1 hour, achieves maximum effect at 2 to 3 hours, and an effect is still seen at 12 hours. There was no evidence of tolerance to these effects after 28 days of dosing.

Histamine skin wheal and flare studies in 7 to 12 year old patients showed that following a single dose of 30 or 60 mg, antihistamine effect was observed at 1 hour and reached a maximum by 3 hours. Greater than 49% inhibition of wheal area, and 74% inhibition of flare area were maintained for 8 hours following the 30 and 60 mg dose.

Effects on QT_C. In dogs (30 mg/kg/orally twice a day), and in rabbits (10 mg/kg, infused intravenously over 1 hour) fexofenadine hydrochloride did not prolong QT_C. In dogs the plasma fexofenadine concentration was approximately 9 times the therapeutic plasma concentrations in adults receiving the maximum recommended daily oral dose. In rabbits, the plasma fexofenadine concentration was approximately 20 times the therapeutic plasma concentration in adults receiving the maximum recommended daily oral dose. No effect was observed on calcium channel current, delayed potassium channel current, or action potential duration in guinea pig myocytes, sodium current in rat neonatal myocytes, or on several delayed rectifier potassium channels cloned from human heart at concentrations up to 1×10^{-5} M of fexofenadine hydrochloride.

No statistically significant increase in mean QT_C interval compared to placebo was observed in 714 seasonal allergic rhinitis patients given fexofenadine hydrochloride capsules in doses of 60 to 240 mg twice daily for two weeks. Pediatric patients from two placebo controlled trials (n=855) treated with up to 60 mg fexofenadine hydrochloride twice daily demonstrated no significant treatment or dose-related increases in QT_C. In addition, no statistically significant increase in mean QT_C interval compared to placebo was observed in 40 healthy volunteers given fexofenadine hydrochloride as an oral solution at doses up to 400 mg twice daily for 6 days, or in 231 healthy volunteers given fexofenadine hydrochloride 240 mg once daily for 1 year.

Clinical Studies

Seasonal Allergic Rhinitis:

Adults. In three, 2-week, multicenter, randomized, double-blind, placebo-controlled trials in patients 12 to 68 years of age with seasonal allergic rhinitis (n=1634), fexofenadine hydrochloride 60 mg twice daily significantly reduced total symptom scores (the sum of the individual scores for sneezing, rhinorrhea, itchy nose/palate/throat, itchy/watery/red eyes) compared to placebo. Statistically significant reductions in symptom scores were observed following the first 60 mg dose, with the effect maintained throughout the 12-hour interval. In these studies, there was no additional reduction in total symptom scores with higher doses of fexofenadine hydrochloride up to 240 mg twice daily.

In one 2-week, multicenter, randomized, double-blind clinical trial in patients 12 to 65 years of age with seasonal allergic rhinitis (n=863), fexofenadine hydrochloride 180 mg once daily significantly reduced total symptom scores (the sum of the individual scores for sneezing, rhinorrhea, itchy nose/palate/throat, itchy/watery/red eyes) compared to placebo. Although the number of patients in some of the subgroups was small, there were no significant differences in the effect of fexofenadine hydrochloride across subgroups of patients defined by gender, age, and race. Onset of action for reduction in total symptom scores, excluding nasal congestion, was observed at 60 minutes compared to placebo following a single 60 mg fexofenadine hydrochloride dose administered to patients with seasonal allergic rhinitis who were exposed to ragweed pollen in an environmental exposure unit. In one clinical trial conducted with ALLEGRA 60 mg capsules, and in one clinical trial conducted with ALLEGRA-D extended release tablets, onset of action was seen within 1 to 3 hours.

Pediatrics. Two 2-week multicenter, randomized, placebo-controlled, double-blind trials in 877 pediatric patients 6 to 11 years of age with seasonal allergic rhinitis were conducted at doses of 15, 30, and 60 mg twice daily. In one of these two studies, conducted in 411 pediatric patients, all three doses of fexofenadine hydrochloride significantly reduced total symptom scores (the sum of the individual scores for sneezing, rhinorrhea, itchy nose/palate/throat, itchy/watery/red eyes) compared to placebo, however a dose response relationship was not seen. The 60 mg twice daily dose did not provide any additional benefit over the 30 mg twice daily dose. Furthermore, exposure in pediatric patients given 30 mg fexofenadine hydrochloride is comparable to adults given 60 mg (see CLINICAL PHARMACOLOGY).

Chronic Idiopathic Urticaria:

Two 4-week multicenter, randomized, double-blind, placebo-controlled clinical trials compared four different doses of fexofenadine hydrochloride tablet (20, 60, 120, and 240 mg twice daily) to placebo in patients aged 12 to 70 years with chronic idiopathic urticaria (n=726). Efficacy was demonstrated by a significant reduction in mean pruritus scores (MPS), mean number of wheals (MNW), and mean total symptom scores (MTSS, the sum of the MPS and MNW score). Although all four doses were significantly superior to placebo, symptom reduction was greater and efficacy was maintained over the entire 4-week treatment period with fexofenadine hydrochloride doses of ≥60 mg twice daily. However, no additional benefit of the 120 or 240 mg fexofenadine hydrochloride twice daily dose was seen over the 60 mg twice daily dose in reducing symptom scores. There were no significant differences in the effect of fexofenadine hydrochloride across subgroups of patients defined by gender, age, weight, and race.

INDICATIONS AND USAGE

Seasonal Allergic Rhinitis

ALLEGRA is indicated for the relief of symptoms associated with seasonal allergic rhinitis in adults and children 6 years of age and older. Symptoms treated effectively were sneezing, rhinorrhea, itchy nose/palate/throat, itchy/watery/red eyes.

Chronic Idiopathic Urticaria

ALLEGRA is indicated for treatment of uncomplicated skin manifestations of chronic idiopathic urticaria in adults and children 6 years of age and older. It significantly reduces pruritus and the number of wheals.

CONTRAINDICATIONS

ALLEGRA is contraindicated in patients with known hypersensitivity to any of its ingredients.

PRECAUTIONS

Drug Interaction with Erythromycin and Ketoconazole

Fexofenadine hydrochloride has been shown to exhibit minimal (ca. 5%) metabolism. However, co-administration of fexofenadine hydrochloride with ketoconazole and erythromycin led to increased plasma levels of fexofenadine hydrochloride. Fexofenadine hydrochloride had no effect on the pharmacokinetics of erythromycin and ketoconazole. In two separate studies, fexofenadine hydrochloride 120 mg twice daily (two times the recommended twice daily dose) was co-administered with erythromycin 500 mg every 8 hours or ketoconazole 400 mg once daily under steady-state conditions to normal, healthy volunteers (n=24, each study). No differences in adverse events or QT_C interval were observed when patients were administered fexofenadine hydrochloride alone or in combination with erythromycin or ketoconazole. The findings of these studies are summarized in the following table:

[See table below]

The changes in plasma levels were within the range of plasma levels achieved in adequate and well-controlled clinical trials.

The mechanism of these interactions has been evaluated in *in vitro, in situ,* and *in vivo* animal models. These studies indicate that ketoconazole or erythromycin co-administration enhances fexofenadine gastrointestinal absorption. *In vivo* animal studies also suggest that in addition to increasing absorption, ketoconazole decreases fexofenadine hydrochloride gastrointestinal secretion, while erythromycin may also decrease biliary excretion.

Drug Interactions with Antacids

Administration of 120 mg of fexofenadine hydrochloride (2 × 60 mg capsule) within 15 minutes of an aluminum and magnesium containing antacid (Maalox®) decreased fexofenadine AUC by 41% and C_{max} by 43%. ALLEGRA should not be taken closely in time with aluminum and magnesium containing antacids.

Carcinogenesis, Mutagenesis, Impairment of Fertility

The carcinogenic potential and reproductive toxicity of fexofenadine hydrochloride were assessed using terfenadine studies with adequate fexofenadine hydrochloride exposure (based on plasma area-under-the-concentration vs. time [AUC] values). No evidence of carcinogenicity was observed in an 18-month study in mice and in a 24-month study in rats at oral doses up to 150 mg/kg of terfenadine (which led to fexofenadine exposures that were respectively approximately 3 and 5 times the exposure from the maximum recommended daily oral dose of fexofenadine hydrochloride in adults and children).

In *in vitro* (Bacterial Reverse Mutation, CHO/HGPRT Forward Mutation, and Rat Lymphocyte Chromosomal Aberration assays) and *in vivo* (Mouse Bone Marrow Micronucleus assay) tests, fexofenadine hydrochloride revealed no evidence of mutagenicity.

In rat fertility studies, dose-related reductions in implants and increases in postimplantation losses were observed at an oral dose of 150 mg/kg of terfenadine (which led to fexofenadine hydrochloride exposures that were approximately 3 times the exposure of the maximum recommended daily oral dose of fexofenadine hydrochloride in adults).

Pregnancy

Teratogenic Effects: Category C. There was no evidence of teratogenicity in rats or rabbits at oral doses of terfenadine up to 300 mg/kg (which led to fexofenadine exposures that were approximately 4 and 31 times, respectively, the exposure from the maximum recommended daily oral dose of fexofenadine in adults).

There are no adequate and well controlled studies in pregnant women. Fexofenadine should be used during pregnancy only if the potential benefit justifies the potential risk to the fetus.

Nonteratogenic Effects. Dose-related decreases in pup weight gain and survival were observed in rats exposed to an oral dose of 150 mg/kg of terfenadine (approximately 3 times the maximum recommended daily oral dose of fexofenadine hydrochloride in adults based on comparison of fexofenadine hydrochloride AUCs).

Nursing Mothers

There are no adequate and well-controlled studies in women during lactation. Because many drugs are excreted in human milk, caution should be exercised when fexofenadine hydrochloride is administered to a nursing woman.

Pediatric Use

The recommended dose in patients 6 to 11 years of age is based on cross-study comparison of the pharmacokinetics of ALLEGRA in adults and pediatric patients and on the safety profile of fexofenadine hydrochloride in both adult and pediatric patients at doses equal to or higher than the recommended doses.

The safety of ALLEGRA tablets at a dose of 30 mg twice daily has been demonstrated in 438 pediatric patients 6 to 11 years of age in two placebo-controlled 2-week seasonal allergic rhinitis trials. The safety of ALLEGRA for the treatment of chronic idiopathic urticaria in patients 6 to 11 years of age is based on cross-study comparison of the pharmacokinetics of ALLEGRA in adult and pediatric patients and on the safety profile of fexofenadine in both adult and pediatric patients at doses equal to or higher than the recommended dose.

The effectiveness of ALLEGRA for the treatment of seasonal allergic rhinitis in patients 6 to 11 years of age was demonstrated in one trial (n=411) in which ALLEGRA tablets 30 mg twice daily significantly reduced total symptom scores compared to placebo, along with extrapolation of demonstrated efficacy in patients ages 12 years and above, and the pharmacokinetic comparisons in adults and children. The effectiveness of ALLEGRA for the treatment of chronic idiopathic urticaria in patients 6 to 11 years of age is based on an extrapolation of the demonstrated efficacy of ALLEGRA in adults with this condition and the likelihood that the disease course, pathophysiology and the drug's effect are substantially similar in children to that of adult patients.

The safety and effectiveness of ALLEGRA in pediatric patients under 6 years of age have not been established.

Geriatric Use

Clinical studies of ALLEGRA tablets and capsules did not include sufficient numbers of subjects aged 65 years and over to determine whether this population responds differently from younger patients. Other reported clinical experience has not identified differences in responses between the geriatric and younger patients. This drug is known to be substantially excreted by the kidney, and the risk of toxic reactions to this drug may be greater in patients with impaired renal function. Because elderly patients are more likely to have decreased renal function, care should be taken in dose selection, and may be useful to monitor renal function. (See CLINICAL PHARMACOLOGY).

ADVERSE REACTIONS

Seasonal Allergic Rhinitis

Adults. In placebo-controlled seasonal allergic rhinitis clinical trials in patients 12 years of age and older, which included 2461 patients receiving fexofenadine hydrochloride capsules at doses of 20 mg to 240 mg twice daily, adverse events were similar in fexofenadine hydrochloride and placebo-treated patients. All adverse events that were reported by greater than 1% of patients who received the recommended daily dose of fexofenadine hydrochloride (60 mg capsules twice daily), and that were more common with fexofenadine hydrochloride than placebo, are listed in Table 1.

In a placebo-controlled clinical study in the United States, which included 570 patients aged 12 years and older receiving fexofenadine hydrochloride tablets at doses of 120 or 180 mg once daily, adverse events were similar in fexofenadine hydrochloride and placebo-treated patients. Table 1 also lists adverse experiences that were reported by greater than 2% of patients treated with fexofenadine hydrochloride tablets at doses of 180 mg once daily and that were more common with fexofenadine hydrochloride than placebo.

The incidence of adverse events, including drowsiness, was not dose-related and was similar across subgroups defined by age, gender, and race.

[See table 1 at top of next page]

Effects on steady-state fexofenadine hydrochloride pharmacokinetics after 7 days of co-administration with fexofenadine hydrochloride 120 mg every 12 hours (two times the recommended twice daily dose) in normal volunteers (n=24)

Concomitant Drug	*C_{maxSS} (Peak plasma concentration)*	*$AUC_{SS(0-12h)}$ (Extent of systemic exposure)*
Erythromycin (500 mg every 8 hrs)	+82%	+109%
Ketoconazole (400 mg once daily)	+135%	+164%

Table 1

Adverse experiences in patients ages 12 years and older reported in placebo-controlled seasonal allergic rhinitis clinical trials in the United States

Twice daily dosing with fexofenadine capsules at rates of greater than 1%

Adverse experience	*Fexofenadine 60 mg Twice Daily (n=679)*	*Placebo Twice Daily (n=671)*
Viral Infection (cold, flu)	2.5%	1.5%
Nausea	1.6%	1.5%
Dysmenorrhea	1.5%	0.3%
Drowsiness	1.3%	0.9%
Dyspepsia	1.3%	0.6%
Fatigue	1.3%	0.9%

Once daily dosing with fexofenadine hydrochloride tablets at rates of greater than 2%

Adverse experience	*Fexofenadine 180 mg once daily (n=283)*	*Placebo (n=293)*
Headache	10.6%	7.5%
Upper Respiratory Tract Infection	3.2%	3.1%
Back Pain	2.8%	1.4%

Table 2

Adverse experiences reported in placebo-controlled seasonal allergic rhinitis studies in pediatric patients ages 6 to 11 in the United States and Canada at rates of greater than 2%

Adverse experience	*Fexofenadine 30 mg twice daily (n=209)*	*Placebo (n=229)*
Headache	7.2%	6.6%
Accidental Injury	2.9%	1.3%
Coughing	3.8%	1.3%
Fever	2.4%	0.9%
Pain	2.4%	0.4%
Otitis Media	2.4%	0.0%
Upper Respiratory Tract Infection	4.3%	1.7%

Table 3

Adverse experiences reported in patients 12 years and older in placebo-controlled chronic idiopathic urticaria studies in the United States and Canada at rates of greater than 2%

Adverse experience	*Fexofenadine 60 mg twice daily (n=186)*	*Placebo (n=178)*
Back Pain	2.2%	1.1%
Sinusitis	2.2%	1.1%
Dizziness	2.2%	0.6%
Drowsiness	2.2%	0.0%

The frequency and magnitude of laboratory abnormalities were similar in fexofenadine hydrochloride and placebo-treated patients.

Pediatric. Table 2 lists adverse experiences in patients aged 6 to 11 years of age which were reported by greater than 2% of patients treated with fexofenadine hydrochloride tablets at a dose of 30 mg twice daily in placebo-controlled seasonal allergic rhinitis studies in the United States and Canada that were more common with fexofenadine hydrochloride than placebo.

[See table 2 above]

Chronic Idiopathic Urticaria

Adverse events reported by patients 12 years of age and older in placebo-controlled chronic idiopathic urticaria studies were similar to those reported in placebo-controlled seasonal allergic rhinitis studies. In placebo-controlled chronic idiopathic urticaria clinical trials, which included 726 patients 12 years of age and older receiving fexofenadine hydrochloride tablets at doses of 20 to 240 mg twice daily, adverse events were similar in fexofenadine hydrochloride and placebo-treated patients. Table 3 lists adverse experiences in patients aged 12 years and older which were reported by greater than 2% of patients treated with fexofenadine hydrochloride 60 mg tablets twice daily in controlled clinical studies in the United States and Canada and that were more common with fexofenadine hydrochloride than placebo. The safety of fexofenadine hydrochloride in the treatment of chronic idiopathic urticaria in pediatric patients 6 to 11 years of age is based on the safety profile of fexofenadine hydrochloride in adults and adolescent patients at doses equal to or higher than the recommended dose (see Pediatric Use).

[See table 3 above]

OVERDOSAGE

Reports of fexofenadine hydrochloride overdose have been infrequent and contain limited information. However, dizziness, drowsiness, and dry mouth have been reported. Single doses of fexofenadine hydrochloride up to 800 mg (six normal volunteers at this dose level), and doses up to 690 mg twice daily for 1 month (three normal volunteers at this dose level) or 240 mg once daily for 1 year (234 normal volunteers at this dose level) were administered without the development of clinically significant adverse events as compared to placebo.

In the event of overdose, consider standard measures to remove any unabsorbed drug. Symptomatic and supportive treatment is recommended.

Hemodialysis did not effectively remove fexofenadine hydrochloride from blood (1.7% removed) following terfenadine administration.

No deaths occurred at oral doses of fexofenadine hydrochloride up to 5000 mg/kg in mice (110 times the maximum recommended daily oral dose in adults and 200 times the maximum recommended daily oral dose in children based on mg/m^2) and up to 5000 mg/kg in rats (230 times the maximum recommended daily oral dose in adults and 400 times the maximum recommended daily oral dose in children based on mg/m^2). Additionally, no clinical signs of toxicity or gross pathological findings were observed. In dogs, no evidence of toxicity was observed at oral doses up to 2000 mg/kg (300 times the maximum recommended daily oral dose in adults and 530 times the maximum recommended daily oral dose in children based on mg/m^2).

DOSAGE AND ADMINISTRATION

Seasonal Allergic Rhinitis

Adults and Children 12 Years and Older. The recommended dose of ALLEGRA is 60 mg twice daily, or 180 mg once daily. A dose of 60 mg once daily is recommended as the starting dose in patients with decreased renal function (see CLINICAL PHARMACOLOGY).

Children 6 to 11 Years. The recommended dose of ALLEGRA is 30 mg twice daily. A dose of 30 mg once daily is recommended as the starting dose in pediatric patients with decreased renal function (see CLINICAL PHARMACOLOGY).

Chronic Idiopathic Urticaria

Adults and Children 12 Years and Older. The recommended dose of ALLEGRA is 60 mg twice daily. A dose of 60 mg once daily is recommended as the starting dose in patients with decreased renal function (see CLINICAL PHARMACOLOGY).

Children 6 to 11 Years. The recommended dose of ALLEGRA is 30 mg twice daily. A dose of 30 mg once daily is recommended as the starting dose in pediatric patients with decreased renal function (see CLINICAL PHARMACOLOGY).

HOW SUPPLIED

ALLEGRA 60 mg capsules are available in: high-density polyethylene (HDPE) bottles of 60 (NDC 0088-1102-41); HDPE bottles of 100 (NDC 0088-1102-47); HDPE bottles of 500 (NDC 0088-1102-55); and aluminum-foil blister packs of 100 (NDC 0088-1102-49).

ALLEGRA capsules have a white opaque cap and a pink opaque body. The capsules are imprinted in black ink, with "ALLEGRA" on the cap and "60 mg" on the body.

ALLEGRA 30 mg tablets are available in: high-density polyethylene (HDPE) bottles of 100 (NDC 0088-1106-47) with a polypropylene screw cap containing a pulp/wax liner with heat-sealed foil inner seal and HDPE bottles of 500 (NDC 0088-1106-55) with a polypropylene screw cap containing a pulp/wax liner with heat-sealed foil inner seal.

ALLEGRA 60 mg tablets are available in: HDPE bottles of 100 (NDC 0088-1107-47) with a polypropylene screw cap containing a pulp/wax liner with heat-sealed foil inner seal; HDPE bottles of 500 (NDC 0088-1107-55) with a polypropylene screw cap containing a pulp/wax liner with heat-sealed foil inner seal; and aluminum foil-backed clear blister packs of 100 (NDC 0088-1107-49).

ALLEGRA 180 mg tablets are available in: HDPE bottles of 100 (NDC 0088-1109-47) with a polypropylene screw cap containing a pulp/wax liner with heat-sealed foil inner seal; and HDPE bottles of 500 (NDC 0088-1109-55) with a polypropylene screw cap containing a pulp/wax liner with heat-sealed foil inner seal.

ALLEGRA tablets are coated with a peach colored film coating. Tablets have the following unique identifiers: 30 mg tablets have 03 on one side and 0088 on the other; 60 mg tablets have 06 on one side and 0088 on the other; and 180 mg tablets have 018 on one side and 0088 on the other.

Store ALLEGRA capsules and tablets at controlled room temperature 20–25°C (68–77°F). (See USP Controlled Room Temperature). Foil-backed blister packs containing ALLEGRA capsules and all tablet packaging should be protected from excessive moisture.

Prescribing Information as of February 2000

Aventis Pharmaceuticals Inc.
(formerly Hoechst Marion Roussel, Inc.)
Kansas City, MO 64137 USA
US Patents 4,254,129; 5,375,693; 5,578,610

Shown in Product Identification Guide, page 306

ALLEGRA-D® ℞

[ə-'lĕgra-D]

(fexofenadine HCl 60 mg and pseudoephedrine HCl 120 mg) Extended-Release Tablets

Prescribing Information as of June 1998A

DESCRIPTION

ALLEGRA-D® (fexofenadine hydrochloride and pseudoephedrine hydrochloride) Extended-Release Tablets for oral administration contain 60 mg fexofenadine hydrochloride for immediate-release and 120 mg pseudoephedrine hydrochloride for extended-release. Tablets also contain as excipients: microcrystalline cellulose, pregelatinized starch, croscarmellose sodium, magnesium stearate, carnauba wax, stearic acid, silicon dioxide, hydroxypropyl methylcellulose and polyethylene glycol.

Fexofenadine hydrochloride, one of the active ingredients of ALLEGRA-D, is a histamine H_1-receptor antagonist with the chemical name (±)-4-[1-hydroxy-4-[4-(hydroxydiphenylmethyl)-1-piperidinyl]-butyl]-α, α-dimethyl benzeneacetic acid hydrochloride and the following chemical structure:

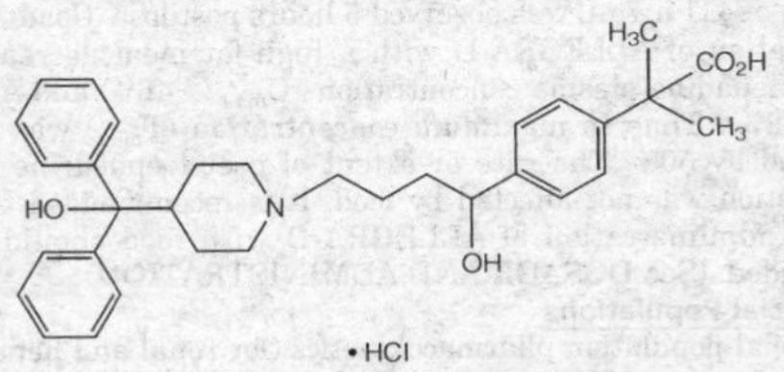

The molecular weight is 538.13 and the empirical formula is $C_{32}H_{39}NO_4$•HCl. Fexofenadine hydrochloride is a white to off-white crystalline powder. It is freely soluble in methanol and ethanol, slightly soluble in chloroform and water, and insoluble in hexane. Fexofenadine hydrochloride is a racemate and exists as a zwitterion in aqueous media at physiological pH.

Pseudoephedrine hydrochloride, the other active ingredient of ALLEGRA-D, is an adrenergic (vasoconstrictor) agent with the chemical name [S-(R*,R*)]-α-[1-(methylamino) ethyl]-benzenemethanol hydrochloride and the following chemical structure:

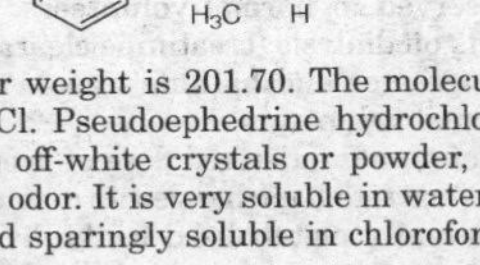

The molecular weight is 201.70. The molecular formula is $C_{10}H_{15}NO$•HCl. Pseudoephedrine hydrochloride occurs as fine, white to off-white crystals or powder, having a faint characteristic odor. It is very soluble in water, freely soluble in alcohol, and sparingly soluble in chloroform.

Continued on next page

Allegra-D—Cont.

CLINICAL PHARMACOLOGY

Mechanism of Action

Fexofenadine hydrochloride, the major active metabolite of terfenadine, is an antihistamine with selective peripheral H_1-receptor antagonist activity. Fexofenadine hydrochloride inhibited antigen-induced bronchospasm in sensitized guinea pigs and histamine release from peritoneal mast cells in rats. In laboratory animals, no anticholinergic or alpha$_1$-adrenergic-receptor blocking effects were observed. Moreover, no sedative or other central nervous system effects were observed. Radiolabeled tissue distribution studies in rats indicated that fexofenadine does not cross the blood-brain barrier.

Pseudoephedrine hydrochloride is an orally active sympathomimetic amine and exerts a decongestant action on the nasal mucosa. Pseudoephedrine hydrochloride is recognized as an effective agent for the relief of nasal congestion due to allergic rhinitis. Pseudoephedrine produces peripheral effects similar to those of ephedrine and central effects similar to, but less intense than, amphetamines. It has the potential for excitatory side effects. At the recommended oral dose, it has little or no pressor effect in normotensive adults.

Pharmacokinetics

The pharmacokinetics of fexofenadine hydrochloride and pseudoephedrine hydrochloride when administered separately have been well characterized. Fexofenadine pharmacokinetics were linear for oral doses of fexofenadine hydrochloride up to 120 mg twice daily. The mean elimination half-life of fexofenadine was 14.4 hours following administration of 60 mg fexofenadine hydrochloride, twice daily, to steady-state in normal volunteers. Human mass balance studies documented a recovery of approximately 80% and 11% of the [^{14}C] fexofenadine hydrochloride dose in the feces and urine, respectively. Approximately 5% of the total dose was metabolized. Because the absolute bioavailability of fexofenadine hydrochloride has not been established, it is unknown if the fecal component is unabsorbed drug or the result of biliary excretion. The pharmacokinetics of fexofenadine hydrochloride in seasonal allergic rhinitis patients were similar to those in healthy subjects. Peak fexofenadine plasma concentrations were similar between adolescent (12–16 years of age) and adult patients. Fexofenadine is 60% to 70% bound to plasma proteins, primarily albumin and α_1-acid glycoprotein.

Pseudoephedrine has been shown to have a mean elimination half-life of 4–6 hours which is dependent on urine pH. The elimination half-life is decreased at urine pH lower than 6 and may be increased at urine pH higher than 8.

The bioavailability of fexofenadine hydrochloride and pseudoephedrine hydrochloride from ALLEGRA-D Extended-Release Tablets is similar to that achieved with separate administration of the components. Coadministration of fexofenadine and pseudoephedrine does not significantly affect the bioavailability of either component.

Fexofenadine hydrochloride was rapidly absorbed following single-dose administration of the 60 mg fexofenadine hydrochloride/120 mg pseudoephedrine hydrochloride tablet with median time to mean maximum fexofenadine plasma concentration of 191 ng/mL occurring 2 hours postdose. Pseudoephedrine hydrochloride produced a mean single-dose pseudoephedrine peak plasma concentration of 206 ng/mL which occurred 6 hours postdose. Following multiple dosing to steady-state, a fexofenadine peak concentration of 255 ng/mL was observed 2 hours postdose. Following multiple dosing to steady-state, a pseudoephedrine peak concentration of 411 ng/mL was observed 5 hours postdose. Coadministration of ALLEGRA-D with a high-fat meal decreased fexofenadine plasma concentrations C_{max} (−46%) and AUC (−42%). Time to maximum concentration (T_{max}) was delayed by 50%. The rate or extent of pseudoephedrine absorption was not affected by food. It is recommended that the administration of ALLEGRA-D with food should be avoided. (See DOSAGE AND ADMINISTRATION).

Special Populations

Special population pharmacokinetics (for renal and hepatic impairment and age), obtained after a single dose of 80 mg fexofenadine hydrochloride, were compared to those from normal subjects in a separate study of similar design. While subject weights were relatively uniform between studies, these special population patients were substantially older than the healthy, young volunteers. Thus, an age effect may be confounding the pharmacokinetic differences observed in some of the special populations.

Effect of Age. In older subjects (≥65 years old), peak plasma levels of fexofenadine were 99% greater than those observed in younger subjects (<65 years old). Mean elimination half-lives were similar to those observed in younger subjects.

Renally Impaired. In patients with mild (creatinine clearance 41–80 mL/min) to severe (creatinine clearance 11–40 mL/min) renal impairment, peak plasma levels of fexofenadine were 87% and 111% greater, respectively, and mean elimination half-lives were 59% and 72% longer, respectively, than observed in normal volunteers. Peak plasma levels in patients on dialysis (creatinine clearance ≤10 mL/min) were 82% greater and half-life was 31% longer than observed in normal volunteers.

About 55–75% of an administered dose of pseudoephedrine hydrochloride is excreted unchanged in the urine; the remainder is apparently metabolized in the liver. Therefore, pseudoephedrine may accumulate in patients with renal insufficiency.

Based on increases in bioavailability and half-life of fexofenadine hydrochloride and pseudoephedrine hydrochloride, a dose of one tablet once daily is recommended as the starting dose in patients with decreased renal function (see DOSAGE AND ADMINISTRATION).

Hepatically Impaired. The pharmacokinetics of fexofenadine hydrochloride in patients with hepatic disease did not differ substantially from that observed in healthy subjects. The effect on pseudoephedrine pharmacokinetics is unknown.

Effect of Gender. Across several trials, no clinically significant gender-related differences were observed in the pharmacokinetics of fexofenadine hydrochloride.

Pharmacodynamics

Wheal and Flare. Human histamine skin wheal and flare studies following single and twice daily doses of 20 mg and 40 mg fexofenadine hydrochloride demonstrated that the drug exhibits an antihistamine effect by 1 hour, achieves maximum effect at 2–3 hours, and an effect is still seen at 12 hours. There was no evidence of tolerance to these effects after 28 days of dosing. The clinical significance of these observations is not known.

Effects on QT_c. In dogs, (10 mg/kg/day, orally for 5 days) and rabbits (10 mg/kg, intravenously over one hour) fexofenadine hydrochloride did not prolong QT_c at plasma concentrations that were at least 28 and 63 times, respectively, the therapeutic plasma concentrations in man (based on a 60 mg twice daily fexofenadine hydrochloride dose). No effect was observed on calcium channel current, delayed K^+ channel current, or action potential duration in guinea pig myocytes, Na^+ current in rat neonatal myocytes, or on the delayed rectifier K^+ channel cloned from human heart at concentrations up to 1×10^{-5} M of fexofenadine. This concentration was at least 32 times the therapeutic plasma concentration in man (based on a 60 mg twice daily fexofenadine hydrochloride dose).

No statistically significant increase in mean QT_c interval compared to placebo was observed in 714 seasonal allergic rhinitis patients given fexofenadine hydrochloride capsules in doses of 60 mg to 240 mg twice daily for two weeks or in 40 healthy volunteers given fexofenadine hydrochloride as an oral solution at doses up to 400 mg twice daily for 6 days.

A one year study designed to evaluate safety and tolerability of 240 mg of fexofenadine hydrochloride (n=240) compared to placebo (n=237) in healthy subjects, did not reveal a statistically significant increase in the mean QT_c interval for the fexofenadine hydrochloride treated group when evaluated pretreatment and after 1, 2, 3, 6, 9, and 12 months of treatment.

Administration of the 60 mg fexofenadine hydrochloride/120 mg pseudoephedrine hydrochloride combination tablet for approximately 2 weeks to 213 patients with seasonal allergic rhinitis demonstrated no statistically significant increase in the mean QT_c interval compared to fexofenadine hydrochloride administered alone (60 mg twice daily, n=215), or compared to pseudoephedrine hydrochloride (120 mg twice daily, n=215) administered alone.

Clinical Studies

In a 2-week, multicenter, randomized, double-blind, active-controlled trial in patients 12–65 years of age with seasonal allergic rhinitis due to ragweed allergy (n=651), the 60 mg fexofenadine hydrochloride/120 mg pseudoephedrine hydrochloride combination tablet administered twice daily significantly reduced the intensity of sneezing, rhinorrhea, itchy nose/palate/throat, itchy/watery/red eyes, and nasal congestion.

In three, 2-week, multicenter, randomized, double-blind, placebo-controlled trials in patients 12–68 years of age with seasonal allergic rhinitis (n=1634), fexofenadine hydrochloride 60 mg twice daily significantly reduced total symptom scores (the sum of the individual scores for sneezing, rhinorrhea, itchy nose/palate/throat, itchy/watery/red eyes) compared to placebo. Statistically significant reductions in symptom scores were observed following the first 60 mg dose, with the effect maintained throughout the 12-hour interval. In general, there was no additional reduction in total symptom scores with higher doses of fexofenadine hydrochloride up to 240 mg twice daily. Although the number of subjects in some of the subgroups was small, there were no significant differences in the effect of fexofenadine hydrochloride across subgroups of patients defined by gender, age, and race. Onset of action for reduction in total symptom scores, excluding nasal congestion, was observed at 60 minutes compared to placebo following a single 60 mg fexofenadine hydrochloride dose administered to patients with seasonal allergic rhinitis who were exposed to ragweed pollen in an environmental exposure unit.

INDICATIONS AND USAGE

ALLEGRA-D is indicated for the relief of symptoms associated with seasonal allergic rhinitis in adults and children 12 years of age and older. Symptoms treated effectively include sneezing, rhinorrhea, itchy nose/palate/ and/or throat, itchy/watery/red eyes, and nasal congestion. ALLEGRA-D should be administered when both the antihistaminic properties of fexofenadine hydrochloride and the nasal decongestant properties of pseudoephedrine hydrochloride are desired (see CLINICAL PHARMACOLOGY).

CONTRAINDICATIONS

ALLEGRA-D is contraindicated in patients with known hypersensitivity to any of its ingredients.

Due to its pseudoephedrine component, ALLEGRA-D is contraindicated in patients with narrow-angle glaucoma or urinary retention, and in patients receiving monoamine oxidase (MAO) inhibitor therapy or within fourteen (14) days of stopping such treatment (see Drug Interactions section). It is also contraindicated in patients with severe hypertension, or severe coronary artery disease, and in those who have shown hypersensitivity or idiosyncrasy to its components, to adrenergic agents, or to other drugs of similar chemical structures. Manifestations of patient idiosyncrasy to adrenergic agents include: insomnia, dizziness, weakness, tremor, or arrhythmias.

WARNINGS

Sympathomimetic amines should be used judiciously and sparingly in patients with hypertension, diabetes mellitus, ischemic heart disease, increased intraocular pressure, hyperthyroidism, renal impairment, or prostatic hypertrophy (see CONTRAINDICATIONS). Sympathomimetic amines may produce central nervous system stimulation with convulsions or cardiovascular collapse with accompanying hypotension.

PRECAUTIONS

General

Due to its pseudoephedrine component, ALLEGRA-D should be used with caution in patients with hypertension, diabetes mellitus, ischemic heart disease, increased intraocular pressure, hyperthyroidism, renal impairment, or prostatic hypertrophy (see WARNINGS and CONTRAINDICATIONS). Patients with decreased renal function should be given a lower initial dose (one tablet per day) because they have reduced elimination of fexofenadine and pseudoephedrine (See CLINICAL PHARMACOLOGY and DOSAGE AND ADMINISTRATION).

Information for Patients

Patients taking ALLEGRA-D tablets should receive the following information: ALLEGRA-D tablets are prescribed for the relief of symptoms of seasonal allergic rhinitis. Patients should be instructed to take ALLEGRA-D tablets only as prescribed. **Do not exceed the recommended dose.** If nervousness, dizziness, or sleeplessness occur, discontinue use and consult the doctor. Patients should also be advised against the concurrent use of ALLEGRA-D tablets with over-the-counter antihistamines and decongestants.

The product should not be used by patients who are hypersensitive to it or to any of its ingredients. Due to its pseudoephedrine component, this product should not be used by patients with narrow-angle glaucoma, urinary retention, or by patients receiving a monoamine oxidase (MAO) inhibitor or within 14 days of stopping use of MAO inhibitor. It also should not be used by patients with severe hypertension or severe coronary artery disease.

Patients should be told that this product should be used in pregnancy or lactation only if the potential benefit justifies the potential risk to the fetus or nursing infant. Patients should be cautioned not to break or chew the tablet. Patients should be directed to swallow the tablet whole. Patients should be instructed not to take the tablet with food. Patients should also be instructed to store the medication in a tightly closed container in a cool, dry place, away from children.

Drug Interactions

Fexofenadine hydrochloride and pseudoephedrine hydrochloride do not influence the pharmacokinetics of each other when administered concomitantly.

Fexofenadine has been shown to exhibit minimal (ca. 5%) metabolism. However, co-administration of fexofenadine with ketoconazole and erythromycin led to increased plasma levels of fexofenadine. Fexofenadine had no effect on the pharmacokinetics of erythromycin and ketoconazole. In two separate studies, fexofenadine HCl 120 mg BID (twice the recommended dose) was co-administered with erythromycin 500 mg every 8 hours or ketoconazole 400 mg once daily under steady-state conditions to normal, healthy volunteers (n=24, each study). No differences in adverse events or QT_c interval were observed when subjects were administered fexofenadine HCl alone or in combination with erythromycin or ketoconazole. The findings of these studies are summarized in the following table:

Effects on Steady-State Fexofenadine Pharmacokinetics After 7 Days of Co-Administration with Fexofenadine Hydrochloride 120 mg Every 12 Hours (twice recommended dose) in Normal Volunteers (n=24)

Concomitant Drug	$C_{max,SS}$ *(Peak plasma concentration)*	$AUC_{SS}(0–12h)$ *(Extent of systemic exposure)*
Erythromycin (500 mg every 8 hrs)	+82%	+109%
Ketoconazole (400 mg once daily)	+135%	+164%

The changes in plasma levels were within the range of plasma levels achieved in adequate and well-controlled clinical trials.

The mechanism of these interactions has been evaluated in *in vitro, in situ* and *in vivo* animal models. These studies indicate that ketoconazole or erythromycin co-administration enhances fexofenadine gastrointestinal absorption. In vivo animal studies also suggest that in addition to enhancing absorption, ketoconazole decreases fexofenadine gastrointestinal secretion, while erythromycin may also decrease biliary excretion.

ALLEGRA-D tablets (pseudoephedrine component) are contraindicated in patients taking monoamine oxidase inhibitors and for 14 days after stopping use of an MAO inhibitor. Concomitant use with antihypertensive drugs which interfere with sympathetic activity (eg, methyldopa, mecamylamine, and reserpine) may reduce their antihypertensive effects. Increased ectopic pacemaker activity can occur when pseudoephedrine is used concomitantly with digitalis.

Care should be taken in the administration of ALLEGRA-D concomitantly with other sympathomimetic amines because combined effects on the cardiovascular system may be harmful to the patient (see WARNINGS).

Carcinogenesis, Mutagenesis, Impairment of Fertility

There are no animal or in vitro studies on the combination product fexofenadine hydrochloride and pseudoephedrine hydrochloride to evaluate carcinogenesis, mutagenesis, or impairment of fertility.

The carcinogenic potential and reproductive toxicity of fexofenadine hydrochloride were assessed using terfenadine studies with adequate fexofenadine exposure (area-under-the plasma concentration versus time curve [AUC]). No evidence of carcinogenicity was observed when mice and rats were given daily oral doses up to 150 mg/kg of terfenadine for 18 and 24 months, respectively. In both species, 150 mg/kg of terfenadine produced AUC values of fexofenadine that were approximately 3 times the human AUC at the maximum recommended daily oral dose in adults.

Two-year feeding studies in rats and mice conducted under the auspices of the National Toxicology Program (NTP) demonstrated no evidence of carcinogenic potential with ephedrine sulfate, a structurally related drug with pharmacological properties similar to pseudoephedrine, at doses up to 10 and 27 mg/kg, respectively (approximately 1/3 and 1/2, respectively, the maximum recommended daily oral dose of pseudoephedrine hydrochloride in adults on a mg/m^2 basis).

In-vitro (Bacterial Reverse Mutation, CHO/HGPRT Forward Mutation, and Rat Lymphocyte Chromosomal Aberration assays) and in vivo (Mouse Bone Marrow Micronucleus assay) tests, fexofenadine hydrochloride revealed no evidence of mutagenicity.

Reproduction and fertility studies with terfenadine in rats produced no effect on male or female fertility at oral doses up to 300 mg/kg/day. However, reduced implants and post implantation losses were reported at 300 mg/kg. A reduction in implants was also observed at an oral dose of 150 mg/kg/day. Oral doses of 150 and 300 mg/kg of terfenadine produced AUC values of fexofenadine that were approximately 3 and 4 times, respectively, the human AUC at the maximum recommended daily oral dose in adults.

Pregnancy

Teratogenic Effects: Category C. Terfenadine alone was not teratogenic in rats and rabbits at oral doses up to 300 mg/kg; 300 mg/kg of terfenadine produced fexofenadine AUC values that were approximately 4 and 30 times, respectively, the human AUC at the maximum recommended daily oral dose in adults.

The combination of terfenadine and pseudoephedrine hydrochloride in a ratio of 1:2 by weight was studied in rats and rabbits. In rats, an oral combination dose of 150/300 mg/kg produced reduced fetal weight and delayed ossification with a finding of wavy ribs. The dose of 150 mg/kg of terfenadine in rats produced an AUC value of fexofenadine that was approximately 3 times the human AUC at the maximum recommended daily oral dose in adults. The dose of 300 mg/kg of pseudoephedrine hydrochloride in rats was approximately 10 times the maximum recommended daily oral dose in adults on a mg/m^2 basis. In rabbits, an oral combination dose of 100/200 mg/kg produced decreased fetal weight. By extrapolation, the AUC of fexofenadine for 100 mg/kg orally of terfenadine was approximately 10 times the human AUC at the maximum recommended daily oral dose in adults. The dose of 200 mg/kg of pseudoephedrine hydrochloride was approximately 15 times the maximum recommended daily oral dose in adults on a mg/m^2 basis.

There are no adequate and well-controlled studies in pregnant women. ALLEGRA-D should be used during pregnancy only if the potential benefit justifies the potential risk to the fetus.

Nonteratogenic Effects. Dose-related decreases in pup weight gain and survival were observed in rats exposed to an oral dose of 150 mg/kg of terfenadine; this dose produced an AUC of fexofenadine that was approximately 3 times the human AUC at the maximum recommended daily oral dose in adults.

Nursing Mothers

It is not known if fexofenadine is excreted in human milk. Because many drugs are excreted in human milk, caution should be used when fexofenadine hydrochloride is administered to a nursing woman. Pseudoephedrine hydrochloride administered alone distributes into breast milk of lactating human females. Pseudoephedrine concentrations in milk are consistently higher than those in plasma. The total amount of drug in milk as judged by AUC is 2 to 3 times greater than the plasma AUC. The fraction of a pseudoephedrine dose excreted in milk is estimated to be 0.4% to 0.7%. A decision should be made whether to discontinue nursing or to discontinue the drug, taking into account the importance of the drug to the mother. Caution should be exercised when ALLEGRA-D is administered to nursing women.

Adverse Experiences Reported in One Active-Controlled Seasonal Allergic Rhinitis Clinical Trial at Rates of Greater than 1%

Adverse Experience	60 mg Fexofenadine Hydrochloride/120 mg Pseudoephedrine Hydrochloride Combination Tablet Twice Daily (n=215)	Fexofenadine Hydrochloride 60 mg Twice Daily (n=218)	Pseudoephedrine Hydrochloride 120 mg Twice Daily (n=218)
Headache	13.0%	11.5%	17.4%
Insomnia	12.6%	3.2%	13.3%
Nausea	7.4%	0.5%	5.0%
Dry Mouth	2.8%	0.5%	5.5%
Dyspepsia	2.8%	0.5%	0.9%
Throat Irritation	2.3%	1.8%	0.5%
Dizziness	1.9%	0.0%	3.2%
Agitation	1.9%	0.0%	1.4%
Back Pain	1.9%	0.5%	0.5%
Palpitation	1.9%	0.0%	0.9%
Nervousness	1.4%	0.5%	1.8%
Anxiety	1.4%	0.0%	1.4%
Upper Respiratory Infection	1.4%	0.9%	0.9%
Abdominal Pain	1.4%	0.5%	0.5%

Pediatric Use

Safety and effectiveness of ALLEGRA-D in pediatric patients under the age of 12 years have not been established.

Geriatric Use

Clinical studies of ALLEGRA-D did not include sufficient numbers of patients aged 65 and older to determine whether they respond differently from younger patients. Other reported clinical experience has not identified differences in responses between the elderly and younger patients, although the elderly are more likely to have adverse reactions to sympathomimetic amines. In general, dose selection for an elderly patient should be cautious, usually starting at the low end of the dosing range, reflecting the greater frequency of decreased hepatic, renal, or cardiac function, and of concomitant disease or other drug therapy. The pseudoephedrine component of ALLEGRA-D is known to be substantially excreted by the kidney, and the risk of toxic reactions to this drug may be greater in patients with impaired renal function. Because elderly patients are more likely to have decreased renal function, care should be taken in dose selection, and it may be useful to monitor renal function.

ADVERSE REACTIONS

ALLEGRA-D

In one clinical trial (n=651) in which 215 patients with seasonal allergic rhinitis received the 60 mg fexofenadine hydrochloride/120 mg pseudoephedrine hydrochloride combination tablet twice daily for up to 2 weeks, adverse events were similar to those reported either in patients receiving fexofenadine hydrochloride 60 mg alone (n=218 patients) or in patients receiving pseudoephedrine hydrochloride 120 mg alone (n=218). A placebo group was not included in this study.

The percent of patients who withdrew prematurely because of adverse events was 3.7% for the fexofenadine hydrochloride/pseudoephedrine hydrochloride combination group, 0.5% for the fexofenadine hydrochloride group, and 4.1% for the pseudoephedrine hydrochloride group. All adverse events that were reported by greater than 1% of patients who received the recommended daily dose of the fexofenadine hydrochloride/pseudoephedrine hydrochloride combination are listed in the following table.

[See table above]

Many of the adverse events occurring in the fexofenadine hydrochloride/pseudoephedrine hydrochloride combination group were adverse events also reported predominately in the pseudoephedrine hydrochloride group, such as insomnia, headache, nausea, dry mouth, dizziness, agitation, nervousness, anxiety, and palpitation.

Fexofenadine Hydrochloride

In placebo-controlled clinical trials, which included 2461 patients receiving fexofenadine hydrochloride at doses of 20 mg to 240 mg twice daily, adverse events were similar in fexofenadine hydrochloride and placebo-treated patients. The incidence of adverse events, including drowsiness, was not dose related and was similar across subgroups defined by age, gender, and race. The percent of patients who withdrew prematurely because of adverse events was 2.2% with fexofenadine hydrochloride vs 3.3% with placebo.

Pseudoephedrine Hydrochloride

Pseudoephedrine hydrochloride may cause mild CNS stimulation in hypersensitive patients. Nervousness, excitability, restlessness, dizziness, weakness, or insomnia may occur. Headache, drowsiness, tachycardia, palpitation, pressor activity, and cardiac arrhythmias have been reported. Sympathomimetic drugs have also been associated with other untoward effects such as fear, anxiety, tenseness, tremor, hallucinations, seizures, pallor, respiratory difficulty, dysuria, and cardiovascular collapse.

OVERDOSAGE

Most reports of fexofenadine hydrochloride overdose contain limited information. However, dizziness, drowsiness, and dry mouth have been reported. For the pseudoephedrine hydrochloride component of ALLEGRA-D, information on acute overdose is limited to the marketing history of pseudoephedrine hydrochloride. Single doses of fexofenadine hydrochloride up to 800 mg (6 normal volunteers at this dose level), and doses up to 690 mg twice daily for one month (3 normal volunteers at this dose level), were administered without the development of clinically significant adverse events.

In large doses, sympathomimetics may give rise to giddiness, headache, nausea, vomiting, sweating, thirst, tachycardia, precordial pain, palpitations, difficulty in micturition, muscular weakness and tenseness, anxiety, restlessness, and insomnia. Many patients can present a toxic psychosis with delusions and hallucinations. Some may develop cardiac arrhythmias, circulatory collapse, convulsions, coma, and respiratory failure.

In the event of overdose, consider standard measures to remove any unabsorbed drug. Symptomatic and supportive treatment is recommended. Hemodialysis did not effectively remove fexofenadine from blood (up to 1.7% removed) following terfenadine administration.

The effect of hemodialysis on the removal of pseudoephedrine is unknown.

No deaths occurred in mature mice and rats at oral doses of fexofenadine hydrochloride up to 5000 mg/kg (approximately 170 and 340 times, respectively, the maximum recommended daily oral dose in adults on a mg/m^2 basis.) The median oral lethal dose in newborn rats was 438 mg/kg (approximately 30 times the maximum recommended daily oral dose in adults on a mg/m^2 basis). In dogs, no evidence of toxicity was observed at oral doses up to 2000 mg/kg (approximately 450 times the maximum recommended human daily oral dose in adults on a mg/m^2 basis). The oral median lethal dose of pseudoephedrine hydrochloride in rats was 1674 mg/kg (approximately 55 times the maximum recommended daily oral dose in adults on a mg/m^2 basis).

DOSAGE AND ADMINISTRATION

The recommended dose of ALLEGRA-D is one tablet twice daily for adults and children 12 years of age and older. It is recommended that the administration of ALLEGRA-D with food should be avoided. A dose of one tablet once daily is recommended as the starting dose in patients with decreased renal function. (See CLINICAL PHARMACOLOGY and PRECAUTIONS.)

HOW SUPPLIED

ALLEGRA-D (fexofenadine hydrochloride and pseudoephedrine hydrochloride) Extended-Release Tablets are available in: high-density polyethylene (HDPE) bottles of 60 (NDC 0088-1090-41) with a polypropylene child-resistant cap containing a pulp/wax liner with heat-sealed foil inner seal; HDPE bottles of 100 (NDC 0088-1090-47) with a polypropylene screw cap containing a pulp/wax liner with heat-sealed foil inner seal; HDPE bottles of 500 (NDC 0088-1090-

Continued on next page

Allegra-D—Cont.

55) with a polypropylene screw cap containing a pulp/wax liner with heat-sealed foil inner seal; and aluminum foil-backed clear blister packs of 100 (NDC 0088-1090-49).
ALLEGRA-D is a two-layer tablet, one white layer and one tan layer with a clear film coating on the tablet. The tablets are engraved with "Allegra-D" on the white layer.
Store ALLEGRA-D Extended-Release Tablets at 20–25°C (68–77°F). (See USP Controlled Room Temperature.)

Prescribing Information as of June 1998A

Hoechst Marion Roussel, Inc.
Kansas City, MO 64137 USA
US Patents 4,254,129; 5,375,693; 5,578,610.
Shown in Product Identification Guide, page 306

AMARYL ℞

[am'-ah-ril]
(glimepiride tablets) 1, 2, and 4 mg

Prescribing Information as of October 1999

DESCRIPTION

AMARYL® (glimepiride tablets) is an oral blood-glucose-lowering drug of the sulfonylurea class. Glimepiride is a white to yellowish-white, crystalline, odorless to practically odorless powder formulated into tablets of 1-mg, 2-mg, and 4-mg strengths for oral administration. AMARYL tablets contain the active ingredient glimepiride and the following inactive ingredients: lactose (hydrous), sodium starch glycolate, povidone, microcrystalline cellulose, and magnesium stearate. In addition, AMARYL 1-mg tablets contain Ferric Oxide Red, AMARYL 2-mg tablets contain Ferric Oxide Yellow and FD&C Blue #2 Aluminum Lake, and AMARYL 4-mg tablets contain FD&C Blue #2 Aluminum Lake.
Chemically, glimepiride is identified as 1-[[p-[2-(3-ethyl-4-methyl-2-oxo-3-pyrroline-1-carboxamido) ethyl]phenyl]-sulfonyl]-3-(trans-4-methylcyclohexyl)urea.
The CAS Registry Number is 93479-97-1
The structural formula is:

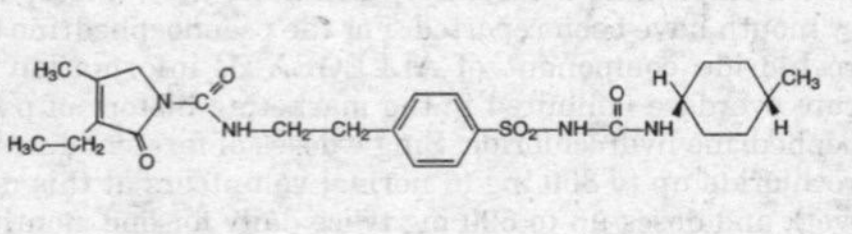

Molecular Formula: $C_{24}H_{34}N_4O_5S$
Molecular Weight: 490.62

Glimepiride is practically insoluble in water.

CLINICAL PHARMACOLOGY

Mechanism Of Action

The primary mechanism of action of glimepiride in lowering blood glucose appears to be dependent on stimulating the release of insulin from functioning pancreatic beta cells. In addition, extrapancreatic effects may also play a role in the activity of sulfonylureas such as glimepiride. This is supported by both preclinical and clinical studies demonstrating that glimepiride administration can lead to increased sensitivity of peripheral tissues to insulin. These findings are consistent with the results of a long-term, randomized, placebo-controlled trial in which AMARYL therapy improved postprandial insulin/C-peptide responses and overall glycemic control without producing clinically meaningful increases in fasting insulin/C-peptide levels. However, as with other sulfonylureas, the mechanism by which glimepiride lowers blood glucose during long-term administration has not been clearly established.
AMARYL is effective as initial drug therapy. In patients where monotherapy with AMARYL or metformin has not produced adequate glycemic control, the combination of AMARYL and metformin may have a synergistic effect, since both agents act to improve glucose tolerance by different primary mechanisms of action. This complementary effect has been observed with metformin and other sulfonylureas, in multiple studies.

Pharmacodynamics

A mild glucose-lowering effect first appeared following single oral doses as low as 0.5–0.6 mg in healthy subjects. The time required to reach the maximum effect (i.e., minimum blood glucose level [T_{min}]) was about 2 to 3 hours. In noninsulin-dependent (Type II) diabetes mellitus (NIDDM) patients, both fasting and 2-hour postprandial glucose levels were significantly lower with glimepiride (1, 2, 4, and 8 mg once daily) than with placebo after 14 days of oral dosing. The glucose-lowering effect in all active treatment groups was maintained over 24 hours.
In larger dose-ranging studies, blood glucose and HbA1c were found to respond in a dose-dependent manner over the range of 1 to 4 mg/day of AMARYL. Some patients, particularly those with higher fasting plasma glucose (FPG) levels, may benefit from doses of AMARYL up to 8 mg once daily. No difference in response was found when AMARYL was administered once or twice daily.
In two 14-week, placebo-controlled studies in 720 subjects, the average net reduction in HbA1c for AMARYL (glimepiride tablets) patients treated with 8 mg once daily was 2.0% in absolute units compared with placebo-treated patients. In a long-term, randomized, placebo-controlled study of NIDDM patients unresponsive to dietary management, AMARYL therapy improved postprandial insulin/C-peptide responses, and 75% of patients achieved and maintained control of blood glucose and HbA1c. Efficacy results were not affected by age, gender, weight, or race.
In long-term extension trials with previously-treated patients, no meaningful deterioration in mean fasting blood glucose (FBG) or HbA1c levels was seen after $2^1/_2$ years of AMARYL therapy.
Combination therapy with AMARYL and insulin (70% NPH/30% regular) was compared to placebo/insulin in secondary failure patients whose body weight was >130% of their ideal body weight. Initially, 5–10 units of insulin were administered with the main evening meal and titrated upward weekly to achieve predefined FPG values. Both groups in this double-blind study achieved similar reductions in FPG levels but the AMARYL/insulin therapy group used approximately 38% less insulin.
AMARYL therapy is effective in controlling blood glucose without deleterious changes in the plasma lipoprotein profiles of patients treated for NIDDM.

Pharmacokinetics

Absorption. After oral administration, glimepiride is completely (100%) absorbed from the GI tract. Studies with single oral doses in normal subjects and with multiple oral doses in patients with NIDDM have shown significant absorption of glimepiride within 1 hour after administration and peak drug levels (C_{max}) at 2 to 3 hours. When glimepiride was given with meals, the mean T_{max} (time to reach C_{max}) was slightly increased (12%) and the mean C_{max} and AUC (area under the curve) were slightly decreased (8% and 9%, respectively).
Distribution. After intravenous (IV) dosing in normal subjects, the volume of distribution (Vd) was 8.8 L (113 mL/kg), and the total body clearance (CL) was 47.8 mL/min. Protein binding was greater than 99.5%.
Metabolism. Glimepiride is completely metabolized by oxidative biotransformation after either an IV or oral dose. The major metabolites are the cyclohexyl hydroxy methyl derivative (M1) and the carboxyl derivative (M2). Cytochrome P450 II C9 has been shown to be involved in the biotransformation of glimepiride to M1. M1 is further metabolized to M2 by one or several cytosolic enzymes. M1, but not M2, possesses about $^1/_3$ of the pharmacological activity as compared to its parent in an animal model; however, whether the glucose-lowering effect of M1 is clinically meaningful is not clear.
Excretion. When ^{14}C-glimepiride was given orally, approximately 60% of the total radioactivity was recovered in the urine in 7 days and M1 (predominant) and M2 accounted for 80–90% of that recovered in the urine. Approximately 40% of the total radioactivity was recovered in feces and M1 and M2 (predominant) accounted for about 70% of that recovered in feces. No parent drug was recovered from urine or feces. After IV dosing in patients, no significant biliary excretion of glimepiride or its M1 metabolite has been observed.
Pharmacokinetic Parameters. The pharmacokinetic parameters of glimepiride obtained from a single-dose, crossover, dose-proportionality (1, 2, 4, and 8 mg) study in normal subjects and from a single- and multiple-dose, parallel, dose-proportionality (4 and 8 mg) study in patients with NIDDM are summarized below.
[See table below]

	Volunteers	Patients with NIDDM	
	Single Dose	Single Dose (Day 1)	Multiple Dose (Day 10)
	Mean ± SD	Mean ± SD	Mean ± SD
C_{max} (ng/mL)			
1 mg	103 ± 34 (12)	___	___
2 mg	177 ± 44 (12)	___	___
4 mg	308 ± 69 (12)	352 ± 222 (12)	309 ± 134 (12)
8 mg	557 ± 152 (12)	591 ± 232 (14)	578 ± 265 (11)
T_{max} (h)	2.4 ± 0.8 (48)	2.5 ± 1.2 (26)	2.8 ± 2.2 (23)
CL/f (mL/min)	52.1 ± 16.0 (48)	48.5 ± 29.3 (26)	52.7 ± 40.3 (23)
Vd/f (L)	21.8 ± 13.9 (48)	19.8 ± 12.7 (26)	37.1 ± 18.2 (23)
$T^1/_2$ (h)	5.3 ± 4.1 (48)	5.0 ± 2.5 (26)	9.2 ± 3.6 (23)

( ) = No. of subjects
CL/f = Total body clearance after oral dosing
Vd/f = Volume of distribution calculated after oral dosing

These data indicate that glimepiride did not accumulate in serum, and the pharmacokinetics of glimepiride were not different in healthy volunteers and in NIDDM patients. Oral clearance of glimepiride did not change over the 1–8-mg dose range, indicating linear pharmacokinetics.
Variability. In normal healthy volunteers, the intra-individual variabilities of C_{max}, AUC, and CL/f for glimepiride were 23%, 17%, and 15%, respectively, and the inter-individual variabilities were 25%, 29%, and 24%, respectively.

Special Populations

Geriatric. Comparison of glimepiride pharmacokinetics in NIDDM patients ≤ 65 years and those > 65 years was performed in a study using a dosing regimen of 6 mg daily. There were no significant differences in glimepiride pharmacokinetics between the two age groups. The mean AUC at steady state for the older patients was about 13% lower than that for the younger patients; the mean weight-adjusted clearance for the older patients was about 11% higher than that for the younger patients.
Pediatric. No studies were performed in pediatric patients.
Gender. There were no differences between males and females in the pharmacokinetics of glimepiride when adjustment was made for differences in body weight.
Race. No pharmacokinetic studies to assess the effects of race have been performed, but in placebo-controlled studies of AMARYL (glimepiride tablets) in patients with NIDDM, the antihyperglycemic effect was comparable in whites (n=536), blacks (n=63), and Hispanics (n=63).
Renal Insufficiency. A single-dose, open-label study was conducted in 15 patients with renal impairment. AMARYL (3 mg) was administered to 3 groups of patients with different levels of mean creatinine clearance (CLcr); (Group I, CLcr = 77.7 mL/min, n=5), (Group II, CLcr = 27.7 mL/min, n=3), and (Group III, CLcr = 9.4 mL/min, n=7). AMARYL was found to be well tolerated in all 3 groups. The results showed that glimepiride serum levels decreased as renal function decreased. However, M1 and M2 serum levels (mean AUC values) increased 2.3 and 8.6 times from Group I to Group III. The apparent terminal half-life ($T_{1/2}$) for glimepiride did not change, while the half-lives for M1 and M2 increased as renal function decreased. Mean urinary excretion of M1 plus M2 as percent of dose, however, decreased (44.4%, 21.9%, and 9.3% for Groups I to III).
A multiple-dose titration study was also conducted in 16 NIDDM patients with renal impairment using doses ranging from 1–8 mg daily for 3 months. The results were consistent with those observed after single doses. All patients with a CLcr less than 22 mL/min had adequate control of their glucose levels with a dosage regimen of only 1 mg daily. The results from this study suggested that a starting dose of 1 mg AMARYL may be given to NIDDM patients with kidney disease, and the dose may be titrated based on fasting blood glucose levels.
Hepatic Insufficiency. No studies were performed in patients with hepatic insufficiency.
Other Populations. There were no important differences in glimepiride metabolism in subjects identified as phenotypically different drug-metabolizers by their metabolism of sparteine.
The pharmacokinetics of glimepiride in morbidly obese patients were similar to those in the normal weight group, except for a lower C_{max} and AUC. However, since neither C_{max} nor AUC values were normalized for body surface area, the lower values of C_{max} and AUC for the obese patients were likely the result of their excess weight and not due to a difference in the kinetics of glimepiride.
Drug Interactions. The hypoglycemic action of sulfonylureas may be potentiated by certain drugs, including nonsteroidal anti-inflammatory drugs and other drugs that are highly protein bound, such as salicylates, sulfonamides, chloramphenicol, coumarins, probenecid, monoamine oxidase inhibitors, and beta adrenergic blocking agents. When these drugs are administered to a patient receiving AMARYL, the patient should be observed closely for hypoglycemia. When these drugs are withdrawn from a patient receiving AMARYL, the patient should be observed closely for loss of glycemic control.
Certain drugs tend to produce hyperglycemia and may lead to loss of control. These drugs include the thiazides and other diuretics, corticosteroids, phenothiazines, thyroid products, estrogens, oral contraceptives, phenytoin, nicotinic acid, sympathomimetics, and isoniazid. When these drugs are administered to a patient receiving AMARYL, the patient should be closely observed for loss of control. When these drugs are withdrawn from a patient receiving AMARYL, the patient should be observed closely for hypoglycemia.
Coadministration of aspirin (1 g tid) and AMARYL led to a 34% decrease in the mean glimepiride AUC and, therefore, a 34% increase in the mean CL/f. The mean C_{max} had a decrease of 4%. Blood glucose and serum C-peptide concentrations were unaffected and no hypoglycemic symptoms were reported. Pooled data from clinical trials showed no evidence of clinically significant adverse interactions with uncontrolled concurrent administration of aspirin and other salicylates.
Coadministration of either cimetidine (800 mg once daily) or ranitidine (150 mg bid) with a single 4-mg oral dose of AMARYL did not significantly alter the absorption and disposition of glimepiride, and no differences were seen in hypoglycemic symptomatology. Pooled data from clinical trials

showed no evidence of clinicallly significant adverse interactions with uncontrolled concurrent administration of H2-receptor antagonists.

Concomitant administration of propranolol (40 mg tid) and AMARYL significantly increased C_{max}, AUC, and $T_{1/2}$ of glimepiride by 23%, 22%, and 15%, respectively, and it decreased CL/f by 18%. The recovery of M1 and M2 from urine, however, did not change. The pharmacodynamic responses to glimepiride were nearly identical in normal subjects receiving propranolol and placebo. Pooled data from clinical trials in patients with NIDDM showed no evidence of clinically significant adverse interactions with uncontrolled concurrent administration of beta-blockers. However, if beta-blockers are used, caution should be exercised and patients should be warned about the potential for hypoglycemia.

Concomitant administration of AMARYL (glimepiride tablets) (4 mg once daily) did not alter the pharmacokinetic characteristics of R- and S-warfarin enantiomers following administration of a single dose (25 mg) of racemic warfarin to healthy subjects. No changes were observed in warfarin plasma protein binding. AMARYL treatment did result in a slight, but statistically significant, decrease in the pharmacodynamic response to warfarin. The reductions in mean area under the prothrombin time (PT) curve and maximum PT values during AMARYL treatment were very small (3.3% and 9.9%, respectively) and are unlikely to be clinically important.

The responses of serum glucose, insulin, C-peptide, and plasma glucagon to 2 mg AMARYL were unaffected by coadministration of ramipril (an ACE inhibitor) 5 mg once daily in normal subjects. No hypoglycemic symptoms were reported. Pooled data from clinical trials in patients with NIDDM showed no evidence of clinically significant adverse interactions with uncontrolled concurrent administration of ACE inhibitors.

A potential interaction between oral miconazole and oral hypoglycemic agents leading to severe hypoglycemia has been reported. Whether this interaction also occurs with the intravenous, topical, or vaginal preparations of miconazole is not known. Potential interactions of glimepiride with other drugs metabolized by cytochrome P450 II C9 also include phenytoin, diclofenac, ibuprofen, naproxen, and mefenamic acid.

Although no specific interaction studies were performed, pooled data from clinical trials showed no evidence of clinically significant adverse interactions with uncontrolled concurrent administration of calcium-channel blockers, estrogens, fibrates, NSAIDS, HMG CoA reductase inhibitors, sulfonamides, or thyroid hormone.

INDICATIONS AND USAGE

AMARYL is indicated as an adjunct to diet and exercise to lower the blood glucose in patients with noninsulin-dependent (Type II) diabetes mellitus (NIDDM) whose hyperglycemia cannot be controlled by diet and exercise alone. AMARYL may be used concomitantly with metformin when diet, exercise, and AMARYL or metformin alone do not result in adequate glycemic control.

AMARYL is also indicated for use in combination with insulin to lower blood glucose in patients whose hyperglycemia cannot be controlled by diet and exercise in conjunction with an oral hypoglycemic agent. Combined use of glimepiride and insulin may increase the potential for hypoglycemia.

In initiating treatment for noninsulin-dependent diabetes, diet and exercise should be emphasized as the primary form of treatment. Caloric restriction, weight loss, and exercise are essential in the obese diabetic patient. Proper dietary management and exercise alone may be effective in controlling the blood glucose and symptoms of hyperglycemia. In addition to regular physical activity, cardiovascular risk factors should be identified and corrective measures taken where possible.

If this treatment program fails to reduce symptoms and/or blood glucose, the use of an oral sulfonylurea or insulin should be considered. Use of AMARYL must be viewed by both the physician and patient as a treatment in addition to diet and exercise and not as a substitute for diet and exercise or as a convenient mechanism for avoiding dietary restraint. Furthermore, loss of blood glucose control on diet and exercise alone may be transient, thus requiring only short-term administration of AMARYL.

During maintenance programs, AMARYL monotherapy should be discontinued if satisfactory lowering of blood glucose is no longer achieved. Judgments should be based on regular clinical and laboratory evaluations. Secondary failures to AMARYL monotherapy can be treated with AMARYL-insulin combination therapy.

In considering the use of AMARYL in asymptomatic patients, it should be recognized that blood glucose control in NIDDM has not definitely been established to be effective in preventing the long-term cardiovascular and neural complications of diabetes. However, the Diabetes Control and Complications Trial (DCCT) demonstrated that control of HbA1c and glucose was associated with a decrease in retinopathy, neuropathy, and nephropathy for insulin-dependent diabetic (IDDM) patients.

CONTRAINDICATIONS

AMARYL is contraindicated in patients with

1. Known hypersensitivity to the drug.
2. Diabetic ketoacidosis, with or without coma. This condition should be treated with insulin.

WARNINGS

SPECIAL WARNING ON INCREASED RISK OF CARDIOVASCULAR MORTALITY

The administration of oral hypoglycemic drugs has been reported to be associated with increased cardiovascular mortality as compared to treatment with diet alone or diet plus insulin. This warning is based on the study conducted by the University Group Diabetes Program (UGDP), a long-term, prospective clinical trial designed to evaluate the effectiveness of glucose-lowering drugs in preventing or delaying vascular complications in patients with non-insulin-dependent diabetes. The study involved 823 patients who were randomly assigned to one of four treatment groups (Diabetes, 19 supp. 2: 747–830, 1970).

UGDP reported that patients treated for 5 to 8 years with diet plus a fixed dose of tolbutamide (1.5 grams per day) had a rate of cardiovascular mortality approximately 2-$^1/_2$ times that of patients treated with diet alone. A significant increase in total mortality was not observed, but the use of tolbutamide was discontinued based on the increase in cardiovascular mortality, thus limiting the opportunity for the study to show an increase in overall mortality. Despite controversy regarding the interpretation of these results, the findings of the UGDP study provide an adequate basis for this warning. The patient should be informed of the potential risks and advantages of AMARYL (glimepiride tablets) and of alternative modes of therapy.

Although only one drug in the sulfonylurea class (tolbutamide) was included in this study, it is prudent from a safety standpoint to consider that this warning may also apply to other oral hypoglycemic drugs in this class, in view of their close similarities in mode of action and chemical structure.

PRECAUTIONS

General

Hypoglycemia: All sulfonylurea drugs are capable of producing severe hypoglycemia. Proper patient selection, dosage, and instructions are important to avoid hypoglycemic episodes. Patients with impaired renal function may be more sensitive to the glucose-lowering effect of AMARYL. A starting dose of 1 mg once daily followed by appropriate dose titration is recommended in those patients. Debilitated or malnourished patients, and those with adrenal, pituitary, or hepatic insufficiency are particularly susceptible to the hypoglycemic action of glucose-lowering drugs. Hypoglycemia may be difficult to recognize in the elderly and in people who are taking beta-adrenergic blocking drugs or other sympatholytic agents. Hypoglycemia is more likely to occur when caloric intake is deficient, after severe or prolonged exercise, when alcohol is ingested, or when more than one glucose-lowering drug is used. Combined use of glimepiride with insulin or metformin may increase the potential for hypoglycemia.

Loss of control of blood glucose: When a patient stabilized on any diabetic regimen is exposed to stress such as fever, trauma, infection, or surgery, a loss of control may occur. At such times, it may be necessary to add insulin in combination with AMARYL or even use insulin monotherapy. The effectiveness of any oral hypoglycemic drug, including AMARYL, in lowering blood glucose to a desired level decreases in many patients over a period of time, which may be due to progression of the severity of the diabetes or to diminished responsiveness to the drug. This phenomenon is known as secondary failure, to distinguish it from primary failure in which the drug is ineffective in an individual patient when first given. Should secondary failure occur with AMARYL or metformin monotherapy, combined therapy with AMARYL and metformin or AMARYL and insulin may result in a response. Should secondary failure occur with combined AMARYL/metformin therapy, it may be necessary to initiate insulin therapy.

Information for Patients

Patients should be informed of the potential risks and advantages of AMARYL and of alternative modes of therapy. They should also be informed about the importance of adherence to dietary instructions, of a regular exercise program, and of regular testing of blood glucose.

The risks of hypoglycemia, its symptoms and treatment, and conditions that predispose to its development should be explained to patients and responsible family members. The potential for primary and secondary failure should also be explained.

Laboratory Tests

Fasting blood glucose should be monitored periodically to determine therapeutic response. Glycosylated hemoglobin should also be monitored, usually every 3 to 6 months, to more precisely assess long-term glycemic control.

Drug Interactions

(See CLINICAL PHARMACOLOGY, Drug Interactions.)

Carcinogenesis, Mutagenesis, and Impairment of Fertility

Studies in rats at doses of up to 5000 ppm in complete feed (approximately 340 times the maximum recommended human dose, based on surface area) for 30 months showed no evidence of carcinogenesis. In mice, administration of glimepiride for 24 months resulted in an increase in benign pancreatic adenoma formation which was dose related and is thought to be the result of chronic pancreatic stimulation. The no-effect dose for adenoma formation in mice in this study was 320 ppm in complete feed, or 46–54 mg/kg body weight/day. This is about 35 times the maximum human recommended dose of 8 mg once daily based on surface area. Glimepiride was non-mutagenic in a battery of *in vitro* and *in vivo* mutagenicity studies (Ames test, somatic cell mutation, chromosomal aberration, unscheduled DNA synthesis, mouse micronucleus test).

There was no effect of glimepiride on male mouse fertility in animals exposed up to 2500 mg/kg body weight (>1,700 times the maximum recommended human dose based on surface area). Glimepiride had no effect on the fertility of male and female rats administered up to 4000 mg/kg body weight (approximately 4,000 times the maximum recommended human dose based on surface area).

Pregnancy

Teratogenic Effects. Pregnancy Category C. Glimepiride did not produce teratogenic effects in rats exposed orally up to 4000 mg/kg body weight (approximately 4,000 times the maximum recommended human dose based on surface area) or in rabbits exposed up to 32 mg/kg body weight (approximately 60 times the maximum recommended human dose based on surface area). Glimepiride has been shown to be associated with intrauterine fetal death in rats when given in doses as low as 50 times the human dose based on surface area and in rabbits when given in doses as low as 0.1 times the human dose based on surface area. This fetotoxicity, observed only at doses inducing maternal hypoglycemia, has been similarly noted with other sulfonylureas, and is believed to be directly related to the pharmacologic (hypoglycemic) action of glimepiride.

There are no adequate and well-controlled studies in pregnant women. On the basis of results from animal studies, AMARYL (glimepiride tablets) should not be used during pregnancy. Because recent information suggests that abnormal blood glucose levels during pregnancy are associated with a higher incidence of congenital abnormalities, many experts recommend that insulin be used during pregnancy to maintain glucose levels as close to normal as possible.

Nonteratogenic Effects. In some studies in rats, offspring of dams exposed to high levels of glimepiride during pregnancy and lactation developed skeletal deformities consisting of shortening, thickening, and bending of the humerus during the postnatal period. Significant concentrations of glimepiride were observed in the serum and breast milk of the dams as well as in the serum of the pups. These skeletal deformations were determined to be the result of nursing from mothers exposed to glimepiride.

Prolonged severe hypoglycemia (4 to 10 days) has been reported in neonates born to mothers who were receiving a sulfonylurea drug at the time of delivery. This has been reported more frequently with the use of agents with prolonged half-lives. Patients who are planning a pregnancy should consult their physician, and it is recommended that they change over to insulin for the entire course of pregnancy and lactation.

Nursing Mothers

In rat reproduction studies, significant concentrations of glimepiride were observed in the serum and breast milk of the dams, as well as in the serum of the pups. Although it is not known whether AMARYL is excreted in human milk, other sulfonylureas are excreted in human milk. Because the potential for hypoglycemia in nursing infants may exist, and because of the effects on nursing animals, AMARYL should be discontinued in nursing mothers. If AMARYL is discontinued, and if diet and exercise alone are inadequate for controlling blood glucose, insulin therapy should be considered. (See above Pregnancy, Nonteratogenic Effects.)

Pediatric Use

Safety and effectiveness in pediatric patients have not been established.

ADVERSE REACTIONS

The incidence of hypoglycemia with AMARYL, as documented by blood glucose values < 60 mg/dL, ranged from 0.9–1.7% in two large, well-controlled, 1-year studies. (See WARNINGS and PRECAUTIONS.)

AMARYL has been evaluated for safety in 2,013 patients in US controlled trials, and in 1,551 patients in foreign controlled trials. More than 1,650 of these patients were treated for at least 1 year.

Adverse events, other than hypoglycemia, considered to be possibly or probably related to study drug that occurred in US placebo-controlled trials in more than 1% of patients treated with AMARYL are shown below.

Adverse Events Occurring in ≥ 1% AMARYL Patients

	AMARYL		Placebo	
	No.	%	No.	%
Total Treated	746	100	294	100
Dizziness	13	1.7	1	0.3
Asthenia	12	1.6	3	1.0
Headache	11	1.5	4	1.4
Nausea	8	1.1	0	0.0

Gastrointestinal Reactions

Vomiting, gastrointestinal pain, and diarrhea have been reported, but the incidence in placebo-controlled trials was less than 1%. In rare cases, there may be an elevation of liver enzyme levels. In isolated instances, impairment of liver function (e.g. with cholestasis and jaundice), as well as hepatitis, which may also lead to liver failure have been reported with sulfonylureas, including AMARYL.

Dermatologic Reactions

Allergic skin reactions, e.g., pruritus, erythema, urticaria, and morbilliform or maculopapular eruptions, occur in less than 1% of treated patients. These may be transient and may disappear despite continued use of AMARYL. If those hypersensitivity reactions persist, the drug should be dis-

Continued on next page

Amaryl—Cont.

continued. Porphyria cutanea tarda, photosensitivity reactions, and allergic vasculitis have been reported with sulfonylureas.

Hematologic Reactions

Leukopenia, agranulocytosis, thrombocytopenia, hemolytic anemia, aplastic anemia, and pancytopenia have been reported with sulfonylureas.

Metabolic Reactions

Hepatic porphyria reactions and disulfiram-like reactions have been reported with sulfonylureas; however, no cases have yet been reported with AMARYL (glimepiride tablets). Cases of hyponatremia have been reported with glimepiride and all other sulfonylureas, most often in patients who are on other medications or have medical conditions known to cause hyponatremia or increase release of antidiuretic hormone. The syndrome of inappropriate antidiuretic hormone (SIADH) secretion has been reported with certain other sulfonylureas, and it has been suggested that these sulfonylureas may augment the peripheral (antidiuretic) action of ADH and/or increase release of ADH.

Other Reactions

Changes in accommodation and/or blurred vision may occur with the use of AMARYL. This is thought to be due to changes in blood glucose, and may be more pronounced when treatment is initiated. This condition is also seen in untreated diabetic patients, and may actually be reduced by treatment. In placebo-controlled trials of AMARYL, the incidence of blurred vision was placebo, 0.7%, and AMARYL, 0.4%.

OVERDOSAGE

Overdosage of sulfonylureas, including AMARYL, can produce hypoglycemia. Mild hypoglycemic symptoms without loss of consciousness or neurologic findings should be treated aggressively with oral glucose and adjustments in drug dosage and/or meal patterns. Close monitoring should continue until the physician is assured that the patient is out of danger. Severe hypoglycemic reactions with coma, seizure, or other neurological impairment occur infrequently, but constitute medical emergencies requiring immediate hospitalization. If hypoglycemic coma is diagnosed or suspected, the patient should be given a rapid intravenous injection of concentrated (50%) glucose solution. This should be followed by a continuous infusion of a more dilute (10%) glucose solution at a rate that will maintain the blood glucose at a level above 100 mg/dL. Patients should be closely monitored for a minimum of 24 to 48 hours, because hypoglycemia may recur after apparent clinical recovery.

DOSAGE AND ADMINISTRATION

There is no fixed dosage regimen for the management of diabetes mellitus with AMARYL or any other hypoglycemic agent. The patient's fasting blood glucose and HbA1c must be measured periodically to determine the minimum effective dose for the patient; to detect primary failure, i.e., inadequate lowering of blood glucose at the maximum recommended dose of medication; and to detect secondary failure, i.e., loss of adequate blood glucose lowering response after an initial period of effectiveness. Glycosylated hemoglobin levels should be performed to monitor the patient's response to therapy.

Short-term administration of AMARYL may be sufficient during periods of transient loss of control in patients usually controlled well on diet and exercise.

Usual Starting Dose

The usual starting dose of AMARYL as initial therapy is 1–2 mg once daily, administered with breakfast or the first main meal. Those patients who may be more sensitive to hypoglycemic drugs should be started at 1 mg once daily, and should be titrated carefully. (See PRECAUTIONS Section for patients at increased risk.)

No exact dosage relationship exists between AMARYL and the other oral hypoglycemic agents. The maximum starting dose of AMARYL should be no more than 2 mg.

Failure to follow an appropriate dosage regimen may precipitate hypoglycemia. Patients who do not adhere to their prescribed dietary and drug regimen are more prone to exhibit unsatisfactory response to therapy.

Usual Maintenance Dose

The usual maintenance dose is 1 to 4 mg once daily. The maximum recommended dose is 8 mg once daily. After reaching a dose of 2 mg, dosage increases should be made in increments of no more than 2 mg at 1–2 week intervals based upon the patient's blood glucose response. Long-term efficacy should be monitored by measurement of HbA1c levels, for example, every 3 to 6 months.

AMARYL-Metformin Combination Therapy

If patients do not respond adequately to the maximal dose of AMARYL monotherapy, addition of metformin may be considered. Published clinical information exists for the use of other sulfonylureas including glyburide, glipizide, chlorpropamide, and tolbutamide in combination with metformin.

With concomitant AMARYL and metformin therapy, the desired control of blood glucose may be obtained by adjusting the dose of each drug. However, attempts should be made to identify the minimum effective dose of each drug to achieve this goal. With concomitant AMARYL and metformin therapy, the risk of hypoglycemia associated with AMARYL therapy continues and may be increased. Appropriate precautions should be taken.

AMARYL-Insulin Combination Therapy

Combination therapy with AMARYL and insulin may also be used in secondary failure patients. The fasting glucose level for instituting combination therapy is in the range of > 150 mg/dL in plasma or serum depending on the patient. The recommended AMARYL dose is 8 mg once daily administered with the first main meal. After starting with low-dose insulin, upward adjustments of insulin can be done approximately weekly as guided by frequent measurements of fasting blood glucose. Once stable, combination-therapy patients should monitor their capillary blood glucose on an ongoing basis, preferably daily. Periodic adjustments of insulin may also be necessary during maintenance as guided by glucose and HbA1c levels.

Specific Patient Populations

AMARYL (glimepiride tablets) is not recommended for use in pregnancy, nursing mothers, or children. In elderly, debilitated, or malnourished patients, or in patients with renal or hepatic insufficiency, the initial dosing, dose increments, and maintenance dosage should be conservative to avoid hypoglycemic reactions (See CLINICAL PHARMACOLOGY, Special Populations and PRECAUTIONS, General).

Patients Receiving Other Oral Hypoglycemic Agents

As with other sulfonylurea hypoglycemic agents, no transition period is necessary when transferring patients to AMARYL. Patients should be observed carefully (1–2 weeks) for hypoglycemia when being transferred from longer half-life sulfonylureas (e.g., chlorpropamide) to AMARYL due to potential overlapping of drug effect.

HOW SUPPLIED

AMARYL tablets are available in the following strengths and package sizes:

1 mg (pink, flat-faced, oblong with notched sides at double bisect, imprinted with "AMA RYL" on one side and the Hoechst logo on both sides of the bisect on the other side)
Bottles of 100 (NDC 0039-0221-10)

2 mg (green, flat-faced, oblong with notched sides at double bisect, imprinted with "AMA RYL" on one side and the Hoechst logo on both sides of the bisect on the other side)
Bottles of 100 (NDC 0039-0222-10)
Unit Dose Cartons (100) (NDC 0039-0222-11)

4 mg (blue, flat-faced, oblong with notched sides at double bisect, imprinted with "AMA RYL" on one side and the Hoechst logo on both sides of the bisect on the other side)
Bottles of 100 (NDC 0039-0223-10)
Unit Dose Cartons (100) (NDC 0039-0223-11)

Store between 59 and 86° F (15 and 30° C).
Dispense in well-closed containers with safety closures.
Caution: Federal law prohibits dispensing without a prescription.
AMARYL® REG TM HOECHST AG
*US Patent 4,379,785

ANIMAL TOXICOLOGY

Reduced serum glucose values and degranulation of the pancreatic beta cells were observed in beagle dogs exposed to 320 mg glimepiride/kg/day for 12 months (approximately 1,000 times the recommended human dose based on surface area). No evidence of tumor formation was observed in any organ. One female and one male dog developed bilateral subcapsular cataracts. Non-GLP studies indicated that glimepiride was unlikely to exacerbate cataract formation. Evaluation of the co-cataractogenic potential of glimepiride in several diabetic and cataract rat models was negative and there was no adverse effect of glimepiride on bovine ocular lens metabolism in organ culture.

HUMAN OPHTHALMOLOGY DATA

Ophthalmic examinations were carried out in over 500 subjects during long-term studies using the methodology of Taylor and West and Laties et al. No significant differences were seen between AMARYL and glyburide in the number of subjects with clinically important changes in visual acuity, intra-ocular tension, or in any of the five lens-related variables examined.

Ophthalmic examinations were carried out during long-term studies using the method of Chylack et al. No significant or clinically meaningful differences were seen between AMARYL and glipizide with respect to cataract progression by subjective LOCS II grading and objective image analysis systems, visual acuity, intraocular pressure, and general ophthalmic examination.

Prescribing Information as of October 1999

Hoechst-Roussel Pharmaceuticals
Division of Hoechst Marion Roussel, Inc.
Kansas City, MO 64137 USA

Shown in Product Identification Guide, page 306

ANZEMET® Injection ℞

[*an-zĕmĕt*]
(dolasetron mesylate injection)

Prescribing Information as of February 1999

DESCRIPTION

ANZEMET (dolasetron mesylate) is an antinauseant and antiemetic agent. Chemically, dolasetron mesylate is (2α,6α,8α,9aβ)-octahydro-3-oxo-2,6-methano-2*H*-quinolizin-8-yl-1*H*-indole-3-carboxylate monomethanesulfonate, monohydrate. It is a highly specific and selective serotonin subtype 3 (5-HT_3) receptor antagonist both in vitro and in vivo. Dolasetron mesylate has the following structural formula:

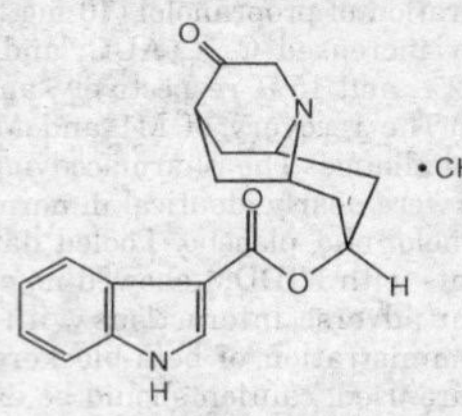

The empirical formula is $C_{19}H_{20}N_2O_3 \cdot CH_3SO_3H \cdot H_2O$, with a molecular weight of 438.50. Approximately 74% of dolasetron mesylate monohydrate is dolasetron base.

Dolasetron mesylate monohydrate is a white to off-white powder that is freely soluble in water and propylene glycol, slightly soluble in ethanol, and slightly soluble in normal saline.

ANZEMET Injection is a clear, colorless, nonpyrogenic, sterile solution for intravenous administration. Each milliliter of ANZEMET Injection contains 20 mg of dolasetron mesylate and 38.2 mg mannitol with an acetate buffer in water for injection. The pH of the resulting solution is 3.2 to 3.8.

CLINICAL PHARMACOLOGY

Dolasetron mesylate and its active metabolite, hydrodolasetron (MDL 74,156), are selective serotonin 5-HT_3 receptor antagonists not shown to have activity at other known serotonin receptors and with low affinity for dopamine receptors. The serotonin 5-HT_3 receptors are located on the nerve terminals of the vagus in the periphery and centrally in the chemoreceptor trigger zone of the area postrema. It is thought that chemotherapeutic agents produce nausea and vomiting by releasing serotonin from the enterochromaffin cells of the small intestine, and that the released serotonin then activates 5-HT_3 receptors located on vagal efferents to initiate the vomiting reflex.

Acute, usually reversible, ECG changes (PR and QT_c prolongation; QRS widening), caused by dolasetron mesylate, have been observed in healthy volunteers and in controlled clinical trials. The active metabolites of dolasetron may block sodium channels, a property unrelated to its ability to block 5-HT_3 receptors. QT_c prolongation is primarily due to QRS widening. Dolasetron appears to prolong both depolarization and, to a lesser extent, repolarization time. The magnitude and frequency of the ECG changes increased with dose (related to peak plasma concentrations of hydrodolasetron but not the parent compound). These ECG interval prolongations usually returned to baseline within 6 to 8 hours, but in some patients were present at 24 hour follow up. Dolasetron mesylate administration has little or no effect on blood pressure.

In healthy volunteers (N=64), dolasetron mesylate in single intravenous doses up to 5 mg/kg produced no effect on pupil size or meaningful changes in EEG tracings. Results from neuropsychiatric tests revealed that dolasetron mesylate did not alter mood or concentration. Multiple daily doses of dolasetron have had no effect on colonic transit in humans. Dolasetron mesylate has no effect on plasma prolactin concentrations.

Pharmacokinetics in Humans

Intravenous dolasetron mesylate is rapidly eliminated ($t_{1/2}$ <10 min) and completely metabolized to the most clinically relevant species, hydrodolasetron.

The reduction of dolasetron to hydrodolasetron is mediated by a ubiquitous enzyme, carbonyl reductase. Cytochrome P-450 (CYP)IID6 is primarily responsible for the subsequent hydroxylation of hydrodolasetron and both CYPIIIA and flavin monooxygenase are responsible for the N-oxidation of hydrodolasetron.

Hydrodolasetron is excreted in the urine unchanged (53.0% of administered intravenous dose). Other urinary metabolites include hydroxylated glucuronides and N-oxide.

Hydrodolasetron appeared rapidly in plasma, with a maximum concentration occurring approximately 0.6 hour after the end of intravenous treatment, and was eliminated with a mean half-life of 7.3 hours (%CV=24) and an apparent clearance of 9.4 mL/min/kg (%CV=28) in 24 adults. Hydrodolasetron is eliminated by multiple routes, including renal excretion and, after metabolism, mainly glucuronidation, and hydroxylation. Hydrodolasetron exhibits linear pharmacokinetics over the intravenous dose range of 50 to 200 mg and they are independent of infusion rate. Doses lower than 50 mg have not been studied. Two thirds of the administered dose is recovered in the urine and one third in the feces. Hydrodolasetron is widely distributed in the body with a mean apparent volume of distribution of 5.8 L/kg (%CV=25, N=24) in adults.

Sixty-nine to 77% of hydrodolasetron is bound to plasma protein. In a study with ^{14}C labeled dolasetron, the distribution of radioactivity to blood cells was not extensive. The binding of hydrodolasetron to α_1-acid glycoprotein is approximately 50%. The pharmacokinetics of hydrodolasetron are linear and similar in men and women.

The pharmacokinetics of hydrodolasetron, in special and targeted patient populations following intravenous administration of ANZEMET Injection, are summarized in Table 1. The pharmacokinetics of hydrodolasetron are similar in adult healthy volunteers and in adult cancer patients receiving chemotherapeutic agents. The apparent clearance of hydrodolasetron in pediatric and adolescent patients is 1.4

times to twofold higher than in adults. The apparent clearance of hydrodolasetron is not affected by age in adult cancer patients. Following intravenous administration, the apparent clearance of hydrodolasetron remains unchanged with severe hepatic impairment and decreases 47% with severe renal impairment. No dose adjustment is necessary for elderly patients or for patients with hepatic or renal impairment.

In a pharmacokinetic study in pediatric cancer patients (ages 3 to 11, N=25; ages 12 to 17, N=21) given a single 0.6, 1.2, 1.8, or 2.4 mg/kg dose of ANZEMET Injection intravenously, apparent clearance values were highest and half-lives were lowest in the youngest age group. For the 3 to 11 and the 12 to 17 year age groups, all receiving doses between 0.6 to 2.4 mg/kg, mean apparent clearances are 2 and 1.3 times greater, respectively, than for healthy adults receiving the same range of doses.

Thirty-two pediatric cancer patients ages 3 to 11 years (N=19) and 12 to 17 years (N=13), received 0.6, 1.2, or 1.8 mg ANZEMET Injection diluted with either apple or apple-grape juice and administered orally. In this study, the mean apparent clearances were 3 times greater in the younger pediatric group and 1.8 times greater in the older pediatric group than those observed in healthy adult volunteers. Across this spectrum of pediatric patients, maximum plasma concentrations were 0.6 to 0.7 times those observed in healthy adults receiving similar doses.

In a pharmacokinetic study in 18 pediatric patients (2 to 11 years of age) undergoing surgery with general anesthesia and administered a single 1.2 mg/kg intravenous dose of ANZEMET Injection, mean apparent clearance was greater (40%) and terminal half-life shorter (36%) for hydrodolasetron than in healthy adults receiving the same dose.

For 12 pediatric patients, ages 2 to 12 years receiving 1.2 mg/kg ANZEMET Injection diluted in apple or apple-grape juice and administered orally, the mean apparent clearance was 34% greater and half-life was 21% shorter than in healthy adults receiving the same dose.

[See table 1 at right]

CLINICAL STUDIES

Prevention of Cancer Chemotherapy-Induced Nausea and Vomiting

ANZEMET Injection administered intravenously at a dose of 1.8 mg/kg gave similar results in preventing nausea and vomiting as the other selective serotonin 5-HT_3 receptor antagonists studied as active comparators. It was more effective than metoclopramide. Efficacy was based on complete response rates (0 emetic episodes and no rescue medication).

Cisplatin Based Chemotherapy

A randomized, double-blind trial compared single intravenous doses of ANZEMET Injection with metoclopramide in 226 (160 men and 66 women) adult cancer patients receiving ≥80 mg/m^2 cisplatin. ANZEMET Injection at a dose of 1.8 mg/kg was significantly more effective than metoclopramide in the prevention of chemotherapy-induced nausea and vomiting in this study (Table 2).

[See table 2 at right]

A second randomized, double-blind trial compared single intravenous doses of ANZEMET Injection with intravenous ondansetron in 609 (377 men and 232 women) adult cancer patients receiving ≥70 mg/m^2 cisplatin. A single intravenous 1.8 mg/kg dose of ANZEMET Injection was shown to be equivalent to a single intravenous 32 mg dose of ondansetron (Table 3).

[See table 3 at right]

Another randomized, double-blind trial compared single IV doses of ANZEMET with a single 3-mg IV dose of granisetron in 474 (315 men and 159 women) patients receiving ≥80 mg/m^2 cisplatin chemotherapy. A single intravenous 1.8-mg/kg dose of ANZEMET gave similar results as those from granisetron.

Cyclophosphamide Based Chemotherapy

In a study of ANZEMET Injection in 309 patients (96 men and 213 women) receiving moderately emetogenic chemotherapy such as cyclophosphamide based regimens, a single intravenous 1.8 mg/kg dose of ANZEMET Injection was equivalent to metoclopramide administered as a 2 mg/kg intravenous bolus followed by 3 mg/kg intravenously over 8 hours. Complete response rates were 63% and 52%, respectively, p=0.12.

Prevention of Postoperative Nausea and Vomiting

ANZEMET Injection administered intravenously at a dose of 12.5 mg approximately 15 minutes before the cessation of general balanced anesthesia (short-acting barbiturate, nitrous oxide, narcotic and analgesic, and skeletal muscle relaxant) was significantly more effective than placebo in preventing postoperative nausea and vomiting. No increased efficacy was seen with higher doses.

One trial compared single intravenous ANZEMET Injection doses of 12.5, 25, 50, and 100 mg with placebo in 635 women surgical patients undergoing laparoscopic procedures. ANZEMET Injection at a dose of 12.5 mg was statistically superior to placebo for complete response (no vomiting, no rescue medication) (p=.0003). Complete response rates were 50% and 31%, respectively.

Another trial compared single intravenous ANZEMET Injection doses of 12.5, 25, 50, and 100 mg with placebo in 1030 (722 women and 308 men) surgical patients. In women, the 12.5 mg dose was statistically superior to placebo for complete response. The complete response rates were 50% and 40%, respectively. However, in men, there was no statistically significant difference in complete response between any ANZEMET dose and placebo.

Table 1. Pharmacokinetic Values for Plasma Hydrodolasetron Following Intravenous Administration of ANZEMET Injection*

	Age (years)	Dose	CL_{app} (mL/min/kg)	$t_{1/2}$ (h)	C_{max} (ng/mL)
Young Healthy Volunteers (N=24)	19–40	100 mg	9.4 (28%)	7.3 (24%)	320 (25%)
Elderly Healthy Volunteers (N=15)	65–75	2.4 mg/kg	8.3 (30%)	6.9 (22%)	620 (31%)
Cancer Patients					
Adults (N=273)	19–87	0.6–3.0 mg/kg	10.2 (34%)†	7.5 (43%)†	505 (26%)‡
Adolescents (N=21)	12–17	0.6–3.0 mg/kg	12.5 (37%)	5.5 (31%)	562 (45%)§
Children (N=25)	3–11	0.6–2.4 mg/kg	19.2 (30%)	4.4 (24%)	505 (100%)‖
Pediatric Surgery Patients (N=18)	2–11	1.2 mg/kg	13.1 (47%)	4.8 (23%)	255 (22%)
Patients with Severe Renal Impairment (N=12) (Creatinine clearance ≤10 mL/min)	28–74	200 mg	5.0 (33%)	10.9 (30%)	867 (31%)
Patients with Severe Hepatic Impairment (N=3)	42–52	150 mg	9.6 (19%)	11.7 (22%)	396 (45%)

CL_{app}: apparent clearance $t_{1/2}$: terminal elimination half-life ( ): coefficient of variation in %
*: mean values
†: results from population kinetic study
‡: results from adult cancer study (dose=1.8 mg/kg, N=8)
§: results from adolescents (dose=1.8 mg/kg, N=7)
‖: results from children (dose=1.8 mg/kg, N=5)

Table 2. Prevention of Chemotherapy-Induced Nausea and Emesis from Cisplatin Chemotherapy*

	ANZEMET Injection 1.8 mg/kg†	Metoclopramide‡	*p*-value
Number of Patients	72	69	
Response Over 24 Hours			
Complete Response§	41 (57%)	24 (35%)	0.0009
Nausea Score‖	4	30	0.0400

*: Dose ≥80 mg/m^2
†: Administered intravenously
‡: 3 mg/kg intravenous bolus and 0.5 mg/kg/h intravenously over 8 h.
§: No emetic episodes and no rescue medication.
‖: Median 24-h change from baseline nausea score using visual analog scale (VAS): Score range 0="none" to 100="nausea as bad as it could be."

Table 3. Prevention of Chemotherapy-Induced Nausea and Emesis from Cisplatin Chemotherapy*

	ANZEMET Injection 1.8 mg/kg†	Ondansetron 32 mg‡	*p*-value
Number of Patients	198	206	
Response Over 24 Hours			
Complete Response§	88 (44%)	88 (43%)	NS
Nausea Score‖	10	16	NS

*: Dose ≥70 mg/m^2
†: Administered intravenously
‡: Includes 12 patients who received 3 doses 0.15 mg/kg of ondansetron intravenously.
§: No emetic episodes and no rescue medication.
‖: Median 24-h change from baseline nausea score using visual analog scale (VAS): Score range 0="none" to 100="nausea as bad as it could be."

Treatment of Postoperative Nausea and/or Vomiting

Two randomized, double-blinded trials compared single intravenous ANZEMET Injection doses of 12.5, 25, 50, and 100 mg with placebo in 124 male and 833 female patients who had undergone surgery with general balanced anesthesia and presented with early postoperative nausea or vomiting requiring antiemetic treatment.

In both studies, the 12.5 mg intravenous dose of ANZEMET was statistically superior to placebo for complete response (no vomiting, no escape medication). No significant increased efficacy was seen with higher doses.

INDICATIONS AND USAGE

ANZEMET Injection is indicated for the following:

(1) the prevention of nausea and vomiting associated with initial and repeat courses of emetogenic cancer chemotherapy, including high dose cisplatin;

(2) the prevention of postoperative nausea and vomiting. As with other antiemetics, routine prophylaxis is not recommended for patients in whom there is little expectation that nausea and/or vomiting will occur postoperatively. In patients where nausea and/or vomiting must be avoided postoperatively, ANZEMET Injection is recommended even where the incidence of postoperative nausea and/or vomiting is low;

(3) the treatment of postoperative nausea and/or vomiting.

CONTRAINDICATIONS

ANZEMET Injection is contraindicated in patients known to have hypersensitivity to the drug.

WARNINGS

ANZEMET can cause ECG interval changes (PR, QT_c, JT prolongation and QRS widening). These changes are related in magnitude and frequency to blood levels of the active metabolite. These changes are self-limiting with declining blood levels. Some patients have interval prolongations for 24 hours or longer. Interval prolongation could lead to cardiovascular consequences, including heart block or cardiac arrhythmias. These have rarely been reported.

A cardiac conduction abnormality observed on an intraoperative cardiac rhythm monitor (interpreted as complete heart block) was reported in a 61-year-old woman who received 200 mg ANZEMET for the prevention of postoperative nausea and vomiting. This patient was also taking verapamil. A similar event also interpreted as complete heart block was reported in one patient receiving placebo.

A 66-year-old man with Stage IV non-Hodgkins lymphoma died suddenly 6 hours after receiving 1.8 mg/kg (119 mg) intravenous ANZEMET Injection. This patient had other potential risk factors including substantial exposure to doxorubicin and concomitant cyclophosphamide.

PRECAUTIONS

General

Dolasetron should be administered with caution in patients who have or may develop prolongation of cardiac

Continued on next page

Anzemet Injection—Cont.

conduction intervals, particularly QT_c. These include patients with hypokalemia or hypomagnesemia, patients taking diuretics with potential for inducing electrolyte abnormalities, patients with congenital QT syndrome, patients taking anti-arrhythmic drugs or other drugs which lead to QT prolongation, and cumulative high dose anthracycline therapy.

Cross hypersensitivity reactions have been reported in patients who received other selective 5-HT_3 receptor antagonists. These reactions have not been seen with dolasetron mesylate.

Drug Interactions

The potential for clinically significant drug-drug interactions posed by dolasetron and hydrodolasetron appears to be low for drugs commonly used in chemotherapy or surgery, because hydrodolasetron is eliminated by multiple routes. See PRECAUTIONS, General for information about potential interaction with other drugs that prolong the QT_c interval. Blood levels of hydrodolasetron increased 24% when dolasetron was coadministered with cimetidine (nonselective inhibitor of cytochrome P-450) for 7 days, and decreased 28% with coadministration of rifampin (potent inducer of cytochrome P-450) for 7 days.

ANZEMET Injection has been safely coadministered with drugs used in chemotherapy and surgery. As with other agents which prolong ECG intervals, caution should be exercised in patients taking drugs which prolong ECG intervals, particularly QT_c.

In patients taking furosemide, nifedipine, diltiazem, ACE inhibitors, verapamil, glyburide, propranolol, and various chemotherapy agents, no effect was shown on the clearance of hydrodolasetron. Clearance of hydrodolasetron decreased by about 27% when dolasetron mesylate was administered intravenously concomitantly with atenolol. ANZEMET did not influence anesthesia recovery time in patients. Dolasetron mesylate did not inhibit the antitumor activity of four chemotherapeutic agents (cisplatin, 5-fluorouracil, doxorubicin, cyclophosphamide) in four murine models.

Carcinogenesis, Mutagenesis, Impairment of Fertility

In a 24-month carcinogenicity study, there was a statistically significant (P<0.001) increase in the incidence of combined hepatocellular adenomas and carcinomas in male mice treated with 150 mg/kg/day and above. In this study, mice (CD-1) were treated orally with dolasetron mesylate 75, 150 or 300 mg/kg/day (225, 450 or 900 mg/m^2/day). For a 50 kg person of average height (1.46 m^2 body surface area), these doses represent 3.4, 6.8 and 13.5 times the recommended clinical dose (66.6 mg/m^2, intravenous) on a body surface area basis. No increase in liver tumors was observed at a dose of 75 mg/kg/day in male mice and at doses up to 300 mg/kg/day in female mice.

In a 24-month rat (Sprague-Dawley) carcinogenicity study, oral dolasetron was not tumorigenic at doses up to 150 mg/kg/day (900 mg/m^2/day, 13.5 times the recommended human dose based on body surface area) in male rats and 300 mg/kg/day (1800 mg/m^2/day, 27 times the recommended human dose based on body surface area) in female rats.

Dolasetron mesylate was not genotoxic in the Ames test, the rat lymphocyte chromosomal aberration test, the Chinese hamster ovary (CHO) cell (HGPRT) forward mutation test, the rat hepatocyte unscheduled DNA synthesis (UDS) test or the mouse micronucleus test.

Dolasetron mesylate was found to have no effect on fertility and reproductive performance at oral doses up to 100 mg/kg/day (600 mg/m^2/day, 9 times the recommended human dose based on body surface area) in female rats and up to 400 mg/kg/day (2400 mg/m^2/day, 36 times the recommended human dose based on body surface area) in male rats.

Pregnancy: Teratogenic Effects, Pregnancy Category B.

Teratology studies have not revealed evidence of impaired fertility or harm to the fetus due to dolasetron mesylate. These studies have been performed in pregnant rats at intravenous doses up to 60 mg/kg/day (5.4 times the recommended human dose based on body surface area) and pregnant rabbits at intravenous doses up to 20 mg/kg/day (3.2 times the recommended human dose based on body surface area). There are, however, no adequate and well-controlled studies in pregnant women. Because animal reproduction studies are not always predictive of human response, this drug should be used during pregnancy only if clearly needed.

Nursing Mothers

It is not known whether dolasetron mesylate is excreted in human milk. Because many drugs are excreted in human milk, caution should be exercised when ANZEMET Injection is administered to a nursing woman.

Pediatric Use

Four open-label, noncomparative pharmacokinetic studies have been performed in a total of 108 pediatric patients receiving emetogenic chemotherapy or undergoing surgery with general anesthesia. These patients received ANZEMET Injection either intravenously or orally in juice. Pediatric patients from 2 to 17 years of age participated in these trials, which included intravenous ANZEMET Injection doses of 0.6, 1.2, 1.8, or 2.4 mg/kg, and oral doses of 0.6, 1.2, or 1.8 mg/kg. There is no experience in pediatric patients under 2 years of age. Overall, ANZEMET Injection was well tolerated in these pediatric patients. Efficacy information collected in pediatric patients receiving cancer chemotherapy are consistent with those obtained in adults. No efficacy information was collected in the pediatric postoperative nausea and vomiting studies.

Table 4. Adverse Events ≥ 2% from Chemotherapy-Induced Nausea and Vomiting Studies

Event	ANZEMET Injection 1.8 mg/kg (n=695)	Ondansetron/ Granisetron* (n=356)
Headache	169 (24.3%)	73 (20.5%)
Diarrhea	86 (12.4%)	25 (7.0%)
Fever	30 (4.3%)	18 (5.1%)
Fatigue	25 (3.6%)	12 (3.4%)
Hepatic Function Abnormal†	25 (3.6%)	12 (3.4%)
Abdominal Pain	22 (3.2%)	7 (2.0%)
Hypertension	20 (2.9%)	9 (2.5%)
Pain	17 (2.4%)	7 (2.0%)
Dizziness	15 (2.2%)	7 (2.0%)
Chills/Shivering	14 (2.0%)	6 (1.7%)

*: Ondansetron 32 mg intravenous, granisetron 3 mg intravenous.
†: Includes events coded as SGOT- and/or SGPT-increased (see also Liver and Biliary System below)

Table 5. Adverse Events ≥ 2% from Placebo-Controlled Postoperative Nausea and Vomiting Studies

Event	ANZEMET Injection 12.5 mg (n=615)	Placebo (n=739)
Headache	58 (9.4%)	51 (6.9%)
Dizziness	34 (5.5%)	23 (3.1%)
Drowsiness	15 (2.4%)	18 (2.4%)
Pain	15 (2.4%)	21 (2.8%)
Urinary Retention	12 (2.0%)	16 (2.2%)

ANZEMET® Injection
(dolasetron mesylate injection)
20 mg/mL

Strength	Description	NDC Number
12.5 mg	0.625-mL single use ampules (Box of 6)	0088-1208-65
100 mg/5 mL	5-mL single-use vial	0088-1206-32

Use in Elderly Patients

Dosage adjustment is not needed in patients over 65. Effectiveness in prevention of nausea and vomiting in elderly patients was no different than in younger age groups.

ADVERSE REACTIONS

Chemotherapy Patients

In controlled clinical trials, 2265 adult patients received ANZEMET Injection. The overall adverse event rates were similar with 1.8 mg/kg ANZEMET Injection and ondansetron or granisetron. Patients were receiving concurrent chemotherapy, predominantly high-dose (≥50 mg/m^2) cisplatin. Following is a combined listing of all adverse events reported in ≥2% of patients in these controlled trials (Table 4).

[See table 4 above]

Postoperative Patients

In controlled clinical trials with 2550 adult patients, headache and dizziness were reported more frequently with 12.5 mg ANZEMET Injection than with placebo. Rates of other adverse events were similar. Following is a listing of all adverse events reported in ≥2% of patients receiving either placebo or 12.5 mg ANZEMET Injection for the prevention or treatment of postoperative nausea and vomiting in controlled clinical trials (Table 5).

[See table 5 above]

In clinical trials, the following infrequently reported adverse events, assessed by investigators as treatment-related or causality unknown, occurred following oral or intravenous administration of ANZEMET to adult patients receiving concomitant cancer chemotherapy or surgery:

Cardiovascular: Hypotension; rarely–edema, peripheral edema. The following events also occurred rarely and with a similar frequency as placebo and/or active comparator: Mobitz I AV block, chest pain, orthostatic hypotension, myocardial ischemia, syncope, severe bradycardia, and palpitations. See PRECAUTIONS section for information on potential effects on ECG.

In addition, the following asymptomatic treatment-emergent ECG changes were seen at rates less than or equal to those for active or placebo controls: bradycardia, tachycardia, T wave change, ST-T wave change, sinus arrhythmia, extrasystole (APCs or VPCs), poor R-wave progression, bundle branch block (left and right), nodal arrhythmia, U wave change, atrial flutter/fibrillation.

Furthermore, severe hypotension, bradycardia and syncope have been reported immediately or closely following IV administration.

Dermatologic: Rash, increased sweating.

Gastrointestinal System: Constipation, dyspepsia, abdominal pain, anorexia; rarely–pancreatitis.

Hearing, Taste and Vision: Taste perversion, abnormal vision; rarely–tinnitus, photophobia.

Hematologic: Rarely–hematuria, epistaxis, prothrombin time prolonged, PTT increased, anemia, purpura/hematoma, thrombocytopenia.

Hypersensitivity: Rarely–anaphylactic reaction, facial edema, urticaria.

Liver and Biliary System: Transient increases in AST (SGOT) and/or ALT (SGPT) values have been reported as adverse events in less than 1% of adult patients receiving ANZEMET in clinical trials. The increases did not appear to be related to dose or duration of therapy and were not associated with symptomatic hepatic disease. Similar increases were seen with patients receiving active comparator. Rarely–hyperbilirubinemia, increased GGT.

Metabolic and Nutritional: Rarely–alkaline phosphatase increased.

Musculoskeletal: Rarely–myalgia, arthralgia.

Nervous System: Flushing, vertigo, paraesthesia, tremor; rarely–ataxia, twitching.

Psychiatric: Agitation, sleep disorder, depersonalization; rarely–confusion, anxiety, abnormal dreaming.

Respiratory System: Rarely–dyspnea, bronchospasm.

Urinary System: Rarely–dysuria, polyuria, acute renal failure.

Vascular (Extracardiac): Local pain or burning on IV administration; rarely–peripheral ischemia, thrombophlebitis/phlebitis.

OVERDOSAGE

A 59-year-old man with metastatic melanoma and no known pre-existing cardiac conditions developed severe hypotension and dizziness 40 minutes after receiving a 15 minute intravenous infusion of 1000 mg (13 mg/kg) of dolasetron mesylate. Treatment for the overdose consisted of infusion of 500 mL of a plasma expander, dopamine, and atropine. The patient had normal sinus rhythm and prolongation of PR, QRS and QT_c intervals on an ECG recorded 2 hours after the infusion. The patient's blood pressure was normal 3 hours after the event and the ECG intervals returned to baseline on follow-up. The patient was released from the hospital 6 hours after the event.

Following a suspected overdose of ANZEMET Injection, a patient found to have second-degree or higher AV conduction block with ECG should undergo cardiac telemetry monitoring.
There is no known specific antidote for dolasetron mesylate, and patients with suspected overdose should be managed with supportive therapy. Individual doses as large as 5 mg/kg intravenously or 400 mg orally have been safely given to healthy volunteers or cancer patients.
It is not known if dolasetron mesylate is removed by hemodialysis or peritoneal dialysis.
A 7-year-old boy received 6 mg/kg dolasetron mesylate orally before surgery. No symptoms occurred and no treatment was required.
Single intravenous doses of dolasetron mesylate at 160 mg/kg in male mice and 140 mg/kg in female mice and rats of both sexes (6.3 to 12.6 times the recommended human dose based on body surface area) were lethal. Symptoms of acute toxicity were tremors, depression and convulsions.

DOSAGE AND ADMINISTRATION

The recommended dose of ANZEMET Injection should not be exceeded.

Prevention of Cancer Chemotherapy-Induced Nausea and Vomiting

Adults: The recommended intravenous dosage of ANZEMET Injection from clinical trial results is 1.8 mg/kg given as a single dose approximately 30 minutes before chemotherapy (see Administration). Alternatively, for most patients, a fixed dose of 100 mg can be administered over 30 seconds.
Pediatric Patients: The recommended intravenous dosage in pediatric patients 2 to 16 years of age is 1.8 mg/kg given as a single dose approximately 30 minutes before chemotherapy, up to a maximum of 100 mg (see Administration). Safety and effectiveness in pediatric patients under 2 years of age have not been established.
ANZEMET Injection mixed in apple or apple-grape juice may be used for oral dosing of pediatric patients. When ANZEMET Injection is administered orally, the recommended dosage in pediatric patients 2 to 16 years of age is 1.8 mg/kg up to a maximum 100 mg dose given within 1 hour before chemotherapy.
The diluted product may be kept up to 2 hours at room temperature before use.
Use in the Elderly, in Renal Failure Patients, or in Hepatically Impaired Patients: No dosage adjustment is recommended.

Prevention or Treatment of Postoperative Nausea and/or Vomiting

Adults: The recommended intravenous dosage of ANZEMET Injection is 12.5 mg given as a single dose approximately 15 minutes before the cessation of anesthesia (prevention) or as soon as nausea or vomiting presents (treatment).
Pediatric Patients: The recommended intravenous dosage in pediatric patients 2 to 16 years of age is 0.35 mg/kg, with a maximum dose of 12.5 mg, given as a single dose approximately 15 minutes before the cessation of anesthesia or as soon as nausea or vomiting presents. Safety and effectiveness in pediatric patients under 2 years of age have not been established.
ANZEMET Injection mixed in apple or apple-grape juice may be used for oral dosing of pediatric patients. When ANZEMET Injection is administered orally, the recommended oral dosage in pediatric patients 2 to 16 years of age is 1.2 mg/kg up to a maximum 100-mg dose given within 2 hours before surgery. The diluted product may be kept up to 2 hours at room temperature before use.
Use in the Elderly, in Renal Failure Patients, or in Hepatically Impaired Patients: No dosage adjustment is recommended.

Administration

ANZEMET Injection can be safely infused intravenously as rapidly as 100 mg/30 seconds or diluted in a compatible intravenous solution (see below) to 50 mL and infused over a period of up to 15 minutes. ANZEMET Injection should not be mixed with other drugs. Flush the infusion line before and after administration of ANZEMET Injection.

Stability

After dilution, ANZEMET Injection is stable under normal lighting conditions at room temperature for 24 hours or under refrigeration for 48 hours with the following compatible intravenous fluids: 0.9% sodium chloride injection, 5% dextrose injection, 5% dextrose and 0.45% sodium chloride injection, 5% dextrose and Lactated Ringer's injection, Lactated Ringer's injection, and 10% mannitol injection. Although ANZEMET Injection is chemically and physically stable when diluted as recommended, sterile precautions should be observed because diluents generally do not contain preservative. After dilution, do not use beyond 24 hours, or 48 hours if refrigerated.
Parenteral drug products should be inspected visually for particulate matter and discoloration before administration whenever solution and container permit.

HOW SUPPLIED

ANZEMET Injection (dolasetron mesylate injection) is supplied in single-use ampuls and vials as a clear, colorless solution.
[See third table on previous page]
Store at controlled room temperature 20–25°C (68–77°F). Protect from light.

Prescribing information as of February 1999

Manufactured for Hoechst Marion Roussel, Inc.
Kansas City, MO 64137 USA

Manufactured by Ben Venue Laboratories, Inc.
Bedford, OH 44146 USA
Shown in Product Identification Guide, page 306

ANZEMET® Tablets ℞

[*an-zĕmĕt*]
(dolasetron mesylate)

Prescribing Information as of February 1999

DESCRIPTION

ANZEMET (dolasetron mesylate) is an antinauseant and antiemetic agent. Chemically, dolasetron mesylate is (2α,6α,8α,9aβ)-octahydro-3-oxo-2,6-methano-2*H*-quinolizin-8-yl-1*H*-indole-3-carboxylate monomethanesulfonate, monohydrate. It is a highly specific and selective serotonin subtype 3 (5-HT_3) receptor antagonist both in vitro and in vivo. Dolasetron mesylate has the following structural formula:

$\cdot CH_3SO_3H \cdot H_2O$

The empirical formula is $C_{19}H_{20}N_2O_3 \cdot CH_3SO_3H \cdot H_2O$, with a molecular weight of 438.50. Approximately 74% of dolasetron mesylate monohydrate is dolasetron base.
Dolasetron mesylate monohydrate is a white to off-white powder that is freely soluble in water and propylene glycol, slightly soluble in ethanol, and slightly soluble in normal saline.
Each ANZEMET Tablet for oral administration contains dolasetron mesylate (as the monohydrate) and also contains the inactive ingredients: carnauba wax, croscarmellose sodium, hydroxypropyl methylcellulose, lactose, magnesium stearate, polyethylene glycol, polysorbate 80, pregelatinized starch, synthetic red iron oxide, titanium dioxide, and white wax. The tablets are printed with black ink, which contains lecithin, pharmaceutical glaze, propylene glycol, and synthetic black iron oxide.

CLINICAL PHARMACOLOGY

Dolasetron mesylate and its active metabolite, hydrodolasetron (MDL 74,156), are selective serotonin 5-HT_3 receptor antagonists not shown to have activity at other known serotonin receptors and with low affinity for dopamine receptors. The serotonin 5-HT_3 receptors are located on the nerve terminals of the vagus in the periphery and centrally in the chemoreceptor trigger zone of the area postrema. It is thought that chemotherapeutic agents produce nausea and vomiting by releasing serotonin from the enterochromaffin cells of the small intestine, and that the released serotonin then activates 5-HT_3 receptors located on vagal efferents to initiate the vomiting reflex.
Acute, usually reversible, ECG changes (PR and QT_c prolongation; QRS widening), caused by dolasetron mesylate, have been observed in healthy volunteers and in controlled clinical trials. The active metabolites of dolasetron may block sodium channels, a property unrelated to its ability to block 5-HT_3 receptors. QT_c prolongation is primarily due to QRS widening. Dolasetron appears to prolong both depolarization and, to a lesser extent, repolarization time. The magnitude and frequency of the ECG changes increased with dose (related to peak plasma concentrations of hydrodolasetron but not the parent compound). These ECG interval prolongations usually returned to baseline within 6 to 8 hours, but in some patients were present at 24 hour follow up. Dolasetron mesylate administration has little or no effect on blood pressure.
In healthy volunteers (N=64), dolasetron mesylate in single intravenous doses up to 5 mg/kg produced no effect on pupil size or meaningful changes in EEG tracings. Results from neuropsychiatric tests revealed that dolasetron mesylate did not alter mood or concentration. Multiple daily doses of dolasetron have had no effect on colonic transit in humans. Dolasetron has no effect on plasma prolactin concentrations.

Pharmacokinetics in Humans

Oral dolasetron is well absorbed, although parent drug is rarely detected in plasma due to rapid and complete metabolism to the most clinically relevant species, hydrodolasetron.
The reduction of dolasetron to hydrodolasetron is mediated by a ubiquitous enzyme, carbonyl reductase. Cytochrome P-450 (CYP)IID6 is primarily responsible for the subsequent hydroxylation of hydrodolasetron and both CYPIIIA and flavin monooxygenase are responsible for the N-oxidation of hydrodolasetron.
Hydrodolasetron is excreted in the urine unchanged (61.0% of administered oral dose). Other urinary metabolites include hydroxylated glucuronides and N-oxide.
Hydrodolasetron appears rapidly in plasma, with a maximum concentration occurring approximately 1 hour after dosing, and is eliminated with a mean half-life of 8.1 hours (%CV=18%) and an apparent clearance of 13.4 mL/min/kg (%CV=29%) in 30 adults. The apparent absolute bioavailability of oral dolasetron, determined by the major active metabolite hydrodolasetron, is approximately 75%. Orally administered dolasetron intravenous solution and tablets are bioequivalent. Food does not affect the bioavailability of dolasetron taken by mouth.
Hydrodolasetron is eliminated by multiple routes, including renal excretion and, after metabolism, mainly, glucuronidation and hydroxylation. Two thirds of the administered dose is recovered in the urine and one third in the feces. Hydrodolasetron is widely distributed in the body with a mean apparent volume of distribution of 5.8 L/kg (%CV=25%, N=24) in adults.
Sixty-nine to 77% of hydrodolasetron is bound to plasma protein. In a study with ^{14}C labeled dolasetron, the distribution of radioactivity to blood cells was not extensive. Approximately 50% of hydrodolasetron is bound to α_1-acid glycoprotein. The pharmacokinetics of hydrodolasetron are linear and similar in men and women.
The pharmacokinetics of hydrodolasetron, in special and targeted patient populations following oral administration of dolasetron, are summarized in Table 1. The pharmacokinetics of hydrodolasetron are similar in adult healthy volunteers and in adult cancer patients receiving chemotherapeutic agents. The apparent clearance following oral administration of hydrodolasetron is approximately 1.6- to 3.4-fold higher in children and adolescents than in adults. The clearance following oral administration of hydrodolasetron is not affected by age in adult cancer patients. The apparent oral clearance of hydrodolasetron decreases 42% with severe hepatic impairment and 44% with severe renal impairment. No dose adjustment is necessary for elderly patients or for patients with hepatic or renal impairment.
The pharmacokinetics of ANZEMET Tablets have not been studied in the pediatric population. However, the following pharmacokinetic data are available on intravenous ANZEMET Injection administered orally to children.
Thirty-two pediatric cancer patients ages 3 to 11 years (N=19) and 12 to 17 years (N=13), received 0.6, 1.2, or 1.8 mg ANZEMET Injection diluted with either apple or apple-grape juice and administered orally. In this study, the mean apparent clearances of hydrodolasetron were 3 times greater in the younger pediatric group and 1.8 times greater in the older pediatric group than those observed in healthy adult volunteers. Across this spectrum of pediatric patients, maximum plasma concentrations were 0.6 to 0.7 times those observed in healthy adults receiving similar doses.
For 12 pediatric patients, ages 2 to 12 years receiving 1.2 mg/kg ANZEMET Injection diluted in apple or apple-grape juice and administered orally, the mean apparent clearance was 34% greater and half-life was 21% shorter than in healthy adults receiving the same dose.
[See table 1 at top of next page]

CLINICAL STUDIES

Prevention of Cancer Chemotherapy-Induced Nausea and Vomiting

Oral ANZEMET at a dose of 100 mg prevents nausea and vomiting associated with moderately emetogenic cancer therapy as shown by 24 hour efficacy data from two double-blind studies. Efficacy was based on complete response (ie, no vomiting, no rescue medication).
The first randomized, double-blind trial compared single oral ANZEMET doses of 25, 50, 100 and 200 mg in 60 men and 259 women cancer patients receiving cyclophosphamide and/or doxorubicin. There was no statistically significant difference in complete response between the 100 mg and 200 mg dose. Results are summarized in Table 2.
[See table 2 on next page]
Another trial also compared single oral ANZEMET doses of 25, 50, 100, and 200 mg in 307 patients receiving moderately emetogenic chemotherapy. In this study, the 100 mg ANZEMET dose gave a 73% complete response rate.

Prevention of Postoperative Nausea and Vomiting

ANZEMET Tablets at a dose of 100 mg administered orally 1–2 hours before surgery and before general balanced anesthesia (short-acting barbiturate, nitrous oxide, narcotic analgesic, and skeletal muscle relaxant) was significantly more effective than placebo in preventing postoperative nausea and vomiting. Efficacy was based on complete response rates (0 emetic episodes and no rescue medication over 24 hours). No increased efficacy was seen with higher doses.
One trial compared single ANZEMET Tablet doses of 25, 50, 100, and 200 mg with placebo in 789 women undergoing gynecological surgery. In this study the 100 mg dose produced a complete response rate statistically superior to placebo. The study results are summarized in Table 3.
[See table 3 on next page]
Another trial also compared single oral ANZEMET doses of 25, 50, 100, and 200 mg with placebo in 373 women undergoing gynecological surgery. In this study, the 100 mg ANZEMET dose gave a 54% complete response rate as compared to the 29% rate of placebo.

INDICATIONS AND USAGE

ANZEMET Tablets are indicated for:

1) **the prevention of nausea and vomiting associated with moderately emetogenic cancer chemotherapy, including initial and repeat courses;**
2) **the prevention of postoperative nausea and vomiting.**

CONTRAINDICATIONS

ANZEMET Tablets are contraindicated in patients known to have hypersensitivity to the drug.

Continued on next page

Table 1. Pharmacokinetic Values for Plasma Hydrodolasetron Following Oral Administration of ANZEMET*

	Age (years)	Dose	CL_{app} (mL/min/kg)	$t_{1/2}$ (h)	C_{max} (ng/mL)
Young Healthy Volunteers (N=30)	19–45	200 mg	13.4 (29%)	8.1 (18%)	556 (28%)
Elderly Healthy Volunteers (N=15)	65–75	2.4 mg/kg	9.5 (36%)	7.2 (32%)	662 (28%)
Cancer Patients					
Adults (N=61)†	24–84	25–200 mg	12.9 (49%)	7.9 (43%)	— ‡
Adolescents (N=13)†	12–17	0.6–1.8 mg/kg	26.5 (67%)	6.4 (30%)	374§ (32%)
Children (N=19)†	3–11	0.6–1.8 mg/kg	44.2 (49%)	5.5 (39%)	217‖ (67%)
Pediatric Surgery Patients (N=11)	2–12	1.2 mg/kg	20.8 (49%)	5.9 (24%)	159 (32%)
Patients with Severe Renal Impairment (N=12) (Creatinine clearance ≤10 mL/min)	28–74	200 mg	7.2 (48%)	10.7 (29%)	701 (21%)
Patients with Severe Hepatic Impairment (N=3)	42–52	150 mg	8.8 (57%)	11.0 (36%)	410 (12%)

CL_{app}: apparent clearance $t_{1/2}$: terminal elimination half-life ( ): coefficient of variation in %
*: mean values
†: analyzed by nonlinear mixed effect modeling with data pooled across dose strengths
‡: sampling times did not allow calculation
§: results from adolescents (dose=1.8 mg/kg, N=3)
‖: results from children (dose=1.8 mg/kg, N=7)

Table 2. Prevention of Chemotherapy-Induced Nausea and Vomiting from Moderately Emetogenic Chemotherapy

	ANZEMET Tablets				
Response Over 24 Hours	25 mg (N=78)	50 mg (N=83)	**100 mg† (N=80)**	200 mg (N=78)	*p*-value for Linear Trend
Complete Response‡	24 (31%)	34 (41%)	**49 (61%)**	46 (59%)	P<.0001
Nausea Score§	49	10	**11**	7	P=.0006

†: The recommended dose
‡: No emetic episodes and no rescue medication.
§: Median 24-h change from baseline nausea score using visual analog scale (VAS): Score range 0="none" to 100="nausea as bad as it could be."

Table 3. Prevention of Postoperative Nausea and Vomiting

	ANZEMET Tablets				
Response Over 24 Hours	25 mg (N=159)	50 mg (N=166)	**100 mg† (N=154)**	200 mg (N=154)	Placebo (N=156)
Complete Response‡	71 (45%)	95 (57%)*	**78 (51%)***	73 (47%)*	55 (35%)
Nausea Score§	5*	4*	**5***	6*	15

*: $p<.05$ vs placebo
†: The recommended dose
‡: No emetic episodes and no rescue medication.
§: Median 24-h change from baseline nausea score using visual analog scale (VAS): Score range 0="none" to 100="nausea as bad as it could be."

ANZEMET®
(dolasetron mesylate)
Tablets

Strength	Quantity	NDC Number	Description
50 mg	5 ct Bottle 10 ct Unit Dose 5 ct Blister Pack	0088-1202-05 0088-1202-43 0088-1202-29	Light pink, film coated, round tablet imprinted with"ANZEMET 50" on one side.
100 mg	5 ct Bottle 10 ct Unit Dose 5 ct Blister Pack	0088-1203-05 0088-1203-43 0088-1203-29	Pink, film coated, elongated oval tablet imprinted with "100" on one side and "ANZEMET" on the other.

Anzemet—Cont.

WARNINGS

ANZEMET can cause ECG interval changes (PR, QT_C, JT prolongation and QRS widening). These changes are related in magnitude and frequency to blood levels of the active metabolite. These changes are self-limiting with declining blood levels. Some patients have interval prolongations for 24 hours or longer. Interval prolongation could lead to cardiovascular consequences, including heart block or cardiac arrhythmias. These have rarely been reported.

A cardiac conduction abnormality observed on an intraoperative cardiac rhythm monitor (interpreted as complete heart block) was reported in a 61-year-old woman who received 200 mg ANZEMET for the prevention of postoperative nausea and vomiting. This patient was also taking verapamil. A similar event also interpreted as complete heart block was reported in one patient receiving placebo.

A 66-year-old man with Stage IV non-Hodgkins lymphoma died suddenly 6 hours after receiving 1.8 mg/kg (119 mg) intravenous ANZEMET Injection. This patient had other potential risk factors including substantial exposure to doxorubicin and concomitant cyclophosphamide.

PRECAUTIONS

General

Dolasetron should be administered with caution in patients who have or may develop prolongation of cardiac conduction intervals, particularly QT_c. These include patients with hypokalemia or hypomagnesemia, patients taking diuretics with potential for inducing electrolyte abnormalities, patients with congenital QT syndrome, patients taking anti-arrhythmic drugs or other drugs which lead to QT prolongation, and cumulative high dose anthracycline therapy.

Cross hypersensitivity reactions have been reported in patients who received other selective $5\text{-}HT_3$ receptor antagonists. These reactions have not been seen with dolasetron mesylate.

Drug Interactions

The potential for clinically significant drug-drug interactions posed by dolasetron and hydrodolasetron appears to be low for drugs commonly used in chemotherapy or surgery, because hydrodolasetron is eliminated by multiple routes. See PRECAUTIONS, General for information about potential interaction with other drugs that prolong the QT_c interval. Blood levels of hydrodolasetron increased 24% when dolasetron was coadministered with cimetidine (nonselective inhibitor of cytochrome P-450) for 7 days, and decreased 28% with coadministration of rifampin (potent inducer of cytochrome P-450) for 7 days.

ANZEMET has been safely coadministered with drugs used in chemotherapy and surgery. As with other agents which prolong ECG intervals, caution should be exercised in patients taking drugs which prolong ECG intervals, particularly QT_c.

In patients taking furosemide, nifedipine, diltiazem, ACE inhibitors, verapamil, glyburide, propranolol, and various chemotherapy agents, no effect was shown on the clearance of hydrodolasetron. Clearance of hydrodolasetron decreased by about 27% when dolasetron mesylate was administered intravenously concomitantly with atenolol. ANZEMET did not influence anesthesia recovery time in patients. Dolasetron mesylate did not inhibit the antitumor activity of four chemotherapeutic agents (cisplatin, 5-fluorouracil, doxorubicin, cyclophosphamide) in four murine models.

Carcinogenesis, Mutagenesis, Impairment of Fertility

In a 24-month carcinogenicity study, there was a statistically significant (P<0.001) increase in the incidence of combined hepatocellular adenomas and carcinomas in male mice treated with 150 mg/kg/day and above. In this study, mice (CD-1) were treated orally with dolasetron mesylate 75, 150, or 300 mg/kg/day (225, 450 or 900 mg/m^2/day). For a 50 kg person of average height (1.46 m^2 body surface area), these doses represent 3, 6, and 12 times the recommended clinical dose (74 mg/m^2) on a body surface area basis. No increase in liver tumors was observed at a dose of 75 mg/kg/day in male mice and at doses up to 300 mg/kg/day in female mice.

In a 24-month rat (Sprague-Dawley) carcinogenicity study, oral dolasetron mesylate was not tumorigenic at doses up to 150 mg/kg/day (900 mg/m^2/day, 12 times the recommended human dose based on body surface area) in male rats and 300 mg/kg/day (1800 mg/m^2/day, 24 times the recommended human dose based on body surface area) in female rats.

Dolasetron mesylate was not genotoxic in the Ames test, the rat lymphocyte chromosomal aberration test, the Chinese hamster ovary (CHO) cell (HGPRT) forward mutation test, the rat hepatocyte unscheduled DNA synthesis (UDS) test or the mouse micronucleus test.

Dolasetron mesylate was found to have no effect on fertility and reproductive performance at oral doses up to 100 mg/kg/day (600 mg/m^2/day, 8 times the recommended human dose based on body surface area) in female rats and up to 400 mg/kg/day (2400 mg/m^2/day, 32 times the recommended human dose based on body surface area) in male rats.

Pregnancy: Teratogenic Effects, Pregnancy Category B.

Teratology studies have not revealed evidence of impaired fertility or harm to the fetus due to dolasetron mesylate. These studies have been performed in pregnant rats at oral doses up to 100 mg/kg/day (8 times the recommended human dose based on body surface area) and pregnant rabbits at oral doses up to 100 mg/kg/day (16 times the recommended human dose based on body surface area). There are, however, no adequate and well-controlled studies in pregnant women. Because animal reproduction studies are not always predictive of human response, this drug should be used during pregnancy only if clearly needed.

Nursing Mothers

It is not known whether dolasetron mesylate is excreted in human milk. Because many drugs are excreted in human milk, caution should be exercised when ANZEMET Tablets are administered to a nursing woman.

Pediatric Use

ANZEMET Tablets are expected to be as safe and effective as when ANZEMET Injection is given orally to pediatric patients. ANZEMET Tablets are recommended for children old enough to swallow tablets (see CLINICAL PHARMACOLOGY, Pharmacokinetics in Humans).

Elderly

Dosage adjustment is not needed in patients over 65. Effectiveness in prevention of nausea and vomiting in elderly patients was no different than in younger age groups.

ADVERSE REACTIONS

Chemotherapy Patients

In controlled clinical trials, 943 adult cancer patients received ANZEMET Tablets. These patients were receiving concurrent chemotherapy, predominantly cyclophosphamide and doxorubicin regimens. The following adverse events were reported in ≥2% of patients receiving either ANZEMET 25 mg or ANZEMET 100 mg tablets for prevention of cancer chemotherapy induced nausea and vomiting in controlled clinical trials (Table 4).

Table 4. Adverse Events ≥ 2% from Chemotherapy-Induced Nausea and Vomiting Studies

	ANZEMET	
Event	25 mg (N=235)	100 mg (N=227)
Headache	42 (17.9%)	52 (22.9%)
Fatigue	6 (2.6%)	13 (5.7%)
Diarrhea	5 (2.1%)	12 (5.3%)
Bradycardia	12 (5.1%)	9 (4.0%)

Dizziness	3 (1.3%)	7 (3.1%)
Pain	0	7 (3.1%)
Tachycardia	7 (3.0%)	6 (2.6%)
Dyspepsia	7 (3.0%)	5 (2.2%)
Chills/Shivering	3 (1.3%)	5 (2.2%)

Postoperative Patients
In controlled clinical trials, 936 adult female patients have received oral ANZEMET for the prevention of postoperative nausea and vomiting. Following is a listing of all adverse events reported in ≥2% of patients receiving either placebo or ANZEMET for prevention of postoperative nausea and vomiting in controlled clinical trials (Table 5).

Table 5. Adverse Events ≥ 2% from Placebo-Controlled Postoperative Nausea and Vomiting Studies

Event	ANZEMET 100 mg (N=228)	Placebo (N=231)
Headache	16 (7.0%)	11 (4.8%)
Hypotension	12 (5.3%)	15 (6.5%)
Dizziness	10 (4.4%)	0 (0.0%)
Fever	8 (3.5%)	7 (3.0%)
Pruritus	7 (3.1%)	8 (3.5%)
Oliguria	6 (2.6%)	3 (1.3%)
Hypertension	5 (2.2%)	7 (3.0%)
Tachycardia	5 (2.2%)	2 (0.9%)

In clinical trials, the following infrequently reported adverse events, assessed by investigators as treatment-related or causality unknown, occurred following oral or intravenous administration of ANZEMET to adult patients receiving concomitant cancer chemotherapy or surgery:
Cardiovascular: Hypotension; rarely–edema, peripheral edema. The following events also occurred rarely and with a similar frequency as placebo and/or active comparator: Mobitz I AV block, chest pain, orthostatic hypotension, myocardial ischemia, syncope, severe bradycardia, and palpitations. See PRECAUTIONS section for information on potential effects on ECG.
In addition, the following asymptomatic treatment-emergent ECG changes were seen at rates less than or equal to those for active or placebo controls: bradycardia, T wave change, ST-T wave change, sinus arrhythmia, extrasystole (APCs or VPCs), poor R-wave progression, bundle branch block (left and right), nodal arrhythmia, U wave change, atrial flutter/fibrillation.
Furthermore, severe hypotension, bradycardia and syncope have been reported immediately or closely following IV administration.
Dermatologic: Rash, increased sweating.
Gastrointestinal System: Constipation, dyspepsia, abdominal pain, anorexia; rarely—pancreatitis.
Hearing, Taste and Vision: Taste perversion, abnormal vision; rarely—tinnitus, photophobia.
Hematologic: Rarely—hematuria, epistaxis, prothrombin time prolonged, PTT increased, anemia, purpura/hematoma, thrombocytopenia.
Hypersensitivity: Rarely—anaphylactic reaction, facial edema, urticaria.
Liver and Biliary System: Transient increases in AST (SGOT) and/or ALT (SGPT) values have been reported as adverse events in less than 1% of adult patients receiving ANZEMET in clinical trials. The increases did not appear to be related to dose or duration of therapy and were not associated with symptomatic hepatic disease. Similar increases were seen with patients receiving active comparator. Rarely—hyperbilirubinemia, increased GGT.
Metabolic and Nutritional: Rarely—alkaline phosphatase increased.
Musculoskeletal: Rarely—myalgia, arthralgia.
Nervous System: Flushing, vertigo, paresthesia, tremor; rarely—ataxia, twitching.
Psychiatric: Agitation, sleep disorder, depersonalization; rarely—confusion, anxiety, abnormal dreaming.
Respiratory System: Rarely—dyspnea, bronchospasm.
Urinary System: Rarely—dysuria, polyuria, acute renal failure.
Vascular (Extracardiac): Local pain or burning on IV administration; rarely—peripheral ischemia, thrombophlebitis/phlebitis.

OVERDOSAGE

A 59-year-old man with metastatic melanoma and no known pre-existing cardiac conditions developed severe hypotension and dizziness 40 minutes after receiving a 15 minute intravenous infusion of 1000 mg (13 mg/kg) of dolasetron mesylate. Treatment for the overdose consisted of infusion of 500 mL of a plasma expander, dopamine, and atropine. The patient had normal sinus rhythm and prolongation of PR, QRS and QT_c intervals on an ECG recorded 2 hours after the infusion. The patient's blood pressure was normal 3 hours after the event and the ECG intervals returned to baseline on follow-up. The patient was released from the hospital 6 hours after the event.
Following a suspected overdose of ANZEMET Injection, a patient found to have second-degree or higher AV conduction block with ECG should undergo cardiac telemetry monitoring.
There is no known specific antidote for dolasetron mesylate, and patients with suspected overdose should be managed with supportive therapy. Individual doses as large as 5 mg/kg intravenously or 400 mg orally have been safely given to healthy volunteers or cancer patients.
It is not known if dolasetron mesylate is removed by hemodialysis or peritoneal dialysis.
A 7-year-old boy received 6 mg/kg of dolasetron mesylate orally before surgery. No symptoms occurred and no treatment was required.
Single intravenous doses of dolasetron mesylate at 160 mg/kg in male mice and 140 mg/kg in female mice and rats of both sexes (6.3 to 12.6 times the recommended human dose based on body surface area) were lethal. Symptoms of acute toxicity were tremors, depression and convulsions.

DOSAGE AND ADMINISTRATION

The recommended doses of ANZEMET Tablets should not be exceeded.
Prevention of Cancer Chemotherapy-Induced Nausea and Vomiting
Adults: The recommended oral dosage of ANZEMET (dolasetron mesylate) is 100 mg given within one hour before chemotherapy.
Pediatric Patients: The recommended oral dosage in pediatric patients 2 to 16 years of age is 1.8 mg/kg given within one hour before chemotherapy, up to a maximum of 100 mg. Safety and effectiveness in pediatric patients under 2 years of age have not been established.
Use in the Elderly, Renal Failure Patients, or Hepatically Impaired Patients: No dosage adjustment is recommended. (See Pharmacokinetics in Humans.)
Prevention of Postoperative Nausea and Vomiting
Adults: The recommended oral dosage of ANZEMET (dolasetron mesylate) is 100 mg within two hours before surgery.
Pediatric Patients: The recommended oral dosage in pediatric patients 2 to 16 years of age is 1.2 mg/kg given within two hours before surgery, up to a maximum of 100 mg. Safety and effectiveness in pediatric patients under 2 years of age have not been established.
Use in the Elderly, Renal Failure Patients, or Hepatically Impaired Patients: No dosage adjustment is recommended. (See Pharmacokinetics in Humans.)

HOW SUPPLIED

[See fourth table on previous page]
Store at controlled room temperature 20–25°C (68–77°F). Protect from light.

Prescribing Information as of February 1999

Hoechst Marion Roussel, Inc.
Kansas City, MO 64137 USA

Shown in Product Identification Guide, page 306

ARAVA™ Tablets ℞
(leflunomide)
10 mg, 20 mg, 100 mg
Prescribing Information as of February 2000

CONTRAINDICATIONS AND WARNINGS
PREGNANCY MUST BE EXCLUDED BEFORE THE START OF TREATMENT WITH ARAVA. ARAVA IS CONTRAINDICATED IN PREGNANT WOMEN, OR WOMEN OF CHILDBEARING POTENTIAL WHO ARE NOT USING RELIABLE CONTRACEPTION. (SEE CONTRAINDICATIONS AND WARNINGS.) PREGNANCY MUST BE AVOIDED DURING ARAVA TREATMENT OR PRIOR TO THE COMPLETION OF THE DRUG ELIMINATION PROCEDURE AFTER ARAVA TREATMENT.

DESCRIPTION

ARAVA™ (leflunomide) is a pyrimidine synthesis inhibitor. The chemical name for leflunomide is N-(4'-trifluoromethylphenyl)-5-methylisoxazole-4-carboxamide. It has an empirical formula $C_{12}H_9F_3N_2O_2$, a molecular weight of 270.2 and the following structural formula:

ARAVA is available for oral administration as tablets containing 10, 20, or 100 mg of active drug. Combined with leflunomide are the following inactive ingredients: colloidal silicon dioxide, crospovidone, hydroxypropyl methylcellulose, lactose monohydrate, magnesium stearate, polyethylene glycol, povidone, starch, talc, titanium dioxide, and yellow ferric oxide (20 mg tablet only).

CLINICAL PHARMACOLOGY

Mechanism of Action
Leflunomide is an isoxazole immunomodulatory agent which inhibits dihydroorotate dehydrogenase (an enzyme involved in de novo pyrimidine synthesis) and has antiproliferative activity. Several *in vivo* and *in vitro* experimental models have demonstrated an anti-inflammatory effect.
Pharmacokinetics
Following oral administration, leflunomide is metabolized to an active metabolite A77 1726 (hereafter referred to as M1) which is responsible for essentially all of its activity *in vivo*. Plasma levels of leflunomide are occasionally seen, at very low levels. Studies of the pharmacokinetics of leflunomide have primarily examined the plasma concentrations of this active metabolite.

A77 1726 (M1)

Absorption
Following oral administration, peak levels of the active metabolite, M1, occurred between 6–12 hours after dosing. Due to the very long half-life of M1 (~2 weeks), a loading dose of 100 mg for 3 days was used in clinical studies to facilitate the rapid attainment of steady-state levels of M1. Without a loading dose, it is estimated that attainment of steady-state plasma concentrations would require nearly two months of dosing. The resulting plasma concentrations following both loading doses and continued clinical dosing indicate that M1 plasma levels are dose proportional.
[See table 1 at top of next page]
Relative to an oral solution, ARAVA tablets are 80% bioavailable. Co-administration of leflunomide tablets with a high fat meal did not have a significant impact on M1 plasma levels.
Distribution
M1 has a low volume of distribution (Vss = 0.13 L/kg) and is extensively bound (>99.3%) to albumin in healthy subjects. Protein binding has been shown to be linear at therapeutic concentrations. The free fraction of M1 is slightly higher in patients with rheumatoid arthritis and approximately doubled in patients with chronic renal failure; the mechanism and significance of these increases are unknown.
Metabolism
Leflunomide is metabolized to one primary (M1) and many minor metabolites. Of these minor metabolites, only 4-trifluoromethylaniline (TFMA) is quantifiable, occurring at low levels in the plasma of some patients. The parent compound is rarely detectable in plasma. At the present time the specific site of leflunomide metabolism is unknown. *In vivo* and *in vitro* studies suggest a role for both the GI wall and the liver in drug metabolism. No specific enzyme has been identified as the primary route of metabolism for leflunomide; however, hepatic cytosolic and microsomal cellular fractions have been identified as sites of drug metabolism.
Elimination
The active metabolite M1 is eliminated by further metabolism and subsequent renal excretion as well as by direct biliary excretion. In a 28 day study of drug elimination (n=3) using a single dose of radiolabeled compound, approximately 43% of the total radioactivity was eliminated in the urine and 48% was eliminated in the feces. Subsequent analysis of the samples revealed the primary urinary metabolites to be leflunomide glucuronides and an oxanilic acid derivative of M1. The primary fecal metabolite was M1. Of these two routes of elimination, renal elimination is more significant over the first 96 hours after which fecal elimination begins to predominate. In a study involving the intravenous administration of M1, the clearance was estimated to be 31 mL/hr.
In small studies using activated charcoal (n=1) or cholestyramine (n=3) to facilitate drug elimination, the *in vivo* plasma half-life of M1 was reduced from >1 week to approximately 1 day (see PRECAUTIONS—General—Need for Drug Elimination). Similar reductions in plasma half-life were observed for a series of volunteers (n=96) enrolled in pharmacokinetic trials who were given cholestyramine. This suggests that biliary recycling is a major contributor to the long elimination half-life of M1. Studies with both hemodialysis and CAPD (chronic ambulatory peritoneal dialysis) indicate that M1 is not dialyzable.
Special Populations
Age and Gender. Neither age nor gender has been shown to cause a consistent change in the *in vivo* pharmacokinetics of M1.
Smoking. A population based pharmacokinetic analysis of the phase III data indicates that smokers have a 38% increase in clearance over non-smokers; however, no difference in clinical efficacy was seen between smokers and nonsmokers.

Continued on next page

Arava—Cont.

Chronic Renal Insufficiency. In single dose studies in patients (n=6) with chronic renal insufficiency requiring either chronic ambulatory peritoneal dialysis (CAPD) or hemodialysis, neither had a significant impact on circulating levels of M1. The free fraction of M1 was almost doubled, but the mechanism of this increase is not known. In light of the fact that the kidney plays a role in drug elimination, and without adequate studies of leflunomide use in subjects with renal insufficiency, caution should be used when ARAVA is administered to these patients.

Hepatic Insufficiency. Studies of the effect of hepatic insufficiency on M1 pharmacokinetics have not been done. Given the need to metabolize leflunomide into the active species, the role of the liver in drug elimination/recycling, and the possible risk of increased hepatic toxicity, the use of leflunomide in patients with hepatic insufficiency is not recommended.

Drug Interactions

In vivo drug interaction studies have demonstrated a lack of a significant drug interaction between leflunomide and triphasic oral contraceptives, and cimetidine.

In vitro studies of protein binding indicated that warfarin did not affect M1 protein binding. At the same time M1 was shown to cause increases ranging from 13–50% in the free fraction of diclofenac, ibuprofen and tolbutamide at concentrations in the clinical range. *In vitro* studies of drug metabolism indicate that M1 inhibits CYP 450 2C9, which is responsible for the metabolism of many NSAIDs. M1 has been shown to inhibit the formation of 4′-hydroxydiclofenac from diclofenac *in vitro*. The clinical significance of these findings is unknown, however, there was extensive concomitant use of NSAIDs in the clinical studies and no differential effect was observed.

Methotrexate. Coadministration, in 30 patients, of ARAVA (100 mg/day × 2 days followed by 10–20 mg/day) with methotrexate (10–25 mg/week, with folate) demonstrated no pharmacokinetic interaction between the two drugs. However, co-administration increased risk of hepatotoxicity (see PRECAUTIONS—Drug Interactions—Hepatotoxic Drugs).

Rifampin. Following concomitant administration of a single dose of ARAVA to subjects receiving multiple doses of rifampin, M1 peak levels were increased (~40%) over those seen when ARAVA was given alone. Because of the potential for ARAVA levels to continue to increase with multiple dosing, caution should be used if patients are to receive both ARAVA and rifampin.

CLINICAL STUDIES

The efficacy of ARAVA in the treatment of rheumatoid arthritis (RA) was demonstrated in three controlled trials. Relief of signs and symptoms was assessed using the ACR20 Responder Index, a composite of clinical, laboratory, and functional measures in rheumatoid arthritis. An "ACR20 Responder" is a patient who had ≥20% improvement in both tender and swollen joint counts and in 3 of the following 5 criteria: physician global assessment, patient global assessment, function/disability measure [Modified Health Assessment Questionnaire (MHAQ)], visual analog pain scale, and erythrocyte sedimentation rate or C-reactive protein. An "ACR20 Responder at Endpoint" is a patient who completed the study and was an ACR20 Responder at the completion of the study. Retardation of structural damage compared to control was assessed using the Sharp Score (Sharp, JT. Scoring Radiographic Abnormalities in Rheumatoid Arthritis, Radiologic Clinics of North America, 1996; vol. 34, pp. 233–241), a composite score of erosions and joint space narrowing in hands/wrists and forefeet.

All leflunomide patients used in initial loading dose of 100 mg/day for 3 days.

Study US301 randomized 482 subjects with active RA of at least 6 months duration to leflunomide 20 mg/day (n=182), methotrexate 7.5 mg/week increasing to 15 mg/week (n=182), or placebo (n=118). All patients received folate 1 mg BID. Treatment duration was 52 weeks.

Study MN301 randomized 358 subjects with active RA to leflunomide 20 mg/day (n=133), sulfasalazine 2.0 g/day (n=133), or placebo (n=92). Treatment duration was 24 weeks. Study MN303 was an optional 6-month blinded continuation of MN301 without the placebo arm, resulting in a 12-month comparison of leflunomide and sulfasalazine.

Study MN302 randomized 999 subjects with active RA to leflunomide 20 mg/day (n=501) or methotrexate at 7.5 mg/week increasing to 15 mg/week (n=498). Folate supplementation was used in 10% of patients. Treatment duration was 52 weeks.

Clinical Trial Data

The ACR20 Responder at Endpoint rates are shown in Figure 1. ARAVA was statistically significantly superior to placebo in reducing the signs and symptoms of RA by the primary efficacy analysis, ACR20 Responder at Endpoint. ACR20 Responder at Endpoint rates with ARAVA treatment were consistent across the 6 and 12 month studies (41–49%). No consistent differences were demonstrated between leflunomide and methotrexate or between leflunomide and sulfasalazine. ARAVA treatment effect was evident by 1 month, stabilized by 3–6 months, and continued throughout the course of treatment as shown in Figure 2.

[See figure 1 next column]

[See figure 2 next column]

ACR 50 and ACR 70 Responders are defined in an analogous manner to the ACR 20 Responder, but use improvements of 50% to 70%, respectively (Table 2). Mean change for the individual components of the ACR Responder Index are shown in Table 3.

[See table 2 above]

[See table 3 at top of next page]

Table 1. Pharmacokinetic Parameters for M1 after Administration of Leflunomide at Doses of 5, 10, and 25 mg/day for 24 Days to Patients (n=54) with Rheumatoid Arthritis (Mean ± SD) (Study YU204)

Maintenance (Loading) Dose			
Parameter	5 mg (50 mg)	10 mg (100 mg)	25 mg (100 mg)
C_{24} (Day 1) (µg/mL)[1]	4.0 ± 0.6	8.4 ± 2.1	8.5 ± 2.2
C_{24} (ss) (µg/mL)[2]	8.8 ± 2.9	18 ± 9.6	63 ± 36
$t_{1/2}$ (DAYS)	15 ± 3	14 ± 5	18 ± 9

[1] Concentration at 24 hours after loading dose
[2] Concentration at 24 hours after maintenance doses at steady state

Table 2. Summary of ACR Response Rates*

Study and Treatment Group	ACR 20%	ACR 50%	ACR 70%
Placebo-Controlled Studies			
US301 (12 months)			
Leflunomide (n=178)†	52.2‡	34.3‡	20.2‡
Placebo (n=118)†	26.3	7.6	4.2
Methotrexate (n=180)†	45.6	22.8	9.4
MN301 (6 months)			
Leflunomide (n=130)†	54.6‡	33.1‡	10.0§
Placebo (n=91)†	28.6	14.3	2.2
Sulfasalazine (n=132)†	56.8	30.3	7.6
Non-Placebo Active-Controlled Studies			
MN302 (12 months)			
Leflunomide (n=495)†	51.1	31.1	9.9
Methotrexate (n=489)†	65.2	43.8	16.4

* Intent to treat (ITT) analysis using last observation carried forward (LOCF) technique for patients who discontinued early.
† N is the number of ITT patients for whom adequate data were available to calculate the indicated rates.
‡ p<0.001 leflunomide vs placebo
§ p<0.02 leflunomide vs placebo

Figure 1

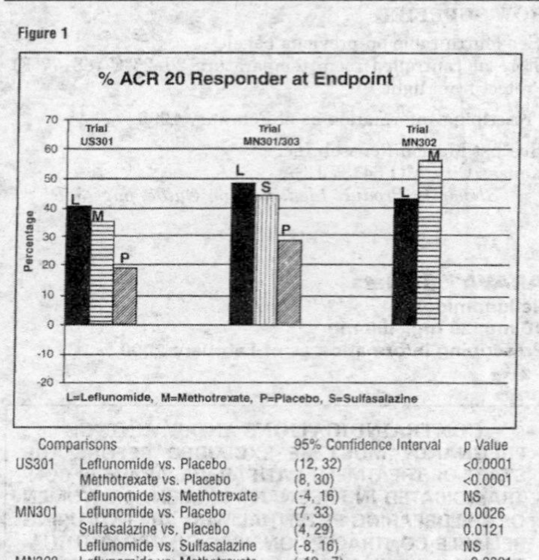

	Comparisons	95% Confidence Interval	p Value
US301	Leflunomide vs. Placebo	(12, 32)	<0.0001
	Methotrexate vs. Placebo	(8, 30)	<0.0001
	Leflunomide vs. Methotrexate	(-4, 16)	NS
MN301	Leflunomide vs. Placebo	(7, 33)	0.0026
	Sulfasalazine vs. Placebo	(4, 29)	0.0121
	Leflunomide vs. Sulfasalazine	(-8, 16)	NS
MN302	Leflunomide vs. Methotrexate	(-19, -7)	<0.0001

Figure 2

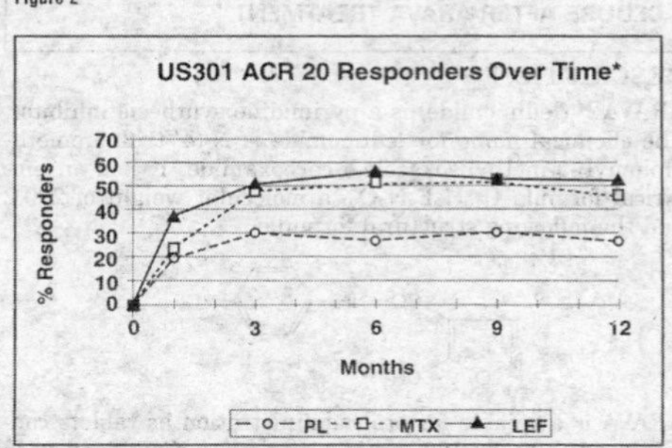

*Last Observation Carried Forward.

The change from baseline to endpoint in progression of structural disease, as measured by the Shart X-ray score, is displayed in Figure 3. ARAVA was statistically significantly superior to placebo in reducing the progression of disease by the Sharp Score. No consistent differences were demonstrated between leflunomide and methotrexate or between leflunomide and sulfasalazine.

Figure 3

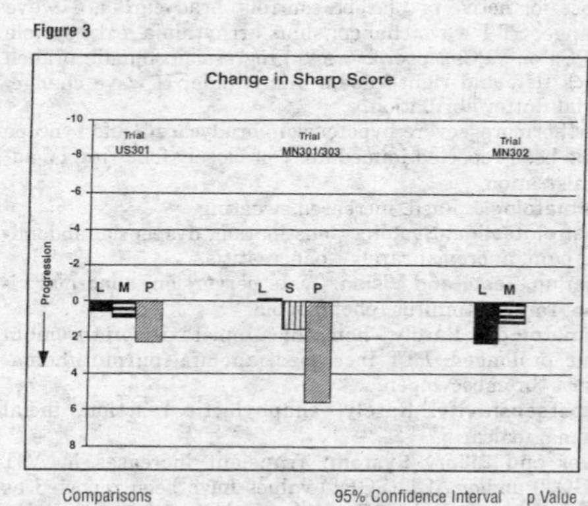

	Comparisons	95% Confidence Interval	p Value
US301	Leflunomide vs. Placebo	(-4.0, -1.1)	0.0007
	Methotrexate vs. Placebo	(-2.6, -0.2)	0.0187
	Leflunomide vs. Methotrexate	(-2.3, 0.0)	0.0494
MN301	Leflunomide vs. Placebo	(-9.0, -1.4)	0.0081
	Sulfasalazine vs. Placebo	(-7.7, 0.0)	NS
	Leflunomide vs. Sulfasalazine	(-5.4, 2.3)	NS
MN302	Leflunomide vs. Methotrexate	(-2.7, 8.0)	NS

INDICATIONS AND USAGE

ARAVA is indicated in adults for the treatment of active rheumatoid arthritis (RA) to reduce signs and symptoms and to retard structural damage as evidenced by X-ray erosions and joint space narrowing (see CLINICAL STUDIES). Aspirin, nonsteroidal anti-inflammatory agents and/or low dose corticosteroids may be continued during treatment with ARAVA (see PRECAUTIONS—Drug Interactions—NSAIDs). The combined use of ARAVA with antimalarials, intramuscular or oral gold, D penicillamine, azathioprine, or methotrexate has not been adequately studied (see WARNINGS—Immunosuppression Potential).

CONTRAINDICATIONS

ARAVA is contraindicated in patients with known hypersensitivity to leflunomide or any of the other components of ARAVA.

ARAVA can cause fetal harm when administered to a pregnant woman. Leflunomide, when administered orally to rats during organogenesis at a dose of 15 mg/kg, was teratogenic (most notably anophthalmia or microphthalmia and internal hydrocephalus). The systemic exposure of rats at this

Table 3. Mean Change in the Components of the ACR Responder Index*

Components	Placebo-Controlled Studies						Non-placebo Controlled Study	
	US301 (12 months)			MN301 Non-US (6 months)			MN302 Non-US (12 months)	
	Leflunomide	Methotrexate	Placebo	Leflunomide	Sulfasalazine	Placebo	Leflunomide	Methotrexate
Tender joint count[1]	−7.7	−6.6	−3.0	−9.7	−8.1	−4.3	−8.3	−9.7
Swollen joint count[1]	−5.7	−5.4	−2.9	−7.2	−6.2	−3.4	−6.8	−9.0
Patient global assessment	−2.1	−1.5	0.1	−2.8	−2.6	−0.9	−2.3	−3.0
Physician global assessment	−2.8	−2.4	−1.0	−2.7	−2.5	−0.8	−2.3	−3.1
Physical function/ disability (MHAQ/HAQ)	−0.29	−0.15	0.07	−0.50	−0.29	−0.04	−0.37	−0.44
Pain intensity[2]	−2.2	−1.7	−0.5	−2.7	−2.0	−0.9	−2.1	−2.9
Erythrocyte Sedimentation rate	−6.26	−6.48	2.56	−7.48	−16.56	3.44	−10.12	−22.18
C-reactive protein	−0.62	−0.50	0.47	−2.26	−1.19	0.16	−1.86	−2.45

* Last Observation Carried Forward; Negative Change Indicates Improvement
1 Based on 28 joint count
2 Visual Analog Scale - 0=Best; 10=Worst

Table 4. Liver Enzyme Elevations >3-fold Upper Limits of Normal (ULN)

	US301			MN301			MN302*	
	LEF	PL	MTX	LEF	PL	SSZ	LEF	MTX
ALT (SGPT)								
>3-fold ULN	8	3	5	2	1	2	13	83
(n %)	(4.4)	(2.5)	(2.7)	(1.5)	(1.1)	(1.5)	(2.6)	(16.7)
Reversed to ≤2-fold ULN:	8	3	5	2	1	2	12	82
Timing of Elevation								
0–3 Months	6	1	1	2	1	2	7	27
4–6 Months	1	1	3	—	—	—	1	34
7–9 Months	1	1	1	—	—	—	—	16
10–12 Months	—	—	—	—	—	—	5	6
AST (SGOT)								
>3-fold ULN	4	2	1	2	0	5	7	29
(n %)	(2.2)	(1.7)	(0.6)	(1.5)	—	(3.8)	(1.4)	(5.8)
Reversed to ≤2-fold ULN:	4	2	1	2	—	4	5	29
Timing of Elevation								
0–3 Months	2	1	—	2	—	4	3	10
4–6 Months	1	1	1	—	—	1	1	11
7–9 Months	1	—	—	—	—	—	—	8
10–12 Months	—	—	—	—	—	—	3	—

* Only 10% of patients in MN302 received folate. All patients in US301 received folate.

dose was approximately 1/10 the human exposure level based on AUC. Under these exposure conditions, leflunomide also caused a decrease in the maternal body weight and an increase in embryolethality with a decrease in fetal body weight for surviving fetuses. In rabbits, oral treatment with 10 mg/kg of leflunomide during organogenesis resulted in fused, dysplastic sternebrae. The exposure level at this dose was essentially equivalent to the maximum human exposure level based on AUC. At a 1 mg/kg dose, leflunomide was not teratogenic in rats and rabbits.

When female rats were treated with 1.25 mg/kg of leflunomide beginning 14 days before mating and continuing until the end of lactation, the offspring exhibited marked (greater than 90%) decreases in postnatal survival. The systemic exposure level at 1.25 mg/kg was approximately 1/100 the human exposure level based on AUC.

ARAVA is contraindicated in women who are or may become pregnant. If this drug is used during pregnancy, or if the patient becomes pregnant while taking this drug, the patient should be apprised of the potential hazard to the fetus.

WARNINGS

Immunosuppression Potential

ARAVA is not recommended for patients with severe immunodeficiency, bone marrow dysplasia, or severe, uncontrolled infections.

There have been rare reports of pancytopenia in patients receiving ARAVA. In most of these cases, patients received concomitant treatment with methotrexate or other immunosuppressive agents, or they had recently discontinued these therapies; in some cases, patients had a prior history of a significant hematologic abnormality. If ARAVA is used in such patients, it should be administered with caution and with frequent clinical and hematologic monitoring. The use of ARAVA in combination therapy with methotrexate has not been adequately studied in a controlled setting.

If evidence of bone marrow suppression occurs in a patient taking ARAVA, treatment with ARAVA should be stopped, and cholestyramine or charcoal should be used to reduce the plasma concentration of leflunomide active metabolite (see PRECAUTIONS—General—Need for Drug Elimination).

In any situation in which the decision is made to switch from ARAVA to another anti-rheumatic agent with a known potential for hematologic suppression, it would be prudent to monitor for hematologic toxicity, because there will be overlap of systemic exposure to both compounds. ARAVA washout with cholestyramine or charcoal may decrease this risk, but also may induce disease worsening if the patient had been responding to ARAVA treatment.

Skin Reactions

Rare cases of Stevens-Johnson syndrome and toxic epidermal necrolysis have been reported in patients receiving ARAVA. If a patient taking ARAVA develops any of these conditions, ARAVA therapy should be stopped, and a drug elimination procedure is recommended (see PRECAUTIONS—General—Need for Drug Elimination).

Hepatotoxicity

In clinical trials, ARAVA treatment was associated with elevations of liver enzymes, primarily ALT and AST, in a significant number of patients; these effects were generally reversible. Most transaminase elevations were mild (≤2-fold ULN) and usually resolved while continuing treatment. Marked elevations (>3-fold ULN) occurred infrequently and reversed with dose reduction or discontinuation of treatment. The following table shows liver enzyme elevations seen with monthly monitoring in clinical trials US301 and MN301. It was notable that the absence of folate use in MN302 was associated with a considerably greater incidence of liver enzyme elevation on methotrexate.

[See table 4 below]

At minimum, ALT (SGPT) should be performed at baseline and monitored initially at monthly intervals then, if stable, at intervals determined by the individual clinical situation.

Guidelines for dose adjustment or discontinuation based on the severity and persistence of ALT elevation are recommended as follows: For confirmed ALT elevations >2-fold ULN, dose reduction to 10 mg/day may allow continued administration of ARAVA. If elevations >2 but ≤3-fold ULN persist despite dose reduction, liver biopsy is recommended if continued treatment is desired. If elevations >3-fold ULN persist despite dose reduction, ARAVA should be discontinued and cholestyramine should be administered (see PRECAUTIONS—General—Need for Drug Elimination) with close monitoring, including retreatment with cholestyramine as indicated.

Rare elevations of alkaline phosphatase and bilirubin have been observed. Trial US301 used ACR Methotrexate Liver Biopsy Guidelines for monitoring therapy. One of 182 patients receiving leflunomide and 1 of 182 patients receiving methotrexate underwent liver biopsy at 106 and 50 weeks respectively. The biopsy for the leflunomide subject was Roegnik Grade IIIA and for the methotrexate subject, Roegnik Grade I.

Pre-existing Hepatic Disease

Given the possible risk of increased hepatotoxicity, and the role of the liver in drug activation, elimination and recycling, the use of ARAVA is not recommended in patients with significant hepatic impairment or evidence of infection with hepatitis B or C viruses.

Malignancy

The risk of malignancy, particularly lymphoproliferative disorders, is increased with the use of some immunosuppression medications. There is a potential for immunosuppression with ARAVA. No apparent increase in the incidence of malignancies and lymphoproliferative disorders was reported in the clinical trials of ARAVA, but larger and longer-term studies would be needed to determine whether there is an increased risk of malignancy or lympho-proliferative disorders with ARAVA.

Use in Women of Childbearing Potential

There are no adequate and well-controlled studies evaluating ARAVA in pregnant women. However, based on animal studies, leflunomide may increase the risk of fetal death or teratogenic effects when administered to a pregnant woman (see CONTRAINDICATIONS). Women of childbearing potential must not be started on ARAVA until pregnancy is excluded and it has been confirmed that they are using reliable contraception. Before starting treatment with ARAVA, patients must be fully counseled on the potential for serious risk to the fetus.

The patient must be advised that if there is any delay in onset of menses or any other reason to suspect pregnancy, they must notify the physician immediately for pregnancy testing and, if positive, the physician and patient must discuss the risk to the pregnancy. It is possible that rapidly lowering the blood level of the active metabolite by instituting the drug elimination procedure described below at the first delay of menses may decrease the risk to the fetus from ARAVA. Upon discontinuing ARAVA, it is recommended that all women of childbearing potential undergo the drug elimination procedure described below. Women receiving ARAVA treatment who wish to become pregnant must discontinue ARAVA and undergo the drug elimination procedure described below which includes verification of M1 metabolite plasma levels less than 0.02 mg/L (0.02 µg/mL). Human plasma levels of the active metabolite (M1) less than 0.02 mg/L (0.02 µg/mL) are expected to have minimal risk based on available animal data.

Drug Elimination Procedure

The following drug elimination procedure is recommended to achieve non-detectable plasma levels (less than 0.02 mg/L or 0.02 µg/mL) after stopping treatment with ARAVA:

1) Administer cholestyramine 8 grams 3 times daily for 11 days. (The 11 days do not need to be consecutive unless there is a need to lower the plasma level rapidly.)
2) Verify plasma levels less than 0.2 mg/L (0.02 µg/mL) by two separate tests at least 14 days apart. If plasma levels are higher than 0.02 mg/L, additional cholestyramine treatment should be considered.

Without the drug elimination procedure, it may take up to 2 years to reach plasma M1 metabolite levels less than 0.02 mg/L due to individual variation in drug clearance.

PRECAUTIONS

General

Need for Drug Elimination

The active metabolite of leflunomide is eliminated slowly from the plasma. In instances of any serious toxicity from ARAVA, including hypersensitivity, use of a drug elimination procedure as described in this section is highly recommended to reduce the drug concentration more rapidly after stopping ARAVA therapy. If hypersensitivity is the suspected clinical mechanism, more prolonged cholestyramine or charcoal administration may be necessary to achieve rapid and sufficient clearance. The duration may be modified based on the clinical status of the patient.

Continued on next page

Arava—Cont.

Cholestyramine given orally at a dose of 8 g three times a day for 24 hours to three healthy volunteers decreased plasma levels of M1 by approximately 40% in 24 hours and by 49 to 65% in 48 hours.

Administration of activated charcoal (powder made into a suspension) orally or via nasogastric tube (50 g every 6 hours for 24 hours) has been shown to reduce plasma concentrations of the active metabolite, M1, by 37% in 24 hours and by 48% in 48 hours.

These drug elimination procedures may be repeated if clinically necessary.

Renal Insufficiency

Single dose studies in dialysis patients show a doubling of the free fraction of M1 in plasma. There is no clinical experience in the use of ARAVA in patients with renal impairment. Caution should be used when administering this drug in this population.

Vaccinations

No clinical data are available on the efficacy and safety of vaccinations during ARAVA treatment. Vaccination with live vaccines is, however, not recommended. The long half-life of ARAVA should be considered when contemplating administration of a live vaccine after stopping ARAVA.

Information for Patients

The potential for increased risk of birth defects should be discussed with female patients of childbearing potential. It is recommended that physicians advise women that they may be at increased risk of having a child with birth defects if they are pregnant when taking ARAVA, become pregnant while taking ARAVA, or do not wait to become pregnant until they have stopped taking ARAVA and followed the drug elimination procedure (as described in WARNINGS—Use In Women of Childbearing Potential—Drug Elimination Procedure).

Patients should be advised of the possibility of rare, serious skin reactions. Patients should be instructed to inform their physicians promptly if they develop a skin rash or mucous membrane lesions.

Patients should be advised of the potential hepatotoxic effects of ARAVA and of the need for monitoring liver enzymes.

Patients who are receiving other immunosuppressive therapy concurrently with ARAVA, who have recently discontinued such therapy before starting treatment with ARAVA, or who have had a history of significant hematologic abnormality, should be advised of the potential for pancytopenia and of the need for frequent hematologic monitoring. They should be instructed to notify their physicians promptly if they notice symptoms of pancytopenia (such as easy bruising, proneness to infections, paleness or unusual tiredness).

Laboratory tests

At minimum, ALT (SGPT) should be performed at baseline and monitored initially at monthly intervals then, if stable, at intervals determined by the individual clinical situation. In patients who are at an increased risk of hematologic toxicity (see WARNINGS—Immunosuppression Potential), more vigilant monitoring, including hematologic monitoring, is warranted.

Due to a specific effect on the brush border of the renal proximal tubule, ARAVA has a uricosuric effect. A separate effect of hypophosphaturia is seen in some patients. These effects have not been seen together, nor have there been alterations in renal function.

Carcinogenesis, Mutagenesis, and Impairment of Fertility

No evidence of carcinogenicity was observed in a 2-year bioassay in rats at oral doses of leflunomide up to the maximally tolerated dose of 6 mg/kg (approximately 1/40 the maximum human M1 systemic exposure based on AUC). However, male mice in a 2-year bioassay exhibited an increased incidence in lymphoma at an oral dose of 15 mg/kg, the highest dose studied (1.7 times the human M1 exposure based on AUC). Female mice, in the same study, exhibited a dose-related increased incidence of bronchoalveolar adenomas and carcinomas combined beginning at 1.5 mg/kg (approximately 1/10 the human M1 exposure based on AUC). The significance of the findings in mice relative to the clinical use of ARAVA is not known.

Leflunomide was not mutagenic in the Ames Assay, the Unscheduled DNA Synthesis Assay, or in the HGPRT Gene Mutation Assay. In addition, leflunomide was not clastogenic in the *in vivo* Mouse Micronucleus Assay nor in the *in vivo* Cytogenetic Test in Chinese Hamster Bone Marrow Cells. However, 4-trifluoromethylaniline (TFMA), a minor metabolite of leflunomide, was mutagenic in the Ames Assay and in the HGPRT Gene Mutation Assay, and was clastogenic in the *in vitro* Assay for Chromosome Aberrations in the Chinese Hamster Cells. TFMA was not clastogenic in the *in vivo* Mouse Micronucleus Assay nor in the *in vivo* Cytogenetic Test in Chinese Hamster Bone Marrow Cells.

Leflunomide had no effect on fertility in either male or female rats at oral doses up to 4.0 mg/kg (approximately 1/30 the human M1 exposure based on AUC).

Pregnancy

Pregnancy Category X. See CONTRAINDICATIONS section. Pregnancy Registry: To monitor fetal outcomes of pregnant women exposed to leflunomide, health care providers are encouraged to register such patients by calling 1-877-311-8972.

Nursing Mothers

ARAVA should not be used by nursing mothers. It is not known whether ARAVA is excreted in human milk. Many drugs are excreted in human milk, and there is a potential for serious adverse reactions in nursing infants from ARAVA. Therefore, a decision should be made whether to proceed with nursing or to initiate treatment with ARAVA, taking into account the importance of the drug to the mother.

Use in Males

Available information does not suggest that ARAVA sould be associated with an increased risk of male-mediated fetal toxicity. However, animal studies to evaluate this specific risk have not been conducted. To minimize any possible risk, men wishing to father a child should consider discontinuing use of ARAVA and taking cholestyramine 8 grams 3 times daily for 11 days.

Drug Interactions

Cholestyramine and Charcoal

Administration of cholestyramine or activated charcoal in patients (n=13) and volunteers (n=96) resulted in a rapid and significant decrease in plasma M1 (the active metabolite of leflunomide) concentration (see PRECAUTIONS—General—Need for Drug Elimination).

Hepatotoxic Drugs

Increased side effects may occur when leflunomide is given concomitantly with hepatotoxic substances. This is also to be considered when leflunomide treatment is followed by such drugs without a drug elimination procedure. In a small (n=30) combination study of ARAVA with methotrexate, a 2- to 3-fold elevation in liver enzymes was seen in 5 of 30 patients. All elevations resolved, 2 with continuation of both drugs and 3 after discontinuation of leflunomide. A >3-fold increase was seen in another 5 patients. All of these also resolved, 2 with continuation of both drugs and 3 after discontinuation of leflunomide. Three patients met "ACR criteria" for liver biopsy (1: Roegnik Grade I, 2: Roegnik Grade IIIa). No pharmacokinetic interaction was identified (see CLINICAL PHARMACOLOGY).

Table 5. Percentage of Patients With Adverse Events ≥3% In Any Leflunomide Treated Group

	All RA Studies	Placebo-Controlled Trials				Active-Controlled Trials	
		MN 301 and US 301				MN 302*	
	LEF (N=1339)[1]	LEF (N=315)	PBO (N=210)	SSZ (N=133)	MTX (N=182)	LEF (N=501)	MTX (N=498)
BODY AS A WHOLE							
Allergic Reaction	2%	5%	2%	0%	6%	1%	2%
Asthenia	3%	6%	4%	5%	6%	3%	3%
Flu Syndrome	2%	4%	2%	0%	7%	0%	0%
Infection	4%	0%	0%	0%	0%	0%	0%
Injury Accident	5%	7%	5%	3%	11%	6%	7%
Pain	2%	4%	2%	2%	5%	1%	<1%
Abdominal Pain	6%	5%	4%	4%	8%	6%	4%
Back Pain	5%	6%	3%	4%	9%	8%	7%
CARDIOVASCULAR							
Hypertension[2]	10%	9%	4%	4%	3%	10%	4%
Chest Pain	2%	4%	2%	2%	4%	1%	2%
GASTROINTESTINAL							
Anorexia	3%	3%	2%	5%	2%	3%	3%
Diarrhea	17%	27%	12%	10%	20%	22%	10%
Dyspepsia	5%	10%	10%	9%	13%	6%	7%
Gastroenteritis	3%	1%	1%	0%	6%	3%	3%
Abnormal Liver Enzymes	5%	10%	2%	4%	10%	6%	17%
Nausea	9%	13%	11%	19%	18%	13%	18%
GI/Abdominal Pain	5%	6%	4%	7%	8%	8%	8%
Mouth Ulcer	3%	5%	4%	3%	10%	3%	6%
Vomiting	3%	5%	4%	4%	3%	3%	3%
METABOLIC AND NUTRITIONAL							
Hypokalemia	1%	3%	1%	1%	1%	1%	<1%
Weight Loss	4%	2%	1%	2%	0%	2%	2%
MUSCULO-SKELETAL SYSTEM							
Arthralgia	1%	4%	3%	0%	9%	<1%	1%
Leg Cramps	1%	4%	2%	2%	6%	0%	0%
Joint Disorder	4%	2%	2%	2%	2%	8%	6%
Synovitis	2%	<1%	1%	0%	2%	4%	2%
Tenosynovitis	3%	2%	0%	1%	2%	5%	1%
NERVOUS SYSTEM							
Dizziness	4%	5%	3%	6%	5%	7%	6%
Headache	7%	13%	11%	12%	21%	10%	8%
Paresthesia	2%	3%	1%	1%	2%	4%	3%
RESPIRATORY SYSTEM							
Bronchitis	7%	5%	2%	4%	7%	8%	7%
Increased Cough	3%	4%	5%	3%	6%	5%	7%
Respiratory Infection	15%	21%	21%	20%	32%	27%	25%
Pharyngitis	3%	2%	1%	2%	1%	3%	3%
Pneumonia	2%	3%	0%	0%	1%	2%	2%
Rhinitis	2%	5%	2%	4%	3%	2%	2%
Sinusitis	2%	5%	5%	0%	10%	1%	1%
SKIN AND APPENDAGES							
Alopecia	10%	9%	1%	6%	6%	17%	10%
Eczema	2%	1%	1%	1%	1%	3%	2%
Pruritus	4%	5%	2%	3%	2%	6%	2%
Rash	10%	12%	7%	11%	9%	11%	10%
Dry Skin	2%	3%	2%	2%	0%	3%	1%
UROGENITAL SYSTEM							
Urinary Tract Infection	5%	5%	7%	4%	2%	5%	6%

* Only 10% of patients in MN302 received folate. All patients in US301 received folate; none in MN301 received folate.

1 Includes all controlled and uncontrolled trials with leflunomide.

2 Hypertension as a preexisting condition was overrepresented in all leflunomide treatment groups in phase III trials. Analysis of new onset hypertension revealed no difference among the treatment groups.

ARAVA™ (leflunomide) Tablets

Strength	Quantity	NDC Number	Description
10 mg	30 count bottle 100 count bottle	0088-2160-30 0088-2160-47	White, round film-coated tablet embossed with "ZBN" on one side.
20 mg	30 count bottle 100 count bottle	0088-2161-30 0088-2161-47	Light yellow, triangular film-coated tablet embossed with "ZBO" on one side.
100 mg	3 count blister pack	0088-2162-03	White, round film-coated tablet embossed with "ZBP" on one side.

NSAIDs
In *in vitro* studies, M1 was shown to cause increases ranging from 13–50% in the free fraction of diclofenac and ibuprofen at concentrations in the clinical range. The clinical significance of this finding is unknown, however, there was extensive concomitant use of NSAIDs in clinical studies and no differential effect was observed.

Tolbutamide
In *in vitro* studies, M1 was shown to cause increases ranging from 13–50% in the free fraction of tolbutamide at concentrations in the clinical range. The clinical significance of this finding is unknown.

Rifampin
Following concomitant administration of a single dose of ARAVA to subjects receiving multiple doses of rifampin, M1 peak levels were increased (~40%) over those seen when ARAVA was given alone. Because of the potential for ARAVA levels to continue to increase with multiple dosing, caution should be used if patients are to be receiving both ARAVA and rifampin.

Pediatric Use
The safety and efficacy of ARAVA in the pediatric population have not been studied. Use of ARAVA in patients less than 18 years of age is not recommended.

Geriatric Use
No dosage adjustment is needed in patients over 65.

ADVERSE REACTIONS

Adverse reactions associated with the use of leflunomide in RA include diarrhea, elevated liver enzymes (ALT and AST), alopecia and rash. In the controlled studies, the following adverse events were reported, regardless of causality. (See Table 5.)

[See table 5 at top of previous page]

In addition, the following adverse events have been reported in 1% to <3% of the RA patients in the leflunomide treatment group in controlled clinical trials.

Body as a Whole: abscess, cyst, fever, hernia, malaise, pain, neck pain, pelvic pain;
Cardiovascular: angina pectoris, migraine, palpitation, tachycardia, varicose vein, vasculitis, vasodilatation;
Gastrointestinal: cholelithiasis, colitis, constipation, esophagitis, flatulence, gastritis, gingivitis, melena, oral moniliasis, pharyngitis, salivary gland enlarged, stomatitis (or aphthous stomatitis), tooth disorder;
Endocrine: diabetes mellitus, hyperthyroidism;
Hemic and Lymphatic System: anemia (including iron deficiency anemia), ecchymosis;
Metabolic and Nutritional: creatinine phosphokinase increased, hyperglycemia, hyperlipidemia, peripheral edema;
Musculo-Skeletal System: arthrosis, bone necrosis, bone pain, bursitis, muscle cramps, myalgia, tendon rupture;
Nervous System: anxiety, depression, dry mouth, insomnia, neuralgia, neuritis, sleep disorder, sweating increased, vertigo;
Respiratory System: asthma, dyspnea, epistaxis, lung disorder;
Skin and Appendages: acne, contact dermatitis, fungal dermatitis, hair discoloration, hematoma, herpes simplex, herpes zoster, maculopapular rash, nail disorder, skin discoloration, skin disorder, skin nodule, subcutaneous nodule, ulcer skin;
Special Senses: blurred vision, cataract, conjunctivitis, eye disorder, taste perversion.
Urogenital System: albuminuria, cystitis, dysuria, hematuria, menstrual disorder, prostate disorder, urinary frequency, vaginal moniliasis.

Other less common adverse events seen in clinical trials include: 1 case of anaphylactic reaction occurred in Phase 2 following rechallenge of drug after withdrawal due to rash (rare); urticaria; eosinophilia; transient thrombocytopenia (rare); and leukopenia <2000 WBC/mm^3 (rare). In postmarketing experience, rare cases of pancytopenia, Stevens-Johnson syndrome, toxic epidermal necrolysis, and erythema multiforme have been reported.

DRUG ABUSE AND DEPENDENCE

ARAVA has no known potential for abuse or dependence.

OVERDOSAGE

There is no human experience regarding leflunomide overdosage. In mouse and rat acute toxicology studies, the minimally toxic dose for oral leflunomide was 200–500 mg/kg and 100 mg/kg, respectively (approximately >350 times the maximum recommended human dose, respectively).

In the event of a significant overdose or toxicity, cholestyramine or charcoal administration is recommended to accelerate elimination (see PRECAUTIONS—General—Need for Drug Elimination).

DOSAGE AND ADMINISTRATION

Loading Dose
Due to the long half-life in patients with RA and recommended dosing interval (24 hours), a loading dose is needed to provide steady-state concentrations more rapidly. It is recommended that ARAVA therapy be initiated with a loading dose of one 100 mg tablet per day for 3 days.

Maintenance Therapy
Daily dosing of 20 mg is recommended for treatment of patients with RA. A small cohort of patients (n=104), treated with 25 mg/day, experienced a greater incidence of side effects; alopecia, weight loss, liver enzyme elevations. Doses higher than 20 mg/day are not recommended. If dosing at 20 mg/day is not well tolerated clinically, the dose may be decreased to 10 mg daily. Liver enzymes should be monitored and dose adjustments may be necessary (see WARNINGS—Hepatotoxicity). Due to the prolonged half-life of the active metabolite of leflunomide, patients should be carefully observed after dose reduction, since it may take several weeks for metabolite levels to decline.

HOW SUPPLIED

ARAVA Tablets in 10 and 20 mg strengths are packaged in bottles. ARAVA Tablets 100 mg strength are packaged in blister packs.
[See table above]
Store at 25°C (77°F); excursions permitted to 15–30°C (59–86°F) [see USP Controlled Room Temperature]. Protect from light.
Rx only.
Prescribing Information as of February 2000
Manufactured by
Upishar, 60200 Compiegne, France
for
Aventis Pharmaceuticals Inc.
(formerly Hoechst Marion Roussel, Inc.)
Kansas City, MO 64137
Made in France

Shown in Product Identification Guide, page 306

AZMACORT® ℞

[*ăz 'ma-kort*]
(triamcinolone acetonide)
Inhalation Aerosol

Rx only
For Oral Inhalation Only
Shake Well Before Using

DESCRIPTION

Triamcinolone acetonide, USP, the active ingredient in **Azmacort®** Inhalation Aerosol, is a corticosteroid with a molecular weight of 434.5 and with the chemical designation 9-Fluoro-11β,16α,17,21-tetrahydroxypregna-1,4-diene-3,20-dione cyclic 16,17-acetal with acetone. ($C_{24}H_{31}FO_6$).

Azmacort Inhalation Aerosol is a metered-dose aerosol unit containing a microcrystalline suspension of triamcinolone acetonide in the propellant dichlorodifluoromethane and dehydrated alcohol USP 1% w/w. Each canister contains 60 mg triamcinolone acetonide. The canister must be primed prior to the first use. After initial priming of 2 actuations, each actuation delivers 200 mcg triamcinolone acetonide from the valve and 100 mcg from the spacer-mouthpiece under defined *in vitro* test conditions. The canister will remain primed for 3 days. If the canister is not used for more than 3 days, then it should be reprimed with 2 actuations. There are at least 240 actuations in one **Azmacort** Inhalation Aerosol canister. **After 240 actuations, the amount delivered per actuation may not be consistent and the unit should be discarded.**

CLINICAL PHARMACOLOGY

Triamcinolone acetonide is a more potent derivative of triamcinolone. Although triamcinolone itself is approximately one to two times as potent as prednisone in animal models of inflammation, triamcinolone acetonide is approximately 8 times more potent than prednisone.

The precise mechanism of the action of glucocorticoids in asthma is unknown. However, the inhaled route makes it possible to provide effective local anti-inflammatory activity with reduced systemic corticosteroid effects. Though highly effective for asthma, glucocorticoids do not affect asthma symptoms immediately. While improvement in asthma may occur as soon as one week after initiation of **Azmacort** Inhalation Aerosol therapy, maximum improvement may not be achieved for 2 weeks or longer.

Based upon intravenous dosing of triamcinolone acetonide phosphate ester, the half-life of triamcinolone acetonide was reported to be 88 minutes. The volume of distribution (Vd) reported was 99.5 L (SD ± 27.5) and clearance was 45.2 L/hour (SD ± 9.1) for triamcinolone acetonide. The plasma half-life of glucocorticoids does not correlate well with the biologic half-life.

The pharmacokinetics of radiolabeled triamcinolone acetonide [^{14}C] were evaluated following a single oral dose of 800 mcg to healthy male volunteers. Radiolabeled triamcinolone acetonide was found to undergo relatively rapid absorption following oral administration with maximum plasma triamcinolone acetonide and [^{14}C]-derived radioactivity occurring between 1.5 and 2 hours. Plasma protein binding of triamcinolone acetonide appears to be relatively low and consistent over a wide plasma triamcinolone acetonide concentration range as a function of time. The overall mean percent fraction bound was approximately 68%.

The metabolism and excretion of triamcinolone acetonide were both rapid and extensive with no parent compound being detected in the plasma after 24 hours post-dose and a low ratio (10.6%) of parent compound $AUC_{0-\infty}$ to total [^{14}C] radioactivity $AUC_{0-\infty}$. Greater than 90% of the oral [^{14}C]-radioactive dose was recovered within 5 days after administration in 5 out of the 6 subjects in the study. Of the recovered [^{14}C]-radioactivity, approximately 40% and 60% were found in the urine and feces, respectively.

Three metabolites of triamcinolone acetonide have been identified. They are 6β-hydroxytriamcinolone acetonide, 21-carboxytriamcinolone acetonide and 21-carboxy-6β-hydroxytriamcinolone acetonide. All three metabolites are expected to be substantially less active than the parent compound due to (a) the dependence of anti-inflammatory activity on the presence of a 21-hydroxyl group, (b) the decreased activity observed upon 6-hydroxylation, and (c) the markedly increased water solubility favoring rapid elimination. There appeared to be some quantitative differences in the metabolites among species. No differences were detected in metabolic pattern as a function of route of administration.

CLINICAL TRIALS

Double-blind, placebo controlled efficacy and safety studies have been conducted in asthma patients with a range of asthma severities, from those patients with mild disease to those with severe disease requiring oral steroid therapy.

The efficacy and safety of **Azmacort** Inhalation Aerosol given twice daily was demonstrated in two placebo-controlled clinical trials. In two separate studies, 222 asthmatic patients were randomized to receive either **Azmacort** Inhalation Aerosol 400 mcg twice daily or matching placebo for a treatment period of 6 weeks. Patients were adult asthmatics who were using inhaled beta$_2$-agonists on more than an occasional basis (at least three times weekly), either without or with inhaled corticosteroids, for control of their asthma symptoms. For the combined studies, 48% (52/109) patients randomized to placebo and 41% (46/113) patients randomized to **Azmacort** treatment were previously treated with inhaled corticosteroids.

Results of weekly lung function tests (FEV$_1$) from one of these trials is presented graphically below. Results of the second study are presented in tabular form as the changes in asthma measures from baseline to the end of the treatment period.

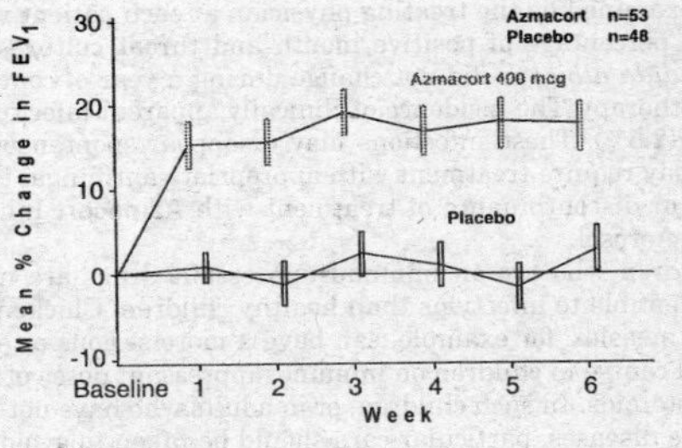

Mean Changes in Asthma Measures from Baseline to Endpoint[a]
All-Treated Patients
Results from a Placebo-Controlled, 6 Week Study

Asthma Measure	Placebo (N=61)	Azmacort 400 mcg bid (N=60)
Percent Change in FEV$_1$(%)	2.8%	17.5%
Increase in Morning Peak Flow Rate (L/min)	6.7	45.9

Azmacort—Cont.

Decrease in Albuterol Use (puffs/day)	0.6	3.4
Decrease in Daily Asthma Symptom Score (units/day)[b]	0.5	2.3

[a] Endpoint Results are obtained from the last evaluable data, regardless of whether the patient completed 6 weeks of treatment.

[b] Scale (0–6) with 0 = no symptom: Maximum Score (AM + PM) = 12

In both studies, treatment with **Azmacort** Inhalation Aerosol (400 mcg twice daily) resulted in significant improvements in all clinical asthma measures (lung functions, asthma symptoms, use of as-needed beta$_2$-agonist medications) when compared to placebo.

INDICATIONS

Azmacort Inhalation Aerosol is indicated in the maintenance treatment of asthma as prophylactic therapy.

Azmacort Inhalation Aerosol is also indicated for asthma patients who require systemic corticosteroid administration, where adding Azmacort may reduce or eliminate the need for the systemic corticosteroids.

Azmacort Inhalation Aerosol is NOT indicated for the relief of acute bronchospasm.

CONTRAINDICATIONS

Azmacort Inhalation Aerosol is contraindicated in the primary treatment of status asthmaticus or other acute episodes of asthma where intensive measures are required.

Hypersensitivity to triamcinolone acetonide or any of the other ingredients in this preparation contraindicates its use.

WARNINGS

Particular care is needed in patients who are transferred from systemically active corticosteroids to **Azmacort** Inhalation Aerosol because deaths due to adrenal insufficiency have occurred in asthmatic patients during and after transfer from systemic corticosteroids to aerosolized steroids in recommended doses. After withdrawal from systemic corticosteroids, a number of months is usually required for recovery of hypothalamic-pituitary-adrenal (HPA) function. For some patients who have received large doses of oral steroids for long periods of time before therapy with **Azmacort** Inhalation Aerosol is initiated, recovery may be delayed for one year or longer. During this period of HPA suppression, patients may exhibit signs and symptoms of adrenal insufficiency when exposed to trauma, surgery, or infections, particularly gastroenteritis or other conditions with acute electrolyte loss. Although **Azmacort** Inhalation Aerosol may provide control of asthmatic symptoms during these episodes, in recommended doses it supplies only normal physiological amounts of corticosteroid systemically and does NOT provide the increased systemic steroid which is necessary for coping with these emergencies.

During periods of stress or a severe asthmatic attack, patients who have been recently withdrawn from systemic corticosteroids should be instructed to resume systemic steroids (in large doses) immediately and to contact their physician for further instruction. These patients should also be instructed to carry a warning card indicating that they may need supplementary systemic steroids during periods of stress or a severe asthma attack.

Localized infections with *Candida albicans* have occurred infrequently in the mouth and pharynx. These areas should be examined by the treating physician at each patient visit. The percentage of positive mouth and throat cultures for *Candida albicans* did not change during a year of continuous therapy. The incidence of clinically apparent infection is low (2.5%). These infections may disappear spontaneously or may require treatment with appropriate antifungal therapy or discontinuance of treatment with **Azmacort** Inhalation Aerosol.

Children who are on immunosuppressant drugs are more susceptible to infections than healthy children. Chickenpox and measles, for example, can have a more serious or even fatal course in children on immunosuppressant doses of corticosteroids. In such children, or in adults who have not had these diseases, particular care should be taken to avoid exposure. If exposed, therapy with varicella zoster immune globulin (VZIG) or pooled intravenous immunoglobulin (IVIG), as appropriate, may be indicated. If chickenpox develops, treatment with antiviral agents may be considered.

Azmacort Inhalation Aerosol is not to be regarded as a bronchodilator and is not indicated for rapid relief of bronchospasm.

As with other inhaled asthma medications, bronchospasm may occur with an immediate increase in wheezing following dosing. If bronchospasm occurs following use of **Azmacort** Inhalation Aerosol, it should be treated immediately with a fast-acting inhaled bronchodilator. Treatment with **Azmacort** Inhalation Aerosol should be discontinued and alternative treatment should be instituted.

Patients should be instructed to contact their physician immediately when episodes of asthma which are not responsive to bronchodilators occur during the course of treatment with **Azmacort** Inhalation Aerosol. During such episodes, patients may require therapy with systemic corticosteroids.

The use of **Azmacort** Inhalation Aerosol with systemic prednisone, dosed either daily or on alternate-days, could increase the likelihood of HPA suppression compared to a therapeutic dose of either one alone. Therefore, **Azmacort** Inhalation Aerosol should be used with caution in patients already receiving prednisone treatment for any disease.

Transfer of patients from systemic steroid therapy to **Azmacort** Inhalation Aerosol may unmask allergic conditions previously suppressed by the systemic steroid therapy, *e.g.,* rhinitis, conjunctivitis, and eczema.

PRECAUTIONS

During withdrawal from oral steroids, some patients may experience symptoms of systemically active steroid withdrawal, *e.g.,* joint and/or muscular pain, lassitude, and depression, despite maintenance or even improvement of respiratory function. (See **DOSAGE AND ADMINISTRATION.**) Although steroid withdrawal effects are usually transient and not severe, severe and even fatal exacerbation of asthma can occur if the previous daily oral corticosteroid requirement had significantly exceeded 10 mg/day of prednisone or equivalent.

In responsive patients, inhaled corticosteroids will often permit control of asthmatic symptoms with less suppression of HPA function than therapeutically equivalent oral doses of prednisone. Since triamcinolone acetonide is absorbed into the circulation and can be systemically active, the beneficial effects of **Azmacort** Inhalation Aerosol in minimizing or preventing HPA dysfunction may be expected only when recommended dosages are not exceeded.

Suppression of HPA function has been reported in volunteers who received 4000 mcg daily of triamcinolone acetonide by oral inhalation. In addition, suppression of HPA function has been reported in some patients who have received recommended doses for as little as 6 to 12 weeks. Since the response of HPA function to inhaled corticosteroids is highly individualized, the physician should consider this information when treating patients.

When used at excessive doses or at recommended doses in a small number of susceptible individuals, systemic corticosteroid effects such as hypercorticoidism and adrenal suppression may appear. If such changes occur, **Azmacort®** (triamcinolone acetonide) Inhalation Aerosol should be discontinued slowly, consistent with accepted procedures for reducing systemic steroid therapy and for management of asthma symptoms.

Azmacort Inhalation Aerosol should be used with caution, if at all, in patients with active or quiescent tuberculosis infection of the respiratory tract; untreated systemic fungal, bacterial, parasitic, or viral infections; or ocular herpes simplex.

The long-term local and systemic effects of **Azmacort** Inhalation Aerosol in human subjects are still not fully known. While there has been no clinical evidence of adverse experiences, the effects resulting from chronic use of **Azmacort** Inhalation Aerosol on developmental or immunologic processes in the mouth, pharynx, trachea, and lung are unknown.

Because of the possibility of systemic absorption of inhaled corticosteroids, patients treated with these drugs should be observed carefully for any evidence of systemic corticosteroid effects including suppression of growth in children. Particular care should be taken in observing patients postoperatively or during periods of stress for evidence of a decrease in adrenal function.

Information for Patients: Patients being treated with **Azmacort** Inhalation Aerosol should receive the following information and instructions. This information is intended to aid them in the safe and effective use of this medication. It is not a complete disclosure of all possible adverse or intended effects.

Patients should use **Azmacort** Inhalation Aerosol at regular intervals as directed. Results of clinical trials indicate that significant improvement in asthma may occur by 1 week, but maximum benefit may not be achieved for 2 weeks or more. The patient should not increase the prescribed dosage but should contact the physician if symptoms do not improve or if the condition worsens.

In clinical studies and post-marketing experience with **Azmacort** Inhalation Aerosol, local infections of the oropharynx with *Candida albicans* have occurred. When such an infection develops, it should be treated with appropriate local or systemic (*i.e.,* oral antifungal) therapy while remaining on treatment with **Azmacort** Inhalation Aerosol. However, at times therapy with **Azmacort** Inhalation Aerosol may need to be interrupted.

Patients should be instructed to track their use of **Azmacort** Inhalation Aerosol and to dispose of the canister after 240 actuations since reliable dose delivery cannot be assured after 240 doses.

Patients who are on immunosuppressant doses of corticosteroids should be warned to avoid exposure to chickenpox or measles and, if exposed, to obtain medical advice.

Carcinogenesis, Mutagenesis, Impairment of Fertility: No evidence of treatment-related carcinogenicity was demonstrated after two years of once daily gavage of triamcinolone acetonide at doses of 0.05, 0.2, and 1.0 mcg/kg (approximately 0.02, 0.07, and 0.4% of the maximum recommended human daily inhalation dose on a mcg/m^2 basis) in the rat and 0.1, 0.6, and 3.0 mcg/kg (approximately 0.02, 0.1, and 0.6% of the maximum recommended human daily inhalation dose on a mcg/m^2 basis) in a mouse.

Mutagenesis studies with triamcinolone acetonide have not been carried out.

No evidence of impaired fertility was manifested when oral doses of up to 15.0 mcg/kg (8% of the maximum recommended human daily inhalation dose on a mcg/m^2 basis) were administered to female and male rats. However, triamcinolone acetonide at oral doses of 8 mcg/kg (approximately 4% of the maximum recommended human daily inhalation dose on a mcg/m^2 basis) caused dystocia and prolonged delivery and at oral doses of 5.0 mcg/kg (approximately 2.5% of the maximum recommended human daily inhalation dose on a mcg/m^2 basis) and above caused increases in fetal resorptions and stillbirths and decreases in pup body weight and survival. At a lower dose of 1.0 mcg/kg (approximately 0.5% of the maximum recommended human daily inhalation dose on a mcg/m^2 basis) it did not induce the above mentioned effects.

Pregnancy: Pregnancy Category C. Triamcinolone acetonide has been shown to be teratogenic at inhalational doses of 20, 40, and 80 mcg/kg in rats (approximately 0.1, 0.2, and 0.4 times the maximum recommended human daily inhalation dose on a mcg/m^2 basis, respectively), in rabbits at the same doses (approximately 0.2, 0.4, and 0.8 times the maximum recommended human daily inhalation dose on a mcg/m^2 basis, respectively) and in monkeys, at an inhalational dose of 500 mcg/kg (approximately 5 times the maximum recommended human daily inhalation dose on a mcg/m^2 basis). Dose related teratogenic effects in rats and rabbits included cleft palate and/or internal hydrocephaly and axial skeletal defects whereas the teratogenic effects observed in the monkey were CNS and/or cranial malformations. There are no adequate and well controlled studies in pregnant women. Triamcinolone acetonide should be used during pregnancy only if the potential benefit justifies the potential risk to the fetus.

Experience with oral glucocorticoids since their introduction in pharmacologic as opposed to physiologic doses suggests that rodents are more prone to teratogenic effects from glucocorticoids than humans. In addition, because there is a natural increase in glucocorticoid production during pregnancy, most women will require a lower exogenous steroid dose and many will not need glucocorticoid treatment during pregnancy.

Nonteratogenic Effects: Hypoadrenalism may occur in infants born of mothers receiving corticosteroids during pregnancy. Such infants should be carefully observed.

Nursing Mothers: It is not known whether triamcinolone acetonide is excreted in human milk. Because other corticosteroids are excreted in human milk, caution should be exercised when **Azmacort** Inhalation Aerosol is administered to nursing women.

Pediatric Use: Safety and effectiveness have not been established in pediatric patients below the age of 6. Oral corticosteroids have been shown to cause growth suppression in children and teenagers, particularly with higher doses over extended periods. If a child or teenager on any corticosteroid appears to have growth suppression, the possibility that they are particularly sensitive to this effect of steroids should be considered.

ADVERSE REACTIONS

The table below describes the incidence of common adverse experiences based upon three placebo-controlled, multicenter US clinical trials of 507 patients (297 female and 210 male adults (age range 18-64)). These trials included asthma patients who had previously received inhaled beta$_2$-agonists alone, as well as those who previously required inhaled corticosteroid therapy for the control of their asthma. The patients were treated with **Azmacort** Inhalation Aerosol (including doses ranging from 200 to 800 mcg twice daily for 6 weeks) or placebo.

[See table at left]

Adverse events that occurred at an incidence of 1-3% in the overall **Azmacort** Inhalation Aerosol treatment group and greater than placebo included:

Adverse Events Occurring at an Incidence of Greater Than 3% and Greater than Placebo

Adverse Event	Azmacort Dose 200 mcg bid (n=57)	400 mcg bid (n=170)	800 mcg bid (n=57)	Placebo (n=167)	Adverse Event	Azmacort Dose 200 mcg bid (n=57)	400 mcg bid (n=170)	800 mcg bid (n=57)	Placebo (n=167)
Sinusitis	5 (9%)	7 (4%)	1 (2%)	6 (4%)	Flu Syndrome	2 (4%)	8 (5%)	1 (2%)	5 (3%)
Pharyngitis	4 (7%)	42 (25%)	10 (18%)	19 (11%)	Back Pain	2 (4%)	3 (2%)	2 (4%)	3 (2%)
Headache	4 (7%)	35 (21%)	7 (12%)	24 (14%)					

Body as a whole:	facial edema, pain, abdominal pain, photosensitivity
Digestive system:	diarrhea, oral monilia, toothache, vomiting
Metabolic and Nutrition:	weight gain
Musculoskeletal system:	bursitis, myalgia, tenosynovitis
Nervous system:	dry mouth
Organs of special sense:	rash
Respiratory system:	chest congestion, voice alteration
Urogenital system:	cystitis, urinary tract infection, vaginal monilia

In older controlled clinical trials of steroid dependent asthmatics, urticaria was reported rarely. Anaphylaxis was not reported in these controlled trials. Typical steroid withdrawal effects including muscle aches, joint aches, and fatigue were noted in clinical trials when patients were transferred from oral steroid therapy to **Azmacort** Inhalation Aerosol. Easy bruisability was also noted in these trials. Hoarseness, dry throat, irritated throat, dry mouth, facial edema, increased wheezing, and cough have been reported. These adverse effects have generally been mild and transient. Cases of oral candidiasis occurring with clinical use have been reported. (See **WARNINGS**.) Anaphylaxis has also been reported from post-marketing surveillance.

OVERDOSAGE

There are no data available on the effects of acute or chronic overdose. However, acute overdosing with **Azmacort** Inhalation Aerosol is unlikely in view of the total amount of active ingredient present and the route of administration. The maximum total daily dose (1600 mcg) has been well tolerated when administered as a single dose of 16 consecutive inhalations to adult asthmatics in a controlled clinical trial. Chronic overdosage may result in signs/symptoms of hypercorticoidism. (See **PRECAUTIONS**.) The risk of candidiasis could also be increased.

DOSAGE AND ADMINISTRATION

Adults: The usual recommended dosage is two inhalations (200 mcg) given three to four times a day or four inhalations (400 mcg) given twice daily. The maximal daily intake should not exceed 16 inhalations (1600 mcg) in adults. Higher initial doses (12 to 16 inhalations per day) may be considered in patients with more severe asthma.

Children 6 to 12 Years of Age: The usual recommended dosage is one or two inhalations (100 to 200 mcg) given three to four times a day or two to four inhalations (200 to 400 mcg) given twice daily. The maximal daily intake should not exceed 12 inhalations (1200 mcg) in children 6 to 12 years of age. Insufficient clinical data exist with respect to the safety and efficacy of the administration of **Azmacort** Inhalation Aerosol to children below the age of 6. The long-term effects of inhaled steroids, including **Azmacort** Inhalation Aerosol, on growth are still not fully known.

Rinsing the mouth after inhalation is advised.

Different considerations must be given to the following groups of patients in order to obtain the full therapeutic benefit of **Azmacort** Inhalation Aerosol:

Note: In all patients, it is desirable to titrate to the lowest effective dose once asthma stability has been achieved.

Patients Not Receiving Systemic Corticosteroids: Patients who require maintenance therapy of their asthma may benefit from treatment with **Azmacort** Inhalation Aerosol at the doses recommended above. In patients who respond to **Azmacort** Inhalation Aerosol, improvement in pulmonary function is usually apparent within one to two weeks after the initiation of therapy.

Patients Maintained on Systemic Corticosteroids: Clinical studies have shown that **Azmacort** Inhalation Aerosol may be effective in the management of asthmatics dependent or maintained on systemic corticosteroids and may permit replacement or significant reduction in the dosage of systemic corticosteroids.

The patient's asthma should be reasonably stable before treatment with **Azmacort** Inhalation Aerosol is started. Initially, **Azmacort** Inhalation Aerosol should be used concurrently with the patient's usual maintenance dose of systemic corticosteroid. After approximately one week, gradual withdrawal of the systemic corticosteroid is started by reducing the daily or alternate daily dose. Reductions may be made after an interval of one or two weeks, depending on the response of the patient. A slow rate of withdrawal is strongly recommended. Generally, these decrements should not exceed 2.5 mg of prednisone or its equivalent. During withdrawal, some patients may experience symptoms of systemic corticosteroid withdrawal, *e.g.*, joint and/or muscular pain, lassitude, and depression, despite maintenance or even improvement in pulmonary function. Such patients should be encouraged to continue with the inhaler but should be monitored for objective signs of adrenal insufficiency. If evidence of adrenal insufficiency occurs, the systemic corticosteroid doses should be increased temporarily and thereafter withdrawal should continue more slowly. Inhaled corticosteroids should be used with caution when used chronically in patients receiving prednisone regimens, either daily or alternate day. (See **WARNINGS**.)

During periods of stress or a severe asthma attack, transfer patients may require supplementary treatment with systemic corticosteroids.

Directions for Use: An illustrated leaflet of patient instructions for proper use accompanies each package of **Azmacort** Inhalation Aerosol.

HOW SUPPLIED

Azmacort Inhalation Aerosol contains 60 mg triamcinolone acetonide in a 20 gram package which delivers at least 240 actuations. It is supplied with a white plastic actuator, a white plastic spacer-mouthpiece and patient's leaflet of instructions: box of one. NDC 0075-0060-37. Each actuation delivers 200 mcg triamcinolone acetonide from the valve and 100 mcg from the spacer-mouthpiece under defined *in vitro* test conditions.

Avoid spraying in eyes.

For best results, the canister should be at room temperature before use.

Shake well before using.

CONTENTS UNDER PRESSURE. Do not puncture. Do not use or store near heat or open flame. Exposure to temperatures above 120°F may cause bursting. Never throw canister into fire or incinerator. Keep out of reach of children unless otherwise prescribed. Store at Controlled Room Temperature 20 to 25°C (68 to 77°F) [see USP].

Note: The indented statement below is required by the Federal government's Clean Air Act for all products containing or manufactured with chlorofluorocarbons (CFCs):

> WARNING: Contains CFC-12, a substance which harms public health and the environment by destroying ozone in the upper atmosphere.

A notice similar to the above WARNING has been placed in the "Information For The Patient" portion of this package insert under the Environmental Protection Agency's (EPA's) regulations. The patient's warning states that the patient should consult his or her physician if there are questions about alternatives.

Aventis Pharmaceuticals Products Inc.
Parsippany, NJ 07054 ©2000
Rev. 3/99 IN-6337D!

Shown in Product Identification Guide, page 306

CARAFATE® Tablets ℞

[*kār 'afāt*]
(sucralfate)

Prescribing Information as of May 1996

DESCRIPTION

CARAFATE Tablets contain sucralfate and sucralfate is an α-D-glucopyranoside, β-D-fructofuranosyl-, octakis-(hydrogen sulfate), aluminum complex.

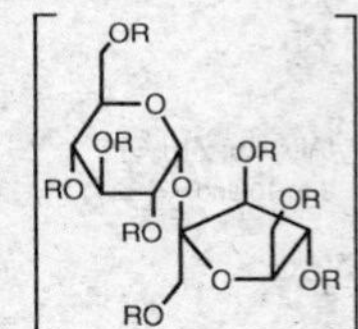

Tablets for oral administration contain 1 g of sucralfate. Also contain: D&C Red #30 Lake, FD&C Blue #1 Lake, magnesium stearate, microcrystalline cellulose, and starch. Therapeutic category: antiulcer.

CLINICAL PHARMACOLOGY

Sucralfate is only minimally absorbed from the gastrointestinal tract. The small amounts of the sulfated disaccharide that are absorbed are excreted primarily in the urine.

Although the mechanism of sucralfate's ability to accelerate healing of duodenal ulcers remains to be fully defined, it is known that it exerts its effect through a local, rather than systemic, action. The following observations also appear pertinent:

1. Studies in human subjects and with animal models of ulcer disease have shown that sucralfate forms an ulcer-adherent complex with proteinaceous exudate at the ulcer site.
2. In vitro, a sucralfate-albumin film provides a barrier to diffusion of hydrogen ions.
3. In human subjects, sucralfate given in doses recommended for ulcer therapy inhibits pepsin activity in gastric juice by 32%.
4. In vitro, sucralfate adsorbs bile salts.

These observations suggest that sucralfate's antiulcer activity is the result of formation of an ulcer-adherent complex that covers the ulcer site and protects it against further attack by acid, pepsin, and bile salts. There are approximately 14 to 16 mEq of acid-neutralizing capacity per 1-g dose of sucralfate.

CLINICAL TRIALS

Acute Duodenal Ulcer

Over 600 patients have participated in well-controlled clinical trials worldwide. Multicenter trials conducted in the United States, both of them placebo-controlled studies with endoscopic evaluation at 2 and 4 weeks, showed:

STUDY 1

Treatment Groups	Ulcer Healing/No. Patients	
	2 wk	4wk (Overall)
Sucralfate	37/105 (35.2%)	82/109 (75.2%)
Placebo	26/106 (24.5%)	68/107 (63.6%)

STUDY 2

Treatment Groups	Ulcer Healing/No. Patients	
	2 wk	4wk (Overall)
Sucralfate	8/24 (33%)	22/24 (92%)
Placebo	4/31 (13%)	18/31 (58%)

The sucralfate-placebo differences were statistically significant in both studies at 4 weeks but not at 2 weeks. The poorer result in the first study may have occurred because sucralfate was given 2 hours after meals and at bedtime rather than 1 hour before meals and at bedtime, the regimen used in international studies and in the second United States study. In addition, in the first study liquid antacid was utilized as needed, whereas in the second study antacid tablets were used.

Maintenance Therapy After Healing of Duodenal Ulcer

Two double-blind randomized placebo-controlled U.S. multicenter trials have demonstrated that sucralfate (1 g bid) is effective as maintenance therapy following healing of duodenal ulcers.

In one study, endoscopies were performed monthly for 4 months. Of the 254 patients who enrolled, 239 were analyzed in the intention-to-treat life table analysis presented below.

Duodenal Ulcer Recurrence Rate (%)

Drug	n	Months of Therapy 1	2	3	4
CARAFATE	122	20*	30*	38†	42†
Placebo	117	33	46	55	63

*$P<0.05$, †$P<0.01$

In this study, prn antacids were not permitted.

In the other study, scheduled endoscopies were performed at 6 and 12 months, but for-cause endoscopies were permitted as symptoms dictated. Median symptom scores between the sucralfate and placebo groups were not significantly different. A life table intention-to-treat analysis for the 94 patients enrolled in the trial had the following results:

Duodenal Ulcer Recurrence Rate (%)

Drug	n	6 months	12 months
CARAFATE	48	19*	27*
Placebo	46	54	65

*$P<0.002$

In this study, prn antacids were permitted.

Data from placebo-controlled studies longer than 1 year are not available.

INDICATIONS AND USAGE

CARAFATE® (sucralfate) is indicated in:

- Short-term treatment (up to 8 weeks) of active duodenal ulcer. While healing with sucralfate may occur during the first week or two, treatment should be continued for 4 to 8 weeks unless healing has been demonstrated by x-ray or endoscopic examination.
- Maintenance therapy for duodenal ulcer patients at reduced dosage after healing of acute ulcers.

CONTRAINDICATIONS

There are no known contraindications to the use of sucralfate.

PRECAUTIONS

Duodenal ulcer is a chronic, recurrent disease. While short-term treatment with sucralfate can result in complete healing of the ulcer, a successful course of treatment with sucralfate should not be expected to alter the posthealing frequency or severity of duodenal ulceration.

Special Populations: Chronic Renal Failure and Dialysis Patients

When sucralfate is administered orally, small amounts of aluminum are absorbed from the gastrointestinal tract. Concomitant use of sucralfate with other products that contain aluminum, such as aluminum-containing antacids, may increase the total body burden of aluminum. Patients with normal renal function receiving the recommended

Continued on next page

Carafate—Cont.

doses of sucralfate and aluminum-containing products adequately excrete aluminum in the urine. Patients with chronic renal failure or those receiving dialysis have impaired excretion of absorbed aluminum. In addition, aluminum does not cross dialysis membranes because it is bound to albumin and transferrin plasma proteins. Aluminum accumulation and toxicity (aluminum osteodystrophy, osteomalacia, encephalopathy) have been described in patients with renal impairment. Sucralfate should be used with caution in patients with chronic renal failure.

Drug Interactions

Some studies have shown that simultaneous sucralfate administration in healthy volunteers reduced the extent of absorption (bioavailability) of single doses of the following: cimetidine, digoxin, fluoroquinolone antibiotics, ketoconazole, l-thyroxine, phenytoin, quinidine, ranitidine, tetracycline, and theophylline. Subtherapeutic prothrombin times with concomitant warfarin and sucralfate therapy have been reported in spontaneous and published case reports. However, two clinical studies have demonstrated no change in either serum warfarin concentration or prothrombin time with the addition of sucralfate to chronic warfarin therapy.

The mechanism of these interactions appears to be nonsystemic in nature, presumably resulting from sucralfate binding to the concomitant agent in the gastrointestinal tract. In all cases studied to date (cimetidine, ciprofloxacin, digoxin, norfloxacin, ofloxacin, and ranitidine), dosing the concomitant medication 2 hours before sucralfate eliminated the interaction. Because of the potential of CARAFATE to alter the absorption of some drugs, CARAFATE should be administered separately from other drugs when alterations in bioavailability are felt to be critical. In these cases, patients should be monitored appropriately.

Carcinogenesis, Mutagenesis, Impairment of Fertility

Chronic oral toxicity studies of 24 months' duration were conducted in mice and rats at doses up to 1 g/kg (12 times the human dose). There was no evidence of drug-related tumorigenicity. A reproduction study in rats at doses up to 38 times the human dose did not reveal any indication of fertility impairment. Mutagenicity studies were not conducted.

Pregnancy

Teratogenic effects. Pregnancy Category B. Teratogenicity studies have been performed in mice, rats, and rabbits at doses up to 50 times the human dose and have revealed no evidence of harm to the fetus due to sucralfate. There are, however, no adequate and well-controlled studies in pregnant women. Because animal reproduction studies are not always predictive of human response, this drug should be used during pregnancy only if clearly needed.

Nursing Mothers

It is not known whether this drug is excreted in human milk. Because many drugs are excreted in human milk, caution should be exercised when sucralfate is administered to a nursing woman.

Pediatric Use

Safety and effectiveness in pediatric patients have not been established.

ADVERSE REACTIONS

Adverse reactions to sucralfate in clinical trials were minor and only rarely led to discontinuation of the drug. In studies involving over 2700 patients treated with sucralfate tablets, adverse effects were reported in 129 (4.7%).

Constipation was the most frequent complaint (2%). Other adverse effects reported in less than 0.5% of the patients are listed below by body system:

Gastrointestinal: diarrhea, nausea, vomiting, gastric discomfort, indigestion, flatulence, dry mouth

Dermatological: pruritus, rash

Nervous System: dizziness, insomnia, sleepiness, vertigo

Other: back pain, headache

Postmarketing reports of hypersensitivity reactions, including urticaria (hives), angioedema, respiratory difficulty, rhinitis, laryngospasm, and facial swelling have been reported in patients receiving sucralfate tablets. Similar events were reported with sucralfate suspension. However, a causal relationship has not been established.

Bezoars have been reported in patients treated with sucralfate. The majority of patients had underlying medical conditions that may predispose to bezoar formation (such as delayed gastric emptying) or were receiving concomitant enteral tube feedings.

Inadvertent injection of insoluble sucralfate and its insoluble excipients has led to fatal complications, including pulmonary and cerebral emboli. Sucralfate is **not** intended for intravenous administration.

OVERDOSAGE

Due to limited experience in humans with overdosage of sucralfate, no specific treatment recommendations can be given. Acute oral toxicity studies in animals, however, using doses up to 12 g/kg body weight, could not find a lethal dose. Sucralfate is only minimally absorbed from the gastrointestinal tract. Risks associated with acute overdosage should, therefore, be minimal. In rare reports describing sucralfate overdose, most patients remained asymptomatic. Those few reports where adverse events were described included symptoms of dyspepsia, abdominal pain, nausea, and vomiting.

DOSAGE AND ADMINISTRATION

Active Duodenal Ulcer: The recommended adult oral dosage for duodenal ulcer is 1 g four times a day on an empty stomach.

Antacids may be prescribed as needed for relief of pain but should not be taken within one-half hour before or after sucralfate.

While healing with sucralfate may occur during the first week or two, treatment should be continued for 4 to 8 weeks unless healing has been demonstrated by x-ray or endoscopic examination.

Maintenance Therapy: The recommended adult oral dosage is 1 g twice a day.

HOW SUPPLIED

CARAFATE (sucralfate) 1-g tablets are supplied in bottles of 100 (NDC 0088-1712-47), 120 (NDC 0088-1712-53), and 500 (NDC 0088-1712-55) and in Unit Dose Identification Paks of 100 (NDC 0088-1712-49). Light pink, scored, oblong tablets are embossed with CARAFATE on one side and 1712 on the other.

Prescribing Information as of May 1996

Hoechst Marion Roussel, Inc.
Kansas City, MO 64137 USA

Shown in Product Identification Guide, page 306

CARAFATE® ℞

[*kār 'afāt*]
(sucralfate)
Suspension

Prescribing Information as of November 1997

DESCRIPTION

CARAFATE Suspension contains sucralfate and sucralfate is an α-D-glucopyranoside, β-D-fructofuranosyl-, octakis-(hydrogen sulfate), aluminum complex.

$[Al(OH)_3]_x [H_2O]_y$
(x = 8 to 10 and y = 22 to 31)

$R = SO_3Al(OH)_2$

CARAFATE Suspension for oral administration contains 1 g of sucralfate per 10 mL.

CARAFATE Suspension also contains: colloidal silicon dioxide NF, FD&C Red #40, flavor, glycerin USP, methylcellulose USP, methylparaben NF, microcrystalline cellulose NF, purified water USP, simethicone USP, and sorbitol solution USP.

Therapeutic category: antiulcer.

CLINICAL PHARMACOLOGY

Sucralfate is only minimally absorbed from the gastrointestinal tract. The small amounts of the sulfated disaccharide that are absorbed are excreted primarily in the urine.

Although the mechanism of sucralfate's ability to accelerate healing of duodenal ulcers remains to be fully defined, it is known that it exerts its effect through a local, rather than systemic, action. The following observations also appear pertinent:

1. Studies in human subjects and with animal models of ulcer disease have shown that sucralfate forms an ulcer-adherent complex with proteinaceous exudate at the ulcer site.
2. In vitro, a sucralfate-albumin film provides a barrier to diffusion of hydrogen ions.
3. In human subjects, sucralfate given in doses recommended for ulcer therapy inhibits pepsin activity in gastric juice by 32%.
4. In vitro, sucralfate adsorbs bile salts.

These observations suggest that sucralfate's antiulcer activity is the result of formation of an ulcer-adherent complex that covers the ulcer site and protects it against further attack by acid, pepsin, and bile salts. There are approximately 14 to 16 mEq of acid-neutralizing capacity per 1-g dose of sucralfate.

CLINICAL TRIALS

In a multicenter, double-blind, placebo-controlled study of CARAFATE Suspension, a dosage regimen of 1 g (10 mL) four times daily was demonstrated to be superior to placebo in ulcer healing.

Results From Clinical Trials
Healing Rates for Acute Duodenal Ulcer

Treatment	n	Week 2 Healing Rates	Week 4 Healing Rates	Week 8 Healing Rates
CARAFATE Suspension	145	23(16%)*	66(46%)†	95(66%)‡
Placebo	147	10(7%)	39(27%)	58(39%)

* P=0.016 †P=0.001 ‡P=0.0001

Equivalence of sucralfate suspension to sucralfate tablets has not been demonstrated.

INDICATIONS AND USAGE

CARAFATE (sucralfate) Suspension is indicated in the short-term (up to 8 weeks) treatment of active duodenal ulcer.

CONTRAINDICATIONS

There are no known contraindications to the use of sucralfate.

PRECAUTIONS

Duodenal ulcer is a chronic, recurrent disease. While short-term treatment with sucralfate can result in complete healing of the ulcer, a successful course of treatment with sucralfate should not be expected to alter the posthealing frequency or severity of duodenal ulceration.

Special Populations: Chronic Renal Failure and Dialysis Patients

When sucralfate is administered orally, small amounts of aluminum are absorbed from the gastrointestinal tract. Concomitant use of sucralfate with other products that contain aluminum, such as aluminum-containing antacids, may increase the total body burden of aluminum. Patients with normal renal function receiving the recommended doses of sucralfate and aluminum-containing products adequately excrete aluminum in the urine. Patients with chronic renal failure or those receiving dialysis have impaired excretion of absorbed aluminum. In addition, aluminum does not cross dialysis membranes because it is bound to albumin and transferrin plasma proteins. Aluminum accumulation and toxicity (aluminum osteodystrophy, osteomalacia, encephalopathy) have been described in patients with renal impairment. Sucralfate should be used with caution in patients with chronic renal failure.

Drug Interactions

Some studies have shown that simultaneous sucralfate administration in healthy volunteers reduced the extent of absorption (bioavailability) of single doses of the following: cimetidine, digoxin, fluoroquinolone antibiotics, ketoconazole, l-thyroxine, phenytoin, quinidine, ranitidine, tetracycline, and theophylline. Subtherapeutic prothrombin times with concomitant warfarin and sucralfate therapy have been reported in spontaneous and published case reports. However, two clinical studies have demonstrated no change in either serum warfarin concentration or prothrombin time with the addition of sucralfate to chronic warfarin therapy.

The mechanism of these interactions appears to be nonsystemic in nature, presumably resulting from sucralfate binding to the concomitant agent in the gastrointestinal tract. In all cases studied to date (cimetidine, ciprofloxacin, digoxin, norfloxacin, ofloxacin, and ranitidine), dosing the concomitant medication 2 hours before sucralfate eliminated the interaction. Because of the potential of CARAFATE to alter the absorption of some drugs, CARAFATE should be administered separately from other drugs when alterations in bioavailability are felt to be critical. In these cases, patients should be monitored appropriately.

Carcinogenesis, Mutagenesis, Impairment of Fertility

Chronic oral toxicity studies of 24 months' duration were conducted in mice and rats at doses up to 1 g/kg (12 times the human dose). There was no evidence of drug-related tumorigenicity. A reproduction study in rats at doses up to 38 times the human dose did not reveal any indication of fertility impairment. Mutagenicity studies were not conducted.

Pregnancy

Teratogenic effects. Pregnancy Category B. Teratogenicity studies have been performed in mice, rats, and rabbits at doses up to 50 times the human dose and have revealed no evidence of harm to the fetus due to sulcralfate. There are, however, no adequate and well-controlled studies in pregnant women. Because animal reproduction studies are not always predictive of human response, this drug should be used during pregnancy only if clearly needed.

Nursing Mothers

It is not known whether this drug is excreted in human milk. Because many drugs are excreted in human milk, caution should be exercised when sucralfate is administered to a nursing woman.

Pediatric Use

Safety and effectiveness in pediatric patients have not been established.

ADVERSE REACTIONS

Adverse reactions to sucralfate tablets in clinical trials were minor and only rarely led to discontinuation of the drug. In studies involving over 2700 patients treated with sucralfate, adverse effects were reported in 129 (4.7%).

Constipation was the most frequent complaint (2%). Other adverse effects reported in less than 0.5% of the patients are listed below by body system:
Gastrointestinal: diarrhea, dry mouth, flatulence, gastric discomfort, indigestion, nausea, vomiting
Dermatological: pruritus, rash
Nervous System: dizziness, insomnia, sleepiness, vertigo
Other: back pain, headache
Postmarketing reports of hypersensitivity reactions, including urticaria (hives), angioedema, respiratory difficulty, rhinitis, laryngospasm, and facial swelling have been reported in patients receiving sucralfate tablets. Similar events were reported with sucralfate suspension. However, a causal relationship has not been established.
Bezoars have been reported in patients treated with sucralfate. The majority of patients had underlying medical conditions that may predispose to bezoar formation (such as delayed gastric emptying) or were receiving concomitant enteral tube feedings.
Inadvertent injection of insoluble sucralfate and its insoluble excipients has led to fatal complications, including pulmonary and cerebral emboli. Sucralfate is **not** intended for intravenous administration.

OVERDOSAGE

Due to limited experience in humans with overdosage of sucralfate, no specific treatment recommendations can be given. Acute oral studies in animals, however, using doses up to 12 g/kg body weight, could not find a lethal dose. Sucralfate is only minimally absorbed from the gastrointestinal tract. Risks associated with acute overdosage should, therefore, be minimal. In rare reports describing sucralfate overdose, most patients remained asymptomatic. Those few reports where adverse events were described included symptoms of dyspepsia, abdominal pain, nausea, and vomiting.

DOSAGE AND ADMINISTRATION

Active Duodenal Ulcer. The recommended adult oral dosage for duodenal ulcer is 1 g (10 mL/2 teaspoonfuls) four times per day. CARAFATE should be administered on an empty stomach.
Antacids may be prescribed as needed for relief of pain but should not be taken within one-half hour before or after sucralfate.
While healing with sucralfate may occur during the first week or two, treatment should be continued for 4 to 8 weeks unless healing has been demonstrated by x-ray or endoscopic examination.

HOW SUPPLIED

CARAFATE (sucralfate) Suspension 1 g/10 mL is a pink suspension supplied in bottles of 14 fl oz (NDC 0088-1700-15).

SHAKE WELL BEFORE USING.

Store at controlled room temperature 20–25°C (68–77°F). [see USP].

Prescribing Information as of November 1997

Hoechst Marion Roussel, Inc.
Kansas City, MO 64137 USA

CARDIZEM® CD ℞

[kar'diz-em]
(diltiazem HCl)
Capsules

Prescribing Information as of May 1999

DESCRIPTION

CARDIZEM® (diltiazem hydrochloride) is a calcium ion influx inhibitor (slow channel blocker or calcium antagonist). Chemically, diltiazem hydrochloride is 1,5-benzothiazepin-4(5H)one,3-(acetyloxy)-5-[2-(dimethylamino)ethyl]-2,3-dihydro-2-(4-methoxyphenyl)-, monohydrochloride,(+)-cis-. The chemical structure is:

Diltiazem hydrochloride is a white to off-white crystalline powder with a bitter taste. It is soluble in water, methanol, and chloroform. It has a molecular weight of 450.98. CARDIZEM CD is formulated as a once-a-day extended release capsule containing either 120 mg, 180 mg, 240 mg, 300 mg, or 360 mg diltiazem hydrochloride. The 120 mg, 180 mg, 240 mg, and 300 mg capsules also contain: black iron oxide, ethylcellulose, FD&C Blue #1, fumaric acid, gelatin-NF, sucrose, starch, talc, titanium dioxide, white wax, and other ingredients. The 360 mg capsule also contains: black iron oxide, diethyl phthalate, FD&C Blue #1, gelatin-NF, povidone K17, sodium lauryl sulfate, starch, sucrose, talc, titanium dioxide, and other ingredients.
For oral administration.

CLINICAL PHARMACOLOGY

The therapeutic effects of CARDIZEM CD are believed to be related to its ability to inhibit the influx of calcium ions during membrane depolarization of cardiac and vascular smooth muscle.

Mechanisms of Action

Hypertension. CARDIZEM CD produces its antihypertensive effect primarily by relaxation of vascular smooth muscle and the resultant decrease in peripheral vascular resistance. The magnitude of blood pressure reduction is related to the degree of hypertension; thus hypertensive individuals experience an antihypertensive effect, whereas there is only a modest fall in blood pressure in normotensives.
Angina. CARDIZEM CD has been shown to produce increases in exercise tolerance, probably due to its ability to reduce myocardial oxygen demand. This is accomplished via reductions in heart rate and systemic blood pressure at submaximal and maximal work loads. Diltiazem has been shown to be a potent dilator of coronary arteries, both epicardial and subendocardial. Spontaneous and ergonovine-induced coronary artery spasm are inhibited by diltiazem.
In animal models, diltiazem interferes with the slow inward (depolarizing) current in excitable tissue. It causes excitation-contraction uncoupling in various myocardial tissues without changes in the configuration of the action potential. Diltiazem produces relaxation of coronary vascular smooth muscle and dilation of both large and small coronary arteries at drug levels which cause little or no negative inotropic effect. The resultant increases in coronary blood flow (epicardial and subendocardial) occur in ischemic and nonischemic models and are accompanied by dose-dependent decreases in systemic blood pressure and decreases in peripheral resistance.

Hemodynamic and Electrophysiologic Effects

Like other calcium channel antagonists, diltiazem decreases sinoatrial and atrioventricular conduction in isolated tissues and has a negative inotropic effect in isolated preparations. In the intact animal, prolongation of the AH interval can be seen at higher doses.
In man, diltiazem prevents spontaneous and ergonovine-provoked coronary artery spasm. It causes a decrease in peripheral vascular resistance and a modest fall in blood pressure in normotensive individuals and, in exercise tolerance studies in patients with ischemic heart disease, reduces the heart rate-blood pressure product for any given work load. Studies to date, primarily in patients with good ventricular function, have not revealed evidence of a negative inotropic effect; cardiac output, ejection fraction, and left ventricular end diastolic pressure have not been affected. Such data have no predictive value with respect to effects in patients with poor ventricular function, and increased heart failure has been reported in patients with preexisting impairment of ventricular function. There are as yet few data on the interaction of diltiazem and beta-blockers in patients with poor ventricular function. Resting heart rate is usually slightly reduced by diltiazem.
In hypertensive patients, CARDIZEM CD produces antihypertensive effects both in the supine and standing positions. In a double-blind, parallel, dose-response study utilizing doses ranging from 90 to 540 mg once daily, CARDIZEM CD lowered supine diastolic blood pressure in an apparent linear manner over the entire dose range studied. The changes in diastolic blood pressure, measured at trough, for placebo, 90 mg, 180 mg, 360 mg, and 540 mg were –2.9, –4.5, –6.1, –9.5, and –10.5 mm Hg, respectively. Postural hypotension is infrequently noted upon suddenly assuming an upright position. No reflex tachycardia is associated with the chronic antihypertensive effects. CARDIZEM CD decreases vascular resistance, increases cardiac output (by increasing stroke volume), and produces a slight decrease or no change in heart rate. During dynamic exercise, increases in diastolic pressure are inhibited, while maximum achievable systolic pressure is usually reduced. Chronic therapy with CARDIZEM CD produces no change or an increase in plasma catecholamines. No increased activity of the renin-angiotensin-aldosterone axis has been observed. CARDIZEM CD reduces the renal and peripheral effects of angiotensin II. Hypertensive animal models respond to diltiazem with reductions in blood pressure and increased urinary output and natriuresis without a change in urinary sodium/potassium ratio.
In a double-blind, parallel dose-response study of doses from 60 mg to 480 mg once daily, CARDIZEM CD increased time to termination of exercise in a linear manner over the entire dose range studied. The improvement in time to termination of exercise utilizing a Bruce exercise protocol, measured at trough, for placebo, 60 mg, 120 mg, 240 mg, 360 mg, and 480 mg was 29, 40, 56, 51, 69, and 68 seconds, respectively. As doses of CARDIZEM CD were increased, overall angina frequency was decreased. CARDIZEM CD, 180 mg once daily, or placebo was administered in a double-blind study to patients receiving concomitant treatment with long-acting nitrates and/or beta-blockers. A significant increase in time to termination of exercise and a significant decrease in overall angina frequency was observed. In this trial the overall frequency of adverse events in the CARDIZEM CD treatment group was the same as the placebo group.
Intravenous diltiazem in doses of 20 mg prolongs AH conduction time and AV node functional and effective refractory periods by approximately 20%. In a study involving single oral doses of 300 mg of CARDIZEM in six normal volunteers, the average maximum PR prolongation was 14% with no instances of greater than first-degree AV block. Diltiazem-associated prolongation of the AH interval is not more pronounced in patients with first-degree heart block. In patients with sick sinus syndrome, diltiazem significantly prolongs sinus cycle length (up to 50% in some cases).
Chronic oral administration of CARDIZEM to patients in doses of up to 540 mg/day has resulted in small increases in PR interval, and on occasion produces abnormal prolongation. (See WARNINGS.)

Pharmacokinetics and Metabolism

Diltiazem is well absorbed from the gastrointestinal tract and is subject to an extensive first-pass effect, giving an absolute bioavailability (compared to intravenous administration) of about 40%. CARDIZEM undergoes extensive metabolism in which only 2% to 4% of the unchanged drug appears in the urine. Drugs which induce or inhibit hepatic microsomal enzymes may alter diltiazem disposition.
Total radioactivity measurement following short IV administration in healthy volunteers suggests the presence of other unidentified metabolites, which attain higher concentrations than those of diltiazem and are more slowly eliminated; half-life of total radioactivity is about 20 hours compared to 2 to 5 hours for diltiazem.
In vitro binding studies show CARDIZEM is 70% to 80% bound to plasma proteins. Competitive in vitro ligand binding studies have also shown CARDIZEM binding is not altered by therapeutic concentrations of digoxin, hydrochlorothiazide, phenylbutazone, propranolol, salicylic acid, or warfarin. The plasma elimination half-life following single or multiple drug administration is approximately 3.0 to 4.5 hours. Desacetyl diltiazem is also present in the plasma at levels of 10% to 20% of the parent drug and is 25% to 50% as potent as a coronary vasodilator as diltiazem. Minimum therapeutic plasma diltiazem concentrations appear to be in the range of 50 to 200 ng/mL. There is a departure from linearity when dose strengths are increased; the half-life is slightly increased with dose. A study that compared patients with normal hepatic function to patients with cirrhosis found an increase in half-life and a 69% increase in bioavailability in the hepatically impaired patients. A single study in nine patients with severely impaired renal function showed no difference in the pharmacokinetic profile of diltiazem compared to patients with normal renal function.
CARDIZEM CD Capsules. When compared to a regimen of CARDIZEM tablets at steady-state, more than 95% of drug is absorbed from the CARDIZEM CD formulation. A single 360-mg dose of the capsule results in detectable plasma levels within 2 hours and peak plasma levels between 10 and 14 hours; absorption occurs throughout the dosing interval. When CARDIZEM CD was coadministered with a high fat content breakfast, the extent of diltiazem absorption was not affected. Dose-dumping does not occur. The apparent elimination half-life after single or multiple dosing is 5 to 8 hours. A departure from linearity similar to that seen with CARDIZEM tablets and CARDIZEM SR capsules is observed. As the dose of CARDIZEM CD capsules is increased from a daily dose of 120 mg to 240 mg, there is an increase in the area-under-the-curve of 2.7 times. When the dose is increased from 240 mg to 360 mg there is an increase in the area-under-the-curve of 1.6 times.

INDICATIONS AND USAGE

CARDIZEM CD is indicated for the treatment of hypertension. It may be used alone or in combination with other antihypertensive medications.
CARDIZEM CD is indicated for the management of chronic stable angina and angina due to coronary artery spasm.

CONTRAINDICATIONS

CARDIZEM is contraindicated in (1) patients with sick sinus syndrome except in the presence of a functioning ventricular pacemaker, (2) patients with second- or third-degree AV block except in the presence of a functioning ventricular pacemaker, (3) patients with hypotension (less than 90 mm Hg systolic), (4) patients who have demonstrated hypersensitivity to the drug, and (5) patients with acute myocardial infarction and pulmonary congestion documented by x-ray on admission.

WARNINGS

1. **Cardiac Conduction.** CARDIZEM prolongs AV node refractory periods without significantly prolonging sinus node recovery time, except in patients with sick sinus syndrome. This effect may rarely result in abnormally slow heart rates (particularly in patients with sick sinus syndrome) or second- or third-degree AV block (13 of 3290 patients or 0.40%). Concomitant use of diltiazem with beta-blockers or digitalis may result in additive effects on cardiac conduction. A patient with Prinzmetal's angina developed periods of asystole (2 to 5 seconds) after a single dose of 60 mg of diltiazem. (See ADVERSE REACTIONS section.)
2. **Congestive Heart Failure.** Although diltiazem has a negative inotropic effect in isolated animal tissue preparations, hemodynamic studies in humans with normal ventricular function have not shown a reduction in cardiac index nor consistent negative effects on contractility (dp/dt). An acute study of oral diltiazem in patients with impaired ventricular function (ejection fraction 24% ± 6%) showed improvement in indices of ventricular function without significant decrease in contractile function (dp/dt). Worsening of congestive heart failure has been reported in patients with preexisting impairment of ventricular function. Experience with the use of CARDIZEM (diltiazem hydrochloride) in combination with beta-blockers in patients with impaired ventricular function is limited. Caution should be exercised when using this combination.

Continued on next page

Cardizem CD—Cont.

3. **Hypotension.** Decreases in blood pressure associated with CARDIZEM therapy may occasionally result in symptomatic hypotension.
4. **Acute Hepatic Injury.** Mild elevations of transaminases with and without concomitant elevation in alkaline phosphatase and bilirubin have been observed in clinical studies. Such elevations were usually transient and frequently resolved even with continued diltiazem treatment. In rare instances, significant elevations in enzymes such as alkaline phosphatase, LDH, SGOT, SGPT, and other phenomena consistent with acute hepatic injury have been noted. These reactions tended to occur early after therapy initiation (1 to 8 weeks) and have been reversible upon discontinuation of drug therapy. The relationship to CARDIZEM is uncertain in some cases, but probable in some. (See PRECAUTIONS.)

PRECAUTIONS

General

CARDIZEM (diltiazem hydrochloride) is extensively metabolized by the liver and excreted by the kidneys and in bile. As with any drug given over prolonged periods, laboratory parameters of renal and hepatic function should be monitored at regular intervals. The drug should be used with caution in patients with impaired renal or hepatic function. In subacute and chronic dog and rat studies designed to produce toxicity, high doses of diltiazem were associated with hepatic damage. In special subacute hepatic studies, oral doses of 125 mg/kg and higher in rats were associated with histological changes in the liver which were reversible when the drug was discontinued. In dogs, doses of 20 mg/kg were also associated with hepatic changes; however, these changes were reversible with continued dosing.

Dermatological events (see ADVERSE REACTIONS section) may be transient and may disappear despite continued use of CARDIZEM. However, skin eruptions progressing to erythema multiforme and/or exfoliative dermatitis have also been infrequently reported. Should a dermatologic reaction persist, the drug should be discontinued.

Drug Interactions

Due to the potential for additive effects, caution and careful titration are warranted in patients receiving CARDIZEM concomitantly with other agents known to affect cardiac contractility and/or conduction. (See WARNINGS.) Pharmacologic studies indicate that there may be additive effects in prolonging AV conduction when using beta-blockers or digitalis concomitantly with CARDIZEM. (See WARNINGS.)

As with all drugs, care should be exercised when treating patients with multiple medications. CARDIZEM undergoes biotransformation by cytochrome P-450 mixed function oxidase. Coadministration of CARDIZEM with other agents which follow the same route of biotransformation may result in the competitive inhibition of metabolism. Especially in patients with renal and/or hepatic impairment, dosages of similarly metabolized drugs, particularly those of low therapeutic ratio, may require adjustment when starting or stopping concomitantly administered diltiazem to maintain optimum therapeutic blood levels.

Beta-blockers. Controlled and uncontrolled domestic studies suggest that concomitant use of CARDIZEM and beta-blockers is usually well tolerated, but available data are not sufficient to predict the effects of concomitant treatment in patients with left ventricular dysfunction or cardiac conduction abnormalities.

Administration of CARDIZEM (diltiazem hydrochloride) concomitantly with propranolol in five normal volunteers resulted in increased propranolol levels in all subjects and bioavailability of propranolol was increased approximately 50%. In vitro, propranolol appears to be displaced from its binding sites by diltiazem. If combination therapy is initiated or withdrawn in conjunction with propranolol, an adjustment in the propranolol dose may be warranted. (See WARNINGS.)

Cimetidine. A study in six healthy volunteers has shown a significant increase in peak diltiazem plasma levels (58%) and area-under-the-curve (53%) after a 1-week course of cimetidine at 1200 mg per day and a single dose of diltiazem 60 mg. Ranitidine produced smaller, nonsignificant increases. The effect may be mediated by cimetidine's known inhibition of hepatic cytochrome P-450, the enzyme system responsible for the first-pass metabolism of diltiazem. Patients currently receiving diltiazem therapy should be carefully monitored for a change in pharmacological effect when initiating and discontinuing therapy with cimetidine. An adjustment in the diltiazem dose may be warranted.

Digitalis. Administration of CARDIZEM with digoxin in 24 healthy male subjects increased plasma digoxin concentrations approximately 20%. Another investigator found no increase in digoxin levels in 12 patients with coronary artery disease. Since there have been conflicting results regarding the effect of digoxin levels, it is recommended that digoxin levels be monitored when initiating, adjusting, and discontinuing CARDIZEM therapy to avoid possible over- or under-digitalization. (See WARNINGS.)

Anesthetics. The depression of cardiac contractility, conductivity, and automaticity as well as the vascular dilation associated with anesthetics may be potentiated by calcium channel blockers. When used concomitantly, anesthetics and calcium blockers should be titrated carefully.

Cyclosporine. A pharmacokinetic interaction between diltiazem and cyclosporine has been observed during studies involving renal and cardiac transplant patients. In renal and cardiac transplant recipients, a reduction of cyclosporine dose ranging from 15% to 48% was necessary to maintain cyclosporine trough concentrations similar to those seen prior to the addition of diltiazem. If these agents are to be administered concurrently, cyclosporine concentrations should be monitored, especially when diltiazem therapy is initiated, adjusted, or discontinued.

The effect of cyclosporine on diltiazem plasma concentrations has not been evaluated.

Carbamazepine. Concomitant administration of diltiazem with carbamazepine has been reported to result in elevated serum levels of carbamazepine (40% to 72% increase), resulting in toxicity in some cases. Patients receiving these drugs concurrently should be monitored for a potential drug interaction.

Carcinogenesis, Mutagenesis, Impairment of Fertility

A 24-month study in rats at oral dosage levels of up to 100 mg/kg/day and a 21-month study in mice at oral dosage levels of up to 30 mg/kg/day showed no evidence of carcinogenicity. There was also no mutagenic response in vitro or in vivo in mammalian cell assays or in vitro in bacteria. No evidence of impaired fertility was observed in a study performed in male and female rats at oral dosages of up to 100 mg/kg/day.

Pregnancy

Category C. Reproduction studies have been conducted in mice, rats, and rabbits. Administration of doses ranging from five to ten times greater (on a mg/kg basis) than the daily recommended therapeutic dose has resulted in embryo and fetal lethality. These doses, in some studies, have been reported to cause skeletal abnormalities. In the perinatal/postnatal studies, there was an increased incidence of stillbirths at doses of 20 times the human dose or greater.

There are no well-controlled studies in pregnant women; therefore, use CARDIZEM in pregnant women only if the potential benefit justifies the potential risk to the fetus.

Nursing Mothers

Diltiazem is excreted in human milk. One report suggests that concentrations in breast milk may approximate serum levels. If use of CARDIZEM is deemed essential, an alternative method of infant feeding should be instituted.

Pediatric Use

Safety and effectiveness in pediatric patients have not been established.

ADVERSE REACTIONS

Serious adverse reactions have been rare in studies carried out to date, but it should be recognized that patients with impaired ventricular function and cardiac conduction abnormalities have usually been excluded from these studies.

The following table presents the most common adverse reactions reported in placebo-controlled angina and hypertension trials in patients receiving CARDIZEM CD up to 360 mg with rates in placebo patients shown for comparison.

CARDIZEM CD Capsule Placebo-Controlled Angina and Hypertension Trials Combined

Adverse Reactions	Cardizem CD (n=607)	Placebo (n=301)
Headache	5.4%	5.0%
Dizziness	3.0%	3.0%
Bradycardia	3.3%	1.3%
AV Block First Degree	3.3%	0.0%
Edema	2.6%	1.3%
ECG Abnormality	1.6%	2.3%
Asthenia	1.8%	1.7%

In clinical trials of CARDIZEM CD capsules, CARDIZEM tablets, and CARDIZEM SR capsules involving over 3200 patients, the most common events (ie, greater than 1%) were edema (4.6%), headache (4.6%), dizziness (3.5%), asthenia (2.6%), first-degree AV block (2.4%), bradycardia (1.7%), flushing (1.4%), nausea (1.4%), and rash (1.2%).

In addition, the following events were reported infrequently (less than 1%) in angina or hypertension trials:

Cardiovascular: Angina, arrhythmia, AV block (second- or third-degree), bundle branch block, congestive heart failure, ECG abnormalities, hypotension, palpitations, syncope, tachycardia, ventricular extrasystoles

Nervous System: Abnormal dreams, amnesia, depression, gait abnormality, hallucinations, insomnia, nervousness, paresthesia, personality change, somnolence, tinnitus, tremor

Gastrointestinal: Anorexia, constipation, diarrhea, dry mouth, dysgeusia, dyspepsia, mild elevations of SGOT, SGPT, LDH, and alkaline phosphatase (see hepatic warnings), thirst, vomiting, weight increase

Dermatological: Petechiae, photosensitivity, pruritus, urticaria

Other: Amblyopia, CPK increase, dyspnea, epistaxis, eye irritation, hyperglycemia, hyperuricemia, impotence, muscle cramps, nasal congestion, nocturia, osteoarticular pain, polyuria, sexual difficulties

The following postmarketing events have been reported infrequently in patients receiving CARDIZEM: allergic reactions, alopecia, angioedema (including facial or periorbital edema), asystole, erythema multiforme (including Stevens-Johnson syndrome, toxic epidermal necrolysis), exfoliative dermatitis, extrapyramidal symptoms, gingival hyperplasia, hemolytic anemia, increased bleeding time, leukopenia, purpura, retinopathy, and thrombocytopenia. In addition, events such as myocardial infarction have been observed which are not readily distinguishable from the natural history of the disease in these patients. A number of well-documented cases of generalized rash, some characterized as leukocytoclastic vasculitis, have been reported. However, a definitive cause and effect relationship between these events and CARDIZEM therapy is yet to be established.

OVERDOSAGE

The oral LD_{50}'s in mice and rats range from 415 to 740 mg/kg and from 560 to 810 mg/kg, respectively. The intravenous LD_{50}'s in these species were 60 and 38 mg/kg, respectively. The oral LD_{50} in dogs is considered to be in excess of 50 mg/kg, while lethality was seen in monkeys at 360 mg/kg.

The toxic dose in man is not known. Due to extensive metabolism, blood levels after a standard dose of diltiazem can vary over tenfold, limiting the usefulness of blood levels in overdose cases.

There have been 29 reports of diltiazem overdose in doses ranging from less than 1 g to 10.8 g. Sixteen of these reports involved multiple drug ingestions.

Twenty-two reports indicated patients had recovered from diltiazem overdose ranging from less than 1 g to 10.8 g. There were seven reports with a fatal outcome; although the amount of diltiazem ingested was unknown, multiple drug ingestions were confirmed in six of the seven reports.

Events observed following diltiazem overdose included bradycardia, hypotension, heart block, and cardiac failure. Most reports of overdose described some supportive medical measure and/or drug treatment. Bradycardia frequently responded favorably to atropine as did heart block, although cardiac pacing was also frequently utilized to treat heart block. Fluids and vasopressors were used to maintain blood pressure, and in cases of cardiac failure, inotropic agents were administered. In addition, some patients received treatment with ventilatory support, gastric lavage, activated charcoal, and/or intravenous calcium. Evidence of the effectiveness of intravenous calcium administration to reverse the pharmacological effects of diltiazem overdose was conflicting.

CARDIZEM® CD (diltiazem hydrochloride) Capsules

Strength	Quantity	NDC Number	Description
120 mg	30 btl 90 btl 100 UDIP®	0088-1795-30 0088-1795-42 0088-1795-49	Light turquoise blue/light turquoise blue capsule imprinted with cardizem CD and 120 mg on one end.
180 mg	30 btl 90 btl 100 UDIP®	0088-1796-30 0088-1796-42 0088-1796-49	Light turquoise blue/blue capsule imprinted with cardizem CD and 180 mg on one end.
240 mg	30 btl 90 btl 100 UDIP®	0088-1797-30 0088-1797-42 0088-1797-49	Blue/blue capsule imprinted with cardizem CD and 240 mg on one end.
300 mg	30 btl 90 btl 100 UDIP®	0088-1798-30 0088-1798-42 0088-1798-49	Light gray/blue capsule imprinted with cardizem CD and 300 mg on one end.
360 mg	90 btl	0088-1799-42	Light blue/white capsule imprinted with cardizem CD and 360 mg on one end.

In the event of overdose or exaggerated response, appropriate supportive measures should be employed in addition to gastrointestinal decontamination. Diltiazem does not appear to be removed by peritoneal or hemodialysis. Limited data suggest that plasmapheresis or charcoal hemoperfusion may hasten diltiazem elimination following overdose. Based on the known pharmacological effects of diltiazem and/or reported clinical experiences, the following measures may be considered:

Bradycardia: Administer atropine (0.60 to 1.0 mg). If there is no response to vagal blockade, administer isoproterenol cautiously.

High-degree AV Block: Treat as for bradycardia above. Fixed high-degree AV block should be treated with cardiac pacing.

Cardiac Failure: Administer inotropic agents (isoproterenol, dopamine, or dobutamine) and diuretics.

Hypotension: Vasopressors (eg, dopamine or levarterenol bitartrate).

Actual treatment and dosage should depend on the severity of the clinical situation and the judgment and experience of the treating physician.

DOSAGE AND ADMINISTRATION

Patients controlled on diltiazem alone or in combination with other medications may be switched to CARDIZEM CD capsules at the nearest equivalent total daily dose. Higher doses of CARDIZEM CD may be needed in some patients. Patients should be closely monitored. Subsequent titration to higher or lower doses may be necessary and should be initiated as clinically warranted. There is limited general clinical experience with doses above 360 mg, but doses to 540 mg have been studied in clinical trials. The incidence of side effects increases as the dose increases with first-degree AV block, dizziness, and sinus bradycardia bearing the strongest relationship to dose.

Hypertension. Dosage needs to be adjusted by titration to individual patient needs. When used as monotherapy, reasonable starting doses are 180 to 240 mg once daily, although some patients may respond to lower doses. Maximum antihypertensive effect is usually observed by 14 days of chronic therapy; therefore, dosage adjustments should be scheduled accordingly. The usual dosage range studied in clinical trials was 240 to 360 mg once daily. Individual patients may respond to higher doses of up to 480 mg once daily.

Angina. Dosages for the treatment of angina should be adjusted to each patient's needs, starting with a dose of 120 or 180 mg once daily. Individual patients may respond to higher doses of up to 480 mg once daily. When necessary, titration may be carried out over a 7- to 14-day period.

Concomitant Use With Other Cardiovascular Agents.

1. **Sublingual NTG.** May be taken as required to abort acute anginal attacks during CARDIZEM CD (diltiazem hydrochloride) therapy.
2. **Prophylactic Nitrate Therapy.** CARDIZEM CD may be safely coadministered with short- and long-acting nitrates.
3. **Beta-blockers.** (See WARNINGS and PRECAUTIONS.)
4. **Antihypertensives.** CARDIZEM CD has an additive antihypertensive effect when used with other antihypertensive agents. Therefore, the dosage of CARDIZEM CD or the concomitant antihypertensives may need to be adjusted when adding one to the other.

HOW SUPPLIED

[See table at top of previous page]

Storage Conditions: Store at 25°C (77°F); excursions permitted to 15–30°C (59–86°F) [see USP Controlled Room Temperature]. Avoid excessive humidity.

Prescribing Information as of May 1999

Hoechst Marion Roussel, Inc.
Kansas City, MO 64137 USA
www.hmri.com

Shown in Product Identification Guide, page 306

CARDIZEM® Injectable ℞

[*kar'diz-em*]
(diltiazem HCl injection)

CARDIZEM® Lyo-Ject® Syringe

(diltiazem HCl)

CARDIZEM® Monovial®

(diltiazem HCl for injection)

Prescribing Information as of June 1997

DESCRIPTION

CARDIZEM® (diltiazem hydrochloride) is a calcium ion influx inhibitor (slow channel blocker or calcium channel antagonist). Chemically, diltiazem hydrochloride is 1,5-benzothiazepin-4(5H)one,3-(acetyloxy)-5-[2-(dimethyl-amino) ethyl]-2, 3-dihydro-2-(4-methoxyphenyl)-, monohydrochloride,(+)-cis-. The chemical structure is:

[See chemical structure at top of next column]

Diltiazem hydrochloride is a white to off-white crystalline powder with a bitter taste. It is soluble in water, methanol, and chloroform. It has a molecular weight of 450.98.

CARDIZEM Injectable (diltiazem hydrochloride injection) is a clear, colorless, sterile, nonpyrogenic solution. It has a pH range of 3.7 to 4.1.

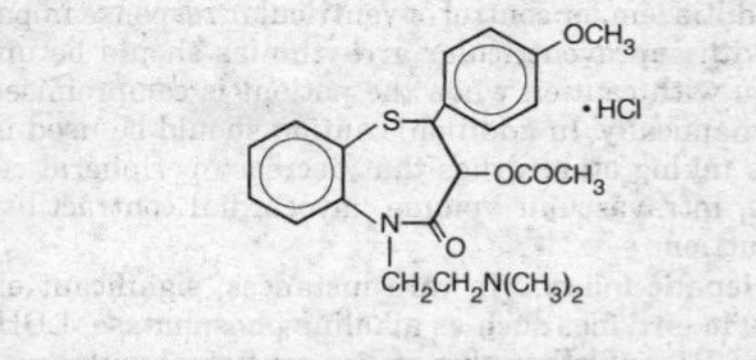

CARDIZEM Injectable is for direct intravenous bolus injection and continuous intravenous infusion.

25-mg, 5-mL vial—each sterile vial contains 25 mg diltiazem hydrochloride, 3.75 mg citric acid USP, 3.25 mg sodium citrate dihydrate USP, 357 mg sorbitol solution USP, and water for injection USP up to 5 mL. Sodium hydroxide or hydrochloric acid is used for pH adjustment.

50-mg, 10-mL vial—each sterile vial contains 50 mg diltiazem hydrochloride, 7.5 mg citric acid USP, 6.5 mg sodium citrate dihydrate USP, 714 mg sorbitol solution USP, and water for injection USP up to 10 mL. Sodium hydroxide or hydrochloric acid is used for pH adjustment.

CARDIZEM Lyo-Ject Syringe (diltiazem hydrochloride) after reconstitution contains a clear, colorless, sterile, nonpyrogenic solution. It has a pH range of 4.0 to 7.0.

CARDIZEM Lyo-Ject Syringe after reconstitution is for direct intravenous bolus injection and continuous intravenous infusion.

CARDIZEM Lyo-Ject Syringe 25-mg syringe is available in a dual chamber, disposable syringe. Chamber 1 contains lyophilized powder comprised of diltiazem hydrochloride 25 mg and mannitol USP 37.5 mg. Chamber 2 contains sterile diluent composed of 5 mL water for injection with 0.5% benzyl alcohol NF, and 0.6% sodium chloride USP.

CARDIZEM Monovial (diltiazem hydrochloride for injection), after reconstitution in an infusion bag, produces a clear, colorless, sterile nonpyrogenic solution.

CARDIZEM Monovial for continuous intravenous infusion is available in a glass vial with transfer needle set. The vial contains lyophilized powder comprised of diltiazem hydrochloride 100 mg and mannitol USP 75 mg.

CLINICAL PHARMACOLOGY

Mechanisms of Action.

CARDIZEM inhibits the influx of calcium (Ca^{2+}) ions during membrane depolarization of cardiac and vascular smooth muscle. The therapeutic benefits of CARDIZEM in supraventricular tachycardias are related to its ability to slow AV nodal conduction time and prolong AV nodal refractoriness. CARDIZEM exhibits frequency (use) dependent effects on AV nodal conduction such that it may selectively reduce the heart rate during tachycardias involving the AV node with little or no effect on normal AV nodal conduction at normal heart rates.

CARDIZEM slows the ventricular rate in patients with a rapid ventricular response during atrial fibrillation or atrial flutter. CARDIZEM converts paroxysmal supraventricular tachycardia (PSVT) to normal sinus rhythm by interrupting the reentry circuit in AV nodal reentrant tachycardias and reciprocating tachycardias, eg, Wolff-Parkinson-White syndrome (WPW).

CARDIZEM prolongs the sinus cycle length. It has no effect on the sinus node recovery time or on the sinoatrial conduction time in patients without SA nodal dysfunction. CARDIZEM has no significant electrophysiologic effects on tissues in the heart that are fast sodium channel dependent, eg, His-Purkinje tissue, atrial and ventricular muscle, and extranodal accessory pathways.

Like other calcium channel antagonists, because of its effect on vascular smooth muscle, CARDIZEM decreases total peripheral resistance resulting in a decrease in both systolic and diastolic blood pressure.

Hemodynamics.

In patients with cardiovascular disease, CARDIZEM Injectable (diltiazem hydrochloride injection) administered intravenously in single bolus doses, followed in some cases by a continuous infusion, reduced blood pressure, systemic vascular resistance, the rate-pressure product, and coronary vascular resistance and increased coronary blood flow. In a limited number of studies of patients with compromised myocardium (severe congestive heart failure, acute myocardial infarction, hypertrophic cardiomyopathy), administration of intravenous diltiazem produced no significant effect on contractility, left ventricular end diastolic pressure, or pulmonary capillary wedge pressure. The mean ejection fraction and cardiac output/index remained unchanged or increased. Maximal hemodynamic effects usually occurred within 2 to 5 minutes of an injection. However, in rare instances, worsening of congestive heart failure has been reported in patients with preexisting impaired ventricular function.

Pharmacodynamics.

The prolongation of PR interval correlated significantly with plasma diltiazem concentration in normal volunteers using the Sigmoidal E_{max} model. Changes in heart rate, systolic blood pressure, and diastolic blood pressure did not correlate with diltiazem plasma concentrations in normal volunteers. Reduction in mean arterial pressure correlated linearly with diltiazem plasma concentration in a group of hypertensive patients.

In patients with atrial fibrillation and atrial flutter, a significant correlation was observed between the percent reduction in HR and plasma diltiazem concentration using the Sigmoidal E_{max} model. Based on this relationship, the mean plasma diltiazem concentration required to produce a 20% decrease in heart rate was determined to be 80 ng/mL. Mean plasma diltiazem concentrations of 130 ng/mL and 300 ng/mL were determined to produce reductions in heart rate of 30% and 40%.

Pharmacokinetics and Metabolism.

Following a single intravenous injection in healthy male volunteers, CARDIZEM appears to obey linear pharmacokinetics over a dose range of 10.5 to 21.0 mg. The plasma elimination half-life is approximately 3.4 hours. The apparent volume of distribution of CARDIZEM is approximately 305 L. CARDIZEM is extensively metabolized in the liver with a systemic clearance of approximately 65 L/h.

After constant rate intravenous infusion to healthy male volunteers, diltiazem exhibits nonlinear pharmacokinetics over an infusion range of 4.8 to 13.2 mg/h for 24 hours. Over this infusion range, as the dose is increased, systemic clearance decreases from 64 to 48 L/h while the plasma elimination half-life increases from 4.1 to 4.9 hours. The apparent volume of distribution remains unchanged (360 to 391 L). In patients with atrial fibrillation or atrial flutter, diltiazem systemic clearance has been found to be decreased compared to healthy volunteers. In patients administered bolus doses ranging from 2.5 mg to 38.5 mg, systemic clearance averaged 36 L/h. In patients administered continuous infusions at 10 mg/h or 15 mg/h for 24 hours, diltiazem systemic clearance averaged 42 L/h and 31 L/h, respectively.

Based on the results of pharmacokinetic studies in healthy volunteers administered different ***oral*** CARDIZEM formulations, constant rate intravenous infusions of CARDIZEM at 3, 5, 7, and 11 mg/h are predicted to produce steady-state plasma diltiazem concentrations equivalent to 120-, 180-, 240-, and 360-mg total daily oral doses of CARDIZEM tablets or CARDIZEM SR capsules.

After oral administration, CARDIZEM undergoes extensive metabolism in man by deacetylation, N-demethylation, and O-demethylation via cytochrome P-450 (oxidative metabolism) in addition to conjugation. Metabolites N-monodesmethyldiltiazem, desacetyldiltiazem, desacetyl-N-monodesmethyldiltiazem, desacetyl-O-desmethyldiltiazem, and desacetyl-N, O-desmethyldiltiazem have been identified in human urine. Following oral administration, 2% to 4% of the unchanged CARDIZEM appears in the urine. Drugs which induce or inhibit hepatic microsomal enzymes may alter diltiazem disposition.

Following single intravenous injection of CARDIZEM, however, plasma concentrations of N-monodesmethyldiltiazem and desacetyldiltiazem, two principal metabolites found in plasma after oral administration, are typically not detected. These metabolites are observed, however, following 24 hour constant rate intravenous infusion. Total radioactivity measurement following short IV administration in healthy volunteers suggests the presence of other unidentified metabolites which attain higher concentrations than those of diltiazem and are more slowly eliminated; half-life of total radioactivity is about 20 hours compared to 2 to 5 hours for diltiazem.

CARDIZEM is 70% to 80% bound to plasma proteins. In vitro studies suggest alpha$_1$-acid glycoprotein binds approximately 40% of the drug at clinically significant concentrations. Albumin appears to bind approximately 30% of the drug, while other constituents bind the remaining bound fraction. Competitive in vitro ligand binding studies have shown that CARDIZEM binding is not altered by therapeutic concentrations of digoxin, phenytoin, hydrochlorothiazide, indomethacin, phenylbutazone, propranolol, salicylic acid, tolbutamide, or warfarin.

Renal insufficiency, or even end-stage renal disease, does not appear to influence diltiazem disposition following ***oral*** administration. Liver cirrhosis was shown to reduce diltiazem's apparent ***oral*** clearance and prolong its half-life.

INDICATIONS AND USAGE

CARDIZEM Injectable, CARDIZEM Lyo-Ject Syringe, or CARDIZEM Monovial (diltiazem hydrochloride for injection) are indicated for the following:

Atrial Fibrillation or Atrial Flutter. Temporary control of rapid ventricular rate in atrial fibrillation or atrial flutter. It should not be used in patients with atrial fibrillation or atrial flutter associated with an accessory bypass tract such as in Wolff-Parkinson-White (WPW) syndrome or short PR syndrome.

In addition, CARDIZEM Injectable or CARDIZEM Lyo-Ject Syringe are indicated for:

Paroxysmal Supraventricular Tachycardia. Rapid conversion of paroxysmal supraventricular tachycardias (PSVT) to sinus rhythm. This includes AV nodal reentrant tachycardias and reciprocating tachycardias associated with an extranodal accessory pathway such as the WPW syndrome or short PR syndrome. Unless otherwise contraindicated, appropriate vagal maneuvers should be attempted prior to administration of CARDIZEM Injectable or CARDIZEM Lyo-Ject Syringe.

The use of CARDIZEM Injectable, CARDIZEM Lyo-Ject Syringe, or CARDIZEM Monovial should be undertaken with caution when the patient is compromised hemodynamically or is taking other drugs that decrease any or all of the following: peripheral resistance, myocardial filling, myocardial contractility, or electrical impulse propagation in the myocardium.

Continued on next page

Cardizem Injectable—Cont.

For either indication and particularly when employing continuous intravenous infusion, the setting should include continuous monitoring of the ECG and frequent measurement of blood pressure. A defibrillator and emergency equipment should be readily available.

In domestic controlled trials in patients with atrial fibrillation or atrial flutter, bolus administration of CARDIZEM Injectable was effective in reducing heart rate by at least 20% in 95% of patients. CARDIZEM Injectable rarely converts atrial fibrillation or atrial flutter to normal sinus rhythm. Following administration of one or two intravenous bolus doses of CARDIZEM Injectable, response usually occurs within 3 minutes and maximal heart rate reduction generally occurs in 2 to 7 minutes. Heart rate reduction may last from 1 to 3 hours. If hypotension occurs, it is generally short-lived, but may last from 1 to 3 hours.

A 24-hour continuous infusion of CARDIZEM Injectable in the treatment of atrial fibrillation or atrial flutter maintained at least a 20% heart rate reduction during the infusion in 83% of patients. Upon discontinuation of infusion, heart rate reduction may last from 0.5 hours to more than 10 hours (median duration 7 hours). Hypotension, if it occurs, may be simply persistent.

In the controlled clinical trials, 3.2% of patients required some form of intervention (typically, use of intravenous fluids or the Trendelenburg position) for blood pressure support following CARDIZEM Injectable.

In domestic controlled trials, bolus administration of CARDIZEM Injectable was effective in converting PSVT to normal sinus rhythm in 88% of patients within 3 minutes of the first or second bolus dose.

Symptoms associated with the arrhythmia were improved in conjunction with decreased heart rate or conversion to normal sinus rhythm following administration of CARDIZEM Injectable.

CONTRAINDICATIONS

Injectable forms of diltiazem are contraindicated in:

1. Patients with sick sinus syndrome except in the presence of a functioning ventricular pacemaker.
2. Patients with second- or third-degree AV block except in the presence of a functioning ventricular pacemaker.
3. Patients with severe hypotension or cardiogenic shock.
4. Patients who have demonstrated hypersensitivity to the drug.
5. Intravenous diltiazem and intravenous beta-blockers should not be administered together or in close proximity (within a few hours).
6. Patients with atrial fibrillation or atrial flutter associated with an accessory bypass tract such as in WPW syndrome or short PR syndrome.

   As with other agents which slow AV nodal conduction and do not prolong the refractoriness of the accessory pathway (eg, verapamil, digoxin), in rare instances patients in atrial fibrillation or atrial flutter associated with an accessory bypass tract may experience a potentially life-threatening increase in heart rate accompanied by hypotension when treated with injectable forms of diltiazem. As such, the initial use of injectable forms of diltiazem should be, if possible, in a setting where monitoring and resuscitation capabilities, including DC cardioversion/defibrillation, are present (see OVERDOSAGE). Once familiarity of the patient's response is established, use in an office setting may be acceptable.
7. Patients with ventricular tachycardia. Administration of other calcium channel blockers to patients with wide complex tachycardia (QRS ≥0.12 seconds) has resulted in hemodynamic deterioration and ventricular fibrillation. It is important that an accurate pretreatment diagnosis distinguish wide complex QRS tachycardia of supraventricular origin from that of ventricular origin prior to administration of injectable forms of diltiazem.
8. In newborns, due to the presence of benzyl alcohol (CARDIZEM Lyo-Ject Syringe only).

WARNINGS

1. **Cardiac Conduction.** Diltiazem prolongs AV nodal conduction and refractoriness that may rarely result in second- or third-degree AV block in sinus rhythm. Concomitant use of diltiazem with agents known to affect cardiac conduction may result in additive effects (see Drug Interactions). If high-degree AV block occurs in sinus rhythm, intravenous diltiazem should be discontinued and appropriate supportive measures instituted (see OVERDOSAGE).
2. **Congestive Heart Failure.** Although diltiazem has a negative inotropic effect in isolated animal tissue preparations, hemodynamic studies in humans with normal ventricular function and in patients with a compromised myocardium, such as severe CHF, acute MI, and hypertrophic cardiomyopathy, have not shown a reduction in cardiac index nor consistent negative effects on contractility (dp/dt). Administration of oral diltiazem in patients with acute myocardial infarction and pulmonary congestion documented by x-ray on admission is contraindicated. Experience with the use of CARDIZEM Injectable in patients with impaired ventricular function is limited. Caution should be exercised when using the drug in such patients.
3. **Hypotension.** Decreases in blood pressure associated with CARDIZEM Injectable therapy may occasionally result in symptomatic hypotension (3.2%). The use of intravenous diltiazem for control of ventricular response in patients with supraventricular arrhythmias should be undertaken with caution when the patient is compromised hemodynamically. In addition, caution should be used in patients taking other drugs that decrease peripheral resistance, intravascular volume, myocardial contractility or conduction.
4. **Acute Hepatic Injury.** In rare instances, significant elevations in enzymes such as alkaline phosphatase, LDH, SGOT, SGPT, and other phenomena consistent with acute hepatic injury have been noted following oral diltiazem. Therefore, the potential for acute hepatic injury exists following administration of intravenous diltiazem.
5. **Ventricular Premature Beats (VPBs).** VPBs may be present on conversion of PSVT to sinus rhythm with CARDIZEM Injectable. These VPBs are transient, are typically considered to be benign, and appear to have no clinical significance. Similar ventricular complexes have been noted during cardioversion, other pharmacologic therapy, and during spontaneous conversion of PSVT to sinus rhythm.

PRECAUTIONS

General

CARDIZEM (diltiazem hydrochloride) is extensively metabolized by the liver and excreted by the kidneys and in bile. The drug should be used with caution in patients with impaired renal or hepatic function (see WARNINGS). High intravenous dosages (4.5 mg/kg tid) administered to dogs resulted in significant bradycardia and alterations in AV conduction. In subacute and chronic dog and rat studies designed to produce toxicity, high oral doses of diltiazem were associated with hepatic damage. In special subacute hepatic studies, oral doses of 125 mg/kg and higher in rats were associated with histological changes in the liver, which were reversible when the drug was discontinued. In dogs, oral doses of 20 mg/kg were also associated with hepatic changes; however, these changes were reversible with continued dosing.

Dermatologic events progressing to erythema multiforme and/or exfoliative dermatitis have been infrequently reported following oral diltiazem. Therefore, the potential for these dermatologic reactions exists following exposure to intravenous diltiazem. Should a dermatologic reaction persist, the drug should be discontinued.

Drug Interactions

Due to potential for additive effects, caution is warranted in patients receiving CARDIZEM Injectable, CARDIZEM Lyo-Ject Syringe, or CARDIZEM Monovial concomitantly with other agent(s) known to affect cardiac contractility and/or SA or AV node conduction (see WARNINGS).

As with all drugs, care should be exercised when treating patients with multiple medications. CARDIZEM undergoes extensive metabolism by the cytochrome P-450 mixed function oxidase system. Although specific pharmacokinetic drug-drug interaction studies have not been conducted with single intravenous injection or constant rate intravenous infusion, coadministration of injectable diltiazem with other agents which primarily undergo the same route of biotransformation may result in competitive inhibition of metabolism.

Digitalis. Intravenous diltiazem has been administered to patients receiving either intravenous or oral digitalis therapy. The combination of the two drugs was well tolerated without serious adverse effects. However, since both drugs affect AV nodal conduction, patients should be monitored for excessive slowing of the heart rate and/or AV block.

Beta-blockers. Intravenous diltiazem has been administered to patients on chronic oral beta-blocker therapy. The combination of the two drugs was generally well tolerated without serious adverse effects. If intravenous diltiazem is administered to patients receiving chronic oral beta-blocker therapy, the possibility for bradycardia, AV block, and/or depression of contractility should be considered (see CONTRAINDICATIONS). ***Oral*** administration of diltiazem with propranolol in five normal volunteers resulted in increased propranolol levels in all subjects and bioavailability of propranolol was increased approximately 50%. In vitro, propranolol appears to be displaced from its binding sites by diltiazem.

Anesthetics. The depression of cardiac contractility, conductivity, and automaticity as well as the vascular dilation associated with anesthetics may be potentiated by calcium channel blockers. When used concomitantly, anesthetics and calcium blockers should be titrated carefully.

Cyclosporine. A pharmacokinetic interaction between diltiazem and cyclosporine has been observed during studies involving renal and cardiac transplant patients. In renal and cardiac transplant recipients, a reduction of cyclosporine dose ranging from 15% to 48% was necessary to maintain cyclosporine trough concentrations similar to those seen prior to the addition of diltiazem. If these agents are to be administered concurrently, cyclosporine concentrations should be monitored, especially when diltiazem therapy is initiated, adjusted or discontinued.

The effect of cyclosporine on diltiazem plasma concentrations has not been evaluated.

Carbamazepine. Concomitant administration of ***oral*** diltiazem with carbamazepine has been reported to result in elevated plasma levels of carbamazepine (by 40 to 72%), resulting in toxicity in some cases. Patients receiving these drugs concurrently should be monitored for a potential drug interaction.

Carcinogenesis, Mutagenesis, Impairment of Fertility

A 24-month study in rats at oral dosage levels of up to 100 mg/kg/day and a 21-month study in mice at oral dosage levels of up to 30 mg/kg/day showed no evidence of carcinogenicity. There was also no mutagenic response in vitro or in vivo in mammalian cell assays or in vitro in bacteria. No evidence of impaired fertility was observed in a study performed in male and female rats at oral dosages of up to 100 mg/kg/day.

Pregnancy

Category C. Reproduction studies have been conducted in mice, rats, and rabbits.

Administration of oral doses ranging from five to ten times greater (on a mg/kg basis) than the daily recommended oral antianginal therapeutic dose has resulted in embryo and fetal lethality. These doses, in some studies, have been reported to cause skeletal abnormalities. In the perinatal/postnatal studies there was some reduction in early individual pup weights and survival rates. There was an increased incidence of stillbirths at doses of 20 times the human oral antianginal dose or greater.

There are no well-controlled studies in pregnant women; therefore, use CARDIZEM in pregnant women only if the potential benefit justifies the potential risk to the fetus.

Nursing Mothers

Diltiazem is excreted in human milk. One report with oral diltiazem suggests that concentrations in breast milk may approximate serum levels. If use of CARDIZEM is deemed essential, an alternative method of infant feeding should be instituted.

Pediatric Use

Safety and effectiveness in pediatric patients have not been established.

ADVERSE REACTIONS

The following adverse reaction rates are based on the use of CARDIZEM Injectable in over 400 domestic clinical trial patients with atrial fibrillation/flutter or PSVT under double-blind or open-label conditions. Worldwide experience in over 1300 patients was similar.

Adverse events reported in controlled and uncontrolled clinical trials were generally mild and transient. Hypotension was the most commonly reported adverse event during clinical trials. Asymptomatic hypotension occurred in 4.3% of patients. Symptomatic hypotension occurred in 3.2% of patients. When treatment for hypotension was required, it generally consisted of administration of saline or placing the patient in the Trendelenburg position. Other events reported in at least 1% of the diltiazem-treated patients were injection site reactions (eg, itching, burning) 3.9%, vasodilation (flushing) 1.7%, and arrhythmia (junctional rhythm or isorhythmic dissociation) 1.0%.

In addition, the following events were reported infrequently (less than 1%):

Cardiovascular: Asystole, atrial flutter, AV block first degree, AV block second degree, bradycardia, chest pain, congestive heart failure, sinus pause, sinus node dysfunction, syncope, ventricular arrhythmia, ventricular fibrillation, ventricular tachycardia

Dermatologic: Pruritus, sweating

Gastrointestinal: Constipation, elevated SGOT or alkaline phosphatase, nausea, vomiting

Nervous System: Dizziness, paresthesia

Other: Amblyopia, asthenia, dry mouth, dyspnea, edema, headache, hyperuricemia

Although not observed in clinical trials with CARDIZEM Injectable, the following events associated with oral diltiazem may occur:

Cardiovascular: AV block (third degree), bundle branch block, ECG abnormality, palpitations, syncope, tachycardia, ventricular extrasystoles

Dermatologic: Alopecia, erythema multiforme (including Stevens-Johnson syndrome, toxic epidermal necrolysis), exfoliative dermatitis, leukocytoclastic vasculitis, petechiae, photosensitivity, purpura, rash, urticaria

Gastrointestinal: Anorexia, diarrhea, dysgeusia, dyspepsia, mild elevations of SGPT and LDH, thirst, weight increase

Nervous System: Abnormal dreams, amnesia, depression, extrapyramidal symptoms, gait abnormality, hallucinations, insomnia, nervousness, personality change, somnolence, tremor

Other: Allergic reactions, angioedema (including facial or periorbital edema), CPK elevation, epistaxis, eye irritation, gingival hyperplasia, hemolytic anemia, hyperglycemia, impotence, increased bleeding time, leukopenia, muscle cramps, nasal congestion, nocturia, osteoarticular pain, polyuria, retinopathy, sexual difficulties, thrombocytopenia, tinnitus

Events such as myocardial infarction have been observed which are not readily distinguishable from the natural history of the disease for the patient.

OVERDOSAGE

Overdosage experience is limited. In the event of overdosage or an exaggerated response, appropriate supportive measures should be employed. The following measures may be considered:

Bradycardia: Administer atropine (0.60 to 1.0 mg). If there is no response to vagal blockade administer isoproterenol cautiously.

High-degree AV Block: Treat as for bradycardia above. Fixed high-degree AV block should be treated with cardiac pacing.

CARDIZEM Injectable or CARDIZEM Lyo-Ject Syringe

Diluent Volume	Quantity of CARDIZEM Injectable or CARDIZEM Lyo-Ject to Add	Final Concentration	Administration	
			Dose*	Infusion Rate
100 mL	125 mg (25 mL) Final Volume 125 mL	1 mg/mL	10 mg/h 15 mg/h	10 mL/h 15 mL/h
250 mL	250 mg (50 mL) Final Volume 300 mL	0.83 mg/mL	10 mg/h 15 mg/h	12 mL/h 18 mL/h
500 mL	250 mg (50 mL) Final Volume 550 mL	0.45 mg/mL	10 mg/h 15 mg/h	22 mL/h 33 mL/h

*5 mg/h may be appropriate for some patients

CARDIZEM Monovial

Diluent Volume	Quantity of CARDIZEM Monovial to Add	Final Concentration	Administration	
			Dose*	Infusion Rate
100 mL	100 mg (1 monovial)	1 mg/mL	10 mg/h 15 mg/h	10 mL/h 15 mL/h
250 mL	200 mg (2 monovials)	0.80 mg/mL	10 mg/h 15 mg/h	12.5 mL/h 18.8 mL/h
500 mL	200 mg (2 monovials)	0.40 mg/mL	10 mg/h 15 mg/h	25 mL/h 37.5 mL/h

*5 mg/h may be appropriate for some patients

Cardiac Failure: Administer inotropic agents (isoproterenol, dopamine, or dobutamine) and diuretics.

Hypotension: Vasopressors (eg, dopamine or levarterenol bitartrate).

Actual treatment and dosage should depend on the severity of the clinical situation and the judgment and experience of the treating physician.

Diltiazem does not appear to be removed by peritoneal or hemodialysis. Limited data suggest that plasmapheresis or charcoal hemoperfusion may hasten diltiazem elimination following overdose.

The intravenous LD_{50}'s in mice and rats were 60 and 38 mg/kg, respectively. The toxic dose in man is not known.

DOSAGE AND ADMINISTRATION

Direct Intravenous Single Injections (Bolus)

The initial dose of CARDIZEM Injectable or CARDIZEM Lyo-Ject Syringe (see instructions for reconstitution of Lyo-Ject Syringe in blister pack) should be 0.25 mg/kg actual body weight as a bolus administered over 2 minutes (20 mg is a reasonable dose for the average patient). If response is inadequate, a second dose may be administered after 15 minutes. The second bolus dose of CARDIZEM Injectable or CARDIZEM Lyo-Ject Syringe should be 0.35 mg/kg actual body weight administered over 2 minutes (25 mg is a reasonable dose for the average patient). Subsequent intravenous bolus doses should be individualized for each patient. Patients with low body weights should be dosed on a mg/kg basis. Some patients may respond to an initial dose of 0.15 mg/kg, although duration of action may be shorter. Experience with this dose is limited.

Continuous Intravenous Infusion

For continued reduction of the heart rate (up to 24 hours) in patients with atrial fibrillation or atrial flutter, an intravenous infusion of CARDIZEM Injectable, CARDIZEM Lyo-Ject Syringe, or CARDIZEM Monovial may be administered. (For reconstitution of CARDIZEM Lyo-Ject Syringe or CARDIZEM Monovial, see instructions contained within packaging.) Immediately following bolus administration of 20 mg (0.25 mg/kg) or 25 mg (0.35 mg/kg) CARDIZEM Injectable or CARDIZEM Lyo-Ject Syringe, and reduction of heart rate, begin an intravenous infusion of CARDIZEM Injectable, CARDIZEM Lyo-Ject Syringe, or CARDIZEM Monovial. The recommended initial infusion rate of CARDIZEM Injectable, CARDIZEM Lyo-Ject Syringe, or CARDIZEM Monovial is 10 mg/h. Some patients may maintain response to an initial rate of 5 mg/h. The infusion rate may be increased in 5 mg/h increments up to 15 mg/h as needed, if further reduction in heart rate is required. The infusion may be maintained for up to 24 hours.

Diltiazem shows dose-dependent, non-linear pharmacokinetics. Duration of infusion longer than 24 hours and infusion rates greater than 15 mg/h have not been studied. Therefore, infusion duration exceeding 24 hours and infusion rates exceeding 15 mg/h are not recommended.

Dilution: To prepare CARDIZEM Injectable, CARDIZEM Lyo-Ject Syringe, or CARDIZEM Monovial for continuous intravenous infusion, aseptically transfer the appropriate quantity (see charts) of CARDIZEM to the desired volume of either Normal Saline, D5W, or D5W/0.45% NaCl. Mix thoroughly. Keep diluted CARDIZEM Injectable refrigerated until use. Diluted CARDIZEM Lyo-Ject Syringe and CARDIZEM Monovial may be stored at room temperature 15–30°C (59–86°F). Use within 24 hours.

[See tables above]

Compatibility: CARDIZEM Injectable, CARDIZEM Lyo-Ject Syringe, and CARDIZEM Monovial were tested for compatibility with three commonly used intravenous fluids at a maximal concentration of 1 mg diltiazem hydrochloride per milliliter. CARDIZEM Injectable, CARDIZEM Lyo-Ject Syringe, and CARDIZEM Monovial were found to be physically compatible and chemically stable in the following parenteral solutions for at least 24 hours when stored in glass (CARDIZEM Injectable/CARDIZEM Lyo-Ject Syringe only) or polyvinylchloride (PVC) bags at controlled room temperature 15–30°C (59–86°F) or under refrigeration 2–8°C (36–46°F).

- dextrose (5%) injection USP
- sodium chloride (0.9%) injection USP
- dextrose (5%) and sodium chloride (0.45%) injection USP.

Physical Incompatibilities:

Because of potential physical incompatibilities, it is recommended that CARDIZEM Injectable, CARDIZEM Lyo-Ject Syringe, or CARDIZEM Monovial not be mixed with any other drugs in the same container. If possible, it is recommended that CARDIZEM Injectable, CARDIZEM Lyo-Ject Syringe, or CARDIZEM Monovial not be co-infused in the same intravenous line. Parenteral drug products should be inspected visually for particulate matter and discoloration prior to administration whenever solution and container permit.

CARDIZEM Injectable/CARDIZEM Lyo-Ject Syringe. Physical incompatibilities (precipitate formation or cloudiness) were observed when CARDIZEM Injectable or CARDIZEM Lyo-Ject Syringe was infused in the same intravenous line with the following drugs: acetazolamide, acyclovir, aminophylline, ampicillin, ampicillin sodium/sulbactam sodium, cefamandole, cefoperazone, diazepam, furosemide, hydrocortisone sodium succinate, insulin, (regular: 100 units/mL), methylprednisolone sodium succinate, mezlocillin, nafcillin, phenytoin, rifampin, and sodium bicarbonate.

NOTE: CARDIZEM Lyo-Ject Syringe was found to be compatible with insulin (regular, 100 units/mL).

CARDIZEM Monovial. Physical incompatibilities (precipitate formation or cloudiness) were observed when CARDIZEM Monovial at a concentration of 1 mg/mL diluted in normal saline was infused in the same intravenous line with the following drugs: acetazolamide, acyclovir, cefoperazone sodium, diazepam, furosemide, phenytoin and rifampin.

NOTE: CARDIZEM Monovial at a concentration of 1 mg/mL diluted in normal saline was infused in the same intravenous line and was found to be compatible with the following drugs: aminophylline, ampicillin sodium, ampicillin sodium/sulbactam sodium, cefamandole, hydrocortisone sodium succinate, regular insulin (100 units/mL), methylprednisolone sodium succinate, mezlocillin sodium, nafcillin sodium and sodium bicarbonate.

Transition to Further Antiarrhythmic Therapy.

Transition to other antiarrhythmic agents following administration of CARDIZEM Injectable is generally safe. However, reference should be made to the respective agent manufacturer's package insert for information relative to dosage and administration.

In controlled clinical trials, therapy with antiarrhythmic agents to maintain reduced heart rate in atrial fibrillation or atrial flutter or for prophylaxis of PSVT was generally started within 3 hours after bolus administration of CARDIZEM Injectable. These antiarrhythmic agents were intravenous or oral digoxin, Class 1 antiarrhythmics (eg, quinidine, procainamide), calcium channel blockers, and oral beta-blockers.

Experience in the use of antiarrhythmic agents following maintenance infusion of CARDIZEM Injectable is limited. Patients should be dosed on an individual basis and reference should be made to the respective manufacturer's package insert for information relative to dosage and administration.

HOW SUPPLIED

CARDIZEM® Injectable (diltiazem hydrochloride injection) is supplied in boxes of six 5-mL vials with each vial containing 25 mg of diltiazem hydrochloride (5 mg/mL) (NDC 0088-1790-32) and boxes of six 10-mL vials with each vial containing 50 mg diltiazem hydrochloride (5 mg/mL) (NDC 0088-1790-33). STORE PRODUCT UNDER REFRIGERATION 2–8°C (36–46°F). DO NOT FREEZE. MAY BE STORED AT ROOM TEMPERATURE FOR UP TO 1 MONTH. DESTROY AFTER 1 MONTH AT ROOM TEMPERATURE. SINGLE-USE CONTAINERS. DISCARD UNUSED PORTION.

CARDIZEM Lyo-Ject 25-mg syringe is supplied in a single molded nonsterile tray in cartons of 6 syringes (NDC 0088-1789-17—formerly NDC 0088-1790-17). PRODUCT IS TO BE STORED AT ROOM TEMPERATURE 15–30°C (59–86°F). DO NOT FREEZE. RECONSTITUTED MATERIAL IS STABLE FOR 24 HOURS AT CONTROLLED ROOM TEMPERATURE. SINGLE-USE CONTAINERS. DISCARD UNUSED PORTION.

CARDIZEM Monovial for continuous infusion (100 mg) is supplied in a glass vial with transfer needle set (NDC 0088-1788-16). PRODUCT IS TO BE STORED AT ROOM TEMPERATURE 15–30°C (59–86°F). DO NOT FREEZE. RECONSTITUTED MATERIAL IS STABLE FOR 24 HOURS AT CONTROLLED ROOM TEMPERATURE. SINGLE-USE VIAL.

Monovial® is a registered trademark of Becton Dickinson S.A.

Cardizem® is a registered trademark of Carderm Capital L.P.

Lyo-Ject® is a registered trademark of Arzneimittel GmbH Apotheker Vetter & Company.

Prescribing Information as of June 1997

Manufactured for:
Hoechst Marion Roussel, Inc.
Kansas City, MO 64137 USA

Shown in Product Identification Guide, page 306

CLAFORAN® ℞

[kla 'fər-an]

Sterile (sterile cefotaxime sodium)
and
Injection (cefotaxime sodium injection)

Prescribing Information as of October 1996

DESCRIPTION

Sterile CLAFORAN® (cefotaxime sodium) is a semisynthetic, broad spectrum cephalosporin antibiotic for parenteral administration. It is the sodium salt of 7-[2-(2-amino-4-thiazolyl) glyoxylamido]-3-(hydroxymethyl)-8-oxo-5-thia-1-azabicyclo [4.2.0] oct-2-ene-2-carboxylate 7^2 (Z)-(o-methyloxime), acetate (ester). CLAFORAN contains approximately 50.5 mg (2.2 mEq) of sodium per gram of cefotaxime activity. Solutions of CLAFORAN range from very pale yellow to light amber depending on the concentration and the diluent used. The pH of the injectable solutions usually ranges from 5.0 to 7.5. The CAS Registry Number is 64485-93-4.

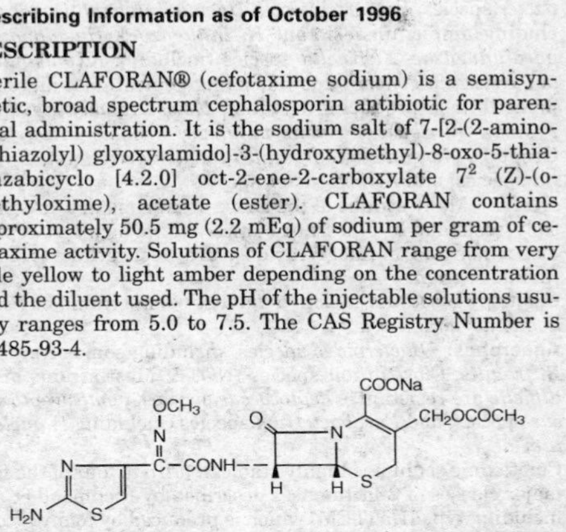

CLAFORAN is supplied as a dry powder in conventional and ADD-Vantage® System compatible vials, infusion bottles, pharmacy bulk package bottles, and as a frozen, premixed, iso-osmotic injection in a buffered diluent solution in plastic containers. CLAFORAN, equivalent to 1 gram and 2 grams cefotaxime, is supplied as frozen, premixed iso-osmotic injections in plastic containers. Solutions range from very pale yellow to light amber. Dextrose Hydrous, USP has been added to adjust osmolality (approximately 1.7 g and 700 mg to the 1 g and 2 g cefotaxime dosages, respectively). The injections are buffered with sodium citrate hydrous, USP. The pH is adjusted with hydrochloric acid and may be adjusted with sodium hydroxide.

The plastic container is fabricated from a specially designed multilayer plastic (PL 2040). Solutions are in contact with the polyethylene layer of this container and can leach out certain chemical components of the plastic in very small amounts within the expiration period. The suitability of the plastic has been confirmed in tests in animals according to the USP biological tests for plastic containers, as well as by tissue culture toxicity studies.

CLINICAL PHARMACOLOGY

Following IM administration of a single 500 mg or 1 g dose of CLAFORAN to normal volunteers, mean peak serum concentrations of 11.7 and 20.5 μg/mL respectively were attained within 30 minutes and declined with an elimination half-life of approximately 1 hour. There was a dose-dependent increase in serum levels after the IV administration of 500 mg, 1 g, and 2 g of CLAFORAN (38.9, 101.7, and 214.4 μg/mL respectively) without alteration in the elimination half-life. There is no evidence of accumulation following repetitive IV infusion of 1 g doses every 6 hours for 14 days as there are no alterations of serum or renal clearance. About 60% of the administered dose was recovered from urine during the first 6 hours following the start of the infusion.

Continued on next page

Claforan—Cont.

Approximately 20–36% of an intravenously administered dose of ^{14}C-cefotaxime is excreted by the kidney as unchanged cefotaxime and 15–25% as the desacetyl derivative, the major metabolite. The desacetyl metabolite has been shown to contribute to the bactericidal activity. Two other urinary metabolites (M_2 and M_3) account for about 20–25%. They lack bactericidal activity.
A single 50 mg/kg dose of CLAFORAN was administered as an intravenous infusion over a 10- to 15-minute period to 29 newborn infants grouped according to birth weight and age. The mean half-life of cefotaxime in infants with lower birth weights (≤1500 grams), regardless of age, was longer (4.6 hours) than the mean half-life (3.4 hours) in infants whose birth weight was greater than 1500 grams. Mean serum clearance was also smaller in the lower birth weight infants. Although the differences in mean half-life values are statistically significant for weight, they are not clinically important. Therefore, dosage should be based solely on age. (See DOSAGE AND ADMINISTRATION section.)
Additionally, no disulfiram-like reactions were reported in a study conducted in 22 healthy volunteers administered CLAFORAN and ethanol.

Microbiology

The bactericidal activity of cefotaxime sodium results from inhibition of cell wall synthesis. Cefotaxime sodium has *in vitro* activity against a wide range of gram-positive and gram-negative organisms. CLAFORAN has a high degree of stability in the presence of beta-lactamases, both penicillinases and cephalosporinases, of gram-negative and gram-positive bacteria. Cefotaxime sodium has been shown to be a potent inhibitor of β-lactamases produced by certain gram-negative bacteria. Cefotaxime sodium is usually active against the following microorganisms both *in vitro* and in clinical infections (see INDICATIONS AND USAGE).

Aerobes, Gram-positive: *Staphylococcus aureus*, including penicillinase and non-penicillinase producing strains, *Staphylococcus epidermidis, Enterococcus* species, *Streptococcus pyogenes* (Group A beta-hemolytic streptococci), *Streptococcus agalactiae* (Group B streptococci), *Streptococcus pneumoniae* (formerly *Diplococcus pneumoniae*).

Aerobes, Gram-negative: *Citrobacter* species, *Enterobacter* species, *Escherichia coli, Haemophilus influenzae* (including ampicillin-resistant *H. influenzae*), *Haemophilus parainfluenzae, Klebsiella* species (including *K. pneumoniae*), *Neisseria gonorrhoeae* (including penicillinase and non-penicillinase producing strains), *Neisseria meningitidis, Proteus mirabilis, Proteus vulgaris, Proteus inconstans* Group B, *Morganella morganii, Providencia rettgeri, Serratia* species, and *Acinetobacter* species.

NOTE: Many strains of the above organisms that are multiply resistant to other antibiotics, e.g. penicillins, cephalosporins, and aminoglycosides, are susceptible to cefotaxime sodium.

Cefotaxime sodium is active against some strains of *Pseudomonas aeruginosa*.

Anaerobes: *Bacteroides* species, including some strains of *B. fragilis, Clostridium* species (NOTE: Most strains of *C. difficile* are resistant.), *Peptococcus* species, *Peptostreptococcus* species, and *Fusobacterium* species (including *F. nucleatum*).

Cefotaxime sodium is highly stable *in vitro* to four of the five major classes of β-lactamases described by Richmond et al., including type IIIa (TEM) which is produced by many gram-negative bacteria. The drug is also stable to β-lactamase (penicillinase) produced by staphylococci. In addition, cefotaxime sodium shows high affinity for penicillin-binding proteins in the cell wall, including PBP: Ib and III.
Cefotaxime sodium also demonstrates *in vitro* activity against the following microorganisms although clinical significance is unknown: *Salmonella* species (including *S. typhi*), *Providencia* species, and *Shigella* species.
Cefotaxime sodium and aminoglycosides have been shown to be synergistic *in vitro* against some strains of *Pseudomonas aeruginosa*.

Susceptibility Tests

Quantitative methods that require measurement of zone diameters give the most precise estimate of antibiotic susceptibility. One such procedure[1] has been recommended for use with discs to test susceptibility to cefotaxime sodium. Interpretation involves correlation of the diameters obtained in the disc test with minimum inhibitory concentration (MIC) values for cefotaxime sodium.
Reports from the laboratory giving results of the standardized single-disc susceptibility test using a 30 µg cefotaxime sodium disc should be interpreted according to the following criteria:

Susceptible organisms produce zones of 20 mm or greater, indicating that the tested organism is likely to respond to therapy.

Organisms that produce zones of 15 to 19 mm are expected to be susceptible if high dosage is used or if the infection is confined to tissues and fluids (e.g. urine) in which high antibiotic levels are attained.

Resistant organisms produce zones of 14 mm or less, indicating that other therapy should be selected.

Organisms should be tested with the cefotaxime sodium disc, since cefotaxime sodium has been shown by *in vitro* tests to be active against certain strains found resistant when other beta lactam discs are used. The cefotaxime sodium disc should not be used for testing susceptibility to other cephalosporins. Organisms having zones of less than 18 mm around the cephalothin disc are not necessarily of intermediate susceptibility or resistant to cefotaxime sodium.
A bacterial isolate may be considered susceptible if the MIC value for cefotaxime sodium is not more than 16 µg/mL. Organisms are considered resistant to cefotaxime sodium if the MIC is equal to or greater than 64 µg/mL. Organisms having an MIC value of less than 64 µg/mL but greater than 16 µg/mL are expected to be susceptible if high dosage is used or if the infection is confined to tissues and fluids (e.g., urine) in which high antibiotic levels are attained.

INDICATIONS AND USAGE

Treatment

CLAFORAN is indicated for the treatment of patients with serious infections caused by susceptible strains of the designated microorganisms in the diseases listed below.

(1) Lower respiratory tract infections, including pneumonia, caused by *Streptococcus pneumoniae* (formerly *Diplococcus pneumoniae*), *Streptococcus pyogenes** (Group A streptococci) and other streptococci (excluding enterococci, e.g., *Streptococcus faecalis*), *Staphylococcus aureus* (penicillinase and non-penicillinase producing), *Escherichia coli, Klebsiella* species, *Haemophilus influenzae* (including ampicillin resistant strains), *Haemophilus parainfluenzae, Proteus mirabilis, Serratia marcescens*, Enterobacter* species, indole positive *Proteus* and *Pseudomonas* species (including *P. aeruginosa*).

(2) Genitourinary infections. Urinary tract infections caused by *Enterococcus* species, *Staphylococcus epidermidis, Staphylococcus aureus**, (penicillinase and non-penicillinase producing), *Citrobacter* species, *Enterobacter* species, *Escherichia coli, Klebsiella* species, *Proteus mirabilis, Proteus vulgaris*, Proteus inconstans* group B, *Morganella morganii*, Providencia rettgeri*, Serratia marcescens* and *Pseudomonas* species (including *P. aeruginosa*). Also, uncomplicated gonorrhea (cervical/urethral and rectal) caused by *Neisseria gonorrhoeae*, including penicillinase producing strains.

(3) Gynecologic infections, including pelvic inflammatory disease, endometritis and pelvic cellulitis caused by *Staphylococcus epidermidis, Streptococcus* species, *Enterococcus* species, *Enterobacter* species*, *Klebsiella* species*, *Escherichia coli, Proteus mirabilis, Bacteroides* species (including *Bacteroides fragilis**), *Clostridium* species, and anaerobic cocci (including *Peptostreptococcus* species and *Peptococcus* species) and *Fusobacterium* species (including *F. nucleatum**).

CLAFORAN, like other cephalosporins, has no activity against *Chlamydia trachomatis*. Therefore, when cephalosporins are used in the treatment of patients with pelvic inflammatory disease and *C. trachomatis* is one of the suspected pathogens, appropriate antichlamydial coverage should be added.

(4) Bacteremia/Septicemia caused by *Escherichia coli, Klebsiella* species, *Serratia marcescens, Staphylococcus aureus*, and *Streptococcus* species (including *S. pneumoniae*).

(5) Skin and skin structure infections caused by *Staphylococcus aureus* (penicillinase and non-penicillinase producing), *Staphylococcus epidermidis, Streptococcus pyogenes* (Group A streptococci) and other streptococci, *Enterococcus* species, *Acinetobacter* species*, *Escherichia coli, Citrobacter* species (including *C. freundii**). *Enterobacter* species, *Klebsiella* species, *Proteus mirabilis, Proteus vulgaris*, Morganella morganii, Providencia rettgeri*, Pseudomonas* species, *Serratia marcescens, Bacteroides* species, and anaerobic cocci (including *Peptostreptococcus** species and *Peptococcus* species).

(6) Intra-abdominal infections including peritonitis caused by *Streptococcus* species*, *Escherichia coli, Klebsiella* species, *Bacteroides* species, and anaerobic cocci (including *Peptostreptococcus** species and *Peptococcus** species), *Proteus mirabilis**, and *Clostridium* species*.

(7) Bone and/or joint infections caused by *Staphylococcus aureus* (penicillinase and non-penicillinase producing strains), *Streptococcus* species (including *S. pyogenes**), *Pseudomonas* species (including *P. aeruginosa**), and *Proteus mirabilis**.

(8) Central nervous system infections, e.g., meningitis and ventriculitis, caused by *Neisseria meningitidis, Haemophilus influenzae, Streptococcus pneumoniae, Klebsiella pneumoniae** and *Escherichia coli**.

(*) Efficacy for this organism, in this organ system, has been studied in fewer than 10 infections.

Although many strains of enterococci (e.g., *S. faecalis*) and *Pseudomonas* species are resistant to cefotaxime sodium *in vitro*, CLAFORAN has been used successfully in treating patients with infections caused by susceptible organisms.
Specimens for bacteriologic culture should be obtained prior to therapy in order to isolate and identify causative organisms and to determine their susceptibilities to CLAFORAN. Therapy may be instituted before results of susceptibility studies are known; however, once these results become available, the antibiotic treatment should be adjusted accordingly.
In certain cases of confirmed or suspected gram-positive or gram-negative sepsis or in patients with other serious infections in which the causative organism has not been identified, CLAFORAN may be used concomitantly with an aminoglycoside. The dosage recommended in the labeling of both antibiotics may be given and depends on the severity of the infection and the patient's condition. Renal function should be carefully monitored, especially if higher dosages of the aminoglycosides are to be administered or if therapy is prolonged, because of the potential nephrotoxicity and ototoxicity of aminoglycoside antibiotics. It is possible that nephrotoxicity may be potentiated if CLAFORAN is used concomitantly with an aminoglycoside.

Prevention

The administration of CLAFORAN preoperatively reduces the incidence of certain infections in patients undergoing surgical procedures (e.g., abdominal or vaginal hysterectomy, gastrointestinal and genitourinary tract surgery) that may be classified as contaminated or potentially contaminated.
In patients undergoing cesarean section, intraoperative (after clamping the umbilical cord) and postoperative use of CLAFORAN may also reduce the incidence of certain postoperative infections. See DOSAGE AND ADMINISTRATION section.
Effective use for elective surgery depends on the time of administration. To achieve effective tissue levels, CLAFORAN should be given $^1/_2$ or $1^1/_2$ hours before surgery. See DOSAGE AND ADMINISTRATION section.
For patients undergoing gastrointestinal surgery, preoperative bowel preparation by mechanical cleansing as well as with a non-absorbable antibiotic (e.g., neomycin) is recommended.
If there are signs of infection, specimens for culture should be obtained for identification of the causative organism so that appropriate therapy may be instituted.

CONTRAINDICATIONS

CLAFORAN is contraindicated in patients who have shown hypersensitivity to cefotaxime sodium or the cephalosporin group of antibiotics.

WARNINGS

BEFORE THERAPY WITH CLAFORAN IS INSTITUTED, CAREFUL INQUIRY SHOULD BE MADE TO DETERMINE WHETHER THE PATIENT HAS HAD PREVIOUS HYPERSENSITIVITY REACTIONS TO CEFOTAXIME SODIUM, CEPHALOSPORINS, PENICILLINS, OR OTHER DRUGS. THIS PRODUCT SHOULD BE GIVEN WITH CAUTION TO PATIENTS WITH TYPE I HYPERSENSITIVITY REACTIONS TO PENICILLIN. ANTIBIOTICS SHOULD BE ADMINISTERED WITH CAUTION TO ANY PATIENT WHO HAS DEMONSTRATED SOME FORM OF ALLERGY, PARTICULARLY TO DRUGS. IF AN ALLERGIC REACTION TO CLAFORAN OCCURS, DISCONTINUE TREATMENT WITH THE DRUG. SERIOUS HYPERSENSITIVITY REACTIONS MAY REQUIRE EPINEPHRINE AND OTHER EMERGENCY MEASURES.
During post-marketing surveillance, a potentially life-threatening arrhythmia was reported in each of six patients who received a rapid (less than 60 seconds) bolus injection of cefotaxime through a central venous catheter. Therefore, cefotaxime should only be administered as instructed in the DOSAGE AND ADMINISTRATION section.
Pseudomembranous colitis has been reported with nearly all antibacterial agents, including cefotaxime, and may range from mild to life threatening. Therefore, it is important to consider its diagnosis in patients with diarrhea subsequent to the administration of antibacterial agents.
Treatment with antibacterial agents alters the normal flora of the colon and may permit overgrowth of Clostridia. Studies indicate that a toxin produced by *Clostridium difficile* is one primary cause of antibiotic-associated colitis.
After the diagnosis of pseudomembranous colitis has been established, appropriate therapeutic measures should be initiated. Mild cases of colitis may respond to drug discontinuance alone. In moderate to severe cases, consideration should be given to management with fluids and electrolytes, protein supplementation, and treatment with an antibacterial drug clinically effective against *Clostridium difficile* colitis.
When the colitis is not relieved by drug discontinuance or when it is severe, oral vancomycin is the treatment of choice for antibiotic-associated pseudomembranous colitis produced by *C. difficile*. Other causes of colitis should also be considered.

PRECAUTIONS

CLAFORAN should be prescribed with caution in individuals with a history of gastrointestinal disease, particularly colitis.
Because high and prolonged serum antibiotic concentrations can occur from usual doses in patients with transient or persistent reduction of urinary output because of renal insufficiency, the total daily dosage should be reduced when CLAFORAN is administered to such patients. Continued dosage should be determined by degree of renal impairment, severity of infection, and susceptibility of the causative organism.
Although there is no clinical evidence supporting the necessity of changing the dosage of cefotaxime sodium in patients with even profound renal dysfunction, it is suggested that, until further data are obtained, the dose of cefotaxime sodium be halved in patients with estimated creatinine clearances of less than 20 mL/min/1.73 m^2.
When only serum creatinine is available, the following formula[2] (based on sex, weight, and age of the patient) may be used to convert this value into creatinine clearance. The serum creatinine should represent a steady state of renal function.

	Weight (kg) × (140 − age)
Males:	72 × serum creatinine
Females:	0.85 × above value

As with other antibiotics, prolonged use of CLAFORAN may result in overgrowth of nonsusceptible organisms. Repeated evaluation of the patient's condition is essential. If superinfection occurs during therapy, appropriate measures should be taken.
As with other beta-lactam antibiotics, granulocytopenia and, more rarely, agranulocytosis may develop during treatment with CLAFORAN, particularly if given over long periods. For courses of treatment lasting longer than 10 days, blood counts should therefore be monitored.
CLAFORAN, like other parenteral anti-infective drugs, may be locally irritating to tissues. In most cases, perivascular extravasation of CLAFORAN responds to changing of the infusion site. In rare instances, extensive perivascular extravasation of CLAFORAN may result in tissue damage and require surgical treatment. To minimize the potential for tissue inflammation, infusion sites should be monitored regularly and changed when appropriate.
Drug Interactions: Increased nephrotoxicity has been reported following concomitant administration of cephalosporins and aminoglycoside antibiotics.
Carcinogenesis, Mutagenesis: Long-term studies in animals have not been performed to evaluate carcinogenic potential. Mutagenic tests included a micronucleus and an Ames test. Both tests were negative for mutagenic effects.
Pregnancy (Category B): Reproduction studies have been performed in mice and rats at doses up to 30 times the usual human dose and have revealed no evidence of impaired fertility or harm to the fetus because of cefotaxime sodium. However, there are no well-controlled studies in pregnant women. Because animal reproductive studies are not always predictive of human response, this drug should be used during pregnancy only if clearly needed.
Nonteratogenic Effects: Use of the drug in women of childbearing potential requires that the anticipated benefit be weighed against the possible risks.
In perinatal and postnatal studies with rats, the pups in the group given 1200 mg/kg of CLAFORAN were significantly lighter in weight at birth and remained smaller than pups in the control group during the 21 days of nursing.
Nursing Mothers: CLAFORAN is excreted in human milk in low concentrations. Caution should be exercised when CLAFORAN is administered to a nursing woman.
Pediatric Use: See Precautions above regarding perivascular extravasation. The potential for toxic effects in pediatric patients from chemicals that may leach from the plastic in single dose Galaxy® containers (premixed CLAFORAN Injection) has not been determined.

ADVERSE REACTIONS

CLAFORAN is generally well tolerated. The most common adverse reactions have been local reactions following IM or IV injection. Other adverse reactions have been encountered infrequently.
The most frequent adverse reactions (greater than 1%) are:
Local (4.3%)—Injection site inflammation with IV administration. Pain, induration, and tenderness after IM injection.
Hypersensitivity (2.4%)—Rash, pruritus, fever, and eosinophilia and less frequently urticaria and anaphylaxis.
Gastrointestinal (1.4%)—Colitis, diarrhea, nausea, and vomiting.
Symptoms of pseudomembranous colitis can appear during or after antibiotic treatment.
Nausea and vomiting have been reported rarely.
Less frequent adverse reactions (less than 1%) are:
Cardiovascular System—Potentially life-threatening arrhythmias following rapid (less than 60 seconds) bolus administration via central venous catheter have been observed.
Hematologic System—Neutropenia, transient leukopenia, eosinophilia, thrombocytopenia and agranulocytosis have been reported. Some individuals have developed positive direct Coombs Tests during treatment with CLAFORAN (cefotaxime sodium injection) and other cephalosporin antibiotics. Rare cases of hemolytic anemia have been reported.
Genitourinary System—Moniliasis, vaginitis.
Central Nervous System—Headache.
Liver—Transient elevations in SGOT, SGPT, serum LDH, and serum alkaline phosphatase levels have been reported.
Kidney—As with some other cephalosporins, interstitial nephritis and transient elevations of BUN and creatinine have been occasionally observed with CLAFORAN.

DOSAGE AND ADMINISTRATION

Adults

Dosage and route of administration should be determined by susceptibility of the causative organisms, severity of the infection, and the condition of the patient (see table for dosage guideline). CLAFORAN may be administered IM or IV after reconstitution. Premixed CLAFORAN Injection is intended for IV administration after thawing. The maximum daily dosage should not exceed 12 grams.
[See first table above]
If *C. trachomatis* is a suspected pathogen, appropriate antichlamydial coverage should be added, because cefotaxime sodium has no activity against this organism.
To prevent postoperative infection in contaminated or potentially contaminated surgery, the recommended dose is a single 1 gram IM or IV administered 30 to 90 minutes prior to start of surgery.

GUIDELINES FOR DOSAGE OF CLAFORAN

Type of Infection	Daily Dose (grams)	Frequency and Route
Gonococcal urethritis/cervicitis in males and females	0.5	0.5 gram IM (single dose)
Rectal gonorrhea in females	0.5	0.5 gram IM (single dose)
Rectal gonorrhea in males	1	1 gram IM (single dose)
Uncomplicated Infections	2	1 gram every 12 hours IM or IV
Moderate to severe infections	3–6	1–2 grams every 8 hours IM or IV
Infections commonly needing antibiotics in higher dosage (e.g., septicemia)	6–8	2 grams every 6–8 hours IV
Life-threatening infections	up to 12	2 grams every 4 hours IV

Strength	Reconstituted Concentration mg/mL	Stability at or below 22° C	Stability under Refrigeration (at or below 5° C) Original Containers	Plastic Syringes
500 mg vial IM	200	12 hours	7 days	5 days
1 g vial IM	300	12 hours	7 days	5 days
2 g vial IM	330	12 hours	7 days	5 days
500 mg vial IV	50	24 hours	7 days	5 days
1 g vial IV	95	24 hours	7 days	5 days
2 g vial IV	180	12 hours	7 days	5 days
1 g infusion bottle	10–20	24 hours	10 days	
2 g infusion bottle	20–40	24 hours	10 days	

Cesarean Section Patients
The first dose of 1 gram is administered intravenously as soon as the umbilical cord is clamped. The second and third doses should be given as 1 gram intravenously or intramuscularly at 6 and 12 hours after the first dose.

Neonates, Infants, and Children
The following dosage schedule is recommended:
Neonates (birth to 1 month):

0–1 week of age	50 mg/kg per dose every 12 hours IV
1–4 weeks of age	50 mg/kg per dose every 8 hours IV

It is not necessary to differentiate between premature and normal-gestational age infants.
Infants and Children (1 month to 12 years): For body weights less than 50 kg, the recommended daily dose is 50 to 180 mg/kg IM or IV body weight divided into four to six equal doses. The higher dosages should be used for more severe or serious infections, including meningitis. For body weights 50 kg or more, the usual adult dosage should be used; the maximum daily dosage should not exceed 12 grams.
Impaired Renal Function — see PRECAUTIONS section.
NOTE: As with antibiotic therapy in general, administration of CLAFORAN should be continued for a minimum of 48 to 72 hours after the patient defervesces or after evidence of bacterial eradication has been obtained; a minimum of 10 days of treatment is recommended for infections caused by Group A beta-hemolytic streptococci in order to guard against the risk of rheumatic fever or glomerulonephritis; frequent bacteriologic and clinical appraisal is necessary during therapy of chronic urinary tract infection and may be required for several months after therapy has been completed; persistent infections may require treatment of several weeks and doses smaller than those indicated above should not be used.

PREPARATION OF CLAFORAN STERILE

CLAFORAN for IM or IV administration should be reconstituted as follows:

Strength	Diluent (mL)	Withdrawable Volume (mL)	Approximate Concentration (mg/mL)
500 mg vial* (IM)	2	2.2	230
1 g vial* (IM)	3	3.4	300
2 g vial* (IM)	5	6.0	330
500 mg vial* (IV)	10	10.2	50
1 g vial* (IV)	10	10.4	95
2 g vial* (IV)	10	11.0	180
1 g infusion	50–100	50–100	20–10
2 g infusion	50–100	50–100	40–20
10 g bottle	47	52.0	200
10 g bottle	97	102.0	100

(*) in conventional vials

Shake to dissolve; inspect for particulate matter and discoloration prior to use. Solutions of CLAFORAN range from very pale yellow to light amber, depending on concentration, diluent used, and length and condition of storage.
For intramuscular use: Reconstitute VIALS with Sterile Water for Injection or Bacteriostatic Water for Injection as described above.
For intravenous use: Reconstitute VIALS with at least 10 mL of Sterile Water for Injection. Reconstitute INFUSION BOTTLES with 50 or 100 mL of 0.9% Sodium Chloride Injection or 5% Dextrose Injection. For other diluents, see COMPATIBILITY AND STABILITY section.

Pharmacy Bulk Package: Reconstitute with 47 mL of diluent for an approximate concentration of 200 mg/mL or 97 mL of diluent for an approximate concentration of 100 mg/mL. Stock solutions may be further diluted for IV infusion with diluents as listed in COMPATIBILITY AND STABILITY section.
NOTE: Solution of CLAFORAN must not be admixed with aminoglycoside solutions. If CLAFORAN and aminoglycosides are to be administered to the same patient, they must be administered separately and not as mixed injection.
A SOLUTION OF 1 G CLAFORAN IN 14 ML OF STERILE WATER FOR INJECTION IS ISOTONIC.
IM Administration: As with all IM preparations, CLAFORAN should be injected well within the body of a relatively large muscle such as the upper outer quadrant of the buttock (i.e., gluteus maximus); aspiration is necessary to avoid inadvertent injection into a blood vessel. Individual IM doses of 2 grams may be given if the dose is divided and is administered in different intramuscular sites.
IV Administration: The IV route is preferable for patients with bacteremia, bacterial septicemia, peritonitis, meningitis, or other severe or life-threatening infections, or for patients who may be poor risks because of lowered resistance resulting from such debilitating conditions as malnutrition, trauma, surgery, diabetes, heart failure, or malignancy, particularly if shock is present or impending.
For intermittent IV administration, a solution containing 1 gram or 2 grams in 10 mL of Sterile Water for Injection can be injected over a period of three to five minutes. Cefotaxime should not be administered over a period of less than three minutes. (See WARNINGS.) With an infusion system, it may also be given over a longer period of time through the tubing system by which the patient may be receiving other IV solutions. However, during infusion of the solution containing CLAFORAN, it is advisable to discontinue temporarily the administration of other solutions at the same site.
For the administration of higher doses by continuous IV infusion, a solution of CLAFORAN may be added to IV bottles containing the solutions discussed below.
DIRECTIONS FOR USE OF CLAFORAN (cefotaxime sodium injection) IN GALAXY CONTAINER (PL 2040 PLASTIC)
CLAFORAN Injection in Galaxy containers (PL 2040 plastic) is for continuous or intermittent infusion using sterile equipment.
Storage
Store in a freezer capable of maintaining a temperature of −20° C / −4° F.
Thawing of Plastic Container
Thaw frozen container at room temperature or under refrigeration (at or below 5° C). [DO NOT FORCE THAW BY IMMERSION IN WATER BATHS OR BY MICROWAVE IRRADIATION.]
Check for minute leaks by squeezing container firmly. If leaks are detected, discard solution as sterility may be impaired.
DO NOT ADD SUPPLEMENTARY MEDICATION.
The container should be visually inspected. Components of the solution may precipitate in the frozen state and will dissolve upon reaching room temperature with little or no agitation. Potency is not affected. Agitate after solution has reached room temperature. If after visual inspection the solution remains cloudy or if an insoluble precipitate is noted or if any seals or outlet ports are not intact, the container should be discarded.
The thawed solution is stable for 10 days under refrigeration (at or below 5° C) or 24 hours at or below 22° C. Do not refreeze thawed antibiotics.

Continued on next page

Claforan—Cont.

CAUTION: Do not use plastic containers in series connections. Such use could result in air embolism due to residual air being drawn from the primary container before administration of the fluid from the secondary container is complete.

Preparation for Intravenous Administration:
1. Suspend container from eyelet support.
2. Remove protector from outlet port at bottom of container.
3. Attach administration set. Refer to complete directions accompanying set.

PREPARATION OF CLAFORAN STERILE IN ADD-VANTAGE® SYSTEM

CLAFORAN Sterile 1 g or 2 g may be reconstituted in 50 mL or 100 mL of 5% Dextrose or 0.9% Sodium Chloride in the ADD-Vantage® diluent container. Refer to enclosed, separate INSTRUCTIONS FOR ADD-VANTAGE SYSTEM.

COMPATIBILITY AND STABILITY

Solutions of CLAFORAN Sterile reconstituted as described above (Preparation of CLAFORAN Sterile) remain chemically stable (potency remains above 90%) as follows when stored in original containers and disposable plastic syringes:

[See second table at top of previous page]

Reconstituted solutions stored in original containers and plastic syringes remain stable for 13 weeks frozen.

For the 10 g bottle withdraw reconstituted contents immediately. However, if it is not possible, aliquoting operations must be completed within four hours of reconstitution. Discard the reconstituted stock solution 4 hours after initial entry.

Reconstituted solutions may be further diluted up to 1000 mL with the following solutions and maintain satisfactory potency for 24 hours at or below 22° C, and at least 5 days under refrigeration (at or below 5° C): 0.9% Sodium Chloride Injection; 5 or 10% Dextrose Injection; 5% Dextrose and 0.9% Sodium Chloride Injection, 5% Dextrose and 0.45% Sodium Chloride Injection; 5% Dextrose and 0.2% Sodium Chloride Injection; Lactated Ringers Solution; Sodium Lactate Injection (M/6); 10% Invert Sugar Injection, 8.5% TRAVASOL® (Amino Acid) Injection without Electrolytes.

Solutions of CLAFORAN Sterile reconstituted in 0.9% Sodium Chloride Injection or 5% Dextrose Injection in Viaflex® plastic containers maintain satisfactory potency for 24 hours at or below 22° C, 5 days under refrigeration (at or below 5° C) and 13 weeks frozen. Solutions of CLAFORAN Sterile reconstituted in 0.9% Sodium Chloride Injection or 5% Dextrose Injection in the ADD-Vantage® flexible containers maintain satisfactory potency for 24 hours at or below 22° C. DO NOT FREEZE.

NOTE: CLAFORAN solutions exhibit maximum stability in the pH 5–7 range. Solutions of CLAFORAN should not be prepared with diluents having a pH above 7.5, such as Sodium Bicarbonate Injection.

HOW SUPPLIED

Sterile CLAFORAN is a dry off-white to pale yellow crystalline powder supplied in vials and bottles containing cefotaxime sodium as follows:

500 mg cefotaxime (free acid equivalent) in vials in packages of 10 (NDC 0039-0017-10).

1 g cefotaxime (free acid equivalent) in vials in packages of 10 (NDC 0039-0018-10), packages of 25 (NDC 0039-0018-25), packages of 50 (NDC 0039-0018-50); infusion bottles in packages of 10 (NDC 0039-0018-11).

2 g cefotaxime (free acid equivalent) in vials in packages of 10 (NDC 0039-0019-10), packages of 25 (NDC 0039-0019-25), packages of 50 (NDC 0039-0019-50); infusion bottles in packages of 10 (NDC 0039-0019-11).

10 g cefotaxime (free acid equivalent) in bottles (NDC 0039-0020-01).

1 g cefotaxime (free acid equivalent) in ADD-Vantage® System vials in packages of 25 (NDC 0039-0023-25) and 50 (NDC 0039-0023-50).

2 g cefotaxime (free acid equivalent) in ADD-Vantage® System vials in packages of 25 (NDC 0039-0024-25) and 50 (NDC 0039-0024-50).

ADD-Vantage® System diluents (5% Dextrose or 0.9% Sodium Chloride) are available from Abbott Laboratories.

NOTE: CLAFORAN in the dry state should be stored below 30° C. The dry material as well as solutions tend to darken depending on storage conditions and should be protected from elevated temperatures and excessive light.

Premixed CLAFORAN Injection is supplied as a frozen, iso-osmotic, sterile, nonpyrogenic solution in 50 mL single dose Galaxy® containers (PL 2040 plastic) as follows:

1 g cefotaxime (free acid equivalent) in packages of 12 (NDC 0039-0037-05) 2G3518.

2 g cefotaxime (free acid equivalent) in packages of 12 (NDC 0039-0038-05) 2G3519.

NOTE: Store Premixed CLAFORAN Injection at or below −20° C / −4° F. [See DIRECTIONS FOR USE OF CLAFORAN (cefotaxime sodium injection) IN GALAXY® CONTAINERS (PL 2040 PLASTIC)].

CLAFORAN Injection supplied as a frozen, iso-osmotic, sterile, nonpyrogenic solution in Galaxy® containers (PL 2040 plastic) is manufactured for Hoechst-Roussel Pharmaceuticals, a Division of Hoechst Marion Roussel, Inc. by Baxter Healthcare Corporation.

REFERENCES

1) Bauer, A.W.; Kirby, W.M.M.; Sherris, J.C.; and Turck, M. Antibiotic Susceptibility Testing by a Standardized Single Disk Method, Am. J. Clin. Pathol., 45:493, 1966; Standardized Disc Susceptibility Test, Federal Register, 39: 19182-4, 1974. National Committee for Clinical Laboratory Standards. Approved Standard: ASM-2, Performance Standards for Antimicrobial Disc Susceptibility Tests. July, 1975.

2) Cockcroft, D.W. and Gault, M.H.: Prediction of Creatinine Clearance from Serum Creatinine. Nephron 16:31-41, 1976.

Sterile cefotaxime sodium US Patents 4,152,432; 4,224,371; 4,298,606; cefotaxime sodium injection US Patents 4,152,432; 4,298,606.

Claforan REG TM ROUSSEL-UCLAF.

Galaxy and PL 2040 REG TM Baxter International Inc.

ADD-Vantage REG TM Abbott Laboratories.

US Patents ADD-Vantage System: 4,614,267; 4,614,515; 4,757,911; 4,703,864; 4,784,658; 4,784,259; 4,948,000; 4,936,445.

Prescribing Information as of October 1996

Hoechst-Roussel Pharmaceuticals
Division of Hoechst Marion Roussel, Inc.
Kansas City, MO 64137 USA

Shown in Product Identification Guide, page 306

CLOMID® ℞

[clo'-mid]

(clomiphene citrate tablets USP)

Prescribing Information as of February 1996

DESCRIPTION

CLOMID (clomiphene citrate tablets USP) is an orally administered, nonsteroidal, ovulatory stimulant designated chemically as 2-[p-(2-chloro-1,2-diphenylvinyl)phenoxy] triethylamine citrate (1:1). It has the molecular formula of $C_{26}H_{28}ClNO \cdot C_6H_8O_7$ and a molecular weight of 598.09. It is represented structurally as:

$(C_2H_5)_2NCH_2CH_2O$–[structure]–$C=C(Cl)$–[structure] $\cdot C_6H_8O_7$

Clomiphene citrate is a white to pale yellow, essentially odorless, crystalline powder. It is freely soluble in methanol; soluble in ethanol; slightly soluble in acetone, water, and chloroform; and insoluble in ether.

CLOMID is a mixture of two geometric isomers [cis (zuclomiphene) and trans (enclomiphene)] containing between 30% and 50% of the cis-isomer.

Each white scored tablet contains 50 mg clomiphene citrate USP. The tablet also contains the following inactive ingredients: corn starch, lactose, magnesium stearate, pregelatinized corn starch, and sucrose.

CLINICAL PHARMACOLOGY

Action

CLOMID is a drug of considerable pharmacologic potency. With careful selection and proper management of the patient, CLOMID has been demonstrated to be a useful therapy for the anovulatory patient desiring pregnancy.

Clomiphene citrate is capable of interacting with estrogen-receptor-containing tissues, including the hypothalamus, pituitary, ovary, endometrium, vagina, and cervix. It may compete with estrogen for estrogen-receptor-binding sites and may delay replenishment of intracellular estrogen receptors. Clomiphene citrate initiates a series of endocrine events culminating in a preovulatory gonadotropin surge and subsequent follicular rupture. The first endocrine event in response to a course of clomiphene therapy is an increase in the release of pituitary gonadotropins. This initiates steroidogenesis and folliculogenesis, resulting in growth of the ovarian follicle and an increase in the circulating level of estradiol. Following ovulation, plasma progesterone and estradiol rise and fall as they would in a normal ovulatory cycle.

Available data suggest that both the estrogenic and antiestrogenic properties of clomiphene may participate in the initiation of ovulation. The two clomiphene isomers have been found to have mixed estrogenic and antiestrogenic effects, which may vary from one species to another. Some data suggest that zuclomiphene has greater estrogenic activity than enclomiphene.

Clomiphene citrate has no apparent progestational, androgenic, or antiandrogenic effects and does not appear to interfere with pituitary-adrenal or pituitary-thyroid function.

Although there is no evidence of a "carryover effect" of CLOMID, spontaneous ovulatory menses have been noted in some patients after CLOMID therapy.

Pharmacokinetics

Based on early studies with ^{14}C-labeled clomiphene citrate, the drug was shown to be readily absorbed orally in humans and excreted principally in the feces. Cumulative urinary and fecal excretion of the ^{14}C averaged about 50% of the oral dose and 37% of an intravenous dose after 5 days. Mean urinary excretion was approximately 8% with fecal excretion of about 42%.

Some ^{14}C label was still present in the feces 6 weeks after administration. Subsequent single-dose studies in normal volunteers showed that zuclomiphene (cis) has a longer half-life than enclomiphene (trans). Detectable levels of zuclomiphene persisted for longer than a month in these subjects. This may be suggestive of stereo-specific enterohepatic recycling or sequestering of the zuclomiphene. Thus, it is possible that some active drug may remain in the body during early pregnancy in women who conceive in the menstrual cycle during CLOMID therapy.

CLINICAL STUDIES

During clinical investigations, 7578 patients received CLOMID, some of whom had impediments to ovulation other than ovulatory dysfunction (see INDICATIONS AND USAGE). In those clinical trials, successful therapy characterized by pregnancy occurred in approximately 30% of these patients.

There were a total of 2635 pregnancies reported during the clinical trial period. Of those pregnancies, information on outcome was only available for 2369 of the cases. Table 1 summarizes the outcome of these cases.

Of the reported pregnancies, the incidence of multiple pregnancies was 7.98%: 6.9% twin, 0.5% triplet, 0.3% quadruplet, and 0.1% quintuplet. Of the 165 twin pregnancies for which sufficient information was available, the ratio of monozygotic to dizygotic twins was about 1:5. Table 1 reports the survival rate of the live multiple births.

A sextuplet birth was reported after completion of original clinical studies; none of the sextuplets survived (each weighed less than 400 g), although each appeared grossly normal.

Table 1. Outcome of Reported Pregnancies in Clinical Trials (n = 2369)

Outcome	Total Number of Pregnancies	Survival Rate
Pregnancy Wastage		
Spontaneous Abortions	483*	
Stillbirths	24	
Live Births		
Single Births	1697	98.16%†
Multiple Births	165	83.26%†

*Includes 28 ectopic pregnancies, 4 hydatiform moles, and 1 fetus papyraceous.

†Indicates percentage of surviving infants from these pregnancies.

The overall survival of infants from multiple pregnancies including spontaneous abortions, stillbirths, and neonatal deaths is 73%.

INDICATIONS AND USAGE

CLOMID is indicated for the treatment of ovulatory dysfunction in women desiring pregnancy. Impediments to achieving pregnancy must be excluded or adequately treated before beginning CLOMID therapy. Those patients most likely to achieve success with clomiphene therapy include patients with polycystic ovary syndrome (see WARNINGS: Ovarian Hyperstimulation Syndrome), amenorrhea-galactorrhea syndrome, psychogenic amenorrhea, post-oral-contraceptive amenorrhea, and certain cases of secondary amenorrhea of undetermined etiology.

Properly timed coitus in relationship to ovulation is important. A basal body temperature graph or other appropriate tests may help the patient and her physician determine if ovulation occurred. Once ovulation has been established, each course of CLOMID should be started on or about the 5th day of the cycle. Long-term cyclic therapy is not recommended beyond a total of about six cycles (including three ovulatory cycles). See DOSAGE AND ADMINISTRATION and PRECAUTIONS.)

CLOMID is indicated only in patients with demonstrated ovulatory dysfunction who meet the conditions described below (see CONTRAINDICATIONS):

1. Patients who are not pregnant.
2. Patients without ovarian cysts. CLOMID should not be used in patients with ovarian enlargement except those with polycystic ovary syndrome. Pelvic examination is necessary prior to the first and each subsequent course of CLOMID treatment.
3. Patients without abnormal vaginal bleeding. If abnormal vaginal bleeding is present, the patient should be carefully evaluated to ensure that neoplastic lesions are not present.
4. Patients with normal liver function.

In addition, patients selected for CLOMID therapy should be evaluated in regard to the following:

1. **Estrogen Levels.** Patients should have adequate levels of endogenous estrogen (as estimated from vaginal smears, endometrial biopsy, assay of urinary estrogen, or from bleeding in response to progesterone). Reduced estrogen levels, while less favorable, do not preclude successful therapy.
2. **Primary Pituitary or Ovarian Failure.** CLOMID therapy cannot be expected to substitute for specific treatment of other causes of ovulatory failure.
3. **Endometriosis and Endometrial Carcinoma.** The incidence of endometriosis and endometrial carcinoma increases with age as does the incidence of ovulatory disorders. Endometrial biopsy should always be performed prior to CLOMID therapy in this population.

4. **Other Impediments to Pregnancy.** Impediments to pregnancy can include thyroid disorders, adrenal disorders, hyperprolactinemia, and male factor infertility.
5. **Uterine Fibroids.** Caution should be exercised when using CLOMID in patients with uterine fibroids due to the potential for further enlargement of the fibroids.

There are no adequate or well-controlled studies that demonstrate the effectiveness of CLOMID in the treatment of male infertility. In addition, testicular tumors and gynecomastia have been reported in males using clomiphene. The cause and effect relationship between reports of testicular tumors and the administration of CLOMID is not known.

Although the medical literature suggests various methods, there is no universally accepted standard regimen for combined therapy (ie, CLOMID in conjunction with other ovulation-inducing drugs). Similarly, there is no standard CLOMID regimen for ovulation induction in *in vitro* fertilization programs to produce ova for fertilization and reintroduction. Therefore, CLOMID is not recommended for these uses.

CONTRAINDICATIONS

Hypersensitivity

CLOMID is contraindicated in patients with a known hypersensitivity or allergy to clomiphene citrate or to any of its ingredients.

Pregnancy

CLOMID should not be administered during pregnancy. CLOMID may cause fetal harm in animals (see Animal Fetotoxicity). Although no causative evidence of a deleterious effect of CLOMID therapy on the human fetus has been established, there have been reports of birth anomalies which, during clinical studies, occurred at an incidence within the range reported for the general population (see Fetal/Neonatal Anomalies and Mortality; ADVERSE REACTIONS).

To avoid inadvertent CLOMID administration during early pregnancy, appropriate tests should be utilized during each treatment cycle to determine whether ovulation occurs. The patient should be evaluated carefully to exclude pregnancy, ovarian enlargement, or ovarian cyst formation between each treatment cycle. The next course of CLOMID therapy should be delayed until these conditions have been excluded.

Fetal/Neonatal Anomalies and Mortality. The following fetal abnormalities have been reported subsequent to pregnancies following ovulation induction therapy with CLOMID during clinical trials. Each of the following fetal abnormalities were reported at a rate of <1% (experiences are listed in order of decreasing frequency): Congenital heart lesions, Down syndrome, club foot, congenital gut lesions, hypospadias, microcephaly, harelip and cleft palate, congenital hip, hemangioma, undescended testicles, polydactyly, conjoined twins and teratomatous malformation, patent ductus arteriosus, amaurosis, arteriovenous fistula, inguinal hernia, umbilical hernia, syndactyly, pectus excavatum, myopathy, dermoid cyst of scalp, omphalocele, spina bifida occulta, ichthyosis, and persistent lingual frenulum. Neonatal death and fetal death/stillbirth in infants with birth defects have also been reported at a rate of <1%. The overall incidence of reported birth anomalies from pregnancies associated with maternal CLOMID ingestion during clinical studies was within the range of that reported for the general population.

In addition, reports of birth anomalies have been received during postmarketing surveillance of CLOMID (see ADVERSE REACTIONS).

Animal Fetotoxicity. Oral administration of clomiphene citrate to pregnant rats during organogenesis at doses of 1 to 2 mg/kg/day resulted in hydramnion and weak, edematous fetuses with wavy ribs and other temporary bone changes. Doses of 8 mg/kg/day or more also caused increased resorptions and dead fetuses, dystocia, and delayed parturition, and 40 mg/kg/day resulted in increased maternal mortality. Single doses of 50 mg/kg caused fetal cataracts, while 200 mg/kg caused cleft palate.

Following injection of clomiphene citrate 2 mg/kg to mice and rats during pregnancy, the offspring exhibited metaplastic changes of the reproduction tract. Newborn mice and rats injected during the first few days of life also developed metaplastic changes in uterine and vaginal mucosa, as well as premature vaginal opening and anovulatory ovaries. These findings are similar to the abnormal reproductive behavior and sterility described with other estrogens and antiestrogens.

In rabbits, some temporary bone alterations were seen in fetuses from dams given oral doses of 20 or 40 mg/kg/day during pregnancy, but not following 8 mg/kg/day. No permanent malformations were observed in those studies. Also, rhesus monkeys given oral doses of 1.5 to 4.5 mg/kg/day for various periods during pregnancy did not have any abnormal offspring.

Liver Disease. CLOMID therapy is contraindicated in patients with liver disease or a history of liver dysfunction (see also INDICATIONS AND USAGE and ADVERSE REACTIONS).

Abnormal Uterine Bleeding. CLOMID is contraindicated in patients with abnormal uterine bleeding of undetermined origin (see INDICATIONS AND USAGE).

Ovarian Cysts. CLOMID is contraindicated in patients with ovarian cysts or enlargement not due to polycystic ovarian syndrome (see INDICATIONS AND USAGE and WARNINGS).

Other. CLOMID is contraindicated in patients with uncontrolled thyroid or adrenal dysfunction or in the presence of an organic intracranial lesion such as pituitary tumor (see INDICATIONS AND USAGE).

WARNINGS

Visual Symptoms

Patients should be advised that blurring or other visual symptoms such as spots or flashes (scintillating scotomata) may occasionally occur during therapy with CLOMID. These visual symptoms increase in incidence with increasing total dose or therapy duration and generally disappear within a few days or weeks after CLOMID is discontinued. Patients should be warned that these visual symptoms may render such activities as driving a car or operating machinery more hazardous than usual, particularly under conditions of variable lighting.

These visual symptoms appear to be due to intensification and prolongation of afterimages. Symptoms often first appear or are accentuated with exposure to a brightly lit environment. While measured visual acuity usually has not been affected, a study patient taking 200 mg CLOMID daily developed visual blurring on the 7th day of treatment, which progressed to severe diminution of visual acuity by the 10th day. No other abnormaltiy was found, and the visual acuity returned to normal on the 3rd day after treatment was stopped.

Ophthalmologically definable scotomata and retinal cell function (electroretinographic) changes have also been reported. A patient treated during clinical studies developed phosphenes and scotomata during prolonged CLOMID administration, which disappeared by the 32nd day after stopping therapy.

Postmarketing surveillance of adverse events has also revealed other visual signs and symptoms during CLOMID therapy (see ADVERSE REACTIONS).

While the etiology of these visual symptoms is not yet understood, patients with any visual symptoms should discontinue treatment and have a complete ophthalmological evaluation carried out promptly.

Ovarian Hyperstimulation Syndrome

The ovarian hyperstimulation syndrome (OHSS) has been reported to occur in patients receiving clomiphene citrate therapy for ovulation induction. In some cases, OHSS occurred following cyclic use of clomiphene citrate therapy or when clomiphene citrate was used in combination with gonadotropins. Transient liver function test abnormalities suggestive of hepatic dysfunction, which may be accompanied by morphologic changes on liver biopsy, have been reported in association with ovarian hyperstimulation syndrome (OHSS).

OHSS is a medical event distinct from uncomplicated ovarian enlargement. The clinical signs of this syndrome in severe cases can include gross ovarian enlargement, gastrointestinal symptoms, ascites, dyspnea, oliguria, and pleural effusion. In addition, the following symptoms have been reported in association with this syndrome: pericardial effusion, anasarca, hydrothorax, acute abdomen, hypotension, renal failure, pulmonary edema, intraperitoneal and ovarian hemorrhage, deep venous thrombosis, torsion of the ovary, and acute respiratory distress. The early warning signs of OHSS are abdominal pain and distention, nausea, vomiting, diarrhea, and weight gain. Elevated urinary steroid levels, varying degrees of electrolyte imbalance, hypovolemia, hemoconcentration, and hypoproteinemia may occur. Death due to hypovolemic shock, hemoconcentration, or thromboembolism has occurred. Due to fragility of enlarged ovaries in severe cases, abdominal and pelvic examination should be performed very cautiously. If conception results, rapid progression to the severe form of the syndrome may occur.

To minimize the hazard associated with occasional abnormal ovarian enlargement associated with CLOMID therapy, the lowest dose consistent with expected clinical results should be used. Maximal enlargement of the ovary, whether physiologic or abnormal, may not occur until several days after discontinuation of the recommended dose of CLOMID. Some patients with polycystic ovary syndrome who are unusually sensitive to gonadotropin may have an exaggerated response to usual doses of CLOMID. Therefore, patients with polycystic ovary syndrome should be started on the lowest recommended dose and shortest treatment duration for the first course of therapy (see DOSAGE AND ADMINISTRATION).

If enlargement of the ovary occurs, additional CLOMID therapy should not be given until the ovaries have returned to pretreatment size, and the dosage or duration of the next course should be reduced. Ovarian enlargement and cyst formation associated with CLOMID therapy usually regress spontaneously within a few days or weeks after discontinuing treatment. The potential benefit of subsequent CLOMID therapy in these cases should exceed the risk. Unless surgical indication for laparotomy exists, such cystic enlargement should always be managed conservatively.

A causal relationship between ovarian hyperstimulation and ovarian cancer has not been determined. However, because a correlation between ovarian cancer and nulliparity, infertility, and age has been suggested, if ovarian cysts do not regress spontaneously, a thorough evaluation should be performed to rule out the presence of ovarian neoplasia.

PRECAUTIONS

General

Careful attention should be given to the selection of candidates for CLOMID therapy. Pelvic examination is necessary prior to CLOMID treatment and before each subsequent course (see CONTRAINDICATIONS and WARNINGS).

Information for Patients

The purpose and risks of CLOMID therapy should be presented to the patient before starting treatment. It should be emphasized that the goal of CLOMID therapy is ovulation for subsequent pregnancy. The physician should counsel the patient with special regard to the following potential risks:

Visual Symptoms: Advise that blurring or other visual symptoms occasionally may occur during or shortly after CLOMID therapy. Warn that visual symptoms may render such activities as driving a car or operating machinery more hazardous than usual, particularly under conditions of variable lighting (see WARNINGS).

The patient should be instructed to inform the physician whenever any unusual visual symptoms occur. If the patient has any visual symptoms, treatment should be discontinued and complete ophthalmologic evaluation performed.

Abdominal/Pelvic Pain or Distention: Ovarian enlargement may occur during or shortly after therapy with CLOMID. To minimize the risks associated with ovarian enlargement, the patient should be instructed to inform the physician of any abdominal or pelvic pain, weight gain, discomfort, or distention after taking CLOMID (see WARNINGS).

Multiple Pregnancy: Inform the patient that there is an increased chance of multiple pregnancy, including bilateral tubal pregnancy and coexisting tubal and intrauterine pregnancy, when conception occurs in relation to CLOMID therapy. The potential complications and hazards of multiple pregnancy should be explained.

Pregnancy Wastage and Birth Anomalies: The physician should explain the assumed risk of any pregnancy, whether ovulation is induced with the aid of CLOMID or occurs naturally. The patient should be informed of the greater risks associated with certain characteristics or conditions of any pregnant woman, eg, age of female and male partner, history of spontaneous abortions, Rh genotype, abnormal menstrual history, infertility history, organic heart disease, diabetes, exposure to infectious agents such as rubella, familial history of birth anomaly, that may be pertinent to the patient for whom CLOMID is being considered. Based upon the evaluation of the patient, genetic counseling may be indicated.

The overall incidence of reported birth anomalies from pregnancies associated with maternal CLOMID ingestion during the investigational studies was within the range of that reported in published references for the general population. (See CONTRAINDICATIONS: Pregnancy.)

During clinical investigation, the experience from patients with known pregnancy outcome (Table 1) shows a spontaneous abortion rate of 20.4% and stillbirth rate of 1.0%. (See CLINICAL PHARMACOLOGY.)

Drug Interactions

Drug interactions with CLOMID have not been documented.

Carcinogenesis, Mutagenesis, Impairment of Fertility

Long-term toxicity studies in animals have not been performed to evaluate the carcinogenic or mutagenic potential of clomiphene citrate.

Oral administration of CLOMID to male rats at doses of 0.3 or 1 mg/kg/day caused decreased fertility, while higher doses caused temporary infertility. Oral doses of 0.1 mg/kg/day in female rats temporarily interrupted the normal cyclic vaginal smear pattern and prevented conception. Doses of 0.3 mg/kg/day slightly reduced the number of ovulated ova and corpora lutea, while 3 mg/kg/day inhibited ovulation.

Pregnancy

Pregnancy Category X. (See CONTRAINDICATIONS.)

Nursing Mothers

It is not known whether CLOMID is excreted in human milk. Because many drugs are excreted in human milk, caution should be exercised if CLOMID is administered to a nursing woman. In some patients, CLOMID may reduce lactation.

Ovarian Cancer

Prolonged use of clomiphene citrate tablets USP may increase the risk of a borderline or invasive ovarian tumor (see ADVERSE REACTIONS).

ADVERSE REACTIONS

Clinical Trial Adverse Events. CLOMID, at recommended dosages, is generally well tolerated. Adverse reactions usually have been mild and transient and most have disappeared promptly after treatment has been discontinued. Adverse experiences reported in patients treated with clomiphene citrate during clinical studies are shown in Table 2.

Table 2. Incidence of Adverse Events In Clinical Studies (Events Greater than 1%) (n = 8029*)

Adverse Event	%
Ovarian Enlargement	13.6
Vasomotor Flushes	10.4
Abdominal-Pelvic Discomfort/ Distention/Bloating	5.5
Nausea and Vomiting	2.2
Breast Discomfort	2.1
Visual Symptoms	1.5
Blurred vision, lights, floaters, waves, unspecified visual complaints, photophobia, diplopia, scotomata, phosphenes	
Headache	1.3

Continued on next page

Clomid—Cont.

Abnormal Uterine Bleeding Intermenstrual spotting, menorrhagia	1.3

* Includes 498 patients whose reports may have been duplicated in the event totals and could not be distinguished as such. Also, excludes 47 patients who did not report symptom data.

The following adverse events have been reported in fewer than 1% of patients in clinical trials: Acute abdomen, appetite increase, constipation, dermatitis or rash, depression, diarrhea, dizziness, fatigue, hair loss/dry hair, increased urinary frequency/volume, insomnia, light-headedness, nervous tension, vaginal dryness, vertigo, weight gain/loss.

Patients on prolonged CLOMID therapy may show elevated serum levels of desmosterol. This is most likely due to a direct interference with cholesterol synthesis. However, the serum sterols in patients receiving the recommended dose of CLOMID are not significantly altered. Ovarian cancer has been infrequently reported in patients who have received fertility drugs. Infertility is a primary risk factor for ovarian cancer; however, epidemiology data suggest that prolonged use of clomiphene may increase the risk of a borderline or invasive ovarian tumor.

Postmarketing Adverse Events

The following adverse experiences were reported spontaneously with CLOMID. The cause and effect relationship of the listed events to the administration of CLOMID is not known.

Dermatologic: Acne, allergic reaction, erythema, erythema multiforme, erythema nodosum, hypertrichosis, pruritus

Central Nervous System: Migraine headache, paresthesia, seizure, stroke, syncope

Psychiatric: Anxiety, irritability, mood changes, psychosis

Visual Disorders: Abnormal accommodation, cataract, eye pain, macular edema, optic neuritis, photopsia, posterior vitreous detachment, retinal hemorrhage, retinal thrombosis, retinal vascular spasm, temporary loss of vision

Cardiovascular: Arrhythmia, chest pain, edema, hypertension, palpitation, phlebitis, pulmonary embolism, shortness of breath, tachycardia, thrombophlebitis

Musculoskeletal: Arthralgia, back pain, myalgia

Hepatic: Transaminases increased, hepatitis

Neoplasms: Liver (hepatic hemangiosarcoma, liver cell adenoma, hepatocellular carcinoma); breast (fibrocystic disease, breast carcinoma); endometrium (endometrial carcinoma); nervous system (astrocytoma, pituitary tumor, prolactinoma, neurofibromatosis, glioblastoma multiforme, brain abscess); ovary (luteoma of pregnancy, dermoid cyst of the ovary, ovarian carcinoma); trophoblastic (hydatiform mole, choriocarcinoma); miscellaneous (melanoma, myeloma, perianal cysts, renal cell carcinoma, Hodgkin's lymphoma, tongue carcinoma, bladder carcinoma); and neoplasms of offspring (neuroectodermal tumor, thyroid tumor, hepatoblastoma, lymphocytic leukemia)

Genitourinary: Endometriosis, ovarian cyst (ovarian enlargement or cysts could, as such, be complicated by adnexal torsion), ovarian hemorrhage, tubal pregnancy, uterine hemorrhage

Body as a Whole: Fever, tinnitus, weakness

Other: Leukocytosis, thyroid disorder

Fetal/Neonatal anomalies. The following fetal abnormalities have also been reported during postmarketing surveillance: delayed development; abnormal bone development including skeletal malformations of the skull, face, nasal passages, jaw, hand, limb (ectromelia including amelia, hemimelia, and phocomelia), foot, and joints; tissue malformations including imperforate anus, tracheoesophageal fistula, diaphragmatic hernia, renal agenesis and dysgenesis, and malformations of the eye and lens (cataract), ear, lung, heart (ventricular septal defect and tetralogy of Fallot), and genitalia; as well as dwarfism, deafness, mental retardation, chromosomal disorders, and neural tube defects (including anencephaly).

DRUG ABUSE AND DEPENDENCE

Tolerance, abuse, or dependence with CLOMID has not been reported.

OVERDOSAGE

Signs and Symptoms

Toxic effects accompanying acute overdosage of CLOMID have not been reported. Signs and symptoms of overdosage as a result of the use of more than the recommended dose during CLOMID therapy include nausea, vomiting, vasomotor flushes, visual blurring, spots or flashes, scotomata, ovarian enlargement with pelvic or abdominal pain. (See CONTRAINDICATIONS: Ovarian Cyst.)

Oral LD_{50}. The acute oral LD_{50} of CLOMID is 1700 mg/kg in mice and 5750 mg/kg in rats. The toxic dose in humans is not known.

Dialysis: It is not known if CLOMID is dialyzable.

Treatment

In the event of overdose, appropriate supportive measures should be employed in addition to gastrointestinal decontamination.

DOSAGE AND ADMINISTRATION

General Considerations

The workup and treatment of candidates for CLOMID therapy should be supervised by physicians experienced in management of gynecologic or endocrine disorders. Patients should be chosen for therapy with CLOMID only after careful diagnostic evaluation (see INDICATIONS AND USAGE). The plan of therapy should be outlined in advance. Impediments to achieving the goal of therapy must be excluded or adequately treated before beginning CLOMID. The therapeutic objective should be balanced with potential risks and discussed with the patient and others involved in the achievement of a pregnancy.

Ovulation most often occurs from 5 to 10 days after a course of CLOMID. Coitus should be timed to coincide with the expected time of ovulation. Appropriate tests to determine ovulation may be useful during this time.

Recommended Dosage

Treatment of the selected patient should begin with a low dose, 50 mg daily (1 tablet) for 5 days. The dose should be increased only in those patients who do not ovulate in response to cyclic 50 mg CLOMID. A low dosage or duration of treatment course is particularly recommended if unusual sensitivity to pituitary gonadotropin is suspected, such as in patients with polycystic ovary syndrome (see WARNINGS: Ovarian Hyperstimulation Syndrome).

The patient should be evaluated carefully to exclude pregnancy, ovarian enlargement, or ovarian cyst formation between each treatment cycle.

If progestin-induced bleeding is planned, or if spontaneous uterine bleeding occurs prior to therapy, the regimen of 50 mg daily for 5 days should be started on or about the 5th day of the cycle. Therapy may be started at any time in the patient who has had no recent uterine bleeding. When ovulation occurs at this dosage, there is no advantage to increasing the dose in subsequent cycles of treatment. If ovulation does not appear to occur after the first course of therapy, a second course of 100 mg daily (two 50 mg tablets given as a single daily dose) for 5 days should be given. This course may be started as early as 30 days after the previous one after precautions are taken to exclude the presence of pregnancy. Increasing the dosage or duration of therapy beyond 100 mg/day for 5 days is not recommended.

The majority of patients who are going to ovulate will do so after the first course of therapy. If ovulation does not occur after three courses of therapy, further treatment with CLOMID is not recommended and the patient should be reevaluated. If three ovulatory responses occur, but pregnancy has not been achieved, further treatment is not recommended. If menses does not occur after an ovulatory response, the patient should be reevaluated. Long-term cyclic therapy is not recommended beyond a total of about six cycles (see PRECAUTIONS).

HOW SUPPLIED

NDC 0068-0226-30: 50 mg tablets in cartons of 30

Tablets are round, white, scored, and debossed CLOMID 50.

Store tablets at controlled room temperature 59–86°F (15–30°C).

Protect from heat, light, and excessive humidity, and store in closed containers.

Prescribing Information as of February 1996

Merrell Pharmaceuticals Inc.
Subsidiary of Hoechst Marion Roussel, Inc.
Kansas City, MO 64137 USA

Shown in Product Identification Guide, page 306

DDAVP®
Injection 4 μg/mL ℞
(desmopressin acetate)

DESCRIPTION

DDAVP® Injection 4 μg/mL (desmopressin acetate) is a synthetic analogue of the natural pituitary hormone 8-arginine vasopressin (ADH), an antidiuretic hormone affecting renal water conservation. It is chemically defined as follows:

Mol. Wt. 1183.34

Empirical Formula: $C_{46}H_{64}N_{14}O_{12}S_2 \bullet C_2H_4O_2 \bullet 3H_2O$

$SCH_2CH_2C(=O)$-Tyr-Phe-Gln-Asn-Cys-Pro-D-Arg-Gly-$NH_2 \cdot CH_3COOH \cdot 3H_2O$
(residues numbered 1 2 3 4 5 6 7 8 9; bridge between 1 and 6)

1-(3-mercaptopropionic acid)-8-D-arginine vasopressin monoacetate (salt) trihydrate.

DDAVP Injection 4 μg/mL is provided as a sterile, aqueous solution for injection.

Each mL provides:

Desmopressin acetate	4.0 μg
Sodium chloride	9.0 mg

Hydrochloric acid to adjust pH to 4

The 10 mL vial contains chlorobutanol as a preservative (5.0 mg/mL).

CLINICAL PHARMACOLOGY

DDAVP Injection 4 μg/mL contains as active substance, desmopressin acetate, a synthetic analogue of the natural hormone arginine vasopressin. One mL (4 μg) of DDAVP (desmopressin acetate) solution has an antidiuretic activity of about 16 IU; 1 μg of DDAVP is equivalent to 4 IU.

DDAVP has been shown to be more potent than arginine vasopressin in increasing plasma levels of factor VIII activity in patients with hemophilia and von Willebrand's disease Type I.

Dose-response studies were performed in healthy persons, using doses of 0.1 to 0.4 μg/kg body weight, infused over a 10-minute period. Maximal dose response occurred at 0.3 to 0.4 μg/kg. The response to DDAVP of factor VIII activity and plasminogen activator is dose-related, with maximal plasma levels of 300 to 400 percent of initial concentrations obtained after infusion of 0.4 μg/kg body weight. The increase is rapid and evident within 30 minutes, reaching a maximum at a point ranging from 90 minutes to two hours. The factor VIII related antigen and ristocetin cofactor activity were also increased to a smaller degree, but still are dose-dependent.

1. The biphasic half-lives of DDAVP were 7.8 and 75.5 minutes for the fast and slow phases, respectively, compared with 2.5 and 14.5 minutes for lysine vasopressin, another form of the hormone. As a result, DDAVP provides a prompt onset of antidiuretic action with a long duration after each administration.
2. The change in structure of arginine vasopressin to DDAVP has resulted in a decreased vasopressor action and decreased actions on visceral smooth muscle relative to the enhanced antidiuretic activity, so that clinically effective antidiuretic doses are usually below threshold levels for effects on vascular or visceral smooth muscle.
3. When administered by injection, DDAVP has an antidiuretic effect about ten times that of an equivalent dose administered intranasally.
4. The bioavailability of the subcutaneous route of administration was determined qualitatively using urine output data. The exact fraction of drug absorbed by that route of administration has not been quantitatively determined.
5. The percentage increase of factor VIII levels in patients with mild hemophilia A and von Willebrand's disease was not significantly different from that observed in normal healthy individuals when treated with 0.3 μg/kg of DDAVP infused over 10 minutes.
6. Plasminogen activator activity increases rapidly after DDAVP infusion, but there has been no clinically significant fibrinolysis in patients treated with DDAVP.
7. The effect of repeated DDAVP administration when doses were given every 12 to 24 hours has generally shown a gradual diminution of the factor VIII activity increase noted with a single dose. The initial response is reproducible in any particular patient if there are 2 or 3 days between administrations.

INDICATIONS AND USAGE

Hemophilia A: DDAVP Injection 4 μg/mL is indicated for patients with hemophilia A with factor VIII coagulant activity levels greater than 5%.

DDAVP will often maintain hemostasis in patients with hemophilia A during surgical procedures and postoperatively when administered 30 minutes prior to scheduled procedure.

DDAVP will also stop bleeding in hemophilia A patients with episodes of spontaneous or trauma-induced injuries such as hemarthroses, intramuscular hematomas or mucosal bleeding.

DDAVP is not indicated for the treatment of hemophilia A with factor VIII coagulant activity levels equal to or less than 5%, or for the treatment of hemophilia B, or in patients who have factor VIII antibodies.

In certain clinical situations, it may be justified to try DDAVP in patients with factor VIII levels between 2% to 5%; however, these patients should be carefully monitored.

von Willebrand's Disease (Type I): DDAVP Injection 4 μg/mL is indicated for patients with mild to moderate classic von Willebrand's disease (Type I) with factor VIII levels greater than 5%. DDAVP will often maintain hemostasis in patients with mild to moderate von Willebrand's disease during surgical procedures and postoperatively when administered 30 minutes prior to the scheduled procedure.

DDAVP will usually stop bleeding in mild to moderate von Willebrand's patients with episodes of spontaneous or trauma-induced injuries such as hemarthroses, intramuscular hematomas or mucosal bleeding.

Those von Willebrand's disease patients who are least likely to respond are those with severe homozygous von Willebrand's disease with factor VIII coagulant activity and factor VIII von Willebrand factor antigen levels less than 1%. Other patients may respond in a variable fashion depending on the type of molecular defect they have. Bleeding time and factor VIII coagulant activity, ristocetin cofactor activity, and von Willebrand factor antigen should be checked during administration of DDAVP to ensure that adequate levels are being achieved.

DDAVP is not indicated for the treatment of severe classic von Willebrand's disease (Type I) and when there is evidence of an abnormal molecular form of factor VIII antigen. (See **WARNINGS**.)

Diabetes Insipidus: DDAVP Injection 4 μg/mL is indicated as antidiuretic replacement therapy in the management of central (cranial) diabetes insipidus and for the management of the temporary polyuria and polydipsia following head trauma or surgery in the pituitary region. DDAVP is ineffective for the treatment of nephrogenic diabetes insipidus.

DDAVP is also available as an intranasal preparation. However, this means of delivery can be compromised by a variety of factors that can make nasal insufflation ineffective or inappropriate. These include poor intranasal absorption, nasal congestion and blockage, nasal discharge, atrophy of nasal mucosa, and severe atrophic rhinitis. Intranasal delivery may be inappropriate where there is an impaired level of consciousness. In addition, cranial surgical procedures, such as transsphenoidal hypophysectomy, create situations where an alternative route of administration is needed as in cases of nasal packing or recovery from surgery.

CONTRAINDICATIONS

DDAVP Injection 4 µg/mL is contraindicated in individuals with known hypersensitivity to desmopressin acetate or to any of the components of **DDAVP Injection 4 µg/mL.**

WARNINGS

Patients who do not have need of antidiuretic hormone for its antidiuretic effect, in particular those who are young or elderly, should be cautioned to ingest only enough fluid to satisfy thirst, in order to decrease the potential occurrence of water intoxication and hyponatremia.

Fluid intake should be adjusted downward, particularly in very young and elderly patients, in order to decrease the potential occurrence of water intoxication and hyponatremia. Particular attention should be paid to the possibility of the rare occurrence of an extreme decrease in plasma osmolality that may result in seizures which could lead to coma.

DDAVP should not be used to treat patients with Type IIB von Willebrand's disease since platelet aggregation may be induced.

PRECAUTIONS

General: For injection use only.

DDAVP® Injection 4 µg/mL (desmopressin acetate) has infrequently produced changes in blood pressure causing either a slight elevation in blood pressure or a transient fall in blood pressure and a compensatory increase in heart rate. The drug should be used with caution in patients with coronary artery insufficiency and/or hypertensive cardiovascular disease.

DDAVP (desmopressin acetate) should be used with caution in patients with conditions associated with fluid and electrolyte imbalance, such as cystic fibrosis, because these patients are prone to hyponatremia.

There have been rare reports of thrombotic events following **DDAVP Injection 4 µg/mL** in patients predisposed to thrombus formation. No causality has been determined, however, the drug should be used with caution in these patients.

Severe allergic reactions have been reported rarely. Fatal anaphylaxis has been reported in one patient who received intravenous DDAVP. It is not known whether antibodies to **DDAVP Injection 4 µg/mL** are produced after repeated injections.

Hemophilia A: Laboratory tests for assessing patient status include levels of factor VIII coagulant, factor VIII antigen and factor VIII ristocetin cofactor (von Willebrand factor) as well as activated partial thromboplastin time. Factor VIII coagulant activity should be determined before giving DDAVP for hemostasis. If factor VIII coagulant activity is present at less than 5% of normal, DDAVP should not be relied on.

von Willebrand's Disease: Laboratory tests for assessing patient status include levels of factor VIII coagulant activity, factor VIII ristocetin cofactor activity, and factor VIII von Willebrand factor antigen. The skin bleeding time may be helpful in following these patients.

Diabetes Insipidus: Laboratory tests for monitoring the patient include urine volume and osmolality. In some cases, plasma osmolality may be required.

Drug Interactions: Although the pressor activity of DDAVP is very low compared with the antidiuretic activity, use of doses as large as 0.3 µg/kg of DDAVP with other pressor agents should be done only with careful patient monitoring.

DDAVP has been used with epsilon aminocaproic acid without adverse effects.

Carcinogenicity, Mutagenicity, Impairment of Fertility: Studies with DDAVP have not been performed to evaluate carcinogenic potential, mutagenic potential or effects on fertility.

Pregnancy Category B: Fertility studies have not been done. Teratology studies in rats and rabbits at doses from 0.05 to 10 µg/kg/day (approximately 0.1 times the maximum systemic human exposure in rats and up to 38 times the maximum systemic human exposure in rabbits based on surface area, mg/m^2) revealed no harm to the fetus due to DDAVP. There are, however, no adequate and well controlled studies in pregnant women. Because animal reproduction studies are not always predictive of human response, this drug should be used during pregnancy only if clearly needed.

Several publications of desmopressin acetate's use in the management of diabetes insipidus during pregnancy are available; these include a few anecdotal reports of congenital anomalies and low birth weight babies. However, no causal connection between these events and desmopressin acetate has been established. A fifteen year, Swedish epidemiologic study of the use of desmopressin acetate in pregnant women with diabetes insipidus found the rate of birth defects to be no greater than that in the general population; however, the statistical power of this study is low. As opposed to preparations containing natural hormones, desmopressin acetate in antidiuretic doses has no uterotonic action and the physician will have to weigh the therapeutic advantages against the possible risks in each case.

Nursing Mothers: There have been no controlled studies in nursing mothers. A single study in postpartum women demonstrated a marked change in plasma, but little if any change in assayable DDAVP in breast milk following an intranasal dose of 10 µg. It is not known whether this drug is excreted in human milk. Because many drugs are excreted in human milk, caution should be exercised when DDAVP is administered to a nursing woman.

Pediatric Use: Use in infants and pediatric patients will require careful fluid intake restriction to prevent possible hyponatremia and water intoxication. **DDAVP Injection 4 µg/mL** *should not be used in infants less than three months of age* in the treatment of hemophilia A or von Willebrand's disease; safety and effectiveness in pediatric patients under 12 years of age with diabetes insipidus have not been established.

ADVERSE REACTIONS

Infrequently, DDAVP has produced transient headache, nausea, mild abdominal cramps and vulval pain. These symptoms disappeared with reduction in dosage. Occasionally, injection of DDAVP has produced local erythema, swelling or burning pain. Occasional facial flushing has been reported with the administration of DDAVP. **DDAVP Injection** has infrequently produced changes in blood pressure causing either a slight elevation or a transient fall and a compensatory increase in heart rate. Severe allergic reactions including anaphylaxis have been reported rarely with **DDAVP Injection.**

See **WARNINGS** for the possibility of water intoxication and hyponatremia.

There have been rare reports of thrombotic events (acute cerebrovascular thrombosis, acute myocardial infarction) following **DDAVP Injection** in patients predisposed to thrombus formation.

OVERDOSAGE

(See **ADVERSE REACTIONS.**) In case of overdosage, the dosage should be reduced, frequency of administration decreased, or the drug withdrawn according to the severity of the condition.

There is no known specific antidote for desmopressin acetate or **DDAVP Injection 4 µg/mL.**

An oral LD_{50} has not been established. An intravenous dose of 2 mg/kg in mice demonstrated no effect.

DOSAGE AND ADMINISTRATION

Hemophilia A and von Willebrand's Disease (Type I): DDAVP Injection 4 µg/mL is administered as an intravenous infusion at a dose of 0.3 µg DDAVP/kg body weight diluted in sterile physiological saline and infused slowly over 15 to 30 minutes. In adults and children weighing more than 10 kg, 50 mL of diluent is recommended; in children weighing 10 kg or less, 10 mL of diluent is recommended. Blood pressure and pulse should be monitored during infusion. If **DDAVP Injection 4 µg/mL** is used preoperatively, it should be administered 30 minutes prior to the scheduled procedure.

The necessity for repeat administration of DDAVP or use of any blood products for hemostasis should be determined by laboratory response as well as the clinical condition of the patient. The tendency toward tachyphylaxis (lessening of response) with repeated administration given more frequently than every 48 hours should be considered in treating each patient.

Diabetes Insipidus: This formulation is administered subcutaneously or by direct intravenous injection. **DDAVP Injection 4 µg/mL** dosage must be determined for each patient and adjusted according to the pattern of response. Response should be estimated by two parameters: adequate duration of sleep and adequate, not excessive, water turnover.

The usual dosage range in adults is 0.5 mL (2.0 µg) to 1 mL (4.0 µg) daily, administered intravenously or subcutaneously, usually in two divided doses. The morning and evening doses should be separately adjusted for an adequate diurnal rhythm of water turnover. For patients who have been controlled on intranasal DDAVP and who must be switched to the injection form, either because of poor intranasal absorption or because of the need for surgery, the comparable antidiuretic dose of the injection is about one-tenth the intranasal dose.

Parenteral drug products should be inspected visually for particulate matter and discoloration prior to administration whenever solution and container permit.

See directions for use of One Point Cut (OPC) ampules for **DDAVP Injection** on back of carton.

HOW SUPPLIED

DDAVP Injection 4 µg/mL is available as a sterile solution in cartons of ten 1 mL single-dose ampules (NDC 0075-2451-01) and in 10 mL multiple-dose vials (NDC 0075-2451-53), each containing 4.0 µg DDAVP per mL.

Store refrigerated 2 to 8°C (36 to 46°F).

Caution: Federal law prohibits dispensing without prescription.

Keep out of the reach of children.

Manufactured for
Aventis Pharmaceuticals Products Inc.
Parsippany, NJ 07054
By Ferring Pharmaceuticals, Malmö, Sweden
Rev. 11/97 IN-4708L!

Shown in Product Identification Guide, page 306

DDAVP® Nasal Spray ℞
(desmopressin acetate)

DESCRIPTION

DDAVP® Nasal Spray (desmopressin acetate) is a synthetic analogue of the natural pituitary hormone 8-arginine vasopressin (ADH), an antidiuretic hormone affecting renal water conservation. It is chemically defined as follows:

Mol. wt. 1183.34

Empirical formula: $C_{46}H_{64}N_{14}O_{12}S_2 \bullet C_2H_4O_2 \bullet 3H_2O$

$SCH_2CH_2C(=O)$-Tyr-Phe-Gln-Asn-Cys-Pro-D-Arg-Gly-NH_2 • CH_3COOH • $3H_2O$
(1 2 3 4 5 6 7 8 9)

1-(3-mercaptopropionic acid)-8-D-arginine vasopressin monoacetate (salt) trihydrate.

DDAVP Nasal Spray is provided as an aqueous solution for intranasal use.

Each mL contains:

Desmopressin acetate	0.1 mg
Sodium Chloride	7.5 mg
Citric acid monohydrate	1.7 mg
Disodium phosphate dihydrate	3.0 mg
Benzalkonium chloride solution (50%)	0.2 mg

The **DDAVP Nasal Spray** compression pump delivers 0.1 mL (10 µg) of DDAVP (desmopressin acetate) per spray.

CLINICAL PHARMACOLOGY

DDAVP contains as active substance desmopressin acetate, a synthetic analogue of the natural hormone arginine vasopressin. One mL (0.1 mg) of intranasal DDAVP has an antidiuretic activity of about 400 IU; 10 µg of desmopressin acetate is equivalent to 40 IU.

1. The biphasic half-lives for intranasal DDAVP were 7.8 and 75.5 minutes for the fast and slow phases, compared with 2.5 and 14.5 minutes for lysine vasopressin, another form of the hormone used in this condition. As a result, intranasal DDAVP provides a prompt onset of antidiuretic action with a long duration after each administration.
2. The change in structure of arginine vasopressin to DDAVP has resulted in a decreased vasopressor action and decreased actions on visceral smooth muscle relative to the enhanced antidiuretic activity, so that clinically effective antidiuretic doses are usually below threshold levels for effects on vascular or visceral smooth muscle.
3. DDAVP administered intranasally has an antidiuretic effect about one-tenth that of an equivalent dose administered by injection.

INDICATIONS AND USAGE

Primary Nocturnal Enuresis: DDAVP Nasal Spray is indicated for the management of primary nocturnal enuresis. It may be used alone or adjunctive to behavioral conditioning or other nonpharmacological intervention. It has been shown to be effective in some cases that are refractory to conventional therapies.

Central Cranial Diabetes Insipidus: DDAVP Nasal Spray is indicated as antidiuretic replacement therapy in the management of central cranial diabetes insipidus and for management of the temporary polyuria and polydipsia following head trauma or surgery in the pituitary region. It is ineffective for the treatment of nephrogenic diabetes insipidus.

The use of **DDAVP Nasal Spray** in patients with an established diagnosis will result in a reduction in urinary output with increase in urine osmolality and a decrease in plasma osmolality. This will allow the resumption of a more normal life-style with a decrease in urinary frequency and nocturia.

There are reports of an occasional change in response with time, usually greater than 6 months. Some patients may show a decreased responsiveness, others a shortened duration of effect. There is no evidence this effect is due to the development of binding antibodies but may be due to a local inactivation of the peptide.

Patients are selected for therapy by establishing the diagnosis by means of the water deprivation test, the hypertonic saline infusion test, and/or the response to antidiuretic hormone. Continued response to intranasal DDAVP can be monitored by urine volume and osmolality.

DDAVP is also available as a solution for injection when the intranasal route may be compromised. These situations include nasal congestion and blockage, nasal discharge, atrophy of nasal mucosa, and severe atrophic rhinitis. Intranasal delivery may also be inappropriate where there is an impaired level of consciousness. In addition, cranial surgical procedures, such as transphenoidal hypophysectomy create situations where an alternative route of administration is needed as in cases of nasal packing or recovery from surgery.

CONTRAINDICATIONS

DDAVP Nasal Spray is contraindicated in individuals with known hypersensitivity to desmopressin acetate or to any of the components of **DDAVP Nasal Spray.**

WARNINGS

1. For intranasal use only.
2. In very young and elderly patients in particular, fluid intake should be adjusted downward in order to decrease the potential occurrence of water intoxication and hyponatremia. Particular attention should be paid to the possibility of the rare occurrence of an extreme decrease in plasma osmolality that may result in seizures which could lead to coma.

Continued on next page

DDAVP Nasal Spray—Cont.

PRECAUTIONS

General: Intranasal DDAVP at high dosage has infrequently produced a slight elevation of blood pressure, which disappeared with a reduction in dosage. The drug should be used with caution in patients with coronary artery insufficiency and/or hypertensive cardiovascular disease because of possible rise in blood pressure.
DDAVP should be used with caution in patients with conditions associated with fluid and electrolyte imbalance, such as cystic fibrosis, because these patients are prone to hyponatremia.
Rare severe allergic reactions have been reported with DDAVP. Anaphylaxis has been reported with intravenous administration of DDAVP Injection, but not with DDAVP intranasal.
Central Cranial Diabetes Insipidus: Since DDAVP is used intranasally, changes in the nasal mucosa such as scarring, edema, or other disease may cause erratic, unreliable absorption in which case intranasal DDAVP should not be used. For such situations, DDAVP Injection should be considered.
Primary Nocturnal Enuresis: If changes in the nasal mucosa have occurred, unreliable absorption may result. **DDAVP Nasal Spray** should be discontinued until the nasal problems resolve.
Information for Patients: Patients should be informed that the **DDAVP Nasal Spray** bottle accurately delivers 50 doses of 10 µg each. Any solution remaining after 50 doses should be discarded since the amount delivered thereafter may be substantially less than 10 µg of drug. No attempt should be made to transfer remaining solution to another bottle. Patients should be instructed to read accompanying directions on use of the spray pump carefully before use.
Laboratory Tests: Laboratory tests for following the patient with central cranial diabetes insipidus or post-surgical or head trauma-related polyuria and polydipsia include urine volume and osmolality. In some cases plasma osmolality measurements may be required. For the healthy patient with primary nocturnal enuresis, serum electrolytes should be checked at least once if therapy is continued beyond 7 days.
Drug Interactions: Although the pressor activity of DDAVP is very low compared to the antidiuretic activity, use of large doses of intranasal DDAVP with other pressor agents should only be done with careful patient monitoring.
Carcinogenesis, Mutagenesis, Impairment of Fertility: Studies with DDAVP have not been performed to evaluate carcinogenic potential, mutagenic potential or effects on fertility.
Pregnancy: *Category B:* Fertility studies have not been done. Teratology studies in rats and rabbits at doses from 0.05 to 10 µg/kg/day (approximately 0.1 times the maximum systemic human exposure in rats and up to 38 times the maximum systemic human exposure in rabbits based on surface area, mg/m^2) revealed no harm to the fetus due to DDAVP (desmopressin acetate). There are, however, no adequate and well controlled studies in pregnant women. Because animal reproduction studies are not always predictive of human response, this drug should be used during pregnancy only if clearly needed.
Several publications of desmopressin acetate's use in the management of diabetes insipidus during pregnancy are available; these include a few anecdotal reports of congenital anomalies and low birth weight babies. However, no causal connection between these events and desmopressin acetate has been established. A fifteen year Swedish epidemiologic study of the use of desmopressin acetate in pregnant women with diabetes insipidus found the rate of birth defects to be no greater than that in the general population; however, the statistical power of this study is low. As opposed to preparations containing natural hormones, desmopressin acetate in antidiuretic doses has no uterotonic action and the physician will have to weigh the therapeutic advantages against the possible risks in each case.
Nursing Mothers: There have been no controlled studies in nursing mothers. A single study in a post-partum woman demonstrated a marked change in plasma, but little if any change in assayable DDAVP in breast milk following an intranasal dose of 10 µg. It is not known whether this drug is excreted in human milk. Because many drugs are excreted in human milk, caution should be exercised when DDAVP is administered to a nursing woman.
Pediatric Use: *Primary Nocturnal Enuresis:*
DDAVP Nasal Spray (desmopressin acetate) has been used in childhood nocturnal enuresis. Short-term (4–8 weeks) **DDAVP Nasal Spray** administration has been shown to be safe and modestly effective in pediatric patients aged 6 years or older with severe childhood nocturnal enuresis. Adequately controlled studies with intranasal DDAVP in primary nocturnal enuresis have not been conducted beyond 4–8 weeks. The dose should be individually adjusted to achieve the best results.
Central Cranial Diabetes Insipidus: DDAVP Nasal Spray has been used in children with diabetes insipidus. Use in infants and children will require careful fluid intake restriction to prevent possible hyponatremia and water intoxication. The dose must be individually adjusted to the patient with attention in the very young to the danger of an extreme decrease in plasma osmolality with resulting convulsions. Dose should start at 0.05 mL or less.
Since the spray cannot deliver less than 0.1 mL (10 µg), smaller doses should be administered using the rhinal tube delivery system. Do not use the nasal spray in pediatric patients requiring less than 0.1 mL (10 µg) per dose.
There are reports of an occasional change in response with time, usually greater than 6 months. Some patients may show a decreased responsiveness, others a shortened duration of effect. There is no evidence this effect is due to the development of binding antibodies but may be due to a local inactivation of the peptide.

ADVERSE REACTIONS

Infrequently, high dosages of intranasal DDAVP have produced transient headache and nausea. Nasal congestion, rhinitis and flushing have also been reported occasionally along with mild abdominal cramps. These symptoms disappeared with reduction in dosage. Nosebleed, sore throat, cough and upper respiratory infections have also been reported.
The following table lists the percentage of patients having adverse experiences without regard to relationship to study drug from the pooled pivotal study data for nocturnal enuresis.

ADVERSE REACTION	PLACEBO (N=59) %	DDAVP 20 µg (N=60) %	DDAVP 40 µg (N=61) %
BODY AS A WHOLE			
Abdominal Pain	0	2	2
Asthenia	0	0	2
Chills	0	0	2
Headache	0	2	5
Throat Pain	2	0	0
NERVOUS SYSTEM			
Depression	2	0	0
Dizziness	0	0	3
RESPIRATORY SYSTEM			
Epistaxis	2	3	0
Nostril Pain	0	2	0
Respiratory Infection	2	0	0
Rhinitis	2	8	3
CARDIOVASCULAR SYSTEM			
Vasodilation	2	0	0
DIGESTIVE SYSTEM			
Gastrointestinal Disorder	0	2	0
Nausea	0	0	2
SKIN & APPENDAGES			
Leg Rash	2	0	0
Rash	2	0	0
SPECIAL SENSES			
Conjunctivitis	0	2	0
Edema Eyes	0	2	0
Lachrymation Disorder	0	0	2

See **WARNINGS** for the possibility of water intoxication and hyponatremia.

OVERDOSAGE

(See **ADVERSE REACTIONS.**) In case of overdosage, the dose should be reduced, frequency of administration decreased, or the drug withdrawn according to the severity of the condition. There is no known specific antidote for desmopressin acetate or **DDAVP Nasal Spray**.
An oral LD_{50} has not been established. An intravenous dose of 2 mg/kg in mice demonstrated no effect.

DOSAGE AND ADMINISTRATION

Primary Nocturnal Enuresis: Dosage should be adjusted according to the individual. The recommended initial dose for those 6 years of age and older is 20 µg or 0.2 mL solution intranasally at bedtime. Adjustment up to 40 µg is suggested if the patient does not respond.
Some patients may respond to 10 µg and adjustment to that lower dose may be done if the patient has shown a response to 20 µg. It is recommended that one-half of the dose be administered per nostril. Adequately controlled studies with intranasal DDAVP in primary nocturnal enuresis have not been conducted beyond 4–8 weeks.
Central Cranial Diabetes Insipidus: DDAVP Nasal Spray dosage must be determined for each individual patient and adjusted according to the diurnal pattern of response. Response should be estimated by two parameters: adequate duration of sleep and adequate, not excessive, water turnover. Patients with nasal congestion and blockage have often responded well to intranasal DDAVP. The usual dosage range in adults is 0.1 to 0.4 mL daily, either as a single dose or divided into two or three doses. Most adults require 0.2 mL daily in two divided doses. The morning and evening doses should be separately adjusted for an adequate diurnal rhythm of water turnover. For children aged 3 months to 12 years, the usual dosage range is 0.05 to 0.3 mL daily, either as a single dose or divided into two doses. About $^1/_4$ to $^1/_3$ of patients can be controlled by a single daily dose of DDAVP administered intranasally.
The nasal spray pump can only deliver doses of 0.1 mL (10 µg) or multiples of 0.1 mL. If doses other than these are required, the rhinal tube delivery system may be used.
The spray pump must be primed prior to the first use. To prime pump, press down four times. The bottle will now deliver 10 µg of drug per spray. Discard **DDAVP Nasal Spray** after 50 sprays since the amount delivered thereafter per spray may be substantially less than 10 µg of drug.

HOW SUPPLIED

DDAVP Nasal Spray is available in a 5-mL bottle with spray pump delivering 50 sprays of 10 µg (NDC 0075-2452-01).
Desmopressin acetate is also available as DDAVP Rhinal Tube, a refrigerated product with 2.5 mL per vial, packaged with two rhinal tube applicators per carton (NDC 0075-2450-01).
Store at Controlled Room Temperature 20 to 25°C (68 to 77°F) [see USP]. STORE BOTTLE IN UPRIGHT POSITION.
Caution: Federal law prohibits dispensing without prescription.
Keep out of the reach of children.
Rev. 2/97 IN-5534B!
Manufactured for:
Aventis Pharmaceuticals Products Inc.
Parsippany, NJ 07054
By: Ferring Pharmaceuticals, Malmö, Sweden
Shown in Product Identification Guide, page 307

DDAVP® Tablets ℞
(desmopressin acetate)

DESCRIPTION

DDAVP® Tablets (desmopressin acetate) are a synthetic analogue of the natural pituitary hormone 8-arginine vasopressin (ADH), an antidiuretic hormone affecting renal water conservation. It is chemically defined as follows:
Mol. Wt. 1183.34 Empirical Formula:
$C_{46}H_{64}N_{14}O_{12}S_2 \bullet C_2H_4O_2 \bullet 3H_2O$

SCH_2CH_2C-Tyr-Phe-Gln-Asn-Cys-Pro-D-Arg-Gly-NH_2 • CH_3COOH • $3H_2O$
1 2 3 4 5 6 7 8 9

1-(3-mercaptopropionic acid)-8-D-arginine vasopressin monoacetate (salt) trihydrate.
DDAVP Tablets contain either 0.1 or 0.2 mg desmopressin acetate. Inactive ingredients include: lactose, potato starch, magnesium stearate and povidone.

CLINICAL PHARMACOLOGY

DDAVP Tablets contain as active substance, desmopressin acetate, a synthetic analogue of the natural hormone arginine vasopressin.
Central Diabetes Insipidus: Dose response studies in patients with diabetes insipidus have demonstrated that oral doses of 0.025 mg to 0.4 mg produced clinically significant antidiuretic effects. In most patients, doses of 0.1 mg to 0.2 mg produced optimal antidiuretic effects lasting up to eight hours. With doses of 0.4 mg, antidiuretic effects were observed for up to 12 hours; measurements beyond 12 hours were not recorded. Increasing oral doses produced dose dependent increases in the plasma levels of DDAVP (desmopressin acetate).
The plasma half-life of DDAVP followed a monoexponential time course with $t_{1/2}$ values of 1.5 to 2.5 hours which was independent of dose.
The bioavailability of DDAVP oral tablets is about 5% compared to intranasal DDAVP, and about 0.16% compared to intravenous DDAVP. The time to reach maximum plasma DDAVP levels ranged from 0.9 to 1.5 hours following oral or intranasal administration, respectively. Following administration of **DDAVP Tablets**, the onset of antidiuretic effect occurs at around 1 hour, and it reaches a maximum at about 4 to 7 hours based on the measurement of increased urine osmolality.
The use of **DDAVP Tablets** in patients with an established diagnosis will result in a reduction in urinary output with an accompanying increase in urine osmolality. These effects usually will allow resumption of a more normal life style, with a decrease in urinary frequency and nocturia.
There are reports of an occasional change in response to the intranasal formulations of DDAVP (DDAVP Nasal Spray and DDAVP Rhinal Tube). Usually, the change occurred over a period of time greater than six months. This change may be due to decreased responsiveness, or to shortened duration of effect. There is no evidence that this effect is due to the development of binding antibodies, but may be due to a local inactivation of the peptide. No lessening of effect was observed in the 46 patients who were treated with **DDAVP Tablets** for 12 to 44 months and no serum antibodies to desmopressin were detected.
The change in structure of arginine vasopressin to desmopressin acetate resulted in less vasopressor activity and decreased action on visceral smooth muscle relative to enhanced antidiuretic activity. Consequently, clinically effective antidiuretic doses are usually below the threshold for effects on vascular or visceral smooth muscle. In the four long-term studies of **DDAVP Tablets**, no increases in blood pressure in 46 patients receiving **DDAVP Tablets** for periods of 12 to 44 months were reported.
In one study, the pharmacodynamic characteristics of **DDAVP Tablets** and intranasal formulation were compared during an 8-hour dosing interval at steady state. The doses administered to 36 hydrated (water loaded) healthy male adult volunteers every 8 hours were 0.1, 0.2, 0.4 mg orally and 0.01 mg intranasally by rhinal tube. The results are shown in the following table:

Mean Changes from Baseline (SE) in Pharmacodynamic Parameters in Normal Healthy Adult Volunteers

Treatment	Total Urine Volume in mL	Maximum Urine Osmolality in mOsm/kg
0.1 mg PO q8h	−3689.3 (149.6)	514.8 (21.9)
0.2 mg PO q8h	−4429.9 (149.6)	686.3 (21.9)
0.4 mg PO q8h	−4998.8 (149.6)	769.3 (21.9)
0.01 mg IN q8h	−4844.9 (149.6)	754.1 (21.9)

(SE) = Standard error of the mean

With respect to the mean values of total urine volume decrease and maximum urine osmolality increase from baseline, the 90% confidence limits estimated that the 0.4 mg and 0.2 mg oral dose produced between 95% and 110% and 84% to 99% of pharmacodynamic activity, respectively, when compared to the 0.01 mg intranasal dose.

While both the 0.2 mg and 0.4 mg oral doses are considered pharmacodynamically similar to the 0.01 mg intranasal dose, the pharmacodynamic data on an inter-subject basis was highly variable and, therefore, individual dosing is recommended.

In another study in diabetes insipidus patients, the pharmacodynamic characteristics of **DDAVP Tablets** and intranasal formulations were compared over a 12-hour period. Ten fluid-controlled patients under age 18 were administered tablet doses of 0.2 mg and 0.4 mg, and intranasal doses of 0.01 mg and 0.02 mg.

Mean Peak Pharmacodynamic Parameters (SD) in Pediatric and Adolescent Diabetes Insipidus Patients

Treatment	Urine Volume in mL/min	Maximum Urine Osmolality in mOsm/kg
0.01 mg IN	0.3 (0.15)	717.0 (224.63)
0.02 mg IN	0.3 (0.25)	761.8 (298.82)
0.2 mg PO	0.3 (0.12)	678.3 (147.91)
0.4 mg PO	0.2 (0.15)	787.2 (73.34)

(SD) = Standard Deviation

All four dose formulations (0.01 mg IN, 0.02 mg IN, 0.2 mg PO and 0.4 mg PO) have a similar, pronounced pharmacodynamic effect on urine volume and urine osmolality. At two hours after study drug administration, mean urine volume was 4 mL/min and urine osmolality was >500 mOsm/kg. Mean plasma osmolality remained relatively constant over the time course recorded (0 to 12 hours). A statistical separation from baseline did not occur at any dose or time point. In these patients, the 0.2 mg tablets and the 0.01 mg intranasal spray exhibited similar pharmacodynamic profiles as did the 0.4 mg tablets and the 0.02 mg intranasal spray formulation. In another study of adult diabetes insipidus patients previously controlled on DDAVP intranasal spray, after one week of self-titration from spray to tablets, patients' diuresis was controlled with 0.1 mg **DDAVP Tablets** three times a day.

Primary Nocturnal Enuresis: Two double-blind, randomized, placebo-controlled studies were conducted in 340 patients with primary nocturnal enuresis. Patients were 5–17 years old, and 72% were males. A total of 329 patients were evaluated for efficacy. Patients were evaluated over a two-week baseline period in which the average number of wet nights was 10 (range 4–14). Patients were then randomized to receive 0.2, 0.4, or 0.6 mg of DDAVP or placebo. The pooled results after two weeks are shown in the following table:

[See table at top right of page]

Response to DDAVP and Placebo at Two Weeks of Treatment Mean (SE) Number of Wet Nights/2 Weeks

	Placebo (n = 85)	0.2 mg/day (n = 79)	0.4 mg/day (n = 82)	0.6 mg/day (n = 83)
Baseline	10 (0.3)	11 (0.3)	10 (0.3)	10 (0.3)
Reduction from Baseline	1 (0.3)	3 (0.4)	3 (0.4)	4 (0.4)
Percent Reduction from Baseline	10%	27%	30%	40%
p-value vs placebo	—	<0.05	<0.05	<0.05

Patients treated with **DDAVP Tablets** showed a statistically significant reduction in the number of wet nights compared to placebo-treated patients. A greater response was observed with increasing doses up to 0.6 mg.

In a six month, open-label extension study, patients completing the placebo-controlled studies were started on 0.2 mg/day DDAVP, and the dose was progressively increased until the optimal response was achieved (maximum dose 0.6 mg/day). A total of 230 patients were evaluated for efficacy; the average number of wet nights/2 weeks during the untreated baseline period was 10 (range 4–14), and the average duration (SD) of treatment was 4.2 (1.8) months. Twenty-five (25) patients (11%) achieved a complete or near complete response (≤2 wet nights/2 weeks) and did not require titration to the 0.6 mg/day dose. The majority of patients (198 of 230, 86%) were titrated to the highest dose. When all dose groups were combined, 128 (56%) showed at least a 50% reduction from baseline in the number of wet nights/2 weeks, while 87 (38%) patients achieved a complete or near complete response.

INDICATIONS AND USAGE

Central Diabetes Insipidus: DDAVP Tablets are indicated as antidiuretic replacement therapy in the management of central diabetes insipidus and for the management of the temporary polyuria and polydipsia following head trauma or surgery in the pituitary region. DDAVP is ineffective for the treatment of nephrogenic diabetes insipidus.

Patients were selected for therapy based on the diagnosis by means of the water deprivation test, the hypertonic saline infusion test, and/or response to antidiuretic hormone. Continued response to DDAVP can be monitored by measuring urine volume and osmolality.

Primary Nocturnal Enuresis: DDAVP® Tablets (desmopressin acetate) are indicated for the management of primary nocturnal enuresis. DDAVP may be used alone or as an adjunct to behavioral conditioning or other non-pharmacologic intervention.

CONTRAINDICATIONS

DDAVP Tablets are contraindicated in individuals with known hypersensitivity to desmopressin acetate or to any of the components of **DDAVP Tablets**.

WARNINGS

In very young and elderly patients, in particular, fluid intake should be adjusted downward to decrease the potential occurrence of water intoxication and hyponatremia. Particular attention should be paid to the possibility of the rare occurrence of an extreme decrease in plasma osmolality that may result in seizures which could lead to coma.

PRECAUTIONS

General: Intranasal formulations of DDAVP at high doses and DDAVP Injection have infrequently produced a slight elevation of blood pressure which disappears with a reduction of dosage. Although this effect has not been observed when single oral doses up to 0.6 mg have been administered, the drug should be used with caution in patients with coronary artery insufficiency and/or hypertensive cardiovascular disease, because of a possible rise in blood pressure.

DDAVP should be used with caution in patients with conditions associated with fluid and electrolyte imbalance, such as cystic fibrosis, since these patients may develop hyponatremia.

Rare severe allergic reactions have been reported with DDAVP. Anaphylaxis has been reported with intravenous administration of DDAVP Injection, but not with **DDAVP Tablets.**

Laboratory Tests: *Central Diabetes Insipidus:* Laboratory tests for monitoring the patient with central diabetes insipidus or post-surgical or head trauma-related polyuria and polydipsia include urine volume and osmolality. In some cases, measurements of plasma osmolality may be useful.

Drug Interactions: Although the pressor activity of DDAVP is very low compared to its antidiuretic activity, large doses of **DDAVP Tablets** should be used with other pressor agents only with careful patient monitoring.

Carcinogenicity, Mutagenicity, Impairment of Fertility: Studies with DDAVP have not been performed to evaluate carcinogenic potential, mutagenic potential or effects on fertility.

Pregnancy: *Category B:* Fertility studies have not been done. Teratology studies in rats and rabbits at doses from 0.05 to 10 µg/kg/day (approximately 0.1 times the maximum systemic human exposure in rats and up to 38 times the maximum systemic human exposure in rabbits based on surface area, mg/m^2) revealed no harm to the fetus due to DDAVP (desmopressin acetate). There are, however, no adequate and well-controlled studies in pregnant women. Because animal studies are not always predictive of human response, this drug should be used during pregnancy only if clearly needed.

Several publications where desmopressin acetate was used in the management of diabetes insipidus during pregnancy are available; these include a few anecdotal reports of congenital anomalies and low birth weight babies. However, no causal connection between these events and desmopressin acetate has been established. A fifteen year Swedish epidemiologic study of the use of desmopressin acetate in pregnant women with diabetes insipidus found the rate of birth defects to be no greater than that in the general population; however, the statistical power of this study is low. As opposed to preparations containing natural hormones, desmopressin acetate in antidiuretic doses has no uterotonic action and the physician will have to weigh the possible therapeutic advantages against the possible risks in each case.

Nursing Mothers: There have been no controlled studies in nursing mothers. A single study in postpartum women demonstrated a marked change in plasma, but little if any change in assayable DDAVP in breast milk following an intranasal dose of 0.01 mg.

It is not known whether the drug is excreted in human milk. Because many drugs are excreted in human milk, caution should be exercised when DDAVP is administered to nursing mothers.

Pediatric Use: *Central Diabetes Insipidus:* **DDAVP Tablets** have been used safely in pediatric patients, age 4 years and older, with diabetes insipidus for periods up to 44 months. In younger pediatric patients the dose must be individually adjusted in order to prevent an excessive decrease in plasma osmolality leading to hyponatremia and possible convulsions; dosing should start at 0.05 mg (1/2 of the 0.1 mg tablet). Use of **DDAVP Tablets** in pediatric patients requires careful fluid intake restrictions to prevent possible hyponatremia and water intoxication.

Primary Nocturnal Enuresis: **DDAVP Tablets** have been safely used in pediatric patients age 6 years and older with primary nocturnal enuresis for up to 6 months. Some patients respond to a dose of 0.2 mg; however, increasing responses are seen at doses of 0.4 mg and 0.6 mg. No increase in the frequency or severity of adverse reactions or decrease in efficacy was seen with an increased dose or duration. The dose should be individually adjusted to achieve the best results.

ADVERSE REACTIONS

Infrequently, large doses of the intranasal formulations of DDAVP and DDAVP Injection have produced transient headache, nausea, flushing and mild abdominal cramps. These symptoms have disappeared with reduction in dosage.

Central Diabetes Insipidus: In long-term clinical studies in which patients with diabetes insipidus were followed for periods up to 44 months of **DDAVP Tablet** therapy, transient increases in AST (SGOT) no higher than 1.5 times the upper limit of normal were occasionally observed. Elevated AST (SGOT) returned to the normal range despite continued use of **DDAVP Tablets.**

Primary Nocturnal Enuresis: The only adverse event occurring in ≥3% of patients in controlled clinical trials with **DDAVP Tablets** that was probably, possibly, or remotely related to study drug was headache (4% DDAVP, 3% placebo).

Other: The following adverse events have been reported; however their relationship to DDAVP has not been established: abnormal thinking, diarrhea, and edema-weight gain.

See **WARNINGS** for the possibility of water intoxication and hyponatremia.

OVERDOSAGE

(See **ADVERSE REACTIONS.**) In case of overdose, the dose should be reduced, frequency of administration decreased, or the drug withdrawn according to the severity of the condition. There is no known specific antidote for DDAVP. The patient should be observed and treated with appropriate symptomatic therapy.

An oral LD_{50} has not been established. Oral doses up to 0.2 mg/kg/day have been administered to dogs and rats for 6 months without any significant drug-related toxicities reported. An intravenous dose of 2 mg/kg in mice demonstrated no effect.

DOSAGE AND ADMINISTRATION

Central Diabetes Insipidus: The dosage of **DDAVP Tablets** must be determined for each individual patient and adjusted according to the diurnal pattern of response. Response should be estimated by two parameters: adequate duration of sleep and adequate, not excessive, water turnover. Patients previously on intranasal DDAVP therapy should begin tablet therapy twelve hours after the last intranasal dose. During the initial dose titration period, patients should be observed closely and appropriate safety parameters measured to assure adequate response. Patients should be monitored at regular intervals during the course of **DDAVP Tablet** therapy to assure adequate antidiuretic response. Modifications in dosage regimen should be implemented as necessary to assure adequate water turnover.

Adults and Children: It is recommended that patients be started on doses of 0.05 mg (1/2 of the 0.1 mg tablet) two times a day and individually adjusted to their optimum therapeutic dose. Most patients in clinical trials found that the optimal dosage range is 0.1 mg to 0.8 mg daily, administered in divided doses. Each dose should be separately adjusted for an adequate diurnal rhythm of water turnover. Total daily dosage should be increased or decreased in the range of 0.1 mg to 1.2 mg divided into two or three daily doses as needed to obtain adequate antidiuresis. See **Pediatric Use** subsection for special considerations when administering desmopressin acetate to pediatric diabetes insipidus patients.

Primary Nocturnal Enuresis: The dosage of **DDAVP Tablets** must be determined for each individual patient and adjusted according to response. Patients previously on intranasal DDAVP therapy can begin tablet therapy the night following (24 hours after) the last intranasal dose. The recommended initial dose for patients age 6 years and older is

Continued on next page

DDAVP Tablets—Cont.

0.2 mg at bedtime. The dose may be titrated up to 0.6 mg to achieve the desired response.

HOW SUPPLIED

Strength	Size	NDC 0075-	Color	Markings
0.1 mg	Bottle of 100	0016-00	White	
0.2 mg	Bottle of 100	0026-00	White	

Store at Controlled Room Temperature 20 to 25°C (68 to 77°F) [see USP]. Avoid exposure to excessive heat or light.
Rx only.
Keep out of the reach of children.
U.S. Patent Nos. 5,500,413, 5,596,078, 5,674,850, 5,047,398
Manufactured for
Aventis Pharmaceuticals Products Inc.
Parsippany, NJ 07054
Rev. 4/98
By Ferring Pharmaceuticals, Malmö, Sweden IN-5547D!
413953

Shown in Product Identification Guide, page 307

DIAβETA® ℞
[*dī "ə-bū 'ta*]
(glyburide USP)
Tablets 1.25, 2.5 and 5 mg

Prescribing Information as of September 1997

DESCRIPTION

Diaβeta (glyburide USP) is an oral blood-glucose-lowering drug of the sulfonylurea class. It is a white, crystalline compound, formulated as tablets of 1.25 mg, 2.5 mg, and 5 mg strengths for oral administration. Diaβeta tablets contain the active ingredient glyburide and the following inactive ingredients: dibasic calcium phosphate USP, magnesium stearate NF, microcrystalline cellulose NF, sodium alginate NF, talc USP. Diaβeta 1.25 mg tablets also contain D&C Yellow #10 Aluminum Lake and FD&C Red #40 Aluminum Lake. Diaβeta 2.5 mg tablets also contain FD&C Red #40 Aluminum Lake. Diaβeta 5 mg tablets also contain D&C Yellow #10 Aluminum Lake, and FD&C Blue #1. Chemically, Diaβeta is identified as 1-[[p-[2-(5-Chloro-*o*-anisamido)ethyl]phenyl]sulfonyl]-3-cyclohexylurea.
The CAS Registry Number is 10238-21-8.
The structural formula is:

Cl
CONHCH$_2$CH$_2$— —SO$_2$NHCONH—
OCH$_3$

The molecular weight is 493.99. The aqueous solubility of Diaβeta increases with pH as a result of salt formation.

CLINICAL PHARMACOLOGY

Diaβeta appears to lower the blood glucose acutely by stimulating the release of insulin from the pancreas, an effect dependent upon functioning beta cells in the pancreatic islets. The mechanism by which Diaβeta lowers blood glucose during long-term administration has not been clearly established.
With chronic administration in Type II diabetic patients, the blood glucose lowering effect persists despite a gradual decline in the insulin secretory response to the drug. Extrapancreatic effects may play a part in the mechanism of action of oral sulfonylurea hypoglycemic drugs.
In addition to its blood glucose lowering actions, Diaβeta produces a mild diuresis by enhancement of renal free water clearance. Clinical experience to date indicates an extremely low incidence of disulfiram-like reactions in patients while taking Diaβeta.

Pharmacokinetics

Single-dose studies with Diaβeta in normal subjects demonstrate significant absorption within 1 hour, peak drug levels at about 4 hours, and low but detectable levels at 24 hours. Mean serum levels of glyburide, as reflected by areas under the serum concentration-time curve, increase in proportion to corresponding increases in dose. Multiple-dose studies with Diaβeta in diabetic patients demonstrate drug level concentration-time curves similar to single-dose studies, indicating no build-up of drug in tissue depots. The decrease of glyburide in the serum of normal healthy individuals is biphasic, the terminal half-life being about 10 hours. In single-dose studies in fasting normal subjects, the degree and duration of blood glucose lowering is proportional to the dose administered and to the area under the drug level concentration-time curve. The blood glucose lowering effect persists for 24 hours following single morning doses in nonfasting diabetic patients. Under conditions of repeated administration in diabetic patients, however, there is no reliable correlation between blood drug levels and fasting blood glucose levels. A one-year study of diabetic patients treated with Diaβeta showed no reliable correlation between administered dose and serum drug level.
The major metabolite of Diaβeta is the 4-trans-hydroxy derivative. A second metabolite, the 3-cis-hydroxy derivative, also occurs. These metabolites contribute no significant hypoglycemic action since they are only weakly active (1/400th and 1/40th, respectively, as glyburide) in rabbits.
Diaβeta is excreted as metabolites in the bile and urine, approximately 50% by each route. This dual excretory pathway is qualitatively different from that of other sulfonylureas, which are excreted primarily in the urine.
Sulfonylurea drugs are extensively bound to serum proteins. Displacement from protein binding sites by other drugs may lead to enhanced hypoglycemic action. *In vitro*, the protein binding exhibited by Diaβeta is predominantly non-ionic, whereas that of other sulfonylureas (chlorpropamide, tolbutamide, tolazamide) is predominantly ionic. Acidic drugs such as phenylbutazone, warfarin, and salicylates displace the ionic-binding sulfonylureas from serum proteins to a far greater extent than the non-ionic binding Diaβeta. It has not been shown that this difference in protein binding will result in fewer drug-drug interactions with Diaβeta in clinical use.

INDICATIONS AND USAGE

Diaβeta is indicated as an adjunct to diet to lower the blood glucose in patients with non-insulin-dependent diabetes mellitus (Type II) whose hyperglycemia cannot be controlled by diet alone.
In initiating treatment for non-insulin-dependent diabetes, diet should be emphasized as the primary form of treatment. Caloric restriction and weight loss are essential in the obese diabetic patient. Proper dietary management alone may be effective in controlling the blood glucose and symptoms of hyperglycemia. The importance of regular physical activity should also be stressed, and cardiovascular risk factors should be identified and corrective measures taken where possible.
If this treatment program fails to reduce symptoms and/or blood glucose, the use of an oral sulfonylurea or insulin should be considered. Use of Diaβeta must be viewed by both the physician and patient as a treatment in addition to diet, and not as a substitute for diet or as a convenient mechanism for avoiding dietary restraint. Furthermore, loss of blood glucose control on diet alone may be transient, thus requiring only short-term administration of Diaβeta.
During maintenance programs, Diaβeta should be discontinued if satisfactory lowering of blood glucose is no longer achieved. Judgments should be based on regular clinical and laboratory evaluations.
In considering the use of Diaβeta in asymptomatic patients, it should be recognized that controlling the blood glucose in non-insulin dependent diabetes has not been definitely established to be effective in preventing the long-term cardiovascular or neural complications of diabetes.

CONTRAINDICATIONS

Diaβeta is contraindicated in patients with:
1. Known hypersensitivity to the drug.
2. Diabetic ketoacidosis, with or without coma.
This condition should be treated with insulin.

WARNINGS

SPECIAL WARNING ON INCREASED RISK OF CARDIOVASCULAR MORTALITY

The administration of oral hypoglycemic drugs has been reported to be associated with increased cardiovascular mortality as compared to treatment with diet alone or diet plus insulin. This warning is based on the study conducted by the University Group Diabetes Program (UGDP), a long-term prospective clinical trial designed to evaluate the effectiveness of glucose-lowering drugs in preventing or delaying vascular complications in patients with non-insulin-dependent diabetes. The study involved 823 patients who were randomly assigned to one of four treatment groups (Diabetes 19 (supp. 2): 747-830, 1970).
UGDP reported that patients treated for 5 to 8 years with diet plus a fixed dose of tolbutamide (1.5 grams per day) had a rate of cardiovascular mortality approximately 2½ times that of patients treated with diet alone. A significant increase in total mortality was not observed, but the use of tolbutamide was discontinued based on the increase in cardiovascular mortality, thus limiting the opportunity for the study to show an increase in overall mortality. Despite controversy regarding the interpretation of these results, the findings of the UGDP study provide an adequate basis for this warning. The patient should be informed of the potential risks and advantages of Diaβeta and of alternative modes of therapy.
Although only one drug in the sulfonylurea class (tolbutamide) was included in this study, it is prudent from a safety standpoint to consider that this warning may also apply to other oral hypoglycemic drugs in this class, in view of their close similarities in mode of action and chemical structure.

PRECAUTIONS

General

Hypoglycemia: All sulfonylurea drugs are capable of producing severe hypoglycemia. Proper patient selection, dosage, and instructions are important to avoid hypoglycemic episodes. Renal or hepatic insufficiency may cause elevated blood levels of Diaβeta and the latter may also diminish gluconeogenic capacity, both of which increase the risk of serious hypoglycemic reactions. Elderly, debilitated or malnourished patients, and those with adrenal or pituitary insufficiency are particularly susceptible to the hypoglycemic action of glucose-lowering drugs. Hypoglycemia may be difficult to recognize in the elderly, and in people who are taking beta-adrenergic blocking drugs or other sympatholytic agents. Hypoglycemia is more likely to occur when caloric intake is deficient, after severe or prolonged exercise, when alcohol is ingested, or when more than one glucose-lowering drug is used.
Loss of control of blood glucose: When a patient stabilized on any diabetic regimen is exposed to stress such as fever, trauma, infection, or surgery, a loss of control may occur. At such times, it may be necessary to discontinue Diaβeta and administer insulin.
The effectiveness of any oral hypoglycemic drug, including Diaβeta, in lowering blood glucose to a desired level decreases in many patients over a period of time, which may be due to progression of the severity of the diabetes or to diminished responsiveness to the drug. This phenomenon is known as secondary failure, to distinguish it from primary failure in which the drug is ineffective in an individual patient when first given.

Information for Patients

Patients should be informed of the potential risks and advantages of Diaβeta and of alternative modes of therapy. They should also be informed about the importance of adherence to dietary instructions, of a regular exercise program, and of regular testing of blood glucose.
The risks of hypoglycemia, its symptoms and treatment, and conditions that predispose to its development should be explained to patients and responsible family members. Primary and secondary failure should also be explained.

Laboratory Tests

Periodic fasting blood glucose measurements should be performed to monitor therapeutic response. A glycosylated hemoglobin determination should also be performed periodically.

Drug Interactions

The hypoglycemic action of sulfonylureas may be potentiated by certain drugs including nonsteroidal anti-inflammatory agents and other drugs that are highly protein bound, salicylates, sulfonamides, chloramphenicol, probenecid, monoamine oxidase inhibitors and beta adrenergic blocking agents. When such drugs are administered to a patient receiving Diaβeta, the patient should be observed closely for hypoglycemia. When such drugs are withdrawn from a patient receiving Diaβeta, the patient should be observed closely for loss of control.
A possible interaction between glyburide and fluoroquinolone antibiotics has been reported resulting in a potentiation of the hypoglycemic action of glyburide. The mechanism for this interaction is not known.
Possible interactions between glyburide and coumarin derivatives have been reported that may either potentiate or weaken the effects of coumarin derivatives. The mechanism of these interactions is not known.
Certain drugs tend to produce hyperglycemia and may lead to loss of control. These drugs include the thiazides and other diuretics, corticosteroids, phenothiazines, thyroid products, estrogens, oral contraceptives, phenytoin, nicotinic acid, sympathomimetics, calcium channel blocking drugs, and isoniazid. When such drugs are administered to a patient receiving Diaβeta, the patient should be closely observed for loss of control. When such drugs are withdrawn from a patient receiving Diaβeta, the patient should be observed closely for hypoglycemia. A potential interaction between oral miconazole and oral hypoglycemic agents leading to severe hypoglycemia has been reported. Whether this interaction also occurs with the intravenous, topical or vaginal preparations of miconazole is not known.

Carcinogenesis, Mutagenesis, and Impairment of Fertility

Diaβeta is non-mutagenic when studied in the Salmonella microsome test (Ames test) and in the DNA damage/alkaline elution assay. Studies in rats at doses up to 300 mg/kg/day for 18 months showed no carcinogenic effects.
No drug related effects were noted in any of the criteria evaluated in the two year oncogenicity study of glyburide in mice.

Pregnancy

Teratogenic Effects: Pregnancy Category C
Diaβeta has been shown to effect the maturation of the long bones (humerus and femur) in rat pups when given in doses 6250 times the maximum recommended human dose. These effects, which were seen during the period of lactation and not during organogenesis, are a shortening of the bones with effects to various structures of the long bones, especially in humerus and femur.
There are no adequate and well-controlled studies in pregnant women. Because animal reproduction studies are not always predictive of human response, Diaβeta should be used during pregnancy only if the potential benefit justifies the risk to the fetus. Because recent information suggests that abnormal blood glucose levels during pregnancy are associated with a higher incidence of congenital abnormalities, many experts recommend that insulin be used during pregnancy to maintain blood glucose levels as close to normal as possible.
Nonteratogenic Effects: Prolonged severe hypoglycemia (4 to 10 days) has been reported in neonates born to mothers who were receiving a sulfonylurea drug at the time of delivery. This has been reported more frequently with the use of agents with prolonged half-lives. If Diaβeta is used during

pregnancy, it should be discontinued at least two weeks before the expected delivery date.

Nursing Mothers

Although it is not known whether Diaβeta (glyburide USP) is excreted in human milk, some sulfonylureas are known to be excreted in human milk. Because the potential for hypoglycemia in nursing infants may exist, a decision should be made whether to discontinue nursing or to discontinue administering the drug, taking into account the importance of the drug to the mother. If Diaβeta is discontinued and if diet alone is inadequate for controlling blood glucose, insulin therapy should be considered.

PEDIATRIC USE

Safety and effectiveness in pediatric patients have not been established.

ADVERSE REACTIONS

Hypoglycemia: See PRECAUTIONS and OVERDOSAGE Sections.

Gastrointestinal Reactions: Cholestatic jaundice and hepatitis may occur rarely; Diaβeta should be discontinued if this occurs. Liver function abnormalities, including isolated transaminase elevations, have been reported. Gastrointestinal disturbances, e.g., nausea, epigastric fullness, and heartburn, are the most common reactions and occur in 1.8% of treated patients. They tend to be dose-related and may disappear when dosage is reduced.

Dermatologic Reactions: Allergic skin reactions, e.g., pruritus, erythema, urticaria, and morbilliform or maculopapular eruptions, occur in 1.5% of treated patients. These may be transient and may disappear despite continued use of Diaβeta; if skin reactions persist, the drug should be discontinued.

Porphyria cutanea tarda and photosensitivity reactions have been reported with sulfonylureas.

Hematologic Reactions: Leukopenia, agranulocytosis, thrombocytopenia, which occasionally may present as purpura, hemolytic anemia, aplastic anemia, and pancytopenia have been reported with sulfonylureas.

Metabolic Reactions: Hepatic porphyria reactions have been reported with sulfonylureas; however, these have not been reported with Diaβeta. Disulfiram-like reactions have been reported very rarely with Diaβeta. Cases of hyponatremia have been reported with glyburide and all other sulfonylureas, most often in patients who are on other medications or have medical conditions known to cause hyponatremia or increase release of antidiuretic hormone. The syndrome of inappropriate antidiuretic hormone (SIADH) secretion has been reported with certain other sulfonylureas, and it has been suggested that these sulfonylureas may augment the peripheral (antidiuretic) action of ADH and/or increase release of ADH.

Other Reactions: Changes in accommodation and/or blurred vision have been reported with glyburide and other sulfonylureas. These are thought to be related to fluctuation in glucose levels.

In addition to dermatologic reactions, allergic reactions such as angioedema, arthralgia, myalgia and vasculitis have been reported.

OVERDOSAGE

Overdosage of sulfonylureas, including Diaβeta, can produce hypoglycemia. Mild hypoglycemic symptoms without loss of consciousness or neurologic findings should be treated aggressively with oral glucose and adjustments in drug dosage and/or meal patterns. Close monitoring should continue until the physician is assured that the patient is out of danger. Severe hypoglycemic reactions with coma, seizure, or other neurological impairment occur infrequently, but constitute medical emergencies requiring immediate hospitalization. If hypoglycemic coma is diagnosed or suspected, the patient should be given a rapid intravenous injection of concentrated (50%) glucose solution. This should be followed by a continuous infusion of a more dilute (10%) glucose solution at a rate that will maintain the blood glucose at a level above 100 mg/mL. Patients should be closely monitored for a minimum of 24 to 48 hours, since hypoglycemia may recur after apparent clinical recovery.

DOSAGE AND ADMINISTRATION

There is no fixed dosage regimen for the management of diabetes mellitus with Diaβeta or any other hypoglycemic agent. The patient's fasting blood glucose must be measured periodically to determine the minimum effective dose for the patient; to detect primary failure, i.e., inadequate lowering of blood glucose at the maximum recommended dose of medication; and to detect secondary failure, i.e., loss of adequate blood glucose lowering response after an initial period of effectiveness. Periodic glycosylated hemoglobin determinations should be performed.

Short-term administration of Diaβeta may be sufficient during periods of transient loss of control in patients usually controlled well on diet.

1. Usual Starting Dose

The usual starting dose of Diaβeta as initial therapy is 2.5 to 5 mg daily, administered with breakfast or the first main meal. Those patients who may be more sensitive to hypoglycemic drugs should be started at 1.25 mg daily. (See PRECAUTIONS Section for patients at increased risk). Failure to follow an appropriate dosage regimen may precipitate hypoglycemia. Patients who do not adhere to their prescribed dietary and drug regimen are more prone to exhibit unsatisfactory response to therapy. Transfer of patients from other oral antidiabetic regimens to Diaβeta should be done conservatively and the initial daily dose should be 2.5 to 5 mg. When transferring patients from oral hypoglycemic agents other than chlorpropamide, to Diaβeta, no transition period and no initial priming dose is necessary. When transferring patients from chlorpropamide, particular care should be exercised during the first 2 weeks because the prolonged retention of chlorpropamide in the body and subsequent overlapping drug effects may provoke hypoglycemia.

Bioavailability studies have demonstrated that Glynase PresTab® Tablets 3 mg are not bioequivalent to Diaβeta Tablets 5 mg. Therefore, these products are not substitutable and patients should be retitrated if transferred.

Some Type II diabetic patients being treated with insulin may respond satisfactorily to Diaβeta. If the insulin dose is less than 20 units daily, substitution of Diaβeta 2.5 to 5 mg as a single daily dose may be tried. If the insulin dose is between 20 and 40 units daily, the patient may be placed directly on Diaβeta 5 mg daily as a single dose. If the insulin dose is more than 40 units daily, a transition period is required for conversion to Diaβeta. In these patients, insulin dosage is decreased by 50% and Diaβeta 5 mg daily is started. Please refer to Usual Maintenance Dose for further explanation.

2. Usual Maintenance Dose

The usual maintenance dose is in the range of 1.25 to 20 mg daily, which may be given as a single dose or in divided doses (See Dosage Interval Section). Dosage increases should be made in increments of no more than 2.5 mg at weekly intervals based upon the patient's blood glucose response.

No exact dosage relationship exists between Diaβeta and the other oral hypoglycemic agents. Although patients may be transferred from the maximum dose of other sulfonylureas, the maximum starting dose of 5 mg of Diaβeta should be observed. A maintenance dose of 5 mg Diaβeta provides approximately the same degree of blood glucose control as 250 to 375 mg chlorpropamide, 250 to 375 mg tolazamide, 500 to 750 mg acetohexamide, or 1000 to 1500 mg tolbutamide.

When transferring patients receiving more than 40 units of insulin daily, they may be started on a daily dose of Diaβeta 5 mg concomitantly with a 50% reduction in insulin dose. Progressive withdrawal of insulin and increase of Diaβeta in increments of 1.25 to 2.5 mg every 2 to 10 days is then carried out. During this conversion period when both insulin and Diaβeta are being used, hypoglycemia may rarely occur. During insulin withdrawal, patients should self-test their blood for glucose and their urine for acetone at least 3 times daily and report results to their physician. Self-testing of urinary glucose is a less desirable alternative. The appearance of persistent acetonuria with glycosuria indicates that the patient is a Type I diabetic who requires insulin therapy.

3. Maximum Dose

Daily doses of more than 20 mg are not recommended.

4. Dosage Interval

Once-a-day therapy is usually satisfactory, based upon usual meal patterns and a 10 hour half-life of Diaβeta. Some patients, particularly those receiving more than 10 mg daily, may have a more satisfactory response with twice-a-day dosage.

In elderly patients, debilitated or malnourished patients, and patients with impaired renal or hepatic function, the initial and maintenance dosing should be conservative to avoid hypoglycemic reactions. (See PRECAUTIONS Section.)

HOW SUPPLIED

Diaβeta (glyburide USP) tablets are available in the following strengths and package sizes:

1.25 mg (peach oblong, scored tablets with beveled edges, imprinted with "Hoechst" on one side and "Dia β" on the other side).

Bottles of 50 (NDC 0039-0053-05)

2.5 mg (pink oblong, scored tablets with beveled edges, imprinted with "Hoechst" on one side and "Dia β" on the other side).

Bottles of 100 (NDC 0039-0051-10)
Bottles of 500 (NDC 0039-0051-50)
Unit Dose Cartons of 100 (NDC 0039-0051-11)

5 mg (green oblong, scored tablets with beveled edges, imprinted with "Hoechst" on one side and "Dia β" on the other side).

Bottles of 100 (NDC 0039-0052-10)
Bottles of 500 (NDC 0039-0052-50)
Bottles of 1000 (NDC 0039-0052-70)
Unit Dose Cartons of 100 (NDC 0039-0052-11)

Store between 59 and 86° F (15 and 30° C).

Dispense in well-closed containers with safety closures.

Prescribing Information as of September 1997.

Glynase and PresTab are registered trademarks of The Upjohn Company

Hoechst-Roussel Pharmaceuticals
Division of Hoechst Marion Roussel, Inc.
Kansas City, MO 64137 USA

Shown in Product Identification Guide, page 307

GLIADEL® Wafer ℞
(polifeprosan 20 with carmustine implant)

DESCRIPTION

GLIADEL® Wafer (polifeprosan 20 with carmustine implant) is a sterile, off-white to pale yellow wafer approximately 1.45 cm in diameter and 1 mm thick. Each wafer contains 192.3 mg of a biodegradable polyanhydride copolymer and 7.7 mg of carmustine [1,3-bis (2-chloroethyl)-1-nitrosourea, or BCNU]. Carmustine is a nitrosourea oncolytic agent. The copolymer, polifeprosan 20, consists of poly[bis(p-carboxyphenoxy) propane: sebacic acid] in a 20:80 molar ratio and is used to control the local delivery of carmustine. Carmustine is homogeneously distributed in the copolymer matrix.

The structural formula for polifeprosan 20 is:

$$\left[-O-\overset{O}{\overset{\|}{C}}-C_6H_4-O(CH_2)_3O-C_6H_4-\overset{O}{\overset{\|}{C}}-\right]_m\left[-O-\overset{O}{\overset{\|}{C}}-CH_2(CH_2)_6CH_2-\overset{O}{\overset{\|}{C}}-\right]_n$$

Ratio m:n = 20:80; random copolymer

The structural formula for carmustine is:

$$Cl-CH_2-CH_2-\underset{NO}{\underset{|}{N}}\overset{O}{\overset{\|}{C}}NHCH_2-CH_2-Cl$$

CLINICAL PHARMACOLOGY

GLIADEL is designed to deliver carmustine directly into the surgical cavity created when a brain tumor is resected. On exposure to the aqueous environment of the resection cavity, the anhydride bonds in the copolymer are hydrolyzed, releasing carmustine, carboxyphenoxypropane, and sebacic acid. The carmustine released from GLIADEL diffuses into the surrounding brain tissue and produces an antineoplastic effect by alkylating DNA and RNA.

Carmustine has been shown to degrade both spontaneously and metabolically. The production of an alkylating moiety, hypothesized to be chloroethyl carbonium ion, leads to the formation of DNA cross-links.

The tumoricidal activity of GLIADEL is dependent on release of carmustine to the tumor cavity in concentrations sufficient for effective cytotoxicity.

More than 70% of the copolymer degrades by three weeks. The metabolic disposition and excretion of the monomers differ. Carboxyphenoxypropane is eliminated by the kidney and sebacic acid, an endogenous fatty acid, is metabolized by the liver and expired as CO_2 in animals.

The absorption, distribution, metabolism, and excretion of the copolymer in humans is unknown. Carmustine concentrations delivered by GLIADEL in human brain tissue have not been determined. Plasma levels of carmustine after GLIADEL wafer implant were not determined. In rabbits implanted with wafers containing 3.85% carmustine, no detectible levels of carmustine were found in the plasma or cerebrospinal fluid.

Following an intravenous infusion of carmustine at doses ranging from 30 to 170 mg/m^2, the average terminal half-life, clearance, and steady-state volume of distribution were 22 minutes, 56 mL/min/kg, and 3.25 L/kg, respectively. Approximately 60% of the intravenous 200 mg/m^2 dose of ^{14}C-carmustine was excreted in the urine over 96 hours and 6% was expired as CO_2.

GLIADEL wafers are biodegradable in human brain when implanted into the cavity after tumor resection. The rate of biodegradation is variable from patient to patient. During the biodegradation process, a wafer remnant may be observed on brain imaging scans or at re-operation even though extensive degradation of all components has occurred. Data obtained from review of CT scans obtained 49 days after implantation of GLIADEL demonstrated that images consistent with wafers were visible to varying degrees in the scans of 11 of 18 patients. Data obtained at re-operation and autopsies have demonstrated wafer remnants up to 232 days after GLIADEL implantation.

Wafer remnants removed at re-operation from two patients with recurrent malignant glioma, one at 64 days and the second at 92 days after implantation, were analyzed for content. The following table presents the results of analyses completed on these remnants.

COMPOSITION OF WAFER REMNANTS REMOVED FROM TWO PATIENTS ON RE-OPERATION

Component	Patient A	Patient B
Days After GLIADEL Implantation	64	92
Anhydride Bonds	None detected	None detected
Water Content (% of wafer remnant weight)	95–97%	74–86%
Carmustine Content (% of initial)	<0.0004%	0.034%
Carboxyphenoxypropane Content (% of initial)	9%	14%
Sebacic Acid Content (% of initial)	4%	3%

The wafer remnants consisted mostly of water and monomeric components with minimal detectable carmustine present.

CLINICAL STUDIES

In a randomized, double-blind, placebo-controlled clinical trial in adults with recurrent malignant glioma, GLIADEL

Continued on next page

Gliadel—Cont.

prolonged survival in patients with glioblastoma multiforme (GBM). Ninety-five percent of the patients treated with GLIADEL had 7–8 wafers implanted.

In 222 patients with recurrent malignant glioma who had failed initial surgery and radiation therapy, the six-month survival rate after surgery increased from 47% (53/112) for patients receiving placebo to 60% (66/110) for patients treated with GLIADEL. Median survival increased by 33%, from 24 weeks with placebo to 32 weeks with GLIADEL treatment. In patients with GBM, the six-month survival rate increased from 36% (26/73) with placebo to 56% (40/72) with GLIADEL treatment. Median survival of GBM patients increased by 41% from 20 weeks with placebo to 28 weeks with GLIADEL treatment. In patients with pathologic diagnoses other than GBM at the time of surgery for tumor recurrence, GLIADEL produced no survival prolongation.

6-MONTH KAPLAN-MEIER SURVIVAL CURVES FOR PATIENTS UNDERGOING SURGERY FOR RECURRENT GBM

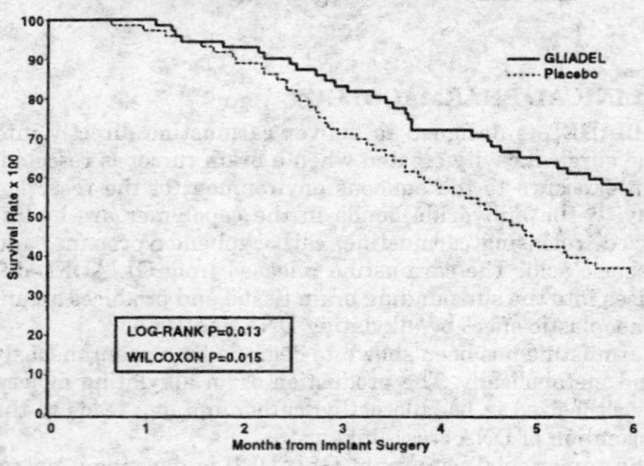

OVERALL KAPLAN-MEIER SURVIVAL CURVES FOR PATIENTS UNDERGOING SURGERY FOR RECURRENT GBM

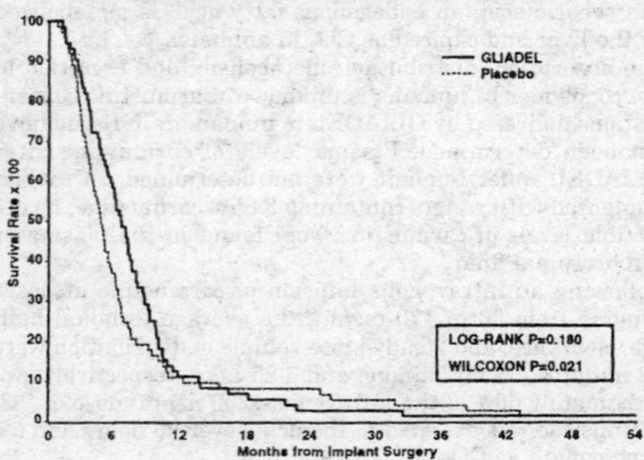

INDICATIONS AND USAGE

GLIADEL is indicated for use as an adjunct to surgery to prolong survival in patients with recurrent glioblastoma multiforme for whom surgical resection is indicated.

CONTRAINDICATIONS

GLIADEL contains carmustine. GLIADEL should not be given to individuals who have demonstrated a previous hypersensitivity to carmustine or any of the components of GLIADEL.

WARNINGS

Patients undergoing craniotomy for malignant glioma and implantation of GLIADEL should be monitored closely for known complications of craniotomy, including seizures, intracranial infections, abnormal wound healing, and brain edema. Cases of intracerebral mass effect unresponsive to corticosteroids have been described in patients treated with GLIADEL, including one case leading to brain herniation.

Pregnancy: There are no studies assessing the reproductive toxicity of GLIADEL. Carmustine, the active component of GLIADEL, can cause fetal harm when administered to a pregnant woman. Carmustine has been shown to be embryotoxic and teratogenic in rats at i.p. doses of 0.5, 1, 2, 4, or 8 mg/kg/day when given on gestation days 6 through 15. Carmustine caused fetal malformations (anophthalmia, micrognathia, omphalocele) at 1.0 mg/kg/day (about 1/6 the recommended human dose (eight wafers of 7.7 mg carmustine/wafer) on a mg/m^2 basis). Carmustine was embryotoxic in rabbits at i.v. doses of 4.0 mg/kg/day (about 1.2 times the recommended human dose on a mg/m^2 basis). Embryotoxicity was characterized by increased embryo-fetal deaths, reduced numbers of litters, and reduced litter sizes.

There are no studies of GLIADEL in pregnant women. If GLIADEL is used during pregnancy, or if the patient becomes pregnant after GLIADEL implantation, the patient must be warned of the potential hazard to the fetus.

PRECAUTIONS

General: Communication between the surgical resection cavity and the ventricular system should be avoided to prevent the wafers from migrating into the ventricular system and causing obstructive hydrocephalus. If a communication exists, it should be closed prior to wafer implantation.

Imaging Studies: Computed tomography and magnetic resonance imaging of the head may demonstrate enhancement in the brain tissue surrounding the resection cavity after implantation of GLIADEL wafers. This enhancement may represent edema and inflammation caused by GLIADEL or tumor progression.

Therapeutic Interactions: Interactions of GLIADEL with other drugs or radiotherapy have not been formally evaluated. In clinical trials, few patients have received systemic chemotherapy within 30 days of GLIADEL (6) or external beam radiation therapy (36). Chemotherapy was withheld at least four weeks (six weeks for nitrosoureas) prior to and two weeks after surgery in patients undergoing re-operation for malignant glioma. External beam radiation therapy was initiated no sooner than three weeks after GLIADEL implantation. Of the 36 patients who received GLIADEL at initial surgery for newly diagnosed, malignant glioma followed by external beam radiation therapy, 3/15 (20%) in one study and 11/21 (52%) in the other study experienced new or worsened seizures. Patients were followed for a maximum of 24 months. The short and long-term toxicity profiles of GLIADEL when given in conjunction with radiation or chemotherapy have not been fully explored.

Carcinogenesis, Mutagenesis, Impairment of Fertility: No carcinogenicity, mutagenicity or impairment of fertility studies have been conducted with GLIADEL. Carcinogenicity, mutagenicity and impairment of fertility studies have been conducted with carmustine, the active component of GLIADEL. Carmustine was given three times a week for six months, followed by 12 months observation, to Swiss mice at i.p. doses of 2.5 and 5.0 mg/kg (about 1/5 and 1/3 the recommended human dose (eight wafers of 7.7 mg carmustine/wafer) on a mg/m^2 basis) and to SD rats at i.p. dose of 1.5 mg/kg (about 1/4 the recommended human dose on a mg/m^2 basis.) There were increases in tumor incidence in all treated animals, predominantly subcutaneous and lung neoplasms. *Mutagenesis:* Carmustine was mutagenic *in vitro* (Ames assay, human lymphoblast HGPRT assay) and clastogenic both *in vitro* (V79 hamster cell micronucleus assay) and *in vivo* (SCE assay in rodent brain tumors, mouse bone marrow micronucleus assay). *Impairment of Fertility:* Carmustine caused testicular degeneration at i.p. doses of 8 mg/kg/week for eight weeks (about 1.3 times the recommended human dose on a mg/m^2 basis) in male rats.

Pregnancy: Pregnancy Category D: see **WARNINGS**.

Nursing Mothers: It is not known if either carmustine, carboxyphenoxypropane, or sebacic acid is excreted in human milk. Because many drugs are excreted in human milk and because of the potential for serious adverse reactions from carmustine in nursing infants, it is recommended that patients receiving GLIADEL discontinue nursing.

Pediatric Use: The safety and effectiveness of GLIADEL in pediatric patients have not been established.

ADVERSE REACTIONS

Data in the following table are based on the experience of 222 patients with recurrent malignant glioma randomized to GLIADEL or placebo (wafer without carmustine).

The spectrum of adverse events observed in patients who received GLIADEL or placebo in clinical studies was consistent with that encountered in patients undergoing craniotomy for malignant gliomas.

GLIADEL was not reported to be the cause of death in any of the GLIADEL clinical trials.

The following post-operative adverse events were observed in 4% or more of the patients receiving GLIADEL in the placebo-controlled clinical trial. Except for nervous system effects, where there is a possibility that the placebo wafers could have been responsible, only events more common in the GLIADEL group are listed. These adverse events were either not present pre-operatively or worsened post-operatively during the follow-up period. The follow-up period in the randomized trial was up to 71 months.

COMMON ADVERSE EVENTS OBSERVED IN ≥4% OF PATIENTS IN THE RANDOMIZED TRIAL

Body System Adverse Event	GLIADEL Wafer with Carmustine [N=110] n (%)	PLACEBO Wafer without Carmustine [N=112] n (%)
Body as a Whole		
Fever	13 (12)	9 (8)
Pain*	8 (7)	1 (1)
Digestive System		
Nausea and Vomiting	9 (8)	7 (6)
Metabolic and Nutritional Disorders		
Healing Abnormal*	15 (14)	6 (5)
Nervous System		
Aphasia	10 (9)	12 (11)
Brain Edema	4 (4)	1 (1)
Confusion	11 (10)	9 (8)
Convulsion	21 (19)	21 (19)
Headache	16 (15)	14 (13)
Hemiplegia	21 (19)	22 (20)
Intracranial Hypertension	4 (4)	7 (6)
Meningitis or Abscess	4 (4)	1 (1)
Somnolence	15 (14)	12 (11)
Stupor	7 (6)	7 (6)
Skin and Appendages		
Rash	6 (5)	4 (4)
Urogenital System		
Urinary Tract Infection	23 (21)	19 (17)

*$p < 0.05$ for comparison of GLIADEL versus placebo groups in the randomized trial (two-sided Fisher's Exact Test)

The following adverse events were also reported in 4–9% of GLIADEL patients but were at least as frequent in the placebo group as in GLIADEL-treated patients: infection, deep thrombophlebitis, pulmonary embolism, nausea, oral moniliasis, anemia, hyponatremia, pneumonia.

The following four categories of adverse events are possibly related to treatment with GLIADEL. The frequency with which they occurred in the randomized trial along with descriptive detail are provided below.

1. Seizures: In the randomized study, the majority of seizures in the placebo and GLIADEL groups were mild or moderate in severity. The incidence of new or worsened seizures was 19% in patients treated with GLIADEL and 19% in patients receiving placebo. Of the patients with new or worsened seizures post-operatively, 12/22 (54%) of patients treated with GLIADEL and 2/22 (9%) of placebo patients experienced the first new or worsened seizure within the first five post-operative days. The median time to onset of the first new or worsened post-operative seizure was 3.5 days in patients treated with GLIADEL and 61 days in placebo patients. The occurrence of seizures did not reduce the survival benefit of GLIADEL.

2. Brain Edema: In the randomized trial, brain edema was noted in 4% of patients treated with GLIADEL and in 1% of patients treated with placebo. Development of brain edema with mass effect (due to tumor recurrence, intracranial infection, or necrosis) may necessitate re-operation and, in some cases, removal of wafer or its remnants.

3. Healing Abnormalities: The majority of these events were mild to moderate in severity. Healing abnormalities occurred in 14% of GLIADEL-treated patients compared to 5% of placebo recipients. These events included cerebrospinal fluid leaks, subdural fluid collections, subgaleal or wound effusions, and wound breakdown.

4. Intracranial Infection: In the randomized trial, intracranial infection (meningitis or abscess) occurred in 4% of patients treated with GLIADEL and in 1% of patients receiving placebo. In GLIADEL-treated patients, there were two cases of bacterial meningitis, one case of chemical meningitis, and one case of meningitis which was not further specified. A brain abscess developed in one placebo-treated patient. The rate of deep wound infection (infection of subgaleal space, bone, meninges, or neural parenchyma) was 6% in both GLIADEL and placebo treated patients.

The following adverse events, not listed in the table above, were reported in less than 4% but at least 1% of patients treated with GLIADEL in all studies (n=273). The events listed were either not present pre-operatively or worsened post-operatively. Whether GLIADEL caused these events cannot be determined.

Body as a Whole: peripheral edema (2%); neck pain (2%); accidental injury (1%); back pain (1%); allergic reaction (1%); asthenia (1%); chest pain (1%); sepsis (1%)

Cardiovascular System: hypertension (3%); hypotension (1%)

Digestive System: diarrhea (2%); constipation (2%); dysphagia (1%); gastrointestinal hemorrhage (1%); fecal incontinence (1%)

Hemic and Lymphatic System: thrombocytopenia (1%); leukocytosis (1%)

Metabolic and Nutritional Disorders: hyponatremia (3%); hyperglycemia (3%); hypokalemia (1%)

Musculoskeletal System: infection (1%)

Nervous System: hydrocephalus (3%); depression (3%); abnormal thinking (2%); ataxia (2%); dizziness (2%); insomnia (2%); monoplegia (2%); coma (1%); amnesia (1%); diplopia (1%); paranoid reaction (1%). In addition, cerebral hemorrhage and cerebral infarct were each reported in less than 1% of patients treated with GLIADEL.

Respiratory System: infection (2%); aspiration pneumonia (1%)

Skin and Appendages: rash (2%)

Special Senses: visual field defect (2%); eye pain (1%)

Urogenital System: urinary incontinence (2%)

OVERDOSAGE

There is no clinical experience with use of more than eight GLIADEL wafers per surgical procedure.

DOSAGE AND ADMINISTRATION

Each GLIADEL wafer contains 7.7 mg of carmustine, resulting in a dose of 61.6 mg when eight wafers are implanted. It is recommended that eight wafers be placed in the resection cavity if the size and shape of it allows. Should the size and shape not accommodate eight wafers, the maximum number of wafers as allowed should be placed. Since there is no clinical experience, no more than eight wafers should be used per surgical procedure.

Handling and Disposal[1–7]: Wafers should only be handled by personnel wearing surgical gloves because exposure to carmustine can cause severe burning and hyperpigmentation of the skin. Use of double gloves is recommended and the outer gloves should be discarded into a biohazard waste container after use. A surgical instrument dedicated to the handling of the wafers should be used for wafer implantation. If repeat neurosurgical intervention is indicated, any wafer or wafer remnant should be handled as a potentially cytotoxic agent.

GLIADEL wafers should be handled with care. The aluminum foil laminate pouches containing GLIADEL should be delivered to the operating room and remain unopened until ready to implant the wafers. **The outside surface of the outer foil pouch is not sterile.**

Instructions for Opening Pouch Containing GLIADEL

Figure 1: To remove the sterile inner pouch from the outer pouch, locate the folded corner and slowly pull in an outward motion.

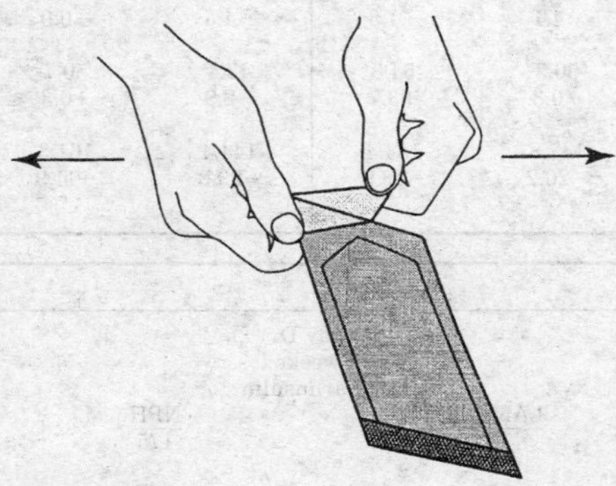

Figure 2: Do NOT pull in a downward motion rolling knuckles over the pouch. This may exert pressure on the wafer and cause it to break.

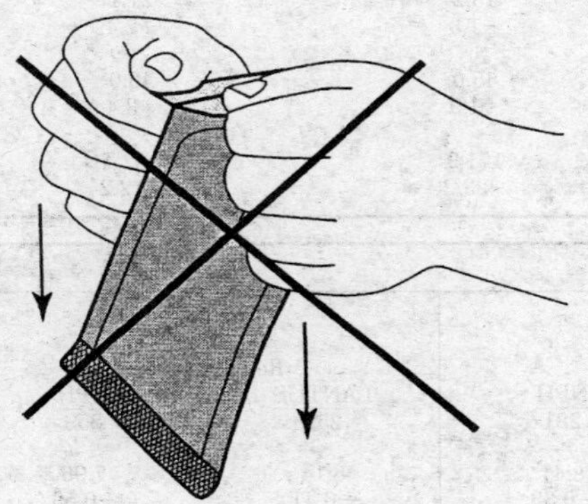

Figure 3: Remove the inner pouch by grabbing hold of the **crimped** edge and pulling upward.

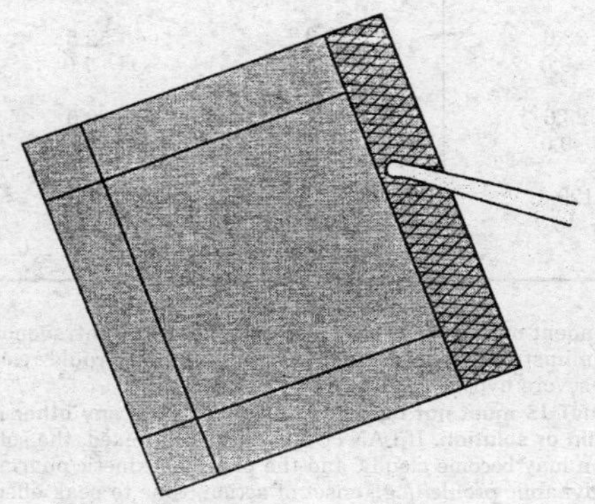

Figure 4: To open the inner pouch, gently hold the crimped edge and cut in an arc-like fashion around the wafer.

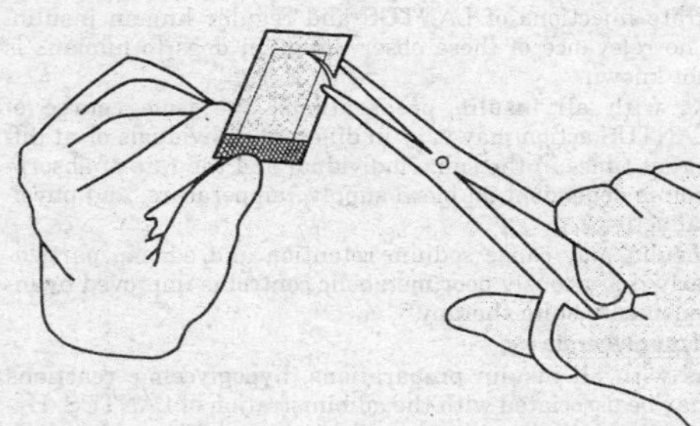

Figure 5: To remove the GLIADEL wafer, gently grasp the wafer with the aid of forceps and place it onto a designated sterile field.

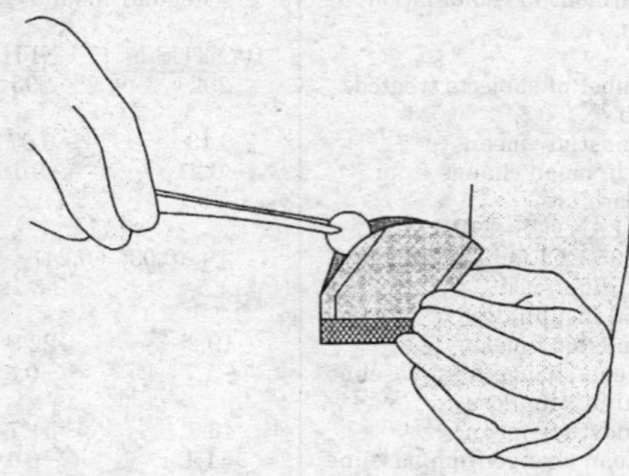

Once the tumor is resected, tumor pathology is confirmed, and hemostasis is obtained, up to eight GLIADEL® Wafers (polifeprosan 20 with carmustine implant) may be placed to cover as much of the resection cavity as possible. Slight overlapping of the wafers is acceptable. Wafers broken in half may be used, but wafers broken in more than two pieces should be discarded in a biohazard container. Oxidized regenerated cellulose (Surgicel®) may be placed over the wafers to secure them against the cavity surface. After placement of the wafers, the resection cavity should be irrigated and the dura closed in a water tight fashion.

Unopened foil pouches may be kept at ambient room temperature for a maximum of six hours at a time.

HOW SUPPLIED

GLIADEL is available in a single dose treatment box containing eight individually pouched wafers. Each wafer contains 7.7 mg of carmustine and is packaged in two aluminum foil laminate pouches. The inner pouch is sterile and is designed to maintain product sterility and protect the product from moisture. The outer pouch is a peelable overwrap. **The outside surface of the outer pouch is not sterile.**

GLIADEL must be stored at or below −20°C (−4°F).

REFERENCES

1. Recommendations for the Safe Handling of Parenteral Antineoplastic Drugs, NIH Publication No. 83-2621. For sale by the Superintendent of Documents, U.S. Government Printing Office, Washington, DC 20402.
2. AMA Council Report, Guidelines for Handling Parenteral Antineoplastics. JAMA, 1985; 253(11):1590-1592.
3. National Study Commission on Cytotoxic Exposure — Recommendations for Handling Cytotoxic Agents. Available from Louis P. Jeffrey, ScD., Chairman, National Study Commission on Cytotoxic Exposure, Massachusetts College of Pharmacy and Allied Health Sciences, 179 Longwood Avenue, Boston, Massachusetts 02115.
4. Clinical Oncological Society of Australia, Guidelines and Recommendations for Safe Handling of Antineoplastic Agents. Med J Australia, 1983; 1:426-428.
5. Jones RB, et al: Safe Handling of Chemotherapeutic Agents: A Report from the Mount Sinai Medical Center. CA — A Cancer Journal for Clinicians, 1983; (Sept/Oct) 258-263.
6. American Society of Hospital Pharmacists Technical Assistance Bulletin on Handling Cytotoxic and Hazardous Drugs. Am J Hosp Pharm, 1990; 47:1033-1049.
7. OSHA Work-Practice Guidelines for Personnel Dealing with Cytotoxic (Antineoplastic) Drugs. Am J Hosp Pharm, 1986; 43:1193-1204.

NDC: 0075-9995-08

CAUTION: FEDERAL LAW PROHIBITS DISPENSING WITHOUT PRESCRIPTION.

U.S. Patent Nos. 4,789,724 and 5,179,189.

Manufactured for
Aventis Pharmaceuticals Products Inc.
Parsippany, NJ 07054
By
Guilford Pharmaceuticals Inc.
Baltimore, MD 21224
Rev. 10/96 IN-2250!

Shown in Product Identification Guide, page 307

LANTUS® ℞

[*lăn' tus*]
(insulin glargine [rDNA origin] injection)
Prescribing Information as of April 2000

LANTUS® must not be diluted or mixed with any other insulin or solution.

DESCRIPTION

LANTUS® (insulin glargine [rDNA origin] injection) is a sterile solution of insulin glargine for use as an injection. Insulin glargine is a recombinant human insulin analog that is a long-acting (up to 24-hour duration of action), parenteral blood-glucose-lowering agent. (See CLINICAL PHARMACOLOGY). LANTUS is produced by recombinant DNA technology utilizing a non-pathogenic laboratory strain of *Escherichia coli* (K12) as the production organism. Insulin glargine differs from human insulin in that the amino acid asparagine at position A21 is replaced by glycine and two arginines are added to the C-terminus of the B-chain. Chemically, it is 21^{A}-Gly-30^{B}a-L-Arg-30^{B}b-L-Arg-human insulin and has the empirical formula $C_{267}H_{404}N_{72}O_{78}S_6$ and a molecular weight of 6063. It has the following structural formula:

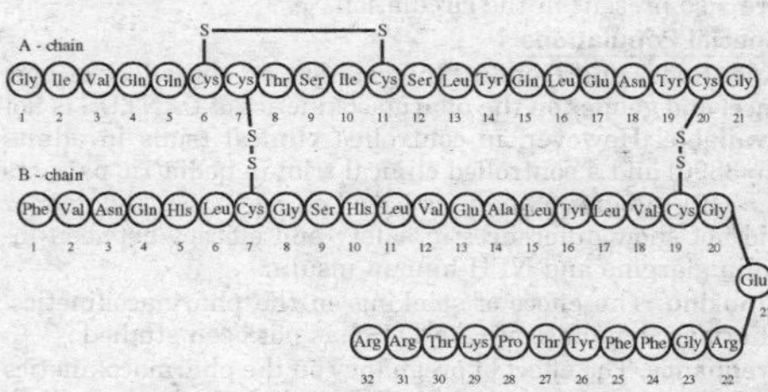

LANTUS consists of insulin glargine dissolved in a clear aqueous fluid. Each milliliter of LANTUS (insulin glargine injection) contains 100 IU (3.6378 mg) insulin glargine, 30 mcg zinc, 2.7 mg m-cresol, 20 mg glycerol 85%, and water for injection. The pH is adjusted by addition of aqueous solutions of hydrochloric acid and sodium hydroxide. LANTUS has a pH of approximately 4.

CLINICAL PHARMACOLOGY

Mechanism of Action

The primary activity of insulin, including insulin glargine, is regulation of glucose metabolism. Insulin and its analogs lower blood glucose levels by stimulating peripheral glucose uptake, especially by skeletal muscle and fat, and by inhibiting hepatic glucose production. Insulin inhibits lipolysis in the adipocyte, inhibits proteolysis, and enhances protein synthesis.

Pharmacodynamics

Insulin glargine is a human insulin analog that has been designed to have low aqueous solubility at neutral pH. At pH 4, as in the LANTUS injection solution, it is completely soluble. After injection into the subcutaneous tissue, the acidic solution is neutralized, leading to formation of microprecipitates from which small amounts of insulin glargine are slowly released, resulting in a relatively constant concentration/time profile over 24 hours with no pronounced peak. This profile allows once-daily dosing as a patient's basal insulin.

In clinical studies, the glucose-lowering effect on a molar basis (i.e., when given at the same doses) of intravenous insulin glargine is approximately the same as human insulin. In euglycemic clamp studies in healthy subjects or in patients with type 1 diabetes, the onset of action of subcutaneous insulin glargine was slower than NPH human insulin. The effect profile of insulin glargine was relatively constant with no pronounced peak and the duration of its effect was prolonged compared to NPH human insulin. *Figure 1* shows results from a study in patients with type 1 diabetes conducted for a maximum of 24 hours after the injection. The median time between injection and the end of pharmacological effect was 14.5 hours (range: 9.5 to 19.3 hours) for NPH human insulin, and 24 hours (range: 10.8 to >24.0 hours) (24 hours was the end of the observation period) for insulin glargine.

Figure 1. Activity Profile in Patients with Type 1 Diabetes†

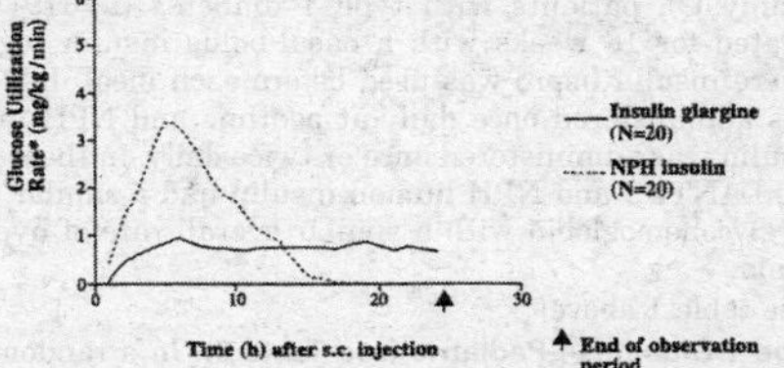

* Determined as amount of glucose infused to maintain constant plasma glucose levels (hourly mean values); indicative of insulin activity.

† Between-patient variability (CV, coefficient of variation); insulin glargine, 84% and NPH, 78%.

The longer duration of action (up to 24 hours) of LANTUS is directly related to its slower rate of absorption and supports once-daily subcutaneous administration. The time course of action of insulins, including LANTUS, may vary between individuals and/or within the same individual.

Pharmacokinetics

Absorption and Bioavailability. After subcutaneous injection of insulin glargine in healthy subjects and in patients with diabetes, the insulin serum concentrations indicated a slower, more prolonged absorption and a relatively constant concentration/time profile over 24 hours with no pronounced peak in comparison to NPH human insulin. Serum insulin concentrations were thus consistent with the time profile of the pharmacodynamic activity of insulin glargine.

After subcutaneous injection of 0.3 IU/kg insulin glargine in patients with type 1 diabetes, a relatively constant concentration/time profile has been demonstrated. The duration of action after abdominal, deltoid, or thigh subcutaneous administration was similar.

Metabolism. A metabolism study in humans indicates that insulin glargine is partly metabolized at the carboxyl terminus of the B chain in the subcutaneous depot to form two

Continued on next page

Lantus—Cont.

active metabolites with in vitro activity similar to that of insulin, M1 (21^A-Gly-insulin) and M2 (21^A-Gly-des-30^B-Thr-insulin). Unchanged drug and these degradation products are also present in the circulation.

Special Populations

Age, Race, and Gender. Information on the effect of age, race, and gender on the pharmacokinetics of LANTUS is not available. However, in controlled clinical trials in adults (n=3890) and a controlled clinical trial in pediatric patients (n=349), subgroup analyses based on age, race, and gender did not show differences in safety and efficacy between insulin glargine and NPH human insulin.

Smoking. The effect of smoking on the pharmacokinetics/pharmacodynamics of LANTUS has not been studied.

Pregnancy. The effect of pregnancy on the pharmacokinetics and pharmacodynamics of LANTUS has not been studied. (See PRECAUTIONS, Pregnancy)

Obesity. In controlled clinical trials, which included patients with Body Mass Index (BMI) up to and including 49.6 kg/m^2, subgroup analyses based on BMI did not show any differences in safety and efficacy between insulin glargine and NPH human insulin.

Renal Impairment. The effect of renal impairment on the pharmacokinetics of LANTUS has not been studied. However, some studies with human insulin have shown increased circulating levels of insulin in patients with renal failure. Careful glucose monitoring and dose adjustments of insulin, including LANTUS, may be necessary in patients with renal dysfunction. (See PRECAUTIONS, Renal Impairment)

Hepatic Impairment. The effect of hepatic impairment on the pharmacokinetics of LANTUS has not been studied. However, some studies with human insulin have shown increased circulating levels of insulin in patients with liver failure. Careful glucose monitoring and dose adjustments of insulin, including LANTUS, may be necessary in patients with hepatic dysfunction (See PRECAUTIONS, Hepatic Impairment)

CLINICAL STUDIES

The safety and effectiveness of insulin glargine given once-daily at bedtime was compared to that of once-daily and twice-daily NPH human insulin in open-label, randomized, active-control, parallel studies of 2327 adult patients and 349 pediatric patients with type 1 diabetes mellitus and 1563 adult patients with type 2 diabetes mellitus (see Tables 1–3). In general, LANTUS achieved a level of glycemic control similar to NPH human insulin as measured by glycated hemoglobin (GHb). The overall rate of hypoglycemia did not differ between patients with diabetes treated with LANTUS compared with NPH human insulin.

Type 1 Diabetes—Adult (see Table 1). In two large, randomized, controlled clinical studies (Studies A and B), patients with type 1 diabetes (Study A; n=585, Study B; n=534) were randomized to basal-bolus treatment with LANTUS once daily or to NPH human insulin once or twice daily and treated for 28 weeks. Regular human insulin was administered before each meal. LANTUS was administered at bedtime. NPH human insulin was administered once daily at bedtime or in the morning and at bedtime when used twice daily. In one large, randomized, controlled clinical study (Study C), patients with type 1 diabetes (n=619) were treated for 16 weeks with a basal-bolus insulin regimen where insulin lispro was used before each meal. LANTUS was administered once daily at bedtime and NPH human insulin was administered once or twice daily. In these studies, LANTUS and NPH human insulin had a similar effect on glycohemoglobin with a similar overall rate of hypoglycemia.

[See table 1 above]

Type 1 Diabetes—Pediatric (see Table 2). In a randomized, controlled clinical study (Study D), pediatric patients (age range 6 to 15 years) with type 1 diabetes (n=349) were treated for 28 weeks with a basal-bolus insulin regimen where regular human insulin was used before each meal. LANTUS was administered once daily at bedtime and NPH human insulin was administered once or twice daily. Similar effects on glycohemoglobin and the incidence of hypoglycemia were observed in both treatment groups.

[See table 2 above]

Type 2 Diabetes—Adult (see Table 3). In a large, randomized, controlled clinical study (Study E) (n=570), LANTUS was evaluated for 52 weeks as part of a regimen of combination therapy with insulin and oral antidiabetic agents (a sulfonylurea, metformin, acarbose, or combinations of these drugs). LANTUS administered once daily at bedtime was as effective as NPH human insulin administered once daily at bedtime in reducing glycohemoglobin and fasting glucose. There was a low rate of hypoglycemia that was similar in LANTUS and NPH human insulin treated patients. In a large, randomized, controlled clinical study (Study F), in patients with type 2 diabetes not using oral antidiabetic agents (n=518), a basal-bolus regimen of LANTUS once daily at bedtime or NPH human insulin administered once or twice daily was evaluated for 28 weeks. Regular human insulin was used before meals as needed. LANTUS had similar effectiveness as either once- or twice-daily NPH human insulin in reducing glycohemoglobin and fasting glucose with a similar incidence of hypoglycemia.

[See table 3 above]

Table 1: Type 1 Diabetes Mellitus—Adult

	Study A		Study B		Study C	
Treatment duration	28 weeks		28 weeks		16 weeks	
Treatment in combination with	Regular insulin		Regular insulin		Insulin lispro	
	LANTUS	NPH	LANTUS	NPH	LANTUS	NPH
Number of subjects treated	292	293	264	270	310	309
GHb						
Endstudy mean	8.13	8.07	7.55	7.49	7.53	7.60
Adj. mean change from baseline	+0.21	+0.10	−0.16	−0.21	−0.07	−0.08
LANTUS—NPH	+0.11		+0.05		+0.01	
95% CI for Treatment difference	(−0.03; +0.24)		(−0.08; +0.19)		(−0.11; +0.13)	
Basal insulin dose						
Endstudy mean	19.2	22.8	24.8	31.3	23.9	29.2
Mean change from baseline	−1.7	−0.3	−4.1	+1.8	−4.5	+0.9
Total insulin dose						
Endstudy mean	46.7	51.7	50.3	54.8	47.4	50.7
Mean change from baseline	−1.1	−0.1	+0.3	+3.7	−2.9	+0.3
Fasting blood glucose (mg/dL)						
Endstudy mean	146.3	150.8	147.8	154.4	144.4	161.3
Adj. mean change from baseline	−21.1	−16.0	−20.2	−16.9	−29.3	−11.9

Table 2: Type 1 Diabetes Mellitus—Pediatric

	Study D	
Treatment duration	28 weeks	
Treatment in combination with	Regular insulin	
	LANTUS	NPH
Number of subjects treated	174	175
GHb		
Endstudy mean	8.91	9.18
Adj. mean change from baseline	+0.28	+0.27
LANTUS—NPH	+0.01	
95% CI for Treatment difference	(−0.24; +0.26)	
Basal insulin dose		
Endstudy mean	18.2	21.1
Mean change from baseline	−1.3	+2.4
Total insulin dose		
Endstudy mean	45.0	46.0
Mean change from baseline	+1.9	+3.4
Fasting blood glucose (mg/dL)		
Endstudy mean	171.9	182.7
Adj. mean change from baseline	−23.2	−12.2

Table 3: Type 2 Diabetes Mellitus—Adult

	Study E		Study F	
Treatment duration	52 weeks		28 weeks	
Treatment in combination with	Oral agents		Regular insulin	
	LANTUS	NPH	LANTUS	NPH
Number of subjects treated	289	281	259	259
GHb				
Endstudy mean	8.51	8.47	8.14	7.96
Adj. mean change from baseline	−0.46	−0.38	−0.41	−0.59
LANTUS—NPH	−0.08		+0.17	
95% CI for Treatment difference	(−0.28; +0.12)		(−0.00; +0.35)	
Basal insulin dose				
Endstudy mean	25.9	23.6	42.9	52.5
Mean change from baseline	+11.5	+9.0	−1.2	+7.0
Total insulin dose				
Endstudy mean	25.9	23.6	74.3	80.0
Mean change from baseline	+11.5	+9.0	+10.0	+13.1
Fasting blood glucose (mg/dL)				
Endstudy mean	126.9	129.4	141.5	144.5
Adj. mean change from baseline	−49.0	−46.3	−23.8	−21.6

INDICATIONS AND USAGE

LANTUS is indicated for once-daily subcutaneous administration at bedtime in the treatment of adult and pediatric patients with type 1 diabetes mellitus or adult patients with type 2 diabetes mellitus who require basal (long-acting) insulin for the control of hyperglycemia.

CONTRAINDICATIONS

LANTUS is contraindicated in patients hypersensitive to insulin glargine or the excipients.

WARNINGS

Hypoglycemia is the most common adverse effect of insulin, including LANTUS. As with all insulins, the timing of hypoglycemia may differ among various insulin formulations. Glucose monitoring is recommended for all patients with diabetes.

Any change of insulin should be made cautiously and only under medical supervision. Changes in insulin strength, manufacturer, type (e.g., regular, NPH, or insulin analogs), species (animal, human), or method of manufacture (recombinant DNA versus animal-source insulin) may result in the need for a change in dosage. Concomitant oral antidiabetic treatment may need to be adjusted.

PRECAUTIONS

General

LANTUS is not intended for intravenous administration. The prolonged duration of activity of insulin glargine is dependent on injection into subcutaneous tissue. Intravenous administration of the usual subcutaneous dose could result in severe hypoglycemia.

LANTUS must not be diluted or mixed with any other insulin or solution. If LANTUS is diluted or mixed, the solution may become cloudy, and the pharmacokinetic/pharmacodynamic profile (e.g., onset of action, time to peak effect) of LANTUS and/or the mixed insulin may be altered in an unpredictable manner. When LANTUS and regular human insulin were mixed immediately before injection in dogs, a delayed onset of action and time to maximum effect for regular human insulin was observed. The total bioavailability of the mixture was also slightly decreased compared to separate injections of LANTUS and regular human insulin. The relevance of these observations in dogs to humans is not known.

As with all insulin preparations, the time course of LANTUS action may vary in different individuals or at different times in the same individual and the rate of absorption is dependent on blood supply, temperature, and physical activity.

Insulin may cause sodium retention and edema, particularly if previously poor metabolic control is improved by intensified insulin therapy.

Hypoglycemia

As with all insulin preparations, hypoglycemic reactions may be associated with the administration of LANTUS. Hypoglycemia is the most common adverse effect of insulins.

Early warning symptoms of hypoglycemia may be different or less pronounced under certain conditions, such as long duration of diabetes, diabetic nerve disease, use of medications such as beta-blockers, or intensified diabetes control. (See PRECAUTIONS, Drug Interactions). Such situations may result in severe hypoglycemia (and, possibly, loss of consciousness) prior to patients' awareness of hypoglycemia. The time of occurrence of hypoglycemia depends on the action profile of the insulins used and may, therefore, change when the treatment regimen is changed. Patients being switched from twice daily NPH insulin to once-daily LANTUS should have their LANTUS dose reduced by 20% from the previous total daily NPH dose to reduce the risk of hypoglycemia. (See DOSAGE AND ADMINISTRATION, Changeover to LANTUS)

The prolonged effect of subcutaneous LANTUS may delay recovery from hypoglycemia.

In a clinical study, symptoms of hypoglycemia or counterregulatory hormone responses were similar after intravenous insulin glargine and regular human insulin both in healthy subjects and patients with type 1 diabetes.

Renal Impairment

Although studies have not been performed in patients with diabetes and renal impairment, LANTUS requirements may be diminished because of reduced insulin metabolism, similar to observations found with other insulins. (See CLINICAL PHARMACOLOGY, Special Populations)

Hepatic Impairment

Although studies have not been performed in patients with diabetes and hepatic impairment, LANTUS requirements may be diminished due to reduced capacity for gluconeogenesis and reduced insulin metabolism, similar to observations found with other insulins. (See CLINICAL PHARMACOLOGY, Special Populations)

Injection Site and Allergic Reactions

As with any insulin therapy, lipodystrophy may occur at the injection site and delay insulin absorption. Other injection site reactions with insulin therapy include redness, pain, itching, hives, swelling, and inflammation. Continuous rotation of the injection site within a given area may help to reduce or prevent these reactions. Most minor reactions to insulins usually resolve in a few days to a few weeks.

Reports of injection site pain were more frequent with LANTUS than NPH human insulin (2.7% insulin glargine versus 0.7% NPH). The reports of pain at the injection site were usually mild and did not result in discontinuation of therapy.

Immediate-type allergic reactions are rare. Such reactions to insulin (including insulin glargine) or the excipients may, for example, be associated with generalized skin reactions, angioedema, bronchospasm, hypotension, or shock and may be life threatening.

Intercurrent Conditions

Insulin requirements may be altered during intercurrent conditions such as illness, emotional disturbances, or stress.

Information for Patients

LANTUS must only be used if the solution is clear and colorless with no particles visible. (See DOSAGE AND ADMINISTRATION, Preparation and Handling)

Patients must be advised that LANTUS must not be diluted or mixed with any other insulin or solution. (See PRECAUTIONS, General)

Patients should be instructed on self-management procedures including glucose monitoring, proper injection technique, and hypoglycemia and hyperglycemia management. Patients must be instructed on handling of special situations such as intercurrent conditions (illness, stress, or emotional disturbances), an inadequate or skipped insulin dose, inadvertent administration of an increased insulin dose, inadequate food intake, or skipped meals. Refer patients to the LANTUS Information for the Patient circular for additional information.

As with all patients who have diabetes, the ability to concentrate and/or react may be impaired as a result of hypoglycemia or hyperglycemia.

Patients with diabetes should be advised to inform their doctor if they are pregnant or are contemplating pregnancy.

Drug Interactions

A number of substances affect glucose metabolism and may require insulin dose adjustment and particularly close monitoring.

The following are examples of substances that may increase the blood-glucose-lowering effect and susceptibility to hypoglycemia: oral antidiabetic products, ACE inhibitors, disopyramide, fibrates, fluoxetine, MAO inhibitors, propoxyphene, salicylates, somatostatin analog (e.g., octreotide), sulfonamide antibiotics.

The following are examples of substances that may reduce the blood-glucose-lowering effect of insulin: corticosteroids, danazol, diuretics, sympathomimetic agents (e.g., epinephrine, albuterol, terbutaline), isoniazid, phenothiazine derivatives, somatropin, thyroid hormones, estrogens, progestogens (e.g., in oral contraceptives).

Beta-blockers, clonidine, lithium salts, and alcohol may either potentiate or weaken the blood-glucose-lowering effect of insulin. Pentamidine may cause hypoglycemia, which may sometimes be followed by hyperglycemia. In addition, under the influence of sympatholytic medicinal products such as beta-blockers, clonidine, guanethidine, and reserpine, the signs of hypoglycemia may be reduced or absent.

Carcinogenesis, Mutagenesis, Impairment of Fertility

In mice and rats, standard two-year carcinogenicity studies with insulin glargine were performed at doses up to 0.455 mg/kg, which is for the rat approximately 10 times and for the mouse approximately 5 times the recommended human subcutaneous starting dose of 10 IU (0.008 mg/kg/day), based on mg/m^2. The findings in female mice were not conclusive due to excessive mortality in all dose groups during the study. Histiocytomas were found at injection sites in male rats (statistically significant) and male mice (not statistically significant) in acid vehicle containing groups. These tumors were not found in female animals, in saline control, or insulin comparator groups using a different vehicle. The relevance of these findings to humans is unknown.

Insulin glargine was not mutagenic in tests for detection of gene mutations in bacteria and mammalian cells (Ames- and HGPRT-test) and in tests for detection of chromosomal aberrations (cytogenetics in vitro in V79 cells and in vivo in Chinese hamsters).

In a combined fertility and prenatal and postnatal study in male and female rats at subcutaneous doses up to 0.36 mg/kg/day, which is approximately 7 times the recommended human subcutaneous starting dose of 10 IU (0.008 mg/kg/day), based on mg/m^2, maternal toxicity due to dose-dependent hypoglycemia, including some deaths, was observed. Consequently, a reduction of the rearing rate occurred in the high-dose group only. Similar effects were observed with NPH human insulin.

Pregnancy

Teratogenic Effects: Pregnancy Category C. Subcutaneous reproduction and teratology studies have been performed with insulin glargine and regular human insulin in rats and Himalayan rabbits. The drug was given to female rats before mating, during mating, and throughout pregnancy at doses up to 0.36 mg/kg/day, which is approximately 7 times the recommended human subcutaneous starting dose of 10 IU (0.008 mg/kg/day), based on mg/m^2. In rabbits, doses of 0.072 mg/kg/day, which is approximately 2 times the recommended human subcutaneous starting dose of 10 IU (0.008 mg/kg/day), based on mg/m^2, were administered during organogenesis. The effects of insulin glargine did not generally differ from those observed with regular human insulin in rats or rabbits. However, in rabbits, five fetuses from two litters of the high-dose group exhibited dilation of the cerebral ventricles. Fertility and early embryonic development appeared normal.

There are no well-controlled clinical studies of the use of insulin glargine in pregnant women. It is essential for patients with diabetes or a history of gestational diabetes to maintain good metabolic control before conception and throughout pregnancy. Insulin requirements may decrease during the first trimester, generally increase during the second and third trimesters, and rapidly decline after delivery. Careful monitoring of glucose control is essential in such patients. Because animal reproduction studies are not always predictive of human response, this drug should be used during pregnancy only if clearly needed.

Nursing Mothers

It is unknown whether insulin glargine is excreted in significant amounts in human milk. Many drugs, including human insulin, are excreted in human milk. For this reason, caution should be exercised when LANTUS is administered to a nursing woman. Lactating women may require adjustments in insulin dose and diet.

Pediatric Use

Safety and effectiveness of LANTUS have been established in the age group 6 to 15 years with type 1 diabetes.

Geriatric Use

In controlled clinical studies comparing insulin glargine to NPH human insulin, 593 of 3890 patients with type 1 and type 2 diabetes were 65 years and older. The only difference in safety or effectiveness in this subpopulation compared to the entire study population was an expected higher incidence of cardiovascular events in both insulin glargine and NPH human insulin-treated patients.

In elderly patients with diabetes, the initial dosing, dose increments, and maintenance dosage should be conservative to avoid hypoglycemic reactions. Hypoglycemia may be difficult to recognize in the elderly. (See PRECAUTIONS, Hypoglycemia)

ADVERSE REACTIONS

The adverse events commonly associated with LANTUS include the following:

Body as a whole: allergic reactions (See PRECAUTIONS)

Skin and appendages: injection site reaction, lipodystrophy, pruritus, rash (See PRECAUTIONS)

Other: hypoglycemia (See WARNINGS and PRECAUTIONS)

In clinical studies in adult patients, there was a higher incidence of treatment-emergent injection site pain in LANTUS-treated patients (2.7%) compared to NPH insulin-treated patients (0.7%). The reports of pain at the injection site were usually mild and did not result in discontinuation of therapy. Other treatment-emergent injection site reactions occurred at similar incidences with both insulin glargine and NPH human insulin.

Retinopathy was evaluated in the clinical studies by means of retinal adverse events reported and fundus photography. The numbers of retinal adverse events reported for LANTUS and NPH treatment groups were similar for patients with type 1 and type 2 diabetes. Progression of retinopathy was investigated by fundus photography using a grading protocol derived from the Early Treatment Diabetic Retinopathy Study (ETDRS). In one clinical study involving patients with type 2 diabetes, a difference in the number of subjects with ≥3-step progression in ETDRS scale over a 6-month period was noted by fundus photography (7.5% in LANTUS group versus 2.7% in NPH treated group). The overall relevance of this isolated finding cannot be determined due to the small number of patients involved, the short follow-up period, and the fact that this finding was not observed in other clinical studies.

OVERDOSAGE

An excess of insulin relative to food intake, energy expenditure, or both may lead to severe and sometimes long-term and life-threatening hypoglycemia. Mild episodes of hypoglycemia can usually be treated with oral carbohydrates. Adjustments in drug dosage, meal patterns, or exercise may be needed.

More severe episodes with coma, seizure, or neurologic impairment may be treated with intramuscular/subcutaneous glucagon or concentrated intravenous glucose. After apparent clinical recovery from hypoglycemia, continued observation and additional carbohydrate intake may be necessary to avoid reoccurrence of hypoglycemia.

DOSAGE AND ADMINISTRATION

LANTUS is a recombinant human insulin analog. Its potency is approximately the same as human insulin. It exhibits a relatively constant glucose-lowering profile over 24 hours that permits once-daily dosing.

LANTUS should be administered subcutaneously once a day at bedtime. LANTUS is not intended for intravenous administration (See PRECAUTIONS). Intravenous administration of the usual subcutaneous dose could result in severe hypoglycemia. The desired blood glucose levels as well as the doses and timing of antidiabetic medications must be determined individually. Blood glucose monitoring is recommended for all patients with diabetes. The prolonged duration of activity of LANTUS is dependent on injection into subcutaneous space.

As with all insulins, injection sites within an injection area (abdomen, thigh or deltoid) must be rotated from one injection to the next.

In clinical studies, there was no relevant difference in insulin glargine absorption after abdominal, deltoid, or thigh subcutaneous administration. As for all insulins, the rate of absorption, and consequently the onset and duration of action, may be affected by exercise and other variables.

LANTUS is not the insulin of choice for the treatment of diabetic ketoacidosis. Intravenous short-acting insulin is the preferred treatment.

Pediatric Use

LANTUS can be safely administered to pediatric patients ≥6 years of age. Administration to pediatric patients <6 years has not been studied. Based on the results of a study in pediatric patients, the dose recommendation for changeover to LANTUS is the same as described for adults in DOSAGE AND ADMINISTRATION, Changeover to LANTUS.

Initiation of LANTUS Therapy

In a clinical study with insulin naïve patients with type 2 diabetes already treated with oral antidiabetic drugs, LANTUS was started at an average dose of 10 IU once daily, and subsequently adjusted according to the patient's need to a total daily dose ranging from 2 to 100 IU.

Changeover to LANTUS

If changing from a treatment regimen with an intermediate- or long-acting insulin to a regimen with LANTUS, the amount and timing of short-acting insulin or fast-acting insulin analog or the dose of any oral antidiabetic drug may need to be adjusted. In clinical studies, when patients were transferred from once-daily NPH human insulin or ultralente human insulin to once-daily LANTUS, the initial dose was usually not changed. However, when patients were transferred from twice-daily NPH human insulin to LANTUS once daily at bedtime, to reduce the risk of hypoglycemia, the initial dose (IU) was usually reduced by approximately 20% (compared to total daily IU of NPH human insulin) within the first week of treatment and then adjusted based on patient response. (See PRECAUTIONS, Hypoglycemia)

A program of close metabolic monitoring under medical supervision is recommended during transfer and in the initial weeks thereafter. The amount and timing of short-acting insulin or fast-acting insulin analog may need to be adjusted. This is particularly true for patients with acquired antibodies to human insulin needing high-insulin doses and occurs with all insulin analogs. Dose adjustment of LANTUS and other insulins or oral antidiabetic drugs may be required; for example, if the patient's weight or lifestyle changes or other circumstances arise that increase susceptibility to hypoglycemia or hyperglycemia. (See PRECAUTIONS, Hypoglycemia)

The dose may also have to be adjusted during intercurrent illness. (See PRECAUTIONS, Intercurrent Conditions)

Preparation and Handling

Parenteral drug products should be inspected visually prior to administration whenever the solution and the container permit. LANTUS must only be used if the solution is clear and colorless with no particles visible.

The syringes must not contain any other medicinal product or residue.

Mixing and diluting. LANTUS must not be diluted or mixed with any other insulin or solution. (See PRECAUTIONS, General)

Cartridge version only: If the OptiPen™ One Insulin Delivery Device malfunctions, LANTUS may be drawn from the cartridge into a U 100 syringe and injected.

Continued on next page

Lantus—Cont.

HOW SUPPLIED

LANTUS 100 units per mL (U 100) is available in the following package sizes:
5 mL vials (NDC 0088-2220-32)
10 mL vials (NDC 0088-2220-33)
3 mL cartridges*, package of 5 (NDC 0088-2220-52)
*Cartridges are for use only in the OptiPen™ One Insulin Delivery Device

Storage

Unopened LANTUS vials and cartridges should be stored in a refrigerator, 36°F - 46°F (2°C - 8°C). LANTUS should not be stored in the freezer and it should not be allowed to freeze.

If refrigeration is not possible, the 10 mL vial or cartridge of LANTUS in use can be kept unrefrigerated for up to 28 days away from direct heat and light, as long as the temperature is not greater than 86°F (30°C). Unrefrigerated 10 mL vials and cartridges must be used within the 28-day period or they must be discarded.

If refrigeration is not possible, 5 mL vials of LANTUS in use can be kept unrefrigerated for up to 14 days away from direct heat and light, as long as the temperature is not greater than 86°F (30°C). Unrefrigerated 5 mL vials must be used within the 14-day period or they must be discarded.

If refrigerated, the 5 mL vial of LANTUS in use can be kept for up to 28 days. Once the cartridge is placed in an OptiPen One, it should not be put in the refrigerator.

Rx only
Prescribing Information as of April 2000
Manufactured by:
Hoechst Marion Roussel Deutschland GmbH
D-65926 Frankfurt am Main
Germany
Manufactured for:
Aventis Pharmaceuticals Inc.
Kansas City, MO 64137 USA
US Patents 5,656,722, 5,370,629, and 5,509,905
Made in Germany
www.aventispharma-us.com

LANTUS®
(insulin glargine [Recombinant DNA origin] injection)

Patient Information for the LANTUS Vial

This leaflet tells you about LANTUS (LAN-tus) and about how to use LANTUS in a vial. At the end of the leaflet is a list of vocabulary words you may find useful. Read this information carefully before you use LANTUS. Read the information you get when you refill your LANTUS prescriptions because there may be new information. This leaflet does not take the place of complete discussions with your health care professional. If you have questions about LANTUS or about diabetes, talk with your health care professional.

What is the most important information I should know about LANTUS?

Do not dilute or mix LANTUS with any other insulin or solution. It will not work as intended, and you may lose blood sugar control, which could be serious.

What is LANTUS?

LANTUS is a long-acting synthetic (man-made) human insulin to treat diabetes. You need a prescription to get LANTUS. Always be sure the pharmacy gives you the right insulin. The carton and vial should look like the ones in this picture.

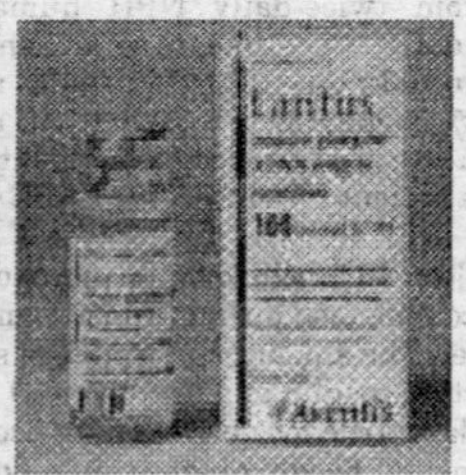

Diabetes is a disease caused when the body cannot produce or use insulin. Insulin is a hormone produced by the pancreas. Your body needs insulin to turn glucose (sugar) from food into energy. If your body does not make enough insulin, you need another source of insulin so you will not have too much sugar in your blood. That is why you must take insulin injections.

LANTUS is similar to the insulin made by your body. It is used once a day to lower blood glucose. Like other insulins, you take LANTUS by injecting it in the fatty layer under the skin (subcutaneously). The dose your health care professional prescribes helps keep the glucose level in your blood close to normal.

You will be able to tell if LANTUS is working by testing your blood and/or urine for glucose.

LANTUS contains active and inactive ingredients. The active ingredient is insulin. It is dissolved in a colorless sterile (germ-free) fluid. The concentration is 100 units/mL (U-100). Inactive ingredients are zinc, glycerol, m-cresol, and water for injection.

Insulin injections play an important role in keeping your diabetes in control. But the way you live—your diet, careful monitoring of your glucose levels, exercise, and planned physical activity—all work with your insulin to help you control your diabetes.

Who should not take LANTUS?

You should not take LANTUS if you are allergic to insulin or any of the inactive ingredients in LANTUS.

How should I take LANTUS?

Inject LANTUS under your skin once a day at bedtime. You do not need to shake the vial before use. You should look at the medicine in the vial. If the medicine is cloudy or has particles in it, throw the vial away and get a new one.

What sort of syringe should I use?

Always use a syringe that is marked for U-100 insulin preparations. If you use the wrong syringe, you may get the wrong dose and develop a blood glucose level that is too low or too high.

Use disposable syringes and needles only once. Throw them away properly. Use a new needle and syringe every time you dose. **Never** share needles and syringes.

How do I draw insulin into the syringe?

Do not dilute or mix LANTUS with any other insulin or solution. The syringe must not contain any other medicine or residue.

Follow these steps:

1. Wash your hands.
2. Check the insulin to make sure it is clear and colorless. Do not use it if it is cloudy or if you see particles.
3. If you are using a new vial, remove the protective cap. **Do not** remove the stopper.
4. Wipe the top of the vial with an alcohol swab.
5. Draw air into the syringe equal to your insulin dose. Put the needle through the rubber top of the vial and push the plunger to inject the air into the vial.
6. Leave the syringe in the vial and turn both upside down. Hold the syringe and vial firmly in one hand.
7. Make sure the tip of the needle is in the insulin. With your free hand, pull the plunger to withdraw the correct dose into the syringe.
8. Before you take the needle out of the vial, check the syringe for air bubbles. If bubbles are in the medicine, hold the syringe straight up and tap the side of the syringe until the bubbles float to the top. Push the bubbles out with the plunger and draw the insulin back in until you have the correct dose.
9. Remove the needle from the vial. Do not let the needle touch anything. You are now ready to inject.

How do I inject LANTUS?

Do not mix or dilute LANTUS with any other insulin or solution or LANTUS will not work as intended, and you may lose blood sugar control, which could be serious. You do not have to shake the vial before use.

Follow these steps:

1. Decide on an injection area—either upper arm, thigh, or abdomen. Injection sites within an injection area must be different from one injection to the next.
2. Use alcohol to clean the skin where you are going to inject.
3. Pinch the skin and hold it. Stick the needle in the way your doctor, nurse, or diabetes educator showed you.
4. Slowly push in the plunger of the syringe all the way, making sure you have injected all the insulin. Leave the needle in the skin for several seconds.
5. Pull the needle straight out and gently press on the spot where you injected yourself for several seconds. **Do not rub the area.**
6. Follow your health care professional's instructions for throwing away the needle and syringe.

If your blood glucose reading is high or low, or if your urine tests show glucose, tell your health care professional so the dose can be adjusted.

What can affect how much insulin I need?

Illness. Illness may change how much insulin you need. It is a good idea to think ahead and make a "sick day" plan with your health care professional so you will be ready when this happens. Be sure to test your blood and urine often and call your health care professional if you are sick.

Pregnancy and nursing. If you are pregnant or nursing, or if you plan to get pregnant, talk with your health care professional before you take LANTUS. Your diabetes may be harder to control when you are pregnant.

It is important for you to monitor your glucose closer than usual during this time.

Medicines. Other medicines can change the way insulin works. Therefore, tell your health care professional about all other medicines you are taking. Your insulin dosage may need to be changed by your health care professional. Do not change your medicine doses yourself.

For example, your body may need more insulin if you take birth control, thyroid, decongestant, or diet pills. Your body may need less insulin if you are taking antidepressants, antidiabetic pills, or ACE inhibitors (used to lower blood pressure and for certain heart conditions).

Exercise. Exercise may change the way your body uses insulin. Be sure to check with your health care professional before you start an exercise program.

Travel. If you travel across time zones, talk with your health care professional about how to time your injections. When you travel, wear your medical alert identification. Take extra insulin and supplies with you.

What if I want to drink alcohol?

Before you drink alcohol, talk to your health care professional about its effect on diabetes.

What are the possible side effects of insulins?

1. Allergic reactions:

In rare cases, a patient may be allergic to an insulin product. Severe insulin allergies may be life-threatening. If you think you are having an allergic reaction, get medical help right away. Signs of insulin allergy are:

- a rash all over your body
- shortness of breath
- wheezing (trouble breathing)
- a fast pulse
- sweating
- low blood pressure

2. Hypoglycemia:

Hypoglycemia is often called an "insulin reaction" or "low blood sugar." It may occur when you do not have enough glucose in your blood. Common causes of hypoglycemia are illness, emotional or physical stress, too much insulin, too little food or missed meals, and too much exercise.

Some of the symptoms of hypoglycemia are:

- sudden cold sweat
- feeling shaky or nervous
- feeling very tired
- feeling sick to your stomach
- feeling dizzy
- blurry vision
- headache
- confusion
- personality changes

Early warning signs of hypoglycemia may be different or less noticeable in some people. That is why it is important to check your glucose as you have been advised by your doctor.

If you have hypoglycemia, your body needs sugar. That is why you should carry sugar, candy mints, or glucose tablets with you. Learn to recognize the signs and eat or drink something that has some sugar in it.

Hypoglycemia can be very dangerous. Severe hypoglycemia can cause confusion, seizures, and loss of consciousness. Someone with hypoglycemia who cannot take sugar by mouth needs medical help fast. Without immediate medical help, serious reactions or even death could occur.

You will have mild hypoglycemia once in a while when a meal is delayed, if you get sick, or if you are late with your insulin injection. But if hypoglycemia happens often or is severe, tell your health care professional about it. Also, if you have trouble recognizing the symptoms of hypoglycemia, talk with your health care professional.

3. Hyperglycemia:

Hyperglycemia occurs when you have too much glucose in your blood. Usually, it means there is not enough insulin to break down the food you eat into energy your body can use. Hyperglycemia can be caused by a fever, an infection, stress, eating more than you should, taking less insulin than prescribed, or it can be part of the natural progression of diabetes. Routine testing of your blood or urine will let you know if you have hyperglycemia. If your tests are often high, tell your health care professional so your dose of medicine can be changed.

If your glucose is often high, you can develop a very serious condition called diabetic ketoacidosis. Ketoacidosis can be life-threatening. If your blood tests show high amounts of glucose or your urine tests show high amounts of glucose or acetone, or if you have signs of ketoacidosis, you need to get medical help quickly. **Do not use LANTUS to treat diabetic ketoacidosis.** Signs of ketoacidosis are:

- sleepiness
- flushed (red) face
- thirst
- loss of appetite
- fruity odor on your breath

Signs of **severe** ketoacidosis are:

- heavy breathing
- fast pulse

4. Possible reactions on the skin at the injection site:

Injecting insulin can cause the following reactions on the skin at the injection site:

- a little depression in the skin (lipoatrophy)
- skin thickening (lipohypertrophy)
- red, swelling, itchy skin (injection site reaction)

An injection site reaction should clear up in a few days or a few weeks. If it does not go away and it continues to occur, tell your health care professional.

You can reduce the chance of getting lipoatrophy and lipohypertrophy if you change the injection site each time. Tell your health care professional if you have these problems. You may need to learn to inject your insulin a different way.

How should I store LANTUS?

Store new LANTUS vials in the refrigerator (not the freezer) between 36°F - 46°F (2°C - 8°C). Do not freeze LANTUS. If a vial freezes, throw it away.

Once a vial is opened, you can keep it in the refrigerator or as cool as possible (below 86°F [30°C]). The 10 mL vial is good for 28 days. The 5 mL vial is good for 14 days if stored in a cool place (below 86°F [30°C]) or 28 days if refrigerated. Keep LANTUS out of direct heat and light. For example, do not leave it in your car on a summer day.

VOCABULARY

Glucose—A form of sugar that the body uses for fuel. It is made when food is broken down in the digestive system. Blood carries glucose to the cells.

Hypoglycemia—Also called insulin reaction. It means that glucose levels in the blood are too low.

Hyperglycemia—Too much glucose in the blood. Usually testing, not symptoms, reveals a too-high level.

Insulin—A hormone that helps the cells in your body use glucose.

LANTUS—A long-acting insulin similar to insulin made by your body. It is used once a day at bedtime to lower blood glucose.
Lipoatrophy (LIP-o-AT-troe-fee)—Loss of fat under the skin. Can be caused by repeated insulin injections in the same place.
Lipohypertrophy (LIP-o-hi-PER-troe-fee)—A lump under the skin caused by an overgrowth of fat cells. Can be caused by repeated insulin injections in the same place.
Ketoacidosis (kee-toe-as-ih-DOE-sis)—A dangerous condition caused when the body does not have enough insulin.
Pancreas (PAN-kree-as)—A gland near the stomach that produces insulin.
Subcutaneous (sub-ku-TAE-nee-us)—The fatty layer under the skin.

ADDITIONAL INFORMATION

DIABETES FORECAST is a national magazine designed especially for patients with diabetes and their families and is available by subscription from the American Diabetes Association, National Service Center, 1701 N. Beauregard Street, Alexandria, Virginia 22311, 1-800-DIABETES (1-800-342-2383).
Another publication, **DIABETES COUNTDOWN**, is available from the Juvenile Diabetes Foundation International (JDF), 120 Wall Street, 19th Floor, New York, New York 10005, 1-800-JDF-CURE (1-800-533-2873). You may also visit the JDF website at www.jdf.org.
To get more information about diabetes, check with your doctor or diabetes educator. To get more information about LANTUS, ask your health care professional or call 1-800-552-3656.
April 2000
Package insert circular number: 50052781
Aventis Pharmaceuticals Inc.
Kansas City, MO 64137 USA
©2000

LOVENOX® ℞
(enoxaparin sodium)
Injection

SPINAL/EPIDURAL HEMATOMAS

When neuraxial anesthesia (epidural/spinal anesthesia) or spinal puncture is employed, patients anticoagulated or scheduled to be anticoagulated with low molecular weight heparins or heparinoids for prevention of thromboembolic complications are at risk of developing an epidural or spinal hematoma which can result in long-term or permanent paralysis.
The risk of these events is increased by the use of indwelling epidural catheters for administration of analgesia or by the concomitant use of drugs affecting hemostasis such as non steroidal anti-inflammatory drugs (NSAIDs), platelet inhibitors, or other anticoagulants. The risk also appears to be increased by traumatic or repeated epidural or spinal puncture.
Patients should be frequently monitored for signs and symptoms of neurological impairment. If neurologic compromise is noted, urgent treatment is necessary.
The physician should consider the potential benefit versus risk before neuraxial intervention in patients anticoagulated or to be anticoagulated for thromboprophylaxis (see also **WARNINGS**, **Hemorrhage**, and **PRECAUTIONS**, **Drug Interactions**).

DESCRIPTION

Lovenox Injection is a sterile solution containing enoxaparin sodium, a low molecular weight heparin. It is available in: prefilled syringes (30 and 40 mg), graduated prefilled syringes (60, 80, and 100 mg), and ampules (30 mg). Each dosage unit contains 10 mg enoxaparin sodium per 0.1 mL Water for Injection. The solution is preservative-free and intended for use only as a single-dose injection. (See **DOSAGE AND ADMINISTRATION** and **HOW SUPPLIED** for dosage unit descriptions.)
The pH of the injection is 5.5 to 7.5, with an approximate anti-Factor Xa activity per dosage unit of 1000 IU per every 10 mg of enoxaparin sodium (with reference to the W.H.O. First International Low Molecular Weight Heparin Reference Standard). Nitrogen is used in the headspace to inhibit oxidation.
Enoxaparin is obtained by alkaline degradation of heparin benzyl ester derived from porcine intestinal mucosa. Its structure is characterized by a 2-O-sulfo-4-enepyranosuronic acid group at the non-reducing end and a 2-N,6-O-disulfo-D-glucosamine at the reducing end of the chain. The substance is the sodium salt. The average molecular weight is about 4500 daltons. The molecular weight distribution is:

<2000 daltons	≤20%
2000 to 8000 daltons	≥68%
>8000 daltons	≤15%

STRUCTURAL FORMULA
[See chemical structure at top of next column]

CLINICAL PHARMACOLOGY

Enoxaparin is a low molecular weight heparin which has antithrombotic properties. In humans, enoxaparin given at a dose of 1.5 mg/kg subcutaneously (SC) is characterized by a higher ratio of anti-Factor Xa to anti-Factor IIa activity (mean±SD, 14.0±3.1) (based on areas under anti-Factor activity versus time curves) compared to the ratios observed for heparin (mean±SD, 1.22±0.13). Increases of up to 1.8 times the control values were seen in the thrombin time (TT) and the activated partial thromboplastin time (aPTT). Enoxaparin at a 1 mg/kg dose, administered SC every 12 hours to patients in a large clinical trial resulted in aPTT values of 45 seconds or less in the majority of patients (n = 1607).
Pharmacodynamics: Maximum anti-Factor Xa and anti-thrombin (anti-Factor IIa) activities occur 3 to 5 hours after SC injection of enoxaparin. Mean peak anti-Factor Xa activity was 0.16 IU/mL (1.58 µg/mL) and 0.38 IU/mL (3.83 µg/mL) after the 20 mg and the 40 mg clinically tested SC doses, respectively. Mean (n = 46) peak anti-Factor Xa activity was 1.1 IU/mL at steady state in patients with unstable angina receiving 1.0 mg/kg SC every 12 hours for 14 days. Mean absolute bioavailability of enoxaparin, given SC, based on anti-Factor Xa activity is 92% in healthy volunteers. The volume of distribution of anti-Factor Xa activity is about 6 L. Following intravenous (i.v.) dosing, the total body clearance of enoxaparin is 26 mL/min. After i.v. dosing of enoxaparin labeled with the gamma-emitter, ^{99m}Tc, 40% of radioactivity and 8 to 20% of anti-Factor Xa activity were recovered in urine in 24 hours. Elimination half-life based on anti-Factor Xa activity was 4.5 hours after SC administration. Following a 40 mg SC once a day dose, significant anti-Factor Xa activity persists in plasma for about 12 hours.
Following SC dosing, the apparent clearance (CL/F) of enoxaparin is approximately 15 mL/min. Apparent clearance and A_{max} derived from anti-Factor Xa values following single SC dosing (40 mg and 60 mg) were slightly higher in males than in females. The source of the gender difference in these parameters has not been conclusively identified, however, body weight may be a contributing factor.
Apparent clearance and A_{max} derived from anti-Factor Xa values following single and multiple SC dosing in elderly subjects were close to those observed in young subjects. Following once a day SC dosing of 40 mg enoxaparin, the Day 10 mean area under anti-Factor Xa activity versus time curve (AUC) was approximately 15% greater than the mean Day 1 AUC value. In subjects with moderate renal impairment (creatinine clearance 30 to 80 mL/min), anti-Factor Xa CL/F values were similar to those in healthy subjects. However, mean CL/F values of subjects with severe renal impairment (creatinine clearance <30 mL/min), were approximately 30% lower than the mean CL/F value of control group subjects. (See **PRECAUTIONS**.)

CLINICAL TRIALS

Hip or Knee Replacement Surgery: Lovenox Injection has been shown to prevent post-operative deep vein thrombosis (DVT) following hip or knee replacement surgery.
In a double-blind study, Lovenox Injection 30 mg every 12 hours SC was compared to placebo in patients with hip replacement. After hemostasis was established, treatment was initiated 12 to 24 hours after surgery and was continued for 10 to 14 days after surgery. The data are provided below.

Efficacy of Lovenox Injection in Hip Replacement Surgery

Indication	Dosing Regimen: Lovenox 30 mg q12h SC n (%)	Placebo q12h SC n (%)
All Treated Hip Replacement Patients	50 (100)	50 (100)
Treatment Failures Total DVT (%)	5 (10)[1]	23 (46)
Proximal DVT (%)	1 (2)[2]	11 (22)

[1]p value versus placebo = 0.0002
[2]p value versus placebo = 0.0134

A double-blind, multicenter study compared three dosing regimens of Lovenox Injection in patients with hip replacement. Treatment was initiated within two days after surgery and was continued for 7 to 11 days after surgery. The data are provided below.
[See first table above]

Efficacy of Lovenox Injection in Hip Replacement Surgery

Indication	Lovenox Dosing Regimen: 10 mg q.d. SC n (%)	30 mg q12h SC n (%)	40 mg q.d. SC n (%)
All Treated Hip Replacement Patients	161 (100)	208 (100)	199 (100)
Treatment Failures Total DVT (%)	40 (25)	22 (11)[1]	27 (14)
Proximal DVT (%)	17 (11)	8 (4)[2]	9 (5)

[1]p value versus Lovenox 10 mg once a day = 0.0008
[2]p value versus Lovenox 10 mg once a day = 0.0168

There was no significant difference between the 30 mg every 12 hours and 40 mg once a day regimens.
Extended Prophylaxis in Hip Replacement Surgery: In a study of extended prophylaxis for patients undergoing hip replacement surgery, patients were treated, while hospitalized, with enoxaparin 40 mg SC, initiated up to 12 hours prior to surgery for the prevention of post-operative deep vein thrombosis. At the end of the peri-operative period, all patients underwent bilateral venography. In a double-blind design, those patients with no venous thromboembolic disease were randomized to a post-discharge regimen of either enoxaparin 40 mg (n = 90) once a day SC or to placebo (n = 89) for 3 weeks. In this population of patients, the incidence of deep vein thrombosis during extended prophylaxis was significantly lower for enoxaparin compared to placebo. The data are provided below.
[See second table above]

Efficacy of Lovenox Injection with Extended Prophylaxis Following Hip Replacement Surgery

Indication (Post-Discharge)	Post-Discharge Dosing Regimen: Lovenox 40 mg q.d. SC n (%)	Placebo q.d. SC n (%)
All Treated Extended Prophylaxis Patients	90 (100)	89 (100)
Treatment Failures Total DVT (%)	6 (7)[1] (95% CI: 3 to 14)	18 (20) (95% CI: 12 to 30)
Proximal DVT (%)	5 (6)[2] (95% CI: 2 to 13)	7 (8) (95% CI: 3 to 16)

[1]p value versus placebo = 0.008
[2]p value versus placebo = 0.537

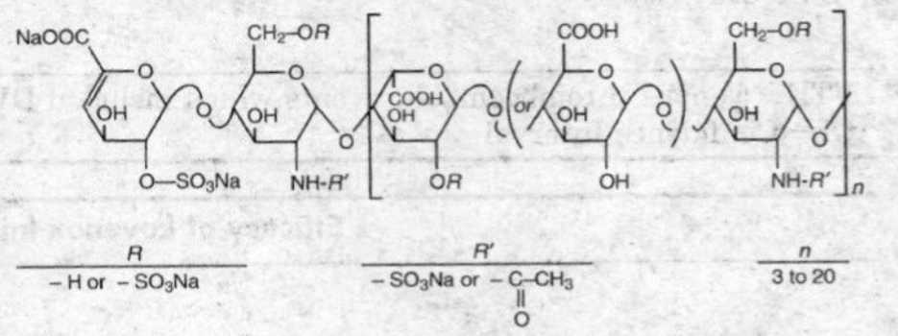

In a second study, patients undergoing hip replacement surgery were treated, while hospitalized, with enoxaparin 40 mg SC, initiated up to 12 hours prior to surgery. All patients were examined for clinical signs and symptoms of venous thromboembolic disease. In a double-blind design, patients without clinical signs and symptoms of venous thromboembolic disease were randomized to a post-discharge regimen of either enoxaparin 40 mg (n = 131) once a day SC or to placebo (n = 131) for 3 weeks. Similar to the first study the incidence of deep vein thrombosis during extended prophylaxis was significantly lower for enoxaparin compared to placebo, with a statistically significant difference in both total DVT (enoxaparin 21 [16%] versus placebo 45 [34%]; p = 0.001) and proximal DVT (enoxaparin 8 [6%] versus placebo 28 [21%]; p = <0.001).
In a double-blind study, Lovenox Injection 30 mg every 12 hours SC was compared to placebo in 99 patients undergoing knee replacement surgery. After hemostasis was established, treatment was initiated 12 to 24 hours after surgery and was continued up to 15 days after surgery. The incidence of proximal and total deep vein thrombosis after surgery was significantly lower for enoxaparin compared to placebo. The data are provided below.

Continued on next page

Lovenox—Cont.

[See first table at right]
Additionally, in an open-label, parallel group, randomized clinical study, Lovenox Injection 30 mg every 12 hours SC in patients undergoing elective knee replacement surgery was compared to heparin 5000 U every 8 hours SC. Treatment was initiated after surgery and continued up to 14 days. The incidence of deep vein thrombosis was significantly lower for enoxaparin compared to heparin.

Abdominal Surgery: In a double-blind, parallel group study of 1115 patients undergoing elective cancer surgery of the gastrointestinal, urological, or gynecological tract, Lovenox Injection 40 mg SC, administered once a day, beginning 2 hours prior to surgery and continuing for a maximum of 12 days after surgery, was comparable to heparin 5000 U every 8 hours SC in preventing deep vein thrombosis (DVT). The data are provided below.
[See second table at right]
In a second double-blind, parallel group study, Lovenox Injection 40 mg SC once a day was compared to heparin 5000 U every 8 hours SC in 1347 patients undergoing colorectal surgery (one-third with cancer). Treatment was initiated approximately 2 hours prior to surgery and continued for approximately 7 to 10 days after surgery. The data are provided below.
[See third table at right]

Treatment of Deep Vein Thrombosis and Pulmonary Embolism: In a multicenter, parallel group study, 900 patients with acute lower extremity deep vein thrombosis (DVT) with or without pulmonary embolism (PE) were randomized to an inpatient (hospital) treatment of either (i) Lovenox Injection 1.5 mg/kg once a day SC, (ii) Lovenox Injection 1.0 mg/kg every 12 hours SC, or (iii) heparin i.v. bolus (5000 IU) followed by a continuous infusion (administered to achieve an aPTT of 55 to 85 seconds). All patients also received warfarin sodium (dose adjusted according to PT to achieve an International Normalization Ratio [INR] of 2.0 to 3.0), commencing within 72 hours of initiation of Lovenox Injection or standard heparin therapy, and continuing for 90 days. Lovenox Injection or standard heparin therapy was administered for a minimum of 5 days and until the targeted warfarin sodium INR was achieved. Both Lovenox Injection regimens were equivalent to standard heparin therapy in the prevention of recurrent venous thromboembolism (DVT and/or PE).
[See first table on next page]
Similarly, in a multicenter, open-label, parallel group study, 501 patients with acute proximal deep vein thrombosis were randomized to enoxaparin or heparin. Patients who could not receive outpatient therapy were excluded from entering the study. Eligible patients could be treated in the hospital, but ONLY enoxaparin patients were permitted to go home on therapy (72%). Patients were randomized to either Lovenox Injection 1 mg/kg every 12 hours SC or heparin i.v. bolus (5000 IU) followed by a continuous infusion administered to achieve an aPTT of 60 to 85 seconds (in-patient treatment). All patients also received warfarin sodium as described in the previous study. Lovenox Injection or standard heparin therapy was administered for a minimum of 5 days. Lovenox Injection was equivalent to standard heparin therapy in the prevention of recurrent venous thromboembolism.
[See second table on next page]

Unstable Angina and Non-Q-Wave Myocardial Infarction: In a multicenter, double-blind, parallel group study, 3171 patients who recently experienced unstable angina or non-Q-wave myocardial infarction were randomized to either Lovenox Injection 1 mg/kg every 12 hours SC or heparin i.v. bolus (5000 U) followed by a continuous infusion (adjusted to achieve an aPTT of 55 to 85 seconds). **All** patients were also treated with aspirin 100 to 325 mg per day. Treatment was initiated within 24 hours of the event and continued until clinical stabilization, revascularization procedures, or hospital discharge, with a maximal duration of 8 days of therapy. The combined incidence of the triple endpoint of death, myocardial infarction, or recurrent angina was lower for Lovenox Injection compared with heparin therapy at 14 days after initiation of treatment. The lower incidence of the triple endpoint was sustained up to 30 days after initiation of treatment. These results were observed in an analysis of both all-randomized and all-treated patients.
Urgent revascularization procedures were performed less frequently in the Lovenox Injection group as compared to the heparin group, 6.3% compared to 8.2% at 30 days ($p = 0.047$).
[See third table on next page]
The combined incidence of death or myocardial infarction at all time points was lower for Lovenox Injection compared to standard heparin therapy, but did not achieve statistical significance. The data are provided below.
[See fourth table on next page]

INDICATIONS AND USAGE

- Lovenox Injection is indicated for the prevention of deep vein thrombosis, which may lead to pulmonary embolism:
  - in patients undergoing hip replacement surgery, during and following hospitalization;
  - in patients undergoing knee replacement surgery;
  - in patients undergoing abdominal surgery who are at risk for thromboembolic complications. Patients at risk include patients who are over 40 years of age, obese, undergoing surgery under general anesthesia lasting longer than 30 minutes or who have additional risk factors such as malignancy or a history of deep vein thrombosis or pulmonary embolism.
- Lovenox Injection is indicated for:
  - the **inpatient treatment** of acute deep vein thrombosis **with and without pulmonary embolism,** when administered in conjunction with warfarin sodium;
  - the **outpatient treatment** of acute deep vein thrombosis **without pulmonary embolism** when administered in conjunction with warfarin sodium.
- Lovenox Injection is indicated for the prevention of ischemic complications of unstable angina and non-Q-wave myocardial infarction, when concurrently administered with aspirin.

See **DOSAGE AND ADMINISTRATION: Adult Dosage** for appropriate dosage regimens.

CONTRAINDICATIONS

Lovenox Injection is contraindicated in patients with active major bleeding, in patients with thrombocytopenia associated with a positive *in vitro* test for anti-platelet antibody in the presence of enoxaparin sodium, or in patients with hypersensitivity to enoxaparin sodium.
Patients with known hypersensitivity to heparin or pork products should not be treated with Lovenox Injection.

WARNINGS

Lovenox Injection is not intended for intramuscular administration.
Lovenox Injection cannot be used interchangeably (unit for unit) with heparin or other low molecular weight heparins as they differ in manufacturing process, molecular weight distribution, anti-Xa and anti-IIa activities, units, and dosage. Each of these medicines has its own instructions for use.
Lovenox Injection should be used with extreme caution in patients with a history of heparin-induced thrombocytopenia.

Hemorrhage: Lovenox Injection, like other anticoagulants, should be used with extreme caution in conditions with increased risk of hemorrhage, such as bacterial endocarditis, congenital or acquired bleeding disorders, active ulcerative and angiodysplastic gastrointestinal disease, hemorrhagic stroke, or shortly after brain, spinal, or ophthalmological surgery, or in patients treated concomitantly with platelet inhibitors.
Cases of epidural or spinal hematomas have been reported with the associated use of enoxaparin and spinal/epidural anesthesia or spinal puncture resulting in long-term or permanent paralysis. The risk of these events is higher with the use of post-operative indwelling epidural catheters or by the concomitant use of additional drugs affecting hemostasis such as NSAIDs (see boxed WARNING; ADVERSE REACTIONS, Ongoing Safety Surveillance; and PRECAUTIONS, Drug Interactions).
Bleeding can occur at any site during therapy with enoxaparin. An unexplained fall in hematocrit or blood pressure should lead to a search for a bleeding site.

Thrombocytopenia: Thrombocytopenia can occur with the administration of Lovenox Injection.
Moderate thrombocytopenia (platelet counts between 100,000/mm^3 and 50,000/mm^3) occurred at a rate of 1.3% in patients given Lovenox Injection, 1.2% in patients given heparin, and 0.6% in patients given placebo in clinical trials.
Platelet counts less than 50,000/mm^3 occurred at a rate of 0.1% in patients given Lovenox Injection, in 0.2% of patients given heparin, and 0% of patients given placebo in the same trials.
Thrombocytopenia of any degree should be monitored closely. If the platelet count falls below 100,000/mm^3, enoxaparin should be discontinued. Rare cases of thrombocytopenia with thrombosis have also been observed in clinical practice. The rate of incidence of this complication in usual medical practice is unknown.

PRECAUTIONS

General: Lovenox Injection should not be mixed with other injections or infusions.
Lovenox Injection should be used with care in patients with a bleeding diathesis, uncontrolled arterial hypertension or a history of recent gastrointestinal ulceration, diabetic retinopathy, and hemorrhage. Elderly patients and patients with renal insufficiency may show delayed elimination of enoxaparin. Enoxaparin should be used with care in these

Efficacy of Lovenox Injection in Knee Replacement Surgery

Indication	Dosing Regimen: Lovenox 30 mg q12h SC n (%)	Placebo q12h SC n (%)
All Treated Knee Replacement Patients	47 (100)	52 (100)
Treatment Failures		
Total DVT (%)	5 (11)[1] (95% CI: 1 to 21)	32 (62) (95% CI: 47 to 76)
Proximal DVT (%)	0 (0)[2] (95% Upper CL: 5)	7 (13) (95% CI: 3 to 24)

[1] p value versus placebo = 0.0001
CI = Confidence Interval
[2] p value versus placebo = 0.013
CL = Confidence Limit

Efficacy of Lovenox Injection in Abdominal Surgery Patients with Cancer

Indication	Dosing Regimen: Lovenox 40 mg q.d. SC n (%)	Heparin 5000 U q8h SC n (%)
All Treated Abdominal Surgery Patients	555 (100)	560 (100)
Treatment Failures		
Total VTE[1] (%)	56 (10.1) (95% CI[2]: 8 to 13)	63 (11.3) (95% CI: 9 to 14)
DVT Only (%)	54 (9.7) (95% CI: 7 to 12)	61 (10.9) (95% CI: 8 to 13)

[1] VTE = Venous thromboembolic events which included DVT, PE, and death considered to be thromboembolic in origin.
[2] CI = Confidence Interval

Efficacy of Lovenox Injection in Colorectal Surgery

Indication	Dosing Regimen: Lovenox 40 mg q.d. SC n (%)	Heparin 5000 U q8h SC n (%)
All Treated Colorectal Surgery Patients	673 (100)	674 (100)
Treatment Failures		
Total VTE[1] (%)	48 (7.1) (95% CI[2]: 5 to 9)	45 (6.7) (95% CI: 5 to 9)
DVT Only (%)	47 (7.0) (95% CI: 5 to 9)	44 (6.5) (95% CI: 5 to 8)

[1] VTE = Venous thromboembolic events which included DVT, PE, and death considered to be thromboembolic in origin.
[2] CI = Confidence Interval

patients. Adjustment of enoxaparin sodium dose may be considered for low weight (<45 kg) patients and/or for patients with severe renal impairment (creatinine clearance <30mL/min).

If thromboembolic events occur despite enoxaparin prophylaxis, appropriate therapy should be initiated.

Laboratory Tests: Periodic complete blood counts, including platelet count, and stool occult blood tests are recommended during the course of treatment with Lovenox Injection. When administered at recommended prophylaxis doses, routine coagulation tests such as Prothrombin Time (PT) and Activated Partial Thromboplastin Time (aPTT) are relatively insensitive measures of Lovenox Injection activity and, therefore, unsuitable for monitoring. Anti-Factor Xa may be used to monitor the anticoagulant effect of Lovenox Injection in patients with significant renal impairment. If during Lovenox Injection therapy abnormal coagulation parameters or bleeding should occur, anti-Factor Xa levels may be used to monitor the anticoagulant effects of Lovenox Injection (see **CLINICAL PHARMACOLOGY: Pharmacodynamics**).

Efficacy of Lovenox Injection in Treatment of Deep Vein Thrombosis and Pulmonary Embolism

Indication	Dosing Regimen[1]		
	Lovenox 1.5 mg/kg q.d. SC n (%)	**Lovenox** 1.0 mg/kg q12h SC n (%)	**Heparin** aPTT Adjusted i.v. Therapy n(%)
All Treated DVT Patients with and without PE	298 (100)	312 (100)	290 (100)
Patient Outcome Total VTE[2] (%)	13 (4.4)[3]	9 (2.9)[3]	12 (4.1)
DVT Only (%)	11 (3.7)	7 (2.2)	8 (2.8)
Proximal DVT (%)	9 (3.0)	6 (1.9)	7 (2.4)
PE (%)	2 (0.7)	2 (0.6)	4 (1.4)

[1] All patients were also treated with warfarin sodium commencing within 72 hours of Lovenox or standard heparin therapy.
[2] VTE = venous thromboembolic event (deep vein thrombosis [DVT] and/or pulmonary embolism [PE]).
[3] The 95% Confidence Intervals for the treatment differences for total VTE were:
Lovenox once a day versus heparin (−3.0 to 3.5)
Lovenox every 12 hours versus heparin (−4.2 to 1.7).

Efficacy of Lovenox Injection in Treatment of Deep Vein Thrombosis

Indication	Dosing Regimen[1]	
	Lovenox 1.0 mg/kg q12h SC n (%)	**Heparin** aPTT Adjusted i.v. Therapy n (%)
All Treated DVT Patients	247 (100)	254 (100)
Patient Outcome Total VTE[2] (%)	13 (5.3)[3]	17 (6.7)
DVT Only (%)	11 (4.5)	14 (5.5)
Proximal DVT (%)	10 (4.0)	12 (4.7)
PE (%)	2 (0.8)	3 (1.2)

[1] All patients were also treated with warfarin sodium commencing on the evening of the second day of Lovenox or standard heparin therapy.
[2] VTE = venous thromboembolic event (deep vein thrombosis [DVT] and/or pulmonary embolism [PE]).
[3] The 95% Confidence Intervals for the treatment difference for total VTE was: Lovenox versus heparin (−5.6 to 2.7).

Efficacy of Lovenox Injection in Unstable Angina and Non-Q-Wave Myocardial Infarction (Combined Endpoint of Death, Myocardial Infarction, or Recurrent Angina)

Indication	Dosing Regimen[1]		Reduction (%)	p Value
	Lovenox 1 mg/kg q12h SC n (%)	**Heparin** aPTT Adjusted i.v. Therapy n (%)		
All Randomized Unstable Angina and Non-Q-Wave MI Patients	1607 (100)	1564 (100)		
Timepoint[2] 48 Hours	99 (6.2)	115 (7.4)	1.2	0.178
14 Days	266 (16.6)	309 (19.8)	3.2	0.019
30 Days	318 (19.8)	364 (23.3)	3.5	0.016

[1] All patients were also treated with aspirin 100 to 325 mg per day.
[2] Evaluation timepoints are after initiation of treatment. Therapy continued for up to 8 days (median duration of 2.6 days).

Efficacy of Lovenox Injection in Unstable Angina and Non-Q-Wave Myocardial Infarction (Combined Endpoint of Death or Myocardial Infarction)

Indication	Dosing Regimen[1]		Reduction (%)	p Value
	Lovenox 1 mg/kg q12h SC n (%)	**Heparin** aPTT Adjusted i.v. Therapy n (%)		
All Randomized Unstable Angina and Non-Q-Wave MI Patients	1607 (100)	1564 (100)		
Timepoint[2] 48 Hours	18 (1.1)	21 (1.3)	0.2	0.119
14 Days	79 (4.9)	96 (6.1)	1.2	0.132
30 Days	99 (6.2)	121 (7.7)	1.5	0.081

[1] All patients were also treated with aspirin 100 to 325 mg per day.
[2] Evaluation timepoints are after initiation of treatment. Therapy continued for up to 8 days (median duration of 2.6 days).

Drug Interactions: Unless really needed, agents which may enhance the risk of hemorrhage should be discontinued prior to initiation of Lovenox Injection therapy. These agents include medications such as: anticoagulants, platelet inhibitors including acetylsalicylic acid, salicylates, NSAIDs (including ketorolac tromethamine), dipyridamole, or sulfinpyrazone. If co-administration is essential, conduct close clinical and laboratory monitoring (see **PRECAUTIONS: Laboratory Tests**).

Carcinogenesis, Mutagenesis, Impairment of Fertility: No long-term studies in animals have been performed to evaluate the carcinogenic potential of enoxaparin. Enoxaparin was not mutagenic in *in vitro* tests, including the Ames test, mouse lymphoma cell forward mutation test, and human lymphocyte chromosomal aberration test, and the *in vivo* rat bone marrow chromosomal aberration test. Enoxaparin was found to have no effect on fertility or reproductive performance of male and female rats at SC doses up to 20 mg/kg/day or 141 mg/m^2/day. The maximum human dose in clinical trials was 2.0 mg/kg/day or 78 mg/m^2/day (for an average body weight of 70 kg, height of 170 cm, and body surface area of 1.8 m^2).

Pregnancy: *Teratogenic Effects:* Pregnancy Category B: Teratology studies have been conducted in pregnant rats and rabbits at SC doses of enoxaparin up to 30 mg/kg/day or 211 mg/m^2/day and 410 mg/m^2/day, respectively. There was no evidence of teratogenic effects or fetotoxicity due to enoxaparin. There are, however, no adequate and well-controlled studies in pregnant women. Because animal reproduction studies are not always predictive of human response, this drug should be used during pregnancy only if clearly needed.

Non-teratogenic Effects: There have been a few spontaneous post-marketing reports of fetal death when pregnant women received enoxaparin. Causality of the cases has not been determined. In one case, placental hemorrhage and detachment were found in association with the fetal death. If enoxaparin is used during pregnancy, or if the patient becomes pregnant while taking this drug, the patient should be apprised of the potential hazard to the fetus.

Nursing Mothers: It is not known whether this drug is excreted in human milk. Because many drugs are excreted in human milk, caution should be exercised when enoxaparin is administered to nursing women.

Pediatric Use: Safety and effectiveness of enoxaparin in pediatric patients have not been established.

ADVERSE REACTIONS

Hemorrhage: The incidence of major hemorrhagic complications during Lovenox Injection treatment has been low. The following rates of major bleeding events have been reported during clinical trials.

[See first table at top of next page]

Injection site hematomas during the extended prophylaxis period after hip replacement surgery occurred in 9% of the enoxaparin patients versus 1.8% of the placebo patients.

Major Bleeding Episodes in Abdominal & Colorectal Surgery[1]

Indications	Dosing Regimen	
	Lovenox 40 mg q.d. SC	**Heparin** 5000 U q8h SC
Abdominal Surgery	n = 555 23 (4%)	n = 560 16 (3%)
Colorectal Surgery	n = 673 28 (4%)	n = 674 21 (3%)

[1] Bleeding complications were considered major: (1) if the hemorrhage caused a significant clinical event, or (2) if accompanied by a hemoglobin decrease ≥2g/dL or transfusion of 2 or more units of blood products. Retroperitoneal, intraocular, and intracranial hemorrhages were always considered major.

[See second table on next page]

Major Bleeding Episodes in Unstable Angina and Non-Q-Wave Myocardial Infarction

Indication	Dosing Regimen	
	Lovenox[1] 1 mg/kg q12h SC	**Heparin**[1] aPTT Adjusted i.v. Therapy
Unstable Angina and Non-Q-Wave MI[2,3]	n = 1578 17 (1%)	n = 1529 18 (1%)

[1] The rates represent major bleeding on study medication up to 12 hours after dose.
[2] Aspirin therapy was administered concurrently (100 to 325 mg per day).
[3] Bleeding complications were considered major: (1) if the

Continued on next page

Lovenox—Cont.

hemorrhage caused a significant clinical event, or (2) if accompanied by a hemoglobin decrease by ≥3g/dL or transfusion of 2 or more units of blood products. Intraocular, retroperitoneal, and intracranial hemorrhages were always considered major.

Thrombocytopenia: see **WARNINGS: Thrombocytopenia.**

Elevations of Serum Aminotransferases: Asymptomatic increases in aspartate (AST [SGOT]) and alanine (ALT [SGPT]) aminotransferase levels greater than three times the upper limit of normal of the laboratory reference range have been reported in up to 6.1% and 5.9% of patients, respectively, during treatment with Lovenox Injection. Similar significant increases in aminotransferase levels have also been observed in patients and healthy volunteers treated with heparin and other low molecular weight heparins. Such elevations are fully reversible and are rarely associated with increases in bilirubin.

Since aminotransferase determinations are important in the differential diagnosis of myocardial infarction, liver disease, and pulmonary emboli, elevations that might be caused by drugs like Lovenox Injection should be interpreted with caution.

Local Reactions: Mild local irritation, pain, hematoma, ecchymosis, and erythema may follow SC injection of Lovenox Injection.

Other: Other adverse effects that were thought to be possibly or probably related to treatment with Lovenox Injection, heparin, or placebo in clinical trials with patients undergoing hip or knee replacement surgery, abdominal or colorectal surgery, or treatment for DVT and that occurred at a rate of at least 2% in the enoxaparin group, are provided below.

[See third table at right]
[See first table at top of next page]
[See second table on next page]

Adverse Events in Lovenox Injection Treated Patients With Unstable Angina or Non-Q-Wave Myocardial Infarction: Non-hemorrhagic clinical events reported to be related to enoxaparin therapy occurred at an incidence of ≤1%.

Non-major hemorrhagic episodes, primarily injection site ecchymoses and hematomas, were more frequently reported in patients treated with SC enoxaparin than in patients treated with i.v. heparin.

Serious adverse events with Lovenox Injection or heparin in a clinical trial in patients with unstable angina or non-Q-wave myocardial infarction that occurred at a rate of at least 0.5% in the enoxaparin group, are provided below (irrespective of relationship to drug therapy).

[See third table on next page]

Ongoing Safety Surveillance: Since 1993, there have been more than 60 reports of epidural or spinal hematoma formation with concurrent use of enoxaparin and spinal/epidural anesthesia or spinal puncture. The majority of patients had a post-operative indwelling epidural catheter placed for analgesia or received additional drugs affecting hemostasis such as NSAIDs. Many of the epidural or spinal hematomas caused neurologic injury, including long-term or permanent paralysis. Because these events were reported voluntarily from a population of unknown size, estimates of frequency cannot be made.

Other reports include: local reactions at the injection site (*i.e.,* skin necrosis, nodules, inflammation, oozing), systemic allergic reactions (*i.e.,* pruritus, urticaria, anaphylactoid reactions), vesiculobullous rash, purpura, and thrombocytosis. Very rare cases of hyperlipidemia have been reported, with one case of hyperlipidemia, with marked hypertriglyceridemia, reported in a diabetic pregnant woman; causality has not been determined.

OVERDOSAGE

Symptoms/Treatment: Accidental overdosage following administration of Lovenox Injection may lead to hemorrhagic complications. Injected Lovenox Injection may be largely neutralized by the slow i.v. injection of protamine sulfate (1% solution). The dose of protamine sulfate should be equal to the dose of Lovenox Injection injected: 1 mg protamine sulfate should be administered to neutralize 1 mg Lovenox Injection. A second infusion of 0.5 mg protamine sulfate per 1 mg of Lovenox Injection may be administered if the aPTT measured 2 to 4 hours after the first infusion remains prolonged. However, even with higher doses of protamine, the aPTT may remain more prolonged than under normal conditions found following administration of heparin. In all cases, the anti-Factor Xa activity is never completely neutralized (maximum about 60%). Particular care should be taken to avoid overdosage with protamine sulfate. Administration of protamine sulfate can cause severe hypotensive and anaphylactoid reactions. Because fatal reactions, often resembling anaphylaxis, have been reported with protamine sulfate, it should be given only when resuscitation techniques and treatment of anaphylactic shock are readily available. For additional information consult the labeling of Protamine Sulfate Injection, USP, products.

A single SC dose of 46.4 mg/kg enoxaparin was lethal to rats. The symptoms of acute toxicity were ataxia, decreased motility, dyspnea, cyanosis, and coma.

DOSAGE AND ADMINISTRATION

All patients should be evaluated for a bleeding disorder before administration of Lovenox Injection, unless the medication is needed urgently. Since coagulation parameters are

Major Bleeding Episodes in Hip or Knee Replacement Surgery[1]

Indications	Dosing Regimen		
	Lovenox 40 mg q.d. SC	**Lovenox** 30 mg q12h SC	**Heparin** 15,000 U/24h SC
Hip Replacement Surgery Without Extended Prophylaxis[2]		n = 786 31 (4%)	n = 541 32 (6%)
Hip Replacement Surgery With Extended Prophylaxis			
Peri-operative Period[3]	n = 288 4 (2%)		
Extended Prophylaxis Period[4]	n = 221 0 (0%)		
Knee Replacement Surgery Without Extended Prophylaxis[2]		n = 294 3 (1%)	n = 225 3 (1%)

[1] Bleeding complications were considered major: (1) if the hemorrhage caused a significant clinical event, or (2) if accompanied by a hemoglobin decrease ≥2g/dL or transfusion of 2 or more units of blood products. Retroperitoneal and intracranial hemorrhages were always considered major. In the knee replacement surgery trials, intraocular hemorrhages were also considered major hemorrhages.

[2] Lovenox 30 mg every 12 hours SC initiated 12 to 24 hours after surgery and continued for up to 14 days after surgery.

[3] Lovenox 40 mg SC once a day initiated up to 12 hours prior to surgery and continued for up to 7 days after surgery.

[4] Lovenox 40 mg SC once a day for up to 21 days after discharge.

NOTE: At no time point were the 40 mg once a day pre-operative and the 30 mg every 12 hours post-operative hip replacement surgery prophylactic regimens compared in clinical trials.

Major Bleeding Episodes in Deep Vein Thrombosis and Pulmonary Embolism Treatment[1]

Indication	Dosing Regimen[2]		
	Lovenox 1.5 mg/kg q.d. SC	**Lovenox** 1.0 mg/kg q12h SC	**Heparin** aPTT Adjusted i.v. Therapy
Deep Vein Thrombosis and Pulmonary Embolism Treatment	n = 298 5 (2%)	n = 559 9 (2%)	n = 554 9 (2%)

[1] Bleeding complications were considered major: (1) if the hemorrhage caused a significant clinical event, or (2) if accompanied by a hemoglobin decrease ≥2 g/dL or transfusion of 2 or more units of blood products. Retroperitoneal, intraocular, and intracranial hemorrhages were always considered major.

[2] All patients also received warfarin sodium (dose-adjusted according to PT to achieve an INR of 2.0 to 3.0) commencing within 72 hours of Lovenox or standard heparin therapy and continuing for up to 90 days.

Adverse Events Occurring at ≥2% Incidence in Lovenox Injection Treated Patients[1] Undergoing Hip or Knee Replacement Surgery

Adverse Event	Dosing Regimen									
	Lovenox 40 mg q.d. SC				**Lovenox** 30 mg q12h SC		**Heparin** 15,000 U/24h SC		**Placebo** q12h SC	
	Peri-operative Period n = 288[2]		Extended Prophylaxis Period n = 131[3]		n = 1080		n = 766		n = 115	
	Severe	**Total**	**Severe**	**Total**	**Severe**	**Total**	**Severe**	**Total**	**Severe**	**Total**
Fever	0%	8%	0%	0%	<1%	5%	<1%	4%	0%	3%
Hemorrhage	<1%	13%	0%	5%	<1%	4%	1%	4%	0%	3%
Nausea					<1%	3%	<1%	2%	0%	2%
Anemia	0%	16%	0%	<2%	<1%	2%	2%	5%	<1%	7%
Edema					<1%	2%	<1%	2%	0%	2%
Peripheral edema	0%	6%	0%	0%	<1%	3%	<1%	4%	0%	3%

[1] Excluding unrelated adverse events.

[2] Data represents Lovenox 40 mg SC once a day initiated up to 12 hours prior to surgery in 288 hip replacement surgery patients who received enoxaparin peri-operatively in an unblinded fashion in one clinical trial.

[3] Data represents Lovenox 40 mg SC once a day given in a blinded fashion as extended prophylaxis at the end of the peri-operative period in 131 of the original 288 hip replacement surgery patients for up to 21 days in one clinical trial.

unsuitable for monitoring Lovenox Injection activity, routine monitoring of coagulation parameters is not required (see **PRECAUTIONS, Laboratory Tests**).

Adult Dosage: *Hip or Knee Replacement Surgery:* In patients undergoing hip or knee replacement surgery, the recommended dose of Lovenox Injection is **30 mg every 12 hours** administered by SC injection. Provided that hemostasis has been established, the initial dose should be given 12 to 24 hours after surgery. Up to 14 days administration (average duration 7 to 10 days) of Lovenox Injection 30 mg every 12 hours has been well tolerated in controlled clinical trials. For hip replacement surgery, a dose of **40 mg once a day** SC, given initially 12 (±3) hours prior to surgery, may be considered. Following the initial phase of thromboprophylaxis in hip replacement surgery patients (Lovenox Injection 30 mg every 12 hours or 40 mg once a day), continued prophylaxis with Lovenox Injection 40 mg once a day administered by SC injection for 3 weeks is recommended.

Abdominal Surgery: In patients undergoing abdominal surgery who are at risk for thromboembolic complications, the recommended dose of Lovenox Injection is **40 mg once a day** administered by SC injection with the initial dose given 2 hours prior to surgery. The usual duration of administration is 7 to 10 days; up to 12 days administration has been well tolerated in clinical trials.

Treatment of Deep Vein Thrombosis and Pulmonary Embolism: In **outpatient treatment,** patients with acute deep vein thrombosis without pulmonary embolism who can be treated at home, the recommended dose of Lovenox Injection is **1.0 mg/kg every 12 hours** administered SC. In **inpatient (hospital) treatment,** patients with acute deep vein thrombosis with pulmonary embolism or patients with acute deep vein thrombosis without pulmonary embolism (who are not candidates for outpatient treatment), the recommended dose of Lovenox Injection is **1.0 mg/kg every 12 hours** administered SC **or 1.5 mg/kg once a day** administered SC at the same time every day. In both outpatient and inpatient (hospital) treatments, warfarin sodium therapy should be initiated when appropriate (usually within 72 hours of Lovenox Injection). Lovenox Injection should be continued for a minimum of 5 days and until a therapeutic oral anticoagulant effect has been achieved (International-Normalization Ratio 2.0 to 3.0). The average duration of administration is 7 days; up to 17 days Lovenox Injection administration has been well tolerated in controlled clinical trials.

Unstable Angina and Non-Q-Wave Myocardial Infarction: In patients with unstable angina or non-Q-wave myocardial

Adverse Events Occurring at ≥2% Incidence in Lovenox Injection Treated Patients[1] Undergoing Abdominal or Colorectal Surgery

	Dosing Regimen			
	Lovenox 40 mg q.d. SC n = 1228		**Heparin** 5000 U q8h SC n = 1234	
Adverse Event	**Severe**	**Total**	**Severe**	**Total**
Hemorrhage	<1%	7%	<1%	6%
Anemia	<1%	3%	<1%	3%
Ecchymosis	0%	3%	0%	3%

[1]Excluding unrelated adverse events.

Adverse Events Occurring at ≥2% Incidence in Lovenox Injection Treated Patients[1] Undergoing Treatment for Deep Vein Thrombosis and Pulmonary Embolism

	Dosing Regimen					
	Lovenox 1.5 mg/kg q.d. SC n = 298		**Lovenox** 1.0 mg/kg q12h SC n = 559		**Heparin** aPTT Adjusted i.v. Therapy n = 544	
Adverse Event	**Severe**	**Total**	**Severe**	**Total**	**Severe**	**Total**
Injection Site Hemorrhage	0%	5%	0%	3%	<1%	<1%
Injection Site Pain	0%	2%	0%	2%	0%	0%
Hematuria	0%	2%	0%	<1%	<1%	2%

[1]Excluding unrelated adverse events.

Serious Adverse Events Occurring at ≥0.5% Incidence in Lovenox Injection Treated Patients With Unstable Angina or Non-Q-Wave Myocardial Infarction

	Dosing Regimen	
Adverse Event	**Lovenox** 1 mg/kg q12h SC n = 1578 n (%)	**Heparin** aPTT Adjusted i.v. Therapy n = 1529 n (%)
Atrial fibrillation	11 (0.70)	3 (0.20)
Heart failure	15 (0.95)	11 (0.72)
Lung edema	11 (0.70)	11 (0.72)
Pneumonia	13 (0.82)	9 (0.59)

Dosage Unit	**Strength[1]**	**Package Size (per carton)**	**Anti-Xa Activity[2]**	**NDC # 0075-**
Ampules	30 mg / 0.3 mL	10 ampules	3000 IU	0624-03
Prefilled Syringes[3]	30 mg / 0.3 mL 40 mg / 0.4 mL	10 syringes 10 syringes	3000 IU 4000 IU	0624-30 0620-40
Graduated Prefilled Syringes[3]	60 mg / 0.6 mL 80 mg / 0.8 mL 100 mg / 1.0 mL	10 syringes 10 syringes 10 syringes	6000 IU 8000 IU 10000 IU	0621-60 0622-80 0623-00

[1] Strength represents the number of milligrams of enoxaparin sodium in Water for Injection. Lovenox ampules and prefilled syringes contain 10 mg enoxaparin sodium per 0.1 mL Water for Injection.
[2] Approximate anti-Factor Xa activity based on reference to the W.H.O. First International Low Molecular Weight Heparin Reference Standard.
[3] Each Lovenox syringe is affixed with a 27 gauge × 1/2 inch needle.

infarction, the recommended dose of Lovenox Injection is **1 mg/kg** administered SC **every 12 hours** in conjunction with oral aspirin therapy (100 to 325 mg once daily). Treatment with Lovenox Injection should be prescribed for a minimum of 2 days and continued until clinical stabilization. The usual duration of treatment is 2 to 8 days. To minimize the risk of bleeding following vascular instrumentation during the treatment of unstable angina, adhere precisely to the intervals recommended between Lovenox Injection doses. The vascular access sheath for instrumentation should remain in place for 6 to 8 hours following a dose of Lovenox Injection. The next scheduled dose should be given no sooner than 6 to 8 hours after sheath removal. The site of the procedure should be observed for signs of bleeding or hematoma formation.

Administration: Enoxaparin injection is a clear, colorless to pale yellow sterile solution, and as with other parenteral drug products, should be inspected visually for particulate matter and discoloration prior to administration.

When using Lovenox Injection ampules, to assure withdrawal of the appropriate volume of drug, the use of a tuberculin syringe or equivalent is recommended.

Lovenox Injection is administered by SC injection. It must not be administered by intramuscular injection.

Subcutaneous Injection Technique: Patients should be lying down and Lovenox Injection administered by deep SC injection. To avoid the loss of drug when using the 30 and 40 mg prefilled syringes, do not expel the air bubble from the syringe before the injection. Administration should be alternated between the left and right anterolateral and left and right posterolateral abdominal wall. The whole length of the needle should be introduced into a skin fold held between the thumb and forefinger; the skin fold should be held throughout the injection. To minimize bruising, do not rub the injection site after completion of the injection. An automatic injector, Lovenox EasyInjector™, is available for patients to administer Lovenox Injection packaged in 30 mg and 40 mg prefilled syringes. Please see directions accompanying the Lovenox EasyInjector™ automatic injection device.

HOW SUPPLIED

Lovenox® (enoxaparin sodium) Injection is available in:

[See fourth table above]

Store at Controlled Room Temperature, 15–25°C (59–77°F) [see USP].

Keep out of the reach of children.

Lovenox Injection prefilled and graduated prefilled syringes manufactured in France.

Lovenox Injection ampules manufactured in England.

RHÔNE-POULENC RORER PHARMACEUTICALS INC.
Collegeville, PA U.S.A. 19426-0107
IN–1107T Rev. 6/99

Shown in Product Identification Guide, page 307

NASACORT® ℞

[*na 'za · cort*]
(triamcinolone acetonide)
Nasal Inhaler
For Intranasal Use Only
Shake Well Before Using

DESCRIPTION

Triamcinolone acetonide, USP, the active ingredient in **Nasacort®** Nasal Inhaler, is a glucocorticosteroid with a molecular weight of 434.5 and with the chemical designation 9-Fluoro-11β,16α,17, 21-tetrahydroxypregna-1, 4-diene-3, 20-dione cyclic 16,17-acetal with acetone. ($C_{24}H_{31}FO_6$).

Nasacort Nasal Inhaler is a metered-dose aerosol unit containing a microcrystalline suspension of triamcinolone acetonide in dichlorodifluoromethane and dehydrated alcohol USP 0.7% w/w. Each canister contains 15 mg triamcinolone acetonide. Each actuation delivers 55 mcg triamcinolone acetonide from the nasal actuator to the patient (estimated from *in vitro* testing). There are at least 100 actuations in one **Nasacort** Nasal Inhaler canister. **After 100 actuations, the amount delivered per actuation may not be consistent and the unit should be discarded.** Patients are provided with a check-off card to track usage as part of the Information for Patients tear-off sheet.

CLINICAL PHARMACOLOGY

Triamcinolone acetonide is a more potent derivative of triamcinolone. Although triamcinolone itself is approximately one to two times as potent as prednisone in animal models of inflammation, triamcinolone acetonide is approximately 8 times more potent than prednisone.

Although the precise mechanism of corticosteroid antiallergic action is unknown, corticosteroids are very effective. However, they do not have an immediate effect on allergic signs and symptoms. When allergic symptoms are very severe, local treatment with recommended doses (microgram) of any available topical corticosteroids are not as effective as treatment with larger doses (milligram) of oral or parenteral formulations. When corticosteroids are prematurely discontinued, symptoms may not recur for several days.

Based upon intravenous dosing of triamcinolone acetonide phosphate ester, the half-life of triamcinolone acetonide was reported to be 88 minutes. The volume of distribution (Vd) reported was 99.5 L (SD ± 27.5) and clearance was 45.2 L/hour (SD ± 9.1) for triamcinolone acetonide. The plasma half-life of corticosteroids does not correlate well with the biologic half-life.

When administered intranasally to man at 440 mcg/day dose, the peak plasma concentration was <1 ng/mL and occurred on average at 3.4 hours (range 0.5 to 8.0 hours) post-dosing. The apparent half-life was 4.0 hours (range 1.0 to 7.0 hours); however, this value probably reflects lingering absorption. Intranasal doses below 440 mcg/day gave sparse data and did not allow for the calculation of meaningful pharmacokinetic parameters.

In animal studies using rats and dogs, three metabolites of triamcinolone acetonide have been identified. They are 6β-hydroxytriamcinolone acetonide, 21-carboxytriamcinolone acetonide and 21-carboxy-6β-hydroxytriamcinolone acetonide. All three metabolites are expected to be substantially less active than the parent compound due to (a) the dependence of anti-inflammatory activity on the presence of a 21-hydroxyl group, (b) the decreased activity observed upon 6-hydroxylation, and (c) the markedly increased water solubility favoring rapid elimination. There appeared to be some quantitative differences in the metabolites among species. No differences were detected in metabolic pattern as a function of route of administration.

CLINICAL TRIALS

In double-blind, parallel, placebo-controlled clinical trials of seasonal and perennial allergic rhinitis, in adults and adolescents in fixed total daily doses of 110, 220 and 440 mcg per day, the responses to aerosolized triamcinolone acetonide demonstrated a statistically significant improvement over placebo. In open label trials where the doses were sometimes adjusted according to patients' signs and symptoms, the daily doses and regimens varied. The most commonly used dose was 110 mcg per day.

Nasacort Nasal Inhaler, at a dose of 220 mcg once daily, has also been studied in two double-blind, placebo-controlled trials of two and four weeks duration in children ages 6 through 11 years with seasonal and perennial allergic rhinitis. These trials included 162 males and 91 females. **Nasacort** administered at a fixed dose of 220 mcg once daily resulted in consistent and statistically significant reductions of allergic rhinitis symptoms over vehicle placebo.

Continued on next page

Nasacort—Cont.

In attempting to determine if systemic absorption played a role in the response to **Nasacort**, a clinical study comparing intranasal and depot intramuscular triamcinolone acetonide was conducted. The doses used were based on bioavailability studies of each formulation. The final doses of **Nasacort** 440 mcg once a day and Kenalog®-40, 4 mg intramuscularly once a week, were chosen to deliver comparable total amounts of weekly triamcinolone acetonide. However, the weekly injection yielded sustained plasma levels throughout the dosing interval while the daily **Nasacort** application resulted in daily peak and trough concentrations, the mean of which was 3.5 times below the Kenalog plasma levels. Both topical **Nasacort** and intramuscular Kenalog-40 were clinically effective. In addition, in some studies there was evidence of improvement of eye symptoms. This suggests that **Nasacort**, at least to some degree is acting by a systemic mechanism.

In order to evaluate the effects of systemic absorption on the Hypothalamic-Pituitary-Adrenal (HPA) axis, **Nasacort** administered to adults in doses of 440 mcg once a day was compared to placebo and 42 days of a single morning dose of prednisone 10 mg. Adrenal response to a six-hour cosyntropin stimulation test suggests that intranasal **Nasacort** 440 mcg/day for six weeks did not measurably affect adrenal activity. Conversely, oral prednisone at 10 mg/day significantly reduced the response to ACTH.

No evidence of adrenal axis suppression was observed in 26 pediatric patients exposed for 6 weeks to systemic levels of triamcinolone acetonide higher than the systemic levels observed following administration of the maximum recommended dose of **Nasacort** Nasal Inhaler.

INDIVIDUALIZATION OF DOSAGE

Individual patients will experience a variable time to onset and degree of symptom relief when using **Nasacort**. It is recommended that dosing be started at 220 mcg once a day and the effect be assessed in four to seven days.

Adults and Children 12 years of age and older: Some relief can be expected in approximately two-thirds of patients within four to seven days. If greater effect is desired an increase of dose to 440 mcg once a day can be tried. If adequate relief has not been obtained by the third week of **Nasacort** treatment, alternate forms of treatment should be considered.

A dose-response between 110 mcg/day (one spray/nostril/day) and 440 mcg/day (four sprays/nostril/day) is not clearly discernible. In general, in the clinical trials the highest dose tended to provide relief sooner. This suggests an alternative approach to starting therapy with **Nasacort**, *e.g.*, starting treatment with 440 mcg (four sprays/nostril/day) and then, depending on the patient's response, decreasing the dose by one spray per day every four to seven days. Although **Nasacort** may be used at 220 mcg/day or 440 mcg/day divided into two or four times a day, the degree of relief does not seem to be significantly different compared to once-a-day dosing. As with other nasal corticosteroids, the vehicle used to deliver the corticosteroid, may cause symptoms that are difficult to distinguish from the patient's rhinitis symptoms. Thus, depending upon the balance between these vehicle side effects and the benefits of treatment, in determining the optimal dose for the relief of symptoms, individual patients may need to have a trial of high and low doses.

Children 6 through 11 years of age: In children 6 through 11 years of age, it is recommended that dosing be started at 220 mcg given as two sprays (55 mcg/spray) in each nostril once a day. In clinical trials, significant relief of rhinitis symptoms in children was observed as early as the fourth day of treatment and generally, it took one to two weeks to achieve maximum benefit. If adequate relief has not been obtained by the third week of **Nasacort** treatment, alternate forms of treatment should be considered.

In general, it is always desirable to titrate an individual patient to the minimum effective dose to reduce the possibility of side effects. In clinical trials, after symptoms have been brought under control at the recommended starting doses, reducing the daily dose to 110 mcg (one spray in each nostril once per day) has been shown to be effective in controlling symptoms in approximately one-half of adult patients being treated long-term for allergic rhinitis. (See **PRECAUTIONS, WARNINGS, Information for Patients** and **ADVERSE REACTIONS** sections).

INDICATIONS AND USAGE

Nasacort Nasal Inhaler is indicated for the nasal treatment of seasonal and perennial allergic rhinitis symptoms in adults and children 6 years of age and older.

CONTRAINDICATIONS

Hypersensitivity to any of the ingredients of this preparation contraindicates its use.

WARNINGS

The replacement of a systemic corticosteroid with a topical corticoid can be accompanied by signs of adrenal insufficiency and, in addition, some patients may experience symptoms of withdrawal, *e.g.*, joint and/or muscular pain, lassitude and depression. Patients previously treated for prolonged periods with systemic corticosteroids and transferred to topical corticoids should be carefully monitored for acute adrenal insufficiency in response to stress. In those patients who have asthma or other clinical conditions requiring long-term systemic corticosteroid treatment, too rapid a decrease in systemic corticosteroids may cause a severe exacerbation of their symptoms.

Children who are on immunosuppressant drugs are more susceptible to infections than healthy children. Chickenpox and measles, for example, can have a more serious or even fatal course in children on immunosuppressant doses of corticosteroids. In such children, or in adults who have not had these diseases, particular care should be taken to avoid exposure. If exposed, therapy with varicella-zoster immune globulin (VZIG) or pooled intravenous immunoglobulin (IVIG), as appropriate, may be indicated. If chickenpox develops, treatment with antiviral agents may be considered.

The use of **Nasacort** Nasal Inhaler with alternate-day systemic prednisone could increase the likelihood of hypothalamic-pituitary-adrenal (HPA) suppression compared to a therapeutic dose of either one alone. Therefore, **Nasacort** Nasal Inhaler should be used with caution in patients already receiving alternate-day prednisone treatment for any disease.

PRECAUTIONS

General: In clinical studies with triamcinolone acetonide administered intranasally, the development of localized infections of the nose and pharynx with *Candida albicans* has rarely occurred. When such an infection develops, it may require treatment with appropriate local therapy and discontinuance of treatment with **Nasacort** Nasal Inhaler.

Triamcinolone acetonide administered intranasally has been shown to be absorbed into the systemic circulation in humans. Patients with active rhinitis showed absorption similar to that found in normal volunteers. **Nasacort** at 440 mcg/day for 42 days did not measurably affect adrenal response to a six hour cosyntropin test. In the same study, prednisone 10 mg/day significantly reduced adrenal response to ACTH over the same period (see **CLINICAL TRIALS** section).

Nasacort Nasal Inhaler should be used with caution, if at all, in patients with active or quiescent tuberculous infections of the respiratory tract or in patients with untreated fungal, bacterial, or systemic viral infections or ocular herpes simplex.

Because of the inhibitory effect of corticosteroids on wound healing in patients who have experienced recent nasal septal ulcers, nasal surgery or trauma, a corticosteroid should be used with caution until healing has occurred. As with other nasally inhaled corticosteroids, nasal septal perforations have been reported in rare instances.

When used at excessive doses, systemic corticosteroid effects such as hypercorticism and adrenal suppression may appear. If such changes occur, **Nasacort** Nasal Inhaler should be discontinued slowly, consistent with accepted procedures for discontinuing oral steroid therapy.

Information for Patients: Patients being treated with **Nasacort** Nasal Inhaler should receive the following information and instructions.

Patients who are on immunosuppressant doses of corticosteroids should be warned to avoid exposure to chickenpox or measles and, if exposed, to obtain medical advice.

Patients should use **Nasacort** Nasal Inhaler at regular intervals since its effectiveness depends on its regular use. A decrease in symptoms may occur as soon as 12 hours after starting steroid therapy and generally can be expected to occur within a few days of initiating therapy in allergic rhinitis. The patient should take the medication as directed and should not exceed the prescribed dosage. The patient should contact the physician if symptoms do not improve after three weeks, or if the condition worsens. Nasal irritation and/or burning or stinging after use of the spray occur only rarely with this product. The patient should contact the physician if they occur.

For the proper use of this unit and to attain maximum improvement, the patient should read and follow the accompanying patient instructions carefully. Spraying triamcinolone acetonide directly onto the nasal septum should be avoided. Because the amount dispensed per puff may not be consistent, it is important to shake the canister well. Also, the canister should be discarded after 100 actuations.

Carcinogenesis, Mutagenesis: No evidence of treatment-related carcinogenicity was demonstrated after 2 years of once daily gavage administration of triamcinolone acetonide at doses of 0.05, 0.2 and 1.0 mcg/kg (approximately 0.1, 0.4 and 1.8% of the recommended clinical dose on a mcg/m^2 basis) in the rat and 0.1, 0.6 and 3.0 mcg/kg (approximately 0.1, 0.6 and 3.0% of the recommended clinical dose on a mcg/m^2 basis) in the mouse.

Mutagenesis studies with triamcinolone acetonide have not been conducted.

Impairment of Fertility: No evidence of impaired fertility was demonstrated when oral doses up to 15 mcg/kg (approximately 28% of the recommended clinical dose on a mcg/m^2 basis) were administered to female and male rats. However, triamcinolone acetonide at oral doses of 8.0 mcg/kg (approximately 15.0% of the recommended clinical dose on a mcg/m^2 basis) caused dystocia and prolonged delivery and at oral doses of 5.0 mcg/kg (approximately 9.0% of the recommended clinical dose on a mcg/m^2 basis) and above produced increases in fetal resorptions and stillbirths as well as decreases in pup body weight and survival. At an oral dose of 1.0 mcg/kg (approximately 2.0% of the recommended clinical dose on a mcg/m^2 basis), it did not manifest the above mentioned effects.

Pregnancy: Pregnancy Category C. Triamcinolone acetonide was teratogenic at inhalational doses of 20, 40 and 80 mcg/kg in rats (approximately 0.4, 0.75 and 1.5 times the recommended clinical dose on a mcg/m^2 basis, respectively) and rabbits (approximately 0.75, 1.5 and 3.0 times the recommended dose on a mcg/m^2 basis, respectively). Triamcinolone acetonide was also teratogenic at an inhalational dose of 500 mcg/kg in monkeys (approximately 18 times the recommended clinical dose on a mcg/m^2 basis). Dose-related teratogenic effects in rats and rabbits included cleft palate, internal hydrocephaly, and axial skeletal defects. Teratogenic effects observed in the monkey were CNS and cranial malformations. There are no adequate and well-controlled studies in pregnant women. Triamcinolone acetonide should be used during pregnancy only if the potential benefits justify the potential risk to the fetus.

Experience with oral corticoids since their introduction in pharmacologic as opposed to physiologic doses suggests that rodents are more prone to teratogenic effects from corticoids than humans. In addition, because there is a natural increase in glucocorticoid production during pregnancy, most women will require a lower exogenous steroid dose and many will not need corticoid treatment during pregnancy.

Nonteratogenic Effects: Hypoadrenalism may occur in infants born of mothers receiving corticosteroids during pregnancy. Such infants should be carefully observed.

Nursing Mothers: It is not known whether triamcinolone acetonide is excreted in human milk. Because other corticosteroids are excreted in human milk, caution should be exercised when **Nasacort** Nasal Inhaler is administered to nursing women.

Pediatric Use: Safety and effectiveness in pediatric patients below the age of 6 have not been established. Oral corticosteroids have been shown to cause growth suppression in children and teenagers, particularly with higher doses over extended periods. If a child or teenager on any corticosteroid appears to have growth suppression, the possibility that they are particularly sensitive to this effect of steroids should be considered.

ADVERSE REACTIONS

Adults and Children 12 years of age and older: In controlled and uncontrolled studies, 1257 adult and adolescent patients received treatment with intranasal triamcinolone acetonide. Adverse reactions are based on the 567 patients who received a product similar to the marketed **Nasacort** canister.

These patients were treated for an average of 48 days (range 1 to 117 days). The 145 patients enrolled in uncontrolled studies received treatment from 1 to 820 days (average 332 days). The most prevalent adverse experience was headache, being reported by approximately 18% of the patients who received **Nasacort**. Nasal irritation was reported by 2.8% of the patients receiving **Nasacort**. Other nasopharyngeal side effects were reported by fewer than 5% of the patients who received **Nasacort** and included: dry mucous membranes, naso-sinus congestion, throat discomfort, sneezing, and epistaxis. The complaints do not usually interfere with treatment and in the controlled and uncontrolled studies approximately 1% of patients have discontinued because of these nasal adverse effects. In the event of accidental overdose, an increased potential for these adverse experiences may be expected, but systemic adverse experiences are unlikely (see **OVERDOSAGE** section).

Children 6 through 11 years of age: Adverse event data in children 6 through 11 years of age are derived from two controlled clinical trials of two and four weeks duration. In these trials, 127 patients received fixed doses of 220 mcg/day of triamcinolone acetonide for an average of 22 days (range 8 to 33 days).

Adverse events occurring at an incidence of 3% or greater and more common among children treated with 220 mcg triamcinolone acetonide daily than vehicle placebo were:

Adverse Events	220 mcg of triamcinolone acetonide daily (n=127)	Vehicle placebo (n=322)
Epistaxis	11.0%	9.3%
Cough	9.4%	9.3%
Fever	7.9%	5.6%
Nausea	6.3%	3.1%
Throat discomfort	5.5%	5.3%
Otitis	4.7%	3.7%
Dyspepsia	4.7%	2.2%

Adverse events occurring at a rate of 3% or greater that were more common in the placebo group were upper respiratory tract infection, headache and concurrent infection.

Only 1.6% of patients discontinued due to adverse experiences. No patient discontinued due to a serious adverse event related to **Nasacort** therapy.

Though not observed in controlled clinical trials of **Nasacort** Nasal Inhaler in children, cases of nasal septum perforation among pediatric users have been reported in post-marketing surveillance of this product.

DOSAGE AND ADMINISTRATION

A decrease in symptoms may occur as soon as 12 hours after starting steroid therapy and generally can be expected to occur within a few days of initiating therapy in allergic rhinitis.

If improvement is not evident after 2 to 3 weeks, the patient should be re-evaluated. (See **INDIVIDUALIZATION OF DOSAGE** section).

Adults and Children 12 years of age and older: The recommended starting dose of **Nasacort** Nasal Inhaler is 220 mcg per day given as two sprays (55 mcg/spray) in each nostril once a day. If needed, the dose may be increased to 440 mcg per day (55 mcg/spray) either as once-a-day dosage or divided up to four times a day, *i.e.,* twice a day (two sprays/nostril), or four times a day (one spray/nostril). After the desired effect is obtained, some patients may be maintained on a dose of as little as one spray (55 mcg) in each nostril once a day (total daily dose 110 mcg per day).

Children 6 through 11 years of age: The recommended starting dose of **Nasacort** Nasal Inhaler is 220 mcg per day given as two sprays (55 mcg/spray) in each nostril once a day. Once the maximal effect has been achieved, it is always desirable to titrate the patient to the minimum effective dose.

Nasacort Nasal Inhaler is not recommended for children below 6 years of age since adequate numbers of patients have not been studied in this age group.

Directions for Use: Illustrated Patient's Instructions for use accompany each package of **Nasacort** Nasal Inhaler.

OVERDOSAGE

Acute overdosage with this dosage form is unlikely. The acute topical application of the entire 15 mg of the canister would most likely cause nasal irritation and headache. It would be unlikely to see acute systemic adverse effects even if the entire 15 mg of triamcinolone acetonide was administered intranasally all at once.

HOW SUPPLIED

Nasacort Nasal Inhaler is supplied as an aerosol canister which will provide 100 metered dose actuations. Each actuation delivers 55 mcg triamcinolone acetonide through the nasal actuator. The **Nasacort** Nasal Inhaler canister and accompanying nasal actuator are designed to be used together. The **Nasacort** Nasal Inhaler canister should not be used with other nasal actuators and the supplied nasal actuator should not be used with other products' canisters.

Nasacort Nasal Inhaler is supplied with a white plastic nasal actuator and patient instructions. Net weight of the canister contents is 10 grams.

NDC 0075-1505-43.

CONTENTS UNDER PRESSURE

Avoid spraying in eyes.

Do not puncture. Do not use or store near heat or open flame. Exposure to temperatures above 120°F may cause bursting. Never throw container into fire or incinerator. Keep out of reach of children. Store at Controlled Room Temperature 20 to 25°C (68 to 77°F) [see USP].

Note: The indented statement below is required by the Federal government's Clean Air Act for all products containing or manufactured with chlorofluorocarbons (CFC's):

> WARNING: Contains CFC-12, a substance which harms public health and the environment by destroying ozone in the upper atmosphere.

A notice similar to the above WARNING has been placed in the "Information For The Patient" portion of this package insert under the Environmental Protection Agency's (EPA's) regulations. The patient's warning states that the patient should consult his or her physician if there are questions about alternatives.

Caution: Federal (U.S.A.) law prohibits dispensing without prescription.

U.S. Pat. No. 4,767,612
Rev. 11/96
IN-0479J!
Marketed by
Aventis Pharmaceuticals Products Inc.
Parsippany, NJ 07054 ©1996

Shown in Product Identification Guide, page 307

NASACORT® AQ ℞

[*na´za · cort*]
(triamcinolone acetonide)
Nasal Spray
For intranasal use only.
Shake Well Before Using

DESCRIPTION

Triamcinolone acetonide, USP, the active ingredient in **Nasacort® AQ** Nasal Spray, is a corticosteroid with a molecular weight of 434.51 and with the chemical designation 9-Fluoro-11β,16α,17,21-tetrahydroxypregna-1,4-diene-3,20-dione cyclic 16,17-acetal with acetone ($C_{24}H_{31}FO_6$).

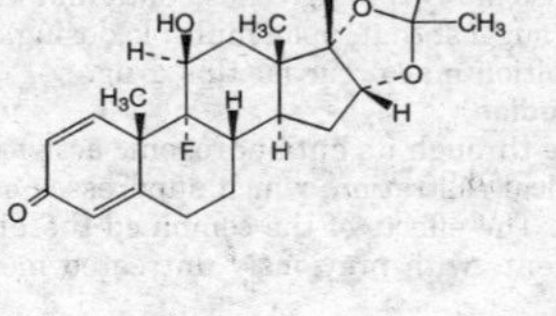

Nasacort AQ Nasal Spray is an unscented, thixotropic, water-based metered-dose pump spray formulation unit containing a microcrystalline suspension of triamcinolone acetonide in an aqueous medium. Microcrystalline cellulose, carboxymethylcellulose sodium, polysorbate 80, dextrose, benzalkonium chloride, and edetate disodium are contained in this aqueous medium; hydrochloric acid or sodium hydroxide may be added to adjust the pH to a target of 5.0 within a range of 4.5 and 6.0.

Each actuation delivers 55 mcg triamcinolone acetonide from the nasal actuator after an initial priming of 5 sprays. It will remain adequately primed for 2 weeks. If the product is not used for more than 2 weeks, then it can be adequately reprimed with one spray. The contents of one 6.5 gram sample bottle provide 30 actuations, and the contents of one 16.5 gram bottle provide 120 actuations. **After either 30 actuations or 120 actuations, the amount of triamcinolone acetonide delivered per actuation may not be consistent and the unit should be discarded.** Each 30 actuation sample bottle contains 3.575 mg of triamcinolone acetonide and each 120 actuation bottle contains 9.075 mg of triamcinolone acetonide.

In the Information for Patients tear-off sheet, patients are provided with a check-off form to track usage.

CLINICAL PHARMACOLOGY

Triamcinolone acetonide is a more potent derivative of triamcinolone. Although triamcinolone itself is approximately one to two times as potent as prednisone in animal models of inflammation, triamcinolone acetonide is approximately 8 times more potent than prednisone.

Although the precise mechanism of corticosteroid antiallergic action is unknown, corticosteroids are very effective. However, when allergic symptoms are very severe, local treatment with recommended doses (microgram) of any available topical corticosteroid are not as effective as treatment with larger doses (milligram) of oral or parenteral formulations.

Based upon intravenous dosing of triamcinolone acetonide phosphate ester in adults, the half-life of triamcinolone acetonide was reported to be 88 minutes. The volume of distribution (Vd) reported was 99.5 L (SD ± 27.5) and clearance was 45.2 L/hour (SD ± 9.1) for triamcinolone acetonide. The plasma half-life of corticosteroids does not correlate well with the biologic half-life.

Pharmacokinetic characterization of the **Nasacort AQ** Nasal Spray formulation was determined in both normal adult subjects and patients with allergic rhinitis. Single dose intranasal administration of 220 mcg of **Nasacort AQ** Nasal Spray in normal adult subjects and patients demonstrated minimal absorption of triamcinolone acetonide. The mean peak plasma concentration was approximately 0.5 ng/mL (range: 0.1 to 1.0 ng/mL) and occurred at 1.5 hours post dose. The mean plasma drug concentration was less than 0.06 ng/mL at 12 hours, and below the assay detection limit at 24 hours. The average terminal half-life was 3.1 hours. The range of mean $AUC_{0-\infty}$ values was 1.4 ng•hr/mL to 4.7 ng•hr/mL between doses of 110 mcg to 440 mcg in both patients and healthy volunteers. Dose proportionality was demonstrated in both normal adult subjects and in allergic rhinitis patients following single intranasal doses of 110 mcg or 220 mcg **Nasacort AQ** Nasal Spray. The C_{max} and AUC of the 440 mcg dose increased less than proportionally when compared to 110 and 220 mcg doses. Following multiple doses in pediatric patients receiving 440 mcg/day, plasma drug concentrations, AUC, C_{max} and T_{max} were similar to those values observed in adult patients.

In animal studies using rats and dogs, three metabolites of triamcinolone acetonide have been identified. They are 6β-hydroxytriamcinolone acetonide, 21-carboxytriamcinolone acetonide and 21-carboxy-6β-hydroxytriamcinolone acetonide. All three metabolites are expected to be substantially less active than the parent compound due to (a) the dependence of anti-inflammatory activity on the presence of a 21-hydroxyl group, (b) the decreased activity observed upon 6-hydroxylation, and (c) the markedly increased water solubility favoring rapid elimination. There appeared to be some quantitative differences in the metabolites among species. No differences were detected in metabolic pattern as a function of route of administration.

In order to determine if systemic absorption plays a role in **Nasacort AQ's** treatment of allergic rhinitis symptoms, a two week double-blind, placebo-controlled clinical study was conducted comparing **Nasacort AQ**, orally ingested triamcinolone acetonide, and placebo in 297 adult patients with seasonal allergic rhinitis. The study demonstrated that the therapeutic efficacy of **Nasacort AQ** Nasal Spray can be attributed to the topical effects of triamcinolone acetonide.

In order to evaluate the effects of systemic absorption on the Hypothalamic-Pituitary-Adrenal (HPA) axis, a clinical study was performed in adults comparing 220 mcg or 440 mcg **Nasacort AQ** per day, or 10 mg prednisone per day with placebo for 42 days. Adrenal response to a six-hour cosyntropin stimulation test showed that **Nasacort AQ** administered at doses of 220 mcg and 440 mcg had no statistically significant effect on HPA activity versus placebo. Conversely, oral prednisone at 10 mg/day significantly reduced the response to ACTH.

A study evaluating plasma cortisol response thirty and sixty minutes after cosyntropin stimulation in 80 pediatric patients who received 220 mcg or 440 mcg (twice the maximum recommended daily dose) daily for six weeks was conducted. No abnormal response to cosyntropin infusion (peak serum cortisol <18 mcg/dL) was observed in any pediatric patient after six weeks of dosing with **Nasacort AQ** at 440 mcg per day.

CLINICAL TRIALS

The safety and efficacy of **Nasacort AQ** Nasal Spray have been evaluated in 10 double-blind, placebo-controlled clinical trials of two- to four-weeks duration in adults and children 12 years and older with seasonal or perennial allergic rhinitis. The number of patients treated with **Nasacort AQ** Nasal Spray in these studies was 1266; of these patients, 675 were males and 591 were females.

Overall, the results of these clinical trials in adults and children 12 years and older demonstrated that **Nasacort AQ** Nasal Spray 220 mcg once daily (2 sprays in each nostril), when compared to placebo, provides statistically significant relief of nasal symptoms of seasonal or perennial allergic rhinitis including sneezing, stuffiness, discharge, and itching.

The safety and efficacy of **Nasacort AQ** Nasal Spray, at doses of 110 mcg or 220 mcg once daily, have also been adequately studied in two double-blind, placebo-controlled trials of two- and twelve-weeks duration in children ages 6 through 12 years with seasonal and perennial allergic rhinitis. These trials included 341 males and 177 females. **Nasacort AQ** administered at either dose resulted in statistically significant reductions in the severity of nasal symptoms of allergic rhinitis.

INDICATIONS AND USAGE

Nasacort AQ Nasal Spray is indicated for the treatment of the nasal symptoms of seasonal and perennial allergic rhinitis in adults and children 6 years of age and older.

CONTRAINDICATIONS

Hypersensitivity to any of the ingredients of this preparation contraindicates its use.

WARNINGS

The replacement of a systemic corticosteroid with a topical corticosteroid can be accompanied by signs of adrenal insufficiency and, in addition, some patients may experience symptoms of withdrawal; *e.g.,* joint and/or muscular pain, lassitude and depression. Patients previously treated for prolonged periods with systemic corticosteroids and transferred to topical corticosteroids should be carefully monitored for acute adrenal insufficiency in response to stress. In those patients who have asthma or other clinical conditions requiring long-term systemic corticosteroid treatment, too rapid a decrease in systemic corticosteroids may cause a severe exacerbation of their symptoms.

Children who are on immunosuppressant drugs are more susceptible to infections than healthy children. Chickenpox and measles, for example, can have a more serious or even fatal course in children on immunosuppressant doses of corticosteroids. In such children, or in adults who have not had these diseases, particular care should be taken to avoid exposure. If exposed, therapy with varicella-zoster immune globulin (VZIG) or pooled intravenous immunoglobulin (IVIG), as appropriate, may be indicated. If chickenpox develops, treatment with antiviral agents may be considered.

PRECAUTIONS

General: In clinical studies with triamcinolone acetonide nasal spray, the development of localized infections of the nose and pharynx with *Candida albicans* has rarely occurred. When such an infection develops it may require treatment with appropriate local or systemic therapy and discontinuance of treatment with **Nasacort AQ** Nasal Spray.

Nasacort AQ Nasal Spray should be used with caution, if at all, in patients with active or quiescent tuberculous infection of the respiratory tract or in patients with untreated fungal, bacterial, or systemic viral infections or ocular herpes simplex.

Because of the inhibitory effect of corticosteroids, in patients who have experienced recent nasal septal ulcers, nasal surgery, or trauma, a corticosteroid should be used with caution until healing has occurred. As with other nasally inhaled corticosteroids, nasal septal perforations have been reported in rare instances.

When used at excessive doses, systemic corticosteroid effects such as hypercorticism and adrenal suppression may appear. If such changes occur, **Nasacort AQ** Nasal Spray should be discontinued slowly, consistent with accepted procedures for discontinuing oral steroid therapy.

Information for Patients: Patients being treated with **Nasacort AQ** Nasal Spray should receive the following information and instructions. Patients who are on immunosuppressant doses of corticosteroids should be warned to avoid exposure to chickenpox or measles and, if exposed, to obtain medical advice.

Patients should use **Nasacort AQ** Nasal Spray at regular intervals since its effectiveness depends on its regular use. (See **DOSAGE AND ADMINISTRATION.**)

An improvement in some patient symptoms may be seen within the first day of treatment, and generally, it takes one week of treatment to reach maximum benefit. Initial assessment for response should be made during this time frame and periodically until the patient's symptoms are stabilized. The patient should take the medication as directed and should not exceed the prescribed dosage. The patient should contact the physician if symptoms do not improve after three weeks, or if the condition worsens. Patients who experience recurrent episodes of epistaxis (nose bleeds) or nasal septum discomfort while taking this medication should contact their physician. For the proper use of this unit and to attain maximum improvement, the patient should read and follow the accompanying patient instructions carefully. It is important to shake the bottle well before each use. **Also, the bottle should be discarded after 120 actuations since the amount of triamcinolone acetonide delivered**

Continued on next page

Nasacort AQ—Cont.

thereafter per actuation may be substantially less than 55 mcg of drug. Do not transfer any remaining suspension to another bottle.

Carcinogenesis, Mutagenesis, and Impairment of Fertility: In a two-year study in rats, triamcinolone acetonide caused no treatment-related carcinogenicity at oral doses up to 1.0 mcg/kg (approximately 1/30 and 1/50 of the maximum recommended daily intranasal dose in adults and children on a mcg/m^2 basis, respectively). In a two-year study in mice, triamcinolone acetonide caused no treatment-related carcinogenicity at oral doses up to 3.0 mcg/kg (approximately 1/12 and 1/30 of the maximum recommended daily intranasal dose in adults and children on a mcg/m^2 basis, respectively). No mutagenicity studies with triamcinolone acetonide have been performed.

In male and female rats, triamcinolone acetonide caused no change in pregnancy rate at oral doses up to 15.0 mcg/kg (approximately 1/2 of the maximum recommended daily intranasal dose in adults on a mcg/m^2 basis). Triamcinolone acetonide caused increased fetal resorptions and stillbirths and decreases in pup weight and survival at doses of 5.0 mcg/kg and above (approximately 1/5 of the maximum recommended daily intranasal dose in adults on a mcg/m^2 basis). At 1.0 mcg/kg (approximately 1/30 of the maximum recommended daily intranasal dose in adults on a mcg/m^2 basis), it did not induce the above mentioned effects.

Pregnancy: *Teratogenic Effects: Pregnancy Category C.* Triamcinolone acetonide was teratogenic in rats, rabbits, and monkeys. In rats, triamcinolone acetonide was teratogenic at inhalation doses of 20 mcg/kg and above (approximately 7/10 of the maximum recommended daily intranasal dose in adults on a mcg/m^2 basis). In rabbits, triamcinolone acetonide was teratogenic at inhalation doses of 20 mcg/kg and above (approximately 2 times the maximum recommended daily intranasal dose in adults on a mcg/m^2 basis). In monkeys, triamcinolone acetonide was teratogenic at an inhalation dose of 500 mcg/kg (approximately 37 times the maximum recommended daily intranasal dose in adults on a mcg/m^2 basis). Dose-related teratogenic effects in rats and rabbits included cleft palate and/or internal hydrocephaly and axial skeletal defects, whereas the effects observed in the monkey were cranial malformations.

There are no adequate and well-controlled studies in pregnant women. Therefore, triamcinolone acetonide should be used in pregnancy only if the potential benefit justifies the potential risk to the fetus. Since their introduction, experience with oral corticosteroids in pharmacologic as opposed to physiologic doses suggests that rodents are more prone to teratogenic effects from corticosteroids than humans. In addition, because there is a natural increase in glucocorticoid production during pregnancy, most women will require a lower exogenous corticosteroid dose and many will not need corticosteroid treatment during pregnancy.

Nonteratogenic Effects: Hypoadrenalism may occur in infants born of mothers receiving corticosteroids during pregnancy. Such infants should be carefully observed.

Nursing Mothers: It is not known whether triamcinolone acetonide is excreted in human milk. Because other corticosteroids are excreted in human milk, caution should be exercised when **Nasacort AQ** Nasal Spray is administered to nursing women.

Pediatric Use: Safety and effectiveness in pediatric patients below the age of 6 years have not been established. Corticosteroids have been shown to cause growth suppression in children and teenagers, particularly with higher doses over extended periods. If a child or teenager on any corticosteroid appears to have growth suppression, the possibility that they are particularly sensitive to this effect of corticosteroids should be considered.

ADVERSE REACTIONS

In placebo-controlled, double-blind, and open-label clinical studies, 1483 adults and children 12 years and older received treatment with triamcinolone acetonide aqueous nasal spray. These patients were treated for an average duration of 51 days. In the controlled trials (2–5 weeks duration) from which the following adverse reaction data are derived, 1394 patients were treated with **Nasacort AQ** Nasal Spray for an average of 19 days. In a long-term, open-label study, 172 patients received treatment for an average duration of 286 days.

Adverse events occurring at an incidence of 2% or greater and more common among **Nasacort AQ**-treated patients than placebo-treated patients in controlled adult clinical trials were:

[See table below]

A total of 602 children 6 to 12 years of age were studied in 3 double-blind, placebo-controlled clinical trials. Of these, 172 received 110 mcg/day and 207 received 220 mcg/day of **Nasacort AQ** Nasal Spray for two, six, or twelve weeks. The longest average durations of treatment for patients receiving 110 mcg/day and 220 mcg/day were 76 days and 80 days, respectively. Only 1% of those patients treated with **Nasacort AQ** were discontinued due to adverse experiences. No patient receiving 110 mcg/day discontinued due to a serious adverse event and one patient receiving 220 mcg/day discontinued due to a serious event that was considered not drug related. Overall, these studies found the adverse experience profile for **Nasacort AQ** to be similar to placebo. A similar adverse event profile was observed in pediatric patients 6–12 years of age as compared to older children and adults with the exception of epistaxis which occurred in less than 2% of the pediatric patients studied.

Adverse events occurring at an incidence of 2% or greater and more common among adult patients treated with placebo than **Nasacort AQ** were: headache, and rhinitis. In children aged 6 to 12 years these events included: asthma, epistaxis, headache, infection, otitis media, sinusitis, and vomiting.

In clinical trials, nasal septum perforation was reported in one adult patient although relationship to **Nasacort AQ** Nasal Spray has not been established.

In the event of accidental overdose, an increased potential for these adverse experiences may be expected, but acute systemic adverse experiences are unlikely. (See **OVERDOSAGE.**)

DOSAGE AND ADMINISTRATION

Recommended Doses: *Adults and children 12 years of age and older:* The recommended starting and maximum dose is 220 mcg per day as two sprays in each nostril once daily.

Children 6 to 12 years of age: The recommended starting dose is 110 mcg per day given as one spray in each nostril once daily. The maximum recommended dose is 220 mcg per day as two sprays per nostril once daily.

Nasacort AQ Nasal Spray is not recommended for children under 6 years of age since adequate numbers of patients have not been studied in this age group.

Individualization of Dosage: It is always desirable to titrate an individual patient to the minimum effective dose to reduce the possibility of side effects. In adults, when the maximum benefit has been achieved and symptoms have been controlled, reducing the dose to 110 mcg per day (one spray in each nostril once a day) has been shown to be effective in maintaining control of the allergic rhinitis symptoms in patients who were initially controlled at 220 mcg/day.

In children six to twelve years of age, the recommended starting dose is 110 mcg per day given as one spray in each nostril once daily. The maximum recommended daily dose in children 6 to 12 years of age is 220 mcg per day (two sprays in each nostril once daily). Some patients who do not achieve maximum symptom control at a dose of 110 mcg per day may benefit from a dose of 220 mcg given as two sprays in each nostril once daily. The minimum effective dose should be used to ensure continued control of symptoms. Once symptoms are controlled, pediatric patients may be able to be maintained on 110 mcg per day (1 spray in each nostril once daily).

An improvement in some patient symptoms may be seen within the first day of treatment, and generally, it takes one week of treatment to reach maximum benefit. Initial assessment for response should be made during this time frame and periodically until the patient's symptoms are stabilized. If adequate relief of symptoms has not been obtained after 3 weeks of treatment, **Nasacort AQ** Nasal Spray should be discontinued. (See **WARNINGS**, **PRECAUTIONS**, **Information for Patients**, and **ADVERSE REACTIONS**.)

Directions For Use: Illustrated Patient's Instructions for use accompany each package of **Nasacort AQ** Nasal Spray.

OVERDOSAGE

Like any other nasally administered corticosteroid, acute overdosing is unlikely in view of the total amount of active ingredient present. In the event that the entire contents of the bottle were administered all at once, via either oral or nasal application, clinically significant systemic adverse events would most likely not result. The patient may experience some gastrointestinal upset.

HOW SUPPLIED

Nasacort AQ Nasal Spray is a nonchlorofluorocarbon (non-CFC) containing metered-dose pump spray. The contents of one 6.5 gram sample bottle provide 30 actuations, and the contents of one 16.5 gram bottle provide 120 actuations. The bottle should be discarded when the labeled number of actuations have been reached even though the bottle is not completely empty.

It is supplied in a white high-density polyethylene container with a metered-dose pump unit, white nasal adapter, and patient instructions.

NDC 0075-1506-16

Caution: Federal law prohibits dispensing without prescription.

Keep out of reach of children.

Store at Controlled Room Temperature, 20 to 25°C (68 to 77°F) [see USP].

Manufactured by Rhône-Poulenc Rorer Puerto Rico Inc.
Aventis Pharmaceuticals Products Inc.
Parsippany, NJ 07054 ©1997

Adverse Events	Patients treated with 220 mcg triamcinolone acetonide (n=857) %	Vehicle Placebo (n=962) %
Pharyngitis	5.1	3.6
Epistaxis	2.7	0.8
Increase in cough	2.1	1.5

Patent Pending Rev. 10/97
IN-6361B!

Shown in Product Identification Guide, page 307

NILANDRON™ ℞
(nilutamide)
Tablets

Prescribing Information as of September 1996

DESCRIPTION

NILANDRON™ tablets contain nilutamide, a nonsteroidal, orally active antiandrogen having the chemical name 5,5-dimethyl 3-[4-nitro 3-(trifluoromethyl) phenyl] 2,4-imidazolidinedione with the following structural formula:

Nilutamide is a microcrystalline, white to practically white powder with a molecular weight of 317.25.

It is freely soluble in ethyl acetate, acetone, chloroform, ethyl alcohol, dichloromethane, and methanol. It is slightly soluble in water [< 0.1% W/V at 25°C (77°F)]. It melts between 153°C and 156°C (307.4°F and 312.8°F).

Each NILANDRON tablet contains 50 mg nilutamide. Other ingredients in NILANDRON tablets are corn starch, lactose, providone, docusate sodium, magnesium stearate, and talc.

CLINICAL PHARMACOLOGY

Mechanism of Action

Prostate cancer is known to be androgen sensitive and responds to androgen ablation. In animal studies, nilutamide has demonstrated antiandrogenic activity without other hormonal (estrogen, progesterone, mineralocorticoid, and glucocorticoid) effects. In vitro, nilutamide blocks the effects of testosterone at the androgen receptor level. In vivo, nilutamide interacts with the androgen receptor and prevents the normal androgenic response.

Pharmacokinetics

Absorption: Analysis of blood, urine, and feces samples following a single oral 150-mg dose of [^{14}C]-nilutamide in patients with metastatic prostate cancer showed that the drug is rapidly and completely absorbed and that it yields high and persistent plasma concentrations.

Distribution: After absorption of the drug, there is a detectable distribution phase. There is moderate binding of the drug to plasma proteins and low binding to erythrocytes. The binding is nonsaturable except in the case of alpha-1-glycoprotein, which makes a minor contribution to the total concentration of proteins in the plasma. The results of binding studies do not indicate any effects that would cause nonlinear pharmacokinetics.

Metabolism: The results of a human metabolism study using ^{14}C-radiolabelled tablets show that nilutamide is extensively metabolized and less than 2% of the drug is excreted unchanged in urine after 5 days. Five metabolites have been isolated from human urine. Two metabolites display an asymmetric center, due to oxidation of a methyl group, resulting in the formation of D- and L-isomers. One of the metabolites was shown, in vitro, to possess 25 to 50% of the pharmacological activity of the parent drug, and the D-isomer of the active metabolite showed equal or greater potency compared to the L-isomer. However, the pharmacokinetics and the pharmacodynamics of the metabolites have not been fully investigated.

Elimination: The majority (62%) of orally administered [^{14}C]-nilutamide is eliminated in the urine during the first 120 hours after a single 150-mg dose. Fecal elimination is negligible, ranging from 1.4% to 7% of the dose after 4 to 5 days. Excretion of radioactivity in urine likely continues beyond 5 days. The mean elimination half-life of nilutamide determined in studies in which subjects received a single dose of 100–300 mg ranged from 38.0 to 59.1 hours with most values between 41 and 49 hours. The elimination of at least one metabolite is generally longer than that of unchanged nilutamide (59–126 hours). During multiple dosing of 3 × 50 mg twice a day, steady state was reached within 2 to 4 weeks for most patients, and mean steady state AUC_{0-12} was 110% higher than the $AUC_{0-\infty}$ obtained from the first dose of 3 × 50 mg. These data and in vitro metabolism data suggest that, upon multiple dosing, metabolic enzyme inhibition may occur for this drug.

Clinical Studies

Nilutamide through its antiandrogenic activity can complement surgical castration, which suppresses only testicular androgens. The effects of the combined therapy were studied in patients with previously untreated metastatic prostate cancer.

In a double-blind, randomized, multicenter study that enrolled 457 patients (225 treated with orchiectomy and NILANDRON, 232 treated with orchiectomy and placebo), the NILANDRON group showed a statistically significant benefit in time to progression and time to death. The results are summarized below.

[See first table at right]

INDICATIONS AND USAGE

Metastatic Prostate Cancer

NILANDRON tablets are indicated for use in combination with surgical castration for the treatment of metastatic prostate cancer (Stage D_2).

For maximum benefit, NILANDRON treatment must begin on the same day as or on the day after surgical castration.

CONTRAINDICATIONS

NILANDRON tablets are contraindicated in patients:

- with severe hepatic impairment (baseline hepatic enzymes should be evaluated prior to treatment)
- with severe respiratory insufficiency
- with hypersensitivity to nilutamide or any component of this preparation.

WARNINGS

Interstitial pneumonitis

Interstitial pneumonitis has been reported in 2% of patients in controlled clinical trials in patients exposed to nilutamide. Patients typically presented with progressive exertional dyspnea, and possibly with cough, chest pain, and fever. X-rays showed interstitial or alveolo-interstitial changes. The suggestive signs of pneumonitis most often occurred within the first three months of NILANDRON treatment.

A routine chest X-ray should be performed before treatment, and patients should be told to report immediately any dyspnea or aggravation of pre-existing dyspnea.

At the onset of dyspnea or worsening of pre-existing dyspnea at any time during treatment, NILANDRON should be interrupted until it can be determined if respiratory symptoms are drug related. A chest X-ray should be obtained, and if there are findings suggestive of interstitial pneumonitis, treatment with NILANDRON should be discontinued. The pneumonitis is almost always reversible when treatment is discontinued.

If the chest X-ray appears normal, pulmonary function tests including DL_{CO} (diffusing capacity of the lung for carbon monoxide) should be performed. If a significant decrease of DL_{CO} and/or a restrictive pattern is observed on pulmonary function testing, NILANDRON treatment should be terminated. In the absence of chest X-ray and pulmonary function test findings consistent with interstitial pneumonitis, treatment with NILANDRON can be restarted under close monitoring of pulmonary symptoms.

Because interstitial pneumonitis was reported in 8 of 47 patients (17%) in a small study performed in Japan, specific caution should be observed in the treatment of Asian patients.

Hepatitis

Hepatitis or marked increases in liver enzymes leading to drug discontinuation occurred in 1% of NILANDRON patients in controlled clinical trials:

Serum hepatic enzyme levels should be measured at baseline and at regular intervals (3 months); if transaminases increase over 2–3 times the upper limit of normal, treatment should be discontinued.

Appropriate laboratory testing should be done at the first symptom/sign of liver injury (e.g., jaundice, dark urine, fatigue, abdominal pain, or unexplained gastrointestinal symptoms) and NILANDRON treatment must be discontinued immediately if transaminases exceed 3 times the upper limit of normal.

There has been a report of elevated hepatic enzymes followed by death in a 65-year-old patient being treated with nilutamide.

Other

Foreign postmarketing surveillance has revealed isolated cases of aplastic anemia in which a causal relationship with NILANDRON could not be ascertained.

PRECAUTIONS

Information for Patients

Patients should be informed that NILANDRON tablets should be started on the day of, or on the day after, surgical castration. They should also be informed that they should not interrupt their dosing of NILANDRON or stop taking this medication without consulting their physician.

Because of the possibility of interstitial pneumonitis, patients should also be told to report immediately any dyspnea or aggravation of pre-existing dyspnea.

Because of the possibility of hepatitis, patients should be told to consult with their physician should nausea, vomiting, abdominal pain, or jaundice occur.

Because of the possibility of an intolerance to alcohol (facial flushes, malaise, hypotension) following ingestion of NILANDRON, it is recommended that intake of alcoholic beverages be avoided by patients who experience this reaction. This effect has been reported in about 5% of patients treated with NILANDRON.

In clinical trials, 13% to 57% of patients receiving NILANDRON reported a delay in adaptation to dark, ranging from seconds to a few minutes, when passing from a lighted area to a dark area. This effect sometimes does not abate as drug treatment is continued. Patients who experience this effect should be cautioned about driving at night or through tunnels. This effect can be alleviated by the wearing of tinted glasses.

Drug Interactions

In vitro, nilutamide has been shown to inhibit the activity of liver cytochrome P-450 isoenzymes and, therefore, may reduce the metabolism of compounds requiring these systems.

	NILANDRON	PLACEBO
Median Survival (months)	27.3	23.6
Progression-Free Survival (months)	21.1	14.9
Complete or Partial Regression	41%	24%
Improvement in Bone Pain	54%	37%

Adverse Experience	NILANDRON + surgical castration (N=225) % All	Placebo + surgical castration (N=232) % All
Cardiovascular System		
Hypertension	5.3	2.6
Digestive System		
Nausea	9.8	6.0
Constipation	7.1	3.9
Endocrine System		
Hot flushes	28.4	22.4
Metabolic and Nutritional System		
Increased AST	8.0	3.9
Increased ALT	7.6	4.3
Nervous System		
Dizziness	7.1	3.4
Respiratory System		
Dyspnea	6.2	7.3
Special Senses		
Impaired adaptation to dark	12.9	1.3
Abnormal vision	6.7	1.7
Urogenital System		
Urinary tract infection	8.0	9.1

Adverse Experience	NILANDRON + leuprolide (N=209) % All	Placebo + leuprolide (N=202) % All
Body as a Whole		
Pain	26.8	27.7
Headache	13.9	10.4
Asthenia	19.1	20.8
Back pain	11.5	16.8
Abdominal pain	10.0	5.4
Chest pain	7.2	4.5
Flu syndrome	7.2	3.0
Fever	5.3	6.4
Cardiovascular System		
Hypertension	9.1	9.9
Digestive System		
Nausea	23.9	8.4
Constipation	19.6	16.8
Anorexia	11.0	6.4
Dyspepsia	6.7	4.5
Vomiting	5.7	4.0
Endocrine System		
Hot flushes	66.5	59.4
Impotence	11.0	12.9
Libido decreased	11.0	4.5
Hemic and Lymphatic System		
Anemia	7.2	6.4
Metabolic and Nutritional System		
Increased AST	12.9	13.9
Peripheral edema	12.4	17.3
Increased ALT	9.1	8.9
Musculo Skeletal System		
Bone Pain	6.2	5.0
Nervous System		
Insomnia	16.3	15.8
Dizziness	10.0	11.4
Depression	8.6	7.4
Hypesthesia	5.3	2.0
Respiratory System		
Dyspnea	10.5	7.4
Upper respiratory infection	8.1	10.9
Pneumonia	5.3	3.5
Skin and Appendages		
Sweating	6.2	3.0
Body hair loss	5.7	0.5
Dry skin	5.3	2.5
Rash	5.3	4.0
Special Senses		
Impaired adaptation to dark	56.9	5.4
Chromatopsia	8.6	0.0
Impaired adaptation to light	7.7	1.0
Abnormal vision	6.2	4.5
Urogenital System		
Testicular atrophy	16.3	12.4
Gynecomastia	10.5	11.9
Urinary tract infection	8.6	21.3
Hematuria	8.1	7.9
Urinary tract disorder	7.2	10.4
Nocturia	6.7	6.4

Consequently, drugs with a low therapeutic margin, such as vitamin K antagonists, phenytoin, and theophylline, could have a delayed elimination and increases in their serum half-life leading to a toxic level. The dosage of these drugs or others with a similar metabolism may need to be modified if they are administered concomitantly with nilutamide. For

Continued on next page

Nilandron—Cont.

example, when vitamin K antagonists are administered concomitantly with nilutamide, prothrombin time should be carefully monitored and, if necessary, the dosage of vitamin K antagonists should be reduced.

Carcinogenesis, Mutagenesis, Impairment of Fertility

Administration of nilutamide to rats for 18 months at doses of 0, 5, 15, or 45 mg/kg/day produced benign Leydig cell tumors in 35% of the high-dose male rats (AUC exposures in high-dose rats were approximately 1–2 times human AUC exposures with therapeutic doses). The increased incidence of Leydig cell tumors is secondary to elevated luteinizing hormone (LH) concentrations resulting from loss of feedback inhibition at the pituitary. Elevated LH and testosterone concentrations are not observed in castrated men receiving NILANDRON. Nilutamide had no effect on the incidence, size, or time of onset of any spontaneous tumor in rats.

Nilutamide displayed no mutagenic effects in a variety of in vitro and in vivo tests (Ames test, mouse micronucleus test, and two chromosomal aberration tests).

In reproduction studies in rats, nilutamide had no effect on the reproductive function of males and females, and no lethal, teratogenic, or growth-suppressive effects on fetuses were found. The maximal dose at which nilutamide did not affect reproductive function in either sex or have an effect on fetuses was estimated to be 45 mg/kg orally (AUC exposures in rats approximately 1–2 times human therapeutic AUC exposures).

Pregnancy

Pregnancy Category C; Animal reproduction studies have not been conducted with nilutamide. It is also not known whether nilutamide can cause fetal harm when administered to a pregnant woman or can affect reproductive capacity. Nilutamide should be given to a pregnant woman only if clearly needed.

Pediatric Use

Safety and effectiveness in pediatric patients have not been determined.

Animal Pharmacology and Toxicology

Administration of NILANDRON to beagle dogs resulted in drug-related deaths at dose levels that produce AUC exposures in dogs much lower than the AUC exposures of men receiving the therapeutic doses of 150 and 300 mg/day. Nilutamide-induced toxicity in dogs was cumulative with progressively lower doses producing death when given for longer durations. Nilutamide given to dogs at 60 mg/kg/day (1–2 times human AUC exposure) for 1 month produced 100% mortality. Administration of 20 and 30 mg/kg/day nilutamide ($^1/_2$–1 times human AUC exposure) for 6 months resulted in 20% and 70% mortality in treated dogs. Administration to dogs of 3, 6, and 12 mg/kg/day nilutamide ($^1/_{10}$–$^1/_2$ human AUC exposure) for 1 year resulted in 8%, 33%, and 50% mortality, respectively. **A "no-effect level" for nilutamide-induced mortality in dogs was not identified.** Pathology data from the one-year oral toxicity study suggest that the deaths in dogs were secondary to liver toxicity. Marked-to-massive hepatocellular swelling and vacuolization were observed in affected dogs. Liver toxicity in dogs was not consistently associated with elevations of liver enzymes.

Administration of nilutamide to rats at a dose level of 45 mg/kg/day (AUC exposure in rats 1–2 times human therapeutic AUC exposures) for 18 months increased the incidence of lung pathology (granulomatous inflammation and chronic alveolitis).

The hepatic and pulmonary adverse effects observed in nilutamide-treated animals and men are similar to effects observed with another nitroaromatic compound, nitrofurantoin. Nilutamide and nitrofurantoin are both metabolized in vitro to nitroanion free-radicals by microsomal NADPH-cytochrome P450 reductase in the lungs and liver of rats and humans.

ADVERSE REACTIONS

The following adverse experiences were reported during a multicenter clinical trial comparing NILANDRON + surgical castration versus placebo + surgical castration. The most frequently reported (greater than 5%) adverse experiences during treatment with NILANDRON tablets in combination with surgical castration are listed below. For comparison, adverse experiences seen with surgical castration and placebo are also listed.

[See second table on previous page]

The overall incidence of adverse experiences was 86% (194/225) for the NILANDRON group and 81% (188/232) for the placebo group.

The following adverse experiences were reported during a multicenter clinical trial comparing NILANDRON + leuprolide versus placebo + leuprolide. The most frequently reported (greater than 5%) adverse experiences during treatment with NILANDRON tablets in combination with leuprolide are listed below. For comparison, adverse experiences seen with leuprolide and placebo are also listed.

[See third table on previous page]

The overall incidence of adverse experiences is 99.5% (208/209) for the NILANDRON group and 98.5% (199/202) for the placebo group.

Some frequently occurring adverse experiences, for example hot flushes, impotence, and decreased libido, are known to be associated with low serum androgen levels and known to occur with medical or surgical castration alone. Notable was the higher incidence of visual disturbances (variously described as impaired adaptation to darkness, abnormal vision, and colored vision), which led to treatment discontinuation in 1% to 2% of patients.

Interstitial pneumonitis occurred in one (<1%) patient receiving NILANDRON in combination with surgical castration and in seven patients (3%) receiving NILANDRON in combination with leuprolide and one patient receiving placebo in combination with leuprolide. Overall, it has been reported in 2% of patients receiving NILANDRON. This included a report of interstitial pneumonitis in 8 of 47 patients (17%) in a small study performed in Japan.

In addition, the following adverse experiences were reported in 2 to 5% of patients treated with NILANDRON in combination with leuprolide or orchiectomy.

Body as a Whole: Malaise (2%).

Cardiovascular System: Angina (2%), heart failure (3%), syncope (2%).

Digestive System: Diarrhea (2%), gastrointestinal disorder (2%), gastrointestinal hemorrhage (2%), melena (2%).

Metabolic and Nutritional System: Alcohol intolerance (5%), edema (2%), weight loss (2%).

Musculoskeletal System: Arthritis (2%).

Nervous System: Dry mouth (2%), nervousness (2%), paresthesia (3%).

Respiratory System: Cough increased (2%), interstitial lung disease (2%), lung disorder (4%), rhinitis (2%).

Skin and Appendages: Pruritus (2%).

Special Senses: Cataract (2%), photophobia (2%).

Laboratory Values: Haptoglobin increased (2%), leukopenia (3%), alkaline phosphatase increased (3%), BUN increased (2%), creatinine increased (2%), hyperglycemia (4%).

OVERDOSAGE

One case of massive overdosage has been published. A 79-year-old man attempted suicide by ingesting 13 g of nilutamide (i.e., 43 times the maximum recommended dose). Despite immediate gastric lavage and oral administration of activated charcoal, plasma nilutamide levels peaked at 6 times the normal range 2 hours after ingestion. There were no clinical signs or symptoms or changes in parameters such as transaminases or chest X-ray. Maintenance treatment (150 mg/day) was resumed 30 days later.

In repeated-dose tolerance studies, doses of 600 mg/day and 900 mg/day were administered to 9 and 4 patients, respectively. The ingestion of these doses was associated with gastrointestinal disorders, including nausea and vomiting, malaise, headache, and dizziness. In addition, a transient elevation in hepatic enzyme levels was noted in one patient. Since nilutamide is protein bound, dialysis may not be useful as treatment for overdose. As in the management of overdosage with any drug, it should be borne in mind that multiple agents may have been taken. If vomiting does not occur spontaneously, it should be induced if the patient is alert. General supportive care, including frequent monitoring of the vital signs and close observation of the patient, is indicated.

DOSAGE AND ADMINISTRATION

The recommended dosage is six tablets (50 mg each) once a day for a total daily dose of 300 mg for 30 days followed thereafter by three tablets (50 mg each) once a day for a total daily dosage of 150 mg. NILANDRON tablets can be taken with or without food.

HOW SUPPLIED

White, biconvex (with a triangular logo on one face and an internal reference number [168] on the other), cylindrical (about 7 mm in diameter) NILANDRON tablets containing 50 mg of nilutamide are available in "child-resistant" PVC blister pack with an aluminum foil backing in

Boxes of 90 tablets (6 blisters of 15 tablets each) NDC 0088-1110-35

Store at room temperature between 15°C and 30°C (59° and 86°F). Protect from light.

Prescribing Information as of September 1996

Manufactured by Usiphar, 60200 Compiegne, France for:
Hoechst Marion Roussel, Inc.
Kansas City, MO 64137 USA

Shown in Product Identification Guide, page 307

NORPRAMIN® ℞

[nor·pram' in]

(desipramine hydrochloride tablets USP)

Prescribing Information as of November 1997

DESCRIPTION

NORPRAMIN® (desipramine hydrochloride USP) is an antidepressant drug of the tricyclic type, and is chemically:

$$\cdot HCl \quad N\text{—}CH_2CH_2CH_2NHCH_3$$

5*H*-Dibenz[*bf*]azepine-5-propanamine, 10,11-dihydro-*N*-methyl-, monohydrochloride.

Inactive Ingredients

The following inactive ingredients are contained in all dosage strengths: acacia, calcium carbonate, corn starch, D&C Red No. 30 and D&C Yellow No. 10 (except 10 mg and 150 mg), FD&C Blue No. 1 (except 50 mg, 75 mg, and 100 mg), hydrogenated soy oil, iron oxide, light mineral oil, magnesium stearate, mannitol, polyethylene glycol 8000, pregelatinized corn starch, sodium benzoate (except 150 mg), sucrose, talc, titanium dioxide, and other ingredients.

CLINICAL PHARMACOLOGY

Mechanism of Action

Available evidence suggests that many depressions have a biochemical basis in the form of a relative deficiency of neurotransmitters such as norepinephrine and serotonin. Norepinephrine deficiency may be associated with relatively low urinary 3-methoxy-4-hydroxyphenyl glycol (MHPG) levels, while serotonin deficiencies may be associated with low spinal fluid levels of 5-hydroxyindoleacetic acid.

While the precise mechanism of action of the tricyclic antidepressants is unknown, a leading theory suggests that they restore normal levels of neurotransmitters by blocking the re-uptake of these substances from the synapse in the central nervous system. Evidence indicates that the secondary amine tricyclic antidepressants, including NORPRAMIN, may have greater activity in blocking the re-uptake of norepinephrine. Tertiary amine tricyclic antidepressants, such as amitriptyline, may have greater effect on serotonin re-uptake.

NORPRAMIN (desipramine hydrochloride) is not a monoamine oxidase (MAO) inhibitor and does not act primarily as a central nervous system stimulant. It has been found in some studies to have a more rapid onset of action than imipramine. Earliest therapeutic effects may occasionally be seen in 2 to 5 days, but full treatment benefit usually requires 2 to 3 weeks to obtain.

Metabolism

Tricyclic antidepressants, such as desipramine hydrochloride, are rapidly absorbed from the gastrointestinal tract. Tricyclic antidepressants or their metabolites are to some extent excreted through the gastric mucosa and reabsorbed from the gastrointestinal tract. Desipramine is metabolized in the liver, and approximately 70% is excreted in the urine. The rate of metabolism of tricyclic antidepressants varies widely from individual to individual, chiefly on a genetically determined basis. Up to a 36-fold difference in plasma level may be noted among individuals taking the same oral dose of desipramine. In general, the elderly metabolize tricyclic antidepressants more slowly than do younger adults.

Certain drugs, particularly the psychostimulants and the phenothiazines, increase plasma levels of concomitantly administered tricyclic antidepressants through competition for the same metabolic enzyme systems. Concurrent administration of cimetidine and tricyclic antidepressants can produce clinically significant increases in the plasma concentrations of the tricyclic antidepressants. Conversely, decreases in plasma levels of the tricyclic antidepressants have been reported upon discontinuation of cimetidine, which may result in the loss of the therapeutic efficacy of the tricyclic antidepressant. Other substances, particularly barbiturates and alcohol, induce liver enzyme activity and thereby reduce tricyclic antidepressant plasma levels. Similar effects have been reported with tobacco smoke.

Research on the relationship of plasma level to therapeutic response with the tricyclic antidepressants has produced conflicting results. While some studies report no correlation, many studies cite therapeutic levels for most tricyclics in the range of 50 to 300 nanograms per milliliter. The therapeutic range is different for each tricyclic antidepressant. For desipramine, an optimal range of therapeutic plasma levels has not been established.

INDICATIONS AND USAGE

NORPRAMIN (desipramine hydrochloride) is indicated for the treatment of depression.

CONTRAINDICATIONS

Desipramine hydrochloride should not be given in conjunction with, or within 2 weeks of, treatment with an MAO inhibitor drug; hyperpyretic crises, severe convulsions, and death have occurred in patients taking MAO inhibitors and tricyclic antidepressants. When NORPRAMIN (desipramie hydrochloride) is substituted for an MAO inhibitor, at least 2 weeks should elapse between treatments. NORPRAMIN should then be started cautiously and should be increased gradually.

The drug is contraindicated in the acute recovery period following myocardial infarction. It should not be used in those who have shown prior hypersensitivity to the drug. Cross-sensitivity between this and other dibenzazepines is a possibility.

WARNINGS

Extreme caution should be used when this drug is given in the following situations:

a. In patients with cardiovascular disease, because of the possibility of conduction defects, arrhythmias, tachycardias, strokes, and acute myocardial infarction.
b. In patients with a history of urinary retention or glaucoma, because of the anticholinergic properties of the drug.
c. In patients with thyroid disease or those taking thyroid medication, because of the possibility of cardiovascular toxicity, including arrhythmias.
d. In patients with a history of seizure disorder, because this drug has been shown to lower the seizure threshold.

This drug is capable of blocking the antihypertensive effect of guanethidine and similarly acting compounds.

The patient should be cautioned that this drug may impair the mental and/or physical abilities required for the performance of potentially hazardous tasks such as driving a car or operating machinery.

In patients who may use alcohol excessively, it should be borne in mind that the potentiation may increase the danger inherent in any suicide attempt or overdosage.

Use in Pregnancy

Safe use of desipramine hydrochloride during pregnancy and lactation has not been established; therefore, if it is to be given to pregnant patients, nursing mothers, or women of childbearing potential, the possible benefits must be weighed against the possible hazards to mother and child. Animal reproductive studies have been inconclusive.

Use in Children

NORPRAMIN (desipramine hydrochloride) is not recommended for use in children since safety and effectiveness in the pediatric age group have not been established. (See ADVERSE REACTIONS, Cardiovascular.)

PRECAUTIONS

General

It is important that this drug be dispensed in the least possible quantities to depressed outpatients, since suicide has been accomplished with this class of drug. Ordinary prudence requires that children not have access to this drug or to potent drugs of any kind; if possible, this drug should be dispensed in containers with child-resistant safety closures. Storage of this drug in the home must be supervised responsibly.

If serious adverse effects occur, dosage should be reduced or treatment should be altered.

NORPRAMIN (desipramine hydrochloride) therapy in patients with manic-depressive illness may induce a hypomanic state after the depressive phase terminates.

The drug may cause exacerbation of psychosis in schizophrenic patients.

Both elevation and lowering of blood sugar levels have been reported.

Leukocyte and differential counts should be performed in any patient who develops fever and sore throat during therapy; the drug should be discontinued if there is evidence of pathologic neutrophil depression.

Clinical experience in the concurrent administration of ECT and antidepressant drugs is limited. Thus, if such treatment is essential, the possibility of increased risk relative to benefits should be considered.

This drug should be discontinued as soon as possible prior to elective surgery because of possible cardiovascular effects. Hypertensive episodes have been observed during surgery in patients taking desipramine hydrochloride.

Drug Interactions

Drugs Metabolized by P450 2D6. The biochemical activity of the drug metabolizing isozyme cytochrome P450 2D6 (debrisoquin hydroxylase) is reduced in a subset of the Caucasian population (about 7% to 10% of Caucasians are so called "poor metabolizers"); reliable estimates of the prevalence of reduced P450 2D6 isozyme activity among Asian, African and other populations are not yet available. Poor metabolizers have higher than expected plasma concentrations of tricyclic antidepressants (TCAs) when given usual doses. Depending on the fraction of drug metabolized by P450 2D6, the increase in plasma concentration may be small, or quite large (8 fold increase in plasma AUC of the TCA).

In addition, certain drugs inhibit the activity of this isozyme and make normal metabolizers resemble poor metabolizers. An individual who is stable on a given dose of TCA may become abruptly toxic when given one of these inhibiting drugs as concomitant therapy. The drugs that inhibit cytochrome P450 2D6 include some that are not metabolized by the enzyme (quinidine; cimetidine) and many that are substrates for P450 2D6 (many other antidepressants, phenothiazines, and the Type IC antiarrhythmics propafenone and flecainide). While all the selective serotonin reuptake inhibitors (SSRIs), e.g., fluoxetine, sertraline, paroxetine, inhibit P450 2D6, they may vary in the extent of inhibition. The extent to which SSRI TCA interactions may pose clinical problems will depend on the degree of inhibition and the pharmacokinetics of the SSRI involved. Nevertheless, caution is indicated in the co-administration of TCAs with any of the SSRIs and also in switching from one class to the other. Of particular importance, sufficient time must elapse before initiating TCA treatment in a patient being withdrawn from fluoxetine, given the long half-life of the parent and active metabolite (at least 5 weeks may be necessary).

Concomitant use of tricyclic antidepressants with drugs that can inhibit cytochrome P450 2D6 may require lower doses than usually prescribed for either the tricyclic antidepressant or the other drug. Furthermore, whenever one of these other drugs is withdrawn from co-therapy, an increased dose of tricyclic antidepressant may be required. It is desirable to monitor TCA plasma levels whenever a TCA is going to be co-administered with another drug known to be an inhibitor of P450 2D6.

Close supervision and careful adjustment of dosage are required when this drug is given concomitantly with anticholinergic or sympathomimetic drugs.

Patients should be warned that while taking this drug their response to alcoholic beverages may be exaggerated.

If NORPRAMIN (desipramine hydrochloride) is to be combined with other psychotropic agents such as tranquilizers or sedative/hypnotics, careful consideration should be given to the pharmacology of the agents employed since the sedative effects of NORPRAMIN and benzodiazepines (e.g., chlordiazepoxide or diazepam) are additive. Both the sedative and anticholinergic effects of the major tranquilizers are also additive to those of NORPRAMIN.

ADVERSE REACTIONS

Included in the following listing are a few adverse reactions that have not been reported with this specific drug. However, the pharmacologic similarities among the tricyclic antidepressant drugs require that each of the reactions be considered when NORPRAMIN (desipramine hydrochloride) is given.

Cardiovascular: hypotension, hypertension, palpitations, heart block, myocardial infarction, stroke, arrhythmias, premature ventricular contractions, tachycardia, ventricular tachycardia, ventricular fibrillation, sudden death

There has been a report of an "acute collapse" and "sudden death" in an 8-year-old (18 kg) male, treated for 2 years for hyperactivity.

There have been additional reports of sudden death in children. (See WARNINGS, Use in Children.)

Psychiatric: confusional states (especially in the elderly) with hallucinations, disorientation, delusions; anxiety, restlessness, agitation; insomnia and nightmares; hypomania; exacerbation of psychosis

Neurologic: numbness, tingling, paresthesias of extremities; incoordination, ataxia, tremors; peripheral neuropathy; extrapyramidal symptoms; seizures; alterations in EEG patterns; tinnitus

Symptoms attributed to Neuroleptic Malignant Syndrome have been reported during desipramine use with and without concomitant neuroleptic therapy.

Anticholinergic: dry mouth, and rarely associated sublingual adenitis; blurred vision, disturbance of accommodation, mydriasis, increased intraocular pressure; constipation, paralytic ileus; urinary retention, delayed micturition, dilation of urinary tract

Allergic: skin rash, petechiae, urticaria, itching, photosensitization (avoid excessive exposure to sunlight), edema (of face and tongue or general), drug fever, cross-sensitivity with other tricyclic drugs

Hematologic: bone marrow depressions including agranulocytosis, eosinophilia, purpura, thrombocytopenia

Gastrointestinal: anorexia, nausea and vomiting, epigastric distress, peculiar taste, abdominal cramps, diarrhea, stomatitis, black tongue, hepatitis, jaundice (simulating obstructive), altered liver function, elevated liver function tests, increased pancreatic enzymes

Endocrine: gynecomastia in the male, breast enlargement and galactorrhea in the female; increased or decreased libido, impotence, painful ejaculation, testicular swelling; elevation or depression of blood sugar levels; syndrome of inappropriate antidiuretic hormone secretion (SIADH)

Other: weight gain or loss; perspiration, flushing; urinary frequency, nocturia; parotid swelling; drowsiness, dizziness, weakness and fatigue, headache; fever; alopecia; elevated alkaline phosphatase

Withdrawal Symptoms: Though not indicative of addiction, abrupt cessation of treatment after prolonged therapy may produce nausea, headache, and malaise.

OVERDOSAGE*

Deaths may occur from overdosage with this class of drugs. Multiple drug ingestion (including alcohol) is common in deliberate tricyclic antidepressant overdose. As the management is complex and changing, it is recommended that the physician contact a poison control center for current information on treatment. Signs and symptoms of toxicity develop rapidly after tricyclic antidepressant overdose; therefore, hospital monitoring is required as soon as possible. There is no specific antidote for desipramine overdosage.

Oral LD_{50}

The oral LD_{50} of desipramine is 290 mg/kg in male mice and 320 mg/kg in female rats.

Manifestations of Overdosage

Critical manifestations of overdose include: cardiac dysrhythmias, severe hypotension, convulsions, and CNS depression, including coma. Changes in the electrocardiogram, particularly in QRS axis or width, are clinically significant indicators or tricyclic antidepressant toxicity.

Other signs of overdose may include: confusion, disturbed concentration, transient visual hallucinations, dilated pupils, agitation, hyperactive reflexes, stupor, drowsiness, muscle rigidity, vomiting, hypothermia, hyperpyrexia, or any of the symptoms listed under ADVERSE REACTIONS.

Management

Aggressive supportive care and serum alkalinization are the mainstays of therapy.

General. Obtain an ECG and immediately initiate cardiac monitoring. Protect the patient's airway, establish an intravenous line, and initiate gastric decontamination. A minimum of 6 hours of observation with cardiac monitoring and observation for signs of CNS or respiratory depression, hypotension, cardiac dysrhythmias and/or conduction blocks, and seizures is necessary. If signs of toxicity occur at any time during this period, extended monitoring is required. Follow ECG, renal function, CPK, and arterial blood gasses as clinically indicated. There are case reports of patients succumbing to fatal dysrhythmias late after overdose; these patients had clinical evidence of significant poisoning prior to death, and most received inadequate gastrointestinal decontamination. Monitoring of plasma drug levels should not guide management of the patient.

Gastrointestinal Decontamination. All patients suspected of tricyclic antidepressant overdose should receive gastrointestinal decontamination. This should include large volume gastric lavage followed by activated charcoal. If consciousness is impaired, the airway should be secured prior to lavage. Emesis is contraindicated.

Cardiovascular. A maximal limb-lead QRS duration of ≥0.10 seconds may be the best indication of the severity of the overdose. Serum alkalinization, to a pH of 7.45 to 7.55, using intravenous sodium bicarbonate and hyperventilation (as needed) should be instituted for patients with dysrhythmias and/or QRS widening. A pH >7.60 or a pCO_2 <20mm Hg is undesirable. Dysrhythmias unresponsive to sodium bicarbonate therapy/hyperventilation may respond to lidocaine, bretylium or phenytoin. Type IA and IC antiarrhythmics are generally contraindicated (eg, quinidine, disopyramide, and procainamide).

In rare instances, hemoperfusion may be beneficial in acute refractory cardiovascular instability in patients with acute toxicity. However, hemodialysis, peritoneal dialysis, exchange transfusions, and forced diuresis generally have been reported as ineffective in tricyclic antidepressant poisoning.

CNS. In patients with CNS depression, early intubation is advised because of the potential for abrupt deterioration. Seizures should be controlled with benzodiazepines. If these are ineffective or seizures recur, other anticonvulsants (eg, phenobarbital, phenytoin) may be used. Physostigmine is not recommended except to treat life-threatening symptoms that have been unresponsive to other therapies, and then only in consultation with a poison control center.

Psychiatric Follow-up. Since overdosage is often deliberate, patients may attempt suicide by other means during the recovery phase. Psychiatric referral may be appropriate.

Pediatric Management. The principles of management of child and adult overdosages are similar. It is strongly recommended that the physician contact the local poison control center for specific pediatric treatment.

* Poisindex®: Toxicologic Management
Topic: Antidepressants, Tricyclic
Micromedex Inc. Vol. 85

DOSAGE AND ADMINISTRATION

Not recommended for use in children (see WARNINGS).

Lower dosages are recommended for elderly patients and adolescents. Lower dosages are also recommended for outpatients compared to hospitalized patients, who are closely supervised. Dosage should be initiated at a low level and increased according to clinical response and any evidence of intolerance. Following remission, maintenance medication may be required for a period of time and should be at the lowest dose that will maintain remission.

Usual Adult Dose

The usual adult dose is 100 to 200 mg per day. In more severely ill patients, dosage may be further increased gradually to 300 mg/day if necessary. Dosages above 300 mg/day are not recommended.

Dosage should be initiated at a lower level and increased according to tolerance and clinical response.

Treatment of patients requiring as much as 300 mg should generally be initiated in hospitals, where regular visits by the physician, skilled nursing care, and frequent electrocardiograms (ECGs) are available.

The best available evidence of impending toxicity from very high doses of NORPRAMIN is prolongation of the QRS or QT intervals on the ECG. Prolongation of the PR interval is also significant, but less closely correlated with plasma levels. Clinical symptoms of intolerance, especially drowsiness, dizziness, and postural hypotension, should also alert the physician to the need for reduction in dosage. Plasma desipramine measurement would constitute the optimal guide to dosage monitoring.

Initial therapy may be administered in divided doses or a single daily dose.

Maintenance therapy may be given on a once-daily schedule for patient convenience and compliance.

Adolescent and Geriatric Dose

The usual adolescent and geriatric dose is 25 to 100 mg daily.

Dosage should be initiated at a lower level and increased according to tolerance and clinical response to a usual maximum of 100 mg daily. In more severely ill patients, dosage may be further increased to 150 mg/day. Doses above 150 mg/day are not recommended in these age groups.

Initial therapy may be administered in divided doses or a single daily dose.

Maintenance therapy may be given on a once-daily schedule for patient convenience and compliance.

HOW SUPPLIED

10 mg blue coated tablets imprinted 68-7
NDC 0068-0007-01: bottles of 100

25 mg yellow coated tablets imprinted NORPRAMIN 25
NDC 0068-0011-01: bottles of 100

50 mg green coated tablets imprinted NORPRAMIN 50
NDC 0068-0015-01: bottles of 100

75 mg orange coated tablets imprinted NORPRAMIN 75
NDC 0068-0019-01: bottles of 100

100 mg peach coated tablets imprinted NORPRAMIN 100
NDC 0068-0020-01: bottles of 100

150 mg white coated tablets imprinted NORPRAMIN 150
NDC 0068-0021-50: bottles of 50

Continued on next page

Norpramin—Cont.

NORPRAMIN tablets should be stored at room temperature, preferably below 86°F (30°C). Protect from excessive heat.

Prescribing Information as of November 1997

Merrell Pharmaceuticals Inc.
Subsidiary of Hoechst Marion Roussel, Inc.
Kansas City, MO 64137 USA

Shown in Product Identification Guide, page 307

ONCASPAR® ℞

[ən ′-cə-spər]

(pegaspargase)

DESCRIPTION

ONCASPAR®, the ENZON trademark for pegaspargase, is a modified version of the enzyme L-asparaginase. It is an oncolytic agent used in combination chemotherapy for the treatment of patients with acute lymphoblastic leukemia who are hypersensitive to native forms of L-asparaginase (as described in **CLINICAL PHARMACOLOGY**).

The generic name for **ONCASPAR®** is **pegaspargase.** The chemical name is monomethoxypolyethylene glycol succinimidyl L-asparaginase. L-asparaginase is modified by covalently conjugating units of monomethoxypolyethylene glycol (PEG), molecular weight of 5,000, to the enzyme, forming the active ingredient PEG-L-asparaginase. The L-asparaginase (L-asparagine amidohydrolase, type EC-2, EC 3.5.1.1) used in the manufacture of **ONCASPAR®** is derived from *Escherichia coli.* ENZON purchases the enzyme L-asparaginase in bulk from Merck, Sharp and Dohme, Division of Merck & Co., Inc., West Point, PA 19486, U.S. License Number 2. Merck & Co., Inc. supplies bulk L-asparaginase as a licensed intermediate for further manufacture by ENZON into PEG-L-asparaginase. Merck & Co., Inc. can only assume responsibility for the bulk intermediate supplied to ENZON.

ONCASPAR® is supplied as an isotonic sterile solution in phosphate buffered saline, pH 7.3, for intramuscular or intravenous administration only. The solution is clear, colorless and contains no preservatives. It is supplied in 5 mL single-dose vials.

ONCASPAR® activity is expressed in International Units (IU) according to the recommendation of the International Union of Biochemistry. One IU of L-asparaginase is defined as that amount of enzyme required to generate 1 μmol of ammonia per minute at pH 7.3 and 37°C.

Each milliliter of **ONCASPAR®** contains:

PEG-L-asparaginase	750 IU ± 20%
Monobasic sodium phosphate, USP	1.20 mg ± 5%
Dibasic sodium phosphate, USP	5.58 mg ± 5%
Sodium chloride, USP	8.50 mg ± 5%
Water for injection, USP	qs to 1.0 mL

The specific activity of **ONCASPAR®** is at least 85 IU per milligram protein.

CLINICAL PHARMACOLOGY

Leukemic cells are unable to synthesize asparagine due to a lack of asparagine synthetase and are dependent on an exogenous source of asparagine for survival. Rapid depletion of asparagine which results from treatment with the enzyme L-asparaginase, kills the leukemic cells. Normal cells, however, are less affected by the rapid depletion due to their ability to synthesize asparagine. This is an approach to therapy based on a specific metabolic defect in some leukemic cells which do not produce asparagine synthetase.[1]

In a study in predominately L-asparaginase naive adult patients with leukemia and lymphoma, initial plasma levels of L-asparaginase following intravenous administration were determined. Plasma half-life did not appear to be influenced by dose levels, and it could not be correlated with age, sex, surface area, renal or hepatic function, diagnosis or extent of disease. Apparent volume of distribution was equal to estimated plasma volume. L-asparaginase was measurable for at least 15 days following the initial treatment with **ONCASPAR®**. The enzyme could not be detected in the urine.[2]

In a study of newly diagnosed pediatric patients with acute lymphoblastic leukemia (ALL) who received either a single intramuscular injection of **ONCASPAR®** (2,500 IU/m^2), *E. coli* L-asparaginase (25,000 IU/m^2), or *Erwinia* L-asparaginase (25,000 IU/m^2), the plasma half-lives for the three forms of L-asparaginase were:[3]

PLASMA HALF-LIVES OF THREE FORMS OF L-ASPARAGINASE

TREATMENT GROUP	NO. OF PATIENTS	MEAN (DAYS)	STANDARD DEVIATION
ONCASPAR®	10	5.73	3.24
E. coli L-asparaginase	17	1.24	0.17
Erwinia L-asparaginase	10	0.65	0.13

In this same study of newly diagnosed pediatric ALL patients, the *in vivo* early leukemic cell kill after a single intramuscular injection of native *E. coli* L-asparaginase (25,000 IU/m^2), *Erwinia* L-asparaginase (25,000 IU/m^2), and **ONCASPAR®** (2,500 IU/m^2) during a five day "investigational window" was studied.[4] Bone marrow aspirates were taken before and five days after a single dose of one of the three different forms of L-asparaginase. Rhodamine-123 (RH-123), a selectively incorporated fluorescent mitochondrial dye, was used in an *in vitro* assay on the bone marrow aspirates to ascertain cell viability. The percent reduction of viable lymphoblasts at day five for each group is presented in the following table:[4]

RHODAMINE-123 (*IN VIVO* CELL KILL)

TREATMENT GROUP	NO. OF PATIENTS	PERCENT REDUCTION OF VIABLE LYMPHOBLASTS AT DAY 5 MEAN ± S.D.
ONCASPAR®	21	55.7 ± 10.2
E. coli L-asparaginase	28	57.8 ± 10.1
Erwinia L-asparaginase	19	57.9 ± 13.8

In three pharmacokinetic studies, 37 relapsed ALL patients received **ONCASPAR®** at 2,500 IU/m^2 every two weeks. The plasma half-life of **ONCASPAR®** was 3.24 ± 1.83 days in nine patients who were previously hypersensitive to native L-asparaginase and 5.69 ± 3.25 days in 28 non-hypersensitive patients. The area under the curve was 9.50 ± 3.95 IU/mL/day in the previously hypersensitive patients, and 9.83 ± 5.94 IU/mL/day in the non-hypersensitive patients.

Hypersensitivity Reactions

Hypersensitivity reactions to *E. coli* L-asparaginase have been reported in the literature in 3% to 73% of patients.[1] Patients in **ONCASPAR®** clinical studies were considered to be previously hypersensitive if they experienced a systemic rash, urticaria, bronchospasm, laryngeal edema, or hypotension following administration of any form of native L-asparaginase. Patients were also considered to be previously hypersensitive if they experienced local erythema, urticaria, or swelling, greater than two centimeters, for at least ten minutes following administration of any form of native L-asparaginase. The National Cancer Institute Common Toxicity Criteria (CTC) were used to classify the severity of the hypersensitivity reactions. These are: grade 1 — transient rash (mild); grade 2 — mild bronchospasm (moderate); grade 3 — moderate bronchospasm and/or serum sickness (severe); grade 4 — hypotension and/or anaphylaxis (life-threatening). Additionally, most transient local urticaria were considered grade 2 hypersensitivity reactions, while most sustained urticaria distant from the injection site were considered grade 3 hypersensitivity reactions. In general, the moderate to life-threatening hypersensitivity reactions were considered dose-limiting; that is, they required L-asparaginase treatment to be discontinued.

In separate studies, **ONCASPAR®** was administered intravenously to 48 patients and intramuscularly to 126 patients. The incidence of hypersensitivity reactions when **ONCASPAR®** was administered intramuscularly was 30% in patients who were previously hypersensitive to native L-asparaginase and 11% in non-hypersensitive patients (p-value of 0.007). The incidence of hypersensitivity reactions when **ONCASPAR®** was administered intravenously was 60% in patients who were previously hypersensitive to native L-asparaginase and 12% in non-hypersensitive patients. Since only five previously hypersensitive patients received **ONCASPAR®** intravenously, no meaningful analysis of the incidence of hypersensitivity reactions was possible between either the previously hypersensitive and non-hypersensitive patients, or between the intravenous and intramuscular routes of administration.

The overall incidence of hypersensitivity reactions in 174 patients who received **ONCASPAR®** in five clinical studies is shown in the table below:

INCIDENCE OF ONCASPAR® HYPERSENSITIVITY REACTIONS

PATIENT STATUS	N	CTC GRADE OF HYPERSENSITIVITY REACTION 1	2	3	4	TOTAL
Previously Hypersensitive Patients	62	7	8	4	1	20 (32%)
Non-Hypersensitive Patients	112	5	4	1	1	11 (10%)
Total Patients	174	12	12	5	2	31 (18%)

The probability of a previously hypersensitive or non-hypersensitive patient completing 8 doses of **ONCASPAR®** therapy without developing a dose-limiting hypersensitivity reaction was 77% and 95%, respectively.

All of the 62 hypersensitive patients treated with **ONCASPAR®** in five clinical studies had previous hypersensitivity reactions to one or more of the native forms of L-asparaginase. Of the 35 patients who had previous hypersensitivity reactions to *E. coli* L-asparaginase only, 5 (14%) had **ONCASPAR®** dose-limiting hypersensitivity reactions. Of the 27 patients who had hypersensitivity reactions to both *E. coli* and *Erwinia* L-asparaginase, 7 (26%) had **ONCASPAR®** dose-limiting hypersensitivity reactions. The overall incidence of dose-limiting hypersensitivity reactions in 174 patients treated with **ONCASPAR®** was 9% (19% in 62 hypersensitive and 3% in 112 non-hypersensitive patients). Of the total of 9% dose-limiting hypersensitivity reactions, 1% were anaphylactic (CTC grade 4) and the other 8% were ≤ CTC grade 3.

Clinical Activity

ONCASPAR® was evaluated as part of combination therapy in four open label studies comprising 42 multiply-relapsed, previously hypersensitive acute leukemia patients [39 (93%) with ALL] at a dose of 2,000 or 2,500 IU/m^2 administered intramuscularly or intravenously every 14 days during induction combination chemotherapy. The reinduction response rate was 50% (36% complete remissions and 14% partial remissions), with a 95% confidence interval of 35% to 65%. This response rate is comparable to that reported in the literature for relapsed patients treated with native L-asparaginase as part of combination chemotherapy.[1]

ONCASPAR® was also shown to have some activity as a single agent in multiply-relapsed hypersensitive ALL patients, the majority of whom were pediatric. Treatment with **ONCASPAR®** resulted in three responses (one complete remission and two partial remissions) in nine previously hypersensitive patients who would not have been able to receive any further L-asparaginase treatment.

ONCASPAR® was also studied in non-hypersensitive, relapsed ALL patients who were randomized to receive two doses of **ONCASPAR®** at 2,500 IU/m^2 every 14 days or twelve doses of *E. coli* L-asparaginase at 10,000 IU/m^2 three times a week during a 28 day induction combination chemotherapy regimen (which included vincristine and prednisone). Although the enrollment in this study was too small to be conclusive, the data showed that for 20 patients there was no significant difference between the overall response rates of 60% and 50%, respectively, or the complete remission rates of 50% and 50%, respectively.

ONCASPAR® was administered during maintenance therapy regimens to 33 previously hypersensitive patients. The average number of doses received during maintenance therapy was 5.8 (range of 1 to 24) and the average duration of maintenance therapy was 126 (range of 1 to 513) days for this patient population.

INDICATIONS AND USAGE

ONCASPAR® is indicated for patients with acute lymphoblastic leukemia who require L-asparaginase in their treatment regimen, but have developed hypersensitivity to the native forms of L-asparaginase **(SEE CLINICAL PHARMACOLOGY). ONCASPAR®,** like native L-asparaginase, is generally used in combination with other chemotherapeutic agents, such as vincristine, methotrexate, cytarabine, daunorubicin, and doxorubicin.[1,5] Use of **ONCASPAR®** as a single agent should only be undertaken when multi-agent chemotherapy is judged to be inappropriate for the patient.

CONTRAINDICATIONS

ONCASPAR® is contraindicated in patients with pancreatitis or a history of pancreatitis. **ONCASPAR®** is contraindicated in patients who have had significant hemorrhagic events associated with prior L-asparaginase therapy. **ONCASPAR®** is also contraindicated in patients who have had previous serious allergic reactions, such as generalized urticaria, bronchospasm, laryngeal edema, hypotension, or other unacceptable adverse reactions to **ONCASPAR®**.

WARNINGS

It is recommended that **ONCASPAR®** be given under the supervision of an individual who is qualified by training and experience to administer cancer chemotherapeutic agents. Especially in patients with known hypersensitivity to the other forms of L-asparaginase, hypersensitivity reactions to **ONCASPAR®,** including life-threatening anaphylaxis, may occur during therapy. As a routine precaution, patients should be kept under observation for one hour with resuscitation equipment and other agents necessary to treat anaphylaxis (epinephrine, oxygen, intravenous steroids, etc.) available.

PRECAUTIONS

General

This drug may be a contact irritant, and the solution must be handled and administered with care. Gloves are recommended. Inhalation of vapors and contact with skin or mucous membranes, especially those of the eyes, must be avoided. In case of contact, wash with copious amounts of water for at least 15 minutes. Anaphylactic reactions require the immediate use of epinephrine, oxygen, intravenous steroids, and antihistamines. Patients taking **ONCASPAR®** are at higher than usual risk for bleeding problems, especially with simultaneous use of other drugs that have anticoagulant properties, such as aspirin, and non-steroidal anti-inflammatories **(SEE DRUG INTERACTIONS). ONCASPAR®** may have immunosuppressive activity. Therefore, it is possible that use of the drug in patients may predispose the patient to infection. Severe hepatic and central nervous system toxicity following multi-agent chemotherapy that includes **ONCASPAR®** may occur. Caution appears warranted when treating patients with **ONCASPAR®** given in combination with hepatotoxic agents, particularly when liver dysfunction is present.

Patients undergoing **ONCASPAR®** therapy must be carefully monitored and the therapeutic regimen adjusted according to response and toxicity. Physicians using a given treatment regimen incorporating **ONCASPAR®** should be thoroughly familiar with its benefits and risks.

Information For Patients

Patients should be informed of the possibility of hypersensitivity reactions, including immediate anaphylaxis, to **ONCASPAR®**. Patients taking **ONCASPAR®** are at higher than usual risk for bleeding problems. Patients should be instructed that the simultaneous use of **ONCASPAR®** with other drugs that may increase the risk of bleeding should be avoided **(SEE DRUG INTERACTIONS). ONCASPAR®** may affect the ability of the liver to function normally in some patients. Therapy with **ONCASPAR®** may increase the toxicity of other medications **(SEE DRUG INTERACTIONS). ONCASPAR®** may have immunosuppressive activity. Therefore, it is possible that use of the drug in patients may predispose the patient to infection. Patients should notify their physicians of any adverse reactions that occur.

Laboratory Tests

A fall in circulating lymphoblasts is often noted after initiating therapy. This may be accompanied by a marked rise in serum uric acid. As a guide to the effects of therapy, the patient's peripheral blood count and bone marrow should be monitored.

Frequent serum amylase determinations should be obtained to detect early evidence of pancreatitis **(SEE CONTRAINDICATIONS).** Blood sugar should be monitored during therapy with **ONCASPAR®** because hyperglycemia may occur. When using **ONCASPAR®** in conjunction with hepatotoxic chemotherapy, patients should be monitored for liver dysfunction.

ONCASPAR® may affect a number of plasma proteins; therefore, monitoring of fibrinogen, PT, and PTT may be indicated.

Drug Interactions

Unfavorable interactions of L-asparaginase with some antitumor agents have been demonstrated.[1] It is recommended, therefore, that **ONCASPAR®** be used in combination regimens only by physicians familiar with the benefits and risks of a given regimen. Depletion of serum proteins by **ONCASPAR®** may increase the toxicity of other drugs which are protein bound. Additionally, during the period of its inhibition of protein synthesis and cell replication, **ONCASPAR®** may interfere with the action of drugs such as methotrexate, which require cell replication for their lethal effects. **ONCASPAR®** may interfere with the enzymatic detoxification of other drugs, particularly in the liver. Physicians using a given treatment regimen should be thoroughly familiar with its benefits and risks.

Imbalances in coagulation factors have been noted with the use of **ONCASPAR®** predisposing to bleeding and/or thrombosis. Caution should be used when administering any concurrent anticoagulant therapy, such as coumadin, heparin, dipyridamole, aspirin, or non-steroidal anti-inflammatories.

Carcinogenesis, Mutagenesis, Impairment of Fertility

Long-term carcinogenic studies in animals have not been performed with **ONCASPAR®** nor have studies been performed on impairment of fertility. **ONCASPAR®** did not exhibit a mutagenic effect when tested against *Salmonella typhimurium* strains in the Ames assay.

Pregnancy

Pregnancy Category C. Animal reproduction studies have not been conducted with **ONCASPAR®**. It is also not known whether **ONCASPAR®** can cause fetal harm when administered to a pregnant woman or can affect reproduction capacity. **ONCASPAR®** should be given to a pregnant woman only if clearly needed.

Nursing Mothers

It is not known whether **ONCASPAR®** is excreted in human milk. Because many drugs are excreted in human milk and because of the potential for serious adverse reactions due to **ONCASPAR®** in nursing infants, a decision should be made to discontinue nursing or discontinue the drug, taking into account the importance of the drug to the mother.

ONCASPAR® ADVERSE REACTIONS

Adverse reactions have been reported in adults and pediatric patients. Overall, the adult patients treated with **ONCASPAR®** had a somewhat higher incidence of known L-asparaginase toxicities, except for hypersensitivity reactions, than the pediatric patients treated with **ONCASPAR®**.

Excluding hypersensitivity reactions, the most frequently occurring known L-asparaginase related toxicities and adverse experiences reported for the 174 patients in clinical studies were chemical hepatotoxicities and coagulopathies, the majority of which did not result in any significant clinical events. The incidence of significant clinical events included clinical pancreatitis (1%), hyperglycemia requiring insulin therapy (3%), and thrombosis (4%).

The following adverse reactions related to **ONCASPAR®** were reported for 174 patients in five clinical studies.

The adverse reactions reported most frequently (greater than 5%) were allergic reactions (which may have included rash, erythema, edema, pain, fever, chills, urticaria, dyspnea, or bronchospasm), SGPT increase, nausea and/or vomiting, fever, and malaise.

The adverse reactions reported occasionally (greater than 1% but less than 5%) were anaphylactic reactions, dyspnea, injection site hypersensitivity, lip edema, rash, urticaria, abdominal pain, chills, pain in the extremities, hypotension, tachycardia, thrombosis, anorexia, diarrhea, jaundice, abnormal liver function test, decreased anticoagulant effect, disseminated intravascular coagulation, decreased fibrinogen, hemolytic anemia, leukopenia, pancytopenia, thrombocytopenia, increased thromboplastin, injection site pain, injection site reaction, bilirubinemia, hyperglycemia, hyperuricemia, hypoglycemia, hypoproteinemia, peripheral edema, increased SGOT, arthralgia, myalgia, convulsion, headache, night sweats, and paresthesia.

The adverse reactions reported rarely (less than 1%) were bronchospasm, petechial rash, face edema, lesional edema, sepsis, septic shock, chest pain, endocarditis, hypertension, constipation, flatulence, gastrointestinal pain, hepatomegaly, increased appetite, liver fatty deposits, coagulation disorder, increased coagulation time, decreased platelet count, purpura, increased amylase, edema, excessive thirst, hyperammonemia, hyponatremia, weight loss, bone pain, joint disorder, confusion, dizziness, emotional lability, somnolence, increased cough, epistaxis, upper respiratory infection, erythema simplex, pruritus, hematuria, increased urinary frequency, and abnormal kidney function.

The following **ONCASPAR®** related adverse reactions have been observed in patients with hematologic malignancies, primarily acute lymphoblastic leukemia (approximately 75%), non-Hodgkins lymphoma (approximately 13%), acute myelogenous leukemia (approximately 3%), and a variety of solid tumors (approximately 9%):

HYPERSENSITIVITY REACTIONS: a variety of hypersensitivity reactions have occurred. These reactions may be acute or delayed, and include acute anaphylaxis, bronchospasm, dyspnea, urticaria, arthralgia, erythema, induration, edema, pain, tenderness, hives, swelling, lip edema, chills, fever, and skin rashes **(SEE WARNINGS AND CONTRAINDICATIONS).**

PANCREATIC FUNCTION: pancreatitis, sometimes fulminant and fatal, has occurred. Increased serum amylase and lipase have also occurred.

LIVER FUNCTION: a variety of liver function abnormalities have been observed, including elevations of SGOT, SGPT, and bilirubin (direct and indirect). Jaundice, ascites, and hypoalbuminemia, which may be associated with peripheral edema, have been observed. These abnormalities usually are reversible on discontinuance of therapy, and some reversal may occur during the course of therapy. Fatty changes in the liver and liver failure have occurred.

HEMATOLOGIC: hypofibrinogenemia, prolonged prothrombin times, prolonged partial thromboplastin times, and decreased antithrombin III have been observed. Superficial and deep venous thrombosis, sagittal sinus thrombosis, venous catheter thrombosis, and atrial thrombosis have occurred. Leukopenia, agranulocytosis, pancytopenia, thrombocytopenia, disseminated intravascular coagulation, severe hemolytic anemia, and anemia have been observed. Clinical hemorrhage, which may be fatal; easy bruisability, and ecchymosis have also been observed.

METABOLIC: mild to severe hyperglycemia has been observed in low incidence, and usually responds to discontinuation of **ONCASPAR®** and the judicious use of intravenous fluid and insulin. Hypoglycemia, increased thirst and hyponatremia, uric acid nephropathy, hyperuricemia, hypoproteinemia, and peripheral edema have also been observed. Hypoalbuminemia, proteinuria, weight loss, and metabolic acidosis have occurred. Therapy with **ONCASPAR®** is associated with an increase in blood ammonia during the conversion of L-asparagine to aspartic acid by the enzyme.

NEUROLOGIC: status epilepticus and temporal lobe seizures, somnolence, coma, malaise, mental status changes, dizziness, emotional lability, headache, lip numbness, finger paresthesia, mood changes, night sweats, and a Parkinson-like syndrome have occurred. Mild to severe confusion, disorientation, and paresthesia have also occurred. These side effects usually have reversed spontaneously after treatment was stopped.

RENAL: increased BUN, increased creatinine, increased urinary frequency, hematuria due to thrombopenia, severe hemorrhagic cystitis, renal dysfunction, and renal failure have been observed.

CARDIOVASCULAR: chest pain, subacute bacterial endocarditis, hypertension, severe hypotension, and tachycardia have occurred.

DIGESTIVE: anorexia, constipation, decreased appetite, diarrhea, indigestion, flatulence, gas, gastrointestinal pain, mucositis, hepatomegaly, elevated gamma-glutamyltranspeptidase, increased appetite, mouth tenderness, severe colitis, and nausea and/or vomiting have been observed.

MUSCULOSKELETAL: diffuse and local musculoskeletal pain, arthralgia, joint stiffness, and cramps have occurred.

RESPIRATORY: cough, epistaxis, severe bronchospasm, and upper respiratory infection have been observed.

SKIN/APPENDAGES: itching, alopecia, fever blister, purpura, hand whiteness and fungal changes, nail whiteness and ridging, erythema simplex, jaundice, and petechial rash have occurred.

GENERAL: localized edema, injection site reactions (including pain, swelling, or redness), malaise, infection, sepsis, fatigue, and septic shock may occur.

OVERDOSAGE

Three patients received 10,000 IU/m^2 of **ONCASPAR®** as an intravenous infusion. One patient experienced a slight increase in liver enzymes. A second patient developed a rash ten minutes after the start of the infusion, which was controlled with the administration of an antihistamine and by slowing down the infusion rate. A third patient did not experience any adverse reactions.

DOSAGE AND ADMINISTRATION

As a component of selected multiple agent regimens, the recommended dose of **ONCASPAR®** is 2,500 IU/m^2 every 14 days by either the intramuscular or intravenous route of administration.

The preferred route of administration, however, is the intramuscular route because of the lower incidence of hepatotoxicity, coagulopathy, and gastrointestinal and renal disorders compared to the intravenous route of administration.

The safety and effectiveness of **ONCASPAR®** have been established in patients with known previous hypersensitivity to L-asparaginase whose ages ranged from 1 to 21 years old. The recommended dose of **ONCASPAR®** for children with a body surface area ≥0.6 m^2 is 2,500 IU/m^2 administered every 14 days. The recommended dose of **ONCASPAR®** for children with a body surface area <0.6 m^2 is 82.5 IU/kg administered every 14 days.

Do not administer ONCASPAR® if there is any indication that the drug has been frozen. Although there may not be an apparent change in the appearance of the drug, ONCASPAR®'s activity is destroyed after freezing.

When administering **ONCASPAR®** intramuscularly, the volume at a single injection site should be limited to 2 mL. If the volume to be administered is greater than 2 mL, multiple injection sites should be used.

When administered intravenously, **ONCASPAR®** should be given over a period of 1 to 2 hours in 100 mL of sodium chloride or dextrose injection 5%, through an infusion that is already running.

Anaphylactic reactions require the immediate use of antihistamines, epinephrine, oxygen, and intravenous steroids.

Use of **ONCASPAR®** as the sole induction agent should be undertaken only in an unusual situation when a combined regimen, which uses other chemotherapeutic agents such as vincristine, methotrexate, cytarabine, daunorubicin, or doxorubicin, is inappropriate because of toxicity or other specific patient-related factors, or in patients refractory to other therapy. When **ONCASPAR®** is to be used as the sole induction agent, the recommended dosage regimen is also 2,500 IU/m^2 every 14 days.

When a remission is obtained, appropriate maintenance therapy may be instituted. **ONCASPAR®** may be used as part of a maintenance regimen.

Parenteral drug products should be inspected visually for particulate matter, cloudiness or discoloration prior to administration, whenever solution and container permit.

HOW SUPPLIED

Dosage Form

ONCASPAR®: Use only one dose per vial; do not re-enter the vial. Discard unused portions. Do not save unused drug for later administration.

Sterile solution for injection in ready to use single-use vials. Preservative free.

Quantity per Individual Container

5 mL per vial containing 750 IU/mL **ONCASPAR®** in a clear, colorless, phosphate buffered saline solution, pH 7.3. Each vial contains 3,750 IU of **ONCASPAR®**.

Handling and Storage

Avoid excessive agitation. DO NOT SHAKE.

Keep refrigerated at +2°C to +8°C (36°F to 46°F).

Do not use if cloudy or if precipitate is present.

Do not use if stored at room temperature for more than 48 hours.

DO NOT FREEZE. Do not use product if it is known to have been frozen. Freezing destroys activity, which cannot be detected visually.

NDC 0075-0640-05

U.S. Patent 4,179,337 and pat. pending

40 Kingsbridge Road

Piscataway, NJ 08854-3998 USA

01/21/94

License No. 1171

REFERENCES

1. Capizzi, RL and Holcenberg, JS. Asparaginase. In: Holland and Frei (eds). *Cancer Med* third edition, Lea and Febiger, Phila. PA, 1993.
2. Ho, DH, et al. Clinical pharmacology of polyethylene glycol-L-asparaginase. *Drug Metab Dispos* 14 (3): 349–352, 1986.
3. Asselin, BL, et al. Comparative Pharmacokinetic Studies of Three L-asparaginase Preparations. *J Clin Oncology* (11): 1780–1786, 1993.
4. Data on File at ENZON.
5. Clavell, LA, et al. Four-agent induction and intensive asparaginase therapy for treatment of childhood acute lymphoblastic leukemia. *N Engl J Med* 315 (11): 657–663, 1986.

IN-1724! Rev. 2/94

Manufactured by:

Enzon, Inc.

40 Kingsbridge Road

Piscataway, NJ 08854 USA

Distributed by: Aventis Pharmaceuticals Products Inc.

Parsippany, NJ 07054

PENETREX® ℞

(enoxacin) Tablets

DESCRIPTION

Penetrex® (enoxacin) is a broad-spectrum azafluoroquinolone antibacterial agent for oral administration. Enoxacin is 1-ethyl-6-fluoro-1,4-dihydro-4-oxo-7-(1-piperazinyl)-1,8-naphthyridine-3-carboxylic acid sesquihydrate. The chemical structure of enoxacin is:

[See chemical structure at top of next column]

Its empirical formula is $C_{15}H_{17}N_4O_3F \cdot 1^1/_2\ H_2O$, and its molecular weight is 320.32 (anhydrous). Enoxacin is an ivory-to-slightly yellow powder. In dilute aqueous solution, it is unstable in strong sunlight.

Penetrex is available in 200 mg and 400 mg film-coated tablets. Each "200" and "400" Penetrex tablet contains enoxa-

Continued on next page

Penetrex—Cont.

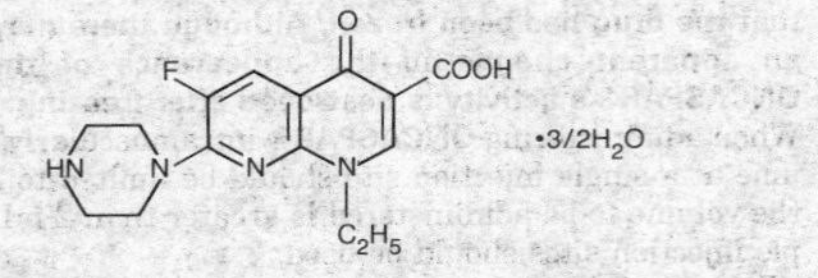

cin sesquihydrate equivalent to 200 mg and 400 mg of anhydrous enoxacin, respectively. Each Penetrex 200 mg and 400 mg tablet contains the following inactive ingredients: cellulose microcrystalline NF, colloidal silicon dioxide NF, croscarmellose sodium NF, FD&C Blue No. 2 aluminum lake, hydroxypropyl cellulose NF, hydroxypropyl methylcellulose, magnesium stearate USP, polyethylene glycol, simethicone, sorbic acid, stearate emulsifiers, and titanium dioxide.

CLINICAL PHARMACOLOGY

Following oral administration to healthy subjects, peak plasma enoxacin concentrations were achieved within 1 to 3 hours. Absolute oral bioavailability of enoxacin is approximately 90%. Maximum plasma concentrations of enoxacin average 0.93 μg/mL and 2.0 μg/mL after single 200 mg and 400 mg doses, respectively. Enoxacin plasma half-life is 3 to 6 hours. Enoxacin is excreted primarily via the kidney. After a single dose, greater than 40% was recovered in urine by 48 hours as unchanged drug. In elderly patients, the mean peak enoxacin plasma concentration was 50% higher than that in young adult volunteers receiving comparable single doses of enoxacin. This appears to correspond to age-associated reduction of renal function in the elderly population. Five metabolites of enoxacin have been identified in human urine and account for 15% to 20% of the administered dose.
Enoxacin diffuses into cervix, fallopian tube, and myometrium at levels approximately 1–2 times those achieved in plasma, and into kidney and prostate at levels approximately 2–4 times those achieved in plasma. Studies have not been conducted to assess the penetration of enoxacin into human cerebrospinal fluid.
Enoxacin is approximately 40% bound to plasma proteins in healthy subjects and is approximately 14% bound to plasma proteins in patients with impaired renal function.
The effect of food on the absorption of enoxacin from the tablet formulation has not been studied.
Some isozymes of the cytochrome P-450 hepatic microsomal enzyme system are inhibited by enoxacin. This inhibition results in significant drug/drug interactions with theophylline and caffeine. Enoxacin interferes with the metabolism of theophylline, resulting in a dose-related decrease in theophylline clearance. Elevated serum theophylline concentrations may increase the risk of theophylline-related adverse reactions. (See **PRECAUTIONS: Drug Interactions.**)
Clearance of enoxacin is reduced in patients with impaired renal function (creatinine clearance ≤30 mL/min/1.73 m^2), and dosage adjustment is necessary. (See **DOSAGE AND ADMINISTRATION.**)

MICROBIOLOGY

Enoxacin is an inhibitor of the bacterial enzyme DNA gyrase and is a bactericidal agent. Enoxacin may be active against pathogens resistant to drugs that act by different mechanisms.
Enoxacin has been shown to be active against most strains of the following organisms both *in vitro* and in clinical infections: (See **INDICATIONS AND USAGE.**)
Gram-positive aerobes: *Staphylococcus epidermidis, Staphylococcus saprophyticus.*
Gram-negative aerobes: *Enterobacter cloacae, Escherichia coli, Klebsiella pneumoniae, Neisseria gonorrhoeae, Proteus mirabilis, Pseudomonas aeruginosa.*
The following *in vitro* data are available but their clinical significance is unknown.
In addition, enoxacin exhibits *in vitro* minimum inhibitory concentrations (MICs) of 2.0 μg/mL or less against most strains of the following organisms; however, the safety and effectiveness of enoxacin in treating clinical infections due to these organisms have not been established in adequate and well-controlled trials.
Gram-negative aerobes: *Aeromonas hydrophila, Citrobacter diversus, Citrobacter freundii, Citrobacter koseri, Enterobacter aerogenes, Haemophilus ducreyi, Klebsiella oxytoca, Klebsiella ozaenae, Morganella morganii, Proteus vulgaris, Providencia stuartii, Providencia alcalifaciens, Serratia marcescens, Serratia proteomaculans* (formerly *S. liquefaciens*)
Many strains of *Streptococcus* species and anaerobes are usually resistant to enoxacin.
The activity of enoxacin against *Treponema pallidum* has not been evaluated; however, other quinolones are not active against *T. pallidum.* (See **WARNINGS.**)
Cross-resistance with other quinolones has been demonstrated.
The addition of human serum has no effect on the *in vitro* MIC values; however, enoxacin activity is decreased in acidic (pH 5.5) environments.

Susceptibility Testing

Diffusion Techniques: Quantitative methods that require measurement of zone diameters give the most precise estimate of susceptibility of bacteria to antimicrobial agents. One such standardized procedure[1] that has been recommended for use with disks to test susceptibility of organisms to enoxacin uses the 10-μg enoxacin disk.
Interpretation involves the correlation of the diameter obtained in the disk test with the minimum inhibitory concentration (MIC) for enoxacin.
Reports from the laboratory giving results of the standard single-disk susceptibility test with a 10-μg enoxacin disk should be interpreted according to the following criteria:

Zone Diameter (mm)	Interpretation
≥18	(S) Susceptible
15–17	(MS) Moderately susceptible
≤14	(R) Resistant

A report of "Susceptible" indicates that the pathogen is likely to be inhibited by generally achievable blood concentrations. A report of "Moderately susceptible" suggests that the organism would be susceptible if high dosage is used or if the infection is confined to tissues or fluids in which high antimicrobial levels are attained. A report of "Resistant" indicates that achievable drug concentrations are unlikely to be inhibitory, and other therapy should be selected.
Standardized susceptibility test procedures require the use of laboratory control organisms. The 10-μg enoxacin disk should give the following zone diameters:

Organism	Zone Diameter (mm)
Escherichia coli (ATCC 25922)	28–36
Neisseria gonorrhoeae (ATCC 49226)	43–51
Pseudomonas aeruginosa (ATCC 27853)	22–28
Staphylococcus aureus (ATCC 25923)	22–28

Other quinolone antibacterial disks should not be substituted when performing susceptibility tests for enoxacin because of spectrum differences. The 10-μg enoxacin disk should be used for all *in vitro* testing of isolates for enoxacin susceptibility using diffusion techniques.
Dilution Techniques: Use a standardized dilution method[2] (broth, agar, or microdilution) or equivalent with enoxacin powder. The MIC values obtained should be interpreted according to the following criteria:

MIC (μg/mL)	Interpretation
≤2	(S) Susceptible
4	(MS) Moderately susceptible
≥8	(R) Resistant

As with standard diffusion methods, dilution procedures require the use of laboratory control organisms. Standard enoxacin powder should give the following MIC values:

Organism	MIC (μg/mL)
Enterococcus faecalis (ATCC 29212)	2–16
Escherichia coli (ATCC 25922)	0.06–0.25
Neisseria gonorrhoeae (ATCC 49226)	0.015–0.06
Pseudomonas aeruginosa (ATCC 27853)	2–8
Staphylococcus aureus (ATCC 29213)	0.5–2

INDICATIONS AND USAGE

Penetrex® (enoxacin) is indicated for the treatment of adults (≥18 years of age) with the following infections caused by susceptible strains of the designated microorganisms:
Sexually Transmitted Diseases (See **WARNINGS.**)
Uncomplicated urethral or cervical gonorrhea due to *Neisseria gonorrhoeae.*
Urinary Tract
Uncomplicated urinary tract infections (cystitis) due to *Escherichia coli, Staphylococcus epidermidis**, or *Staphylococcus saprophyticus**.
Complicated urinary tract infections due to *Escherichia coli, Klebsiella pneumoniae, Proteus mirabilis, Pseudomonas aeruginosa, Staphylococcus epidermidis,* or *Enterobacter cloacae**.
*Efficacy for this organism in this organ system at the recommended dose was studied in fewer than ten infections. The dosage regimens for complicated and uncomplicated urinary tract infections are different. (See **DOSAGE AND ADMINISTRATION.**)
Penicillinase production should have no effect on enoxacin activity.
Appropriate culture and susceptibility tests should be performed before treatment in order to isolate and identify organisms causing the infection and to determine their susceptibility to enoxacin. Therapy with enoxacin may be initiated while awaiting the results of these studies; therapy should be adjusted if necessary once the results are known. Culture and susceptibility testing performed periodically during therapy will provide information not only on the therapeutic effect of the antimicrobial agent but also on the possible emergence of bacterial resistance.

CONTRAINDICATIONS

Penetrex is contraindicated in persons with a history of hypersensitivity, tendinitis, or tendon rupture associated with the use of enoxacin or any member of the quinolone group of antimicrobial agents.

WARNINGS

THE SAFETY AND EFFECTIVENESS OF ENOXACIN IN PEDIATRIC PATIENTS AND ADOLESCENTS (UNDER THE AGE OF 18 YEARS), PREGNANT WOMEN, AND LACTATING WOMEN HAVE NOT BEEN ESTABLISHED. (See **PRECAUTIONS: Pediatric Use, Pregnancy,** and **Nursing Mothers** subsections.) Enoxacin has been shown to cause arthropathy in immature rats and dogs when given in oral doses approximately 1.5 and 3.8 times, respectively, the highest human clinical dose based on a mg/m^2 basis after a four-week dosage regimen. Gross and histopathological examination of the weight-bearing joints of the dogs revealed lesions of the cartilage. Other quinolones also produce erosions of cartilage of weight-bearing joints and other signs of arthropathy in immature animals of various species. (See **ANIMAL PHARMACOLOGY.**)
Convulsions and abnormal electroencephalograms have been reported in some patients receiving enoxacin. Increased intracranial pressure, and toxic psychoses have been reported in patients receiving drugs in this class. Quinolones may also cause central nervous system stimulation which may lead to: tremors, restlessness/agitation, nervousness/anxiety, lightheadedness, confusion, hallucinations, paranoia, depression, nightmares, insomnia, and, rarely, suicidal thoughts or acts. These reactions may occur following the first dose. If these reactions occur in patients receiving enoxacin, the drug should be discontinued and appropriate measures instituted. As with all quinolones, enoxacin should be used with caution in patients with known or suspected CNS disorder that may predispose to seizures or lower the seizure threshold (*e.g.*, severe cerebral arteriosclerosis, epilepsy) or in the presence of other risk factors that may predispose to seizures or lower the seizure threshold (*e.g.*, certain drug therapy, renal dysfunction). (See **PRECAUTIONS: General, Information for Patients, Drug Interactions** and **ADVERSE REACTIONS.**)
Enoxacin is a potent inhibitor of the hepatic microsomal enzyme system, resulting in significant drug/drug interactions with theophylline and caffeine. (See **PRECAUTIONS: Drug Interactions.**)
Serious and occasionally fatal hypersensitivity (anaphylactoid or anaphylactic) reactions, some following the first dose, have been reported in patients receiving quinolone therapy. Some reactions were accompanied by cardiovascular collapse, loss of consciousness, tingling, pharyngeal or facial edema, dyspnea, urticaria, or itching. Only a few patients had a history of previous hypersensitivity reactions. Serious hypersensitivity reactions have also been reported following treatment with enoxacin. If an allergic reaction to enoxacin occurs, discontinue the drug. Serious acute hypersensitivity reactions may require immediate treatment with epinephrine. Oxygen, intravenous fluids, antihistamines, corticosteroids, pressor amines, and airway management, including intubation, should be administered as indicated.
Pseudomembranous colitis has been reported with nearly all antibacterial agents, including enoxacin, and may range in severity from mild to life-threatening. Therefore, it is important to consider this diagnosis in patients who present with diarrhea subsequent to the administration of antibacterial agents.
Treatment with broad-spectrum antibacterial agents alters the normal flora of the colon and may permit overgrowth of clostridia. Studies indicate that a toxin produced by *Clostridium difficile* is a primary cause of "antibiotic-associated colitis."
After the diagnosis of pseudomembranous colitis has been established, therapeutic measures should be initiated.
Mild cases of pseudomembranous colitis usually respond to discontinuation of the drug alone. In moderate to severe cases, consideration should be given to management with fluids and electrolytes, protein supplementation, and treatment with an antibacterial drug clinically effective against *C. difficile* colitis.
Ruptures of the shoulder, hand and Achilles tendons that required surgical repair or resulted in prolonged disability have been reported with fluoroquinolone antimicrobials. Enoxacin should be discontinued if the patient experiences pain, inflammation or rupture of a tendon. Patients should rest and refrain from exercise until the diagnosis of tendinitis or tendon rupture has been confidently excluded. Tendon rupture can occur at anytime during or after therapy with enoxacin.
Enoxacin has not been shown to be effective in the treatment of syphilis. Antimicrobial agents used in high doses for short periods of time to treat gonorrhea may mask or delay the symptoms of incubating syphilis. All patients with gonorrhea should have a serologic test for syphilis at the time of diagnosis. Patients treated with enoxacin should have a follow-up serologic test for syphilis after 3 months.

PRECAUTIONS

General: Alteration of the dosage regimen is necessary for patients with impaired renal function (creatinine clearance ≤30 mL/min/1.73 m^2). (See **DOSAGE AND ADMINISTRATION.**)
As with other quinolones, enoxacin should be used with caution in patients with a known or suspected CNS disorder that may predispose to seizures or lower the seizure thresh-

old (*e.g.*, severe cerebral arteriosclerosis, epilepsy) or in the presence of other risk factors that may predispose to seizures or lower the seizure threshold (*e.g.*, certain drug therapy, renal dysfunction). (See **WARNINGS** and **PRECAUTIONS: Drug Interactions.**)

Moderate-to-severe phototoxicity reactions have been observed in patients exposed to direct sunlight while receiving enoxacin or some other drugs in this class. Excessive sunlight should be avoided. Therapy should be discontinued if phototoxicity occurs.

Ophthalmologic abnormalities, including cataracts and multiple punctate lenticular opacities, have been noted in patients undergoing treatment with enoxacin, as well as with some other quinolones, but have also been observed in patients receiving placebo in comparative trials. In clinical trials using multiple-dose therapy, ophthalmic tissue levels of enoxacin and other quinolones were significantly higher than respective plasma concentrations. The causal relationship, if any, of quinolones to lenticular abnormalities has not been established.

Decreased spermatogenesis and subsequent decreased fertility were noted in rats and dogs treated with doses of enoxacin that produced plasma levels in the animals three times higher than those produced in humans at the recommended therapeutic dosage. The potential for enoxacin to affect spermatogenesis in male patients is unknown.

Information for Patients:

Patients should be advised:

- not to take magnesium-, aluminum-, or calcium-containing antacids, bismuth subsalicylate, products containing iron, or multivitamins containing zinc for 8 hours prior to enoxacin or for 2 hours after enoxacin administration (see **PRECAUTIONS: Drug Interactions**);
- to drink fluids liberally;
- to avoid consumption of caffeine-containing products (certain drugs, coffee, tea, chocolate, certain carbonated beverages) during enoxacin therapy (see **PRECAUTIONS: Drug Interactions**);
- that convulsions have been reported in patients taking quinolones, including enoxacin, and to notify their physicians before taking this drug if there is a history of this condition;
- to discontinue treatment and inform their physician if they experience pain, inflammation, or rupture of a tendon, and to rest and refrain from exercise until the diagnosis of tendinitis or tendon rupture has been confidently excluded;
- that enoxacin may cause dizziness and lightheadedness and, therefore, patients should know how they react to enoxacin before they operate an automobile or machinery or engage in activities requiring mental alertness and coordination;
- that enoxacin may be associated with hypersensitivity reaction, even following the first dose, and to discontinue the drug at the first sign of a skin rash or other allergic reaction;
- to avoid undue exposure to excessive sunlight while receiving enoxacin and to discontinue therapy if phototoxicity occurs.

Drug Interactions:

Bismuth: Bismuth subsalicylate, given concomitantly with enoxacin or 60 minutes following enoxacin administration, decreased enoxacin bioavailability by approximately 25%. Thus, concomitant administration of enoxacin and bismuth subsalicylate should be avoided.

Caffeine: Enoxacin is a potent inhibitor of the cytochrome P-450 isozymes responsible for the metabolism of methylxanthines. In a multiple-dose study, enoxacin caused a dose-related increase in the mean elimination half-life of caffeine, thereby decreasing the clearance of caffeine by up to 80% and leading to a five-fold increase in the AUC and the half-life of caffeine. Trough plasma enoxacin levels were also 20% higher when caffeine and enoxacin were administered concomitantly. Caffeine-related adverse effects have occurred in patients consuming caffeine while on therapy with enoxacin. (See **WARNINGS.**)

Cyclosporine: Elevated serum levels of cyclosporine have been reported with concomitant use of cyclosporine with other members of the quinolone class.

Digoxin: Enoxacin may raise serum digoxin levels in some individuals. If signs and symptoms suggestive of digoxin toxicity occur when enoxacin and digoxin are given concomitantly, physicians are advised to obtain serum digoxin levels and adjust digoxin doses appropriately.

Non-steroidal anti-inflammatory agents: Seizures have been reported in patients taking enoxacin concomitantly with the nonsteroidal anti-inflammatory drug fenbufen. Animal studies also suggest an increased potential for seizures when these two drugs are given concomitantly. Fenbufen is not approved in the United States at this time.

Sucralfate and antacids: Quinolones form chelates with metal cations. Therefore, administration of quinolones with antacids containing calcium, magnesium, or aluminum; with sucralfate; with divalent or trivalent cations such as iron; or with multivitamins containing zinc may substantially interfere with drug absorption and result in insufficient plasma and tissue quinolone concentrations. Antacids containing aluminum hydroxide and magnesium hydroxide reduce the oral absorption of enoxacin by 75%. The oral bioavailability of enoxacin is reduced by 60% with coadministration of ranitidine. These agents should not be taken for 8 hours before or for 2 hours after enoxacin administration.

Theophylline: Enoxacin is a potent inhibitor of the cytochrome P-450 isozymes responsible for the metabolism of methylxanthines. Enoxacin interferes with the metabolism of theophylline resulting in a 42% to 74% dose-related decrease in theophylline clearance and a subsequent 260% to 350% increase in serum theophylline levels. Theophylline-related adverse effects have occurred in patients when theophylline and enoxacin were coadministered. (See **WARNINGS.**)

Warfarin: Quinolones, including enoxacin, decrease the clearance of R-warfarin, the less active isomer of racemic warfarin. Enoxacin does not affect the clearance of the active S-isomer, and changes in clotting time have not been observed when enoxacin and warfarin were coadministered. Nevertheless, the prothrombin time or other suitable coagulation test should be monitored when warfarin or its derivatives and enoxacin are given concomitantly.

Carcinogenesis, Mutagenesis, Impairment of Fertility: Long-term studies in animals to determine the carcinogenic potential of enoxacin have not been conducted.

Genetic toxicology tests included *in vitro* mutagenicity and cytogenetic assays and *in vivo* cytogenetic and micronucleus tests. Enoxacin did not induce point mutations in bacterial cells or mitotic gene conversion in yeast cells, with or without metabolic activation. Enoxacin did not induce sister chromatid exchanges or structural chromosomal aberrations in mammalian cells *in vitro*, with or without metabolic activation. In addition, enoxacin did not induce chromosomal aberrations in mice.

There was a minimal, dose-related, statistically significant increase in micronuclei at high doses in mice. The significance of these findings, in the absence of effects in other test systems, is not established.

Enoxacin produced no consistent effects on fertility and reproductive parameters in female rats given oral doses of enoxacin at levels up to 1000 mg/kg. Decreased spermatogenesis and subsequent impaired fertility was noted in male rats given oral doses of 1000 mg/kg. This dose is approximately 13-fold greater than the highest human clinical daily oral dose of 16 mg/kg, assuming a 50 kg person and based on a mg/m^2 basis.

Pregnancy: *Teratogenic effects.* Pregnancy Category C. Studies with enoxacin given orally to mice and rats have shown no evidence of teratogenic potential. The intravenous infusion of enoxacin into pregnant rabbits at doses of 10 to 50 mg/kg caused dose-related maternal toxicity (venous irritation, body weight loss, and reduced food intake) and, at 50 mg/kg, fetal toxicity (increased post-implantation loss and stunted fetuses).

At 50 mg/kg, the incidence of fetal malformations was significantly increased in the presence of overt maternal and fetal toxicity. There are no adequate and well-controlled studies in pregnant women. Enoxacin should be used during pregnancy only if the potential benefit justifies the potential risk to the fetus. (See **WARNINGS.**)

Nursing Mothers: It is not known whether enoxacin is excreted in human milk. Enoxacin is excreted in the milk of lactating rats. Because drugs of this class are excreted in human milk and because of the potential for serious adverse reactions from enoxacin in nursing infants, a decision should be made whether to discontinue nursing or to discontinue the drug, taking into account the importance of the drug to the mother.

Pediatric Use: Safety and effectiveness in pediatric patients and adolescents below the age of 18 years have not been established. Enoxacin causes arthropathy in juvenile animals. (See **WARNINGS** and **ANIMAL PHARMACOLOGY.**)

Geriatric Use: In multiple-dose clinical trials of enoxacin, elderly patients (≥65 years of age) experienced significantly more overall adverse events than patients under 65 years of age. However, the incidence of drug-related adverse reactions was comparable between age groups.

ADVERSE REACTIONS

Single-Dose Studies

During clinical trials, approximately 9% of patients treated with a single dose of 400 mg of enoxacin for uncomplicated urethral or endocervical gonorrhea reported adverse events.

The most frequently reported events in single-dose trials, without regard to drug relationship, were nausea and vomiting (2%). Events that occurred in less than 1% of patients are listed below.

CENTRAL NERVOUS SYSTEM: headache, dizziness, somnolence; GASTROINTESTINAL: abdominal pain; GYNECOLOGIC: vaginal moniliasis; SKIN/HYPERSENSITIVITY: rash; LABORATORY ABNORMALITIES: increased AST (SGOT), decreased hemoglobin, decreased hematocrit, eosinophilia, leukocytosis, leukopenia, thrombocytosis, increased urinary protein, increased alkaline phosphatase, increased ALT (SGPT), increased bilirubin, hyperkalemia.

Multiple-Dose Studies

The incidence of adverse events reported by patients in multiple-dose clinical trials, without regard to drug relationship, was 23%. The incidence of drug-related adverse reactions in multiple-dose clinical trials was 16%. Among patients receiving multiple-dose therapy, enoxacin was discontinued because of an adverse event in 3.8% of patients.

The following events were considered likely to be drug-related in patients receiving multiple doses of enoxacin in clinical trials: nausea and/or vomiting 6%, dizziness 2%, headache 1%, abdominal pain 1%, diarrhea 1%, dyspepsia 1%.

The most frequently reported events in all multiple-dose clinical trials, without regard to drug relationship, were as follows: nausea and/or vomiting 8%, dizziness and/or vertigo 3%, headache 2%, diarrhea 2%, abdominal pain 2%, insomnia 1%, dyspepsia 1%, rash 1%, nervousness and/or anxiety 1%, unusual taste 1%, pruritus 1%.

Additional events that occurred in less than 1% of patients but >0.1% of patients are listed below.

BODY AS A WHOLE: asthenia, fatigue, fever, malaise, back pain, chest pain, edema, chills; GASTROINTESTINAL: flatulence, constipation, dry mouth/throat, stomatitis, anorexia, gastritis, bloody stools; CENTRAL NERVOUS SYSTEM: somnolence, tremor, convulsions, paresthesia, confusion, agitation, depression, syncope, myoclonus, depersonalization, hypertonia; SKIN/HYPERSENSITIVITY: photosensitivity reaction, urticaria, hyperhidrosis, mycotic infection, erythema multiforme, toxic epidermal necrolysis, Stevens-Johnson syndrome; SPECIAL SENSES: tinnitus, conjunctivitis, visual disturbances including amblyopia; MUSCULOSKELETAL: myalgia, arthralgia; CARDIOVASCULAR: palpitations, tachycardia, vasodilation; RESPIRATORY: dyspnea, cough, epistaxis; HEMIC AND LYMPHATIC: purpura; UROGENITAL: vaginal moniliasis, vaginitis, urinary incontinence, renal failure.

The following adverse events occurred in less than 0.1% of patients in multiple-dose clinical trials but were considered significant: pseudomembranous colitis, hyperkinesia, amnesia, ataxia, hypotonia, psychosis, emotional lability, hallucination, schizophrenic reaction.

LABORATORY CHANGES: The following laboratory abnormalities appeared in ≥1.0% of patients receiving multiple doses of enoxacin: elevated AST (SGOT), elevated ALT (SGPT). It is not known whether these abnormalities were caused by the drug or the underlying conditions.

Worldwide Post-Marketing Experience

The most frequent spontaneously-reported adverse events in the worldwide post-marketing experience with multiple- and single-dose enoxacin use have been rashes, seizures/convulsions, and photosensitivity reactions; however, there is no evidence that the incidences of these events were larger than those observed in the clinical trials population.

Quinolone-class adverse reactions: Although not reported in completed clinical studies with enoxacin, a variety of adverse events have been reported with other quinolones.

Clinical adverse events include: erythema nodosum, hepatic necrosis, possible exacerbation of myasthenia gravis, nystagmus, intestinal perforation, hyperpigmentation, interstitial nephritis, polyuria, urinary retention, renal calculi, cardiopulmonary arrest, cerebral thrombosis, and laryngeal or pulmonary edema.

Laboratory adverse events include: agranulocytosis, elevation of serum triglycerides and/or serum cholesterol, prolongation of the prothrombin time, candiduria, and crystalluria.

OVERDOSAGE

In the event of acute overdosage, the stomach should be emptied by inducing vomiting or by gastric lavage and the patient carefully observed and given supportive treatment. Enoxacin is poorly removed (<5% over 4 hours) by hemodialysis.

DOSAGE AND ADMINISTRATION

Penetrex® (enoxacin) should be taken at least one hour before or at least two hours after a meal.

See **INDICATIONS AND USAGE** for information on appropriate pathogens and patient populations.

Sexually Transmitted Diseases

Uncomplicated urethral or cervical gonorrhea: 400 mg single dose

Urinary Tract Infections

Uncomplicated urinary tract infections: 200 mg q12h for 7 days

Complicated urinary tract infections: 400 mg q12h for 14 days

Dosage Adjustment for Renal Impairment: Dosage should be adjusted in patients with a creatinine clearance value of 30 mL/min/1.73 m^2 or less. After a normal initial dose, the dosing interval should be adjusted as follows:

Continued on next page

Strength	Size	NDC 0075-	Color	Markings
200 mg	Bottles of 50	5100-50	light blue	5100
400 mg	Bottles of 50	5140-50	dark blue	5140

Penetrex—Cont.

Creatinine Clearance	Dosage Adjustment	Dosage Interval
>30 mL/min/1.73 m^2	None	12 hours
≤30 mL/min/1.73 m^2	1/2 recommended dose	12 hours

When only the serum creatinine is known, the following formula may be used to estimate creatinine clearance.

Men:

$$\text{creatinine clearance (mL/min)} = \frac{\text{Weight (kg)} \times (140-\text{age})}{72 \times \text{serum creatinine (mg/dL)}}$$

Women: 0.85 × the value calculated for men.

The serum creatinine should represent a steady state of renal function.

Dosage adjustment is not necessary in elderly patients with normal renal function, but dose should be adjusted according to the previous guidelines in elderly patients with compromised renal function.

HOW SUPPLIED

[See table at bottom of previous page]

Store at Controlled Room Temperature, 20° to 25°C (68° to 77°F) [see USP].

This product should be dispensed in a container with a child-resistant cap.

Keep out of the reach of children.

ANIMAL PHARMACOLOGY

Enoxacin and other members of the quinolone class have been shown to cause arthropathy in immature animals of most species tested. (See **WARNINGS.**)

REFERENCES

1. National Committee for Clinical Laboratory Standards, Performance Standards for Antimicrobial Disk Susceptibility Tests—Fourth Edition. Approved Standard NCCLS Document M2-A4, Vol. 10, No. 7, NCCLS, Villanova, PA, 1990.
2. National Committee for Clinical Laboratory Standards, Methods for Dilution Antimicrobial Susceptibility Tests for Bacteria that Grow Aerobically—Second Edition. Approved Standard NCCLS Document M7-A2, Vol. 10, No. 8, NCCLS, Villanova, PA, 1990.

Rx only

Rev. 7/98 IN-5391D!

Aventis Pharmaceuticals Products Inc.
Parsippany, NJ 07054

PRIFTIN® ℞

[*prĭf-tĭn*]

(rifapentine)

150 mg Tablets

Prescribing Information as of June 1998

DESCRIPTION

PRIFTIN® (rifapentine) for oral administration contains 150 mg of the active ingredient rifapentine per tablet.

The 150 mg tablets also contain, as inactive ingredients: calcium stearate, disodium EDTA, FD&C Blue No. 2 aluminum lake, hydroxypropyl cellulose, hydroxypropyl methylcellulose, microcrystalline cellulose, polyethylene glycol, pregelatinized starch, propylene glycol, sodium ascorbate, sodium lauryl sulfate, sodium starch glycolate, synthetic red iron oxide, and titanium dioxide.

Rifapentine is a rifamycin derivative antibiotic and has a similar profile of microbiological activity to rifampin (rifampicin). The molecular weight is 877.04.

The molecular formula is $C_{47}H_{64}N_4O_{12}$.

The chemical name for rifapentine is rifamycin, 3-[[(4-cyclopentyl-1-piperazinyl)imino]methyl]-

or

3-[N-(4-Cyclopentyl - 1-piperazinyl)formimidoyl] rifamycin or 5,6,9,17,19,21-hexahydroxy-23-methoxy-2,4,12,16,18, 20, 22-heptamethyl- 8 -[N-(4-cyclopentyl-l-piperazinyl)-formimidoyl]- 2,7 -(epoxy-pentadeca[1,11,13]trienimino) naphtho[2, 1-b]furan-1,11 (2H)-dione 21-acetate. It has the following structure:

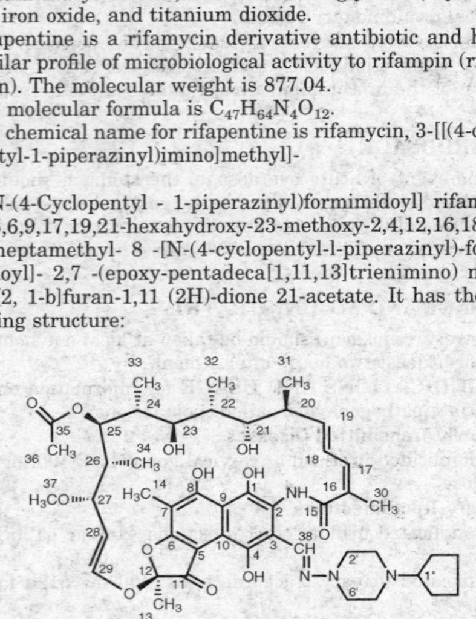

ACTIONS/CLINICAL PHARMACOLOGY

Pharmacokinetics

Absorption

The absolute bioavailability of rifapentine has not been determined. The relative bioavailability (with an oral solution as a reference) of rifapentine after a single 600 mg dose to healthy adult volunteers was 70%. The maximum concentrations were achieved from 5 to 6 hours after administration of the 600 mg rifapentine dose. Food (850 total calories: 33 g protein, 55 g fat and 58 g carbohydrate) increased AUC (0–∞) and C_{max} by 43% and 44%, respectively over that observed when administered under fasting conditions. When oral doses of rifapentine were administered once daily or once every 72 hours to healthy volunteers for 10 days, single dose AUC (0–∞) value of rifapentine was similar to its steady-state AUC_{ss} (0–24h) or AUC_{ss} (0–72h) values, suggesting no significant auto-induction effect on steady-state pharmacokinetics of rifapentine. Steady-state conditions were achieved by day 10 following daily administration of rifapentine 600 mg. The pharmacokinetic characteristics of rifapentine and 25-desacetyl rifapentine (active metabolite) on day 10 following oral administration of 600 mg rifapentine every 72 hours to healthy volunteers are contained in the following table.

[See first table above]

Parameter	Rifapentine	25-desacetyl Rifapentine
	Mean ± SD (n=12)	
C_{max} (µg/mL)	15.05 ± 4.62	6.26 ± 2.06
AUC (0–72h) (µg*h/mL)	319.54 ± 91.52	215.88 ± 85.96
$T_{1/2}$ (h)	13.19 ± 1.38	13.35 ± 2.67
T_{max} (h)	4.83 ± 1.80	11.25 ± 2.73
Clpo (L/h)	2.03 ± 0.60	–

Table 2-1. Dose of Rifapentine, Rifampin, Isoniazid, Pyrazinamide, and Ethambutol

	Rifapentine Combination Treatment			
Intensive Phase	*Rifapentine (mg) Twice Weekly*	*Isoniazid (mg) Daily*	*Pyrazinamide (mg) Daily*	*Ethambutol* (mg) Daily*
Patient Weight				
<50 kg	600	300	1500	800
≥50 kg	600	300	2000	1200
Continuation Phase	*Rifapentine (mg) Once Weekly*	*Isoniazid (mg) Once Weekly*		
Patient Weight				
<50 kg	600	600		
≥50 kg	600	900		
	Rifampin Combination Treatment			
Intensive Phase	*Rifampin (mg) Daily*	*Isoniazid (mg) Daily*	*Pyrazinamide (mg) Daily*	*Ethambutol (mg) Daily*
Patient Weight				
<50 kg	450	300	1500	800
≥50 kg	600	300	2000	1200
Continuation Phase	*Rifampin (mg) Twice Weekly*	*Isoniazid (mg) Twice Weekly*		
Patient Weight				
<50 kg	450	600		
≥50 kg	600	900		

*Ethambutol was to be discontinued once baseline susceptibility test results were available

Distribution

In a population pharmacokinetic analysis in 351 tuberculosis patients who received 600 mg rifapentine in combination with isoniazid, pyrazinamide and ethambutol, the estimated apparent volume of distribution was 70.2 ± 9.1 L. In healthy volunteers, rifapentine and 25-desacetyl rifapentine were 97.7% and 93.2% bound to plasma proteins, respectively. Rifapentine was mainly bound to albumin. Similar extent of protein binding was observed in healthy volunteers, asymptomatic HIV-infected subjects and hepatically impaired subjects.

Metabolism/Excretion

Following a single 600 mg oral dose of radiolabelled rifapentine to healthy volunteers (n=4), 87% of the total ^{14}C rifapentine was recovered in the urine (17%) and feces (70%). Greater than 80% of the total ^{14}C rifapentine dose was excreted from the body within 7 days. Rifapentine was hydrolyzed by an esterase enzyme to form a microbiologically active 25-desacetyl rifapentine. Rifapentine and 25-desacetyl rifapentine accounted for 99% of the total radioactivity in plasma. Plasma AUC(0-∞) and C_{max} values of the 25-desacetyl rifapentine metabolite were one-half and one-third those of the rifapentine, respectively. Based upon relative in vitro activities and AUC(0-∞) values, rifapentine and 25-desacetyl rifapentine potentially contributes 62% and 38% to the clinical activities against *M. tuberculosis*, respectively.

Special Populations

Gender: In a population pharmacokinetics analysis of sparse blood samples obtained from 351 tuberculosis patients who received 600 mg rifapentine in combination with isoniazid, pyrazinamide and ethambutol, the estimated apparent oral clearance of rifapentine for males and females was 2.51 ± 0.14 L/h and 1.69 ± 0.41 L/h, respectively. The clinical significance of the difference in the estimated apparent oral clearance is not known.

Elderly: Following oral administration of a single 600 mg dose of rifapentine to elderly (≥65 years) male healthy volunteers (n=14), the pharmacokinetics of rifapentine and 25-desacetyl metabolite were similar to that observed for young (18 to 45 years) healthy male volunteers (n=20).

Pediatric (Adolescents): In a pharmacokinetics study of rifapentine in healthy adolescents (age 12 to 15), 600 mg rifapentine was administered to those weighing ≥45 kg (n=10) and 450 mg was administered to those weighing <45 kg (n=2). The pharmacokinetics of rifapentine were similar to those observed in healthy adults.

Renal Impaired Patients: The pharmacokinetics of rifapentine have not been evaluated in renal impaired patients. Although only about 17% of an administered dose is excreted via the kidneys, the clinical significance of impaired renal function on the disposition of rifapentine and its 25-desacetyl metabolite is not known.

Hepatic Impaired Patients: Following oral administration of a single 600 mg dose of rifapentine to mild to severe hepatic impaired patients (n=15), the pharmacokinetics of rifapentine and 25-desacetyl metabolite were similar in patients with various degrees of hepatic impairment and to that observed in another study for healthy volunteers (n=12). Since the elimination of these agents are primarily via the liver, the clinical significance of impaired hepatic function on the disposition of rifapentine and its 25-desacetyl metabolite is not known.

Asymptomatic HIV-Infected Volunteers: Following oral administration of a single 600 mg dose of rifapentine to asymptomatic HIV-infected volunteers (n=15) under fasting conditions, mean C_{max} and AUC(0–∞) of rifapentine were lower (20–32%) than that observed in other studies in healthy volunteers (n=55). In a cross-study comparison, mean C_{max} and AUC values of the 25-desacetyl metabolite of rifapentine, when compared to healthy volunteers were higher (6–21%) in one study (n=20), but lower (15–16%) in a different study (n=40). The clinical significance of this observation is not known. Food (850 total calories: 33 g protein, 55 g fat, and 58 g carbohydrate) increases the mean AUC and C_{max} of rifapentine observed under fasting conditions in asymptomatic HIV-infected volunteers by about 51% and 53%, respectively.

Microbiology

Mechanism of Action

Rifapentine, a cyclopentyl rifamycin, inhibits DNA-dependent RNA polymerase in susceptible strains of *Mycobacterium tuberculosis* but not in mammalian cells. At therapeutic levels, rifapentine exhibits bactericidal activity against both intracellular and extracellular *M. tuberculosis* organisms. Both rifapentine and the 25-desacetyl metabolite accumulate in human monocyte-derived macrophages with intracellular/extracellular ratios of approximately 24:1 and 7:1, respectively.

Resistance Development

In the treatment of tuberculosis (see INDICATIONS AND USAGE), a small number of resistant cells present within large populations of susceptible cells can rapidly become predominant. Rifapentine resistance development in *M. tuberculosis* strains is principally due to one of several single point mutations that occur in the rpoB portion of the gene coding for the beta subunit of the DNA-dependent RNA polymerase. The incidence of rifapentine resistant mutants in an otherwise susceptible population of *M. tuberculosis* strains is approximately one in 10^7 to 10^8 bacilli. Due to the potential for resistance development to rifapentine, appropriate susceptibility tests should be performed in the event of persistently positive cultures.

M. tuberculosis organisms resistant to other rifamycins are likely to be resistant to rifapentine. A high level of cross resistance between rifampin and rifapentine has been demonstrated with *M. tuberculosis* strains. Cross resistance does not appear between rifapentine and non-rifamycin antimycobacterial agents such as isoniazid and streptomycin.

In Vitro Activity of Rifapentine against *M. tuberculosis*

Rifapentine and its 25-desacetyl metabolite have demonstrated in vitro activity against rifamycin-susceptible strains of *Mycobacterium tuberculosis* including cidal activity against phagocytized *M. tuberculosis* organisms grown in activated human macrophages.

In vitro results indicate that rifapentine MIC values for *M. tuberculosis* organisms are influenced by study conditions. Rifapentine MIC values were substantially increased employing egg-based medium compared to liquid or agar-based solid media. The addition of Tween 80 in these assays has been shown to lower MIC values for rifamycin compounds. In mouse infection studies a therapeutic effect, in terms of enhanced survival time or reduction of organ bioburden, has been observed in *M. tuberculosis*-infected animals treated with various intermittent rifapentine-containing regimens. Animal studies have shown that the activity of rifapentine is influenced by dose and frequency of administration.

Susceptibility testing for *Mycobacterium tuberculosis*

Breakpoints to determine whether clinical isolates of *M. tuberculosis* are susceptible or resistant to rifapentine have not been established. The clinical relevance of rifapentine in vitro susceptibility test results for other mycobacterial species has not been determined.

CLINICAL TRIALS

A total of 722 patients were enrolled in Clinical Study 008, an open label, prospective, randomized, parallel group, active controlled trial, for the treatment of pulmonary tuberculosis. This population was mostly comprised of Black (>60%) or Multiracial (>31%) patients and the mean ± standard deviation age was 37 ± 11 years. Treatment groups were comparable with respect to age and race. The percentage of male patients was higher in the rifapentine combination group (80%) than in the rifampin combination group (73%). The study was divided into two phases on the basis of dosing frequency. For the first phase, designated as the Intensive Phase, 361 patients were randomized to receive rifapentine, isoniazid, pyrazinamide, and ethambutol for 60 days and 361 patients were randomized to receive rifampin, isoniazid, pyrazinamide, and ethambutol for 60 days. (Ethambutol was to be discontinued once baseline susceptibility test results were available.) Rifapentine and isoniazid were each administered at a fixed dose regardless of body weight. Rifampin, pyrazinamide, and ethambutol were administered based on body weight according to Table 2-1. **Note:** All drugs were administered ***daily*** in the Intensive Phase **except for rifapentine** which was administered twice weekly. During the second phase, designated as the Continuation Phase, 317 patients who had received rifapentine in the Intensive Phase continued to receive rifapentine and isoniazid once weekly for up to 120 days. Three hundred four patients who had received rifampin in the Intensive Phase continued to receive rifampin and isoniazid during the Continuation Phase twice weekly for up to 120 days. Rifampin and isoniazid were administered based on body weight according to Table 2-1.

Patients in either treatment group were scheduled to receive study drug over a 180-day period with a subsequent 24-month follow-up. Additionally, both treatment groups received pyridoxine (Vitamin B_6) over the 180-day treatment period.

The indication for treatment of pulmonary tuberculosis with PRIFTIN is based on the 6 month follow-up treatment outcome observed in Clinical Study 008 as a surrogate for the 2 year follow-up generally accepted as evidence of efficacy in the treatment of pulmonary tuberculosis.

[See table 2-1 at top of previous page]

Table 2-2 presents clinical outcome in Study 008.

[See table 2-2 above]

Table 2-2. Clinical Outcome in Study 008*

	Rifapentine Combination	Rifampin Combination
Status at End of Treatment		
Converted	87% (249/286)	81% (229/284)
Not Converted	1% (4/286)	3% (8/284)
Lost to Follow-up	12% (33/286)	17% (47/284)
Status in Follow-up:		
Relapsed	10% (25/249)	5% (11/229)
Sputum negative, Still being followed	81% (201/249)	90% (205/229)
Lost to Follow-up	9% (23/249)	6% (13/229)

* All data through 8 July 1997 for patients with confirmed susceptible MTB (rifapentine combination, n=286; rifampin combination, n=284).

Risk of relapse was higher in the rifapentine regimen. During the Intensive Phase of treatment the rate of noncompliance with companion medications was somewhat higher for the rifapentine regimen than for the rifampin regimen. Most of the relapses occurred among those with poor compliance with these companion medications and this group also had the largest risk of relapse for the rifapentine regimen relative to the rifampin regimen. This factor appears to explain most, but not all, of the higher relapse rate observed in the rifapentine arm. Failure to convert sputum after two months of treatment (ie, end of Intensive Phase) was associated with a greater risk of relapse for both treatment regimens. Relapse rates were also higher for males in both regimens. Relapse in the rifapentine group was not associated with development of mono-resistance to rifampin.

In vitro susceptibility testing was conducted against initial and subsequent *M. tuberculosis* isolates recovered from 620 patients enrolled in the study. Rifapentine and rifampin MIC values were determined employing the radiometric susceptibility testing method utilizing 7H12 broth at pH 6.8 (NCCLS procedure M24-T). Six hundred and fourteen patients with rifampin susceptible (MIC ≤0.5 µg/ml) strains of *M. tuberculosis* had rifapentine MICs of ≤0.125 µg/ml. The remaining six patients with rifampin resistant (MIC > 8.0 µg/ml) *M. tuberculosis* isolates had rifapentine MICs of >8.0 µg/ml). Four of these represented baseline values for patients with multiresistant tuberculosis. One rifampin resistant isolate was from a rifapentine relapse patient while the remaining isolate was from a rifampin relapse patient. Restriction fragment length polymorphism (RFLP) studies showed the rifapentine relapse isolate to be genetically different from the baseline strain while RFLP data on the matched rifampin isolate is pending. This information is provided for comparative purposes only as rifapentine breakpoints have not been established.

INDICATIONS AND USAGE

PRIFTIN is indicated for the treatment of pulmonary tuberculosis. This indication is based on the 6 month follow-up treatment outcome observed in the controlled clinical trial as a surrogate for the 2 year follow-up generally accepted as evidence of efficacy in the treatment of pulmonary tuberculosis. PRIFTIN must always be used in conjunction with at least one other antituberculosis drug to which the isolate is susceptible. In the intensive phase of the short-course treatment of pulmonary tuberculosis, **PRIFTIN should be administered twice weekly for two months,** with an interval of no less than 3 days (72 hours) between doses, as part of an appropriate regimen which includes daily companion drugs (Table 2-1). It may also be necessary to add either streptomycin or ethambutol until the results of susceptibility testing are known. ***Compliance with all drugs in the Intensive Phase (ie, PRIFTIN, isoniazid, pyrazinamide, ethambutol or streptomycin) is imperative to assure early sputum conversion and protection against relapse.*** Following the intensive phase, Continuation Phase treatment should be continued with PRIFTIN for 4 months. **During this phase, PRIFTIN should be administered on a once-weekly basis** in combination with an appropriate antituberculous agent for susceptible organisms (Table 2-1) (see DOSAGE AND ADMINISTRATION section).

In the treatment of tuberculosis, the small number of resistant cells present within large populations of susceptible cells can rapidly become the predominant type. Consequently, clinical samples for mycobacterial culture and susceptibility testing should be obtained prior to the initiation of therapy, as well as during treatment to monitor therapeutic response. The susceptibility of *M. tuberculosis* organisms to isoniazid, rifampin, pyrazinamide, ethambutol, rifapentine and other appropriate agents should be measured. If test results show resistance to any of these drugs and the patient is not responding to therapy, the drug regimen should be modified.

CONTRAINDICATIONS

This product is contraindicated in patients with a history of hypersensitivity to any of the rifamycins (eg, rifampin and rifabutin).

WARNINGS

Poor compliance with the dosage regimen, particularly the daily administered non-rifamycin drugs in the Intensive Phase, was associated with late sputum conversion and a high relapse rate in the rifapentine arm of Clinical Study 008. Therefore, compliance with the full course of therapy must be emphasized, and the importance of not missing any doses must be stressed. (See PRECAUTIONS and DOSAGE AND ADMINISTRATION.)

Since antituberculosis multidrug treatments, including the rifamycin class, are associated with serious hepatic events, patients with abnormal liver tests and/or liver disease should only be given rifapentine in cases of necessity and then with caution and under strict medical supervision. In these patients, careful monitoring of liver tests (especially serum transaminases) should be carried out prior to therapy and then every 2 to 4 weeks during therapy. If signs of liver disease occur or worsen, rifapentine should be discontinued.

Hyperbilirubinemia resulting from competition for excretory pathways between rifapentine and bilirubin cannot be excluded since competition between the related drug rifampin and bilirubin can occur. An isolated report showing a moderate rise in bilirubin and/or transaminase level is not in itself an indication for interrupting treatment; rather, the decision should be made after repeating the tests, noting trends in the levels and considering them in conjunction with the patient's clinical condition. Pseudomembranous colitis has been reported to occur with various antibiotics, including other rifamycins. Diarrhea, particularly if severe and/or persistent, occurring during treatment or in the initial weeks following treatment may be symptomatic of *Clostridium difficile*-associated disease, the most severe form of which is pseudomembranous colitis. If pseudomembranous colitis is suspected, rifapentine should be stopped immediately and the patient should be treated with supportive and specific treatment without delay (eg, oral vancomycin). Products inhibiting peristalsis are contraindicated in this clinical situation.

Experience in HIV-infected patients is limited. In an ongoing CDC TB trial, five out of 30 HIV-infected patients randomized to once weekly rifapentine (plus INH) in the Continuation Phase who completed treatment, relapsed. Four of these patients developed rifampin mono-resistant (RMR) TB. Each RMR patient had late-stage HIV infection, low CD4 counts and extrapulmonary disease, and documented co-administration of antifungal azoles. These findings are consistent with the literature in which an emergence of RMR TB in HIV-infected TB patients has been reported in recent years. Further study in this sub-population is warranted. As with other antituberculous treatments, when rifapentine is used in HIV-infected patients, a more aggressive regimen should be employed (eg, more frequent dosing). Based on results to date of the CDC trial (see above), once weekly dosing during the Continuation Phase of treatment is not recommended at this time.

Because rifapentine has been shown to increase indinavir metabolism (see DRUG INTERACTIONS), it should be used with extreme caution, if at all, in patients who are also taking protease inhibitors.

PRECAUTIONS

General

Rifapentine may produce a predominately red-orange discoloration of body tissues and/or fluids (eg, skin, teeth, tongue, urine, feces, saliva, sputum, tears, sweat, and cerebrospinal fluid).

Contact lenses may become permanently stained.

Information for Patients

The patient should be told that PRIFTIN may produce a reddish coloration of the urine, sweat, sputum, and tears, and the patient should be forewarned that contact lenses may be permanently stained. The patient should be advised that the reliability of oral or other systemic hormonal contraceptives may be affected; consideration should be given to using alternative contraceptive measures. For those patients with a propensity to nausea, vomiting, or gastrointestinal upset, administration of PRIFTIN with food may be useful. Patients should be instructed to notify their physician promptly if they experience any of the following: fever, loss of appetite, malaise, nausea and vomiting, darkened urine, yellowish discoloration of the skin and eyes, and pain or swelling of the joints.

Compliance with the full course of therapy must be emphasized, and the importance of not missing any doses of the daily administered companion medications in the Intensive Phase must be stressed. (See DOSAGE AND ADMINISTRATION and WARNINGS).

Laboratory Tests

Adults treated for tuberculosis with rifapentine should have baseline measurements of hepatic enzymes, bilirubin, a complete blood count, and a platelet count (or estimate).

Patients should be seen at least monthly during therapy and should be specifically questioned concerning symptoms associated with adverse reactions. All patients with abnormalities should have follow-up, including laboratory testing, if necessary. Routine laboratory monitoring for toxicity in people with normal baseline measurements is generally not necessary.

Therapeutic concentrations of rifampin have been shown to inhibit standard microbiological assays for serum folate and Vitamin B_{12}. Similar drug-laboratory interactions should be considered for rifapentine; thus, alternative assay methods should be considered.

Drug Interaction

Rifapentine-Indinavir Interaction: In a study in which 600 mg rifapentine was administered twice weekly for 14 days followed by rifapentine twice weekly plus 800 mg indinavir 3 times a day for an additional 14 days, indinavir C_{max} decreased by 55% while AUC reduced by 70%. Clearance of indinavir increased by 3-fold in the presence of rifapentine while half-life did not change. But when indinavir was administered for 14 days followed by coadministration with

Continued on next page

Priftin—Cont.

rifapentine for an additional 14 days, indinavir did not affect the pharmacokinetics of rifapentine. **Rifapentine should be used with extreme caution, if at all, in patients who are also taking protease inhibitors.** (See WARNINGS and DOSAGE AND ADMINISTRATION.) (See Reference 1.)
Rifapentine is an inducer of cytochromes P4503A4 and P4502C8/9. Therefore, rifapentine may increase the metabolism of other coadministered drugs that are metabolized by these enzymes. Induction of enzyme activities by rifapentine occurred within 4 days after the first dose. Enzyme activities returned to baseline levels 14 days after discontinuing rifapentine. In addition, the magnitude of enzyme induction by rifapentine was dose and dosing frequency dependent; less enzyme induction occurred when 600 mg oral doses of rifapentine were given once every 72 hours versus daily. In vitro and in vivo enzyme induction studies have suggested rifapentine induction potential may be less than rifampin but more potent than rifabutin. Rifampin has been reported to accelerate the metabolism and may reduce the activity of the following drugs; hence, rifapentine may also increase the metabolism and decrease the activity of these drugs. Dosage adjustments of the following drugs or of drugs metabolized by cytochrome P4503A4 or P4502C8/9 may be necessary if they are given concurrently with rifapentine. Patients using oral or other systemic hormonal contraceptives should be advised to change to nonhormonal methods of birth control.
Anticonvulsants: eg, phenytoin
Antiarrhythmics: eg, disopyramide, mexiletine, quinidine, tocainide
Antibiotics: eg, chloramphenicol, clarithromycin, dapsone, doxycycline, fluoroquinolones (such as ciprofloxacin)
Oral anticoagulants: eg, warfarin
Antifungals: eg, fluconazole, itraconazole, ketoconazole
Barbiturates
Benzodiazepines: eg, diazepam
Beta-blockers, calcium channel blockers: eg, diltiazem, nifedipine, verapamil
Corticosteroids
Cardiac glycoside preparations
Clofibrate
Oral or other systemic hormonal contraceptives
Haloperidol
HIV protease inhibitors: eg, indinavir, ritonavir, nelfinavir, saquinavir (see Rifapentine-Indinavir Interaction above)
Oral hypoglycemic agents: eg, sulfonylureas
Immunosuppressants: eg, cyclosporine, tacrolimus
Levothyroxine
Narcotic analgesics: eg, methadone
Progestins
Quinine
Reverse transcriptase inhibitors: eg, delavirdine, zidovudine
Sildenafil
Theophylline
Tricyclic antidepressants: eg, amitriptyline, nortriptyline
The conversion of rifapentine to 25-desacetyl rifapentine is mediated by an esterase enzyme. There is minimal potential for rifapentine metabolism to be inhibited or induced by another drug, or for rifapentine to inhibit the metabolism of another drug based upon the characteristics of the esterase enzymes. Rifapentine does not induce its own metabolism. Since rifapentine is highly bound to albumin, drug displacement interactions may also occur.
In Clinical Study 008 patients were advised to take rifapentine at least 1 hour before or 2 hours after ingestion of antacids.

Carcinogenesis, Mutagenesis, Impairment of Fertility
Carcinogenicity studies with rifapentine have not been completed. Rifapentine was negative in the following genotoxicity tests: in vitro gene mutation assay in bacteria (Ames test); in vitro point mutation test in *Aspergillus nidulans*; in vitro gene conversion assay in *Saccharomyces cerevisiae*; host-mediated (mouse) gene conversion assay with *Saccharomyces cerevisiae*; in vitro Chinese hamster ovary cell/hypoxanthine-guanine-phosphoribosyl transferase (CHO/HGPRT) forward mutation assay; in vitro chromosomal aberration assay utilizing rat lymphocytes; and in vivo mouse bone marrow micronucleus assay. Fertility and reproductive performance were not affected by oral administration of rifapentine to male and female rats at doses of up to one-third of the human dose (based on body surface area conversions).

Pregnancy Category C
Teratogenic Effects
Rifapentine has been shown to be teratogenic in rats and rabbits. In rats, when given in doses 0.6 times the human dose (based on body surface area comparisons) during the period of organogenesis, pups showed cleft palates, right aortic arch and increased incidence of delayed ossification and increased number of ribs. Rabbits treated with drug at doses between 0.3 and 1.3 times the human dose (based on body surface area comparison) displayed major malformations including ovarian agenesis, pes varus, arhinia, microphthalmia and irregularities of the ossified facial tissues (4 of 321 examined fetuses).
Nonteratogenic Effects
In rats, rifapentine administration was associated with increased resorption rate and post implantation loss, decreased mean fetus weight, increased number of stillborn pups and slightly increased mortality during lactation. Rabbits given 1.3 times the human dose (based on body surface area comparisons) showed higher post-implantation losses and an increased incidence of stillborn pups.
When rifapentine was administered at 0.3 times the human dose (based on body surface area comparisons) to mated female rats late in gestation (from day 15 of gestation to day 21 postpartum), pup weights and gestational survival (live pups born/pups born) were reduced compared to controls.
Pregnancy—Human Experience
There are no adequate and well-controlled studies in pregnant women. In Clinical Study 008, six patients randomized to rifapentine became pregnant; two had normal deliveries; two had first trimester spontaneous abortions, one had an elective abortion and one patient was lost to follow-up. Of the two patients who spontaneously aborted, co-morbid conditions of ethanol abuse in one and HIV infection in the other were noted.
When administered during the last few weeks of pregnancy, rifampin can cause postnatal hemorrhages in the mother and infant for which treatment with Vitamin K may be indicated. Thus, patients and infants who receive rifapentine during the last few weeks of pregnancy should have appropriate clotting parameters evaluated.
Rifapentine should be used during pregnancy only if the potential benefit justifies the potential risk to the fetus.

Nursing Mothers
It is not known whether rifapentine is excreted in human milk. Because many drugs are excreted in human milk and because of the potential for serious adverse reactions in nursing infants, a decision should be made whether to discontinue nursing or discontinue the drug, taking into account the importance of the drug to the mother.

Pediatric Use
The safety and effectiveness of rifapentine in pediatric patients under the age of 12 have not been established. A pharmacokinetic study was conducted in 12- to 15-year-old healthy volunteers. (See ACTIONS/CLINICAL PHARMACOLOGY Special Populations for pharmacokinetic information).

ADVERSE REACTIONS

The investigators in the tuberculosis treatment clinical trial (Study 008) assessed the causality of adverse events as definitely, probably, possibly, unlikely or not related to one of the two drug regimens tested. The following table (Table 2-3) presents treatment-related adverse events deemed by the investigators to be at least possibly related to any of the four drugs in the regimens (rifapentine/rifampin, isoniazid, pyrazinamide, or ethambutol) which occurred in ≥1% of patients. Hyperuricemia was the most frequently reported event that was assessed as treatment related and was most likely related to the pyrazinamide since no cases were reported in the Continuation Phase when this drug was no longer included in the treatment regimen.
[See table 2-3 at left]
Treatment-related adverse events of moderate or severe intensity in <1% of the rifapentine combination therapy patients in Study 008 are presented below by body system.

Table 2-3. Treatment-Related Adverse Events Occurring in ≥1% of the Patients in Study 008

	Intensive Phase[1]		*Continuation Phase*[2]		*Total*	
Preferred Term	*Rifapentine Combination (N=361) N (%)*	*Rifampin Combination (N=361) N (%)*	*Rifapentine Combination (N=321) N (%)*	*Rifampin Combination (N=306) N (%)*	*Rifapentine Combination (N=361) N (%)*	*Rifampin Combination (N=361) N (%)*
Hyperuricemia	77 (21.3)	55 (15.2)	0	0	77 (21.3)	55 (15.2)
ALT increased	14 (3.9)	17 (4.7)	5 (1.6)	7 (2.3)	19 (5.3)	24 (6.6)
AST increased	12 (3.3)	16 (4.4)	5 (1.6)	7 (2.3)	16 (4.4)	23 (6.4)
Neutropenia	7 (1.9)	9 (2.5)	12 (3.7)	9 (2.9)	18 (5.0)	18 (5.0)
Pyuria	12 (3.3)	10 (2.8)	6 (1.9)	2 (0.7)	15 (4.2)	12 (3.3)
Proteinuria	15 (4.2)	10 (2.8)	2 (0.6)	1 (0.3)	17 (4.7)	11 (3.0)
Hematuria	10 (2.8)	11 (3.0)	4 (1.2)	3 (1.0)	13 (3.6)	14 (3.9)
Lymphopenia	14 (3.9)	13 (3.6)	3 (0.9)	1 (0.3)	16 (4.4)	14 (3.9)
Urinary casts	11 (3.0)	3 (0.8)	4 (1.2)	0	14 (3.9)	3 (0.8)
Rash	9 (2.5)	20 (5.5)	4 (1.2)	3 (1.0)	13 (3.6)	22 (6.1)
Pruritus	8 (2.2)	15 (4.2)	1 (0.3)	1 (0.3)	9 (2.5)	16 (4.4)
Acne	5 (1.4)	3 (0.8)	2 (0.6)	1 (0.3)	7 (1.9)	4 (1.1)
Anorexia	6 (1.7)	8 (2.2)	3 (0.9)	4 (1.3)	8 (2.2)	10 (2.8)
Anemia	7 (1.9)	9 (2.5)	2 (0.6)	1 (0.3)	9 (2.5)	10 (2.8)
Leukopenia	4 (1.1)	4 (1.1)	3 (0.9)	5 (1.6)	7 (1.9)	8 (2.2)
Arthralgia	9 (2.5)	7 (1.9)	0	0	9 (2.5)	7 (1.9)
Pain	7 (1.9)	5 (1.4)	0	1 (0.3)	7 (1.9)	6 (1.7)
Nausea	7 (1.9)	2 (0.6)	0	1 (0.3)	7 (1.9)	3 (0.8)
Vomiting	4 (1.1)	6 (1.7)	1 (0.3)	1 (0.3)	5 (1.4)	7 (1.9)
Headache	3 (0.8)	4 (1.1)	1 (0.3)	3 (1.0)	4 (1.1)	7 (1.9)
Dyspepsia	3 (0.8)	5 (1.4)	2 (0.6)	3 (1.0)	4 (1.1)	8 (2.2)
Hypertension	3 (0.8)	0 (0.0)	1 (0.3)	1 (0.3)	4 (1.1)	1 (0.3)
Dizziness	4 (1.1)	0	0	1 (0.3)	4 (1.1)	1 (0.3)
Thrombocytosis	4 (1.1)	2 (0.6)	0	0	4 (1.1)	2 (0.6)
Diarrhea	4 (1.1)	0	0	0	4 (1.1)	0
Rash maculopapular	4 (1.1)	3 (0.8)	0	0	4 (1.1)	3 (0.8)
Hemoptysis	2 (0.6)	0	2 (0.6)	0	4 (1.1)	0

Note: ≥1% refers to rifapentine in the TOTAL column.

Note: A patient may have experienced the same adverse event more than once during the course of the study, therefore, patient counts across the columns may not equal the patient counts in the TOTAL column.

1 Intensive Phase consisted of therapy with either rifapentine or rifampin combined with isoniazid, pyrazinamide, and ethambutol administered daily (rifapentine twice weekly) for 60 days.

2 Continuation Phase consisted of therapy with either rifapentine or rifampin combined with isoniazid for 120 days. Rifapentine patients were dosed once weekly; rifampin patients were dosed twice weekly. Events recorded in this phase includes those reported up to 3 months after Continuation Phase therapy was completed.

Hepatic & Biliary: bilirubinemia, hepatitis
Dermatologic: urticaria, skin discoloration
Hematologic: thrombocytopenia, neutrophilia, leukocytosis, purpura, hematoma
Metabolic & Nutritional: hyperkalemia, hypovolemia, alkaline phosphatase increased, LDH increased
Body as a Whole – General: peripheral edema, fatigue
Gastrointestinal: constipation, esophagitis, gastritis, pancreatitis
Musculoskeletal: gout, arthrosis
Psychiatric: aggressive reaction

Three patients (two rifampin combination therapy patients and one rifapentine combination therapy patient) were discontinued in the Intensive Phase as a result of hepatitis with increased liver function tests (ALT, AST, LDH, and bilirubin). Concomitant medications for all three patients included isoniazid, pyrazinamide, ethambutol, and pyridoxine. The two rifampin patients and one rifapentine patient recovered without sequelae.

Eighteen deaths occurred in Study 008 (nine in the rifampin combination therapy group and nine in the rifapentine combination therapy group). None of the deaths were attributed to study medication. In the study, 18/361 (5.0%) rifampin combination therapy patients discontinued the study due to an adverse event compared to 9/361 (2.5%) rifapentine combination therapy patients.

The overall occurrence rate of treatment-related adverse events was higher in males with the rifapentine combination regimen (50%) versus the rifampin combination regimen (43%), while in females the overall rate was greater in the rifampin combination group (68%) compared to the rifapentine combination group (59%). However, there were higher frequencies of treatment-related hematuria and ALT increases for female patients in both treatment groups compared to those for male patients.

Adverse events associated with rifampin may occur with rifapentine: effects of enzyme induction to increase metabolism resulting in decreased concentration of endogenous substrates, including adrenal hormones, thyroid hormones, and vitamin D.

OVERDOSAGE

There is no experience with the treatment of acute overdose with rifapentine at doses exceeding 1200 mg per dose.

In a pharmacokinetic study involving healthy volunteers (n=9), single oral doses up to 1200 mg have been administered without serious adverse events. The only adverse events reported with the 1200 mg dose were heartburn (3/8), headache (2/8) and increased urinary frequency (1/8). In clinical trials, tuberculosis patients ranging in age from 20 to 74 years accidentally received continuous daily doses of rifapentine 600 mg. Some patients received continuous daily dosing for up to 20 days without evidence of serious adverse effects. One patient experienced a transient elevation in SGPT and glucose (the latter attributed to pre-existing diabetes); a second patient experienced slight pruritis. While there is no experience with the treatment of acute overdose with rifapentine, clinical experience with rifamycins suggests that gastric lavage to evacuate gastric contents (within a few hours of overdose), followed by instillation of an activated charcoal slurry into the stomach, may help adsorb any remaining drug from the gastrointestinal tract.

Rifapentine and 25-desacetyl rifapentine are 97.7% and 93.2% plasma protein bound, respectively. Rifapentine and related compounds excreted in urine account for only 17% of the administered dose, therefore, neither hemodialysis nor forced diuresis is expected to enhance the systemic elimination of unchanged rifapentine from the body of a patient with PRIFTIN overdose.

DOSAGE AND ADMINISTRATION

PRIFTIN should not be used alone, in initial treatment or in retreatment of pulmonary tuberculosis. In the intensive phase of short-course therapy which is to continue for 2 months, 600 mg **(four 150 mg tablets)** of PRIFTIN should be given twice weekly with an interval of not less than 3 days (72 hours) between doses. For those patients with propensity to nausea, vomiting or gastrointestinal upset, administration of PRIFTIN with food may be useful. In the Intensive Phase, PRIFTIN must be administered in combination as part of an appropriate regimen which includes daily companion drugs. *Compliance with all drugs in the Intensive Phase (ie, PRIFTIN, isoniazid, pyrazinamide, ethambutol, or streptomycin), especially on days when rifapentine is not administered, is imperative to assure early sputum conversion and protection against relapse.* The Advisory Council for the Elimination of Tuberculosis, the American Thoracic Society and the Centers for Disease Control and Prevention also recommend that either streptomycin or ethambutol be added to the regimen unless the likelihood of isoniazid resistance is very low. The need for streptomycin or ethambutol should be reassessed when the results of susceptibility testing are known. An initial treatment regimen with less than four drugs may be considered if there is little possibility of drug resistance (that is, less than 4% primary resistance to isoniazid in the community, and the patient has had no previous treatment with antituberculosis medications, is not from a country with a high prevalence of drug resistance, and has no known exposure to a drug-resistant case) (see Reference 2).

Following the intensive phase, treatment should be continued with PRIFTIN once weekly for 4 months in combination with isoniazid or an appropriate agent for susceptible organisms. If the patient is still sputum smear or culture positive, if resistant organisms are present, or if the patient is HIV positive, follow the ATS/CDC treatment guidelines (see Reference 2).

Concomitant administration of pyridoxine (Vitamin B_6) is recommended in the malnourished, in those predisposed to neuropathy (eg, alcoholics and diabetics), and in adolescents.

The above recommendations apply to patients with drug-susceptible organisms. Patients with drug-resistant organisms may require longer duration treatment with other drug regimens.

HOW SUPPLIED

PRIFTIN (rifapentine) 150 mg pink film-coated tablets are packaged in aluminum foil blisters in cartons of 32 tablets (NDC 0088-2100-03).

Store at 25°C (77°F); excursions permitted 15–30°C (59–86°F) (see USP Controlled Room Temperature). Protect from excessive heat and humidity.

Prescribing Information as of June 1998

Manufactured by:
Gruppo Lepitit S.p.A.
20020 Lainate, Italy
Manufactured for:
Hoechst Marion Roussel, Inc.
Kansas City, MO 64137 USA
MADE IN ITALY

References:
1. Update on US Public Health Service (USPHS) Study 22: A trial of once weekly isoniazid (INH) & rifapentine (RPT) in the continuation phase of TB treatment. The USPHS Rifapentine Trial Group, A Vernon, et al. Am J Respir Crit Care Med. 157: (suppl) A467 (abstract), March 1998.
2. American Thoracic Society, CDC. Treatment of tuberculosis and tuberculosis infection in adults and children. Am J Respir Crit Care Med. 149:1359–1374, 1994.

REFLUDAN® ℞

[rĕ-flu'-dăn]
[lepirudin (rDNA) for injection]

Prescribing Information as of October 1998

DESCRIPTION

REFLUDAN [lepirudin (rDNA) for injection] is a highly specific direct inhibitor of thrombin. Lepirudin (chemical designation: [Leu[1], Thr[2]]-63-desulfohirudin) is a recombinant hirudin derived from yeast cells. The polypeptide composed of 65 amino acids has a molecular weight of 6979.5 daltons. Natural hirudin is produced in trace amounts as a family of highly homologous isopolypeptides by the leech *Hirudo medicinalis*. The biosynthetic molecule (lepirudin) is identical to natural hirudin except for substitution of leucine for isoleucine at the N-terminal end of the molecule and the absence of a sulfate group on the tyrosine at position 63.

The activity of lepirudin is measured in a chromogenic assay. One antithrombin unit (ATU) is the amount of lepirudin that neutralizes one unit of World Health Organization preparation 89/588 of thrombin. The specific activity of lepirudin is approximately 16,000 ATU/mg. Its mode of action is independent of antithrombin III. Platelet factor 4 does not inhibit lepirudin. One molecule of lepirudin binds to one molecule of thrombin and thereby blocks the thrombogenic activity of thrombin. As a result, all thrombin-dependent coagulation assays are affected, eg, activated partial thromboplastin time (aPTT) values increase in a dose-dependent fashion (*Roethig 1991*).

REFLUDAN is supplied as a sterile, white, freeze-dried powder for injection or infusion and is freely soluble in Sterile Water for Injection USP or 0.9% Sodium Chloride Injection USP.

Each vial of REFLUDAN contains 50 mg lepirudin. Other ingredients are 40 mg mannitol and sodium hydroxide for adjustment of pH to approximately 7.

CLINICAL PHARMACOLOGY

Pharmacokinetic Properties

The pharmacokinetic properties of lepirudin following intravenous administration are well described by a two-compartment model. Distribution is essentially confined to extracellular fluids and is characterized by an initial half-life of approximately 10 minutes. Elimination follows a first-order process and is characterized by a terminal half-life of about 1.3 hours in young healthy volunteers. As the intravenous dose is increased over the range of 0.1 to 0.4 mg/kg, the maximum plasma concentration and the area-under-the-curve increase proportionally.

Lepirudin is thought to be metabolized by release of amino acids via catabolic hydrolysis of the parent drug. However, conclusive data are not available. About 48% of the administered dose is excreted in the urine which consists of unchanged drug (35%) and other fragments of the parent drug. The systemic clearance of lepirudin is proportional to the glomerular filtration rate or creatinine clearance. Dose adjustment based on creatinine clearance is recommended (see DOSAGE AND ADMINISTRATION: Monitoring and Adjusting Therapy; Use in Renal Impairment). In patients with marked renal insufficiency (creatinine clearance below 15 mL/min) and on hemodialysis, elimination half-lives are prolonged up to 2 days.

The systemic clearance of lepirudin in women is about 25% lower than in men. In elderly patients, the systemic clearance of lepirudin is 20% lower than in younger patients. This may be explained by the lower creatinine clearance in elderly patients compared to younger patients.

Table 1 summarizes systemic clearance (Cl) and volume of distribution at steady state (Vss) of lepirudin for various study populations.

Table 1: Systemic clearance (Cl) and volume of distribution at steady state (Vss) of lepirudin

	Cl (mL/min) Mean (% CV*)	Vss (L) Mean (% CV*)
Healthy young subjects (n = 18, age 18–60 years)	164 (19.3%)	12.2 (16.4%)
Healthy elderly subjects (n = 10, age 65–80 years)	139 (22.5%)	18.7 (20.6%)
Renally impaired patients (n = 16, creatinine clearance below 80 mL/min)	61 (89.4%)	18.0 (41.1%)
HIT† patients (n = 73)	114 (46.8%)	32.1 (98.9%)

* CV: Coefficient of variation
†HIT: Heparin-induced thrombocytopenia

Pharmacodynamic Properties

The pharmacodynamic effect of REFLUDAN on the proteolytic activity of thrombin was routinely assessed as an increase in aPTT. This was observed with increasing plasma concentrations of lepirudin, with no saturable effect up to the highest tested dose (0.5 mg/kg body weight intravenous bolus). Thrombin time (TT) frequently exceeded 200 seconds even at low plasma concentrations of lepirudin, which renders this test unsuitable for routine monitoring of REFLUDAN therapy.

The pharmacodynamic response defined by the aPTT ratio (aPTT at a time after REFLUDAN administration over an aPTT reference value, usually median of the laboratory normal range for aPTT) depends on plasma drug levels which in turn depend on the individual patient's renal function (see CLINICAL PHARMACOLOGY: Pharmacokinetic Properties). For patients undergoing additional thrombolysis, elevated aPTT ratios were already observed at low lepirudin plasma concentrations, and further response to increasing plasma concentrations was relatively flat. In other populations, the response was steeper. At plasma concentrations of 1500 ng/mL, aPTT ratios were nearly 3.0 for healthy volunteers, 2.3 for patients with heparin-induced thrombocytopenia, and 2.1 for patients with deep venous thrombosis.

CLINICAL TRIAL DATA

Heparin-induced thrombocytopenia (HIT) is described as an allergy-like adverse reaction to heparin. It can be found in about 1% to 2% of patients treated with heparin for more than 4 days. The clinical picture of HIT is characterized by thrombocytopenia alone or in combination with thromboembolic complications (TECs). These complications comprise the entire spectrum of venous and arterial thromboembolism including deep venous thrombosis, pulmonary embolism, myocardial infarction, ischemic stroke, and occlusion of limb arteries, which may ultimately result in necroses requiring amputation. Furthermore, there is evidence to suggest that warfarin-induced venous limb gangrene may be associated with HIT. Without further treatment, the mortality in HIT patients with new TECs is about 20% to 30% (*Fondu 1995; Greinacher 1995; Warkentin, Chong, et al., Warkentin, Elavathil, et al. 1997*).

The conclusion that REFLUDAN is an effective treatment for HIT is based upon the data of two prospective, historically controlled clinical trials ("HAT-1" study and "HAT-2" study). The trials were comparable with regard to study design, primary and secondary objectives, and dosing regimens, as well as general study outline and organization. They both used the same historical control group for comparison. This historical control was mainly compiled from a recent retrospective registry of HIT patients.

Overall, 198 (HAT-1: 82, HAT-2: 116) patients were treated with REFLUDAN and 182 historical control patients were treated with other therapies. All except 5 (HAT-1: 1, HAT-2: 4) prospective patients and all historical control patients were diagnosed with HIT using the heparin-induced platelet activation assay (HIPAA) or equivalent assays for testing. In total, 113 (HAT-1: 54, HAT-2: 59) prospective patients ("REFLUDAN") and 91 historical control patients ("historical control") presented with TECs at baseline (day of positive test result) and qualified for direct comparison of clinical endpoints.

The gender distribution was found to be similar in REFLUDAN patients and historical control patients. Overall, REFLUDAN patients tended to be younger than histor-

Continued on next page

Refludan—Cont.

ical control patients. Table 2 summarizes the demographic baseline characteristics of patients presenting with TECs at baseline.

Table 2: Demographic baseline characteristics of patients presenting with TECs

	REFLUDAN		Historical Control
	HAT-1 (n = 54)	HAT-2 (n = 59)	(n = 91)
Males	27.8%	44.1%	35.2%
Females	72.2%	55.9%	64.8%
Age <65 years	63.0%	67.8%	44.0%
Age ≥65 years	37.0%	32.2%	56.0%
Mean age ± SD (years)	57 ± 17	58 ± 12	64 ± 14

The key criteria of efficacy from a laboratory standpoint (n = 115 evaluable patients) were platelet recovery (increase in platelet count by at least 30% of nadir to values >100,000) and effective anticoagulation (aPTT ratio >1.5 with a maximum total 40% increase in the initial infusion rate). The proportions of REFLUDAN patients presenting with TECs at baseline who showed platelet recovery, effective anticoagulation, or both (laboratory responders) are shown in Table 3. Comparable rates for the historical control group cannot be given, because (1) platelet counts were not monitored as closely as in the REFLUDAN group, and (2) most historical control patients did not receive therapies affecting aPTT.

Table 3: Proportions of laboratory responders among REFLUDAN patients presenting with TECs

	HAT-1	HAT-2
Number of evaluable patients	55	60
Platelet recovery	90.9%	95.0%
Effective anticoagulation	81.8%	75.0%
Both	72.7%	71.7%

Comparisons of clinical efficacy were made between REFLUDAN patients and historical control patients with regard to the combined and individual incidences of death, limb amputation, or new TEC.

The original main analyses included all events that occurred after laboratory confirmation of HIT. This approach was revealed to be substantially confounded by the relative contribution of the pretreatment period (time between laboratory confirmation of HIT and start of treatment). Although short in duration (mean length 1.5 days in HAT-1 and 2.0 days in HAT-2), the pretreatment period accounted for 45% and 26% of events observed in the main analyses of HAT-1 REFLUDAN patients and HAT-2 REFLUDAN patients, respectively. Therefore, initiation of treatment was set as the starting point for the analyses. For the historical control group, the first treatment selected within 2 days of laboratory confirmation of HIT was used for reference.

Seven days after start of treatment, the cumulative risk of death, limb amputation, or new TEC was 3.7% in the HAT-1 REFLUDAN patients and 16.9% in the HAT-2 REFLUDAN patients, as compared to 24.9% in the historical control group. At 35 days, when approximately 10% of patients were still at risk, the cumulative risk was 13.0% in the HAT-1 REFLUDAN patients and 28.9% in the HAT-2 REFLUDAN patients, as compared to 47.8% in the historical control group.

In an additional meta-analysis, the pooled REFLUDAN patients of the HAT-1 and HAT-2 studies who presented with TECs at baseline were compared to the respective historical control patients. Seven and 35 days after start of treatment, the cumulative risks of death were 4.4% and 8.9% in the REFLUDAN group, as compared to 1.4% and 17.6% in the historical control group. The cumulative risks of limb amputation were 2.7% and 6.5% in the REFLUDAN group, as compared to 2.6% and 10.4% in the historical control group. Most importantly, the cumulative risks of new TEC were 6.3% and 10.1% in the REFLUDAN group, as compared to 22.2% and 27.2% in the historical control group. As shown in Fig 1, the differences in the cumulative risk of death, limb amputation, or new TEC between the groups were statistically significant in favor of REFLUDAN in the analysis of time to event (P = 0.004 according to log-rank test).

[See figure 1 below]

The immediate impact of treatment on the combined risk of death, limb amputation, or new TEC is demonstrated by comparing pretreatment period and treatment period in regard to average combined event rates per patient day. In the pretreatment period, these rates were found to be 0.075 in the HAT-1 REFLUDAN patients, 0.052 in the HAT-2 REFLUDAN patients, and 0.040 in the historical control group. In the treatment period, the rates showed a marked reduction in the REFLUDAN patients, where they dropped to 0.005 (HAT-1) and to 0.018 (HAT-2), while there was only a moderate decrease to 0.030 in the historical control group. In conclusion, REFLUDAN substantially reduced the risk of serious sequelae of HIT in comparison to a historical control group.

INDICATIONS AND USAGE

REFLUDAN is indicated for anticoagulation in patients with heparin-induced thrombocytopenia (HIT) and associated thromboembolic disease in order to prevent further thromboembolic complications.

CONTRAINDICATIONS

REFLUDAN is contraindicated in patients with known hypersensitivity to hirudins.

WARNINGS

Hemorrhagic Events

Intracranial bleeding following concomitant thrombolytic therapy with rt-PA or streptokinase may be life-threatening (see also ADVERSE REACTIONS: Adverse Events Reported in Other Populations; Intracranial Bleeding).

For patients with increased risk of bleeding, a careful assessment weighing the risk of REFLUDAN administration vs its anticipated benefit has to be made by the treating physician.

In particular, this includes the following conditions:

- **Recent puncture of large vessels or organ biopsy**
- **Anomaly of vessels or organs**
- **Recent cerebrovascular accident, stroke, intracerebral surgery, or other neuraxial procedures**
- **Severe uncontrolled hypertension**
- **Bacterial endocarditis**
- **Advanced renal impairment (see also WARNINGS: Renal Impairment)**
- **Hemorrhagic diathesis**
- **Recent major surgery**
- **Recent major bleeding (eg, intracranial, gastrointestinal, intraocular, or pulmonary bleeding)**

Renal Impairment

With renal impairment, relative overdose might occur even with standard dosage regimen. Therefore, the bolus dose and the rate of infusion must be reduced in patients with known or suspected renal insufficiency (see CLINICAL PHARMACOLOGY: Pharmacokinetic Properties and DOSAGE AND ADMINISTRATION: Monitoring and Adjusting Therapy; Use in Renal Impairment).

PRECAUTIONS

General

Antibodies. Formation of antihirudin antibodies was observed in about 40% of HIT patients treated with REFLUDAN. This may increase the anticoagulant effect of REFLUDAN possibly due to delayed renal elimination of active lepirudin-antihirudin complexes (see also PRECAUTIONS: Animal Pharmacology and Toxicology). Therefore, strict monitoring of aPTT is necessary also during prolonged therapy (see also PRECAUTIONS: Laboratory Tests and DOSAGE AND ADMINISTRATION: Monitoring and Adjusting Therapy; Standard Recommendations). No evidence of neutralization of REFLUDAN or of allergic reactions associated with positive antibody test results was found.

Liver Injury. Serious liver injury (eg, liver cirrhosis) may enhance the anticoagulant effect of REFLUDAN due to coagulation defects secondary to reduced generation of vitamin K-dependent coagulation factors.

Reexposure. Clinical trials have provided limited information to support any recommendations for reexposure to REFLUDAN. A total of 13 patients were reexposed in the HAT-1 and HAT-2 studies. One of these patients experienced a mild allergic skin reaction during the second treatment cycle. No further adverse experience was observed in relation to reexposure.

Laboratory Tests

In general, the dosage (infusion rate) should be adjusted according to the aPTT ratio (patient aPTT at a given time over an aPTT reference value, usually median of the laboratory normal range for aPTT); for full information, see DOSAGE AND ADMINISTRATION: Monitoring and Adjusting Therapy; Standard Recommendations. Other thrombin-dependent coagulation assays are changed by REFLUDAN (see also DESCRIPTION).

Drug Interactions

Concomitant treatment with thrombolytics (eg, rt-PA or streptokinase) may:

- increase the risk of bleeding complications
- considerably enhance the effect of REFLUDAN on aPTT prolongation

(See also WARNINGS: Hemorrhagic Events, ADVERSE REACTIONS: Adverse Events Reported in Other Populations; Intracranial Bleeding and DOSAGE AND ADMINISTRATION: Monitoring and Adjusting Therapy; Concomitant Use With Thrombolytic Therapy)

Concomitant treatment with coumarin derivatives (vitamin K antagonists) and drugs that affect platelet function may also increase the risk of bleeding (see also DOSAGE AND ADMINISTRATION: Monitoring and Adjusting Therapy; Use in Patients Scheduled for a Switch to Oral Anticoagulation).

Animal Pharmacology and Toxicology

General Toxicity. Lepirudin caused bleeding in animal toxicity studies. Antibodies against hirudin which appeared in several monkeys treated with lepirudin resulted in a prolongation of the terminal half-life and an increase of AUC plasma values of lepirudin.

Carcinogenesis, Mutagenesis, Impairment of Fertility. Long-term animal studies to evaluate the potential for carcinogenesis have not been performed with lepirudin. Lepirudin was not genotoxic in the Ames test, the Chinese hamster cell (V79/HGPRT) forward mutation test, the A549 human cell line unscheduled DNA synthesis (UDS) test, the Chinese hamster V79 cell chromosome aberration test, or the mouse micronucleus test. An effect on fertility and reproductive performance of male and female rats was not seen with lepirudin at intravenous doses up to 30 mg/kg/day (180 mg/m^2/day, 1.2 times the recommended maximum human total daily dose based on body surface area of 1.45m^2 for a 50 kg subject).

Pregnancy

Teratogenic Effects: Category B. Teratology studies with lepirudin performed in pregnant rats at intravenous doses up to 30 mg/kg/day (180 mg/m^2/day, 1.2 times the recommended maximum human total daily dose based on body surface area) and in pregnant rabbits at intravenous doses up to 30 mg/kg/day (360 mg/m^2/day, 2.4 times the recommended maximum human total daily dose based on body surface area) have revealed no evidence of harm to the fetus due to lepirudin. There are, however, no adequate and well-controlled studies in pregnant women. Because animal reproduction studies are not always predictive of human response, this drug should be used during pregnancy only if clearly needed.

Lepirudin (1 mg/kg) by intravenous administration crosses the placental barrier in pregnant rats. It is not known whether the drug crosses the placental barrier in humans. Following intravenous administration of lepirudin at 30 mg/kg/day (180 mg/m^2/day, 1.2 times the recommended maximum human total daily dose based on body surface area) during organogenesis and perinatal-postnatal periods, pregnant rats showed an increased maternal mortality due to undetermined causes.

Nursing Mothers

It is not known whether REFLUDAN is excreted in human milk. Because many drugs are excreted in human milk and because of the potential for serious adverse reactions in nursing infants from REFLUDAN, a decision should be made whether to discontinue nursing or to discontinue the drug, taking into account the importance of the drug to the mother.

Pediatric Use

Safety and effectiveness in pediatric patients have not been established. In the HAT-2 study, two children, an 11-year-old girl and a 12-year-old boy, were treated with REFLUDAN. Both children presented with TECs at baseline. REFLUDAN doses given ranged from 0.15 mg/kg/h to 0.22 mg/kg/h for the girl, and from 0.1 mg/kg/h (in conjunction with urokinase) to 0.7 mg/kg/h for the boy. Treatment

Fig 1: Cumulative risk of death, limb amputation, or new thromboembolic complication after start of treatment

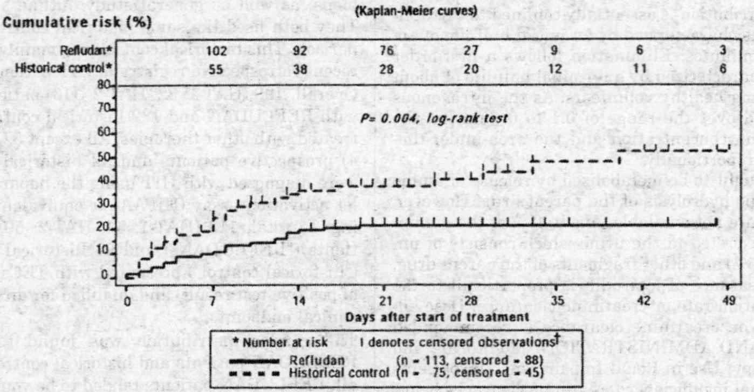

with REFLUDAN was completed after 8 and 58 days, respectively, without serious adverse events (*Schiffmann 1997*).

ADVERSE REACTIONS

Adverse Events Reported in HIT Patients

The following safety information is based on all 198 patients treated with REFLUDAN in the HAT-1 and HAT-2 studies. The safety profile of 113 REFLUDAN patients from these studies who presented with TECs at baseline is compared to 91 such patients in the historical control.

Hemorrhagic Events. Bleeding was the most frequent adverse event observed in patients treated with REFLUDAN. Table 4 gives an overview of all hemorrhagic events which occurred in at least two patients.

Table 4: Hemorrhagic Events*

	HAT-1 HAT-2 (All patients) (n = 198)	Patients with TECs	
		REFLUDAN (n = 113)	Historical control (n = 91)
Bleeding from puncture sites and wounds	14.1%	10.6%	4.4%
Anemia or isolated drop in hemoglobin	13.1%	12.4%	1.1%
Other hematoma and unclassified bleeding	11.1%	10.6%	4.4%
Hematuria	6.6%	4.4%	0
Gastrointestinal and rectal bleeding	5.1%	5.3%	6.6%
Epistaxis	3.0%	4.4%	1.1%
Hemothorax	3.0%	0	1.1%
Vaginal bleeding	1.5%	1.8%	0
Intracranial bleeding	0	0	2.2%

***Patients may have suffered more than one event.**

Other hemorrhagic events (hemoperitoneum, hemoptysis, liver bleeding, lung bleeding, mouth bleeding, retroperitoneal bleeding) each occurred in one individual among all 198 patients treated with REFLUDAN.

Nonhemorrhagic events. Table 5 gives an overview of the most frequently observed nonhemorrhagic events.

Table 5: Nonhemorrhagic adverse events*

	HAT-1 HAT-2 (All patients) (n = 198)	Patients with TECs	
		REFLUDAN (n = 113)	Historical control (n = 91)
Fever	6.1%	4.4%	8.8%
Abnormal liver function	6.1%	5.3%	0
Pneumonia	4.0%	4.4%	5.5%
Sepsis	4.0%	3.5%	5.5%
Allergic skin reactions	3.0%	3.5%	1.1%
Heart failure	3.0%	1.8%	2.2%
Abnormal kidney function	2.5%	1.8%	4.4%
Unspecified infections	2.5%	1.8%	1.1%
Multiorgan failure	2.0%	3.5%	0
Pericardial effusion	1.0%	0	1.1%
Ventricular fibrillation	1.0%	0	0

***Patients may have suffered more than one event.**

Adverse Events Reported in Other Populations

The following safety information is based on a total of 2302 individuals who were treated with REFLUDAN in clinical pharmacology studies (n = 323) or for clinical indications other than HIT (n = 1979).

Intracranial Bleeding. Intracranial bleeding was the most serious adverse reaction found in populations other than HIT patients. However, it only occurred in patients with acute myocardial infarction who were started on both REFLUDAN and thrombolytic therapy with rt-PA or streptokinase. The overall frequency of this potentially life-threatening complication among patients receiving both REFLUDAN and thrombolytic therapy was 0.6% (7 out of 1134 patients). No intracranial bleeding was observed in 1168 subjects or patients who did not receive concomitant thrombolysis.

Allergic Reactions. Allergic reactions or suspected allergic reactions in populations other than HIT patients include (in descending order of frequency*):

- Airway reactions (cough, bronchospasm, stridor, dyspnea): common
- Unspecified allergic reactions: uncommon
- Skin reactions (pruritus, urticaria, rash, flushes, chills): uncommon
- General reactions (anaphylactoid or anaphylactic reactions): uncommon
- Edema (facial edema, tongue edema, larynx edema, angioedema): rare

* The CIOMS (Council for International Organization of Medical Sciences) III standard categories are used for classification of frequencies:

very common	10% or more
common (frequent)	1 to <10%
uncommon (infrequent)	0.1 to <1%
rare	0.01 to <0.1%
very rare	0.01% or less

About 53% (n = 46) of all allergic reactions or suspected allergic reactions occurred in patients who concomitantly received thrombolytic therapy (eg, streptokinase) for acute myocardial infarction and/or contrast media for coronary angiography.

OVERDOSAGE

In case of overdose (eg, suggested by excessively high aPTT values) the risk of bleeding is increased.

No specific antidote for REFLUDAN is available. If life-threatening bleeding occurs and excessive plasma levels of lepirudin are suspected, the following steps should be followed:

- Immediately STOP REFLUDAN administration
- Determine aPTT and other coagulation levels as appropriate
- Determine hemoglobin and prepare for blood transfusion
- Follow the current guidelines for treating patients with shock

Individual clinical case reports and in vitro data suggest that either hemofiltration or hemodialysis (using high-flux dialysis membranes with a cutoff point of 50,000 daltons, eg, AN/69) may be useful in this situation.

In studies in pigs, the application of von Willebrand Factor (vWF, 66 IU/kg body weight) markedly reduced the bleeding time. The clinical significance of this data is unknown.

DOSAGE AND ADMINISTRATION

Initial Dosage

Anticoagulation in adult patients with HIT and associated thromboembolic disease:

- 0.4 mg/kg body weight (up to 110 kg) slowly intravenously (eg, over 15 to 20 seconds) as a bolus dose,
- followed by 0.15 mg/kg body weight (up to 110 kg)/hour as a continuous intravenous infusion for 2 to 10 days or longer if clinically needed.

Normally the initial dosage depends on the patient's body weight. This is valid up to a body weight of 110 kg. In patients with a body weight exceeding 110 kg, the initial dosage should not be increased beyond the 110 kg body weight dose (maximal initial bolus dose of 44 mg, maximal initial infusion dose of 16.5 mg/h; see also DOSAGE AND ADMINISTRATION: Administration; Initial Intravenous Bolus, Table 7 and DOSAGE AND ADMINISTRATION: Administration; Intravenous Infusion, Table 8).

In general, therapy with REFLUDAN is monitored using the aPTT ratio (patient aPTT at a given time over an aPTT reference value, usually median of the laboratory normal range for aPTT, see DOSAGE AND ADMINISTRATION: Monitoring and Adjusting Therapy; Standard Recommendations). A patient baseline aPTT should be determined prior to initiation of therapy with REFLUDAN, since REFLUDAN should not be started in patients presenting with a baseline aPTT ratio of 2.5 or more, in order to avoid initial overdosing.

Monitoring and Adjusting Therapy

Standard Recommendations.

Monitoring.

- **In general, the dosage (infusion rate) should be adjusted according to the aPTT ratio (patient aPTT at a given time over an aPTT reference value, usually median of the laboratory normal range for aPTT).**
- **The target range for the aPTT ratio during treatment (therapeutic window) should be 1.5 to 2.5. Data from clinical trials in HIT patients suggest that with aPTT ratios higher than this target range, the risk of bleeding increases, while there is no incremental increase in clinical efficacy.**
- **As stated in DOSAGE AND ADMINISTRATION: Initial Dosage, REFLUDAN should not be started in patients presenting with a baseline aPTT ratio of 2.5 or more, in order to avoid initial overdosing.**
- **The first aPTT determination for monitoring treatment should be done 4 hours after start of the REFLUDAN infusion.**
- **Follow-up aPTT determinations are recommended at least once daily, as long as treatment with REFLUDAN is ongoing.**
- **More frequent aPTT monitoring is highly recommended in patients with renal impairment or serious liver injury (see DOSAGE AND ADMINISTRATION: Monitoring and Adjusting Therapy; Use in Renal Impairment) or with an increased risk of bleeding.**

Dose Modifications.

- **Any aPTT ratio out of the target range is to be confirmed at once before drawing conclusions with respect to dose modifications, unless there is a clinical need to react immediately.**
- **If the confirmed aPTT ratio is above the target range, the infusion should be stopped for two hours. At restart, the infusion rate should be decreased by 50% (no additional intravenous bolus should be administered). The aPTT ratio should be determined again 4 hours later.**
- **If the confirmed aPTT ratio is below the target range, the infusion rate should be increased in steps of 20%. The aPTT ratio should be determined again 4 hours later.**
- **In general, an infusion rate of 0.21 mg/kg/h should not be exceeded without checking for coagulation abnormalities which might be preventive of an appropriate aPTT response.**

Use in Renal Impairment.

As REFLUDAN is almost exclusively excreted in the kidneys (see also CLINICAL PHARMACOLOGY: Pharmacokinetic Properties), individual renal function should be considered prior to administration. In case of renal impairment, relative overdose might occur even with the standard dosage regimen. Therefore, the bolus dose and the infusion rate must be reduced in case of known or suspected renal insufficiency (creatinine clearance below 60 mL/min or serum creatinine above 1.5 mg/dL).

There is only limited information on the therapeutic use of REFLUDAN in HIT patients with significant renal impairment. The following dosage recommendations are mainly based on single-dose studies in a small number of patients with renal impairment. Therefore, these recommendations are only tentative.

Dose adjustments should be based on creatinine clearance values, whenever available, as obtained from a reliable method (24 h urine sampling). If creatinine clearance is not available, the dose adjusments should be based on the serum creatinine.

In all patients with renal insufficiency, the bolus dose is to be reduced to 0.2 mg/kg body weight.

The standard initial infusion rate given in DOSAGE AND ADMINISTRATION: Initial Dosage and DOSAGE AND ADMINISTRATION: Administration; Intravenous Infusion, Table 8 must be reduced according to the recommendations given in Table 6. Additional aPTT monitoring is highly recommended.

Table 6: Reduction of infusion rate in patients with renal impairment

Creatinine clearance [mL/min]	Serum creatinine [mg/dL]	Adjusted infusion rate [% of standard initial infusion rate]	[mg/kg/h]
45–60	1.6–2.0	50%	0.075
30–44	2.1–3.0	30%	0.045
15–29	3.1–6.0	15%	0.0225
below 15*	above 6.0*	avoid or STOP infusion!*	

*In hemodialysis patients or in case of acute renal failure (creatinine clearance below 15 mL/min or serum creatinine above 6.0 mg/dL), infusion of REFLUDAN is to be avoided or stopped. Additional intravenous bolus doses of 0.1 mg/kg body weight should be considered every other day only if the aPTT ratio falls below the lower therapeutic limit of 1.5 (see also DOSAGE AND ADMINISTRATION: Monitoring and Adjusting Therapy; Standard Recommendations).

Concomitant Use With Thrombolytic Therapy.

Clinical trials in HIT patients have provided only limited information on the combined use of REFLUDAN and thrombolytic agents. The following dosage regimen of REFLUDAN was used in a total of 9 HIT patients in the HAT-1 and HAT-2 studies who presented with TECs at baseline and were started on both REFLUDAN and thrombolytic therapy (rt-PA, urokinase or streptokinase):

- Initial intravenous bolus: 0.2 mg/kg body weight
- Continuous intravenous infusion: 0.1 mg/kg body weight/h

The number of patients receiving combined therapy was too small to identify differences in clinical outcome of patients who were started on both REFLUDAN and thrombolytic therapy as compared to those who were started on REFLUDAN alone. The combined incidences of death, limb amputation, or new TEC were 22.2% and 20.7%, respectively. While there was a 47% relative increase in the over-

Continued on next page

Refludan—Cont.

all bleeding rate in patients who were started on both REFLUDAN and thrombolytic therapy (55.6% vs 37.9%), there were no differences in the rates of serious bleeding events (fatal or life-threatening bleeds, bleeds that were permanently or significantly disabling, overt bleeds requiring transfusion of 2 or more units of packed red blood cells, bleeds necessitating surgical intervention, intracranial bleeds) between the groups (11.1% vs 11.2%). Although no intracranial bleeding has been observed in any of these patients, the risk of this potentially life-threatening complication may be increased in conjunction with thrombolytic agents (see ADVERSE REACTIONS: Adverse Events Reported in Other Populations; Intracranial Bleeding).

Special attention should be paid to the fact that thrombolytic agents per se may increase the aPTT ratio. Therefore, aPTT ratios with a given plasma level of lepirudin are usually higher in patients who receive concomitant thrombolysis than in those who do not (see also CLINICAL PHARMACOLOGY: Pharmacodynamic Properties).

Use in Patients Scheduled for a Switch to Oral Anticoagulation.

If a patient is scheduled to receive coumarin derivatives (vitamin K antagonists) for oral anticoagulation after REFLUDAN therapy, the dose of REFLUDAN should first be gradually reduced in order to reach an aPTT ratio just above 1.5 before initiating oral anticoagulation. As soon as an international normalized ratio (INR) of 2.0 is reached, REFLUDAN therapy should be stopped.

Administration

Directions on Preparation and Dilution.

REFLUDAN should not be mixed with other drugs except for Sterile Water for Injection USP, 0.9% Sodium Chloride Injection USP or 5% Dextrose Injection.

Use REFLUDAN before the expiration date given on the carton and container.

Reconstitution and further dilution are to be carried out under sterile conditions:

- For reconstitution, Sterile Water for Injection USP or 0.9% Sodium Chloride Injection USP are to be used.
- For further dilution, 0.9% Sodium Chloride Injection USP or 5% Dextrose Injection are suitable.
- For rapid, complete reconstitution, inject 1 mL of diluent into the vial and shake it gently. After reconstitution a clear, colorless solution is usually obtained in a few seconds, but definitely in less than 3 minutes.
- Parenteral drug products should be inspected visually for particulate matter and discoloration prior to administration whenever solution and container permit. Do not use solutions that are cloudy or contain particles.
- The reconstituted solution is to be used immediately. It remains stable for up to 24 hours at room temperature (eg, during infusion).
- The preparation should be warmed to room temperature before administration.
- Discard any unused solution appropriately.

Initial Intravenous Bolus.

For intravenous bolus injection, use a solution with a concentration of 5 mg/mL.

Preparation of a REFLUDAN solution with a concentration of 5 mg/mL:

- Reconstitute one vial (50 mg of lepirudin) with 1 mL of Sterile Water for Injection USP or 0.9% Sodium Chloride Injection USP.
- The final concentration of 5 mg/mL is obtained by transferring the contents of the vial into a sterile, single-use syringe (of at least 10 mL capacity) and diluting the solution to a total volume of 10 mL, using Sterile Water for Injection USP, 0.9% Sodium Chloride Injection USP or 5% Dextrose Injection.
- The final solution is to be administered according to body weight (see Table 7 below and DOSAGE AND ADMINISTRATION: Initial Dosage).

Intravenous injection of the bolus is to be carried out slowly (eg, over 15 to 20 seconds).

Table 7: Standard bolus injection volumes according to body weight for a 5 mg/mL concentration

Body Weight [kg]	Injection volume	
	Dosage 0.4 mg/kg	Dosage 0.2 mg/kg*
50	4.0 mL	2.0 mL
60	4.8 mL	2.4 mL
70	5.6 mL	2.8 mL
80	6.4 mL	3.2 mL
90	7.2 mL	3.6 mL
100	8.0 mL	4.0 mL
≥110	8.8 mL	4.4 mL

*Dosage recommended for all patients with renal insufficiency (see DOSAGE AND ADMINISTRATION: Monitoring and Adjusting Therapy; Use in Renal Impairment)

Intravenous Infusion

For continuous intravenous infusion, solutions with concentration of 0.2 mg/mL or 0.4 mg/mL may be used.

Preparation of a REFLUDAN solution with a concentration of 0.2 or 0.4 mg/mL:

- Reconstitute two vials (each containing 50 mg of lepirudin) with 1 mL each using either Sterile Water for Injection USP or 0.9% Sodium Chloride Injection USP.
- The final concentrations of 0.2 mg/mL or 0.4 mg/mL are obtained by transferring the contents of both vials into an infusion bag containing 500 mL or 250 mL of 0.9% Sodium Chloride Injection USP or 5% Dextrose Injection.

The infusion rate [mL/h] is to be set according to body weight (see Table 8 below and DOSAGE AND ADMINISTRATION: Initial Dosage).

Table 8: Standard infusion rates according to body weight

Body Weight [kg]	Infusion rate at 0.15 mg/kg/h	
	500-mL infusion bag 0.2 mg/mL	250-mL infusion bag 0.4 mg/mL
50	38 mL/h	19 mL/h
60	45 mL/h	23 mL/h
70	53 mL/h	26 mL/h
80	60 mL/h	30 mL/h
90	68 mL/h	34 mL/h
100	75 mL/h	38 mL/h
≥110	83 mL/h	41 mL/h

HOW SUPPLIED

REFLUDAN [lepirudin (rDNA) for injection] is supplied in boxes of 10 vials, each vial containing 50 mg lepirudin (NDC 0088-2150-57). STORE UNOPENED VIALS AT 2 to 25°C (36 to 77°F). USE REFLUDAN BEFORE THE EXPIRATION DATE GIVEN ON THE CARTON AND CONTAINER. ONCE RECONSTITUTED, USE REFLUDAN IMMEDIATELY.

REFERENCES

1. Fondu P. Heparin associated thrombocytopenia: an update. *Acta Clinica Belgica. 1995;50(6):343–357.*
2. Greinacher A. Antigen generation in heparin-associated thrombocytopenia: the nonimmunologic type and the immunologic type are closely linked in their pathogenesis. *Seminars Thromb Hemost. 1995;21:106–116.*
3. Roethig HJ, Maree JS, Meyer BH. Clinical pharmacology of hirudin (HBW 023). In: Reidenberg, MM ed. *The clinical pharmacology of biotechnology products.* Elsevier Publishers; 1991:227–236.
4. Schiffmann H, Unterhalt M, Harms K, Figula HR, Voelpel H, Greinacher A. Successful treatment of heparin-induced thrombocytopenia (HIT) type II in childhood with recombinant hirudin. *Monatsschr Kinderheilkd.* 1997; 145:606–612.
5. Warkentin TE, Chong BH, Greinacher A. Heparin-induced thrombocytopenia: towards consensus. *Thromb Haemostas.* 1998; 79:1–7.
6. Warkentin TE, Elavathil LJ, Hayward CPM, Johnston MA, Russett JI, Kelton JG. The pathogenesis of venous limb gangrene associated with heparin-induced thrombocytopenia. *Ann Intern Med. 1997; 127:804–812.*

Prescribing Information as of October 1998

Manufactured by:
Hoechst Marion Roussel
Deutschland GmbH
D-65926 Frankfurt am Main
Germany

Manufactured for:
Hoechst Marion Roussel, Inc.
Kansas City, MO 64137
www.hmri.com

RIFADIN® ℞

[*rĭf' uh-din*]
(rifampin capsules USP)
and
RIFADIN® IV
(rifampin for injection USP)

Prescribing Information as of June 1999

DESCRIPTION

RIFADIN (rifampin capsules USP) for oral administration contain 150 mg or 300 mg of rifampin per capsule. The 150 mg and 300 mg capsules also contain, as inactive ingredients: corn starch, D&C Red No. 28, FD&C Blue No. 1, FD&C Red No. 40, gelatin, magnesium stearate, and titanium dioxide.

RIFADIN IV (rifampin for injection USP) contains rifampin 600 mg, sodium formaldehyde sulfoxylate 10 mg, and sodium hydroxide to adjust pH.

Rifampin is a semisynthetic antibiotic derivative of rifamycin SV. Rifampin is a red-brown crystalline powder very slightly soluble in water at neutral pH, freely soluble in chloroform, soluble in ethyl acetate and in methanol. Its molecular weight is 822.95 and its chemical formula is $C_{43}H_{58}N_4O_{12}$. The chemical name for rifampin is either:

3-[[(4-Methyl-1-piperazinyl)imino]methyl]rifamycin

or

5,6,9,17,19,21-hexahydroxy-23-methoxy-2,4,12,16,20,22-heptamethyl-8-[N-(4-methyl-1-piperazinyl)formimidoyl]-2,7-(epoxypentadeca [1,11,13]trienimino)naphtho[2,1-*b*] furan-1,11(2H)-dione 21-acetate.

Its structural formula is:

CLINICAL PHARMACOLOGY

Oral Administration

Rifampin is readily absorbed from the gastrointestinal tract. Peak serum concentrations in healthy adults and pediatric populations vary widely from individual to individual. Following a single 600 mg oral dose of rifampin in healthy adults, the peak serum concentration averages 7 µg/mL but may vary from 4 to 32 µg/mL. Absorption of rifampin is reduced by about 30% when the drug is ingested with food.

Rifampin is widely distributed throughout the body. It is present in effective concentrations in many organs and body fluids, including cerebrospinal fluid. Rifampin is about 80% protein bound. Most of the unbound fraction is not ionized and, therefore, diffuses freely into tissues.

In healthy adults, the mean biological half-life of rifampin in serum averages 3.35 ± 0.66 hours after a 600 mg oral dose, with increases up to 5.08 ± 2.45 hours reported after a 900 mg dose. With repeated administration, the half-life decreases and reaches average values of approximately 2 to 3 hours. The half-life does not differ in patients with renal failure at doses not exceeding 600 mg daily, and consequently, no dosage adjustment is required. Following a single 900 mg oral dose of rifampin in patients with varying degrees of renal insufficiency, the mean half-life increased from 3.6 hours in healthy adults to 5.0, 7.3, and 11.0 hours in patients with glomerular filtration rates of 30 to 50 mL/min, less than 30 mL/min, and in anuric patients, respectively. Refer to the WARNINGS section for information regarding patients with hepatic insufficiency.

Rifampin is rapidly eliminated in the bile, and an enterohepatic circulation ensues. During this process, rifampin undergoes progressive deacetylation so that nearly all the drug in the bile is in this form in about 6 hours. This metabolite is microbiologically active. Intestinal reabsorption is reduced by deacetylation, and elimination is facilitated. Up to 30% of a dose is excreted in the urine, with about half of this being unchanged drug.

Intravenous Administration

After intravenous administration of a 300 or 600 mg dose of rifampin infused over 30 minutes to healthy male volunteers (n=12), mean peak plasma concentrations were 9.0 ± 3.0 and 17.5 ± 5.0 µg/mL, respectively. Total body clearance after the 300 and 600 mg IV doses were 0.19 ± 0.06 and 0.14 ± 0.03 L/hr/kg, respectively. Volumes of distribution at steady state were 0.66 ± 0.14 and 0.64 ± 0.11 L/kg for the 300 and 600 mg IV doses, respectively. After intravenous administration of 300 or 600 mg doses, rifampin plasma concentrations in these volunteers remained detectable for 8 and 12 hours, respectively (see Table).

[See table at bottom of next page]

Plasma concentrations after the 600 mg dose, which were disproportionately higher (up to 30% greater than expected) than those found after the 300 mg dose, indicated that the elimination of larger doses was not as rapid.

After repeated once-a-day infusions (3 hr duration) of 600 mg in patients (n=5) for 7 days, concentrations of IV rifampin decreased from 5.81 ± 3.38 µg/mL 8 hours after the infusion on day 1 to 2.6 ± 1.88 µg/mL 8 hours after the infusion on day 7.

Rifampin is widely distributed throughout the body. It is present in effective concentrations in many organs and body fluids, including cerebrospinal fluid. Rifampin is about 80% protein bound. Most of the unbound fraction is not ionized and therefore diffuses freely into tissues.

Rifampin is rapidly eliminated in the bile and undergoes progressive enterohepatic circulation and deacetylation to the primary metabolite, 25-desacetyl-rifampin. This metabolite is microbiologically active. Less than 30% of the dose is excreted in the urine as rifampin or metabolites. Serum concentrations do not differ in patients with renal failure at a studied dose of 300 mg and consequently, no dosage adjustment is required.

Pediatrics

Oral Administration. In one study, pediatric patients 6 to 58 months old were given rifampin suspended in simple syrup or as dry powder mixed with applesauce at a dose of 10 mg/kg body weight. Peak serum concentrations of 10.7 ± 3.7 and 11.5 ± 5.1 µg/mL were obtained 1 hour after preprandial ingestion of the drug suspension and the applesauce mixture, respectively. After the administration of either preparation, the $t_{1/2}$ of rifampin averaged 2.9 hours. It should be noted that in other studies in pediatric populations, at doses of 10 mg/kg body weight, mean peak serum concentrations of 3.5 μg/mL to 15 μg/mL have been reported.

Intravenous Administration. In pediatric patients 0.25 to 12.8 years old (n=12), the mean peak serum concentration of rifampin at the end of a 30 minute infusion of approximately 300 mg/m² was 25.9 ± 1.3 μg/mL; individual peak concentrations 1 to 4 days after initiation of therapy ranged from 11.7 to 41.5 μg/mL; individual peak concentrations 5 to 14 days after initiation of therapy were 13.6 to 37.4 μg/mL. The individual serum half-life of rifampin changed from 1.04 to 3.81 hours early in therapy to 1.17 to 3.19 hours 5 to 14 days after therapy was initiated.

Microbiology

Rifampin inhibits DNA-dependent RNA polymerase activity in susceptible cells. Specifically, it interacts with bacterial RNA polymerase but does not inhibit the mammalian enzyme. Rifampin at therapeutic levels has demonstrated bactericidal activity against both intracellular and extracellular *Mycobacterium tuberculosis* organisms.

Organisms resistant to rifampin are likely to be resistant to other rifamycins.

Rifampin has bactericidal activity against slow and intermittently growing *M tuberculosis* organisms. It also has significant activity against *Neisseria meningitidis* isolates (see INDICATIONS AND USAGE).

In the treatment of both tuberculosis and the meningococcal carrier state (see INDICATIONS AND USAGE), the small number of resistant cells present within large populations of susceptible cells can rapidly become predominant. In addition, resistance to rifampin has been determined to occur as single-step mutations of the DNA-dependent RNA polymerase. Since resistance can emerge rapidly, appropriate susceptibility tests should be performed in the event of persistent positive cultures.

Rifampin has been shown to be active against most strains of the following microorganisms, both in vitro and in clinical infections as described in the INDICATIONS AND USAGE section.

Aerobic Gram-Negative Microorganisms:
Neisseria meningitidis

"Other" Microorganisms:
Mycobacterium tuberculosis

The following in vitro data are available, but their clinical significance is unknown.

Rifampin exhibits in vitro activity against most strains of the following microorganisms; however, the safety and effectiveness of rifampin in treating clinical infections due to these microorganisms have not been established in adequate and well-controlled trials.

Aerobic Gram-Positive Microorganisms:
Staphylococcus aureus (including Methicillin-Resistant *S. aureus*/MRSA)
Staphylococcus epidermidis

Aerobic Gram-Negative Microorganisms:
Haemophilus influenzae

"Other" Microorganisms:
Mycobacterium leprae

β-lactamase production should have no effect on rifampin activity.

Susceptibility Tests

Prior to initiation of therapy, appropriate specimens should be collected for identification of the infecting organism and in vitro susceptibility tests.

In vitro testing for *Mycobacterium tuberculosis* isolates:

Two standardized in vitro susceptibility methods are available for testing rifampin against *M tuberculosis* organisms. The agar proportion method (CDC or NCCLS[1] M24-P) utilizes Middlebrook 7H10 medium impregnated with rifampin at a final concentration of 1.0 μg/mL to determine drug resistance. After three weeks of incubation MIC_{99} values are calculated by comparing the quantity of organisms growing in the medium containing drug to the control cultures. Mycobacterial growth in the presence of drug, of at least 1% of the growth in the control culture, indicates resistance.

The radiometric broth method employs the BACTEC 460 machine to compare the growth index from untreated control cultures to cultures grown in the presence of 2.0 μg/mL of rifampin. Strict adherence to the manufacturer's instructions for sample processing and data interpretation is required for this assay.

Susceptibility test results obtained by the two different methods can only be compared if the appropriate rifampin concentration is used for each test method as indicated above. Both procedures require the use of *M tuberculosis* H37Rv ATCC 27294 as a control organism.

The clinical relevance of in vitro susceptibility test results for mycobacterial species other than *M tuberculosis* using either the radiometric or the proportion method has not been determined.

In vitro testing for *Neisseria meningitidis* isolates:

Dilution Techniques: Quantitative methods that are used to determine minimum inhibitory concentrations provide reproducible estimates of the susceptibility of bacteria to antimicrobial compounds. One such standardized procedure uses a standardized dilution method[2,4] (broth, agar, or microdilution) or equivalent with rifampin powder. The MIC values obtained should be interpreted according to the following criteria for *Neisseria meningitidis:*

MIC (μg/mL)	Interpretation
≤1	(S) Susceptible
2	(I) Intermediate
≥4	(R) Resistant

A report of "susceptible" indicates that the pathogen is likely to be inhibited by usually achievable concentrations of the antimicrobial compound in the blood. A report of "intermediate" indicates that the result should be considered equivocal, and if the microorganism is not fully susceptible to alternative, clinically feasible drugs, the test should be repeated. This category implies possible clinical applicability in body sites where the drug is physiologically concentrated or in situations where the maximum acceptable dose of drug can be used. This category also provides a buffer zone that prevents small uncontrolled technical factors from causing major discrepancies in interpretation. A report of "resistant" indicates that usually achievable concentrations of the antimicrobial compound in the blood are unlikely to be inhibitory and that other therapy should be selected.

Measurement of MIC or minimum bactericidal concentrations (MBC) and achieved antimicrobial compound concentrations may be appropriate to guide therapy in some infections. (See CLINICAL PHARMACOLOGY section for further information on drug concentrations achieved in infected body sites and other pharmacokinetic properties of this antimicrobial drug product.)

Standardized susceptibility test procedures require the use of laboratory control microorganisms. The use of these microorganisms does not imply clinical efficacy (see INDICATIONS AND USAGE); they are used to control the technical aspects of the laboratory procedures. Standard rifampin powder should give the following MIC values:

Microorganism		MIC (μg/mL)
Staphylococcus aureus	ATCC 29213	0.008–0.06
Enterococcus faecalis	ATCC 29212	1–4
Escherichia coli	ATCC 25922	8–32
Pseudomonas aeruginosa	ATCC 27853	32–64
Haemophilus influenzae	ATCC 49247	0.25–1

Diffusion Techniques: Quantitative methods that require measurement of zone diameters provide reproducible estimates of the susceptibility of bacteria to antimicrobial compounds. One such standardized procedure[3,4] that has been recommended for use with disks to test the susceptibility of microorganisms to rifampin uses the 5 μg rifampin disk. Interpretation involves correlation of the diameter obtained in the disk test with the MIC for rifampin.

Reports from the laboratory providing results of the standard single-disk susceptibility test with a 5 μg rifampin disk should be interpreted according to the following criteria for *Neisseria meningitidis*:

Zone Diameter (mm)	Interpretation
≥20	(S) Susceptible
17–19	(I) Intermediate
≤16	(R) Resistant

Interpretation should be as stated above for results using dilution techniques.

As with standard dilution techniques, diffusion methods require the use of laboratory control microorganisms. The use of these microorganisms does not imply clinical efficacy (see INDICATIONS AND USAGE); they are used to control the technical aspects of the laboratory procedures. The 5 μg rifampin disk should provide the following zone diameters in these quality control strains:

Microorganism		Zone Diameter (mm)
S. aureus	ATCC 25923	26–34
E. coli	ATCC 25922	8–10
H. influenzae	ATCC 49247	22–30

INDICATIONS AND USAGE

In the treatment of both tuberculosis and the meningococcal carrier state, the small number of resistant cells present within large populations of susceptible cells can rapidly become the predominant type. Bacteriologic cultures should be obtained before the start of therapy to confirm the susceptibility of the organism to rifampin and they should be repeated throughout therapy to monitor the response to treatment. Since resistance can emerge rapidly, susceptibility tests should be performed in the event of persistent positive cultures during the course of treatment. If test results show resistance to rifampin and the patient is not responding to therapy, the drug regimen should be modified.

Tuberculosis

Rifampin is indicated in the treatment of all forms of tuberculosis.

A three-drug regimen consisting of rifampin, isoniazid, and pyrazinamide (eg, RIFATER®) is recommended in the initial phase of short-course therapy which is usually continued for 2 months. The Advisory Council for the Elimination of Tuberculosis, the American Thoracic Society, and Centers for Disease Control and Prevention recommend that either streptomycin or ethambutol be added as a fourth drug in a regimen containing isoniazid (INH), rifampin, and pyrazinamide for initial treatment of tuberculosis unless the likelihood of INH resistance is very low. The need for a fourth drug should be reassessed when the results of susceptibility testing are known. If community rates of INH resistance are currently less than 4%, an initial treatment regimen with less than four drugs may be considered.

Following the initial phase, treatment should be continued with rifampin and isoniazid (eg, RIFAMATE®) for at least 4 months. Treatment should be continued for longer if the patient is still sputum or culture positive, if resistant organisms are present, or if the patient is HIV positive.

RIFADIN IV is indicated for the initial treatment and retreatment of tuberculosis when the drug cannot be taken by mouth.

Meningococcal Carriers

Rifampin is indicated for the treatment of asymptomatic carriers of *Neisseria meningitidis* to eliminate meningococci from the nasopharynx. **Rifampin is not indicated for the treatment of meningococcal infection because of the possibility of the rapid emergence of resistant organisms.** (See WARNINGS.)

Rifampin should not be used indiscriminately, and therefore, diagnostic laboratory procedures, including serotyping and susceptibility testing, should be performed for establishment of the carrier state and the correct treatment. So that the usefulness of rifampin in the treatment of asymptomatic meningococcal carriers is preserved, the drug should be used only when the risk of meningococcal disease is high.

CONTRAINDICATIONS

Rifampin is contraindicated in patients with a history of hypersensitivity to any of the rifamycins. (See WARNINGS.)

WARNINGS

Rifampin has been shown to produce liver dysfunction. Fatalities associated with jaundice have occurred in patients with liver disease and in patients taking rifampin with other hepatotoxic agents. Patients with impaired liver function should be given rifampin only in cases of necessity and then with caution and under strict medical supervision. In these patients, careful monitoring of liver function, especially SGPT/ALT and SGOT/AST should be carried out prior to therapy and then every 2 to 4 weeks during therapy. If signs of hepatocellular damage occur, rifampin should be withdrawn.

In some cases, hyperbilirubinemia resulting from competition between rifampin and bilirubin for excretory pathways of the liver at the cell level can occur in the early days of treatment. An isolated report showing a moderate rise in bilirubin and/or transaminase level is not in itself an indication for interrupting treatment; rather, the decision should be made after repeating the tests, noting trends in the levels, and considering them in conjunction with the patient's clinical condition.

Rifampin has enzyme-inducing properties, including induction of delta amino levulinic acid synthetase. Isolated reports have associated porphyria exacerbation with rifampin administration.

The possibility of rapid emergence of resistant meningococci restricts the use of RIFADIN to short-term treatment of the asymptomatic carrier state. **RIFADIN is not to be used for the treatment of meningococcal disease.**

PRECAUTIONS

General

For the treatment of tuberculosis, rifampin is usually administered on a daily basis. Doses of rifampin greater than 600 mg given once or twice weekly have resulted in a higher incidence of adverse reactions, including the "flu syndrome" (fever, chills and malaise), hematopoietic reactions (leukopenia, thrombocytopenia, or acute hemolytic anemia), cutaneous, gastrointestinal, and hepatic reactions, shortness of breath, shock, anaphylaxis, and renal failure. Recent studies indicate that regimens using twice-weekly doses of rifampin 600 mg plus isoniazid 15 mg/kg are much better tolerated.

Intermittent therapy may be used if the patient cannot (or will not) self-administer drugs on a daily basis. Patients on intermittent therapy should be closely monitored for compliance and cautioned against intentional or accidental interruption of prescribed therapy, because of the increased risk of serious adverse reactions.

Rifampin has enzyme induction properties that can enhance the metabolism of endogenous substrates including adrenal hormones, thyroid hormones, and vitamin D. Rifampin and isoniazid have been reported to alter vitamin D metabolism. In some cases, reduced levels of circulating 25-hydroxy vi-

Plasma Concentrations (mean ± standard deviation, μg/mL)

Rifampin Dosage IV	30 min	1 hr	2 hr	4 hr	8 hr	12 hr
300 mg	8.9±2.9	4.9±1.3	4.0±1.3	2.5±1.0	1.1±0.6	<0.4
600 mg	17.4±5.1	11.7±2.8	9.4±2.3	6.4±1.7	3.5±1.4	1.2±0.6

Continued on next page

Rifadin—Cont.

tamin D and 1,25-dihydroxy vitamin D have been accompanied by reduced serum calcium and phosphate, and elevated parathyroid hormone.

RIFADIN IV

For intravenous infusion only. Must not be administered by intramuscular or subcutaneous route. Avoid extravasation during injection: local irritation and inflammation due to extravascular infiltration of the infusion have been observed. If these occur, the infusion should be discontinued and restarted at another site.

Information for Patients

The patient should be told that rifampin may produce a reddish coloration of the urine, sweat, sputum, and tears, and the patient should be forewarned of this. Soft contact lenses may be permanently stained.

The patients should be advised that the reliability of oral or other systemic hormonal contraceptives may be affected; consideration should be given to using alternative contraceptive measures.

Patients should be instructed to take rifampin either 1 hour before or 2 hours after a meal with a full glass of water.

Patients should be instructed to notify their physicians promptly if they experience any of the following: fever, loss of appetite, malaise, nausea and vomiting, darkened urine, yellowish discoloration of the skin and eyes, and pain or swelling of the joints.

Compliance with the full course of therapy must be emphasized, and the importance of not missing any doses must be stressed.

Laboratory Tests

Adults treated for tuberculosis with rifampin should have baseline measurements of hepatic enzymes, bilirubin, serum creatinine, a complete blood count, and a platelet count (or estimate). Baseline tests are unnecessary in pediatric patients unless a complicating condition is known or clinically suspected.

Patients should be seen at least monthly during therapy and should be specifically questioned concerning symptoms associated with adverse reactions. All patients with abnormalities should have follow-up, including laboratory testing, if necessary. Routine laboratory monitoring for toxicity in people with normal baseline measurements is generally not necessary.

Drug Interactions

ENZYME INDUCTION: Rifampin is known to induce certain cytochrome P-450 enzymes. Administration of rifampin with drugs that undergo biotransformation through these metabolic pathways may accelerate elimination of coadministered drugs. To maintain optimum therapeutic blood levels, dosages of drugs metabolized by these enzymes may require adjustment when starting or stopping concomitantly administered rifampin.

Rifampin has been reported to accelerate the metabolism of the following drugs: anticonvulsants (eg, phenytoin), antiarrhythmics (eg, disopyramide, mexiletine, quinidine, tocainide), oral anticoagulants, antifungals (eg, fluconazole, itraconazole, ketoconazole), barbiturates, beta-blockers, calcium channel blockers (eg, diltiazem, nifedipine, verapamil), chloramphenicol, clarithromycin, corticosteroids, cyclosporine, cardiac glycoside preparations, clofibrate, oral or other systemic hormone contraceptives, dapsone, diazepam, doxycycline, fluoroquinolones (eg ciprofloxacin), haloperidol, oral hypoglycemic agents (sulfonylureas), levothyroxine, methadone, narcotic analgesics, nortriptyline, progestins, quinine, tacrolimus, theophylline tricyclic antidepressants (eg, amitriptyline, nortriptyline), and zidovudine. It may be necessary to adjust the dosages of these drugs if they are given concurrently with rifampin.

Patients using oral or other systemic hormonal contraceptives should be advised to change to nonhormonal methods of birth control during rifampin therapy.

Rifampin has been observed to increase the requirements for anticoagulant drugs of the coumarin type. In patients receiving anticoagulants and rifampin concurrently, it is recommended that the prothrombin time be performed daily or as frequently as necessary to establish and maintain the required dose of anticoagulant.

Diabetes may become more difficult to control.

OTHER INTERACTIONS: When the two drugs were taken concomitantly, decreased concentrations of atovaquone and increased concentrations of rifampin were observed.

Concurrent use of ketoconazole and rifampin has resulted in decreased serum concentrations of both drugs. Concurrent use of rifampin and enalapril has resulted in decreased concentrations of enalaprilat, the active metabolite of enalapril. Dosage adjustments should be made if indicated by the patient's clinical condition.

Concomitant antacid administration may reduce the absorption of rifampin. Daily doses of rifampin should be given at least 1 hour before the ingestion of antacids.

Probenecid and cotrimoxazole have been reported to increase the blood level of rifampin.

When rifampin is given concomitantly with either halothane or isoniazid, the potential for hepatotoxicity is increased. The concomitant use of rifampin and halothane should be avoided. Patients receiving both rifampin and isoniazid should be monitored close for hepatotoxicity.

Plasma concentrations of sulfapyridine may be reduced following the concomitant administration of sulfasalazine and rifampin. This finding may be the result of alteration in the colonic bacteria responsible for the reduction of sulfasalazine to sulfapyridine and mesalamine.

Drug/Laboratory Interactions

Cross-reactivity and false-positive urine screening tests for opiates have been reported in patients receiving rifampin when using the KIMS (Kinetic Interaction of Microparticles in Solution) method (eg, Abuscreen OnLine opiates assay; Roche Diagnostic Systems). Confirmatory tests, such as gas chromatography/mass spectrometry, will distinguish rifampin from opiates.

Therapeutic levels of rifampin have been shown to inhibit standard microbiological assays for serum folate and vitamin B_{12}. Thus, alternate assay methods should be considered. Transient abnormalities in liver function tests (eg, elevation in serum bilirubin, alkaline phosphatase, and serum transaminases) and reduced biliary excretion of contrast media used for visualization of the gallbladder have also been observed. Therefore, these tests should be performed before the morning dose of rifampin.

Carcinogenesis, Mutagenesis, Impairment of Fertility

There are no known human data on long-term potential for carinogenicity, mutagenicity, or impairment of fertility. A few cases of accelerated growth of lung carcinoma have been reported in man, but a causal relationship with the drug has not been established. An increase in the incidence of hepatomas in female mice (of a strain known to be particularly susceptible to the spontaneous development of hepatomas) was observed when rifampin was administered in doses 2 to 10 times the average daily human dose for 60 weeks, followed by an observation period of 46 weeks. No evidence of carcinogenicity was found in male mice of the same strain, mice of a different strain, or rats under similar experimental conditions.

Rifampin has been reported to possess immunosuppressive potential in rabbits, mice, rats, guinea pigs, human lymphocytes in vitro, and humans. Antitumor activity in vitro has also been shown with rifampin.

There was no evidence of mutagenicity in bacteria, *Drosophila melanogaster*, or mice. An increase in chromotid breaks was noted when whole blood cell cultures were treated with rifampin. Increased frequency of chromosomal aberrations was observed in vitro in lymphocytes obtained from patients treated with combinations of rifampin, isoniazid, and pyrazinamide and combinations of streptomycin, rifampin, isoniazid, and pyrazinamide.

Pregnancy—Teratogenic Effects

Category C. Rifampin has been shown to be teratogenic in rodents given oral doses of rifampin 15 to 25 times the human dose. Although rifampin has been reported to cross the placental barrier and appear in cord blood, the effect of RIFADIN, alone or in combination with other antituberculosis drugs, on the human fetus is not known. Neonates of rifampin-treated mothers should be carefully observed for any evidence of adverse effects. Isolated cases of fetal malformations have been reported; however, there are no adequate and well-controlled studies in pregnant women. Rifampin should be used during pregnancy only if the potential benefit justifies the potential risk to the fetus. Rifampin in oral doses of 150 to 250 mg/kg produced teratogenic effects in mice and rats. Malformations were primarily cleft palate in the mouse and spina bifida in the rat. The incidence of these anomalies was dose-dependent. When rifampin was given to pregnant rabbits in doses up to 20 times the usual daily human dose, imperfect osteogenesis and embryotoxicity were reported.

Pregnancy—Non-Teratogenic Effects

When administered during the last few weeks of pregnancy, rifampin can cause post-natal hemorrhages in the mother and infant for which treatment with vitamin K may be indicated.

Nursing Mothers

Because of the potential for tumorigenicity shown for rifampin in animal studies, a decision should be made whether to discontinue nursing or discontinue the drug, taking into account the importance of the drug to the mother.

Pediatric Use

See CLINICAL PHARMACOLOGY—Pediatrics; see also DOSAGE AND ADMINISTRATION.

ADVERSE REACTIONS

Gastrointestinal

Heartburn, epigastric distress, anorexia, nausea, vomiting, jaundice, flatulence, cramps, and diarrhea have been noted in some patients. Although *Clostridium difficile* has been shown in vitro to be sensitive to rifampin, pseudomembranous colitis has been reported with the use of rifampin (and other broad spectrum antibiotics). Therefore, it is important to consider this diagnosis in patients who develop diarrhea in association with antibiotic use. Rarely, hepatitis or a shock-like syndrome with hepatic involvement and abnormal liver function tests has been reported.

Hematologic

Thrombocytopenia has occurred primarily with high dose intermittent therapy, but has also been noted after resumption of interrupted treatment. It rarely occurs during well supervised daily therapy. This effect is reversible if the drug is discontinued as soon as purpura occurs. Cerebral hemorrhage and fatalities have been reported when rifampin administration has been continued or resumed after the appearance of purpura.

Rare reports of disseminated intravascular coagulation have been observed.

Transient leukopenia, hemolytic anemia, and decreased hemoglobin have been observed.

Central Nervous System

Headache, fever, drowsiness, fatigue, ataxia, dizziness, inability to concentrate, mental confusion, behavioral changes, pain in extremities, and generalized numbness have been observed.

Psychoses has been rarely reported.

Ocular

Visual disturbances have been observed.

Endocrine

Menstrual disturbances have been observed.

Rare reports of adrenal insufficiency in patients with compromised adrenal function have been observed.

Renal

Elevations in BUN and serum uric acid have been reported. Rarely, hemolysis, hemoglobinuria, hematuria, interstitial nephritis, acute tubular necrosis, renal insufficiency, and acute renal failure have been noted. These are generally considered to be hypersensitivity reactions. They usually occur during intermittent therapy or when treatment is resumed following intentional or accidental interruption of a daily dosage regimen, and are reversible when rifampin is discontinued and appropriate therapy instituted.

Dermatologic

Cutaneous reactions are mild and self-limiting and do not appear to be hypersensitivity reactions. Typically, they consist of flushing and itching with or without a rash. More serious cutaneous reactions which may be due to hypersensitivity occur but are uncommon.

Hypersensitivity Reactions

Occasionally, pruritus, urticaria, rash, pemphigoid reaction, erythema multiforme including Stevens-Johnson Syndrome, toxic epidermal necrolysis, vasculitis, eosinophilia, sore mouth, sore tongue, and conjunctivitis have been observed.

Anaphylaxis has been reported rarely.

Miscellaneous

Rare reports of myopathy and muscular weakness have also been observed.

Edema of the face and extremities has been reported. Other reactions reported to have occurred with intermittent dosage regimens include "flu syndrome" (such as episodes of fever, chills, headache, dizziness, and bone pain), shortness of breath, wheezing, decrease in blood pressure and shock. The "flu syndrome" may also appear if rifampin is taken irregularly by the patient or if daily administration is resumed after a drug free interval.

OVERDOSAGE

Signs and Symptoms

Nausea, vomiting, abdominal pain, pruritus, headache, and increasing lethargy will probably occur within a short time after ingestion; unconsciousness may occur when there is severe hepatic disease. Transient increases in liver enzymes and/or bilirubin may occur. Brownish-red or orange discoloration of the skin, urine, sweat, saliva, tears, and feces will occur, and its intensity is proportional to the amount ingested.

Facial or periorbital edema has also been reported in pediatric patients. Hypotension, sinus tachycardia, ventricular arrhythmias, seizures and cardiac arrest were reported in some fatal cases.

Acute Toxicity

The LD_{50} of rifampin is approximately 885 mg/kg in the mouse, 1720 mg/kg in the rat, and 2120 mg/kg in the rabbit. The minimum acute lethal or toxic dose is not well established. However, nonfatal acute overdoses in adults have been reported with doses ranging from 9 to 12 gm rifampin. Fatal acute overdoses in adults have been reported with doses ranging from 14 to 60 gm. Alcohol or a history of alcohol abuse was involved in some of the fatal and nonfatal reports. Nonfatal overdoses in pediatric patients ages 1 to 4 years old of 100 mg/kg for one to two doses has been reported.

Treatment

Intensive support measures should be instituted and individual symptoms treated as they arise. Since nausea and vomiting are likely to be present, gastric lavage is probably preferable to induction of emesis. Following evacuation of the gastric contents, the instillation of activated charcoal slurry into the stomach may help absorb any remaining drug from the gastrointestinal tract. Antiemetic medication may be required to control severe nausea and vomiting. Active diuresis (with measured intake and output) will help promote excretion of the drug. Hemodialysis may be of value in some patients.

DOSAGE AND ADMINISTRATION

Rifampin can be administered by the oral route or by IV infusion (see INDICATIONS AND USAGE). IV doses are the same as those for oral.

See CLINICAL PHARMACOLOGY for dosing information in patients with renal failure.

Tuberculosis

Adults: 10 mg/kg, in a single daily administration, not to exceed 600 mg/day, oral or IV

Pediatric Patients: 10–20 mg/kg, not to exceed 600 mg/day, oral or IV

It is recommended that oral rifampin be administered once daily, either 1 hour before or 2 hours after a meal with a full glass of water.

Rifampin is indicated in the treatment of all forms of tuberculosis. A three-drug regimen consisting of rifampin, isoniazid, and pyrazinamide (eg, RIFATER®) is recommended in the initial phase of short-course therapy which is usually continued for 2 months. The Advisory Council for the Elimination of Tuberculosis, the American Thoracic Society, and the Centers for Disease Control and Prevention recommend that either streptomycin or ethambutol be added as a fourth drug in a regimen containing isoniazid (INH), rifampin and pyrazinamide for initial treatment of tuberculosis unless the likelihood of INH resistance is very low. The need for a fourth drug should be reassessed when the results of susceptibility testing are known. If community rates of INH resistance are currently less than 4%, an initial treatment regimen with less than four drugs may be considered.

Following the initial phase, treatment should be continued with rifampin and isoniazid (eg, RIFAMATE®) for at least 4 months. Treatment should be continued for longer if the patient is still sputum or culture positive, if resistant organisms are present, or if the patient is HIV positive.

Preparation of Solution for IV Infusion: Reconstitute the lyophilized powder by transferring 10 mL of sterile water for injection to a vial containing 600 mg of rifampin for injection. Swirl vial gently to completely dissolve the antibiotic. The reconstituted solution contains 60 mg rifampin per mL and is stable at room temperature for 24 hours. Prior to administration, withdraw from the reconstituted solution a volume equivalent to the amount of rifampin calculated to be administered and add to 500 mL of infusion medium. Mix well and infuse at a rate allowing for complete infusion within 3 hours. Alternatively, the amount of rifampin calculated to be administered may be added to 100 mL of infusion medium and infused in 30 minutes.

Dilutions in dextrose 5% for injection (D5W) are stable at room temperature for up to 4 hours and should be prepared and used within this time. Precipitation of rifampin from the infusion solution may occur beyond this time. Dilutions in normal saline are stable at room temperature for up to 24 hours and should be prepared and used within this time. Other infusion solutions are not recommended.

Incompatibilities: Physical incompatibility (precipitate) was observed with undiluted (5 mg/mL) and diluted (1 mg/mL in normal saline) diltiazem hydrochloride and rifampin (6 mg/mL in normal saline) during simulated Y-site administration.

Meningococcal Carriers

Adults: For adults, it is recommended that 600 mg rifampin be administered twice daily for two days.

Pediatric Patients: Pediatric patients 1 month of age or older: 10 mg/kg (not to exceed 600 mg per dose) every 12 hours for two days.

Pediatric patients under 1 month of age: 5 mg/kg every 12 hours for two days.

Preparation of Extemporaneous Oral Suspension

For pediatric and adult patients in whom capsule swallowing is difficult or where lower doses are needed, a liquid suspension may be prepared as follows:

RIFADIN 1% w/v suspension (10 mg/mL) can be compounded using one of four syrups—Simple Syrup (Syrup NF), Simple Syrup (Humco Laboratories), Syrpalta® Syrup (Emerson Laboratories), or Raspberry Syrup (Humco Laboratories).

1. Empty the contents of four RIFADIN 300 mg capsules or eight RIFADIN 150 mg capsules onto a piece of weighing paper.
2. If necessary, gently crush the capsule contents with a spatula to produce a fine powder.
3. Transfer the rifampin powder blend to a 4-ounce amber glass or plastic (high density polyethylene [HDPE], polypropylene, or polycarbonate) prescription bottle.
4. Rinse the paper and spatula with 20 mL of one of the above-mentioned syrups, and add the rinse to the bottle. Shake vigorously.
5. Add 100 mL of syrup to the bottle and shake vigorously.

This compounding procedure results in a 1% w/v suspension containing 10 mg rifampin/mL. Stability studies indicate that the suspension is stable when stored at room temperature (25 ± 3°C) or in a refrigerator (2–8°C) for four weeks. This extemporaneously prepared suspension must be shaken well prior to administration.

HOW SUPPLIED

150 mg maroon and scarlet capsules imprinted "RIFADIN 150."

Bottles of 30 (NDC 0068-0510-30)

300 mg maroon and scarlet capsules imprinted "RIFADIN 300."

Bottles of 30 (NDC 0068-0508-30)
Bottles of 60 (NDC 0068-0508-60)
Bottles of 100 (NDC 0068-0508-61)

Storage: Keep tightly closed. Store in a dry place. Avoid excessive heat.

RIFADIN IV (rifampin for injection USP) is available in glass vials containing 600 mg rifampin (NDC 0068-0597-01).

Storage: Avoid excessive heat (temperatures above 40°C or 104°F). Protect from light.

References:

1. National Committee for Clinical Laboratory Standards. Antimycobacterial Susceptibility Testing. Proposed Standard NCCLS Document M24-P, Vol. 10, No. 10, NNCLS, Villanova, PA, 1990.
2. National Committee for Clinical Laboratory Standards. Methods for Dilution Antimicrobial Susceptibility Tests for Bacteria that Grow Aerobically—Third Edition. Approved Standard NCCLS Document M7-A3, Vol. 13, No. 25, NCCLS, Villanova, PA, December 1993.
3. National Committee for Clinical Laboratory Standards. Performance Standards for Antimicrobial Disk Susceptibility Tests—Fifth Edition. Approved Standard NCCLS Document M2-A5, Vol. 13, No. 24, NCCLS, Villanova, PA, December 1993.
4. National Committee for Clinical Laboratory Standards. Performance Standards for Antimicrobial Susceptibility Testing; Fifth Informational Supplement, NCCLS Document M100-S5, Vol. 14, No. 16, NCCLS, Villanova, PA, December 1994.

Prescribing Information as of June 1999

Merrell Pharmaceuticals Inc.
Subsidiary of Hoechst Marion Roussel, Inc.
Kansas City, MO 64137 USA

Rifadin IV (rifampin for injection USP) is manufactured by:
GRUPPO LEPETIT S.p.A.
20020 Lainate, Italy

Shown in Product Identification Guide, page 307

RIFAMATE® ℞
[*rĭf 'uh-māt*]
(rifampin and isoniazid capsules USP)

Prescribing Information as of September 1999

WARNING

Severe and sometimes fatal hepatitis associated with isoniazid therapy may occur and may develop even after many months of treatment. The risk of developing hepatitis is age related. Approximate case rates by age are: 0 per 1,000 for persons under 20 years of age, 3 per 1,000 for persons in the 20–34 year age group, 12 per 1,000 for persons in the 35–49 year age group, 23 per 1,000 for persons in the 50–64 year age group, and 8 per 1,000 for persons over 65 years of age. The risk of hepatitis is increased with daily consumption of alcohol. Precise data to provide a fatality rate for isoniazid-related hepatitis is not available; however, in a U.S. Public Health Service Surveillance Study of 13,838 persons taking isoniazid, there were 8 deaths among 174 cases of hepatitis.

Therefore, patients given isoniazid should be carefully monitored and interviewed at monthly intervals. Serum transaminase concentration becomes elevated in about 10–20 percent of patients, usually during the first few months of therapy, but it can occur at any time. Usually enzyme levels return to normal despite continuance of drug, but in some cases progressive liver dysfunction occurs. Patients should be instructed to report immediately any of the prodromal symptoms of hepatitis, such as fatigue, weakness, malaise, anorexia, nausea, or vomiting. If these symptoms appear or if signs suggestive of hepatic damage are detected, isoniazid should be discontinued promptly, since continued use of the drug in these cases has been reported to cause a more severe form of liver damage.

Patients with tuberculosis should be given appropriate treatment with alternative drugs. If isoniazid must be reinstituted, it should be reinstituted only after symptoms and laboratory abnormalities have cleared. The drug should be restarted in very small and gradually increasing doses and should be withdrawn immediately if there is any indication of recurrent liver involvement. Treatment should be deferred in persons with acute hepatic diseases.

DESCRIPTION

RIFAMATE is a combination capsule containing 300 mg rifampin and 150 mg isoniazid. The capsules also contain as inactive ingredients: colloidal silicon dioxide, FD&C Blue No. 1, FD&C Red No. 40, gelatin, magnesium stearate, sodium starch glycolate, and titanium dioxide.

Rifampin is a semisynthetic antibiotic derivative of rifamycin B. The chemical name for rifampin is 3-(4-methyl-1-piperazinyliminomethyl) rifamycin SV.

Isoniazid is the hydrazide of isonicotinic acid. It exists as colorless or white crystals or as a white, crystalline powder that is water soluble, odorless, and slowly affected by exposure to air and light.

ACTIONS

Rifampin

Rifampin inhibits DNA-dependent RNA polymerase activity in susceptible cells. Specifically, it interacts with bacterial RNA polymerase but does not inhibit the mammalian enzyme. This is the mechanism of action by which rifampin exerts its therapeutic effect. Rifampin cross resistance has only been shown with other rifamycins.

In a study of 14 normal human adult males, peak blood levels of rifampin occured $1^1/_2$ to 3 hours following oral administration of two RIFAMATE capsules. The peaks ranged from 6.9 to 14 mcg/ml with an average of 10 mcg/ml.

In normal subjects the $T^1/_2$ (biological half-life) of rifampin in blood is approximately 3 hours. Elimination occurs mainly through the bile and, to a much lesser extent, the urine.

Isoniazid

Isoniazid acts against actively growing tubercle bacilli.

After oral administration isoniazid produces peak blood levels within 1 to 2 hours which decline to 50% or less within 6 hours. It diffuses readily into all body fluids (cerebrospinal, pleural, and ascitic fluids), tissues, organs, and excreta (saliva, sputum, and feces). The drug also passes through the placental barrier and into milk in concentrations comparable to those in the plasma. From 50 to 70% of a dose of isoniazid is excreted in the urine in 24 hours.

Isoniazid is metabolized primarily by acetylation and dehydrazination. The rate of acetylation is genetically determined. Approximately 50% of Blacks and Caucasians are "slow inactivators"; the majority of Eskimos and Orientals are "rapid inactivators."

The rate of acetylation does not significantly alter the effectiveness of isoniazid. However, slow acetylation may lead to higher blood levels of the drug, and thus an increase in toxic reactions.

Pyridoxine deficiency (B_6) is sometimes observed in adults with high doses of isoniazid and is considered probably due to its competition with pyridoxal phosphate for the enzyme apotryptophanase.

INDICATIONS

For pulmonary tuberculosis in which organisms are susceptible, and when the patient has been titrated on the individual components and it has therefore been established that this fixed dosage is therapeutically effective.

This fixed-dosage combination drug is not recommended for initial therapy of tuberculosis or for preventive therapy.

In the treatment of tuberculosis, small numbers of resistant cells, present within large populations of susceptible cells, can rapidly become the predominating type. Since rapid emergence of resistance can occur, culture and susceptibility tests should be performed in the event of persistent positive cultures.

This drug is not indicated for the treatment of meningococcal infections or asymptomatic carriers of *N. meningitidis* to eliminate meningococci from the nasopharynx.

CONTRAINDICATIONS

Previous isoniazid-associated hepatic injury; severe adverse reactions to isoniazid, such as drug fever, chills, and arthritis; acute liver disease of any etiology. A history of previous hypersensitivity reaction to any of the rifamycins or to isoniazid, including drug-induced hepatitis.

WARNINGS

RIFAMATE (rifampin and isoniazid capsules USP) is a combination of two drugs, each of which has been associated with liver dysfunction. Liver function tests should be performed prior to therapy with RIFAMATE and periodically during treatment.

Rifampin

Rifampin has been shown to produce liver dysfunction. There have been fatalities associated with jaundice in patients with liver disease or receiving rifampin concomitantly with other hepatoxic agents. Since an increased risk may exist for individuals with liver disease, benefits must be weighed carefully against the risk of further liver damage.

Several studies of tumorigenicity potential have been done in rodents. In one strain of mice known to be particularly susceptible to the spontaneous development of hepatomas, rifampin given at a level 2–10 times the maximum dosage used clinically resulted in a significant increase in the occurrence of hepatomas in female mice of this strain after one year of administration.

There was no evidence of tumorigenicity in the males of this strain, in males or females of another mouse strain, or in rats.

Isoniazid

See the boxed warning.

PRECAUTIONS

Rifampin

Rifampin is not recommended for intermittent therapy; the patient should be cautioned against intentional or accidental interruption of the daily dosage regimen since rare renal hypersensitivity reactions have been reported when therapy was resumed in such cases.

Rifampin has been observed to increase the requirements for anticoagulant drugs of the coumarin type. The cause of the phenomenon is unknown. In patients receiving anticoagulants and rifampin concurrently, it is recommended that the prothrombin time be performed daily or as frequently as necessary to establish and maintain the required dose of anticoagulant.

Urine, feces, saliva, sputum, sweat, and tears may be colored red-orange by rifampin and its metabolites. Soft contact lenses may be permanently stained. Individuals to be treated should be made aware of these possibilities.

It has been reported that the reliability of oral contraceptives may be affected in some patients being treated for tuberculosis with rifampin in combination with at least one other antituberculosis drug. In such cases, alternative contraceptive measures may need to be considered.

It has also been reported that rifampin given in combination with other antituberculosis drugs may decrease the pharmacologic activity of methadone, oral hypoglycemics, digitoxin, quinidine, disopyramide, dapsone, and corticosteroids. In these cases, dosage adjustment of the interacting drugs is recommended.

Therapeutic levels of rifampin have been shown to inhibit standard microbiological assays for serum folate and vitamin B_{12}. Alternative methods must be considered when determining folate and vitamin B_{12} concentrations in the presence of rifampin.

Continued on next page

Rifamate—Cont.

Since rifampin has been reported to cross the placental barrier and appear in cord blood and in maternal milk, neonates and newborns of rifampin-treated mothers should be carefully observed for any evidence of untoward effects.

Isoniazid

All drugs should be stopped and an evaluation of the patient should be made at the first sign of a hypersensitivity reaction.

Use of isoniazid should be carefully monitored in the following:

1. Patients who are receiving phenytoin (diphenylhydantoin) concurrently. Isoniazid may decrease the excretion of phenytoin or may enhance its effects. To avoid phenytoin intoxication, appropriate adjustment of the anticonvulsant dose should be made.
2. Daily users of alcohol. Daily ingestion of alcohol may be associated with a higher incidence of isoniazid hepatitis.
3. Patients with current chronic liver disease or severe renal dysfunction.

Periodic ophthalmoscopic examination during isoniazid therapy is recommended when visual symptoms occur.

Usage in Pregnancy and Lactation

Rifampin

Although rifampin has been reported to cross the placental barrier and appear in cord blood, the effect of rifampin, alone or in combination with other antituberculosis drugs, on the human fetus is not known. An increase in congenital malformations, primarily spina bifida and cleft palate, has been reported in the offspring of rodents given oral doses of 150–250 mg/kg/day of rifampin during pregnancy.

The possible teratogenic potential in women capable of bearing children should be carefully weighed against the benefits of therapy.

Isoniazid

It has been reported that in both rats and rabbits, isoniazid may exert an embryocidal effect when administered orally during pregnancy, although no isoniazid-related congenital anomalies have been found in reproduction studies in mammalian species (mice, rats, and rabbits). Isoniazid should be prescribed during pregnancy only when therapeutically necessary. The benefit of preventive therapy should be weighed against a possible risk to the fetus. Preventive treatment generally should be started after delivery because of the increased risk of tuberculosis for new mothers.

Since isoniazid is known to cross the placental barrier and to pass into maternal breast milk, neonates and breast-fed infants of isoniazid treated mothers should be carefully observed for any evidence of adverse effects.

Carcinogenesis: Isoniazid has been reported to induce pulmonary tumors in a number of strains of mice.

ADVERSE REACTIONS

Rifampin

Nervous system reactions: headache, drowsiness, fatigue, ataxia, dizziness, inability to concentrate, mental confusion, visual disturbances, muscular weakness, pain in extremities, and generalized numbness

Gastrointestinal disturbances: in some patients heartburn, epigastric distress, anorexia, nausea, vomiting, gas, cramps, and diarrhea

Hepatic reactions: transient abnormalities in liver function tests (e.g., elevations in serum bilirubin, BSP, alkaline phosphatase, serum transaminases) have been observed. Rarely, hepatitis or a shocklike syndrome with hepatic involvement and abnormal liver function tests.

Renal reactions: elevations in BUN and serum uric acid have been reported. Rarely, hemolysis, hemoglobinuria, hematuria, interstitial nephritis, renal insufficiency, and acute renal failure have been noted. These are generally considered to be hypersensitivity reactions. They usually occur during intermittent therapy or when treatment is resumed following intentional or accidental interruption of a daily dosage regimen, and are reversible when rifampin is discontinued and appropriate therapy instituted.

Hematologic reactions: thrombocytopenia, transient leukopenia, hemolytic anemia, eosinophilia, and decreased hemoglobin have been observed. Thrombocytopenia has occurred when rifampin and ethambutol were administered concomitantly according to an intermittent dose schedule twice weekly and in high doses.

Allergic and immunological reactions: occasionally pruritus, urticaria, rash, pemphigoid reaction, eosinophilia, sore mouth, sore tongue, and exudative conjunctivitis. Rarely, hemolysis, hemoglobinuria, hematuria, renal insufficiency or acute renal failure have been reported which are generally considered to be hypersensitivity reactions. These have usually occurred during intermittent therapy or when treatment was resumed following intentional or accidental interruption of a daily dosage regimen and were reversible when rifampin was discontinued and appropriate therapy instituted.

Although rifampin has been reported to have an immunosuppressive effect in some animal experiments, available human data indicate that this has no clinical significance.

Metabolic reactions: elevations in BUN and serum uric acid have occurred.

Miscellaneous reactions: fever and menstrual disturbances have been noted.

Isoniazid

The most frequent reactions are those affecting the nervous system and the liver.

Nervous system reactions: peripheral neuropathy is the most common toxic effect. It is dose-related, occurs most often in the malnourished and in those predisposed to neuritis (e.g., alcoholics and diabetics), and is usually preceded by paresthesias of the feet and hands. The incidence is higher in "slow inactivators."

Other neurotoxic effects, which are uncommon with conventional doses, are convulsions, toxic encephalopathy, optic neuritis and atrophy, memory impairment, and toxic psychosis.

Gastrointestinal reactions: nausea, vomiting, and epigastric distress

Hepatic reactions: elevated serum transaminases (SGOT; SGPT), bilirubinemia, bilirubinuria, jaundice, and occasionally severe and sometimes fatal hepatitis. The common prodromal symptoms are anorexia, nausea, vomiting, fatigue, malaise, and weakness. Mild and transient elevations of serum transaminase levels occurs in 10 to 20 percent of persons taking isoniazid. The abnormality usually occurs in the first 4 to 6 months of treatment but can occur at any time during therapy. In most instances, enzyme levels return to normal with no necessity to discontinue medication. In occasional instances, progressive liver damage occurs, with accompanying symptoms. In these cases, the drug should be discontinued immediately. The frequency of progressive liver damage increases with age. It is rare in persons under 20, but occurs in up to 2.3 percent of those over 50 years of age.

Hematologic reactions: agranulocytosis, hemolytic sideroblastic or aplastic anemia, thrombocytopenia, and eosinophilia

Hypersensitivity reactions: fever, skin eruptions (morbilliform, maculopapular, purpuric, or exfoliative), lymphadenopathy, and vasculitis

Metabolic and endocrine reactions: pyridoxine deficiency, pellagra, hyperglycemia, metabolic acidosis, and gynecomastia

Miscellaneous reactions: rheumatic syndrome and systemic lupus erythematosus-like syndrome

OVERDOSAGE

Rifampin

Signs and Symptoms

Nausea, vomiting, and increasing lethargy will probably occur within a short time after ingestion; actual unconsciousness may occur with severe hepatic involvement. Brownish-red or orange discoloration of the skin, urine, sweat, saliva, tears, and feces is proportional to amount ingested.

Liver enlargement, possibly with tenderness, can develop within a few hours after severe overdosage, and jaundice may develop rapidly. Hepatic involvement may be more marked in patients with prior impairment of hepatic function. Other physical findings remain essentially normal.

Direct and total bilirubin levels may increase rapidly with severe overdosage; hepatic enzyme levels may be affected, especially with prior impairment of hepatic function. A direct effect upon hemopoietic system, electrolyte levels, or acid-base balance is unlikely.

Isoniazid

Signs and Symptoms

Isoniazid overdosage produces signs and symptoms within 30 minutes to 3 hours. Nausea, vomiting, dizziness, slurring of speech, blurring of vision, visual hallucinations (including bright colors and strange designs), are among the early manifestations. With marked overdosage, respiratory distress and CNS depression, progressing rapidly from stupor to profound coma, are to be expected, along with severe, intractable seizures. Severe metabolic acidosis, acetonuria, and hyperglycemia are typical laboratory findings.

RIFAMATE (rifampin and isoniazid capsules USP)

Treatment

The airway should be secured and adequate respiratory exchange established. Only then should gastric emptying (lavage-aspiration) be attempted; this may be difficult because of seizures. Since nausea and vomiting are likely to be present, gastric lavage is probably preferable to induction of emesis.

Activated charcoal slurry instilled into the stomach following evacuation of gastric contents can help absorb any remaining drug in the GI tract. Antiemetic medication may be required to control severe nausea and vomiting.

Blood samples should be obtained for immediate determination of gases, electrolytes, BUN, glucose, etc. Blood should be typed and crossmatched in preparation for possible hemodialysis.

Rapid control of metabolic acidosis is fundamental to management. Intravenous sodium bicarbonate should be given at once and repeated as needed, adjusting subsequent dosage on the basis of laboratory findings (i.e., serum sodium, pH, etc.). At the same time, anticonvulsants should be given intravenously (i.e., barbiturates, diphenylhydantoin, diazepam) as required, and large doses of intravenous pyridoxine.

Forced osmotic diuresis must be started early and should be continued for some hours after clinical improvement to hasten renal clearance of drug and help prevent relapse. Fluid intake and output should be monitored.

Bile drainage may be indicated in presence of serious impairment of hepatic function lasting more than 24–48 hours. Under these circumstances and for severe cases, extracorporeal hemodialysis may be required; if this is not available, peritoneal dialysis can be used along with forced diuresis.

Along with measures based on initial and repeated determination of blood gases and other laboratory tests as needed, meticulous respiratory and other intensive care should be utilized to protect against hypoxia, hypotension, aspiration, pneumonitis, etc.

In patients with previously adequate hepatic function, reversal of liver enlargement and impaired hepatic excretory function probably will be noted within 72 hours, with rapid return toward normal thereafter.

Untreated or inadequately treated cases of gross isoniazid overdosage can terminate fatally, but good response has been reported in most patients brought under adequate treatment within the first few hours after drug ingestion.

DOSAGE AND ADMINISTRATION

In general, therapy should be continued until bacterial conversion and maximal improvement have occurred.

Adults: Two RIFAMATE (rifampin and isoniazid capsules USP) capsules (600 mg rifampin, 300 mg isoniazid) once daily, administered one hour before or two hours after a meal.

Concomitant administration of pyridoxine (B_6) is recommended in the malnourished, in those predisposed to neuropathy (e.g., diabetic), and in adolescents.

Susceptibility Testing

Rifampin

Rifampin susceptibility powders are available for both direct and indirect methods of determining the susceptibility of strains of mycobacteria. The MIC's of susceptible clinical isolates when determined in 7H10 or other non-egg-containing media have ranged from 0.1 to 2 mcg/ml.

Quantitative methods that require measurement of zone diameters give the most precise estimates of antibiotic susceptibility. One such procedure has been recommended for use with discs for testing susceptibility to rifampin. Interpretations correlate zone diameters from the disc test with MIC (minimal inhibitory concentration) values for rifampin.

HOW SUPPLIED

Capsules (opaque red), imprinted "RIFAMATE" on both ends of the capsule, containing 300 mg rifampin and 150 mg isoniazid; bottles of 60 (NDC 0068-0509-60).

Prescribing Information as of September 1999

Merrell Pharmaceuticals Inc.
Subsidiary of
Hoechst Marion Roussel, Inc.
Kansas City, MO 64137 USA

Shown in Product Identification Guide, page 307

RIFATER® ℞

[rĭf' uh-ter]

(rifampin, isoniazid and pyrazinamide)
Tablets

Prescribing Information as of December 1995

> **WARNING**
>
> Severe and sometimes fatal hepatitis associated with isoniazid therapy may occur and may develop even after many months of treatment. The risk of developing hepatitis is age related. Approximate case rates by age are: 0 per 1,000 for persons under 20 years of age, 3 per 1,000 for persons in the 20 to 34 year age group, 12 per 1,000 for persons in the 35 to 49 year age group, 23 per 1,000 for persons in the 50 to 64 year age group, and 8 per 1,000 for persons over 65 years of age. The risk of hepatitis is increased with daily consumption of alcohol. Precise data to provide a fatality rate for isoniazid-related hepatitis is not available; however, in a U.S. Public Health Service Surveillance Study of 13,838 persons taking isoniazid, there were 8 deaths among 174 cases of hepatitis.
>
> Therefore, patients given isoniazid should be carefully monitored and interviewed at monthly intervals. Serum transaminase concentration becomes elevated in about 10% to 20% of patients, usually during the first few months of therapy, but it can occur at any time. Usually enzyme levels return to normal despite continuance of drug, but in some cases progressive liver dysfunction occurs. Patients should be instructed to report immediately any of the prodromal symptoms of hepatitis, such as fatigue, weakness, malaise, anorexia, nausea, or vomiting. If these symptoms appear or if signs suggestive of hepatic damage are detected, isoniazid should be discontinued promptly since continued use of the drug in these cases has been reported to cause a more severe form of liver damage.
>
> Patients with tuberculosis should be given appropriate treatment with alternative drugs. If isoniazid must be reinstituted, it should be reinstituted only after symptoms and laboratory abnormalities have cleared. The drug should be restarted in very small and gradually increasing doses and should be withdrawn immediately if there is any indication of recurrent liver involvement. Treatment should be deferred in persons with acute hepatic diseases.

DESCRIPTION

RIFATER (rifampin/isoniazid/pyrazinamide) tablets are combination tablets containing 120 mg rifampin, 50 mg iso-

niazid, and 300 mg pyrazinamide for use in antibacterial therapy. The tablets also contain as inactive ingredients: povidone, carboxymethylcellulose sodium, calcium stearate, sodium lauryl sulfate, sucrose, talc, acacia, titanium dioxide, kaolin, magnesium carbonate, colloidal silicon dioxide, dried aluminum hydroxide gel, ferric oxide, black iron oxide, carnauba wax, white beeswax, colophony, hard paraffin, lecithin, shellac, and propylene glycol. The RIFATER triple therapy combinaion was developed for dosing convenience.
Rifampin is a semisynthetic antibiotic derivative of rifamycin SV. Rifampin is a red-brown crystalline powder very slightly soluble in water at neutral pH, freely soluble in chloroform, soluble in ethyl acetate and methanol. Its molecular weight is 822.95 and its chemical formula is $C_{43}H_{58}N_4O_{12}$. The chemical name for rifampin is either:
3-[[(4-methyl-1-piperazinyl) imino]-methyl]-rifamycin;
or
5, 6, 9, 17, 19, 21-hexahydroxy-23methoxy-2,4,12,16,18,-20,22 heptamethyl-8-[N-(4-methyl-1-piperazinyl) formimidoyl]-2,7-(epoxypentadeca [1,11,13]trienimino)naphtho-[2,1-b]furan-1,11 (2H)-dione 21-acetate.
Its structural formula is:

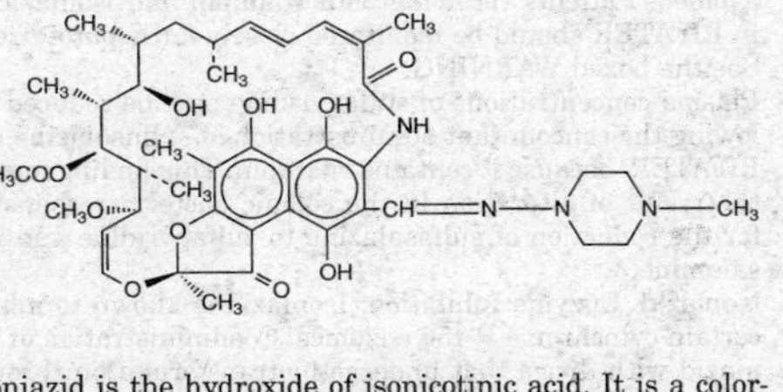

Isoniazid is the hydroxide of isonicotinic acid. It is a colorless or white crystalline powder or white crystals. It is odorless and slowly affected by exposure to air and light. It is freely soluble in water, sparingly soluble in alcohol and slightly soluble in chloroform and in ether. Its molecular weight is 137.14 and its chemical formula is $C_6H_7N_3O$. The chemical name for isoniazid is 4-pyridinecarboxylic acid, hydrazide and its structural formula is:

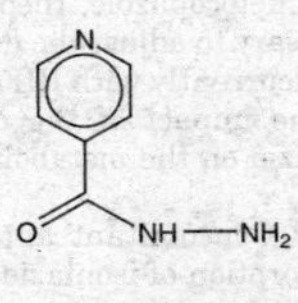

Pyrazinamide, the pyrazine analogue of nicotinamide, is a white, crystalline powder, stable at room temperature, and sparingly soluble in water. The chemical name for pyrazinamide is pyrazinecarboxamide and its molecular weight is 123.11. Its chemical formula is $C_5H_5N_3O$ and its structural formula is:

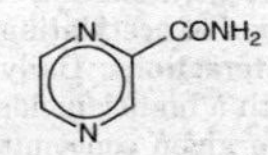

CLINICAL PHARMACOLOGY

General

Rifampin. Rifampin is readily absorbed from the gastrointestinal tract. Peak serum levels in normal adults and pediatric populations vary widely from individual to individual. Following a single 600 mg oral dose of rifampin in healthy adults, the peak serum level averages 7 µg/mL but may vary from 4 to 32 µg/mL. Absorption of rifampin is reduced when the drug is ingested with food.
In normal subjects, the biological half-life of rifampin in serum averages about 3 hours after a 600 mg oral dose, with increases up to 5.1 hours reported after a 900 mg dose. With repeated administration, the half-life decreases and reaches average values of approximately 2 to 3 hours. The half-life dos not differ in patients with renal failure at doses not exceeding 600 mg daily and, consequently, no dosage adjustment is required. The half-life of rifampin at a dose of 720 mg daily has not been established in patients with renal failure. Following a single 900 mg oral dose of rifampin in patients with varying degrees of renal insufficiency, the half-life increased from 3.6 hours in normal subjects to 5.0, 7.3, and 11.0 hours in patients with glomerular filtration rates of 30–50 mL/min, less than 30 mL/min, and in anuric patients, respectively. Refer to the WARNINGS section for information regarding patients with hepatic insufficiency.
After absorption, rifampin is rapidly eliminated in the bile, and an enterohepatic circulation ensues. During this process, rifampin undergoes progressive deacetylation so that nearly all the drug in the bile is in this form in about 6 hours. This metabolite has antibacterial activity. Intestinal reabsorption is reduced by deacetylation, and elimination is facilitated. Up to 30% of a dose is excreted in the urine, with about half as unchanged drug.
Rifampin is widely distributed throughout the body. It is present in effective concentration in many organs and body fluids, including cerebrospinal fluid. Rifampin is about 80% protein bound. Most of the unbound fraction is not ionized and therefore is diffused freely in tissues.
Isoniazid. After oral administration, isoniazid is readily absorbed from the GI tract and produces peak blood levels within 1 to 2 hours. It diffuses readily into all body fluids (cerebrospinal, pleural, and ascitic fluids), tissues, organs, and excreta (saliva, sputum, and feces). Isoniazid is not substantially bound to plasma proteins. The drug also passes through the placental barrier and into milk in concentrations comparable to those in the plasma. The plasma half-life of isoniazid in patients with normal renal and hepatic function ranges from 1–4 hours, depending on the rate of metabolism. From 50% to 70% of a dose of isoniazid is excreted in the urine within 24 hours, mostly as metabolites.
Isoniazid is metabolized in the liver mainly by acetylation and dehydrazination. The rate of acetylation is genetically determined. Approximately 50% of African Americans and Caucasians are "slow inactivators" and the rest are "rapid inactivators"; the majority of Eskimos and Asians are "rapid inactivators." The rate of acetylation does not significantly alter the effectiveness of isoniazid. However, slow acetylation may lead to higher blood levels of the drug, and thus, an increase in toxic reactions.
Pyridoxin (B_6) deficiency is sometimes observed in adults with high doses of isoniazid and is probably due to its competition with pyridoxal phosphate for the enzyme apotryptophanase.
Pyrazinamide. Pyrazinamide is well absorbed from the gastrointestinal tract and attains peak plasma concentrations within 2 hours. Plasma concentrations generally range from 30 to 50 µg/mL with doses of 20 to 25 mg/kg. It is widely distributed in body tissues and fluids including the liver, lungs, and cerebrospinal fluid (CSF). The CSF concentration is approximately equal to concurrent steady-state plasma concentrations in patients with inflamed meninges. Pyrazinamide is approximately 10% bound to plasma proteins. The plasma half-life of pyrazinamide is 9 to 10 hours in patients with normal renal and hepatic function. The half-life of the drug may be prolonged in patients with impaired renal or hepatic function. Pyrazinamide is hydrolyzed in the liver to its major active metabolite, pyrazinoic acid. Pyrazinoic acid is hydroxylated to the main excretory product, 5-hydroxypyrazinoic acid.
Within 24 hours, approximately 70% of an oral dose of pyrazinamide is excreted in urine, mainly by glomerular filtration. About 4% to 14% of the dose is excreted as unchanged drug; the remainder is excreted as metabolites.

RIFATER

In a single-dose bioavailabilty study of five RIFATER tablets (Treatment A, n=23) versus RIFADIN 600 mg, isoniazid 250 mg, and pyrazinamide 1500 mg (Treatment B, n=24) administered concurrently in normal subjects, there was no difference in extent of absorption, as measured by the area under the plasma concentration versus time curve (AUC), of all three components. However, the mean peak plasma concentration of rifampin was approximately 18% lower following the single-dose administration of RIFATER tablets as compared to RIFADIN administered in combination with pyrazinamide and isoniazid. Mean (±SD) pharmacokinetic parameters are summarized in the following table.

Parameter	C_{max} (µg/mL)		Half-life (hr)		Apparent Oral Clearance (L/hr)		Bioavailability (%)
Treatment	A	B	A	B	A	B	A
Isoniazid	3.09 ± 0.88	3.14 ± 0.92	2.80 ± 1.02	2.80 ± 1.11	24.02 ± 15.29	25.72 ± 18.38	100.6 ± 16.6
Rifampin	11.04 ± 3.08	13.61 ± 3.96	3.19 ± 0.63	3.41 ± 0.86	9.62 ± 3.00	8.30 ± 2.50	88.8 ± 16.5
Pyrazinamide	28.02 ± 4.52	29.21 ± 4.35	10.04 ± 1.54	10.08 ± 1.29	3.82 ± 0.65	3.70 ± 0.59	96.8 ± 7.6

Dose of Isoniazid, Rifampin and Pyrazinamide Administered as Separate Drugs

Patient Weight	Isoniazid (mg)	Rifampin (mg)	Pyrazinamide (mg)
<50 kg	300	450	1500
≥50 kg	300	600	2000

Dose of Isoniazid, Rifampin and Pyrazinamide Administered as RIFATER

Patient Weight	Number of Tablets	Isoniazid (mg)	Rifampin (mg)	Pyrazinamide (mg)
≤44 kg	4	200	480	1200
45 to 54 kg	5	250	600	1500
≥55 kg	6	300	720	1800

[See first table above]
The effect of food on the pharmacokinetics of RIFATER tablets was not studied.

Microbiology

Rifampin, isoniazid, and pyrazinamide at therapeutic levels have demonstrated bactericidal activity against both intracellular and extracellular *Mycobacterium tuberculosis* organisms.

Mechanism of Action

Rifampin. Rifampin inhibits DNA-dependent RNA polymerase activity in susceptible *Mycobacterium tuberculosis* organisms. Specifically, it interacts with bacterial RNA polymerase, but does not inhibit the mammalian enzyme. Organisms resistant to rifampin are likely to be resistant to other rifamycins.
Isoniazid. Isoniazid kills actively growing tubercle bacilli by inhibiting the biosynthesis of mycolic acids which are major components of the cell wall of *Mycobacterium tuberculosis*.
Pyrazinamide. The exact mechanism of action by which pyrazinamide inhibits the growth of *Mycobacterium tuberculosis* organisms is unknown. *In vitro* and *in vivo* studies have demonstrated that pyrazinamide is only active at a slightly acidic pH (pH 5.5).

Susceptibility Testing

Prior to initiation of therapy, appropriate specimens should be collected for identification of the infecting organism and *in vitro* susceptibility tests
Two standardized *in vitro* susceptibility methods are available for testing isoniazid, rifampin, and pyrazinamide against *Mycobacterium tuberculosis* organisms. The agar proportion method (CDC or NCCLS M24-P) utilizes Middlebrook 7H10 medium impregnated with isoniazid at 0.2 and 1.0 µg/mL for the final concentrations of drug. The final concentration for pyrazinamide is 25.0 µg/mL at pH 5.5. After 3 weeks of incubation MIC_{99} values are calculated by comparing the quantity of organisms growing in the medium containing drug to the control cultures. Mycobacterial growth in the presence of drug ≥1% of the control indicates resistance.
The radiometric broth method employs the BACTEC 460 machine to compare the growth index from untreated control cultures to cultures grown in the presence of 0.2 and 1.0 µg/mL of isoniazid and 2.0 µg/mL of rifampin. Strict adherence to the manufacturer's instructions for sample processing and data interpretation is required for this assay. The radiometric broth method has not been approved for the testing of pyrazinamide.
Susceptibility test results obtained by the two different methods can only be compared if the appropriate rifampin or isoniazid concentrations are used for each test method as indicated above. Both test procedures require the use of *Mycobacterium tuberculosis* H37Rv, ATCC 27294, as a control organism.
The clinical relevance of *in vitro* susceptibility test results for mycobacterial species other than *Mycobacterium tuberculosis* using either the radiometric broth method or the proportion method has not been determined.

CLINICAL TRIALS

A total of 250 patients were enrolled in an open label, prospective, randomized, parallel group, active controlled trial, for the treatment of pulmonary tuberculosis. There were 241 patients evaluable for efficacy, 123 patients received isoniazid, rifampin and pyrazinamide as separate tablets and capsules for 56 days, and 118 patients received 4 to 6 RIFATER tablets based on body weight for 56 days. RIFATER tablets and the drugs dosed as separate tablets and capsules were administered based on body weight during the intensive phase of treatment according to the following table.
[See second table above]
During the continuation phase, both treatment groups received 450 mg of rifampin and 300 mg of isoniazid per day for 4 months if the patient weighed <50 kg or 600 mg of rifampin and 300 mg of isoniazid per day for 4 months if the patient weighed ≥50 kg. Patients were followed for occurrence of relapses for up to 30 months after the end of therapy.

Continued on next page

Rifater—Cont.

There were no significant differences in the negative bacteriological sputum results (available in a subset of patients) between the two treatments at 2 and 6 months during the trial and during the follow-up period. See table below.
[See table at right]
For adverse events, see ADVERSE REACTIONS section.

	Negative Sputums/No. of Patients (Percent Negative)		
Treatment	2 Months	6 Months	Follow-up Period*
RIFATER	91/96 (95%)	100/104 (96%)	99/101 (98%)
Separate†	99/108 (92%)	95/96 (99%)	105/106 (99%)

* The median follow-up time for all the RIFATER patients was 756 days with a range of 42 to 1325 days and 745 days with a range of 50 to 1427 days for the patients dosed with separate tablets and capsules.
† Isoniazid, rifampin, and pyrazinamide dosed as separate tablets and capsules.

INDICATIONS AND USAGE

RIFATER is indicated in the initial phase of the short-course treatment of pulmonary tuberculosis. During this phase, which should last 2 months, RIFATER should be administered on a daily, continuous basis (see DOSAGE AND ADMINISTRATION section).
Following the initial phase and treatment with RIFATER, treatment should be continued with rifampin and isoniazid (eg, RIFAMATE) for at least 4 months. Treatment should be continued for a longer period of time if the patient is still sputum or culture positive, if resistant organisms are present, or if the patient is HIV positive.
In the treatment of tuberculosis, the small number of resistant cells present within large populations of susceptible cells can rapidly become the predominant type. Since resistance can emerge rapidly, susceptibility tests should be performed in the event of persistent positive cultures during the course of treatment. Bacteriologic smears or cultures should be obtained before the start of therapy to confirm the susceptibility of the organism to rifampin, isoniazid, and pyrazinamide and they should be repeated throughout therapy to monitor response to the treatment. If test results show resistance to any of the components of RIFATER and the patient is not responding to therapy, the drug regimen should be modified.

CONTRAINDICATIONS

RIFATER is contraindicated in patients with a history of hypersensitivity to rifampin, isoniazid, pyrazinamide, or any of the components. Other contraindications include patients with severe hepatic damage; severe adverse reactions to isoniazid, such as drug fever, chills, and arthritis; patients with acute liver disease of any etiology; and patients with acute gout.

WARNINGS

RIFATER is a combination of the three drugs, rifampin, isoniazid, and pyrazinamide. Each of these individual drugs has been associated with liver dysfunction.
Rifampin. Rifampin has been shown to produce liver dysfunction. Fatalities associated with jaundice have occurred in patients with liver disease and in patients taking rifampin with other hepatoxic agents. Because RIFATER contains both rifampin and isoniazid, it should only be given with caution and under strict medical supervision to patients with impaired liver function. In these patients, careful monitoring of liver function, especially serum glutamic pyruvic transaminase (SGPT) and serum glutamic oxaloacetic transaminase (SGOT) should be carried out prior to therapy and then every 2 to 4 weeks during therapy. If signs of hepatocellular damage occur, RIFATER should be withdrawn.
In some cases, hyperbilirubinemia resulting from competition between rifampin and bilirubin for excretory pathways of the liver at the cell level can occur in the early days of treatment. An isolated report showing a moderate rise in bilirubin and/or transminase level is not in itself an indication for interrupting treatment; rather, the decision should be made after repeating the tests, noting trends in the levels, and considering them in conjunction with the patient's clinical condition.
Rifampin has enzyme-inducing properties, including induction of delta amino levulinic acid synthetase. Isolated reports have associated porphyria exacerbation with rifampin administration.
Isoniazid. See the boxed WARNING.
Since RIFATER contains isoniazid, ophthalmologic examinations (including ophthalmoscopy) should be done before treatment is started and periodically thereafter, even without occurrence of visual symptoms.
Pyrazinamide. Since RIFATER contains pyrazinamide, patients started on RIFATER should have baseline serum uric acid and liver function determinations. Patients with preexisting liver disease or those patients at increased risk for drug related hepatitis (eg, alcohol abusers) should be followed closely.
Because it contains pyrazinamide, RIFATER should be discontinued and not be resumed if signs of hepatocellular damage or hyperuricemia accompanied by an acute gouty arthritis appear. If hyperuricemia accompanied by an acute gouty arthritis occurs without liver dysfunction, the patient should be transferred to a regimen not containing pyrazinamide.

PRECAUTIONS

General

RIFATER should be used with caution in patients with a history of diabetes mellitus, as diabetes management may be more difficult.
Rifampin. For treatment of tuberculosis, rifampin is usually administered on a daily basis. Doses of rifampin (>600 mg) given once or twice weekly have resulted in a higher incidence of adverse reactions, including the "flu syndrome" (fever, chills and malaise); hematopoietic reactions (leukopenia, thrombocytopenia, or acute hemolytic anemia); cutaneous, gastrointestinal, and hepatic reactions; shortness of breath; shock and renal failure.
The patient should be advised that the reliability of oral contraceptives may be affected; consideration should be given to using alternative contraceptive measures.
Isoniazid. All drugs should be stopped and an evaluation of the patient should be made at the first sign of a hypersensitivity reaction. Use of RIFATER, because it contains isoniazid, should be carefully monitored in the following:

1. Patients who are receiving phenytoin (diphenylhydantoin) concurrently. Isoniazid may decrease the excretion of phenytoin or may enhance its effects. To avoid phenytoin intoxication, appropriate adjustment of the anticonvulsant dose should be made.
2. Daily users of alcohol. Daily ingestion of alcohol may be associated with a higher incidence of isoniazid hepatitis.
3. Patients with current chronic liver disease or severe renal dysfunction.

Pyrazinamide. Pyrazinamide inhibits renal excretion of urates, frequently resulting in hyperuricemia which is usually asymptomatic. If hyperuricemia is accompanied by acute gouty arthritis, RIFATER, because it contains pyrazinamide, should be discontinued.

Information for Patients

Food Interactions: Because isoniazid has some monoamine oxidase inhibiting activity, an interaction with tyramine-containing foods (cheese, red wine) may occur. Diamine oxidase may also be inhibited, causing exaggerated response (eg, headache, sweating, palpitations, flushing, hypotension) to foods containing histamine (eg, skipjack, tuna, other tropical fish). Tyramine- and histamine-containing foods should be avoided in patients receiving RIFATER.
RIFATER, because it contains rifampin, may produce a reddish coloration of the urine, sweat, sputum, and tears, and the patient should be forewarned of this. Soft contact lenses may be permanently stained.
Patients should be instructed to take RIFATER either 1 hour before or 2 hours after a meal.
Patients should be instructed to notify their physicians promptly if they experience any of the following: fever, loss of appetite, malaise, nausea and vomiting, darkened urine, yellowish discoloration of the skin and eyes, pain or swelling of the joints.
Compliance with the full course of therapy must be emphasized, and the importance of not missing any doses must be stressed.

Laboratory Tests

A complete blood count (CBC), liver function tests, and blood uric acid determinations should be obtained prior to instituting therapy and periodically throughout the course of therapy. Because of a possible transient rise in transaminase and bilirubin values, blood for baseline clinical chemistries should be obtained before RIFATER dosing.

Drug Interactions

Rifampin. Enzyme Induction: Rifampin is known to induce certain cytochrome P-450 enzymes. Coadministration of RIFATER, because it contains rifampin, with drugs that undergo biotransformation through these metabolic pathways may accelerate elimination. To maintain optimum therapeutic blood levels, dosages of drugs metabolized by these enzymes may require adjustment when starting or stopping concomitantly administered rifampin.
Rifampin has been reported to accelerate the metabolism of the following drugs: anticonvulsants (eg, phenytoin), antiarrythmics (eg, disopyramide, mexiletine, quinidine, tocainide), anticoagulants, antifungals (eg, fluconazole, itraconazole, ketoconazole), barbiturates, beta-blockers, calcium channel blockers (eg, diltiazem, nifedipine, verapamil), chloramphenicol, ciprofloxacin, corticosteroids, cyclosporine, cardiac glycoside preparations, clofibrate, oral contraceptives, dapsone, diazepam, haloperidol, oral hypoglycemic agents (sulfonylureas), methadone, narcotic analgesics, nortriptyline, progestins, and theophylline. It may be necessary to adjust dosages of these drugs if they are given concurrently with RIFATER since it contains rifampin.
Rifampin has been observed to increase the requirements for anticoagulant drugs of the coumarin type. In patients receiving anticoagulants and RIFATER concurrently, it is recommended that the prothrombin time be performed daily or as frequently as necessary to establish and maintain the required dose of anticoagulant.
Concurrent use of ketoconazole and rifampin has resulted in decreased serum concentration of both drugs. Concurrent use of rifampin and enalapril has resulted in decreased concentrations of enalaprilat, the active metabolite of enalapril. Since RIFATER contains rifampin, dosage adjustments should be made if RIFATER is concurrently administered with ketoconazole or enalapril if indicated by the patient's clinical condition.
Other Interactions: Concomitant antacid administration may reduce the absorption of rifampin. Daily doses of RIFATER, because it contains rifampin, should be given at least 1 hour before the ingestion of antacids.
Probenecid and cotrimoxazole have been reported to increase the blood level of rifampin.
When rifampin is given concomitantly with either halothane or isoniazid the potential for hepatotoxicity is increased. The concomitant use of RIFATER, because it contains both rifampin and isoniazid, and halothane should be avoided. Patients receiving both rifampin and isoniazid as in RIFATER should be monitored closely for hepatotoxicity. See the boxed WARNING.
Plasma concentrations of sulfapyridine may be reduced following the concomitant administration of sulfasalazine and RIFATER, because it contains rifampin. This finding may be the result of alteration in the colonic bacteria responsible for the reduction of sulfasalazine to sulfapyridine and mesalamine.
Isoniazid. Enzyme Inhibition: Isoniazid is known to inhibit certain cytochrome P-450 enzymes. Coadministration of isoniazid with drugs that undergo biotransformation through these metabolic pathways may decrease elimination. Consequently, dosages of drugs metabolized by these enzymes may require adjustment when starting or stopping concomitantly administered RIFATER, because it contains isoniazid, to maintain optimum therapeutic blood levels.
Isoniazid has been reported to inhibit the metabolism of the following drugs: anticonvulsants (eg, carbamazepine, phenytoin, primidone, valproic acid), benzodiazepines (eg, diazepam), haloperidol, ketoconazole, theophylline, and warfarin. It may be necessary to adjust the dosages of these drugs if they are given concurrently with RIFATER because it contains isoniazid. The impact of the competing effects of rifampin and isoniazid on the metabolism of these drugs is unknown.
Other Interactions: Concomitant antacid administration may reduce the absorption of isoniazid. Ingestion with food may also reduce the absorption of isoniazid. Daily doses of RIFATER, because it contains isoniazid, should be given on an empty stomach at least 1 hour before the ingestion of antacids or food.
Corticosteroids (eg, prednisolone) may decrease the serum concentration of isoniazid by increasing acetylation rate and/or renal clearance. Para-aminosalicylic acid may increase the plasma concentration and elimination half-life of isoniazid by competition of acetylating enzymes.
Pharmacodynamic Interactions: Daily ingestion of alcohol may be associated with a higher incidence of isoniazid hepatitis. Isoniazid, when given concomitantly with rifampin, has been reported to increase the hepatotoxicity of both drugs. Patients receiving both rifampin and isoniazid as in RIFATER should be monitored closely for hepatotoxicity.
The CNS effects of meperidine (drowsiness), cycloserine (dizziness, drowsiness), and disulfiram (acute behavioral and coordination changes) may be exaggerated when concomitant RIFATER, because it contains isoniazid, is given.
Concurrent RIFATER, because it contains isoniazid, and levodopa administration may produce symptoms of excess catecholamine stimulation (agitation, flushing, palpitations) or lack of levodopa effect.
Isoniazid may produce hyperglycemia and lead to loss of glucose control in patients on oral hypoglycemics.
Fast acetylation of isoniazid may produce high concentrations of hydrazine which facilitate deflorination of enflurane. Renal function should be monitored in patients receiving both RIFATER and enflurane.
Food Interactions: Because isoniazid has some monoamine oxidase inhibiting activity, an interaction with tyramine-containing foods (cheese, red wine) may occur. Diamine oxidase may also be inhibited, causing exaggerated response (eg, headache, sweating, palpitations, flushing, hypotension) to foods containing histamine (eg, skipjack, tuna, other tropical fish). Tyramine- and histamine-containing foods should be avoided by patients receiving RIFATER.

Drug/Laboratory Tests Interaction

Rifampin. Therapeutic levels of rifampin have been shown to inhibit standard microbiological assays for serum folate and vitamin B_{12}. Therefore, alternative assay methods should be considered. Transient abnormalities in liver function tests (eg, elevation in serum bilirubin, abnormal bromsulphalein [BSP] excretion, alkaline phosphatase and serum transaminases), and reduced biliary excretion of contrast media used for visualization of the gallbladder have also been observed. Therefore, these tests should be performed before the morning dose of RIFATER.
Rifampin and isoniazid have been reported to alter vitamin D metabolism. In some cases, reduced levels of circulating 25-hydroxy vitamin D and 1,25-dihydroxy vitamin D have been accompanied by reduced serum calcium and phosphate, and elevated parathyroid hormone.

Pyrazinamide. Pyrazinamide has been reported to interfere with ACETEST® and KETOSTIX® urine tests to produce a pink-brown color.

Carcinogenesis, Mutagenesis, Impairment of Fertility

Increased frequency of chromosomal aberrations was observed *in vitro* in lymphocytes obtained from patients treated with combinations of rifampin, isoniazid, and pyrazinamide and combinations of streptomycin, rifampin, isoniazid, and pyrazinamide.

Rifampin. There are no known human data on long-term potential for carcinogenicity, mutagenicity, or impairment of fertility. A few cases of accelerated growth of lung carcinoma have been reported in man, but a causal relationship with the drug has not been established. An increase in the incidence of hepatomas in female mice (of a strain known to be particularly susceptible to the spontaneous development of hepatomas) was observed when rifampicin was administered in doses two to ten times the average daily human dose for 60 weeks followed by an observation period of 46 weeks. No evidence of carcinogenicity was found in male mice of the same strain, mice of a different strain, or rats under similar experimental conditions.

Rifampin has been reported to possess immunosuppressive potential in rabbits, mice, rats, guinea pigs, human lymphocytes *in vitro*, and humans. Antitumor activity *in vitro* has also been shown with rifampin.

There was no evidence of mutagenicity in bacteria, *Drosophila melanogaster*, or mice. An increase in chromatid breaks was noted when whole blood cell cultures were treated with rifampin.

Isoniazid. Isoniazid has been reported to induce pulmonary tumors in a number of strains of mice.

Pyrazinamide. In lifetime bioassays in rats and mice, pyrazinamide was administered in the diet at concentrations of up to 10,000 ppm. This resulted in estimated daily doses of 2 g/kg for the mouse, or 40 times the maximum human dose, and 0.5 g/kg for the rat, or 10 times the maximum human dose. Pyrazinamide was not carcinogenic in rats or male mice and no conclusion was possible for female mice.

Pyrazinamide was not mutagenic in the Ames bacterial test, but induced chromosomal aberrations in human lymphocyte cell cultures.

Pregnancy – Teratogenic Effects

Category C. Animal reproduction studies have not been conducted with RIFATER. It is also not known whether RIFATER can cause fetal harm when administered to a pregnant woman. RIFATER should be given to a pregnant woman only if clearly needed.

Rifampin. Although rifampin has been reported to cross the placental barrier and appear in cord blood, the effect of rifampin, alone or in combination with other antituberculosis drugs, on the human fetus is not known. An increase in congenital malformations, primarily spina bifida and cleft palate, has been reported in the offspring of rodents given oral doses of 150 to 250 mg/kg/day of rifampin during pregnancy. The possible teratogenic potential in women capable of bearing children should be carefully weighed against the benefits of RIFATER therapy.

Isoniazid. It has been reported that in both rats and rabbits, isoniazid may exert an embryocidal effect when administered orally during pregnancy, although no isoniazid-related congenital anomalies have been found in reproduction studies in mammalian species (mice, rats, and rabbits). RIFATER, because it contains isoniazid, should be prescribed during pregnancy only when therapeutically necessary. The benefit of preventive therapy should be weighed against a possible risk to the fetus. Preventive treatment generally should be started after delivery because of the increased risk of tuberculosis for new mothers.

Pyrazinamide. Animal reproduction studies have not been conducted with pyrazinamide. It is also not known whether pyrazinamide can cause fetal harm when administered to a pregnant woman. RIFATER, because it contains pyrazinamide, should be given to a pregnant women only if clearly needed.

Pregnancy – Non-Teratogenic Effects

It is not known whether RIFATER can affect reproduction capacity.

Rifampin. When administered during the last few weeks of pregnancy, rifampin can cause postnatal hemorrhages in the mother and infant. In this case, treatment with vitamin K may be indicated for postnatal hemorrhage.

Nursing Mothers

Since rifampin, isoniazid, and pyrazinamide are known to pass into maternal breast milk, a decision should be made whether to discontinue nursing or to discontinue RIFATER, taking into account the importance of the drug to the mother.

Pediatric Use

Safety and effectiveness in pediatric patients under the age of 15 have not been established.

ADVERSE REACTIONS

Adverse Experiences During the Clinical Trial

Adverse event data reported for the RIFATER and the separate drug treatment groups during the first 2 months of the trial are shown in the table below.

Adverse Events Reported During the Clinical Study

Adverse Events by Body Systems During First 2 Months of Trial	Number of Patients With Adverse Events* RIFATER n = 122‡	Separate† n = 123‡
Cutaneous (rash, erythrodema, erythema, exfoliative dermatitis, Lyell syndrome, urticaria, localized skin rash, diffuse skin rash, pruritus, generalized hypersensitivity)	8 (7%)	21 (17%)
Gastrointestinal (nausea, vomiting, digestive pain, diarrhea)	8 (7%)	14 (11%)
Musculoskeletal (arthralgia, long bones pain, phlebitis, localized joint pain, diffuse joint pain, edema of the legs)	5 (4%)	8 (7%)
Hearing and Vestibular(tinnitus, vertigo, vertigo with loss of equilibrium)	3 (2%)	6 (5%)
Liver and Biliary (hepatitis with conjunctival jaundice, hepatitis with deep jaundice)	0 (0%)	2 (2%)
Central and Peripheral Nervous System (sweating, headache, insomnia, diffuse paresthesia of the legs, anxiety, diabetic coma)	5 (4%)	4 (3%)
Total Body (spiking fever, persistent fever)	2 (2%)	4 (3%)
Cardiorespiratory (tightness in chest, coughing, diffuse chest pain, hemoptysis, angina, palpitation, total pneumothorax)	8 (7%)	3 (2%)
Total number of patients with one or more adverse events	29	43

* A given patient may have experienced ≥1 adverse event.

† Isoniazid, rifampin and pyrazinamide dosed as separate tablets and capsules.

‡ A total of 250 patients (124 RIFATER; 126 separate) were originally enrolled in the study. Five patients (2 RIFATER; 3 separate) were excluded due to admission errors.

No serious adverse events were reported in the patients receiving RIFATER tablets. Three serious adverse events were reported in the patients given isoniazid, rifampin, and pyrazinamide as separate tablets and capsules. The three serious adverse events were two general hypersensitivity reactions and one jaundice reaction.

There were no significant differences between the two treatment groups in standard liver function, renal function and hematological laboratory test values measured at baseline and after 8 weeks of treatment. As would be expected for these drugs, there were alterations in liver enzymes (SGOT, SGPT) and serum uric acid levels. The adverse reactions reported during therapy with RIFATER are consistent with those described below for the individual components.

Adverse Reactions Reported for Individual Components

Rifampin, Gastrointestinal: Heartburn, epigastric distress, anorexia, nausea, vomiting, jaundice, flatulence, cramps, and diarrhea have been noted in some patients. Although *Clostridium difficile* has been shown *in vitro* to be sensitive to rifampin, pseudomembranous colitis has been reported with the use of rifampin (and other broad spectrum antibiotics). Therefore, it is important to consider this diagnosis in patients who develop diarrhea in association with antibiotic use. Rarely, hepatitis or a shocklike syndrome with hepatic involvement and abnormal liver function tests has been reported.

Hematologic: Thrombocytopenia has occurred primarily with high dose intermittent therapy, but has also been noted after resumption of interrupted treatment. It rarely occurs during well-supervised daily therapy. This effect is reversible if the drug is discontinued as soon as purpura occurs. Cerebral hemorrhage and fatalities have been reported when rifampin administration has been continued or resumed after the appearance of purpura.

Transient leukopenia, hemolytic anemia, and decreased hemoglobin have been observed.

Central Nervous System: Headache, fever, drowsiness, fatigue, ataxia, dizziness, inability to concentrate, mental confusion, behavioral changes, muscular weakness, pains in extremities, and generalized numbness have been observed. Rare reports of myopathy have also been observed.

Ocular: Visual disturbances have been observed.

Endocrine: Menstrual disturbances have been observed.

Renal: Elevations in BUN and serum uric acid have been reported. Rarely, hemolysis, hemoglobinuria, hematuria, interstitial nephritis, renal insufficiency, and acute renal failure have been noted. These are generally considered to be hypersensitivity reactions. They usually occur during intermittent therapy or when treatment is resumed following intentional or accidental interruption of a daily dosage regimen, and are reversible when rifampin is discontinued and appropriate therapy instituted.

Dermatologic: Cutaneous reactions are mild and self-limiting and do not appear to be hypersensitivity reactions. Typically, they consist of flushing and itching with or without a rash. More serious cutaneous reactions which may be due to hypersensitivity occur but are uncommon.

Hypersensitivity Reactions: Occasionally pruritus, urticaria, rash, pemphigoid reaction, eosinophilia, sore mouth, sore tongue and conjunctivitis have been observed.

Miscellaneous: Edema of the face and extremities have been reported. Other reactions which have occurred with intermittent dosage regimens include "flu" syndrome (such as episodes of fever, chills, headache, dizziness, and bone pain), shortness of breath, wheezing, decrease in blood pressure and shock. The "flu" syndrome may also appear if rifampin is taken irregularly by the patient or if daily administration is resumed after a drug free interval.

Isoniazid. The most frequent reactions are those affecting the nervous system and the liver. See the boxed WARNING.

Nervous System: Peripheral neuropathy is the most common toxic effect. It is dose-related, occurs most often in the malnourished and in those predisposed to neuritis (eg, alcoholics and diabetics), and is usually preceded by paresthesias of the feet and hands. The incidence is higher in "slow inactivators."

Other neurotoxic effects, which are uncommon with conventional doses, are convulsions, toxic encephalopathy, optic neuritis and atrophy, memory impairment, and toxic psychosis.

Gastrointestinal: Nausea, vomiting, and epigastric distress.

Hepatic: Elevated serum transaminases (SGOT, SGPT), bilirubinemia, bilirubinuria, jaundice, and occasionally severe and sometimes fatal hepatitis. The common prodromal symptoms are anorexia, nausea, vomiting, fatigue, malaise, and weakness. Mild and transient elevation of serum transaminase levels occurs in 10 to 20% of persons taking isoniazid. The abnormality usually occurs in the first 4 to 6 months of treatment but can occur at any time during therapy. In most instances, enzyme levels return to normal with no necessity to discontinue medication. In occasional instances, progressive liver damage occurs, with accompanying symptoms. In these cases, the drug should be discontinued immediately. The frequency of progressive liver damage increases with age. It is rare in persons under 20, but occurs in up to 2.3% of those over 50 years of age.

Hematologic: Agranulocytosis; hemolytic, sideroblastic, or aplastic anemia; thrombocytopenia; and eosinophilia.

Hypersensitivity Reactions: Fever, skin eruptions (morbilliform, maculopapular, purpuric, or exfoliative), lymphadenopathy, and vasculitis.

Metabolic and Endocrine: Pyridoxine deficiency, pellagra, hyperglycemia, metabolic acidosis, and gynecomastia.

Miscellaneous: Rheumatic syndrome and systemic lupus erythematosus-like syndrome.

Pyrazinamide. The principal adverse effect is a hepatic reaction (see WARNINGS). Hepatotoxicity appears to be dose related and may appear at any time during therapy. Pyrazinamide can cause hyperuricemia and gout (see PRECAUTIONS).

Gastrointestinal: GI disturbances including nausea, vomiting, and anorexia have also been reported.

Hematologic and Lymphatic: Thrombocytopenia and sideroblastic anemia with erythroid hyperplasia, vacuolation of erythrocytes and increased serum concentration have occurred rarely with this drug. Adverse effects on blood clotting mechanisms have also been rarely reported.

Other: Mild arthralgia and myalgia have been reported frequently. Hypersensitivity reactions including rashes, urticaria, and pruritus have been reported. Fever, acne, photosensitivity, porphyria, dysuria, and interstitial nephritis have been reported rarely.

OVERDOSAGE

RIFATER. There is no human experience with RIFATER overdosage.

Rifampin. Non-fatal overdoses with as high as 12 g of rifampin have been reported.

One case of fatal overdose is known: A 26-year-old man died after self-administering 60 g of rifampin.

Isoniazid. Untreated or inadequately treated cases of gross isoniazid overdosage can be fatal, but good response has been reported in most patients treated within the first few hours after drug ingestion.

Ingested acutely, as little as 1.5 g isoniazid may cause toxicity in adults. Doses of 35 to 40 mg/kg have resulted in seizures. Ingestion of 80 to 150 mg/kg isoniazid has been associated with severe toxicity and, if untreated, significant mortality.

Pyrazinamide. Overdosage experience with pyrazinamide is limited.

Signs and Symptoms

The following signs and symptoms have been seen with each individual component in an overdosage situation.

Rifampin. Nausea, vomiting, and increasing lethargy will probably occur within a short time after rifampin overdosage; unconsciousness may occur when there is severe hepatic disease. Brownish red or orange discoloration of the skin, urine, sweat, saliva, tears, and feces will occur, and its intensity is proportional to the amount ingested.

Continued on next page

Rifater—Cont.

Liver enlargement, possibly with tenderness, can develop within a few hours after severe overdosage; bilirubin levels may increase and jaundice may develop rapidly. Hepatic involvement may be more marked in patients with prior impairment of hepatic function. Other physical findings remain essentially normal. A direct effect upon the hematopoietic system, electrolyte levels, or acid-base balance is unlikely.

Isoniazid. Isoniazid overdosage produces signs and symptoms within 30 minutes to 3 hours. Nausea, vomiting, dizziness, slurring of speech, blurring of vision, and visual hallucinations (including bright colors and strange designs) are among the early manifestations. With marked overdosage, respiratory distress and CNS depression progressing rapidly from stupor to profound coma, are to be expected along with severe, intractable seizures. Severe metabolic acidosis, acetonuria, and hyperglycemia are typical laboratory findings.

Pyrazinamide. In one case of pyrazinamide overdosage, abnormal liver function tests developed. These spontaneously reverted to normal when the drug was stopped.

Treatment

The airway should be secured and adequate respiratory exchange should be established in cases of overdosage with RIFATER.

Obtain blood samples for immediate determination of gases, electrolytes, BUN, glucose, etc; type and cross-match blood in preparation for possible hemodialysis.

Gastric lavage within the first 2 to 3 hours after ingestion is advised, but it should not be attempted until convulsions are under control. To treat convulsions, administer IV diazepam or short-acting barbiturates, and IV pyridoxine (usually 1 mg/1 mg isoniazid ingested). Following evacuation of gastric contents, the instillation of activated charcoal slurry into the stomach may help absorb any remaining drug from the gastrointestinal tract. Antiemetic medication may be required to control severe nausea and vomiting.

RAPID CONTROL OF METABOLIC ACIDOSIS IS FUNDAMENTAL TO MANAGEMENT. Give IV sodium bicarbonate at once and repeat as needed, adjusting subsequent dosage on the basis of laboratory findings (ie, serum sodium, pH, etc).

Forced osmotic diuresis must be started early and should be continued for some hours after clinical improvement to hasten renal clearance of drug and help prevent relapse; monitor fluid intake and output.

Hemodialysis is advised for severe cases; if this is not available, peritoneal dialysis can be used along with forced diuresis.

Along with measures based on initial and repeated determination of blood gases and other laboratory tests as needed, utilize meticulous respiratory and other intensive care to protect against hypoxia, hypotension, aspiration pneumonitis, etc.

DOSAGE AND ADMINISTRATION

Adults: Patients should be given the following single daily dose of RIFATER either 1 hour before or 2 hours after a meal with a full glass of water.

Patients weighing ≤44 kg – 4 tablets
Patients weighing between 45–54 kg – 5 tablets
Patients weighing ≥55 kg – 6 tablets

Pediatric Patients: The ratio of the drugs in RIFATER may not be appropriate in pediatric patients under the age of 15 (eg, higher mg/kg doses of isoniazid are usually given in pediatric patients than adults).

RIFATER is recommended in the initial phase of short-course therapy which is usually continued for 2 months. The Advisory Council for the Elimination of Tuberculosis, the American Thoracic Society, and the Centers for Disease Control and Prevention recommend that either streptomycin or ethambutol be added as a fourth drug in a regimen containing isoniazid (INH), rifampin and pyrazinamide for initial treatment of tuberculosis unless the likelihood of INH or rifampin resistance is very low. The need for a fourth drug should be reassessed when the results of susceptibility testing are known. If community rates of INH resistance are currently less than 4%, an initial treatment regimen with less than four drugs may be considered.

Following the initial phase, treatment should be continued with rifampin and isoniazid (eg, RIFAMATE®) for at least 4 months. Treatment should be continued for longer if the patient is still sputum or culture positive, if resistant organisms are present, or if the patient is HIV positive.

Concomitant administration of pyridoxine (B_6) is recommended in the malnourished, in those predisposed to neuropathy (eg, alcoholics and diabetics), and in adolescents.

See CLINICAL PHARMACOLOGY: General for dosing information in patients with renal failure.

HOW SUPPLIED

RIFATER tablets are light beige, smooth, round, and shiny sugar-coated tablets imprinted with "RIFATER" in black ink and contain 120 mg rifampin, 50 mg isoniazid, and 300 mg pyrazinamide, and are supplied as:

Bottles of 60 tablets (NDC 0088-0576-41).

Storage Conditions: Store at controlled room temperature 59–86°F (15–30°C). Protect from excessive humidity.

REFERENCE 1. National Committee for Clinical Laboratory Standards. 1990. Antimycobacterial Susceptibility Testing (Proposed Standard). Document M24-P.

Prescribing Information as of December 1995

Merrell Pharmaceuticals Inc.
Subsidiary of Hoechst Marion Roussel, Inc.
Kansas City, MO 64137 USA
Rifater Tablets are manufactured by:
GRUPPO LEPETIT S.p.A.
20020 Lainate, Italy

Shown in Product Identification Guide, page 307

RILUTEK® ℞
(riluzole) Tablets
[rĭl-ū-tĕk]
Rx only

DESCRIPTION

RILUTEK® (riluzole) is a member of the benzothiazole class. Chemically, riluzole is 2-amino-6-(trifluoromethoxy) benzothiazole. Its molecular formula is $C_8H_5F_3N_2OS$ and its molecular weight is 234.2. Its structural formula is as follows:

Riluzole is a white to slightly yellow powder that is very soluble in dimethylformamide, dimethylsulfoxide and methanol, freely soluble in dichloromethane, sparingly soluble in 0.1 N HCl and very slightly soluble in water and in 0.1 N NaOH. RILUTEK is available as a capsule-shaped, white, film-coated tablet for oral administration containing 50 mg of riluzole. Each tablet is engraved with "RPR 202" on one side.

Inactive Ingredients: Core: anhydrous dibasic calcium phosphate, USP; microcrystalline cellulose, NF; anhydrous colloidal silica, NF; magnesium stearate, NF; croscarmellose sodium, NF. **Film coating:** hydroxypropyl methylcellulose, USP; polyethylene glycol 6000; titanium dioxide, USP.

CLINICAL PHARMACOLOGY

Mechanism of Action

The etiology and pathogenesis of amyotrophic lateral sclerosis (ALS) are not known, although a number of hypotheses have been advanced. One hypothesis is that motor neurons, made vulnerable through either genetic predisposition or environmental factors, are injured by glutamate. In some cases of familial ALS the enzyme superoxide dismutase has been found to be defective.

The mode of action of RILUTEK is unknown. Its pharmacological properties include the following, some of which may be related to its effect: 1) an inhibitory effect on glutamate release, 2) inactivation of voltage-dependent sodium channels, and 3) ability to interfere with intracellular events that follow transmitter binding at excitatory amino acid receptors.

Riluzole has also been shown, in a single study, to delay median time to death in a transgenic mouse model of ALS. These mice express human superoxide dismutase bearing one of the mutations found in one of the familial forms of human ALS.

It is also neuroprotective in various *in vivo* experimental models of neuronal injury involving excitotoxic mechanisms. In *in vitro* tests, riluzole protected cultured rat motor neurons from the excitotoxic effects of glutamic acid and prevented the death of cortical neurons induced by anoxia.

Due to its blockade of glutamatergic neurotransmission, riluzole also exhibits myorelaxant and sedative properties in animal models at doses of 30 mg/kg (about 20 times the recommended human daily dose) and anticonvulsant properties at a dose of 2.5 mg/kg (about 2 times the recommended human daily dose).

Pharmacokinetics

Riluzole is well-absorbed (approximately 90%), with average absolute oral bioavailability of about 60% (CV=30%). Pharmacokinetics are linear over a dose range of 25–100 mg given every 12 hours. A high fat meal decreases absorption, reducing AUC by about 20% and peak blood levels by about 45%. The mean elimination half-life of riluzole is 12 hours (CV=35%) after repeated doses. With multiple-dose administration, riluzole accumulates in plasma by about twofold and steady-state is reached in less than 5 days. Riluzole is 96% bound to plasma proteins, mainly to albumin and lipoproteins over the clinical concentration range.

The 50 mg market tablet was equivalent, with respect to AUC, to the tablet used in the dose ranging clinical trials, while the C_{max} was approximately 30% higher. Both tablets have been used in clinical trials. However, if doses greater than those recommended are given, it is likely that higher plasma levels will be achieved, the safety of which has not been established (see DOSAGE AND ADMINISTRATION).

Metabolism and Elimination

Riluzole is extensively metabolized to six major and a number of minor metabolites, not all of which have been identified. Some metabolites appear pharmacologically active in *in vitro* assays. The metabolism of riluzole is mostly hepatic and consists of cytochrome P450-dependent hydroxylation and glucuronidation.

There is marked inter-individual variability in the clearance of riluzole, probably attributable to variability of CYP 1A2 activity, the principal isozyme involved in N-hydroxylation.

In vitro studies using liver microsomes show that hydroxylation of the primary amine group producing N-hydroxyriluzole is the main metabolic pathway in human, monkey, dog and rabbit. In humans, cytochrome P450 1A2 is the principal isozyme involved in N-hydroxylation. *In vitro* studies predict that CYP 2D6, CYP 2C19, CYP 3A4 and CYP 2E1 are unlikely to contribute significantly to riluzole metabolism in humans. Whereas direct glucuroconjugation of riluzole (involving the glucurotransferase isoform UGT-HP4) is very slow in human liver microsomes, N-hydroxyriluzole is readily conjugated at the hydroxylamine group resulting in the formation of O- (>90%) and N-glucuronides.

Following a single 150 mg dose of ^{14}C-riluzole to 6 healthy males, 90% and 5% of the radioactivity was recovered in the urine and feces respectively over a period of 7 days. Glucuronides accounted for more than 85% of the metabolites in urine. Only 2% of a riluzole dose was recovered in the urine as unchanged drug.

Special Populations

The pharmacokinetics of riluzole have not been studied in renally and hepatically impaired subjects, nor is there information about the effects of smoking, age and gender on the pharmacokinetics of riluzole but certain differences in population subsets should be anticipated (see PRECAUTIONS).

Hepatic and Renal Disease: Since riluzole is extensively metabolized and subsequently excreted in the urine, it is likely that functional hepatic and renal impairment will reduce the clearance of riluzole and its metabolites and give higher plasma levels (see PRECAUTIONS and WARNINGS).

Age: Age-related decreased renal function would be expected to give higher plasma levels of riluzole and metabolites. However, in controlled clinical trials, in which approximately 30% of patients were over 65, there were no differences in adverse events between younger and older patients (see PRECAUTIONS).

Gender: CYP 1A2 activity has been reported to be lower in women than in men. Therefore, a gender effect on riluzole kinetics may be expected in women, resulting in higher blood concentrations of riluzole and its metabolites (see PRECAUTIONS). No gender effect on favorable or adverse effects of riluzole was seen in controlled trials, however.

Smoking: Cigarette smoking is known to induce CYP 1A2. Patients who smoke cigarettes would be expected to eliminate riluzole faster. There is no information, however, on the effect of, or need for, dosage adjustment in these patients.

Race: Clearance of riluzole in Japanese subjects native to Japan was found to be 50% lower as compared to Caucasians after normalizing for body weight. Although it is not clear if this difference is due to genetic or environmental factors (*e.g.,* smoking, alcohol, coffee, and dietary preferences), it is possible that Japanese subjects may possess a lower capacity (oxidative and/or conjugative) for metabolizing riluzole. There are no studies, however, of lower doses in Japanese subjects (see PRECAUTIONS).

Clinical Trials

The efficacy of RILUTEK as a treatment of ALS was established in two adequate and well-controlled trials in which the time to tracheostomy or death was longer for patients randomized to RILUTEK than for those randomized to placebo.

These studies admitted patients with either familial or sporadic ALS, a disease duration of less than 5 years, and a baseline forced vital capacity greater than or equal to 60%.

In one study, performed in France and Belgium, 155 ALS patients were followed for at least 13 months (maximum duration 18 months) after being randomized to either 100 mg/day (given 50 mg BID) of RILUTEK or placebo.

Figure 1, which follows, displays the survival curves for time to death or tracheostomy. The vertical axis represents the proportion of individuals alive without tracheostomy at various times following treatment initiation (horizontal axis). Although these survival curves were not statistically significantly different when evaluated by the analysis specified in the study protocol (Logrank test p=0.12), the difference was found to be significant by another appropriate analysis (Wilcoxon test p=0.05). As seen, the study showed an early increase in survival in patients given riluzole. Among the patients in whom treatment failed during the study (tracheostomy or death) there was a difference between the treatment groups in median survival of approximately 90 days. There was no statistically significant difference in mortality at the end of the study.

[See figure 1 at top of next column]

In the second study, performed in both Europe and North America, 959 ALS patients were followed for at least 1 year (North American centers) and up to 18 months (European centers) after being randomized to either 50, 100, 200 mg/day of RILUTEK or placebo.

Figure 2, which follows, displays the survival curves for time to death or tracheostomy for patients randomized to either 100 mg/day of RILUTEK or placebo. Although these survival curves were not statistically significantly different when evaluated by the analysis specified in the study protocol (Logrank test p = 0.076), the difference was found to be significant by another appropriate analysis (Wilcoxon test p = 0.05). Not displayed in Figure 2 are the results of 50 mg/day of RILUTEK which could not be statistically distin-

Figure 1: Kaplan-Meier Survival Curves

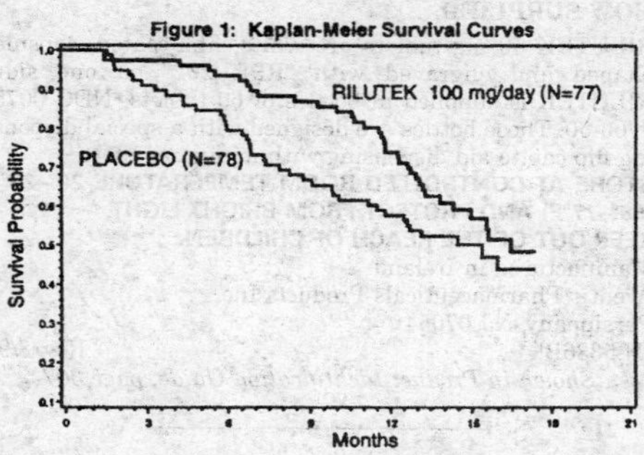

guished from placebo and the results of 200 mg/day which are essentially identical to 100 mg/day. As seen, the study showed an early increase in survival in patients given riluzole. Among the patients in whom treatment failed during the study (tracheostomy or death) there was a difference between the treatment groups in median survival of approximately 60 days. There was no statistically significant difference in mortality at the end of the study.

Figure 2: Kaplan-Meier Survival Curves

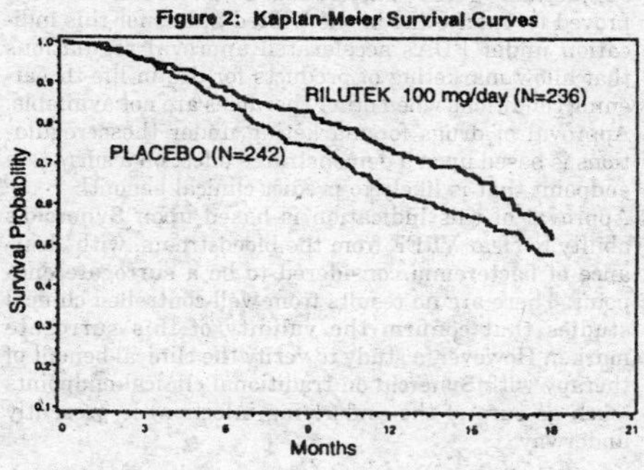

Although riluzole improved early survival in both studies, measures of muscle strength and neurological function did not show a benefit.

INDICATIONS AND USAGE

RILUTEK is indicated for the treatment of patients with amyotrophic lateral sclerosis (ALS). Riluzole extends survival and/or time to tracheostomy.

CONTRAINDICATIONS

RILUTEK is contraindicated in patients who have a history of severe hypersensitivity reactions to riluzole or any of the tablet components.

WARNINGS

Liver Injury/Monitoring Liver Chemistries

RILUTEK should be prescribed with care in patients with current evidence or history of abnormal liver function indicated by significant abnormalities in serum transaminase (ALT/SGPT; AST/SGOT), bilirubin, and/or gamma-glutamate transferase (GGT) levels (see PRECAUTIONS and DOSAGE AND ADMINISTRATION sections). Baseline elevations of several LFTs (especially elevated bilirubin) should preclude the use of RILUTEK.

RILUTEK, even in patients without a prior history of liver disease, causes serum aminotransferase elevations. Experience in almost 800 ALS patients indicates that about 50% of riluzole-treated patients will experience at least one ALT/SGPT level above the upper limit of normal, about 8% will have elevations > 3 × ULN, and about 2% of patients will have elevations > 5 × ULN. A single non-ALS patient with epilepsy treated with concomitant carbamazepine and phenobarbital experienced marked, rapid elevations of liver enzymes with jaundice (ALT 26 × ULN, AST 17 × ULN, and bilirubin 11 × ULN) four months after starting RILUTEK; these returned to normal 7 weeks after treatment discontinuation.

Maximum increases in serum ALT usually occurred within 3 months after the start of riluzole therapy and were usually transient when < 5 times ULN. In trials, if ALT levels were <5 times ULN, treatment continued and ALT levels usually returned to below 2 times ULN within 2 to 6 months. Treatment in studies was discontinued, however, if ALT levels exceeded 5 × ULN, so that there is no experience with continued treatment of ALS patients once ALT values exceed 5 times ULN (see PRECAUTIONS: Laboratory Tests). There were rare instances of jaundice.

Liver chemistries should be monitored (see PRECAUTIONS).

Neutropenia

Among approximately 4000 patients given riluzole for ALS, there were three cases of marked neutropenia (absolute neutrophil count less than 500/mm^3), all seen within the first 2 months of riluzole treatment. In one case, neutrophil counts rose on continued treatment. In a second case, counts rose after therapy was stopped. A third case was more complex, with marked anemia as well as neutropenia and the etiology of both is uncertain. Patients should be warned to report any febrile illness to their physicians. The report of a febrile illness should prompt treating physicians to check white blood cell counts.

PRECAUTIONS

Use in Patients with Concomitant Disease

RILUTEK should be used with caution in patients with concomitant liver and/or renal insufficiency (see WARNINGS, CLINICAL PHARMACOLOGY). In particular, in cases of RILUTEK-induced hepatic injury manifested by elevated liver enzymes, the effect of the hepatic injury on RILUTEK metabolism is unknown.

Special Populations

Riluzole should be used with caution in elderly patients whose hepatic or renal functions may be compromised due to age. Also, females and Japanese patients may possess a lower metabolic capacity to eliminate riluzole compared to males and Caucasian subjects, respectively (see CLINICAL PHARMACOLOGY: Special Populations).

Information for the Patient

Patients should be advised to report any febrile illness to their physicians (see WARNINGS: Neutropenia).

Patients and caregivers should be advised that RILUTEK should be taken on a regular basis and at the same time of the day (*e.g.*, in the morning and evening) each day. If a dose is missed, take the next tablet as originally planned (see DOSAGE AND ADMINISTRATION).

Patients should be warned about the potential for dizziness, vertigo, or somnolence and advised not to drive or operate machinery until they have gained sufficient experience on RILUTEK to gauge whether or not it affects their mental and/or motor performance adversely.

Whether alcohol increases the risk of serious hepatotoxicity with RILUTEK is unknown; therefore, patients being treated with RILUTEK should be discouraged from drinking excessive amounts of alcohol.

Patients should also be made aware that RILUTEK should be stored at temperatures between 20°–25°C (68°–77°F) and protected from bright light.

RILUTEK must be kept out of the reach of children.

Laboratory Tests

It is recommended that serum aminotransferases including ALT levels be measured before and during riluzole therapy. Serum ALT levels should be evaluated every month during the first 3 months of treatment, every 3 months during the remainder of the first year, and periodically thereafter. Serum ALT levels should be evaluated more frequently in patients who develop elevations (see WARNINGS).

As noted in the WARNINGS Section, there is no experience with continued treatment of patients once ALT exceeds 5 × ULN. If a decision is made to continue to treat these patients, frequent monitoring (at least weekly) of complete liver function is recommended. Treatment should be discontinued if ALT exceeds 10 × ULN or if clinical jaundice develops. Because there is no experience with rechallenge of patients who have had RILUTEK discontinued for ALT > 5 × ULN, no recommendations about restarting RILUTEK can be made.

In the two controlled trials in patients with ALS, the frequency with which values for hemoglobin, hematocrit, and erythrocyte counts fell below the lower limit of normal was greater in RILUTEK-treated patients than in placebo-treated patients; however, these changes were mild and transient. The proportions of patients observed with abnormally low values for these parameters showed a dose-response relationship. Only one patient was discontinued from treatment because of severe anemia. The significance of this finding is unknown.

Drug Interactions

There have been no clinical studies designed to evaluate the interaction of riluzole with other drugs.

As with all drugs, the potential for interaction by a variety of mechanisms is a possibility.

Hepatotoxic Drugs: The clinical trials in ALS excluded patients on concomitant medications which were potentially hepatotoxic, (*e.g.*, allopurinol, methyldopa, sulfasalazine). Accordingly, there is no information about the safety of administering RILUTEK in conjunction with such medications. If the practitioner chooses to prescribe such a combination, caution should be exercised.

Drugs Highly Bound To Plasma Proteins: Riluzole is highly bound (96%) to plasma proteins, binding mainly to serum albumin and to lipoproteins. The effect of riluzole (up to 5 mcg/mL) on warfarin (5 mcg/mL) binding did not show any displacement of warfarin. Conversely, riluzole binding was unaffected by the addition of warfarin, digoxin, imipramine and quinine at high therapeutic concentrations.

Effect of Other Drugs On Riluzole Metabolism: *In vitro* studies using human liver microsomal preparations suggest that CYP 1A2 is the principal isozyme involved in the initial oxidative metabolism of riluzole and, therefore, potential interactions may occur when riluzole is given concurrently with agents that affect CYP 1A2 activity. Potential inhibitors of CYP 1A2 (*e.g.*, caffeine, phenacetin, theophylline, amitriptyline, and quinolones) could decrease the rate of riluzole elimination, while inducers of CYP 1A2 (*e.g.*, cigarette smoke, charcoal-broiled food, rifampicin, and omeprazole) could increase the rate of riluzole elimination.

Effect of Riluzole On the Metabolism of Other Drugs: CYP 1A2 is the principal isoenzyme involved in the initial oxidative metabolism of riluzole; potential interactions may occur when riluzole is given concurrently with other agents which are also metabolized primarily by CYP 1A2 (*e.g.*, theophylline, caffeine, and tacrine). Currently, it is not known whether riluzole has any potential for enzyme induction in humans.

Drug Laboratory Test Interactions: None known

Carcinogenesis, Mutagenesis, Impairment of Fertility

Long-term studies to determine the carcinogenic potential of riluzole have not yet been completed.

The genotoxic potential of riluzole was evaluated in the bacterial mutagenicity (Ames) test, the mouse lymphoma mutation assay in L5178Y cells, the *in vitro* chromosomal aberration assay in human lymphocytes and the *in vivo* rat cytogenetic assay and *in vivo* mouse micronucleus assay in bone marrow. There was no evidence of mutagenic or clastogenic potential in the Ames test, the mouse lymphoma assay, or the *in vivo* assays in the mouse and rat. There was an equivocal clastogenic response in the *in vitro* lymphocyte chromosomal aberration assay.

Riluzole impaired fertility when administered to male and female rats prior to and during mating at an oral dose of 15 mg/kg or 1.5 times the maximum daily dose on a mg/m^2 basis (see PRECAUTIONS: "Pregnancy" for effects on fertility).

Pregnancy

Pregnancy category C:

Oral administration of riluzole to pregnant animals during the period of organogenesis caused embryotoxicity in rats and rabbits at doses of 27 mg/kg and 60 mg/kg, respectively, or 2.6 and 11.5 times, respectively, the recommended maximum human daily dose on a mg/m^2 basis. Evidence of maternal toxicity was also observed at these doses.

When administered to rats prior to and during mating (males and females) and throughout gestation and lactation (females), riluzole produced adverse effects on pregnancy (decreased implantations, increased intrauterine death) and offspring viability and growth at an oral dose of 15 mg/kg or 1.5 times the maximum daily dose on a mg/m^2 basis.

There are no adequate and well-controlled studies in pregnant women. Riluzole should be used during pregnancy only if the potential benefit justifies the potential risk to the fetus.

Nursing Women

In rat studies, ^{14}C-riluzole was detected in maternal milk. It is not known whether riluzole is excreted in human breast milk. Because many drugs are excreted in human milk, and because the potential for serious adverse reactions in nursing infants from RILUTEK® is unknown, women should be advised not to breast-feed during treatment with RILUTEK.

Use in the Elderly

Age-related compromised renal and hepatic function may cause a decrease in clearance of riluzole (see CLINICAL PHARMACOLOGY: Special Populations). In controlled clinical trials, about 30% of patients were over 65. There were no differences in adverse effects between younger and older patients.

Pediatric Use

The safety and the effectiveness of RILUTEK in pediatric patients have not been established.

ADVERSE REACTIONS

The most commonly observed AEs associated with the use of RILUTEK more frequently than placebo treated patients were: asthenia, nausea, dizziness, decreased lung function, diarrhea, abdominal pain, pneumonia, vomiting, vertigo, circumoral paresthesia, anorexia, and somnolence. Asthenia, nausea, dizziness, diarrhea, anorexia, vertigo, somnolence, and circumoral paresthesia were dose related.

Approximately 14% (n=141) of the 982 individuals with ALS who received RILUTEK in pre-marketing clinical trials discontinued treatment because of an adverse experience. Of those patients who discontinued due to adverse events, the most commonly reported were: nausea, abdominal pain, constipation, and ALT elevations. In a dose response study in ALS patients, the rates of discontinuation of RILUTEK for asthenia, nausea, abdominal pain, and ALT elevation were dose related.

Incidence in Controlled ALS Clinical Studies

Table 1 lists treatment-emergent signs and symptoms that occurred in at least 2% of patients with ALS treated with RILUTEK (n=794) participating in placebo-controlled trials and were numerically greater in the patients treated with RILUTEK 100 mg/day than with placebo or for which a dose response relationship is suggested.

The prescriber should be aware that these figures cannot be used to predict the frequency of adverse experiences in the course of usual medical practice where patient characteristics and other factors may differ from those prevailing during clinical studies. Inspection of these frequencies, however, does provide the prescriber with one basis to estimate the relative contribution of drug and non-drug factors to the AE incidences in the population studied.

Table 1
Adverse Events Occurring in Placebo-Controlled Clinical Trials

	Percentage of patients reporting events†			
Body System/ Adverse Event†	**Riluzole 50 mg/day** (N=237)	**Riluzole 100 mg/day** (N=313)	**Riluzole 200 mg/day** (N=244)	**Placebo** (N=320)
Body as a Whole				
Asthenia	14.8	19.2	20.1	12.2
Headache	8.0	7.3	7.0	6.6
Abdominal pain	6.8	5.1	7.8	3.8
Back pain	1.7	3.2	4.1	2.5

Continued on next page

Rilutek—Cont.

Aggravation reaction	0.4	1.3	2.0	0.9
Malaise	0.4	0.6	1.2	0.0
Digestive				
Nausea	12.2	16.3	20.5	10.6
Vomiting	4.2	4.2	4.5	1.6
Dyspepsia	2.5	3.8	6.1	5.0
Anorexia	3.8	3.2	8.6	3.8
Diarrhea	5.5	2.9	9.0	3.1
Flatulence	2.5	2.6	2.0	1.9
Stomatitis	0.8	1.0	1.2	0.0
Tooth disorder	0.0	1.0	1.2	0.3
Oral Moniliasis	0.4	0.6	1.2	0.3
Nervous				
Hypertonia	5.9	6.1	5.3	5.9
Depression	4.2	4.5	6.1	5.0
Dizziness	5.1	3.8	12.7	2.5
Dry mouth	3.0	3.5	2.0	3.4
Insomnia	2.1	3.5	2.9	3.4
Somnolence	0.8	1.9	4.1	1.3
Vertigo	2.5	1.9	4.5	0.9
Circumoral paresthesia	1.3	1.6	3.3	0.0
Skin and Appendages				
Pruritus	3.8	3.8	2.5	3.1
Eczema	0.8	1.6	1.6	0.6
Alopecia	0.0	1.0	1.2	0.6
Exfoliative dermatitis	0.0	0.6	1.2	0.0
Respiratory				
Decreased lung function	13.1	10.2	16.0	9.4
Rhinitis	8.9	6.4	7.8	6.3
Increased cough	2.1	2.6	3.7	1.6
Sinusitis	0.4	1.0	1.6	0.9
Cardiovascular				
Hypertension	6.8	5.1	3.3	4.1
Tachycardia	1.3	2.6	2.0	1.3
Phlebitis	0.4	1.0	0.8	0.3
Palpitation	0.4	0.6	1.2	0.9
Postural hypotension	0.8	0.0	1.6	0.6
Metabolic and Nutritional Disorders				
Weight loss	4.6	4.8	3.7	4.7
Peripheral edema	4.2	2.9	3.3	2.2
Musculoskeletal System				
Arthralgia	5.1	3.5	1.6	3.4
Urogenital System				
Urinary tract infection	2.5	2.6	4.5	2.2
Dysuria	0.0	1.0	1.2	0.3

Other Adverse Events Observed

Other events which occurred in more than 2% of patients treated with RILUTEK 100 mg/day but equally or more frequently in the placebo group included: accidental injury, apnea, bronchitis, constipation, death, dysphagia, dyspnea, flu syndrome, heart arrest, increased sputum, pneumonia, and respiratory disorder.

The overall adverse event profile for RILUTEK was similar between females and males, and was independent of age. Because the largest non-white racial subgroup was only 2% of patients exposed to RILUTEK (18/794) in placebo-controlled trials, there are insufficient data to support a statement regarding the distribution of adverse experience reports by race. In ALS studies, dizziness did occur more commonly in females (11%) than in males (4%). There was not a difference between females and males in the rates of discontinuation of RILUTEK for individual adverse experiences.

Other Adverse Events Observed During All Clinical Trials

RILUTEK has been administered to 1713 individuals during all clinical trials, some of which were placebo-controlled. During these trials, all adverse events were recorded by the clinical investigators using terminology of their own choosing. To provide a meaningful estimate of the proportion of individuals having adverse events, similar types of events were grouped into a smaller number of standardized categories using modified COSTART dictionary terminology. The frequencies presented represent the proportion of the 1713 individuals exposed to RILUTEK who experienced an event of the type cited on at least one occasion while receiving RILUTEK. All reported events are included except those already listed in the previous table, those too general to be informative, and those not reasonably associated with the use of the drug.

Events are further classified within body system categories and enumerated in order of decreasing frequency using the following definitions: *frequent* adverse events are defined as those occurring in at least 1/100 patients; *infrequent* adverse events are those occurring in 1/100 to 1/1000 patients; *rare* adverse events are those occurring in fewer than 1/1000 patients.

***=AE frequency ≤to placebo**

Body as a Whole: *Frequent:* Hostility*. *Infrequent:* Abscess*, sepsis*, photosensitivity reaction*, cellulitis, face edema*, hernia, peritonitis, attempted suicide, injection site reaction, chills*, flu syndrome, intentional injury, enlarged abdomen, neoplasm. *Rare:* Acrodynia, hypothermia, moniliasis*, rheumatoid arthritis.

Digestive System: *Infrequent:* Increased appetite, intestinal obstruction*, fecal impaction, gastrointestinal hemorrhage, gastrointestinal ulceration, gastritis*, fecal incontinence, jaundice, hepatitis, glossitis, gum hemorrhage*, pancreatitis, tenesmus, esophageal stenosis. *Rare:* Cheilitis*, cholecystitis, hematemesis, melena*, biliary pain, proctitis, pseudomembranous enterocolitis, enlarged salivary gland, tongue discoloration, tooth caries.

Nervous System: *Frequent:* Agitation*, tremor. *Infrequent:* Hallucinations, personality disorder*, abnormal thinking*, coma, paranoid reaction*, manic reaction, ataxia, extrapyramidal syndrome, hypokinesia, urinary retention, emotional lability, delusions, apathy, hypesthesia, incoordination, confusion*, convulsion, leg cramps, amnesia, dysarthria, increased libido, stupor, subdural hematoma, abnormal gait, delirium, depersonalization, facial paralysis, hemiplegia, decreased libido, myoclonus. *Rare:* Abnormal dreams, acute brain syndrome, CNS depression, dementia, cerebral embolism, euphoria*, hypotonia, ileus*, peripheral neuritis, psychosis*, psychotic depression, schizophrenic reaction, trismus, wristdrop.

Skin and Appendages: *Infrequent:* Skin ulceration, urticaria, psoriasis, seborrhea*, skin disorder, fungal dermatitis*. *Rare:* Angioedema, contact dermatitis, erythema multiforme, furunculosis*, skin moniliasis, skin granuloma, skin nodule.

Respiratory System: *Infrequent:* Hiccup, pleural disorder*, asthma, epistaxis, hemoptysis, yawn, hyperventilation*, lung edema*, hypoventilation*, lung carcinoma, hypoxia, laryngitis, pleural effusion, pneumothorax*, respiratory moniliasis, stridor.

Cardiovascular System: *Infrequent:* Syncope*, hypotension, heart failure, migraine, peripheral vascular disease, angina pectoris*, myocardial infarction*, ventricular extrasystoles, cerebral hemorrhage, atrial fibrillation*, bundle branch block, congestive heart failure, pericarditis, lower extremity embolus, myocardial ischemia*, shock*. *Rare:* Bradycardia, cerebral ischemia, hemorrhage, mesenteric artery occlusion, subarachnoid hemorrhage, supraventricular tachycardia*, thrombosis, ventricular fibrillation, ventricular tachycardia.

Metabolic and Nutritional Disorders: *Infrequent:* Gout*, respiratory acidosis, edema, thirst*, hypokalemia, hyponatremia, weight gain*. *Rare:* Generalized edema, hypercalcemia, hypercholesteremia.

Endocrine System: *Infrequent:* Diabetes mellitus, thyroid neoplasia. *Rare:* Diabetes insipidus, parathyroid disorder.

Hemic and Lymphatic System: *Infrequent:* Anemia*, leukocytosis, leukopenia, ecchymosis. *Rare:* Neutropenia, aplastic anemia, cyanosis, hypochromic anemia, iron deficiency anemia, lymphadenopathy, petechiae*, purpura.

Musculoskeletal System: *Infrequent:* Arthrosis, myasthenia*, bone neoplasm. *Rare:* Bone necrosis, osteoporosis, tetany.

Special Senses: *Infrequent:* Amblyopia, ophthalmitis. *Rare:* Blepharitis, cataract, deafness, diplopia*, ear pain, glaucoma, hyperacusis, photophobia, taste loss, vestibular disorder.

Urogenital System: *Infrequent:* Urinary urgency, urine abnormality, urinary incontinence, kidney calculus, hematuria, impotence, prostate carcinoma, kidney pain, metrorrhagia, priapism. *Rare:* Amenorrhea, breast abscess, breast pain, nephritis*, nocturia, pyelonephritis, enlarged uterine fibroids, uterine hemorrhage, vaginal moniliasis.

Laboratory Tests: *Infrequent:* Increased gamma glutamyl transferase, abnormal liver function/tests, increased alkaline phosphatase, positive direct Coombs test, increased gamma globulins. *Rare:* increased lactic dehydrogenase.

OVERDOSAGE

No specific antidote or information on treatment of overdosage with RILUTEK is available. In the event of overdose, RILUTEK therapy should be discontinued immediately. Treatment should be supportive and directed toward alleviating symptoms.

Experience with riluzole overdose in humans is limited. Methemoglobinemia of undetermined origin has been reported in association with a riluzole overdose many times the recommended daily dose. This was rapidly reversible after treatment with methylene blue.

The estimated oral median lethal dose is 94 mg/kg and 39 mg/kg for male mice and rats, respectively.

DOSAGE AND ADMINISTRATION

The recommended dose for RILUTEK is 50 mg every 12 hours. No increased benefit can be expected from higher daily doses, but adverse events are increased.

RILUTEK tablets should be taken at least an hour before, or two hours after, a meal to avoid a food-related decrease in bioavailability.

Special Populations

Patients with Impaired Renal or Hepatic Function: Studies have not yet been completed in these populations (see WARNINGS, PRECAUTIONS, CLINICAL PHARMACOLOGY).

HOW SUPPLIED

RILUTEK 50 mg tablets are white, film-coated, capsule-shaped and engraved with "RPR 202" on one side. RILUTEK is supplied in bottles of 60 tablets, NDC 0075-7700-60. These bottles are designed with a special dispensing flip cap to aid dispensing with minimum effort.

STORE AT CONTROLLED ROOM TEMPERATURE 20°–25°C (68°–77°F) AND PROTECT FROM BRIGHT LIGHT.

KEEP OUT OF THE REACH OF CHILDREN.

Manufactured in Ireland
Aventis Pharmaceuticals Products Inc.
Parsippany, NJ 07054
IN-5336B! Rev. 8/99

Shown in Product Identification Guide, page 307

SYNERCID® I.V. ℞

quinupristin/dalfopristin for injection
Rx only

One of **Synercid's** approved indications is for the treatment of patients with serious or life-threatening infections associated with vancomycin-resistant *Enterococcus faecium* (VREF) bacteremia. **Synercid** has been approved for marketing in the United States for this indication under FDA's accelerated approval regulations that allow marketing of products for use in life-threatening conditions when other therapies are not available. Approval of drugs for marketing under these regulations is based upon a demonstrated effect on a surrogate endpoint that is likely to predict clinical benefit. Approval of this indication is based upon **Synercid's** ability to clear VREF from the bloodstream, with clearance of bacteremia considered to be a surrogate endpoint. There are no results from well-controlled clinical studies that confirm the validity of this surrogate marker. However, a study to verify the clinical benefit of therapy with **Synercid** on traditional clinical endpoints (such as cure of the underlying infection) is presently underway.

DESCRIPTION

Synercid® (quinupristin and dalfopristin powder for injection) I.V., a streptogramin antibacterial agent for intravenous administration, is a sterile lyophilized formulation of two semisynthetic pristinamycin derivatives, quinupristin (derived from pristinamycin I) and dalfopristin (derived from pristinamycin IIA) in the ratio of 30:70 (w/w).

Quinupristin is a white to very slightly yellow, hygroscopic powder. It is a combination of three peptide macrolactones. The main component of quinupristin (>88.0%) has the following chemical name: N- [(6*R*,9*S*,10*R*,13*S*,15a*S*,18*R*,22*S*,24a*S*)-22-[*p*-(dimethylamino)benzyl]-6-ethyldocosahydro-10,23-dimethyl-5,8,12,15,17,21,24-heptaoxo-13-phenyl-18-[[(3*S*)-3-quinuclidinylthio]methyl]-12*H*-pyrido[2,1-*f*]pyrrolo-[2,1-*l*][1,4,7,10,13,16] oxapentaazacyclononadecin-9-yl]-3-hydroxypicolinamide.

The main component of quinupristin has an empirical formula of $C_{53}H_{67}N_9O_{10}S$, a molecular weight of 1022.24 and the following structural formula:

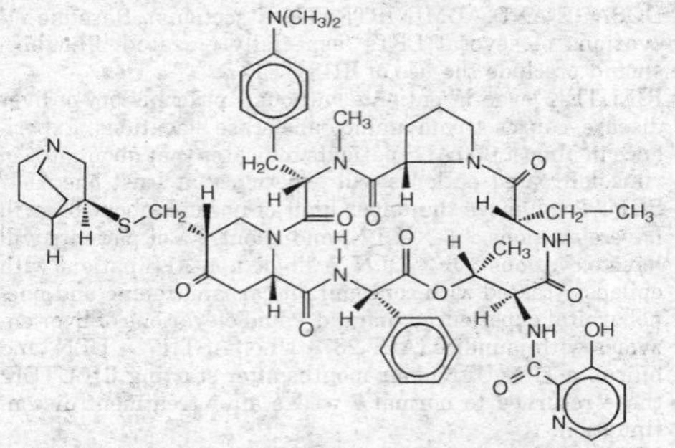

Dalfopristin is a slightly yellow to yellow, hygroscopic, powder. The chemical name for dalfopristin is: (3*R*,4*R*,5*E*,10*E*,12*E*,14*S*,26*R*,26a*S*)-26-[[2-(diethylamino)ethyl]sulfonyl]-8,9,14,15,24,25,26,26a-octahydro-14-hydroxy-3-isopropyl-4, 12-dimethyl-3*H*-21,18-nitrilo-1*H*,22*H*-pyrrolo[2,1-c][1,8,4,19]-dioxadiazacyclotetracosine-1,7,16,22(4*H*,17*H*)-tetrone.

Dalfopristin has an empirical formula of $C_{34}H_{50}N_4O_9S$, a molecular weight of 690.85 and the following structural formula:

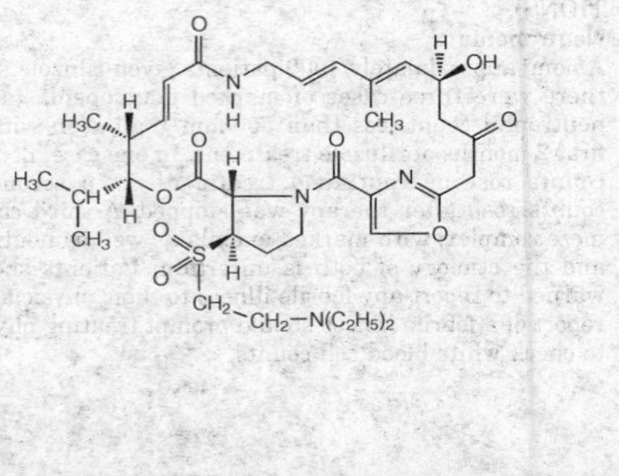

CLINICAL PHARMACOLOGY

Pharmacokinetics: Quinupristin and dalfopristin are the main active components circulating in plasma in human subjects. Quinupristin and dalfopristin are converted to several active major metabolites: two conjugated metabolites for quinupristin (one with glutathione and one with cysteine) and one non-conjugated metabolite for dalfopristin (formed by drug hydrolysis).

Pharmacokinetic profiles of quinupristin and dalfopristin in combination with their metabolites were determined using a bioassay following multiple 60-minute infusions of **Synercid** in two groups of healthy young adult male volunteers. Each group received 7.5 mg/kg of **Synercid** intravenously q12h or q8h for a total of 9 or 10 doses, respectively. The pharmacokinetic parameters were proportional with q12h and q8h dosing; those of the q8h regimen are shown in the following table:

Mean Steady-State Pharmacokinetic Parameters of Quinupristin and Dalfopristin in Combination with their Metabolites (±SD[1]) (dose = 7.5 mg/kg q8h; n=10)

	C_{max}[2] (µg/mL)	AUC[3] (µg.h/mL)	$t^1/_2$[4] (hr)
Quinupristin and metabolites	3.20 ± 0.67	7.20 ± 1.24	3.07 ± 0.51
Dalfopristin and metabolite	7.96 ± 1.30	10.57 ± 2.24	1.04 ± 0.20

[1] SD = Standard Deviation
[2] C_{max} = Maximum drug plasma concentration
[3] AUC = Area under the drug plasma concentration-time curve
[4] $t^1/_2$ = Half-life

The clearances of unchanged quinupristin and dalfopristin are similar (0.72 L/h/kg), and the steady-state volume of distribution for quinupristin is 0.45 L/kg and for dalfopristin is 0.24 L/kg. The elimination half-life of quinupristin and dalfopristin is approximately 0.85 and 0.70 hours, respectively. The protein binding of **Synercid** is moderate.

Penetration of unchanged quinupristin and dalfopristin in noninflammatory blister fluid corresponds to about 19% and 11% of that estimated in plasma, respectively. The penetration into blister fluid of quinupristin and dalfopristin in combination with their major metabolites was in total approximately 40% compared to that in plasma.

In vitro, the transformation of the parent drugs into their major active metabolites occurs by non-enzymatic reactions and is not dependent on cytochrome-P450 or glutathione-transferase enzyme activities.

Synercid has been shown to be a major inhibitor (*in vitro* inhibits 70% cyclosporin A biotransformation at 10 µg/mL of **Synercid**) of the activity of cytochrome P450 3A4 isoenzyme. (See **WARNINGS**.)

Synercid can interfere with the metabolism of other drug products that are associated with QTc prolongation. However, electrophysiologic studies confirm that **Synercid** does not itself induce QTc prolongation. (See **WARNINGS**.)

Fecal excretion constitutes the main elimination route for both parent drugs and their metabolites (75 to 77% of dose). Urinary excretion accounts for approximately 15% of the quinupristin and 19% of the dalfopristin dose. Preclinical data in rats have demonstrated that approximately 80% of the dose is excreted in the bile and suggest that in man, biliary excretion is probably the principal route for fecal elimination.

Special Populations

Elderly: The pharmacokinetics of quinupristin and dalfopristin were studied in a population of elderly individuals (range 69 to 74 years). The pharmacokinetics of the drug products were not modified in these subjects.

Gender: The pharmacokinetics of quinupristin and dalfopristin are not modified by gender.

Renal Insufficiency: In patients with creatinine clearance 6 to 28 mL/min, the AUC of quinupristin and dalfopristin in combination with their major metabolites increased about 40% and 30%, respectively.

In patients undergoing Continuous Ambulatory Peritoneal Dialysis, dialysis clearance for quinupristin, dalfopristin and their metabolites is negligible. The plasma AUC of unchanged quinupristin and dalfopristin increased about 20% and 30%, respectively. The high molecular weight of both components of **Synercid** suggests that it is unlikely to be removed by hemodialysis.

Hepatic Insufficiency: In patients with hepatic dysfunction (Child-Pugh scores A and B), the terminal half-life of quinupristin and dalfopristin was not modified. However, the AUC of quinupristin and dalfopristin in combination with their major metabolites increased about 180% and 50%, respectively. (See **DOSAGE AND ADMINISTRATION** and **PRECAUTIONS**.)

Obesity (body mass index ≥ 30): In obese patients the C_{max} and AUC of quinupristin increased about 30% and those of dalfopristin about 40%.

Pediatric Patients: The pharmacokinetics of **Synercid** in patients less than 16 years of age have not been studied.

Microbiology: The streptogramin components of **Synercid,** quinupristin and dalfopristin, are present in a ratio of 30 parts quinupristin to 70 parts dalfopristin. These two components act synergistically so that **Synercid's** microbiologic *in vitro* activity is greater than that of the components individually. Quinupristin's and dalfopristin's metabolites also contribute to the antimicrobial activity of **Synercid**. *In vitro* synergism of the major metabolites with the complementary parent compound has been demonstrated.

Synercid is bacteriostatic against *Enterococcus faecium* and bactericidal against strains of methicillin-susceptible and methicillin-resistant staphylococci.

The site of action of quinupristin and dalfopristin is the bacterial ribosome. Dalfopristin has been shown to inhibit the early phase of protein synthesis while quinupristin inhibits the late phase of protein synthesis.

In vitro combination testing of **Synercid** with aztreonam, cefotaxime, ciprofloxacin, and gentamicin against *Enterobacteriaceae* and *Pseudomonas aeruginosa* did not show antagonism.

In vitro combination testing of **Synercid** with prototype drugs of the following classes: aminoglycosides (gentamicin), β-lactams (cefepime, ampicillin, and amoxicillin), glycopeptides (vancomycin), quinolones (ciprofloxacin), tetracyclines (doxycycline) and also chloramphenicol against enterococci and staphylococci did not show antagonism.

The mode of action differs from that of other classes of antibacterial agents such as β-lactams, aminoglycosides, glycopeptides, quinolones, macrolides, lincosamides and tetracyclines. There is no cross resistance between **Synercid** and these agents when tested by the minimum inhibitory concentration (MIC) method.

In non-comparative studies, emerging resistance to **Synercid** during treatment of VREF infections occurred. Resistance to **Synercid** is associated with resistance to both components (*i.e.,* quinupristin and dalfopristin).

Synercid has been shown to be active against most strains of the following microorganisms, both *in vitro* and in clinical infections, as described in the **INDICATIONS AND USAGE** section.

Aerobic gram-positive microorganisms

Enterococcus faecium **(Vancomycin-resistant and multi-drug resistant strains only)**
Staphylococcus aureus (methicillin-susceptible strains only)
Streptococcus pyogenes

NOTE: Synercid is **not active** against *Enterococcus faecalis.* Differentiation of enterococcal species is important to avoid misidentification of *Enterococcus faecalis* as *Enterococcus faecium.*

The following *in vitro* data are available, **but their clinical significance is unknown.**

The combination of quinupristin and dalfopristin (**Synercid**) exhibits *in vitro* minimum inhibitory concentrations (MIC's) of ≤1.0µg/mL against most (≥90%) isolates of the following microorganisms; however, the safety and effectiveness of **Synercid** in treating clinical infections due to these microorganisms have not been established in adequate and well-controlled clinical trials.

Aerobic gram-positive microorganisms

Corynebacterium jeikeium
Staphylococcus aureus (methicillin-resistant strains)
Staphylococcus epidermidis (including methicillin-resistant strains)
Streptococcus agalactiae

SUSCEPTIBILITY TESTING

Dilution Techniques

Quantitative methods are used to determine antimicrobial minimum inhibitory concentrations (MICs). These MICs provide estimates of the susceptibility of microorganisms to antimicrobial compounds. The MICs should be determined using a standardized procedure. Standardized procedures are based on a dilution[1] method (broth or agar) or equivalent using standardized inoculum concentrations, and standardized concentrations of quinupristin/dalfopristin (**Synercid**) in a 30:70 ratio made from powder of known potency. The MIC values should be interpreted according to the following criteria:

For Susceptibility Testing of *Enterococcus Faecium, Staphylococcus* SPP., and *Streptococcus* SPP. (excluding *Streptococcus pneumoniae*)[a]

MIC (µg/mL)	Interpretation
≤1.0	Susceptible (S)
2.0	Intermediate (I)
≥4.0	Resistant (R)

[a] The interpretive values for *Streptococcus* spp. are applicable only to broth microdilution susceptibility testing using cation-adjusted Mueller-Hinton broth with 2 to 5% lysed horse blood.

A report of "Susceptible" indicates that the pathogen is likely to be inhibited if the concentration of the antimicrobial compound in the blood reaches usually achievable levels. A report of "Intermediate" indicates that the result should be considered equivocal, and if the microorganism is not fully susceptible to alternative, clinically feasible drugs, the test should be repeated. This category implies possible clinical applicability in body sites where the drug is physiologically concentrated or in situations where high dosage of drug can be used. This category provides a buffer zone which prevents small uncontrolled technical factors from causing major discrepancies in interpretation. A report of "Resistant" indicates that the pathogen is not likely to be inhibited if the antimicrobial compound in the blood reaches the concentrations usually achievable; other therapy should be selected.

Quality Control

A standardized susceptibility test procedure requires the use of laboratory control organisms to control the technical aspects of the laboratory procedures. Standard quinupristin/dalfopristin powder in a 30:70 ratio should provide the following MIC values with the indicated quality control strains:

Microorganism (ATCC®#)	MIC (µg/mL)
Enterococcus faecalis (29212)	2.0 to 8.0
Staphylococcus aureus (29213)	0.25 to 1.0

Diffusion Techniques

Quantitative methods that require measurement of zone diameters also provide reproducible estimates of the susceptibility of bacteria to antimicrobial compounds. One such standardized procedure[2] requires the use of standardized inoculum concentrations. This procedure uses paper disks impregnated with 15 µg quinupristin/dalfopristin in a ratio of 30:70 (**Synercid**) to test the susceptibility of microorganisms to quinupristin/dalfopristin. Reports from the laboratory providing results of the standard single-disk susceptibility test with a 15 µg quinupristin/dalfopristin disk should be interpreted according to the following criteria:

For Susceptibility Testing of *Enterococcus Faecium, Staphylococcus* SPP., and *Streptococcus* SPP. (excluding *Streptococcus pneumoniae*)[b]

Zone Diameter (mm)	Interpretation
≥19	Susceptible (S)
16 to 18	Intermediate (I)
≤15	Resistant (R)

[b] The zone diameter for *Streptococcus* spp. are applicable only to tests performed using Mueller-Hinton agar supplemented with 5% sheep blood when incubated in 5% CO_2.

These zone diameters are applicable only to tests performed using Mueller-Hinton agar supplemented with 5% sheep blood when incubated in 5% CO_2.

Interpretation should be as stated above for results using dilution techniques. Interpretation involves correlation of the diameter obtained in the disk test with the MIC for quinupristin/dalfopristin.

Quality Control

As with standardized dilution techniques, diffusion methods require the use of laboratory control microorganisms that are used to control the technical aspects of the laboratory procedures. For the diffusion technique, the 15-µg quinupristin/dalfopristin (30:70 ratio) disk should provide the following zone diameter with the quality control strain listed below:

Microorganism (ATCC®#)	Zone Diameter Range (mm)
Staphylococcus aureus (25923)	23 to 29

ATCC® is a registered trademark of the American Type Culture Collection

INDICATIONS AND USAGE

Synercid is indicated in adults for the treatment of the following infections when caused by susceptible strains of the designated microorganisms.

Vancomycin-resistant *Enterococcus faecium* (VREF)

Synercid is indicated for the treatment of patients with serious or life-threatening infections associated with vancomycin-resistant *Enterococcus faecium* (VREF) bacteremia. (See **CLINICAL STUDIES**.)

One of **Synercid's** approved indications is for the treatment of patients with serious or life-threatening infections associated with vancomycin-resistant *Enterococcus faecium* (VREF) bacteremia. **Synercid** has been approved for marketing in the United States for this indication under FDA's accelerated approval regulations that allow marketing of products for use in life-threatening conditions when other therapies are not available. Approval of drugs for marketing under these regulations is based upon a demonstrated effect on a surrogate endpoint that is likely to predict clinical benefit.

Approval of this indication is based upon **Synercid's** ability to clear VREF from the bloodstream, with clearance of bacteremia considered to be a surrogate endpoint. There are no results from well-controlled clinical studies that confirm the validity of this surrogate marker. However, a study to verify the clinical benefit of therapy with **Synercid** on traditional clinical endpoints (such as cure of the underlying infection) is presently underway.

Continued on next page

Synercid—Cont.

Complicated skin and skin structure infections caused by *Staphylococcus aureus* (methicillin susceptible) or *Streptococcus pyogenes.* (See **CLINICAL STUDIES.**)

CONTRAINDICATIONS

Synercid is contraindicated in patients with known hypersensitivity to **Synercid**, or with prior hypersensitivity to other streptogramins (*e.g.*, pristinamycin or virginiamycin).

WARNINGS

Drug Interactions: *In vitro* drug interaction studies have demonstrated that **Synercid** significantly inhibits cytochrome P450 3A4 metabolism of cyclosporin A, midazolam, nifedipine and terfenadine. In addition, 24 subjects given **Synercid** 7.5 mg/kg q8h for 2 days and 300 mg of cyclosporine on day 3 showed an increase of 63% in the AUC of cyclosporine, an increase of 30% in the C_{max} of cyclosporine, a 77% increase in the $t^1/_2$ of cyclosporine, and, a decrease of 34% in the clearance of cyclosporine. **Therapeutic level monitoring of cyclosporine should be performed when cyclosporine must be used concomitantly with Synercid.**

It is reasonable to expect that the concomitant administration of Synercid and other drugs primarily metabolized by the cytochrome P450 3A4 enzyme system may likely result in increased plasma concentrations of these drugs that could increase or prolong their therapeutic effect and/or increase adverse reactions. (See Table below.) Therefore, coadministration of Synercid with drugs which are cytochrome P450 3A4 substrates and possess a narrow therapeutic window requires caution and monitoring of these drugs (*e.g.*, cyclosporine), whenever possible. Concomitant medications metabolized by the cytochrome P450 3A4 enzyme system that may prolong the QTc interval should be avoided.

Concomitant administration of **Synercid** and nifedipine (repeated oral doses) and midazolam (intravenous bolus dose) in healthy volunteers led to elevated plasma concentrations of these drugs. The C_{max} increased by 18% and 14% (median values) and the AUC increased by 44% and 33% for nifedipine and midazolam, respectively.

Table of Selected Drugs That Are Predicted to Have Plasma Concentrations Increased by Synercid†

Antihistamines: astemizole, terfenadine
Anti-HIV (NNRTIs and Protease inhibitors): delavirdine, nevirapine, indinavir, ritonavir
Antineoplastic agents: vinca alkaloids (*e.g.*, vinblastine), docetaxel, paclitaxel
Benzodiazepines: midazolam, diazepam
Calcium channel blockers: dihydropyridines (*e.g.*, nifedipine), verapamil, diltiazem
Cholesterol-lowering agents: HMG-CoA reductase inhibitors (*e.g.*, lovastatin)
GI motility agents: cisapride
Immunosuppressive agents: cyclosporine, tacrolimus
Steroids: methylprednisolone
Other: carbamazepine, quinidine, lidocaine, disopyramide

†This list of drugs is not all inclusive.

Pseudomembranous colitis has been reported with nearly all antibacterial agents, including Synercid, and may range in severity from mild to life-threatening. Therefore, it is important to consider this diagnosis in patients who present with diarrhea subsequent to the administration of antibacterial agents.

Treatment with antibacterial agents alters the normal flora of the colon and may permit overgrowth of clostridia. Studies indicate that a toxin produced by *Clostridium difficile* is one primary cause of "antibiotic-associated colitis".

After the diagnosis of pseudomembranous colitis has been established, therapeutic measures should be initiated. Mild cases usually respond to drug discontinuation alone. In moderate to severe cases, consideration should be given to management with fluids and electrolytes, protein supplementation and treatment with an antibacterial drug clinically effective against *C. difficile* colitis.

PRECAUTIONS

General: *Venous Irritation:* Following completion of a peripheral infusion, the vein should be flushed with 5% Dextrose in Water solution to minimize venous irritation. **DO NOT FLUSH** with saline or heparin **after Synercid** administration because of incompatibility concerns.

If moderate to severe venous irritation occurs following peripheral administration of **Synercid** diluted in 250 mL of Dextrose 5% in water, consideration should be given to increasing the infusion volume to 500 or 750 mL, changing the infusion site, or infusing by a peripherally inserted central catheter (PICC) or a central venous catheter. In clinical trials, concomitant administration of hydrocortisone or diphenhydramine did not appear to alleviate venous pain or inflammation.

Rate of Infusion: In animal studies toxicity was higher when **Synercid** was administered as a bolus compared to slow infusion. However, the safety of an intravenous bolus of **Synercid** has not been studied in humans. Clinical trial experience has been exclusively with an intravenous duration of 60 minutes and, thus, other infusion rates cannot be recommended.

Arthralgias/Myalgias: Episodes of arthralgia and myalgia, some severe, have been reported in patients treated with **Synercid.** In some patients, improvement has been noted with a reduction in dose frequency to q12h. In those patients available for follow-up, treatment discontinuation has been followed by resolution of symptoms. The etiology of these myalgias and arthralgias is under investigation.

Superinfections: The use of antibiotics may promote the overgrowth of nonsusceptible organisms. Should superinfection occur during therapy, appropriate measures should be taken.

Hyperbilirubinemia: Elevations of total bilirubin greater than 5 times the upper limit of normal were noted in approximately 25% of patients in the non-comparative studies (see **CLINICAL STUDIES: Non-Comparative Trials**). In some patients, isolated hyperbilirubinemia (primarily conjugated) can occur during treatment, possibly resulting from competition between **Synercid** and bilirubin for excretion. Of note, in the comparative trials, elevations in ALT and AST occurred at a similar frequency in both the **Synercid** and comparator groups.

Drug Interactions: *In vitro* drug interaction studies have shown that **Synercid** significantly inhibits cytochrome P450 3A4. (See **WARNINGS.**)

Synercid does not significantly inhibit human cytochrome P450 1A2, 2A6, 2C9, 2C19, 2D6, or 2E1. Therefore, clinical interactions with drugs metabolized by these cytochrome P450 isoenzymes are not expected.

A drug interaction between **Synercid** and digoxin cannot be excluded but is unlikely to occur via CYP3A4 enzyme inhibition. **Synercid** has shown *in vitro* activity (MICs of 0.25 mcg/mL when tested on two strains) against *Eubacterium lentum.* Digoxin is metabolized in part by bacteria in the gut and as such, a drug interaction based on **Synercid's** inhibition of digoxin's gut metabolism (by *Eubacterium lentum*) may be possible.

In vitro combination testing of **Synercid** with aztreonam, cefotaxime, ciprofloxacin, and gentamicin, against *Enterobacteriaceae* and *Pseudomonas aeruginosa* did not show antagonism.

In vitro combination testing of **Synercid** with prototype drugs of the following classes: aminoglycosides (gentamicin), β-lactams (cefepime, ampicillin, and amoxicillin), glycopeptides (vancomycin), quinolones (ciprofloxacin), tetracyclines (doxycycline) and also chloramphenicol against enterococci and staphylococci did not show antagonism.

Carcinogenesis, Mutagenesis, Impairment of Fertility: Long-term carcinogenicity studies in animals have not been conducted with **Synercid.** Five genetic toxicity tests were performed. **Synercid,** dalfopristin, and quinupristin were tested in the bacterial reverse mutation assay, the Chinese hamster ovary cell HGPRT gene mutation assay, the unscheduled DNA synthesis assay in rat hepatocytes, the Chinese hamster ovary cell chromosome aberration assay, and the mouse micronucleus assay in bone marrow. Dalfopristin was associated with the production of structural chromosome aberrations when tested in the Chinese hamster ovary cell chromosome aberration assay. **Synercid** and quinupristin were negative in this assay. **Synercid,** dalfopristin, and quinupristin were all negative in the other four genetic toxicity assays.

No impairment of fertility or perinatal/postnatal development was observed in rats at doses up to 12 to 18 mg/kg (approximately 0.3 to 0.4 times the human dose based on body-surface area).

Pregnancy: Teratogenic Effects: *Pregnancy Category B:* Reproductive studies have been performed in mice at doses up to 40 mg/kg/day (approximately half the human dose based on body-surface area), in rats at doses up to 120 mg/kg/day (approximately 2.5 times the human dose based on body-surface area), and in rabbits at doses up to 12 mg/kg/day (approximately half the human dose based on body-surface area) and have revealed no evidence of impaired fertility or harm to the fetus due to **Synercid.**

There are, however, no adequate and well-controlled studies with **Synercid** in pregnant women. Because animal reproduction studies are not always predictive of the human response, this drug should be used during pregnancy only if clearly needed.

Nursing Mothers: In lactating rats, **Synercid** was excreted in milk. It is not known whether **Synercid** is excreted in human breast milk. Because many drugs are excreted in human milk, caution should be exercised when **Synercid** is administered to a nursing woman.

Hepatic Insufficiency: Following a single 1-hour infusion of **Synercid** (7.5 mg/kg) to patients with hepatic insufficiency, plasma concentrations were significantly increased. (See **CLINICAL PHARMACOLOGY: Special Populations.**) However, the effect of dose reduction or increase in dosing interval on the pharmacokinetics of **Synercid** in these patients has not been studied. Therefore, no recommendations can be made at this time regarding the appropriate dose modification.

Pediatric Use: **Synercid** has been used in a limited number of pediatric patients under emergency-use conditions at a dose of 7.5 mg/kg q8h or q12h. However, the safety and effectiveness of **Synercid** in patients under 16 years of age have not been established.

Geriatric Use: In phase 3 comparative trials of **Synercid,** 37% of patients (n=404) were ≥65 years of age, of which 145 were ≥75 years of age. In the phase 3 non-comparative trials, 29% of patients (n=346) were ≥65 years of age, of which 112 were ≥75 years of age. There were no apparent differences in the frequency, type, or severity of related adverse reactions including cardiovascular events between elderly and younger individuals.

ADVERSE REACTIONS

The safety of **Synercid** was evaluated in 1099 patients enrolled in 5 comparative clinical trials. Additionally, 4 non-comparative clinical trials (3 prospective and 1 retrospective in design) were conducted in which 1199 patients received **Synercid** for infections due to Gram-positive pathogens for which no other treatment option was available. In non-comparative trials, the patients were severely ill, often with multiple co-morbidities or physiological impairments, and may have been intolerant to or failed other antibacterial therapies.

COMPARATIVE TRIALS

ADVERSE REACTION SUMMARY—ALL COMPARATIVE STUDIES

Safety data are available from five comparative clinical studies (n=1099 **Synercid**; n=1095 comparator). One of the deaths in the comparative studies was assessed as possibly related to **Synercid.** The most frequent reasons for discontinuation due to drug-related adverse reactions were as follows:

% of patients discontinuing therapy by reaction type

Type	Synercid	Comparator
Venous	9.2	2.0
Non-venous	9.6	4.3
-Rash	1.0	0.5
-Nausea	0.9	0.6
-Vomiting	0.5	0.5
-Pain	0.5	0.0
-Pruritus	0.5	0.3

CLINICAL REACTIONS—ALL COMPARATIVE STUDIES

Adverse reactions with an incidence of ≥1% and possibly or probably related to **Synercid** administration include:

Adverse Reactions	% of patients with adverse reactions	
	Synercid	Comparator
Inflammation at infusion site	42.0	25.0
Pain at infusion site	40.0	23.7
Edema at infusion site	17.3	9.5
Infusion site reaction	13.4	10.1
Nausea	4.6	7.2
Thrombophlebitis	2.4	0.3
Diarrhea	2.7	3.2
Vomiting	2.7	3.8
Rash	2.5	1.4
Headache	1.6	0.9
Pruritus	1.5	1.1
Pain	1.5	0.1

Additional adverse reactions that were possibly or probably related to **Synercid** with an incidence less than 1% within each body system are listed below:

Body as a Whole: abdominal pain, worsening of underlying illness, allergic reaction, chest pain, fever, infection;
Cardiovascular: palpitation, phlebitis;
Digestive: constipation, dyspepsia, oral moniliasis, pancreatitis, pseudomembranous enterocolitis, stomatitis;
Metabolic: gout, peripheral edema;
Musculoskeletal: arthralgia, myalgia, myasthenia;
Nervous: anxiety, confusion, dizziness, hypertonia, insomnia, leg cramps, paresthesia, vasodilation;
Respiratory: dyspnea, pleural effusion;
Skin and Appendages: maculopapular rash, sweating, urticaria;
Urogenital: hematuria, vaginitis

CLINICAL REACTIONS—SKIN AND SKIN STRUCTURE STUDIES

In two of the five comparative clinical trials **Synercid** (n=450) and comparator regimens (*e.g.*, oxacillin/vancomycin or cefazolin/vancomycin; n=443) were studied for safety and efficacy in the treatment of complicated skin and skin structure infections. The adverse event profile seen in the **Synercid** patients in these two studies differed significantly from that seen in the other comparative studies. What follows is safety data from these two studies.

Discontinuation of therapy was most frequently due to the following drug related events:

% of patients discontinuing therapy by reaction type

Type	Synercid	Comparator
Venous	12.0	2.0
Non-venous	11.8	4.0
-Rash	2.0	0.9
-Nausea	1.1	0.0
-Vomiting	0.9	0.0
-Pain	0.9	0.0
-Pruritus	0.9	0.5

Venous adverse events were seen predominately in patients who had peripheral infusions. The most frequently reported venous and non-venous adverse reactions possibly or probably related to study drug were:

	% of patients with adverse reactions	
	Synercid	Comparator
Venous	68.0	32.7
-Pain at infusion site	44.7	17.8
-Inflammation at infusion site	38.2	14.7
-Edema at infusion site	18.0	7.2
-Infusion site reaction	11.6	3.6
Non-venous	24.7	13.1
-Nausea	4.0	2.0
-Vomiting	3.7	1.0
-Rash	3.1	1.3
-Pain	3.1	0.2

There were eight (1.7%) episodes of thrombus or thrombophlebitis in the **Synercid** arms and none in the comparator arms.

LABORATORY EVENTS—ALL COMPARATIVE STUDIES

The following table shows the number (%) of patients exhibiting laboratory values above or below the clinically relevant "critical" values during treatment phase (with an incidence of 0.1% or greater in either treatment group).
[See first table at right]

NON-COMPARATIVE TRIALS

CLINICAL ADVERSE REACTIONS

Approximately one-third of patients discontinued therapy in these trials due to adverse events. However, the discontinuation rate due to adverse reactions assessed by the investigator as possibly or probably related to **Synercid** therapy was approximately 5.0%.

There were three prospectively designed non-comparative clinical trials in patients (n – 972) treated with **Synercid**. One of these studies (301), had more complete documentation than the other two (398 and 398B). The most common events probably or possibly related to therapy were:
[See second table at right]

The percentage of patients who experienced severe related arthralgia and myalgia was 3.3% and 3.1%, respectively. The percentage of patients who discontinued treatment due to related arthralgia and myalgia was 2.3% and 1.8%, respectively.

LABORATORY EVENTS

The most frequently observed abnormalities in laboratory studies were in total and conjugated bilirubin, with increases greater than 5 times upper limit of normal, irrespective of relationship to **Synercid**, reported in 25.0% and 34.6% of patients, respectively. The percentage of patients who discontinued treatment due to increased total and conjugated bilirubin was 2.7% and 2.3%, respectively. Of note, 46.5% and 59.0% of patients had high baseline total and conjugated bilirubin levels before study entry.

OTHER

Serious adverse reactions in clinical trials, including non-comparative studies, considered possibly or probably related to **Synercid** administration with an incidence <0.1% include: acidosis, anaphylactoid reaction, apnea, arrhythmia, bone pain, cerebral hemorrhage, cerebrovascular accident, coagulation disorder, convulsion, dysautonomia, encephalopathy, grand mal convulsion, hemolysis, hemolytic anemia, heart arrest, hepatitis, hypoglycemia, hyponatremia, hypoplastic anemia, hypoventilation, hypovolemia, hypoxia, jaundice, mesenteric arterial occlusion, neck rigidity, neuropathy, pancytopenia, paraplegia, pericardial effusion, pericarditis, respiratory distress syndrome, shock, skin ulcer, supraventricular tachycardia, syncope, tremor, ventricular extrasystoles and ventricular fibrillation. Cases of hypotension and gastrointestinal hemorrhage were reported in less than 0.2% of patients.

OVERDOSAGE

There are four reports of patients receiving **Synercid** doses at up to three times that recommended (7.5 mg/kg). No adverse events were considered possibly or probably related to **Synercid** overdose. Signs of acute overdosage may include dyspnea, emesis, tremors, and ataxia as seen in animals given extremely high doses (50 mg/kg) of **Synercid**. Patients who receive an overdose should be carefully observed and given supportive treatment. **Synercid** is not removed by peritoneal dialysis or by hemodialysis.

DOSAGE AND ADMINISTRATION

Synercid should be administered by intravenous infusion in 5% Dextrose in Water solution over a 60-minute period. (See **WARNINGS.**) The recommended dosage for the treatment of infections is described in the table below. An infusion pump or device may be used to control the rate of infusion. If necessary, central venous access (*e.g.,* PICC) can be used to administer **Synercid** to decrease the incidence of venous irritation.

	Dose
Vancomycin-Resistant *Enterococcus faecium*	7.5 mg/kg q8h
Complicated Skin and Skin Structure Infection	7.5 mg/kg q12h

The minimum recommended treatment duration for Complicated Skin and Skin Structure Infections is seven days.

Parameter	Critically High or Low Value	Synercid Critically High or Low	Comparator Critically High or Low
AST	> 10 × ULN	9 (0.9)	2 (0.2)
ALT	> 10 × ULN	4 (0.4)	4 (0.4)
Total Bilirubin	> 5 × ULN	9 (0.9)	2 (0.2)
Conjugated Bilirubin	> 5 × ULN	29 (3.1)	12 (1.3)
LDH	> 5 × ULN	10 (2.6)	8 (2.1)
Alk Phosphatase	> 5 × ULN	3 (0.3)	7 (0.7)
Gamma-GT	> 10 × ULN	19 (1.9)	10 (1.0)
CPK	> 10 × ULN	6 (1.6)	5 (1.4)
Creatinine	>=440 μmol/L	1 (0.1)	1 (0.1)
BUN	>=35.5 mmol/L	2 (0.3)	9 (1.2)
Blood Glucose	> 22.2 mmol/L	11 (1.3)	11 (1.3)
	< 2.2 mmol/L	1 (0.1)	1 (0.1)
Bicarbonates	>40 mmol/L	2 (0.3)	3 (0.5)
	< 10 mmol/L	3 (0.5)	3 (0.5)
CO_2	> 50 mmol/L	0 (0.0)	0 (0.0)
	< 15 mmol/L	1 (0.2)	0 (0.0)
Sodium	> 160 mmol/L	0 (0.0)	0 (0.0)
	< 120 mmol/L	5 (0.5)	3 (0.3)
Potassium	> 6.0 mmol/L	3 (0.3)	6 (0.6)
	< 2.0 mmol/L	0 (0.0)	1 (0.1)
Hemoglobin	< 8 g/dL	25 (2.6)	16 (1.6)
Hematocrit	> 60%	2 (0.2)	0 (0.0)
Platelets	> 1,000,000/mm^3	2 (0.2)	2 (0.2)
	< 50,000/mm^3	6 (0.6)	7 (0.7)

	% of patients with adverse reaction		
Adverse Reactions	Study 301	Study 398A	Study 398B
Arthralgia	7.8	5.2	4.3
Myalgia	5.1	0.95	3.1
Arthralgia and Myalgia	7.4	3.3	6.8
Nausea	3.8	2.8	4.9

	Cured or Improved	
Infection Type	Synercid	Comparator
	(n/N) (%)	(n/N) (%)
Erysipelas (cellulitis)	52/82 (63.4)	43/77 (55.8)
Post-operative infections	14/38 (36.8)	24/42 (57.1)
Traumatic wound infection	33/55 (60.0)	33/55 (60.0)

For Vancomycin-Resistant *Enterococcus faecium* infection, the treatment duration should be determined based on the site and severity of the infection.

Special Populations: *Elderly:* No dosage adjustment of **Synercid** is required for use in the elderly. (See **CLINICAL PHARMACOLOGY: Pharmacokinetics** and **PRECAUTIONS: Geriatric Use.**)

Renal Insufficiency: No dosage adjustment of **Synercid** is required for use in patients with renal impairment or patients undergoing peritoneal dialysis. (See **CLINICAL PHARMACOLOGY: Pharmacokinetics.**)

Hepatic Insufficiency: Data from clinical trials of **Synercid** suggest that the incidence of adverse effects in patients with chronic liver insufficiency or cirrhosis was comparable to that in patients with normal hepatic function. Pharmacokinetic data in patients with hepatic cirrhosis (Child Pugh A or B) suggest that dosage reduction may be necessary but exact recommendations cannot be made at this time. (See **CLINICAL PHARMACOLOGY: Special Populations** and **PRECAUTIONS: General:** *Hepatic Insufficiency* sections.)

Pediatric Patients (less than 16 years of age): Based on a limited number of pediatric patients treated under emergency-use conditions, no dosage adjustment of **Synercid** is required. (See **PRECAUTIONS: Pediatric Use.**)

Preparation and administration of solution:

1. Reconstitute the single dose vial by slowly adding 5 mL of 5% Dextrose in Water or Sterile Water for injection.
2. **GENTLY** swirl the vial by manual rotation without shaking to ensure dissolution of contents while **LIMITING FOAM FORMATION.**
3. Allow the solution to sit for a few minutes until all the foam has disappeared. The resulting solution should be clear. Vials reconstituted in this manner will give a solution of 100 mg/mL. **CAUTION: FURTHER DILUTION REQUIRED BEFORE INFUSION.**
4. According to the patient's weight, the reconstituted **Synercid solution** should be added to 250 mL of 5% Dextrose solution (approximately 2 mg/mL). An infusion volume of 100 mL may be used for central line infusions.
5. If moderate to severe venous irritation occurs following peripheral administration of **Synercid** diluted in 250 mL of Dextrose 5% in water, consideration should be given to increasing the infusion volume to 500 or 750 mL, changing the infusion site, or infusing by a peripherally inserted central catheter (PICC) or a central venous catheter.
6. The desired dose should be administered by intravenous infusion over 60 minutes.

NOTE: As for other parenteral drug products, **Synercid** should be inspected visually for particulate matter prior to administration.

COMPATIBILITY:

DO NOT DILUTE WITH SALINE SOLUTIONS BECAUSE SYNERCID IS NOT COMPATIBLE WITH THESE AGENTS.

Synercid should not be mixed with, or physically added to, other drugs except for the following drugs where compatibility by Y-site injection has been established:

Y-Site Injection Compatibility of Synercid at 2 mg/mL Concentration

Admixture and Concentration	IV Infusion Solutions for Admixture
Aztreonam 20 mg/mL	D5W
Ciprofloxacin 1 mg/mL	D5W
Fluconazole 2 mg/mL	Used as the undiluted solution
Haloperidol 0.2 mg/mL	D5W
Metoclopramide 5 mg/mL	D5W
Potassium Chloride 40 mEq/L	D5W

D5W = 5% Dextrose Injection

If **Synercid** is to be given concomitantly with another drug, each drug should be given separately in accordance with the recommended dosage and route of administration for each drug.

With intermittent infusion of **Synercid** and other drugs through a common intravenous line, the line should be flushed before and after administration with 5% Dextrose in Water solution.

Stability and Storage: Before Reconstitution: The unopened vials should be stored in a refrigerator at 2 to 8°C (36 to 46°F).

Reconstituted and Infusions Solutions: Because **Synercid** contains no antibacterial preservative, it should be reconstituted under strict aseptic conditions (*e.g.,* Laminar Air Flow Hood). The reconstituted solution should be diluted within 30 minutes. Vials are for single use. The storage time of the diluted solution should be as short as possible to minimize the risk of microbial contamination. Stability of the diluted solution prior to the infusion is established as 5 hours at room temperature or 54 hours if stored under refrigeration 2 to 8°C (36 to 46°F). The solution should not be frozen.

HOW SUPPLIED

Synercid is supplied as a sterile lyophilized pyrogen-free preparation in single-dose 10 mL type 1 glass vials with gray elastomeric closure, and aluminum seal with a dark blue flip-off cap.

Each 10 mL vial contains sufficient quinupristin/dalfopristin to deliver 500 mg (150 mg of quinupristin and 350 mg of dalfopristin) for intravenous administration:

NDC 0075-9051-10 in trays of 10 vials.

Continued on next page

Synercid—Cont.

CLINICAL STUDIES

Non-comparative Trials

In the non-comparative trials, patients often presented with multiple co-morbidities and/or physiologic impairments, and may have been intolerant to or failed other antibacterial therapies.

Vancomycin-Resistant *Enterococcus Faecium*

Results are available from four non-comparative studies of **Synercid** (7.5 mg/kg q8h) for the treatment of vancomycin-resistant *Enterococcus faecium* (VREF) (N=1222). Three of these studies were prospective, the fourth consisted of a collection of individual emergency-use requests.

Of the 1222 patients, 27% did not have a specific site of infection identified, but presented with pure growth of VREF in two or more blood cultures. Ninety percent (90%) of these patients had clearance of their VREF bacteremia within the first 48 to 72 hours of therapy.

Because of the emergency use nature of the VREF trials and the variability in data collection in these severely ill patients, the percentage of patients found to be evaluable was 24.4%. The overall efficacy rate (defined as clinical success and eradication of the initial pathogen) in the evaluable patients (n=298) was 52.3%. The most common sites of infection included intra-abdominal, skin and skin structure, and the urinary tract. In these subgroups, the efficacy rates for the evaluable patients having the most complete documentation were 46.3% (n=67), 66.7% (n=15), and 73.9% (n=23), respectively.

The most common adverse reactions considered related to **Synercid** use were myalgias and arthralgias. (See **ADVERSE REACTIONS**.) All-cause mortality in the 4 studies ranged from 49.5% to 54.0%.

COMPARATIVE TRIALS

Complicated Skin and Skin Structure Infections

Two randomized, open-label, controlled clinical trials of **Synercid** (7.5 mg/kg q12h intravenously [iv]) in the treatment of complicated skin and skin structure infections were performed. The comparator drug was oxacillin (2g q6h iv) in the first study (JRV 304) and cefazolin (1g q8h iv) in the second study (JRV 305); however, in both studies vancomycin (1g q12h iv) could be substituted for the specified comparator if the causative pathogen was suspected or confirmed methicillin-resistant staphylococcus or if the patient was allergic to penicillins, cephalosporins or carbapenems. Study JRV 304 enrolled 450 patients (n = 229 **Synercid**; n = 221 Comparator) and Study JRV 305 enrolled 443 patients (n = 221 **Synercid**; n = 222 Comparator).

In the first study, 105 patients (45.9%) and 106 patients (48.0%) in the **Synercid** and Comparator arms, respectively, were found to be clinically evaluable. For the second study, these values were 113 (51.1%) and 120 (54.1%) patients in the **Synercid** and Comparator arms, respectively. Patients were found not to be clinically evaluable for reasons such as: wrong diagnosis, lower extremity infection in patients with diabetes or peripheral vascular disease since these infections were assumed to include aerobic gram-negative and anaerobic organisms, no specimen for culture obtained, insufficient therapy, no test of cure assessment, etc.

For the patients found to be clinically evaluable, in Study JRV 304 the success rate was 49.5% in the **Synercid** arm and 51.9% in the Comparator arm. In Study JRV 305, the success rates were 66.4% and 64.2% in the **Synercid** and Comparator arms, respectively.

The following table shows the clinical success rate (combined results from two clinical trials) in the clinically evaluable population. Due to the small numbers of patients in the subsets, statistical conclusions could not be reached.

[See third table on previous page]

SAFETY

Discontinuations of therapy because of adverse reactions which were probably or possibly due to drug therapy occurred more than four times as often in the **Synercid** group than in the comparator group. Approximately half of the discontinuations in the **Synercid** arm were due to venous adverse events. (See **ADVERSE REACTIONS: Clinical Reactions: Skin and Skin Structure Studies.**)

Keep out of the reach of children.

REFERENCES

1. National Committee for Clinical Laboratory Standards, *Methods for Dilution Antimicrobial Susceptibility Tests for Bacteria that Grow Aerobically*—Fourth Edition; Approved Standard. NCCLS Document M7-A4 (ISBN 1-56238-309-4). NCCLS, 940 West Valley Road, Suite 1400, Wayne, PA 19087-1898, 1997.
2. National Committee for Clinical Laboratory Standards, *Performance Standards for Antimicrobial Disk Susceptibility Tests*—Sixth Edition; Approved Standard. NCCLS document M2-A6 (ISBN 1-56238-308-6). NCCLS, 940 West Valley Road, Suite 1400, Wayne, PA 19087-1898, 1997.

Manufactured for
AVENTIS PHARMACEUTICALS PRODUCTS INC.
Parsippany, NJ 07054
by
CATALYTICA PHARMACEUTICALS, INC.
GREENVILLE, NC 27834 USA
IN-1300! Revised 7/99

Shown in Product Identification Guide, page 307

TAXOTERE® ℞

[*tax-ō-tĕr*]
(docetaxel)
for Injection Concentrate
Rx only

WARNING

TAXOTERE® (docetaxel) for Injection Concentrate should be administered under the supervision of a qualified physician experienced in the use of antineoplastic agents. Appropriate management of complications is possible only when adequate diagnostic and treatment facilities are readily available.

The incidence of treatment-related mortality associated with TAXOTERE therapy is increased in patients with abnormal liver function, in patients receiving higher doses, and in patients with non-small cell lung carcinoma and a history of prior treatment with platinum-based chemotherapy who receive TAXOTERE at a dose of 100 mg/m^2 (see **WARNINGS**).

TAXOTERE should generally not be given to patients with bilirubin > upper limit of normal (ULN), or to patients with SGOT and/or SGPT >1.5 × ULN concomitant with alkaline phosphatase > 2.5 × ULN. Patients with elevations of bilirubin or abnormalities of transaminase concurrent with alkaline phosphatase are at increased risk for the development of grade 4 neutropenia, febrile neutropenia, infections, severe thrombocytopenia, severe stomatitis, severe skin toxicity, and toxic death. Patients with isolated elevations of transaminase > 1.5 × ULN also had a higher rate of febrile neutropenia grade 4 but did not have an increased incidence of toxic death. Bilirubin, SGOT or SGPT, and alkaline phosphatase values should be obtained prior to each cycle of TAXOTERE therapy and reviewed by the treating physician.

TAXOTERE therapy should not be given to patients with neutrophil counts of < 1500 cells/mm^3. In order to monitor the occurrence of neutropenia, which may be severe and result in infection, frequent blood cell counts should be performed on all patients receiving TAXOTERE.

Severe hypersensitivity reactions characterized by hypotension and/or bronchospasm, or generalized rash/erythema occurred in 2.2% (2/92) of patients who received the recommended 3-day dexamethasone premedication. Hypersensitivity reactions requiring discontinuation of the TAXOTERE infusion were reported in five patients who did not receive premedication. These reactions resolved after discontinuation of the infusion and the administration of appropriate therapy. TAXOTERE must not be given to patients who have a history of severe hypersensitivity reactions to TAXOTERE or to other drugs formulated with polysorbate 80 (see **WARNINGS**).

Severe fluid retention occurred in 6.5% (6/92) of patients despite use of a 3-day dexamethasone premedication regimen. It was characterized by one or more of the following events: poorly tolerated peripheral edema, generalized edema, pleural effusion requiring urgent drainage, dyspnea at rest, cardiac tamponade, or pronounced abdominal distention (due to ascites) (see **PRECAUTIONS**).

DESCRIPTION

Docetaxel is an antineoplastic agent belonging to the taxoid family. It is prepared by semisynthesis beginning with a precursor extracted from the renewable needle biomass of yew plants. The chemical name for docetaxel is (2R,3S)-N-carboxy-3-phenylisoserine,N-*tert*-butyl ester, 13-ester with 5β-20-epoxy-1,2α,4,7β,10β,13α-hexahydroxytax-11-en-9-one 4-acetate 2-benzoate, trihydrate. Docetaxel has the following structural formula:

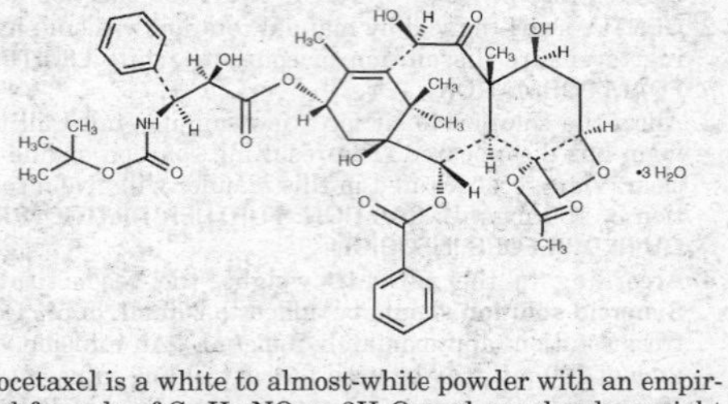

Docetaxel is a white to almost-white powder with an empirical formula of $C_{43}H_{53}NO_{14} \bullet 3H_2O$, and a molecular weight of 861.9. It is highly lipophilic and practically insoluble in water. TAXOTERE (docetaxel) for Injection Concentrate is a clear yellow to brownish-yellow viscous solution. TAXOTERE is sterile, non-pyrogenic, and is available in single-dose vials containing 20 mg (0.5 mL) or 80 mg (2.0 mL) docetaxel (anhydrous). Each mL contains 40 mg docetaxel (anhydrous) and 1040 mg polysorbate 80.

TAXOTERE for Injection Concentrate requires dilution prior to use. A sterile, non-pyrogenic, single-dose diluent is supplied for that purpose. The diluent for TAXOTERE contains 13% ethanol in Water for Injection, and is supplied in 1.5 mL (to be used with 20 mg TAXOTERE for Injection Concentrate) and 6.0 mL (to be used with 80 mg TAXOTERE for Injection Concentrate) vials.

CLINICAL PHARMACOLOGY

Docetaxel is an antineoplastic agent that acts by disrupting the microtubular network in cells that is essential for mitotic and interphase cellular functions. Docetaxel binds to free tubulin and promotes the assembly of tubulin into stable microtubules while simultaneously inhibiting their disassembly. This leads to the production of microtubule bundles without normal function and to the stabilization of microtubules, which results in the inhibition of mitosis in cells. Docetaxel's binding to microtubules does not alter the number of protofilaments in the bound microtubules, a feature which differs from most spindle poisons currently in clinical use.

HUMAN PHARMACOKINETICS

The pharmacokinetics of docetaxel have been evaluated in cancer patients after administration of 20–115 mg/m^2 in phase I studies. The area under the curve (AUC) was dose proportional following doses of 70–115 mg/m^2 with infusion times of 1 to 2 hours. Docetaxel's pharmacokinetic profile is consistent with a three-compartment pharmacokinetic model, with half-lives for the α, β, and γ phases of 4 min, 36 min, and 11.1 hr, respectively. The initial rapid decline represents distribution to the peripheral compartments and the late (terminal) phase is due, in part, to a relatively slow efflux of docetaxel from the peripheral compartment. Mean values for total body clearance and steady state volume of distribution were 21 L/h/m^2 and 113 L, respectively. Mean total body clearance for Japanese patients dosed at the range of 10–90 mg/m^2 was similar to that of European/American populations dosed at 100 mg/m^2, suggesting no significant difference in the elimination of docetaxel in the two populations.

A study of ^{14}C-docetaxel was conducted in three cancer patients. Docetaxel was eliminated in both the urine and feces following oxidative metabolism of the *tert*-butyl ester group, but fecal excretion was the main elimination route. Within 7 days, urinary and fecal excretion accounted for approximately 6% and 75% of the administered radioactivity, respectively. About 80% of the radioactivity recovered in feces is excreted during the first 48 hours as 1 major and 3 minor metabolites with very small amounts (less than 8%) of unchanged drug.

A population pharmacokinetic analysis was carried out after TAXOTERE treatment of 535 patients dosed at 100 mg/m^2. Pharmacokinetic parameters estimated by this analysis were very close to those estimated from phase I studies. The pharmacokinetics of docetaxel were not influenced by age or gender and docetaxel total body clearance was not modified by pretreatment with dexamethasone. In patients with clinical chemistry data suggestive of mild to moderate liver function impairment (SGOT and/or SGPT >1.5 times the upper limit of normal [ULN] concomitant with alkaline phosphatase >2.5 times ULN), total body clearance was lowered by an average of 27%, resulting in a 38% increase in systemic exposure (AUC). This average, however, includes a substantial range and there is, at present, no measurement that would allow recommendation for dose adjustment in such patients. Patients with combined abnormalities of transaminase and alkaline phosphatase should, in general, not be treated with TAXOTERE.

In vitro studies showed that docetaxel is about 94% protein bound, mainly to α_1–acid glycoprotein, albumin, and lipoproteins. In three cancer patients, the *in vitro* binding to plasma proteins was found to be approximately 97%. Dexamethasone does not affect the protein binding of docetaxel.

In vitro drug interaction studies revealed that docetaxel is metabolized by the CYP3A4 isoenzyme, and its metabolism can be inhibited by CYP3A4 inhibitors, such as ketoconazole, erythromycin, troleandomycin, and nifedipine. Based on *in vitro* findings, it is likely that CYP3A4 inhibitors and/or substrates may lead to substantial increases in docetaxel blood concentrations. No clinical studies have been performed to evaluate this finding (see **PRECAUTIONS**).

CLINICAL STUDIES

Breast Cancer: The efficacy and safety of TAXOTERE have been evaluated in locally advanced or metastatic breast cancer after failure of previous chemotherapy (alkylating agent-containing regimens or anthracycline-containing regimens), primarily at a dose of 100 mg/m^2 given as a 1-hour infusion every 3 weeks, but with some experience at 60 mg/m^2, in two large randomized trials and a number of smaller single arm studies.

Randomized Trials: In one randomized trial, patients with a history of prior treatment with an anthracycline-containing regimen were assigned to treatment with TAXOTERE or the combination of mitomycin (12 mg/m^2 every 6 weeks) and vinblastine (6 mg/m^2 every 3 weeks). 203 patients were randomized to TAXOTERE and 189 to the comparator arm. Most patients had received prior chemotherapy for metastatic disease; only 27 patients on the TAXOTERE arm and 33 patients on the comparator arm entered the study following relapse after adjuvant therapy. Three-quarters of patients had measurable, visceral metastases. The primary endpoint was time to progression. The following table summarizes the study results:

[See first table at top of next page]

In a second randomized trial, patients previously treated with an alkylating-containing regimen were assigned to treatment with TAXOTERE or doxorubicin (75 mg/m^2 every 3 weeks). 161 patients were randomized to TAXOTERE and 165 patients to doxorubicin. Approximately one-half of patients had received prior chemotherapy for metastatic disease, and one-half entered the study following relapse after adjuvant therapy. Three-quarters of patients had measurable, visceral metastases. The primary endpoint was time to progression. The study results are summarized below:

[See second table on next page]

Efficacy of TAXOTERE in the Treatment of Breast Cancer Patients Previously Treated with an Anthracycline-Containing Regimen (Intent-to-Treat Analysis)

Efficacy Parameter	Docetaxel (n=203)	Mitomycin/ Vinblastine (n=189)	p-value
Median Survival	11.4 months	8.7 months	p=0.01 Log Rank
Risk Ratio*, Mortality (Docetaxel: Control)	0.73		
95% CI (Risk Ratio)	0.58–0.93		
Median Time to Progression	4.3 months	2.5 months	p=0.01 Log Rank
Risk Ratio*, Progression (Docetaxel: Control)	0.75		
95% CI (Risk Ratio)	0.61–0.94		
Overall Response Rate Complete Response Rate	28.1% 3.4%	9.5% 1.6%	p<0.0001 Chi Square

*For the risk ratio, a value less than 1.00 favors docetaxel.

Efficacy of TAXOTERE in the Treatment of Breast Cancer Patients Previously Treated with an Alkylating-Containing Regimen (Intent-to-Treat Analysis)

Efficacy Parameter	Docetaxel (n=161)	Doxorubicin (n=165)	p-value
Median Survival	14.7 months	14.3 months	p=0.39 Log Rank
Risk Ratio*, Mortality (Docetaxel: Control)	0.89		
95% CI (Risk Ratio)	0.68–1.16		
Median Time to Progression	6.5 months	5.3 months	p=0.45 Log Rank
Risk Ratio*, Progression (Docetaxel: Control)	0.93		
95% CI (Risk Ratio)	0.71–1.16		
Overall Response Rate Complete Response Rate	45.3% 6.8%	29.7% 4.2%	p=0.004 Chi Square

*For the risk ratio, a value less than 1.00 favors docetaxel.

Hematologic Adverse Events in Breast Cancer Patients Previously Treated with Chemotherapy Treated at TAXOTERE 100 mg/m² with Normal or Elevated Liver Function Tests or 60 mg/m² with Normal Liver Function Tests

Adverse Event	TAXOTERE 100 mg/m² Normal LFTs* n=730 %	TAXOTERE 100 mg/m² Elevated LFTs** n=18 %	TAXOTERE 60 mg/m² Normal LFTs* n=174 %
Neutropenia			
Any <2000 cells/mm³	98.4	100	95.4
Grade 4 <500 cells/mm³	84.4	93.8	74.9
Thrombocytopenia			
Any <100,000 cells/mm³	10.8	44.4	14.4
Grade 4 <20,000 cells/mm³	0.6	16.7	1.1
Anemia <11 g/dL	94.6	94.4	64.9
Infection***			
Any	22.5	38.9	1.1
Grade 3 and 4	7.1	33.3	0
Febrile Neutropenia****			
By Patient	11.8	33.3	0
By Course	2.4	8.6	0
Septic Death	1.5	5.6	1.1
Non-Septic Death	1.1	11.1	0

***Normal Baseline LFTs: Transaminases ≤ 1.5 times ULN or alkaline phosphatase ≤ 2.5 times ULN or isolated elevations of transaminases or alkaline phosphatase up to 5 times ULN**
**** Elevated Baseline LFTs: SGOT and/or SGPT >1.5 times ULN concurrent with alkaline phosphatase >2.5 times ULN**
***** Incidence of infection requiring hospitalization and/or intravenous antibiotics was 8.5% (n=62) among the 730 patients with normal LFTs at baseline; 7 patients had concurrent grade 3 neutropenia, and 46 patients had grade 4 neutropenia.**
****** Febrile Neutropenia: For 100 mg/m², ANC grade 4 and fever > 38°C with IV antibiotics and/or hospitalization; for 60 mg/m², ANC grade 3/4 and fever > 38.1°C**

Single Arm Studies: TAXOTERE at a dose of 100 mg/m² was studied in six single arm studies involving a total of 309 patients with metastatic breast cancer in whom previous chemotherapy had failed. Among these, 190 patients had anthracycline-resistant breast cancer, defined as progression during an anthracycline-containing chemotherapy regimen for metastatic disease, or relapse during an anthracycline-containing adjuvant regimen. In anthracycline-resistant patients, the overall response rate was 37.9% (72/190; 95% C.I.: 31.0–44.8) and the complete response rate was 2.1%.

TAXOTERE was also studied in three single arm Japanese studies at a dose of 60 mg/m², in 174 patients who had received prior chemotherapy for locally advanced or metastatic breast cancer. Among 26 patients whose best response to an anthracycline had been progression, the response rate was 34.6% (95% C.I.: 17.2–55.7), similar to the response rate in single arm studies of 100 mg/m².

Hematologic and Other Toxicity: Relation to dose and baseline liver chemistry abnormalities. Hematologic and other toxicity is increased at higher doses and in patients with elevated baseline liver function tests (LFTs). In the following tables, adverse drug reactions are compared for three populations: 730 patients with normal LFTs given TAXOTERE at 100 mg/m² in the randomized and single arm studies of metastatic breast cancer after failure of previous chemotherapy; 18 patients in these studies who had abnormal baseline LFTs (defined as SGOT and/or SGPT > 1.5 times ULN concurrent with alkaline phosphatase > 2.5 times ULN); and 174 patients in Japanese studies given TAXOTERE at 60 mg/m² who had normal LFTs.

[See third table at left]

[See first table at top of next page]

Non-Small Cell Lung Cancer (NSCLC): The efficacy and safety of TAXOTERE in non-small cell lung cancer have been evaluated in patients with locally advanced or metastatic disease and a history of prior treatment with a platinum-based chemotherapy regimen. Two randomized, controlled trials established that a TAXOTERE dose of 75 mg/m² was tolerable and yielded a favorable outcome (see below). TAXOTERE at a dose of 100 mg/m², however, was associated with unacceptable hematologic toxicity, infections, and treatment-related mortality and this dose should not be used (see **BOXED WARNING**, **WARNINGS**, and **DOSAGE AND ADMINISTRATION** sections).

One trial (TAX317), randomized patients with locally advanced or metastatic non-small cell lung cancer, a history of prior platinum-based chemotherapy, no history of taxane exposure, and an ECOG performance status ≤2 to TAXOTERE or best supportive care. The primary endpoint of the study was survival. Patients were initially randomized to TAXOTERE 100 mg/m² or best supportive care, but early toxic deaths at this dose led to a dose reduction to TAXOTERE 75 mg/m². A total of 104 patients were randomized in this amended study to either TAXOTERE 75 mg/m² or best supportive care.

In a second randomized trial (TAX320), 373 patients with locally advanced or metastatic non-small cell lung cancer, a history of prior platinum-based chemotherapy, and an ECOG performance status ≤2 were randomized to TAXOTERE 75 mg/m², TAXOTERE 100 mg/m² and a treatment in which the investigator chose either vinorelbine 30 mg/m² days 1, 8, and 15 repeated every 3 weeks <u>or</u> ifosfamide 2 g/m² days 1–3 repeated every 3 weeks. Forty percent of the patients in this study had a history of prior paclitaxel exposure. The primary endpoint was survival in both trials. The efficacy data for the TAXOTERE 75 mg/m² arm and the comparator arms are summarized in the table below and in figures 1 and 2 showing the survival curves for the two studies.

[See second table on next page]

Only one of the two trials (TAX317) showed a clear effect on survival, the primary endpoint; that trial also showed an increased rate of survival to one year. In the second study (TAX320) the rate of survival at one year favored TAXOTERE 75 mg/m².

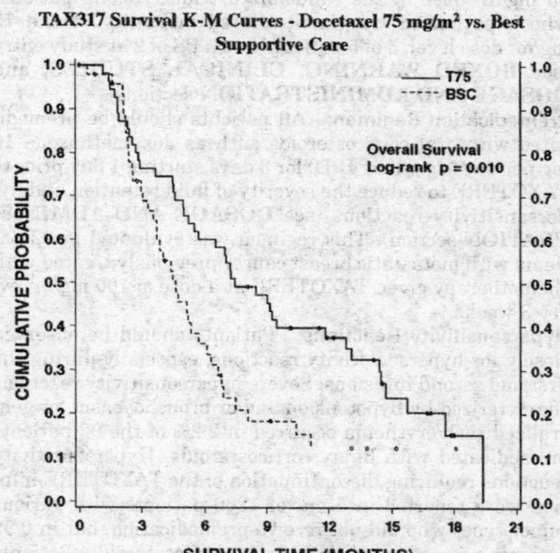

[See figure at top of next column]

Patients treated with TAXOTERE at a dose of 75 mg/m² experienced no deterioration in performance status and body weight relative to the comparator arms used in these trials.

INDICATIONS AND USAGE

Breast Cancer: TAXOTERE is indicated for the treatment of patients with locally advanced or metastatic breast cancer after failure of prior chemotherapy.

Continued on next page

Taxotere—Cont.

TAX320 Survival K-M Curves - Docetaxel 75 mg/m² vs. Vinorelbine or Ifosfamide Control

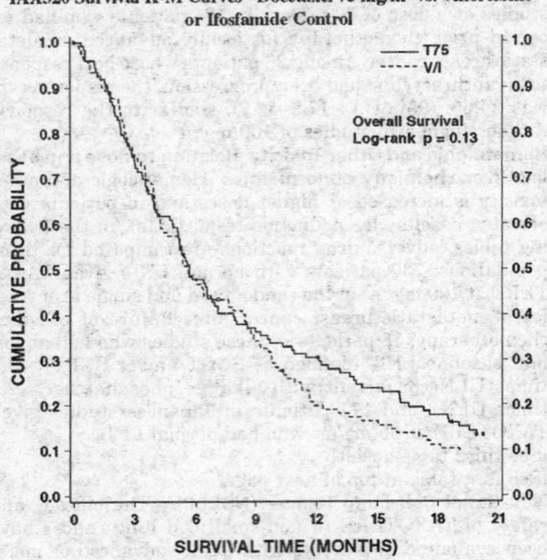

Non-Small Cell Lung Cancer: TAXOTERE is indicated for the treatment of patients with locally advanced or metastatic non-small cell lung cancer after failure of prior platinum-based chemotherapy.

CONTRAINDICATIONS

TAXOTERE is contraindicated in patients who have a history of severe hypersensitivity reactions to docetaxel or to other drugs formulated with polysorbate 80.

TAXOTERE should not be used in patients with neutrophil counts of <1500 cells/mm³.

WARNINGS

TAXOTERE should be administered under the supervision of a qualified physician experienced in the use of antineoplastic agents. Appropriate management of complications is possible only when adequate diagnostic and treatment facilities are readily available.

Toxic Deaths

Breast Cancer: TAXOTERE administered at 100 mg/m² was associated with deaths considered possibly or probably related to treatment in 2.0% (19/965) of metastatic breast cancer patients, both previously treated and untreated, with normal baseline liver function and in 11.5% (7/61) of patients with various tumor types who had abnormal baseline liver function (SGOT and/or SGPT > 1.5 times ULN together with AP > 2.5 times ULN). Among patients dosed at 60 mg/m², mortality related to treatment occurred in 0.6% (3/481) of patients with normal liver function, and in 3 of 7 patients with abnormal liver function. Approximately half of these deaths occurred during the first cycle. Sepsis accounted for the majority of the deaths.

Non-Small Cell Lung Cancer: TAXOTERE administered at a dose of 100 mg/m² in patients with locally advanced or metastatic non-small cell lung cancer who had a history of prior platinum-based chemotherapy was associated with increased treatment-related mortality (14% and 5% in two randomized, controlled studies). There were 2.8% treatment-related deaths among the 176 patients treated at the 75 mg/m² dose in the randomized trials. Among patients who experienced treatment-related mortality at the 75 mg/m² dose level, 3 of 5 patients had a PS of 2 at study entry (see **BOXED WARNING, CLINICAL STUDIES,** and **DOSAGE AND ADMINISTRATION** sections).

Premedication Regimen: All patients should be premedicated with oral corticosteroids such as dexamethasone 16 mg per day (*e.g.,* 8 mg BID) for 3 days starting 1 day prior to TAXOTERE to reduce the severity of fluid retention and hypersensitivity reactions (see **DOSAGE AND ADMINISTRATION** section). This regimen was evaluated in 92 patients with metastatic breast cancer previously treated with chemotherapy given TAXOTERE at a dose of 100 mg/m² every 3 weeks.

Hypersensitivity Reactions: Patients should be observed closely for hypersensitivity reactions, especially during the first and second infusions. Severe hypersensitivity reactions characterized by hypotension and/or bronchospasm, or generalized rash/erythema occurred in 2.2% of the 92 patients premedicated with 3-day corticosteroids. Hypersensitivity reactions requiring discontinuation of the TAXOTERE infusion were reported in 5 out of 1260 patients with various tumor types who did not receive premedication, but in 0/92 patients premedicated with 3-day corticosteroids. Patients with a history of severe hypersensitivity reactions should not be rechallenged with TAXOTERE.

Hematologic Effects: Neutropenia (< 2000 neutrophils/mm³) occurs in virtually all patients given 60–100 mg/m² of TAXOTERE and grade 4 neutropenia (< 500 cells/mm³) occurs in 85% of patients given 100 mg/m² and 75% of patients given 60 mg/m². Frequent monitoring of blood counts is, therefore, essential so that dose can be adjusted. TAXOTERE should not be administered to patients with neutrophils < 1500 cells/mm³.

Febrile neutropenia occurred in about 12% of patients given 100 mg/m² but was very uncommon in patients given 60 mg/m². Hematologic responses, febrile reactions and infections, and rates of septic death for different regimens are dose related and are described in **CLINICAL STUDIES**.

Three breast cancer patients with severe liver impairment (bilirubin > 1.7 times ULN) developed fatal gastrointestinal bleeding associated with severe drug-induced thrombocytopenia.

Hepatic Impairment: (see **BOXED WARNING**).

Fluid Retention: (see **BOXED WARNING**).

Pregnancy: TAXOTERE can cause fetal harm when administered to pregnant women. Studies in both rats and rabbits at doses ≥ 0.3 and 0.03 mg/kg/day, respectively (about 1/50 and 1/300 the daily maximum recommended human dose on a mg/m² basis), administered during the period of organogenesis, have shown that TAXOTERE is embryotoxic and fetotoxic (characterized by intrauterine mortality, increased resorption, reduced fetal weight, and fetal ossification delay). The doses indicated above also caused maternal toxicity.

There are no adequate and well-controlled studies in pregnant women using TAXOTERE. If TAXOTERE is used during pregnancy, or if the patient becomes pregnant while re-

Non-Hematologic Adverse Events in Breast Cancer Patients Previously Treated with Chemotherapy Treated at TAXOTERE 100 mg/m² with Normal or Elevated Liver Function Tests or 60 mg/m² with Normal Liver Function Tests

Adverse Event	TAXOTERE 100 mg/m² Normal LFTs* n=730 %	TAXOTERE 100 mg/m² Elevated LFTs** n=18 %	TAXOTERE 60 mg/m² Normal LFTs* n=174 %
Acute Hypersensitivity Reaction Regardless of Premedication			
Any	13.0	5.6	0.6
Severe	1.2	0	0
Fluid Retention* Regardless of Premedication**			
Any	56.2	61.1	12.6
Severe	7.9	16.7	0
Neurosensory			
Any	56.8	50	19.5
Severe	5.8	0	0
Myalgia	22.7	33.3	3.4
Cutaneous			
Any	44.8	61.1	30.5
Severe	4.8	16.7	0
Asthenia			
Any	65.2	44.4	65.5
Severe	16.6	22.2	0
Diarrhea			
Any	42.2	27.8	NA
Severe	6.3	11.1	
Stomatitis			
Any	53.3	66.7	19.0
Severe	7.8	38.9	0.6

***Normal Baseline LFTs: Transaminases ≤ 1.5 times ULN or alkaline phosphatase ≤ 2.5 times ULN or isolated elevations of transaminases or alkaline phosphatase up to 5 times ULN**

**** Elevated Baseline Liver Function: SGOT and/or SGPT >1.5 times ULN concurrent with alkaline phosphatase >2.5 times ULN**

***** Fluid Retention includes (by COSTART): edema (peripheral, localized, generalized, lymphedema, pulmonary edema, and edema otherwise not specified) and effusion (pleural, pericardial, and ascites); no premedication given with the 60 mg/m² dose**

NA = not available

Efficacy of TAXOTERE in the Treatment of Non-Small Cell Lung Cancer Patients Previously Treated with a Platinum-Based Chemotherapy Regimen (Intent-to-Treat Analysis)

	TAX317		TAX320	
	Docetaxel 75 mg/m² n=55	Best Supportive Care/75 n=49	Docetaxel 75 mg/m² n=125	Control (V/I) n=123
Overall Survival Log-rank Test	p=0.01		p=0.13	
Risk Ratio††, Mortality (Docetaxel: Control)	0.56		0.82	
95% CI (Risk Ratio)	(0.35, 0.88)		(0.63, 1.06)	
Median Survival	7.5 months*	4.6 months	5.7 months	5.6 months
95% CI	(5.5, 12.8)	(3.7, 6.1)	(5.1, 7.1)	(4.4, 7.9)
% 1-year Survival	37%*†	12%	30%*†	20%
95% CI	(24, 50)	(2, 23)	(22, 39)	(13, 27)
Time to Progression	12.3 weeks*	7.0 weeks	8.3 weeks	7.6 weeks
95% CI	(9.0, 18.3)	(6.0, 9.3)	(7.0, 11.7)	(6.7, 10.1)
Response Rate	5.5%	Not Applicable	5.7%	0.8%
95% CI	(1.1, 15.1)		(2.3, 11.3)	(0.0, 4.5)

* p≤0.05; † uncorrected for multiple comparisons; †† a value less than 1.00 favors docetaxel.

ceiving this drug, the patient should be apprised of the potential hazard to the fetus or potential risk for loss of the pregnancy. Women of childbearing potential should be advised to avoid becoming pregnant during therapy with TAXOTERE.

PRECAUTIONS

General: Responding patients may not experience an improvement in performance status on therapy and may experience worsening. The relationship between changes in performance status, response to therapy, and treatment-related side effects has not been established.

Hematologic Effects: In order to monitor the occurrence of myelotoxicity, it is recommended that frequent peripheral blood cell counts be performed on all patients receiving TAXOTERE. Patients should not be retreated with subsequent cycles of TAXOTERE until neutrophils recover to a level > 1500 cells/mm^3 and platelets recover to a level > 100,000 cells/mm^3.

A 25% reduction in the dose of TAXOTERE® (docetaxel) for Injection Concentrate is recommended during subsequent cycles following severe neutropenia (< 500 cells/mm^3) lasting 7 days or more, febrile neutropenia, or a grade 4 infection in a TAXOTERE cycle (see **DOSAGE AND ADMINISTRATION** section).

Hypersensitivity Reactions: Hypersensitivity reactions may occur within a few minutes following initiation of a TAXOTERE infusion. If minor reactions such as flushing or localized skin reactions occur, interruption of therapy is not required. More severe reactions, however, require the immediate discontinuation of TAXOTERE and aggressive therapy. All patients should be premedicated with an oral corticosteroid prior to the initiation of the infusion of TAXOTERE (see **BOXED WARNING** and **WARNINGS: Premedication Regimen**).

Cutaneous: Localized erythema of the extremities with edema followed by desquamation has been observed. In case of severe skin toxicity, an adjustment in dosage is recommended (see **DOSAGE AND ADMINISTRATION** section). The discontinuation rate due to skin toxicity was 1.6% (15/965) for metastatic breast cancer patients. Among 92 breast cancer patients premedicated with 3-day corticosteroids, there were no cases of severe skin toxicity reported and no patient discontinued TAXOTERE due to skin toxicity.

Fluid Retention: Severe fluid retention has been reported following TAXOTERE therapy (see **BOXED WARNING** and **WARNINGS: Premedication Regimen**). Patients should be premedicated with oral corticosteroids prior to each TAXOTERE administration to reduce the incidence and severity of fluid retention (see **DOSAGE AND ADMINISTRATION** section). Patients with pre-existing effusions should be closely monitored from the first dose for the possible exacerbation of the effusions.

When fluid retention occurs, peripheral edema usually starts in the lower extremities and may become generalized with a median weight gain of 2 kg.

Among 92 breast cancer patients premedicated with 3-day corticosteroids, moderate fluid retention occurred in 27.2% and severe fluid retention in 6.5%. The median cumulative dose to onset of moderate or severe fluid retention was 819 mg/m^2. 9.8% (9/92) of patients discontinued treatment due to fluid retention: 4 patients discontinued with severe fluid retention; the remaining 5 had mild or moderate fluid retention. The median cumulative dose to treatment discontinuation due to fluid retention was 1021 mg/m^2. Fluid retention was completely, but sometimes slowly, reversible with a median of 16 weeks from the last infusion of TAXOTERE to resolution (range: 0 to 42+ weeks). Patients developing peripheral edema may be treated with standard measures, *e.g.,* salt restriction, oral diuretic(s).

Neurologic: Severe neurosensory symptoms (paresthesia, dysesthesia, pain) were observed in 5.5% (53/965) of metastatic breast cancer patients, and resulted in treatment discontinuation in 6.1%. When these symptoms occur, dosage must be adjusted. If symptoms persist, treatment should be discontinued (see **DOSAGE AND ADMINISTRATION** section). Patients who experienced neurotoxicity in clinical trials and for whom follow-up information on the complete resolution of the event was available had spontaneous reversal of symptoms with a median of 9 weeks from onset (range: 0 to 106 weeks). Severe peripheral motor neuropathy mainly manifested as distal extremity weakness occurred in 4.4% (42/965).

Asthenia: Severe asthenia has been reported in 14.9% (144/965) of metastatic breast cancer patients but has led to treatment discontinuation in only 1.8%. Symptoms of fatigue and weakness may last a few days up to several weeks and may be associated with deterioration of performance status in patients with progressive disease.

Information for Patients: For additional information, see the accompanying Patient Information Leaflet.

Drug Interactions: There have been no formal clinical studies to evaluate the drug interactions of TAXOTERE with other medications. *In vitro* studies have shown that the metabolism of docetaxel may be modified by the concomitant administration of compounds that induce, inhibit, or are metabolized by cytochrome P450 3A4, such as cyclosporine, terfenadine, ketoconazole, erythromycin, and troleandomycin. Caution should be exercised with these drugs when treating patients receiving TAXOTERE as there is a potential for a significant interaction.

Carcinogenicity, Mutagenicity, Impairment of Fertility: No studies have been conducted to assess the carcinogenic potential of TAXOTERE. TAXOTERE has been shown to be clastogenic in the *in vitro* chromosome aberration test in CHO-K$_1$ cells and in the *in vivo* micronucleus test in the mouse, but it did not induce mutagenicity in the Ames test or the CHO/HGPRT gene mutation assays. TAXOTERE produced no impairment of fertility in rats when administered in multiple IV doses of up to 0.3 mg/kg (about 1/50 the recommended human dose on a mg/m^2 basis), but decreased testicular weights were reported. This correlates with findings of a 10-cycle toxicity study (dosing once every 21 days for 6 months) in rats and dogs in which testicular atrophy or degeneration was observed at IV doses of 5 mg/kg in rats and 0.375 mg/kg in dogs (about 1/3 and 1/15 the recommended human dose on a mg/m^2 basis, respectively). An increased frequency of dosing in rats produced similar effects at lower dose levels.

Pregnancy: Pregnancy Category D (see **WARNINGS** section).

Nursing Mothers: It is not known whether TAXOTERE is excreted in human milk. Because many drugs are excreted in human milk, and because of the potential for serious adverse reactions in nursing infants from TAXOTERE, mothers should discontinue nursing prior to taking the drug.

Pediatric Use: The safety and effectiveness of TAXOTERE in pediatric patients have not been established.

ADVERSE REACTIONS

The adverse reactions are described separately for TAXOTERE 100 mg/m^2, the maximum dose approved for breast cancer, and 75 mg/m^2, the dose approved for advanced non-small cell lung carcinoma after prior platinum-based chemotherapy.

TAXOTERE 100 mg/m^2: Adverse drug reactions occurring in at least 5% of patients are compared for three populations who received TAXOTERE administered at 100 mg/m^2 as a 1-hour infusion every 3 weeks: 2045 patients with various tumor types and normal baseline liver function tests; the subset of 965 patients with locally advanced or metastatic breast cancer, both previously treated and untreated with chemotherapy, who had normal baseline liver function tests; and an additional 61 patients with various tumor types who had abnormal liver function tests at baseline. These reactions were described using COSTART terms and were considered possibly or probably related to TAXOTERE. At least 95% of these patients did not receive hematopoietic support. The safety profile is generally similar in patients receiving TAXOTERE for the treatment of breast cancer and in patients with other tumor types.

[See table at top of next page]

Hematologic: (see **WARNINGS**). Reversible marrow suppression was the major dose-limiting toxicity of TAXOTERE. The median time to nadir was 7 days, while the median duration of severe neutropenia (<500 cells/mm^3) was 7 days. Among 2045 patients with solid tumors and normal baseline LFTs, severe neutropenia occurred in 75.4% and lasted for more than 7 days in 2.9% of cycles.

Febrile neutropenia (<500 cells/mm^3 with fever > 38°C with IV antibiotics and/or hospitalization) occurred in 11% of patients with solid tumors, in 12.3% of patients with metastatic breast cancer, and in 9.8% of 92 breast cancer patients premedicated with 3-day corticosteroids.

Severe infectious episodes occurred in 6.1% of patients with solid tumors, in 6.4% of patients with metastatic breast cancer, and in 5.4% of 92 breast cancer patients premedicated with 3-day corticosteroids.

Thrombocytopenia (<100,000 cells/mm^3) associated with fatal gastrointestinal hemorrhage has been reported.

Hypersensitivity Reactions: Severe hypersensitivity reactions are discussed in the **BOXED WARNING, WARNINGS,** and **PRECAUTIONS** sections. Minor events, including flushing, rash with or without pruritus, chest tightness, back pain, dyspnea, drug fever, or chills, have been reported and resolved after discontinuing the infusion and appropriate therapy.

Fluid Retention: (see **BOXED WARNING, WARNINGS: Premedication Regimen,** and **PRECAUTIONS** sections).

Cutaneous: Severe skin toxicity is discussed in **PRECAUTIONS**. Reversible cutaneous reactions characterized by a rash including localized eruptions, mainly on the feet and/or hands, but also on the arms, face, or thorax, usually associated with pruritus, have been observed. Eruptions generally occurred within 1 week after TAXOTERE infusion, recovered before the next infusion, and were not disabling.

Severe nail disorders were characterized by hypo- or hyperpigmentation, and occasionally by onycholysis (in 0.8% of patients with solid tumors) and pain.

Neurologic: (see **PRECAUTIONS**).

Gastrointestinal: Gastrointestinal reactions (nausea and/or vomiting and/or diarrhea) were generally mild to moderate. Severe reactions occurred in 3–5% of patients with solid tumors and to a similar extent among metastatic breast cancer patients. The incidence of severe reactions was 1% or less for the 92 breast cancer patients premedicated with 3-day corticosteroids.

Severe stomatitis occurred in 5.5% of patients with solid tumors, in 7.4% of patients with metastatic breast cancer, and in 1.1% of the 92 breast cancer patients premedicated with 3-day corticosteroids.

Cardiovascular: Hypotension occurred in 2.8% of patients with solid tumors; 1.2% required treatment. Clinically meaningful events such as heart failure, sinus tachycardia, atrial flutter, dysrhythmia, unstable angina, pulmonary edema, and hypertension occurred rarely. 8.1% (7/86) of metastatic breast cancer patients receiving TAXOTERE 100 mg/m^2 in a randomized trial and who had serial left ventricular ejection fractions assessed developed deterioration of LVEF by ≥ 10% associated with a drop below the institutional lower limit of normal.

Infusion Site Reactions: Infusion site reactions were generally mild and consisted of hyperpigmentation, inflammation, redness or dryness of the skin, phlebitis, extravasation, or swelling of the vein.

Hepatic: In patients with normal LFTs at baseline, bilirubin values greater than the ULN occurred in 8.9% of patients. Increases in SGOT or SGPT > 1.5 times the ULN, or alkaline phosphatase > 2.5 times ULN, were observed in 18.9% and 7.3% of patients, respectively. While on TAXOTERE, increases in SGOT and/or SGPT > 1.5 times ULN concomitant with alkaline phosphatase > 2.5 times ULN occurred in 4.3% of patients with normal LFTs at baseline. (Whether these changes were related to the drug or underlying disease has not been established.)

TAXOTERE 75 mg/m^2: Treatment emergent adverse drug reactions are shown below. Included in this table are safety data for a total of 176 patients with non-small cell lung carcinoma and a history of prior treatment with platinum-based chemotherapy who were treated in two randomized, controlled trials. These reactions were described using NCI Common Toxicity Criteria regardless of relationship to study treatment, except for the hematologic toxicities or otherwise noted.

[See table on page 753]

Ongoing Evaluation: The following serious adverse events of uncertain relationship to TAXOTERE have been reported:

Body as a whole: abdominal pain, diffuse pain, chest pain, radiation recall phenomenon

Cardiovascular: atrial fibrillation, deep vein thrombosis, ECG abnormalities, thrombophlebitis, pulmonary embolism, syncope, tachycardia, myocardial infarction

Digestive: constipation, duodenal ulcer, esophagitis, gastrointestinal hemorrhage, intestinal obstruction, ileus, gastrointestinal perforation, neutropenic enterocolitis, dehydration in relation to digestive disorders

Nervous: confusion, seizures

Respiratory: dyspnea, acute pulmonary edema, acute respiratory distress syndrome, interstitial pneumonia

Urogenital: renal insufficiency

OVERDOSAGE

There is no known antidote for TAXOTERE overdosage. In case of overdosage, the patient should be kept in a specialized unit where vital functions can be closely monitored. Anticipated complications of overdosage include: bone marrow suppression, peripheral neurotoxicity, and mucositis. Patients should receive therapeutic G-CSF as soon as possible after discovery of overdose. Other appropriate symptomatic measures should be taken, as needed.

In two reports of overdose, one patient received 150 mg/m^2 and the other received 200 mg/m^2 as 1-hour infusions. Both patients experienced severe neutropenia, mild asthenia, cutaneous reactions, and mild paresthesia, and recovered without incident.

In mice, lethality was observed following single IV doses that were ≥154 mg/kg (about 4.5 times the recommended human dose on a mg/m^2 basis); neurotoxicity associated with paralysis, non-extension of hind limbs, and myelin degeneration was observed in mice at 48 mg/kg (about 1.5 times the recommended human dose on a mg/m^2 basis). In male and female rats, lethality was observed at a dose of 20 mg/kg (comparable to the recommended human dose on a mg/m^2 basis) and was associated with abnormal mitosis and necrosis of multiple organs.

DOSAGE AND ADMINISTRATION

Breast Cancer: The recommended dose of TAXOTERE is 60–100 mg/m^2 administered intravenously over 1 hour every 3 weeks.

Non-Small Cell Lung Cancer: The recommended dose of TAXOTERE is 75 mg/m^2 administered intravenously over 1 hour every 3 weeks. A dose of 100 mg/m^2 in patients previously treated with chemotherapy was associated with increased hematologic toxicity, infection, and treatment-related mortality in randomized, controlled trials (see **BOXED WARNING, WARNINGS** and **CLINICAL STUDIES** sections).

Premedication Regimen: All patients should be premedicated with oral corticosteroids such as dexamethasone 16 mg per day (*e.g.,* 8 mg BID) for 3 days starting 1 day prior to TAXOTERE administration in order to reduce the incidence and severity of fluid retention as well as the severity of hypersensitivity reactions (see **BOXED WARNING, WARNINGS,** and **PRECAUTIONS** sections).

Dosage Adjustments During Treatment

Breast Cancer: Patients who are dosed initially at 100 mg/m^2 and who experience either febrile neutropenia, neutrophils < 500 cells/mm^3 for more than 1 week, or severe or cumulative cutaneous reactions during TAXOTERE therapy should have the dosage adjusted from 100 mg/m^2 to 75 mg/m^2. If the patient continues to experience these reactions, the dosage should either be decreased from 75 mg/m^2 to 55 mg/m^2 or the treatment should be discontinued. Conversely, patients who are dosed initially at 60 mg/m^2 and who do not experience febrile neutropenia, neutrophils <500 cells/mm^3 for more than 1 week, severe or cumulative cutaneous reactions, or severe peripheral neuropathy during TAXOTERE therapy may tolerate higher doses. Pa-

Continued on next page

Taxotere—Cont.

tients who develop ≥ grade 3 peripheral neuropathy should have TAXOTERE treatment discontinued entirely.

Non-Small Cell Lung Cancer: Patients who are dosed initially at 75 mg/m^2 and who experience either febrile neutropenia, neutrophils <500 cells/mm^3 for more than one week, severe or cumulative cutaneous reactions, or other grade 3/4 non-hematological toxicities during TAXOTERE treatment should have treatment withheld until resolution of the toxicity and then resumed at 55 mg/m^2. Patients who develop ≥ grade 3 peripheral neuropathy should have TAXOTERE treatment discontinued entirely.

Special Populations:

Hepatic Impairment: Patients with bilirubin > ULN should generally not receive TAXOTERE. Also, patients with SGOT and/or SGPT > 1.5 × ULN concomitant with alkaline phosphatase > 2.5 × ULN should generally not receive TAXOTERE.

Children: The safety and effectiveness of docetaxel in pediatric patients below the age of 16 years have not been established.

Elderly: No dosage adjustments are required for use in elderly.

PREPARATION AND ADMINISTRATION PRECAUTIONS

TAXOTERE is a cytotoxic anticancer drug and, as with other potentially toxic compounds, caution should be exercised when handling and preparing TAXOTERE solutions. The use of gloves is recommended. Please refer to **Handling and Disposal** section.

If TAXOTERE concentrate, initial diluted solution, or final dilution for infusion should come into contact with the skin, immediately and thoroughly wash with soap and water. If TAXOTERE concentrate, initial diluted solution, or final dilution for infusion should come into contact with mucosa, immediately and thoroughly wash with water.

TAXOTERE for Injection Concentrate requires two dilutions prior to administration. Please follow the preparation instructions provided below. **Note:** Both the TAXOTERE for Injection Concentrate and the diluent vials contain an overfill.

A. Preparation of the Initial Diluted Solution

1. Remove the appropriate number of vials of TAXOTERE for Injection Concentrate and diluent (13% Ethanol in Water for Injection) from the refrigerator. Allow the vials to stand at room temperature for approximately 5 minutes.
2. Aseptically withdraw the contents of the appropriate diluent vial into a syringe and transfer it to the appropriate vial of TAXOTERE for Injection Concentrate. **If the procedure is followed as described, an initial diluted solution of 10mg docetaxel/mL will result.**
3. Gently rotate the initial diluted solution for approximately 15 seconds to assure full mixture of the concentrate and diluent.
4. The initial diluted TAXOTERE solution (10 mg docetaxel/mL) should be clear; however, there may be some foam on top of the solution due to the polysorbate 80. Allow the solution to stand for a few minutes to allow any foam to dissipate. It is not required that all foam dissipate prior to continuing the preparation process.

   The initial diluted solution may be used immediately or stored either in the refrigerator or at room temperature for a maximum of 8 hours.

B. Preparation of the Final Dilution for Infusion

1. Aseptically withdraw the required amount of initial diluted TAXOTERE solution (10 mg docetaxel/mL) with a calibrated syringe and inject into a 250 mL infusion bag or bottle of either 0.9% Sodium Chloride solution or 5% Dextrose solution to produce a final concentration of 0.3 to 0.74 mg/mL.

   If a dose greater than 200 mg of TAXOTERE is required, use a larger volume of the infusion vehicle so that a concentration of 0.74 mg/mL TAXOTERE is not exceeded.
2. Thoroughly mix the infusion by manual rotation.
3. As with all parenteral products, TAXOTERE should be inspected visually for particulate matter or discoloration prior to administration whenever the solution and container permit. If the TAXOTERE for Injection initial diluted solution or final dilution for infusion is not clear or appears to have precipitation, these should be discarded.

The final TAXOTERE dilution for infusion should be administered intravenously as a 1-hour infusion under ambient room temperature and lighting conditions.

Contact of the TAXOTERE concentrate with plasticized PVC equipment or devices used to prepare solutions for infusion is not recommended. In order to minimize patient exposure to the plasticizer DEHP (di-2-ethylhexyl phthalate), which may be leached from PVC infusion bags or sets, the final TAXOTERE dilution for infusion should be stored in bottles (glass, polypropylene) or plastic bags (polypropylene, polyolefin) and administered through polyethylene-lined administration sets.

Stability: TAXOTERE infusion solution, if stored between 2 and 25°C (36 and 77°F) is stable for 4 hours. Fully prepared TAXOTERE infusion solution (in either 0.9% Sodium Chloride solution or 5% Dextrose solution) should be used within 4 hours (including the 1 hour i.v. administration).

HOW SUPPLIED

TAXOTERE for Injection Concentrate is supplied in a single-dose vial as a sterile, pyrogen-free, non-aqueous, viscous

Summary of Adverse Events in Patients Receiving TAXOTERE at 100 mg/m^2

Adverse Event	All Tumor Types Normal LFTs* n=2045 %	All Tumor Types Elevated LFTs** n=61 %	Breast Cancer Normal LFTs* n=965 %
Hematologic			
Neutropenia			
<2000 cells/mm^3	95.5	96.4	98.5
<500 cells/mm^3	75.4	87.5	85.9
Leukopenia			
<4000 cells/mm^3	95.6	98.3	98.6
<1000 cells/mm^3	31.6	46.6	43.7
Thrombocytopenia			
<100,000 cells/mm^3	8.0	24.6	9.2
Anemia			
<11 g/dL	90.4	91.8	93.6
<8 g/dL	8.8	31.1	7.7
Febrile Neutropenia***	11.0	26.2	12.3
Septic Death	1.6	4.9	1.4
Non-Septic Death	0.6	6.6	0.6
Infections			
Any	21.6	32.8	22.2
Severe	6.1	16.4	6.4
Fever in Absence of Infection			
Any	31.2	41.0	35.1
Severe	2.1	8.2	2.2
Hypersensitivity Reactions			
Regardless of Premedication			
Any	21.0	19.7	17.6
Severe	4.2	9.8	2.6
With 3-day Premedication	n=92	n=3	n=92
Any	15.2	33.3	15.2
Severe	2.2	0	2.2
Fluid Retention			
Regardless of Premedication			
Any	47.0	39.3	59.7
Severe	6.9	8.2	8.9
With 3-day Premedication	n=92	n=3	n=92
Any	64.1	66.7	64.1
Severe	6.5	33.3	6.5
Neurosensory			
Any	49.3	34.4	58.3
Severe	4.3	0	5.5
Cutaneous			
Any	47.6	54.1	47.0
Severe	4.8	9.8	5.2
Nail Changes			
Any	30.6	23.0	40.5
Severe	2.5	4.9	3.7
Gastrointestinal			
Nausea	38.8	37.7	42.1
Vomiting	22.3	23.0	23.4
Diarrhea	38.7	32.8	42.6
Severe	4.7	4.9	5.5
Stomatitis			
Any	41.7	49.2	51.7
Severe	5.5	13.0	7.4
Alopecia	75.8	62.3	74.2
Asthenia			
Any	61.8	52.5	66.3
Severe	12.8	24.6	14.9
Myalgia			
Any	18.9	16.4	21.1
Severe	1.5	1.6	1.8
Arthralgia	9.2	6.6	8.2
Infusion Site Reactions	4.4	3.3	4.0

***Normal Baseline LFTs: Transaminases ≤ 1.5 times ULN or alkaline phosphatase ≤ 2.5 times ULN or isolated elevations of transaminases or alkaline phosphatase up to 5 times ULN**

**** Elevated Baseline LFTs: SGOT and/or SGPT >1.5 times ULN concurrent with alkaline phosphatase >2.5 times ULN**

***** Febrile Neutropenia: ANC grade 4 with fever > 38°C with IV antibiotics and/or hospitalization**

solution with an accompanying sterile, non-pyrogenic, diluent (13% ethanol in Water for Injection) vial. The following strengths are available:

TAXOTERE 80 MG (NDC 0075-8001-80)

TAXOTERE (docetaxel) 80 mg Concentrate for Infusion: 80 mg docetaxel in 2 mL polysorbate 80 and diluent for TAXOTERE 80 mg. 13% (w/w) ethanol in Water for Injection. Both items are in a blister pack in one carton.

TAXOTERE 20 MG (NDC 0075-8001-20)

TAXOTERE (docetaxel) 20 mg Concentrate for Infusion: 20 mg docetaxel in 0.5 mL polysorbate 80 and diluent for TAXOTERE 20 mg. 13% (w/w) ethanol in Water for Injection. Both items are in a blister pack in one carton.

Storage: Store between 2 and 25°C (36 and 77°F). Retain in the original package to protect from bright light. Freezing does not adversely affect the product.

Handling and Disposal: Procedures for proper handling and disposal of anticancer drugs should be considered. Several guidelines on this subject have been published[1–7]. There is no general agreement that all of the procedures recommended in the guidelines are necessary or appropriate.

REFERENCES

1. OSHA Work-Practice Guidelines for Controlling Occupational Exposure to Hazardous Drugs. *Am J Health-Syst Pharm.* 1996; 53: 1669–1685.

2. American Society of Hospital Pharmacists Technical Assistance Bulletin on Handling Cytotoxic and Hazardous Drugs. *Am J Hosp Pharm.* 1990; 47(95): 1033–1049.
3. AMA Council Report. Guidelines for Handling Parenteral Antineoplastics. *JAMA* 1985; 253 (11): 1590–1592.
4. Recommendations for the Safe Handling of Parenteral Antineoplastic Drugs. NIH Publication No. 83-2621. For sale by the Superintendent of Documents, US Government Printing Office, Washington, DC 20402.
5. National Study Commission on Cytotoxic Exposure—Recommendations for Handling Cytotoxic Agents. Available from Louis P. Jeffry, Chairman, National Study Commission on Cytotoxic Exposure. Massachusetts College of Pharmacy and Allied Health Sciences, 179 Longwood Avenue, Boston, MA 02115.
6. Clinical Oncological Society of Australia. Guidelines and Recommendations for Safe Handling of Antineoplastic Agents. *Med J Austr.* 1983; 426–428.
7. Jones, RB, et al. Safe Handling of Chemotherapeutic Agents: A Report from the Mt. Sinai Medical Center. *CA-A Cancer Journal for Clinicians* 1983; Sept/Oct: 258–263.

Treatment Emergent Adverse Events in Non-Small Cell Lung Cancer Patients Receiving TAXOTERE Regardless of Relationship to Treatment*

Adverse Event	TAXOTERE 75 mg/m² n=176 %	Best Supportive Care n=49 %	Vinorelbine/ Ifosfamide n=119 %
Neutropenia			
Any	84.1	14.3	83.2
Grade 3/4	65.3	12.2	57.1
Leukopenia			
Any	83.5	6.1	89.1
Grade 3/4	49.4	0	42.9
Thrombocytopenia			
Any	8.0	0	7.6
Grade 3/4	2.8	0	1.7
Anemia			
Any	91.0	55.1	90.8
Grade 3/4	9.1	12.2	14.3
Febrile Neutropenia**	6.3	NA†	0.8
Infection			
Any	33.5	28.6	30.3
Grade 3/4	10.2	6.1	9.2
Treatment Related Mortality	2.8	NA†	3.4
Hypersensitivity Reactions			
Any	5.7	0	0.8
Grade 3/4	2.8	0	0
Fluid Retention			
Any	33.5	ND††	22.7
Severe	2.8		3.4
Neurosensory			
Any	23.3	14.3	28.6
Grade 3/4	1.7	6.1	5.0
Neuromotor			
Any	15.9	8.2	10.1
Grade 3/4	4.5	6.1	3.4
Skin			
Any	19.9	6.1	16.8
Grade 3/4	0.6	2.0	0.8
Gastrointestinal			
Nausea			
Any	33.5	30.6	31.1
Grade 3/4	5.1	4.1	7.6
Vomiting			
Any	21.6	26.5	21.8
Grade 3/4	2.8	2.0	5.9
Diarrhea			
Any	22.7	6.1	11.8
Grade 3/4	2.8	0	4.2
Alopecia	56.3	34.7	49.6
Asthenia			
Any	52.8	57.1	53.8
Severe***	18.2	38.8	22.7
Stomatitis			
Any	26.1	6.1	7.6
Grade 3/4	1.7	0	0.8
Pulmonary			
Any	40.9	49.0	45.4
Grade 3/4	21.0	28.6	18.5
Nail Disorder			
Any	11.4	0	1.7
Severe***	1.1	0	0
Myalgia			
Any	6.3	0	2.5
Severe***	0	0	0
Arthralgia			
Any	3.4	2.0	1.7
Severe***	0	0	0.8
Taste Perversion			
Any	5.7	0	0
Severe***	0.6	0	0

***Normal Baseline LFTs: Transaminases ≤ 1.5 times ULN or alkaline phosphatase ≤ 2.5 times ULN or isolated elevations of transaminases or alkaline phosphatase up to 5 times ULN**
**** Febrile Neutropenia: ANC grade 4 with fever > 38°C with IV antibiotics and/or hospitalization**
***** COSTART term and grading system**
† Not Applicable; †† Not Done

Aventis Pharmaceuticals Products Inc.
Parsippany, NJ 07054
IN-5493H! Rev. 1/00
Shown in Product Identification Guide, page 307

TRENTAL® ℞

[tren 'tal]
(pentoxifylline)*
Tablets, 400 mg

Prescribing Information as of January 1998

DESCRIPTION

TRENTAL® (pentoxifylline) tablets for oral administration contain 400 mg of the active drug and the following inactive ingredients: D&C Red No. 27 Aluminum Lake or FD&C Red No. 3, hydroxypropyl methylcellulose USP, magnesium stearate NF, polyethylene glycol NF, povidone USP, talc USP, titanium dioxide USP, and other ingredients in a controlled-release formulation. Trental is a tri-substituted xanthine derivative designated chemically as 1-(5-oxohexyl)-3, 7-dimethylxanthine that, unlike theophylline, is a hemorrheologic agent, i.e. an agent that affects blood viscosity. Pentoxifylline is soluble in water and ethanol, and sparingly soluble in toluene. The CAS Registry Number is 6493-05-6. The chemical structure is:

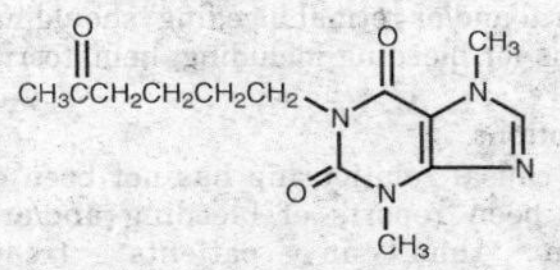

CLINICAL PHARMACOLOGY

Mode of Action

Pentoxifylline and its metabolites improve the flow properties of blood by decreasing its viscosity. In patients with chronic peripheral arterial disease, this increases blood flow to the affected microcirculation and enhances tissue oxygenation. The precise mode of action of pentoxifylline and the sequence of events leading to clinical improvement are still to be defined. Pentoxifylline administration has been shown to produce dose-related hemorrheologic effects, lowering blood viscosity, and improving erythrocyte flexibility. Leukocyte properties of hemorrheologic importance have been modified in animal and *in vitro* human studies. Pentoxifylline has been shown to increase leukocyte deformability and to inhibit neutrophil adhesion and activation. Tissue oxygen levels have been shown to be significantly increased by therapeutic doses of pentoxifylline in patients with peripheral arterial disease.

Pharmacokinetics and Metabolism

After oral administration in aqueous solution pentoxifylline is almost completely absorbed. It undergoes a first-pass effect and the various metabolites appear in plasma very soon after dosing. Peak plasma levels of the parent compound and its metabolites are reached within 1 hour. The major metabolites are Metabolite I (1-[5-hydroxyhexyl]-3,7-dimethylxanthine) and Metabolite V (1-[3-carboxypropyl]-3,7-dimethylxanthine), and plasma levels of these metabolites are 5 and 8 times greater, respectively, than pentoxifylline. Following oral administration of aqueous solutions containing 100 to 400 mg of pentoxifylline, the pharmacokinetics of the parent compound and Metabolite I are dose-related and not proportional (non-linear), with half-life and area under the blood-level time curve (AUC) increasing with dose. The elimination kinetics of Metabolite V are not dose-dependent. The apparent plasma half-life of pentoxifylline varies from 0.4 to 0.8 hours and the apparent plasma half-lives of its metabolites vary from 1 to 1.6 hours. There is no evidence of accumulation or enzyme induction (Cytochrome P450) following multiple oral doses.

Excretion is almost totally urinary; the main biotransformation product is Metabolite V. Essentially no parent drug is found in the urine. Despite large variations in plasma levels of parent compound and its metabolites, the urinary recovery of Metabolite V is consistent and shows dose proportionality. Less than 4% of the administered dose is recovered in feces. Food intake shortly before dosing delays absorption of an immediate-release dosage form but does not affect total absorption. The pharmacokinetics and metabolism of TRENTAL have not been studied in patients with renal

Continued on next page

Trental—Cont.

and/or hepatic dysfunction, but AUC was increased and elimination rate decreased in an older population (60–68 years) compared to younger individuals (22–30 years).
After administration of the 400 mg controlled-release TRENTAL tablet, plasma levels of the parent compound and its metabolites reach their maximum within 2 to 4 hours and remain constant over an extended period of time. Coadministration of TRENTAL tablets with meals resulted in an increase in mean C_{max} and AUC by about 28% and 13% for pentoxifylline, respectively. C_{max} for Metabolite 1 also increased by about 20%. The controlled release of pentoxifylline from the tablet eliminates peaks and troughs in plasma levels for improved gastrointestinal tolerance.

INDICATIONS AND USAGE

TRENTAL is indicated for the treatment of patients with intermittent claudication on the basis of chronic occlusive arterial disease of the limbs. TRENTAL can improve function and symptoms but is not intended to replace more definitive therapy, such as surgical bypass, or removal of arterial obstructions when treating peripheral vascular disease.

CONTRAINDICATIONS

TRENTAL should not be used in patients with recent cerebral and/or retinal hemorrhage or in patients who have previously exhibited intolerance to this product or methylxanthines such as caffeine, theophylline, and theobromine.

PRECAUTIONS

General

Patients with chronic occlusive arterial disease of the limbs frequently show other manifestations of arteriosclerotic disease. TRENTAL has been used safely for treatment of peripheral arterial disease in patients with concurrent coronary artery and cerebrovascular diseases, but there have been occasional reports of angina, hypotension, and arrhythmia. Controlled trials do not show that TRENTAL causes such adverse effects more often than placebo, but, as it is a methylxanthine derivative, it is possible some individuals will experience such responses. Patients on Warfarin should have more frequent monitoring of prothrombin times, while patients with other risk factors complicated by hemorrhage (e.g., recent surgery, peptic ulceration, cerebral and/or retinal bleeding) should have periodic examinations for bleeding including, hematocrit and/or hemoglobin.

Drug Interactions

Although a causal relationship has not been established, there have been reports of bleeding and/or prolonged prothrombin time in patients treated with TRENTAL with and without anticoagulants or platelet aggregation inhibitors. Patients on Warfarin should have more frequent monitoring of prothrombin times, while patients with other risk factors complicated by hemorrhage (e.g., recent surgery, peptic ulceration) should have periodic examinations for bleeding including hematocrit and/or hemoglobin. Concomitant administration of TRENTAL and theophylline-containing drugs leads to increased theophylline levels and theophylline toxicity in some individuals. Such patients should be closely monitored for signs of toxicity and have their theophylline dosage adjusted as necessary. TRENTAL has been used concurrently with antihypertensive drugs, beta blockers, digitalis, diuretics, antidiabetic agents, and antiarrhythmics, without observed problems. Small decreases in blood pressure have been observed in some patients treated with TRENTAL; periodic systemic blood pressure monitoring is recommended for patients receiving concomitant antihypertensive therapy. If indicated, dosage of the antihypertensive agents should be reduced.

Carcinogenesis, Mutagenesis and Impairment of Fertility

Long-term studies of the carcinogenic potential of pentoxifylline were conducted in mice and rats by dietary administration of the drug at doses up to 450 mg/kg (approximately 19 times the maximum recommended human daily dose (MRHD) in both species when based on body weight; 1.5 times the MRHD in the mouse and 3.3 times the MRHD in the rat when based on body surface area). In mice, the drug was administered for 18 months, whereas in rats, the drug was administered for 18 months followed by an additional 6 months without drug exposure. In the rat study, there was a statistically significant increase in benign mammary fibroadenomas in females of the 450 mg/kg group. The relevance of this finding to human use is uncertain. Pentoxifylline was devoid of mutagenic activity in various strains of *Salmonella* (Ames test) and in cultured mammalian cells (unscheduled DNA synthesis test) when tested in the presence and absence of metabolic activation. It was also negative in the in vivo mouse micronucleus test.

Pregnancy

Category C. Teratogenic studies have been performed in rats and rabbits using oral doses up to 576 and 264 mg/kg, respectively. On a weight basis, these doses are 24 and 11 times the maximum recommended human daily dose (MRHD); on a body-surface-area basis, they are 4.2 and 3.5 times the MRHD. No evidence of fetal malformation was observed. Increased resorption was seen in rats of the 576 mg/kg group.
There are no adequate and well controlled studies in pregnant women. TRENTAL (pentoxifylline) should be used during pregnancy only if the potential benefit justifies the potential risk to the fetus.

Nursing Mothers

Pentoxifylline and its metabolites are excreted in human milk. Because of the potential for tumorigenicity shown for pentoxifylline in rats, a decision should be made whether to discontinue nursing or discontinue the drug, taking into account the importance of the drug to the mother.

Pediatric Use

Safety and effectiveness in pediatric patients have not been established.

ADVERSE REACTIONS

Clinical trials were conducted using either controlled-release TRENTAL tablets for up to 60 weeks or immediate-release TRENTAL capsules for up to 24 weeks. Dosage ranges in the tablet studies were 400 mg bid to tid and in the capsule studies, 200–400 mg tid. The table summarizes the incidence (in percent) of adverse reactions considered drug related, as well as the numbers of patients who received controlled-release TRENTAL tablets, immediate-release TRENTAL capsules, or the corresponding placebos. The incidence of adverse reactions was higher in the capsule studies (where dose related increases were seen in digestive and nervous system side effects) than in the tablet studies. Studies with the capsule include domestic experience, whereas studies with the controlled-release tablets were conducted outside the U.S.
The table indicates that in the tablet studies few patients discontinued because of adverse effects.
[See table below]
TRENTAL been marketed in Europe and elsewhere since 1972. In addition to the above symptoms, the following have been reported spontaneously since marketing or occurred in other clinical trials with an incidence of less than 1%; the causal relationship was uncertain:

Cardiovascular—dyspnea, edema, hypotension.
Digestive—anorexia, cholecystitis, constipation, dry mouth/thirst.
Nervous—anxiety, confusion, depression, seizures.
Respiratory—epistaxis, flu-like symptoms, laryngitis, nasal congestion.
Skin and Appendages—brittle fingernails, pruritus, rash, urticaria, angioedema.
Special Senses—blurred vision, conjunctivitis, earache, scotoma.
Miscellaneous—bad taste, excessive salivation, leukopenia, malaise, sore throat/swollen neck glands, weight change.

A few rare events have been reported spontaneously worldwide since marketing in 1972. Although they occurred under circumstances in which a causal relationship with pentoxifylline could not be established, they are listed to serve as information for physicians: "Cardiovascular—angina, arrhythmia, tachycardia, anaphylactoid reactions." Digestive—hepatitis, jaundice, increased liver enzymes; and Hemic and Lymphatic—decreased serum fibrinogen, pancytopenia, aplastic anemia, leukemia, purpura, thrombocytopenia.

OVERDOSAGE

Overdosage with TRENTAL has been reported in pediatric patients and adults. Symptoms appear to be dose related. A report from a poison control center on 44 patients taking overdoses of enteric-coated pentoxifylline tablets noted that symptoms usually occurred 4–5 hours after ingestion and lasted about 12 hours. The highest amount ingested was 80 mg/kg; flushing, hypotension, convulsions, somnolence, loss of consciousness, fever, and agitation occurred. All patients recovered. In addition to symptomatic treatment and gastric lavage, special attention must be given to supporting respiration, maintaining systemic blood pressure, and controlling convulsions. Activated charcoal has been used to absorb pentoxifylline in patients who have overdosed.

DOSAGE AND ADMINISTRATION

The usual dosage of TRENTAL in controlled-release tablet form is one tablet (400 mg) three times a day with meals.
While the effect of TRENTAL may be seen within 2 to 4 weeks, it is recommended that treatment be continued for at least 8 weeks. Efficacy has been demonstrated in double-blind clinical studies of 6 months duration.
Digestive and central nervous system side effects are dose related. If patients develop these side effects it is recommended that the dosage be lowered to one tablet twice a day (800 mg/day). If side effects persist at this lower dosage, the administration of TRENTAL should be discontinued.

HOW SUPPLIED

TRENTAL (pentoxifylline) is available for oral administration as 400 mg pink film-coated oblong tablets imprinted Trental®; supplied in bottles of 100 (NDC 0039-0078-10), Bulk Pack 5000 (NDC 0039-0078-80), and Unit Dose Packs of 100 (NDC 0039-0078-11).
Store between 59 and 86° F (15 and 30° C).
Dispense in well-closed, light-resistant containers.

Protect blisters from light.

Prescribing Information as of January 1998

*US Patents 3,737,433 & 4,189,469
US Patent 3,737,433 patent term has been extended.

Hoechst-Roussel Pharmaceuticals
Division of Hoechst Marion Roussel, Inc.
Kansas City, MO 64137 USA

Shown in Product Identification Guide, page 307

INCIDENCE (%) OF SIDE EFFECTS

	Controlled-Release Tablets		Immediate-Release Capsules	
	Commercially Available		Used only for Controlled Clinical Trials	
	TRENTAL	**Placebo**	**TRENTAL**	**Placebo**
(Numbers of Patients at Risk)	(321)	(128)	(177)	(138)
Discontinued for Side Effect	3.1	0	9.6	7.2
CARDIOVASCULAR SYSTEM				
Angina/Chest pain	0.3	—	1.1	2.2
Arrhythmia/Palpitation	—	—	1.7	0.7
Flushing	—	—	2.3	0.7
DIGESTIVE SYSTEM				
Abdominal Discomfort	—	—	4.0	1.4
Belching/Flatus/Bloating	0.6	—	9.0	3.6
Diarrhea	—	—	3.4	2.9
Dyspepsia	2.8	4.7	9.6	2.9
Nausea	2.2	0.8	28.8	8.7
Vomiting	1.2	—	4.5	0.7
NERVOUS SYSTEM				
Agitation/Nervousness	—	—	1.7	0.7
Dizziness	1.9	3.1	11.9	4.3
Drowsiness	—	—	1.1	5.8
Headache	1.2	1.6	6.2	5.8
Insomnia	—	—	2.3	2.2
Tremor	0.3	0.8	—	—
Blurred Vision	—	—	2.3	1.4

Aventis Behring L.L.C.

1020 FIRST AVENUE
KING OF PRUSSIA, PA 19406-1310

Direct Inquiries to:
(610) 878-4000

For Medical Information Contact:
(800) 504-5434

Sales and Ordering:
Customer Support Center
(800) 683-1288
Fax: (610) 878-4888

PRESCRIBING INFORMATION ℞
ALBUMINAR®-5

ALBUMIN (HUMAN) U.S.P., 5%
Rx only

DESCRIPTION

Albumin (Human) 5%, Albuminar®-5 is a sterile solution of albumin obtained from large pools of adult human venous plasma by low temperature controlled fractionation according to the Cohn process. It is heated at 60°C for 10 hours and stabilized with 0.004 M sodium acetyltryptophanate and 0.004 M sodium caprylate.
The plasma used in the manufacture of this product has been tested and found negative for HBV, HCV, and HIV-1 by an investigational test procedure referred to as Nucleic Acid Testing (NAT) using Polymerase Chain Reaction (PCR) Technology. Investigational testing is being performed to determine the effectiveness of NAT to detect low levels of viral material. The significance of a negative result is unknown since the effectiveness of the test has not been established. Each 50 mL bottle of 5% solution contains 2.5 grams of albumin in normal saline. Each 250 mL bottle of 5% solution contains 12.5 grams of albumin in normal saline. Each 500

mL bottle of 5% solution contains 25 grams of albumin in normal saline. Each 1000 mL bottle of 5% solution contains 50 grams of albumin in normal saline. The 5% solution is osmotically equivalent with citrated plasma. The pH of the solution is adjusted to 6.9 ± 0.5 with sodium bicarbonate, sodium hydroxide, or acetic acid. Approximate concentrations of significant electrolytes per liter are: sodium 130 - 160 mEq; and potassium-n.m.t. 1mEq. The solution contains no preservative. This product has been prepared in accordance with the requirements established by the Food and Drug Administration and is in compliance with the standards of the United States Pharmacopeia.
Albumin (Human) 5%, Albuminar®-5, is to be administered by the intravenous route.
The heat treatment step employed in the manufacture of Albumin (Human) 5%, Albuminar®-5, pasteurization of the final container at 60°C for 10 hours, has been validated in a series of *in vitro* experiments for its capacity to inactivate Human Immunodeficiency Virus type 1 (HIV-1), and the following model viruses: Bovine Viral Diarrhea Virus (BVDV - an enveloped virus used as a model for hepatitis C virus), Pseudorabies (PrV - a large, enveloped virus), and Encephalomyocarditis Virus (EMC - a small non-enveloped virus). For each virus studied, three independent experiments were conducted using Albumin (Human) 5%, Albuminar®-5 and Albumin (Human) 25%, Albuminar®-25 with the following results.[1]
[See table above]

Pasteurization (60°C for 10 hours) Viral Reduction Studies ($\log_{10}$ reduction)

Virus	Albumin (Human) 5%, Albuminar®-5	Albumin (Human) 25%, Albuminar®-25
HIV-1	>5.44, >6.38 and >6.31	>5.50, >6.57 and >6.64
BVDV	>6.01, >6.76 and >6.55	>5.99, >5.81 and >5.32
PrV	>7.30, >7.68 and >7.63	>7.32, >7.20 and >7.42
EMC	>7.38, >7.97 and >7.97	>7.10, >7.89 and >7.87

CLINICAL PHARMACOLOGY

Albumin (Human) 5%, Albuminar®-5, being active osmotically, is useful in regulating the volume of circulating blood. It is a valuable therapeutic aid for the treatment of conditions that will be benefited by its marked osmotic effect. When the circulating blood volume has been depleted, the hemodilution following albumin administration persists for many hours. In individuals with normal blood volume, it usually lasts only a few hours.
Albumin (Human), unlike whole blood or plasma, is considered free of the danger of viral hepatitis because it is heated at 60°C for 10 hours. It is convenient to use since no cross-matching is required and the absence of cellular elements removes the danger of sensitization with repeated infusions.

INDICATIONS AND USAGE

SHOCK - Albumin (Human) 5%, Albuminar®-5 is indicated in the emergency treatment of shock due to burns, trauma, operations and infections, in the treatment of severe injuries, and in other similar conditions where the restoration of blood volume is urgent. The primary function is maintenance of colloid osmotic pressure. If there has been considerable loss of red blood cells, transfusion with packed red blood cells is indicated.
BURNS - Albumin (Human) 5%, Albuminar®-5 is indicated in conjunction with adequate infusions of crystalloid to counteract hemoconcentration and the loss of protein, electrolytes and water that usually follow severe burns. Because of changes in permeability, little administered albumin is likely to be retained intravenously in the first 12 hours after a major burn. However, an optimum regimen for the use of colloid, electrolytes and water in the treatment of burns has not been established.
HYPOPROTEINEMIA - Albumin (Human) 5%, Albuminar®-5 may be used in acutely hypoproteinemic patients, provided sodium restriction is not a problem.

CONTRAINDICATIONS

Albumin (Human) 5%, Albuminar®-5 is contraindicated in patients with severe anemia or cardiac failure and in patients with a history of allergic reactions to human albumin.

WARNINGS

Do not use if the solution is turbid or if there is a sediment in the bottle. Since the product contains no antimicrobial preservative, do not begin administration more than 4 hours after the container has been entered. Destroy unused portions to prevent the possibility of subsequent use of a solution that may have become contaminated.
Albumin (Human) U.S.P., 5%, Albuminar®-5 is made from human plasma. Products made from human plasma may contain infectious agents such as viruses, that can cause disease. The risk that such products will transmit an infectious agent has been reduced by screening plasma donors for prior exposure to certain viruses, by testing for the presence of certain current virus infections, and by inactivating and/or removing certain viruses during manufacture. The manufacturing procedure for Albumin (Human) 5%, Albuminar®-5 includes processing steps designed to reduce further the risk of viral transmission. Stringent procedures utilized at plasma collection centers, plasma testing laboratories, and fractionation facilities are designed to reduce the risk of viral transmission. Albuminar®-5 is pasteurized in the final container at 60.0 +/− 0.5°C for 10 - 11 hours. Virus elimination/inactivation is also achieved by the cold alcohol fractionation process. (See **DESCRIPTION** section for further information on viral reduction measures.) Despite these measures, such products may still potentially contain human pathogenic agents, including those not yet known or identified. Thus the risk of transmission of infectious agents cannot be totally eliminated. Any infections thought by a physician possibly to have been transmitted by this product should be reported by the physician or other healthcare provider to Aventis Behring at 800-504-5434. The physician should discuss the risks and benefits of this product with the patient.

PRECAUTIONS

GENERAL
Administration of large quantities of albumin should be supplemented with red blood cells or replaced by whole blood to combat the relative anemia which would follow such use. The quick response of blood pressure, which may follow the rapid administration of albumin, necessitates careful observation of the injured patient to detect bleeding points which failed to bleed at lower blood pressure. Albumin (Human) 5%, Albuminar®-5 should be administered with caution to patients with low cardiac reserve or with no albumin deficiency because a rapid increase in plasma volume may cause circulatory compromise (e.g. hypertension, hypotension, or pulmonary edema.) In cases of hypertension, a slower rate of administration is desired. Albumin (Human) 5%, Albuminar® -5 may be administered at a rate of 10 grams of albumin (200 mL) per hour.
If anaphylactic or severe anaphylactoid reactions occur, discontinue infusion immediately. Infusion rates and the patient's clinical state should be monitored closely during infusion.
INFORMATON FOR PATIENT - Some viruses, such as parvovirus B19 or hepatitis A are particularly difficult to remove or inactivate at this time. Parvovirus B19 may most seriously affect pregnant women, or immune-compromised individuals. The majority of parvovirus B19 and hepatitis A infections are acquired by environmental (community acquired) sources.
PREGNANCY CATEGORY C - Animal reproduction studies have not been conducted with Albumin (Human) 5%, Albuminar®-5. It is also not known whether Albuminar®-5 can cause fetal harm when administered to a pregnant woman or can affect reproduction capacity. Albuminar®-5 should be given to a pregnant woman only if clearly needed.
PEDIATRIC USE - No clinical studies using Albumin (Human) 5%, Albuminar®-5 have been conducted in pediatric patients. Safety and effectiveness in pediatric patients have not been established. However, extensive experience in patients suggests that children respond to Albumin (Human) 5%, Albuminar®-5 in the same manner as adults.

ADVERSE REACTIONS

The incidence of untoward reactions to Albumin (Human) 5% is low. Reports have been received of anaphylaxis, which may be severe, and hypersensitivity reactions (including urticaria, skin rash, pruritus, edema, erythema, hypotension and bronchospasm.) Nausea, vomiting, increased salivation, chills and febrile reactions have also been reported (see also **PRECAUTIONS**).

DOSAGE AND ADMINISTRATION

Albumin (Human) 5%, Albuminar®-5 may be given intravenously without further dilution. This concentration is approximately isotonic and iso-osmotic with citrated plasma. Albumin (Human) in this concentration provides additional fluid for plasma volume expansion. Therefore, when it is administered to patients with normal blood volume, the rate of infusion should be slow enough to prevent too rapid expansion of plasma volume.
In the treatment of shock in an adult patient an initial dose of 500 mL of the 5% albumin solution is given as rapidly as tolerated. If response within 30 minutes is inadequate, an additional 500 mL of 5% albumin solution may be given. The 50 mL dosage form would be appropriate for pediatric use, with a dose of 10–20 mL per kg of body weight infused intravenously at a rate up to 5 - 10 mL per minute. Therapy should be guided by the clinical response, blood pressure and an assessment of relative anemia. If more than 1000 mL are given, or if hemorrhage has occurred, the administration of packed red blood cells may be desirable.
In severe burns, immediate therapy should include large volumes of crystalloid with lesser amounts of 5% albumin solution to maintain an adequate plasma volume. After the first 24 hours, the ratio of albumin to crystalloid may be increased to establish and maintain a plasma albumin level of about 2.5 g/100 mL - or a total serum protein level of about 5.2 g/100 mL. However, an optimal regimen for the use of colloids, electrolytes and water after severe burns has not been established.
The infusion of Albumin (Human) as a nutrient in the treatment of chronic hypoproteinemia is not recommended. In acute hypoproteinemia, 5% albumin may be used in replacing the protein lost in hypoproteinemic conditions. However, if edema is present or if large amounts of albumin are lost, Albumin (Human) 25% is preferred because of the greater amount of protein in the concentrated solution.
Parenteral drug products should be inspected visually for particulate matter and discoloration prior to administration, whenever solution and container permit.

HOW SUPPLIED

Albumin (Human) 5%, Albuminar®-5 is supplied as a 5% solution in:
NDC 0053-7670-06
50 mL bottles containing 2.5 grams of albumin;
NDC 0053-7670-01
250 mL bottles containing 12.5 grams of albumin;
NDC 0053-7670-02
500 mL bottles containing 25.0 grams of albumin;
NDC 0053-7670-03
1000 mL bottles containing 50.0 grams of albumin.
The packaging of this product contains dry natural rubber.
Store at controlled room temperature - between 15°-30°C (59°-86°F).

REFERENCES

1. Data on file.

BIBLIOGRAPHY

Finlayson, J.S.: Albumin Products.
Seminars in Thrombosis and Hemostasis 6:85 - 120, 1980.
Tullis, J.L.: Albumin. JAMA 237:355-360 and 460 - 463, 1977.
Rudolf, A.M.: Pediatrics. 18th ED., p. 1839, Appleton and Lange, 1987.

12602–01

PRESCRIBING INFORMATION
ALBUMINAR®-25 ℞
ALBUMIN (HUMAN) U.S.P., 25%
Rx only

DESCRIPTION

Albumin (Human) 25%, Albuminar®-25 is a sterile aqueous solution of albumin obtained from large pools of adult human venous plasma by low temperature controlled fractionation according to the Cohn process. It is stabilized with 0.02 M sodium acetyltryptophanate and 0.02 M sodium caprylate and pasteurized at 60°C for 10 hours.
The plasma used in the manufacture of this product has been tested and found negative for HBV, HCV, and HIV-1 by an investigational test procedure referred to as Nucleic Acid Testing (NAT) using Polymerase Chain Reaction (PCR) Technology. Investigational testing is being performed to determine the effectiveness of NAT to detect low levels of viral material. The significance of a negative result is unknown since the effectiveness of the test has not been established.
Albumin (Human) 25%, Albuminar®-25 is a solution containing in each 100 mL, 25 grams of serum albumin, osmotically equivalent to 500 mL of normal human plasma. The pH of the solution is adjusted with sodium bicarbonate, sodium hydroxide, or acetic acid. Approximate concentrations of significant electrolytes per liter are: sodium-130-160 mEq; and potassium-n.m.t. 1 mEq. The solution contains no preservative. This product has been prepared in accordance with the requirements established by the Food and Drug Administration and is in compliance with the standards of the United States Pharmacopeia.
Albumin (Human) 25%, Albuminar®-25, is to be administered by the intravenous route.
The heat treatment step employed in the manufacture of Albumin (Human) 25%, Albuminar®-25, pasteurization of the final container at 60°C for 10 hours, has been validated in a series of in vitro experiments for its capacity to inactivate Human Immunodeficiency Virus type 1 (HIV-1), and the following model viruses: Bovine Viral Diarrhea Virus (BVDV- an enveloped virus used as a model for hepatitis C virus), Pseudorabies (PrV-a large, enveloped virus), and Encephalomyocarditis Virus (EMC - a small non-enveloped virus). For each virus studied, three independent experiments were conducted using Albumin (Human) 5%, Albuminar®-5 and Albumin (Human) 25%, Albuminar®-25 with the following results.[1]
[See table at bottom of next page]

CLINICAL PHARMACOLOGY

Albumin (Human) 25%, Albuminar®-25 is active osmotically and is therefore important in regulating the volume of circulating blood. When injected intravenously, 50 mL of 25% albumin draws approximately 175 mL of additional fluid into the circulation within 15 minutes, except in the presence of marked dehydration. This extra fluid reduces hemoconcentration and blood viscosity. The degree of volume expansion is dependent on the initial blood volume. When the circulating blood volume has been depleted, the

Continued on next page

Albuminar-25—Cont.

hemodilution following albumin administration persists for many hours. In individuals with normal blood volume, it usually lasts only a few hours.
Albumin, unlike whole blood or plasma, is considered free of the danger of homologous serum hepatitis. Albumin (Human) 25%, Albuminar®-25 may be given in conjunction with other parenteral fluids - such as saline, dextrose or sodium lactate. It is convenient to use since no crossmatching is required and the absence of cellular elements removes the danger of sensitization with repeated infusions.

INDICATIONS AND USAGE

SHOCK - Albumin is indicated in the emergency treatment of shock and in other similar conditions where the restoration of blood volume is urgent. If there has been considerable loss of red blood cells, transfusion with packed red blood cells is indicated.
BURNS - Albumin or Albumin in either normal saline or dextrose is indicated to prevent marked hemoconcentration and to maintain appropriate electrolyte balance.
HYPOPROTEINEMIA with or without edema - Albumin is indicated in those clinical situations usually associated with a low concentration of plasma protein and a resulting decreased circulating blood volume. Although diuresis may occur soon after albumin administration has been instituted, best results are obtained if albumin is continued until the normal serum protein level is regained.

CONTRAINDICATIONS

Albumin (Human) 25%, Albuminar®-25 may be contraindicated in patients with severe anemia or cardiac failure and in patients with a history of allergic reactions to human albumin.

WARNING

Infusion of protein-containing solutions such as Albuminar®-25 that have been excessively or inappropriately diluted with hypotonic solutions such as sterile water for injection may result in severe hemolysis and acute renal failure. Please refer to the **DOSAGE AND ADMINISTRATION** section for information about the recommended diluents for Albuminar®-25, which are normal saline and 5% dextrose.
Do not use if the solution is turbid. Since this product contains no antimicrobial preservative, do not begin administration more than 4 hours after the container has been entered.
Albumin (Human) U.S.P., 25%, Albuminar®-25 is made from human plasma. Products made from human plasma may contain infectious agents such as viruses, that can cause disease. The risk that such products will transmit an infectious agent has been reduced by screening plasma donors for prior exposure to certain viruses, by testing for the presence of certain current virus infections, and by inactivating and/or removing certain viruses during manufacture. The manufacturing procedure for Albumin (Human) 25%, Albuminar®-25 includes processing steps designed to reduce further the risk of viral transmission. Stringent procedures utilized at plasma collection centers, plasma testing laboratories, and fractionation facilities are designed to reduce the risk of viral transmission. Albuminar®-25 is pasteurized in the final container at 60.0 +/− 0.5°C for 10 - 11 hours. Virus elimination/inactivation is also achieved by the cold alcohol fractionation process. (See **DESCRIPTION** section for further information on viral reduction measures.) Despite these measures, such products may still potentially contain human pathogenic agents, including those not yet known or identified. Thus the risk of transmission of infectious agents cannot be totally eliminated. Any infections thought by a physician possibly to have been transmitted by this product should be reported by the physician or other healthcare provider to Aventis Behring at 800-504-5434. The physician should discuss the risks and benefits of this product with the patient.

PRECAUTIONS

GENERAL

If dehydration is present additional fluids must accompany or follow the administration of albumin. Administration of large quantities of albumin should be supplemented with or replaced by packed red blood cells to combat the relative anemia which would follow such use. The quick response of blood pressure which may follow the rapid administration of concentrated albumin necessitates careful observation of the injured patient to detect bleeding points which failed to bleed at lower blood pressure. Albumin (Human) 25%, Albuminar®-25 should be administered with caution to patients with low cardiac reserve or with no albumin deficiency because a rapid increase in plasma volume may cause circulatory compromise (e.g. hypertension, hypotension, or pulmonary edema.) In cases of hypertension, a slower rate of administration is desired - 200 mL of albumin solution may be mixed with 300 mL of 10% dextrose solution and administered at a rate of 10 grams of albumin (100 mL) per hour. If anaphylactic or severe anaphylactoid reactions occur, discontinue infusion immediately. Infusion rates and the patient's clinical state should be monitored closely during infusion.
INFORMATION FOR PATIENT - Some viruses, such as parvovirus B19 or hepatitis A are particularly difficult to remove or inactivate at this time. Parvovirus B19 may most seriously affect pregnant women, or immune-compromised individuals. The majority of parvovirus B19 and hepatitis A infections are acquired by environmental (community acquired) sources.
PREGNANCY CATEGORY C - Animal reproduction studies have not been conducted with Albumin (Human) 25%, Albuminar®-25. It is also not known whether Albuminar®-25 can cause fetal harm when administered to a pregnant woman or can affect reproduction capacity. Albuminar®-25 should be given to a pregnant woman only if clearly needed.
PEDIATRIC USE - No clinical studies using Albumin (Human) 25%, Albuminar®-25 have been conducted in pediatric patients. Safety and effectiveness in pediatric patients have not been established. However, extensive experience in patients suggests that children respond to Albumin (Human) 25%, Albuminar®-25 in the same manner as adults.

ADVERSE REACTIONS

The incidence of untoward reactions to Albumin (Human) 25% is low. Reports have been received of anaphylaxis, which may be severe, and hypersensitivity reactions (including urticaria, skin rash, pruritus, edema, erythema, hypotension and bronchospasm.) Nausea, vomiting, increased salivation, chills and febrile reactions have also been reported (see also **PRECAUTIONS**).

DOSAGE AND ADMINISTRATION

Albumin (Human) 25%, Albuminar®-25 may be given intravenously without dilution or it may be diluted with normal saline or 5% dextrose before administration. Two hundred mL-per liter gives a solution which is approximately isotonic and iso-osmotic with citrated plasma.
When undiluted albumin solution is administered in patients with normal blood volume, the rate of infusion should be slow enough (1 mL per minute) to prevent too rapid expansion of plasma volume.
In the treatment of shock the amount of albumin and duration of therapy must be based on the responsiveness of the patient as indicated by blood pressure, degree of pulmonary congestion, and hematocrit. The initial dose may be followed by additional albumin within 15 - 30 minutes if the response is deemed inadequate. If there is continued loss of protein, it also may be desirable to give packed red blood cells.
In the treatment of burns an optimal regimen involving use of albumin, crystalloids, electrolytes and water has not been established. Suggested therapy during the first 24 hours includes administration of large volumes of crystalloid solution to maintain an adequate plasma volume. Continuation of therapy beyond 24 hours usually requires more albumin and less crystalloid solution to prevent marked hemoconcentration and maintain electrolyte balance. Duration of treatment varies depending upon the extent of protein loss through renal excretion, denuded areas of skin and decreased albumin synthesis. Attempts to raise the albumin level above 4.0 g/100 mL may only result in an increased rate of catabolism.
In the treatment of hypoproteinemia, 200 to 300 mL of 25% albumin may be required to reduce edema and to bring serum protein values to normal. Since such patients usually have approximately normal blood volume, doses of more than 100 mL of 25% albumin should not be given faster than 100 mL in 30 to 45 minutes to avoid circulatory embarrassment. If slower administration is desired, 200 mL of 25% albumin may be mixed with 300 mL of 10% dextrose solution and administered by continuous drip at a rate of 100 mL of this dextrose solution an hour.
Parenteral drug products should be inspected visually for particulate matter and discoloration prior to administration, whenever solution and container permit.

HOW SUPPLIED

Albumin (Human), Albuminar®-25 is supplied as a 25% solution in:
NDC 0053-7680-01
20 mL vials containing 5.0 grams of albumin;
NDC 0053-7680-02
50 mL vials containing 12.5 grams of albumin;
NDC 0053-7680-03
100 mL vials containing 25.0 grams of albumin.
The packaging of this product contains dry natural rubber.
Store at controlled room temperature—between 15° - 30°C (59° - 86°F).

REFERENCES

1. Data on file.

BIBLIOGRAPHY

Finlayson, J.S.: Albumin Products. Seminars in Thrombosis and Hemostasis 6:85 - 120, 1980.
Tullis, J.L.: Albumin. JAMA 237:355–360 and 460–463, 1977.
Rudolf, A.M.: Pediatrics. 18th ED., p. 1839, Appleton and Lange, 1987.

12522-01

Pasteurization (60°C for 10 hours) Viral Reduction Studies (log_{10} reduction)

Virus	Albumin (Human) 5%, Albuminar®-5	Albumin (Human) 25%, Albuminar®-25
HIV-1	>5.44, >6.38 and >6.31	>5.50, >6.57 and >6.64
BVDV	>6.01, >6.76 and >6.55	>5.99, >5.81 and >5.32
PrV	>7.30, >7.68 and >7.63	>7.32, >7.20 and >7.42
EMC	>7.38, >7.97 and >7.97	>7.10, >7.89 and >7.87

PRESCRIBING INFORMATION
GAMMAR®-P I.V. ℞
IMMUNE GLOBULIN INTRAVENOUS (HUMAN)
℞ only

DESCRIPTION

Immune Globulin Intravenous (Human), Gammar®-P I.V., is a sterile, lyophilized preparation of intact, unmodified, immunoglobulin, primarily IgG, stabilized with Albumin (Human) and sucrose. The distribution of IgG subclasses is similar to that present in normal human plasma. It is prepared by cold alcohol fractionation of pooled plasma and is not chemically altered or enzymatically degraded.
The plasma used in the manufacture of this product has been tested and found negative for HBV, HCV, and HIV-1 by an investigational test procedure referred to as Nucleic Acid Testing (NAT) using Polymerase Chain Reaction (PCR) Technology. Investigational testing is being performed to determine the effectiveness of NAT to detect low levels of viral material. The significance of a negative result is unknown since the effectiveness of the test has not been established.
When reconstituted with the appropriate volume of Sterile Water for Injection, USP, Gammar®-P I.V. contains 5% IgG, 3% Albumin (Human), 5% sucrose, and 0.5% sodium chloride. The pH of the solution has been adjusted to 6.8 ± 0.4 with citric acid and/or sodium carbonate. Gammar®-P I.V. contains no preservative. This product is intended for intravenous administration.
The heat treatment step employed in the manufacture of Immune Globulin Intravenous (Human), Gammar®-P I.V., pasteurization at 60°C for 10 hours in aqueous solution form with stabilizers, has been validated in a series of *in vitro* experiments for its capacity to inactivate Human Immunodeficiency Virus (HIV) and the following model viruses: Sindbis, Vesicular Stomatitis (VSV), Bovine Viral Diarrhea Virus (BVD), Vaccinia, Pseudorabies and Murine Encephalomyocarditis (EMC), a non-lipid enveloped model virus. HIV was reduced by 6.0 and 5.4 log_{10} to an undetectable level after 0.5 hours of heating in two independent experiments. For each of the model viruses studied, two independent experiments were also conducted with the following results: Sindbis was reduced by 7.5 and 7.9 log_{10} to an undetectable level after two hours of heating, VSV was reduced by 6.8 and 7.2 log_{10} to an undetectable level after 0.5 hours of heating, BVD, a model for hepatitis C virus, was reduced by 6.4 and 6.5 log_{10} to an undetectable level after four hours of heating, Vaccinia was reduced by 5.6 and 5.6 log_{10} to an undetectable level after two hours of heating, Pseudorabies was reduced by 4.9 and 3.6 log_{10} to an undetectable level after six hours of heating and EMC, a non-lipid enveloped model virus, was reduced by 4.5 and 4.8 log_{10} after ten hours of heating.[1]
The viral reduction capacity of the purification procedures used in the manufacture of Immune Globulin Intravenous (Human), Gammar®-P I.V., exclusive of heat treatment, was also studied in a series of *in vitro* experiments using HIV and the model virus EMC, a non-lipid enveloped virus. EMC was reduced by 4.9 log_{10} and 3.4 log_{10} by two independent purification steps which are conducted before and after heat treatment, respectively. HIV was reduced by at least 6.7 log_{10} by the processing steps employed to isolate Cohn Fraction II from pooled plasma during the initial purification of Gammar®-P I.V. The total viral reduction capacity for HIV and EMC attributable to the Gammar®-P I.V. manufacturing procedure, inclusive of both the heat treatment protocol and the fractionation steps studied, is, therefore, $\geq$12.1 log_{10} for HIV and $\geq$12.8 log_{10} for EMC.[1]

CLINICAL PHARMACOLOGY

The half-life of Immune Globulin Intravenous (Human), Gammar®-P I.V., was evaluated in a double blind clinical study in which it was compared to Gammar® I.V. The mean half-life of Gammar®-P I.V. in nine patients was determined to be approximately 40 days and was not statistically different from the mean half-life of 34 days found for Gammar® I.V. in seven patients. Furthermore, there do not appear to be any clinically relevant differences between children, adolescents, and adults with respect to the mean half-life of IgG. The half-life of IgG, however, can vary considerably from patient to patient.[1]
Immune Globulin Intravenous (Human), Gammar®-P I.V., is a native, non-chemically modified IgG fractionated from pooled human donor plasma. The distribution of IgG subclasses (IgG_1, IgG_2, IgG_3, IgG_4) is similar to that present in Cohn Fraction II. Since the IgG concentrate is prepared from a large pool of at least 1000 donors, it represents the expected diversity of antibodies in that population. In a

study of an unheated version of this product, Gammar® I.V., it was found that Gammar® I.V. provided a broad range of antibodies, capable of opsonization and neutralization of microbes and toxins, against bacterial and viral antigens for prevention or attenuation of infectious diseases.[2] In *in vitro* testing, Gammar®-P I.V. has been shown to provide equivalent levels of a broad range of antibodies when compared to Gammar® I.V.[1]

Albumin (Human) and sucrose are added to the formulation in order to provide adequate stabilization of the IgG molecules and the reconstituted product. Because sucrose, when given intravenously, is excreted unchanged in the urine, Immune Globulin Intravenous (Human), Gammar®-P I.V., may be given to diabetics without compensatory changes in insulin dosage regimen.[3] **[SEE BOXED WARNING.]**

INDICATIONS AND USAGE

Gammar®-P I.V. is indicated for adults, children and adolescents with primary defective antibody synthesis such as agammaglobulinemia or hypogammaglobulinemia, who are at increased risk of infection. When high levels or rapid elevation of circulating gamma globulins are desired, intravenous administration is more desirable than intramuscular therapy. The safety and efficacy of Gammar®-P I.V. in neonates and infants with primary defective antibody synthesis has not been established.

CONTRAINDICATIONS

Gammar®-P I.V. is contraindicated in individuals with a history of anaphylactic or severe systemic response to immune globulin intramuscular or intravenous preparations or in individuals with a history of allergic reactions to human albumin.

Immune Globulin Intravenous (Human), Gammar®-P I.V., should not be given to persons with isolated immunoglobulin A (IgA) deficiency. Such persons have the potential for developing antibodies to IgA and could have anaphylactic reactions to subsequent administration of blood products that contain IgA.[4]

WARNINGS

Immune Globulin Intravenous (Human) products have been reported to be associated with renal dysfunction, acute renal failure, osmotic nephrosis, and death.(12) Patients predisposed to acute renal failure include patients with any degree of pre-existing renal insufficiency, diabetes mellitus, age greater than 65, volume depletion, sepsis, paraproteinemia, or patients receiving known nephrotoxic drugs. Especially in such patients, IGIV products should be administered at the minimum concentration available and the minimum rate of infusion practicable. While these reports of renal dysfunction and acute renal failure have been associated with the use of many of the licensed IGIV products, those containing sucrose as a stabilizer accounted for a disproportionate share of the total number. See PRECAUTIONS and DOSAGE AND ADMINISTRATION sections for important information intended to reduce the risk of acute renal failure.

If anaphylactic or severe anaphylactoid reactions occur, discontinue infusion immediately. Epinephrine should be available for the treatment of any acute anaphylactoid reactions.

Patients with agammaglobulinemia or extreme hypogammaglobulinemia who have never received immunoglobulin substitution therapy before or who have not received immunoglobulin therapy within the preceding 8 weeks may be at risk of developing inflammatory reactions upon the infusion of human immunoglobulins. These reactions are manifested by a rise in temperature, chills, nausea and vomiting, and appear to be related to the rate of infusion.

Infusion rates and the patient's clinical state should be monitored closely during infusion. (See **Administration** section under **DOSAGE AND ADMINISTRATION**.)

PRECAUTIONS

GENERAL - Assure that patients are not volume depleted prior to the initiation of the infusion of IGIV.

Periodic monitoring of renal function tests and urine output is particularly important in patients judged to have a potential increased risk for developing acute renal failure. Renal function, including measurement of blood urea nitrogen (BUN)/serum creatinine, should be assessed prior to the initial infusion of Gammar®-P I.V. and again at appropriate intervals thereafter. If renal function deteriorates, discontinuation of the product should be considered.

For patients judged to be at risk for developing renal dysfunction, it may be prudent to reduce the amount of product (and sucrose stabilizer) infused per unit time by infusing Gammar®-P I.V. at a rate less than 3.0 mg IG/kg/min (0.06 mL/kg/min).

Epinephrine should be available for treatment of acute allergic reactions. See **DOSAGE AND ADMINISTRATION** section for product compatibility information.

INFORMATION FOR PATIENTS - Patients should be instructed to immediately report symptoms of decreased urine output, sudden weight gain, fluid retention/edema, and/or shortness of breath (which may suggest kidney damage) to their physicians.

DRUG INTERACTIONS - It is reported that antibodies in immune globulin preparations may interfere with the response to live viral vaccines such as measles, mumps and rubella. Immunizing physicians should be informed of recent therapy with Immune Globulin Intravenous (Human) so that appropriate precautions may be taken.

PREGNANCY CATEGORY C - Animal reproduction studies have not been performed with Immune Globulin Intravenous (Human), Gammar®-P I.V. It is also not known whether Immune Globulin Intravenous (Human), Gammar®-P I.V., can cause fetal harm when administered to a pregnant woman or can affect reproduction capacity. Gammar®-P I.V. should be given to a pregnant woman only if clearly needed.

PEDIATRIC USE - The safety and efficacy of Gammar®-P I.V. has not been established in neonates and infants with primary defective antibody synthesis.

ASEPTIC MENINGITIS SYNDROME - An aseptic meningitis syndrome (AMS) has been reported to occur infrequently in association with Immune Globulin Intravenous (Human) (IGIV) treatment. The syndrome usually begins within several hours to two days following IGIV treatment. It is characterized by symptoms and signs including severe headache, nuchal rigidity, drowsiness, fever, photophobia, painful eye movements, and nausea and vomiting. Cerebrospinal fluid (CSF) studies are frequently positive with pleocytosis up to several thousand cells per cubic millimeter, predominantly from the granulocytic series, and elevated protein levels up to several hundred mg/dL. Patients exhibiting such symptoms and signs should receive a thorough neurological examination, including CSF studies, to rule out other causes of meningitis. AMS may occur more frequently in association with high dose (2 g/kg) IGIV treatment. Discontinuation of IGIV treatment has resulted in remission of AMS within several days without sequelae.[5-8]

ADVERSE REACTIONS

Increases in creatinine and blood urea nitrogen (BUN) have been observed as soon as one to two days following infusion. Progression to oliguria and anuria requiring dialysis has been observed, although some patients have improved spontaneously following cessation of treatment.[10] Types of severe renal adverse reactions that have been seen following IGIV therapy include: acute renal failure, acute tubular necrosis[11], proximal tubular nephropathy, and osmotic nephrosis[12, 13-15].

Potential reactions for all Immune Globulin Intravenous (Human) products are often related to infusion rate and may include: nausea, vomiting, abdominal cramps, chills, pyrexia, chest tightness, palpitations, tachycardia, blood pressure changes, edema, flushing, diaphoresis, rash, erythema, pruritus, cyanosis, dizziness, headache, backache or other body aches, anxiety, wheezing (and other respiratory events), myalgia, shaking, fatigue, malaise and arthralgia, usually beginning within one hour of the start of the infusion.

A double blind study comparing Gammar® I.V. and Gammar®-P I.V. as replacement therapy was conducted in 19 patients (108 infusions) with primary defective antibody synthesis, such as common variable or X-linked hypogammaglobulinemia. The types of infusion related adverse reactions noted were similar in frequency and nature. For the ten patients receiving only Gammar®-P I.V. (56 infusions), all of the infusion-related adverse reactions were characterized as mild and of short duration. These included the following most frequent reactions: Chills 8.9% (5/56), Headache 5.4% (3/56), and Pain: Back/Neck 3.6% (2/56). The overall incidence of infusions associated with an adverse reaction was 16% (9/56 infusions) for Gammar®-P I.V. which compared favorably to the overall incidence of infusions associated with an adverse reaction for Gammar® I.V. (25%; 13/52 infusions).[1]

True anaphylactic reactions may occur in patients with a history of prior systemic allergic reactions or seizure following administration of human immunoglobulin preparations. Very rarely an anaphylactoid reaction may occur in patients with no prior history of severe allergic reactions to human immunoglobulin preparations. Patients previously sensitized to certain antigens, including IgA, may be at risk of immediate anaphylactoid and hypersensitivity reactions.[4] Epinephrine should be available for the treatment of any acute anaphylactoid reaction (See **WARNINGS** and **CONTRAINDICATIONS**.)

Infusion rates and clinical state should be monitored closely during infusion. If an adverse reaction occurs, the infusion rate should be reduced or the infusion stopped until the symptoms have subsided (See **DOSAGE AND ADMINISTRATION**.)

DOSAGE AND ADMINISTRATION

For treatment of primary defective antibody synthesis in adults, adolescents and children, Immune Globulin Intravenous (Human), Gammar®-P I.V., is administered to restore the patient's circulating IgG level to near-normal levels. Starting doses of 200 mg/kg body weight every three to four weeks are recommended in children and adolescents. Slightly higher doses of 200 mg/kg to 400 mg/kg body weight given every three to four weeks are recommended in adults. The clinical management of adult, children and adolescent patients is optimized by adjusting doses to maintain desired IgG blood levels and clinical results.

PRODUCT COMPATIBILITY - It is recommended that Immune Globulin Intravenous (Human), Gammar®-P I.V., be administered by a separate infusion line without admixture with other drugs or medications which the patient may be receiving. However, based upon compatibility studies, Gammar®-P I.V. may be infused sequentially into a primary i.v. line containing either 0.9% sodium chloride injection or 5% dextrose injection or flushed with 0.9% sodium chloride injection or 5% dextrose injection. Do not mix Immune Globulin Intravenous (Human) products of differing formulations. If several doses of Immune Globulin Intravenous (Human), Gammar®-P I.V. are to be administered, several reconstituted vials of identical formulation and diluent may be pooled, using proper aseptic technique. As described under **Reconstitution**, below, do not shake or cause excessive foaming. Swirl gently to mix. Filtration is acceptable but not required; pore sizes of greater than or equal to 15 microns will be less likely to slow infusion.

Reconstitution

CAUTION: Reconstitution instructions must be followed exactly. Please read the following instructions in their entirety before attempting to reconstitute product.

1) Bring both product vial and diluent vial to room temperature prior to reconstitution.
2) Examine product vial to ensure no product powder or cake is wedged in the neck of the vial. If so, gently tap the vial to dislodge the product.
3) Remove plastic flip-off caps from both vials.
4) Treat rubber stoppers with antiseptic solution and allow to dry.

CAUTION: The double ended vented transfer spike (see diagram below), provided in the package is comprised of a white (diluent) end, which has a double orifice, and a green (product) end, which has a single orifice. Incorrect use of the transfer spike will result in loss of vacuum, and prevent transfer of diluent thereby preventing reconstitution of the product.

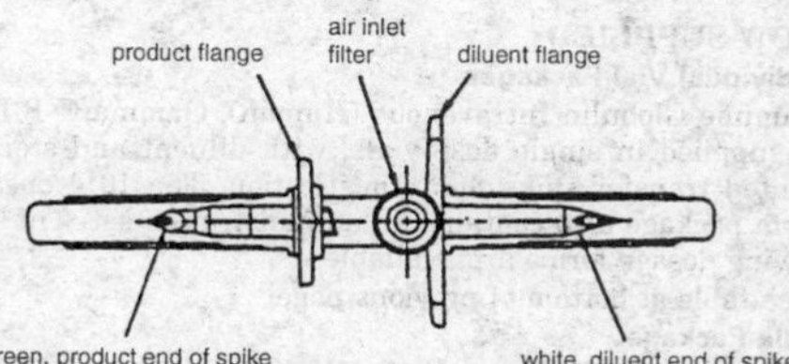

The transfer spike is sterile. Do not touch the exposed ends of the spike after removing the guards.

5) Remove the guard from the white (diluent) end of the transfer spike. Insert the white end of the transfer spike into the center of the stopper of the upright diluent vial first.
6) Remove the guard from the green (product) end of the transfer spike. Invert the diluent vial with the attached transfer spike and, using minimum force, insert the green end into the center of the stopper of the upright product vial. The flange of the transfer spike should rest on the surface of the stopper and the diluent will begin to transfer into the product vial.
7) Allow the vacuum in the product vial to pull the diluent into the product vial.
8) During diluent transfer, wet the lyophilized cake completely by gently tilting the product vial. Do not allow the air inlet filter to face downward. Care should be taken not to lose the vacuum, as this will prolong reconstitution of the product.
9) After diluent transfer is complete, the transfer spike will allow filtered air into the product vial through the air filter. Additional venting of the product vial after diluent transfer is complete, is not required. When diluent transfer is complete, withdraw and properly discard transfer spike and diluent bottle.
10) Allow the product vial to remain undisturbed for 5 minutes after diluent addition. Do not touch or mix during this time.
11) After 5 minutes, mix the product vial by gently swirling the vial without creating excessive foam. Never shake the product vial.

Note: A syrup-like layer may remain on the bottom of the vial following reconstitution. Swirl gently to disperse this layer until a homogenous solution is obtained.

12) Examine solution. All unreconstituted product should dissolve with gentle swirling and the solution should be clear and ready to administer in 20 minutes or less.
13) Product contains no preservative. Infusion must be initiated within 3 hours of reconstitution. If not used within this time frame, it should be properly disposed of and not administered.
14) Reconstituted product does not need to be filtered. If a filter is used, it should be a 15 micron filter or larger.

Continued on next page

	Product	Diluent
NDC 0053-7486-01	1 g immune globulin/vial	20 mL
NDC 0053-7486-02	2.5 g immune globulin/vial	50 mL
NDC 0053-7486-05	5 g immune globulin/vial	100 mL
NDC 0053-7486-10	10 g immune globulin/vial	200 mL

Gammar-P I.V.—Cont.

15) If several doses of Immune Globulin Intravenous (Human), Gammar®-P I.V., are to be pooled aseptically for administration, avoid excessive formation of foam in the pooling container and gently swirl the pooling container to mix. **DO NOT SHAKE THE POOLING CONTAINER.**

Administration

CAUTION: When entering the product stopper with an IV set spike for administration, care should be taken to follow the path made by the transfer spike (see **Reconstitution**).

Immune Globulin Intravenous (Human), Gammar®-P I.V., is to be administered by intravenous infusion. The infusion should begin at a rate of 0.01 mL/kg/min, increasing to 0.02 mL/kg/min after 15 to 30 minutes. Most patients tolerate a gradual increase to 0.03-0.06 mL/kg/min. For the average 70 kg person this is equivalent to 2 to 4 mL/min. If adverse reactions develop, slowing the infusion rate will usually eliminate the reaction. Discard any unused solution.

For patients judged to be at increased risk for developing renal dysfunction, it may be prudent to reduce the amount of product (and sucrose stabilizer) infused per unit time by infusing Gammar®-P I.V. at a rate less than 3.0 mg IG/kg/min (= 3.0 mg sucrose/kg/min) (0.06 mL/kg/min).

No prospective data are presently available to identify a maximum safe dose, concentration, and rate of infusion in patients determined to be at an increased risk of acute renal failure. In the absence of prospective data, recommended doses should not be exceeded and the concentration and infusion rate selected should be the minimum level practicable. Reduction in dose, concentration, and/or rate of administration in patients at risk of acute renal failure has been proposed in the literature in order to reduce the risk of acute renal failure.[9]

Parenteral drug products should be inspected visually for particulate matter and discoloration prior to administration whenever solution and container permit.

HOW SUPPLIED

Individual Vial Packages

Immune Globulin Intravenous (Human), Gammar®-P I.V., is supplied in single dose vials, with diluent and sterile, vented transfer spike for reconstitution. The 10 g dosage form package also contains an administration set. The following dosage forms are available:

[See table at bottom of previous page]

Bulk Package

Immune Globulin Intravenous (Human), Gammar®-P I.V., 5 g immune globulin/vial is supplied in a bulk pack (NDC 0053-7486-06) of six (6) single dose vials. Each single dose vial should be reconstituted with 100 mL Sterile Water for Injection, USP (not supplied).

STORAGE

When stored at temperatures not exceeding 25°C (77°F), Immune Globulin Intravenous (Human), Gammar®-P I.V., is stable for the period indicated by the expiration date on its label. Avoid freezing which may damage container for the diluent.

REFERENCES

1. Data on File: Aventis Behring L.L.C. 2. Steele RW, Augustine RA, Tannenbaum AS, Marmer DJ. Intravenous Immune Globulin for Hypogammaglobulinemia: A Comparison of Opsonizing Capacity in Recipient Sera. *Clin. Immunol. Immunopathol.* 1985; 34:275 - 283. 3. Martindale. *The Extra Pharmacopoeia* 27th ed. Edited by Wade A. London: The Pharmaceutical Press. 1979; 65. 4. Fudenberg HH. Sensitization to Immunoglobulins and Hazards of Gamma Globulin Therapy. Immunoglobulins, Biologic Aspects and Clinical Uses. 1970; 211 - 220. Edited by Merler E. National Academy of Sciences, Washington, D.C. 5. Sekul EA, Cupler EJ, Dalakas, MC. Aseptic Meningitis Associated with High Dose Intravenous Immunoglobulin Therapy: Frequency and Risk Factors. *Ann Int Med* 1994; 121:4, 259 - 262. 6. Kato E, Shindo S, Eto Y, et al. Administration of Immune Globulin Associated with Aseptic Meningitis. *JAMA* 1988; 259:3269 - 3271. 7. Casteels-Van Daele M, Wijndaele L, Hunninck K, Gillis P, Ziekenhuis V. Intravenous Immune Globulin and Acute Aseptic Meningitis. *N Engl J Med* 1990; 323:614 - 615. 8. Scribner C, Kapit R, Phillips E, Rickels N. Aseptic Meningitis and Intravenous Immunoglobulin Therapy. *Ann Int Med* 1994; 121:305 - 306. 9. Tan E, *et al.* Acute Renal Failure Resulting from Intravenous Immunoglobulin Therapy. *Arch Neurol.* 1993; 50(2):137 - 139. 10. Winward DB, Brophy MT: Acute renal failure after administration of intravenous immunoglobulin: review of the literature and case report. 1995; *Pharmacotherapy* 15:765 - 772. 11. Phillips AO: Renal failure and intravenous immunoglobulin [letter; comment]. 1992; *Clin Nephrol* 36:83 - 86. 12. Cayco AV, Perazella MA, Hayslett JP: Renal insufficiency after intravenous immune globulin therapy: A Report of Two Cases and an Analysis of the Literature. 1997; *J Amer Soc Nephrology* 8:1788 - 1793. 13. Anderson W, Bethea W: Renal lesion following administration of hypertonic solutions of sucrose. 1940; *JAMA* 114:1983–1987. 14. Lindberg H, Wald A: Renal changes following the administration of hypertonic solutions. 1939; *Arch Intern Med* 63:907 - 918. 15. Rigdon RH, Cardwell ES: Renal lesions following the intravenous injection of hypertonic solution of sucrose: A clinical and experimental study. 1942; *Arch Intern Med* 69:670-690.

BIBLIOGRAPHY

Polley MJ, Fischetti VA, Landaburu PH. Native Intravenous IgG Exhibits Greater Biological Activity than Modified IgG. From the *XX Cong. Int. Soc. of Hematology*; 1984.

12173-01

PRESCRIBING INFORMATION
HELIXATE® FS ℞
Antihemophilic Factor (Recombinant)
Formulated with Sucrose

DESCRIPTION

Helixate® FS Antihemophilic Factor (Recombinant) is a sterile, stable, purified, nonpyrogenic, dried concentrate that has been manufactured using recombinant DNA technology. Helixate® FS is intended for use in the treatment of classical hemophilia (hemophilia A), and is produced by Baby Hamster Kidney (BHK) cells into which the human factor VIII (FVIII) gene has been introduced.[1] The cell culture medium contains Human Plasma Protein Solution (HPPS) and recombinant insulin, but does not contain any proteins derived from animal sources. Helixate FS is a highly purified glycoprotein consisting of multiple peptides including an 80 kD and various extensions of the 90 kD subunit. It has the same biological activity as FVIII derived from human plasma. Compared to its predecessor product HELIXATE® Antihemophilic Factor (Recombinant), Helixate FS incorporates a revised purification and formulation process that eliminates the addition of Albumin (Human).

The purification process includes an effective solvent/detergent virus inactivation step in addition to the use of the classical purification methods of ion exchange chromatography, monoclonal antibody immunoaffinity chromatography, along with other chromatographic steps designed to purify recombinant FVIII and remove contaminating substances. Helixate FS is formulated with sucrose (0.9-1.3%), glycine (21–25 mg/mL), and histidine (18-23 mM) as stabilizers in the final container in place of Albumin (Human) as used in HELIXATE, and is then lyophilized. The final product also contains calcium chloride (2–3 mM), sodium (27–36 mEq/L), chloride (32–40 mEq/L), polysorbate 80 (not more than [NMT] 35 µg/mL), imidazole (NMT 20 µg/1000 IU), tri-n-butyl phosphate (NMT 5 µg/1000 IU), and copper (NMT 0.6 µg/1000 IU). The product contains no preservatives. The amount of sucrose in each vial is 28 mg. Intravenous administration of sucrose contained in Helixate FS will not affect blood glucose levels.

Each vial of Helixate FS contains the labeled amount of recombinant FVIII in international units (IU). One IU, as defined by the World Health Organization standard for blood coagulation FVIII, human, is approximately equal to the level of FVIII activity found in 1 mL of fresh pooled human plasma.

Helixate FS must be administered by the intravenous route.

CLINICAL PHARMACOLOGY

Pharmacokinetic studies were conducted in 20 patients with severe hemophilia A in North America. In this comparative pharmacokinetic study, Helixate® FS Antihemophilic Factor (Recombinant) was shown to be similar to its predecessor product HELIXATE® Antihemophilic Factor (Recombinant) (rFVIII). Mean FVIII recovery measured 10 minutes following infusion was 2.1 ± 0.3 %/IU/kg for Helixate FS and 2.4 ± 0.7 %/IU/kg for HELIXATE. The two recoveries were not statistically different (confidence interval 0.815-1.01). The mean biological half-life of recombinant FVIII formulated with sucrose (rFVIII-FS) is similar to HELIXATE with a mean of approximately 13 hours, which has previously been shown to be similar to plasma-derived Antihemophilic Factor (AHF). The activated partial thromboplastin time shortened appropriately with both rFVIII and rFVIII-FS. The recovery and half-life data for rFVIII-FS were unchanged after 24 weeks of exclusive treatment indicating continued efficacy and no evidence of FVIII inhibition. The mean FVIII recovery measured 10 minutes following a dose of rFVIII-FS in 37 patients (after 24 weeks of treatment with rFVIII-FS) was 2.1%/IU/kg, which was unchanged from FVIII recovery determined at baseline and at weeks 4 and 12.

Seventy-one patients with severe hemophilia A, ages 12–59, who had been previously treated with other recombinant and with plasma-derived AHF products, were enrolled in 6-month studies of home therapy with rFVIII-FS in Europe and North America. A total of 3995 infusions have been administered under this portion of the study, or 7.4 million units of rFVIII-FS. Treatment of 659 bleeding episodes during the study period required 951 infusions of rFVIII-FS. The majority of bleeding episodes (89.5%) were treated successfully with one or two infusions, using a mean dosage of approximately 28 IU/kg per treatment infusion. Regularly scheduled treatment accounted for 76% of infusions administered on study. Nine patients have received rFVIII-FS on 11 occasions for surgical procedures. The procedures included removal of a brain tumor, two total knee replacements, two joint synovectomies (one with Achilles tendon lengthening), two circumcisions, a hernia repair, and three teeth extractions. Hemostasis was satisfactory in all cases. In clinical studies, Helixate FS has been used in the treatment of bleeding episodes in previously untreated patients (PUPs) and minimally treated (MTP) pediatric patients. In ongoing studies, 61 PUPs/MTPs have been treated with Helixate FS. Bleeding episodes were treated effectively with one or two infusions of rFVIII-FS. Ten patients have developed inhibitors. In these trials, approximately half of the patients have achieved 20 or more exposure days, and the incidence of inhibitor formation (16%) is consistent with that observed in other pediatric studies using plasma-derived and recombinant factor VIII products.[2–5]

INDICATIONS AND USAGE

Helixate FS is indicated for the treatment of classical hemophilia (hemophilia A) in which there is a demonstrated deficiency of activity of the plasma clotting factor FVIII. Helixate FS provides a means of temporarily replacing the missing clotting factor in order to correct or prevent bleeding episodes, or in order to perform emergency or elective surgery in hemophiliacs.

In clinical studies with the predecessor product HELIXATE, some patients who developed inhibitors on study continued to manifest a clinical response when inhibitor titers were less than 10 Bethesda Units (BU) per mL. When an inhibitor is present, the dosage requirement for FVIII is variable. The dosage can be determined only by clinical response, and by monitoring circulating FVIII levels after treatment (see **DOSAGE AND ADMINISTRATION**). Because Helixate FS has similar biological activity to HELIXATE it can be used in the same manner.

Helixate® FS Antihemophilic Factor (Recombinant) does not contain von Willebrand's factor and therefore is not indicated for the treatment of von Willebrand's disease.

CONTRAINDICATIONS

Known intolerance of allergic reactions to constituents of the preparation.

Known hypersensitivity to mouse or hamster protein may be a contraindication to the use of Helixate FS.

WARNINGS

None.

PRECAUTIONS

General

Helixate FS is intended for the treatment of bleeding disorders arising from a deficiency in FVIII. This deficiency should be proven prior to administering Helixate FS.

The development of circulating neutralizing antibodies to FVIII may occur during the treatment of patients with hemophilia A. Inhibitor formation is especially common in young children with severe hemophilia during their first years of treatment, or in patients of any age who have received little previous treatment with FVIII. Nonetheless, inhibitor formation may occur at any time in the treatment of a patient with hemophilia A. Patients treated with any AHF preparation, including Helixate FS, should be carefully monitored for the development of antibodies to FVIII by appropriate clinical observation and laboratory tests, according to the recommendation of the patient's hemophilia treatment center.

Formation of Antibodies to Mouse and Hamster Protein

Assays to detect seroconversion to mouse and hamster protein were conducted on all patients on study. No patient has developed specific antibodies to these proteins after commencing study, and no allergic reactions have been associated with rFVIII-FS infusions. Although no reactions were observed, patients should be made aware of the theoretical possibility of a hypersensitivity reaction, and alerted to the early signs of such a reaction (e.g., hives, localized or generalized urticaria, wheezing, and hypotension). Patients should be advised to discontinue use of the product and contact their physician if such symptoms occur.

Carcinogenesis, Mutagenesis, and Impairment of Fertility

In vitro evaluation of the mutagenic potential of rFVIII failed to demonstrate reverse mutation or chromosomal aberrations at doses substantially greater than the maximum expected clinical dose. In vivo evaluation of rFVIII in animals using doses ranging between 10 and 40 times the expected clinical maximum also indicated that rFVIII does not possess a mutagenic potential. Long-term investigations of carcinogenic potential in animals have not been performed.

Pediatric Use

Helixate FS is appropriate for use in pediatric patients of all ages, including neonates, infants, children, and adolescents. Safety and efficacy studies have been performed in previously untreated and minimally treated pediatric patients (n=62). Helixate FS is similar to HELIXATE® Antihemophilic Factor (Recombinant) in its biological activity and may be used in pediatric patients in the same manner as HELIXATE.

Geriatric Use

Clinical studies with Helixate FS did not include sufficient numbers of patients aged 65 and over to be able to determine whether they respond differently from younger patients. However, clinical experience with HELIXATE and other AHF products has not identified differences between the elderly and younger patients. As with any patient receiving Helixate FS, dose selection for an elderly patient should be individualized.

Pregnancy Category C

Animal reproduction studies have not been conducted with Helixate® FS Antihemophilic Factor (Recombinant). It is also not known whether Helixate FS can cause fetal harm when administered to a pregnant woman or affect reproduction capacity. Helixate FS should be used during pregnancy and lactation only if clearly indicated.

ADVERSE REACTIONS

During the clinical studies conducted in previously treated patients (PTPs), 109 adverse events were reported in the course of 4160 infusions (2.6%). Only 13 events were reported by the investigator as at least remotely related to study drug. Another 7 events were nonassessable. Thus 20 events in 11 patients were considered to be either nonassessable or at least remotely related to Helixate FS administration, for an incidence of 0.5% relative to the number of infusions administered. Events that were at least remotely drug-related included: local injection site reactions (2), dizziness (2), rash (2), unusual taste in the mouth (1), mild increase in blood pressure (1), pruritus (1), depersonalization (1), nausea (1), and rhinitis (1). No FVIII inhibitors have developed in the 72 PTPs with severe hemophilia A who have received Helixate FS for a mean of 54 exposure days.

In clinical studies with previously untreated patients (PUPs) and minimally treated (MTP) pediatric patients, 18 adverse events were reported by the clinical investigators as at least possibly related to the study drug including the expected complication of inhibitor development in 8 patients (included in the 10 patients discussed under **CLINICAL PHARMACOLOGY**), a forearm bleed following venipuncture, constipation, adenopathy, rash, anemia and pallor in one inhibitor patient with gastroenteritis, and serious otitis media.

DOSAGE AND ADMINISTRATION

Each bottle of Helixate FS has the rFVIII potency in international units stated on the label based on the one-stage assay methodology. The reconstituted product must be administered within 3 hours after reconstitution. It is recommended to use the administration set provided.

GENERAL APPROACH TO TREATMENT AND ASSESSMENT OF TREATMENT EFFICACY

The dosages described below are presented as general guidance. It should be emphasized that the dosage of Helixate FS required for hemostasis must be individualized according to the needs of the patient, the severity of the deficiency, the severity of the hemorrhage, the presence of inhibitors, and the FVIII level desired. It is often critical to follow the course of therapy with FVIII level assays. The clinical effect of FVIII is the most important element in evaluating the effectiveness of treatment. It may be necessary to administer more FVIII than estimated in order to attain satisfactory clinical results. If the calculated dose fails to attain the expected FVIII levels, or if bleeding is not controlled after administration of the calculated dosage, the presence of a circulating inhibitor in the patient should be suspected. Its presence should be substantiated and the inhibitor level quantitated by appropriate laboratory tests. When an inhibitor is present, the dosage requirement for FVIII could be extremely variable among different patients, and the optimal treatment can be determined only by the clinical response.

Some patients with low-titer inhibitors (<10 BU) can be successfully treated with FVIII preparations without a resultant anamnestic rise in inhibitor titer.[6] FVIII levels and clinical response to treatment must be assessed to insure adequate response. Use of alternative treatment products, such as Factor IX Complex concentrates, Antihemophilic Factor (Porcine), recombinant Factor VIIa or Anti-Inhibitor Coagulant Complex, may be necessary for patients with anamnestic responses to FVIII treatment and/or high-titer inhibitors.

Calculation of Dosage

The in vivo percent elevation in FVIII level can be estimated by multiplying the dose of Helixate® FS Antihemophilic Factor (Recombinant) per kilogram of body weight (IU/kg) by 2% per IU per kg. This method of calculation is based on clinical findings with the use of plasma-derived and recombinant AHF products[7–9] and is illustrated in the following examples:

[See first table above]
[See second table above]
or
[See third table above]
[See fourth table above]

The dosage necessary to achieve hemostasis depends upon the type and severity of the bleeding episode, according to the following general guidelines:

[See fifth table above]

Prophylaxis

AHF concentrates may also be administered on a regular schedule for prophylaxis of bleeding, as reported by Nilsson et al.[10]

Instructions for Use

Reconstitution, product administration, and handling of the administration set and needles must be done with caution. Percutaneous puncture with a needle contaminated with blood can transmit infectious viruses including HIV (AIDS) and hepatitis. Obtain immediate medical attention if injury occurs. Place needles in a sharps container after single use. Discard all equipment, including any reconstituted Helixate® FS Antihemophilic Factor (Recombinant) product, in accordance with biohazard procedures.

Reconstitution

Always wash your hands before performing the following procedures:

Vacuum Transfer

1. Warm the unopened diluent and the concentrate to a temperature not to exceed 37°C, 99°F.

$$\text{Expected \% factor VIII increase} = \frac{\text{\# units administered} \times 2\%/\text{IU/kg}}{\text{body weight (kg)}}$$

$$\text{Example for a 70 kg adult: } \frac{1400 \text{ IU} \times 2\%/\text{IU/kg}}{70 \text{ kg}} = 40\%$$

$$\text{Dosage required (IU)} = \frac{\text{body weight (kg)} \times \text{desired \% FVIII increase}}{2\%/\text{IU/kg}}$$

$$\text{Example for a 15 kg child: } \frac{15 \text{ kg} \times 100\%}{2\%/\text{IU/kg}} = 750 \text{ IU required}$$

Hemorrhagic event	Therapeutically necessary plasma level of FVIII activity	Dosage necessary to maintain the therapeutic plasma level
Minor hemorrhage (superficial, early hemorrhages, hemorrhages into joints)	20–40%	10–20 IU per kg Repeat dose if evidence of further bleeding.
Moderate to major hemorrhage (hemorrhages into muscles, hemorrhages into the oral cavity, definite hemarthroses, known trauma) **Surgery** (minor surgical procedures)	30–60%	15–30 IU per kg Repeat one dose at 12–24 hours if needed.
Major to life-threatening hemorrhage (intracranial, intraabdominal or intrathoracic hemorrhages, gastrointestinal bleeding, central nervous system bleeding, bleeding in the retropharyngeal or retroperitoneal spaces, or iliopsoas sheath) **Fractures** **Head trauma**	80–100%	Initial dose 40-50 IU per kg Repeat dose 20-25 IU per kg every 8-12 hours.
Surgery Major surgical procedures	~100%	Preoperative dose 50 IU/kg Verify ~100% activity prior to surgery. Repeat as necessary after 6 to 12 hours initially, and for 10 to 14 days until healing is complete.

2. After removing the plastic flip-top caps (Fig. A), aseptically cleanse the rubber stoppers of both bottles with alcohol, being careful not to handle the rubber stopper.
3. Remove the protective cover from *one end* of the plastic transfer needle cartridge and penetrate the stopper of the diluent bottle (Fig. B).
4. Remove the remaining portion of the *protective cover*, invert the diluent bottle and penetrate the rubber seal on the concentrate bottle (Fig. C) with the needle at an angle.
[Alternate method of transferring sterile water: With a sterile needle and syringe, withdraw the appropriate volume of diluent and transfer to the bottle of lyophilized concentrate.]
5. The vacuum will draw the diluent into the concentrate bottle. Hold the diluent bottle at an angle to the concentrate bottle in order to direct the jet of diluent against the wall of the concentrate bottle (Fig. C). Avoid excessive foaming.
6. After removing the diluent bottle and transfer needle (Fig. D), swirl until completely dissolved without creating excessive foaming (Fig. E).
7. Re-swab top of reconstituted Helixate FS bottle with alcohol. Allow the stopper to air dry.
8. After the concentrate powder is completely dissolved, withdraw solution into the syringe through the filter needle that is supplied in the package (Fig. F). Replace the filter needle with the administration set provided and inject intravenously. NOTE: Firmly grasp one or both wings to perform venipuncture; do not use the post-use needle shield for this purpose.
9. After infusion, lock post-use needle shield in place using one of the following methods:
   a) One-hand technique: Hold tubing in hand and advance needle shield with thumb and index finger until locked over needle tip (Fig. G).
   b) Two-hand technique: Hold wing stationary and slide needle shield forward with other hand until locked over needle tip (Fig. H).
10. If the same patient is to receive more than one bottle, the contents of two bottles may be drawn into the same syringe through a separate unused filter needle before attaching the vein needle.
11. Parenteral drug products should be inspected visually for particulate matter and discoloration prior to administration, whenever solution and container permit.

Rate of Administration

The rate of administration should be adapted to the response of the individual patient, but administration of the entire dose in 5 to 10 minutes or less is well tolerated.

[See figures A-H in next column]

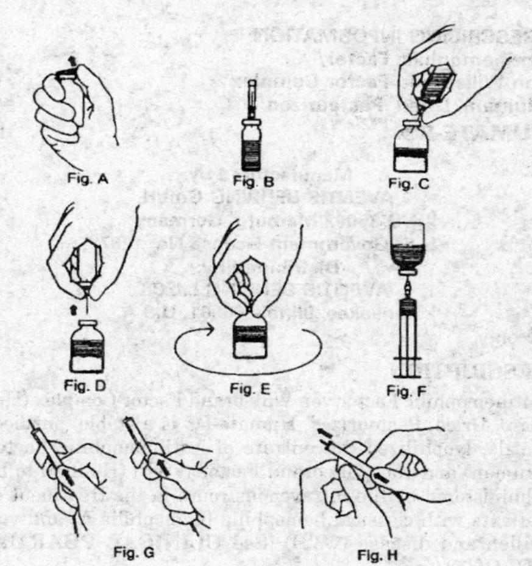

HOW SUPPLIED

Helixate® FS Antihemophilic Factor (Recombinant) is supplied in the following single use bottles. A suitable volume of Sterile Water for Injection, USP, a sterile double-ended transfer needle, a sterile filter needle, and a sterile administration set are provided.

NDC Number	Approximate FVIII Activity (IU)	Diluent (mL)
0053-8130-01	250	2.5
0053-8130-02	500	2.5
0053-8130-04	1000	2.5

STORAGE

Helixate FS should be stored under refrigeration (2–8°C; 36–46°F). Storage of lyophilized powder at room temperature (up to 25°C or 77°F) for 2 months, such as in home treatment situations, may be done. Freezing must be avoided. Do not use beyond the expiration date indicated on the bottle. Protect from extreme exposure to light and store the lyophilized powder in the carton prior to use.

CAUTION

℞ only

Continued on next page

Helixate—Cont.

REFERENCES

1. Lawn RM, Vehar GA: The molecular genetics of hemophilia. *Sci Am* 254(3): 48–54, 1986.
2. Scharrer I, Bray GL, Neutzling O: Incidence of inhibitors in haemophilia A patients - a review of recent studies of recombinant and plasma-derived factor VIII concentrates. *Haemophilia* 5(3): 145–154, 1999.
3. Lusher JM, Arkin S, Abildgaard CF, et al: Recombinant factor VIII for the treatment of previously untreated patients with hemophilia A: safety, efficacy, and development of inhibitors. *N Engl J Med* 328(7): 453–459, 1993.
4. Schwarzinger I, Pabinger I, Korninger C, et al: Incidence of inhibitors in patients with severe and moderate hemophilia A treated with factor VIII concentrates. *Am J Hematol* 24(3): 241–5, 1987.
5. Ehrenforth S, Kreuz W, Scharrer I, et al: Incidence of development of factor VIII and factor IX inhibitors in hemophiliacs. *Lancet* 339(8793): 594–8, 1992.
6. Kasper CK: Complications of hemophilia A treatment: factor VIII inhibitors. *Ann NY Acad Sci* 614:97–105, 1991.
7. Abildgaard CF, Simone JV, Corrigan JJ, et al: Treatment of hemophilia with glycine-precipitated Factor VIII. *N Engl J Med* 275(9): 471–5, 1966.
8. Schwartz RS, Abildgaard CF, Aledort LM, et al: Human recombinant DNA-derived antihemophilic factor (factor VIII) in the treatment of hemophilia A. Recombinant Factor VIII Study Group. *N Engl J Med* 323(26): 1800–5, 1990.
9. White GC 2nd, Courter S, Bray GL, et al: A multicenter study of recombinant factor VIII (Recombinate) in previously treated patients with hemophilia A. The Recombinate Previously Treated Patient Study Group. *Thromb Haemost* 77(4): 660–667, 1997.
10. Nilsson IM, Berntorp E, Löfqvist T, et al: Twenty-five years' experience of prophylactic treatment in severe hemophilia A and B. *J Intern Med* 232(1): 25–32, 1992.

14-7372-210 (Issued June 2000)

Aventis Behring
Manufactured by:
Bayer Corporation
Pharmaceutical Division
Elkhart, IN 46515 USA
U.S. License No. 8
Distributed by:
Aventis Behring L.L.C.
Kankakee, Illinois 60901, USA

PRESCRIBING INFORMATION
Antihemophilic Factor/
von Willebrand Factor Complex
(Human), Dried, Pasteurized
HUMATE-P® ℞

Manufactured by:
AVENTIS BEHRING GmbH
D-35002 Marburg, Germany
U.S. Government License No. 1287
Distributed by:
AVENTIS BEHRING L.L.C.
Kankakee, Illinois 60901, U.S.A.

℞ only

DESCRIPTION

Antihemophilic Factor/von Willebrand Factor Complex (Human), Dried, Pasteurized, Humate-P® is a stable, purified, sterile, lyophilized concentrate of Antihemophilic Factor (Human) and von Willebrand Factor (vWF) (Human) to be administered by the intravenous route in the treatment of patients with classical hemophilia (hemophilia A) and von Willebrand disease (vWD) (See **CLINICAL PHARMACOLOGY**).

Humate-P® is purified from the cold insoluble fraction of pooled human fresh-frozen plasma and contains highly purified and concentrated Antihemophilic Factor/von Willebrand Factor Complex (Human). Humate-P® has a high degree of purity with a low amount of non-factor proteins. Fibrinogen is less than or equal to 0.1 mg/mL. Humate-P® has a higher Factor potency than cryoprecipitate preparations. Each vial of Humate-P® contains the labeled amount of Factor VIII activity in international units. Additionally, each vial of Humate-P® also contains the labeled amount of von Willebrand factor: Ristocetin Cofactor (vWF:RCof) activity expressed in IU (See **DOSAGE AND ADMINISTRATION**). An international unit (IU) is defined by the current international standard established by the World Health Organization. One IU Factor VIII or 1 IU vWF:RCof is approximately equal to the level of Factor VIII or vWF:RCof found in 1.0 mL of fresh-pooled human plasma.

Upon reconstitution with the volume of diluent provided (Sterile Water for Injection, USP), each mL of Humate-P® contains 20 to 40 IU Factor VIII activity, 50 to 100 IU vWF:RCof activity, 15 to 33 mg of glycine, 3.5 to 9.3 mg of sodium citrate, 2 to 5.3 mg of sodium chloride, 4 to 8 mg of Albumin (Human), 1 to 7 mg of other proteins and 5 to 15 mg of total proteins.

This product is prepared from pooled human plasma collected from U.S. licensed facilities in the U.S.

Humate-P® is heat-treated in aqueous solution at 60°C for 10 hours.[1] This pasteurization protocol has been shown *in vitro* to inactivate both enveloped (e.g., Human Immunodeficiency Virus [HIV], Herpes Simplex Virus [HSV-1], Bovine Viral Diarrhea Virus [BVDV], and Cytomegalovirus [CMV]) and non-enveloped (e.g., Poliovirus) viruses. However, no procedure has been shown to be totally effective in removing the risk of viral infectivity from coagulant factor concentrates (See **CLINICAL PHARMACOLOGY** and **WARNINGS**).

Humate-P® has been demonstrated in several studies to contain the high molecular weight multimers of vWF. This component is considered to be important for correcting the coagulation defect in patients with vWD (See **CLINICAL PHARMACOLOGY**).

Humate-P® contains anti-A and anti-B blood group isoagglutinins (see **PRECAUTIONS**).

Viral Reduction Capacity

The pasteurization process (10 hours at 60° C in aqueous solution) used in the manufacture of this concentrate has been shown to inactivate *in vitro* HIV and several model viruses. In each experiment, inactivation to undetectable levels was achieved in considerably less than 10 hours. In replicate studies, HIV was reduced by ≥5.6, ≥6.3 and ≥6.8 $\log_{10}$, respectively, to undetectable levels. In addition to HIV, studies were also performed using three lipid enveloped model viruses (HSV-1, BVDV and CMV), and one non-enveloped virus (Poliovirus). HSV-1 was reduced by ≥5.8, ≥7.2 and ≥7.3 $\log_{10}$, respectively, to undetectable levels in three replicate experiments; BVDV was reduced by ≥4.8 and ≥5.4 $\log_{10}$ to undetectable levels in two replicate experiments; and CMV was reduced by ≥6.0 $\log_{10}$ to an undetectable level in one experiment. In the case of Poliovirus, a non-enveloped virus, reduction by ≥7.1 and ≥7.3 $\log_{10}$ to undetectable levels in two replicate experiments was observed.

The viral reduction capacity of the purification and preparative steps employed in the production of Humate-P®, exclusive of the pasteurization protocol, has also been evaluated in *in vitro* experiments using HIV, HSV-1 and Poliovirus. In duplicate experiments, the mean cumulative reduction capacity for the processing steps evaluated was found to be the following: ≥10.8 $\log_{10}$ for HIV, ≥11.1 $\log_{10}$ for HSV-1 and ≥9.1 $\log_{10}$ for the non-enveloped virus Poliovirus.

The results of the validation studies described above document a mean cumulative total process viral reduction capacity of ≥17.0 $\log_{10}$ for HIV, ≥17.8 $\log_{10}$ for HSV-1 and ≥16.3 $\log_{10}$ for Poliovirus for the manufacturing steps evaluated (inclusive of pasteurization).

In vivo experiments of infectivity on chimpanzees[2] have confirmed the reliability of the manufacturing process, including the pasteurization method, in reducing the risk of transmission of hepatitis. Two chimpanzee studies were used to evaluate the efficacy of the manufacturing process in inactivating experimentally added hepatitis B virus, and one chimpanzee study evaluated the efficacy of the manufacturing process in inactivating experimentally added hepatitis C virus, as represented by agents of non-A, non-B (NANB) hepatitis from the Hutchinson pool.[2] In the first two studies, cryoprecipitate infected with hepatitis B virus, to yield a concentration of 3000 infectious units/mL, was injected into chimpanzees followed for six months or longer. All chimpanzees injected with either cryoprecipitate (n=4) or non-pasteurized Antihemophilic Factor/von Willebrand Factor Complex (Human) (n=4) developed hepatitis B markers (HBsAg, Anti-HBs, Anti-HBc). None of the seven chimpanzees injected with the pasteurized product became sero-positive. In an equivalent study of hepatitis C that utilized agents of NANB hepatitis from the Hutchinson pool[2] as the viral inoculum, four chimpanzees injected with pasteurized Antihemophilic Factor/von Willebrand Factor Complex (Human) product consistently remained serologically negative.

CLINICAL PHARMACOLOGY

General

The Antihemophilic Factor/vWF complex consists of two different noncovalently bound proteins (Factor VIII and von Willebrand factor). Factor VIII is an essential cofactor in activation of Factor X leading ultimately to formation of thrombin and fibrin. The vWF promotes platelet aggregation and platelet adhesion on damaged vascular endothelium; it also serves as a stabilizing carrier protein for the procoagulant protein Factor VIII.[3,4] The activity of vWF is measured as vWF:RCof.

Pharmacokinetics in Hemophilia A

After intravenous injection of Antihemophilic Factor/von Willebrand Factor Complex (Human), Dried, Pasteurized, Humate-P® in humans, there is a rapid increase of plasma Factor VIII activity (FVIII:C) followed by a rapid decrease in activity and a subsequent slower rate of decrease in activity. Studies with Humate-P® in hemophilic patients have demonstrated a mean half-life of 12.2 hours (range: 8.4 to 17.4 hours).

Pharmacokinetics in von Willebrand disease

Humate-P® has been demonstrated in several studies to contain the high-molecular-weight multimers of vWF. This component is reported to be important for correcting the coagulation defect in patients with vWD.[5-9]

When administered to patients with vWD (types 1, 2 [A, B, C], or 3)[13], bleeding time decreased.[6, 9, 10, 11, 12] This effect was correlated with the presence of a multimeric composition of vWF similar to that found in normal plasma.[6,8,9,10,12]

The pharmacokinetics of Humate-P® have been evaluated in 8 vWD patients [type 1, n=1; type 2, n=1; type 2A, n=4; type 3, n=2] in the non-bleeding state. The median half-life of vWF:RCof was 10.3 hours (range: 6.4 to 13.3 hours.) The median *in vivo* recovery for vWF:RCof activity was 1.89 (IU/dL)/(IU/kg) [range: 1.10 to 2.74 (IU/dL)/(IU/kg)]. In all patients, the administration of Humate-P® resulted in a transient shortening of the bleeding time. Humate-P® was effective in improving the vWF multimer pattern in vWD patients and in most cases this improvement was sustained through 22 to 26 hours postinfusion.

Clinical Studies

Clinical efficacy of Humate-P® in the control of bleeding in patients with vWD was determined by a retrospective review of clinical safety and efficacy data obtained from 97 Canadian vWD patients who were provided with product under an Emergency Drug Release Program. Dosage schedule and duration of therapy were determined by the judgment of the medical practitioner.

There were 514 requests for product use for surgery, bleeding or prophylaxis in the 97 Canadian patients. Of these, product was not used in 151 cases, and follow-up safety and/or efficacy information was available for 303 (83%) of the remaining 363 requests. In many cases, product from one request was used for several treatment courses in one patient. Therefore, there are more reported treatment courses than requests.

Humate-P® was administered to 97 patients, in 530 treatment courses: 73 for surgery, 344 for treatment of bleeding and 20 for prophylaxis of bleeding. For 93 "other" uses, the majority involved dental procedures, diagnostic procedures, prophylaxis prior to a procedure, or a test dose.

A summary of the number of patients and bleeding episodes treated, by vWD type, and corresponding efficacy rating is provided in Table 1. The efficacy rating was excellent/good in 100% of bleeding episodes treated in type 1, 2A and 2B patients. In type 3 patients, 95% of the bleeding episodes were rated as excellent/good and a poor (or no) response was observed in the remaining 5% of bleeding episodes treated.

[See table 1 below]

For pediatric patients a summary of the number of patients and bleeding episodes treated, by vWD type, and corresponding efficacy rating is provided in Table 2. The efficacy rating was excellent/good in 100% of bleeding episodes treated in infants (types 2A, 3), children (types 1, 2A, 2B) and adolescents (types 1, 2B). In type 3 children and adolescents, 90% and 96% of the bleeding episodes were rated as excellent/good and a poor/none response was observed in the remaining 10% and 4% of the bleeding episodes, respectively.

[See 2 table on next page]

The dosing information (all patients) for bleeding events is summarized in Table 3.

[See table 3 on next page]

Clinical evidence of the viral safety of Humate-P® was obtained in additional studies. In one study, all evaluable patients (31 of 67) who received Humate-P® remained HBs-antigen negative. None of the 31 patients developed hepatitis B infection or showed clinical signs of NANB hepatitis infection.[14]

In an additional study, a total of 32 lots of Humate-P® were administered to a cohort of 26 hemophilic or vWD patients who had not previously received any blood products. Markers for hepatitis B virus and liver enzymes (ALT and AST) were tested at regular intervals as recommended by the International Committee on Thrombosis and Hemostasis. The study showed no significant elevation in liver enzyme levels over an observation period ranging from 2 months to 12 months. The 10 patients not previously vaccinated remained seronegative for markers of hepatitis B infection as well as for markers of infection with hepatitis A virus, CMV, Epstein-Barr virus and HIV. No patient developed any signs of an infectious disease.[15]

In a retrospective study, all 155 patients evaluated remained negative for the presence of HIV-1 antibody for time periods ranging from four months to nine years from initial administration of product. Sixty-seven of these patients were also tested for HIV-2 antibodies and all remained seronegative.[16]

Table 1: Summary of efficacy for bleeding episodes – all patients

	Diagnosis							
	Type 1 vWD		Type 2A vWD		Type 2B vWD		Type 3 vWD	
NUMBER OF PATIENTS	13		2		10		21	
Excellent/good Poor/none	13 —	100 % —	2 —	100 % —	10 —	100 % —	18 3	86 % 14 %
NUMBER OF EVENTS	32		17		60		208	
Excellent/good Poor/none	32 —	100 % —	17 —	100 % —	60 —	100 % —	198 10	95 % 5 %

INDICATIONS AND USAGE

Antihemophilic Factor/von Willebrand Factor Complex (Human), Dried, Pasteurized, Humate-P® is indicated (1) in adult patients for treatment and prevention of bleeding in hemophilia A (classical hemophilia) and (2) in adult and pediatric patients for treatment of spontaneous and trauma-induced bleeding episodes in severe von Willebrand disease, and in mild and moderate von Willebrand disease where use of desmopressin is known or suspected to be inadequate.

Controlled clinical trials to evaluate the safety and efficacy of prophylactic dosing with Humate-P® to prevent spontaneous bleeding and to prevent excessive bleeding related to surgery have not been evaluated in von Willebrand disease patients. Adequate data are not presently available on which to evaluate or to base dosing recommendations in either of these settings.

CONTRAINDICATIONS

None known.

WARNINGS

Antihemophilic Factor/von Willebrand Factor Complex (Human), Dried, Pasteurized, Humate-P® is made from human plasma. Products made from human plasma may contain infectious agents, such as viruses, that can cause disease. The risk that such products will transmit an infectious agent has been reduced by screening plasma donors for prior exposure to certain viruses, by testing for the presence of certain current viral infections and by inactivating and/or removing certain viruses during manufacture (see **DESCRIPTION** section for viral reduction measures). The manufacturing procedure for Humate-P® includes processing steps designed to reduce further the risk of viral transmission. Stringent procedures, utilized at plasma collection centers, plasma testing laboratories, and fractionation facilities are designed to reduce the risk of viral transmission. The primary viral reduction step of the Humate-P® manufacturing process is the heat treatment of the purified, stabilized aqueous solution at 60.0 +/- 1° C for 10 hours. In addition, the purification procedure (several precipitation steps) used in the manufacture of Humate-P® also provides viral reduction capacity. Despite these measures, such products may still potentially contain human pathogenic agents, including those not yet known or identified. Thus the risk of transmission of infectious agents cannot be totally eliminated. Any infections thought by a physician possibly to have been transmitted by this product should be reported by the physician or other healthcare provider to Aventis Behring at 800-504-5434 (in the U.S. and Canada). The physician should discuss the risks and benefits of this product with the patient.

PRECAUTIONS

It is important to determine that the coagulation disorder is caused by factor VIII or vWF deficiency, since no benefit in treating other deficiencies can be expected.

This Antihemophilic Factor/von Willebrand Factor (Human), Dried, Pasteurized, Humate-P® preparation contains blood group isoagglutinins (anti-A and anti-B). When very large or frequently repeated doses are needed, as when inhibitors are present or when pre- and post- surgical care is involved, patients of blood groups A, B and AB should be monitored for signs of intravascular hemolysis and decreasing hematocrit values and be treated appropriately as required.

The replacement therapy should be monitored with the aid of coagulation tests, especially in cases of major surgery.

Other precautions are as follows:

- The sterile filter spike should only be used to transfer solution from the preparation vial to a syringe or infusion bottle or bag. The sterile filter spike must not be used for injection.
- The administration equipment and any unused Humate-P® should be discarded.

Pregnancy Category C

Animal reproduction studies have not been conducted with Antihemophilic Factor/von Willebrand Factor (Human). It is also not known whether Humate-P® can cause fetal harm when administered to a pregnant woman or can affect reproduction capacity. Humate-P® should be given to a pregnant woman only if clearly needed.

Pediatric Use

Adequate and well-controlled studies with long term evaluation of joint damage have not been done in pediatric patients. Joint damage may result from suboptimal treatment of hemarthroses. For immediate control of bleeding for Hemophilia A, the general recommendations for dosing and administration for adults, found in the **DOSAGE AND ADMINISTRATION**, section may be referenced.

The safety and effectiveness of Humate-P® for the treatment of von Willebrand's disease was demonstrated in 26 pediatric patients, including infants, children and adolescents but has not yet been evaluated in neonates. As in adults, pediatric patients should be dosed based upon weight (kg) in accordance to information in the **DOSAGE AND ADMINISTRATION** section.

Information for Patients - Some viruses, such as parvovirus B19 or hepatitis A, are particularly difficult to remove or inactivate at this time. Parvovirus B19 may most seriously affect pregnant women, or immune-compromised individuals.

Although the overwhelming number of hepatitis A and parvovirus B19 cases are community acquired, there have been reports of these infections associated with the use of some plasma-derived products. Therefore, physicians should be alert to the potential symptoms of parvovirus B19 and hepatitis A infections and inform patients under their supervision receiving plasma-derived products to report potential symptoms promptly.

Symptoms of parvovirus B19 may include low-grade fever, rash, arthralgias and transient symmetric, nondestructive arthritis. Diagnosis is often established by measuring B19 specific IgM and IgG antibodies. Symptoms of hepatitis A include low grade fever, anorexia, nausea, vomiting, fatigue and jaundice. A diagnosis may be established by determination of specific IgM antibodies.

ADVERSE REACTIONS

Antihemophilic Factor/von Willebrand Factor (Human), Dried, Pasteurized, Humate-P® is usually tolerated without reaction. Rare cases of allergic reaction and rise in temperature have been observed. Anaphylactic reactions can occur in rare instances. If allergic/anaphylactic reactions occur, the infusion should be discontinued and appropriate treatment given as required.

In some cases, inhibitors of Factor VIII may occur.

Allergic symptoms, including allergic reaction, urticaria, chest tightness, rash, pruritus, and edema, were reported in 6 of 97 (6%) of patients in a Canadian retrospective study. Two of 97 (2%) experienced other adverse events that were considered to have a possible or probable relationship to the product. These included chills, phlebitis, vasodilatation, and paresthesia. All adverse events were mild or moderate in intensity.

DOSAGE AND ADMINISTRATION

GENERAL - Physicians should strongly consider administration of hepatitis A and hepatitis B vaccines to individuals receiving plasma derivatives. Potential risks and benefits of vaccination should be carefully weighed by the physician and discussed with the patient.

Antihemophilic Factor/von Willebrand Factor (Human), Dried, Pasteurized, Humate-P® is for intravenous administration only.

Each vial of Humate-P® contains the labeled amount of Factor VIII activity in IU for the treatment of hemophilia A. Additionally, each vial of Humate-P® also contains vWF:RCof activity in IU for the treatment of vWD.

THERAPY FOR HEMOPHILIA A - As a general rule, 1 IU of Factor VIII activity per kg body weight will increase the circulating Factor VIII level by approximately 2 IU/dL. Adequacy of treatment must be judged by the clinical effects; thus, the dosage may vary with individual cases. Although dosage must be individualized according to the needs of the patient (weight, severity of hemorrhage, presence of inhibitors), the following general dosages are recommended for adult patients: [After 17]

[See table 4 at top of next page]

In all cases, the dose should be adjusted individually by clinical judgement of the potential for compromise of a vital structure, and by frequent monitoring of factor VIII activity in the patient's plasma.

Pediatric Use for Hemophilia A:

See **PRECAUTIONS**.

THERAPY FOR VON WILLEBRAND DISEASE - The dosage should be adjusted according to the extent and location of bleeding. As a rule, 40-80 IU vWF:RCof (corresponding to 16 to 32 IU factor VIII in Humate-P®) per kg body weight are given every 8 to 12 hours. Repeat doses are administered for as long as needed based on repeat monitoring of appropriate clinical and laboratory measures. Expected levels of vWF:RCof are based on an expected *in vivo* recovery of 1.5 IU/dL rise per IU/kg vWF:RCof administered. The administration of 1 IU of Factor VIII per kg body weight can be expected to lead to a rise in circulating vWF:RCof of approximately 3.5 to 4 IU/dL. The following table provides dosing guidelines for adult patients. [After 18]

[See table 5 on next page]

Table 2: Summary of efficacy for bleeding episodes – pediatric patients

	Diagnosis							
	Type 1 vWD		Type 2A wWD		Type 2B vWB		Type 3 vWD	
NUMBER OF PATIENTS	4		2		5		12	
Excellent/good Poor/none	4	100%	2	100%	5 —	100%	9 3	75% 25%
NUMBER OF EVENTS	8		17		22		138	
Excellent/good Poor/none	8 —	100% —	17 —	100% —	22 —	100% —	128 10	93% 7%

Table 3: Summary of dosing information for bleeding events

		Type/location				
		Digestive System	Nose + Mouth + Pharynx	Integument System	Female Genital System	Musculo-skeletal
No. of Patients		14	29	11	4	22
Loading Dose (IU vWF:RCof/kg)	Loading Doses[1]	37	127	22	7	107
	Mean	62.1	66.9	73.4	88.5	50.2
	SD	31.1	24.3	37.7	28.3	24.9
Maintenance Dose (IU vWF:RCof/kg)	Maintenance Doses[1]	250	55	4	15	121
	Mean	61.5	67.5	56.5	74.5	63.8
	SD	38.0	22.4	63.3	17.7	28.8
No. of Treatment Days per Event	No. of Events	49	130	22	9	108
	Mean	4.6	1.4	1.1	2.8	2.0
	SD	3.6	1.2	0.4	2.9	1.9
No. of Infusions/day						
Day 1	No. of Patients	14	29	11	4	22
Day 1	No. of Events	49	130	22	9	108
	Mean (# of infusions)	1.2	1.1	1.0	1.0	1.0
	SD	0.4	0.2	0.2	0.0	0.1
Day 2	No. of Patients	13	9	3	1	15
Day 2	No. of Events	41	12	3	1	26
	Mean (# of infusions)	1.2	1.3	1.0	1.0	1.2
	SD	0.6	0.5	0.0	—	0.5
Day 3	No. of Patients	12	6	—	2	10
Day 3	No. of Events	25	9	—	3	18
	Mean (# of infusions)	1.5	1.4	—	1.0	1.2
	SD	0.8	0.7	—	0.0	0.4

Day 1 = First treatment day ([1] Number of infusions where the dose per kg body weight was available)

Continued on next page

Humate-P—Cont.

Reconstitution

1. Warm both diluent and Humate-P® in unopened vials to room temperature [not above 37°C (98°F)].
2. Remove caps from both vials to expose central portions of the rubber stoppers.
3. Treat surface of rubber stoppers with the alcohol swab provided and allow to dry.
4. Using aseptic technique, pierce the double needle of the transfer set into the diluent vial. Remove the protective cap and insert the exposed (longer) needle into the upright Humate-P® vial. The diluent will be transferred into the Humate-P® by vacuum.
5. Remove the diluent vial, and the transfer set and discard.
6. Gently rotate the vial. DO NOT SHAKE VIAL. Vigorous shaking will prolong the reconstitution time. Continue swirling until the powder is dissolved and the solution is ready for administration. To assure product sterility, Humate-P® should be administered within three hours after reconstitution.
7. Parenteral drug products should be inspected visually for particulate matter and discoloration prior to administration, whenever solution and container permit.

Administration

INTRAVENOUS INJECTION

Plastic disposable syringes are recommended for administration of Humate-P® solution. The ground glass surface of all-glass syringes tend to adhere protein solutions of this type.

Use sterile technique, for the following steps:

1. Remove the paper cover from the package containing the disposable filter spike. Attach the filter spike to a sterile disposable syringe and take the filter spike out of the package.
2. Remove the protective cap and - without touching the tip of the filter spike - insert the disposable filter spike into the stopper of the Humate-P® vial; inject air.
3. Draw up the solution slowly (when using several syringes leave the filter spike in the vial). Separate the syringe from the filter spike and attach the syringe to an infusion kit or a suitable injection needle. Discard the filter spike.
4. Slowly inject the solution (maximally 4 mL/minute) intravenously with an infusion kit or with a suitable injection needle.

HOW SUPPLIED

Antihemophilic Factor/von Willebrand Factor Complex (Human), Dried, Pasteurized, Humate-P® is supplied in a single dose vial with a vial of diluent (Sterile Water for Injection, USP), a sterile transfer set for reconstitution, a sterile filter spike for withdrawal and alcohol swabs. International unit activity of Factor VIII and vWF:RCof is stated on the carton and label of each vial.

STORAGE

When stored at refrigerator temperature, 2 - 8°C (36 - 46°F), Antihemophilic Factor/von Willebrand Factor Complex (Human), Dried, Pasteurized, Humate-P® is stable for the period indicated by the expiration date on its label. Within this period, Humate-P® may be stored at room temperature not to exceed 30°C (86°F), for up to six months. Avoid freezing, which may damage the diluent container.

Table 4: Dosage recommendations for the treatment of Hemophilia A

Hemorrhagic event	Dosage (IU FVIII:C/kg body weight)
Minor hemorrhage: • Early joint or muscle bleed • Severe epistaxis	Loading dose 15 IU FVIII:C/kg to achieve FVIII:C plasma level of approximately 30% of normal; one infusion may be sufficient. If needed, half of the loading dose may be given once or twice daily for 1 - 2 days
Moderate hemorrhage: • Advanced joint or muscle bleed • Neck, tongue or pharyngeal hematoma (without airway compromise) • Tooth extraction • Severe abdominal pain	Loading dose 25 IU FVIII:C/kg to achieve FVIII:C plasma level of approximately 50% of normal, followed by 15 IU FVIII:C/kg every 8 - 12 hours for first 1 - 2 days to maintain FVIII:C plasma level at 30% of normal, and then the same dose once or twice a day for a total of up to 7 days, or until adequate wound healing
Life-threatening hemorrhage: • Major operations • Gastrointestinal bleeding • Neck, tongue or pharyngeal hematoma with potential for airway compromise • Intracranial, intraabdominal or intrathoracic bleeding • Fractures	Initially 40 to 50 IU FVIII:C/kg, followed by 20 - 25 IU FVIII:C/kg every 8 hours to maintain FVIII:C plasma level at 80 - 100% of normal for 7 days, then continue the same dose once or twice a day for another 7 days in order to maintain the FVIII:C level at 30 - 50% of normal

Table 5: Dosing recommendations for the treatment of von Willebrand disease

Classification of vWD	Hemorrhage	Dosage (IU vWF:RCof/kg body weight)
Type 1 • mild, if desmopressin is inappropriate (Baseline vWF:RCoF activity typically >30%)	Major (e.g. severe or refractory epistaxis, GI bleeding, CNS trauma, or traumatic hemorrhage)	Loading dose 40 to 60 IU/kg, then 40 to 50 IU/kg every 8 to 12 hours for 3 days to keep the nadir level of vWF:RCof >50%; then 40 to 50 IU/kg daily for a total of up to 7 days of treatment
• moderate or severe (Baseline vWF:RCoF activity typically <30%)	Minor (e.g. epistaxis, oral bleeding, menorrhagia)	40 to 50 IU/kg (1 or 2 doses)
	Major (e.g. severe or refractory epistaxis, GI bleeding, CNS trauma, hemarthrosis or traumatic hemorrhage	Loading dose 50 to 75 IU/kg, then 40 to 60 IU/kg every 8 to 12 hours for 3 days to keep the nadir level of vWF:RCof >50%; then 40 to 60 IU/kg daily for a total of up to 7 days of treatment. Factor VIII:C levels should be monitored and maintained according to the guidelines for hemophilia A therapy, Table 4
Types 2 (all variants) and 3	Minor (clinical indications above)	40 to 50 IU/kg (1 or 2 doses)
	Major (clinical indications above)	Loading dose of 60 to 80 IU/kg, then 40 to 60 IU/kg every 8 to 12 hours for 3 days to keep the nadir level of vWF:RCof >50%, then 40 to 60 IU/kg daily for a total of up to 7 days of treatment Factor VIII:C levels should be monitored and maintained according to the guidelines for hemophilia A therapy, Table 4

REFERENCES

1. Heimburger N, Schwinn H, Gratz P, *et al.* Factor VIII Concentrate-highly purified and heated in solution. *Arzneim Forsch* 31(1): 619–22, 1981.
2. Mauler R, Merkle W, Hilfenhaus, J. Inactivation of HTLV-III/LAV, Hepatitis B and Non-A/Non-B Viruses by Pasteurization in Human Plasma Protein Preparations. *Develop. biol. Standard.*, 67: 337–351, 1987.
3. Hoyer LW. The Factor VIII complex: Structure and function. *Blood* 58: 1–13, 1981.
4. Meyer D, and Girma J-P. von Willebrand factor: Structure and function. *Thromb Haemostas.* 70:99–104, 1993.
5. Berntorp E, Nilsson IM. Biochemical and *in vivo* properties of commercial virus-inactivated factor VIII concentrates. *Eur J Haematol.* 40: 205–214, 1988.
6. Berntorp E, and Nilsson IM: Use of a high-purity Factor VIII Concentrate (Humate-P) in von Willebrand disease. *Vox Sang* 56: 212–217, 1989.
7. Mannucci PM, Tenconi PM, Castaman G, Rodeghiero F. Comparison of four virus-inactivated plasma concentrates for treatment of severe von Willebrand disease: A cross-over randomized trial. *Blood* 79: 3130–3137, 1992.
8. Berntorp E. Plasma product treatment in various types of von Willebrand's disease. *Haemostasis* 24: 289–297, 1994.
9. Scharrer I, Vigh T, Aygörn-Pürsün E. Experience with Haemate-P in von Willebrand's disease in adults. *Haemostasis* 24: 298–303, 1994.
10. Fukui H, Nishino M, Terada S, et al: Hemostatic effect of 2 heat-treated factor VIII concentrate (Haemate-P) in von Willebrand disease. *Blut* 56: 171–178, 1988.
11. Rose E, Forster A and Aledort LM: Correction of prolonged bleeding time in von Willebrand's disease with Humate-P®. *Transfusion* 30(4): 381, 1990.
12. Kreuz W, Mentzer D, Becker S, Scharrer I, Kornhuber B. Haemate P in children with von Willebrand's disease. *Haemostasis* 24: 304–310, 1994.
13. Sadler JE. For the Subcommittee on von Willebrand Factor of the Scientific and Standardization Committee of the International Society on Thrombosis and Haemostasis. *Thrombosis and Hemostasis* 71(4): 520–525, 1994.
14. Heimburger N, Karges HE, Mauler R, Nováková-Banet A, Hilfenhaus J, Wiedmann E. Factor VIII concentrate: Hepatitis-safe preparation, virus inactivation and clinical experience. *Proc. 4th Int. Symp. Hemophilia Treatment*, Tokyo 1984, pp. 107–115.
15. Schimpf K, *et al*: Absence of hepatitis after treatment with a pasteurized Factor VIII concentrate in patients with hemophilia and no previous transfusions. *New Engl J Med* 316: 918 - 922, 1987.
16. Schimpf K, *et al*: Absence of anti-human immunodeficiency virus types 1 and 2 seroconversion after treatment of hemophilia or von Willebrand disease with pasteurized Factor VIII concentrates. *New Engl J Med* 321: 1148 - 1152, 1989.
17. Levine PH, Brettler DB. Clinical aspects and therapy for hemophilia A. In: Hoffman R, Benz JB, Shattil SJ, Furie B, Cohen HJ, eds. *Hematology - Basic Principles and Practice*, Churchill Livingstone Inc.; 1991, pp.1296–1297.
18. Scott JP, Montgomery RT. Therapy of von Willebrand Disease. *Seminars in Thrombosis and Hemostasis* 19(1): 37–47, 1993.

Revised: February 1999 OBKC G46 00450 (11829)

PRESCRIBING INFORMATION

ANTIHEMOPHILIC FACTOR (HUMAN) ℞
MONOCLATE-P®
FACTOR VIII:C PASTEURIZED, MONOCLONAL ANTIBODY PURIFIED

℞ only

DESCRIPTION

Antihemophilic Factor (Human), Monoclate-P®, Factor VIII:C Pasteurized, Monoclonal Antibody Purified, is a sterile, stable, lyophilized concentrate of Factor VIII:C with reduced amounts of vWf:Ag and purified of extraneous plasma-derived protein by use of affinity chromatography. A murine monoclonal antibody to vWf:Ag is used as an affinity ligand to first isolate the Factor VIII Complex. Factor VIII:C is then dissociated from vWf:Ag, recovered, formulated and provided as a sterile lyophilized powder.[1,2,3] The concentrate as formulated contains Albumin (Human) as a stabilizer, resulting in a concentrate with a specific activity between 5 and 10 units/mg of total protein. In the absence of this added Albumin (Human) stabilizer, specific activity has been determined to exceed 3000 units/mg of protein.[4] Monoclate-P® has been prepared from pooled human plasma and is intended for use in therapy of classical hemophilia (hemophilia A).

The plasma used in the manufacture of this product has been tested and found negative for HBV, HCV, and HIV-1 by an investigational test procedure referred to as Nucleic Acid Testing (NAT) using Polymerase Chain Reaction (PCR) Technology. Investigational testing is being performed to determine the effectiveness of NAT to detect low levels of viral material. The significance of a negative result is unknown since the effectiveness of the test has not been established.

This concentrate has been pasteurized by heating at 60°C for 10 hours in aqueous solution form during its manufacture in order to further reduce the risk of viral transmission.[5] However, no procedure has been shown to be totally effective in removing viral infectivity from coagulant factor concentrates. (See **CLINICAL PHARMACOLOGY** and **WARNINGS**.)

Monoclate-P® is a highly purified preparation of Factor VIII:C. When stored as directed, it will maintain its labeled potency for the period indicated on the container and package labels.[8,9]

Upon reconstitution, a clear, colorless solution is obtained, containing 50 to 150 times as much Factor VIII:C as does an equal volume of plasma.

Each vial contains the labeled amount of antihemophilic factor (AHF) activity as expressed in terms of International Units of antihemophilic activity. One unit of antihemophilic activity is equivalent to that quantity of AHF present in one mL of normal human plasma. When reconstituted as recommended, the resulting solution contains approximately 300 to 450 millimoles of sodium ions per liter and has 2 to 3 times the tonicity of saline. It contains approximately 2–5 millimoles of calcium ions per liter, contributed as calcium chloride, approximately 1 to 2% Albumin (Human), 0.8% mannitol, and 1.2 mM histidine. The pH is adjusted with hydrochloric acid and/or sodium hydroxide. Monoclate-P® also contains trace amounts (≤ 50 ng per 100 I.U. of AHF) of the murine monoclonal antibody used in its purification (see **CLINICAL PHARMACOLOGY**).

Monoclate-P® is to be administered only intravenously.

CLINICAL PHARMACOLOGY

Factor VIII:C is the coagulant portion of the Factor VIII complex circulating in plasma. It is noncovalently associated with the von Willebrand protein responsible for von Willebrand factor activity. These two proteins have distinct biochemical and immunological properties and are under separate genetic control. Factor VIII:C acts as a cofactor for Factor IX to activate Factor X in the intrinsic pathway of blood coagulation.[6] Hemophilia A, a hereditary disorder of blood coagulation due to decreased levels of Factor VIII:C, results in profuse bleeding into joints, muscles or internal organs as a result of a trauma. Antihemophilic Factor (Human), Monoclate-P®, Factor VIII:C Pasteurized, Monoclonal Antibody Purified, provides an increase in plasma levels of AHF, thereby enabling temporary correction of hemophilia A bleeding.

Clinical evaluation of Monoclate-P®, Factor VIII:C Pasteurized, Monoclonal Antibody Purified concentrate for its half-life characteristics in hemophilic patients showed it to be comparable to other commercially available Antihemophilic Factor (Human) concentrates. The mean half-life obtained from six patients was 17.5 hours with a mean recovery of 1.9 units/dL rise/U/kg.

The pasteurization process used in the manufacture of this concentrate has demonstrated *in vitro* inactivation of human immunodeficiency virus (HIV) and several model viruses. In two separate studies, HIV was reduced by $\geq$7.0 $\log_{10}$ to an undetectable level and by 10.5 $\log_{10}$, respectively. In addition to HIV, studies were also performed using three lipid containing model viruses and one non-lipid, encapsulated model virus. Vesicular stomatitis (VSV) was reduced by $\geq$6.79 $\log_{10}$ to undetectable, Sindbis was reduced by $\geq$6.48 $\log_{10}$ to undetectable and Vaccinia was reduced by $\geq$5.36 $\log_{10}$ to undetectable. Murine encephalomyocarditis (EMC), a non-lipid, encapsulated model virus, was reduced by $\geq$7.1 $\log_{10}$ to undetectable.

Evidence of the capability of the purification and preparative steps used in the production of Antihemophilic Factor (Human), Monoclate-P®, Factor VIII:C Pasteurized, Monoclonal Antibody Purified to reduce viral bioburden was obtained in studies involving the addition of known quantities of virus to cryoprecipitate. These studies were conducted using an earlier form of the concentrate which had not undergone liquid pasteurization (Antihemophilic Factor (Human), Monoclate®, Monoclonal Antibody Purified, Factor VIII:C, Heat-Treated). These studies provide evidence of the viral removal potential of the purification and preparative steps of the manufacturing process (exclusive of heat treatment) which are common to both concentrates. In one study, the viruses used were human immunodeficiency virus (HIV), Sindbis virus, vesicular stomatitis virus (VSV) and pseudorabies virus (PsRV). A comparison of the cumulative mean reductions for all viruses tested with the individual values obtained in each experiment indicates that the combined effects of the manufacturing steps, which purify the Factor VIII:C and prepare the concentrate in a final sterile container as a lyophilized powder, contribute viral reduction capabilities of approximately 5 to 6 logs. In a separate study, aluminum hydroxide treatment followed by antibody affinity chromatography reduced vaccinia virus infectivity by 4.81 logs. These studies indicate that the purification and preparative steps of the manufacturing process are capable of providing a non-specific, viral reduction of approximately 5 to 6 logs, independent of the pasteurization process.

Monoclate-P® contains trace amounts of mouse protein[7] ($\leq$ 50 ng per 100 I.U. of AHF). In a study using an earlier form of the concentrate which had not undergone pasteurization (Monoclate®), a number of patients seronegative for Anti-HIV-1 were monitored to determine whether they would develop antibody or experience adverse reactions as a result of repeated exposure. These patients were treated on multiple occasions. Pre-study serum measurements of 27 patients for human anti-mouse lgG showed that, prior to treatment, 6 of them had either detectable antibody to mouse proteins or cross-reactive proteins. These patients continued to demonstrate similar or lower antibody levels during the study. Of the remaining 21 patients, 6 were shown to have low antibody levels on one or more occasions. In no case was observance of low antibody level associated with an anamnestic response or with any clinical adverse reaction. Patients were observed for time periods ranging from 2 to 30 months.

INDICATIONS AND USAGE

Antihemophilic Factor (Human), Monoclate-P®, Factor VIII:C Pasteurized, Monoclonal Antibody Purified is indicated for treatment of classical hemophilia (hemophilia A). Affected individuals frequently require therapy following minor accidents. Surgery, when required in such individuals, must be preceded by temporary corrections of the clotting abnormality. Presurgical correction of severe AHF deficiency can be accomplished with a small volume of Monoclate-P®.

Monoclate-P® is not effective in controlling the bleeding of patients with von Willebrand's disease.

CONTRAINDICATIONS

Known hypersensitivity to mouse protein is a contraindication to Antihemophilic Factor (Human), Monoclate-P®, Factor VIII:C Pasteurized, Monoclonal Antibody Purified.

WARNINGS

This product is prepared from pooled human plasma which may contain the causative agents of hepatitis and other viral diseases. Prescribed manufacturing procedures utilized at the plasma collection centers, plasma testing laboratories, and the fractionation facilities are designed to reduce the risk of transmitting viral infection. However, the risk of viral infectivity from this product cannot be totally eliminated. Accordingly, the benefits and risks of treatment with this concentrate should be carefully assessed prior to use.

Individuals who receive infusions of blood or plasma products may develop signs and/or symptoms of some viral infections, particularly nonA, nonB hepatitis.

Number of AHF I.U. Required	=	Body weight (in kg)	×	desired Factor VIII increase (% normal)	×	0.5[10]

PRECAUTIONS

General—Most Antihemophilic Factor (Human) concentrates contain naturally occurring blood group specific antibodies. However, the processing of Monoclate-P® significantly reduces the presence of blood group specific antibodies in the final product. Nevertheless, when large or frequently repeated doses of product are needed, patients should be monitored by means of hematocrit and direct Coombs tests for signs of progressive anemia.

Formation of Antibodies to Mouse Protein - Although no hypersensitivity reactions have been observed, because Monoclate-P® contains trace amounts of mouse protein ($\leq$ 50 ng per 100 I.U. of AHF), the possibility exists that patients treated with Monoclate-P® may develop hypersensitivity to the mouse proteins.

Information For Patients - Patients should be informed of the early signs of hypersensitivity reactions including hives, generalized urticaria, tightness of the chest, wheezing, hypotension, and anaphylaxis, and should be advised to discontinue use of the concentrate and contact their physician if these symptoms occur.

Pregnancy Category C - Animal reproduction studies have not been conducted with Antihemophilic Factor (Human), Monoclate-P®, Factor VIII:C Pasteurized, Monoclonal Antibody Purified. It is also not known whether Monoclate-P® can cause fetal harm when administered to a pregnant woman or can affect reproduction capacity. Monoclate-P® should be given to a pregnant woman only if clearly needed.

GERIATRIC USE

Clinical studies of Monoclate-P® did not include sufficient numbers of subjects aged 65 and over to determine whether they respond differently from younger subjects. Other reported clinical experience has not identified differences in responses between the elderly and younger patients. In general, dose selection for an elderly patient should be cautious, reflecting the greater frequency of decreased hepatic, renal, or cardiac function, and of concomitant disease or other drug therapy. Dosing should be appropriate to the clinical situation.

ADVERSE REACTIONS

Products of this type are known to cause allergic reactions, mild chills, nausea or stinging at the infusion site.

DOSAGE AND ADMINISTRATION

Antihemophilic Factor (Human), Monoclate-P®, Factor VIII:C Pasteurized, Monoclonal Antibody Purified is for intravenous administration only. As a general rule 1 unit of AHF activity per kg will increase the circulating AHF level by 2%.[10] The following formula provides a guide of dosage calculations:

[See table above]

Although dosage must be individualized according to the needs of the patient (weight, severity of hemorrhage, presence of inhibitors), the following general dosages are suggested.[11]

1. MILD HEMORRHAGES - Minor hemorrhagic episodes will generally subside with a single infusion if a level of 30% or more is attained.
2. MODERATE HEMORRHAGE AND MINOR SURGERY - For more serious hemorrhages and minor surgical procedures, the patient's Factor VIII level should be raised to 30-50% of normal, which usually requires an initial dose of 15-25 I.U. per kg. If further therapy is required a maintenance dose is 10-15 I.U. per kg every 8 - 12 hours.
3. SEVERE HEMORRHAGE - In hemorrhages near vital organs (neck, throat, subperitoneal) it may be desirable to raise the Factor VIII level to 80-100% of normal which can be achieved with an initial dose of 40-50 I.U. per kg and a maintenance dose of 20-25 I.U. per kg every 8 - 12 hours.
4. MAJOR SURGERY - For surgical procedures a dose of AHF sufficient to achieve a level 80-100% of normal should be given an hour prior to surgery. A second dose, half the size of the priming dose, should be given five hours after the first dose. Factor VIII levels should be maintained at a daily minimum of at least 30% for a period of 10-14 days postoperatively. Close laboratory control to maintain AHF plasma levels deemed appropriate to maintain hemostasis is recommended.

Reconstitution

1. Warm both the diluent and Antihemophilic Factor (Human), Monoclate-P®, Factor VIII:C Pasteurized, Monoclonal Antibody Purified in unopened vials to room temperature [not above 37°C (98°F)].
2. Remove the caps from both vials to expose the central portions of the rubber stoppers.
3. Treat the surface of the rubber stoppers with antiseptic solution and allow them to dry.
4. Using aseptic technique, insert one end of the double-end needle into the rubber stopper of the diluent vial. Invert the diluent vial and insert the other end of the double-end needle into the rubber stopper of the Monoclate-P® vial. Direct the diluent, which will be drawn in by vacuum, over the entire surface of the Monoclate-P® cake. (In order to assure transfer of all the diluent, adjust the position of the tip of the needle in the diluent vial to the inside edge of the diluent stopper.) Rotate the vial to ensure complete wetting of the cake during the transfer process.
5. Remove the diluent vial to release the vacuum, then remove the double-end needle, from the Monoclate-P® vial.
6. Gently swirl the vial until the powder is dissolved and the solution is ready for administration. The concentrate routinely and easily reconstitutes within one minute. To assure sterility, Monoclate-P® should be administered within three hours after reconstitution.
7. Parenteral drug preparations should be inspected visually for particulate matter and discoloration prior to administration, whenever solution and container permit.

Administration

CAUTION: This kit contains two devices, a stainless steel 5 micron filter needle, individually labeled as a 5 micron filter needle and contained in a separate blister pack, and an all plastic 5 micron vented filter spike which is supplied with the four-item administration components blister pack, either of which may be used to withdraw the reconstituted product for administration. The withdrawal directions specific for each of these alternate devices must be followed exactly for whichever device is chosen for use as described below. Product loss or inability to withdraw product will result if the improper instructions are followed.

A. Administration using the Stainless Steel Filter Needle for Withdrawal
(This item is individually packaged in a separate, labeled blister pack.)

Intravenous Injection

Plastic disposable syringes are recommended with Antihemophilic Factor (Human), Monoclate-P®, Factor VIII:C Pasteurized, Monoclonal Antibody Purified solution. The ground glass surfaces of all-glass syringes tend to stick with solutions of this type.

1. Using aseptic technique, attach the filter needle to a sterile disposable syringe.
2. Draw air into the syringe equal to or greater than the contents of the vial.
3. Insert the filter needle into the stopper of the Monoclate-P® vial, invert the vial, position the filter needle above the level of the liquid and inject all of the air into the vial.
4. Pull the filter needle back down below the level of the liquid until the tip is at the inside edge of the stopper.
5. Withdraw the reconstituted solution into the syringe being careful to always keep the tip of the needle below the level of the liquid.
   CAUTION: Failure to inject air into the vial, or allowing air to pass through the filter needle while filling the syringe with reconstituted solution, may cause the needle to clog.
6. Discard the filter needle. Perform venipuncture using the enclosed winged needle with microbore tubing. Attach the syringe to the luer end of the tubing.
   CAUTION: Use of other winged needles without microbore tubing, although compatible with the concentrate, will result in a larger retention of solution within the winged infusion set.
7. **Administer solution intravenously at a rate (approximately 2 mL/minute) comfortable to the patient.**

B. Administration using the all plastic vented filter spike for withdrawal
(This spike is supplied in the four-item Administration Components pack.)

Intravenous Injection

Plastic disposable syringes are recommended with Antihemophilic Factor (Human), Monoclate-P®, Factor VIII:C Pasteurized, Monoclonal Antibody Purified solution. The ground glass surfaces of all-glass syringes tend to stick with solutions of this type.

1. Using aseptic technique, attach the vented filter spike to a sterile disposable syringe.
   CAUTION: DO NOT INJECT AIR INTO THE MONOCLATE-P® VIAL. The self-venting feature of the vented filter spike precludes the need to inject air in order to facilitate withdrawal of the reconstituted solution. The injection of air could cause partial product loss through the vent filter.
   CAUTION: The use of other, non-vented filter needles or spikes without the proper procedure may result in an air lock and prevent the complete transfer of the concentrate.
2. Insert the vented filter spike into the stopper of the Monoclate-P® vial, invert the vial, and position the filter spike so that the orifice is at the inside edge of the stopper.
3. Withdraw the reconstituted solution into the syringe.
4. Discard the filter spike. Perform venipuncture using the enclosed winged needle with microbore tubing. Attach the syringe to the luer end of the tubing.
   CAUTION: Use of other winged needles without microbore tubing, although compatible with the concentrate, will result in a larger retention of solution within the winged infusion set.
5. **Administer solution intravenously at a rate (approximately 2 mL/minute) comfortable to the patient.**

STORAGE

When stored at refrigerator temperature, 2 - 8°C (36 - 46°F), Antihemophilic Factor (Human), Monoclate-P®, Factor VIII:C Pasteurized, Monoclonal Antibody Purified, is stable for the period indicated by the expiration date on its label.

Continued on next page

Monoclate-P—Cont.

Within this period, Monoclate-P® may be stored at room temperature not to exceed 30°C (86°F), for up to 6 months. Avoid freezing which may damage container for the diluent.

HOW SUPPLIED

Monoclate-P® is supplied in a single dose vial with diluent, double-ended needle for reconstitution, vented filter spike for withdrawal, filter needle for withdrawal, winged infusion set and alcohol swabs. I.U. activity is stated on the label of each vial.

REFERENCES

1. W. Terry, A. Schreiber, C. Tarr, M. Hrinda, W. Curry, and F. Feldman, Human Factor VIII:C Produced Using Monoclonal Antibodies, in *Research in Clinic and Laboratory*, Vol. XVI, (#1), 202 (1986) from the XVIIth International Congress of the World Federation of Hemophilia. **2.** A.B. Schreiber, The Preclinical Characterization of Monoclate Factor VIII C Antihemophilic Factor Human, *Semin Hematol*, 25 (2 Suppl. 1), 1988, pp. 27–32. **3.** E. Berntorp and I.M. Nilsson, Biochemical Properties of Human Factor VIII C Monoclate Purified Using Monoclonal Antibody to VWF, *Thromb Res* O (Suppl. 7), 1987, p. 60, from the Satellite Symposia of the XIth International Congress on Thrombosis and Haemostasis, Brussels, Belgium, July 11, 1987. **4.** S. Chandra, C.C. Huang, R.L. Weeks, K. Beatty and F. Feldman, Purity of a Factor VIII:C Preparation (Monoclate) Manufactured by Monoclonal Immunoaffinity Chromatography Technique, from the XVIII International Congress of the World Federation of Hemophilia, May 1988. **5.** B. Spire, D. Dormont, F. Barre-Sinousii, L. Montagnier, and J.C. Chermann, Inactivation of Lymphadenopathy Associated Virus by Heat, Gamma Rays, and Ultraviolet Light, *Lancet*, Jan. 26, 1985, p. 188. **6.** L.W. Hoyer, The Factor VIII Complex: Structure and Function, *Blood*, 58 (1981), p. 1. **7.** F. Feldman, S. Chandra, R. Kleszynski, C.C. Huang and R.L. Weeks, Measurement of Murine Protein Levels in Monoclonal Antibody Purified Coagulation Factor, from the XVIII International Congress of the World Federation of Hemophilia, May 1988. **8.** F. Feldman, R. Kleszynski, L. Ho, R. Kling, S. Chandra and C.C. Huang, Validation of Coagulation Test Methods for Evaluation of Monoclate (Factor VIII:C) Potencies, from the XVIII International Congress of the World Federation of Hemophilia, May 1988. **9.** S. Chandra, C.C. Huang, L. Ho, R. Kling, R.L. Weeks and F. Feldman, Studies on the Stability of Factor VIII:C (Monoclate) in Lyophilized and Solution Form, from the XVIII International Congress of the World Federation of Hemophilia, May 1988. **10.** C.F. Abilgaard, J.V. Simone, J.J. Corrigan, *et al.*, Treatment of Hemophilia with Glycine—Precipitated Factor VIII, *New Eng J Med*, 275 (1966), p. 471. **11.** C.K. Kasper, Hematologic Care, Comprehensive Management of Hemophilia, ed. Boone, D.C., Philadelphia, F.A. Davis Co., (1976) pp. 2–20.

BIBLIOGRAPHY

Hershman, R.J., Naconti, S.B., and Shulman, N.R. Prophylactic Treatment of Factor VIII Deficiency. *Blood*, 35 (1970), p. 189. Kasper, C.K., Dietrich, S.I. and Rapaport, S.K. Hemophilia Prophylaxis in Factor VIII Concentrate. *Arch. Int. Med.*, 125 (1970), p. 1004. Biggs, R., ed. The Treatment of Hemophilia A and B and von Willebrands Disease. Oxford: Blackwell, 1978. Fulcher, C.A., Zimmerman, T.S., Characterization of the Human Factor VIII Procoagulant Protein With a Heterologous Precipitating Antibody. *Proc. Natl. Acad. Sci.*, 79 (1982), pp. 1648 - 1652. Levine, P.H., Factor VIII C Purified from Plasma Via Monoclonal Antibodies Human Studies. *Semin Hematol*, 25 (2 Suppl. 1), 1988, pp. 38–41.

12810-01

PRESCRIBING INFORMATION

COAGULATION FACTOR IX (HUMAN) MONONINE®

MONOCLONAL ANTIBODY PURIFIED

Rx only ℞

DESCRIPTION

Coagulation Factor IX (Human), Mononine®, is a sterile, stable, lyophilized concentrate of Factor IX prepared from pooled human plasma and is intended for use in therapy of Factor IX deficiency, known as hemophilia B or Christmas disease. Coagulation Factor IX (Human), Mononine®, is purified of extraneous plasma-derived proteins, including Factors II, VII and X, by use of immunoaffinity chromatography. A murine monoclonal antibody to Factor IX is used as an affinity ligand to isolate Factor IX from the source material. Factor IX is then dissociated from the monoclonal antibody, recovered, purified further, formulated and provided as a sterile, lyophilized powder. The immunoaffinity protocol utilized results in a highly pure Factor IX preparation. It shows predominantly a single component by SDS polyacrylamide electrophoretic evaluation and has a specific activity of not less than 190 Factor IX units per mg total protein.

The plasma used in the manufacture of this product has been tested and found negative for HBV, HCV, and HIV-1 by an investigational test procedure referred to as Nucleic Acid Testing (NAT) using Polymerase Chain Reaction (PCR) Technology. Investigational testing is being performed to determine the effectiveness of NAT to detect low levels of viral material. The significance of a negative result is unknown since the effectiveness of the test has not been established.

This concentrate has been processed by monoclonal antibody immunoaffinity chromatography during its manufacture which has been shown to be capable of reducing the risk of viral transmission. Additionally, a chemical treatment protocol and two sequential ultrafiltration steps used in its manufacture have also been shown to be capable of significant viral reductions. However, no procedure has been shown to be totally effective in removing the risk of viral infectivity from coagulation factor concentrates (see **CLINICAL PHARMACOLOGY** and **WARNINGS**).

Mononine® is a highly purified preparation of Factor IX. When stored as directed, it will maintain its labeled potency for the period indicated on the container label.

Each vial contains the labeled amount of Factor IX activity expressed in International Units (IU). One IU represents the activity of Factor IX present in 1 mL of normal, pooled plasma. When reconstituted as recommended, the resulting solution is a clear, colorless, isotonic preparation of neutral pH, containing approximately 100 times the Factor IX potency found in an equal volume of plasma. Each mL of the reconstituted concentrate contains approximately 100 IU of Factor IX and non-detectable levels of Factors II, VII and X (<0.0025 IU per Factor IX unit using standard coagulation assays). It also contains histidine (approx. 10mM), sodium chloride (approx. 0.066M) and mannitol (approx. 3%). Hydrochloric acid and/or sodium hydroxide may have been used to adjust pH. Mononine® also contains trace amounts (≤ 50 ng mouse protein/100 Factor IX activity units) of the murine monoclonal antibody used in its purification (see **CLINICAL PHARMACOLOGY**).

Mononine® is to be administered only intravenously.

CLINICAL PHARMACOLOGY

Hemophilia B, or Christmas disease, is an X-linked recessively inherited disorder of blood coagulation characterized by insufficient or abnormal synthesis of the clotting protein Factor IX. Factor IX is a vitamin K-dependent coagulation factor, which is synthesized in the liver. Factor IX is activated by Factor XIa in the intrinsic coagulation pathway. Activated Factor IX (IXa), in combination with Factor VIII:C, activates Factor X to Xa, resulting ultimately in the conversion of prothrombin to thrombin and the formation of a fibrin clot. The infusion of exogenous Factor IX to replace the deficiency present in hemophilia B temporarily restores hemostasis. Depending upon the patient's level of biologically active Factor IX, clinical symptoms range from moderate skin bruising or excessive hemorrhage after trauma or surgery to spontaneous hemorrhage into joints, muscles or internal organs including the brain. Severe or recurring hemorrhages can produce death, organ dysfunction or orthopedic deformity.

Infusion of Factor IX Complex concentrates that contain varying but significant amounts of the other liver-dependent blood coagulation proteins, Factors II, VII and X, into patients with hemophilia B results in Factor IX recoveries ranging from approximately 0.57–1.1 IU/dL rise per IU/kg body weight infused with plasma half-lives for Factor IX ranging from approximately 23 hours to 31 hours.[1,2] Infusion of Coagulation Factor IX (Human), Mononine®, into ten patients with severe or moderate hemophilia B has shown a mean recovery of 0.67 IU/dL rise per IU/kg body weight infused and a mean half-life of 22.6 hours.[3] After six months of experience with repeated infusions performed on the nine patients who remained in the study, it was shown that the half-life and recovery was maintained at a level comparable to that found with the initial infusion. The six-month data showed a mean recovery of 0.68 IU/dL rise per IU/kg body weight infused and a mean half-life of 25.3 hours.[3] The data show no statistically significant differences between the initial and six-month values.

Two studies were conducted to provide Mononine® for compassionate treatment of hemophilia B patients who required extensive Factor IX replacement for surgery, trauma, or spontaneous bleeding (73 unique patients and eight patients enrolled twice for a total of 81 patients), as well as to evaluate the safety and efficacy of Mononine®. The overall mean recovery during treatment was determined to be 1.23 ± 0.42 IU/dL rise/IU/kg (K) (range = 0.59 to 2.92 K) among the 55 patients included in recovery analyses in the one study and to be 1.12 ± 0.52 K (range = 0.61 to 2.08 K) among 10 patients included in these analyses in the second study. Five (5/81, 6%) patients reported adverse events attributed to Mononine® across the two studies. In these studies, 100 doses of Mononine® were administered at what are considered high doses for a Factor IX concentrate, a range of 71 to 161 IU/kg to a total of 36 patients. Sixty-seven (67) of these infusions were the subject of recovery analyses. Mean recovery tended to decrease as the dose of Mononine® increased: 1.09 ± 0.52 K at doses > 75–95 IU/kg (n=38), 0.98 ± 0.45 K at doses >95–115 IU/kg (n = 21), 0.70 ± 0.38 K at doses >115–135 IU/kg (n = 2), 0.67 K at doses >135–155 IU/kg (n = 1), and 0.73 ± 0.34 K at doses >155 IU/kg (n = 5). Among the 36 patients who received these high doses, only one (2.8%) reported an adverse experience with a possible relationship to Mononine® ("difficulty in concentrating"; patient recovered). In no patients were thrombogenic complications observed or reported.[4]

The manufacturing procedure for Coagulation Factor IX (Human), Mononine®, includes multiple processing steps that have been designed to reduce the risk of viral transmission. Validation studies of the monoclonal antibody (MAb) immunoaffinity chromatography/chemical treatment steps and two sequential ultrafiltration steps used in the production of Mononine® document the viral reduction capacity of the processes employed. These studies were conducted using the Human Immunodeficiency Virus (HIV) and four model viruses representing a broad range of viral characteristics, *i.e.*, Sindbis, Vaccinia, Vesicular Stomatitis (VSV) and Murine Encephalomyocarditis (EMC), a non-lipid encapsulated model virus. The results of these validation studies (see Table 1 below) document cumulative viral reduction capacities of ≥11.56 log_{10} for HIV, 10.24 log_{10} for Sindbis, 11.64 log_{10} for EMC, ≥14.23 log_{10} for VSV, and ≥10.90 log_{10} for Vaccinia.

[See table at bottom of page]

Similar viral reduction studies were conducted using porcine parvovirus (used as a model for human parvovirus B19). The results for these validation studies (see Table 2 below) document cumulative viral reduction capacity of ≥11.64 log_{10} for porcine parvovirus.

Viral Reduction Studies Table 2
(Log_{10} Reduction)

Processing Step	Porcine Parvovirus
Combined MAb Chromatography and Sodium Thiocyanate Chemical Treatment	>4.28
AH Sepharose Chromatography	2.26
Ultrafiltration	5.10
Total Log_{10} Reduction	≥11.64

CLINICAL STUDIES

The viral safety of Coagulation Factor IX (Human), Mononine®, has been studied in clinical trials of two cohorts of hemophilia B patients previously unexposed to blood or blood products.[5] One cohort of patients included those with moderate to severe factor IX deficiency requiring chronic replacement therapy (36 patients dosed thus far); the second cohort included patients with a mild deficiency requiring factor IX replacement for surgical procedures (nine patients dosed thus far).

These patients were followed for serum ALT elevations, as well as for a range of viral serologies. Thirty-two (32) patients (25 with a moderate to severe deficiency and seven with a mild deficiency) were evaluable for assessment of viral hepatitis safety by ISTH-SSC criteria. None of these patients showed evidence of transmission of hepatitis B, hepatitis C, or HIV. In two of the evaluable patients, ALT elevations were attributed to causes other than Mononine®. In addition, one patient considered unevaluable for assessment of viral safety was found to have persistent and significant ALT elevations after infusion. This patient received hepatitis B hyperimmune immunoglobulin and his first injection of hepatitis B vaccine approximately three days after his first infusion. As a result, definitive conclusions regarding the occurrence of hepatitis B in this patient cannot be made.

Coagulation Factor IX (Human), Mononine®, contains trace amounts of the murine monoclonal antibody (MAb) used in

Viral Reduction Studies Table 1
(Log_{10} Reduction)

Processing Step	HIV	Sindbis	EMC	VSV	Vaccinia
MAb Chromatography	*	2.76	3.89	≥7.18**	≥3.60
Sodium Thiocyanate Chemical Treatment	≥4.16	0	0	**	0
Ultrafiltration***	≥7.4	7.48	7.75	7.05	≥7.30
Total Log_{10} Reduction	≥11.56	10.24	11.64	≥14.23	≥10.90

* MAb Chromatography not studied.
** Results are for combined MAb chromatography/sodium thiocyanate step.
*** For VSV and Vaccinia these data are results for a single ultrafiltration; the data for HIV, Sindbis, and EMC are results for double ultrafiltration.

its purification (≤50 ng mouse protein/100 IU). While the levels of mouse protein are extremely low, infusion of such proteins might theoretically induce human anti-mouse antibody (HAMA) responses. To test this possibility, human IgG, IgM, and IgE antibodies to mouse IgG were assessed by immunoradiometric assay (IRMA) in 11 hemophilia B patients who received Mononine® and were previously untreated with other blood products. HAMAs were evaluated prior to the first infusion and at 2 to 42 months after initial treatment. Human IgE antibodies to mouse IgG were below the level of detectability at all time points for all patients, and there were no statistically significant increases in either human IgG antibodies or human IgM antibodies to mouse protein. In addition, an analysis of clinical data shows that no replacement factor-related adverse events occurred that might have been considered as allergic or anaphylactoid reactions.[6]

In clinical studies of Coagulation Factor IX (Human), Mononine®, patients were monitored for evidence of disseminated intravascular coagulation. In six patients evaluated after infusion, fibrinogen levels and platelet counts were unchanged, and fibrin degradation products did not appear.[3]

In further clinical evaluations of Coagulation Factor IX (Human), Mononine®, in a crossover study with a Factor IX Complex concentrate, Mononine® was not associated with the formation of prothrombin activation fragment (F_{1+2}) whereas the Factor IX Complex was associated with the formation of prothrombin activation fragment (F_{1+2}).[3,7] Prothrombin activation fragment (F_{1+2}) is indicative of activation of prothrombin.

INDICATIONS AND USAGE

Coagulation Factor IX (Human), Mononine®, is indicated for the prevention and control of bleeding in Factor IX deficiency, also known as hemophilia B or Christmas disease.

Mononine® is not indicated in the treatment or prophylaxis of hemophilia A patients with inhibitors to Factor VIII.

Coagulation Factor IX (Human), Mononine®, contains non-detectable levels of Factors II, VII and X (<0.0025 IU per Factor IX unit using standard coagulation assays) and is, therefore, not indicated for replacement therapy of these clotting factors.

Mononine® is also not indicated in the treatment or reversal of coumarin-induced anticoagulation or in a hemorrhagic state caused by hepatitis-induced lack of production of liver dependent coagulation factors.

CONTRAINDICATIONS

Known hypersensitivity to mouse protein is a contraindication to Coagulation Factor IX (Human), Mononine®.

WARNINGS

Coagulation Factor IX (Human), Mononine®, is derived from human plasma that may contain human pathogenic agents, including those not yet known or identified. Thus, the risk of transmission of infectious agents can not be totally eliminated. Stringent procedures, designed to reduce the risk of adventitious agent transmission, have been employed in the manufacture of this product from the collection and testing of plasma, through to the application of viral elimination/reduction steps. As with any pharmaceutical, the physician should weigh the risks and benefits of administration.

Individuals who receive infusions of blood or plasma products may develop signs and/or symptoms of some viral infections, particularly nonA, nonB hepatitis.

Since the use of Factor IX Complex concentrates has historically been associated with the development of thromboembolic complications, the use of Factor IX-containing products may be potentially hazardous in patients with signs of fibrinolysis and in patients with disseminated intravascular coagulation (DIC).

PRECAUTIONS

Extensive clinical experience suggests that there is a lower risk of thromboembolic complications with the use of Mononine® than with prothrombin complex concentrates. However, as with all products containing Factor IX, caution should be exercised when administering Mononine® to patients with liver disease, to patients post-operatively, to neonates, or to patients at risk of thromboembolic phenomena or DIC.[8,9] In each of these situations, the potential benefit of treatment with Mononine® should be weighed against the potential risk of these complications.

Coagulation Factor IX (Human), Mononine®, should be administered intravenously at a rate that will permit observation of the patient for any immediate reaction. Rates of infusion of up to 225 IU per minute have been regularly tolerated with no adverse reactions. If any reaction takes place that is thought to be related to the administration of Mononine®, the rate of infusion should be decreased or the infusion stopped, as dictated by the response of the patient.

During the course of treatment, determination of daily Factor IX levels is advised to guide the dose to be administered and the frequency of repeated infusions. Individual patients may vary in their response to Mononine®, achieving different levels of *in vivo* recovery and demonstrating different half-lives.

The use of high doses of Factor IX Complex concentrates has been reported to be associated with instances of myocardial infarction, disseminated intravascular coagulation, venous thrombosis and pulmonary embolism. Generally a Factor IX level of 25% to 50% is considered adequate for hemostasis, including major hemorrhages and surgery. Attempting to maintain Factor IX levels of >75% to 100% during treatment is not routinely recommended nor required. To achieve Factor IX levels that will remain above 25% between once a day administrations, each daily dose should attempt to raise the level to 50 - 60% (see **DOSAGE AND ADMINISTRATION**).

No controlled studies have been available regarding the use of ϵ-amino caproic acid or other antifibrinolytic agents following an initial infusion of Mononine® for the prevention or treatment of oral bleeding following trauma or dental procedures such as extractions.

Information For Patients

Patients should be informed of the early signs of hypersensitivity reactions including hives, generalized urticaria, tightness of the chest, wheezing, hypotension, and anaphylaxis, and should be advised to discontinue use of the concentrate and contact their physician if these symptoms occur.

Pregnancy Category C - Animal reproduction studies have not been conducted with Coagulation Factor IX (Human), Mononine®. It is also not known whether Mononine® can cause fetal harm when administered to a pregnant woman or can affect reproduction capacity. Mononine® should be given to a pregnant woman only if clearly needed.

Pediatric Use

Evaluation of the safety and effectiveness of Mononine® treatment in 51 pediatric patients between the ages of 1 day and 20 years, as a part of viral safety trials and trials for surgery, trauma or spontaneous bleeding, showed that excellent hemostasis was acheived with no thrombotic complications.[10] Included in the experience with patients aged birth to 20 years are two long-term viral safety studies demonstrating lack of viral transmission. Dosing in children is based on body weight and is generally based on the same guidelines as for adults (see below).

Geriatric Use

Clinical studies of mononine® did not include sufficient numbers of patients aged 65 and over to determine whether they respond differently from younger patients. Other reported clinical experience has not identified differences in responses between the elderly and younger patients. As for all patients, dosing for geriatric patients should be appropriate to their overall situation.

ADVERSE REACTIONS

As with the administration of any product intravenously, the following reactions may be observed following administration: headache, fever, chills, flushing, nausea, vomiting, tingling, lethargy, hives, stinging or burning at the infusion site or other manifestations of allergic reactions including anaphylaxis.

There is a potential risk of thromboembolic episodes following the administration of Mononine® (see **WARNINGS** and **PRECAUTIONS**).

The patient should be monitored closely during the infusion of Mononine® to observe for the development of any reaction. If any reaction takes place that is thought to be related to the administration of Mononine®, the rate of infusion should be decreased or the infusion stopped, as dictated by the response of the patient.

DOSAGE AND ADMINISTRATION

Coagulation Factor IX (Human), Mononine®, is intended for intravenous administration only. It should be reconstituted with the volume of Sterile Water for Injection, USP supplied with the lot, and administered within three hours of reconstitution. Do not refrigerate after reconstitution. After administration, any unused solution and the administration equipment should be discarded. As a general rule, 1 IU of Factor IX activity per kg can be expected to increase the circulating level of Factor IX by 1% of normal. The following formula provides a guide to dosage calculations:

[See first table above]

Number of Factor IX IU required	=	Body Weight (in kg)	×	desired Factor IX increase (% normal)	×	1.0 IU/kg

The amount of Coagulation Factor IX (Human), Mononine®, to be infused, as well as the frequency of infusions, will vary with each patient and with the clinical situation.[11,12]

As a general rule, the level of Factor IX required for treatment of different conditions is as follows:

[See second table above]

	Minor Spontaneous Hemorrhage, Prophylaxis	Major Trauma or Surgery
Desired levels of Factor IX for Hemostasis	15 - 25%	25 - 50%
Initial loading dose to achieve desired level	up to 20 - 30 IU/kg	up to 75 IU/kg
Frequency of dosing	once; repeated in 24 hours if necessary	every 18 - 30 hours, depending on $T_{1/2}$ and measured Factor IX levels
Duration of treatment	once; repeated if necessary	up to ten days, depending upon nature of insult

Recovery of the loading dose varies from patient to patient. Doses administered should be titrated to the patient's response. Mononine® administered in doses of ≥ 75 IU/kg were well tolerated (see **CLINICAL PHARMACOLOGY**). In the presence of an inhibitor to Factor IX, higher doses of Mononine® might be necessary to overcome the inhibitor (See **PRECAUTIONS**). No data on the treatment of patients with inhibitors to Factor IX with Mononine® are available.

For information on rate of administration, see **Rate of Administration**, below.

Reconstitution

1. Warm both the diluent and Coagulation Factor IX (Human), Mononine®, in unopened vials to room temperature [not above 37°C (98°F)].
2. Remove the caps from both vials to expose the central portions of the rubber stoppers.
3. Treat the surface of the rubber stoppers with antiseptic solution and allow them to dry.
4. Using aseptic technique, insert one end of the double-end needle into the rubber stopper of the diluent vial. Invert the diluent vial and insert the other end of the double-end needle into the rubber stopper of the Mononine® vial. Direct the diluent, which will be drawn in by vacuum, over the entire surface of the Mononine® cake. (In order to assure transfer of all the diluent, adjust the position of the tip of the needle in the diluent vial to the inside edge of the diluent stopper.) Rotate the vial to ensure complete wetting of the cake during the transfer process.
5. Remove the diluent vial to release the vacuum, then remove the double-end needle from the Mononine® vial.
6. Gently swirl the vial until the powder is dissolved and the solution is ready for administration. The concentrate routinely and easily reconstitutes within one minute. To assure sterility, Mononine® should be administered within three hours after reconstitution.
7. Product should be filtered prior to use as described under **Administration**. Parenteral drug preparations should be inspected visually for particulate matter and discoloration prior to administration, whenever solution and container permit.

Administration

Intravenous Injection

Parenteral drug products should be inspected visually for particulate matter and discoloration prior to administration, whenever solution and container permit.

Plastic disposable syringes are recommended with Coagulation Factor IX (Human), Mononine® solution. The ground glass surfaces of all-glass syringes tend to stick with solutions of this type. Please note, this concentrate is supplied with a SELF-VENTING filter spike.

1. Using aseptic technique, attach the vented filter spike to a sterile disposable syringe.
   CAUTION: The use of other, non-vented filter needles or spikes without the proper procedure may result in an air lock and prevent the complete transfer of the concentrate.
   CAUTION: DO NOT INJECT AIR INTO THE MONONINE® VIAL. The self-venting feature of the vented filter spike precludes the need to inject air in order to facilitate withdrawal of the reconstituted solution. The injection of air could cause partial product loss through the vent filter.
2. Insert the vented filter spike into the stopper of the Mononine® vial, invert the vial, and position the filter spike so that the orifice is at the inside edge of the stopper.
3. Withdraw the reconstituted solution into the syringe.
4. Discard the filter spike. Perform venipuncture using the enclosed winged needle with microbore tubing. Attach the syringe to the luer end of the tubing.
   CAUTION: Use of other winged needles without microbore tubing, although compatible with the concentrate, will result in a larger retention of solution within the winged infusion set.

Rate of Administration

The rate of administration should be determined by the response and comfort of the patient; intravenous dosage administration rates of up to 225 IU/minute have been regularly tolerated without incident. When reconstituted as directed, i.e., to approximately 100 IU/mL, Mononine® should be administered at a rate of approximately 2.0 mL per minute.

STORAGE

When stored at refrigerator temperature, 2° - 8°C (36° - 46°F), Coagulation Factor IX (Human), Mononine®, is stable for the period indicated by the expiration date on its label. Within this period, Mononine® may be stored at room temperature not to exceed 30°C (86°F), for up to one month. Avoid freezing, which may damage container for the diluent.

Continued on next page

Mononine—Cont.

HOW SUPPLIED

Mononine® is supplied in a single dose vial with diluent, double-ended needle for reconstitution, vented filter spike for withdrawal, winged infusion set and alcohol swabs. Factor IX activity in IU is stated on the label of each vial.

The following dosage forms are available:

NDC 0053-7668-01 in 10 mL vials containing approximately 250 IU

NDC 0053-7668-02 in 10 mL vials containing approximately 500 IU

NDC 0053-7668-04 in 20 mL vials containing approximately 1,000 IU

REFERENCES

1. Zauber NP, Levin J. Factor IX levels in patients with hemophilia B (Christmas disease) following transfusion with concentrates of Factor IX or fresh frozen plasma (FFP). *Medicine* (Baltimore) 56(3): 213 - 24, 1977.
2. Smith KJ, Thompson AR. Labeled Factor IX Kinetics in Patients with Hemophilia-B. *Blood* 58(3): 625 - 629, 1981.
3. Kim HC, McMillan CW, White GC, Bergman GE, Horton MW, Saidi P. Purified Factor IX Using Monoclonal Immunoaffinity Technique: Clinical Trials in Hemophilia B and Comparison to Prothrombin Complex Concentrates. *Blood* 79(3):568 - 575, 1992.
4. Warrier I, Kasper CK, White II GC, Shapiro AD, Bergman GE, the Mononine® Study Group. Safety of high doses of a monoclonal antibody-purified factor IX concentrate. *Am J Hematol.* 49:92 - 94, 1995.
5. Shapiro AD, Ragni MV, Lusher JM, Culbert S, Koerper MA, Bergman GE, Hannan MM. Safety and Efficacy of Monoclonal Antibody Purified Factor IX Concentrate in Previously Untreated Patients with Hemophilia B. *Thrombosis and Haemostasis* 75:30 - 35, 1996.
6. Davis HM, Nash DW, Clymer MD, Frigo ML, Bergman GE. Lack of immune response to mouse IgG in previously untreated haemophilia A and haemophilia B patients treated with monoclonal antibody purified factor VIII and factor IX preparations. *Haemophilia* 3(2):102 - 107, April 1997.
7. Kim HC, Matts L, Eisele J, Czachur M, Saidi P. Monoclonal Antibody Purified Factor IX - Comparative Thrombogenicity to Prothrombin Complex Concentrate. *Seminars in Hematology* 28(Suppl.6 to no. 3):15 - 20, July 1991.
8. Aledort LM. Factor IX and Thrombosis. *Scand. J. Haematology* Suppl. 30:40, 1977.
9. Cederbaum AI, Blatt PM, Roberts HR. Intravascular coagulation with use of human prothrombin complex concentrates. *Ann. Intern. Med.* 84: 683 - 687, 1976.
10. Kurczynski E, Lusher JM, Pitel P, Shapiro AD, Bergman GE, the Mononine® Study Group. Safety and efficacy of monoclonal antibody-purified factor IX concentrate for management of bleeding and surgical prophylaxis in previously treated children with hemophilia B. *Int J Ped Hemat/Oncol.* 2:211 - 216, 1995.
11. Kasper CK, Dietrich SL. Comprehensive Management of Hemophilia. *Clin. Haematol.* 14(2):489 - 512, 1985.
12. Johnson AJ, Aronson DL, Williams WJ. Preparation and clinical use of plasma and plasma fractions. Chap 167 in *Hematology* 3rd Edition, Williams WJ, Beutler E, Erslev AJ, Lichtman MA (Eds.), McGraw Hill Book Co., New York: 1563 - 1583, 1983.

12835-01

PRESCRIBING INFORMATION

STIMATE™

(DESMOPRESSIN ACETATE)

NASAL SPRAY, 1.5 MG/ML

Manufactured for
AVENTIS BEHRING L.L.C.
KING OF PRUSSIA, PA 19406-1310
By Ferring Pharmaceuticals, Malmö, Sweden

Rx only

DESCRIPTION

Stimate™ (desmopressin acetate) is a synthetic analogue of the natural pituitary hormone 8-arginine vasopressin (ADH), an antidiuretic hormone affecting renal water conservation. **Stimate™ Nasal Spray** contains 1.5 mg/mL desmopressin acetate in a pH-adjusted aqueous solution with chlorobutanol and sodium chloride as inactive ingredients. **Stimate™ Nasal Spray's** compression pump delivers 0.1 mL (150 µg) of solution per spray. It is chemically defined as follows:

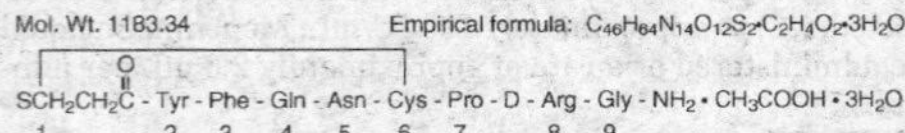

1-(3-mercaptopropionic acid)-8-D-arginine vasopressin monoacetate (salt) trihydrate. **Stimate™ Nasal Spray** is provided as an aqueous solution for intranasal use.

Each mL contains:

Desmopressin acetate	1.5 mg
Chlorobutanol	5.0 mg
Sodium Chloride	9.0 mg

Hydrochloric acid to adjust pH to approximately 4

CLINICAL PHARMACOLOGY

Stimate™ Nasal Spray contains as active substance, desmopressin acetate, which is a synthetic analogue of the natural hormone arginine vasopressin. One spray or 0.1 mL (150 µg) of **Stimate™ Nasal Spray** solution has an antidiuretic activity of about 600 IU.

Desmopressin acetate has been shown to be more potent than arginine vasopressin in increasing plasma levels of Factor VIII activity in patients with hemophilia and von Willebrand's disease Type I.

Dose-response studies were performed in healthy persons using doses of 150 to 450 µg, administered as one to three sprays. The response to **Stimate™ Nasal Spray** is dose-related, with maximal plasma levels of 150 to 250 percent of initial concentrations achieved for both Factor VIII and von Willebrand factor [1]. The increase is rapid and evident within 30 minutes, reaching a maximum at about 1.5 hours [1].

The percentage increase of Factor VIII and von Willebrand factor levels in patients with mild hemophilia A and von Willebrand's disease was not notably different from that observed in normal healthy individuals when treated with 300 µg of **Stimate™ Nasal Spray** [1-4]. In patients with von Willebrand's disease, levels of Factor VIII coagulant activity and von Willebrand factor antigen remained greater than 30 U/dL for 8 hours after a 300 µg dose of **Stimate™ Nasal Spray** [7]. After 300 µg of **Stimate™ Nasal Spray**, the percentage increase of Factor VIII and von Willebrand factor levels in patients with mild hemophilia A and von Willebrand's disease was less than observed after 0.3 µg/kg of intravenous desmopressin acetate [2-4].

Plasminogen activator activity increases rapidly after intravenous desmopressin acetate infusion, but there has been no clinically significant fibrinolysis in patients treated with desmopressin acetate.

The effect of repeated intravenous desmopressin acetate administration when doses were given every 12 to 24 hours has generally shown a diminution of the Factor VIII activity increase noted after a single dose. It is possible to reproduce the initial response in some patients after an interval of one week, but other patients may require as long as 6 weeks [2,4,6].

The half-life of **Stimate™ Nasal Spray** was between 3.3 and 3.5 hours, over the range of intranasal doses, 150 to 450 µg [1]. Plasma concentrations of **Stimate™ Nasal Spray** were maximal approximately 40 to 45 minutes after dosing [1].

The bioavailability of **Stimate™ Nasal Spray** when administered by the intranasal route as a 1.5 mg/mL solution is between 3.3 and 4.1 percent [1].

The change in structure of arginine vasopressin to desmopressin acetate has resulted in a decreased vasopressor action and decreased actions on visceral smooth muscle relative to the enhanced antidiuretic activity, so that clinically effective antidiuretic doses are usually below threshold levels for effects on vascular or visceral smooth muscle.

INDICATIONS AND USAGE

Before the initial therapeutic administration of **Stimate™ Nasal Spray**, the physician should establish that the patient shows an appropriate change in the coagulation profile following a test dose of intranasal administration of **Stimate™ Nasal Spray** [2-4].

Desmopressin acetate is also available as a solution for injection (DDAVP® Injection) when the intranasal route may be compromised. These situations include nasal congestion and blockage, nasal discharge, atrophy of nasal mucosa, and severe atrophic rhinitis. Intranasal delivery may also be inappropriate where there is an impaired level of consciousness.

Hemophilia A

Stimate™ Nasal Spray is indicated for patients with hemophilia A with Factor VIII coagulant activity levels greater than 5%.

Desmopressin acetate will also stop bleeding in patients with hemophilia A with episodes of spontaneous or trauma-induced injuries such as hemarthroses, intramuscular hematomas or mucosal bleeding [2,3].

In the outpatient setting during two clinical trials where patients recorded bleeding episodes, **Stimate™ Nasal Spray** provided effective hemostasis 100% of the time in 2 of the 5 patients. For those patients not responding in 100% of bleeding occasions, 45% (14 of 31) of bleeding episodes were effectively controlled with **Stimate™ Nasal Spray**.

Desmopressin acetate is not indicated for the treatment of hemophilia A with Factor VIII coagulant activity levels equal to or less than 5%, or for the treatment of hemophilia B, or in patients who have Factor VIII antibodies.

von Willebrand's Disease (Type I)

Stimate™ Nasal Spray is indicated for patients with mild to moderate classic von Willebrand's disease (Type I) with Factor VIII levels greater than 5%.

Desmopressin acetate will also stop bleeding in mild to moderate von Willebrand's disease patients with episodes of spontaneous or trauma-induced injuries such as hemarthroses, intramuscular hematomas, mucosal bleeding or menorrhagia [2,3].

In the outpatient setting during two clinical trials where patients recorded bleeding episodes, **Stimate™ Nasal Spray** provided effective hemostasis 100% of the time in 75% of the patients (n=16). For those patients not responding in 100% of bleeding occasions, 78% (64 of 82) of bleeding episodes were effectively controlled with **Stimate™ Nasal Spray**.

Patients may respond in a variable fashion depending on the type of molecular defect they have. Bleeding time and Factor VIII coagulant activity, ristocetin cofactor activity, and von Willebrand factor antigen should be checked after initial administration of **Stimate™ Nasal Spray** to ensure that adequate levels have been achieved.

Stimate™ Nasal Spray is not indicated for the treatment of severe classic von Willebrand's disease (Type I) and when there is evidence of an abnormal molecular form of Factor VIII antigen. See WARNING.

CONTRAINDICATIONS

Stimate™ Nasal Spray is contraindicated in individuals with known hypersensitivity to desmopressin acetate or to any of the components of **Stimate™ Nasal Spray**.

WARNINGS

For intranasal use only.

Patients who do not have need of antidiuretic hormone for its antidiuretic effect, in particular those who are young or elderly, should be cautioned to ingest only enough fluid to satisfy thirst, in order to decrease the potential occurrence of water intoxication and hyponatremia.

Fluid intake should be adjusted downward, particularly in very young and elderly patients, in order to decrease the potential occurrence of water intoxication and hyponatremia [1]. Particular attention should be paid to the possibility of the rare occurrence of an extreme decrease in plasma osmolality that may result in seizures which could lead to coma.

Stimate™ Nasal Spray should not be used to treat patients with Type IIB von Willebrand's disease since platelet aggregation may be induced.

PRECAUTIONS

General

Desmopressin acetate has infrequently produced changes in blood pressure causing either a slight elevation in blood pressure or a transient fall in blood pressure and a compensatory increase in heart rate. The drug should be used with caution in patients with coronary artery insufficiency and/or hypertensive cardiovascular disease.

Stimate™ Nasal Spray should be used with caution in patients with conditions associated with fluid and electrolyte imbalance, such as cystic fibrosis, because these patients are prone to hyponatremia.

There have been rare reports of thrombotic events (thrombosis [9], acute cerebrovascular thrombosis, acute myocardial infarction) following desmopressin acetate injection in patients predisposed to thrombus formation. No causality has been determined; however, the drug should be used with caution in these patients.

Severe allergic reactions have been reported rarely [2,11–13]. Fatal anaphylaxis has been reported in one patient who received intravenous DDAVP® (desmopressin acetate). It is not known whether antibodies to desmopressin acetate are produced after repeated administration.

Since **Stimate™ Nasal Spray** is used intranasally, changes in the nasal mucosa such as scarring, edema, or other disease may cause erratic, unreliable absorption in which case **Stimate™ Nasal Spray** should be discontinued until the nasal problems resolve. For such situations, DDAVP® Injection should be considered.

Information for Patients: Patients should be informed that the bottle accurately delivers 25 doses of 150 µg each. Any solution remaining after 25 doses should be discarded since the amount delivered thereafter may be substantially less than 150 µg of drug. No attempt should be made to transfer remaining solution to another bottle. Patients should be instructed to read accompanying directions on use of the spray pump carefully before use.

Patients should also be advised that if bleeding is not controlled, the physician should be contacted [2,3].

Hemophilia A

Laboratory tests for assessing patient status include levels of Factor VIII coagulant, Factor VIII antigen and Factor VIII ristocetin cofactor (von Willebrand factor) as well as activated partial thromboplastin time. Factor VIII coagulant activity should be determined before giving **Stimate™ Nasal Spray** for hemostasis. If Factor VIII coagulant activity is present at less than 5% of normal, **Stimate™ Nasal Spray** should not be relied on.

von Willebrand's Disease

Laboratory tests for assessing patient status include levels of Factor VIII coagulant activity, Factor VIII ristocetin cofactor activity, and Factor VIII von Willebrand factor antigen. The skin bleeding time may be helpful in following these patients.

Drug Interactions

Although the pressor activity of desmopressin acetate is very low, its use with other pressor agents should be done only with careful patient monitoring.

DDAVP® Injection has been used with epsilon aminocaproic acid without adverse effects.

Carcinogenicity, Mutagenicity, Impairment of Fertility: There have been no long-term studies in animals to assess the carcinogenic, mutagenic or impairment of fertility potential of **Stimate™ Nasal Spray**.

Pregnancy Category B: Reproduction studies performed in rats and rabbits by the subcutaneous route at doses up to 10 µg/kg/day have revealed no evidence of harm to the fetus due to desmopressin acetate. This dose is equivalent to 10 times (for Factor VIII stimulation) or 38 times (for diabetes insipidus) the systemic human dose based on a mg/M^2 surface area.

There are no adequate and well-controlled studies in pregnant women. Several publications of desmopressin acetate's use in the management of diabetes insipidus during pregnancy are available; these include a few anecdotal reports of congenital anomalies and low birth weight babies. However, no causal connection between these events and desmopressin acetate has been established. A 15-year, Swedish epidemiologic study of the use of desmopressin acetate in pregnant women with diabetes insipidus found the rate of birth defects to be no greater than that in the general population. As opposed to preparations containing natural hormones, desmopressin acetate in antidiuretic doses has no uterotonic action and the physician will have to weigh the therapeutic advantages against the possible risks in each case.

Nursing Mothers: There have been no controlled studies in nursing mothers. A single study in postpartum women demonstrated a marked change in plasma, but little if any change in assayable DDAVP in breast milk following an intranasal dose of 10 µg. It is not known whether this drug is excreted in human milk. Because many drugs are excreted in human milk, caution should be exercised when **Stimate™ Nasal Spray** is administered to a nursing woman.

Pediatric Use: Use in infants and children will require careful fluid intake restriction to prevent possible hyponatremia and water intoxication. **Stimate™ Nasal Spray** should not be used in infants younger than 11 months in the treatment of hemophilia A or von Willebrand's disease; safety and effectiveness in children between 11 months and 12 years of age has been demonstrated [2-4].

ADVERSE REACTIONS

Infrequently, DDAVP® Injection has produced transient headache, nausea, mild abdominal cramps and vulval pain. These symptoms disappeared with reduction in dosage. Occasional facial flushing has been reported with the administration of DDAVP® Injection. Infrequently, high doses of intranasal DDAVP® have produced transient headache and nausea. Nasal congestion, rhinitis and flushing have also been reported occasionally along with mild abdominal cramps. These symptoms disappeared with reduction in dosage. Nosebleed, sore throat, cough and upper respiratory infections have also been reported.

In addition to those listed above, the following have also been reported in clinical trials with **Stimate™ Nasal Spray**: Somnolence, dizziness, itchy or light-sensitive eyes, insomnia, chills, warm feeling, pain, chest pain, palpitations, tachycardia, dyspepsia, edema, vomiting, agitation and balanitis [1-4].

DDAVP® Injection (desmopressin acetate) has infrequently produced changes in blood pressure causing either a slight elevation or a transient fall and a compensatory increase in heart rate. Severe allergic reactions including anaphylaxis have been reported rarely with DDAVP® Injection.

See WARNING for the possibility of water intoxication, hyponatremia and coma [10].

OVERDOSAGE

See ADVERSE REACTIONS above. In cases of overdosage, the dosage should be reduced, frequency of administration decreased, or the drug withdrawn according to the severity of the condition.

There is no known specific antidote for desmopressin acetate or **Stimate™ Nasal Spray**.

An oral LD_{50} has not been established. An intravenous dose of 2 mg/kg in mice demonstrated no effect.

DOSAGE AND ADMINISTRATION

Hemophilia A and von Willebrand's Disease (Type I)

Stimate™ Nasal Spray is administered by nasal insufflation, one spray per nostril, to provide a total dose of 300 µg. In patients weighing less than 50 kg, 150 µg administered as a single spray provided the expected effect on Factor VIII coagulant activity, Factor VIII ristocetin cofactor activity and skin bleeding time [3,4]. If **Stimate™ Nasal Spray** is used preoperatively, it should be administered 2 hours prior to the scheduled procedure [5,8].

The necessity for repeat administration of **Stimate™ Nasal Spray** or use of any blood products for hemostasis should be determined by laboratory response as well as the clinical condition of the patient. The tendency toward tachyphylaxis (lessening of response) with repeated administration given more frequently than every 48 hours should be considered in treating each patient.

The nasal spray pump can only deliver doses of 0.1 mL (150 µg) or multiples of 0.1 mL. If doses other than these are required, DDAVP® Injection may be used.

The spray pump must be primed prior to the first use. To prime pump, press down 4 times. The bottle should be discarded after 25 doses since the amount delivered thereafter per spray may be substantially less than 150 µg of drug.

HOW SUPPLIED

A 2.5 mL bottle with spray pump capable of delivering 25 doses of 150 µg (NDC 0053-2453-00).

KEEP REFRIGERATED AT 2°-8°C (36°-46°F). When traveling, product will maintain stability for up to 3 weeks when stored at room temperature, 22°C (72°F).

REFERENCES

1. RHÔNE-POULENC RORER STUDY RG-83884-141: An Open-Label Pharmacokinetic Comparison of Desmopressin Acetate Administration by Intranasal (1.5 mg/mL) and Intravenous Routes: A Dose-Proportionality Trial. 2. RHÔNE-POULENC RORER STUDY RG-83884-142: Nasal Spray Desmopressin (DDAVP). A simple Technique for Treatment of Mild Hemophilia A and von Willebrand's disease. 3. RHÔNE-POULENC RORER STUDY RG-83884-143: Intranasal Desmopressin (DDAVP) by spray in Mild Hemophilia A and von Willebrand's disease Type I. 4. RHÔNE-POULENC RORER STUDY RG-83884-144: Evaluation of Intranasal Spray DDAVP in Patients with Mild or Moderate Hemophilia A or von Willebrand's disease: Inpatient Trial. 5. Chistolini A, Dragoni F, Ferrari A, La Verde G, Arcieri R, Mohamud AE and Mazzucconi MG: Intranasal DDAVP: Biological and clinical evaluation in mild Factor VIII deficiency. Haemostasis, 21: 273-277, 1991. 6. Lethagen S, Harris AS, Sjörin E and Nilsson IM: Intranasal and intravenous administration of desmopressin: Effect on FVIII/vWF, pharmacokinetics and reproducibility. Thromb. Haemost., 58:1033-1036, 1987. 7. Lethagen S, Harris AS and Nilsson IM: Intranasal desmopressin (DDAVP) by spray in mild hemophilia A and von Willebrand's disease type I. Blut, 60: 187-191, 1990. 8. Rose EH and Aledort LM: Nasal spray desmopressin (DDAVP) for mild hemophilia A and von Willebrand's disease. Ann. Int. Med., 114: 563-568, 1991. 9. Viron B, Michel C, Serrato T and Verdy E: Risque thrombogène du D.D.A.V.P. dans l'insuffisance rénale chronique (Thrombogenic risk of DDAVP in chronic renal failure). Néphrologie, 8: 225, 1987. 10. RHÔNE-POULENC RORER PHARMACEUTICALS INC. ADVERSE REACTION REPORT No. 01-003827; Coma, grand mal seizure, etc. 11. RHÔNE-POULENC RORER PHARMACEUTICALS INC. ADVERSE REACTION REPORT No. 01-000657; Anaphylaxis, etc. 12. RHÔNE-POULENC RORER PHARMACEUTICALS INC. ADVERSE REACTION REPORT No. 01-001182; Anaphylactoid reaction. 13. RHÔNE-POULENC RORER PHARMACEUTICALS INC. ADVERSE REACTION REPORT No. US-870671; Erythema, rash.

Adapted from IN-8155B, Rev. 3/95 Issued: August 1999

Aventis Pasteur Inc.

SWIFTWATER, PA 18370

For Medical Information Contact:

Generally:
Medical Affairs
(800) VACCINE
(800) 822-2463

Adverse Drug Experiences:
Medical Director
(570) 839-7187
(800) 822-2463

Sales and Ordering:
Aventis Pasteur Inc.
Customer Service
(800) VACCINE
(800) 822-2463
(570) 839-7187

ActHIB® ℞
HAEMOPHILUS b CONJUGATE VACCINE
(Tetanus Toxoid Conjugate)
℞ only

Caution: Federal (USA) law prohibits dispensing without prescription.

NOTE: Haemophilus b Conjugate Vaccine (Tetanus Toxoid Conjugate)—ActHIB® is identical to Haemophilus b Conjugate Vaccine (Tetanus Toxoid Conjugate)—OmniHIB® (distributed by SmithKline Beecham Pharmaceuticals); and is manufactured by Aventis Pasteur SA.

DESCRIPTION

ActHIB®, Haemophilus b Conjugate Vaccine (Tetanus Toxoid Conjugate), produced by Aventis Pasteur SA, is a sterile, lyophilized powder which is reconstituted at the time of use with either saline diluent (0.4% Sodium Chloride) or Aventis Pasteur Inc. (AvP) Diphtheria and Tetanus Toxoids and Pertussis Vaccine Adsorbed (whole-cell pertussis vaccine DTP) or Tripedia®, AvP Diphtheria and Tetanus Toxoids and Acellular Pertussis Vaccine Adsorbed (DTaP) (when reconstituted known as TriHIBit®) for intramuscular use only. The vaccine consists of the Haemophilus b capsular polysaccharide (polyribosyl-ribitol-phosphate, PRP), a high molecular weight polymer prepared from the *Haemophilus influenzae* type b strain 1482 grown in a semi-synthetic medium, covalently bound to tetanus toxoid.[1] The lyophilized ActHIB® powder and saline diluent contain no preservative. The tetanus toxoid is prepared by extraction, ammonium sulfate purification, and formalin inactivation of the toxin from cultures of *Clostridium tetani* (Harvard strain) grown in a modified Mueller and Miller medium.[2] The toxoid is filter sterilized prior to the conjugation process. Potency of ActHIB® is specified on each lot by limits on the content of PRP polysaccharide and protein in each dose and the proportion of polysaccharide and protein in the vaccine which is characterized as high molecular weight conjugate.

When ActHIB® is reconstituted with saline diluent, each single dose of 0.5 mL is formulated to contain 10 µg of purified capsular polysaccharide conjugated to 24 µg of inactivated tetanus toxoid, and 8.5% of sucrose.

When ActHIB® is combined with AvP DTP vaccine by reconstitution, each single dose (0.5 mL) is formulated to contain 10 µg of purified capsular polysaccharide conjugated to 24 µg of inactivated tetanus toxoid, 8.5% of sucrose, 6.7 Lf of diphtheria toxoid, 5 Lf of tetanus toxoid and an estimate of 4 protective units of pertussis vaccine. Thimerosal (mercury derivative) 1:10,000 is added as a preservative to AvP DTP vaccine. ***(Refer to product insert for AvP whole-cell DTP.)***

When ActHIB® is combined with Tripedia® (TriHIBit®) by reconstitution **for booster dose**, each single dose (0.5 mL) is formulated to contain 10 µg of purified capsular polysaccharide conjugated to 24 µg of inactivated tetanus toxoid, 8.5% of sucrose, 6.7 Lf of diphtheria toxoid, 5 Lf of tetanus toxoid and 46.8 µg of pertussis antigens. Thimerosal (mercury derivative) 1:10,000 is added as a preservative to Tripedia®. ***(Refer to product insert for Tripedia®.)***

The reconstituted vaccine, using saline diluent, appears clear and colorless. The reconstituted vaccine, using AvP DTP vaccine, appears whitish in color. TriHIBit®, the reconstituted vaccine, using Tripedia®, is a homogenous white suspension.

CLINICAL PHARMACOLOGY

NOTE: Haemophilus b Conjugate Vaccine (Tetanus Toxoid Conjugate)—ActHIB® is identical to Haemophilus b Conjugate Vaccine (Tetanus Toxoid Conjugate)—OmniHIB® (distributed by SmithKline Beecham Pharmaceuticals); and is manufactured by Aventis Pasteur SA.

H influenzae type b was the leading cause of invasive bacterial disease among children in the United States prior to licensing of Haemophilus b conjugate vaccines. Based on its active surveillance areas, the Centers for Disease Control and Prevention (CDC) now estimate that *H influenzae* type b disease in children under the age of 5 years has been reduced by 95%.[3] Before effective vaccines were introduced, it was estimated that one in 200 children developed invasive *H influenzae* type b disease by the age of 5 years. In children less than 5 years of age, the mortality rate for invasive *H influenzae* type b disease ranged between 3% and 6%.[3] In more than 60% of these children, meningitis was the clinical syndrome and permanent sequelae ranging from mild hearing loss to mental retardation affecting 20% to 30% of all survivors.[3] Ninety-five percent of the cases of invasive *H influenzae* disease among children < 5 years of age were caused by organisms with the type b polysaccharide capsule. Approximately two-thirds of all cases of invasive *H influenzae* type b disease affected infants and children < 15 months of age, a group for which a vaccine was not available until late 1990.[4,5]

Incidence rates of invasive *H influenzae* type b disease have been shown to be increased in certain high-risk groups, such as native Americans (both American Indians and Eskimos), blacks, individuals of lower socioeconomic status, and patients with asplenia, sickle cell disease, Hodgkin's disease, and antibody deficiency syndromes.[5,6] Studies also have suggested that the risk of acquiring primary invasive *H influenzae* type b disease for children under 5 years of age appears to be greater for those who attend day-care facilities.[7,8,9,10]

The potential for person to person transmission of the organism among susceptible individuals has been recognized. Studies of secondary spread of disease in household contacts of index patients have shown a substantially increased risk among exposed household contacts under 4 years of age.[11] Adults can be colonized with *H influenzae* type b from children infected with the organism.[12]

The response to ActHIB® is typical of a T-dependent immune response to antigen. The prominent isotype of anticapsular PRP antibody induced by ActHIB® is IgG.[13] A substantial booster response has been demonstrated in children 12 months of age or older who previously received two or three doses. Bactericidal activity against *H influenzae* type b is demonstrated in serum after immunization and statistically correlates with the anti-PRP antibody response induced by ActHIB®.[14]

Antibody to *H influenzae* capsular polysaccharide (anti-PRP) titers of > 1.0 µg/mL following vaccination with unconjugated PRP vaccine correlated with long-term protection against invasive *H influenzae* type b disease in children older than 24 months of age.[15] Although the relevance of this threshold to clinical protection after immunization with conjugate vaccines is not known, particularly in light of the induced, immunologic memory, this level continues to be considered as indicative of long-term protection.[4] The immunogenicity and safety of ActHIB® has been demonstrated in the United States and worldwide. ActHIB® induced, on average anti-PRP levels ≥ 1.0 µg/mL in 90% of infants after the primary series and in more than 98% of infants after a booster dose.[14]

Two clinical trials supported by the National Institutes of Health (NIH) have compared the anti-PRP antibody responses to three Haemophilus b conjugate vaccines in racially mixed populations of children. These studies were done in Tennessee[16] (Table 1) and in Minnesota, Missouri and Texas[17] (Table 2) in infants immunized with ActHIB® and other Haemophilus b conjugate vaccines at 2, 4 and 6 months of age. All Haemophilus b conjugate vaccines were administered concomitantly with Poliovirus Vaccine Live Oral and DTP vaccines at separate sites.

[See table 1 at top of next page]

[See table 2 on next page]

Native American populations have had high rates of *H influenzae* type b disease and have been observed to have low immune responses to Haemophilus b conjugate vaccines. Following three doses of ActHIB® at six weeks, four and six months of age, 75% of Native Americans in Alaska showed an anti-PRP antibody titer of ≥ 1.0 µg/mL.[18]

Continued on next page

ActHIB—Cont.

Children 12 to 24 months of age who had not previously received Haemophilus b conjugate vaccination were immunized with a single dose of ActHIB®. GMT anti-PRP antibody responses were 5.12 μg/mL (90% responding with ≥ 1.0 μg/mL) for children 12 to 15 months of age and 4.4 μg/mL (82% responding with ≥ 1.0 μg/mL) for children 17 to 24 months of age.[18]

These trials demonstrated that ActHIB® consistently conferred an anti-PRP antibody response previously shown to correlate with protection, when administered either as a regimen of three doses at least four to eight weeks apart in infants 2 to 6 months of age or as a single dose in children 12 months of age and older.[18]

ActHIB® has been found to be immunogenic in children with sickle cell anemia, a condition which may cause increased susceptibility to Haemophilus b disease. Two doses of ActHIB® given at two-month intervals induced anti-PRP antibody titers of 1.0 μg/mL in 89% of these children with a mean age of 11 months. This is comparable to anti-PRP antibody levels demonstrated in normal children of similar age following two doses of ActHIB®.[19]

ActHIB® COMBINED WITH WHOLE-CELL PERTUSSIS VACCINE (DTP) BY RECONSTITUTION FOR PRIMARY IMMUNIZATION

Comparative clinical trials demonstrated that a similar anti-PRP response was achieved in infants as young as 2 months old when one dose of AvP whole-cell DTP vaccine was used to reconstitute lyophilized ActHIB® (Table 3).[14,18]

[See table 3 at right]

Antibody responses to diphtheria, tetanus and pertussis antigens were also measured in this trial. Post dose three antibody responses to all measured vaccine antigens were similar, within each study, when infants who received the combined vaccine were compared to infants who received whole-cell DTP and ActHIB® separately. Interference with the antibody response to the pertussis component has been suggested with a DTP vaccine unlicensed in the US.[20] Percentages of subjects achieving antibody titers over 1 μg/mL and GMT to PRP in 2-month-old infants following immunization with ActHIB® combined with AvP DTP by reconstitution was similar when compared to infants who received DTP and ActHIB® separately (84% versus 85% and 4.3 μg/mL versus 4.8 μg/mL).[14,18]

TriHIBit®, ActHIB® COMBINED WITH TRIPEDIA® VACCINE BY RECONSTITUTION FOR BOOSTER DOSE

Randomized comparative clinical trials demonstrated that the anti-PRP response achieved in 15 to 20-month-old children after one dose of TriHIBit®, Tripedia® and ActHIB® combination vaccine, was similar to that achieved when the two vaccines were given concomitantly at different sites with separate needles and syringes (Table 4).[18] All children had received three doses of a Haemophilus b conjugate vaccine (HibTITER® or ActHIB®) and three doses of a whole-cell DTP vaccine prior to entry into this clinical trial.

[See table 4 at top of next page]

Geometric mean titers in response to diphtheria, tetanus and pertussis (PT and FHA) were also similar between groups. ***(Refer to product insert for Tripedia®.)*** A difference in four-fold antibody response to FHA was noted in this trial. However, the clinical significance of this difference is not known at present.

INDICATIONS AND USAGE

NOTE: Haemophilus b Conjugate Vaccine (Tetanus Toxoid Conjugate)—ActHIB® is identical to Haemophilus b Conjugate Vaccine (Tetanus Toxoid Conjugate)—OmniHIB® (distributed by SmithKline Beecham Pharmaceuticals); and is manufactured by Aventis Pasteur SA.

ActHIB® or ActHIB® combined with AvP DTP vaccine by reconstitution is indicated for the active immunization of infants and children 2 through 18 months of age for the prevention of invasive disease caused by *H influenzae* type b and/or diphtheria, tetanus and pertussis.

TriHIBit®, ActHIB® combined with Tripedia® by reconstitution, is indicated for the active immunization of children 15 to 18 months of age for prevention of invasive disease caused by *H influenzae* type b and diphtheria, tetanus and pertussis.

Antibody levels associated with protection may not be achieved earlier than two weeks following the last recommended dose.

***Only AvP whole-cell DTP, Tripedia® or 0.4% Sodium Chloride diluent may be used for reconstitution of lyophilized ActHIB®.* TriHIBit®, ActHIB® combined with Tripedia® by reconstitution, should not be administered to infants younger than 15 months of age.**

As with any vaccine, vaccination with ActHIB® reconstituted with AvP DTP or ActHIB® reconstituted with Tripedia® (TriHIBit®) or 0.4% Sodium Chloride diluent may not protect 100% of susceptible individuals.

A single injection containing diphtheria, tetanus, pertussis and Haemophilus b conjugate antigens may be more acceptable to parents and may increase compliance with vaccination programs. Therefore, in these situations it may be the judgment of the physician that it is of benefit to administer a single injection of whole-cell DTP or DTaP Haemophilus b conjugate vaccines.

CONTRAINDICATIONS

ActHIB® IS CONTRAINDICATED IN CHILDREN WITH A HISTORY OF HYPERSENSITIVITY TO ANY COMPONENT OF THE VACCINE AND TO ANY COMPONENT OF DTP OR Tripedia® WHEN COMBINED BY RECONSTITUTION WITH THESE VACCINES. ANY CONTRAINDICATION FOR DTP IS A CONTRAINDICATION FOR ActHIB® RECONSTITUTED WITH DTP. ANY CONTRAINDICATION FOR Tripedia® IS A CONTRAINDICATION FOR TriHIBit®, ActHIB® RECONSTITUTED WITH Tripedia®. ***(Refer to product inserts for AvP whole-cell DTP and Tripedia®.)***

TABLE 1[16] ANTI-PRP ANTIBODY RESPONSES IN 2-MONTH-OLD INFANTS NIH TRIAL IN TENNESSEE

VACCINE	N*	GEOMETRIC MEAN TITER (GMT) (μg/mL) Pre-Immunization	Post Second Immunization	Post Third Immunization	Post Third Immunization % 1.0 μg/mL
PRP-T† (ActHIB®)	65	0.10	0.30	3.64	83%
PRP-OMP¶ (PedvaxHIB®)	64	0.11	0.84	N/A	50%**
HbOC‡(HibTITER®)	61	0.07	0.13	3.08	75%

TABLE 2[17] ANTI-PRP ANTIBODY RESPONSES IN 2-MONTH-OLD INFANTS NIH TRIAL IN MINNESOTA, MISSOURI AND TEXAS

VACCINE	N*	GEOMETRIC MEAN TITER (GMT) (μg/mL) Pre-Immunization	Post Second Immunization	Post Third§ Immunization	Post Third§ Immunization % 1.0 μg/mL
PRP-T† (ActHIB®)	142	0.25	1.25	6.37	97%
PRP-OMP¶ (PedvaxHIB®)	149	0.18	4.00	N/A	85%**
HbOC‡(HibTITER®)	167	0.17	0.45	6.31	90%

* N = Number of Children

§ Sera were obtained after the third dose from 86 to 110 infants, in PRP-T and HbOC vaccine groups, respectively.

† Haemophilus b Conjugate Vaccine (Tetanus Toxoid Conjugate)

¶ Haemophilus b Conjugate Vaccine (Meningococcal Protein Conjugate)

** Seroconversion after the recommended 2-dose primary immunization series is shown.

‡ Haemophilus b Conjugate Vaccine (Diphtheria CRM_{197} Protein Conjugate)

N/A Not applicable in this comparison trial although third dose data have been published.[16,17]

TABLE 3[18] ANTI-PRP RESPONSES IN 2-MONTH-OLD INFANTS FOLLOWING IMMUNIZATION WITH ActHIB® COMBINED WITH CONNAUGHT LABORATORIES, INC. DTP BY RECONSTITUTION

STUDY SITE	N*	GEOMETRIC MEAN TITER (GMT) (μg/mL) Pre-Immunization	Post Second Immunization	Post Third Immunization	Post Third Immunization % 1.0 μg/mL
US	45	0.13	0.55	4.49	91
US	135	0.12	0.43	4.46	85
Chile	94	0.09	4.31	6.94	96

* N = Number of Children

WARNINGS

This product contains dry natural latex rubber as follows: The stopper to the diluent vial contains dry natural latex rubber. The lyophilized vaccine vial contains no rubber of any kind.

If ActHIB® or ActHIB® reconstituted with AvP DTP or ActHIB® reconstituted with Tripedia® (TriHIBit®) is administered to immunosuppressed persons or persons receiving immunosuppressive therapy, the expected antibody responses may not be obtained. This includes patients with asymptomatic or symptomatic HIV-infection,[21] severe combined immunodeficiency, hypogammaglobulinemia, or agammaglobulinemia; altered immune states due to diseases such as leukemia, lymphoma, or generalized malignancy; or an immune system compromised by treatment with corticosteroids, alkylating drugs, antimetabolites or radiation.[22] ***(Refer to product inserts for AvP whole-cell DTP and Tripedia®.)***

TriHIBit®, ActHIB® combined with Tripedia® by reconstitution, should not be administered to infants younger than 15 months of age.

PRECAUTIONS

GENERAL

Care is to be taken by the health-care provider for the safe and effective use of this vaccine.

EPINEPHRINE INJECTION (1:1000) MUST BE IMMEDIATELY AVAILABLE SHOULD AN ANAPHYLACTIC OR OTHER ALLERGIC REACTIONS OCCUR DUE TO ANY COMPONENT OF THE VACCINE.

Prior to an injection of any vaccine, all known precautions should be taken to prevent adverse reactions. This includes a review of the patient's history with respect to possible sensitivity and any previous adverse reactions to the vaccine or similar vaccines, and to possible sensitivity to dry natural latex rubber, previous immunization history, current health status (see **CONTRAINDICATIONS; WARNINGS** sections), and a current knowledge of the literature concerning the use of the vaccine under consideration. ***(Refer to product inserts for AvP whole-cell DTP and Tripedia®.)***

The health-care provider should ask the parent or guardian about the recent health status of the infant or child to be immunized including the infant's or child's previous immunization history prior to administration of ActHIB®, AvP DTP and Tripedia®.

Minor illnesses such as upper respiratory infection with or without low-grade fever are not contraindications for use of ActHIB®.[23]

As reported with Haemophilus b polysaccharide vaccines,[24] cases of *H influenzae* type b disease may occur subsequent to vaccination and prior to the onset of protective effects of the vaccine.[18] (See **INDICATIONS AND USAGE** section.)

The evidence favors rejection of a causal relation between immunization with Hib conjugate vaccines and early-onset of Hib disease.[25]

Antigenuria has been detected in some instances following receipt of ActHIB®; therefore, urine antigen detection may not have definitive diagnostic value in suspected *H influenzae* type b disease within one week of immunization.[26]

Special care should be taken to ensure that ActHIB® reconstituted with AvP DTP or Tripedia® or saline diluent (0.4% Sodium Chloride) is not injected into a blood vessel.

Administration of ActHIB® reconstituted with AvP DTP or ActHIB® reconstituted with Tripedia® (TriHIBit®) or saline diluent (0.4% Sodium Chloride) is not contraindicated in individuals with HIV infection.[22]

A separate, sterile syringe and needle or a sterile disposable unit should be used for each patient to prevent transmission of hepatitis or other infectious agents from person to person. Needles should not be recapped and should be properly disposed.

INFORMATION FOR PATIENT

The health-care provider should inform the parent or guardian of the benefits and risks of the vaccine.

Prior to administration of ActHIB® reconstituted with AvP DTP or ActHIB® reconstituted with Tripedia® (TriHIBit®) or saline diluent (0.4% Sodium Chloride), the parent or guardian should be asked about the recent health status of the infant or child to be immunized.

The physician should inform the parent or guardian about the significant adverse reactions that have been temporally associated with the administration of ActHIB® reconstituted with saline or DTP, or ActHIB® reconstituted with Tripedia® (TriHIBit®). The parent or guardian should be instructed to report any serious adverse reactions to their health-care provider.

As part of the child's immunization record, the date, lot number and manufacturer of the vaccine administered should be recorded.[27,28,29]

TABLE 4[18] **ANTI-PRP RESPONSES IN 15 TO 20-MONTH-OLD CHILDREN FOLLOWING IMMUNIZATION WITH TriHIBit® COMPARED TO ActHIB® AND TRIPEDIA® GIVEN CONCOMITANTLY AT SEPARATE SITES**

IMMUNOGENICITY	Pre-Dose		Post-Dose	
	TriHIBit®	Separate Injections	TriHIBit®	Separate Injections
N*	88	94	93	98
Anti-PRP (μg/mL)	0.89	1.15	90.30	80.90
% > 1 μg/mL	45.50	53.20	100.00	100.00

* N = Number of Children

TABLE 5[14] **PERCENTAGE OF INFANTS PRESENTING WITH LOCAL OR SYSTEMIC REACTIONS AT 6, 24, AND 48 HOURS OF IMMUNIZATION WITH ActHIB® ADMINISTERED SIMULTANEOUSLY, AT SEPARATE SITES, WITH AvP DTP VACCINE**

REACTION	AGE AT IMMUNIZATION								
	2 Months (n=365)			4 Months (n=364)			6 Months (n=365)		
	6 Hrs.	24 Hrs.	48 Hrs.	6 Hrs.	24 Hrs.	48 Hrs.	6 Hrs.	24 Hrs.	48 Hrs.
Local§									
Tenderness	46.3%	11.5%	2.2%	23.4%	7.4%	1.1%	19.2%	6.0%	1.1%
Erythema	14.3%	4.1%	0.3%	8.8%	5.8%	0.6%	11.5%	6.9%	1.6%
Induration	22.5%	6.3%	1.9%	12.4%	4.7%	0.8%	9.6%	3.8%	1.1%
Systemic*									
Fever >100.8°F†	20.1%	1.3%	0.6%	14.6%	6.6%	1.4%	15.7%	8.8%	0.8%
Irritability	72.6%	21.9%	12.6%	48.4%	25.0%	13.2%	44.1%	25.2%	10.1%
Drowsiness	57.5%	29.9%	10.4%	44.2%	18.1%	7.4%	32.6%	13.4%	2.5%
Anorexia	15.3%	5.8%	4.9%	8.0%	5.0%	3.0%	5.5%	4.9%	2.2%
Diarrhea	4.4%	6.6%	5.2%	5.0%	4.7%	4.7%	4.7%	6.3%	3.6%
Vomiting	2.7%	4.1%	2.7%	2.5%	3.3%	2.8%	2.2%	2.7%	1.9%
Persistent Crying	Percentage of infants within 72 hours after immunization was 1.6% after dose one, 0.6% after dose two, and 0.3% after dose three.								

§Local reactions were evaluated at the ActHIB® injection site.
*The adverse reaction profile is defined by the concomitant use of AvP DTP vaccine.
†The number of individuals observed at each time point for fever varied from 357 to 363.

The US Department of Health and Human Services has established a new Vaccine Adverse Event Reporting System (VAERS) to accept all reports of suspected adverse events after the administration of any vaccine, including but not limited to the reporting of events required by the National Childhood Vaccine Injury Act of 1986.[27] The toll-free number for VAERS forms and information is 1-800-822-7967.

The National Vaccine Injury Compensation Program, established by the National Childhood Vaccine Injury Act of 1986, requires physicians and other health-care providers who administer vaccines to maintain permanent vaccination records and to report occurrences of certain adverse events to the US Department of Health and Human Services. Reportable events include those listed in the Act for each vaccine and events specified in the package insert as contraindications to further doses of the vaccine.[28,29]

The health-care provider should inform the parent or guardian of the importance of completing the immunization series.

The health-care provider should provide the Vaccine Information Materials (VIMs) which are required to be given with each immunization.

DRUG INTERACTIONS

When AvP DTP is used to reconstitute ActHIB® or Tripedia® is used to reconstitute ActHIB® (TriHIBit®) and administered to immunosuppressed persons or persons receiving immunosuppressive therapy, the expected antibody response may not be obtained.

Immunosuppressive therapies, including irradiation, antimetabolites, alkylating agents, cytotoxic drugs, and corticosteroids (used in greater than physiologic doses), may reduce the immune response to vaccines. Short-term (< 2 weeks) corticosteroid therapy or intra-articular, bursal, or tendon injections with corticosteroids should not be immunosuppressive. Although no specific studies with pertussis vaccine are available, if immunosuppressive therapy will be discontinued shortly, it is reasonable to defer vaccination until the patient has been off therapy for one month; otherwise, the patient should be vaccinated while still on therapy.[23]

If ActHIB® reconstituted with AvP DTP or ActHIB® reconstituted with Tripedia® (TriHIBit®) has been administered to persons receiving immunosuppressive therapy, a recent injection of immunoglobulin or having an immunodeficiency disorder, an adequate immunologic response may not be obtained.

In clinical trials, ActHIB® was administered, at separate sites, concomitantly with one or more of the following vaccines: DTP, DTaP, Poliovirus Vaccine Live Oral (OPV), Measles, Mumps and Rubella vaccine (MMR), Hepatitis B vaccine and occasionally Inactivated Poliovirus Vaccine (IPV). No impairment of the antibody response to the individual antigens, diphtheria, tetanus and pertussis, was demonstrated when ActHIB® was given at the same time, at separate sites, with IPV or MMR.[18] In addition, more than 47,000 infants in Finland have received a third dose of ActHIB® concomitantly with MMR vaccine with no increase in serious or unexpected adverse events.[18]

No significant impairment of antibody response to Measles, Mumps and Rubella was noted in 15- to 20-month-old children who received TriHIBit®, ActHIB® reconstituted with Tripedia®, concomitantly with MMR. No data are available to the manufacturer concerning the effects of immune response of OPV, IPV or Hepatitis B vaccine when given concurrently with ActHIB® reconstituted with 0.4% Sodium Chloride or AvP DTP or ActHIB® reconstituted with Tripedia® (TriHIBit®).[18]

As with other intramuscular injections, use with caution in patients on anticoagulant therapy.

CARCINOGENESIS, MUTAGENESIS, IMPAIRMENT OF FERTILITY

ActHIB® reconstituted with AvP DTP or ActHIB® reconstituted with Tripedia® (TriHIBit®) has not been evaluated for its carcinogenic, mutagenic potential or impairment of fertility.

PREGNANCY

REPRODUCTIVE STUDIES—PREGNANCY CATEGORY C

Animal reproduction studies have not been conducted with ActHIB® reconstituted with AvP DTP or ActHIB® reconstituted with Tripedia® (TriHIBit®) or saline diluent (0.4% Sodium Chloride). It is also not known whether ActHIB® reconstituted with AvP DTP or ActHIB® reconstituted with Tripedia® (TriHIBit®) or saline diluent (0.4% Sodium Chloride) can cause fetal harm when administered to a pregnant woman or can affect reproduction capacity. ActHIB® reconstituted with AvP DTP or ActHIB® reconstituted with Tripedia® (TriHIBit®) or saline diluent (0.4% Sodium Chloride) is NOT recommended for use in a pregnant woman and is not approved for use in children 5 years of age or older.

PEDIATRIC USE

SAFETY AND EFFECTIVENESS OF TriHIBit®, ActHIB® RECONSTITUTED WITH Tripedia®, IN INFANTS BELOW THE AGE OF 15 MONTHS HAVE NOT BEEN ESTABLISHED. (See **DOSAGE AND ADMINISTRATION** section.)

SAFETY AND EFFECTIVENESS OF ActHIB® RECONSTITUTED WITH AvP DTP OR SALINE DILUENT (0.4% SODIUM CHLORIDE) IN INFANTS BELOW THE AGE OF SIX WEEKS HAVE NOT BEEN ESTABLISHED. (See **DOSAGE AND ADMINISTRATION** section.)

ADVERSE REACTIONS

NOTE: Haemophilus b Conjugate Vaccine (Tetanus Toxoid Conjugate)—ActHIB® is identical to Haemophilus b Conjugate Vaccine (Tetanus Toxoid Conjugate)—OmniHIB® (distributed by SmithKline Beecham Pharmaceuticals); and is manufactured by Aventis Pasteur SA.

More than 7,000 infants and young children (≤ 2 years of age) have received at least one dose of ActHIB® during US clinical trials. Of these, 1,064 subjects 12 to 24 months of age who received ActHIB® alone reported no serious or life threatening adverse reactions.

Adverse reactions commonly associated with a first ActHIB® immunization of children 12 to 15 months of age who were previously unimmunized with any Haemophilus b conjugate vaccine, include local pain, redness and swelling at the injection site. Systemic reactions include fever, irritability and lethargy.[14,18]

In a multicenter trial, ActHIB® was administered to US infants at 2, 4, and 6 months of age concomitantly, at separate sites, with AvP DTP. The adverse events observed are summarized in Table 5.

[See table 5 at left]

In general, the rates of minor systemic reactions after ActHIB® and DTP immunization were comparable to those usually reported after DTP vaccine alone.[30,31,32,33]

When ActHIB® reconstituted with AvP whole-cell DTP was administered in infants at 2, 4, and 6 months of age, the systemic adverse experience profile (Table 6) was comparable to that observed when the two vaccines were given separately (Table 5). An increase in the rates of local reactions was observed within the 24-hour period after immunization.[18]

[See table 6 at top of next page]

In a third US trial when ActHIB® was combined with DTP by reconstitution, approximately 1,450 doses were administered to infants starting at 2 months of age. Adverse reactions observed at 6 and 24 hours respectively after the first immunization (n = 498) were tenderness 66.9% and 30.7%; erythema (> 1") 8.6% and 2.2%; induration 38.2% and 21.7%; irritability 77.9% and 35.7%; drowsiness 63.7% and 34.1%; anorexia 26.1% and 12.9%; diarrhea 6.8% and 9.0%; and vomiting 3.4% and 3.8%.[18] One hypotonic/hyporesponsive episode (HHE) was seen in an infant following the second dose in this trial. This is consistent with the HHE incidence rate observed with DTP vaccination alone.[4]

Adverse reactions associated with ActHIB® generally subsided after 24 hours and usually do not persist beyond 48 hours after immunization.

No data are available on the safety of a booster dose of ActHIB® combined with AvP DTP vaccine by reconstitution given in 15 to 20-month-old children.

In a US trial, safety of TriHIBit®, ActHIB® combined with Tripedia® by reconstitution, in 110 children aged 15 to 20 months was compared to ActHIB® given with Tripedia® at separate sites to 110 children. All children received three doses of Haemophilus b conjugate vaccine (ActHIB® or HibTITER®) and three doses of whole-cell DTP at approximately 2, 4 and 6 months of age.

[See table 7 on next page]

TriHIBit®, ActHIB® combined with Tripedia® by reconstitution, and administered to approximately 850 children, aged 15 to 20 months. All children received three doses of a Haemophilus b conjugate vaccine (ActHIB® or HibTITER®) and three doses of whole-cell DTP at approximately 2, 4, and 6 months of age. Local reactions were typically mild and usually resolved within the 24 to 48 hour period after immunization. The most common local reactions were pain and tenderness at the injection site. Systemic reactions occurring were usually mild and resolved within 72 hours of immunization. The reaction rates were similar to those observed in Table 7 when TriHIBit®, ActHIB® reconstituted with Tripedia® was administered and when Tripedia® was administered alone as a booster.[18]

In a randomized, double-blind US clinical trial, ActHIB® was given concomitantly with DTP to more than 5,000 infants and hepatitis B vaccine was given with DTP to a similar number. In this large study, deaths due to sudden infant death syndrome (SIDS) and other causes were observed but were not different in the two groups. In the first 48 hours following immunization, two definite and three possible seizures were observed after ActHIB® and DTP in comparison with none after Hepatitis B vaccine and DTP.[18] This rate of seizures following ActHIB® and DTP was not greater than previously reported in infants receiving DTP alone. **(Refer to product insert for AvP DTP.)** Other adverse reactions reported with administration of other Haemophilus b conjugate vaccines include urticaria, seizures, hives, renal failure and Guillain-Barré syndrome (GBS).[18,34] A cause and effect relationship among any of these events and the vaccination has not been established.

When ActHIB® was given with DTP and inactivated poliovirus vaccine to more than 100,000 Finnish infants, the rate and extent of serious adverse reactions were not different from those seen when other Haemophilus b conjugate vaccines were evaluated in Finland (i.e. HibTITER®, ProHIBit®).[18]

However, the number of subjects studied with TriHIBit®, ActHIB® combined with Tripedia® by reconstitution, was inadequate to detect rare serious adverse events.

Reporting of Adverse Events

Reporting by the parent or guardian of all adverse events occurring after vaccine administration should be encouraged. Adverse events following immunization with vaccine should be reported by the health-care provider to the US Department of Health and Human Services (DHHS) Vaccine Adverse Event Reporting System (VAERS). Reporting forms and information about reporting requirements or completion of the form can be obtained from VAERS through a toll-free number 1-800-822-7967.[26,27,28]

Continued on next page

ActHIB—Cont.

Health-care providers also should report these events to the Director of Scientific and Medical Affairs, Aventis Pasteur Inc., Discovery Drive, Swiftwater, PA 18370 or call 1-800-822-2463.

DOSAGE AND ADMINISTRATION

NOTE: Haemophilus b Conjugate Vaccine (Tetanus Toxoid Conjugate)—ActHIB® is identical to Haemophilus b Conjugate Vaccine (Tetanus Toxoid Conjugate)—OmniHIB® (distributed by SmithKline Beecham Pharmaceuticals); and is manufactured by Aventis Pasteur SA.

Parenteral drug products should be inspected visually for particulate matter and/or discoloration prior to administration, whenever solution and container permit. If these conditions exist, the vaccine should not be administered.

RECONSTITUTION:

Using Aventis Pasteur Inc. DTP, cleanse both the DTP and ActHIB® vial rubber stoppers with a suitable germicide prior to reconstitution. Thoroughly agitate the vial of AvP DTP then withdraw a 0.6 mL dose and inject into the vial of lyophilized ActHIB®. After reconstitution and thorough agitation, the combined vaccines will appear whitish in color. Withdraw and administer 0.5 mL dose of the combined vaccines intramuscularly. Vaccine should be used within 24 hours after reconstitution. Refer to Figures 1, 2, 3, 4, and 5.

To prepare TriHIBit®, cleanse both the Tripedia® and ActHIB® vial rubber stoppers with a suitable germicide prior to reconstitution. Thoroughly agitate the vial of AvP Tripedia® then withdraw a 0.6 mL dose and inject into the vial of lyophilized ActHIB®. After reconstitution and thorough agitation, the combined vaccines will appear whitish in color. Withdraw and administer 0.5 mL dose of the combined vaccines intramuscularly. Vaccine should be used immediately **(within 30 minutes)** after reconstitution. Refer to Figures 1, 2, 3, 4, and 5.

Using saline diluent (0.4% Sodium Chloride) cleanse the vaccine vial rubber stopper with a suitable germicide and inject the entire volume of diluent contained in the vial or syringe into the vial of lyophilized vaccine. Thorough agitation is advised to ensure complete reconstitution. The entire volume of reconstituted vaccine is then drawn back into the syringe before injecting one 0.5 mL dose intramuscularly. The vaccine will appear clear and colorless. Vaccine should be used within 24 hours after reconstitution. Refer to Figures 1, 2, 3, 4, and 5.

INSTRUCTIONS FOR RECONSTITUTION OF ActHIB® WITH AvP DTP OR RECONSTITUTION OF ActHIB® WITH TRIPEDIA® (TriHIBit®) OR SALINE DILUENT (0.4% SODIUM CHLORIDE):

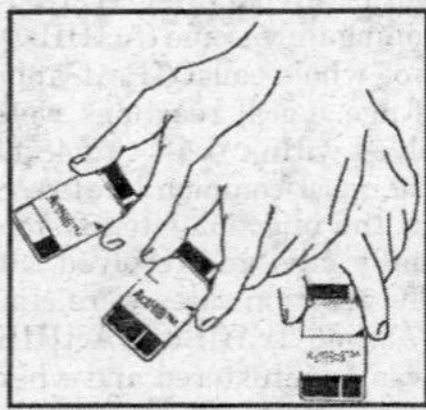

Figure 1. Cleanse stopper and agitate the vial of DTP, Tripedia®, or 0.4% Sodium Chloride used to reconstitute ActHIB®.

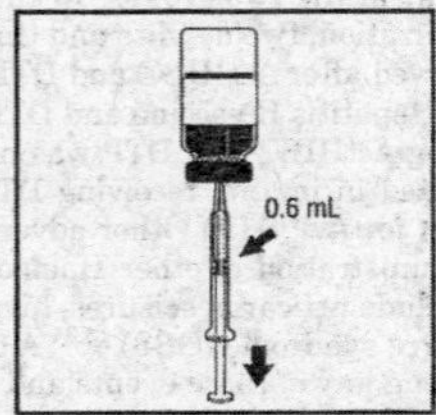

Figure 2. Withdraw volume of DTP, Tripedia®, or 0.4% Sodium Chloride as indicated.

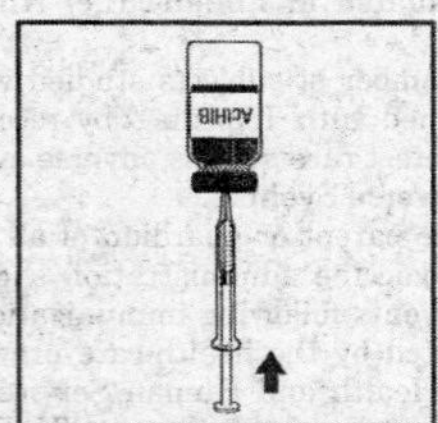

Figure 3. Cleanse the ActHIB® stopper, insert syringe needle through the rubber stopper and inject volume as directed.

[See figure 4 in next column]

TABLE 6[18] **PERCENTAGE OF INFANTS PRESENTING WITH LOCAL OR SYSTEMIC REACTIONS AT 6, 24, AND 48 HOURS OF IMMUNIZATION WITH ActHIB® COMBINED WITH AvP DTP VACCINE BY RECONSTITUTION**

REACTION	AGE AT IMMUNIZATION								
	2 Months (n=204)			4 Months (n=199)			6 Months (n=200)		
	6 Hrs.	24 Hrs.	48 Hrs.	6 Hrs.	24 Hrs.	48 Hrs.	6 Hrs.	24 Hrs.	48 Hrs.
Local									
Tenderness	47.1%	18.6%	3.4%	33.2%	17.6%	4.0%	25.0%	17.0%	3.5%
Erythema > 1″	11.8%	2.5%	0.0%	11.6%	9.1%	2.5%	10.5%	13.5%	3.5%
Induration	31.4%	17.2%	3.9%	26.1%	20.1%	7.5%	28.5%	22.5%	10.0%
Systemic									
Fever >100.4°F	24.6%	2.0%	0.5%	15.8%	6.1%	3.6%	13.0%	10.3%	3.1%
Irritability	70.6%	22.1%	12.8%	56.8%	31.2%	19.1%	40.5%	28.2%	15.9%
Drowsiness	60.3%	23.5%	11.3%	42.2%	20.6%	9.6%	30.3%	12.3%	5.6%
Anorexia	17.7%	6.4%	2.9%	10.1%	7.5%	5.5%	5.1%	4.6%	4.1%
Diarrhea	2.5%	5.4%	1.5%	3.5%	3.5%	2.5%	2.6%	4.1%	5.6%
Vomiting	2.9%	5.4%	2.9%	3.0%	5.0%	3.0%	3.6%	3.6%	1.5%
Persistent Crying	Percentage of infants within 72 hours after immunization was 0.0% after dose one, 0.0% after dose two, and 0.005% after dose three.								

TABLE 7[18] **PERCENTAGE OF 15 TO 20-MONTH-OLD CHILDREN PRESENTING WITH LOCAL OR SYSTEMIC REACTIONS AT 6, 24 AND 48 HOURS OF IMMUNIZATION WITH TriHIBit® COMPARED TO ActHIB® AND TRIPEDIA® GIVEN CONCOMITANTLY AT SEPARATE SITES**

REACTION	6 Hrs. Post-dose		24 Hrs. Post-dose		48 Hrs. Post-dose	
	Separate Injections*	TriHIBit®	Separate Injections*	TriHIBit®	Separate Injections*	TriHIBit®
Local	n=110	n=110	n=110	n=110	n=110	n=110
Tenderness	17.3/20.0	19.1	8.2/8.2	10.0	1.8/0.9	1.8
Erythema > 1″	0.9/0.0	3.6	2.7/0.9	3.6	0.9/0.0	1.8
Induration**	3.6/5.5	2.7	2.7/3.6	8.2	4.5/0.9	3.6
Swelling	3.6/3.6	3.6	2.7/1.8	5.5	0.9/0.0	4.5
Systemic	n=103–110	n=102–109	n=105–110	n=103–108	n=104–110	n=103–109
Fever > 102.2°F	0	2.0	1.0	1.9	1.9	0
Irritability	27.3	22.9	20.9	17.6	12.7	10.1
Drowsiness	36.4	30.3	17.3	13.9	12.7	11.0
Anorexia	12.7	9.2	10.0	6.5	6.4	2.8
Vomiting	0.9	1.8	0.9	1.9	0.9	2.8
Persistent Cry	0	0	0	0	0	0
Unusual Cry	0	0	0	0	0	0.9

* Tripedia® injection site/ActHIB® injection site.
** Induration is defined as hardness with or without swelling

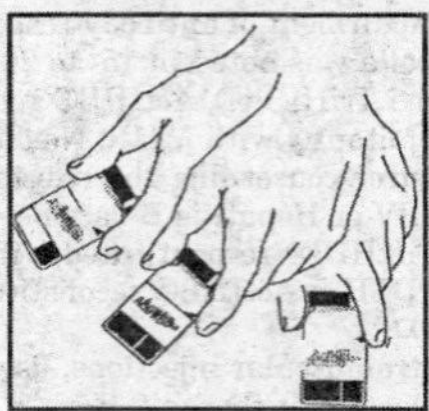

Figure 4. Agitate vial thoroughly.

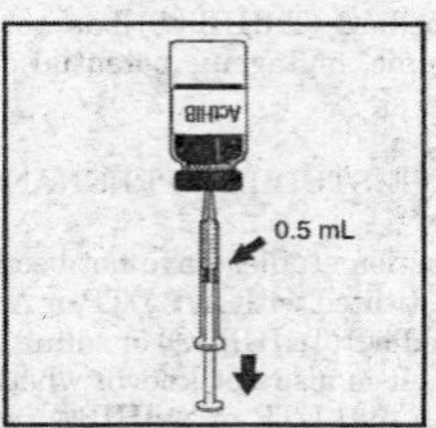

Figure 5. After reconstitution with either DTP, or reconstitution with Tripedia® (TriHIBit®) or 0.4% Sodium Chloride withdraw 0.5 mL of reconstituted vaccine and administer **intramuscularly.**

Before injection, the skin over the site to be injected should be cleansed with a suitable germicide. After insertion of the needle, aspirate to ensure that the needle has not entered a blood vessel.

DO NOT INJECT INTRAVENOUSLY.

Each dose of ActHIB® reconstituted with AvP DTP or ActHIB® reconstituted with Tripedia® (TriHIBit®) or saline diluent (0.4% Sodium Chloride) is administered intramuscularly in the outer aspect of the vastus lateralis (midthigh) or deltoid. The vaccine should not be injected into the gluteal area or areas where there may be a nerve trunk. During the course of primary immunizations, injections should not be made more than once at the same site.

When ActHIB® is reconstituted with AvP DTP, the combined vaccines are indicated for infants and children 2 through 18 months of age for intramuscular administration in accordance with the schedule indicated in Table 8.[14]

When ActHIB® is reconstituted with Tripedia® (TriHIBit®), the combined vaccines are indicated for children 15 to 18 months of age for intramuscular administration in accordance with the schedule in Table 8.[14]

[See table 8 at top of next page]

For Previously Unvaccinated Children

The number of doses of Haemophilus b Conjugate Vaccine indicated depends on the age at which immunization is begun. A child 7 to 11 months of age should receive 2 doses of Haemophilus b Conjugate Vaccine at 8-week intervals and a booster dose at 15 to 18 months of age. A child 12 to 14 months of age should receive 1 dose of Haemophilus b Conjugate Vaccine followed by a booster 2 months later.

Preterm infants should be vaccinated according to their chronological age from birth.[35]

Interruption of the recommended schedule with a delay between doses should not interfere with the final immunity achieved with ActHIB® reconstituted with AvP DTP or ActHIB® reconstituted with Tripedia® (TriHIBit®) or saline diluent (0.4% Sodium Chloride). There is no need to start the series over again, regardless of the time elapsed between doses.

It is acceptable to administer a booster dose of TriHIBit®, ActHIB® reconstituted with Tripedia®, following a primary series of Haemophilus b conjugate and whole-cell DTP vaccines, or a primary series of a combination vaccine containing whole-cell DTP.

HOW SUPPLIED

ActHIB® RECONSTITUTED WITH WHOLE-CELL DTP

Vial, 1 Dose, lyophilized vaccine (10 × 1 Dose vials per package), packaged with one 7.5 mL vial of Aventis Pasteur Inc. Diphtheria and Tetanus Toxoids and Pertussis Vaccine as Diluent—Product No. 49281-549-10

ActHIB® RECONSTITUTED WITH 0.4% SODIUM CHLORIDE DILUENT

Vial, 1 Dose, lyophilized vaccine (5 × 1 Dose vials per package), packaged with 0.6 mL vial containing diluent (5 × 0.6 mL vials per package)—Product No. 49281-545-05

Administer vaccine within 24 hours after reconstitution.

TriHIBit®, ActHIB® RECONSTITUTED WITH TRIPEDIA®

Vial, 1 Dose, lyophilized vaccine (10 × 1 Dose vials per package), packaged with one 7.5 mL vial of Tripedia® as Diluent—Product No. 49281-557-10

Vial, 1 Dose, lyophilized vaccine (5 × 1 Dose vials per package), packaged with five 1 Dose vials of Tripedia® as Diluent—Product No. 49281-557-05

Administer vaccine immediately (within 30 minutes) after reconstitution.

STORAGE

Store lyophilized vaccine packaged with saline diluent, Diphtheria and Tetanus Toxoids and Pertussis or Tripedia® between 2°–8°C (35°–46°F). DO NOT FREEZE.

REFERENCES

1. Chu CY, et al. Further studies on the immunogenicity of *Haemophilus influenzae* type b and pneumococcal type 6A polysaccharide-protein conjugate. Infect Immun 40:245–246, 1983

TABLE 8[14] **RECOMMENDED IMMUNIZATION SCHEDULE FOR ActHIB® AND DTP OR TRIPEDIA®**
For Previously Unvaccinated Children

DOSE	AGE	IMMUNIZATION
First, Second and Third	At 2, 4 and 6 months	ActHIB® /reconstituted with DTP or with saline diluent (0.4% Sodium Chloride)
Fourth	At 15 to 18 months	ActHIB® reconstituted with DTP or with Tripedia® (TriHIBit®) or with saline diluent (0.4% Sodium Chloride)
Fifth	At 4 to 6 years	DTP or Tripedia®

2. Mueller JH et al. Production of diphtheria toxin of high potency (100 Lf) on a reproducible medium. J Immunol 40: 21–32, 1941
3. Adams WG, et al. Decline of Childhood *Haemophilus influenzae* Type b (Hib) Disease in the Hib Vaccine Era. JAMA 269: 221–226, 1993
4. Recommendations of the Immunization Practices Advisory Committee (ACIP). Haemophilus b conjugate vaccines for prevention of *Haemophilus influenzae* type b disease among infants and children two months of age and older. MMWR 40: No. RR-1, 1991
5. Broome CV. Epidemiology of *Haemophilus influenzae* type b infections in the United States. Pediatr Infect Dis J 6: 779–782, 1987
6. ACIP. Polysaccharide vaccine for prevention of *Haemophilus influenzae* type b disease. MMWR 34: 201–205, 1985
7. Istre GR, et al. Risk factors for primary invasive *Haemophilus influenzae* disease: Increased risk from day care attendance and school-aged household members. J Pediatr 106: 190–195, 1985
8. Redmond SR, et al. *Haemophilus influenzae* type b disease. An epidemiologic study with special reference to day-care centers. JAMA 252: 2581–2584, 1984
9. Murphy TV, et al. County-wide surveillance of invasive Haemophilus infections: Risk of associated cases in Child Care Programs (CCPs). Twenty-third Interscience Conference on Antimicrobial Agents and Chemotherapy (Abstract #788) 229, 1983
10. Fleming D, et al. *Haemophilus influenzae* b (Hib) disease—secondary spread in day care. Twenty-fourth Interscience Conference on Antimicrobial Agents and Chemotherapy (Abstract #967) 261, 1984
11. CDC. Prevention of secondary cases of *Haemophilus influenzae* type b disease. MMWR 31: 672–680, 1982
12. Michaels RH, et al. Pharyngeal colonization with *Haemophilus influenzae* type b: A longitudinal study of families with a child with meningitis or epiglottitis due to *H. influenzae* type b. J Infec Dis 136: 222–227, 1977
13. Holmes SJ, et al. Immunogenicity of four *Haemophilus influenzae* type b conjugate vaccines in 17- to 19-month-old children. J Pediatr 118: 364–371, 1991
14. Data on file, Aventis Pasteur Inc.
15. Peltola H, et al. Prevention of *Haemophilus influenzae* type b bacteremic infections with the capsular polysaccharide vaccine. N Engl J Med 310: 1561–1566, 1984
16. Decker MD, et al. Comparative trial in infants of four conjugate *Haemophilus influenzae* type b vaccines. J Pediatr 120: 184–189, 1992
17. Granoff DM, et al. Differences in the immunogenicity of three *Haemophilus influenzae* type b conjugate vaccines in infants. J Pediatr 121: 187–194, 1992
18. Data on file, Aventis Pasteur Inc.
19. Kaplan SL, et al. Immunogenicity of *Haemophilus influenzae* type b polysaccharide-tetanus protein conjugate vaccine in children with sickle hemoglobinopathy or malignancies, and after systemic *Haemophilus influenzae* type b infection. J Pediatr 120: 367–370, 1992
20. Clemens JD, et al. Impact of *Haemophilus influenzae* Type b Polysaccharide-Tetanus Protein Conjugate Vaccine on responses to concurrently administered Diphtheria-Tetanus-Pertussis Vaccine. JAMA 267: 673–678, 1992
21. Steinhoff MC, et al. Antibody responses to *Haemophilus influenzae* type b vaccines in men with human immunodeficiency virus infection. N Engl J Med 325 (26): 1837–1842, 1991
22. ACIP. General recommendations on immunization. MMWR 38: 205–227, 1989
23. ACIP. Diphtheria, Tetanus, and Pertussis: Recommendations for Vaccine Use and Other Preventive Measures. MMWR 40: No. RR-10, 1991
24. FDA Workshop on Haemophilus b Polysaccharide Vaccine—A Preliminary Report. MMWR 36: 529–531, 1987
25. IOM. Adverse Events Associated with Childhood Vaccines: Evidence Bearing on Causality. *Haemophilus Influenzae* Type b Vaccines. In: Stratton KR, Howe CJ, Johnston Jr. RB, eds. 1993. National Academy Press. Washington DC, pp. 236–273, 1993
26. Rothstein EP, et al. Comparison antigenuria after immunization with three *Haemophilus influenzae* type b conjugate vaccines. Pediatr Infect Dis J 10: 311–314, 1991
27. Vaccine Adverse Event Reporting System—United States. MMWR 39: 730–733, 1990
28. CDC. National Childhood Vaccine Injury Act: Requirements for permanent vaccination records and for reporting of selected events after vaccination. MMWR 37: 197–200, 1988
29. National Childhood Vaccine Injury Act of 1986 (Amended 1987)
30. Cody CL, et al. Nature and rates of adverse reactions associated with DTP and DT immunizations in infants and children. Pediatr 68: 650–660, 1981
31. Barkin RM, et al. Diphtheria-tetanus-pertussis vaccine: reactogenicity of commercial products. Pediatr 63: 256–260, 1979
32. Baraff LJ, et al. DTP-associated reactions: an analysis by injection site, manufacturer, prior reactions and dose. Pediatr 73: 31–39, 1984
33. Long SS, et al. Longitudinal study of adverse reactions following diphtheria-tetanus-pertussis vaccine in infancy. Pediatr 85: 294–302, 1990
34. D'Cruz OF, et al. Acute inflammatory demyelinating polyradiculoneuropathy (Guillain-Barré Syndrome) after immunization with *Haemophilus influenzae* type b conjugate vaccine. J Pediatr 115: 743–746, 1989
35. American Academy of Pediatrics. Immunization in Special Clinical Circumstances. In: Peter G, ed. 1994 Red Book: Report of the Committee on Infectious Diseases. 23rd ed. Elk Grove Village, IL 51–52, 1994

Product information as of September 1996

Manufactured by:
Aventis Pasteur SA
Lyon France
US Govt License #1279
Distributed by:
Aventis Pasteur Inc.
Swiftwater, PA 18370 USA
1-800-VACCINE (1-800-822-2463) 4187

ActHIB for reconstitution with Connaught DTP vaccine Haemophilus b Conjugate Vaccine (Tetanus Toxoid Conjugate) packaged with Diphtheria and Tetanus Toxoids and Pertussis Vaccine Adsorbed USP (For Pediatric Use)
See package inserts for each component product.

Influenza Virus Vaccine USP
Trivalent Types A and B
(Zonal Purified, Subvirion)
2000–2001 Formula—For 6 Months and Older
FLUZONE® ℞
Rx only
SPECIAL NOTICE: *FOR USE IN IMMUNIZATION BY OR UNDER THE DIRECTION OF A PHYSICIAN.*
Caution: Federal (USA) law prohibits dispensing without prescription.

DESCRIPTION

Fluzone®, Influenza Virus Vaccine USP, (Zonal Purified, Subvirion) for intramuscular use, is a sterile suspension prepared from influenza viruses propagated in chicken embryos. The virus-containing fluids are harvested and inactivated with formaldehyde. Influenza virus is concentrated and purified in a linear sucrose density gradient solution using a continuous flow centrifuge. The virus is then chemically disrupted using Polyethylene Glycol p-Isooctylphenyl Ether (Triton® X-100—A registered trademark of Rohm and Haas, Co.) producing a "split-antigen." The split-antigen is then further purified by chemical means and suspended in sodium phosphate-buffered isotonic sodium chloride solution. Fluzone has been standardized according to USPHS requirements for the 2000–2001 influenza season and is formulated to contain 45 micrograms (µg) hemagglutinin (HA) per 0.5 mL dose, in the recommended ratio of 15 µg HA each, representative of the following three prototype strains: A/New Caledonia/20/99 (H1N1), A/Panama/2007/99 (H3N2) (an A/Moscow/10/99-like strain) and B/Yamanashi/166/98 (a B/Beijing/184/93-like strain).[1] Gelatin 0.05% is added as a stabilizer and thimerosal (mercury derivative) 1:10,000 is added as a preservative. Fluzone, after shaking syringe/vial well, is essentially clear and slightly opalescent in color.

ANTIBIOTICS ARE NOT USED IN THE MANUFACTURE OF FLUZONE.

CLINICAL PHARMACOLOGY

Epidemics of influenza occur during the winter months nearly every year and are responsible for an average of approximately 20,000 deaths per year in the United States (US).[1,2,3] Influenza viruses also can cause global epidemics of disease, known as pandemics, during which rates of illness and death from influenza-related complications can increase dramatically. Influenza viruses cause disease in all age groups.[1,4–6] Rates of infection are highest among children, but rates of serious illness and death are highest among persons greater than or equal to 65 years of age and persons of any age who have medical conditions that place them at high-risk for complications from influenza.[1,4,7–9]

Influenza vaccine is the primary method for preventing influenza and its more severe complications. The primary target group for influenza vaccination includes persons who are at high-risk for serious complications from influenza, including approximately 35 million persons greater than or equal to 65 years of age and approximately 33 to 39 million persons less than 65 years of age who have chronic underlying medical conditions.[1]

Beginning with the 2000–2001 influenza season, the Advisory Committee on Immunization Practices (ACIP) has added persons 50 to 64 years of age to the primary target group for annual influenza vaccination. This age group was added because a substantial proportion of persons 50 to 64 years of age (24% to 32%) have one or more chronic medical conditions that place them at high-risk for influenza-related hospitalization and death.[1,10–13] Further, 50 years is an age when other preventive services begin and when routine assessment of vaccination and other preventive services has been recommended.[1,14]

Among persons greater than or equal to 65 years of age, influenza vaccination levels increased from 33% in 1989[1,15] to 63% in 1997.[1,16] Although influenza vaccination coverage increased in black, Hispanic, and white populations, vaccination levels among blacks and Hispanics continue to lag behind those among whites.[1,16,17]

Increasing vaccination coverage among persons at high-risk less than 65 years of age now is the highest priority for expanding influenza vaccine use.[1]

Vaccination of health-care workers has been associated with reduced work absenteeism,[1,11] and decreased deaths among nursing home patients.[1,18,19] Efforts should be made to educate health-care workers about the benefits of vaccination and the potential health consequences of influenza illness for themselves and their patients.[1]

Influenza A and B are the two types of influenza viruses that cause epidemic human disease.[1,20] Influenza A viruses are further categorized into subtypes based on two surface antigens: hemagglutinin (H) and neuraminidase (N). Influenza B viruses are not categorized into subtypes. Both influenza A and B viruses are further separated into groups based on antigenic characteristics. New influenza virus variants result from frequent antigenic change (i.e., antigenic drift), resulting from point mutations that occur during viral replication. Influenza B viruses undergo antigenic drift less rapidly than influenza A viruses. Since 1977, influenza A (H1N1) viruses, influenza A (H3N2) viruses, and influenza B viruses have been in global circulation. A person's immunity to the surface antigens, especially hemagglutinin, reduces the likelihood of infection and the severity of disease if infection occurs.[1,21] However, antibody against one influenza virus type or subtype confers little or no protection against another virus type or subtype. Furthermore, antibody to one antigenic variant of influenza virus might not protect against a new antigenic variant of the same type or subtype.[1,22] The frequent development of antigenic variants through antigenic drift is the virologic basis for seasonal epidemics and the reason for the incorporation of one or more new strains in each year's influenza vaccine.[1]

Formal subclassification utilizing neuraminidase antigens has not been done for influenza B viruses.

The incubation period for influenza is one to four days with an average of two days.[1,23] Persons can be infectious starting the day before symptoms begin through approximately five days after illness onset; children can be infectious for a longer period. Uncomplicated influenza illness is characterized by the abrupt onset of constitutional and respiratory signs and symptoms (e.g., fever, myalgia, headache, severe malaise, nonproductive cough, sore throat, and rhinitis).[1,24]

Illness typically resolves after several days in most persons, although cough and malaise can persist for two or more weeks. In some persons, influenza can exacerbate underlying medical conditions (e.g., pulmonary or cardiac disease) or lead to secondary bacterial pneumonia or primary influenza viral pneumonia.[1,25]

The risks for complications, hospitalization, and deaths from influenza are higher among persons greater than or equal to 65 years of age, very young children, and persons of any age with some underlying health conditions than among healthy older children and younger adults.[1–3,25–27]

Estimated rates of influenza-associated hospitalizations have varied substantially by age group in studies conducted during different influenza epidemics:[1]

- Among children 0 to 4 years of age, rates have ranged from approximately 500 per 100,000 population for those with high-risk conditions to 100 per 100,000 population for those without high-risk conditions.[1,28] Among children without high-risk conditions, rates differ substantially within the 0- to four-year age group: babies less than 6 months of age have the highest hospitalization rate at approximately 1,040 per 100,000 population, and children 2 to 4 years of age are hospitalized at a rate of approximately 8 to 136 per 100,000 population.[1,29,30]
- Among children 5 to 14 years of age, rates have ranged from approximately 200 per 100,000 population for those with high-risk conditions to 20 to 40 per 100,000 population for those without high-risk conditions.[1,28,30]

Continued on next page

Fluzone—Cont.

- Among persons 15 to 44 years of age, rates have ranged from approximately 40 to 60 per 100,000 population for those with high-risk conditions to approximately 20 to 30 per 100,000 population for those without high-risk conditions.[1,7,8]
- Among persons 45 to 64 years of age, rates have ranged from approximately 80 to 400 per 100,000 population for those with high-risk medical conditions to approximately 20 to 40 per 100,000 population for those without high-risk conditions.[1,8,28]
- Among persons greater than or equal to 65 years of age, rates have ranged from approximately 200 to greater than 1,000 per 100,000 population.[1,8,28,31]

During influenza epidemics from 1969–1970 through 1993–1994, the estimated overall number of influenza-associated hospitalizations in the US has ranged from approximately 20,000 to greater than 300,000 per epidemic. An analysis of national hospital discharge data indicate an average of approximately 114,000 excess hospitalizations per year are related to influenza. Since the 1968 influenza A (H3N2) virus pandemic, the greatest numbers of influenza-associated hospitalizations have occurred during epidemics caused by type A (H3N2) viruses, with an estimated average of 142,000 influenza-associated hospitalizations per year.[1,32]

During influenza epidemics, deaths can increase from influenza and pneumonia as well as from exacerbations of cardiopulmonary conditions and other chronic diseases. In studies of influenza epidemics occurring from 1972–1973 through 1994–1995, excess deaths (i.e., the number of influenza-related deaths above a projected baseline of expected deaths) occurred during 19 of 23 influenza epidemics.[1,33] During those 19 influenza seasons, estimated rates of influenza-associated deaths ranged from approximately 30 to greater than 150 deaths per 100,000 persons greater than or equal to 65 years of age. These older adults currently account for more than 90% of the deaths attributed to pneumonia and influenza.[1,34] From 1972–1973 through 1994–1995, more than 20,000 influenza-associated deaths were estimated to occur during each of 11 different US epidemics, and more than 40,000 influenza-associated deaths were estimated for each of six of these 11 epidemics.[1,33] In the US, pneumonia and influenza deaths might be increasing in part because the number of elderly persons is increasing.[1,35]

Vaccinating persons at high-risk for complications before the influenza season each year is the most effective means of reducing the impact of influenza. Vaccination coverage can be increased by administering vaccine to persons during hospitalizations or routine health-care visits before the influenza season, making special visits to physicians' offices or clinics unnecessary. When vaccine and epidemic strains of virus are well matched, achieving high vaccination rates among persons living in closed settings (e.g., nursing homes and other chronic-care facilities) and among the staff can reduce the risk for outbreaks by inducing herd immunity.[1,36] Vaccination of health-care workers and other persons in close contact with persons in high-risk groups also can reduce transmission of influenza and subsequent influenza-related complications.[1]

Influenza vaccine contains three virus strains (two type A and one type B), representing the influenza viruses likely to circulate in the US in the upcoming winter. The vaccine is made from highly purified, egg-grown viruses that have been made noninfectious (inactivated).[1,37]

Most vaccinated children and young adults develop high postvaccination hemagglutination-inhibition antibody titers.[1,38,39] These antibody titers are protective against illness caused by strains similar to those in the vaccine.[1,39–41] The effectiveness of influenza vaccine depends primarily on the age and immunocompetence of the vaccine recipient and the degree of similarity between the viruses in the vaccine and those in circulation. When the antigenic match between vaccine and circulating viruses is close, influenza vaccine prevents illness in approximately 70% to 90% of healthy persons younger than 65 years of age.[1,42] Vaccination of healthy adults also has resulted in decreased work absenteeism and decreased use of health-care resources when the vaccine and circulating viruses are well matched.[1,11–13,43] Other studies suggest that the use of trivalent inactivated influenza vaccine or live attenuated influenza vaccine decreases the incidence of otitis media and the use of antibiotics among children.[1,44–46]

Elderly persons and persons with certain chronic diseases might develop lower post-vaccination antibody titers than healthy young adults and thus can remain susceptible to influenza-related upper-respiratory-tract infection.[1,47–49] However, among such persons, the vaccine can be effective in preventing secondary complications and reducing the risk for influenza-related hospitalization and death.[1,36,50,51] Among elderly persons living outside of nursing homes or similar chronic-care facilities, influenza vaccine is 30% to 70% effective in preventing hospitalization for pneumonia and influenza.[1,10,51] Among elderly persons residing in nursing homes, influenza vaccine is most effective in preventing severe illness, secondary complications, and deaths. In this population, the vaccine can be 50% to 60% effective in preventing hospitalization or pneumonia and 80% effective in preventing death, even though the effectiveness in preventing influenza illness often ranges from 30% to 40%.[1,52,53]

INDICATIONS AND USAGE

Fluzone is indicated only for immunization against the selected virus strains contained in the vaccine (see **PRECAUTIONS** section).

The optimal time to vaccinate persons in high-risk groups is usually from the beginning of October through mid-November, because influenza activity in the US generally peaks between late December and early March. Although vaccine generally becomes available in August or September, in some years, vaccine for the upcoming influenza season might not be available in some locations until later in the fall. Administering vaccine before October should generally be avoided in facilities such as nursing homes, because antibody levels can begin to decline within a few months after vaccination.[1,54,55]

Influenza vaccine (subvirion) is strongly recommended for any person greater than or equal to 6 months of age who—because of age or underlying medical condition—is at increased risk for complications of influenza. In addition, health-care workers and other individuals (including household members) in close contact with persons in high-risk groups should be vaccinated to decrease the risk of transmitting influenza to persons at high-risk. Influenza vaccine also can be administered to any person greater than or equal to 6 months of age to reduce the chance of becoming infected with influenza.[1]

Dosage recommendations for the 2000–2001 season are given in Table 1. Guidelines for the use of vaccine among certain patient populations are given below.[1]

REMAINING 1999–2000 VACCINE SHOULD NOT BE USED TO PROVIDE PROTECTION FOR THE 2000–2001 INFLUENZA SEASON.[1]

Beginning each September, influenza vaccine should be offered to persons at high-risk when they are seen by health-care providers for routine care or are hospitalized. If regional influenza activity is expected to begin earlier than December, vaccination programs also can be undertaken as early as September. Health-care providers should offer vaccine to unvaccinated persons even after influenza virus activity is documented in a community and should continue to offer vaccine throughout the influenza season.[1] (For information on vaccination of travelers, see **Travelers** section.)

Dosage recommendations vary according to age group (Table 1). Among previously unvaccinated children younger than 9 years of age, two doses administered at least one month apart are recommended for satisfactory antibody responses. If possible, the second dose should be administered before December. Among adults, studies have indicated little or no improvement in antibody response when a second dose is administered during the same season.[1,56–59] Even when the current influenza vaccine contains one or more of the antigens administered in previous years, annual vaccination with the current vaccine is necessary because immunity declines during the year following vaccination.[1,54,55] Vaccine prepared for a previous influenza season should not be administered to provide protection for the current season.[1]

During recent decades, data on influenza vaccine immunogenicity and side effects have been obtained for intramuscularly administered vaccine. Because recent influenza vaccines have not been adequately evaluated when administered by other routes, the intramuscular route is recommended. Adults and older children should be vaccinated in the deltoid muscle; *a needle length greater than or equal to 1 inch can be considered for these age groups.* Infants and young children should be vaccinated in the anterolateral aspect of the thigh.[1,60]

SAFETY AND EFFECTIVENSS OF FLUZONE (SUBVIRION) IN INFANTS BELOW THE AGE OF 6 MONTHS HAVE NOT BEEN ESTABLISHED.

TARGET GROUPS FOR VACCINATION

Groups at Increased Risk for Complications

Vaccination is recommended for the following groups of persons who are at increased risk for complications from influenza or who have a higher prevalence of chronic medical conditions that place them at risk for influenza-related complications:[1]

- persons greater than or equal to 50 years of age;[1]
- residents of nursing homes and other chronic-care facilities that house persons of any age who have chronic medical conditions;[1]
- adults and children who have chronic disorders of the pulmonary or cardiovascular systems, including asthma;[1]
- adults and children who have required regular medical follow-up or hospitalization during the preceding year because of chronic metabolic diseases (including diabetes mellitus), renal dysfunction, hemoglobinopathies, or immunosuppression (including immunosuppression caused by medications or by human immunodeficiency virus [HIV]);[1]
- infants, children and teenagers (6 months to 18 years of age) who are receiving long-term aspirin therapy and therefore might be at risk for developing Reye syndrome after influenza infection; and[1]
- women who will be in the second or third trimester of pregnancy during the influenza season.[1]

Also, persons who smoke tobacco products are at increased risk for influenza-related complications and therefore should receive influenza vaccine.[61–63]

Persons Who Can Transmit Influenza to Those at High-Risk:[1]

Persons who are clinically or subclinically infected can transmit influenza virus to persons at high-risk for complications from influenza. Decreasing transmission of influenza from care-givers to persons at high-risk might reduce influenza-related deaths among persons at high-risk. Evidence from two studies suggest that vaccination of health-care workers is associated with decreased deaths among nursing home patients.[1,15,16] Vaccination of health-care workers and others in close contact with persons at high-risk is recommended. The following groups should be vaccinated:[1]

- physicians, nurses, and other personnel in both hospital and outpatient-care settings, including emergency response workers;
- employees of nursing homes and chronic-care facilities who have contact with patients or residents;
- employees of assisted living and other residences for persons in high-risk groups;
- persons who provide home care to persons in high-risk groups; and
- household members (including children) of persons in high-risk groups.

General Population

Physicians should administer influenza vaccine to any person who wishes to reduce the likelihood of becoming ill with influenza (the vaccine can be administered to children as young as 6 months of age). Persons who provide essential community services should be considered for vaccination to minimize disruption of essential activities during influenza outbreaks. Students or other persons in institutional settings (e.g., those who reside in dormitories) should be encouraged to receive vaccine to minimize the disruption of routine activities during epidemics.[1]

Pregnant Women

Influenza-associated excess deaths among pregnant women were documented during the pandemics of 1918–1919 and 1957–1958.[1,64–67] Case reports and limited studies also suggest that pregnancy can increase the risk for serious medical complications of influenza as a result of increases in heart rate, stroke volume, and oxygen consumption; decreases in lung capacity; and changes in immunologic function.[1,68–71] A study of the impact of influenza during 17 interpandemic influenza seasons demonstrated that the relative risk for hospitalization for selected cardiorespiratory conditions among pregnant women increased from 1.4 during weeks 14 to 20 of gestation to 4.7 during weeks 37 to 42 in comparison with women who were 1 to 6 months postpartum.[1,72] The risk during the third trimester was comparable to the risk for non-pregnant women with high-risk medical conditions for whom influenza vaccine has traditionally been recommended. It was estimated that immunizing 1,000 women who would be in their third trimester during influenza season would prevent one hospitalization.[1]

In view of these and other data which suggest that influenza infection may cause increased morbidity in women during the second and third trimesters of pregnancy, the ACIP recommends that health-care workers who provide care for pregnant women should consider administering influenza vaccine.[1] **(Refer to Pregnancy Category C statement.)**

Breastfeeding Mothers

Influenza vaccine does not affect the safety of mothers who are breastfeeding or their infants. Breastfeeding does not adversely affect immune response and is not a contraindication for vaccination.[1]

Persons Infected with Human Immunodeficiency Virus (HIV)

Limited information is available regarding the frequency and severity of influenza illness or the benefits of influenza vaccination among persons with HIV infection.[1,73,74] However, a recent retrospective study of young and middle-aged women found that the attributable risk for cardiopulmonary hospitalizations among women with HIV infection was higher during influenza seasons than in the peri-influenza periods. The risk of hospitalization for HIV-infected women was higher than the risk for women with other well-recognized high-risk conditions for influenza complications, including chronic heart and lung diseases.[1,75] Other reports suggest that influenza symptoms might be prolonged and the risk for complications from influenza increased for some HIV-infected persons.[1,76,77]

Influenza vaccination has been shown to produce substantial antibody titers against influenza in vaccinated HIV-infected persons who have minimal acquired immunodeficiency syndrome-related symptoms and high CD4+ T-lymphocyte cell counts.[1,78–81] A small, randomized, placebo-controlled trial found that influenza vaccine was highly effective in preventing symptomatic, laboratory-confirmed influenza infection among HIV-infected persons with a mean of 400 CD4+ T-lymphocyte cells/mm^3; few persons with CD4+ T-lymphocyte cell counts of less than 200 were included in this study.[1,74] In patients who have advanced HIV disease and low CD4+ T-lymphocyte cell counts, influenza vaccine might not induce protective antibody titers;[1,80,81] a second dose of vaccine does not improve the immune response in these persons.[1,81,82]

One study found that HIV RNA levels increased transiently in one HIV-infected patient after influenza infection.[1,83] Some studies have demonstrated a transient (i.e., 2- to 4-week) increase in replication of HIV-1 in the plasma or peripheral blood mononuclear cells of HIV-infected persons after vaccine administration.[1,80–84] Other studies using similar laboratory techniques have not documented a substantial increase in replication of HIV.[1,85–87] Deterioration of CD4+ T-lymphocyte cell counts or progression of HIV disease have not been demonstrated among HIV-infected persons following influenza vaccination. The effect of antiretroviral therapy on potential increases in HIV RNA levels following either natural influenza infection or influenza vaccination is unknown.[1,73] Because influenza can result in serious illness and complications and because influenza vaccination can result in the production of protective antibody titers, vaccination will benefit many HIV-infected patients, including HIV-infected pregnant women.[1]

Travelers

The risk of exposure to influenza during travel depends on the time of year and destination. In the tropics, influenza can occur throughout the year. In the temperate regions of the Southern Hemisphere, most influenza activity occurs from April through September. In temperate climate zones of the Northern and Southern Hemispheres, travelers also can be exposed to influenza during the summer, especially when traveling as part of large organized tourist groups that includes persons from areas of the world where influenza viruses are circulating.[1] Persons at high-risk for complications of influenza who were not vaccinated with influenza vaccine during the preceding fall or winter should consider receiving influenza vaccine before travel if they plan to:[1]

- travel to the tropics;
- travel with large organized tourist groups at any time of year; or
- travel to the Southern Hemisphere from April through September.

No information is available regarding the benefits of revaccinating persons before summer travel who were already vaccinated in the preceding fall. Persons at high-risk who received the previous season's vaccine before travel should be revaccinated with the current vaccine in the following fall or winter. Persons greater than or equal to 50 years of age and others at high-risk might wish to consult with their physicians before embarking on travel during the summer to discuss the symptoms and risks of influenza and the advisability of carrying antiviral medications for either prophylaxis or treatment of influenza.[1]

SIMULTANEOUS ADMINISTRATION OF OTHER VACCINES, INCLUDING CHILDHOOD VACCINES

CONCURRENT USE WITH PNEUMOCOCCAL VACCINE.

Fluzone has been shown in clinical studies to be acceptable for concurrent use with pneumococcal vaccine using separate syringes at different sites. Although Influenza Virus Vaccine is recommended for annual use, the pneumococcal vaccine should only be given once.[1,88,89] Children at high-risk for influenza-related complications can receive influenza vaccine at the same time they receive other routine vaccinations.[1]

CONTRAINDICATIONS

INFLUENZA VIRUS IS PROPAGATED IN EGGS FOR THE PREPARATION OF INFLUENZA VIRUS VACCINE. THEREFORE, FLUZONE SHOULD NOT BE ADMINISTERED TO ANYONE WITH A HISTORY OF HYPERSENSITIVITY (ALLERGY), ESPECIALLY ANAPHYLACTIC REACTIONS, TO EGGS OR EGG PRODUCTS. IT IS ALSO A CONTRAINDICATION TO ADMINISTER FLUZONE TO INDIVIDUALS KNOWN TO BE SENSITIVE TO THIMEROSAL. EPINEPHRINE INJECTION (1:1000) MUST BE IMMEDIATELY AVAILABLE SHOULD AN ACUTE ANAPHYLACTIC REACTION OCCUR DUE TO ANY COMPONENT OF FLUZONE.

Fluzone should not be administered to patients with acute respiratory or other active infections or illnesses.

Immunization should be delayed in a patient with an active neurologic disorder, but should be considered when the disease process has been stabilized.

WARNINGS

This product contains dry natural rubber latex as follows: The stopper to the vial contains dry natural rubber latex. In the case of the syringe, the needle cover contains dry natural rubber latex, but the plunger for the syringe contains no dry natural rubber latex.

Fluzone should not be administered to individuals who have a prior history of Guillain-Barré syndrome (GBS).

If Fluzone is administered to immunosuppressed persons, the expected antibody response may not be obtained.

As with any vaccine, vaccination with Fluzone may not protect 100% of susceptible individuals.

PRECAUTIONS

GENERAL

Care is to be taken by the health-care provider for the safe and effective use of this vaccine.

EPINEPHRINE INJECTION (1:1000) MUST BE IMMEDIATELY AVAILABLE SHOULD AN ACUTE ANAPHYLACTIC REACTION OCCUR DUE TO ANY COMPONENT OF THIS VACCINE.

Influenza virus is remarkably capricious in that significant antigenic changes may occur from time-to-time. *It is known definitely that Influenza Virus Vaccine, as now constituted, is not effective against all possible strains of influenza virus. Protection is limited to those strains of virus from which the vaccine is prepared or against closely related strains.*

During the course of any febrile respiratory illness or other active infection, use of Influenza Virus Vaccine should be delayed.

Since the likelihood of febrile convulsions is greater in children 6 months through 35 months of age, special care should be taken in weighing relative risks and benefits of vaccination.

Prior to an injection of any vaccine, all known precautions should be taken to prevent side reactions. This includes a review of the patient's history with respect to possible sensitivity to the vaccine or similar vaccine, to possible sensitivity to dry natural rubber latex, previous immunization history, current health status (see CONTRAINDICATIONS and WARNINGS sections) and a knowledge of the current literature concerning the use of the vaccine under consideration.

TABLE 1[1]—Influenza Vaccine Dosage by Age Group 2000–2001 Season

Age Group	Vaccine†	Dosage	No. of Doses
6–35 months	Split virus only	0.25 mL	1 or 2*
3–8 years	Split virus only	0.50 mL	1 or 2*
9–12 years	Split virus only	0.50 mL	1
> 12 years	Whole or split virus	0.50 mL	1

† Because of decreased potential for causing febrile reactions, only split-virus (subvirion) vaccines should be used for children. Immunogenicity and side effects of split- and whole-virus vaccines are similar among adults when vaccines are administered at the recommended dosage.

* Two doses administered at least one month apart are recommended for children less than 9 years of age who are receiving influenza vaccine for the first time.

Special care should be taken to prevent injection into a blood vessel.

A separate, sterile syringe and needle or a sterile disposable unit should be used for each patient to prevent transmission of hepatitis or other infectious agents from person to person. Needles should not be recapped and should be disposed of according to biohazard waste guidelines.

INFORMATION FOR PATIENT

Patients, parents or guardians should be fully informed by their health-care provider of the benefits and risks of immunization with Influenza Virus Vaccine.

Patients, parents or guardians should be instructed to report any serious adverse reactions to their health-care provider.

Drug Interaction:

Although influenza vaccination can inhibit the clearance of warfarin, theophylline, phenytoin, and aminopyrine therapy, studies have failed to show any adverse clinical effects attributable to these drugs in patients receiving influenza vaccine.[90–96]

If Fluzone is administered to immunosuppressed persons or persons receiving immunosuppressive therapy, the expected antibody response may not be obtained. This includes patients with asymptomatic HIV infection, AIDS or AIDS-Related Complex, severe combined immunodeficiency, hypogammaglobulinemia, aggammaglobulinemia; altered immune states due to diseases such as leukemia, lymphoma, or generalized malignancy; or an immune system compromised by treatment with corticosteroids, alkylating drugs, antimetabolites or radiation.[97]

PREGNANCY

REPRODUCTIVE STUDIES—PREGNANCY CATEGORY C

Animal reproduction studies have not been conducted with Influenza Virus Vaccine USP Trivalent, Types A and B. It is not known whether Influenza Virus Vaccine can cause fetal harm when administered to a pregnant woman or can affect reproduction capacity. Influenza Virus Vaccine should be given to a pregnant women only if clearly needed (see **INDICATIONS AND USAGE** section).

PEDIATRIC USE

SAFETY AND EFFECTIVENESS OF FLUZONE (SUBVIRION) IN INFANTS BELOW THE AGE OF 6 MONTHS HAVE NOT BEEN ESTABLISHED.

ADVERSE REACTIONS

When educating patients about potential side effects, clinicians should emphasize that a) inactivated influenza vaccine contains noninfectious killed viruses and cannot cause influenza; and b) coincidental respiratory disease unrelated to influenza vaccine can occur after vaccination.[1]

Local Reactions

In placebo-controlled blinded studies, the most frequent side effect of vaccination is soreness at the vaccination site (affecting 10% to 64% of patients) that lasts up to 2 days.[1,98–100] These local reactions generally are mild and rarely interfere with the person's ability to conduct usual daily activities.[1]

Systemic Reactions

Fever, malaise, myalgia, and other systemic symptoms can occur following vaccination and most often affect persons who have had no exposure to the influenza virus antigens in the vaccine (e.g., young children).[1,101,102] These reactions begin 6 to 12 hours after vaccination and can persist for 1 to 2 days. Recent placebo-controlled trials suggest that among elderly persons and healthy young adults, administration of split-virus vaccine is not associated with higher rates of systemic symptoms (e.g., fever, malaise, myalgia, and headache) when compared with placebo injections.[1,98–100]

Immediate—presumably allergic—reactions (e.g., hives, angioedema, allergic asthma, and systemic anaphylaxis) rarely occur after influenza vaccination.[1,103] These reactions probably result from hypersensitivity to some vaccine component; most reactions likely are caused by residual egg protein. Although current influenza vaccines contain only a small quantity of egg protein, this protein can induce immediate hypersensitivity reactions among persons who have severe egg allergy. Persons who have developed hives, have had swelling of the lips or tongue, or have experienced acute respiratory distress or collapse after eating eggs should consult a physician for appropriate evaluation to help determine if vaccine should be administered. Persons who have documented immunoglobulin E (IgE)-mediated hypersensitivity to eggs—including those who have had occupational asthma or other allergic responses to egg protein—also might be at increased risk for allergic reactions to influenza vaccine, and consultation with a physician should be considered. Protocols have been published for safely administering influenza vaccine to persons with egg allergies.[1,104,105]

The 1976 swine influenza vaccine was associated with an increased frequency of Guillain-Barré syndrome (GBS).[1,106,107] Among persons who received the swine influenza vaccine in 1976, the rate of GBS that exceeded the background rate was slightly less than 10 cases per million persons vaccinated. Evidence for a causal relationship of GBS with subsequent vaccines prepared from other influenza viruses is less clear. Obtaining strong epidemiologic evidence for a possible small increase in risk is difficult for a rare condition such as GBS, which has an annual incidence of only 10 to 20 cases per million adults,[1,108] and stretches the limits of epidemiologic investigation.[1]

During three of four influenza seasons studied from 1977 through 1991, the overall relative risk estimates for GBS after influenza vaccination were slightly elevated but were not statistically significant in any of these studies.[1,109–111] However, in a study of the 1992–1993 and 1993–1994 seasons, the overall relative risk for GBS was 1.7 (95% confidence interval = 1.0–2.8; p = 0.04) during the six weeks following vaccination, representing an excess of slightly more than one additional case of GBS per million persons vaccinated; the combined number of GBS cases peaked two weeks after vaccination.[1,112] Thus, investigations to date suggest that there is no large increase in GBS associated with influenza vaccines (other than the swine influenza vaccine in 1976) and that if influenza vaccine does pose a risk, it is probably quite small—slightly more than one additional case per million persons vaccinated.[1]

Even if GBS were a true side effect of vaccination in the years after 1976, the estimated risk for GBS of slightly more than one additional case per million persons vaccinated is substantially less than the risk for severe influenza, which could be prevented by vaccination in all age groups, especially persons greater than or equal to 65 years of age and those who have medical indications for influenza vaccination. During different epidemics occurring from 1972 through 1981, estimated rates of influenza-associated hospitalization have ranged from approximately 200 to 300 hospitalizations per million population for previously healthy persons 5 to 44 years of age and from 2,000 to greater than 10,000 hospitalizations per million population for persons greater than or equal to 65 years of age.[1,7,8,28,31] During epidemics from 1972–1973 through 1994–1995, estimates rates of influenza-associated deaths have ranged from approximately 300 to greater than 1,500 per million persons greater than or equal to 65 years of age, who account for more than 90% of all influenza-associated deaths. The potential benefits of influenza vaccination in preventing serious illness, hospitalization, and death greatly outweigh the possible risks for developing vaccine-associated GBS. The average case-fatality ratio for GBS is 6% and increases with age.[1,108,113] However, no evidence indicates that the case-fatality ratio for GBS differs among vaccinated persons and those not vaccinated.[1]

The incidence of GBS in the general population is very low, but persons with a history of GBS have a substantially greater likelihood of subsequently developing GBS than persons without such a history.[1,109,114] Thus, the likelihood of coincidently developing GBS after influenza vaccination is expected to be greater among persons with a history of GBS than among persons with no history of this syndrome. Whether influenza vaccination specifically might increase the risk for recurrence of GBS is not known.[1]

Neurological disorders temporally associated with influenza vaccination such as encephalopathy, optic neuritis/neuropathy,[115,116] partial facial paralysis, and brachial plexus neuropathy have been reported. However, no cause and effect has been established.[117,118] Almost all persons affected were adults, and the described clinical reactions began as soon as a few hours and as late as 2 weeks after vaccination. Full recovery was almost always reported.[102,119,120]

Microscopic polyangitis (vasculitis) has been reported temporally associated with influenza vaccination. However, no cause and effect has been established.[121]

Reporting of Adverse Events

Reporting by patients, parents or guardians of all adverse events occurring after vaccine administration should be encouraged. Adverse events following immunization with vaccine should be reported by the health-care provider to the US Department of Health and Human Services (DHHS) Vaccine Adverse Event Reporting Systems (VAERS). Reporting forms and information about reporting requirements or completion of the form can be obtained from VAERS through a toll-free number 1-800-822-7967.[122]

Continued on next page

Fluzone—Cont.

The health-care provider also should report these events to the Director of Scientific and Medical Affairs, Aventis Pasteur Inc., Discovery Drive, Swiftwater, PA 18370 or call 1-800-822-2463.

DOSAGE AND ADMINISTRATION

Parenteral drug products should be inspected visually for particulate matter and/or discoloration prior to administration whenever solution and container permit. If either of these conditions exist, the vaccine should not be administered.

The syringe or vial should be well shaken before withdrawing each 0.5 mL dose.

Do NOT inject intravenously.

Injections of Influenza Virus Vaccine should be administered intramuscularly, preferably in the region of the deltoid muscle, in adults and older children. The preferred site for infants and young children is the anterolateral aspect of the thigh. Before injection, the skin over the site to be injected should be cleansed with a suitable germicide. After insertion of the needle, aspirate to assure that the needle has not entered a blood vessel.

Influenza vaccine should be offered beginning in September (see **INDICATIONS AND USAGE** section).

Children less than 9 years of age who have not previously been vaccinated should receive two doses of vaccine at least one month apart to maximize the likelihood of a satisfactory antibody response to all three vaccine antigens. The second dose should be administered before December, if possible.[1] Fluzone (Subvirion) is to be used for persons 6 months of age and older. Fluzone (Subvirion) is NOT approved for infants under 6 months of age. The dosage is as follows:

[See table 1 at top of previous page]

HOW SUPPLIED

Syringe with 1" needle, 0.5 mL (Shake syringe well before administering.) **(Do not use for administering 0.25 mL)**—Product No. 49281-366-11

Vial, 5 mL, for administration with needle and syringe (Shake vial well before withdrawing each dose.)—Product No. 49281-366-15

STORAGE

Store between 2°–8°C (35°–46°F). Potency is destroyed by freezing. **DO NOT USE FLUZONE IF IT HAS BEEN FROZEN.**

REFERENCES

1. Recommendations of the Advisory Committee on Immunization Practices (ACIP). MMWR 49: (RR03): 1–38, 2000. **2.** Simonsen L, et al. Elsevier Science BV. 26–33, 1996. **3.** Lui K-J, et al. Am J Public Health 77: 712–716, 1987 **4.** Monto AS, et al. Am J Epidemiol 102: 553–563, 1975. **5.** Glezen WP, et al. N Engl J Med 298: 587–592, 1978. **6.** Glezen WP, et al. JAMA 283: 499–505, 2000. **7.** Barker WH, et al. Am J Public Health 76: 761–765, 1986. **8.** Barker WH, et al. Am J Epidemiol 112: 798–813, 1980. **9.** Glezen WP. Epidemiol Rev 4: 25–44, 1982. **10.** Nichol KL, et al. N Engl J Med 331: 778–784, 1994. **11.** Wilde JA, et al. JAMA 281: 908–913, 1999. **12.** Campbell DS, et al. J Occup Environ Med 39: 408–414, 1997. **13.** Smith JWG, et al. J Hygiene 83: 157–170, 1979. **14.** Centers for Disease Control and Prevention (CDC). MMWR 44: 561–563, 1995. **15.** CDC. MMWR 44: 506–507, 513–515, 1995. **16.** Singleton JA, et al. In: Abstracts of the 34th National Immunization Conference. Atlanta, GA: CDC, 2000 (in press). **17.** CDC. MMWR 47: 797–802, 1998. **18.** Potter J, et al. J Infect Dis 175: 1–6, 1997. **19.** Carman WF, et al. Lancet 355: 93–97, 2000. **20.** Murphy BR, et al. In: Fields BN, Knipe DM, Howley PM, et al. Third edition. Philadelphia, PA: Lippincott-Raven Publishers, 1397–1445, 1996. **21.** Clements ML, et al. J Clin Microbiol 24: 157–160, 1986. **22.** Couch RB, et al. Annu Rev Microbiol 37: 529–549, 1983. **23.** Cox NJ, et al. The Lancet 354: 1277–1282, 1999. **24.** Nicholson KG. Semin Respir Infect 7: 26–37, 1992. **25.** Noble GR. In: Beare AS, ed. Boca Raton, FL: CRC Press, 11–50, 1982. **26.** Eickhoff TC, et al. JAMA 176: 776–782, 1961. **27.** Barker WH, et al. Arch Intern Med 142: 85–89, 1982. **28.** Glezen WP, et al. Am Rev Resp Dis 136: 550–555, 1987. **29.** Izurieta HS, et al. N Engl J Med 342: 232–239, 2000. **30.** Neuzil KM, et al. N Engl J Med 342: 225–231, 2000. **31.** Glezen WP. Can J Infect Dis 4: 272–274, 1993. **32.** Simonsen L, et al. J Infect Dis 2000 (in press). **33.** Simonsen L, et al. Am J Public Health 87: 1944–1950, 1997. **34.** Simonsen L, et al. J Infect Dis 178: 53–60, 1998. **35.** National Center for Health Statistics. Health, United States, 1998, Hyattsville, MD: National Center for Health Statistics, 1998. **36.** Patriarca PA, et al. Am J Epidemiol 124: 114–119, 1986. **37.** Kilbourne ED. Influenza. New York, NY: Plenum Medical Book Company, 1987. **38.** La Montagne JR, et al. Rev Infect Dis 5: 723–735, 1983. **39.** Oxford JS, et al. J Hygiene 82: 51–61, 1979. **40.** Potter CW, et al. Br Med Bull 35: 69–75, 1979. **41.** Hirota Y, et al. Vaccine 15: 962–967, 1997. **42.** Palache AM. Drugs 54: 841–856, 1997. **43.** Nichol KL, et al. N Engl J Med 333: 889–893, 1995. **44.** Belshe RB, et al. N Engl J Med 338: 1405–1412, 1998. **45.** Clements DA, et al. Arch Pediatr Adolesc Med 149: 1113–1117, 1995. **46.** Heikkinen T, et al. Am J Dis Child 145: 445–448, 1991. **47.** Blumberg EA, et al. Clin Infect Dis 22: 295–302, 1996. **48.** Dorrell L, et al. Inst J STD AIDS 8: 776–779, 1997. **49.** McElhaney JE, et al. J Am Geriatr Soc 38: 652–658, 1990. **50.** Gross PA, et al. Ann Intern Med 123: 518–527, 1995. **51.** Mullooly JP, et al. Ann Intern Med 121: 947–952, 1994. **52.** Patriarca PA, et al. JAMA 253: 1136–1139, 1985. **53.** Arden NH, et al. In: Kendal AP, Patriarca PA, eds. New York, NY: Alan R. Liss Inc. 155–168, 1986. **54.** Cate TR, et al. Rev Infect Dis 5: 737–747, 1983. **55.** Kunzel W, et al. Vaccine 14: 1108–1110, 1996. **56.** Gross PA, et al. J Clin Microbiol 25: 1763–1765, 1987. **57.** Iorio AM, et al. Vaccine 15: 97–102, 1997. **58.** Feery BJ, et al. Med J Aust 1: 186, 188–189, 1976. **59.** Howells CHL, et al. Lancet 1: 1436–1438, 1973. **60.** CDC. MMWR 43: No. RR-1, 1–36, 1994. **61.** Mulloy E. Ir Med J Vol 89 (6): 202, 204, 1996. **62.** Zimmerman RK, et al. Am Fam Physician 51 (4): 859–867, 1995. **63.** Rothbarth PH, et al. Am J Respir Crit Care Med 151: 1682–1686, 1995. **64.** Noble GR. In: Beare AS, ed. Boca Raton, FL: CRC Press: 41–42, 1982. **65.** Harris JW. JAMA 72: 978–980, 1919. **66.** Widelock D, et al. Public Health Rep 78: 1–11, 1963. **67.** Freeman DW, et al. Am J Obstet Gynecol 78: 1172–1175, 1959. **68.** Shahab SZ, et al. In: Gonik B, ed. New York, NY: Springer-Veriag. 215–223, 1994. **69.** Schoenbaum SC, et al. Clin Obstet Gynecol 22: 293–300, 1979. **70.** Kirshon B, et al. J Reprod Med 33: 399–401, 1988. **71.** Kort BA, et al. Am J Perinatol 3: 179–182, 1986. **72.** Neuzil KM, et al. Am J Epidemiol 148: 1094–1102, 1998. **73.** Couch RB, Clin Infect Dis 28: 548–551, 1999. **74.** Tasker SA, et al. Ann Intern Med 131: 430–433, 1999. **75.** Neuzil KM, et al. JAMA 281: 901–907, 1999. **76.** Safrin S, et al. Chest 98: 33–37, 1990. **77.** Radwan H, et al. Infectious Diseases Society of America, 1998. **78.** Chadwick EG, et al. Pediatr Infect Dis J 13: 206–211, 1994. **79.** Huang K-L, et al. JAMA 257: 2047–2050, 1987. **80.** Staprans SI, et al. J Exp Med 182: 1727–1737, 1995. **81.** Kroon FP, et al. AIDS 8: 469–476, 1994. **82.** Miotti PG, et al. JAMA 262: 779–783, 1989. **83.** Ho DD. Lancet 339: 1549, 1992. **84.** O'Brien WA, et al. Blood 86: 1082–1089, 1995. **85.** Glesby MJ, et al. J Infect Dis 174: 1332–1336, 1996. **86.** Fowke KR, et al. AIDS 11: 1013–1021, 1997. **87.** Fuller JD, et al. Clin Infect Dis 28: 541–547, 1999. **88.** Grilli G, et al. Eur J Epidemiol 13: 287–291, 1997. **89.** Fletcher TJ, et al. BMJ 314: 1663–1665, 1997. **90.** Renton KW, et al. Can Med Assoc J 123: 288–290, 1980. **91.** Fischer RG, et al. Can Med Assoc J 126: 1312–1313, 1982. **92.** Lipsky BA, et al. Ann Intern Med 100: 6: 835–837, 1984. **93.** Kramer P, et al. Clin Pharmacol Ther Vol 35, #3: 416–418, 1984. **94.** Patriarca PA, et al. New Engl J Med 308: 1601–1602, 1983. **95.** Levine M, et al. Clin Pharm 3: 505–509, 1984. **96.** Kilbourne ED. Vaccines (Plotkin and Mortimer eds.) Saunders Company: 429, 1988. **97.** ACIP. MMWR 35: 595–606, 1986. **98.** Govaert ME, et al. BMJ 307: 988–990, 1993. **99.** Margolis KL, et al. JAMA 254: 1139–1141, 1990. **100.** Nichol KL, et al. Arch Intern Med 156: 1546–1550, 1996. **101.** Scheifele DW, et al. Can Med Assoc J 142: 127–130, 1990. **102.** Barry DW, et al. Am J Epidemiol 104: 47–59, 1976. **103.** Bierman CW, et al. J Infect Dis 236: S652–S655, 1997. **104.** James JM, et al. J Pediatr 133: 624–628, 1998. **105.** Murphy KR, et al. J Pediatr 106: 931–933, 1985. **106.** Schonberger LB, et al. Am J Epidemiol 110: 105–123, 1979. **107.** Safranek TJ, et al. Am J Epidemiol 133: 940–951, 1991. **108.** Ropper AH. N Engl J Med 326: 1130–1136, 1992. **109.** Hurwitz ES, et al. N Engl J Med 304: 1557–1561, 1981. **110.** Kaplan JE, et al. JAMA 248: 698–700, 1982. **111.** Chen R, et al. Post Marketing Surveillance 6: 5–6, 1992. **112.** Lasky T, et al. N Engl J Med 339: 1797–1802, 1998. **113.** Prevots DR, et al. J Infect Dis 175 (Suppl 1): S151–S155, 1997. **114.** Barohn RJ, et al. Semin Neurol 18: 49–61, 1998. **115.** Hull TP, et al. Am J Opthalmol 703–704, 1997. **116.** Kawasaki A, et al. J Neuro-Opthalmol: 18 (1), 57–59, 1998. **117.** CDC. Surveillance Report No. 3, 1985–1986, Issued February 1989. **118.** Aventis Pasteur Inc., Data on File. MKT5720, 1994. **119.** Retaillaiu HF, et al. Am J Epid III (3): 270–278, 1980. **120.** Guerrero IC, et al. N Engl J Med 300 (10): 565, 1979. **121.** Kelsall JT, et al. J Rheumatol 1198–1202, 1997. **122.** CDC. MMWR 39: 730–733, 1990.

Product information as of April 2000

Manufactured by:
Aventis Pasteur Inc.
Swiftwater PA 18370 USA

4354/4362

Rabies Immune Globulin (Human) USP

IMOGAM® RABIES – HT ℞

℞ only

[Im 'o-gam]

Caution: Federal (USA) law prohibits dispensing without prescription.

DESCRIPTION

Rabies Immune Globulin (Human) USP, Imogam® Rabies – HT, is a sterile solution of antirabies immunoglobulin (10–18% protein) for intramuscular administration. It is prepared by cold alcohol fractionation from pooled venous plasma of individuals immunized with Rabies Vaccine prepared from human diploid cells (HDCV). The product is stabilized with 0.3 M glycine. The globulin solution has a pH of 6.8 ± 0.4 adjusted with sodium hydroxide or hydrochloric acid. No preservatives are added. Imogam® Rabies – HT is a colorless to light opalescent liquid.

A heat-treatment process step (58° to 60°C, 10 hours) to inactivate viruses has been added to further reduce any risk of blood-borne viral transmission. The inactivation and removal of model and laboratory strains of enveloped and non-enveloped viruses during the manufacturing and heat treatment processes for Imogam® Rabies – HT has been validated by spiking experiments. Human immunodeficiency virus, type 1 (HIV-1) and type 2 (HIV-2) were selected as relevant viruses for plasma derived products. Bovine viral diarrhea virus and Sindbis virus were chosen to model hepatitis C virus. Porcine pseudorabies virus was selected to model hepatitis B virus and herpes virus. Avian reovirus was used to model non-enveloped RNA viruses and for its relative resistance to inactivation by chemical and physical methods. Finally, porcine parvovirus was selected to model human parvovirus B19 and its notable resistance to inactivation by heat treatment.

Removal and/or inactivation of the studied enveloped and non-enveloped model viruses was demonstrated at the precipitation III stage of manufacturing. In addition, inactivation was demonstrated to occur during the 10-hour (58° to 60°C) heat treatment process for the studied enveloped and non-enveloped viruses.

The product is standardized against the United States (US) Standard Rabies Immune Globulin. The US unit of potency is equivalent to the International Unit (IU) for Rabies antibody. The average potency is 150 IU/mL.

CLINICAL PHARMACOLOGY

Following the marked decrease of rabies cases among domestic animals in the US in the 1940s and 1950s, indigenously acquired rabies among humans decreased to fewer than two cases per year in the 1960s and 1970s and fewer than one case per year during the 1980s.[1,2] In 1950, for example, 4,979 cases of rabies were reported among dogs and 18 were reported among human populations; in 1989, 160 cases were reported among dogs and one was reported among humans. Thus, the likelihood of human exposure to a rabid domestic animal has decreased greatly; however, the many possible exposures that result from frequent contact between domestic dogs and humans continue to be the basis of most antirabies treatments.[1,3]

Rabies among wild animals—especially skunks, raccoons, and bats—has become more prevalent since the 1950s accounting for > 85% of all reported cases of animal rabies every year since 1976.[1,2] Rabies among animals occurs throughout the continental US; only Hawaii remains consistently rabies-free. Wild animals now constitute the most important potential source of infection for both humans and domestic animals in the US. In much of the rest of the world, including most of Asia, Africa, and Latin America, the dog remains the major species with rabies and the major source of rabies among humans. Nine of the 13 human rabies deaths reported to CDC from 1980 through 1990 appear to have been related to exposure to rabid animals outside of the US.[1,4-10]

Although rabies among humans is rare in the US, every year approximately 18,000 persons receive rabies pre-exposure prophylaxis and an additional 10,000 receive postexposure prophylaxis. Appropriate management of persons possibly exposed to rabies depends on the interpretation of the risk of infection. Decisions about management must be made immediately. All available methods of systemic prophylactic treatment are complicated by occasional adverse reactions, but these are rarely severe.[1,11-15]

Data on the efficacy of active and passive rabies immunization have come from both human and animal studies. Evidence from laboratory and field experience in many areas of the world indicates that postexposure prophylaxis combining local wound treatment, passive immunization, and vaccination is uniformly effective when appropriately applied.[1,16-21]

Although no postexposure vaccine failures have occurred in the US during the 10 years that HDCV has been licensed, seven persons have contracted rabies after receiving postexposure treatment with both HRIG and HDCV outside the US. An additional six persons have contracted the disease after receiving postexposure prophylaxis with other cell culture-derived vaccines and HRIG or ARS (equine antirabies serum). However, in each of these cases, there was some deviation from the recommended postexposure treatment protocol.[1,22-24] Specifically, patients who contracted rabies after postexposure prophylaxis did not have their wounds cleansed with soap and water or other antiviral agents, did not receive their rabies vaccine injections in the deltoid area (i.e., vaccine was administered in the gluteal area), or did not receive passive vaccination around the wound site.[1]

Rabies antibody provides passive protection when given immediately to individuals exposed to rabies virus.[25,26] Rabies Immune Globulin (Human) [RIG(H)] of adequate potency[27] was used in conjunction with Rabies Vaccine of duck embryo origin.[27,28] When a globulin dose of 20 IU/kg of rabies antibody was given simultaneously with the first dose of vaccine, levels of passive rabies antibody were detected 24 hours after injection in all individuals. There was minimal or no interference with the immune response to the initial and subsequent doses of vaccine, including booster doses.

Studies of Rabies Immune Globulin (Human)[29] Imogam® Rabies given with the first of five doses of Aventis Pasteur SA HDCV[1] confirmed that passive immunization with 20 IU/kg of Rabies Immune Globulin (Human) provides maximum circulating antibody with minimum interference of active immunization by HDCV.

A double-blind randomized trial[30] was conducted to compare the safety and antibody levels achieved following intramuscular injection of Imogam® Rabies – HT (heat treated) and Rabies Immune Globulin (Human), Imogam® Rabies (non-heat treated). Each immune globulin was administered on day 0, either alone or in combination with the human diploid cell Rabies Vaccine (Imovax® Rabies) using the standard post-exposure prophylactic schedule of day 0, 3, 7, 14, and 28.

Sixty-four healthy veterinary student volunteers were randomized into four parallel groups of 16 each to receive the following immune globulin and vaccine regimens.

Imogam® Rabies – HT	+	Imovax®
Imogam® Rabies	+	Imovax®
Imogam® Rabies – HT	+	placebo
Imogam® Rabies	+	placebo

The dosage corresponded to the post-exposure recommended dose of 20 IU/kg of rabies immune globulin and was administered in three, equally divided IM injections of under 5 mL in either gluteus. Serum rabies antibody levels were assessed before treatment and on days 3, 7, 14, 28, 35, and 42 by the Rabies Fluorescent Focus Inhibition Test (RFFIT).

Serum antibody levels were similar in the Imogam® Rabies – HT and Imogam® Rabies groups. By day three, 60% of each group had detectable antibody titers of ≥ 0.05 IU/mL. By day 14, the geometric mean titers (with 95% confidence interval) were 19 IU/mL (11–38) in the Imogam® Rabies – HT + vaccine group and 31 IU/mL (20–48) in the Imogam® Rabies + vaccine group. These differences were not statistically different.

Two subjects reported severe headaches, one in the Imogam® Rabies – HT + placebo group and one in the Imogam® Rabies + Imovax® Rabies group. One third of the volunteers had moderate systemic (headache and malaise) reactions. These were equally distributed among the 4 treatment groups with no significant differences between the groups.

Both Imogam® Rabies – HT + Imogam® Rabies were safe and without serious adverse events or allergic reactions. The safety profile did not differ between groups, although Imogam® Rabies – HT produced fewer and milder local reactions such as pain or tenderness at the injection site.

INDICATIONS AND USAGE

Rabies Immune Globulin (Human) Imogam® Rabies – HT is indicated for individuals suspected of exposure to rabies, particularly severe exposure, with one exception: persons who have been previously immunized with HDCV Rabies Vaccine in a pre or postexposure treatment series should receive only vaccine. Persons who have received Rabies Vaccines other than HDCV or RVA vaccines should have confirmed adequate rabies antibody titers if they are to receive only vaccine.[1]

Imogam® Rabies – HT should be injected as promptly as possible after exposure along with the first dose of vaccine. If initiation of treatment is delayed for any reason, Imogam® Rabies – HT and the first dose of vaccine should still be given, regardless of the interval between exposure and treatment Imogam® Rabies – HT may be given up to eight days after the first dose of vaccine was given.

Rabies virus is usually transmitted by the bite of a rabid animal but can occasionally penetrate abraded skin contaminated with the saliva of infected animals. Progress of the virus after exposure is believed to follow a neural pathway and the time between exposure and clinical rabies is a function of the proximity of the bite (or abrasion) to the central nervous system and the dose of virus injected. The incubation is usually 2 to 6 weeks but can be longer. After severe bites about the face and neck and arms, it may be as short as 10 days. After initiation of the vaccine series (human diploid cell origin), it takes approximately one week for development of immunity to rabies; therefore, the value of immediate passive immunization with rabies antibodies in the form of Rabies Immune Globulin (Human) cannot be overemphasized.

Recommendations for passive and/or active immunization after exposure to an animal suspected of having rabies have been outlined by the WHO[31] and by the United States Public Health Service Advisory Committee on Immunization Practices (ACIP).[1]

I. Rationale of Treatment

In the United States and Canada the following factors should be considered before specific antirabies treatment is indicated:

1. Species of Biting Animal

Carnivorous animals (especially skunks, foxes, coyotes, raccoons, dogs, bobcats, and cats) and bats are more likely to be infected with rabies than other animals. Rats, mice, squirrels, hamsters, guinea pigs, gerbils, chipmunks and other rodents or rabbits and hares are rarely infected with rabies and have not been known to cause human rabies in the United States. Their bites almost never call for antirabies prophylaxis; therefore, before initiating antirabies prophylaxis, the local state health department should be consulted. **Because some bat bites may be less severe, and therefore more difficult to recognize, than bites inflicted by larger mammalian carnivores, rabies postexposure treatment should be considered for any physical contact with bats when bite or mucous membrane contact cannot be excluded.[32,33]**

2. Circumstances of Biting Incident

An UNPROVOKED attack is more likely than a provoked attack to indicate that the animal is rabid. Bites inflicted on a person attempting to feed or handle an apparently healthy animal should generally be regarded as PROVOKED.

TABLE 1 RABIES POSTEXPOSURE PROPHYLAXIS GUIDE, UNITED STATES, 1991[1]

Animal Type	Evaluation and disposition of animal	Postexposure Prophylaxis Recommendations
Dogs and cats	Healthy and available for 10 days observation	Should not begin prophylaxis unless animal develops symptoms of rabies*
	Rabid or suspected rabid	Immediate vaccination
	Unknown (escaped)	Consult public health officials
Skunks, raccoons, bats, foxes, and most other carnivores; woodchucks	Regarded as rabid unless geographic area is known to be free of rabies or until animal proven negative by laboratory tests†	Immediate vaccination
Livestock, rodents, and lagomorphs (rabbits and hares)	Consider individually	Consult public health officials. Bites of squirrels, hamsters, guinea pigs gerbils, chipmunks, rats, mice, other rodents, rabbits, and hares almost never require antirabies treatment

*During the 10-day holding period, begin treatment with HRIG and HDCV or RVA at first sign of rabies in a dog or cat that has bitten someone. The symptomatic animal should be killed immediately and tested.

† The animal should be killed and tested as soon as possible. Holding for observation is not recommended. Discontinue vaccine if immunofluorescence test results of the animal are negative.

3. Type of Exposure

Rabies is commonly transmitted by inoculation with infectious saliva. The likelihood that rabies infection will result from exposure to a rabid animal varies with the nature and extent of the exposure. Two categories of exposure should be considered:

Bite: Any penetration of the skin by teeth.

Nonbite: Scratches, abrasions, open wounds or mucous membranes contaminated with saliva or other potentially infectious material such as brain tissue from a rabid animal.

In addition, two cases of rabies have been attributed to airborne exposures in laboratories and two cases of rabies have been attributed to probable exposures to a bat-infested cave (Frio Cave, Texas).[1,34-36] Casual contact with a rabid animal, such as petting the animal (without a bite or nonbite exposure as described above) does not constitute an exposure and is not an indication for prophylaxis.

The only documented cases of rabies due to human-to-human transmission occurred in patients who received corneas transplanted from persons who died of rabies undiagnosed at the time of death.[1,37]

Each exposure to possible rabies infection must be individually evaluated. Local or state public health officials should be consulted if questions arise about the need for rabies prophylaxis.

4. Vaccination Status of Biting Animal

A properly immunized animal has only a minimal chance of developing rabies and transmitting the virus.

II. Postexposure Treatment of Rabies

1. Local Treatment of Wounds

Immediate and thorough local treatment of all bite wounds and scratches is perhaps the most effective preventive measure. The wound should be thoroughly cleansed immediately with soap and water. Tetanus prophylaxis and measures to control bacterial infection should be given as indicated.

2. Specific Treatment

Postexposure antirabies treatment should always include both passive (preferably Rabies Immune Globulin—Human) and active (preferably Rabies Vaccine prepared from human diploid cells) immunization with one exception: persons who have been previously immunized with HDCV Rabies Vaccine in a pre or postexposure treatment series should receive only vaccine. Persons who have received Rabies Vaccines other than HDCV or RVA vaccines should have confirmed adequate rabies antibody titers if they are to receive only vaccine.[1] The combination of globulin and vaccine is recommended for both bite exposures and nonbite exposures (as described under "Rationale of Treatment") and regardless of the interval between exposure and treatment. The sooner treatment is begun after exposure, the better.

3. Postexposure Treatment Guide

The following recommendations are only a guide. They should be applied in conjunction with knowledge of the animal species involved, circumstances of the bite or other exposure, vaccination status of the animal, and presence of rabies in the region. Local and state public health officials should be consulted if questions arise about the need for rabies prophylaxis.

[See table 1 above]

CONTRAINDICATIONS

Imogam® Rabies – HT should NOT be administered in repeated doses once vaccine treatment has been initiated. Repeating the dose may interfere with maximum active immunity expected from the vaccine.

WARNINGS

Rabies Immune Globulin (Human) USP, Imogam® Rabies – HT, is made from human plasma. Products made from human plasma may contain infectious agents, such as viruses, that can cause disease. The risk that such products will transmit an infectious agent has been reduced by screening plasma donors for prior exposure to certain viruses, by testing for the presence of certain current virus infections, and by inactivating and/or removing certain viruses. An alcohol fractionation procedure used to purify the immunoglobulin component removes and/or inactivates both enveloped and non-enveloped viruses. An added heat treatment process (60°C, 10 hours) further inactivates both enveloped and non-enveloped viruses. Despite these measures, it is still theoretically possible that known or unknown infectious agents may be present. All infections thought by a physician possibly to have been transmitted by this product should be reported by the physician or other health-care provider to the Director of Scientific and Medical Affairs, Aventis Pasteur Inc., telephone 1-800-822-2463. The physician should discuss the risks and benefits of this product with the patient.

Imogam® Rabies – HT should be given with caution to patients with a history of prior systemic allergic reactions following the administration of human immune globulin.

Persons with specific IgA deficiency have increased potential for developing antibodies to IgA and could have anaphylactic reactions to subsequent administration of blood products containing IgA.[38,39]

PRECAUTIONS

GENERAL

Care is to be taken by the health-care provider for the safe and effective use of this product.

EPINEPHRINE INJECTION (1:1000) MUST BE IMMEDIATELY AVAILABLE SHOULD AN ACUTE ANAPHYLACTIC REACTION OCCUR DUE TO ANY COMPONENT OF THIS PRODUCT.

Imogam® Rabies – HT should not be administered intravenously because of the potential for serious reactions. Injection should be made intramuscularly and care should be taken to draw back on the plunger of the syringe before injection in order to be certain that the needle is not in a blood vessel. Although systemic reactions to immunoglobulin preparations are rare, epinephrine should be available for treatment of acute anaphylactoid reactions. As with all preparations given intramuscularly, bleeding complications may be encountered in patients with bleeding disorders.

HRIG should never be administered in the same syringe or into the same anatomical site as vaccine. Because HRIG may partially suppress active production of antibody, no more than the recommended dose should be given.[1]

A separate, sterile syringe and needle or a sterile disposable unit should be used for each patient to prevent transmission of hepatitis or other infectious agents from person to person. Needles should not be recapped and should be disposed of according to biohazard waste guidelines.

INFORMATION FOR PATIENT

Patients, parents or guardians should be fully informed by their health-care provider of the benefits and risks of administration of Imogam® Rabies – HT.

Patients, parents or guardians should be instructed to report any serious adverse reactions to their health-care provider.

DRUG INTERACTIONS

Live virus vaccine such as measles vaccines should not be given close to the time of Imogam® Rabies – HT administration because antibodies in the globulin preparation may interfere with the immune response to the vaccination. Immunization with live vaccines should not be given within three months after Imogam® Rabies – HT administration.

PREGNANCY

REPRODUCTIVE STUDIES—PREGNANCY CATEGORY C

Animal reproduction studies have not been conducted with Imogam® Rabies – HT. It is also not known whether Imogam® Rabies – HT can cause fetal harm when administered to a pregnant woman or can affect reproductive capacity. Imogam® Rabies – HT should be given to a pregnant woman only if clearly needed.

ADVERSE REACTIONS

In a recent clinical trial involving 16 volunteers in 4 treatment groups, two subjects reported severe headaches, one in the Imogam® Rabies – HT + placebo group and one in the Imogam® Rabies + Imovax® Rabies group, and one third of the volunteers reported moderate systemic (headache and

Continued on next page

Imogam Rabies—Cont.

malaise) reactions. These were equally distributed among the 4 treatment groups with no significant differences between the groups.[30]

Local adverse reactions such as tenderness, pain, soreness or stiffness of the muscles may occur at the injection site and may persist for several hours after injection. These may be treated symptomatically. Mild systemic adverse reactions to the globulin after intramuscular injection are uncommon.[30,40,41]

Although not reported specifically for HRIG, angioneurotic edema, nephrotic syndrome, and anaphylaxis have been reported after injection of immune globulin (IG). These reactions occur so rarely that a causal relationship between IG and these reactions is not clear.[1]

Reporting of Adverse Events

The National Vaccine Injury Compensation Program, established by the National Childhood Vaccine Injury Act of 1986, requires physicians and other health-care providers who administer vaccines to maintain permanent vaccination records and to report occurrences of certain adverse events to the US Department of Health and Human Services. Reportable events include those listed in the Act for each vaccine and events specified in the package insert as contraindications to further doses of that vaccine.[42,43,44]

Reporting by patients, parents or guardians of all adverse events occurring after HRIG administration should be encouraged. Adverse events following treatment with HRIG should be reported by the health-care provider to the US Department of Health and Human Services (DHHS) Vaccine Adverse Event Reporting Systems (VAERS). Reporting forms and information about reporting requirements or completion of the form can be obtained from VAERS through a toll-free number 1-800-822-7967.[42,43,44]

The health-care provider also should report these events to the Director of Scientific and Medical Affairs, Aventis Pasteur Inc., Discovery Drive, Swiftwater, PA 18370 or call 1-800-822-2463.

DOSAGE AND ADMINISTRATION

Parenteral drug products should be inspected visually for particulate matter and/or discoloration prior to administration, whenever solution and container permit. If either of these conditions exist, the vaccine should not be administered.

Imogam® Rabies – HT should be used in conjunction with Rabies Vaccine such as Rabies Vaccine Imovax® Rabies, for intramuscular immunization, vaccine prepared from human diploid cell cultures. The recommended dose of Imogam® Rabies – HT is 20 IU/kg (0.133 mL/kg) or 9 IU/lb (0.06 mL/lb) of body weight administered at time of the first vaccine dose.[27,28] As much as possible of the recommended dose should be infiltrated around the wound if anatomically feasible and the remaining HRIG should be administered intramuscularly in the gluteal region.[45] Two injections would be given in the gluteal region if the volume is greater than 5 mL.

HRIG should never be administered in the same syringe or into the same anatomical site as vaccine. Because HRIG may partially suppress active production of antibody, no more than the recommended dose should be given.[1]

HOW SUPPLIED

Imogam® Rabies – HT is supplied in 2 mL and 10 mL vials with average potency of 150 International Units per milliliter (IU/mL). The 2 mL vial contains 300 IU which is sufficient for a child weighing 15 kg (33 lb). Product No. 49281-190-20. The 10 mL vial contains a total of 1,500 IU which is sufficient for an adult weighing 75 kg (165 lb). Product No. 49281-190-10

STORAGE

Imogam® Rabies – HT should be stored in the refrigerator between 2° and 8°C (35° and 46°F). Do not freeze.

Imogam® Rabies – HT CONTAINS NO PRESERVATIVE AND UNUSED PORTION MUST BE DISCARDED IMMEDIATELY.

REFERENCES

1. Recommendation of the Advisory Committee on Immunization Practices (ACIP). Rabies prevention—United States, 1991. MMWR 40: No. RR-3, 1991
2. Reid-Sanden FL, et al. Rabies surveillance, United States during 1989. J Am Vet Med Assoc 197: 1571–1583, 1990
3. Helmick CG. The epidemiology of human rabies postexposure prophylaxis, 1980–1981. JAMA 250: 1990–1996, 1983
4. CDC. Human rabies diagnosed 2 months postmortem—Texas. MMWR 34: 700, 705–707, 1985
5. CDC. Human rabies acquired outside the United States. MMWR 34: 235–236, 1985
6. CDC. Human rabies—California, 1987. MMWR 37: 305–308, 1988
7. CDC. Human rabies—Oregon, 1989. MMWR 38: 335–337, 1989
8. CDC. Human rabies—Texas. MMWR 33: 469–470, 1984
9. CDC. Imported human rabies. MMWR 32: 78–80, 85–86, 1983
10. CDC. Human rabies acquired outside the United States from a dog bite. MMWR 30: 537–540, 1981
11. Bernard, KW, et al. Neuroparalytic illness and human diploid cell rabies vaccine. JAMA 248: 3136–3138, 1982
12. CDC. Systemic allergic reactions following immunization with human diploid cell rabies vaccine. MMWR 33: 185–187, 1984
13. Dreesen EW, et al. Immune complex-like disease in 23 persons following a booster dose of rabies human diploid cell vaccine. Vaccine 4: 45–49, 1986
14. Aoki FY, et al. Immunogenicity and acceptability of a human diploid-cell culture rabies vaccine in volunteers. Lancet 1: 660–662, 1975
15. Cox JH, et al. Prophylactic immunization of humans against rabies by intradermal inoculation of human diploid cell culture vaccine. J Clin Microbiol 3: 96–101, 1976
16. Anderson LJ, et al. Postexposure trial of a human diploid cell strain rabies vaccine. J Infect Dis 142: 133–138, 1980
17. Bahmanyar M, et al. Successful protection of humans exposed to rabies infection. Postexposure treatment with the new human diploid cell rabies vaccine and antirabies serum. JAMA 236: 2751–2754, 1976
18. Hattwick MAW. Human rabies. Public Health Rev 3: 229–274, 1974
19. Wiktor TJ, et al. Development and clinical trials of the new human rabies vaccine of tissue culture (human diploid cell) origin. Dev. Biol Stand 40: 3–9, 1978
20. World Health Organization. WHO expert committee on rabies. WHO Tech Rep Ser 709: 1–104, 1984
21. Kuwert EK, et al. Immunization against rabies with rabies immune globulin, human (RIGH) and a human diploid cell strain (HDCS) rabies vaccine. J Biol Stand 6: 211–219, 1978
22. CDC. Human rabies despite treatment with rabies immune globulin and human diploid cell rabies vaccine – Thailand. MMWR 36: 759–760, 765, 1987
23. Shill M, et al. Fatal rabies encephalitis despite appropriate post-exposure prophylaxis. A case report. N Engl J Med 316: 1257–1258, 1987
24. Wilde H, et al. Failure of rabies postexposure treatment in Thailand. Vaccine 7: 49–52, 1989
25. Baltazard M, et al. Essai pratique du serum antirabique chez les mordus par loups enragés. Bull WHO 13: 747–772, 1955
26. Habel K, et al. Laboratory data supporting clinical trial of antirabies serum in persons bitten by rabid wolf. Bull WHO 13: 773–779, 1955
27. Cabasso VJ, et al. Rabies immune globulin of human origin: preparation and dosage determination in non-exposed volunteer subjects. Bull WHO 45: 303–315, 1971
28. Loofbourow JC, et al. Rabies immune globulin (human). Clinical trials and dose determination. JAMA 217:1825–1831, 1971
29. Helmick CG, et al. A clinical study of Mérieux human rabies immune globulin. J Biol Stand 10:357–367 1982
30. Lang J, et al. A clinical evaluation of a new heat treated Rabies Immune Globulin (Human). VII Annual International Meeting on Research Advances & Rabies Control in the Americas. Centers for Disease Control & Prevention, Atlanta, Georgia, December 9–13, 1996
31. WHO Expert Committee on Rabies. WHO Tech Rep Ser 523: 50–51, 1973
32. ACIP. Human Rabies—California, 1994. MMWR 43: 455–457, 1994
33. Wilde H, et al. Failure of Postexposure Treatment of Rabies in Children. Clin Infect Dis 22: 228–232, 1996
34. Afshar A. A review of non-bite transmission of rabies virus infection. Br Vet J 135: 142–148, 1979
35. Winkler WG, et al. Airborne rabies transmission in a laboratory worker. JAMA 226: 1219–1221, 1973
36. CDC. Rabies in a laboratory worker—New York. MMWR 26: 183–184, 1977
37. Gode GR, et al. Two rabies deaths after corneal grafts from one donor (letter). Lancet 2: 791, 1988
38. Fudenberg HH. Sensitization to immunoglobulins and hazards of gamma globulin therapy, pp 211–220 in Merler E, Editor Immunoglobulins: biologic aspects and clinical uses. National Academy of Sciences, Wash., DC. 1970
39. Pineda AA, et al. Transfusion reactions associated with anti-IgA antibodies: report of four cases and review of the literature. Transfusion 15:10–15, 1975
40. Janeway CA, et al. The gamma globulins. IV. Therapeutic uses of gamma globulins. N Engl J Med 275: 826–831, 1966
41. Kjellman H. Adverse reactions to human immune serum globulin in Sweden (1969–1978). pp 143–150. Immunoglobulins: characteristics and uses of intravenous preparations. Alving BM and Finlayson JS, Editors. US Dept. Health & Human Services, DHHS Publ. No. (FDA) 80–9005, Wash., DC. 1980
42. CDC. Vaccine Adverse Event Reporting System—United States. MMWR 39: 730–733, 1990
43. CDC. National Childhood Vaccine Injury Act. Requirements for permanent vaccination records and for reporting of selected events after vaccination. MMWR 37: 197–200, 1988
44. Food and Drug Administration. New Reporting Requirements for Vaccine Adverse Events. FDA Drug Bull 18(2), 16–18, 1988
45. World Health Organization. WHO expert committee on rabies. WHO Tech Rep Ser 824: 1992

Product Information
as of April 1997

Manufactured by:
Aventis Pasteur SA
Lyon France
US Govt License #1279

Distributed by:
Aventis Pasteur Inc.
Swiftwater PA 18370 USA
1-800-VACCINE (1-800-822-2463)

4210

Rabies Vaccine
IMOVAX® RABIES ℞

[Im 'o-vaks]

WISTAR RABIES VIRUS STRAIN PM-1503-3M GROWN IN HUMAN DIPLOID CELL CULTURES

Rx only

DESCRIPTION

The Imovax® Rabies Vaccine produced by Aventis Pasteur is a sterile, stable, freeze-dried suspension of rabies virus prepared from strain PM-1503-3M obtained from the Wistar Institute, Philadelphia, PA.

The virus is harvested from infected human diploid cells, MRC-5 strain, concentrated by ultrafiltration and is inactivated by beta propiolactone. One dose of reconstituted vaccine contains less than 100 mg albumin, less than 150 µg neomycin sulfate and 20 µg of phenol red indicator. This vaccine must only be used intramuscularly and as a single dose vial.

The vaccine contains no preservative or stabilizer. It should be used immediately after reconstitution, and if not administered promptly, discard contents.

The potency of one dose (1.0 mL) Aventis Imovax Rabies Vaccine is equal to or greater than 2.5 international units of rabies antigen.

CLINICAL PHARMACOLOGY

Pre-exposure immunization

High titer antibody responses of the Aventis Imovax Rabies Vaccine made in human diploid cells have been demonstrated in trials conducted in England[1], Germany[2,3] France[4] and Belgium.[5] Seroconversion was often obtained with only one dose. With two doses one month apart, 100% of the recipients developed specific antibody and the geometric mean titer of the group was approximately 10 international units. In the US, Aventis Imovax Rabies Vaccine resulted in geometric mean titers (GMT) of 12.9 IU/mL at Day 49 and 5.1 IU/mL at Day 90 when three doses were given intramuscularly during the course of one month. The range of antibody responses was 2.8 to 55.0 IU/mL at Day 49 and 1.8 to 12.4 IU at Day 90.[6] The definition of a minimally accepted antibody titer varies among laboratories and is influenced by the type of test conducted. CDC currently specifies a 1:5 titer (complete inhibition) by the rapid fluorescent focus inhibition test (RFFIT) as acceptable. The World Health Organization (WHO) specifies a titer of 0.5 IU.

Postexposure immunization

Postexposure efficacy of Aventis Imovax Rabies Vaccine was successfully proven during clinical experience in Iran[7] in conjunction with antirabies serum. Forty-five persons severely bitten by rabid dogs and wolves received Aventis vaccine within hours of and up to 14 days after the bites. All individuals were fully protected against rabies.

There have been reports of possible vaccine failure when the vaccine has been administered in the gluteal area. Presumably subcutaneous fat in the gluteal area may interfere with the immunogenicity of human diploid cell rabies vaccine (HDCV).[26,29] For adults and children, Rabies Vaccine should be administered in the deltoid muscle. (See DOSAGE AND ADMINISTRATION).

INDICATIONS AND USAGE

1. Rationale of treatment

Physicians must evaluate each possible rabies exposure. Local or state public health officials should be consulted if questions arise about the need for prophylaxis.[8]

In the United States and Canada, the following factors should be considered before antirabies treatment is initiated.

Species of biting animal

Carnivorous wild animals (especially skunks, raccoons, foxes, coyotes, and bobcats) and bats are the animals most commonly infected with rabies and have caused most of the indigenous cases of human rabies in the United States since 1960. Unless an animal is tested and shown not to be rabid, postexposure prophylaxis should be initiated upon bite or nonbite exposure to the animals. (See definition in "Type of Exposure" below.) If treatment has been initiated and subsequent testing in a competent laboratory shows the exposing animal is not rabid, treatment can be discontinued.[8]

The likelihood that a domestic dog or cat is infected with rabies varies from region to region; hence the need for postexposure prophylaxis also varies.[8]

Rodents (such as squirrels, hamsters, guinea pigs, gerbils, chipmunks, rats and mice) and lagomorphs (including rabbits and hares) are rarely found to be infected with rabies and have not been known to cause human rabies in the United States. In these cases, the state or local health department should be consulted before a decision is made to initiate postexposure antirabies prophylaxis.[8]

Circumstances of biting incident

An UNPROVOKED attack is more likely than a provoked attack to indicate the animal is rabid. Bites inflicted on a person attempting to feed or handle an apparently healthy animal should generally be regarded as PROVOKED.

Type of exposure
Rabies is transmitted by introducing the virus into open cuts or wounds in skin or via mucous membranes. The likelihood of rabies infection varies with the nature and extent of exposure. Two categories of exposure should be considered.
Bite: Any penetration of the skin by teeth.
Nonbite: Scratches, abrasions, open wounds, or mucous membranes contaminated with saliva or other potentially infectious material, such as brain tissue, from a rabid animal. Casual contact, such as petting a rabid animal (without a bite or nonbite exposure as described above), does not constitute an exposure and is not an indication for prophylaxis. There have been two instances of airborne rabies acquired in laboratories and two probable airborne rabies cases acquired in a bat-infested cave in Texas.[8,9]
The only documented cases for rabies from human-to-human transmission occurred in four patients in the United States and overseas who received corneas transplanted from persons who died of rabies undiagnosed at the time of death.[9,10] Stringent guidelines for acceptance of donor cornea should reduce this risk. Bite and nonbite exposure from humans with rabies theoretically could transmit rabies, although no cases of rabies acquired this way have been documented. Each potential exposure to human rabies should be carefully evaluated to minimize unnecessary rabies prophylaxis.[8,11]

2. Pre- and postexposure treatment of rabies

A. Pre-exposure—See Table 1
Pre-exposure immunization may be offered to persons in high risk groups, such as veterinarians, animal handlers, certain laboratory workers, and persons spending time (e.g. 1 month or more) in foreign countries where rabies is a constant threat. Persons whose vocational or avocational pursuits bring them into contact with potentially rabid dogs, cats, foxes, skunks, bats, or other species at risk of having rabies should also be considered for pre-exposure prophylaxis.[8]
Vaccination is recommended for children living in or visiting countries where exposure to rabid animals is a constant threat. Worldwide statistics indicate children are more at risk than adults.
Pre-exposure prophylaxis is given for several reasons. First, it may provide protection to persons with inapparent exposure to rabies. Secondly, it may protect persons whose postexposure therapy might be expected to be delayed. Finally, although it does not eliminate the need for additional therapy after a rabies exposure, it simplifies therapy by eliminating the need for globulin and decreasing the number of doses of vaccine needed. This is of particular importance for persons at high risk of being exposed in countries where the available rabies immunizing products may carry a higher risk of adverse reactions.
Pre-exposure immunization does not eliminate the need for prompt prophylaxis following an exposure. It only reduces the postexposure treatment regimen.[8]

PRE-EXPOSURE RABIES TREATMENT GUIDE

1. Pre-exposure immunization: Consists of the three doses of HDCV, 1.0 mL, intramuscularly (deltoid area), one each on Days 0, 7 and 21 or 28. Administration of routine booster doses of vaccine depends on exposure risk category as noted in Table 1. Pre-exposure immunization of immunosuppressed persons is not recommended.[8]
[See table 1 above]

B. Postexposure—See Table 2
The essential components of rabies postexposure prophylaxis are local treatment of wounds and immunization, including administration, in most instances, of both globulin and vaccine (Table 2).[8,13]
1. Local treatment of wounds: Immediate and thorough washing of all bite wounds and scratches with soap and water is perhaps the most effective measure for preventing rabies. In experimental animals, simple local wound cleansing has been shown to reduce markedly the likelihood of rabies.[8,11]
Tetanus prophylaxis and measures to control bacterial infection should be given as indicated.
2. Specific treatment: Postexposure antirabies immunization should always include administration of both antibody (preferably RIG) and vaccine, with one exception: persons who have been previously immunized with the recommended pre-exposure or postexposure regimens with HDCV or who have been immunized with other types of vaccines and have a history of documented adequate rabies antibody titer should receive only vaccine. The combination of globulin and vaccine is recommended for both bite exposures and nonbite exposures regardless of the interval between exposure and treatment.[14,15] The sooner treatment is begun after exposure, the better. However, there have been instances in which the decision to begin treatment was made as late as 6 months or longer after the exposure due to delay in recognition that an exposure had occurred.[8,13]
3. Treatment outside the United States: If postexposure is begun outside the United States with locally produced biologics, it may be desirable to provide additional treatment when the patient reaches the US. State health departments should be contacted for specific advice in such cases.[8]

POSTEXPOSURE TREATMENT GUIDE

The following recommendations are only a guide. In applying them, take into account the animal species involved, the circumstances of the bite or other exposure, the vaccination status of the animal, and presence of rabies in the region. Local or state public health officials should be consulted if questions arise about the need for rabies prophylaxis.[8]
[See table 2 above]

TABLE 1[8]

CRITERIA FOR PRE-EXPOSURE IMMUNIZATION

Risk category	Nature of risk	Typical populations	Pre-exposure regimen
Continuous	Virus present continuously often in high concentrations. Aerosol, mucus membrane, bite or nonbite exposure possible. Specific exposures may go unrecognized.	Rabies research lab workers.* Rabies biologics production workers.	Primary pre-exposure immunization course. Serology every 6 months. Booster immunization when antibody titer falls below acceptable level.*
Frequent	Exposure usually episodic, with source recognized, but exposure may also be unrecognized. Aerosol, mucous membrane, bite or nonbite exposure.	Rabies diagnostic lab workers*, spelunkers, veterinarians, and animal control and wildlife workers in rabies epizootic areas.	Primary pre-exposure immunization course. Booster immunization or serology every 2 years.†
Infrequent (greater than population-at-large)	Exposure nearly always episodic with source recognized. Mucous membrane, bite or nonbite exposure.	Veterinarians and animal control and wildlife workers in areas of low rabies endemicity. Certain travelers to foreign rabies epizootic areas. Veterinary students.	Primary pre-exposure immunization course. No routine booster immunization or serology.
Rare (population-at-large)	Exposure always episodic, mucous membrane, or bite with source recognized.	U.S. population-at-large, including individuals in rabies epizootic areas.	No pre-exposure immunization.

* Judgement of relative risk and extra monitoring of immunization status of laboratory workers is the responsibility of the laboratory supervisor (see U.S. Department of Health and Human Service's Biosafety in Microbiological and Biomedical Laboratories, 1984).
† Pre-exposure booster immunization consists of one dose of HDCV, 1.0 ml/dose, IM (deltoid area). Acceptable antibody level is 1:5 titer (complete inhibition in RFFIT at 1:5 dilution). See CLINICAL PHARMACOLOGY. Boost if titer falls below 1:5.

TABLE 2[8]

Animal species	Condition of animal at time of attack	Treatment of exposed person*
DOMESTIC: Dog and cat	Healthy and available for 10 days of observation. Rabid or suspected rabid. Unknown (escaped).	None unless animal develops rabies.† RIG§ and HDCV. Consult public health officials. If treatment is indicated, give RIG§ and HDCV.
WILD: Skunk, bat, fox, coyote, raccoon, bobcat and other carnivores	Regard as rabid unless proven negative by laboratory tests. £	RIG§ and HDCV.
OTHER: Livestock, rodents and lagomorphs (rabbits and hares)	Consider individually. Local and state public health officials should be consulted on questions about the need for rabies prophylaxis. Bites of squirrels, hamsters, guinea pigs, gerbils, chipmunks, rats, mice, other rodents, rabbits and hares, almost never call for antirabies prophylaxis.	

* All bites and wounds should immediately be thoroughly cleansed with soap and water. If antirabies treatment is indicated, both rabies immune globulin (RIG) and human diploid cell rabies vaccine (HDCV) should be given as soon as possible regardless of the interval from exposure. Local reactions to vaccines are common and do not contraindicate continuing treatment. Discontinue vaccine if fluorescent antibody tests of the animal are negative.
† During the usual holding period of 10 days, begin treatment with RIG and HDCV at first sign of rabies in a dog or cat that has bitten someone. The symptomatic animal should be killed immediately and tested.
§ If RIG is not available, use antirabies serum, equine (ARS). Do not use more than the recommended dosage.
£ The animal should be killed and tested as soon as possible. Holding for observation is not recommended.

CONTRAINDICATIONS

For postexposure treatment, there are no known specific contraindications to the use of Aventis Imovax Rabies Vaccine. In cases of pre-exposure immunization, there are no known specific contraindications other than situations such as developing febrile illness, etc.

WARNINGS

Rabies Vaccine in this package is a unit dose to be delivered intramuscularly in the deltoid area.[8]
This vaccine must not be used intradermally or as a multiple dose dispensing unit. In both pre-exposure and postexposure immunization, the full 1.0 mL dose should be given intramuscularly.
In the case of pre-exposure immunization, recently a significant increase has been noted in "immune complex-like" reactions in persons receiving booster doses of HDCV.[16] The illness characterized by onset 2–21 days post-booster, presents with a generalized urticaria and may also include arthralgia, arthritis, angioedema, nausea, vomiting, fever, and malaise. In no cases were the illnesses life-threatening. Preliminary data suggest this "immune complex-like" illness may occur in up to 6% of persons receiving booster vaccines and much less frequently in persons receiving primary immunization. Additional experience with this vaccine is needed to define more clear the risk of these adverse reactions.[8,17]
Two cases of neurologic illness resembling Guillain-Barré syndrome[18,19] transient neuroparalytic illness, that resolved without sequelae in 12 weeks and a focal subacute central nervous system disorder temporally associated with HDCV, have been reported.[20]
All serious systemic neuroparalytic reactions to a rabies vaccine should be immediately reported to the state health department or Aventis Pasteur Inc., 1-800-VACCINE/1-800-822-2463.[8]

PRECAUTIONS

IN ADULTS AND CHILDREN THE VACCINE SHOULD BE INJECTED INTO THE DELTOID MUSCLE. IN INFANTS AND SMALL CHILDREN THE MID-LATERAL ASPECT OF THE THIGH MAY BE PREFERABLE.

General
When a person with a history of hypersensitivity must be given rabies vaccine, antihistamines may be given; epinephrine (1:1000) should be readily available to counteract anaphylactic reactions, and the person should be carefully observed after immunization.
While the concentration of antibiotics in each dose of vaccine is extremely small, persons with known hypersensitivity to any of these agents could manifest an allergic reaction. While the risk is small, it should be weighed in light of the potential risk of contracting rabies.

Drug interactions
Corticosteroids, other immunosuppressive agents, and immunosuppressive illnesses can interfere with the development of active immunity and predispose the patient to developing rabies. Immunosuppressive agents should not be administered during postexposure therapy, unless essential for the treatment of other conditions. When rabies postexposure prophylaxis is administered to persons receiving steroids or other immunosuppressive therapy, it is especially important that serum be tested for rabies antibody to ensure that an adequate response has developed.[8]

Usage in pregnancy
Pregnancy Category C. Animal reproduction studies have not been conducted with Imovax Rabies Vaccine. It is also not known whether the product can cause fetal harm when administered to a pregnant woman or can affect reproductive capacity. Rabies vaccine should be given to a pregnant woman only if clearly needed.
Because of the potential consequences of inadequately treated rabies exposure and limited data that indicate that fetal abnormalities have not been associated with rabies vaccination, pregnancy is not considered a contraindication

Continued on next page

Imovax Rabies—Cont.

to postexposure prophylaxis.[8,21] If there is substantial risk of exposure to rabies, pre-exposure prophylaxis may also be indicated during pregnancy.[8]

Pediatric use

Both safety and efficacy in children have been established.

ADVERSE REACTIONS

ALSO SEE WARNINGS AND CONTRAINDICATIONS SECTIONS FOR ADDITIONAL STATEMENTS.

Once initiated, rabies prophylaxis should not be interrupted or discontinued because of local or mild systemic adverse reactions to rabies vaccine. Usually such reactions can be successfully managed with anti-inflammatory and antipyretic agents (e.g. aspirin).

Reactions after vaccination with HDCV are less common than with previously available vaccines.[12,16,17] In a study using five doses of HDCV, local reactions, such as pain, erythema, and swelling or itching at the injection site were reported in about 25% of recipients of HDCV, and mild systemic reactions such as headache, nausea, abdominal pain, muscle aches and dizziness were reported in about 20% of recipients.[8] Serious systemic anaphylactic or neuroparalytic reactions occurring during the administration of rabies vaccines pose a dilemma for the attending physician. A patient's risk of developing rabies must be carefully considered before deciding to discontinue vaccination. Moreover, the use of corticosteroids to treat life-threatening neuroparalytic reactions carries the risk of inhibiting the development of active immunity to rabies. It is especially important in these cases that the serum of the patient be tested for rabies antibodies. Advice and assistance on the management of serious adverse reactions in persons receiving rabies vaccines may be sought from the state health department.[8]

DOSAGE AND ADMINISTRATION

Parenteral drug products should be inspected visually for particulate matter and discoloration prior to administration, whenever solution and container permit. Reconstitute the freeze-dried vaccine in its vial with the 1.0 mL of diluent supplied in the disposable syringe using the longer of the two needles. Gently swirl the contents until completely dissolved and withdraw the total amount of dissolved vaccine into the syringe by setting the vial in an upright position on the table. Remove the reconstitution needle and replace it with the smaller needle.

The reconstituted vaccine should be used immediately.

After preparation of the injection site, immediately inject the vaccine intramuscularly. For adults and children, the vaccine should be injected into the deltoid muscle.[22–27,29] In adults and small children, the mid lateral aspect of the thigh may be preferable. Care should be taken to avoid injection into or near blood vessels and nerves. After aspiration, if blood or any suspicious discoloration appears in the syringe, do not inject but discard contents and repeat procedure using a new dose of vaccine, at a different site.

NOTE: The freeze-dried vaccine is creamy white to orange. After reconstitution it is pink to red.

A. Pre-exposure dosage

1. Primary vaccination: In the United States, the Immunization Practices Advisory Committee (ACIP) recommends three injections of 1.0 mL each, one injection on Day 0 and one on Day 7 and one either on Day 21 or 28.[8]

2. Booster dose: Persons working with live rabies virus in research laboratories and in vaccine production facilities should have rabies antibody titers checked every six months and boosters given as needed to maintain an adequate titer. (For definition of adequate titer, see CLINICAL PHARMACOLOGY.) Only laboratory workers, such as those doing rabies diagnostic tests, spelunkers and veterinarians, animal control and wildlife officers in areas where rabies is epizootic should have boosters every 2 years or have their serum tested for rabies antibody every 2 years and, if the titer is inadequate, have a booster dose. Veterinarians and animal control and wildlife officers, if working in areas of low rabies endemicity, do not require routine booster doses of HDCV after completion of primary pre-exposure immunization (Table 1).[8]

Persons who have experienced "immune complex-like" hypersensitivity reactions should receive no further doses of HDCV unless they are exposed to rabies or they are truly likely to be inapparently and/or unavoidably exposed to rabies virus and have unsatisfactory antibody titers.

B. Postexposure dosage

The World Health Organization established a recommendation for six intramuscular doses of human diploid cell vaccine (HDCV) based on studies in Germany and Iran.[3,7] Used in this way, a total of 6 injections of a 1.0 mL dose of vaccine are given according to the following schedule: on Day 0, 3, 7, 14, 30 and 90. The first dose should be accompanied by Rabies Immune Globulin (RIG) or Antirabies Serum (ARS). If possible, up to half the dose of RIG or ARS should be used to infiltrate the wound, and the rest administered intramuscularly, in a different site from the rabies vaccine, preferably in the gluteal region.

Studies conducted at the CDC in the United States have shown that a regimen of 1 dose of Rabies Immune Globulin (RIG) and 5 doses of HDCV induced an excellent antibody response in all recipients. Of 511 persons bitten by proven rabid animals and so treated, none developed rabies.[8]

Based on these data, the ACIP recommends a 5-dose regimen for postexposure situations. Five 1.0 mL doses are given intramuscularly on Day 0, 3, 7, 14 and 28 in conjunction with RIG on Day 0.[8]

Because the antibody response following the recommended vaccination regimen with HDCV has been so satisfactory, routine postvaccination serologic testing is not recommended. Serologic testing is indicated in unusual circumstances, as when the patient is known to be immunosuppressed. Contact state health department or CDC for recommendations.[8,28]

C. Postexposure therapy of previously immunized persons

When an immunized person who was vaccinated by the recommended regimen with HDCV or who had previously demonstrated rabies antibody is exposed to rabies, that person should receive two IM doses (1.0 mL each) of HDCV, one immediately and one 3 days later. RIG should not be given in these cases. If the immune status of a previously vaccinated person who did not receive the recommended HDCV regimen is not known, full primary postexposure antirabies treatment (RIG plus 5 doses of HDCV) may be necessary. In such cases, if antibody can be demonstrated in a serum sample collected before vaccine is given, treatment can be discontinued after at least two doses of HDCV.[8]

HOW SUPPLIED

Imovax Rabies Vaccine is supplied in a tamperproof unit dose plastic box with:

—One vial of freeze-dried vaccine containing a single dose.

—One disposable needle and syringe containing diluent for reconstitution.

—One smaller disposable needle for administration.

Product No. 49281-250-10

STORAGE

The freeze-dried vaccine is stable if stored in the refrigerator between 2°C and 8°C (35°F to 46°F). Do not freeze.

REFERENCES

1. Aoki FY, Tyrell DAJ, Hill LE. Immunogenicity and acceptability of a human diploid cell culture rabies vaccine in volunteers. The Lancet, March 22, pp. 660–2 (1975).
2. Cox JH, Schneider LG. Prophylactic immunization of humans against rabies by intradermal inoculation of human diploid cell culture vaccine. J Clin Microbiol 3: 96–101 (1976).
3. Kuwert EK, Marcus 1, Werner J, Iwand A, Thraenhart O. Some experiences with human diploid cell strain—(HDCS) rabies vaccine in pre-and postexposure vaccinated humans. Develop Biol Standard 40: 79–88 (1978).
4. Ajjan N, Soulebot J-P, Stellmann C, Biron G, Charbonnier C, Triau R, Mérieux C. Resultats de la vaccination antirabique préventive par le vaccin inactivé concentré souche rabies PM/W138-1503-3M cultivés sur cellules diploïdes humaines. Develop Biol Standard 40:89–199 (1978).
5. Costy-Berger F. Vaccination antirabique préventive par du vaccin préparé sur cellules diploïdes humaines. Develop Biol Standard 40: 101–4 (1978).
6. Bernard KW, Roberts MA, Sumner J, Winkler WG, Mallonee J, Baer GM, Chaney R. Human diploid cell rabies vaccine JAMA 247:1138–42 (1982).
7. Bahmanyar M, Fayaz A, Nour-Salehi S, Mohammadi M, Koprowski H. Successful protection of humans exposed to rabies infection. JAMA 236: 2751–4 (1976).
8. CDC. Recommendations of the Immunization Practices Advisory Committee (ACIP). Rabies Prevention—United States, 1984, MMWR 33: 393–402, 407–8 (1984).
9. Anderson LJ, Nicholson KG, Tauxe RV, Winkler WG. Human rabies in the United States, 1960 to 1979, epidemiology, diagnosis and prevention. Ann Intern Med 100: 728–35 (1984).
10. WHO. Sixth report of the Expert Committee on Rabies. Geneva Switzerland: World Health Organization. (WHO technical report No. 523) (1973).
11. Baer GM, ed. The natural history of rabies. New York: Academic Press. (1975).
12. Greenberg M, Childress J. Vaccination against rabies with duck-embryo and Semple vaccines JAMA 173: 333–7 (1960).
13. Helmick CG. The Epidemiology of Human rabies postexposure prophylaxis. JAMA 250:1990–6 (1983).
14. Devriendt J, Staroukine M, Costy F, Vanderhaegen, JJ. Fatal encephalitis apparently due to rabies. JAMA 248: 2304–6 (1982).
15. CDC. Human Rabies—Rwanda MMWR 31:135 (1982).
16. CDC. Systemic allergic reactions following immunization with human diploid cell rabies vaccine. MMWR 33: 185–7 (1984).
17. Rubin RH, Hattwick MAW, Jones S, Gregg MB, Schwartz VD. Adverse reactions to duck embryo rabies vaccine. Ann Intern Med 78:643–9 (1973).
18. Boe E, Nyland H. Guillain-Barré syndrome after vaccination with human diploid cell rabies vaccine. Scand J Infect Dis 12: 231–2 (1980).
19. CDC. Adverse reactions to human diploid cell rabies vaccine. MMWR 29: 609–10 (1980).
20. Bernard KW, Smith PW, Kader FJ, Moran MJ. Neuroparalytic illness and human diploid cell rabies vaccine. JAMA 248: 3136–8 (1982).
21. Varner MW, McGuinness GA, Galask RP. Rabies vaccination in pregnancy. Am J of Obst and Gyn 143:717–18 (1982).
22. Cockshott WP, Thompson GT, Howlett LJ, Seely ET. Intramuscular or intralipomatous injections? N Eng J Med 307: 356–58 (1982).
23. CDC. General Recommendations on Immunization, ACIP. MMWR 32: 1–8, 13–17 (1983).
24. Committee on Immunization Council of Medical Societies, American College of Physicians. Guide for Adult Immunizations. (1985).
25. CDC. Rabies postexposure prophylaxis with HDCV: Lower neutralizing antibody titers with Wyeth vaccine. MMWR 34: 90–92 (1985).
26. Shill M, Baynes RD, Miller SD. Fatal rabies encephalitis despite appropriate postexposure prophylaxis. N Engl J Med 316: 1257–58 (1987).
27. Baer GM, Fishbein DB. Rabies postexposure prophylaxis. N Engl J Med 316: 1270–72 (1987).
28. CDC. Recommendations of the Immunization Practices Advisory Committee (ACIP). Supplementary statement on rabies vaccine and serologic testing. MMWR 30: 535–6 (1981).
29. CDC. Human rabies despite treatment with Rabies Immune Globulin and Human Diploid Cell Rabies Vaccine—Thailand. MMWR 36: 759–765 (1987).

Manufactured by:
Aventis Pasteur SA
Lyon France US Govt License #1279
Distributed by:
Aventis Pasteur Inc.
Swiftwater PA 18370 USA
1-800-VACCINE (1-800-822-2463)
Revised: July 1991 4313

IPOL® ℞

Poliovirus Vaccine Inactivated

Rx only

Caution: Federal (USA) law prohibits dispensing without prescription.

DESCRIPTION

IPOL®, Poliovirus Vaccine Inactivated, produced by Aventis Pasteur SA, is a sterile suspension of three types of poliovirus: Type 1 (Mahoney), Type 2 (MEF-1), and Type 3 (Saukett). IPOL® is a highly purified, inactivated poliovirus vaccine produced by microcarrier culture.[1,2] This culture technique and improvements in purification, concentration and standardization of poliovirus antigen produce a more potent and consistent immunogenic vaccine than the IPV available in the US prior to 1988. The viruses are grown in cultures of VERO cells, a continuous line of monkey kidney cells, by the microcarrier technique. The cells are grown in Eagle MEM modified medium, supplemented with newborn calf serum tested for adventitious agents prior to use, originated from countries free of bovine spongiform encephalopathy. For viral growth the culture medium is replaced by M-199, without calf serum.

After clarification and filtration, viral suspensions are concentrated by ultrafiltration, and purified by three liquid chromatography steps; one column of anion exchanger, one column of gel filtration and again one column of anion exchanger. After re-equilibration of the purified viral suspension, with Medium M-199 and adjustment of the antigen titer, the monovalent viral suspensions are inactivated at + 37°C for at least 12 days with 1:4000 formalin.

Each sterile immunizing dose (0.5 mL) of trivalent vaccine is formulated to contain 40 D antigen units of Type 1, 8 D antigen units of Type 2, and 32 D antigen units of Type 3 poliovirus. For each lot of IPOL®, D-antigen content is determined *in vitro* using the D-antigen ELISA assay and immunogenicity is determined by *in vivo* testing in animals. IPOL® is produced from vaccine concentrates diluted with M-199 medium. Also present are 0.5% of 2-phenoxyethanol and a maximum of 0.02% of formaldehyde per dose as preservatives. Neomycin, streptomycin and polymyxin B are used in vaccine production, and although purification procedures eliminate measurable amounts, less than 5 ng neomycin, 200 ng streptomycin and 25 ng polymyxin B per dose may still be present. The residual calf serum protein is less than 1 ppm in the final vaccine.

The vaccine is clear and colorless and should be administered intramuscularly or subcutaneously.

CLINICAL PHARMACOLOGY

Poliomyelitis is caused by poliovirus Types 1, 2, or 3. It is primarily spread by the fecal-oral route of transmission but may also be spread by the pharyngeal route.

Approximately 90% to 95% of poliovirus infections are asymptomatic. Nonspecific illness with low-grade fever and sore throat (minor illness) occurs in 4% to 8% of infections. Aseptic meningitis occurs in 1% to 5% of patients a few days after the minor illness has resolved. Rapid onset of asymmetric acute flaccid paralysis occurs in 0.1% to 2% of infections, and residual paralytic disease involving motor neurons (paralytic poliomyelitis) occurs in approximately 1 per 1,000 infections.[3]

Prior to the introduction of conventional (non-enhanced) inactivated poliovirus vaccines in 1955, large outbreaks of poliomyelitis occurred each year in the United States (US). The annual incidence of paralytic disease of 11.4 cases/100,000 population declined to 0.5 cases by the time oral poliovirus vaccine (OPV) was introduced in 1961. Incidence continued to decline thereafter to its present rate of 0.002 to 0.005 cases per 100,000 population. Of the 127 cases of paralytic poliomyelitis reported in the US between 1980 and 1994, six were imported cases (caused by wild polioviruses), two were "intermediate" cases, and 119 were vaccine associated paralytic poliomyelitis (VAPP) cases associated with the use of live, attenuated oral poliovirus vaccine (OPV).[4]

TABLE 1 **US STUDIES WITH IPOL® ADMINISTERED USING IPV ONLY OR SEQUENTIAL IPV-OPV SCHEDULES**

Age (months) for				Post Dose 2				Post Dose 3				Pre Booster				Post Booster			
2 Dose 1	4 Dose 2	6 Dose 3	12 to 18 Booster	N*	Type 1 %DA**	Type 2 %DA	Type 3 %DA	N*	Type 1 %DA	Type 2 %DA	Type 3 %DA	N*	Type 1 %DA	Type 2 %DA	Type 3 %DA	N*	Type 1 %DA	Type 2 %DA	Type 3 %DA
STUDY 1[11¶]																			
I(s)	I(s)	NA†	I(s)	56	97	100	97		—	—	—	53	91	97	93	53	97	100	100
O	O	NA	O	22	100	100	100		—	—	—	22	78	91	78	20	100	100	100
I(s)	O	NA	O	17	95	100	95		—	—	—	17	95	100	95	17	100	100	100
I(s)	I(s)	NA	O	17	100	100	100		—	—	—	16	100	100	94	16	100	100	100
STUDY 2[10§]																			
I(c)	I(c)	NA	I(s)	94	98	97	96		—	—	—	100	92	95	88	97	100	100	100
I(s)	I(s)	NA	I(s)	68	99	100	99		—	—	—	72	100	100	94	75	100	100	100
I(c)	I(c)	NA	O	75	95	99	96		—	—	—	77	86	97	82	78	100	100	97
I(s)	I(s)	NA	O	101	99	99	95		—	—	—	103	99	97	89	107	100	100	100
STUDY 3[10§]																			
I(c)	I(c)	I(c)	O	91	98	99	100	91	100	100	100	41	100	100	100	40	100	100	100
I(c)	I(c)	O	O	96	100	98	99	94	100	100	99	47	100	100	100	45	100	100	100
I(c)	I(c)	I(c) + O	O	91	96	97	100	85	100	100	100	47	100	100	100	46	100	100	100

* N = Number of children from whom serum was available
** Detectable antibody (neutralizing titer ≥ 1:4)
† NA—No poliovirus vaccine administered
¶ IPOL® given subcutaneously
§ IPOL® given intramuscularly
I IPOL® given either separately in association with DTP in two sites (s) or combined (c) with DTP in a dual chambered syringe
O OPV

Poliovirus Vaccine Inactivated induces the production of neutralizing antibodies against each type of virus which are related to protective efficacy and induces antibody responses in most children after administering fewer doses[5] than the vaccine available in the United States prior to 1988.

Studies in developed[5] and developing[6,7] countries with a similar enhanced inactivated poliovirus vaccine produced by the same technology with the use of different cell substrate (primary kidney cells) have shown that a direct relationship exists between the antigenic content of the vaccine, the frequency of seroconversion, and resulting antibody titer. Approval in the US was based upon demonstration of immunogenicity and safety in US children.[8]

In the US, 219 infants received three doses of IPV at two, four and eighteen months of age manufactured by the same process as IPOL® except the cell substrate for IPV was primary monkey kidney cells. Seroconversion to all three types of poliovirus was demonstrated in 99% of these infants after two doses of vaccine given at 2 and 4 months of age. Following the third dose of vaccine at 18 months of age, neutralizing antibodies were present at a level of ≥ 1:10 in 99.1% of children to Type 1 and 100% of children to Types 2 and 3 polioviruses.[9]

IPOL® was administered to more than 700 infants between 2 to 18 months of age during three clinical studies conducted in the US using IPV only schedules and sequential IPV-OPV schedules.[10,11] Seroprevalence rates for detectable serum neutralizing antibody (DA) at a ≥ 1:4 dilution were 95% to 100% (Type 1); 97% to 100% (Type 2) and 96% to 100% (Type 3) after two doses of IPOL® depending on studies.

[See table 1 above]

In one study,[11] the persistence of DA in infants receiving two doses of IPOL® at 2 and 4 months of age was 91% to 100% (Type 1), 97% to 100% (Type 2), and 93% to 94% (Type 3) at twelve months of age. In another study,[10] 86% to 100% (Type 1), 95% to 100% (Type 2), and 82% to 94% (Type 3) of infants still had DA at 18 months of age.

In trials and field studies conducted outside the US, IPOL®, or a combination vaccine containing IPOL® and DTP, was administered to more than 3,000 infants between 2 to 18 months of age using IPV only schedules and immunogenicity data are available from 1,485 infants. After two doses of vaccine given during the first year of life, seroprevalence rates for detectable serum neutralizing antibody (neutralizing titer ≥ 1:4) were 88% to 100% (Type 1); 84% to 100% (Type 2) and 94% to 100% (Type 3) of infants, depending on studies. When three doses were given during the first year of life, post-dose 3 DA ranged between 93% to 100% (Type 1); 89% to 100% (Type 2) and 97% to 100% (Type 3) and reached 100% for Types 1, 2, and 3 after the fourth dose given during the second year of life (12 to 18 months of age).[12]

In infants immunized with three doses of an unlicensed combination vaccine containing IPOL® and DTP given during the first year of life, and a fourth dose given during the second year of life, the persistence of detectable neutralizing antibodies was 96%, 96% and 97% against poliovirus Types 1, 2, and 3, respectively, at six years of age. DA reached 100% for all types after a booster dose of IPOL® combined with DTP vaccine.[8] A survey of Swedish children and young adults given a Swedish IPV only schedule demonstrated persistence of detectable serum neutralizing antibody for at least 10 years to all three types of poliovirus.[13]

IPV is able to induce secretory antibody (IgA) produced in the pharynx and gut and reduces pharyngeal excretion of poliovirus Type 1 from 75% in children with neutralizing antibodies at levels less than 1:8 to 25% in children with neutralizing antibodies at levels more than 1:64.[12,14,15–21] There is also evidence of induction of herd immunity with IPV, [13,22–25] and that this herd immunity is sufficiently maintained in a population vaccinated only with IPV.[25]

Paralytic polio and VAPP have not been reported in association with administration of IPOL®. It is expected that an IPV only schedule will eliminate the risk of VAPP in both recipients and contacts compared to a schedule that included OPV.[26]

INDICATIONS AND USAGE

IPOL® is indicated for active immunization of infants (as young as 6 weeks of age), children and adults for the prevention of poliomyelitis caused by poliovirus Types 1, 2, and 3.[27]

INFANTS, CHILDREN AND ADOLESCENTS

General Recommendations

It is recommended that all infants (as young as 6 weeks of age), unimmunized children and adolescents not previously immunized be vaccinated routinely against paralytic poliomyelitis.[28] Following the eradication of poliomyelitis caused by wild poliovirus from the Western Hemisphere (including North and South America)[29] VAPP is the only cause of paralytic poliomyelitis in the US.[30] The use of IPV has been suggested as a way to reduce VAPP incidence.[30]

All children should receive four doses of IPV at ages 2, 4, 6 to 18 months and 4 to 6 years. OPV is no longer recommended for routine immunization.[26] In the special circumstances that OPV is acceptable, please refer to the manufacturer's latest package insert for the appropriate administration schedule and all other issues related to the use of OPV.

Previous clinical poliomyelitis (usually due to only a single poliovirus type) or incomplete immunization with OPV are not contraindications to completing the primary series of immunization with IPOL®.

Children Incompletely Immunized

Children of all ages should have their immunization status reviewed and be considered for supplemental immunization as follows for adults. Time intervals between doses longer than those recommended for routine primary immunization do not necessitate additional doses as long as a final total of four doses is reached (see **DOSAGE AND ADMINISTRATION** section).

ADULTS

General Recommendations

Routine primary poliovirus vaccination of adults (generally those 18 years of age or older) residing in the US is not recommended. Unimmunized adults residing in a household when a child is receiving OPV and/or adults who have increased risk of exposure to either oral vaccine or wild poliovirus and have not been adequately immunized should receive polio vaccination in accordance with the schedule given in the **DOSAGE AND ADMINISTRATION** section.[27]

Persons with previous wild poliovirus disease who are incompletely immunized or unimmunized should be given additional doses of IPOL® if they fall into one or more categories listed previously.

The following categories of adults are at an increased risk of exposure to wild polioviruses:[27,31]

- Travelers to regions or countries where poliomyelitis is endemic or epidemic.
- Health-care workers in close contact with patients who may be excreting polioviruses.
- Laboratory workers handling specimens that may contain polioviruses.
- Members of communities or specific population groups with disease caused by wild polioviruses.
- Incompletely vaccinated or unvaccinated adults in a household (or other close contacts) with children given OPV. The adult should be informed of the risk of VAPP associated with contact of those receiving OPV.

IMMUNODEFICIENCY AND ALTERED IMMUNE STATUS

Patients with recognized immunodeficiency are at greater risk of developing paralysis when exposed to live poliovirus than persons with a normal immune system. Under no circumstances should oral poliovirus vaccine be used in such patients or introduced into a household where such a patient resides.[27]

IPOL® should be used in all patients with immunodeficiency diseases and members of such patients' households when vaccination of such persons is indicated. This includes patients with asymptomatic HIV infection, AIDS or AIDS-Related Complex, severe combined immunodeficiency, hypogammaglobulinemia, or agammaglobulinemia; altered immune states due to disease such as leukemia, lymphoma, or generalized malignancy; or an immune system compromised by treatment with corticosteroids, alkylating drugs, antimetabolites or radiation. Immunogenicity of IPOL® in individuals receiving immunoglobulin could be impaired and patients with an altered immune state may or may not develop a protective response against paralytic poliomyelitis after administration of IPV.[32]

As with any vaccine, vaccination with IPOL® may not protect 100% of susceptible individuals.

Use with other vaccines: refer to **DOSAGE AND ADMINISTRATION** section for this information.

CONTRAINDICATIONS

IPOL® is contraindicated in persons with a history of hypersensitivity to any component of the vaccine, including 2-phenoxyethanol, formaldehyde, neomycin, streptomycin and polymyxin B.

No further doses should be given if anaphylaxis or anaphylactic shock occurs within 24 hours of administration of one dose of vaccine.

Vaccination of persons with an acute, febrile illness should be deferred until after recovery; however, minor illness, such as mild upper respiratory infection, with or without low grade fever, are not reasons for postponing vaccine administration.

WARNINGS

This product contains dry natural latex rubber as follows: The stopper to the vial contains no rubber of any kind. In the case of the syringe, the needle cover contains dry natural latex rubber, but the plunger for the syringe contains no rubber of any kind.

Neomycin, streptomycin, polymyxin B, 2-phenoxyethanol, and formaldehyde are used in the production of this vaccine. Although purification procedures eliminate measurable amounts of these substances, traces may be present (see **DESCRIPTION** section) and allergic reactions may occur in persons sensitive to these substances (see **CONTRAINDICATIONS** section).

Systemic adverse reactions reported in infants receiving IPV concomitantly at separate sites or combined with DTP have been similar to those associated with administration of DTP alone.[8] Local reactions are usually mild and transient in nature.

Although no causal relationship between IPOL® and Guillain-Barré Syndrome (GBS) has been established,[27] GBS has been temporally related to administration of another inactivated poliovirus vaccine. Deaths have been reported in temporal association with the administration of IPV (see **ADVERSE REACTIONS** section).

PRECAUTIONS

GENERAL

Prior to an injection of any vaccine, all known precautions should be taken to prevent side reactions. This includes a review of the patient's history with respect to possible sensitivity to the vaccine or similar vaccines and to possible sensitivity to dry natural latex rubber.

Health-care providers should question the patient, parent or guardian about reactions to a previous dose of this product, or similar product.

Epinephrine Injection (1:1000) and other appropriate agents should be available to control immediate allergic reactions.

Health-care providers should obtain the previous immunization history of the vaccinee, and inquire about the current health status of the vaccinee.

Continued on next page

Ipol—Cont.

Immunodeficient patients or patients under immunosuppressive therapy may not develop a protective immune response against paralytic poliomyelitis after administration of IPV.

Administration of IPOL® is not contraindicated in individuals infected with HIV.[33,34,35]

Special care should be taken to ensure that the injection does not enter a blood vessel.

A separate, sterile syringe and needle or a sterile disposable unit must be used for each patient to prevent transmission of hepatitis or other infectious agents from person to person. Needles should not be recapped and should be disposed of according to biohazard waste guidelines.

INFORMATION FOR PATIENTS

Patients, parents, or guardians should be instructed to report any serious adverse reactions to their health-care provider.

The health-care provider should inform the patient, parent, or guardian of the benefits and risks of the vaccine.

The health-care provider should inform the patient, parent, or guardian of the importance of completing the immunization series.

The health-care provider should provide the Vaccine Information Materials (VIMs) which are required to be given with each immunization.

DRUG INTERACTIONS

There are no known interactions of IPOL® with drugs or foods. Simultaneous administration, with separate syringes at separate sites, of other parenteral vaccines is not contraindicated. The first two doses of IPOL® may be administered at separate sites using separate syringes concomitantly with DTP, acellular pertussis, *Haemophilus influenzae* type b (Hib), and hepatitis B vaccines. From historical data on the antibody responses to diphtheria, tetanus, whole-cell or acellular pertussis, Hib, or hepatitis B vaccines used concomitantly or in combination with IPOL®, no interferences have been observed on the immunological end points accepted for clinical protection.[8,14,36] (See **DOSAGE AND ADMINISTRATION** section.)

If IPOL® has been administered to persons receiving immunosuppressive therapy, an adequate immunologic response may not be obtained. (See **PRECAUTIONS—GENERAL** section.)

CARCINOGENESIS, MUTAGENESIS, IMPAIRMENT OF FERTILITY

Long-term studies in animals to evaluate carcinogenic potential or impairment of fertility have not been conducted.

PREGNANCY

REPRODUCTIVE STUDIES—PREGNANCY CATEGORY C

Animal reproduction studies have not been conducted with IPOL®. It is also not known whether IPOL® can cause fetal harm when administered to a pregnant woman or can affect reproduction capacity. IPOL® should be given to a pregnant woman only if clearly needed.

NURSING MOTHERS

It is not known whether IPOL® is excreted in human milk. Because many drugs are excreted in human milk, caution should be exercised when IPOL® is administered to a nursing woman.

PEDIATRIC USE

SAFETY AND EFFECTIVENESS OF IPOL® IN INFANTS BELOW SIX WEEKS OF AGE HAVE NOT BEEN ESTABLISHED.[10,19] (See **DOSAGE AND ADMINISTRATION** section.)

In the US, infants receiving two doses of IPV at 2 and 4 months of age, the seroprevalence to all three types of poliovirus was demonstrated in 95% to 100% of these infants after two doses of vaccine.[10,11]

ADVERSE REACTIONS

BODY SYSTEM AS A WHOLE

In earlier studies with the vaccine grown in primary monkey kidney cells, transient local reactions at the site of injection were observed.[9] Erythema, induration and pain occurred in 3.2%, 1% and 13%, respectively, of vaccinees within 48 hours post-vaccination. Temperatures of ≥ 39°C (≥ 102°F) were reported in 38% of vaccinees. Other symptoms included irritability, sleepiness, fussiness, and crying. Because IPV was given in a different site but concurrently with Diphtheria and Tetanus Toxoids and Pertussis Vaccine Adsorbed (DTP), these systemic reactions could not be attributed to a specific vaccine. However, these systemic reactions were comparable in frequency and severity to that reported for DTP given alone without IPV[10] Although no causal relationship has been established, deaths have occurred in temporal association after vaccination of infants with IPV.[37]

Four additional US studies using IPOL® in more than 1,300 infants,[10] between 2 to 18 months of age administered with DTP at the same time at separate sites or combined have demonstrated that local and systemic reactions were similar when DTP was given alone.

[See table 2 below]

DIGESTIVE SYSTEM

Anorexia and vomiting occurred with frequencies not significantly different as reported when DTP was given alone without IPV or OPV.[10]

NERVOUS SYSTEM

Although no causal relationship between IPOL® and GBS has been established,[27] GBS has been temporally related to administration of another inactivated poliovirus vaccine.

Reporting of Adverse Events

The National Vaccine Injury Compensation Program, established by the National Childhood Vaccine Injury Act of 1986, requires physicians and other health-care providers who administer vaccines to maintain permanent vaccination records and to report occurrences of certain adverse events to the US Department of Health and Human Services. Reportable events include those listed in the Act for each vaccine and events specified in the package insert as contraindications to further doses of that vaccine.[38,39,40]

Reporting by parents or guardians of all adverse events after vaccine administration should be encouraged. Adverse events following immunization with vaccine should be reported by health-care providers to the US Department of Health and Human Services (DHHS) Vaccine Adverse Event Reporting System (VAERS). Reporting forms and information about reporting requirements or completion of the form can be obtained from VAERS through a toll-free number 1-800-822-7967.[38,39,40]

Health-care providers also should report these events to the Director of Scientific and Medical Affairs, Aventis Pasteur Inc., Discovery Drive, Swiftwater, PA 18370 or call 1-800-822-2463.

DOSAGE AND ADMINISTRATION

Parenteral drug products should be inspected visually for particulate matter and/or discoloration prior to administration whenever solution and container permit. If these conditions exist, the vaccine should not be administered.

After preparation of the injection site, immediately administer IPOL® intramuscularly or subcutaneously. In infants and small children, the mid-lateral aspect of the thigh is the preferred site. In older children and adults IPOL® should be administered intramuscularly or subcutaneously in the deltoid area.

Care should be taken to avoid administering the injection into or near blood vessels and nerves. After aspiration, if blood or any suspicious discoloration appears in the syringe, do not inject but discard contents and repeat procedures using a new dose of vaccine administered at a different site.

TABLE 2[10] PERCENTAGE OF INFANTS PRESENTING WITH LOCAL OR SYSTEMIC REACTIONS AT 6, 24, AND 48 HOURS OF IMMUNIZATION WITH IPOL® ADMINISTERED INTRAMUSCULARLY CONCOMITANTLY AT SEPARATE SITES WITH AvP¶ WHOLE-CELL DTP VACCINE AT 2 AND 4 MONTHS OF AGE AND WITH AvP ACELLULAR PERTUSSIS VACCINE (TRIPEDIA®) AT 18 MONTHS OF AGE

REACTION	AGE AT IMMUNIZATION								
	2 Months (n=211)			4 Months (n=206)			18 Months† (n=74)		
	6 Hrs.	24 Hrs.	48 Hrs.	6 Hrs.	24 Hrs.	48 Hrs.	6 Hrs.	24 Hrs.	48 Hrs.
Local, IPOL® alone§									
Erythema > 1″	0.5%	0.5%	0.5%	1.0%	0.0%	0.0%	1.4%	0.0%	0.0%
Swelling	11.4%	5.7%	0.9%	11.2%	4.9%	1.9%	2.7%	0.0%	0.0%
Tenderness	29.4%	8.5%	2.8%	22.8%	4.4%	1.0%	13.5%	4.1%	0.0%
Systemic*									
Fever > 102.2°F	1.0%	0.5%	0.5%	2.0%	0.5%	0.0%	0.0%	0.0%	4.2%
Irritability	64.5%	24.6%	17.5%	49.5%	25.7%	11.7%	14.7%	6.7%	8.0%
Tiredness	60.7%	31.8%	7.1%	38.8%	18.4%	6.3%	9.3%	5.3%	4.0%
Anorexia	16.6%	8.1%	4.3%	6.3%	4.4%	2.4%	2.7%	1.3%	2.7%
Vomiting	1.9%	2.8%	2.8%	1.9%	1.5%	1.0%	1.3%	1.3%	0.0%
Persistent Crying	Percentage of infants within 72 hours after immunization was 0.0% after dose one, 1.4% after dose two, and 0.0% after dose three.								

¶AvP (Aventis Pasteur Inc.) formerly known as Connaught Laboratories, Inc.

§Data are from the IPOL® administration site, given intramuscularly.

*The adverse reaction profile includes the concomitant use of AvP whole-cell DTP vaccine or Tripedia® with IPOL®. Rates are comparable in frequency and severity to that reported for whole-cell DTP given alone.

†Children vaccinated with Tripedia® vaccine.

DO NOT ADMINISTER VACCINE INTRAVENOUSLY.

Children

The primary series of IPOL® consists of three 0.5 mL doses administered intramuscularly or subcutaneously, preferably eight or more weeks apart and usually at ages 2, 4, and 6 to 18 months. Under no circumstances should the vaccine be given more frequently than four weeks apart. The first immunization may be administered as early as six weeks of age. For this series, a booster dose of IPOL® is administered at 4 to 6 years of age.[41]

Use with Other Vaccines

From historical data on the antibody responses to diphtheria, tetanus, whole-cell or acellular pertussis, Hib, or hepatitis B vaccines used concomitantly with IPOL®, no interferences have been observed on the immunological end points accepted for clinical protection.[8,14,36] (See DRUG INTERACTIONS section.) If the third dose of IPOL® is given between 12 to 18 months of age, it may be desirable to administer this dose with Measles, Mumps, and Rubella (MMR) and/or other vaccines using separate syringes at separate sites,[27] but no data on the immunological interference between IPOL® and these vaccines exist.

Use in Previously Vaccinated Children

Children and adolescents with a previously incomplete series of IPOL®/OPV or IPOL® only should receive sufficient additional doses of IPOL® to complete the series. OPV is no longer recommended for routine immunization and is recommended only in special circumstances[26] (see **General Recommendations** section).

Interruption of the recommended schedule with a delay between doses does not interfere with the final immunity. There is no need to start either series over again, regardless of the time elapsed between doses.

The need to routinely administer additional doses is unknown at this time.[27]

Adults

Unvaccinated Adults

A primary series of IPOL® is recommended for unvaccinated adults at increased risk of exposure to poliovirus. While the responses of adults to primary series have not been studied, the recommended schedule for adults is two doses given at a 1 to 2 month interval and a third dose given 6 to 12 months later. If less than 3 months but more than 2 months are available before protection is needed, three doses of IPOL® should be given at least 1 month apart. Likewise, if only 1 or 2 months are available, two doses of IPOL® should be given at least 1 month apart. If less than 1 month is available, a single dose of IPOL® is recommended.[27]

Incompletely Vaccinated Adults

Adults who are at an increased risk of exposure to poliovirus and who have had at least one dose of OPV, fewer than three doses of conventional IPV or a combination of conventional IPV or OPV totaling fewer than three doses should receive at least one dose of IPOL®. Additional doses needed to complete a primary series should be given if time permits.[27]

Completely Vaccinated Adults

Adults who are at an increased risk of exposure to poliovirus and who have previously completed a primary series with one or a combination of polio vaccines can be given a dose of IPOL®.

The preferred injection site of IPOL® for adults is in the tissue of the deltoid area.

HOW SUPPLIED

Syringe, 0.5 mL with integrated needle (1 × 1 Dose package—Product No. 49281-860-51) (10 × 1 Dose package Product No. 49281-860-52)

Vial, 10 Dose—Product No. 49281-860-10

STORAGE

The vaccine is stable if stored in the refrigerator between 2°C and 8°C (35°F and 46°F). The vaccine must not be frozen.

REFERENCES

1. van Wezel AL, et al. Inactivated poliovirus vaccine: Current production methods and new developments. Rev Infect Dis 6 (Suppl 2): S335–S340, 1984
2. Montagnon BJ, et al. Industrial scale production of inactivated poliovirus vaccine prepared by culture of Vero cells on microcarrier. Rev Infect Dis 6 (Suppl 2): S341–S344, 1984
3. Sabin AB. Poliomyelitis. In Brande Al, Davis CE, Fierer J (eds) International Textbook of Medicine, Vol II. Infectious Diseases and Medical Microbiology. 2nd ed. Philadelphia, WBSaunders, 1986
4. Prevots DR, et al. Vaccine-associated paralytic poliomyelitis in the United States, 1980–1994: current risk and potential impact of a proposed sequential schedule of IPV followed by OPV (Abstract #H90). In: Abstracts of the 36th Interscience Conference on Antimicrobial Agents and Chemotherapy. Washington, DC. American Society for Microbiology, 179, 1996
5. Salk J, et al. Antigen content of inactivated poliovirus vaccine for use in a one- or two-dose regimen. Ann Clin Res 14: 204–212, 1982
6. Salk J, et al. Killed poliovirus antigen titration in humans. Develop Biol Standard 41: 119–132, 1978
7. Salk J, et al. Theoretical and practical considerations in the application of killed poliovirus vaccine for the control of paralytic poliomyelitis. Develop Biol Standard 47: 181–198, 1981
8. Unpublished data available from Aventis Pasteur SA

9. McBean AM, et al. Serologic response to oral polio vaccine and enhanced-potency inactivated polio vaccines. Am J Epidemiol 128: 615–628, 1988
10. Unpublished data available from Aventis Pasteur Inc.
11. Faden H, et al. Comparative evaluation of immunization with live attenuated and enhanced potency inactivated trivalent poliovirus vaccines in childhood: Systemic and local immune responses. J Infect Dis 162: 1291–1297, 1990
12. Vidor E, et al. The place of DTP/eIPV vaccine in routine paediatric vaccination. Rev Med Virol 4: 261–277, 1994
13. Bottiger M. Long-term immunity following vaccination with killed poliovirus vaccine in Sweden, a country with no circulating poliovirus. Rev Infect Dis 6 (Suppl 2): S548–S551, 1984
14. Plotkin SA, et al. Inactivated polio vaccine for the United States: a missed vaccination opportunity. Pediatr Infect Dis J 14: 835–839, 1995
15. Murdin AD, et al. Inactivated poliovirus vaccine: past and present experience. Vaccine 8: 735–746, 1996
16. Marine WM, et al. Limitation of fecal and pharyngeal poliovirus excretion in Salk-vaccinated children. A family study during a Type 1 poliomyelitis epidemic. Amer J Hyg 76: 173–195, 1962
17. Bottiger M, et al. Vaccination with attenuated Type 1 poliovirus, the Chat strain. II. Transmission of virus in relation to age. Acta Paed Scand 55: 416–421, 1966
18. Dick GWA, et al. Vaccination against poliomyelitis with live virus vaccines. Effect of previous Salk vaccination on virus excretion. Brit Med J 2: 266–269, 1961
19. Wehrle PF, et al. Transmission of poliovirus; III. Prevalence of polioviruses in pharyngeal secretions of infected household contacts of patients with clinical disease. Pediatrics 27: 762–764, 1961
20. Adenyi-Jones SC, et al. Systemic and local immune responses to enhanced-potency inactivated poliovirus vaccine in premature and term infants. J Pediatr 120: No 5, 686–689, 1992
21. Chin TDY. Immunity induced by inactivated poliovirus vaccine and excretion of virus. Rev Infect Dis 6 (Suppl 2): S369–S370, 1984
22. Salk D. Herd effect and virus eradication with use of killed poliovirus vaccine. Develop Biol Standard 47: 247–255, 1981
23. Bijerk H. Surveillance and control of poliomyelitis in the Netherlands. Rev Infect Dis 6 (Suppl 2): S451–S456, 1984
24. Lapinleimu K. Elimination of poliomyelitis in Finland. Rev Infect Dis 6 (Suppl 2): S457–S460, 1984
25. Conyn van Spaendonck M, et al. Circulation of Poliovirus during the poliomyelitis outbreak in the Netherlands in 1992–1993. Amer J Epidemiology 143: 929–935, 1996
26. ACIP. Recommendations of the Advisory Committee on Immunization Practices: Revised recommendations for routine poliomyelitis vaccination. MMWR 48(27), 590, 1999
27. ACIP. Poliomyelitis prevention in the United States: introduction of a sequential vaccination schedule of Inactivated Poliovirus Vaccine followed by Oral Poliovirus Vaccine. MMWR 46: No. RR-3, 1997
28. WHO. Weekly Epidemiology Record 54: 82–83, 1979
29. Certification of poliomyelitis eradication—the Americas, 1994. MMWR 43: 720–722, 1994
30. Strebel PM, et al. Epidemiology of poliomyelitis in the United States one decade after the last reported case of indigenous wild virus associated disease. Clin Infect Dis 14: 568–579, 1992
31. Institute of Medicine. An evaluation of poliomyelitis vaccine policy options. Washington, DC. National Academy of Sciences, 1988
32. ACIP. Immunization of children infected with human T-lymphotropic virus type III/lymphadenopathy-associated virus. MMWR 35: 595–606, 1986
33. ACIP. General recommendations on immunization. MMWR 43: No. RR-1, 1994
34. Barbi M, et al. Antibody response to inactivated polio vaccine (eIPV) in children born to HIV positive mothers. Eur J Epidemiol 8: 211–216, 1992
35. Varon D, et al. Response to hemophilic patients to poliovirus vaccination: Correlation with HIV serology and with immunological parameters. J Med Virol 40: 91–95, 1993
36. Vidor E, et al. Fifteen-years experience with vero-produced enhanced potency inactivated poliovirus vaccine (eIPV). Ped Infect Dis J, 312–322, 1997
37. Stratton, R. et al. Adverse Events Associated with Childhood Vaccines. Polio Vaccines. National Academy Press, 295–299, 1994
38. CDC. Vaccine Adverse Event Reporting System—United States. MMWR 39: 730–733, 1990
39. CDC. National Childhood Vaccine Injury Act. Requirements for permanent vaccination records and for reporting of selected events after vaccination. MMWR 37: 197–200, 1988.
40. Food & Drug Administration. New Reporting Requirements for Vaccine Adverse Events. FDA Drug Bull 18 (2), 16–18, 1988
41. Recommended childhood immunization schedule—United States, 1999. MMWR 48: 12–16, 1999

Product information as of December 1999

Manufactured by:
Aventis Pasteur SA
Lyon France
US Govt License #1279
Distributed by:
Aventis Pasteur Inc.
Swiftwater PA 18370 USA
1-800-VACCINE (1-800-822-2463)

4305/4308

Japanese Encephalitis Virus Vaccine Inactivated
JE-VAX® ℞
Rx only
CAUTION: Federal (USA) law prohibits dispensing without prescription.

DESCRIPTION

JE-VAX®, Japanese Encephalitis Virus Vaccine Inactivated, is a sterile, lyophilized vaccine for subcutaneous use, prepared by inoculating mice intracerebrally with Japanese encephalitis (JE) virus, "Nakayama-NIH" strain, manufactured by The Research Foundation for Microbial Diseases of Osaka University ("BIKEN®"). Infected brains are harvested and homogenized in phosphate buffered saline, pH 8.0. The homogenate is centrifuged and the supernatant inactivated with formaldehyde, then processed to yield a partially purified, inactivated virus suspension. This is further purified by ultra-centrifugation through 40% w/v sucrose. The suspension is then lyophilized in final containers and sealed under dry nitrogen atmosphere. Thimerosal (mercury derivative) is added as a preservative to a final concentration of 0.007%. The diluent, Sterile Water for Injection, contains no preservative. Each 1.0 mL dose contains approximately 500 µg of gelatin, less than 100 µg of formaldehyde, less than 0.0007% v/v Polysorbate 80, and less than 50 ng of mouse serum protein. No myelin basic protein can be detected at the detection threshold of the assay (< 2 ng/mL). Prior to reconstitution, the vaccine is a white caked powder, and after reconstitution the vaccine is a colorless transparent liquid. The potency of JE vaccine is determined by immunizing mice with either the test vaccine or the JE reference vaccine. Neutralizing antibodies are measured in a plaque neutralization assay performed on sera from the immunized mice. The potency of the test vaccine must be no less than that of the reference vaccine.

CLINICAL PHARMACOLOGY

Japanese encephalitis (JE), a mosquito-borne arboviral Flavivirus infection, is the leading cause of viral encephalitis in Asia.

Infection leads to overt encephalitis in 1 of 20 to 1000 cases. Encephalitis, usually is severe, resulting in a fatal outcome in 25% of cases and residual neuropsychiatric sequelae in 50% of cases. JE acquired during the first or second trimesters of pregnancy may cause intrauterine infection and miscarriage. Infections that occur during the third trimester of pregnancy have not been associated with adverse outcomes in newborns.[1]

The virus is transmitted in an enzootic cycle among mosquitoes and vertebrate amplifying hosts, chiefly domestic pigs and, in some areas, wild Ardeid (wading) birds. Viral infection rates in mosquitoes range from < 1% to 3%. These species are prolific in rural areas where their larvae breed in ground pools and flooded rice fields. Thus all elements of the transmission cycle are prevalent in rural areas of Asia and human infections occur principally in this setting. Because vertebrate amplifying hosts and agricultural activities may be situated within and at the periphery of cities, human cases occasionally are reported from urban locations.[1]

JE virus is transmitted seasonally in most areas of Asia. The seasonal patterns of viral transmission are correlated with the abundance of vector mosquitoes and of vertebrate amplifying hosts. Although the abundance of vector mosquitoes fluctuates with the amount of rainfall, and with the impact of the rainy season, in some tropical locations, irrigation associated with agricultural practices is a more important factor affecting vector abundance, and transmission may occur year-round. Thus the periods of greatest risk for JE viral transmission vary regionally and within countries, and from year to year.[1]

In areas where JE is endemic, annual incidence ranges from 1 to 10 per 10,000 people. Cases occur primarily in children under 10 years of age. Seroprevalence studies in these endemic areas indicate nearly universal exposure by adulthood (calculating from a ratio of asymptomatic to symptomatic infections of 200 to 1, approximately 10% of the susceptible population is infected per year). In addition to children < 10 years, an increase in JE incidence has been observed in the elderly.[1]

Challenge experiments in passively protected mice have defined the levels of neutralizing antibody that may be protective for humans.[2] Mice passively immunized to achieve a neutralizing antibody titer of 1:10 were protected from a JE virus challenge of $10^5 LD_{50}$, a viral dose thought to be transmitted by an infected mosquito.[2]

The efficacy of the BIKEN Nakayama-NIH strain Japanese Encephalitis Virus Vaccine Inactivated was demonstrated in a placebo-controlled, randomized clinical trial in Thai children, sponsored by the US Army.[3] In this trial, children between 1 and 14 years of age received BIKEN monovalent Nakayama-NIH strain (n = 21,628) or a bivalent vaccine containing the Nakayama-NIH and Beijing JE virus strains (n = 22,080) or tetanus toxoid as a placebo (n = 21,516). Immunization consisted of two (2) subcutaneous 1.0 mL doses of vaccine, *except in children under 3 years of age who received two 0.5 mL doses.* One case (5 cases/100,000) of JE occurred in the monovalent vaccine group, one case (5 cases/100,000) in the bivalent vaccine group, and 11 cases (51 cases/100,000) in the placebo group. The observed efficacy of both monovalent and bivalent vaccines was 91% (95% confidence interval, 54% to 98%). Side effects of vaccination, including headache, sore arm, rash, and swelling are reported at rates similar to those in the placebo group, usually less than 1%. Symptoms did not increase after the second dose. It should be noted that a schedule of two doses, separated by seven days, as employed in this trial, may be appropriate for use in residents of endemic or epidemic areas, where preexisting exposure to Flaviviruses may contribute to the immune response.[3]

A three-dose vaccination schedule is recommended for US travelers and military personnel, based on the Centers for Disease Control and Prevention (CDC) experience and on a controlled immunogenicity trial performed in US military personnel.[4,5] The CDC experience demonstrated that neutralizing antibody was produced in fewer than 80% of vaccinees following two doses of vaccine in US travelers and antibody levels declined substantially in most vaccinees within six months. The US Army studied the immunogenicity of JE-VAX in 538 volunteers. Two three-dose regimens were evaluated (Day 0, 7, and 14 or Day 0, 7, and 30). All vaccine recipients demonstrated neutralizing antibodies at 2 months and 6 months after initiation of vaccination. The schedule of Day 0, 7, and 30 produced higher antibody responses than the Day 0, 7, and 14 schedule. Two hundred and seventy-three of the original study participants were tested at 12 months post-vaccination and there was no longer a statistical difference in antibody titers between the two vaccination regimens.[5]

The full duration of protection is unknown. Of US Army volunteers completing a three-dose regimen, 252 agreed to receive a booster dose of vaccine one year after the primary series. All boosted participants still had antibody 12 months after the booster. Protective levels of neutralizing antibody persisted for 24 months (2 years) in all 21 persons who had not received a booster.[5] Definitive recommendations cannot be given on the timing of booster doses at this time.

INDICATIONS AND USAGE

JE-VAX is indicated for active immunization against JE for persons one year of age and older. For recommended primary immunization series see **DOSAGE AND ADMINISTRATION** section.

JE-VAX should be considered for use in persons who plan to reside in or travel to areas where JE is endemic or epidemic during a transmission season. ***JE-VAX is NOT recommended for all persons traveling to or residing in Asia.*** The incidence of JE in the location of intended stay, the conditions of housing, nature of activities, duration of stay, and the possibility of unexpected travel to high-risk areas are factors that should be considered in the decision to administer vaccine. In general, vaccine should be considered for use in persons spending a month or longer in epidemic or endemic areas during the transmission season, especially if travel will include rural areas. Depending on the epidemic circumstances, vaccine should be considered for persons spending less than 30 days whose activities, such as extensive outdoor activities in rural areas, place them at particularly high risk for exposure.[1]

In all instances, travelers are advised to take personal precautions to reduce exposure to mosquito bites. (See INFORMATION FOR PATIENTS section.)

Current CDC advisories should be consulted with regard to JE epidemicity in specific locales.[1]

The decision to use JE-VAX should balance the risks for exposure to the virus and for developing illness, the availability and acceptability of repellents and other alternative measures, and the side effects of vaccination. Assessments should be interpreted cautiously because risk can vary within areas and from year to year and available data are incomplete. Estimates suggest that risk of JE in highly endemic areas during the transmission season can reach 1 per 5,000 per month of exposure; risk for most short-term travelers may be 1 per million or less. Although JE vaccine is reactogenic, rates of serious allergic reactions (generalized urticaria and/or angioedema) are low (approximately 1–104 per 10,000).[1]

Advanced age may be a risk factor for developing symptomatic illness after infection. JE acquired during pregnancy carries the potential for intrauterine infection and fetal death. These factors should be considered when advising elderly persons and pregnant women who plan visits to JE endemic areas.

There are no data on the safety and efficacy of JE vaccine in infants under one year of age. Whenever possible, immunization of infants should be deferred until they are one year of age or older.[1]

Research laboratory workers:

Laboratory acquired JE has been reported in 22 cases. JE virus may be transmitted in a laboratory setting through needle sticks and other accidental exposures. Vaccine-derived immunity presumably protects against exposure through these percutaneous routes. Exposure to aerosolized JE virus, and particularly to high concentrations of virus, such as may occur during viral purfication, potentially could

Continued on next page

Je-Vax—Cont.

lead to infection through mucous membranes and possibly directly into the central nervous system through the olfactory mucosa. It is unknown whether vaccine-derived immunity protects against such exposures, but immunization is recommended for all laboratory workers with a potential for exposure to infectious JE virus.[1]

As with any vaccine, vaccination with JE-VAX may not result in protection in all individuals. Long-term protection, as demonstrated by persistence of neutralizing antibody for more than two years, has not yet been shown.

CONTRAINDICATIONS

Adverse reactions to a prior dose of JE vaccine manifesting as generalized urticaria and angioedema are considered to be contraindications to further vaccination.

Patients who developed allergic or unusual adverse events after vaccination should be reported through the Vaccine Adverse Event Reporting System (VAERS) 1-800-822-7967.[1]

JE vaccine is produced in mouse brains and should not be administered to persons with a proven or suspected hypersensitivity to proteins of rodent or neural origin. ***HYPERSENSITIVITY TO THIMEROSAL IS A CONTRAINDICATION TO VACCINATION.***[1]

WARNINGS

Adverse reactions to JE vaccine manifesting as generalized urticaria or angioedema may occur within minutes following vaccination. A possibly related reaction has occurred as late as 17 days after vaccination. Most reactions occur within 10 days with the majority occurring within 48 hours.[1] (See ADVERSE REACTIONS section)

Vaccinees should be observed for 30 minutes after vaccination and warned about the possibility of delayed generalized urticaria, often in a generalized distribution or angioedema of the extremities, face and oropharynx, especially of the lips.[1]

Vaccinees should be advised to remain in areas where they have ready access to medical care for 10 days after receiving a dose of JE vaccine. *Vaccinees should be instructed to seek medical attention immediately upon onset of any reaction.*[1]

***Persons should not embark on international travel within 10 days of JE-VAX immunization because of the possibility of delayed allergic reactions.*[1]**

Persons with a past history of urticaria after hymenoptera envenomation, drugs, physical or other provocations, or of idiopathic cause appear to have a greater risk of developing reactions to JE vaccine (relative risk 9.1, 95% confidence interval 1.8 to 50.9).[6] This history should be considered when weighing risks and benefits of the vaccine for an individual patient. When patients with such a history are offered JE vaccine, they should be alerted to their increased risk for reaction and monitored appropriately. There are no data supporting the efficacy of prophylactic antihistamines or steroids in preventing JE vaccine-related allergic reactions.[1]

Another case control study consisting of 5 cases and 15 controls identified an increased risk of hypersensitivity reactions to JE vaccine in individuals who had unusual alcohol consumption during the two days following vaccination (p=0.005).[7] **Recipients should be advised to avoid more than the usual alcohol intake during the 48 hours following JE vaccination.**

In the same study an increased risk for hypersensitivity reactions was seen in individuals who received other vaccines within the 7-day period prior to receipt of JE vaccine. **Where possible JE vaccine should be administered concurrently with other vaccines.[7]**

Epinephrine and other medications and equipment to treat anaphylaxis should be available at vaccine administration centers.

PRECAUTIONS

GENERAL

Epinephrine Injection (1:1000) must be immediately availabe should an acute anaphylactic reaction occur due to any component of the vaccine.

Prior to injection of any vaccine, all known precautions should be taken to prevent adverse reactions. This includes a review of the patient's history with respect to possible sensitivity to this vaccine, a similar vaccine or allergic disorders in general (see **CONTRAINDICATIONS** section).

A separate, sterile syringe and needle or a disposable unit should be used for each patient to prevent transmission of infectious agents from person to person. Needles should not be recapped and should be disposed of according to biohazard waste guidelines.

Although substantial neutralizing antibody titers are elicited by JE-VAX in more than 90% of US travelers without history of prior JE immunization or of prior exposure to JE, the precise relationship between antibody level and efficacy has not been established even though these titers persisted for at least two years after immunization.[8]

The decision to administer JE vaccine should balance the risks for exposure to the virus and for developing illness, the availability and acceptability of repellents and other alternative protective measures, and the side effects of vaccination.

INFORMATION FOR PATIENTS

Patients should be advised of the following:

- JE-VAX is given to provide immunization against Japanese encephalitis virus.
- A three-dose immunizing series should be completed, except in unusual circumstances. (See **CONTRAINDICATIONS** and **DOSAGE AND ADMINISTRATION** sections)
- JE-VAX should be given to a pregnant woman only if, in the opinion of a physician, withholding the vaccine entails even greater risk.
- Any adverse events following JE-VAX should be reported through the Vaccine Adverse Event Reporting System (VAERS) 1-800-822-7967 after contacting the physician immediately.
- If the patient has a past history of urticaria (hives) (following hymenoptera envenomation, drugs, physical or other provocation or of idiopathic origin), adverse effects are more likely.
- Adverse events consisting of arm soreness and local redness can occur shortly after vaccination.
- Adverse events consisting of headache, rash, edema and generalized urticaria or angioedema may occur shortly after vaccination or up to 17 days (usually within 10 days) following vaccination.
- International travel should not be initiated within 10 days of JE-VAX vaccination because of the possibility of delayed adverse reactions. Patients should be instructed to seek medical attention immediately upon onset of any adverse reaction.
- Personal precautions should be taken to avoid exposure to mosquito bites by the use of insect repellents, and protective clothing. Avoiding outdoor activity, especially during twilight periods and in the evening, will reduce risk even further.

DRUG INTERACTIONS

There are no data on the effect of concurrent administration of other vaccines, drugs (e.g. chloroquine, mefloquine) or biologicals on the safety and immunogenicity of JE vaccine.

CARCINOGENESIS, MUTAGENESIS, IMPAIRMENT OF FERTILITY

No studies have been performed to evaluate carcinogenicity, mutagenic potential, or impact on fertility.

PREGNANCY

REPRODUCTIVE STUDIES - PREGNANCY CATEGORY C

Animal reproduction studies have not been conducted with Japanese Encephalitis Virus Vaccine. It is not known whether Japanese Encephalitis Virus Vaccine can cause fetal harm when administered to a pregnant woman or can affect reproductive capacity. Pregnant women who must travel to an area where risk of JE is high should be immunized when the theoretical risks of immunization are outweighed by the risk of infection to the mother and developing fetus. Japanese Encephalitis Virus Vaccine should be given to a pregnant woman only if clearly needed.

NURSING MOTHERS

It is not known whether JE-VAX is excreted in human milk. Because many drugs are excreted in human milk, caution should be exercised when JE-VAX is administered to a nursing woman.

PEDIATRIC USE

SAFETY AND EFFECTIVENESS OF JE-VAX IN INFANTS UNDER ONE YEAR OF AGE HAVE NOT BEEN ESTABLISHED. (See **DOSAGE AND ADMINISTRATION** section.)

ADVERSE REACTIONS

JE vaccine is associated with a moderate frequency of local and mild systemic adverse effects.[3,4,5,9,10,11,12] Tenderness, redness, swelling and other local effects have been reported in about 20% of vaccinees (< 1% to 31%). Systemic side effects, principally fever, headache, malaise, rash, and other reactions, such as chills, dizziness, myalgia, nausea, vomiting and abdominal pain have been reported in approximately 10% of vaccinees.

In a study conducted by the CDC less than 5% of the 1,756 US travelers immunized with a three-dose regimen of the vaccine reported headache, flu-like symptoms, fever, and other systemic complaints. Hives and facial swelling were reported in 0.2% and 0.1% of vaccinees, respectively. Local soreness occurred in 5.9% and local redness in 2.9%. There was no increase in the number or severity of reactions with increasing numbers of doses.[8]

The US Army studied 4,034 personnel from 1987 to 1989.[11] Using a two- or three-dose regimen of JE vaccine, arm soreness was described in 22.7%, local redness in 4.8%, headache in 15.2%, and a febrile episode in 5.5%. In another trial evaluating the safety and immunogenicity of a three-dose immunizing series (Day 0, 7, and 30 or Day 0, 7, and 14), performed in 538 adult volunteers in 1990, the Army determined that local soreness and redness occurred in 21% of vaccinees after the first dose, then decreased with subsequent injections ($p < 0.0001$, Chi-square for downward trend). Systemic symptoms including feverishness, headache and rash occurred in 5% of vaccinees after the first dose, then decreased with subsequent injections ($p < 0.001$, Chi-square for downward trend).[5] Participants who received the third dose on Day 14 reported more side effects than those who received the injection on Day 30. Among these volunteers, 252 received a booster injection of vaccine one year after receiving the first dose of the primary series. Side effects reported after the booster injections included local symptoms of soreness (24.5%) and redness (6.1%) at the injection site and systemic complaints of headache (4.9%), fever (1.6%), and rash (0.8%). Less than 1% of all reported symptoms was graded as severe. No generalized urticaria or anaphylaxis was reported.

Since 1989, an apparently new pattern of adverse reactions has been reported among vaccinees in Europe, North America, and Australia.[12,13,14] The reactions have been characterized by urticaria, often in a generalized distribution, or angioedema of the extremities, face, especially of the lips and oropharynx. Three vaccine recipients developed respiratory distress. Distress or collapse due to hypotension or other causes led to hospitalization in several cases. Most reactions were treated successfully with antihistamines or oral steroids; however some patients were hospitalized for parenteral steroid therapy. Three patients developed an erythema multiforme or erythema nodosum and some patients have had joint swelling. Some vaccinees complained of generalized itching without objective evidence of a rash.

An important feature of the reactions has been the interval between vaccination and onset of symptoms. Reactions after a first vaccine dose occurred after a median of 12 hours after immunization (88% of reactions occurred within 3 days). The interval between administration of a second dose and onset of symptoms generally was longer, (median 3 days and possibly as long as 2 weeks). Reactions have occurred after a second or third dose, when preceding doses were received uneventfully.

Between November 1991 and May 1992, the US Navy immunized 35,253 US personnel (marines, other military and dependents) with JE-VAX on Okinawa. The overall reaction rate, 62.4 per 10,000 vaccinees (95% confidence interval 54.2 to 70.6) includes persons reporting urticaria, angioedema, generalized itching and wheezing. The reaction rate per 10,000 vaccinees was 26.7 (95% confidence interval 21.3 to 32.1), 30.8 (95% confidence interval 24.6 to 37.0) or 12.2 (95% confidence interval 7.9 to 16.5) after the first, second or third dose, respectively.[6] These reactions were generally mild to moderate in severity. Nine out of 35,253 persons immunized were hospitalized (2.6 per 10,000 vaccinees) primarily to allow administration of intravenous steroids for refractory urticaria. None of these reactions were considered life-threatening.

A case-control study conducted as part of the JE immunization campaign in Okinawa found that persons developing these reactions after JE vaccination were more likely to have had a past history of urticaria after hymenoptera envenomation, drugs, physical or other provocations or of idiopathic origins (relative risk 9.1, 95% confidence interval 1.8 to 50.9).[6] The vaccine constituents responsible for these adverse reactions have not been identified.

Other serious adverse events reported following vaccination including (1) one case of Guillain-Barré syndrome after JE vaccination has been reported in the United States since 1984 (this patient was diagnosed as having mononucleosis three weeks before the onset of weakness); (2) one case of urticaria, hepatitis and respiratory failure one week after dose 2 (this person showed effusion and infiltrate on chest x-ray and eosinophilia); (3) one case of respiratory and renal failure one week after a dose (this 26-month-old male had infiltrate on chest x-ray and acid fast bacilli in sputum); and (4) one case of newly diagnosed hypertension in a young adult male presenting with a headache several hours after receiving dose one. The relationship of JE-VAX to the etiology of these adverse events is unknown.

Optic neuritis has been reported for one patient. In addition to JE-VAX, this patient concurrently received a number of other vaccines.[15]

Fatal myocarditis has been reported in a patient who had recently been given meningococcal vaccine and at least one dose of JE vaccine. Any causal role for the vaccines is unclear.[15]

Sudden death occurred approximately 60 hours after receiving the first dose of JE vaccine in a 21-year-old US military person with a history of recurrent hypersensitivity and an episode of possible anaphylaxis. This person also received the third dose of plague vaccine approximately 12 to 15 hours prior to the death. There was no evidence of urticaria or angioedema. Cause of death was not established at autopsy.

Surveillance of JE vaccine related complications in Japan from 1965 to 1973 disclosed neurologic events (primarily encephalitis, encephalopathy, seizures, and peripheral neuropathy) in 1 to 2.3 per million vaccinees.[16,17] Very rarely, deaths occurred with vaccine-associated encephalitis. Between 1987 and 1989, two cases of neurologic dysfunction were reported from Japan; one of these was a transverse myelitis, while the second included seizures, cranial nerve paresis, cerebellar ataxia, and behavior disorder.[17] In 1992, two cases of acute disseminated encephalomyelitis were reported from Japan; one occurred 14 days after the second dose and the second occurred 17 days after a booster dose of JE vaccine. Both cases recovered.[18] One case of Bell's Palsy was reported from Thailand.

Reporting of Adverse Events

The National Vaccine Injury Compensation Program, established by the National Childhood Vaccine Injury Act of 1986, requires physicians and other health-care providers who administer vaccines to maintain permanent vaccination records and to report occurrences of certain adverse events to the US Department of Health and Human Services. Reportable events include those listed in the Act for each vaccine and events specified in the package insert as contraindications to further doses of that vaccine.[19,20,21]

Reporting by parents and patients of all adverse events occurring after antigen administration should be encouraged. Adverse events following immunization with vaccine should be reported by the health-care provider to the US Department of Health and Human Services (DHHS) Vaccine Adverse Event Reporting System (VAERS). Reporting forms and information about reporting requirements or completion of the form can be obtained from VAERS through a toll-free number 1-800-822-7967.[19,20,21]

Health-care providers also should report these events to the Director of Scientific and Medical Affairs, Aventis Pasteur Inc., Discovery Drive, Swiftwater, PA 18370 or call 1-800-822-2463.

DOSAGE AND ADMINISTRATION

Parenteral drug products should be inspected visually for extraneous particulate matter and/or discoloration prior to administration whenever solution and container permit. If either of these conditions exist, the vaccine should not be administered.

For persons 3 years of age and older, a single dose is 1.0 mL of vaccine. *For children 1 year to 3 years of age, a single dose is 0.5 mL of vaccine.* (See PRIMARY IMMUNIZATION SCHEDULE below.)

Single-Dose vial of lyophilized vaccine: Remove plastic tab of flip-off cap. DO NOT REMOVE RUBBER STOPPER. Cleanse stopper with a suitable disinfectant. Reconstitute only with the supplied 1.3 mL of diluent (Sterile Water for Injection). Shake vial thoroughly. After reconstitution the vaccine should be stored between 2° – 8°C (35° – 46°F) and used within 8 hours. DO NOT FREEZE RECONSTITUTED VACCINE.

10-Dose vial of lyophilized vaccine: Remove plastic tab of flip-off cap. DO NOT REMOVE RUBBER STOPPER. Cleanse stopper with a suitable disinfectant. Reconstitute only with the supplied 11 mL of diluent (Sterile Water for Injection). Shake vial thoroughly. After reconstitution the vaccine should be stored between 2° – 8°C (35° – 46°F) and used within 8 hours. DO NOT FREEZE RECONSTITUTED VACCINE.

The vaccine is to be given by subcutaneous administration only.

A separate, sterile syringe and needle or a sterile disposable unit should be used for each patient to prevent transmission of infectious agents from person to person. Needles should not be recapped and should be disposed of according to biohazard waste guidelines.

SHAKE VIAL WELL.

PRIMARY IMMUNIZATION SCHEDULE[1]

The recommended primary immunization series is three doses of 1.0 mL each for individuals > 3 years of age given subcutaneously on days 0, 7, and 30. *For children 1 to 3 years of age a series of three doses of 0.5 mL each should be given subcutaneously on days 0, 7, and 30.* An abbreviated schedule of days 0, 7, and 14 can be used when the longer schedule is impractical because of time constraints. (When it is impossible to follow one of the above recommended schedules, two doses given a week apart will induce antibodies in approximately 80% of vaccinees; however, this two-dose regimen should not be used except under unusual circumstances.) The last dose should be given at least 10 days before the commencement of international travel to ensure an adequate immune response and access to medical care in the event of delayed adverse reactions.

A booster dose of 1.0 mL *(0.5 mL for children from 1 to 3 years of age)* may be given after two years. In the absence of firm data on the persistence of antibody after primary immunization, a definite recommendation cannot be made on the spacing of boosters beyond two years.

There are no data on the safety and efficacy of JE vaccine in infants under one year of age. Whenever possible, immunization of infants should be deferred until they are one year of age or older.[1]

The skin at the site of injection first should be cleansed and disinfected. Shake vial thoroughly before each use. Cleanse top of rubber stopper of the vial with a suitable antiseptic and wipe away all excess before withdrawing vaccine.

When JE-VAX and any other vaccines are given concurrently, separate syringes and separate sites should be used.

HOW SUPPLIED

Vial, Single Dose (3 per package) with vial of Diluent (3 per package) – Product No. 49281-680-30

Vial, 10 Dose with vial of Diluent – Product No. 49281-680-20

For persons 3 years of age and older, a single dose is 1.0 mL of vaccine. *For children 1 year to 3 years of age, a single dose is 0.5 mL of vaccine.* (See PRIMARY IMMUNIZATION SCHEDULE above.)

STORAGE

The vaccine should be stored between 2° – 8°C (35° – 46°F). DO NOT FREEZE. After reconstitution the vaccine should be stored between 2° – 8°C (35° – 46°F) and used within 8 hours. DO NOT FREEZE RECONSTITUTED VACCINE.

REFERENCES

1. Recommendations of the Advisory Committee on Immunization Practices (ACIP). Inactivated Japanese Encephalitis Virus Vaccine. MMWR 42: 1–15, 1993
2. Oya A. Japanese Encephalitis Vaccine. Acta Paediatr Jpn 30: 175–184, 1988
3. Hoke CH, et al. Protection Against Japanese Encephalitis by Inactivated Vaccines. N Eng J Med 319: 608–614, 1988
4. Poland JD, et al. Evaluation of the Potency and Safety of Inactivated Japanese Encephalitis Vaccine in US Inhabitants. J Infect Dis 161: 878–882, 1990
5. DeFraites RF. Immunogenicity and Safety of Japanese Encephalitis Vaccine (Inactivated: Nakayama/BIKEN) in U.S. Army Soldiers: Evaluation of Three Consecutively Manufactured Lots of Vaccine Administered in Two Dosing Regimens. April 30, 1991, and November 12, 1992. Unpublished Data, on file with BIKEN and with Walter Reed Army Institute of Research, Washington, DC
6. Berg WS. Systemic Reactions in U.S. Marine Corps Personnel Who Received Japanese Encephalitis Vaccine. Clin Infect Dis 24: 265–266, 1997
7. Robinson P, et al. Australian Case-Control Study of Adverse Reactions to Japanese Encephalitis Vaccine. J Travel Med 2: 159–164, 1995
8. Unpublished data on file with "BIKEN" and CDC
9. Rojanasuphot S. et al. A field trial of Japanese encephalitis vaccine produced in Thailand. Southeast Asian J Trop Med Publ Health 20: 653–654, 1989
10. Rao Bhau LN, et al. Safety and efficacy of Japanese encephalitis vaccine produced in India. Indian J Med Res 88: 301–307, 1988
11. Sanchez JL, et al. Further Experience with Japanese Encephalitis Vaccine. Lancet 335: 972–973, 1990
12. Japanese Encephalitis Vaccine and Adverse Effects among Travelers. Canada Diseases Weekly Report. Vol. 17–32: 173–177, 1991
13. Andersen MM, et al. Side-Effects with Japanese Encephalitis Vaccine. Lancet 337: 1044, 1991
14. Ruff TA, et al. Adverse Reactions to Japanese Encephalitis Vaccine. Lancet 338: 881–882, 1991
15. Unpublished data on file with Aventis Pasteur Inc.
16. Kitaoka M. Follow-up on use of vaccine in children in Japan, in McD Hammon W, Kitaoka M, Downs WG eds. Immunization for Japanese encephalitis. Excerpta Medica, Amsterdam 275–277, 1972
17. Unpublished data on file with "BIKEN"
18. Ohtaki E, et al. Acute disseminated encephalomyelitis after Japanese B Encephalitis Vaccination. Pediatric Neurology Vol. 8 No. 2: 137–139, 1992
19. CDC. Vaccine Adverse Event Reporting System – United States. MMWR 39: 730–733, 1990
20. CDC. National Childhood Vaccine Injury Act. Requirements for permanent vaccination records and for reporting of selected events after vaccination. MMWR 37: 197–200, 1988
21. Food and Drug Administration. New Reporting Requirements for Vaccine Adverse Events. FDA Drug Bull 18(2), 16–18, 1988

Manufactured by:
The Research Foundation for Microbial Diseases of Osaka University
Suita, Osaka, Japan
"BIKEN®"

Distributed by:
Aventis Pasteur Inc.
Swiftwater PA 18370 USA
1-800-VACCINE (1-800-822-2463)

Product Information
as of February 1997

4345

MENOMUNE®—A/C/Y/W-135 ℞

[*mĕn-ō-mūne*]
Meningococcal Polysaccharide Vaccine Groups A, C, Y and W-135 Combined
Rx only

Caution: Federal (USA) law prohibits dispensing without prescription.

DESCRIPTION

Menomune®—A/C/Y/W-135, Meningococcal Polysaccharide Vaccine, Groups A, C, Y and W-135 Combined, for subcutaneous use, is a freeze-dried preparation of the group-specific polysaccharide antigens from *Neisseria meningitidis*, Group A, Group C, Group Y and Group W-135. *N. meningitidis* are cultivated with Mueller Hinton agar[1] and Watson Scherp[2] media. The purified polysaccharide is extracted from the *Neisseria meningitidis* cells and separated from the media by procedures which include centrifugation, detergent precipitation, alcohol precipitation, solvent or organic extraction and diafiltration. No preservative is added during manufacture.

The 0.78 mL vial of diluent contains sterile, preservative-free, pyrogen-free distilled water and is used for reconstitution of product supplied in 1 mL vials. The 6 mL vial of diluent contains sterile, pyrogen-free distilled water to which thimerosal (mercury derivative) 1:10,000 is added as a preservative. The 6 mL vial is for reconstitution of product supplied in 10 mL vials. After reconstitution with diluent as indicated on the label, the 0.5 mL dose is formulated to contain 50 µg of "isolated product" from each of Groups A, C, Y and W-135 in an isotonic sodium chloride solution.

Each dose of vaccine also is formulated to contain 2.5 mg to 5 mg of lactose added as a stabilizer.[3] The vaccine when reconstituted is a clear colorless liquid.

Potency is evaluated by measuring the molecular size of each polysaccharide component using a column chromatography method as standardized by the US Food and Drug Administration (FDA) and the World Health Organization (WHO)[4] for Meningococcal Polysaccharide Vaccine.

THIS VACCINE CONFORMS TO THE WORLD HEALTH ORGANIZATION (WHO) REQUIREMENTS.

CLINICAL PHARMACOLOGY

N. meningitidis causes both endemic and epidemic disease, principally meningitis and meningococcemia. As a result of the control of *Haemophilus influenzae* type b infections, *N. meningitidis* has become the leading cause of bacterial meningitis in children and young adults in the United States (US), with an estimated 2,600 cases each year.[5,6] The case-fatality rate is 13% for meningitis disease (defined as the isolation of *N. meningitidis* from cerebrospinal fluid) and 11.5% for persons who have *N. meningitidis* isolated from blood,[5,6] despite therapy with antimicrobial agents (e.g., penicillin) to which US strains remain clinically sensitive.[5] The incidence of meningococcal disease peaks in late winter to early spring. Based on multistate surveillance conducted during 1989 to 1991, serogroup B organisms accounted for 46% of all cases and serogroup C for 45%; serogroups W-135 and Y and strains that could not be serotyped accounted for most of the remaining cases.[5,6] Recent data indicate that the proportion of cases caused by serogroup Y strains is increasing.[5] In 1995, among the 30 states reporting supplemental data on culture-confirmed cases of meningococcal disease, serogroup Y accounted for 21% of cases.[7] Because of the success of *H. influenzae* type b vaccinations, the median age of persons with bacterial meningitis increased from 15 months in 1986 to 25 years in 1995.[8] The predominate organism causing meningitis in children 2 to 18 years of age is *N. meningitidis* based on 1995 surveillance data.[8] Serogroup A, which rarely causes disease in the US, is the most common cause of epidemics in Africa and Asia. A statewide serogroup B epidemic has been reported in the US.[9] Within the US, a vaccine for serogroup B is not yet available.

Outbreaks of serogroup C meningococcal disease (SCMD) have been occurring more frequently in the US since the early 1990s, and the use of vaccine to control these outbreaks has increased.[5] During 1980–1993, 21 outbreaks of SCMD were identified; eight of these occurred during 1992–1993.[10] Each of these 21 outbreaks involved from three to 45 cases of SCMD, and most outbreaks had attack rates exceeding 10 cases per 100,000 population, which is approximately 20 times higher than rates of endemic SCMD.[5] During 1981–1988, only 7,600 doses of meningococcal vaccine were used to control four outbreaks; whereas, from January 1992 through June 1993, 180,000 doses of vaccine were used in response to eight outbreaks.[5]

Several discoveries impacted the future of meningococcal polysaccharide vaccines and demonstrated the significance of anti-capsular antibodies in protection.[11] In the late 1930s, serogroup-specific antigens of meningococcal serogroups A and C were identified as polysaccharides.[9] During the mid 1940s, investigators demonstrated that the protection of mice by anti-serogroup A meningococcal horse serum was directly related to its content of anti-polysaccharide antibodies.[11] Meningococcal polysaccharide vaccines were first demonstrated to be immunogenic in humans by Gotschlich and his co-workers in the 1960s when immunization of US Army recruits with serogroup A and C polysaccharides induced protective antibodies.[11] The investigators recorded a significantly reduced acquisition rate of serogroup C carriage among vaccinated recruits compared with unvaccinated individuals.[11]

Persons who have certain medical conditions are at increased risk for developing meningococcal infection. Meningococcal disease is particularly common among persons who have component deficiencies in the terminal common complement pathway (C3, C5–C9); many of these persons experience multiple episodes of infection.[5] Asplenic persons also may be at increased risk for acquiring meningococcal disease with particularly severe infections.[5] Persons who have other diseases associated with immunosuppression (e.g., human immunodeficiency virus [HIV] and *Streptococcus pneumoniae*) may be at higher risk for developing meningococcal disease and for disease caused by some other encapsulated bacteria.[5] Evidence suggests that HIV-infected persons are not at substantially increased risk for epidemic serogroup A meningococcal disease;[5] however, such patients may be at increased risk for sporadic meningococcal disease or disease caused by other meningococcal serogroups.[5] Previously, military recruits had high rates of meningococcal disease, particularly serogroup C disease; however, since the initiation of routine vaccination of recruits with bivalent A/C meningococcal vaccine in 1971, the high rates of meningococcal disease caused by those serogroups have decreased substantially and cases occur infrequently.[5]

A retrospective, epidemiological study was conducted in Maryland to compare the incidence of invasive meningococcal infection in college students with that of the general population of the same age. For the years 1992 to 1997, the incidence of meningococcal infection in Maryland college students was similar to the incidence of the general Maryland population of the same age. However, college students residing on-campus appeared to be at higher risk than those residing off campus.[12]

Vaccine efficacy. The immunogenicity and clinical efficacy of serogroups A and C meningococcal vaccines have been well established.[5] The serogroup A polysaccharide induces antibody in some children as young as 3 months of age, although a response comparable with that among adults is not achieved until 4 or 5 years of age; the serogroup C component is poorly immunogenic in recipients who are less than 18 to 24 months of age.[5] The serogroups A and C vaccines have demonstrated estimated clinical efficacies of 85% to 100% in older children and adults and are useful in controlling epidemics.[5] Serogroups Y and W-135 polysaccharides are safe and immunogenic in adults and in children greater than 2 years of age.[5] Although clinical protection

Continued on next page

Menomune-A/C/Y/W-135—Cont.

has not been documented, vaccination with these polysaccharides induces bactericidal antibody. The antibody responses to each of the four polysaccharides in the quadrivalent vaccine are serogroup-specific and independent.[5]

Efficacy of serogroup A meningococcal vaccines was demonstrated in the 1970s in Africa and Finland. Egyptian school children aged 6 to 15 years showed 90% or greater protection during the first year after immunization with two different molecular sizes of serogroup A polysaccharide.[11] The higher molecular weight vaccine provided protection for at least three years.[11] In Finland, a randomized controlled mass immunization trial with serogroup A vaccine was conducted in response to a serogroup A epidemic. Results indicated 90 to 100% protection for three years.[11] In Rwanda, vaccination with bivalent A/C polysaccharide vaccine was performed in response to a serogroup A epidemic. A complete cessation of meningococcal disease was observed within two weeks of vaccination, yet the serogroup A carrier rate remained unchanged.[11]

Efficacy of serogroup C meningococcal vaccines was demonstrated in a field trial involving 20,000 troops in the US Army. Results suggested 90% efficacy under epidemic conditions which existed in basic training centers.[13] In Brazil, young children were vaccinated with serogroup C polysaccharide in response to a serogroup C epidemic. Results indicated that the vaccine was not effective in children under 24 months of age and only 52% effective in children aged 24 to 36 months.[11] However, studies suggested that the vaccine used in this trial was less immunogenic than other batches of similar vaccine that were used in US children; also, it was shown that the molecular size of the vaccine was smaller than the serogroup C polysaccharide in the present vaccine.[13] Thus, it is quite probable that the current serogroup C polysaccharide vaccine is more effective.[11]

A study performed using 4 lots of Menomune®—A/C/Y/W-135 in 150 adults showed at least a 4-fold increase in bactericidal antibodies to all groups in greater than 90 percent of the subjects.[14,15]

A study was conducted in 73 children 2 to 12 years of age. Post-immunization sera were not obtained on four children; seroconversion rates were calculated on 69 paired samples. Seroconversion rates as measured by bactericidal antibody were: Group A—72%, Group C—58%, Group Y—90% and Group W-135—82%. Seroconversion rates as measured by a 2-fold rise in antibody titers based on Solid Phase Radioimmunoassay were: Group A—99%, Group C—99%, Group Y—97% and Group W-135—89%.[16]

Duration of efficacy. Measurable levels of antibodies against the group A and C polysaccharides decrease markedly during the first 3 years following a single dose of vaccine.[5] This decrease in antibody occurs more rapidly in infants and young children than in adults. Similarly, although vaccine-induced clinical protection probably persists in schoolchildren and adults for at least 3 years, the efficacy of the group A vaccine in young children may decrease markedly with the passage of time. In a 3-year study, efficacy declined from greater than 90% to less than 10% among children who were less than 4 years of age at the time of vaccination, whereas among children who were greater than or equal to 4 years of age when vaccinated, efficacy was 67% 3 years later.[5,17] In a New Zealand study, children 2 to 13 years of age received a single dose of monovalent group A vaccine, 26% of children 3 to 23 months of age in this study received two doses of the vaccine, given approximately 3 months apart. After 2-1/2 years of active surveillance (1987 to 1989) there were no cases of invasive group A disease in children vaccinated at 2 years of age and older.[18]

INDICATIONS AND USAGE

Meningococcal Polysaccharide Vaccine, Groups A, C, Y and W-135 Combined, is indicated for active immunization against invasive meningococcal disease caused by these serogroups.[5]

Meningococcal Polyscaccharide Vaccine, Groups A, C, Y and W-135 Combined may be used to prevent and control outbreaks of serogroup C meningococcal disease.[5]

For evaluation and management of suspected outbreaks, it is recommended that the health-care workers consult the MMWR for guidance.[5]

Routine vaccination is recommended for the following high-risk groups:[5]

1. Deficiencies in late Complement components (C3, C5-C9).
2. Functional or actual asplenia.
3. Persons with laboratory or industrial exposure to *N. meningitidis* aerosols.
4. Travelers to, and residents of, hyperendemic areas such as sub-Saharan Africa. For information concerning geographic areas for which vaccination is recommended, contact CDC at 404-332-4559.

The American College Health Association (ACHA) also recommends that college students consider vaccination to reduce the risk for potentially fatal meningococcal disease.[19]

Vaccinations also should be considered for household or institutional contacts of persons with meningococcal disease and for medical and laboratory personnel at risk of exposure to meningococcal disease.

This vaccine will not stimulate protection against infections caused by organisms other than Groups A, C, Y and W-135 meningococci.

Protective antibody levels may be achieved within 7 to 10 days after vaccination.[5]

Menomune®—A/C/Y/W-135 vaccine is not to be used for treatment of actual infection.

Menomune®—A/C/Y/W-135 vaccine will not protect against other etiologic agents, including *N. meningitidis* serogroup B, that cause meningitis.

Menomune®—A/C/Y/W-135 vaccine is not indicated for infants and children younger than 2 years of age except as short-term protection of infants 3 months and older against Group A.[11]

As with any vaccine, vaccination with Menomune®—A/C/Y/W-135 may not protect 100% of susceptible individuals.

For persons remaining at high-risk, especially children who were first vaccinated at < 4 years of age, revaccination may be indicated.[5] (See **DOSAGE AND ADMINISTRATION** section.)

CONTRAINDICATIONS

Immunization should be deferred during the course of any acute illness.

IT IS A CONTRAINDICATION TO ADMINISTER MENOMUNE®—A/C/Y/W-135 TO INDIVIDUALS KNOWN TO BE SENSITIVE TO THIMEROSAL OR ANY OTHER COMPONENT OF THE VACCINE. FOR INDIVIDUALS SENSITIVE TO THIMEROSAL, ADMINISTER THE ONE DOSE PACKAGE SIZE AND RECONSTITUTE WITH THE 0.78 ML VIAL OF DILUENT THAT CONTAINS NO PRESERVATIVE.

WARNING

This product contains dry natural latex rubber as follows: The stopper to the vial contains dry natural latex rubber.

If the vaccine is used in persons receiving immunosuppressive therapy, the expected immune response may not be obtained.

Menomune®—A/C/Y/W-135 should NOT be given at the same time as whole-cell pertussis or whole-cell typhoid vaccines due to combined endotoxin content.[20,21]

PRECAUTIONS

GENERAL

Care is to be taken by the health-care provider for the safe and effective use of Menomune®—A/C/Y/W-135.

EPINEPHRINE INJECTION (1:1000) MUST BE IMMEDIATELY AVAILABLE TO COMBAT UNEXPECTED ANAPHYLACTIC OR OTHER ALLERGIC REACTIONS.

Prior to an injection of any vaccine, all known precautions should be taken to prevent adverse reactions. This includes a review of the patient's history with respect to possible sensitivity to the vaccine or similar vaccines and to possible sensitivity to dry natural latex rubber.

Special care should be taken to avoid injecting the vaccine intradermally, intramuscularly, or intravenously since clinical studies have not been done to establish safety and efficacy of the vaccine using these routes of administration.

Health-care providers should obtain the previous immunization history of the vaccinee, and inquire about the current health status of the vaccinee.

A separate, sterile syringe and needle or a sterile disposable unit should be used for each patient to prevent transmission of hepatitis and other infectious agents from person to person. Needles should not be recapped and should be disposed of according to biohazard waste guidelines.

INFORMATION FOR PATIENT

Patients, parents or guardians should be fully informed of the benefits and risks of immunization with Menomune®—A/C/Y/W-135.

Patients, parents or guardians should be instructed to report any serious adverse reactions to their health-care provider.

As part of the patient's immunization record, the date, lot number and manufacturer of the vaccine administered should be recorded.[22,23,24]

DRUG INTERACTIONS

If Menomune®—A/C/Y/W-135 is administered to immunosuppressed persons or persons receiving immunosuppressive therapy, an adequate immunologic response may not be obtained.

CARCINOGENESIS, MUTAGENESIS, IMPAIRMENT OF FERTILITY

Menomune®—A/C/Y/W-135 has not been evaluated in animals for its carcinogenic, mutagenic potentials or impairment of fertility.

PREGNANCY

REPRODUCTIVE STUDIES—PREGNANCY CATEGORY C

Animal reproduction studies have not been conducted with Meningococcal Polysaccharide Vaccine, Groups A, C, Y and W-135. It is also not known whether Meningococcal Polysaccharide Vaccine, Groups A, C, Y and W-135 can cause fetal harm when administered to a pregnant woman or can affect reproduction capacity. Meningococcal Polysaccharide Vaccine, Groups A, C, Y and W-135 should be given to a pregnant woman only if clearly needed.

Although there is limited data, studies to date have found no evidence of teratogenicity of the polysaccharide quadrivalent meningococcal vaccine when given to pregnant women.[25]

NURSING MOTHERS

It is not known whether this drug is excreted in human milk. Because many drugs are excreted in human milk, caution should be exercised when Menomune®-A/C/Y/W-135 is administered to a nursing woman.

PEDIATRIC USE

SAFETY AND EFFECTIVENESS OF MENOMUNE®—A/C/Y/W-135 IN CHILDREN BELOW THE AGE OF 2 YEARS HAVE NOT BEEN ESTABLISHED.

ADVERSE REACTIONS

Adverse reactions to meningococcal vaccine are mild and consist principally of pain and redness at the injection site for 1 to 2 days. Pain at the site of injection is the most commonly reported adverse reaction, and a transient fever might develop in less than or equal to 2% of young children.[5]

Adverse events reported by 150 adults following vaccination with Menomune®—A/C/Y/W-135 are shown in Table 1.[14] The subjects were observed for three weeks following vaccination. Local reactions resolved within 48 hours and no significant systemic reactions were reported.[14]

[See table 1 below]

In a clinical study involving 73 children 2 to 12 years of age, who received Menomune®—A/C/Y/W-135, local reactions consisting of erythema or tenderness were seen in approximately 40% of the children.[15] In another clinical study involving 53 children 4 to 6 years of age, who received Menomune®—A/C/Y/W-135, erythema was seen in 89% of the children, swelling in 92% and tenderness in 64%. None of these reactions were considered serious or necessitated medical intervention.[26]

On rare occasions, IgA nephropathy has occurred following vaccination with Menomune®—A/C/Y/W-135. However, a cause and effect relationship has not been established.[16]

Menomune®—A/C/Y/W-135 should NOT be given at the same time as whole-cell pertussis or whole-cell typhoid vaccines due to combined endotoxin content.[20,21]

As with the administration of any vaccine, vaccine components can cause hypersensitivity reactions in some recipients.

Reporting of Adverse Events

The National Vaccine Injury Compensation Program, established by the National Childhood Vaccine Injury Act of 1986, requires physicians and other health-care providers who administer vaccines to maintain permanent vaccination records and to report occurrences of certain adverse events to the US Department of Health and Human Services. Reportable events include those listed in the Act for each vaccine and events specified in the package insert as contraindications to further doses of that vaccine.[22,23,24]

Reporting by patients, parents or guardians of all adverse events occurring after vaccine administration should be encouraged. Adverse events following immunization with vaccine should be reported by the health-care provider to the US Department of Health and Human Services (DHHS) Vaccine Adverse Event Reporting System (VAERS). Reporting forms and information about reporting requirements or completion of the form can be obtained from VAERS through a toll-free number 1-800-822-7967.[24]

Health-care providers also should report these events to the Director of Scientific and Medical Affairs, Aventis Pasteur Inc., Discovery Drive, Swiftwater, PA 18370 or call 1-800-822-2463.

DOSAGE AND ADMINISTRATION

Parenteral drug products should be inspected visually for extraneous particulate matter and/or discoloration prior to administration whenever solution and container permit. If either of these conditions exist, the vaccine should not be administered.

Reconstitute the vaccine using only the diluent supplied for this purpose. Draw the volume of diluent shown on the diluent label into a suitable size syringe and inject into the vial containing the vaccine. Shake vial until the vaccine is dissolved.

The immunizing dose is a single injection of 0.5 mL administered **subcutaneously.**

TABLE 1[14] ADVERSE EVENTS (%) FOLLOWING VACCINATION OF 150 ADULTS WITH MENOMUNE®—A/C/Y/W-135

REACTIONS	MILD	MODERATE
Local		
Pain	2.6	2.0
Tenderness	36.0	9.0
Diameter	<2 in.	≥ 2 in.
Erythema	3.8	1.2
Induration	4.4	1.2
Systemic		
Headaches	5.2	1.8
Malaise	2.5	0
Chills	2.5	0
Oral Temperature (°F)	2.6 (100–101)	0.6 (>101)

Special care should be taken to avoid injecting the vaccine intradermally, intramuscularly, or intravenously since clinical studies have not been done to establish safety and efficacy of the vaccine using these routes of administration.

Primary Immunization

For both adults and children, vaccine is administered subcutaneously as a single 0.5 mL dose. Protective antibody levels may be achieved within 7 to 10 days after vaccination.[5]

REVACCINATION

Revaccination of a single 0.5 mL dose administered subcutaneously may be indicated for individuals at high-risk of infection, particularly children who were first vaccinated when they were less than 4 years of age; such children should be considered for revaccination after 2 or 3 years if they remain at high-risk. Although the need for revaccination in older children and adults has not been determined, antibody levels decline rapidly over 2 to 3 years, and if indications still exist for immunization, revaccination may be considered within 3 to 5 years.[5,18]

Simultaneous administration of Menomune®—A/C/Y/W-135 can be given concurrently with other vaccines at separate sites and separate syringes.[27] However, due to the combined endotoxin content, the vaccine should NOT be administered at the same time as whole-cell pertussis or whole-cell typhoid vaccines.[20,21] (See **WARNINGS** section.)

HOW SUPPLIED

Vial, 1 Dose, with 0.78 mL vial of diluent (contains NO preservative). Product No. 49281-489-01

Vial, 1 Dose (5 per package) with 0.78 mL vial of diluent (5 per package) (contains NO preservative). Product No. 49281-489-05

Vial, 10 Dose, with 6 mL vial of diluent (contains preservative), for administration with needle and syringe (NOT to be used with jet injector). Product No. 49281-489-91

STORAGE

Store freeze-dried vaccine and reconstituted vaccine, when not in use, between 2°–8°C (35°–46°F). Discard remainder of multidose vials of vaccine within 5 days after reconstitution. The single dose vial should be used within 30 minutes after reconstitution.

REFERENCES

1. Mueller, H, et al. A protein-free medium for primary isolation of the gonococcus and meningococcus. Proc Soc Exp Biol Med 48: 330, 1941
2. Watson, RG, et al. The specific hapten of group C (group IIa) meningococcus. II. Chemical nature. J Immunol. 81: 337, 1958
3. Tiesjema, RH, et al: Enhanced stability of meningococcal polysaccharide vaccines by using lactose as a menstruum for lyophilization. Bull WHO 55: 43–48, 1977
4. WHO Technical Report Series, No. 658, 1981
5. Recommendation of the Advisory Committee on Immunization Practices (ACIP). Control and prevention of meningococcal disease and control and prevention of serogroup C meningococcal disease: evaluation and management of suspected outbreaks. MMWR 46: No. RR-5, 1997
6. CDC. Laboratory-based surveillance for meningococcal disease in selected areas—United States, 1989–1991. MMWR 42: No SS-2, 1993
7. CDC. Serogroup Y Meningococcal Disease—Illinois, Connecticut, and Selected Areas, United States, 1989–1996. MMWR 46: Vol. 45, 1010–1013, 1996
8. Schuchat, A, et al. Bacterial Meningitis in the United States in 1995. N Eng J Med 337: 970–976, 1997
9. CDC. Serogroup B meningococcal disease—Oregon 1994. MMWR 44: 121–124, 1995
10. Jackson, LA, et al. Serogroup C meningococcal outbreaks in the United States: an emerging threat. JAMA 273: 383–389, 1995
11. Frasch, CE. Meningococcal vaccines; past, present and future, in Meningococcal Disease, ed. K. Cartwright. John Wiley and Sons Ltd, 1995
12. Harrison LH, et al. Risk of meningococcal infection in college students. JAMA 281: 1906–1910, 1999
13. Lepow, ML. Meningococcal vaccines, in Vaccines, ed. SA Plotkin and EA Mortimer. WB Saunders Co., 1994
14. Hankins, WA, et al: Clinical and serological evaluation of a Meningococcal Polysaccharide Vaccine Groups A, C, Y and W-135. Proc Soc Exper Biol Med 169: 54–57, 1982
15. Lepow, ML, et al: Reactogenicity and immunogenicity of a quadrivalent combined meningococcal polysaccharide vaccine in children. J Infect Dis 154: 1033–1036, 1986
16. Unpublished data available from Aventis Pasteur Inc.
17. Reingold, AL, et al: Age-specific differences in duration of clinical protection after vaccination with meningococcal polysaccharide A vaccine. Lancet. No. 8447: 114–118, 1985
18. Lennon, D, et al: Successful intervention in a Group A meningococcal outbreak in Auckland, New Zealand. Pediatr Infect Dis J 11: 617–623, 1992
19. Collins, MJ, et al. Student Health Centers urged to alert students to danger of the disease and provide campus vaccination programs. American College Health Association (ACHA), Baltimore, MD, Press Release 1997
20. Kuronen, T, et al. Adverse reactions and endotoxin content of polysaccharide vaccines. Develop Biol Standard, Vol. 34: 117–125, 1977
21. Peltola, H., et al. Meningococcus group A vaccine in children three months to five years of age: adverse reactions and immunogenicity related to endotoxin content and molecular weight of the polysaccharide. J Pediatr Vol 92: No 5, 818–822, 1978
22. CDC. National Childhood Vaccine Injury Act: requirements for permanent vaccination records and for reporting of selected events after vaccination. MMWR 37: 197–200, 1988
23. Food and Drug Administration. New reporting requirements for vaccine adverse events. FDA Drug Bull 18 (2), 16–18, 1988
24. CDC. Vaccine Adverse Event Reporting System—United States. MMWR 39: 730–733, 1990
25. Letson, GW, et al. Meningococcal vaccine in pregnancy: an assessment of infant risk. Pediatr Infect Dis J 17(3), 261–263, 1998
26. Scheifele, DW, et al. Local adverse effects of meningococcal vaccine. Can Med Assoc J 150: 14–15, 1994
27. American Academy of Pediatrics, Meningococcal infections. In: Peter G, ed. 1997 Red Book: Report of the Committee on Infectious Diseases. 24th ed. Elk Grove Village, IL: American Academy of Pediatrics; 361, 1997

Product information
as of August 1999

Manufactured by:
Aventis Pasteur Inc.
Swiftwater PA 18370 USA

4050/4051

TETANUS AND DIPHTHERIA ℞

TOXOIDS ADSORBED FOR ADULT USE

Rx only

Caution: Federal (USA) law prohibits dispensing without prescription.

DESCRIPTION

Tetanus and Diphtheria Toxoids Adsorbed for Adult Use, for intramuscular use, is a sterile suspension of alum-precipitated (aluminum potassium sulfate) toxoid in an isotonic sodium chloride solution containing sodium phosphate buffer to control pH. The vaccine, after shaking, is a turbid liquid, whitish-gray in color.

Clostridium tetani culture is grown in a peptone-based medium. *Corynebacterium diphtheriae* culture is grown in a modified Mueller and Miller medium.[1] Both toxins are detoxified with formaldehyde. The detoxified materials are then separately purified by serial ammonium sulfate fractionation and diafiltration. Thimerosal (a mercury derivative) 1:10,000 is added as a preservative.

Each 0.5 mL dose is formulated to contain 5 Lf of tetanus toxoid, 2 Lf of diphtheria toxoid, and not more than 0.28 mg of aluminum by assay. The tetanus and diphtheria toxoids induce as least 2 units and 0.5 units of antitoxin per mL, respectively, in the guinea pig potency test.

CLINICAL PHARMACOLOGY

TETANUS

Tetanus is an intoxication manifested primarily by neuromuscular dysfunction caused by a potent exotoxin elaborated by *Clostridium tetani*.

The occurrence of tetanus in the United States (US) has decreased dramatically from 560 reported cases in 1947 to a record low of 48 reported cases in 1987. Tetanus in the US is primarily a disease of older adults. Of 99 tetanus patients with complete information reported to the Centers for Disease Control and Prevention (CDC) during 1987 and 1988, 68% were ≥ 50 years of age, while only six were < 20 years of age. Overall, the case-fatality rate was 21%. The age distribution of recent cases and the results of serosurveys indicate that many US adults are not protected against tetanus. Serosurveys undertaken since 1977 indicate that 6% to 11% of adults 18 to 39 years of age and 49% to 66% of those ≥ 60 years of age may lack protective levels of circulating tetanus antitoxin.[2] In 1992, 45 cases were reported of which 82% were ≥ 50 years of age.[3] The disease continues to occur almost exclusively among persons who are unvaccinated or inadequately vaccinated or whose vaccination histories are unknown or uncertain.[2]

In 4% of tetanus cases reported during 1987 and 1988, no wound or other condition was implicated. Non-acute skin lesions, such as ulcers, or medical conditions such as abscesses, were reported in association with 14% of cases.[2]

Neonatal tetanus occurs among infants born under unhygienic conditions to inadequately vaccinated mothers. Vaccinated mothers confer protection to their infants through transplacental transfer of maternal antibody. From 1972 through 1984, 29 cases of neonatal tetanus were reported in the US. No cases of neonatal tetanus were reported in the period 1985 to 1989.[2]

Spores of *C. tetani* are ubiquitous. Serologic tests indicate that naturally acquired immunity to tetanus toxin does not occur in the US.[2] Thus, universal primary vaccination, with subsequent maintenance of adequate antitoxin levels by means of appropriately timed boosters, is necessary to protect persons among all age-groups. Tetanus toxoid is a highly effective antigen, and a completed primary series generally induces protective levels of neutralizing antibodies to tetanus toxin that persists for ≥ 10 years.[2]

DIPHTHERIA

Corynebacterium diphtheriae may cause both localized and generalized disease. The systemic intoxication is caused by diphtheria exotoxin, an extracellular protein metabolite of toxigenic strains of *C. diphtheriae*. Protection against disease is due to the development of neutralizing antibodies to diphtheria toxin.

At one time, diphtheria was common in the US. More than 200,000 cases, primarily among young children, were reported in 1921. Approximately 5% to 10% of cases were fatal; the highest case-fatality ratios were recorded for the very young and the elderly. Reported cases of diphtheria of all types declined from 306 in 1975 to 59 in 1979; most were cutaneous diphtheria reported from a single state. After 1979, cutaneous diphtheria was no longer a notifiable disease. From 1980 to 1989, only 24 cases of respiratory diphtheria were reported; two cases were fatal, and 18 (75%) occurred among persons 20 years of age or older.[2]

Diphtheria is currently a rare disease in the US primarily because of the high level of appropriate vaccination among children (97% of children entering school have received ≥ three doses of diphtheria and tetanus toxoids and pertussis vaccine adsorbed [DTP]) and because of an apparent reduction in the prevalence of toxigenic strains of *C. diphtheriae*. Most cases occur among unvaccinated or inadequately vaccinated persons.[2]

Both toxigenic and nontoxigenic strains of *C. diphtheriae* can cause disease, but only strains that produce toxin cause myocarditis and neuritis. Toxigenic strains are more often associated with severe or fatal illness in noncutaneous (respiratory or other mucosal surface) infections and are more commonly recovered in association with respiratory than from cutaneous infections.[2]

A complete vaccination series substantially reduces the risk of developing diphtheria, and vaccinated persons who develop disease have milder illness. Protection lasts at least 10 years. Vaccination does not, however, eliminate carriage of *C. diphtheriae* in the pharynx or nose or on the skin.[2]

The potency of tetanus and diphtheria toxoids was determined on the basis of immunogenicity studies, with a comparison to a serological correlate of protection (0.01 antitoxin units/mL) established by the Panel on Review of Bacterial Vaccines & Toxoids.[4]

A clinical study to evaluate the serological responses and adverse reactions was performed in 58 individuals 6 years of age and older. The results indicated protective levels of antibody were achieved in greater than 90% of the study population after primary immunization with both components. Booster effects were achieved in 100% of the individuals with pre-existing antibody responses.[5]

INDICATIONS AND USAGE

Tetanus and Diphtheria Toxoids Adsorbed for Adult Use (Td) is indicated for active immunization of children 7 years of age or older, and adults, against tetanus and diphtheria. Td is the preparation of choice for vaccination of all persons 7 years of age or older because side effects from higher doses of diphtheria toxoid are more common in this group than they are among younger children. Diphtheria and Tetanus Toxoids Adsorbed (For Pediatric Use) (DT) is indicated for active immunization of children up to age 7 years against diphtheria and tetanus.[2]

The Advisory Committee on Immunization Practices (ACIP) recommends the following: *A previously unvaccinated pregnant woman whose child might be born under unhygienic circumstances (without sterile technique) should receive two doses of Td 4 to 8 weeks apart before delivery, preferably during the last two trimesters. Pregnant woman in similar circumstances who have not had a complete vaccination series should complete the three-dose series. Those vaccinated more than 10 years previously should have a booster dose. No evidence exists to indicate that tetanus and diphtheria toxoids administered during pregnancy are teratogenic.*[2] (See **PREGNANCY** section)

This vaccine is not to be used for the treatment of tetanus or diphtheria infection.

This vaccine should not be used for immunizing children below 7 years of age. In children below 7 years of age, either Diphtheria and Tetanus Toxoids and Acellular Pertussis Vaccine Adsorbed (DTaP)—Tripedia®, or Diphtheria and Tetanus Toxoids and Pertussis Vaccine Adsorbed USP (For Pediatric Use) (DTP) is recommended. If a contraindication to pertussis immunization exists, the recommended vaccine is Diphtheria and Tetanus Toxoids Adsorbed (For Pediatric Use) (DT).[2]

As with any vaccine, vaccination with Td may not protect 100% of susceptible individuals.

If passive immunization is required, Tetanus Immune Globulin (Human) (TIG) and/or equine Diphtheria Antitoxin are the products of choice for tetanus and diphtheria, respectively (see **DRUG INTERACTIONS** and **DOSAGE AND ADMINISTRATION** sections).

CONTRAINDICATIONS

HYPERSENSITIVITY TO ANY COMPONENT OF THE VACCINE, INCLUDING THIMEROSAL, A MERCURY DERIVATIVE, IS A CONTRAINDICATION FOR FURTHER USE OF THIS VACCINE.

It is a contraindication to use this or any other related vaccine after a serious adverse reaction temporally associated with a previous dose including an anaphylactic reaction.

A history of systemic allergic or neurologic reactions following a previous dose of Td is an *absolute contraindication* for further use.[2]

If a contraindication to using tetanus toxoid-containing preparations exists in a person who has not completed a pri-

Continued on next page

Tetanus and Diphtheria—Cont.

mary immunizing course of tetanus toxoid and other than a clean, minor wound is sustained, *only* passive immunization should be given using TIG (Human).[2]

Immunization should be deferred during the course of an acute illness. Vaccination of persons with severe, febrile illness should generally be deferred until these persons have recovered. However, the presence of minor illnesses such as mild upper respiratory infections with or without fever should not preclude vaccination.[2]

Elective immunization procedures should be deferred during an outbreak of poliomyelitis.[6]

WARNINGS

This product contains dry natural latex rubber as follows: The stopper to the vial contains dry natural latex rubber. In the case of the syringe, the needle cover and plunger contain dry natural latex rubber.

Persons who experienced Arthus-type hypersensitivity reactions or a temperature of > 103°F (> 39.4°C) following a prior dose of tetanus toxoid usually have high serum tetanus antitoxin levels and should not be given even emergency doses of Td more frequently than every 10 years, even if they have a wound that is neither clean nor minor.[2]

Intramuscular injections should be given with great care in patients suffering from thrombocytopenia or other coagulation disorders.[2]

A routine booster should not be given more frequently than every ten years. (This guideline should not preclude wound management considerations.)

Deaths have been reported in temporal association with the administration of Td vaccine; however, no causal relationship was proven[7] (see **ADVERSE REACTIONS** section).

PRECAUTIONS

GENERAL

Care is to be taken by the health-care provider for the safe and effective use of Td.

EPINEPHRINE INJECTION (1:1000) MUST BE IMMEDIATELY AVAILABLE SHOULD AN ACUTE ANAPHYLACTIC REACTION OCCUR DUE TO ANY COMPONENT OF THE VACCINE.

There is an increased incidence of local and systemic reactions to booster doses of tetanus toxoid when given to previously immunized persons. (Refer to **DOSAGE AND ADMINISTRATION** section for timing of recall injections).

Prior to an injection of any vaccine, all known precautions should be taken to prevent adverse reactions. This should include review of the patient's history with respect to possible sensitivity and any previous adverse reactions (see **CONTRAINDICATIONS** section) to the vaccine or similar vaccine, to possible sensitivity to dry natural latex rubber, and a current knowledge of the literature concerning the use of the vaccine under consideration.

Special care should be taken to ensure that the injection does not enter a blood vessel.

Immunosuppressive therapies including radiation, corticosteroids, antimetabolites, alkylating agents, and cytotoxic drugs may reduce the immune response to vaccines. Therefore, routine vaccination should be deferred, if possible, while patients are receiving such therapy.[2] If Td has been administered to persons receiving immunosuppressive therapy, or having an immunodeficiency disorder, an adequate antibody response may not be obtained.[2] When possible, immunosuppressive treatment should be interrupted when immunization is required due to a tetanus-prone wound.

Administration of Td is not contraindicated in individuals with HIV infection.[8]

It is advisable to use Td (For Adult Use—7 years of age and older) in wound prophylaxis instead of tetanus toxoid alone in order to maintain adequate levels of diphtheria immunity.[2]

A separate, sterile syringe and needle or a sterile disposable unit must be used for each patient to prevent transmission of hepatitis or other infectious agents from person to person. Needles should not be recapped and should be disposed of according to biohazard waste guidelines.

INFORMATION FOR PATIENTS

Prior to administration of Td, health-care personnel should inform the parent, guardian or adult patient the benefits and risks of immunization, and also inquire about the recent health status of the patient to be injected.

As part of the child's or adult's permanent immunization record, the date, lot number and manufacturer of the vaccine administered MUST be recorded.[9,10,11]

The health-care provider should inform the parent, guardian or adult patient about the potential for adverse reactions that have been temporally associated with Td administration. The parent, guardian or adult patient should be instructed to report any serious adverse reactions to their health-care provider.

IT IS EXTREMELY IMPORTANT WHEN THE PARENT GUARDIAN OR ADULT PATIENT RETURNS FOR THE NEXT DOSE IN THE SERIES, THE PARENT, GUARDIAN, OR ADULT PATIENT SHOULD BE QUESTIONED CONCERNING OCCURRENCE OF ANY SYMPTOMS AND/OR SIGNS OF AN ADVERSE REACTION AFTER THE PREVIOUS DOSE (SEE **CONTRAINDICATIONS; ADVERSE REACTIONS** SECTIONS).

The health-care provider should inform the parent, guardian or adult patient of the importance of completing the immunization series.

Table 1[2] SUMMARY GUIDE TO TETANUS PROPHYLAXIS IN ROUTINE WOUND MANAGEMENT, 1991*

History of Adsorbed Tetanus Toxoid (doses)	Clean, Minor Wounds		All Other Wounds**	
	Td	TIG	Td	TIG
Unknown or < three	Yes	No	Yes	Yes
≥ Three	No†	No	No§	No

* Important details are in the text of the insert.
** Such as, but not limited to, wounds contaminated with dirt, feces, soil, and saliva; puncture wounds; avulsions; and wounds resulting from missiles, crushing, burns, and frostbite.
† Yes, if > 10 years since last dose.
§ Yes, if > 5 years since last dose. (More frequent boosters are not needed and can accentuate side effects.)

The health-care provider should provide the Vaccine Information Materials (VIMs) which are required to be given with each immunization.

DRUG INTERACTIONS

If passive immunization for tetanus is needed, TIG (Human) is the product of choice for tetanus. It provides longer protection than antitoxin of animal origin and causes few adverse reactions. The currently recommended prophylactic dose of TIG (Human) for wounds of average severity is 250 units intramuscularly. When tetanus toxoid and TIG (Human) are given concurrently, separate syringes and different sites should be used. The ACIP recommends the use of only adsorbed toxoid in this situation.[2]

Diphtheria Antitoxin (equine) is available for treatment of the acute phases of diphtheria. When Td and Diphtheria Antitoxin are used together, they must be given at different sites using separate needles and syringes.

As with other intramuscular injections, use with caution in patients on anticoagulant therapy.

Immunosuppressive therapies may reduce the response to vaccines (see **PRECAUTIONS**—GENERAL section).

CARCINOGENESIS, MUTAGENESIS, IMPAIRMENT OF FERTILITY

No studies have been performed to evaluate carcinogenicity, mutagenic potential, or impact on fertility.

PREGNANCY

REPRODUCTIVE STUDIES—PREGNANCY CATEGORY C

Animal reproduction studies have not been conducted with Tetanus and Diphtheria Toxoids Adsorbed For Adult Use vaccine. It is also not known whether Tetanus and Diphtheria Toxoids Adsorbed For Adult Use vaccine can cause fetal harm when administered to a pregnant woman or can affect reproduction capacity. Tetanus and Diphtheria Toxoids Adsorbed For Adult Use vaccine should be given to a pregnant woman only if clearly needed.

Adequate immunization by routine boosters in non-pregnant women of child-bearing age can obviate the need to vaccinate women during pregnancy (see **DOSAGE AND ADMINISTRATION** section).

Physicians generally avoid prescribing unnecessary drugs and biologics for pregnant women.

However, the ACIP recommends, the following: *A previously unvaccinated pregnant woman whose child might be born under unhygienic circumstances (without sterile technique) should receive two doses of Td 4 to 8 weeks apart before delivery, preferably during the last two trimesters. Pregnant women in similar circumstances who have not had a complete vaccination series should complete the three-dose series. Those vaccinated more than 10 years previously should have a booster dose. No evidence exists to indicate that tetanus and diphtheria toxoids administered during pregnancy are teratogenic.*[2]

It has been reported that tetanus toxoid administered to pregnant women prevents neonatal tetanus in newborns.[12,13] However, the data reported on the safety of tetanus toxoid when so used is inconclusive because the incidence of neonatal deaths in New Guinea was significantly higher than in the United States.[12] A prospective study in the United States has not been done to confirm these reports.

PEDIATRIC USE

SAFETY AND EFFECTIVENESS OF TETANUS AND DIPHTHERIA TOXOIDS ADSORBED FOR ADULT USE VACCINE BELOW 7 YEARS OF AGE HAVE NOT BEEN ESTABLISHED.

In children below 7 years of age, either Diphtheria and Tetanus Toxoids and Acellular Pertussis Vaccine Adsorbed (DTaP)—Tripedia®, or Diphtheria and Tetanus Toxoids and Pertussis Vaccine Adsorbed USP (For Pediatric Use) (DTP) is recommended. If a contraindication to pertussis immunization exists, the recommended vaccine is Diphtheria and Tetanus Toxoids Adsorbed (For Pediatric Use) (DT).[2]

ADVERSE REACTIONS

BODY SYSTEM AS A WHOLE

Adverse reactions may be local and include redness, warmth, edema, induration with or without tenderness as well as urticaria, and rash. Malaise, transient fever, pain hypotension, nausea and arthralgia may develop in some patients after the injection. Arthus-type hypersensitivity reactions, characterized by severe local reactions (generally starting 2 to 8 hours after an injection) may occur, particularly in persons who have received multiple prior boosters.[2]

Rarely, an anaphylactic reaction (i.e., hives, swelling of the mouth, difficulty breathing, hypotension, or shock) and death have been reported after receiving preparations containing tetanus and diphtheria antigens.[2]

In a clinical study involving 58 individuals 6 years of age and older, 19% of the individuals noted local reactions consisting of erythema, tenderness, and induration at the injection site and 2% systemic reactions consisting of headache, malaise and temperature elevations.[5]

Deaths have been reported in temporal association with the administration of tetanus toxoid containing vaccines. On rare occasions, anaphylaxis has been reported following administration of products containing tetanus toxoid. Upon review, a report by the Institute of Medicine (IOM) concluded the evidence established a causal relationship between tetanus toxoid and anaphylaxis.[7]

NERVOUS SYSTEM

The following neurologic illnesses have been reported as temporally associated with vaccines containing tetanus toxoid: neurological complications[14] including cochlear lesion,[15] brachial plexus neuropathies,[14,16] paralysis of the radial nerve,[17] paralysis of the recurrent nerve,[15] accommodation paresis, Guillain-Barré syndrome (GBS), and EEG disturbances with encephalopathy. The IOM following review of the reports of neurologic events following vaccination with tetanus toxoid, Td or DT, concluded the evidence favored acceptance of a causal relationship between tetanus toxoid and brachial neuritis and GBS.[7,18]

CARDIOVASCULAR SYSTEM

Acute anaphylatic reactions may occur rarely following administration of tetanus and diphtheria antigens which may cause acute hives and cardiovascular collapse.

Adverse reactions to diphtheria toxoid in adults are minimized by the small amount of the antigen (not more than 2 Lf units per dose), contained in Td.[19–23]

EPINEPHRINE INJECTION (1:1000) MUST BE IMMEDIATELY AVAILABLE SHOULD AN ACUTE ANAPHYLACTIC REACTION OCCUR DUE TO ANY COMPONENT OF THE VACCINE.

Reporting of Adverse Events

The National Vaccine Injury Compensation Program, established by the National Childhood Vaccine Injury Act of 1986, requires physicians and other health-care providers who administer vaccines to maintain permanent vaccination records and to report occurrences of certain adverse events to the US Department of Health and Human Services. Reportable events include those listed in the Act for each vaccine and events specified in the package insert as contraindications to further doses of the vaccine.[9,10,11]

Reporting by parents, guardians or adult patients of all adverse events occurring after vaccine administration should be encouraged. Patients experiencing adverse events following immunization who require a visit to a health-care provider should be reported by health-care providers to the US Department of Health and Human Services (DHHS) Vaccine Adverse Event Reporting System (VAERS). Reporting forms and information about reporting requirements or completion of the form can be obtained from VAERS through a toll-free number 1-800-822-7967.[9,10,11]

Health-care providers also should report these events to Director of Scientific and Medical Affairs, Aventis Pasteur Inc., Discovery Drive, Swiftwater, PA 18370 or call 1-800-822-2463.

DOSAGE AND ADMINISTRATION

Parenteral drug products should be inspected visually for extraneous particulate matter and/or discoloration prior to administration whenever solution and container permit. If these conditions exist, the vaccine should not be administered.

SHAKE VIAL WELL *before withdrawing each dose*. Discard vial if it cannot be resuspended.

Inject 0.5 mL intramuscularly in the area of the vastus lateralis (mid-thigh laterally) or deltoid. The vaccine should not be injected into the gluteal area or areas where there may be a major nerve trunk.

The following guidelines are derived from the Advisory Committee on Immunization Practices (ACIP).[2]

Primary Immunization for Children over 7 Years of Age and Adults:

A series of three doses of 0.5 mL each of Td should be given intramuscularly; the second dose of 0.5 mL is given 4 to 8 weeks after the first dose; and the third dose of 0.5 mL is given 6 to 12 months after the second dose. Td is the agent of choice for immunization of all individuals 7 years of age and older, because side effects from higher doses of diphtheria toxoid are more common in older children and adults.

Children who remain incompletely immunized after their seventh birthday should be counted as having prior exposure to tetanus and diphtheria toxoids (e.g., a child who previously received two doses of DTP needs only one dose of Td to complete the primary series for tetanus and diphtheria).

Interruption of the recommended schedule with a delay between doses does not interfere with the final immunity achieved with Td. There is no need to start the series over again, regardless of the time elapsed between doses.

Routine Recall Injections:

To maintain adequate protection a booster dose of 0.5 mL every 10 years thereafter is recommended.

Recall Injection After Injury:

A thorough attempt must be made to determine whether a patient has completed primary immunization. Patients with unknown or uncertain previous immunization histories should be considered to have no previous tetanus toxoid doses. Persons who had military service since 1941 can be considered to have received at least one dose. Although most people in the military since 1941 may have completed a primary series of tetanus toxoid, this cannot be assumed for each individual. Patients who have not completed a primary series may require tetanus toxoid and passive immunization at the time of wound cleaning and debridement (Table 1).[2]

Available evidence indicates that complete primary vaccination with tetanus toxoid provides long-lasting protection ≥ 10 years for most recipients. Consequently, after complete primary tetanus vaccination, boosters, even for wound management, need to be given only every 10 years when wounds are minor and uncontaminated. For other wounds, a booster is appropriate if the patient has not received tetanus toxoid within the preceding five years. Persons who have received at least two doses of tetanus toxoid rapidly develop antitoxin antibodies.[2]

Td is the preferred preparation for active tetanus immunization in wound management of patients ≥ 7 years of age. Because a large proportion of adults are susceptible, this plan enhances diphtheria protection. Thus, by taking advantage of acute health-care visits, such as for wound management, some patients can be protected who otherwise would remain susceptible. For inadequately vaccinated patients of all ages, completion of primary vaccination at the time of discharge or at follow-up visits should be ensured.[2]

[See table 1 at top of previous page]

If passive immunization for tetanus is needed, TIG (Human) is the product of choice. It provides longer protection than antitoxin of animal origin and causes few adverse reactions. The currently recommended prophylactic dose of TIG (Human) for wounds of average severity is 250 units intramuscularly. When tetanus toxoid and TIG (Human) are given concurrently, separate syringes and separate sites should be used. The ACIP recommends the use of only adsorbed toxoid in this situation.[2]

HOW SUPPLIED

Syringe, 0.5 mL (10 × 0.5 mL syringes per package)—Product No. 49281-271-10

Vial, 5 mL—Product No. 49281-271-83

STORAGE

Store between 2°–8°C (35°–46°F). DO NOT FREEZE.

1. Mueller JH, et al. Production of diphtheria toxin of high potency (100 Lf) on a reproducible medium. J Immunol 40:21–32, 1941
2. Recommendations of the Immunization Practices Advisory Committee (ACIP). Diphtheria, Tetanus, and Pertussis: Recommendations for vaccine use and other preventive measures. MMWR 40: No. RR-10, 1991
3. Centers for Disease Control and Prevention (CDC). Summary of Notifiable Disease, United States 1992. MMWR 41: No. 55, 1993
4. Department of Health and Human Services, Food and Drug Administration. Biologicals Products; Bacterial Vaccines and Toxoids; Implementation of Efficacy Review; Proposed Rule. Federal Register Vol 50 No 240, pp 51002–51117, 1985
5. Myers MG, et al. Primary immunization with tetanus and diphtheria toxoids. JAMA 248:2478–2480, 1982
6. Wilson GS. The Hazards of Immunization. Provocation poliomyelitis. 270–274, 1967
7. Stratton KR, et al. *Adverse events associated with childhood vaccines. Evidence Bearing on Causality*. National Academy Press, Washington, DC, 1994
8. ACIP. General recommendations on immunization. MMWR 38: 205–207, 1989
9. CDC. Vaccine Adverse Event Reporting System—United States. MMWR 39: 730–733, 1990
10. CDC. National Childhood Vaccine Injury Act: requirements for permanent vaccination records and for reporting of selected events after vaccination. MMWR 37: 197–200, 1988
11. Food and Drug Administration. New reporting requirements for vaccine adverse events. FDA Drug Bull 18 (2), 16–18, 1988
12. MacLennan R, et al. Immunization against neonatal tetanus in New Guinea. Antitoxin response of pregnant women to adjuvant and plain toxoids. Bull WHO 32: 683–697, 1965
13. Newell KW, et al. The use of toxoid for the prevention of tetanus neonatorium. Bull WHO 35: 863–871, 1966
14. Rutledge SL, et al. Neurological complications of immunizations. J Pediatr 109: 917–924, 1986
15. Wilson GS. The Hazards of Immunization. Allergic manifestations: Post-vaccinal neuritis. pp 153–156, 1967
16. Tsairis P, et al. Natural history of brachial plexus neuropathy. Arch Neurol 27:109–117, 1972.
17. Blumstein GI, et al. Peripheral neuropathy following Tetanus toxoid administration. JAMA 198: 1030–1031, 1966
18. Pollard JD, et al. Relapsing neuropathy due to tetanus toxoid: report of a case. J Neurol Sci 37: 113–125, 1978
19. Edsall G, et al. Combined tetanus-diphtheria immunization of adults: Use of small doses of diphtheria toxoid. Am J Public Health 44: 1537–1545, 1954
20. Scheibel L, et al. Immunization of adults against diphtheria. Acta Pathol Microbiol Scand 27: 69–77, 1950
21. Sellers AH, et al. The use of a combined antigen-TABTD. Can J Public Health 41: 141, 1950
22. Ipsen J Jr. Immunization of adults against diphtheria and tetanus. N Engl J Med 251: 459–466, 1954
23. Middaugh JP. Side effects of diphtheria-tetanus toxoid in adults. Am J Public Health 69:246–249, 1979

Product information
as of June 1996

Manufactured by:
Aventis Pasteur Inc.
Swiftwater PA 18370 USA

4152/4153

TRIHIBIT® ℞

ActHIB® Haemophilus b Conjugate Vaccine (Tetanus Toxoid Conjugate) reconstituted with Tripedia® Diphtheria and Tetanus Toxoids and Acellular Pertussis Vaccine Adsorbed.

See package inserts for Acthib® and Tripedia®

TRIPEDIA® ℞

Diphtheria and Tetanus Toxoids and Acellular Pertussis Vaccine Adsorbed

Rx only

CAUTION: Federal (USA) law prohibits dispensing without prescription.

DESCRIPTION

Tripedia®, Diphtheria and Tetanus Toxoids and Acellular Pertussis Vaccine Adsorbed (DTaP), for intramuscular use, is a sterile preparation of diphtheria and tetanus toxoids adsorbed, with acellular pertussis vaccine in an isotonic sodium chloride solution containing thimerosal as a preservative and sodium phosphate to control pH. After shaking, the vaccine is a homogeneous white suspension. Tripedia® vaccine is distributed by Aventis Pasteur Inc. (AvP).

The acellular pertussis vaccine components are isolated from culture fluids of Phase 1 *Bordetella pertussis* grown in a modified Stainer-Scholte medium.[1] After purification by salt precipitation, ultracentrifugation, and ultrafiltration, preparations containing varying amounts of both pertussis toxin (PT) and filamentous hemagglutinin (FHA) are combined to obtain a 1:1 ratio and treated with formaldehyde to inactivate PT. Thimerosal (mercury derivative) 1:10,000 is added as a preservative.

Corynebacterium diphtheriae cultures are grown in a modified Mueller and Miller medium.[2] *Clostridium tetani* cultures are grown in a peptone-based medium. Both toxins are detoxified with formaldehyde. The detoxified materials are then separately purified by serial ammonium sulfate fractionation and diafiltration.

The toxoids are adsorbed using aluminum potassium sulfate (alum). The adsorbed diphtheria and tetanus toxoids are combined with acellular pertussis concentrate, and diluted to a final volume using sterile phosphate-buffered physiological saline. Thimerosal (mercury derivative) 1:10,000 is added as a preservative. Each 0.5 mL dose contains, by assay, not more than 0.170 mg of aluminum and not more than 100 µg (0.02%) of residual formaldehyde. The vaccine contains gelatin and polysorbate 80 (Tween-80) which are used in the production of the pertussis concentrate.

Each 0.5 mL dose is formulated to contain 6.7 Lf of diphtheria toxoid and 5 Lf of tetanus toxoid (both toxoids induce at least 2 units of antitoxin per mL in the guinea pig potency test), and 46.8 µg of pertussis antigens. This is represented in the final vaccine as approximately 23.4 µg of inactivated PT (also referred to as lymphocytosis promoting factor or LPF) and 23.4 µg of FHA. The inactivated acellular pertussis component contributes not more than 50 endotoxin units (EU) to the endotoxin content of 1 mL of DTaP. The potency of the pertussis components is evaluated by measuring the antibody response to PT and FHA in immunized mice using an ELISA system.

Acellular Pertussis Vaccine Concentrates (For Further Manufacturing Use) are produced by The Research Foundation for Microbial Diseases of Osaka University (BIKEN), Osaka, Japan under United States (US) license, and are combined with diphtheria and tetanus toxoids manufactured by AvP. The Tripedia® vaccine is filled, labeled, packaged, and released by AvP.

TriHIBit®, when Tripedia® vaccine is used to reconstitute ActHIB® **for the fourth dose only**, each single dose of combined vaccine (0.5 mL) is formulated to contain 6.7 Lf of diphtheria toxoid, 5 Lf of tetanus toxoid (both toxoids induce at least 2 units of antitoxin per mL in the guinea pig potency test), 46.8 µg of pertussis antigens (approximately 23.4 µg of inactivated PT and 23.4 µg of FHA), 10 µg of purified *Haemophilus influenzae* type b capsular polysaccharide conjugated to 24 µg of inactivated tetanus toxoid, and 8.5% sucrose.

CLINICAL PHARMACOLOGY

Simultaneous immunization against diphtheria, tetanus, and pertussis, using a conventional "whole-cell" pertussis DTP vaccine (Diphtheria and Tetanus Toxoids and Pertussis Vaccine Adsorbed—For Pediatric Use), has been a routine practice during infancy and childhood in the US since the late 1940s. This practice has played a major role in markedly reducing the incidence rates of cases and deaths from each of these diseases.[3]

Tripedia® vaccine combines AvP's diphtheria and tetanus toxoids with purified pertussis antigens (inactivated PT and FHA). These pertussis antigens have been used routinely for childhood vaccination in Japan since 1981[4,5,6,7] and have been used for investigational purposes in Sweden,[1,8,9,10,11] as well as in the US and Germany.[1,12,13,14,15] In the US, since 1992, Tripedia® vaccine has been indicated for immunization of children 15 months to 7 years of age (prior to the seventh birthday) who have previously been immunized with three or four doses of whole-cell pertussis DTP.

DIPHTHERIA

Corynebacterium diphtheriae may cause both localized and generalized disease. The systemic intoxication is caused by diphtheria exotoxin, an extracellular protein metabolite of toxigenic strains of *C. diphtheriae*. Protection against disease is due to the development of neutralizing antibody to diphtheria toxin.

Both toxigenic and nontoxigenic strains of *C. diphtheriae* can cause disease, but only strains that produce diphtheria toxin cause severe manifestations, such as myocarditis and neuritis. Diphtheria remains a serious disease, with the highest case-fatality rates among infants and the elderly.[3]

At one time, diphtheria was common in the US. More than 200,000 cases, primarily among children, were reported in 1921. Approximately 5% to 10% of cases were fatal; the highest case-fatality rates were in the very young and the elderly. Reported cases of diphtheria of all types declined from 306 in 1975 to 59 in 1979; most were cutaneous diphtheria reported from a single state. After 1979, cutaneous diphtheria was no longer reportable.[3] From 1980 to 1989, only 24 cases of respiratory diphtheria were reported in the US; 2 cases were fatal and 18 (75%) occurred among persons ≥20 years of age.[3] From 1990 through 1994, 15 cases were reported.[16]

Diphtheria is currently a rare disease in the US primarily because of the high level of appropriate vaccination among children (97% of children entering school have received three doses of diphtheria and tetanus toxoids and pertussis vaccine adsorbed [DTP]) and because of an apparent reduction in the circulation of toxigenic strains of *C. diphtheriae*.[3]

Most cases occur among unvaccinated or inadequately vaccinated persons.[3] Diphtheria remains a serious disease in some areas of the world as evidenced by the recent outbreak in the former Soviet Union.[17]

Complete immunization significantly reduces the risk of developing diphtheria, and immunized persons who develop disease have milder illness. Protection is thought to last at least 10 years. Immunization does not, however, eliminate carriage of *C. diphtheriae* in the pharynx, nose or on the skin.[3]

Efficacy of AvP's diphtheria toxoid used in Tripedia® vaccine was determined on the basis of immunogenicity studies, with a comparison to a serological correlate of protection (0.01 antitoxin units/mL) established by the Panel on Review of Bacterial Vaccines & Toxoids.[18]

TETANUS

Tetanus is an intoxication manifested primarily by neuromuscular dysfunction caused by a potent exotoxin elaborated by *Clostridium tetani*.

The occurrence of tetanus in the US has decreased dramatically from 560 reported cases in 1947 to an average of 57 cases reported annually from 1985-1994.[16] Tetanus in the US is primarily a disease of older adults. Of 99 tetanus patients with complete information reported to the Centers for Disease Control and Prevention (CDC) during 1987 and 1988, 68% were ≥ 50 years of age, while only six were < 20 years of age. Overall, the case-fatality rate was 21%. The disease continues to occur almost exclusively among persons who are unvaccinated or inadequately vaccinated or whose vaccination histories are unknown or uncertain.[3]

In 4% of tetanus cases reported during 1987 and 1988, no wound or other condition was implicated. Non-acute skin lesions, such as ulcers, or medical conditions, such as abscesses, were reported in 14% of cases.[3]

Spores of *C. tetani* are ubiquitous. Serological tests indicate that naturally acquired immunity to tetanus toxin does not occur in the US. Thus, universal primary immunization, with subsequent maintenance of adequate antitoxin levels by means of appropriately timed boosters, is necessary to protect all age groups. Tetanus toxoid is a highly effective antigen, and a completed primary series generally induces protective levels of serum antitoxin that persist for 10 or more years.[3]

Efficacy of AvP's tetanus toxoid used in Tripedia® vaccine was determined on the basis of immunogenicity studies, with a comparison to a serological correlate of protection (0.01 antitoxin units/mL) established by the Panel on Review of Bacterial Vaccines & Toxoids.[18]

PERTUSSIS

Since pertussis became a nationally reportable disease in 1922, the highest number of pertussis cases (approximately 266,000) was reported in 1934. Following the licensure of

Continued on next page

Tripedia—Cont.

whole-cell pertussis DTP vaccine in 1949 and the widespread use of DTP among infants and children, the incidence of reported pertussis declined to a historical low of 1,010 cases in 1976. However, since the early 1980s, reported pertussis incidence has increased with cyclical peaks occurring in 1983, 1986, 1990, and 1993. Following the peak in reported cases in 1993, the number declined during 1994 and the first 2 quarters of 1995, a pattern consistent with the previously observed 3–4 year periodicity in pertussis incidence. National pertussis surveillance data for January 1992-December 1994 during which an average of 5,095 cases were reported annually, demonstrate the continued effectiveness of the current pertussis vaccination program.[19]
Pertussis (whooping cough) is a disease of the respiratory tract caused by *Bordetella pertussis*. This gram-negative coccobacillus produces a variety of biologically active components. The role of the different components produced by *B pertussis* in either the pathogenesis of, or the immunity to, pertussis is not well understood. However, efficacy has been demonstrated for this vaccine that contained both inactivated PT and FHA.
Pertussis is highly communicable (attack rates of > 90% have been reported among unvaccinated household contacts[20]) and can cause severe disease, particularly among very young children. Of 10,749 patients < 1 year of age reported nationally as having pertussis during the period 1980 to 1989, 69% were hospitalized, 22% had pneumonia, 3.0% had one or more seizures, 0.9% had encephalopathy, and 0.6% died.[21]
In older children and adults, including some who were previously immunized, infection may result in nonspecific symptoms of bronchitis or an upper respiratory tract infection, and pertussis may not be diagnosed because classic signs, especially the inspiratory whoop, may be absent. Older preschool-aged children and school-aged siblings who are not fully immunized and develop pertussis may be important sources of infection for young infants, the group at highest risk of clinical disease and severe pertussis.[3] The infected adult may play a role in the transmission of pertussis.[22,23]
General use of whole-cell pertussis DTP vaccines has resulted in a substantial reduction in cases and deaths from pertussis disease.[20,24] The use of Tripedia® vaccine as a primary series evokes an antibody response with respect to PT and FHA and has been shown to be effective in clinical studies.[1]
Acellular pertussis vaccines have been used in Japan since 1981, mostly in 2-year-old children. Evidence for the efficacy of these vaccines, as a group, is demonstrated by the decline in pertussis disease with their routine use in that country.[4,20] In addition, a review of epidemiological studies of the Japanese acellular pertussis vaccines estimated that these vaccines, as a group, were 88% efficacious in protecting against clinical pertussis on household exposure, with a 95% confidence interval (CI) of 79% to 93%.[25]
Two clinical studies were conducted to assess the protective efficacy of these acellular pertussis components of Tripedia® vaccine. A randomized, controlled clinical trial in Sweden assessed efficacy after only two doses of the pertussis component in children 5 to 11 months of age.[10] A second study was conducted in Germany using a three-dose schedule to evaluate the protective efficacy of the Tripedia® vaccine in younger infants.
In 1986-1987, a double-blind, randomized, placebo-controlled efficacy trial of two BIKEN acellular pertussis vaccines was conducted in Sweden. One of the vaccines was a two-component vaccine comparable to the acellular pertussis components contained in Tripedia® vaccine. This prospective trial used a standardized case definition and active case ascertainment. In this trial, 1,389 children, 5 to 11 months of age (median 8.5 months), received two doses of the acellular pertussis vaccine 7 to 13 weeks apart and 954 received a placebo control. During the 15 months of follow-up from 30 days after the second dose, culture-confirmed whooping cough (cough of any duration and a positive culture of *B pertussis*) occurred in 40 placebo and 18 acellular pertussis vaccine recipients. The point estimate of protective efficacy for two doses of vaccine was 69% (95% CI; 47% to 82%) for all cases of culture-confirmed pertussis with any cough 1 day or longer and 79% (95% CI; 57% to 90%) using a secondary case definition of culture-confirmed cases with cough of over 30 days duration.[10] In a reanalysis of the Swedish data efficacy estimates increased with duration of coughing spasms and when the case definition included whoops and whoops plus at least nine coughing spasms a day.[26] Using a case definition of cough of 21 days or more of coughing spasms, confirmed by positive culture resulted in an efficacy estimate of 81% (95% CI; 61% to 90%).[26]
Using a passive reporting system, three-year unblinded follow-up of vaccine and placebo recipients from the above Swedish study has shown a post-trial efficacy of 77% (95% CI; 65% to 85%) for all culture-proven cases of pertussis, and an efficacy of 92% (95% CI; 84% to 96%) for culture-proven cases with a cough of over 30 days duration.[27]
A case-control study to evaluate the efficacy of Tripedia® vaccine was conducted in Germany. The study population consisted of patients in 63 pediatric practices who had no contraindications to pertussis immunization and were enrolled in the study between the ages of 6 and 17 weeks (actual range of age at first visit was up to 20 weeks for the DT group). By parental choice, infants received Tripedia® vaccine or whole-cell pertussis DTP (Behringwerke, Germany) at approximately 3, 5, and 7 months of age, or DT, or no vaccine. Cases of pertussis were identified by obtaining cultures for *B pertussis* from all patients between the ages of 2 and 24 months who presented to the physician's office with 7 or more days of cough. Identification of presumptive cases of pertussis was made by primary care physicians who were not blinded to the vaccine status of subjects. Cases were confirmed by positive culture in the subject or positive culture in a subject's household contact. Duration of cough in study subjects was determined at an office visit, by telephone, or by home visit 21–24 days after the onset of cough. Four aged-matched controls were selected for each case from the same pediatric practice. Selection of controls was done without knowledge of vaccination status. The vaccine (or no vaccine) and number of doses which each case and control subjects received subsequently was determined from medical records.
In order to adjust for potentially confounding variables, information on sex, race, day-care attendance, well-baby visits, sick-child visits, pertussis vaccination status of siblings, age of siblings, number of siblings, day-care attendance of siblings, and parental employment status was obtained through interview of parents. Information on erythromycin use was not obtained for the study population.
A total of 16,780 infants were enrolled in the study, of whom 74.6% received Tripedia® vaccine and 10.9%, 12.5%, and 2.1% received DTP, DT, or no vaccine, respectively, by nonrandom parental choice. A total of 11,017 cultures for *B pertussis* was obtained and 140 cases were identified using a primary case definition of cough ≥ 21 days, plus positive culture for *B pertussis* or household contact with a person with culture-positive pertussis. Of the 140 cases, 130 cases were diagnosed on the basis of a positive culture and 10 on the basis of household contact with a culture-positive case. For the 140 cases, 543 controls were selected. Of the 140 cases, 29 (20.7%) received three doses of DTaP, 5 (3.6%) received two doses of DTaP, 44 (31.4%) received two or three doses of DT vaccine, 44 (31.4%) received one dose of either DTaP, whole-cell pertussis DTP or DT, and 18 (13%) received no vaccine. Of the 543 controls, 175 (32.2%) received three doses of DTaP, 67 (12.3%) received two doses of DTaP, 45 (8.3%) received two or three doses of whole-cell pertussis DTP, 73 (13.4%) received DT vaccine, 153 (28.2%) received one dose of either DT, DTP, or DTaP, and 30 (5.5%) received no vaccine. Adjusting for sibling age, sibling pertussis immunization by age group, siblings in day care, number of siblings in day care, and father's employment status, the vaccine efficacy of three doses of Tripedia® vaccine compared to two or three doses of DT was 80% (95% CI; 59% to 90%).[1]
In a clinical study conducted in 65 US and 89 German infants, a single lot of Tripedia® vaccine was administered at 2, 4 and 6 months of age for the purpose of comparing immune responses to PT and FHA. This study showed that US and German infants, who received three doses of Tripedia® vaccine, expressed similar antibody responses to these antigens. The percentage of infants demonstrating a four-fold or greater antibody response, was also similar for PT and FHA in both groups.[1]
In a clinical study, US infants received Tripedia®, ActHIB®, OPV, and hepatitis B vaccines simultaneously. In one of the study groups, Tripedia®, ActHIB® and OPV were administered at 2, 4, and 6 months of age and hepatitis B was given at 2 and 4 months of age. One hundred percent of the 69 children who received ActHIB® simultaneously with Tripedia® vaccine demonstrated anti-PRP antibodies ≥1 µg/mL. Sera from a subset of 12 infants who received hepatitis B simultaneously at 2 and 4 months of age showed that 93% had anti-HBs titers of > 10 mIU/mL. Sera from a subset of 20 infants who received OPV simultaneously at 2, 4, and 6 months of age showed that 100% had protective neutralizing antibody responses to all three polio virus types.

TRIPEDIA® COMBINED WITH ActHIB®, TriHIBit®, BY RECONSTITUTION

Clinical studies examined the immune response in 15- to 20-month-old children when Tripedia® vaccine was used to reconstitute one lyophilized single dose vial of ActHIB® (TriHIBit®). All children received three doses of Haemophilus b Conjugate Vaccine (ActHIB® or HibTITER®) and three doses of whole-cell DTP at approximately 2, 4, and 6 months of age. Table 1 shows the diphtheria, tetanus and pertussis responses when Tripedia® vaccine was used to reconstitute ActHIB® (TriHIBit®) compared to the two vaccines given concomitantly but at different sites. In children who received the vaccines separately or combined, 100% had an antibody response to the PRP component ≥1.0 µg/mL.[1]
[See table 1 below]
In clinical studies evaluating simultaneous administration of Tripedia® and ActHIB® with MMR vaccine to 15- to 20-month-old children, the data suggest that the combination vaccine does not interfere with the immunogenicity of the MMR vaccine. Overall seroconversion rates in children who received ActHIB® reconstituted with Tripedia® (TriHIBit®) vaccine were 98% (46/47), 98% (42/43) and 96% (43/45) for measles, mumps and rubella, respectively.

INDICATIONS AND USAGE

Tripedia® vaccine is indicated for active immunization against diphtheria, tetanus and pertussis (whooping cough) simultaneously in infants and children 6 weeks to 7 years of age (prior to seventh birthday). Because of the substantial risks of complications of the disease, completion of a primary series of pertussis vaccine early in life is strongly recommended.[3] However, in instances where the pertussis vaccine component is contraindicated, Diphtheria and Tetanus Toxoids Adsorbed (For Pediatric Use) (DT) should be used for each of the remaining doses. (See **CONTRAINDICATIONS** section.)
When Tripedia® vaccine is used to reconstitute ActHIB® (TriHIBit®), the combined vaccines are indicated for the active immunization of children 15 to 18 months of age who have previously been immunized against diphtheria, tetanus and pertussis with three doses consisting of either whole-cell pertussis DTP or acellular pertussis vaccine and three or fewer doses of ActHIB® (OmniHIB®) within the first year of life for the prevention of invasive diseases caused by *H influenzae* type b and caused by diphtheria, tetanus, and pertussis.[1] ***(Refer to ActHIB® package insert.)***
If passive immunization is required, Tetanus Immune Globulin (Human) (TIG) and/or equine Diphtheria Antitoxin should be used.
Persons who have recovered from culture-confirmed pertussis do not need additional doses of Tripedia® vaccine but should receive additional doses of DT to complete the series.
Tripedia® vaccine is not to be used for treatment of *B. pertussis, C. diphtheriae, or C. tetani* infections.
As with any vaccine, vaccination with Tripedia® vaccine may not protect 100% of susceptible individuals.

CONTRAINDICATIONS

Hypersensitivity to any component of the vaccine, including thimerosal and gelatin, is a contraindication.
It is a contraindication to use this vaccine after an immediate anaphylactic reaction temporally associated with a previous dose. Because of uncertainty as to which component of the vaccine might be responsible, no further vaccination with diphtheria, tetanus, or pertussis components should be carried out. Alternatively, because of the importance of tetanus vaccination, such individuals may be referred for evaluation by an allergist.[3]
Immunization should be deferred during the course of an acute febrile illness. The decision to administer or delay vaccination because of a current or recent febrile illness depends on the severity of symptoms and on the etiology of the disease. All vaccines can be administered to persons with mild illness such as diarrhea, mild upper-respiratory infection with or without low-grade fever, or other low grade febrile illness.[28]
Elective immunization procedures should be deferred during an outbreak of poliomyelitis.[29]
Encephalopathy not due to an identifiable cause, occurring within 7 days of a prior whole-cell pertussis DTP or DTaP immunization and consisting of major alterations of con-

TABLE 1[1] IMMUNE RESPONSES IN 15- TO 20-MONTH-OLD CHILDREN WHEN TRIPEDIA® VACCINE IS COMBINED WITH ActHIB® BY RECONSTITUTION (TriHIBit®) COMPARED TO THE VACCINES ADMINISTERED SEPARATELY

VACCINE GROUP N*	PRE-DOSE TriHIBit® 92–93	 Separate 102–103	POST-DOSE TriHIBit® 93	 Separate 98
Anti-LPF				
GMT (ELISA units/mL)	26.30	24.56	471.00	363.90
% 4-Fold Rise	–	–	87.0	85.7
Anti-LPF				
GMT (CHO CELL)	33.48	31.78	806.70	701.60
% 4-Fold Rise	–	–	92.3	90.6
Anti-FHA				
GMT (ELISA units/mL)	3.83	3.61	44.68	38.81
% 4-Fold Rise	–	–	68.5**	80.6
Diphtheria Antitoxin				
GMT (units/mL)	0.15	0.16	6.31	6.65
> 0.01 u/mL	–	–	100.00	100.00
Tetanus Antitoxin				
GMT (equivalents/mL)	0.05	0.06	1.10	1.15
> 0.01 u/mL	–	–	100.00	100.00

* N = number of children
**The clinical significance of the difference in 4-fold rise of anti-FHA is unknown at present.

sciousness, unresponsiveness, generalized or focal seizures that persist for more than a few hours and failure to recover within 24 hours should be considered a contraindication to further use; this includes severe alterations in consciousness with generalized or focal neurologic signs. Even though causation cannot be established, no subsequent doses of pertussis vaccine should be given.[3]

WARNINGS

This product contains dry natural latex rubber as follows: The stopper to the vial contains dry natural latex rubber.

If any of the following events occurs in temporal relation with the receipt of either whole-cell pertussis DTP or DTaP, the decision to administer subsequent doses of vaccine containing the pertussis component should be carefully considered. Although these events were once considered contraindications to whole-cell pertussis DTP, there may be circumstances, such as high incidence of pertussis, in which the potential benefits outweigh the possible risks, particularly since the following events have not been proven to cause permanent sequelae:[3,30]

1. Temperature of ≥40.5°C (105°F) within 48 hours, not due to another identifiable cause.
2. Collapse or shock-like state (hypotonic-hyporesponsive episode) within 48 hours.
3. Persistent, inconsolable crying lasting ≥3 hours, occurring within 48 hours.
4. Convulsions with or without fever, occurring within 3 days.

A recent clinical study suggests that persistent, inconsolable crying lasting at least 3 hours following vaccination with Tripedia® vaccine may occur less frequently than has been observed historically for DTP vaccine.[1,31]

When a decision is made to withhold the pertussis component, immunization with DT should be continued.

Tripedia® vaccine should not be given to children with any coagulation disorder, including thrombocytopenia, that would contraindicate intramuscular injection unless the potential benefit clearly outweighs the risk of administration.

In the opinion of the manufacturer, seizure disorder in children before or after any immunization with Tripedia® is considered a warning against further immunization with this vaccine. Recent studies suggest that infants and children with a history of convulsions in first-degree family members (i.e., siblings and parents) have a 3.2-fold increased risk for neurologic events compared with those without such histories when given DTP.[25,32] However, the ACIP has concluded that a family history of convulsions in parents and siblings is not a contraindication to pertussis vaccination and that children with such family histories should receive pertussis vaccine according to the recommended schedule.[3,20,28]

In children with a history of febrile or non-febrile convulsions, acetaminophen should be given at the time of Tripedia® vaccination according to acetaminophen package insert recommended dosage to reduce the possibility of post-vaccination fever.[3,20,28]

A committee of the Institute of Medicine (IOM) has concluded that evidence is consistent with a causal relationship between DTP and acute neurologic illness, and under special circumstances, between DTP and chronic neurologic disease in the context of the NCES report.[33,34] However, the IOM committee concluded that the evidence was insufficient to indicate whether or not DTP increased the overall risk of chronic neurologic disease.[34] Acute encephalopathy or permanent neurological injury, have not been reported in temporal association after administration of Tripedia® vaccine but the experience with this vaccine is insufficient to rule this out. (See **ADVERSE REACTIONS** section).

Infants and children with recognized possible or potential underlying neurologic conditions seem to be at enhanced risk for the appearance of manifestations of the underlying neurologic disorder within two or three days following whole-cell pertussis vaccination.[3] Whether to administer Tripedia® vaccine to children with proven or suspected underlying neurologic disorders must be decided on an individual basis. Important considerations include the current local incidence of pertussis.[3]

Tripedia® vaccine should not be combined through reconstitution with any vaccine for administration to infants younger than 15 months of age. Tripedia® vaccine should not be reconstituted with any vaccine other than ActHIB® (OmniHIB®) for children 15 months of age or older.

PRECAUTIONS

GENERAL

Care is to be taken by the health-care provider for the safe and effective use of this vaccine.

EPINEPHRINE INJECTION (1:1000) MUST BE IMMEDIATELY AVAILABLE SHOULD AN ACUTE ANAPHYLACTIC REACTION OCCUR DUE TO ANY COMPONENT OF THE VACCINE.

Prior to an injection of any vaccine, all known precautions should be taken to prevent adverse reactions. This includes a review of the patient's history with respect to possible sensitivity and any previous adverse reactions to the vaccine or similar vaccines, and to possible sensitivity to dry natural latex rubber, previous immunization history, current health status (see **CONTRAINDICATIONS** section), and a current knowledge of the literature concerning the use of the vaccine under consideration. Immunosuppressed patients may not respond. Tripedia® vaccine is not contraindicated in patients with HIV infection.[3]

Special care should be taken to ensure that the injection does not enter a blood vessel.

TABLE 2[1] ADVERSE EVENTS OCCURRING WITHIN 72 HOURS FOLLOWING DIPHTHERIA AND TETANUS TOXOIDS AND ACELLULAR PERTUSSIS VACCINE ADSORBED (TRIPEDIA®) IMMUNIZATIONS GIVEN TO INFANTS 2 TO 6 MONTHS OF AGE

	FREQUENCY					
EVENT	**TRIPEDIA® REACTION %**			**WHOLE-CELL PERTUSSIS DTP REACTION %**		
	Dose 1	Dose 2	Dose 3	Dose 1	Dose 2	Dose 3
No. of Infants†	505	499	490	167	159	152
Local						
Erythema*	9.0	9.8	16.9	28.3	32.9	32.9
Erythema > 1″*	1.2	1.8	2.2	7.8	8.4	7.4
Swelling*	6.4	4.5	6.5	28.3	23.9	27.5
Swelling > 1″*	1.4	0.6	1.0	12.7	11.0	11.4
Tenderness*	11.8	6.7	7.1	50.6	44.2	42.6
Systemic						
Fever > 101°F (rectal)*	0.4	1.6	3.5	3.6	7.5	11.2
Irritability*	35.3	30.1	27.1	72.9	71.8	57.7
Drowsiness*	39.4	17.6	15.9	59.6	45.2	25.5
Anorexia*	6.0	5.3	5.7	26.5	20.0	18.8
Vomiting	6.0**	5.5	3.7	10.8	7.1	2.7
High-pitched cry	2.4	1.0	1.4	10.8	5.8	3.4
Persistent cry	0.2	0.2	0.8	3.0	1.3	2.0

* $p < 0.01$ when compared to whole-cell pertussis DTP for all doses.
** $p < 0.05$ when compared to whole-cell pertussis DTP.
† For certain adverse events information was not available for a small number of infants.

A separate, sterile syringe and needle or a sterile disposable unit should be used for each patient to prevent transmission of hepatitis or other infectious agents from person to person. Needles should not be recapped but should be disposed of properly.

INFORMATION FOR PATIENT

Parents should be fully informed of the benefits and risks of immunization with Tripedia® vaccine.

The physician should inform the parents or guardians about the potential for adverse reactions that have been temporally associated with Tripedia® and other pertussis vaccine administration. The health-care provider should provide the Vaccine Information Materials (VIMs) which are required by the National Childhood Vaccine Injury Act of 1986 to be given with each immunization. Parents or guardians should be instructed to report any serious adverse reactions to their health-care provider.

IT IS EXTREMELY IMPORTANT WHEN A CHILD IS RETURNED FOR THE NEXT DOSE IN THE SERIES THAT THE PARENT SHOULD BE QUESTIONED CONCERNING OCCURRENCE OF ANY SYMPTOMS AND/OR SIGNS OF AN ADVERSE REACTION AFTER THE PREVIOUS DOSE OF THE SAME VACCINE (SEE **CONTRAINDICATIONS** AND **ADVERSE REACTIONS** SECTIONS).

The health-care provider should inform the parent or guardian of the importance of completing the pertussis immunization series, unless a contraindication to further immunization exists.

The US Department of Health and Human Services has established a Vaccine Adverse Event Reporting System (VAERS) to accept all reports of suspected adverse events after the administration of any vaccine, including but not limited to the reporting of events required by the National Childhood Vaccine Injury Act of 1986.[35] The toll-free number for VAERS forms and information is 1-800-822-7967.

The National Vaccine Injury Compensation Program, established by the National Childhood Vaccine Injury Act of 1986, requires physicians and other health-care providers who administer vaccines to maintain permanent vaccination records and to report occurrences of certain adverse events to the US Department of Health and Human Services. Reportable events include those listed in the Act (i.e. those listed in the vaccine injury table) for each vaccine and events specified in the package insert as contraindications to further doses of the vaccine.[36,37]

DRUG INTERACTIONS

As with other IM injections use with caution in patients on anticoagulant therapy.

Immunosuppressive therapies, including irradiation, antimetabolites, alkylating agents, cytotoxic drugs, and corticosteroids (used in greater than physiologic doses), may reduce the immune response to vaccines. Although no specific studies with pertussis vaccine are available, if immunosuppressive therapy will be discontinued shortly, it would be reasonable to defer immunization until the patient has been off therapy for one month; otherwise, the patient should be vaccinated while still on therapy.[3]

For information regarding simultaneous administration with other vaccines refer to **DOSAGE AND ADMINISTRATION** section.

If Tripedia® vaccine has been administered to persons receiving immunosuppressive therapy, a recent injection of immune globulin or having an immunodeficiency disorder, an adequate immunologic response may not be obtained.

Tetanus Immune Globulin, or Diphtheria Antitoxin, if used, should be given in a separate site, with a separate needle and syringe.

The combination of Tripedia® vaccine with other vaccines has not been evaluated for safety and immunogenicity in infants younger than 15 months of age. The combination of Tripedia® vaccine with any vaccine other than ActHIB® (OmniHIB®) has not been evaluated for safety and immunogenicity in infants 15 months of age or older.

CARCINOGENESIS, MUTAGENESIS, IMPAIRMENT OF FERTILITY

Tripedia® vaccine has not been evaluated for its carcinogenic or mutagenic potentials or impairment of fertility.

PREGNANCY

REPRODUCTIVE STUDIES—PREGNANCY CATEGORY C

Animal reproduction studies have not been conducted with Tripedia® vaccine. It is not known whether Tripedia® vaccine can cause fetal harm when administered to a pregnant woman or can affect reproductive capacity. Tripedia® vaccine is NOT recommended for use in a pregnant woman.

PEDIATRIC USE

SAFETY AND EFFECTIVENESS OF TRIPEDIA® VACCINE IN INFANTS BELOW SIX WEEKS OF AGE HAVE NOT BEEN ESTABLISHED. (SEE **DOSAGE AND ADMINISTRATION** SECTION.)

THIS VACCINE IS NOT RECOMMENDED FOR PERSONS 7 YEARS OF AGE AND OLDER. Tetanus and Diphtheria Toxoids Adsorbed For Adult Use (Td) is to be used in individuals 7 years of age or older.

Tripedia® vaccine should **not** be combined through reconstitution with any vaccine for administration to infants younger than 15 months of age. Tripedia® vaccine can only be combined with ActHIB® (OmniHIB®) by reconstitution for children 15 months of age or older.

ADVERSE REACTIONS

A total of 11,400 doses of Tripedia® vaccine has been administered in US clinical trials in children 2 to 6 months, 15 to 20 months of age or 4 to 6 years of age. When compared to CLI's whole-cell pertussis DTP vaccine, Tripedia® vaccine produced fewer local reactions such as erythema, swelling, and tenderness at the injection site and fewer systemic reactions such as fever, irritability, drowsiness, vomiting, anorexia and high-pitched unusual cry.[1] In a double-blind, comparative US trial, 673 infants were randomized to receive either 3 doses of Tripedia® vaccine or CLI's DTP vaccine (Table 2).[1] Safety data are available for 672 infants. Rates for all reported local reactions and other reactions such as fever > 101°F, irritability, drowsiness, and anorexia were significantly less in Tripedia® vaccine recipients. In contrast to whole-cell pertussis DTP, no hypotonic-hyporesponsive episodes occurred in Tripedia® vaccine recipients. Reaction rates generally peaked within the first 24 hours, and decreased substantially over the next two days.[1,14,15]

[See table 2 above]

Adverse event data for Tables 2–6 were actively collected using patient diaries, phone call follow-up and/or by questioning the parent(s) at clinic visits. All data were recorded on standardized case report forms.

A similar reduction in adverse events was seen in a randomized, double-blind, comparative trial conducted in the US by the National Institutes of Health (NIH) when Tripedia® vaccine was compared to Lederle Laboratories whole-cell pertussis DTP vaccine (Table 3).[38] Each data point presented in Table 3 is a summary of the frequency of reactions following any of the three primary immunizing doses. Local adverse reactions which include pain, erythema, swelling, and systemic reactions such as fever, anorexia, vomiting, drowsiness and fussiness may occur following any of the three primary vaccinations.

[See table 3 at top of next page]

The frequency of adverse reactions following each dose in children who received only Tripedia® vaccine is shown in Table 4.[1,38] Of the 135 infants who received Tripedia® vaccine at 2, 4, and 6 months of age, a subset of 82 received a fourth dose of Tripedia® vaccine and a subset of 18 received a fifth dose of Tripedia® vaccine.

[See table 4 on next page]

In an open label US study additional data are available in 15- to 20-month-old children who had previously received

Continued on next page

Tripedia—Cont.

three doses of either Tripedia® vaccine (n = 109) or whole-cell pertussis DTP (n = 30).[39] Reaction rates are presented in Table 5. Data on 738 children (a subset of the German case control study) receiving a fourth dose of Tripedia® vaccine in an open label study showed local and systemic reaction rates in the day following vaccination as follows: erythema (36.7%), erythema > 1 inch (12.5%), swelling (20.2%), pain (14%), temperature ≥ 100.4°F (10.6%), irritability (14.6%), anorexia (8.4%), and persistent crying > 3 hours (0.4%).[1]

[See table 5 at right]

Table 6 lists the frequency of adverse reactions in 372 US children who received Tripedia® vaccine at 15 to 20 months of age and 240 US children who received Tripedia® vaccine at 4 to 6 years of age in a study conducted from 1989-1990. These children had previously received three or four doses of whole-cell pertussis DTP vaccine at approximately 2, 4, 6, and 18 months of age.[1]

[See table 6 on next page]

The results of an open label, non-controlled clinical study, of 2,457 US children and targeted to evaluate less common and more severe adverse events following three doses of Tripedia® vaccine in the primary series are shown in Table 7.[1] Data were collected by parental interview at subsequent immunizations, chart review and telephone calls to the parents 60 days after the third dose.

[See table 7 on next page]

Adverse experiences that are more serious and less common than those reported in Table 7 are not known at this time. In the large German efficacy study that enrolled 16,780 infants, 12,514 of whom received 41,615 doses of Tripedia® vaccine, hospitalization rates and death rates were similar between Tripedia® vaccine and DT recipients.[1] Adverse events were monitored by spontaneous reporting by parents and a medical history obtained at each subsequent vaccination. Adverse events (rates per 1,000 doses) occurring within 7 days including those events interpreted by the investigator as related as well as those interpreted as unrelated to vaccination included; unusual cry (0.96), persistent cry > 3 hours (0.12), febrile seizure (0.05), afebrile seizure (0.02) and hypotonic/hyporesponsive episodes (0.05). In contrast to the first Swedish pertussis efficacy trial conducted in 1986-87,[10] no deaths due to invasive bacterial infections were reported.

Rarely, an anaphylactic reaction (i.e., hives, swelling of the mouth, difficulty breathing, hypotension, or shock) has been reported after receiving preparations containing diphtheria, tetanus, and/or pertussis antigens.[3]

Arthus-type hypersensitivity reactions, characterized by severe local reactions (generally starting 2 to 8 hours after an injection), may follow receipt of tetanus toxoid. A few cases of peripheral neuropathy have been reported following tetanus toxoid administration, although the evidence is inadequate to accept or reject a causal relation.[40]

Whole-cell pertussis DTP has been associated with acute encephalopathy.[33] A 10-year follow-up to the National Childhood Encephalopathy Study (NCES) of children who experienced acute neurologic disorders in infancy concluded that serious acute neurologic illness increased the risk of chronic neurologic disease or death.[41] A committee of the Institute of Medicine (IOM) has concluded that, because DTP may cause acute neurologic illness, DTP may also cause chronic neurologic disease in the context of the NCES report.[34] However the IOM committee concluded that the evidence was insufficient to indicate whether or not DTP increased the overall risk of chronic neurologic disease.[34]

Sudden Infant Death Syndrome (SIDS) has occurred in infants following administration of whole-cell pertussis DTP and DTaP. Large case-control studies of SIDS in the US have shown that receipt of whole-cell pertussis DTP was not causally related to SIDS.[42,43,44] It should be recognized that the first three primary immunizing doses of whole-cell pertussis DTP and DTaP are usually administered to infants 2 to 6 months old and that approximately 85% of SIDS cases occur at ages 1 to 6 months, with the peak incidence occurring at 6 weeks to 4 months of age. By chance alone, some cases of SIDS can be expected to follow receipt of whole-cell pertussis DTP[44] and DTaP. A review by a committee of the IOM concluded that available evidence did not indicate a causal relation between DTP vaccine and SIDS.[33]

Onset of infantile spasms has occurred in infants who have recently received DTP or DT. Analysis of data from the NCES on children with infantile spasms showed that receipt of DT or DTP was not causally related to infantile spasms.[45] The incidence of onset of infantile spasms increases at 3 to 9 months of age, the time period in which the second and third doses of DTP are generally given. Therefore, some cases of infantile spasms can be expected to be related by chance alone to recent receipt of DTP.[3]

A bulging fontanelle associated with increased intracranial pressure which occurred within 24 hours following DTP immunization has been reported, although a causal relationship has not been established.[33,46,47,48]

The above findings regarding possible association of unusual neurologic events and SIDS relate only to DTP vaccine containing whole-cell pertussis. At this time there are insufficient data to determine their relevance to Tripedia® vaccine.

A review by the IOM found a causal relation between tetanus toxoid and brachial neuritis and Guillain-Barré syndrome.[40] The following illnesses have been reported as temporally associated with vaccine containing tetanus toxoid: neurological complications[49,50] including cochlear lesion,[51] brachial plexus neuropathies,[51,52] paralysis of the radial nerve,[53] paralysis of the recurrent nerve,[51] accommodation paresis, and EEG disturbances with encephalopathy.[17] In the differential diagnosis of polyradiculoneuropathies following administration of a vaccine containing tetanus toxoid, tetanus toxoid should be considered as a possible etiology.[54,55]

TABLE 3[38] PERCENT OF INFANTS WHO WERE REPORTED TO HAVE HAD THE INDICATED REACTION BY THE THIRD EVENING AFTER ANY OF THE FIRST THREE DOSES OF WHOLE-CELL PERTUSSIS DTP OR DTaP

	N¶	ERYTHEMA	SWELLING	PAIN†	FEVER* >101°F	ANOREXIA	VOMITING	DROWSINESS	FUSSINESS‡
Tripedia®	135	32.6**	20.0**	9.6**	5.2**	22.2**	7.4	41.5**	19.3**
Whole-Cell Pertussis DTP	371	72.7	60.9	40.2	15.9	35.0	13.7	62.0	41.5

* Rectal Temperatures
** $p < 0.01$ when compared to whole-cell pertussis DTP.
† Moderate or severe = cried or protested to touch or when leg moved.
‡ Moderate or severe = prolonged or persistent crying that could not be comforted and refusal to play.
¶ N = Number of infants

TABLE 4[1,38] ADVERSE EVENTS (%) OCCURRING WITHIN 72 HOURS FOLLOWING EACH DOSE OF DIPHTHERIA AND TETANUS TOXOID AND ACELLULAR PERTUSSIS VACCINE (TRIPEDIA®) VACCINATION IN CHILDREN IN WHICH ALL DOSES WERE TRIPEDIA® VACCINE

EVENT	PRIMARY (N = 135 INFANTS)			BOOSTER (N = 82 CHILDREN)	(N = 18 CHILDREN)
	DOSE 1 2 Months	DOSE 2 4 Months	DOSE 3 6 Months	DOSE 4 15 to 20 Months	DOSE 5 4 to 6 Years
Local					
Erythema	12.6	12.7	19.1	17.1	33.3
Swelling	8.8	8.2	10.7	15.9	27.8
Pain*	8.1	3.7	2.3	7.3	11.1
Systemic					
Fever > 101°F†	0.7	1.4	3.1	2.4	0
Anorexia	8.1	9.7	9.9	8.5	0
Vomiting	5.2	1.5	2.3	2.4	0
Drowsiness	28.9	17.9	4.6	6.1	5.6
Fussiness**	8.1	7.4	7.6	3.7	0

* Moderate or severe = cried or protested to touch or when leg moved.
** Moderate or severe = prolonged or persistent crying that could not be comforted and refusal to play.
† Rectal temperatures for primary series, oral temperatures for Dose 4 and Dose 5.

TABLE 5[1,39] COMPARISON OF ADVERSE EVENTS (%) OCCURRING WITHIN 72 HOURS FOLLOWING VACCINATION WITH TRIPEDIA® VACCINE IN CHILDREN WHO HAD RECEIVED THREE PREVIOUS DOSES OF TRIPEDIA® VACCINE OR THREE DOSES OF WHOLE-CELL PERTUSSIS DTP

	N	ERYTHEMA ≥ INCH	SWELLING ≥ INCH	PAIN	TEMPERATURE ≥ 101°F	IRRITABILITY
Tripedia® Primed	109	30.3	29.4	19.3	5.5	19.3
Whole-Cell pertussis DTP Primed	30	23.3	20.0	10.3	3.3	13.3

In the German case-control study and US open-label safety study in which 14,971 infants received Tripedia® vaccine, 13 deaths in Tripedia® vaccine recipients were reported to study investigators. Causes of deaths included, seven SIDS, and one of each of the following; enteritis, Leigh Syndrome, adrenogenital syndrome, cardiac arrest, motor vehicle accident and accidental drowning. None of these events were determined to be vaccine-related and all occurred more than two weeks past immunization.[1] The rate of SIDS observed in the German case-control study was 0.4/1,000 vaccinated infants. The rate of SIDS observed in the US open-label safety study was 0.8/1,000 vaccinated infants and the reported rate of SIDS in the US from 1985-1991 was 1.5/1,000 live births.[56] By chance alone, some cases of SIDS can be expected to follow receipt of whole-cell pertussis DTP[44] and DTaP.

In the Swedish efficacy trial where 1,419 recipients received the pertussis components in Tripedia® vaccine, three deaths due to invasive bacterial infections occurred. Further investigation revealed no evidence for a causal relation between vaccination and altered resistance to invasive disease caused by encapsulated bacteria.[11] While the hypothesis that the two variables are related cannot be ruled out in the Swedish trial, deaths due to invasive bacterial infections have been monitored in other trials. In contrast to the Swedish trial, in the German case-control study and US open-label safety study, 14,971 infants received Tripedia® vaccine and no deaths due to invasive bacterial infections were reported.

When Tripedia® vaccine was used to reconstitute ActHIB® (TriHIBit®) and administered to children 15 to 20 months of age, the systemic adverse experience profile was comparable to that observed when the two vaccines were given separately. An increase in rates of minor local reactions was observed within the 24-hour period after immunization when compared to the Tripedia® and ActHIB® (OmniHIB®) vaccines administered separately. However, local adverse event rates of the combined vaccines were comparable when taking into consideration reactions observed at the ActHIB® site.[1] ***(Refer to ActHIB® package insert; Table 7.)***

Reporting of Adverse Events

Reporting by parents and patients of all adverse events occurring after vaccine administration should be encouraged. Adverse events following immunization with vaccine should be reported by the health-care provider to the US Department of Health and Human Services (DHHS) Vaccine Adverse Events Reporting System (VAERS). Reporting forms and information about reporting requirements or completion of the form can be obtained from VAERS through a toll-free number 1-800-822-7967.[35,36,37]

The health-care provider also should report these events to the Director of Scientific and Medical Affairs, Aventis Pasteur Inc., Discovery Drive, Swiftwater, PA 18370 or call 1-800-822-2463.

DOSAGE AND ADMINISTRATION

Parenteral drug products should be inspected visually for extraneous particulate matter and/or discoloration prior to administration whenever solution and container permit. If these conditions exist, the vaccine should not be administered.

SHAKE VIAL WELL *before withdrawing each dose.* Inject 0.5 mL of Tripedia® vaccine intramuscularly only. The preferred injection sites are the anterolateral aspect of the thigh and the deltoid muscle of the upper arm. The vaccine should not be injected into the gluteal area or areas where there may be a major nerve trunk.

The primary series for children less than 7 years of age is three intramuscular doses of 0.5 mL. The customary age for the first dose is 2 months of age but may be given as early as 6 weeks of age and up to the seventh birthday.

Before injection, the skin over the site to be injected should be cleansed with a suitable germicide. After insertion of the needle, aspirate to ensure that the needle has not entered a blood vessel.

Fractional doses (doses < 0.5 mL) should not be given. The effect of fractional doses on the frequency of serious adverse events and on efficacy has not been determined.

Do NOT administer this product subcutaneously.

PRIMARY IMMUNIZATION

The primary series consists of three doses administered at intervals of 4 to 8 weeks. It is recommended that Tripedia® vaccine be given for all three doses since no interchangeability data on DTaP vaccines exist for the primary series.

Tripedia® vaccine may be used to complete the primary series in infants who have received one or two doses of whole-cell pertussis DTP. However, the safety and efficacy of Tripedia® vaccine in such infants has not been evaluated.

Tripedia® vaccine should not be combined through reconstitution with any other vaccine for administration to infants younger than 15 months of age. There are insufficient data at this time to support the use of Tripedia® vaccine to reconstitute ActHIB® (TriHIBit®) for primary immunization.

BOOSTER IMMUNIZATION

When Tripedia® vaccine is given for the primary series, a fourth dose is recommended at 15 to 20 months of age. The interval between the third and fourth dose should be at least 6 months. At this time, data are insufficient to establish frequencies of adverse events following a fifth dose of Tripedia® vaccine in children who have previously received 4 doses of Tripedia® vaccine. (See **ADVERSE REACTIONS** section.)

If a child receives whole-cell pertussis DTP for one or more doses, Tripedia® vaccine may be given to complete the five-dose series. A fourth dose is recommended at 15 to 20 months of age. The interval between the third and fourth dose should be at least 6 months. Children four to six years of age (up to the seventh birthday) who received all four doses by the fourth birthday, including one or more doses of whole-cell pertussis DTP, should receive a single dose of Tripedia® vaccine before entering kindergarten or elementary school. This dose is not needed if the fourth dose was given on or after the fourth birthday.

Tripedia® vaccine combined with ActHIB® (TriHIBit®) by reconstitution, may be administered at 15 to 18 months of age for the fourth dose. ***(Refer to ActHIB® package insert.)***

Tripedia® vaccine may be administered according to any of the following schedules for infants and children 6 weeks through 6 years of age (up to the 7th birthday).

Primary series
- Three doses administered at intervals of 4 to 8 weeks, beginning at 6 weeks of age
- To complete the primary series for infants who have received one or two doses of DTP

Booster doses
- As a 4th and/or 5th dose following a primary series of three doses of DTP
- As a 4th dose following a primary series of Tripedia® vaccine*
- As a 4th dose when used to reconstitute ActHIB® (TriHIBit®)**

* Data are insufficient to establish frequencies of adverse events following a fifth dose of Tripedia® vaccine in children who have previously received four doses of Tripedia® vaccine.

** Tripedia® vaccine should not be combined through reconstitution with any other vaccine.

If any recommended dose of pertussis vaccine cannot be given, DT (For Pediatric Use) should be given as needed to complete the series.

PERSONS 7 YEARS OF AGE AND OLDER SHOULD NOT BE IMMUNIZED WITH TRIPEDIA® VACCINE.[28]

Preterm infants should be vaccinated according to their chronological age from birth.[20]

Interruption of the recommended schedule with a delay between doses should not interfere with the final immunity achieved with Tripedia® vaccine. There is no need to start the series over again, regardless of the time between doses.

Routine simultaneous administration of DTaP, OPV (or IPV), Haemophilus b conjugate vaccine, MMR, and hepatitis B vaccine is encouraged for children who are the recommended age to receive these vaccines and for whom no specific contraindications exist at the time of the visit, unless, in the judgment of the provider, complete vaccination of the child will not be compromised by administering different vaccines at different visits. Simultaneous administration is particularly important if the child might not return for subsequent vaccinations (see **CLINICAL PHARMACOLOGY** section).[28]

Data are unavailable to the manufacturer concerning the effects on immune response of IPV when given concurrently with ActHIB® reconstituted with Tripedia® (TriHIBit®).

If passive immunization is needed for tetanus prophylaxis, Tetanus Immune Globulin (Human) (TIG) is the product of choice. It provides longer protection than antitoxin of animal origin and causes few adverse reactions. The currently recommended prophylactic dose of TIG for wounds of average severity is 250 units intramuscularly. When tetanus toxoid and TIG are administered concurrently, separate syringes and separate sites should be used. The ACIP recommends the use of only adsorbed toxoid in this situation.

HOW SUPPLIED

Vial, 1 Dose (10 per package) – Product No. 49281-288-10
Vial, 15 Dose (7.5 mL) – Product No. 49281-288-15
TriHIBit®, One 7.5 mL vial of Tripedia® vaccine as Diluent packaged with Ten 1 Dose vials of lyophilized ActHIB®—Product No. 49281-557-10
TriHIBit®, Five 0.6 mL vials of Tripedia® vaccine as Diluent packaged with Five 1 Dose vials of lyophilized ActHIB®—Product No. 49281-557-05

STORAGE

Store between 2°–8°C (35°–46°F). DO NOT FREEZE. Temperature extremes may adversely affect resuspendability of this vaccine.

REFERENCES

1. Unpublished data available from Aventis Pasteur Inc.
2. Mueller JH, et al. Production of diphtheria toxin of high potency (100 Lf) on a reproducible medium. J Immunol 40: 21–32, 1941
3. Recommendations of the Advisory Committee of Immunization Practices (ACIP). Diphtheria, Tetanus, and Pertussis: Recommendations for vaccine use and other preventive measures. MMWR 40: No RR-10, 1991
4. Kimura M, et al. Developments in pertussis immunisation in Japan. The Lancet: 30–32, 1990
5. Kimura M, et al. Current epidemiology of pertussis in Japan. Pediatr Infect Dis J 9: 705–709, 1990
6. Aoyama T, et al. Efficacy and immunogenicity of acellular pertussis vaccine by manufacturer and patient age. Amer J Dis Child 143: 655–659, 1989
7. Aoyama T, et al. Efficacy of an acellular pertussis vaccine in Japan. J Pediatr 107: 180–183, 1985
8. Blennow M, et al. Preliminary data from a clinical trial (phase 2) of an Acellular Pertussis Vaccine, J NIH-6. Develop Biol Standard 65: 185–190, 1986
9. Blennow M, et al. Primary immunization of infants with an Acellular Pertussis Vaccine in a double-blind randomized clinical trial. Pediatr 82: 293–299, 1988
10. Kallings LO, et al. Placebo-controlled trial of two Acellular Pertussis Vaccines in Sweden—protective efficacy and adverse events. Lancet: 955–960, 1988
11. Storsaeter J, et al. Mortality and morbidity from invasive bacterial infections during a clinical trial of acellular pertussis vaccines in Sweden. Pediatr Infect Dis J 7: 637–645, 1988
12. Bernstein H, et al. Clinical reactions and immunogenicity of the BIKEN Acellular Diphtheria and Tetanus Toxoids and Pertussis Vaccine in 4- through 6-year-old US children. Amer J Dis Child 146: 556–559, 1992
13. Feldman S, et al. Comparison of acellular (B-Type) and whole-cell pertussis-component diphtheria-tetanus-pertussis vaccines as the first booster immunization in 15- to 24-month old children. J Pediatr 121: 857–861, 1992
14. Feldman S, et al. Comparison of two-component acellular and standard whole-cell pertussis vaccines, combined with diphtheria-tetanus toxoids, as the primary immunization series in infants. South Med J 86: 269–275, 284, 1993
15. Pichichero ME, et al. Acellular pertussis vaccination of 2-month-old infants in the United States. J Pediatr 89: 882–887, 1992
16. CDC. Summary of Notifiable Disease, United States, 1994. MMWR 43: No. 53, 1995
17. CDC. Diphtheria Epidemic – New Independent States of the Former Soviet Union, 1990-1994. MMWR 44: 177–181, 1995
18. Department of Health and Human Services, Food and Drug Administration. Biological Products; Bacterial Vaccines and Toxoids; Implementation of Efficacy Review; Proposed Rule. Federal Register Vol 50 No 240, pp 51002–51117, 1985
19. CDC—Pertussis—United States, January 1992–June 1995. MMWR 44: 525–529, 1995
20. Report of the Committee on Infectious Diseases. American Academy of Pediatrics, Evanston, Illinois. Twenty-third Edition, 1994
21. Farizo KM, et al. Epidemiologic features of pertussis in the United States, 1980-1989. Clin Infect Dis 14: 708–719, 1992
22. Nennig ME, et al. Prevalence and Incidence of Adult Pertussis in an Urban Population. JAMA (21) 275: 1672–1674, 1996
23. Linnemann CC, et al. Pertussis in the adult. Ann Rev Med 28: 179–185, 1977
24. CDC. Pertussis Surveillance—United States, 1986 and 1988. MMWR 39: 57–66, 1990
25. Noble GR, et al. Acellular and whole-cell pertussis vaccines in Japan. JAMA 257: 1351–1356, 1987
26. Blackwelder WC, et al., Acellular Pertussis Vaccines. Efficacy and evaluation of clinical case definitions. Am J Dis Child: 145 (11): 1285–1289, 1991
27. Olin P, et al. Relative efficacy of two acellular pertussis vaccines during three years of passive surveillance. Vaccine 10: pp 142–144, 1992
28. ACIP. General recommendations on immunization. MMWR 43: No. RR-1, 1994
29. Wilson GS. The Hazards of Immunization. Provocation poliomyelitis. pp 270–274, 1967
30. ACIP. Pertussis Vaccination: Acellular Pertussis Vaccine for Reinforcing and Booster Use—Supplementary ACIP Statement. MMWR 41: No. RR-1, 1992
31. Cody CL, et al. Nature and rates of adverse reactions associated with DTP and DT immunizations in infants and children. Pediatr 68: 650–660, 1981
32. ACIP. Pertussis immunization: Family history of convulsions and use of antipyretics—Supplementary ACIP statement. MMWR 36: 281–282, 1987
33. Howson CP, et al. Adverse Effects of Pertussis and Rubella Vaccines, Pertussis Vaccines and CNS Disorders. Institute of Medicine (IOM). National Academy Press, Washington, DC, 1991
34. IOM. DTP vaccine and chronic nervous system dysfunction: a new analysis. National Academy Press, Washington, DC, 1994 (Supplement)
35. CDC. Vaccine Adverse Event Reporting System—United States. MMWR 39: 730–733, 1990
36. CDC. National Childhood Vaccine Injury Act: requirements for permanent vaccination records and for reporting of selected events after vaccination. MMWR 37: 197–200, 1988
37. Food and Drug Administration. New reporting requirements for vaccine adverse events. FDA Drug Bull 18 (2), 16–18, 1988
38. Decker MD, et al. Comparison of 13 Acellular Pertussis Vaccines: Adverse Reactions. Pediatr 96: 557–566, 1995
39. Pichichero ME, et al. Safety and immunogenicity of an acellular pertussis vaccine booster in 15- to 20-month-old children previously immunized with acellular or whole-cell pertussis vaccine as infants. Pediatr 91: 756–760, 1993
40. Stratton KR, et al. Adverse Events Associated with Childhood Vaccines. Evidence Bearing on Causality. IOM. National Academy Press. Washington, DC, 1994
41. Miller D, et al. Pertussis immunization and serious acute neurological illnesses in children. Academic Department of Public Health, St Mary's Hospital Medical School, University of London, 1993
42. Griffin MR, et al. Risk of sudden infant death syndrome after immunization with Diphtheria-Tetanus-Pertussis Vaccine. N Engl J Med 618–623, 1988
43. Hoffman HJ, et al. Diphtheria-tetanus-pertussis immunization and sudden infant death: Results of the National Institute of Child Health and Human Devel-

Continued on next page

TABLE 6[1] ADVERSE EVENTS (%) OCCURRING WITHIN 72 HOURS FOLLOWING DIPHTHERIA AND TETANUS TOXOIDS AND ACELLULAR PERTUSSIS VACCINE ADSORBED (TRIPEDIA®) IMMUNIZATIONS GIVEN AT 15 TO 20 MONTHS AND 4 TO 6 YEARS OF AGE IN CHILDREN WHO HAD RECEIVED THREE OR FOUR DOSES OF DTP

EVENT	15 TO 20 MONTHS THREE PREVIOUS DTP DOSES REACTION % (N = 372 CHILDREN)	4 TO 6 YEARS FOUR PREVIOUS DTP DOSES REACTION % (N = 240 CHILDREN)
Local		
Erythema*	18.3	31.3
Swelling**	10.8	27.9
Tenderness	14.2	46.2
Systemic		
Fever > 101°F	4.7	4.8
Diarrhea	6.3	0.8
Vomiting	2.2	1.7
Anorexia	7.8	5.4
Drowsiness	12.4	15.0
Irritability	21.2	15.8
High-pitched unusual cry	1.1	NA

* Includes all occurrences of erythema.
** Includes all occurrences of swelling.
NA Data not collected in this age group.

TABLE 7[1] MODERATELY SEVERE ADVERSE EVENTS OCCURRING WITHIN 48 HOURS FOLLOWING VACCINATION WITH TRIPEDIA® AT 2, 4, OR 6 MONTHS OF AGE (N = 7,102 DOSES)

EVENT	NUMBER	RATE/1,000 DOSES
Fever ≥ 105°F	2	0.28
Hypotonic/Hyporesponsive Episode	1	0.14
Persistent cry ≥ 3 hours	4	0.56
Convulsions*	0	0

*One seizure episode was noted between 48 and 72 hours.

Tripedia—Cont.

opment Cooperative Epidemiological Study of Sudden Infant Death Syndrome Risk Factors. Pediatr 79: 598–611, 1987

44. Walker AM, et al. Diphtheria-tetanus-pertussis immunization and sudden infant death syndrome. Am J Public Health 77: 945–951, 1987
45. Bellman MH, et al. Infantile spasms and pertussis immunization. Lancet, i: 1031–1034, 1983
46. Jacob J, et al. Increased intracranial pressure after diphtheria, tetanus and pertussis immunization. Am J Dis Child Vol 133: 217–218, 1979
47. Mathur R, et al. Bulging fontanel following triple vaccine. Indian Pediatr 18 (6): 417–418, 1981
48. Shendurnikar N, et al. Bulging fontanel following DTP vaccine. Indian Pediatr 23 (11): 960, 1986
49. Rutledge SL, et al. Neurological complications of immunizations. J Pediatr 109: 917–924, 1986
50. Walker AM, et al. Neurologic events following diphtheria-tetanus-pertussis immunization. Pediatr 81: 345–349, 1988
51. Wilson GS. The Hazards of Immunization. Allergic manifestations: Post-vaccinal neuritis. pp 153–156, 1967
52. Tsairis P, et al. Natural history of brachial plexus neuropathy. Arch Neurol 27: 109–117, 1972
53. Blumstein GI, et al. Peripheral neuropathy following tetanus toxoid administration. JAMA 198: 1030–1031, 1966
54. CDC. *Adverse events following immunization.* Surveillance Report No. 3, 1985–1986, Issued February 1989
55. Schlenska GK. Unusual neurological complications following tetanus toxoid administration. J Neurol 215: 299–302, 1977
56. Willinger M, et al. Infant Sleep Position and Risk for Sudden Infant Death Syndrome: Report of Meeting Held January 13 and 14, 1994, National Institutes of Health, Bethesda, MD. Pediatr 93: 814–819, 1994

Product information
as of September 1996

Manufactured by:
Aventis Pasteur Inc.
Swiftwater, Pa 18370 USA
and
The Research Foundation for Microbial
Diseases of Osaka University ("BIKEN®")
Suita, Osaka, Japan

4196/4268

ProHIBiT® ℞
HAEMOPHILUS b CONJUGATE VACCINE
(Diphtheria Toxoid-Conjugate)

Caution: Federal (U.S.A.) law prohibits dispensing without prescription.

DESCRIPTION

ProHIBiT®, Haemophilus b Conjugate Vaccine (Diphtheria Toxoid-Conjugate), for intramuscular use, is a sterile solution, prepared from the purified capsular polysaccharide, a polymer of ribose, ribitol and phosphate (PRP) of the Eagen *Haemophilus influenzae* type b strain covalently bound to diphtheria toxoid (D) and dissolved in sodium phosphate buffered isotonic sodium chloride solution. The polysaccharide-protein conjugate molecule is referred to as PRP-D. Thimerosal (mercury derivative) 1:10,000 is added as a preservative. The vaccine is a clear, colorless solution. Each single dose of 0.5 mL is formulated to contain 25 µg of purified capsular polysaccharide and 18 µg of diphtheria toxoid protein.

HOW SUPPLIED

Vial, 1 Dose (5 per package)—Product No. 49281-541-01
Vial, 5 Dose—Product No. 49281-541-05
Vial, 10 Dose—Product No. 49281-541-10

THERACYS® ℞
BCG LIVE (INTRAVESICAL)
Rx only

WARNING
TheraCys® [BCG Live (Intravesical)] contains live, attenuated mycobacteria. Because of the potential risk for transmission, it should be prepared, handled, and disposed of as a biohazard material (see PRECAUTIONS and DOSAGE AND ADMINISTRATION).
BCG infections have been reported in health care workers, primarily from exposures resulting from accidental needle sticks or skin lacerations during the preparation of BCG for administration. Nosocomial infections have been reported in immunosuppressed patients receiving parenteral drugs which were prepared in areas in which BCG was prepared. BCG is capable of dissemination when administered by the intravesical route, and serious infections, including fatal infections, have been reported in patients receiving intravesical BCG (see WARNINGS, PRECAUTIONS, and ADVERSE REACTIONS).

DESCRIPTION

TheraCys®-BCG Live (intravesical) is a freeze-dried preparation made from the Connaught strain of *Bacillus Calmette and Guérin,* which is an attenuated strain of *Mycobacterium bovis.*

The BCG organisms in the product are grown on media containing potatoes, glycerine, asparagine, citric acid, potassium phosphate, magnesium sulfate, ferric ammonium citrate, calcium chloride, copper sulfate and zinc sulfate. Monosodium glutamate is added to the BCG organisms prior to freeze-drying.

Each vial of TheraCys® contains 81 mg of freeze-dried BCG. Prior to use, each vial is reconstituted with the accompanying diluent (3 mL), which contains sodium chloride, sodium phosphate and Tween 80. Neither the freeze dried BCG nor the diluent contain preservative.

One dose of TheraCys® consists of one 81 mg vial of reconstituted material further diluted in 50 mL sterile, preservative-free saline.

The BCG organisms are viable upon reconstitution. *In vitro* potency is determined by an assay of the number of colonies grown on solid medium. The reconstituted product contains $10.5 \pm 8.7 \times 10^8$ colony forming units (CFU) per vial when resuspended in the diluent provided.

CLINICAL PHARMACOLOGY

BCG Live (Intravesical) promotes a local acute inflammatory and sub-acute granulomatous reaction with macrophage and lymphocyte infiltration in the urothelium and lamina propria of the urinary bladder.[1] The exact mechanism of action is unknown, but the anti-tumor effect appears to be T-lymphocyte-dependent.[1]

CLINICAL STUDIES

In a multicenter randomized clinical trial conducted by the Southwest Oncology Group (SWOG), TheraCys® was compared to doxorubicin hydrochloride (Adriamycin®) in patients with carcinoma *in situ* (CIS) of the urinary bladder, recurrent Ta/T1 papillary tumors of the urinary bladder, or both[2]. Patients were stratified by the presence or absence of CIS, and analyzed separately. All papillary tumors were completely resected prior to study entry. The study endpoints were disease-free survival and 2-year disease-free survival. TheraCys® was administered intravesically weekly for 6 weeks, with an additional single instillation at 3, 6, 12, 18 and 24 months following the initiation of treatment (total of 11 instillations over 2 years). The initial treatment with doxorubicin was given within 3 days of TUR, followed by 4 weekly treatments and then by 11 monthly treatments (total of 16 instillations over 1 year). Cytology and cystoscopy were obtained every 3 months for 2 years. A total of 285 patients were randomized: 142 to treatment with doxorubicin (69 CIS and 73 non-CIS) and 143 to treatment with TheraCys® (70 CIS and 73 non-CIS). An intent-to-treat analysis was performed.

For patients with CIS, the complete response rate (*i.e.,* negative biopsies and urine cytology) within 6 months of the initiation of treatment was 33% with doxorubicin and 71% with TheraCys® (p<0.001, Fisher's Exact Test). The probability of being disease-free at 2 years was 23% with doxorubicin and 51% with TheraCys® (p<0.001, Z Test). The median disease-free survival was 4.9 months for doxorubicin and 30 months for TheraCys® (p<0.001, Long Rand Test).

For patients with Ta/T1 papillary tumors only, the 2-year disease-free survival was 29% with doxorubicin and 50% with TheraCys® (p=0.008, Z Test). The median disease-free survival was 10.5 months with doxorubicin and 22.5 months with TheraCys® (p=0.001, Log Rank Test).

The results are summarized in Table 1.
[See table 1 below]

INDICATIONS AND USAGE

TheraCys® is indicated for the treatment and prophylaxis of carcinoma *in situ* (CIS) of the urinary bladder, and for the prophylaxis of primary or recurrent stage Ta and/or T1 papillary tumors following transurethral resection (TUR). TheraCys® is not recommended for stage TaG1 papillary tumors, unless they are judged to be at high risk of tumor recurrence.

TheraCys® is not indicated as an immunizing agent for the prevention of tuberculosis.

CONTRAINDICATIONS

TheraCys® should not be used in immunosuppressed patients or persons with congenital or acquired immune deficiencies, whether due to concurrent disease (*e.g.,* AIDS, leukemia, lymphoma), cancer therapy (*e.g.,* cytoxotic drugs, radiation), or immunosuppressive therapy (*e.g.,* corticosteroids).

Treatment should be postponed until resolution of a concurrent febrile illness, urinary tract infection, or grass hematuria. Seven to 14 days should elapse before BCG is administered following biopsy, TUR, or traumatic catheterization. TheraCys® should not be administered to persons with active tuberculosis. Active tuberculosis should be ruled out in individuals who are PPD positive before starting treatment with TheraCys®.

WARNINGS

TheraCys® is not a vaccine for the prevention of cancer.
TheraCys® is an infectious agent. Physicians using this product should be familiar with the literature on the prevention and treatment of BCG-related complications, and should be prepared in such emergencies to contact an infectious disease specialist with experience in treating the infectious complications of infectious complications of BCG. The treatment of the infectious complications of BCG requires long-term, multiple-drug antibiotic therapy. Special culture media are required for mycobacteria and physicians administering intravesical BCG should have these media readily available.

Intravesical instillation of TheraCys® into a patient with an actively bleeding urinary mucosa may promote systemic BCG infection. Treatment should be postponed for at least 1 week following transurethral section, biopsy, traumatic catheterization, or gross hematuria.

Deaths have been reported as a result of systemic BCG infection and sepsis. Patients should be monitored for the presence of symptoms and signs of toxicity after each intravesical treatment. Febrile episodes with flu-like symptoms lasting more than 72 hours, fever ≥ 103°F (39.4°C), systemic manifestations increasing in intensity with repeated instillations, or persistent abnormalities of liver function tests suggest systemic BCG infection and may require antituberculous therapy. Local symptoms (prostatitis, epididymitis, orchitis) lasting more than 2–3 days may also suggest active infection (See Management of Serious BCG Complications subsection of Warnings).

The use of TheraCys® may cause tuberculin sensitivity. Since this is a valuable aid in the diagnosis of tuberculosis, it may be advisable to determine the tuberculin reactivity by PPD skin testing before treatment.

Intravesical instillations of BCG should be postponed during treatment with antibiotics, since antimicrobial therapy may interfere with the effectiveness of TheraCys® (see DRUG INTERACTIONS). TheraCys® should not be used in individuals with concurrent infections.

Small bladder capacity has been associated with increased risk of severe local reactions and should be considered in deciding to use TheraCys® therapy.

BCG infection of aneurysms and prosthetic devices (including arterial grafts, cardiac devices, and artificial joints) have been reported following intravesical administration of BCG. The risk of these ectopic BCG infections has not been determined, but is considered to be very small. The benefits of BCG therapy must be carefully weighed against the possibility of an ectopic BCG infection in patients with preexisting arterial aneurysms or prosthetic devices of any kind.

Caution: the stopper of the vial for this product contains natural rubber latex which may cause allergic reactions.

Management of Serious BCG Complications Acute, localized irritative toxicities of TheraCys® may be accompanied by systemic manifestations, consistent with a "flu-like" syndrome. Systemic adverse effects of 1–2 days' duration such as malaise, fever, and chills often reflect hypersensitivity reactions. However, **symptoms such as fever of ≥ 101.3°F (38.5°C), or acute localized inflammation such as epididymitis, prostatitis, or orchitis persisting longer than 2–3 days suggest active infection, and evaluation for serious infectious complications should be considered.**

In patients who develop persistent fever or experience an acute febrile illness consistent with BCG infection, two or more antimycobacterial agents should be administered while diagnostic evaluation, including cultures, is conducted. **BCG treatment should be discontinued.** Negative cultures do not necessarily rule out infection. Physicians using product should be familiar with the literature on prevention, diagnosis, and treatment of BCG-related complications and, when appropriate, should consult an infectious disease specialist or other physician with experience in the diagnosis and treatment of mycobacterial infections.

TheraCys® is sensitive to the most commonly used antituberculous agents (isoniazid, rifampin and ethambutol). **TheraCys® is not sensitive to pyrazinamide.**

PRECAUTIONS

General
TheraCys® contains live mycobacteria and should be prepared and handled using aseptic technique (See Prepara-

Table No. 1: SWOG Study 8216—Efficacy

	Carcinoma *in situ* Doxorubicin N = 69	TheraCys® N = 70	Ta/T1 Papillary Tumors Doxorubicin N=73	TheraCys® N=73
Complete Response	23 (33%)	50 (71%)	—	—
Median Disease-free Survival†	4.9 Months	30 Months	10.5 Months	22.5 Months
2-Year Disease-free Survival†	23%	51%	29%	50%
95% Confidence Interval	(15%, 35%)	(41%, 65%)	(20%, 41%)	(39%, 63%)

† Based upon Kaplan-Meier estimates.

tion of Agent subsection of Dosage and Administration). BCG infections have been reported in health care workers preparing BCG for administration. Needle stick injuries should be avoided during the handling and mixing of TheraCys®. Nosocomial infections have been reported in immunosuppressed patients receiving parenteral drugs which were prepared in areas in which BCG was prepared.[3] BCG is capable is dissemination when administered by intravesical route and serious infections, including fatal infections, have been reported in patients receiving intravesical BCG.[4] Care should be taken not to traumatize the urinary tract or to introduce contaminants into the urinary system. Seven to 14 days should elapse before TheraCys® is administered following TUR, biopsy, or traumatic catheterization. TheraCys® should be administered with caution to persons in groups at high risk for HIV infection.

The use of TheraCys® may cause tuberculin sensitivity. It may therefore be advisable to determine the tuberculin reactivity by PPD skin testing before treatment.

Information For Patients: TheraCys® is retained in the bladder for 2 hours and then voided. Patients should void while seated in order to avoid splashing of urine. For the 6 hours after treatment, voided urine should be disinfected for 15 minutes with an equal volume of household bleach before flushing. Patients should be instructed to increase fluid intake in order to "flush" the bladder in the hours following BCG treatment. Patients may experience burning with the first void after treatment.

Patients should be attentive to side effects, such as fever, chills, malaise, flu-like symptoms, or increased fatigue. If the patient experiences severe urinary side effects, such as burning or pain on urination, urgency, frequency of urination, blood in urine, or other symptoms such as joint pain, cough, or skin rash, the physician should be notified.

Drug Interaction: Drug combinations containing immunosuppressants and/or bone marrow depressants and/or radiation interfere with the development of the immune response and should not be used in combination with TheraCys®. Antimicrobial therapy for other infections may interfere with the effectiveness of TheraCys®. There are no data to suggest that the acute, local urinary tract toxicity common with BCG is due to mycobacterial infection, and **antituberculosis drugs (*e.g.,* isoniazid) should not be used to prevent or treat the local, irritative toxicities of TheraCys®.**

For patients with a condition that may in the future require mandatory immunosuppression (e.g., awaiting an organ transplant, myasthenia gravis) the decision to treat with TheraCys® should be considered carefully.

Pregnancy Category C: Animal reproduction studies have not been conducted with TheraCys®. It is also not known whether TheraCys® can cause fetal harm when administered to a pregnant woman or can affect reproduction capacity. TheraCys® should not be given to a pregnant woman unless clearly needed. Women should be advised not to become pregnant while on therapy.

Nursing Mothers: It is not known whether TheraCys® is excreted in human milk. Because many drugs are excreted in human milk and because of the potential for serious adverse reactions from TheraCys® in nursing infants, it is advisable to discontinue nursing or to discontinue the drug, taking into account the importance of the drug to the mother.

Pediatric Use: Safety and effectiveness of TheraCys® for the treatment of superficial bladder cancer in pediatric patients have not been established.

ADVERSE EVENTS

Symptoms of bladder irritability, related to the inflammatory response induced, are reported in approximately 50% of patients receiving TheraCys® (refer to Table No. 2). The symptoms typically begin 4–6 hours after instillation and last 24–72 hours. The irritative side effects are usually seen following the third instillation, and tend to increase in severity after each administration.

The irritative bladder adverse effects can usually be managed symptomatically with products such as pyridium, propantheline bromide, oxybutynin chloride and acetaminophen. The mechanism of action of the irritative side effect has not been studied, but is most consistent with an immunological mechanism. There is no evidence that dose reduction or antituberculous drug therapy can prevent or lessen the irritative toxicity of TheraCys®.

The "flu-like" symptoms (malaise, fever, and chills) which may accompany the localized, irritative toxicities often reflect hypersensitivity reactions which can be treated symptomatically. Antihistamines have also been used.

Adverse reactions to TheraCys® tend to be progressive in frequency and severity with subsequent instillation. Delay or postponement of treatment may or may not reduce the severity of a reaction during subsequent instillation.

Ocular symptoms (including uveitis, conjunctivitis, iritis, keratitis, granulomatous choreoretinitis) alone, or in combination with joint symptoms (arthritis or arthralgia), urinary symptoms and/or skin rash, have been reported following administration of intravesical BCG. The risk appears to be elevated among patients who are positive for HLA-B27.[5]

Although uncommon, serious infectious complications of intravesical BCG have been reported. The most serious infectious complication of BCG is disseminated sepsis with associated mortality. In addition, *M. bovis* infections have been reported in lung, liver, bone, bone marrow, kidney, regional lymph nodes, and prostate in patients who have received

Table No. 2: SWOG Sutdy 8216—Toxicity

Adverse Event	Percent of Patients Overall (Grade ≥ 3)	Adverse Event	Percent of Patients Overall (Grade ≥ 3)
Dysuria	52% (4%)	Arthralgia/Myalgia	7% (1%)
Urinary Frequency	40% (2%)	Urinary Incontinence	6% (0%)
Malaise	40% (2%)	Cramps/Pain	6% (0%)
Hematuria	39% (7%)	Diarrhea	6% (0%)
Fever (>38 C)	38% (3%)	Contracted Bladder	5% (0%)
Chills	34% (3%)	Leucopenia	5% (0%)
Cystitis	29% (0%)	Coagulopathy	3% (0%)
Anemia	21% (0%)	Abdominal Pain	3% (0%)
Urinary tract Infection	18% (1%)	Liver Involvement	3% (0%)
Urgency	18% (0%)	Systemic Infection	3% (0%)
Nausea/Vomiting	16% (0%)	Pulmonary Infection	3% (0%)
Anorexia	11% (0%)	Cardiac (Unclassified)	3% (0%)
Renal Toxicity (NOS)	10% (2%)	Headache	2% (0%)
Genital Pain	10% (0%)	Skin Rash	2% (0%)

Table No. 3 SWOG Study 8216—Comparative Toxicity

	Study Arm			
	TheraCys® (N=112)		Doxorubicin (N=119)	
	All Grades	Grade ≥ 3	All Grades	Grade ≥ 3
Dysuria	58 (52%)	4 (4%)	48 (40%)	7 (6%)
Frequency	45 (40%)	2 (2%)	34 (29%)	5 (4%)
Malaise	45 (40%)	2 (2%)	17 (14%)	0
Hematuria	44 (39%)	8 (7%)	33 (28%)	8 (7%)
Fever (>38 C)	43 (38%)	3 (3%)	11 (9%)	0
Chills	38 (34%)	3 (3%)	7 (6%)	0
Cystitis	33 (29%)	0	23 (19%)	1 (<1%)
Urgency	20 (18%)	1 (<1%)	14 (12%)	3 (2%)
Nausea/Vomiting	18 (16%)	0	10 (8%)	1 (<1%)
Bladder Cramps/Pain	7 (6%)	0	6 (5%)	2 (1%)

intravesical BCG. Some male genitourinary tract infections (orchitis/epididymitis) have been refractory to mulitple drug antituberculous therapy and required orchiectomy.

If a patient develops persistent fever or experiences an acute febrile illness consistent with BCG infection, BCG treatment should be discontinued and the patient immediately evaluated and treated for BCG infection (See Warnings).

In SWOG study 8216, 112 patients received TheraCys®.[2] The incidence of adverse reactions associated with intravesical TheraCys® is given below.

[See table 2 above]

The following adverse events were reported in ≥ 1% of patients: tissue in urine, local infection, constipation, dizziness, fatigue, thrombocytopenia, and flank pain.

In this study, local irritative symptoms were more common with TheraCys® than with doxorubicin; however, grade ≥ 3 irritative toxicity was similar, occurring ~2–7% of patients. Systemic symptoms (fever, chills, malaise, *etc.*) were also more common with TheraCys®. Overall, grade ≥ 3 toxicities were seen in 26 patients (23%) treated with TheraCys® and 25 patients (21%) treated with doxorubicin. "Systemic infection" was reported to occur in three patients treated with TheraCys® (one grade 2 and two grade 3) and one patient treated with doxorubicin (grade 2). In four patients, treatment was discontinued because of toxicity (two with irritative symptoms, one with severe hematuria, and one with possible BCG infection). In addition, six patients refused further treatment because of severe local toxicity and/or chills. Six of these ten patients received TheraCys®. Table 3 compares the common adverse events reported in SWOG Study 8216.

[See table 3 above]

Reporting of Adverse Reactions

Patients should be encouraged to report all adverse events after treatment with TheraCys®. Adverse events should be reported by health care providers to MEDWATCH (call 1-800-FDA-1088). Physicians, physician assistants, nurses and pharmacists should report adverse occurrences temporally related to the administration of the product to the Director of Medical Affairs, Aventis Pasteur Inc., Discovery Drive, Swiftwater PA 18370 or call 1-800-822-2463.

OVERDOSAGE

Overdosage occurs if more than one vial of TheraCys® is administered per instillation. If overdosage occurs, the patient should be closely monitored for signs of active local or systemic infection. For acute local or systemic reactions suggesting active infection, an infectious disease specialist experienced in BCG complications should be consulted.

DOSAGE AND ADMINISTRATION

One dose of TheraCys® [BCG Live (Intravesical)] consists of the intravesical instillation of 81 mg (dry weight) BCG. This dose is prepared by reconstituting the vial containing freeze-dried BCG with the contents of the vial containing diluent. The vial of reconstituted BCG is further diluted in 50 mL of sterile, preservative-free saline, for a total of 53 mL instillation volume (see reconstitution instructions).

Do not injection subcutaneously or intravenously.

A urethral catheter is inserted into the bladder under aseptic conditions, the bladder is drained, and then 53 mL suspension of TheraCys® is instilled slowly by gravity, following which the catheter is withdrawn.

The patient retains the suspension for as long possible for a total of up to two hours. During the first 15 minutes following instillation, the patient should lie prone. Thereafter, the patient is allowed to be up. At the end of 2 hours, all patients should void in a seated position for safety reasons. Patients should be instructed to maintain adequate hydration.

Preparation of Agent: The preparation of the TheraCys® suspension should be done using aseptic technique. To avoid cross-contamination, parenteral drugs should not be prepared in areas where BCG has been prepared. A separate area for the preparation of the TheraCys® suspension is recommended. All equipment, supplies and receptacles in contact with TheraCys® should be handled and disposed of as biohazardous. The pharmacist or individual responsible for mixing the agent should wear gloves and eye protection, and take precautions to avoid contact of BCG with broken skin. If the preparation cannot be performed in a biocontainment hood, then a mask and gown may be worn to avoid inhalation of BCG organisms and inadvertent exposure to broken skin.

TheraCys® should not be handled by persons with an immunologic deficiency.

Do not remove the rubber stopper from the vial.

Apply a sterile piece of cotton moistened with a suitable antiseptic to the surface of the rubber stoppers of the vial of diluent and vial of TheraCys®. Reconstitute the freeze-dried material with the total 3 mL volume of diluent. Shake the vial gently until a fine, even suspension results. Avoid foaming since this will prevent withdrawal of the proper dose. Withdraw the entire contents (approximately 3 mL) of the reconstituted material into the syringe.

TheraCys® should be reconstituted only with the diluent provided to ensure proper dispersion of the organisms.

The reconstituted material from the vial (1 dose) is further diluent in an additional 50 mL of sterile, preservative-free saline to a final volume of 53 mL for intravesical instillation.

TheraCys® should be used immediately after reconstitution. However, if there is an unavoidable delay between reconstitution and administration, this delay must not exceed 2 hours. Any reconstituted product which exhibits flocculation or clumping that cannot be dispersed with gentle shaking should not be used.

Treatment Schedule: Intravesical treatment of the urinary bladder should begin 7 to 14 days after biopsy or transuretheral resection, and consists of induction and maintenance therapy. For the induction therapy, one dose of TheraCys® is administered each week for 6 consecutive weeks. Induction therapy should be followed by maintenance therapy, consisting of one dose given 3, 6, 12, 18 and 24 months following the initial dose.

HOW SUPPLIED

TheraCys® is supplied in packages containing one vial of the freeze-dried product, containing 81 mg (dry weight) ($10.5 \pm 8.7 \times 10^8$ (CFU) and one vial containing 3 mL of diluent–Product No. 49281-880-01.

STORAGE

TheraCys® [BCG Live (Intravesical)] and the accompanying diluent should be kept in a refrigerator at a temperature between 2°–8°C (35°–46°F). It should not be used after the expiration date marked on the vial, otherwise it may be inactive.

Continued on next page

Theracys BCG Live—Cont.

At no time should the freeze-fried TheraCys® be exposed to sunlight, direct or indirect. Exposure to artificial light should be kept to a minimum.

REFERENCES

1. O'Donnell MA, DeWolf WC. BCG immunotherapy for superficial bladder cancer. New prospects for an old warehouse. *Surg Oncol Clin North Amer* 1995; 4:189–202.
2. Lamm DL, et al. A randomized trial of intravesical doxorubicin and immunotherapy with Bacille Calmette-Guérin for transitional-cell carcinoma of the bladder. *N Eng J Med* 1991;325:1205–1209.
3. Stone MM, et al. Brief report: Meningitis due to iatrogenic BCG infection in two immunocompromised children. *N Engl J Med* 1995,333:561–563.
4. Lamm DL, et al. Incidence and treatment of complications of Bacillus Calmette-Guérin intravesical therapy in superficial bladder cancer. *J Urol* 1992; 147:596–600.
5. Wittes RC, et al. Characterization of BCG-associated sterile arthritis and Reiter's syndrome. New Delhi, India: 10th International Congress of Immunology. 1998:1245–1249.

Product Information as of October 1999.
Manufactured by:
Aventis Pasteur Limited
Toronto, Ontario, Canada
Distributed by:
Aventis Pasteur Inc.
Swiftwater PA 18370 USA

R2-1099 USA 4296
D55
2001457

TYPHIM VI® ℞

Typhoid Vi Polysaccharide Vaccine
Rx only
Caution: Federal (USA) law prohibits dispensing without prescription.

DESCRIPTION

Typhim Vi®, Typhoid Vi Polysaccharide Vaccine, produced by Aventis Pasteur SA, for intramuscular use, is a sterile solution containing the cell surface Vi polysaccharide extracted from *Salmonella typhi* Ty2 strain. The organism is grown in a semi-synthetic medium without animal proteins. The capsular polysaccharide is precipitated from the concentrated culture supernatant by the addition of hexadecyltrimethylammonium bromide and the product is purified by differential centrifugation and precipitation. The potency of the purified polysaccharide is assessed by molecular size and O-acetyl content. Phenol, 0.25%, is added as a preservative. The vaccine contains residual polydimethylsiloxane or fatty-acid ester-based antifoam. The vaccine is a clear, colorless solution. Each single-dose of 0.5 mL is formulated to contain 25 µg of purified Vi polysaccharide in a colorless isotonic phosphate buffered saline (pH 7 ± 0.3), 4.150 mg of Sodium Chloride, 0.065 mg of Disodium Phosphate ($2H_2O$), 0.023 mg of Monosodium Phosphate and 0.5 mL of Sterile Water for Injection.

CLINICAL PHARMACOLOGY

Typhoid fever is an infectious disease caused by *S. typhi*. Humans are the only natural host and reservoir for *S. typhi*; infections result from the consumption of food or water that has been contaminated by the excretions of an acute case or a carrier. *S. typhi* organisms efficiently invade the human intestinal mucosae ultimately leading to bacteremia; following a typical 10- to 14-day incubation period, a systemic illness occurs. The clinical presentation of typhoid fever exhibits a broad range of severity and can be debilitating. Classical cases have fever, myalgia, anorexia, abdominal discomfort and headaches; the fever increases step-wise over a period of days and then may remain at 102°F to 106°F over 10 to 14 days before decreasing in a step-wise manner. Skin lesions known as rose spots may be present. Constipation is common in older children and adults, while diarrhea may occur in younger children. Among the less common but most severe complications are intestinal perforation and hemorrhage, and death. The course is typically more severe without appropriate antimicrobial therapy. The case fatality rate was reported to be approximately 10% to 20% in the pre-antibiotic era.[1,2,3] During the period of 1983 to 1991 in the US, the case fatality rate reported to the Centers for Disease Control and Prevention (CDC) was 0.2% (9/4010).[4] Infection of the gallbladder can lead to the chronic carrier state.

Typhoid fever is still epidemic in many countries of the world where it is predominantly a disease of school-age children and may be a major public health problem. Most cases of typhoid fever in the US are thought to be acquired during foreign travel. During the periods of 1975 to 1984 and 1983 to 1984, respectively, 62% and 70% of the cases of typhoid fever reported to the CDC were acquired during foreign travel; this compares to 33% of cases during 1967–1972.[5]

In 1992, 414 cases of typhoid fever were reported to the CDC. Of these 414 cases, 1 (0.2%) case occurred in an infant under one year of age; 77 (18.6%) cases occurred in persons one to nine years of age; 81 (19.6%) cases occurred in persons 10 to 19 years of age; 251 (60.6%) cases occurred in individuals ≥ 20 years of age; the age was not available for 4 (1%) cases. One death was reported in 1991.[4] Domestic surveillance could underestimate the risk of typhoid fever in travelers since the disease is unlikely to be reported for persons who received diagnosis and treatment overseas.[6]

Approximately 2% to 4% of acute typhoid fever cases develop into a chronic carrier state. The chronic carrier state occurs more frequently with advanced age, and among females than males.[2,7] These non-symptomatic carriers are the natural reservoir for *S. typhi* and can serve to maintain the disease in its endemic state or to directly infect new individuals. Outbreaks of typhoid fever are often traced to food handlers who are asymptomatic carriers.[8]

Other vaccines used for the prevention of typhoid fever in selected populations include a parenteral vaccine containing killed *S. typhi* bacteria and an oral vaccine with live, attenuated *S. typhi*. Typhim Vi, consisting of purified *S. typhi* Vi capsular polysaccharide, is a different type of vaccine. Two formulations were utilized in studies of the typhoid Vi polysaccharide vaccine. These include the liquid formulation which is identical to Typhim Vi and a lyophilized formulation.

The protective efficacy of each of these formulations of the typhoid Vi polysaccharide vaccine was assessed independently in two trials conducted in areas where typhoid fever is endemic. A single intramuscular dose of 25 µg was used in these efficacy studies. A randomized double-blind controlled trial with Typhim Vi (liquid formulation) was conducted in five villages west of Katmandu, Nepal. There were 6,908 vaccinated subjects: 3,454 received Typhim Vi and 3,454 in the control group received a 23-valent pneumococcal polysaccharide vaccine. Of the 6,908 subjects, 6,439 subjects were in the target population of 5 to 44 years of age. In addition, 165 children ages 2 to 4 years and 304 adults over 44 years of age were included in the study. The overall protective efficacy of Typhim Vi was 74% (95% confidence interval (CI): 49% to 87%) for blood culture confirmed cases of typhoid fever during 20 months of post-vaccination follow-up.[9,10,11]

The protective efficacy of the typhoid Vi polysaccharide vaccine, lyophilized formulation, was evaluated in a randomized double-blind controlled trial conducted in South Africa. There were 11,384 vaccinated children 5 to 15 years of age; 5,692 children received the Vi capsular polysaccharide vaccine and 5,692 in the control group received meningococcal polysaccharide (Groups A+C) vaccine. The protective efficacy for the Vi capsular polysaccharide (lyophilized formulation) group for blood culture confirmed cases of typhoid fever was 55% (95% CI: 30% to 70%) overall during 3 years of post-vaccination follow-up, and was 61%, 52% and 50%, respectively, for years 1, 2, and 3. Vaccination was associated with an increase in anti-Vi antibodies as measured by radioimmunoassay (RIA) and enzyme-linked immunosorbent assay. Antibody levels remained elevated at 6 and 12 months post-vaccination.[11,12]

Because of the very low incidence of typhoid fever in the US, efficacy studies are not currently feasible in this population. Controlled comparative efficacy studies of Typhim Vi and other types of typhoid vaccines have not been performed.

An increase in serum anti-capsular antibodies is thought to be the basis of protection provided by Typhim Vi. However, a specific correlation of post-vaccination antibody levels with subsequent protection is not available and the level of Vi antibody that will provide protection has not been determined. Also, limitations exist for comparing immunogenicity results from subjects in endemic areas, where some subjects have baseline serological evidence of prior *S. typhi* exposure, to naive populations such as most American travelers.

In endemic regions (Nepal, South Africa, Indonesia) where trials were conducted, pre-vaccination geometric mean antibody levels suggest that infection with *S. typhi* has previously occurred in a large percentage of the vaccinees. In these populations, specific antibody levels increased four-fold or greater in 68% to 87.5% of older children and adult subjects following vaccination. For 43 persons 15 to 44 years of age in the Nepal pilot study, geometric mean specific antibody levels pre- and 3 weeks post-vaccination were, respectively, 0.38 and 3.68 µg antibody/mL by RIA; 79% had a four-fold or greater rise in Vi antibody levels.[9,12]

Immunogenicity and safety trials were conducted in a racially mixed US population. A single dose of Typhim Vi vaccine induced a four-fold or greater increase in antibody levels in 88% and 96% of this adult population for 2 studies, respectively, following vaccination (see TABLE 1).[10,13]

[See table 1 above]

TABLE 1.[10,13] **Vi ANTIBODY LEVELS IN US ADULTS 18 TO 40 YEARS OF AGE GIVEN TYPHIM Vi**

	N	GEOMETRIC MEAN ANTIBODY LEVELS (µg antibody/mL by RIA) Pre (95% CI)	Post (4 weeks)	% ≥4 FOLD INCREASE (95% CI)
Trial 1 (1 lot)	54	0.16 (0.13 to 0.21)	3.23 (2.59 to 4.03)	96% (52/54) (87% to 100%)
Trial 2 (2 lots combined)	97	0.17 (0.14 to 0.21)	2.86 (2.26 to 3.62)	88% (85/97) (81% to 94%)

No studies of safety and immunogenicity have been conducted in US children. A double-blind randomized controlled trial testing the safety and immunogenicity of Typhim Vi was performed in 175 Indonesian children. The percentage of 2- to 5-year-old children achieving a four-fold or greater increase in antibody levels at 4 weeks post-vaccination was 96.3% (52/54) (95% CI: 87.3% to 99.6%), and in the study subset of 2-year-old children was 94.4% (17/18) (95% CI: 72.7% to 99.9%). The geometric mean levels (µg antibody/mL by RIA) for the 2- to 5-year-old children and the subset of 2-year-olds were, respectively, 5.81 (4.36 to 7.77) and 5.76 (3.48 to 9.53).[10,11]

In the US Reimmunization Study, adults previously immunized with Typhim Vi in other studies were reimmunized with a 25 µg dose at 27 or 34 months after the primary dose. Data on antibody response to primary immunization, decline following primary immunization, and response to reimmunization are presented in TABLE 2. Antibody levels attained following reimmunization at 27 or 34 months after the primary dose were similar to levels attained following the primary immunization.[10,13] This response is typical for a T-cell independent polysaccharide vaccine in that reimmunization does not elicit higher antibody levels than primary immunization. The safety of reimmunization was also evaluated in this study (see **ADVERSE REACTIONS** section).

[See table 2 above]

TABLE 2.[10,13] **US STUDIES IN 18- TO 40-YEAR-OLD ADULTS: KINETICS AND PERSISTENCE OF Vi ANTIBODY* RESPONSE TO PRIMARY IMMUNIZATION WITH TYPHIM Vi, AND RESPONSE TO REIMMUNIZATION AT 27 OR 34 MONTHS**

	PRE-DOSE 1	1 MONTH	11 MONTHS	18 MONTHS	27 MONTHS	34 MONTHS	1 MONTH POST-REIMMUNIZATION[e]
GROUP 1[a]							
N	43	43	39	ND[c]	43	ND	43
Level*	0.19	3.01	1.97		1.07[d]		3.04
95% CI	(0.14–0.26)	(2.22–4.06)	(1.31–3.00)		(0.71–1.62)		(2.17–4.26)
GROUP 2[b]							
N	12	12	ND	10	ND	12	12
Level	0.14	3.78		1.21		0.76[d]	3.31
95% CI	(0.11–0.18)	(2.18–6.56)		(0.63–2.35)		(0.37–1.55)	(1.61–6.77)

*µg antibody/mL by RIA
[a] Group 1: Reimmunized at 27 months following primary immunization.
[b] Group 2: Reimmunized at 34 months following primary immunization.
[c] Not Done
[d] Antibody levels pre-reimmunization.
[e] Includes available data from all reimmunized subjects (subjects initially randomized to Typhim Vi, and subjects initially randomized to placebo who received open label Typhim Vi two weeks later).

INDICATIONS AND USAGE

Typhim Vi vaccine is indicated for active immunization against typhoid fever for persons two years of age or older. Immunization with Typhim Vi should occur at least two weeks prior to expected exposure to *S. typhi*.

Routine immunization against typhoid fever is not recommended in the United States.[14]

Selective immunization against typhoid fever is recommended under the following circumstances: 1) travelers to areas where a recognized risk of exposure to typhoid exists, particularly ones who will have prolonged exposure to potentially contaminated food and water, 2) persons with intimate exposure (i.e., continued household contact) to a documented typhoid carrier, and 3) workers in microbiology laboratories who frequently work with *S. typhi*.[14]

Typhoid vaccination is not required for international travel, but is recommended for travelers to areas where there is a recognized risk of exposure to *S. typhi. S typhi* is prevalent in many countries of Africa, Asia, and Central and South America. Current CDC advisories should be consulted with regard to specific locales. Vaccination is particularly recommended for travelers who will have prolonged exposure to potentially contaminated food and water. However, even travelers who have been vaccinated should use caution in selecting food and water.[15]

Based on the available efficacy data, vaccination with Typhim Vi may not be expected to protect 100% of susceptible individuals.

There is no evidence to support the use of typhoid vaccine to control common source outbreaks, disease following natural disaster or in persons attending rural summer camps.[16]

An optimal reimmunization schedule has not been established. Reimmunization every two years under conditions of repeated or continued exposure to the *S. typhi* organism is recommended at this time.

Typhim Vi has efficacy against typhoid fever caused by *S. typhi* infection but will not afford protection against species of *Salmonella* other than *S. typhi* or other bacteria that cause enteric disease.

For recommended primary immunization and reimmunization see **DOSAGE AND ADMINISTRATION** section.

Typhim Vi should not be used to treat a patient with typhoid fever or a chronic typhoid carrier.

CONTRAINDICATIONS

TYPHIM Vi IS CONTRAINDICATED IN PATIENTS WITH A HISTORY OF HYPERSENSITIVITY TO ANY COMPONENT OF THIS VACCINE.

WARNINGS

This product contains dry natural latex rubber as follows: The stopper to the vial contains no rubber of any kind. In the case of the syringe, the needle cover contains dry natural latex rubber, but the plunger for the syringe contains no rubber of any kind.

Allergic reactions have been reported rarely in the French post-marketing experience (see **ADVERSE REACTIONS** section).

If Typhim Vi is administered to immunosuppressed persons or persons receiving immunosuppressive therapy, the expected immune response may not be obtained. This includes patients with asymptomatic or symptomatic HIV-infection, severe combined immunodeficiency, hypogammaglobulinemia, or agammaglobulinemia; altered immune states due to diseases such as leukemia, lymphoma, or generalized malignancy; or an immune system compromised by treatment with corticosteroids, alkylating drugs, antimetabolites or radiation.[17]

As with any intramuscular injection, Typhim Vi should be given with caution to individuals with thrombocytopenia or any coagulation disorder that would contraindicate intramuscular injection (see **DRUG INTERACTIONS** section).

PRECAUTIONS

GENERAL

Care is to be taken by the health-care provider for the safe and effective use of Typhim Vi.

EPINEPHRINE INJECTION (1:1000) MUST BE IMMEDIATELY AVAILABLE FOLLOWING IMMUNIZATION SHOULD AN ANAPHYLACTIC OR OTHER ALLERGIC REACTIONS OCCUR DUE TO ANY COMPONENT OF THE VACCINE.

Prior to an injection of any vaccine, all known precautions should be taken to prevent adverse reactions. This includes a review of the patient's history with respect to possible hypersensitivity to the vaccine or similar vaccines, and to possible sensitivity to dry natural latex rubber.

Acute infection or febrile illness may be reason for delaying use of Typhim Vi except when in the opinion of the physician, withholding the vaccine entails a greater risk.

A separate, sterile syringe and needle or a sterile disposable unit must be used for each patient to prevent the transmission of infectious agents from person to person. Needles should not be recapped and should be properly disposed.

Special care should be taken to ensure that Typhim Vi is not injected into a blood vessel.

Safety and immunogenicity data from controlled trials are not available for Typhim Vi following previous immunization with whole-cell typhoid or live, oral typhoid vaccine (See **ADVERSE REACTIONS** section).

INFORMATION FOR PATIENTS

Patients, parents or guardians should be fully informed of the benefits and risks of immunization with Typhim Vi.

Prior to administration of Typhim Vi, patients, parents and guardians should be asked about the recent health status of the patient to be immunized.

Typhim Vi is indicated in persons traveling to endemic or epidemic areas. Current CDC advisories should be consulted with regard to specific locales.

Travelers should take all necessary precautions to avoid contact with or ingestion of contaminated food and water.

One dose of vaccine should be given at least 2 weeks prior to expected exposure.

An optimal reimmunization schedule has not been established. Reimmunization consisting of a single-dose for US travelers every two years under conditions of repeated or continued exposure to the *S. typhi* organism is recommended at this time.

As part of the child's or adult's immunization record, the date, lot number and manufacturer of the vaccine administered should be recorded.[18]

The US Department of Health and Human Services has established a new Vaccine Adverse Event Reporting System (VAERS) to accept reports of suspected adverse events after the administration of any vaccine, including but not limited to the reporting of events required by the National Childhood Vaccine Injury Act of 1986.[19,20] The toll-free number for VAERS forms and information is 1-800-822-7967.[18]

DRUG INTERACTIONS

There are no known interactions of Typhim Vi with drugs or foods.

No studies have been conducted in the US to evaluate interactions or immunological interference between the concurrent use of Typhim Vi and drugs (including antibiotics and antimalarial drugs), immune globulins or common traveler's vaccines (e.g., vaccines for tetanus, poliomyelitis, yellow fever and meningococcus). (See **ADVERSE REACTIONS** section.)

As with other intramuscular injections, Typhim Vi should be given with caution to individuals on anticoagulant therapy.

CARCINOGENESIS, MUTAGENESIS, IMPAIRMENT OF FERTILITY

Typhim Vi has not been evaluated for its carcinogenic potential, mutagenic potential or impairment of fertility.

PREGNANCY

REPRODUCTIVE STUDIES – PREGNANCY CATEGORY C

Animal reproduction studies have not been conducted with Typhim Vi. It is not known whether Typhim Vi can cause fetal harm when administered to a pregnant woman or can affect reproduction capacity. Typhim Vi should be given to a pregnant woman only if clearly needed.[21]

When possible, delaying vaccination until the second or third trimester to minimize the possibility of teratogenicity is a reasonable precaution.[14]

NURSING MOTHERS

It is not known if Typhim Vi is excreted in human milk. There is no data to warrant the use of this product in nursing mothers for passive antibody transfer to an infant.

PEDIATRIC USE

Safety and effectiveness of Typhim Vi have been established in children 2 years of age and older.[10,11] (See **DOSAGE AND ADMINISTRATION** section.) FOR CHILDREN BELOW THE AGE OF 2 YEARS, SAFETY AND EFFECTIVENESS HAVE NOT BEEN ESTABLISHED.

ADVERSE REACTIONS

Safety of Typhim Vi, the US licensed liquid formulation, has been assessed in clinical trials in more than 4,000 subjects both in countries of high and low endemicity. In addition, the safety of the lyophilized formulation has been assessed in more than 6,000 individuals. The adverse reactions were predominately minor and transient local reactions. Local reactions such as injection site pain, erythema and induration almost always resolved within 48 hours of vaccination. Elevated oral temperature, above 38°C (100.4°F), was observed in approximately 1% of vaccinees in all studies. No serious or life-threatening systemic events were reported in these clinical trials.[10,11]

Adverse reactions from two trials evaluating Typhim Vi lots in the US (18- to 40-year-old adults) are summarized in TABLE 3. No severe or unusual side effects were observed.

TABLE 3.[10,11] **PERCENTAGE OF 18- TO 40-YEAR-OLD US ADULTS PRESENTING WITH LOCAL OR SYSTEMIC REACTIONS WITHIN 48 HOURS AFTER THE FIRST IMMUNIZATION WITH TYPHIM Vi**

REACTION	Trial 1 Placebo N = 54	Trial 1 Typhim Vi N = 54 (1 Lot)	Trial 2 Typhim Vi N = 98 (2 Lots combined)
Local			
Tenderness	7 (13.0%)	53 (98.0%)	95 (96.9%)
Pain	4 (7.4%)	22 (40.7%)	26 (26.5%)
Induration	0	8 (14.8%)	5 (5.1%)
Erythema	0	2 (3.7%)	5 (5.1%)
Systemic			
Malaise	8 (14.8%)	13 (24.0%)	4 (4.1%)
Headache	7 (13.0%)	11 (20.4%)	16 (16.3%)
Myalgia	0	4 (7.4%)	3 (3.1%)
Nausea	2 (3.7%)	1 (1.9%)	8 (8.2%)
Diarrhea	2 (3.7%)	0	3 (3.1%)
Feverish (subjective)	0	6 (11.1%)	3 (3.1%)
Fever ≥100°F	0	1 (1.9%)	0
Vomiting	0	1 (1.9%)	0

TABLE 4.[10,11] **PERCENTAGE OF INDONESIAN CHILDREN ONE TO TWELVE YEARS OF AGE PRESENTING WITH LOCAL OR SYSTEMIC REACTIONS WITHIN 48 HOURS AFTER THE FIRST IMMUNIZATION WITH TYPHIM Vi**

REACTIONS	N=175
Local	
Soreness	23 (13.0%)
Pain	25 (14.3%)
Erythema	12 (6.9%)
Induration	5 (2.9%)
Impaired Limb Use	0
Systemic	
Feverishness*	5 (2.9%)
Headache	0
Decreased Activity	3 (1.7%)

* Subjective feeling of fever.

TABLE 5.[10,11,13] **U. S. REIMMUNIZATION STUDY, SUBJECTS PRESENTING WITH LOCAL AND SYSTEMIC REACTIONS WITHIN 48 HOURS AFTER IMMUNIZATION WITH TYPHIM Vi**

REACTIONS	PLACEBO (N=32)	FIRST IMMUNIZATION (N=30)	REIMMUNIZATION (N=45*)
Local			
Tenderness	2 (6%)	28 (93%)	44 (98%)
Pain	1 (3%)	13 (43%)	25 (56%)
Induration	0	5 (17%)	8 (18%)
Erythema	0	1 (3%)	5 (11%)
Systemic			
Malaise	1 (3%)	11 (37%)	11 (24%)
Headache	5 (16%)	8 (27%)	5 (11%)
Myalgia	0	2 (7%)	1 (2%)
Nausea	0	1 (3%)	1 (2%)
Diarrhea	0	0	1 (2%)
Feverish (subjective)	0	3 (10%)	2 (4%)
Fever ≥100°F	1 (3%)	0	1 (2%)
Vomiting	0	0	0

* At 27 or 34 months following a previous dose given in different studies.

Continued on next page

Typhim Vi—Cont.

Most subjects reported pain and/or tenderness (pain upon direct pressure). Local adverse experiences were generally limited to the first 48 hours.[10,11]

[See table 3 at top of previous page]

No studies were conducted in US children. Adverse reactions from a trial in Indonesia in children one to twelve years of age are summarized in TABLE 4.[10,11] No severe or unusual side effects were observed.

[See table 4 on previous page]

In the US Reimmunization Study, subjects who had received Typhim Vi 27 or 34 months earlier, and subjects who had never previously received a typhoid vaccination, were randomized to placebo or Typhim Vi, in a double-blind study. Safety data from the US Reimmunization Study are presented in TABLE 5.[10,11,13] In this study 5/30 (17%) primary immunization subjects and 10/45 (22%) reimmunization subjects had an objective local reaction. No severe or unusual side effects were observed. Most subjects reported pain and/or tenderness (pain upon direct pressure). Local adverse experiences were generally limited to the first 48 hours.[10,11,13]

[See table 5 on previous page]

Post-marketing data from foreign countries are available. During the first 5.5 years following approval of Typhim Vi in France, approximately 3.89 million doses were distributed in France. An additional 10.8 million doses have been distributed to other countries worldwide. Reports of adverse events were received either by the French post-marketing surveillance system, which utilizes spontaneous reporting of adverse events, or directly by Aventis Pasteur; 56 and 16 reports were received, respectively, from French and other foreign distribution. Local events reported included erythema, induration and/or pain at the injection site and lymphadenopathy. Systemic events reported included fever, flu-like episode, headache, cervical pain, vomiting, diarrhea, abdominal pain, tremor, hypotension, loss of consciousness, allergic type reactions including urticaria, and other events described below.[10,11]

In the French post-marketing experience, there was one report of diffuse arthralgias and fever two weeks post-vaccination in a 44-year-old female who had also received Hepatitis B vaccine simultaneously; one report of glomerulonephritis seven days post-vaccination in a 23-year-old male who had also received BCG vaccine; one report of neutropenia in a 29-year-old female two days post-vaccination who had also received yellow fever vaccine; one report of bilateral retinitis three weeks post-vaccination in a 26-year-old male who had also received Hepatitis B vaccine; and one report of polyarthritis four days post-vaccination in an 18-year-old male who had also received Meningococcal Groups A + C vaccine and and DT Polio (Diphtheria Tetanus Poliomyelitis) vaccine combination manufactured by Aventis Pasteur.[10,11]

In the French post-marketing experience, the most severe allergic-type reaction occurred in a 24-year-old female with known multiple allergies who had previously received two complete series with a whole-cell typhoid vaccine; she experienced sweats, myalgia and difficulty breathing starting two hours after an IM injection (deltoid) of Typhim Vi. She received 10 mg hydrocortisone and did not require hospitalization.[10,11]

Reporting of Adverse Events

Reporting by parents and patients of all adverse events occurring after vaccine administration should be encouraged. Adverse events following immunization with vaccine should be reported by the health-care provider to the US Department of Health and Human Services (DHHS) Vaccine Adverse Event Reporting System (VAERS). Reporting forms and information about reporting requirements or completion of the form can be obtained from VAERS through a toll-free number 1-800-822-7967.[18]

Health-care providers also should report these events to the Director of Scientific and Medical Affairs, Aventis Pasteur Inc., Discovery Drive, Swiftwater, PA 18370, or call 1-800-822-2463.

DOSAGE AND ADMINISTRATION

Parenteral drug products should be inspected visually for particulate matter and/or discoloration prior to administration. If either of these conditions exist, the vaccine should not be administered.

For intramuscular use only. Do NOT inject intravenously.

Typhim Vi vaccine is indicated for persons two years of age and older.

The immunizing dose for adults and children is a single injection of 0.5 mL. The dose for adults is given intramuscularly in the deltoid, and the dose for children is given IM either in the deltoid or the vastus lateralis. The vaccine should not be injected into the gluteal area or areas where there may be a nerve trunk.

A reimmunizing dose is 0.5 mL. An optimal reimmunization schedule has not been established. Reimmunization consisting of a single dose for US travelers every two years under conditions of repeated or continued exposure to the *S. typhi* organism is recommended at this time.

The skin at the site of injection first should be cleansed and disinfected. Tear off upper aluminum seal of cap. Cleanse top of rubber stopper of the vial with a suitable antiseptic and wipe away all excess antiseptic before withdrawing vaccine.

For single dose syringes, thread the plunger rod into stopper until the plunger rod bottoms out against the stopper and resistance is felt. Do not over tighten the plunger rod.

A separate, sterile syringe and needle or a sterile disposable unit should be used for each patient to prevent transmission of infectious agents from person to person. Needles should not be recapped and should be properly disposed.

There are no data on the safety and efficacy of Typhim Vi administered with any jet injector apparatus and this method of delivery is not recommended.

HOW SUPPLIED

Syringe, 0.5 mL – Product No. 49281-790-01

Vial, 20 Dose (Available on special contract basis only.) – Product No. 49281-790-20

Vial, 50 Dose (Available on special contract basis only.) – Product No. 49281-790-50

STORAGE

Store between 2°–8°C (35°–45°F). DO NOT FREEZE.

REFERENCES

1. Levine MM, et al. New knowledge on pathogenesis of bacterial enteric infections as applied to vaccine development. Microbiol. Rev. 47: 510–550, 1983
2. Levine MM. Typhoid Fever Vaccines. p 333–361. In Vaccines, Plotkin SA, Mortimer EA, eds. W.B. Saunders, 1988
3. Levine MM, et al. Typhoid Fever Chapter 5, In: *Vaccines and Immunotherapy.* Stanley J. Cryz, Jr., Editor. pp 59–72, 1991
4. CDC. Summary of Notifiable Diseases, United States 1992. MMWR 41: No. 55, 1993
5. Ryan CA, et al. *Salmonella typhi* infections in the United States, 1975–1984: Increasing Role of Foreign Travel. Rev Infect Dis 11:1–8, 1989
6. Woodruff BA, et al. A new look at typhoid vaccination. Information for the practicing physician. JAMA 265: 756–759, 1991
7. Ames WR, et al. Age and sex as factors in the development of the typhoid carrier state, and a method for estimating carrier prevalence. Am J Public Health 33: 221–230, 1943
8. CDC. Typhoid fever – Skagit County, Washington. MMWR 39: 749–751, 1990
9. Acharya IL, et al. Prevention of typhoid fever in Nepal with the Vi capsular polysaccharide of *Salmonella typhi.* N Engl J Med 317: 1101–1104, 1987
10. Unpublished data available from Aventis Pasteur Inc., compiled 1991
11. Unpublished data available from Aventis Pasteur SA
12. Klugman KP, et al. Protective activity of Vi capsular polysaccharide vaccine against typhoid fever. The Lancet, 1165–1169, 1987
13. Keitel WA, et al. Clinical and serological responses following primary and booster immunization with *Salmonella typhi* Vi capsular polysaccharide vaccines. Vaccine 12: 195–199, 1994
14. Recommendations of the Advisory Committee on Immunization Practices (ACIP): Update on Adult Immunization. MMWR 40: No. RR-12, 1991
15. CDC. Health Information for International Travel 1992. U. S. Department of Health and Human Services, Public Health Service
16. Recommendations of the Immunization Practices Advisory Committee (ACIP). Typhoid Immunization. MMWR 39: No. RR-10, 1990
17. ACIP: Use of vaccines and immune globulins in persons with altered immunocompetence. MMWR 42: No. RR-4, 1993
18. CDC. Vaccine Adverse Event Reporting System – United States. MMWR 39: 730–733, 1990
19. National Childhood Vaccine Injury Act: Requirements for permanent vaccination records and for reporting of selected events after vaccination. MMWR 37: 197–200, 1988
20. National Childhood Vaccine Injury Act of 1986 (Amended 1987)
21. Recommendations of the ACIP. General recommendations on immunization. MMWR 43: No. RR-14, 1994

Product Information as of June 1995

Manufactured by:
Aventis Pasteur SA
Lyon France Us Gov't License #1279
Distributed by:
Aventis Pasteur Inc.
Swiftwater PA 18370 USA
1-800-VACCINE (1-800-822-2463)

4327/4331

YF-VAX®
YELLOW FEVER VACCINE
Rx only ℞

Caution: Federal (USA) law prohibits dispensing without prescription.

DESCRIPTION

YF-VAX®, Yellow Fever Vaccine, for subcutaneous use, is prepared by culturing the 17D strain of yellow fever virus in living avian leukosis virus-free (ALV-free) chicken embryos. The vaccine, containing sorbitol and gelatin as a stabilizer, is lyophilized, and hermetically sealed under nitrogen. No preservative is added. The vaccine must be reconstituted immediately before use with the sterile diluent provided (Sodium Chloride Injection USP—contains no preservative). YF-VAX® is formulated to contain not less than 5.04 Log_{10} Plaque Forming Units (PFU) per 0.5 mL dose. The vaccine appears slightly opalescent and light orange in color after reconstitution.

YF-VAX® complies with official potency tests and other requirements of the US Food and Drug Administration (FDA) and the World Health Organization (WHO).

CLINICAL PHARMACOLOGY

A clinical study to evaluate the serological responses and adverse reactions of Aventis' YF-VAX® was performed on healthy young adults. One group of six received yellow fever vaccine non-ALV-free (manufactured by Aventis Pasteur Inc.) and another group of 18 received an immunization with YF-VAX®.[1]

Immunologic protection was measured utilizing a serum neutralizing antibody assay. No neutralizing antibody was detected prior to immunization. Both groups demonstrated a 100% conversion in the post-immunization sera. The incidence and severity of adverse reactions in each group were comparable.[1]

In a study involving 101 Nigerian women in various stages of pregnancy, it was concluded that vaccinating pregnant women with the 17D vaccines was not associated with adverse effects on the fetus or with risk of fetal infection. However, the percentage of pregnant women without neutralizing antibodies, who sero-converted, was significantly less than a non-pregnant control group (38.6% vs. 81.5%).[2] Following a mass immunization campaign in Trinidad, congenital infection based on the observation of virus specific IgM in the blood of one infant exposed through maternal immunization with the 17D strain has been reported.[3] This infant appeared normal at delivery.

One case of fatal vaccine-associated encephalitis occurred after 17D yellow fever vaccine was administered to an apparently healthy 39-month-old girl.[4]

INDICATIONS AND USAGE

YF-VAX® is recommended for active immunization of all persons ≥ 9 months of age traveling to or living in areas of South America and Africa where yellow fever infection is officially reported or to countries which require a certificate of vaccination against yellow fever.[5,6]

Vaccination is also recommended for travel outside the urban areas of countries that do not officially report the disease but that lie in the yellow fever endemic zone. In recent years, fatal cases of yellow fever have occurred among unvaccinated tourists visiting rural areas within the yellow fever endemic zone.[5]

Laboratory personnel who might be exposed to virulent yellow fever virus by direct or indirect contact or by aerosols also should be vaccinated.[5]

For simultaneous administration of other vaccines see **DOSAGE AND ADMINISTRATION** section.

Infants < 9 months of age and pregnant women should be considered for vaccination if traveling to areas experiencing ongoing epidemic yellow fever when travel cannot be postponed and a high level of prevention against mosquito exposure is not feasible. *However, in no instance should infants < 4 months of age receive yellow fever vaccine because of the risk of encephalitis.*[5] (See **CONTRAINDICATIONS, WARNINGS** and **PRECAUTIONS** sections.)

United States vaccination certificates are valid for a period of 10 years commencing 10 days after initial vaccination or revaccination.[6] (See **DOSAGE AND ADMINISTRATION** section.)

As with any vaccine, vaccination with YF-VAX® may not protect 100% of susceptible individuals.

CONTRAINDICATIONS

Since the yellow fever virus is propagated in chicken embryos, it should not be administered to an individual with a history of hypersensitivity to egg, chicken protein, or to any other component of the vaccine. Generally, persons who are able to eat eggs or egg products may receive the vaccine. (See **PRECAUTIONS** section for sensitivity testing.)[5]

Infection with yellow fever vaccine virus poses a theoretical risk of encephalitis to patients with immunosuppression in association with acquired immunodeficiency syndrome (AIDS) or other manifestations of human immunodeficiency virus (HIV) infection, leukemia, lymphoma, generalized malignancy, or to those whose immunologic responses are suppressed by corticosteroids, alkylating drugs, antimetabolites, or radiation. Such patients should not be vaccinated. If travel to a yellow fever-infected zone is necessary, patients should be advised of the risk, instructed in methods for avoiding vector mosquitoes, and supplied with vaccination waiver letters by their physicians.[5,6]

Low-dose (10 mg prednisone or equivalent) or short-term (< 2 weeks) corticosteroid therapy or intra-articular, bursal, or tendon injections with corticosteroids should not be immunosuppressive and constitute no increased hazard to recipients of yellow fever vaccine. Persons who have had previously diagnosed asymptomatic HIV infections and who cannot avoid potential exposure to yellow fever virus should be offered the choice of vaccination. Vaccinees should be monitored for possible adverse effects. Since the vaccination of such persons may be less effective than that for non-HIV-infected persons, their neutralizing antibody response to vaccination may be desired before travel. For such determinations, the appropriate state health department or Centers for Disease Control and Prevention (CDC) (303-221-

6400) may be contacted. Family members of immunosuppressed persons, who themselves have no contraindications, may receive yellow fever vaccine.[5]

Infants < 4 months of age should not be immunized because they are more susceptible to encephalitis temporally associated with yellow fever vaccination than older children.[5,6,7] (See **INDICATIONS AND USAGE** and **WARNINGS** sections.)

WARNINGS

This product contains dry natural latex rubber as follows: The stopper to the vial contains dry natural latex rubber.

Infants < 9 months of age and pregnant women should not be vaccinated. *The decision to immunize infants between 4 and 9 months of age and pregnant women should be based upon estimates of the risk of exposure.*[5,6,7]

Anaphylaxis may occur following the use of YF-VAX®, even in individuals with no prior history of hypersensitivity to the vaccine components.

The clinical judgment of the responsible physician should prevail.

PRECAUTIONS

GENERAL

Care is to be taken by the health-care provider for the safe and effective use of YF-VAX®.

EPINEPHRINE INJECTION (1:1000) ALWAYS MUST BE IMMEDIATELY AVAILABLE TO COMBAT UNEXPECTED ANAPHYLACTIC OR OTHER ALLERGIC REACTIONS.

Prior to an injection of any vaccine, all known precautions should be taken to prevent side reactions. This includes a review of the patient's history with respect to possible sensitivity to the vaccine or similar vaccines and to possible sensitivity to dry natural latex rubber.

Health-care providers should obtain the previous immunization history of the vaccinee, and inquire about the current health status of the vaccinee.

Administration of YF-VAX® is not contraindicated in individuals infected with HIV.[7]

A separate, sterile syringe and needle should be used for each patient to prevent transmission of hepatitis or other infectious agents from person to person. Needles should not be recapped and should be properly disposed (e.g., sterilized or disposed in red hazardous waste containers).

INFORMATION FOR PATIENTS

Patients, parents or guardians should be fully informed of the benefits and risks of immunization with YF-VAX®.

Prior to administration of YF-VAX®, patients, parents or guardians should be asked about the recent health status of the patient to be immunized.

The health-care provider, at an approved yellow fever vaccination center, should inform the patients, parents or guardians about the significant adverse reactions that have been temporally associated with YF-VAX® administration and obtain informed consent. Patients, parents or guardians should be instructed to report any serious adverse reactions to their health-care provider.

As part of the patient's immunization record, the date, lot number and manufacturer of the vaccine administered should be recorded.[8,9,10]

Vaccinees should receive an International Certificate of Vaccination completed, signed, and validated with the center's stamp where the vaccine was given.

The US Department of Health and Human Services has established a Vaccine Adverse Event Reporting System (VAERS) to accept all reports of suspected adverse events after the administration of any vaccine, including but not limited to the reporting of events required by the National Childhood Vaccine Injury Act of 1986.[7,8] The VAERS toll-free number for forms and information is 1-800-822-7967.[8]

HYPERSENSITIVITY REACTIONS

Since the yellow fever virus is propagated in chicken embryos, it should not be administered to an individual with a history of hypersensitivity to egg or chicken protein. In some instances, although symptoms appear soon after a vaccine is administered, differentiation between allergic reaction to the vaccine and reaction to an environmental allergen is impossible.[11]

Four types of hypersensitivity reactions are:[11]

1. allergic reactions to egg or egg-related antigens,
2. mercury sensitivity in some recipients of immune globulins or vaccines,
3. antibiotic-induced allergic reactions, and
4. hypersensitivity to some component of the infectious agent or other vaccine components.

Less severe or localized manifestations of allergy to egg or to feathers are not contraindications to vaccine administration and do not usually warrant vaccine skin testing.[11]

An egg-sensitive individual can be tested with the vaccine before it is used in the following manner:[11]

1. Scratch, prick, or puncture test: a drop of 1:10 dilution of the vaccine in physiologic saline is applied at the site of a superficial scratch, prick, or puncture on the volar surface of the forearm. Positive (histamine) and negative (physiologic saline) control tests should also be used. The test is read after 15 to 20 minutes. A positive test is a wheal 3 mm larger than that of the saline control, usually with surrounding erythema. The histamine control must be positive for valid interpretation. If the result of this test is negative, an intradermal (ID) test is performed.
2. Intradermal test: a dose of 0.02 mL of a 1:100 dilution of the vaccine in physiologic saline is injected; positive and negative control skin tests are performed concurrently. A wheal 5 mm or larger than the negative control with surrounding erythema is considered a positive reaction.

STABILITY OF YF-VAX® (FREEZE-DRIED) AT ELEVATED TEMPERATURES[1]

The following information is provided for those countries or areas of the world where an adequate cold chain is a problem and inadvertent exposure to abnormal temperatues has occurred.

Temperature °C	Test	Number of Lots Tested	Computed Half-Life (Days)
35°–37°C	Mouse Assay	3	14.0
35°–37°C	Vero Cell Assay	3	13.9
45°–47°C	Mouse Assay	3	3.3
45°–47°C	Vero Cell Assay	3	4.5

EPINEPHRINE INJECTION (1:1000) ALWAYS MUST BE IMMEDIATELY AVAILABLE TO COMBAT UNEXPECTED ANAPHYLACTIC OR OTHER ALLERGIC REACTIONS.

DESENSITIZATION[11]

If the individual has a history of severe egg sensitivity and has a positive skin test to the vaccine, the individual may be given the vaccine using a "desensitization" procedure if immunization is imperative. The following successive doses should be administered subcutaneously at 15- to 20-minute intervals:

1. 0.05 mL of 1:10 dilution
2. 0.05 mL of full strength
3. 0.10 mL of full strength
4. 0.15 mL of full strength
5. 0.20 mL of full strength

This type of skin testing and "desensitization" should be undertaken only if supervised by a physician experienced in the management of anaphylaxis and with necessary emergency equipment immediately available.

DRUG INTERACTIONS

In a prospective study of persons given yellow fever vaccine and 5 cc of commercially available immune globulin, no alteration of the immunologic response to yellow fever vaccine was detected when compared with controls.[5,11,12]

Studies have shown that the serologic response to yellow fever vaccine is not inhibited by the administration of certain other vaccines concurrently at separate sites or at various intervals of a few days to one month. Measles and yellow fever vaccines have been administered in combination with full efficacy of each of the components; Bacillus Calmette Guérin (BCG) and yellow fever vaccines have been administered simultaneously without interference. Additionally, severity of reactions to vaccination has not been amplified by the concurrent administration of yellow fever and other live virus vaccines. If life virus vaccines are not given concurrently, four weeks should elapse between sequential vaccinations.[5]

Some data have indicated that persons given yellow fever and cholera vaccines simultaneously or 1 to 3 weeks apart had lower than normal antibody responses to both vaccines.[5] Unless there are time constraints, cholera and yellow fever vaccines should be administered at a minimal interval of 3 weeks. If the vaccines cannot be administered at least 3 weeks apart, the vaccines can be given simultaneously at separate sites or at any time within the 3-week interval.[5]

Hepatitis B and yellow fever vaccine may be given concurrently at separate sites.[5] No data exist on possible interference between yellow fever and typhoid, paratyphoid, typhus, plague, rabies or Japanese encephalitis vaccines.[5]

Although chloroquine inhibits replication of yellow fever virus in vitro, it does not adversely affect antibody responses to yellow fever vaccine in humans receiving antimalaria prophylaxis.[5,13] (See **DOSAGE AND ADMINISTRATION** section.)

Usually, YF-VAX® should be administered at least one month apart from other live-virus vaccines. However, field observations and clinical data indicate that simultaneous administration of the most widely used live-virus vaccines have not resulted in impaired antibody response or increased adverse reactions.[7] Thus, if time is a critical factor for required vaccinations, the clinical judgment of the responsible physician should prevail.

CARCINOGENESIS, MUTAGENESIS, IMPAIRMENT OF FERTILITY

YF-VAX® has not been evaluated for its carcinogenic, mutagenic potentials or impairment of fertility.

PREGNANCY

REPRODUCTIVE STUDIES—PREGNANCY CATEGORY C

Animal reproduction studies have not been conducted with YF-VAX®. It is also not known whether YF-VAX® can cause fetal harm when administered to a pregnant woman or can affect reproduction capacity. YF-VAX® should be given to a pregnant woman only if clearly needed.

NURSING MOTHERS

Yellow fever virus is not excreted in breast milk following vaccination, and there is no contraindication for vaccinating breastfeeding mothers with yellow fever vaccine.[6]

PEDIATRIC USE

Safety and effectiveness of Yellow Fever Vaccine in infants below the age of 9 months have not been established. Therefore, *YF-VAX® is NOT recommended for infants < 9 months of age unless they live in or are traveling to a high-risk area.* ***In NO instance should infants < 4 months of age receive yellow fever vaccine because of the risk of encephalitis.***[5] (See **INDICATIONS AND USAGE** and **WARNINGS** sections.)

ADVERSE REACTIONS

Adverse reactions to 17D yellow fever vaccine are generally mild. After vaccination, 2% to 5% of vaccinees have mild headaches, myalgia, low-grade fevers, or other minor symptoms for 5 to 10 days. Fewer than 0.2% of the vaccinees curtail regular activities. Immediate hypersensitivity reactions, characterized by rash, urticaria, and/or asthma, are uncommon (incidence <1/1,000,000) and occur principally among persons with histories of egg allergy.[5]

Two cases of encephalitis temporally associated with vaccinations have been reported in the United States; in one fatal case, 17D virus was isolated from the brain.[4,5]

Anaphylaxis may occur following the use of YF-VAX®, even in individuals with no prior history of hypersensitivity to the vaccine components.

EPINEPHRINE INJECTION (1:1000) ALWAYS MUST BE IMMEDIATELY AVAILABLE TO COMBAT UNEXPECTED ANAPHYLACTIC OR OTHER ALLERGIC REACTIONS.

Reporting of Adverse Events

Reporting by patients, parents or guardians of all adverse events occurring after vaccine administration should be encouraged. Adverse events following immunization with vaccine should be reported by the health-care provider to the US Department of Health and Human Services (DHHS) Vaccine Adverse Event Reporting System (VAERS). Reporting forms and information about reporting requirements or completion of the form can be obtained from VAERS through a toll-free number 1-800-822-7967.[8]

Health-care providers also should report these events to the Director of Scientific and Medical Affairs, Aventis Pasteur Inc., Discovery Drive, Swiftwater, PA 18370 or call 1-800-822-2463.

DOSAGE AND ADMINISTRATION

Parenteral drug products should be inspected visually for extraneous particulate matter and/or discoloration prior to administration whenever solution and container permit. If these conditions exist, the vaccine should not be administered.

Reconstitute the vaccine using only the diluent supplied (Sodium Chloride Injection USP). The vaccine appears slightly opalescent and light orange in color after reconstitution. Draw the volume of the diluent, shown on the diluent label, into a suitable size syringe and inject into the vial containing the vaccine. Slowly add diluent to vaccine, let set for one to two minutes and then carefully swirl mixture until a uniform suspension is achieved. Avoid vigorous shaking as this tends to cause foaming of the suspension. Use vaccine within 60 minutes following reconstitution. *All reconstituted vaccine and containers which remain unused after one hour must be properly disposed (e.g., sterilized or disposed in red hazardous waste containers).*[5] *Do not dilute reconstituted vaccine.*

SWIRL VACCINE WELL before withdrawing each dose. *Administer the single immunizing dose of 0.5 mL subcutaneously at once.*

If immunization is imperative to an individual with a history of severe egg sensitivity and a positive skin test to the vaccine, see **DESENSITIZATION** section.

Primary vaccination. For persons of all ages, a single subcutaneous injection of 0.5 mL of reconstituted vaccine (formulated to contain not less than 5.04 Log_{10} Plaque Forming Units [PFU]) is administered.[5] Immunity develops by the 10th day after primary vaccination.[6]

Booster doses. The International Health Regulations require revaccination at intervals of 10 years. Revaccination boosts antibody titer; however, evidence from several studies suggests that yellow fever vaccine immunity persists for at least 30 to 35 years and probably for life.[5]

SIMULTANEOUS ADMINISTRATION OF OTHER VACCINES

Studies have shown that the serologic response to yellow fever vaccine is not inhibited by the administration of certain other vaccines concurrently at separate sites or at various intervals of a few days to one month. Measles and yellow fever vaccines have been administered in combination with full efficacy of each of the components; Bacillus Calmette Guérin (BCG) and yellow fever vaccines have been administered simultaneously without interference. Additionally, severity of reactions to vaccination has not been amplified by the concurrent administration of yellow fever and other live virus vaccines. If the live virus vaccines are not given concurrently, four weeks should elapse between sequential vaccinations.[5]

Continued on next page

YF-Vax—Cont.

Some data have indicated that persons given yellow fever and cholera vaccines simultaneously or 1 to 3 weeks apart had lower than normal antibody responses to both vaccines.[5] Unless there are time constraints, cholera and yellow fever vaccines should be administered at a minimal interval of 3 weeks. If the vaccines cannot be administered at least 3 weeks apart, the vaccines can be given simultaneously at separate sites or at any time within the 3-week interval.[5]

Hepatitis B and yellow fever vaccine may be given concurrently at separate sites.[5] No data exist on possible interference between yellow fever and typhoid, paratyphoid, typhus, plague, rabies or Japanese encephalitis vaccines.[5]

HOW SUPPLIED

Vial, 1 Dose (5 per package) with vial of diluent (5 per package) for administration with needle and syringe. Product No. 49281-915-01

Vial, 5-Dose, with vial of diluent, for administration with needle and syringe. Product No. 49281-915-05

Vial, 20-Dose, with vial of diluent, for administration with needle and syringe (NOT to be used with jet injector). Product No. 49281-915-20

YF-VAX® (Yellow Fever Vaccine) in the United States is supplied only to designated Yellow Fever Vaccination Centers authorized to issue valid certificates of Yellow Fever Vaccination. Location of the nearest Yellow Fever Vaccination Centers may be obtained from the Centers for Disease Control and Prevention, Atlanta, GA 30333, state or local health departments, or the USPHS booklet "Immunization Information for International Travel" (obtainable from the Superintendent of Documents, US Government Printing Office, Washington, DC 20402).

STORAGE

Storage Temperature

Freeze-dried vaccine must be maintained continuously at a temperature between 0°–5°C (32°–41°F).

YF-VAX® does not contain a preservative, therefore all reconstituted vaccine and containers which remain unused after one hour must be properly disposed (e.g., sterilized or disposed in red hazardous waste containers).[5]

Shipping Temperatures

YF-VAX® is shipped in a container with solid carbon dioxide; use is not recommended unless the shipping case contains some dry ice upon arrival.

STABILITY STUDIES

[See table at top of previous page]

YF-VAX® is formulated to satisfy the current US potency requirements of not less than 5.04 Log_{10} Plaque Forming Units (PFU) per 0.5 mL dose and meets the minimum requirements of WHO.[14]

REFERENCES

1. Unpublished data available from Aventis Pasteur Inc.
2. Nasidi A, et al. Yellow fever vaccination and pregnancy: a four-year prospective study. Transactions of the Royal Society of Tropical Medicine and Hygiene 87: 337–339, 1993
3. Tsai TF, et al. Congenital yellow fever virus infection after immunization in pregnancy. J Infect Dis 168: 1520–1523, 1993
4. Jennings AD, et al. Analysis of a yellow fever virus isolated from a fatal case of vaccine-associated human encephalitis. J Infect Dis 169: 512–518, 1994
5. Recommendations of the Advisory Committee on Immunization Practices (ACIP). Yellow Fever Vaccine. MMWR 39: No. RR-6, 1990
6. Vaccination Certificate Requirements. Health information for international travel. US Department of Health and Human Services. June 1991
7. ACIP. General recommendations on immunization. MMWR 38: 205–227, 1989
8. CDC. Vaccine Adverse Event Reporting System—United States. MMWR 39: 730–733, 1990
9. CDC. National Childhood Vaccine Injury Act: requirements for permanent vaccination records and for reporting of selected events after vaccination. MMWR 37: 197–200, 1988
10. Food and Drug Administration. New reporting requirements for vaccine adverse events. FDA Drug Bull 18 (2), 16–18, 1988
11. American Academy of Pediatrics. Report of the Committee on Infectious Diseases. 23rd ed. Elk Grove Village, IL, 1994
12. Kaplan JE, et al. The effect of immune globulin on the response to trivalent oral poliovirus and yellow fever vaccinations. Bull WHO Vol 62: 585–590, 1984
13. Tsai TF, et al. Chloroquine does not adversely affect the antibody response to yellow fever vaccine. J Infect Dis 154: 726, 1986
14. Requirements for yellow fever vaccine. WHO Technical Report Series 594, 1976

Product information as of May 1996

Manufactured by:
Aventis Pasteur Inc.
Swiftwater PA 18370 USA 4283/4290

Axcan Scandipharm Inc.

22 INVERNESS PARKWAY
BIRMINGHAM, AL 35242

Direct Inquiries to:
Customer Service
(800) 950-8085
Fax: (205) 991-8426

For Medical Information Contact:
John S. Cipriano, M.S., R.Ph.
(205) 991-8085
Fax: (205) 991-8047

PHOTOFRIN® ℞
(porfimer sodium)
for Injection

DESCRIPTION

PHOTOFRIN® (porfimer sodium) for Injection is a photosensitizing agent used in the photodynamic therapy (PDT) of tumors. Following reconstitution of the freeze-dried product with 5% Dextrose Injection (USP) or 0.9% Sodium Chloride Injection (USP), it is injected intravenously. This is followed 40–50 hours later by illumination of the tumor with laser light (630 nm wavelength). PHOTOFRIN® is not a single chemical entity; it is a mixture of oligomers formed by ether and ester linkages of up to eight porphyrin units. It is a dark red to reddish brown cake or powder. Each vial of PHOTOFRIN® contains 75 mg of porfimer sodium as a sterile freeze-dried cake or powder. Hydrochloric Acid and/or Sodium Hydroxide may be added during manufacture to adjust pH. There are no preservatives or other additives. The structural formula below is representative of the components present in PHOTOFRIN®.

[See chemical structure below]

CLINICAL PHARMACOLOGY

Pharmacology

The cytotoxic and antitumor actions of PHOTOFRIN® are light and oxygen dependent. Photodynamic therapy (PDT) with PHOTOFRIN® is a two-stage process. The first stage is the intravenous injection of PHOTOFRIN®. Clearance from a variety of tissues occurs over 40–72 hours, but tumors, skin, and organs of the reticuloendothelial system (including liver and spleen) retain PHOTOFRIN® for a longer period. Illumination with 630 nm wavelength laser light constitutes the second stage of therapy. Tumor selectivity in treatment occurs through a combination of selective retention of PHOTOFRIN® and selective delivery of light. Cellular damage caused by PHOTOFRIN® PDT is a consequence of the propagation of radical reactions. Radical initiation may occur after PHOTOFRIN® absorbs light to form a porphyrin excited state. Spin transfer from PHOTOFRIN® to molecular oxygen may then generate singlet oxygen. Subsequent radical reactions can form superoxide and hydroxyl radicals. Tumor death also occurs through ischemic necrosis secondary to vascular occlusion that appears to be partly mediated by thromboxane A_2 release. The laser treatment induces a photochemical, not a thermal, effect. The necrotic reaction and associated inflammatory responses may evolve over several days.

Pharmacokinetics

Following a 2 mg/kg dose of porfimer sodium to 4 male cancer patients, the average peak plasma concentration was 15 ± 3 mcg/mL, the elimination half-life was 250 ± 285 hours, the steady-state volume of distribution was 0.49 ± 0.28 L/kg, and the total plasma clearance was 0.051 ± 0.035 mL/min/kg. The mean plasma concentration at 48 hours was 2.6 ± 0.4 mcg/mL. The influence of impaired hepatic function on PHOTOFRIN® disposition has not been evaluated.

PHOTOFRIN® was approximately 90% protein bound in human serum, studied in vitro. The binding was independent of concentration over the concentration range of 20–100 mcg/mL.

Clinical Studies

Clinical studies of PDT with PHOTOFRIN® were conducted in patients with obstructing esophageal and endobronchial nonsmall cell lung cancers and in patients with early-stage radiologically occult endobronchial cancer. In all clinical studies, the method of PDT administration was essentially identical. A course of therapy consisted of one injection of PHOTOFRIN® (2 mg/kg administered as a slow intravenous injection over 3–5 minutes) followed by up to two nonthermal applications of 630 nm laser light. Doses of 300 J/cm of tumor length were used in esophageal cancer. Doses of 200 J/cm were used in endobronchial cancer for both palliation of obstructing cancer and treatment of superficial lesions. The first application of light occurred 40–50 hours after injection. Debridement of residua was performed via endoscopy/bronchoscopy 96–120 hours after injection, after which any residual tumor could be retreated with a second laser light application at the same dose used for the initial treatment. Additional courses of PDT with PHOTOFRIN® were allowed after 1 month, up to a maximum of three courses.

Esophageal Cancer

PDT with PHOTOFRIN® was utilized in a multicenter, single-arm study in 17 patients with completely obstructing esophageal carcinoma. Assessments were made at 1 week and 1 month after the last treatment procedure. As shown in Table 1, after a single course of therapy, 94% of patients obtained an objective tumor response and 76% of patients experienced some palliation of their dysphagia. On average, before treatment these patients had difficulty swallowing liquids, even saliva. After one course of therapy, there was a statistically significant improvement in mean dysphagia grade (1.5 units, $p < 0.05$) and 13 of 17 patients could swal-

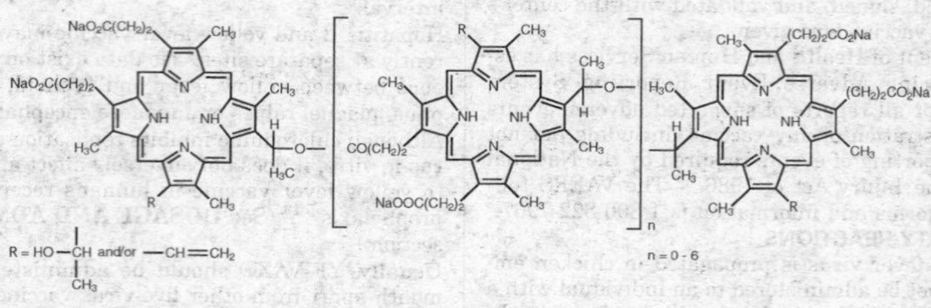

TABLE 1. Course 1 Efficacy Results in Patients with Completely Obstructing Esophageal Cancer

EFFICACY PARAMETER	PDT n=17
OBJECTIVE TUMOR RESPONSE[a]	
Week 1	82%
Month 1	35%[b]
Any assessment[c]	94%
IMPROVEMENT[d] IN DYSPHAGIA	
Week 1	71%
Month 1	47%
Any assessment[c]	76%
MEAN DYSPHAGIA GRADE[e] AT BASELINE	4.6
MEAN IMPROVEMENT[e] IN DYSPHAGIA GRADE (units)	
Week 1	1.4
Month 1	1.5
MEAN NUMBER OF LASER APPLICATIONS	1.4

[a] CR+PR, CR = complete response (absence of endoscopically visible tumor), PR = partial response (appearance of a visible lumen)
[b] Eight of the 17 treated patients did not have assessments at Month 1.
[c] Week 1 or Month 1
[d] Patients with at least a one-grade improvement in dysphagia grade
[e] Dysphagia Scale: Grade 1 = normal swallowing, Grade 2 = difficulty swallowing some hard solids; can swallow semisolids, Grade 3 = unable to swallow any solids; can swallow liquids, Grade 4 = difficulty swallowing liquids, Grade 5 = unable to swallow saliva.

low liquids without difficulty 1 week and/or 1 month after treatment. Based on all courses, three patients achieved a complete tumor response (CR). In two of these patients, the CR was documented only at Week 1 as they had no further assessments. The third patient achieved a CR after a second course of therapy, which was supported by negative histopathology and maintained for the entire follow-up of 6 months.
Of the 17 treated patients, 11 (65%) received clinically important benefit from PDT. Clinically important benefit was defined hierarchically as a complete tumor response (3 patients), achievement of normal swallowing (2 patients went from Grade 5 dysphagia to Grade 1), or achievement of a marked improvement of two or more grades of dysphagia with minimal adverse reactions (6 patients). The median duration of benefit in these patients was 69+ days. Duration of benefit was calculated only for the period with documented evidence of improvement. All of these patients were still in response at their last assessment and, therefore, the estimate of 69 days is conservative. The median survival for these 11 patients was 115 days.
[See table 1 on previous page]

Endobronchial Cancer

Two randomized multicenter Phase 3 studies were conducted to compare the safety and efficacy of PHOTOFRIN® PDT versus Nd:YAG laser therapy for reduction of obstruction and palliation of symptomatic patients with partially or completely obstructing endobronchial nonsmall cell lung cancer. Assessments were made at 1 week and at monthly intervals after treatment. Table 2 shows the results from all randomized patients in the two studies combined. Objective tumor response rates (CR + PR), which demonstrate reduction of obstruction, were 59% for PDT and 58% for Nd:YAG at Week 1. The response rate at 1 month or later was 60% for PDT and 41% for Nd:YAG.
[See table 2 above]

TABLE 2. Efficacy Results from Studies in Late-stage Obstructing Endobronchial Cancer—All Randomized Patients[a]

EFFICACY PARAMETER (% of Patients)	PDT n=102	Nd:YAG n=109
OBJECTIVE TUMOR RESPONSE[b]		
Week 1	59%	58%
Month 1 or later	60%	41%[a]
ATELECTASIS IMPROVEMENT[c]	n=60	n=71
Week 1	35%	18%
Month 1 or later	35%	20%

[a] Statistical comparisons were precluded by the amount of missing data at Month 1 or later (e.g. for tumor response, PDT 28% missing, Nd:YAG 38%).
[b] CR+PR, CR = complete response (absence of bronchoscopically visible tumor), PR = partial response (increase of ≥50% in the smallest luminal diameter); for completely obstructing tumors, any appearance of a lumen).
[c] In patients with atelectasis at baseline

Patient symptoms were evaluated using a 5- or 6-grade pulmonary symptoms severity rating scale for dyspnea, cough, and hemoptysis. Patients with moderate to severe symptoms are those most in need of palliation. Improvements of 2 or more grades are considered to be clinically significant. Table 3 shows the percentages of patients with moderate to severe symptoms at baseline who demonstrated a 2-grade improvement at any time during the interval evaluated.
[See table 3 above]

TABLE 3. Efficacy Results from Studies in Late-stage Obstructing Endobronchial Cancer—Clinically Significant Improvements in Patients with Moderate to Severe Symptoms at Baseline[a]

CLINICALLY SIGNIFICANT SYMPTOM IMPROVEMENT[b] (% of Patients)	PDT	Nd:YAG
ANY SYMPTOM	n=89	n=89
Week 1	25%	29%
Month 1 or later	40%	27%[a]
DYSPNEA	n=60	n=68
Week 1	15%	18%
Month 1 or later	23%	13%
COUGH	n=63	n=65
Week 1	6%	9%
Month 1 or later	24%	8%
HEMOPTYSIS	n=24	n=31
Week 1	58%	29%
Month 1 or later	79%	35%

[a] Statistical comparisons were precluded by the amount of missing data at Month 1 or later.
[b] Dyspnea was graded on a 6-point severity rating scale; cough and hemoptysis on 5-point scales. Clinically significant improvement was defined as a change of at least two grades from baseline.

In a separate retrospective analysis, patients were individually evaluated to identify those patients whose benefit to risk ratio was most favorable, i.e., those who obtained clinically important benefit with minimal adverse reactions. Clinically important benefit was defined as one of the following:

1. a substantial improvement in pulmonary symptoms at Month 1 or later (dyspnea ≥2 grades, hemoptysis ≥3 grades, cough ≥3 grades or increase in FEV_1 ≥40%);
2. a moderate improvement in symptoms at Month 2 or later (dyspnea 1 grade, cough 2 grades, hemoptysis 2 grades or increase in FEV_1 ≥20%); or
3. a durable objective tumor response (CR or PR maintained to Month 2 or longer).

Thirty-six (36) of the 99 PDT-treated patients (36%) and 23 of the 99 Nd:YAG-treated patients (23%) received clinically important benefit with only minimal or moderate toxicities of short duration. 34 of 99 PDT-treated patients demonstrated improvements in 2 or more efficacy endpoints (dyspnea, cough, hemoptysis, sputum, atelectasis, pulmonary function tests of FEV1 or FVC, Karnofsky Performance Score or tumor response) and 29 patients had improvements in 3 or more. The median duration of documented benefit in the 36 patients was 63 days. In these patients with late-stage obstructing lung cancer, median survival was 174 days in PDT-treated patients and 161 days in Nd:YAG-treated patients.
The efficacy of PHOTOFRIN® PDT was also evaluated in the treatment of microinvasive endobronchial tumors in 62 inoperable patients in three noncomparative studies. Microinvasive lung cancer is defined histologically as disease which invades beyond the basement membrane but not through or into the cartilage. For 11 of the 62 patients, it was clearly documented that surgery and radiotherapy were not indicated. These 11 patients were all inoperable for medical or technical reasons. Radiotherapy was not indicated due to prior high-dose radiotherapy (7 patients), poor pulmonary function (2 patients), multifocal multilobar disease (1 patient), and poor medical condition (1 patient). As shown in Table 4, the complete tumor response rate, biopsy-proven at least 3 months after treatment, was 50%, median time to tumor recurrence was more than 2.7 years, median survival was 2.9 years and disease-specific survival was 4.1 years.
[See table 4 above]

TABLE 4. Overall Efficacy Results in Patients with Superficial Endobronchial Tumors

EFFICACY PARAMETER	PDT n=11	PDT n=62
COMPLETE TUMOR RESPONSE, BIOPSY-PROVEN AT 3 MONTHS		
Number of Patients (%)	3 (27%)	31 (50%)[a]
TIME TO TUMOR RECURRENCE IN PATIENTS WITH COMPLETE RESPONSE		
Number of Patients (%) with Recurrences	1 (33%)	11 (35%)
Median Time to Tumor Recurrence		>2.7 years
[95% Confidence Interval]		[1.6,—[b]]
SURVIVAL		
Number of Patients (%) who Died of Any Cause	4 (36%)	32 (52%)
Median Survival		2.9 years
[95% Confidence Interval]		[2.1, 5.7]
DISEASE-SPECIFIC SURVIVAL		
Number of Patients (%) who Died of Lung Cancer	3 (27%)	22 (35%)
Median Disease-Specific Survival		4.1 years
[95% Confidence Interval]		[2.5,—[b]]

[a] Not included are an additional 18 patients (6 patients not eligible for surgery or radiotherapy) who had complete tumor responses which were documented earlier than 3 months after treatment.
[b] The upper limit of the confidence interval could not be estimated due to an insufficient number of patients whose tumors recurred (Time to Tumor Recurrence) or who died (Survival).

INDICATIONS AND USAGE

Photodynamic therapy with PHOTOFRIN® is indicated for:

— palliation of patients with completely obstructing esophageal cancer, or of patients with partially obstructing esophageal cancer who, in the opinion of their physician, cannot be satisfactorily treated with Nd:YAG laser therapy.
— reduction of obstruction and palliation of symptoms in patients with completely or partially obstructing endobronchial nonsmall cell lung cancer (NSCLC).
— treatment of microinvasive endobronchial NSCLC in patients for whom surgery and radiotherapy are not indicated.

CONTRAINDICATIONS

PHOTOFRIN® is contraindicated in patients with porphyria or in patients with known allergies to porphyrins.
PDT is contraindicated in patients with an existing tracheoesophageal or bronchoesophageal fistula.
PDT is contraindicated in patients with tumors eroding into a major vessel.

WARNINGS

Following injection with PHOTOFRIN® precautions must be taken to avoid exposure of skin and eyes to direct sunlight or bright indoor light (see PRECAUTIONS, General Precautions and Information for Patients).

Esophageal Cancer

If the esophageal tumor is eroding into the trachea or bronchial tree, the likelihood of tracheoesophageal or bronchoesophageal fistula resulting from treatment is sufficiently high that PDT is not recommended.
Patients with esophageal varices should be treated with extreme caution. Light should not be given directly to the variceal area because of the high risk of bleeding.

Endobronchial Cancer

Patients should be assessed for the possibility that a tumor may be eroding into a pulmonary blood vessel (see CONTRAINDICATIONS). Patients at high risk for fatal hemoptysis include those with large, centrally located tumors, those with cavitating tumors or those with extensive tumor extrinsic to the bronchus.
If the endobronchial tumor invades deeply into the bronchial wall, the possibility exists for fistula formation upon resolution of tumor.
PDT should be used with extreme caution for endobronchial tumors in locations where treatment-induced inflammation could obstruct the main airway, e.g., long or circumferential tumors of the trachea, tumors of the carina that involve both mainstem bronchi circumferentially, or circumferential tumors in the mainstem bronchus in patients with prior pneumonectomy.

PRECAUTIONS

General Precautions and Information for Patients

Photosensitivity

All patients who receive PHOTOFRIN® will be photosensitive and must observe precautions to avoid exposure of skin and eyes to direct sunlight or bright indoor light (from examination lamps, including dental lamps, operating room lamps, unshaded light bulbs at close proximity, etc.) for at least 30 days. Some patients may remain photosensitive for up to 90 days or more. The photosensitivity is due to residual drug which will be present in all parts of the skin. Exposure of the skin to ambient indoor light is, however, beneficial because the remaining drug will be inactivated gradually and safely through a photobleaching reaction. Therefore, patients should not stay in a darkened room during this period and should be encouraged to expose their skin to ambient indoor light. The level of photosensitivity will vary for different areas of the body, depending on the extent of previous exposure to light. Before exposing any area of skin to direct sunlight or bright indoor light, the patient should test it for residual photosensitivity. A small area of skin should be exposed to sunlight for 10 minutes. If no photosensitivity reaction (erythema, edema, blistering) occurs within 24 hours, the patient can gradually resume normal outdoor activities, initially continuing to exercise caution and gradually allowing increased exposure. If some photosensitivity reaction occurs with the limited skin test, the patient should continue precautions for another 2 weeks before retesting. The tissue around the eyes may be more

Continued on next page

Photofrin—Cont.

sensitive, and therefore, it is not recommended that the face be used for testing. If patients travel to a different geographical area with greater sunshine, they should retest their level of photosensitivity. **UV (ultraviolet) sunscreens are of no value in protecting against photosensitivity reactions because photoactivation is caused by visible light.**

Ocular Sensitivity

Ocular discomfort, commonly described as sensitivity to sun, bright lights, or car headlights, has been reported in patients who received PHOTOFRIN®. For 30 days, when outdoors, patients should wear dark sunglasses which have an average white light transmittance of <4%.

Use Before or After Radiotherapy

If PDT is to be used before or after radiotherapy, sufficient time should be allotted between the two therapies to ensure that the inflammatory response produced by the first treatment has subsided before commencing the second treatment. The inflammatory response from PDT will depend on tumor size and extent of surrounding normal tissue that receives light. It is recommended that 2 to 4 weeks be allowed after PDT before commencing radiotherapy. Similarly, if PDT is to be given after radiotherapy, the acute inflammatory reaction from radiotherapy usually subsides within 4 weeks after completing radiotherapy, after which PDT may be given.

Chest Pain

As a result of PDT treatment, patients may complain of substernal chest pain because of inflammatory responses within the area of treatment. Such pain may be of sufficient intensity to warrant the short-term prescription of opiate analgesics.

Respiratory Distress

Patients with endobronchial lesions must be closely monitored between the laser light therapy and the mandatory debridement bronchoscopy for any evidence of respiratory distress. Inflammation, mucositis, and necrotic debris may cause obstruction of the airway. If respiratory distress occurs, the physician should be prepared to carry out immediate bronchoscopy to remove secretions and debris to open the airway.

Avoidance of Pregnancy

Women of childbearing potential should practice an effective method of contraception during therapy (see Pregnancy).

Drug Interactions

There have been no formal interaction studies of PHOTOFRIN® and any other drugs. However, it is possible that concomitant use of other photosensitizing agents (e.g., tetracyclines, sulfonamides, pnenothiazines, sulfonylurea hypoglycemic agents, thiazide diuretics, and griseofulvin) could increase the photosensitivity reaction.

PHOTOFRIN® PDT causes direct intracellular damage by initiating radical chain reactions that damage intracellular membranes and mitochondria. Tissue damage also results from ischemia secondary to vasoconstriction, platelet activation and aggregation and clotting. Research in animals and in cell culture has suggested that many drugs could influence the effects of PDT, possible examples of which are described below. There are no human data that support or rebut these possibilities.

Compounds that quench active oxygen species or scavenge radicals, such as dimethyl sulfoxide, b-carotene, ethanol, formate and mannitol would be expected to decrease PDT activity. Preclinical data also suggest that tissue ischemia, allopurinol, calcium channel blockers and some prostaglandin synthesis inhibitors could interfere with PHOTOFRIN® PDT. Drugs that decrease clotting, vasoconstriction or platelet aggregation, e.g., thromboxane A_2 inhibitors, could decrease the efficacy of PDT. Glucocorticoid hormones given before or concomitant with PDT may decrease the efficacy of the treatment.

Carcinogenesis, Mutagenesis, Impairment of Fertility

No long-term studies have been conducted to evaluate the carcinogenic potential of PHOTOFRIN®. In vitro, PHOTOFRIN® PDT did not cause mutations in the Ames test, nor did it cause chromosome aberrations or mutations (HGPRT locus) in Chinese hamster ovary (CHO) cells. PHOTOFRIN® caused <2-fold, but significant, increases in sister chromatid exchange in CHO cells irradiated with visible light and a 3-fold increase in Chinese hamster lung fibroblasts irradiated with near UV light. PHOTOFRIN® PDT caused an increase in thymidine kinase mutants and DNA-protein cross-links in mouse L5178Y cells, but not mouse LYR83 cells. PHOTOFRIN® PDT caused a light-dose dependant increase in DNA-strand breaks in malignant human cervical carcinoma cells, but not in normal cells. The mutagenicity of PHOTOFRIN® without light has not been adequately determined. In vivo, PHOTOFRIN® did not cause chromosomal aberrations in the mouse micronucleus test.

PHOTOFRIN® given to male and female rats intravenously, at 4 mg/kg/d (0.32 times the clinical dose on a mg/m^2 basis) before conception and through Day 7 of pregnancy caused no impairment of fertility. In this study, long-term dosing with PHOTOFRIN® caused discoloration of testes and ovaries and hypertrophy of the testes. PHOTOFRIN® also caused decreased body weight in the parent rats.

Pregnancy: Pregnancy Category C

There are no adequate and well-controlled studies in pregnant women. PHOTOFRIN® should be used during pregnancy only if the potential benefit justifies the potential risk to the fetus.

PHOTOFRIN® given to rat dams during fetal organogenesis intravenously at 8 mg/kg/d (0.64 times the clinical dose on a mg/m^2 basis) for 10 days caused no major malformations or developmental changes. This dose caused maternal and fetal toxicity resulting in increased resorptions, decreased litter size, delayed ossification, and reduced fetal weight. PHOTOFRIN® caused no major malformations when given to rabbits intravenously during organogenesis at 4 mg/kg/d (0.65 times the clinical dose on a mg/m^2 basis) for 13 days. This dose caused maternal toxicity resulting in increased resorptions, decreased litter size, and reduced fetal body weight.

PHOTOFRIN® given to rats during late pregnancy through lactation intravenously at 4 mg/kg/d (0.32 times the clinical dose on a mg/m^2 basis) for at least 42 days caused a reversible decrease in growth of offspring. Parturition was unaffected.

Nursing Mothers

It is not known whether this drug is excreted in human milk. Because many drugs are excreted in human milk and because of the potential for serious adverse reactions in nursing infants from PHOTOFRIN®, women receiving PHOTOFRIN® must not breast feed.

Pediatric Use

Safety and effectiveness in children have not been established.

Use in Elderly Patients

Approximately 70% of the patients treated with PDT using PHOTOFRIN® in clinical trials were over 60 years of age. There was no apparent difference in effectiveness or safety in these patients compared to younger people. Dose modification based upon age is not required.

ADVERSE REACTIONS

Systemically induced effects associated with PDT with PHOTOFRIN® consist of photosensitivity and mild constipation. All patients who receive PHOTOFRIN® will be photosensitive and must observe precautions to avoid sunlight and bright indoor light (see PRECAUTIONS). Photosensitivity reactions occurred in approximately 20% of patients treated with PHOTOFRIN® in clinical studies. Typically these reactions were mostly mild to moderate erythema but they also included swelling, itching, burning sensations, feeling hot, or blisters. In a single study of 24 healthy subjects, some evidence of photosensitivity reactions occurred in all subjects. Other less common skin manifestations were also reported in areas where photosensitivity reactions had occurred, such as increased hair growth, skin discoloration, skin nodules, increased wrinkles and increased skin fragility. These manifestations may be attributable to a pseudoporphyria state (temporary drug-induced cutaneous porphyria).

Most toxicities associated with this therapy are local effects seen in the region of illumination and occasionally in surrounding tissues. The local adverse reactions are characteristic of an inflammatory response induced by the photodynamic effect.

Esophageal Carcinoma

The following adverse events were reported over the entire follow-up period in at least 5% of patients treated with PHOTOFRIN® PDT, who had completely or partially obstructing esophageal cancer. Table 5 presents data from 88 patients who received the currently marketed formulation. The relationship of many of these adverse events to PDT with PHOTOFRIN® is uncertain.

[See table 5 at left]

TABLE 5. Adverse Events Reported in 5% or More of Patients[a] with Obstructing Esophageal Cancer

BODY SYSTEM/ Adverse Event	Number (%) of Patients n=88	
Patients with at Least One Adverse Event	84	(95%)
AUTONOMIC NERVOUS SYSTEM		
Hypertension	5	(6%)
Hypotension	6	(7%)
BODY AS A WHOLE		
Asthenia	5	(6%)
Back pain	10	(11%)
Chest pain	19	(22%)
Chest pain (substernal)	4	(5%)
Edema generalized	4	(5%)
Edema peripheral	6	(7%)
Fever	27	(31%)
Pain	19	(22%)
Surgical complication	4	(5%)
CARDIOVASCULAR		
Cardiac failure	6	(7%)
GASTROINTESTINAL		
Abdominal pain	18	(20%)
Constipation	21	(24%)
Diarrhea	4	(5%)
Dyspepsia	5	(6%)
Dysphagia	9	(10%)
Eructation	4	(5%)
Esophageal edema	7	(8%)
Esophageal tumor bleeding	7	(8%)
Esophageal stricture	5	(6%)
Esophagitis	4	(5%)
Hematemesis	7	(8%)
Melena	4	(5%)
Nausea	21	(24%)
Vomiting	15	(17%)
HEART RATE/RHYTHM		
Atrial fibrillation	9	(10%)
Tachycardia	5	(6%)
METABOLIC & NUTRITIONAL		
Dehydration	6	(7%)
Weight decrease	8	(9%)
PSYCHIATRIC		
Anorexia	7	(8%)
Anxiety	6	(7%)
Confusion	7	(8%)
Insomnia	12	(14%)
RED BLOOD CELL		
Anemia	28	(32%)
RESISTANCE MECHANISM		
Moniliasis	8	(9%)
RESPIRATORY		
Coughing	6	(7%)
Dyspnea	18	(20%)
Pharyngitis	10	(11%)
Pleural effusion	28	(32%)
Pneumonia	16	(18%)
Respiratory insufficiency	9	(10%)
Tracheoesophageal fistula	5	(6%)
SKIN & APPENDAGES		
Photosensitivity reaction	17	(19%)
URINARY		
Urinary tract infection	6	(7%)

[a] Based on adverse events reported at any time druing the entire period of follow-up.

Location of the tumor was a prognostic factor for three adverse events: upper-third of the esophagus (esophageal edema), middle-third (atrial fibrillation), and lower-third, the most vascular region (anemia). Also, patients with large tumors (>10 cm) were more likely to experience anemia. Two of 17 patients with complete esophageal obstruction from tumor experienced esophageal perforations which were considered to be possibly treatment associated; these perforations occurred during subsequent endoscopies.

Serious and other notable adverse events observed in less than 5% of PDT-treated patients with obstructing esophageal cancer in the clinical studies include the following; their relationship to therapy is uncertain. In the gastrointestinal system, esophageal perforation, gastric ulcer, ileus, jaundice, and peritonitis have occurred. Sepsis has been reported occasionally. Cardiovascular events have included angina pectoris, bradycardia, myocardial infarction, sick sinus syndrome, and supraventricular tachycardia. Respiratory events of bronchitis, bronchospasm, laryngotracheal edema, pneumonitis, pulmonary hemorrhage, pulmonary edema, respiratory failure, and stridor have occurred. The temporal relationship of some gastrointestinal, cardiovascular and respiratory events to the administration of light was suggestive of mediastinal inflammation in some patients. Vision-related events of abnormal vision, diplopia, eye pain and photophobia have been reported.

Obstructing Endobronchial Cancer

Table 6 presents adverse events that were reported over the entire follow-up period in at least 5% of patients with obstructing endobronchial cancers treated with PHOTOFRIN® PDT or Nd:YAG. These data are based on the 86 patients who received the currently marketed formulation. Since it seems likely that most adverse events caused by these acute acting therapies would occur within 30 days of treatment, Table 6 presents those events occurring within 30 days of a treatment procedure, as well as those occurring over the entire follow-up period. It should be noted that follow-up was 33% longer for the PDT group than for the Nd:YAG group, thereby introducing a bias against PDT when adverse event rates are compared for the entire follow-up period. The extent of follow-up in the 30-day period following treatment was comparable between groups (only 9% more for PDT).

[See table 6 above]

TABLE 6. Adverse Events Reported in 5% or More of Patients with Obstructing Endobronchial Cancers

BODY SYSTEM/ Adverse Event	Number (%) of Patients: Within 30 Days of Treatment				Entire Follow-up Period[a]			
	PDT n=86		Nd:YAG n=86		PDT n=86		Nd:YAG n=86	
Patients with at Least One Adverse Event	43	(50%)	33	(38%)	62	(72%)	48	(56%)
BODY AS A WHOLE								
Back pain	3	(3%)	1	(1%)	3	(3%)	5	(6%)
Chest pain	6	(7%)	6	(7%)	7	(8%)	8	(9%)
Edema peripheral	3	(3%)	3	(3%)	4	(5%)	3	(3%)
Fever	7	(8%)	7	(8%)	14	(16%)	8	(9%)
Pain	1	(1%)	4	(5%)	4	(5%)	8	(9%)
CENTRAL NERVOUS SYSTEM								
Dysphonia	3	(3%)	2	(2%)	4	(5%)	2	(2%)
GASTROINTESTINAL								
Constipation	4	(5%)	1	(1%)	4	(5%)	2	(2%)
Dyspepsia	1	(1%)	4	(5%)	2	(2%)	5	(6%)
PSYCHIATRIC								
Anxiety	3	(3%)	0	(0%)	5	(6%)	0	(0%)
Insomnia	4	(5%)	2	(2%)	4	(5%)	3	(4%)
RESPIRATORY								
Bronchitis	9	(10%)	2	(2%)	9	(10%)	2	(2%)
Coughing	5	(6%)	8	(9%)	13	(15%)	11	(13%)
Dyspnea	15	(17%)	7	(8%)	26	(30%)	13	(15%)
Hemoptysis	6	(7%)	5	(6%)	14	(16%)	7	(8%)
Pleural effusion	0	(0%)	0	(0%)	4	(5%)	1	(1%)
Pneumonia	5	(6%)	4	(5%)	10	(12%)	5	(6%)
Pneumothorax	0	(0%)	0	(0%)	0	(0%)	4	(5%)
Respiratory insufficiency	0	(0%)	0	(0%)	5	(6%)	1	(1%)
Sputum increased	4	(5%)	5	(6%)	7	(8%)	6	(7%)
SKIN & APPENDAGES								
Photosensitivity reaction	16	(19%)	0	(0%)	18	(21%)	0	(0%)

[a] Follow-up was 33% longer for the PDT group than for the Nd:YAG group, introducing a bias against PDT when adverse events are compared for the entire follow-up period.

Transient inflammatory reactions in PDT-treated patients occur in about 10% of patients and manifest as fever, bronchitis, chest pain and dyspnea. The incidences of bronchitis and dyspnea were higher with PDT than with Nd:YAG. Most cases of bronchitis occurred within 1 week of treatment and all but one were mild or moderate in intensity. The events usually resolved within 10 days with antibiotic therapy. Treatment-related worsening of dyspnea is generally transient and self-limiting. Debridement of the treated area is mandatory to remove exudate and necrotic tissue. Life-threatening respiratory insufficiency likely due to therapy occurred in 3% of PDT-treated patients and 2% of Nd:YAG-treated patients (see WARNINGS AND PRECAUTIONS).

There was a trend toward a higher rate of fatal hemoptysis (FMH) occurring on the PDT arm (10%) versus the Nd:YAG arm (5%), however, the rate of FMH occurring within 30 days of treatment was the same for PDT and Nd:YAG (4% total events, 3% treatment-associated events). Patients who have received radiation therapy have a higher incidence of FMH after treatment with PDT and after other forms of local therapy than patients who have not received radiation therapy, but analyses suggest that this increased risk may be due to associated prognostic factors such as having a centrally located tumor. The incidence of FMH in patients previously treated with radiotherapy was 21% (6/29) in the PDT group and 10% (3/29) in the Nd:YAG group. In patients with no prior radiotherapy, the overall incidence of FMH was less than 1%. Characteristics of patients at high risk for FMH are described in WARNINGS and CONTRAINDICATIONS.

Other serious or notable adverse events were observed in less than 5% of PDT-treated patients with endobronchial cancer; their relationship to therapy is uncertain. In the respiratory system, pulmonary thrombosis, pulmonary embolism and lung abscess have occurred. Cardiac failure, sepsis and possible cerebrovascular accident have also been reported in one patient each.

Superficial Endobronchial Tumors

The following adverse events were reported over the entire follow-up period in at least 5% of patients with superficial tumors (microinvasive or carcinoma in situ) who received the currently marketed formulation.

[See table 7 above]

TABLE 7. Adverse Events Reported in 5% or More of Patients[a] with Superficial Endobronchial Tumors

Adverse Event	Number (%) of Patients n=90	
Patients with at Least One Adverse Event	44	(49%)
Photosensitivity reaction	20	(22%)
Coughing	8	(9%)
Dyspnea	6	(7%)
Edema	16	(18%)
Exudate	20	(22%)
Obstruction	19	(21%)
Stricture	10	(11%)
Ulceration	8	(9%)

[a] Based on adverse events reported at any time during the entire period of follow-up.

In patients with superficial endobronchial tumors, 44 of 90 patients (49%) experienced an adverse event, two-thirds of which were related to the respiratory system. The most common reaction to therapy was a mucositis reaction in one-fifth of the patients which manifested as edema, exudate, and obstruction. The obstruction (mucus plug) is easily removed with suction or forceps. Mucositis can be minimized by avoiding exposure of normal tissue to excessive light (see PRECAUTIONS). Three patients experienced life-threatening dyspnea: one was given a double dose of light, one was treated concurrently in both mainstem bronchi and the other had had prior pneumonectomy and was treated in the sole remaining main airway (see WARNINGS). Stent placement was required in 3% of the patients due to endobronchial stricture. Fatal hemoptysis occurred within 30 days of treatment in one patient with superficial tumors (1%).

Laboratory Abnormalities

In patients with esophageal cancer, PDT with PHOTOFRIN® may result in anemia due to tumor bleeding. No consistent effects were observed for other parameters or in patients with endobronchial carcinoma.

OVERDOSAGE

PHOTOFRIN® Overdose

There is no information on overdosage situations involving PHOTOFRIN®. Higher than recommended drug doses of two 2 mg/kg doses given two days apart (10 patients) and three 2 mg/kg doses given within two weeks (1 patient), were tolerated without notable adverse reactions. Effects of overdosage on the duration of photosensitivity are unknown. Laser treatment should not be given if an overdose of PHOTOFRIN® is administered. In the event of an overdose, patients should protect their eyes and skin from direct sunlight or bright indoor lights for 30 days. At this time, patients should test for residual photosensitivity (see PRECAUTIONS). PHOTOFRIN® is not dialyzable.

Overdose of Laser Light Following PHOTOFRIN® Injection

Light doses of two to three times the recommended dose have been administered to a few patients with superficial endobronchial tumors. One patient experienced life-threatening dyspnea and the others had no notable complications. Increased symptoms and damage to normal tissue might be expected following an overdose of light.

DOSAGE AND ADMINISTRATION

Photodynamic therapy with PHOTOFRIN® is a two-stage process requiring administration of both drug and light. The first stage of PDT is the intravenous injection of PHOTOFRIN® at 2 mg/kg. Illumination with laser light 40–50 hours following injection with PHOTOFRIN® constitutes the second stage of therapy. A second laser light application may be given 96–120 hours after injection, preceded by gentle debridement of residual tumor (see Administration of Laser Light). In clinical studies, debridement via endoscopy was required 2 days after the initial light application. Standard endoscopic techniques are used for light administration and debridement. Practitioners should be fully familiar with the patient's condition and trained in the safe and efficacious treatment of esophageal or endobronchial cancer using photodynamic therapy with PHOTOFRIN® and associated light delivery devices.

Patients may receive a second course of PDT a minimum of 30 days after the initial therapy; up to three courses of PDT (each separated by a minimum of 30 days) can be given. Before each course of treatment, patients with esophageal cancer should be evaluated for the presence of a tracheoesophageal or bronchoesophageal fistula (see CONTRAINDICATIONS). In patients with endobronchial lesions who have recently undergone radiotherapy, sufficient time (approximately 4 weeks) should be allowed between the therapies to ensure that the acute inflammation produced by radiotherapy has subsided prior to PDT (see PRECAUTIONS, Use Before or After Radiotherapy). All patients should be evaluated for the possibility that the tumor may be eroding into a major blood vessel (see CONTRAINDICATIONS).

PHOTOFRIN® Administration

PHOTOFRIN® should be administered as a single slow intravenous injection over 3 to 5 minutes at 2 mg/kg body weight. Reconstitute each vial of PHOTOFRIN® with 31.8 mL of either 5% Dextrose Injection (USP) or 0.9% Sodium Chloride Injection (USP), resulting in a final concentration of 2.5 mg/mL. Shake well until dissolved. Do not mix PHOTOFRIN® with other drugs in the same solution. PHOTOFRIN®, reconstituted with 5% Dextrose Injection (USP) or with 0.9% Sodium Chloride Injection (USP), has a pH in the range of 7 to 8. PHOTOFRIN® has been formulated with an overage to deliver the 75 mg labeled quantity. **The reconstituted product should be protected from bright light and used immediately.** Reconstituted PHOTOFRIN® is an opaque solution, in which detection of particulate matter by visual inspection is extremely difficult. Reconstituted PHOTOFRIN®, however, like all parenteral drug products, should be inspected visually for particulate matter and discoloration prior to administration whenever solution and container permit.

Precautions should be taken to prevent extravasation at the injection site. If extravasation occurs, care must be taken to protect the area from light. There is no known benefit from injecting the extravasation site with another substance.

Administration of Laser Light

Initiate 630 nm wavelength laser light delivery to the patient 40–50 hours following injection with PHOTOFRIN®. A second laser light treatment may be given as early as 96

Continued on next page

Photofrin—Cont.

hours or as late as 120 hours after the initial injection with PHOTOFRIN®. No further injection of PHOTOFRIN® should be given for such retreatment with laser light. Before providing a second laser light treatment, the residual tumor should be debrided. Vigorous debridement may cause tumor bleeding. For endobronchial tumors, debridement of necrotic tissue should be discontinued when the volume of bleeding increases, as this may indicate that debridement has gone beyond the zone of the PDT treatment effect.

The laser system must be approved for delivery of a stable power output at a wavelength of 630 ± 3 nm. Light is delivered to the tumor by cylindrical OPTIGUIDE™ fiber optic diffusers passed through the operating channel of an endoscope/bronchoscope. Instructions for use of the fiber optic and the selected laser system should be read carefully before use. OPTIGUIDE™ cylindrical diffusers are available in several lengths. The choice of diffuser tip length depends on the length of the tumor. Diffuser length should be sized to avoid exposure of nonmalignant tissue to light and to prevent overlapping of previously treated malignant tissue.

Photoactivation of PHOTOFRIN® is controlled by the total light dose delivered:

In the treatment of esophageal cancer, a light dose of 300 joules/cm of tumor length should be delivered. The total power output at the fiber tip is set to deliver the appropriate light dose using exposure times of 12 minutes and 30 seconds.

In the treatment of endobronchial cancer, the light dose should be 200 joules/cm of tumor length. The total power output at the fiber tip is set to deliver the appropriate light dose using exposure times of 8 minutes and 20 seconds. For noncircumferential endobronchial tumors that are soft enough to penetrate, interstitial fiber placement is preferred to intraluminal activation, since this method produces better efficacy and results in less exposure of the normal bronchial mucosa to light. It is important to perform a debridement 2 to 3 days after each light administration to minimize the potential for obstruction caused by necrotic debris (see PRECAUTIONS).

Refer to the OPTIGUIDE™ instructions for use for complete instructions concerning the fiber optic diffuser.

HOW SUPPLIED

PHOTOFRIN® (porfimer sodium) for Injection is supplied as a freeze-dried cake or powder as follows:

NDC 0024-1550-01—75 mg vial

PHOTOFRIN® freeze-dried cake or powder should be stored at Controlled Room Temperature 20–25°C (68–77°F) [see USP].

Spills and Disposal

Spills of PHOTOFRIN® should be wiped up with a damp cloth. Skin and eye contact should be avoided due to the potential for photosensitivity reactions upon exposure to light; use of rubber gloves and eye protection is recommended. All contaminated materials should be disposed of in a polyethylene bag in a manner consistent with local regulations.

Accidental Exposure

PHOTOFRIN® is neither a primary ocular irritant nor a primary dermal irritant. However, because of its potential to induce photosensitivity, PHOTOFRIN® might be an eye and/or skin irritant in the presence of bright light. It is important to avoid contact with the eyes and skin during preparation and/or administration. As with therapeutic overdosage, any overexposed person must be protected from bright light.

Manufactured by
LEDERLE PARENTERALS, INC.
Carolina, Puerto Rico 00987
for
Axcan Scandipharm Inc.
Birmingham, AL 35242

ULTRASE® ℞

[*ul 'trāce*]
(pancrelipase) Capsules
Enteric-Coated Microspheres

Prescribing Information

DESCRIPTION

ULTRASE® (pancrelipase) Capsules are orally administered capsules containing enteric-coated microspheres of porcine pancreatic enzyme concentrate, predominantly pancreatic lipase, amylase, and protease.

Each ULTRASE ® capsule contains:

Lipase	4,500 U.S.P. Units
Amylase	20,000 U.S.P. Units
Protease	25,000 U.S.P. Units

Inactive ingredients: povidone, talc, sugar, methacrylic acid copolymer (Type C), triethyl citrate, simethicone emulsion.

CLINICAL PHARMACOLOGY

ULTRASE® (pancrelipase) Capsules are designed to prevent inactivation by gastric acid thereby resulting in the delivery of high levels of biologically active enzymes into the duodenum. The enzymes catalyze the hydrolysis of fats into glycerol and fatty acids, starch into dextrins and sugars, and protein into proteoses and derived substances.

INDICATIONS AND USAGE

ULTRASE® (pancrelipase) Capsules are indicated for patients with partial or complete exocrine pancreatic insufficiency caused by:

- Cystic fibrosis (CF)
- Chronic pancreatitis due to alcohol use or other causes
- Surgery (pancreatico-duodenectomy or Whipple's procedure, with or without Wirsung duct injection, total pancreatectomy)
- Obstruction (pancreatic and biliary duct lithiasis, pancreatic and duodenal neoplasms, ductal stenosis)
- Other pancreatic disease (hereditary, post traumatic and allograft pancreatitis, hemochromatosis, Shwachman's Syndrome, lipomatosis, hyperparathyroidism)
- Poor mixing (Billroth II gastrectomy, other types of gastric bypass surgery, gastrinoma)

Pancrelipase capsules are effective in controlling steatorrhea.[1–9]

CONTRAINDICATIONS

Pancrelipase capsules are contraindicated in patients known to be hypersensitive to pork protein. Pancrelipase capsules are contraindicated in patients with acute pancreatitis or with acute exacerbations of chronic pancreatic diseases.

WARNINGS

Should hypersensitivity occur, discontinue medication and treat symptomatically.

PRECAUTIONS

General

TO PROTECT ENTERIC COATING, MICROSPHERES MUST NOT BE CRUSHED OR CHEWED. Where swallowing of capsules is difficult, they may be opened and the microspheres added to a small quantity of a soft food (e.g. applesauce, gelatin, etc.) that does not require chewing, and swallowed immediately. Contact of the microsphere with foods having a pH greater than 5.5 can dissolve the protective enteric shell.

Carcinogenesis, Mutagenesis, Impairment of Fertility

Long-term studies in animals have not been performed to evaluate carcinogenic potential. Methacrylic acid, a minor component of the methacrylic acid copolymer enteric-coating contained in ULTRASE® (pancrelipase) Capsules, has been reported to act as a teratogen in rat embryo cultures. However, the copolymer enteric-coating of ULTRASE® (pancrelipase) Capsules was not mutagenic by the Ames test, and it did not produce chromosome damage in a test for unscheduled DNA synthesis in rat hepatocytes.

Pregnancy: Category C.

Animal reproduction studies have not been conducted with ULTRASE® (pancrelipase) Capsules. It is not known whether ULTRASE® (pancrelipase) Capsules can cause fetal harm when administered to a pregnant woman or can affect reproduction capacity. ULTRASE® (pancrelipase) Capsules should be given to a pregnant woman only if the potential benefit outweighs the potential risk to the fetus.

Nursing Mothers

It is not known whether ULTRASE® (pancrelipase) is excreted in human milk. Because many drugs are excreted in human milk, caution should be exercised when ULTRASE® (pancrelipase) Capsules are administered to a nursing mother.

ADVERSE REACTIONS

The most frequently reported adverse reactions to products containing pancrelipase are gastrointestinal in nature. Less frequently, allergic-type reactions have also been observed. Extremely high doses of exogenous pancreatic enzymes have been associated with hyperuricosuria and hyperuricemia when the preparations given were pancrelipase in powdered or capsule form, or pancreatin in tablet form.

Colonic strictures have been reported in cystic fibrosis patients treated with both high- and lower-strength enzyme supplements.[10] A causal relationship has not been established. The possibility of bowel stricture should be considered if symptoms suggestive of gastrointestinal obstruction occur. Since impaired fluid secretion may be a factor in the development of intestinal obstruction, care should be taken to maintain adequate hydration, particularly in warm weather.[11]

"Fibrosing colonopathy" is a term used to describe a condition seen in patients with CF who have taken high amounts of pancreatic enzyme supplements (>6,000 lipase U/kg/meal). At its most advanced, this condition leads to colonic strictures.

1. In whom should one consider the diagnosis of fibrosing colonopathy?

a. Patients with cystic fibrosis who have evidence of partial or complete obstruction, bloody diarrhea or chylous ascites.

b. Patients who have two of the following three symptoms:
- abdominal pain
- ongoing diarrhea
- poor weight gain

ESPECIALLY if they have:
- taken >6,000 lipase U/kg/meal
- age less than twelve years
- history of meconium ileus
- prior intestinal surgery
- history of recurrent DIOS
- "inflammatory bowel disease"[12]

DOSAGE AND ADMINISTRATION

The enzymatic activity of ULTRASE® (pancrelipase) Capsules is expressed in U.S.P. units. The smallest effective dose should be used. Dosage should be adjusted according to the severity of the exocrine pancreatic insufficiency. Begin therapy with one or two capsules with meals or snacks and adjust dosage according to symptoms.

The number of capsules or capsule strength given with meals and/or snacks should be estimated by assessing which dose minimizes steatorrhea and maintains good nutritional status. Dosages should be adjusted according to the response of the patient. Where swallowing of capsules is difficult, they may be opened and the microspheres added to a small quantity of a soft food (e.g. applesauce, gelatin, etc.) that does not require chewing, and swallowed immediately.

It is recommended that the total dose of pancrelipase being ingested for a meal or snack be dispersed equally (with fluids) before, during, and after the meal or snack.

SUGGESTION FOR THE USE OF PANCREATIC ENZYMES IN CYSTIC FIBROSIS [12]

1. Patients should be receiving optimal diet for age and clinical status, recognizing that those with failure to thrive or malnutrition require additional calories and other nutrients for catch-up growth.
2. Nutrition assessment should be a part of routine clinical evaluations.
3. Initial dosing of pancreatic enzyme supplements should begin with 500 lipase U/kg/meal using enteric-coated microsphere products.
4. Patients should be reassessed 2–4 weeks after initiation of therapy. The following items should be assessed:
   Clinical status, e.g. abdominal symptoms and exam;
   Nutritional intake and growth (height, weight, head circumference);
   Character of stools—greasy, oily (for information, not for decision making);
   Quantitative 72-hour fecal fat when indicated but not less than annually (perform on a normal diet for age);
   Fat soluble vitamin measures.
5. Corollaries to dosing suggestions:
   a. Dose may be altered in a stepwise fashion according to the response of the patient (see 4. above).
   b. Dose approaching 2,000 lipase U/kg/meal would indicate the need for further investigation (see below). Patients presently on higher doses should be reevaluated; either immediately decrease the dose or titrate down to a lower dose range at, or below, 2,000 lipase U/kg/meal. Doses >6,000 lipase U/kg/meal have been associated with colonic strictures.
   c. Pancreatic supplements mixed with applesauce or other acidic food substances should be administered immediately, not stored.
   d. Enteric-coated microspheres should not be crushed.
   e. Enzyme doses (as lipase U/kg/meal) tend to decrease with advancing age.
   f. Patients should accept only product brands prescribed by their physician.
   g. Adjustment of dosage is the responsibility of the physician. Patients should be advised not to adjust doses without consulting their physician. Changes in product or dosage may require an adjustment period.
   h. Complaints transmitted by phone should be investigated thoroughly before dose is adjusted. If indicated, this investigation should include 72-hour fecal fat testing.
   i. Pancreatic supplements should be stored in a cool, dry place and checked regularly for expiration date.

HOW SUPPLIED

ULTRASE ® (pancrelipase) Capsules

Gelatin capsules (opaque white and opaque white), imprinted "ULTRASE". Bottles of 100 (NDC 58914-045-10).

Store at controlled room temperature, between 15°C and 25°C (59°F and 77°F), in a dry place. Do not refrigerate.

REFERENCES

1. Delchier JC, Vidon N. *et al.* Fate of orally ingested enzymes in pancreatic insufficiency: comparison of two pancreatic enzyme preparations. *Aliment Pharmacol Therap.* 1991;5:365-378.
2. Duhamel JP, Vidailhet M, *et al.* Étude multicentrique comparative d'une nouvelle présentation de pancréatine en microgranules gastrorésistants dans l'insuffisance pancréatique exocrine de la mucoviscidose chez l'enfant. *Ann Pediatr.* 1988;35:69-74.
3. Dutta SK, Tilley DK. The pH-sensitive enteric-coated pancreatic enzyme preparations: an evaluation of therapeutic efficacy in adult patients with pancreatic insufficiency. *J Clin Gastroenterol.* 1983;5:51-54.
4. Dutta SK, Rubin J, Harvey J. Comparative evaluation of the therapeutic efficacy of a pH-sensitive enteric-coated pancreatic enzyme preparation with conventional pancreatic enzyme therapy in the treatment of exocrine pancreatic insufficiency. *Gastroenterol.* 1983;84:476-482.
5. Gouerou H, Dain MP, *et al.* Alipase versus nonenteric-coated enzymes in pancreatic insufficiency. *Int J Pancreatol.* 1989;5:45-50.
6. Mischler EH, Parrell S, *et al.* Comparison of effectiveness of pancreatic enzyme preparations in cystic fibrosis. *Am J Dis Child:* 1982;136:1060-1063.
7. Salen G, Prakash A. Evaluation of enteric-coated microspheres for enzyme replacement therapy in adults with pancreatic insufficiency. *Cur Ther Res.* 1979;25:650-656.

8. Schneider MU, Knoll-Ruzicka ML, *et al.* Pancreatic enzyme replacement therapy: comparative effects of conventional and enteric-coated microspheric pancreatin and acid-stable fungal enzyme preparations on steatorrhea in chronic pancreatitis. *Hepatogastroenterol.* 1985;32:97-102.
9. Halgreen H, Thorsgaard Pedersen N, Worning H. Symptomatic effect of pancreatic enzyme therapy in patients with chronic pancreatitis. *Scand J Gastroenterol.* 1986;21:104-108.
10. Smyth RL, van Velzen D, *et al.* Strictures of ascending colon in cystic fibrosis and high-strength pancreatic enzymes. *The Lancet.* 1994;343:85-86.
11. Lands L, Zinman R, *et al.* Pancreatic function testing in meconium disease in CF: two case reports. *J Ped Gastroenterol and Nut.* 1988;7:276-279.
12. Cystic Fibrosis Foundation Conference on Pancreatic Enzyme Supplementation in the Context of Fibrosing Colonopathy; Washington, D.C., March 23-24, 1995.

Marketed as ULTRASE® by:
Axcan Scandipharm Inc.
22 Inverness Center Parkway
Birmingham, AL 35242
U.S.A.
Rx only
Rev. 4/00. Printed in U.S.A.
ULTRASE® is a registered trademark of Axcan Scandipharm Inc. Manufactured by Eurand International, Milan, Italy, using its DIFFUCAPS® technology for Axcan Scandipharm Inc.

Shown in Product Identification Guide, page 307

ULTRASE® MT ℞

[ul 'trāce]
(pancrelipase) Capsules
Enteric-Coated Minitablets

Prescribing Information

DESCRIPTION

ULTRASE® MT (pancrelipase) Capsules are orally administered capsules containing enteric-coated minitablets of porcine pancreatic enzyme concentrate, predominantly pancreatic lipase, amylase, and protease.

Each ULTRASE ® MT12 Capsule contains:

Lipase	12,000 U.S.P. Units
Amylase	39,000 U.S.P. Units
Protease	39,000 U.S.P. Units

Each ULTRASE ® MT18 Capsule contains:

Lipase	18,000 U.S.P. Units
Amylase	58,500 U.S.P. Units
Protease	58,500 U.S.P. Units

Each ULTRASE ® MT20 Capsule contains:

Lipase	20,000 U.S.P. Units
Amylase	65,000 U.S.P. Units
Protease	65,000 U.S.P. Units

ULTRASE® MT (pancrelipase) Capsules contain an amount of pancrelipase equivalent to but not more than 125% of the labeled lipase activity expressed in U.S.P. Units.

Inactive ingredients: hydrogenated castor oil, silicon dioxide, sodium carboxymethylcellulose, magnesium stearate, microcrystalline cellulose, methacrylic acid copolymer (Type C), talc, simethicone, triethyl citrate, iron oxides and titanium oxide.

CLINICAL PHARMACOLOGY

ULTRASE® MT (pancrelipase) Capsules are designed to prevent inactivation by gastric acid thereby resulting in the delivery of high levels of biologically active enzymes into the duodenum. The enzymes catalyze the hydrolysis of fats into glycerol and fatty acids, starch into dextrins and sugars, and protein into proteoses and derived substances.

INDICATIONS AND USAGE

ULTRASE® MT (pancrelipase) Capsules are indicated for patients with partial or complete exocrine pancreatic insufficiency caused by:

- Cystic fibrosis (CF)
- Chronic pancreatitis due to alcohol use or other causes
- Surgery (pancreatico-duodenectomy or Whipple's procedure, with or without Wirsung duct injection, total pancreatectomy)
- Obstruction (pancreatic and biliary duct lithiasis, pancreatic and duodenal neoplasms, ductal stenosis)
- Other pancreatic disease (hereditary, post traumatic and allograft pancreatitis, hemochromatosis, Shwachman's Syndrome, lipomatosis, hyperparathyroidism)
- Poor mixing (Billroth II gastrectomy, other types of gastric bypass surgery, gastrinoma)

Pancrelipase capsules are effective in controlling steatorrhea.[1–9]

CONTRAINDICATIONS

Pancrelipase capsules are contraindicated in patients known to be hypersensitive to pork protein. Pancrelipase capsules are contraindicated in patients with acute pancreatitis or with acute exacerbations of chronic pancreatic diseases.

WARNINGS

Should hypersensitivity occur, discontinue medication and treat symptomatically.

PRECAUTIONS

General

TO PROTECT ENTERIC COATING, MINITABLETS MUST NOT BE CRUSHED OR CHEWED. Where swallowing of capsules is difficult, they may be opened and the minitablets added to a small quantity of a soft food (e.g. applesauce, gelatin, etc.) that does not require chewing, and swallowed immediately. Contact of the minitablet with foods having a pH greater than 5.5 can dissolve the protective enteric shell.

Carcinogenesis, Mutagenesis, Impairment of Fertility

Long-term studies in animals have not been performed to evaluate carcinogenic potential. Methacrylic acid, a minor component of the methacrylic acid copolymer enteric-coating contained in ULTRASE® MT (pancrelipase) Capsules, has been reported to act as a teratogen in rat embryo cultures. However, ULTRASE® MT (pancrelipase) Capsules have been shown to contain <0.001% of methacrylic acid, and the mammalian teratology studies in the rat and rabbit were negative.

The copolymer enteric-coating of ULTRASE® MT (pancrelipase) Capsules was not mutagenic by the Ames test, and it did not produce chromosome damage in a test for unscheduled DNA synthesis in rat hepatocytes.

Pregnancy : Category C.

Animal reproduction studies have not been conducted with ULTRASE® MT (pancrelipase) Capsules. It is not known whether ULTRASE® MT (pancrelipase) Capsules can cause fetal harm when administered to a pregnant woman or can affect reproduction capacity. ULTRASE® MT (pancrelipase) Capsules should be given to a pregnant woman only if the potential benefit outweighs the potential risk to the fetus.

Nursing Mothers

It is not known whether ULTRASE® MT (pancrelipase) is excreted in human milk. Because many drugs are excreted in human milk, caution should be exercised when ULTRASE® MT (pancrelipase) Capsules are administered to a nursing mother.

ADVERSE REACTIONS

The most frequently reported adverse reactions to products containing pancrelipase are gastrointestinal in nature. Less frequently, allergic-type reactions have also been observed. Extremely high doses of exogenous pancreatic enzymes have been associated with hyperuricosuria and hyperuricemia when the preparations given were pancrelipase in powdered or capsule form, or pancreatin in tablet form.

In two clinical studies with ULTRASE® MT in 193 patients with cystic fibrosis, the adverse events described were all gastrointestinal in nature and may actually represent symptoms of the underlying disease, such as abdominal pain/cramps (5.7%), diarrhea (3.6%), and greasy stools and flatulence (1.5% each). In a postmarketing trial with another enteric-coated formulation, 160 adverse events occurred in the 15,711 patients (0.97%) evaluated.[10] The most frequent events reported were diarrhea, skin reaction, and abdominal discomfort (0.2% each).

Colonic strictures have been reported in cystic fibrosis patients treated with both high- and lower-strength enzyme supplements.[11] A causal relationship has not been established. The possibility of bowel stricture should be considered if symptoms suggestive of gastrointestinal obstruction occur. Since impaired fluid secretion may be a factor in the development of intestinal obstruction, care should be taken to maintain adequate hydration, particularly in warm weather.[12]

"Fibrosing colonopathy" is a term used to describe a condition seen in patients with CF who have taken high amounts of pancreatic enzyme supplements (>6,000 lipase U/kg/meal). At its most advanced, this condition leads to colonic strictures.

1. In whom should one consider the diagnosis of fibrosing colonopathy?

a. Patients with cystic fibrosis who have evidence of partial or complete obstruction, bloody diarrhea or chylous ascites.

b. Patients who have two of the following three symptoms:
- abdominal pain
- ongoing diarrhea
- poor weight gain

ESPECIALLY if they have:
- taken >6,000 lipase U/kg/meal
- age less than twelve years
- history of meconium ileus
- prior intestinal surgery
- history of recurrent DIOS
- "inflammatory bowel disease"[13]

DOSAGE AND ADMINISTRATION

The enzymatic activity of ULTRASE® MT (pancrelipase) Capsules is expressed in U.S.P. units. Each capsule contains the labeled amount of lipase activity and an overage of not more than 25%.

The smallest effective dose should be used. Dosage should be adjusted according to the severity of the exocrine pancreatic insufficiency. Begin therapy with one or two capsules with meals or snacks and adjust dosage according to symptoms. The number of capsules or capsule strength given with meals and/or snacks should be estimated by assessing which dose minimizes steatorrhea and maintains good nutritional status. Dosages should be adjusted according to the response of the patient. Where swallowing of capsules is difficult, they may be opened and the minitablets added to a small quantity of a soft food (e.g. applesauce, gelatin, etc.) that does not require chewing, and swallowed immediately. It is recommended that the total dose of pancrelipase being ingested for a meal or snack be dispersed equally (with fluids) before, during, and after the meal or snack.

SUGGESTIONS FOR THE USE OF PANCREATIC ENZYMES IN CYSTIC FIBROSIS[13]

1. Patients should be receiving optimal diet for age and clinical status, recognizing that those with failure to thrive or malnutrition require additional calories and other nutrients for catch-up growth.
2. Nutrition assessment should be a part of routine clinical evaluations.
3. Initial dosing of pancreatic enzyme supplements should begin with 500 lipase U/kg/meal using enteric-coated minitablet products.
4. Patients should be reassessed 2–4 weeks after initiation of therapy.
   The following items should be assessed:
   Clinical status, e.g. abdominal symptoms and exam;
   Nutritional intake and growth (height, weight, head circumference);
   Character of stools—greasy, oily (for information, not for decision making);
   Quantitative 72-hour fecal fat when indicated but not less than annually (perform on a normal diet for age);
   Fat soluble vitamin measures.
5. Corollaries to dosing suggestions:
   a. Dose may be altered in a stepwise fashion according to the response of the patient (see 4. above).
   b. Dose approaching 2,000 lipase U/kg/meal would indicate the need for further investigation (see below). Patients presently on higher doses should be reevaluated; either immediately decrease the dose or titrate down to a lower dose range at, or below, 2,000 lipase U/kg/meal. Doses >6,000 lipase U/kg/meal have been associated with colonic strictures.
   c. Pancreatic supplements mixed with applesauce or other acidic food substances should be administered immediately, not stored.
   d. Enteric-coated minitablets should not be crushed.
   e. Enzyme doses (as lipase U/kg/meal) tend to decrease with advancing age.
   f. Patient should accept only product brands prescribed by their physician.
   g. Adjustment of dosage is the responsibility of the physician. Patients should be advised not to adjust doses without consulting their physician. Changes in product or dosage may require an adjustment period.
   h. Complaints transmitted by phone should be investigated thoroughly before dose is adjusted. If indicated, this investigation should include 72-hour fecal fat testing.
   i. Pancreatic supplements should be stored in a cool, dry place and checked regularly for expiration date.

HOW SUPPLIED

ULTRASE ® MT12 (pancrelipase) Capsules
Gelatin capsules (white and yellow), imprinted "ULTRASE MT12". Bottles of 100 (NDC 58914-002-10).

ULTRASE ® MT18 (pancrelipase) Capsules
Gelatin capsules (gray and white), imprinted "ULTRASE MT18". Bottles of 100 (NDC 58914-018-10).

ULTRASE ® MT20 (pancrelipase) Capsules
Gelatin capsules (light gray and yellow), imprinted "ULTRASE MT20". Bottles of 100 (NDC 58914-004-10), and bottles of 500 (NDC 58914-004-50).

Store at controlled room temperature, between 15°C and 25°C (59°F and 77°F), in a dry place. Do not refrigerate.

REFERENCES

1. Delchier JC, Vidon N, *et al.* Fate of orally ingested enzymes in pancreatic insufficiency: comparison of two pancreatic enzyme preparations. *Aliment Pharmacol Therap.* 1991;5:365–378.
2. Duhamel JP, Vidailhet M, *et al.* Étude multicentrique comparative d'une nouvelle présentation de pancréatine en microgranules gastrorésistants dans l'insuffisance pancréatique exocrine de la mucoviscidose chez l'enfant. *Ann Pediatr.* 1988;35:69–74.
3. Dutta SK, Tilley DK. The pH-sensitive enteric-coated pancreatic enzyme preparations: an evaluation of therapeutic efficacy in adult patients with pancreatic insufficiency. *J Clin Gastroenterol.* 1983;5:51–54.
4. Dutta SK, Rubin J, Harvey J. Comparative evaluation of the therapeutic efficacy of a pH-sensitive enteric-coated pancreatic enzyme preparation with conventional pancreatic enzyme therapy in the treatment of exocrine pancreatic insufficiency. *Gastroenterol.* 1983;84:476–482.
5. Gouerou H, Dain MP, *et al.* Alipase versus nonenteric-coated enzymes in pancreatic insufficiency. *Int J Pancreatol.* 1989;5:45–50.
6. Mischler EH, Parrell S, *et al.* Comparison of effectiveness of pancreatic enzyme preparations in cystic fibrosis. *Am J Dis Child.* 1982;136:1060–1063.
7. Salen G, Prakash A. Evaluation of enteric-coated microspheres for enzyme replacement therapy in adults with pancreatic insufficiency. *Cur Ther Res.* 1979;25: 650–656.
8. Schneider MU, Knoll-Ruzicka ML, *et al.* Pancreatic enzyme replacement therapy: comparative effects of

Continued on next page

Ultrase MT—Cont.

conventional and enteric-coated microspheric pancreatin and acid-stable fungal enzyme preparations on steatorrhea in chronic pancreatitis. *Hepatogastroenterol.* 1985;32:97–102.

9. Halgreen H, Thorsgaard Pedersen N, Worning H. Symptomatic effect of pancreatic enzyme therapy in patients with chronic pancreatitis. *Scand J Gastroenterol.* 1986;21:104–108.
10. Gretzmacher I, Rüther HG. Maldigestion. *Therapiewoche.* 1983;33:6776–6782.
11. Smyth RL, van Velzen D, *et al.* Strictures of ascending colon in cystic fibrosis and high-strength pancreatic enzymes. *The Lancet.* 1994;343:85–86.
12. Lands L, Zinman R, *et al.* Pancreatic function testing in meconium disease in CF: two case reports. *J Ped Gastroenterol and Nut.* 1988;7:276–279.
13. Cystic Fibrosis Foundation Conference on Pancreatic Enzyme Supplementation in the Context of Fibrosing Colonopathy; Washington, D.C., March 23–24, 1995.

Marketed as ULTRASE® MT by:

Axcan Scandipharm Inc.
22 Inverness Center Parkway
Birmingham, AL 35242
U.S.A.

Rx only

Rev. 4/00. Printed in U.S.A.

ULTRASE® is a registered trademark of Axcan Scandipharm Inc. Manufactured by Eurand International, Milan, Italy, using its EURAND MINITABS® technology for Axcan Scandipharm Inc.

Shown in Product Identification Guide, page 307

URSO® ℞

[*ūr-so*]
Ursodiol Tablets 250 mg
Rx only

DESCRIPTION

URSO® is a bile acid available as 250 mg film-coated tablets for oral administration.

URSO® is ursodiol (ursodeoxycholic acid), a naturally occurring bile acid found in small quantities in normal human bile and in larger quantities in the biles of certain species of bears. It is a bitter-tasting white powder consisting of crystalline particles freely soluble in ethanol and glacial acetic acid, slightly soluble in chloroform, sparingly soluble in ether, and practically insoluble in water. The chemical name of ursodiol is 3α,7β-dihydroxy-5β-cholan-24-oic ($C_{24}H_{40}O_4$). Ursodiol has a molecular weight of 392.56. Its structure is shown below.

Inactive ingredients: microcrystalline cellulose, povidone, sodium starch glycolate, magnesium stearate, ethylcellulose, dibutyl sebacate, carnauba wax, hydroxypropyl methylcellulose, PEG 3350, PEG 8000, cetyl alcohol, sodium lauryl sulfate and hydrogen peroxide.

CLINICAL PHARMACOLOGY

Ursodiol (UDCA) is normally present as a minor fraction of the total bile acids in humans (about 5%). Following oral administration, the majority of ursodiol is absorbed by passive diffusion and its absorption is incomplete. Once absorbed, ursodiol undergoes hepatic extraction to the extent of about 50% in the absence of liver disease. As the severity of liver disease increases, the extent of extraction decreases. In the liver, ursodiol is conjugated with glycine or taurine, then secreted into bile. These conjugates of ursodiol are absorbed in the small intestine by passive and active mechanisms. The conjugates can also be deconjugated in the ileum by intestinal enzymes, leading to the formation of free ursodiol that can be reabsorbed and reconjugated in the liver. Nonabsorbed ursodiol passes into the colon where it is mostly 7-dehydroxylated to lithocholic acid. Some ursodiol is epimerized to chenodiol (CDCA) via a 7-oxo intermediate. Chenodiol also undergoes 7-dehydroxylation to form lithocholic acid. These metabolites are poorly soluble and excreted in the feces. A small portion of lithocholic acid is reabsorbed, conjugated in the liver with glycine, or taurine and sulfated at the 3 position. The resulting sulfated lithocholic acid conjugates are excreted in bile and then lost in feces.

Lithocholic acid, when administered chronically to animals, causes cholestatic liver injury that may lead to death from liver failure in certain species unable to form sulfate conjugates. Ursodiol is 7-dehydroxylated more slowly than chenodiol. For equimolar doses of ursodiol and chenodiol, steady state levels of lithocholic acid in biliary bile acids are lower during ursodiol administration than with chenodiol administration. Humans and chimpanzees can sulfate lithocholic acid. Although liver injury has not been associated with ursodiol therapy, a reduced capacity to sulfate may exist in some individuals. Nonetheless, such a deficiency has not yet been clearly demonstrated and must be extremely rare, given the several thousand patient-years of clinical experience with ursodiol.

In healthy subjects, at least 70% of ursodiol (unconjugated) is bound to plasma protein. No information is available on the binding of conjugated ursodiol to plasma protein in healthy subjects or primary biliary cirrhosis (PBC) patients. Its volume of distribution has not been determined, but is expected to be small since the drug is mostly distributed in the bile and small intestine. Ursodiol is excreted primarily in the feces. With treatment, urinary excretion increases, but remains less than 1% except in severe cholestatic liver disease.

During chronic administration of ursodiol, it becomes a major biliary and plasma bile acid. At a chronic dose of 13–15 mg/kg/day, ursodiol constitutes 30–50% of biliary and plasma bile acids.

CLINICAL STUDIES

A U.S., multicenter, randomized, double-blind, placebo-controlled study was conducted to evaluate the efficacy of ursodeoxycholic acid at a dose of 13–15 mg/kg/day, administered in 4 divided doses in 180 patients with PBC. Upon completion of the double-blind portion, all patients entered an open-label active treatment extension phase.

Treatment failure, the main efficacy end point measured during this study, was defined as death, need for liver transplantation, histologic progression by two stages or to cirrhosis, development of varices, ascites or encephalopathy, marked worsening of fatigue or pruritus, inability to tolerate the drug, doubling of serum bilirubin and voluntary withdrawal. After two years of double-blind treatment, the incidence of treatment failure was significantly reduced in the URSO® group (n=89) as compared to the placebo group (n=91). Time to treatment failure was also significantly delayed in the URSO® treated group regardless of either histologic stage or baseline bilirubin levels (>1.8 or ≤1.8 mg/dl).

Using a definition of treatment failure which excluded doubling of serum bilirubin and voluntary withdrawal, time to treatment failure was significantly delayed in the URSO® group. In comparison with placebo, treatment with URSO® resulted in a significant improvement in the following serum hepatic biochemistries when compared to baseline: total bilirubin, SGOT, alkaline phosphatase and IgM.

A second study conducted in Canada randomized 222 PBC patients to ursodiol, 14 mg/kg/day or placebo, in a double-blind manner during a two-year period. At two years, a statistically significant difference between the two treatments, in favor of ursodiol, was demonstrated in the following: reduction in the proportion of patients exhibiting a more than 50% increase in serum bilirubin; median percent decrease in bilirubin, transaminases and alkaline phosphatase; incidence of treatment failure; and time to treatment failure. The definition of treatment failure included: discontinuing the study for any reason; a total serum bilirubin level greater than or equal to 1.5 mg/dl or increasing to a level equal to or greater than two times the baseline level; and the development of ascites or encephalopathy.

INDICATIONS AND USAGE

URSO® (ursodiol) tablets are indicated for the treatment of patients with primary biliary cirrhosis.

CONTRAINDICATIONS

Hypersensitivity or intolerance to ursodiol or any of the components of the formulation.

PRECAUTIONS

Patients with variceal bleeding, hepatic encephalopathy, ascites or in need of an urgent liver transplant, should receive appropriate specific treatment.

Drug Interactions

Bile acid sequestering agents such as cholestyramine and colestipol may interfere with the action of **URSO®** by reducing its absorption. Aluminum-based antacids have been shown to adsorb bile acids *in vitro* and may be expected to interfere with **URSO®** in the same manner as the bile acid sequestering agents. Estrogens, oral contraceptives, and clofibrate (and perhaps other lipid-lowering drugs) increase hepatic cholesterol secretion, and encourage cholesterol gallstone formation and hence may counteract the effectiveness of **URSO®**.

Carcinogenicity, Mutagenicity and Impairment of Fertility

In two 24-month oral carcinogenicity studies in mice, ursodiol at doses up to 1,000 mg/kg/day (3,000 mg/m²/day) was not tumorigenic. Based on body surface area, for a 50 kg person of average height (1.46 m² body surface area), this dose represents 5.4 times the recommended maximum clinical dose of 15 mg/kg/day (555 mg/m²/day).

In a two-year oral carcinogenicity study in Fischer 344 rats, ursodiol at doses up to 300 mg/kg/day (1,800 mg/m²/day, 3.2 times the recommended maximum human dose based on body surface area) was not tumorigenic.

In a life-span (126–138 weeks) oral carcinogenicity study, Sprague-Dawley rats were treated with doses of 33 to 300 mg/kg/day, 0.4 to 3.2 times the recommended maximum human dose based on body surface area. Ursodiol produced a significantly ($p \leq 0.5$, Fisher's exact test) increased incidence of pheochromocytomas of the adrenal medulla in females of the highest dose group.

In 103-week oral carcinogenicity studies of lithocholic acid, a metabolite of ursodiol, doses up to 250 mg/kg/day in mice and 500 mg/kg/day in rats did not produce any tumors. In a 78-week rat study, intrarectal instillation of lithocholic acid (1 mg/kg/day) for 13 months did not produce colorectal tumors. A tumor-promoting effect was observed when it was administered after a single intrarectal dose of a known carcinogen N-methyl-N'-nitro-N-nitrosoguanidine. On the other hand, in a 32-week rat study, ursodiol at a daily dose of 240 mg/kg (1,440 mg/m², 2.6 times the maximum recommended human dose based on body surface area) suppressed the colonic carcinogenic effect of another known carcinogen azoxymethane.

Ursodiol was not genotoxic in the Ames test, the mouse lymphoma cell (L5178Y, $TK^{+/-}$) forward mutation test, the human lymphocyte sister chromatid exchange test, the mouse spermatogenia chromosome aberration test, the Chinese hamster micronucleus test and the Chinese hamster bone marrow cell chromosome aberration test.

Ursodiol at oral doses of up to 2,700 mg/kg/day (16,200 mg/m²/day, 29 times the recommended maximum human dose based on body surface area) was found to have no effect on fertility and reproductive performance of male and female rats.

Pregnancy, Teratogenic Effects. Pregnancy Category B

Teratology studies have been performed in pregnant rats at oral doses up to 2,000 mg/kg/day (12,000 mg/m²/day, 22 times the recommended maximum human dose based on body surface area) and in pregnant rabbits at oral doses up to 300 mg/kg/day (3,600 mg/m²/day, 7 times the recommended maximum human dose based on body surface area) and have revealed no evidence of impaired fertility or harm to the fetus due to ursodiol.

There are no adequate or well-controlled studies in pregnant women. Because animal reproduction studies are not always predictive of human response, this drug should be used during pregnancy only if clearly needed.

Nursing Mothers

It is not known whether ursodiol is excreted in human milk. Because many drugs are excreted in human milk, caution should be exercised when **URSO®** is administered to a nursing mother.

Pediatric Use

The safety and effectiveness of **URSO®** in pediatric patients have not been established.

[See table at left]

ADVERSE EVENTS (AEs)

ADVERSE EVENTS	*VISIT AT 12 MONTHS*		*VISIT AT 24 MONTHS*	
	UDCA n (%)	Placebo n (%)	UDCA n (%)	Placebo n (%)
Diarrhea	—	—	1 (1.32)	—
Elevated creatinine	—	—	1 (1.32)	—
Elevated blood glucose	1 (1.18)	—	1 (1.32)	—
Leukopenia	—	—	2 (2.63)	—
Peptic ulcer	—	—	1 (1.32)	—
Skin rash	—	—	2 (2.63)	—

Note: Those AEs occurring at the same or higher incidence in the placebo as in the UDCA group have been deleted from this table (this includes diarrhea and thrombocytopenia at 12 months, nausea/vomiting, fever and other toxicity).

UDCA = Ursodeoxycholic acid = Ursodiol

Adverse events are reported regardless of attribution to the test medication.

OVERDOSE

Accidental or intentional overdosage with ursodiol has not been reported. The most severe manifestation of overdosage would likely consist of diarrhea which should be treated symptomatically.

Single oral doses of ursodiol at 10, 5 and 10 g/kg in mice, rats and dogs, respectively were not lethal. A single oral dose of ursodiol at 1.5 g/kg was lethal in hamsters. Symptoms of acute toxicity were salivation and vomiting in dogs, and ataxia, dyspnea, ptosis, agonal convulsions and coma in hamsters.

DOSAGE AND ADMINISTRATION

The recommended adult dosage for **URSO®** in the treatment of PBC is 13–15 mg/kg/day administered in four divided doses with food.

HOW SUPPLIED

Each URSO® film-coated tablet, white, engraved with "URS785", contains 250 mg of ursodiol. Available in bottles of 500 tablets (NDC 58914-785-50) and in bottles of 100's (NDC 58914-785-10). Store at 20°C to 25°C (68°F to 77°F). Dispense in a tight container.

Caution: Federal law prohibits dispensing without a prescription.

Manufactured by:
GLOBAL PHARM INC.
Toronto, Ontario M3B 1Y5
Canada
for:
Axcan Scandipharm, Inc.
Birmingham, AL 35242
USA
®Reg. TM of Axcan Pharma US Inc., used under license by Axcan Scandipharm Inc.
April 2000

Shown in Product Identification Guide, page 307

VIOKASE® ℞

[*vī'ō-kās*]
Pancrelipase, USP
Tablets, Powder
Rx only

For product information please call 1-800-742-6706.

DESCRIPTION

VIOKASE® (pancrelipase, USP) is a pancreatic enzyme concentrate of porcine origin containing standardized lipase, protease, and amylase as well as other pancreatic enzymes. VIOKASE® is available in tablet and powder dosage form for oral administration.

The enzyme potencies of the tablets and powder are:
[See first table below]

Inactive Ingredients: VIOKASE® 8 Tablet: Lactose, magnesium stearate, sodium chloride, stearic acid.
VIOKASE® 16 Tablet: Lactose, croscarmellose sodium, microcrystalline cellulose, silicon dioxide, stearic acid, talc.
Powder: Lactose, sodium chloride.

CLINICAL PHARMACOLOGY

The natural digestive enzymes in VIOKASE® hydrolyze fats into fatty acids and glycerol, split protein into amino acids, and convert carbohydrates to dextrins and short chain sugars.

Under conditions of the USP test method (in vitro) VIOKASE® has the following total digestive capacity.
[See second table below]

VIOKASE® 8 and 16 Tablets are immediate release and are not enteric coated.

The digestive capacity of a pancreatic enzyme concentrate depends on the amount that passes through the stomach unchanged and is available at the site of action in the small intestine.

INDICATIONS

VIOKASE® (Pancrelipase, USP) is indicated in the treatment of exocrine pancreatic insufficiency as associated with but not limited to cystic fibrosis, chronic pancreatitis, pancreatectomy, or obstruction of the pancreas ducts.

CONTRAINDICATIONS

Should not be used in patients hypersensitive to pork protein.

PRECAUTIONS

General: Individuals previously sensitized to trypsin, pancreatin or pancrelipase may have allergic manifestations.

Information for Patients: VIOKASE® should not be held in the mouth as the proteolytic action may cause irritation of the mucosa.

Avoid inhalation of the powder when administering VIOKASE®.

Carcinogenesis, Mutagenesis: Long-term studies in animals have not been performed to evaluate the carcinogenic potential.

Pregnancy Category C: Animal reproduction studies have not been conducted with VIOKASE®. It is also not known whether VIOKASE® can cause fetal harm when administered to a pregnant woman or can affect reproduction capacity. VIOKASE® should be given to a pregnant woman only if clearly needed.

Nursing Mothers: It is not known whether this drug is excreted in human milk. Because many drugs are excreted in human milk, caution should be exercised when pancrelipase is administered to a nursing mother.

ADVERSE EFFECTS

The dust or finely powdered pancreatic enzyme concentrate is irritating to the nasal mucosa and the respiratory tract. It has been documented that inhalation of the airborne powder can precipitate an asthma attack. The literature also contains several references to asthma due to inhalation in patients sensitized to pancreatic enzyme concentrates. Extremely high doses of exogenous pancreatic enzymes have been associated with hyperuricemia and hyperuricosuria. Overdosage of pancreatic enzyme concentrate may cause diarrhea or transient intestinal upset.

OVERDOSE

Acute toxicity determinations in animals have not been possible since the maximum dose that could be given orally produced no toxic reaction. In chronic feeding tests rats developed swollen salivary glands. This is believed due to the proteolytic activity and the mucosal irritation caused by tissue digestion.

No acute toxic reactions have been reported.

DOSAGE AND ADMINISTRATION

Powder: Dosage for patients with cystic fibrosis: 1/4 teaspoonful (0.7g) with meals.

Tablets: Dosage range for patients with cystic fibrosis or chronic pancreatitis is from 8,000 to 32,000 Lipase USP Units taken with meals, i.e., one to four VIOKASE® 8 tablets or one to two VIOKASE® 16 with meals or as directed by a physician.

In patients with pancreatectomy or obstruction of pancreatic ducts: one to two VIOKASE® 8 tablets or one VIOKASE® 16 tablet taken at 2-hour intervals or as directed by a physician.

HOW SUPPLIED

VIOKASE® 8 Tablets: Tan, round, compressed tablets engraved VIOKASE® on one side and 9111 on the other side in bottles of 100 (NDC 58914-111-10) and 500 (NDC 58914-111-50).

VIOKASE® 16 Tablets: Tan, oval, biconvex tablets engraved V^{16} on one side and 9116 on the other side in bottles of 100 (NDC 58914-116-10) and 500 (NDC 58914-116-50).

Powder: Tan powder in bottles of 8 oz (227 g) (NDC 58914-115-08).

Store in tightly closed container in a dry place at a temperature not exceeding 25°C (77°F).

Dispense tablets and powder in tight container, preferably with a desiccant.

REFERENCES

1. Regan PT, Malagelada J-R, DiMagno EP, Gianzman SL, Go VLW. Comparative effects of antacids, cimetidine and enteric coating on the therapeutic response to oral enzymes in severe pancreatic insufficiency. N Engl J Med 1997;297:854–8.
2. Graham DY. Enzyme replacement therapy of exocrine pancreatic insufficiency in man. N Eng J Med 1977;296:1314–7.

® Reg. TM of Axcan Pharma US Inc.,
used under license by
Axcan Scandipharm Inc.

Rev. April 2000

Manufactured for:
Axcan Scandipharm Inc.
Birmingham, AL 35242

Shown in Product Identification Guide, page 307

For information on over-the-counter drugs, consult **PDR For Nonprescription Drugs.**

	VIOKASE® 8 Tablet	VIOKASE® 16 Tablet	Each 0.7 g Powder (1/4 Teaspoonful)
Lipase, USP units	8,000	16,000	16,800
Protease, USP units	30,000	60,000	70,000
Amylase, USP units	30,000	60,000	70,000

	VIOKASE® 8 Tablet	VIOKASE® 16 Tablet	Each 0.7 g Powder (1/4 Teaspoonful)
Dietary fat, grams	28	56	59
Dietary protein, grams	30	60	70
Dietary starch, grams	30	60	70

Ayerst Laboratories Inc.

A Wyeth-Ayerst Company

See listing under Wyeth-Ayerst Laboratories for prescription products and Whitehall-Robins for nonprescription products.

Baxter Healthcare Corporation

Hyland Division
550 NORTH BRAND BLVD.
GLENDALE, CA 91203

Direct Inquiries to:
Product Management
(800) 423-2090

For Medical Information Contact:
In Emergencies:
Edward Gomperts, M.D.
Medical Director,
Baxter Healthcare Corporation:
(818) 956-3200

ALBUMIN (HUMAN) 5% SOLUTION ℞

DESCRIPTION

Albumin (Human) 5% is a sterile aqueous solution for intravenous use containing the albumin component human plasma. The solution is approximately isotonic and isooncotic with human plasma. The effective oncotic pressure of the solution depends largely on its albumin content. Sodium bicarbonate is used to adjust the pH to 6.9 ± 0.5. The sodium content of the solution ranges between 130 and 160 meq/L. 0.08 millimole sodium caprylate/g albumin and 0.08 millimole sodium N- acetyltryptophanate/g albumin are added as stabilizers to prevent denaturation during heating. The solution has been heat-treated at 60°C for 10 hours for inactivation of hepatitis viruses.

CLINICAL PHARMACOLOGY

Albumin is a very soluble, globular protein (MW 66,500) accounting for 70–80% of the colloid osmotic pressure of plasma. Albumin (Human) 5% is an effective and long acting agent for plasma volume expansion. The rationale for this is the Starling concept of the capillary balance of hydrostatic and oncotic pressure gradients across the capillary walls as the determinant of the fluid-i.e., volume-distribution between the intravascular and interstitial compartments (10). Albumin is distributed throughout the extracellular water; more than 60% of the body albumin pool is located in the extravascular fluid compartment. The total body albumin in a 70 kg man is approximately 320 g. Albumin has a half life of 15–20 days in the circulation (2,7) with a turnover of approximately 15 g per day.

When injected intravenously, Albumin (Human) 5% will increase the circulating plasma volume by an amount approximately equal to the amount infused. The additional fluid will reduce the hemoconcentration and decrease blood viscosity. The degree and duration of volume expansion depend upon the initial blood volume. In patients with diminished blood volume, the effect of infused Albumin (Human) may persist many hours. The hemodilution lasts for a much shorter time when albumin is administered to individuals with normal blood volume.

Albumin is a transport protein which binds naturally occurring therapeutic and toxic materials in the circulation. The binding properties of albumin may, in special circumstances, provide an indication for its clinical use. For such purposes, however, Albumin (Human) 25% should be used.

INDICATIONS AND USAGE

Conditions For Which Albumin (Human) 5% Is Recommended:

Shock

The definitive treatment of major hemorrhage is the transfusion of red blood cells for restoring the normal oxygen transport capacity of the blood. Since, however, the life-threatening event in major hemorrhage is the loss of blood volume and not the erythrocyte deficit, the blood volume should, as an emergency measure, be supported by Albumin (Human) 5% or another rapidly acting plasma substitute if blood is not immediately available. This will restore cardiac output and abolish circulatory failure with tissue anoxia. In the presence of dehydration, electrolyte solutions such as Ringer's lactate should be administered in conjunction with Albumin (Human).

Burns

Apart from damage to the respiratory tract, the development of burn shock is the most life-threatening event in the immediate care of the burned patient. An optimum regimen for the use of Albumin (Human), electrolytes, and fluid in the treatment of burns has not been established. Therapy

Continued on next page

Albumin (Human) 5%—Cont.

during the first 24 hours after a severe burn is usually directed at the administration of large volumes of crystalloid solutions and lesser amounts of Albumin (Human) to maintain an adequate plasma volume. For continuation of therapy beyond 24 hours, larger amounts of Albumin (Human) and lesser amounts of crystalloid are generally used (12).

Conditions For Which Albumin (Human) 5% May Be Useful:

Pancreatitis and Peritonitis

Albumin (Human) 5% may be useful in the early therapy of shock associated with acute hemorrhagic pancreatitis and peritonitis. It has been found that the correction of the blood volume deficit and adequate fluid therapy are mandatory in the acute stage of pancreatitis and peritonitis when there is loss of fluid into the peritoneal cavity or the retroperitoneal space (1).

Conditions For Which Albumin (Human) 5% Is Usually Not Recommended:

Postoperative albumin loss

It is now recognized that intraoperative damage to capillary walls, e.g., by blunt handling and sharp dissection of tissue, leads to substantial postoperative losses of circulating albumin, over and above those due to bleeding. However, this internal redistribution rarely causes clinically significant hypovolemia or adversely affects wound healing, and treatment of this condition with Albumin (Human) 5% is usually not indicated.

Hypoproteinemia with an oncotic deficit

In subacute or chronic hypoproteinemia, efforts should always be made to determine the underlying cause and to improve circulating protein levels by dietary means. Most commonly, such states are due to protein-calorie malnutrition, defective absorption in gastrointestinal disorders, faulty albumin synthesis in chronic hepatic failure, increased protein catabolism after operation or in sepsis, and abnormal renal losses of albumin in chronic kidney disease. In all these situations, the circulating plasma volume is usually maintained by the renal retention of sodium and water, but this is associated with tissue edema due to the hypoalbuminemia and with an oncotic deficit. Though relief of the basic pathology is the definitive therapy for restoration of the plasma protein level, Albumin (Human) is effective in the rapid correction of an oncotic deficit occurring in the aforementioned acute complications of chronic hypoproteinemia. For this purpose, however, Albumin (Human) 25% is the preferable therapeutic agent, possibly in conjunction with a diuretic. It is emphasized that whereas Albumin (Human) may be needed to treat the acute complications of chronic hypoproteinemia, it is NOT indicated for treatment of the chronic disease itself.

CONTRAINDICATIONS

The use of Albumin (Human) is contraindicated in patients with a history of an incompatibility reaction to such preparations (see Adverse Reactions). In addition, the Albumin (Human) may be contraindicated in patients with cardiac failure, pulmonary edema or severe anemia because of the risk of acute circulatory overload. Also, Albumin (Human) has been reported to contain trace amounts of aluminum (4,5). Accumulations of aluminum in patients with chronic renal insufficiencies has led to toxic manifestations such as hypercalcemia, vitamin D-refractory osteodystrophy, anemia, and severe progressive encephalopathy (5,6,13). Therefore, when large volumes of Albumin (Human) are contemplated for administration to such patients, serious consideration of these potential risks relative to the anticipated benefits should be given.

WARNINGS

Albumin (Human) is made from human plasma. Products made from human plasma may contain infectious agents, such as viruses, that can cause disease. The risk that such products will transmit an infectious agent has been reduced by screening plasma donors for prior exposure to certain viruses, by testing for the presence of certain current virus infections, and by inactivating and/or removing certain viruses. Despite these measures, such products can still potentially transmit disease. There is also the possibility that unknown infectious agents may be present in such products. ALL infections thought by a physician possibly to have been transmitted by this product should be reported by the physician or other healthcare provider to our U.S. distributor at (800) 423-2862. The physician should discuss the risks and benefits of this product with the patient.

ALBUMIN (HUMAN) 5% MUST NOT BE USED IF THE SOLUTION IS TURBID.

ALBUMIN (HUMAN) 5% MUST BE INFUSED IMMEDIATELY AND WITHOUT INTERRUPTION AFTER PERFORATION OF THE R/C BOTTLE. DO NOT BEGIN ADMINISTRATION MORE THAN 4 HOURS AFTER THE CONTAINER HAS BEEN ENTERED. PARTIALLY USED BOTTLES MUST BE DISCARDED. ALBUMIN (HUMAN) 5% MUST NOT BE GIVEN THROUGH INFUSION SETS WHICH HAVE ALREADY BEEN USED OR ARE INTENDED FOR SIMULTANEOUS INFUSION OF PROTEIN HYDROSYLATE OR SOLUTIONS CONTAINING ALCOHOL.

PRECAUTIONS

Adequate precautions should be taken against circulatory overload; this can be done, for example, by measurement of the pulmonary wedge pressure. Special caution is indicated in patients with stabilized chronic anemia or renal insufficiency.

The rapid rise in blood pressure following infusion necessitates careful observation of injured or postoperative patients to detect and treat severed blood vessels that may not have bled at the lower blood pressure.

Certain components used in the packaging of this product contain natural rubber latex.

PREGNANCY CATEGORY C. Albumin (Human) 5% — Animal reproduction studies have not been conducted with Albumin (Human) 5%. It is also not known whether Albumin (Human) 5% can cause fetal harm when administered to a pregnant woman or can affect reproduction capacity. Albumin (Human) 5% should be given to a pregnant woman only if clearly needed.

ADVERSE REACTIONS

Though very rare, adverse reactions such as chills, fever, tachycardia, hypotension, urticaria, skin rash and nausea may occur (3,8,9,11). These symptoms may disappear if the infusion is slowed or stopped for a short period of time. If necessary, the intravenous administration of 50 to 200 mg of prednisolone may be useful (9).

DOSAGE AND ADMINISTRATION

Upon administration of Albumin (Human) 5% there is a rapid increase of the plasma volume about equal to the volume infused. The initial dose for adults is 250 to 500 mL. The quantity given may be increased to a total of 0.5 g albumin per pound of body weight (i.e., 10 mL/pound), but administration should be monitored by careful observation of the patient. The rate of infusion and the total volume administered are determined by the condition and the response of the patient. A rate of 1–2 mL per minute is usually suitable in the absence of overt shock, whereas the capacity of the administration set is the only limit in the exsanguinated patient. During resuscitation, constant monitoring of the patient provides the guidelines for treatment. For children, a dose of 10 to 15 mL per pound of body weight is usually adequate and close surveillance of the small patient is essential. In severely injured or septic patients, administration of Albumin (Human) 5% should always be guided by an appropriate hemodynamic monitoring of the patient.

Parenteral drug products should be inspected visually for particulate matter and discoloration prior to administration, whenever solution and container permit.

To prepare Albumin (Human) 5% for administration, remove outer seal to expose central portion of rubber stopper, cleanse stopper with germicidal solution and follow directions for use of intravenous injection set.

Albumin (Human) 5% must be administered INTRAVENOUSLY. The venipuncture site should not be infected or traumatized, and should be prepared with standard aseptic technique. The solution is compatible with whole blood or packed red blood cells as well as the usual electrolyte and carbohydrate solutions intended for intravenous use. By contrast, it should not be mixed with protein hydrolysates, amino acid mixtures, or solutions containing alcohol. It is ready for use as contained in the bottle and may be given without regard to the blood group of the recipient.

Only clear solutions of a light yellowish color should be administered.

HOW SUPPLIED

Puncture vial containing 50 mL of Albumin (Human) 5%.
Puncture vial containing 250 mL of Albumin (Human) 5%.
Puncture vial containing 500 mL of Albumin (Human) 5%.
The package may be supplied with an intravenous injection set.

STORAGE

Albumin (Human) 5% can be stored for 3 years at a temperature not exceeding 30°C (86°F).

Protect from freezing.

REFERENCES

1. CLOWES, G.H.A., Jr., VUCINIC, M., and WEIDNER, M.G.: Ann. Surg. 163, 866 (1996).
2. JANEWAY, C.A. In: Sgouris, J.T. and Rene A. (eds.): Proceedings of the Workshop on Albumin, DHEW Publication No. (NIH) 76–925, U.S. Government Printing Office, Washington, D.C., p. 3–21 (1976).
3. LOWENSTEIN, E. In: Sgouris, J.T. and Rene A. (eds.): Proceedings of the Workshop on Albumin, DHEW Publication No. (NIH) 76–925, U.S. Government Printing Office, Washington, D.C., p. 302 (1976).
4. MAHARAJ, D., FELL, G.S., BOYCE, B.F., NG, J.P., SMITHE, G.D., BOULTON-JONES, J.M., CUMMING, R.L., and DAVIDSON, J.F.: Brit. Med. J. 295, 693–696 (1987).
5. MILLINER, D.S., SHINABERGER, J.H., SHUMAN, P., and COBURN, J.W.: N. Engl. J. Med. 312, 165–167 (1985).
6. OTT, S.M., MALONEY, N.A., KLEIN, G.L., ALFREY, A.C., AMENT, M.E., COBURN, J.W., and SHERRAND, D.J.: Ann. of Inter. Med. 98, 910–914 (1983).
7. PETERS, T., Jr., In: Putnam, F.W. (ed.): Plasma Proteins, 2nd Edition, Vol. 1, Academic Press, New York, p. 133–181 (1975).
8. RING, J. and MESSMER, K.: Lancet 1, 466 (1977).
9. RING, J., SEIFERT, J., LOB, G., COULIN, K., and BRENDEL, W.: W. Klin, Wschr. 52, 595 (1974).
10. STARLING, E.H.: J. Physiol. (London) 19, 312 (1896).
11. TULLIS, J.L.: J.A.M.A. 237, 355 (1977).
12. TULLIS, J.L.: J.A.M.A. 237, 460 (1977).
13. WILLIS, M.R., and SAVORY, J.A.: Lancet 2, 29–34 (1983).

IMMUNO-U.S., INC.
1200 Parkdale Road
Rochester, MI 48307 USA
Distributed in Canada By:
IMMUNO (Canada) LTD.
U.S. License No. 850 Canadian License No. 227
Rev. April, 1998

ALBUMIN (HUMAN) 25% SOLUTION ℞

DESCRIPTION

Albumin (Human) 25% is a sterile aqueous solution for intravenous use, mainly containing the albumin component of human plasma. The effective oncotic pressure of the 25% solution largely depends on its albumin content and is approximately five times that of human plasma. Sodium bicarbonate is used to adjust the pH to 6.9 ± 0.5. The sodium content of the solution ranges between 130 and 160 meq/L. 0.08 millimole sodium caprylate and 0.08 millimole sodium N-acetyltryptophanate per gram albumin are added as stabilizers or prevent denaturation during heating. The solution is heat-treated at 60°C for 10 hours for inactivation of hepatitis viruses.

CLINICAL PHARMACOLOGY

Albumin is a very soluble, globular protein (MW 66,500) accounting for 70–80% of the colloid osmotic pressure of plasma which is the predominant reason for its clinical use. The rationale for this is the Starling concept of the capillary balance of hydrostatic and oncotic pressure gradients across the capillary walls as the determinant of the fluid - i.e., volume - distribution between the intravascular and the interstitial compartments (12). Albumin is distributed throughout the extracellular water; more than 60% of the body albumin pool is located in the extravascular fluid compartment. The total body albumin in a 70 kg man is approximately 320 g. Albumin has a half life of 15–20 days in the circulation (2,8), with a turnover of approximately 15 g per day.

When injected intravenously, Albumin (Human) 25% will draw approximately 3.5 times its volume of additional fluid into the circulation within 15 minutes, if the recipient is adequately hydrated. The additional fluid will reduce the hemoconcentration and decrease blood viscosity. The degree and duration of volume expansion depends upon the initial blood volume. In patients with diminished blood volume, the effect of infused Albumin (Human) may persist many hours. The hemodilution lasts for a much shorter time when Albumin (Human) is administered to individuals with normal blood volume. The minimum plasma albumin level necessary to prevent or reverse peripheral edema is unknown. Although it varies from patient to patient, there is some evidence that it is approximately 2.5 g/dL. This concentration provides a plasma oncotic pressure of 20 mm Hg (the equivalent of a total protein concentration of 5.2 g/dL).

Albumin is a transport protein which binds naturally occurring therapeutic and toxic materials in the circulation. The binding properties of albumin may provide an indication for its use in severe hemolytic disease of the newborn, where it may lower the plasma concentration of free bilirubin pending or in conjunction with an exchange transfusion (14). This effect may also be relevant in certain cases of acute liver failure with rapidly increasing levels of serum bilirubin, particularly in the presence of severe hypoproteinemia. Albumin (Human) 25% offers minimal risk of hemorrhagic diathesis or blockage of the reticuloendothelial system. It does not impair coagulation or platelet function. Antibodies, including isoagglutinins, have been removed, thus enabling the product to be used without regard to the patient's blood group or blood factors.

INDICATIONS AND USAGE

General Principles

The two main indications for the use of Albumin (Human) 25% - are a plasma or blood volume deficit and the oncotic deficit resulting from hypoproteinemia.

Volume Deficit

Since the oncotic pressure of Albumin (Human) 25% solution is about five times that of normal human serum, it will expand the plasma volume if interstitial water is available for an inflow through the capillary walls. However, many patients suffering from an acute volume deficit also have some degree of interstitial dehydration. If the absence of overhydration, the treatment of an acute volume deficit with Albumin (Human) 25% should, therefore, include isotonic electrolyte solutions with an albumin: electrolyte ratio of 1:3 or 1:4. By contrast, chronic volume deficits have usually been at least partially compensated for by the renal retention of sodium and water with some degree of tissue edema, and in these circumstances a trial with Albumin (Human) 25% only is indicated.

Oncotic Deficit

The common causes of hypoproteinemia are protein-calorie malnutrition, defective absorption in gastrointestinal disorders, faulty albumin synthesis (e.g., in chronic hepatic failure), increased protein catabolism after operation or in sepsis, and abnormal renal losses of albumin in chronic kidney disease. In these situations, the circulating plasma volume is usually maintained by the renal retention of sodium and water, but this is associated with tissue edema and an oncotic deficit. Though relief of the underlying pathology is the definitive therapy for the restoration of the plasma protein level, this process takes time to become effective and the rapid correction of an oncotic deficit by the administration of Albumin (Human) 25%, possibly in conjunction with a diuretic, may be indicated.

It is emphasized that whereas Albumin (Human) may be necessary to prevent or treat the aforementioned acute complication of hypoproteinemia, it is NOT indicated for treatment of the chronic condition itself.

SPECIFIC INDICATIONS

Acute Circumstances In Which Albumin (Human) 25% Use Is Usually Appropriate:

Shock

The definitive treatment of major hemorrhage is the transfusion of red blood cells restoring a normal oxygen transport capacity of the blood. However, the life-threatening event in major hemorrhage is the loss of blood volume and not the erythrocyte deficit. Therefore, the blood volume should, as an emergency measure, be supported by Albumin (Human) 5% or another rapidly acting plasma substitute if blood is not immediately available. This will restore cardiac output and abolish circulatory failure with tissue anoxia. If Albumin (Human) 5% is not available, Albumin (Human) 5% can be prepared by diluting Albumin (Human) 25% with 4 volumes of an appropriate electrolyte solution, such as Ringer's lactate. Alternatively, the two solutions may be administered concurrently. If the patient is severely dehydrated, additional electrolyte solutions may be required.

Burns

An optimal regimen for the use of Albumin (Human), electrolytes, and water in the treatment of burns has not been established. Therapy during the first 24 hours after a severe burn is usually directed at the administration of crystalloid solutions in order to maintain an adequate plasma volume. For continuation of therapy beyond 24 hours, larger amounts of Albumin (Human) and lesser amounts of crystalloid are generally used (14).

Adult Respiratory Distress Syndrome

Several factors are usually involved in the development of the state now commonly called the adult respiratory distress syndrome, one of these being a hypoproteinemic fluid overload. In its initial phase, this may be corrected by the use of Albumin (Human) 25% and a diuretic (11, 14) along with careful hemodynamic and respiratory monitoring of the patient. It must be recognized, however, that the beneficial effects of Albumin (Human) in this condition depend on the integrity of the pulmonary microvasculature. Increased permeability to albumin can negate these beneficial effects, and in such circumstances Albumin (Human) could actually contribute to the respiratory distress.

Cardiopulmonary Bypass

An adequate blood volume during cardiopulmonary bypass can be maintained with crystalloids or colloids (albumin). A commonly employed program is an Albumin (Human) and crystalloid pump prime adjusted so as to achieve a hematocrit of 20% and a plasma albumin level of 2.5 g/100 mL in the patient, but the level to which either may be lowered safely has not yet bet been defined (14).

Hemolytic Disease of the Newborn

Albumin (Human) 25% may be indicated in order to bind and thus detoxify free serum bilirubin in severely hemolytic infants pending an exchange transfusion (14). Caution is recommended in hypervolemic infants.

Acute Nephrosis

Patients with acute nephrosis may prove refractory to cyclophosphamide or steroid therapy and their edema may even be aggravated initially by steroids. In such cases, a response may be elicited by combining Albumin (Human) 25% with an appropriate diuretic, after which the patient may react satisfactorily to drug therapy (14).

Circumstances In Which Albumin (Human) 25% Is Usually Not Justified:

Postoperative Hypoproteinemia

Intraoperative damage of capillary walls, e.g., by blunt dissection, leads to substantial losses of circulating albumin over and above those due to bleeding. However, this redistribution of albumin in the body rarely causes clinically significant hypovolemia, and treatment of the resultant plasma oncotic defect with Albumin (Human) 25% is not usually indicated.

Red Cell Resuspension Media

As a rule, the use of Albumin (Human) for resuspending red cells can be dispensed with. However, in exceptional circumstances such as certain types of exchange transfusions and the use of very large volumes of erythrocyte concentrates and frozen or washed red cells, the addition of Albumin (Human) to the resuspension medium may be indicated in order to provide sufficient volume and/or avoid excessive hypoproteinemia during the subsequent transfusion. If necessary, 20–25 g or more of albumin per liter of red cells should be added as a concentrated solution to the isotonic electrolyte suspension of erythrocytes immediately before transfusion.

Renal Dialysis

Patients undergoing long-term hemodialysis may need Albumin (Human) for the treatment of a volume or an oncotic deficit. The patients should be carefully observed for signs of a circulatory overload to which they are particularly sensitive.

Acute Liver Failure

In acute liver failure, Albumin (Human) may serve the triple purpose of stabilizing the circulation, correcting an oncotic deficit and binding excessive serum bilirubin. The therapeutic approach is guided by the individual circumstances (14).

Ascites

The use of Albumin (Human) for blood volume support may be indicated if circulatory instability follows the withdrawal of large amounts (>1500 mL) of ascitic fluid.

Third Space Problems of Infectious Origin

The sequestration of protein-rich fluid during acute peritonitis, pancreatitis, mediastinitis or extensive cellulitis will very rarely be of sufficient magnitude to require the treatment of a volume of an oncotic deficit with Albumin (Human)(1).

There is no valid reason for the use of Albumin (Human) as an intravenous nutrient.

CONTRAINDICATIONS

The use of Albumin (Human) is contraindicated in patients with a history of an incompatibility reaction to such preparations (see Adverse Reactions). In addition, the Albumin (Human) may be contraindicated in patients with cardiac failure, pulmonary edema or severe anemia because of the risk of acute circulatory overload. Also, Albumin (Human) has been reported to contain trace amounts of aluminum (5,6). Accumulations of aluminum in patients with chronic renal insufficiencies has led to toxic manifestations such as hypercalcemia, vitamin D-refractory osteodystrophy, anemia, and severe progressive encephalopathy (6,7,15). Therefore, when large volumes of Albumin (Human) are contemplated for administration to such patients, serious consideration of these potential risks relative to the anticipated benefits should be given.

WARNINGS

Albumin (Human) is made from human plasma. Products made from human plasma may contain infectious agents, such as viruses, that can cause disease. The risk that such products will transmit an infectious agent has been reduced by screening plasma donors for prior exposure to certain viruses, by testing for the presence of certain current virus infections, and by inactivating and/or removing certain viruses. Despite these measures, such products can still potentially transmit disease. There is also the possibility that unknown infectious agents may be present in such products. ALL infections thought by a physician possibly to have been transmitted by this product should be reported by the physician or other healthcare provider to our U.S. distributor at (800) 423-2862. The physician should discuss the risks and benefits of this product with the patient.

THERE EXISTS A RISK OF POTENTIALLY FATAL HEMOLYSIS AND ACUTE RENAL FAILURE FROM THE INAPPROPRIATE USE OF STERILE WATER-FOR-INJECTION AS A DILUENT FOR ALBUMIN (HUMAN) 25%. ACCEPTABLE DILUENTS INCLUDE 0.9% SODIUM CHLORIDE OR 5% DEXTROSE IN WATER.

ALBUMIN (HUMAN) 25% MUST NOT BE USED IF THE SOLUTION IS TURBID.

ALBUMIN (HUMAN) 25% MUST BE INFUSED IMMEDIATELY AND WITHOUT INTERRUPTION AFTER PERFORATION OF THE R/C BOTTLE. DO NOT BEGIN ADMINISTRATION MORE THAN 4 HOURS AFTER THE CONTAINER HAS BEEN ENTERED. PARTIALLY USED BOTTLES MUST BE DISCARDED.

ALBUMIN (HUMAN) 25% MUST NOT BE GIVEN THROUGH INFUSION SETS WHICH HAVE ALREADY BEEN USED OR ARE INTENDED FOR SIMULTANEOUS INFUSION OF PROTEIN HYDROLYSATE OR SOLUTIONS CONTAINING ALCOHOL.

PRECAUTIONS

Adequate precautions should be taken against circulatory overload; this can be done, for example, by the measurement of the pulmonary wedge pressure. Special caution is indicated in patients with stabilized chronic anemia or renal insufficiency. A rapid rise in blood pressure following infusion necessitates careful observation of injured or postoperative patients to detect and treat severed blood vessels that may not have bled at a lower blood pressure.

Certain components used in the packaging of this product contain natural rubber latex.

PREGNANCY CATEGORY C. Albumin (Human) 25% - Animal reproduction studies have not been conducted with Albumin (Human) 25%. It is also not known whether Albumin (Human) 25% can cause fetal harm when administered to a pregnant woman or can affect reproduction capacity. Albumin (Human) 25% should be given to a pregnant woman only if clearly needed.

ADVERSE REACTIONS

Though very rare, adverse reactions such as chills, fever, tachycardia, hypotension, urticaria, skin rash and nausea may occur (4,9,10,13).

The symptoms may disappear if the infusion is slowed or stopped for a short period of time. If necessary, the intravenous administration of 50 to 200 mg of prednisolone may be useful (10).

DOSAGE AND ADMINISTRATION

The dosage of Albumin (Human) 25% is based on the principles outlined in the section of Indications and Usage but should always be adapted to the individual situation. The quantities required may be underestimated because of hidden extravascular deficits, and the effect of Albumin (Human) infusion on the serum protein level should, therefore, be checked by laboratory analysis.

The appropriate Albumin (Human) 25% dose for the treatment of a volume deficit should be estimated from the recipient's hemodynamic response (3) and precautions taken to safeguard against circulatory overload. In the absence of active hemorrhage, the total dose should not exceed the normal circulating albumin mass, i.e., 2 g per kg body weight. Patients with acute nephrosis may respond to a combination of 100 mL of Albumin (Human) 25% and an appropriate diuretic, repeated daily for about one week. For hemolytic disease of the newborn, the dosage is 4 mL of Albumin (Human) 25% /kg body mass, to be given about one hour prior to ordering exchange transfusion. If Albumin (Human) is considered necessary for a renal dialysis patient, the initial dose should not exceed 100 mL of the 25% solution.

Parenteral drug products should be inspected visually for particulate matter and discoloration prior to administration, whenever solution and container permit.

To prepare Albumin (Human) 25% for administration, remove outer seal to expose central portion of rubber stopper and cleanse stopper with germicidal solution before use in syringes. Follow directions for use if the solution is administered by an intravenous injection set.

Albumin (Human) 25% must be administered INTRAVENOUSLY. The venipuncture site should not be infected or traumatized, and should be prepared with standard aseptic technique. The solution is compatible with whole blood or packed red cells as well as the usual electrolyte and carbohydrate solutions intended for intravenous use. By contrast, it should not be mixed with protein hydrolysates, amino acid mixtures, or solutions containing alcohol. It is ready for use as contained in the bottle and may be given without regard to the blood group of the recipient.

Only clear solutions of a light yellowish or amber color should be administered.

HOW SUPPLIED

Puncture vial containing 20 mL of Albumin (Human) 25%.
Puncture vial containing 50 mL of Albumin (Human) 25%.
Puncture vial containing 100 mL of Albumin (Human) 25%.
The package may be supplied with an intravenous injection set.

STORAGE

Albumin (Human) 25% can be stored for 3 years at a temperature not exceeding 30°C (86°F).

Protect from freezing.

REFERENCES

1. CLOWES, G.H.A., Jr., VUCINIC, M., and WEIDNER, M.G.: Ann. Surg. 163, 866 (1966).
2. JANEWAY, C.A.: In: Sgouris, J.T. and Rene A. (eds.): Proceedings of the Workshop on Albumin, DHEW Publication No. (NIH) 76-925, U.S. Government Printing Office, Washington, D.C., p. 3–21 (1976).
3. KINNEY, J.M., EGDAHL, R.H., and ZUIDEMA, G.D.: Manual of Preoperative and Postoperative Care, American College of Surgeons, W.B. Saunders Co., Philadelphia (1971).
4. LOWENSTEIN, E. In: Sgouris, J.T. and Rene A. (eds.): Proceedings of the Workshop on Albumin, DHEW Publication No. (NIH) 76–925, U.S. Government Printing Office, Washington, D.C., p. 302 (1976).
5. MAHARAJ, D., FELL, G.S., BOYCE, B.F., NG, J.P., SMITHE, G.D., BOULTON-JONES, J.M., CUMMING, R.L., and DAVIDSON, J.F.: Brit. Med. J. 295, 693–696 (1987).
6. MILLINER, D.S., SHINABERGER, J.H., SHUMAN, P., and COBURN, J.W.: N. Engl. J. Med. 312, 165–167 (1985).
7. OTT, S.M., MALONEY, N.A., KLEIN, G.L., ALFREY, A.C., AMENT, M.E., COBURN, J.W., and SHERRAND, D.J.: Ann. of Inter. Med. 98, 910–914 (1983).
8. PETERS, T., Jr., In: Putnam, F.W. (ed.): Plasma Proteins, 2nd Edition, Vol. 1, Academic Press, New York, p. 133–181 (1975).
9. RING, J. and MESSMER, K.: Lancet 1, 466 (1977).
10. RING, J., SEIFERT, J., LOB, G., COULIN, K., and BRENDEL, W.: W. Klin, Wschr. 52, 595 (1974).
11. SKILLMAN, J.J., PARIKH, B.M., and TANENBAUM, B.J.: Amer. J. Surg. 119, 440 (1970).
12. STARLING, E.H.: J. Physiol. (London) 19, 312 (1896).
13. TULLIS, J.L.: J.A.M.A. 237, 355 (1977).
14. TULLIS, J.L.: J.A.M.A. 237, 460 (1977).
15. WILLIS, M.R., and SAVORY, J.A.: Lancet 2, 29–34 (1983).

IMMUNO-U.S., INC.
1200 Parkdale Road
Rochester, MI 48307 USA
Distributed in Canada By:
IMMUNO (Canada) LTD.
U.S. License No. 850 Canadian License No. 227
Rev. July, 1998

BEBULIN® VH IMMUNO ℞
FACTOR IX COMPLEX,
VAPOR HEATED

DESCRIPTION

FACTOR IX COMPLEX, VAPOR HEATED, BEBULIN VH IMMUNO is a purified, sterile, stable, freeze-dried concentrate of the coagulation Factors IX (Christmas Factor) as well as II (Prothrombin) and X (Stuart Prower Factor) and

Continued on next page

Bebulin VH—Cont.

low amounts of Factor VII. In addition, the product contains small amounts of heparin (≤0.15 I.U. heparin per I.U. Factor IX).

FACTOR IX COMPLEX, VAPOR HEATED, BEBULIN VH IMMUNO is standardized in terms of Factor IX content and each vial is labeled for the Factor IX content indicated in International Units (I.U.). One International Unit of Factor IX (according to the current International Standard for Human Blood Coagulation Factors II, IX, and X in Concentrates, Code 84/681) corresponds to the activity of Factor IX in 1 mL of fresh normal human plasma.

CLINICAL PHARMACOLOGY

FACTOR IX COMPLEX, VAPOR HEATED, BEBULIN VH IMMUNO is a combination of vitamin K-dependent clotting factors found in normal plasma. The administration of FACTOR IX COMPLEX, VAPOR HEATED, BEBULIN VH IMMUNO provides an increase in plasma levels of Factor IX and can temporarily correct the coagulation defect of patients with Factor IX deficiency. Plasma levels of Factors II and X will also be increased. However, no clinical studies have been conducted to show benefit from this product for treating deficiencies other than Factor IX deficiency.

In vivo recovery of FACTOR IX COMPLEX, VAPOR HEATED, BEBULIN VH IMMUNO was determined by investigators in Germany, Japan, and the United States using the former International Standard, WHO 72/32 and found to be 53.3% ±9.6%, 57.5% ±21.8%, and 53.24% ±16.95%, respectively. In the same studies, using different methodologies, half-lives were determined to be 19.4 hrs ±3.8 hrs, 24.6 hrs ±3.2 hrs, and 19.97 hrs ±8.24 hrs, respectively (1,2, 3).

The product has been subjected to virus inactivation by vapor heating where vapor is first applied for 10 hours at 60°C ±0.5°C and an excess pressure of 190 ±25 mbar followed by 1 hour at 80°C ±0.5°C and an excess pressure of 375 ±35 mbar (4). The effectiveness of vapor heating was evaluated in vitro using Human Immunodeficiency Virus (HIV-1) and Sindbis Virus. Lyophilization followed by vapor heat treatment at 60°C inactivated >5.8 logs of HIV-1 and 4.0 logs of Sindbis Virus within 3 hours. Lyophilization with vapor heating at 60°C for 10 hours resulted in no detectable Sindbis Virus (>4.5 log reduction). Vapor heating at 80°C inactivated >3.5 logs of HIV-1 and >4.4 logs of Sindbis Virus within one hour.

In the context of two prospective clinical studies (5, 6) and a retrospective survey (7) FACTOR IX COMPLEX, VAPOR HEATED, BEBULIN VH IMMUNO was followed up for the risk of transfusion-transmitted viral infections. All patients received blood products for the first time. Using criteria established by the ICTH, 16 patients could be followed up for nonA, nonB hepatitis, 9 for HCV seroconversion, 3 for hepatitis B, and 24 for HIV seroconversion. None tested positive for any of these infections. An additional 3 patients with 2 or more consecutive test samples missing tested negative for nonA, nonB hepatitis for all samples available. Three studies using ICTH criteria for testing (5, 6, 8), a retrospective survey (7), and a case report (9) on other vapor heated factors of the prothrombin complex that were subjected to the same inactivation process as BEBULIN VH gave the following results: 27 patients tested negative for nonA, nonB hepatitis, 15 for HCV seroconversion, 25 for hepatitis B, and 75 for HIV seroconversion.

INDICATIONS AND USAGE

FACTOR IX COMPLEX, VAPOR HEATED, BEBULIN VH IMMUNO is indicated for the prevention and control of hemorrhagic episodes in hemophilia B patients.

FACTOR IX COMPLEX, VAPOR HEATED, BEBULIN VH IMMUNO is not indicated for use in the treatment of Factor VII deficiency. No clinical studies have been conducted to show benefit from this product for treating deficiencies other than Factor IX deficiency.

CONTRAINDICATIONS

None known.

WARNINGS

This product is prepared from pooled human plasma which may contain the causative agents of hepatitis and other viral diseases. Prescribed manufacturing procedures utilized at the plasma collection centers, plasma testing laboratories, and the fractionation facilities are designed to reduce the risk of transmitting viral infection. However, the risk of viral infectivity from this product cannot be totally eliminated.

Individuals who receive infusions of blood or plasma products may develop signs and/or symptoms of some viral infections, particularly nonA, nonB hepatitis. Hepatitis B vaccination is essential for patients with hemophilia and it is recommended that this be done at birth or diagnosis.

The risk of thromboembolic complications including DIC and hyperfibrinolysis is present with the administration of Factor IX Complex, particularly in the postoperative period and in patients with risk factors predisposing to thrombosis.

PRECAUTIONS

In patients with risk factors predisposing to thrombosis the Factor IX level should not be raised to more than approximately 60% of normal (10). In addition, it is recommended that such patients as well as patients who require high doses of Factor IX because of major surgical interventions be monitored for the possible development of DIC and/or thrombosis. In case changes occur in blood pressure or pulse rate or symptoms such as respiratory distress, chest pain or cough, treatment should be stopped immediately.

Information for Patients

Patients should be informed of the early signs of hypersensitivity reactions such as fever, urticaria, rashes, nausea or retching and should be advised to discontinue use of the product and contact their physician if these symptoms occur.

Pregnancy Category C.

Animal reproduction studies have not been conducted with FACTOR IX COMPLEX, VAPOR HEATED, BEBULIN VH IMMUNO. It is also not known whether FACTOR IX COMPLEX, VAPOR HEATED, BEBULIN VH IMMUNO can cause fetal harm when administered to a pregnant woman or can affect reproduction capacity. FACTOR IX COMPLEX, VAPOR HEATED, BEBULIN VH IMMUNO should be given to a pregnant woman only if clearly needed.

ADVERSE REACTIONS

As with any other infused plasma derivatives, anaphylactoid or anaphylactic reactions may occur in rare cases. The occurrence of these reactions (e.g. fever, urticarial rashes, nausea, retching, dyspnea, anaphylactic shock) necessitates the interruption of replacement therapy. Mild reactions can be managed with antihistamines; severe hypotensive reactions require immediate intervention using current principles of shock therapy.

DOSAGE AND ADMINISTRATION

General

FACTOR IX COMPLEX, VAPOR HEATED, BEBULIN VH IMMUNO is intended for intravenous administration only. As a general rule, 1 International Unit of Factor IX activity/kg will increase the plasma level of Factor IX by 0.8%. Accordingly, the following formula is provided for dosage calculations:

$$\text{Number of Factor IX I.U. required} = \text{bodyweight (kg)} \times \text{desired Factor IX increase (\% of normal)} \times 1.2$$

It must, however, be emphasized that the response to treatment will vary from patient to patient and that occasionally larger doses than those derived from the above formula will be required, particularly if treatment is delayed. Exact dosage determination should be based on localization and extent of hemorrhage, and the level of Factor IX to be achieved.

It must be emphasized that particularly with severe hemorrhage and major surgery close laboratory monitoring of the Factor IX level is required to determine proper dosage.

Management of Specific Types of Bleeding (10, 11, 12, 13, 14)

Approximate Factor IX levels, typical initial doses, and the average duration of treatment are suggested in the table below. For minor bleeding a single dose will usually be sufficient, otherwise a second dose may be given after 24 hours. More severe hemorrhage will require the administration of several doses at approximately 24 hour intervals. For maintenance therapy usually two thirds of the initial dose is infused.

Type of Bleeding	Approximate Factor IX Level (% Normal)	Typical Initial Dose (I.U./kg)	Average Duration of Treatment Days
Minor early hemarthrosis, minor epistaxis, and gingival bleeding, mild hematuria	20	25–35	1
Moderate severe joint bleeding, early hematoma, major open bleeding, minor trauma, minor hemoptysis hematemesis, and melena, major hematuria	40	40–55	2 or until adequate wound healing
Major severe hematoma, major trauma, severe hemoptysis, hematemesis, and melena	≥60*	60–70	2–3 or until adequate wound healing

* For patients predisposing to thrombosis see "PRECAUTIONS" section.

Management of Surgical Procedures (10, 11, 12, 13, 14)

Dosage guidelines for surgical procedures are suggested below. The preoperative loading dose should be administered one hour prior to surgery. Depending on the type of surgery replacement therapy has to be continued over one to several weeks until adequate wound healing is achieved. The average treatment interval will initially be 12 hours, while in the later postoperative period 24 hours are generally adequate.

[See table at top of page]

Type of Surgery	Day of Operation: Approx. Level F IX (% Normal)	Day of Operation: Dose (I.U./kg)	Init. Postop. Period (1st to 2nd Week): Approx. Level F IX (% Normal)	Init. Postop. Period (1st to 2nd Week): Dose (I.U./kg)	Late Postop. Period (from 3rd Week Onwards): Approx. Level F IX (% Normal)	Late Postop. Period (from 3rd Week Onwards): Dose (I.U./kg)
Major	≥60*	70–95	60→20	70→35	20	35→25
Minor	40–60	50–60	40→20	55→25		

* For patients predisposing to thrombosis see "PRECAUTIONS" section.

For tooth extraction the same initial dose as for minor surgery is recommended. Generally, one infusion will be sufficient. In case of extraction of several teeth, replacement therapy for up to one week may be necessary using the same doses as for minor surgery (12, 13, 14).

Long-Term Prophylactic Treatment

Prophylactic doses of 20–30 I.U./kg administered once, or preferably up to twice a week have been shown to significantly reduce the frequency of spontaneous hemorrhage (12, 15). It is, however, recommended that prophylactic dosage regimens be tailored to individual needs.

Reconstitution

FACTOR IX COMPLEX, VAPOR HEATED, BEBULIN VH IMMUNO should be reconstituted immediately before application. The solution does not contain a preservative and must be used within 3 hours of reconstitution.

For reconstitution proceed as follows:

1. Warm both diluent and concentrate in unopened vials to room temperature (not above 37°C, 98°F).
2. Remove caps from both vials to expose central portions of the rubber stoppers.
3. Cleanse exposed surface of the rubber stoppers with germicidal solution and allow to dry.
4. Using aseptic technique, remove protective covering from one end of the double-ended needle, and insert the exposed end through the diluent vial stopper.
5. Remove protective covering from the other end of the double-ended needle, taking care not to touch the exposed end. Invert diluent vial over the concentrate vial, then insert free end of the needle through the concentrate vial stopper. Diluent will be drawn into the concentrate vial by vacuum.
6. Disconnect the two vials by removing needle from the concentrate vial stopper. Gently agitate or rotate the concentrate vial until all material is dissolved.

Do not refrigerate after reconstitution!

Administration

Parenteral drug products should be inspected for particulate matter and discoloration prior to administration, whenever solution and container permit.

Intravenous Injection:

1. After reconstituting the concentrate as described above attach the enclosed filter needle to a sterile disposable syringe using aseptic technique. Insert filter needle through the concentrate vial stopper.
2. Inject air and withdraw solution into the syringe.
3. Remove and discard filter needle. Attach a suitable intravenous needle or infusion set with winged adapter.
4. Administer the solution intravenously at a rate comfortable to the patient (maximum rate 2 ml per minute).

HOW SUPPLIED

FACTOR IX COMPLEX, IMMUNO, VAPOR HEATED, BEBULIN VH is supplied in single dose vials with Sterile Water for Injection, U.S.P. (This Product Contains Dry Natural Rubber.), double-ended needle, and filter needle for reconstitution and withdrawal.

FACTOR IX activity in International Units is stated on the label of each vial.

Rx only

STORAGE

When stored at refrigerator temperature (2°C–8°C, 35°F–46°F), FACTOR IX COMPLEX, VAPOR HEATED, BEBULIN VH IMMUNO is stable for the period indicated by the expiration date on its label.

Avoid freezing, which may damage the diluent vial.

REFERENCES

1. H.H. Brackmann: A Study to Investigate the In Vivo Recovery and Half-Life Time of Factor IX Concentrate S-TIM 4. Unpublished Report, 1985.

2. T. Abe et al.: Clinical Study with BENOBIL TIM 4, Steam-Treated Factor IX Complex, Single Administration. Jap. Pharm. & Ther., 14, 1986, 1, pp. 19–31.
3. C. Kasper, A. Andes, L.M. Aledort: Clinical Study of Recovery and Half-Life of Factor IX Complex (Human) IMMUNO, Vapor Heated, Bebulin VH. Unpublished Report, 1990.
4. F. Elsinger, G. Wöber, F. Dorner, J. Eibl, Y. Linnau, A. Philapitsch, O. Schwarz: Steam Treatment of Freeze-Dried Plasma Fractions. In: N.L. Ciavarella, Z.M. Ruggeri, Th.S. Zimmermann (Eds.): Factor VII/von Willebrand Factor–Biological and Clinical Advances. Milano: Wichtig Editore srl, 1986, pp. 297–302.
5. Kl. Schimpf: Klinische Studien zur Infektiosität von konventionellen und virusinaktivierten Gerinnungsfaktorenkonzentraten. In: G. Landbeck, Kl. Schimpf (Eds.): 3. Rundtischgespräch über aktuelle Probleme der Substitutionstherapie Hämophiler. Berlin: Springer Verlag, 1986, pp. 69–79.
6. A Study to Determine the Safety of Virus Inactivated Factor Concentrates in Hemophiliacs Naive to Blood Product Administration. Data on file.
7. Kl. Schimpf: Substitutionstherapie bei angeborenen Gerinnungsstörungen. In: O. H. Just, C. Krier (Eds.): Haemostasis in Anaesthesia and Intensive Medicine. Berlin: Springer Verlag, 1988, pp. 17–31.
8. D. U. Preiss, B. Eberspächer, D. Abdullah, I. Rosner: Safety of Vapour Heated Prothrombin Complex Concentrate (PCC) Prothromplex S-TIM 4. Thrombosis Research, 63, 1991, pp. 651–659.
9. M. Köhler, P. Hellstern, G. Pindur, E. Wenzel, G. v. Blohn: Factor VII Half-Life after Transfusion of a Steam-Treated Prothrombin Complex Concentrate in a Patient with Homozygous Factor VII Deficiency. Vox Sang., 56, 1989, pp. 200–201.
10. P.H. Levine: Clinical Manifestations and Therapy of Hemophilias A and B. In: R.W. Colman, J. Hirsh, V.J. Marder, E.W. Salzman (Eds.): Hemostasis and Thrombosis. Philadelphia: J.B. Lippincott Company, 1987, pp. 97–111.
11. C. R. Rizza, P. Jones: Management of patients with inherited blood coagulation defects. In: A.L. Bloom, D.P. Thomas (Eds.): Hemostasis and Thrombosis. Edinburgh: Churchill Livingstone, 1987, pp. 465–493.
12. T. Abe, M. Kazama: An International Survey on the Appropriate Dosage of Hemophilias and Related Congenital Coagulopathies. In: Proceedings of the 3rd International Symposion on Haemostasis and Thrombosis, 1982, pp. 273–304.
13. I.M. Nilsson Å. Ahlberg, G. Björlin: Clinical Experience with a Swedish Factor IX Concentrate. Acta Med. Scand., 190, 1971, pp. 257–266.
14. J.N. George, R. T. Breckenridge: The Use of Factor VIII and Factor IX Concentrates During Surgery. JAMA, 214, 1970, 9, pp. 1673–1676.
15. E. Ludwig, K. Lechner. Prophylaktische Behandlung bei schwerer Hämophilie B mit einem Faktor-IX-Konzentrat. Dtsch. Med. Wschr., 99 1974 25 pp. 1355–1361.

Manufactured by
ÖSTERREICHISCHES INSTITUT FÜR HAEMODERIVATE GES.M.B.H.
Subsidiary of **IMMUNO AG**
A-1220 Vienna, Austria
U.S. Establishment Licence 258
U.S. Pat. Nos. 4,640,834 and 4,388,232
Distributed by
IMMUNO U.S., Inc.
1200 Parkdale Road
Rochester, Michigan 48307

Issued April 1998
6205212EH03

BUMINATE® 5% ℞
Albumin (Human), USP, 5% Solution

DESCRIPTION
Albumin (Human), 5% Solution, Buminate® 5% is a sterile, nonpyrogenic preparation of albumin in a single dosage form for intravenous administration. Each 100 mL contains 5 g of albumin and was prepared from human venous plasma using the Cohn cold ethanol fractionation process. It has been adjusted to physiological pH with sodium bicarbonate and/or sodium hydroxide and has been stabilized with 0.004 M sodium acetyltryptophanate and 0.004 M sodium caprylate. The sodium content is 145 ± 15 mEq/L. The solution contains no preservative and none of the coagulation factors found in fresh whole blood or plasma. Albumin (Human), 5% Solution, Buminate 5% is a transparent or slightly opalescent solution which may have a greenish tint or may vary from a pale straw to an amber color.

The likelihood of the presence of viable hepatitis viruses has been reduced by heating the product for 10 hours at 60 °C. This procedure has been shown to be an effective method of inactivating hepatitis virus in albumin solutions even when those solutions were prepared from plasma known to be infective.[1–3]

Albumin (Human), 5% Solution, Buminate 5% contains no blood group isoagglutinins thereby permitting its administration without regard to the recipient's blood group.

CLINICAL PHARMACOLOGY
Albumin is responsible for 70–80% of the colloid osmotic pressure of normal plasma, thus making it useful in regulating and increasing blood volume.[4,5,6] It is also a transport protein and binds naturally occurring, therapeutic and toxic materials in the circulation.[5,6] Albumin (Human), 5% Solution, Buminate 5% is osmotically equivalent to an equal volume of normal human plasma and will increase circulating plasma volume by an amount approximately equal to the volume infused. The degree and duration of volume expansion depends upon the initial blood volume. With patients treated for diminished blood volume, the effect of infused albumin may last for many hours. In patients with normal blood volumes, the hemodilution lasts for a shorter period.[7,8]

Total body albumin is estimated to be 350 g for a 70 kg man and is distributed throughout the extracellular compartments. The half-life of albumin is 15 to 20 days with a turnover of approximately 15 g per day.[5]

The minimum plasma albumin level necessary to prevent or reverse peripheral edema is unknown. Some investigators recommend that plasma albumin levels be maintained at approximately 2.5 g/dL. This concentration provides a plasma oncotic pressure value of 20 mm Hg.[4]

INDICATIONS AND USAGE
1. Hypovolemia

Hypovolemia is a possible indication for use of Albumin (Human), 5% Solution, Buminate 5%. Its effectiveness in reversing hypovolemia depends largely upon its colloid osmotic pressure. Although crystalloid solutions and colloid-containing plasma substitutes can be used in emergency treatment of shock, Albumin (Human) has a longer intravascular half-life than crystalloid solutions.[9]

When the hypovolemia is long-standing and hypoalbuminemia exists accompanied by adequate hydration or edema, treatment with Albumin (Human), 25% Solution is preferable.[4,6]

When blood volume deficit is the result of hemorrhage, compatible red blood cells or whole blood should be administered as quickly as possible.

2. Hypoalbuminemia

A. General

Hypoalbuminemia is another possible indication for use of Albumin (Human), 5% Solution, Buminate 5%. Hypoalbuminemia can result from one or more of the following:[5]

(1) Inadequate production (malnutrition, burns, major injury, infections, etc.)
(2) Excessive catabolism (burns, major injury, pancreatitis, etc.)
(3) Loss from the body (hemorrhage, excessive renal excretion, burn exudates, etc.)
(4) Redistribution within the body (major surgery, various inflammatory conditions, etc.)

When albumin deficit is the result of excessive protein loss, the effect of administration of albumin will be temporary unless the underlying disorder is reversed. In most cases, increased nutritional replacement of amino acids and/or protein with concurrent treatment of the underlying disorder will restore normal plasma albumin levels more effectively than administration of albumin solutions. Occasionally hypoalbuminemia accompanying severe injuries, infections or severe pancreatitis cannot be quickly reversed and nutritional supplements may fail to restore adequate plasma albumin levels. In these cases, Albumin (Human), 5% Solution, Buminate 5% may be useful.

B. Burns

In conjunction with appropriate crystalloid therapy, Albumin (Human), 5% Solution, Buminate 5% may be useful for treatment of protein deficits after the initial 24 hour period following extensive burns.[4]

3. Miscellaneous Indications

Albumin (Human), 5% Solution, Buminate 5% may be indicated prior to or during cardiopulmonary bypass surgery,[4,6,10] though the data do not indicate a clear-cut advantage over crystalloid solutions.

There is no valid reason for use of albumin as an intravenous nutrient.

CONTRAINDICATIONS
A history of allergic reactions to albumin is a specific contraindication to the use of this product.

Albumin (Human), 5% Solution, Buminate 5% is also contraindicated in severely anemic patients and in patients with cardiac failure.

WARNINGS
Do not use if turbid. Do not begin administration more than 4 hours after the container has been entered.

PRECAUTIONS
Certain components used in the packaging of this product contain natural rubber latex.

Albumin (Human), 5% Solution, Buminate 5% may be given rapidly to individuals with reduced plasma volume with the following exception: if a patient has a history of cardiac or circulatory disease, Albumin (Human), 5% Solution, Buminate 5% should be administered slowly (5 to 10 mL per minute) to avoid too rapid a rise in the blood pressure.

Patients should always be carefully monitored in order to guard against the possibility of circulatory overload.

When Albumin (Human), 5% Solution, Buminate 5% is used following injuries or surgery, the quick rise in blood pressure which follows administration makes it necessary to monitor the patient to detect and treat severed blood vessels that may not have bled at a lower blood pressure.

Pregnancy—Category C

Animal reproduction studies have not been conducted with Albumin (Human), 5% Solution. It is not known whether Albumin (Human), 5% Solution can cause fetal harm when administered to a pregnant woman or can affect reproductive capacity. Albumin (Human), 5% Solution should be given to a pregnant woman only if clearly needed.

Pediatric Use

The use of Albumin (Human), 5% Solution in children has not been associated with any special or specific hazard, if the dose is appropriate for the child's body weight.

ADVERSE REACTIONS
Untoward reactions to Albumin (Human), 5% Solution are extremely rare, although nausea, fever, chills or urticaria may occasionally occur. Such symptoms usually disappear when the infusion is slowed or stopped for a short period of time.

DOSAGE AND ADMINISTRATION
Albumin (Human), 5% Solution, Buminate 5% must be administered intravenously. It may be administered either in conjunction with or combined with other parenterals such as whole blood, plasma, saline, glucose or sodium lactate.

The volume of the total dose and the rate of infusion depends on the patient's condition and response.

Recommended Dosages

1. Hypovolemia

Although the volume of Albumin (Human), 5% Solution, Buminate 5% administered must be individualized, the initial dose should be 250 to 500 mL for older children and adults and 12 to 20 mL per kilogram of body weight for infants and young children. It may be repeated after 30 minute intervals if the response is not adequate.

2. Hypoalbuminemia

Hypoalbuminemia is usually accompanied by a hidden extravascular albumin deficiency of equal magnitude. This total body albumin deficit must be considered when determining the amount of albumin necessary to reverse the hypoalbuminemia. When using the patient's serum albumin concentration to estimate the deficit, the body albumin compartment should be calculated to be 80 to 100 mL per kilogram of body weight.[5,6] Daily dose should not exceed 2 g of albumin per kilogram of body weight.

3. Burns

When Albumin (Human), 5% Solution, Buminate 5% is administered after the first 24 hours following burns, an initial dose of 500 mL is recommended.

Preparation for Administration

Parenteral drug products should be inspected visually for particulate matter and discoloration prior to administration, whenever solution and container permit.

1. Remove cap from bottle to expose center portion of rubber stopper.
2. Clean stopper with germicidal solution.

Administration

Follow directions for use printed on the administration set container. Make certain that the administration set contains an adequate filter.

HOW SUPPLIED
Albumin (Human), 5% Solution, Buminate 5% is supplied in 250 mL and 500 mL bottles.

STORAGE

Store Albumin (Human), 5% Solution, Buminate 5% at room temperature, not to exceed 30 °C (86 °F). Avoid freezing to prevent damage to the bottle.

REFERENCES
1. Gellis SS, Neefe JR, Stokes J Jr, *et al:* Chemical, clinical and immunological studies on the products of human plasma fractionation. XXXVI. Inactivation of the virus of homologous serum hepatitis in solutions of normal human serum albumin by means of heat. **J Clin Invest 27**: 239–244, 1948.
2. Gerety RJ, Aronson DL: Plasma derivatives and viral hepatitis. **Transfusion 22**: 347–351, 1982.
3. Murray R, Diefenbach WCL, Geller H, *et al:* Problem of reducing danger of serum hepatitis from blood and blood products. **NY State J Med 55**: 1145–1150, 1955.
4. Tullis JL: Albumin, 1. Background and use, and 2. Guidelines for clinical use. **JAMA 237**: 355–360, 460–463, 1977.
5. Peters T Jr: Serum Ablumin, in **The Plasma Proteins, 2nd ed. Vol 1.** Putnam FW (ed). New York, Academic Press. 1975, pp 133–181.
6. Finlayson JS: Albumin products. **Sem Thromb Hemostas 6**: 85–120, 1980.
7. Janeway CA, Berenberg W, Hutchins G: Indications and uses of blood, blood derivatives and blood substitutes. **Med Clin N Amer 29**: 1069–1094, 1945.
8. Janeway CA, Gibson ST, Woodruff LM, *et al:* Chemical, clinical, and immunological studies on the products of human plasma fractionation. VII. Concentrated human serum albumin. **J Clin Invest 23**: 465–490, 1944.
9. Shoemaker WC, Schluchter M, Hopkins JA, *et al:* Comparison of the relative effectiveness of colloids and crystalloids in emergency resuscitation. **Am J Surg 142**: 73–83, 1981.

Continued on next page

Buminate 5%—Cont.

10. Lowenstein E, Hallowell P, Bland JHL: Use of colloid and crystalloid solutions in open heart surgery: Physiological basis and clinical results, in **Proceedings of the Workshop on Albumin.** Sgouris JT, Rene A (eds.) DHEW Publication No. (NIH) 76-925, Washington DC, U.S. Government Printing Office, 1976, pp. 195–210.

Baxter Healthcare Corporation
Hyland Division
Glendale, CA 91203 USA
U.S. License No. 140 Revised January 1998

BUMINATE® 25% ℞
Albumin (Human), USP, 25% Solution

DESCRIPTION

Albumin (Human), 25% Solution, Buminate® 25% is a sterile, nonpyrogenic preparation of albumin in a single dosage form for intravenous administration. Each 100 mL contains 25 g of albumin and was prepared from human venous plasma using the Cohn cold ethanol fractionation process. Source material for fractionation may be obtained from another U.S. licensed manufacturer. It has been adjusted to physiological pH with sodium bicarbonate and/or sodium hydroxide and stabilized with 0.02 M sodium acetyltryptophanate and 0.02 M sodium caprylate. The sodium content is 145 ± 15 mEq/L. This solution contains no preservative and none of the coagulation factors found in fresh whole blood or plasma. Albumin (Human), 25% Solution, Buminate 25% is a transparent or slightly opalescent solution which may have a greenish tint or may vary from a pale straw to an amber color.

The likelihood of the presence of viable hepatitis viruses has been minimized by heating the product for 10 hours at 60°C. This procedure has been shown to be an effective method of inactivating hepatitis virus in albumin solutions even when those solutions were prepared from plasma known to be infective.[1–3]

CLINICAL PHARMACOLOGY

Albumin is responsible for 70–80% of the colloid osmotic pressure of normal plasma, thus making it useful in regulating the volume of circulating blood.[4–6] Albumin is also a transport protein and binds naturally occurring, therapeutic and toxic materials in the circulation.[5,6]

Albumin (Human), 25% Solution, Buminate 25% is osmotically equivalent to approximately five times its volume of human plasma. When injected intravenously, 25% albumin will draw about 3.5 times its volume of additional fluid into the circulation within 15 minutes, except when the patient is markedly dehydrated. This extra fluid reduces hemoconcentration and blood viscosity. The degree and duration of volume expansion depends upon the initial blood volume. With patients treated for diminished blood volume, the effect of infused albumin may persist for many hours; however, in patients with normal volume, the duration will be shorter.[7,8]

Total body albumin is estimated to be 350 g for a 70 kg man and is distributed throughout the extracellular compartments; more than 60% is located in the extravascular fluid compartment. The half-life of albumin is 15 to 20 days with a turnover of approximately 15 g per day.[5]

The minimum plasma albumin level necessary to prevent or reverse peripheral edema is unknown. Some investigators recommend that plasma albumin levels be maintained at approximately 2.5 g/dL. This concentration provides a plasma oncotic value of 20 mm Hg.[4]

INDICATIONS AND USAGE

1. Hypovolemia

Hypovolemia is a possible indication for Albumin (Human), 25% Solution, Buminate 25%. Its effectiveness in reversing hypovolemia depends largely upon its ability to draw interstitial fluid into the circulation. It is most effective with patients who are well hydrated.

When hypovolemia is long standing and hypoalbuminemia exists accompanied by adequate hydration or edema, 25% albumin is preferable to 5% protein solutions.[4,6] However, in the absence of adequate or excessive hydration, 5% protein solutions should be used or 25% albumin should be diluted with crystalloid.

Although crystalloid solutions and colloid-containing plasma substitutes can be used in emergency treatment of shock, Albumin (Human) has a prolonged intravascular half-life.[9] When blood volume deficit is the result of hemorrhage, compatible red blood cells or whole blood should be administered as quickly as possible.

2. Hypoalbuminemia

A. General

Hypoalbuminemia is another possible indication for use of Albumin (Human), 25% Solution, Buminate 25%. Hypoalbuminemia can result from one or more of the following:[5]

(1) Inadequate production (malnutrition, burns, major injury, infections, etc.)
(2) Excessive catabolism (burns, major injury, pancreatitis, etc.)
(3) Loss from the body (hemorrhage, excessive renal excretion, burn exudates, etc.)
(4) Redistribution within the body (major surgery, various inflammatory conditions, etc.)

When albumin deficit is the result of excessive protein loss, the effect of administration of albumin will be temporary unless the underlying disorder is reversed. In most cases, increased nutritional replacement of amino acids and/or protein with concurrent treatment of the underlying disorder will restore normal plasma albumin levels more effectively than albumin solutions. Occasionally hypoalbuminemia accompanying severe injuries, infections or pancreatitis cannot be quickly reversed and nutritional supplements may fail to restore serum albumin levels. In these cases, Albumin (Human), 25% Solution, Buminate 25% might be a useful therapeutic adjunct.

B. Burns

An optimum regimen for the use of albumin, electrolytes and fluid in the early treatment of burns has not been established, however, in conjunction with appropriate crystalloid therapy, Albumin (Human), 25% Solution, Buminate 25% may be indicated for treatment of oncotic deficits after the initial 24 hour period following extensive burns and to replace the protein loss which accompanies any severe burn.[4,6]

C. Adult Respiratory Distress Syndrome (ARDS)

A characteristic of ARDS is a hypoproteinemic state which may be causally related to the interstitial pulmonary edema. Although uncertainty exists concerning the precise indication of albumin infusion in these patients, if there is a pulmonary overload accompanied by hypoalbuminemia, 25% albumin solution may have a therapeutic effect when used with a diuretic.[4]

D. Nephrosis

Albumin (Human), 25% Solution may be a useful aid in treating edema in patients with severe nephrosis who are receiving steroids and/or diuretics.

3. Cardiopulmonary Bypass Surgery

Albumin (Human), 25% Solution, Buminate 25% has been recommended prior to or during cardiopulmonary bypass surgery, although no clear data exist indicating its advantage over crystalloid solutions.[4,6,10]

4. Hemolytic Disease of the Newborn (HDN)

Albumin (Human), 25% Solution, Buminate 25% may be administered in an attempt to bind and detoxify unconjugated bilirubin in infants with severe HDN.

There is no valid reason for use of albumin as an intravenous nutrient.

CONTRAINDICATIONS

A history of allergic reactions to albumin is a specific contraindication to the use of this product.

Albumin (Human), 25% Solution, Buminate 25% is also contraindicated in severely anemic patients and in patients with cardiac failure.

WARNINGS

Do not use if turbid. Do not begin administration more than 4 hours after the container has been entered. Discard unused portion.

PRECAUTIONS

Certain components used in the packaging of this product contain natural rubber latex.

Albumin (Human), 25% Solution, Buminate 25% must be administered intravenously at a rate not to exceed 1 mL/min to patients with normal blood volume. More rapid administration might cause circulatory overload and pulmonary edema.

A rise in blood pressure after 25% albumin infusion necessitates careful observation of the injured or post-operative patient in order to detect and treat severed blood vessels that may not have bled at a lower blood pressure.

Pregnancy—Category C

Animal reproduction studies have not been conducted with Albumin (Human), 25% Solution. It is not known whether Albumin (Human), 25% Solution can cause fetal harm when administered to a pregnant woman or can affect reproductive capacity. Albumin (Human) 25% Solution should be given to a pregnant woman only if clearly needed.

Pediatric Use

The use of Albumin (Human), 25% Solution in children has not been associated with any special or specific hazard, if the dose is appropriate for the child's body weight.

ADVERSE REACTIONS

Untoward reactions to Albumin (Human), 25% Solution are extremely rare, although nausea, fever, chills or urticaria may occasionally occur. Such symptoms usually disappear when the infusion is slowed or stopped for a short period of time.

DOSAGE AND ADMINISTRATION

Albumin (Human), 25% Solution, Buminate 25% must be administered intravenously.

This solution may be administered in conjunction with or combined with other parenterals such as whole blood, plasma, saline, glucose or sodium lactate. The addition of four volumes of normal saline or 5% glucose to 1 volume of Albumin (Human), 25% Solution, Buminate 25% gives a solution which is approximately isotonic and isosmotic with citrated plasma.

Albumin solutions should not be mixed with protein hydrolysates or solutions containing alcohol.

Recommended Dosages

1. Hypovolemic Shock

The dosage of Albumin (Human), 25% Solution, Buminate 25% must be individualized. As a guideline, the initial treatment should be in the range of 100 to 200 mL for adults and 2.5 to 5 mL per kilogram body weight for children. This may be repeated after 15 to 30 minutes, if the response is not adequate. For patients with significant plasma volume deficits, albumin replacement is best administered in the form of 5% Albumin (Human).

Upon administration of additional albumin or if hemorrhage has occurred, hemodilution and a relative anemia will follow. This condition should be controlled by the supplemental administration of compatible red blood cells or compatible whole blood.

2. Burns

The optimal therapeutic regimen for administration of crystalloid and colloid solutions after extensive burns has not been established. When Albumin (Human), 25% Solution, Buminate 25% is administered after the first 24 hours following burns, the dose should be determined according to the patient's condition and response to treatment.

3. Hypoalbuminemia

Hypoalbuminemia is usually accompanied by a hidden extravascular albumin deficiency of equal magnitude. This total body albumin deficit must be considered when determining the amount of albumin necessary to reverse the hypoalbuminemia. When using patient's serum albumin concentration to estimate the deficit, the body albumin compartment should be calculated to be 80 to 100 mL per kg of body weight.[5,6] Daily dose should not exceed 2 g of albumin per kilogram of body weight.

4. Hemolytic Disease of the Newborn

Albumin (Human), 25% Solution, Buminate 25% may be administered prior to or during exchange transfusion in a dose of 1 g per kilogram body weight.[11]

Preparation for Administration

Parenteral drug products should be inspected visually for particulate matter and discoloration prior to administration, whenever solution and container permit.

1. Remove cap from bottle to expose center portion of rubber stopper.
2. Clean stopper with germicidal solution.

Administration

Follow directions for use printed on the administration set container. Make certain that the administration set contains an adequate filter.

HOW SUPPLIED

Albumin (Human), 25% Solution, Buminate 25% is supplied in 20 mL, 50 mL and 100 mL bottles

Storage

Store Albumin (Human), 25% Solution, Buminate 25% at room temperature, not to exceed 30°C (86°F). Avoid freezing to prevent damage to the bottle.

REFERENCES

1. Gellis SS, Neefe JR, Stokes J Jr, *et al:* Chemical, clinical and immunological studies on the products of human plasma fractionation. XXXVI. Inactivation of the virus of homologous serum hepatitis in solutions of normal human serum albumin by means of heat. **J Clin Invest 27**:239–244, 1948
2. Gerety RJ, Aronson DL: Plasma derivatives and viral hepatitis. **Transfusion 22**:347–351, 1982
3. Murray R, Diefenbach WCL, Geller H, *et al:* Problem of reducing danger of serum hepatitis from blood and blood products. **NY State J Med 55**:1145–1150, 1955
4. Tullis JL: Albumin, 1. Background and use, and 2. Guidelines for clinical use. **JAMA 237**:355–360, 460–463, 1977
5. Peters T Jr: Serum albumin, in **The Plasma Proteins, 2nd ed, Vol 1.** Putnam FW (ed). New York, Academic Press, 1975, pp 133–181
6. Finlayson JS: Albumin products. **Semin Thromb Hemostas 6**:85–120, 1980
7. Janeway CA, Berenberg W, Hutchins G: Indications and uses of blood, blood derivatives and blood substitutes. **Med Clin N Amer 29**:1069–1094, 1945
8. Janeway CA, Gibson ST, Woodruff LM, *et al:* Chemical, clinical and immunological studies on the products of human plasma fractionation. VII. Concentrated human serum albumin. **J Clin Invest 23**:465–490, 1944
9. Shoemaker WC, Schluchter M, Hopkins JA, *et al:* Comparison of the relative effectiveness of colloids and crystalloids in emergency resuscitation. **Am J Surg 142**:73–83, 1981
10. Lowenstein E, Hallowell P, Bland JHL: Use of colloid and crystalloid solutions in open heart surgery: Physiological basis and clinical results, in **Proceedings of the Workshop on Albumin.** Sgouris JT, Rene A (eds). DHEW Publication No. (NIH) 76–925, Washington, DC, US Government Printing Office 1976, pp 195–210
11. Tsao YC, Yu VYH; Albumin in management of neonatal hyperbilirubinaemia. **Arch Dis Childhood 47**:250–256, 1972

Revised October 1999

FEIBA® VH IMMUNO ℞
ANTI-INHIBITOR, COAGULANT COMPLEX, VAPOR HEATED

DESCRIPTION

Anti-Inhibitor Coagulant Complex, Vapor Heated, FEIBA® VH IMMUNO, is a freeze-dried sterile human plasma fraction with Factor VIII inhibitor bypassing activity. In vitro, FEIBA® VH IMMUNO shortens the activated partial thromboplastin time (APTT) of plasma containing Factor VIII inhibitor. Factor VIII inhibitor bypassing activity is expressed in arbitrary units. One IMMUNO Unit of activity is defined as that amount of Anti-Inhibitor Coagulant Complex, Vapor Heated, FEIBA® VH IMMUNO which shortens the APTT of a high titer Factor VIII inhibitor reference plasma to 50% of the blank value. The product is intended for intravenous administration.

Anti-Inhibitor Coagulant Complex, Vapor Heated, FEIBA® VH IMMUNO contains Factors II, IX, and X, mainly nonactivated, and Factor VII[1–3] mainly in the activated form. The product contains approximately equal unitages of Factor VIII inhibitor bypassing activity and Prothrombin Complex Factors. In addition, 1–6 units of Factor VIII coagulant antigen (F VIII C: Ag) per mL are present. The preparation contains only traces of factors of the kinin generating system. It contains no heparin.

Reconstituted Anti-Inhibitor Coagulant Complex, Vapor Heated, FEIBA® VH IMMUNO contains 4 mg of trisodium citrate and 8 mg of sodium chloride per mL.

Anti-Inhibitor Coagulant Complex, Vapor Heated, FEIBA® VH IMMUNO has been prepared from Source Plasma and/or Plasma.

The produce has been subjected to in-process virus inactivation where vapor is first applied for 10 hours at 60° ± 0.5°C and an excess pressure of 190 ± 20 mbar followed by 1 hour at 80° ± 0.5°C and an excess pressure of 370 ± 30 mbar. (Refer to Clinical Pharmacology and Warnings sections.)

CLINICAL PHARMACOLOGY

In a preclinical study to determine the virus inactivating efficacy of vapor heating, samples of bulk Anti-Inhibitor Coagulant Complex, FEIBA® IMMUNO were spiked with 2×10^6/mL infectious units of HIV and subjected to vapor heat treatment. The residual virus titer was found to be less than 1 infectious unit/0.5 mL. A clinical study[4] testing Antihemophilic Factor treated by a similar vapor heating procedure has shown none of 4 lots used in the study to produce nonA, nonB hepatitis in intensively followed patients naive to blood product administration.

The safety and efficacy of Anti-Inhibitor Coagulant Complex, FEIBA® IMMUNO has been demonstrated by two prospective clinical trials[5–7]. The first, conducted by Sixma and collaborators during 1979 and early 1980, was a randomized double-blind study comparing the effect of Anti-Inhibitor Coagulant Complex, FEIBA® IMMUNO, and PROTHROMPLEX IMMUNO (a non-activated prothrombin complex concentrate) in 15 patients with hemophilia A and inhibitors to Factor VIII. A total of 150 bleeding episodes (primarily joint and musculoskeletal plus a few mucocutaneous) were treated. A single dose of 88 IMMUNO Units per kg of body weight was used uniformly for treatments with Anti-Inhibitor Coagulant Complex, FEIBA® IMMUNO. The study showed that, based on subjective patient evaluation, FEIBA® IMMUNO was fully effective in 41.0% and partly effective in 24.6% of episodes (i.e. combined effectiveness of 65.6%), while PROTHROMPLEX IMMUNO was rated fully effective in 25.0% and partly effective in 21.4% of episodes (i.e. combined effectiveness of 46.4%).

The second study with FEIBA® IMMUNO was a multiclinic study conducted by Hilgartner et al. It was designed to evaluate the efficacy of FEIBA® IMMUNO in the treatment of joint, mucous membrane, musculocutaneous and emergency bleeding episodes such as central nervous system hemorrhages and surgical bleedings. In 49 patients with inhibitor titers of greater than 5 Bethesda Units (from nine cooperating hemophilia centers), 489 single doses were given for the treatment of 165 bleeding episodes. The usual dosage was 50 IMMUNO Units per kg of body weight, repeated at 12-hour intervals (6-hour intervals in mucous membrane bleedings), if necessary. Bleeding was controlled in 153 episodes (93%). In 130 (78%) of the episodes hemostasis was achieved with one or more infusions within 36 hours. Of these 36% were controlled with one infusion within 12 hours. An additional 14% of episodes responded after more than 36 hours.

Of the 489 single doses only 18 (3.7%) caused minor transient reactions in recipients. 10 out of 49 patients (20%) showed a rise in their inhibitor titers. In 5 of these patients (10%) the rise was tenfold or more. However, of these 10 patients 3 had received Factor VIII or Factor IX concentrates within 2 weeks prior to treatment with FEIBA® IMMUNO. These anamnestic rises have not been observed to interfere with the efficacy of Anti-Inhibitor Coagulant Complex, FEIBA® IMMUNO.

INDICATIONS AND USAGE

Anti-Inhibitor Coagulant Complex, Vapor Heated, FEIBA® VH IMMUNO is indicated for the control of spontaneous bleeding episodes or to cover surgical interventions in hemophilia A and B patients with inhibitors.

In addition, the use of Anti-Inhibitor Coagulant Complex, FEIBA® IMMUNO has been described in a few non-hemophiliacs with acquired inhibitors to Factors VIII, XI, and XII[8–12]. One case has been reported where Anti-Inhibitor Coagulant Complex, FEIBA® IMMUNO was effective in a patient with von Willebrand's disease with an inhibitor[16].

Clinical experience suggests that patients with a Factor VIII inhibitor titer of less than 5 B.U. may be successfully treated with Antihemophilic Factor. Patients with titers ranging between 5 and 10 B.U. may either be treated with Antihemophilic Factor or Anti-Inhibitor Coagulant Complex, Vapor Heated, FEIBA® VH IMMUNO. Cases with Factor VIII inhibitor titers greater than 10 B.U. have generally been refractory to treatment with Antihemophilic Factor.

Guidelines to First and Second Choice Treatment:

AICC = Anti-Inhibitor Coagulant Complex, Vapor Heated, FEIBA® VH IMMUNO

AHF = Antihemophilic Factor

Patient's Inhibitor Titer	Clinical Situation		
	Minor Bleeding	Major Bleeding	Surgery (Emergency)
less than 5 B.U.	AHF	AHF	AHF
5 to 10 B.U.	AHF AICC	AHF AICC	AHF AICC
more than 10 B.U.	AICC	AICC	AICC

Inadequate response to treatment may result from an abnormal platelet count or impaired platelet function[13–15] which were present before treatment with Anti-Inhibitor Coagulant Complex, Vapor Heated, FEIBA® VH IMMUNO.

CONTRAINDICATIONS

The use of Anti-Inhibitor Coagulant Complex, Vapor Heated, FEIBA® VH IMMUNO is contraindicated in patients who are known to have a normal coagulation mechanism.

WARNINGS

Anti-Inhibitor Coagulant Complex, Vapor Heated, FEIBA® VH IMMUNO must be used only in patients with circulating inhibitors to one or more coagulation factors and should not be used for the treatment of bleeding episodes resulting from coagulation factor deficiencies. It should not be given to patients with significant signs of disseminated intravascular coagulation (DIC) or fibrinolysis.

In the course of treatment with preparations containing the prothrombin complex thromboembolic events may occur, particularly following the administration of high doses and/or in patients with thrombotic risk factors.

Single doses of 100 units per kg of body weight of FEIBA® VH IMMUNO and daily doses of 200 units per kg of body weight of FEIBA® VH IMMUNO should not be exceeded. Patients receiving more than 100 units per kg of body weight of Anti-Inhibitor Coagulant Complex, Vapor Heated, FEIBA® VH IMMUNO must be monitored for the development of DIC and/or symptoms of acute coronary ischemia (see Adverse Reactions section).

High doses of FEIBA® VH IMMUNO should be given only as long as absolutely necessary to stop bleeding.

It has been reported that Anti-Inhibitor Coagulant Complex, Vapor Heated, FEIBA® VH IMMUNO and antifibrinolytics have been given simultaneously without complications. It is, however, recommended not to use antifibrinolytics until 12 hours after the administration of Anti-Inhibitor Coagulant Complex, Vapor Heated, FEIBA® VH IMMUNO.

Anamnestic responses with rise in Factor VIII inhibitor titer have been observed in 20% of the cases (see Clinical Pharmacology section).

This product is prepared from pooled human plasma which may contain the causative agents of hepatitis and other viral diseases. Prescribed manufacturing procedures utilized at the plasma collection centers, plasma testing laboratories, and the fractionation facilities are designed to reduce the risk of transmitting viral infection. However, the risk of viral infectivity from this product cannot be totally eliminated.

Individuals who receive infusions of blood or plasma products may develop signs and/or symptoms of some viral infections, particularly nonA, nonB hepatitis.

PRECAUTIONS

Monitoring of Therapy

If clinical signs of intravascular coagulation occur, which include changes in blood pressure, pulse rate, respiratory distress, chest pain and cough, the infusion should be stopped promptly and appropriate diagnostic and therapeutic measures are to be initiated.

Laboratory indications of DIC are decreased fibrinogen, decreased platelet count, and/or presence of fibrin-fibrinogen degradation products (FDP). Other indications of DIC include significantly prolonged thrombin time, prothrombin time, or partial thromboplastin time.

Non Hemophilic Patients

Non hemophilic patients with acquired inhibitors against Factors VIII, IX or XII may have both a bleeding tendency and an increased risk of thrombosis at the same time.

Laboratory Tests and Clinical Efficacy

Tests used to control efficacy such as APTT, WBCT, and TEG do not correlate with clinical improvement. For this reason, attempts at normalizing these values by increasing the dose of Anti-Inhibitor Coagulant Complex, Vapor Heated, FEIBA® VH IMMUNO may not be successful and are strongly discouraged because of the potential hazard of producing DIC by overdosage.

Pregnancy Category C. Animal reproduction studies have not been conducted with Anti-Inhibitor Coagulant Complex, Vapor Heated, FEIBA® VH IMMUNO. It is also not known whether Anti-Inhibitor Coagulant Complex, Vapor Heated, FEIBA® VH IMMUNO can cause fetal harm when administered to a pregnant woman or can affect reproduction capacity. Anti-Inhibitor Coagulant Complex, Vapor Heated, FEIBA® VH IMMUNO should be given to a pregnant woman only if clearly needed.

Pediatric Use

No data are available regarding the use of Anti-Inhibitor Coagulant Complex, Vapor Heated, FEIBA® VH IMMUNO in newborns.

ADVERSE REACTIONS

In the course of treatment with preparations containing the prothrombin complex thromboembolic events may occur, particularly after high doses and/or in patients with thrombotic risk factors.

After application of high doses (single infusion of beyond 100 units per kg of body weight, and daily doses of 200 units per kg of body weight) of Anti-Inhibitor Coagulant Complex, Vapor Heated, FEIBA® VH IMMUNO laboratory and/or clinical signs of DIC have occasionally been observed.

In individual instances myocardial infarction was found to occur after high doses and/or prolonged administration and/or in the presence of risk factors predisposing to myocardial infarction.

As will all human plasma products, any kind of allergic reaction may be seen, ranging from mild, short-term urticarial rashes to severe anaphylactoid reactions.

Administration of Anti-Inhibitor Coagulant Complex, Vapor Heated, FEIBA® VH IMMUNO should be discontinued immediately, if such signs appear. Allergic reactions should be treated with antihistamines and glucocorticoids. Shock should be treated in the usual way.

DOSAGE AND ADMINISTRATION

Parenteral drug products should be inspected visually for particulate matter and discoloration prior to administration, whenever solution and container permit.

Clinical trials[5–7] have demonstrated that the response to treatment with Anti-Inhibitor Coagulant Complex, FEIBA® IMMUNO, may differ from patient to patient with no correlation to the patient's inhibitor titer. Response may also vary between different types of hemorrhage (e.g. joint hemorrhage vs. CNS hemorrhage).

As a general guideline a dosage range of 50 to 100 IMMUNO Units of Anti-Inhibitor Coagulant Complex, Vapor Heated, FEIBA® VH IMMUNO per kg of body weight is recommended. However, care should be taken to distinguish between the following four indications, all of which have undergone careful clinical evaluation:

Joint Hemorrhage

In joint hemorrhage, a dose of 50 units per kg of body weight is recommended at 12-hour intervals, which may be increased to doses of 100 units per kg of body weight at 12-hour intervals.

Treatment should be continued until clear signs of clinical improvement appear, such as relief of pain, reduction of swelling or mobilization of the joint.

Mucous Membrane Bleeding

A dose of 50 units per kg of body weight is recommended to be given at 6-hour intervals under careful monitoring (visible bleeding site, repeated measurements of the patient's hematocrit). Again, if hemorrhage does not stop, the dose may be increased to 100 units per kg of body weight at 6-hour intervals. However, 2 such administrations or 200 units per kg of body weight a day should not be exceeded.

Soft Tissue Hemorrhage

For serious soft tissue bleeding, such as retroperitoneal bleeding, doses of 100 units per kg of body weight at 12-hour intervals are recommended. A daily dosage of 200 units per kg of body weight should not be exceeded.

Other Severe Hemorrhages

Severe hemorrhages, such as CNS bleedings have been effectively treated with doses of 100 units per kg of body weight at 12-hour intervals. Sometimes, Anti-Inhibitor Coagulant Complex, Vapor Heated, FEIBA® VH IMMUNO may be indicated at 6-hour intervals until clear clinical improvement is achieved.

Reconstitution

1. Warm the unopened bottle containing Sterile Water for Injection (diluent) to room temperature (not above 37°C, 98°F).
2. Remove caps from the concentrate and diluent bottles to expose central portions of the rubber stoppers.
3. Cleanse exposed surface of the rubber stoppers with germicidal solution and allow to dry.
4. Using aseptic technique, remove protective covering from one end of the double-ended needle, and completely insert the exposed end through the diluent bottle stopper.
5. Remove protective covering from the other end of the double-ended needle, taking care not to touch the exposed end. Invert diluent bottle over the concentrate bottle, then rapidly insert free end of the needle to its full length through the concentrate bottle stopper. Diluent will be drawn into the concentrate bottle by vacuum.
6. Disconnect the two bottles by removing needle from the concentrate bottle stopper. Gently agitate or rotate the concentrate bottle until all material is dissolved.

Do not refrigerate after reconstitution!

After complete reconstitution of Anti-Inhibitor Coagulant Complex, Vapor Heated, FEIBA® VH IMMUNO, its injection or infusion should be commenced as promptly as practicable, but must be completed within three hours following reconstitution.

Continued on next page

Feiba VH—Cont.

The solution must be given by intravenous injection or intravenous drip infusion and the **maximum injection or infusion rate must not exceed 2 units per kg of body weight per minute.** In a patient with a body weight of 75 kg, this corresponds to an infusion rate of 2.5–7.5 mL per minute depending on the number of units per vial (see label on vial).

For Intravenous Injection:

1. After reconstituting the concentrate as described under **Reconstitution,** attach the enclosed filter needle to a sterile disposable syringe. Insert filter needle through the concentrate bottle stopper.
2. Inject air and withdraw solution into the syringe.
3. Remove and discard the filter needle. Attach a suitable intravenous needle or infusion set with winged adapter, and inject solution intravenously.

For Intravenous Infusion:

Prepare a solution of Anti-Inhibitor Coagulant Complex, Vapor Heated, FEIBA® VH IMMUNO as described under **Reconstitution.**

Follow manufacturer's instructions for the administration set used. Make sure that the set contains an adequate filter.

HOW SUPPLIED

Anti-Inhibitor Coagulant Complex, Vapor Heated, FEIBA® VH IMMUNO is supplied as freeze-dried powder, accompanied by a suitable volume of Sterile Water for Injection, U.S.P. (This Product Contains Dry Natural Rubber.), a sterile double-ended needle, and a sterile filter needle.

The number of IMMUNO Units of Factor VIII inhibitor bypassing activity is stated on the label of each bottle.

STORAGE

Store at refrigerator temperature (2° to 8°C, 35° to 46°F).

Avoid freezing, which may damage the diluent bottle.

REFERENCES

1. ELSINGER F.: Aktivierter Faktor VII in Prothrombinkomplex-Konzentraten, 23rd Annual Meeting of "Deutsche Arbeitsgemeinschaft für Blutgerinnungsforschung" (DAB), Heidelberg, 1979. F. K. Schattauer Verlag, Stuttgart-New York, 367, 1980.
2. SELIGSOHN U., ØSTERUD B., RAPAPORT S.I.: Coupled Amidolytic Assay for Factor VII: Its Use With a Clotting Assay to Determine the Activity State of Factor VII. Blood 52: 978, 1978.
3. SELIGSOHN U., KASPER C. K., ØSTERUD B., RAPAPORT S.I.: Activated Factor VII: Presence in Factor IX Concentrates and Persistence in the Circulation After Infusion. Blood 53: 828, 1979.
4. MANNUCCI P. M.: Personal communication.
5. SJAMSOEDIN L. J. M., HEIJNEN L., MAUSER-BUNSCHOTEN E. P., van GEIJLSWIJK J. L., van HOUWELINGEN H., van ASTEN P., SIXMA J. J.: The Effect of Activated Prothrombin-Complex Concentrate (FEIBA) on Joint and Muscle Bleeding in Patients with Hemophilia A and Antibodies to Factor VIII. The New England. J. of Med. 305: 717, 1981.
6. ROBERTS H. R.: Hemophiliacs with inhibitors. Therapeutic Options. The New Engl. J. of Med. 305: 757, 1981.
7. HILGARTNER M. W., KNATTERUD G. AND THE FEIBA STUDY GROUP: The Use of Factor-Eight-Inhibitor-By-Passing-Activity (FEIBA Immuno) Product for Treatment of Bleeding Episodes in Hemophiliacs with Inhibitors. Blood 61: 36, 1983.
8. THOMAS T., WILLIAMS H., WILLIAMS Y., HUNT J.: FEIBA in Haemophiliacs with Factor VIII Inhibitor. Brit. Med. J. 1: 52, 1977.
9. ROLOVIC Z., ELEZOVIC I., OBRENOVIC B.: Life-Threatening Bleeding Due to an Acquired Inhibitor to Factor XII–XI Successfully Treated with FEIBA. Proceedings of Joint Meeting of the 18th Congress of the International Society of Hematology and 16th Congress of the International Society of Blood Transfusion, Montreal. Abstract 703, 1980.
10. DORMANDY K.: Unpublished data.
11. VINAZZER H.: Personal communication.
12. PRESTON F. E.: A Review of Cases Treated with FEIBA in 1977/78. Presentation at the Second Workshop on Factor VIII Inhibitor Patients, Vienna, 1979.
13. VERMYLEN J., SCHETZ J., SEMERARO N., MERTENS F., VERSTRAETE M.: Evidence that 'Activated' Prothrombin Concentrates Enhance Platelet Coagulant Activity. Brit. J. Haematol. 38: 235, 1978.
14. SEMERARO N., VERMYLEN J.: Evidence that Washed Human Platelets Possess Factor-X Activator Activity. Brit. J. Haematol 36: 107, 1977.
15. WENSLEY R. T.: General Summary of the Use of FEIBA in Haemophiliacs with Inhibitors to F VIII. Presentation at the Second Workshop on Factor VIII Inhibitor Patients, Vienna, 1979.
16. HILGARTNER M. W.: Personal communication.

Issued April 1998

Manufactured by
ÖSTERREICHISCHES INSTITUT FÜR HAEMODERIVATE GES.M.B.H.
Subsidiary of **IMMUNO AG**
A-1220 Vienna, Austria
U.S. Establishment Licence 258
U.S. Pat. Nos. 4,364,861, 4,391,746, 4,395,396, and 4,640,834

Distributed by
IMMUNO-U.S., Inc.
1200 Parkdale Road
Rochester, Michigan 48307

6205820EH15

GAMMAGARD S/D ℞

Immune Globulin Intravenous (Human)
Solvent/Detergent Treated

DESCRIPTION

Immune Globulin Intravenous (Human) [IGIV] *Gammagard S/D* is a solvent/detergent treated, sterile, freeze-dried preparation of highly purified immunoglobulin G (IgG) derived from large pools of human plasma. The product is manufactured by the Cohn-Oncley cold ethanol fractionation process followed by ultrafiltration and ion exchange chromatography. Source material for fractionation may be obtained from another U.S. licensed manufacturer. The manufacturing process includes treatment with an organic solvent/detergent mixture,[1,2] composed of tri-n-butyl phosphate, octoxynol 9 and polysorbate 80.[3] The *Gammagard S/D IGIV* manufacturing process provides a significant viral reduction in *in vitro* studies.[3] These studies, summarized in Table 1, demonstrate virus clearance during *Gammagard S/D* manufacturing using infectious Human Immunodeficiency virus, Types 1 and 2 (HIV-1, HIV-2); Bovine Viral Diarrhea virus (BVD), a model virus for Hepatitis C virus; Sindbis virus (SIN), a model virus for lipid enveloped viruses; Pseudorabies virus (PRV), a model virus for lipid-enveloped DNA viruses such as Herpes; Vesicular stomatitis virus (VSV), a model virus for lipid-enveloped RNA viruses; and Encephalomyocarditis virus (EMC), a model virus for non-lipid enveloped viruses.[3] These reductions are achieved through a combination of process chemistry, partitioning and/or inactivation during cold ethanol fractionation and the solvent/detergent treatment.[3]

[See table 1 below]

When reconstituted with the total volume of diluent (Sterile Water for Injection, USP) supplied, this preparation contains approximately 50 mg of protein per mL (5%), of which at least 90% is gamma globulin. The product, reconstituted to 5%, contains a physiological concentration of sodium chloride (approximately 8.5 mg/mL) and has a pH of 6.8 ± 0.4. Stabilizing agents and additional components are present in the following maximum amounts for a 5% solution: 3 mg/mL Albumin (Human), 22.5 mg/mL glycine, 20 mg/mL glucose, 2 mg/mL polyethylene glycol (PEG), µg/mL tri-n-butyl phosphate, 1 µg/mL octoxynol 9, and 100 µg/mL polysorbate 80. If it is necessary to prepare a 10% (100 mg/mL) solution for infusion, half the volume of diluent should be added, as described in the Dosage and Administration section. In this case, the stabilizing agents and other components will be present at double the concentrations given for the 5% solution.

The manufacturing process for *Gammagard S/D IGIV* isolates IgG without additional chemical or enzymatic modification, and the Fc portion is maintained intact. *Gammagard S/D IGIV* contains all of the IgG antibody activities which are present in the donor population. On the average, the distribution of IgG subclasses present in this product is similar to that in normal plasma.[3] *Gammagard S/D IGIV* contains only trace amounts of IgA (< 3.7 µg/mL in a 5% solution). IgM is also present in trace amounts.

Immune Globulin Intravenous (Human), *Gammagard S/D IGIV* contains no preservative.

CLINICAL PHARMACOLOGY

Immune Globulin Intravenous (Human), *Gammagard S/D*, contains a broad spectrum of IgG antibodies against bacterial and viral agents that are capable of opsonization and neutralization of microbes and toxins. Peak levels of IgG are reached immediately after infusion of *Gammagard S/D IGIV* S/D. It has been shown that, after infusion, exogenous IgG is distributed relatively rapidly between plasma and extravascular fluid until approximately half is partitioned in the extravascular space. Therefore a rapid initial drop in serum IgG levels is to be expected.[4]

As a class, IgG survives longer *in vivo* than other serum proteins.[4,5] Studies show that the half-life of *Gammagard S/D IGIV* is approximately 37.7 ± 15 days.[3] Previous studies reported IgG half-life values of 21 to 25 days.[4,5,6] The half-life of IgG can vary considerably from person to person, however. In particular, high concentrations of IgG and hypermetabolism associated with fever and infection have been seen to coincide with a shortened half-life of IgG.[4–7]

INDICATIONS AND USAGE

Primary Immunodeficiency Diseases

Gammagard S/D IGIV is indicated for the treatment of primary immunodeficient states, such as: congenital agammaglobulinemia, common variable immunodeficiency, Wiskott-Aldrich syndrome, and severe combined immunodeficiencies.[6,7] This indication was supported by a clinical trial of 17 patients with primary immunodeficiency who received a total of 341 infusions. *Gammagard S/D IGIV* is especially useful when high levels or rapid elevation of circulating IgG are desired or when intramuscular injections are contraindicated (e.g., small muscle mass).

B-cell Chronic Lymphocytic Leukemia (CLL)

Gammagard S/D IGIV is indicated for prevention of bacterial infections in patients with hypogammaglobulinemia and/or recurrent bacterial infections associated with B-cell Chronic Lymphocytic Leukemia (CLL). In a study of 81 patients, 41 of whom where treated with Immune Globulin Intravenous (Human), *Gammagard S/D IGIV,* bacterial infections were significantly reduced in the treatment group.[8,9] In this study, the placebo group had approximately twice as many bacterial infections as the IGIV group. The median time to first bacterial infection for the IGIV group was greater than 365 days. By contrast, the time to first bacterial infection in the placebo group was 192 days. The number of viral and fungal infections, which were for the most part minor, was not statistically different between the two groups.

Idiopathic Thrombocytopenic Purpura (ITP)

When a rapid rise in platelet count is needed to prevent and/or to control bleeding in a patient with Idiopathic Thrombocytopenic Purpura, the administration of *Gammagard S/D IGIV,* should be considered.

The efficacy of *Gammagard S/D IGIV* has been demonstrated in a clinical study involving 16 patients. Of these 16 patients, 13 had chronic ITP (11 adults, 2 children), and three patients had acute ITP (one adult, two children). All 16 patients (100%) demonstrated a clinically significant rise in platelet count to a level greater than 40,000/mm³ following the administration of *Gammagard S/D IGIV.* Ten of the 16 patients (62.5%) exhibited a significant rise to greater

Table 1: *In Vitro* Virus Clearance During *Gammagard S/D IGIV* Manufacturing

Process Step No.	Process Step Evaluated	Virus Clearance, log10						
		HIV-1	HIV-2	SIN	BVD	PRV	VSV	EMC
1A	Fraction I+II+III Wash to Fraction I+III Centrifugate	8.2*†	N.T.•	5.2*	1.7	2.9	N.D.**	2.4
1B	Fraction I+II+III Wash to Fraction I+III Filter Press Filtrate	8.2*†	N.T.•	N.D.**	1.3	3.7	N.D.**	3.7
2A	Fraction I+III Centrifugate to Fraction I+III Filtrate	8.2*†	N.T.•	4.6*	N.D.**	N.D.**	N.D.**	N.D.**
2B	Fraction I+III Filter Press Filtrate to Fraction I+III Filtrate	8.2*†	N.T.•	N.D.**	0.7	4.5	N.D.**	3.0
3	Fraction I+III Filtrate to Fraction II Precipitate	8.1*†	N.T.•	N.A.***	N.A.***	N.A.***	N.D.**	N.A.***
4	Treatment of Resuspended Fraction II Precipitate with Solvent/Detergent Mixture	8.3*	5.7*	5.1*	4.9*	4.1*	6.0*	N.A.‡

Note: Centrifugation (steps 1A and 2A) **or** Filtration by Filter Press (steps 1B and 2B) is used in the IGIV manufacturing process.
* Minimum log reduction due to detection limit of the assay.
** Not determined.
*** Not applicable. Virus co-precipitates with Fraction II proteins.
• Not tested. HIV-1 serves as a model for HIV-2.
† Inactivation soley by ethanol.
‡ Not applicable. Solvent/Detergent inactivates only lipid enveloped viruses.

than 80,000 platelets/mm^3. Of these ten patients, seven had chronic ITP (five adults, two children), and three patients had acute ITP (one adult, two children).

The rise in platelet count to greater than 40,000/mm^3 occurred after a single 1 g/kg infusion of *Gammagard S/D IGIV* in eight patients with chronic ITP (six adults, two children), and in two patients with acute ITP (one adult, one child). A similar response was observed after two 1 g/kg infusions in three adult patients with chronic ITP, and one child with acute ITP. The remaining two adult patients with chronic ITP received more than two 1 g/kg infusions before achieving a platelet count greater than 40,000/mm^3. The rise in platelet count was generally rapid, occurring within five days. However, this rise was transient and not considered curative. Platelet count rises lasted two to three weeks, with a range of 12 days to six months. It should be noted that childhood ITP may resolve spontaneously without treatment.

Kawasaki Syndrome

Gammagard S/D IGIV is indicated for the prevention of coronary artery aneurysms associated with Kawasaki syndrome. The percentage incidence of coronary artery aneurysm in patients with Kawasaki syndrome receiving *Gammagard S/D IGIV* either at a single dose of 1 g/kg (n=22) or at a dose of 400 mg/kg for four consecutive days (n=22), beginning within seven days of onset of fever, was 3/44 (6.8%). This was significantly different (p=0.008) from a comparable group of patients that received aspirin only in previous trials and of whom 42/185 (22.7%) experienced coronary arter aneurysms.[19, 22, 23] All patients in the *Gammagard S/D IGIV* trial received concomitant aspirin therapy and none experienced hypersensitivity-type reactions (urticaria, bronchospasm or generalized anaphylaxis).[18]

Several studies have documented the efficacy of intravenous gammaglobulin in reducing the incidence of coronary artery abnormalities resulted from Kawasaki syndrome.[19–25]

CONTRAINDICATIONS

None known.

WARNINGS

Warnings

Immune Globulin Intravenous (Human) products have been reported to be associated with renal dysfunction, acute renal failure, osmotic nephrosis, and death.[24,26] Patients predisposed to acute renal failure include patients with any degree of pre-existing renal insufficiency, diabetes mellitus, age greater than 65, volume depletion, sepsis, paraproteinemia, or patients receiving known nephrotoxic drugs. Especially in such patients, IGIV products should be administered at the minimum concentration available and the minimum rate of infusion practicable. While these reports of renal dysfunction and acute renal failure have been associated with the use of many of the licensed IGIV products, those containing sucrose as a stabilizer accounted for a disproportionate share of the total number.* See Precautions and Dosage and Administration sections for important information intended to reduce the risk of acute renal failure.

***Gammagard S/D IGIV* does not contain sucrose**

Immune Globulin Intravenous (Human), *Gammagard S/D*, should only be administered intravenously. Other routes of administration have not been evaluated.

Immediate anaphylactic and hypersensitivity reactions are a remote possibility. Epinephrine should be available for treatment of any acute anaphylactoid reactions.

Gammagard S/D IGIV contains only trace amounts of IgA (< 3.7 µg/mL in a 5% solution). Nonetheless, it should be given with caution to patients with antibodies to IgA or selective IgA deficiencies.[7,10]

PRECAUTIONS

General

There is clinical evidence of a possible association between Immune Globulin Intravenous (Human) (IGIV) administration and thrombotic events. The exact cause of this is unknown; therefore, caution should be exercised in the prescribing and infusion of IGIV in patients with a history of cardiovascular disease or thrombotic episodes.[12–17]

As aseptic meningitis syndrome (AMS) has been reported to occur infrequently in association with Immune Globulin Intravenous (Human) (IGIV) treatment. Discontinuation of IGIV treatment has resulted in remission of AMS within several days without sequelae. The syndrome usually begins within several hours to two days following IGIV treatment. It is characterized by symptoms and signs including severe headache, nuchal rigidity, drowsiness, fever, photophobia, painful eye movements, and nausea and vomiting. Cerebrospinal fluid (CSF) studies are frequently positive with pleocytosis up to several thousand cells per cu.mm., predominantly from the granulocytic series, and elevated protein levels up to several hundred mg/dL. Patients exhibiting such symptoms and signs should receive a thorough neurological examination, including CSF studies, to rule out other causes of meningitis. AMS may occur more frequently in association with high dose (2 g/kg) IGIV treatment.

Assure that patients are not volume depleted prior to the initiation of the infusion of IGIV.

Periodic monitoring of renal function tests and urine output is particularly important in patients judged to have a potential increased risk for developing acute renal failure. Renal function, including measurement of blood urea nitrogen (BUN)/serum creatinine, should be assessed prior to the initial infusion of *Gammagard S/D IGIV* and again at appropriate intervals thereafter. If renal function deteriorates, discontinuation of the product should be considered.

For patients judged to be at risk for developing renal dysfunction, it may be prudent to reduce the amount of product infused per unit time by infusing *Gammagard S/D IGIV* at a rate less than 13.3 mg IG/kg/min.

Certain components used in the packaging of this product contain natural rubber latex.

INFORMATION FOR PATIENTS

Patients should be instructed to immediately report symptoms of decreased urine output, sudden weight gain, fluidretention/edema, and/or shortness of breath (which may suggest kidney damage) to their physician.

Drug Interactions

See Dosage and Administration Section.

Pregnancy Category C

Animal reproduction studies have not been conducted with Immune Globulin Intravenous (Human), *Gammagard S/D IGIV*. It is also not known whether *Gammagard S/D IGIV* can cause fetal harm when administered to a pregnant woman or can affect reproduction capacity. *Gammagard S/D IGIV* should be given to a pregnant woman only if clearly needed.

ADVERSE REACTIONS

Increases in creatinine and blood urea nitogen (BUN) have been observed as soon as one to two days following infusion. Progressionn to oliguria and anuria requiring dialysis has been observed, although some patients have improved spontaneously following cessation of treatment.[27]

Types of severe renal adverse reactions that have been seen following IGIV therapy include:

- acute renal failure
- acute tubular necrosis[28]
- proximal tubular nephropathy
- osmotic nephrosis[29–31 (see also 29–31]

In general, reported adverse reactions to *Gammagard S/D IGIV* in patients with either congenital or acquired immunodeficiencies are similar in kind and frequency. Various minor reactions, such as headache, fatigue, chills, backache, leg cramps, lightheadedness, fever, urticaria, flushing, slight elevation of blood pressure, nausea and vomiting may occasionally occur. Slowing or stopping the infusion usually allows the symptoms to disappear promptly. Immediate anaphylactic and hypersensitivity reactions are a remote possibility. Epinephrine should be available for treatment of any acute anaphylactoid reaction (See **Warnings**).

Primary Immunodeficiency Diseases

Twenty-one adverse reactions occurred in 341 infusions (6%), when using *Gammagard S/D IGIV* (5% solution). in a clinical trial of 17 patients with primary immunodeficiency.[11] Of the 17 patients, 12 (71%) were adults, and 5 (29%) were children (16 years or younger).

In a cross-over study comparing *Gammagard S/D IGIV* and *Gammard* (5% solutions) conducted in a small number (n=10) of primary immunodeficient patients, no unusual or unexpected adverse reactions were observed in the *Gammagard S/D IGIV* group. The adverse reactions experienced in the *Gammagard S/D IGIV* group were similar in frequency and nature to those observed in the control group consisting of patients receiving *Gammagard S/D IGIV*.

Gammagard S/D IGIV reconstituted to a concentration of 10%, was administered intravenously at rates varying from 2–11 mL/kg/Hr. Systemic reactions occurred in 23 (10.5%) of 219 infusions. This compares with an adverse reaction incidence of 6% (only systemic reactions reported) for primary immunodeficient patients previously treated with a 5% solution at infusion rates varying between 2 and 8 mL/kg/Hr, as described above (also, see reference 11). Local pain or irritation was experienced during 35 (16%) of 219 infusions. Application of a warm compress to the infusion site alleviated local symptoms.

These local reactions tended to be associated with hand vein infusions and their incidence may be reduced by infusions via the antecubital vein.

B-cell Chronic Lymphocytic Leukemia (CLL)

In the study of patients with B-cell Chronic Lymphocytic Leukemia, the incidence of adverse reactions associated with *Gammagard S/D IGIV* infusions was approximately 1.3% while that associated with placebo (normal saline) infusions was 0.6%.[9]

Idiopathic Thrombocytopenic Purpura (ITP)

During the clinical study of *Gammagard S/D IGIV* for the treatment of Idiopathic Thrombocytopenic Purpura, the only adverse reaction reported was headache which occurred in 12 of 16 patients (75%). Of these 12 patients, 11 had chronic ITP (9 adults, 2 children), and one child had acute ITP. Oral antihistamines and analgesics alleviated the symptoms and were used as pretreatment for those patients requiring additional IGIV therapy. The remaining four patients did not report any side effects and did not require pretreatment.

Kawasaki Syndrome

In a study of patients (n=51) with Kawasaki syndrome, no hypersensitivity type reactions (urticaria, bronchospasm or generalized anaphylaxis) were reported in patients receiving either a single 1 g/kg dose of IGIV. *Gammagard S/D IGIV*, or 400 mg/kg of IGIV, *Gammagard S/D IGIV*, for four consecutive days. 12 Mild adverse reactions, including chills, flushing, cramping, headache, hypotension, nausea, rash, and wheezing, were reported with both dose regimens. These adverse reactions occurred in 7/51 (13.7%) patients and in association with 7/129 (5.4%) infusions. Of the 25 patients who received a single 1g/kg dose, four patients experienced adverse reactions for an incidence of 16%. Of the 26 patients who received 400 mg/kgday over four days, three experienced a single adverse reaction for an incidence of 11.5%.[3]

DOSAGE AND ADMINISTRATION

Primary Immunodeficiency Diseases

For patients with primary immunodeficiencies, monthly doses of at least 100 mg/kg are recommended. Initially, patients may receive 200–400 mg/kg. As there are significant differences in the half-life of IgG among patients with primary immunodeficiencies, the frequency and amount of immunoglobulin therapy may vary from patient to patient. The proper amount can be determined by monitoring clinical response. The minimum serum concentration of IgG necessary for protection has not been established.

B-cell Chronic Lymphocytic Leukemia (CLL)

For patients with hypogammaglobulinemia and/or recurrent bacterial infrections due to B-cell Chronic Lymphocytic Leukemia, a dose of 400 mg/kg every three to four weeks is recommended.

Kawasaki Syndrome

For patients with Kawasaki syndrome, either a single 1 g/kg dose or a dose of 400 mg/kg for four consecutive days beginning within seven days of the onset of fever, administered concomitantly with appropriate aspirin therapy (80–100 mg/kg/day in four divided doses) is recommended.

Idiopathic Thrombocytopenic Purpura (ITP)

For patients with acute or chronic Idiopathic Thrombocytopenic Purpura, a dose of 1 g/kg is recommended. The need for additional doses can be determined by clinical response and platelet count. Up to three separate doses may be given on alternate days, if required.

No prospective data are presently available to identify a maximum safe dose, concentration, and rate of infusion in patients determined to be at increased risk of acute renal failure. In the absence of prospective data, the recommended doses should not be exceeded and the concentration and infusion rate selected should be the minimum level practicable. Reduction in dose, concentration, and/or rate of administration in patients at risk of acute renal failure has been proposed in the literature in order to reduce the risk of acute renal failure.[32]

Reconstitution: Use Aseptic Technique

When reconstitution is performed aspetically outside of a sterile laminar air flow hood, administration should begin as soon as possible, but not more than two hours after reconstitution.

When reconstitution is performed aseptically in a sterile laminar air flow hood, the reconstituted product may be either maintained in the original glass container or pooled into Viaflex® bags and stored under constant refrigeration (2–8°C), for up to 24 hours. (The data and time of reconstitution/pooling should be recorded). If these conditions are not met, sterility of the reconstituted product cannot be maintained. Partially used vials should be discarded.

A. 5-Solution

1. **Note: Reconstitute immediately before use.**
2. If refrigerated, warm the Sterile Water for Injection, USP (diluent) and Immune Globulin Intravenous (Human), *Gammagard S/D* (dried concentrate), to room temperature.
3. Remove caps from concentrate and diluent bottles to expose central portion of rubber stoppers.
4. Cleanse stoppers with germicidal solution.
5. Remove protective covering from the spike at one end of the transfer device (Figure 1).

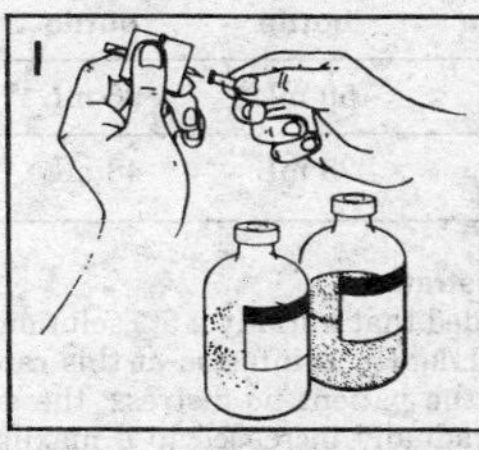

1. Place the diluent bottle on a flat surface and, while holding the bottle to prevent slipping, insert the spike of the transfer device **perpendicularly through the center** of the bottle stopper.
2. Press down firmly so that the transfer device fits snugly against the diluent bottle (Figure 2).

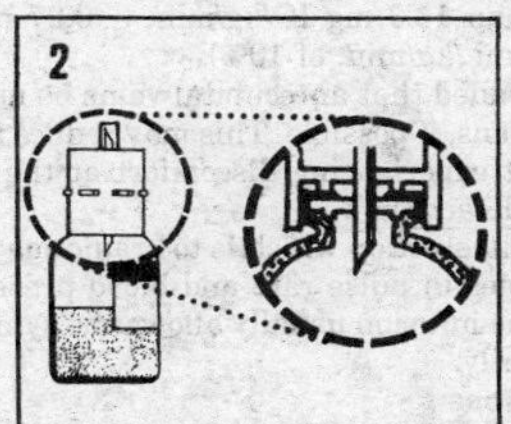

Continued on next page

Gammagard S/D—Cont.

Caution: Failure to use center of stopper may result in dislodging the stopper.

1. Remove the protective convering from the other end of the transfer device. Hold diluent bottle to prevent slipping.
2. Hold concentrate bottle firmly and at an angle of approximately 45 degrees. Invert the diluent bottle with the transfer device at an angle complementary to the concentrate bottle (approximately 45 degrees) and firmly insert the transfer device into the concentrate bottle through the center of the rubber stopper (Figure 3).

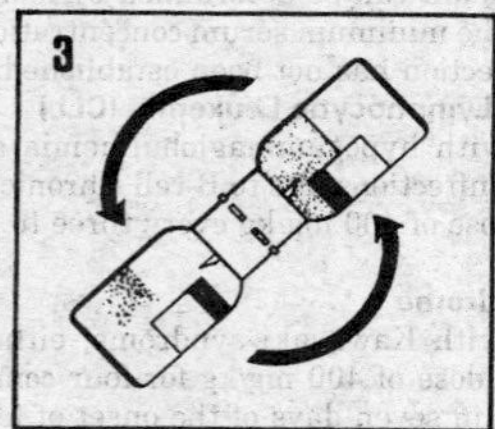

Note: Invert the diluent bottle with attached transfer device rapidly into the concentrate bottle in order to avoid loss of diluent.

Caution: Failure to use center of stopper may result in dislodging the stopper and loss of vacuum.

1. The diluent will flow into the concentrate bottle quickly. When diluent transfer is complete, remove empty diluent bottle and transfer device from concentrate bottle. Discard transfer device after single use.
2. Thoroughly wet the dried material by tilting or inverting and gently rotating the bottle (Figure 4). Do not shake. Avoid foaming.

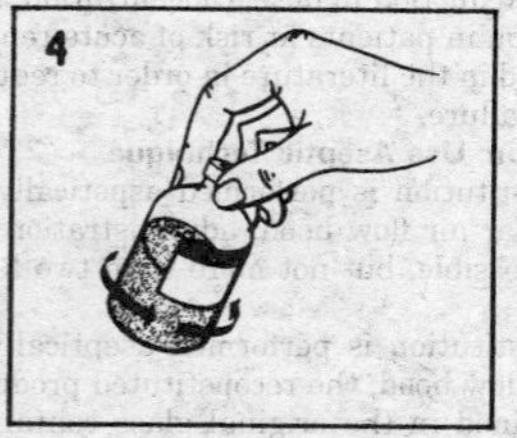

1. Repeat gentle rotation as long as undissolved product is observed.

B. 10% Solution

Follow steps 1–4 as previously described in **A.**

5. To prepare a 10% solution, reconstitute with the appropriate volume of diluent as indicated in Table 2, which indicates the volume of diluent required for a 5% or 10% concentration. Using aseptic technique, draw required volume into a sterile hypodermic syringe and needle. Discard the filled syringe.

6. Using the residual diluent in the diluent vial, follow steps 5–12 as previously described in **A.**

Table 2: Required Diluent Volume

Concentration	2.5 g bottle	5 g bottle	10 g bottle
5%	50 mL	96 mL	192 mL
10%	25 mL	48 mL	96 mL

Rate of Administration

It is recommended that initially a 5% solution be infused at a rate of 0.5 mL/kg/Hr. If infusion at this rate and concentration causes the patient no distress, the administration rate may be gradually increased to a maximum rate of 4 mL/kg/Hr. Patients who tolerate the 5% concentration at 4 mL/kg/Hr can be infused with the 10% concentration starting a 0.5 mL/kg/Hr. If no adverse effects occur, the rate can be increased gradually up to a maximum of 8 mL/kg/Hr.

For patients judged to be at risk for developing renal dysfunction, it may be prudent to reduce the amount of product infused per unit time by infusing *Gammagard S/D IGIV* at a rate less than 13.3 mg IG/kg/min. (<0.27 mL/kg/min. of 5% or <0.13 mL/kg/min. of 10%).

It is recommended that antecubital veins be used especially for 10% solutions, if possible. This may reduce the likelihood of the patient experiencing discomfort at the infusion site (see Adverse Reactions).

A rate of administration which is too rapid may cause flushing and changes in pulse rate and blood pressure. Slowing or stopping the infusion usually allows the symptoms to disappear promptly.

Drug Interactions

Admixtures of Immune Globulin Intravenous (Human), *Gammagard S/D*, with other drugs and intravenous solutions have not been evaluated. It is recommended that *Gammagard S/D IGIV*, be administered separately from other drugs or medications which the patient may be receiving. The product should not be mixed with Immune Globulin Intravenous (Human) from other manufacturers.

Antibodies in immune globulin preparations may interfere with patient responses to live vaccines, such as those for measles, mumps, and rubella. The immunizing physician should be informed of recent therapy with Immune Globulin Intravenous (Human) so that appropriate precautions can be taken.

Administration

Gammagard S/D IGIV should be administered as soon after reconstitution as possible or as described in the Dosage and Administration section. The reconstituted material should be at room temperature during administration. Parenteral drug products should be inspected visually for particulate matter and discoloration prior to administration, whenever solution and container permit. Do not use if particulate matter and/or discoloration is observed.

Follow directions for use which accompany the administration set provided. If another administration set is used, ensure that the set contains a similar filter.

How Supplied

Gammagard S/D IGIV is supplied in 0.5 g, 2.5 g, 5 g, or 10 g single use bottles. Each bottle of Gammagard S/D IGIV is furnished with a suitable volume of Sterile Water for Injection, USP, a transfer device and an administration set which contains an integral airway and a 15 micron filter.

Storage

Gammagard S/D IGIV, is to be stored at a temperature not to exceed 25°C (77°F). Freezing should be avoided to prevent the diluent bottle from breaking.

REFERENCES

1. Prince AM, Horowitz B, Brotman B: Sterilisation of hepatitis and HTLV-III viruses by exposure to tri-n-butyl phosphate and sodium cholate. **Lancet 1**:706–710, 1986
2. Horowitz B, Wiebe ME, Lippin A, *et al*: Inactivation of viruses in labile blood derivatives: I. Disruption of lipid enveloped viruses by tri-n-butyl phosphate detergent combinations. **Transfusion 25**:516–522, 1985
3. Unpublished data in the files of Baxter health-care Corporation
4. Waldmann TA, Storber W: Metabolism of immunoglobulins. **Prog Allergy 13**:1–110, 1969
5. Morell A, Riesen W: Structure, function and catabolism of immuno globulins in **Immunohemotherapy**. Nydegger UE (ed), London, Academic Press, 1981, pp 17–26
6. Stiehm ER: Standard and special human immune serum globulins as therapeutic agents. **Pediatrics 63**: 301–319, 1979
7. Buckley RH: Immunoglobulin replacement therapy: Indications and contraindications for use and variable IgG levels achieved in **Immunoglobulins: Characteristics and Use of Intravenous Preparations**. Alving BM, Finlayson JS (eds), Washington, DC, U.S. Department of Health and Human Services, 1979, pp 3–8.
8. Bunch C, Chapel HM, Rai K, *et al*:: Intravenous Immune Globulin reduces bacterial infections in Chronic Lymphocytic Leukemia: A controlled randomized clinical trial. **Blood 70 Suppl 1**:753, 1987
9. Cooperative Group for the Study of Immunoglobulin in Chronic Lymphocytic Leukemia: Intravenous immunoglobulin for the prevention of infection in Chronic Lymphocytic Leukemia: A randomized, controlled clinical trial. **N Eng J Med 319**:902–907, 1988
10. Burks AW, Sampson HA, Buckley RH: Anaphylactic reactions after gammaglobulin administration in patients with hypogammaglobulinemia: Detection of IgE antibodies to IgA. **N Eng J Med 314**:560–564, 1986
11. Ochs HD, Lee ML, Fischer SH, *et al*: Efficacy of a New Intravenous Immunoglobulin Preparation in Primary Immunodeficient Patients. **Clinical Therapeutics 9**:512–522, 1987
12. Reinhart WH, Berchtold PE: Effect of high-dose intravenous immunoglobulin therapy on blood rheology. **Lancet 339**: 662–664, 1992
13. Dalakas MC: High-dose intravenous immunoglobulin and serum viscosity: Risk of precipitating thromboembolic events. **Neurology 44**:223–226, 1994
14. Harkness K, Howell SJL, Davies-Jones GAB: Encephalopathy associated with intravenous immunoglobulin treatment for Guillain-Barre syndrome. **Journal of Neurology 60**:586–598, 1996
15. Woodruff RK, Grigg AP, Firkin FC, Smith IL: Fatal thrombotic events during treatment of autoimmune thrombocytopenia with intravenous immunoglobulin in elderly patients. **Lancet ii**:217–218, 1986
16. Silbert PL, Knezevic WV, Bridge DT: Cerebral infarction complicating intravenous immunoglobulin therapy for polyneuritis cranialis. **Neurology 42**:257–258, 1992
17. Duhem C, Dicato MA, Ries F: Side effects of intravenous immune globulins. **Clin Exp Immunol 97: (Suppl 1)** 70–83, 1994
18. Data in the files of Baxter Healthcare Corporation
19. Newburger J, Takahashi M, Burns JG, *et al*: The Treatment of Kawasaki Syndrome with Intravenous Gamma Globulin. **New England Journal of Medicine 315**:341–347, 1986
20. Furusho K, Hroyuki N, Shinomiya K, *et al*: High Dose Intravenous Gammaglobulin for Kawasaki Disease. **Lancet 2**:1055–1058, 1984
21. Engle MA, Fatica NS, Bussel JB, O'Laughlin JE, Snyder MS, Lesser ML: Clinical Trial of Single-Dose Intravenous Gammaglobulin in Acute Kawasaki Disease. **AJDC143**:1300–1304, 1989
22. Furusho K, Sato K, Soeda T, *et al*: High Dose Intravenous Gammaglobulin for Kawasaki Disease [letter]. **Lancet 2**:1359, 1983
23. Nagashima M, Matsushima M, Matsucka H, Ogawa A, Okumura N: High Dose Gammaglobulin Therapy for Kawasaki Disease. **Journal of Pediatrics 110**:710–712, 1987
24. Isawa M, Sugiyama K, Kawase A, *et al*: Prevention of Coronary Artery Involvement in Kawasaki Disease by Early Intravenous High Dose Gammaglobulin. In: Doyle EF, Engle MA, Gersony WM, Rashkind EJ, Talner NS, eds. **Pediatric Cardiology**. New York: Springer-Verlag, 1986:1083–1085
25. Okuri M, Harada K, Yamaguchi H, *et al*: Intravenous Gammaglobulin Therapy in Kawasaki Disease: Trial of Low-Dose Gammaglobulin. In: Shulman ST, ed. **Kawasaki Disease**. New York: Alan R. Liss, 1987:433–439
26. Cayco AV, Perazella MA, Hayslett JP: Renal insufficiency after intravenous immune globulin therapy: A Report of Two Cases and an Analysis of the Literature. 1997; **J Amer Soc Nephrology 8**: 1788–1793
27. Winward DB, Brophy MT: Acute renal failure after administration of intravenous immunoglobulin: review of the literature and case report. 1995; **Pharmacotherapy 15**:765?
28. Phillips AO: Renal failure and intravenous immunoglobulin [letter, comment]. 1992; **Clin Nephrol 36**: 83–86
29. Anderson W, Bethea W: Renal lesions following administration of hypertonic solutions of sucrose. 1940; **JAMA 114**:1983–1987
30. Lindberg H, Wald A: Renal changes following the administration of hypertonic solutions. 1939; **Arch Intern Med 63**: 907–918
31. Rigdon RH, Cardwell ES: Renal lesions following the intravenous injection of hypertonic solution of sucrose: A clinical and experimental study. 1942; **Arch Intern Med 69**:670–690
32. Tan E, Hajinazarian M, Bay, *et al*: Acute renal failure resulting from intravenous immunoglobulin therapy. 1993; **Arch Neurology 50**:137–139

BIBLIOGRAPHY

Bussel JB, Kimberly RP, Inman RD, *et al*: Intravenous gammaglobulin treatment of chronic idiopathic thrombocytopenic purpura. **Blood 62**:480–486, 1983

* Manufactured Under U.S. Patent No. 4,439,421.

Baxter Healthcare Corporation
Hyland Division
Glendale, CA 91203 USA
U.S. License No. 140 Revised May 1999
30-5K-03-120

HEMOFIL M ℞

Antihemophilic Factor (Human)
Method M, Monoclonal Purified

DESCRIPTION

Antihemophilic Factor (Human) (AHF), Hemofil M, Method M, Monoclonal Purified, is a sterile, nonpyrogenic, dried preparation of antihemophilic factor (Factor VIII, Factor VIII:C, AHF) in concentrated form with a specific activity range of 2 to 15 AHF International Units/mg of total protein. When reconstituted with the appropriate volume of diluent, it contains approximately 12.5 mg/mL Albumin (Human), 1.5 mg/mL polyethylene glycol (3350), 0.055 M histidine and 0.030 M glycine as stabilizing agents. In the absence of the added Albumin (Human), the specific activity is approximately 2,000 AHF International Units/mg of protein. It also contains, per AHF International Unit, not more than 0.1 ng mouse protein, 18 ng organic solvent (tri-n-butyl phosphate) and 50 ng detergent (octoxynol 9). See **Clinical Pharmacology.**

Hemofil M AHF is prepared by the Method M process from pooled human plasma by immunoaffinity chromatography utilizing a murine monoclonal antibody to Factor VIII:C, followed by an ion exchange chromatography step for further purification. Source material may be provided by other US licensed manufacturers. Hemofil M AHF also includes an organic solvent (tri-n-butyl phosphate) and detergent (octoxynol 9) virus inactivation step designed to reduce the risk of transmission of hepatitis and other viral diseases. However, no procedure has been shown to be totally effective in removing viral infectivity from coagulation factor products.

Each bottle of Hemofil M AHF is labeled with the AHF activity expressed in International Units per bottle, which is referenced to the WHO International Standard.

Hemofil M AHF is to be administered only intravenously.

CLINICAL PHARMACOLOGY

Antihemophilic factor (AHF) is a protein found in normal plasma which is necessary for clot formation.

The administration of Hemofil M AHF provides an increase in plasma levels of AHF and can temporarily correct the coagulation defect of patients with hemophilia A (classical hemophilia). The administration of Hemofil M AHF will also correct deficiencies caused by circulating inhibitors when the inhibitor level does not exceed 10 Bethesda Units per mL.

The half-life of Antihemophilic Factor (Human) (AHF), Hemofil M, Method M, Monoclonal Purified, administered to Factor VIII deficient patients has been shown to be 14.8 ± 3.0 hours.

Use of an organic solvent (tri-n-butyl phosphate; TNBP) in the manufacture of Antihemophilic Factor (Human) has little or no effect on AHF activity, while lipid enveloped viruses, such as hepatitis B and human immunodeficiency virus (HIV) are inactivated.[1] Prince, *et al*, report inactivation of at least 10,000 Chimpanzee Infectious Doses (CID-50) of hepatitis B virus, 10,000 CID-50 of hepatitis non A, non B virus, and 30,000 Tissue Culture Infectious Doses of HIV with TNBP/detergent treatment during manufacture of an Antihemophilic Factor (Human) concentrate[2]

In vitro studies demonstrate that the Hemofil M AHF, manufacturing process provides for significant viral reduction. These studies, summarized in Table 1, demonstrate virus clearance during the Hemofil M AHF manufacturing process using Human Immunodeficiency virus, Type 1 (HIV-1); Bovine Viral Diarrhea virus (BVD), a model for lipid enveloped RNA viruses, such as hepatitis C virus (HCV); Pseudorabies virus (PRV), a model for lipid enveloped DNA viruses, such as herpes; Porcine Parvovirus (PPV), a model for non-lipid enveloped DNA viruses, such as human parvovirus B19; and hepatitis A virus (HAV), a model for non-lipid enveloped RNA viruses. These reductions are achieved through a combination of process chemistry, partitioning and/or inactivation during solvent/detergent treatment, immunoaffinity chromatography, Q-Sepharose column chromatography and lyophilization.

[See table 1 above]

Hemofil M AHF was administered to 11 patients previously untreated with Antihemophilic Factor (Human). They have shown no signs of hepatitis or HIV infection following three to nine months of evaluation.

A study of 25 patients treated with Hemofil M AHF, and monitored for three to six months has demonstrated no evidence of antibody response to mouse protein. More than 1,000 infusions of Antihemophilic Factor (Human) (AHF), Hemofil M, Method M, Monoclonal Purified, have been administered during the clinical trials with no significant reactions. Reported events included a single episode each of chest tightness, fuzziness and dizziness, and one patient reported an unusual taste after each infusion.

INDICATIONS AND USAGE

The use of Hemofil M AHF is indicated in hemophilia A (classical hemophilia) for the prevention and control of hemorrhagic episodes.

Hemofil M AHF can be of significant therapeutic value in patients with acquired Factor VIII inhibitors not exceeding 10 Bethesda Units per mL.[3] However, in such uses, the dosage should be controlled by frequent laboratory determinations of circulating AHF.

Hemofil M AHF is not indicated in von Willebrand's disease.

CONTRAINDICATIONS

Known hypersensitivity to mouse protein is a contraindication to the use of Antihemophilic Factor (Human) (AHF), Hemofil M, Method M, Monoclonal Purified.

WARNINGS

Antihemophilic Factor (Human) (AHF), Hemofil M, Method M, Monoclonal Purified, is made from human plasma. Products made from human plasma may contain infectious agents, such as viruses, that can cause disease. The risk that such products will transmit an infectious agent has been reduced by screening plasma donors for prior exposure to certain viruses, by testing for the presence of certain current virus infections, and by inactivating and/or removing certain viruses. Despite these measures, such products can still potentially transmit disease. There is also the possibility that unknown infectious agents may be present in such products. ALL infections thought by a physician possibly to have been transmitted by this product should be reported by the physician or other healthcare provider to Baxter Healthcare Corporation, Hyland Immuno at 1-800-423-2862 (in the U.S.). The physician should discuss the risks and benefits of this product with the patient.

Individuals who receive infusions of blood or plasma products may develop signs and/or symptoms of some viral infections, particularly non A, non B hepatitis. As indicated under **Clinical Pharmacology**, however, a group of such patients treated with Hemofil M AHF did not demonstrate signs or symptoms of non A, non B hepatitis over observation periods ranging from three to nine months.

PRECAUTIONS

General

Certain components used in the packaging of this product contain natural rubber latex.

Identification of the clotting defect as a Factor VIII deficiency is essential before the administration of Antihemophilic Factor (Human) (AHF), Hemofil M, Method M, Monoclonal Purified, is initiated.

Table 1
***In Vitro* Virus Clearance During the Manufacture of Hemofil M AHF**

Process Step Evaluated	Virus Clearance, $\log_{10}$				
	Lipid-enveloped			Non-Lipid enveloped	
	HIV-1	BVD	PRV	PPV	HAV
Solvent/Detergent Treatment	10.3	3.8	4.3	*	*
Immunoaffinity Chromatography	N.A.**	N.A.**	N.A.**	4.2	5.3
Q-Sepharose Column Chromatography	N.T.†	2.3	1.1	1.4	<0.9‡
Lyophilization	N.T.†	N.T.†	N.T.†	N.T.†	1.9
Cumulative Total, $\log_{10}$	10.3	6.1	5.4	5.6	7.2

* Solvent/Detergent treatment inactivates only lipid enveloped viruses. PV and HAV are non-lipid enveloped viruses.
** Not Applicable for lipid enveloped viruses due to the presence of solvent/detergent in the starting material.
† Not Tested.
‡ Value not included in cumulative total.

HEMORRHAGE		
Degree of hemorrhage	**Required peak post-infusion AHF activity in the blood (as % of normal or IU/dL plasma)**	**Frequency of infusion**
Early hemarthrosis or muscle bleed or oral bleed	20–40	Begin infusion every 12 to 24 hours for one-three days until the bleeding episode as indicated by pain is resolved or healing is achieved.
More extensive hemarthrosis, muscle bleed, or hematoma	30–60	Repeat infusion every 12 to 24 hours for usually three days or more until pain and disability are resolved
Life threatening bleeds such as head injury, throat bleed, severe abdominal pain.	60–100	Repeat infusion every 8 to 24 hours until threat is resolved.
SURGERY		
Type of operation		
Minor surgery, including tooth extraction	60–80	A single infusion plus oral antifibrinoytic therapy within one hour is sufficient in approximately 70% of cases.
Major surgery	80–100 (pre- and post-operative)	Repeat infusion every 8 to 24 hours depending on state of healing.

No benefit may be expected from this product in treating other deficiencies.

The processing of Hemofil M AHF significantly reduces the presence of blood group specific antibodies in the final product.

Formation of Antibodies to Mouse Protein

Although no hypersensitivity reactions have been observed, because Hemofil M AHF contains trace amounts of mouse protein (less than 0.1 ng/AHF activity units), the possibility exists that patients treated with this product may develop hypersensitivity to the mouse proteins.

The pulse rate should be determined before and during administration of Hemofil M AHF. Should a significant increase occur, reducing the rate of administration or temporarily halting the injection usually allows the symptoms to disappear promptly.

Information for Patients

Some viruses, such as parvovirus B19 or hepatitis A, are particularly difficult to remove or inactivate at this time. Parvovirus B19 most seriously affects pregnant women, or immune-compromised individuals. Symptoms of parvovirus B19 infection include fever, drowsiness, chills, and runny nose followed about two weeks later by a rash, and joint pain. Evidence of hepatitis A may include several days to weeks of poor appetite, tiredness, and low-grade fever followed by nausea, vomiting, and pain in the belly. Dark urine and a yellowed complexion are also common symptoms. Patients should be encouraged to consult their physician if such symptoms appear.

Patients should be informed of the early signs of hypersensitivity reactions including hives, generalized urticaria, tightness of the chest, wheezing, hypotension, and anaphylaxis, and should be advised to discontinue use of the product and contact their physician if these symptoms occur.

Laboratory Tests

Although dosage can be estimated by the calculations which follow, it is strongly recommended that whenever possible, appropriate laboratory tests be performed on the patient's plasma at suitable intervals to assure that adequate AHF levels have been reached and are maintained.

If the AHF content of the patient's plasma fails to reach expected levels or if bleeding is not controlled after apparently adequate dosage, the presence of inhibitor should be suspected. By appropriate laboratory procedures, the presence of inhibitor can be demonstrated and quantified in terms of AHF units neutralized by each mL of plasma or by the total estimated plasma volume. If the inhibitor is at low levels (i.e., <10 Bethesda Units/mL), after administration of sufficient AHF units to neutralize the inhibitor, additional AHF units will elicit the predicted response.

Pregnancy

Pregnancy Category C. Animal reproduction studies have not been conducted with Antihemophilic Factor (Human) (AHF), Hemofil M, Method M, Monoclonal Purified. It is not known whether Hemofil M AHF can cause fetal harm when administered to a pregnant woman or can affect reproduction capacity. Hemofil M AHF should be given to a pregnant woman only if clearly needed.

ADVERSE REACTIONS

Allergic reactions may be encountered from the use of Antihemophilic Factor (Human) preparations. See **Information for Patients.**

The protein in greatest concentration in Hemofil M AHF is Albumin (Human). Reactions associated with albumin are extremely rare, although nausea, fever, chills or urticaria have been reported.

DOSAGE AND ADMINISTRATION

Each bottle of Antihemophilic Factor (Human) (AHF), Hemofil M AHF, Method M, Monoclonal Purified, is labeled with the AHF activity expressed in IU per bottle. This potency assignment is referenced to the World Health Organization International Standard.

The high purity of Hemofil M AHF has been thought to influence the difficulty of producing an accurate potency measurement. Experiments have shown that to achieve accurate activity levels, such a potency assay should be conducted using plastic test tubes and pipets as well as substrate containing normal levels of von Willebrand's Factor.

The expected *in vivo* peak AHF level, expressed as IU/dL of plasma or % (percent) of normal, can be calculated by multiplying the dose administered per kg body weight (IU/kg) by two. This calculation is based on the clinical finding by Abildgaard, *et al*,[4] which is supported by data from the collaborative study of *in vivo* recovery and survival with 15 different lots of Hemofil M AHF on 56 hemophiliacs that demonstrated a mean peak recovery point above the mean pre-infusion baseline of about 2.0 IU/dL per infused IU/kg body weight.[5]

Example:

(1) A dose of 1750 IU AHF administered to a 70 kg patient, i.e. 25 IU/kg (1750/70), should be expected to cause a peak post-infusion AHF increase of $25 \times 2 = 50$ IU/dL (50% of normal).

Continued on next page

Hemofil M—Cont.

(2) A peak level of 70% is required in a 40 kg child. In this situation the dose would be 70/2 × 40 = 1400 IU.

Reconstitution: Use Aseptic Technique

1. Bring Hemofil M AHF (dry concentrate) and Sterile Water for Injection, USP, (diluent) to room temperature.
2. Remove caps from concentrate and diluent bottles to expose central portion of rubber stoppers.
3. Cleanse stoppers with germicidal solution.
4. Remove protective covering from one end of double-ended needle and insert exposed needle through diluent stopper.
5. Remove protective covering from other end of double-ended needle. Invert diluent bottle over upright Hemofil M AHF bottle, then rapidly insert free end of the needle through the Hemofil M AHF bottle stopper at its center. The vacuum in the Hemofil M AHF bottle will draw in the diluent.
6. Disconnect the two bottles by removing needle from diluent bottle stopper, then remove needle from Hemofil M AHF bottle. Swirl gently until all material is dissolved. Be sure that Hemofil M AHF is completely dissolved, otherwise active material will be removed by the filter.

Note: Do not refrigerate after reconstitution.

Administration: Use Aseptic Technique

Administer at room temperature.

Antihemophilic Factor (Human) (AHF), Hemofil M, Method M, Monoclonal Purified, should be administered not more than three hours after reconstitution.

Intravenous Syringe Injection

Parenteral drug products should be inspected for particulate matter and discoloration prior to administration, whenever solution and container permit.

Plastic syringes are recommended for use with this product. The ground glass surface of all-glass syringes tend to stick with solutions of this type.

1. Attach filter needle to a disposable syringe and draw back plunger to admit air into syringe.
2. Insert needle into reconstituted Hemofil M AHF.
3. Inject air into bottle and then withdraw the reconstituted material into the syringe.
4. Remove and discard the filter needle from the syringe; attach a suitable needle and inject intravenously as instructed under **Rate of Administration.**
5. If a patient is to receive more than one bottle of Hemofil M AHF the contents of two bottles may be drawn into the same syringe by drawing up each bottle through a separate unused filter needle. This practice lessens the loss of Hemofil M AHF. Please note, filter needles are intended to filter the contents of a single bottle of Hemofil M AHF only.

Rate of Administration

Preparations of Hemofil M AHF can be administered at a rate of up to 10 mL per minute with no significant reactions. The pulse rate should be determined before and during administration of Hemofil M AHF. Should a significant increase occur, reducing the rate of administration or temporarily halting the injection usually allows the symptoms to disappear promptly.

HOW SUPPLIED

Hemofil M AHF is available as single dose bottles. Each bottle is labeled with the potency in International Units, and is packaged together with 10 mL of Sterile Water for Injection, USP, a double-ended needle, and a filter needle.

STORAGE

Store Antihemophilic Factor (Human) (AHF), Hemofil M, Method M, Monoclonal Purified at 2–8°C (36–46°F) until the expiration date noted on the package. Within this period (indicated by the expiration date), the product may be stored at room temperature, not to exceed 30°C (86°F), for up to twelve months. Avoid freezing to prevent damage to the diluent bottle.

REFERENCES

1. Horowitz B, Wiebe ME, Lippin A, *et al:* Inactivation of viruses in labile blood derivatives: 1. Disruption of lipid enveloped viruses by tri(n-butyl)phosphate detergent combinations. **Transfusion 25**:516–522, 1985
2. Prince AM, Horowitz B, Brotman B: Sterilisation of hepatitis and HTLV-III viruses by exposure to tri(n-butyl)phosphate and sodium cholate. **Lancet 1**:706–710, 1986
3. Kessler CM: An Introduction to Factor VIII Inhibitors: The Detection and Quantitation. **Am J Med 91 (Suppl 5A)**:1S–5S, 1991
4. Abildgaard CF, Simone JV, Corrigan JJ, *et al:* Treatment of hemophilia with glycine-precipitated Factor VIII. **New Eng J Med 275**:471–475, 1966
5. Addiego, Jr. JE, Gomperts E, Liu S. *et al:* Treatment of hemophilia A with a highly purified Factor VIII concentrate prepared by Anti-FVIIIc immunoaffinity chromatography. **Thrombosis and Haemostasis 67**:19–27, 1992
6. Schimpf K, Rothmann P, Zimmermann K: Factor VIII dosis in prophylaxis of hemophilia A; A further controlled study, in **Proc XIth Cong W.F.H.** Kyoto, Japan, Academic Press, 1976, pp 363–366

RECOMMENDED DOSAGE SCHEDULE

Physician supervision of the dosage is required. The following dosage schedule may be used as a guide.

[See second table on previous page]

The careful control of the substitution therapy is especially important in cases of major surgery or life threatening hemorrhages.

Although dosage can be estimated by the calculations above, it is strongly recommended that whenever possible, appropriate laboratory tests including serial AHF assays be performed on the patient's plasma at suitable intervals to assure that adequate AHF levels have been reached and are maintained.

Other dosage regimens have been proposed such as that of Schimpf, *et al*, which describes continuous maintenance therapy.[6]

To enroll in the confidential, industry-wide Patient Notification System, call 1-888-UPDATE U (1-888-873-2838)

Baxter, Hyland Immuno, and Hemofil are trademarks of Baxter International, Inc.

Baxter and Hemofil are registered in the U.S. Patent and Trademark office.

Baxter Healthcare Corporation
Hyland Immuno
Glendale, CA 91203 USA
U.S. License No. 140
Printed in USA
Part No. 7260
Revised February 2000

IVEEGAM® EN IGIV
IMMUNE GLOBULIN INTRAVENOUS (HUMAN) ℞

DESCRIPTION

Immune Globulin Intravenous (Human) [IGIV], *IVEEGAM EN*, is a sterile freeze-dried concentrate of immunoglobulin G (IgG). Reconstitution of the freeze-dried powder with the accompanying quantity of Sterile Water for Injection, U.S.P. gives a 5% protein solution suitable for intravenous administration. This final solution contains, per mL, 50±5 mg of IgG, 50 mg of glucose as a stabilizer, and 3 mg of sodium chloride. Trace amounts of IgM and IgA are also present. The reconstituted solution is clear, colorless, and free of detectable aggregates. It contains no preservative.

IVEEGAM EN is prepared from large pools of human plasma. The pooled plasma is fractionated by a modified cold ethanol process. Cohn Fraction II is subjected to treatment with immobilized trypsin and purified by sequential precipitation steps with polyethylene glycol. (PEG) Polyethylene glycol may be present in the final product at levels below 0.5 g/dL. The *IVEEGAM EN* manufacturing process provides a significant viral reduction in in vitro studies. These studies, summarized in Table 1, demonstrate virus clearance during *IVEEGAM EN* manufacturing using infectious Human Immunodeficiency virus, Type 1 (HIV-1); Tick Born Encephalitis virus (TBEV), a model virus for Hepatitis C virus; Pseudorabies virus (PRV), a model virus for lipid-enveloped DNA viruses; Equine Rhinovirus, Type 1 (ERV-1), a model virus for non-lipid enveloped RNA viruses; Mouse Murine virus (MMV), a model virus for B19 Parvovirus; and infectious Hepatitis A virus (HAV). These reductions are achieved through a combination of precipitation of Cohn Fraction II + III, 12% alcohol precipitation, DEAE-Sephadex adsorption, incubation with immobilized hydrolases and PEG precipitation.

[See table below]

CLINICAL PHARMACOLOGY

Patients with primary humoral immunodeficiency are at high risk for the development of acute and chronic bacterial infections because of their low levels of circulation IgG [1,2]. Immune Globulin Intravenous (Human), *IVEEGAM EN* provides a broad spectrum of IgG antibodies [43]. The opsonizing, neutralizing, and complement binding activities of these antibodies help prevent or attenuate a multiplicity of infectious diseases. When administered intravenously, 100% of the IgG antibodies are available in the circulation immediately. The distribution of the intravenously administered preparation between intra- and extravascular compartments requires several days to reach an equilibrium. The serum IgG level therefore drops to approximately 40–50% of the peak level during the first week postinfusion.[4,5]. *IVEEGAM EN* has a half-life of approximately three to four weeks, which is in agreement with that reported for intramuscular immunoglobulin [4,6]. In six agamma-globulinemic patients, the half-life of *IVEEGAM* was determined by measuring the activity of tetanus antibody during a four week period after infusion of 150 mg/kg body mass. The half-life ranged from 23 to 29 days[6]. Variation in half-life has been observed among patients and is important in determining the dosage regimen for each patient.

IgG serum levels were measured in 21 patients with primary immunodeficiencies treated with *IVEEGAM* with an average monthly dose of 225 mg/kg body mass for approximately 16 months. Serum levels increased from an average preinfusion level of 406 mg IgG/dL to an average of 762 mg IgG/dL postinfusion. The average increase in individual patients' serum IgG levels calculated per 100 mg IgG/kg body mass varied from 44 to 309 mg/dl.

Infections were evaluated in 12 primary immunodeficient children receiving one of two dose levels of *IVEEGAM*: 150 mg/kg (low dose) or 500 mg/kg (high dose). Eight children had been previously treated with fresh plasma for up to two years. The number of days with infections was reduced when comparing low dose *IVEEGAM* to plasma and when comparing high dose to low dose *IVEEGAM*. The geometric means and ranges (mg/dL) of serum IgG levels for eight patients were: plasma: 169 (62–435), low dose *IVEEGAM*: 212 (68–425), and high dose *IVEEGAM*: 557 (315–810) [7]. Studies were performed to monitor for the presence of antibody to Human Immunodeficiency Virus (HIV) and markers for viral hepatitis. No evidence of viral transmission has been observed in more than 30 patients on various dosage regimens followed for periods of 4 to 12 months and tested at intervals ranging from 3 to 6 weeks.

Reports of adverse reactions from clinical trials and clinical experience in Europe and Canada have been infrequent and no serious adverse reactions have been observed [7,8]. See Adverse Reaction Section.

In order to evaluate the efficacy and safety of *IVEEGAM* in the treatment of Kawasaki syndrome (KS), two controlled, multi-center, randomized studies were performed. The first study compared the efficacy and safety of *IVEEGAM* plus aspirin with that of aspirin alone in reducing the frequency of coronary artery abnormalities in children with acute KS[9]. Children randomly assigned to the immune globulin group received *IVEEGAM*, 400 mg/kg body mass per day, for four consecutive days. Both treatment groups received aspirin, 100 mg/kg body mass each day through the fourteenth day of illness, and 3 to 5 mg/kg each day thereafter for approximately five weeks. Two weeks after enrollment, coronary artery abnormalities were present in 18 (23%) of 78 children in the aspirin only group as compared to 6 (8%) of 75 in the *IVEEGAM* group ($p<0.01$). Seven weeks after enrollment, abnormalities were present in 14 (18%) of 79 patients in the aspirin only group and 3 (4%) of 79 in the *IVEEGAM* group ($p<0.005$). It was concluded that high-dose *IVEEGAM* is safe and effective in reducing the prevalence of coronary artery abnormalities when administered early in the course of KS. The second clinical trial was a multi-center, randomized trial involving 549 children with acute KS [10]. Children were randomly assigned to receive *IVEEGAM* either in a single infusion of 2 g/kg over 10 hours or in daily infusions of 400 mg/kg for four consecutive days. Both treatment groups received aspirin, 100 mg/kg each day through the fourteenth day of illness, then 3 to 5 mg/kg each day thereafter. Results showed that at two weeks after enrollment coronary artery abnormalities were present in 24 (9.1%) of 263 children in the four-day group as compared to 12 (4.6%) of 260 in the single-infusion group ($p <0.05$). Seven weeks after enrollment abnormalities were present

***In Vitro* Virus Clearance During *IVEEGAM EN* Manufacturing**

Manufacturing Step	Virus Clearance, $\log_{10}$					
	HIV-1	TBEV[1]	PRV[1]	ERV-1[3]	MMV[4]	HAV
Precipitation of Cohn Fraction II+ III	2.2	1.6	1.2	4.2	ND	ND
12% Alcohol	> 4.9	> 4.8	4.7	> 5.0	ND	ND
DEAE Sephadex	> 4.3	5.0	1.5	> 5.1	> 6.6	> 5.4
Hydrolase Incubation	4.1	4.8	> 5.4	5.6	< 1.0	ND
PEG Precipitation	4.1	> 4.4	> 5.1	4.6	ND	ND
Cumulative Reduction	> 19.6	> 20.6	> 18.9	> 24.5	> 6.6	> 5.4

ND = Not Done; [1]Model virus for Hepatitis C virus (HCV); [2] Model virus for lipid enveloped DNA viruses; [3]Model virus for non-lipid enveloped RNA viruses; [4] Model virus for B19 Parvovirus

in 7.2% of the four-day group and in 3.9% of the single-infusion group ($p<0.1$). The two groups had a similar incidence of adverse effects, occurring in approximately 3% of children overall.

The second study thus supports the efficacy of *IVEEGAM EN* in treating acute KS, and further demonstrates that a single dose of 2 g/kg of *IVEEGAM EN* infused over 10 hours is at least as effective as four conservative daily doses of 400 mg/kg.

INDICATIONS AND USAGE

Immunodeficiency Syndromes

Immune Globulin Intravenous (Human), *IVEEGAM EN* is indicated for replacement therapy in patients with primary immunodeficiency syndromes such as congenital agammaglobulinemia, common variable immunodeficiency, x-linked agammaglobulinemia (with or without hyper IgM) and Wiskott-Aldrich syndrome [2].

Patients with severe combined immunodeficiency have, in addition to a T-cell defect, an impairment of antibody production. They may benefit from replacement therapy with *IVEEGAM EN* even though this therapy will not correct the cellular immune defect. *IVEEGAM EN* is especially useful when high levels or rapid elevation of circulating antibodies are desired or when intramuscular injections are contraindicated.

Kawasaki Syndrome

IVEEGAM EN is indicated in the treatment of Kawasaki syndrome. When administered in conjunction with aspirin, within ten days of onset of disease, treatment with either a single dose of 2000 mg *IVEEGAM*/kg body mass given over a ten hour period, or 400 mg *IVEEGAM*/kg body mass on four consecutive days resulted in a 65% to 78% decrease in the incidence of coronary artery abnormalities compared to treatment with aspirin alone [9,10].

CONTRAINDICATIONS

IVEEGAM EN is contraindicated in individuals who are known to have had an anaphylactic or severe systemic response to Immune Globulin (Human).

Individuals with selective IgA deficiency should not receive *IVEEGAM EN* since these patients may experience severe reactions to the IgA which may be present.

WARNINGS

Warnings

Immune Globulin Intravenous (Human) products have been reported to be associated with renal dysfunction, acute renal failure, osmotic nephrosis, and death [15]. Patients predisposed to acute renal failure include patients with any degree of pre-existing renal insufficiency, diabetes mellitus, age greater than 65, volume depletion, sepsis, paraproteinemia, or patients receiving known nephrotoxic drugs. Especially in such patients, IGIV products should be administered at the minimum concentration available and the minimum rate of infusion practicable. While these reports of renal dysfunction and acute renal failure have been associated with the use of many of the licensed IGIV products, those containing sucrose as a stabilizer accounted for a disproportionate share of the total number.*

See **Precautions** and **Dosage and Administration** sections for important information intended to reduce the risk of acute renal failure.

IVEEGAM EN IGIV does not contain sucrose*

IVEEGAM EN should be administered only intravenously as the intramuscular and subcutaneous routes have not been evaluated.

Although not observed in the clinical studies with this product, severe anaphylactic reactions have been observed following administration of other immunoglobulin preparations [11, 12, 13, 14]. These reactions have been attributed to the presence of immunoglobulin A in certain preparations, and in certain instances, to antigen-antibody interactions, if patients had antigenemia and the respective antibodies were present in the product[12].

IF ANAPHYLACTIC OR SEVERE ANAPHYLACTOID REACTIONS OCCUR, THE INFUSION IS TO BE DISCONTINUED IMMEDIATELY. Whenever *IVEEGAM* is administered, appropriate therapy should be available to treat a severe anaphylactic reaction, e.g. epinephrine.

IVEEGAM EN is made from human plasma. Products made from human plasma may contain infectious agents, such as viruses, that can cause disease. The risk that such products will transmit an infectious agent has been reduced by screening plasma donors for prior exposure to certain viruses, by testing for the presence of certain current virus infections, and by inactivating and/or removing certain viruses (see **Description**). Despite these measures, such products can still potentially transmit disease. There is also possibility that unknown infectious agents may be present in such products. ALL infections thought by a physician possibly to have been transmitted by this product should be reported by the physician or other healthcare provider to Baxter Healthcare, Hyland Division, at 1-800-423-2862. The physician should discuss the risks and benefits of this product with the patient.

PRECAUTIONS

General

Assure that patients are not volume depleted prior to the initiation of the infusion of IGIV.

Periodic monitoring of renal function tests and urine output is particularly important in patients judged to have a potential increased risk for developing acute renal failure. Renal function, including measurement of blood urea nitrogen (BUN)/serum creatinine, should be assessed prior to the initial infusion of *IVEEGAM EN* and again at appropriate intervals thereafter. If renal function deteriorates, discontinuation of the product should be considered.

For patients judged to be at risk for developing renal dysfunction, it may be prudent to reduce the amount of product infused per unit time by infusing *IVEEGAM EN* at a rate less than 1.5 mg lg per kg body weight per minute (0.03 mL/kg/minute). Any vial which has been reconstituted should be used promptly. Partially used vials should be discarded.

Patients with severe antibody deficiency syndromes are more likely to react adversely to the initial infusions of homologous IGIV. Modified dosage regimens have been used to prevent such reactions. See **Dosage and Administration** Section.

In isolated cases and mostly with the use of high doses, administration of IGIV from different manufacturers has been associated with the development of aseptic meningitis manifesting as neck rigidity with severe headache, nausea, vomiting, fevew, drowsiness, photophobia, pain when moving the eyes, and dizziness[15]. These symptoms can begin within hours or a few days after the infusion. These symptoms were reversible with or without therapy, and disappeared completely within a few hours or days.

Information For Patient

Patients should be instructed to immediately report symptoms of decreased urine output, sudden weight gain, fluid retention/edema, and/or shortness of breath (which may suggest kidney damage) to their physicians.

Some viruses, such as parvovirus B19, are particularly difficult to remove or inactivate at this time. Parvovirus B19 most seriously affects pregnant women, or immune compromised individuals.

Symptoms of parvovirus B19 infection include fever, drowsiness, chills and runny nose followed about two weeks later by a rash and joint pain. Patients should be encouraged to consult their physician if such symptoms appear.

Drug Interactions

For compatibility issues see **Dosage and Administration** Section.

It is reported that antibodies in immune globulin preparations may interfere with the responses by patients to live viral vaccines such as measles, mumps, and rubella. Immunizing physicians should be informed of recent therapy with Immune Globulin Intravenous (Human), so that appropriate precautions may be taken.

Pregnancy Category C

Animal reproduction studies have not been carried out with Immune Globulin Intravenous (Human), *IVEEGAM EN*. It is also not known whether *IVEEGAM EN* can cause fetal harm when administered to a pregnant woman or can affect reproduction capacity. *IVEEGAM EN* should be given to a pregnant woman only if clearly needed.

ADVERSE REACTIONS

Increses in creatinine and blood urea nitrogen (BUN) have been observed as soon as one to two days following infusion. Progression to oliguria and anuria requiring dialysis has been observed, although some patients have improved spontaneously following cessation of treatment[16].

Types of severe renal adverse reactions that have been seen following IGIV therapy include:

- acute renal failure
- acute tubular necrosis[17]
- proximal tubular nephropathy
- osmotic nephrosis ([15] see also [18–20])

Reported reactions to *IVEEGAM* in patients with primary humoral immunodeficiency have been mild and transient in nature, and have included flushing, increased blood pressure, malaise, headache, nausea, vomiting, low-grade fever, and rash. In clinical trials involving more than 1300 infusions, adverse reaction rates have ranged from 0.3% to 0.8% [4–8]. Although not observed in clinical trials with *IVEEGAM*, severe anaphylactic reactions have been reported with other immunoglobulin preparations. In the first clinical trial of *IVEEGAM* in the treatment of Kawasaki syndrome, mild congestive heart failure developed with comparable frequency in the aspirin only group (5%) and in the aspirin plus *IVEEGAM* group (4%). In each of the latter cases, the child tolerated subsequent infusions without difficulty. After the first infusion, one child had shaking chills and itching, which resolved after treatment with diphenhydramine. These symptoms did not recur with subsequent infusions. One child had sepsis secondary to an intravenous line. One child treated with *IVEEGAM* had neutropenia and splenomegaly for several months after treatment; one child in the aspirin group also had neutropenia.

In the second Kawasaki syndrome clinical trial, 3.3% of children overall had possible complications attributable to *IVEEGAM*. Two children (0.36%) had hypotension, two (0.36%) had pruritus, nine (1.6%) had mild worsening of congestive heart failure, and five (0.91%) had other events, including infiltrates at the site of the i.v. line and skin slough[1], generalized edema without congestive heart failure [2], acute onset of nasal congestion and cough without urticaria, pruritus, or hypotension, responding to Benadryl Diphenhyramine HCl without interruption of infusion [1], and probable auto-immune hemolytic anemia [1]. There were no life-threatening complications in either study.

No long-term hematological or biochemical changes attributable to *IVEEGAM* therapy were detected during the course of either study. No evidence for the transmission of non-A/non-B hepatitis or human immunodeficiency virus was associated with the use of *IVEEGAM*.

DOSAGE AND ADMINISTRATION

Parenteral drug products should be inspected visually for particulate matter and discoloration prior to administration whenever solution and container permit. Reconstituted vials found to contain particles or to be discolored should not be used. Reconstitute Immune Globulin Intravenous (Human), *IVEEGAM EN* with Sterile Water for Injection, U.S.P. only. The reconstituted product may be diluted with 5% dextrose or saline.

Interactions or incompatibilities with other drugs have not been evaluated.

Do not mix *IVEEGAM EN* with other brands of intravenous immunoglobulins in preparing a large dose.

If administered with other preparations, always use separate infusion lines. When using primary infusion lines, rinse with saline prior to the infusion of *IVEEGAM EN*. Immune Globulin Intravenous (Human), *IVEEGAM EN* must be administered intravenously after reconstitution. The usual rate of administration is 1 mL per minute up to a maximum of 2 mL per minute for the 5% solution..

For patients judged to be at risk for developing renal dysfunciton, it may be prudent to reduce the amount of product infused per unit time by infusing *IVEEGAM EN* at a rate less than 1.5 mg lg per kg body weight per minute (0.03 mL/kg/minute).

No prospective data are presently available to identify a maximum safe dose, conentration, and rate of infusion in patients determined to be at increased risk of acute renal failure. In the absene of prospective data, the recommended doses should not be exceeded and the concentration and infusion rate selected should be the minimum level practicable. Reduction in dose, concentration, and/or rate of administration in patients at risk of acute renal failure has been proposed in the literature in order to reduce the risk of acute renal failure [21].

Immunodeficiency Syndromes

A dose of 200 mg/kg per month is recommended for treatment of primary humoral immunodeficiency syndromes.

If the desired clinical results are not obtained, the dose may be increased up to 4-fold or intervals between infusions shortened. Doses of Immune Globulin Intravenous (Human), *IVEEGAM EN* up to 800 mg/kg body mass per month were tolerated by immunodeficient patients [6].

If adequate doses are given at regular intervals, pre-infusion IgG levels may be expected to rise steadily over a period of 6–12 months until a plateau is reached. The minimum serum concentration of IgG necessary for protection has not been established.

Dose regimens have been modified in an attempt to prevent adverse reactions in previously untreated, severe, immunodeficient patients. In a limited number of such patients, treatment has been initiated with lower doses of *IVEEGAM* diluted with saline or 5% dextrose. With gradually increasing dose levels and protein concentrations (up to 5% protein) adverse reactions were not observed[6].

Kawasaki Syndrome

Treatment with *IVEEGAM EN* should be initiated within ten days of onset of the disease. Either a dose of 400 mg/kg body mass daily for four consecutive days or a single dose of 2000 mg/kg given over a ten hour period may be used. Because all studies of this product, to date, have involved concurrent administration of aspirin, the treatment regimen should include aspirin, 100 mg/kg each day through the fourteenth day of illness, then 3 to 5 mg/kg each day thereafter for a period of five weeks.

Reconstitution

Reconstitution with the Sterile Water for Injection, U.S.P. provided in each package results in a 5% solution.

1. Remove protective caps from the concentrate and solvent bottles (Fig. 1) and disinfect rubber stoppers of both bottles. Remove protective covering from one end of the accompanying double-ended spike and insert the exposed spike through the diluent bottle stopper Fig. 2.
2. Remove protective cap from the other end of the double-ended spike. Do not touch exposed spike end!
3. Turn diluent bottle upside down and insert free end of the spike into the concentrate bottle stopper to its full length, then invert the connected bottles (Fig. 3). Diluent will be drawn into the concentrate bottle by vacuum.
4. Disconnect the two bottles leaving the spike on the solvent bottle (Fig. 4). Accelerate reconstitution by agitating or rotating the concentrate bottle. DO NOT SHAKE VIGOROUSLY! Either draw up the clear solution into a syringe using the accompanying filter needle Fig. 5, 500 mg and 1000 mg sizes) or administer the solution directly using the accompanying infusion set with filter (2500 mg and 5000 mg sizes).

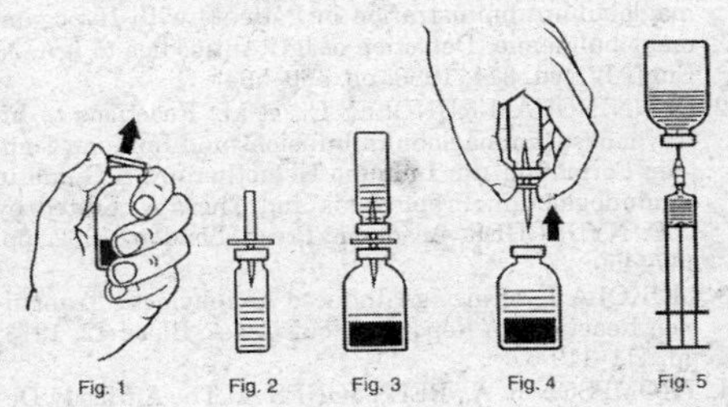

Continued on next page

Iveegam—Cont.

HOW SUPPLIED

Immune Globulin Intravenous (Human), *IVEEGAM EN* 500 mg:
1 vial containing 500 mg of freeze-dried Immune Globulin Intravenous (Human), *IVEEGAM EN*
1 vial containing 10 ml of Sterile Water for Injection, U.S.P.,
(This Product Contains Dry Natural Rubber.)
1 double-ended spike,
1 filter needle.

Immune Globulin Intravenous (Human), *IVEEGAM EN* 1000 mg:
1 vial containing 1000 mg of freeze-dried Immune globulin Intravenous (Human), *IVEEGAM EN*
1 vial containing 20 ml of Sterile Water for Injection, U.S.P.,
(This Product Contains Dry Natural Rubber.)
1 double-ended spike,
1 filter needle.

Immune Globulin Intravenous (Human), *IVEEGAM EN* 2500 mg:
1 infusion bottle containing 2500 mg of freeze-dried Immune Globulin Intravenous (Human), *IVEEGAM EN*
1 vial containing 50 ml of Sterile Water for Injection, U.S.P.,
(This Product Contains Dry Natural Rubber.)
1 double-ended spike.
1 infusion set with filter.

Immune globulin Intravenous (Human), *IVEEGAM EN* 5000 mg:
1 infusion bottle containing 5000 mg of freeze-dried Immune Globulin Intravenous (Human), *IVEEGAM EN*
1 vial containing 100 ml of Sterile Water for Injection, U.S.P.,
(This Product Contains Dry Natural Rubber.)
1 double-ended spike,
1 infusion set with filter.

Rx only

Storage

Store at +2°C to +8°C (+35°F to +46°F).
Avoid freezing, which may damage the diluent bottle.
Do not use after expiration date.

REFERENCES

1. JANEWAY C. A., ROSEN F. S.: The Gamma Globulins: IV. Therapeutic Uses of Gamma Globulin, N. Engl. J. Med. 275, 1966, pp. 826–831
2. ROSEN F. S., WEDGWOOD R. J., EIBL M.: Primary Immunodeficiency Diseases. Report of a WHO Scientific Group. Clin. Immunol. Immunopathol. 40, 1986, pp. 166–196
3. EIBL M.: Treatment of Defect of Humoral Immunity. In: Primary Immunodeficiency Diseases; Birth Defects: Original Article Series. Edited by R. J. WEDGWOOD and F. S. ROSEN. Alan R. Liss, Inc. New York, Vol. 19, No. 3, 1983, pp. 193–200
4. EIBL M.: Intravenous Immunoglobulins: Clinical and Experimental Studies. In: Immunoglobulins: Characteristics and Uses of Intravenous Preparations. Edited by B. M. ALVING and J. S. FINLAYSON. U.S. Department of Health and Human Services, Public Health Service, FDA, DHHS Publication No. (FDA)-80-9005, 1979, pp. 23–30
5. WALDMANN T. A., et al.: Metabolism of Immunoglobulins. In: Progress in Allergy. Edited by P. KALLOS and B. H. WAKSMAN, Karger, Basel, Vol. 13, 1969, pp. 1–110
6. Data on File, IMMUNO AG, Vienna.
7. BERNATOWSKA E., et al: Results of a Prospective Controlled Two-Dose Crossover Study with Intravenous Immunoglobulin and Comparison (Retrospective) with Plasma Treatment. Clin. Immunol. Immuno-pathol. 43, 1987, pp. 153–162
8. EIBL M., et al.: Safety and Efficacy of a Monomeric, Functionally Intact Intravenous IgG Preparation in Patients with Primary Immunodeficiency Syndromes. Clin. Immunol. Immunopathol. 31, 1984, pp. 151–160
9. NEWBURGER J. W., et al.: The Treatment of Kawasaki Syndrome with Intravenous Gamma Globulin. N. Engl. J. Med., 315, 1986, pp. 341–347
10. NEWBURGER J. W., et al.: A Single Intravenous Infusion of Gamma Globulin as Compared with Four Infusions in the Treatment of Acute Kawasaki Syndrome. N. Engl. J. Med., 324, 1991, pp. 1633–1639
11. BURKS A.W., et al.: Anaphylactic Reactions after Gammaglobulin Administration in Patients with Hypogammaglobulinemia. Detection of IgG Antibodies to IgA. N. Engl. J. Med. 314, 1986, pp. 560–564
12. CUNNINGHAM-RUNDLES C., et al.: Reactions to Intravenous Gammaglobulin Infusions and Immune Complex Formation. In: Immuno Hemotherapy. A Guide to Immunoglobulin Prophylaxis and Therapy. Edited by U.E. NYDEGGER. Academic Press, London, 1982, pp. 447–450
13. LEIKOLA J., et al.: IgA-Induced Anaphylactic Transfusion Reactions: A Report of Four Cases. Blood 42, 1973, pp. 111–119
14. THOMPSON R. A., REES-JONES A.: The Antibody Deficiency Syndrome: A Report on Current Management. J. Infect. 1, 1979, pp. 49–60
15. CAYCO A. V. PERAZELLA M. A., HAYSLETT J.P.: Renal insufficiency after intravenous immune globulin therapy: A Report of Two Cases and an Analysis of the Literature, 1997; J Amer Soc Nephrology 8: 1788–1793
16. WINWARD D.B., BROPHY M.T.: Acute renal failure after administration of intravenous immunoglobulin: review of the literature and case report. 1995; Pharmacotherapy 15: 765–772
17. PHILLIPS A.O.: Renal failure and intravenous immunoglobulin (letter, comment). 1992; Clin Nephrol 36: 83D86
18. ANDERSON W., BETHEA W.: Renal lesions following administration of hypertonic solutions of sucrose. 1940; JAMA 114: 1983–1987
19. LINDBERG H., WALD A., Renal changes following the administration of hypertonic solutions. 1939; Arch Intern Med 63: 907–918
20. RIGDON R.H., CARDWELL E.S.: Renal lesions following the intravenous injection of hypertonic solution of sucrose: A clinical and experimental study. 1942; Arch Intern Med 60: 670–690
21. TAN E., HAJINAZARIAN M., BAY, et al.: Acute renal failure resulting from intravenous immunoglobulin therapy. 1993; Arch Neurology 50: 137–139

BIBLIOGRAPHY

ALVING B. M., FINLAYSON J. S. (Eds.): Immunoglobulins: Characteristics and Uses of Intravenous Preparations. U.S. Department of Health and Human Services, Public Health Service, DHHS Publication No. (FDA)-80-9005, 1979

AMMANN A. J., ASHMAN R. F., BUCKLEY R. H., HARDIE W. R., KRANTMANN H. J., NELSON J., OCHS H., STIEHM E. R., TILLER T., WARA D. W., WEDGWOOD R.: Use of Intravenous g-Globulin in Antibody Immunodeficiency: Results of a Multicenter Controlled Trial. Clin. Immunol. Immunopathol. 22, 1982, pp. 60–67

BARANDUN S., SKVARIL F., MORELL A.: Prophylaxe und Therapie mit g-Globulin. Allgemeine Charakterisie-rung und klinische Anwendung von g-Globulin-Präparaten. Schweiz, med. Wschr. 106, 1976, pp. 533–542 BARANDUN S., MORELL A., SKVARIL F.: Clinical Use of Intravenous Gamma-Globulin. Biblthca haemat. 46, 1980, pp. 170–174

BUCKLEY R. H.: Long Term Use of Intravenous Immune Globulin in Patients with Primary Immunodeficiency Diseases: Inadequacy of Current Dosage Practices and Approaches to the Problem. J. Clin. Immunol. 2 (Suppl.) 1982, pp. 15S–21S

EIBL., M.: Treatment of Defects of Humoral Immunity. In: Primary Immunodeficiency Diseases: Birth Defects.: Original Articles Series, Edited by R. J. WEDGWOOD and F. S. ROSEN, Alan R. Liss, Inc. New York, Vol. 19, No. 3, 1983, pp. 193–200

KISHIMOTO S.: The Application of Immunoglobulin Preparations. Proc. Symp. Immunoglob., 1979, pp. 24–29

KOBAYASHI M.: Replacement Therapy for Immunodeficiency Syndrome. Proc. Symp. on Immunoglobulin Therapy (Ed.: K. Mashimo) Tokyo, 1979, pp. 94–100

LITMAN G. W., GOOD R. A. (Eds.): Immunoglobulins. Comprehensive Immunology 5. (Series editors: R. A. Good, S. B. Day). Plenum Medical Book Company, New York and London, 1978

MAGILAVY D. B., CASSIDY J. T., TUBERGEN D. G., PETTY R. E., CHISHOLM R. McCALL K.: Intravenous Gamma Globulin in the Management of Patients with Hypogammaglobulinemia. J. Allergy Clin. Immunol. 61, 1978, pp. 378–383

MAZZUCCONI M. G., MELONI G., BOTTINI F., ROMOLI D.: Sperimentazione Clinica e Tollerabilità di un Nuovo Preparato di Immunoglobuline per Uso Endovenoso. Quaderni di Medicina e Chirurgia, 43; Suppl. a Malattie del Torace e Cardiovascolari, Vol. VII, 1975

MORELL A., SCHÜRCH B., RYSER D., HOFER F., SKVARIL F., BARANDUN S.: In vivo Behaviour of Gamma Globulin Preparations. Vox Sang. 38, 1980, pp. 272–283

MORELL A., BARANDUN S.: Substitution mit Immunglobulinen bei primärem Antikörpermangelsyndrom. Beitr. Infusionstherapie klin. Ernähr. 9, 1982, pp. 16–24

NOLTE M. T., PIROFSKY B., GERRITZ G. A., GOLDING B.: Intravenous Immunoglobulin Therapy for Anti-body Deficiency. Clin. Exp. Immunol. 36, 1979, pp. 237–243

RÖMER J., MORGENTHALER J.-J., SCHERZ R., SKVARIL F.: Characterization of Various Immunoglobulin Preparations for Intravenous Application. I. Protein Composition and Antibody Content. Vox. Sang. 42, 1982, pp. 62–73

RÖMER J., SPÄTH P. J., SKVARIL F., NYDEGGER U.E.: Characterization of Various Immunoglobulin Preparations for Intravenous Application. II. Complement Activation and Binding to Staphylococcus Protein A. Vox. Sang. 42, 1982, pp. 74–80

ROSEN F. S.: The Immunodeficiency Syndromes. In: Immunological Diseases. (Ed.: M. Samter). Third Edition, Vol. 1, Little, Brown and Comp., Boston, 1978, pp. 472–498

ROSEN F. S. in: Panel Discussion on Indications and Limitations of Immunoglobulin Prophylaxis and Therapy. In: Immuno Hemotherapy. A Guide to Immunoglobulin Prophylaxis and Therapy, 1981, pp. 451–460

SKVARIL F., PROBST M., AUDRAN R., STEINBUCH M.: Distribution of IgG Subclasses in Commercial and Some Experimental g-Globulin Preparations. Vox Sang. 32, 1977, pp. 335–338

Benadryl is a trademark of Warner Lambert Consumer Healthcare

Manufactured by
ÖSTERREICHISCHES INSTITUT FÜR HAEMODERIVATE GES.M.B.H.
Subsidiary of IMMUNO AG, A-1220 Vienna, Austria
U.S. Establishment License 258
U.S. Pat. Nos. 4,814,277, 4,886,758, 5,094,949, 5,122,373, 5,234,685, and 5,324,638
Distributed by
IMMUNO U.S., Inc.
1200 Parkdale Road, Rochester, Michigan 48307
Revised August 1999© 1999 IMMUNO AG

6224000EH10

PROPLEX® T ℞

Factor IX Complex, Heat Treated

Warning: This is a potent drug with potential hazards. For maximal safety and efficacy, carefully read and follow directions below.

DESCRIPTION

Factor IX Complex, Heat Treated, Proplex® T*, is a sterile product prepared from pooled normal human plasma. It contains, in concentrated form, clotting Factors II (prothrombin), VII (proconvertin), IX (PTC, antihemophilic factor B), and X (Stuart-Prower factor). Other proteins are also present in minimal amounts. The product also contains a small amount of heparin, 1.5 units or less per mL of reconstituted material, as a stabilizing agent. This amount does not affect the clinical usefulness of the complex in moderate dosage.

Factor IX Complex **must** be administered intravenously.

During the manufacturing process, this product was heated for 144 hours at 60°C. This heating step was designed to reduce the risk of transmission of hepatitis and other viral infections. No procedure has been shown to be totally effective in removing viral infectivity from Factor IX Complex.

CLINICAL PHARMACOLOGY

Factor IX Complex is a combination of vitamin K-dependent clotting factors found in normal plasma. The administration of Factor IX Complex, Proplex® T, provides an increase in plasma levels of Factor VII and Factor IX and can temporarily correct the coagulation defect of patients with deficiencies in these factors. Plasma levels of Factors II and X will also be increased.

The half-life of Factor VII in non-treated Factor IX Complex administered to Factor VII deficient patients has been found to range from 3 to 6 hours.[1,2]

The half-life of Factor IX in non-treated Factor IX Complex administered to Factor IX deficient patients has been found to range from 24 to 32 hours.[3,4]

The effectiveness of the heating step in reducing viral infectivity was assessed by *in vitro* viral inactivation studies using, as markers, viruses not commonly found in plasma. When known quantities of these viruses were added to the product, the heat treatment employed inactivated the following quantities of virus:

Sindbis	10.5 Log_{10}
Vesicular Stomatitis	5.6 Log_{10}
Pseudorabies	1.4 Log_{10}

In addition, it has been shown that Cytomegalovirus does not survive the manufacturing process. As these data indicate, all viruses are not equally affected by the heat treatment. Work by Colombo, *et al* with first-exposure hemophiliacs who received heat treated Antihemophilic Factor (Human) shows that while some reduction of hepatitis infectivity may have been achieved by heat treatment, a substantial portion of the patients who had not previously received blood products developed signs and/or symptoms of hepatitis.[5] (See **Warnings**.)

It has been reported that HIV is heat labile and that it is inactivated by treatment with 19–20% alcohol.[6,7,8] Lengthy exposure to 20% ethanol occurs in the Cohn cold ethanol fractionation procedure from which this product is derived.

In a retrospective study conducted with patients receiving Anti-Inhibitor Coagulant Complex, Autoplex®, which is also derived from the Cohn process, none of the patients who received Anti-Inhibitor Coagulant Complex, Autoplex, exclusively seroconverted for HIV antibodies, while 56% of those patients who received other treatment modalities seroconverted during the three year study.[9] Heat treatment has also been shown to be an effective means of inactivating HIV.[10] In a study comparing heat treated Antihemophilic Factor (Human), Hemofil® T to untreated Antihemophilic Factor (Human) products, none of the patients receiving the heat treated product developed antibodies to HIV, while 17% of the patients receiving untreated products did seroconvert by the end of the study.[11]

INDICATIONS AND USAGE

Factor IX Complex, Proplex® T, is indicated for:

1. Factor IX deficiency (hemophilia B, Christmas disease). The intravenous administration of Factor IX Complex, Proplex® T, is intended to prevent or control bleeding episodes in patients with this deficiency. Factor IX Complex should not be used in patients with mild Factor IX deficiency for whom fresh frozen plasma is effective.

2. Bleeding episodes in patients with inhibitors to Factor VIII. Lusher, *et al*,[12] have described the use of Factor IX Complex in hemarthroses occurring in hemophiliacs with inhibitors to Factor VIII.
3. Factor VII deficiency. The Factor VII content present in Factor IX Complex, Proplex® T, has been shown to be effective in prevention or control of bleeding episodes in patients with Factor VII deficiency.[13]

CONTRAINDICATIONS

None known.

WARNINGS

The use of Factor IX Complex is potentially hazardous in patients with signs of fibrinolysis and in patients with disseminated intravascular coagulation (DIC).

This product is prepared from pooled human plasma which may contain the causative agents of hepatitis and other viral diseases. Prescribed manufacturing procedures utilized at the plasma collection centers, plasma testing laboratories, and the fractionation facilities are designed to reduce the risk of transmitting viral infection. However, the risk of viral infectivity from this product cannot be totally eliminated.

Individuals who receive infusions of blood or plasma products may develop signs and/or symptoms of some viral infections, particularly non A, non B hepatitis.

PRECAUTIONS

General

Identification of the deficiency as one of either Factor IX, Factor VII or Factor VIII with inhibitors is essential before administration of the Factor IX Complex, Proplex® T, is initiated.

With the exception of its use in treating hemarthroses occurring in Factor VIII-inhibitor patients, no benefit may be expected from this product in treating deficiencies other than those of Factor IX or Factor VII.

Caution: It is important that the dosage regimen chosen is carefully evaluated with respect to the entire spectrum of factors present in this product. Levels of Factors II, IX and X should be monitored during therapy to prevent unnecessarily high levels of these factors, which may increase the risk of intravascular coagulation. Factor IX Complex, Proplex® T, is prepared by calcium phosphate absorption of cold ethanol precipitated material and therefore, contains higher ratios of Factor VII and Factor X to Factor IX than products prepared by Sephadex exchange.[14]

The use of high doses of prothrombin complex concentrates has been reported to be associated with instances of myocardial infarction, disseminated intravascular coagulation, venous thrombosis and pulmonary embolism.[1,12,15,16]

If signs of intravascular coagulation, thrombosis, or emboli occur, which include changes in blood pressure and pulse rate, respiratory distress, chest pain and cough, the infusion should be stopped promptly. In general, the risk of enhancing DIC may be reduced by raising the patient's Factor VII or Factor IX level to not more than about 50% of normal. If the need exists to raise the patient's Factor IX or Factor VII level higher than 50% of normal, the physician should monitor infusion of material to detect signs and symptoms of DIC.

Special caution should be taken in the use of this concentrate in newborns, where a higher morbidity and mortality may be associated with hepatitis, and in individuals with pre-existing liver disease.

Laboratory Tests

Since the dosage of Factor IX Complex, Proplex® T is calculated on the basis of its potency, frequent laboratory tests to monitor the effectiveness of treatment usually are unnecessary. This is particularly true for single dose treatment of an uncomplicated hemarthrosis. However, if a major bleeding episode is being treated in the hospital, or if adequate hemostatic levels of Factor VII or Factor IX are needed to permit performance of surgery, Factor VII or Factor IX assays should be performed at least once a day, prior to infusion, to ensure that the daily dose of Factor IX Complex is sufficient to maintain adequate levels of the desired clotting factor.

Pregnancy

Pregnancy Category C. Animal reproduction studies have not been conducted with Factor IX Complex. It is also not known whether Factor IX Complex can cause fetal harm when administered to a pregnant woman or can affect reproduction capacity. Factor IX Complex should be given to a pregnant woman only if clearly needed.

ADVERSE REACTIONS

As with other plasma preparations, reactions manifested by chills and fever may occasionally be seen,[17,18] particularly when large doses of Factor IX Complex, Proplex® T, are administered.

A rate of infusion that is too rapid may cause headache, flushing, and changes in pulse rate and blood pressure. In such instances, stopping the infusion allows the symptoms to disappear promptly. With all but the most reactive individuals, the infusion may be resumed at a slower rate. (See **Rate of Administration**.)

The risk of thrombosis is present with the administration of Factor IX Complex.

DOSAGE AND ADMINISTRATION

Each bottle of Factor IX Complex, Proplex® T, is labeled with both the Factor IX and Factor VII content. The Factor IX concent is expressed in International Units per bottle and is traceable to the World Health Organization International Standard through a secondary concentrate standard. The Factor VII content is expressed in units per bottle and is traceable to pooled normal plasma through a secondary standard.

The amount of Factor IX Complex, Proplex® T, required to restore normal hemostasis varies with the circumstances and with the patient. Dosage depends on the degree of deficiency and the desired hemostatic level of the deficient factor. As a guide to calculation of dosage, experience[4,19] indicates that the following formulas may be used:

Factor IX Deficiency

Units required to raise blood level percentages:
1.0 unit/kg × body weight (in kg) × desired increase (% of normal)

If a 70 kg (154 lb) patient with a Factor IX level of 0% needs to be elevated to 25%, give 1.0 unit/kg × 70 kg × 25 = 1750 units.

In preparation for and following surgery, levels above 25%, maintained for at least a week after surgery, are suggested. Laboratory control to assure such levels is recommended. To maintain levels above 25% for a reasonable time, each dose should be calculated to raise the level to 40 to 60% of normal (See **Precautions.**)

The preceding dosage formula for Factor IX deficiency is presented as a reference and a guideline. Exact dosage determinations should be made based on the medical judgment of the physician regarding circumstances, condition of patient, degree of deficiency, and the desired level of Factor IX to be achieved. If inhibitors to Factor IX appear to be present, sufficient additional dosage to overcome the inhibitor would be needed.

For maintenance of an elevated level of the deficient factor, dosage may be repeated as often as needed. Clinical studies suggest that relatively high levels may be maintained by daily or twice-daily doses, while the lower effective levels may require injections only once every two or three days. A single dose may be sufficient to stop a minor bleeding episode.[20,21]

Factor VIII Inhibitor

In using Factor IX Complex in the treatment of hemarthroses occurring in hemophiliacs with inhibitors to Factor VIII, dosage levels approximating 75 Factor IX units per kg of body weight have been employed.[12]

Anti-Inhibitor Coagulant Complex, Autoplex®T, is recommended when hemarthroses occurring in hemophiliacs with inhibitors to Factor VIII cannot be resolved by administration of Factor IX Complex, and in other types of bleeding episodes in Factor VIII-inhibitor patients.

Factor VII Deficiency

Units required to raise blood level percentages:
0.5 unit/kg × body weight (in kg) × desired increase (% of normal)

Repeat dose every 4 to 6 hours as needed.

If a 70 kg (154 lb) patient with a Factor VII level of 0% needs to be elevated to 25%, give 0.5 unit/kg × 70 kg × 25 = 875 units.

In preparation for and following surgery, levels above 25%, maintained for at least a week after surgery, are suggested. Laboratory control to assure such levels is recommended. To maintain levels above 25% for a reasonable time, each dose should be calculated to raise the level to 40 to 60% of normal. (See **Precautions.**)

The preceding dosage formula for Factor VII deficiency is presented as a reference and a guideline. Exact dosage determinations should be made based on the medical judgment of the physician regarding circumstances, condition of patient, degree of deficiency, and the desired level of Factor VII to be achieved. If inhibitors to Factor VII appear to be present, sufficient additional dosage to overcome the inhibitor would be needed.[22,23]

Reconstitution: Use Aseptic Technic

1. Bring Factor IX Complex, Proplex® T, (dry concentrate) and Sterile Water for Injection, USP, (diluent) to room temperature.
2. Remove caps from concentrate and diluent bottles to expose central portions of rubber stoppers.
3. Cleanse stoppers with germicidal solution.
4. Remove protective covering from one end of double-ended needle and insert exposed needle through diluent stopper.
5. Remove protective covering from other end of double-ended needle. Invert diluent bottle over the upright concentrate bottle, then rapidly insert free end of the needle through the concentrate bottle stopper at its center. The vacuum in the concentrate bottle with draw in the diluent.
6. Disconnect the two bottles by removing needle from diluent bottle stopper, then remove needle from concentrate bottle. Swirl or rotate bottle until all material is dissolved. Be sure that the material is completely dissolved, otherwise active material will be removed by the filter.

Note: Do not refrigerate after reconstitution.

Rate of Administration

Factor IX Complex should be infused slowly, at a rate of approximately two to three mL per minute. If headache, flushing, changes in pulse rate or blood pressure appear, the infusion rate should be decreased. In such instances it is advisable, initially, to stop the infusion until the symptoms disappear, then resume the infusion at a slower rate.

Administration: Use Aseptic Technic

When reconstitution of Factor IX Complex, Proplex® T, is complete, its infusion should commence within three hours. However, it is recommended that the infusion begin as promptly as is practical.

The reconstituted material should be at room temperature during infusion.

Parenteral drug products should be inspected visually for particulate matter and discoloration prior to administration, whenever solution and container permit.

A. Intravenous Drip Infusion

When a Hyland administration set is used, follow directions for use printed on the administration set container. When an administration set from another source is used, follow directions accompanying that set where necessary. The use of a Hyland administration set is recommended as it contains a suitable filter.

B. Intravenous Syringe Injection

1. Attach filter needle to syringe and draw back plunger to admit air into the syringe.
2. Insert needle into the reconstituted Factor IX Complex.
3. Inject air into bottle and then withdraw the reconstituted material into the syringe.
4. Remove and discard the filter needle from the syringe; attach a suitable needle and inject intravenously at a rate **not exceeding 3 ml per minute.**
5. If a patient is to receive more than one bottle of concentrate, the contents of two bottles may be drawn into the same syringe, by drawing up each bottle through a separate unused filter needle. This practice lessens the loss of concentrate. Please note, filter needles are intended to filter single bottles of Factor IX Complex only.

HOW SUPPLIED

Factor IX Complex, Proplex® T, is furnished with a suitable volume of Sterile Water for Injection, USP; a double-ended needle; and a filter needle.

Storage

Factor IX Complex, Proplex® T, should be stored under ordinary refrigeration (2 to 8 °C, 36 to 46 °F). Avoid freezing to prevent damage to the diluent bottle.

REFERENCES

1. White GC, Lundblad RL, Kingdon HS: Prothrombin complex concentrates: Preparation, properties and clinical uses. **Curr Top Hematol 2**:203–244, 1979
2. Marder VJ, Shulman NR: Clinical aspects of congenital Factor VII deficiency. **Am J Med 37**:182–192, 1964
3. Mollison PL: The transfusion of platelets, leucocytes and plasma components (Ch 3) in **Blood Transfusion in Clinical Medicine, Sixth Ed.** Oxford, Blackwell Scientific Publications, 1979, pp 103–113
4. Zauber NP, Levin J: Factor IX levels in patients with hemophilia B (Christmas disease) following transfusion with concentrates of Factor IX or fresh frozen plasma (FFP). **Medicine 56**:213–224, 1977
5. Colombo M, Carnelli V, Gazengel C, *et al:* Transmission of non-A, non-B hepatitis by heat-treated Factor VIII concentrate. **Lancet 2**:1–4, 1985
6. Update: Acquired immune deficiency syndrome (AIDS) in persons with hemophilia. **Morbidity and Mortality Weekly Report 33**:589–591, October 26, 1984
7. Spire B, Barre-Sinoussi F, Montagnier L, *et al:* Inactivation of lymphadenopathy associated virus by chemical disinfectants. **Lancet 2**:899–901, 1984
8. Piszkiewicz D, Kingdon H, Apfelzweig R, *et al:* Inactivation of HTLV-III/LAV during plasma fractionation. **Lancet 2**:1188–1189, 1985
9. Gazengel C, Larrieu MJ: Lack of seroconversion for LAV/HTLV-III in patients exclusively given unheated activated prothrombin complex prepared with ethanol step. **Lancet 2**:1189, 1985
10. Petricciani J, McDougal JS, Evatt BL: Case for concluding that heat-treated, licensed anti-haemophilic factor is free from HTLV-III. **Lancet 2**:890–891, 1985
11. Rouzioux C, Chamaret S, Montagnier L, *et al:* Absence of antibodies to AIDS virus in haemophiliacs treated with heat-treated Factor VIII concentrate. **Lancet 1**:271–272, 1985
12. Lusher JM, Shapiro SS, Palascak JE, *et al:* Efficiency of prothrombin-complex concentrates in hemophiliacs with antibodies to Factor VIII. A multicenter therapeutic trial. **New Engl J Med 303**:421–425, 1980
13. Ragni MV, Lewis JH, Spero JA, *et al:* Factor VII deficiency. **Am J Hemotology 10**:79–88, 1981
14. Aronson DL: Factor IX complex. **Semin Thromb Hemostas VI**:28–43, 1979
15. Fuerth JH, Mahrer P: Myocardial infarction after Factor IX therapy. **JAMA 214**:1445–1456, 1981
16. Abildgaard CF: Hazards of prothrombin-complex concentrates in treatment of hemophilia. **New Eng J Med 304**:670, 1981
17. Hutchinson JL, Freedman SO, Richards BA, *et al:* Plasma volume expansion and reactions after infusion of autologous and nonautologous plasma in man. **J Lab Clin Med 56**:734–746, 1960
18. Mollison PL: Some unfavourable effects of transfusion (Ch 15) in **Blood Transfusions in Clinical Medicine, Sixth Edition.** Oxford, Blackwell Scientific Publications, 1979, p 626
19. Levine PH: Hemophilia and allied conditions, in **Current Therapy, 1979.** Conn HF (ed), Philadelphia, W.B. Saunders Co., 1979, pp 268–275
20. Nilsson IM: Clinical experience with a Swedish Factor IX concentrate, in **Haemophilia.** Ala F, Denson KWE (eds), Amsterdam, Excerpta Medica, 1973, pp 249–253

Continued on next page

Proplex T—Cont.

21. Owen CA Jr, Bowie EJW: Infusion therapy in hemophilia A and B, in **Handbook of Hemophilia.** Brinkhous KM, Hemker HC (eds), Amsterdam, Excerpta Medica, 1975, pp 449–473
22. Hoag MS, Aggeler PM, Fowell AH: Disappearance rate of concentrated proconvertin extracts in congenital and acquired hypoproconvertinemia. **J Clin Invest 39**:554–563, 1960
23. Bedizel M, Albers R: Hereditary Factor VII deficiency in newborns. **Clinical Pediatrics 22**:774–775, 1983

*Manufactured under U.S. Patent No. 4,495,278.

Baxter Healthcare Corporation
Hyland Division
Glendale, CA 91203 USA
U.S. License No. 140
4153 Revised November 1990

RECOMBINATE™ ℞
Antihemophilic Factor (Recombinant)

DESCRIPTION

Antihemophilic Factor (Recombinant) Recombinate™ is a glycoprotein synthesized by a genetically engineered Chinese Hamster Ovary (CHO) cell line. In culture the CHO cell line secretes recombinant antihemophilic factor (rAHF) into the cell culture medium. The rAHF is purified from the culture medium utilizing a series of chromatography columns. A key step in the purification process is an immunoaffinity chromatography methodology in which a purification matrix, prepared by immobilization of a monclonal antibody directed to factor VIII, is utilized to selectively isolate the rAHF in the medium. The synthesized rAHF produced by the CHO cells has the same biological effects as Antihemophilic Factor (Human) [AHF (Human)] and structurally has a similar combination of heterogenous heavy and light chains as found in AHF (Human).
Recombinate™ is formulated as a sterile, nonpyrogenic, off-white to faint yellow, lyophilized powder preparation of concentrated recombinant AHF for intravenous injection and is available in single-dose bottles which contain nominally 250, 500 and 1000 International Units per bottle. When reconstituted with the appropriate volume of diluent, it contains the following stabilizers in maximum amounts: 12.5 mg/mL Albumin (Human), 0.20 mg/mL calcium, 1.5 mg/mL polyethylene glycol (3350), 180 mEq/L sodium, 55 mM histidine, 1.5 µg/AHF International Unit (IU) polysorbate-80. Von Willebrand Factor (vWF) is coexpressed with the Antihemophilic Factor (Recombinant) and helps to stabilize it. The final product contains not more than 2 ng vWF/IU rAHF which will not have any clinically relevant effect in patients with von Willebrand's disease. The product contains no preservative.
Manufacturing of Recombinate™ is shared by Baxter Healthcare Corporation, Hyland Division and Genetics Institute, Inc. The Antihemophilic Factor Concentrate (Recombinant), is produced by Baxter Healthcare Corporation, Hyland Division and Genetics Institute (For Further Manufacturing Use) and subsequently formulated and packaged at Baxter Healthcare Corporation, Hyland Division.
Each bottle of Recombinate™ is labeled with the AHF activity expressed in IU per bottle. Biological potency is determined by an *in vitro* assay which is referenced to the World Health Organization (WHO) International Standard for Factor VIII:C Concentrate.

CLINICAL PHARMACOLOGY

AHF is the specific clotting factor deficient in patients with hemophilia A (classical hemophilia). Hemophilia A is a genetic bleeding disorder characterized by hemorrhages which may occur spontaneously or after minor trauma. The administration of Recombinate™ provides an increase in plasma levels of AHF and can temporarily correct the coagulation defect in these patients. Pharmacokinetic studies on sixty-six (66) patients revealed the circulating mean half-life for rAHF to be 14.4 ± 4.9 hours, which was not statistically significantly different from plasma-derived Antihemophilic Factor (Human), Hemofil® M, (pdAHF), which had a mean half-life of 14.0 ± 3.9 hours (n=59). Mean highest *in vivo* recovery in plasma was also similar at 2.18 ± 0.72 (n=19) IU/dL per IU/kg body weight compared to the mean highest recovery point above the pre-infusion baseline for Hemofil® M of 1.97 ± 0.66 (n=57) IU/dL per IU/kg.
The clinical study of rAHF in previously treated patients (individuals with hemophilia A who had been treated with plasma derived AHF) was based on observations made on a study group of 67 patients. These individuals received 18,451 to 1,110,111 IU over the 58.2 month study period, 13,394 infusions for a total of 21,437,195 IU rAHF.
These patients were successfully treated for bleeding episodes on a demand basis and also for the prevention of bleeds (prophylaxis). Spontaneous bleeding episodes successfully managed include hemarthroses, soft tissue and muscle bleeds. Management of hemostasis was also evaluated in surgeries. A total of 24 procedures on 13 patients were performed during this study. These included minor (e.g. tooth extraction) and major (e.g. bilateral osteotomies, thoracotomy and liver transplant) procedures. Hemostasis was maintained perioperatively and postoperatively with individualized AHF replacement.

Hemorrhage		
Degree of hemorrhage	**Required peak post-infuson AHF activity in the blood (as % of normal or IU/dL plasma)**	**Frequency of infusion**
Early hemarthrosis or muscle bleed or oral bleed	20–40	Begin infusion every 12 to 24 hours for one-three days until the bleeding episode as indicated by pain is resolved or healing is achieved.
More extensive hemarthrosis, muscle bleed, or hematoma	30–60	Repeat infusion every 12 to 24 hours for usually three days or more until pain and disability are resolved.
Life threatening bleeds such as head injury, throat bleed, severe abdominal pain	60–100	Repeat infusion every 8 to 24 hours until threat is resolved.
Surgery		
Type of operation		
Minor surgery, including tooth extraction	60–80	A single infusion plus oral antifibrinolytic therapy within one hour is sufficient in approximately 70% of cases.
Major surgery	80–100 (pre- and post-operative)	Repeat infusion every 8 to 24 hours depending on state of healing.

A study of rAHF in previously untreated patients was also performed. The study group comprised seventy-nine (79) patients, of whom seventy-five (75) had received at least one infusion of rAHF. In total, this cohort has been given 1,054 infusions totaling 437,126 IU rAHF. Hemostasis was appropriately managed in spontaneous bleeding episodes, intracranial hemorrhage and surgical procedures.

INDICATIONS AND USAGE

The use of Antihemophilic Factor (Recombinant), Recombinate™ is indicated in hemophilia A (classical hemophilia) for the prevention and control of hemorrhagic episodes.[1] Recombinate™ is also indicated in the perioperative management of patients with hemophilia A (classical hemophilia). Recombinate™ can be of significant therapeutic value in patients with acquired AHF inhibitors not exceeding 10 Bethesda Units per mL[2]. In clinical studies with Recombinate™, patients with inhibitors who were entered into the previously treated patient trial and those previously untreated children who have developed inhibitor activity on study, showed clinical hemostatic response when the titer of inhibitor was less than 10 Bethesda Units per mL. However, in such uses, the dosage of Recombinate™ should be controlled by frequent laboratory determinations of circulating AHF levels.
Recombinate™ is not indicated in von Willebrand's disease.

CONTRAINDICATIONS

Known hypersensitivity to mouse, hamster or bovine protein may be a contraindication to the use of Antihemophilic Factor (Recombinant) (see **Precautions**).

WARNINGS

None.

PRECAUTIONS

General
Certain components used in the packaging of this product contain natural rubber latex.
Identification of the clotting defect as a Factor VIII deficiency is essential before the administration of Antihemophilic Factor (Recombinant), Recombinate™ is initiated. No benefit may be expected from this product in treating other deficiencies.
The formation of neutralizing antibodies, inhibitors to factor VIII, is a known complication in the management of individuals with hemophilia A. The reported prevalence of these antibodies in patients receiving plasma derived AHF is 10–20%[3,4,5,6,7,10,11,12]. These inhibitors are invariably IgG immunoglobulins, the factor VIII procoagulant inhibitory activity of which is expressed as Bethesda Units (B.U.) per mL of plasma or serum[3,4,5,6,7]. Over the investigational period, none of the 65 previously treated individuals, without an inhibitor at entry into the study, developed an inhibitor. In the previously untreated patient group there were 66 patients with factor VIII levels less than or equal to 2% who were tested for inhibitor after treatment with Recombinate™ rAHF. Of this group 12 individuals developed detectable inhibitor and of these, 3 patients showed a titer greater than 10 B.U. Patients treated with rAHF should be carefully monitored for the development of antibodies to rAHF by appropriate clinical observations and laboratory tests.
Formation of Antibodies to Mouse, Hamster or Bovine Protein
As Antihemophilic Factor (Recombinant), Recombinate™ contains trace amounts of mouse protein (maximum of 0.1 ng/IU rAHF), hamster protein (maximum of 1.5 ng CHO protein/IU rAHF), and bovine protein (maximum of 1 ng BSA/IU rAHF), the remote possibility exists that patients treated with this product may develop hypersensitivity to these non-human mammalian proteins.
Information for Patients
Although allergic type hypersensitivity reactions were not observed in any patient receiving Recombinate™ on study, such reactions are theoretically possible. Patients should be informed of the early signs of hypersensitivity reactions including hives, generalized urticaria, tightness of the chest, wheezing, hypotension, and anaphylaxis. Patients should be advised to discontinue use of the product and contact their physician if these symptoms occur.
Laboratory Tests
Although dosage can be estimated by the calculations which follow, it is strongly recommended that whenever possible, appropriate laboratory tests be performed on the patient's plasma at suitable intervals to assure that adequate AHF levels have been reached and are maintained.
If the patient's plasma AHF fails to reach expected levels or if bleeding is not controlled after adequate dosage, the presence of inhibitor should be suspected. By performing appropriate laboratory procedures, the presence of an inhibitor can be demonstrated and quantified in terms of AHF International Units neutralized by each mL of plasma or by the total estimated plasma volume. If the inhibitor is present at levels less than 10 Bethesda Units per mL, administration of additional AHF may neutralize the inhibitor.
Thereafter, the administration of additional AHF International Units should elicit the predicted response. The control of AHF levels by laboratory assay is necessary in this situation.
Inhibitor titers above 10 Bethesda Units per mL may make hemostasis control with AHF either impossible or impractical because of the very large dose required. In addition, the inhibitor titer may rise following AHF infusion because of an anamnestic response to the AHF antigen.
Carcinogenesis, Mutagenesis, Impairment of Fertility
Recombinate™ was tested for mutagenicity at doses considerably exceeding plasma concentrations of rAHF *in vitro* and at doses up to ten times the expected maximum clinical dose *in vivo*, and did not cause reverse mutations, chromosomal aberrations, or an increase in micronuclei in bone marrow polychromatic erythrocytes. Long term studies in animals have not been performed to evaluate carcinogenic potential.
Pediatric Use
Recombinate™ is appropriate for use in children of all ages, including the newborn. Safety and efficacy studies have been performed in both previously treated (n=23) and previously untreated (n=75) children. (See **Clinical Pharmacology** and **Precautions**).
Pregnancy
Pregnancy Category C. Animal reproduction studies have not been conducted with Antihemophilic Factor (Recombinant). It is not known whether Antihemophilic Factor (Recombinant) can cause fetal harm when administered to a pregnant woman or can affect reproductive capacity. Antihemophilic Factor (Recombinant) should be given to a pregnant woman only if clearly needed.

ADVERSE REACTIONS

During the clinical studies conducted in the previously treated patient group, there were 13 infusion related minor adverse reactions reported out of 13,394 infusions (0.097%). One patient experienced flushing and nausea during his first infusion which abated on decreasing the infusion rate. A second patient experienced mild fatigue during and following one infusion and a third patient had a series of eleven nose bleeds with a periodicity associated with the infusions.
The protein in greatest concentration in Antihemophilic Factor (Recombinant) Recombinate™ is Albumin (Human). Reactions associated with intravenous administration of albumin are extremely rare, although nausea, fever, chills or

urticaria have been reported. Other allergic reactions could theoretically be encountered in the use of this Antihemophilic Factor preparation. See **Information for Patients.**

DOSAGE AND ADMINISTRATION

Each bottle of Recombinate™ is labeled with the AHF activity expressed in IU per bottle. This potency assignment is referenced to the World Health Organization International Standard for Factor VIII:C Concentrate and is evaluated by appropriate methodology to ensure accuracy of the results.

The expected *in vivo* peak increase in AHF level expressed as IU/dL of plasma or % (percent) of normal can be estimated by multiplying the dose administered per kg body weight (IU/kg) by two. This calculation is based on the clinical findings of Abildgaard *et al*[8] and is supported by the data generated by 419 clinical pharmacokinetic studies with rAHF in 67 patients over time. This pharmacokinetic data demonstrated a peak recovery point above the pre-infusion baseline of approximately 2.0 IU/dL per IU/kg body weight.

Example (Assuming patient's baseline AHF level is at <1%):

(1) A dose of 1750 IU AHF administered to a 70 kg patient, *i.e.* 25 IU/kg (1750/70), should be expected to cause a peak post-infusion AHF increase of 25 × 2 = 50 IU/dL (50% or normal).

(2) A peak level of 70% is required in a 40 kg child. In this situation the dose would be 70/2 × 40 = 1400 IU.

Recommended Dosage Schedule

Physician supervision of the dosage is required. The following dosage schedule may be used as a guide.

[See table at top of previous page]

The careful control of the substitution therapy is especially important in cases of major surgery or life threatening hemorrhages.

Although dosage can be estimated by the calculations above, it is strongly recommended that whenever possible, appropriate laboratory tests including serial AHF assays be performed on the patient's plasma at suitable intervals to assure that adequate AHF levels have been reached and are maintained.

Other dosage regimens have been proposed such as that of Schimpf, *et al*, which describes continuous maintenance therapy.[9]

Reconstitution: Use Aseptic Technique

1. Bring Antihemophilic Factor (Recombinant), Recombinate™ (dry concentrate) and Sterile Water for Injection, USP, (diluent) to room temperature.
2. Remove caps from concentrate and diluent bottles.
3. Cleanse stoppers with germicidal solution and allow to dry prior to use.
4. Remove protective covering from one end of double-ended needle and insert exposed needle through the center of the stopper.
5. Remove protective covering from other end of double-ended needle. Invert diluent bottle over the upright Recombinate™ bottle, then rapidly insert free end of the needle through the Recombinate™ bottle stopper at its center. The vacuum in the bottle will draw in the diluent.
6. Disconnect the two bottles by removing needle from diluent bottle stopper, then remove needle from Recombinate™ bottle. Swirl gently until all material is dissolved. Be sure that Recombinate™ is completely dissolved, otherwise active material will be removed by the filter needle.

NOTE: Do not refrigerate after reconstitution. See **Administration.**

Administration:

Use Aseptic Technique

Administer at room temperature.

Recombinate™ should be administered not more than 3 hours after reconstitution.

Intravenous Syringe Injection

Parenteral drug products should be inspected for particulate matter and discoloration prior to administration, whenever solution and container permit. A colorless to faint yellow appearance is acceptable for Antihemophilic Factor (Recombinant), Recombinate™.

Plastic syringes are recommended for use with this product since proteins such as AHF tend to stick to the surface of all-glass syringes.

1. Attach filter needle to a disposable syringe and draw back plunger to admit air into the syringe.
2. Insert needle into reconstituted Recombinate™.
3. Inject air into bottle and then withdraw the reconstituted material into the syringe.
4. Remove and discard the filter needle from the syringe; attach a suitable needle and inject intravenously as instructed under **Rate of Administration.**
5. If a patient is to receive more than one bottle of Recombinate™, the contents of multiple bottles may be drawn into the same syringe by drawing up each bottle through separate unused filter needle. Please note filter needles are intended to filter the contents of a single bottle of Recombinate™ only.

Rate of Administration

Preparations of Recombinate™ can be administered at a rate of up to 10 mL per minute with no significant reactions. The pulse rate should be determined before and during administration of Recombinate™. Should a significant increase in pulse rate occur, reducing the rate of administration or temporarily halting the injection usually allow the symptoms to disappear promptly.

HOW SUPPLIED

Antihemophilic Factor (Recombinant), Recombinate™ is available in single-dose bottles which contain nominally 250, 500 and 1000 International Units per bottle. Recombinate™ is packaged with 10 mL of Sterile Water for Injection, USP, a double-ended needle, a filter needle, and a package insert.

Storage

Recombinate™ can be stored under refrigeration [2–8°C (36–46°F)] or at room temperature, not to exceed 30°C (86°F). Avoid freezing to prevent damage to the diluent bottle. Do not use beyond the expiration date printed on the bottle.

REFERENCES

1. White GC, McMillan CW, Kingdon HS, *et al:* Use of recombinant antihemophilic factor in the treatment of two patients with classic hemophilia. **New Eng J Med 320:** 166–170, 1989
2. Kessler CM: An Introduction to Factor VIII Inhibitors: The Detection and Quantitation. **Am J Med 91 (Suppl 5A):** 1S–5S, 1991
3. Schwarzinger I, Pabinger I, Korninger C, Haschke F, Kundi M, Niessner H, Lechner K: Incidence of inhibitors in patients with severe and moderate hemophilia A treated with factor VIII concentrates. **Am J Hematology 24:**241–245, 1987
4. Penner JA, Kelly PE: Management of patients with factor VIII or IX inhibitors. **Sem Thromb Hemostasis 1:**386–399, 1975
5. Ehrenforth S, Kreuz W, Scharrer I, *et al:* Incidence of development of factor VIII and factor IX inhibitors in hemophiliacs. **Lancet 339:**594–598, 1992
6. McMillan CW, Shapiro SS, Whitehurst D, *et al:* The natural history of factor VIII inhibitors in patients with hemophilia A: a national cooperative study. II. Observations on the initial development of factor VIII:C inhibitors. **Blood 71:** 344–348, 1988
7. Addiego JE Jr., Gomperts E, Liu S, *et al:* Treatment of hemophilia A with a highly purified Factor VIII concentrate prepared by Anti-FVIIIc immunoaffinity chromatography. **Thrombosis and Haemostasis 67:**19–27, 1992
8. Abildgaard CF, Simone JV, Corrigan JJ, *et al:* Treatment of hemophilia with glycine-precipitated Factor VIII. **New Eng J Med 275:**471–475, 1966
9. Schimpf K, Rothman P, Zimmermann K: Factor VIII dosis in prophylaxis of hemophilia A; A further controlled study in **Proc XIth Cong W.F.H.** Kyoto, Japan, Academic Press, 1976, pp 363–366
10. Gill FM: The Natural History of Factor VIII Inhibitors in Patients with Hemophilia A. Hoyer LW (ed), Factor VIII Inhibitors, **N.Y. AR Liss,** 1984, pp 19–29
11. Rasi V, Ikkala E: Haemophiliacs with factor VIII inhibitors in Finland: prevalence, incidence and outcome. **Br J Haemotol 76:**369–371, 1990
12. Lusher JM, Salzman PM: Viral Safety and Inhibitor Development Associated with Factor VIIIC Ultra-Purified From Plasma in Hemophiliacs Previously Unexposed to Factor VIIIC Concentrates. **Seminars in Hematology 27:**1–7, 1990

Baxter Healthcare Corporation
Hyland Division
Glendale, CA 91203 USA
U.S. License No. 140
6891 Revised August 1998

Baxter Pharmaceutical Products Inc.

95 SPRING ST
NEW PROVIDENCE, NJ 07974

Direct Inquiries to:
Professional Services Department
(800) ANA DRUG
(800) 262-3784

For Medical Information Contact:
In Emergencies:
Kent Allenby
VP Clinical Research & Medical Affairs
(800) ANA-DRUG
(800) 262-3784

Sales and Ordering:
To place an order, call or fax:
(800) 667-0959
Fax 877-702-3580

ALFENTANIL HCl Injection Ⓒ℞

DESCRIPTION

Alfentanil Hydrochloride Injection is an opioid analgesic chemically designated as N-[1-[2-(4-ethyl-4,5-dihydro-5-oxo-1H-tetrazol-1-yl)ethyl]-4-(methoxymethyl)-4-piperidinyl]-N-phenylpropanamide monohydrochloride (1:1) with a molecular weight of 452.98 and an n-octanol:water partition coefficient of 128:1 at pH 7.4. The structural formula of alfentanil hydrochloride is:

Alfentanil hydrochloride is a sterile, non-pyrogenic, preservative free aqueous solution containing alfentanil hydrochloride equivalent to 500 µg per mL of alfentanil base for intravenous injection. The solution, which contains sodium chloride for isotonicity, has a pH range of 4–6.

HOW SUPPLIED

Each mL of Alfentanil Hydrochloride Injection for intravenous use contains alfentanil hydrochloride equivalent to 500 µg of alfentanil base.

Alfentanil Hydrochloride Injection is available as:
NDC 10019-060-01, 2 mL ampuls in packages of 10
NDC 10019-060-02, 5 mL ampuls in packages of 10
NDC 10019-060-03, 10 mL ampuls in packages of 5
NDC 10019-060-04, 20 mL ampuls in packages of 5

PROTECT FROM LIGHT. Store at controlled room temperature (59°–77°F/15°–25°C).

ATIVAN® Ⓒ℞
(lorazepam) Injection

DESCRIPTION

Lorazepam, a benzodiazepine with antianxiety, sedative, and anticonvulsant effects, is intended for the intramuscular or intravenous routes of administration. It has the chemical formula: 7-chloro-5(2-chlorophenyl)-1,3-dihydro-3-hydroxy-2*H*-1,4-benzodiazepin-2-one. The molecular weight is 321.16, and the C.A.S. No. is [846-49-1]. The structural formula is:

Lorazepam is a nearly white powder almost insoluble in water. Each mL of sterile injection contains either 2.0 or 4.0 mg of lorazepam, and 0.18 mL polyethylene glycol 400 in propylene glycol with 2.0% benzyl alcohol as preservative.

HOW SUPPLIED

Ativan® (lorazepam) Injection is available in the following dosage strengths in single-dose and multiple-dose vials:
2 mg per mL, NDC 10019-102-01, 25 × 1 mL vial
NDC 10019-102-10, 10 × 10 mL vial
4 mg per mL, NDC 10019-103-01, 25 × 1 mL vial
NDC 10019-103-10, 10 × 10 mL vial

For IM or IV injection.
Store in a refrigerator.
PROTECT FROM LIGHT.
Use carton to protect contents from light.

Also Available

TUBEX® Sterile Cartridge-Needle Units (22 gauge × 1 1/4 in needle), in boxes of 10 **TUBEX®** in the following dosage strengths:
2 mg per mL, NDC 10019-102-46, 1 mL fill in 2 mL size
4 mg per mL, NDC 10019-103-46, 1 mL fill in 2 mL size

TUBEX® Sterile Cartridge-Needle Units (22 gauge × 1 1/4 inch needle), packaged in boxes of 10 **TUBEX®** in TAMP-R-TEL® tamper-resistant packages in the following dosage strengths:
2 mg per mL, NDC 10019-102-47, 1 mL fill in 2 mL size
4 mg per mL, NDC 10019-103-47, 1 mL fill in 2 mL size

Ativan®, **TUBEX®**, and TAMP-R-TEL® are registered trademarks of Wyeth-Ayerst Laboratories.

ATRACURIUM BESYLATE ℞
[ătră-cŭr-ē-ŭm -bĕ-syl-āte]
Injection

This drug should be used only by adequately trained individuals familiar with its actions, characteristics, and hazards.

DESCRIPTION

Atracurium Besylate Injection is an intermediate-duration, nondepolarizing, skeletal muscle relaxant for intravenous administration. Atracurium besylate is designated as 2,2'-[1,5-pentanediylbis [oxy (3-oxo-3,1-propanediyl)]] bis [1-[(3,4-dimethoxyphenyl) methyl] - 1,2,3,4 - tetrahydro - 6,7-dimethoxy-2-methylisoquinolinium] dibenzenesulfonate. It

Continued on next page

Atracurium Besylate—Cont.

has a molecular weight of 1243.49, and its molecular formula is $C_{65}H_{82}N_2O_{18}S_2$. The structural formula is:

Atracurium besylate is a complex molecule containing four sites at which different stereochemical configurations can occur. The symmetry of the molecule, however, results in only ten, instead of sixteen, possible different isomers. The manufacture of atracurium besylate results in these isomers being produced in unequal amounts but with a consistent ratio. Those molecules in which the methyl group attached to the quarternary nitrogen projects on the opposite side to the adjacent substituted-benzyl moiety predominate by approximately 3:1.

Atracurium Besylate Injection is a sterile, non-pyrogenic aqueous solution for intravenous administration. Each mL contains 10 mg atracurium besylate. The pH is adjusted to 3.25–3.65 with benzenesulfonic acid. The multiple dose vial contains 0.9% benzyl alcohol added as a preservative. Atracurium Besylate Injection slowly loses potency with time at the rate of approximately 6% per *year* under refrigeration (5°C). Atracurium Besylate Injection should be refrigerated at 2° to 8°C (36° to 46°F) to preserve potency. Rate of loss in potency increases to approximately 5% per *month* at 25°C (77°F). Upon removal from refrigeration to room temperature storage conditions (25°C/77°F), use Atracurium Besylate Injection within 14 days even if rerefrigerated.

HOW SUPPLIED

Atracurium Besylate Injection, 10 mg atracurium besylate in each mL.

5 mL *Single Dose* Vial (50 mg per vial) – Packaged in 10s (NDC 10019-002-05).

10 mL *Multiple Dose* Vial (100 mg per vial). Contains benzyl alcohol (see WARNINGS in full prescribing information). Packaged in 10s (NDC 10019-001-10).

STORAGE: Atracurium Besylate Injection should be refrigerated at 2° to 8°C (36° to 46°F) to preserve potency. DO NOT FREEZE. Upon removal from refrigeration to room temperature storage conditions (25°C/77°F), use Atracurium Besylate Injection within 14 days even if rerefrigerated.

ATROPINE ℞

[*a 'troe-peen*]
Sulfate Injection, USP
For IM, IV or SC Use

DESCRIPTION

Atropine Sulfate Injection, USP is a sterile solution of atropine sulfate in water for injection. Each mL contains Atropine Sulfate 0.4 mg or 1.0 mg; Sodium Chloride 9 mg; Benzyl Alcohol 9 mg; Water for injection qs; pH may be adjusted with H_2SO_4 if necessary. pH: 3.0–6.5.

Atropine Sulfate Injection, USP may be given intramuscularly, intravenously or subcutaneously.

Atropine is a white crystalline alkaloid which may be extracted from belladonna root or may be produced synthetically. It is used as atropine sulfate because this compound has much greater solubility.

Atropine sulfate is an anticholinergic drug. The empirical formula of atropine sulfate is $(C_{17}H_{23}NO_3)_2 \cdot H_2SO_4 \cdot H_2O$.

The structural formula is:

$\cdot H_2SO_4 \cdot H_2O$

HOW SUPPLIED

NDC Number	Atropine Sulfate per mL	Volume
10019-250-12	0.4 mg/mL	1 mL in a 2 mL vial
10019-251-12	1 mg/mL	1 mL in a 2 mL vial
10019-250-20	0.4 mg/mL	20 mL in a 20 mL vial

2 mL vials packaged 25 per shelf pack.
20 mL multiple dose vials packaged 10 per shelf pack.
Use only if solution is clear and seal intact.

BREVIBLOC® INJECTION ℞

[*brĕv ə-blŏc*]
(esmolol hydrochloride)
10 mL Ampul—2500 mg

NOT FOR DIRECT INTRAVENOUS INJECTION. AMPUL MUST BE DILUTED PRIOR TO ITS INFUSION - SEE DOSAGE AND ADMINISTRATION.

10 mL Single Dose Vial—100 mg

DESCRIPTION

BREVIBLOC® (esmolol HCl) is a beta$_1$-selective (cardioselective) adrenergic receptor blocking agent with a very short duration of action (elimination half-life is approximately 9 minutes). Esmolol HCl is:

(±)-Methyl p-[2-hydroxy-3-(isopropylamino) propoxy] hydrocinnamate hydrochloride and has the following structure:

$CH_3O_2CCH_2CH_2-C_6H_4-OCH_2CHOHCH_2NHCH(CH_3)_2 \cdot HCl$

Esmolol HCl has the empirical formula $C_{16}H_{26}NO_4Cl$ and a molecular weight of 331.8. It has one asymmetric center and exists as an enantiomeric pair.

Esmolol HCl is a white to off-white crystalline powder. It is a relatively hydrophilic compound which is very soluble in water and freely soluble in alcohol. Its partition coefficient (octanol/water) at pH 7.0 is 0.42 compared to 17.0 for propranolol.

BREVIBLOC® INJECTION is a clear, colorless to light yellow, sterile, nonpyrogenic solution.

2500 mg, 10 mL Ampul—Each mL contains 250 mg esmolol HCl in 25% Propylene Glycol, USP, 25% Alcohol, USP and Water for Injection, USP; buffered with 17.0 mg Sodium Acetate, USP, and 0.00715 mL Glacial Acetic Acid, USP. Sodium hydroxide and/or hydrochloric acid added, as necessary, to adjust pH to 3.5–5.5.

100 mg, 10 mL Single Dose Vial—Each mL contains 10 mg esmolol HCl and Water for Injection, USP; buffered with 2.8 mg Sodium Acetate, USP and 0.546 mg Glacial Acetic Acid, USP. Sodium hydroxide and/or hydrochloric acid added, as necessary to adjust pH to 4.5–5.5.

CLINICAL PHARMACOLOGY

BREVIBLOC® (esmolol HCl) is a beta$_1$-selective (cardioselective) adrenergic receptor blocking agent with rapid onset, a very short duration of action, and no significant intrinsic sympathomimetic or membrane stabilizing activity at therapeutic dosages. Its elimination half-life after intravenous infusion is approximately 9 minutes. BREVIBLOC® inhibits the beta$_1$ receptors located chiefly in cardiac muscle, but this preferential effect is not absolute and at higher doses it begins to inhibit beta$_2$ receptors located chiefly in the bronchial and vascular musculature.

Pharmacokinetics and Metabolism

BREVIBLOC® (esmolol HCl) is rapidly metabolized by hydrolysis of the ester linkage, chiefly by the esterases in the cytosol of red blood cells and not by plasma cholinesterases or red cell membrane acetylcholinesterase. Total body clearance in man was found to be about 20 L/kg/hr, which is greater than cardiac output; thus the metabolism of BREVIBLOC® is not limited by the rate of blood flow to metabolizing tissues such as the liver or affected by hepatic or renal blood flow. BREVIBLOC® has a rapid distribution half-life of about 2 minutes and an elimination half-life of about 9 minutes.

Using an appropriate loading dose, steady-state blood levels of BREVIBLOC® for dosages from 50–300 mcg/kg/min (0.05–0.3 mg/kg/min) are obtained within five minutes. (Steady-state is reached in about 30 minutes without the loading dose.) Steady-state blood levels of BREVIBLOC® increase linearly over this dosage range and elimination kinetics are dose-independent over this range. Steady-state blood levels are maintained during infusion but decrease rapidly after termination of the infusion. Because of its short half-life, blood levels of BREVIBLOC® can be rapidly altered by increasing or decreasing the infusion rate and rapidly eliminated by discontinuing the infusion.

Consistent with the high rate of blood-based metabolism of BREVIBLOC®, less than 2% of the drug is excreted unchanged in the urine. Within 24 hours of the end of infusion, approximately 73–88% of the dosage has been accounted for in the urine as the acid metabolite of BREVIBLOC®.

Metabolism of BREVIBLOC® results in the formation of the corresponding free acid and methanol. The acid metabolite has been shown in animals to have about 1/1500th the activity of esmolol and in normal volunteers its blood levels do not correspond to the level of beta blockade. The acid metabolite has an elimination half-life of about 3.7 hours and is excreted in the urine with a clearance approximately equivalent to the glomerular filtration rate. Excretion of the acid metabolite is significantly decreased in patients with renal disease, with the elimination half-life increased to about ten-fold that of normals, and plasma levels considerably elevated.

Methanol blood levels, monitored in subjects receiving BREVIBLOC® for up to 6 hours at 300 mcg/kg/min (0.3 mg/kg/min) and 24 hours at 150 mcg/kg/min (0.15 mg/kg/min), approximated endogenous levels and were less than 2% of levels usually associated with methanol toxicity.

BREVIBLOC® has been shown to be 55% bound to human plasma protein, while the acid metabolite is only 10% bound.

Pharmacodynamics

Clinical pharmacology studies in normal volunteers have confirmed the beta blocking activity of BREVIBLOC® (esmolol HCl), showing reduction in heart rate at rest and during exercise, and attenuation of isoproterenol-induced increases in heart rate. Blood levels of BREVIBLOC® have been shown to correlate with extent of beta blockade. After termination of infusion, substantial recovery from beta blockade is observed in 10–20 minutes.

In human electrophysiology studies, BREVIBLOC® produced effects typical of a beta blocker; a decrease in the heart rate, increase in sinus cycle length, prolongation of the sinus node recovery time, prolongation of the AH interval during normal sinus rhythm and during atrial pacing, and an increase in antegrade Wenckebach cycle length.

In patients undergoing radionuclide angiography, BREVIBLOC®, at dosages of 200 mcg/kg/min (0.2 mg/kg/min), produced reductions in heart rate, systolic blood pressure, rate pressure product, left and right ventricular ejection fraction and cardiac index at rest, which were similar in magnitude to those produced by intravenous propranolol (4 mg). During exercise, BREVIBLOC® produced reductions in heart rate, rate pressure product and cardiac index which were also similar to those produced by propranolol, but produced a significantly larger fall in systolic blood pressure. In patients undergoing cardiac catheterization, the maximum therapeutic dose of 300 mcg/kg/min (0.3 mg/kg/min) of BREVIBLOC® produced similar effects and, in addition, there were small, clinically insignificant increases in the left ventricular end diastolic pressure and pulmonary capillary wedge pressure. At thirty minutes after the discontinuation of BREVIBLOC® infusion, all of the hemodynamic parameters had returned to pretreatment levels.

The relative cardioselectivity of BREVIBLOC® was demonstrated in 10 mildly asthmatic patients. Infusions of BREVIBLOC® [100, 200 and 300 mcg/kg/min (0.1, 0.2 and 0.3 mg/kg/min)] produced no significant increases in specific airway resistance compared to placebo. At 300 mcg/kg/min (0.3 mg/kg/min), BREVIBLOC® produced slightly enhanced bronchomotor sensitivity to dry air stimulus. These effects were not clinically significant, and BREVIBLOC® was well tolerated by all patients. Six of the patients also received intravenous propranolol, and at a dosage of 1 mg, two experienced significant, symptomatic bronchospasm requiring bronchodilator treatment. One other propranolol-treated patient also experienced dry air-induced bronchospasm. No adverse pulmonary effects were observed in patients with COPD who received therapeutic dosages of BREVIBLOC® for treatment of supraventricular tachycardia (51 patients) or in perioperative settings (32 patients).

Supraventricular Tachycardia

In two multicenter, randomized, double-blind, controlled comparisons of BREVIBLOC® (esmolol HCl) with placebo and propranolol, maintenance doses of 50 to 300 mcg/kg/min (0.05 to 0.3 mg/kg/min) of BREVIBLOC® were found to be more effective than placebo and about as effective as propranolol, 3–6 mg given by bolus injections, in the treatment of supraventricular tachycardia, principally atrial fibrillation and atrial flutter. The majority of these patients developed their arrhythmias postoperatively. About 60–70% of the patients treated with BREVIBLOC® had a desired therapeutic effect (either a 20% reduction in heart rate, a decrease in heart rate to less than 100 bpm, or, rarely, conversion to NSR) and about 95% of those who responded did so at a dosage of 200 mcg/kg/min (0.2 mg/kg/min) or less. The average effective dosage of BREVIBLOC® was approximately 100–115 mcg/kg/min (0.1–0.115 mg/kg/min) in the two studies. Other multicenter baseline-controlled studies gave essentially similar results. In the comparison with propranolol, about 50% of patients in both the BREVIBLOC® and propranolol groups were on concomitant digoxin. Response rates were slightly higher with both beta blockers in the digoxin-treated patients.

In all studies significant decreases of blood pressure occurred in 20–50% of patients, identified either as adverse reaction reports by investigators, or by observation of systolic pressure less than 90 mmHg or diastolic pressure less than 50 mmHg. The hypotension was symptomatic (mainly diaphoresis or dizziness) in about 12% of patients, and therapy was discontinued in about 11% of patients, about half of whom were symptomatic. In comparison to propranolol, hypotension was about three times as frequent with BREVIBLOC®, 53% vs. 17%. The hypotension was rapidly reversible with decreased infusion rate or after discontinuation of therapy with BREVIBLOC®. For both BREVIBLOC® and propranolol, hypotension was reported less frequently in patients receiving concomitant digoxin.

INDICATIONS AND USAGE

Supraventricular Tachycardia

BREVIBLOC® (esmolol HCl) is indicated for the rapid control of ventricular rate in patients with atrial fibrillation or atrial flutter in perioperative, postoperative, or other emergent circumstances where short term control of ventricular rate with a short-acting agent is desirable. BREVIBLOC® is also indicated in noncompensatory sinus tachycardia where, in the physician's judgment, the rapid heart rate requires specific intervention. BREVIBLOC® is not intended for use in chronic settings where transfer to another agent is anticipated.

Intraoperative and Postoperative Tachycardia and/or Hypertension

BREVIBLOC® (esmolol HCl) is indicated for the treatment of tachycardia and hypertension that occur during induction and tracheal intubation, during surgery, on emergence from anesthesia, and in the postoperative period, when in the physician's judgment such specific intervention is considered indicated.

Use of BREVIBLOC® to prevent such events is not recommended.

CONTRAINDICATIONS

BREVIBLOC® (esmolol HCl) is contraindicated in patients with sinus bradycardia, heart block greater than first degree, cardiogenic shock or overt heart failure (see WARNINGS).

WARNINGS

Hypotension: In clinical trials 20–50% of patients treated with BREVIBLOC® (esmolol HCl) have experienced hypotension, generally defined as systolic pressure less than 90 mmHg and/or diastolic pressure less than 50 mmHg. About 12% of the patients have been symptomatic (mainly diaphoresis or dizziness). Hypotension can occur at any dose but is dose-related so that doses beyond 200 mcg/kg/min (0.2 mg/kg/min) are not recommended. Patients should be closely monitored, especially if pretreatment blood pressure is low. Decrease of dose or termination of infusion reverses hypotension, usually within 30 minutes.

Cardiac Failure: Sympathetic stimulation is necessary in supporting circulatory function in congestive heart failure, and beta blockade carries the potential hazard of further depressing myocardial contractility and precipitating more severe failure. Continued depression of the myocardium with beta blocking agents over a period of time can, in some cases, lead to cardiac failure. At the first sign or symptom of impending cardiac failure, BREVIBLOC® (esmolol HCl) should be withdrawn. Although withdrawal may be sufficient because of the short elimination half-life of BREVIBLOC®, specific treatment may also be considered (see OVERDOSAGE). The use of BREVIBLOC® for control of ventricular response in patients with supraventricular arrhythmias should be undertaken with caution when the patient is compromised hemodynamically or is taking other drugs that decrease any or all of the following: peripheral resistance, myocardial filling, myocardial contractility, or electrical impulse propagation in the myocardium. Despite the rapid onset and offset of the effects of BREVIBLOC®, several cases of death have been reported in complex clinical states where BREVIBLOC® was presumably being used to control ventricular rate.

Intraoperative and Postoperative Tachycardia and/or Hypertension: BREVIBLOC® (esmolol HCl) should not be used as the treatment for hypertension in patients in whom the increased blood pressure is primarily due to the vasoconstriction associated with hypothermia.

Bronchospastic Diseases: PATIENTS WITH BRONCHOSPASTIC DISEASES SHOULD, IN GENERAL, NOT RECEIVE BETA BLOCKERS. Because of its relative $beta_1$ selectivity and titratability, BREVIBLOC® (esmolol HCl) may be used with caution in patients with bronchospastic diseases. However, since $beta_1$ selectivity is not absolute, BREVIBLOC® should be carefully titrated to obtain the lowest possible effective dose. In the event of bronchospasm, the infusion should be terminated immediately; a $beta_2$ stimulating agent may be administered if conditions warrant but should be used with particular caution as patients already have rapid ventricular rates.

Diabetes Mellitus and Hypoglycemia: BREVIBLOC® (esmolol HCl) should be used with caution in diabetic patients requiring a beta blocking agent. Beta blockers may mask tachycardia occurring with hypoglycemia, but other manifestations such as dizziness and sweating may not be significantly affected.

PRECAUTIONS

General

Infusion concentrations of 20 mg/mL were associated with more serious venous irritation, including thrombophlebitis, than concentrations of 10 mg/mL. Extravasation of 20 mg/mL may lead to a serious local reaction and possible skin necrosis. Concentrations greater than 10 mg/mL or infusion into small veins or through a butterfly catheter should be avoided.

Because the acid metabolite of BREVIBLOC® is primarily excreted unchanged by the kidney, BREVIBLOC® (esmolol HCl) should be administered with caution to patients with impaired renal function. The elimination half-life of the acid metabolite was prolonged ten-fold and the plasma level was considerably elevated in patients with end-stage renal disease.

Care should be taken in the intravenous administration of BREVIBLOC® as sloughing of the skin and necrosis have been reported in association with infiltration and extravasation of intravenous infusions.

Drug Interactions

Catecholamine-depleting drugs, e.g., reserpine, may have an additive effect when given with beta blocking agents. Patients treated concurrently with BREVIBLOC® (esmolol HCl) and a catecholamine depletor should therefore be closely observed for evidence of hypotension or marked bradycardia, which may result in vertigo, syncope, or postural hypotension.

A study of interaction between BREVIBLOC® and warfarin showed that concomitant administration of BREVIBLOC® and warfarin does not alter warfarin plasma levels. BREVIBLOC® concentrations were equivocally higher when given with warfarin, but this is not likely to be clinically important.

When digoxin and BREVIBLOC® were concomitantly administered intravenously to normal volunteers, there was a 10–20% increase in digoxin blood levels at some time points. Digoxin did not affect BREVIBLOC® pharmacokinetics. When intravenous morphine and BREVIBLOC® were concomitantly administered in normal subjects, no effect on morphine blood levels was seen, but BREVIBLOC® steady-state blood levels were increased by 46% in the presence of morphine. No other pharmacokinetic parameters were changed.

The effect of BREVIBLOC® on the duration of succinylcholine-induced neuromuscular blockade was studied in patients undergoing surgery. The onset of neuromuscular blockade by succinylcholine was unaffected by BREVIBLOC®, but the duration of neuromuscular blockade was prolonged from 5 minutes to 8 minutes.

Although the interactions observed in these studies do not appear to be of major clinical importance, BREVIBLOC® should be titrated with caution in patients being treated concurrently with digoxin, morphine, succinylcholine or warfarin.

While taking beta blockers, patients with a history of severe anaphylactic reaction to a variety of allergens may be more reactive to repeated challenge, either accidental, diagnostic, or therapeutic. Such patients may be unresponsive to the usual doses of epinephrine used to treat allergic reaction.

Caution should be exercised when considering the use of BREVIBLOC® and verapamil in patients with depressed myocardial function. Fatal cardiac arrests have occurred in patients receiving both drugs. Additionally, BREVIBLOC® should not be used to control supraventricular tachycardia in the presence of agents which are vasoconstrictive and inotropic such as dopamine, epinephrine, and norepinephrine because of the danger of blocking cardiac contractility when systemic vascular resistance is high.

Carcinogenesis, Mutagenesis, Impairment of Fertility

Because of its short term usage no carcinogenicity, mutagenicity or reproductive performance studies have been conducted with BREVIBLOC® (esmolol HCl).

Pregnancy Category C

Teratogenicity studies in rats at intravenous dosages of BREVIBLOC® (esmolol HCl) up to 3000 mcg/kg/min (3 mg/kg/min) (ten times the maximum human maintenance dosage) for 30 minutes daily produced no evidence of maternal toxicity, embryotoxicity or teratogenicity, while a dosage of 10,000 mcg/kg/min (10 mg/kg/min) produced maternal toxicity and lethality. In rabbits, intravenous dosages up to 1000 mcg/kg/min (1 mg/kg/min) for 30 minutes daily produced no evidence of maternal toxicity, embryotoxicity or teratogenicity, while 2500 mcg/kg/min (2.5 mg/kg/min) produced minimal maternal toxicity and increased fetal resorptions.

Although there are no adequate and well-controlled studies in pregnant women, use of esmolol in the last trimester of pregnancy or during labor or delivery has been reported to cause fetal bradycardia, which continued after termination of drug infusion. BREVIBLOC® should be used during pregnancy only if the potential benefit justifies the potential risk to the fetus.

Nursing Mothers

It is not known whether BREVIBLOC® (esmolol HCl) is excreted in human milk; however, caution should be exercised when BREVIBLOC® is administered to a nursing woman.

Pediatric Use

The safety and effectiveness of BREVIBLOC® (esmolol HCl) in pediatric patients have not been established.

ADVERSE REACTIONS

The following adverse reaction rates are based on use of BREVIBLOC® (esmolol HCl) in clinical trials involving 369 patients with supraventricular tachycardia and over 600 intraoperative and postoperative patients enrolled in clinical trials. Most adverse effects observed in controlled clinical trial settings have been mild and transient. The most important adverse effect has been hypotension (see WARNINGS). Deaths have been reported in post-marketing experience occurring during complex clinical states where BREVIBLOC® was presumably being used simply to control ventricular rate (see WARNINGS/Cardiac Failure).

Cardiovascular—Symptomatic hypotension (diaphoresis, dizziness) occurred in 12% of patients, and therapy was discontinued in about 11%, about half of whom were symptomatic. Asymptomatic hypotension occurred in about 25% of patients. Hypotension resolved during BREVIBLOC® (esmolol HCl) infusion in 63% of these patients and within 30 minutes after discontinuation of infusion in 80% of the remaining patients. Diaphoresis accompanied hypotension in 10% of patients. Peripheral ischemia occurred in approximately 1% of patients. Pallor, flushing, bradycardia (heart rate less than 50 beats per minute), chest pain, syncope, pulmonary edema and heart block have each been reported in less than 1% of patients. In two patients without supraventricular tachycardia but with serious coronary artery disease (post inferior myocardial infarction or unstable angina), severe bradycardia/sinus pause/asystole has developed, reversible in both cases with discontinuation of treatment.

Central Nervous System—Dizziness has occurred in 3% of patients; somnolence in 3%; confusion, headache, and agitation in about 2%; and fatigue in about 1% of patients. Paresthesia, asthenia, depression, abnormal thinking, anxiety, anorexia, and lightheadedness were reported in less than 1% of patients. Seizures were also reported in less than 1% of patients, with one death.

Respiratory—Bronchospasm, wheezing, dyspnea, nasal congestion, rhonchi, and rales have each been reported in less than 1% of patients.

Gastrointestinal—Nausea was reported in 7% of patients. Vomiting has occurred in about 1% of patients. Dyspepsia, constipation, dry mouth, and abdominal discomfort have each occurred in less than 1% of patients. Taste perversion has also been reported.

Skin (Infusion Site)—Infusion site reactions including inflammation and induration were reported in about 8% of patients. Edema, erythema, skin discoloration, burning at the infusion site, thrombophlebitis, and local skin necrosis from extravasation have each occurred in less than 1% of patients.

Miscellaneous—Each of the following has been reported in less than 1% of patients: Urinary retention, speech disorder, abnormal vision, midscapular pain, rigors, and fever.

OVERDOSAGE

Acute Toxicity

Overdoses of BREVIBLOC® (esmolol HCl) can cause cardiac arrest. In addition, overdoses can produce bradycardia, hypotension, electromechanical dissociation and loss of consciousness. Cases of massive accidental overdoses of BREVIBLOC® have occurred due to dilution errors. Some of these overdoses have been fatal while others resulted in permanent disablility. Bolus doses in the range of 625 mg to 2.5 g (12.5–50 mg/kg) have been fatal. Patients have recovered completely from overdoses as high as 1.75 g given over one minute or doses of 7.5 g given over one hour for cardiovascular surgery. The patients who survived appear to be those whose circulation could be supported until the effects of BREVIBLOC® resolved.

Because of its approximately 9-minute elimination half-life, the first step in the management of toxicity should be to discontinue the BREVIBLOC® infusion. Then, based on the observed clinical effects, the following general measures should also be considered.

Bradycardia: Intravenous administration of atropine or another anticholinergic drug.

Bronchospasm: Intravenous administration of $beta_2$ stimulating agent and/or a theophylline derivative.

Cardiac Failure: Intravenous administration of a diuretic and/or digitalis glycoside. In shock resulting from inadequate cardiac contractility, intravenous administration of dopamine, dobutamine, isoproterenol, or amrinone may be considered.

Symptomatic Hypotension: Intravenous administration of fluids and/or pressor agents.

DOSAGE AND ADMINISTRATION

2500 mg AMPUL

THE 2500 mg AMPUL IS NOT FOR DIRECT INTRAVENOUS INJECTION. THIS DOSAGE FORM IS A CONCENTRATED, POTENT DRUG WHICH MUST BE DILUTED PRIOR TO ITS INFUSION. BREVIBLOC® SHOULD NOT BE ADMIXED WITH SODIUM BICARBONATE. BREVIBLOC® SHOULD NOT BE MIXED WITH OTHER DRUGS PRIOR TO DILUTION IN A SUITABLE INTRAVENOUS FLUID.

(See Compatability Section below.)

Dilution: Aseptically prepare a 10 mg/mL infusion by adding two 2500 mg ampuls to a 500 mL container or one 2500 mg ampul to a 250 mL container of a compatible intravenous solution listed below. (Remove overage prior to dilution as appropriate.) This yields a final concentration of 10 mg/mL. The diluted solution is stable for at least 24 hours at room temperature. Note: Concentrations of BREVIBLOC® (esmolol HCl) greater than 10 mg/mL are likely to produce irritation on continued infusion (see PRECAUTIONS). BREVIBLOC® has, however, been well tolerated when administered via a central vein.

100 mg VIAL

This dosage form is prediluted to provide a ready-to-use 10 mg/mL concentration recommended for BREVIBLOC® intravenous administration. It may be used to administer the appropriate BREVIBLOC® (esmolol HCl) loading dosage infusions by hand-held syringe while the maintenance infusion is being prepared.

When using the 100 mg vial, a loading dose of 0.5 mg/kg/min for a 70 kg patient would be 3.5 mL.

Supraventricular Tachycardia

In the treatment of supraventricular tachycardia, responses to BREVIBLOC® (esmolol HCl) usually (over 95%) occur within the range of 50 to 200 mcg/kg/min (0.05 to 0.2 mg/kg/min). The average effective dosage is approximately 100 mcg/kg/min (0.1 mg/kg/min) although dosages as low as 25 mcg/kg/min (0.025 mg/kg/min) have been adequate in some patients. Dosages as high as 300 mcg/kg/min (0.3 mg/kg/min) have been used, but these provide little added effect and an increased rate of adverse effects, and are not recommended. Dosage of BREVIBLOC® in supraventricular tachycardia must be individualized by titration in which each step consists of a loading dosage followed by a maintenance dosage.

To initiate treatment of a patient with supraventricular tachycardia, administer a loading infusion of 500 mcg/kg/min (0.5 mg/kg/min) over one minute followed by a four-minute maintenance infusion of 50 mcg/kg/min (0.05 mg/kg/min). If an adequate therapeutic effect is observed over the five minutes of drug administration, maintain the maintenance infusion dosage with periodic adjustments up or down as needed. If an adequate therapeutic effect is not ob-

Continued on next page

Brevibloc—Cont.

served, the same loading dosage is repeated over one minute followed by an increased maintenance infusion rate of 100 mcg/kg/min (0.1 mg/kg/min).

Continue titration procedure as above, repeating the original loading infusion of 500 mcg/kg/min (0.5 mg/kg/min) over 1 minute, but increasing the maintenance infusion rate over the subsequent four minutes by 50 mcg/kg/min (0.05 mg/kg/min) increments. As the desired heart rate or blood pressure is approached, omit subsequent loading doses and titrate the maintenance dosage up or down to endpoint. Also, if desired, increase the interval between steps from 5 to 10 minutes.

Time	Loading Dose (over 1 minute)		Maintenance Dose (over 4 minutes)	
(minutes)	mcg/kg/min	mg/kg/min	mcg/kg/min	mg/kg/min
0–1	500	0.5		
1–5			50	0.05
5–6	500	0.5		
6–10			100	0.1
10–11	500	0.5		
11–15			150	0.15
15–16	•	•		
16–20			*200	*0.2
20–(24 hrs)			Maintenance dose titrated to heart rate or other clinical endpoint.	

*As the desired heart rate or endpoint is approached, the loading infusion may be omitted and the maintenance infusion titrated to 300 mcg/kg/min (0.3 mg/kg/min) or downward as appropriate. Maintenance dosages above 200 mcg/kg/min (0.2 mg/kg/min) have not been shown to have significantly increased benefits. The interval between titration steps may be increased.

This specific dosage regimen has not been studied intraoperatively and, because of the time required for titration, may not be optimal for intraoperative use.

The safety of dosages above 300 mcg/kg/min (0.3 mg/kg/min) has not been studied.

In the event of an adverse reaction, the dosage of BREVIBLOC® may be reduced or discontinued. If a local infusion site reaction develops, an alternate infusion site should be used and caution should be taken to prevent extravasation. The use of butterfly needles should be avoided.

Abrupt cessation of BREVIBLOC® in patients has not been reported to produce the withdrawal effects which may occur with abrupt withdrawal of beta blockers following chronic use in coronary artery disease (CAD) patients. However, caution should still be used in abruptly discontinuing infusions of BREVIBLOC® in CAD patients.

After achieving an adequate control of the heart rate and a stable clinical status in patients with supraventricular tachycardia, transition to alternative antiarrhythmic agents such as propranolol, digoxin, or verapamil, may be accomplished. A recommended guideline for such a transition is given below but the physician should carefully consider the labeling instructions for the alternative agent selected.

Alternative Agent	Dosage
Propranolol hydrochloride	10–20 mg q 4–6 hrs
Digoxin	0.125–0.5 mg q 6 hrs (p.o. or i.v.)
Verapamil	80 mg q 6 hrs

The dosage of BREVIBLOC® (esmolol HCl) should be reduced as follows:

1. Thirty minutes following the first dose of the alternative agent, reduce the infusion rate of BREVIBLOC® by one-half (50%).
2. Following the second dose of the alternative agent, monitor the patient's response and if satisfactory control is maintained for the first hour, discontinue BREVIBLOC®.

The use of infusions of BREVIBLOC® up to 24 hours has been well documented; in addition, limited data from 24–48 hrs (N=48) indicate that BREVIBLOC® is well tolerated up to 48 hours.

Intraoperative and Postoperative Tachycardia and/or Hypertension

In the intraoperative and postoperative settings it is not always advisable to slowly titrate the dose of BREVIBLOC® (esmolol HCl) to a therapeutic effect. Therefore, two dosing options are presented: immediate control dosing and a gradual control when the physician has time to titrate.

1. Immediate Control
   For intraoperative treatment of tachycardia and/or hypertension give an 80 mg (approximately 1 mg/kg) bolus dose over 30 seconds followed by a 150 mcg/kg/min infusion, if necessary. Adjust the infusion rate as required up to 300 mcg/kg/min to maintain desired heart rate and/or blood pressure.
2. Gradual Control
   For postoperative tachycardia and hypertension, the dosing schedule is the same as that used in supraventricular tachycardia. To initiate treatment, administer a loading dosage infusion of 500 mcg/kg/min of BREVIBLOC® for one minute followed by a four-minute maintenance infusion of 50 mcg/kg/min. If an adequate therapeutic effect is not observed within five minutes, repeat the same loading dosage and follow with a maintenance infusion increased to 100 mcg/kg/min (see above Supraventricular Tachycardia).

Note: Higher dosages (250–300 mcg/kg/min) may be required for adequate control of blood pressure than those required for the treatment of atrial fibrillation, flutter and sinus tachycardia. One third of the postoperative hypertensive patients required these higher doses.

Compatibility with Commonly Use Intravenous Fluids

BREVIBLOC® INJECTION was tested for compatibility with ten commonly used intravenous fluids at a final concentration of 10 mg esmolol HCl per mL. BREVIBLOC® INJECTION was found to be compatible with the following solutions and was stable for at least 24 hours at controlled room temperature or under refrigeration:

Dextrose (5%) Injection, USP
Dextrose (5%) in Lactated Ringer's Injection
Dextrose (5%) in Ringer's Injection
Dextrose (5%) and Sodium Chloride (0.45%) Injection, USP
Dextrose (5%) and Sodium Chloride (0.9%) Injection, USP
Lactated Ringer's Injection, USP
Potassium Chloride (40 mEq/liter) in Dextrose (5%) Injection, USP
Sodium Chloride (0.45%) Injection, USP
Sodium Chloride (0.9%) Injection, USP

BREVIBLOC® INJECTION was NOT compatible with Sodium Bicarbonate (5%) Injection, USP.

Note: Parenteral drug products should be inspected visually for particulate matter and discoloration prior to administration, whenever solution and container permit.

HOW SUPPLIED

NDC 10019-015-71, 100 mg—10 mL vial, Box of 20
NDC 10019-025-18, 2500 mg—10 mL ampul, Box of 10
STORE AT CONTROLLED ROOM TEMPERATURE (59°–86° F, 15°–30° C). Freezing does not adversely affect the product, but exposure to elevated temperatures should be avoided.

BAXTER
Mfd. for an affiliate of
Baxter Healthcare Corporation
Deerfield, IL 60015 USA
by: Faulding Puerto Rico, Inc.
P.O.Box 471 Aguadilla, PR 00604 USA
For Product Inquiry 1 800 ANA DRUG
Revised: June 1998 400-277-04

BUMETANIDE Injection, USP ℞

[*bŭmĕ-tanide*]

WARNING: Bumetanide is a potent diuretic which, if given in excessive amounts, can lead to a profound diuresis with water and electrolyte depletion. Therefore, careful medical supervision is required, and dose and dosage schedule have to be adjusted to the individual patient's needs. (See **DOSAGE AND ADMINISTRATION** in full prescribing information.)

DESCRIPTION

Bumetanide is a loop diuretic, available as 2 mL vials, 4 mL vials and 10 mL vials (0.25 mg/mL) for intravenous or intramuscular injection as a sterile solution.

Each mL contains: Bumetanide 0.25 mg, Sodium Chloride 8.5 mg and Ammonium Acetate 4.0 mg as buffers, Disodium Edetate 0.1 mg, Benzyl Alcohol 10 mg as preservative, Water for Injection q.s. pH adjusted with Sodium Hydroxide. pH 6.8–7.8

Chemically, bumetanide is 3-(butylamino)-4-phenoxy-5-sulfamoylbenzoic acid. It is a practically white powder, slightly soluble in water; soluble in alkaline solutions, having the following structural formula:

COOH
$CH_3(CH_2)_3HN$ SO_2NH_2
OC_6H_5
$C_{17}H_{20}N_2O_5S$ 364.42

HOW SUPPLIED

Bumetanide Injection, USP 0.25 mg/mL is supplied in amber vials as follows:

NDC Number	Size
10019-506-02	2 mL
10019-506-45	4 mL
10019-506-10	10 mL Mutliple Dose Vial

Packaged 10 per shelf pack.
Store at controlled room temperature 15°–30°C (59°–86°F).

BUTORPHANOL TARTRATE INJECTION, USP Ⓒ℞

DESCRIPTION

Butorphanol tartrate is a synthetically derived opioid agonist-antagonist analgesic of the phenanthrene series. The chemical name is (-)-17-(cylcobutylmethyl)morphinan-3,14-diol D-(-)-tartrate(1:1)(salt). The molecular formula is $C_{21}H_{29}NO_2 \cdot C_4H_6O_6$, which corresponds to a molecular weight of 477.56 and the following structural formula:

H_2C N CH_2 HO CH_2 HO COOH HO—C—H H—C—OH COOH

Butorphanol tartrate is a white powder. Its solutions are slightly acidic. It melts between 102.8°C (217°F) and 103.9°C (219°F), with decomposition. It is sparingly soluble in water; slightly soluble in methanol; insoluble in alcohol and chloroform; soluble in dilute acids. The dose is expressed as the tartrate salt. One milligram of the salt is equivalent to 0.68 mg of the free base. The n-octanol/aqueous buffer partition coefficient of butorphanol is 180:1 at pH 7.5.

Butorphanol tartrate injection is a sterile, parenteral, aqueous solution of butorphanol tartrate for intravenous or intramuscular administration. Each mL of solution contains 1 or 2 mg of butorphanol tartrate. In addition, each mL contains 3.3 mg citric acid, 6.4 mg sodium citrate, and 6.4 mg sodium chloride. The pH range is 3.0 to 5.5.

HOW SUPPLIED

Butorphanol Tartrate Injection, USP 1 mg/1 mL
Carton of ten 1 mL single dose vials (NDC 10019-461-01)
Butorphanol Tartrate Injection, USP 2 mg/1 mL
Carton of ten 1 mL single dose vials (NDC 10019-462-01)

STORAGE CONDITIONS

Store at controlled room temperature between 15°–30°C (59°–86°F).

CISPLATIN ℞

[*sĭs-plă̆tin*]
Injection
℞ only

WARNINGS

CISplatin should be administered under the supervision of a qualified physician experienced in the use of cancer chemotherapeutic agents. Appropriate management of therapy and complications is possible only when adequate diagnostic and treatment facilities are readily available.

Cumulative renal toxicity associated with **CIS**platin is severe. Other major dose-related toxicities are myelosuppression, nausea, and vomiting.

Ototoxicity, which may be more pronounced in children, and is manifested by tinnitus, and/or loss of high frequency hearing and occasionally deafness is significant.

Anaphylactic-like reactions to **CIS**platin have been reported. Facial edema, bronchoconstriction, tachycardia, and hypotension may occur within minutes of **CIS**platin administration. Epinephrine, corticosteroids, and antihistamines have been effectively employed to alleviate symptoms (see **"WARNINGS"** and **"ADVERSE REACTIONS"** sections of full prescribing information).

Exercise caution to prevent inadvertent CISplatin overdose. Doses greater than 100 mg/m²/cycle once every 3 to 4 weeks are rarely used. Care must be taken to avoid inadvertent **CIS**platin overdose due to confusion with carboplatin or prescribing practices that fail to differentiate daily doses from total dose per cycle.

DESCRIPTION

CISplatin (cis-diamminedichloroplatinum) is a heavy metal complex containing a central atom of platinum surrounded by two chloride atoms and two ammonia molecules in the cis position. It is a white powder with the molecular formula $PtCl_2H_6N_2$ and a molecular weight of 300.1. It is soluble in water or saline at 1 mg/mL and in dimethylformamide at 24 mg/mL. It has a melting point of 207°C. **CIS**platin Injection is a sterile aqueous solution, each mL containing 1 mg **CIS**platin and 9 mg sodium chloride. HCl and/or sodium hydroxide added to adjust pH (3.2–4.4).

Cl NH_3 Pt Cl NH_3

Store at 15°C–25°C (59°F–77°F). Do not refrigerate. Protect unopened container from light. The **CIS**platin remaining in the amber vial following initial entry is stable for 28 days protected from light or for 7 days under fluorescent room light.

Procedures for proper handling and disposal of anticancer drugs should be considered. Several guidelines on this subject have been published.[1–7] [See full prescribing information for references]. There is no general agreement that all of the procedures recommended in the guidelines are necessary or appropriate.

HOW SUPPLIED

CISplatin Injection, 1 mg/mL, is supplied in multiple dose vials containing 50 mL and 100 mL.

- (NDC 10019-910-01)—Each multiple dose vial contains 50 mg in 50 mL of **CIS**platin.
- (NDC 10019-910-02)—Each multiple dose vial contains 100 mg in 100 mL of **CIS**platin.

DIAZEPAM Injection, USP ℂ ℞

DESCRIPTION

Each mL of Diazepam Injection, USP, an anxiolytic, contains diazepam 5 mg, propylene glycol 0.4 mL, alcohol 0.1 mL, benzyl alcohol 0.015 mL and sodium benzoate/ benzoic acid, a total of 50 mg, in Water for Injection. pH 6.2–6.9. Sealed under nitrogen.

NOTE: Solution may appear colorless to light yellow.

Diazepam is a benzodiazepine derivative, identified chemically as 7-Chloro-1,3-dihydro-1-methyl-5-phenyl-2*H*-1,4-benzodiazepin-2-one. It is a colorless crystalline compound, insoluble in water and has the following structural formula:

$C_{16}H_{13}ClN_2O$ MW 284.75

HOW SUPPLIED

Diazepam Injection, USP 5 mg/mL

1 mL (5 mg) DOSETTE® Cartridge-Needle Units (22 gauge, 1¼ inch) packaged in 10s (NDC 10019-004-55)
2 mL (10 mg) DOSETTE® Cartridge-Needle Units (22 gauge, 1¼ inch) packaged in 10s (NDC 10019-005-70)
2 mL (10 mg) DOSETTE® amber ampuls packaged in 10s (NDC 10019-005-67)
1 mL (5 mg) DOSETTE® amber vials packaged in 25s (NDC 10019-004-44)
2 mL (10 mg) DOSETTE® amber vials packaged in 25s (NDC 10019-005-42)
10 mL amber Multiple Dose vials packaged individually (NDC 10019-004-62)

STORAGE

Store at controlled room temperature 15°–30°C (59°–86°F). PROTECT FROM LIGHT.

DOSETTE® is a registered trademark of A.H. Robins Company.

DILTIAZEM HYDROCHLORIDE INJECTION ℞

[*dĭl'tia-zem*]

DESCRIPTION

Diltiazem hydrochloride is a calcium ion influx inhibitor (slow channel blocker or calcium channel antagonist). Chemically, diltiazem hydrochloride is (+)-5-[2-(Dimethylamino)ethyl]-*cis*-2,3-dihydro-3-hydroxy-2-(*p*-methoxyphenyl)-1,5-benzothiazepin-4(5*H*)-one acetate(ester) monohydrochloride. The structural formula is:

$C_{22}H_{26}N_2O_4S \cdot HCl$

Diltiazem hydrochloride is a white to off-white crystalline powder with a bitter taste. It is soluble in water, methanol, and chloroform. It has a molecular weight of 450.99.

Diltiazem Hydrochloride Injection is a clear, colorless, sterile, nonpyrogenic solution. It has a pH range of 3.5 to 4.3.

Dilitiazem Hydrochloride Injection is for direct intravenous bolus injection and continuous intravenous infusion.

Each mL contains: 5 mg Diltiazem Hydrochloride, 0.75 mg Citric Acid USP, 0.65 mg Sodium Citrate Dihydrate USP, 50 mg Sorbitol NF, and Water for Injection USP q.s. Sodium Hydroxide or Hydrochloric Acid is used to adjust pH. The pH range is 3.5 to 4.3.

HOW SUPPLIED

Diltiazem Hydrochloride Injection 5 mg/mL is supplied as follows:

NDC Number		
10019-510-01	25 mg	5 mL vials packaged 10 vials per shelfpack
10019-510-02	50 mg	10 mL vials packaged 10 vials per shelfpack

SINGLE-DOSE CONTAINERS. DISCARD UNUSED PORTION.

Store Diltiazem Hydrochloride Injection under refrigeration 2°–8°C (36°–46°F). DO NOT FREEZE. May be stored at room temperature for up to 1 month. Destroy after 1 month at room temperature.

DOBUTAMINE ℞

[*dō-bū-tā-mēn*]

Hydrochloride Injection

DESCRIPTION

Dobutamine Hydrochloride Injection is a synthetic catecholamine. The chemical name for dobutamine hydrochloride is (±)-4-[2-[[3-(*p*-Hydroxyphenyl)-1-methylpropyl]amino]-ethyl]-pyrocatechol hydrochloride, and it has the following structural formula:

$C_{18}H_{23}NO_3 \cdot HCl$ MW 337.85

The clinical formulation is supplied in a sterile form for intravenous use only. Each mL contains dobutamine hydrochloride equivalent to 12.5 mg (41.5 μmol) dobutamine and sodium metabisulfite 0.24 mg in Water for Injection. Sodium hydroxide and/or hydrochloric acid added, if needed, for pH adjustment to pH 2.5–5.5.

HOW SUPPLIED

Dobutamine Hydrochloride Injection equivalent to 12.5 mg dobutamine per mL is available in the following:

20 mL (250 mg) SINGLE DOSE vial packaged in 25s (NDC 10019-184-20).

STORAGE

Store at controlled room temperature 15°–30°C (59°–86°F).

DOXORUBICIN Hydrochloride for Injection, USP ℞

[*dŏx-ō-rubĭcĭn*]

FOR INTRAVENOUS USE ONLY

Rx only

WARNINGS

1. Severe local tissue necrosis will occur if there is extravasation during administration (See **DOSAGE AND ADMINISTRATION** in full prescribing information). Doxorubicin must not be given by the intramuscular or subcutaneous route.
2. Myocardial toxicity manifested in its most severe form by potentially fatal congestive heart failure may occur either during therapy or months to years after termination of therapy. The probability of developing impaired myocardial function based on a combined index of signs, symptoms and decline in left ventricular ejection fraction (LVEF) is estimated to be 1 to 2% at a total cumulative dose of 300 mg/m^2 of doxorubicin, 3 to 5% at a dose of 400 mg/m^2, 5 to 8% at 450 mg/m^2 and 6 to 20% at 500 mg/m^2 (Data on file are available at Pharmacia & Upjohn). The risk of developing CHF increases rapidly with increasing total cumulative doses of doxorubicin in excess of 450 mg/m^2. This toxicity may occur at lower cumulative doses in patients with prior mediastinal irradiation or on concurrent cyclophosphamide therapy or with pre-existing heart disease. Pediatric patients are at increased risk for developing delayed cardiotoxicity.
3. Dosage should be reduced in patients with impaired hepatic function.
4. Severe myelosuppression may occur.
5. Doxorubicin should be administered only under the supervision of a physician who is experienced in the use of cancer chemotherapeutic agents.

DESCRIPTION

Doxorubicin is a cytotoxic anthracycline antibiotic isolated from cultures of *Streptomyces peucetius* var. *caesius*.

Doxorubicin consists of a naphthacenequinone nucleus linked through a glycosidic bond at ring atom 7 to an amino sugar, daunosamine.

Chemically, doxorubicin hydrochloride is: (8S, 10S)-10-[(3-Amino-2,3,6-trideoxy-α-L-*lyxo*-hexopyranosyl)-oxy]-8-glycoloyl - 7,8,9,10 - tetrahydro - 6,8,11 - trihydroxy -1- methoxy-5,12-naphthacenedione hydrochloride [*25316-40-9*].

The structural formula is as follows:

[See chemical structure at top of next column]

Doxorubicin binds to nucleic acids, presumably by specific intercalation of the planar anthracycline nucleus with the DNA double helix. The anthracycline ring is lipophilic, but the saturated end of the ring system contains abundant hydroxyl groups adjacent to the amino sugar, producing a hydrophilic center. The molecule is amphoteric, containing acidic functions in the ring phenolic groups and a basic function in the sugar amino group. It binds to cell membranes as well as plasma proteins.

Doxorubicin Hydrochloride for Injection, USP, a sterile red lyophilized powder for intravenous use only, is available in

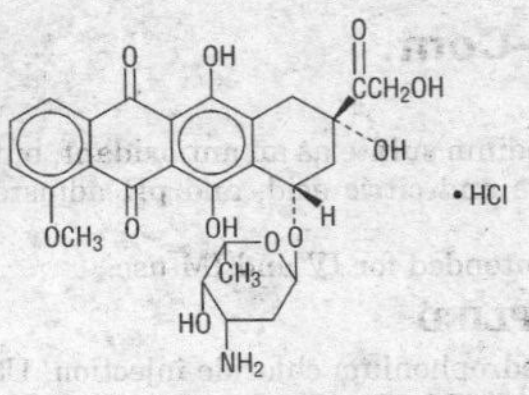

$C_{27}H_{29}NO_{11}.HCl$ M.W. = 579.99

10 mg and in 50 mg single dose vials. Each single dose vial contains 10 or 50 mg doxorubicin hydrochloride and 50 mg or 250 mg lactose monohydrate respectively, as a sterile red lyophilized powder.

HOW SUPPLIED

Doxorubicin Hydrochloride for Injection, USP is available as follows:

SINGLE DOSE VIALS:
NDC 10019-920-01, 10 mg, single dose vial, box of 1.
NDC 10019-921-02, 50 mg, single dose vial, box of 1.

Store at controlled room temperature, 15°C–30°C (59°F–86°F). Protect from light.

Retain in carton until time of use. Contains no preservatives.

Discard unused portion.

DURAMORPH® Ⓒ ℞

[*dŭrā-morph*]

PRESERVATIVE-FREE

(morphine sulfate injection, USP)

DESCRIPTION

Morphine is the most important alkaloid of opium and is a phenanthrene derivative. It is available as the sulfate salt, having the following structural formula:

7,8-Didehydro-4,5-epoxy-17-methyl-(5α,6α)-morphinan-3,6-diol sulfate (2:1) (salt), pentahydrate

$(C_{17}H_{19}NO_3)_2 \cdot H_2SO_4 \cdot 5H_2O$ Molecular weight is 758.83

Preservative-free DURAMORPH® (morphine sulfate injection, USP) is a sterile, nonpyrogenic, isobaric solution of morphine sulfate, free of antioxidants, preservatives or other potentially neurotoxic additives and is intended for intravenous, epidural or intrathecal administration as a narcotic analgesic. Each milliliter contains morphine sulfate 0.5 mg or 1 mg and sodium chloride 9 mg in Water for Injection. pH range is 2.5–6.5. Ampuls are sealed under nitrogen. Each 10 mL DOSETTE® ampul of DURAMORPH® is intended for **SINGLE USE ONLY**. *Discard any unused portion.* DO NOT HEAT-STERILIZE.

HOW SUPPLIED

Preservative-free DURAMORPH® (morphine sulfate injection, USP) is available in amber DOSETTE® ampuls for intravenous, epidural and intrathecal administration:

5 mg/10 mL (0.5 mg/mL) packaged in 10s (NDC 10019-006-73)
10 mg/10 mL (1 mg/1 mL) packaged in 10s (NDC 10019-007-73)

STORAGE

PROTECT FROM LIGHT. Store in carton at controlled room temperature 15°–30°C (59°–86°F) until ready to use. DO NOT FREEZE. DURAMORPH® contains no preservative or antioxidant. DISCARD ANY UNUSED PORTION. DO NOT HEAT-STERILIZE.

Duramorph® and DOSETTE® are registered trademarks of A.H. Robins Company.

ENLON® ℞

[*ĕn 'lon*]

(edrophonium chloride injection, USP)

DESCRIPTION

Enlon® is a short and rapid-acting cholinergic drug. Chemically, edrophonium chloride is ethyl(m-hydroxyphenyl) dimethylammonium chloride and its structural formula is:

Each mL contains, in a sterile solution, 10 mg edrophonium chloride compounded with 0.45% phenol as a preservative,

Continued on next page

Enlon—Cont.

and 0.2% sodium sulfite as an antioxidant, buffered with sodium citrate and citric acid, and pH adjusted to approximately 5.4.
Enlon® is intended for IV and IM use.

HOW SUPPLIED

ENLON® (edrophonium chloride injection, USP):
NDC 10019-873-15 15 mL vials
ENLON® (edrophonium chloride injection, USP) should be stored at controlled room temperature 15°–30°C (59°–86°F).

ENLON-PLUS® ℞

[ĕn '-lon ' plus]
(edrophonium chloride, USP and atropine sulfate, USP) Injection

DESCRIPTION

Enlon-Plus® (edrophonium chloride, USP and atropine sulfate, USP) Injection, for intravenous use, is a sterile, nonpyrogenic, nondepolarizing neuromuscular relaxant antagonist. Enlon-Plus® is a combination drug containing a rapid acting acetylcholinesterase inhibitor, edrophonium chloride, and an anticholinergic, atropine sulfate. Chemically, edrophonium chloride is ethyl (m-hydroxyphenyl) dimethylammonium chloride; its structural formula is:

Molecular Formula: $C_{10}H_{16}ClNO$
Molecular Weight: 201.70
Chemically, atropine sulfate is:
endo- (±) -alpha- (hydroxymethyl) -8-methyl-8-azabicyclo [3.2.1]oct-3-yl benzeneacetate sulfate (2:1) monohydrate. Its structural formula is:

Molecular Formula: $(C_{17}H_{23}NO_3)_2.H_2SO_4.H_2O$
Molecular Weight: 694.84
Enlon-Plus® contains in each mL of sterile solution:
5 mL Ampuls: 10 mg edrophonium chloride and 0.14 mg atropine sulfate compounded with 2.0 mg sodium sulfite as a preservative and buffered with sodium citrate and citric acid. The pH is adjusted in the range of 4.4–4.6.
15 mL Multidose Vials: 10 mg edrophonium chloride and 0.14 mg atropine sulfate compounded with 2.0 mg sodium sulfite and 4.5 mg phenol as a preservative and buffered with sodium citrate and citric acid. The pH is adjusted in the range of 4.4–4.6.

HOW SUPPLIED

Enlon-Plus® (edrophonium chloride, USP and atropine sulfate, USP) Injection should be stored between 15°–26°C (59°–78°F)
NDC 10019-180-05 5 mL ampuls, boxes of 10
NDC 10019-195-15 15 mL multidose vials

ĔTHRANE® ℞

[ē 'thrān]
(enflurane, USP)
Liquid For Inhalation

DESCRIPTION

Ēthrane® (enflurane, USP), a nonflammable liquid administered by vaporizing, is a general inhalation anesthetic drug. It is 2-chloro-1,1,2-trifluoroethyl difluoromethyl ether (CHF_2OCF_2CHFCl). The boiling point is 56.5° C at 760 mm Hg, and the vapor pressure (in mm Hg) is 175 at 20° C, 218 at 25° C, and 345 at 36° C. Vapor pressures can be calculated using the equation:

$$\log_{10}P_{vap} = A + \frac{B}{T} \qquad A = 7.967,\; B = -1678.4,\; T = °C + 273.16 \text{ (Kelvin)}$$

The specific gravity (25°/25° C) is 1.517. The refractive index at 20° C is 1.3026–1.3030. The blood/gas coefficient is 1.91 at 37° C and the oil/gas coefficient is 98.5 at 37° C.
Enflurane is a clear, colorless, stable liquid whose purity exceeds 99.9% (area percent by gas chromatography). No stabilizers are added as these have been found, through controlled laboratory tests, to be unnecessary even in the presence of ultraviolet light. Enflurane is stable to strong base, does not decompose in contact with soda lime (at normal operating temperatures), and does not react with aluminum, tin, brass, iron or copper. The partition coefficients of enflurane at 25° C are 74 in conductive rubber and 120 in polyvinyl chloride.

HOW SUPPLIED

Ēthrane® (enflurane, USP) is packaged in 125 and 250 mL amber-colored bottles.
125 mL—NDC 10019-350-50
250 mL—NDC 10019-350-60
Storage: Store at room temperature 15°–30° C (59°–86° F). Enflurane contains no additives and has been demonstrated to be stable at room temperature for periods in excess of five years.

ETOPOSIDE ℞

[ē tōpō-side]
Injection

WARNINGS
Etoposide should be administered under the supervision of a qualified physician experienced in the use of cancer chemotherapeutic agents. Severe myelosuppression with resulting infection or bleeding may occur.

DESCRIPTION

Etoposide (also commonly known as VP-16) is a semisynthetic derivative of podophyllotoxin used in the treatment of certain neoplastic diseases. It is 4'-demethylepipodophyllotoxin 9-[4,6-O-(R)-ethylidene-β-D-glucopyranoside]. It is very soluble in methanol and chloroform, slightly soluble in ethanol, and sparingly soluble in water and ether. It is made more miscible with water by means of organic solvents. It has a molecular weight of 588.56 and a molecular formula of $C_{29}H_{32}O_{13}$.
Etoposide injection is available for intravenous use as 20 mg/mL (100 mg/5 mL and 500 mg/25 mL) in 5 mL and in 25 mL multiple dose vials. The pH of the clear yellow solution is 3.0 to 4.0. Each mL contains 20 mg etoposide, 2 mg citric acid, 30 mg benzyl alcohol, 80 mg polysorbate 80, 650 mg polyethylene glycol 300, and 30.5 percent (v/v) alcohol.
The structural formula is:

HOW SUPPLIED

Etoposide Injection is supplied as a sterile, clear, yellow solution, in a 5 mL and 25 mL multi-dose vial.
NDC 10019-930-01, 100 mg (20 mg/mL).
NDC 10019-930-02, 500 mg (20 mg/mL).
Store at controlled room temperature 15°C–30°C (59°F–86°F).

FENTANYL Citrate Injection, USP Ⓒ ℞

[fĕn tăn-ill]

DESCRIPTION

Fentanyl Citrate Injection is a sterile, non-pyrogenic solution for intravenous or intramuscular use as a potent narcotic analgesic. Each mL contains fentanyl citrate equivalent to 50 mcg (0.05 mg) fentanyl base in Water for Injection. pH 4.0–7.5; sodium hydroxide and/or hydrochloric acid added, if needed, for pH adjustment. Contains no preservative.
Fentanyl citrate is chemically identified as N-(1-phenethyl-4-piperidyl)propionanilide citrate (1:1) with the following structural formula:

$C_{22}H_{28}N_2O \cdot C_6H_8O_7$ MW 528.60

HOW SUPPLIED

Fentanyl Citrate Injection, USP, equivalent to 50 mcg (0.05 mg) fentanyl base per mL, is available as follows:
2 mL DOSETTE® ampuls packaged in 10s (NDC 10019-038-67)
5 mL DOSETTE® ampuls packaged in 10s (NDC 10019-033-72)
For Intravenous Use by Hospital Personnel Specifically Trained in the Use of Narcotic Analgesics:
10 mL DOSETTE® ampuls packaged in 5s (NDC 10019-034-73)
20 mL DOSETTE® ampuls packaged in 5s (NDC 10019-035-74)
30 mL *SINGLE DOSE* vials packaged individually (NDC 10019-036-82)
50 mL *SINGLE DOSE* vials packaged individually (NDC 10019-037-83)
STORAGE
PROTECT FROM LIGHT
Keep covered in carton until time of use. Store at controlled room temperature 15°–30°C (59°–86°F).
DOSETTE® is a registered trademark of A.H. Robins Company.

FLUOROURACIL ℞

Injection, USP
℞ only

WARNING
It is recommended that fluorouracil be given only by or under the supervision of a qualified physician who is experienced in cancer chemotherapy and who is well versed in the use of potent antimetabolites. Because of the possibility of severe toxic reactions, it is recommended that patients be hospitalized at least during the initial course of therapy.

DESCRIPTION

Fluorouracil Injection, USP, an antineoplastic antimetabolite, is a sterile, nonpyrogenic injectable solution for intravenous administration. Each vial contains 250 mg or 500 mg of fluorouracil. Sodium hydroxide and if necessary hydrochloric acid may be added to adjust pH to 9.0–9.2 during manufacture.
Chemically, fluorouracil, a fluorinated pyrimidine, is 5-fluoro-2,4(1*H*,3*H*)-pyrimidinedione. It is a white to practically white crystalline powder which is sparingly soluble in water.
The molecular weight of fluorouracil is 130.08.
Molecular formula of fluorouracil is: $C_4H_3FN_2O_2$
The structural formula is:

HOW SUPPLIED

Fluorouracil Injection is available for intravenous use in 10 mL and 5 mL vials. Each 10 mL contains 500 mg fluorouracil in a colorless to faint yellow aqueous solution. Each 5 mL contains 250 mg fluorouracil in a colorless to faint yellow aqueous solution. Sodium hydroxide and if necessary hydrochloric acid may be added to adjust pH to 9.0–9.2 during manufacture.
5 mL single-dose vials, boxes of 10 - NDC 10019-950-01
10 mL single-dose vials, boxes of 10 - NDC 10019-950-02

STORAGE

Store at room temperature 15°–30°C (59°–86°F).
PROTECT FROM LIGHT. Retain in carton until contents are used. Discard any unused portion.

FORANE® ℞

[for 'ān]
(isoflurane, USP)
Liquid For Inhalation

DESCRIPTION

FORANE® (isoflurane, USP), a nonflammable liquid administered by vaporizing, is a general inhalation anesthetic drug. It is 1-chloro-2,2,2-trifluoroethyl difluoromethyl ether, and its structural formula is:

Some physical constants are:

Molecular weight		184.5
Boiling point at 760 mm Hg		48.5 °C (uncorr.)
Refractive index n_D^{20}		1.2990–1.3005
Specific gravity 25 °/25 °C		1.496
Vapor pressure in mm Hg**	20 °C	238
	25 °C	295
	30 °C	367
	35 °C	450

**Equation for vapor pressure calculation:

$$\log_{10}P_{vap} = A + \frac{B}{T} \quad \text{where: } A = 8.056,\; B = -1664.58,\; T = °C + 273.16 \text{ (Kelvin)}$$

Partition coefficients at 37 °C	
Water/gas	0.61
Blood/gas	1.43
Oil/gas	90.8

Partition coefficients at 25 °C—rubber and plastic	
Conductive rubber/gas	62.0

Butyl rubber/gas	75.0
Polyvinyl chloride/gas	110.0
Polyethylene/gas	~2.0
Polyurethane/gas	~1.4
Polyolefin/gas	~1.1
Butyl acetate/gas	~2.5
Purity by gas chromatography	>99.9%
Lower limit of flammability in oxygen or nitrous oxide at 9 joules/sec. and 23°C	None
Lower limit of flammability in oxygen or nitrous oxide at 900 joules/sec. and 23°C	Greater than useful concentration in anesthesia.

Isoflurane is a clear, colorless, stable liquid containing no additives or chemical stabilizers. Isoflurane has a mildly pungent, musty, ethereal odor. Samples stored in indirect sunlight in clear, colorless glass for five years, as well as samples directly exposed for 30 hours to a 2 amp, 115 volt, 60 cycle long wave U.V. light were unchanged in composition as determined by gas chromatography. Isoflurane in one normal sodium methoxide-methanol solution, a strong base, for over six months consumed essentially no alkali, indicative of strong base stability. Isoflurane does not decompose in the presence of soda lime (at normal operating temperatures), and does not attack aluminum, tin, brass, iron or copper.

HOW SUPPLIED

FORANE® (isoflurane, USP) is packaged in 100 mL and 250 mL amber-colored bottles.
100 mL – NDC 10019-360-40
250 mL – NDC 10019-360-60

Storage: Store at room temperature 15°–30° C (59°–86° F). Isoflurane contains no additives and has been demonstrated to be stable at room temperature for periods in excess of five years.

FUROSEMIDE INJECTION, USP ℞

[*fūr-o-sĕmīde*]

WARNING

Furosemide is a potent diuretic which, if given in excessive amounts, can lead to a profound diuresis with water and electrolyte depletion. Therefore, careful medical supervision is required and dose and dosage schedule have to be adjusted to individual patient's needs. (See DOSAGE AND ADMINISTRATION in full prescribing information.)

DESCRIPTION

Furosemide is a diuretic which is an anthranilic acid derivative, chemically known as 4-chloro-*N*-furfuryl-5-sulfamoylanthranilic acid. Furosemide is a white to off-white odorless crystalline powder. It is practically insoluble in water, sparingly soluble in alcohol, freely soluble in dilute alkali solutions and insoluble in dilute acids. The structural formula is as follows:

$C_{12}H_{11}ClN_2O_5S$ MW 330.74

Furosemide Injection, for intramuscular or slow intravenous use, is a sterile, non-pyrogenic solution of furosemide in Water for Injection prepared with the aid of sodium hydroxide. Each mL contains furosemide 10 mg and sodium chloride for isotonicity. pH adjusted to 8.0–9.3 with sodium hydroxide; hydrochloric acid used, if needed. The preparation contains no antimicrobial preservatives.

HOW SUPPLIED

Furosemide Injection, USP is available in the following:
10 mg/mL DOSETTE® Ampuls
20 mg/2 mL packaged in 25s (NDC 10019-009-67)
40 mg/4 mL packaged in 25s (NDC 10019-010-76)
10 mg/mL DOSETTE® SINGLE USE Vials
20 mg/2 mL packaged in 25s (NDC 10019-009-75)
40 mg/4 mL packaged in 25s (NDC 10019-010-77)
100 mg/10 mL packaged in 25s (NDC 10019-011-78)

STORAGE

Protect from light. Store at controlled room temperature 15°–30°C (59°–86°F). Do not use if solution is discolored.
DOSETTE® is a registered trademark of A.H. Robins Company.

6% HETASTARCH in 0.9% Sodium Chloride Injection ℞

DESCRIPTION

6% Hetastarch in 0.9% Sodium Chloride Injection (Hetastarch Injection) is a sterile, nonpyrogenic solution for intravenous administration. The composition of each 100 mL is as follows:

Hetastarch	6 g
Sodium Chloride, USP	0.9 g
Water for Injection, USP	qs

pH adjusted with Sodium Hydroxide, NF if necessary
Concentration of Electrolytes (mEq/L): Sodium 154, Chloride 154
pH: approximately 5.5 with negligible buffering capacity
Calculate Osmolarity: approximately 309 mOsM

Hetastarch is an artificial colloid derived from a waxy starch composed almost entirely of amylopectin. Hydroxyethyl ether groups are introduced into the glucose units of the starch, and the resultant material is hydrolyzed to yield a product with a molecular weight suitable for use as a plasma volume expander and erythrocyte sedimenting agent. Hetastarch is characterized by its molar substitution and also by its molecular weight. The molar substitution is approximately 0.75 which means hetastarch has an average of approximately 75 hydroxyethyl groups for every 100 glucose units. The weight average molecular weight is approximately 600,000 with a range of 450,000 to 800,000 and with at least 80% of the polymers falling within the range of 20,000 to 2,500,000. Hydroxyethyl groups are attached by ether linkage primarily at C-2 of the glucose unit and to a lesser extent at C-3 and C-6. The polymer resembles glycogen, and the polymerized D-glucose units are joined primarily by α-1,4 linkages with occasional α-1,6 branching linkages. The degree of branching is approximately 1:20 which means that there is an average of approximately one α-1,6 branch for every 20 glucose monomer units.
The chemical name for hetastarch is hydroxyethyl starch.
The structural formula is as follows:

Amylopectin derivative in which R_2 and R_3 are H or CH_2CH_2OH and R_6 is H, CH_2CH_2OH, or a branching point in the starch polymer connected through an α-1,6 link to additional D-glucopyranosyl units.
Hetastarch Injection is a clear, pale yellow to amber solution. Exposure to prolonged adverse storage conditions may result in a change to a turbid deep brown or the formation of a crystalline precipitate. Do not use the solution if these conditions are evident.
The flexible plastic container is fabricated from a specially formulated polyvinylchloride. Solutions in contact with the plastic container may leach out certain chemical components from the plastic in very small amounts; however, biological testing was supportive of the safety of the plastic container materials. The container solution unit is a closed system and is not dependent upon entry of external air during administration. The container is overwrapped to provide protection from the physical environment and to provide an additional moisture barrier when necessary.
The closure system has two ports: the one for the administration set has a tamper evident plastic protector.

HOW SUPPLIED

6% Hetastarch in 0.9% Sodium Chloride Injection is supplied sterile and nonpyrogenic in 500 mL intravenous plastic infusion containers.

NDC 10019-999-59	12-Pack	500 mL bags

Exposure of pharmaceutical products to heat should be minimized. Avoid excessive heat. Protect from freezing. It is recommended that the product be stored at room temperature (25°C); however, brief exposure up to 40°C does not adversely affect the product.

KETOROLAC Tromethamine ℞

[*kĕ tōrō-lăc*]
Injection, USP
Rx only

WARNING

Ketorolac tromethamine, a nonsteroidal anti-inflammatory drug (NSAID), is indicated for the short-term (up to 5 days) management of moderately severe acute pain that requires analgesia at the opioid level. It is NOT indicated for minor or chronic painful conditions. Ketorolac tromethamine is a potent NSAID analgesic, and its administration carries many risks. The resulting NSAID-related adverse events can be serious in certain patients for whom ketorolac tromethamine is indicated, especially when the drug is used inappropriately. Increasing the dose of ketorolac tromethamine beyond the label recommendations will not provide better efficacy but will result in increasing the risk of developing serious adverse events.

GASTROINTESTINAL EFFECTS

- Ketorolac tromethamine can cause peptic ulcers, gastrointestinal bleeding and/or perforation. Therefore, ketorolac tromethamine is CONTRAINDICATED in patients with active peptic ulcer disease, in patients with recent gastrointestinal bleeding or perforation, and in patients with a history of peptic ulcer disease or gastrointestinal bleeding.

RENAL EFFECTS

- Ketorolac tromethamine is CONTRAINDICATED in patients with advanced renal impairment and in patients at risk for renal failure due to volume depletion (see **WARNINGS** in full prescribing information).

RISK OF BLEEDING

- Ketorolac tromethamine inhibits platelet function and is, therefore, CONTRAINDICATED in patients with suspected or confirmed cerebrovascular bleeding, patients with hemorrhagic diathesis, incomplete hemostasis and those at high risk of bleeding (see **WARNINGS** and **PRECAUTIONS** in full prescribing information).

Ketorolac tromethamine is CONTRAINDICATED as prophylactic analgesic before any major surgery and is CONTRAINDICATED intra-operatively when hemostasis is critical because of the increased risk of bleeding.

HYPERSENSITIVITY

- Hypersensitivity reactions, ranging from bronchospasm to anaphylactic shock, have occurred and appropriate counteractive measures must be available when administering the first dose of Ketorolac Tromethamine Injection (see **CONTRAINDICATIONS** and **WARNINGS** in full prescribing information). Ketorolac tromethamine is CONTRAINDICATED in patients with previously demonstrated hypersensitivity to ketorolac tromethamine or allergic manifestations to aspirin or other nonsteroidal anti-inflammatory drugs (NSAIDs).

INTRATHECAL OR EPIDURAL ADMINISTRATION

- Ketorolac tromethamine is CONTRAINDICATED for intrathecal or epidural administration due to its alcohol content.

LABOR, DELIVERY AND NURSING

- The use of ketorolac tromethamine in labor and delivery is CONTRAINDICATED because it may adversely affect fetal circulation and the uterus.
- The use of ketorolac tromethamine is CONTRAINDICATED in nursing mothers because of the potential adverse effects of prostaglandin-inhibiting drugs on neonates.

CONCOMITANT USE WITH NSAIDs

- Ketorolac tromethamine is CONTRAINDICATED in patients currently receiving ASA or NSAIDs because of the cumulative risk of inducing serious NSAID-related side effects.

DOSAGE AND ADMINISTRATION

Ketorolac Tromethamine Tablets

- Ketorolac tromethamine tablets are indicated only as continuation therapy to Ketorolac Tromethamine Injection, and the combined duration of use of Ketorolac Tromethamine Injection and ketorolac tromethamine tablets is not to exceed five (5) days because of the increased risk of serious adverse events.
- The recommended total daily dose of ketorolac tromethamine tablets (maximum 40 mg) is significantly lower than for Ketorolac Tromethamine Injection (maximum 120 mg) (see **DOSAGE AND ADMINISTRATION** in full prescribing information).

Special Populations

- Dosage should be adjusted for patients 65 years or older, for patients under 50 kg (110 lbs) of body weight (see **DOSAGE AND ADMINISTRATION** in full prescribing information) and for patients with moderately elevated serum creatinine (see **WARNINGS** in full prescribing information). Doses of Ketorolac Tromethamine Injection are not to exceed 60 mg (total dose per day) in these patients.

DESCRIPTION

Ketorolac tromethamine is a member of the pyrrolo-pyrrole group of nonsteroidal anti-inflammatory drugs (NSAIDs). The chemical name for ketorolac tromethamine is (±)-5-benzoyl- 2,3-dihydro-1H-pyrrolizine-1-carboxylic acid, compound with 2-amino- 2-(hydroxymethyl)-1,3-propanediol.

Ketorolac tromethamine is a racemic mixture of [-]S and [+]R ketorolac tromethamine. Ketorolac tromethamine may exist in three crystal forms. All forms are equally soluble in water. Ketorolac tromethamine has a pK_a of 3.5 and an n-octanol/water partition coefficient of 0.26. The molecular weight of ketorolac tromethamine is 376.41.
Ketorolac tromethamine is available for intravenous (IV) or intramuscular (IM) administration as: 15 mg in 1 mL (1.5%) and 30 mg in 1 mL (3%) in sterile solution; 60 mg in 2 mL (3%) of ketorolac tromethamine in sterile solution is available for IM administration only. The solutions contain 10% (w/v) alcohol, USP, and 6.68 mg, 4.35 mg and 8.70 mg, respectively, of sodium chloride in sterile water. The pH is adjusted with sodium hydroxide and/or hydrochloric acid, and the solutions are packaged with nitrogen. The sterile solutions are clear and slightly yellow in color.

Continued on next page

Ketorolac Tromethamine—Cont.

HOW SUPPLIED

Ketorolac Tromethamine Injection, USP is available in prefilled syringes as follows:

For IV or IM Single-Dose use:

A syringe containing 1 mL of 15 mg/mL Ketorolac Tromethamine, USP, NDC 10019-021-09, available in boxes of 10.

A syringe containing 1 mL of 30 mg/mL Ketorolac Tromethamine, USP, NDC 10019-022-09, available in boxes of 10.

For IM Single-Dose use only:

A syringe containing 2 mL of 30 mg/mL Ketorolac Tromethamine, USP, (60 mg), NDC 10019-022-17, available in boxes of 10.

Each disposable syringe is supplied with an individually wrapped 22 gauge, 1 1/4 inch needle.

Directions for use: Peel back needle wrapping and expose needle hub; avoid touching hub. Aseptically remove rubber protective cap from the syringe. Attach needle to syringe hub with a twist, keeping needle sheath intact. Remove needle sheath and inject medication. To prevent needle-stick injuries, needles should not be recapped, purposely bent, or broken by hand. Dispose of used syringe in accordance with applicable medical waste regulations and guidelines.

Store at controlled room temperature 15°–30°C (59°–86°F).
PROTECT FROM LIGHT
Retain in carton until time of use.

LABETALOL HYDROCHLORIDE ℞
Injection, USP
Rx only

DESCRIPTION

Labetalol Hydrochloride is an adrenergic receptor blocking agent that has both selective $alpha_1$- and non-selective beta-adrenergic receptor blocking agents in a single substance.

Labetalol HCl is a racemate, chemically designated as 5-[1-hydroxy-2-[(1-methyl-3-phenylpropyl) amino] ethyl]salicylamide monohydrochloride, and has the following structural formula:

CONH₂ OH • HCl CH₂CH₂CHNHCH₂CH CH₃ OH

Labetalol HCl has the molecular formula $C_{19}H_{24}N_2O_3 \bullet HCl$ and a molecular weight of 364.87. It has two asymmetric centers and therefore exists as a molecular complex of two diastereoisomeric pairs. Dilevalol, the R,R' stereoisomer, makes up 25% of racemic labetalol.

Labetalol HCl is a white or off-white crystalline powder, soluble in water.

Labetalol Hydrochloride Injection is a clear, colorless to light yellow aqueous sterile isotonic solution for intravenous injection. It has a pH range of 3.0 to 4.0. Each mL contains 5 mg labetalol HCl, USP, 45 mg anhydrous dextrose, 0.10 mg edetate disodium; 0.80 mg methylparaben and 0.10 mg propylparaben as preservatives; citric acid anhydrous and sodium hydroxide, as necessary, to bring the solution into the pH range.

HOW SUPPLIED

Labetalol HCl Injection, 5 mg/mL, is supplied in:
20 mL (100 mg) (NDC 10019-210-02) multi-dose vial, pack of 10 individually boxed vials
40 mL (200 mg) (NDC 10019-210-04) multi-dose vial, pack of 10 individually boxed vials

Store between 15° and 25°C (59° and 77°F). Protect from freezing. PROTECT FROM LIGHT.

LIDOCAINE HCl Injection, USP ℞
[līdō' caīne]
FOR INFILTRATION AND NERVE BLOCK

(Preservative-Free and Preserved. See HOW SUPPLIED section.)
Do Not Use Solutions Containing Preservatives for Spinal or Epidural Anesthesia.

DESCRIPTION

Lidocaine Hydrochloride Injection is a sterile solution of Lidocaine Hydrochloride 1% or 2% in Water for Injection. Each mL of the available solutions of Lidocaine Hydrochloride Injection contains the ingredients listed in Table 1. [See table below]

pH 5.0–7.0; sodium hydroxide and/or hydrochloric acid added, if needed, for pH adjustment.

Lidocaine hydrochloride is a local anesthetic that is administered parenterally by injection and is chemically designated as 2-(diethylamino)-*N*-(2,6-dimethylphenyl) acetamide monohydrochloride. The molecular weight is 270.80 and the molecular formula is $C_{14}H_{22}N_2O \bullet HCl$. The structural formula is:

CH₃ —NHCOCH₂N(C₂H₅)₂ • HCl CH₃

Lidocaine Hydrochloride Injection is available with and without epinephrine. Lidocaine Hydrochloride Injection without epinephrine may be reautoclaved if necessary.

HOW SUPPLIED

Lidocaine Hydrochloride Injection, USP, with preservative, is available as:

Preservative-Free

1% (10 mg/mL)
5 mL DOSETTE® vials packaged in 25s (NDC 10019-018-79)
2% (20 mg/mL)
5 mL DOSETTE® vials packaged in 25s (NDC 10019-020-79)

With Preservative

1% (10 mg/mL)
30 mL Multiple Dose vials packaged in 25s (NDC 10019-017-56)
50 mL Multiple Dose vials packaged in 25s (NDC 10019-017-57)
2% (20 mg/mL)
30 mL Multiple Dose vials packaged in 25s (NDC 10019-019-56)
50 mL Multiple Dose vials packaged in 25s (NDC 10019-019-57)

STERILIZATION, STORAGE AND TECHNICAL PROCEDURES
Store at controlled room temperature 15°–30°C (59°–86°F).

Disinfecting agents containing heavy metals, which cause release of respective ions (mercury, zinc, copper, etc), should not be used for skin or mucous membrane disinfection as they have been related to incidents of swelling and edema. When chemical disinfection of the rubber stopper of multiple dose vials is desired, either isopropyl alcohol (91%) or 70% ethyl alcohol is recommended. Many commercially available brands of rubbing alcohol, as well as solutions of ethyl alcohol not of USP grade, contain denaturants which are injurious to rubber and, therefore, are not to be used.

It is recommended that chemical disinfection be accomplished by wiping the vial thoroughly with cotton or gauze that has been moistened with the recommended alcohol just prior to use.

If sterilization of vial exterior is desired, it may be done only by steam autoclaving at 121°C (250°F), 15 psi for 15 minutes.

DO NOT STERILIZE WITH ETHYLENE OXIDE.

DOSETTE® is a registered trademark of A.H. Robins Company.

LIDOCAINE HCl

TABLE 1
Composition of Available Solutions

Product	Composition: Lidocaine HCl (mg/mL)	Sodium Chloride (mg/mL)	Methylparaben (mg/mL)
Lidocaine Hydrochloride Injection 1%, unpreserved	10	7	—
Lidocaine Hydrochloride Injection 2%, unpreserved	20	6	—
Lidocaine Hydrochloride Injection 1%, preserved	10	7	1
Lidocaine Hydrochloride Injection 2%, preserved	20	6	1

MEPERIDINE Ⓒ℞
[mĕ'pĕr-ĭdīne]
Hydrochloride Injection, USP

DESCRIPTION

Meperidine Hydrochloride Injection, USP is a sterile solution for intramuscular, subcutaneous or slow intravenous use as a narcotic analgesic.

Each mL of the DOSETTE® vial contains meperidine hydrochloride, either 25 mg, 50 mg, 75 mg or 100 mg, sodium metabisulfite 1.5 mg and phenol 5 mg in Water for Injection. Buffered with acetic acid-sodium acetate. pH 3.5–6.0. Sealed under nitrogen.

Meperidine hydrochloride is ethyl 1-methyl-4-phenylisonipecotate hydrochloride, a white crystalline substance with a melting point of 186°–189°C. It is readily soluble in water and has a slightly bitter taste.

Its structural formula is as follows:

CH₃ N • HCl COOC₂H₅

$C_{15}H_{21}NO_2 \bullet HCl$ MW 283.80

HOW SUPPLIED

Meperidine Hydrochloride Injection, USP is available in the following packages:
25 mg/mL, 1 mL DOSETTE® vials packaged in 25s (NDC 10019-151-44)
50 mg/mL, 1 mL DOSETTE® vials packaged in 25s (NDC 10019-152-44)
75 mg/mL, 1 mL DOSETTE® vials packaged in 25s (NDC 10019-153-44)
100 mg/mL, 1 mL DOSETTE® vials packaged in 25s (NDC 10019-154-44)

STORAGE
Store at controlled room temperature 15°–30°C (59°–86°F).

DOSETTE® is a registered trademark of A.H. Robins Company.

MEPERIDINE Ⓒ℞
Hydrochloride Injection, USP

DESCRIPTION

Meperidine hydrochloride is ethyl 1-methyl-4-phenylisonipecotate hydrochloride, a white, crystalline compound with a melting point of 186°–189° C. It has a slightly bitter taste and is readily soluble in water. Aqueous solutions may be boiled for short periods without decomposition.

In addition to the stated concentration of meperidine hydrochloride (see **HOW SUPPLIED**), each mL of the product in **TUBEX®** Sterile Cartridge-Needle Units for parenteral administration contains sodium acetate buffer. The parenteral products are intended for intramuscular, subcutaneous or slow intravenous* use. (*See **DOSAGE AND ADMINISTRATION** section of full prescribing information.)

HOW SUPPLIED

For Parenteral Use

Meperidine HCl Injection, USP, is available in **TUBEX®** Sterile Cartridge-Needle Units, boxes of 10 **TUBEX®** TAMP-R-TEL® tamper-resistant packages in the following dosage strengths:
25 mg per mL, NDC 10019-151-47, 1 mL fill in 2 mL size (22 gauge × 1 1/4 inch needle)
50 mg per mL, NDC 10019-152-47, 1 mL fill in 2 mL size (22 gauge × 1 1/4 inch needle)
75 mg per mL, NDC 10019-153-47, 1 mL fill in 2 mL size (22 gauge × 1 1/4 inch needle)
100 mg per mL, NDC 10019-154-47, 1 mL fill in 2 mL size (22 gauge × 1 1/4 inch needle)

Store at room temperature, 15°–25° C (59°–77° F).
Do not use if solution is discolored or contains a precipitate.

TUBEX® and TAMP-R-TEL® are registered trademarks of Wyeth-Ayerst Laboratories

---

METHOTREXATE ℞
[meth-ō-trexāte]
Injection, USP
PRESERVED AND PRESERVATIVE FREE
Rx Only

WARNINGS

METHOTREXATE SHOULD BE USED ONLY BY PHYSICIANS WHOSE KNOWLEDGE AND EXPERIENCE INCLUDE THE USE OF ANTIMETABOLITE THERAPY.

BECAUSE OF THE POSSIBILITY OF SERIOUS TOXIC REACTIONS (WHICH CAN BE FATAL):

METHOTREXATE SHOULD BE USED ONLY IN LIFE THREATENING NEOPLASTIC DISEASES, OR IN PATIENTS WITH PSORIASIS OR RHEUMATOID ARTHRITIS WITH SEVERE, RECALCITRANT, DISABLING DISEASE WHICH IS NOT ADEQUATELY RESPONSIVE TO OTHER FORMS OF THERAPY.

DEATHS HAVE BEEN REPORTED WITH THE USE OF METHOTREXATE IN THE TREATMENT OF MALIGNANCY, PSORIASIS, AND RHEUMATOID ARTHRITIS.

PATIENTS SHOULD BE CLOSELY MONITORED FOR BONE MARROW, LIVER, LUNG AND KIDNEY TOXICITIES. (See **PRECAUTIONS** in full prescribing information.)

PATIENTS SHOULD BE INFORMED BY THEIR PHYSICIAN OF THE RISKS INVOLVED AND BE UNDER A PHYSICIAN'S CARE THROUGHOUT THERAPY.

THE USE OF METHOTREXATE HIGH DOSE REGIMENS RECOMMENDED FOR OSTEOSARCOMA REQUIRES METICULOUS CARE. (See **DOSAGE AND ADMINISTRATION** in full prescribing information.)

HIGH DOSE REGIMENS FOR OTHER NEOPLASTIC DISEASES ARE INVESTIGATIONAL AND A THERAPEUTIC ADVANTAGE HAS NOT BEEN ESTABLISHED.

METHOTREXATE FORMULATIONS AND DILUENTS CONTAINING PRESERVATIVES MUST NOT BE USED FOR INTRATHECAL OR HIGH DOSE METHOTREXATE THERAPY.

1. Methotrexate has been reported to cause fetal death and/or congenital anomalies. Therefore, it is not recommended for women of childbearing potential unless there is clear medical evidence that the benefits can be expected to outweigh the considered risks. Pregnant women with psoriasis or rheumatoid arthritis should not receive methotrexate. (See **CONTRAINDICATIONS** in full prescribing information.)

2. Methotrexate elimination is reduced in patients with impaired renal functions, ascites, or pleural effusions. Such patients require especially careful monitoring for toxicity, and require dose reduction or, in some cases, discontinuation of methotrexate administration.

3. Unexpectedly severe (sometimes fatal) bone marrow suppression and gastrointestinal toxicity have been reported with concomitant administration of methotrexate (usually in high dosage) along with some nonsteroidal anti-inflammatory drugs (NSAIDs). (See **PRECAUTIONS, Drug Interactions** in full prescribing information.)

4. Methotrexate causes hepatotoxicity, fibrosis and cirrhosis, but generally only after prolonged use. Acutely, liver enzyme elevations are frequently seen. These are usually transient and asymptomatic, and also do not appear predictive of subsequent hepatic disease. Liver biopsy after sustained use often shows histologic changes, and fibrosis and cirrhosis have been reported; these latter lesions may not be preceded by symptoms or abnormal liver function tests in the psoriasis population. For this reason, periodic liver biopsies are usually recommended for psoriatic patients who are under long-term treatment. Persistent abnormalities in liver function tests may precede appearance of fibrosis or cirrhosis in the rheumatoid arthritis population. (See **PRECAUTIONS, Organ System Toxicity,** HEPATIC in full prescribing information.)

5. Methotrexate-induced lung disease is a potentially dangerous lesion, which may occur acutely at any time during therapy and which has been reported at doses as low as 7.5 mg/week. It is not always fully reversible. Pulmonary symptoms (especially a dry, nonproductive cough) may require interruption of treatment and careful investigation.

6. Diarrhea and ulcerative stomatitis require interruption of therapy; otherwise, hemorrhagic enteritis and death from intestinal perforation may occur.

7. Malignant lymphomas, which may regress following withdrawal of methotrexate, may occur in patients receiving low dose methotrexate and, thus, may not require cytotoxic treatment. Discontinue methotrexate first and, if the lymphoma does not regress, appropriate treatment should be instituted.

8. Like other cytoxic drugs, methotrexate may induce "tumor lysis syndrome" in patients with rapidly growing tumors. Appropriate supportive and pharmacologic measures may prevent or alleviate this complication.

9. Severe, occasionally fatal, skin reactions have been reported following single or multiple doses of methotrexate. Reactions have occurred within days of oral, intramuscular, intravenous, or intrathecal methotrexate administration. Recovery has been reported with discontinuation of therapy. (See **PRECAUTIONS, Organ System Toxicity,** SKIN in full prescribing information.)

10. Potentially fatal opportunistic infections, especially *Pneumocystis carinii* pneumonia, may occur with methotrexate therapy.

11. Methotrexate given concomitantly with radiotherapy may increase the risk of soft tissue necrosis and osteonecrosis.

DESCRIPTION

Methotrexate (formerly Amethopterin) is an antimetabolite used in the treatment of certain neoplastic diseases and severe psoriasis.

Chemically methotrexate is *N*-[4[[(2,4-diamino-6-pteridinyl) methyl] methylamino]benzoyl]-L-glutamic acid.

The structural formula is:

$C_{20}H_{22}N_8O_5$
Molecular Weight: 454.45

Methotrexate Injection, USP is sterile and non-pyrogenic and may be given by the intramuscular, intravenous, intra-arterial or intrathecal route. (See **DOSAGE AND ADMINISTRATION** in full prescribing information.)

However, the preservative formulation contains Benzyl Alcohol and must not be used for intrathecal or high dose therapy.

Methotrexate Injection, USP, Isotonic Liquid, Contains Preservative is available in 25 mg/mL, 2 mL (50 mg) and 10 mL (250 mg) vials.

Each 25 mg/mL, 2 mL and 10 mL vial contains methotrexate sodium equivalent to 50 mg and 250 mg methotrexate respectively, 0.90% w/v of Benzyl Alcohol as a preservative, and the following inactive ingredients: Sodium Chloride 0.260% w/v and Water for Injection qs ad 100% v. Sodium Hydroxide and, if necessary, Hydrochloric Acid are added to adjust the pH during manufacture to 8.5–8.7.

Methotrexate Injection, USP Isotonic Liquid, Preservative Free, for single use only, is available in 25 mg/mL, 2 mL (50 mg), 4 mL (100 mg), 8 mL (200 mg) and 10 mL (250 mg) vials.

Each 25 mg/mL, 2 mL, 4 mL, 8 mL, and 10 mL vial contains methotrexate sodium equivalent to 50 mg, 100 mg, 200 mg, and 250 mg methotrexate respectively, and the following inactive ingredients: Sodium Chloride 0.490% w/v and Water for Injection qs ad 100 % v. Sodium Hydroxide and/or Hydrochloric Acid are added to adjust the pH during manufacture to 8.5–8.7. The 2 mL, 4 mL, 8 mL, and 10 mL solutions contain approximately 0.43 mEq, 0.86 mEq, 1.72 mEq, and 2.15 mEq of Sodium per vial, respectively, and are isotonic solutions.

HOW SUPPLIED

Methotrexate Injection, USP, Isotonic Liquid, Contains Preservative

Each mL contains methotrexate sodium equivalent to 25 mg methotrexate.

NDC No.	Contents	Packaging
10019-941-01	2 mL—50 mg	Packaged individually
10019-941-03	10 mL—250 mg	Packaged individually

Methotrexate Injection, USP, Isotonic Liquid, Preservative Free, for Single Use Only

Each mL contains methotrexate sodium equivalent to 25 mg methotrexate.

NDC No.	Contents	Packaging
10019-940-01	2 mL—50 mg	Packaged individually
10019-940-02	4 mL—100 mg	Packaged individually
10019-940-03	8 mL—200 mg	Packaged individually
10019-940-04	10 mL—250 mg	Packaged individually

Store at controlled room temperature 15°–30°C (59°–86°F). PROTECT FROM LIGHT. RETAIN IN CARTON UNTIL CONTENTS ARE USED.

METOCLOPRAMIDE ℞

[*mĕtō clō-pra-mide*]
Injection, USP

DESCRIPTION

Metoclopramide Injection, USP is a clear, colorless, sterile solution with a pH of 2.5–6.5 for intravenous or intramuscular administration.

Each mL contains Metoclopramide 5 mg (present as the hydrocloride); Sodium Chloride 8.5 mg; Water for Injection qs; pH is adjusted with Hydrochloric Acid and/or Sodium Hydroxide if necessary. pH 2.5–6.5.

Metoclopramide hydrochloride is a white or practically white, crystalline, odorless or practically odorless powder. It is very soluble in water, freely soluble in alcohol, sparingly soluble in chloroform, practically insoluble in ether. Chemically, it is 4-amino-5-chloro-**N**-[2-(diethylamino)ethyl]-2-methoxy benzamide monohydrochloride monohydrate. Molecular weight, 354.3, with the following structural formula:

$C_{14}H_{22}ClN_3O_2 \bullet HCl \bullet H_2O$

HOW SUPPLIED

Metoclopramide Injection, USP, is supplied in 2 mL vials packaged 25 per shelf pack.

NDC Number	Metoclopramide Injection USP	Volume
10019-450-02	5 mg/mL	2 mL in a 2 mL vial

PROTECT FROM LIGHT. Store in shelf pack until time of use.

Store at controlled room temperature 15°–30°C (59°–86°F). Do not freeze. Do not store open single dose vials for later use as they contain no preservative. Discard unused portion.

MIDAZOLAM Ⓒ ℞

[*mĭdă-zōlăm*]
HCl Injection
℞ only

WARNING

Adults and Pediatrics: Intravenous midazolam HCl has been associated with respiratory depression and respiratory arrest, especially when used for sedation in noncritical care settings. In some cases, where this was not recognized promptly and treated effectively, death or hypoxic encephalopathy has resulted. Intravenous midazolam HCl should be used only in hospital or ambulatory care settings, including physicians' and dental offices, that provide for continuous monitoring of respiratory and cardiac function, ie, pulse oximetry. Immediate availability of resuscitative drugs and age- and size-appropriate equipment for bag/valve/mask ventilation and intubation, and personnel trained in their use and skilled in airway management should be assured (see **WARNINGS** in full prescribing information). For deeply sedated pediatric patients, a dedicated individual, other than the practitionar performing the procedure, should monitor the patient throughout the procedure.

The initial intravenous dose for sedation in adult patients may be as little as 1 mg, but should not exceed 2.5 mg in a normal healthy adult. Lower doses are necessary for older (over 60 years) or debilitated patients and in patients receiving concomitant narcotics or other central nervous system (CNS) depressants. The initial dose and all subsequent doses should always be titrated slowly; administer over at least 2 minutes and allow an additional 2 or more minutes to fully evaluate the sedative effect. The use of the 1 mg/mL formulation or dilution of the 1 mg/mL or 5 mg/mL formulation is recommended to facilitate slower injection. Doses of sedative medications in pediatric patients must be calculated on a mg/kg basis, and initial doses and all subsequent doses should always be titrated slowly. The initial pediatric dose of midazolam HCl for sedation/anxiolysis/amnesia is age, procedure, and route dependent (see **DOSAGE AND ADMINISTRATION** in full prescribing information for complete dosing information).

Neonates: Midazolam HCl should not be administered by rapid injection in the neonatal population. Severe hypotension and seizures have been reported following rapid IV administration, particularly with concomitant use of fentanyl (see **DOSAGE AND ADMINISTRATION** in full prescribing information for complete information).

DESCRIPTION

Midazolam HCl is a water-soluble benzodiazepine available as a sterile, nonpyrogenic parenteral dosage form for intravenous or intramuscular injection. Each mL contains midazolam hydrochloride equivalent to 1 mg or 5 mg midazolam compounded with 0.8% sodium chloride and 0.01% edetate disodium, with 1% benzyl alcohol as preservative; the pH is adjusted to 2.9–3.7 with hydrochloric acid and, if necessary, sodium hydroxide.

Midazolam is a white to light yellow crystalline compound, insoluble in water. The hydrochloride salt of midazolam, which is formed *in situ,* is soluble in aqueous solutions. Chemically, midazolam HCl is 8-chloro-6-(2-fluorophenyl)-1-methyl-4*H*-imidazo[1,5-a][1,4] benzodiazepine hydrochloride. Midazolam hydrochloride has the molecular formula $C_{18}H_{13}ClFN_3 \bullet HCl$, a calculated molecular weight of 362.25 and the following structural formula:

HOW SUPPLIED

Package configurations containing midazolam hydrochloride equivalent to 5 mg midazolam/mL:

1-mL vials (5 mg)—boxes of 10 (NDC 10019-027-01)
2-mL vials (10 mg)—boxes of 10 (NDC 10019-027-02)
5-mL vials (25 mg)—boxes of 10 (NDC 10019-027-05)
10-mL vials (50 mg)—boxes of 10 (NDC 10019-027-10)

Package configurations containing midazolam hydrochloride equivalent to 1 mg midazolam/mL:

2-mL vials (2 mg)—boxes of 10 (NDC 10019-028-02)
5-mL vials (5 mg)—boxes of 10 (NDC 10019-028-05)
10-mL vials (10 mg)—boxes of 10 (NDC 10019-028-10)

Store at 15°–30°C (59°–86°F).

Continued on next page

MORPHINE Sulfate Injection, USP Ⓒ℞

[*mōre-phēne*]

FOR SUBCUTANEOUS, INTRAMUSCULAR OR SLOW INTRAVENOUS ADMINISTRATION NOT FOR EPIDURAL OR INTRATHECAL ADMINISTRATION

DESCRIPTION

Chemistry

Morphine Sulfate Injection, USP is a sterile solution for subcutaneous, intramuscular or intravenous injection. Each mL contains morphine sulfate, either 5 mg, 8 mg, 10 mg or 15 mg, monobasic sodium phosphate, monohydrate 10 mg, dibasic sodium phosphate, anhydrous 2.8 mg, sodium formaldehyde sulfoxylate 3 mg and phenol 2.5 mg in Water for Injection; sulfuric acid added, if needed, for pH adjustment. The pH range is 2.5–6.5. Sealed under nitrogen.

Because of the presence and nature of the preservative and antioxidant, the product may have a characteristic odor.

Morphine is a phenanthrene-derivative opiate agonist. It is the principal alkaloid of opium and is considered to be the prototype of the opiate agonists.

Morphine sulfate occurs as white, feathery, silky crystals; cubical masses of crystals; or a white, crystalline powder. The drug contains five molecules of water of hydration and is soluble in water, having an aqueous solubility of approximately 62.5 mg/mL at 25°C, and slightly soluble in alcohol. The chemical name of morphine sulfate is 7,8-didehydro-4,5α-epoxy-17-methylmorphinan-3,6α-diol sulfate (2:1) (salt) pentahydrate, with the following structural formula:

$(C_{17}H_{19}NO_3)_2 \cdot H_2SO_4 \cdot 5H_2O$ MW 758.83

HOW SUPPLIED

Morphine Sulfate Injection, USP is available in the following:

5 mg/mL

1 mL DOSETTE® vials packaged in 25s (NDC 10019-176-44)

8 mg/mL

1 mL DOSETTE® vials packaged in 25s (NDC 10019-177-44)

1 mL DOSETTE® ampuls packaged in 25s (NDC 10019-177-68)

10 mg/mL

1 mL DOSETTE® vials packaged in 25s (NDC 10019-178-44)

1 mL DOSETTE® ampuls packaged in 25s (NDC 10019-178-68)

10 mL Multiple Dose amber vials packaged individually (NDC 10019-178-62)

15 mg/mL

1 mL DOSETTE® vials packaged in 25s (NDC 10019-179-44)

1 mL DOSETTE® ampuls packaged in 25s (NDC 10019-179-68)

20 mL Multiple Dose amber vials packaged individually (NDC 10019-179-63)

STORAGE

PROTECT FROM LIGHT: Keep covered in carton. Store at controlled room temperature 15°–30°C (59°–86°F).

Avoid freezing. Do not use if the color is darker than pale yellow, if it is discolored in any other way or if it contains a precipitate.

DOSETTE® is a registered trademark of A.H. Robins Company.

MORPHINE Ⓒ℞
Sulfate Injection, USP

FOR SUBCUTANEOUS, INTRAMUSCULAR OR SLOW INTRAVENOUS ADMINISTRATION NOT FOR EPIDURAL OR INTRATHECAL ADMINISTRATION

DESCRIPTION

Morphine Sulfate Injection, USP is a sterile solution for subcutaneous, intramuscular, or intravenous injection. Each mL contains 2 mg, 4 mg, 8 mg, 10 mg, or 15 mg morphine sulfate in Water for Injection, with not more than 5 mg chlorobutanol and 1 mg edetate disodium.

The pH range is 2.5 to 6.5. Sealed under nitrogen. The 2 mg and 4 mg strengths are available in a 1 mL size **TUBEX®** Sterile Cartridge-Needle Unit. The 8 mg, 10 mg, and 15 mg are available as a 1 mL fill in a 2 mL size **TUBEX®**. This provides excess space of approximately 1 mL to permit mixture with other compatible medications immediately prior to injection.

Morphine is a phenanthrene-derivative opiate agonist. It is the principal alkaloid of opium and considered to be the prototype of the opiate agonists.

Morphine sulfate occurs as white, feathery, silky crystals; cubical masses of crystals; or a white, crystalline powder. The drug contains live molecules of water of hydration and is soluble in water, having an aqueous solubility of approximately 62.5 mg/mL at 25°C, and slightly soluble in alcohol. The chemical name of morphine sulfate is 7,8-didehydro-4,5α-epoxy-17-methylmorphinan-3,6α-diol sulfate (2:1) (salt) pentahydrate, with the following structural formula:

$(C_{17}H_{19}NO_3)_2 \cdot H_2SO_4 \cdot 5H_2O$ MW 758.83

HOW SUPPLIED

Morphine Sulfate Injection, USP is available in the following dosage strengths in **TUBEX®** Sterile Cartridge-Needle Units, packaged in boxes of 10 cartridges in TAMP-R-TEL® tamper-resistant packages:

2 mg per mL, NDC 10019-182-65, 1 mL size (25 gauge × 5/8 inch needle).

4 mg per mL, NDC 10019-183-65, 1 mL size (25 gauge × 5/8 inch needle).

8 mg per mL, NDC 10019-177-47, 1 mL fill in 2 mL size (22 gauge × 1 1/4 inch needle).

10 mg per mL, NDC 10019-178-47, 1 mL fill in 2 mL size (22 gauge × 1 1/4 inch needle).

15 mg per mL, NDC 10019-179-47, 1 mL fill in 2 mL size (22 gauge × 1 1/4 inch needle).

Store at room temperature, approximately 25°C (77°F).

PROTECT FROM LIGHT. Use carton to protect contents from light.

Do not use if solution is discolored or contains a precipitate.

NALOXONE HCl Injection, USP ℞

[*nă-lō xōne*]

DESCRIPTION

Naloxone hydrochloride, a narcotic antagonist, is a synthetic congener of oxymorphone. In structure it differs from oxymorphone in that the methyl group on the nitrogen atom is replaced by an allyl group.

The structure for naloxone hydrochloride is as follows:

(-)-17-Allyl-4, 5α-epoxy-3,14-dihydroxymorphinan-6-one hydrochloride

$C_{19}H_{21}NO_4 \cdot HCl$ MW 363.84

Naloxone hydrochloride occurs as a white to slightly off-white powder, and is soluble in water, in dilute acids, and in strong alkali; slightly soluble in alcohol; practically insoluble in ether and in chloroform.

Naloxone Hydrochloride Injection is a sterile solution intended for intramuscular, subcutaneous or intravenous use. Each mL contains naloxone hydrochloride 400 micrograms (0.4 mg), sodium chloride 8.6 mg, methylparaben 1.8 mg and propylparaben 0.2 mg in Water for Injection. pH 3.0–4.5; hydrochloric acid and/or sodium hydroxide used, if needed, for pH adjustment. Sealed under nitrogen.

HOW SUPPLIED

Naloxone Hydrochloride Injection is available in the following packages:

0.4 mg/mL

1 mL DOSETTE® ampuls packaged in 10s (NDC 10019-039-68)

1 mL DOSETTE® vials packaged in 10s (NDC 10019-039-44)

10 mL Multiple Dose Vials packaged individually (NDC 10019-039-62)

STORAGE

PROTECT FROM LIGHT. Store at controlled room temperature 15°–30°C (59°–86°F).

DOSETTE® is a registered trademark of A.H. Robins Company

NEOSTIGMINE ℞

[*nē-ō-stĭg-mēn*]

Methylsulfate Injection, USP

DESCRIPTION

Neostigmine methylsulfate is the dimethylcarbamate of (m-hydroxyphenyl) trimethylammonium methylsulfate.

The chemical structure is:

Neostigmine methylsulfate, an anticholinesterase agent, is a bitter tasting, white crystalline powder and is very soluble in water and soluble in alcohol. Neostigmine Methylsulfate Injection is a sterile solution intended for intramuscular, subcutaneous or slow intravenous use. Each mL of the 1:1000 concentration contains neostigmine methylsulfate 1 mg, methylparaben 1.8 mg and propylparaben 0.2 mg in water for injection qs; pH adjusted with NaOH if necessary. pH: 5.0–6.5. Each mL of the 1:2000 concentration contains neostigmine methylsulfate 0.5 mg, methylparaben 1.8 mg, propylparaben 0.2 mg, water for injection qs; pH adjusted with NaOH if necessary. pH: 5.0–6.5.

HOW SUPPLIED

[See table below]

10 mL multiple dose and 1 mL vials packaged in 10 per shelf pack.

Storage

Store at controlled room temperature 15°–30°C (59°–86°F). PROTECT FROM LIGHT. Store in shelf pack until time of use.

NEOSTIGMINE

NDC Number	Neostigmine Methylsulfate per mL	Volume
NDC 10019-271-02	1:2000 (0.5 mg/mL)	1 mL in a 2 mL Vial
NDC 10019-271-10	1:2000 (0.5 mg/mL)	10 mL in a 10 mL Vial
NDC 10019-270-10	1:1000 (1 mg/mL)	10 mL in a 10 mL Vial

PANCURONIUM BROMIDE ℞

[*pan 'cū-rō-nē-ūm brō 'mīde*]

Injection

This drug should be administered by adequately trained individuals familiar with its actions, characteristics, and hazards.

DESCRIPTION

Pancuronium bromide is a nondepolarizing, neuromuscular blocking agent chemically designated as the aminosteroid 2β, 16β-dipiperidino-5α-androstane-3α, 17-β diol diacetate dimethobromide. The structural formula is:

Each mL contains: pancuronium bromide 1 mg or 2 mg; sodium acetate, anhydrous, 2 mg; sodium chloride, 4 mg to make isotonic; benzyl alcohol 10 mg (as preservative); water for injection qs; pH is adjusted with acetic acid and/or sodium hydroxide if necessary. pH: 3.8–4.2

HOW SUPPLIED

NDC Number	Pancuronium Bromide	
NDC 10019-281-02	2 mg/mL	2 mL in a 2 mL vial
NDC 10019-281-05	2 mg/mL	5 mL in a 5 mL vial
NDC 10019-280-10	1 mg/mL	10 mL in a 10 mL vial

2 mL vials packaged 25 per shelf pack.

5 mL multiple dose vials packaged 25 per shelf pack.

10 mL multiple dose vials packaged 10 per shelf pack.

STORAGE

Both concentrations of Pancuronlum Bromide Injection will maintain full clinical potency for six months if kept at room temperature of 18° to 22°C (65° to 72°F); or for 36 months when refrigerated at 2° to 8°C (36° to 46°F).

PHENYLEPHRINE ℞

[*phē-nyl-eph-rĭn*]

Hydrochloride Injection, USP

CONTAINS NO ANTIMICROBIAL PRESERVATIVE

WARNING: Physicians should completely familiarize themselves with the complete contents of the full prescribing information before prescribing Phenylephrine Hydrochloride Injection, USP.

DESCRIPTION

Phenylephrine hydrochloride is a vasoconstrictor and pressor drug chemically related to epinephrine and ephedrine. Phenylephrine hydrochloride is a synthetic sympathomi-

NDC 10019-163-12	1 mL fill in 2 mL vial	Packaged in 25s
NDC 10019-163-01	5 mL vial*	Packaged in 25s

* FOR PHARMACY USE ONLY

metic agent in sterile form for parenteral injection. Chemically, phenylephrine hydrochloride is (-)-*m*-Hydroxy-α-[(methylamino)methyl]benzyl alcohol hydrochloride, and has the following structural formula:

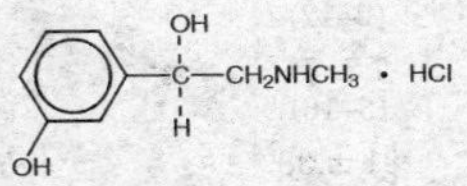

Each mL contains: Phenylephrine Hydrochloride 10 mg; Sodium Chloride 3.5 mg; Sodium Citrate Dihydrate 4.56 mg; Citric Acid Monohydrate 1 mg; Sodium Metabisulfite not more than 2 mg; Water for Injection q.s. Air replaced with Nitrogen. pH adjusted with Sodium Hydroxide and/or Hydrochloric Acid if necessary. pH 3.0–6.5

HOW SUPPLIED

Phenylephrine Hydrochloride Injection, USP 1% (10 mg/mL) is supplied as follows:
[See table above]

Store at controlled room temperature 15°–30°C (59°–86°F). PROTECT FROM LIGHT. Keep covered in carton until time of use. FOR SINGLE USE ONLY. DISCARD UNUSED PORTION.

PROPOFOL ℞

Injectable Emulsion 1%
10 mg/mL propofol
Contains a Sulfite
For IV Administration

DESCRIPTION

Propofol injectable emulsion is a sterile, nonpyrogenic emulsion containing 10 mg/mL of propofol suitable for intravenous administration. Propofol is chemically described as 2, 6-diisopropylphenol and has a molecular weight of 178.27. The structural and molecular formulas are:

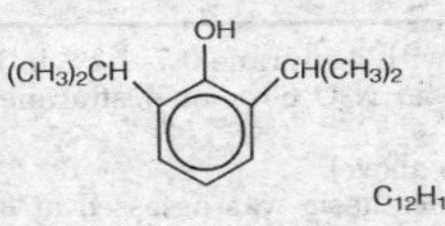

$C_{12}H_{18}O$

Propofol is very slightly soluble in water and, thus, is formulated in a white, oil-in-water emulsion. The pKa is 11. The octanol/water partition coefficient for propofol is 6761:1 at a pH of 6-8.5. In addition to the active component, propofol, the formulation also contains soybean oil (100 mg/mL), glycerol (22.5 mg/mL), egg yolk phospholipid (12 mg/mL), and sodium metabisulfite (0.25 mg/mL); with sodium hydroxide to adjust pH. The propofol injectable emulsion is isotonic and has a pH of 4.5-6.4.

STRICT ASEPTIC TECHNIQUE MUST ALWAYS BE MAINTAINED DURING HANDLING. PROPOFOL INJECTABLE EMULSION IS A SINGLE-USE PARENTERAL PRODUCT WHICH CONTAINS SODIUM METABISULFITE (0.25 MG/ML) TO RETARD THE RATE OF GROWTH OF MICROORGANISMS IN THE EVENT OF ACCIDENTAL EXTRINSIC CONTAMINATION. HOWEVER, PROPOFOL INJECTABLE EMULSION CAN STILL SUPPORT THE GROWTH OF MICROORGANISMS AS IT IS NOT AN ANTIMICROBIALLY PRESERVED PRODUCT UNDER USP STANDARDS. ACCORDINGLY, STRICT ASEPTIC TECHNIQUE MUST STILL BE ADHERED TO. DO NOT USE IF CONTAMINATION IS SUSPECTED. DISCARD UNUSED PORTIONS AS DIRECTED WITHIN THE REQUIRED TIME LIMITS (SEE DOSAGE AND ADMINISTRATION, HANDLING PROCEDURES IN FULL PRESCRIBING INFORMATION). THERE HAVE BEEN REPORTS IN WHICH FAILURE TO USE ASEPTIC TECHNIQUE WHEN HANDLING PROPOFOL INJECTABLE EMULSION WAS ASSOCIATED WITH MICROBIAL CONTAMINATION OF THE PRODUCT AND WITH FEVER, INFECTION/SEPSIS, OTHER LIFE-THREATENING ILLNESS, AND/OR DEATH.

HOW SUPPLIED

Propofol injectable emulsion is available in ready-to-use 20 mL vials, 50 mL infusion vials, and 100 mL infusion vials containing 10 mg/mL of propofol.

NDC Number	Propofol	Available Packaging
10019-013-01	20 mL vial	25 vials/shelf tray
10019-013-02	50 mL infusion vial	20 vials/shelf tray
10019-013-03	100 mL infusion vial	10 vials/shelf tray

Propofol undergoes oxidative degradation in the presence of oxygen, and is, therefore, packaged under nitrogen to eliminate this degradation path. **Store between 4°–22°C (40°–72°F). Do not freeze.** Shake well before use.

REVEX® ℞

[*Rē-vĕx*]
(nalmefene hydrochloride injection)

DESCRIPTION

REVEX® (nalmefene hydrochloride injection), an opioid antagonist, is a 6-methylene analogue of naltrexone. The chemical structure is shown below:

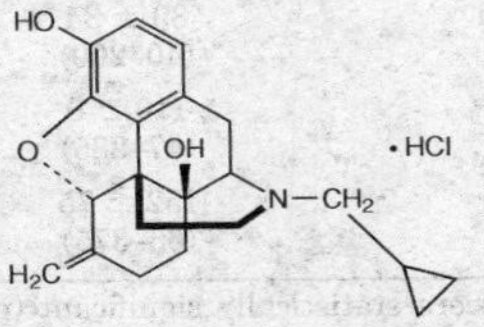

Molecular Formula: $C_{21}H_{25}NO_3 \cdot HCl$
Molecular Weight: 375.9, CAS # 58895-64-0
Chemical Name: 17-(Cyclopropylmethyl)-4,5α-epoxy-6-methylenemorphinan-3,14-diol, hydrochloride salt.

Nalmefene hydrochloride is a white to off-white crystalline powder which is freely soluble in water up to 130 mg/mL and slightly soluble in chloroform up to 0.13 mg/mL, with a pK_a of 7.6.

REVEX® is available as a sterile solution for intravenous, intramuscular, and subcutaneous administration in two concentrations, containing 100 µg or 1.0 mg of nalmefene free base per mL. The 100 µg/mL concentration contains 110.8 µg of nalmefene hydrochloride and the 1.0 mg/mL concentration contains 1.108 mg of nalmefene hydrochloride per mL. Both concentations contain 9.0 mg of sodium chloride per mL and the pH is adjusted to 3.9 with hydrochloric acid.

Concentrations and dosages of REVEX® are expressed as the free base equivalent of nalmefene.

HOW SUPPLIED

REVEX® (nalmefene hydrochloride injection) is available in the following presentations:
An ampul containing 1 mL of 100 µg/mL nalmefene base (Blue Label) Box of 10 (NDC 10019-315-21)
An ampul containing 2 mL of 1 mg/mL nalmefene base (Green Label) Box of 10 (NDC 10019-311-22)
Store at controlled room temperature.
REVEX® is a registered trademark of Baker Norton Pharmaceuticals, Inc.

ROBINUL® Injectable ℞

(glycopyrrolate injection, USP)

DESCRIPTION

Robinul (glycopyrrolate) is a synthetic anticholinergic agent. Each 1 mL contains:

Glycopyrrolate, USP	0.2 mg
Water for Injection, USP	q.s.
Benzyl Alcohol, NF (preservative)	0.9%

pH adjusted, when necessary, with hydrochloric acid and/or sodium hydroxide.

FOR INTRAMUSCULAR OR INTRAVENOUS ADMINISTRATION.

Glycopyrrolate is a quaternary ammonium compound with the following chemical structure:

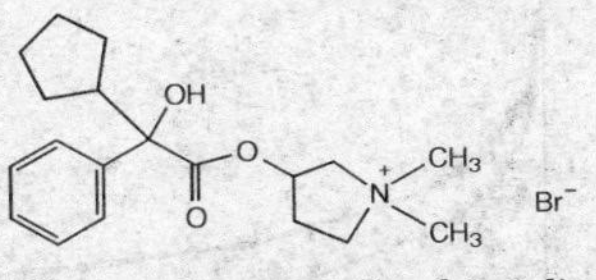

3[(cyclopentylhydroxyphenylacetyl)oxy]-1, 1-dimethyl pyrrolidinium bromide.

Unlike atropine, glycopyrrolate is completely ionized at physiological pH values.

Robinul Injectable is a clear, colorless, sterile liquid; pH 2.0–3.0.

HOW SUPPLIED

Robinul® (glycopyrrolate) Injectable, 0.2 mg/mL, is available in
1 mL single dose vials packaged in 25s (NDC 10019-016-81)
2 mL single dose vials packaged in 25s (NDC 10019-016-17)
5 mL multiple dose vials packaged in 25s (NDC 10019-016-54)
20 mL multiple dose vials packaged in 6s (NDC 10019-016-63).

Store at controlled room temperature, between 20°C and 25°C (68°F and 77°F).

Robinul® is a registered trademark of A.H. Robins Company.

SODIUM NITROPRUSSIDE ℞

[*sōdĭum nitrō 'prussĭde*]
Injection

Sodium Nitroprusside Injection is not suitable for direct injection. The solution must be further diluted in 5% Dextrose Injection before infusion.
Sodium Nitroprusside Injection can cause precipitous decreases in blood pressure (*see* **DOSAGE AND ADMINISTRATION** in full prescribing information). In patients not properly monitored, these decreases can lead to irreversible ischemic injuries or death. Sodium nitroprusside should be used only when available equipment and personnel allow blood pressure to be continuously monitored.
Except when used briefly or at low (< 2 µg/kg/min) infusion rates, sodium nitroprusside gives rise to important quantities of cyanide ion, which can reach toxic, potentially lethal levels (*see* **WARNINGS** in full prescribing information). The usual dose rate is 0.5–10 µg/kg/min, but infusion at the maximum dose rate should never last more than 10 minutes. If blood pressure has not been adequately controlled after 10 minutes of infusion at the maximum rate, administration of sodium nitroprusside should be terminated immediately.
Although acid-base balance and venous oxygen concentration should be monitored and may indicate cyanide toxicity, these laboratory tests provide imperfect guidance.
The full prescribing information should be thoroughly reviewed before administration of Sodium Nitroprusside Injection.

DESCRIPTION

Sodium nitroprusside is disodium pentacyanonitrosylferrate (2-)dihydrate, an inorganic hypotensive agent whose structural formula is

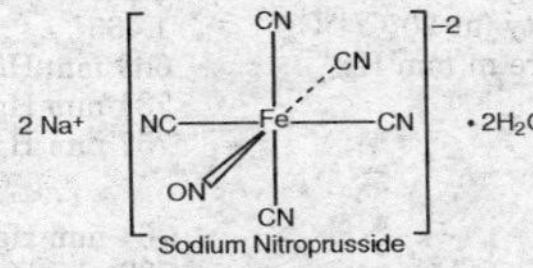

Sodium Nitroprusside

whose molecular formula is $Na_2[Fe(CN)_5NO] \cdot 2H_2O$, and whose molecular weight is 297.95. Dry sodium nitroprusside is a reddish-brown powder, soluble in water. In an aqueous solution infused intravenously, sodium nitroprusside is a rapid-acting vasodilator, active on both arteries and veins.

Sodium nitroprusside solution is rapidly degraded by trace contaminants, often with resulting color changes. (*See* **DOSAGE AND ADMINISTRATION** section of full prescribing information.) The solution is also sensitive to certain wavelengths of light, and it must be protected from light in clinical use.

Each 2 mL of Sodium Nitroprusside Injection contains the equivalent of 50 mg Sodium Nitroprusside Dihydrate in Sterile Water for Injection.

HOW SUPPLIED

Sodium Nitroprusside Injection is supplied as follows in amber-colored, single-dose 50 mg/2mL containers:

NDC 10019-082-02	25 mg/mL vials packaged individually

PROTECT FROM LIGHT. Store in carton until time of use. Light-protective covering enclosed. Avoid excessive heat. Protect from freezing.
Store at controlled room temperature 15°–30°C (59°–86°F).

SUFENTANIL CITRATE Injection, USP Ⓒ ℞

[*sū'fĕn-tănĭl*]

DESCRIPTION

Sufentanil Citrate Injection, USP is a sterile, nonpyrogenic, aqueous solution for intravenous and epidural injection. Each mL contains sufentanil citrate equivalent to 50 mcg (0.05 mg) of sufentanil in Water for Injection. pH 3.5–6.0; citric acid added, if needed, for pH adjustment. Contains no preservative. Sufentanil Citrate is a potent opioid analgesic chemically designated as N-[4-(methoxymethyl)-1-[2-(2-thienyl)ethyl]-4-piperidinyl]-N-phenylpropanamide 2-hydroxy-1,2,3-propanetricarboxylate (1:1) with the following structural formula:

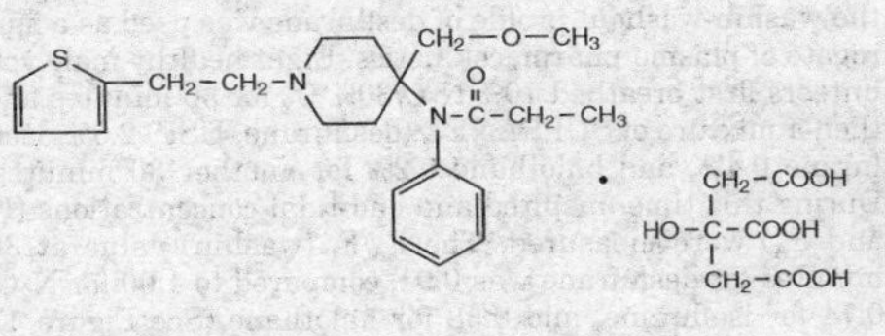

$C_{22}H_{30}N_2O_2S \cdot C_6H_8O_7$ MW 578.68

HOW SUPPLIED

Sufentanil Citrate Injection, USP, equivalent to 50 mcg (0.05 mg) sufentanil per mL, is available in the following:

Continued on next page

Sufentanil Citrate—Cont.

1 mL (50 mcg) DOSETTE® ampuls packaged in 10s (NDC 10019-050-43)
2 mL (100 mcg) DOSETTE® ampuls packaged in 10s (NDC 10019-050-21)
5 mL (250 mcg) DOSETTE® ampuls packaged in 10s (NDC 10019-050-06)

STORAGE

PROTECT FROM LIGHT: Keep covered in carton until time of use.

Store at controlled room temperature 15°–30°C (59°–86°F).

DOSETTE® is a registered trademark of A.H. Robins Company.

SUPRANE® ℞

[sū 'prān]
(desflurane, USP)
Volatile Liquid for Inhalation

DESCRIPTION

SUPRANE® (desflurane, USP), a nonflammable liquid administered via vaporizer, is a general inhalation anesthetic. It is (±)1,2,2,2-tetrafluoroethyl difluoromethyl ether:

```
   F  H  F
   |  |  |
F—C—C—O—C—H
   |  |     |
   F  F     F
```

Some physical constants are:

Molecular weight	168.04
Specific gravity (at 20°C/4°C)	1.465
Vapor pressure in mm Hg	669 mm Hg @ 20°C
	731 mm Hg @ 22°C
	757 mm Hg @ 22.8°C (boiling point; 1atm)
	764 mm Hg @ 23°C
	798 mm Hg @ 24°C
	869 mm Hg @ 26°C

Partition coefficients at 37°C:

Blood/Gas	0.424
Olive Oil/Gas	18.7
Brain/Gas	0.54

Mean Component/Gas Partition Coefficients:

Polypropylene (Y piece)	6.7
Polyethylene (circuit tube)	16.2
Latex rubber (bag)	19.3
Latex rubber (bellows)	10.4
Polyvinylchloride (endotracheal tube)	34.7

Desflurane is nonflammable as defined by the requirements of International Electrotechnical Commission 601-2-13.

Desflurane is a colorless, volatile liquid below 22.8°C. Data indicate that desflurane is stable when stored under normal room lighting conditions according to instructions.

Desflurane is chemically stable. The only known degradation reaction is through prolonged direct contact with soda lime producing low levels of fluoroform (CHF_3). The amount of CHF_3 obtained is similar to that produced with MAC-equivalent doses of isoflurane. No discernible degradation occurs in the presence of strong acids.

Desflurane does not corrode stainless steel, brass, aluminum, anodized aluminum, nickel plated brass, copper, or beryllium.

CLINICAL PHARMACOLOGY

SUPRANE® (desflurane, USP) is a volatile liquid inhalation anesthetic minimally biotransformed in the liver in humans. Less than 0.02% of the SUPRANE® absorbed can be recovered as urinary metabolites (compared to 0.2% for isoflurane).

Minimum alveolar concentration (MAC) of desflurane in oxygen for a 25 year-old adult is 7.3%. The MAC of SUPRANE® (desflurane, USP) decreases with increasing age and with addition of depressants such as opioids or benzodiazepines. (See DOSAGE AND ADMINISTRATION for details).

Pharmacokinetics

Due to the volatile nature of desflurane in plasma samples, the washin-washout profile of desflurane was used as a surrogate of plasma pharmacokinetics. Eight healthy male volunteers first breathed 70% N_2O/30% O_2 for 30 minutes and then a mixture of SUPRANE® (desflurane, USP) 2.0%, isoflurane 0.4%, and halothane 0.2% for another 30 minutes. During this time, inspired and end-tidal concentrations (F_I and F_A) were measured. The F_A/F_I (washin) value at 30 minutes for desflurane was 0.91, compared to 1.00 for N_2O, 0.74 for isoflurane, and 0.58 for halothane (See Figure 1). The washin rates for halothane and isoflurane were similar to literature values. The washin was faster for desflurane than for isoflurane and halothane at all time points. The F_A/F_{AO} (washout) value at 5 minutes was 0.12 for desflurane, 0.22 for isoflurane, and 0.25 for halothane (See Figure 2). The washout for SUPRANE® was more rapid than that for isoflurane and halothane at all elimination time points. By 5 days, the F_A/F_{AO} for desflurane is 1/20th of that for halothane or isoflurane.

EMERGENCE AND RECOVERY AFTER OUTPATIENT LAPAROSCOPY
178 FEMALES, AGES 20-47
TIMES IN MINUTES: MEAN ± SD (RANGE)

Induction:	Propofol	Propofol	Desflurane/N_2O	Desflurane/O_2
Maintenance:	Propofol/N_2O	Desflurane/N_2O	Desflurane/N_2O	Desflurane/O_2
Number of Pts:	N = 48	N = 44	N = 43	N = 43
Median age	30 (20–43)	26 (21–47)	29 (21–42)	30 (20–40)
Anesthetic Time	49 ± 53 (8–336)	45 ± 35 (11–178)	44 ± 29 (14–149)	41 ± 26 (19–126)
Time to open eyes	7 ± 3 (2–19)	5 ± 2* (2–10)	5 ± 2* (2–12)	4 ± 2* (1–11)
Time to state name	9 ± 4 (4–22)	8 ± 3 (3–18)	7 ± 3* (3–16)	7 ± 3* (2–15)
Time to stand	80 ± 34 (40–200)	86 ± 55 (30–320)	81 ± 38 (35–190)	77 ± 38 (35–200)
Time to walk	110 ± 6 (47–285)	122 ± 85 (37–375)	108 ± 59 (48–220)	108 ± 66 (49–250)
Time to fit for discharge	152 ± 75 (66–375)	157 ± 80 (73–385)	150 ± 66 (68–310)	155 ± 73 (69–325)

*Differences were statistically significant ($p < 0.05$) by Dunnett's procedure comparing all treatments to the propofol-propofol/N_2O (induction and maintenance) group. Results for comparisons greater than one hour after anesthesia show no differences between groups and considerable variability within groups.

EMERGENCE AND RECOVERY TIMES IN OUTPATIENT SURGERY
46 MALES, 42 FEMALES, AGES 19-70
TIMES IN MINUTES: MEAN ± SD (RANGE)

Induction:	Thiopental	Thiopental	Thiopental	Desflurane/O_2
Maintenance:	Isoflurane/N_2O	Desflurane/N_2O	Desflurane/O_2	Desflurane/O_2
Number of Pts:	N = 23	N = 21	N = 23	N = 21
Median age	43 (20–70)	40 (22–67)	43 (19–70)	41 (21–64)
Anesthetic Time	49 ± 23 (11–94)	50 ± 19 (16–80)	50 ± 27 (16–113)	51 ± 23 (19–117)
Time to open eyes	13 ± 7 (5–33)	9 ± 3* (4–16)	12 ± 8 (4–39)	8 ± 2* (4–13)
Time to state name	17 ± 10 (6–44)	11 ± 4* (6–19)	15 ± 10 (6–46)	9 ± 3* (5–14)
Time to walk	195 ± 67 (124–365)	176 ± 60 (101–315)	168 ± 34 (119–258)	181 ± 42 (92–252)
Time to fit for discharge	205 ± 53 (153–365)	202 ± 41 (144–315)	197 ± 35 (155–280)	194 ± 37 (134–288)

*Differences were statistically significant ($p < 0.05$) by Dunnett's procedure comparing all treatments to the thiopental-isoflurane/N_2O (induction and maintenance) group. Results for comparisons greater than one hour after anesthesia show no differences between groups and considerable variability within groups.

Figure 1.
Desflurane Washin

Figure 2.
Desflurane Washout

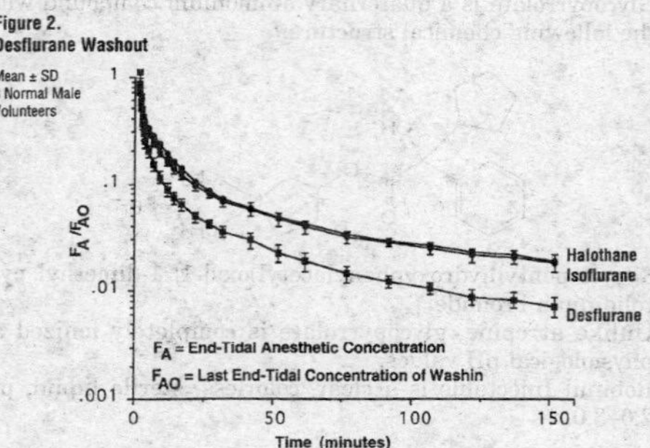

Pharmacodynamics

Changes in the clinical effects of SUPRANE® (desflurane, USP) rapidly follow changes in the inspired concentration. The duration of anesthesia and selected recovery measures for SUPRANE® are given in the following tables:

In 178 female outpatients undergoing laparoscopy, premedicated with fentanyl (1.5–2.0 µg/kg), anesthesia was initiated with propofol 2.5 mg/kg, desflurane/N_2O 60% in O_2 or desflurane/O_2 alone. Anesthesia was maintained with either propofol 1.5–9.0 mg/kg/hr, desflurane 2.6–8.4% in N_2O 60% in O_2, or desflurane 3.1–8.9% in O_2.

[See first table above]

In 88 unpremedicated outpatients, anesthesia was initiated with thiopental 3–9 mg/kg or desflurane in O_2. Anesthesia was maintained with isoflurane 0.7–1.4% in N_2O 60%, desflurane 1.8–7.7% in N_2O 60%, or desflurane 4.4–11.9% in O_2.

[See second table above]

Recovery from anesthesia was assessed at 30, 60, and 90 minutes following 0.5 MAC desflurane (3%) or isoflurane (0.6%) in N_2O 60% using subjective and objective tests. At 30 minutes after anesthesia, only 43% of the isoflurane group were able to perform the psychometric tests compared to 76% in the desflurane group ($p < 0.05$).

[See first table at top of next page]

SUPRANE® (desflurane, USP) was studied in twelve volunteers receiving no other drugs. Hemodynamic effects during controlled ventilation ($PaCO_2$ 38mm Hg) were:

[See second table at top of next page]

When the same volunteers breathed spontaneously during desflurane anesthesia, systemic vascular resistance and mean arterial blood pressure decreased; cardiac index, heart rate, stroke volume, and central venous pressure (CVP) increased compared to values when the volunteers were conscious. Cardiac index, stroke volume, and CVP were greater during spontaneous ventilation than during controlled ventilation.

During spontaneous ventilation in the same volunteers, increasing the concentration of SUPRANE® (desflurane, USP) from 3% to 12% decreased tidal volume and increased arterial carbon dioxide tension and respiratory rate. The combination of N_2O 60% with a given concentration of desflurane gave results similar to those with desflurane alone. Respiratory depression produced by desflurane is similar to that produced by other potent inhalation agents.

The use of desflurane concentrations higher than 1.5 MAC may produce apnea.

Figure 3. PaCO, During Spontaneous Ventilation in Unstimulated Volunteers

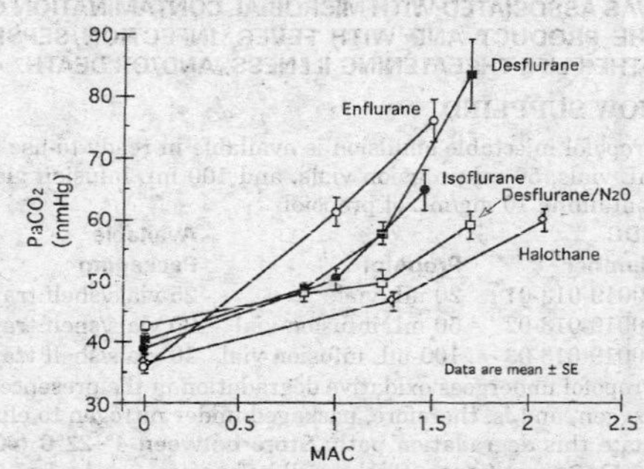

NOTE: Data for enflurane, halothane and isoflurane are from earlier studies

CLINICAL TRIALS

SUPRANE® (desflurane, USP) was evaluated in 1,843 patients including ambulatory (N=1,061), cardiovascular (N=277), geriatric (N=103), neurosurgical (N=40), and pediatric (N=235) patients. Clinical experience with these patients and with 1,087 control patients in these studies not receiving desflurane are described below. Although desflurane can be used in adults for the inhalation induction of anesthesia via mask, it produces a high incidence of respiratory irritation (coughing, breathholding, apnea, increased secretions, laryngospasm). For incidence, see ADVERSE REACTIONS. Oxyhemoglobin saturation below 90% occurred in 6% of patients (from pooled data, N = 370 adults).

Ambulatory Surgery

SUPRANE® (desflurane, USP) plus N_2O was compared to isoflurane plus N_2O in multicenter studies (21 sites) of 792 ASA physical status I, II, or III patients aged 18–76 years (median 32).

INDUCTION: Anesthetic induction begun with thiopental and continued with desflurane was associated with a 7% incidence of oxyhemoglobin saturation of 90% or less (from pooled data, N = 307) compared with 5% in patients in whom anesthesia was induced with thiopental and isoflurane (from pooled data, N = 152).

MAINTENANCE & RECOVERY: SUPRANE® (desflurane, USP) with or without N_2O or other anesthetics was generally well tolerated. There were no differences between desflurane and the other anesthetics studied in the times that patients were judged fit for discharge.

In one outpatient study, patients received a standardized anesthetic consisting of thiopental 4.2–4.4 mg/kg, fentanyl 3.5–4.0 µg/kg, vecuronium 0.05–0.07 mg/kg, and N_2O 60% in oxygen with either desflurane 3% or isoflurane 0.6%. Emergence times were significantly different; but times to sit up and discharge were not different (see Table).

RECOVERY PROFILES AFTER DESFLURANE 3% IN N_2O 60% vs ISOFLURANE 0.6% IN N_2O 60% IN OUTPATIENTS
16 MALES, 22 FEMALES, AGES 20-65
MEAN ± SD

	Isoflurane	Desflurane
Number	21	17
Anesthetic time (min)	127 ± 80	98 ± 55
Recovery time to:		
Follow commands (min)	11.1 ± 7.9	6.5 ± 2.3*
Sit up (min)	113 ± 27	95 ± 56
Fit for discharge (min)	231 ± 40	207 ± 54

* Difference was statistically significant from the isoflurane group ($p < 0.05$), unadjusted for multiple comparisons.

Cardiovascular Surgery

Desflurane was compared to isoflurane, sufentanil or fentanyl for the anesthetic management of coronary artery bypass graft (CABG), abdominal aortic aneurysm, peripheral vascular and carotid endarterectomy surgery in 7 studies at 15 centers involving a total of 558 patients. In all patients except the desflurane vs sufentanil study, the volatile anesthetics were supplemented with intravenous opioids, usually fentanyl. Blood pressure and heart rate were controlled by changes in concentration of the volatile anesthetics or opioids and cardiovascular drugs if necessary. Oxygen (100%) was the carrier gas in 253 of 277 desflurane cases (24 of 277 received N_2O/O_2).

[See third table above]

No differences were found in cardiovascular outcome (death, myocardial infarction, ventricular tachycardia or fibrillation, heart failure) among desflurane and the other anesthetics.

INDUCTION: Desflurane should not be used as the sole agent for anesthetic induction in patients with coronary artery disease or any patients where increases in heart rate or blood pressure are undesirable. In the desflurane vs sufentanil study, anesthetic induction with desflurane without opioids was associated with new transient ischemia in 14 patients vs 0 in the sufentanil group. In the desflurane group, mean heart rate, arterial pressure, and pulmonary blood pressure increased and stroke volume decreased in contrast to no change in the sufentanil group. Cardiovascular drugs were used frequently in both groups: especially esmolol in the desflurane group (56% vs 0%) and phenylephrine in the sufentanil group (43% vs 27%). When 10 µg/kg of fentanyl was used to supplement induction of anesthesia at one other center, continuous 2-lead ECG analysis showed a low incidence of myocardial ischemia and no difference between desflurane and isoflurane. If desflurane is to be used in patients with coronary artery disease, it should be used in combination with other medications for induction of anesthesia, preferably intravenous opioids and hypnotics.

MAINTENANCE & RECOVERY: In studies where desflurane or isoflurane anesthesia was supplemented with fentanyl, there were no differences in hemodynamic variables or the incidence of myocardial ischemia in the patients anesthetized with desflurane compared to those anesthetized with isoflurane.

During the precardiopulmonary bypass period, in the desflurane vs sufentanil study where the desflurane patients received no intravenous opioid, more desflurane patients required cardiovascular adjuvants to control hemodynamics than the sufentanil patients. During this period, the incidence of ischemia detected by ECG or echocardiography was not statistically different between desflurane (18 of 99) and sufentanil (9 of 98) groups. However, the duration and severity of ECG-detected myocardial ischemia was significantly less in the desflurane group. The incidence of myocardial ischemia after cardiopulmonary bypass and in the ICU did not differ between groups.

RECOVERY TESTS: PERCENT OF PREOPERATIVE BASELINE VALUES
16 MALES, 22 FEMALES, AGES 20-65
PERCENT: MEAN ± SD

	60 minutes After Anesthesia		90 minutes After Anesthesia	
Maintenance:	Desflurane/N_2O	Isoflurane/N_2O	Desflurane/N_2O	Isoflurane/N_2O
Confusion Δ	66±6	47±8	75±7*	56±8
Fatigue Δ	70±9*	33±6	89±12*	47±8
Drowsiness Δ	66±5*	36±8	76±7*	49±9
Clumsiness Δ	65±5	49±8	80±7*	57±9
Comfort Δ	59±7*	30±6	60±8*	31±7
DSST† score	74±4*	50±9	75±4*	55±7
Trieger Tests††	67±5	74±6	90±6	83±7

Δ Visual analog scale (values from 0-100; 100=baseline)
† DSST = Digit Symbol Substitution Test
†† Trieger Test = Dot Connecting Test
* Differences were statistically significant ($p < 0.05$) using a two-sample t-test

HEMODYNAMIC EFFECTS OF DESFLURANE DURING CONTROLLED VENTILATION
12 MALE VOLUNTEERS, AGES 16-26
MEAN ± SD (RANGE)

			Heart Rate (beats/min)		Mean Arterial Pressure (mmHg)		Cardiac Index (L/min/m^2)	
Total MAC Equivalent	End-Tidal % Des/O_2	End-Tidal %Des/N_2O	O_2	N_2O	O_2	N_2O	O_2	N_2O
0	0%/21%	0%/0%	69 ± 4 (63–76)	70 ± 6 (62–85)	85 ± 9 (74–102)	85 ± 9 (74–102)	3.7 ± 0.4 (3.0–4.2)	3.7 ± 0.4 (3.0–4.2)
0.8	6%/94%	3%/60%	73 ± 5 (67–80)	77 ± 8 (67–97)	61 ± 5* (55–70)	69 ± 5* (62–80)	3.2 ± 0.5 (2.6–4.0)	3.3 ± 0.5 (2.6–4.1)
1.2	9%/91%	6%/60%	80 ± 5* (72–84)	77 ± 7 (67–90)	59 ± 8* (44–71)	63 ± 8* (47–74)	3.4 ± 0.5 (2.6–4.1)	3.1 ± 0.4* (2.6–3.8)
1.7	12%/88%	9%/60%	94 ± 14* (78–109)	79 ± 9 (61–91)	51 ± 12* (31–66)	59 ± 6* (46–68)	3.5 ± 0.9 (1.7–4.7)	3.0 ± 0.4* (2.4–3.6)

*Differences were statistically significant ($p<0.05$) compared to awake values, Newman-Keul's method of multiple comparison.

CARDIOVASCULAR PATIENTS BY AGENT AND TYPE OF SURGERY
418 MALES, 140 FEMALES, AGES 27-87 (MEDIAN 64)

Type of Surgery	13 Centers Isoflurane	13 Centers Desflurane	1 Center Sufentanil	1 Center Desflurane	1 Center Fentanyl	1 Center Desflurane
CABG	58	57	100	100	25	25
Abd Aorta	29	25	-	-	-	-
Periph Vasc	24	24	-	-	-	-
Carotid Art	45	46	-	-	-	-
Total	156	152	100	100	25	25

Geriatric Surgery

SUPRANE® (desflurane, USP) plus N_2O was compared to isoflurane plus N_2O in a multicenter study (6 sites) of 203 ASA physical status II or III elderly patients, aged 57–91 years (median 71).

INDUCTION: Most patients were premedicated with fentanyl (mean 2 µg/kg), preoxygenated, and received thiopental (mean 4.3 mg/kg IV) or thiamylal (mean 4 mg/kg IV) followed by succinylcholine (mean 1.4 mg/kg IV) for intubation.

MAINTENANCE & RECOVERY: Heart rate and arterial blood pressure remained within 20% of preinduction baseline values during administration of SUPRANE® (desflurane, USP) 0.5–7.7% (average 3.6%) with 50–60% N_2O. Induction, maintenance, and recovery cardiovascular measurements did not differ from those during isoflurane/N_2O administration nor did the postoperative incidence of nausea and vomiting differ. The most common cardiovascular adverse event was hypotension occurring in 8% of the SUPRANE® patients and 6% of the isoflurane patients.

Neurosurgery

SUPRANE® (desflurane, USP) was studied in 38 patients aged 26–76 years (median 48 years), ASA physical status II or III undergoing neurosurgical procedures for intracranial lesions.

INDUCTION: Induction consisted of standard neuroanesthetic techniques including hyperventilation and thiopental.

MAINTENANCE: No change in cerebrospinal fluid pressure (CSFP) was observed in 8 patients who had intracranial tumors when the dose of desflurane was 0.5 MAC in N_2O 50%. In another study of 9 patients with intracranial tumors, 0.8 MAC desflurane/air/O_2 did not increase CSFP above postinduction baseline values. In a different study of 10 patients receiving 1.1 MAC desflurane/air/O_2, CSFP increased 7mm Hg (range 3–13 mm Hg increase, with final values of 11–26 mm Hg) above the predrug values.

All volatile anesthetics may increase intracranial pressure in patients with intracranial space occupying lesions. In such patients, desflurane should be administered at 0.8 MAC or less, and in conjunction with a barbiturate induction and hyperventilation (hypocapnia) in the period before cranial decompression. Appropriate attention must be paid to maintain cerebral perfusion pressure. The use of a lower dose of desflurane and the administration of a barbiturate and mannitol would be predicted to lessen the effect of desflurane on CSFP.

Under hypocapnic conditions ($PaCO_2$ 27 mm Hg) desflurane 1 and 1.5 MAC did not increase cerebral blood flow (CBF) in 9 patients undergoing craniotomies. CBF reactivity to increasing $PaCO_2$ from 27 to 35 mm Hg was also maintained at 1.25 MAC desflurane/air/O_2.

Pediatric Surgery

SUPRANE® (desflurane, USP) or halothane with or without N_2O was used to anesthetize 235 patients aged 2 weeks-12 years (median 2 years), ASA physical status I or II.

INDUCTION: SUPRANE® (desflurane, USP) is not recommended for induction of general anesthesia in infants or pediatric patients because of a high incidence of moderate to severe laryngospasm, coughing, breathholding, and secretions. The occurrence of oxyhemoglobin desaturation was 26%. For incidence, see ADVERSE REACTIONS.

MAINTENANCE & RECOVERY: The concentration of SUPRANE® (desflurane, USP) required for maintenance of general anesthesia is age-dependent (see INDIVIDUALIZATION OF DOSE). Changes in blood pressure during maintenance of and recovery from anesthesia with desflurane/N_2O/O_2 are similar to those observed with halothane/N_2O/O_2. Heart rate during maintenance of anesthesia is approximately 10 beats per minute faster with desflurane than with halothane. Patients were judged fit for discharge from post-anesthesia care units within one hour with both desflurane and halothane. There were no differences in the incidence of nausea and vomiting between patients receiving desflurane or halothane.

INDIVIDUALIZATION OF DOSE

(Also see DOSAGE AND ADMINISTRATION)

Preanesthetic Medication: Issues such as whether or not to premedicate and the choice of premedicant(s) must be individualized. In clinical studies, patients scheduled to be anesthetized with desflurane frequently received IV preanesthetic medication, such as opioid and/or benzodiazepine.

INDUCTION: In adults, some premedicated with opioid, a frequent starting concentration was 3% desflurane, increased in 0.5–1.0% increments every 2 to 3 breaths. End-tidal concentrations of 4–11% SUPRANE® (desflurane, USP) with and without N_2O, produced anesthesia within 2

Continued on next page

Suprane—Cont.

to 4 minutes. When desflurane was tested as the primary anesthetic induction agent, the incidence of upper airway irritation (apnea, breathholding, laryngospasm, coughing and secretions) was high (see ADVERSE REACTIONS). During induction in adults, the overall incidence of oxyhemoglobin desaturation ($SpO_2 < 90\%$) was 6%.
After induction in adults with an intravenous drug such as thiopental or propofol, desflurane can be started at approximately 0.5–1 MAC, whether the carrier gas is O_2 or N_2O/O_2.
MAINTENANCE: Surgical levels of anesthesia in adults may be maintained with concentrations of 2.5–8.5% SUPRANE® (desflurane, USP) with or without the concomitant use of nitrous oxide. In children, surgical levels of anesthesia may be maintained with concentrations of 5.2–10% SUPRANE® with or without the concomitant use of nitrous oxide.
During the maintenance of anesthesia, increasing concentrations of SUPRANE® (desflurane, USP) produce dose-dependent decreases in blood pressure. Excessive decreases in blood pressure may be due to depth of anesthesia and in such instances may be corrected by decreasing the inspired concentration of SUPRANE®.
Concentrations of desflurane exceeding 1 MAC may increase heart rate. Thus with this drug, an increased heart rate may not serve reliably as a sign of inadequate anesthesia. SUPRANE® (desflurane, USP) decreases the doses of neuromuscular blocking agents required (see PRECAUTIONS, Drug Interactions).

INDICATIONS AND USAGE

SUPRANE® (desflurane, USP) is indicated as an inhalation agent for induction and/or maintenance of anesthesia for inpatient and outpatient surgery in adults (see PRECAUTIONS).
SUPRANE® (desflurane, USP) is not recommended for induction of anesthesia in pediatric patients because of a high incidence of moderate to severe upper airway adverse events (see WARNINGS). After induction of anesthesia with agents other than SUPRANE®, and tracheal intubation, SUPRANE® is indicated for maintenance of anesthesia in infants and children.

CONTRAINDICATIONS

SUPRANE® (desflurane, USP) should not be used in patients with a known or suspected genetic susceptibility to malignant hyperthermia.
Known sensitivity to SUPRANE® (desflurane, USP) or to other halogenated agents.

WARNINGS

Pediatric Use: SUPRANE® (desflurane, USP) is not recommended for induction of general anesthesia via mask in infants or children because of the high incidence of moderate to severe laryngospasm in 50% of patients, coughing 72%, breathholding 68%, increase in secretions 21% and oxyhemoglobin desaturation 26%.
SUPRANE® (desflurane, USP) should be administered only by persons trained in the administration of general anesthesia, using a vaporizer specifically designed and designated for use with desflurane. Facilities for maintenance of a patent airway, artificial ventilation, oxygen enrichment, and circulatory resuscitation must be immediately available. Hypotension and respiratory depression increase as anesthesia is deepened.

PRECAUTIONS

During the maintenance of anesthesia, increasing concentrations of SUPRANE® (desflurane, USP) produce dose-dependent decreases in blood pressure. Excessive decreases in blood pressure may be related to depth of anesthesia and in such instances may be corrected by decreasing the inspired concentration of SUPRANE®.
Concentrations of desflurane exceeding 1 MAC may increase heart rate. Thus an increased heart rate may not be a sign of inadequate anesthesia.
In patients with intracranial space occupying lesions, SUPRANE® (desflurane, USP) should be administered at 0.8 MAC or less, in conjunction with a barbiturate induction and hyperventilation (hypocapnia). Appropriate measures should be taken to maintain cerebral perfusion pressure (see CLINICAL STUDIES, Neurosurgery).
In patients with coronary artery disease, maintenance of normal hemodynamics is important to the avoidance of myocardial ischemia. Desflurane should not be used as the sole agent for anesthetic induction in patients with coronary artery disease or patients where increases in heart rate or blood pressure are undesirable. It should be used with other medications, preferably intravenous opioids and hypnotics (see CLINICAL STUDIES, Cardiovascular Surgery).
Inspired concentrations of SUPRANE® (desflurane, USP) greater than 12% have been safely administered to patients, particularly during induction of anesthesia. Such concentrations will proportionately dilute the concentration of oxygen; therefore, maintenance of an adequate concentration of oxygen may require a reduction of nitrous oxide or air if these gases are used concurrently.
The recovery from general anesthesia should be assessed carefully before patients are discharged from the post anesthesia care unit (PACU).
SUPRANE® (desflurane, USP), like some other inhalational anesthetics, can react with desiccated carbon dioxide (CO_2) absorbents to produce carbon monoxide which may result in elevated levels of carboxyhemoglobin in some patients. Case reports suggest that barium hydroxide lime and soda lime become desiccated when fresh gases are passed through the CO_2 absorber cannister at high flow rates over many hours or days. When a clinician suspects that CO_2 absorbent may be desiccated, it should be replaced before the administration of SUPRANE® (desflurane, USP).
As with other halogenated anesthetic agents, SUPRANE® (desflurane, USP) may cause sensitivity hepatitis in patients who have been sensitized by previous exposure to halogenated anesthetics (see **CONTRAINDICATIONS**).

Drug Interactions
No clinically significant adverse interactions with commonly used preanesthetic drugs, or drugs used during anesthesia (muscle relaxants, intravenous agents, and local anesthetic agents) were reported in clinical trials. The effect of desflurane on the disposition of other drugs has not been determined.
Like isoflurane, desflurane does not predispose to premature ventricular arrhythmias in the presence of exogenously infused epinephrine in swine.
BENZODIAZEPINES AND OPIOIDS (MAC REDUCTION): Benzodiazepines (midazolam 25–50 μg/kg) decrease the MAC of desflurane by 16% as do the opioids (fentanyl 3–6 μg/kg) by 50% (see DOSAGE AND ADMINISTRATION).
NEUROMUSCULAR BLOCKING AGENTS:
Anesthetic concentrations of desflurane at equilibrium (administered for 15 or more minutes before testing) reduced the ED_{95} of succinylcholine by approximately 30% and that of atracurium and pancuronium by approximately 50% compared to N_2O/opioid anesthesia. The effect of desflurane on duration of nondepolarizing neuromuscular blockade has not been studied.

DOSAGE OF MUSCLE RELAXANT CAUSING 95% DEPRESSION IN NEUROMUSCULAR BLOCKADE

Desflurane Concentration	Mean ED_{95} (μg/kg) Pancuronium	Atracurium	Succinylcholine
0.65 MAC 60% N_2O/O_2	26	123	-
1.25 MAC 60% N_2O/O_2	18	91	-
1.25 MAC O_2	22	120	362

Dosage reduction of neuromuscular blocking agents during induction of anesthesia may result in delayed onset of conditions suitable for endotracheal intubation or inadequate muscle relaxation, because potentiation of neuromuscular blocking agents requires equilibration of muscle with the delivered partial pressure of desflurane.
Among nondepolarizing drugs, only pancuronium and atracurium interactions have been studied. In the absence of specific guidelines:
1. For endotracheal intubation, do not reduce the dose of nondepolarizing muscle relaxants or succinylcholine.
2. During maintenance of anesthesia, the dose of nondepolarizing muscle relaxants is likely to be reduced compared to that during N_2O/opioid anesthesia. Administration of supplemental doses of muscle relaxants should be guided by the response to nerve stimulation.

Malignant Hyperthermia: In susceptible individuals, potent inhalation anesthetic agents may trigger a skeletal muscle hypermetabolic state leading to high oxygen demand and the clinical syndrome known as malignant hyperthermia. In genetically susceptible pigs, desflurane induced malignant hyperthermia. The clinical syndrome is signalled by hypercapnia, and may include muscle rigidity, tachycardia, tachypnea, cyanosis, arrhythmias, and/or unstable blood pressure. Some of these nonspecific signs may also appear during light anesthesia: acute hypoxia, hypercapnia, and hypovolemia.
Treatment of malignant hyperthermia includes discontinuation of triggering agents, administration of intravenous dantrolene sodium, and application of supportive therapy. (Consult prescribing information for dantrolene sodium intravenous for additional information on patient management.) Renal failure may appear later, and urine flow should be monitored and sustained if possible.

Renal or Hepatic Insufficiency
Nine patients receiving SUPRANE® (desflurane, USP) (N=9) were compared to 9 patients receiving isoflurane, all with chronic renal insufficiency (serum creatinine 1.5–6.9 mg/dL). No differences in hematological or biochemical tests, including renal function evaluation, were seen between the two groups. Similarly, no differences were found in a comparison of patients receiving either SUPRANE® (desflurane, USP) (N=28) or isoflurane (N=30) undergoing renal transplant.
Eight patients receiving SUPRANE® (desflurane, USP) were compared to six patients receiving isoflurane, all with chronic hepatic disease (viral hepatitis, alcoholic hepatitis, or cirrhosis). No differences in hematological or biochemical tests, including hepatic enzymes and hepatic function evaluation, were seen.

Carcinogenesis, Mutagenesis, Impairment of Fertility
Animal carcinogenicity studies have not been performed with SUPRANE® (desflurane, USP). *In vitro* and *in vivo* genotoxicity studies did not demonstrate mutagenicity or chromosomal damage by SUPRANE®. Tests for genotoxicity included the Ames mutation assay, the metaphase analysis of human lymphocytes, and the mouse micronucleus assay.
Fertility was not affected after 1 MAC-Hour per day exposure (cumulative 63 and 14 MAC-Hours for males and females, respectively). At higher doses, parental toxicity (mortalities and reduced weight gain) was observed which could affect fertility.

Teratogenic Effects: No teratogenic effect was observed at approximately 10 and 13 cumulative MAC-Hour exposures at 1 MAC-Hour per day during organogenesis in rats or rabbits. At higher doses increased incidences of post-implantation loss and maternal toxicity were observed. However, at 10 MAC-Hours cumulative exposure in rats, about 6% decrease in the weight of male pups was observed at preterm caesarean delivery.

Pregnancy Category B: There are no adequate and well-controlled studies in pregnant women. SUPRANE® (desflurane, USP) should be used during pregnancy only if the potential benefit justifies the potential risk to the fetus.
Rats exposed to desflurane at 1 MAC-hour per day from gestation day 15 to lactation day 21, did not show signs of dystocia. Body weight of pups delivered by these dams at birth and during lactation were comparable to that of control pups. No treatment related behavioral changes were reported in these pups during lactation.

Labor and Delivery: The safety of desflurane during labor or delivery has not been demonstrated.

Nursing Mothers: The concentrations of desflurane in milk are probably of no clinical importance 24 hours after anesthesia. Because of rapid washout, desflurane concentrations in milk are predicted to be below those found with other volatile potent anesthetics.

Geriatric Use: The average MAC for SUPRANE® (desflurane, USP) in a 70 year old patient is two-thirds the MAC for a 20 year old patient (see DOSAGE AND ADMINISTRATION).

Pediatric Use: SUPRANE® (desflurane, USP) is not recommended for induction of general anesthesia via mask in infants or children because of the high incidence of moderate to severe laryngospasm, coughing, breathholding and increase in secretions and oxyhemoglobin desaturation (see WARNINGS).

Neurosurgical Use: SUPRANE® (desflurane, USP) may produce a dose-dependent increase in cerebrospinal fluid pressure (CSFP) when administered to patients with intracranial space occupying lesions. Desflurane should be administered at 0.8 MAC or less, and in conjunction with a barbiturate induction and hyperventilation (hypocapnia) until cerebral decompression in patients with known or suspected increases in CSFP. Appropriate attention must be paid to maintain cerebral perfusion pressure (see CLINICAL STUDIES, Neurosurgery).

ADVERSE REACTIONS

Adverse event information is derived from controlled clinical trials, the majority of which were conducted in the United States. The studies were conducted using a variety of premedications, other anesthetics, and surgical procedures of varying length. Most adverse events reported were mild and transient, and may reflect the surgical procedures, patient characteristics (including disease) and/or medications administered.
Of the 1,843 patients exposed to SUPRANE® (desflurane, USP) in clinical trials, 370 adults and 152 children were induced with desflurane alone and 687 patients were maintained principally with desflurane. The frequencies given reflect the percent of patients with the event. Each patient was counted once for each type of adverse event. They are presented in alphabetical order according to body system.

PROBABLY CAUSALLY RELATED: Incidence greater than 1%.

Induction (use as a mask inhalation agent):

ADULT PATIENTS (N=370):	Coughing 34%, breathholding 30%, apnea 15%, increased secretions*, laryngospasm* oxyhemoglobin desaturation (SpO_2<90%)* pharyngitis*
PEDIATRIC PATIENTS (N=152):	Coughing 72%, breathholding 68%, laryngospasm 50%, oxyhemoglobin desaturation (SpO_2<90%) 26%, increased secretions 21%, bronchospasm* (See WARNINGS)

Maintenance or Recovery
ADULT AND PEDIATRIC PATIENTS (N=687):

Body as a Whole:	Headache.
Cardiovascular:	Bradycardia, hypertension, nodal arrhythmia, tachycardia.
Digestive:	Nausea 27%, vomiting 16%.
Nervous system:	Increased Salivation.
Respiratory:	Apnea*, breathholding, cough increased* laryngospasm*, pharyngitis.
Special Senses:	Conjunctivitis (conjunctival hyperemia)

* Incidence of events: 3%–10%

PROBABLY CAUSALLY RELATED: Incidence less than 1% and reported in 3 or more patients, regardless of severity (N=1,843) Adverse reactions reported only from postmarketing experience or in the literature, not seen in clinical trials, are considered rare and are italicized.

Cardiovascular:	Arrhythmia, bigeminy, abnormal electrocardiogram, myocardial ischemia, vasodilation.
Digestive:	*Hepatitis.*
Nervous System:	Agitation, dizziness.
Respiratory:	Asthma, dyspnea, hypoxia.

CAUSAL RELATIONSHIP UNKNOWN: Incidence less than 1% and reported in 3 or more patients, regardless of severity (N=1,843)

Body as a Whole:	Fever.
Cardiovascular:	Hemorrhage, myocardial infarct.
Metabolic and Nutrition:	Increased creatinine phosphokinase.
Musculoskeletal System:	Myalgia.
Skin and Appendages:	Pruritis.

See PRECAUTIONS for information regarding pediatric use and malignant hyperthermia.

Laboratory Findings: Transient elevations in glucose and white blood cell count may occur as with use of other anesthetic agents.

DRUG ABUSE AND DEPENDENCE

The potential drug abuse liability, and dependence associated with SUPRANE® (desflurane, USP) have not been studied.

OVERDOSAGE

In the event of overdosage, or suspected overdosage, take the following actions: discontinue administration of SUPRANE® (desflurane, USP), maintain a patent airway, initiate assisted or controlled ventilation with oxygen, and maintain adequate cardiovascular function.

DOSAGE AND ADMINISTRATION

Deliver SUPRANE® (desflurane, USP) from a vaporizer specifically designed and designated for use with desflurane.

The administration of general anesthesia must be individualized based on the patient's response (see INDIVIDUALIZATION OF DOSE). The following two tables provide mean relative potency based upon age and drug interaction studies in predominately ASA physical status I or II patients.

EFFECT OF AGE ON MAC OF DESFLURANE
MEAN ± SD (percent atmospheres)

Age	N	O_2 100%	N	N_2O 60%
2 weeks	6	9.2 ± 0.0	-	-
10 weeks	5	9.4 ± 0.4	-	-
9 months	4	10.0 ± 0.7	5	7.5 ± 0.8
2 years	3	9.1 ± 0.6	-	-
3 years	-	-	5	6.4 ± 0.4
4 years	4	8.6 ± 0.6	-	-
7 years	5	8.1 ± 0.6	-	-
25 years	4	7.3 ± 0.0	4	4.0 ± 0.3
45 years	4	6.0 ± 0.3	6	2.8 ± 0.6
70 years	6	5.2 ± 0.6	6	1.7 ± 0.4

N = number of crossover pairs (using up-and-down method of quantal response)

Opioids or benzodiazepines decrease the amounts of SUPRANE® (desflurane, USP) required to produce anesthesia. The following table is based on studies of drug interaction (MAC reduction).

SUPRANE® (desflurane, USP) MAC WITH FENTANYL OR MIDAZOLAM
MEAN ± SD (percent reduction)

Dose	18-30 years	31-65 years
No fentanyl	6.4 ± 0.0	6.3 ± 0.4
3 µg/kg fentanyl	3.5 ± 1.9 (46%)	3.1 ± 0.6 (51%)
6 µg/kg fentanyl	3.0 ± 1.2 (53%)	2.3 ± 1.0 (64%)
No midazolam	6.9 ± 0.1	5.9 ± 0.6
25 µg/kg midazolam		4.9 ± 0.9 (16%)
50 µg/kg midazolam	-	4.9 ± 0.5 (17%)

SUPRANE® (desflurane, USP) decreases the doses of neuromuscular blocking agents required (see PRECAUTIONS, Drug Interactions).

During the maintenance of anesthesia with inflow rates of 2 L/min or more, the alveolar concentration of desflurane will usually be within 10% of the inspired concentration. (F_A/F_I, see Figure 1 in Pharmacokinetics section.)

HOW SUPPLIED

SUPRANE® (desflurane, USP), NDC 10019-641-24, is packaged in amber-colored bottles containing 240 mL desflurane.

THIOPENTAL SODIUM

Cat/Kit Number	Thiopental Sodium for Injection, USP	Diluent Volume	Reconstituted Concentration (%)	NDC Number
Syringe Kits[1]				
2580-0101	500 mg	20 mL	2.5	10019-258-96
Injection Kits[2]				
2530-0101	1 g	40 mL	2.5	10019-253-99
2540-0101	2.5 g	100 mL	2.5	10019-252-97
2550-0101	5 g	200 mL	2.5	10019-255-98

[1] Syringe Kits contain 1 vial of Thiopental Sodium for Injection, USP; 1 vial of 0.9% Sodium Chloride Injection, USP; 1 sterile syringe and needle.

[2] Injection Kits contain 1 vial of Thiopental Sodium for Injection, USP; 1 vial of Sterile Water for Injection, USP; sterile transfer spikes.

SAFETY AND HANDLING

Occupational Caution: There is no specific work exposure limit established for SUPRANE® (desflurane, USP). However, the National Institute for Occupational Safety and Health Administration has recommended an 8-hr, time-weighted average limit of 2 ppm for halogenated anesthetic agents in general (0.5 ppm when coupled with exposure to N_2O).

The predicted effects of acute overexposure by inhalation of SUPRANE® (desflurane, USP) include headache, dizziness or (in extreme cases) unconsciousness.

There are no documented adverse effects of chronic exposure to halogenated anesthetic vapors (Waste Anesthetic Gases or WAGs) in the workplace. Although results of some epidemiological studies suggest a link between exposure to halogenated anesthetics and increased health problems (particularly spontaneous abortion), the relationship is not conclusive. Since exposure to WAGs is one possible factor in the findings for these studies, operating room personnel, and pregnant women in particular, should minimize exposure. Precautions include adequate general ventilation in the operating room, the use of a well-designated and well-maintained scavenging system, work practices to minimize leaks and spills while the anesthetic agent is in use, and routine equipment maintenance to minimize leaks.

STORAGE

Store at room temperature, 15°–30°C (59°–86°F). SUPRANE® (desflurane, USP) has been demonstrated to be stable for the period defined by the expiration dating on the label.

Rx only

BAXTER
Mfd. and Mktd. by affiliates of
Baxter Healthcare Corporation
Deerfield, IL 60015 USA
Revised: June 1998
For Product Inquiry 1 800 ANA DRUG
400-447-05

THIOPENTAL SODIUM Ⓒ℞

[*thī-ō-pent-ăl sō-dē-ŭm*]
For Injection, USP

DESCRIPTION

Thiopental Sodium for Injection, USP is a thiobarbiturate, the sulfur analogue of sodium pentobarbital.

The drug is prepared as a sterile lyophilized powder and, after reconstitution with an appropriate diluent, is administered by the intravenous route.

Thiopental Sodium, USP is chemically designated sodium 5-ethyl-5-(1-methylbutyl)-2-thiobarbiturate and has the following structural formula:

The drug is a yellowish, hygroscopic powder, stabilized with anhydrous sodium carbonate as a buffer (60 mg/g of Thiopental Sodium).

HOW SUPPLIED

Thiopental Sodium for Injection, USP, (Lyophilized) is available as follows:
[See table above]

Syringe Kits and Injection Kits are individually packaged. Store product prior to reconstitution at controlled room temperature 15°–30°C (59°–86°F).

Store reconstituted solution in a cool place and use within 24 hours of mixing. Administer only clear solution.

VECURONIUM BROMIDE ℞

for Injection
℞ only

THIS DRUG SHOULD BE ADMINISTERED BY ADEQUATELY TRAINED INDIVIDUALS FAMILIAR WITH ITS ACTIONS, CHARACTERISTICS, AND HAZARDS.

DESCRIPTION

Vecuronium Bromide for Injection is a nondepolarizing neuromuscular blocking agent of intermediate duration, chemically designated as piperidinium, 1-[(2β, 3α, 5α, 16β, 17β)-3, 17-bis(acetyloxy)-2-(1-piperidinyl)androstan-16-yl]-1-methyl-, bromide. The structural formula is:

Its molecular formula is $C_{34}H_{57}BrN_2O_4$ with molecular weight 637.74.

Vecuronium Bromide for Injection is supplied as a sterile nonpyrogenic freeze-dried buffered cake of very fine microscopic crystalline particles for intravenous injection only.

Each 10 mL vial contains:
Vecuronium Bromide 10 mg; Citric Acid Anhydrous 20.75 mg; Sodium Phosphate Dibasic Anhydrous 16.25 mg; Mannitol (to adjust tonicity) 97 mg. pH is adjusted with sodium hydroxide and/or phosphoric acid if necessary. pH: 3.5–4.5.

Each 20 mL vial contains: Vecuronium Bromide 20 mg; Citric Acid Anhydrous 41.5 mg; Sodium Phosphate Dibasic Anhydrous 32.5 mg; Mannitol (to adjust tonicity) 194 mg. pH is adjusted with sodium hydroxide and/or phosphoric acid if necessary. pH: 3.5–4.5. When reconstituted with Bacteriostatic Water for Injection, USP, CONTAINS 0.9% w/v BENZYL ALCOHOL WHICH IS NOT FOR USE IN NEWBORNS.

HOW SUPPLIED

Vecuronium Bromide for Injection is supplied as follows:

NDC Number	Packaging Configuration	Vial Size
10019-481-01	Vecuronium Bromide for Injection 10 mg (diluent not supplied) Shelf pack carton of 10 individual vials.	10 mL
10019-482-02	Vecuronium Bromide for Injection 20 mg (diluent not supplied) Shelf pack carton of 10 individual vials.	20 mL

Store at controlled room temperature 15°–30°C (59°–86°F). PROTECT FROM LIGHT.

EDUCATIONAL MATERIAL

Educational Resources

Baxter Pharmaceutical Products Inc offers a wide range of educational materials free of charge to physicians, nurse-anesthetists, post-anesthesia nurses and hospital pharmacists. They are available from Baxter PPI sales representatives or by writing to: Baxter Pharmaceutical Products Inc, 95 Spring Street, New Providence, NJ 07974, or by calling (800) 262-3784.

For information on over-the-counter drugs, consult **PDR For Nonprescription Drugs.**

Bayer Corporation
Pharmaceutical Division
400 MORGAN LANE
WEST HAVEN, CT 06516

For Medical Information Contact:
Director, Medical Services
(800) 468-0894
(203) 812-2000

ADALAT® CAPSULES ℞
(nifedipine)
For Oral Use

DESCRIPTION

ADALAT® (nifedipine) is an antianginal drug belonging to a class of pharmacological agents, the calcium channel blockers. Nifedipine is 3,5-pyridinedicarboxylic acid, 1,4-dihydro-2,6-dimethyl-4-(2-nitrophenyl)-, dimethyl ester, $C_{17}H_{18}N_2O_6$, and has the structural formula:

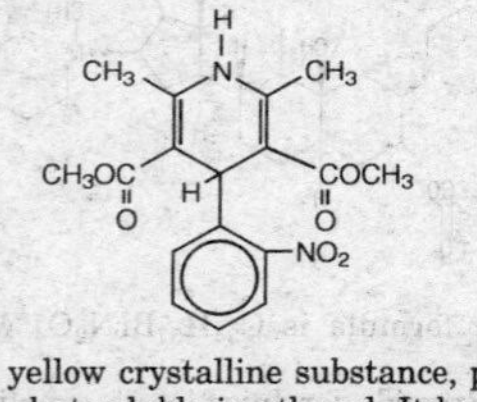

Nifedipine is a yellow crystalline substance, practically insoluble in water but soluble in ethanol. It has a molecular weight of 346.3. ADALAT® CAPSULES are formulated as soft gelatin capsules for oral administration each containing 10 mg or 20 mg of nifedipine.

Inert ingredients in the formulations are: glycerin, peppermint oil, polyethylene glycol 400; soft gelatin capsules (which contain FD&C Yellow No. 6, Red Ferric Oxide and other inert ingredients), and water. The 10 mg capsules also contain saccharin sodium.

CLINICAL PHARMACOLOGY

ADALAT® is a calcium ion influx inhibitor (slow channel blocker or calcium ion antagonist) and inhibits the transmembrane influx of calcium ions into cardiac muscle and smooth muscle. The contractile processes of cardiac muscle and vascular smooth muscle are dependent upon the movement of extracellular calcium ions into these cells through specific ion channels. ADALAT® selectively inhibits calcium ion influx across the cell membrane of cardiac muscle and vascular smooth muscle without changing serum calcium concentrations.

Mechanism of Action

The precise means by which this inhibition relieves angina has not been fully determined, but includes at least the following two mechanisms:

1) Relaxation and Prevention of Coronary Artery Spasm

ADALAT® dilates the main coronary arteries and coronary arterioles, both in normal and ischemic regions, and is a potent inhibitor of coronary artery spasm, whether spontaneous or ergonovine-induced. This property increases myocardial oxygen delivery in patients with coronary artery spasm, and is responsible for the effectiveness of ADALAT® in vasospastic (Prinzmetal's or variant) angina. Whether this effect plays any role in classical angina is not clear, but studies of exercise tolerance have not shown an increase in the maximum exercise rate-pressure product, a widely accepted measure of oxygen utilization. This suggests that, in general, relief of spasm or dilation of coronary arteries is not an important factor in classical angina.

2) Reduction of Oxygen Utilization

ADALAT® regularly reduces arterial pressure at rest and at a given level of exercise by dilating peripheral arterioles and reducing the total peripheral resistance (afterload) against which the heart works. This unloading of the heart reduces myocardial energy consumption and oxygen requirements and probably accounts for the effectiveness of ADALAT® in chronic stable angina.

Pharmacokinetics and Metabolism

ADALAT® is rapidly and fully absorbed after oral administration. The drug is detectable in serum 10 minutes after oral administration, and peak blood levels occur in approximately 30 minutes. Bioavailability is proportional to dose from 10 to 30 mg; half-life does not change significantly with dose. There is little difference in relative bioavailability when ADALAT® capsules are given orally and swallowed whole, bitten and swallowed, or bitten and held sublingually. However, biting through the capsule prior to swallowing does result in slightly earlier plasma concentrations (27 ng/mL 10 minutes after 10 mg) than if capsules are swallowed intact. It is highly bound by serum proteins. ADALAT® is extensively converted to inactive metabolites and approximately 80 percent of ADALAT® and metabolites are eliminated via the kidneys. The half-life of nifedipine in plasma is approximately two hours. Since hepatic biotransformation is the predominant route for the disposition of nifedipine, the pharmacokinetics may be altered in patients with chronic liver disease. Patients with hepatic impairment (liver cirrhosis) have a longer disposition half-life and higher bioavailability of nifedipine than healthy volunteers. The degree of serum protein binding of nifedipine is high (92–98%). Protein binding may be greatly reduced in patients with renal or hepatic impairment.

In healthy subjects, the elimination half-life of a sustained release nifedipine formulation was longer in elderly subjects (6.7 h) compared to young subjects (3.8 h) following oral administration. A decreased clearance was also observed in the elderly (348 mL/min) compared to young subjects (519 mL/min) following intravenous administration.

Co-administration of nifedipine with grapefruit juice results in up to a 2-fold increase in AUC and C_{max}, due to inhibition of CYP3A4 related first-pass metabolism.

Hemodynamics

Like other slow channel blockers, ADALAT® exerts a negative inotropic effect on isolated myocardial tissue. This is rarely, if ever, seen in intact animals or man, probably because of reflex responses to its vasodilating effects. In man, ADALAT® causes decreased peripheral vascular resistance and a fall in systolic and diastolic pressure, usually modest (5–10mm Hg systolic), but sometimes larger. There is usually a small increase in heart rate, a reflex response to vasodilation. Measurements of cardiac function in patients with normal ventricular function have generally found a small increase in cardiac index without major effects on ejection fraction, left ventricular end diastolic pressure (LVEDP) or volume (LVEDV). In patients with impaired ventricular function, most acute studies have shown some increase in ejection fraction and reduction in left ventricular filling pressure.

Electrophysiologic Effects

Although like other members of its class, ADALAT® decreases sinoatrial node function and atrioventricular conduction in isolated myocardial preparations, such effects have not been seen in studies in intact animals or in man. In formal electrophysiologic studies, predominantly in patients with normal conduction system, ADALAT® has had no tendency to prolong atrioventricular conduction, prolong sinus node recovery time, or slow sinus rate.

INDICATIONS AND USAGE

I. Vasospastic Angina

ADALAT® (nifedipine) is indicated for the management of vasospastic angina confirmed by any of the following criteria: 1) classical pattern of angina at rest accompanied by ST segment elevation, 2) angina or coronary artery spasm provoked by ergonovine, or 3) angiographically demonstrated coronary artery spasm. In those patients who have had angiography, the presence of significant fixed obstructive disease is not incompatible with the diagnosis of vasospastic angina, provided that the above criteria are satisfied. ADALAT® may also be used where the clinical presentation suggests a possible vasospastic component but where vasospasm has not been confirmed, e.g., where pain has a variable threshold on exertion or when angina is refractory to nitrates and/or adequate doses of beta blockers.

II. Chronic Stable Angina
(Classical Effort-Associated Angina)

ADALAT® is indicated for the management of chronic stable angina (effort-associated angina) without evidence of vasospasm in patients who remain symptomatic despite adequate dose of beta blockers and/or organic nitrates or who cannot tolerate those agents.

In chronic stable angina (effort-associated angina) ADALAT® has been effective in controlled trials of up to eight weeks duration in reducing angina frequency and increasing exercise tolerance, but confirmation of sustained effectiveness and evaluation of long term safety in these patients are incomplete.

Controlled studies in small numbers of patients suggest concomitant use of ADALAT® and beta blocking agents may be beneficial in patients with chronic stable angina, but available information is not sufficient to predict with confidence the effects of concurrent treatment, especially in patients with compromised left ventricular function or cardiac conduction abnormalities. When introducing such concomitant therapy, care must be taken to monitor blood pressure closely since severe hypotension can occur from the combined effects of the drugs (See **WARNINGS**).

CONTRAINDICATIONS

Known hypersensitivity reaction to ADALAT®.

WARNINGS

Excessive Hypotension

Although in most patients, the hypotensive effect of ADALAT® CAPSULES is modest and well tolerated, occasional patients have had excessive and poorly tolerated hypotension. These responses have usually occurred during initial titration or at the time of subsequent upward dosage adjustment, and may be more likely in patients on concomitant beta blockers.

Although not approved for this purpose, ADALAT® CAPSULES and other immediate-release nifedipine capsules have been used (orally and sublingually) for acute reduction of blood pressure. Several well-documented reports describe profound hypotension, myocardial infarction, and death when immediate-release nifedipine capsules were used in this way. **ADALAT® CAPSULES should not be used for acute reduction of blood pressure.**

ADALAT® CAPSULES and other immediate-release nifedipine capsules have also been used for the long-term control of essential hypertension although no properly-controlled studies have been conducted to define an appropriate dose or dose interval for such treatment. **ADALAT® CAPSULES should not be used for the control of essential hypertension.**

Several well-controlled, randomized trials studied the use of immediate-release nifedipine capsules in patients who had just sustained myocardial infarctions. In none of these trials did immediate-release nifedipine appear to provide any benefit. In some of the trials, patients who received immediate-release nifedipine had significantly worse outcomes than patients who received placebo. **ADALAT® CAPSULES should not be administered for 1 week after myocardial infarction, and it should also be avoided in the setting of acute coronary syndrome (when infarction may be imminent).**

Severe hypotension and/or increased fluid volume requirements have been reported in patients receiving ADALAT® together with a beta blocking agent who underwent coronary artery bypass surgery using high dose fentanyl anesthesia. The interaction with high dose fentanyl appears to be due to the combination of ADALAT® and a beta blocker, but the possibility that it may occur with ADALAT® alone, with low doses of fentanyl, in other surgical procedures, or with other narcotic analgesics cannot be ruled out. In ADALAT® treated patients where surgery using high dose fentanyl anesthesia is contemplated, the physician should be aware of these potential problems and, if the patient's condition permits, sufficient time (at least 36 hours) should be allowed for ADALAT® to be washed out of the body prior to surgery.

Increased Angina and/or Myocardial Infarction

Rarely, patients, particularly those who have severe obstructive coronary artery disease, have developed well documented increased frequency, duration, and/or severity of angina or acute myocardial infarction on starting ADALAT® or at the time of dosage increase. The mechanism of this effect is not established.

Beta Blocker Withdrawal

Patients recently withdrawn from beta blockers may develop a withdrawal syndrome with increased angina, probably related to increased sensitivity to catecholamines. Initiation of ADALAT® treatment will not prevent this occurrence and might be expected to exacerbate it by provoking reflex catecholamine release. There have been occasional reports of increased angina in a setting of beta blocker withdrawal and ADALAT® initiation. It is important to taper beta blockers if possible, rather than stopping them abruptly before beginning ADALAT®.

Congestive Heart Failure

Rarely, patients (usually those receiving a beta blocker) have developed heart failure after beginning ADALAT®. Patients with tight aortic stenosis may be at greater risk for such an event since the unloading effect of ADALAT® would be expected to be of less benefit to these patients, owing to the fixed impedance to flow across the aortic valve.

PRECAUTIONS

General: Hypotension: Because ADALAT® decreases peripheral vascular resistance, careful monitoring of blood pressure during the initial administration and titration of ADALAT® is suggested. Close observation is especially recommended for patients already taking medications that are known to lower blood pressure (See **WARNINGS**).

Peripheral Edema: Mild to moderate peripheral edema, typically associated with arterial vasodilation and not due to left ventricular dysfunction, occurs in about one in ten patients treated with ADALAT® (nifedipine). This edema occurs primarily in the lower extremities and usually responds to diuretic therapy. With patients whose angina is complicated by congestive heart failure, care should be taken to differentiate this peripheral edema from the effects of increasing left ventricular dysfunction.

Laboratory Tests: Rare, usually transient, but occasionally significant elevations of enzymes such as alkaline phosphatase, CPK, LDH, SGOT, and SGPT have been noted. The relationship to ADALAT® therapy is uncertain in most cases, but probable in some. These laboratory abnormalities have rarely been associated with clinical symptoms, however, cholestasis with or without jaundice has been reported. Rare instances of allergic hepatitis have been reported.

ADALAT®, like other calcium channel blockers, decreases platelet aggregation *in vitro*. Limited clinical studies have demonstrated a moderate but statistically significant decrease in platelet aggregation and increase in bleeding time in some ADALAT® patients. This is thought to be a function of inhibition of calcium transport across the platelet membrane. No clinical significance for these findings has been demonstrated.

Positive direct Coombs test with/without hemolytic anemia has been reported.

Although ADALAT® has been used safely in patients with renal dysfunction and has been reported to exert a beneficial effect in certain cases, rare reversible elevations in BUN and serum creatinine have been reported in patients with pre-existing chronic renal insufficiency. The relationship to ADALAT® therapy is uncertain in most cases but probable in some.

Drug Interactions: *Beta-adrenergic blocking agents*: (See **INDICATIONS** and **WARNINGS**). Experience in over 1400 patients in a non-comparative clinical trial has shown that concomitant administration of ADALAT® and beta blocking agents is usually well tolerated, but there have been occasional literature reports suggesting that the combination may increase the likelihood of congestive heart failure, severe hypotension or exacerbation of angina.

Long acting nitrates: ADALAT® may be safely co-administered with nitrates, but there have been no controlled studies to evaluate the antianginal effectiveness of this combination.

Digitalis: Since there have been isolated reports of patients with elevated digoxin levels, and there is a possible interaction between digoxin and nifedipine, it is recommended that digoxin levels be monitored when initiating, adjusting and discontinuing nifedipine to avoid possible over- or under-digitalization.

Coumarin anticoagulants: There have been rare reports of increased prothrombin time in patients taking coumarin anticoagulants to whom ADALAT® was administered. However, the relationship to ADALAT® therapy is uncertain.

Cimetidine: A study in six healthy volunteers has shown a significant increase in peak nifedipine plasma levels (80%) and area-under-the-curve (74%) after a one week course of cimetidine at 1000 mg per day and nifedipine at 40 mg per day. Ranitidine produced smaller, non-significant increases. The effect may be mediated by the known inhibition of cimetidine on hepatic cytochrome P-450, the enzyme system probably responsible for the first-pass metabolism of nifedipine. If nifedipine therapy is initiated in a patient currently receiving cimetidine, cautious titration is advised.

Quinidine: There have been rare reports of an interaction between quinidine and nifedipine (with a decreased plasma level of quinidine).

Other Interactions:

Grapefruit Juice: Co-administration of nifedipine with grapefruit juice results in up to a 2-fold increase in AUC and C_{max}, due to inhibition of CYP3A4 related first-pass metabolism. Co-administration of nifedipine with grapefruit juice is to be avoided.

Carcinogenesis, Mutagenesis, Impairment of Fertility: Nifedipine was administered orally to rats for two years and was not shown to be carcinogenic. When given to rats prior to mating, nifedipine caused reduced fertility at a dose approximately 30 times the maximum recommended human dose. ***There is a literature report of reversible reduction in the ability of human sperm obtained from a limited number of infertile men taking recommended doses of nifedipine to bind to and fertilize an ovum in vitro.*** *In vivo* mutagenicity studies were negative.

Pregnancy: Pregnancy Category C. In rodents, rabbits, and monkeys, nifedipine has been shown to have a variety of embryotoxic, placentoxic, and fetotoxic effects, including stunted fetuses (rats, mice, and rabbits), digital anomalies (rats and rabbits), rib deformities (mice), cleft palate (mice), small placentas and underdeveloped chorionic villi (monkeys), embryonic and fetal deaths (rats, mice, and rabbits), prolonged pregnancy (rats; not evaluated in other species), and decreased neonatal survival (rats; not evaluated in other species). On a mg/kg or mg/m^2 basis, some of the doses associated with these various effects are higher than the maximum recommended human dose and some are lower, but all are within one order of magnitude of it.

The digital anomalies seen in nifedipine-exposed rabbit pups are strikingly similar to those seen in pups exposed to phenytoin, and these are in turn similar to the phalangeal deformities that are the most common malformation seen in human children with *in utero* exposure to phenytoin.

There are no adequate and well-controlled studies in pregnant women. ADALAT® should be used during pregnancy only if the potential benefit justifies the potential risk to the fetus.

Nursing Mothers: Nifedipine is excreted in human milk. Therefore, a decision should be made to discontinue nursing or to discontinue the drug, taking into account the importance of the drug to the mother.

Geriatric Use: Although small pharmacokinetic studies have identified an increased half-life and increased C_{max} and AUC (See **CLINICAL PHARMACOLOGY: Pharmacokinetics and Metabolism**), clinical studies of nifedipine did not include sufficient numbers of subjects aged 65 and over to determine whether they respond differently from younger subjects. Other reported clinical experience has not identified differences in responses between the elderly and younger patients. In general, dose selection for an elderly patient should be cautious, usually starting at the low end of the dosing range, reflecting the greater frequency of decreased hepatic, renal, or cardiac function, and of concomitant disease or other drug therapy.

ADVERSE REACTION

In multiple-dose U.S. and foreign controlled studies in which adverse reactions were reported spontaneously, adverse effects were frequent but generally not serious and rarely required discontinuation of therapy or dosage adjustment. Most were expected consequences of the vasodilator effects of ADALAT®.

Adverse Effect	ADALAT® (%) (N = 226)	Placebo (%) (N = 235)
Dizziness, lightheadedness, giddiness	27	15
Flushing, heat sensation	25	8
Headache	23	20
Weakness	12	10
Nausea, heartburn	11	8
Muscle cramps, tremor	8	3
Peripheral edema	7	1
Nervousness, mood changes	7	4
Palpitation	7	5
Dyspnea, cough, wheezing	6	3
Nasal congestion, sore throat	6	8

There is also a large uncontrolled experience in over 2100 patients in the United States. Most of the patients had vasospastic or resistant angina pectoris, and about half had concomitant treatment with beta-adrenergic blocking agents. The most common adverse events were:

Incidence Approximately 10%

Cardiovascular: peripheral edema
Central Nervous System: dizziness or lightheadedness
Gastrointestinal: nausea
Systemic: headache and flushing, weakness.

Incidence Approximately 5%

Cardiovascular: transient hypotension.

Incidence 2% or Less:

Cardiovascular: palpitation
Respiratory: nasal and chest congestion, shortness of breath
Gastrointestinal: diarrhea, constipation, cramps, flatulence
Musculoskeletal: inflammation, joint stiffness, muscle cramps
Central Nervous System: shakiness, nervousness, jitteriness, sleep disturbances, blurred vision, difficulties in balance
Other: dermatitis, pruritus, urticaria, fever, sweating, chills, sexual difficulties.

Incidence Approximately 0.5%

Cardiovascular: syncope. Syncopal episodes occurred mostly with initial dose and/or increase of dosage.

Incidence Less Than 0.5%

Hematologic: thrombocytopenia, anemia, leukopenia, purpura
Gastrointestinal: allergic hepatitis
Face and Throat: angioedema (mostly oropharyngeal edema with breathing difficulty in a few patients), gingival hyperplasia
CNS: depression, paranoid syndrome
Musculoskeletal: myalgia
Special Senses: transient blindness at the peak of plasma level
Urogenital: nocturia, polyuria
Other: erythromelalgia, arthritis with ANA (+), gynecomastia, exfoliative dermatitis, Stevens-Johnson syndrome, toxic epidermal necrolysis.

Several of these side effects appear to be dose related. Peripheral edema occurred in about one in 25 patients at doses less than 60 mg per day and in about one patient in eight at 120 mg per day or more. Transient hypotension, generally mild to moderate severity and seldom requiring discontinuation of therapy, occurred in one of 50 patients at less than 60 mg per day and in one of 20 patients at 120 mg per day or more. Very rarely, introduction of ADALAT® therapy was associated with an increase in anginal pain, possibly due to associated hypotension.

In addition, more serious adverse events were observed, not readily distinguishable from the natural history of the disease in these patients. It remains possible, however, that some or many of these events were drug related. Myocardial infarction occurred in about 4% of patients and congestive heart failure or pulmonary edema in about 2%. Ventricular arrhythmias or conduction disturbances each occurred in fewer than 0.5% of patients.

In a subgroup of over 1000 patients receiving ADALAT® with concomitant beta blocker therapy, the pattern and incidence of adverse experiences were not different from that of the entire group of ADALAT® (nifedipine) treated patients (See **PRECAUTIONS**).

In a subgroup of approximately 250 patients with a diagnosis of congestive heart failure as well as angina, dizziness or lightheadedness, peripheral edema, headache or flushing each occurred in one in eight patients. Hypotension occurred in about one in 20 patients. Syncope occurred in approximately one patient in 250. Myocardial infarction or symptoms of congestive heart failure each occurred in about one patient in 15. Atrial or ventricular dysrhythmias each occurred in about one patient in 150.

OVERDOSAGE

Experience with nifedipine overdosage is limited. Generally, overdosage with nifedipine leading to pronounced hypotension calls for active cardiovascular support including monitoring of cardiovascular and respiratory function, elevation of extremities, judicious use of calcium infusion, pressor agents and fluids. Clearance of nifedipine would be expected to be prolonged in patients with impaired liver function. Since nifedipine is highly protein bound, dialysis is not likely to be of any benefit; however, plasmapheresis may be beneficial.

DOSAGE AND ADMINISTRATION

The dosage of ADALAT® needed to suppress angina and that can be tolerated by the patient must be established by titration. Excessive doses can result in hypotension.

Therapy should be initiated with the 10 mg capsule. The starting dose is one 10 mg capsule, swallowed whole, 3 times/day. The usual effective dose range is 10–20 mg three times daily. Some patients, especially those with evidence of coronary artery spasm, respond only to higher doses, more frequent administration, or both. In such patients, doses of 20–30 mg three or four times daily may be effective. Doses above 120 mg daily are rarely necessary. More than 180 mg per day is not recommended.

In most cases, ADALAT® titration should proceed over a 7–14 day period so that the physician can assess the response to each dose level and monitor the blood pressure before proceeding to higher doses.

If symptoms so warrant, titration may proceed more rapidly provided that the patient is assessed frequently. Based on the patient's physical activity level, attack frequency, and sublingual nitroglycerin consumption, the dose of ADALAT® CAPSULES may be increased from 10 mg t.i.d. to 20 mg t.i.d. and then to 30 mg t.i.d. over a three-day period.

In hospitalized patients under close observation, the dose may be increased in 10 mg increments over four to six-hour periods as required to control pain and arrhythmias due to ischemia. A single dose should rarely exceed 30 mg.

No "rebound effect" has been observed upon discontinuation of ADALAT®. However, if discontinuation of ADALAT® is necessary, sound clinical practice suggests that the dosage should be decreased gradually with close physician supervision.

Co-administration of nifedipine with grapefruit juice is to be avoided (See **CLINICAL PHARMACOLOGY** and **PRECAUTIONS**).

Co-Administration with Other Antianginal Drugs

Sublingual nitroglycerin may be taken as required for the control of acute manifestations of angina, particularly during ADALAT® titration. See **PRECAUTIONS, Drug Interactions**, for information on co-administration of ADALAT® with beta blockers or long acting nitrates.

HOW SUPPLIED

ADALAT® soft gelatin capsules are supplied in:

Bottles of 100:	10 mg (NDC 0026-8811-51) orange
	20 mg (NDC 0026-8821-51) orange and light brown
Bottles of 300:	10 mg (NDC 0026-8811-18) orange
	20 mg (NDC 0026-8821-18) orange and light brown
Unit dose packages of 100:	10 mg (NDC 0026-8811-48) orange
	20 mg (NDC 0026-8821-48) orange and light brown

The capsules are identified as follows: 10 mg (Adalat 10), 20 mg (Adalat 20).

The capsules should be protected from light and moisture and stored at controlled room temperature 59° to 77°F (15° to 25°C). Dispense in tight, light resistant containers (USP).

Bayer Corporation
Pharmaceutical Division
400 Morgan Lane
West Haven, CT 06516 USA

Encapsulated by
R. P. Scherer N.A., Clearwater, FL 33518
Rx Only

PZ500138 6/00 BAY a 1040 9749 ©2000 Bayer Corporation

Shown in Product Identification Guide, page 307

ADALAT® CC ℞

(nifedipine)
Extended Release Tablets
For Oral Use

DESCRIPTION

ADALAT® CC is an extended release tablet dosage form of the calcium channel blocker nifedipine. Nifedipine is 3,5-pyridinedicarboxylic acid, 1,4-dihydro-2,6-dimethyl-4-(2-nitrophenyl)-dimethyl ester, $C_{17}H_{18}N_2O_6$, and has the structural formula:

Nifedipine is a yellow crystalline substance, practically insoluble in water but soluble in ethanol. It has a molecular weight of 346.3. ADALAT CC tablets consist of an external coat and an internal core. Both contain nifedipine, the coat as a slow release formulation and the core as a fast release formulation. ADALAT CC tablets contain either 30, 60, or 90 mg of nifedipine for once-a-day oral administration.

Inert ingredients in the formulation are: hydroxypropylcellulose, lactose, corn starch, crospovidone, microcrystalline cellulose, silicon dioxide, and magnesium stearate. The inert ingredients in the film coating are: hydroxypropylmethylcellulose, polyethylene glycol, ferric oxide, and titanium dioxide.

CLINICAL PHARMACOLOGY

Nifedipine is a calcium ion influx inhibitor (slow-channel blocker or calcium ion antagonist) which inhibits the transmembrane influx of calcium ions into vascular smooth muscle and cardiac muscle. The contractile processes of vascular

Continued on next page

Adalat CC—Cont.

smooth muscle and cardiac muscle are dependent upon the movement of extracellular calcium ions into these cells through specific ion channels. Nifedipine selectively inhibits calcium ion influx across the cell membrane of vascular smooth muscle and cardiac muscle without altering serum calcium concentrations.

Mechanism of Action: The mechanism by which nifedipine reduces arterial blood pressure involves peripheral arterial vasodilatation and consequently, a reduction in peripheral vascular resistance. The increased peripheral vascular resistance that is an underlying cause of hypertension results from an increase in active tension in the vascular smooth muscle. Studies have demonstrated that the increase in active tension reflects an increase in cytosolic free calcium.

Nifedipine is a peripheral arterial vasodilator which acts directly on vascular smooth muscle. The binding of nifedipine to voltage-dependent and possibly receptor-operated channels in vascular smooth muscle results in an inhibition of calcium influx through these channels. Stores of intracellular calcium in vascular smooth muscle are limited and thus dependent upon the influx of extracellular calcium for contraction to occur. The reduction in calcium influx by nifedipine causes arterial vasodilation and decreased peripheral vascular resistance which results in reduced arterial blood pressure.

Pharmacokinetics and Metabolism: Nifedipine is completely absorbed after oral administration. The bioavailability of nifedipine as ADALAT CC relative to immediate release nifedipine is in the range of 84%–89%. After ingestion of ADALAT CC tablets under fasting conditions, plasma concentrations peak at about 2.5–5 hours with a second small peak or shoulder evident at approximately 6–12 hours post dose. The elimination half-life of nifedipine administered as ADALAT CC is approximately 7 hours in contrast to the known 2 hour elimination half-life of nifedipine administered as an immediate release capsule.

When ADALAT CC is administered as multiples of 30 mg tablets over a dose range of 30 mg to 90 mg, the area under the curve (AUC) is dose proportional; however, the peak plasma concentration for the 90 mg dose given as 3 × 30 mg is 29% greater than predicted from the 30 mg and 60 mg doses.

Two 30 mg ADALAT CC tablets may be interchanged with a 60 mg ADALAT CC tablet. Three 30 mg ADALAT CC tablets, however, result in substantially higher C_{max} values than those after a single 90 mg ADALAT CC tablet. Three 30 mg tablets should, therefore, not be considered interchangeable with a 90 mg tablet.

Once daily dosing of ADALAT CC under fasting conditions results in decreased fluctuations in the plasma concentration of nifedipine when compared to t.i.d. dosing with immediate release nifedipine capsules. The mean peak plasma concentration of nifedipine following a 90 mg ADALAT CC tablet, administered under fasting conditions, is approximately 115 ng/mL. When ADALAT CC is given immediately after a high fat meal in healthy volunteers, there is an average increase of 60% in the peak plasma nifedipine concentration, a prolongation in the time to peak concentration, but no significant change in the AUC. Plasma concentrations of nifedipine when ADALAT CC is taken after a fatty meal result in slightly lower peaks compared to the same daily dose of the immediate release formulation administered in three divided doses. This may be, in part, because ADALAT CC is less bioavailable than the immediate release formulation.

Nifedipine is extensively metabolized to highly water soluble, inactive metabolites accounting for 60% to 80% of the dose excreted in the urine. Only traces (less than 0.1% of the dose) of the unchanged form can be detected in the urine. The remainder is excreted in the feces in metabolized form, most likely as a result of biliary excretion.

No studies have been performed with ADALAT CC in patients with renal failure; however, significant alterations in the pharmacokinetics of nifedipine immediate release capsules have not been reported in patients undergoing hemodialysis or chronic ambulatory peritoneal dialysis. Since the absorption of nifedipine from ADALAT CC could be modified by renal disease, caution should be exercised in treating such patients.

Because hepatic biotransformation is the predominant route for the disposition of nifedipine, its pharmacokinetics may be altered in patients with chronic liver disease. ADALAT CC has not been studied in patients with hepatic disease; however, in patients with hepatic impairment (liver cirrhosis) nifedipine has a longer elimination half-life and higher bioavailability than in healthy volunteers.

The degree of protein binding of nifedipine is high (92%–98%). Protein binding may be greatly reduced in patients with renal or hepatic impairment.

After administration of ADALAT CC to healthy elderly men and women (age > 60 years), the mean C_{max} is 36% higher and the average plasma concentration is 70% greater than in younger patients.

In healthy subjects, the elimination half-life of a different sustained release nifedipine formulation was longer in elderly subjects (6.7 h) compared to young subjects (3.8 h) following oral administration. A decreased clearance was also observed in the elderly (348 mL/min) compared to young subjects (519 mL/min) following intravenous administration.

Co-administration of nifedipine with grapefruit juice results in up to a 2-fold increase in AUC and C_{max}, due to inhibition of CYP3A4 related first-pass metabolism.

Clinical Studies: ADALAT CC produced dose-related decreases in systolic and diastolic blood pressure as demonstrated in two double-blind, randomized, placebo-controlled trials in which over 350 patients were treated with ADALAT CC 30, 60 or 90mg once daily for 6 weeks. In the first study, ADALAT CC was given as monotherapy and in the second study, ADALAT CC was added to a beta-blocker in patients not controlled on a beta-blocker alone. The mean trough (24 hours post-dose) blood pressure results from these studies are shown below:

MEAN REDUCTIONS IN TROUGH SUPINE BLOOD PRESSURE (mmHG) SYSTOLIC/DIASTOLIC

ADALAT CC DOSE	N	MEAN TROUGH REDUCTION*
STUDY 1		
30 MG	60	5.3/2.9
60 MG	57	8.0/4.1
90 MG	55	12.5/8.1
STUDY 2		
30 MG	58	7.6/3.8
60 MG	63	10.1/5.3
90 MG	62	10.2/5.8

*Placebo response subtracted.

The trough/peak ratios estimated from 24 hour blood pressure monitoring ranged from 41%–78% for diastolic and 46%–91% for systolic blood pressure.

Hemodynamics: Like other slow-channel blockers, nifedipine exerts a negative inotropic effect on isolated myocardial tissue. This is rarely, if ever, seen in intact animals or man, probably because of reflex responses to its vasodilating effects. In man, nifedipine decreases peripheral vascular resistance which leads to a fall in systolic and diastolic pressures, usually minimal in normotensive volunteers (less than 5–10 mm Hg systolic), but sometimes larger. With ADALAT CC, these decreases in blood pressure are not accompanied by any significant change in heart rate. Hemodynamic studies of the immediate release nifedipine formulation in patients with normal ventricular function have generally found a small increase in cardiac index without major effects on ejection fraction, left ventricular end-diastolic pressure (LVEDP) or volume (LVEDV). In patients with impaired ventricular function, most acute studies have shown some increase in ejection fraction and reduction in left ventricular filling pressure.

Electrophysiologic Effects: Although, like other members of its class, nifedipine causes a slight depression of sinoatrial node function and atrioventricular conduction in isolated myocardial preparations, such effects have not been seen in studies in intact animals or in man. In formal electrophysiologic studies, predominantly in patients with normal conduction systems, nifedipine administered as the immediate release capsule has had no tendency to prolong atrioventricular conduction or sinus node recovery time, or to slow sinus rate.

INDICATION AND USAGE

ADALAT CC is indicated for the treatment of hypertension. It may be used alone or in combination with other antihypertensive agents.

CONTRAINDICATIONS

Known hypersensitivity to nifedipine.

WARNINGS

Excessive Hypotension: Although in most patients the hypotensive effect of nifedipine is modest and well tolerated, occasional patients have had excessive and poorly tolerated hypotension. These responses have usually occurred during initial titration or at the time of subsequent upward dosage adjustment, and may be more likely in patients using concomitant beta-blockers.

Severe hypotension and/or increased fluid volume requirements have been reported in patients who received immediate release capsules together with a beta-blocking agent and who underwent coronary artery bypass surgery using high dose fentanyl anesthesia. The interaction with high dose fentanyl appears to be due to the combination of nifedipine and a beta-blocker, but the possibility that it may occur with nifedipine alone, with low doses of fentanyl, in other surgical procedures, or with other narcotic analgesics cannot be ruled out. In nifedipine-treated patients where surgery using high dose fentanyl anesthesia is contemplated, the physician should be aware of these potential problems and, if the patient's condition permits, sufficient time (at least 36 hours) should be allowed for nifedipine to be washed out of the body prior to surgery.

Increased Angina and/or Myocardial Infarction: Rarely, patients, particularly those who have severe obstructive coronary artery disease, have developed well documented increased frequency, duration and/or severity of angina or acute myocardial infarction upon starting nifedipine or at the time of dosage increase. The mechanism of this effect is not established.

Beta-Blocker Withdrawal: When discontinuing a beta-blocker it is important to taper its dose, if possible, rather than stopping abruptly before beginning nifedipine. Patients recently withdrawn from beta blockers may develop a withdrawal syndrome with increased angina, probably related to increased sensitivity to catecholamines. Initiation of nifedipine treatment will not prevent this occurrence and on occasion has been reported to increase it.

Congestive Heart Failure: Rarely, patients (usually while receiving a beta-blocker) have developed heart failure after beginning nifedipine. Patients with tight aortic stenosis may be at greater risk for such an event, as the unloading effect of nifedipine would be expected to be of less benefit to these patients, owing to their fixed impedance to flow across the aortic valve.

PRECAUTIONS

General—Hypotension: Because nifedipine decreases peripheral vascular resistance, careful monitoring of blood pressure during the initial administration and titration of ADALAT CC is suggested. Close observation is especially recommended for patients already taking medications that are known to lower blood pressure (See **WARNINGS**).

Peripheral Edema: Mild to moderate peripheral edema occurs in a dose-dependent manner with ADALAT CC. The placebo subtracted rate is approximately 8% at 30 mg, 12% at 60 mg and 19% at 90 mg daily. This edema is a localized phenomenon, thought to be associated with vasodilation of dependent arterioles and small blood vessels and not due to left ventricular dysfunction or generalized fluid retention. With patients whose hypertension is complicated by congestive heart failure, care should be taken to differentiate this peripheral edema from the effects of increasing left ventricular dysfunction.

Information for Patients: ADALAT CC is an extended release tablet and should be swallowed whole and taken on an empty stomach. It should not be administered with food. Do not chew, divide or crush tablets.

Laboratory Tests: Rare, usually transient, but occasionally significant elevations of enzymes such as alkaline phosphatase, CPK, LDH, SGOT, and SGPT have been noted. The relationship to nifedipine therapy is uncertain in most cases, but probable in some. These laboratory abnormalities have rarely been associated with clinical symptoms; however, cholestasis with or without jaundice has been reported. A small increase (<5%) in mean alkaline phosphatase was noted in patients treated with ADALAT CC. This was an isolated finding and it rarely resulted in values which fell outside the normal range. Rare instances of allergic hepatitis have been reported with nifedipine treatment. In controlled studies, ADALAT CC did not adversely affect serum uric acid, glucose, cholesterol or potassium.

Nifedipine, like other calcium channel blockers, decreases platelet aggregation *in vitro*. Limited clinical studies have demonstrated a moderate but statistically significant decrease in platelet aggregation and increase in bleeding time in some nifedipine patients. This is thought to be a function of inhibition of calcium transport across the platelet membrane. No clinical significance for these findings has been demonstrated.

Positive direct Coombs' test with or without hemolytic anemia has been reported but a causal relationship between nifedipine administration and positivity of this laboratory test, including hemolysis, could not be determined.

Although nifedipine has been used safely in patients with renal dysfunction and has been reported to exert a beneficial effect in certain cases, rare reversible elevations in BUN and serum creatinine have been reported in patients with pre-existing chronic renal insufficiency. The relationship to nifedipine therapy is uncertain in most cases but probable in some.

Drug Interactions: Beta-adrenergic blocking agents: (See **WARNINGS**).

ADALAT CC was well tolerated when administered in combination with a beta blocker in 187 hypertensive patients in a placebo-controlled clinical trial. However, there have been occasional literature reports suggesting that the combination of nifedipine and beta-adrenergic blocking drugs may increase the likelihood of congestive heart failure, severe hypotension, or exacerbation of angina in patients with cardiovascular disease.

Digitalis: Since there have been isolated reports of patients with elevated digoxin levels, and there is a possible interaction between digoxin and ADALAT CC, it is recommended that digoxin levels be monitored when initiating, adjusting, and discontinuing ADALAT CC to avoid possible over- or under-digitalization.

Coumarin Anticoagulants: There have been rare reports of increased prothrombin time in patients taking coumarin anticoagulants to whom nifedipine was administered. However, the relationship to nifedipine therapy is uncertain.

Quinidine: There have been rare reports of an interaction between quinidine and nifedipine (with a decreased plasma level of quinidine).

Cimetidine: Both the peak plasma level of nifedipine and the AUC may increase in the presence of cimetidine. Ranitidine produces smaller non-significant increases. This effect of cimetidine may be mediated by its known inhibition of hepatic cytochrome P-450, the enzyme system probably responsible for the first-pass metabolism of nifedipine. If nifedipine therapy is initiated in a patient currently receiving cimetidine, cautious titration is advised.

Other Interactions:

Grapefruit Juice: Co-administration of nifedipine with grapefruit juice results in up to a 2-fold increase in AUC and C_{max}, due to inhibition of CYP3A4 related first-pass metabolism. Co-administration of nifedipine with grapefruit juice is to be avoided.

Carcinogenesis, Mutagenesis, Impairment of Fertility: Nifedipine was administered orally to rats for two years and was not shown to be carcinogenic. When given to rats prior to mating, nifedipine caused reduced fertility at a dose approximately 30 times the maximum recommended human dose. ***There is a literature report of reversible reduction in the ability of human sperm obtained from a limited number of infertile men taking recommended doses of nifedipine to bind to and fertilize an ovum in vitro.*** *In vivo* mutagenicity studies were negative.

Pregnancy: Pregnancy Category C. In rodents, rabbits and monkeys, nifedipine has been shown to have a variety of embryotoxic, placentotoxic and fetotoxic effects, including stunted fetuses (rats, mice and rabbits), digital anomalies (rats and rabbits), rib deformities (mice), cleft palate (mice), small placentas and underdeveloped chorionic villi (monkeys), embryonic and fetal deaths (rats, mice and rabbits), prolonged pregnancy (rats; not evaluated in other species), and decreased neonatal survival (rats; not evaluated in other species). On a mg/kg or mg/m^2 basis, some of the doses associated with these various effects are higher than the maximum recommended human dose and some are lower, but all are within an order of magnitude of it.

The digital anomalies seen in nifedipine-exposed rabbit pups are strikingly similar to those seen in pups exposed to phenytoin, and these are in turn similar to the phalangeal deformities that are the most common malformation seen in human children with *in utero* exposure to phenytoin.

There are no adequate and well-controlled studies in pregnant women. ADALAT CC should be used during pregnancy only if the potential benefit justifies the potential risk to the fetus.

Nursing Mothers: Nifedipine is excreted in human milk. Therefore, a decision should be made to discontinue nursing or to discontinue the drug, taking into account the importance of the drug to the mother.

Geriatric Use: Although small pharmacokinetic studies have identified an increased half-life and increased C_{max} and AUC (See **CLINICAL PHARMACOLOGY: Pharmacokinetics and Metabolism**), clinical studies of nifedipine did not include sufficient numbers of subjects aged 65 and over to determine whether they respond differently from younger subjects. Other reported clinical experience has not identified differences in responses between the elderly and younger patients. In general, dose selection for an elderly patient should be cautious, usually starting at the low end of the dosing range, reflecting the greater frequency of decreased hepatic, renal, or cardiac function, and of concomitant disease or other drug therapy.

ADVERSE EXPERIENCES

The incidence of adverse events during treatment with ADALAT® CC in doses up to 90 mg daily were derived from multi-center placebo-controlled clinical trials in 370 hypertensive patients. Atenolol 50 mg once daily was used concomitantly in 187 of the 370 patients on ADALAT CC and in 64 of the 126 patients on placebo. All adverse events reported during ADALAT CC therapy were tabulated independently of their causal relationship to medication.

The most common adverse event reported with ADALAT CC was peripheral edema. This was dose related and the frequency was 18% on ADALAT CC 30 mg daily, 22% on ADALAT CC 60 mg daily and 29% on ADALAT CC 90 mg daily versus 10% on placebo.

Other common adverse events reported in the above placebo-controlled trials include:

Adverse Event	ADALAT CC (%) (n=370)	PLACEBO (%) (n=126)
Headache	19	13
Flushing/heat sensation	4	0
Dizziness	4	2
Fatigue/asthenia	4	4
Nausea	2	1
Constipation	1	0

Where the frequency of adverse events with ADALAT CC and placebo is similar, causal relationship cannot be established.

The following adverse events were reported with an incidence of 3% or less in daily doses up to 90 mg:

Body as a Whole/Systemic: chest pain, leg pain
Central Nervous System: paresthesia, vertigo
Dermatologic: rash
Gastrointestinal: constipation
Musculoskeletal: leg cramps
Respiratory: epistaxis, rhinitis
Urogenital: impotence, urinary frequency

Other adverse events reported with an incidence of less than 1.0% were:

Body as a Whole/Systemic: cellulitis, chills, facial edema, neck pain, pelvic pain, pain
Cardiovascular: atrial fibrillation, bradycardia, cardiac arrest, extrasystole, hypotension, palpitations, phlebitis, postural hypotension, tachycardia, cutaneous angiectases
Central Nervous System: anxiety, confusion, decreased libido, depression, hypertonia, insomnia, somnolence
Dermatologic: pruritus, sweating
Gastrointestinal: abdominal pain, diarrhea, dry mouth, dyspepsia, esophagitis, flatulence, gastrointestinal hemorrhage, vomiting
Hematologic: lymphadenopathy
Metabolic: gout, weight loss
Musculoskeletal: arthralgia, arthritis, myalgia
Respiratory: dyspnea, increased cough, rales, pharyngitis
Special Senses: abnormal vision, amblyopia, conjunctivitis, diplopia, tinnitus
Urogenital/Reproductive: kidney calculus, nocturia, breast engorgement

The following adverse events have been reported rarely in patients given nifedipine in other formulations: allergenic hepatitis, alopecia, anemia, arthritis with ANA (+), depression, erythromelalgia, exfoliative dermatitis, fever, gingival hyperplasia, gynecomastia, leukopenia, mood changes, muscle cramps, nervousness, paranoid syndrome, purpura, shakiness, sleep disturbances, Stevens-Johnson syndrome, syncope, taste perversion, thrombocytopenia, toxic epidermal necrolysis, transient blindness at the peak of plasma level, tremor and urticaria.

OVERDOSAGE

Experience with nifedipine overdosage is limited. Generally, overdosage with nifedipine leading to pronounced hypotension calls for active cardiovascular support including monitoring of cardiovascular and respiratory function, elevation of extremities, judicious use of calcium infusion, pressor agents and fluids. Clearance of nifedipine would be expected to be prolonged in patients with impaired liver function. Since nifedipine is highly protein bound, dialysis is not likely to be of any benefit; however, plasmapheresis may be beneficial.

There has been one reported case of massive overdosage with tablets of another extended release formulation of nifedipine. The main effects of ingestion of approximately 4800 mg of nifedipine in a young man attempting suicide as a result of cocaine-induced depression was initial dizziness, palpitations, flushing, and nervousness. Within several hours of ingestion, nausea, vomiting, and generalized edema developed. No significant hypotension was apparent at presentation, 18 hours post ingestion. Blood chemistry abnormalities consisted of a mild, transient elevation of serum creatinine, and modest elevations of LDH and CPK, but normal SGOT. Vital signs remained stable, no electrocardiographic abnormalities were noted and renal function returned to normal within 24 to 48 hours with routine supportive measures alone. No prolonged sequelae were observed.

The effect of a single 900 mg ingestion of nifedipine capsules in a depressed anginal patient on tricyclic antidepressants was loss of consciousness within 30 minutes of ingestion, and profound hypotension, which responded to calcium infusion, pressor agents, and fluid replacement. A variety of ECG abnormalities were seen in this patient with a history of bundle branch block, including sinus bradycardia and varying degrees of AV block. These dictated the prophylactic placement of a temporary ventricular pacemaker, but otherwise resolved spontaneously. Significant hyperglycemia was seen initially in this patient, but plasma glucose levels rapidly normalized without further treatment.

A young hypertensive patient with advanced renal failure ingested 280 mg of nifedipine capsules at one time, with resulting marked hypotension responding to calcium infusion and fluids. No AV conduction abnormalities, arrhythmias, or pronounced changes in heart rate were noted, nor was there any further deterioration in renal function.

DOSAGE AND ADMINISTRATION

Dosage should be adjusted according to each patient's needs. It is recommended that ADALAT CC be administered orally once daily on an empty stomach. ADALAT CC is an extended release dosage form and tablets should be swallowed whole, not bitten or divided. In general, titration should proceed over a 7–14 day period starting with 30 mg once daily. Upward titration should be based on therapeutic efficacy and safety. The usual maintenance dose is 30 mg to 60 mg once daily. Titration to doses above 90 mg daily is not recommended.

If discontinuation of ADALAT CC is necessary, sound clinical practice suggests that the dosage should be decreased gradually with close physician supervision.

Co-administration of nifedipine with grapefruit juice is to be avoided (See **CLINICAL PHARMACOLOGY** and **PRECAUTIONS**).

Care should be taken when dispensing ADALAT CC to assure that the extended release dosage form has been prescribed.

HOW SUPPLIED

ADALAT CC extended release tablets are supplied as 30 mg, 60 mg, and 90 mg round film coated tablets. The different strengths can be identified as follows:

Strength	Color	Markings
30 mg	Pink	30 on one side and ADALAT CC on the other side
60 mg	Salmon	60 on one side and ADALAT CC on the other side
90 mg	Dark Red	90 on one side and ADALAT CC on the other side

ADALAT® CC Tablets are supplied in:

	Strength	NDC Code
Bottles of 100	30 mg	0026-8841-51
	60 mg	0026-8851-51
	90 mg	0026-8861-51
Unit Dose Packages of 100	30 mg	0026-8841-48
	60 mg	0026-8851-48
	90 mg	0026-8861-48

The tablets should be protected from light and moisture and stored below 86°F (30°C). Dispense in tight, light-resistant containers.

Bayer Corporation
Pharmaceutical Division
400 Morgan Lane
West Haven, CT 06516 USA

℞ Only

PZ500161 5/00 © 2000 Bayer Corporation 9709

Shown in Product Identification Guide, page 307

AVELOX™ ℞

(moxifloxacin hydrochloride)
Tablets

DESCRIPTION

AVELOX™ (moxifloxacin hydrochloride) is a synthetic broad spectrum antibacterial agent for oral administration. Moxifloxacin, a fluoroquinolone, is available as the monohydrochloride salt of 1-cyclopropyl-7-[(S,S)-2,8-diazabicyclo[4.3.0]non-8-yl]-6-fluoro-8-methoxy-1,4-dihydro-4-oxo-3-quinoline carboxylic acid. It is a slightly yellow to yellow crystalline substance with a molecular weight of 437.9. Its empirical formula is $C_{21}H_{24}FN_3O_4$ *HCl and its chemical structure is as follows:

Moxifloxacin differs from other quinolones in that it has a methoxy function at the 8-position, and an S,S—configured diazabicyclononyl ring moiety at the 7-position.

AVELOX is available in 400 mg (moxifloxacin equivalent) film-coated tablets. The inactive ingredients are microcrystalline cellulose, lactose monohydrate, croscarmellose sodium, magnesium stearate, hydroxypropyl methylcellulose, titanium dioxide, polyethylene glycol and ferric oxide.

CLINICAL PHARMACOLOGY

Absorption

Moxifloxacin, given as an oral tablet, is well absorbed from the gastrointestinal tract. The absolute bioavailability of moxifloxacin is approximately 90 percent. Co-administration with a high fat meal (i.e., 500 calories from fat) does not affect the absorption of moxifloxacin.

Consumption of 1 cup of yogurt with moxifloxacin does not significantly affect the extent or rate of systemic absorption (AUC).

The mean (± SD) C_{max} and AUC values at steady-state with a 400 mg once daily dosage regimen are 4.5 ± 0.53 µg/mL and 48 ± 2.7 µg*h/mL, respectively. C_{max} is attained 1 to 3 hours after oral dosing. The mean (± SD) trough concentration is 0.95 ± 0.10 µg/mL. Plasma concentrations increase proportionately with dose up to the highest dose tested (800 mg single dose). The mean (± SD) elimination half-life from plasma is 12 ± 1.3 hours; steady-state is achieved after at least three days with a 400 mg once daily regimen. The figure below illustrates the time course of plasma concentrations of moxifloxacin following a 400 mg dose administered at steady-state.

Steady-State Plasma Concentrations of Moxifloxacin Obtained With Once Daily Dosing of 400 mg (mean;SD) (n=10)

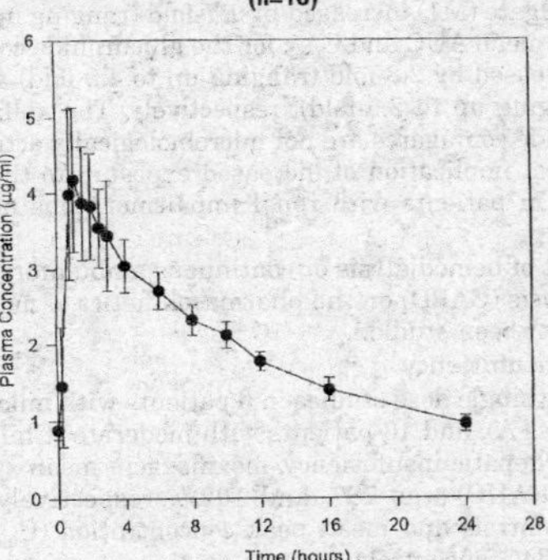

Distribution

Moxifloxacin is approximately 50% bound to serum proteins, independent of drug concentration. The volume of distribution of moxifloxacin ranges from 1.7 to 2.7 L/kg. Moxifloxacin is widely distributed throughout the body, with tissue concentrations often exceeding plasma concentrations. Moxifloxacin has been detected in the saliva, nasal and bronchial secretions, mucosa of the sinuses, skin blister fluid, and subcutaneous tissue, and skeletal muscle following oral administration of 400 mg. Concentrations measured at 3 hours post-dose are summarized in the following table. The rates of elimination of moxifloxacin from tissues generally parallel the elimination from plasma.

Continued on next page

Avelox—Cont.

[See table at right]

Metabolism

Moxifloxacin is metabolized via glucuronide and sulfate conjugation. The cytochrome P450 system is not involved in moxifloxacin metabolism, and is not affected by moxifloxacin. The sulfate conjugate (M1) accounts for approximately 38% of the dose, and is eliminated primarily in the feces. Approximately 14% of an oral or intravenous dose is converted to a glucuronide conjugate (M2), which is excreted exclusively in the urine. Peak plasma concentrations of M2 are approximately 40% those of the parent drug, while plasma concentrations of M1 are generally less than 10% those of moxifloxacin.

Excretion

Approximately 45% of an oral or intravenous dose of moxifloxacin is excreted as unchanged drug (~20% in urine and ~25% in feces). A total of 96% ± 4% of an oral dose is excreted as either unchanged drug or known metabolites. The mean (± SD) apparent total body clearance and renal clearance are 12 ± 2.0 L/hr and 2.6 ± 0.5 L/hr, respectively.

Special Populations

Geriatric

In 16 healthy elderly male and female volunteers (66–81 years of age) given a single 200 mg dose of moxifloxacin, the extent of systemic exposure (AUC and C_{max}) was not statistically different between young and elderly males and elimination half-life was unchanged. No dosage adjustment is necessary based on age.

Whether pharmacokinetic differences exist between young and elderly females is unknown. The pharmacokinetics of moxifloxacin with repeated 400 mg administration in elderly subjects has not been studied.

Pediatric

The pharmacokinetics of moxifloxacin in pediatric subjects have not been studied.

Gender

Following a single 200 mg dose of moxifloxacin to 16 healthy elderly subjects, the mean AUC and C_{max} were 29% and 24% higher, respectively, in healthy elderly females compared to healthy elderly males. There are no significant differences in moxifloxacin pharmacokinetics between elderly male and female subjects when differences in body weight are taken into consideration.

A 400 mg single dose study was conducted in 18 young males and females. The comparison of moxifloxacin pharmacokinetics in this study (9 young females and 9 young males) showed no differences in AUC or C_{max} due to gender. Dosage adjustments based on gender are not necessary.

Race

Steady state moxifloxacin pharmacokinetics in male Japanese subjects were similar to those determined in Caucasians, with a mean C_{max} of 4.1 µg/mL, an AUC_{24} of 47 µg*h/mL, and an elimination half-life of 14 hours.

Renal Insufficiency

The pharmacokinetic parameters of moxifloxacin are not significantly altered by mild, moderate, or severe renal impairment. No dosage adjustment is necessary in patients with renal impairment.

In a single-dose study of 24 patients with varying degrees of renal function from normal to severely impaired, the mean peak concentrations (C_{max}) of moxifloxacin were reduced by 22% and 21% in the patients with moderate ($CL_{CR} \geq 30$ and ≤ 60 mL/min) and severe ($CL_{CR} < 30$ mL/min) renal impairment, respectively. The mean systemic exposure (AUC) in these patients was increased by 13%. In the moderate and severe renally impaired patients, the mean AUC for the sulfate conjugate (M1) increased by 1.7-fold (ranging up to 2.8-fold) and mean AUC and C_{max} for the glucuronide conjugate (M2) increased by 2.8-fold (ranging up to 4.8-fold) and 1.4-fold (ranging up to 2.5-fold), respectively. The sulfate and glucuronide conjugates are not microbiologically active, and the clinical implication of increased exposure to these metabolites in patients with renal impairment has not been studied.

The effect of hemodialysis or continuous ambulatory peritoneal dialysis (CAPD) on the pharmacokinetics of moxifloxacin has not been studied.

Hepatic Insufficiency

In 400 mg single dose studies in 6 patients with mild (Child Pugh Class A), and 10 patients with moderate (Child Pugh Class B), hepatic insufficiency, moxifloxacin mean systemic exposure (AUC) was 78% and 102%, respectively, of 18 healthy controls and mean peak concentration (C_{max}) was 79% and 84% of controls.

The mean AUC of the sulfate conjugate of moxifloxacin (M1) increased by 3.9-fold (ranging up to 5.9-fold) and 5.7-fold (ranging up to 8.0-fold) in the mild and moderate groups, respectively. The mean C_{max} of M1 increased by approximately 3-fold in both groups (ranging up to 4.7- and 3.9-fold). The mean AUC of the glucuronide conjugate of moxifloxacin (M2) increased by 1.5-fold (ranging up to 2.5-fold) in both groups. The mean C_{max} of M2 increased by 1.6- and 1.3-fold (ranging up to 2.7- and 2.1-fold), respectively. The clinical significance of increased exposure to the sulfate and glucuronide conjugates has not been studied. No dosage adjustment is recommended for mild or moderate hepatic insufficiency (Child Pugh Classes A and B). The pharmacokinetics of moxifloxacin in severe hepatic insufficiency (Child Pugh Class C) have not been studied. (See **DOSAGE AND ADMINISTRATION**.)

Moxifloxacin Concentrations (mean ± SD) in Plasma and Tissues Measured 3 Hours After Dosing with 400 mg§

Tissue or Fluid	N	Plasma Concentration (µg/mL)	Tissue or Fluid Concentration (µg/mL or µg/g)	Tissue: Plasma Ratio
Respiratory				
Alveolar Macrophages	5	3.3 ± 0.7	61.8 ± 27.3	21.2 ± 10.0
Bronchial Mucosa	8	3.3 ± 0.7	5.5 ± 1.3	1.7 ± 0.3
Epithelial Lining Fluid	5	3.3 ± 0.7	24.4 ± 14.7	8.7 ± 6.1
Sinus				
Maxillary Sinus Mucosa	4	3.7 ± 1.1†	7.6 ± 1.7	2.0 ± 0.3
Anterior Ethmoid Mucosa	3	3.7 ± 1.1†	8.8 ± 4.3	2.2 ± 0.6
Nasal Polyps	4	3.7 ± 1.1†	9.8 ± 4.5	2.6 ± 0.6

§ all moxifloxacin concentrations were measured after a single 400 mg dose, except the sinus concentrations which were measured after 5 days of dosing.

† N = 5

Photosensitivity Potential

A study of the skin response to ultraviolet (UVA and UVB) and visible radiation conducted in 32 healthy volunteers (8 per group) demonstrated that moxifloxacin does not show phototoxicity in comparison to placebo. The minimum erythematous dose (MED) was measured before and after treatment with moxifloxacin (200 mg or 400 mg once daily), lomefloxacin (400 mg once daily), or placebo. In this study, the MED measured for both doses of moxifloxacin were not significantly different from placebo, while lomefloxacin significantly lowered the MED. (See **PRECAUTIONS, Information for Patients.**)

Drug-drug interactions

The potential for pharmacokinetic drug interactions between moxifloxacin and theophylline, warfarin, digoxin, probenecid, ranitidine, glyburide, iron, and antacids has been evaluated. There was no clinically significant effect of moxifloxacin on theophylline, warfarin, digoxin, or glyburide kinetics. Theophylline, digoxin, probenecid, and ranitidine did not affect the pharmacokinetics of moxifloxacin. However, as with all other quinolones, iron and antacids significantly reduced the bioavailability of moxifloxacin.

Theophylline: No significant effect of moxifloxacin (200 mg every twelve hours for 3 days) on the pharmacokinetics of theophylline (400 mg every twelve hours for 3 days) was detected in a study involving 12 healthy volunteers. In addition, theophylline was not shown to affect the pharmacokinetics of moxifloxacin. The effect of co-administration of a 400 mg dose of moxifloxacin with theophylline has not been studied, but it is not expected to be clinically significant based on *in vitro* metabolic data showing that moxifloxacin does not inhibit the CYP1A2 isoenzyme.

Warfarin: No significant effect of moxifloxacin (400 mg once daily for eight days) on the pharmacokinetics of R- and S-warfarin (25 mg single dose of warfarin sodium on the fifth day) was detected in a study involving 24 healthy volunteers. No significant change in prothrombin time was observed. (See **PRECAUTIONS, Drug Interactions.**)

Digoxin: No significant effect of moxifloxacin (400 mg once daily for two days) on digoxin (0.6 mg as a single dose) AUC was detected in a study involving 12 healthy volunteers. The mean digoxin C_{max} increased by about 50% during the distribution phase of digoxin. This transient increase in digoxin C_{max} is not viewed to be clinically significant. Moxifloxacin pharmacokinetics were similar in the presence or absence of digoxin. No dosage adjustment for moxifloxacin or digoxin is required when these drugs are administered concomitantly.

Probenecid: Probenecid (500 mg twice daily for two days) did not alter the renal clearance and total amount of moxifloxacin (400 mg single dose) excreted renally in a study of 12 healthy volunteers.

Ranitidine: No significant effect of ranitidine (150 mg twice daily for three days as pretreatment) on the pharmacokinetics of moxifloxacin (400 mg single dose) was detected in a study involving 10 healthy volunteers.

Antidiabetic agents: In diabetics, glyburide (2.5 mg once daily for two weeks pretreatment and for five days concurrently) mean AUC and C_{max} were 12% and 21% lower, respectively, when taken with moxifloxacin (400 mg once daily for five days) in comparison to placebo. Nonetheless, blood glucose levels were decreased slightly in patients taking glyburide and moxifloxacin in comparison to those taking glyburide alone, suggesting no interference by moxifloxacin on the activity of glyburide. These interaction results are not viewed as clinically significant.

Antacids: When moxifloxacin (single 400 mg dose) was administered two hours before, concomitantly, or 4 hours after an aluminum/magnesium-containing antacid (900 mg aluminum hydroxide and 600 mg magnesium hydroxide as a single oral dose) to 12 healthy volunteers there was a 26%, 60% and 23% reduction in the mean AUC of moxifloxacin, respectively. Moxifloxacin should be taken at least 4 hours before or 8 hours after antacids containing magnesium or aluminum, as well as sucralfate, metal cations such as iron, and multivitamin preparations with zinc, or Videx® (didanosine) chewable/buffered tablets or the pediatric powder for oral solution. (See **PRECAUTIONS, Drug Interactions** and **DOSAGE AND ADMINISTRATION.**)

Iron: When moxifloxacin was administered concomitantly with iron (ferrous sulfate 100 mg once daily for two days), the mean AUC and C_{max} of moxifloxacin was reduced by 39% and 59%, respectively. Moxifloxacin should only be taken more than 4 hours before or 8 hours after iron products. (See **PRECAUTIONS, Drug Interactions** and **DOSAGE AND ADMINISTRATION.**)

There is limited information available on the potential for a pharmacodynamic interaction in humans between moxifloxacin and other drugs that prolong the QTc interval of the electrocardiogram. Sotalol, a Class III antiarrhythmic, has been shown to further increase the QTc interval when combined with high doses of intravenous (IV) moxifloxacin in dogs. Therefore, moxifloxacin should be avoided with Class IA and Class III antiarrhythmics. (See **ANIMAL PHARMACOLOGY, WARNINGS,** and **PRECAUTIONS.**)

MICROBIOLOGY

Moxifloxacin has *in vitro* activity against a wide range of Gram-positive and Gram-negative microorganisms. The bactericidal action of moxifloxacin results from inhibition of the topoisomerase II (DNA gyrase) and topoisomerase IV required for bacterial DNA replication, transcription, repair, and recombination. It appears that the C8-methoxy moiety contributes to enhanced activity and lower selection of resistant mutants of Gram-positive bacteria compared to the C8-H moiety.

The mechanism of action for quinolones, including moxifloxacin, is different from that of macrolides, beta-lactams, aminoglycosides, or tetracyclines; therefore, microorganisms resistant to these classes of drugs may be susceptible to moxifloxacin and other quinolones. There is no known cross-resistance between moxifloxacin and other classes of antimicrobials.

Cross-resistance has been observed between moxifloxacin and other fluoroquinolones against Gram-negative bacteria. Gram-positive bacteria resistant to other fluoroquinolones may, however, still be susceptible to moxifloxacin.

Moxifloxacin has been shown to be active against most strains of the following microorganisms, both *in vitro* and in clinical infections as described in the **INDICATIONS AND USAGE** section.

Aerobic Gram-positive microorganisms

Staphylococcus aureus (methicillin-susceptible strains only)
Streptococcus pneumoniae (penicillin-susceptible strains)

Aerobic Gram-negative microorganisms

Haemophilus influenzae
Haemophilus parainfluenzae
Klebsiella pneumoniae
Moraxella catarrhalis

Other microorganisms

Chlamydia pneumoniae
Mycoplasma pneumoniae

The following *in vitro* data are available, **but their clinical significance is unknown.**

Moxifloxacin exhibits *in vitro* minimum inhibitory concentrations (MICs) of 2 µg/mL or less against most (≥90%) strains of the following microorganisms; however, the safety and effectiveness of moxifloxacin in treating clinical infections due to these microorganisms have not been established in adequate and well-controlled clinical trials.

Aerobic Gram-positive microorganisms

Streptococcus pneumoniae (penicillin-resistant strains)
Streptococcus pyogenes

Aerobic Gram-negative microorganisms

Citrobacter freundii
Enterobacter cloacae
Escherichia coli
Klebsiella oxytoca
Legionella pneumophila
Proteus mirabilis

Anaerobic microorganisms

Fusobacterium species
Peptostreptococcus species
Prevotella species

Susceptibility Tests

Dilution Techniques: Quantitative methods are used to determine antimicrobial minimum inhibitory concentrations (MICs). These MICs provide estimates of the susceptibility of bacteria to antimicrobial compounds. The MICs should be determined using a standardized procedure. Standardized procedures are based on a dilution method[1] (broth or agar) or equivalent with standardized inoculum concentrations and standardized concentrations of moxifloxacin powder. The MIC values should be interpreted according to the following criteria:

For testing Enterobacteriaceae and *Staphylococcus* species:

MIC (µg/mL)	Interpretation	
≤ 2.0	Susceptible	(S)
4.0	Intermediate	(I)
≥ 8.0	Resistant	(R)

For testing *Haemophilus influenzae* and *Haemophilus parainfluenzae*[a]:

MIC (µg/mL)	Interpretation	
≤ 1.0	Susceptible	(S)

[a] This interpretive standard is applicable only to broth microdilution susceptibility tests with *Haemophilus influenzae* and *Haemophilus parainfluenzae* using *Haemophilus* Test Medium[1].

The current absence of data on resistant strains precludes defining any results other than "Susceptible". Strains yielding MIC results suggestive of a "nonsusceptible" category should be submitted to a reference laboratory for further testing.

For testing *Streptococcus pneumoniae*[b]:

MIC (µg/mL)	Interpretation	
≤ 1.0	Susceptible	(S)
2.0	Intermediate	(I)
≥ 4.0	Resistant	(R)

[b] This interpretive standard is applicable only to broth microdilution susceptibility tests using cation-adjusted Mueller-Hinton broth with 2–5% lysed horse blood.

A report of "Susceptible" indicates that the pathogen is likely to be inhibited if the antimicrobial compound in the blood reaches the concentrations usually achievable. A report of "Intermediate" indicates that the result should be considered equivocal, and, if the microorganism is not fully susceptible to alternative, clinically feasible drugs, the test should be repeated. This category implies possible clinical applicability in body sites where the drug is physiologically concentrated or in situations where a high dosage of drug can be used. This category also provides a buffer zone which prevents small uncontrolled technical factors from causing major discrepancies in interpretation. A report of "Resistant" indicates that the pathogen is not likely to be inhibited if the antimicrobial compound in the blood reaches the concentrations usually achievable; other therapy should be selected.

Standardized susceptibility test procedures require the use of laboratory control microorganisms to control the technical aspects of the laboratory procedures. Standard moxifloxacin powder should provide the following MIC values:

Microorganism		MIC (µg/mL)
Enterococcus faecalis	ATCC 29212	0.06–0.5
Escherichia coli	ATCC 25922	0.008–0.06
Haemophilus influenzae	ATCC 49247[c]	0.008–0.03
Staphylococcus aureus	ATCC 29213	0.015–0.06
Streptococcus pneumoniae	ATCC 49619[d]	0.06–0.25

[c] This quality control range is applicable to only *H. influenzae* ATCC 49247 tested by a broth microdilution procedure using *Haemophilus* Test Medium (HTM)[1].

[d] This quality control range is applicable to only *S. pneumoniae* ATCC 49619 tested by a broth microdilution procedure using cation-adjusted Mueller-Hinton broth with 2–5% lysed horse blood.

Diffusion Techniques: Quantitative methods that require measurement of zone diameters also provide reproducible estimates of the susceptibility of bacteria to antimicrobial compounds. One such standardized procedure[2] requires the use of standardized inoculum concentrations. This procedure uses paper disks impregnated with 5-µg moxifloxacin to test the susceptibility of microorganisms to moxifloxacin. Reports from the laboratory providing results of the standard single-disk susceptibility test with a 5-µg moxifloxacin disk should be interpreted according to the following criteria:

The following zone diameter interpretive criteria should be used for testing Enterobacteriaceae and *Staphylococcus* species:

Zone Diameter (mm)	Interpretation	
≥ 19	Susceptible	(S)
16–18	Intermediate	(I)
≤ 15	Resistant	(R)

For testing *Haemophilus influenzae* and *Haemophilus parainfluenzae*[e]:

Zone Diameter (mm)	Interpretation	
≥ 18	Susceptible	(S)

[e] This zone diameter standard is applicable only to tests with *Haemophilus influenzae* and *Haemophilus parainfluenzae* using *Haemophilus* Test Medium (HTM) [2].

The current absence of data on resistant strains precludes defining any results other than "Susceptible". Strains yielding zone diameter results suggestive of a "nonsusceptible" category should be submitted to a reference laboratory for further testing.

For testing *Streptococcus pneumoniae*[f]:

Zone Diameter (mm)	Interpretation	
≥ 18	Susceptible	(S)
15–17	Intermediate	(I)
≤ 14	Resistant	(R)

[f] These interpretive standards are applicable only to disk diffusion tests using Mueller-Hinton agar supplemented with 5% sheep blood incubated in 5% CO_2.

Interpretation should be as stated above for results using dilution techniques. Interpretation involves correlation of the diameter obtained in the disk test with the MIC for moxifloxacin.

As with standardized dilution techniques, diffusion methods require the use of laboratory control microorganisms that are used to control the technical aspects of the laboratory procedures. For the diffusion technique, the 5-µg moxifloxacin disk should provide the following zone diameters in these laboratory test quality control strains:

Microorganism		Zone Diameter (mm)
Escherichia coli	ATCC 25922	28–35
Haemophilus influenzae	ATCC 49247[g]	31–39
Staphylococcus aureus	ATCC 25923	28–35
Streptococcus pneumoniae	ATCC 49619[h]	25–31

[g] These quality control limits are applicable to only *H. influenzae* ATCC 49247 testing using *Haemophilus* Test Medium (HTM)[2].

[h] These quality control limits are applicable only to tests conducted with *S. pneumoniae* ATCC 49619 performed by disk diffusion using Mueller-Hinton agar supplemented with 5% defibrinated sheep blood.

INDICATIONS AND USAGE

AVELOX Tablets are indicated for the treatment of adults (≥ 18 years of age) with infections caused by susceptible strains of the designated microorganisms in the conditions listed below. Please see **DOSAGE AND ADMINISTRATION** for specific recommendations.

Acute Bacterial Sinusitis caused by *Streptococcus pneumoniae, Haemophilus influenzae*, or *Moraxella catarrhalis*.

Acute Bacterial Exacerbation of Chronic Bronchitis caused by *Streptococcus pneumoniae, Haemophilus influenzae, Haemophilus parainfluenzae, Klebsiella pneumoniae, Staphylococcus aureus*, or *Moraxella catarrhalis*.

Community Acquired Pneumonia (of mild to moderate severity) caused by *Streptococcus pneumoniae, Haemophilus influenzae, Mycoplasma pneumoniae, Chlamydia pneumoniae*, or *Moraxella catarrhalis*.

Appropriate culture and susceptibility tests should be performed before treatment in order to isolate and identify organisms causing infection and to determine their susceptibility to moxifloxacin. Therapy with AVELOX may be initiated before results of these tests are known; once results become available, appropriate therapy should be continued.

CONTRAINDICATIONS

Moxifloxacin is contraindicated in persons with a history of hypersensitivity to moxifloxacin or any member of the quinolone class of antimicrobial agents.

WARNINGS

THE SAFETY AND EFFECTIVENESS OF MOXIFLOXACIN IN PEDIATRIC PATIENTS, ADOLESCENTS (LESS THAN 18 YEARS OF AGE), PREGNANT WOMEN, AND LACTATING WOMEN HAVE NOT BEEN ESTABLISHED. (SEE PRECAUTIONS-PEDIATRIC USE, PREGNANCY AND NURSING MOTHERS SUBSECTIONS.)

MOXIFLOXACIN HAS BEEN SHOWN TO PROLONG THE QT INTERVAL OF THE ELECTROCARDIOGRAM IN SOME PATIENTS. THE DRUG SHOULD BE AVOIDED IN PATIENTS WITH KNOWN PROLONGATION OF THE QT INTERVAL, PATIENTS WITH UNCORRECTED HYPOKALEMIA AND PATIENTS RECEIVING CLASS IA (E.G. QUINIDINE, PROCAINAMIDE) OR CLASS III (E.G. AMIODARONE, SOTALOL) ANTIARRHYTHMIC AGENTS, DUE TO THE LACK OF CLINICAL EXPERIENCE WITH THE DRUG IN THESE PATIENT POPULATIONS.

Pharmacokinetic studies between moxifloxacin and other drugs that prolong the QT interval such as cisapride, erythromycin, antipsychotics, and tricyclic antidepressants have not been performed. An additive effect of moxifloxacin and these drugs cannot be excluded, therefore moxifloxacin should be used with caution when given concurrently with these drugs.

The effect of moxifloxacin on patients with congenital prolongation of the QT interval has not been studied, however, it is expected that these individuals may be more susceptible to drug-induced QT prolongation. Because of limited clinical experience, moxifloxacin should be used with caution in patients with ongoing proarrhythmic conditions, such as clinically significant bradycardia, acute myocardial ischemia.

The magnitude of QT prolongation may increase with increasing concentrations of the drug, therefore the recommended dose should not be exceeded. QT prolongation may lead to an increased risk for ventricular arrhythmias including torsade de pointes. In 787 patients with paired valid ECGs in Phase III clinical trials, the mean ± SD effect of moxifloxacin 400 mg on the QTc interval was 6 ± 26 msec. No cardiovascular morbidity or mortality attributable to QTc prolongation occurred with moxifloxacin treatment in over 4000 patients, however certain predisposing conditions may increase the risk for ventricular arrhythmias.

The oral administration of moxifloxacin caused lameness in immature dogs. Histopathological examination of the weight-bearing joints of these dogs revealed permanent lesions of the cartilage. Related quinolone-class drugs also produce erosions of cartilage of weight-bearing joints and other signs of arthropathy in immature animals of various species. (See **ANIMAL PHARMACOLOGY**.)

Convulsions have been reported in patients receiving quinolones. Quinolones may also cause central nervous system (CNS) events including: dizziness, confusion, tremors, hallucinations, depression, and, rarely, suicidal thoughts or acts. These reactions may occur following the first dose. If these reactions occur in patients receiving moxifloxacin, the drug should be discontinued and appropriate measures instituted. As with all quinolones, moxifloxacin should be used with caution in patients with known or suspected CNS disorders (e.g. severe cerebral arteriosclerosis, epilepsy) or in the presence of other risk factors that may predispose to seizures or lower the seizure threshold. (See **PRECAUTIONS: General, Information for Patients**, and **ADVERSE REACTIONS**.)

Serious and occasionally fatal hypersensitivity (anaphylactic) reactions, some following the first dose, have been reported in patients receiving quinolone therapy. Some reactions were accompanied by cardiovascular collapse, loss of consciousness, tingling, pharyngeal or facial edema, dyspnea, urticaria, and itching. Serious anaphylactic reactions require immediate emergency treatment with epinephrine. Moxifloxacin should be discontinued at the first appearance of a skin rash or any other sign of hypersensitivity. Oxygen, intravenous steroids, and airway management, including intubation, may be administered as indicated.

Severe and sometimes fatal events, some due to hypersensitivity, and some of uncertain etiology, have been reported in patients receiving therapy with all antibiotics. These events may be severe and generally occur following the administration of multiple doses. Clinical manifestations may include one or more of the following: rash, fever, eosinophilia, jaundice, and hepatic necrosis.

Pseudomembranous colitis has been reported with nearly all antibacterial agents and may range in severity from mild to life-threatening. Therefore, it is important to consider this diagnosis in patients who present with diarrhea subsequent to the administration of antibacterial agents.

Treatment with antibacterial agents alters the normal flora of the colon and may permit overgrowth of clostridia. Studies indicate that a toxin produced by *Clostridium difficile* is one primary cause of "antibiotic-associated colitis."

After the diagnosis of pseudomembranous colitis has been established, therapeutic measures should be initiated. Mild cases of pseudomembranous colitis usually respond to drug discontinuation alone. In moderate to severe cases, consideration should be given to management with fluids and electrolytes, protein supplementation, and treatment with an antibacterial drug clinically effective against *C. difficile* colitis.

Although not observed in moxifloxacin clinical trials, Achilles and other tendon ruptures that required surgical repair or resulted in prolonged disability have been reported with quinolones. Moxifloxacin should be discontinued if the patient experiences pain, inflammation, or rupture of a tendon.

PRECAUTIONS

General: Quinolones may cause central nervous system (CNS) events, including: nervousness, agitation, insomnia, anxiety, nightmares or paranoia. (See **WARNINGS** and **Information for Patients**.)

Information for Patients:

To assure safe and effective use of moxifloxacin, the following information and instructions should be communicated to the patient when appropriate:

Patients should be advised:

- that moxifloxacin may produce changes in the electrocardiogram (QTc interval prolongation).
- that moxifloxacin should be avoided in patients receiving Class IA (e.g. quinidine, procainamide) or Class III (e.g. amiodarone, sotalol) antiarrhythmic agents.
- that moxifloxacin may add to the QTc prolonging effects of other drugs such as cisapride, erythromycin, antipsychotics, and tricyclic antidepressants.
- to inform their physician of any personal or family history of QTc prolongation or proarrhythmic conditions such as recent hypokalemia, significant bradycardia, acute myocardial ischemia.

Continued on next page

Avelox—Cont.

- to inform their physician of any other medications when taken concurrently with moxifloxacin, including over-the-counter medications.
- to contact their physician if they experience palpitations or fainting spells while taking moxifloxacin.
- that moxifloxacin may be taken with or without meals, and to drink fluids liberally.
- that moxifloxacin should be taken at least 4 hours before or 8 hours after multivitamins (containing iron or zinc), antacids (containing magnesium, calcium, or aluminum), sucralfate, or Videx® (didanosine) chewable/buffered tablets or the pediatric powder for oral solution. (See **CLINICAL PHARMACOLOGY, Drug Interactions** and **PRECAUTIONS, Drug Interactions.**)
- that moxifloxacin may be associated with hypersensitivity reactions, even following a single dose, and to discontinue the drug at the first sign of a skin rash or other signs of an allergic reaction.
- to discontinue treatment; rest and refrain from exercise; and inform their physician if they experience pain, inflammation, or rupture of a tendon.
- that moxifloxacin may cause dizziness and lightheadedness; therefore, patients should know how they react to this drug before they operate an automobile or machinery or engage in activities requiring mental alertness or coordination.
- that phototoxicity has been reported in patients receiving certain quinolones. There was no phototoxicity seen with moxifloxacin at the recommended dose. In keeping with good medical practice, avoid excessive sunlight or artificial ultraviolet light (e.g. tanning beds). If sunburn-like reaction or skin eruptions occur, contact your physician. (See **CLINICAL PHARMACOLOGY, Photosensitivity Potential.**)
- that convulsions have been reported in patients receiving quinolones, and they should notify their physician before taking this drug if there is a history of this condition.

Drug Interactions:

Antacids, Sucralfate, Metal Cations, Multivitamins: Quinolones form chelates with alkaline earth and transition metal cations. Administration of quinolones with antacids containing aluminum, magnesium, or calcium, with sucralfate, with metal cations such as iron, or with multivitamins containing iron or zinc, or with formulations containing divalent and trivalent cations such as Videx® (didanosine) chewable/buffered tablets or the pediatric powder for oral solution, may substantially interfere with the absorption of quinolones, resulting in systemic concentrations considerably lower than desired. Therefore, moxifloxacin should be taken at least 4 hours before or 8 hours after these agents. (See **CLINICAL PHARMACOLOGY, Drug Interactions** and **DOSAGE AND ADMINISTRATION.**)

No clinically significant drug-drug interactions between theophylline, warfarin, digoxin, or glyburide have been observed with moxifloxacin. Theophylline, digoxin, probenecid, and ranitidine have been shown not to alter the pharmacokinetics of moxifloxacin. (See **CLINICAL PHARMACOLOGY.**)

Warfarin: No significant effect of moxifloxacin on R- and S-warfarin was detected in a clinical study involving 24 healthy volunteers. No significant changes in prothrombin time were noted in the presence of moxifloxacin. However, since some quinolones have been reported to enhance the anticoagulant effects of warfarin or its derivatives in the patient population, the prothrombin time or other suitable coagulation test should be closely monitored if a quinolone antimicrobial is administered concomitantly with warfarin or its derivatives.

Drugs metabolized by Cytochrome P450 enzymes: *In vitro* studies with cytochrome P450 isoenzymes (CYP) indicate that moxifloxacin does not inhibit CYP3A4, CYP2D6, CYP2C9, CYP2C19, or CYP1A2, suggesting that moxifloxacin is unlikely to alter the pharmacokinetics of drugs metabolized by these enzymes (e.g. midazolam, cyclosporine, warfarin, theophylline).

Nonsteroidal anti-inflammatory drugs (NSAIDs): Although not observed with moxifloxacin in preclinical and clinical trials, the concomitant administration of a nonsteroidal anti-inflammatory drug with a quinolone may increase the risks of CNS stimulation and convulsions. (See **WARNINGS.**)

Carcinogenesis, Mutagenesis, Impairment of Fertility:

Long term studies in animals to determine the carcinogenic potential of moxifloxacin have not been performed.

Moxifloxacin was not mutagenic in 4 bacterial strains (TA 98, TA 100, TA 1535, TA 1537) used in the Ames *Salmonella* reversion assay. As with other quinolones, the positive response observed with moxifloxacin in strain TA 102 using the same assay may be due to the inhibition of DNA gyrase. Moxifloxacin was not mutagenic in the CHO/HGPRT mammalian cell gene mutation assay. An equivocal result was obtained in the same assay when v79 cells were used. Moxifloxacin was clastogenic in the v79 chromosome aberration assay, but it did not induce unscheduled DNA synthesis in cultured rat hepatocytes. There was no evidence of genotoxicity *in vivo* in a micronucleus test or a dominant lethal test in mice.

Moxifloxacin had no effect on fertility in male and female rats at oral doses as high as 500 mg/kg/day, approximately 12 times the maximum recommended human dose based on body surface area (mg/m^2). At 500 mg/kg there were slight effects on sperm morphology (head-tail separation) in male rats and on the estrous cycle in female rats.

Pregnancy: Teratogenic Effects. Pregnancy Category C:

Moxifloxacin was not teratogenic when administered to pregnant rats during organogenesis at oral doses as high as 500 mg/kg/day or 0.24 times the maximum recommended human dose based on systemic exposure (AUC), but decreased fetal body weights and slightly delayed fetal skeletal development (indicative of fetotoxicity) were observed. Intravenous administration of 20 mg/kg/day (approximately equal to the maximum recommended human oral dose based upon systemic exposure) to pregnant rabbits during organogenesis resulted in decreased fetal body weights and delayed fetal skeletal ossification. When rib and vertebral malformations were combined, there was an increased fetal and litter incidence of these effects. Signs of maternal toxicity in rabbits at this dose included mortality, abortions, marked reduction of food consumption, decreased water intake, body weight loss and hypoactivity. There was no evidence of teratogenicity when pregnant Cynomolgus monkeys were given oral doses as high as 100 mg/kg/day (2.5 times the maximum recommended human dose based upon systemic exposure). An increased incidence of smaller fetuses was observed at 100 mg/kg/day. In an oral pre- and postnatal development study conducted in rats, effects observed at 500 mg/kg/day included slight increases in duration of pregnancy and prenatal loss, reduced pup birth weight and decreased neonatal survival. Treatment-related maternal mortality occurred during gestation at 500 mg/kg/day in this study.

Since there are no adequate or well-controlled studies in pregnant women, moxifloxacin should be used during pregnancy only if the potential benefit justifies the potential risk to the fetus.

Nursing Mothers: Moxifloxacin is excreted in the breast milk of rats. Moxifloxacin may also be excreted in human milk. Because of the potential for serious adverse reactions in infants nursing from mothers taking moxifloxacin, a decision should be made whether to discontinue nursing or to discontinue the drug, taking into account the importance of the drug to the mother.

Pediatric Use: Safety and effectiveness in pediatric patients and adolescents less than 18 years of age have not been established. Moxifloxacin causes arthropathy in juvenile animals. (See **WARNINGS.**)

Geriatric Use: In controlled multiple-dose clinical trials, 23% of patients receiving moxifloxacin were greater than or equal to 65 years of age and 9% were greater than or equal to 75 years of age. The clinical trial data demonstrate that there is no difference in the safety and efficacy of moxifloxacin in patients aged 65 or older compared to younger adults.

ADVERSE REACTIONS

Clinical efficacy trials enrolled over 4900 moxifloxacin treated patients, of whom over 4300 patients received the 400 mg dose. Most adverse events reported in moxifloxacin trials were described as mild to moderate in severity and required no treatment. Moxifloxacin was discontinued due to adverse reactions thought to be drug-related in 3.8% of patients.

Adverse reactions, judged by investigators to be at least possibly drug-related, occurring in greater than or equal to 1% of moxifloxacin treated patients were: nausea (8%), diarrhea (6%), dizziness (3%), headache (2%), abdominal pain (2%), vomiting (2%), taste perversion (1%), abnormal liver function test (1%), and dyspepsia (1%).

Additional events, judged by investigators to be at least possibly drug-related, that occurred in greater than 0.05% and less than 1% of moxifloxacin treated patients were:

BODY AS A WHOLE: asthenia, moniliasis, pain, malaise, lab test abnormal (not specified), allergic reaction, leg pain, pelvic pain, abdominal pain, back pain, chills, infection, chest pain, hand pain

CARDIOVASCULAR: palpitation, vasodilatation, tachycardia, hypertension, peripheral edema, hypotension

CENTRAL NERVOUS SYSTEM: insomnia, nervousness, anxiety, confusion, hallucinations, depersonalization, hypertonia, incoordination, somnolence, tremor, vertigo, paresthesia

DIGESTIVE: dry mouth, constipation, oral moniliasis, anorexia, stomatitis, gastritis, glossitis, gastrointestinal disorder, cholestatic jaundice, GGTP increased

HEMIC AND LYMPHATIC: prothrombin time decrease, prothrombin time increase, thrombocythemia, thrombocytopenia, eosinophilia, leukopenia

METABOLIC AND NUTRITIONAL: amylase increased, hyperglycemia, hyperlipidemia, lactic dehydrogenase increased

MUSCULOSKELETAL: arthralgia, myalgia

RESPIRATORY: asthma, dyspnea, cough increased, pneumonia, pharyngitis, rhinitis, sinusitis

SKIN/APPENDAGES: rash, pruritus, sweating, urticaria, dry skin,

SPECIAL SENSES: tinnitus, amblyopia

UROGENITAL: vaginal moniliasis, vaginitis,cystitis, kidney function abnormal

LABORATORY CHANGES

Changes in laboratory parameters, without regard to drug relationship, which are not listed above and which occurred in ≥ 2% of patients and at an incidence greater than in controls included: increases in MCH, neutrophils, WBCs, PT ratio, ionized calcium, chloride, albumin, globulin, bilirubin; decreases in hemoglobin, RBCs, neutrophils, eosinophils, basophils, PT ratio, glucose, pO_2, bilirubin and amylase. It cannot be determined if any of the above laboratory abnormalities were caused by the drug or the underlying condition being treated.

OVERDOSAGE

In the event of acute overdosage, the stomach should be emptied and ECG monitoring is recommended due to the possible prolongation of the QT interval. The patient should be carefully observed and given supportive treatment. Adequate hydration must be maintained. It is not known whether moxifloxacin is dialyzable.

Single oral moxifloxacin doses of 2000, 500, and 1500 mg/kg were lethal to rats, mice, and cynomolgus monkeys, respectively. The minimum lethal intravenous dose in mice and rats was 100 mg/kg. Toxic signs after administration of a single high dose of moxifloxacin to these animals included CNS and gastrointestinal effects such as decreased activity, somnolence, tremor, convulsions, vomiting and diarrhea.

DOSAGE AND ADMINISTRATION

The dose of AVELOX Tablets is one 400 mg tablet taken orally every 24 hours. The duration of therapy depends on the type of infection as described below.

Infection*	Daily Dose	Duration
Acute Bacterial Sinusitis	400 mg	10 days
Acute Bacterial Exacerbation of Chronic Bronchitis	400 mg	5 days
Community Acquired Pneumonia	400 mg	10 days

* due to the designated pathogens (See **INDICATIONS AND USAGE.**)

Oral doses of moxifloxacin should be administered at least 4 hours before or 8 hours after antacids containing magnesium or aluminum, as well as sucralfate, metal cations such as iron, and multivitamin preparations with zinc, or Videx® (didanosine) chewable/buffered tablets or the pediatric powder for oral solution. (See **CLINICAL PHARMACOLOGY, Drug Interactions** and **PRECAUTIONS, Drug Interactions.**)

Impaired Renal Function

No dosage adjustment is required in renally impaired patients. Moxifloxacin has not been studied in patients on hemodialysis or continuous ambulatory peritoneal dialysis (CAPD).

Impaired Hepatic Function

No dosage adjustment is required in patients with mild or moderate hepatic insufficiency (Child Pugh Classes A and B). The pharmacokinetics of moxifloxacin in patients with severe hepatic insufficiency (Child Pugh Class C) have not been studied. (See **CLINICAL PHARMACOLOGY, Hepatic Insufficiency.**)

HOW SUPPLIED

AVELOX (moxifloxacin hydrochloride) Tablets are available as oblong, dull red film-coated tablets containing 400 mg moxifloxacin. The tablet is coded with the word "BAYER" on one side and "M400" on the reverse side.

Package	NDC Code
Bottles of 30:	0026-8581-69
ABC Pack of 5:	0026-8581-41

Store at 25°C (77°F); excursions permitted to 15–30°C (59–86°F) [see USP Controlled Room Temperature]. Avoid high humidity.

ANIMAL PHARMACOLOGY

Quinolones have been shown to cause arthropathy in immature animals. In studies in juvenile dogs oral doses of moxifloxacin ≥ 30 mg/kg/day (approximately 1.5 times the maximum recommended human dose based upon systemic exposure) for 28 days resulted in arthropathy. There was no evidence of arthropathy in mature monkeys and rats at oral doses up to 135 and 500 mg/kg, respectively.

Unlike some other members of the quinolone class, crystalluria was not observed in 6 month repeat dose studies in rats and monkeys with moxifloxacin.

Ocular toxicity was not observed in 6 month repeat dose studies in rats and monkeys. In beagle dogs, electroretinographic (ERG) changes were observed in a 2 week study at doses of 60 and 90 mg/kg. Histopathological changes were observed in the retina from one of four dogs at 90 mg/kg, a dose associated with mortality in this study.

Some quinolones have been reported to have proconvulsant activity that is exacerbated with concomitant use of non-steroidal anti-inflammatory drugs (NSAIDs). Moxifloxacin at an oral dose of 300 mg/kg did not show an increase in acute toxicity or potential for CNS toxicity (e.g. seizures) in mice when used in combination with NSAIDs such as diclofenac, ibuprofen, or fenbufen.

In animal studies, at plasma concentrations about five times the human therapeutic level, a QT-prolonging effect of moxifloxacin was found. Electrophysiological *in vitro* studies suggested an inhibition of the rapid activating component of the delayed rectifier potassium current (I_{Kr}) as an underlying mechanism. In dogs, the combined infusion of sotalol, a Class III antiarrhythmic agent, with moxifloxacin induced a higher degree of QTc prolongation than that induced by the same dose (30mg/kg) of moxifloxacin alone.

CLINICAL STUDIES

Acute Bacterial Exacerbation of Chronic Bronchitis

AVELOX Tablets (400 mg once daily for five days) were evaluated for the treatment of acute bacterial exacerbation of chronic bronchitis in a large, randomized, double-blind, controlled clinical trial conducted in the US. This study compared AVELOX with clarithromycin (500 mg twice daily for 10 days) and enrolled 629 patients. The primary endpoint for this trial was clinical success at 7–17 days post-therapy. The clinical success for AVELOX was 89% (222/250) compared to 89% (224/251) for clarithromycin.

The following outcomes are the clinical success rates at the follow-up visit for the clinically evaluable patient groups by pathogen:

PATHOGEN	AVELOX	Clarithromycin
Streptococcus pneumoniae	100% (16/16)	87% (20/23)
Haemophilus influenzae	89% (33/37)	88% (36/41)
Haemophilus parainfluenzae	100% (16/16)	100% (14/14)
Moraxella catarrhalis	85% (29/34)	100% (24/24)
Staphylococcus aureus	94% (15/16)	75% (6/8)
Klebsiella pneumoniae	90% (18/20)	91% (10/11)

The microbiological eradication rates (eradication plus presumed eradication) in AVELOX treated patients were *Streptococcus pneumoniae* 100%, *Haemophilus influenzae* 89%, *Haemophilus parainfluenzae* 100%, *Moraxella catarrhalis* 85%, *Staphylococcus aureus* 94%, and *Klebsiella pneumoniae* 85%.

Community Acquired Pneumonia

A large, randomized, double-blind, controlled clinical trial was conducted in the US to compare the efficacy of AVELOX Tablets (400 mg once daily) to that of high-dose clarithromycin (500 mg twice daily) in the treatment of patients with clinically and radiologically documented community acquired pneumonia. This study enrolled 474 patients (382 of which were valid for the primary efficacy analysis conducted at the 14–35 day follow-up visit). Clinical success for clinically evaluable patients was 95% (184/194) for AVELOX and 95% (178/188) for high dose clarithromycin.

In addition to the trial described above, a noncomparative trial of AVELOX (400 mg once daily for ten days) was also conducted in the US in patients with community acquired pneumonia. The combined moxifloxacin clinical success rates by pathogen for the two studies were as follows:

PATHOGEN	14–35 DAY FOLLOW-UP
Streptococcus pneumoniae	97% (30/31)
Haemophilus influenzae	92% (33/36)
Mycoplasma pneumoniae	96% (51/53)
Chlamydia pneumoniae	93% (106/114)
Moraxella catarrhalis	91% (10/11)

The microbiological eradication rates (eradication plus presumed eradication) in AVELOX treated patients were *Streptococcus pneumoniae* 97%, *Haemophilus influenzae* 92%, and *Moraxella catarrhalis* 91%.

Acute Bacterial Sinusitis

In a large, controlled double-blind study conducted in the US, AVELOX (400 mg once daily for ten days) was compared with cefuroxime axetil (250 mg twice daily for ten days) for the treatment of acute bacterial sinusitis. The trial included 457 patients valid for the primary efficacy determination. Clinical success (cure plus improvement) at the 7 to 21 day post-therapy test of cure visit was 90% for AVELOX and 89% for cefuroxime.

An additional non-comparative study was conducted to gather bacteriological data and to evaluate microbiological eradication in adult patients treated with AVELOX 400 mg once daily for seven days. All patients (n = 336) underwent antral puncture in this study. Clinical success rates and eradication/presumed eradication rates at the 21 to 37 day follow-up visit were 97% (29 out of 30) for *Streptococcus pneumoniae*, 83% (15 out of 18) for *Moraxella catarrhalis*, and 80% (24 out of 30) for *Haemophilus influenzae*.

REFERENCES:

1. National Committee for Clinical Laboratory Standards, Methods for Dilution Antimicrobial Susceptibility Tests for Bacteria That Grow Aerobically-Fourth Edition. Approved Standard NCCLS Document M7-A4, Vol. 17, No. 2, NCCLS, Wayne, PA, January 1997.

2. National Committee for Clinical Laboratory Standards, Performance Standards for Antimicrobial Disk Susceptibility Tests-Sixth Edition. Approved Standard NCCLS Document M2-A6, Vol. 17, No. 1, NCCLS, Wayne, PA, January, 1997.

Bayer Corporation
Pharmaceutical Division
400 Morgan Lane
West Haven, CT 06516
Made in Germany

Rx Only

Patient Information About:
AVELOX™
(moxifloxacin hydrochloride)
400 mg Tablets

This section contains important patient information about AVELOX (moxifloxacin hydrochloride), and should be read completely before you begin treatment. This section does not take the place of discussions with your doctor or health care professional about your medical condition or your treatment. This section does not list all benefits and risks of AVELOX. The medicine described here can be prescribed only by a licensed health care professional. If you have any questions about AVELOX talk with your health care professional. Only your health care professional can determine if AVELOX is right for you.

What is AVELOX?

AVELOX is an antibiotic used to treat lung or sinus infections caused by certain germs called bacteria. AVELOX kills many of the types of bacteria that can infect the lungs and sinuses and has been shown in a large number of clinical trials to be safe and effective for the treatment of bacterial infections.

Sometimes viruses rather than bacteria may infect the lungs and sinuses (for example the common cold). AVELOX, like all other antibiotics, does not kill viruses.

You should contact your doctor if you think your condition is not improving while taking AVELOX. AVELOX Tablets are red and contain 400 mg of active drug.

How and when should I take AVELOX?

AVELOX should be taken once a day for 5 or 10 days depending on your prescription. It should be swallowed and may be taken with or without food. Try to take the tablet at the same time each day.

You may begin to feel better quickly; however, in order to make sure that all bacteria are killed, you should complete the full course of medication. Do not take more than the prescribed dose of AVELOX even if you missed a dose by mistake. You should not take a double dose.

Who should not take AVELOX?

You should not take AVELOX if you have ever had a severe allergic reaction to any of the group of antibiotics known as "quinolones" such as ciprofloxacin or levofloxacin.

You should avoid AVELOX if you have a rare condition known as congenital prolongation of the QT interval. If you or any of your family members have this condition you should inform your health care professional. You should avoid AVELOX if you are being treated for heart rhythm disturbances with certain medicines such as quinidine, procainamide, amiodarone, or sotalol. Inform your health care professional if you are taking a heart rhythm drug.

You should also avoid AVELOX if the amount of potassium in your blood is low. Low potassium can sometimes be caused by medicines called diuretics such as furosemide and hydrochlorothiazide. If you are taking a diuretic medicine you should speak with your health care professional.

If you are pregnant or planning to become pregnant while taking AVELOX, talk to your doctor before taking this medication. AVELOX is not recommended for use during pregnancy or nursing, as the effects on the unborn child or nursing infant are unknown.

AVELOX is not recommended for children.

What are the possible side effects of AVELOX?

AVELOX is generally well tolerated. The most common side effects caused by AVELOX, which are usually mild, include nausea, vomiting, stomach pain, diarrhea, dizziness and headache. You should be careful about driving or operating machinery until you are sure AVELOX is not causing dizziness. If you notice any side effects not mentioned in this section or you have any concerns about the side effects you are experiencing, please inform your health care professional.

In some people, AVELOX, as with some other antibiotics, may produce a small effect on the heart that is seen on an electrocardiogram test. Although this has not caused any serious problems in more than 4000 patients who have already taken the medication, in theory it could result in extremely rare cases of abnormal heartbeat which may be dangerous. Contact your health care professional if you develop heart palpitations (fast beating), or have fainting spells.

Which medicines should not be used with AVELOX?

You should avoid taking AVELOX with certain medicines used to treat abnormal heartbeat. These include quinidine, procainamide, amiodarone and sotalol.

Some medicines also produce an effect on the electrocardiogram test, including cisapride, erythromycin, some antidepressants and some antipsychotic drugs. These may increase the risk of heart beat problems when taken with AVELOX. For this reason it is important to let your health care provider know all of the medicines that you are using.

Many antacids and multivitamins may interfere with the absorption of AVELOX and may prevent it from working properly. You should take AVELOX either 4 hours before or 8 hours after taking these products.

Remember

Take your dose of AVELOX once a day.

Complete the course of medication even if you are feeling better.

Keep this medication out of the reach of children.

This information does not take the place of discussions with your doctor or health care professional about your medical condition or your treatment.

Bayer Corporation
Pharmaceutical Division
400 Morgan Lane
West Haven, CT 06516
Made in Germany

Rx Only

BAYCOL® ℞
(cerivastatin sodium tablets)

DESCRIPTION

Cerivastatin sodium is sodium [S-[R*,S*-(E)]]-7-[4-(4-fluorophenyl) -5-methoxymethyl) -2,6bis (1-methylethyl) -3-pyridinyl]-3,5-dihydroxy-6-heptenoate. The empirical formula for cerivastatin sodium is $C_{26}H_{33}FNO_5Na$ and its molecular weight is 481.5. It has the following chemical structure:

Cerivastatin sodium is a white to off-white hygroscopic amorphous powder that is soluble in water, methanol, and ethanol, and very slightly soluble in acetone.

Cerivastatin sodium is an entirely synthetic, enantiomerically pure inhibitor of 3-hydroxy-3-methylglutaryl-coenzyme A (HMG-CoA) reductase. HMG-CoA reductase catalyzes the conversion of HMG-CoA to mevalonate, which is an early and rate-limiting step in the biosynthesis of cholesterol.

BAYCOL® (cerivastatin sodium tablets) is supplied as tablets containing 0.2, 0.3, 0.4 or 0.8 mg of cerivastatin sodium, for oral administration. Active Ingredient: cerivastatin sodium. Inactive Ingredients: mannitol, magnesium stearate, sodium hydroxide, crospovidone, povidone, iron oxide yellow, methylhydroxypropylcellulose, polyethylene glycol, and titanium dioxide.

CLINICAL PHARMACOLOGY

Cholesterol and triglycerides circulate as part of lipoprotein complexes throughout the bloodstream. These complexes can be separated via ultracentrifugation into high-density lipoprotein (HDL), intermediate-density lipoprotein (IDL), low-density lipoprotein (LDL) and very-low-density lipoprotein (VLDL) fractions. In the liver, cholesterol and triglycerides (TG) are synthesized, incorporated into VLDL, and released into the plasma for delivery to peripheral tissues.

A variety of clinical studies have demonstrated that elevated levels of total cholesterol (total-C), LDL-C, and apolipoprotein B (apo-B, a membrane complex for LDL-C) promote human atherosclerosis. Similarly, decreased levels of HDL-C (and its transport complex, apolipoprotein A) are associated with the development of atherosclerosis. Epidemiologic investigations have established that cardiovascular morbidity and mortality vary directly with the level of total-C and LDL-C and inversely with the level of HDL-C.

Like LDL, cholesterol-enriched triglyceride-rich lipoproteins, including VLDL, IDL and remnants, can also promote atherosclerosis. Elevated plasma triglycerides are frequently found in a triad with low HDL-C levels and small LDL particles, as well as in association with nonlipid metabolic risk factors for coronary heart disease. As such, total plasma TG has not consistently been shown to be an independent risk factor for CHD. Furthermore, the independent effect of raising HDL or lowering TG on the risk of coronary and cardiovascular morbidity and mortality has not been determined.

In patients with hypercholesterolemia, BAYCOL® (cerivastatin sodium tablets) has been shown to reduce plasma total cholesterol, LDL-C, and apolipoprotein B. In addition, it also reduces VLDL-C and plasma triglycerides and increases plasma HDL-C and apolipoprotein A-1. The agent has no consistent effect on plasma Lp(a). The effect of BAYCOL® on cardiovascular morbidity and mortality has not been determined.

Mechanism of Action: Cerivastatin is a competitive inhibitor of HMG-CoA reductase, which is responsible for the conversion of 3-hydroxy-3-methyl-glutaryl-coenzyme A (HMG-CoA) to mevalonate, a precursor of sterols, including cholesterol. The inhibition of cholesterol biosynthesis by cerivastatin reduces the level of cholesterol in hepatic cells, which stimulates the synthesis of LDL receptors, thereby increasing the uptake of cellular LDL particles. The end result of these biochemical processes is a reduction of the plasma cholesterol concentration.

Pharmacokinetics:

Absorption: BAYCOL® (cerivastatin sodium tablets) is administered orally in the active form. The mean absolute bioavailability of cerivastatin following a 0.2-mg tablet oral dose is 60% (range 39 - 101%). In general, the coefficient of variation (based on the inter-subject variability) for both systemic exposure (area under the curve, AUC) and C_{max} is in the 20% to 40% range. The bioavailability of cerivastatin sodium tablets is equivalent to that of a solution of cerivastatin sodium. No unchanged cerivastatin is excreted in feces. Cerivastatin exhibits linear kinetics over the dose range of 0.2 to 0.8-mg daily. In male and female patients at steady-state, the mean maximum concentrations (C_{max}) following evening cerivastatin tablet doses of 0.2, 0.3, 0.4, and 0.8-mg are 2.8, 5.1, 6.2, and 12.7 µg/L, respectively. AUC values are also dose-proportional over this dose range and the mean time to maximum concentration (t_{max}) is approximately 2 hours for all dose strengths. Following oral administration, the terminal elimination half-life ($t_{1/2}$) for cerivastatin is 2 to 4 hours. Steady-state plasma concentrations show no evidence of cerivastatin accumulation following administration of up to 0.8 mg daily.

Results from an overnight pharmacokinetic evaluation following single-dose administration of cerivastatin with the

Continued on next page

Baycol—Cont.

evening meal or 4 hours after the evening meal showed that administration of cerivastatin with the evening meal did not significantly alter either AUC or C_{max} compared to dosing the drug 4 hours after the evening meal. In patients given 0.2 mg cerivastatin sodium once daily for 4 weeks, either at mealtime or at bedtime, there were no differences in the lipid-lowering effects of cerivastatin. Both regimens of 0.2 mg once daily were slightly more efficacious than 0.1 mg twice daily.

Distribution: The volume of distribution (VD_{ss}) is calculated to be 0.3 L/kg. More than 99% of the circulating drug is bound to plasma proteins (80% to albumin). Binding is reversible and independent of drug concentration up to 100 mg/L.

Metabolism: Biotransformation pathways for cerivastatin in humans include the following: demethylation of the pyridilic methyl ether to form M1 and hydroxylation of the methyl group in the 6'-isopropyl moiety to form M23. The combination of both reactions leads to formation of metabolite M24. The major circulating blood components are cerivastatin and the pharmacologically active M1 and M23 metabolites. The relative potencies of metabolites M1 and M23 are comparable to, but do not exceed, the potency of the parent conpound. Following a 0.8-mg dose of cerivastatin to male and female patients, mean steady state C_{max} values for cerivastatin, M1, and M23 were 12.7, 0.55, and 1.4 μg/L, respectively. Therefore, the cholesterol-lowering effect is due primarily to the parent compound, cerivastatin.

Excretion: Cerivastatin itself is not found in either urine or feces; M1 and M23 are the major metabolites excreted by these routes. Following an oral dose of 0.4 mg ^{14}C-cerivastatin to healthy volunteers, excretion of radioactivity is about 24% in the urine and 70% in the feces. The parent compound, cerivastatin, accounts for less than 2% of the total radioactivity excreted. The plasma clearance for cerivastatin in humans after intravenous dosing is 12 to 13 liters per hour.

Special Populations

Geriatric: Plasma concentrations of cerivastatin are similar in healthy elderly male subjects (>65 years) and in young males (<40 years).

Gender: Plasma concentrations of cerivastatin in females are slightly higher than in males (approximately 12% higher for C_{max} and 16% higher for AUC).

Pediatric: Cerivastatin pharmacokinetics have not been studied in pediatric patients.

Race: Cerivastatin pharmacokinetics were compared across studies in Caucasian, Japanese and Black subjects. No significant differences in AUC, C_{max}, t_{max}, and $t_{1/2}$ were found.

Renal: Steady-state plasma concentrations of cerivastatin are similar in healthy volunteers (Cl_{cr}>90 mL/min/1.73m^2) and in patients with mild renal impairment (Cl_{cr} 61-90 mL/min/1.73m^2). In patients with moderate (Cl_{cr} 31-60 mL/min/1.73m^2) or severe ($Cl_{cr} \leq 30$ mL/min/1.73m^2) renal impairment, AUC is up to 60% higher, C_{max} up to 23% higher, and $t_{1/2}$ up to 47% longer compared to subjects with normal renal function.

Hemodialysis: While studies have not been conducted in patients with end-stage renal disease, hemodialysis is not expected to significantly enhance clearance of cerivastatin since the drug is extensively bound to plasma proteins.

Hepatic: Cerivastatin has not been studied in patients with active liver disease (see **CONTRAINDICATIONS**). Caution should be exercised when BAYCOL® (cerivastatin sodium tablets) is administered to patients with a history of liver disease or heavy alcohol ingestion (see **WARNINGS**).

Clinical Studies: BAYCOL® (cerivastatin sodium tablets) has been studied in controlled trials in North America, Europe, Israel, and South Africa and has been shown to be effective in reducing plasma Total-C, LDL-C, VLDL-C, apo B, and TG and increasing HDL-C and apo A1 in patients with heterozygous familial and non-familial forms of hypercholesterolemia and in mixed dyslipidemia. Over 5,000 patients with Type IIa and IIb hypercholesterolemia were treated in trials of 4 to 104 weeks duration.

The effectiveness of BAYCOL® in lowering plasma cholesterol has been shown in men and women, in patients with and without elevated triglycerides, and in the elderly. In four large, multicenter, placebo-controlled dose response studies in patients with primary hypercholesterolemia, BAYCOL® given as a single daily dose over 8 weeks, significantly reduced Total-C, LDL-C, apo B, TG, total cholesterol/HDL cholesterol (Total-C/HDL-C) ratio and LDL cholesterol/HDL cholesterol (LDL-C/HDL-C) ratio. Significant increases in HDL-C were also observed. The median (25th and 75th percentile) percent changes from baseline in HDL-C for Baycol 0.2, 0.3, 0.4, and 0.8 mg were +8 (+1, +15), +8 (+1, +14), +7 (0, +14), and +9 (+2, +16), respectively. Significant reductions in mean total-C and LDL-C were evident after one week, peaked at four weeks, and were maintained for the duration of the trial. (Pooled results at week 8 are presented in Table 1).

[See table 1 below]

In a pool of eight studies in patients with hypercholesterolemia and TG levels ranging from 250 mg/dL to 500 mg/dL who were treated for at least eight weeks, the following reductions in TG and increases in HDL-C were observed at Week 8 as shown in Table 2 below:

[See table 2 on next page]

In a large clinical study, the number of patients meeting their National Cholesterol Education Program-Adult Treatment Panel (NCEP-ATP) II target LDL-C levels on BAYCOL® 0.4 and 0.8 mg daily was assessed. The results up to 24 weeks are shown in Table 3 below:

[See table 3 on next page]

INDICATIONS AND USAGE

BAYCOL® (cerivastatin sodium tablets) is indicated as an adjunct to diet to reduce elevated Total-C, LDL-C, apo B, and TG and to increase HDL-C levels in patients with primary hypercholesterolemia and mixed dyslipidemia (Fredrickson Types IIa and IIb) when the response to dietary restriction of saturated fat and cholesterol and other non-pharmacological measures alone has been inadequate.

Therapy with lipid-altering drugs should be a component of multiple risk factor intervention in those patients at significantly high risk for atherosclerotic vascular disease due to hypercholesterolemia.

Before considering therapy with lipid-altering agents, secondary causes of hypercholesterolemia, e.g., poorly controlled diabetes mellitus, hypothyroidism, nephrotic syndrome, dysproteinemias, obstructive liver disease, other drug therapy, alcoholism, should be excluded and a lipid profile performed to measure Total-C, HDL-C, and triglycerides (TG). For patients with TG of 400 mg/dL or less, LDL-C can be estimated using the following equation:

$$\text{LDL-C} = [\text{Total-C}] \text{ minus } [\text{HDL-C} + \text{TG}/5]$$

For TG levels > 400 mg/dL, this equation is less accurate and LDL-C concentrations should be directly measured by preparative ultracentrifugation. In many hypertriglyceridemic patients, LDL-C may be low or normal despite elevated Total-C. In such cases, BAYCOL® (cerivastatin sodium tablets) is not indicated.

Lipid determinations should be performed at intervals of no less than four weeks.

The National Cholesterol Education Program (NCEP) Treatment Guidelines are summarized in Table 4.

[See table 4 on next page]

At the time of hospitalization for an acute coronary event, consideration can be given to initiating drug therapy at discharge if the LDL-C level is ≥ 130 mg/dL (NCEP-ATP II).

Since the goal of treatment is to lower LDL-C, the NCEP recommends that LDL-C levels be used to initiate and assess treatment response. Only if LDL-C levels are not available, should the Total-C be used to monitor therapy.

Although BAYCOL® may be useful to reduce elevated LDL-cholesterol levels in patients with combined hypercholesterolemia and hypertriglyceridemia where hypercholesterolemia is the major abnormality (Type IIb hyperlipoproteinemia), it has not been studied in conditions where the major abnormality is elevation of chylomicrons, VLDL, or IDL (i.e., hyperlipoproteinemia types I, III, IV, or V).[1]

CONTRAINDICATIONS

Active liver disease or unexplained persistent elevations of serum transaminases (see **WARNINGS**).

Concurrent treatment with gemfibrozil due to a risk for rhabdomyolysis (see WARNINGS: Skeletal Muscle).

Pregnancy and lactation: Atherosclerosis is a chronic process, and the discontinuation of lipid-lowering drugs during pregnancy should have little impact on the outcome of long-term therapy of primary hypercholesterolemia. Moreover, cholesterol and other products of the cholesterol biosynthesis pathway are essential components for fetal development, including synthesis of steroids and cell membranes. Since HMG-CoA reductase inhibitors decrease cholesterol synthesis and possibly the synthesis of other biologically active substances derived from cholesterol, they may cause fetal harm when administered to pregnant women. Therefore, HMG-CoA reductase inhibitors are contraindicated during pregnancy and in nursing mothers. **Cerivastatin sodium should be administered to women of child-bearing age only when such patients are highly unlikely to conceive and have been informed of the potential hazards.** If the patient becomes pregnant while taking this drug, cerivastatin sodium should be discontinued and the patient should be apprised of the potential hazard to the fetus.

Hypersensitivity to any component of this medication.

WARNINGS

Liver Enzymes: HMG-CoA reductase inhibitors have been associated with biochemical abnormalities of liver function. Persistent increases of serum transaminase (ALT, AST) values to more than 3 times the upper limit of normal (occurring on two or more not necessarily sequential occasions, regardless of baseline status) have been reported in 0.5% of patients treated with cerivastatin sodium in the US over an average period of 11 months. The incidence of these abnormalities was 0.1%, 0.4%, 0.9% and 0.6% for BAYCOL® 0.2, 0.3, 0.4, and 0.8 mg respectively. These abnormalities usually occurred within the first 6 months of treatment, usually resolved after discontinuation of the drug, and were not associated with cholestasis. In most cases, these biochemical abnormalities were asymptomatic.

It is recommended that liver function tests be performed before the initiation of treatment, at 6 and 12 weeks after initiation of therapy or elevation in dose, and periodically thereafter, e.g., semiannually. Patients who develop increased transaminase levels should be monitored with a second liver function evaluation to confirm the finding and be followed thereafter with frequent liver function tests until the abnormality(ies) return to normal. Should an increase in AST or ALT of three times the upper limit of normal or greater persist, withdrawal of cerivastatin sodium therapy is recommended.

Active liver disease or unexplained transaminase elevations are contraindications to the use of BAYCOL® (cerivastatin sodium tablets) (see **CONTRAINDICATIONS**). Caution should be exercised when cerivastatin sodium is administered to patients with a history of liver disease or heavy alcohol ingestion (see **CLINICAL PHARMACOLOGY: Pharmacokinetics/Metabolism**). Such patients should be started at the low end of the recommended dosing range and closely monitored.

Skeletal Muscle: **Cases of rhabdomyolysis, some with acute renal failure secondary to myoglobinuria, have been reported with cerivastatin and other drugs in this class.** Myopathy, defined as muscle aching or muscle weakness, associated with increases in plasma creatine kinase (CK) values to greater than 10 times the upper limit of normal, was seen in 0.4% of patients in U.S. cerivastatin clinical trials. In one clinical study using BAYCOL 0.8 mg as the starting dose, women over 65 years of age, especially those with low body weight, were observed to be at an increased risk of myopathy. Myopathy should be considered in any patient with diffuse myalgias, muscle tenderness or weakness, and/or marked elevation of CK. Patients should be advised to report promptly unexplained muscle pain, tenderness, or weakness, particularly if accompanied by malaise or fever. BAYCOL® (cerivastatin sodium tablets) therapy should be discontinued if markedly elevated CK levels occur or myopathy is diagnosed or suspected. **BAYCOL® (cerivastatin sodium tablets) should be temporarily withheld in any patient experiencing an acute or serious condition predisposing to the development of renal failure secondary to rhabdomyolysis, e.g., sepsis; hypotension; major surgery; trauma; severe metabolic, endocrine or electrolyte disorders; or uncontrolled epilepsy.**

The risk of myopathy during treatment with HMG-CoA reductase inhibitors is increased with concurrent administration of cyclosporine, fibric acid derivatives, erythromycin, azole antifungals or lipid-lowering doses of niacin.

The combined use of HMG-CoA inhibitors and fibrates generally should be avoided. The use of fibrates alone may be associated with myopathy including rhabdomyolysis and associated renal failure. **The combined use of cerivastatin and gemfibrozil is contraindicated due to a risk for rhabdomyolysis** (see **Contraindications**).

PRECAUTIONS

General: Before instituting therapy with BAYCOL® (cerivastatin sodium tablets), an attempt should be made to control hypercholesterolemia with appropriate diet, exercise, weight reduction in obese patients, and treatment of underlying medical problems (see **INDICATIONS AND USAGE**).

Cerivastatin sodium may elevate creatine kinase and transaminase levels (see **ADVERSE REACTIONS**). This should be considered in the differential diagnosis of chest pain in a patient on therapy with cerivastatin sodium.

Homozygous Familial Hypercholesterolemia: Cerivastatin sodium has not been evaluated in patients with rare homozygous familial hypercholesterolemia. HMG-CoA reductase inhibitors have been reported to be less effective in these patients because they lack functional LDL receptors.

Table 1
Response in Patients with Primary Hypercholesterolemia
Mean Percent Change from Baseline to Week 8
Intent-To-Treat Population

Dosage	N[1]	Total-C	LDL-C	Apo-B	TG[2]	HDL-C	LDL-C/ HDL-C	Total-C/ HDL-C
Placebo	608–620	+1	0	+1	0	+2	−1	0
BAYCOL® qd								
0.2 mg	150–151	−18	−25	−19	−16	+9	−31	−24
0.3 mg	494–497	−22	−31	−24	−16	+8	−35	−27
0.4 mg	754–758	−24	−34	−27	−16	+7	−38	−29
0.8 mg	731–735	−30	−42	−33	−22	+9	−46	−35

1 - N given as a range since test results for each lipid vairable were not available in every patient
2 - Median percent change from baseline

Information for Patients: Patients should be advised to report promptly unexplained muscle pain, tenderness, or weakness, particularly if accompanied by malaise or fever.

DRUG INTERACTIONS:

Immunosuppressive Drugs, Fibric Acid Derivatives, Niacin (Nicotinic Acid), Erythromycin, Azole Antifungals: see **WARNINGS: Skeletal Muscle.**

ANTACID (Magnesium-Aluminum Hydroxide): Cerivastatin plasma concentrations were not affected by co-administration of antacid.

CIMETIDINE: Cerivastatin plasma concentrations were not affected by co-administration of cimetidine.

CHOLESTYRAMINE: The influence of the bile-acid-sequestering agent cholestyramine on the pharmacokinetics of cerivastatin sodium was evaluated in 12 healthy males in 2 separate randomized crossover studies. In the first study, concomitant administration of 0.2 mg cerivastatin sodium and 12 g cholestyramine resulted in decreases of more than 22% for AUC and 40% for C_{max} when compared to dosing cerivastatin sodium alone. However, in the second study, administration of 12 g cholestyramine 1 hour before the evening meal and 0.3 mg cerivastatin sodium approximately 4 hours after the same evening meal resulted in a decrease in the cerivastatin AUC of less than 8%, and a decrease in C_{max} of about 30% when compared to dosing cerivastatin sodium alone. Therefore, it would be expected that a dosing schedule of cerivastatin sodium given at bedtime and cholestyramine given before the evening meal would not result in a significant decrease in the clinical effect of cerivastatin sodium.

DIGOXIN: Plasma digoxin levels and digoxin clearance at steady-state were not affected by co-administration of 0.2 mg cerivastatin sodium. Cerivastatin plasma concentrations were also not affected by co-administration of digoxin.

WARFARIN: Co-administration of warfarin and cerivastatin to healthy volunteers did not result in any changes in prothrombin time or clotting factor VII when compared to co-administration of warfarin and placebo. The AUC and C_{max} of both the (R) and (S) isomers of warfarin were unaffected by concurrent dosing of 0.3 mg cerivastatin sodium. Co-administration of warfarin and cerivastatin did not alter the pharmacokinetics of cerivastatin sodium.

ERYTHROMYCIN: In hypercholesterolemic patients, steady-state cerivastatin AUC and C_{max} increased approximately 50% and 24% respectively after 10 days with co-administration of erythromycin, a known inhibitor of cytochrome P450 3A4.

ITRACONAZOLE: In hypercholesterolemic patients, following a 0.3 mg dose of cerivastatin, steady-state cerivastatin AUC and C_{max} increased 38% and 12%, respectively after 10 days with co-administration of 200 mg itraconazole, a potent inhibitor of cytochrome P450 3A4. Cerivastatin half-life was approximately 5 hours (a 64% increase) following co-administration with itraconazole, which would not lead to accumulation of cerivastatin upon multiple dosing. The administration of 0.3 mg of cerivastatin concomitantly with itraconazole has no effect on itraconazole pharmacokinetics. In a single dose crossover study using 0.8 mg cerivastatin, the AUC and C_{max} of cerivastatin were increased 27% and 25% respectively during concomitant itraconazole treatment.

Endocrine Function: HMG-CoA reductase inhibitors interfere with cholesterol synthesis and lower cholesterol levels and, as such, might theoretically blunt adrenal or gonadal steroid hormone production.

Clinical studies have shown that cerivastatin sodium has no adverse effect on sperm production and does not reduce basal plasma cortisol concentration, impair adrenal reserve or have an adverse effect on thyroid metabolism as assessed by TSH. Results of clinical trials with drugs in this class have been inconsistent with regard to drug effect on basal and reserve steroid levels. The effects of HMG-CoA reductase inhibitors on male fertility have not been studied in adequate numbers of male patients. The effects, if any, on the pituitary-gonadal axis in pre-menopausal women are unknown.

Patients treated with cerivastatin sodium who develop clinical evidence of endocrine dysfunction should be evaluated appropriately. Caution should be exercised if an HMG-CoA reductase inhibitor or other agent used to lower cholesterol levels is administered to patients also receiving other drugs that may decrease the levels or activity of endogenous steroid hormones, e.g., ketoconazole, spironolactone, or cimetidine.

GEMFIBROZIL: The potential for clinically relevant interaction between gemfibrozil and cerivastatin has not been assessed in clinical trials. However, during postmarketing surveillance, patients on cerivastatin who experienced rhabdomyolysis and associated renal failure, were in most cases also taking gemfibrozil. (See **CONTRAINDICATIONS** and **WARNINGS: Skeletal Muscle)**

CNS and other Toxicities: Chronic administration of cerivastatin to rodent and non-rodent species demonstrated the principal toxicologic targets and effects observed with other HMG-CoA reductase inhibitors: Hemorrhage and edema in multiple organs and tissues including CNS (dogs); cataracts (dogs); degeneration of muscle fibers (dogs, rats, and mice); hyperkeratosis in the non-glandular stomach (rats and mice, this organ has no human equivalent); liver lesions (dogs, rats, and mice).

Table 2
Median Percent Change from Baseline to Week 8 in Patients with Baseline TG between 250–500 mg/dL

	Placebo	BAYCOL® 0.2 mg	BAYCOL® 0.3 mg	BAYCOL® 0.4 mg	BAYCOL® 0.8 mg
N[1]	135–138	127–129	156–157	139	125
Triglycerides	−3.3	−22.6	−22.4	−26.2	−30.7
HDL-C	3.1	7.3	9.2	10.7	13.3

1 - N given as a range since test results for each lipid variable were not available in every patient

Table 3
Percent of Patients Reaching NCEP-ATP II Goal Up to 24 Weeks of Treatment with BAYCOL® 0.4 mg and 0.8 mg

NCEP-ATP II Treatment Guidelines			Patients Reaching LDL-C Target Up to 24 Weeks			
Risk Factors for CHD	Baseline LDL-C (mg/dL)	Target LDL-C (mg/dL)	BAYCOL® 0.4 mg		BAYCOL® 0.8 mg	
			Baseline LDL-C Mean (mg/dL)	Percent To Goal	Baseline LDL-C Mean (mg/dL)	Percent To Goal
< 2 risk factors	≥ 190	< 160	234 (n=33)	79%	224 (n=156)	79%
≥ 2 risk factors	≥ 160	< 130	204 (n=43)	65%	201 (n=186)	72%
CHD	≥ 130	≤ 100	188 (n=34)	24%	187 (n=99)	53%

Table 4
National Cholesterol Education Program (NCEP) Treatment Guidelines LDL-Cholesterol mg/dL (mmol/L)

Definite Atherosclerotic Disease*	Two or More Other Risk Factors**	Initiation Level***	Goal
NO	NO	≥ 190 (≥ 4.9)	< 160 (< 4.1)
NO	YES	≥ 160 (≥ 4.1)	< 130 (< 3.4)
YES	YES or NO	≥ 130 (≥ 3.4)	≤ 100 (≤ 2.6)

* Coronary heart disease or peripheral vascular disease (including symptomatic carotid artery disease).

** Other risk factors for coronary heart disease (CHD) include the following: age (males: ≥ 45 years; females: ≥ 55 years or premature menopause without estrogen replacement therapy); family history of permature CHD; current cigarette smoking; hypertension; confirmed HDL-C < 35 mg/dL (< 0.91 mmol/L); and diabetes mellitus. Subtract one risk factor if HDL-C is ≥ 60 mg/dL (≥ 1.6 mmol/L).

*** In CHD patients with LDL-C levels 100–129 mg/dL, the physician should exercise clinical judgment in deciding whether to initiate drug treatment.

CNS lesions were characterized by multifocal bleeding with fibrinoid degeneration of vessel walls in the plexus chorioideus of the brain stem and in the ciliary body of the eye at 0.1 mg/kg/day in the dog. This dose resulted in plasma levels of cerivastatin (C_{max}, measured as free drug), that were about 17 times higher than the mean values in humans taking 0.8 mg/day. No CNS lesions were observed after chronic treatment with cerivastatin for up to two years in the mouse (up to 6 times human $C_{max\ free}$ drug levels) and rat (in the range of human $C_{max\ free}$ drug levels).

Carcinogenesis, Mutagenesis, Impairment of Fertility: A 2-year study was conducted in rats with dietary administration resulting in average daily doses of cerivastatin of 0.007, 0.034, or 0.158 mg/kg. The high dosage level corresponded to plasma free drug levels (AUC) of approximately 2 times those in humans following a 0.8-mg oral dose. Tumor incidences of treated rats were comparable to controls in all treatment groups. In a 2-year carcinogenicity study conducted in mice with dietary administration resulting in average daily doses of cerivastatin of 0.4, 1.8, 9.1, or 55 mg/kg hepatocellular adenomas were significantly increased in male and female mice at ≥ 9.1 mg/kg (AUC_{free} values about 3 times human at 0.8 mg/day). Hepatocellular carcinomas were significantly increased in male mice at ≥ 1.8 mg/k (AUC_{free} values in the range of human exposure at 0.8 mg/day).

No evidence of genotoxicity was observed *in vitro* with or without metabolic activation in the following assays: microbial mutagen tests using mutant strains of *S. typhimurium* or *E. coli*, Chinese Hamster Ovary Forward Mutation Assay, Unscheduled DNA Synthesis in rat primary hepatocytes, chromosome aberrations in Chinese Hamster Ovary cells, and spindle inhibition in human lymphocytes. In addition, there was no evidence of genotoxicity *in vivo* in a mouse Micronucleus Test; there was equivocal evidence of mutagenicity in a mouse Dominant Lethal Test.

In a combined male and female rat fertility study, cerivastatin had no adverse effects on fertility or reproductive performance at doses up to 0.1 mg/kg/day (in the range of human $C_{max\ free}$ drug levels). At a dose of 0.3 mg/kg/day (about 3 times human $C_{max\ free}$ drug levels), the length of gestation was marginally prolonged, stillbirths were increased, and the survival rate up to day 4 postpartum was decreased. In the fetuses (F1), a marginal reduction in fetal weight and delay in bone development was observed. In the mating of the F1 generation, there was a reduced number of female rats that littered.

In the testicles of dogs treated chronically with cerivastatin at a dose of 0.008 mg/kg/day (in the range of human $C_{max\ free}$ drug levels), atrophy, vacuolization of the germinal epithelium, spermatidic giant cells, and focal oligospermia were observed. In another 1-year study in dogs treated with 0.1 mg/kg/day (approximately 17-fold the human exposure at doses of 0.8 mg based on $C_{max\ free}$), ejaculate volume was small and libido was decreased. Semen analysis revealed an increased number of morphologically altered spermatozoa indicating disturbances of epididymal sperm maturation that was reversible when drug administration was discontinued.

Pregnancy: Pregnancy Category X: (See **CONTRAINDICATIONS**): Cerivastatin caused a significant increase in incomplete ossification of the lumbar center of the vertebrae in rats at an oral dose of 0.72 mg/kg. Cerivastatin did not cause any anomalies or malformations in rabbits at oral doses up to 0.75 mg/kg. These doses resulted in plasma levels about 6 times the human exposure ($C_{max\ free}$) for rats and 3 times the human exposure for rabbits ($C_{max\ free}$) at a human dose of 0.8 mg. Cerivastatin crossed the placenta and was found in fetal liver, gastrointestinal tract, and kidneys when pregnant rats were given a single oral dose of 2 mg/kg.

Safety in pregnant women has not been established. Cerivastatin should be administered to women of child-bearing potential only when such patients are highly unlikely to conceive and have been informed of the potential hazards. Rare reports of congenital anomalies have been received following intrauterine exposure to other HMG-CoA reductase inhibitors. In a review of approximately 100 prospectively followed pregnancies in women exposed to simvastatin or lovastatin, the incidences of congenital anomalies, spontaneous abortions and fetal deaths/stillbirths did not exceed what would be expected in the general population. The number of cases is adequate only to exclude a three- to four-fold increase in congenital anomalies over the background incidence. In 89% of the prospectively followed pregnancies, drug treatment was initiated prior to pregnancy and was discontinued at some point in the first trimester when pregnancy was identified. As safety in pregnant women has not been established and there is no apparent benefit to therapy with BAYCOL® during pregnancy (see **CONTRAINDICATIONS**), treatment should be immediately discontinued as soon as pregnancy is recognized. If a women becomes pregnant while taking cerivastatin, the drug should be discontinued and the patient advised again as to potential hazards to the fetus.

Nursing Mothers: Based on preclinical data, cerivastatin is present in breast milk in a 1.3:1 ratio (milk:plasma). Because of the potential for serious adverse reactions in nursing infants, nursing women should not take cerivastatin (see **CONTRAINDICATIONS**).

Continued on next page

Baycol—Cont.

Pediatric Use: Safety and effectiveness in pediatric patients have not been established.
Geriatric Use: In clinical pharmacology studies, there were no clinically relevant effects of age on the pharmacokinetics of cerivastatin sodium. In one clinical study using BAYCOL 0.8 mg as the starting dose, women over 65 years of age, especially those with low body weight, were observed to be at an increased risk of myopathy. Caution should be exercised when titrating such patients to the 0.8 mg dose of BAYCOL.
Renal Insufficiency: Patients with significant renal impairment ($Cl_{cr} \leq 60$ mL/min/1.73m^2) have increased AUC (up to 60%) and C_{max} (up to 23%) and should be administered BAYCOL® with caution.
Hepatic Insufficiency: Safety and effectiveness in hepatically impaired patients have not been established. Cerivastatin should be used with caution in patients who have a history of liver disease and/or consume substantial quantities of alcohol (see **CONTRAINDICATIONS** and **WARNINGS**).

ADVERSE REACTIONS

Cerivastatin sodium has been evaluated for adverse events in more than 5,000 patients worldwide. In the U.S. placebo-controlled clinical studies, discontinuations due to adverse events occurred in 3.1% of cerivastatin sodium treated patients and in 2.0% of patients treated with placebo. Adverse reactions have usually been mild and transient.
Clinical Adverse Experiences: Adverse experiences occurring with a frequency ≥2% for marketed doses of cerivastatin sodium, regardless of causality assessment, in U.S. placebo-controlled clinical studies, are shown in Table 5 below:

Table 5
Adverse Experiences occurring in ≥2% Patients in U.S. Placebo Controlled Clinical Studies

Adverse Event	BAYCOL® (n = 2231)	Placebo (n = 702)
Any event	63.2%	63.0%
Pharyngitis	9.6%	12.1%
Headache	8.5%	9.5%
Rhinitis	8.3%	10.1%
Sinusitis	4.7%	5.0%
Accidental injury	4.4%	5.6%
Arthralgia	4.3%	3.4%
Dyspepsia	3.8%	4.8%
Flu syndrome	3.7%	6.3%
Back pain	3.4%	5.0%
Asthenia	3.4%	2.1%
Diarrhea	3.3%	3.3%
Rash	3.0%	4.4%
Myalgia	2.5%	2.3%
Abdominal pain	2.5%	3.0%
Nausea	2.4%	3.1%
Leg pain	2.2%	1.4%
Constipation	2.2%	2.0%
Dizziness	2.1%	2.4%
Flatulence	2.1%	2.7%
Chest pain	2.0%	1.8%
Bronchitis	1.3%	2.1%

The following effects have been reported with drugs in this class; not all effects listed below have necessarily been associated with cerivastatin therapy.
Skeletal: myopathy, muscle cramps, rhabdomyolysis, arthralgias, myalgia.
Neurological: dysfunction of certain cranial nerves (including alteration of taste, impairment of extra-ocular movement, facial paresis), tremor, dizziness, memory loss, vertigo, paresthesia, peripheral neuropathy, peripheral nerve palsy, anxiety, insomnia, depression, psychic disturbances.
Hypersensitivity Reactions: An apparent hypersensitivity syndrome has been reported that included one or more of the following features: anaphylaxis, angioedema, lupus erythematous-like syndrome, polymyalgia rheumatica, dermatomyositis, vasculitis, purpura, thrombocytopenia, leukopenia, hemolytic anemia, positive ANA, ESR increase, eosinophilia, arthritis, arthralgia, urticaria, asthenia, photosensitivity, fever, chills, flushing, malaise, dyspnea, toxic epidermal necrolysis, erythema multiforme, including Stevens-Johnson syndrome.
Gastrointestinal: pancreatitis, hepatitis, including chronic active hepatitis, cholestatic jaundice, fatty change in liver, cirrhosis, fulminant hepatic necrosis, and hepatoma; anorexia, vomiting.
Skin: alopecia, pruritus. A variety of skin changes, (e.g., nodules, discoloration, dryness of skin/mucous membranes, changes to hair/nails), have been reported.
Reproductive: gynecomastia, loss of libido, erectile dysfunction.
Eye: progression of cataracts (lens opacities), ophthalmoplegia.
Laboratory Abnormalities: elevated transaminases, creatine kinase, alkaline phosphatase, γ-glutamyl transpeptidase, and bilirubin; thyroid function abnormalities.
Post-Marketing Adverse Event Reports: The following events have been reported since market introduction. While these events were generally associated with the use of BAYCOL®, a casual relationship to the use of BAYCOL® cannot be readily determined due to the spontaneous nature of reporting of medical events, and the lack of controls.

Body as a Whole: Asthenia, fever, headache, anorexia, abdominal pain, epistaxis, edema.
Cardiovascular System: Hypertension, angina pectoris.
Digestive System: Colitis, constipation, diarrhea, duodenal ulcer, dyspepsia, flatulance, gastrointestinal disorder, gastrointestinal hemorrhage, hepatitis, nausea.
Hemolytic and Lymphatic System: Anemia, leukopenia.
Hypersensitivity Reaction: Allergic reaction, anaphylactoid reaction, angioedema, urticaria.
Nervous System: Paralysis, somnolence.
Musculoskeletal System: Myalgia, myasthenia, myopathy, myositis, rhabdomyolysis, hypertonia, hyperkinesia.
Respiratory System: Cough increase.
Urogenital System: Acute renal failure secondary to myoglobinuria.
Special Senses: Cataract specified, visual disturbance, blurred vision.
Laboratory Abnormalities: Amylase increase, elevated transaminases, laboratory tests abnormal, kidney function abnormal, creatine phosphokinase increase.
Concomitant Therapy: In studies where cerivastatin sodium has been administered concomitantly with cholestyramine, no adverse reactions unique to this combination or in addition to those previously reported for this class of drugs were reported. Myopathy and rhabdomyolysis (with or without acute renal failure) have been reported when HMG-CoA reductase inhibitors are used in combination with immunosuppressive drugs, fibric acid derivatives, erythromycin, azole antifungals or lipid-lowering doses of nicotinic acid. Concomitant therapy with HMG-CoA reductase inhibitors and these agents is generally not recommended (see **WARNINGS: Skeletal Muscle**). Concurrent treatment with gemfibrozil is contraindicated (see **CONTRAINDICATIONS** and **WARNINGS: Skeletal Muscle**).

OVERDOSAGE

No specific recommendations concerning the treatment of an overdosage can be made. Should an overdose occur, it should be treated symptomatically and supportive measures should be undertaken as required.
Dialysis of cerivastatin sodium is not expected to significantly enhance clearance since the drug is extensively (>99%) bound to plasma proteins.

DOSAGE AND ADMINISTRATION

The patient should be placed on a standard cholesterol-lowering diet before receiving cerivastatin sodium and should continue on this diet during treatment with cerivastatin sodium. (See NCEP Treatment Guidelines for details on dietary therapy.)
The recommended starting-dose of BAYCOL® is 0.4 mg once daily in the evening. The dosage range is 0.2 mg to 0.8 mg. Cerivastatin sodium may be taken with or without food. In patients with significant renal impairment (creatinine clearance ≤60 mL/min/1.73m^2) the lower doses are recommended.
Since the maximal effect of cerivastatin sodium is seen within 4 weeks, lipid determinations should be performed at this time and dose adjusted as necessary.
Concomitant Therapy: The lipid-lowering effects on LDL-C and Total-C are additive when cerivastatin sodium is combined with a bile-acid-binding resin. When co-administering cerivastatin sodium and a bile-acid-exchange resin, e.g., cholestyramine, cerivastatin sodium should be given at least 2 hours after the resin (see also **ADVERSE REACTIONS: Concomitant Therapy**).
Dosage in Patients with Renal Insufficiency: No dose adjustment is necessary for patients with mild renal dysfunction (Cl_{cr} 61-90 mL/min/1.73m^2). For patients with moderate or severe renal dysfunction, a starting dose of 0.2 mg or 0.3 mg is recommended (see **CLINICAL PHARMACOLOGY - Special Populations - Renal**).

HOW SUPPLIED

BAYCOL® (cerivastatin sodium tablets) is supplied as 0.2-mg, 0.3-mg, 0.4-mg and 0.8-mg tablets. The different tablet strengths can be identified as follows:

Strength	Color	Markings Front	Markings Back
0.2 mg	light yellow	283	200 MCG
0.3 mg	yellow brown	284	300 MCG
0.4 mg	ocher	285	400 MCG
0.8 mg	brown orange	286	800 MCG

BAYCOL® (cerivastatin sodium tablets) is supplied as follows:

Bottles of 30:	0.4 mg	(NDC 0026-2885-69)
	0.8 mg	(NDC 0026-2886-69)
Bottles of 90:	0.2 mg	(NDC 0026-2883-86)
	0.3 mg	(NDC 0026-2884-86)
	0.4 mg	(NDC 0026-2885-86)
	0.8 mg	(NDC 0026-2886-86)
Bottles of 100:	0.2 mg	(NDC 0026-2883-51)
	0.3 mg	(NDC 0026-2884-51)
	0.4 mg	(NDC 0026-2885-51)

The tablets should be protected from moisture and stored below 77°F (25°C). Dispense in tight containers.

References:

[1] **Classification of Hyperlipoproteinemias**

Type	Lipoproteins Elevated	Lipid Elevations major	Lipid Elevations minor
I (rare)	chylomicrons	TG	↑→C
IIa	LDL	C	–
IIb	LDL,VLDL	C	TG
III (rare)	IDL	C/TG	–
IV	VLDL	TG	↑→C
V (rare)	chylomircons, VLDL	TG	↑→C

C=cholesterol, TG=triglycerides, LDL=low-density lipoprotein, VLDL=very-low-density lipoprotein, IDL=intermediate-density lipoprotein.

Bayer Corporation
Pharmaceutical Division
400 Morgan Lane
West Haven, CT 06516 USA
Made in Germany
Rx Only
PZ500148 7/00 ©2000 Bayer Corporation 9787
Shown in Product Identification Guide, page 307

BILTRICIDE® Tablets ℞
(praziquantel)

DESCRIPTION

BILTRICIDE® (praziquantel) is a trematodicide provided in tablet form for the oral treatment of schistosome infections and infections due to liver fluke.
BILTRICIDE® (praziquantel) is 2-(cyclohexylcarbonyl)-1,2,3,6,7, 11b-hexahydro-4H-pyrazino [2, 1-a] isoquinolin-4-one with the molecular formula; $C_{19}H_{24}N_2O_2$. The structural formula is as follows:

Praziquantel is a white to nearly white crystalline powder of bitter taste. The compound is stable under normal conditions and melts at 136–140°C with decomposition. The active substance is hygroscopic. Praziquantel is easily soluble in chloroform and dimethylsulfoxide, soluble in ethanol and very slightly soluble in water.
BILTRICIDE® tablets contain 600 mg of praziquantel. Inactive ingredients: corn starch, magnesium stearate, microcrystalline cellulose, povidone, sodium lauryl sulfate, polyethylene glycol, titanium dioxide and HPM cellulose.

CLINICAL PHARMACOLOGY

BILTRICIDE® induces a rapid contraction of schistosomes by a specific effect on the permeability of the cell membrane. The drug further causes vacuolization and disintegration of the schistosome tegument.
After oral administration BILTRICIDE® is rapidly absorbed (80%), subjected to a first pass effect, metabolized and eliminated by the kidneys. Maximal serum concentration is achieved 1–3 hours after dosing. The half-life of praziquantel in serum is 0.8–1.5 hours.

INDICATIONS AND USAGE

BILTRICIDE® is indicated for the treatment of infections due to: all species of schistosoma (e.g. *Schistosoma mekongi, Schistosoma japonicum, Schistosoma mansoni* and *Schistosoma hematobium),* and infections due to the liver flukes, *Clonorchis sinensis/Opisthorchis viverrini* (approval of this indication was based on studies in which the two species were not differentiated).

CONTRAINDICATIONS

BILTRICIDE® should not be given to patients who previously have shown hypersensitivity to the drug. Since parasite destruction within the eye may cause irreparable lesions, ocular cysticercosis should not be treated with this compound.

PRECAUTIONS

Information for the patient: Patients should be warned not to drive a car and not to operate machinery on the day of BILTRICIDE® treatment and the following day.
Minimal increases in liver enzymes have been reported in some patients.
When schistosomiasis or fluke infection is found to be associated with cerebral cysticercosis it is advised to hospitalize the patient for the duration of treatment.
Drug Interactions: No data are available regarding interaction of BILTRICIDE® with other drugs.
Mutagenesis, Carcinogenesis: Mutagenic effects in Salmonella tests found by one laboratory have not been confirmed in the same tested strain by other laboratories. Long term carcinogenicity studies in rats and golden hamsters did not reveal any carcinogenic effect.
Pregnancy Category B: Reproduction studies have been performed in rats and rabbits at doses up to 40 times the

human dose and have revealed no evidence of impaired fertility or harm to the fetus due to BILTRICIDE®. There are, however, no adequate and well-controlled studies in pregnant women. An increase of the abortion rate was found in rats at three times the single human therapeutic dose. While animal reproduction studies are not always predictive of human response, this drug should be used during pregnancy only if clearly needed.

Nursing mothers: BILTRICIDE® appeared in the milk of nursing women at a concentration of about 1/4 that of maternal serum. Women should not nurse on the day of BILTRICIDE® treatment and during the subsequent 72 hours.

Pediatric use: Safety in children under 4 years of age has not been established.

ADVERSE EFFECTS

In general BILTRICIDE® is very well tolerated. Side effects are usually mild and transient and do not require treatment. The following side effects were observed generally in order of severity: malaise, headache, dizziness, abdominal discomfort with or without nausea, rise in temperature and, rarely, urticaria. Such symptoms can, however, also result from the infection itself. Such side effects may be more frequent and/or serious in patients with a heavy worm burden. In patients with liver impairment caused by the infection, no adverse effects of BILTRICIDE® have occurred which would necessitate restriction in use.

OVERDOSAGE

In rats and mice the acute LD_{50} was about 2,500 mg/kg. No data are available in humans. In the event of overdose a fast-acting laxative should be given.

DOSAGE AND ADMINISTRATION

The dosage recommended for the treatment of schistosomiasis is: 3 × 20 mg/kg bodyweight as a one day treatment. The recommended dose for clonorchiasis and opisthorchiasis is: 3 × 25 mg/kg as a one day treatment. The tablets should be washed down unchewed with some liquid during meals. Keeping the tablets or segments thereof in the mouth can reveal a bitter taste which can promote gagging or vomiting. The interval between the individual doses should not be less than 4 and not more than 6 hours.

HOW SUPPLIED

BILTRICIDE® is supplied as a 600 mg white to orange tinged, filmcoated, oblong tablets with three scores. The tablet is coded with "BAYER" on one side and "LG" on the reverse side. When broken each of the four segments contain 150 mg of active ingredient so that the dosage can be easily adjusted to the patient's bodyweight.

Segments are broken off by pressing the score (notch) with thumbnails. If 1/4 of a tablet is required, this is best achieved by breaking the segment from the outer end.

BILTRICIDE® is available in bottles of 6 tablets.

	Strength	NDC
Bottles of 6:	600 mg	0026-2521-06

Store below 86°F (30°C).

Bayer Corporation
Pharmaceutical Division
400 Morgan Lane
West Haven, CT 06516 USA
Made in Germany

Caution: Federal (USA) law prohibits dispensing without a prescription.

PD500021 10/96 EMBAY 8440 6750

Shown in Product Identification Guide, page 307

CIPRO® ℞
(ciprofloxacin hydrochloride)
TABLETS

CIPRO® ℞
(ciprofloxacin)
5% and 10% ORAL SUSPENSION

DESCRIPTION

CIPRO® (ciprofloxacin hydrochloride) Tablets and CIPRO® (ciprofloxacin) Oral Suspension are synthetic broad spectrum antimicrobial agents for oral administration. Ciprofloxacin hydrochloride, USP, a fluoroquinolone, is the monohydrochloride monohydrate salt of 1-cyclopropyl-6-fluoro-1,4-dihydro-4-oxo-7-(1-piperazinyl)-3-quinolinecarboxylic acid. It is a faintly yellowish to light yellow crystalline substance with a molecular weight of 385.8. Its empirical formula is $C_{17}H_{18}FN_3O_3 \bullet HCl \bullet H_2O$ and its chemical structure is as follows:

Ciprofloxacin is 1-cyclopropyl-6-fluoro-1, 4-dihydro-4-oxo-7-(1-piperazinyl)-3-quinolinecarboxylic acid. Its empirical formula is $C_{17}H_{18}FN_3O_3$ and its molecular weight is 331.4. It is a faintly yellowish to light yellow crystalline substance and its chemical structure is as follows:

Steady-state Pharmacokinetic Parameter Following Multiple Oral and I.V. Doses

Parameters	500 mg q12h, P.O.	400 mg q12h, I.V.	750 mg q12h, P.O.	400 mg q8h, I.V.
AUC (μg•hr/mL)	13.7[a]	12.7[a]	31.6[b]	32.9[c]
C_{max} (μg/mL)	2.97	4.56	3.59	4.07

[a]AUC_{0-12h}
[b]AUC 24h=AUC_{0-12h} × 2
[c]AUC 24h=AUC_{0-8h} × 3

Ciprofloxacin differs from other quinolones in that it has a fluorine atom at the 6-position, a piperazine moiety at the 7-position, and a cyclopropyl ring at the 1-position.

CIPRO® film-coated tablets are available in 100-mg, 250-mg, 500-mg and 750-mg (ciprofloxacin equivalent) strengths. The inactive ingredients are starch, microcrystalline cellulose, silicon dioxide, crospovidone, magnesium stearate, hydroxypropyl methylcellulose, titanium dioxide, polyethylene glycol and water.

Ciprofloxacin Oral Suspension is available in 5% (5 g ciprofloxacin in 100 mL) and 10% (10 g ciprofloxacin in 100 mL) strengths. Ciprofloxacin Oral Suspension is a white to slightly yellowish suspension with strawberry flavor which may contain yellow-orange droplets. It is composed of ciprofloxacin microcapsules and diluent which are mixed prior to dispensing (See instructions for USE/HANDLING). The components of the suspension have the following compositions:

Microcapsules—ciprofloxacin, polyvinylpyrrolidone, methacrylic acid copolymer, hydroxypropyl methylcellulose, magnesium stearate, and Polysorbate 20.

Diluent—medium-chain triglycerides, sucrose, lecithin, water, and strawberry flavor.

CLINICAL PHARMACOLOGY

Ciprofloxacin given as an oral tablet is rapidly and well absorbed from the gastrointestinal tract after oral administration. The absolute bioavailability is approximately 70% with no substantial loss by first pass metabolism. Ciprofloxacin maximum serum concentrations and area under the curve are shown in the chart for the 250-mg to 1000-mg dose range.

Dose (mg)	Maximum Serum Concentration (μg/mL)	Area Under Curve (AUC) (μg•hr/mL)
250	1.2	4.8
500	2.4	11.6
750	4.3	20.2
1000	5.4	30.8

Maximum serum concentrations are attained 1 to 2 hours after oral dosing. Mean concentrations 12 hours after dosing with 250, 500, or 750-mg are 0.1, 0.2, and 0.4 μg/mL, respectively. The serum elimination half-life in subjects with normal renal function is approximately 4 hours. Serum concentrations increase proportionately with doses up to 1000-mg.

A 500-mg oral dose given every 12 hours has been shown to produce an area under the serum concentration time curve (AUC) equivalent to that produced by an intravenous infusion of 400 mg ciprofloxacin given over 60 minutes every 12 hours. A 750-mg oral dose given every 12 hours has been shown to produce an AUC at steady-state equivalent to that produced by an intravenous infusion of 400 mg over 60 minutes every 8 hours. A 750-mg oral dose results in a C_{max} similar to that observed with a 400-mg I.V. dose. A 250-mg oral dose given every 12 hours produces an AUC equivalent to that produced by an infusion of 200 mg ciprofloxacin given every 12 hours.

[See table at top of page]

The serum elimination half-life in subjects with normal renal function is approximately 4 hours. Approximately 40 to 50% of an orally administered dose is excreted in the urine as unchanged drug. After a 250-mg oral dose, urine concentrations of ciprofloxacin usually exceed 200 μg/mL during the first two hours and are approximately 30 μg/mL at 8 to 12 hours after dosing. The urinary excretion of ciprofloxacin is virtually complete within 24 hours after dosing. The renal clearance of ciprofloxacin, which is approximately 300 mL/minute, exceeds the normal glomerular filtration rate of 120 mL/minute. Thus, active tubular secretion would seem to play a significant role in its elimination. Co-administration of probenecid with ciprofloxacin results in about a 50% reduction in the ciprofloxacin renal clearance and a 50% increase in its concentration in the systemic circulation. Although bile concentrations of ciprofloxacin are several fold higher than serum concentrations after oral dosing, only a small amount of the dose administered is recovered from the bile as unchanged drug. An additional 1 to 2% of the dose is recovered from the bile in the form of metabolites. Approximately 20 to 35% of an oral dose is recovered from the feces within 5 days after dosing. This may arise from either biliary clearance or transintestinal elimination. Four metabolites have been identified in human urine which together account for approximately 15% of an oral dose. The metabolites have antimicrobial activity, but are less active than unchanged ciprofloxacin.

With oral administration, a 500-mg dose, given as 10 mL of the 5% CIPRO® Suspension (containing 250-mg ciprofloxacin/5mL) is bioequivalent to the 500-mg tablet. A 10 mL volume of the 5% CIPRO® Suspension (containing 250-mg ciprofloxacin/5mL) is bioequivalent to a 5 mL volume of the 10% CIPRO® Suspension (containing 500-mg ciprofloxacin/5mL).

When CIPRO® Tablet is given concomitantly with food, there is a delay in the absorption of the drug, resulting in peak concentrations that occur closer to 2 hours after dosing rather than 1 hour whereas there is no delay observed when CIPRO® Suspension is given with food. The overall absorption of CIPRO® Tablet or CIPRO® Suspension, however, is not substantially affected. The pharmacokinetics of ciprofloxacin given as the suspension are also not affected by food. Concurrent administration of antacids containing magnesium hydroxide or aluminum hydroxide may reduce the bioavailability of ciprofloxacin by as much as 90%. (See **PRECAUTIONS**.)

The serum concentrations of ciprofloxacin and metronidazole were not altered when these two drugs were given concomitantly.

Concomitant administration of ciprofloxacin with theophylline decreases the clearance of theophylline resulting in elevated serum theophylline levels and increased risk of a patient developing CNS or other adverse reactions. Ciprofloxacin also decreases caffeine clearance and inhibits the formation of paraxanthine after caffeine administration. (See **PRECAUTIONS**.)

Pharmacokinetic studies of the oral (single dose) and intravenous (single and multiple dose) forms of ciprofloxacin indicate that plasma concentrations of ciprofloxacin are higher in elderly subjects (>65 years) as compared to young adults. Although the C_{max} is increased 16–40%, the increase in mean AUC is approximately 30%, and can be at least partially attributed to decreased renal clearance in the elderly. Elimination half-life is only slightly (~20%) prolonged in the elderly. These differences are not considered clinically significant. (See **PRECAUTIONS: Geriatric Use.**)

In patients with reduced renal function, the half-life of ciprofloxacin is slightly prolonged. Dosage adjustments may be required. (See **DOSAGE AND ADMINISTRATION.**)

In preliminary studies in patients with stable chronic liver cirrhosis, no significant changes in ciprofloxacin pharmacokinetics have been observed. The kinetics of ciprofloxacin in patients with acute hepatic insufficiency, however, have not been fully elucidated.

The binding of ciprofloxacin to serum proteins is 20 to 40% which is not likely to be high enough to cause significant protein binding interactions with other drugs.

After oral administration, ciprofloxacin is widely distributed throughout the body. Tissue concentrations often exceed serum concentrations in both men and women, particularly in genital tissue including the prostate. Ciprofloxacin is present in active form in the saliva, nasal and bronchial secretions, mucosa of the sinuses, sputum, skin blister fluid, lymph, peritoneal fluid, bile, and prostatic secretions. Ciprofloxacin has also been detected in lung, skin, fat, muscle, cartilage, and bone. The drug diffuses into the cerebrospinal fluid (CSF); however, CSF concentrations are generally less than 10% of peak serum concentrations. Low levels of the drug have been detected in the aqueous and vitreous humors of the eye.

Microbiology: Ciprofloxacin has *in vitro* activity against a wide range of gram-negative and gram-positive organisms. The bactericidal action of ciprofloxacin results from interference with the enzyme DNA gyrase which is needed for the synthesis of bacterial DNA. Ciprofloxacin does not cross-react with other antimicrobial agents such as beta-lactams or aminoglycosides; therefore, organisms resistant to these drugs may be susceptible to ciprofloxacin. *In vitro* studies have shown that additive activity often results when ciprofloxacin is combined with other antimicrobial agents such as beta-lactams, aminoglycosides, clindamycin, or metronidazole. Synergy has been reported particularly with the combination of ciprofloxacin and a beta-lactam; antagonism is observed only rarely.

Ciprofloxacin has been shown to be active against most strains of the following microorganisms, both *in vitro* and in clinical infections as described in the **INDICATIONS AND USAGE** section of the package insert for CIPRO® (ciprofloxacin hydrochloride) Tablets and CIPRO® (ciprofloxacin) 5% and 10% Oral Suspension.

Continued on next page

Cipro—Cont.

Aerobic gram-positive microorganisms
Enterococcus faecalis
(Many strains are only moderately susceptible.)
Staphylococcus aureus (methicillin susceptible)
Staphylococcus epidermidis
Staphylococcus saprophyticus
Streptococcus pneumoniae
Streptococcus pyogenes
Aerobic gram-negative microorganisms
Campylobacter jejuni
Citrobacter diversus
Citrobacter freundii
Enterobacter cloacae
Escherichia coli
Haemophilus influenzae
Haemophilus parainfluenzae
Klebsiella pneumoniae
Moraxella catarrhalis
Morganella morganii
Neisseria gonorrhoeae
Proteus mirabilis
Proteus vulgaris
Providencia rettgeri
Providencia stuartii
Pseudomonas aeruginosa
Salmonella typhi
Serratia marcescens
Shigella boydii
Shigella dysenteriae
Shigella flexneri
Shigella sonnei

Ciprofloxacin has been shown to be active against most strains of the following microorganisms, both *in vitro* and in clinical infections as described in the **INDICATIONS AND USAGE** section of the package insert for CIPRO® I.V. (ciprofloxacin for intravenous infusion).

Aerobic gram-positive microorganisms
Enterococcus faecalis
(Many strains are only moderately susceptible.)
Staphylococcus aureus (methicillin susceptible)
Staphylococcus epidermidis
Staphylococcus saprophyticus
Streptococcus pneumoniae
Streptococcus pyogenes
Aerobic gram-negative microorganisms
Citrobacter diversus
Citrobacter freundii
Enterobacter cloacae
Escherichia coli
Haemophilus influenzae
Haemophilus parainfluenzae
Klebsiella pneumoniae
Morganella morganii
Proteus mirabilis
Proteus vulgaris
Providencia rettgeri
Providencia stuartii
Pseudomonas aeruginosa
Serratia marcescens

The following *in vitro* data are available, **but their clinical significance in unknown.**

Ciprofloxacin exhibits *in vitro* minimum inhibitory concentrations (MICs) of 1 µg/mL or less against most (≥90%) strains of the following microorganisms; however, the safety and effectiveness of ciprofloxacin in treating clinical infections due to these microorganisms have not been established in adequate and well-controlled clinical trials.

Aerobic gram-positive microorganisms
Staphylococcus haemolyticus
Staphylococcus hominis
Aerobic gram-negative microorganisms
Acinetobacter lwoffi
Aeromonas hydrophila
Edwardsiella tarda
Enterobacter aerogenes
Klebsiella oxytoca
Legionella pneumophilia
Pasteurella multocida
Salmonella enteritidis
Vibrio cholerae
Vibrio parahaemolyticus
Vibrio vulnificus
Yersinia enterocolitica

Most strains of *Burkholderia cepacia* and some strains of *Stenotrophomonas maltophilia* are resistant to ciprofloxacin as are most anaerobic bacteria, including *Bacteroides fragilis* and *Clostridium difficile*.

Ciprofloxacin is slightly less active when tested at acidic pH. The inoculum size has little effect when tested *in vitro*. The minimal bactericidal concentration (MBC) generally does not exceed the minimal inhibitory concentration (MIC) by more than a factor of 2. Resistance to ciprofloxacin *in vitro* develops slowly (multiple-step mutation).

Susceptibility Tests

Dilution Techniques: Quantitative methods are used to determine antimicrobial minimum inhibitory concentrations (MICs). These MICs provide estimates of the susceptibility of bacteria to antimicrobial compounds. The MICs should be determined using a standardized procedure. Standardized procedures are based on a dilution method[1] (broth or agar) or equivalent with standardized inoculum concentrations and standardized concentrations of ciprofloxacin powder. The MIC values should be interpreted according to the following criteria:

For testing aerobic microorganisms other than *Haemophilus influenzae, Haemophilus parainfluenzae,* and *Neisseria gonorrhoeae*[a]:

MIC (µg/mL)	Interpretation
≤1	Susceptible (S)
2	Intermediate (I)
≥4	Resistant (R)

[a] These interpretive standards are applicable only to broth microdilution susceptibility tests with streptococci using cation-adjusted Mueller-Hinton broth with 2–5% lysed horse blood.

For testing *Haemophilus influenzae* and *Haemophilus parainfluenzae*[b]:

MIC (µg/mL)	Interpretation
≤1	Susceptible (S)

[b] This interpretive standard is applicable only to broth microdilution susceptibility tests with *Haemophilus influenzae* and *Haemophilus parainfluenzae* using *Haemophilus* Test Medium[1].

The current absence of data on resistant strains precludes defining any results other than "Susceptible". Strains yielding MIC results suggestive of a "nonsusceptible" category should be submitted to a reference laboratory for further testing.

For testing *Neisseria gonorrhoeae*[c]:

MIC (µg/mL)	Interpretation
≤0.06	Susceptible (S)

[c] This interpretive standard is applicable only to agar dilution test with GC agar base and 1% defined growth supplement.

The current absence of data on resistant strains precludes defining any results other than "Susceptible". Strains yielding MIC results suggestive of a "nonsusceptible" category should be submitted to a reference laboratory for further testing.

A report of "Susceptible" indicates that the pathogen is likely to be inhibited if the antimicrobial compound in the blood reaches the concentrations usually achievable. A report of "Intermediate" indicates that the result should be considered equivocal, and, if the microorganism is not fully susceptible to alternative, clinically feasible drugs, the test should be repeated. This category implies possible clinical applicability in body sites where the drug is physiologically concentrated or in situations where high dosage of drug can be used. This category also provides a buffer zone which prevents small uncontrolled technical factors from causing major discrepancies in interpretation. A report of "Resistant" indicates that the pathogen is not likely to be inhibited if the antimicrobial compound in the blood reaches the concentrations usually achievable; other therapy should be selected.

Standardized susceptibility test procedures require the use of laboratory control microorganisms to control the technical aspects of the laboratory procedures. Standard ciprofloxacin powder should provide the following MIC values:

Organism		MIC (µg/mL)
E. faecalis	ATCC 29212	0.25 – 2.0
E. coli	ATCC 25922	0.004 – 0.015
H. influenzae[a]	ATCC 49247	0.004 – 0.03
N. gonorrhoeae[b]	ATCC 49226	0.001 – 0.008
P. aeruginosa	ATCC 27853	0.25 – 1.0
S. aureus	ATCC 29213	0.12 – 0.5

[a] This quality control range is applicable to only *H. influenzae* ATCC 49247 tested by a broth microdilution procedure using *Haemophilus* Test Medium (HTM)[1].
[b] This quality control range is applicable to only *N. gonorrhoeae* ATCC 49226 tested by an agar dilution procedure using GC agar base and 1% defined growth supplement.

Diffusion Techniques: Quantitative methods that require measurement of zone diameters also provide reproducible estimates of the susceptibility of bacteria to antimicrobial compounds. One such standardized procedure[2] requires the use of standardized inoculum concentrations. This procedure uses paper disks impregnated with 5-µg ciprofloxacin to test the susceptibility of microorganisms to ciprofloxacin. Reports from the laboratory providing results of the standard single-disk susceptibility test with a 5-µg ciprofloxacin disk should be interpreted according to the following criteria:

For testing aerobic microorganisms other than *Haemophilus influenzae, Haemophilus parainfluenzae,* and *Neisseria gonorrhoeae*[a]:

Zone Diameter (mm)	Interpretation
≥21	Susceptible (S)
16–20	Intermediate (I)
≤15	Resistant (R)

[a] These zone diameter standards are applicable only to tests performed for streptococci using Mueller-Hinton agar supplemented with 5% sheep blood incubated in 5% CO_2.

For testing *Haemophilus influenzae* and *Haemophilus parainfluenzae*[b]:

Zone Diameter (mm)	Interpretation
≥21	Susceptible (S)

[b] This zone diameter standard is applicable only to tests with *Haemophilus influenzae* and *Haemophilus parainfluenzae* using *Haemophilus* Test Medium (HTM)[2].

The current absence of data on resistant strains precludes defining any results other than "Susceptible". Strains yielding zone diameter results suggestive of a "nonsusceptible" category should be submitted to a reference laboratory for further testing.

For testing *Neisseria gonorrhoeae*[c]:

Zone Diameter (mm)	Interpretation
≥36	Susceptible (S)

[c] This zone diameter standard is applicable only to disk diffusion tests with GC agar base and 1% defined growth supplement.

The current absence of data on resistant strains precludes defining any results other than "Susceptible". Strains yielding zone diameter results suggestive of a "nonsusceptible" category should be submitted to a reference laboratory for further testing.

Interpretation should be as stated above for results using dilution techniques. Interpretation involves correlation of the diameter obtained in the disk test with the MIC for ciprofloxacin.

As with standardized dilution techniques, diffusion methods require the use of laboratory control microorganisms that are used to control the technical aspects of the laboratory procedures. For the diffusion technique, the 5-µg ciprofloxacin disk should provide the following zone diameters in these laboratory test quality control strains:

Organism		Zone Diameter (mm)
E. coli	ATCC 25922	30 – 40
H. influenzae[a]	ATCC 49247	34 – 42
N. gonorrhoeae[b]	ATCC 49226	48 – 58
P. aeruginosa	ATCC 27853	25 – 33
S. aureus	ATCC 25923	22 – 30

[a] These quality control limits are applicable to only *H. influenzae* ATCC 49247 testing using *Haemophilus* Test Medium (HTM)[2].
[b] These quality control limits are applicable only to tests conducted with *N. gonorrhoeae* ATCC 49226 performed by disk diffusion using GC agar base and 1% defined growth supplement.

INDICATIONS AND USAGE

CIPRO® is indicated for the treatment of infections caused by susceptible strains of the designated microorganisms in the conditions listed below. Please see **DOSAGE AND ADMINISTRATION** for specific recommendations.

Acute Sinusitis caused by *Haemophilus influenzae, Streptococcus pneumoniae*, or *Moraxella catarrhalis*.

Lower Respiratory Tract Infections caused by *Escherichia coli, Klebsiella pneumoniae, Enterobacter cloacae, Proteus mirabilis, Pseudomonas aeruginosa, Haemophilus influenzae, Haemophilus parainfluenzae*, or *Streptococcus pneumoniae*. Also, *Moraxella catarrhalis* for the treatment of acute exacerbations of chronic bronchitis.

NOTE: Although effective in clinical trials, ciprofloxacin is not a drug of first choice in the treatment of presumed or confirmed pneumonia secondary to *Streptococcus pneumoniae*.

Urinary Tract Infections caused by *Escherichia coli, Klebsiella pneumoniae, Enterobacter cloacae, Serratia marcescens, Proteus mirabilis, Providencia rettgeri, Morganella morganii, Citrobacter diversus, Citrobacter freundii, Pseudomonas aeruginosa, Staphylococcus epidermidis, Staphylococcus saprophyticus*, or *Enterococcus faecalis*.

Acute Uncomplicated Cystitis in females caused by *Escherichia coli* or *Staphylococcus saprophyticus*. (See **DOSAGE AND ADMINISTRATION.)**

Chronic Bacterial Prostatitis caused by *Escherichia coli* or *Proteus mirabilis*.

Complicated Intra-Abdominal Infections (used in combination with metronidazole) caused by *Escherichia coli, Pseudomonas aeruginosa, Proteus mirabilis, Klebsiella pneumoniae*, or *Bacteroides fragilis*. (See **DOSAGE AND ADMINISTRATION.)**

Skin and Skin Structure Infections caused by *Escherichia coli, Klebsiella pneumoniae, Enterobacter cloacae, Proteus mirabilis, Proteus vulgaris, Providencia stuartii, Morganella morganii, Citrobacter freundii, Pseudomonas aeruginosa, Staphylococcus aureus* (methicillin susceptible), *Staphylococcus epidermidis*, or *Streptococcus pyogenes*.

Bone and Joint Infections caused by *Enterobacter cloacae, Serratia marcescens*, or *Pseudomonas aeruginosa*.

Infectious Diarrhea caused by *Escherichia coli* (enterotoxigenic strains), *Campylobacter jejuni, Shigella boydii*, Shigella dysenteriae, Shigella flexneri* or *Shigella sonnei** when antibacterial therapy is indicated.

Typhoid Fever (Enteric Fever) caused by *Salmonella typhi*.

NOTE: The efficacy of ciprofloxacin in the eradication of the chronic typhoid carrier state has not been demonstrated.

Uncomplicated cervical and urethral gonorrhea due to *Neisseria gonorrhoeae.*

*Although treatment of infections due to this organism in this organ system demonstrated a clinically significant outcome, efficacy was studied in fewer than 10 patients.

If anaerobic organisms are suspected of contributing to the infection, appropriate therapy should be administered.

Appropriate culture and susceptibility tests should be performed before treatment in order to isolate and identify organisms causing infection and to determine their susceptibility to ciprofloxacin. Therapy with CIPRO® may be initiated before results of these tests are known; once results become available appropriate therapy should be continued. As with other drugs, some strains of *Pseudomonas aeruginosa* may develop resistance fairly rapidly during treatment with ciprofloxacin. Culture and susceptibility testing performed periodically during therapy will provide information not only on the therapeutic effect of the antimicrobial agent but also on the possible emergence of bacterial resistance.

CONTRAINDICATIONS

CIPRO® (ciprofloxacin hydrochloride) is contraindicated in persons with a history of hypersensitivity to ciprofloxacin or any member of the quinolone class of antimicrobial agents.

WARNINGS

THE SAFETY AND EFFECTIVENESS OF CIPROFLOXACIN IN PEDIATRIC PATIENTS AND ADOLESCENTS (LESS THAN 18 YEARS OF AGE), PREGNANT WOMEN, AND LACTATING WOMEN HAVE NOT BEEN ESTABLISHED. (See **PRECAUTIONS: Pediatric Use, Pregnancy** and **Nursing Mothers** subsections.) The oral administration of ciprofloxacin caused lameness in immature dogs. Histopathological examination of the weight-bearing joints of these dogs revealed permanent lesions of the cartilage. Related quinolone-class drugs also produce erosions of cartilage of weight-bearing joints and other signs of arthropathy in immature animals of various species. (See **ANIMAL PHARMACOLOGY**.)

Convulsions, increased intracranial pressure, and toxic psychosis have been reported in patients receiving quinolones, including ciprofloxacin. Ciprofloxacin may also cause central nervous system (CNS) events including: dizziness, confusion, tremors, hallucinations, depression, and, rarely, suicidal thoughts or acts. These reactions may occur following the first dose. If these reactions occur in patients receiving ciprofloxacin, the drug should be discontinued and appropriate measures instituted. As with all quinolones, ciprofloxacin should be used with caution in patients with known or suspected CNS disorders that may predispose to seizures or lower the seizure threshold (e.g. severe cerebral arteriosclerosis, epilepsy), or in the presence of other risk factors that may predispose to seizures or lower the seizure threshold (e.g. certain drug therapy, renal dysfunction). (See **PRECAUTIONS**: **General, Information for Patients, Drug Interactions** and **ADVERSE REACTIONS**.)

SERIOUS AND FATAL REACTIONS HAVE BEEN REPORTED IN PATIENTS RECEIVING CONCURRENT ADMINISTRATION OF CIPROFLOXACIN AND THEOPHYLLINE. These reactions have included cardiac arrest, seizure, status epilepticus, and respiratory failure. Although similar serious adverse effects have been reported in patients receiving theophylline alone, the possibility that these reactions may be potentiated by ciprofloxacin cannot be eliminated. If concomitant use cannot be avoided, serum levels of theophylline should be monitored and dosage adjustments made as appropriate.

Serious and occasionally fatal hypersensitivity (anaphylactic) reactions, some following the first dose, have been reported in patients receiving quinolone therapy. Some reactions were accompanied by cardiovascular collapse, loss of consciousness, tingling, pharyngeal or facial edema, dyspnea, urticaria, and itching. Only a few patients had a history of hypersensitivity reactions. Serious anaphylactic reactions require immediate emergency treatment with epinephrine. Oxygen, intravenous steroids, and airway management, including intubation, should be administered as indicated.

Severe hypersensitivity reactions characterized by rash, fever, eosinophilia, jaundice, and hepatic necrosis with fatal outcome have also been rarely reported in patients receiving ciprofloxacin along with other drugs. The possibility that these reactions were related to ciprofloxacin cannot be excluded. Ciprofloxacin should be discontinued at the first appearance of a skin rash or any other sign of hypersensitivity.

Pseudomembranous colitis has been reported with nearly all antibacterial agents, including ciprofloxacin, and may range in severity from mild to life-threatening. Therefore, it is important to consider this diagnosis in patients who present with diarrhea subsequent to the administration of antibacterial agents.

Treatment with antibacterial agents alters the normal flora of the colon and may permit overgrowth of clostridia. Studies indicate that a toxin produced by *Clostridium difficile* is one primary cause of "antibiotic-associated colitis."

After the diagnosis of pseudomembranous colitis has been established, therapeutic measures should be initiated. Mild cases of pseudomembranous colitis usually respond to drug discontinuation alone. In moderate to severe cases, consideration should be given to management with fluids and electrolytes, protein supplementation, and treatment with an antibacterial drug clinically effective against *C. difficile* colitis.

Achilles and other tendon ruptures that required surgical repair or resulted in prolonged disability have been reported with ciprofloxacin and other quinolones. Ciprofloxacin should be discontinued if the patient experiences pain, inflammation, or rupture of a tendon.

Ciprofloxacin has not been shown to be effective in the treatment of syphilis. Antimicrobial agents used in high dose for short periods of time to treat gonorrhea may mask or delay the symptoms of incubating syphilis. All patients with gonorrhea should have a serologic test for syphilis at the time of diagnosis. Patients treated with ciprofloxacin should have a follow-up serologic test for syphilis after three months.

PRECAUTIONS

General: Crystals of ciprofloxacin have been observed rarely in the urine of human subjects but more frequently in the urine of laboratory animals, which is usually alkaline. (See **ANIMAL PHARMACOLOGY**.) Crystalluria related to ciprofloxacin has been reported only rarely in humans because human urine is usually acidic. Alkalinity of the urine should be avoided in patients receiving ciprofloxacin. Patients should be well hydrated to prevent the formation of highly concentrated urine.

Quinolones, including ciprofloxacin, may also cause central nervous system (CNS) events, including: nervousness, agitation, insomnia, anxiety, nightmares or paranoia. (See **WARNINGS, Information for Patients**, and **Drug Interactions**.)

Alteration of the dosage regimen is necessary for patients with impairment of renal function. (See **DOSAGE AND ADMINISTRATION**.)

Moderate to severe phototoxicity manifested as an exaggerated sunburn reaction has been observed in patients who are exposed to direct sunlight while receiving some members of the quinolone class of drugs. Excessive sunlight should be avoided. Therapy should be discontinued if phototoxicity occurs.

As with any potent drug, periodic assessment of organ system functions, including renal, hepatic, and hematopoietic function, is advisable during prolonged therapy.

Information for Patients:

Patients should be advised:

- that ciprofloxacin may be taken with or without meals and to drink fluids liberally. As with other quinolones, concurrent administration of ciprofloxacin with magnesium/aluminum antacids, or sucralfate, Videx® (didanosine) chewable/buffered tablets or pediatric powder, or with other products containing calcium, iron or zinc should be avoided. These products may be taken two hours after or six hours before ciprofloxacin. Ciprofloxacin should not be taken concurrently with milk or yogurt alone, since absorption of ciprofloxacin may be significantly reduced. Dietary calcium as part of a meal, however, does not significantly affect ciprofloxacin absorption.
- that ciprofloxacin may be associated with hypersensitivity reactions, even following a single dose, and to discontinue the drug at the first sign of a skin rash or other allergic reaction.
- to avoid excessive sunlight or artificial ultraviolet light while receiving ciprofloxacin and to discontinue therapy if phototoxicity occurs.
- to discontinue treatment; rest and refrain from exercise; and inform their physician if they experience pain, inflammation, or rupture of a tendon.
- that ciprofloxacin may cause dizziness and lightheadedness; therefore, patients should know how they react to this drug before they operate an automobile or machinery or engage in activities requiring mental alertness or coordination.
- that ciprofloxacin may increase the effects of theophylline and caffeine. There is a possibility of caffeine accumulation when products containing caffeine are consumed while taking quinolones.
- that convulsions have been reported in patients taking quinolones, including ciprofloxacin, and to notify their physician before taking the drug if there is a history of this condition.

Drug Interactions: As with some other quinolones, concurrent administration of ciprofloxacin with theophylline may lead to elevated serum concentrations of theophylline and prolongation of its elimination half-life. This may result in increased risk of theophylline-related adverse reactions. (See **WARNINGS**.) If concomitant use cannot be avoided, serum levels of theophylline should be monitored and dosage adjustments made as appropriate.

Some quinolones, including ciprofloxacin, have also been shown to interfere with the metabolism of caffeine. This may lead to reduced clearance of caffeine and a prolongation of its serum half-life.

Concurrent administration of a quinolone, including ciprofloxacin, with multivalent cation-containing products such as magnesium/aluminum antacids, sucralfate, Videx® (didanosine) chewable/buffered tablets or pediatric powder, or products containing calcium, iron, or zinc may substantially decrease its absorption, resulting in serum and urine levels considerably lower than desired. (See **DOSAGE AND ADMINISTRATION** for concurrent administration of these agents with ciprofloxacin.)

Histamine H_2-receptor antagonists appear to have no significant effect on the bioavailability of ciprofloxacin.

Altered serum levels of phenytoin (increased and decreased) have been reported in patients receiving concomitant ciprofloxacin.

The concomitant administration of ciprofloxacin with the sulfonylurea glyburide has, on rare occasions, resulted in severe hypoglycemia.

Some quinolones, including ciprofloxacin, have been associated with transient elevations in serum creatinine in patients receiving cyclosporine concomitantly.

Quinolones have been reported to enhance the effects of the oral anticoagulant warfarin or its derivatives. When these products are administered concomitantly, prothrombin time or other suitable coagulation tests should be closely monitored.

Probenecid interferes with renal tubular secretion of ciprofloxacin and produces an increase in the level of ciprofloxacin in the serum. This should be considered if patients are receiving both drugs concomitantly.

As with other broad spectrum antimicrobial agents, prolonged use of ciprofloxacin may result in overgrowth of nonsusceptible organisms. Repeated evaluation of the patient's condition and microbial susceptibility testing is essential. If superinfection occurs during therapy, appropriate measures should be taken.

Carcinogenesis, Mutagenesis, Impairment of Fertility: Eight *in vitro* mutagenicity tests have been conducted with ciprofloxacin, and the test results are listed below:

Salmonella/Microsome Test (Negative)
E. coli DNA Repair Assay (Negative)
Mouse Lymphoma Cell Forward Mutation Assay (Positive)
Chinese Hamster V_{79} Cell HGPRT Test (Negative)
Syrian Hamster Embryo Cell Transformation Assay (Negative)
Saccharomyces cerevisiae Point Mutation Assay (Negative)
Saccharomyces cerevisiae Mitotic Crossover and Gene Conversion Assay (Negative)
Rat Hepatocyte DNA Repair Assay (Positive)

Thus, 2 of the 8 tests were positive, but results of the following 3 *in vivo* test systems gave negative results:

Rat Hepatocyte DNA Repair Assay
Micronucleus Test (Mice)
Dominant Lethal Test (Mice)

Long-term carcinogenicity studies in mice and rats have been completed. After daily oral doses of 750 mg/kg (mice) and 250 mg/kg (rats) were administered for up to 2 years, there was no evidence that ciprofloxacin had any carcinogenic or tumorigenic effects in these species.

Results from photo co-carcinogenicity testing indicate that ciprofloxacin does not reduce the time to appearance of UV-induced skin tumors as compared to vehicle control. Hairless (Skh-1) mice were exposed to UVA light for 3.5 hours five times every two weeks for up to 78 weeks while concurrently being administered ciprofloxacin. The time to development of the first skin tumors was 50 weeks in mice treated concomitantly with UVA and ciprofloxacin (mouse dose approximately equal to maximum recommended human dose based upon mg/m^2), as opposed to 34 weeks when animals were treated with both UVA and vehicle. The times to development of skin tumors ranged from 16–32 weeks in mice treated concomitantly with UVA and other quinolones.[3]

In this model, mice treated with ciprofloxacin alone did not develop skin or systemic tumors. There are no data from similar models using pigmented mice and/or fully haired mice. The clinical significance of these findings to humans is unknown.

Fertility studies performed in rats at oral doses of ciprofloxacin up to 100 mg/kg (0.8 times the highest recommended human dose of 1200 mg based upon body surface area) revealed no evidence of impairment.

Pregnancy: Teratogenic Effects. Pregnancy Category C: Reproduction studies have been performed in rats and mice using oral doses up to 100 mg/kg (0.6 and 0.3 times the maximum daily human dose based upon body surface area, respectively) and have revealed no evidence of harm to the fetus due to ciprofloxacin. In rabbits, ciprofloxacin (30 and 100 mg/kg orally) produced gastrointestinal disturbances resulting in maternal weight loss and an increased incidence of abortion, but no teratogenicity was observed at either dose. After intravenous administration of doses up to 20 mg/kg, no maternal toxicity was produced in the rabbit, and no embryotoxicity or teratogenicity was observed. There are, however, no adequate and well-controlled studies in pregnant women. Ciprofloxacin should be used during pregnancy only if the potential benefit justifies the potential risk to the fetus. (See **WARNINGS**.)

Nursing Mothers: Ciprofloxacin is excreted in human milk. Because of the potential for serious adverse reactions in infants nursing from mothers taking ciprofloxacin, a decision should be made whether to discontinue nursing or to discontinue the drug, taking into account the importance of the drug to the mother.

Pediatric Use: Safety and effectiveness in pediatric patients and adolescents less than 18 years of age have not been established. Ciprofloxacin causes arthropathy in juvenile animals. (See **WARNINGS**.)

Short-term safety data from a single trial in pediatric cystic fibrosis patients are available. In a randomized, double-blind clinical trial for the treatment of acute pulmonary exacerbations in cystic fibrosis patients (ages 5–17 years), 67 patients received ciprofloxacin I.V. 10 mg/kg/dose q8h for one week followed by ciprofloxacin tablets 20 mg/kg/dose q12h to complete 10–21 days treatment and 62 patients received the combination of ceftazidime I.V. 50 mg/kg/dose q8h and tobramycin I.V. 3 mg/kg/dose q8h for a total of

Continued on next page

Cipro—Cont.

10–21 days. Patients less than 5 years of age were not studied. Safety monitoring in the study included periodic range of motion examinations and gait assessments by treatment-blinded examiners. Patients were followed for an average of 23 days after completing treatment (range 0–93 days). This study was not designed to determine long term effects and the safety of repeated exposure to ciprofloxacin.

In the study, injection site reactions were more common in the ciprofloxacin group (24%) than in the comparison group (8%). Other adverse events were similar in nature and frequency between treatment arms. Musculoskeletal adverse events were reported in 22% of the patients in the ciprofloxacin group and 21% in the comparison group. Decreased range of motion was reported in 12% of the subjects in the ciprofloxacin group and 16% in the comparison group. Arthralgia was reported in 10% of the patients in the ciprofloxacin group and 11% in the comparison group. One of sixty-seven patients developed arthritis of the knee nine days after a ten day course of treatment with ciprofloxacin. Clinical symptoms resolved, but an MRI showed knee effusion without other abnormalities eight months after treatment. However, the relationship of this event to the patient's course of ciprofloxacin can not be definitively determined, particularly since patients with cystic fibrosis may develop arthralgias/arthritis as part of their underlying disease process.

Geriatric Use: In a retrospective analysis of 23 multiple-dose controlled clinical trials of ciprofloxacin encompassing over 3500 ciprofloxacin treated patients, 25% of patients were greater than or equal to 65 years of age and 10% were greater than or equal to 75 years of age. No overall differences in safety or effectiveness were observed between these subjects and younger subjects, and other reported clinical experience has not identified differences in responses between the elderly and younger patients, but greater sensitivity of some older individuals on any drug therapy cannot be ruled out. Ciprofloxacin is known to be substantially excreted by the kidney, and the risk of adverse reactions may be greater in patients with impaired renal function. No alteration of dosage is necessary for patients greater than 65 years of age with normal renal function. However, since some older individuals experience reduced renal function by virtue of their advanced age, care should be taken in dose selection for elderly patients, and renal function monitoring may be useful in these patients (See **CLINICAL PHARMACOLOGY** and **DOSAGE AND ADMINISTRATION**.)

ADVERSE REACTIONS

During clinical investigation with the tablet, 2,799 patients received 2,868 courses of the drug. Adverse events that were considered likely to be drug related occurred in 7.3% of patients treated, possibly related in 9.2% (total of 16.5% thought to be possibly or probably related to drug therapy), and remotely related in 3.0%. Ciprofloxacin was discontinued because of an adverse event in 3.5% of patients treated, primarily involving the gastrointestinal system (1.5%), skin (0.6%), and central nervous system (0.4%).

The most frequently reported events, drug related or not, were nausea (5.2%), diarrhea (2.3%), vomiting (2.0%), abdominal pain/discomfort (1.7%), headache (1.2%), restlessness (1.1%), and rash (1.1%).

Additional events that occurred in less than 1% of ciprofloxacin patients are listed below.

CARDIOVASCULAR: palpitation, atrial flutter, ventricular ectopy, syncope, hypertension, angina pectoris, myocardial infarction, cardiopulmonary arrest, cerebral thrombosis

CENTRAL NERVOUS SYSTEM: dizziness, lightheadedness, insomnia, nightmares, hallucinations, manic reaction, irritability, tremor, ataxia, convulsive seizures, lethargy, drowsiness, weakness, malaise, anorexia, phobia, depersonalization, depression, paresthesia (See above.) (See **PRECAUTIONS**.)

GASTROINTESTINAL: painful oral mucosa, oral candidiasis, dysphagia, intestinal perforation, gastrointestinal bleeding (See above.) Cholestatic jaundice has been reported.

MUSCULOSKELETAL: arthralgia or back pain, joint stiffness, achiness, neck or chest pain, flare up of gout

RENAL/UROGENITAL: interstitial nephritis, nephritis, renal failure, polyuria, urinary retention, urethral bleeding, vaginitis, acidosis

RESPIRATORY: dyspnea, epistaxis, laryngeal or pulmonary edema, hiccough, hemoptysis, bronchospasm, pulmonary emoblism

SKIN/HYPERSENSITIVITY: pruritus, urticaria, photosensitivity, flushing, fever, chills, angioedema, edema of the face, neck, lips, conjunctivae or hands, cutaneous candidiasis, hyperpigmentation, erythema nodosum (See above.)

Allergic reactions ranging from urticaria to anaphylactic reactions have been reported. (See **WARNINGS**.)

SPECIAL SENSES: blurred vision, disturbed vision (change in color perception, overbrightness of lights), decreased visual acuity, diplopia, eye pain, tinnitus, hearing loss, bad taste

Most of the adverse events reported were described as only mild or moderate in severity, abated soon after the drug was discontinued, and required no treatment.

In several instances nausea, vomiting, tremor, irritability, or palpitation were judged by investigators to be related to elevated serum levels of theophylline possibly as a result of drug interaction with ciprofloxacin.

DOSAGE GUIDELINES

Infection	Type or Severity	Unit Dose	Frequency	Usual Durations†
Acute Sinusitis	Mild/Moderate	500-mg	q 12 h	10 Days
Lower Respiratory Tract	Mild/Moderate Severe/Complicated	500-mg 750-mg	q 12 h q 12 h	7 to 14 Days 7 to 14 Days
Urinary Tract	Acute Uncomplicated Mild/Moderate Severe/Complicated	100-mg or 250-mg 250-mg 500-mg	q 12 h q 12 h q 12 h	3 Days 7 to 14 Days 7 to 14 Days
Chronic Bacterial Prostatitis	Mild/Moderate	500-mg	q 12 h	28 Days
Intra-Abdominal*	Complicated	500-mg	q 12 h	7 to 14 Days
Skin and Skin Structure	Mild/Moderate Severe/Complicated	500-mg 750-mg	q 12 h q 12 h	7 to 14 Days 7 to 14 Days
Bone and Joint	Mild/Moderate Severe/Complicated	500-mg 750-mg	q 12 h q 12 h	≥4 to 6 weeks ≥4 to 6 weeks
Infectious Diarrhea	Mild/Moderate/Severe	500-mg	q 12 h	5 to 7 Days
Typhoid Fever	Mild/Moderate	500-mg	q 12 h	10 Days
Urethral and Cervical Gonococcal Infections	Uncomplicated	250-mg	single dose	single dose

* used in conjunction with metronidazole

† Generally ciprofloxacin should be continued for at least 2 days after the signs and symptoms of infection have disappeared.

$$\text{Men: Creatinine clearance (mL/min)} = \frac{\text{Weight (kg)} \times (140 - \text{age})}{72 \times \text{serum creatinine (mg/dL)}}$$

Women: 0.85 × the value calculated for men.

In domestic clinical trials involving 214 patients receiving a single 250-mg oral dose, approximately 5% of patients reported adverse experiences without reference to drug relationship. The most common adverse experiences were vaginitis (2%), headache (1%), and vaginal pruritus (1%). Additional reactions, occurring in 0.3%–1% of patients, were abdominal discomfort, lymphadenopathy, foot pain, dizziness, and breast pain. Less than 20% of these patients had laboratory values obtained, and these results were generally consistent with the pattern noted for multi-dose therapy.

In randomized, double-blind controlled clinical trials comparing ciprofloxacin tablets (500 mg BID) to cefuroxime axetil (250 mg – 500 mg BID) and to clarithromycin (500 mg BID) in patients with respiratory tract infections, ciprofloxacin demonstrated a CNS adverse event profile comparable to the control drugs.

Post-Marketing Adverse Events: Additional adverse events, regardless of relationship to drug, reported from worldwide marketing experience with quinolones, including ciprofloxacin, are:

BODY AS A WHOLE: change in serum phenytoin

CARDIOVASCULAR: postural hypotension, vasculitis

CENTRAL NERVOUS SYSTEM: agitation, confusion, delirium, dysphasia, myoclonus, nystagmus, toxic psychosis

GASTROINTESTINAL: constipation, dyspepsia, flatulence, hepatic necrosis, jaundice, pancreatitis, pseudomembranous colitis (The onset of pseudomembranous colitis symptoms may occur during or after antimicrobial treatment.)

HEMIC/LYMPHATIC: agranulocytosis, hemolytic anemia, methemoglobinemia, prolongation of prothrombin time

METABOLIC/NUTRITIONAL: elevation of serum triglycerides, cholesterol, blood glucose, serum potassium

MUSCULOSKELETAL: myalgia, possible exacerbation of myasthenia gravis, tendinitis/tendon rupture

RENAL/UROGENITAL: albuminuria, candiduria, renal calculi, vaginal candidiasis

SKIN/HYPERSENSITIVITY: anaphylactic reactions, erythema multiforme/Stevens-Johnson syndrome, exfoliative dermatitis, toxic epidermal necrolysis

SPECIAL SENSES: anosmia, taste loss (See **PRECAUTIONS**.)

Adverse Laboratory Changes: Changes in laboratory parameters listed as adverse events without regard to drug relationship are listed below:

Hepatic — Elevations of ALT (SGPT) (1.9%), AST (SGOT) (1.7%), alkaline phosphatase (0.8%), LDH (0.4%), serum bilirubin (0.3%).

Hematologic— Eosinophilia (0.6%), leukopenia (0.4%), decreased blood platelets (0.1%), elevated blood platelets (0.1%), pancytopenia (0.1%).

Renal — Elevations of serum creatinine (1.1%), BUN (0.9%), CRYSTALLURIA, CYLINDRURIA, AND HEMATURIA HAVE BEEN REPORTED.

Other changes occurring in less than 0.1% of courses were: elevation of serum gammaglutamyl transferase, elevation of serum amylase, reduction in blood glucose, elevated uric acid, decrease in hemoglobin, anemia, bleeding diathesis, increase in blood monocytes, leukocytosis.

OVERDOSAGE

In the event of acute overdosage, the stomach should be emptied by inducing vomiting or by gastric lavage. The patient should be carefully observed and given supportive treatment. Adequate hydration must be maintained. Only a small amount of ciprofloxacin (<10%) is removed from the body after hemodialysis or peritoneal dialysis.

In mice, rats, rabbits and dogs, significant toxicity including tonic/clonic convulsions was observed at intravenous doses of ciprofloxacin between 125 and 300 mg/kg.

Single doses of ciprofloxacin were relatively non-toxic via the oral route of administration in mice, rats, and dogs. No deaths occurred within a 14-day post treatment observation period at the highest oral doses tested; up to 5000 mg/kg in either rodent species, or up to 2500 mg/kg in the dog. Clinical signs observed included hypoactivity and cyanosis in both rodent species and severe vomiting in dogs. In rabbits, significant mortality was seen at doses of ciprofloxacin > 2500 mg/kg. Mortality was delayed in these animals, occurring 10–14 days after dosing.

DOSAGE AND ADMINISTRATION

The recommended adult dosage for acute sinusitis is 500-mg every 12 hours.

Lower respiratory tract infections may be treated with 500-mg every 12 hours. For more severe or complicated infections, a dosage of 750-mg may be given every 12 hours.

Severe/complicated urinary tract infections or urinary tract infections caused by organisms not highly susceptible to ciprofloxacin may be treated with 500-mg every 12 hours. For other mild/moderate urinary infections, the usual adult dosage is 250-mg every 12 hours.

In acute uncomplicated cystitis in females, the usual dosage is 100-mg or 250-mg every 12 hours. For acute uncomplicated cystitis in females, 3 days of treatment is recommended while 7 to 14 days is suggested for other mild/moderate, severe or complicated urinary tract infections.

The recommended adult dosage for chronic bacterial prostatitis is 500-mg every 12 hours.

The recommended adult dosage for oral sequential therapy of complicated intra-abdominal infections is 500-mg every 12 hours. (To provide appropriate anaerobic activity, metronidazole should be given according to product labeling.) (See CIPRO® I.V. package insert.)

Skin and skin structure infections and bone and joint infections may be treated with 500-mg every 12 hours. For more severe or complicated infections, a dosage of 750-mg may be given every 12 hours.

The recommended adult dosage for infectious diarrhea or typhoid fever is 500-mg every 12 hours. For the treatment of uncomplicated urethral and cervical gonococcal infections, a single 250-mg dose is recommended.

See Instructions To The Pharmacist for Use/Handling of CIPRO® Oral Suspension.

[See first table above]

One teaspoonful (5 mL) of 5% ciprofloxacin oral suspension = 250-mg of ciprofloxacin.

One teaspoonful (5 mL) of 10% ciprofloxacin oral suspension = 500-mg of ciprofloxacin.

See Instructions for USE/HANDLING.

	Volume (mL) of Oral Suspension	
Dosage	**5%**	**10%**
250-mg	5 mL	2.5 mL
500-mg	10 mL	5 mL
750-mg	15 mL	7.5 mL

	Strength	NDC Code	Tablet Identification
Bottles of 50:	750-mg	NDC 0026-8514-50	CIPRO 750
Bottles of 100:	250-mg	NDC 0026-8512-51	CIPRO 250
	500-mg	NDC 0026-8513-51	CIPRO 500
Unit Dose Package of 100:	250-mg	NDC 0026-8512-48	CIPRO 250
	500-mg	NDC 0026-8513-48	CIPRO 500
	750-mg	NDC 0026-8514-48	CIPRO 750
Cystitis Package of 6:	100-mg	NDC 0026-8511-06	CIPRO 100

Drug Regimen	Clinical Response Resolution n (%)	Bacteriological Response By Organism (Eradication Rate) *E. coli* n (%)	*S. saprophyticus* n (%)
STUDY 1			
CIPRO 100-mg BID × 3 days	82/94 (87)	64/70 (91)	8/8 (100)
CIPRO 250-mg BID × 7 days	81/86 (94)	67/69 (97)	4/4 (100)
STUDY 2			
CIPRO 100-mg BID × 3 days	134/141 (95)	117/123 (95)	8/8 (100)
Control (3 days)	128/133 (96)	103/105 (98)	10/10 (100)

CIPRO (ciprofloxacin) 5% and 10% Oral Suspension should not be administered through feeding tubes due to its physical characteristics.

Complicated Intra-Abdominal Infections: Sequential therapy [parenteral to oral - 400-mg CIPRO® I.V. q 12 h (plus I.V. metronidazole) → 500-mg CIPRO® Tablets q 12 h (plus oral metronidazole)] can be instituted at the discretion of the physician.

The determination of dosage for any particular patient must take into consideration the severity and nature of the infection, the susceptibility of the causative organism, the integrity of the patient's host-defense mechanisms, and the status of renal function and hepatic function.

The duration of treatment depends upon the severity of infection. Generally ciprofloxacin should be continued for at least 2 days after the signs and symptoms of infection have disappeared. The usual duration is 7 to 14 days; however, for severe and complicated infections more prolonged therapy may be required. Bone and joint infections may require treatment for 4 to 6 weeks or longer. Chronic Bacterial Prostatitis should be treated for 28 days. Infectious diarrhea may be treated for 5–7 days. Typhoid fever should be treated for 10 days.

Ciprofloxacin should be administered at least 2 hours before or 6 hours after magnesium/aluminum antacids, or sucralfate Videx® (didanosine) chewable/buffered tablets or pediatric powder for oral solution, or other products containing calcium, iron or zinc.

Impaired Renal Function: Ciprofloxacin is eliminated primarily by renal excretion; however, the drug is also metabolized and partially cleared through the biliary system of the liver and through the intestine. These alternate pathways of drug elimination appear to compensate for the reduced renal excretion in patients with renal impairment. Nonetheless, some modification of dosage is recommended, particularly for patients with severe renal dysfunction. The following table provides dosage guidelines for use in patients with renal impairment; however, monitoring of serum drug levels provides the most reliable basis for dosage adjustment:

RECOMMENDED STARTING AND MAINTENANCE DOSES FOR PATIENTS WITH IMPAIRED RENAL FUNCTION

Creatinine Clearance (mL/min)	Dose
>50	See Usual Dosage.
30–50	250–500 mg q 12 h
5–29	250–500 mg q 18 h
Patients on hemodialysis or Peritoneal dialysis	250–500 mg q 24 h (after dialysis)

When only the serum creatinine concentration is known, the following formula may be used to estimate creatinine clearance.

[See second table at top of previous page]

The serum creatinine should represent a steady state of renal function.

In patients with severe infections and severe renal impairment, a unit dose of 750-mg may be administered at the intervals noted above; however, patients should be carefully monitored and the serum ciprofloxacin concentration should be measured periodically. Peak concentrations (1–2 hours after dosing) should generally range from 2 to 4 µg/mL.

For patients with changing renal function or for patients with renal impairment and hepatic insufficiency, measurement of serum concentration of ciprofloxacin will provide additional guidance for adjusting dosage.

HOW SUPPLIED

CIPRO® (ciprofloxacin hydrochloride) Tablets are available as round, slightly yellowish film-coated tablets containing 100-mg or 250-mg ciprofloxacin. The 100-mg tablet is coded with the word "CIPRO" on one side and "100" on the reverse side. The 250-mg tablet is coded with the word "CIPRO" on one side and "250" on the reverse side. CIPRO® is also available as capsule shaped, slightly yellowish film-coated tablets containing 500-mg or 750-mg ciprofloxacin. The 500-mg tablet is coded with the word "CIPRO" on one side and "500" on the reverse side. The 750-mg tablet is coded with the word "CIPRO" on one side and "750" on the reverse side. CIPRO® 250-mg, 500-mg, and 750-mg are available in bottles of 50, 100, and Unit Dose packages of 100. The 100-mg strength, is available only as CIPRO® Cystitis pack containing 6 tablets for use only in female patients with acute uncomplicated cystitis.

[See first table above]

Store below 30°C (86°F).

CIPRO® Oral Suspension is supplied in 5% (5g ciprofloxacin in 100 mL) and 10% (10g ciprofloxacin in 100 mL) strengths. The drug product is composed of two components (microcapsules and diluent) which are mixed prior to dispensing. See Instructions To The Pharmacist For Use/Handling.

Total volume after reconstitution	Ciprofloxacin contents after reconstitution	Ciprofloxacin contents per bottle	NDC Code
100 mL	250 mg/5 mL	5,000 mg	0026-8551-36
100 mL	500 mg/5 mL	10,000 mg	0026-8553-36

Microcapsules and diluent should be stored below 25°C (77°F) and protected from freezing.

Reconstituted product may be stored below 30°C (86°F) Protect from freezing. A teaspoon is provided for the patient.

ANIMAL PHARMACOLOGY

Ciprofloxacin and other quinolones have been shown to cause arthropathy in immature animals of most species tested. (See **WARNINGS.**) Damage of weight bearing joints was observed in juvenile dogs and rats. In young beagles, 100 mg/kg ciprofloxacin, given daily for 4 weeks, caused degenerative articular changes of the knee joint. At 30 mg/kg, the effect on the joint was minimal. In a subsequent study in beagles, removal of weight bearing from the joint reduced the lesions but did not totally prevent them.

Crystalluria, sometimes associated with secondary nephropathy, occurs in laboratory animals dosed with ciprofloxacin. This is primarily related to the reduced solubility of ciprofloxacin under alkaline conditions, which predominate in the urine of test animals; in man, crystalluria is rare since human urine is typically acidic. In rhesus monkeys, crystalluria without nephropathy has been noted after single oral doses as low as 5 mg/kg. After 6 months of intravenous dosing at 10 mg/kg/day, no nephropathological changes were noted; however, nephropathy was observed after dosing at 20 mg/kg/day for the same duration.

In dogs, ciprofloxacin at 3 and 10 mg/kg by rapid IV injection (15 sec.) produces pronounced hypotensive effects. These effects are considered to be related to histamine release, since they are partially antagonized by pyrilamine, an antihistamine. In rhesus monkeys, rapid IV injection also produced hypotension but the effect in this species is inconsistent and less pronounced.

In mice, concomitant administration of nonsteroidal anti-inflammatory drugs such as phenylbutazone and indomethacin with quinolones has been reported to enhance the CNS stimulatory effect of quinolones.

Ocular toxicity seen with some related drugs has not been observed in ciprofloxacin-treated animals.

CLINICAL STUDIES

Acute Sinusitis Studies

Ciprofloxacin tablets (500-mg BID) were evaluated for the treatment of acute sinusitis in two randomized, double-blind, controlled clinical trials conducted in the United States. Study 1 compared ciprofloxacin with cefuroxime axetil (250-mg BID) and enrolled 501 patients (400 of which were valid for the primary efficacy analysis). Study 2 compared ciprofloxacin with clarithromycin (500-mg BID) and enrolled 560 patients (418 of whom were valid for the primary efficacy analysis). The primary test of cure endpoint was a follow-up visit performed approximately 30 days after the completion of treatment with study medication. Clinical response data from these studies are summarized below:

Drug Regimen	Clinical Response Resolution at 30 Day Follow-up n (%)
STUDY 1	
CIPRO 500-mg BID × 10 days	152/197 (77)
Cefuroxime Axetil 250-mg BID × 10 days	145/203 (71)
STUDY 2	
CIPRO 500-mg BID × 10 days	168/212 (79)
Clarithromycin 500-mg BID × 14 days	169/206 (82)

In ciprofloxacin-treated patients enrolled in controlled and uncontrolled acute sinusitis studies, all of which included antral puncture, bacteriological eradication/presumed eradication was documented at the 30 day follow-up visit in 44 of 50 (88%) *H. influenzae*, 17 of 21 (80.9%) *M. catarrhalis*, and 42 of 51 (82.3%) *S. pneumoniae*. Patients infected with *S. pneumoniae* strains whose baseline susceptibilities were intermediate or resistant to ciprofloxacin had a lower success rate than patients infected with susceptible strains.

Uncomplicated Cystitis Studies

Efficacy: Two U.S. double-blind, controlled clinical studies of acute uncomplicated cystitis in women compared ciprofloxacin 100-mg BID for 3 days to ciprofloxacin 250-mg BID for 7 days or control drug. In these two studies, using strict evaluability criteria and microbiologic and clinical response criteria at the 5–9 day post-therapy follow-up, the following clinical resolution and bacterial eradication rates were obtained:

[See second table above]

Instructions To The Pharmacist For Use/Handling of CIPRO® Oral Suspension:

Preparation of the suspension:

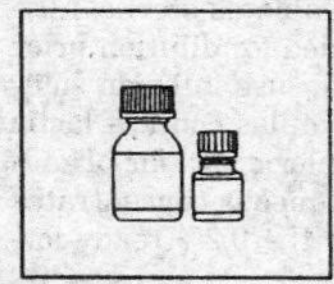

1. The small bottle contains the microcapsules, the large bottle contains the diluent.

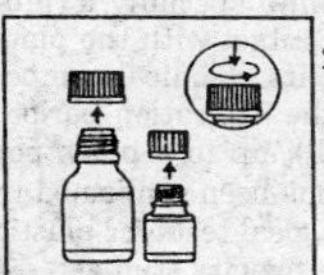

2. Open both bottles. Child-proof cap: Press down according to instructions on the cap while turning to the left.

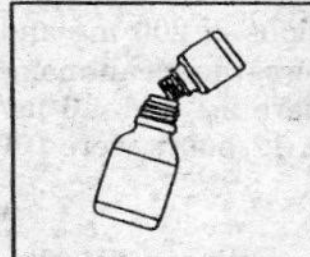

3. Pour the microcapsules completely into the large bottle of diluent. **Do not add water to the suspension.**

4. Remove the top layer of the diluent bottle label (to reveal the CIPRO® Oral Suspension label).

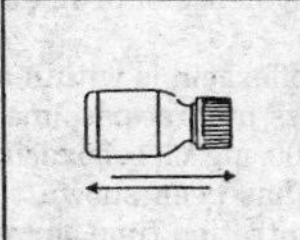

5. Close the large bottle completely according to the directions on the cap and shake vigorously for about 15 seconds. The suspension is ready for use.

Instructions To The Patient For Taking CIPRO® ORAL Suspension:

Shake vigorously each time before use for approximately 15 seconds.

Swallow the prescribed amount of suspension. Do not chew the microcapsules. Reclose the bottle completely after use according to the instructions on the cap. Shake vigorously each time before use for approximately 15 seconds. The product can be used 14 days when stored in a refrigerator or at room temperature (below 86°F). After treatment has been completed, any remaining suspension should not be reused.

REFERENCES

1. National Committee for Clinical Laboratory Standards, Methods for Dilution Antimicrobial Susceptibility Tests for Bacteria That Grow Aerobically-Fourth Edition. Approved Standard NCCLS Document M7–A4, Vol. 17, No. 2, NCCLS, Wayne, PA, January, 1997. **2.** National Committee for Clinical Laboratory Standards, Performance Standards for Antimicrobial Disk Susceptibility Tests-Sixth Edition. Approved Standard NCCLS Document M2–A6, Vol. 17, No. 1,

Continued on next page

Cipro—Cont.

NCCLS, Wayne, PA, January, 1997. **3.** Report presented at the FDA's Anti-Infective Drug and Dermatological Drug Product's Advisory Committee meeting, March 31, 1993, Silver Spring, MD. Report available from FDA, CDER, Advisors and Consultants Staff, HFD-21, 1901 Chapman Avenue, Room 200, Rockville, MD 20852, USA

Bayer Corporation
Pharmaceutical Division
400 Morgan Lane
West Haven, CT 06516 USA

℞ **Only**

PZ500167 7/00 Bay o 9867 5202-2-A-U.S.-10

CIPRO® (ciprofloxacin) 5% and 10% ORAL SUSPENSION

Made in Italy Printed in U.S.A.

CIPRO® I.V. ℞

(ciprofloxacin)
For Intravenous Infusion

DESCRIPTION

CIPRO® I.V. (ciprofloxacin) is a synthetic broad-spectrum antimicrobial agent for intravenous (I.V.) administration. Ciprofloxacin, a fluoroquinolone, is 1-cyclopropyl-6-fluoro-1, 4-dihydro-4-oxo-7-(1-piperazinyl) -3- quinolinecarboxylic acid. Its empirical formula is $C_{17}H_{18}FN_3O_3$ and its chemical structure is:

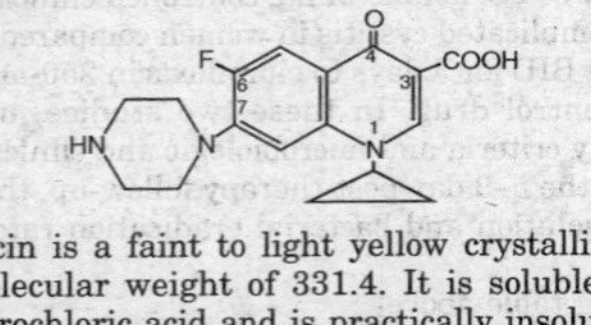

Ciprofloxacin is a faint to light yellow crystalline powder with a molecular weight of 331.4. It is soluble in dilute (0.1N) hydrochloric acid and is practically insoluble in water and ethanol. Ciprofloxacin differs from other quinolones in that it has a fluorine atom at the 6-position, a piperazine moiety at the 7-position, and a cyclopropyl ring at the 1-position. CIPRO® I.V. solutions are available as sterile 1.0% aqueous concentrates, which are intended for dilution prior to administration, and as 0.2% ready-for-use infusion solutions in 5% Dextrose Injection. All formulas contain lactic acid as a solubilizing agent and hydrochloric acid for pH adjustment. The pH range for the 1.0% aqueous concentrates in vials is 3.3 to 3.9. The pH range for the 0.2% ready-for-use infusion solutions is 3.5 to 4.6.

The plastic container is fabricated from a specially formulated polyvinyl chloride. Solutions in contact with the plastic container can leach out certain of its chemical components in very small amounts within the expiration period, e.g., di(2-ethylhexyl) phthalate (DEHP), up to 5 parts per million. The suitability of the plastic has been confirmed in tests in animals according to USP biological tests for plastic containers as well as by tissue culture toxicity studies.

CLINICAL PHARMACOLOGY

Following 60-minute intravenous infusions of 200 mg and 400 mg ciprofloxacin to normal volunteers, the mean maximum serum concentrations achieved were 2.1 and 4.6 μg/mL, respectively; the concentrations at 12 hours were 0.1 and 0.2 μg/mL, respectively.

[See first table above]

Steady-state Ciprofloxacin Serum Concentrations (μg/mL) After 60-minute I.V. Infusions q 12 h.

	Time after starting the infusion					
Dose	**30 min**	**1 hr**	**3 hr**	**6 hr**	**8 hr**	**12 hr**
200 mg	1.7	2.1	0.6	0.3	0.2	0.1
400 mg	3.7	4.6	1.3	0.7	0.5	0.2

The pharmacokinetics of ciprofloxacin are linear over the dose range of 200 to 400 mg administered intravenously. The serum elimination half-life is approximately 5–6 hours and the total clearance is around 35 L/hr. Comparison of the pharmacokinetic parameters following the 1st and 5th I.V. dose on a q 12 h regimen indicates no evidence of drug accumulation.

The absolute bioavailability of oral ciprofloxacin is within a range of 70–80% with no substantial loss by first pass metabolism. An intravenous infusion of 400 mg ciprofloxacin given over 60 minutes every 12 hours has been shown to produce an area under the serum concentration time curve (AUC) equivalent to that produced by a 500-mg oral dose given every 12 hours. An intravenous infusion of 400 mg ciprofloxacin given over 60 minutes every 8 hours has been shown to produce an AUC at steady-state equivalent to that produced by a 750-mg oral dose given every 12 hours. A 400-mg I.V. dose results in a C_{max} similar to that observed with a 750-mg oral dose. An infusion of 200 mg ciprofloxacin given every 12 hours produces an AUC equivalent to that produced by a 250-mg oral dose given every 12 hours.

[See second table above]

Steady-state Pharmacokinetic Parameter Following Multiple Oral and I.V. Doses

Parameters	500 mg q12h, P.O.	400 mg q12h, I.V.	750 mg q12h, P.O.	400 mg q8h, I.V.
AUC (μg•hr/mL)	13.7[a]	12.7[a]	31.6[b]	32.9[c]
C_{max} (μg/mL)	2.97	4.56	3.59	4.07

[a]AUC_{0-12h}
[b]AUC 24h=AUC_{0-12h} × 2
[c]AUC 24h=AUC_{0-8h} × 3

After intravenous administration, approximately 50% to 70% of the dose is excreted in the urine as unchanged drug. Following a 200-mg I.V. dose, concentrations in the urine usually exceed 200 μg/mL 0–2 hours after dosing and are generally greater than 15 μg/mL 8–12 hours after dosing. Following a 400-mg I.V. dose, urine concentrations generally exceed 400 μg/mL 0–2 hours after dosing and are usually greater than 30 μg/mL 8–12 hours after dosing. The renal clearance is approximately 22 L/hr. The urinary excretion of ciprofloxacin is virtually complete by 24 hours after dosing.

The serum concentrations of ciprofloxacin and metronidazole were not altered when these two drugs were given concomitantly.

Co-administration of probenecid with ciprofloxacin results in about a 50% reduction in the ciprofloxacin renal clearance and a 50% increase in its concentration in the systemic circulation. Although bile concentrations of ciprofloxacin are severalfold higher than serum concentrations after intravenous dosing, only a small amount of the administered dose (<1%) is recovered from the bile as unchanged drug. Approximately 15% of an I.V. dose is recovered from the feces within 5 days after dosing.

After I.V. administration, three metabolites of ciprofloxacin have been identified in human urine which together account for approximately 10% of the intravenous dose.

Pharmacokinetic studies of the oral (single dose) and intravenous (single and multiple dose) forms of ciprofloxacin indicate that plasma concentrations of ciprofloxacin are higher in elderly subjects (>65 years) as compared to young adults. Although the C_{max} is increased 16–40%, the increase in mean AUC is approximately 30%, and can be at least partially attributed to decreased renal clearance in the elderly. Elimination half-life is only slightly (~20%) prolonged in the elderly. These differences are not considered clinically significant. (See **PRECAUTIONS: Geriatric Use.**)

In patients with reduced renal function, the half-life of ciprofloxacin is slightly prolonged and dosage adjustments may be required. (See **DOSAGE AND ADMINISTRATION.**)

In preliminary studies in patients with stable chronic liver cirrhosis, no significant changes in ciprofloxacin pharmacokinetics have been observed. However, the kinetics of ciprofloxacin in patients with acute hepatic insufficiency have not been fully elucidated.

Following infusion of 400 mg I.V. ciprofloxacin every eight hours in combination with 50 mg/kg I.V. piperacillin sodium every 4 hours, mean serum ciprofloxacin concentrations were 3.02 μg/mL ½ hour and 1.18 μg/mL between 6–8 hours after the end of infusion.

The binding of ciprofloxacin to serum proteins is 20 to 40%. After intravenous administration, ciprofloxacin is present in saliva, nasal and bronchial secretions, sputum, skin blister fluid, lymph, peritoneal fluid, bile, and prostatic secretions. It has also been detected in the lung, skin, fat, muscle, cartilage, and bone. Although the drug diffuses into cerebrospinal fluid (CSF), CSF concentrations are generally less than 10% of peak serum concentrations. Levels of the drug in the aqueous and vitreous chambers of the eye are lower than in serum.

Microbiology: Ciprofloxacin has *in vitro* activity against a wide range of gram-negative and gram-positive microorganisms. The bactericidal action of ciprofloxacin results from interference with the enzyme DNA gyrase which is needed for the synthesis of bacterial DNA.

Ciprofloxacin has been shown to be active against most strains of the following microorganisms, both *in vitro* and in clinical infections as described in the **INDICATIONS AND USAGE** section of the package insert for CIPRO® I.V. (ciprofloxacin for intravenous infusion).

Aerobic gram-positive microorganisms
Enterococcus faecalis
(Many strains are only moderately susceptible.)
Staphylococcus aureus
(methicillin susceptible)
Staphylococcus epidermidis
Staphylococcus saprophyticus
Streptococcus pneumoniae
Streptococcus pyogenes

Aerobic gram-negative microorganisms
Citrobacter diversus
Citrobacter freundii
Enterobacter cloacae
Escherichia coli
Haemophilus influenzae
Haemophilus parainfluenzae
Klebsiella pneumoniae
Moraxella catarrhalis
Morganella morganii
Proteus mirabilis
Proteus vulgaris
Providencia rettgeri
Providencia stuartii
Pseudomonas aeruginosa
Serratia marcescens

Ciprofloxacin has been shown to be active against most strains of the following microorganisms, both *in vitro* and in clinical infections as described in the **INDICATIONS AND USAGE** section of the package insert for CIPRO® (ciprofloxacin hydrochloride) Tablets.

Aerobic gram-positive microorganisms
Enterococcus faecalis
(Many strains are only moderately susceptible.)
Staphylococcus aureus
(methicillin susceptible)
Staphylococcus epidermidis
Staphylococcus saprophyticus
Streptococcus pneumoniae
Streptococcus pyogenes

Aerobic gram-negative microorganisms
Campylobacter jejuni
Citrobacter diversus
Citrobacter freundii
Enterobacter cloacae
Escherichia coli
Haemophilus influenzae
Haemophilus parainfluenzae
Klebsiella pneumoniae
Moraxella catarrhalis
Morganella morganii
Neisseria gonorrhoeae
Proteus mirabilis
Proteus vulgaris
Providencia rettgeri
Providencia stuartii
Pseudomonas aeruginosa
Salmonella typhi
Serratia marcescens
Shigella boydii
Shigella dysenteriae
Shigella flexneri
Shigella sonnei

The following *in vitro* data are available, **but their clinical significance is unknown.**

Ciprofloxacin exhibits *in vitro* minimum inhibitory concentrations (MICs) of 1 μg/mL or less against most (≥90%) strains of the following microorganisms; however, the safety and effectiveness of ciprofloxacin in treating clinical infections due to these microorganisms have not been established in adequate and well-controlled clinical trials.

Aerobic gram-positive microorganisms
Staphylococcus haemolyticus
Staphylococcus hominis

Aerobic gram-negative microorganisms
Acinetobacter iwoffi
Aeromonas hydrophila
Edwardsiella tarda
Enterobacter aerogenes
Klebsiella oxytoca
Legionella pneumophila
Pasteurella multocida
Salmonella enteritidis
Vibrio cholerae
Vibrio parahaemolyticus
Vibrio vulnificus
Yersinia enterocolitica

Most strains of *Burkholderia cepacia* and some strains of *Stenotrophomonas maltophilia* are resistant to ciprofloxacin as are most anaerobic bacteria, including *Bacteroides fragilis* and *Clostridium difficile*.

Ciprofloxacin is slightly less active when tested at acidic pH. The inoculum size has little effect when tested *in vitro*. The minimum bactericidal concentration (MBC) generally does not exceed the minimum inhibitory concentration (MIC) by more than a factor of 2. Resistance of ciprofloxacin *in vitro* usually develops slowly (multiple-step mutation).

Ciprofloxacin does not cross-react with other antimicrobial agents such as beta-lactams or aminoglycosides; therefore, organisms resistant to these drugs may be susceptible to ciprofloxacin.

In vitro studies have shown that additive activity often results when ciprofloxacin is combined with other antimicrobial agents such as beta-lactams, aminoglycosides, clindamycin, or metronidazole. Synergy has been reported particularly with the combination of ciprofloxacin and a beta-lactam; antagonism is observed only rarely.

Susceptibility Tests

Dilution Techniques: Quantitative methods are used to determine antimicrobial minimum inhibitory concentrations (MICs). These MICs provide estimates of the susceptibility of bacteria to antimicrobial compounds. The MICs should be determined using a standardized procedure. Standardized procedures are based on a dilution method[1] (broth or agar) or equivalent with standardized inoculum concentrations and standardized concentrations of ciprofloxacin powder. The MIC values should be interpreted according to the following criteria:

For test aerobic microorganisms other than *Haemophilus influenzae, Haemophilus parainfluenzae*, and *Neisseria gonorrhoeae*[a]:

MIC (μg/mL)	Interpretation
≤ 1	Susceptible (S)
2	Intermediate (I)
≥ 4	Resistant (R)

[a] These interpretive standards are applicable only to broth microdilution susceptibility tests with streptococci using cation-adjusted Mueller-Hinton broth with 2–5% lysed horse blood.

For testing *Haemophilus influenzae* and *Haemophilus parainfluenzae*[b]:

MIC (μg/mL)	Interpretation
≤ 1	Susceptible (S)

[b] This interpretive standard is applicable only to broth microdilution susceptibility tests with *Haemophilus influenzae* and *Haemophilus parainfluenzae* using *Haemophilus* Test Medium[1].

The current absence of data on resistant strains precludes defining any results other than "Susceptible". Strains yielding MIC results suggestive of a "nonsusceptible" category should be submitted to a reference laboratory for further testing.

For testing *Neisseria gonorrhoeae*[c]:

MIC (μg/mL)	Interpretation
≤0.06	Susceptible (S)

[c] This interpretive standard is applicable only to agar dilution test with GC agar base and 1% defined growth supplement.

The current absence of data on resistant strains precludes defining any results other than "Susceptible". Strains yielding MIC results suggestive of a "nonsusceptible" category should be submitted to a reference laboratory for further testing.

A report of "Susceptible" indicates that the pathogen is likely to be inhibited if the antimicrobial compound in the blood reaches the concentrations usually achievable. A report of "Intermediate" indicates that the result should be considered equivocal, and, if the microoganism is not fully susceptible to alternative, clinically feasible drugs, the test should be repeated. This category implies possible clinical applicability in body sites where the drug is physiologically concentrated or in situations where high dosage of drug can be used. This category also provides a buffer zone which prevents small uncontrolled technical factors from causing major discrepancies in interpretation. A report of "Resistant" indicates that the pathogen is not likely to be inhibited if the antimicrobial compound in the blood reaches the concentrations usually achievable; other therapy should be selected.

Standardized susceptibility test procedures require the use of laboratory control microorganisms to control the technical aspects of the laboratory procedures. Standard ciprofloxacin powder should provide the following MIC values:

[See first table above]

Diffusion Techniques: Quantitative methods that require measurement of zone diameters also provide reproducible estimates of the susceptibility of bacteria to antimicrobial compounds. One such standardized procedure[2] requires the use of standardized inoculum concentrations. This procedure uses paper disks impregnated with 5-μg ciprofloxacin to test the susceptibility of microorganisms to ciprofloxacin. Reports from the laboratory providing results of the standard single-disk susceptibility test with a 5-μg ciprofloxacin disk should be interpreted according to the following criteria:

For testing aerobic microorganisms other than *Haemophilus influenzae, Haemophilus parainfluenzae*, and *Neisseria gonorrhoeae*[a]:

Zone Diameter (mm)	Interpretation
≥ 21	Susceptible (S)
16–20	Intermediate (I)
≤ 15	Resistant (R)

[a] These zone diameter standards are applicable only to tests performed for streptococci using Mueller-Hinton agar supplemented with 5% sheep blood incubated in 5% CO_2.

For testing *Haemophilus influenzae* and *Haemophilus parainfluenzae*[b]:

Zone Diameter (mm)	Interpretation
≥ 21	Susceptible (S)

[b] This zone diameter standard is applicable only to tests with *Haemophilus influenzae* and *Haemophilus parainfluenzae* using *Haemophilus* Test Medium (HTM)[2].

The current absence of data on resistant strains precludes defining any results other than "Susceptible". Strains yield-

Organism		MIC (μg/mL)
E. faecalis	ATCC 29212	0.25–2.0
E. coli	ATCC 25922	0.004–0.015
H. influenzae[a]	ATCC 49247	0.004–0.03
N. gonorrhoeae[b]	ATCC 49226	0.001–0.008
P. aeruginosa	ATCC 27853	0.25–1.0
S. aureus	ATCC 29213	0.12–0.5

[a] This quality control range is applicable to only *H. influenzae* ATCC 49247 tested by a broth microdilution procedure using *Haemophilus* Test Medium (HTM)[1].

[b] This quality control range is applicable to only *N. gonorrhoeae* ATCC 49226 tested by an agar dilution procedure using GC agar base and 1% defined growth supplement.

Organism		Zone Diameter (mm)
E. coli	ATCC 25922	30–40
H. influenzae[a]	ATCC 49247	34–42
N. gonorrhoeae[b]	ATCC 49226	48–58
P. aeruginosa	ATCC 27853	25–33
S. aureus	ATCC 25923	22–30

[a] These quality control limits are applicable to only *H. influenzae* ATCC 49247 testing using *Haemophilus* Test Medium (HTM)[2].

[b] These quality control limits are applicable only to tests conducted with *N. gonorrhoeae* ATCC 49226 performed by disk diffusion using GC agar base and 1% defined growth supplement.

Total	Ciprofloxacin/Piperacillin N = 233		Tobramycin/Piperacillin N = 237	
Median Age (years)	47.0	(range 19–84)	50.0	(range 18–81)
Male	114	(48.9%)	117	(49.4%)
Female	119	(51.1%)	120	(50.6%)
Leukemia/Bone Marrow Transplant	165	(70.8%)	158	(66.7%)
Solid Tumor/Lymphoma	68	(29.2%)	79	(33.3%)
Medial Duration of Neutropenia (days)	15.0	(range 1–61)	14.0	(range 1–89)

ing zone diameter results suggestive of a "nonsusceptible" category should be submitted to a reference laboratory for further testing.

For testing *Neisseria gonorrhoeae*[c]:

Zone Diameter (mm)	Interpretation
≥36	Susceptible (S)

[c] This zone diameter standard is applicable only to disk diffusion tests with GC agar base and 1% defined growth supplement.

The current absence of data on resistant strains precludes defining any results other than "Susceptible". Strains yielding zone diameter results suggestive of a "nonsusceptible" category should be submitted to a reference laboratory for further testing.

Interpretation should be as stated above for results using dilution techniques. Interpretation involves correlation of the diameter obtained in the disk test with the MIC for ciprofloxacin.

As with standardized dilution techniques, diffusion methods require the use of laboratory control microorganisms that are used to control the technical aspects of the laboratory procedures. For the diffusion technique, the 5-μg ciprofloxacin disk should provide the following zone diameters in these laboratory test quality control strains:

[See second table above]

INDICATIONS AND USAGE

CIPRO® I.V. is indicated for the treatment of infections caused by susceptible strains of the designated miroorganisms in the conditions listed below when the intravenous administration offers a route of administration advantageous to the patient. Please see **DOSAGE AND ADMINISTRATION** for specific recommendations.

Urinary Tract Infections caused by *Escherichia coli* (including cases with secondary bacteremia), *Klebsiella pneumoniae* subspecies *pneumoniae, Enterobacter cloacae, Serratia marcescens, Proteus mirabilis, Providencia rettgeri, Morganella morganii, Citrobacter diversus, Citrobacter freundii, Pseudomonas aeruginosa, Staphylococcus epidermidis, Staphylococcus saprophyticus*, or *Enterococcus faecalis*.

Lower Respiratory Infections caused by *Escherichia coli, Klebsiella pneumoniae* subspecies *pneumoniae, Enterobacter cloacae, Proteus mirabilis, Pseudomonas aeruginosa, Haemophilus influenzae, Haemophilus parainfluenzae*, or *Streptococcus pneumoniae*.

NOTE: Although effective in clinical trials, ciprofloxacin is not a drug of first choice in the treatment of presumed or confirmed pneumonia secondary to *Streptococcus pneumoniae*.

Nosocomial Pneumonia caused by *Haemophilus influenzae* or *Klebsiella pneumoniae*.

Skin and Skin Structure Infections caused by *Escherichia coli, Klebsiella pneumoniae* subspecies *pneumoniae, Enterobacter cloacae, Proteus mirabilis, Proteus vulgaris, Providencia stuartii, Morganella morganii, Citrobacter freundii, Pseudomonas aeruginosa, Staphylococcus aureus* (methicillin susceptible), *Staphylococcus epidermidis*, or *Streptococcus pyogenes*.

Bone and Joint Infections caused by *Enterobacter cloacae, Serratia marcescens*, or *Pseudomonas aeruginosa*.

Complicated Intra-Abdominal Infections (used in conjunction with metronidazole) caused by *Escherichia coli, Pseudomonas aeruginosa, Proteus mirabilis, Klebsiella pneumonia*, or *Bacteroides fragilis*. (See **DOSAGE AND ADMINISTRATION.**)

Acute Sinusitis caused by *Haemophilus influenzae, Streptococcus pneumoniae*, or *Moraxella catarrhalis*.

Chronic Bacterial Prostatitis caused by *Escherichia coli* or *Proteus mirabilis*.

Empirical Therapy for Febrile Neutropenic Patients in combination with piperacillin sodium. (See **DOSAGE AND ADMINISTRATION** and **CLINICAL STUDIES.**)

If anaerobic organisms are suspected of contributing to the infection, appropriate therapy should be administered.

Appropriate culture and susceptibility tests should be performed before treatment in order to isolate and identify organisms causing infection and to determine their susceptibility to ciprofloxacin. Therapy with CIRPO® I.V. may be initiated before results of these tests are known; once results become available, appropriate therapy should be continued.

As with other drugs, some strains of *Pseudomonas aeruginosa* may develop resistance fairly rapidly during treatment with ciprofloxacin. Culture and susceptibility testing performed periodically during therapy will provide information not only on the therapeutic effect of the antimicrobial agent but also on the possible emergence of bacterial resistance.

CLINICAL STUDIES

EMPIRICAL THERAPY IN FEBRILE NEUTROPENIC PATIENTS

The safety and efficacy of ciprofloxacin, 400 mg I.V. q 8h, in combination with piperacillin sodium, 50 mg/kg I.V. q 4h, for the empirical therapy of febrile neutropenic patients were studied in one large multicenter, randomized trial and were compared to those of tobramycin, 2 mg/kg I.V. q 8h, in combination with piperacilin sodium, 50 mg/kg I.V. q 4h.

The demographics of the evaluable patients were as follows:

[See third table above]

Clinical response rates observed in this study were as follows:

[See table at top of next page]

CONTRAINDICATIONS

CIPRO® I.V. (ciprofloxacin) is contraindicated in persons with a history of hypersensitivity to ciprofloxacin or any member of the quinolone class of antimicrobial agents.

WARNINGS

THE SAFETY AND EFFECTIVENESS OF CIPROFLOXACIN IN PEDIATRIC PATIENTS AND ADOLESCENTS (LESS THAN 18 YEARS OF AGE), PREGNANT WOMEN, AND LACTATING WOMEN HAVE NOT BEEN ESTABLISHED. (See **PRECAUTIONS: Pediatric Use, Pregnancy,** and **Nursing Mothers** subsections.) Ciprofloxacin causes lameness in immature dogs. Histopathological examination of the weight-bearing joints of these dogs revealed permanent lesions of the cartilage. Related quinolone-class drugs also produce erosions of cartilage of weight-bearing joints and other signs of arthropathy in immature animals of various species. (See **ANIMAL PHARMACOLOGY.**)

Continued on next page

Cipro I.V.—Cont.

Convulsions, increased intracranial pressure, and toxic psychosis have been reported in patients receiving quinolones, including ciprofloxacin. Ciprofloxacin may also cause central nervous system (CNS) events including: dizziness, confusion, tremors, hallucinations, depression, and, rarely, suicidal thoughts or acts. These reactions may occur following the first dose. If these reactions occur in patients receiving ciprofloxacin, the drug should be discontinued and appropriate measures instituted. As with all quinolones, ciprofloxacin should be used with caution in patients with known or suspected CNS disorders that may predispose to seizures or lower the seizure threshold (e.g. severe cerebral arteriosclerosis, epilepsy), or in the presence of other risk factors that may predispose to seizures or lower the seizure threshold (e.g. certain drug therapy, renal dysfunction). (See **PRECAUTIONS: General, Information for Patients, Drug Interactions** and **ADVERSE REACTIONS.**)

SERIOUS AND FATAL REACTIONS HAVE BEEN REPORTED IN PATIENTS RECEIVING CONCURRENT ADMINISTRATION OF INTRAVENOUS CIPROFLOXACIN AND THEOPHYLLINE. These reactions have included cardiac arrest, seizure, status epilepticus, and respiratory failure. Although similar serious adverse events have been reported in patients receiving theophylline alone, the possibility that these reactions may be potentiated by ciprofloxacin cannot be eliminated. If concomitant use cannot be avoided, serum levels of theophylline should be monitored and dosage adjustments made as appropriate.

Serious and occasionally fatal hypersensitivity (anaphylactic) reactions, some following the first dose, have been reported in patients receiving quinolone therapy. Some reactions were accompanied by cardiovascular collapse, loss of consciousness, tingling, pharyngeal or facial edema, dyspnea, urticaria, and itching. Only a few patients had a history of hypersensitivity reactions. Serious anaphylactic reactions require immediate emergency treatment with epinephrine and other resuscitation measures, including oxygen, intravenous fluids, intravenous antihistamines, corticosteroids, pressor amines, and airway management, as clinically indicated.

Severe hypersensitivity reactions characterized by rash, fever, eosinophilia, jaundice, and hepatic necrosis with fatal outcome have also been reported extremely rarely in patients receiving ciprofloxacin along with other drugs. The possibility that these reactions were related to ciprofloxacin cannot be excluded. Ciprofloxacin should be discontinued at the first appearance of a skin rash or any other sign of hypersensitivity.

Pseudomembranous colitis has been reported with nearly all antibacterial agents, including ciprofloxacin, and may range in severity from mild to life-threatening. Therefore, it is important to consider this diagnosis in patients who present with diarrhea subsequent to the administration of antibacterial agents.

Treatment with antibacterial agents alters the normal flora of the colon and may permit overgrowth of clostridia. Studies indicate that a toxin produced by *Clostridium difficile* is one primary cause of "antibiotic-associated colitis".

After the diagnosis of pseudomembranous colitis has been established, therapeutic measures should be initiated. Mild cases of pseudomembranous colitis usually respond to drug discontinuation alone. In moderate to severe cases, consideration should be given to management with fluids and electrolytes, protein supplementation and treatment with an antibacterial drug clinically effective against *C. difficile* colitis.

Achilles and other tendon ruptures that required surgical repair or resulted in prolonged disability have been reported with ciprofloxacin and other quinolones. Ciprofloxacin should be discontinued if the patient experiences pain, inflammation, or rupture of a tendon.

PRECAUTIONS

General: INTRAVENOUS CIPROFLOXACIN SHOULD BE ADMINISTERED BY SLOW INFUSION OVER A PERIOD OF 60 MINUTES. Local I.V. site reactions have been reported with the intravenous administration of ciprofloxacin. These reactions are more frequent if infusion time is 30 minutes or less or if small veins of the hand are used. (See **ADVERSE REACTIONS.**)

Quinolones, including ciprofloxacin, may also cause central nervous system (CNS) events, including nervousness, agitation, insomnia, anxiety, nightmares or paranoia. (See **WARNINGS, Information for Patients,** and **Drug Interactions.**)

Crystals of ciprofloxacin have been observed rarely in the urine of human subjects but more frequently in the urine of laboratory animals, which is usually alkaline. (See **ANIMAL PHARMACOLOGY.**) Crystalluria related to ciprofloxacin has been reported only rarely in humans because human urine is usually acidic. Alkalinity of the urine should be avoided in patients receiving ciprofloxacin. Patients should be well hydrated to prevent the formation of highly concentrated urine.

Alteration of the dosage regimen is necessary for patients with impairment of renal function. (See **DOSAGE AND ADMINISTRATION.**)

Moderate to severe phototoxicity manifested as an exaggerated sunburn reaction has been observed in some patients who were exposed to direct sunlight while receiving some members of the quinolone class of drugs. Excessive sunlight should be avoided.

Outcomes	Ciprofloxacin/Piperacillin N = 233 Success (%)		Tobramycin/Piperacillin N = 237 Success (%)	
Clinical Resolution of Initial Febrile Episode with No Modifications of Empirical Regimen*	63	(27.0%)	52	(21.9%)
Clinical Resolution of Initial Febrile Episode Including Patients with Modifications of Empirical Regimen	187	(80.3%)	185	(78.1%)
Overall Survival	224	(96.1%)	223	(94.1%)

* To be evaluated as a clinical resolution, patients had to have: (1) resolution of fever; (2) microbiological eradication of infection (if an infection was microbiologically documented); (3) resolution of signs/symptoms of infection; and (4) no modification of empirical antibiotic regimen.

As with any potent drug, periodic assessment of organ system functions, including renal, hepatic, and hematopoietic, is advisable during prolonged therapy.

Information for Patients: Patients should be advised that ciprofloxacin may be associated with hypersensitivity reactions, even following a single dose, and to discontinue the drug at the first sign of a skin rash or other allergic reaction.

Ciprofloxacin may cause dizziness and lightheadedness; therefore, patients should know how they react to this drug before they operate an automobile or machinery or engage in activities requiring mental alertness or coordination.

Patients should be advised that ciprofloxacin may increase the effects of theophylline and caffeine. There is a possibility of caffeine accumulation when products containing caffeine are consumed while taking ciprofloxacin.

Patients should be advised to discontinue treatment; rest and refrain from exercise; and inform their physician if they experience pain, inflammation, or rupture of a tendon.

Patients should be advised that convulsions have been reported in patients taking quinolones, including ciprofloxacin, and to notify their physician before taking the drug if there is a history of this condition.

Drug Interactions: As with some other quinolones, concurrent administration of ciprofloxacin with theophylline may lead to elevated serum concentrations of theophylline and prolongation of its elimination half-life. This may result in increased risk of theophylline-related adverse reactions. (See **WARNINGS.**) If concomitant use cannot be avoided, serum levels of theophylline should be monitored and dosage adjustments made as appropriate.

Some quinolones, including ciprofloxacin, have also been shown to interfere with the metabolism of caffeine. This may lead to reduced clearance of caffeine and prolongation of its serum half-life.

Some quinolones, including ciprofloxacin, have been associated with transient elevations in serum creatinine in patients receiving cyclosporine concomitantly.

Altered serum levels of phenytoin (increased and decreased) have been reported in patients receiving concomitant ciprofloxacin.

The concomitant administration of ciprofloxacin with the sulfonylurea has, in some patients, resulted in severe hypoglycemia. Fatalities have been reported.

Quinolones have been reported to enhance the effects of the oral anticoagulant warfarin or its derivatives. When these products are administered concomitantly, prothrombin time or other suitable coagulation tests should be closely monitored.

Probenecid interferes with renal tubular secretion of ciprofloxacin and produces an increase in the level of ciprofloxacin in the serum. This should be considered if patients are receiving both drugs concomitantly.

As with other broad-spectrum antimicrobial agents, prolonged use of ciprofloxacin may result in overgrowth of nonsusceptible organisms. Repeated evaluation of the patient's condition and microbial susceptibility testing are essential. If superinfection occurs during therapy, appropriate measures should be taken.

Carcinogenesis, Mutagenesis, Impairment of Fertility: Eight *in vitro* mutagenicity tests have been conducted with ciprofloxacin. Test results are listed below:

- Salmonella/Microsome Test (Negative)
- *E. coli* DNA Repair Assay (Negative)
- Mouse Lymphoma Cell Forward Mutation Assay (Positive)
- Chinese Hamster V_{79} Cell HGPRT Test (Negative)
- Syrian Hamster Embryo Cell Transformation Assay (Negative)
- *Saccharomyces cerevisiae* Point Mutation Assay (Negative)
- *Saccharomyces cerevisiae* Mitotic Crossover and Gene Conversion Assay (Negative)
- Rat Hepatocyte DNA Repair Assay (Positive)

Thus, two of the eight tests were positive, but results of the following three *in vivo* test systems gave negative results:

- Rat Hepatocyte DNA Repair Assay
- Micronucleus Test (Mice)
- Dominant Lethal Test (Mice)

Long-term carcinogenicity studies in mice and rats have been completed. After daily oral doses of 750 mg/kg (mice) and 250 mg/kg (rats) were administered for up to 2 years, there was no evidence that ciprofloxacin had any carcinogenic or tumorigenic effects in these species.

Results from photo co-carcinogenicity testing indicate that ciprofloxacin dose not reduce the time to appearance of UV-induced skin tumors as compared to vehicle control. Hairless (Skh-1) mice were exposed to UVA light for 3.5 hours five times every two weeks for up to 78 weeks while concurrently being administered ciprofloxacin. The time to development of the first skin tumors was 50 weeks in mice treated concomitantly with UVA and ciprofloxacin (mouse dose approximately equal to maximum recommended human dose based upon mg/m^2), as opposed to 34 weeks when animals were treated with both UVA and vehicle. The times to development of skin tumors ranged from 16–32 weeks in mice treated concomitantly with UVA and other quinolones.[3]

In this model, mice treated with ciprofloxacin alone did not develop skin or systemic tumors. There are no data from similar models using pigmented mice and/or fully haired mice. The clinical significance of these findings to humans in unknown.

Fertility studies performed in rats at oral doses of ciprofloxacin up to 100 mg/kg (0.8 times the highest recommended human dose of 1200 mg based upon body surface area) revealed no evidence of impairment.

Pregnancy: Teratogenic Effects. Pregnancy Category C: Reproduction studies have been performed in rats and mice using oral doses of up to 100 mg/kg (0.8 and 0.4 times the maximum daily human dose based upon body surface area, respectively) and I.V. doses of up to 30 mg/kg (0.24 and 0.12 times the maximum daily human dose based upon body surface area, respectively) and have revealed no evidence of harm to the fetus due to ciprofloxacin. In rabbits, ciprofloxacin (30 and 100 mg/kg orally) produced gastrointestinal disturbances resulting in maternal weight loss and an increased incidence of abortion, but no teratogenicity was observed at either dose. After intravenous administration of doses up to 20 mg/kg, no maternal toxicity was produced in the rabbit, and no embryotoxicity or teratogenicity was observed. There are, however, no adequate and well-controlled studies in pregnant women. Ciprofloxacin should be used during pregnancy only if the potential benefit justifies the potential risk to the fetus. (See **WARNINGS.**)

Nursing Mothers: Ciprofloxacin is excreted in human milk. Because of the potential for serious adverse reactions in infants nursing from mothers taking ciprofloxacin, a decision should be made whether to discontinue nursing or to discontinue the drug, taking into account the importance of the drug to the mother.

Pediatric Use: Safety and effectiveness in pediatric patients and adolescents less than 18 years of age have not been established. Ciprofloxacin causes arthropathy in juvenile animals. (See **WARNINGS.**)

Short-term safety data from a single trial in pediatric cystic fibrosis patients are available. In a randomized, double-blind clinical trial for the treatment of acute pulmonary exacerbations in cystic fibrosis patients (ages 5–17 years), 67 patients received ciprofloxacin I.V. 10 mg/kg/dose q8h for one week followed by ciprofloxacin tablets 20 mg/kg/dose q12h to complete 10–21 days treatment and 62 patients received the combination of ceftazidime I.V. 50 mg/kg/dose q8h and tobramycin I.V. 3 mg/kg/dose q8h for a total of 10–21 days. Patients less than 5 years of age were not studied. Safety monitoring in the study included periodic range of motion examinations and gait assessments by treatment-blinded examiners. Patients were followed for an average of 23 days after completing treatment (range 0–93 days). This study was not designed to determine long term effects and the safety of repeated exposure to ciprofloxacin.

In the study, injection site reactions were more common in the ciprofloxacin group (24%) than in the comparison group (8%). Other adverse events were similar in nature and frequency between treatment arms. Musculoskeletal adverse events were reported in 22% of the patients in the ciprofloxacin group and 21% in the comparison group. Decreased range of motion was reported in 12% of the subjects in the ciprofloxacin group and 16% in the comparison group. Arthralgia was reported in 10% of the patients in the ciprofloxacin group and 11% in the comparison group. One of sixty-seven patients developed arthritis of the knee nine days after a ten day course of treatment with ciprofloxacin. Clinical symptoms resolved, but an MRI showed knee effusion without other abnormalities eight months after treatment. However, the relationship of this event to the patient's course of ciprofloxacin can not be definitively determined, particularly since patients with cystic fibrosis may develop arthralgias/arthritis as part of their underlying disease process.

Geriatric Use: In a retrospective analysis of 23 multiple-dose controlled clinical trials of ciprofloxacin encompassing over 3500 ciprofloxacin treated patients, 25% of patients were greater than or equal to 65 years of age and 10% were greater than or equal to 75 years of age. No overall differences in safety or effectiveness were observed between these subjects and younger subjects, and other reported clinical experience has not identified differences in responses between the elderly and younger patients, but greater sensitivity of some older individuals on any drug therapy cannot be ruled out. Ciprofloxacin is known to be substantially excreted by the kidney, and the risk of adverse reactions may be greater in patients with impaired renal function. No alteration of dosage is necessary for patients greater than 65 years of age with normal renal function. However, since some older individuals experience reduced renal function by virtue of their advanced age, care should be taken in dose selection for elderly patients, and renal function monitoring may be useful in these patients. (See **CLINICAL PHARMACOLOGY** and **DOSAGE AND ADMINISTRATION.**

ADVERSE REACTIONS

The most frequently reported events, without regard to drug relationship, among patients treated with intravenous ciprofloxacin were nausea, diarrhea, central nervous system disturbance, local I.V. site reactions, abnormalities of liver associated enzymes (hepatic enzymes), and eosinophilia. Headache, restlessness, and rash were also noted in greater than 1% of patients treated with the most common doses of ciprofloxacin.

Local I.V. site reactions have been reported with the intravenous administration of ciprofloxacin. These reactions are more frequent if the infusion time is 30 minutes or less. These may appear as local skin reactions which resolve rapidly upon completion of the infusion. Subsequent intravenous administration is not contraindicated unless the reactions recur or worsen.

Additional events, without regard to drug relationship or route of administration, that occurred in 1% or less of ciprofloxacin patients are listed below:

CARDIOVASCULAR: cardiovascular collapse, cardiopulmonary arrest, myocardial infarction, arrhythmia, tachycardia, palpitation, cerebral thrombosis, syncope, cardiac murmur, hypertension, hypotension, angina pectoris

CENTRAL NERVOUS SYSTEM: convulsive seizures, paranoia, toxic psychosis, depression, dysphasia, phobia, depersonalization, manic reaction, unresponsiveness, ataxia, confusion, hallucinations, dizziness, lightheadedness, paresthesia, anxiety, tremor, insomnia, nightmares, weakness, drowsiness, irritability, malaise, lethargy

GASTROINTESTINAL: ileus, jaundice, gastrointestinal bleeding, *C. difficile* associated diarrhea, pseudomembranous colitis, pancreatitis, hepatic necrosis, intestinal perforation, dyspepsia, epigastric or abdominal pain, vomiting, constipation, oral ulceration, oral candidiasis, mouth dryness, anorexia, dysphagia, flatulence

I.V. INFUSION SITE: thrombophlebitis, burning, pain, pruritus, paresthesia, erythema, swelling

MUSCULOSKELETAL: arthralgia, jaw, arm or back pain, joint stiffness, neck and chest pain, achiness, flare up of gout

RENAL/UROGENITAL: renal failure, interstitial nephritis, hemorrhage cystitis, renal calculi, frequent urination, acidosis, urethral bleeding, polyuria, urinary retention, gynecomastia, candiduria, vaginitis. Crystalluria, cylindruria, hematuria, and albuminuria have also been reported.

RESPIRATORY: respiratory arrest, pulmonary embolism, dyspnea, pulmonary edema, respiratory distress, pleural effusion, hemoptysis, epistaxis, hiccough

SKIN/HYPERSENSITIVITY: anaphylactic reactions, erythema multiforme/Stevens-Johnson syndrome, exfoliative dermatitis, toxic epidermal necrolysis, vasculitis, angioedema, edema of the lips, face, neck, cojunctivae, hands or lower extremities, purpura, fever, chills, flushing, pruritus, urticaria, cutaneous candidiasis, vesicles, increased perspiration, hyperpigmentation, erythema nodosum, photosensitivity (See **WARNINGS.**)

SPECIAL SENSES: decreased visual acuity, blurred vision, disturbed vision (flashing lights, change in color perception, overbrightness of lights, diplopia), eye pain, anosmia, hearing loss, tinnitus, nystagmus, a bad taste

Also reported were agranulocytosis, prolongation of prothrombin time, and possible exacerbation of myasthenia gravis.

Many of these events were described as only mild to moderate in severity, abated soon after the drug was discontinued, and required no treatment.

In several instances, nausea, vomiting, tremor, irritability, or palpitation were judged by investigators to be related to elevated serum levels of theophylline possibly as a result of drug interaction with ciprofloxacin.

In randomized, double-blind controlled clinical trials comparing ciprofloxacin (I.V. and I.V. P.O. sequential) with intravenous beta-lactam control antibiotics, the CNS adverse event profile of ciprofloxacin was comparable to that of the control drugs.

Post-Marketing Adverse Events: Additional adverse events, regardless of relationship to drug, reported from worldwide marketing experience with quinolones, including ciprofloxacin, are:

BODY AS A WHOLE: change in serum phenytoin

CARDIOVASCULAR: postural hypotension, vasculitis

DOSAGE GUIDELINES

Intravenous

Infection†	Type or Severity	Unit Dose	Frequency	Daily Dose
Urinary tract	Mild/Moderate Severe/Complicated	200 mg 400 mg	q 12h q 12h	400 mg 800 mg
Lower Respiratory Tract	Mild/Moderate Severe/Complicated	400 mg 400 mg	q 12h q 8h	800 mg 1200 mg
Nosocomial Pneumonia	Mild/Moderate/Severe	400 mg	q 8h	1200 mg
Skin and Skin Structure	Mild/Moderate Severe/Complicated	400 mg 400 mg	q 12h q 8h	800 mg 1200 mg
Bone and Joint	Mild/Moderate Severe/Complicated	400 mg 400 mg	q 12h q 8h	800 mg 1200 mg
Intra-Abdominal*	Complicated	400 mg	q 12h	800 mg
Acute Sinusitis	Mild/Moderate	400 mg	q 12h	800 mg
Chronic Bacterial Prostatitis	Mild/Moderate	400 mg	q 12h	800 mg
Empirical Therapy in Febrile Neutropenic Patients	Severe Ciprofloxacin + Piperacillin	 400 mg 50 mg/kg	 q 8h q 4h	 1200 mg Not to exceed 24 g/day

* used in conjunction with metronidazole. (See product labeling for prescribing information.)
† DUE TO THE DESIGNATED PATHOGENS (See **INDICATIONS AND USAGE.**)

RECOMMENDED STARTING AND MAINTENANCE DOSES FOR PATIENTS WITH IMPAIRED RENAL FUNCTION

Creatinine Clearance (mL/min)	Dosage
> 30	See usual dosage.
5 – 29	200 – 400 mg q 18–24 hr

Men: Creatinine clearance (mL/min) = $\frac{\text{Weight (kg)} \times (140 - \text{age})}{72 \times \text{serum creatinine (mg/dL)}}$

Women: 0.85 × the value calculated for men.

SIZE	STRENGTH	NDC NUMBER
100 mL 5% dextrose	200 mg, 0.2%	0026-8552-36
200 mL 5% dextrose	400 mg, 0.2%	0026-8554-63

CENTRAL NERVOUS SYSTEM: agitation, delirium, myoclonus, toxic psychosis

HEMIC/LYMPHATIC: hemolytic anemia, methemoglobinemia

METABOLIC/NUTRITIONAL: elevation of serum triglycerides, cholesterol, blood glucose, serum potassium

MUSCULOSKELETAL: myalgia, tendinitis/tendon rupture

RENAL/UROGENITAL: vaginal candidiasis

(See **PRECAUTIONS.**)

Adverse Laboratory Changes: The most frequently reported changes in laboratory parameters with intravenous ciprofloxacin therapy, without regard to drug relationship are listed below:

Hepatic—	elevations of AST (SGOT), ALT (SGPT), alkaline phosphatase, LDH, and serum bilirubin;
Hematologic—	elevated eosinophil and platelet counts, decreased platelet counts, hemoglobin and/or hematocrit;
Renal—	elevations of serum creatinine, BUN, and uric acid;
Other—	elevations of serum creatinine, phosphokinase, serum theophylline (in patients receiving theophylline concomitantly), blood glucose, and triglycerides.

Other changes occurring infrequently were: decreased leukocyte count, elevated atypical lymphocyte count, immature WBCs, elevated serum calcium, elevation of serum gamma-glutamyl transpeptidase (γ GT), decreased BUN, decreased uric acid, decreased total serum protein, decreased serum albumin, decreased serum potassium, elevated serum potassium, elevated serum cholesterol.

Other changes occurring rarely during administration of ciprofloxacin were: elevation of serum amylase, decrease of blood glucose, pancytopenia, leukocytosis, elevated sedimentation rate, change in serum phenytoin, decreased prothrombin time, hemolytic anemia, and bleeding diathesis.

OVERDOSAGE

In the event of acute overdosage, the patient should be carefully observed and given supportive treatment. Adequate hydration must be maintained. Only a small amount of ciprofloxacin (<10%) is removed from the body after hemodialysis or peritoneal dialysis.

In mice, rats, rabbits and dogs, significant toxicity including tonic/clonic convulsions was observed at intravenous doses of ciprofloxacin between 125 and 300 mg/kg.

DOSAGE AND ADMINISTRATION

The recommended adult dosage for urinary tract infections of mild to moderate severity is 200 mg I.V. every 12 hours. For severe or complicated urinary tract infections, the recommended dosage is 400 mg I.V. every 12 hours.

The recommended adult dosage for lower respiratory tract infections, skin and skin structure infections, and bone and joint infections of mild to moderate severity is 400 mg I.V. every 12 hours.

For severe/complicated infections of the lower respiratory tract, skin and skin structure, and bone and joint, the recommended adult dosage is 400 mg I.V. every 8 hours.

The recommended adult dosage for mild, moderate, and severe nosocomial pneumonia is 400 mg I.V. every 8 hours.

Complicated Intra-Abdominal Infections: Sequential therapy [parenteral to oral—400 mg CIPRO® I.V. q 12 h (plus I.V. metronidazole) → 500 mg CIPRO® Tablets q 12 h (plus oral metronidazole)] can be instituted at the discretion of the physician. Metronidazole should be given according to product labeling to provide appropriate anaerobic coverage.

The recommended dosage for mild to moderate Acute Sinusitis and Chronic Bacterial Prostatitis is 400 mg I.V. every 12 hours.

The recommended adult dosage for empirical therapy of febrile neutropenic patients is 400 mg I.V. every 8 hours in combination with piperacillin sodium 50 mg/kg I.V. q 4 hours, not to exceed 24 g/day (300 mg/kg/day), for 7–14 days.

The determination of dosage for any particular patients must take into consideration the severity and nature of the infection, the susceptibility of the causative microorganism, the integrity of the patient's host-defense mechanisms and the status of renal and hepatic function.

[See first table above]

CIPRO® I.V. should be administered by intravenous infusion over a period of 60 minutes.

Parenteral drug products should be inspected visually for particulate matter and discoloration prior to administration.

Ciprofloxacin hydrochloride (CIPRO® Tablets) for oral administration are available. Parenteral therapy may be changed to oral CIPRO® Tablets when the condition warrants, at the discretion of the physician. For complete dosage and administration information, see CIPRO® Tablets package insert.

Impaired Renal Function: The following table provides dosage guidelines for use in patients with renal impair-

Continued on next page

Cipro I.V.—Cont.

ment; however, monitoring of serum drug levels provides the most reliable basis for dosage adjustment.
[See second table on previous page]
When only the serum creatinine concentration is known, the following formula may be used to estimate creatinine clearance:
[See third table on previous page]
The serum creatinine should represent a steady state of renal function.
For patients with changing renal function or for patients with renal impairment and hepatic insufficiency, measurement of serum concentrations of ciprofloxacin will provide additional guidance for adjusting dosage.

INTRAVENOUS ADMINISTRATION
CIPRO® I.V. should be administered by intravenous infusion over a period of 60 minutes. Slow infusion of a dilute solution into a large vein will minimize patient discomfort and reduce the risk of venous irritation.
Vials (Injection Concentrate): THIS PREPARATION MUST BE DILUTED BEFORE USE. The intravenous dose should be prepared by aseptically withdrawing the concentrate from the vial of CIPRO® I.V. This should be diluted with a suitable intravenous solution to a final concentration of 1–2 mg/mL. (See **COMPATIBILITY AND STABILITY.**) The resulting solution should be infused over a period of 60 minutes by direct infusion or through a Y-type intravenous infusion set which may already be in place.
If this method or the "piggyback" method of administration is used, it is advisable to discontinue temporarily the administration of any other solutions during the infusion of CIPRO® I.V.
Flexible Containers: CIPRO® I.V. is also available as a 0.2% premixed solution in 5% dextrose in flexible containers of 100 mL or 200 mL. The solutions in flexible containers may be infused as described above.

COMPATIBILITY AND STABILITY
Ciprofloxacin injection 1% (10 mg/mL), when diluted with the following intravenous solutions to concentrations of 0.5 to 2.0 mg/mL, is stable for up to 14 days at refrigerated or room temperature storage.

0.9% Sodium Chloride Injection, USP
5% Dextrose Injection, USP
Sterile Water for Injection
10% Dextrose for Injection
5% Dextrose and 0.225% Sodium Chloride for Injection
5% Dextrose and 0.45% Sodium Chloride for Injection
Lactated Ringer's for Injection

If CIPRO® I.V. is to be given concomitantly with another drug, each drug should be given separately in accordance with the recommended dosage and route of administration for each drug.

HOW SUPPLIED

CIPRO® I.V. (ciprofloxacin) is available as a clear, colorless to slightly yellowish solution. CIPRO® I.V. is available in 200 mg and 400 mg strengths. The concentrate is supplied in vials while the premixed solution is supplied in flexible containers as follows:

VIAL:	SIZE	STRENGTH	NDC NUMBER
	20 mL	200 mg, 1%	0026-8562-20
	40 mL	400 mg, 1%	0026-8564-64

FLEXIBLE CONTAINER: manufactured for Bayer Corporation by Abbott Laboratories, North Chicago, IL 60064.
[See fourth table on previous page]
FLEXIBLE CONTAINER: manufactured for Bayer Corporation by Baxter Healthcare Corporation, Deerfield, IL 60015.
[See table below]

STORAGE
Vial: Store between 5–30°C (41–86°F).
Flexible Container: Store between 5–25°C (41–77°F).
Protect from light, avoid excessive heat, protect from freezing.
CIPRO® I.V. (ciprofloxacin) is also available in a 120 mL Pharmacy Bulk Package.
Ciprofloxacin is also available as CIPRO® (ciprofloxacin HCl) Tablets 100, 250, 500, and 750 mg and CIPRO® (ciprofloxacin) 5% and 10% Oral Suspension.

ANIMAL PHARMACOLOGY

Ciprofloxacin and other quinolones have been shown to cause arthropathy in immature animals of most species tested. (See **WARNINGS.**) Damage of weight-bearing joints was observed in juvenile dogs and rats. In young beagles, 100 mg/kg ciprofloxacin given daily for 4 weeks caused degenerative articular changes of the knee joint. At 30 mg/kg, the effect on the joint was minimal. In a subsequent study in beagles, removal of weight-bearing from the joint reduced the lesions but did not totally prevent them.
Crystalluria, sometimes associated with secondary nephropathy, occurs in laboratory animals dosed with ciprofloxacin. This is primarily related to the reduced solubility of ciprofloxacin under alkaline conditions, which predominate in the urine of test animals; in man, crystalluria is rare since human urine is typically acidic. In rhesus monkeys, crystalluria without nephropathy has been noted after intravenous doses as low as 5 mg/kg. After 6 months of intravenous dosing at 10 mg/kg/day, no nephropathological changes were noted; however, nephropathy was observed after dosing at 20 mg/kg/day for the same duration.
In dogs, ciprofloxacin administered at 3 and 10 mg/kg by rapid intravenous injection (15 sec.) produces pronounced hypotensive effects. These effects are considered to be related to histamine release because they are partially antagonized by pyrilamine, an antihistamine. In rhesus monkeys, rapid intravenous injection also produces hypotension, but the effect in this species is inconsistent and less pronounced.
In mice, concomitant administration of nonsteroidal anti-inflammatory drugs, such as phenylbutazone and indomethacin, with quinolones has been reported to enhance the CNS stimulatory effect of quinolones.
Ocular toxicity, seen with some related drugs, has not been observed in ciprofloxacin-treated animals.

REFERENCES

1. National Committee for Clinical Laboratory Standards, Methods for Dilution Antimicrobial Susceptibility Tests for Bacteria That Grow Aerobically—Fourth Edition. Approved Standard NCCLS Document M7–A4, Vol. 17, No.2, NCCLS, Wayne, PA, January, 1997. **2.** National Committee for Clinical Laboratory Standards, Performance Standards for Antimicrobial Disk Susceptibility Tests—Sixth Edition. Approved Standard NCCLS Document M2–A6, Vol. 17, No. 1, NCCLS, Wayne, PA, January, 1997. **3.** Report presented at the FDA's Anti-Infective Drug and Dermatological Drug Products Advisory Committee Meeting, March 31, 1993, Silver Spring MD. Report available from FDA, CDER, Advisors and Consultants Staff, HFD-21, 1901 Chapman Avenue, Room 200, Rockville, MD 20852, USA.

Manufactured for:
Bayer Corporation
Pharmaceutical Division
400 Morgan Lane
West Haven, CT 06516 USA
Rx Only
PZ500169
8/00
BAY q 3939
5202-4-A-U.S.-7

9803
Shown in Product Identification Guide, page 307

CIPRO® I.V. ℞
(ciprofloxacin)
For Intravenous Infusion

PHARMACY BULK PACKAGE—NOT FOR DIRECT INFUSION

DESCRIPTION

The pharmacy bulk package is a single-entry container of a sterile preparation for parenteral use that contains many single doses. It contains ciprofloxacin as a 1% aqueous solution concentrate. The contents are intended for use in a pharmacy admixture program and are restricted to the preparation of admixtures for intravenous infusion.
CIPRO® I.V. (ciprofloxacin) is a synthetic broad-spectrum antimicrobial agent for intravenous (I.V.) administration. Ciprofloxacin, a fluoroquinolone, is 1-cyclopropyl-6-fluoro-1,4-dihydro-4-oxo-7-(1-piperazinyl)-3-quinolinecarboxylic acid. Its empirical formula is $C_{17}H_{18}FN_3O_3$ and its chemical structure is:

Ciprofloxacin is a faint to light yellow crystalline powder with a molecular weight of 331.4. It is soluble in dilute (0.1N) hydrochloric acid and is practically insoluble in water and ethanol. Ciprofloxacin differs from other quinolones in that it has a fluorine atom at the 6-position, a piperazine moiety at the 7-position, and a cyclopropyl ring at the 1-position. CIPRO® I.V. solution is available as sterile 1.0% aqueous concentrate, which is intended for dilution prior to administration. Ciprofloxacin solution contains lactic acid as a solubilizing agent and hydrochloric acid for pH adjustment. The pH range for the 1.0% aqueous concentrate is 3.3 to 3.9.

CLINICAL PHARMACOLOGY

Following 60-minute intravenous infusions of 200 mg and 400 mg ciprofloxacin to normal volunteers, the mean maximum serum concentrations achieved were 2.1 and 4.6 μg/mL, respectively; the concentrations at 12 hours were 0.1 and 0.2 μg/mL, respectively.

Steady-state Ciprofloxacin Serum Concentrations (μg/mL) After 60-minute I.V. Infusions q 12 h.

	Time after starting the infusion					
Dose	**30 min**	**1 hr**	**3 hr**	**6 hr**	**8 hr**	**12 hr**
200 mg	1.7	2.1	0.6	0.3	0.2	0.1
400 mg	3.7	4.6	1.3	0.7	0.5	0.2

The pharmacokinetics of ciprofloxacin are linear over the dose range of 200 to 400 mg administered intravenously. The serum elimination half-life is approximately 5–6 hours and the total clearance is around 35 L/hr. Comparison of the pharmacokinetic parameters following the 1st and 5th I.V. dose on a q 12 h regimen indicates no evidence of drug accumulation.
The absolute bioavailability of oral ciprofloxacin is within a range of 70–80% with no substantial loss by first pass metabolism. An intravenous infusion of 400 mg ciprofloxacin given over 60 minutes every 12 hours has been shown to produce an area under the serum concentration time curve (AUC) equivalent to that produced by a 500-mg oral dose given every 12 hours. An intravenous infusion of 400 mg ciprofloxacin given over 60 minutes every 8 hours has been shown to produce an AUC at steady-state equivalent to that produced by a 750-mg oral dose given every 12 hours. A 400-mg I.V. dose results in a C_{max} similar to that observed with a 750-mg oral dose. An infusion of 200 mg ciprofloxacin given every 12 hours produces an AUC equivalent to that produced by a 250-mg oral dose given every 12 hours.
[See table at bottom of next page]
After intravenous administration, approximately 50% to 70% of the dose is excreted in the urine as unchanged drug. Following a 200-mg I.V. dose, concentrations in the urine usually exceed 200 μg/mL 0–2 hours after dosing and are generally greater than 15 μg/mL 8–12 hours after dosing. Following a 400-mg I.V. dose, urine concentrations generally exceed 400 μg/mL 0–2 hours after dosing and are usually greater than 30 μg/mL 8–12 hours after dosing. The renal clearance is approximately 22 L/hr. The urinary excretion of ciprofloxacin is virtually complete by 24 hours after dosing.
The serum concentrations of ciprofloxacin and metronidazole were not altered when these two drugs were given concomitantly.
Co-administration of probenecid with ciprofloxacin results in about a 50% reduction in the ciprofloxacin renal clearance and a 50% increase in its concentration in the systemic circulation. Although bile concentrations of ciprofloxacin are severalfold higher than serum concentrations after intravenous dosing, only a small amount of the administered dose (<1%) is recovered from the bile as unchanged drug. Approximately 15% of an I.V. dose is recovered from the feces within 5 days after dosing.
After I.V. administration, three metabolites of ciprofloxacin have been identified in human urine which together account for approximately 10% of the intravenous dose.
Pharmacokinetic studies of the oral (single dose) and intravenous (single and multiple dose) forms of ciprofloxacin indicate that plasma concentrations of ciprofloxacin are higher in elderly subjects (>65 years) as compared to young adults. Although the C_{max} is increased 16–40%, the increase in mean AUC is approximately 30%, and can be at least partially attributed to decreased renal clearance in the elderly. Elimination half-life is only slightly (~20%) prolonged in the elderly. These differences are not considered clinically significant. (See **PRECAUTIONS: Geriatric Use.**)
In patients with reduced renal function, the half-life of ciprofloxacin is slightly prolonged and dosage adjustments may be required. (See **DOSAGE AND ADMINISTRATION.**)
In preliminary studies in patients with stable chronic liver cirrhosis, no significant changes in ciprofloxacin pharmacokinetics have been observed. However, the kinetics of ciprofloxacin in patients with acute hepatic insufficiency have not been fully elucidated.
Following infusion of 400 mg I.V. ciprofloxacin every eight hours in combination with 50 mg/kg I.V. piperacillin sodium every 4 hours, mean serum ciprofloxacin concentrations were 3.02 μg/mL ½ hour and 1.18 μg/mL between 6–8 hours after the end of infusion.
The binding of ciprofloxacin to serum proteins is 20 to 40%.
After intravenous administration, ciprofloxacin is present in saliva, nasal and bronchial secretions, sputum, skin blister fluid, lymph, peritoneal fluid, bile, and prostatic secretions. It has also been detected in the lung, skin, fat, muscle, cartilage, and bone. Although the drug diffuses into cerebrospinal fluid (CSF), CSF concentrations are generally less than 10% of peak serum concentrations. Levels of the drug in the aqueous and vitreous chambers of the eye are lower than in serum.
Microbiology: Ciprofloxacin has *in vitro* activity against a wide range of gram-negative and gram-positive microorganisms. The bactericidal action of ciprofloxacin results from interference with the enzyme DNA gyrase which is needed for the synthesis of bacterial DNA.
Ciprofloxacin has been shown to be active against most strains of the following microorganisms, both *in vitro* and in clinical infections as described in the **INDICATIONS AND USAGE** section of the package insert for CIPRO® I.V. (ciprofloxacin for intravenous infusion).

Aerobic gram-positive microorganisms
Enterococcus faecalis
(Many strains are only moderately susceptible.)

SIZE	STRENGTH	NDC NUMBER
100 mL 5% dextrose	200 mg, 0.2%	0026-8527-36
200 mL 5% dextrose	400 mg, 0.2%	0026-8527-63

Staphylococcus aureus (methicillin susceptible)
Staphylococcus epidermidis
Staphylococcus saprophyticus
Streptococcus pneumoniae
Streptococcus pyogenes

Aerobic gram-negative microorganisms
Citrobacter diversus
Citrobacter freundii
Enterobacter cloacae
Escherichia coli
Haemophilus influenzae
Haemophilus parainfluenzae
Klebsiella pneumoniae
Moraxella catarrhalis
Morganella morganii
Proteus mirabilis
Proteus vulgaris
Providencia rettgeri
Providencia stuartii
Pseudomonas aeruginosa
Serratia marcescens

Ciprofloxacin has been shown to be active against most strains of the following microorganisms, both *in vitro* and in clinical infections as described in the **INDICATIONS AND USAGE** section of the package insert for CIPRO® (ciprofloxacin hydrochloride) Tablets.

Aerobic gram-positive microorganisms
Enterococcus faecalis
(Many strains are only moderately susceptible.)
Staphylococcus aureus (methicillin susceptible)
Staphylococcus epidermidis
Staphylococcus saprophyticus
Streptococcus pneumoniae
Streptococcus pyogenes

Aerobic gram-negative microorganisms
Campylobacter jejuni
Citrobacter diversus
Citrobacter freundii
Enterobacter cloacae
Escherichia coli
Haemophilus influenzae
Haemophilus parainfluenzae
Klebsiella pneumoniae
Moraxella catarrhalis
Morganella morganii
Neisseria gonorrhoeae
Proteus mirabilis
Proteus vulgaris
Providencia rettgeri
Providencia stuartii
Pseudomonas aeruginosa
Salmonella typhi
Serratia marcescens
Shigella boydii
Shigella dysenteriae
Shigella flexneri
Shigella sonnei

The following *in vitro* data are available, **but their clinical significance is unknown.**

Ciprofloxacin exhibits *in vitro* minimum inhibitory concentrations (MICs) of 1 μg/mL or less against most (≥ 90%) strains of the following microorganisms; however, the safety and effectiveness of ciprofloxacin in treating clinical infections due to these microorganisms have not been established in adequate and well-controlled clinical trials.

Aerobic gram-positive microorganisms
Staphylococcus haemolyticus
Staphylococcus hominis

Aerobic gram-negative microorganisms
Acinetobacter lwoffi
Aeromonas hydrophila
Edwardsiella tarda
Enterobacter aerogenes
Klebsiella oxytoca
Legionella pneumophila
Pasteurella multocida
Salmonella enteritidis
Vibrio cholerae
Vibrio parahaemolyticus
Vibrio vulnificus
Yersinia enterocolitica

Most strains of *Burkholderia cepacia* and some strains of *Stenotrophomonas maltophilia* are resistant to ciprofloxacin as are most anaerobic bacteria, including *Bacteroides fragilis* and *Clostridium difficile*.

Ciprofloxacin is slightly less active when tested at acidic pH. The inoculum size has little effect when tested *in vitro*. The minimum bactericidal concentration (MBC) generally does not exceed the minimum inhibitory concentration (MIC) by more than a factor of 2. Resistance of ciprofloxacin *in vitro* usually develops slowly (multiple-step mutation).

Ciprofloxacin does not cross-react with other antimicrobial agents such as beta-lactams or aminoglycosides; therefore, organisms resistant to these drugs may be susceptible to ciprofloxacin.

In vitro studies have shown that additive activity often results when ciprofloxacin is combined with other antimicrobial agents such as beta-lactams, aminoglycosides, clindamycin, or metronidazole. Synergy has been reported particularly with the combination of ciprofloxacin and a beta-lactam; antagonism is observed only rarely.

Susceptibility Tests

Dilution Techniques: Quantitative methods are used to determine antimicrobial minimum inhibitory concentrations (MICs). These MICs provide estimates of the susceptibility of bacteria to antimicrobial compounds. The MICs should be determined using a standardized procedure. Standardized procedures are based on a dilution method[1] (broth or agar) or equivalent with standardized inoculum concentrations and standardized concentrations of ciprofloxacin powder. The MIC values should be interpreted according to the following criteria:

For testing aerobic microorganisms other than *Haemophilus influenzae, Haemophilus parainfluenzae*, and *Neisseria gonorrhoeae*[a]:

MIC (μg/mL)	Interpretation
≤1	Susceptible (S)
2	Intermediate (I)
≥4	Resistant (R)

[a] These interpretive standards are applicable only to broth microdilution susceptibility tests with streptococci using cation-adjusted Mueller-Hinton broth with 2–5% lysed horse blood.

For testing *Haemophilus influenzae* and *Haemophilus parainfluenzae*[b]:

MIC (μg/mL)	Interpretation
≤1	Susceptible (S)

[b] This interpretive standard is applicable only to broth microdilution susceptibility tests with *Haemophilus influenzae* and *Haemophilus parainfluenzae* using *Haemophilus* Test Medium[1].

The current absence of data on resistant strains precludes defining any results other than "Susceptible". Strains yielding MIC results suggestive of a "nonsusceptible" category should be submitted to a reference laboratory for further testing.

For testing *Neisseria gonorrhoeae*[c]:

MIC (μg/mL)	Interpretation
≤0.06	Susceptible (S)

[c] This interpretive standard is applicable only to agar dilution test with GC agar base and 1% defined growth supplement.

The current absence of data on resistant strains precludes defining any results other than "Susceptible". Strains yielding MIC results suggestive of a "nonsusceptible" category should be submitted to a reference laboratory for further testing.

A report of "Susceptible" indicates that the pathogen is likely to be inhibited if the antimicrobial compound in the blood reaches the concentrations usually achievable. A report of "Intermediate" indicates that the result should be considered equivocal, and, if the microorganism is not fully susceptible to alternative, clinically feasible drugs, the test should be repeated. This category implies possible clinical applicability in body sites where the drug is physiologically concentrated or in situations where high dosage of drug can be used. This category also provides a buffer zone which prevents small uncontrolled technical factors from causing major discrepancies in interpretation. A report of "Resistant" indicates that the pathogen is not likely to be inhibited if the antimicrobial compound in the blood reaches the concentrations usually achievable; other therapy should be selected.

Standardized susceptibility test procedures require the use of laboratory control microorganisms to control the technical aspects of the laboratory procedures. Standard ciprofloxacin powder should provide the following MIC values:

Organism		MIC (μg/mL)
E. faecalis	ATCC 29212	0.25 –2.0
E. coli	ATCC 25922	0.004–0.015
H. influenzae[a]	ATCC 49247	0.004–0.03
N. gonorrhoeae[b]	ATCC 49226	0.001–0.008
P. aeruginosa	ATCC 27853	0.25 –1.0
S. aureus	ATCC 29213	0.12 –0.5

[a] This quality control range is applicable to only *H. influenzae* ATCC 49247 tested by a broth microdilution procedure using *Haemophilus* Test Medium (HTM)[1].

[b] This quality control range is applicable to only *N. gonorrhoeae* ATCC 49226 tested by an agar dilution procedure using GC agar base and 1% defined growth supplement.

Diffusion Techniques: Quantitative methods that require measurement of zone diameters also provide reproducible estimates of the susceptibility of bacteria to antimicrobial compounds. One such standardized procedure[2] requires the use of standardized inoculum concentrations. This procedure uses paper disks impregnated with 5-μg ciprofloxacin to test the susceptibility of microorganisms to ciprofloxacin. Reports from the laboratory providing results of the standard single-disk susceptibility test with a 5-μg ciprofloxacin disk should be interpreted according to the following criteria:

For testing aerobic microorganisms other than *Haemophilus influenzae, Haemophilus parainfluenzae*, and *Neisseria gonorrhoeae*[a]:

Zone Diameter (mm)	Interpretation
≥21	Susceptible (S)
16–20	Intermediate (I)
≤ 15	Resistant (R)

[a] These zone diameter standards are applicable only to tests performed for streptococci using Mueller-Hinton agar supplemented with 5% sheep blood incubated in 5% CO_2.

For testing *Haemophilus influenzae* and *Haemophilus parainfluenzae*[b]:

Zone Diameter (mm)	Interpretation
≥21	Susceptible (S)

[b] This zone diameter standard is applicable only to tests *with Haemophilus influenzae* and *Haemophilus parainfluenzae* using *Haemophilus* Test Medium (HTM)[2].

The current absence of data on resistant strains precludes defining any results other than "Susceptible". Strains yielding zone diameter results suggestive of a "nonsusceptible" category should be submitted to a reference laboratory for further testing.

For testing *Neisseria gonorrhoeae*[c]:

Zone Diameter (mm)	Interpretation
≥36	Susceptible (S)

[c] This zone diameter standard is applicable only to disk diffusion tests with GC agar base and 1% defined growth supplement.

The current absence of data on resistant strains precludes defining any results other than "Susceptible". Strains yielding zone diameter results suggestive of a "nonsusceptible" category should be submitted to a reference laboratory for further testing.

Interpretation should be as stated above for results using dilution techniques. Interpretation involves correlation of the diameter obtained in the disk test with the MIC for ciprofloxacin.

As with standardized dilution techniques, diffusion methods require the use of laboratory control microorganisms that are used to control the technical aspects of the laboratory procedures. For the diffusion technique, the 5-μg ciprofloxacin disk should provide the following zone diameters in these laboratory test quality control strains:

Organism		Zone Diameter (mm)
E. coli	ATCC 25922	30–40
H. influenzae[a]	ATCC 49247	34–42
N. gonorrhoeae[b]	ATCC 49226	48–58
P. aeruginosa	ATCC 27853	25–33
S. aureus	ATCC 25923	22–30

[a] These quality control limits are applicable to only *H. influenzae* ATCC 49247 testing using *Haemophilus* Test Medium (HTM)[2].

[b] These quality control limits are applicable only to tests conducted with *N. gonorrhoeae* ATCC 49226 performed by disk diffusion using GC agar base and 1% defined growth supplement.

Steady-state Pharmacokinetic Parameter Following Multiple Oral and I.V. Doses

Parameters	500 mg q12h, P.O.	400 mg q12h, I.V.	750 mg q12h, P.O.	400 mg q8h, I.V.
AUC (μg·hr/mL)	13.7[a]	12.7[a]	31.6[b]	32.9[c]
C_{max} (μg/mL)	2.97	4.56	3.59	4.07

[a] AUC_{0-12h}
[b] AUC 24h=$AUC_{0-12h} \times 2$
[c] AUC 24h=$AUC_{0-8h} \times 3$

INDICATIONS AND USAGE

CIPRO® I.V. is indicated for the treatment of infections caused by susceptible strains of the designated microorganisms in the conditions listed below when the intravenous administration offers a route of administration advantageous to the patient. Please see **DOSAGE AND ADMINISTRATION** for specific recommendations.

Continued on next page

Cipro I.V. Pharm Bulk—Cont.

Urinary Tract Infections caused by *Escherichia coli* (including cases with secondary bacteremia), *Klebsiella pneumoniae* subspecies *pneumoniae, Enterobacter cloacae, Serratia marcescens, Proteus mirabilis, Providencia rettgeri, Morganella morganii, Citrobacter diversus, Citrobacter freundii, Pseudomonas aeruginosa, Staphylococcus epidermidis, Staphylococcus saprophyticus*, or *Enterococcus faecalis*.
Lower Respiratory Infections caused by *Escherichia coli, Klebsiella pneumoniae* subspecies *pneumoniae, Enterobacter cloacae, Proteus mirabilis, Pseudomonas aeruginosa, Haemophilus influenzae, Haemophilus parainfluenzae*, or *Streptococcus pneumoniae*.
NOTE: Although effective in clinical trials, ciprofloxacin is not a drug of first choice in the treatment of presumed or confirmed pneumonia secondary to *Streptococcus pneumoniae*.
Nosocomial Pneumonia caused by *Haemophilus influenzae* or *Klebsiella pneumoniae*.
Skin and Skin Structure Infections caused by *Escherichia coli, Klebsiella pneumoniae* subspecies *pneumoniae, Enterobacter cloacae, Proteus mirabilis, Proteus vulgaris, Providencia stuartii, Morganella morganii, Citrobacter freundii, Pseudomonas aeruginosa, Staphylococcus aureus* (methicillin susceptible), *Staphylococcus epidermidis*, or *Streptococcus pyogenes*.
Bone and Joint Infections caused by *Enterobacter cloacae, Serratia marcescens*, or *Pseudomonas aeruginosa*.
Complicated Intra-Abdominal Infections (used in conjunction with metronidazole) caused by *Escherichia coli, Pseudomonas aeruginosa, Proteus mirabilis, Klebsiella pneumoniae*, or *Bacteroides fragilis*. (See **DOSAGE AND ADMINISTRATION.**)
Acute Sinusitis caused by *Haemophilus influenzae, Streptococcus pneumoniae*, or *Moraxella catarrhalis*.
Chronic Bacterial Prostatitis caused by *Escherichia coli* or *Proteus mirabilis*.
Empirical Therapy for Febrile Neutropenic Patients in combination with piperacillin sodium. (See **DOSAGE AND ADMINISTRATION** and **CLINICAL STUDIES.**)
If anaerobic organisms are suspected of contributing to the infection, appropriate therapy should be administered.
Appropriate culture and susceptibility tests should be performed before treatment in order to isolate and identify organisms causing infection and to determine their susceptibility to ciprofloxacin. Therapy with CIPRO® I.V. may be initiated before results of these tests are known; once results become available, appropriate therapy should be continued.
As with other drugs, some strains of *Pseudomonas aeruginosa* may develop resistance fairly rapidly during treatment with ciprofloxacin. Culture and susceptibility testing performed periodically during therapy will provide information not only on the therapeutic effect of the antimicrobial agent but also on the possible emergence of bacterial resistance.

CLINICAL STUDIES

EMPIRICAL THERAPY IN FEBRILE NEUTROPENIC PATIENTS
The safety and efficacy of ciprofloxacin, 400 mg I.V. q 8h, in combination with piperacillin sodium, 50 mg/kg I.V. q 4h, for the empirical therapy of febrile neutropenic patients were studied in one large pivotal multicenter, randomized trial and were compared to those of tobramycin, 2 mg/kg I.V. q 8h, in combination with piperacillin sodium, 50 mg/kg I.V. q 4h.
The demographics of the evaluable patients were as follows:
[See first table above]
Clinical response rates observed in this study were as follows:
[See second table above]

Total	Ciprofloxacin/Piperacillin N = 233	Tobramycin/Piperacillin N = 237
Median Age (years)	47.0 (range 19–84)	50.0 (range 18–81)
Male	114 (48.9%)	117 (49.4%)
Female	119 (51.1%)	120 (50.6%)
Leukemia/Bone Marrow Transplant	165 (70.8%)	158 (66.7%)
Solid Tumor/Lymphoma	68 (29.2%)	79 (33.3%)
Median Duration of Neutropenia (days)	15.0 (range 1–61)	14.0 (range 1–89)

Outcomes	Ciprofloxacin/Piperacillin N = 233 Success (%)	Tobramycin/Piperacillin N = 237 Success (%)
Clinical Resolution of Initial Febrile Episode with No Modification of Empirical Regimen*	63 (27.0%)	52 (21.9%)
Clinical Resolution of Initial Febrile Episode Including Patients with Modifications of Empirical Regimen	187 (80.3%)	185 (78.1%)
Overall Survival	224 (96.1%)	223 (94.1%)

* To be evaluated as a clinical resolution, patients had to have: (1) resolution of fever; (2) microbiological eradication of infection (if an infection was microbiologically documented); (3) resolution of signs/symptoms of infection; and (4) no modification of empirical antibiotic regimen.

CONTRAINDICATIONS

CIPRO® I.V. (ciprofloxacin) is contraindicated in persons with a history of hypersensitivity to ciprofloxacin or any member of the quinolone class of antimicrobial agents.

WARNINGS

THE SAFETY AND EFFECTIVENESS OF CIPROFLOXACIN IN PEDIATRIC PATIENTS AND ADOLESCENTS (LESS THAN 18 YEARS OF AGE), PREGNANT WOMEN, AND LACTATING WOMEN HAVE NOT BEEN ESTABLISHED. (See **PRECAUTIONS: Pediatric Use, Pregnancy** and **Nursing Mothers** subsections.) Ciprofloxacin causes lameness in immature dogs. Histopathological examination of the weight-bearing joints of these dogs revealed permanent lesions of the cartilage. Related quinolone-class drugs also produce erosions of cartilage of weight-bearing joints and other signs of arthropathy in immature animals of various species. (See **ANIMAL PHARMACOLOGY.**)
Convulsions, increased intracranial pressure, and toxic psychosis have been reported in patients receiving quinolones, including ciprofloxacin. Ciprofloxacin may also cause central nervous system (CNS) events including: dizziness, confusion, tremors, hallucinations, depression, and, rarely, suicidal thoughts or acts. These reactions may occur following the first dose. If these reactions occur in patients receiving ciprofloxacin, the drug should be discontinued and appropriate measures instituted. As with all quinolones, ciprofloxacin should be used with caution in patients with known or suspected CNS disorders that may predispose to seizures or lower the seizure threshold (e.g. severe cerebral arteriosclerosis, epilepsy), or in the presence of other risk factors that may predispose to seizures or lower the seizure threshold (e.g. certain drug therapy, renal dysfunction). (See **PRECAUTIONS: General, Information for Patients, Drug Interactions** and **ADVERSE REACTIONS.**)
SERIOUS AND FATAL REACTIONS HAVE BEEN REPORTED IN PATIENTS RECEIVING CONCURRENT ADMINISTRATION OF INTRAVENOUS CIPROFLOXACIN AND THEOPHYLLINE. These reactions have included cardiac arrest, seizure, status epilepticus, and respiratory failure. Although similar serious adverse events have been reported in patients receiving theophylline alone, the possibility that these reactions may be potentiated by ciprofloxacin cannot be eliminated. If concomitant use cannot be avoided, serum levels of theophylline should be monitored and dosage adjustments made as appropriate.
Serious and occasionally fatal hypersensitivity (anaphylactic) reactions, some following the first dose, have been reported in patients receiving quinolone therapy. Some reactions were accompanied by cardiovascular collapse, loss of consciousness, tingling, pharyngeal or facial edema, dyspnea, urticaria, and itching. Only a few patients had a history of hypersensitivity reactions. Serious anaphylactic reactions require immediate emergency treatment with epinephrine and other resuscitation measures, including oxygen, intravenous fluids, intravenous antihistamines, corticosteroids, pressor amines, and airway management, as clinically indicated.
Severe hypersensitivity reactions characterized by rash, fever, eosinophilia, jaundice, and hepatic necrosis with fatal outcome have also been reported extremely rarely in patients receiving ciprofloxacin along with other drugs. The possibility that these reactions were related to ciprofloxacin cannot be excluded. Ciprofloxacin should be discontinued at the first appearance of a skin rash or any other sign of hypersensitivity.
Pseudomembranous colitis has been reported with nearly all antibacterial agents, including ciprofloxacin, and may range in severity from mild to life-threatening. Therefore, it is important to consider this diagnosis in patients who present with diarrhea subsequent to the administration of antibacterial agents.
Treatment with antibacterial agents alters the normal flora of the colon and may permit overgrowth of clostridia. Studies indicate that a toxin produced by *Clostridium difficile* is one primary cause of "antibiotic-associated colitis".
After the diagnosis of pseudomembranous colitis has been established, therapeutic measures should be initiated. Mild cases of pseudomembranous colitis usually respond to drug discontinuation alone. In moderate to severe cases, consideration should be given to management with fluids and electrolytes, protein supplementation and treatment with an antibacterial drug clinically effective against *C. difficile* colitis.
Achilles and other tendon ruptures that required surgical repair or resulted in prolonged disability have been reported with ciprofloxacin and other quinolones. Ciprofloxacin should be discontinued if the patient experiences pain, inflammation, or rupture of a tendon.

PRECAUTIONS

General: INTRAVENOUS CIPROFLOXACIN SHOULD BE ADMINISTERED BY SLOW INFUSION OVER A PERIOD OF 60 MINUTES. Local I.V. site reactions have been reported with the intravenous administration of ciprofloxacin. These reactions are more frequent if infusion time is 30 minutes or less or if small veins of the hand are used. (See **ADVERSE REACTIONS.**)
Quinolones, including ciprofloxacin, may also cause central nervous system (CNS) events, including nervousness, agitation, insomnia, anxiety, nightmares or paranoia. (See **WARNINGS, Information for Patients,** and **Drug Interactions.**)
Crystals of ciprofloxacin have been observed rarely in the urine of human subjects but more frequently in the urine of laboratory animals, which is usually alkaline. (See **ANIMAL PHARMACOLOGY.**) Crystalluria related to ciprofloxacin has been reported only rarely in humans because human urine is usually acidic. Alkalinity of the urine should be avoided in patients receiving ciprofloxacin. Patients should be well hydrated to prevent the formation of highly concentrated urine.
Alteration of the dosage regimen is necessary for patients with impairment of renal function. (See **DOSAGE AND ADMINISTRATION.**)
Moderate to severe phototoxicity manifested as an exaggerated sunburn reaction has been observed in some patients who were exposed to direct sunlight while receiving some members of the quinolone class of drugs. Excessive sunlight should be avoided.
As with any potent drug, periodic assessment of organ system functions, including renal, hepatic, and hematopoietic, is advisable during prolonged therapy.
Information For Patients: Patients should be advised that ciprofloxacin may be associated with hypersensitivity reactions, even following a single dose, and to discontinue the drug at the first sign of a skin rash or other allergic reaction.
Ciprofloxacin may cause dizziness and lightheadedness; therefore, patients should know how they react to this drug before they operate an automobile or machinery or engage in activities requiring mental alertness or coordination.
Patients should be advised that ciprofloxacin may increase the effects of theophylline and caffeine. There is a possibility of caffeine accumulation when products containing caffeine are consumed while taking ciprofloxacin.
Patients should be advised to discontinue treatment; rest and refrain from exercise; and inform their physician if they experience pain, inflammation, or rupture of a tendon.
Patients should be advised that convulsions have been reported in patients taking quinolones, including ciprofloxacin, and to notify their physician before taking this drug if there is a history of this condition.
Drug Interactions: As with some other quinolones, concurrent administration of ciprofloxacin with theophylline may lead to elevated serum concentrations of theophylline and prolongation of its elimination half-life. This may result in increased risk of theophylline-related adverse reactions. (See **WARNINGS.**) If concomitant use cannot be avoided, serum levels of theophylline should be monitored and dosage adjustments made as appropriate.
Some quinolones, including ciprofloxacin, have also been shown to interfere with the metabolism of caffeine. This may lead to reduced clearance of caffeine and prolongation of its serum half-life.
Some quinolones, including ciprofloxacin, have been associated with transient elevations in serum creatinine in patients receiving cyclosporine concomitantly.
Altered serum levels of phenytoin (increased and decreased) have been reported in patients receiving concomitant ciprofloxacin.
The concomitant administration of ciprofloxacin with the sulfonylurea glyburide has, in some patients, resulted in severe hypoglycemia. Fatalities have been reported.
Quinolones have been reported to enhance the effects of the oral anticoagulant warfarin or its derivatives. When these products are administered concomitantly, prothrombin time or other suitable coagulation tests should be closely monitored.
Probenecid interferes with renal tubular secretion of ciprofloxacin and produces an increase in the level of ciprofloxacin in the serum. This should be considered if patients are receiving both drugs concomitantly.
As with other broad-spectrum antimicrobial agents, prolonged use of ciprofloxacin may result in overgrowth of nonsusceptible organisms. Repeated evaluation of the patient's

condition and microbial susceptibility testing are essential. If superinfection occurs during therapy, appropriate measures should be taken.

Carcinogenesis, Mutagenesis, Impairment of Fertility: Eight *in vitro* mutagenicity tests have been conducted with ciprofloxacin. Test results are listed below:

Salmonella/Microsome Test (Negative)
E. coli DNA Repair Assay (Negative)
Mouse Lymphoma Cell Forward Mutation Assay (Positive)
Chinese Hamster V_{79} Cell HGPRT Test (Negative)
Syrian Hamster Embryo Cell Transformation Assay (Negative)
Saccharomyces cerevisiae Point Mutation Assay (Negative)
Saccharomyces cerevisiae Mitotic Crossover and Gene Conversion Assay (Negative)
Rat Hepatocyte DNA Repair Assay (Positive)

Thus, two of the eight tests were positive, but results of the following three *in vivo* test systems gave negative results:

Rat Hepatocyte DNA Repair Assay
Micronucleus Test (Mice)
Dominant Lethal Test (Mice)

Long-term carcinogenicity studies in mice and rats have been completed. After daily oral doses of 750 mg/kg (mice) and 250 mg/kg (rats) were administered for up to 2 years, there was no evidence that ciprofloxacin had any carcinogenic or tumorigenic effects in these species.

Results from photo co-carcinogenicity testing indicate that ciprofloxacin does not reduce the time to appearance of UV-induced skin tumors as compared to vehicle control. Hairless (Skh-1) mice were exposed to UVA light for 3.5 hours five times every two weeks for up to 78 weeks while concurrently being administered ciprofloxacin. The time to development of the first skin tumors was 50 weeks in mice treated concomitantly with UVA and ciprofloxacin (mouse dose approximately equal to maximum recommended human dose based upon mg/m^2), as opposed to 34 weeks when animals were treated with both UVA and vehicle. The times to development of skin tumors ranged from 16–32 weeks in mice treated concomitantly with UVA and other quinolones.[3]

In this model, mice treated with ciprofloxacin alone did not develop skin or systemic tumors. There are no data from similar models using pigmented mice and/or fully haired mice. The clinical significance of these findings to humans is unknown.

Fertility studies performed in rats at oral doses of ciprofloxacin up to 100 mg/kg (0.8 times the highest recommended human dose of 1200 mg based upon body surface area) revealed no evidence of impairment.

Pregnancy: Teratogenic Effects. Pregnancy Category C: Reproduction studies have been performed in rats and mice using oral doses of up to 100 mg/kg (0.8 and 0.4 times the maximum daily human dose based upon body surface area, respectively) and I.V. doses of up to 30 mg/kg (0.24 and 0.12 times the maximum daily human dose based upon body surface area, respectively) and have revealed no evidence of harm to the fetus due to ciprofloxacin. In rabbits, ciprofloxacin (30 and 100 mg/kg orally) produced gastrointestinal disturbances resulting in maternal weight loss and an increased incidence of abortion, but no teratogenicity was observed at either dose. After intravenous administration of doses up to 20 mg/kg, no maternal toxicity was produced in the rabbit, and no embryotoxicity or teratogenicity was observed. There are, however, no adequate and well-controlled studies in pregnant women. Ciprofloxacin should be used during pregnancy only if the potential benefit justifies the potential risk to the fetus. (See **WARNINGS**.)

Nursing Mothers: Ciprofloxacin is excreted in human milk. Because of the potential for serious adverse reactions in infants nursing from mothers taking ciprofloxacin, a decision should be made whether to discontinue nursing or to discontinue the drug, taking into account the importance of the drug to the mother.

Pediatric Use: Safety and effectiveness in pediatric patients and adolescents less than 18 years of age have not been established. Ciprofloxacin causes arthropathy in juvenile animals. (See **WARNINGS**.)

Short-term safety data from a single trial in pediatric cystic fibrosis patients are available. In a randomized, double-blind clinical trial for the treatment of acute pulmonary exacerbations in cystic fibrosis patients (ages 5–17 years), 67 patients received ciprofloxacin I.V. 10 mg/kg/dose q8h for one week followed by ciprofloxacin tablets 20 mg/kg/dose q12h to complete 10–21 days treatment and 62 patients received the combination of ceftazidime I.V. 50 mg/kg/dose q8h and tobramycin I.V. 3 mg/kg/dose q8h for a total of 10–21 days. Patients less than 5 years of age were not studied. Safety monitoring in the study included periodic range of motion examinations and gait assessments by treatment-blinded examiners. Patients were followed for an average of 23 days after completing treatment (range 0–93 days). This study was not designed to determine long term effects and the safety of repeated exposure to ciprofloxacin.

In the study, injection site reactions were more common in the ciprofloxacin group (24%) than in the comparison group (8%). Other adverse events were similar in nature and frequency between treatment arms. Musculoskeletal adverse events were reported in 22% of the patients in the ciprofloxacin group and 21% in the comparison group. Decreased range of motion was reported in 12% of the subjects in the ciprofloxacin group and 16% in the comparison group. Arthralgia was reported in 10% of the patients in the ciprofloxacin group and 11% in the comparison group. One of sixty-seven patients developed arthritis of the knee nine days after a ten day course of treatment with ciprofloxacin. Clinical symptoms resolved, but an MRI showed knee effusion without other abnormalities eight months after treatment. However, the relationship of this event to the patient's course of ciprofloxacin can not be definitively determined, particularly since patients with cystic fibrosis may develop arthralgias/arthritis as part of their underlying disease process.

Geriatric Use: In a retrospective analysis of 23 multiple-dose controlled clinical trials of ciprofloxacin encompassing over 3500 ciprofloxacin treated patients, 25% of patients were greater than or equal to 65 years of age and 10% were greater than or equal to 75 years of age. No overall differences in safety or effectiveness were observed between these subjects and younger subjects, and other reported clinical experience has not identified differences in responses between the elderly and younger patients, but greater sensitivity of some older individuals on any drug therapy cannot be ruled out. Ciprofloxacin is known to be substantially excreted by the kidney, and the risk of adverse reactions may be greater in patients with impaired renal function. No alteration of dosage is necessary for patients greater than 65 years of age with normal renal function. However, since some older individuals experience reduced renal function by virtue of their advanced age, care should be taken in dose selection for elderly patients, and renal function monitoring may be useful in these patients. (See **CLINICAL PHARMACOLOGY** and **DOSAGE AND ADMINISTRATION**.)

ADVERSE REACTIONS

The most frequently reported events, without regard to drug relationship, among patients treated with intravenous ciprofloxacin were nausea, diarrhea, central nervous system disturbance, local I.V. site reactions, abnormalities of liver associated enzymes (hepatic enzymes), and eosinophilia. Headache, restlessness, and rash were also noted in greater than 1% of patients treated with the most common doses of ciprofloxacin.

Local I.V. site reactions have been reported with the intravenous administration of ciprofloxacin. These reactions are more frequent if the infusion time is 30 minutes or less. These may appear as local skin reactions which resolve rapidly upon completion of the infusion. Subsequent intravenous administration is not contraindicated unless the reactions recur or worsen.

Additional events, without regard to drug relationship or route of administration, that occurred in 1% or less of ciprofloxacin patients are listed below:

CARDIOVASCULAR: cardiovascular collapse, cardiopulmonary arrest, myocardial infarction, arrhythmia, tachycardia, palpitation, cerebral thrombosis, syncope, cardiac murmur, hypertension, hypotension, angina pectoris

CENTRAL NERVOUS SYSTEM: convulsive seizures, paranoia, toxic psychosis, depression, dysphasia, phobia, depersonalization, manic reaction, unresponsiveness, ataxia, confusion, hallucinations, dizziness, lightheadedness, paresthesia, anxiety, tremor, insomnia, nightmares, weakness, drowsiness, irritability, malaise, lethargy

GASTROINTESTINAL: ileus, jaundice, gastrointestinal bleeding, *C. difficile* associated diarrhea, pseudomembranous colitis, pancreatitis, hepatic necrosis, intestinal perforation, dyspepsia, epigastric or abdominal pain, vomiting, constipation, oral ulceration, oral candidiasis, mouth dryness, anorexia, dysphagia, flatulence

I.V. INFUSION SITE: thrombophlebitis, burning, pain, pruritus, paresthesia, erythema, swelling

MUSCULOSKELETAL: arthralgia, jaw, arm or back pain, joint stiffness, neck and chest pain, achiness, flare up of gout

RENAL/UROGENITAL: renal failure, interstitial nephritis, hemorrhagic cystitis, renal calculi, frequent urination, acidosis, urethral bleeding, polyuria, urinary retention, gynecomastia, candiduria, vaginitis. Crystalluria, cylindruria, hematuria, and albuminuria have also been reported.

RESPIRATORY: respiratory arrest, pulmonary embolism, dyspnea, pulmonary edema, respiratory distress, pleural effusion, hemoptysis, epistaxis, hiccough

SKIN/HYPERSENSITIVITY: anaphylactic reactions, erythema multiforme/Stevens-Johnson syndrome, exfoliative dermatitis, toxic epidermal necrolysis, vasculitis, angioedema, edema of the lips, face, neck, conjunctivae, hands or lower extremities, purpura, fever, chills, flushing, pruritus, urticaria, cutaneous candidiasis, vesicles, increased perspiration, hyperpigmentation, erythema nodosum, photosensitivity (See **WARNINGS**.)

SPECIAL SENSES: decreased visual acuity, blurred vision, disturbed vision (flashing lights, change in color perception, overbrightness of lights, diplopia), eye pain, anosmia, hearing loss, tinnitus, nystagmus, a bad taste

Also reported were agranulocytosis, prolongation of prothrombin time, and possible exacerbation of myasthenia gravis.

Many of these events were described as only mild or moderate in severity, abated soon after the drug was discontinued, and required no treatment.

In several instances, nausea, vomiting, tremor, irritability, or palpitation were judged by investigators to be related to elevated serum levels of theophylline possibly as a result of drug interaction with ciprofloxacin.

In randomized, double-blind controlled clinical trials comparing ciprofloxacin (I.V. and I.V. P.O. sequential) with intravenous beta-lactam control antibiotics, the CNS adverse event profile of ciprofloxacin was comparable to that of the control drugs.

Post-Marketing Adverse Events: Additional adverse events, regardless of relationship to drug, reported from worldwide marketing experience with quinolones, including ciprofloxacin, are:

BODY AS A WHOLE: change in serum phenytoin
CARDIOVASCULAR: postural hypotension, vasculitis
CENTRAL NERVOUS SYSTEM: agitation, delirium, myoclonus, toxic psychosis
HEMIC/LYMPHATIC: hemolytic anemia, methemoglobinemia
METABOLIC/NUTRITIONAL: elevation of serum triglycerides, cholesterol, blood glucose, serum potassium
MUSCULOSKELETAL: myalgia, tendinitis/tendon rupture
RENAL/UROGENITAL: vaginal candidiasis
(See **PRECAUTIONS**.)

Adverse Laboratory Changes: The most frequently reported changes in laboratory parameters with intravenous ciprofloxacin therapy, without regard to drug relationship are listed below:

DOSAGE GUIDELINES
Intravenous

Infection†	Type or Severity	Unit Dose	Frequency	Daily Dose
Urinary tract	Mild/Moderate	200 mg	q12h	400 mg
	Severe/Complicated	400 mg	q12h	800 mg
Lower Respiratory Tract	Mild/Moderate	400 mg	q12h	800 mg
	Severe/Complicated	400 mg	q8h	1200 mg
Nosocomial Pneumonia	Mild/Moderate/Severe	400 mg	q8h	1200 mg
Skin and Skin Structure	Mild/Moderate	400 mg	q12h	800 mg
	Severe/Complicated	400 mg	q8h	1200 mg
Bone and Joint	Mild/Moderate	400 mg	q12h	800 mg
	Severe/Complicated	400 mg	q8h	1200 mg
Intra-Abdominal*	Complicated	400 mg	q12h	800 mg
Acute Sinusitis	Mild/Moderate	400 mg	q12h	800 mg
Chronic Bacterial Prostatitis	Mild/Moderate	400 mg	q12h	800 mg
Empirical Therapy in Febrile Neutropenic Patients	Severe Ciprofloxacin	400 mg	q8h	1200 mg
	+ Piperacillin	50 mg/kg	q4h	Not to exceed 24 g/day

* used in conjunction with metronidazole. (See product labeling for prescribing information.)
† DUE TO THE DESIGNATED PATHOGENS (See **INDICATIONS AND USAGE**.)

$$\text{Men: Creatinine clearance (mL/min)} = \frac{\text{Weight (kg)} \times (140 - \text{age})}{72 \times \text{serum creatinine (mg/dL)}}$$

Women: 0.85 × the value calculated for men.

Continued on next page

Cipro I.V. Pharm Bulk—Cont.

CONTAINER	SIZE	STRENGTH	NDC NUMBER
Pharmacy Bulk Package:	120 mL	1200-mg, 1%	0026-8566-65

VIAL:	SIZE	STRENGTH	NDC NUMBER
	20 mL	200 mg, 1%	0026-8562-20
	40 mL	400 mg, 1%	0026-8564-64

FLEXIBLE CONTAINER: manufactured for Bayer Corporation by Abbott Laboratories, North Chicago, IL 60064.

SIZE	STRENGTH	NDC NUMBER
100 mL 5% dextrose	200 mg, 0.2%	0026-8552-36
200 mL 5% dextrose	400 mg, 0.2%	0026-8554-63

FLEXIBLE CONTAINER: manufactured for Bayer Corporation by Baxter Healthcare Corporation, Deerfield, IL 60015.

SIZE	STRENGTH	NDC NUMBER
100 mL 5% dextrose	200 mg, 0.2%	0026-8527-36
200 mL 5% dextrose	400 mg, 0.2%	0026-8527-63

Hepatic—elevations of AST (SGOT), ALT (SGPT), alkaline phosphatase, LDH, and serum bilirubin;
Hematologic—elevated eosinophil and platelet counts, decreased platelet counts, hemoglobin and/or hematocrit;
Renal—elevations of serum creatinine, BUN, and uric acid;
Other—elevations of serum creatinine, phosphokinase, serum theophylline (in patients receiving theophylline concomitantly), blood glucose, and triglycerides.

Other changes occurring infrequently were: decreased leukocyte count, elevated atypical lymphocyte count, immature WBCs, elevated serum calcium, elevation of serum gammaglutamyl transpeptidase (γ GT), decreased BUN, decreased uric acid, decreased total serum protein, decreased serum albumin, decreased serum potassium, elevated serum potassium, elevated serum cholesterol.

Other changes occurring rarely during administration of ciprofloxacin were: elevation of serum amylase, decrease of blood glucose, pancytopenia, leukocytosis, elevated sedimentation rate, change in serum phenytoin, decreased prothrombin time, hemolytic anemia, and bleeding diathesis.

OVERDOSAGE

In the event of acute overdosage, the patient should be carefully observed and given supportive treatment. Adequate hydration must be maintained. Only a small amount of ciprofloxacin (<10%) is removed from the body after hemodialysis or peritoneal dialysis.

In mice, rats, rabbits and dogs, significant toxicity including tonic/clonic convulsions was observed at intravenous doses of ciprofloxacin between 125 and 300 mg/kg.

DOSAGE AND ADMINISTRATION

The recommended adult dosage for urinary tract infections of mild to moderate severity is 200 mg I.V. every 12 hours. For severe or complicated urinary tract infections, the recommended dosage is 400 mg I.V. every 12 hours.

The recommended adult dosage for lower respiratory tract infections, skin and skin structure infections, and bone and joint infections of mild to moderate severity is 400 mg I.V. every 12 hours.

For severe/complicated infections of the lower respiratory tract, skin and skin structure, and bone and joint, the recommended adult dosage is 400 mg I.V. every 8 hours.

The recommended adult dosage for mild, moderate, and severe nosocomial pneumonia is 400 mg I.V. every 8 hours.

Complicated Intra-Abdominal Infections: Sequential therapy [parenteral to oral—400 mg CIPRO® I.V. q 12 h (plus I.V. metronidazole) → 500 mg CIPRO® Tablets q 12 h (plus oral metronidazole)] can be instituted at the discretion of the physician. Metronidazole should be given according to product labeling to provide appropriate anaerobic coverage.

The recommended dosage for mild to moderate Acute Sinusitis and Chronic Bacterial Prostatitis is 400 mg I.V. every 12 hours.

The recommended adult dosage for empirical therapy of febrile neutropenic patients is 400 mg I.V. every 8 hours in combination with piperacillin sodium 50 mg/kg I.V. q 4 hours, not to exceed 24 g/day (300 mg/kg/day), for 7–14 days.

The determination of dosage for any particular patient must take into consideration the severity and nature of the infection, the susceptibility of the causative microorganism, the integrity of the patient's host-defense mechanisms and the status of renal and hepatic function.

[See first table at top of previous page]

After dilution CIPRO® I.V. should be administered by intravenous infusion over a period of 60 minutes.

Parenteral drug products should be inspected visually for particulate matter and discoloration prior to administration.

CIPRO® (ciprofloxacin hydrochloride) Tablets for oral administration are available. Parenteral therapy may be changed to oral CIPRO® Tablets when the condition warrants, at the discretion of the physician. For complete dosage and administration information, see CIPRO® Tablets package insert.

Impaired Renal Function: The following table provides dosage guidelines for use in patients with renal impairment; however, monitoring of serum drug levels provides the most reliable basis for dosage adjustment.

RECOMMENDED STARTING AND MAINTENANCE DOSES FOR PATIENTS WITH IMPAIRED RENAL FUNCTION

Creatinine Clearance (mL/min)	Dosage
>30	See usual dosage.
5–29	200–400 mg q 18–24 hr

When only the serum creatinine concentration is known, the following formula may be used to estimate creatinine clearance:

[See second table at top of previous page]

The serum creatinine should represent a steady state of renal function.

For patients with changing renal function or for patients with renal impairment and hepatic insufficiency, measurement of serum concentrations of ciprofloxacin will provide additional guidance for adjusting dosage.

INTRAVENOUS ADMINISTRATION

After dilution, CIPRO® I.V. should be administered by intravenous infusion over a period of 60 minutes. Slow infusion of a dilute solution into a large vein will minimize patient discomfort and reduce the risk of venous irritation.

PHARMACY BULK PACKAGE: The pharmacy bulk package is a single-entry container of a sterile preparation for parenteral use that contains many single doses. It contains ciprofloxacin as a 1% aqueous solution concentrate. The contents are intended for use in a pharmacy admixture program and are restricted to the preparation of admixtures for intravenous infusion. **THE CLOSURE SHALL BE PENETRATED ONLY ONE TIME** with a suitable sterile transfer set or dispensing device which allows measured dispensing of the contents.

The pharmacy bulk package is to be used only in a suitable work area such as laminar flow hood or an equivalent clean air or compounding area. **THIS PREPARATION MUST BE DILUTED BEFORE USE.** The intravenous dose should be prepared by aseptically withdrawing the CIPRO® I.V. concentrate from the pharmacy bulk package and diluting the appropriate volume with a suitable intravenous solution to a final concentration of 0.5–2 mg/mL. (See **COMPATIBILITY AND STABILITY**.) The resulting solution should be infused over a period of 60 minutes by direct infusion or through a Y-type intravenous set which may already be in place. If this method or the "piggyback" method of administration is used, it is advisable to discontinue the administration of any other intravenous solutions during the infusion of CIPRO® I.V.

COMPATIBILITY AND STABILITY

Ciprofloxacin injection 1% (10 mg/mL), when diluted with the following intravenous solutions to concentrations of 0.5 to 2.0 mg/mL, is stable for up to 14 days at refrigerated or room temperature storage.

- 0.9% Sodium Chloride Injection, USP
- 5% Dextrose Injection, USP
- Sterile Water for Injection
- 10% Dextrose for Injection
- 5% Dextrose and 0.225% Sodium Chloride for Injection
- 5% Dextrose and 0.45% Sodium Chloride for Injection
- Lactated Ringer's for Injection

If CIPRO® I.V. is to be given concomitantly with another drug, each drug should be given separately in accordance with the recommended dosage and route of administration for each drug.

HOW SUPPLIED

CIPRO® I.V. (ciprofloxacin) is available as a clear, colorless to slightly yellowish solution supplied in the pharmacy bulk package as follows:

[See first table above]

STORAGE

Store between 5–30°C (41–86°F). Protect from light, avoid excessive heat, protect from freezing.

CIPRO® I.V. (ciprofloxacin) is also available as follows:

[See second table above]

Ciprofloxacin is also available as CIPRO® (ciprofloxacin HCl) Tablets 100, 250, 500, and 750 mg and as CIPRO® (ciprofloxacin) 5% and 10% Oral Suspension.

ANIMAL PHARMACOLOGY

Ciprofloxacin and other quinolones have been shown to cause arthropathy in immature animals of most species tested. (See **WARNINGS**.) Damage of weight-bearing joints was observed in juvenile dogs and rats. In young beagles, 100 mg/kg ciprofloxacin given daily for 4 weeks caused degenerative articular changes of the knee joint. At 30 mg/kg, the effect on the joint was minimal. In a subsequent study in beagles, removal of weight-bearing from the joint reduced the lesions but did not totally prevent them.

Crystalluria, sometimes associated with secondary nephropathy, occurs in laboratory animals dosed with ciprofloxacin. This is primarily related to the reduced solubility of ciprofloxacin under alkaline conditions, which predominate in the urine of test animals; in man, crystalluria is rare since human urine is typically acidic. In rhesus monkeys, crystalluria without nephropathy has been noted after intravenous doses as low as 5 mg/kg. After 6 months of intravenous dosing at 10 mg/kg/day, no nephropathological changes were noted; however, nephropathy was observed after dosing at 20 mg/kg/day for the same duration.

In dogs, ciprofloxacin administered at 3 and 10 mg/kg by rapid intravenous injection (15 sec.) produces pronounced hypotensive effects. These effects are considered to be related to histamine release because they are partially antagonized by pyrilamine, an antihistamine. In rhesus monkeys, rapid intravenous injection also produces hypotension, but the effect in this species is inconsistent and less pronounced.

In mice, concomitant administration of nonsteroidal anti-inflammatory drugs, such as phenylbutazone and indomethacin, with quinolones has been reported to enhance the CNS stimulatory effect of quinolones.

Ocular toxicity, seen with some related drugs, has not been observed in ciprofloxacin-treated animals.

REFERENCES

1. National Committee for Clinical Laboratory Standards, Methods for Dilution Antimicrobial Susceptibility Tests for Bacteria That Grow Aerobically—Fourth Edition. Approved Standard NCCLS Document M7-A4, Vol. 17, No. 2, NCCLS, Wayne, PA, January, 1997. **2.** National Committee for Clinical Laboratory Standards, Performance Standards for Antimicrobial Disk Susceptibility Tests—Sixth Edition. Approved Standard NCCLS Document M2-A6, Vol. 17, No. 1, NCCLS, Wayne, PA, January, 1997. **3.** Report presented at the FDA's Anti-Infective Drug and Dermatological Drug Products Advisory Committee Meeting, March 31, 1993, Silver Spring, MD. Report available from FDA, CDER, Advisors and Consultants Staff, HFD-21, 1901 Chapman Avenue, Room 200, Rockville, MD 20852, USA.

Bayer Corporation
Pharmaceutical Division
400 Morgan Lane
West Haven, CT 06516 USA

Rx Only

PD500170 8/00 BAY q 3939 5202-4-A-U.S.-6 ©2000 Bayer Corporation Printed in USA 9804

Shown in Product Identification Guide, page 307

DTIC-Dome® ℞
(dacarbazine)
Sterile

> **WARNING**
> It is recommended that DTIC-Dome (dacarbazine) be administered under the supervision of a qualified physician experienced in the use of cancer chemotherapeutic agents.
> 1. Hemopoietic depression is the most common toxicity with DTIC-Dome (See Warnings).
> 2. Hepatic necrosis has been reported (See Warnings).
> 3. Studies have demonstrated this agent to have a carcinogenic and teratogenic effect when used in animals.
> 4. In treatment of each patient, the physician must weigh carefully the possibility of achieving therapeutic benefit against the risk of toxicity.

DESCRIPTION

DTIC-Dome Sterile (dacarbazine) is a colorless to an ivory colored solid which is light sensitive. Each vial contains 100 mg of dacarbazine, or 200 mg of dacarbazine (the active ingredient), anhydrous citric acid and mannitol. DTIC-Dome is reconstituted and administered intravenously (pH 3–4). DTIC-Dome is an anticancer agent. Chemically, DTIC-Dome is 5-(3,3-dimethyl-1-triazeno)-imidazole-4-carboxamide (DTIC) with the following structural formula:

$(CH_3)_2N{-}N{=}N$ … H_2N … $C_6H_{10}N_6O$

CLINICAL PHARMACOLOGY

After intravenous administration of DTIC-Dome, the volume of distribution exceeds total body water content suggesting localization in some body tissue, probably the liver. Its disappearance from the plasma is biphasic with initial half-life of 19 minutes and a terminal half-life of 5 hours.[1] In a patient with renal and hepatic dysfunctions, the half-lives were lengthened to 55 minutes and 7.2 hours.[1] The average cumulative excretion of unchanged DTIC in the urine is 40% of the injected dose in 6 hours.[1] DTIC is subject to renal tubular secretion rather than glomerular filtration. At therapeutic concentrations DTIC is not appreciably bound to human plasma protein.

In man, DTIC is extensively degraded. Besides unchanged DTIC, 5-aminoimidazole -4 carboxamide (AIC) is a major metabolite of DTIC excreted in the urine. AIC is not derived endogenously but from the injected DTIC, because the administration of radioactive DTIC labeled with ^{14}C in the imidazole portion of the molecule (DTIC-2-^{14}C) gives rise to AIC-2-^{14}C.[1]

Although the exact mechanism of action of DTIC-Dome is not known, three hypotheses have been offered:

1. inhibition of DNA synthesis by acting as a purine analog
2. action as an alkylating agent
3. interaction with SH groups

INDICATIONS AND USAGE

DTIC-Dome is indicated in the treatment of metastatic malignant melanoma. In addition, DTIC-Dome is also indicated for Hodgkin's disease as a secondary-line therapy when used in combination with other effective agents.

CONTRAINDICATIONS

DTIC-Dome is contraindicated in patients who have demonstrated a hypersensitivity to it in the past.

WARNINGS

Hemopoietic depression is the most common toxicity with DTIC-Dome and involves primarily the leukocytes and platelets, although, anemia may sometimes occur. Leukopenia and thrombocytopenia may be severe enough to cause death. The possible bone marrow depression requires careful monitoring of white blood cells, red blood cells, and platelet levels. Hemopioetic toxicity may warrant temporary suspension or cessation of therapy with DTIC-Dome.

Hepatic toxicity accompanied by hepatic vein thrombosis and hepatocellular necrosis resulting in death, has been reported. The incidence of such reactions has been low; approximately 0.01% of patients treated. This toxicity has been observed mostly when DTIC-Dome has been administered concomitantly with other anti-neoplastic drugs; however, it has also been reported in some patients treated with DTIC-Dome alone.

Anaphylaxis can occur following the administration of DTIC-Dome.

PRECAUTIONS

Hospitalization is not always necessary but adequate laboratory study capability must be available. Extravasation of the drug subcutaneously during intravenous administration may result in tissue damage and severe pain. Local pain, burning sensation, and irritation at the site of injection may be relieved by locally applied hot packs.

Carcinogenicity of DTIC was studied in rats and mice. Proliferative endocardial lesions, including fibrosarcomas and sarcomas were induced by DTIC in rats. In mice, administration of DTIC resulted in the induction of angiosarcomas of the spleen.

Pregnancy Category C. DTIC-Dome has been shown to be teratogenic in rats when given in doses 20 times the human daily dose on day 12 of gestation. DTIC when administered in 10 times the human daily dose to male rats (twice weekly for 9 weeks) did not affect the male libido, although female rats mated to male rats had higher incidence of resorptions than controls. In rabbits, DTIC daily dose 7 times the human daily dose given on Days 6–15 of gestation resulted in fetal skeletal anomalies. There are no adequate and well controlled studies in pregnant women. DTIC-Dome should be used during pregnancy only if the potential benefit justifies the potential risk to the fetus.

It is not known whether this drug is excreted in human milk. Because many drugs are excreted in human milk and because of the potential for tumorigenicity shown for DTIC-Dome in animal studies, a decision should be made whether to discontinue nursing or to discontinue the drug, taking into account the importance of the drug to the mother.

ADVERSE REACTIONS

Symptoms of anorexia, nausea, and vomiting are the most frequently noted of all toxic reactions. Over 90% of patients are affected with the initial few doses. The vomiting lasts 1–12 hours and is incompletely and unpredictably palliated with phenobarbital and/or prochlorperazine. Rarely, intractable nausea and vomiting have necessitated discontinuance of therapy with DTIC-Dome. Rarely, DTIC-Dome has caused diarrhea. Some helpful suggestions include restricting the patient's oral intake of food for 4–6 hours prior to treatment. The rapid toleration of these symptoms suggests that a central nervous system mechanism may be involved, and usually these symptoms subside after the first 1 or 2 days.

There are a number of minor toxicities that are infrequently noted. Patients have experienced an influenza-like syndrome of fever to 39°C, myalgias and malaise. These symptoms occur usually after large single doses, may last for several days, and they may occur with successive treatments. Alopecia has been noted as has facial flushing and facial paresthesia. There have been few reports of significant liver or renal function test abnormalities in man. However, these abnormalities have been observed more frequently in animal studies.

Erythematous and urticarial rashes have been observed infrequently after administration of DTIC-Dome. Rarely, photosensitivity reactions may occur.

OVERDOSAGE

Give supportive treatment and monitor blood cell counts.

DOSAGE AND ADMINISTRATION

Malignant Melanoma: The recommended dosage is 2 to 4.5mg/kg/day for 10 days. Treatment may be repeated at 4 week intervals.[2]

An alternate recommended dosage is 250mg/square meter body surface/day I.V. for 5 days. Treatment may be repeated every 3 weeks.[3,4]

Hodgkin's Disease: The recommended dosage of DTIC-Dome in the treatment of Hodgkin's disease is 150mg/square meter body surface/day for 5 days, in combination with other effective drugs. Treatment may be repeated every 4 weeks.[5] An alternative recommended dosage is 375mg/square meter body surface on day 1, in combination with other effective drugs, to be repeated every 15 days.[6]

DTIC-Dome (dacarbazine) 100mg/vial and 200mg/vial are reconstituted with 9.9 mL and 19.7 mL, respectively, of Sterile Water for Injection, U.S.P. The resulting solution contains 10mg/mL of dacarbazine having a pH of 3.0 to 4.0. The calculated dose of the resulting solution is drawn into a syringe and administered *only* intravenously.

The reconstituted solution may be further diluted with 5% dextrose injection, U.S.P. or sodium chloride injection, U.S.P. and administered as an intravenous infusion.

After reconstitution and prior to use, the solution in the vial may be stored at 4°C for up to 72 hours or at normal room conditions (temperature and light) for up to 8 hours. If the reconstituted solution is further diluted in 5% dextrose, injection, U.S.P. or sodium chloride injection, U.S.P., the resulting solution may be stored at 4°C for up to 24 hours or at normal room conditions for up to 8 hours.

Procedures for proper handling and disposal of anticancer drugs should be considered. Several guidelines on this subject have been published.[7–12] There is no general agreement that all of the procedures recommended in the guidelines are necessary or appropriate.

HOW SUPPLIED

10 mL vials containing 100 mg or 20 mL vials containing 200 mg of DTIC-Dome as sterile dacarbazine in boxes of 12. Store in a refrigerator 2°C to 8°C (36°F to 46°F).

REFERENCES

1. Loo, T.J., *et al.*: Mechanism of action and pharmacology studies with DTIC (NSC-45388). Cancer Treatment Reports 60: 149–152, 1976.
2. Nathanson, L., *et al.*: Characteristics of prognosis and response to an imidazole carboxamide in malignant melanoma. Clinical Pharmacology and Therapeutics 12: 955–962, 1971.
3. Costanza, M.E., *et al.*: Therapy of malignant melanoma with an imidazole carboxamide and bischloroethyl nitrosourea. Cancer 30: 1457–1461, 1972.
4. Luce, J.K., *et al.*: Clinical trials with the antitumor agent 5-(3, 3-dimethyl-l-triazeno) imidazole-4-carboxamide (NSC-45388). Cancer Chemotherapy Reports 54: 119–124, 1970.
5. Bonadonna, G., *et al.*: Combined Chemotherapy (MOPP or ABVD)—radiotherapy approach in advanced Hodgkin's disease. Cancer Treatment Reports 61: 769–777, 1977.
6. Santoro, A., and Bonadonna, G.: Prolonged disease-free survival in MOPP-resistant Hodgkin's disease after treatment with adriamycin, bleomycin, vinblastine and dacarbazine (ABVD). Cancer Chemotherapy Pharmacol. 2: 101–105, 1979.
7. Recommendations for the Safe Handling of Parenteral Antineoplastic Drugs. NIH Publication No. 83-2621. For sale by the Superintendent of Documents, U.S. Government Printing Office, Washington, D.C. 20402.
8. AMA Council Report. Guidelines for Handling Parenteral Antineoplastics. JAMA, March 15, 1985.
9. National Study Commission on Cytotoxic Exposure—Recommendations for Handling Cytotoxic Agents. Available from Louis P. Jeffrey, Sc. D., Director of Pharmacy Services, Rhode Island Hospital, 593 Eddy Street, Providence, Rhode Island 02902.
10. Clinical Oncological Society of Australia: Guidelines and recommendations for safe handling of antineoplastic agents. Med. J. Australia 1: 426–428, 1983.
11. Jones, R.B., *et al.*: Safe handling of chemotherapeutic agents: A report from the Mount Sinai Medical Center. Ca-A Cancer Journal for Clinicians Sept./Oct. 258–263, 1983.
12. American Society of Hospital Pharmacists technical assistance bulletin on handling cytotoxic drugs in hospitals. Am. J. Hosp. Pharm. 42: 131–137, 1985.

Manufactured by:
Ben Venue Laboratories
Bedford, Ohio 44146
Distributed by:
Bayer Corporation
Pharmaceutical Division
400 Morgan Lane
West Haven, CT 06516 USA
PD500102 9/98 ©1998 Bayer Corporation 8675

MITHRACIN® ℞

(plicamycin)

FOR INTRAVENOUS USE

WARNING

IT IS RECOMMENDED THAT MITHRACIN (plicamycin) BE ADMINISTERED ONLY TO HOSPITALIZED PATIENTS BY OR UNDER THE SUPERVISION OF A QUALIFIED PHYSICIAN WHO IS EXPERIENCED IN THE USE OF CANCER CHEMOTHERAPEUTIC AGENTS, BECAUSE OF THE POSSIBILITY OF SEVERE REACTIONS. FACILITIES FOR THE DETERMINATION OF NECESSARY LABORATORY STUDIES MUST BE AVAILABLE.

SEVERE THROMBOCYTOPENIA, A HEMORRHAGIC TENDENCY AND EVEN DEATH MAY RESULT FROM THE USE OF MITHRACIN. ALTHOUGH SEVERE TOXICITY IS MORE APT TO OCCUR IN PATIENTS WHO HAVE FAR-ADVANCED DISEASE OR ARE OTHERWISE CONSIDERED POOR RISKS FOR THERAPY, SERIOUS TOXICITY MAY ALSO OCCASIONALLY OCCUR EVEN IN PATIENTS WHO ARE IN RELATIVELY GOOD CONDITION.

IN THE TREATMENT OF EACH PATIENT, THE PHYSICIAN MUST WEIGH CAREFULLY THE POSSIBILITY OF ACHIEVING THERAPEUTIC BENEFIT VERSUS THE RISK OF TOXICITY WHICH MAY OCCUR WITH MITHRACIN THERAPY. THE FOLLOWING DATA CONCERNING THE USE OF MITHRACIN IN THE TREATMENT OF TESTICULAR TUMORS, HYPERCALCEMIC AND/OR HYPERCALCIURIC CONDITIONS ASSOCIATED WITH VARIOUS ADVANCED MALIGNANCIES, SHOULD BE THOROUGHLY REVIEWED BEFORE ADMINISTERING THIS COMPOUND.

DESCRIPTION

Mithracin (plicamycin) is a yellow crystalline compound which is produced by a microorganism, *Streptomyces plicatus*. Mithracin is available in vials as a freeze-dried, sterile preparation for intravenous administration. Each vial contains 2500 mcg (2.5 mg) of Mithracin with 100 mg of mannitol and sufficient disodium phosphate to adjust to pH 7. After reconstitution with sterile water for injection, the solution has a pH of 7. The drug is unstable in acid solutions with a pH below 4.

Mithracin is an antineoplastic agent. It has an empirical formula of $C_{52}H_{76}O_{24}$. The following structural formula has been proposed for this compound.

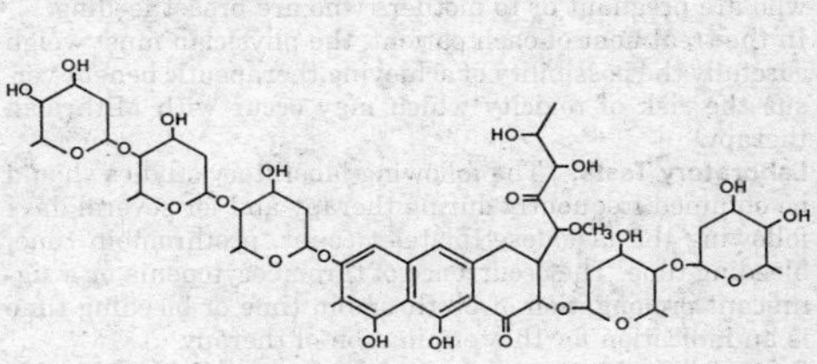

CLINICAL PHARMACOLOGY

Although the exact mechanism by which Mithracin causes tumor inhibition is not yet known, studies have indicated that this compound forms a complex with deoxyribonucleic acid (DNA) and inhibits cellular ribonucleic acid (RNA) and enzymic RNA synthesis. The binding of Mithracin to DNA in the presence of Mg^{++} (or other divalent cations) is responsible for the inhibition of DNA-dependent or DNA-directed RNA synthesis. This action presumably accounts for the biological properties of Mithracin.

Mithracin shows potent cytotoxicity against malignant cells of human origin (Hela cells) growing in tissue culture. Mithracin is lethal to Hela cells in 48 hours at concentrations as low as 0.5 micrograms per milliliter of tissue culture medium. Mithracin has shown significant anti-tumor activity against experimental leukemia in mice when administered intraperitoneally.

Plicamycin may lower serum calcium levels; the exact mechanism (or mechanisms) by which the drug exerts this effect is unknown. It appears that plicamycin may block the hypercalcemic action of pharmacologic doses of vitamin D. It has also been suggested that plicamycin may lower calcium serum levels by inhibiting the effect of parathyroid hormone upon osteoclasts. Plicamycin's inhibition of DNA-dependent RNA synthesis appears to render osteoclasts unable to fully respond to parathyroid hormone with the biosynthesis necessary for osteolysis. Decreases in serum phosphate levels and urinary calcium excretion accompany the lowering of serum calcium concentrations.

Radioautography studies[1] with ^{3}H-labeled plicamycin in C3H mice show that the greatest concentrations of the isotope are in the Kupffer cells of the liver and cells of the renal tubules. Plicamycin is rapidly cleared from the blood within the first 2 hours and excretion is also rapid. Sixty-seven percent of measured excretion occurs within 4 hours, 75% within 8 hours, and 90% is recovered in the first 24 hours after injection. There is no evidence of protein binding, nor is there any evidence of metabolism of the carbohydrate moiety of the drug to carbon dioxide and water with loss through respiration. Plicamycin crosses the blood-brain barrier; the concentration found in brain tissue is low but it persists longer than in other tissues. The experimental results in animals correlate closely with results achieved in man.[2]

INDICATIONS

Mithracin is a potent antineoplastic agent which has been shown to be useful in the treatment of carefully selected hospitalized patients with malignant tumors of the testis in whom successful treatment by surgery and/or radiation is impossible. Also, on the basis of limited clinical experience to date, it may be considered in the treatment of certain symptomatic patients with hypercalcemia and hypercalciuria associated with a variety of advanced neoplasms.

The use of Mithracin in other types of neoplastic disease is not recommended at the present time.

CONTRAINDICATIONS

Mithracin (plicamycin) is contraindicated in patients with thrombocytopenia, thrombocytopathy, coagulation disorder

Continued on next page

Mithracin—Cont.

or an increased susceptibility to bleeding due to other causes. Mithracin should not be administered to any patient with impairment of bone marrow function.
Mithracin may cause fetal harm when administered to a pregnant woman. Mithracin is contraindicated in women who are or may become pregnant. If this drug is used during pregnancy, or if the patient becomes pregnant while taking this drug, the patient should be apprised of the potential hazard to the fetus.

PRECAUTIONS

General: Mithracin should be administered only to patients who are hospitalized and who can be observed carefully and frequently during and after therapy.
Severe thrombocytopenia, a hemorrhagic tendency and even death may result from the use of Mithracin. Although severe toxicity is more apt to occur in patients who have far-advanced disease or are otherwise considered poor risks for therapy, serious toxicity may also occasionally occur even in patients who are in relatively good condition.
Electrolyte imbalance, especially hypocalcemia, hypokalemia, and hypophosphatemia, should be corrected with appropriate electrolyte therapy prior to treatment with Mithracin.
Mithracin should be used with extreme caution in patients with significant impairment of renal or hepatic function.
Mithracin should not normally be administered to patients who are pregnant or to mothers who are breast feeding.
In the treatment of each patient, the physician must weigh carefully the possibility of achieving therapeutic benefit versus the risk of toxicity which may occur with Mithracin therapy.
Laboratory Tests: The following laboratory studies should be obtained frequently during therapy and for several days following the last dose: platelet count, prothrombin time, bleeding time. The occurrence of thrombocytopenia or a significant prolongation of prothrombin time or bleeding time is an indication for the termination of therapy.
Carcinogenesis, mutagenesis, impairment of fertility: No long-term studies in animals have been performed to evaluate the carcinogenic potential of Mithracin. Histologic evidence of inhibition of spermatogenesis was observed in a substantial number of male rats receiving doses of 0.6 mg/kg/day and above.
Pregnancy Category X: See "Contraindications" section.
Nursing Mothers: It is not known whether this drug is excreted in human milk. Because many drugs are excreted in human milk and because of the potential for serious adverse reactions in nursing infants from Mithracin, a decision should be made whether to discontinue nursing or to discontinue the drug, taking into account the importance of the drug to the mother.

ADVERSE REACTIONS

THE MOST IMPORTANT FORM OF TOXICITY ASSOCIATED WITH THE USE OF MITHRACIN CONSISTS OF A BLEEDING SYNDROME WHICH USUALLY BEGINS WITH AN EPISODE OF EPISTAXIS. This bleeding tendency may only consist of a single or several episodes of epistaxis and progress no further. However, in some cases, this hemorrhagic syndrome can start with an episode of hematemesis which may progress to more widespread hemorrhage in the gastrointestinal tract or to a more generalized bleeding tendency. This hemorrhagic diathesis is most likely due to abnormalities in multiple clotting factors.
A detailed analysis of the clinical data in 1,160 patients treated with Mithracin indicates that the hemorrhagic syndrome is dose related. With doses of 30 mcg/kg/day or less for 10 or fewer doses, the incidence of bleeding episodes has been 5.4% with an associated drug-related mortality rate of 1.6%. With doses greater than 30 mcg/kg/day and/or for more than 10 doses, a significantly larger number of bleeding episodes occurred (11.9%) and the associated drug-related mortality rate was also significantly higher (5.7%).
The most common side effects reported with the use of Mithracin consist of gastrointestinal symptoms: anorexia, nausea, vomiting, diarrhea, and stomatitis. Other less frequently reported side effects include fever, drowsiness, weakness, lethargy, malaise, headache, depression, phlebitis, facial flushing, and skin rash.

The following laboratory abnormalities have been reported during therapy with Mithracin and in most instances were reversible following cessation of treatment:
Hematologic Abnormalities: Depression of platelet count, white count, hemoglobin and prothrombin content; elevation of clotting time and bleeding time; abnormal clot retraction.
Thrombocytopenia may be rapid in onset and may occur at any time during therapy or within several days following the last dose. With the occurrence of severe thrombocytopenia, the infusion of platelet concentrates of platelet-rich plasma may be helpful in elevating the platelet count.
The occurrence of leukopenia with the use of Mithracin is relatively uncommon, occurring only in approximately 6% of patients.
It has been uncommon for abnormalities in clotting time or clot retraction to be demonstrated prior to the onset of an overt bleeding episode noted in some patients treated with Mithracin. Nevertheless, the performance of these tests periodically is recommended because in a few instances, an abnormality in one of these studies may have served as a warning to terminate therapy because of impending serious toxicity.
Abnormal Liver Function Tests: Increased levels of serum glutamic oxalacetic transaminase, serum glutamic pyruvic transaminase, lactic dehydrogenase, alkaline phosphatase, serum bilirubin, ornithine carbamyl transferase, isocitric dehydrogenase, and increased retention of bromsulphalein.
Abnormal Renal Function Tests: Increased blood urea nitrogen and serum creatinine; proteinuria.
Abnormalities in Electrolyte Concentrations: Depression of serum calcium, phosphorus, and potassium.

OVERDOSAGE

Generally, adverse effects following the use of Mithracin, especially the hemorrhagic syndrome, are dose related. Therefore, following administration of an overdose, patients can be expected to experience an exaggeration of the usual adverse effects. Close monitoring of the hematologic picture, including factors involved in the clotting mechanism, hepatic and renal functions, and serum electrolytes, is necessary. No specific antidote for Mithracin is known. Management of overdosage would include general supportive measures to sustain the patient through the period of toxicity.

DOSAGE AND ADMINISTRATION

The daily dose of Mithracin is based on the patient's body weight. If a patient has abnormal fluid retention such as edema, hydrothorax or ascites, the patient's ideal weight rather than actual body weight should be used to calculate the dose.
Treatment of Testicular Tumors: In the treatment of patients with testicular tumors the recommended daily dose of Mithracin (plicamycin) is 25 to 30 mcg (0.025–0.030 mg) per kilogram of body weight. Therapy should be continued for a period of 8 to 10 days unless significant side effects or toxicity occur during therapy. A course of therapy consisting of more than 10 daily doses is not recommended. Individual daily doses should not exceed 30 mcg (0.030 mg) per kilogram of body weight.
In those patients with responsive tumors, some degree of tumor regression is usually evident within 3 or 4 weeks following the initial course of therapy. If tumor masses remain unchanged following an initial course of therapy, additional courses of therapy at monthly intervals are warranted.
When a significant tumor regression is obtained, it is suggested that additional courses of therapy be given at monthly intervals until a complete regression of tumor masses is achieved or until definite tumor progression or new tumor masses occur in spite of continued courses of therapy.
Treatment of Hypercalcemia and Hypercalciuria: Reversal of hypercalcemia and hypercalciuria can usually be achieved with Mithracin at doses considerably lower than those recommended for use in the treatment of testicular tumors.
In hypercalcemia and hypercalciuria associated with advanced malignancy the recommended course of treatment with Mithracin is 25 mcg (0.025 mg) per kilogram of body weight per day for 3 or 4 days.
If the desired degree of reversal of hypercalcemia or hypercalciuria is not achieved with the initial course of therapy, additional courses of therapy may then be administered at intervals of one week or more to achieve the desired result or to maintain serum calcium and urinary calcium excretion at normal levels. It may be possible to maintain normal calcium balance with single, weekly doses or with a schedule of 2 or 3 doses per week.

NOTE: BECAUSE OF THE DRUG'S TOXICITY AND THE LIMITED CLINICAL EXPERIENCE TO DATE IN THESE INDICATIONS, THE FOLLOWING RECOMMENDATIONS SHOULD BE KEPT IN MIND BY THE PHYSICIAN.

1. **CONSIDER CASES OF HYPERCALCEMIA AND HYPERCALCIURIA NOT RESPONSIVE TO CONVENTIONAL TREATMENT.**
2. **APPLY SAME CONTRAINDICATIONS AND PRECAUTIONARY MEASURES AS IN ANTITUMOR TREATMENT.**
3. **RENAL FUNCTION SHOULD BE CAREFULLY MONITORED BEFORE, DURING, AND AFTER TREATMENT.**
4. **BENEFITS OF USE DURING PREGNANCY OR IN WOMEN OF CHILDBEARING AGE SHOULD BE WEIGHED AGAINST POTENTIAL TOXICITY TO EMBRYO OR FETUS.**

ADMINISTRATION

By IV administration only. The appropriate daily dose of Mithracin should be diluted in one liter of 5% Dextrose Injection, USP or Sodium Chloride Injection, USP and administered by slow intravenous infusion over a period of 4 to 6 hours. Rapid direct intravenous injection of Mithracin should be avoided as it may be associated with a higher incidence and greater severity of gastrointestinal side effects. Extravasation of solutions of Mithracin may cause local irritation and cellulitis at injection sites. Should thrombophlebitis or perivascular cellulitis occur, the infusion should be terminated and reinstituted at another site. The application of moderate heat to the site of extravasation may help to disperse the compound and minimize discomfort and local tissue irritation. The use of antiemetic compounds prior to and during treatment with Mithracin may be helpful in relieving nausea and vomiting.
Procedures for proper handling and disposal of anti-cancer drugs should be considered. Several guidelines on this subject have been published.[3–8] There is no general agreement that all of the procedures recommended in the guidelines are necessary or appropriate.

HOW SUPPLIED

Mithracin is available in vials as a freeze-dried preparation for intravenous administration. Each vial contains 2500 mcg (2.5 mg) of Mithracin with 100 mg of mannitol and sufficient disodium phosphate to adjust to pH 7. These vials should be stored at refrigerator temperatures between 2°C to 8°C (36°F to 46°F).
To reconstitute, add aseptically 4.9 mL of Sterile Water for Injection to the contents of the vial and shake to dissolve. Each mL of the resulting solution will then contain 500 mcg (0.5 mg) of Mithracin. NOTE: 1 mg (milligram)=1000 mcg (micrograms). AFTER REMOVAL OF THE APPROPRIATE DOSE, THE REMAINING UNUSED SOLUTION MUST BE DISCARDED, FRESH SOLUTIONS MUST BE PREPARED IN THE ABOVE MANNER EACH DAY OF THERAPY.

ANIMAL PHARMACOLOGY AND TOXICOLOGY

In mice the average intravenous LD_{50} of Mithracin is 2,000 mcg/kg of body weight. When administered orally, it is not toxic to mice even at doses 100 times greater than the intravenous LD_{50}. In rats the average intravenous LD_{50} of Mithracin is 1,700 mcg/kg of body weight. It is not toxic to rats when administered orally at doses 17 times greater than the intravenous LD_{50}. In dogs and monkeys Mithracin is essentially non-toxic when administered intravenously for 24 days at daily doses as high as 50 and 24 mcg/kg of body weight, respectively. However, at higher doses of 100 mcg/kg/day intravenously it is lethal to dogs and monkeys. Signs of toxicity in dogs and monkeys included anorexia, vomiting, listlessness, melena, anemia, lymphopenia, elevated alkaline phosphatase, serum glutamic oxalacetic transaminase, serum glutamic pyruvic transaminase values, hypochloremia, and azotemia. Dogs also showed marked thrombocytopenia, hyponatremia, hypokalemia, hypocalcemia, and decreased prothrombin consumption. Necropsy findings consisted of necrosis of lymphoid tissue and multiple generalized hemorrhages. Mithracin (plicamycin) was only mildly irritating when injected intramuscularly in rabbits and subcutaneously in guinea pigs. Histologic evidence of inhibition of spermatogenesis was observed in a substantial number of male rats receiving doses of 0.6 mg/kg/day and above. This preclinical finding of selective drug effect constituted the scientific rationale for clinical trials in testicular tumors.

CLINICAL REPORTS

Treatment of Patients with Inoperable Testicular Tumors: In a combined series of 305 patients with inoperable testicular tumors treated with Mithracin, 33 patients (10.8%) showed a complete disappearance of tumor masses and an additional 80 patients (26.2%) responded with significant partial regression of tumor masses. The longest duration of a continuing complete response is now over $8^{1}/_{2}$ years. The therapeutic responses in this series of patients have been summarized by type of testicular tumor in the accompanying table.
[See table at left]

MITHRACIN
RESULTS IN 305 TESTICULAR TUMOR CASES BY TUMOR TYPE

TYPE OF TESTICULAR TUMOR	TOTAL	COMPLETE RESPONSE	PARTIAL RESPONSE	NO RESPONSE
EMBRYONAL CELL	173	26	42	105
TERATOMA	5	0	1	4
TERATOCARCINOMA	23	0	5	18
SEMINOMA	18	0	7	11
CHORIOCARCINOMA	13	1	6	6
MIXED TUMOR	73	6	19	48
TOTALS	305	33	80	192

Mithracin may be useful in the treatment of patients with testicular tumors which are resistant to other chemotherapeutic agents. Prior radiation therapy or prior chemotherapy did not alter the response rate with Mithracin. This suggests that there is no significant cross resistance between Mithracin and other chemotherapeutic agents.

Treatment of Patients with Hypercalcemia and Hypercalciuria: A limited number of patients with hypercalcemia (range: 12.0–25.8 mg%) and patients with hypercalciuria (range 215–492 mg/day) associated with malignant disease were treated with Mithracin. Hypercalcemia and hypercalciuria were promptly reversed in all patients. In some patients, the primary malignancy was of non-testicular origin.

REFERENCES

1. Kennedy, B.D., et al: Cancer Res. *27* :1534, 1967.
2. Ransohoff, J., et al: Cancer Chemother. Rep. *49* :51, 1965.
3. Recommendations for the Safe Handling of Parenteral Antineoplastic Drugs. NIH Publication No. 83-2621. For sale by the Superintendent of Documents, U.S. Government Printing Office, Washington, D.C. 20402.
4. AMA Council Report. Guidelines for Handling Parenteral Antineoplastics. JAMA, March 15, 1985.
5. National Study Commission on Cytotoxic Exposure—Recommendations for Handling Cytotoxic Agents. Available from Louis P. Jeffrey, Sc.D., Director of Pharmacy Services, Rhode Island Hospital, 593 Eddy Street, Providence, Rhode Island 02902.
6. Clinical Oncological Society of Australia: Guidelines and recommendations for safe handling of antineoplastic agents. Med J Australia *1* :426–428, 1983.
7. Jones, R.B., et al: Safe handling of chemotherapeutic agents: A report from the Mount Sinai Medical Center. Ca—A Cancer Journal for Clinicians, Sept/Oct. 258–263, 1983.
8. American Society of Hospital Pharmacists technical assistance bulletin on handling cytotoxic drugs in hospitals. Am J Hosp Pharm *42* :131–137, 1985.

Manufactured for
Bayer Corporation
Pharmaceutical Division
400 Morgan Lane
West Haven, CT 06516
by Ben Venue Laboratories
Bedford, Ohio 44146
PD100654—60-4178-81-5 Revised Feb. 1995

MYCELEX®-G 500 mg ℞
Brand of clotrimazole
Vaginal Tablets

PRODUCT OVERVIEW

KEY FACTS

Mycelex®-G 500 mg is an effective antifungal containing 500 mg of clotrimazole (the active ingredient). Clotrimazole is a broad spectrum antifungal which exhibits fungicidal activity *in vitro* against *Candida albicans* and other species of the genus *Candida.* No single-step or multiple-step resistance to clotrimazole has developed during successive passages of *Candida albicans.*

MAJOR USES

Mycelex®-G 500 mg has proved to be clinically effective for local treatment of vulvovaginal candidiasis when one day therapy is felt warranted. In the case of severe vulvovaginal candidiasis longer antimycotic therapy such as Mycelex®-G 100 mg tablets or Mycelex®-G Cream is recommended.

SAFETY INFORMATION

Mycelex®-G 500 Vaginal Tablets are contraindicated in women who have shown hypersensitivity to any components of the compound. If there is a lack of response to treatment with Mycelex®-G 500 mg, appropriate microbiological studies should be performed to confirm the diagnosis and rule out other pathogens before instituting another course of antimycotic therapy. There are, however, no adequate and well-controlled studies in pregnant women during the first trimester of pregnancy.

PRESCRIBING INFORMATION

MYCELEX®-G 500 mg ℞
Brand of clotrimazole
Vaginal Tablets

DESCRIPTION

Each Mycelex®-G 500 mg Vaginal Tablet contains 500 mg clotrimazole (the active ingredient) dispersed in lactose, microcrystalline cellulose, lactic acid, corn starch, crospovidone, calcium lactate, magnesium stearate, silicon dioxide and hydroxypropyl methylcellulose. Chemically, clotrimazole is [1-(o-Chloro-α, α-diphenylbenzyl) imidazole], a synthetic antifungal agent having the chemical formula $C_{22}H_{17}ClN_2$; a molecular weight of 344.84; and the following chemical structure:

[See chemical structure at top of next column]

Clotrimazole is an odorless, white crystalline substance, practically insoluble in water, sparingly soluble in ether, soluble in carbon tetrachloride, and very soluble in ethanol and chloroform.

CLINICAL PHARMACOLOGY

Serum levels and levels in vaginal secretions of clotrimazole were measured in six healthy volunteers who had one 500

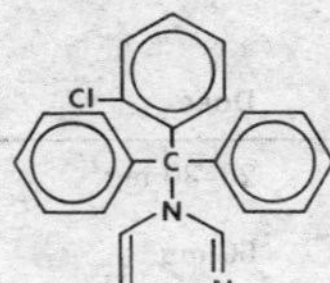

mg vaginal tablet inserted. Although serum levels of clotrimazole were higher than those in other volunteers given 100 mg and 200 mg vaginal tablets these levels did not exceed 10 nanograms/mL. It has been estimated that three to ten percent of a vaginal dose of clotrimazole may be absorbed, but the drug rapidly and efficiently degrades to microbiologically inactive metabolites. The clotrimazole concentrations remaining in vaginal secretions were still in the mg/mL range for 48 hours and in two of the six subjects at 72 hours.

The findings of high clotrimazole concentrations in vaginal secretions for up to 72 hours and low concentrations in the serum suggest that nearly all the clotrimazole given in the 500 mg vaginal tablet remains in the vagina for 48 hours, and in some cases 72 hours, in fungicidal concentrations.

Clotrimazole is a broad-spectrum antifungal agent. It has been postulated that the compound affects the permeability characteristics of the membrane allowing the leakage of essential intracellular components with a consequent inhibition of the synthesis of such macromolecules as protein, lipid, DNA, and polysaccharides.

At concentrations as low as 2–5 µg/mL, clotrimazole exhibits its fungicidal activity *in vitro* against *Candida albicans* and other species of the genus *Candida.*

No single-step or multiple-step resistance to clotrimazole has developed during successive passages of *Candida albicans.*

INDICATIONS

Mycelex-G 500 mg Vaginal Tablets are indicated for the local treatment of vulvovaginal candidiasis when one day therapy is felt warranted. In the case of severe vulvovaginitis due to candidiasis, longer antimycotic therapy is recommended. The diagnosis should be confirmed by KOH smears and/or cultures. Other pathogens commonly associated with vulvovaginitis, *Trichomonas* and *Gardnerella (Haemophilus) vaginalis,* should be ruled out by appropriate laboratory methods.

CONTRAINDICATIONS

Mycelex-G 500 mg Vaginal Tablets are contraindicated in women who have shown hypersensitivity to any components of the preparation.

WARNINGS

None.

PRECAUTIONS

If there is a lack of response to Mycelex-G 500 mg Vaginal Tablets, appropriate microbiological studies should be repeated to confirm the diagnosis and rule out other pathogens before instituting another course of antimycotic therapy.

CARCINOGENESIS

No long term studies in animals have been performed to evaluate the carcinogenic potential of Mycelex-G 500 mg Vaginal Tablets intravaginally. A long term study in rats (Wistar strains) where clotrimazole was administered orally provided no indication of carcinogenicity.

USAGE IN PREGNANCY

Pregnancy Category B: The disposition of ^{14}C-clotrimazole has been studied in humans and animals. Clotrimazole is poorly absorbed following intravaginal administration to humans, whereas it is rather well absorbed after oral administration.

In clinical trials, use of vaginally applied clotrimazole in pregnant women in their second and third trimesters has not been associated with ill effects. There are, however, no adequate and well-controlled studies in pregnant women during the first trimester of pregnancy.

Studies in pregnant rats given repeated intravaginal doses up to 100 mg/kg/day have revealed no evidence of harm to the fetus due to clotrimazole.

Repeated high oral doses of clotrimazole in rats and mice ranging from 50 to 120 mg/kg resulted in embryotoxicity (possibly secondary to maternal toxicity), impairment of mating, decreased litter size and number of viable young and decreased pup survival to weaning. However, clotrimazole was not teratogenic in mice, rabbits and rats at oral doses up to 200, 180 and 100 mg/kg, respectively. Oral absorption in the rat amounts to approximately 90% of the administered dose.

Because animal reproduction studies are not always predictive of human response, this drug should be used only if clearly indicated during the first trimester of pregnancy.

ADVERSE REACTIONS

Of 297 patients in double-blind studies with the 500 mg vaginal tablet, 3 of 149 patients treated with active drug and 3 of 148 patients treated with placebo reported complaints during therapy that were possibly drug related. In the active drug group, vomiting occurred in one patient, vaginal soreness with coitus in another, and complaints of vaginal irritation, itching, burning and dyspareunia in the third patient. In the placebo group, clitoral irritation occurred in one patient and dysuria, described as remotely related to drug, in the other. A third patient in the placebo group developed bacterial vaginitis which the investigator classed as possibly related to drug.

Eighteen (1.6%) of the 1116 patients treated with Mycelex-G in other formulations in double-blind studies reported complaints during therapy that were possibly drug-related. Mild burning occurred in six patients while other complaints such as skin rash, itching, vulval irritation, lower abdominal cramps and bloating, slight cramping, slight urinary frequency, and burning or irritation in the sexual partner, occurred rarely.

OVERDOSAGE

No data available.

DRUG ABUSE AND DEPENDENCE

Drug abuse and dependence with Mycelex-G 500 mg Vaginal Tablets has not been reported.

DOSAGE AND ADMINISTRATION

The recommended dose is one tablet inserted intravaginally one time only, preferably at bedtime. In the event of treatment failure, that is, persistence of signs and symptoms of vaginitis after five days, other pathogens commonly responsible for vaginitis should be ruled out before instituting another course of antimycotic therapy.

HOW SUPPLIED

Mycelex-G 500 mg Vaginal Tablets are white, bullet shaped, uncoated tablets, coded with Mycelex on one side and 500 on the other, supplied as a single 500 mg tablet with plastic applicator and patient instructions, or in twin pack with Mycelex 1% cream 7g tube.

Store Below 30°C (86°F).

U.S. Patent Numbers 3,660,577; 3,705,172; 3,839,573; 4,457,938.

Manufactured by
Bayer Corporation
Pharmaceutical Division
400 Morgan Lane
West Haven, CT 06516 USA
PD500056 5/95 BAY 5097

 5213

Shown in Product Identification Guide, page 307

NIMOTOP® ℞
(nimodipine)
CAPSULES
For Oral Use

DESCRIPTION

Nimotop® (nimodipine) belongs to the class of pharmacological agents known as calcium channel blockers. Nimodipine is isopropyl (2 - methoxyethyl) 1, 4 - dihydro - 2, 6 - dimethyl - 4 - (3 - nitrophenyl) - 3, 5 - pyridine - dicarboxylate. It has a molecular weight of 418.5 and a molecular formula of $C_{21}H_{26}N_2O_7$. The structural formula is:

Nimodipine is a yellow crystalline substance, practically insoluble in water.

NIMOTOP® capsules are formulated as soft gelatin capsules for oral administration. Each liquid filled capsule contains 30 mg of nimodipine in a vehicle of glycerin, peppermint oil, purified water and polyethylene glycol 400. The soft gelatin capsule shell contains gelatin, glycerin, purified water and titanium dioxide.

CLINICAL PHARMACOLOGY

Mechanism of Action: Nimodipine is a calcium channel blocker. The contractile processes of smooth muscle cells are dependent upon calcium ions, which enter these cells during depolarization as slow ionic transmembrane currents. Nimodipine inhibits calcium ion transfer into these cells and thus inhibits contractions of vascular smooth muscle. In animal experiments, nimodipine had a greater effect on cerebral arteries than on arteries elsewhere in the body perhaps because it is highly lipophilic, allowing it to cross the blood-brain barrier; concentrations of nimodipine as high as 12.5 ng/mL have been detected in the cerebrospinal fluid of nimodipine treated subarachnoid hemorrhage (SAH) patients. Based on animal experiments, it was hoped that nimodipine would prevent cerebral arterial spasm in SAH patients. While the clinical studies described below demonstrate a favorable effect by nimodipine on the severity of neurological deficits caused by cerebral vasospasm following SAH, there is no arteriographic evidence that the drug either prevents or relieves the spasm of these arteries. The actual mechanism of action in humans is, therefore, unknown.

Continued on next page

Nimotop—Cont.

Pharmacokinetics and Metabolism: In man, nimodipine is rapidly absorbed after oral administration, and peak concentrations are generally attained within one hour. The terminal elimination half-life is approximately 8 to 9 hours but earlier elimination rates are much more rapid, equivalent to a half-life of 1–2 hours; a consequence is the need for frequent (every 4 hours) dosing. There were no signs of accumulation when nimodipine was given three times a day for seven days. Nimodipine is over 95% bound to plasma proteins. The binding was concentration independent over the range of 10 ng/mL to 10 µg/mL. Nimodipine is eliminated almost exclusively in the form of metabolites and less than 1% is recovered in the urine as unchanged drug. Numerous metabolites, all of which are either inactive or considerably less active than the parent compound, have been identified. Because of a high first-pass metabolism, the bioavailability of nimodipine averages 13% after oral administration. The bioavailability is significantly increased in patients with hepatic cirrhosis, with C_{max} approximately double that in normals which necessitates lowering the dose in this group of patients (see Dosage and Administration). In a study of 24 healthy male volunteers, administration of nimodipine capsules following a standard breakfast resulted in a 68% lower peak plasma concentration and 38% lower bioavailability relative to dosing under fasted conditions.

Clinical Trials: Nimodipine has been shown, in 4 randomized, placebo-controlled trials, to reduce the severity of neurological deficits resulting from vasospasm in patients who have had a recent subarachnoid hemorrhage (SAH). The trials used doses ranging from 20–30 mg to 90 mg every 4 hours, with drug given for 21 days in 3 studies, and for at least 18 days in the other. Three of the four trials followed patients for 3–6 months. Three of the trials studied relatively well patients, with all or most patients in Hunt and Hess Grades I–II (essentially free of focal deficits after the initial bleed); the fourth studied much sicker patients, Hunt and Hess Grades III–V. Two studies, one domestic, one French, were similar in design, with relatively unimpaired SAH patients randomized to nimodipine or placebo. In each, a judgment was made as to whether any late-developing deficit was due to spasm or other causes, and the deficits were graded. Both studies showed significantly fewer severe deficits due to spasm in the nimodipine group; the second (French) study showed fewer spasm-related deficits of all severities. No effect was seen on deficits not related to spasm.

[See first table above]

A Canadian study entered much sicker patients, who had a high rate of death and disability, and used a dose of 90 mg every 4 hours, but was otherwise similar to the first two studies. Analysis of delayed ischemic deficits, many of which result from spasm, showed a significant reduction in spasm-related deficits. Among analyzed patients (72 nimodipine, 82 placebo), there were the following outcomes.

[See second table above]

A fourth, large, study was performed in the United Kingdom in SAH patients with all grades of severity (but about 90% were in Grades I–III). Outcomes were not defined as spasm related or not but there was a significant reduction in the overall rate of infarction and severely disabling neurological outcome at 3 months:

	Nimodipine	Placebo
Total patients	278	276
Good recovery	199*	169
Moderate disability	24	16
Severe disability	12**	31
Death	43***	60

* p = 0.0444—good and moderate vs severe and dead
** p = 0.001—severe disability
*** p = 0.056—death

A dose-ranging study comparing 30, 60 and 90 mg doses found a generally low rate of spasm-related neurological deficits but no significant relation of response to dose.

The effect of nimodipine on mortality is not yet clear. The large United Kingdom study showed near-significantly improved survival. The two smaller studies (domestic, French) had too few deaths to contribute to this question. The Canadian study, despite showing markedly decreased spasm-related deficits, showed overall (all patients randomized) greater 90 day mortality, 49/91 (54%) on nimodipine vs 38/97 (39%) on placebo, a significant difference. Most of the deaths appeared, in this very severely ill group (Hunt and Hess Grades III–V), to be consequences of SAH, but a drug effect cannot be ruled out. In this study 90 mg every 4 hours was the dose used, perhaps too high for the very ill population studied. The 90 mg dose is not recommended nor is treatment of Hunt and Hess Grades IV–V patients.

INDICATIONS AND USAGE

Nimotop® (nimodipine) is indicated for the improvement of neurological outcome by reducing the incidence and severity of ischemic deficits in patients with subarachnoid hemorrhage from ruptured congenital aneurysms who are in good neurological condition post-ictus (e.g., Hunt and Hess Grades I–III).

CONTRAINDICATIONS

None known.

Study	Dose	Grade*	Patients: Number Analyzed	Patients: Any Deficit Due to Spasm	Patients: Numbers With Severe Deficit
1.	20–30 mg	I–III	Nimodipine 56	13	1
			Placebo 60	16	8**
2.	60 mg	I–III	Nimodipine 31	4	2
			Placebo 39	11	10**

* Hunt and Hess Grade
** p = 0.03

	Delayed Ischemic Deficits (DID)		Permanent Deficits	
	Nimodipine n (%)	Placebo n (%)	Nimodipine n (%)	Placebo n (%)
DID Spasm Alone	8 (11)*	25 (31)	5 (7) *	22 (27)
DID Spasm Contributing	18 (25)	21 (26)	16 (22)	17 (21)
DID Without Spasm	7 (10)	8 (10)	6 (8)	7 (9)
No DID	39 (54)	28 (34)	45 (63)	36 (44)

* P = 0.001, nimodipine vs placebo

DOSE q4h

Number of Patients (%)

Sign/Symptom	Nimodipine 0.35 mg/kg (n = 82)	Nimodipine 30 mg (n = 71)	Nimodipine 60 mg (n = 494)	Nimodipine 90 mg (n = 172)	Nimodipine 120 mg (n = 4)	Placebo (n = 479)
Decreased Blood Pressure	1 (1.2)	0	19 (3.8)	14 (8.1)	2 (50.0)	6 (1.2)
Abnormal Liver Function Test	1 (1.2)	0	2 (0.4)	1 (0.6)	0	7 (1.5)
Edema	0	0	2 (0.4)	2 (1.2)	0	3 (0.6)
Diarrhea	0	3 (4.2)	0	3 (1.7)	0	3 (0.6)
Rash	2 (2.4)	0	3 (0.6)	2 (1.2)	0	3 (0.6)
Headache	0	1 (1.4)	6 (1.2)	0	0	1 (0.2)
Gastrointestinal Symptoms	2 (2.4)	0	0	2 (1.2)	0	0
Nausea	1 (1.2)	1 (1.4)	6 (1.2)	1 (0.6)	0	0
Dyspnea	1 (1.2)	0	0	0	0	0
EKG Abnormalities	0	1 (1.4)	0	1 (0.6)	0	0
Tachycardia	0	1 (1.4)	0	0	0	0
Bradycardia	0	0	5 (1.0)	1 (0.6)	0	0
Muscle Pain/Cramp	0	1 (1.4)	1 (0.2)	1 (0.6)	0	0
Acne	0	1 (1.4)	0	0	0	0
Depression	0	1 (1.4)	0	0	0	0

PRECAUTIONS

General: Blood Pressure: Nimodipine has the hemodynamic effects expected of a calcium channel blocker, although they are generally not marked. However, intravenous administration of the contents of Nimotop Capsules has resulted in serious adverse consequences including hypotension, cardiovascular collapse, and cardiac arrest. In patients with subarachnoid hemorrhage given Nimotop® in clinical studies, about 5% were reported to have had lowering of the blood pressure and about 1% left the study because of this (not all could be attributed to nimodipine). Nevertheless, blood pressure should be carefully monitored during treatment with Nimotop® based on its known pharmacology and the known effects of calcium channel blockers.

Hepatic Disease: The metabolism of Nimotop® is decreased in patients with impaired hepatic function. Such patients should have their blood pressure and pulse rate monitored closely and should be given a lower dose (see Dosage and Administration).

Intestinal pseudo-obstruction and ileus have been reported rarely in patients treated with nimodipine. A causal relationship has not been established. The condition has responded to conservative management.

Laboratory Test Interactions: None known.

Drug Interaction: It is possible that the cardiovascular action of other calcium channel blockers could be enhanced by the addition of Nimotop®.

In Europe, Nimotop® was observed to occasionally intensify the effect of antihypertensive compounds taken concomitantly by patients suffering from hypertension; this phenomenon was not observed in North American clinical trials.

A study in eight healthy volunteers has shown a 50% increase in mean peak nimodipine plasma concentrations and a 90% increase in mean area under the curve, after a one-week course of cimetidine at 1,000 mg/day and nimodipine at 90 mg/day. This effect may be mediated by the known inhibition of hepatic cytochrome P-450 by cimetidine, which could decrease first-pass metabolism of nimodipine.

Carcinogenesis, Mutagenesis, Impairment of Fertility: In a two-year study, higher incidences of adenocarcinoma of the uterus and Leydig-cell adenoma of the testes were observed in rats given a diet containing 1800 ppm nimodipine (equivalent to 91 to 121 mg/kg/day nimodipine) than in placebo controls. The differences were not statistically significant, however, and the higher rates were well within historical control range for these tumors in the Wistar strain. Nimodipine was found not to be carcinogenic in a 91-week mouse study but the high dose of 1800 ppm nimodipine-in-feed (546 to 774 mg/kg/day) shortened the life expectancy of the animals. Mutagenicity studies, including the Ames, micronucleus and dominant lethal tests were negative.

Nimodipine did not impair the fertility and general reproductive performance of male and female Wistar rats following oral doses of up to 30 mg/kg/day when administered daily for more than 10 weeks in the males and 3 weeks in the females prior to mating and continued to day 7 of pregnancy. This dose in a rat is about 4 times the equivalent clinical dose of 60 mg q4h in a 50 kg patient.

Pregnancy: Pregnancy Category C. Nimodipine has been shown to have a teratogenic effect in Himalayan rabbits. Incidences of malformations and stunted fetuses were increased at oral doses of 1 and 10 mg/kg/day administered (by gavage) from day 6 through day 18 of pregnancy but not at 3.0 mg/kg/day in one of two identical rabbit studies. In the second study an increased incidence of stunted fetuses was seen at 1.0 mg/kg/day but not at higher doses. Nimodipine was embryotoxic, causing resorption and stunted growth of fetuses, in Long Evans rats at 100 mg/kg/day administered by gavage from day 6 through day 15 of pregnancy. In two other rat studies, doses of 30 mg/kg/day nimodipine administered by gavage from day 16 of gestation and continued until sacrifice (day 20 of pregnancy or day 21 post partum) were associated with higher incidences of skeletal variation, stunted fetuses and stillbirths but no malformations. There are no adequate and well controlled studies in pregnant women to directly assess the effect on human fetuses. Nimodipine should be used during pregnancy only if the potential benefit justifies the potential risk to the fetus.

Nursing Mothers: Nimodipine and/or its metabolites have been shown to appear in rat milk at concentrations much higher than in maternal plasma. It is not known whether the drug is excreted in human milk. Because many drugs are excreted in human milk, nursing mothers are advised not to breast feed their babies when taking the drug.

Pediatric Use: Safety and effectiveness in children have not been established.

Geriatric Use: A review of controlled clinical trials conducted with Nimotop revealed that there were too few geriatric patients exposed to this product to determine any difference in response between elderly and younger patients.

ADVERSE REACTIONS

Adverse experiences were reported by 92 of 823 patients with subarachnoid hemorrhage (11.2%) who were given nimodipine. The most frequently reported adverse experience was decreased blood pressure in 4.4% of these patients. Twenty-nine of 479 (6.1%) placebo treated patients also reported adverse experiences. The events reported with a frequency greater than 1% are displayed below by dose.

[See third table on previous page]

There were no other adverse experiences reported by the patients who were given 0.35 mg/kg q4h, 30 mg q4h or 120 mg q4h. Adverse experiences with an incidence rate of less than 1% in the 60 mg q4h dose group were: hepatitis; itching; gastrointestinal hemorrhage; thrombocytopenia; anemia; palpitations; vomiting; flushing; diaphoresis; wheezing; phenytoin toxicity; lightheadedness; dizziness; rebound vasospasm; jaundice; hypertension; hematoma.

Adverse experiences with an incidence rate less than 1% in the 90 mg q4h dose group were: itching, gastrointestinal hemorrhage; thrombocytopenia; neurological deterioration; vomiting; diaphoresis; congestive heart failure; hyponatremia; decreasing platelet count; disseminated intravascular coagulation; deep vein thrombosis.

As can be seen from the table, side effects that appear related to nimodipine use based on increased incidence with higher dose or a higher rate compared to placebo control, included decreased blood pressure, edema and headaches which are known pharmacologic actions of calcium channel blockers. It must be noted, however, that SAH is frequently accompanied by alterations in consciousness which lead to an under reporting of adverse experiences. Patients who received nimodipine in clinical trials for other indications reported flushing (2.1%), headache (4.1%) and fluid retention (0.3%), typical responses to calcium channel blockers. As a calcium channel blocker, nimodipine may have the potential to exacerbate heart failure in susceptible patients or to interfere with A-V conduction, but these events were not observed.

No clinically significant effects on hematologic factors, renal or hepatic function or carbohydrate metabolism have been causally associated with oral nimodipine. Isolated cases of non-fasting elevated serum glucose levels (0.8%), elevated LDH levels (0.4%), decreased platelet counts (0.3%), elevated alkaline phosphatase levels (0.2%) and elevated SGPT levels (0.2%) have been reported rarely.

DRUG ABUSE AND DEPENDENCE

There have been no reported instances of drug abuse or dependence with Nimotop®.

OVERDOSAGE

There have been no reports of overdosage from the oral administration of Nimotop®. Symptoms of overdosage would be expected to be related to cardiovascular effects such as excessive peripheral vasodilation with marked systemic hypotension. Clinically significant hypotension due to Nimotop® overdosage may require active cardiovascular support. Norepinephrine or dopamine may be helpful in restoring blood pressure. Since Nimotop® is highly protein-bound, dialysis is not likely to be of benefit.

DOSAGE AND ADMINISTRATION

Nimotop is given orally in the form of ivory colored, soft gelatin 30 mg capsules for subarachnoid hemorrhage.

The oral dose is 60 mg (two 30 mg capsules) every 4 hours for 21 consecutive days, preferably not less than one hour before or two hours after meals. Oral Nimotop® therapy should commence within 96 hours of the subarachnoid hemorrhage.

If the capsule cannot be swallowed, e.g., at the time of surgery, or if the patient is unconscious, a hole should be made in both ends of the capsule with an 18 gauge needle, and the contents of the capsule extracted into a syringe. The contents should then be emptied into the patient's *in situ* nasogastric tube and washed down the tube with 30 mL of normal saline (0.9%).

The contents of Nimotop Capsules must not be administered by intravenous injection or other parenteral routes.

Patients with hepatic cirrhosis have substantially reduced clearance and approximately doubled C_{max}. Dosage should be reduced to 30 mg every 4 hours, with close monitoring of blood pressure and heart rate.

HOW SUPPLIED

Each ivory colored, soft gelatin NIMOTOP® capsule is imprinted with the word Nimotop and contains 30 mg of nimodipine. The 30 mg capsules are packaged in unit dose foil pouches and supplied in cartons containing 100 capsules. The product is also available in child resistant unit dose safety pak foil pouches containing 30 capsules per carton. The capsules should be stored in the manufacturer's original foil package at a controlled room temperature of 59°F to 86°F (15°C to 30°C).

Capsules should be protected from light and freezing.

	Strength	NDC Code	Capsule Identification
Unit Dose Package of 100:	30 mg	0026-2855-48	Nimotop
Unit Dose Package of 30:	30 mg	0026-2855-70	Nimotop

Manufactured by:
Bayer Corporation
Pharmaceutical Division
400 Morgan Lane
West Haven, CT 06516

Encapsulated by:
R.P. Scherer North America
Division of R.P. Scherer Corp.
Clearwater, FL 33518

Rx Only

PZ500105 10/98 BAY e 9736 5202-7-A-U.S.-6 8767

Shown in Product Identification Guide, page 308

Otic DOMEBORO® ℞

Acetic Acid 2% in Aqueous Aluminum Acetate Otic Solution

DESCRIPTION

Otic Domeboro® solution contains 2% acetic acid as the active ingredient, in modified Burow's solution (water, aluminum acetate, and sodium acetate) with boric acid as a stabilizer. Otic Domeboro® solution is instilled in the external auditory canal. Acetic acid is an astringent and antimicrobial agent. The pH range is from 4.5 to 6.0.

Chemically, acetic acid is $C_2H_4O_2$ and has the following structural formula:

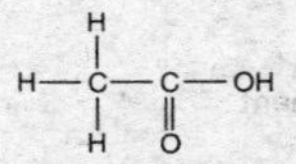

Molecular weight of acetic acid is 60.05.

CLINICAL PHARMACOLOGY

Acetic acid is antibacterial and antifungal; and is effective against microorganisms (bacteria and fungi) that infect the ears of patients with acute diffuse external otitis. In *in vitro* tests, minimum lethal-time was less than 0.25 minutes when bacteria and fungi isolated from patients with otitis externa were exposed to 2% acetic acid. Quantitative absorption of acetic acid 2% from external auditory canal is not known.

INDICATIONS AND USAGE

Otic Domeboro® solution is indicated for the treatment of superficial infections of the external auditory canal caused by organisms susceptible to the action of the antimicrobial.

CONTRAINDICATIONS

Hypersensitivity to acetic acid or any of the ingredients of this product. Perforated tympanic membrane is considered a contraindication to the use of any medication in the external ear canal.

WARNINGS

Avoid use or use with caution in patients with perforated tympanic membrane (see CONTRAINDICATIONS).
NOT FOR OPHTHALMIC USE.

PRECAUTIONS

General

Care should be taken to assure that the Otic Domeboro® solution gets into the ear canal and stays in contact with the affected area long enough for the drug to act.

Discontinue promptly if sensitization or irritation occurs.

Carcinogenesis, Mutagenesis, Impairment of Fertility: No long term studies in animals have been performed to evaluate the carcinogenic potential of Otic Domeboro® solution.

ADVERSE REACTIONS

Irritation may occur.

OVERDOSAGE

No toxic effect has been reported with overdosage of Otic Domeboro® solution.

DOSAGE AND ADMINISTRATION

Patient should lie on his side with affected ear uppermost. Instill 4 to 6 drops into the external auditory canal and maintain this position for five minutes. Repeat the procedure every 2 to 3 hours.

HOW SUPPLIED

Otic Domeboro® solution (Acetic Acid 2% in Aqueous Aluminum Acetate Otic solution) is supplied in 2 fl. oz. dropper bottle.

Store below (30°C), 86°F, avoid freezing.

Otic Domeboro® Solution is a clear colorless liquid.

	NDC
2 fl. oz.	0026-4312-02

Bayer Corporation
Pharmaceutical Division
400 Morgan Lane
West Haven, CT 06516 USA

CAUTION: Federal (USA) law prohibits dispensing without prescription.

PD500003 2/95 4787

PRECOSE® ℞

(acarbose tablets)

DESCRIPTION

PRECOSE® (acarbose tablets) is an oral alpha-glucosidase inhibitor for use in the management of type 2 diabetes mellitus. Acarbose is an oligosaccharide which is obtained from fermentation processes of a microorganism, *Actinoplanes utahensis,* and is chemically known as *O*-4,6-dideoxy-4-[[(1*S*,4*R*,5*S*,6*S*)-4,5,6-trihydroxy-3-(hydroxymethyl)-2-cyclohexen-1-yl]amino]-α-D-glucopyranosyl-(1 → 4)-*O*-α-D-glucopyranosyl-(1 → 4)-D-glucose. It is a white to off-white powder with a molecular weight of 645.6. Acarbose is soluble in water and has a pK_a of 5.1. Its empirical formula is $C_{25}H_{43}NO_{18}$ and its chemical structure is as follows:

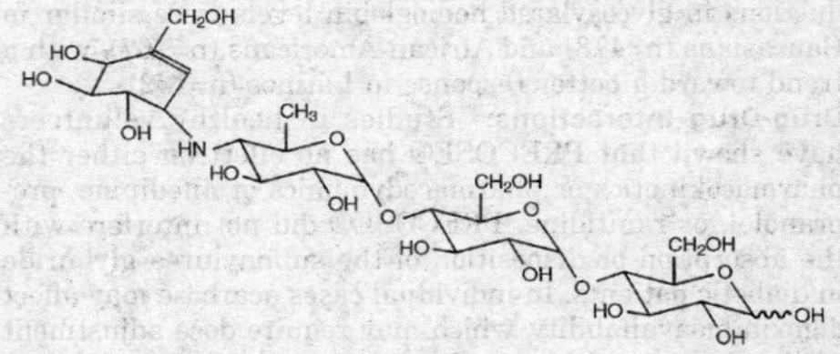

PRECOSE® is available as 25 mg, 50 mg and 100 mg tablets for oral use. The inactive ingredients are starch, microcrystalline cellulose, magnesium stearate, and colloidal silicon dioxide.

CLINICAL PHARMACOLOGY

Acarbose is a complex oligosaccharide that delays the digestion of ingested carbohydrates, thereby resulting in a smaller rise in blood glucose concentration following meals. As a consequence of plasma glucose reduction, PRECOSE® reduces levels of glycosylated hemoglobin in patients with type 2 diabetes mellitus. Systemic non-enzymatic protein glycosylation, as reflected by levels of glycosylated hemoglobin, is a function of average blood glucose concentration over time.

Mechanism of Action: In contrast to sulfonylureas, PRECOSE® does not enhance insulin secretion. The antihyperglycemic action of acarbose results from a competitive, reversible inhibition of pancreatic alpha-amylase and membrane-bound intestinal alpha-glucoside hydrolase enzymes. Pancreatic alpha-amylase hydrolyzes complex starches to oligosaccharides in the lumen of the small intestine, while the membrane-bound intestinal alpha-glucosidases hydrolyze oligosaccharides, trisaccharides, and disaccharides to glucose and other monosaccharides in the brush border of the small intestine. In diabetic patients, this enzyme inhibition results in a delayed glucose absorption and a lowering of postprandial hyperglycemia.

Because its mechanism of action is different, the effect of PRECOSE® to enhance glycemic control is additive to that of sulfonylureas, insulin or metformin when used in combination. In addition, PRECOSE® diminishes the insulinotropic and weight-increasing effects of sulfonylureas.

Acarbose has no inhibitor activity against lactase and consequently would not be expected to induce lactose intolerance.

Pharmacokinetics:

Absorption: In a study of 6 healthy men, less than 2% of an oral dose of acarbose was absorbed as active drug, while approximately 35% of total radioactivity from a ^{14}C-labeled oral dose was absorbed. An average of 51% of an oral dose was excreted in the feces as unabsorbed drug-related radioactivity within 96 hours of ingestion. Because acarbose acts locally within the gastrointestinal tract, this low systemic bioavailability of parent compound is therapeutically desired. Following oral dosing of healthy volunteers with ^{14}C-labeled acarbose, peak plasma concentrations of radioactivity were attained 14–24 hours after dosing, while peak plasma concentrations of active drug were attained at approximately 1 hour. The delayed absorption of acarbose-related radioactivity reflects the absorption of metabolites that may be formed by either intestinal bacteria or intestinal enzymatic hydrolysis.

Metabolism: Acarbose is metabolized exclusively within the gastrointestinal tract, principally by intestinal bacteria, but also by digestive enzymes. A fraction of these metabolites (approximately 34% of the dose) was absorbed and subsequently excreted in the urine. At least 13 metabolites have been separated chromatographically from urine specimens. The major metabolites have been identified as 4-methylpyrogallol derivatives (i.e., sulfate, methyl, and glucuronide conjugates). One metabolite (formed by cleavage of a glucose molecule from acarbose) also has alpha-glucosidase inhibitory activity. This metabolite, together with the parent compound, recovered from the urine, accounts for less than 2% of the total administered dose.

Excretion: The fraction of acarbose that is absorbed as intact drug is almost completely excreted by the kidneys. When acarbose was given *intravenously,* 89% of the dose was recovered in the urine as active drug within 48 hours. In contrast, less than 2% of an *oral dose* was recovered in the urine as active (i.e., parent compound and active metabolite) drug. This is consistent with the low bioavailability of the parent drug. The plasma elimination half-life of acarbose activity is approximately 2 hours in healthy volunteers. Consequently, drug accumulation does not occur with three times a day (t.i.d.) oral dosing.

Special Populations: The mean steady-state area under the curve (AUC) and maximum concentrations of acarbose were approximately 1.5 times higher in elderly compared to young volunteers; however, these differences were not statistically significant. Patients with severe renal impairment (Clcr<25 mL/min/1.73m^2) attained about 5 times higher

Continued on next page

Precose—Cont.

peak plasma concentrations of acarbose and 6 times larger AUCs than volunteers with normal renal function. No studies of acarbose pharmacokinetic parameters according to race have been performed. In U.S. controlled clinical studies of PRECOSE® in patients with type 2 diabetes mellitus, reductions in glycosylated hemoglobin levels were similar in Caucasians (n=478) and African-Americans (n=167), with a trend toward a better response in Latinos (n=132).

Drug-Drug Interactions: Studies in healthy volunteers have shown that PRECOSE® has no effect on either the pharmacokinetics or pharmacodynamics of nifedipine, propranolol, or ranitidine. PRECOSE® did not interfere with the absorption or disposition of the sulfonylurea glyburide in diabetic patients. In individual cases acarbose may affect digoxin bioavailability, which may require dose adjustment of digoxin.

The amount of metformin absorbed while taking PRECOSE was bioequivalent to the amount absorbed when taking placebo, as indicated by the plasma AUC values. However, the peak plasma level of metformin was reduced by approximately 20% when taking PRECOSE due to a slight delay in the absorption of metformin. There is little if any clinically significant interaction between PRECOSE and metformin.

CLINICAL TRIALS

Clinical Experience from Dose Finding Studies in Type 2 Diabetes Mellitus Patients on Dietary Treatment Only: Results from six controlled, fixed-dose, monotherapy studies of PRECOSE® in the treatment of type 2 diabetes mellitus, involving 769 PRECOSE®-treated patients, were combined and a weighted average of the difference from placebo in the mean change from baseline in glycosylated hemoglobin (HbA1c) was calculated for each dose level as presented below:

[See table 1 above]

Results from these six fixed-dose, monotherapy studies were also combined to derive a weighted average of the difference from placebo in mean change from baseline for one-hour postprandial plasma glucose levels as shown in the following figure:

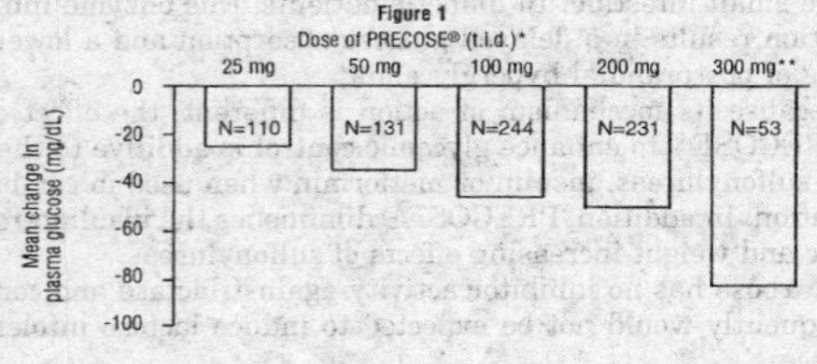

* PRECOSE® was statistically significantly different from placebo at all doses with respect to effect on one-hour postprandial plasma glucose.

**The 300 mg t.i.d. PRECOSE® regimen was superior to lower doses, but there were no statistically significant differences from 50 to 200 mg t.i.d.

Clinical Experience in Type 2 Diabetes Mellitus Patients on Monotherapy, or in Combination with Sulfonylureas, Metformin or Insulin: PRECOSE® was studied as monotherapy and as combination therapy to sulfonylurea, metformin, or insulin treatment. The treatment effects on HbA1c levels and one-hour postprandial glucose levels are summarized for four placebo-controlled, double-blind, randomized studies conducted in the United States in Tables 2 and 3 respectively. The placebo-subtracted treatment differences, which are summarized below, were statistically significant for both variables in all of these studies.

Study 1 (n=109) involved patients on background treatment with diet only. The mean effect of the addition of PRECOSE® to diet therapy was a change in HbA1c of −0.78%, and an improvement of one-hour postprandial glucose of −74.4 mg/dL.

In Study 2 (n=137), the mean effect of the addition of PRECOSE® to maximum sulfonylurea therapy was a change in HbA1c of −0.54%, and an improvement of one-hour postprandial glucose of −33.5 mg/dL.

In Study 3 (n=147), the mean effect of the addition of PRECOSE® to maximum metformin therapy was a change in HbA1c of −0.65%, and an improvement of one-hour postprandial glucose of −34.3 mg/dL.

Study 4 (n=145) demonstrated that PRECOSE® added to patients on background treatment with insulin resulted in a mean change in HbA1c of −0.69%, and an improvement of one-hour postprandial glucose of −36.0 mg/dL.

A one year study of PRECOSE® as monotherapy or in combination with sulfonylurea, metformin or insulin treatment was conducted in Canada in which 316 patients were included in the primary efficacy analysis (Figure 2). In the diet, sulfonylurea and metformin groups, the mean decrease in HbA1c produced by the addition of PRECOSE® was statistically significant at six months, and this effect was persistent at one year. In the PRECOSE®-treated patients on insulin, there was a statistically significant reduction in HbA1c at six months, and a trend for a reduction at one year.

[See table 2 above]
[See table 3 above]
[See figure 2 at top of next page]

Table 1

Mean Placebo-Subtracted Change in HbA1c in Fixed-Dose Monotherapy Studies

Dose of PRECOSE*	N	Change in HbA1c %	p-Value
25 mg t.i.d.	110	−0.44	0.0307
50 mg t.i.d.	131	−0.77	0.0001
100 mg t.i.d.	244	−0.74	0.0001
200 mg t.i.d.**	231	−0.86	0.0001
300 mg t.i.d.**	53	−1.00	0.0001

* PRECOSE® was statistically significantly different from placebo at all doses. Although there were no statistically significant differences among the mean results for doses ranging from 50 to 300 mg t.i.d., some patients may derive benefit by increasing the dosage from 50 to 100 mg t.i.d.

**Although studies utilized a maximum dose of 200 or 300 mg t.i.d., the maximum recommended dose for patients < 60 kg is 50 mg t.i.d.; the maximum recommended dose for patients > 60 kg is 100 mg t.i.d.

Table 2: Effect of Precose® on HbA1c

Study	Treatment	HbA1c(%)[a] Mean Baseline	Mean Change from baseline[b]	Treatment Difference	p-Value
1	Placebo Plus Diet	8.67	+0.33	—	—
	PRECOSE 100 mg t.i.d. Plus Diet	8.69	−0.45	−0.78	0.0001
2	Placebo Plus SFU[c]	9.56	+0.24	—	—
	PRECOSE 50–300[d] mg t.i.d. Plus SFU[c]	9.64	−0.30	−0.54	0.0096
3	Placebo Plus Metformin[e]	8.17	+0.08[g]	—	—
	PRECOSE 50–100 mg t.i.d. Plus Metformin[e]	8.46	−0.57[g]	−0.65	0.0001
4	Placebo Plus Insulin[f]	8.69	+0.11	—	—
	PRECOSE 50–100 mg t.i.d. Plus Insulin[f]	8.77	−0.58	−0.69	0.0001

[a] HbA1c Normal Range: 4–6%
[b] After four months treatment in Study 1, and six months in Studies 2, 3, and 4
[c] SFU, sulfonylurea, maximum dose
[d] Although studies utilized a maximum dose of up to 300 mg t.i.d., the maximum recommended dose for patients ≤ 60 kg is 50 mg t.i.d.; the maximum recommended dose for patients > 60 kg is 100 mg t.i.d.
[e] Metformin dosed at 2000 mg/day of 2500 mg/day
[f] Mean dose of insulin 61 U/day
[g] Results are adjusted to a common baseline of 8.33%

Table 3: Effect of Precose® on Postprandial Glucose

Study	Treatment	One-Hour Postprandial Glucose (mg/dL) Mean Baseline	Mean Change from baseline[a]	Treatment Difference	p-Value
1	Placebo Plus Diet	297.1	+31.8	—	—
	PRECOSE 100 mg t.i.d. Plus Diet	299.1	−42.6	−74.4	0.0001
2	Placebo Plus SFU[b]	308.6	+6.2	—	—
	PRECOSE 50–300[c] mg t.i.d. Plus SFU[b]	311.1	−27.3	−33.5	0.0017
3	Placebo Plus Metformin[d]	263.9	+3.3[f]	—	—
	PRECOSE 50–100 mg t.i.d. Plus Metformin[d]	283.0	−31.0[f]	−34.3	0.0001
4	Placebo Plus Insulin[e]	279.2	+8.0	—	—
	PRECOSE 50–100 mg t.i.d. Plus Insulin[e]	277.8	−28.0	−36.0	0.0178

[a] After four months treatment in Study 1, and six months in Studies 2, 3, and 4
[b] SFU, sulfonylurea, maximum dose
[c] Although studies utilized a maximum dose of up to 300 mg t.i.d., the maximum recommended dose for patients ≤ 60 kg is 50 mg t.i.d.; the maximum recommended dose for patients > 60 kg is 100 mg t.i.d.
[d] Metformin dosed at 2000 mg/day of 2500 mg/day
[e] Mean dose of insulin 61 U/day
[f] Results are adjusted to a common baseline of 273 mg/dL

INDICATIONS AND USAGE

PRECOSE®, as monotherapy, is indicated as an adjunct to diet to lower blood glucose in patients with type 2 diabetes mellitus whose hyperglycemia cannot be managed on diet alone. PRECOSE® may also be used in combination with a sulfonylurea when diet plus either PRECOSE® or a sulfonylurea do not result in adequate glycemic control. Also, PRECOSE® may be used in combination with insulin or metformin. The effect of PRECOSE® to enhance glycemic control is additive to that of sulfonylureas, insulin, or metformin when used in combination, presumably because its mechanism of action is different.

In initiating treatment for type 2 diabetes mellitus, diet should be emphasized as the primary form of treatment. Caloric restriction and weight loss are essential in the obese diabetic patient. Proper dietary management alone may be effective in controlling blood glucose and symptoms of hyperglycemia. The importance of regular physical activity when appropriate should also be stressed. If this treatment program fails to result in adequate glycemic control, the use of PRECOSE® should be considered. The use of PRECOSE® must be viewed by both the physician and patient as a treatment in addition to diet, and not as a substitute for diet or as a convenient mechanism for avoiding dietary restraint.

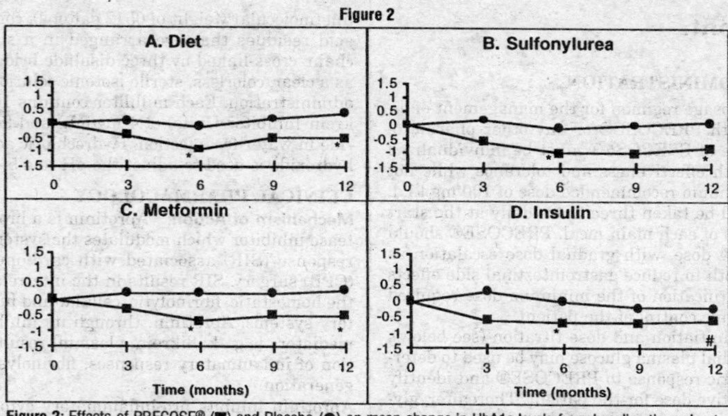

Figure 2: Effects of PRECOSE® (■) and Placebo (●) on mean change in HbA1c levels from baseline throughout a one-year study in patients with type 2 diabetes mellitus when used in combination with: (A) diet alone; (B) sulfonylurea; (C) metformin; or (D) insulin. Treatment differences at 6 and 12 months were tested: * p < 0.01; # p = 0.077.

	Strength	NDC	Tablet Identification
Bottles of 100:	25 mg	0026-2863-51	PRECOSE 25
	50 mg	0026-2861-51	PRECOSE 50
	100 mg	0026-2862-51	PRECOSE 100
Unit Dose Packages of 100:	50 mg	0026-2861-48	PRECOSE 50

CONTRAINDICATIONS

PRECOSE® is contraindicated in patients with known hypersensitivity to the drug and in patients with diabetic ketoacidosis or cirrhosis. PRECOSE® is also contraindicated in patients with inflammatory bowel disease, colonic ulceration, partial intestinal obstruction or in patients predisposed to intestinal obstruction. In addition, PRECOSE® is contraindicated in patients who have chronic intestinal diseases associated with marked disorders of digestion or absorption and in patients who have conditions that may deteriorate as a result of increased gas formation in the intestine.

PRECAUTIONS

General

Hypoglycemia: Because of its mechanism of action, PRECOSE® when administered alone should not cause hypoglycemia in the fasted or postprandial state. Sulfonylurea agents or insulin may cause hypoglycemia. Because PRECOSE® given in combination with a sulfonylurea or insulin will cause a further lowering of blood glucose, it may increase the potential for hypoglycemia. Hypoglycemia does not occur in patients receiving metformin alone under usual circumstances of use, and no increased incidence of hypoglycemia was observed in patients when PRECOSE® was added to metformin therapy. Oral glucose (dextrose), whose absorption is not inhibited by PRECOSE®, should be used instead of sucrose (cane sugar) in the treatment of mild to moderate hypoglycemia. Sucrose, whose hydrolysis to glucose and fructose is inhibited by PRECOSE®, is unsuitable for the rapid correction of hypoglycemia. Severe hypoglycemia may require the use of either intravenous glucose infusion or glucagon injection.

Elevated Serum Transaminase Levels: In long-term studies (up to 12 months, and including PRECOSE® doses up to 300 mg t.i.d.) conducted in the United States, treatment-emergent elevations of serum transaminases (AST and/or ALT) above the upper limit of normal (ULN), greater than 1.8 times the ULN, and greater than 3 times the ULN occurred in 14%, 6%, and 3%, respectively, of PRECOSE®-treated patients as compared to 7%, 2%, and 1%, respectively, of placebo-treated patients. Although these differences between treatments were statistically significant, these elevations were asymptomatic, reversible, more common in females, and, in general, were not associated with other evidence of liver dysfunction. In addition, these serum transaminase elevations appeared to be dose related. In US studies including PRECOSE® doses up to the maximum approved dose of 100 mg t.i.d., treatment-emergent elevations of AST and/or ALT at any level of severity were similar between PRECOSE®-treated patients and placebo-treated patients ($p \geq 0.496$).

In approximately 3 million patient-years of international post-marketing experience with PRECOSE®, 62 cases of serum transaminase elevations >500 IU/L (29 of which were associated with jaundice) have been reported. Forty-one of these 62 patients received treatment with 100 mg t.i.d. or greater and 33 of 45 patients for whom weight was reported weighed <60 kg. In the 59 cases where follow-up was recorded, hepatic abnormalities improved or resolved upon discontinuation of PRECOSE® in 55 and were unchanged in two. A few cases of fulminant hepatitis with fatal outcome have been reported; the relationship to acarbose is unclear.

Loss of Control of Blood Glucose: When diabetic patients are exposed to stress such as fever, trauma, infection, or surgery, a temporary loss of control of blood glucose may occur. At such times, temporary insulin therapy may be necessary.

Information for Patients: Patients should be told to take PRECOSE® orally three times a day at the start (with the first bite) of each main meal. It is important that patients continue to adhere to dietary instructions, a regular exercise program, and regular testing of urine and/or blood glucose.

PRECOSE® itself does not cause hypoglycemia even when administered to patients in the fasted state. Sulfonylurea drugs and insulin, however, can lower blood sugar levels enough to cause symptoms or sometimes life-threatening hypoglycemia. Because PRECOSE® given in combination with a sulfonylurea or insulin will cause a further lowering of blood sugar, it may increase the hypoglycemic potential of these agents. Hypoglycemia does not occur in patients receiving metformin alone under usual circumstances of use, and no increased incidence of hypoglycemia was observed in patients when PRECOSE® was added to metformin therapy. The risk of hypoglycemia, its symptoms and treatment, and conditions that predispose to its development should be well understood by patients and responsible family members. Because PRECOSE® prevents the breakdown of table sugar, patients should have a readily available source of glucose (dextrose, D-glucose) to treat symptoms of low blood sugar when taking PRECOSE® in combination with a sulfonylurea or insulin.

If side effects occur with PRECOSE®, they usually develop during the first few weeks of therapy. They are most commonly mild-to-moderate gastrointestinal effects, such as flatulence, diarrhea, or abdominal discomfort, and generally diminish in frequency and intensity with time.

Laboratory Tests: Therapeutic response to PRECOSE® should be monitored by periodic blood glucose tests. Measurement of glycosylated hemoglobin levels is recommended for the monitoring of long-term glycemic control.

PRECOSE®, particularly at doses in excess of 50 mg t.i.d., may give rise to elevations of serum transaminases and, in rare instances, hyperbilirubinemia. It is recommended that serum transaminase levels be checked every 3 months during the first year of treatment with PRECOSE® and periodically thereafter. If elevated transaminases are observed, a reduction in dosage or withdrawal of therapy may be indicated, particularly if the elevations persist.

Renal Impairment: Plasma concentrations of PRECOSE® in renally impaired volunteers were proportionally increased relative to the degree of renal dysfunction. Long-term clinical trials in diabetic patients with significant renal dysfunction (serum creatinine >2.0 mg/dL) have not been conducted. Therefore, treatment of these patients with PRECOSE® is not recommended.

Drug Interactions: Certain drugs tend to produce hyperglycemia and may lead to loss of blood glucose control. These drugs include the thiazides and other diuretics, corticosteroids, phenothiazines, thyroid products, estrogens, oral contraceptives, phenytoin, nicotinic acid, sympathomimetics, calcium channel-blocking drugs, and isoniazid. When such drugs are administered to a patient receiving PRECOSE®, the patient should be closely observed for loss of blood glucose control. When such drugs are withdrawn from patients receiving PRECOSE® in combination with sulfonylureas or insulin, patients should be observed closely for any evidence of hypoglycemia.

Intestinal adsorbents (e.g., charcoal) and digestive enzyme preparations containing carbohydrate-splitting enzymes (e.g., amylase, pancreatin) may reduce the effect of PRECOSE® and should not be taken concomitantly.

Carcinogenesis, Mutagenesis, and Impairment of Fertility: Eight carcinogenicity studies were conducted with acarbose. Six studies were performed in rats (two strains, Sprague-Dawley and Wistar) and two studies were performed in hamsters.

In the first rat study, Sprague-Dawley rats received acarbose in feed at high doses (up to approximately 500 mg/kg body weight) for 104 weeks. Acarbose treatment resulted in a significant increase in the incidence of renal tumors (adenomas and adenocarcinomas) and benign Leydig cell tumors. This study was repeated with a similar outcome. Further studies were performed to separate direct carcinogenic effects of acarbose from indirect effects resulting from the carbohydrate malnutrition induced by the large doses of acarbose employed in the studies. In one study using Sprague-Dawley rats, acarbose was mixed with feed but carbohydrate deprivation was prevented by the addition of glucose to the diet. In a 26-month study of Sprague-Dawley rats, acarbose was administered by daily postprandial gavage so as to avoid the pharmacologic effects of the drug. In both of these studies, the increased incidence of renal tumors found in the original studies did not occur. Acarbose was also given in food and by postprandial gavage in two separate studies in Wistar rats. No increased incidence of renal tumors was found in either of these Wistar rat studies. In two feeding studies of hamsters, with and without glucose supplementation, there was also no evidence of carcinogenicity. Acarbose did not induce any DNA damage *in vitro* in the CHO chromosomal aberration assay, bacterial mutagenesis (Ames) assay, or a DNA binding assay. *In vivo*, no DNA damage was detected in the dominant lethal test in male mice, or the mouse micronucleus test.

Fertility studies conducted in rats after oral administration produced no untoward effect on fertility or on the overall capability to reproduce.

Pregnancy:

Teratogenic Effects: Pregnancy Category B. The safety of PRECOSE® in pregnant women has not been established. Reproduction studies have been performed in rats at doses up to 480 mg/kg (corresponding to 9 times the exposure in humans, based on drug blood levels) and have revealed no evidence of impaired fertility or harm to the fetus due to acarbose. In rabbits, reduced maternal body weight gain, probably the result of the pharmacodynamic activity of high doses of acarbose in the intestines, may have been responsible for a slight increase in the number of embryonic losses. However, rabbits given 160 mg/kg acarbose (corresponding to 10 times the dose in man, based on body surface area) showed no evidence of embryotoxicity and there was no evidence of teratogenicity at a dose 32 times the dose in man (based on body surface area). There are, however, no adequate and well-controlled studies of PRECOSE® in pregnant women. Because animal reproduction studies are not always predictive of the human response, this drug should be used during pregnancy only if clearly needed. Because current information strongly suggests that abnormal blood glucose levels during pregnancy are associated with a higher incidence of congenital anomalies as well as increased neonatal morbidity and mortality, most experts recommend that insulin be used during pregnancy to maintain blood glucose levels as close to normal as possible.

Nursing Mothers: A small amount of radioactivity has been found in the milk of lactating rats after administration of radiolabeled acarbose. It is not known whether this drug is excreted in human milk. Because many drugs are excreted in human milk, PRECOSE® should not be administered to a nursing woman.

Pediatric Use: Safety and effectiveness of PRECOSE® in pediatric patients have not been established.

Geriatric Use: Of the total number of subjects in clinical studies of PRECOSE® in the United States, 27 percent were 65 and over, while 4 percent were 75 and over. No overall differences in safety and effectiveness were observed between these subjects and younger subjects. The mean steady-state area under the curve (AUC) and maximum concentrations of acarbose were approximately 1.5 times higher in elderly compared to young volunteers; however, these differences were not statistically significant.

ADVERSE REACTIONS

Digestive Tract: Gastrointestinal symptoms are the most common reactions to PRECOSE®. In U.S. placebo-controlled trials, the incidences of abdominal pain, diarrhea, and flatulence were 19%, 31%, and 74% respectively in 1255 patients treated with PRECOSE® 50–300 mg t.i.d., whereas the corresponding incidences were 9%, 12%, and 29% in 999 placebo-treated patients. In a one-year safety study, during which patients kept diaries of gastrointestinal symptoms, abdominal pain and diarrhea tended to return to pretreatment levels over time, and the frequency and intensity of flatulence tended to abate with time. The increased gastrointestinal tract symptoms in patients treated with PRECOSE® are a manifestation of the mechanism of action of PRECOSE® and are related to the presence of undigested carbohydrate in the lower GI tract. Rarely, these gastrointestinal events may be severe and might be confused with paralytic ileus.

Elevated Serum Transaminase Levels: See PRECAUTIONS

Other Abnormal Laboratory Findings: Small reductions in hematocrit occurred more often in PRECOSE®-treated patients than in placebo-treated patients but were not associated with reductions in hemoglobin. Low serum calcium and low plasma vitamin B_6 levels were associated with PRECOSE® therapy but are thought to be either spurious or of no clinical significance.

Hypersensitive Skin Reactions: Rarely, hypersensitive skin reactions such as rash may occur.

Edema: In rare instances edema has been reported.

OVERDOSAGE

Unlike sulfonylureas or insulin, an overdose of PRECOSE® will not result in hypoglycemia. An overdose may result in transient increases in flatulence, diarrhea, and abdominal discomfort which shortly subside.

Continued on next page

Precose—Cont.

DOSAGE AND ADMINISTRATION

There is no fixed dosage regimen for the management of diabetes mellitus with PRECOSE® or any other pharmacologic agent. Dosage of PRECOSE® must be individualized on the basis of both effectiveness and tolerance while not exceeding the maximum recommended dose of 100 mg t.i.d. PRECOSE® should be taken three times daily at the start (with the first bite) of each main meal. PRECOSE® should be started at a low dose, with gradual dose escalation as described below, both to reduce gastrointestinal side effects and to permit identification of the minimum dose required for adequate glycemic control of the patient.

During treatment initiation and dose titration (see below), one-hour postprandial plasma glucose may be used to determine the therapeutic response to PRECOSE® and identify the minimum effective dose for the patient. Thereafter, glycosylated hemoglobin should be measured at intervals of approximately three months. The therapeutic goal should be to decrease both postprandial plasma glucose and glycosylated hemoglobin levels to normal or near normal by using the lowest effective dose of PRECOSE®, either as monotherapy or in combination with sulfonylureas, insulin or metformin.

Initial Dosage: The recommended starting dosage of PRECOSE® is 25 mg given orally three times daily at the start (with the first bite) of each main meal. However, some patients may benefit from more gradual dose titration to minimize gastrointestinal side effects. This may be achieved by initiating treatment at 25 mg once per day and subsequently increasing the frequency of administration to achieve 25 mg t.i.d.

Maintenance Dosage: Once a 25 mg t.i.d. dosage regimen is reached, dosage of PRECOSE® should be adjusted at 4–8 week intervals based on one-hour postprandial glucose or glycosylated hemoglobin levels, and on tolerance. The dosage can be increased from 25 mg t.i.d. to 50 mg t.i.d. Some patients may benefit from further increasing the dosage to 100 mg t.i.d. The maintenance dose ranges from 50 mg t.i.d. to 100 mg t.i.d. However, since patients with low body weight may be at increased risk for elevated serum transaminases, only patients with body weight > 60 kg should be considered for dose titration above 50 mg t.i.d. (see PRECAUTIONS). If no further reduction in postprandial glucose or glycosylated hemoglobin levels is observed with titration to 100 mg t.i.d., consideration should be given to lowering the dose. Once an effective and tolerated dosage is established, it should be maintained.

Maximum Dosage: The maximum recommended dose for patients ≤ 60 kg is 50 mg t.i.d. The maximum recommended dose for patients > 60 kg is 100 mg t.i.d.

Patients Receiving Sulfonylureas or Insulin: Sulfonylurea agents or insulin may cause hypoglycemia. PRECOSE® given in combination with a sulfonylurea or insulin will cause a further lowering of blood glucose and may increase the potential for hypoglycemia. If hypoglycemia occurs, appropriate adjustments in the dosage of these agents should be made.

HOW SUPPLIED

PRECOSE® is available as 25 mg, 50 mg or 100 mg round, unscored tablets. Each tablet strength is white to yellow-tinged in color. The 25 mg tablet is coded with the word "PRECOSE" on one side and "25" on the other side. The 50 mg tablet is coded with the word "PRECOSE" and "50" on the same side. The 100 mg tablet is coded with the word "PRECOSE" and "100" on the same side. PRECOSE is available in bottles of 100 and 50 mg strength in unit dose packages of 100.

[See second table at top of previous page]

Do not store above 25°C (77°F). Protect from moisture. For bottles, keep container tightly closed.

Bayer Corporation
Pharmaceutical Division
400 Morgan Lane
West Haven, CT 06516 USA

℞ Only

PZ500146 10/99 Bay g 5421
PRECOSE®/5202/0/8/USA-9

Shown in Product Identification Guide, page 308

TRASYLOL® ℞
(aprotinin injection)

Anaphylactic or anaphylactoid reactions are possible when Trasylol® is administered. Hypersensitivity reactions are rare in patients with no prior exposure to aprotinin. The risk of anaphylaxis is increased in patients who are re-exposed to aprotinin-containing products. The benefit of Trasylol® to patients undergoing primary CABG surgery should be weighed against the risk of anaphylaxis should a second exposure to aprotinin be required. (See WARNINGS and PRECAUTIONS).

DESCRIPTION

Trasylol® (aprotinin injection), $C_{284}H_{432}N_{84}O_{79}S_7$, is a natural proteinase inhibitor obtained from bovine lung. Aprotinin (molecular weight of 6512 daltons), consists of 58 amino acid residues that are arranged in a single polypeptide chain, cross-linked by three disulfide bridges. It is supplied as a clear, colorless, sterile isotonic solution for intravenous administration. Each milliliter contains 10,000 KIU (Kallikrein Inhibitor Units) (1.4 mg/mL) and 9 mg sodium chloride in water for injection. Hydrochloric acid and/or sodium hydroxide is used to adjust the pH to 4.5–6.5.

CLINICAL PHARMACOLOGY

Mechanism of Action: Aprotinin is a broad spectrum protease inhibitor which modulates the systemic inflammatory response (SIR) associated with cardiopulmonary bypass (CPB) surgery. SIR results in the interrelated activation of the hemostatic, fibrinolytic, cellular and humoral inflammatory systems. Aprotinin, through its inhibition of multiple mediators [e.g., kallikrein, plasmin] results in the attenuation of inflammatory responses, fibrinolysis, and thrombin generation.

Aprotinin inhibits pro-inflammatory cytokine release and maintains glycoprotein homeostasis. In platelets, aprotinin reduces glycoprotein loss (e.g., GpIb, GpIIb/IIIa), while in granulocytes it prevents the expression of pro-inflammatory adhesive glycoproteins (e.g., CD11b).

The effects of aprotinin use in CPB involves a reduction in inflammatory response which translates into a decreased need for allogeneic blood transfusions, reduced bleeding, and decreased mediastinal re-exploration for bleeding.

Pharmacokinetics: The studies comparing the pharmacokinetics of aprotinin in healthy volunteers, cardiac patients undergoing surgery with cardiopulmonary bypass, and women undergoing hysterectomy suggest linear pharmacokinetics over the dose range of 50,000 KIU to 2 million KIU. After intravenous (IV) injection, rapid distribution of aprotinin occurs into the total extracellular space, leading to a rapid initial decrease in plasma aprotinin concentration. Following this distribution phase, a plasma half-life of about 150 minutes is observed. At later time points, (i.e., beyond 5 hours after dosing) there is a terminal elimination phase with a half-life of about 10 hours.

Average steady state intraoperative plasma concentrations were 137 KIU/mL (n=10) after administration of the following dosage regimen: 1 million KIU IV loading dose, 1 million KIU into the pump prime volume, 250,000 KIU per hour of operation as continuous intravenous infusion (Regimen B). Average steady state intraoperative plasma concentrations were 250 KIU/mL in patients (n=20) treated with aprotinin during cardiac surgery by administration of Regimen A (exactly double Regimen B): 2 million KIU IV loading dose, 2 million KIU into the pump prime volume, 500,000 KIU per hour of operation as continuous intravenous infusion.

Following a single IV dose of radiolabelled aprotinin, approximately 25–40% of the radioactivity is excreted in the urine over 48 hours. After a 30 minute infusion of 1 million KIU, about 2% is excreted as unchanged drug. After a larger dose of 2 million KIU infused over 30 minutes, urinary excretion of unchanged aprotinin accounts for approximately 9% of the dose. Animal studies have shown that aprotinin is accumulated primarily in the kidney. Aprotinin, after being filtered by the glomeruli, is actively reabsorbed by the proximal tubules in which it is stored in phagolysosomes. Aprotinin is slowly degraded by lysosomal enzymes. The physiological renal handling of aprotinin is similar to that of other small proteins, e.g., insulin.

CLINICAL TRIALS

Repeat Coronary Artery Bypass Graft Patients:

Four placebo-controlled, double-blind studies of Trasylol® were conducted in the United States; of 540 randomized patients undergoing repeat coronary artery bypass graft (CABG) surgery, 480 were valid for efficacy analysis. The following treatment regimens were used in the studies: Trasylol® Regimen A (2 million KIU IV loading dose, 2 million KIU into the pump prime volume, and 500,000 KIU per hour of surgery as a continuous intravenous infusion); Trasylol® Regimen B (1 million KIU IV loading dose, 1 million KIU into the pump prime volume, and 250,000 KIU per hour of surgery as a continuous intravenous infusion); a pump prime regimen (2 million KIU into the pump prime volume only); and a placebo regimen (normal saline). All patients valid for efficacy in the above studies were pooled by treatment regimen for analyses of efficacy.

In this pooled analysis, fewer patients receiving Trasylol®, either Regimen A or Regimen B, required any donor blood compared to the pump prime only or placebo regimens. The number of units of donor blood required by patients, the volume (milliliters) of donor blood transfused, the number of units of donor blood products transfused, the thoracic drainage rate, and the total thoracic drainage volumes were also reduced in patients receiving Trasylol® as compared to placebo.

[See table below]

Primary Coronary Artery Bypass Graft Patients:

Four placebo-controlled, double-blind studies of Trasylol® were conducted in the United States; of 1745 randomized patients undergoing primary CABG surgery, 1599 were valid for efficacy analysis. The dosage regimens used in these studies were identical to those used in the repeat CABG studies described above (Regimens A, B, pump prime, and placebo). All patients valid for efficacy were pooled by treatment regimen.

In this pooled analysis, fewer patients receiving Trasylol® Regimens A, B, and pump prime required any donor blood in comparison to the placebo regimen. The number of units of donor blood required by patients, the volume of donor blood transfused, the number of units of donor blood products transfused, the thoracic drainage rate, and total thoracic drainage volumes were also reduced in patients receiving Trasylol® as compared to placebo.

[See first table at top of next page]

Additional subgroup analyses showed no diminution in benefit with increasing age. Male and female patients benefited from Trasylol® with a reduction in the average number of units of donor blood transfused. Although male patients did better than female patients in terms of the percentage of patients who required any donor blood transfusions, the number of female patients studied was small.

A double-blind, randomized, Canadian study compared Trasylol® Regimen A (n=28) and placebo (n=23) in primary cardiac surgery patients (mainly CABG) requiring cardiopulmonary bypass who were treated with aspirin within 48 hours of surgery. The mean total blood loss (1209.7 mL vs. 2532.3 mL) and the mean number of units of packed red blood cells transfused (1.6 units vs 4.3 units) were significantly less ($p<0.008$) in the Trasylol® group compared to the placebo group.

In a U.S. randomized study of Trasylol® Regimen A and Regimen B versus the placebo regimen in 212 patients un-

Efficacy Variables: Repeat CABG Patients
Mean (S.D.) or % of Patients

VARIABLE	PLACEBO REGIMEN N=156	Trasylol® PUMP PRIME REGIMEN† N=68	Trasylol® REGIMEN B** N=113	Trasylol® REGIMEN A** N=143
% OF REPEAT CABG PATIENTS WHO REQUIRED DONOR BLOOD	76.3%	72.1%	48.7%	46.9%
UNITS OF DONOR BLOOD TRANSFUSED	3.7 (4.4)	2.5 (2.4)	2.2 (5.0)*	1.6 (2.9)*
mL OF DONOR BLOOD TRANSFUSED	1132 (1443)	756 (807)	723 (1779)*	515 (999)*
PLATELETS TRANSFUSED (Donor Units)	5.0 (10.0)	2.1 (4.6)*	1.3 (4.6)*	0.9 (4.3)*
CRYOPRECIPITATE TRANSFUSED (Donor Units)	0.9 (3.5)	0.0 (0.0)*	0.5 (4.0)	0.1 (0.8)*
FRESH FROZEN PLASMA TRANSFUSED (Donor Units)	1.3 (2.5)	0.5 (1.4)*	0.3 (1.1)*	0.2 (0.9)*
THORACIC DRAINAGE RATE (mL/hr)	89 (77)	73 (69)	66 (244)	40 (36)*
TOTAL THORACIC DRAINAGE VOLUME (mL)[a]	1659 (1226)	1561 (1370)	1103 (2001)*	960 (849)*
REOPERATION FOR DIFFUSE BLEEDING	1.9%	2.9%	0%	0%

† The pump prime regimen was evaluated in only one study in patients undergoing repeat CABG surgery. Note: The pump prime only regimen is not an approved dosage regimen.

* Significantly different from placebo, $p<0.05$
(Transfusion variables analyzed via ANOVA on ranks)

** Differences between Regimen A (high dose) and Regimen B (low dose) in efficacy and safety are not statistically significant.

[a] Excludes patients who required reoperation

dergoing primary aortic and/or mitral valve replacement or repair, no benefit was found for Trasylol® in terms of the need for transfusion or the number of units of blood required.

INDICATIONS AND USAGE

Trasylol is indicated for prophylactic use to reduce perioperative blood loss and the need for blood transfusion in patients undergoing cardiopulmonary bypass in the course of coronary artery bypass graft surgery.

CONTRAINDICATIONS

Hypersensitivity to aprotinin.

WARNINGS

Anaphylactic or anaphylactoid reactions are possible when Trasylol® is administered. Hypersensitivity reactions are rare in patients with no prior exposure to aprotinin. Hypersensitivity reactions can range from skin eruptions, itching, dyspnea, nausea and tachycardia to fatal anaphylactic shock with circulatory failure. If a hypersensitivity reaction occurs during injection or infusion of Trasylol®, administration should be stopped immediately and emergency treatment should be initiated. It should be noted that severe (fatal) hypersensitivity/anaphylactic reactions can also occur in connection with application of the test dose. Even when a second exposure to aprotinin has been tolerated without symptoms, a subsequent administration may result in severe hypersensitivity/anaphylactic reactions.

Re-exposure to aprotinin: In a retrospective review of 387 European patient records with documented re-exposure to Trasylol®, the incidence of hypersensitivity/anaphylactic reactions was 2.7%. Two patients who experienced hypersensitivity/anaphylactic reactions subsequently died, 24 hours and 5 days after surgery, respectively. The relationship of these 2 deaths to Trasylol® is unclear. This retrospective review also showed that the incidence of a hypersensitivity or anaphylactic reaction following re-exposure is increased when the re-exposure occurs within 6 months of the initial administration (5.0% for re-exposure within 6 months and 0.9% for re-exposure greater than 6 months). Other smaller studies have shown that in case of re-exposure, the incidence of hypersensitivity/anaphylactic reactions may reach the five percent level.

Before initiating treatment with Trasylol® in a patient with a history of prior exposure to aprotinin or products containing aprotinin, the recommendations below should be followed to manage a potential hypersensitivity or anaphylactic reaction: 1) Have standard emergency treatments for hypersensitivity or anaphylactic reactions readily available in the operating room (e.g., epinephrine, corticosteroids). 2) Administration of the test dose and loading dose should be done only when the conditions for rapid cannulation (if necessary) are present. 3) Delay the addition of Trasylol® into the pump prime solution until after the loading dose has been safely administered. Additionally, administration of H1 and H2 blockers 15 minutes before the test dose may be considered.

PRECAUTIONS

General: _Test Dose:_ All patients treated with Trasylol® should first receive a test dose to assess the potential for allergic reactions. The test dose of 1 mL Trasylol® should be administered intravenously at least 10 minutes prior to the loading dose. However, even after the uneventful administration of the initial 1 mL test-dose, the therapeutic dose may cause an anaphylactic reaction. If this happens the infusion of aprotinin should immediately be stopped, and standard emergency treatment for anaphylaxis be applied. It should be noted that hypersensitivity/anaphylactic reactions can also occur in connection with application of the test-dose. (see WARNINGS)

Allergic Reactions: Patients with a history of allergic reactions to drugs or other agents may be at greater risk of developing a hypersensitivity or anaphylactic reaction upon exposure to Trasylol®. (see WARNINGS)

Loading Dose: The loading dose of Trasylol® should be given intravenously to patients in the supine position over a 20–30 minute period. Rapid intravenous administration of Trasylol® can cause a transient fall in blood pressure. (see DOSAGE AND ADMINISTRATION).

Use of Trasylol® in patients undergoing deep hypothermic circulatory arrest: Two U.S. case control studies have reported contradictory results in patients receiving Trasylol® while undergoing deep hypothermic circulatory arrest in connection with surgery of the aortic arch.

The first study showed an increase in both renal failure and mortality compared to age-matched historical controls. Similar results were not observed, however, in a second case control study. The strength of this association is uncertain because there are no data from randomized studies to confirm or refute these findings.

Drug Interactions: Trasylol® is known to have antifibrinolytic activity and, therefore, may inhibit the effects of fibrinolytic agents.

In study of nine patients with untreated hypertension, Trasylol® infused intravenously in a dose of 2 million KIU over two hours blocked the acute hypotensive effect of 100mg of captopril.

Trasylol®, in the presence of heparin, has been found to prolong the activated clotting time (ACT) as measured by a celite surface activation method. The kaolin activated clotting time appears to be much less affected. However, Trasylol® should not be viewed as a heparin sparing agent. (see Laboratory Monitoring of Anticoagulation During Cardiopulmonary Bypass).

Efficacy Variables: Primary CABG Patients
Mean (S.D.) or % of Patients

VARIABLE	PLACEBO REGIMEN N=624	Trasylol® PUMP PRIME REGIMEN† N=159	Trasylol® REGIMEN B** N=175	Trasylol® REGIMEN A** N=641
% OF PRIMARY CABG PATIENTS WHO REQUIRED DONOR BLOOD	53.5%	32.7%*	37.1%*	36.8%*
UNITS OF DONOR BLOOD TRANSFUSED	1.7 (2.4)	0.9 (1.6)*	1.0 (1.6)*	0.9 (1.4)*
mL OF DONOR BLOOD TRANSFUSED	584 (840)	286 (518)*	313 (505)*	295 (503)*
PLATELETS TRANSFUSED (Donor Units)	1.3 (3.7)	0.5 (2.4)*	0.3 (1.6)*	0.3 (1.5)*
CRYOPRECIPITATE TRANSFUSED (Donor Units)	0.5 (2.2)	0.0 (0.0)*	0.1 (0.8)*	0.0 (0.0)*
FRESH FROZEN PLASMA TRANSFUSED (Donor Units)	0.6 (1.7)	0.2 (1.7)*	0.2 (0.8)*	0.2 (0.9)*
THORACIC DRAINAGE RATE (mL/hr)	87 (67)	51 (36)*	45 (31)*	39 (32)*
TOTAL THORACIC DRAINAGE VOLUME (mL)	1232 (711)	852 (653)*	792 (465)*	705 (493)*
REOPERATION FOR DIFFUSE BLEEDING	1.4%	0.6%	0%	0%*

† The pump prime regimen was evaluated in only one study in patients undergoing primary CABG surgery. Note: The pump prime only regimen is not an approved dosage regimen.

* Significantly different from placebo, $p<0.05$
(Transfusion variables analyzed via ANOVA on ranks)

** Differences between Regimen A (high dose) and Regimen B (low dose) in efficacy and safety are not statistically significant.

INCIDENCE RATES OF ADVERSE EVENTS (> = 2%) BY BODY SYSTEM AND TREATMENT FOR ALL PATIENTS FROM US PLACEBO-CONTROLLED CLINICAL TRIALS

Adverse Event	Aprotinin (n = 2002) values in %	Placebo (n = 1084) values in %
Any Event	76	77
Body as a Whole		
Fever	15	14
Infection	6	7
Chest Pain	2	2
Asthenia	2	2
Cardiovascular		
Atrial Fibrillation	21	23
Hypotension	8	10
Myocardial Infarct	6	6
Atrial Flutter	6	5
Ventricular Extrasystoles	6	4
Tachycardia	6	7
Ventricular Tachycardia	5	4
Heart Failure	5	4
Pericarditis	5	5
Peripheral Edema	5	5
Hypertension	4	5
Arrhythmia	4	3
Supraventricular Tachycardia	4	3
Atrial Arrhythmia	3	3
Digestive		
Nausea	11	9
Constipation	4	5
Vomiting	3	4
Diarrhea	3	2
Liver Function Tests Abnormal	3	2
Hemic and Lymphatic		
Anemia	2	8
Metabolic & Nutritional		
Creatine Phosphokinase Increased	2	1
Musculoskeletal		
Any Event	2	3
Nervous		
Confusion	4	4
Insomnia	3	4
Respiratory		
Lung Disorder	8	8
Pleural Effusion	7	9
Atelectasis	5	6
Dyspnea	4	4
Pneumothorax	4	4
Asthma	2	3
Hypoxia	2	1
Skin and Appendages		
Rash	2	2
Urogenital		
Kidney Function Abnormal	3	2
Urinary Retention	3	3
Urinary Tract Infection	2	2

Carcinogenesis, Mutagenesis, Impairment of Fertility: Long-term animal studies to evaluate the carcinogenic potential of Trasylol® or studies to determine the effect of Trasylol® on fertility have not been performed.

Results of microbial *in vitro* tests using *Salmonella typhimurium* and *Bacillus subtilis* indicate that Trasylol® is not a mutagen.

Pregnancy: Teratogenic Effects: Pregnancy Category B: Reproduction studies have been performed in rats at intravenous doses up to 200,000 KIU/kg/day for 11 days, and in rabbits at intravenous doses up to 100,000 KIU/kg/day for 13 days, 2.4 and 1.2 times the human dose on a mg/kg basis and 0.37 and 0.36 times the human mg/m^2 dose. They have revealed no evidence of impaired fertility or harm to the fetus due to Trasylol®. There are, however, no adequate and well-controlled studies in pregnant women. Because animal reproduction studies are not always predictive of human response, this drug should be used during pregnancy only if clearly needed.

Nursing Mother: Not applicable.

Pediatric Use: Safety and effectiveness in pediatric patient(s) have not been established.

Geriatric Use: Of the total 3083 subjects in clinical studies of Trasylol®, 1100 (35.7 percent) were 65 and over, while 297 (9.6 percent) were 75 and over. Of patients 65 years and older, 479 (43.5 percent) received Regimen A and 237 (21.5 percent) received Regimen B. No overall differences in safety or effectiveness were observed between these subjects and younger subjects for either dose regimen, and other reported clinical experience has not identified differences in responses between the elderly and younger patients.

Laboratory Monitoring of Anticoagulation during Cardiopulmonary Bypass: Trasylol® prolongs whole blood clotting times by a different mechanism than heparin. In the presence of aprotinin, prolongation is dependent on the type of whole blood clotting test employed. If an activated clotting time (ACT) is used to determine the effectiveness of heparin anticoagulation, the prolongation of the ACT by aprotinin may lead to an overestimation of the degree of anticoagulation, thereby leading to inadequate anticoagulation. During extended extracorporeal circulation, patients may require additional heparin, even in the presence of ACT levels that appear adequate.

In patients undergoing CPB with Trasylol® therapy, one of the following methods may be employed to maintain adequate anticoagulation:

1) ACT - An ACT is not a standardized coagulation test, and different formulations of the assay are affected differently by the presence of aprotinin. The test is further influenced by variable dilution effects and the temperature experienced during cardiopulmonary bypass. It has been observed that Kaolin-based ACTs are not increased to the same degree by aprotinin as are diatomaceous earth-based (celite) ACTs. While protocols vary, a minimal celite ACT of 750 seconds or kaolin-ACT of 480 seconds, independent of the effects of hemodilution and hypothermia, is recommended in the presence of aprotinin. Consult the manufacturer of the ACT test regarding the interpretation of the assay in the presence of Trasylol®.

2) Fixed Heparin Dosing - A standard loading dose of heparin, administered prior to cannulation of the heart, plus the quantity of heparin added to the prime volume of the CPB circuit, should total at least 350 IU/kg. Additional heparin should be administered in a fixed-dose regimen based on patient weight and duration of CPB.

Continued on next page

Trasylol—Cont.

3) Heparin Titration - Protamine titration, a method that is not affected by aprotinin, can be used to measure heparin levels. A heparin dose response, assessed by protamine titration, should be performed prior to administration of aprotinin to determine the heparin loading dose. Additional heparin should be administered on the basis of heparin levels measured by protamine titration. Heparin levels during bypass should not be allowed to drop below 2.7 U/mL (2.0 mg/kg) or below the level indicated by heparin dose response testing performed prior to administration of aprotinin.

Protamine Administration - In patients treated with Trasylol®, the amount of protamine administered to reverse heparin activity should be based on the actual amount of heparin administered, and not on the ACT values.

ADVERSE REACTIONS

Studies of patients undergoing CABG surgery, either primary or repeat, indicate that Trasylol® is generally well tolerated. The adverse events reported are frequent sequelae of cardiac surgery and are not necessarily attributable to Trasylol® therapy. Adverse events reported, up to the time of hospital discharge, from patients in US placebo-controlled trials are listed in the following table. The table lists only those events that were reported in 2% or more of the Trasylol® treated patients without regard to causal relationship.

[See second table on previous page]

In comparison to the placebo group, no increase in mortality in patients treated with Trasylol® was observed. Additional events of particular interest from controlled US trials with an incidence of less than 2%, are listed below:

EVENT	Percentage of patients treated with Trasylol N = 2002	Percentage of patients treated with Placebo N = 1084
Thrombosis	1.0	0.6
Shock	0.7	0.4
Cerebrovascular Accident	0.7	2.1
Thrombophlebitis	0.2	0.5
Deep Thrombophlebitis	0.7	1.0
Lung Edema	1.3	1.5
Pulmonary Embolus	0.3	0.6
Kidney Failure	1.0	0.6
Acute Kidney Failure	0.5	0.6
Kidney Tubular Necrosis	0.8	0.4

Listed below are additional events, from controlled US trials with an incidence between 1 and 2%, and also from uncontrolled, compassionate use trials and spontaneous post-marketing reports. Estimates of frequency cannot be made for spontaneous post-marketing reports *(italicized)*.

Body as a Whole: Sepsis, death, multi-system organ failure, immune system disorder, *hemoperitoneum.*

Cardiovascular: Ventricular fibrillation, heart arrest, bradycardia, congestive heart failure, hemorrhage, bundle branch block, myocardial ischemia, ventricular tachycardia, heart block, pericardial effusion, ventricular arrhythmia, shock, pulmonary hypertension.

Digestive: Dyspepsia, gastrointestinal hemorrhage, jaundice, hepatic failure.

Hematologic and Lymphatic: Although thrombosis was not reported more frequently in aprotinin versus placebo-treated patients in controlled trials, it has been reported in uncontrolled trials, compassionate use trials, and spontaneous post-marketing reporting. These reports of thrombosis encompass the following terms: thrombosis, occlusion, arterial thrombosis, *pulmonary thrombosis*, coronary occlusion, embolus, pulmonary embolus, thrombophlebitis, deep thrombophlebitis, cerebrovascular accident, cerebral embolism. Other hematologic events reported include leukocytosis, thrombocytopenia, coagulation disorder (which includes disseminated intravascular coagulation), decreased prothrombin.

Metabolic and Nutritional: Hyperglycemia, hypokalemia, hypervolemia, acidosis.

Musculoskeletal: Arthralgia.

Nervous: Agitation, dizziness, anxiety, convulsion.

Respiratory: Pneumonia, apnea, increased cough, lung edema.

Skin: *Skin discoloration.*

Urogenital: Oliguria, kidney failure, acute kidney failure, kidney tubular necrosis.

Myocardial Infarction: In the pooled analysis of all patients undergoing CABG surgery, there was no significant difference in the incidence of investigator-reported myocardial infarction (MI) in Trasylol® treated patients as compared to placebo treated patients. However, because no uniform criteria for the diagnosis of myocardial infarction were utilized by investigators, this issue was addressed prospectively in three later studies (two studies evaluated Regimen A, Regimen B and Pump Prime Regimen; one study evaluated only Regimen A), in which data were analyzed by a blinded consultant employing an algorithm for possible, probable or definite MI. Utilizing this method, the incidence of definite myocardial infarction was 5.9% in the aprotinin-treated patients versus 4.7% in the placebo treated patients. This difference in the incidence rates was not statistically significant. Data from these three studies are summarized below.

Incidence of Graft Closure, Myocardial Infarction and Death by Treatment Group

	Overall Closure Rates*		Incidence of MI**	Incidence of Death***
	All Centers n = 703 %	U.S. Centers n = 381 %	All Centers n = 831 %	All Centers n = 870 %
Trasylol®	15.4	9.4	2.9	1.4
Placebo	10.9	9.5	3.8	1.6
Cl for the Difference (%) (Drug - Placebo)	(1.3, 9.6)†	(−3.8, 5.9)†	−3.3 to 1.5‡	−1.9 to 1.4‡

* Population: all patients with assessable saphenous vein grafts
** Population: all patients assessable by blinded consultant
*** All patients
† 90%; per protocol
‡ 95%; not specified in protocol

	TEST DOSE	LOADING DOSE	"PUMP PRIME" DOSE	CONSTANT INFUSION DOSE
TRASYLOL® REGIMEN A	1 mL (1.4 mg, or 10,000 KIU)	200 mL (280 mg, or 2.0 million KIU)	200 mL (280 mg, or 2.0 million KIU)	50 mL/hr (70 mg/hr, or 500,000 KIU/hr)
TRASYLOL® REGIMEN B	1 mL (1.4 mg, or 10,000 KIU)	100 mL (140 mg, or 1.0 million KIU)	100 mL (140 mg, or 1.0 million KIU)	25 mL/hr (35 mg/hr, or 250,000 KIU/hr)

Incidence of Myocardial Infarctions by Treatment Group
Population: All CABG Patients Valid for Safety Analysis

Treatment	Definite MI %	Definite or Probable MI %	Definite, Probable or Possible MI %
Pooled Data from Three Studies that Evaluated Regimen A			
Trasylol® Regimen A n = 646	4.6	10.7	14.1
Placebo n = 661	4.7	11.3	13.4
Pooled Data from Two Studies that Evaluated Regimen B and Pump Prime Regimen			
Trasylol® Regimen B n = 241	8.7	15.9	18.7
Trasylol® Pump Prime Regimen n = 239	6.3	15.7	18.1
Placebo n = 240	6.3	15.1	15.8

Graft Patency: In a recently completed multi-center, multinational study to determine the effects of Trasylol® Regimen A vs. placebo on saphenous vein graft patency in patients undergoing primary CABG surgery, patients were subjected to routine postoperative angiography. Of the 13 study sites, 10 were in the United States and three were non-U.S. centers (Denmark (1), Israel (2)). The results of this study are summarized below.

[See first table above]

Although there was a statistically significantly increased risk of graft closure for Trasylol® treated patients compared to patients who received placebo (p=0.035), further analysis showed a significant treatment by site interaction for one of the non-U.S. sites vs. the U.S. centers. When the analysis of graft closures was repeated for U.S. centers only, there was no statistically significant difference in graft closure rates in patients who received Trasylol® vs. placebo. These results are the same whether analyzed as the proportion of patients who experienced at least one graft closure postoperatively or as the proportion of grafts closed. There were no differences between treatment groups in the incidence of myocardial infarction as evaluated by the blinded consultant (2.9% Trasylol® vs. 3.8% placebo) or of death (1.4% Trasylol® vs. 1.6% placebo) in this study.

Hypersensitivity and Anaphylaxis: See WARNINGS.

Hypersensitivity and anaphylactic reactions during surgery were rarely reported in U.S. controlled clinical studies in patients with no prior exposure to Trasylol® (1/1424 patients or <0.1% on Trasylol® vs. 1/861 patients or 0.1% on placebo). In case of re-exposure the incidence of hypersensitivity/anaphylactic reactions has been reported to reach the 5% level. A review of 387 European patient records involving re-exposure to Trasylol® showed that the incidence of hypersensitivity or anaphylactic reactions was 5.0% for re-exposure within 6 months and 0.9% for re-exposure greater than 6 months.

Laboratory Findings

Serum Creatinine: Data pooled from all patients undergoing CABG surgery in U.S. placebo-controlled trials showed no statistically or clinically significant increase in the incidence of postoperative renal dysfunction in patients treated with Trasylol®. The incidence of serum creatinine elevations > 0.5 mg/dL above pre-treatment levels was 9% in the Trasylol® group vs. 8% in the placebo group (p=0.248), while the incidence of elevations >2.0 mg/dL above baseline was only 1% in each group (p=0.883). In the majority of instances, postoperative renal dysfunction was not severe and was reversible. Patients with baseline elevations in serum creatinine were not at increased risk of developing postoperative renal dysfunction following Trasylol® treatment.

Serum Transaminases: Data pooled from all patients undergoing CABG surgery in U.S. placebo-controlled trials showed no evidence of an increase in the incidence of postoperative hepatic dysfunction in patients treated with Trasylol®. The incidence of treatment-emergent increases in ALT (formerly SGPT) > 1.8 times the upper limit of normal was 14% in both the Trasylol® and placebo-treated patients (p=0.687), while the incidence of increases > 3 times the upper limit of normal was 5% in both groups (p=0.847).

Other Laboratory Findings: The incidence of treatment-emergent elevations in plasma glucose, AST (formerly SGOT), LDH, alkaline phosphatase, and CPK-MB was not notably different between Trasylol® and placebo treated patients undergoing CABG surgery. Significant elevations in the partial thromboplastin time (PTT) and celite Activated Clotting Time (celite ACT) are expected in Trasylol® treated patients in the hours after surgery due to circulating concentrations of Trasylol®, which are known to inhibit activation of the intrinsic clotting system by contact with a foreign material (e.g., celite), a method used in these tests. (see Laboratory Monitoring of Anticoagulation During Cardiopulmonary Bypass).

OVERDOSAGE

The maximum amount of Trasylol® that can be safely administered in single or multiple doses has not been determined. Doses up to 17.5 million KIU have been administered within a 24 hour period without any apparent toxicity. There is one poorly documented case, however, of a patient who received a large, but not well determined, amount of Trasylol® (in excess of 15 million KIU) in 24 hours. The patient, who had pre-existing liver dysfunction, developed hepatic and renal failure postoperatively and died. Autopsy showed hepatic necrosis and extensive renal tubular and glomerular necrosis. The relationship of these findings to Trasylol® therapy is unclear.

DOSAGE AND ADMINISTRATION

Trasylol® given prophylactically in both Regimen A and Regimen B (half Regimen A) to patients undergoing CABG surgery significantly reduced the donor blood transfusion requirement relative to placebo treatment. In low risk patients there is no difference in efficacy between regimen A and B. Therefore, the dosage used (A vs. B) is at the discretion of the practitioner.

Trasylol® is supplied as a solution containing 10,000 KIU/mL, which is equal to 1.4 mg/mL. All intravenous doses of Trasylol® should be administered through a central line. **DO NOT ADMINISTER ANY OTHER DRUG USING THE SAME LINE.** Both regimens include a 1 mL test dose, a loading dose, a dose to be added while recirculating the priming fluid of the cardiopulmonary bypass circuit ("pump prime" dose), and a constant infusion dose. To avoid physical incompatibility of Trasylol® and heparin when adding to the pump prime solution, each agent must be added **during recirculation** of the pump prime to assure adequate dilution prior to admixture with the other component. Regimens A and B (both incorporating a 1 mL test dose) are described in the table below:

[See second table above]

The 1 mL test dose should be administered intravenously at least 10 minutes before the loading dose. With the patient in a supine position, the loading dose is given slowly over 20–30 minutes, after induction of anesthesia but prior to sternotomy. In patients with known previous exposure to Trasylol®, the loading dose should be given just prior to cannulation. When the loading dose is complete, it is followed by the constant infusion dose, which is continued until surgery is complete and the patient leaves the operating room. The "pump prime" dose is added to the **recirculating** priming fluid of the cardiopulmonary bypass circuit, by replacement of an aliquot of the priming fluid, prior to the institution of cardiopulmonary bypass. Total doses of more than 7 million KIU have not been studied in controlled trials.

Parenteral drug products should be inspected visually for particulate matter and discoloration prior to administration whenever solution and container permit. Discard any unused portion.

Renal and Hepatic Impairment: No formal studies of the pharmacokinetics of aprotinin in patients with pre-existing renal insufficiency have been conducted. However, in the placebo-controlled clinical trials conducted in the United States, patients with mildly elevated pretreatment serum creatinine levels did not have a notably higher incidence of clinically significant post-treatment elevations in serum creatinine following either Trasylol® Regimen A or Regimen B compared to administration of the placebo regimen. Changes in aprotinin pharmacokinetics with age or impaired renal function are not great enough to require any dose adjustment. No pharmacokinetic data from patients with pre-existing hepatic disease treated with Trasylol® are available.

HOW SUPPLIED

Size	Strength	NDC
100 mL vials	1,000,000 KIU	0026-8196-36
200 mL vials	2,000,000 KIU	0026-8197-63

STORAGE

Trasylol® should be stored between 2° and 25°C (36° - 77°F).

Protect from freezing.

Bayer Corporation
Pharmaceutical Division
400 Morgan Lane
West Haven, CT 06516
Made in Germany

Rx Only

PZ500155 2/00 ©2000 Bayer Corporation 9498

Bayer Corporation Pharmaceutical Division Biological Products

400 MORGAN LANE
WEST HAVEN, CT 06516

For Medical Information Contact:
Director, Medical Services
(800) 468-0894
(203) 937-2000

BAYGAM® ℞

[*bāy-găm*]
Immune Globulin (Human)
Solvent/Detergent Treated

DESCRIPTION

Immune Globulin (Human)—BayGam® treated with solvent/detergent is a sterile solution of immune globulin for intramuscular administration; it contains no preservative. BayGam is prepared by cold ethanol fractionation from human plasma. The immune globulin is isolated from solubilized Cohn fraction II. The fraction II solution is adjusted to a final concentration of 0.3% tri-n-butyl phosphate (TNBP) and 0.2% sodium cholate. After the addition of solvent (TNBP) and detergent (sodium cholate), the solution is heated to 30°C and maintained at that temperature for not less than 6 hours. After the viral inactivation step, the reactants are removed by precipitation, filtration and finally ultrafiltration and diafiltration. BayGam is formulated as a 15–18% protein solution at a pH of 6.4–7.2 in 0.21–0.32 M glycine. BayGam is then incubated in the final container for 21–28 days at 20–27°C.

The removal and inactivation of spiked model enveloped and non-enveloped viruses during the manufacturing process for BayGam has been validated in laboratory studies. Human Immunodeficiency Virus, Type 1 (HIV-1), was chosen as the relevant virus for blood products; Bovine Viral Diarrhea Virus (BVDV) was chosen to model Hepatitis C virus; Pseudorabies virus (PRV) was chosen to model Hepatitis B virus and the Herpes viruses; and Reo virus type 3 (Reo) was chosen to model non-enveloped viruses and for its resistance to physical and chemical inactivation. Significant removal of model enveloped and non-enveloped viruses is achieved at two steps in the Cohn fractionation process leading to the collection of Cohn Fraction II: the precipitation and removal of Fraction III in the processing of Fraction II + IIIW suspension to Effluent III and the filtration step in the processing of Effluent III to Filtrate III. Significant inactivation of enveloped viruses is achieved at the time of treatment of solubilized Cohn Fraction II with TNBP/sodium cholate.

CLINICAL PHARMACOLOGY

Peak levels of immunoglobulin G are obtained approximately 2 days after intramuscular injection of BayGam.[1] The half-life of IgG in the circulation of individuals with normal IgG levels is 23 days.[2]

Passive immunization with BayGam modifies hepatitis A, prevents or modifies measles, and provides replacement therapy in persons with hypogammaglobulinemia or agammaglobulinemia. BayGam is not standardized with respect to antibody titers against hepatitis B surface antigen (HBsAg) and should not be used for prophylaxis of viral hepatitis type B. Prophylactic treatment to prevent hepatitis B can best be accomplished with use of Heptitis B Immune Globulin (Human), often in combination with Hepatitis B Vaccine.[3]

BayGam may be of benefit in women who have been exposed to rubella in the first trimester of pregnancy and who will not consider a therapeutic abortion.[4] BayGam may also be considered for use in immunocompromised patients for passive immunization against varicella if Varicella-Zoster Immune Globulin (Human) is not available.[5]

Immune Globulin (Human) is not indicated for routine prophylaxis or treatment of rubella, poliomyelitis, mumps, or varicella. It is not indicated for allergy or asthma in patients who have normal levels of immunoglobulin.[6]

In a clinical study in eight healthy human adults receiving another hyperimmune immune globulin product treated with solvent/detergent, Rabies Immune Globulin (Human), BayRab™, prepared by the same manufacturing process, detectable passive antibody titers were observed in the serum of all subjects by 24 hours post injection and persisted through the 21 day study period. These results suggest that passive immunization with immune globulin products is not affected by the solvent/detergent treatment.

INDICATIONS AND USAGE

Hepatitis A

The prophylactic value of BayGam is greatest when given before or soon after exposure to hepatitis A. BayGam is not indicated in persons with clinical manifestations of hepatitis A or in those exposed more than 2 weeks previously.

Measles (Rubeola)

BayGam should be given to prevent or modify measles in a susceptible person exposed fewer than 6 days previously.[7] A susceptible person is one who has not been vaccinated and has not had measles previously. BayGam may be especially indicated for susceptible household contacts of measles patients, particularly contacts under 1 year of age, for whom the risk of complications is highest.[7] **BayGam and measles vaccine should not be given at the same time.**[7] If a child is older than 12 months and has received BayGam, he should be given measles vaccine about 3 months later when the measles antibody titer will have disappeared.

If a susceptible child exposed to measles is immunocompromised, BayGam should be given immediately.[8] Children who are immunocompromised should not receive measles vaccine or any other live viral vaccine.

Varicella

Passive immunization against varicella in immunosuppressed patients is best accomplished by use of Varicella-Zoster Immune Globulin (Human) [VZIG]. If VZIG is unavailable, BayGam, promptly given, may also modify varicella.[5]

Rubella

The routine use of BayGam for prophylaxis of rubella in early pregnancy is of dubious value and cannot be justified.[6] Some studies suggest that the use of BayGam in exposed, susceptible women can lessen the likelihood of infection and fetal damage; therefore, BayGam may benefit those women who will **not** consider a therapeutic abortion.[4]

Immunoglobulin Deficiency

In patients with immunoglobulin deficiencies, BayGam may prevent serious infection. However, BayGam may not prevent chronic infections of the external secretory tissues such as the respiratory and gastrointestinal tract.

Prophylactic therapy, especially against infections due to encapsulated bacteria, is effective in Bruton-type, sex-linked, congenital agammaglobulinemia, agammaglobulinemia associated with thymoma, and acquired agammaglobulinemia.

CONTRAINDICATIONS

BayGam should not be given to persons with isolated immunoglobulin A (IgA) deficiency. Such persons have the potential for developing antibodies to IgA and could have anaphylactic reactions to subsequent administration of blood products that contain IgA.[9]

BayGam should not be administered to patients who have severe thrombocytopenia or any coagulation disorder that would contraindicate intramuscular injections.

WARNINGS

BayGam is made from human plasma. Products made from human plasma may contain infectious agents, such as viruses, that can cause disease. The risk that such products will transmit an infectious agent has been reduced by screening plasma donors for prior exposure to certain viruses, by testing for the presence of certain current virus infections, and by inactivating and/or removing certain viruses. Despite these measures, such products can still potentially transmit disease. There is also the possibility that unknown infectious agents may be present in such products. Individuals who receive infusions of blood or plasma products may develop signs and/or symptoms of some viral infections, particularly hepatitis C. ALL infections thought by a physician possibly to have been transmitted by this product should be reported by the physician or other healthcare provider to Bayer Corporation [1-888-765-3203].

The physician should discuss the risks and benefits of this product with the patient, before prescribing or administering it to the patient.

BayGam should be given with caution to patients with a history of prior systemic allergic reactions following the administration of human immunoglobulin preparations.[9]

PRECAUTIONS

General

Immune Globulin (Human) should not be administered intravenously because of the potential for serious reactions. Injections should be made intramuscularly, and care should be taken to draw back on the plunger of the syringe before injection in order to be certain that the needle is not in a blood vessel.

Skin tests should not be done. In most human beings the intradermal injection of concentrated gamma globulin solution with its buffers causes a localized area of inflammation which can be misinterpreted as a positive allergic reaction. In actuality, this does not represent an allergy; rather, it is localized tissue irritation of a chemical nature. Misinterpretation of the results of such tests can lead the physician to withhold badly needed human immunoglobulin from a patient who is not actually allergic to this material. True allergic responses to human gamma globulin given in the prescribed intramuscular manner are rare.

Although systemic reactions to intramuscular administered immunoglobulin preparations are rare, epinephrine should be available for treatment of acute allergic symptoms.

Clinical and Laboratory Tests

None required.

Clinically Significant Product Interactions

Antibodies in the globulin preparation may interfere with the response to live viral vaccines such as measles, mumps, polio and rubella. Therefore, use of such vaccines should be deferred until approximately 3 months after Immune Globulin (Human)—BayGam® administration.

No interactions with other products are known.

Pregnancy Category C

Animal reproduction studies have not been conducted with BayGam. It is also not known whether BayGam can cause fetal harm when administered to a pregnant woman or can affect reproduction capacity. BayGam should be given to a pregnant woman only if clearly needed.

Pediatric Use

Safety and effectiveness in the pediatric population have not been established.

ADVERSE REACTIONS

Local pain and tenderness at the injection site, urticaria, and angioedema may occur. Anaphylactic reactions, although rare, have been reported following the injection of human immune globulin preparations.[6,9] Anaphylaxis is more likely to occur if BayGam is given intravenously; therefore, BayGam must be administered only intramuscularly.

DOSAGE AND ADMINISTRATION

BayGam is administered **intramuscularly** (see PRECAUTIONS), preferably in the anterolateral aspects of the upper thigh and the deltoid muscle of the upper arm. The gluteal region should not be used routinely as an injection site because of the risk of injury to the sciatic nerve. Doses over 10 mL should be divided and injected into several muscle sites to reduce local pain and discomfort. An individual decision as to which muscle is injected must be made for each patient based on the volume of material to be administered. If the gluteal region is used when very large volumes are to be injected or multiple doses are necessary, the central region MUST be avoided; only the upper, outer quadrant should be used.[10]

Parenteral drug products should be inspected visually for particulate matter and discoloration prior to administration, whenever solution and container permit.

Hepatitis A

BayGam in a dose of 0.01 mL/lb (0.02 mL/kg) is recommended for household and institutional hepatitis A case contacts.

The following doses of BayGam are recommended for persons who plan to travel in areas where hepatitis A is common.[3]

Length of Stay	Dose Volume
Less than 3 months	0.02 mL/kg
3 months or longer	0.06 mL/kg (repeat every 4–6 months)

Measles (Rubeola)

BayGam should be given in a dose of 0.11 mL/lb (0.2 mL/kg) to prevent or modify measles in a susceptible person exposed fewer than 6 days previously.[7]

A susceptible child who is exposed to measles and who is immunocompromised should receive a dose of 0.5 mL/kg (maximum dose, 15 mL) of BayGam immediately.[8]

Continued on next page

BayGam—Cont.

Varicella
If Varicella-Zoster Immune Globulin (Human) is unavailable, BayGam at a dose of 0.6 to 1.2 mL/kg, promptly given, may also modify varicella.[8]

Rubella
Some studies suggest that the use of BayGam in exposed, susceptible women can lessen the likelihood of infection and fetal damage; therefore, BayGam at a dose of 0.55 mL/kg may benefit those women who will not consider a therapeutic abortion.[4]

Immunoglobulin Deficiency
BayGam may prevent serious infection in patients with immunoglobulin deficiencies if circulating IgG levels of approximately 200 mg/100 mL plasma are maintained. The recommended dosage is 0.66 mL/kg (at least 100 mg/kg) given every 3 to 4 weeks.[6] A double dose is given at onset of therapy; some patients may require more frequent injections.

HOW SUPPLIED

BayGam is supplied in 2 mL and 10 mL single dose vials.

NDC Number	Size
0026-0635-02	2 mL vial (10 pack)
0026-0635-04	2 mL vial
0026-0635-10	10 mL vial (10 pack)
0026-0635-12	10 mL vial

STORAGE
Store at 2–8°C (36–48°F). Do not freeze. Do not use after expiration date.

CAUTION
U.S. federal law prohibits dispensing without prescription.

LIMITED WARRANTY
A number of factors beyond our control could reduce the efficacy of this product or even result in an ill effect following its use. These include improper storage and handling of the product after it leaves our hands, diagnosis, dosage, method of administration, and biological differences in individual patients. Because of these factors, it is important that this product be stored properly and that the directions be followed carefully during use.
No warranty, express or implied, including any warranty of merchantability or fitness is made. Representatives of the Company are not authorized to vary the terms or the contents of the printed labeling, including the package insert for this product, except by printed notice from the Company's headquarters. The prescriber and user of this product must accept the terms hereof.

REFERENCES

1. Smith GN, Griffiths B, Mollison D, et al: Uptake of IgG after intramuscular and subcutaneous injection. *Lancet* 1(7762): 1208–12, 1972.
2. Waldmann TA, Strober W, Blaese RM: Variations in the metabolism of immunoglobulins measured by turnover rates. In Merler E (ed.): Immunoglobulins: biologic aspects and clinical uses. Washington DC, Nat Acad Sci, 1970, pp 33–51.
3. Recommendation of the Immunization Practices Advisory Committee (ACIP): Postexposure prophylaxis of hepatitis B. *MMWR* 33(21): 285–90, 1984.
4. American Academy of Pediatrics, Committee on Infectious Diseases: Report. ed. 19. Evanston, 1982, p 231.
5. Gershon AA, Piomelli S, Karpatkin M, et al: Antibody to varicella-zoster virus after passive immunization against chicken-pox. *J Clin Microbiol* 8(6): 733–5, 1978.
6. American Academy of Pediatrics, Committee on Infectious Diseases: Report. ed. 19. Evanston, 1982, pp 134–5.
7. Recommendation of the Public Health Service Advisory Committee on Immunization Practices: Measles prevention. *MMWR* 27(44): 427–30; 435–7, 1978.
8. American Academy of Pediatrics, Committee on Infectious Diseases: Report. ed. 19. Evanston, 1982, pp 34–6.
9. Fudenberg HH: Sensitization to immunoglobulins and hazards of gamma globulin therapy. In: Merler E (ed.): Immunoglobulins: biologic aspects and clinical uses. Washington DC, Nat Acad Sci, 1970, pp 211–20.
10. Recommendations of the Immunization Practices Advisory Committee (ACIP): General recommendations on immunization. *MMWR* 38(13): 205–14; 219–27, 1989.

Bayer Corporation
Pharmaceutical Division
Elkhart, IN 46515 USA
U.S. License No. 8 14-7635-001 (Rev. April 1998)

BAYHEP B® ℞
[bāy-hep"]
Hepatitis B Immune Globulin (Human)

DESCRIPTION

Hepatitis B Immune Globulin (Human)—BayHep B® treated with solvent/detergent is a sterile solution of hepatitis B hyperimmune immune globulin for intramuscular administration; it contains no preservative. BayHep B is prepared by cold ethanol fractionation from the plasma of donors with high titers of antibody to the hepatitis B surface antigen (anti-HBs). The immune globulin is isolated from solubilized Cohn Fraction II. The Fraction II solution is adjusted to a final concentration of 0.3% tri-n-butyl phosphate (TNBP) and 0.2% sodium cholate. After the addition of solvent (TNBP) and detergent (sodium cholate), the solution is heated to 30°C and maintained at that temperature for not less than 6 hours. After the viral inactivation step, the reactants are removed by precipitation, filtration and finally ultrafiltration and diafiltration. BayHep B is formulated as a 15–18% protein solution at a pH of 6.4–7.2 in 0.21–0.32 M glycine. BayHep B is then incubated in the final container for 21–28 days at 20–27°C. Each vial contains anti-HBs antibody equivalent to or exceeding the potency of anti-HBs in a U.S. reference hepatitis B immune globulin (Center for Biologics Evaluation and Research, FDA). The U.S. reference has been tested against the World Health Organization standard Hepatitis B Immune Globulin and found to be equal to 217 international units (IU) per mL.
The removal and inactivation of spiked model enveloped and non-enveloped viruses during the manufacturing process for BayHep B has been validated in laboratory studies. Human Immunodeficiency Virus, Type 1 (HIV-1), was chosen as the relevant virus for blood products; Bovine Viral Diarrhea Virus (BVDV) was chosen to model Hepatitis C virus; Pseudorabies virus (PRV) was chosen to model Hepatitis B virus and the Herpes viruses; and Reo virus type 3 (Reo) was chosen to model non-enveloped viruses and for its resistance to physical and chemical inactivation. Significant removal of model enveloped and non-enveloped viruses is achieved at two steps in the Cohn fractionation process leading to the collection of Cohn Fraction II: the precipitation and removal of Fraction III in the processing of Fraction II + IIIW suspension to Effluent III and the filtration step in the processing of Effluent III to Filtrate III. Significant inactivation of enveloped viruses is achieved at the time of treatment of solubilized Cohn Fraction II with TNBP/sodium cholate.

CLINICAL PHARMACOLOGY

Hepatitis B Immune Globulin (Human) provides passive immunization for individuals exposed to the hepatitis B virus (HBV) as evidenced by a reduction in the attack rate of hepatitis B following its use.[1-6] The administration of the usual recommended dose of this immune globulin generally results in a detectable level of circulating anti-HBs which persists for approximately 2 months or longer. The highest antibody (IgG) serum levels were seen in the following distribution of subjects studied:[7]

DAY	% OF SUBJECTS
3	38%
7	41.7%
14	11.1%
21	8.3%

Mean values for half-life were between 17.5 and 25 days, with the shortest being 5.9 days and the longest 35 days.[7]
Cases of type B hepatitis are rarely seen following exposure to HBV in persons with pre-existing anti-HBs. No confirmed instance of transmission of hepatitis B has been associated with this product.
In a clinical study in eight healthy human adults receiving another hyperimmune immune globulin product treated with solvent/detergent, Rabies Immune Globulin (Human), BayRab®, prepared by the same manufacturing process, detectable passive antibody titers were observed in the serum of all subjects by 24 hours post injection and persisted through the 21 day study period. These results suggest that passive immunization with immune globulin products is not affected by the solvent/detergent treatment.

INDICATIONS AND USAGE

Recommendations on post-exposure prophylaxis are based on available efficacy data and on the likelihood of future HBV exposure for the person requiring treatment. In all exposures, a regimen combining Hepatitis B Immune Globulin (Human) with hepatitis B vaccine will provide both short-and long-term protection, will be less costly than the two-dose Hepatitis B Immune Globulin (Human) treatment alone, and is the treatment of choice.[8]
BayHep B is indicated for post-exposure prophylaxis in the following situations:

Acute Exposure to Blood Containing HBsAg
After either parenteral exposure, e.g., by accidental "needlestick" or direct mucous membrane contact (accidental splash), or oral ingestion (pipetting accident) involving HBsAg-positive materials such as blood, plasma or serum. For inadvertent percutaneous exposure, a regimen of two doses of Hepatitis B Immune Globulin (Human), one given after exposure and one a month later, is about 75% effective in preventing hepatitis B in this setting.

Perinatal Exposure of Infants Born to HBsAg-positive Mothers
Infants born to HBsAg-positive mothers are at risk of being infected with hepatitis B virus and becoming chronic carriers.[5,8,9,10] This risk is especially great if the mother is HBeAg-positive.[11,12,13] For an infant with perinatal exposure to an HBsAg-positive and HBeAg-positive mother, a regimen combining one dose of Hepatitis B Immune Globulin (Human) at birth with the hepatitis B vaccine series started soon after birth is 85%–95% effective in preventing development of the HBV carrier state.[8,14] Regimens involving either multiple doses of Hepatitis B Immune Globulin (Human) alone or the vaccine series alone have 70%–90% efficacy, while a single dose of Hepatitis B Immune Globulin (Human) alone has only 50% efficacy.[8,15]

Sexual Exposure to an HBsAg-positive Person
Sex partners of HBsAg-positive persons are at increased risk of acquiring HBV infection. For sexual exposure to a person with acute hepatitis B, a single dose of Hepatitis B Immune Globulin (Human) is 75% effective if administered within 2 weeks of last sexual exposure.[8]

Household Exposure to Persons with Acute HBV Infection
Since infants have close contact with primary care-givers and they have a higher risk of becoming HBV carriers after acute HBV infection, prophylaxis of an infant less than 12 months of age with Hepatitis B Immune Globulin and hepatitis B vaccine is indicated if the mother or primary care-giver has acute HBV infection.[8]
Administration of Hepatitis B Immune Globulin (Human) either preceding or concomitant with the commencement of active immunization with Hepatitis B Vaccine provides for more rapid achievement of protective levels of hepatitis B antibody, than when the vaccine alone is administered.[16] Rapid achievement of protective levels of antibody to hepatitis B virus may be desirable in certain clinical situations, as in cases of accidental inoculations with contaminated medical instruments.[16] Administration of Hepatitis B Immune Globulin (Human) either 1 month preceding or at the time of commencement of a program of active vaccination with Hepatitis B Vaccine has been shown not to interfere with the active immune response to the vaccine.[16]

CONTRAINDICATIONS

None known.

WARNINGS

BayHep B is made from human plasma. Products made from human plasma may contain infectious agents, such as viruses, that can cause disease. The risk that such products will transmit an infectious agent has been reduced by screening plasma donors for prior exposure to certain viruses, by testing for the presence of certain current virus infections, and by inactivating and/or removing certain viruses. Despite these measures, such products can still potentially transmit disease. There is also the possibility that unknown infectious agents may be present in such products. Individuals who receive infusions of blood or plasma products may develop signs and/or symptoms of some viral infections, particularly hepatitis C. ALL infections thought by a physician possibly to have been transmitted by this product should be reported by the physician or other healthcare provider to Bayer Corporation [1-888-765-3203].
The physician should discuss the risks and benefits of this product with the patient, before prescribing or administering it to the patient.
BayHep B should be given with caution to patients with a history of prior systemic allergic reactions following the administration of human immune globulin preparations. Epinephrine should be available.
In patients who have severe thrombocytopenia or any coagulation disorder that would contraindicate intramuscular injections, Hepatitis B Immune Globulin (Human) should be given only if the expected benefits outweigh the risks.

PRECAUTIONS

General
Hepatitis B Immune Globulin (Human)—BayHep B® should **not** be administered intravenously because of the potential for serious reactions. Injections should be made intramuscularly, and care should be taken to draw back on the plunger of the syringe before injection in order to be certain that the needle is not in a blood vessel.
Intramuscular injections are preferably administered in the anterolateral aspects of the upper thigh and the deltoid muscle of the upper arm. The gluteal region should not be used routinely as an injection site because of the risk of injury to the sciatic nerve. An individual decision as to which muscle is injected must be made for each patient based on the volume of material to be administered. If the gluteal region is used when very large volumes are to be injected or multiple doses are necessary, the central region MUST be avoided; only the upper, outer quadrant should be used.[17]

Laboratory Tests
None required.

Drug Interactions
Although administration of Hepatitis B Immune Globulin (Human) did not interfere with measles vaccination,[18] it is not known whether Hepatitis B Immune Globulin (Human) may interfere with other live virus vaccines. Therefore, use of such vaccines should be deferred until approximately three months after Hepatitis B Immune Globulin (Human) administration. Hepatitis B Vaccine may be administered at the same time, but at a different injection site, without interfering with the immune response.[16] No interactions with other products are known.

Pregnancy Category C
Animal reproduction studies have not been conducted with BayHep B. It is also not known whether BayHep B can cause fetal harm when administered to a pregnant woman or can affect reproduction capacity. BayHep B should be given to a pregnant woman only if clearly needed.

Pediatric Use
Safety and effectiveness in the pediatric population have not been established.

ADVERSE REACTIONS

Local pain and tenderness at the injection site, urticaria and angioedema may occur; anaphylactic reactions, although rare, have been reported following the injection of human immune globulin preparations.[19]

OVERDOSAGE

Although no data are available, clinical experience with other immunoglobulin preparations suggests that the only manifestations would be pain and tenderness at the injection site.

DOSAGE AND ADMINISTRATION

Acute Exposure to Blood Containing HBsAg[15]

Table 1 summarizes prophylaxis for percutaneous (needle stick or bite), ocular, or mucous-membrane exposure to blood according to the source of exposure and vaccination status of the exposed person. For greatest effectiveness, passive prophylaxis with Hepatitis B Immune Globulin (Human) should be given as soon as possible after exposure (its value beyond 7 days of exposure is unclear). If Hepatitis B Immune Globulin (Human) is indicated (see Table 1 below), an injection of 0.06 mL/kg of body weight should be administered intramuscularly (see PRECAUTIONS) as soon as possible after exposure and within 24 hours, if possible. Consult Hepatitis B Vaccine package insert for dosage information regarding that product.

[See table 1 at right]

For persons who refuse Hepatitis B Vaccine, a second dose of Hepatitis B Immune Globulin (Human)—BayHep B® should be given 1 month after the first dose.

Table 1. (adapted from[20])
Recommendations for Hepatitis B Prophylaxis Following Percutaneous or Permucosal Exposure

Source	Exposed Person: Unvaccinated	Exposed Person: Vaccinated
HBsAg-Positive	1. Hepatitis B Immune Globulin (Human)×1 immediately* 2. Initiate HB Vaccine series†	1. Test exposed person for anti-HBs. 2. If inadequate antibody,‡ Hepatitis B Immune Globulin (Human) (×1) immediately plus HB Vaccine booster dose, or 2 doses of HBIG,* one as soon as possible after exposure and the second 1 month later.
Known Source (High Risk)	1. Initiate HB Vaccine series 2. Test source for HBsAg. If positive, Hepatitis B Immune Globulin (Human)×1	1. Test Source for HBsAg only if exposed is vaccine nonresponder; if source is HBsAg-positive, give Hepatitis B Immune Globulin (Human)×1 immediately plus HB Vaccine booster dose, or 2 doses of HBIG,* one as soon as possible after exposure and the second 1 month later.
Low Risk HBsAg-Positive	Initiate HB Vaccine series.	Nothing required.
Unknown Source	Initiate HB Vaccine series within 7 days of exposure.	Nothing required.

* Hepatitis B Immune Globulin (Human), dose 0.06 mL/kg IM.
† HB Vaccine dose 20 µg IM for adults; 10 µg IM for infants or children under 10 years of age. First dose within 1 week; second and third doses, 1 and 6 months later.
‡ Less than 10 sample ratio units (SRU) by radioimmunoassay (RIA), negative by enzyme immunoassay (EIA).

Prophylaxis of Infants Born to HBsAg and HBeAg Positive Mothers

Efficacy of prophylactic Hepatitis B Immune Globulin (Human) in infants at risk depends on administering Hepatitis B Immune Globulin (Human) on the day of birth. It is therefore vital that HBsAg-positive mothers be identified before delivery.

Hepatitis B Immune Globulin (Human) (0.5 mL) should be administered intramuscularly (IM) to the newborn infant after physiologic stabilization of the infant and preferably within 12 hours of birth. Hepatitis B Immune Globulin (Human) efficacy decreases markedly if treatment is delayed beyond 48 hours. Hepatitis B Vaccine should be administered IM in three doses of 0.5 mL of vaccine (10 µg) each. The first dose should be given within 7 days of birth and may be given concurrently with Hepatitis B Immune Globulin (Human) but at a separate site. The second and third doses of vaccine should be given 1 month and 6 months, respectively, after the first. If administration of the first dose of Hepatitis B Vaccine is delayed for as long as 3 months, then a 0.5 mL dose of Hepatitis B Immune Globulin (Human)—HyperHep® should be repeated at 3 months. If Hepatitis B Vaccine is refused, the 0.5 mL dose of Hepatitis B Immune Globulin (Human) should be repeated at 3 and 6 months. Hepatitis B Immune Globulin (Human) administered at birth should not interfere with oral polio and diphtheria-tetanus-pertussis vaccines administered at 2 months of age.[15]

Sexual Exposure to an HBsAg-positive Person

All susceptible persons whose sex partners have acute hepatitis B infection should receive a single dose of HBIG (0.06 mL/kg) and should begin the hepatitis B vaccine series if prophylaxis can be started within 14 days of the last sexual contact or if sexual contact with the infected person will continue (see Table 2 below). Administering the vaccine with HBIG may improve the efficacy of postexposure treatment. The vaccine has the added advantage of conferring long-lasting protection.[8]

[See table 2 above]

Table 2. (adapted from [21])
Recommendations for Postexposure Prophylaxis for Sexual Exposure to Hepatitis B

HBIG*: Dose	HBIG*: Recommended timing	Vaccine: Dose	Vaccine: Recommended timing
0.06 mL/kg IM†	Single dose within 14 days of last sexual contact	1.0 mL IM†	First dose at time of HBIG* treatment¶

* HBIG = Hepatitis B Immune Globulin (Human)
† IM = intramuscularly
¶ The first dose can be administered the same time as the HBIG dose but at a different site; subsequent doses should be administered as recommended for specific vaccine.

Household Exposure to Persons with Acute HBV Infection

Prophylactic treatment with a 0.5 mL dose of Hepatitis B Immune Globulin (Human) and hepatitis B vaccine is indicated for infants < 12 months of age who have been exposed to a primary care-giver who has acute hepatitis B. Prophylaxis for other household contacts of persons with acute HBV infection is not indicated unless they have had identifiable blood exposure to the index patient, such as by sharing toothbrushes or razors. Such exposures should be treated like sexual exposures. If the index patient becomes an HBV carrier, all household contacts should receive hepatitis B vaccine.[8]

Hepatitis B Immune Globulin (Human) may be administered at the same time (but at a different site), or up to 1 month preceding Hepatitis B Vaccination without impairing the active immune response from Hepatitis B Vaccination.[16]

Parenteral drug products should be inspected visually for particulate matter and discoloration prior to administration, whenever solution and container permit.

Administer intramuscularly. Do not inject intravenously.

Directions for Syringe Usage

1. Remove the prefilled syringe from the package. Lift syringe by barrel, **not** by plunger.
2. Twist the plunger rod clockwise until the threads are seated.
3. With the rubber needle shield secured on the syringe tip, push the plunger rod foward a few millimeters to break any friction seal between the rubber stopper and the glass syringe barrel.
4. Remove the needle shield and expel air bubbles.
5. Proceed with hypodermic needle puncture.
6. Aspirate prior to injection to confirm that the needle is not in a vein or artery.
7. Inject the medication.
8. Withdraw the needle and dispose or destroy it.

HOW SUPPLIED

Hepatitis B Immune Globulin (Human)—BayHep B® is supplied in a 0.5 mL neonatal single dose syringe with attached needle, a 1 mL and a 5 mL single dose vial.

NDC Number	Size
0026-0636-00	0.5 mL syringe
0026-0636-01	1 mL vial
0016-0636-05	5 mL vial

STORAGE

Store at 2°–8°C (36°–46°F). Do not freeze. Do not use after expiration date.

CAUTION

U.S. federal law prohibits dispensing without prescription.

LIMITED WARRANTY

A number of factors beyond our control could reduce the efficacy of this product or even result in an ill effect following its use. These include improper storage and handling of the product after it leaves our hands, diagnosis, dosage, method of administration and biological differences in individual patients. Because of these factors, it is important that this product be stored properly and that the directions be followed carefully during use.

No warranty, express or implied, including any warranty of merchantability or fitness is made. Representatives of the Company are not authorized to vary the terms or the contents of the printed labeling, including the package insert for this product, except by printed notice from the Company's headquarters. The prescriber and user of this product must accept the terms hereof.

REFERENCES

1. Grady GF, Lee VA: Hepatitis B immune globulin—prevention of hepatitis from accidental exposure among medical personnel. *N Engl J Med* 293(21): 1067-70, 1975.
2. Seeff LB, Zimmerman HJ, Wright EC, et al: Efficacy of hepatitis B immune serum globulin after accidental exposure. *Lancet* 2(7942):939-41, 1975.
3. Krugman S, Giles JP: Viral hepatitis, type B (MS-2-strain). Further observations on natural history and prevention. *N Engl J Med* 288(15):755-60, 1973.
4. Current trends: Health status of Indochinese refugees: malaria and hepatitis B. *MMWR* 28(39):463-4; 469-70, 1979.
5. Jhaveri R, Rosenfeld W, Salazar JD, et al: High titer multiple dose therapy with HBIG in newborn infants of HBsAg positive mothers. *J Pediatr* 97(2):305-8, 1980.
6. Hoofnagle JH, Seeff LB, Bales ZB, et al: Passive-active immunity from hepatitis B immune globulin. *Ann Intern Med* 91(6):813-8, 1979.
7. Scheiermann N, Kuwert EK: Uptake and elimination of hepatitis B immunoglobulins after intramuscular application in man. *Dev Biol Stand* 54:347-55, 1983.
8. Recommendations of the Immunization Practices Advisory Committee (ACIP): Hepatitis B Virus: A Comprehensive Strategy for Eliminating Transmission in the United States Through Universal Childhood Vaccination. Appendix A: Post-exposure Prophylaxis for Hepatitis B. *MMWR* 40(RR-13):21-25, 1991.
9. Stevens CE, Beasley RP, Tsui J, et al: Vertical transmission of hepatitis B antigen in Taiwan. *N Engl J Med* 292(15):771-4, 1975.
10. Shiraki K, Yoshihara N, Kawana T, et al: Hepatitis B surface antigen and chronic hepatitis in infants born to asymptomatic carrier mothers. *Am J Dis Child* 131(6): 644-7, 1977.
11. Recommendation of the Immunization Practices Advisory Committee (ACIP): Immune globulins for protection against viral hepatitis. *MMWR* 30(34):423-8; 433-5, 1981.
12. Okada K, Kamiyama I, Inomata M, et al: e antigen and anti-e in the serum of asymptomatic carrier mothers as indicators of positive and negative transmission of hepatitis B virus to their infants. *N Engl J Med* 294(14): 746-9, 1976.
13. Beasley RP, Trepo C, Stevens CE, et al: The e antigen and vertical transmission of hepatitis B surface antigen. *Am J Epidemiol* 105(2):94-8, 1977.
14. Beasley RP, Hwang LY, Lee GCY, et al: Prevention of perinatally transmitted hepatitis B virus infections with hepatitis B immune globulin and hepatitis B vaccine. *Lancet* 2(8359):1099-102, 1983.
15. Recommendation of the Immunization Practices Advisory Committee (ACIP): Recommendations for protection against viral hepatitis. *MMWR* 34(22):313-35, 1985.
16. Szmuness W, Stevens CE, Olesko WR, et al: Passive-active immunisation against hepatitis B: Immunogenicity studies in adult Americans. *Lancet* 1:575-77, 1981.

Continued on next page

BayHep B—Cont.

17. Recommendations of the Immunization Practices Advisory Committee (ACIP): General recommendations on immunization. *MMWR* 38(13):205-14; 219-27, 1989.
18. Beasley RP, Hwang LY: Measles vaccination not interfered with by hepatitis B immune globulin. *Lancet* 1:161, 1982.
19. Ellis EF, Henney CS: Adverse reactions following administration of human gamma globulin. *J Allerg* 43(1): 45-54, 1969.
20. Recommendations of the Immunization Practices Advisory Committee (ACIP): Update on Adult Immunization. Table 9. Recommendations for postexposure prophylaxis for percutaneous or permucosal exposure to hepatitis B, United States. *MMWR* 40(RR-12):70, 1991.
21. Recommendations of the Immunization Practices Advisory Committee (ACIP): Update on Adult Immunization. Table 10. Recommendations for postexposure prophylaxis for perinatal and sexual exposure to hepatitis B, United States. *MMWR* 40(RR-12):71, 1991.

BAYRAB® ℞

[*bāy - rab* "]

Rabies Immune Globulin (Human)

DESCRIPTION

Rabies Immune Globulin (Human) — BayRab® treated with solvent/detergent is a sterile solution of antirabies immune globulin for intramuscular administration; it contains no preservative. BayRab is prepared by cold ethanol fractionation from the plasma of donors hyperimmunized with rabies vaccine. The immune globulin is isolated from solubilized Cohn Fraction II. The Fraction II solution is adjusted to a final concentration of 0.3% tri-n-butyl phosphate (TNBP) and 0.2% sodium cholate. After the addition of solvent (TNBP) and detergent (sodium cholate), the solution is heated to 30°C and maintained at that temperature for not less than 6 hours. After the viral inactivation step, the reactants are removed by precipitation, filtration and finally ultrafiltration and diafiltration. BayRab is formulated as a 15–18% protein solution at a pH of 6.4–7.2 in 0.21–0.32 M glycine. BayRab is then incubated in the final container for 21–28 days at 20–27°C. The product is standardized against the U.S. Standard Rabies Immune Globulin to contain an average potency value of 150 IU/mL. The U.S. unit of potency is equivalent to the international unit (IU) for rabies antibody.

The removal and inactivation of spiked model enveloped and non-enveloped viruses during the manufacturing process for BayRab has been validated in laboratory studies. Human Immunodeficiency Virus, Type 1 (HIV-1), was chosen as the relevant virus for blood products; Bovine Viral Diarrhea Virus (BVDV) was chosen to model Hepatitis C virus; Pseudorabies virus (PRV) was chosen to model Hepatitis B virus and the Herpes viruses; and Reo virus type 3 (Reo) was chosen to model non-enveloped viruses and for its resistance to physical and chemical inactivation. Significant removal of model enveloped and non-enveloped viruses is achieved at two steps in the Cohn fractionation process leading to the collection of Cohn Fraction II: the precipitation and removal of Fraction III in the processing of Fraction II + IIIW suspension to Effluent III and the filtration step in the processing of Effluent III to Filtrate III. Significant inactivation of enveloped viruses is achieved at the time of treatment of solubilized Cohn Fraction II with TNBP/sodium cholate.

CLINICAL PHARMACOLOGY

The usefulness of prophylactic rabies antibody in preventing rabies in man when administered immediately after exposure was dramatically demonstrated in a group of persons bitten by a rabid wolf in Iran.[1,2] Similarly, beneficial results were later reported from the U.S.S.R.[3] Studies coordinated by WHO helped determine the optimal conditions under which antirabies serum of equine origin and rabies vaccine can be used in man.[4–7] These studies showed that serum can interfere to a variable extent with the active immunity induced by the vaccine, but could be minimized by booster doses of vaccine after the end of the usual dosage series.

Preparation of rabies immune globulin of human origin with adequate potency was reported by Cabasso et al.[8] In carefully controlled clinical studies, this globulin was used in conjunction with rabies vaccine of duck-embryo origin (DEV).[8,9] These studies determined that a human globulin dose of 20 IU/kg of rabies antibody, given simultaneously with the first DEV dose, resulted in amply detectable levels of passive rabies antibody 24 hours after injection in all recipients. The injections produced minimal, if any, interference with the subject's endogenous antibody response to DEV.

More recently, human diploid cell rabies vaccines (HDCV) prepared from tissue culture fluids containing rabies virus have received substantial clinical evaluation in Europe and the United States.[10–16] In a study in adult volunteers, the administration of Rabies Immune Globulin (Human) did not interfere with antibody formation induced by HDCV when given in a dose of 20 IU per kilogram body weight simultaneously with the first dose of vaccine.[15]

Rabies Postexposure Prophylaxis Guide[19]

Animal species	Condition of animal at time of exposure/attack	Treatment of exposed person [1]
Dog and cat	Healthy and available for 10 days of observation	None, unless animal develops rabies [2]
	Rabid or suspected rabid	RIGH [3] and HDCV
	Unknown (escaped)	Consult public health officials
Skunk, bat, fox, coyote, raccoon, bobcat, and other carnivores; woodchuck	Regard as rabid unless animal proven negative by laboratory tests (4).	RIGH [3] and HDCV
Livestock, rodents, and lagomorphs (rabbits and hares)	Consider individually. Local and state public health officials should be consulted on questions about the need for rabies prophylaxis. In most geographical areas bites of squirrels, hamsters, guinea pigs, gerbils, chipmunks, rats, mice, other rodents, rabbits, and hares almost never call for antirabies prophylaxis.	

[1] ALL POSTEXPOSURE PROPHYLAXIS SHOULD BEGIN WITH IMMEDIATE THOROUGH CLEANSING OF THE WOUND (IF ONE CAN BE DETECTED) WITH SOAP AND WATER. If antirabies treatment is indicated, both Rabies Immune Globulin (Human) [RIGH] and human diploid cell rabies vaccine (HDCV) should be given as soon as possible, REGARDLESS of the interval from exposure.
[2] During the usual holding period of 10 days, begin postexposure prophylaxis at first sign of rabies in a dog or cat that has bitten someone. If the animal exhibits clinical signs of rabies, it should be euthanized immediately and tested.
[3] If RIGH is not available, use antirabies serum, equine (ARS). Do not use more than the recommended dosage.
[4] The animal should be euthanized and tested as soon as possible. Holding for observation is not recommended. Discontinue vaccine if immunofluorescence test results of the animal are negative.

In a clinical study in eight healthy human adults receiving a 20 IU/kg intramuscular dose of Rabies Immune Globulin (Human) treated with solvent/detergent, BayRab™, detectable passive rabies antibody titers were observed in the serum of all subjects by 24 hours post injection and persisted through the 21 day study period. These results are consistent with prior studies[17,18] with non-solvent/detergent treated product.

INDICATIONS AND USAGE

Rabies vaccine and Rabies Immune Globulin (Human), BayRab® should be given to all persons suspected of exposure to rabies with one exception: persons who have been previously immunized with rabies vaccine and have a confirmed adequate rabies antibody titer should receive only vaccine. BayRab should be administered as promptly as possible after exposure, but can be administered up to the eighth day after the first dose of vaccine is given.

Recommendations for use of passive and active immunization after exposure to an animal suspected of having rabies have been detailed by the U.S. Public Health Service Advisory Committee on Immunization Practices (ACIP).[19]

Every exposure to possible rabies infection must be individually evaluated. The following factors should be considered before specific antirabies treatment is initiated:

1. Species of Biting Animal

Carnivorous wild animals (especially skunks, foxes, coyotes, raccoons, and bobcats) and bats are the animals most commonly infected with rabies and have caused most of the indigenous cases of human rabies in the United States since 1960.[20] Unless the animal is tested and shown not to be rabid, postexposure prophylaxis should be initiated upon bite or nonbite exposure to these animals (see item 3 below). If treatment has been initiated and subsequent testing in a competent laboratory shows the exposing animal is not rabid, treatment can be discontinued.

In the United States, the likelihood that a domestic dog or cat is infected with rabies varies from region to region; hence, the need for postexposure prophylaxis also varies. However, in most of Asia and all of Africa and Latin America, the dog remains the major source of human exposure; exposures to dogs in such countries represent a special threat. Travelers to those countries should be aware that >50% of the rabies cases among humans in the United States result from exposure to dogs outside the United States.

Rodents (such as squirrels, hamsters, guinea pigs, gerbils, chipmunks, rats, and mice) and lagomorphs (including rabbits and hares) are rarely found to be infected with rabies and have not been known to cause human rabies in the United States. However, from 1971 through 1988, woodchucks accounted for 70% of the 179 cases of rabies among rodents reported to CDC.[21] In these cases, the state or local health department should be consulted before a decision is made to initiate postexposure antirabies prophylaxis.

2. Circumstances of Biting Incident

An unprovoked attack is more likely to mean that the animal is rabid. (Bites during attempts to feed or handle an apparently healthy animal may generally be regarded as provoked.)

3. Type of Exposure

Rabies is transmitted only when the virus is introduced into open cuts or wounds in skin or mucous membranes. If there has been no exposure (as described in this section), postexposure treatment is not necessary. Thus, the likelihood that rabies infection will result from exposure to a rabid animal varies with the nature and extent of the exposure. Two categories of exposure should be considered:

Bite: any penetration of the skin by teeth. Bites to the face and hands carry the highest risk, but the site of the bite should not influence the decision to begin treatment.[22]

Bat-associated strains of rabies can be transmitted to humans either directly through a bat's bite or indirectly through the bite of an animal previously infected by a bat. Because some bat bites may be less severe, and can go completely undetected, unlike bites inflicted by larger animals, especially mammalian carnivores, rabies postexposure treatment should be considered for any physical contact with bats when bite or mucous membrane contact cannot be excluded.[23]

Nonbite: scratches, abrasions, open wounds or mucous membranes contaminated with saliva or any potentially infectious material, such as brain tissue, from a rabid animal constitute nonbite exposures. If the material containing the virus is dry, the virus can be considered noninfectious. Casual contact, such as petting a rabid animal and contact with the blood, urine, or feces (e.g., guano) of a rabid animal, does not constitute an exposure and is not an indication for prophylaxis. Instances of airborne rabies have been reported rarely. Adherence to respiratory precautions will minimize the risk of airborne exposure.[24]

The only documented cases of rabies from human-to-human transmission have occurred in patients who received corneas transplanted from persons who died of rabies undiagnosed at the time of death. Stringent guidelines for acceptance of donor corneas have reduced this risk.

Bite and nonbite exposures from humans with rabies theoretically could transmit rabies, although no cases of rabies acquired this way have been documented.

4. Vaccination Status of Biting Animal

A properly immunized animal has only a minimal chance of developing rabies and transmitting the virus.

5. Presence of Rabies in Region

If adequate laboratory and field records indicate that there is no rabies infection in a domestic species within a given region, local health officials are justified in considering this in making recommendations on antirabies treatment following a bite by that particular species. Such officials should be consulted for current interpretations.

Rabies Postexposure Prophylaxis

The following recommendations are only a guide. In applying them, take into account the animal species involved, the circumstances of the bite or other exposure, the vaccination status of the animal, and presence of rabies in the region. Local or state public health officials should be consulted if questions arise about the need for rabies prophylaxis.

Local Treatment of Wounds: Immediate and thorough washing of all bite wounds and scratches with soap and water is perhaps the most effective measure for preventing rabies. In experimental animals, simple local wound cleansing has been shown to reduce markedly the likelihood of rabies.

Tetanus prophylaxis and measures to control bacterial infection should be given as indicated.

Active Immunization: Active immunization should be initiated as soon as possible after exposure. Many dosage schedules have been evaluated for the currently available rabies vaccines and their respective manufacturers' literature should be consulted.

Passive Immunization: A combination of active and passive immunization (vaccine and immune globulin) is considered the acceptable postexposure prophylaxis except for those persons who have been previously immunized with rabies vaccine and who have documented adequate rabies antibody titer. These individuals should receive vaccine only. For passive immunization, Rabies Immune

Globulin (Human) is preferred over antirabies serum, equine.[16,17] It is recommended both for treatment of all bites by animals suspected of having rabies and for non-bite exposure inflicted by animals suspected of being rabid. Rabies Immune Globulin (Human) should be used in conjunction with rabies vaccine and can be administered through the seventh day after the first dose of vaccine is given. Beyond the seventh day, Rabies Immune Globulin (Human) is not indicated since an antibody response to cell culture vaccine is presumed to have occurred.

[See table at top of previous page]

CONTRAINDICATIONS

None known.

WARNINGS

Rabies Immune Globulin (Human)—BayRab® is made from human plasma. Products made from human plasma may contain infectious agents, such as viruses, that can cause disease. The risk that such products will transmit an infectious agent has been reduced by screening plasma donors for prior exposure to certain viruses, by testing for the presence of certain current virus infections, and by inactivating and/or removing certain viruses. Despite these measures, such products can still potentially transmit disease. There is also the possibility that unknown infectious agents may be present in such products. Individuals who receive infusions of blood or plasma products may develop signs and/or symptoms of some viral infections, particularly hepatitis C. ALL infections thought by a physician possibly to have been transmitted by this product should be reported by the physician or other healthcare provider to Bayer Corporation [1-800-765-3203].

The physician should discuss the risks and benefits of this product with the patient, before prescribing or administering it to the patient.

Rabies Immune Globulin (Human) - BayRab® should be given with caution to patients with a history of prior systemic allergic reactions following the administration of human immunoglobulin preparations.

The attending physician who wishes to administer BayRab to persons with isolated immunoglobulin A (IgA) deficiency must weigh the benefits of immunization against the potential risks of hypersensitivity reactions. Such persons have increased potential for developing antibodies to IgA and could have anaphylactic reactions to subsequent administration of blood products that contain IgA.[25]

As with all preparations administered by the intramuscular route, bleeding complications may be encountered in patients with thrombocytopenia or other bleeding disorders.

PRECAUTIONS

General

BayRab should **not** be administered intravenously because of the potential for serious reactions. Although systemic reactions to immunoglobulin preparations are rare, epinephrine should be available for treatment of acute anaphylactoid symptoms.

Drug Interactions

Repeated doses of Rabies Immune Globulin (Human) - BayRab® should not be administered once vaccine treatment has been initiated as this could prevent the full expression of active immunity expected from the rabies vaccine.

Other antibodies in the BayRab preparation may interfere with the response to live vaccines such as measles, mumps, polio or rubella. Therefore, immunization with live vaccines should not be given within 3 months after BayRab administration.

Pregnancy Category C

Animal reproduction studies have not been conducted with BayRab. It is also not known whether BayRab can cause fetal harm when administered to a pregnant woman or can affect reproduction capacity. BayRab should be given to a pregnant woman only if clearly needed.

Pediatric Use

Safety and effectiveness in the pediatric population have not been established.

ADVERSE REACTIONS

Soreness at the site of injection and mild temperature elevations may be observed at times. Sensitization to repeated injections has occurred occasionally in immunoglobulin-deficient patients. Angioneurotic edema, skin rash, nephrotic syndrome, and anaphylactic shock have rarely been reported after intramuscular injection, so that a causal relationship between immunoglobulin and these reactions is not clear.

DOSAGE AND ADMINISTRATION

The recommended dose for BayRab is 20 IU/kg (0.133 mL/kg) of body weight given preferably at the time of the first vaccine dose.[8,9] If anatomically feasible, up to the full dose of BayRab should be thoroughly infiltrated in the area around the wound and the rest should be administered intramuscularly in the gluteal area. Because of risk of injury to the sciatic nerve, the central region of the gluteal area MUST be avoided; only the upper, outer quadrant should be used.[26] BayRab should never be administered in the same syringe or into the same anatomical site as vaccine.

Parenteral drug products should be inspected visually for particulate matter and discoloration prior to administration, whenever solution and container permit.

[See table above]

Rabies postexposure prophylaxis schedule—United States, 1999[19]

Vaccination status	Treatment	Regimen*
Not previously vaccinated	Wound cleansing	All postexposure treatment should begin with immediate thorough cleansing of all wounds with soap and water. If available, a virucidal agent such as povidone-iodine solution should be used to irrigate the wounds.
	RIG	Administer 20 IU/kg body weight. If anatomically feasible, the full dose should be infiltrated around the wound(s) and any remaining volume should be administered IM at an anatomical site distant from vaccine administration. Also, RIG should not be administered in the same syringe as vaccine. Because RIG might partially suppress active production of antibody, no more than the recommended dose should be given.
	Vaccine	HDCV, RVA, or PCEC 1.0 mL, IM (deltoid area†), one each on days 0 §, 3, 7, 14, and 28.
Previously vaccinated¶	Wound cleansing	All postexposure treatment should begin with immediate thorough cleansing of all wounds with soap and water. If available, a virucidal agent such as a povidone-iodine solution should be used to irrigate the wounds.
	RIG	RIG should **not** be administered.
	Vaccine	HDCV, RVA, or PCEC 1.0 mL, IM (deltoid area†), one each on days 0 §and 3.

HDCV = human diploid cell vaccine; PCEC = purified chick embryo cell vaccine; RIG = rabies immune globulin; RVA = rabies vaccine adsorbed; IM, intramuscular

* These regimens are applicable for all age groups, including children.

† The deltoid area is the only acceptable site of vaccination for adults and older children. For younger children, the outer aspect of the thigh may be used. Vaccine should never be administered in the gluteal area.

§ Day 0 is the day the first dose of vaccine is administered.

¶ Any person with a history of preexposure vaccination with HDCV, RVA, or PCEC; prior postexposure prophylaxis with HDCV, RVA, or PCEC; or previous vaccination with any other type of rabies vaccine and a documented history of antibody response to the prior vaccination.

HOW SUPPLIED

BayRab is packaged in 2 mL and 10 mL single dose vials with an average potency value of 150 International Units per mL (IU/ mL). The 2 mL vial contains a total of 300 IU which is sufficient for a child weighing 15 kg. The 10 mL vial contains a total of 1500 IU which is sufficient for an adult weighing 75 kg.

NDC Number	Size
0026-0618-02	2 mL vial
0026-0618-10	10 mL vial

STORAGE

BayRab should be stored under refrigeration (2°–8°C, 36°–46°F). Solution that has been frozen should not be used.

CAUTION

Rx only

U.S. federal law prohibits dispensing without prescription.

LIMITED WARRANTY

A number of factors beyond our control could reduce the efficacy of this product or even result in an ill effect following its use. These include improper storage and handling of the product after it leaves our hands, diagnosis, dosage, method of administration, and biological differences in individual patients. Because of these factors, it is important that this product be stored properly and that the directions be followed carefully during use.

No warranty, express or implied, including any warranty of merchantability or fitness is made. Representatives of the Company are not authorized to vary the terms or the contents of the printed labeling, including the package insert for this product, except by printed notice from the Company's headquarters. The prescriber and user of this product must accept the terms hereof.

REFERENCES

1. Baltazard M, Bahmanyar M, Ghodssi M, et al: Essai pratique du sérum antirabique chez les mordus par loups enragés. *Bull WHO* 13:747–72, 1955.
2. Habel K, Koprowski H: Laboratory data supporting the clinical trial of antirabies serum in persons bitten by a rabid wolf. *Bull WHO* 13:773–9, 1955.
3. Selimov M, Boltucij L, Semenova E, et al: [The use of antirabies gamma globulin in subjects severely bitten by rabid wolves or other animals.] *J Hyg Epidemiol Microbiol Immunol (Praha)* 3:168–80, 1959.
4. Atanasiu P, Bahmanyar M, Baltazard M, et al: Rabies neutralizing antibody response to different schedules of serum and vaccine inoculations in non-exposed persons. *Bull WHO* 14:593–611, 1956.
5. Atanasiu P, Bahmanyar M, Baltazard M, et al: Rabies neutralizing antibody response to different schedules of serum and vaccine inoculations in non-exposed persons: Part II. *Bull WHO* 17:911–32, 1957.
6. Atanasiu P, Cannon DA, Dean DJ, et al: Rabies neutralizing antibody response to different schedules of serum and vaccine inoculations in non-exposed persons: Part 3. *Bull WHO* 25:103–14, 1961.
7. Atanasiu P, Dean DJ, Habel K, et al: Rabies neutralizing antibody response to different schedules of serum and vaccine inoculations in non-exposed persons: Part 4. *Bull WHO* 36:361–5, 1967.
8. Cabasso VJ, Loofbourow JC, Roby RE, et al: Rabies immune globulin of human origin: preparation and dosage determination in non-exposed volunteer subjects. *Bull WHO* 45:303–15, 1971.
9. Loofbourow JC, Cabasso VJ, Roby RE, et al: Rabies immune globulin (human): clinical trials and dose determination. *JAMA* 217(13): 1825–31, 1971.
10. Plotkin SA: New rabies vaccine halts disease — without severe reactions. *Mod Med* 45(20):45–8, 1977.
11. Plotkin SA, Wiktor TJ, Koprowski H, et al: Immunization schedules for the new human diploid cell vaccine against rabies. *Am J Epidemiol* 103(1):75–80, 1976.
12. Hafkin B, Hattwick MA, Smith JS, et al: A comparison of a WI-38 vaccine and duck embryo vaccine for preexposure rabies prophylaxis. *Am J Epidemiol* 107(5):439–43, 1978.
13. Kuwert EK, Marcus I, Höher PG; Neutralizing and complement-fixing antibody responses in pre- and post-exposure vaccinees to a rabies vaccine produced in human diploid cells. *J Biol Stand* 4(4):249–62, 1976.
14. Grandien M: Evaluation of tests for rabies antibody and analysis of serum responses after administration of three different types of rabies vaccines. *J Clin Microbiol* 5(3):263–7, 1977.
15. Kuwert EK, Marcus I, Werner J, et al: Postexpositionelle Schutzimpfung des Menschen gegen Tollwut mit einer neuentwickelten Gewebekulturvakzine (HDCS-Impfstoff). *Zentralbl Bakteriol [A]* 239(4):437–58, 1977.
16. Bahmanyar M, Fayaz A, Nour-Salehi S, et al: Successful protection of humans exposed to rabies infection: postexposure treatment with the new human diploid cell rabies vaccine and antirabies serum. *JAMA* 236(24): 2751–4, 1976.
17. American Hospital Formulary Services Drug Information Section 80:04 Rabies Immune Globulin, Bethesda. American Society for Health System Pharmacy 1997, P2545–47.
18. Rubin Rh, Sikes RK, Gregg MB: Human rabies immune globulin. Clinical trials and effects on serum anti-globulins. *JAMA*224:871–4, 1973.
19. Recommendations of the Immunization Practices Advisory Committee (ACIP): Rabies prevention—United States, 1999. *MMWR* 48(RR-1):1–21, 1999.
20. Reid-Sanden FL, Dobbins JG, Smith JS, et al: Rabies surveillance in the United States during 1989. *J Am Vet Med Assoc* 197(12):1571–83, 1990.
21. Fishbein DB, Belotto AJ, Pacer RE, et al: Rabies in rodents and lagomorphs in the United States, 1971–1984: increased cases in the woodchuck (*Marmota monax*) in mid-Atlantic states. *J Wildl Dis* 22(2):151–5, 1986.
22. Hattwick MAW: Human rabies. *Public Health Rev* 3(3): 229–74, 1974.
23. Epidemiologic Notes and Reports: Human Rabies—California, 1994. *MMWR* 43(25):455–457, 1994.
24. Garner JS, Simmons BP: Guideline for isolation precautions in hospitals. *Infect Control.* 4 (4 Suppl): 245–325, 1983.
25. Fudenberg HH: Sensitization to immunoglobulins and hazards of gamma globulin therapy. In: Merler E (ed.): Immunoglobulins: biologic aspects and clinical uses. Washington, DC, Nat Acad Sci, 1970, pp 211–20.

Continued on next page

BayRab—Cont.

26. Recommendations of the Immunization Practices Advisory Committee (ACIP): General recommendations on immunization. *MMWR* 38(13):205–14; 219–27, 1989.

BAYRHO-D® Mini-Dose ℞

[*bāy "rō-d*]

Rh_o(D) Immune Globulin (Human)

DESCRIPTION

Rh_o(D) Immune Globulin (Human) — BayRho-D® Mini-Dose treated with solvent/detergent is a sterile solution of immune globulin containing antibodies to Rh_o(D) for intramuscular administration; it contains no preservative. BayRho-D Mini-Dose is prepared by cold ethanol fractionation from human plasma. The immune globulin is isolated from solubilized Cohn Fraction II. The Fraction II solution is adjusted to a final concentration of 0.3% tri-n-butyl phosphate (TNBP) and 0.2% sodium cholate. After the addition of solvent (TNBP) and detergent (sodium cholate), the solution is heated to 30°C and maintained at that temperature for not less than 6 hours. After the viral inactivation step, the reactants are removed by precipitation, filtration and finally ultrafiltration and diafiltration. BayRho-D Mini-Dose is then incubated in the final container for 21–28 days at 20–27°C. BayRho-D Mini-Dose is formulated as a 15–18% protein solution at a pH of 6.4–7.2 in 0.21–0.32 M glycine. One dose of BayRho-D Mini-Dose contains not less than one-sixth the quantity of Rh_o(D) antibody contained in one standard dose of Rh_o(D) Immune Globulin (Human), and it will suppress the immunizing potential of 2.5 mL of Rh_o(D) positive packed red blood cells or the equivalent of whole blood (5 mL). The quantity of Rh_o(D) antibody in BayRho-D Mini-Dose is not less than one-sixth of that contained in 1 mL of the U.S. Food and Drug Administration Reference Rh_o(D) Immune Globulin (Human).

The removal and inactivation of spiked model enveloped and non-enveloped viruses during the manufacturing process for BayRho-D Mini-Dose has been validated in laboratory studies. Human Immunodeficiency Virus, Type 1 (HIV-1), was chosen as the relevant virus for blood products; Bovine Viral Diarrhea Virus (BVDV) was chosen to model Hepatitis C virus; Pseudorabies virus (PRV) was chosen to model Hepatitis B virus and the Herpes viruses; and Reo virus type 3 (Reo) was chosen to model non-enveloped viruses and for its resistance to physical and chemical inactivation. Significant removal of model enveloped and non-enveloped viruses is achieved at two steps in the Cohn fractionation process leading to the collection of Cohn Fraction II: the precipitation and removal of Fraction III in the processing of Fraction II + IIIW suspension to Effluent III and the filtration step in the processing of Effluent III to Filtrate III. Significant inactivation of enveloped viruses is achieved at the time of treatment of solubilized Cohn Fraction II with TNBP/sodium cholate.

CLINICAL PHARMACOLOGY

Rh sensitization may occur in nonsensitized Rh_o(D) negative women following transplacental hemorrhage resulting from spontaneous or induced abortions.[1–2] The risk of sensitization is higher in women undergoing induced abortions than in those aborting spontaneously.[1–3]

BayRho-D Mini-Dose is used to prevent the formation of anti-Rh_o(D) antibody in Rh_o(D) negative women who are exposed to the Rh_o(D) antigen at the time of spontaneous or induced abortion (up to 12 weeks' gestation).[3–5] BayRho-D Mini-Dose suppresses the stimulation of active immunity by Rh_o(D) positive fetal erythrocytes that may enter the maternal circulation at the time of termination of the pregnancy. The amount of anti-Rh_o(D) in BayRho-D Mini-Dose has been shown to effectively prevent maternal isosensitization to the Rh_o(D) antigens following spontaneous or induced abortion occurring up to the 12th week of gestation.[6–8] After the 12th week of gestation, a standard dose of BayRho-D™ Full Dose is indicated.

In a clinical study in eight healthy human adults receiving another hyperimmune immune globulin product treated with solvent/detergent, Rabies Immune Globulin (Human), BayRab™, prepared by the same manufacturing process, detectable passive antibody titers were observed in the serum of all subjects by 24 hours post injection and persisted through the 21 day study period. These results suggest that passive immunization with immune globulin products is not affected by the solvent/detergent treatment.

INDICATIONS AND USAGE

Rh_o(D) Immune Globulin (Human)—BayRho-D® Mini-Dose is recommended to prevent the isoimmunization of Rh_o(D) negative women at the time of spontaneous or induced abortion of up to 12 weeks' gestation provided the following criteria are met:

1. The mother must be Rh_o(D) negative and must not already be sensitized to the Rh_o(D) antigen.
2. The father is not known to be Rh_o(D) negative.
3. Gestation is not more than 12 weeks at termination.

Note: Rh_o(D) Immune Globulin (Human) prophylaxis is not indicated if the fetus or father can be determined to be Rh negative. If the Rh status of the fetus is unknown, the fetus must be assumed to be Rh_o(D) positive, and BayRho-D Mini-Dose should be administered to the mother.

FOR ABORTIONS OR MISCARRIAGES OCCURRING AFTER 12 WEEKS' GESTATION, A STANDARD DOSE OF RH_O(D) IMMUNE GLOBULIN (HUMAN), IS INDICATED.

BayRho-D Mini-Dose should be administered within 3 hours or as soon as possible after spontaneous passage or surgical removal of the products of conception. However, if BayRho-D Mini-Dose is not given within this time period, consideration should still be given to its administration since clinical studies in male volunteers have demonstrated the effectiveness of Rh_o(D) Immune Globulin (Human), in preventing isoimmunization as long as 72 hours after infusion of Rh_o(D) positive red cells.[9]

CONTRAINDICATIONS

None known.

WARNINGS

BayRho-D Mini-Dose is made from human plasma. Products made from human plasma may contain infectious agents, such as viruses, that can cause disease. The risk that such products will transmit an infectious agent has been reduced by screening plasma donors for prior exposure to certain viruses, by testing for the presence of certain current virus infections, and by inactivating and/or removing certain viruses. Despite these measures, such products can still potentially transmit disease. There is also the possibility that unknown infectious agents may be present in such products. Individuals who receive infusions of blood or plasma products may develop signs and/or symptoms of some viral infections, particularly hepatitis C. ALL infections thought by a physician possibly to have been transmitted by this product should be reported by the physician or other healthcare provider to Bayer Corporation [1-888-765-3203].

The physician should discuss the risks and benefits of this product with the patient, before prescribing or administering it to the patient.

NEVER ADMINISTER BAYRHO-D MINI-DOSE INTRAVENOUSLY. INJECT ONLY INTRAMUSCULARLY. ADMINISTER ONLY TO WOMEN POST-ABORTION OR POST-MISCARRIAGE OF UP TO 12 WEEKS' GESTATION. NEVER ADMINISTER TO THE NEONATE.

BayRho-D Mini-Dose should be given with caution to patients with a history of prior systemic allergic reactions following the administration of human immune globulin preparations.

The attending physician who wishes to administer BayRho-D Mini-Dose to persons with isolated immunoglobulin A (IgA) deficiency must weigh the benefits of immunization against the potential risks of hypersensitivity reactions. Such persons have increased potential for developing antibodies to IgA and could have anaphylactic reactions to subsequent administration of blood products that contain IgA.

As with all preparations administered by the intramuscular route, bleeding complications may be encountered in patients with thrombocytopenia or other bleeding disorders.

PRECAUTIONS

General

Although systemic reactions to immunoglobulin preparations are rare, epinephrine should be available for treatment of acute anaphylactic symptoms.

Drug Interactions

Other antibodies in the Rh_o(D) Immune Globulin (Human)—BayRho-D® Mini-Dose preparation may interfere with the response to live vaccines such as measles, mumps, polio or rubella. Therefore, immunization with live vaccines should not be given within 3 months after BayRho-D Mini-Dose administration.

Pregnancy Category C

Animal reproduction studies have not been conducted with BayRho-D Mini-Dose. It is also not known whether BayRho-D Mini-Dose can cause fetal harm when administered to a pregnant woman or can affect reproduction capacity.

It should be again noted, however, that BayRho-D Mini-Dose is **not** indicated for use during pregnancy and it should be administered only post-abortion or post-miscarriage.

Pediatric Use

Safety and effectiveness in the pediatric population have not been established.

ADVERSE REACTIONS

Reactions to $BayRh_o$-D Mini-Dose are infrequent in Rh_o (D) negative individuals and consist primarily of slight soreness at the site of injection and slight temperature elevation. While sensitization to repeated injections of human globulin is extremely rare, it has occurred.

DOSAGE AND ADMINISTRATION

One syringe of BayRho-D Mini-Dose provides sufficient antibody to prevent Rh sensitization to 2.5 mL Rh_o(D) positive packed red cells or the equivalent (5 mL) of whole blood. This dose is sufficient to provide protection against maternal Rh sensitization for women undergoing spontaneous or induced abortion of up to 12 weeks' gestation.

BayRho-D Mini-Dose should be administered within 3 hours or as soon as possible following spontaneous or induced abortion. If prompt administration is not possible, BayRho-D Mini-Dose should be given within 72 hours following termination of the pregnancy.

BayRho-D Mini-Dose is administered **intramuscularly**, preferably in the anterolateral aspects of the upper thigh and the deltoid muscle of the upper arm. The gluteal region should not be used routinely as an injection site because of the risk of injury to the sciatic nerve. If the gluteal region is used, the central region must be avoided; only the upper, outer quadrant should be used.[10]

Parenteral drug products should be inspected visually for particulate matter and discoloration prior to administration, whenever solution and container permit.

Directions for Syringe Usage

1. Remove the prefilled syringe from the package. Lift syringe by barrel, **not** by plunger.
2. Twist the plunger rod clockwise until the threads are seated.
3. With the rubber needle shield secured on the syringe tip, push the plunger rod forward a few millimeters to break any friction seal between the rubber stopper and the glass syringe barrel.
4. Remove the needle shield and expel air bubbles.
5. Proceed with hypodermic needle puncture.
6. Aspirate prior to injection to confirm that the needle is not in a vein or artery.
7. Inject the medication.
8. Withdraw the needle and dispose or destroy it.

HOW SUPPLIED

BayRho-D Mini-Dose package contains 10 single dose syringes

NDC Number	Size
0026-0631-05	Syringe (10 pack)

STORAGE

Store at 2°–8°C (36°–46°F). Do not freeze.

CAUTION

U.S. federal law prohibits dispensing without prescription.

LIMITED WARRANTY

A number of factors beyond our control could reduce the efficacy of this product or even result in an ill effect following its use. These include improper storage and handling of the product after it leaves our hands, diagnosis, dosage, method of administration, and biological differences in individual patients. Because of these factors, it is important that this product be stored properly and that the directions be followed carefully during use.

No warranty, express or implied, including any warranty of merchantability or fitness is made. Representatives of the Company are not authorized to vary the terms or the contents of the printed labeling, including the package insert for this product, except by printed notice from the Company's headquarters. The prescriber and user of this product must accept the terms hereof.

REFERENCES

1. Queenan JT, Shah S, Kubarych SF, *et al:* Role of induced abortion in rhesus immunisation. *Lancet* 1(7704): 815–7, 1971.
2. Goldman JA, Eckerling B: Prevention of Rh immunization after abortion with anti-Rh_o(D)-immunoglobulin. *Obstet Gynecol* 40(3):366–70, 1972.
3. The selective use of Rho(D) immune globulin (RhIG). *ACOG Tech Bull* 61, 1981.
4. Prevention of Rh sensitization. *WHO Tech Rep Ser* 468, 1971.
5. Recommendation of the Public Health Service Advisory Committee on Immunization Practices: Rh immune globulin. *MMWR* 21(15):126–7, 1972.
6. Stewart FH, Burnhill MS, Bozorgi N: Reduced dose of Rh immunoglobulin following first trimester pregnancy termination. *Obstet Gynecol* 51(3):318–22, 1978.
7. McMaster conference on prevention of Rh immunization, 28-30 September, 1977. *Vox Sang* 36(1):50–64, 1979.
8. Simonovits I: Efficiency of anti-D IgG prevention after induced abortion. *Vox Sang* 26(4):361–7, 1974.
9. Freda VJ, Gorman JG, Pollack W: Prevention of Rh-hemolytic disease with Rh-immune globulin. *Am J Obstet Gynecol* 128(4):456–60, 1977.
10. Recommendations of the Immunization Practices Advisory Committee (ACIP): General recommendations on immunization. *MMWR* 38(13):205–14; 219–27, 1989.

BAYRHO-D® Full Dose ℞

[*bāy "rhō-d*]

Rh_o(D) Immune Globulin (Human)

DESCRIPTION

Rh_o(D) Immune Globulin (Human) — BayRho-D® Full Dose treated with solvent/detergent is a sterile solution of immune globulin containing antibodies to Rh_o(D) for intramuscular administration; it contains no preservative. BayRho-D Full Dose is prepared by cold ethanol fractionation from human plasma. The immune globulin is isolated from solubilized Cohn fraction II. The fraction II solution is adjusted to a final concentration of 0.3% tri-n-butyl phosphate (TNBP) and 0.2% sodium cholate. After the addition of solvent (TNBP) and detergent (sodium cholate), the solution is heated to 30°C and maintained at that temperature for not less than 6 hours. After the viral inactivation step, the reactants are removed by precipitation, filtration and finally ultrafiltration and diafiltration. BayRho-D Full Dose is formulated as a 15–18% protein solution at a pH of 6.4–7.2 in 0.21–0.32 M glycine. BayRho-D Full Dose is then incubated in the final container for 21–28 days at 20–27°C. The potency is equal to or greater than that of the U.S. Food and Drug Administration Reference $Rh_o(D)$ Immune Globulin. Each single dose vial or syringe contains sufficient anti-$Rh_o(D)$ (approximately 300 µg*) to effectively suppress the immunizing potential of 15 mL of $Rh_o(D)$ positive red blood cells.[2–4]

The removal and inactivation of spiked model enveloped and non-enveloped viruses during the manufacturing process for BayRho-D Full Dose has been validated in laboratory studies. Human Immunodeficiency Virus, Type 1 (HIV-1), was chosen as the relevant virus for blood products; Bovine Viral Diarrhea Virus (BVDV) was chosen to model Hepatitis C virus; Pseudorabies virus (PRV) was chosen to model Hepatitis B virus and the Herpes viruses; and Reo virus type 3 (Reo) was chosen to model non-enveloped viruses and for its resistance to physical and chemical inactivation. Significant removal of model enveloped and non-enveloped viruses is achieved at two steps in the Cohn fractionation process leading to the collection of Cohn Fraction II: the precipitation and removal of Fraction III in the processing of Fraction II + IIIW suspension to Effluent III and the filtration step in the processing of Effluent III to Filtrate III. Significant inactivation of enveloped viruses is achieved at the time of treatment of solubilized Cohn Fraction II with TNBP/sodium cholate.

---

*A full dose of $Rh_o(D)$ Immune Globulin (Human), has traditionally been referred to as a "300 µg" dose and this usage is employed here for convenience in terminology. **It should not be construed as the actual anti-D content.** Each full dose of $Rh_o(D)$ Immune Globulin (Human), must contain at least as much anti-D as 1 mL of the U.S. Reference $Rh_o(D)$ Immune Globulin. Studies performed at the FDA have shown that the U.S. Reference contains 820 international units (IU) of anti-D per mL. When the conversion factor determined for the International (WHO) Reference Preparation[1] is used, 820 IU per mL is equivalent to 164 µg per mL of anti-D.

CLINICAL PHARMACOLOGY

BayRho-D Full Dose is used to prevent isoimmunization in the $Rh_o(D)$ negative individual exposed to $Rh_o(D)$ positive blood as a result of a fetomaternal hemorrhage occurring during a delivery of an $Rh_o(D)$ positive infant, abortion (either spontaneous or induced), or following amniocentesis or abdominal trauma. Similarly, immunization resulting in the production of anti-$Rh_o(D)$ following transfusion of Rh positive red cells to an $Rh_o(D)$ negative recipient may be prevented by administering $Rh_o(D)$ Immune Globulin (Human).[5,6]

Rh hemolytic disease of the newborn is the result of the active immunization of an $Rh_o(D)$ negative mother by $Rh_o(D)$ positive red cells entering the maternal circulation during a previous delivery, abortion, amniocentesis, abdominal trauma, or as a result of red cell transfusion.[7,8] BayRho-D Full Dose acts by suppressing the immune response of $Rh_o(D)$ negative individuals to $Rh_o(D)$ positive red blood cells. The mechanism of action of BayRho-D Full Dose is not fully understood.

The administration of $Rh_o(D)$ Immune Globulin (Human), within 72 hours of a full-term delivery of an $Rh_o(D)$ positive infant by an $Rh_o(D)$ negative mother reduces the incidence of Rh isoimmunization from 12%–13% to 1%–2%.[9]

The 1%–2% treatment failures are probably due to isoimmunization occurring during the latter part of pregnancy or following delivery.[10] Bowman and Pollock[11] have reported that the incidence of isoimmunization can be further reduced from approximately 1.6% to less than 0.1% by administering $Rh_o(D)$ Immune Globulin (Human) in two doses, one antenatal at 28 weeks' gestation and another following delivery.

In a clinical study in eight healthy human adults receiving another hyperimmune immune globulin product treated with solvent/detergent, Rabies Immune Globulin (Human), BayRab®, prepared by the same manufacturing process, detectable passive antibody titers were observed in the serum of all subjects by 24 hours post injection and persisted through the 21 day study period. These results suggest that passive immunization with immune globulin products is not affected by the solvent/detergent treatment.

INDICATIONS AND USAGE

Pregnancy and Other Obstetric Conditions

$Rh_o(D)$ Immune Globulin (Human), BayRho-D® Full Dose is recommended for the prevention of Rh hemolytic disease of the newborn by its administration to the $Rh_o(D)$ negative mother within 72 hours after birth of an $Rh_o(D)$ positive infant,[12] providing the following criteria are met:

1. The mother must be $Rh_o(D)$ negative, and must not already be sensitized to the $Rh_o(D)$ factor.
2. Her child must be $Rh_o(D)$ positive, and should have a negative direct antiglobulin test (see PRECAUTIONS).

If BayRho-D Full Dose is administered antepartum, it is essential that the mother receive another dose of BayRho-D Full Dose after delivery of an $Rh_o(D)$ positive infant.

If the father can be determined to be $Rh_o(D)$ negative, BayRho-D Full Dose need not be given.

BayRho-D Full Dose should be administered within 72 hours to all nonimmunized $Rh_o(D)$ negative women who have undergone spontaneous or induced abortion, following ruptured tubal pregnancy, amniocentesis or abdominal trauma unless the blood group of the fetus or the father is known to be $Rh_o(D)$ negative.[7,8] If the fetal blood group cannot be determined, one must assume that it is $Rh_o(D)$ positive,[2] and BayRho-D Full Dose should be administered to the mother.

Transfusion

BayRho-D Full Dose may be used to prevent isoimmunization in $Rh_o(D)$ negative individuals who have been transfused with $Rh_o(D)$ positive red blood cells or blood components containing red blood cells.[5,13]

CONTRAINDICATIONS

None known.

WARNINGS

$Rh_o(D)$ Immune Globulin (Human)—BayRho-D® full dose is made from human plasma. Products made from human plasma may contain infectious agents, such as viruses, that can cause disease. The risk that such products will transmit an infectious agent has been reduced by screening plasma donors for prior exposure to certain viruses, by testing for the presence of certain current virus infections, and by inactivating and/or removing certain viruses. Despite these measures, such products can still potentially transmit disease. There is also the possibility that unknown infectious agents may be present in such products. Individuals who receive infusions of blood or plasma products may develop signs and/or symptoms of some viral infections, particularly hepatitis C. ALL infections thought by a physician possibly to have been transmitted by this product should be reported by the physician or other healthcare provider to Bayer Corporation [1-888-765-3203].

The physician should discuss the risks and benefits of this product with the patient, before prescribing or administering it to the patient.

NEVER ADMINISTER BAYRHO-D FULL DOSE INTRAVENOUSLY. INJECT ONLY INTRAMUSCULARLY. NEVER ADMINISTER TO THE NEONATE.

$Rh_o(D)$ Immune Globulin (Human) should be given with caution to patients with a history of prior systemic allergic reactions following the administration of human immunoglobulin preparations.

The attending physician who wishes to administer $Rh_o(D)$ Immune Globulin (Human) to persons with isolated immunoglobulin A (IgA) deficiency must weigh the benefits of immunization against the potential risks of hypersensitivity reactions. Such persons have increased potential for developing antibodies to IgA and could have anaphylactic reactions to subsequent administration of blood products that contain IgA.

As with all preparations administered by the intramuscular route, bleeding complications may be encountered in patients with thrombocytopenia or other bleeding disorders.

PRECAUTIONS

General

A large fetomaternal hemorrhage late in pregnancy or following delivery may cause a weak mixed field positive D^u test result. If there is any doubt about the mother's Rh type, she should be given $Rh_o(D)$ Immune Globulin (Human). A screening test to detect fetal red blood cells may be helpful in such cases.

If more than 15 mL of D-positive fetal red blood cells are present in the mother's circulation, more than a single dose of $Rh_o(D)$ Immune Globulin (Human), BayRho-D® Full Dose is required. Failure to recognize this may result in the administration of an inadequate dose.

Although systemic reactions to human immunoglobulin preparations are rare, epinephrine should be available for treatment of acute anaphylactic reactions.

Drug Interactions

Other antibodies in the $Rh_o(D)$ Immune Globulin (Human) preparation may interfere with the response to live vaccines such as measles, mumps, polio or rubella. Therefore, immunization with live vaccines should not be given within 3 months after $Rh_o(D)$ Immune Globulin (Human) administration.

Drug/Laboratory Interactions

Babies born of women given $Rh_o(D)$ Immune Globulin (Human) antepartum may have a weakly positive direct antiglobulin test at birth.

Passively acquired anti-$Rh_o(D)$ may be detected in maternal serum if antibody screening tests are performed subsequent to antepartum or postpartum administration of $Rh_o(D)$ Immune Globulin (Human).

Pregnancy Category C

Animal reproduction studies have not been conducted with BayRho-D Full Dose. It is also not known whether BayRho-D Full Dose can cause fetal harm when administered to a pregnant woman or can affect reproduction capacity. BayRho-D Full Dose should be given to a pregnant woman only if clearly needed.

Pediatric Use

Safety and effectiveness in the pediatric population have not been established.

ADVERSE REACTIONS

Reactions to $Rh_o(D)$ Immune Globulin (Human) are infrequent in $Rh_o(D)$ negative individuals and consist primarily of slight soreness at the site of injection and slight temperature elevation. While sensitization to repeated injections of human immune globulin is extremely rare, it has occurred. Elevated bilirubin levels have been reported in some individuals receiving multiple doses of $Rh_o(D)$ Immune Globulin (Human) following mismatched tranfusions. This is believed to be due to a relatively rapid rate of foreign red cell destruction.

DOSAGE AND ADMINISTRATION

NEVER ADMINISTER BAYRHO-D FULL DOSE INTRAVENOUSLY. INJECT ONLY INTRAMUSCULARLY. NEVER ADMINISTER TO THE NEONATE.

Pregnancy and Other Obstetric Conditions

1. For postpartum prophylaxis, administer one vial or syringe of BayRho-D Full Dose (300 µg*), preferably within 72 hours of delivery. Although a lesser degree of protection is afforded if Rh antibody is administered beyond the 72-hour period, BayRho-D Full Dose may still be given.[7,14] Full-term deliveries can vary in their dosage requirements depending on the magnitude of the fetomaternal hemorrhage. One 300 µg* vial or syringe of BayRho-D Full Dose provides sufficient antibody to prevent Rh sensitization if the volume of red blood cells that has entered the circulation is 15 mL or less.[2–4] In instances where a large (greater than 30 mL of whole blood or 15 mL red blood cells) fetomaternal hemorrhage is suspected, a fetal red cell count by an approved laboratory technique (e.g., modified Kleihauer-Betke acid elution stain technique) should be performed to determine the dosage of immune globulin required.[8,15] The red blood cell volume of the calculated fetomaternal hemorrhage is divided by 15 mL to obtain the number of vials or syringes of $Rh_o(D)$ Immune Globulin (Human), BayRho-D® Full Dose for administration.[3,8,13] If more than 15 mL of red cells is suspected or if the dose calculation results in a fraction, administer the next higher whole number of vials or syringes (e.g., if 1.4, give 2 vials or syringes).
2. For antenatal prophylaxis, one 300 µg* vial or syringe of BayRho-D Full Dose is administered at approximately 28 weeks' gestation. This **must** be followed by another 300 µg* dose, preferably within 72 hours following delivery, if the infant is Rh positive.
3. Following threatened abortion at any stage of gestation with continuation of pregnancy, it is recommended that 300 µg* of BayRho-D Full Dose be given. If more than 15 mL of red cells is suspected due to fetomaternal hemorrhage, the same dose modification in No. 1 above applies.
4. Following miscarriage, abortion, or termination of ectopic pregnancy at or beyond 13 weeks' gestation, it is recommended that 300 µg* of BayRho-D Full Dose be given. If more than 15 mL of red blood cells is suspected due to fetomaternal hemorrhage, the same dose modification in No. 1 above applies. If pregnancy is terminated prior to 13 weeks' gestation, a single dose of BayRho-D Mini-Dose (approximately 50 µg*) may be used instead of BayRho-D Full Dose.
5. Following amniocentesis at either 15 to 18 weeks' gestation or during the third trimester, or following abdominal trauma in the second or third trimester, it is recommended that 300 µg* of BayRho-D Full Dose be administered. If there is a fetomaternal hemorrhage in excess of 15 mL of red cells, the same dose modification in No. 1 applies.

If abdominal trauma, amniocentesis, or other adverse event requires the administration of BayRho-D Full Dose at 13 to 18 weeks'gestation, another 300 µg* dose should be given at 26 to 28 weeks. To maintain protection throughout pregnancy, the level of passively acquired anti-$Rh_o(D)$ should not be allowed to fall below the level required to prevent an immune response to Rh positive red cells. The half-life of IgG is 23 to 26 days. In any case, a dose of BayRho-D Full Dose should be given within 72 hours after delivery if the baby is Rh positive. If delivery occurs within 3 weeks after the last dose, the postpartum dose may be withheld unless there is a fetomaternal hemorrhage in excess of 15 mL of red blood cells.[16]

*See footnote under DESCRIPTION.

Transfusion

In the case of a transfusion of $Rh_o(D)$ positive red cells to an $Rh_o(D)$ negative recipient, the volume of Rh positive whole blood administered is multiplied by the hematocrit of the donor unit giving the volume of red blood cells transfused. The volume of red blood cells is divided by 15 mL which provides the number of vials or syringes of BayRho-D Full Dose to be administered.

If the dose calculated results in a fraction, the next higher whole number of vials or syringes should be administered (e.g., if 1.4, give 2 vials or 2 syringes). BayRho-D Full Dose should be administered within 72 hours after an incompatible transfusion, but preferably as soon as possible.

Injection Procedure

DO NOT INJECT INTRAVENOUSLY. DO NOT INJECT NEONATE. $Rh_o(D)$ Immune Globulin (Human), BayRho-D® Full Dose is administered **intramuscularly,** preferably in the anterolateral aspects of the upper thigh and the deltoid muscle of the upper arm. The gluteal region should not be used routinely as an injection site because of the risk of injury to the sciatic nerve. If the gluteal region is used, the central region MUST be avoided; only the upper, outer quadrant should be used.[17]

Continued on next page

BayRho-D Full-Dose—Cont.

A. Single Vial or Syringe Dose
INJECT ENTIRE CONTENTS OF THE VIAL OR SYRINGE INTO THE INDIVIDUAL INTRAMUSCULARLY.

B. Multiple Vial or Syringe Dose
1. Calculate the number of vials or syringes of BayRho-D Full Dose to be given (see Dosage section above).
2. The total volume of BayRho-D Full Dose can be given in divided doses at different sites at one time or the total dose may be divided and injected at intervals, provided the total dosage is given within 72 hours of the fetomaternal hemorrhage or transfusion. USING STERILE TECHNIQUE, INJECT THE ENTIRE CONTENTS OF THE CALCULATED NUMBER OF VIALS OR SYRINGES INTRAMUSCULARLY INTO THE PATIENT.

Parenteral drug products should be inspected visually for particulate matter and discoloration prior to administration, whenever solution and container permit.

Directions for syringe Usage
1. Remove the prefilled syringe from the package. Lift syringe by barrel, **not** by plunger.
2. Twist the plunger rod clockwise until the threads are seated.
3. With the rubber needle shield secured on the syringe tip, push the plunger rod forward a few millimeters to break any friction seal between the rubber stopper and the glass syringe barrel.
4. Remove the needle shield and expel air bubbles.
5. Proceed with hypodermic needle puncture.
6. Aspirate prior to injection to confirm that the needle is not in a vein or artery.
7. Inject the medication.
8. Withdraw the needle and destroy it.

HOW SUPPLIED

BayRho-D Full Dose is available in individual and multiple-pack single dose syringes with attached needles and vials.

NDC Number	Size
0026-0631-01	Syringe
0026-0631-10	Vial (10 pack)
0026-0631-15	Vial
0026-0631-22	Syringe (10 pack)

STORAGE

Store at 2°–8°C (36°–46°F). Do not freeze.

CAUTION

U.S. federal law prohibits dispensing without prescription.

LIMITED WARRANTY

A number of factors beyond our control could reduce the efficacy of this product or even result in an ill effect following its use. These include improper storage and handling of the product after it leaves our hands, diagnosis, dosage, method of administration, and biological differences in individual patients. Because of these factors, it is important that this product be stored properly and that the directions be followed carefully during use.

No warranty, express or implied, including any warranty of merchantability or fitness is made. Representatives of the Company are not authorized to vary the terms or the contents of any printed labeling, including the package insert for this product, except by printed notice from the Company's headquarters. The prescriber and user of this product must accept the terms hereof.

REFERENCES

1. Gunson HH, Bowell PJ, Kirkwood TBL: Collaborative study to recalibrate the International Reference Preparation of Anti-D Immunoglobulin. *J Clin Pathol* 33:249–53, 1980.
2. Rh_o(D) immune globulin (human). *Med Lett Drugs Ther* 16(1):3–4, 1974.
3. Pollack W, Ascari WQ, Kochesky RJ, et al: Studies on Rh prophylaxis I. Relationship between doses of anti-Rh and size of antigenic stimulus. *Transfusion* 11(6):333–9, 1971.
4. Unpublished data in files of Bayer Corporation.
5. Pollack W, Asceri WQ, Crispen JF, et al: Studies on Rh prophylaxis. II. Rh immune prophylaxis after transfusion with Rh-positive blood. *Transfusion* 11 (6):340–4, 1971.
6. Keith LG, Houser GH: Anti-Rh immune globulin after a massive transfusion accident. *Transfusion* 11(3):176, 1971.
7. The selective use of Rh_o(D) Immune Globulin (RhIG). *ACOG Tech Bull* 61, 1981.
8. Current uses of Rh_o immune globulin and detection of antibodies. *ACOG Tech Bull* 35, 1976.
9. Pollack W: Rh hemolytic disease of the newborn; its cause and prevention. *Prog Clin Biol Res* 70:185–203, 1981.
10. Bowman JM, Chown B, Lewis M, et al: Rh isoimmunization during pregnancy: antenatal prophylaxis. *Can Med Assoc J* 118(6):623–7, 1978.
11. Bowman JM, Pollock JM: Antenatal prophylaxis of Rh isommunization: 28-weeks'-gestation service program. *Can Med Assoc J* 118(6):627–30, 1978.
12. Ascari WQ, Allen AE, Baker WJ, et al: Rh_o(D) immune globulin (human): evaluation in women at risk of Rh immunization. *JAMA* 205(1): 1–4, 1968.
13. Prevention of Rh sensitization, *WHO Tech Rep Ser* 468: 25, 1971.
14. Samson D, Mollison PL: Effect on primary Rh immunization of delayed administration of anti-Rh. *Immunology* 28:349–57, 175.
15. Finn R, Harper DT, Stallings, SA, et al: Transplacental hemorrhage. *Transfusion* 3(2):114–24, 1963.
16. Garraty G (ed): Hemolytic disease of the newborn. Arlington, VA, American Association of Blood Banks, 1984, p 78.
17. Recommendations of the Immunization Practices Advisory Committee (ACIP): General recommendations on immunization. *MMWR* 38(13):205–14; 219–27, 1989.

BAYTET® ℞

[*bāy 'tet "*]
Tetanus Immune Globulin (Human)
250 Units

DESCRIPTION

Tetanus Immune Globulin (Human) — BayTet® treated with solvent/detergent is a sterile solution of tetanus hyperimmune immune globulin for intramuscular administration; it contains no preservative. BayTet is prepared by cold ethanol fractionation from the plasma of donors immunized with tetanus toxoid. The immune globulin is isolated from solubilized Cohn Fraction II. The Fraction II solution is adjusted to a final concentration of 0.3% tri-n-butyl phosphate (TNBP) and 0.2% sodium cholate. After the addition of solvent (TNBP) and detergent (sodium cholate), the solution is heated to 30°C and maintained at that temperature for not less than 6 hours. After the viral inactivation step, the reactants are removed by precipitation, filtration and finally ultrafiltration and diafiltration. BayTet is formulated as a 15–18% protein solution at a pH of 6.4–7.2 in 0.21–0.32 M glycine. BayTet is then incubated in the final container for 21–28 days at 20–27°C. The product is standardized against the U.S. Standard Antitoxin and the U.S. Control Tetanus Toxin and contains not less than 250 tetanus antitoxin units per container.

The removal and inactivation of spiked model enveloped and non-enveloped viruses during the manufacturing process for BayTet has been validated in laboratory studies. Human Immunodeficiency Virus, Type 1 (HIV-1), was chosen as the relevant virus for blood products; Bovine Viral Diarrhea Virus (BVDV) was chosen to model Hepatitis C virus; Pseudorabies virus (PRV) was chosen to model Hepatitis B and the Herpes viruses; and Reo virus type 3 (Reo) was chosen to model non-enveloped viruses and for its resistance to physical and chemical inactivation. Significant removal of model enveloped and non-enveloped viruses is achieved at two steps in the Cohn fractionation process leading to the collection of Cohn Fraction II: the precipitation and removal of Fraction III in the processing of Fraction II + IIIW suspension to Effluent III and the filtration step in the processing of Effluent III to Filtrate III. Significant inactivation of enveloped viruses is achieved at the time of treatment of solubilized Cohn Fraction II with TNBP/sodium cholate.

CLINICAL PHARMACOLOGY

The occurrence of tetanus in the United States has decreased dramatically from 560 reported cases in 1947, when national reporting began, to a record low of 48 reported cases in 1987.[1] The decline has resulted from widespread use of tetanus toxoid and improved wound management, including use of tetanus prophylaxis in emergency rooms.[2]

BayTet supplies passive immunity to those individuals who have low or no immunity to the toxin produced by the tetanus organism, *Clostridium tetani*. The antibodies act to neutralize the free form of the powerful exotoxin produced by this bacterium. Historically, such passive protection was provided by antitoxin derived from equine or bovine serum; however, the foreign protein in these heterologous products often produced severe allergic manifestations, even in individuals who demonstrated negative skin and/or conjunctival tests prior to administration. Estimates of the frequency of these foreign protein reactions following antitoxin of equine origin varied from 5%–30%.[3–6] If passive immunization is needed, human tetanus immune globulin (TIG) is the product of choice. It provides protection longer than antitoxin of animal origin and causes few adverse reactions.[2]

Several studies suggest the value of human tetanus antitoxin in the treatment of active tetanus.[7,8] In 1961 and 1962, Nation et al,[7] using Hyper-Tet® treated 20 patients with tetanus using single doses of 3,000 to 6,000 antitoxin units in combination with other accepted clinical and nursing procedures. Six patients, all over 45 years of age, died of causes other than tetanus. The authors felt that the mortality rate (30%) compared favorably with their previous experience using equine antitoxin in larger doses and that the results were much better than the 60% national death rate for tetanus reported from 1951 to 1954.[9] Blake et al,[10] however, found in a data analysis of 545 cases of tetanus reported to the Centers for Disease Control from 1965 to 1971 that survival was no better with 8,000 units of human tetanus immune globulin (TIG) than with 500 units; however, an optimal dose could not be determined.

Serologic tests indicate that naturally acquired immunity to tetanus toxin does not occur in the United States. Thus, universal primary vaccination, with subsequent maintenance of adequate antitoxin levels by means of appropriately timed boosters, is necessary to protect persons among all age groups. Tetanus toxoid is a highly effective antigen; a completed primary series generally induces protective levels of serum antitoxin that persist for ≥10 years.[2]

Passive immunization with BayTet may be undertaken concomitantly with active immunization using tetanus toxoid in those persons who must receive an immediate injection of tetanus antitoxin and in whom it is desirable to begin the process of active immunization. Based on the work of Rubbo,[11] McComb and Dwyer,[12] and Levine et al, [13] the physician may thus supply immediate passive protection against tetanus, and at the same time begin formation of active immunization in the injured individual which upon completion of a **full toxoid series** will preclude future need for antitoxin.

Peak blood levels of IgG are obtained approximately 2 days after intramuscular injection. The half-life of IgG in the circulation of individuals with normal IgG levels is approximately 23 days.[14]

In a clinical study in eight healthy human adults receiving another hyperimmune immune globulin product treated with solvent/detergent, Rabies Immune Globulin (Human), BayRab™, prepared by the same manufacturing process, detectable passive antibody titers were observed in the serum of all subjects by 24 hours post injection and persisted through the 21 day study period. These results suggest that passive immunization with immune globulin products is not affected by the solvent/detergent treatment.

INDICATIONS AND USAGE

BayTet is indicated for prophylaxis against tetanus following injury in patients whose immunization is incomplete or uncertain (see below). It is also indicated, although evidence of effectiveness is limited, in the regimen of treatment of active cases of tetanus.[7,8,15]

A thorough attempt must be made to determine whether a patient has completed primary vaccination. Patients with unknown or uncertain previous vaccination histories should be considered to have had no previous tetanus toxoid doses. Persons who had military service since 1941, can be considered to have received at least one dose, and although most of them may have completed a primary series of tetanus toxoid, this cannot be assumed for each individual. Patients who have not completed a primary series may require tetanus toxoid and passive immunization at the time of wound cleaning and debridement.[2]

The following table is a summary guide to tetanus prophylaxis in wound management:
[See table below]

CONTRAINDICATIONS

None known.

WARNINGS

BayTet is made from human plasma. Products made from human plasma may contain infectious agents, such as viruses, that can cause disease. The risk that such products will transmit an infectious agent has been reduced by screening plasma donors for prior exposure to certain viruses, by testing for the presence of certain current virus infections, and by inactivating and/or removing certain viruses. Despite these measures, such products can still potentially transmit disease. There is also the possibility that unknown infectious agents may be present in such products. Individuals who receive infusions of blood or plasma products may develop signs and/or symptoms of some viral

Guide to Tetanus Prophylaxis in Wound Management[2]

History of Tetanus Immunization (Doses)	Clean, Minor Wounds		All Other Wounds*	
	Td†	TIG‡	Td	TIG
Uncertain or less than 3	Yes	No	Yes	Yes
3 or more§	No‖	No	No¶	No

* Such as, but not limited to, wounds contaminated with dirt, feces, soil, and saliva; puncture wounds; avulsions; and wounds resulting from missiles, crushing, burns and frostbite.
† Adult type tetanus and diphtheria toxoids. If the patient is less than 7 years old, DT or DTP is preferred to tetanus toxoid alone. For persons ≥ 7 years of age, Td is preferred to tetanus toxoid alone. (See Dosage and Administration)
‡ Tetanus Immune Globulin (Human).
§ If only three doses of fluid tetanus toxoid have been received, a fourth dose of toxoid, preferably an adsorbed toxoid, should be given.
‖ Yes if more than 10 years since the last dose.
¶ Yes if more than 5 years since the last dose. (More frequent boosters are not needed and can accentuate side effects).

infections, particularly hepatitis C. ALL infections thought by a physician possibly to have been transmitted by this product should be reported by the physician or other health-care provider to Bayer Corporation [1-888-765-3203].

The physician should discuss the risks and benefits of this product with the patient, before prescribing or administering it to the patient.

BayTet should be given with caution to patients with a history of prior systemic allergic reactions following the administration of human immunoglobulin preparations.

In patients who have severe thrombocytopenia or any coagulation disorder that would contraindicate intramuscular injections, BayTet should be given only if the expected benefits outweigh the risks.

PRECAUTIONS

General

BayTet should not be given intravenously. Intravenous injection of immunoglobulin intended for intramuscular use can, on occasion, cause a precipitous fall in blood pressure, and a picture not unlike anaphylaxis. Injections should only be made **intramuscularly** and care should be taken to draw back on the plunger of the syringe before injection in order to be certain that the needle is not in a blood vessel. Intramuscular injections are preferably administered in the anterolateral aspects of the upper thigh and the deltoid muscle of the upper arm. The gluteal region should not be used routinely as an injection site because of the risk of injury to the sciatic nerve. If the gluteal region is used, the central region MUST be avoided; only the upper, outer quadrant should be used.[16]

Chemoprophylaxis against tetanus is neither practical nor useful in managing wounds. Wound cleaning, debridement when indicated, and proper immunization are important. The need for tetanus toxoid (active immunization), with or without TIG (passive immunization), depends on both the condition of the wound and the patient's vaccination history. Rarely has tetanus occurred among persons with documentation of having received a primary series of toxoid injections.[2] See table under INDICATIONS AND USAGE.

Skin tests should not be done. The intradermal injection of concentrated IgG solutions often causes a localized area of inflammation which can be misinterpreted as a positive allergic reaction. In actuality, this does not represent an allergy; rather, it is localized tissue irritation. Misinterpretation of the results of such tests can lead the physician to withhold needed human antitoxin from a patient who is not actually allergic to this material. True allergic responses to human IgG given in the prescribed intramuscular manner are rare.

Although systemic reactions to human immunoglobulin preparations are rare, epinephrine should be available for treatment of acute anaphylactic reactions.

Drug Interactions

Antibodies in immunoglobulin preparations may interfere with the response to live viral vaccines such as measles, mumps, polio, and rubella. Therefore, use of such vaccines should be deferred until approximately 3 months after Tetanus Immune Globulin (Human), BayTet® administration. No interactions with other products are known.

Pregnancy Category C

Animal reproduction studies have not been conducted with BayTet. It is also not known whether BayTet can cause fetal harm when administered to a pregnant woman or can affect reproduction capacity. BayTet should be given to a pregnant woman only if clearly needed.

Pediatric Use

Safety and effectiveness in the pediatric population have not been established.

ADVERSE REACTIONS

Slight soreness at the site of injection and slight temperature elevation may be noted at times. Sensitization to repeated injections of human immunoglobulin is extremely rare.

In the course of routine injections of large numbers of persons with immunoglobulin there have been a few isolated occurrences of angioneurotic edema, nephrotic syndrome, and anaphylactic shock after injection.

OVERDOSAGE

Although no data are available, clinical experience with other immunoglobulin preparations suggests that the only manifestations would be pain and tenderness at the injection site.

DOSAGE AND ADMINISTRATION

Routine prophylactic dosage schedule:

Adults and children 7 years and older: BayTet, 250 units should be given by deep intramuscular injection (see PRECAUTIONS). At the same time, but in a different extremity and with a separate syringe, Tetanus and Diphtheria Toxoids Adsorbed (For Adult Use) (Td) should be administered according to the manufacturer's package insert. Adults with uncertain histories of a complete primary vaccination series should receive a primary series using the combined Td toxoid. To ensure continued protection, booster doses of Td should be given every 10 years.[2]

Children less than 7 years old: In small children the routine prophylactic dose of BayTet may be calculated by the body weight (4.0 units/kg). However, it may be advisable to administer the entire contents of the vial or syringe of BayTet (250 units) regardless of the child's size, since theoretically the same amount of toxin will be produced in the child's body by the infecting tetanus organism as it will in an adult's body. At the same time but in a different extremity and with a different syringe, Diphtheria and Tetanus Toxoids and Pertussis Vaccine Adsorbed (DTP) or Diphtheria and Tetanus Toxoids Adsorbed (For Pediatric Use) (DT), if pertussis vaccine is contraindicated, should be administered per the manufacturer's package insert.

Note: The single injection of tetanus toxoid only initiates the series for producing active immunity in the recipient. The physician must impress upon the patient the need for further toxoid injections in 1 month and 1 year. Without such, the active immunization series is incomplete. If a contraindication to using tetanus toxoid-containing preparations exists for a person who has not completed a primary series of tetanus toxoid immunization and that person has a wound that is neither clean nor minor, *only* passive immunization should be given using tetanus immune globulin.[2] See table under INDICATIONS AND USAGE.

Available evidence indicates that complete primary vaccination with tetanus toxoid provides long lasting protection ≥10 years for most recipients. Consequently, after complete primary tetanus vaccination, boosters–even for wound management–need be given only every 10 years when wounds are minor and uncontaminated. For other wounds, a booster is appropriate if the patient has not received tetanus toxoid within the preceding 5 years. Persons who have received at least two doses of tetanus toxoid rapidly develop antibodies.[2]

The prophylactic dosage schedule for these patients and for those with incomplete or uncertain immunity is shown on the table in INDICATIONS AND USAGE.

Since tetanus is actually a local infection, proper initial wound care is of paramount importance. The use of antitoxin is adjunctive to this procedure. However, in approximately 10% of recent tetanus cases, no wound or other breach in skin or mucous membrane could be implicated.[17]

Treatment of active cases of tetanus:

Standard therapy for the treatment of active tetanus including the use of BayTet must be implemented immediately. The dosage should be adjusted according to the severity of the infection.[7,8]

Parenteral drug products should be inspected visually for particulate matter and discoloration prior to administration, whenever solution and container permit. They should not be used if particulate matter and/or discoloration are present.

Directions for syrings Usage

1. Remove the prefilled syringe from the package. Lift syringe by barrel, **not** by plunger.
2. Twist the plunger rod clockwise until the threads are seated.
3. With the rubber needle shield secured on the syringe tip, push the plunger rod forward a few millimeters to break any friction seal between the rubber stopper and glass syringe barrel.
4. Remove the needle shield and expel air bubbles.
5. Proceed with hypodermic needle puncture.
6. Aspirate prior to injection to confirm that the needle is not in a vein or artery.
7. Inject the medication.
8. Withdraw the needle and dispose or destroy it.

HOW SUPPLIED

BayTet is supplied in 250 unit prefilled disposable syringes with attached needles and 250 unit single dose vials.

NDC Number	Size
0026-0634-01	250 unit syringe
0026-0634-70	250 unit syringe (10 pack)
0026-0634-86	250 unit vial (10 pack)

Tetanus Immune Globulin (Human) —BayTet® is supplied in 250 unit prefilled disposable syringes and 250 unit single dose vials.

STORAGE

Store at 2°–8°C (36°–46°F). Solution that has been frozen should not be used.

CAUTION

U.S. federal law prohibits dispensing without prescription.

LIMITED WARRANTY

A number of factors beyond our control could reduce the efficacy of this product or even result in an ill effect following its use. These include improper storage and handling of the product after it leaves our hands, diagnosis, dosage, method of administration, and biological differences in individual patients. Because of these factors it is important that this product be stored properly and that the directions be followed carefully during use.

No warranty, express or implied, including any warranty of merchantability or fitness is made. Representatives of the Company are not authorized to vary the terms or the contents of the printed labeling, including the package insert for this product, except by printed notice from the Company's headquarters. The prescriber and user of this product must accept the terms hereof.

REFERENCES

1. Tetanus — United States, 1987 and 1988, *MMWR* 39(3): 37–41, 1990.
2. Diphtheria, Tetanus, and Pertussis: Recommendations for Vaccine Use and Other Preventive Measures. Recommendations of the Immunization Practices Advisory Committee (ACIP). *MMWR* 40 (RR-10): 1–28, 1991.
3. Moynihan NH: Tetanus prophylaxis and serum sensitivity tests. *Br Med J* 1:260–4, 1956.
4. Scheibel I: The uses and results of active tetanus immunization. *Bull WHO* 13:381–94, 1955.
5. Edsall G: Specific prophylaxis of tetanus. *JAMA* 171(4): 417–27, 1959.
6. Bardenwerper HW: Serum neuritis from tetanus antitoxin. *JAMA* 179(10):763–6, 1962.
7. Nation NS, Pierce NF, Adler SJ, et al: Tetanus: the use of human hyperimmune globulin in treatment. *Calif Med* 98(6):305–6, 1963.
8. Ellis M: Human antitetanus serum in the treatment of tetanus. *Br Med J* 1(5338):1123–6, 1963.
9. Axnick NW, Alexander ER: Tetanus in the United States: A review of the problem. *Am J Public Health* 47(12):1493–1501, 1957.
10. Blake PA, Feldman RA, Buchanan TM, et al: Serologic therapy of tetanus in the United States, 1965–1971. *JAMA* 235(1):42–4, 1976.
11. Rubbo SD: New approaches to tetanus prophylaxis. *Lancet* 2(7461):449–53, 1966.
12. McComb JA, Dwyer RC: Passive-active immunization with tetanus immune globulin (human). *N Engl J Med* 268(16):857–62, 1963.
13. Levine L, McComb JA, Dwyer RC, et al: Active-passive tetanus immunization; choice of toxoid, dose of tetanus immune globulin and timing of injections. *N Engl J Med* 274(4);186–90, 1966.
14. Waldmann TA, Strober W, Blaese RM: Variations in the metabolism of immunoglobulins measured by turnover rates. In Merler E (ed.): Immunoglobulins: biologic aspects and clinical uses. Washington, DC, Nat Acad Sci, 1970, p 33–51.
15. McCracken GH Jr., Dowell DL, Marshall FN: Double-blind trial of equine antitoxin and human immune globulin in tetanus neonatorum. *Lancet* 1(7710):1146–9, 1971.
16. Recommendations of the Immunization Practices Advisory Committee (ACIP): General recommendations on immunization. *MMWR* 38(13): 205–14; 219–27, 1989.
17. Tetanus-Rates by year, United States, 1955–1984. Annual Summary 1984. *MMWR* 33 (54):61, 1986.

GAMIMUNE® N, 5% ℞

Immune Globulin Intravenous (Human), 5%
Solvent/Detergent Treated

DESCRIPTION

Immune Globulin Intravenous (Human), 5%—Gamimune® N, 5% treated with solvent/detergent is a sterile 4.5%–5.5% solution of human protein in 9%–11% maltose; it contains no preservative. Each milliliter (mL) contains approximately 50 mg of protein, not less than 98% of which has the electrophoretic mobility of gamma globulin. Not less than 90% of the IgG is monomer. Also present are traces of IgA and of IgM. The distribution of IgG subclasses is similar to that found in normal serum. Gamimune N, 5% has a buffer capacity of 16.5 mEq/L of solution (~0.33 mEq/g of protein). The calculated osmolality is 309 milliosmoles per kilogram of solvent (water) and the calculated osmolarity is 278 milliosmoles per liter of solution.

The product is made by cold ethanol fractionation of large pools of human plasm. Part of the fractionation may be performed by another licensed manufacturer. The immunoglobulin is isolated from Cohn Effluent III after limited diafiltration and ultrafiltration. The solution is adjusted to 0.3% tri-n-butyl phosphate (TNBP) and 0.2% sodium cholate. After addition of the solvent (TNBP) and the detergent (sodium cholate), the solution is heated to 30°C and maintained at that temperature for not less than 6 hours. After the viral inactivation step, the reactants are removed by precipitation, filtration, and finally diafiltration and ultrafiltration. The protein is stabilized during the process by adjusting the pH of the solution to 4.0–4.5.[1] Isotonicity is achieved by the addition of maltose. Gamimune N, 5% treated with solvent/detergent is then incubated in the final container (at the low pH of 4.25), for a minimum of 21 days at 20°C. The product is intended for intravenous administration.

The removal and inactivation of spiked model enveloped and non-enveloped viruses during the manufacturing process for Gamimune N, 5% has been validated in laboratory studies. Human Immunodeficiency Virus, Type 1 (HIV-1) was chosen as the relevant virus for blood products; Bovine Viral Diarrhea Virus (BVDV) was chosen to model for Hepatitis C virus; Pseudorabies virus (PRV) was chosen to model for Hepatitis B and the Herpes viruses; and Reo virus type 3 (Reo) was chosen to model non-enveloped viruses and for its resistance to physical and chemical inactivation. Significant removal of model enveloped and non-enveloped viruses is seen between the Fraction II + IIIW and Effluent III steps and between the Effluent III and Filtrate III steps. Significant inactivation of enveloped viruses is achieved at the time of treatment of Filtrate III with TNBP/sodium cholate and also at the time of low pH incubation in the final container.

CLINICAL PHARMACOLOGY

Primary Humoral Immunodeficiency

Gamimune N, 5% supplies a broad spectrum of opsonic and neutralizing IgG antibodies for the prevention or attenua-

Continued on next page

Gamimune N, 5%—Cont.

tion of a wide variety of infectious diseases. As Gamimune N, 5% is administered intravenously, essentially 100% of the infused IgG antibodies are immediately available in the recipient's circulation.[2] Studies using a modified intravenous immunoglobulin at pH 6.8 have shown that approximately 30% of the infused IgG disappeared from the circulation in the first 24 hours, due primarily to equilibration of the IgG between the plasma and the extravascular space.[2–5] A further decline to about 40% of the peak level found immediately post-infusion is to be expected during the first week.[2–5] The in vivo half-life of Gamimune N, 5% equals or exceeds the 3-week half-life reported for IgG in the literature, but individual patient variation in half-life has been observed.[2] Thus, this variable as well as the amount of immune globulin administered per dose is important in determining the frequency of administration of the drug for each individual patient. A comparative study of Gamimune N, 5% treated with solvent/detergent and Gamimune N, 5% in 16 subjects demonstrated bioequivalence.

Idiopathic Thrombocytopenic Purpura

While Gamimune N, 5% has been shown to be effective in some cases of idiopathic thrombocytopenic purpura (ITP) (see INDICATIONS AND USAGE), the mechanism of action has not been fully elucidated.

Bone Marrow Transplantation

Gamimune N, 5% has been shown to be effective in bone marrow transplant patients ≥20 years of age in the first 100 days posttransplant for the following: prevention of systemic and local infections, interstitial pneumonia of infectious and idiopathic etiologies and acute graft-versus-host disease (AGVHD)[6] (see INDICATIONS AND USAGE). Administration of Gamimune N, 5% to bone marrow transplant patients significantly increased IgG and IgG subclass levels while those seen in the control group fell below predicted levels. The mechanism of action of Gamimune N, 5% in reducing the incidence of AGVHD is presently unknown.

Pediatric HIV Infection

Children infected with human immunodeficiency virus (HIV) may display defects in both cellular and humoral immunity.[7–10] As a result, some children with HIV-1 infection experience serious, potentially life-threatening recurrent bacterial infections.[11–13] In one retrospective report, among 71 HIV-infected children observed over 3.5 years, 27 (37%) experienced serious documented bacterial infections.[12] The types of bacterial and viral infections observed in HIV-infected children are similar to those seen in children with primary hypogammaglobulinemia.[14] The replacement of opsonic and neutralizing IgG antibodies has been shown to reduce serious and minor bacterial infection in HIV-infected children.[15–16]

In a randomized, double-blind, placebo-controlled, multicenter study performed between March 7, 1988 and January 15, 1991, the efficacy of Gamimune N, 5% in pediatric HIV disease to decrease the frequency of serious and minor bacterial infections and the frequency of hospitalization, and to increase the time free of serious bacterial infection was documented in children with clinical or immunologic evidence of HIV disease (see INDICATIONS AND USAGE). The primary endpoint of this study was prospectively defined as a significant reduction in the proportion of subjects who develop at least one serious bacterial infection when compared to the control group of HIV-infected children who received placebo. Serious bacterial infections were defined as laboratory-proven and clinically diagnosed (i.e., radiologically proven acute pneumonia and sinusitis) infections. The Data Safety and Monitoring Board (DSMB) recommended early termination of the study based on data presented to them from an interim analysis in December 1990 which showed that treatment with Gamimune N, 5% increased the time free from serious infections in children with CD4+ counts ≥200/mm^3.

General

The intravenous administration of solutions of maltose has been studied by several investigators.[17–21] Healthy subjects tolerated the infusions well, and no adverse effects were observed at a rate of 0.25 g maltose/kg body weight per hour.[18] In safety studies conducted by Bayer Corporation, infusions of 10% maltose administered at 0.27–0.62 g maltose/kg per hour[21] to normal subjects produced either mild side effects (e.g., headache) or no adverse reaction.[2] Following intravenous administrations of maltose, maltose was detected in the peripheral blood; there was a dose-dependent excretion of maltose and glucose in the urine and a mild diuretic effect.[2] These alterations were well-tolerated without significant adverse effects.[2] The highest recommended infusion rate, 0.08 mL/kg body weight per minute (see DOSAGE AND ADMINISTRATION), is equivalent to 0.48 g maltose/kg body weight per hour.

The buffer capacity of Gamimune N, 5% is 16.5 mEq/L (~0.33 mEq/g protein); a dose of 1000 mg/kg body weight therefore represents an acid load of 0.33 mEq/kg body weight. The total buffering capacity of whole blood in a normal individual is 45–50 mEq/L of blood, or 3.6 mEq/kg body weight.[22] Thus, the acid load delivered with a dose of 1000 mg/kg of Gamimune N, 5% would be neutralized by the buffering capacity of whole blood alone, even if the dose were infused instantaneously. (An infusion usually lasts several hours.)

In Phase I human studies, no change in arterial blood pH measurements was detected following the intravenous administration of Gamimune N, 5% at a dose of 150 mg/kg body weight;[2] following a dose of 400 mg/kg body weight in 37 patients, there were no clinically important differences in mean venous pH or bicarbonate measurements in patients who received Gamimune N, 5% compared with those who received a chemically modified intravenous immunoglobulin preparation with a pH of 6.8.[2]

In patients with limited or compromised acid-base compensatory mechanisms, consideration should be given to the effect of the additional acid load Gamimune N, 5% might present.

INDICATIONS AND USAGE

Primary Humoral Immunodeficiency

Gamimune N, 5% is efficacious in the treatment of primary immunodeficiency states in which severe impairment of antibody forming capacity has been shown, such as: congenital agammaglobulinemias, common variable immunodeficiency. Wiskott-Aldrich syndrome, x-linked immunodeficiency with hyper IgM, and severe combined immunodeficiencies.[5,23–25] Gamimune N, 5% is especially useful when high levels or rapid elevation of circulating antibodies are desired or when intramuscular injections are contraindicated.

Idiopathic Thrombocytopenic Purpura (ITP)

In clinical situations in which a rapid rise in platelet count is needed to control bleeding or to allow a patient with ITP to undergo surgery, administration of Gamimune N, 5% should be considered; in patients in whom a response is achieved, the rise of platelets is generally rapid (within 1–5 days), transient (most often lasting from several days to several weeks) and should not be considered curative. It is presently not possible to predict which patients with ITP will respond to therapy, although the increase in platelet counts in children seems to be better than that of adults. Childhood ITP may, however, respond spontaneously without treatment.

Two different dosing regimens of Gamimune N, 5% have been studied in clinical investigations: a regimen consisting of 400 mg/kg body weight daily for 5 consecutive days, and a high dose treatment regimen consisting of 1,000 mg/kg body weight administered on either 1 day or 2 consecutive days.

In clinical studies of Gamimune N, 5% five of six (83.3%) children and 12 of 16 (75%) adults with acute or chronic ITP treated with 400 mg/kg body weight for 5 consecutive days demonstrated clinically significant platelet increments of ≥30,000/mm^3 over baseline. The mean platelet count in children with ITP rose from 27,800/mm^3 at baseline to 297,000/mm^3 (range 50,000–455,000/mm^3) and the mean platelet counts in adults with ITP rose from 27,900/mm^3 at baseline to 124,900/mm^3 (range 11,000–341,000/mm^3). Two of three children with acute ITP rapidly went into complete remission.

Thirteen of 14 children (92.9%) and 26 of 29 adults (89.7%) with acute or chronic ITP treated with Gamimune N, 5% 1,000 mg/kg body weight administered on either 1 day or 2 consecutive days responded to treatment with clinically significant platelet increments of ≥30,000/mm^3 over baseline. This included three of three patients with ITP that were human immunodeficiency virus (HIV) antibody positive and two of two patients with ITP that were pregnant. The mean platelet count in children with ITP treated with Gamimune N, 5% 1,000 mg/kg body weight on 1 day or 2 consecutive days rose from 44,400/mm^3 at baseline to 285,600/mm^3 (range 89,000–473,000/mm^3) and the mean platelet count in adults with ITP treated with the regimen rose from 23,400/mm^3 at baseline to 173,100/mm^3 (range 28,000–709,000/mm^3.

Two patients, one each with acute adult and chronic childhood ITP, entered complete remission with treatment.

Six of the 29 adult patients with ITP received Gamimune N, 5% 1,000 mg/kg on 1 day or 2 consecutive days to increase the platelet count prior to splenectomy. Mean platelet counts rose from 14,500/mm^3 at baseline to 129,300/mm^3 (range 51,000–242,000/mm^3) prior to surgery.

The duration of the platelet rise following treatment of ITP with either treatment regimen of Gamimune N, 5% was variable, ranging from several days to 12 months or more. Some ITP patients have demonstrated continuing responsiveness over many months to intermittent infusions of Gamimune N, 5% 400–1,000 mg/kg body weight, administered as a single maintenance dose, at intervals as indicated by the platelet count.

Bone Marrow Transplantation (BMT)

Gamimune N, 5% should be considered for use in bone marrow transplant patients ≥20 years of age to decrease the risk of septicemia and other infections, interstitial pneumonia of infectious or idiopathic etiologies and acute graft-versus-host disease (AGVHD) in the first 100 days post-transplant. Gamimune N, 5% is not indicated in bone marrow transplant patients below 20 years of age. In a controlled study of 369 evaluable BMT patients (184 treated and 185 controls) who either did or did not receive Gamimune N, 5% in doses of 500 mg/kg body weight on days −7 and −2 pretransplant, then weekly through day 90 post-transplant, posttransplant complications were evaluated in the entire study group and in patients under age 20 and age 20 or older. For patients ≥20 years of age (128 patients in the control group and 119 patients in the treated group), there was a statistically significant reduction in interstitial pneumonia from 21% in the control group to 9% in the treated group (p = 0.0032) during the first 100 days post-transplant. Also significantly reduced in this age group were: overall septicemia from 53 infections in the 128 patient control group to 26 infections in the 119 patient treated group (relative risk control:treated [RR] 2.36, p = 0.0025); gram-negative septicemia from 24 infections in the 128 patient control group to 9 infections in the 119 patient treated group (RR 2.53, p = 0.015); gram-positive septicemia from 16 infections in the 128 patient control group to 8 infections in the 119 patient treated group (RR 2.73, p = 0.046); and Grade II to IV AGVHD from an incidence of 58 of 110 in the control group to 38 of 108 in the treated group (p = 0.0051).

The given p-values do not take into account multiple endpoints and subset analyses. Therefore, some of the p-values could occur by chance alone. There was no significant improvement in overall mortality in this study.

In patients below age 20, there appeared to be no benefit from treatment with Gamimune N, 5%, either in reducing the incidence of infections or the incidence of AGVHD.

Pediatric HIV Infection

Gamimune N, 5% 400 mg/kg every 28 days significantly decreased the frequency of serious and minor bacterial infections (laboratory-proven and clinically diagnosed) and the frequency of hospitalization, and increased the time free of serious bacterial infection. The effect of Gamimune N, 5% in preventing serious bacterial infections was especially apparent in preventing primary bacteremia (including *Streptococcus pneumoniae* bacteremia) and acute pneumonia.

In a randomized, double-blind, placebo-controlled, multicenter study, 394 HIV-infected, non-hemophilic, children less than 13 years of age were randomized. Of the children randomized, 369 were included in the efficacy analysis and 376 in the safety analysis. The study population had 1) a mean age of 40 months (range 2.4–136.8 months), 2) acquired HIV primarily through vertical transmission (91%), 3) a majority (87%) of CDC Class P-2 (symptomatic), and 4) had a median CD4+ count of 937 cells/mm^3 (range 0–6660 cells/mm^3). At the time of study entry, 14% (52 of 369) were receiving *Pneumocystis carinii* pneumonia (PCP) prophylaxis. During the course of the study, 51% (189 of 369) received PCP prophylaxis and 44% (164 of 369) received zidovudine (ZDV). Children with HIV-1 infection were initially stratified into two groups based upon CD4+ count (<200 cells/mm^3 versus ≥ 200 cells/mm^3) and CDC classification of pediatric HIV disease (history of opportunistic infections [P-2-D-1] and recurrent serious bacterial infections [P-2-D-2] versus others). Subjects received Gamimune N, 5% (400 mg/kg = 8mL/kg) (n=185) or an equivalent volume of placebo (0.1% Albumin [Human]) (n = 184) every 28 days. The mean follow-up for subjects receiving Gamimune N, 5% was 17.9 months and 17.8 months for patients on placebo. The number of subjects who had at least one serious bacterial infection was 86 of 184 (47%) in the placebo group and 55 of 185 (30%) in the Gamimune N, 5% group (p = 0.0009). All p-values reported are two-sided. Treatment with Gamimune N, 5% compared to placebo was also associated with a significant reduction in both the number of subjects with at least one laboratory-proven infection (36 of 184 vs. 18 of 185, p = 0.0081), and the number of subjects with at least one clinically diagnosed infection (71 of 184 vs. 45 of 185, p = 0.0036). Efficacy in patients with CDR+ counts < 200/mm^3 was not established, possibly because of the small number of subjects in this category.

The 2-year treatment period defined in the protocol was truncated for some patients by the DSMB based on data from the interim analysis. Rates of serious bacterial infections per 100 patient-years were computed and analyzed to take into account both the unequal duration of treatment and follow-up, as well as recurrent infections in individual subjects. Children treated with Gamimune N, 5% experienced a 50.5% lower frequency of laboratory-proven serious bacterial infection compared to the group treated with placebo (9.1 vs. 18.2 infections per 100 patient-years, p = 0.031), a 36.0% lower frequency of clinically diagnosed serious infections (24.0 vs. 37.5 infections per 100 patient-years, p = 0.013), a 40.6% reduction in total serious infections (laboratory-proven and clinically diagnosed) (33.1 vs. 55.7 infections per 100 patient-years, p = 0.003), a 60% lower frequency of primary bacteremias (5.8 vs. 14.5 infections per 100 patient-years, p = 0.009), a 75.6% lower frequency of *Streptococcus pneumoniae* bacteremia (1.1 vs. 4.5 bacteremias per 100 patient-years, p = 0.026), a 54.3% lower frequency of clinically diagnosed pneumonia (12.7 vs. 27.8 infections per 100 patient-years, p = 0.001), and a 22.5% lower frequency of minor bacterial infections (including otitis media, skin and soft tissue infections, and upper respiratory tract infections) (123.6 vs. 159.5 infections per 100 patient-years, p = 0.033).

In addition to a reduced frequency of infection, children treated with Gamimune N, 5% had a 36.8% lower number of hospitalizations per 100 patient-years (72 vs. 114 per 100 patient-years, p = 0.002) and a reduced number of hospital days (6.9 vs. 10.5 per patient-year, p = 0.030) than patients treated with placebo. Patients treated with Gamimune N, 5% had a higher probability of remaining free of laboratory-proven infections (p = 0.0093) and combined laboratory-proven and clinically diagnosed infections (p = 0.0015) for 24 months than the group of children treated with placebo. At 24 months, the estimated probabilities of remaining infection-free for the Gamimune N, 5% and placebo arms were 87.8% vs. 76.1%, respectively, for laboratory-proven infections and 63.5% vs. 44.5%, respectively, for combined laboratory-proven and clinically diagnosed infections.

There was no effect of Gamimune N, 5% therapy on mortality, which was low in both treatment groups (17%), or on the frequency of opportunistic or viral infections during the period of study.

Since antibacterial prophylaxis could also account for the observed reduction in the rate of serious bacterial infections, further analysis was performed to evaluate the role of *Pneumocystis carinii* pneumonia (PCP) prophylaxis on the efficacy of Gamimune N, 5%. PCP prophylaxis consisted primarily (96%) of trimethoprim/sulfamethoxazole given 3 successive days each week. This antibiotic combination could be active against the bacteria commonly encountered in this patient population. In the subgroup of patients receiving PCP prophylaxis at study entry, treatment with Gamimune N, 5% was associated with 44.0 infections per 100 patient-years, whereas placebo recipients had 64.7 infections per 100 patient-years (p = 0.047). In the subgroup of patients not receiving PCP prophylaxis at study entry, treatment with Gamimune N, 5% was associated with 22.1 infections per 100 patient-years, whereas placebo recipients had 44.9 infections per 100 patient-years on placebo (p = 0.024). Thus, Gamimune N, 5% benefited patients by reducing the rate of serious bacterial infections whether or not they were receiving PCP prophylactic treatment at study entry. However, it should be noted that the use of PCP prophylactic treatment in this study was not randomized and specific guidelines for its administration were not identified.

CONTRAINDICATION

Immune Globulin Intravenous (Human), 5%—Gamimune® N, 5% is contraindicated in individuals who are known to have had an anaphylactic or severe systemic response to Immune Globulin (Human). Individuals with selective IgA deficiencies who have known antibody against IgA (anti-IgA antibody) should not receive Gamimune N, 5% since these patients may experience severe reactions to the IgA which may be present.[23]

WARNINGS

Immune Globulin Intravenous (Human) products have been reported to be associated with renal dysfunction, acute renal failure, osmotic nephrosis and death.[24] Patients predisposed to acute renal failure include patients with any degree of pre-existing renal insufficiency, diabetes mellitus, age greater than 65, volume depletion, sepsis, paraproteinemia, or patients receiving known nephrotoxic drugs. Especially in such patients, IGIV products should be administered at the minimum concentration available and the minimum rate of infusion practicable. While these reports of renal dysfunction and acute renal failure have been associated with the use of many of the licensed IGIV products, those containing sucrose as a stabilizer accounted for a disproportionate share of the total number. See PRECAUTIONS and DOSAGE AND ADMINISTRATION sections for important information intended to reduce the risk of acute renal failure.

Gamimune N, 5% is made from human plasma. Products made from human plasma may contain infectious agents, such as viruses, that can cause disease. The risk that such products will transmit an infectious agent has been reduced by screening plasma donors for prior exposure to certain viruses, by testing for the presence of certain current virus infections, and by inactivating and/or removing certain viruses. Despite these measures, such products can still potentially transmit disease. There is also the possibility that unknown infectious agents may be present in such products. Individuals who receive infusions of blood or plasma products may develop signs and/or symptoms of some viral infections, particularly hepatitis C. ALL infections thought by a physician possibly to have been transmitted by this product should be reported by the physician or other healthcare provider to Bayer Corporation [1-888-765-3203].

The physician should discuss the risks and benefits of this product with the patient, before prescribing or administering it to the patient.

Gamimune N, 5% should be administered only intravenously as the intramuscular and subcutaneous routes have not been evaluated.

Gamimune N, 5% may, on rare occasions, cause a precipitous fall in blood pressure and a clinical picture of anaphylaxis, even when the patient is not known to be sensitive to immune globulin preparations. These reactions may be related to the rate of infusion. Accordingly, the infusion rate given under DOSAGE AND ADMINISTRATION should be closely followed, at least until the physician has had sufficient experience with a given patient. The patient's vital signs should be monitored continuously and careful observation made for any symptoms throughout the entire infusion. Epinephrine should be available for the treatment of an acute anaphylactic reaction.

PRECAUTIONS

General

Any vial that has been entered should be used promptly. Partially used vials should be discarded. Do not use if turbid. Solution which has been frozen should not be used.

An aseptic meningitis syndrome (AMS) has been reported to occur infrequently in association with Immune Globulin Intravenous (Human) treatment. The syndrome usually begins within several hours to two days following Immune Globulin Intravenous (Human) treatment. It is characterized by symptoms and signs including severe headache, nuchal rigidity, drowsiness, fever, photophobia, painful eye movements, and nausea and vomiting. Cerebrospinal fluid studies are frequently positive with pleocytosis up to several thousand cells per mm^3, predominantly from the granulocytic series, and elevated protein levels up to several hundred mg/dL. Patients exhibiting such symptoms and signs should receive a thorough neurological examination, including CSF studies, to rule out other causes of meningitis. AMS may occur more frequently in association with high dose (2 g/kg) Immune Globulin Intravenous (Human) treatment. Discontinuation of Immune Globulin Intravenous (Human) treatment has resulted in remission of AMS within several days without sequelae.[26–29]

Assure that patients are not volume depleted prior to the initiation of the infusion of IGIV. Periodic monitoring of renal function tests and urine output is particularly important in patients judged to have a potential increased risk for developing acute renal failure. Renal function, including measurement of blood urea nitrogen (BUN)/serum creatinine, should be assessed prior to the initial infusion of Gamimune N, 5% and again at appropriate intervals thereafter. If renal function deteriorates, discontinuation of the product should be considered. For patients judged to be at risk for developing renal dysfunction, it may be prudent to reduce the amount of product infused per unit time by infusing Gamimune N, 5% at a rate less than 8 mg IG/kg/min (0.08 mL/kg/min).

Information for Patients

Patients should be instructed to immediately report symptoms of decreased urine output, sudden weight gain, fluid retention/edema, and/or shortness of breath (which may suggest kidney damage) to their physicians.

Drug Interactions

Antibodies in Gamimune N, 5% may interfere with the response to live viral vaccines such as measles, mumps and rubella. Therefore, use of such vaccines should be deferred until approximately 6 months after Gamimune N, 5% administration.

Please see DOSAGE AND ADMINISTRATION for other drug interactions.

Pregnancy Category C

Animal reproduction studies have not been conducted with Gamimune N, 5%. It is not known whether Gamimune N, 5% can cause fetal harm when administered to a pregnant woman or can affect reproduction capacity. Gamimune N, 5% should be given to a pregnant woman only if clearly needed.

ADVERSE REACTIONS

General

Increases in creatinine and blood urea nitrogen (BUN) have been observed as soon as one to two days following infusion. Progression to oliguria and anuria requiring dialysis has been observed, although some patients have improved spontaneously following cessation of treatment.[34] Types of severe renal adverse reactions that have been seen following IGIV therapy include: acute renal failure, acute tubular necrosis,[35] proximal tubular nephropathy, and osmotic nephrosis.[33, also see 36–38] In the studies undertaken to date, other types of reactions have not been reported with Gamimune N, 5% or Gamimune N, 10%. It may be, however, that adverse effects will be similar to those previously reported with intravenous and intramuscular immunoglobulin administration. Potential reactions, therefore, may also include anxiety, flushing, wheezing, abdominal cramps, myalgias, arthralgia, and dizziness; rash has been reported only rarely. Reactions to intravenous immunoglobulin tend to be related to the rate of infusion. True anaphylactic reactions to Gamimune N, 10% may occur in recipients with documented prior histories of severe allergic reactions to intramuscular immunoglobulin, but some patients may tolerate cautiously administered intravenous immunoglobulin without adverse effects.[34] Very rarely an anaphylactoid reaction may occur in patients with no prior history of severe allergic reactions to either intramuscular or intravenous immunoglobulin.[2]

Primary Humoral Immunodeficiency

In a study of 37 patients with immunodeficiency syndromes receiving Gamimune N, 5% at a monthly dose of 400 mg/kg body weight, reactions were seen in 5.2% of the infusions of Gamimune N, 5%. Symptoms reported with Gamimune N, 5% included malaise, a feeling of faintness, fever, chills, headache, nausea, vomiting, chest tightness, dyspnea and chest, back or hip pain. In addition, mild erythema following infiltration of Gamimune N, 5% at the infusion site was reported in some cases.

A safety study has been conducted in 16 adult and adolescent subjects with primary immunodeficiency syndrome, comparing side effects and bioequivalency of Gamimune N, 5% with those of Gamimune N, 5% treated with solvent/detergent. The incidence, nature and severity of reactions with Gamimune N, 5% treated with solvent/detergent were not different from those observed with Gamimune N, 5%.

Idiopathic Thrombocytopenic Purpura

In studies of Gamimune N, 5% administered at a dose of 400 mg/kg body weight in the treatment of adult and pediatric patients with ITP, systemic reactions were noted in only 4 of 154 (2.6%) infusions, and all but one occurred at rates of infusion greater than 0.04 mL/kg body weight per minute. The symptoms reported included chest tightness, a sense of tachycardia (pulse was 84 beats per minute), and a burning sensation in the head; these symptoms were all mild and transient.

In studies of Gamimune N, 5% administered at a dose of 1,000 mg/kg body weight either as a single dose or as two doses on consecutive days in the treatment of adult and pediatric patients with ITP, adverse reactions were noted in only 25 of 251 (10%) infusions. Symptoms reported included headache, nausea, fever, chills, back pain, chest tightness, and shortness of breath. In children, the high dose regimen has been well-tolerated at the highest rates of infusion. In adults, however, the frequency of adverse reactions tended to increase with infusion rates in excess of 0.06 mL/kg per minute. In general, reactions reported with infusion of Gamimune N, 5% in these studies were reported as mild or moderate, and responded to slowing of the infusion rate.

Bone Marrow Transplantation

In studies of Gamimune N, 5% administered to 185 bone marrow transplant recipients at doses of 500 mg/kg (10 mL/kg) body weight on day -7 and day -2 pretransplant, then weekly through day 90 posttransplant, adverse reactions were noted in 12 (6.5%) of the 185 patients that received Gamimune N, 5% and in 14 (0.6%) of 2,176 infusions. All reactions reported were rate-related and classified as mild. Chills were the most common symptom reported, occurring in nine patients. The other symptoms reported included headache, flushing, fever, pruritus and slight back discomfort. All reactions resolved satisfactorily, usually without treatment or decreasing the infusion rate.

Pediatric HIV Infection

Three hundred seventy-six (376) patients, 187 treated with Gamimune N, 5% and 189 treated with placebo (0.1% Albumin [Human]), were included in the safety analysis. Adverse reactions occurred during or within 24 hours of an infusion in 50 of 3,451 (1.4%) infusions of Gamimune N, 5% and 62 of 3,447 (1.8%) infusions of placebo. Fever was the most common adverse reaction and occurred in 30 of 105 (28.6%) patients receiving placebo and 19 of 78 (24.4%) patients treated with Gamimune N, 5%. Irritability was the second most common symptom reported, with 10 of 105 (9.5%) reports for the placebo group and 9 of 78 (11.5%) for the group treated with Gamimune N, 5%. A large number of diverse adverse reactions accounted for the remaining adverse reactions reported in both study groups. In general, the number of adverse events reported was comparable in both the placebo and Gamimune N, 5% treated groups. Three serious adverse reactions were reported. One patient experienced a hypersensitivity reaction and did not receive further Gamimune N, 5% treatment. A second patient developed tachycardia and was admitted to an intensive care unit, but later continued treatment with Gamimune N, 5%. A third patient had skin infiltration during infusion and developed a full thickness skin slough over the dorsum of the hand that required skin grafting.

DOSAGE AND ADMINISTRATION

General

Dosages for specific indications are indicated below, but in general, it is recommended that Gamimune N, 5% be administered by itself at a rate of 0.01 to 0.02 mL/kg body weight per minute for 30 minutes; if well-tolerated, the rate may be **gradually** increased to a maximum of 0.08 mL/kg body weight per minute. Investigations indicate that Gamimune N, 5% is well-tolerated and less likely to produce side effects when infused at the indicated rate. If side effects occur, the rate may be reduced, or the infusion interrupted until symptoms subside. The infusion may then be resumed at the rate which is comfortable for the patient. Parenteral drug products should be inspected visually for particulate matter and discoloration prior to administration, whenever solution and container permit.

It is recommended that infusion of Gamimune N, 5% be given by a separate line, by itself, without mixing with other intravenous fluids or medications the patient might be receiving. Gamimune N, 5% should not be mixed with Immune Globulin Intravenous (Human) from another manufacturer. Gamimune N, 5% is not compatible with saline. If dilution is required, Gamimune N, 5% may be diluted with 5% dextrose in water (D5/W). No other drug interactions or compatibilities have been evaluated.

For patients judged to be at increased risk for developing renal dysfunction, it may be prudent to reduce the amount of product infused per unit time by infusing Gamimune N, 10% at a rate less than 8 mg IG/kg/min (0.08 mL/kg/min). No prospective data are presently available to identify a maximum safe dose, concentration, and rate of infusion in patients determined to be at increased risk of acute renal failure. In the absence of prospective data, recommended doses should not be exceeded and the concentration and infusion rate should be the minimum level practicable. Reduction in dose, concentration, and/or rate of administration in patients at risk of acute renal failure has been proposed in the literature in order to reduce the risk of acute renal failure.[39]

A number of factors beyond our control could reduce the efficacy of this product or even result in an ill effect following its use. These include improper storage and handling of the product after it leaves our hands, diagnosis, dosage, method of administration, and biological differences in individual patients. Because of these factors, it is important that this product be stored properly and that the directions be followed carefully during use .

Primary Humoral Immunodeficiency

The usual dosage of Gamimune N, 5% for prophylaxis in primary immunodeficiency syndromes is 100–200 mg/kg (2–4 mL/kg) of body weight administered approximately once a month by intravenous infusion. The dosage may be given more frequently or increased as high as 400 mg/kg (8 mL/kg) body weight, if the clinical response is inadequate, or the level of IgG achieved in the circulation is felt to be insufficient. The minimum level of IgG required for protection has not been determined.

Continued on next page

Gamimune N, 5%—Cont.

Idiopathic Thrombocytopenic Purpura (ITP)

Induction: An increase in platelet count has been observed in children and some adults with acute or chronic ITP receiving Gamimune N, 5% 400 mg/kg body weight daily for 5 days, or alternatively, 1,000 mg/kg body weight daily for 1 day or 2 consecutive days. In the latter treatment regimen, if an adequate increase in the platelet count is observed at 24 hours, the second dose of 1,000 mg/kg body weight may be withheld. The high dose regimen (1,000 mg/kg x 1–2 days) is not recommended for individuals with expanded fluid volumes or where fluid volume may be a concern. With both treatment regimens, a response usually occurs within several days and is maintained for a variable period of time. In general, a response is seen less often in adults than in children.

Maintenance: In adults and children with ITP, if after induction therapy the platelet count falls to less than 30,000/mm^3 and/or the patient manifests clinically significant bleeding, Gamimune N, 5% 400 mg/kg body weight may be given as a single infusion. If an adequate response does not result, the dose can be increased to 800–1,000 mg/kg of body weight given as a single infusion. Maintenance infusions may be administered intermittently as clinically indicated to maintain a platelet count greater than 30,000/mm^3

Bone Marrow Transplantation

Gamimune N, 5% should be administered in doses of 500 mg/kg (10 mL/kg) body weight beginning on days −7 and −2 pretransplant (or at the time conditioning therapy for transplantation is begun), then weekly through day 90 posttransplant. Gamimune N, 5% should be administered by itself through a Hickman line while it is in place, and thereafter through a peripheral vein. Please see DOSAGE AND ADMINISTRATION for other drug interactions.

Pediatric HIV Infection

A reduction in bacterial infections has been observed in children infected with HIV-1 receiving Gamimune N, 5% 400 mg/kg (8 mL/kg) body weight every 28 days.

HOW SUPPLIED

Gamimune N, 5% is supplied in the following sizes:

NDC Number	Size	Grams Protein
0026-0646-12	10 mL	0.5
0026-0646-20	50 mL	2.5
0026-0646-71	100 mL	5.0
0026-0646-24	200 mL	10.0
0026-0646-25	250 mL	12.5

STORAGE

Store at 2–8°C (36–46°F). Do not freeze. Do not use after expiration date.

CAUTION

U.S. federal law prohibits dispensing without prescription.

REFERENCES

1. Tenold RA, inventor; Cutter Laboratories, assignee. Intravenously injectable immune serum globulin. U.S. Patent 4,396,608, August 2, 1983
2. Data on file at Bayer Corporation
3. Pirofsky B, Campbell SM, Montanaro A: Individual patient variations in the kinetics of intravenous immune globulin administration. *J Clin Immunol* 2 (2): 7S-14S, 1982.
4. Pirofsky B: Intravenous immune globulin therapy in hypogammaglobulinemia. *Am J Med* 76 (3A): 53–60, 1984.
5. Pirofsky B, Anderson CJ, Bardana EJ Jr: Therapeutic and detrimental effects of intravenous immunoglobulin therapy. In: Alving BM (ed.): *Immunoglobulins: characteristics and uses of Intravenous preparations.* Washington, D.C., U.S. Government Printing Office, (1980), pp 15–22.
6. Sullivan KM, Kopecky KJ, Jocom J, et al: Immunomodulatory and antimicrobial efficacy of intravenous immunoglobulin in bone marrow transplantation, *N Engl J Med* 323(11):705–12, 1990.
7. Bernstein LJ, Ochs HD, Wedgwood RJ, et al; Defective humoral immunity in pediatric acquired immune deficiency syndrome. *J Pediatr* 107(3):352–7, 1985
8. Borkowsky W, Steele CJ, Grubman S. et al: Antibody responses to bacterial toxoids in children infected with human immunodeficiency virus. *J Pediatr* 110(4):563–6, 1987
9. Blanche S, Le Deist F, Fischer A, et al: Longitudinal study of 18 children with perinatal LAV/HTLV III infection: attempt at prognostic evaluation. *J Pediatr* 109(6): 965–70, 1986.
10. Pahwa S, Fikrig S, Menez R, et al: Pediatric acquired immunodeficiency syndrome demonstration of B-lymphocyte defects in vitro. *Diagn Immunol* 4(1):24–30, 1986.
11. Bernstein, LJ, Krieger BZ, Novick B, et al: Bacterial infections in the acquired immunodeficiency syndrome of children. *Pediatr Infect Dis* 4(5):472–5, 1985.
12. Krasinski K, Borkowsky W, Bonk S, et al: Bacterial infections in human immunodeficiency virus-infected children. *Pediatr Infect Dis J* 4(5):323–8, 1988.
13. Scott GB, Buck BE, Leterman JG, et al: Acquired immunodeficiency syndrome in infants. *N Engl J Med* 310(2): 76–81, 1984.
14. Mofenson LM, Willoughby A. Passive immunization. In: Pizzo PA, Wilfert CM, (eds.) *Pediatric AIDS: the challenge of HIV infection in infants, children and adolescents.* Baltimore: Williams & Wilkins (1991) pp 633–50.
15. National Institute of Child Health and Human Development Intravenous Immunoglobulin Study Group. Intravenous immune globulin for the prevention of bacterial infections in children with symptomatic human immunodeficiency virus infection. *N Engl J Med* 325(2):73–80, 1991.
16. Mofenson LM, Moye J Jr, Bethel J, et al: Prophylactic intravenous immunoglobulin in HIV-infected children with CD4+ counts of 0.20 × 10^9/L or more. Effect on viral, opportunistic, and bacterial infections. *JAMA* 268(4):483–88, 1992.
17. Berg G, Matzkies F: Wirkung von Maltose nach intravenöser Dauerinfusion auf den Stoffwechsel. *Z Ernährungswiss* 15:255–62, 1976.
18. Förster H, Hoos I, Boecker S: Versuche mit Probanden zur parenteralen Verwertung von Maltose. *Z Ernährungswiss* 15(3):284–93, 1976.
19. Finke C, Reinauer H: Utilization of maltose and oligosaccharides after intravenous infusion in man. *Nutr Metab* 21(Suppl 1):115–7, 1977.
20. Young EA, Drummond A, Cioletti L, et al: Metabolism of continuously infused intravenous maltose. [abstract] 25(3):543A, 1977.
21. Soroff HS, Hansen LM, Sasvary D, et al: Clinical pharmacology and metabolism of maltose in normal human volunteers, [abstract] *Clin Res* 26(3):286A, 1978.
22. Guyton AC: *Textbook of Medical Physiology.* 5th ed. Philadelphia, W.B. Saunders, 1976, pp 499–500.
23. Buckley RH: Immunoglobulin replacement therapy: Indications and contraindications for use and variable IgG levels achieved. In: Alving BM (ed): *immunoglobulins: characteristics and uses of intravenous preparations.* Washington, D.C., U.S. Government Printing Office, (1980), pp 3–8.
24. Nolte MT, Pirofsky B, Gerritz GA, et. al: Intravenous immunoglobulin therapy for antibody deficiency *Clin Exp Immunol* 36:237–43, 1979.
25. Ochs HD: Intravenous immunoglobulin therapy of patients with primary immunodeficiency syndromes: efficacy and safety of a new modified immune globulin preparation in: Alving BM (ed.): *Immunoglobulins: characteristics and uses of intravenous preparations.* Washington, D.C., U.S. Government printing office, (1980), pp 9–14
26. Sekul E, Cupler E, Dalakas M. Aseptic meningitis associated with high-dose intravenous immunoglobulin therapy: Frequency and risk factors. *Ann Int Med* 121: 259–262, 1994.
27. Kato E, Shindo S, Eto Y, et al: Administration of Immune Globulin Associated with Aseptic Meningitis. *JAMA* 259(22):3269–3270, 1988.
28. Casteels-Van Daele M, Wijndaele L, Hunninck K, et al: Intravenous immune globulin and acute aseptic meningitis. *N Engl J Med* 323(9):614–615, 1990.
29. Scribner C, Kapit R, Phillips E, et al: Aseptic meningitis and Intravenous immunoglobulin therapy. *Ann Intern Med* 121(4):305–306, 1994.
30. Schiavotto C, Ruggeri M, Rodeghiero F. Adverse reactions after high-dose intravenous immunoglobulin: incidence in 83 patients treated for idiopathic thrombocytopenic purpura (ITP) and review of the literature. *Haematologica* 78(6:Suppl 2):35–40, 1993.
31. Pasatiempo AM, Kroser JA, Rudnick M, et al: Acute renal failure after intravenous immunoglobulin therapy. *J Rheumatol* 21(2):347–9, 1994.
32. Peerless AG, Stiehm ER: intravenous gammaglobulin for reaction to intramuscular preparation. [letter] *Lancet* 2(8347):461, 1983.
33. Cayco AV, Perazella MA, Hayslett JP. Renal insufficiency after intravenous immune globulin therapy: A Report of Two Cases and an Analysis of the Literature. *J Amer Soc Nephrology* 8:1788–1793, 1997.
34. Winward DB, Brophy MT: Acute renal failure after administration of intravenous immunoglobulin: review of the literature and case report. *Pharmacotherapy* 15: 765–772, 1995.
35. Phillips, AO: Renal failure and intravenous immunoglobulin [letter; comment]. *Clin Nephrol* 36:83–86, 1992.
36. Anderson W, Bethea W: Renal lesions following administration of hypertonic solutions of sucrose. *JAMA* 114: 1983–1987, 1940.
37. Lindberg H, Wald A: Renal changes following the administration of hypertonic solutions. *Arch Intern Med* 63:907–918, 1939.
38. Ridgon RH, Caldwell ES: Renal lesions following the intravenous injection of hypertonic solution of sucrose: A clinical and experimental study. *Arch Intern Med* 69: 670–690. 1942.
39. Tan E, Hajinazarian M, Bay, et al. Acute renal failure resulting from intravenous immunoglobulin therapy. *Arch Neurology* 50:137–139, 1993.

Bayer Corporation
Pharmaceutical Division
Elkhart, IN 46515 USA
U.S. License No. 8 14-7646-003
(Rev. June 1999)

Shown in Product Identification Guide, page 308

GAMIMUNE® N, 10% ℞

Immune Globulin Intravenous (Human), 10%
Solvent/Detergent Treated

DESCRIPTION

Immune Globulin Intravenous (Human), 10%—Gamimune® N, 10% treated with solvent/detergent is a sterile solution of human protein containing no preservative. Gamimune N, 10% consists of 9%–11% protein in 0.16–0.24 M glycine. Not less than 98% of the protein has the electrophoretic mobility of gamma globulin. Not less than 90% of the IgG is monomer. Also present are traces of IgA and of IgM. The distribution of IgG subclasses is similar to that found in normal serum. The measured buffer capacity is 35 mEq/L and the osmolality is 274 mOsmol/kg solvent. The product is made by cold ethanol fractionation of large pools of human plasma. Part of the fractionation may be performed by another licensed manufacturer. The immunoglobulin is isolated from Cohn Effluent III after limited diafiltration and ultrafiltration. The solution is adjusted to 0.3% tri-n-butyl phosphate (TNBP) and 0.2% sodium cholate. After addition of the solvent (TNBP) and the detergent (sodium cholate), the solution is heated to 30°C and maintained at that temperature for not less than 6 hours. After the viral inactivation step, the reactants are removed by precipitation, filtration, and finally diafiltration and ultrafiltration. The protein is stabilized during the process by adjusting the pH of the solution to 4.0–4.5.[1] Isotonicity is achieved by the addition of glycine. Gamimune N, 10% treated with solvent/detergent is then incubated in the final container (at the low pH of 4.25), for a minimum of 21 days at 20°C. The product is intended for intravenous administration.

The removal and inactivation of spiked model enveloped and non-enveloped viruses during the manufacturing process for Gamimune N, 10% has been validated in laboratory studies. Human Immunodeficiency Virus, Type 1 (HIV-1) was chosen as the relevant virus for blood products; Bovine Viral Diarrhea Virus (BVDV) was chosen to model for Hepatitis C virus; Pseudorabies virus (PRV) was chosen to model for Hepatitis B and the Herpes viruses; and Reo virus type 3 (Reo) was chosen to model non-enveloped viruses and for its resistance to physical and chemical inactivation. Significant removal of model enveloped and non-enveloped viruses is seen between the Fraction II + IIIW and Effluent III steps and between the Effluent III and Filtrate III steps. Significant inactivation of enveloped viruses is achieved at the time of treatment of Filtrate III with TNBP/sodium cholate and also at the time of low pH incubation in the final container.

CLINICAL PHARMACOLOGY

Primary Humoral Immunodeficiency

Gamimune N, 10% supplies a broad spectrum of opsonic and neutralizing IgG antibodies for the prevention or attenuation of a wide variety of infectious diseases. Since Gamimune N, 10% is administered intravenously, essentially 100% of the infused IgG antibodies are immediately available in the recipient's circulation.[2] Studies using a modified intravenous immunoglobulin at pH 6.8 have shown that approximately 30% of the infused IgG disappeared from the circulation in the first 24 hours, due primarily to equilibration of the IgG between the plasma and the extravascular space.[2–5] A further decline to about 40% of the peak level found immediately post-infusion is to be expected during the first week.[2–5] The in vivo half-life of Immune Globulin Intravenous (Human), 5%—Gamimune® N, 5% equals or exceeds the 3-week half-life reported for IgG in the literature, but individual patient variation in half-life has been observed.[2] Thus, this variable as well as the amount of immune globulin administered per dose is important in determining the frequency of administration of the drug for each individual patient. A comparative study of Gamimune N, 10% with Gamimune N, 5% (in 10% maltose) in 18 subjects demonstrated equivalent post-infusion recovery for the two preparations. A comparative study of Gamimune N, 10% treated with solvent/detergent and Gamimune N, 10% in 17 subjects demonstrated bioequivalence.

Idiopathic Thrombocytopenic Purpura

While Gamimune N, 10% has been shown to be effective in some cases of idiopathic thrombocytopenic purpura (ITP) (see INDICATIONS AND USAGE), the mechanism of action has not been fully elucidated.

Bone Marrow Transplantation

Clinical studies with Gamimune N, 5% have shown that it is effective in bone marrow transplant patients ≥20 years of age in the first 100 days posttransplant for the following: prevention of systemic and local infections, interstitial pneumonia of infectious and idiopathic etiologies and acute graft-versus-host disease (AGVHD)[6] (see INDICATIONS AND USAGE). Administration of Gamimune N, 5% to bone marrow transplant patients significantly increased IgG and IgG subclass levels while those seen in the control group fell below predicted levels. The mechanism of action of Gamimune N, 5% in reducing the incidence of AGVHD is presently unknown.

Pediatric HIV Infection

Children infected with human immunodeficiency virus (HIV) may display defects in both cellular and humoral immunity.[7–10] As a result, some children with HIV-1 infection experience serious, potentially life-threatening recurrent bacterial infections.[11–13] In one retrospective report, among 71 HIV-infected children observed over 3.5 years, 27 (37%) experienced serious documented bacterial infections.[12] The types of bacterial and viral infections observed in HIV-infected children are similar to those seen in children with primary hypogammaglobulinemia.[14] The replacement of opsonic and neutralizing IgG antibodies has been shown to reduce serious and minor bacterial infection in HIV-infected children.[15,16]

In a randomized, double-blind, placebo-controlled, multicenter study performed between March 7, 1988 and January 15, 1991, the efficacy of Gamimune N, 5% in pediatric HIV disease to decrease the frequency of serious and minor bacterial infections and the frequency of hospitalization, and to increase the time free of serious bacterial infection was documented in children with clinical or immunologic evidence of HIV disease (see INDICATIONS AND USAGE). The primary endpoint of this study was prospectively defined as a significant reduction in the proportion of subjects who develop at least one serious bacterial infection when compared to the control group of HIV-infected children who received placebo. Serious bacterial infections were defined as laboratory-proven and clinically diagnosed (i.e., radiologically proven acute pneumonia and sinusitis) infections. The Data Safety and Monitoring Board (DSMB) recommended early termination of the study based on data presented to them from an interim analysis in December 1990 which showed that treatment with Gamimune N, 5% increased the time free from serious infections in children with CD4 + counts ≥ 200/mm^3.

General

Glycine (aminoacetic acid) is a nonessential amino acid normally present in the body.[17] Glycine is a major ingredient in amino acid solutions employed in intravenous alimentation.[18] While toxic effects of glycine administration have been reported,[19] the doses and rates of administration were 3 – 4-fold greater than those for Gamimune N, 10%.

The buffer capacity of Gamimune N, 10% is 35.0 mEq/L (~0.35 mEq/g protein). A dose of 1000 mg/kg body weight therefore represents an acid load of 0.35 mEq/kg body weight. The total buffering capacity of whole blood in a normal individual is 45–50 mEq/L of blood, or 3.6 mEq/kg body weight.[20] Thus, the acid load delivered with a dose of 1000 mg/kg of Gamimune N, 10% would be neutralized by the buffering capacity of whole blood alone, even if the dose was infused instantaneously.

In Phase I human studies comparing Gamimune N, 10% with Gamimune N, 5% (in 10% maltose), venous blood measurements were taken following the intravenous administration of 400 mg/kg body weight in 18 patients. There were no clinically important changes in mean venous pH, bicarbonate, or base excess measurements in these patients receiving either preparation.[2]

In a similar, earlier Phase I study Gamimune N, 5% (in 10% maltose) was compared with a chemically modified 5% intravenous immunoglobulin preparation with a pH of 6.8. No clinically important changes in mean venous pH and bicarbonate measurements were detected following infusions of either preparation at doses of 400 mg/kg body weight in 37 patients.

In patients with limited or compromised acid-base compensatory mechanisms, consideration should be given to the effect of the additional acid load Gamimune N, 10% might present.

INDICATIONS AND USAGE

Primary Humoral Immunodeficiency

Gamimune N, 10% is efficacious in the treatment of primary immunodeficiency states in which severe impairment of antibody forming capacity has been shown, such as: congenital agammaglobulinemias, common variable immunodeficiency, Wiskott-Aldrich syndrome, x-linked immunodeficiency with hyper IgM, and severe combined immunodeficiencies.[5,21–23] Gamimune N, 10% is especially useful when high levels or rapid elevation of circulating antibodies are desired or when intramuscular injections are contraindicated.

Idiopathic Thrombocytopenic Purpura (ITP)

In clinical situations in which a rapid rise in platelet count is needed to control bleeding or to allow a patient with ITP to undergo surgery, administration of Gamimune N, 10% should be considered. Studies with Gamimune N, 5% demonstrate that in patients in whom a response was achieved, the rise of platelets was generally rapid (within 1–5 days), transient (most often lasting from several days to several weeks) and were not considered curative. It is presently not possible to predict which patients with ITP will respond to therapy, although the increase in platelet counts in children seems to be better than that in adults. Childhood ITP may, however, respond spontaneously without treatment.

Gamimune N, 10% has been studied in 31 adult and pediatric subjects with ITP using a dosage of 1,000 mg/kg body weight on either 1 day or 2 consecutive days. Fourteen of 16 children (87.5%) and 9 of 10 adults with platelet follow-up (90%) responded to treatment with clinically significant platelet increments of ≥ 30,000/mm^3. In the 12 children with acute ITP, there was an average increase in platelet count above baseline of 274,000/mm^3 (range 33,000–529,000/mm^3).

Two different dosing regimens of Gamimune N, 5% have been studied in clinical investigations: a regimen consisting of 400 mg/kg body weight daily for 5 consecutive days, and a high dose treatment regimen consisting of 1,000 mg/kg body weight administered on either 1 day or 2 consecutive days (these studies are summarized below).

In clinical studies of Gamimune N, 5%, five of six (83.3%) children and 12 of 16 (75%) adults with acute or chronic ITP treated with 400 mg/kg body weight for 5 consecutive days demonstrated clinically significant platelet increments of ≥ 30,000/mm^3 over baseline. The mean platelet count in children with ITP rose from 27,800/mm^3 at baseline to 297,000/mm^3 (range 50,000–455,000/mm^3) and the mean platelet count in adults with ITP rose from 27,900/mm^3 at baseline to 124,900/mm^3 (range 11,000–341,000/mm^3). Two of three children with acute ITP rapidly went into complete remission.

Thirteen of 14 children (92.9%) and 26 of 29 adults (89.7%) with acute or chronic ITP treated with Gamimune N, 5% 1,000 mg/kg body weight administered on either 1 day or 2 consecutive days responded to treatment with clinically significant platelet increments of ≥ 30,000/mm^3 over baseline. This included three of three patients with ITP that were human immunodeficiency virus (HIV) antibody positive and two of two patients with ITP that were pregnant. The mean platelet count in children with ITP treated with Gamimune N, 5% 1,000 mg/kg body weight on 1 day or 2 consecutive days rose from 44,400/mm^3 at baseline to 285,600/mm^3 (range 89,000–473,000/mm^3) and the mean platelet count in adults with ITP treated with the regimen rose from 23,400/mm^3 at baseline to 173,100/mm^3 (range 28,000–709,000/mm^3). Two patients, one each with acute adult and chronic childhood ITP, entered complete remission with treatment.

Six of the 29 adult patients with ITP received Gamimune N, 5% 1,000 mg/kg on 1 day or 2 consecutive days to increase the platelet count prior to splenectomy. Mean platelet counts rose from 14,500/mm^3 at baseline to 129,300/mm^3 (range 51,000–242,000/mm^3) prior to surgery.

The duration of the platelet rise following treatment of ITP with either treatment regimen of Gamimune N, 5% was variable, ranging from several days to 12 months or more. Some ITP patients have demonstrated continuing responsiveness over many months to intermittent infusions of Gamimune N, 5% 400–1,000 mg/kg body weight, administered as a single maintenance dose, at intervals as indicated by the platelet count.

Bone Marrow Transplantation (BMT)

In clinical studies in bone marrow transplant patients ≥ 20 years of age, Gamimune N, 5% decreased the risk of septicemia and other infections, interstitial pneumonia of infectious or idiopathic etiologies and acute graft-versus-host disease (AGVHD) in the first 100 days posttransplant. Gamimune N, 5% is not indicated in bone marrow transplant patients below 20 years of age. In a controlled study of 369 evaluable BMT patients (184 treated and 185 controls) who either did or did not receive Gamimune N, 5% in doses of 500 mg/kg body weight on days –7 and –2 pretransplant, then weekly through day 90 posttransplant, posttransplant complications were evaluated in the entire study group and in patients under age 20 and age 20 or older. For patients ≥ 20 years of age (128 patients in the control group and 119 patients in the treated group), there was a statistically significant reduction in interstitial pneumonia from 21% in the control group to 9% in the treated group (p = 0.0032) during the first 100 days posttransplant. Also significantly reduced in this age group were: overall septicemia from 53 infections in the 128 patient control group to 26 infections in the 119 patient treated group (relative risk-control:treated [RR] 2.36, p = 0.0025); gram-negative septicemia from 24 infections in the 128 patient control group to 9 infections in the 119 patient treated group (RR 2.53, p = 0.015); gram-positive septicemia from 16 infections in the 128 patient control group to 8 infections in the 119 patient treated group (RR 2.73, p = 0.046); and Grade II to IV AGVHD from an incidence of 58 of 110 in the control group to 38 of 108 in the treated group (p = 0.0051).

The given p-values do not take into account multiple endpoints and subset analyses. Therefore, some of the p-values could occur by chance alone. There was no significant improvement in overall mortality in this study.

In patients below age 20, there appeared to be no benefit from treatment with Gamimune N, 5%, either in reducing the incidence of infections or the incidence of AGVHD.

Pediatric HIV Infection

Gamimune N, 5% 400 mg/kg every 28 days significantly decreased the frequency of serious and minor bacterial infections (laboratory-proven and clinically diagnosed) and the frequency of hospitalization, and increased the time free of serious bacterial infection. The effect of Gamimune N, 5% in preventing serious bacterial infections was especially apparent in preventing primary bacteremia (including *Streptococcus pneumoniae* bacteremia) and acute pneumonia.

In a randomized, double-blind, placebo-controlled, multicenter study, 394 HIV-infected, non-hemophilic, children less than 13 years of age were randomized. Of the children randomized, 369 were included in the efficacy analysis and 376 in the safety analysis. The study population had 1) a mean age of 40 months (range 2.4–136.8 months), 2) acquired HIV primarily through vertical transmission (91%), 3) a majority (87%) of CDC Class P-2 (symptomatic), and 4) had a median CD4 + count of 937 cells/mm^3 (range 0–6660 cells/mm^3). At the time of study entry, 14% (52 of 369) were receiving *Pneumocystis carinii* pneumonia (PCP) prophylaxis. During the course of the study, 51% (189 of 369) received PCP prophylaxis and 44% (164 of 369) received zidovudine (ZDV). Children with HIV-1 infection were initially stratified into two groups based upon CD4 + count (< 200 cells/mm^3 versus ≥ 200 cells/mm^3) and CDC classification of pediatric HIV disease (history of opportunistic infections [P-2-D-1] and recurrent serious bacterial infections [P-2-D-2] versus others). Subjects received Gamimune N, 5% (400 mg/kg = 8 mL/kg) (n = 185) or an equivalent volume of placebo (0.1% Albumin [Human]) (n = 184) every 28 days. The mean follow-up for subjects receiving Gamimune N, 5% was 17.9 months and 17.8 months for patients on placebo. The number of subjects who had at least one serious bacterial infection was 86 of 184 (47%) in the placebo group and 55 of 185 (30%) in the Gamimune N, 5% group (p = 0.0009). All p-values reported are two-sided. Treatment with Gamimune N, 5% compared to placebo was also associated with a significant reduction in both the number of subjects with at least one laboratory-proven infection (36 of 184 vs. 18 of 185, p = 0.0081), and the number of subjects with at least one clinically diagnosed infection (71 of 184 vs. 45 of 185, p = 0.0036). Efficacy in patients with CD4 + counts < 200/mm^3 was not established, possibly because of the small number of subjects in this category.

The 2-year treatment period defined in the protocol was truncated for some patients by the DSMB based on data from the interim analysis. Rates of serious bacterial infections per 100 patient-years were computed and analyzed to take into account both the unequal duration of treatment and follow-up, as well as recurrent infections in individual subjects. Children treated with Gamimune N, 5% experienced a 50.5% lower frequency of laboratory-proven serious bacterial infection compared to the group treated with placebo (9.1 vs. 18.2 infections per 100 patient-years, p = 0.031), a 36.0% lower frequency of clinically diagnosed serious infections (24.0 vs. 37.5 infections per 100 patient-years, p = 0.013), a 40.6% reduction in total serious infections (laboratory-proven and clinically diagnosed) (33.1 vs. 55.7 infections per 100 patient-years, p = 0.003), a 60% lower frequency of primary bacteremias (5.8 vs. 14.5 infections per 100 patient-years, p = 0.009), a 75.6% lower frequency of *Streptococcus pneumoniae* bacteremia (1.1 vs. 4.5 bacteremias per 100 patient-years, p = 0.026), a 54.3% lower frequency of clinically diagnosed pneumonia (12.7 vs. 27.8 infections per 100 patient-years, p = 0.001), and a 22.5% lower frequency of minor bacterial infections (including otitis media, skin and soft tissue infections, and upper respiratory tract infections) (123.6 vs. 159.5 infections per 100 patient-years, p = 0.033).

In addition to a reduced frequency of infection, children treated with Gamimune N, 5% had a 36.8% lower number of hospitalizations per 100 patient-years (72 vs. 114 per 100 patient-years, p = 0.002) and a reduced number of hospital days (6.9 vs. 10.5 per patient-year, p = 0.030) than patients treated with placebo. Patients treated with Gamimune N, 5% had a higher probability of remaining free of laboratory-proven infections (p = 0.0093) and combined laboratory-proven and clinically diagnosed infections (p = 0.0015) for 24 months than the group of children treated with placebo. At 24 months, the estimated probabilities of remaining infection-free for the Gamimune N, 5% and placebo arms were 87.8% vs. 76.1%, respectively, for laboratory-proven infections and 63.5% vs. 44.5%, respectively, for combined laboratory-proven and clinically diagnosed infections.

There was no effect of Gamimune N, 5% therapy on mortality, which was low in both treatment groups (17%), or on the frequency of opportunistic or viral infections during the period of study.

Since antibacterial prophylaxis could also account for the observed reduction in the rate of serious bacterial infections, further analysis was performed to evaluate the role of *Pneumocystis carinii* pneumonia (PCP) prophylaxis on the efficacy of Gamimune N, 5%. PCP prophylaxis consisted primarily (96%) of trimethoprim/sulfamethoxazole given 3 successive days each week. This antibiotic combination could be active against the bacteria commonly encountered in this patient population. In the subgroup of patients receiving PCP prophylaxis at study entry, treatment with Gamimune N, 5% was associated with 44.0 infections per 100 patient-years, whereas placebo recipients had 64.7 infections per 100 patient-years (p = 0.047). In the subgroup of patients not receiving PCP prophylaxis at study entry, treatment with Gamimune N, 5% was associated with 22.1 infections per 100 patient-years, whereas placebo recipients had 44.9 infections per 100 patient-years on placebo (p = 0.024). Thus, Gamimune N, 5% benefited patients by reducing the rate of serious bacterial infections whether or not they were receiving PCP prophylactic treatment at study entry. However, it should be noted that the use of PCP prophylactic treatment in this study was not randomized and specific guidelines for its administration were not identified.

CONTRAINDICATIONS

Gamimune N, 10% is contraindicated in individuals who are known to have had an anaphylactic or severe systemic response to Immune Globulin (Human). Individuals with selective IgA deficiencies who have known antibody against IgA (anti-IgA antibody) should not receive Gamimune N, 10% since these patients may experience severe reactions to the IgA which may be present.[22]

WARNINGS

Immune Globulin Intravenous (Human) products have been reported to be associated with renal dysfunction, acute renal failure, osmotic nephrosis and death.[24] Patients predisposed to acute renal failure include patients with any degree of pre-existing renal insufficiency, diabetes mellitus, age greater than 65, volume depletion, sepsis, paraproteinemia, or patients receiving known nephrotoxic drugs. Especially in such patients, IGIV products should be administered at the minimum concentration available and the minimum rate of infusion practicable. While these reports of renal dysfunction and acute renal failure have been associated with the use of many of the licensed IGIV products, those containing sucrose as a stabilizer accounted for a disproportionate share of the total number. See PRECAUTIONS and DOSAGE AND ADMINISTRATION sections for important information intended to reduce the risk of acute renal failure.

Continued on next page

Gamimune N, 10%—Cont.

Gamimune® N, 10% is made from human plasma. Products made from human plasma may contain infectious agents, such as viruses, that can cause disease. The risk that such products will transmit an infectious agent has been reduced by screening plasma donors for prior exposure to certain viruses, by testing for the presence of certain current virus infections, and by inactivating and/or removing certain viruses. Despite these measures, such products can still potentially transmit disease. There is also the possibility that unknown infectious agents may be present in such products. Individuals who receive infusions of blood or plasma products may develop signs and/or symptoms of some viral infections, particularly hepatitis C. ALL infections thought by a physician possibly to have been transmitted by this product should be reported by the physician or other healthcare provider to Bayer Corporation [1-888-765-3203].

The physician should discuss the risks and benefits of this product with the patient, before prescribing or administering it to the patient.

Gamimune N, 10% should be administered only intravenously as the intramuscular and subcutaneous routes have not been evaluated.

Immune Globulin Intravenous (Human), 5%—Gamimune® N, 5% has, on rare occasions, caused a precipitous fall in blood pressure and a clinical picture of anaphylaxis, even when the patient is not known to be sensitive to immune globulin preparations. These reactions may be related to the rate of infusion. Accordingly, the infusion rate given under DOSAGE AND ADMINISTRATION for Gamimune N, 10% should be closely followed, at least until the physician has had sufficient experience with a given patient. The patient's vital signs should be monitored continuously and careful observation made for any symptoms throughout the entire infusion. Epinephrine should be available for the treatment of an acute anaphylactic reaction.

PRECAUTIONS

General

Any vial that has been entered should be used promptly. Partially used vials should be discarded. Do not use if turbid. Solution which has been frozen should not be used.

An aseptic meningitis syndrome (AMS) has been reported to occur infrequently in association with Immune Globulin Intravenous (Human) treatment. The syndrome usually begins within several hours to two days following Immune Globulin Intravenous (Human) treatment. It is characterized by symptoms and signs including severe headache, nuchal rigidity, drowsiness, fever, photophobia, painful eye movements, and nausea and vomiting. Cerebrospinal fluid (CSF) studies are frequently positive with pleocytosis up to several thousand cells per mm^3, predominantly from the granulocytic series, and elevated protein levels up to several hundred mg/dL. Patients exhibiting such symptoms and signs should receive a thorough neurological examination, including CSF studies, to rule out other causes of meningitis. AMS may occur more frequently in association with high dose (2 g/kg) Immune Globulin Intravenous (Human) treatment. Discontinuation of Immune Globulin Intravenous (Human) treatment has resulted in remission of AMS within several days without sequelae.[25,26]

Assure that patients are not volume depleted prior to the initiation of the infusion of IGIV.

Periodic monitoring of renal function tests and urine output is particularly important in patients judged to have a potential increased risk for developing acute renal failure. Renal function, including measurement of blood urea nitrogen (BUN)/serum creatinine, should be assessed prior to the initial infusion of Gamimune N, 10% and again at appropriate intervals thereafter. If renal function deteriorates, discontinuation of the product should be considered. For patients judged to be at risk for developing renal dysfunction, it may be prudent to reduce the amount of product infused per unit time by infusing Gamimune N, 10% at a rate less than 8 mg IG/kg/min (0.08 mL/kg/min).

Information For Patients

Patients should be instructed to immediately report symptoms of decreased urine output, sudden weight gain, fluid retention/edema, and/or shortness of breath (which may suggest kidney damage) to their physicians.

Drug Interactions

Antibodies in Gamimune N, 10% may interfere with the response to live viral vaccines such as measles, mumps and rubella. Therefore, use of such vaccines should be deferred until approximately 6 months after Gamimune N, 10% administration.

Please see DOSAGE AND ADMINISTRATION for other drug interactions.

Pregnancy Category C

Animal reproduction studies have not been conducted with Gamimune N, 10%. It is not known whether Gamimune N, 10% can cause fetal harm when administered to a pregnant woman or can affect reproduction capacity. Gamimune N, 10% should be given to a pregnant woman only if clearly needed.

ADVERSE REACTIONS

General

Increases in creatinine and blood urea nitrogen (BUN) have been observed as soon as one to two days following infusion. Progression to oliguria and anuria requiring dialysis has been observed, although some patients have improved spontaneously following cessation of treatment.[32] Types of severe renal adverse reactions that have been seen following IGIV therapy include: acute renal failure, acute tubular necrosis,[33] proximal tubular nephropathy, and osmotic nephrosis.[24, see also 34–36] In the studies undertaken to date, other types of reactions have not been reported with Gamimune N, 5% or Gamimune N, 10%. It may be, however, that adverse effects will be similar to those previously reported with intravenous and intramuscular immunoglobulin administration. Potential reactions, therefore, may also include anxiety, flushing, wheezing, abdominal cramps, myalgias, arthralgia, and dizziness; rash has been reported only rarely. Reactions to intravenous immunoglobulin tend to be related to the rate of infusion. True anaphylactic reactions to Gamimune N, 10% may occur in recipients with documented prior histories of severe allergic reactions to intramuscular immunoglobulin, but some patients may tolerate cautiously administered intravenous immunogobulin without adverse effects.[32] Very rarely an anaphylactoid reaction may occur in patients with no prior history of severe allergic reactions to either intramuscular or intravenous immunoglobulin.[2]

Primary Humoral Immunodeficiency

A safety study has been conducted in 20 adult and pediatric subjects with primary immunodeficiency syndrome comparing side effects of Gamimune N, 5% with those of Gamimune N, 10%. The incidence, nature, or severity of reactions with Gamimune N, 10% were not different from those observed with Gamimune N, 5%, and were consistent with those observed in previous studies with Gamimune N, 5%. Symptoms related to the infusion of Gamimune N, 10% were observed in 9 (3.5%) of 255 infusions. These symptoms were all mild to moderate in severity and included chills, fever, headache and emesis.

In a study of 37 patients with immunodeficiency syndromes receiving Gamimune N, 5% in a monthly dose of 400 mg/kg body weight, reactions were seen in 5.2% of the infusions. Symptoms reported included malaise, a feeling of faintness, fever, chills, headache, nausea, vomiting, chest tightness, dyspnea and chest, back or hip pain. Mild erythema following infiltration of Gamimune N, 5% at the infusion site was reported in some cases.

A safety study has been conducted in 17 adult and adolescent subjects with primary immunodeficiency syndrome, comparing side effects and bioequivalency of Gamimune N, 10% with those of Gamimune N, 10% treated with solvent/detergent. The incidence, nature and severity of reactions with Gamimune N, 10% treated with solvent/detergent were not different from those observed with Gamimune N, 10%.

Idiopathic Thrombocytopenic Purpura

An investigation of Gamimune N, 10% in 31 adult and pediatric subjects with ITP encountered side effects in 17 of 119 (14.3%) infusions. The dosage in these studies was 1,000 mg/kg body weight for 1 day or 2 consecutive days. However, in the adult study, an induction dosage of 500 mg/kg body weight for 1 day or 2 consecutive days was associated with 17 of these infusions. Of those 17 infusions, three had adverse events. Overall, side effects included mild chest pain, mild and moderate emesis, moderate fever, mild or moderate headache (severe on one occasion) and a single incidence of hives, pruritus and rash. At least 17 of the 50 infusions in the pediatric study were given at rates of ≥ 0.1 mL/kg body weight per minute as part of a rate escalation investigation. Maximum infusion rates obtained were not limited by or interrupted due to adverse effects.

In studies of Gamimune N, 5% administered at a dose of 400 mg/kg body weight in the treatment of adult and pediatric patients with ITP, systemic reactions were noted in only 4 of 154 (2.6%) infusions, and all but one occurred at rates of infusion greater than 0.04 mL/kg body weight per minute. The symptoms reported included chest tightness, a sense of tachycardia (pulse was 84 beats per minute), and a burning sensation in the head; these symptoms were all mild and transient.

In studies of Gamimune N, 5% administered at a dose of 1,000 mg/kg body weight either as a single dose or as two doses on consecutive days in the treatment of adult and pediatric patients with ITP, adverse reactions were noted in 25 of 251 (10%) infusions. Symptoms reported included headache, nausea, fever, chills, back pain, chest tightness, and shortness of breath. In children, the high dose regimen has been well-tolerated at the highest rates of infusion. In adults, however, the frequency of adverse reactions tended to increase with infusion rates in excess of 0.06 mL/kg body weight per minute. In general, reactions reported with infusion of Gamimune N, 5% in these studies were reported as mild or moderate, and responded to slowing of the infusion rate.

Bone Marrow Transplantation

In studies of Gamimune N, 5% administered to 185 bone marrow transplant recipients at doses of 500 mg/kg (10 mL/kg) body weight on day −7 and day −2 pretransplant, then weekly through day 90 posttransplant, adverse reactions were noted in 12 (6.5%) of the 185 patients that received Gamimune N, 5% and in 14 (0.6%) of 2,176 infusions. All reactions reported were rate-related and classified as mild. Chills were the most common symptom reported, occurring in nine patients. The other symptoms reported included headache, flushing, fever, pruritus and slight back discomfort. All reactions resolved satisfactorily, usually without treatment or decreasing the infusion rate.

Pediatric HIV Infection

Three hundred seventy-six (376) patients, 187 treated with Gamimune N, 5% and 189 treated with placebo (0.1% Albumin [Human]), were included in the safety analysis. Adverse reactions occurred during or within 24 hours of an infusion in 50 of 3,451 (1.4%) infusions of Gamimune N, 5% and 62 of 3,447 (1.8%) infusions of placebo. Fever was the most common adverse reaction and occurred 30 of 105 (28.6%) patients receiving placebo and 19 of 78 (24.4%) patients treated with Gamimune N, 5%. Irritability was the second most common symptom reported, with 10 of 105 (9.5%) reports for the placebo group and 9 of 78 (11.5%) for the group treated with Gamimune N, 5%. A large number of diverse adverse reactions accounted for the remaining adverse reactions reported in both study groups. In general, the number of adverse events reported was comparable in both the placebo and Gamimune N, 5% treated groups. Three serious adverse reactions were reported. One patient experienced a hypersensitivity reaction and did not receive further Gamimune N, 5% treatment. A second patient developed tachycardia and was admitted to an intensive care unit, but later continued treatment with Gamimune N, 5%. A third patient had skin infiltration during infusion and developed a full thickness skin slough over the dorsum of the hand that required skin grafting.

DOSAGE AND ADMINISTRATION

General

Dosages for specific indications are indicated below, but in general, it is recommended that Gamimune N, 10% be infused by itself at a rate of 0.01 to 0.02 mL/kg body weight per minute for 30 minutes; if well-tolerated, the rate may be **gradually** increased to a maximum of 0.08 mL/kg body weight per minute. Investigations indicate that Gamimune N, 10% is well-tolerated and less likely to produce side effects when infused at the indicated rate. If side effects occur, the rate may be reduced, or the infusion interrupted until symptoms subside. The infusion may then be resumed at the rate which is comfortable for the patient. Parenteral drug products should be inspected visually for particulate matter and discoloration prior to administration, whenever solution and container permit.

It is recommended that infusion of Gamimune N, 10% be given by a separate line, by itself, without mixing with other intravenous fluids or medications the patient might be receiving. Gamimune N, 10% should not be mixed with Immune Globulin Intravenous (Human) from another manufacturer. Gamimune N, 10% is not compatible with saline. If dilution is required, Gamimune N, 10% may be diluted with 5% dextrose in water (D5/W). No other drug interactions or compatibilities have been evaluated.

For patients judged to be at increased risk for developing renal dysfunction, it may be prudent to reduce the amount of product infused per unit time by infusing Gamimune N, 10% at a rate less than 8 mg IG/kg/min (0.08 mL/kg/min). No prospective data are presently available to identify a maximum safe dose, concentration, and rate of infusion in patients determined to be at increased risk of acute renal failure. In the absence of prospective data, recommended doses should not be exceeded and the concentration and infusion rate should be the minimum level practicable. Reduction in dose, concentration, and/or rate of administration in patients at risk of acute renal failure has been proposed in the literature in order to reduce the risk of acute renal failure.[37]

A number of factors beyond our control could reduce the efficacy of this product or even result in an ill effect following its use. These include improper storage and handling of the product after it leaves our hands, diagnosis, dosage, method of administration, and biological differences in individual patients. Because of these factors, it is important that this product be stored properly and that the directions be followed carefully during use.

Primary Humoral Immunodeficiency

The usual dosage of Gamimune N, 10% of prophylaxis in primary immunodeficiency syndromes is 100–200 mg/kg of body weight administered approximately once a month by intravenous infusion. The dosage may be given more frequently or increased as high as 400 mg/kg body weight, if the clinical response is inadequate, or the level of IgG achieved in the circulation is felt to be insufficient. The minimum level of IgG required for protection has not been determined.

Idiopathic Thrombocytopenic Purpura (ITP)

Induction: An increase in platelet count has been observed in children and some adults with acute or chronic ITP receiving Gamimune N, 5% 400 mg/kg body weight daily for 5 days. Alternatively, studies in adults and children with Gamimune N, 5% and Gamimune N, 10% using a dose of 1,000 mg/kg body weight daily for 1 day or 2 consecutive days have also shown increases in platelet count. In the latter treatment regimen, if an adequate increase in the platelet count is observed at 24 hours, the second dose of 1,000 mg/kg body weight may be withheld. The high dose regimen (1,000 mg/kg × 1–2 days) is not recommended for individuals with expanded fluid volumes or where fluid volume may be a concern. With both treatment regimens, a response usually occurs within several days and is maintained for a variable period of time. In general, a response is seen less often in adults than in children.

Maintenance: In adults and children with ITP, if after induction therapy the platelet count falls to less than 30,000/mm^3 and/or the patient manifests clinically significant bleeding, Gamimune N, 10% 400 mg/kg body weight may be given as a single infusion. If an adequate response does not result, the dose can be increased to 800–1,000 mg/kg of body weight given as a single infusion. Maintenance infusions may be administered intermittently as clinically indicated to maintain a platelet count greater than 30,000/mm^3.

Bone Marrow Transplantation

A reduction in posttransplant complications has been observed in bone marrow transplant patients ≥ 20 years of age receiving Gamimune N, 5%. An equivalent dosage of

Gamimune N, 10% is recommended in doses of 500 mg/kg (5 mL/kg) body weight beginning on days –7 and –2 pretransplant (or at the time conditioning therapy for transplantation is begun), then weekly through day 90 posttransplant. Gamimune N, 10% should be administered by itself through a Hickman line while it is in place, and thereafter through a peripheral vein. Please see DOSAGE AND ADMINISTRATION for other drug interactions.

Pediatric HIV Infection

A reduction in bacterial infections has been observed in children infected with HIV-1 receiving Gamimune N, 5%. An equivalent dosage of Gamimune N, 10% is recommended in doses of 400 mg/kg (4 mL/kg) body weight every 28 days.

HOW SUPPLIED

Gamimune N, 10% is supplied in the following sizes:

NDC Number	Size	Grams Protein
0026-0648-12	10 mL	1.0
0026-0648-20	50 mL	5.0
0026-0648-71	100 mL	10.0
0026-0648-24	200 mL	20.0

STORAGE

Store at 2–8°C (36–46°F). Do not freeze. Do not use after expiration date.

CAUTION

Rx only

U.S. federal law prohibits dispensing without prescription.

REFERENCES

1. Tenold RA, Inventor: Cutter Laboratories, assignee, Intravenously injectable immune serum globulin. U.S. Patent 4,396,608, Aug. 2, 1983.
2. Data on file at Bayer Corporation.
3. Pirofsky B, Campbell SM, Montanaro A: Individual patient variations in the kinetics of intravenous immunoglobulin administration. *J Clin Immunol* 2(2): 7S-14S, 1982.
4. Pirofsky B: Intravenous immune globulin therapy in hypogammaglobulinemia. *Amer J Med* 76(3A):53–60, 1984.
5. Pirofsky B, Anderson CJ, Bardana EJ Jr.: Therapeutic and detrimental effects of intravenous immunoglobulin therapy. In: Alving BM (ed.): *Immunoglobulins: characteristics and uses of intravenous preparations.* Washington, D.C., U.S. Government Printing Office, (1980), pp 15–22.
6. Sullivan KM, Kopecky KJ, Jocom J, et al: Immunomodulatory and antimicrobial efficacy of intravenous immunoglobulin in bone marrow transplantation. *N Engl J Med* 323(11):705–12, 1990.
7. Bernstein LJ, Ochs HD, Wedgwood RJ, et al: Defective humoral immunity in pediatric acquired immune deficiency syndrome. *J Pediatr* 107(3):352–7, 1985.
8. Borlowsky W, Steele CJ, Grubman S, et al: Antibody responses to bacterial toxoids in children infected with human immunodeficiency virus. *J Pediatr* 110(4):563–6, 1987.
9. Blanche S, Le Deist F, Fischer A, et al: Longitudinal study of 18 children with perinatal LAV/HTLV III infection: attempt at prognostic evaluation. *J Pediatr* 109(6): 965–70, 1986.
10. Pahwa S, Fikrig S, Menez R, et al: Pediatric acquired immunodeficiency syndrome demonstration of B-lymphocyte defects in vitro. *Diagn Immunol* 4(1):24–30, 1986.
11. Bernstein LJ, Krieger BZ, Novick B, et al: Bacterial infections in the acquired immunodeficiency syndrome of children. *Pediatr Infect Dis* 4(5):472–5, 1985.
12. Krasinski K, Borkowsky W, Bonk S, et al: Bacterial infections in human immunodeficiency virus-infected children. *Pediatr Infect Dis J* 7(5):323–8, 1988.
13. Scott GB, Buck BE, Leterman JG, et al: Acquired immunodeficiency syndrome in infants. *N Engl J Med* 310(2): 76–81, 1984.
14. Mofenson LM, Willoughby A. Passive immunization. In: Pizzo PA, Wilfert CM, (eds.) *Pediatric AIDS: the challenge of HIV infection in infants, children and adolescents.* Baltimore: Williams & Wilkins (1991) pp 633–50.
15. National Institute of Child Health and Human Development Intravenous Immunoglobulin Study Group. Intravenous immune globulin for the prevention of bacterial infections in children with symptomatic human immunodeficiency virus infection. *N Engl J Med* 325(2):73–80, 1991.
16. Mofenson LM, Moye J Jr, Bethel J, et al: Prophylactic intravenous immunoglobulin in HIV-infected children with CD4 + counts of 0.20 × 10^9/L or more. Effect on viral, opportunistic, and bacterial infections. *JAMA* 268(4):483–88, 1992.
17. Glycine. In: Budavari S, O'Neil MJ, Smith A, et al, eds.: *Merck Index.* 11th ed. Rahway NJ, Merck & Co., 1989, p. 706.
18. Wretlind, A: Complete intravenous nutrition: theoretical and experimental background. *Nutr Metab* 14(Suppl):1–57, 1972.
19. Hahn RG, Stalberg HP, Gustafsson SA: Intravenous infusion of irrigating fluids containing glycine or mannitol with and without ethanol. *J Urol* 142(4):1102–1105, 1989.
20. Guyton AC: *Textbook of Medical Physiology.* 5th ed. Philadelphia, W.B. Saunders, 1976, pp 499–500.
21. Nolte MT, Pirofsky B, Gerritz GA, et al: Intravenous immunoglobulin therapy for antibody deficiency. *Clin Exp Immunol* 36: 237–43, 1979.
22. Buckley RH: Immunoglobulin replacement therapy: Indications and contraindications for use and variable IgG levels achieved. In: Alving BM (ed): *Immunoglobulins: characteristics and uses of intravenous preparations.* Washington, D.C., U.S. Government Printing Office, (1980), pp 3–8.
23. Ochs HD: Intravenous immunoglobulin therapy of patients with primary immunodeficiency syndromes: efficacy and safety of a new modified immune globulin preparation. In: Alving BM (ed.): *Immunoglobulins: characteristics and uses of intravenous preparations.* Washington, D.C., U.S. Government Printing Office, (1980), pp 9–14.
24. Cayco AV, Perazella MA, Hayslett JP: Renal insufficiency after intravenous immune globulin therapy: A Report of Two Cases and an Analysis of the Literature. *J Amer Soc Nephrology* 8:1788–1793, 1997.
25. Sekul E, Cupler E, Dalakas M. Aseptic meningitis associated with high-dose intravenous immunoglobulin therapy: Frequency and risk factors. *Ann Int Med* 121: 259–262, 1994.
26. Kato E, Shindo S, Eto Y, et al: Administration of Immune Globulin Associated with Aseptic Meningitis. *JAMA* 259(22):3269–3270, 1988.
27. Casteels-Van Daele M, Wijndaele L, Hunninck K, et al: Intravenous immune globulin and acute aseptic meningitis. *N Engl J Med* 323(9):614–615, 1990.
28. Scribner C, Kapit R, Phillips E, et al: Aseptic meningitis and Intravenous immunoglobulin therapy. *Ann Intern Med* 121(4):305–306, 1994.
29. Schiavotto C, Ruggeri M. Rodeghiero F. Adverse reactions after high-dose intravenous immunoglobulin: incidence in 83 patients treated for idiopathic thrombocytopenic purpura (ITP) and review of the literature. *Haematologica* 78(6:Suppl 2):35–40, 1993.
30. Pasatiempo AM, Kroser JA, Rudnick M, et al: Acute renal failure after intravenous immunoglobulin therapy. *J Rheumatol* 21(2):347–9, 1994.
31. Peerless AG, Stiehm ER: intravenous gammaglobulin for reaction to intramuscular preparation. [letter] *Lancet* 2(8347):461, 1983.
32. Winward DB, Brophy MT: Acute renal failure after administration of intravenous immunoglobulin: review of the literature and case report. *Pharmacotherapy* 15: 765–772, 1995.
33. Phillips AO: Renal failure and intravenous immunoglobulin [letter; comment]. *Clin Nephrol* 36:83–86, 1992.
34. Anderson W, Bethea W: Renal lesions following administration of hypertonic solutions of sucrose. *JAMA* 114: 1983–1987, 1940.
35. Lindberg H, Wald A: Renal changes following the administration of hypertonic solutions. *Arch Intern Med* 63:907–918, 1939.
36. Ridgon RH, Cardwell ES: Renal lesions following the intravenous injection of hypertonic solution of sucrose: A clinical and experimental study. *Arch Intern Med* 69: 670–690, 1942.
37. Tan E, Hajinazarian M, Bay, et al. Acute renal failure resulting from intravenous immunoglobulin therapy. *Arch Neurology* 50:137–139, 1993.

Bayer Corporation
Pharmaceutical Division
Elkhart, IN 46515 USA 14-7648-002
U.S. License No. 8 (Rev. May 1999)

Shown in Product Identification Guide, page 308

KOĀTE®-DVI

[*kō 'ate*]

Antihemophilic Factor (Human)
Double Viral Inactivation
Solvent/Detergent Treated and Heated in Final Container at 80°C

DESCRIPTION

Antihemophilic Factor (Human), Koāte®-DVI, is a sterile, stable, purified, dried concentrate of human Antihemophilic Factor (AHF, factor VIII, AHG) which has been treated with tri-n-butyl phosphate (TNBP) and polysorbate 80 and heated in lyophilized form in the final container at 80°C for 72 hours. Koāte-DVI is intended for use in therapy of classical hemophilia (hemophilia A).

Koāte-DVI is purified from the cold insoluble fraction of pooled fresh-frozen plasma by modification and refinements of the methods first described by Hershgold, Pool, and Pappanhagen.[1] Koāte-DVI contains purified and concentrated factor VIII. The factor VIII is 300–1000 times purified over whole plasma. Part of the fractionation may be performed by another licensed manufacturer. When reconstituted as directed, Koāte-DVI contains approximately 50–150 times as much factor VIII as an equal volume of fresh plasma. The specific activity, after addition of Albumin (Human), is in the range of 9–22 IU/mg protein. **Koāte-DVI must be administered by the intravenous route.**

Each bottle of Koāte-DVI contains the labeled amount of antihemophilic factor activity in international units (IU). One IU, as defined by the World Health Organization standard for blood coagulation factor VIII, human, is approximately equal to the level of AHF found in 1.0 mL of fresh pooled human plasma. The final product when reconstituted as directed contains not more than (NMT) 1500 µg/mL polyethylene glycol (PEG). NMT 0.05 M glycine, NMT 25 µg/mL polysorbate 80, NMT 5 µg/g tri-n-butyl phosphate (TNBP), NMT 3 mM calcium, NMT 1 µg/mL aluminum, NMT 0.06 M histidine, and NMT 10 mg/mL Albumin (Human).

CLINICAL PHARMACOLOGY

Hemophilia A is a hereditary bleeding disorder characterized by deficient coagulant activity of the specific plasma protein clotting factor, factor VIII. In afflicted individuals, hemorrhages may occur spontaneously or after only minor trauma. Surgery on such individuals is not feasible without first correcting the clotting abnormality. The administration of Koāte-DVI provides an increase in plasma levels of factor VIII and can temporarily correct the coagulation defect in these patients.

After infusion of Antihemophilic Factor (Human), there is usually an instantaneous rise in the coagulant level followed by an initial rapid decrease in activity, and then a subsequent much slower rate of decrease in activity.[2–4] The early rapid phase may represent the time of equilibration with the extravascular compartment, and the second or slow phase of the survival curve presumably is the result of degradation and reflects the true biologic half-life of the infused Antihemophilic Factor (Human).[3]

The removal and inactivation of spiked relevant and model enveloped and non-enveloped viruses during the manufacturing process for Koāte-DVI have been validated in laboratory studies at Bayer Corporation. Studies performed with the model enveloped viruses indicated that the greatest reduction was achieved by TNBP/polysorbate 80 treatment and 80°C heat. For this reason, VSV (Vesicular Stomatitis Virus, model for RNA enveloped viruses) and HIV-I (Human Immunodeficiency Virus Type I) were studied only at these two steps of the manufacturing process. The efficacy of the dry heat treatment was studied using all of the viruses, including BVDV (Bovine Viral Diarrheal Virus, model for hepatitis C virus) and Reo (Reovirus Type 3, model for viruses resistant to physical and chemical agents, such as hepatitis A), and the effect of moisture content on the inactivation of HAV (Hepatitis A Virus), PPV (Porcine Parvovirus, model for parvovirus B19), and PRV (Pseudorabies Virus, model for hepatitis B virus) was investigated.

[See table 1 at top of next page]

Similar studies have shown that a terminal 80°C heat incubation for 72 hours inactivates non-lipid enveloped viruses such as hepatitis A and canine parvovirus in vitro, as well as lipid enveloped viruses such as hepatitis C.[7]

Koāte-DVI is purified by a gel permeation chromatography step serving the dual purpose of reducing the amount of TNBP and polysorbate 80 as well as increasing the purity of the factor VIII.

A two-stage clinical study using Koāte-DVI was performed in individuals with hemophilia A who had been previously treated with other plasma-derived AHF concentrates. In Stage 1 of the pharmacokinetic study with 19 individuals, statistical comparisons demonstrated that Koāte-DVI is bioequivalent to the unheated product, Koāte®-HP. The incremental in vivo recovery ten minutes after infusion of Koāte-DVI was 1.90% IU/kg (Koāte-HP 1.82% IU/kg). Mean biologic half-life of Koāte-DVI was 16.12 hours (Koāte-HP 16.13 hours). In Stage II of the study, participants received Koāte-DVI treatments for six months on home therapy with a median of 54 days (range 24–93). No evidence of inhibitor formation was observed, either in the clinical study or in the preclinical investigations.[2]

INDICATIONS AND USAGE

Koāte-DVI is indicated for the treatment of classical hemophilia (hemophilia A) in which there is a demonstrated deficiency of activity of the plasma clotting factor, factor VIII. Koāte-DVI provides a means of temporarily replacing the missing clotting factor in order to control or prevent bleeding episodes, or in order to perform emergency and elective surgery on individuals with hemophilia.

Koāte-DVI contains naturally occurring von Willebrand's factor, which is co-purified as part of the manufacturing process.

Koāte-DVI has not been investigated for efficacy in the treatment of von Willebrand's disease, and hence is not approved for such usage.

CONTRAINDICATIONS

None known.

WARNINGS

Koāte-DVI is made from human plasma. Products made from human plasma may contain infectious agents, such as viruses, that can cause disease. The risk that such products will transmit an infectious agent has been reduced by screening plasma donors for prior exposure to certain viruses, by testing for the presence of certain current virus infections, and by inactivating and/or removing certain viruses. Despite those measures, such products can still potentially transmit disease. There is also the possibility that unknown infectious agents may be present in such products. ALL infections thought by a physician possibly to have been transmitted by this product should be reported by the physician or other healthcare provider to Bayer Corporation [1-888-765-3203]. The physician should discuss the risks and benefits of this product with the patient, before prescribing it to a patient.

Continued on next page

Koāte-DVI—Cont.

Individuals who receive infusions of blood or plasma products may develop signs and/or symptoms of some viral infections, particularly hepatitis C. It is emphasized that hepatitis B vaccination is essential for patients with hemophilia and it is recommended that this be done at birth or diagnosis.[8,9] Hepatitis A vaccination is also recommended for hemophilic patients who are hepatitis A seronegative.

PRECAUTIONS

General

1. Koāte-DVI is intended for treatment of bleeding disorders arising from a deficiency in factor VIII. This deficiency should be proven prior to administering Koāte-DVI.
2. Administer within 3 hours after reconstitution. Do not refrigerate after reconstitution.
3. **Administer only by the intravenous route.**
4. Filter needle should be used prior to administering.
5. Koāte-DVI contains levels of blood group isoagglutinins which are not clinically significant when controlling relatively minor bleeding episodes. When large or frequently repeated doses are required, patients of blood groups A, B, or AB should be monitored by means of hematocrit for signs of progressive anemia, as well as by direct Coombs' tests.
6. Product administration and handling of the infusion set and needles must be done with caution. Percutaneous puncture with a needle contaminated with blood can transmit infectious viruses including HIV (AIDS) and hepatitis. Obtain immediate medical attention if injury occurs.
   Place needles in sharps container after single use. Discard all equipment including any reconstituted Koāte-DVI product in accordance with biohazard procedures.

Pregnancy Cateogry C

Animal reproduction studies have not been conducted with Koāte-DVI. It is also not known whether Koāte-DVI can cause fetal harm when administered to a pregnant woman or can affect reproduction capacity. Koāte-DVI should be given to a pregnant woman only if clearly needed.

Pediatric Use

Koāte-DVI has not been studied in pediatric patients. Koāte-HP, solvent/detergent treated Antihemophilic Factor (Human), has been used extensively in pediatric patients. Spontaneous adverse event reports with Koāte-HP for pediatric use were within the experience of those reports for adult use.

Information for Patient

Some viruses, such as parvovirus B19 or hepatitis A, are particularly difficult to remove or inactivate at this time. Parvovirus B19 most seriously affects pregnant women, or immune-compromised individuals.

Symptoms of parvovirus B19 infection include fever, drowsiness, chills and runny nose followed about 2 weeks later by a rash and joint pain. Evidence of hepatitis A may include several days to weeks of poor appetite, tiredness, and low-grade fever followed by nausea, vomiting, and pain in the belly. Dark urine and a yellowed complexion are also common symptoms. Patients should be encouraged to consult their physician if such symptoms appear.

ADVERSE REACTIONS

Allergic-type reactions may result from the administration of Antihemophilic Factor (Human) preparations.[10,11]

Ten adverse reactions related to 7 infusions were observed during a total of 1053 infusions performed during the clinical study of Koāte-DVI, for a frequency of 0.7% infusions associated with adverse reactions. All reactions were mild and included tingling in the arm, ear, and face, blurred vision, headache, nausea, stomach ache, and jittery feeling.[2]

DOSAGE AND ADMINISTRATION

Each bottle of Koāte-DVI has the AHF(H) content in international units per bottle stated on the label of the bottle. The reconstituted product must be administered intravenously by either direct syringe injection or drip infusion. The product must be administered within 3 hours after reconstitution.

General Approach to Treatment and Assessment of Treatment Efficacy

The dosages described below are presented as general guidance. It should be emphasized that the dosage of Koāte-DVI required for hemostatis must be individualized according to the needs of the patient, the severity of the deficiency, the severity of the hemorrrhage, the presence of inhibitors, and the factor VIII level desired. It is often critical to follow the course of therapy with factor VIII level assays.

The clinical effect of Koāte-DVI is the most important element in evaluating the effectiveness of treatment. It may be necessary to administer more Koāte-DVI than would be estimated in order to attain satisfactory clinical results. If the calculated dose fails to attain the expected factor VIII levels, or if bleeding is not controlled after administration of the calculated dosage, the presence of a circulating inhibitor in the patient should be suspected. Its presence should be substantiated and the inhibitor level quantitated by appropriate laboratory tests.

When an inhibitor is present, the dosage requirement for AHF(H) is extremely variable and the dosage can be determined only by the clinical response. Some patients with low titer inhibitors, (10 Bethesda units) can be successfully treated with factor VIII without a resultant anamnestic rise in inhibitor titer.[12] Factor VIII levels and clinical response to treatment must be assessed to insure adequate response. Use of alternative treatment products, such as Factor IX Complex concentrates, Antihemophilic Factor (Porcine) or Anti-Inhibitor Coagulant Complex, may be necessary for patients with high titer inhibitors. Immune tolerance therapy using repeated doses of FVIII concentrate administered frequently on a predetermined schedule may result in eradication of the FVIII inhibitor.[13,14] Most successful regimens have employed high doses of FVIII administered at least once daily, but no single dosage regimen has been universally accepted as the most effective. Consultation with a hemophilia expert experienced with the management of immune tolerance regimens is also advisable.

Table I. Summary of In Vitro Log_{10} Viral Reduction Studies

	Enveloped Model Viruses				Non-enveloped Model Viruses		
	HIV-I	BVDV	PRV	VSV	Reo	HAV	PPV
Model for	HIV-1/2	HCV	HBV	RNA enveloped viruses	HAV and viruses resistant to chemical and physical agents	HAV	B19
Global Reduction Factor	9.4	10.3	9.5	10.9	9	4.5	3.7

Calculation of Dosage

The in vivo percent elevation in factor VIII can be estimated by multiplying the dose of AHF(H) per kilogram of body weight (IU/kg) by 2%. This method of calculation is based on clinical findings by Abildgaard et al,[15] and is illustrated in the following examples:

[See second table above]

Expected % factor VIII increase = $\frac{\text{\# units administered} \times 2\%/\text{IU/kg}}{\text{body weight (kg)}}$

Example for a 70 kg adult: $\frac{1\,400 \text{ IU} \times 2\%/\text{IU/kg} = 40\%}{70 \text{ kg}}$

or

Dosage required (IU) = $\frac{\text{body weight (kg)} \times \text{desired \% factor VIII increase}}{2\%/\text{IU/kg}}$

Example for a 15 kg child: $\frac{15 \text{ kg} \times 100\% = 750 \text{ IU required}}{2\%/\text{IU/kg}}$

The dosage necessary to achieve hemostasis depends upon the type and severity of the bleeding episode, according to the following general guidelines:

Mild Hemorrhage

Mild superficial or early hemorrhages may respond to a single dose of 10 IU per kg,[16] leading to an in vivo rise of approximately 20% in the factor VIII level. Therapy need not be repeated unless there is evidence of further bleeding.

Moderate Hemorrhage

For more serious bleeding episodes (e.g., definite hemarthroses, known trauma), the factor VIII level should be raised to 30%–50% by administering approximately 15–25 IU per kg. If further therapy is required, repeated doses of 10–15 IU per kg every 8–12 hours may be given.[17]

Severe Hemorrhage

In patients with life-threatening bleeding or possible hemorrhage involving vital structures (e.g., central nervous system, retropharyngeal and retroperitoneal spaces, iliopsoas sheath), the factor VIII level should be raised to 80%–100% of normal in order to achieve hemostasis. This may be achieved in most patients with an initial AHF [Antihemophilic Factor (Human), Koāte®-DVI] dose of 40–50 IU per kg and a maintenance dose of 20–25 IU per kg every 8–12 hours.[18,19] For major surgical procedures, Factor VIII levels should be checked throughout the perioperative course to ensure adequate replacement therapy.

Surgery

For major surgical procedures, the factor VIII level should be raised to approximately 100% by giving a preoperative dose of 50 IU/kg. The factor VIII level should be checked to assure that the expected level is achieved before the patient goes to surgery in order to maintain hemostatic levels, repeat infusions may be necessary every 6 to 12 hours initially, and for a total of 10 to 14 days until healing is complete. The intensity of factor VIII replacement therapy required depends on the type of surgery and postoperative regimen employed. For minor surgical procedures, less intensive treatment schedules may provide adequate hemostatis.[18,19]

Prophylaxis

Factor VIII concentrates may also be administered on a regular schedule for prophylaxis of bleeding, as reported by Nilsson et al.[20]

Incorrect diagnosis, inappropriate dosage, method of administration, and biological differences in individual patients, could reduce the efficacy of this product or even result in an ill effect following its use. It is important that this product be stored properly, the directions for use be followed carefully during use, the risk of transmitting viruses be carefully weighed before the product is prescribed, and that plasma factor VIII levels be measured in initial treatment situations or if clinical response appears inadequate.

NDC Number	Approximate Factor VIII Activity	Diluent
0026-0665-20	250 IU	5 mL
0026-0665-30	500 IU	5 mL
0026-0665-50	1000 IU	10 mL

Reconstitution

Vacuum Transfer

1. Warm the unopened diluent and the concentrate to room temperature (NMT 37°C, 99°F).
2. After removing the plastic flip-top caps (Fig. A), aseptically cleanse the rubber stoppers of both bottles.
3. Remove the protective cover from the plastic transfer-needle cartridge with tamper-proof seal and penetrate the stopper of the diluent bottle (Fig. B).
4. Remove the remaining portion of the plastic cartridge, invert the diluent bottle and penetrate the rubber seal on the concentrate bottle (Fig. C) with the needle at an angle.
   Alternate method of transferring sterile water: With a sterile needle and syringe, withdraw the appropriate volume of diluent and transfer to the bottle of lyophilized concentrate.
5. The vacuum will draw the diluent into the concentrate bottle. Hold the diluent bottle at an angle to the concentrate bottle in order to direct the jet of diluent against the wall of the concentrate bottle (Fig. C). Avoid excessive foaming.
6. After removing the diluent bottle and transfer needle (Fig. D), swirl vigorously until completely dissolved without creating excessive foaming (Fig. E).
7. After the concentrate powder is completely dissolved, withdraw solution into the syringe through the filter needle which is supplied in the package (Fig. F). Replace the filter needle with the administration set provided and inject intravenously.
8. If a patient is to receive more than one bottle, the contents of two bottles may be drawn into the same syringe; a separate unused filter needle should be used for each bottle, then the needle for intravenous injection should be attached to the syringe.

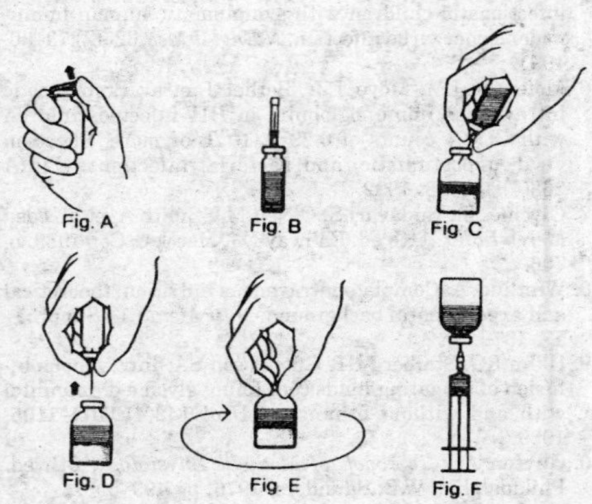

Rate of Administration

The rate of administration should be adapted to the response of the individual patient, but administration of the entire dose in 5 to 10 minutes is generally well-tolerated.

Parenteral drug products should be inspected visually for particulate matter and discoloration prior to administration, whenever solution and container permit.

HOW SUPPLIED

Koāte-DVI is supplied in the following single dose bottles with the total units of factor VIII activity stated on the label of each bottle. A suitable volume of Sterile Water for Injection, USP, is a sterile double-ended transfer needle, a sterile filter needle, and a sterile administration set are provided.

[See third table on previous page]

STORAGE

Koāte-DVI should be stored under refrigeration (2–8°C; 36–46°F). Storage of lyophilized powder at room temperature (up to 25°C or 77°F) for 6 months, such as in home treatment situations, may be done without loss of factor VIII activity. Freezing should be avoided as breakage of the diluent bottle might occur.

CAUTION

Rx only

U.S. federal law prohibits dispensing without prescription.

LIMITED WARRANTY

A number of factors beyond our control could reduce the efficacy of this product or even result in an ill effect following its use. These include improper storage and handling of the product after it leaves our hands, diagnosis, dosage, method of administration, and biological differences in individual patients. Because of these risk factors, it is important that this product be stored properly, that the directions be followed carefully during use, and that the risk of transmitting viruses be carefully weighed before the product is prescribed.

No warranty, express or implied, including any warranty of merchantability or fitness is made. Representatives of the Company are not authorized to vary the terms or the contents of the printed labeling, including the package insert for this product, except by printed notice from the Company's headquarters. The prescriber and user of this product must accept the terms hereof.

REFERENCES

1. Hershgold EJ, Pool JG, Pappenhagen AR: The potent antihemophilic globulin concentrate derived from a cold insoluble fraction of human plasma: characterization and further data on preparation and clinical trial. *J Lab Clin Med* 67(1):23–32, 1966.
2. Data on file at Bayer Corporation.
3. Aronson DL: Factor VIII (antihemophilic globulin). *Semin Thromb Hemostas* 6(1):12–27, 1979.
4. Britton M, Harrison J, Abildgaard CF: Early treatment of hemophilic hemarthroses with minimal dose of new factor VIII concentrate. *J Pediatr* 85(2):245–7, 1974.
5. Winkelman L, Feldman PA, Evan DR: Severe heat treatment of lyophilized coagulation factors in Virus Inactivation in Plasma Products. *Curr Stud Hematol Blood Transfus*, Morgenthaler J-J (ed.). Basel, Karger, 1989 No 56, pp. 55–69.
6. Skidmore SJ, Pasi KJ, Mawson SJ, et al: Serological evidence that dry heating of clotting factor concentrates prevents transmission of non-A, non-B hepatitis. *J. Med Virol* 30(1):50–2, 1990.
7. Hart HF, Hart WG, Crossley J, et al: Effect of terminal (dry) heat treatment on non-enveloped viruses in coagulation factor concentrates. *Vox Sang* 67(4):345–50, 1994.
8. National Hemophilia Foundation Medical and Scientific Advisory Council. Hemophilia Information; Exchange—AIDS Update: Recommendations concernng AIDS and the treatment of hemophilia HIV infection. Section I.G. (Rev. Jan, 1988).
9. Safety of therapeutic products used for hemophilia patients. *MMWR* 37(29):441–4, 449–50, 1988.
10. Eyster ME, Bowman HS, Haverstick JN: Adverse reactions to factor VIII infusions. [letter] *Ann Intern Med* 87(2):248, 1977.
11. Prager D, Djerassi I, Eyster ME, et al: Pennsylvania state-wide hemophilia program: summary of immediate reactions with the use of factor VIII and factor IX concentrate. *Blood* 53(5):1012–3, 1979.
12. Kasper CK: Complications of hemophilia A treatment: factor VIII inhibitors. *Ann NY Acad Sci* 614:97–105, 1991.
13. Mariani G, Hilgartner M, Thompson AR, et al: Immune Tolerance to Factor VIII: International Registry Data. *Adv Exp Med Biol* 386:201–8, 1995.
14. DiMichele D: Hemophilia 1996, New Approach to an Old Disease. *Pediatr Clin North Am* 43:(3) 709–35, Jun 1995.
15. Abildgaard CF, Simone JV, Corrigan JJ, et al: Treatment of hemophilia with glycine-precipitated factor VIII. *N Engl J Med* 275(9):471–5, 1966.
16. Britton M, Harrison J, Abildgaard CF: Early treatment of hemophilic hemarthroses with minimal dose of new factor VIII concentrate. *J Pediatr* 85(2):245–7, 1974.
17. Abildgaard CF: current concepts in the management of hemophilia. *Semin Hematol* 12(3):223–32, 1975.
18. Hilgartner MW: Factor replacement therapy. In: Hilgartner MW, Pochedly C, eds.: Hemophilia in the child and adult. New York, Raven Press, 1989, pp 1–26.
19. Kasper CK, Dietrich SL: Comprehensive management of haemophilia. *Clin Haematol* 14(2):489–512, 1985.
20. Nilsson IM, Berntorp E, Löfquist T, et al: Twenty five years' experience of prophylactic treatment in severe haemophilia A and B. *J Intern Med* 232(1):25–32, 1992.

Bayer Corporation
Pharmaceutical Division
Elkhart, IN 46515 USA
U.S. License No. 8

14-7665-000
(Issued May 1999)

KOĀTE®-HP ℞

[*kō 'ate*]

Antihemophilic Factor (Human)
(Factor VIII, AHF, AHG)

DESCRIPTION

Antihemophilic Factor (Human), Koāte®-HP, is a sterile, stable, purified, dried concentrate of human Antihemophilic Factor (AHF, factor VIII, AHG) which has been treated with tri-n-butyl phosphate (TNBP) and polysorbate 80 and is intended for use in therapy of classical hemophilia (hemophilia A).

Koāte-HP is purified from the cold insoluble fraction of pooled fresh-frozen plasma by modification and refinements of the methods first described by Hershgold, Pool, and Pappenhagen.[1] Koāte-HP contains purified and concentrated factor VIII. The factor VIII is 300-1000 times purified over whole plasma. Part of the fractionation may be performed by another licensed manufacturer. When reconstituted as directed, Koāte-HP contains approximately 50-150 times as much factor VIII as an equal volume of fresh plasma. The specific activity, after addition of Albumin (Human), is in the range of 9-22 IU/mg protein. Koāte-HP must be administered by the intravenous route.

Each bottle of Koāte-HP contains the labeled amount of antihemophilic factor activity in International Units (IU). One IU, as defined by the World Health Organization Standard for blood coagulation factor VIII, human, is approximately equal to the level of AHF found in 1.0 mL of fresh pooled human plasma. The final product when reconstituted as directed contains not more than (NMT) 5 units heparin/mL, NMT 1500 ppm polyethylene glycol (PEG), NMT 0.05 M glycine, NMT 25 ppm polysorbate 80, NMT 5 ppm tri-n-butyl phosphate (TNBP), NMT 3 mM calcium chloride, NMT 1 ppm aluminum, NMT 0.06 M histidine, and NMT 10 mg/mL Albumin (Human).

CLINICAL PHARMACOLOGY

Hemophilia A is a hereditary bleeding disorder characterized by deficient coagulant activity of the specific plasma protein clotting factor, factor VIII. In afflicted individuals, hemorrhages may occur spontaneously or after only minor trauma. Surgery on such individuals is not feasible without first correcting the clotting abnormality. The administration of Koāte-HP provides an increase in plasma levels of factor VIII and can temporarily correct the coagulation defect in these patients.

After infusion of Koāte-HP, there is usually an instantaneous rise in the coagulant level followed by an initial rapid decrease in activity, and then a subsequent much slower rate of decrease in activity.[2–4] The early rapid phase may represent the time of equilibration with the extravascular compartment, and the second or slow phase of the survival curve presumably is the result of degradation and reflects the true biologic half-life of the infused Antihemophilic Factor (Human).[3] Studies with Koāte-HP in hemophilic patients have demonstrated a biologic half-life of approximately 9 to 14 hours.[2]

In 1984, Prince, et al[5] described the susceptibility of hepatitis B virus (HBV) and the Hutchinson strain of non-A, non-B hepatitis virus to inactivation by ether and polysorbate 80. This method is known to disrupt lipid-containing enveloped viruses. Subsequently, others[6,7] using tri-n-butyl phosphate as an alternative organic solvent to the hazardous ethyl ether in combination with a number of different detergents including polysorbate 80, sodium deoxycholate, sodium cholate, or Triton x-100, showed these forms of chemical treatment to be rapidly effective in inactivating certain lipid-enveloped viruses. These viruses included vesicular stomatitis virus (VSV), sindbis virus, and sendai virus[6] as well as, in a later study,[7] human immunodeficiency virus (HIV), HBV and non-A, non-B virus. Similar studies undertaken at Bayer Corporation using TNBP and polysorbate 80 treatment of factor VIII concentrate immediately prior to a gel permeation chromatography purifying/concentrating procedure have confirmed the inactivation of VSV, visna, and sindbis viruses.

Antihemophilic Factor (Human), Koāte®-HP is purified by virtue of a gel permeation chromatography step serving the dual purpose of removing the TNBP and polysorbate 80 as well as increasing the purity of the Factor VIII. Recently, concerns have been expressed concerning alterations to immune function occurring in asymptomatic hemophiliacs,[8–15] with some of the abnormalities being independent of HIV exposure. It has been suggested that the underlying mechanisms might include repeated exposure to viral agents, repeated allostimulation and/or possible contaminants in factor VIII preparations (e.g., lgG aggregates). More highly purified preparations which have minimized risks of viral transmission may therefore be desirable.[6]

INDICATIONS AND USAGE

Koāte-HP is indicated for the treatment of classical hemophilia (hemophilia A) in which there is a demonstrated deficiency of activity of the plasma clotting factor, factor VIII. Koāte-HP provides a means of temporarily replacing the missing clotting factor in order to correct or prevent bleeding episodes, or in order to perform emergency and elective surgery on hemophiliacs.

Koāte-HP has not been investigated for efficacy in the treatment of von Willebrand's disease, and hence is not approved for such usage.

CONTRAINDICATIONS

None known.

WARNINGS

Koāte-HP is made from human plasma. Products made from human plasma may contain infectious agents, such as viruses, that can cause disease. The risk that such products will transmit an infectious agent has been reduced by screening plasma donors for prior exposure to certain viruses, by testing for the presence of certain current virus infections, and by inactivating and/or removing certain viruses. Despite these measures, such products can still potentially transmit disease. There is also the possibility that unknown infectious agents may be present in such products. ALL infections thought by a physician possibly to have been transmitted by this product should be reported by the physician or other healthcare provider to Bayer Corporation [1-888-765-3203]. The physician should discuss the risks and benefits of this product with the patient, before prescribing or administering it to the patient.

Individuals who receive infusions of blood or plasma products may develop signs and/or symptoms of some viral infections, particularly hepatitis C. It is emphasized that hepatitis B vaccination is essential for patients with hemophilia and it is recommended that this be done at birth or diagnosis.[16,17] Hepatitis A vaccination is also recommended for hemophilic patients who are hepatitis A seronegative.

No studies of CD4 cell count surveillance have been done in HIV seropositive patients treated exclusively with Koāte-HP; however, there have been several reports of increased rates of CD4 cell count decline in HIV seropositive hemophilia patients treated with conventionally purified FVIII concentrates compared to those treated with immunoaffinity purified products.[18–20] The clinical significance of these CD4 cell count findings remains uncertain.

PRECAUTIONS

General

1. Antihemophilic Factor (Human), Koāte-HP is intended for treatment of bleeding disorders arising from a deficiency in factor VIII. This deficiency should be proven prior to administering Koāte-HP.
2. Administer within 3 hours after reconstitution. Do not refrigerate after reconstitution.
3. Administer only by the intravenous route.
4. Filter needle should be used prior to administering.
5. Koāte-HP contains levels of blood group isoagglutinins which are not clinically significant when controlling relatively minor bleeding episodes. When large or frequently repeated doses are required, patients of blood groups A, B, or AB should be monitored by means of hematocrit for signs of progressive anemia, as well as by direct Coombs' tests.
6. Product administration and handling of the infusion set and needles must be done with caution. Percutaneous puncture with a needle contaminated with blood can transmit infectious viruses including HIV (AIDS) and hepatitis. Obtain immediate medical attention if injury occurs.

   Place needles in sharps container after single use. Discard all equipment including any reconstituted Koāte-HP product in accordance with biohazard procedures.

Pregnancy Category C

Animal reproduction studies have not been conducted with Koāte-HP. It is also not known whether Koāte-HP can cause fetal harm when administered to a pregnant woman or can affect reproduction capacity. Koāte-HP should be given to a pregnant woman only if clearly needed.

Information for Patient

Some viruses, such as parvovirus B19 or hepatitis A, are particularly difficult to remove or inactivate at this time. Parvovirus B19 most seriously affects pregnant women, or immune-compromised individuals.

Symptoms of parvovirus B19 infection include fever, drowsiness, chills and runny nose followed about 2 weeks later by a rash and joint pain. Evidence of hepatitis A may include several days to weeks of poor appetite, tiredness, and low-grade fever followed by nausea, vomiting, and pain in the belly. Dark urine and a yellowed complexion are also common symptoms. Patients should be encouraged to consult their physician if such symptoms appear.

ADVERSE REACTIONS

Allergic-type reactions may result from the administration of Antihemophilic Factor (Human) preparations.[21,22]

Continued on next page

Koate-HP—Cont.

DOSAGE AND ADMINISTRATION

Each bottle of Koāte-HP has the Antihemophilic Factor (Human) content in International Units per bottle stated on the label of the bottle. The reconstituted product must be administered intravenously by either direct syringe injection or drip infusion.

Shanbrom et al,[23] based upon studies in hemophiliacs, have suggested a linear dose-response relation with an approximate rise of 2.5% in Factor VIII activity for each unit of Antihemophilic Factor (Human) transfused per kg of body weight. Abildgaard et al,[24] in work with hemophilic children 8 months to 14 years of age, reported a response factor of 0.5 units/kg. Clinical experience with Koāte-HP has demonstrated a similar dose-response relationship.[2] The following formulas can provide a guide for dosage calculations:

Expected factor VIII increase (% of normal) =

$$\frac{\text{IU administered}}{\text{body weight (kg)} \times 0.4\ \text{IU/kg}}$$

Example:

$$\frac{840\ \text{IU}}{70\ \text{kg} \times 0.4\ \text{IU/kg}} = 30\%$$

or

IU required = body weight (kg) × desired factor VIII increase (% normal) × 0.4 IU/kg

Example: 70 kg × 0.4 IU/kg × 30% = 840 IU

All efforts should be made to follow the course of therapy with factor VIII level assays. It may be dangerous to assume any certain level has been reached unless direct evidence is obtained.

Prophylaxis of Spontaneous Hemorrhage

The level of factor VIII required to prevent spontaneous hemorrhage is approximately 5% of normal, while a level of 30% of normal is the minimum required for hemostasis following trauma and surgery.[25–27] Mild superficial or early hemorrhages may respond to a single dose of 10 IU per kg,[4,28] leading to an in vivo rise of approximately 20% in the factor VIII level. In patients with early hemarthrosis (mild pain, minimal or no swelling, erythema, warmth, and minimal or no joint limitation), if treated promptly, even smaller doses may be adequate.[28–30]

Mild Hemorrhage

In cases of mild hemorrhage, therapy need not be repeated unless there is evidence of further bleeding.

Moderate Hemorrhage and Minor Surgery

For more serious hemorrhages and for minor surgical procedures, the patient's plasma factor VIII level should be raised to 30%–50% of normal for optimum hemostasis.[28,31] This usually requires an initial dose of 15–25 IU per kg; and if further therapy is required, a maintenance dose of 10–15 IU per kg every 8–12 hours.

Severe Hemorrhage

In patients with life-threatening bleeding, or hemorrhage involving vital structures (central nervous system, retropharyngeal and retroperitoneal spaces, iliopsoas sheath), it may be desirable to raise the factor VIII level to 80%–100% of normal in order to achieve hemostasis.[28,31–33] This may be achieved with an initial Antihemophilic Factor (Human) Koāte®-HP dose of 40–50 IU per kg and a maintenance dose of 20–25 IU per kg every 8–12 hours.

Major Surgery

For major surgical procedures, Kasper[31] recommends that a dose of Antihemophilic Factor (Human) sufficient to achieve a level of 80%–100% of normal be given an hour before the procedure. It is recommended that the factor VIII level be checked prior to going to surgery to assure the expected level is achieved. A second dose, half the size of the priming dose, should be given about 5 hours after the first dose. The factor VIII level should be maintained at a daily minimum of at least 30% for a healing period of 10–14 days, depending on the nature of the operative procedure.

The above discussion is presented as a reference and a guideline. It should be emphasized that the dosage of Antihemophilic Factor (Human), Koāte®-HP required for normalizing hemostasis must be individualized according to the needs of the patient. Factors to be considered include the weight of the patient, the severity of the deficiency, the severity of the hemorrhage, the presence of inhibitors, and the factor VIII level desired. All efforts should be made to follow the course of therapy with factor VIII level assays.

The clinical effect of Koāte-HP is the most important element in evaluating the effectiveness of treatment. It may be necessary to administer more Koāte-HP than would be estimated in order to attain satisfactory clinical results. If the calculated dose fails to attain the expected factor VIII levels, or if bleeding is not controlled after adequate calculated dosage, the presence of a factor VIII inhibitor should be suspected. Its presence should be substantiated and the inhibitor level quantitated by appropriate laboratory procedure. When an inhibitor is present, the dosage requirement for Koāte-HP is extremely variable and the dosage can be determined only by the clinical response.

Parenteral drug products should be inspected visually for particulate matter and discoloration prior to administration, whenever solution and container permit.

Reconstitution

Vacuum Transfer

1. Warm the unopened diluent and the concentrate to room temperature (NMT 37°C, 99°F).
2. After removing the plastic flip-top caps (Fig. A), aseptically cleanse the rubber stoppers of both bottles.
3. Remove the protective cover from the plastic transfer-needle cartridge with tamper-proof seal and penetrate the stopper of the diluent bottle (Fig. B).
4. Remove the remaining portion of the plastic cartridge, invert the diluent bottle and penetrate the rubber seal on the concentrate bottle (Fig. C) with the needle at an angle.

   Alternate method of transferring sterile water: With a sterile needle and syringe, withdraw the appropriate volume of diluent and transfer to the bottle of lyophilized concentrate.
5. The vacuum will draw the diluent into the concentrate bottle. Hold the diluent bottle at an angle to the concentrate bottle in order to direct the jet of diluent against the wall of the concentrate bottle (Fig. C). Avoid excessive foaming.
6. After removing the diluent bottle and transfer needle (Fig. D), swirl continuously until completely dissolved (Fig. E).
7. After the concentrate powder is completely dissolved, withdraw solution into the syringe through the filter needle which is supplied in the package (Fig. F). Replace the filter needle with the administration set provided and inject intravenously.
8. If the same patient is to receive more than one bottle, the contents of two bottles may be drawn into the same syringe through a separate unused filter needle before attaching the vein needle.

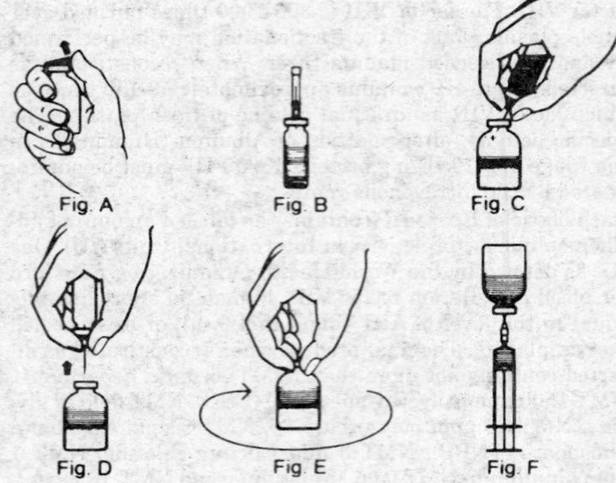

Rate of Administration

The rate of administration should be adapted to the response of the individual patient, but administration of the entire dose in 5 to 10 minutes is generally well-tolerated.

HOW SUPPLIED

Antihemophilic Factor (Human), Koāte®-HP is supplied in the following single dose bottles with the total units of factor VIII activity stated on the label of each bottle. A suitable volume of Sterile Water for Injection, USP, a sterile double-ended transfer needle, a sterile filter needle, and a sterile administration set are provided.

NDC Number	Approximate Factor VIII Activity	Diluent
0026-0664-20	250 IU	5 mL
0026-0664-30	500 IU	5 mL
0026-0664-50	1000 IU	10 mL
0026-0664-60	1500 IU	10 mL

STORAGE

Antihemophilic Factor (Human) Koāte®-HP should be stored under refrigeration (2–8°C; 36–46°F). Storage of lyophilized powder at room temperature (up to 25°C or 77°F) for 6 months, such as in home treatment situations, may be done without loss of factor VIII activity. Freezing should be avoided as breakage of the diluent bottle might occur.

CAUTION

U.S. federal law prohibits dispensing without prescription.

LIMITED WARRANTY

A number of factors beyond our control could reduce the efficacy of this product or even result in an ill effect following its use. These include improper storage and handling of the product after it leaves our hands, diagnosis, dosage, method of administration, and biological differences in individual patients. Because of these factors, it is important that this product be stored properly, that the directions be followed carefully during use, and that the risk of transmitting viruses be carefully weighed before the product is prescribed. No warranty, express or implied, including any warranty of merchantability or fitness is made. Representatives of the Company are not authorized to vary the terms or the contents of the printed labeling, including the package insert for this product, except by printed notice from the Company's headquarters. The prescriber and user of this product must accept the terms hereof.

REFERENCES

1. Hershgold EJ, Pool JG, Pappenhagen AR: The potent antihemophilic globulin concentrate derived from a cold insoluble fraction of human plasma: characterization and further data on preparation and clinical trial. *J Lab Clin Med* 67(1):23–32, 1966.
2. Unpublished data in files of Bayer Corporation.
3. Aronson DL: Factor VIII (antihemophilic globulin). *Semin Thromb Hemostas* 6(1):12–27, 1979.
4. Britton M, Harrison J, Abildgaard CF: Early treatment of hemophilic hemarthroses with minimal dose of new factor VIII concentrate. *J Pediatr* 85(2):245–7, 1974.
5. Prince AM, Horowitz B, Brotman B, et al: Inactivation of hepatitis B and Hutchinson strain non-A, non-B hepatitis viruses by exposure to Tween 80 and ether. *Vox Sang* 46:36–43, 1984.
6. Horowitz B, Wiebe ME, Lippin A, et al: Inactivation of viruses in labile blood derivatives. I. Distruption of lipid-enveloped viruses by tri(n-butyl) phosphate detergent combinations. *Transfusion* 25(6):516–22, 1985.
7. Piet MPJ, Chin S, Prince AM, et al: Inactivtion of viruses in plasma on treatment with tri(n-butyl) phosphate (TNBP) detergent mixtures. [abstract] *Thromb Haemost* 58(1):370, 1987.
8. Lederman MM, Ratnoff OD, Scillian JJ, et al: Impaired cell-mediated immunity in patients with classic hemophilia. *N Engl J Med* 308(2):79–83, 1983.
9. Weintrub PS, Koerper MA, Addiego JE Jr, et al: Immunologic abnormalities in patients with hemophilia A. *J Pediatr* 103(5):692–5, 1983.
10. Goldsmith JC, Moseley PL, Monick M, et al: T-lymphocyte subpopulation abnormalities in apparently healthy patients with hemophilia. *Ann Intern Med* 98:294–6, 1983.
11. Saidi P, Kim HC, Raska K Jr: T-cell subsets in hemophilia. [letter] *N Engl J Med* 308(21):1291–3, 1983.
12. Landay A, Poon MC, Abo T, et al: Immunologic studies in asymptomatic hemophilia patients: relationship to acquired immune deficiency syndrome (AIDS). *J Clin Invest* 71(5):1500–4, 1983.
13. Jones P, Proctor S, Dickinson A, et al: Altered immunology in haemophilia. [letter] *Lancet* 1:120–1, 1983.
14. Mannhalter JW, Zlabinger GJ, Ahmad R, et al: A functional defect in the early phase of the immune response observed in patients with hemophilia A. *Clin Immunol Immunopathol* 38:390–7, 1986.
15. Frydecka I, Kowalewska B, Lesiecki A, et al: Immunologic studies in asymptomatic hemophiliac patients. *Folia Haematol* 113(5):708–15, 1986.
16. National Hemophilia Foundation Medical and Scientific Advisory Council. Hemophilia Information Exchange—AIDS Update: Recommendations concerning HIV infection, AIDS and the treatment of hemophilia. Section I.G. (Rev. Jan., 1988).
17. Safety of therapeutic products used for hemophilia patients. *MMWR* 37(29):441–4, 449–50, 1988.
18. Madhok R, Gracie A, Lowe GDO, et al: Impaired cell mediated immunity in haemophilia in the absence of infection with human immunodeficiency virus. *Br Med J* 239(6553):978–80, 1986.
19. Goldsmith JM, Deutsche J, Tang M, et al: CD4 cells in HIV-1 infected hemophiliacs: effect of factor VIII concentrates. *Thromb Haemost* 66(4):415–9, 1991.
20. Hilgartner MW, Buckley JD, Operskalski EA, et al: Purity of factor VIII concentrates and serial CD4 counts. *Lancet* 341(8857):1373–4, 1993.
21. Eyster ME, Bowman HS, Haverstick JN: Adverse reactions to factor VIII infusions. [letter] *Ann Intern Med* 87(2):248, 1977.
22. Prager D, Djerassi I, Eyster ME, et al: Pennsylvania state-wide hemophilia program: summary of immediate reactions with the use of factor VIII and factor IX concentrate. *Blood* 53(5):1012–3, 1979.
23. Shanbrom E, Thelin GM: Experimental prophylaxis of severe hemophilia with a factor VIII concentrate. *JAMA* 208(10):1853–6, 1969.
24. Abildgaard CF, Simone JV, Corrigan JJ, et al: Treatment of hemophilia with glycine-precipitated factor VIII. *N Engl J Med* 275(9):471–5, 1966.
25. Biggs R, MacFarlane RG: Haemophilia and related conditions: a survey of 187 cases. *Br J Haematol* 4(1):1–27, 1958.
26. Langdell RD, Wagner RH, Brinkhous KM: Antihemophilic factor (AHF) levels following transfusions of blood, plasma and plasma fractions. *Proc Soc Exp Biol Med* 88(2):212–5, 1955.
27. Shulman NR, Cowan DH, Libre EP, et al: The physiologic basis for therapy of classic hemophilia (factor VIII deficiency) and related disorders. *Ann Intern Med* 67(4): 856–82, 1967.
28. Abildgaard CF: Current concepts in the management of hemophilia. *Semin Hematol* 12(3):223–32, 1975.
29. Penner JA, Kelly PE: Low doses of factor VIII for hemophilia. [letter] *N Engl J Med* 297(7):401, 1977.
30. Ashenhurst JB, Langehennig PL, Seller RA: Early treatment of bleeding episodes with 10 U/kg of factor VIII. [letter] *Blood* 50(1):181–2, 1977.
31. Kasper CK: Hematologic care. In: Boone DC (ed.): Comprehensive management of hemophilia. Philadelphia, Davis, 1976, pp 3–17.
32. Edson JR: Hemophilia and related conditions. In: Conn HF (ed): Current therapy. Philadelphia, Saunders, 1980, pp 264–9.
33. Hilgartner MW; Management of hemophilia: the routine and the crises. *Drug Ther* 8(2):141–54, 1978.

KOGENATE® ℞
Antihemophilic Factor (Recombinant)

DESCRIPTION

Antihemophilic Factor (Recombinant), KOGENATE®, is a sterile, stable, purified, dried concentrate which has been manufactured by recombinant DNA technology. KOGENATE is intended for use in therapy of classical hemophilia (hemophilia A). KOGENATE is produced by Baby Hamster Kidney (BHK) cells into which the human factor VIII (FVIII) gene has been introduced.[1] KOGENATE is a highly purified glycoprotein consisting of multiple peptides including an 80 kD and various extensions of the 90 kD subunit. It has the same biological activity as FVIII derived from human plasma. In addition to the use of the classical purification methods of ion exchange chromatography and size exclusion chromatography, monoclonal antibody immunoaffinity chromatography is utilized along with other steps designed to purify recombinant factor VIII (rAHF) and remove contaminating substances. The final preparation is stabilized with Albumin (Human) and lyophilized. The concentration of KOGENATE is approximately 100 IU/mL. The product contains no preservatives.

Each vial of KOGENATE contains the labeled amount of rAHF in international units (IU). One IU, as defined by the World Health Organization standard for blood coagulation factor VIII, human, is approximately equal to the level of factor VIII activity found in 1.0 mL of fresh pooled human plasma. The final product when reconstituted as directed contains the following excipients: 10–30 mg glycine/mL, not more than (NMT) 500 µg imidazole/1000 IU, NMT 600 µg polysorbate 80/1000 IU, 2–5 mM calcium chloride, 100–130 mEq/L sodium, 100–130 mEq/L chloride and 4–10 mg Albumin (Human)/mL. KOGENATE must be administered by the intravenous route.

CLINICAL PHARMACOLOGY

The clinical trial of KOGENATE has included 168 patients, enrolled over a 55-month period. A total of 16,186 infusions have been utilized in this trial. The study was conducted in several stages.

Initial pharmacokinetic studies were conducted in 17 asymptomatic hemophilic patients, comparing pharmacokinetics of plasma-derived Antihemophilic Factor (Human) (pdAHF) and KOGENATE.[2] The mean biologic half-life of rAHF was 15.8 hours. The mean biologic half-life of pdAHF in the same individuals was 13.9 hours. A similar degree of shortening of the activated partial thromboplastin time was seen with both rAHF and pdAHF. The mean *in vivo* recovery of rAHF was similar to pdAHF, with a linear dose-response relationship. The recovery and half-life of rAHF was consistent with initial results following 13 weeks of exclusive treatment with KOGENATE. Subsequently, 826 recovery studies were conducted in 58 hemophilic patients participating in later clinical studies. Mean recovery from this group was 2.48% per IU/kg infused.

Fourteen (14) subjects from initial pharmacokinetic studies commenced home treatment with rAHF. Forty-four (44) additional subjects were then enrolled who treated themselves at home exclusively with rAHF. A total of 12,730 infusions have been administered under this portion of the study, of which 1,021 were given in clinic for recovery studies, 7,339 were given for treatment of bleeds, 4,361 were given as prophylaxis, 5 for minor surgery not requiring hospitalization, and 4 for unspecified reason.

Forty-eight (48) patients have received rAHF on 63 occasions for surgical procedures or in-hospital treatment of serious hemorrhage. Eleven (11) received rAHF for the first time in this study, while 37 were already on study or study participants under an investigation of previously untreated patients. Hemostatis has been satisfactory in all cases, with no adverse reactions.

In a study of previously untreated patients, a total of 3,254 infusions have been administered to 96 patients over a 48-month enrollment period. Hemostasis was successfully achieved in all cases.

During the analytical characterization of Antihemophilic Factor (Recombinant), KOGENATE®, analyses for carbohydrate structure revealed the presence of terminal galactose $\alpha 1 \rightarrow 3$ galactose residues. Since naturally occurring antibody to this structure has been reported in humans, a trial in 18 patients was performed in which the half-life and recovery of rAHF with high levels on this carbohydrate residue was compared to that with KOGENATE, which contains low levels of this structure. As in the normal population, all patients had preexisting endogenous antibody to galactose $\alpha 1 \rightarrow 3$ galactose in titers ranging from 1:320 to 1:5120 and no significant change in antibody level was noted during the study. While the mean recovery for KOGENATE in the study, 2.76%/IU/kg (N=43), was significantly different from that of rAHF with high levels of residues, 2.43%/IU/kg (N=155; p=0.0001), the recovery for rAHF with high levels of galactose $\alpha 1 \rightarrow 3$ galactose is not significantly different from the 2.48%/IU/kg recovery obtained in the larger study from the 58 patients treated with KOGENATE mentioned above. Based on these results, the galactose $\alpha 1 \rightarrow 3$ galactose residue appears to have no clinical significance.

INDICATIONS AND USAGE

KOGENATE is indicated for the treatment of classical hemophilia (hemophilia A) in which there is a demonstrated deficiency of activity of the plasma clotting factor, factor VIII. KOGENATE provides a means of temporarily replacing the missing clotting factor in order to correct or prevent bleeding episodes, or in order to perform emergency and elective surgery in hemophiliacs.

KOGENATE can also be used for treatment of hemophilia A in certain patients with inhibitors to factor VIII. In clinical studies of KOGENATE, patients who developed inhibitors on study continued to manifest a clinical response when inhibitor titers were less than 10 Bethesda Units (B.U.) per mL. When an inhibitor is present, the dosage requirement for factor VIII is variable. The dosage can be determined only by clinical response, and by monitoring of circulating factor VIII levels after treatment (see **DOSAGE AND ADMINISTRATION.**)

KOGENATE does not contain von Willebrand's factor and therefore is not indicated for the treatment of von Willebrand's disease.

CONTRAINDICATIONS

Due to the fact that Antihemophilic Factor (Recombinant) contains trace amounts of mouse protein (maximum 0.03 ng/IU rAHF) and hamster protein (maximum 0.04 ng/IU rAHF), KOGENATE should be administered with caution to individuals with previous hypersensitivity to pdAHF or known hypersensitivity to biologic preparations with trace amounts of murine or hamster proteins.

Assays to detect seroconversion to mouse and hamster protein were conducted on all patients on study. No patient has developed specific antibody titers against these proteins after commencing study, and no allergic reactions have been associated with rAHF infusions. Although no reactions were observed, patients should be warned of the theoretical possibility of a hypersensitivity reaction, and alerted to the early signs of such a reaction (e.g., hives, generalized urticaria, wheezing and hypotension). Patients should be advised to discontinue use of the product and contact their physician if such symptoms occur.

WARNINGS

None.

PRECAUTIONS

General

KOGENATE is intended for the treatment of bleeding disorders arising from a deficiency in factor VIII. This deficiency should be proven prior to administering KOGENATE.

The development of circulating neutralizing antibodies to factor VIII may occur during the treatment of patients with hemophilia A. In a study of previously untreated patients, inhibitor antibodies have developed in 17 of the 92 patients (18.5%) who have had at least one follow-up titer. The incidence of antibodies is 15/56 (26.7%) in patients with severe disease (<2% factor VIII), 2/18 (11%) in patients with moderate disease (2–5% factor VIII) and 0/18 in patients with mild disease (>5% factor VIII). Ten of the antibodies were high titer (>10 Bethesda Units), three were low titer, and four were low titer and transient. Studies most closely resembling the design of the study of inhibitor development with KOGENATE have reported incidences of inhibitor formation ranging between 18.4 and 52% for patients treated with pdAHF.[3–6] The incidence of inhibitor formation in previously untreated patients treated with Antihemophilic Factor (Recombinant), KOGENATE®, appears to be consistent with that reported in the literature, however the true immunogenicity of KOGENATE is not known at present. Patients treated with rAHF should be carefully monitored for the development of antibodies to rAHF by appropriate clinical observation and laboratory tests.

Product administration and handling of the infusion set and needles must be done with caution. Percutaneous puncture with a needle contaminated with blood can transmit infectious virus including HIV (AIDS) and hepatitis. Obtain immediate medical attention if injury occurs.

Place needles in sharps container after single use. Discard all equipment including any reconstituted KOGENATE product in accordance with biohazard procedures.

Carcinogenesis, Mutagenesis, Impairment of Fertility

In vitro evaluation of the mutagenic potential of KOGENATE failed to demonstrate reverse mutation or chromosomal aberrations at doses substantially greater than the maximum expected clinical dose. *In vivo* evaluation of rAHF using doses ranging between 10 and 40 times the expected clinical maximum also indicated that KOGENATE does not possess a mutagenic potential. Long-term investigations of carcinogenic potential in animals have not been performed.

Pediatric Use

KOGENATE has been proven to be safe and efficacious in newborns and the pediatric population while under investigation as previously treated (n=21) and previously untreated patients (n=96) (see **CLINICAL PHARMACOLOGY** and **PRECAUTIONS**).

Pregnancy Category C

Animal reproduction studies have not been conducted with KOGENATE. It is also not known whether KOGENATE can cause fetal harm when administered to a pregnant woman or can affect reproduction capacity. KOGENATE should be given to a pregnant woman only if clearly needed.

ADVERSE REACTIONS

During the clinical studies conducted in previously treated patients, 47 out of 12,932 infusions (0.36%) were associated with 58 reported minor adverse reactions. Of these, 19 reactions were local to the injection site (e.g., burning, pruritus, erythema); and 39 were systemic complaints (dizziness, nausea, chest discomfort, sore throat, cold feet, unusual taste in mouth, and slight decrease in blood pressure). In the study with previously untreated patients, 3,254 infusions have been associated with 11 minor adverse reactions (0.34%): two reports of erythema at the injection site, one of facial flushing related to the infusion, one report of diarrhea, two reports of nonspecific rash, two reports of fever, and three reports of emesis. No serious reactions have been reported, and all reactions have been self-limited.

DOSAGE AND ADMINISTRATION

Each bottle of KOGENATE has the rAHF content in international units per bottle stated on the label of the bottle. The reconstituted product must be administered intravenously by either direct syringe injection or drip infusion. The product must be administered within 3 hours after reconstitution.

General Approach to Treatment and Assessment of Treatment Efficacy

The dosages described below are presented as general guidance. It should be emphasized that the dosage of KOGENATE required for hemostasis must be individualized according to the needs of the patient, the severity of the deficiency, the severity of the hemorrhage, the presence of inhibitors, and the factor VIII level desired. It is often critical to follow the course of therapy with factor VIII level assays.

The clinical effect of KOGENATE is the most important element in evaluating the effectiveness of treatment. It may be necessary to administer more KOGENATE than would be estimated in order to attain satisfactory clinical results. If the calculated dose fails to attain the expected factor VIII levels, or if bleeding is not controlled after administration of the calculated dosage, the presence of a circulating inhibitor in the patient should be suspected. Its presence should be substantiated and the inhibitor level quantitated by appropriate laboratory tests. When an inhibitor is present, the dosage requirement for rAHF is extremely variable and the dosage can be determined only by the clinical response.

Some patients with low titer inhibitors (<10 B.U.) can be successfully treated with factor VIII without a resultant anamnestic rise in inhibitor titer.[7] Factor VIII levels and clinical response to treatment must be assessed to insure adequate response. Use of alternative treatment products, such as Factor IX Complex concentrates, Antihemophilic Factor (Porcine) or Anti-Inhibitor Coagulant Complex, may be necessary for patients with anamnestic responses to factor VIII treatment and/or high titer inhibitors.

Calculation of Dosage

The *in vivo* percent elevation in factor VIII level can be estimated by multiplying the dose of rAHF per kilogram of body weight (IU/kg) by 2%. This method of calculation is based on clinical findings by Abildgaard *et al.*,[8] and is illustrated in the following examples:

$$\text{Expected \% factor VIII increase} = \frac{\text{\# units administered} \times 2\%/\text{IU/kg}}{\text{body weight (kg)}}$$

Example for a 70 kg adult:

$$\frac{1400\ \text{IU} \times 2\%/\text{IU/kg}}{70\ \text{kg}} = 40\%$$

or

$$\text{Dosage required (IU)} = \frac{\text{body weight (kg)} \times \text{desired \% factor VIII increase}}{2\%/\text{IU/kg}}$$

Example for a 15 kg child:

$$\frac{15\ \text{kg} \times 100\%}{2\%/\text{IU/kg}} = 750\ \text{IU required}$$

The dosage necessary to achieve hemostasis depends upon the type and severity of the bleeding episode, according to the following general guidelines:

Mild Hemorrhage

Mild superficial or early hemorrhages may respond to a single dose of 10 IU per kg,[9] leading to an *in vivo* rise of approximately 20% in the factor VIII level. Therapy need not be repeated unless there is evidence of further bleeding.

Moderate Hemorrhage

For more serious bleeding episodes (e.g., definite hemarthroses, known trauma), the factor VIII level should be raised to 30–50% by administering approximately 15–25 IU per kg. If further therapy is required, a repeat infusion can be given at 12–24 hours.[10]

Severe Hemorrhage

In patients with life-threatening bleeding or possible hemorrhage involving vital structures (e.g., central nervous system, retropharyngeal and retroperitoneal spaces, iliopsoas sheath), the factor VIII level should be raised to 80–100% of normal in order to achieve hemostasis. This may be achieved with an initial rAHF (Antihemophilic Factor (Recombinant), KOGENATE®) dose of 40–50 IU per kg and a maintenance dose of 20–25 IU per kg every 8–12 hours.[11,12]

Surgery

For major surgical procedures, the factor VIII level should be raised to approximately 100% by giving a preoperative dose of 50 IU/kg. The factor VIII level should be checked to assure that the expected level is achieved before the patient goes to surgery. In order to maintain hemostatic levels, repeat infusions may be necessary every 6 to 12 hours initially, and for a total of 10 to 14 days until healing is complete. The intensity of factor VIII replacement therapy required depends on the type of surgery and postoperative regimen employed. For minor surgical procedures, less intensive treatment schedules may provide adequate hemostasis.[11,12]

Continued on next page

Kogenate—Cont.

Prophylaxis
Factor VIII concentrates may also be administered on a regular schedule for prophylaxis of bleeding, as reported by Nilsson, *et al.*[13]

Reconstitution
Vacuum Transfer

1. Warm the unopened diluent and the concentrate to room temperature (NMT 37°C, 99°F).
2. After removing the plastic flip-top caps (Fig. A), aseptically cleanse the rubber stoppers of both bottles.
3. Remove the protective cover from the plastic transfer-needle cartridge with tamper-proof seal and penetrate the stopper of the diluent bottle (Fig. B).
4. Remove the remaining portion of the plastic cartridge, invert the diluent bottle and penetrate the rubber seal on the concentrate bottle (Fig. C) with the needle at an angle.
   Alternate method of transferring sterile water: With a sterile needle and syringe, withdraw the appropriate volume of diluent and transfer to the bottle of lyophilized concentrate.
5. The vacuum will draw the diluent into the concentrate bottle. Hold the diluent bottle at an angle to the concentrate bottle in order to direct the jet of diluent against the wall of the concentrate bottle (Fig. C). Avoid excessive foaming.
6. After removing the diluent bottle and transfer needle (Fig. D), swirl continuously until completely dissolved (Fig. E).
7. After the concentrate powder is completely dissolved, withdraw solution into the syringe through the filter needle which is supplied in the package (Fig. F). Replace the filter needle with the administration set provided and inject intravenously. NOTE: Firmly grasp one or both wings to perform venipuncture; do not use the post-use needle shield for this purpose.
8. After infusion, lock post-use needle shield in place using one of the following methods:
   a. One-hand technique: Hold tubing in hand and advance needle shield with thumb and index finger until locked over needle tip (Fig. G).
   b. Two-hand technique: Hold wing stationary and slide needle shield forward with other hand until locked over needle tip (Fig. H).
9. If the same patient is to receive more than one bottle, the contents of two bottles may be drawn into the same syringe through a separate unused filter needle before attaching the vein needle.

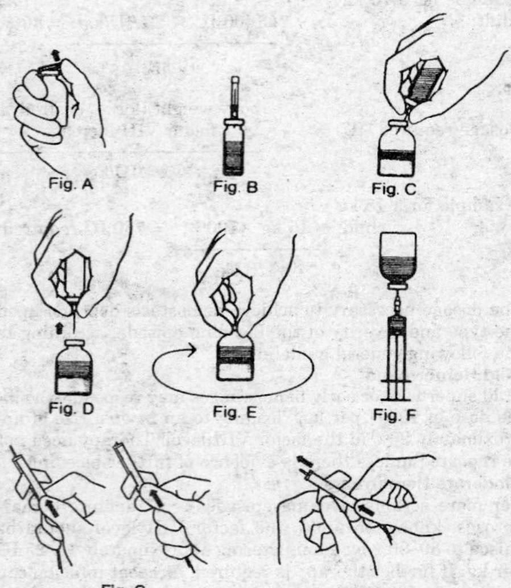

Rate of Administration
The rate of administration should be adapted to the response of the individual patient, but administration of the entire dose in 5 to 10 minutes or less is well-tolerated.
Parenteral drug products should be inspected visually for particulate matter and discoloration prior to administration, whenever solution and container permit.

HOW SUPPLIED
Antihemophilic Factor (Recombinant), KOGENATE®, is supplied in the following single use bottles with the total units of factor VIII activity stated on the label of each bottle. A suitable volume of Sterile Water for Injection, USP, a sterile double-ended transfer needle, a sterile filter needle, and a sterile administration set are provided.

Product Code	Approximate Factor VIII Activity	Diluent
670-20	250 IU	2.5 mL
670-30	500 IU	5 mL
670-50	1000 IU	10 mL

STORAGE
KOGENATE should be stored under refrigeration (2–8°C; 36–46°F). Storage of lyophilized powder at room temperature (up to 25°C or 77°F) for 3 months, such as in home treatment situations, may be done without loss of factor VIII activity. Freezing should be avoided, as breakage of the diluent bottle might occur. Do not use beyond the expiration date indicated on the bottle.

CAUTION
U.S. federal law prohibits dispensing without prescription.

LIMITED WARRANTY
A number of factors beyond our control could reduce the efficacy of this product or even result in an ill effect following its use. These include improper storage and handling of the product after it leaves our hands, diagnosis, dosage, method of administration, and biological differences in individual patients. Because of these factors, it is important that this product be stored properly, and that the directions be followed carefully during use.
No warranty, express or implied, including any warranty of merchantability or fitness is made. Representatives of the Company are not authorized to vary the terms or the contents of the printed labeling, including the package insert for this product, except by printed notice from the Company's headquarters. The prescriber and user of this product must accept the terms hereof.

REFERENCES

1. Lawn RM, Vehar GA: The molecular genetics of hemophilia. *Sci Am* 254(3):48–54, 1986.
2. Schwartz RS, Abildgaard CF, Aledort LM, et al: Human recombinant DNA-derived antihemophilic factor (factor VIII) in the treatment of hemophilia A. *N Engl J Med* 323(26):1800–5, 1990.
3. Lusher JM: Viral safaety and inhibitor development associated with monoclonal antibody-purified FVIIIc. *Ann Hematol* 63(3):138–41, 1991.
4. Addiego JE Jr, Gomperts E, Liu S-L, et al: Treatment of hemophilia A with a highly purified factor VIII concentrate prepared by anti-FVIIIc immunoaffinity chromatography. *Thromb Haemost* 67(1):19–27, 1992.
5. Schwarzinger I, Pabinger I, Korninger C, et al: Incidence of inhibitors in patients with severe and moderate hemophilia A treated with factor VIII concentrates. *Am J Hematol* 24(3):241–5, 1987.
6. Ehrenforth S, Kreuz W. Scharrer I, et al: Incidence of development of factor VIII and factor IX inhibitors in hemophiliacs. *Lancet* 339(8793):594–8, 1992.
7. Kasper CK: Complications of hemophilia A treatment: factor VIII inhibitors, *Ann NY Acad Sci* 614:97–105, 1991.
8. Abildgaard CF, Simone JV, Corrigan JJ, et al: Treatment of hemophilia with glycine-precipitated Factor VIII, *N Engl J Med* 275(9):471–5, 1966.
9. Britton M, Harrison J, Abildgaard CF: Early treatment of hemophilic hemarthroses with minimal dose of new factor VIII concentrate, *J Pediatr* 85(2):245–7, 1974.
10. Abildgaard CF: Current concepts in the management of hemophilia. *Semin Hematol* 12(3):223–32, 1975.
11. Hilgartner MW: Factor replacement therapy. In: Hilgartner MW, Pochedly C, eds.: Hemophilia in the child and adult. New York, Raven Press, 1989, pp 1–26.
12. Kasper CK, Dietrich SL: Comprehensive management of haemophilia. *Clin Haematol* 14(2):489–512, 1985.
13. Nilsson IM, Berntorp E, Lofqvist T, et al: Twenty-five years' experience of prophylactic treatment in severe haemophilia A and B. *J Intern Med* 232(1):25–32, 1992.

KOGENATE® FS ℞
Antihemophilic Factor
(Recombinant)
Formulated with Sucrose

DESCRIPTION
Kogenate® FS Antihemophilic Factor (Recombinant) is a sterile, stable, purified, nonpyrogenic, dried concentrate that has been manufactured using recombinant DNA technology. Kogenate FS is intended for use in the treatment of classical hemophilia (hemophilia A), and is produced by Baby Hamster Kidney (BHK) cells into which the human factor VIII (FVIII) gene has been introduced.[1] The cell culture medium contains Human Plasma Protein Solution (HPPS) and recombinant insulin, but does not contain any proteins derived from animal sources. Kogenate FS is a highly purified glycoprotein consisting of multiple peptides including an 80 kD and various extensions of the 90 kD subunit. It has the same biological activity as FVIII derived from human plasma. Compared to its predecessor product KOGENATE® Antihemophilic Factor (Recombinant), Kogenate FS incorporates a revised purification and formulation process that eliminates the addition of Albumin (Human).
The purification process includes an effective solvent/detergent virus inactivation step in addition to the use of the classical purification methods of ion exchange chromatography, monoclonal antibody immunoaffinity chromatography, along with other chromatographic steps designed to purify recombinant FVIII and remove contaminating substances. Kogenate FS is formulated with sucrose (0.9–1.3%), glycine (21–25 mg/mL), and histidine (18–23 mM) as stabilizers in the final container in place of Albumin (Human) as used in KOGENATE, and is then lyophilized. The final product also contains calcium chloride (2–3 mM), sodium (27–36 mEq/L), chloride (32–40 mEq/L), polysorbate 80 (not more than [NMT] 35 μg/mL), imidazole (NMT 20 μg/1000 IU), tri-n-butyl phosphate (NMT 5 μg/1000 IU), and copper (NMT 0.6 μg/1000 IU). The product contains no preservatives. The amount of sucrose in each vial is 28 mg. Intravenous administration of sucrose contained in Kogenate FS will not affect blood glucose levels.
Each vial of Kogenate FS contains the labeled amount of recombinant FVIII in international units (IU). One IU, as defined by the World Health Organization standard for blood coagulation FVIII, human, is approximately equal to the level of FVIII activity found in 1 mL of fresh pooled human plasma.
Kogenate FS must be administered by the intravenous route.

CLINICAL PHARMACOLOGY
Pharmacokinetic studies were conducted in 20 patients with severe hemophilia A in North America. In this comparative pharmacokinetic study, Kogenate® FS Antihemophilic Factor (Recombinant) was shown to be similar to its predecessor product KOGENATE® Antihemophilic Factor (Recombinant) (rFVIII). Mean FVIII recovery measured 10 minutes following infusion was 2.1 ± 0.3 %/IU/kg for Kogenate FS and 2.4 ± 0.7 %/IU/kg for KOGENATE. The two recoveries were not statistically different (confidence interval 0.815–1.01). The mean biological half-life of recombinant FVIII formulated with sucrose (rFVIII-FS) is similar to KOGENATE with a mean of approximately 13 hours, which has previously been shown to be similar to plasma-derived Antihemophilic Factor (AHF). The activated partial thromboplastin time shortened appropriately with both rFVIII and rFVIII-FS. The recovery and half-life data for rFVIII-FS were unchanged after 24 weeks of exclusive treatment indicating continued efficacy and no evidence of FVIII inhibition. The mean FVIII recovery measured 10 minutes following a dose of rFVIII-FS in 37 patients (after 24 weeks of treatment with rFVIII-FS) was 2.1%/IU/kg, which was unchanged from FVIII recovery determined at baseline and at weeks 4 and 12.
Seventy-one patients with severe hemophilia A, ages 12–59, who had been previously treated with other recombinant and with plasma-derived AHF products, were enrolled in 6-month studies of home therapy with rFVIII-FS in Europe and North America. A total of 3995 infusions have been administered under this portion of the study, or 7.4 million units of rFVIII-FS. Treatment of 659 bleeding episodes during the study period required 951 infusions of rFVIII-FS. The majority of bleeding episodes (89.5%) were treated successfully with one or two infusions, using a mean dosage of approximately 28 IU/kg per treatment infusion. Regularly scheduled treatment accounted for 76% of infusions administered on study. Nine patients have received rFVIII-FS on 11 occasions for surgical procedures. The procedures included removal of a brain tumor, two total knee replacements, two joint synovectomies (one with Achilles tendon lengthening), two circumcisions, a hernia repair, and three teeth extractions. Hemostasis was satisfactory in all cases.
In clinical studies, Kogenate FS has been used in the treatment of bleeding episodes in previously untreated patients (PUPs) and minimally treated (MTP) pediatric patients. In ongoing studies, 61 PUPs/MTPs have been treated with Kogenate FS. Bleeding episodes were treated effectively with one or two infusions of rFVIII-FS. Ten patients have developed inhibitors. In these trials, approximately half of the patients have achieved 20 or more exposure days, and the incidence of inhibitor formation (16%) is consistent with that observed in other pediatric studies using plasma-derived and recombinant factor VIII products.[2–5]

INDICATIONS AND USAGE
Kogenate FS is indicated for the treatment of classical hemophilia (hemophilia A) in which there is a demonstrated deficiency of activity of the plasma clotting factor FVIII. Kogenate FS provides a means of temporarily replacing the missing clotting factor in order to correct or prevent bleeding episodes, or in order to perform emergency or elective surgery in hemophiliacs.
In clinical studies with the predecessor product KOGENATE, some patients who developed inhibitors on study continued to manifest a clinical response when inhibitor titers were less than 10 Bethesda Units (BU) per mL. When an inhibitor is present, the dosage requirement for FVIII is variable. The dosage can be determined only by clinical response, and by monitoring circulating FVIII levels after treatment (see DOSAGE AND ADMINISTRATION).
Because Kogenate FS has similar biological activity to KOGENATE it can be used in the same manner.
Kogenate® FS Antihemophilic Factor (Recombinant) does not contain von Willebrand's factor and therefore is not indicated for the treatment of von Willebrand's disease.

CONTRAINDICATIONS
Known intolerance or allergic reactions to constituents of the preparation.
Known hypersensitivity to mouse or hamster protein may be a contraindication to the use of Kogenate FS.

WARNINGS
None.

PRECAUTIONS
General
Kogenate FS is intended for the treatment of bleeding disorders arising from a deficiency in FVIII. This deficiency should be proven prior to administering Kogenate FS.

The development of circulating neutralizing antibodies to FVIII may occur during the treatment of patients with hemophilia A. Inhibitor formation is especially common in young children with severe hemophilia during their first years of treatment, or in patients of any age who have received little previous treatment with FVIII. Nonetheless, inhibitor formation may occur at any time in the treatment of a patient with hemophilia A. Patients treated with any AHF preparation, including Kogenate FS, should be carefully monitored for the development of antibodies to FVIII by appropriate clinical observation and laboratory tests, according to the recommendation of the patient's hemophilia treatment center.

Formation of Antibodies to Mouse and Hamster Protein

Assays to detect seroconversion to mouse and hamster protein were conducted on all patients on study. No patient has developed specific antibodies to these proteins after commencing study, and no allergic reactions have been associated with rFVIII-FS infusions. Although no reactions were observed, patients should be made aware of the theoretical possibility of a hypersensitivity reaction, and alerted to the early signs of such a reaction (e.g., hives, localized or generalized urticaria, wheezing, and hypotension). Patients should be advised to discontinue use of the product and contact their physician if such symptoms occur.

Carcinogenesis, Mutagenesis, and Impairment of Fertility

In vitro evaluation of the mutagenic potential of rFVIII failed to demonstrate reverse mutation or chromosomal aberrations at doses substantially greater than the maximum expected clinical dose. In vivo evaluation of rFVIII in animals using doses ranging between 10 and 40 times the expected clinical maximum also indicated that rFVIII does not possess a mutagenic potential. Long-term investigations of carcinogenic potential in animals have not been performed.

Pediatric Use

Kogenate FS is appropriate for use in pediatric patients of all ages, including neonates, infants, children, and adolescents. Safety and efficacy studies have been performed in previously untreated and minimally treated pediatric patients (n=62). Kogenate FS is similar to KOGENATE® Antihemophilic Factor (Recombinant) in its biological activity and may be used in pediatric patients in the same manner as KOGENATE.

Geriatric Use

Clinical studies with Kogenate FS did not include sufficient numbers of patients aged 65 and over to be able to determine whether they respond differently from younger patients. However, clinical experience with KOGENATE and other AHF products has not identified differences between the elderly and younger patients. As with any patient receiving Kogenate FS, dose selection for an elderly patient should be individualized.

Pregnancy Category C

Animal reproduction studies have not been conducted with Kogenate® FS Antihemophilic Factor (Recombinant). It is also not known whether Kogenate FS can cause fetal harm when administered to a pregnant woman or affect reproduction capacity. Kogenate FS should be used during pregnancy and lactation only if clearly indicated.

ADVERSE REACTIONS

During the clinical studies conducted in previously treated patients (PTPs), 109 adverse events were reported in the course of 4160 infusions (2.6%). Only 13 events were reported by the investigator as at least remotely related to study drug. Another 7 events were nonassessable. Thus 20 events in 11 patients were considered to be either nonassessable or at least remotely related to Kogenate FS administration, for an incidence of 0.5% relative to the number of infusions administered. Events that were at least remotely drug-related included: local injection site reactions (2), dizziness (2), rash (2), unusual taste in the mouth (1), mild increase in blood pressure (1), pruritus (1), depersonalization (1), nausea (1), and rhinitis (1). No FVIII inhibitors have developed in the 72 PTPs with severe hemophilia A who have received Kogenate FS for a mean of 54 exposure days.

In clinical studies with previously untreated patients (PUPs) and minimally treated (MTP) pediatric patients, 18 adverse events were reported by the clinical investigators as at least possibly related to the study drug including the expected complication of inhibitor development in 8 patients (included in the 10 patients discussed under CLINICAL PHARMACOLOGY), a forearm bleed following venipuncture, constipation, adenopathy, rash, anemia and pallor in one inhibitor patient with gastroenteritis, and serous otitis media.

DOSAGE AND ADMINISTRATION

Each bottle of Kogenate FS has the rFVIII potency in international units stated on the label based on the one-stage assay methodology. The reconstituted product must be administered within 3 hours after reconstitution. It is recommended to use the administration set provided.

GENERAL APPROACH TO TREATMENT AND ASSESSMENT OF TREATMENT EFFICACY

The dosages described below are presented as general guidance. It should be emphasized that the dosage of Kogenate FS required for hemostasis must be individualized according to the needs of the patient, the severity of the deficiency, the severity of the hemorrhage, the presence of inhibitors, and the FVIII level desired. It is often critical to follow the course of therapy with FVIII level assays. The clinical effect of FVIII is the most important element in evaluating the

Expected % factor VIII increase = $\dfrac{\text{\# units administered} \times 2\%/\text{IU/kg}}{\text{body weight (kg)}}$

Example for a 70 kg adult: $\dfrac{1400 \text{ IU} \times 2\%/\text{IU/kg} = 40\%}{70 \text{ kg}}$

or

Dosage required (IU) = $\dfrac{\text{body weight (kg)} \times \text{desired \% FVIII increase}}{2\%/\text{IU/kg}}$

Example for a 15 kg child: $\dfrac{15 \text{ kg} \times 100\% = 750 \text{ IU required}}{2\%/\text{IU/kg}}$

Hemorrhagic event	Therapeutically necessary plasma level of FVIII activity	Dosage necessary to maintain the therapeutic plasma level
Minor hemorrhage (superficial, early hemorrhages, hemorrhages into joints)	20–40%	10–20 IU per kg Repeat dose if evidence of further bleeding.
Moderate to major hemorrhage(hemorrhages into muscles, hemorrhages into the oral cavity, definite hemarthroses, known trauma) Surgery (minor surgical procedures)	30–60%	15–30 IU per kg Repeat one dose at 12–24 hours if needed.
Major to life-threatening hemorrhage(intracranial, intra-abdominal or intrathoracic hemorrhages, gastrointestinal bleeding, central nervous system bleeding, bleeding in the retropharyngeal or retroperitoneal spaces, or iliopsoas sheath) Fractures Head trauma	80–100%	Initial dose 40–50 IU per kg Repeat dose 20–25 IU per kg every 8–12 hours.
Surgery Major surgical procedures	~100%	Preoperative dose 50 IU/kg Verify ~100% activity prior to surgery. Repeat as necessary after 6 to 12 hours initially, and for 10 to 14 days until healing is complete.

effectiveness of treatment. It may be necessary to administer more FVIII than estimated in order to attain satisfactory clinical results. If the calculated dose fails to attain the expected FVIII levels, or if bleeding is not controlled after administration of the calculated dosage, the presence of a circulating inhibitor in the patient should be suspected. Its presence should be substantiated and the inhibitor level quantitated by appropriate laboratory tests. When an inhibitor is present, the dosage requirement for FVIII could be extremely variable among different patients, and the optimal treatment can be determined only by the clinical response.

Some patients with low-titer inhibitors (< 10 BU) can be successfully treated with FVIII preparations without a resultant anamnestic rise in inhibitor titer.[6] FVIII levels and clinical response to treatment must be assessed to insure adequate response. Use of alternative treatment products, such as Factor IX Complex concentrates, Antihemophilic Factor (Porcine), recombinant Factor VIIa or Anti-Inhibitor Coagulant Complex, may be necessary for patients with anamnestic responses to FVIII treatment and/or high-titer inhibitors.

Calculation of Dosage

The in vivo percent elevation in FVIII level can be estimated by multiplying the dose of Kogenate® FS Antihemophilic Factor (Recombinant) per kilogram of body weight (IU/kg) by 2% per IU per kg. This method of calculation is based on clinical findings with the use of plasma-derived and recombinant AHF products[7–9] and is illustrated in the following examples:

[See first table above]

The dosage necessary to achieve hemostasis depends upon the type and severity of the bleeding episode, according to the following general guidelines:

Prophylaxis

AHF concentrates may also be administered on a regular schedule for prophylaxis of bleeding, as reported by Nilsson et al.[10]

Instructions for Use

Reconstitution, product administration, and handling of the administration set and needles must be done with caution. Percutaneous puncture with a needle contaminated with blood can transmit infectious viruses including HIV (AIDS) and hepatitis. Obtain immediate medical attention if injury occurs. Place needles in a sharps container after single use. Discard all equipment, including any reconstituted Kogenate® FS Antihemophilic Factor (Recombinant) product, in accordance with biohazard procedures.

[See second table above]

Reconstitution

Always wash your hands before performing the following procedures:

Vacuum Transfer

1. Warm the unopened diluent and the concentrate to a temperature not to exceed 37°C, 99°F.
2. After removing the plastic flip-top caps (Fig. A), aseptically cleanse the rubber stoppers of both bottles with alcohol, being careful not to handle the rubber stopper.
3. Remove the protective cover from one end of the plastic transfer needle cartridge and penetrate the stopper of the diluent bottle (Fig. B).
4. Remove the remaining portion of the protective cover, invert the diluent bottle and penetrate the rubber seal on the concentrate bottle (Fig. C) with the needle at an angle.
   [Alternate method of transferring sterile water: With a sterile needle and syringe, withdraw the appropriate volume of diluent and transfer to the bottle of lyophilized concentrate.]
5. The vacuum will draw the diluent into the concentrate bottle. Hold the diluent bottle at an angle to the concentrate bottle in order to direct the jet of diluent against the wall of the concentrate bottle (Fig. C). Avoid excessive foaming.
6. After removing the diluent bottle and transfer needle (Fig. D), swirl until completely dissolved without creating excessive foaming (Fig. E).
7. Re-swab top of reconstituted Kogenate FS bottle with alcohol. Allow the stopper to air dry.
8. After the concentrate powder is completely dissolved, withdraw solution into the syringe through the filter needle that is supplied in the package (Fig. F). Replace the filter needle with the administration set provided and inject intravenously. NOTE: Firmly grasp one or both wings to perform venipuncture; do not use the post-use needle shield for this purpose.
9. After infusion, lock post-use needle shield in place using one of the following methods:
   a. One-hand technique: Hold tubing in hand and advance needle shield with thumb and index finger until locked over needle tip (Fig. G).
   b. Two-hand technique: Hold wing stationary and slide needle shield forward with other hand until locked over needle tip (Fig. H).
10. If the same patient is to receive more than one bottle, the contents of two bottles may be drawn into the same syringe through a separate unused filter needle before attaching the vein needle.
11. Parenteral drug products should be inspected visually for particulate matter and discoloration prior to administration, whenever solution and container permit.

Rate of Administration

The rate of administration should be adapted to the response of the individual patient, but administration of the entire dose in 5 to 10 minutes or less is well tolerated.

[See figures A-H at top of next column]

HOW SUPPLIED

Kogenate® FS Antihemophilic Factor (Recombinant) is supplied in the following single use bottles. A suitable volume of

Continued on next page

Kogenate FS—Cont.

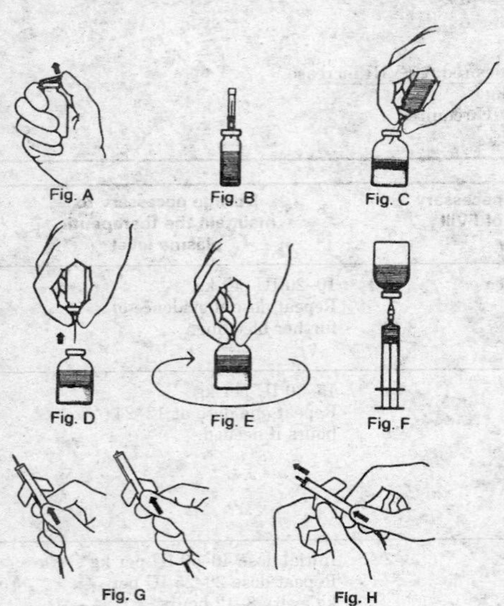

Sterile Water for Injection, USP, a sterile double-ended transfer needle, a sterile filter needle, and a sterile administration set are provided.

NDC Number	Approximate FVIII Activity (IU)	Diluent (mL)
0026-0372-20	250	2.5
0026-0372-30	500	2.5
0026-0372-50	1000	2.5

STORAGE

Kogenate FS should be stored under refrigeration (2–8°C; 36–46°F). Storage of lyophilized powder at room temperature (up to 25°C or 77°F) for 2 months, such as in home treatment situations, may be done. Freezing must be avoided. Do not use beyond the expiration date indicated on the bottle. Protect from extreme exposure to light and store the lyophilized powder in the carton prior to use.

CAUTION

Rx only

U.S. federal law prohibits dispensing without prescription.

REFERENCES

1. Lawn RM, Vehar GA: The molecular genetics of hemophilia. Sci Am 254(3):48–54, 1986.
2. Scharrer I, Bray GL, Neutzling O: Incidence of inhibitors in haemophilia A patients—a review of recent studies of recombinant and plasma-derived factor VIII concentrates. Haemophilia 5(3):145–154, 1999.
3. Lusher JM, Arkin S, Abildgaard CF, et al: Recombinant factor VIII for the treatment of previously untreated patients with hemophilia A: safety, efficacy, and development of inhibitors. N Engl J Med 328(7):453–459, 1993.
4. Schwarzinger I, Pabinger I, Korninger C, et al: Incidence of inhibitors in patients with severe and moderate hemophilia A treated with factor VIII concentrates. Am J Hematol 24(3):241–5, 1987.
5. Ehrenforth S, Kreuz W, Scharrer I, et al: Incidence of development of factor VIII and factor IX inhibitors in hemophiliacs. Lancet 339(8793):594–8, 1992.
6. Kasper CK: Complications of hemophilia A treatment: factor VIII inhibitors. Ann NY Acad Sci 614:97–105, 1991.
7. Abildgaard CF, Simone JV, Corrigan JJ, et al: Treatment of hemophilia with glycine-precipitated Factor VIII. N Engl J Med 275(9):471–5, 1966.
8. Schwartz RS, Abildgaard CF, Aledort LM, et al: Human recombinant DNA-derived antihemophilic factor (factor VIII) in the treatment of hemophilia A. Recombinant Factor VIII Study Group. N Engl J Med 323(26):1800–5, 1990.
9. White GC 2nd, Courter S, Bray GL, et al: A multicenter study of recombinant factor VIII (Recombinate) in previously treated patients with hemophilia A. The Recombinate Previously Treated Patient Study Group.Thromb Haemost 77(4):660–667, 1997.
10. Nilsson IM, Berntorp E, Löfqvist T, et al: Twenty-five years' experience of prophylactic treatment in severe haemophilia A and B. J Intern Med 232(1):25–32, 1992.

14-7372-000 (Issued June 2000)

Bayer Corporation
Pharmaceutical Division
Elkhart, IN 46515 USA
U.S. License No. 8

Factor IX Complex ℞
KONŸNE® 80
Heat-Treated at 80°C

DESCRIPTION

Factor IX Complex, Konÿne® 80, heat-treated at 80°C for 72 hours, is a sterile, dried, plasma fraction comprising coagulation factors II, IX, X and low levels of factor VII.

Factor:	Nomenclature Synonyms:
II	prothrombin
VII	proconvertin
IX	plasma thromboplastin component, PTC, Christmas factor
X	Stuart-Prower factor

Konÿne 80 is standardized in terms of factor IX content and each vial of Konÿne 80 is labeled for factor IX. One international unit (IU) of factor IX as defined by the World Health Organization standard for blood coagulation factor IX is approximately equal to the level of factor IX found in 1.0 mL of fresh, normal plasma.

The factor IX content is approximately 50 times purified over whole plasma, and when reconstituted as directed, Konÿne 80 contains 25 times as much factor IX as an equal volume of fresh plasma. Konÿne 80, containing approximately 1000 IU of factor IX administered in 40 mL, contains the factor IX content of 1 liter of fresh plasma. Konÿne 80 must be administered intravenously.

CLINICAL PHARMACOLOGY

Factor IX Complex raises the plasma level of factor IX and restores hemostasis in patients with factor IX deficiency. In general, a level of factor IX less than 5% of normal will give rise to spontaneous hemorrhage, while levels greater than 20% of normal will lead to satisfactory hemostasis even in the face of trauma or surgery. Approximately 30% to 50% of the factor IX activity can be detected in a hemophilia B (factor IX deficiency) recipient's plasma immediately after infusion.[1,2] The biological activity of the infused factor IX disappears from the plasma with a half-life of approximately 24 hours.[2] A pharmacokinetic study in six patients found similar recoveries and half-lives for Konÿne® 80 as for Konÿne®-HT. It must be noted that administration of Factor IX Complex causes an increase in blood levels of factors II, VII, IX and X.

Factors II, VII, IX and X are the vitamin K dependent coagulation factors and are synthesized in the liver. Congenital deficiencies of each of the four factors do occur and may result in a bleeding tendency. Naturally low levels of the vitamin K dependent factors may also be found in vitamin K deficiency and in severe liver disease.

This product has been heated at 80°C for 72 hours and there is no evidence of adverse effects upon the product. In a study[3] designed to assess the effectiveness of heat treatment at 68°C for 72 hours, hepatitis naive chimpanzees were inoculated with heated Antihemophilic Factor (Human) and Factor IX Complex preparations to which had been previously added non-A, non-B hepatitis Hutchinson Strain[4] to a total level of 2500 chimpanzee infectious doses (CID). The chimpanzees receiving heated preparations failed to exhibit any symptoms of non-A, non-B hepatitis. In contrast, one chimpanzee receiving Antihemophilic Factor (Human) concentrate which was not heated after the non-A, non-B inoculum was added, developed abnormally elevated alanine aminotransferase (ALT) levels beginning 10 weeks postinoculation and liver histopathology at 6 weeks. From these results, it was concluded that the heat treatment employed inactivated a known quantity of non-A, non-B hepatitis: at least 2500 CID.

Additional in vitro studies[5] on the effect of heating Factor IX Complex, Konÿne® 80, in a dried state at 80°C for 72 hours, on virus inactivation were carried out with a number of viruses, including human immunodeficiency virus (HIV), added to Factor IX Complex prior to heating. The following table shows the amount of each model virus inactivated by the process:

Virus	Starting Amount Logs*	Logs Inactivated
Vesicular Stomatitis Virus	8.0	≥7.5
Vaccinia Virus	5.75	1.0
Sindbis Virus	7.25	≥6.75
Bovine Parvovirus	4.5	3.5
Human Immunodeficiency Virus (HIV), HIV-1	4.8	≥4.3

* $\log_{10}$ $TCID_{50}$/mL (for HIV-1, $\log_{10}$ $TCID_{50}$)

INDICATIONS AND USAGE

Factor IX Complex, Konÿne® 80 is indicated for the prevention and control of bleeding caused by Factor IX deficiency due to hemophilia B.

Konÿne 80 is not indicated for use in the treatment of factor VII deficiency.

Konÿne 80 is appropriate for use in:

1. Hemophilia B (Christmas disease); demonstrated factor IX deficiency in children or adults with real or impending bleeding episodes. Spontaneous bleeding can occur even in the absence of any trauma.
2. Reversal of coumarin anticoagulant induced hemorrhage; in situations where prompt reversal is required (e.g., preceding emergency surgery, trauma, etc.), administration of fresh-frozen plasma should be initially considered as treatment; however, Konÿne 80 may be considered as a secondary approach if the risk of transmitting hepatitis is considered justifiable in the face of a life-threatening situation.[6–8]
3. Treatment of bleeding episodes in patients with hemophilia A (factor VIII deficiency) who have inhibitors to factor VIII.[9]

In addition to coumarin anticoagulant induced deficiencies, low levels of factors II, VII, IX and X may be found in vitamin K deficiency, in patients with gut sterilization due to oral antibiotics, in patients with liver disease, and in those with nephrotic syndrome. However, Factor IX Complex, Konÿne 80® is not indicated in these situations and treatment should be aimed at correcting the primary condition.

Note: For publications on the clinical use of Konÿne®, please refer to references 1,2, 6–17.

CONTRAINDICATIONS

None known.

WARNINGS

1. Hepatitis and Viral Diseases

Konÿne 80 is made from human plasma. Products made from human plasma may contain infectious agents, such as viruses, that can cause disease. The risk that such products will transmit an infectious agent has been reduced by screening plasma donors for prior exposure to certain viruses, by testing for the presence of certain current virus infections, and by inactivating certain viruses. Despite these measures, such products can still potentially transmit disease. There is also the possibility that unknown infectious agents may be present in such products. ALL infections thought by a physician possibly to have been transmitted by this product should be reported by the physician or other healthcare provider to Bayer Corporation [1-888-765-3203]. The physician should discuss the risks and benefits of this product with the patient, before prescribing or administering it to the patient.

Individuals who receive infusions of blood or plasma products may develop signs and/or symptoms of some viral infections, particularly hepatitis C. It is emphasized that hepatitis B vaccination is essential for patients with hemophilia and it is recommended that this be done at birth or diagnosis.[19,20] Hepatitis A vaccination is also recommended for hemophilic patients who are hepatitis A seronegative.

2. Thrombosis

Cases of patients developing postoperative thrombosis after treatment with Factor IX Complex have been described. Although thrombosis is a well-known risk of the postoperative period, it is found to be greater in these patients.[13–15] No other data are presently available. Until further surveys and more conclusive studies are available, Konÿne 80 is only advised for patients undergoing elective surgery where the expected beneficial effects of its use outweigh the increased risk of the possibility of thrombosis. This applies especially to those who may be predisposed to thrombosis. Do not use in cases of known liver disease where there is any suspicion of intravascular coagulation or fibrinolysis.

PRECAUTIONS

General

1. Reconstitute only with Sterile Water for Injection, USP.
2. Administer within 3 hours after reconstitution. Do not refrigerate after reconstitution.
3. Administer only by the intravenous route.
4. The administration equipment and any reconstituted Factor IX Complex, Konÿne® 80 not immediately used should be discarded.
5. E-aminocaproic acid should not be administered with Factor IX Complex as this may increase the risk of thrombosis.
6. Patients who receive Konÿne 80 either postoperatively or with known liver disease should be kept under close observation for signs and symptoms of intravascular coagulation or thrombosis. Any suspicious findings of this nature indicate the dosage should be markedly decreased if the patient's conditions are such that the treatment cannot be discontinued entirely. In the event of thrombohemorrhagic disorders occurring, reduction in dosage should be considered, and treatment with heparin may be warranted. Although this preparation does not contain heparin, it has been suggested that reconstitution with heparin in a concentration of 2–5 IU per mL may reduce the risk of development of thrombosis.[17] However, thrombosis can occur even in the presence of heparin.
7. Patients receiving Konÿne 80 for prolonged periods should be continually monitored at least for levels of factors II, IX and X. The same comments as in No. 6 above are indicated. Half-lives of factors II and X are considerably longer than the half-life of factor IX. Hence frequent repeated high-dose administration may result in build-up of factors II and X, with increasing risk of thrombotic side effects.
8. Product administration and handling of the needles must be done with caution. Percutaneous puncture with a needle contaminated with blood can transmit infectious viruses including HIV (AIDS) and hepatitis. Obtain immediate medical attention if injury occurs.

   Place needles in sharps container after single use. Discard all equipment including any reconstituted Konÿne 80 product in accordance with biohazard procedures.

Pregnancy Category C

Animal reproduction studies have not been conducted with Konÿne 80. It is also not known whether Konÿne 80 can cause fetal harm when administered to a pregnant woman or can affect reproduction capacity. Konÿne 80 should be given to a pregnant woman only if clearly needed.

Information for Patient

Some viruses, such as parvovirus B19 or hepatitis A, are particularly difficult to remove or inactivate at this time. Parvovirus B19 most seriously affects pregnant women, or immune-compromised individuals.

Symptoms of parvovirus B19 infection include fever, drowsiness, chills and runny nose followed about 2 weeks later by a rash and joint pain. Evidence of hepatitis A may include several days to weeks of poor appetite, tiredness, and low-grade fever followed by nausea, vomiting, and pain in the belly. Dark urine and a yellowed complexion are also common symptoms. Patients should be encouraged to consult their physician if such symptoms appear.

ADVERSE REACTIONS

In some patients the rapid administration of Konÿne 80 can cause transient fever, chills, headache, flushing or tingling.

DOSAGE AND ADMINISTRATION

Each bottle of Konÿne 80 has the factor IX activity, in IU, stated on the bottle label. One IU is defined as the activity present in 1 mL of fresh, normal plasma. The potency is standardized in terms of factor IX content.

The amount of Konÿne 80 required for normalizing hemostasis will depend upon the patient and upon the circumstances. Sufficient Konÿne 80 should be administered to achieve and maintain a plasma level of at least 20% until hemostasis is achieved.

Levels of factor IX of 30 to 40 percent are considered effective in stopping hemorrhages.[1] Bleeds in life- or limb-threatening areas require factor IX levels of 50 to 80 percent which should be maintained at 30 to 40 percent for a few days.[1] The desired hemostatic plasma level in surgical patients for minor procedures or invasive dental surgery is between 30 and 40 percent of normal.[1] This can be achieved by a dosage not exceeding 30 to 40 units per kg body weight. In major hemorrhage, as during surgery or severe accidental trauma, plasma levels of 60 to 80 percent just prior to surgery, maintained above 30 percent for a further 5 to 7 days and then above 15 to 20 percent for 7 to 10 additional days, until healing occurs, are required.[1]

While the range of values in normal clinical practice is likely to vary depending upon differences between patients, their clinical condition and the type of assay employed, it is again stressed that high dosages, especially if frequently repeated (e.g., more than once per day) are hazardous. Such regimens can induce major thrombotic complications and hence must be avoided.

The following formulas may be used as guidelines to calculate an appropriate dose or to estimate the expected percentage increase obtained from a given dose.:

$$\text{Expected factor IX increase (in \% of normal)} = \frac{\text{IU administered} \times 1.0}{\text{body weight (in kg)}}$$

IU required = body weight (kg) × desired factor IX increase (% normal) × 1.0

Thus, in order to bring a 70 kg patient from 0% to 50% of normal, the patient would require 70 × 50 × 1.0 = 3500 IU or 50 IU/kg body weight.

Prophylaxis

The ideal treatment for proven congenital deficiency of procoagulants is prophylactic administration. For prophylaxis against hemorrhage during times of extensive physical activity, the plasma factor IX levels should be raised to 15 to 30 percent. Maintenance dosage should be adapted to the individual patient's needs. Additional Factor IX Complex, Konÿne® 80 should be administered when a patient on prophylaxis is exposed to trauma or surgery.

Maintenance Dose

Maintenance dosage should be administered according to the clinical response and the factor IX level achieved. Such dosage is usually about 10–20 IU per kg body weight per day.

Inhibitor Patients

For treatment of bleeding episodes in patients with hemophilia A (factor VIII deficiency) who have inhibitors to factor VIII, the recommended dose should be 75 IU/kg. A second dose may be administered after 12 hours if necessary.[9]

Reconstitution

Vacuum Transfer

1. Warm the unopened diluent and concentrate to room temperature (NMT 37°C, 99°F).
2. After removing the plastic flip-top caps (Fig. A) aseptically cleanse the rubber stoppers of both bottles.
3. Remove the protective cover from the plastic transfer-needle cartridge with tamper-proof seal and penetrate the stopper of the diluent bottle (Fig. B).
4. Remove the remaining portion of the plastic cartridge. Invert the diluent bottle and penetrate the rubber seal on the concentrate bottle (Fig. C) with the needle at an angle.

   Alternate method of transferring sterile water: With a sterile needle and syringe, withdraw the appropriate volume of diluent and transfer to the bottle of lyophilized concentrate.
5. Hold the diluent bottle at an angle to the concentrate bottle in order to direct the jet of diluent against the wall of the concentrate bottle. The vacuum will draw the diluent into the concentrate bottle. Avoid excessive foaming. Do not shake the concentrate bottle.
6. After removing the diluent bottle and transfer-needle (Fig. D), optimal reconstitution time is achieved by swirling continuously until completely dissolved (Fig. E). Reconstitution can also be achieved by very gently agitating until dissolved.

   Parenteral drug products should be inspected visually for particulate matter and discoloration prior to administration, whenever solution and container permit.
7. After the concentrate powder is completely dissolved, withdraw the Factor IX Complex, Konÿne® 80 solution into the syringe through the filter needle which is supplied in the package (Fig. F). Replace the filter needle with an appropriate sterile injection needle, e.g., 21 gauge × 1 inch, and inject intravenously.
8. If the same patient is to receive more than one bottle of Konÿne 80, the contents of two bottles may be drawn into the same syringe through filter needles before attaching the vein needle.

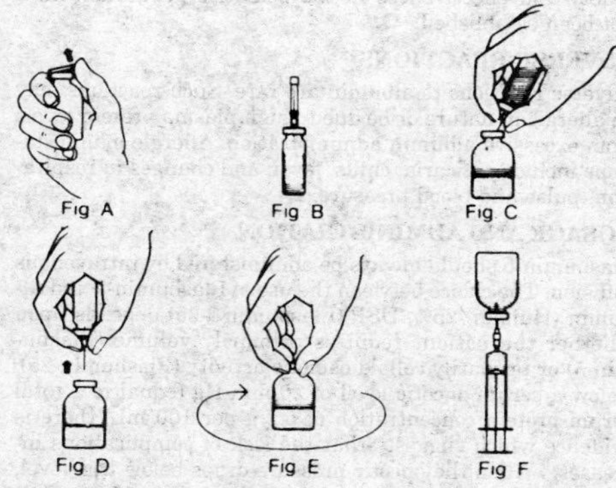

Rate of Administration

The rate of administration should be adapted to the response of the individual patient, but is generally well-tolerated at a rate of approximately 100 IU per minute.

HOW SUPPLIED

Factor IX Complex, Konÿne® 80 is supplied in single dose bottles with the total IU of factor IX activity stated on the label of each bottle. A suitable volume of Sterile Water for Injection, USP, a sterile double-ended transfer needle, and a sterile filter needle are provided.

NDC Number	Approximate Factor IX Activity	Diluent
0026-0626-20	500 IU	20 mL
0026-0626-50	1000 IU	40 mL

STORAGE

Konÿne 80 should be stored under refrigeration (2–8°C; 36–46°F). Freezing should be avoided as breakage of the diluent bottle might occur.

Konÿne 80 concentrate may be stored for a period of up to 1 month at temperatures not to exceed 25°C (77°F) during travel.

CAUTION

U.S. federal law prohibits dispensing without prescription.

LIMITED WARRANTY

A number of factors beyond our control could reduce the efficacy of this product or even result in an ill effect following its use. These include improper storage and handling of the product after it leaves our hands, diagnosis, dosage, method of administration, and biological differences in individual patients. Because of these factors it is important that this product be stored properly, that the directions be followed carefully during use, and that the risk of transmitting viruses be carefully weighed before the product is prescribed. No warranty, express or implied, including any warranty of merchantability or fitness is made. Representatives of the Company are not authorized to vary the terms or the contents of the printed labeling, including the package insert, for this product except by printed notice from the Company's headquarters. The prescriber and user of this product must accept the terms hereof.

REFERENCES

1. Johnson AJ, Aronson DL, Williams WJ: Preparation and clinical use of plasma and plasma fractions. In: Williams WJ (ed): *Hematology,* 4th ed, New York, McGraw-Hill, 1990, ch 170, pp 1659–1673.
2. Zauber NP, Levin J: Factor IX levels in patients with hemophilia B (Christmas disease) following transfusion with concentrates of factor IX or fresh frozen plasma (FFP). *Medicine* (Baltimore) 56(3): 213–24, 1977.
3. Mozen MM, Louie RE, Mitra G: Heat inactivation of viruses in antihemophilic factor concentrates. Abstracts, XVIth International Congress of the World Federation of Hemophilia, Rio de Janeiro, Aug. 24–28, 1984. Number 240.
4. Feinstone SM, Alter HJ, Dienes HP, et al: Non-A, non-B hepatitis in chimpanzees and marmosets. *J Infect Dis* 144(6):588–98, 1981.
5. Unpublished data in files of Bayer Corporation.
6. Taberner DA, Thompson JM, Poller L: Comparison of prothrombin complex concentrate and vitamin K_1 in oral anticoagulant reversal. *Br Med J* 2(6027):83–5, 1976.
7. Menache D, Roberts HR: Summary report and recommendations of the task force members and consultants. *Thromb Diath Haemorrh* 33:645–7, 1975.
8. Aronson DL: Factor IX Complex. *Semin Thromb Hemostas* 6(1):28–43, 1979.
9. Lusher JM, Shapiro SS, Palascak JE, et al: Efficacy of prothrombin-complex concentrates in hemophiliacs with antibodies to factor VIII: a multicenter therapeutic trial. *N Engl J Med* 303(8):421–5, 1980.
10. Hoag MS, Johnson FF, Robinson AJ, et al: Treatment of hemophilia B with a new clotting-factor concentrate. *N Engl J Med* 280(11):581–6, 1969.
11. Hoag MS, Johnson FF, Robinson AJ, et al: Use of plasma concentrate in congenital factor VII and IX deficiencies. *Clin Res* 17:152, 1969.
12. Breen FA Jr, Tullis JL: Prothrombin concentrates in treatment of Christmas disease and allied disorders. *JAMA* 208(10):1848–52, 1969.
13. Kasper CK: Postoperative thrombosis in hemophilia. *N Engl J Med* 289(3):160, 1973.
14. Kasper CK: Surgical operation in hemophilia B. Use of factor IX concentrate. *Calif Med* 113(1):4–8, 1970.
15. George JN, Breckenridge RT: The use of factor VIII and factor IX concentrates during surgery. *JAMA* 214(9): 1673–6, 1970.
16. Gunay U, Choi HS, Maurer HS, et al: Commercial preparations of prothrombin complex. A clinical comparison. *Am J Dis Child* 126(6):775–7, 1973.
17. White GC 2d, Lundblad RL, Kingdon HS: Prothrombin complex concentrates: preparation, properties, and clinical uses. *Curr Top Hematol* 2:203–44, 1979.
18. Colombo M, Mannucci PM, Carnelli V, et al: Transmission of non-A, non-B hepatitis by heat-treated factor VIII concentrate. *Lancet* 2(8445):1–4, 1985.
19. National Hemophilia Foundation Medical and Scientific Advisory Council. Hemophilia Information Exchange—AIDS Update: Recommendations concerning AIDS and the treatment of hemophilia. HIV infection, Section I.G. (Rev. Jan., 1988).

PLASBUMIN®-5 ℞

[*plăs-būmin*]

Albumin (Human) 5%, USP

DESCRIPTION

Albumin (Human) 5%, USP (Plasbumin®-5) is made from pooled human venous plasma using the Cohn cold ethanol fractionation process. Part of the fractionation may be performed by another licensed manufacturer. It is prepared in accordance with the applicable requirements established by the U.S. Food and Drug Administration.

Plasbumin-5 is a 5% sterile solution of albumin in an aqueous diluent. The preparation is stabilized with 0.004 M sodium caprylate and 0.004 M acetyltryptophan. The approximate sodium content of the product is 145 mEq/L. It contains no preservative. Plasbumin-5 must be administered intravenously.

Each vial of Plasbumin-5 is heat-treated at 60°C for 10 hours against the possibility of transmitting the hepatitis viruses.

CLINICAL PHARMACOLOGY

Plasbumin-5 is oncotically equivalent volume for volume to normal human plasma.

When administered intravenously to an adequately hydrated subject, the oncotic (colloid osmotic) effect of Plasbumin-5 is to expand the circulating blood volume by an amount approximately equal to the volume infused. It is primarily used in the treatment of shock associated with hemorrhage, surgery, trauma, burns, bacteremia, renal failure, and cardiovascular collapse.[1]

Albumin is a transport protein and it may be useful in severe jaundice in hemolytic disease of the newborn.[2] This could also be of importance in acute liver failure where albumin might serve the dual role of supporting plasma oncotic pressure, as well as binding excessive plasma bilirubin.[1]

INDICATIONS AND USAGE

Emergency Treatment of Hypovolemic Shock

Plasbumin-5 is iso-oncotic with normal plasma and on intravenous infusion will expand the circulating blood volume by an amount approximately equal to the volume infused. In conditions associated mainly with a volume deficit, albumin is best administered as a 5% solution (Plasbumin-5); but where there is an oncotic deficit, Albumin (Human) 25%, USP (Plasbumin®-25) may be preferred. This is also an important consideration where the treatment of the shock state has been delayed. If Plasbumin-25 is used, appropriate additional crystalloid should be administered.[1]

Crystalloid solutions in volumes several times greater than that of Plasbumin-5 may be effective in treating shock in younger individuals who have no preexisting illness at the

Continued on next page

Plasbumin-5—Cont.

time of the incident. Older patients, especially those with preexisting debilitating conditions, or those in whom the shock is caused by a medical disorder, or where the state of shock has existed for some time before active therapy could be instituted, may not tolerate hypoalbuminemia as well.[1] Removal of ascitic fluid from a patient with cirrhosis may cause changes in cardiovascular function and even result in hypovolemic shock. In such circumstances, the use of albumin infusion may be required to support the blood volume.[1]

Burn Therapy

An optimal therapeutic regimen with respect to the administration of colloids, crystalloids, and water following extensive burns has not been established. During the first 24 hours after sustaining thermal injury, large volumes of crystalloids are infused to restore the depleted extracellular fluid volume. Beyond 24 hours, albumin can be used to maintain plasma colloid osmotic pressure. Plasbumin-25 may be preferred for this purpose.[1]

Cardiopulmonary Bypass[1]

With the relatively small priming volume required with modern pumps, preoperative dilution of the blood using albumin and crystalloid has been shown to be safe and well-tolerated. Although the limit to which the hematocrit and plasma protein concentration can be safely lowered has not been defined, it is common practice to adjust the albumin and crystalloid pump prime to achieve a hematocrit of 20% and a plasma albumin concentration of 2.5 g per 100 mL in the patient.

Acute Liver Failure[1]

In the uncommon situation of rapid loss of liver function, with or without coma, administration of albumin may serve the double purpose of supporting the colloid osmotic pressure of the plasma as well as binding excess plasma bilirubin.

Sequestration of Protein Rich Fluids[2]

This occurs in such conditions as acute peritonitis, pancreatitis, mediastinitis, and extensive cellulitis. The magnitude of loss into the third space may require treatment of reduced volume or oncotic activity with an infusion of albumin.

Situations in Which Albumin Administration is Not Warranted[1]

In chronic nephrosis, infused albumin is promptly excreted by the kidneys with no relief of the chronic edema or effect on the underlying renal lesion. It is of occasional use in the rapid "priming" diuresis of nephrosis. Similarly, in hypoproteinemic states associated with chronic cirrhosis, malabsorption, protein losing enteropathies, pancreatic insufficiency, and undernutrition, the infusion of albumin as a source of protein nutrition is not justified.

CONTRAINDICATIONS

Certain patients, e.g., those with a history of congestive cardiac failure, renal insufficiency or stabilized chronic anemia, are at special risk of developing circulatory overload. A history of allergic reaction to albumin is a specific contraindication for usage.

WARNINGS

Plasbumin-5 is made from human plasma. Products made from human plasma may contain infectious agents, such as viruses, that can cause disease. The risk that such products will transmit an infectious agent has been reduced by screening plasma donors for prior exposure to certain viruses, by testing for the presence of certain current virus infections, and by inactivating and/or removing certain viruses. Despite these measures, such products can still potentially transmit disease. There is also the possibility that unknown infectious agents may be present in such products. Individuals who receive infusions of blood or plasma products may develop signs and/or symptoms of some viral infections, particularly hepatitis C. ALL infections thought by a physician possibly to have been transmitted by this product should be reported by the physician or other healthcare provider to Bayer Corporation [1-888-765-3203].

The physician should discuss the risks and benefits of this product with the patient, before prescribing or administering it to the patient.

Solutions which have been frozen should not be used. Do not use if turbid. Do not begin administration more than 4 hours after the container has been entered. Partially used vials must be discarded. Vials which are cracked or which have been previously entered or damaged should not be used, as this may have allowed the entry of microorganisms. Plasbumin-5 contains no preservative.

General

Patients should always be monitored carefully in order to guard against the possibility of circulatory overload. Albumin (Human) 5%, USP (Plasbumin®-5) is iso-oncotic with normal plasma and will not tend to aggravate tissue dehydration. Appropriate additional crystalloids should be administered, if required by the patient, to maintain normal fluid balance.

In hemorrhage, the administration of albumin should be supplemented by the transfusion of whole blood to treat the relative anemia associated with hemodilution.[3] When circulating blood volume has been reduced, hemodilution following the administration of albumin persists for many hours. In patients with a normal blood volume, hemodilution lasts for a much shorter period.[4–6] The rapid rise in blood pressure, which may follow the administration of a colloid with positive oncotic activity, necessitates careful observation to detect and treat severed blood vessels which may not have bled at the lower blood pressure.

Drug Interactions

Plasbumin-5 is compatible with whole blood and packed red cells, as well as the standard carbohydrate and electrolyte solutions intended for intravenous use. It should not be mixed with protein hydrolysates, amino acid solutions nor those containing alcohol.

Pregnancy Category C

Animal reproduction studies have not been conducted with Plasbumin-5. It is also not known whether Plasbumin-5 can cause fetal harm when administered to a pregnant woman or can affect reproduction capacity. Plasbumin-5 should be given to a pregnant woman only if clearly needed.

Pediatric Use

Safety and effectiveness in the pediatric population have not been established.

ADVERSE REACTIONS

Adverse reactions to albumin are rare. Such reactions may be allergic in nature or be due to high plasma protein levels from excessive albumin administration. Allergic manifestations include urticaria, chills, fever, and changes in respiration, pulse and blood pressure.

DOSAGE AND ADMINISTRATION

Plasbumin-5 should always be administered by intravenous infusion. The choice between the use of Plasbumin-5 and Albumin (Human) 25%, USP (Plasbumin®-25) depends upon whether the patient requires primarily volume (Plasbumin-5) or primarily colloid osmotic activity (Plasbumin-25). Below a serum oncotic level of 20 mm Hg (equal to a total serum protein concentration of 5.2 g per 100 mL) there is evidence which suggests that the risk of complications increases.[1] When the oncotic pressure drops below this level, the patient should be treated with Plasbumin-25 together with diuretics. This is especially important in high risk patients who have undergone abdominal, cardiovascular, thoracic or urologic surgery or who have acute bacteremia.

The volume administered and the speed of administration should be adapted to the response of the individual patient.

Hypovolemic Shock

The volume infused should be related to the estimated volume deficit and the speed of administration adapted to the response of the patient.

In neonates or infants, Plasbumin-5 may be given in large amounts.[7] The recommended dose is 10 to 20 mL/kg equivalent to 0.5 to 1.0 g albumin/kg body weight.

Burns

After a burn injury (usually beyond 24 hours) there is a close correlation between the amount of albumin infused and the resultant increase in plasma colloid osmotic pressure. The aim should be to maintain the plasma albumin concentration in the region of 2.5 ± 0.5 g per 100 mL with a plasma oncotic pressure of 20 mm Hg (equivalent to a total plasma protein concentration of 5.2 g per 100 mL).[1] This is best achieved by the intravenous administration of Plasbumin, usually as Plasbumin-25. The duration of therapy is decided by the loss of protein from burned areas and in the urine. In addition, oral or parenteral feeding with amino acids should be initiated, as the long-term administration of albumin should not be considered as a source of nutrition.

Other dosage recommendations are given under the specific indications referred to above.

Preparation for Administration

Remove seal to expose stopper. Always swab stopper top immediately with suitable antiseptic prior to entering vial.

Parenteral drug products should be inspected visually for particulate matter and discoloration prior to administration, whenever solution and container permit.

HOW SUPPLIED

Plasbumin-5 is available in 50 mL, 250 mL and 500 mL rubber-stoppered vials. Each single dose vial contains albumin in the following approximate amounts:

NDC Number	Size	Grams Protein
0026-0685-20	50 mL	2.5
0026-0685-25	250 mL	12.5
0026-0685-27	500 mL	25.0

STORAGE

Store at room temperature not exceeding 30°C (86°F). Do not freeze. Do not use after expiration date.

CAUTION

U.S. federal law prohibits dispensing without prescription.

LIMITED WARRANTY

A number of factors beyond our control could reduce the efficacy of this product or even result in an ill effect following its use. These include improper storage and handling of the product after it leaves our hands, diagnosis, dosage, method of administration, and biological differences in individual patients. Because of these factors, it is important that this product be stored properly and that the directions be followed carefully during use.

No warranty, express or implied, including any warranty of merchantability or fitness is made. Representatives of the Company are not authorized to vary the terms or the contents of the printed labeling, including the package insert for this product, except by printed notice from the Company's headquarters. The prescriber and user of this product must accept the terms hereof.

REFERENCES

1. Tullis JL: Albumin. 1. Background and use. 2. Guidelines for clinical use. *JAMA* 237:355–60; 460-3, 1977.
2. Clowes GHA Jr, Vucinic M, Weidner MG: Circulatory and metabolic alterations associated with survival or death in peritonitis: clinical analysis of 25 cases. *Ann Surg* 163(6): 866–85, 1966.
3. Heyl JT, Janeway CA: The use of human albumin in military medicine. I. The theoretical and experimental basis for its use. *US Navy Med Bull* 40:785–91, 1942.
4. Janeway CA, Gibson ST, Woodruff LM, et al: Chemical, clinical, and immunological studies on the products of human plasma fractionation. VII. Concentrated human serum albumin, *J Clin Invest* 23:465–90, 1944.
5. Woodruff LM, Gibson ST: The clinical evaluation of human albumin. *US Navy Med Bull* 40:791–6, 1942.
6. Janeway CA, Berenberg W, Hutchins G: Indications and uses of blood, blood derivatives and blood substitutes. *Med Clin North Am* 29:1069–94, 1945.
7. Bennett EJ: Fluid balance in the newborn. *Anesthesiology* 43:210–24, 1975.

Bayer Corporation
Pharmaceutical Division
Elkhart, IN 46515 USA 14-7685-003
U.S. License No. 8 (Rev. April 1998)

Albumin (Human) 20%, USP PLASBUMIN®-20 ℞

[*plăs-bū̆min*]

DESCRIPTION

Albumin (Human) 20%, USP (Plasbumin®-20) is made from pooled human venous plasma using the Cohn cold ethanol fractionation process. Part of the fractionation may be performed by another licensed manufacturer. It is prepared in accordance with the applicable requirements established by the U.S. Food and Drug Administration.

Plasbumin-20 is a 20% sterile solution of albumin in an aqueous diluent. The preparation is stabilized with 0.016 M sodium caprylate and 0.016 M acetyltryptophan. The approximate sodium content of the product is 145 mEq/L. It contains no preservative. Plasbumin-20 must be administered intravenously.

Each vial of Plasbumin-20 is heat-treated at 60°C for 10 hours against the possibility of transmitting the hepatitis viruses.

CLINICAL PHARMACOLOGY

Each 50 mL vial of Plasbumin-20 supplies the oncotic equivalent of approximately 200 mL citrated plasma.

When administered intravenously to an adequately hydrated subject, the oncotic (colloid osmotic) effect of 50 mL Plasbumin-20 is such that it will draw approximately a further 125 mL of fluid from the extravascular tissues into the circulation within 15 minutes,[1] thus increasing the total blood volume and reducing both hemoconcentration and whole blood viscosity. Accordingly, the main clinical indications are for hypoproteinemic states involving reduced oncotic pressure, with or without accompanying edema.[2] Plasbumin-20 can also be used as a plasma volume expander.

Albumin is a transport protein and it may be useful in severe hemolytic disease in the neonate who is awaiting exchange transfusion. The infused albumin may reduce the level of free bilirubin in the blood.[3]

This could also be of importance in acute liver failure where albumin might serve the dual role of supporting plasma oncotic pressure, as well as binding excessive plasma bilirubin.[2]

INDICATIONS AND USAGE

Emergency Treatment of Hypovolemic Shock

Plasbumin-20 is hyperoncotic and on intravenous infusion will expand the plasma volume by an additional amount, three to four times the volume actually administered, by withdrawing fluid from the interstitial spaces, provided the patient is normally hydrated interstitially or there is interstitial edema.[1] If the patient is dehydrated, additional crystalloids must be given,[4] or alternatively, Albumin (Human) 5%, USP (Plasbumin®-5) should be used. The patient's hemodynamic response should be monitored and the usual precautions against circulatory overload observed. The total dose should not exceed the level of albumin found in the normal individual, i.e., about 2 g per kg body weight in the absence of active bleeding. Although Plasbumin-5 is to be preferred for the usual volume deficits, Plasbumin-20 with appropriate crystalloids may offer therapeutic advantages in oncotic deficits or in long-standing shock where treatment has been delayed.[2]

Removal of ascitic fluid from a patient with cirrhosis may cause changes in cardiovascular function and even result in hypovolemic shock. In such circumstances, the use of an albumin infusion may be required to support the blood volume.[2]

Burn Therapy

An optimal therapeutic regimen with respect to the administration of colloids, crystalloids, and water following extensive burns has not been established. During the first 24 hours after sustaining thermal injury, large volumes of crystalloids are infused to restore the depleted extracellular fluid volume. Beyond 24 hours Plasbumin-20 can be used to maintain plasma colloid osmotic pressure.

Hypoproteinemia With or Without Edema
During major surgery, patients can lose over half of their circulating albumin with the attendant complications of oncotic deficit,[2,4,5] A similar situation can occur in sepsis or intensive care patients. Treatment with Plasbumin-20 may be of value in such cases.[2]

Adult Respiratory Distress Syndrome (ARDS)[2,5]
This is characterized by deficient oxygenation caused by pulmonary interstitial edema complicating shock and postsurgical conditions. When clinical signs are those of hypoproteinemia with a fluid volume overload, Plasbumin-20 together with a diuretic may play a role in therapy.

Cardiopulmonary Bypass[2,6]
With the relatively small priming volume required with modern pumps, preoperative dilution of the blood using albumin and crystalloid has been shown to be safe and well-tolerated. Although the limit to which the hematocrit and plasma protein concentration can be safely lowered has not been defined, it is common practice to adjust the albumin and crystalloid pump prime to achieve a hematocrit of 20% and a plasma albumin concentration of 2.5 g per 100 mL in the patient.

Acute Liver Failure[2]
In the uncommon situation of rapid loss of liver function with or without coma, administration of albumin may serve the double purpose of supporting the colloid osmotic pressure of the plasma as well as binding excess plasma bilirubin.

Neonatal Hemolytic Disease[2,3]
The administration of Plasbumin-20 may be indicated prior to exchange transfusion, in order to bind free bilirubin, thus lessening the risk of kernicterus. A dosage of 1 g/kg body weight is given about 1 hour prior to exchange transfusion. Caution must be observed in hypervolemic infants.

Sequestration of Protein Rich fluids[7]
This occurs in such conditions as acute peritonitis, pancreatitis, mediastinitis, and extensive cellulitis. The magnitude of loss into the third space may require treatment of reduced volume or oncotic activity with an infusion of albumin.

Erythrocyte Resuspension[2]
Albumin may be required to avoid excessive hypoproteinemia during certain types of exchange transfusion, or with the use of very large volumes of previously frozen or washed red cells. About 25 g of albumin per liter of erythrocytes is commonly used, although the requirements in preexistent hypoproteinemia or hepatic impairment can be greater. Plasbumin-20 is added to the isotonic suspension of washed red cells immediately prior to transfusion.

Acute Nephrosis[2]
Certain patients may not respond to cyclophosphamide or steroid therapy. The steroids may even aggravate the underlying edema. In this situation a loop diuretic and 100 mL Plasbumin-20 repeated daily for 7 to 10 days may be helpful in controlling the edema and the patient may then respond to steroid treatment.

Renal Dialysis[2]
Although not part of the regular regimen of renal dialysis, Plasbumin-20 may be of value in the treatment of shock or hypotension in these patients. The usual volume administered is about 100 mL, taking particular care to avoid fluid overload as these patients are often fluid overloaded and cannot tolerate substantial volumes of salt solution.

Situations in Which Albumin Administration is Not Warranted[2]
In chronic nephrosis, infused albumin is promptly excreted by the kidneys with no relief of the chronic edema or effect on the underlying renal lesion. It is of occasional use in the rapid "priming" diuresis of nephrosis. Similarly, in hypoproteinemic states associated with chronic cirrhosis, malabsorption, protein-losing enteropathies, pancreatic insufficiency, and undernutrition, the infusion of albumin as a source of protein nutrition is not justified.

CONTRAINDICATIONS

Certain patients, e.g., those with a history of congestive cardiac failure, renal insufficiency or stabilized chronic anemia, are at special risk of developing circulatory overload. A history of an allergic reaction to albumin is a specific contraindication to usage.

WARNINGS

Plasbumin-20 is made from human plasma. Products made from human plasma may contain infectious agents, such as viruses, that can cause disease. The risk that such products will transmit an infectious agent has been reduced by screening plasma donors for prior exposure to certain viruses, by testing for the presence of certain current virus infections, and by inactivating and/or removing certain viruses. Despite these measures, such products can still potentially transmit disease. There is also the possibility that unknown infectious agents may be present in such products. Individuals who receive infusions of blood or plasma products may develop signs and/or symptoms of some viral infections, particularly hepatitis C. ALL infections thought by a physician possibly to have been transmitted by this product should be reported by the physician or other healthcare provider to Bayer Corporation [1-888-765-3203].

The physician should discuss the risks and benefits of this product with the patient, before prescribing or administering it to the patient.

Solutions which have been frozen should not be used. Do not use if turbid. Do not begin administration more than 4 hours after the container has been entered. Partially used vials must be discarded. Vials which are cracked or which have been previously entered or damaged should not be used, as this may have allowed the entry of microorganisms. Albumin (Human) 20%, USP (Plasbumin®-20) contains no preservative.

PRECAUTIONS

General
Patients should always be monitored carefully in order to guard against the possibility of circulatory overload. Plasbumin-20 is hyperoncotic; therefore, in the presence of dehydration, albumin must be given with or followed by addition of fluids.[4]

In hemorrhage the administration of albumin should be supplemented by the transfusion of whole blood to treat the relative anemia associated with hemodilution.[8] When circulating blood volume has been reduced, hemodilution following the administration of albumin persists for many hours. In patients with a normal blood volume, hemodilution lasts for a much shorter period.[4,9,10]

The rapid rise in blood pressure which may follow the administration of a colloid with positive oncotic activity necessitates careful observation to detect and treat severed blood vessels which may not have bled at the lower blood pressure.

Drug Interactions
Plasbumin-20 is compatible with whole blood, packed red cells, as well as the standard carbohydrate and electrolyte solutions intended for intravenous use. It should, however, not be mixed with protein hydrolysates, amino acid solutions nor those containing alcohol.

Pregnancy Category C
Animal reproduction studies have not been conducted with Plasbumin-20. It is also not known whether Plasbumin-20 can cause fetal harm when administered to a pregnant women or can affect reproduction capacity. Plasbumin-20 should be given to a pregnant woman only if clearly needed.

Pediatric Use
Safety and effectiveness in the pediatric population have not been established.

ADVERSE REACTIONS

Adverse reactions to albumin are rare. Such reactions may be allergic in nature or due to high plasma protein levels from excessive albumin administration. Allergic manifestations include urticaria, chills, fever, and changes in respiration, pulse and blood pressure.

DOSAGE AND ADMINISTRATION

Plasbumin-20 should always be administered by intravenous infusion. If sodium restriction is required, Plasbumin-20 may be administered either undiluted or diluted in a sodium-free carbohydrate solution such as 5% dextrose in water.

Hypovolemic Shock—For treatment of hypovolemic shock, the volume administered and the speed of infusion should be adapted to the response of the individual patient.

Burns—After a burn injury (usually beyond 24 hours) there is a close correlation between the amount of albumin infused and the resultant increase in plasma colloid osmotic pressure. The aim should be to maintain the plasma albumin concentration in the region of 2.5 ± 0.5 g per 100 mL with a plasma oncotic pressure of 20 mm Hg (equivalent to a total plasma protein concentration of 5.2 g per 100 mL).[2] This is best achieved by the intravenous administration of Plasbumin-20. The duration of therapy is decided by the loss of protein from the burned areas and in the urine. In addition, oral or parenteral feeding with amino acids should be initiated, as the long-term administration of albumin should not be considered as a source of nutrition.

Hypoproteinemia With or Without Edema—Unless the underlying pathology responsible for the hypoproteinemia can be corrected, the intravenous administration of Plasbumin-20 must be considered purely symptomatic or supportive (see section **Situations in Which Albumin Administration is Not Warranted**).[2] The usual daily dose of albumin for adults is 50 to 75 g and for children 25 g. Patients with severe hypoproteinemia who continue to lose albumin may require larger quantities. Since hypoproteinemic patients usually have approximately normal blood volumes, the rate of administration of Plasbumin-20 should not exceed 2 mL per minute, as more rapid injection may precipitate circulatory embarrassment and pulmonary edema.

Other dosage recommendations are given under the specific indications referred to above.

Preparation for Administration
Remove seal to expose stopper. Always swab stopper top immediately with a suitable antiseptic prior to entering vial. Parenteral drug products should be inspected visually for particulate matter and discoloration prior to administration, whenever solution and container permit.

HOW SUPPLIED

Plasbumin-20 is available in 50 mL and 100 mL rubber-stoppered vials. Each single dose vial contains albumin in the following approximate amounts:

NDC Number	Size	Grams Albumin
0026-0683-20	50 mL	10.0
0026-0683-71	100 mL	20.0

STORAGE
Store at room temperature not exceeding 30°C (86°F). Do not freeze. Do not use after expiration date.

CAUTION
U.S. federal law prohibits dispensing without prescription.

LIMITED WARRANTY
A number of factors beyond our control could reduce the efficacy of this product or even result in an ill effect following its use. These include improper storage and handling of the product after it leaves our hands, diagnosis, dosage, method of administration, and biological differences in individual patients. Because of these factors, it is important that this product be stored properly and that the directions be followed carefully during use.

No warranty, express or implied, including any warranty of merchantability or fitness is made. Representatives of the Company are not authorized to vary the terms or the contents of the printed labeling, including the package insert for this product, except by printed notice from the Company's headquarters. The prescriber and user of this product must accept the terms hereof.

REFERENCES

1. Heyl JT, Gibson JG II, Janeway CA: Studies on the plasma proteins. V. The effect of concentrated solutions of human and bovine serum albumin on blood volume after acute blood loss in man. *J Clin Invest* 22:763–73, 1943.
2. Tullis JL; Albumin. 1. Background and use. 2, Guidelines for clinical use. *JAMA* 237:355–60; 460–3, 1977.
3. Comley A, Wood B; Albumin administration in exchange transfusion for hyperbilirubinaemia. *Arch Dis Child* 43: 151–4, 1968
4. Janeway CA, Gibson ST, Woodruff LM, et al: Chemical, clinical, and immunological studies on the products of human plasma fractionation, VII. Concentrated human serum albumin. *J Clin Invest* 23:465–90, 1944.
5. Skillman JJ, Tanenbaum BJ: Unrecognized losses of albumin, plasma, and red cells during abdominal vascular operations. *Curr Top Surg Res* 2:523–33, 1970.
6. Zubiate P, Kay JH, Mendez AM, et al: Coronary artery surgery: a new technique with use of little blood, if any. *J Thorac Cardiovasc Surg* 68(2):263–7, 1974.
7. Clowes GHA Jr, Vucinic M, Weidner MG: Circulatory and metabolic alterations associated with survival or death in peritonitis: clinical analysis of 25 cases. *Ann Surg* 163:866–85, 1966.
8. Heyl JT, Janeway CA: The use of human albumin in military medicine. I. The theoretical and experimental basis for its use. *US Naval Med Bull* 40:785–91, 1942.
9. Woodruff LM, Gibson ST: The clinical evaluation of human albumin. *US Naval Med Bull* 40:791–6, 1942.
10. Janeway CA, Berenberg W, Hutchins G: Indications and uses of blood, blood derivatives and blood substitutes. *Med Clin North Am* 29:1069–94, 1945.

Bayer Corporation
Pharmaceutical Division
Elkhart, IN 46515 USA 14-7683-007
U.S. License No. 8 (Rev. October 1998)

PLASBUMIN®-25 ℞

[*plăs -bū̆min*]
Albumin (Human) 25%, USP

DESCRIPTION

Albumin (Human) 25%, USP (Plasbumin®-25) is made from pooled human venous plasma using the Cohn cold ethanol fractionation process. Part of the fractionation may be performed by another licensed manufacturer. It is prepared in accordance with the applicable requirements established by the U.S. Food and Drug Administration.

Plasbumin-25 is a 25% sterile solution of albumin in an aqueous diluent. The preparation is stabilized with 0.02 M sodium caprylate and 0.02 M acetyltryptophan. The approximate sodium content of the product is 145 mEq/L. It contains no preservative. Plasbumin-25 must be administered intravenously.

Each vial of Plasbumin-25 is heat-treated at 60°C for 10 hours against the possibility of transmitting the hepatitis viruses.

CLINICAL PHARMACOLOGY

Each 20 mL vial of Plasbumin-25 supplies the oncotic equivalent of approximately 100 mL citrated plasma; 50 mL supplies the oncotic equivalent of approximately 250 mL citrated plasma.

When administered intravenously to an adequately hydrated subject, the oncotic (colloid osmotic) effect of 20 mL Plasbumin-25 is such that it will draw approximately a further 70 mL of fluid from the extravascular tissues into the circulation within 15 minutes,[1] thus increasing the total blood volume and reducing both hemoconcentration and whole blood viscosity. Accordingly, the main clinical indications are for hypoproteinemic states involving reduced oncotic pressure, with or without accompanying edema.[2] Plasbumin-25 can also be used as a plasma volume expander.

Albumin is a transport protein and it may be useful in severe hemolytic disease in the neonate who is awaiting exchange transfusion. The infused albumin may reduce the level of free bilirubin in the blood.[3]

This could also be of importance in acute liver failure where albumin might serve the dual role of supporting plasma oncotic pressure, as well as binding excessive plasma bilirubin.[2]

Continued on next page

Plasbumin-25—Cont.

INDICATIONS AND USAGE

Emergency Treatment of Hypovolemic Shock

Plasbumin-25 is hyperoncotic and on intravenous infusion will expand the plasma volume by an additional amount, three to four times the volume actually administered, by withdrawing fluid from the interstitial spaces, provided the patient is normally hydrated interstitially or there is interstitial edema.[1] If the patient is dehydrated, additional crystalloids must be given,[4] or alternatively, Albumin (Human) 5%, USP (Plasbumin®-5) should be used. The patient's hemodynamic response should be monitored and the usual precautions against circulatory overload observed. The total dose should not exceed the level of albumin found in the normal individual, i.e., about 2 g per kg body weight in the absence of active bleeding. Although Plasbumin-5 is to be preferred for the usual volume deficits, Plasbumin-25 with appropriate crystalloids may offer therapeutic advantages in oncotic deficits or in long-standing shock where treatment has been delayed.[2]

Removal of ascitic fluid from a patient with cirrhosis may cause changes in cardiovascular function and even result in hypovolemic shock. In such circumstances, the use of an albumin infusion may be required to support the blood volume.[2]

Burn Therapy

An optimal therapeutic regimen with respect to the administration of colloids, crystalloids, and water following extensive burns has not been established. During the first 24 hours after sustaining thermal injury, large volumes of crystalloids are infused to restore the depleted extracellular fluid volume. Beyond 24 hours Plasbumin-25 can be used to maintain plasma colloid osmotic pressure.

Hypoproteinemia With or Without Edema

During major surgery, patients can lose over half of their circulating albumin with the attendant complications of oncotic deficit.[2,4,5] A similar situation can occur in sepsis or intensive care patients. Treatment with Plasbumin-25 may be of value in such cases.[2]

Adult Respiratory Distress Syndrome (ARDS)[2,5]

This is characterized by deficient oxygenation caused by pulmonary interstitial edema complicating shock and postsurgical conditions. When clinical signs are those of hypoproteinemia with a fluid volume overload, Plasbumin-25 together with a diuretic may play a role in therapy.

Cardiopulmonary Bypass[2,6]

With the relatively small priming volume required with modern pumps, preoperative dilution of the blood using albumin and crystalloid has been shown to be safe and well-tolerated. Although the limit to which the hematocrit and plasma protein concentration can be safely lowered has not been defined, it is common practice to adjust the albumin and crystalloid pump prime to achieve a hematocrit of 20% and a plasma albumin concentration of 2.5 g per 100 mL in the patient.

Acute Liver Failure[2]

In the uncommon situation of rapid loss of liver function with or without coma, administration of albumin may serve the double purpose of supporting the colloid osmotic pressure of the plasma as well as binding excess plasma bilirubin.

Neonatal Hemolytic Disease[2,3]

The administration of Plasbumin-25 may be indicated prior to exchange transfusion, in order to bind free bilirubin, thus lessening the risk of kernicterus. A dosage of 1 g/kg body weight is given about 1 hour prior to exchange transfusion. Caution must be observed in hypervolemic infants.

Sequestration of Protein Rich Fluids[7]

This occurs in such conditions as acute peritonitis, pancreatitis, mediastinitis, and extensive cellulitis. The magnitude of loss into the third space may require treatment of reduced volume or oncotic activity with an infusion of albumin.

Erythrocyte Resuspension[2]

Albumin may be required to avoid excessive hypoproteinemia, during certain types of exchange transfusion, or with the use of very large volumes of previously frozen or washed red cells. About 25 g of albumin per liter of erythrocytes is commonly used, although the requirements in preexistent hypoproteinemia or hepatic impairment can be greater. Plasbumin-25 is added to the isotonic suspension of washed red cells immediately prior to transfusion.

Acute Nephrosis[2]

Certain patients may not respond to cyclophosphamide or steroid therapy. The steroids may even aggravate the underlying edema. In this situation a loop diuretic and 100 mL Plasbumin-25 repeated daily for 7 to 10 days may be helpful in controlling the edema and the patient may then respond to steroid treatment.

Renal Dialysis[2]

Although not part of the regular regimen of renal dialysis, Plasbumin-25 may be of value in the treatment of shock or hypotension in these patients. The usual volume administered is about 100 mL, taking particular care to avoid fluid overload as those patients are often fluid overloaded and cannot tolerate substantial volumes of salt solution.

Situations in Which Albumin Administration is Not Warranted[2]

In chronic nephrosis, infused albumin is promptly excreted by the kidneys with no relief of the chronic edema or effect on the underlying renal lesion. It is of occasional use in the rapid "priming" diuresis of nephrosis. Similarly, in hypoproteinemic states associated with chronic cirrhosis, malabsorption, protein losing enteropathies, pancreatic insufficiency, and undernutrition, the infusion of albumin as a source of protein nutrition is not justified.

CONTRAINDICATIONS

Certain patients, e.g., those with a history of congestive cardiac failure, renal insufficiency or stabilized chronic enemia, are at special risk of developing circulatory overload. A history of an allergic reaction to albumin is a specific contraindication to usage.

WARNINGS

Plasbumin-25 is made from human plasma. Products made from human plasma may contain infectious agents, such as viruses, that can cause disease. The risk that such products will transmit an infectious agent has been reduced by screening plasma donors for prior exposure to certain viruses, by testing for the presence of certain current virus infections, and by inactivating and/or removing certain viruses. Despite these measures, such products can still potentially transmit disease. There is also the possibility that unknown infectious agents may be present in such products. Individuals who receive infusions of blood or plasma products may develop signs and/or symptoms of some viral infections, particularly hepatitis C. ALL infections thought by a physician possibly to have been transmitted by this product should be reported by the physician or other healthcare provider to Bayer Corporation [1-888-765-3203]. The physician should discuss the risks and benefits of this product with the patient, before prescribing or administering it to the patient.

Solutions which have been frozen should not be used. Do not use if turbid. Do not begin administration more than 4 hours after the container has been entered. Partially used vials must be discarded. Vials which are cracked or which have been previously entered or damaged should not be used, as this may have allowed the entry of microorganisms. Albumin (Human) 25%, USP (Plasbumin®-25) contains no preservatives.

PRECAUTIONS

General

Patients should always be monitored carefully in order to guard against the possibility of circulatory overload. Plasbumin-25 is hyperoncotic, therefore, in the presence of dehydration, albumin must be given with or followed by addition of fluids.[4]

In hemorrhage the administration of albumin should be supplemented by the transfusion of whole blood to treat the relative anemia associated with hemodilution.[8] When circulating blood volume has been reduced, hemodilution following the administration of albumin persists for many hours. In patients with a normal blood volume, hemodilution lasts for a much shorter period.[4,9,10]

The rapid rise in blood pressure which may follow the administration of a colloid with positive oncotic activity necessitates careful observation to defect and treat severed blood vessels which may not have bled at the lower blood pressure.

Drug Interactions

Plasbumin-25 is compatible with whole blood, packed red cells, as well as the standard carbohydrate and electrolyte solutions intended for intravenous use. It should, however, not be mixed with protein hydrolysates, amino acid solutions nor those containing alcohol.

Pregnancy Category C

Animal reproduction studies have not been conducted with Plasbumin-25. It is also not known whether Plasbumin-25 can cause fetal harm when administered to a pregnant woman or can affect reproduction capacity. Plasbumin-25 should be given to a pregnant woman only if clearly needed.

Pediatric Use

Safety and effectiveness in the pediatric population have not been established.

ADVERSE REACTIONS

Adverse reactions to albumin are rare. Such reactions may be allergic in nature or due to high plasma protein levels from excessive albumin administration. Allergic manifestations include urticaria, chills, fever, and changes in respiration, pulse and blood pressure.

DOSAGE AND ADMINISTRATION

Plasbumin-25 should always be administered by intravenous infusion. If sodium restriction is required, Plasbumin-25 may be administered either undiluted or diluted in a sodium-free carbohydrate solution such as 5% dextrose in water.

Hypovolemic Shock—For treatment of hypovolemic shock, the volume administered and the speed of infusion should be adapted to the response of the individual patient.

Burns—After a burn injury (usually beyond 24 hours) there is a close correlation between the amount of albumin infused and the resultant increase in plasma colloid osmotic pressure. The aim should be to maintain the plasma albumin concentration in the region of 2.5 ± 0.5 g per 100 mL with a plasma oncotic pressure of 20 mm Hg (equivalent to a total plasma protein concentration of 5.2 g per 100 mL).[2] This is best achieved by the intravenous administration of Plasbumin-25. The duration of therapy is decided by the loss of protein from the burned areas and in the urine. In addition, oral or parenteral feeding with amino acids should be initiated, as the long-term administration of albumin should not be considered as a source of nutrition.

Hypoproteinemia With or Without Edema—Unless the underlying pathology responsible for the hypoproteinemia can be corrected, the intravenous administration of Plasbumin-25 must be considered purely symptomatic or supportive (see section **Situations in Which Albumin Administration is Not Warranted**).[2] The usual daily dose of albumin for adults is 50 to 75 g and for children 25 g. Patients with severe hypoproteinemia who continue to lose albumin may require larger quantities. Since hypoproteinemic patients usually have approximately normal blood volumes, the rate of administration of Plasbumin-25 should not exceed 2 mL per minute, as more rapid injection may precipitate circulatory embarassment and pulmonary edema.

Other dosage recommendations are given under the specific indications referred to above.

Preparation for Administration

Remove seal to expose stopper. Always swab stopper top immediately with a suitable antiseptic prior to entering vial. Parenteral drug products should be inspected visually for particulate matter and discoloration prior to administration, whenever solution and container permit.

HOW SUPPLIED

Plasbumin-25 is available in 20 mL, 50 mL, and 100 mL rubber-stoppered vials. Each single dose vial contains albumin in the following approximate amounts:

NDC Number	Size	Grams Protein
0026-0684-16	20 mL	5.0
0026-0684-20	50 mL	12.5
0026-0684-71	100 mL	25.0

STORAGE

Store at room temperature not exceeding 30°C (86°F). Do not freeze. Do not use after expiration date.

CAUTION

U.S. federal law prohibits dispensing without prescription.

LIMITED WARRANTY

A number of factors beyond our control could reduce the efficacy of this product or even result in an ill effect following its use. These include improper storage and handling of the product after it leaves our hands, diagnosis, dosage, method of administration, and biological differences in individual patients. Because of these factors, it is important that this product be stored properly and that the directions be followed carefully during use.

No warranty, express or implied, including any warranty of merchantability or fitness is made. Representatives of the Company are not authorized to vary the terms or the contents of the printed labeling, including the package insert for this product, except by printed notice from the Company's headquarters. The prescriber and user of this product must accept the terms hereof.

REFERENCES

1. Heyl JT, Gibson JG II, Janeway CA: Studies on the plasma proteins, V. The effect of concentrated solutions of human and bovine serum albumin on blood volume after acute blood loss in man. *J Clin Invest* 22:763–73, 1943.
2. Tullis JL: Albumin. 1. Background and use. 2. Guidelines for clinical use. *JAMA* 237:355–60; 460–3, 1977.
3. Comley A, Wood B: Albumin administration in exchange transfusion for hyperbilirubinaemia. *Arch Dis Child* 43: 151–4, 1968.
4. Janeway CA, Gibson ST, Woodruff LM, et al: Chemical, clinical, and immunological studies on the products of human plasma fractionation, VII. Concentrated human serum albumin. *J Clin Invest* 23:465–90, 1944.
5. Skillman JJ, Tanenbaum BJ: Unrecognized losses of albumin, plasma, and red cells during abdominal vascular operations. *Curr Top Surg Res* 2:523–33, 1970.
6. Zubiate P, Kay JH, Mendez AM, et al: Coronary artery surgery: a new technique with use of little blood, if any. *J Thorac Cardiovasc Surg* 68(2):263–7, 1974.
7. Clowes GHA Jr, Vucinic M, Weidner MG: Circulatory and metabolic alterations associated with survival or death in peritonitis: clinical analysis of 25 cases. *Ann Surg* 163:866–85, 1966.
8. Heyl JT, Janeway CA: The use of human albumin in military medicine, I. The theoretical and experimental basis for its use. *US Navy Med Bull* 40:785–91, 1942.
9. Woodruff LM, Gibson ST: The clinical evaluation of human albumin. *US Navy Med Bull* 40:791–6, 1942.
10. Janeway CA, Berenberg W, Hutchins G: Indications and uses of blood, blood derivatives and blood substitutes. *Med Clin North Am* 29;1069–94, 1945.

Bayer Corporation
Pharmaceutical Division
Elkhart, IN 46515 USA 14-7684-001
U.S. License No. 8 (Rev. October 1998)

PLASMANATE® ℞

[*plăs'măn-ate*]

Plasma Protein Fraction (Human) 5%, USP

DESCRIPTION

This product has been prepared from large pools of human plasma. Each 100 mL of Plasma Protein Fraction (Human) 5%, USP—Plasmanate® contains 5 g selected plasma proteins buffered with sodium carbonate and stabilized with 0.004 M sodium caprylate and 0.004 M acetyltryptophan. The plasma proteins consist of approximately 88% normal human albumin, 12% alpha and beta globulins and not more than 1% gamma globulin as determined by electrophoresis.[1] The concentration of these proteins is such that this solution is iso-oncotic with normal human plasma and is isotonic. The approximate concentrations of the significant electrolytes in Plasmanate are: sodium 145 mEq/L, potassium 0.25 mEq/L, and chloride 100 mEq/L. Plasmanate must be administered intravenously.

This product is designed to bring to the medical profession a preparation derived from human blood and similar to human plasma. Each vial of Plasmanate is sterile and heat-treated at 60°C for 10 hours against the possibility of transmitting the hepatitis viruses.

The blood group agglutinins and agglutinogens A and B are at such a low level in Plasmanate solution that its use has no effect on routine blood typing procedures. No chemical or microscopic alterations of the urine have been observed with its use.

CLINICAL PHARMACOLOGY

In normal human volunteers, Plasmanate has resulted in an increased blood volume which has lasted up to 48 hours.[2] Clinical experience has indicated that it is an adequate replacement for human plasma in the treatment of shock and is a suitable means of providing human proteins for their osmotic effect.

INDICATIONS AND USAGE

Treatment of Shock—Plasmanate is indicated in the treatment of shock due to burns, crushing injuries, abdominal emergencies, and any other cause where there is a predominant loss of plasma fluids and not red blood cells. It is also effective in the emergency treatment of shock due to hemorrhage.[3,4] Following the emergency phase of therapy, blood transfusions may be indicated depending on the severity of the blood loss.

In infants and small children, Plasmanate has been found to be very useful in the initial therapy of shock due to dehydration and infection.

CONTRAINDICATIONS

Plasmanate is contraindicated for use in patients on cardiopulmonary bypass. Severe hypotension has been reported in such patients when given Plasma Protein Fraction.[4]

Plasma Protein Fraction is contraindicated in patients with severe anemia, congestive heart failure, or increased blood volume.

WARNINGS

Plasmanate is made from human plasma. Products made from human plasma may contain infectious agents, such as viruses, that can cause disease. The risk that such products will transmit an infectious agent has been reduced by screening plasma donors for prior exposure to certain viruses, by testing for the presence of certain current virus infections, and by inactivating and/or removing certain viruses. Despite these measures, such products can still potentially transmit disease. There is also the possibility that unknown infectious agents may be present in such products. Individuals who receive infusions of blood or plasma products may develop signs and/or symptoms of some viral infections, particularly hepatitis C. ALL infections thought by a physician possibly to have been transmitted by this product should be reported by the physician or other healthcare provider to Bayer Corporation [1-888-765-3203].

The physician should discuss the risks and benefits of this product with the patient, before prescribing or administering it to the patient.

Solutions which are turbid or which have been frozen should not be used. Do not use if turbid. Do not begin administration more than 4 hours after the container has been entered. Partially used vials must be discarded. Vials which are cracked or which have been previously entered or damaged should not be used, as this may have allowed the entry of microorganisms. Plasmanate contains no preservative.

PRECAUTIONS

General

Rapid infusion of Plasmanate (greater than 10mL/minute) has produced hypotension in patients undergoing surgery or in the preoperative or postoperative period. Blood pressure should be monitored during use and infusion slowed or ceased if sudden hypotension occurs.

Plasmanate does not provide coagulation factors and therefore does not correct coagulation disorders.

Drug Interactions

Plasma Protein Fraction (Human) 5%, USP—Plasmanate® is compatible with whole blood, packed red cells as well as the standard carbohydrate and electrolyte solutions intended for intravenous use, it should, however, not be mixed with protein hydrolysates or solutions containing alcohol.

Pregnancy Category C

Animal reproduction studies have not been conducted with Plasmanate. It is also not known if Plasmanate can cause fetal harm when administered to a pregnant woman or can affect reproduction capacity. Plasmanate should be given to a pregnant woman only if clearly needed.

Pediatric Use

Safety and effectiveness in the pediatric population have not been established.

ADVERSE REACTIONS

Hypotension may occur, particularly following rapid infusion or intra-arterial administration to patients on cardiopulmonary bypass. The blood pressure may normalize spontaneously after the slowing or discontinuation of the infusion. Vasopressors will also correct the hypotension.

Flushing, urticaria, back pain, nausea and headache have been occasionally reported by conscious patients.

DOSAGE AND ADMINISTRATION

Dosage is based almost entirely on the nature of the individual case and response to therapy. The usual minimum effective dose in adults is 250–500 mL. As with any plasma expander, the rate should be adjusted or slowed according to the clinical response and rising blood pressure.

Administration should be by vein and preferably through an area of skin at some distance from any site of infection or trauma. Plasmanate is compatible with the usual carbohydrate and electrolyte solutions.

We recommend the following procedure: First swab the stopper with Iodine Tincture, USP followed by a sterile antiseptic swab.

Parenteral drug products should be inspected visually for particulate matter and discoloration prior to administration, whenever solution and container permit.

HOW SUPPLIED

Plasmanate is available in 50 mL pediatric size, 250 mL and 500 mL rubber-stoppered vials. Each single dose vial contains plasma protein in the following approximate amounts:

NDC Number	Size	Grams Protein
0026-0613-20	50 mL	2.5
0026-0613-25	250 mL	12.5
0026-0613-27	500 mL	25.0

STORAGE

Store at room temperature not exceeding 30°C (86°F). Solution that has been frozen should not be used. Do not use after expiration date.

CAUTION

U.S. federal law prohibits dispensing without prescription.

LIMITED WARRANTY

A number of factors beyond our control could reduce the efficacy of this product or even result in an ill effect following its use. These include improper storage and handling of the product after it leaves our hands, diagnosis, dosage, method of administration, and biological differences in individual patients. Because of these factors, it is important that this product be stored properly and that the directions be followed carefully during use.

No warranty, express or implied, including any warranty of merchantability or fitness is made. Representatives of the Company are not authorized to vary the terms or the contents of the printed labeling, including the package insert for this product, except by printed notice from the Company's headquarters. The prescriber and user of this product must accept the terms hereof.

REFERENCES

1. Hink JH Jr, Hidalgo J, Seeberg VP, et al: Preparation and properties of a heat-treated human plasma protein fraction. *Vox Sang* 2:174–86, 1957.
2. Bertrand JJ, Feichtmeir TV, Kolomeyer N, et al: Clinical investigations with a heat-treated plasma protein fraction—Plasmanate® *Vox Sang* 4:385–402, 1959.
3. Tullis JL: Albumin, 1. Background and use, 2. Guidelines for clinical use. *JAMA* 237:355–60; 460–3, 1977.
4. Bland JHL, Laver MB, Lowenstein E: Vasodilator effect of commercial 5% plasma protein fraction solutions. *JAMA* 224:1721–4, 1973.

Bayer Corporation
Pharmaceutical Division
Elkhart, IN 46515 USA
U.S. License No. 8 14-7613-008
(Rev. April 1998)

PROLASTIN® ℞

Alpha$_1$–Proteinase Inhibitor
(HUMAN)
[pro-las 'tin]

DESCRIPTION

Alpha$_1$-Proteinase Inhibitor (Human), Prolastin®, is a sterile, stable, lyophilized preparation of purified human Alpha$_1$-Proteinase Inhibitor (alpha$_1$-PI), also known as alpha$_1$-antitrypsin. Prolastin is intended for use in therapy of congenital alpha$_1$-antitrypsin deficiency.

Prolastin is prepared from pooled human plasma of normal donors by modification and refinements of the cold ethanol method of Cohn.[1] Part of the fractionation may be performed by another licensed manufacturer. In order to reduce the potential risk of transmission of infectious agents, Prolastin has been heat-treated in solution at 60±0.5°C for not less than 10 hours. However, no procedure has been found to be totally effective in removing viral infectivity from plasma fractionation products.

The specific activity of Prolastin is ≥0.35 mg functional alpha$_1$-PI/mg protein and when reconstituted as directed, the concentration of alpha$_1$-PI is ≥20 mg/mL. When reconstituted, Prolastin has a pH of 6.6–7.4, a sodium content of 100–210 mEq/L, a chloride content of 60–180 mEq/L, a sodium phosphate content of 0.015–0.025 M, a polyethylene glycol content of not more than (NMT) 5 ppm, NMT 0.1% sucrose. Prolastin contains small amounts of other plasma proteins including alpha$_2$-plasmin inhibitor, alpha$_1$-antichymotrypsin, C$_1$-esterase inhibitor, haptoglobin, antithrombin III, alpha$_1$-lipoprotein, albumin, and IgA.[1]

Each vial of Prolastin contains the labeled amount of functionally active alpha$_1$-PI in milligrams per vial (mg/vial), as determined by capacity to neutralize porcine pancreatic elastase.[1] Prolastin contains no preservative and must be administered by the intravenous route.

CLINICAL PHARMACOLOGY

Alpha$_1$-antitrypsin deficiency is a chronic, hereditary, usually fatal, autosomal recessive disorder in which a low concentration of alpha$_1$-PI (alpha$_1$-antitrypsin) is associated with slowly progressive, severe, panacinar emphysema that most often manifests itself in the third to fourth decades of life.[2–9][Although the terms "Alpha$_1$-Proteinase Inhibitor" and "alpha$_1$-antitrypsin" are used interchangeably in the scientific literature, the hereditary disorder associated with a reduction in the serum level of alpha$_1$-PI is conventionally referred to as "alpha$_1$-antitrypsin deficiency" while the deficient protein is referred to as "Alpha$_1$-Proteinase Inhibitor"[10]]. The emphysema is typically worse in the lower lung zones.[4,8,9] The pathogenesis of development of emphysema in alpha$_1$-antitrypsin deficiency is not well understood at this time. It is believed, however, to be due to a chronic biochemical imbalance between elastase (an enzyme capable of degrading elastin tissues, released by inflammatory cells, primarily neutrophils, in the lower respiratory tract) and alpha$_1$-PI (the principal inhibitor of neutrophil elastase) which is deficient in alpha$_1$-antitrypsin disease.[11–15] As a result, it is believed that alveolar structures are unprotected from chronic exposure to elastase released from a chronic, low level burden of neutrophils in the lower respiratory tract, resulting in progressive degradation of elastin tissues.[11–15] The eventual outcome is the development of emphysema. Neonatal hepatitis with cholestatic jaundice appears in approximately 10% of newborns with alpha$_1$-antitrypsin deficiency.[15] In some adults, alpha$_1$-antitrypsin deficiency is complicated by cirrhosis.[15]

A large number of phenotypic variants of alpha$_1$-antitrypsin deficiency exists.[15] The most severely affected individuals are those with the PiZZ variant, typically characterized by alpha$_1$-PI serum levels <35% normal.[15] Epidemiologic studies of individuals with various phenotypes of alpha$_1$-antitrypsin deficiency have demonstrated that individuals with endogenous serum levels of alpha$_1$-PI ≤50 mg/dL (based on commercial standards) have a risk of >80% of developing emphysema over a lifetime.[3–6,8,9,16] However, individuals with endogenous alpha$_1$-PI levels >80 mg/dL, in general, do not manifest an increased risk for development of emphysema above the general population background risk.[5,15] From these observations, it is believed that the "threshold" level of alpha$_1$-PI in the serum required to provide adequate anti-elastase activity in the lung of individuals with alpha$_1$-antitrypsin deficiency is about 80 mg/dL (based on commercial standards for immunologic assay of alpha$_1$-PI).[12,15,17]

In clinical studies of Alpha$_1$-Proteinase Inhibitor (Human), Prolastin®, 23 subjects with the PiZZ variant of congenital deficiency of alpha$_1$-antitrypsin deficiency and documented destructive lung disease participated in a study of acute and/or chronic replacement therapy with Prolastin.[18] The mean in vivo recovery of alpha$_1$-PI was 4.2 mg (immunologic)/dL per mg (functional)/kg body weight administered.[18,19] The half-life of alpha$_1$-PI in vivo was approximately 4.5 days.[18,19] Based on these observations, a program of chronic replacement therapy was developed. Nineteen of the subjects in these studies received Prolastin replacement therapy, 60 mg/kg body weight, once weekly for up to 26 weeks (average 24 weeks of therapy). With this schedule of replacement therapy, blood levels of alpha$_1$-PI were maintained above 80 mg/dL (based on the commercial standards for alpha$_1$-PI immunologic assay).[18–20]. Within a few weeks of commencing this program, bronchoalveolar lavage studies demonstrated significantly increased levels of alpha$_1$-PI and functional antineutrophil elastase capacity in the epithelial lining fluid of the lower respiratory tract of the lung, as compared to levels prior to commencing the program of chronic replacement therapy with Alpha$_1$-Proteinase Inhibitor (Human), Prolastin®.[18–20].

All 23 individuals who participated in the investigations were immunized with Hepatitis B Vaccine and received a single dose of Hepatitis B Immune Globulin (Human) on entry into the investigation. Although no other steps were taken to prevent hepatitis, neither hepatitis B nor non-A, non-B hepatitis occurred in any of the subjects.[18,19] All subjects remained seronegative for HIV antibody. None of the subjects developed any detectable antibody to alpha$_1$-PI or other serum protein.

Long-term controlled clinical trials to evaluate the effect of chronic replacement therapy with Prolastin® on the development of or progression of emphysema in patients with congenital alpha$_1$-antitrypsin deficiency have not been performed. Estimates of the sample size required of this rare disorder and the slow, progressive nature of the clinical course have been considered impediments in the ability to conduct such a trial.[21] Studies to monitor the long-term effects will continue as part of the postapproval process.

INDICATIONS AND USAGE

Congenital Alpha$_1$-Antitrypsin Deficiency

Prolastin is indicated for chronic replacement therapy of individuals having congenital deficiency of alpha$_1$-PI (alpha$_1$-antitrypsin deficiency) with clinically demonstrable panacinar emphysema. Clinical and biochemical studies have demonstrated that with such therapy, it is possible to increase plasma levels of alpha$_1$-PI, and that levels of functionally active alpha$_1$-PI in the lung epithelial lining fluid are increased proportionately.[18–20]. As some individuals

Continued on next page

Prolastin—Cont.

with alpha$_1$-antitrypsin deficiency will not go on to develop panacinar emphysema, only those with early evidence of such disease should be considered for chronic replacement therapy with Prolastin.[22] Subjects with the PiMZ or PiMS phenotypes of alpha$_1$-antitrypsin deficiency should not be considered for such treatment as they appear to be at small risk for panacinar emphysema.[22] Clinical data are not available as to the long-term effects derived from chronic replacement therapy of individuals with alpha$_1$-antitrypsin deficiency with Prolastin. Only adult subjects have received Prolastin to date.

Prolastin is not indicated for use in patients other than those with PiZZ, PiZ(null), or Pi(null)(null) phenotypes.

CONTRAINDICATIONS

Individuals with selective IgA deficiencies who have known antibody against IgA (anti-IgA antibody) should not receive Prolastin, since these patients may experience severe reactions, including anaphylaxis, to IgA which may be present.

WARNINGS

Alpha$_1$-Proteinase Inhibitor (Human), Prolastin® is made from human plasma. Products made from human plasma may contain infectious agents, such as viruses, that can cause disease. The risk that such products will transmit an infectious agent has been reduced by screening plasma donors for prior exposure to certain viruses, by testing for the presence of certain current virus infections, and by inactivating and/or removing certain viruses. Despite these measures, such products can still potentially transmit disease. There is also the possibility that unknown infectious agents may be present in such products. Individuals who receive infusions of blood or plasma products may develop signs and/or symptoms of some viral infections, particularly hepatitis C. ALL infections thought by a physician possibly to have been transmitted by this product should be reported by the physician or other healthcare provider to Bayer Corporation [1-888-765-3203].

The physician should discuss the risks and benefits of this product with the patient, before prescribing or administering it to a patient.

Prolastin has been heat-treated in solution at 60°C for 10 hours in order to reduce the potential for transmission of infectious agents.[1] No cases of hepatitis, either hepatitis B or hepatitis C, have been recorded to date in individuals receiving Prolastin.[18] However, as all individuals received prophylaxis against hepatitis B, no conclusion can be drawn at this time regarding potential transmission of hepatitis B virus.

PRECAUTIONS

General

1. Administer within 3 hours after reconstitution. Do not refrigerate after reconstitution.
2. Administer only by the intravenous route.
3. As with any colloid solution, there will be an increase in plasma volume following intravenous administration of Prolastin.[23] Caution should therefore be used in patients at risk for circulatory overload.
4. It is recommended that in preparation for receiving Prolastin, recipients be immunized against hepatitis B using a licensed Hepatitis B Vaccine according to the manufacturer's recommendations. Should it become necessary to treat an individual with Prolastin, and time is insufficient for adequate antibody response to vaccination, individuals should receive a single dose of Hepatitis B Immune Globulin (Human), 0.06 mL/kg body weight, intramuscularly, at the time of administration of the initial dose of Hepatitis B Vaccine.
5. Prolastin should be given alone, without mixing with other agents or diluting solutions.
6. Product administration and handling of the needles must be done with caution. Percutaneous puncture with a needle contaminated with blood can transmit infectious virus including HIV (AIDS) and hepatitis. Obtain immediate medical attention if injury occurs.
   Place needles in sharps container after single use. Discard all equipment including any reconstituted Prolastin product in accordance with biohazard procedures.

Carcinogenesis, Mutagenesis, Impairment of Fertility

Long-term studies in animals to evaluate carcinogenesis, mutagenesis or impairment of fertility have not been conducted.

Pregnancy Category C

Animal reproduction studies have not been conducted with Prolastin. It is also not known whether Prolastin can cause fetal harm when administered to a pregnant woman or can affect reproduction capacity. Prolastin should be given to a pregnant woman only if clearly needed.

Nursing Mothers

It is not known whether Prolastin is excreted in human milk. Because many drugs are excreted in human milk, caution should be exercised when Prolastin is administered to a nursing woman.

Pediatric Use

Safety and effectiveness in the pediatric population have not been established.

ADVERSE REACTIONS

Therapeutic administration of Prolastin, 60 mg/kg weekly, has been demonstrated to be well-tolerated. In clinical studies, six reactions were observed with 517 infusions of Prolastin, or 1.16%. None of the reactions was severe.[18] The adverse reactions reported included delayed fever (maximum temperature rise was 38.9°C, resolving spontaneously over 24 hours) occurring up to 12 hours following treatment (0.77%), light-headedness (0.19%), and dizziness (0.19%).[18] Mild transient leukocytosis and dilutional anemia several hours after infusion have also been noted.[18] Since market entry, occasional reports of other flu-like symptoms, allergic-like reactions, chills, dyspnea, rash, tachycardia, and, rarely, hypotension have also been received.

DOSAGE AND ADMINISTRATION

Each bottle of Prolastin has the functional activity, as determined by inhibition of porcine pancreatic elastase,[1] stated on the label of the bottle.

The "threshold" level of alpha$_1$-PI in the serum believed to provide adequate anti-elastase activity in the lung of individuals with alpha$_1$-antitrypsin deficiency is 80 mg/dL (based on commercial standards for alpha$_1$-PI immunologic assay).[12,15,17] However, assays of alpha$_1$-PI based on commercial standards measure antigenic activity of alpha$_1$-PI, whereas the labeled potency value of alpha$_1$-PI is expressed as actual functional activity, i.e., actual capacity to neutralize porcine pancreatic elastase. As functional activity may be less than antigenic activity, serum levels of alpha$_1$-PI determined using commercial immunologic assays may not accurately reflect actual functional alpha$_1$-PI levels. Therefore, although it may be helpful to monitor serum levels of alpha$_1$-PI in individuals receiving Prolastin®, using currently available commercial assays of antigenic activity, results of these assays should not be used to determine the required therapeutic dosage.

The recommended dosage of Prolastin is 60 mg/kg body weight administered once weekly. This dose is intended to increase and maintain a level of functional alpha$_1$-PI in the epithelial lining of the lower respiratory tract, providing adequate anti-elastase activity in the lung of individuals with alpha$_1$-antitrypsin deficiency.

Prolastin may be given at a rate of 0.08 mL/kg/min or greater and must be administered intravenously. The recommended dosage of 60 mg/kg takes approximately 30 minutes to infuse.

Parenteral drug products should be inspected visually for particulate matter and discoloration prior to administration, whenever solution and container permit.

Reconstitution

1. Warm the unopened diluent and concentrate to room temperature (NMT 37°C, 99°F).
2. After removing the plastic flip-top caps (Fig. A), aseptically cleanse rubber stoppers of both bottles.
3. Remove the protective cover from the plastic transfer needle cartridge with tamper-proof seal and penetrate the stopper of the diluent bottle (Fig. B).
4. Remove the remaining portion of the plastic cartridge. Invert the diluent bottle and penetrate the rubber seal on the concentrate bottle (Fig. C) with the needle at an angle.
   Alternate method of transferring sterile water: With a sterile needle and syringe, withdraw the appropriate volume of diluent and transfer to the bottle of lyophilized concentrate.
5. The vacuum will draw the diluent into the concentrate bottle. For best results, and to avoid foaming, hold the diluent bottle at an angle to the concentrate bottle in order to direct the jet of diluent against the wall of the concentrate bottle (Fig. C).
6. After removing the diluent bottle and transfer needle (Fig. D), gently swirl the concentrate bottle until the powder is completely dissolved (Fig. E).
7. Swab top of reconstituted bottle of Prolastin® again.
8. Attach the sterile filter needle provided to syringe. With filter needle in place, insert syringe into reconstituted bottle of Prolastin and withdraw Prolastin solution into syringe (Fig. F).
9. To administer Prolastin, replace filter needle with appropriate injection needle and follow procedure for I.V. administration.
10. The contents of more than one bottle of Prolastin may be drawn into the same syringe before administration. If more than one bottle of Prolastin is used, withdraw contents from bottles using aseptic technique. Place contents into an administration container (plastic minibag or glass bottle) using a syringe.* Avoid pushing an I.V. administration set spike into the product container stopper as this has been known to force the stopper into the vial, with a resulting loss of sterility.

*For a patient of average weight (about 70 kg), the volume needed will exceed the limit of one syringe.

[See figure at top of next column]

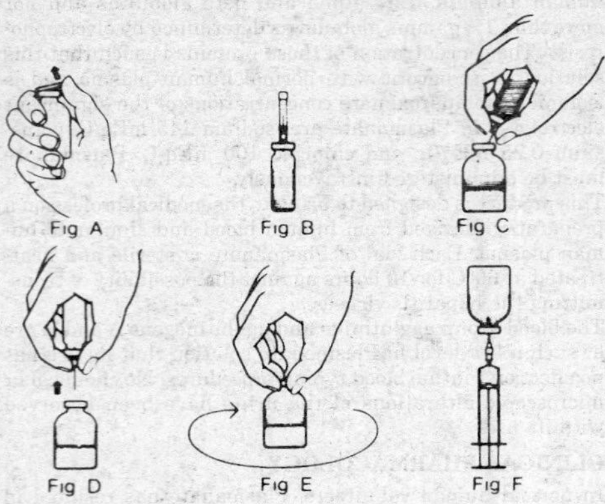

HOW SUPPLIED

Alpha$_1$-Proteinase Inhibitor (Human), Prolastin®, is supplied in the following single use vials with the total alpha$_1$-PI functional activity, in milligrams, stated on the label of each vial. A suitable volume of Sterile Water for Injection, USP, is provided.

NDC Number	Approximate Alpha$_1$-PI Functional Activity	Diluent
0026-0601-30	500 mg	20 mL
0026-0601-35	1000 mg	40 mL

STORAGE

Prolastin should be stored under refrigeration (2°–8°C; 36°–46°F) or at temperatures not to exceed 25°C (77°F). Freezing should be avoided as breakage of the diluent bottle might occur.

CAUTION

U.S. federal law prohibits dispensing without prescription.

LIMITED WARRANTY

A number of factors beyond our control could reduce the efficacy of this product or even result in an ill effect following its use. These include improper storage and handling of the product after it leaves our hands, diagnosis, dosage, method of administration, and biological differences in individual patients. Because of these factors, it is important that this product be stored properly, that the directions be followed carefully during use, and that the risk of transmitting viruses be carefully weighed before the product is prescribed. No warranty, express or implied, including any warranty of merchantability or fitness is made. Representatives of the Company are not authorized to vary the terms or the contents of the printed labeling, including the package insert for this product, except by printed notice from the Company's headquarters. The prescriber and user of this product must accept the terms hereof.

REFERENCES

1. Coan MH, Brockway WJ, Eguizabal H, et al: Preparation and properties of alpha$_1$-proteinase inhibitor concentrate from human plasma. *Vox Sang* 48(6):333–42, 1985.
2. Laurell CB, Eriksson S: The electrophoretic alpha$_1$-globulin pattern of serum in alpha$_1$-antitrypsin deficiency. *Scand J Clin Lab Invest* 15:132–40, 1963.
3. Eriksson S: Pulmonary emphysema and alpha$_1$-antitrypsin deficiency. *Acta Med Scand* 175(2):197–205, 1964.
4. Eriksson S: Studies in alpha$_1$-antitrypsin deficiency. *Acta Med Scand* Suppl 432:1–85, 1965.
5. Kueppers F, Black LF: Alpha$_1$-antitrypsin and its deficiency. *Am Rev Respir Dis* 110(2):176–94, 1974.
6. Morse JO: Alpha$_1$-antitrypsin deficiency. *N Engl J Med* 299:1045–8; 1099–105, 1978.
7. Black LF, Kueppers F: Alpha$_1$-antitrypsin deficiency in nonsmokers. *Am Rev Respir Dis* 117(3):421–8, 1978.
8. Tobin JM, Cook PJ, Hutchison DC: Alpha$_1$-antitrypsin deficiency: the clinical and physiological features of pulmonary emphysema in subjects homozygous for Pi type Z. A survey by the British Thoracic Association. *Br J Dis Chest* 77(1):14–27, 1983.
9. Larsson C. Natural history and life expectancy in severe alpha$_1$-antitrypsin deficiency, Pi Z. *Acta Med Scand* 204(5):345–51, 1978.
10. Pannell R, Johnson D, Travis J: Isolation and properties of human plasma alpha$_1$-proteinase inhibitor. *Biochemistry* 13(26):5439–45, 1974.
11. Lieberman J: Elastase, collagenase, emphysema, and alpha$_1$-antitrypsin deficiency. *Chest* 70(1):62–7, 1976.
12. Gadek JE, Fells GA, Zimmerman RL, et al: Antielastases of the human alveolar structures: implications for the protease-antiprotease theory of emphysema. *J Clin Invest* 68(4):889–98, 1981.
13. Beatty K, Bieth J, Travis J: Kinetics of association of serine proteinases with native and oxidized alpha-1-proteinase inhibitor and alpha-1-antichymotrypsin. *J Biol Chem* 255(9):3931–4, 1980.
14. Janoff A, White R, Carp H, et al: Lung injury induced by leukocytic proteases. *Am J Pathol* 97(1):111–36, 1979.
15. Gadek JE, Crystal RG: Alpha$_1$-antitrypsin deficiency. In: Stanbury JB, Wyngaarden JB, Frederickson DS, et al, eds.: *The Metabolic Basis of Inherited Disease* 5th ed. New York, McGraw-Hill, 1983, p. 1450–67.
16. Larsson C, Dirksen H, Sundstrom G, et al: Lung function studies in asymptomatic individuals with moderately (Pi SZ) and severely (Pi Z) reduced levels of alpha$_1$-antitrypsin. *Scand J Respir Dis* 57(6):267–80, 1976.
17. Gadek JE, Klein HG, Holland PV, et al: Replacement therapy of alpha$_1$-antitrypsin deficiency: reversal of protease-antiprotease imbalance within the alveolar structures of PiZ subjects. *J Clin Invest* 68(5):1158–65, 1981.
18. Data on file, Bayer Corporation.
19. Wewers MD, Casolaro MA, Sellers SE, et al: Replacement therapy for alpha$_1$-antitrypsin deficiency associated with emphysema. *N Engl J Med* 316(17):1055–62, 1987.
20. Wewers MD, Casolaro MA, Crystal RG: Comparison of alpha-1-antitrypsin levels and antineutrophil elastase capacity of blood and lung in a patient with the alpha-

1-antitrypsin phenotype null-null before and during alpha-1-antitrypsin augmentation therapy. *Am Rev Respir Dis* 135(3):539–43, 1987.
21. Burrows B: A clinical trial of efficacy of antiproteolytic therapy: can it be done? *Am Rev Respir Dis* 127(2:2): S42–3, 1983.
22. Cohen AB: Unraveling the mysteries of alpha$_1$-antitrypsin deficiency. *N Engl J Med* 314(12):778–9, 1986.
23. Finlayson JS: Albumin products. *Semin Thromb Hemost* 6(2);85-120, 1980.

Bayer Corporation
Pharmaceutical Division
Elkhart, IN 46515 USA 14-7601-000
U.S. License No. 8 (Rev. April 1998)

ANTITHROMBIN III (HUMAN) ℞
THROMBATE III®

DESCRIPTION

Antithrombin III (Human), THROMBATE III®, is a sterile, nonpyrogenic, stable, lyophilized preparation of purified human antithrombin III.

THROMBATE III is prepared from pooled units of human plasma from normal donors by modifications and refinements of the cold ethanol method of Cohn.[1] When reconstituted with sterile water for injection, USP, THROMBATE III has a pH of 6.0–7.5, a sodium content of 110–210 mEq/L, a chloride content of 110–210 mEq/L, an alanine content of 0.075–0.125 M and a heparin content of not more than 0.004 unit/IU AT-III. THROMBATE III contains no preservative and must be administered by the intravenous route. In addition, THROMBATE III has been heat-treated in solution at 60°C ± 0.5°C for not less than 10 hours.

Each vial of THROMBATE III contains the labeled amount of antithrombin III in international units (IU) per vial. The potency assignment has been determined with a standard calibrated against a World Health Organization (WHO) antithrombin III reference preparation.

CLINICAL PHARMACOLOGY

Antithrombin III (AT-III), an alpha$_2$-glycoprotein of molecular weight 58,000, is normally present in human plasma at a concentration of approximately 12.5 mg/dL[2,3] and is the major plasma inhibitor of thrombin.[4] Inactivation of thrombin by AT-III occurs by formation of a covalent bond resulting in an inactive 1:1 stoichiometric complex between the two, involving an interaction of the active serine of thrombin and an arginine reactive site on AT-III.[4] AT-III is also capable of inactivating other components of the coagulation cascade including factors IXa, Xa, XIa, and XIIa, as well as plasmin.[4]

The neutralization rate of serine proteases by AT-III proceeds slowly in the absence of heparin, but is greatly accelerated in the presence of heparin.[4] As the therapeutic antithrombotic effect in vivo of heparin is mediated by AT-III, heparin is ineffective in the absence or near absence of AT-III.[4–8]

The prevalence of the hereditary deficiency of AT-III is estimated to be one per 2000 to 5000 in the general population.[4,7] The pattern of inheritance is autosomal dominant. In affected individuals, spontaneous episodes of thrombosis and pulmonary embolism may be associated with AT-III levels of 40%–60% of normal.[7] These episodes usually appear after the age of 20, the risk increasing with age and in association with surgery, pregnancy and delivery. The frequency of thromboembolic events in hereditary antithrombin III (AT-III) deficiency during pregnancy has been reported to be 70%, and several studies of the beneficial use of Antithrombin III (Human) concentrates during pregnancy in women with hereditary deficiency have been reported.[9–11] In many cases, however, no precipitating factor can be identified for venous thrombosis or pulmonary embolism.[7] Greater than 85% of individuals with hereditary AT-III deficiency have had at least one thrombotic episode by the age of 50 years.[7] In about 60% of patients thrombosis is recurrent. Clinical signs of pulmonary embolism occur in 40% of affected individuals.[7] In some individuals, treatment with oral anticoagulants leads to an increase of the endogenous levels of AT-III, and treatment with oral anticoagulants may be effective in the prevention of thrombosis in such individuals.[6,7]

In clinical studies of Antithrombin III (Human), THROMBATE III® conducted in 10 asymptomatic subjects with hereditary deficiency of AT-III, the mean in vivo recovery of AT-III was 1.6% per unit per kg administered based on immunologic AT-III assays, and 1.4% per unit per kg administered based on functional AT-III assays.[12] The mean 50% disappearance time (the time to fall to 50% of the peak plasma level following an initial administration) was approximately 22 hours and the biologic half-life was 2.5 days based on immunologic assays and 3.8 days based on functional assays of AT-III.[12] These values are similar to the half-life for radiolabeled Antithrombin III (Human) reported in the literature of 2.8–4.8 days.[13–15]

In clinical studies of THROMBATE III, none of the 13 patients with hereditary AT-III deficiency and histories of thromboembolism treated prophylactically on 16 separate occasions with THROMBATE III for high thrombotic risk situations (11 surgical procedures, 5 deliveries) developed a thrombotic complication. Heparin was also administered in 3 of the 11 surgical procedures and all 5 deliveries. Eight patients with hereditary AT-III deficiency were treated therapeutically with THROMBATE III as well as heparin for major thrombotic or thromboembolic complications, with seven patients recovering. Treatment with THROMBATE III reversed heparin resistance in two patients with hereditary AT-III deficiency being treated for thrombosis or thromboembolism.

During clinical investigation of THROMBATE III, none of 12 subjects monitored for a median of 8 months (range 2–19 months) after receiving THROMBATE III, became antibody positive to human immunodeficiency virus (HIV-1). None of 14 subjects monitored for ≥ 3 months demonstrated any evidence of hepatitis, either non-A, non-B hepatitis or hepatitis B.

INDICATIONS AND USAGE

THROMBATE III is indicated for the treatment of patients with hereditary antithrombin III deficiency in connection with surgical or obstetrical procedures or when they suffer from thromboembolism.

Subjects with AT-III deficiency should be informed about the risk of thrombosis in connection with pregnancy and surgery and about the inheritance of the disease.

The diagnosis of hereditary antithrombin III (AT-III) deficiency should be based on a clear family history of venous thrombosis as well as decreased plasma AT-III levels, and the exclusion of acquired deficiency.

AT-III in plasma may be measured by amidolytic assays using synthetic chromogenic substrates, by clotting assays, or by immunoassays. The latter does not detect all hereditary AT-III deficiencies.[16]

The AT-III level in neonates of parents with hereditary AT-III deficiency should be measured immediately after birth. (Fatal neonatal thromboembolism, such as aortic thrombi in children of women with hereditary antithrombin III deficiency, has been reported.)[17]

Plasma levels of AT-III are lower in neonates than adults, averaging approximately 60% in normal term infants.[18,19] AT-III levels in premature infants may be much lower.[18,19] Low plasma AT-III levels, especially in a premature infant, therefore, do not necessarily indicate hereditary deficiency. It is recommended that testing and treatment with Antithrombin III (Human), THROMBATE III® of neonates be discussed with an expert on coagulation.[11]

CONTRAINDICATIONS

None known.

WARNINGS

THROMBATE III is made from human plasma. Products made from human plasma may contain infectious agents, such as viruses, that can cause disease. The risk that such products will trasmit an infectious agent has been reduced by screening plasma donors for prior exposure to certain viruses, by testing for the presence of certain current virus infections, and by inactivating and/or removing certain viruses. Despite these measures, such products can still potentially transmit disease. There is also the possibility that unknown infectious agents may be present in such products. Individuals who receive infusions of blood or plasma products may develop signs and/or symptoms of some viral infections, particularly hepatitis C. ALL infections thought by a physician possibly to have been transmitted by this product should be reported by the physician or other healthcare provider to Bayer Corporation [1-888-765-3203].

The physician should discuss the risks and benefits of this product with the patient, before prescribing or administering it to a patient.

The anticoagulant effect of heparin is enhanced by concurrent treatment with THROMBATE III in patients with hereditary AT-III deficiency. Thus, in order to avoid bleeding, reduced dosage of heparin is recommended during treatment with THROMBATE III.

PRECAUTIONS

General

1. Administer within 3 hours after reconstitution. Do not refrigerate after reconstitution.
2. Administer only by the intravenous route.
3. THROMBATE III, once reconstituted, should be given alone, without mixing with other agents or diluting solutions.
4. Product administration and handling of the needles must be done with caution. Percutaneous puncture with a needle contaminated with blood can transmit infectious virus including HIV (AIDS) and hepatitis. Obtain immediate medical attention if injury occurs.
   Place needles in sharps container after single use. Discard all equipment including any reconstituted THROMBATE III product in accordance with biohazard procedures.

The diagnosis of hereditary antithrombin III (AT-III) deficiency should be based on a clear family history of venous thrombosis as well as decreased plasma AT-III levels, and the exclusion of acquired deficiency.

Laboratory Tests

It is recommended that AT-III plasma levels be monitored during the treatment period. Functional levels of AT-III in plasma may be measured by amidolytic assays using chromogenic substrates or by clotting assays.

Drug Interactions

The anticoagulant effect of heparin is enhanced by concurrent treatment with THROMBATE III in patients with hereditary AT-III deficiency. Thus, in order to avoid bleeding, reduced dosage of heparin is recommended during treatment with THROMBATE III.

Pregnancy Category B

Reproduction studies have been performed in rats and rabbits at doses up to four times the human dose and have revealed no evidence of impaired fertility or harm to the fetus due to THROMBATE III. It is not known whether THROMBATE III can cause fetal harm when administered to a pregnant woman or can affect reproduction capacity. Because animal reproduction studies are not always predictive of human response, this drug should be used during pregnancy only if clearly needed.

Pediatric Use

Safety and effectiveness in the pediatric population have not been established. The AT-III level in neonates of parents with hereditary AT-III deficiency should be measured immediately after birth. (Fatal neonatal thromboembolism, such as aortic thrombi in children of women with hereditary antithrombin III deficiency, has been reported.)[17]

Plasma levels of AT-III are lower in neonates than adults, averaging approximately 60% in normal term infants.[18,19] AT-III levels in premature infants may be much lower.[18,19] Low plasma AT-III levels, especially in a premature infant, therefore, do not necessarily indicate hereditary deficiency. It is recommended that testing and treatment with Antithrombin III (Human), THROMBATE III® of neonates be discussed with an expert on coagulation.[11]

ADVERSE REACTIONS

In clinical studies involving THROMBATE III, adverse reactions were reported in association with 17 of the 340 infusions during the clinical studies. Included were dizziness (7), chest tightness (3), nausea (3), foul taste in mouth (3), chills (2), cramps (2), shortness of breath (1), chest pain (1), film over eye (1), light-headedness (1), bowel fullness (1), hives (1), fever (1), and oozing and hematoma formation (1). If adverse reactions are experienced, the infusion rate should be decreased, or if indicated, the infusion should be interrupted until symptoms abate.

DOSAGE AND ADMINISTRATION

Each bottle of THROMBATE III has the functional activity, in international units (IU), stated on the label of the bottle. The potency assignment has been determined with a standard calibrated against a World Health Organization antithrombin III reference preparation.

Dosage should be determined on an individual basis based on the pre-therapy plasma antithrombin III (AT-III) level, in order to increase plasma AT-III levels to the level found in normal human plasma (100%). Dosage of THROMBATE III can be calculated from the following formula:

$$\text{units required (IU)} = \frac{[\text{desired - baseline AT-III level*}] \times \text{weight (kg)}}{1.4}$$

*expressed as % normal level based on functional AT-III assay

The above formula is based on an expected incremental in vivo recovery above baseline levels for THROMBATE III of 1.4% per IU per kg administered.[12] Thus, if a 70 kg individual has a baseline AT-III level of 57%, in order to increase plasma AT-III to 120%, the initial THROMBATE III dose would be [(120−57) × 70]/1.4 = 3150 IU total.

However, recovery may vary, and initially levels should be drawn at baseline and 20 minutes postinfusion. Subsequent doses can be calculated based on the recovery of the first dose. These recommendations are intended only as a guide for therapy. The exact loading dose and maintenance intervals should be individualized for each patient.

It is recommended that following an initial dose of THROMBATE III, plasma levels of AT-III be initially monitored at least every 12 hours and before the next infusion of THROMBATE III to maintain plasma AT-III levels greater than 80%. In some situations, e.g., following surgery,[20] hemorrhage or acute thrombosis, and during intravenous heparin administration,[13,21–23] the half-life of Antithrombin III (Human) has been reported to be shortened. In such conditions, plasma AT-III levels should be monitored more frequently, and Antithrombin III (Human), THROMBATE III® administered as necessary.

When an infusion of THROMBATE III is indicated for a patient with hereditary deficiency to control an acute thrombotic episode or prevent thrombosis following surgical or obstetrical procedures, it is desirable to raise the AT-III level to normal and maintain this level for 2 to 8 days, depending on the indication for treatment, type and extent of surgery, patient's medical condition, past history and physician's judgment. Concomitant administration of heparin in each of these situations should be based on the medical judgment of the physician.

As a general recommendation, the following therapeutic program may be utilized as a starting program for treatment, modifying the program based on the actual plasma AT-III levels achieved:

a) An initial loading dose of THROMBATE III calculated to elevate the plasma AT-III level to 120%, assuming an expected rise over the baseline plasma AT-III level of 1.4% (functional activity) per IU per kg of THROMBATE III administered. Thus, if an individual has a baseline AT-III level of 57%, the initial THROMBATE III dose would be (120−57)/1.4 = 45 IU/kg.
b) Measure preinfusion and 20 minutes postinfusion (peak) plasma antithrombin III levels following the initial dose, plasma antithrombin III level after 12 hours, then pre-

Continued on next page

Thrombate III—Cont.

ceding the next infusion (trough level). Subsequently measure antithrombin III levels preceding and 20 minutes after each infusion until predictable peak and trough levels have been achieved, generally between 80%–120%. Plasma levels between 80%–120% may be maintained by administration of maintenance doses of 60% of the initial loading dose, administered every 24 hours. Adjustments in the maintenance dose and/or interval between doses should be made based on actual plasma AT-III levels achieved.

The above recommendations for dosing are provided as a general guideline for therapy only. The exact loading and maintenance dosages and dosing intervals should be individualized for each subject, based on the individual clinical conditions, response to therapy, and actual plasma AT-III levels achieved. In some situations, e.g., following surgery,[20] with hemorrhage or acute thrombosis and during intravenous heparin administration,[13,21–23] in vivo survival of infused THROMBATE III has been reported to be shortened, resulting in the need to administer THROMBATE III more frequently.

THROMBATE III should be reconstituted with Sterile Water for Injection, USP and brought to room temperature prior to administration. THROMBATE III should be filtered through a sterile filter needle as supplied in the package prior to use, and should be administered within 3 hours following reconstitution. THROMBATE III may be infused over 10–20 minutes. THROMBATE III must be administered intravenously.

Parenteral drug products should be inspected visually for particulate matter and discoloration prior to administration, whenever solution and container permit.

Reconstitution

Vacuum Transfer

1. Warm the unopened diluent and the concentrate to room temperature (NMT 37°C, 99°F).
2. After removing the plastic flip-top caps (Fig. A), aseptically cleanse the rubber stoppers of both bottles.
3. Remove the protective cover from the plastic transfer needle cartridge with tamper-proof seal and penetrate the stopper of the diluent bottle (Fig. B).
4. Remove the remaining portion of the plastic cartridge, invert the diluent bottle and penetrate the rubber seal on the concentrate bottle (Fig. C) with the needle at an angle.
   Alternate method of transferring sterile water: With a sterile needle and syringe, withdraw the appropriate volume of diluent and transfer to the bottle of lyophilized concentrate.
5. The vacuum will draw the diluent into the concentrate bottle. Hold the diluent bottle at an angle to the concentrate bottle in order to direct the jet of diluent against the wall of the concentrate bottle (Fig. C). Avoid excessive foaming.
6. After removing the diluent bottle and transfer needle (Fig. D), swirl continuously until completely dissolved (Fig. E).
7. After the concentrate powder is completely dissolved, withdraw solution into the syringe through the filter needle which is supplied in the package (Fig. F). Replace the filter needle with an administration set (not provided) and inject intravenously.
8. If the same patient is to receive more than one bottle, the contents of two bottles may be drawn into the same syringe through a separate unused filter needle before attaching the vein needle.

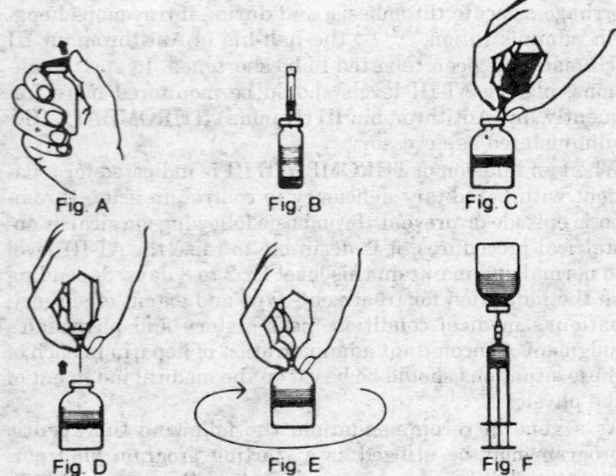

Rate of Administration

The rate of administration should be adapted to the response of the individual patient, but administration of the entire dose in 10 to 20 minutes is generally well-tolerated.

HOW SUPPLIED

Antithrombin III (Human), THROMBATE III® is supplied in the following single use vials with the potency in international units stated on the label of each vial. A suitable volume of Sterile Water for Injection, USP, a sterile double-ended transfer needle, and a sterile filter needle are provided.

NDC Number	Approximate Antithrombin III Potency	Diluent
0026-0603-20	500 IU	10 mL
0026-0603-30	1000 IU	20 mL

STORAGE

Antithrombin III (Human), THROMBATE III® should be stored under refrigeration (2–8°C; 36–46°F). Freezing should be avoided as breakage of the diluent bottle might occur.

CAUTION

U.S. federal law prohibits dispensing without prescription.

LIMITED WARRANTY

A number of factors beyond our control could reduce the efficacy of this product or even result in an ill effect following its use. These include improper storage and handling of the product after it leaves our hands, diagnosis, dosage, method of administration, and biological differences in individual patients. Because of these factors, it is important that this product be stored properly, that the directions be followed carefully during use, and that the risk of transmitting viruses be carefully weighed before the product is prescribed. No warranty, express or implied, including any warranty of merchantability or fitness is made. Representatives of the Company are not authorized to vary the terms or the contents of the printed labeling, including the package insert for this product, except by printed notice from the Company's headquarters. The prescriber and user of this product must accept the terms hereof.

REFERENCES

1. Cohn EJ, Strong LE, Hughes WL Jr, et al: Preparation and properties of serum and plasma proteins. IV. A system for the separation into fractions of the protein and lipoprotein components of biological tissues and fluids. *J Am Chem Soc* 68(3):459–75, 1946.
2. Rosenberg RD, Bauer KA, Marcum JA: Antithrombin III "the heparin-antithrombin system." *Rev Hematol* 2:351–416, 1986.
3. Murano G, Williams L, Miller-Andersson M: Some properties of antithrombin-III and its concentration in human plasma. *Thromb Res* 18(1–2):259–62, 1980.
4. Rosenberg RD: Action and interactions of antithrombin and heparin. *N Engl J Med* 292(3):146–51, 1975.
5. Winter JH, Fenech A, Ridley W, et al: Familial antithrombin III deficiency. *Q J Med* 51(204):373–95, 1982.
6. Marciniak E, Farley CH, DeSimone PA: Familial thrombosis due to antithrombin III deficiency. *Blood* 43(2):219–31, 1974.
7. Thaler E, Lechner K: Antithrombin III deficiency and thromboembolism. *Clin Haematol* 10(2):369–90, 1981.
8. Blauhut B, Necek S, Kramar H, et al: Activity of antithrombin III and effect of heparin on coagulation in shock. *Thromb Res* 19(6):775–82, 1980.
9. Samson D, Stirling Y, Woolf L, et al: Management of planned pregnancy in a patient with congenital antithrombin III deficiency. *Br J Haematol* 56(2):243–9, 1984.
10. Brandt P: Observations during the treatment of antithrombin-III deficient women with heparin and antithrombin concentrate during pregnancy, parturition, and abortion. *Thromb Res* 22(1–2):15–24, 1981.
11. Hellgren M, Tengborn L, Abildgaard U: Pregnancy in women with congenital antithrombin III deficiency; experience of treatment with heparin and antithrombin. *Gynecol Obstet Invest* 14(2):127–41, 1982.
12. Schwartz RS, Bauer KA, Rosenberg RD, et al: Clinical experience with antithrombin III concentrate in treatment of congenital and acquired deficiency of antithrombin. *Am J Med* 87 (Suppl 3B): 53S–60S, 1989.
13. Collen D, Schetz J, de Cock F, et al: Metabolism of antithrombin III (heparin cofactor) in man; effects of venous thrombosis and of heparin administration. *Eur J Clin Invest* 7(1):27–35, 1977.
14. Knot EAR, de Jong E, ten Cate JW, et al: Purified radiolabeled antithrombin III metabolism in three families with hereditary AT III deficiency: application of a three-compartment model. *Blood* 67(1):93–8, 1986.
15. Tengborn L, Frohm B, Nilsson LE, et al: Antithrombin III concentrate; its catabolism in health and in antithrombin III deficiency. *Scand J Clin Lab Invest* 41(5):469–77, 1981.
16. Sas G, Blasko G, Banhegyi D, et al: Abnormal antithrombin III (antithrombin III "Budapest") as a cause of familial thrombophilia. *Thromb Diath Haemorrh* 32(1):105–15, 1974.
17. Bjarke B, Herin P, Blomback M: Neonatal aortic thrombosis. A possible clinical manifestation of congenital antithrombin III deficiency. *Acta Paediatr Scand* 63:297–301, 1974.
18. Hathaway WE, Bonnar J: Perinatal coagulation, New York, Grune & Stratton, 1978, p.68.
19. Peters M, Jansen E, ten Cate JW, et al: Neonatal antithrombin III. *Br J Haematol* 58(4):579–87, 1984.
20. Mannucci PM, Boyer C, Wolf M, et al: Treatment of congenital antithrombin III deficiency with concentrates. *Br J Haematol* 50(3):531–5, 1982.
21. Marciniak E, Gockerman JP: Heparin-induced decrease in circulating antithrombin-III. *Lancet* 2(8038):581–4, 1977.
22. O'Brien JR, Etherington MD: Effect of heparin and warfarin on antithrombin III. *Lancet* 2(8050):1232, 1977.
23. Kakkar VV, Bentley PG, Scully MF, et al: Antithrombin III and heparin. *Lancet* 1(8159):103–4, 1980.

Bayer Corporation
Elkhart, IN 46515 USA 14-7603-006
U.S. License No. 8 (Rev. May 1998)

Beach Pharmaceuticals

Division of Beach Products, Inc.
5220 SOUTH MANHATTAN AVE.
TAMPA, FL 33611

Direct Inquiries to:
Richard Stephen Jenkins
(813) 839-6565
FAX (813) 837-2511

BEELITH Tablets **OTC**
MAGNESIUM SUPPLEMENT
with PYRIDOXINE HCL
Each tablet supplies 362 mg (30 mEq) of magnesium and 25 mg of pyridoxine hydrochloride.

DESCRIPTION

Each tablet contains magnesium oxide 600 mg and pyridoxine hydrochloride (Vitamin B_6) 25 mg equivalent to Vitamin B_6 20 mg. Each tablet yields 362 mg of magnesium and supplies 90% of the Adult U.S. Recommended Daily Allowance (RDA) for magnesium and 1000% of the Adult RDA for Vitamin B_6.

INDICATIONS

As a dietary supplement for patients with magnesium and/or Vitamin B_6 deficiencies resulting from malnutrition, alcoholism, magnesium depleting drugs, chemotherapy, and inadequate nutritional intake or absorption. Also, increases urinary magnesium levels.

DOSAGE

One tablet daily or as directed by a physician.

DRUG INTERACTION PRECAUTION

Do not take this product if you are presently taking a prescription drug without consulting your physician or other health professional.

WARNINGS

If you have kidney disease, take only under the supervision of a physician. Excessive dosage may cause laxation. **KEEP OUT OF THE REACH OF CHILDREN.** As with any drug, if you are pregnant or nursing a baby, seek the advice of a health professional before using this product.

HOW SUPPLIED

Golden yellow, film-coated tablet with the letters **BP** and the number **132** imprinted on each tablet. Packaged in bottles of 100 (NDC 0486-1132-01) tablets.

Shown in Product Identification Guide, page 308

K–PHOS® M.F. ℞
K–PHOS® No.2 ℞

DESCRIPTION

K-PHOS® M.F.: Each tablet contains potassium acid phosphate 155 mg and sodium acid phosphate, anhydrous 350 mg. Each tablet yields approximately 125.6 mg of phosphorus, 44.5 mg of potassium or 1.1 mEq and 67 mg of sodium or 2.9 mEq. **K-PHOS® No.2:** Each tablet contains potassium acid phosphate 305 mg and sodium acid phosphate, anhydrous, 700 mg. Each tablet yields approximately 250 mg of phosphorus, 88 mg of potassium or 2.3 mEq and 134 mg of sodium or 5.8 mEq.

Shown in Product Identification Guide, page 308

K–PHOS® NEUTRAL ℞
Supplies 250 mg of phosphorus per tablet.

DESCRIPTION

Each tablet contains 852 mg dibasic sodium phosphate anhydrous, 155 mg monobasic potassium phosphate, and 130 mg monobasic sodium phosphate monohydrate. Each tablet yields approximately 250 mg of phosphorus, 298 mg of sodium (13.0 mEq) and 45 mg of potassium (1.1 mEq).

CLINICAL PHARMACOLOGY

Phosphorus has a number of important functions in the biochemistry of the body. The bulk of the body's phosphorus is located in the bones, where it plays a key role in osteoblastic and osteoclastic activities. Enzymatically catalyzed phosphate-transfer reactions are numerous and vital in the metabolism of carbohydrate, lipid and protein, and a proper concentration of the anion is of primary importance in assuring an orderly biochemical sequence. In addition, phosphorus plays an important role in modifying steady-state

tissue concentrations of calcium. Phosphate ions are important buffers of the intracellular fluid, and also play a primary role in the renal excretion of hydrogen ion.
Oral administration of inorganic phosphates increases serum phosphate levels. Phosphates lower urinary calcium levels in idiopathic hypercalciuria.
In general, in adults, about two thirds of the ingested phosphate is absorbed from the bowel, most of which is rapidly excreted into the urine.

INDICATIONS AND USAGE

K-PHOS® NEUTRAL increases urinary phosphate and pyrophosphate. As a phosphorus supplement, each tablet supplies 25% of the U.S. Recommended Daily Allowance (U.S. RDA) of phosphorus for adults and children over 4 years of age.

CONTRAINDICATIONS

This product is contraindicated in patients with infected phosphate stones, in patients with severely impaired renal function (less than 30% of normal) and in the presence of hyperphosphatemia.

PRECAUTIONS

General: This product contains potassium and sodium and should be used with caution if regulation of these elements is desired. Occasionally, some individuals may experience a mild laxative effect during the first few days of phosphate therapy. If laxation persists to an unpleasant degree, reduce the daily dosage until this effect subsides or, if necessary, discontinue the use of this product.
Caution should be exercised when prescribing this product in the following conditions: Cardiac disease (particularly in digitalized patients); severe adrenal insufficiency (Addison's disease); acute dehydration; severe renal insufficiency; renal function impairment or chronic renal disease; extensive tissue breakdown (such as severe burns); myotonia congenita; cardiac failure; cirrhosis of the liver or severe hepatic disease; peripheral or pulmonary edema; hypernatremia; hypertension; toxemia of pregnancy; hypoparathyroidism; and acute pancreatitis. Rickets may benefit from phosphate therapy, but caution should be exercised. High serum phosphate levels may increase the incidence of extra-skeletal calcification.
Information for Patients: Patients with kidney stones may pass old stones when phosphate therapy is started and should be warned of this possibility. Patients should be advised to avoid the use of antacids containing aluminum, magnesium, or calcium which may prevent the absorption of phosphate.
Laboratory Tests: Careful monitoring of renal function and serum calcium, phosphorus, potassium, and sodium may be required at periodic intervals during phosphate therapy. Other tests may be warranted in some patients, depending on conditions.
Drug Interactions: The use of antacids containing magnesium, aluminum, or calcium in conjunction with phosphate preparations may bind the phosphate and prevent its absorption. Concurrent use of antihypertensives, especially diazoxide, guanethidine, hydralazine, methyldopa, or rauwolfia alkaloid; or corticosteroids, especially mineralocorticoids or corticotropin, with sodium phosphate may result in hypernatremia. Calcium-containing preparations and/or Vitamin D may antagonize the effects of phosphates in the treatment of hypercalcemia. Potassium-containing medications or potassium-sparing diuretics may cause hyperkalemia. Patients should have serum potassium level determinations at periodic intervals.
Carcinogenesis, Mutagenesis, Impairment of Fertility: No long term or reproduction studies in animals or humans have been performed with **K-PHOS® NEUTRAL** to evaluate its carcinogenic, mutagenic, or impairment of fertility potential.
Pregnancy: Teratogenic Effects: Pregnancy Category C. Animal reproduction studies have not been conducted with **K-PHOS® NEUTRAL**. It is also not known whether this product can cause fetal harm when administered to a pregnant woman or can affect reproductive capacity. This product should be given to a pregnant woman only if clearly needed.
Nursing Mothers: It is not known whether this drug is excreted in human milk. Because many drugs are excreted in human milk, caution should be exercised when this product is administered to a nursing woman.
Pediatric Use: See **DOSAGE AND ADMINISTRATION**.

ADVERSE REACTIONS

Gastrointestinal upset (diarrhea, nausea, stomach pain, and vomiting) may occur with phosphate therapy. Also, bone and joint pain (possible phosphate-induced osteomalacia) could occur. The following adverse effects may be observed (primarily from sodium or potassium): headaches; dizziness; mental confusion; seizures; weakness or heaviness of legs; unusual tiredness or weakness; muscle cramps; numbness, tingling, pain, or weakness of hands or feet; numbness or tingling around lips; fast or irregular heartbeat; shortness of breath or troubled breathing; swelling of feet or lower legs; unusual weight gain; low urine output; unusual thirst.

DOSAGE AND ADMINISTRATION

K-PHOS® NEUTRAL tablets should be taken with a full glass of water, with meals and at bedtime. Adults: One or two tablets four times daily; Pediatric Patients over 4 years of age: One tablet four times daily. For Pediatric Patients under 4 years of age, use only as directed by a physician.

HOW SUPPLIED

White, film-coated, capsule-shaped tablet with the name **BEACH** and number **1125** imprinted on each tablet. Bottles of 100 (NDC 0486-1125-01) and 500 (NDC 0486-1125-05) tablets.
Rx ONLY
Shown in Product Identification Guide, page 308

K–PHOS® ORIGINAL (Sodium Free) ℞
(Potassium Acid Phosphate)
Urinary Acidifier
Supplies 114 mg of phosphorus per tablet.

DESCRIPTION

Each tablet contains potassium acid phosphate 500 mg. Each tablet yields approximately 114 mg of phosphorus and 144 mg of potassium or 3.7 mEq.

ACTIONS

K-PHOS® ORIGINAL (Sodium Free) is a highly effective urinary acidifier.

INDICATIONS AND USAGE

For use in patients with elevated urinary pH. Helps keep calcium soluble and reduces odor and rash caused by ammoniacal urine. Also, by acidifying the urine, it increases the antibacterial activity of methenamine mandelate and methenamine hippurate.

CONTRAINDICATIONS

This product is contraindicated in patients with infected phosphate stones; in patients with severely impaired renal function (less than 30% of normal) and in the presence of hyperphosphatemia and hyperkalemia.

PRECAUTIONS

General: This product contains potassium and should be used with caution if regulation of this element is desired. Occasionally, some individuals may experience a mild laxative effect during the first few days of phosphate therapy. If laxation persists to an unpleasant degree, reduce the daily dosage until this effect subsides or, if necessary, discontinue the use of this product.
Caution should be exercised when prescribing this product in the following conditions: Cardiac disease (particularly in digitalized patients); severe adrenal insufficiency (Addison's disease); acute dehydration; severe renal insufficiency or chronic renal disease; extensive tissue breakdown (such as severe burns); myotonia congenita; hypoparathyroidism; and acute pancreatitis. Rickets may benefit from phosphate therapy, but caution should be exercised. High serum phosphate levels may increase the incidence of extraskeletal calcification.
Information for Patients: Patients with kidney stones may pass old stones when phosphate therapy is started and should be warned of this possibility. Patients should be advised to avoid the use of antacids containing aluminum, calcium, or magnesium which may prevent the absorption of phosphate. To assure against gastrointestinal injury associated with oral ingestion of concentrated potassium salt preparations, patients should be instructed to dissolve tablets completely in an appropriate amount of water before taking.
Laboratory Tests: Careful monitoring of renal function and serum electrolytes (calcium, phosphorus, potassium) may be required at periodic intervals during potassium phosphate therapy. Other tests may be warranted in some patients, depending on conditions.
Drug Interactions: The use of antacids containing magnesium, calcium, or aluminum in conjunction with phosphate preparations may bind the phosphate and prevent its absorption. Potassium-containing medications or potassium-sparing diuretics may cause hyperkalemia when used concurrently with potassium salts. Patients should have serum potassium level determinations at periodic intervals. Concurrent use of salicylates may lead to increased serum salicylate levels since excretion of salicylates is reduced in acidified urine. Serum salicylate levels should be closely monitored to avoid toxicity.
Carcinogenesis, Mutagenesis, Impairment of Fertility: There have been no studies in animals or humans to evaluate the carcinogenesis, mutagenesis, or impairment of fertility for this product.
Pregnancy: Pregnancy Category C. Animal reproduction studies have not been conducted with this product. It is also not known whether this product can cause fetal harm when administered to a pregnant woman or can affect reproductive capacity. This product should be given to a pregnant woman only if clearly needed.
Nursing Mothers: It is not known whether this drug is excreted in human milk. Because many drugs are excreted in human milk, caution should be exercised when this product is administered to a nursing woman.

ADVERSE REACTIONS

Gastrointestinal upset (diarrhea, nausea, stomach pain, and vomiting) may occur with the use of potassium phosphate. Also, bone and joint pain (possible phosphate-induced osteomalacia) could occur. The following adverse effects may be observed with potassium administration: irregular heartbeat; dizziness; mental confusion; weakness or heaviness of legs; unusual tiredness; muscle cramps; numbness, tingling, pain, or weakness in hands or feet; numbness or tingling around lips; shortness of breath or troubled breathing.

DOSAGE AND ADMINISTRATION

Two tablets dissolved in 6–8 oz. of water 4 times daily with meals and at bedtime. For best results, let the tablets soak in water for 2 to 5 minutes, or more if necessary, and stir. If any tablet particles remain undissolved, they may be crushed and stirred vigorously to speed dissolution.

HOW SUPPLIED

White scored tablet with the name **BEACH** and the number **1111** imprinted on each tablet. Bottles of 100 (NDC 0486-1111-01) and bottles of 500 (NDC 0486-1111-05) tablets.
Rx ONLY
Shown in Product Identification Guide, page 308

UROQID-Acid® No.2 Tablets ℞

DESCRIPTION

Each **UROQID-Acid® No.2** tablet contains methenamine mandelate 500 mg and sodium acid phosphate, monohydrate 500 mg.

CLINICAL PHARMACOLOGY

Methenamine mandelate is rapidly absorbed and excreted in the urine. Formaldehyde is released by acid hydrolysis from methenamine with bactericidal levels rapidly reached at pH 5.0–5.5. Proportionally less formaldehyde is released as urinary pH approaches 6.0 and insufficient quantities are released above this level for therapeutic response. In acid urine, mandelic acid exerts its antibacterial action and also contributes to the acidification of the urine. Mandelic acid is excreted by both glomerular filtration and tubular excretion. In acid urine, there is equally effective antibacterial activity against both gram-positive and gram-negative organisms, since the antibacterial action of mandelic acid and formaldehyde is nonspecific. With Proteus vulgaris and urea splitting strains of Pseudomonas and Aerobacter, results may be discouraging and particular attention is required in monitoring urinary pH and overall management.

INDICATIONS AND USAGE

For the suppression or elimination of bacteriuria associated with chronic and recurrent infections of the urinary tract, including pyelitis, pyelonephritis, cystitis, and infected residual urine accompanying neurogenic bladder. When used as recommended, **UROQID-Acid® No.2** is particularly suitable for long-term therapy because of its relative safety and because resistance to the nonspecific bactericidal action of formaldehyde does not develop. Pathogens resistant to other antibacterial agents may respond because of the nonspecific effect of formaldehyde formed in an acid urine.
Prophylactic Use Rationale: Urine is a good culture medium for many urinary pathogens. Inoculation by a few organisms (relapse or reinfection) may lead to bacteriuria in susceptible individuals. Thus, the rationale of management in recurring urinary tract infection (bacteriuria) is to change the urine from a growth-supporting to a growth-inhibiting medium. There is a growing body of evidence that long-term administration of methenamine can prevent recurrence of bacteriuria in patients with chronic pyelonephritis.
Therapeutic Use Rationale: Helps to sterilize the urine and, in some situations in which underlying pathologic conditions prevent sterilization by any means, can help to suppress bacteriuria. As part of the overall management of the urinary tract infection, a thorough diagnostic evaluation should accompany the use of this product.

CONTRAINDICATIONS

UROQID-Acid® No.2 is contraindicated in patients with renal insufficiency, severe hepatic disease, severe dehydration, hyperphosphatemia, and in patients who have exhibited hypersensitivity to any components of this product.

PRECAUTIONS

General
This product should not be used as the sole therapeutic agent in acute parenchymal infections causing systemic symptoms such as chills and fever.
UROQID-Acid® No.2 contains approximately 83 mg of sodium per tablet and should be used with caution in patients on a sodium-restricted diet.
Sodium phosphates should be used with caution in the following conditions: cardiac failure; peripheral or pulmonary edema; hypernatremia; hypertension; toxemia of pregnancy; hypoparathyroidism; and acute pancreatitis. High serum phosphate levels increase the incidence of extraskeletal calcification.
Large doses of methenamine (8 grams daily for 3 to 4 weeks) have caused bladder irritation, painful and frequent micturition, albuminuria and gross hematuria. Dysuria may occur, although usually at higher than recommended doses, and can be controlled by reducing the dosage. This product contains a urinary acidifier and can cause metabolic acidosis.
Care should be taken to maintain an acidic urinary pH (below 5.5), especially when treating infections due to urea-splitting organisms such as Proteus and strains of Pseudomonas.
Drugs and/or foods which produce an alkaline urine should be restricted. Frequent urine pH tests are essential. If acidification of the urine is contraindicated or unattainable, use of this product should be discontinued.

Continued on next page

Uroqid-Acid—Cont.

Information For Patients: To assure an acidic pH, patients should be instructed to restrict or avoid most fruits, milk and milk products, and antacids containing sodium carbonate or bicarbonate.
Laboratory Tests: As with all urinary tract infections, the efficacy of therapy should be monitored by repeated urine cultures. During long-term therapy, careful monitoring of renal function, serum phosphorus and sodium may be required at periodic intervals.
Drug Interactions: Formaldehyde and sulfamethizole form an insoluble precipitate in acid urine and increase the risk of crystalluria; therefore, these products should not be used concurrently. Thiazide diuretics, carbonic anhydrase inhibitors, antacids, or urinary alkalinizing agents should not be used concurrently since they may cause the urine to become alkaline and reduce the effectiveness of methenamine by inhibiting its conversion to formaldehyde. Concurrent use of antihypertensives, especially diazoxide, guanethidine, hydralazine, methyldopa, or rauwolfia alkaloids; or corticosteroids, especially mineralocorticoids or corticotropin, with sodium phosphates may result in hypernatremia. Concurrent use of salicylates may lead to increased serum salicylate levels since excretion of salicylates is reduced in acidified urine. Serum salicylate levels should be closely monitored to avoid toxicity.
Laboratory Test Interactions: Formaldehyde interferes with fluorometric procedures for determination of urinary catecholamines and vanilmandelic acid (VMA) causing erroneously high results. Formaldehyde also causes falsely decreased urine estriol levels by reacting with estriol when acid hydrolysis techniques are used; estriol determinations which use enzymatic hydrolysis are unaffected by formaldehyde. Formaldehyde causes falsely elevated 17-hydroxycorticosteroid levels when the Porter-Silber method is used and falsely decreased 5-hydroxyindoleacetic acid (5HIAA) levels by inhibiting color development when nitrosonaphthol methods are used.
Carcinogenesis, Mutagenesis, Impairment Of Fertility: Long-term animal studies to evaluate the carcinogenic, mutagenic, or impairment of fertility potential of this product have not been performed.
Pregnancy: Teratogenic Effects. Pregnancy Category C. Animal reproduction studies have not been conducted with **UROQID-Acid® No.2**. It is also not known whether this product can cause fetal harm when administered to a pregnant woman or can affect reproductive capacity. Since methenamine is known to cross the placental barrier, this product should be given to a pregnant woman only if clearly needed.
Nursing Mothers: Methenamine is excreted in breast milk. Caution should be exercised when this product is administered to a nursing woman.

ADVERSE REACTIONS

Gastrointestinal disturbances (nausea, stomach upset), generalized skin rash, dysuria, painful or difficult urination may occur occasionally with the use of methenamine preparations. Microscopic and rarely, gross hematuria have also been reported.
Gastrointestinal upset (diarrhea, nausea, stomach pain, and vomiting) may occur with the use of sodium phosphates. Also, bone or joint pain (possible phosphate induced osteomalacia) could occur. The following adverse effects may be observed (primarily from sodium): headaches; dizziness; mental confusion; seizures; weakness or heaviness of legs; unusual tiredness or weakness; muscle cramps; numbness, tingling, pain, or weakness of hands or feet; numbness or tingling around lips; fast or irregular heartbeat; shortness of breath or troubled breathing; swelling of feet or lower legs; unusual weight gain; low urine output, unusual thirst.

DOSAGE AND ADMINISTRATION

UROQID-Acid® No.2: *Adults:* Initially, 2 tablets 4 times daily with a full glass of water. For maintenance, 2 to 4 tablets daily, in divided doses with a full glass of water.

HOW SUPPLIED

UROQID-Acid® No.2 is a yellow, film-coated, capsule-shaped tablet with the name **BEACH** and the number **1114** imprinted on each tablet. Packaged in bottles of 100 tablets (NDC 0486-1114-01).
Rx ONLY
Shown in Product Identification Guide, page 308

For information on over-the-counter drugs, consult **PDR For Nonprescription Drugs**.

Bedford Laboratories

**A Division of Ben Venue Laboratories, Inc.
300 NORTHFIELD ROAD
BEDFORD, OH 44146**

Direct Inquiries to:
Customer Service: (800) 562-4797
FAX: (440) 232-6264
Professional Services: (800) 521-5169

CERUBIDINE® ℞

[sy-rew″bĭ ′dēan]
**(Daunorubicin HCl)
FOR INJECTION
Rx ONLY.**

WARNING

1. Cerubidine must be given into a rapidly flowing intravenous infusion. It must *never* be given by the intramuscular or subcutaneous route. Severe local tissue necrosis will occur if there is extravasation during administration.
2. Myocardial toxicity manifested in its most severe form by potentially fatal congestive heart failure may occur either during therapy or months to years after termination of therapy. The incidence of myocardial toxicity increases after a total cumulative dose exceeding 400 to 550 mg/m^2 in adults, 300 mg/m^2 in children more than 2 years of age, or 10 mg/kg in children less than 2 years of age.
3. Severe myelosuppression occurs when used in therapeutic doses; this may lead to infection or hemorrhage.
4. It is recommended that Cerubidine be administered only by physicians who are experienced in leukemia chemotherapy and in facilities with laboratory and supportive resources adequate to monitor drug tolerance and protect and maintain a patient compromised by drug toxicity. The physician and institution must be capable of responding rapidly and completely to severe hemorrhagic conditions and/or overwhelming infection.
5. Dosage should be reduced in patients with impaired hepatic or renal function.

DESCRIPTION

Cerubidine (daunorubicin hydrochloride) is the hydrochloride salt of an anthracycline cytotoxic antibiotic produced by a strain of *Streptomyces coeruleorubidus*. It is provided as a sterile reddish lyophilized powder in vials for intravenous administration only. Each vial contains 21.4 mg daunorubicin hydrochloride, (equivalent to 20 mg of daunorubicin), and 100 mg mannitol. It is soluble in water when adequately agitated and produces a reddish solution. It has the following structural formula which may be described with the chemical name of (1*S*,3*S*)-3-Acetyl-1,2,3,4,6,11-hexahydro-3,5,12-trihydroxy-10-methoxy-6,11-dioxo-1-naphthacenyl 3-amino-2,3,6-trideoxy-α-L-*lyxo* -hexopyranoside hydrochloride. Its molecular formula is $C_{27}H_{29}NO_{10}$ •HCl with a molecular weight of 563.99. It is a hygroscopic crystalline powder. The pH of a 5 mg/mL aqueous solution is 4.5 to 6.5. The structural formula is as follows.

CLINICAL PHARMACOLOGY

Mechanism of Action: Cerubidine has antimitotic and cytotoxic activity through a number of proposed mechanisms of action. Cerubidine forms complexes with DNA by intercalation between base pairs. It inhibits topoisomerase II activity by stabilizing the DNA-topoisomerase II complex, preventing the religation portion of the ligation-religation reaction that topoisomerase II catalyzes. Single strand and double strand DNA breaks result.
Cerubidine may also inhibit polymerase activity, affect regulation of gene expression, and produce free radical damage to DNA.
Cerubidine possesses an antitumor effect against a wide spectrum of animal tumors, either grafted or spontaneous.
Pharmacokinetics
General: Following intravenous injection of Cerubidine, plasma levels of daunorubicin decline rapidly, indicating rapid tissue uptake and concentration. Thereafter, plasma levels decline slowly with a half-life of 45 minutes in the initial phase and 18.5 hours in the terminal phase. By 1 hour after drug administration, the predominant plasma species is daunorubicinol, and active metabolite, which disappears with a half-life of 26.7 hours.
Distribution: Cerubidine is rapidly and widely distributed in tissues, with highest levels in the spleen, kidneys, liver, lungs, and heart. The drug binds to many cellular components, particularly nucleic acids. There is no evidence that Cerubidine crosses the blood-brain barrier, but the drug apparently crosses the placenta.
Metabolism and Elimination: Cerubidine is extensively metabolized in the liver and other tissues, mainly by cytoplasmic aldo-keto reductases, producing daunorubicinol, the major metabolite which has antineoplastic activity. Approximately 40% of the drug in the plasma is present as daunorubicinol within 30 minutes and 60% in 4 hours after a dose of daunorubicin. Further metabolism via reduction cleavage of the glycosidic bond, 4-O demethylation, and conjugation with both sulfate and glucuronide have been demonstrated. Simple glycosidic cleavage of daunorubicin or daunorubicinol is not a significant metabolic pathway in man. Twenty-five percent of an administered dose of Cerubidine is eliminated in an active form by urinary excretion and an estimated 40% by biliary excretion.
Special Populations
Pediatric Patients: Although appropriate studies with Cerubidine have not been performed in the pediatric population, cardiotoxicity may be more frequent and occur at lower cumulative doses in children.
Geriatric Patients: Although appropriate studies with Cerubidine have not been performed in the geriatric population, cardiotoxicity may be more frequent in the elderly. Caution should also be used in patients who have inadequate bone marrow reserves due to old age. In addition, elderly patients are more likely to have age-related renal function impairment, which may require reduction of dosage in patients receiving Cerubidine.
Renal and Hepatic Impairment: Doses of Cerubidine should be reduced in patients with hepatic and renal impairment. Patients with serum bilirubin concentrations of 1.2 to 3 mg/dL should receive 75% of the usual daily dose and patients with serum bilirubin concentrations greater than 3 mg/dL should receive 50% of the usual daily dose. Patients with serum creatinine concentrations of greater than 3 mg/dL should receive 50% of the usual daily dose. (See **WARNINGS, Evaluation of Hepatic and Renal Function**).
Clinical Studies: In the treatment of adult acute nonlymphocytic leukemia, Cerubidine, used as a single agent, has produced complete remission rates of 40 to 50%, and in combination with cytarabine, has produced complete remission rates of 53 to 65%.
The addition of Cerubidine to the two-drug induction regimen of vincristine-prednisone in the treatment of childhood acute lymphocytic leukemia does not increase the rate of complete remission. In children receiving identical CNS prophylaxis and maintenance therapy (without consolidation), there is prolongation of complete remission duration (statistically significant, $p < 0.02$) in those children induced with the three drug (Cerubidine-vincristine-prednisone) regimen as compared to two drugs. There is no evidence of any impact of Cerubidine on the duration of complete remission when a consolidation (intensification) phase is employed as part of a total treatment program.
In adult acute lymphocytic leukemia, in contrast to childhood acute lymphocytic leukemia, Cerubidine during induction significantly increases the rate of complete remission, but not remission duration, compared to that obtained with vincristine, prednisone, and L-asparaginase alone. The use of Cerubidine in combination with vincristine, prednisone, and L-asparaginase has produced complete remission rates of 83% in contrast to a 47% remission in patients not receiving Cerubidine.

INDICATIONS AND USAGE

Cerubidine in combination with other approved anticancer drugs is indicated for remission induction in acute nonlymphocytic leukemia (myelogenous, monocytic, erythroid) of adults and for remission induction in acute lymphocytic leukemia of children and adults.

CONTRAINDICATIONS

Cerubidine is contraindicated in patients who have shown a hypersensitivity to it.

WARNINGS

Bone Marrow: Cerubidine is a potent bone marrow suppressant. Suppression will occur in all patients given a therapeutic dose of this drug. Therapy with Cerubidine should not be started in patients with pre-existing drug-induced bone marrow suppression unless the benefit from such treatment warrants the risk. Persistent, severe myelosuppression may result in superinfection or hemorrhage.
Cardiac Effects: Special attention must be given to the potential cardiac toxicity of Cerubidine, particularly in infants and children. Pre-existing heart disease and previous therapy with doxorubicin are co-factors of increased risk of Cerubidine-induced cardiac toxicity and the benefit-to-risk ratio of Cerubidine therapy in such patients should be weighed before starting Cerubidine. In adults, at total cumulative doses less than 550 mg/m^2, acute congestive heart failure is seldom encountered. However, rare instances of pericarditis-myocarditis, not dose-related, have been reported.
In adults, at cumulative doses exceeding 550 mg/m^2, there is an increased incidence of drug-induced congestive heart failure. Based on prior clinical experience with doxorubicin, this limit appears lower, namely 400 mg/m^2, in patients who received radiation therapy that encompassed the heart.
In infants and children, there appears to be a greater susceptibility to anthracycline-induced cardiotoxicity compared

to that in adults, which is more clearly dose-related. Anthracycline therapy (including daunorubicin) in pediatric patients has been reported to produce impaired left ventricular systolic performance, reduced contractility, congestive heart failure or death. These conditions may occur months to years following cessation of chemotherapy. This appears to be dose-dependent and aggravated by thoracic irradiation. Long-term periodic evaluation of cardiac function in such patients should, thus, be performed. In both children and adults, the total dose of Cerubidine administered should also take into account any previous or concomitant therapy with other potentially cardiotoxic agents or related compounds such as doxorubicin.

There is no absolutely reliable method of predicting the patients in whom acute congestive heart failure will develop as a result of the cardiac toxic effect of Cerubidine. However, certain changes in the electrocardiogram and a decrease in the systolic ejection fraction from pre-treatment baseline may help to recognize those patients at greatest risk to develop congestive heart failure. On the basis of the electrocardiogram, a decrease equal to or greater than 30% in limb lead QRS voltage has been associated with a significant risk of drug-induced cardiomyopathy. Therefore, an electrocardiogram and/or determination of systolic ejection fraction should be performed before each course of Cerubidine. In the event that one or the other of these predictive parameters should occur, the benefit of continued therapy must be weighed against the risk of producing cardiac damage.

Early clinical diagnosis of drug-induced congestive heart failure appears to be essential for successful treatment.

Evaluation of Hepatic and Renal Function: Significant hepatic or renal impairment can enhance the toxicity of the recommended doses of Cerubidine; therefore, prior to administration, evaluation of hepatic function and renal function using conventional clinical laboratory tests is recommended (See **DOSAGE AND ADMINISTRATION** section).

Pregnancy: Cerubidine may cause fetal harm when administered to a pregnant woman. An increased incidence of fetal abnormalities (parieto-occipital cranioschisis, umbilical hernias, or rachischisis) and abortions was reported in rabbits at doses of 0.05 mg/kg/day or approximately 1/100th of the highest recommended human dose on a body surface area basis. Rats showed an increased incidence of esophageal, cardiovascular and urogenital abnormalities as well as rib fusions at doses of 4 mg/kg/day or approximately 1/2 the human dose on a body surface area basis. Decreases in fetal birth weight and post-delivery growth rate were observed in mice. There are no adequate and well-controlled studies in pregnant women. If this drug is used during pregnancy, or if the patient becomes pregnant while taking this drug, the patient should be apprised of the potential hazard to the fetus. Women of childbearing potential should be advised to avoid becoming pregnant.

Secondary leukemias: There have been reports of secondary leukemias in patients exposed to topoisomerase II inhibitors when used in combination with other antineoplastic agents or radiation therapy.

Extravasation at Injection Site: Extravasation of Cerubidine at the site of intravenous administration can cause severe local tissue necrosis. (See **ADVERSE REACTIONS** section.)

PRECAUTIONS

General: Therapy with Cerubidine requires close patient observation and frequent complete blood-count determinations. Cardiac, renal, and hepatic function should be evaluated prior to each course of treatment.

Appropriate measures must be taken to control any systemic infection before beginning therapy with Cerubidine.

Cerubidine may transiently impart a red coloration to the urine after administration, and patients should be advised to expect this.

Laboratory Tests: Cerubidine may induce hyperuricemia secondary to rapid lysis of leukemic cells. As a precaution, allopurinol administration is usually begun prior to initiating antileukemic therapy. Blood uric acid levels should be monitored and appropriate therapy initiated in the event that hyperuricemia develops.

Carcinogenesis, Mutagenesis, Impairment of Fertility: Cerubidine, when injected subcutaneously into mice, causes fibrosarcomas to develop at the injection site. When administered to mice thrice weekly intraperitoneally, no carcinogenic effect was noted after 18 months of observation. In male rats administered Cerubidine thrice weekly for 6 months, at 1/70th the recommended human dose on a body surface area basis, peritoneal sarcomas were found at 18 months. A single IV dose of Cerubidine administered to rats at 1.6 fold the recommended human dose on a body surface area basis caused mammary adenocarcinomas to appear at 1 year. Cerubidine was mutagenic *in vitro* (Ames assay, V79 hamster cell assay), and clastogenic *in vitro* (CCRFCEM human lymphoblasts) and in vivo (SCE assay in mouse bone marrow) tests.

In male dogs at a daily dose of 0.25 mg/kg administered intravenously, testicular atrophy was noted at autopsy. Histologic examination revealed total aplasia of the spermatocyte series in the seminiferous tubules with complete aspermatogenesis.

Pregnancy: Teratogenic Effects — Pregnancy Category D (See **WARNINGS** section.)

Nursing Mothers: It is not known whether this drug is excreted in human milk. Because many drugs are excreted in human milk and because of the potential for serious adverse reactions in nursing infants from Cerubidine, mothers should be advised to discontinue nursing during Cerubidine therapy.

Elderly: See **CLINICAL PHARMACOLOGY, Special Populations, Geriatric Patients** section.

Pediatric Use: See **CLINICAL PHARMACOLOGY, Special Populations, Pediatric Patients** section and **WARNINGS, Cardiac Effects** section.

Drug Interactions: Use of Cerubidine in a patient who has previously received doxorubicin increases the risk of cardiotoxicity. Cerubidine should not be used in patients who have previously received the recommended maximum cumulative doses of doxorubicin or Cerubidine. Cyclophosphamide used concurrently with Cerubidine may also result in increased cardiotoxicity.

Dosage reduction of Cerubidine may be required when used concurrently with other myelosuppressive agents.

Hepatotoxic medications, such as high-dose methotrexate, may impair liver function and increase the risk of toxicity.

ADVERSE REACTIONS

Dose-limiting toxicity includes myelosuppression and cardiotoxicity (See **WARNINGS** section). Other reactions include:

Cutaneous: Reversible alopecia occurs in most patients. Rash, contact dermatitis and urticaria have occurred rarely.

Gastrointestinal: Acute nausea and vomiting occur but are usually mild. Antiemetic therapy may be of some help. Mucositis may occur 3 to 7 days after administration. Diarrhea and abdominal pain have occasionally been reported.

Local: If extravasation occurs during administration, severe local tissue necrosis, severe cellulitis, thrombophlebitis, or painful induration can result.

Acute Reactions: Rarely, anaphylactoid reaction, fever, and chills can occur. Hyperuricemia may occur, especially in patients with leukemia, and serum uric acid levels should be monitored.

DOSAGE AND ADMINISTRATION

Parenteral drug products should be inspected visually for particulate matter prior to administration, whenever solution and container permit.

Principles: In order to eradicate the leukemic cells and induce a complete remission, a profound suppression of the bone marrow is usually required. Evaluation of both the peripheral blood and bone marrow is mandatory in the formulation of appropriate treatment plans.

It is recommended that the dosage of Cerubidine be reduced in instances of hepatic or renal impairment. For example, using serum bilirubin and serum creatinine as indicators of liver and kidney function, the following dose modifications are recommended:

Serum Bilirubin	Serum Creatinine	Dose Reduction
1.2 to 3.0 mg%		25%
>3 mg%		50%
	>3 mg%	50%

Representative Dose Schedules and Combination for the Approved Indication of Remission Induction in Adult Acute Nonlymphocytic Leukemia:

In Combination: For patients under age 60, Cerubidine 45 mg/m^2/day IV on days 1, 2, and 3 of the first course and on days 1, 2 of subsequent courses AND cytosine arabinoside 100 mg/m^2/day IV infusion daily for 7 days for the first course and for 5 days for subsequent courses.

For patients 60 years of age and above, Cerubidine 30 mg/m^2/day IV on days 1, 2, and 3 of the first course and on days 1, 2 of subsequent courses AND cytosine arabinoside 100 mg/m^2/day IV infusion daily for 7 days for the first course and for 5 days for subsequent courses. This Cerubidine dose-reduction is based on a single study and may not be appropriate if optimal supportive care is available.

The attainment of a normal-appearing bone marrow may require up to three courses of induction therapy. Evaluation of the bone marrow following recovery from the previous course of induction therapy determines whether a further course of induction treatment is required.

Representative Dose Schedule and Combination for the Approved Indication of Remission Induction in Pediatric Acute Lymphocytic Leukemia:

In Combination: Cerubidine 25 mg/m^2 IV on day 1 every week, vincristine 1.5 mg/m^2 IV on day 1 every week, prednisone 40 mg/m^2 PO daily. Generally, a complete remission will be obtained within four such courses of therapy; however, if after four courses the patient is in partial remission, an additional one or, if necessary, two courses may be given in an effort to obtain a complete remission.

In children less than 2 years of age or below 0.5 m^2 body surface area, it has been recommended that the Cerubidine dosage calculation should be based on weight (1 mg/kg) instead of body surface area.

Representative Dose Schedules and Combination for the Approved Indication of Remission Induction in Adult Acute Lymphocytic Leukemia:

In Combination: Cerubidine 45 mg/m^2/day IV on days 1, 2, and 3 AND vincristine 2 mg IV on days 1, 8, and 15; prednisone 40 mg/m^2/day PO on days 1 through 22, then tapered between days 22 to 29; L-asparaginase 500 IU/kg/day x 10 days IV on days 22 through 32.

The contents of a vial should be reconstituted with 4 mL of Sterile Water for Injection and agitated gently until the material has completely dissolved. The sterile vial contents provide 20 mg of daunorubicin, with 5 mg of daunorubicin per mL. The desired dose is withdrawn into a syringe containing 10 mL to 15 mL of 0.9% Sodium Chloride Injection, USP and then injected into the tubing or sidearm in a rapidly flowing IV infusion of 5% Dextrose Injection, USP or 0.9% Sodium Chloride Injection, USP. Cerubidine should not be administered mixed with other drugs or heparin.

Storage and Handling: Store unreconstituted powder at controlled room temperature, 15° to 30° C (59° to 86° F). The reconstituted solution is stable for 24 hours at room temperature and 48 hours under refrigeration. It should be protected from exposure to sunlight. **Protect from light.** Retain in carton until time of use.

If Cerubidine contacts the skin or mucosae, the area should be washed thoroughly with soap and water. Procedures for proper handling and disposal of anticancer drugs should be considered. Several guidelines on this subject have been published.[1–7] There is no general agreement that all of the procedures recommended in the guidelines are necessary or appropriate.

HOW SUPPLIED

Cerubine (daunorubicin HCl) for Injection, is available in butyl-rubber-stoppered vials, each containing 21.4 mg Daunorubicin hydrochloride equivalent to 20 mg of daunorubicin and 100 mg of mannitol, as a sterile reddish lyophilized powder. When reconstituted with 4 mL of Sterile Water for Injection, USP, each mL contains 5 mg daunorubicin activity.

NDC 55390-281-10 20 mg, single dose vials; carton of 10.

REFERENCES

1. Recommendations for the Safe Handling of Parenteral Antineoplastic Drugs. NIH Publication No. 83-2621. For sale by the Superintendent of Documents, U.S. Government Printing Office, Washington, D.C. 20402.
2. AMA Council Report. Guidelines for Handling Parenteral Antineoplastics. *JAMA*, March 15, 1985.
3. National Study Commission on Cytotoxic Exposure Recommendations for Handling Cytotoxic Agents. Available from Louis R Jeffrey, Sc.D., Chairman, National Study Commission on Cytotoxic Exposure, Massachusetts College of Pharmacy and Allied Health Sciences, 179 Longwood Avenue, Boston, Massachusetts 02115.
4. Clinical Oncological Society of Australia: Guidelines and recommendations for safe handling of antineoplastic agents. *Med J Australia* 1:426–428, 1983.
5. Jones RB, et al: Safe handling of chemotherapeutic agents: A report from the Mount Sinai Medical Center, Ca *A Cancer Journal for Clinicians* Sept/Oct, 258–263, 1983.
6. American Society of Hospital Pharmacists technical assistance bulletin on handling cytotoxic and hazardous drugs. *Am J Hosp Pharm* 47:1033–1049, 1990.
7. OSHA Work Practice Guidelines for Personnel Dealing with Cyotoxic (Antineoplastic) Drugs. *Am J Hosp Pharm* 43:1193–1204, 1986.

Manufactured by:
Ben Venue Laboratories, Inc.
Bedford, OH 44146
Manufactured for:
Bedford Laboratories
Bedford, OH 44146
April 1999 CRD-P02

GLUCAGEN® ℞

[glōō 'ka-gĭn]

[Glucagon (rDNA origin) for injection]

Rx ONLY

DESCRIPTION

GlucaGen® [glucagon (rDNA origin) for injection] manufactured by Novo Nordisk A/S is produced by expression of recombinant DNA in a saccharomyces cerevisiae vector with subsequent purification.

The chemical structure of the glucagon in GlucaGen® is identical to naturally occurring human glucagon and to glucagon extracted from beef and pork pancreas. Glucagon with the empirical formula of $C_{153}H_{225}N_{43}O_{49}S$, and a molecular weight of 3483, is a single-chain polypeptide containing 29 amino acid residues. The structure of glucagon is:

His-Ser-Gln-Gly-Thr-Phe-Thr-Ser-Asp-Tyr-Ser-
1 2 3 4 5 6 7 8 9 10 11

Lys-Tyr-Leu-Asp-Ser-Arg-Arg-Ala-Gln-Asp-Phe-
12 13 14 15 16 17 18 19 20 21 22

Val-Gln-Trp-Leu-Met-Asn-Thr
23 24 25 26 27 28 29

GlucaGen® 1 mg (1 IU) is supplied as a sterile, lyophilized white powder in a 2 ml vial, accompanied by Sterile Water for Reconstitution (1 ml) also in a 2 ml vial. Glucagon, as supplied at pH 2.5–3.5, is soluble in water.

Active Ingredient in each vial

Glucagon as hydrochloride 1 mg (corresponding to 1 IU).

Other Ingredients

Lactose monohydrate (107 mg)

When the glucagon powder is reconstituted with Sterile Water for Reconstitution, it forms a solution of 1 mg (1 IU)/ml glucagon for subcutaneous (sc), intramuscular (im), or intravenous (iv) injection.

GlucaGen® is an antihypoglycemic agent, and a gastrointestinal motility inhibitor.

Continued on next page

Glucagen—Cont.

CLINICAL PHARMACOLOGY

Intramuscular (IM) injection of GlucaGen® resulted in a mean C_{max} (CV%) of 1686 pg/ml (43%) and a median T_{max} of 12.5 minutes. The mean apparent half-life of 45 minutes after IM injection probably reflects prolonged absorption from the injection site. Glucagon is degraded in the liver, kidney, and plasma.[1]

Antihypoglycemic Action: Glucagon induces liver glycogen breakdown, releasing glucose from the liver. Blood glucose concentration rises within 10 minutes of injection and maximal concentrations are attained at approximately a half hour after injection (see Figure). Hepatic stores of glycogen are necessary for glucagon to produce an antihypoglycemic effect.

Recovery from insulin induced hypoglycemia (mean blood glucose) after i.m. injection of 1 mg GlucaGen® in Type I diabetic men

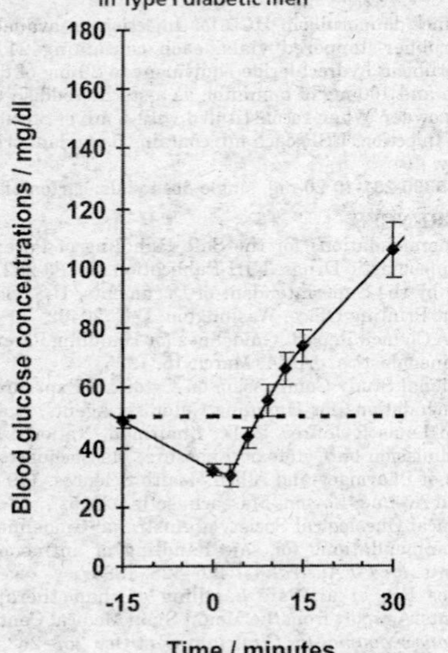

Gastrointestinal Motility Inhibition: Extra hepatic effects of glucagon include relaxation of the smooth muscle of the stomach, duodenum, small bowel, and colon.

INDICATIONS AND USAGE

For the treatment of hypoglycemia: GlucaGen® is used to treat severe hypoglycemic (low blood sugar) reactions which may occur in patients with diabetes treated with insulin.

Because GlucaGen® depletes glycogen stores, the patient should be given supplemental carbohydrates as soon as he/she awakens and is able to swallow, especially children or adolescents.

Medical evaluation is recommended for all patients who experience severe hypoglycemia.

For use as a diagnostic aid: GlucaGen® is indicated for use during radiologic examinations to temporarily inhibit movement of the gastrointestinal tract. Glucagon is as effective for this examination as are the anticholinergic drugs. However, the addition of the anticholinergic agent may result in increased side effects.

CONTRAINDICATIONS

Glucagon is contraindicated in patients with known hypersensitivity to glucagon or any constituent in GlucaGen® and in patients with pheochromocytoma or with insulinoma.

WARNINGS

GlucaGen® should be administered cautiously to patients suspected of having pheochromocytoma of insulinoma. Secondary hypoglycemia may occur and should be countered by adequate carbohydrate intake following glucagon treatment.

Glucagon may release catecholamines from pheochromocytomas and is contraindicated in patients with this condition. Allergic reactions may occur and include generalized rash, and in rare cases anaphylactic shock with breathing difficulties, and hypotension. The anaphylactic reactions have generally occurred in association with endoscopic examination during which patients often received other agents including contrast media and local anesthetics. The patients should be given standard treatment for anaphylaxis including an injection of epinephrine if they encounter respiratory difficulties after GlucaGen® injection.

PRECAUTIONS

General—In order for GlucaGen® treatment to reverse hypoglycemia, adequate amounts of glucose must be stored in the liver (as glycogen). Therefore, GlucaGen® should be used with caution in patients with conditions such as prolonged fasting, starvation, adrenal insufficiency or chronic hypoglycemia because these conditions result in low levels of releasable glucose in the liver and an inadequate reversal of hypoglycemia by GlucaGen® treatment. Caution should be observed when glucagon is used in diabetic patients or in elderly patients with known cardiac disease to inhibit gastrointestinal motility.

Information for Patients—Refer patients and family members to the Information for Patients for instructions describing the method of preparing and injecting GlucaGen®. Advise the patient and family members to become familiar with the technique of preparing glucagon before an emergency arises. Instruct patients to use 1 mg for adults or ½ the adult dose (0.5 mg) for children weighing less than 55 lb (25 kg). To prevent severe hypoglycemia, patients and family members should be informed of the symptoms of mild hypoglycemia and how to treat it appropriately. Family members should be informed to arouse the patient as quickly as possible because prolonged hypoglycemia may result in damage to the central nervous system. Patients should be advised to inform their physician when hypoglycemic reactions occur so that the treatment regimen may be adjusted if necessary.

Laboratory Tests—Blood glucose measurements may be considered to monitor the patient's response.

Carcinogenesis, Mutagenesis, Impairment of Fertility—Long term studies in animals to evaluate carcinogenic potential have not been performed. Several studies have been conducted to evaluate the mutagenic potential of glucagon. The mutagenic potential tested in the Ames and human lymphocyte assays, was borderline positive under certain conditions for both glucagon (pancreatic) and glucagon (rDNA) origin. *In vivo*, very high doses (100 and 200 mg/kg) of glucagon (both origins) gave a slightly higher incidence of micronucleus formation in male mice but there was no effect in females. The weight of evidence indicates that GlucaGen® is not different from glucagon pancreatic origin and does not pose a genotoxic risk to humans.

GlucaGen® was not tested in animal fertility studies. Studies in rats have shown that pancreatic glucagon does not cause impaired fertility.[1]

Pregnancy—Pregnancy Category B—Reproduction studies were performed in rats and rabbits at GlucaGen® doses of 0.4, 2.0, and 10 mg/kg. These doses represent exposures of up to 100 and 200 times the human dose based on mg/m^2 for rats and rabbits, respectively, and revealed no evidence of harm to the fetus. There are, however, no adequate and well-controlled studies in pregnant women. Because animal reproduction studies are not always predictive of human response, this drug should be used during pregnancy only if clearly needed.

Nursing Mothers—It is not known whether this drug is excreted in human milk. Because many drugs are excreted in human milk, caution should be exercised when GlucaGen® is administered to a nursing woman.

No clinical studies have been performed in nursing mothers, however, GlucaGen® is a peptide and intact glucagon is not absorbed from the GI tract. Therefore, even if the infant ingested glucagon it would be unlikely to have any effect on the infant. Additionally, GlucaGen® has a short plasma half life thus limiting amounts available to the child.

Pediatric Use—For the treatment of hypoglycemia: The use of glucagon in pediatric patients has been reported to be safe and effective.[2,3,4,5]

For use as a diagnostic aid: Safety and effectiveness in pediatric patients have not been established.

ADVERSE REACTIONS

Severe side effects are very rare, although nausea and vomiting may occur occasionally especially with doses above 1 mg or with rapid injection (less than 1 minute).[1] Glucagon exerts positive inotropic and chronotropic effects (tachycardia). Adverse reactions indicating toxicity of GlucaGen® have not been reported. A transient increase in both blood pressure and pulse rate may occur following the administration of glucagon. Patients taking β-blockers might be expected to have a greater increase in both pulse and blood pressure, an increase of which will be transient because of glucagon's short half-life. The increase in blood pressure and pulse rate may require therapy in patients with pheochromocytoma or coronary artery disease. (see OVERDOSAGE).

Allergic reactions may occur in rare cases (See WARNINGS).

OVERDOSAGE

Signs and Symptoms—No reports of overdosage with GlucaGen® have been reported. It is expected, if overdosage occurred, that the patient may experience nausea, vomiting, inhibition of GI tract motility, increase in blood pressure and pulse rate.[1] In case of suspected overdosing, the serum potassium may decrease and should be monitored and corrected if needed.

The IV and SC LD_{50} for GlucaGen® in rats and mice ranges from 100 to greater than 200 mg/kg body weight.

Treatment—Standard symptomatic treatment may be undertaken if overdosage occurs. If the patient develops a dramatic increase in blood pressure, 5 to 10 mg of phentolamine mesylate has been shown to be effective in lowering blood pressure for the short time that control would be needed. It is unknown whether GlucaGen® is dialyzable, but such a procedure is unlikely to provide any benefit given the short half-life and nature of the symptoms of overdose.

DOSAGE AND ADMINISTRATION

GlucaGen® should be reconstituted with the supplied 1 ml of Sterile Water for Reconstitution.

Draw up all of the Sterile Water for Reconstitution with syringe and inject into the GlucaGen® vial. Roll the vial gently until powder is completely dissolved and no particles remain in the fluid. The reconstituted fluid should be clear and of water-like consistency. The reconstituted GlucaGen® gives a concentration of approximately 1 mg/ml Glucagon. The reconstituted GlucaGen® should be used immediately after reconstitution. Discard any unused portion.

For the treatment of hypoglycemia: For adults and for pediatric patients weighing 55 lb (25 kg) or more, administer 1 mg by subcutaneous, intramuscular, or intravenous injection.[1,6] According to the literature, ½ adult dose (0.5 mg) is recommended for pediatric patients weighing less than 55 lb (25 kg) or younger than 6–8 years old.[2,3,4,5,6] Emergency assistance should be sought if the patient fails to respond within 15 minutes after subcutaneous or intramuscular injection of glucagon. The glucagon injection may be repeated while waiting for emergency assistance.[1] Intravenous glucose MUST be administered if the patient fails to respond to glucagon. When the patient has responded to the treatment, give oral carbohydrate to restore the liver glycogen and prevent recurrence of hypoglycemia.

Directions for Use as a Diagnostic Aid: Reconstitute as indicated above. Discard any unused portion.

Time of maximal glucose concentration
Intravenous: 5 to 20 minutes
Intramuscular: 30 minutes
Subcutaneous: 30 to 45 minutes

Time for GI smooth muscle relaxation[1]
Intravenous: 0.25 to 2 mg (IU)—45 seconds.
Intramuscular:
1 mg (IU)—8 to 10 minutes
2 mg (IU)—4 to 7 minutes

Duration of action—
Hyperglycemic action—60 to 90 minutes
Smooth muscle relaxation—[1]
Intravenous:
0.25 to 0.5 mg (IU)—9 to 17 minutes
2 mg (IU)—22 to 25 minutes
Intramuscular:
1 mg (IU)—12 to 27 minutes
2 mg (IU)—21 to 32 minutes

Stability and storage

Before Reconstitution: The GlucaGen® package should be kept refrigerated between 2° and 8°C (36° and 46°F) until the expiration date. Avoid freezing and protect from light. The GlucaGen® package may be stored up to 12 months at room temperature 20° to 25°C (68° to 77°F) prior to reconstitution. GlucaGen® should not be used after the expiry date on the vials.

After Reconstitution: Reconstituted GlucaGen® should be used immediately. Discard any unused portion. If the solution shows any sign of gel formation or particles, it should be discarded.

HOW SUPPLIED

GlucaGen® Diagnostic Kit includes:
1 vial containing 1 mg (1 IU) GlucaGen® [glucagon (rDNA origin) for injection]
1 vial containing 1 ml Sterile Water for Reconstitution
NDC 55390-004-01
Edition Date: July 1999

REFERENCES

1. *Drug Information for the Health Care Professional*. 17th ed. Rockville, Maryland: The United States Pharmacopeial Convention, Inc; 1997; Vol. 1, IA:1516–1518.
2. Gibbs et al: Use of Glucagon to terminate insulin reactions in diabetic children. *Nebr Med J* 1958;43:56–57.
3. Carson MJ, Koch R, Clinical studies with glucagon in children. *J Pediatr* 1955;47:161–170.
4. Shipp JC, et al: Treatment of insulin hypoglycemia in diabetic campers. *Diabetes* 1964; 13:645–648.
5. Aman J, Wranne L: Hypoglycemia in childhood diabetes II: Effect of subcutaneous or intramuscular injection of different doses of glucagon. Acta Pediatr Scand 1988;77: 548–553.
6. Aynsley-Green AS, Eyre JA, and Soltesz G, Hypoglycaemia in diabetic children. In: Frier BM and Fisher BM, eds Hypoglycaemia and Diabetes, Edward Arnold, 1993; 237–238.

Bedford Laboratories™
Bedford, OH 44146

NOTICE
Before prescribing or administering any product described in PHYSICIANS' DESK REFERENCE check the **PDR Supplements** for revised information.

Berlex Laboratories
300 FAIRFIELD ROAD
WAYNE, NJ 07470

Direct Inquiries to:
(973) 694-4100

For Medical Information and to report drug adverse events Contact:
Department of Epidemiology and Medical Affairs
300 Fairfield Road
Wayne, NJ 07470
(888) BERLEX-4

BETAPACE® ℞
[bā ′-tăh-pāce″]
(sotalol HCl)

DESCRIPTION
BETAPACE® (sotalol hydrochloride), is an antiarrhythmic drug with Class II (beta-adrenoreceptor blocking) and Class III (cardiac action potential duration prolongation) properties. It is supplied as a light-blue, capsule-shaped tablet for oral administration. Sotalol hydrochloride is a white, crystalline solid with a molecular weight of 308.8. It is hydrophilic, soluble in water, propylene glycol and ethanol, but is only slightly soluble in chloroform. Chemically, sotalol hydrochloride is d,l-N-[4-[l-hydroxy-2-[(l-methyl ethyl)amino] ethyl]phenyl]methane-sulfonamide monohydrochloride. The molecular formula is $C_{12}H_{20}N_2O_3S{\cdot}HCl$ and is represented by the following structural formula:

CH_3SO_2NH—⟨benzene ring⟩—$CH(OH){-}CH_2NHCH(CH_3)_2{\bullet}HCl$

BETAPACE® Tablets contain the following inactive ingredients: microcrystalline cellulose, lactose, starch, stearic acid, magnesium stearate, colloidal silicon dioxide, and FD&C blue color #2 (aluminum lake, conc.).

CLINICAL PHARMACOLOGY
Mechanism of Action: BETAPACE® (sotalol hydrochloride) has both beta-adrenoreceptor blocking (Vaughan Williams Class II) and cardiac action potential duration prolongation (Vaughan Williams Class III) antiarrhythmic properties. BETAPACE® (sotalol hydrochloride) is a racemic mixture of d- and l-sotalol. Both isomers have similar Class III antiarrhythmic effects, while the l-isomer is responsible for virtually all of the beta-blocking activity. The beta-blocking effect of sotalol is non-cardioselective, half maximal at about 80 mg/day and maximal at doses between 320 and 640 mg/day. Sotalol does not have partial agonist or membrane stabilizing activity. Although significant beta-blockade occurs at oral doses as low as 25 mg, Class III effects are seen only at daily doses of 160 mg and above.

Electrophysiology: Sotalol hydrochloride prolongs the plateau phase of the cardiac action potential in the isolated myocyte, as well as in isolated tissue preparations of ventricular or atrial muscle (Class III activity). In intact animals it slows heart rate, decreases AV nodal conduction and increases the refractory periods of atrial and ventricular muscle and conduction tissue.

In man, the Class II (beta-blockade) electrophysiological effects of BETAPACE® are manifested by increased sinus cycle length (slowed heart rate), decreased AV nodal conduction and increased AV nodal refractoriness. The Class III electrophysiological effects in man include prolongation of the atrial and ventricular monophasic action potentials, and effective refractory period prolongation of atrial muscle, ventricular muscle, and atrio-ventricular accessory pathways (where present) in both the anterograde and retrograde directions. With oral doses of 160 to 640 mg/day, the surface ECG shows dose-related mean increases of 40–100 msec in QT and 10–40 msec in QT_c. (See **WARNINGS** for description of relationship between QT_c and torsade de pointes type arrhythmias). No significant alteration in QRS interval is observed.

In a small study (n=25) of patients with implanted defibrillators treated concurrently with BETAPACE®, the average defibrillatory threshold was 6 joules (range 2–15 joules) compared to a mean of 16 joules for a non-randomized comparative group primarily receiving amiodarone.

Hemodynamics: In a study of systemic hemodynamic function measured invasively in 12 patients with a mean LV ejection fraction of 37% and ventricular tachycardia (9 sustained and 3 non-sustained), a median dose of 160 mg twice daily of BETAPACE® produced a 28% reduction in heart rate and a 24% decrease in cardiac index at 2 hours post dosing at steady-state. Concurrently, systemic vascular resistance and stroke volume showed non-significant increases of 25% and 8%, respectively. Pulmonary capillary wedge pressure increased significantly from 6.4 mmHg to 11.8 mmHg in the 11 patients who completed the study. One patient was discontinued because of worsening congestive heart failure. Mean arterial pressure, mean pulmonary artery pressure and stroke work index did not significantly change. Exercise and isoproterenol induced tachycardia are antagonized by BETAPACE®, and total peripheral resistance increases by a small amount.

In hypertensive patients, BETAPACE® (sotalol hydrochloride) produces significant reductions in both systolic and diastolic blood pressures. Although BETAPACE® (sotalol hydrochloride) is usually well-tolerated hemodynamically, caution should be exercised in patients with marginal cardiac compensation as deterioration in cardiac performance may occur. (See **WARNINGS: Congestive Heart Failure**.)

Clinical Actions: BETAPACE® (sotalol hydrochloride) has been studied in life-threatening and less severe arrhythmias. In patients with frequent premature ventricular complexes (VPC), BETAPACE® (sotalol hydrochloride) was significantly superior to placebo in reducing VPCs, paired VPCs and non-sustained ventricular tachycardia (NSVT); the response was dose-related through 640 mg/day with 80–85% of patients having at least a 75% reduction of VPCs. BETAPACE® (sotalol hydrochloride) was also superior, at the doses evaluated, to propranolol (40–80 mg TID) and similar to quinidine (200–400 mg QID) in reducing VPCs. In patients with life-threatening arrhythmias [sustained ventricular tachycardia/fibrillation (VT/VF)], BETAPACE® (sotalol hydrochloride) was studied acutely [by suppression of programmed electrical stimulation (PES) induced VT and by suppression of Holter monitor evidence of sustained VT] and, in acute responders, chronically.

In a double-blind, randomized comparison of BETAPACE® and procainamide given intravenously (total of 2 mg/kg BETAPACE® vs. 19 mg/kg of procainamide over 90 minutes), BETAPACE® suppressed PES induction in 30% of patients vs. 20% for procainamide (p=0.2).

In a randomized clinical trial [Electrophysiologic Study Versus Electrocardiographic Monitoring (ESVEM) Trial] comparing choice of antiarrhythmic therapy by PES suppression vs. Holter monitor selection (in each case followed by treadmill exercise testing) in patients with a history of sustained VT/VF who were also inducible by PES, the effectiveness acutely and chronically of BETAPACE® (sotalol hydrochloride) was compared with 6 other drugs (procainamide, quinidine, mexiletine, propafenone, imipramine and pirmenol). Overall response, limited to first randomized drug, was 39% for sotalol and 30% for the pooled other drugs. Acute response rate for first drug randomized using suppression of PES induction was 36% for BETAPACE® vs. a mean of 13% for the other drugs. Using the Holter monitoring endpoint (complete suppression of sustained VT, 90% suppression of NSVT, 80% suppression of VPC pairs, and at least 70% suppression of VPCs), BETAPACE® yielded 41% response vs. 45% for the other drugs combined. Among responders placed on long-term therapy identified acutely as effective (by either PES or Holter), BETAPACE®, when compared to the pool of other drugs, had the lowest two-year mortality (13% vs. 22%), the lowest two-year VT recurrence rate (30% vs. 60%), and the lowest withdrawal rate (38% vs. about 75–80%). The most commonly used doses of BETAPACE® (sotalol hydrochloride) in this trial were 320–480 mg/day (66% of patients), with 16% receiving 240 mg/day or less and 18% receiving 640 mg or more.

It cannot be determined, however, in the absence of a controlled comparison of BETAPACE® vs. no pharmacologic treatment (e.g., in patients with implanted defibrillators) whether BETAPACE® response causes improved survival or identifies a population with a good prognosis.

In a large double-blind, placebo controlled secondary prevention (post-infarction) trial (n=1,456), BETAPACE® (sotalol hydrochloride) was given as a non-titrated initial dose of 320 mg once daily. BETAPACE® did not produce a significant increase in survival (7.3% mortality on BETAPACE® vs 8.9% on placebo, p=0.3), but overall did not suggest an adverse effect on survival. There was, however, a suggestion of an early (i.e., first 10 days) excess mortality (3% on sotalol vs. 2% on placebo). In a second small trial (n=17 randomized to sotalol) where sotalol was administered at high doses (e.g., 320 mg twice daily) to high-risk post-infarction patients (ejection fraction <40% and either >10 VPC/hr or VT on Holter), there were 4 fatalities and 3 serious hemodynamic/electrical adverse events within two weeks of initiating sotalol.

Pharmacokinetics: In healthy subjects, the oral bioavailability of BETAPACE® (sotalol hydrochloride) is 90–100%. After oral administration, peak plasma concentrations are reached in 2.5 to 4 hours, and steady-state plasma concentrations are attained within 2–3 days (i.e., after 5–6 doses when administered twice daily). Over the dosage range 160–640 mg/day BETAPACE® (sotalol hydrochloride) displays dose proportionality with respect to plasma concentrations. Distribution occurs to a central (plasma) and to a peripheral compartment, with a mean elimination half-life of 12 hours. Dosing every 12 hours results in trough plasma concentrations which are approximately one-half of those at peak.

BETAPACE® (sotalol hydrochloride) does not bind to plasma proteins and is not metabolized. BETAPACE® (sotalol hydrochloride) shows very little intersubject variability in plasma levels. The pharmacokinetics of the d and l enantiomers of sotalol are essentially identical. BETAPACE® (sotalol hydrochloride) crosses the blood brain barrier poorly. Excretion is predominantly via the kidney in the unchanged form, and therefore lower doses are necessary in conditions of renal impairment (see **DOSAGE AND ADMINISTRATION**). Age per se does not significantly alter the pharmacokinetics of BETAPACE®, but impaired renal function in geriatric patients can increase the terminal elimination half-life, resulting in increased drug accumulation. The absorption of BETAPACE® (sotalol hydrochloride) was reduced by approximately 20% compared to fasting when it was administered with a standard meal. Since BETAPACE® (sotalol hydrochloride) is not subject to first-pass metabolism, patients with hepatic impairment show no alteration in clearance of BETAPACE®.

INDICATIONS AND USAGE
Oral BETAPACE® (sotalol hydrochloride) is indicated for the treatment of documented ventricular arrhythmias, such as sustained ventricular tachycardia, that in the judgment of the physician are life-threatening. Because of the proarrhythmic effects of BETAPACE® (See **WARNINGS**), including a 1.5 to 2% rate of torsade de pointes or new VT/VF in patients with either NSVT or supraventricular arrhythmias, its use in patients with less severe arrhythmias, even if the patients are symptomatic, is generally not recommended. Treatment of patients with asymptomatic ventricular premature contractions should be avoided.

Initiation of BETAPACE® treatment or increasing doses, as with other antiarrhythmic agents used to treat life-threatening arrhythmias, should be carried out in the hospital. The response to treatment should then be evaluated by a suitable method (e.g., PES or Holter monitoring) prior to continuing the patient on chronic therapy. Various approaches have been used to determine the response to antiarrhythmic therapy, including BETAPACE®.

In the ESVEM Trial, response by Holter monitoring was tentatively defined as 100% suppression of ventricular tachycardia, 90% suppression of non-sustained VT, 80% suppression of paired VPCs, and 75% suppression of total VPCs in patients who had at least 10 VPCs/hour at baseline; this tentative response was confirmed if VT lasting 5 or more beats was not observed during treadmill exercise testing using a standard Bruce protocol. The PES protocol utilized a maximum of three extrastimuli at three pacing cycle lengths and two right ventricular pacing sites. Response by PES was defined as prevention of induction of the following: 1) monomorphic VT lasting over 15 seconds; 2) non-sustained polymorphic VT containing more than 15 beats of monomorphic VT in patients with a history of monomorphic VT; 3) polymorphic VT or VF greater than 15 beats in patients with VF or a history of aborted sudden death without monomorphic VT; and 4) two episodes of polymorphic VT or VF of greater than 15 beats in a patient presenting with monomorphic VT. Sustained VT or NSVT producing hypotension during the final treadmill test was considered a drug failure.

In a multicenter open-label long-term study of BETAPACE® in patients with life-threatening ventricular arrhythmias which had proven refractory to other antiarrhythmic medications, response by Holter monitoring was defined as in ESVEM. Response by PES was defined as non-inducibility of sustained VT by at least double extrastimuli delivered at a pacing cycle length of 400 msec. Overall survival and arrythmia recurrence rates in this study were similar to those seen in ESVEM, although there was no comparative group to allow a definitive assessment of outcome.

Antiarrhythmic drugs have not been shown to enhance survival in patients with ventricular arrhythmias.

CONTRAINDICATIONS
BETAPACE® (sotalol hydrochloride) is contraindicated in patients with bronchial asthma, sinus bradycardia, second and third degree AV block, unless a functioning pacemaker is present, congenital or acquired long QT syndromes, cardiogenic shock, uncontrolled congestive heart failure, and previous evidence of hypersensitivity to BETAPACE®.

WARNINGS
Mortality: The National Heart, Lung, and Blood Institute's Cardiac Arrhythmia Suppression Trial I (CAST I) was a long-term, multi-center, double-blind study in patients with asymptomatic, non-life-threatening ventricular arrhythmias, 1 to 103 weeks after acute myocardial infarction. Patients in CAST I were randomized to receive placebo or individually optimized doses of encainide, flecainide, or moricizine. The Cardiac Arrhythmia Suppression Trial II (CAST II) was similar, except that the recruited patients had had their index infarction 4 to 90 days before randomization, patients with left ventricular ejection fractions greater than 40% were not admitted, and the randomized regimens were limited to placebo and moricizine.

CAST I was discontinued after an average time-on-treatment of 10 months, and CAST II was discontinued after an average time-on-treatment of 18 months. As compared to placebo treatment, all three active therapies were associated with increases in short-term (14-day) mortality, and encainide and flecainide were associated with significant increases in longer-term mortality as well. The longer-term mortality rate associated with moricizine treatment could not be statistically distinguished from that associated with placebo.

Continued on next page

Information on the Berlex products appearing here is based on the most current information available at the time of publication closing. Further information for these and other products may be obtained from the Medical Affairs Department, Berlex Laboratories, 300 Fairfield Road, Wayne, New Jersey 07470, 1-888-BERLEX-4. Information on Betaseron and Fludara may be obtained from Berlex Laboratories, 15049 San Pablo Avenue, Richmond, California 94804-0016, 1-800-888-4112.

Betapace—Cont.

The applicability of these results to other populations (e.g., those without recent myocardial infarction) and to other than Class I antiarrhythmic agents is uncertain. BETAPACE® (sotalol hydrochloride) is devoid of Class I effects, and in a large (n=1,456) controlled trial in patients with a recent myocardial infarction, who did not necessarily have ventricular arrhythmias, BETAPACE® did not produce increased mortality at doses up to 320 mg/day (see **Clinical Actions**). On the other hand, in the large post-infarction study using a non-titrated initial dose of 320 mg once daily and in a second small randomized trial in high-risk post-infarction patients treated with high doses (320 mg BID), there have been suggestions of an excess of early sudden deaths.

Proarrhythmia: Like other antiarrhythmic agents, BETAPACE® can provoke new or worsened ventricular arrhythmias in some patients, including sustained ventricular tachycardia or ventricular fibrillation, with potentially fatal consequences. Because of its effect on cardiac repolarization (QT_c interval prolongation), torsade de pointes, a polymorphic ventricular tachycardia with prolongation of the QT interval and a shifting electrical axis is the most common form of proarrhythmia associated with BETAPACE®, occurring in about 4% of high risk (history of sustained VT/VF) patients. The risk of torsade de pointes progressively increases with prolongation of the QT interval, and is worsened also by reduction in heart rate and reduction in serum potassium (See **Electrolyte Disturbances.**)

Because of the variable temporal recurrence of arrhythmias, it is not always possible to distinguish between a new or aggravated arrhythmic event and the patient's underlying rhythm disorder. (Note, however, that torsade de pointes is usually a drug-induced arrhythmia in people with an initially normal QT_c.) Thus, the incidence of drug-related events cannot be precisely determined, so that the occurrence rates provided must be considered approximations. Note also that drug-induced arrhythmias may often not be identified, particularly if they occur long after starting the drug, due to less frequent monitoring. It is clear from the NIH-sponsored CAST (see **WARNINGS: Mortality**) that some antiarrhythmic drugs can cause increased sudden death mortality, presumably due to new arrhythmias or asystole, that do not appear early in treatment but that represent a sustained increased risk.

Overall in clinical trials with sotalol, 4.3% of 3257 patients experienced a new or worsened ventricular arrhythmia. Of this 4.3%, there was new or worsened sustained ventricular tachycardia in approximately 1% of patients and torsade de pointes in 2.4%. Additionally, in approximately 1% of patients, deaths were considered possibly drug-related; such cases, although difficult to evaluate, may have been associated with proarrhythmic events. **In patients with a history of sustained ventricular tachycardia, the incidence of torsade de pointes was 4% and worsened VT in about 1%; in patients with other, less serious, ventricular arrhythmias and supraventricular arrhythmias, the incidence of torsade de pointes was 1% and 1.4%, respectively.**

Torsade de pointes arrhythmias were dose related, as is the prolongation of QT (QT_c) interval, as shown in the table below.

Percent Incidence of Torsade de Pointes and Mean QT_c Interval by Dose For Patients With Sustained VT/VF

Daily Dose (mg)	Incidence of Torsade de pointes	Mean QT_c* (msec)
80	0 (69)	463 (17)
160	0.5 (832)	467 (181)
320	1.6 (835)	473 (344)
480	4.4 (459)	483 (234)
640	3.7 (324)	490 (185)
>640	5.8 (103)	512 (62)

( ) Number of patients assessed
*Highest on-therapy value

In addition to dose and presence of sustained VT, other risk factors for torsade de pointes were gender (females had a higher incidence), excessive prolongation of the QT_c interval (see table below) and history of cardiomegaly or congestive heart failure. Patients with sustained ventricular tachycardia and a history of congestive heart failure appear to have the highest risk for serious proarrhythmia (7%). Of the patients experiencing torsade de pointes, approximately two-thirds spontaneously reverted to their baseline rhythm. The others were either converted electrically (D/C cardioversion or overdrive pacing) or treated with other drugs (see **OVERDOSAGE**). It is not possible to determine whether some sudden deaths represented episodes of torsade de pointes, but in some instances sudden death did follow a documented episode of torsade de pointes. Although BETAPACE® therapy was discontinued in most patients experiencing torsade de pointes, 17% were continued on a lower dose. Nonetheless, BETAPACE® should be used with particular caution if the QT_c is greater than 500 msec on-therapy and serious consideration should be given to reducing the dose or discontinuing therapy when the QT_c exceeds 550 msec. Due to the multiple risk-factors associated with torsade de pointes, however, caution should be exercised regardless of the QT_c interval. The table below relates the incidence of torsade de pointes to on-therapy QT_c and change in QT_c from baseline. It should be noted, however, that the highest on-therapy QT_c was in many cases the one obtained at the time of the torsade de pointes event, so that the table overstates the predictive value of a high QT_c.

[See table below]

Relationship Between QT_c Interval Prolongation and Torsade de Pointes

On-Therapy QT_c Interval (msec)	Incidence of Torsade de pointes	Change in QT_c Interval From Baseline (msec)	Incidence of Torsade de pointes
less than 500	1.3% (1787)	less than 65	1.6% (1516)
500–525	3.4% (236)	65–80	3.2% (158)
525–550	5.6% (125)	80–100	4.1% (146)
>550	10.8% (157)	100–130	5.2% (115)
		>130	7.1% (99)

( ) Number of patients assessed

Proarrhythmic events must be anticipated not only on initiating therapy, but with every upward dose adjustment. Proarrhythmic events most often occur within 7 days of initiating therapy or of an increase in dose; 75% of serious proarrhythmias (torsade de pointes and worsened VT) occurred within 7 days of initiating BETAPACE® therapy, while 60% of such events occurred within 3 days of initiation or a dosage change. Initiating therapy at 80 mg BID with gradual upward dose titration and appropriate evaluations for efficacy (e.g., PES or Holter) and safety (e.g., QT interval, heart rate and electrolytes) prior to dose escalation, should reduce the risk of proarrhythmia. Avoiding excessive accumulation of sotalol in patients with diminished renal function, by appropriate dose reduction, should also reduce the risk of proarrhythmia (see **DOSAGE AND ADMINISTRATION**).

Congestive Heart Failure: Sympathetic stimulation is necessary in supporting circulatory function in congestive heart failure, and beta-blockade carries the potential hazard of further depressing myocardial contractility and precipitating more severe failure. In patients who have congestive heart failure controlled by digitalis and/or diuretics, BETAPACE® should be administered cautiously. Both digitalis and sotalol slow AV conduction. As with all beta-blockers, caution is advised when initiating therapy in patients with any evidence of left ventricular dysfunction. In premarketing studies, new or worsened congestive heart failure (CHF) occurred in 3.3% (n=3257) of patients and led to discontinuation in approximately 1% of patients receiving BETAPACE®. The incidence was higher in patients presenting with sustained ventricular tachycardia/fibrillation (4.6%, n=1363), or a prior history of heart failure (7.3%, n=696). Based on a life-table analysis, the one-year incidence of new or worsened CHF was 3% in patients without a prior history and 10% in patients with a prior history of CHF. NYHA Classification was also closely associated to the incidence of new or worsened heart failure while receiving BETAPACE® (1.8% in 1395 Class I patients, 4.9% in 1254 Class II patients and 6.1% in 278 Class III or IV patients).

Electrolyte Disturbances: BETAPACE® should not be used in patients with hypokalemia or hypomagnesemia prior to correction of imbalance, as these conditions can exaggerate the degree of QT prolongation, and increase the potential for torsade de pointes. Special attention should be given to electrolyte and acid-base balance in patients experiencing severe or prolonged diarrhea or patients receiving concomitant diuretic drugs.

Conduction Disturbances: Excessive prolongation of the QT interval (>550 msec) can promote serious arrhythmias and should be avoided (see **Proarrhythmias** above). Sinus bradycardia (heart rate less than 50 bpm) occurred in 13% of patients receiving BETAPACE® in clinical trials, and led to discontinuation in about 3% of patients. Bradycardia itself increases the risk of torsade de pointes. Sinus pause, sinus arrest and sinus node dysfunction occur in less than 1% of patients. The incidence of 2nd- or 3rd-degree AV block is approximately 1%.

Recent Acute MI: BETAPACE® can be used safely and effectively in the long-term treatment of life-threatening ventricular arrhythmias following a myocardial infarction. However, experience in the use of BETAPACE® to treat cardiac arrhythmias in the early phase of recovery from acute MI is limited and at least at high initial doses is not reassuring. (See **WARNINGS: Mortality**.) In the first 2 weeks post-MI caution is advised and careful dose titration is especially important, particularly in patients with markedly impaired ventricular function.

The following warnings are related to the beta-blocking activity of BETAPACE®.

Abrupt Withdrawal: Hypersensitivity to catecholamines has been observed in patients withdrawn from beta-blocker therapy. Occasional cases of exacerbation of angina pectoris, arrhythmias and, in some cases, myocardial infarction have been reported after abrupt discontinuation of beta-blocker therapy. Therefore, it is prudent when discontinuing chronically administered BETAPACE®, particularly in patients with ischemic heart disease, to carefully monitor the patient and consider the temporary use of an alternate beta-blocker if appropriate. If possible, the dosage of BETAPACE® should be gradually reduced over a period of one to two weeks. If angina or acute coronary insufficiency develops, appropriate therapy should be instituted promptly. Patients should be warned against interruption or discontinuation of therapy without the physician's advice. Because coronary artery disease is common and may be unrecognized in patients receiving BETAPACE®, abrupt discontinuation in patients with arrhythmias may unmask latent coronary insufficiency.

Non-Allergic Bronchospasm (e.g., chronic bronchitis and emphysema): **PATIENTS WITH BRONCHOSPASTIC DISEASES SHOULD IN GENERAL NOT RECEIVE BETA-BLOCKERS.** It is prudent, if BETAPACE® (sotalol hydrochloride) is to be administered, to use the smallest effective dose, so that inhibition of bronchodilation produced by endogenous or exogenous catecholamine stimulation of $beta_2$ receptors may be minimized.

Anaphylaxis: While taking beta-blockers, patients with a history of anaphylactic reaction to a variety of allergens may have a more severe reaction on repeated challenge, either accidental, diagnostic or therapeutic. Such patients may be unresponsive to the usual doses of epinephrine used to treat the allergic reaction.

Anesthesia: The management of patients undergoing major surgery who are being treated with beta-blockers is controversial. Protracted severe hypotension and difficulty in restoring and maintaining normal cardiac rhythm after anesthesia have been reported in patients receiving beta-blockers.

Diabetes: In patients with diabetes (especially labile diabetes) or with a history of episodes of spontaneous hypoglycemia, BETAPACE® should be given with caution since beta-blockade may mask some important premonitory signs of acute hypoglycemia; e.g., tachycardia.

Sick Sinus Syndrome: BETAPACE® should be used only with extreme caution in patients with sick sinus syndrome associated with symptomatic arrhythmias, because it may cause sinus bradycardia, sinus pauses or sinus arrest.

Thyrotoxicosis: Beta-blockade may mask certain clinical signs (e.g., tachycardia) of hyperthyroidism. Patients suspected of developing thyrotoxicosis should be managed carefully to avoid abrupt withdrawal of beta-blockade which might be followed by an exacerbation of symptoms of hyperthyroidism, including thyroid storm.

PRECAUTIONS

RENAL IMPAIRMENT: BETAPACE® (sotalol hydrochloride) is mainly eliminated via the kidneys through glomerular filtration and to a small degree by tubular secretion. There is a direct relationship between renal function, as measured by serum creatinine or creatinine clearance, and the elimination rate of BETAPACE®. Guidance for dosing in conditions of renal impairment can be found under "DOSAGE AND ADMINISTRATION."

DRUG INTERACTIONS

Antiarrhythmics: Class Ia antiarrhythmic drugs, such as disopyramide, quinidine and procainamide and other Class III drugs (e.g., amiodarone) are not recommended as concomitant therapy with BETAPACE®, because of their potential to prolong refractoriness (see **WARNINGS**). There is only limited experience with the concomitant use of Class Ib or Ic antiarrhythmics. Additive Class II effects would also be anticipated with the use of other beta-blocking agents concomitantly with BETAPACE®.

Digoxin: Single and multiple doses of BETAPACE® do not substantially affect serum digoxin levels. Proarrhythmic events were more common in BETAPACE® treated patients also receiving digoxin; it is not clear whether this represents an interaction or is related to the presence of CHF, a known risk factor for proarrhythmia, in the patients receiving digoxin.

Calcium blocking drugs: BETAPACE® should be administered with caution in conjunction with calcium blocking drugs because of possible additive effects on atrioventricular conduction or ventricular function. Additionally, concomitant use of these drugs may have additive effects on blood pressure, possibly leading to hypotension.

Catecholamine-depleting agents: Concomitant use of catecholamine-depleting drugs, such as reserpine and guanethidine, with a beta-blocker may produce an excessive reduction of resting sympathetic nervous tone. Patients treated with BETAPACE® plus a catecholamine depletor should therefore be closely monitored for evidence of hypotension and or marked bradycardia which may produce syncope.

Insulin and oral antidiabetics: Hyperglycemia may occur, and the dosage of insulin or antidiabetic drugs may require adjustment. Symptoms of hypoglycemia may be masked.

Beta-2-receptor stimulants: Beta-agonists such as salbutamol, terbutaline and isoprenaline may have to be administered in increased dosages when used concomitantly with BETAPACE®.

Clonidine: Beta-blocking drugs may potentiate the rebound hypertension sometimes observed after discontinuation of clonidine; therefore, caution is advised when discontinuing clonidine in patients receiving BETAPACE®.

Other: No pharmacokinetic interactions were observed with hydrochlorothiazide or warfarin.

Antacids: Administration of BETAPACE® within 2 hours of antacids containing aluminum oxide and magnesium hydroxide should be avoided because it may result in a reduction in Cmax and AUC of 26% and 20%, respectively and consequently in a 25% reduction in the bradycardic effect at rest. Administration of the antacid two hours after BETAPACE® has no effect on the pharmacokinetics or pharmacodynamics of sotalol.

Drugs prolonging the QT interval: BETAPACE® should be administered with caution in conjunction with other drugs known to prolong the QT interval such as Class I antiarrhythmic agents, phenothiazines, tricyclic antidepressants, terfenadine and astemizole (see **WARNINGS**).

DRUG/Laboratory Test Interactions

The presence of sotalol in the urine may result in falsely elevated levels of urinary metanephrine when measured by fluorimetric or photometric methods. In screening patients suspected of having a pheochromocytoma and being treated with sotalol, a specific method, such as a high performance liquid chromatographic assay with solid phase extraction (e.g., J. Chromatogr. 385:241, 1987) should be employed in determining levels of catecholamines.

Carcinogenesis, Mutagenesis, Impairment of Fertility: No evidence of carcinogenic potential was observed in rats during a 24-month study at 137–275 mg/kg/day (approximately 30 times the maximum recommended human oral dose (MRHD) as mg/kg or 5 times the MRHD as mg/m^2) or in mice, during a 24-month study at 4141–7122 mg/kg/day (approximately 450–750 times the MRHD as mg/kg or 36–63 times the MRHD as mg/m^2).

Sotalol has not been evaluated in any specific assay of mutagenicity or clastogenicity.

No significant reduction in fertility occurred in rats at oral doses of 1000 mg/kg/day (approximately 100 times the MRHD as mg/kg or 9 times the MRHD as mg/m^2) prior to mating, except for a small reduction in the number of offspring per litter.

Pregnancy Category B: Reproduction studies in rats and rabbits during organogenesis at 100 and 22 times the MRHD as mg/kg (9 and 7 times the MRHD as mg/m^2), respectively, did not reveal any teratogenic potential associated with sotalol HCl. In rabbits, a high dose of sotalol HCl (160 mg/kg/day) at 16 times the MRHD as mg/kg (6 times the MRHD as mg/m^2) produced a slight increase in fetal death likely due to maternal toxicity. Eight times the maximum dose (80 mg/kg/day or 3 times the MRHD as mg/m^2) did not result in an increased incidence of fetal deaths. In rats, 1000 mg/kg/day sotalol HCl, 100 times the MRHD (18 times the MRHD as mg/m^2), increased the number of early resorptions, while at 14 times the maximum dose (2.5 times the MRHD as mg/m^2), no increase in early resorptions was noted. However, animal reproduction studies are not always predictive of human response.

Although there are no adequate and well-controlled studies in pregnant women, sotalol HCl has been shown to cross the placenta, and is found in amniotic fluid. There has been a report of subnormal birth weight with BETAPACE®. Therefore, BETAPACE® should be used during pregnancy only if the potential benefit outweighs the potential risk.

Nursing Mothers: Sotalol is excreted in the milk of laboratory animals and has been reported to be present in human milk. Because of the potential for adverse reactions in nursing infants from BETAPACE®, a decision should be made whether to discontinue nursing or to discontinue the drug, taking into account the importance of the drug to the mother.

Pediatric Use: The safety and effectiveness of BETAPACE® in children have not been established.

ADVERSE REACTIONS

During premarketing trials, 3186 patients with cardiac arrhythmias (1363 with sustained ventricular tachycardia) received oral BETAPACE®, of whom 2451 received the drug for at least two weeks. The most important adverse effects are torsade de pointes and other serious new ventricular arrhythmias (see **WARNINGS**), occurring at rates of almost 4% and 1%, respectively, in the VT/VF population. Overall, discontinuation because of unacceptable side-effects was necessary in 17% of all patients in clinical trials, and in 13% of patients treated for at least two weeks. The most common adverse reactions leading to discontinuation of BETAPACE® are as follows: fatigue 4%, bradycardia (less than 50 bpm) 3%, dyspnea 3%, proarrhythmia 3%, asthenia 2%, and dizziness 2%.

Occasional reports of elevated serum liver enzymes have occurred with BETAPACE® therapy but no cause and effect relationship has been established. One case of peripheral neuropathy which resolved on discontinuation of

Incidence (%) of Adverse Events and Discontinuations
DAILY DOSE

Body System	160mg (n=832)	240mg (n=263)	320mg (n=835)	480mg (n=459)	640mg (n=324)	Any Dose* (n=1292)	% Patients Discontinued (n=1292)
Body as a whole							
infection	1	2	2	2	3	4	<1
fever	1	2	3	2	2	4	<1
localized pain	1	1	2	2	2	3	<1
Cardiovascular							
dyspnea	5	8	11	15	15	21	2
bradycardia	8	8	9	7	5	16	2
chest pain	4	3	10	10	14	16	<1
palpitation	3	3	8	9	12	14	<1
edema	2	2	5	3	5	8	1
ECG abnormal	4	2	4	2	2	7	1
hypotension	3	4	3	2	3	6	2
proarrhythmia	<1	<1	2	4	5	5	3
syncope	1	1	3	2	5	5	1
heart failure	2	3	2	2	2	5	1
presyncope	1	2	2	4	3	4	<1
peripheral vascular disorder	1	2	1	1	2	3	<1
cardiovascular disorder	1	<1	2	2	2	3	<1
vasodilation	1	<1	1	2	1	3	<1
AICD Discharge	<1	2	2	2	2	3	<1
hypertension	<1	1	1	1	2	2	<1
Nervous							
fatigue	5	8	12	12	13	20	2
dizziness	7	6	11	11	14	20	1
asthenia	4	5	7	8	10	13	1
light-headed	4	3	6	6	9	12	1
headache	3	2	4	4	4	8	<1
sleep problem	1	1	5	5	6	8	<1
perspiration	1	2	3	4	5	6	<1
altered consciousness	2	3	1	2	3	4	<1
depression	1	2	2	2	3	4	<1
paresthesia	1	1	2	3	2	4	<1
anxiety	2	2	2	3	2	4	<1
mood change	<1	<1	1	3	2	3	<1
appetite disorder	1	2	2	1	3	3	<1
stroke	<1	<1	1	1	<1	1	<1
Digestive							
nausea/vomiting	5	4	4	6	6	10	1
diarrhea	2	3	3	3	5	7	<1
dyspepsia	2	3	3	3	3	6	<1
abdominal pain	<1	<1	2	2	2	3	<1
colon problem	2	1	1	<1	2	3	<1
flatulence	1	<1	1	1	2	2	<1
Respiratory							
pulmonary problem	3	3	5	3	4	8	<1
upper respiratory tract problem	1	1	3	4	3	5	<1
asthma	1	<1	1	1	1	2	<1
Urogenital							
genitourinary disorder	1	0	1	1	2	3	<1
sexual dysfunction	<1	1	1	1	3	2	<1
Metabolic							
abnormal lab value	1	2	3	2	1	4	<1
weight change	1	1	1	<1	2	2	<1
Musculoskeletal							
extremity pain	2	2	4	5	3	7	<1
back pain	1	<1	2	2	2	3	<1
Skin and Appendages							
rash	2	3	2	3	4	5	<1
Hematologic							
bleeding	1	<1	1	<1	2	2	<1
Special Senses							
visual problem	1	1	2	4	5	5	<1

* Because patients are counted at each dose level tested, the Any Dose column cannot be determined by adding across the doses.

BETAPACE® and recurred when the patient was rechallenged with the drug was reported in an early dose tolerance study. Elevated blood glucose levels and increased insulin requirements can occur in diabetic patients.

The following table lists as a function of dosage the most common (incidence of 2% or greater) adverse events, regardless of relationship to therapy and the percent of patients discontinued due to the event, as collected from clinical trials involving 1292 patients with sustained VT/VF.

[See table above]

Potential Adverse Effects: Foreign marketing experience with sotalol hydrochloride shows an adverse experience profile similar to that described above from clinical trials. Voluntary reports since introduction include rare reports (less than one report per 10,000 patients) of: emotional lability, slightly clouded sensorium, incoordination, vertigo, paralysis, thrombocytopenia, eosinophilia, leukopenia, photosensitivity reaction, fever, pulmonary edema, hyperlipidemia, myalgia, pruritis, alopecia.

The oculomucocutaneous syndrome associated with the beta-blocker practolol has not been associated with BETAPACE® during investigational use and foreign marketing experience.

OVERDOSAGE

Intentional or accidental overdosage with BETAPACE® (sotalol hydrochloride) has rarely resulted in death.

Symptoms and Treatment of Overdosage: The most common signs to be expected are bradycardia, congestive heart failure, hypotension, bronchospasm and hypoglycemia. In cases of massive intentional overdosage (2–16 grams) of BETAPACE® the following clinical findings were seen: hypotension, bradycardia, cardiac asystole, prolongation of QT interval, torsade de pointes, ventricular tachycardia, and premature ventricular complexes. If overdosage occurs, therapy with BETAPACE® should be discontinued and the patient observed closely. Because of the lack of protein binding, hemodialysis is useful for reducing sotalol plasma concentrations. Patients should be carefully observed until QT intervals are normalized and the heart rate returns to levels >50 bpm. In addition, if required, the following therapeutic measures are suggested:

Bradycardia or Cardiac Asystole: Atropine, another anticholinergic drug, a beta-adrenergic agonist or transvenous cardiac pacing.

Continued on next page

Information on the Berlex products appearing here is based on the most current information available at the time of publication closing. Further information for these and other products may be obtained from the Medical Affairs Department, Berlex Laboratories, 300 Fairfield Road, Wayne, New Jersey 07470, 1-888-BERLEX-4. Information on Betaseron and Fludara may be obtained from Berlex Laboratories, 15049 San Pablo Avenue, Richmond, California 94804-0016, 1-800-888-4112.

Betapace—Cont.

Heart Block: (second and third degree) transvenous cardiac pacemaker.
Hypotension: (depending on associated factors) epinephrine rather than isoproterenol or norepinephrine may be useful.
Bronchospasm: Aminophylline or aerosol beta-2-receptor stimulant.
Torsade de pointes: DC cardioversion, transvenous cardiac pacing, epinephrine, magnesium sulfate.

DOSAGE AND ADMINISTRATION

As with other antiarrhythmic agents, BETAPACE® should be initiated and doses increased in a hospital with facilities for cardiac rhythm monitoring and assessment (see **INDICATIONS AND USAGE**). BETAPACE® should be administered only after appropriate clinical assessment (see **INDICATIONS AND USAGE**), and the dosage of BETAPACE® must be individualized for each patient on the basis of therapeutic response and tolerance. Proarrhythmic events can occur not only at initiation of therapy, but also with each upward dosage adjustment.
Dosage of BETAPACE® should be adjusted gradually, allowing 2–3 days between dosing increments in order to attain steady-state plasma concentrations, and to allow monitoring of QT intervals. Graded dose adjustment will help prevent the usage of doses which are higher than necessary to control the arrhythmia. The recommended initial dose is 80 mg twice daily. This dose may be increased, if necessary, after appropriate evaluation to 240 or 320 mg/day (120–160 mg twice daily). In most patients, a therapeutic response is obtained at a total daily dose of 160 to 320 mg/day, given in two or three divided doses. Some patients with life-threatening refractory ventricular arrhythmias may require doses as high as 480–640 mg/day; however, these doses should only be prescribed when the potential benefit outweighs the increased risk of adverse events, in particular proarrhythmia. Because of the long terminal elimination half-life of BETAPACE®, dosing on more than a BID regimen is usually not necessary.

DOSAGE IN RENAL IMPAIRMENT

Because sotalol is excreted predominantly in urine and its terminal elimination half-life is prolonged in conditions of renal impairment, the dosing interval (time between divided doses) of sotalol should be modified (when creatinine clearance is lower than 60 mL/min) according to the following table.

Creatinine Clearance mL/min	Dosing* Interval (hours)
>60	12
30–59	24
10–29	36–48
<10	Dose should be individualized

*The initial dose of 80 mg and subsequent doses should be administered at these intervals. See following paragraph for dosage escalations.

Since the terminal elimination half-life of BETAPACE® (sotalol hydrochloride) is increased in patients with renal impairment, a longer duration of dosing is required to reach steady-state. Dose escalations in renal impairment should be done after administration of at least 5–6 doses at appropriate intervals (see table above).
Extreme caution should be exercised in the use of sotalol in patients with renal failure undergoing hemodialysis. The half-life of sotalol is prolonged (up to 69 hours) in anuric patients. Sotalol, however, can be partly removed by dialysis with subsequent partial rebound in concentrations when dialysis is completed. Both safety (heart rate, QT interval) and efficacy (arrhythmia control) must be closely monitored.

Transfer to BETAPACE®

Before starting BETAPACE®, previous antiarrhythmic therapy should generally be withdrawn under careful monitoring for a minimum of 2–3 plasma half-lives if the patient's clinical condition permits (see **DRUG INTERACTIONS**). Treatment has been initiated in some patients receiving I.V. lidocaine without ill effect. After discontinuation of amiodarone, BETAPACE® should not be initiated until the QT interval is normalized (see **WARNINGS**).

HOW SUPPLIED

BETAPACE® (sotalol hydrochloride); capsule-shaped light-blue scored tablets imprinted with the strength and "BETAPACE", are available as follows:

NDC 50419–105–10	80 mg strength, bottle of 100
NDC 50419–105–11	80 mg strength, carton of 100 unit dose
NDC 50419–109–10	120 mg strength, bottle of 100
NDC 50419–109–11	120 mg strength, carton of 100 unit dose
NDC 50419–106–10	160 mg strength, bottle of 100
NDC 50419–106–11	160 mg strength, carton of 100 unit dose
NDC 50419–107–10	240 mg strength, bottle of 100
NDC 50419–107–11	240 mg strength, carton of 100 unit dose

Store at controlled room temperature, between 15° to 30°C (59° to 86°F).
Rx only

Manufactured by:
BERLEX Laboratories, Wayne, NJ 07470
6063802 Rev. 12/98
Shown in Product Identification Guide, page 308

BETAPACE AF™ ℞

[*bā-tăh pāce AF*]
(SOTALOL HCl)

> **To minimize the risk of induced arrhythmia, patients initiated or re-initiated on BETAPACE AF™ should be placed for a minimum of three days (on their maintenance dose) in a facility that can provide cardiac resuscitation, continuous electrocardiographic monitoring and calculations of creatinine clearance. For detailed instructions regarding dose selection, and special cautions for people with renal impairment, see DOSAGE AND ADMINISTRATION.** Sotalol is also indicated for the treatment of documented life-threatening ventricular arrhythmias and is marketed under the brand name BETAPACE.® BETAPACE® however, should not be substituted for BETAPACE AF™ because of significant differences in labeling (i.e. patient package insert, dosing administration and safety information).

DESCRIPTION

BETAPACE AF,™ (sotalol hydrochloride), is an antiarrhythmic drug with Class II (beta-adrenoreceptor blocking) and Class III (cardiac action potential duration prolongation) properties. It is supplied as a white, capsule-shaped tablet for oral administration. Sotalol hydrochloride is a white, crystalline solid with a molecular weight of 308.8. It is hydrophilic, soluble in water, propylene glycol and ethanol, but is only slightly soluble in chloroform. Chemically, sotalol hydrochloride is d,l-*N*-[4-[1-hydroxy-2-[(1-methylethyl)amino]ethyl]-phenyl]methane-sulfonamide monohydrochloride. The molecular formula is $C_{12}H_{20}N_2O_3S \bullet HCl$ and is represented by the following structural formula:

CH_3SO_2NH–(C₆H₄)–$CH(OH)$-$CH_2NHCH(CH_3)_2 \bullet HCl$

BETAPACE AF™ tablets contain the following inactive ingredients: microcrystalline cellulose, lactose, starch, stearic acid, magnesium stearate, and colloidal silicon dioxide.

CLINICAL PHARMACOLOGY

Mechanism of Action: BETAPACE AF™ (sotalol hydrochloride) has both beta-adrenoreceptor blocking (Vaughan Williams Class II) and cardiac action potential duration prolongation (Vaughan Williams Class III) antiarrhythmic properties. BETAPACE AF™ (sotalol hydrochloride) is a racemic mixture of d- and l-sotalol. Both isomers have similar Class III antiarrhythmic effects, while the l-isomer is responsible for virtually all of the beta-blocking activity. The beta-blocking effect of sotalol is non-cardioselective, half maximal at about 80 mg/day and maximal at doses between 320 and 640 mg/day. Sotalol does not have partial agonist or membrane stabilizing activity. Although significant beta-blockade occurs at oral doses as low as 25 mg, significant Class III effects are seen only at daily doses of 160 mg and above.
Electrophysiology: Sotalol hydrochloride prolongs the plateau phase of the cardiac action potential in the isolated myocyte, as well as in isolated tissue preparations of ventricular or atrial muscle (Class III activity). In intact animals it slows heart rate, slows AV nodal conduction and increases refractory periods of atrial and ventricular muscle and conduction tissue.
In man, the Class II (beta-blockade) electrophysiological effects of BETAPACE AF™ are manifested by increased sinus cycle length (slowed heart rate), decreased AV nodal conduction and increased AV nodal refractoriness. The Class III electrophysiological effects in man include prolongation of the atrial and ventricular monophasic action potentials, and effective refractory period prolongation of atrial muscle, ventricular muscle, and atrio-ventricular accessory pathways (where present) in both the anterograde and retrograde directions. With oral doses of 160 to 640 mg/day, the surface ECG shows dose-related mean increases of 40–100 msec in QT and 10–40 msec in QT_c. In a study of patients with atrial fibrillation (AFIB)/flutter (AFIB/AFL) receiving three different oral doses of BETAPACE AF™ given q12h (or q24h in patients with a reduced creatinine clearance), mean increases in QT intervals measured from 12-lead ECGs of 25 msec, 40 msec and 54 msec were found in the 80 mg, 120 mg, and 160 mg dose groups, respectively. (See **WARNINGS** for description of relationship between QT_c and torsade de pointes type arrhythmias.) No significant alteration in QRS interval is observed.
In a small study (n=25) of patients with implanted defibrillators treated concurrently with sotalol, the average defibrillatory threshold was 6 joules (range 2–15 joules) compared to a mean of 16 joules for a non-randomized comparative group primarily receiving amiodarone.
In a dose-response trial comparing three dose levels of BETAPACE AF,™ 80 mg, 120 mg, and 160 mg with placebo given q12h (or q24h in patients with a reduced renal creatinine clearance) for the prevention of recurrence of symptomatic atrial fibrillation (AFIB)/flutter (AFL), the mean ventricular rate during recurrence of AFIB/AFL was 125, 107, 110 and 99 beats/min in the placebo, 80 mg, 120 mg and 160 mg dose groups, respectively ($p<0.017$ for each sotalol dose group versus placebo). In another placebo controlled trial in which BETAPACE AF™ was titrated to a dose between 160 and 320 mg/day in patients with chronic AFIB, the mean ventricular rate during recurrence of AFIB was 107 and 84 beats/min in the placebo and BETAPACE AF™ groups, respectively ($p<0.001$).
Hemodynamics: In a study of systemic hemodynamic function measured invasively in 12 patients with a mean LV ejection fraction of 37% and ventricular tachycardia (9 sustained and 3 non-sustained), a median dose of 160 mg twice daily of sotalol produced a 28% reduction in heart rate and a 24% decrease in cardiac index at 2 hours post dosing at steady-state. Concurrently, systemic vascular resistance and stroke volume showed non-significant increases of 25% and 8%, respectively. Pulmonary capillary wedge pressure increased significantly from 6.4 mmHg to 11.8 mmHg in the 11 patients who completed the study. One patient was discontinued because of worsening congestive heart failure. Mean arterial pressure, mean pulmonary artery pressure and stroke work index did not significantly change. Exercise and isoproterenol induced tachycardia are antagonized by sotalol, and total peripheral resistance increases by a small amount.
In hypertensive patients, sotalol produces significant reductions in both systolic and diastolic blood pressures. Although sotalol is usually well-tolerated hemodynamically, caution should be exercised in patients with marginal cardiac compensation as deterioration in cardiac performance may occur. (See **WARNINGS: Congestive Heart Failure.**)

Clinical Studies:

Prolongation of Time to Recurrence of Symptomatic Atrial Fibrillation/Flutter

BETAPACE AF™ has been studied in patients with symptomatic AFIB/AFL in two principal studies, one in patients with primarily paroxysmal AFIB/AFL, the other in patients with primarily chronic AFIB.
In one study, a U.S. multicenter, randomized, placebo-controlled, double-blind, dose-response trial of patients with symptomatic primary paroxysmal AFIB/AFL, three fixed dose levels of BETAPACE AF™ (80 mg, 120 mg and 160 mg) twice daily and placebo were compared in 253 patients. In patients with reduced creatinine clearance (40–60 mL/min) the same doses were given once daily. Patients were not randomized for the following reasons: QT > 450 msec; creatinine clearance < 40 mL/min; intolerance to beta-blockers; bradycardia-tachycardia syndrome in the absence of an implanted pacemaker; AFIB/AFL was asymptomatic or was associated with syncope, embolic CVA or TIA; acute myocardial infarction within the previous 2 months; congestive heart failure; bronchial asthma or other contraindications to beta-blocker therapy; receiving potassium losing diuretics without potassium replacement or without concurrent use of ACE-inhibitors; uncorrected hypokalemia (serum potassium < 3.5 meq/L) or hypomagnesemia (serum magnesium < 1.5 meq/L); received chronic oral amiodarone therapy for > 1 month within previous 12 weeks; congenital or acquired long QT syndromes; history of torsade de pointes with other antiarrhythmic agents which increase the duration of ventricular repolarization; sinus rate < 50 bpm during waking hours; unstable angina pectoris; receiving treatment with other drugs that prolong the QT interval; and AFIB/AFL associated with the Wolff-Parkinson-White (WPW) syndrome. If the QT interval increased to ≥ 520 msec (or JT ≥ 430 msec if QRS > 100 msec) the drug was discontinued. The patient population in this trial was 64% male, and the mean age was 62 years. No structural heart disease was present in 43% of the patients. Doses were administered once daily in 20% of the patients because of reduced creatinine clearance.
BETAPACE AF™ was shown to prolong the time to the first symptomatic, ECG-documented recurrence of AFIB/AFL, as well as to reduce the risk of such recurrence at both 6 and 12 months. The 120 mg dose was more effective than 80 mg, but 160 mg did not appear to have an added benefit. Note that these doses were given twice or once daily, depending on renal function. The results are shown in Figure 1 and Tables 1 and 2.

Figure 1: Study 1 - Time to First ECG-Documented Recurrence of Symptomatic AFIB/AFL Since Randomization

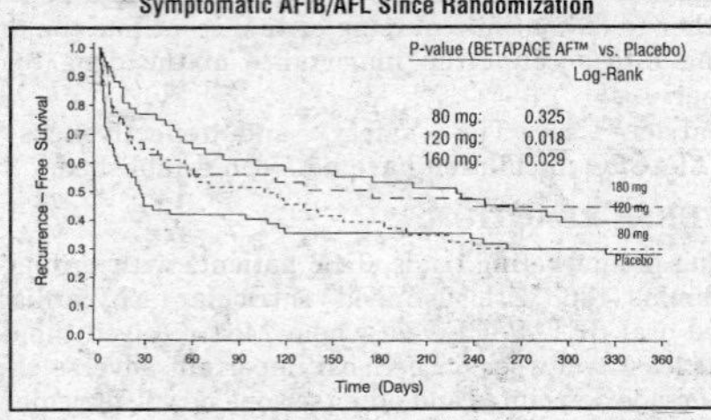

[See table 1 at top of next page]
[See table 2 at top of next page]

Discontinuation because of adverse events was dose related.
In a second multicenter, randomized, placebo-controlled, double-blind study of 6 months duration in 232 patients with chronic AFIB, BETAPACE AF™ was titrated over a dose range from 80 mg/day to 320 mg/day. The patient population of this trial was 70% male with a mean age of 65 years. Structural heart disease was present in 49% of the patients. All patients had chronic AFIB for >2 weeks but <1 year at entry with a mean duration of 4.1 months. Patients were excluded if they had significant electrolyte imbalance,

Table 1: Study 1—Patient Status At 12 Months

		Betapace AF Dose		
	Placebo	80 mg	120 mg	160 mg
Randomized	69	59	63	62
On treatment in NSR at 12 months without recurrance[a]	23%	22%	29%	23%
Recurrence[a,b]	67%	58%	49%	42%
D/C for AEs	6%	12%	18%	29%

[a] Symptomatic AFIB/AFL
[b] Efficacy endpoint of Study 1; study treatment stopped.
Please note that columns do not add up to 100% due to discontinuations (D/C) for "other" reasons.

Table 2: Study 1—Median Time to Recurrence of Symptomatic AFIB/AFL and Relative Risk (vs. Placebo) at 12 Months

		Betapace AF Dose		
	Placebo	80 mg	120 mg	160 mg
p-value vs placebo		p=0.325	p=0.018	p=0.029
Relative Risk (RR) to placebo		0.81	0.59	0.59
Median time to recurrence (days)	27	106	229	175

Table 5
Incidence of Torsade de Pointes in Controlled Trials of AFIB and Other Supraventricular Arrhythmias

	BETAPACE AF™ (Daily Dose)				
	Any Dose (N=659)	>320 mg/day (N=62)	≤320 mg/day (N=597)	≤240 mg/day (N=340)	Placebo (N=358)
	n(%)	n(%)	n(%)	n(%)	n(%)
Torsade de Pointes	4(0.6%)	2(3.2%)	2(0.3%)	1(0.3%)	0

QTc >460 msec, QRS >140 msec, any degree of AV block or functioning pacemaker, uncompensated cardiac failure, asthma, significant renal disease (estimated creatinine clearance <50 mL/min), heart rate < 50 bpm, myocardial infarction or open heart surgery in past 2 months, unstable angina, infective endocarditis, active pericarditis or myocarditis, ≥ 3 DC cardioversions in the past, medications that prolonged QT interval, and previous amiodarone treatment. After successful cardioversion patients were randomized to receive placebo (n=114) or BETAPACE AF™ (n=118), at a starting dose of 80 mg twice daily. If the initial dose was not tolerated it was decreased to 80 mg once daily, but if it was tolerated it was increased to 160 mg twice daily. During the maintenance period 67% of treated patients received a dose of 160 mg twice daily, and the remainder received doses of 80 mg once daily (17%) and 80 mg twice daily (16%).

Figure 2 and Tables 3 and 4 show the results of the trial. There was a longer time to ECG-documented recurrence of AFIB and a reduced risk of recurrence at 6 months compared to placebo.

Figure 2: Study 2 - Time to First ECG-Documented Recurrence of Symptomatic AFIB/AFL/Death Since Randomization

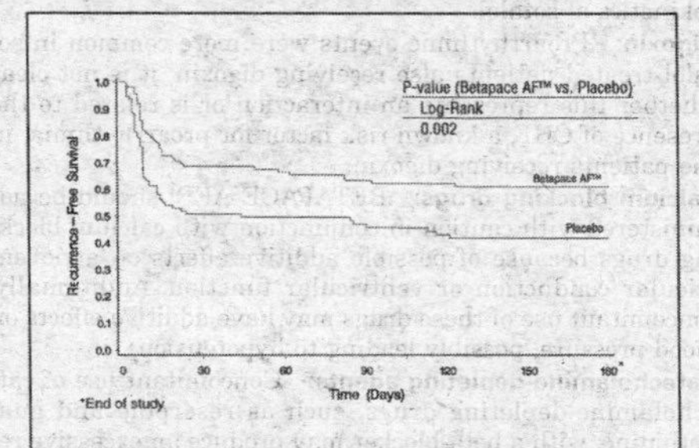

Table 3: Study 2—Patient Status At 6 Months

	Betapace AF	Placebo
Randomized	118	114
On treatment in NSR at 6 months without recurrence[a]	45%	29%
Recurrence[a,b]	49%	67%
D/C for AEs	6%	3%
Death		1%

[a]Symptomatic or asymptomatic AFIB/AFL
[b]Efficacy endpoint of Study 2; study treatment stopped.

Table 4: Study 2—Median Time to Recurrence of Symptomatic AFIB/AFL/Death and Relative Risk (vs. Placebo) at 6 Months

	Betapace AF	Placebo
p-value vs placebo	p=0.002	
Relative Risk (RR) to placebo	0.55	
Median time to recurrence (days)	>180	44

Safety in Patients with Structural Heart Disease:
In a multicenter double-blind randomized study reported by D. Julian et al, the effect of sotalol 320 mg once daily was compared with that of placebo in 1456 patients (randomized 3:2, sotalol to placebo) surviving an acute myocardial infarction (MI). Treatment was started 5–14 days after infarction. Patients were followed for 12 months. The mortality rate was 7.3% in the sotalol group and 8.9% in the placebo group, not a statistically significant difference. Although the results do not show evidence of a benefit of sotalol in this population, they do not show an added risk in post MI patients receiving sotalol.

Pharmacokinetics: In healthy subjects, the oral bioavailability of sotalol is 90–100%. After oral administration, peak plasma concentrations are reached in 2.5 to 4 hours, and steady-state plasma concentrations are attained within 2–3 days (i.e., after 5–6 doses when administered twice daily). Over the dosage range 160–640 mg/day sotalol displays dose proportionality with respect to plasma concentrations. Distribution occurs to a central (plasma) and to a peripheral compartment, with a mean elimination half-life of 12 hours. Dosing every 12 hours results in trough plasma concentrations which are approximately one-half of those at peak.

Sotalol does not bind to plasma proteins and is not metabolized. Sotalol shows very little intersubject variability in plasma levels. The pharmacokinetics of the d and l enantiomers of sotalol are essentially identical. Sotalol crosses the blood brain barrier poorly. Excretion is predominantly via the kidney in the unchanged form, and therefore lower doses are necessary in conditions of renal impairment (See **DOSAGE AND ADMINISTRATION**). Age per se does not significantly alter the pharmacokinetics of sotalol, but impaired renal function in geriatric patients can increase the terminal elimination half-life, resulting in increased drug accumulation. The absorption of sotalol was reduced by approximately 20% compared to fasting when it was administered with a standard meal. Since sotalol is not subject to first-pass metabolism, patients with hepatic impairment show no alteration in clearance of sotalol.

INDICATIONS AND USAGE

BETAPACE AF™ is indicated for the maintenance of normal sinus rhythm [delay in time to recurrence of atrial fibrillation/atrial flutter (AFIB/AFL)] in patients with symptomatic AFIB/AFL who are currently in sinus rhythm. Because BETAPACE AF™ can cause life-threatening ventricular arrhythmias, it should be reserved for patients in whom AFIB/AFL is highly symptomatic. Patients with paroxysmal AFIB whose AFIB/AFL that is easily reversed (by Valsalva maneuver, for example) should usually not be given BETAPACE AF™ (**See WARNINGS**).

In general, antiarrhythmic therapy for AFIB/AFL aims to prolong the time in normal sinus rhythm. Recurrence is expected in some patients (See **CLINICAL STUDIES**).

Sotalol is also indicated for the treatment of documented life-threatening ventricular arrhythmias and is marketed under the brand name **BETAPACE® (sotalol hydrochloride)**. **BETAPACE®**, however, must not be substituted for BETAPACE AF™ because of significant differences in labeling (i.e. patient package insert, dosing administration and safety information).

CONTRAINDICATIONS

BETAPACE AF™ (sotalol hydrochloride) is contraindicated in patients with sinus bradycardia (<50 bpm during waking hours), sick sinus syndrome or second and third degree AV block (unless a functioning pacemaker is present), congenital or acquired long QT syndromes, baseline QT interval >450 msec, cardiogenic shock, uncontrolled heart failure, hypokalemia (<4 meq/L), creatinine clearance <40 mL/min, bronchial asthma and previous evidence of hypersensitivity to sotalol.

WARNINGS

Ventricular Arrhythmia: BETAPACE AF™ (sotalol) can cause serious ventricular arrhythmias, primarily torsade de pointes (TdP) type ventricular tachycardia, a polymorphic ventricular tachycardia associated with QT interval prolongation. QT interval prolongation is directly related to the dose of BETAPACE AF.™ Factors such as reduced creatinine clearance, gender (female) and larger doses increase the risk of TdP. The risk of TdP can be reduced by adjustment of the BETAPACE AF™ dose according to creatinine clearance and by monitoring the ECG for excessive increases in the QT interval.

Treatment with BETAPACE AF™ must therefore be started only in patients observed for a minimum of three days on their maintenance dose in a facility that can provide electrocardiographic monitoring and in the presence of personnel trained in the management of serious ventricular arrhythmias. Calculation of the creatinine clearance must precede administration of the first dose of BETAPACE AF™. For detailed instructions regarding dose selection, see DOSAGE AND ADMINISTRATION.

Proarrhythmia in Atrial Fibrillation/Atrial Flutter Patients:
In eight controlled trials of patients with AFIB/AFL and other supraventricular arrhythmias (N=659) there were four cases of torsade de pointes reported (0.6%) during the controlled phase of treatment with BETAPACE AF.™ The incidence of torsade de pointes was significantly lower in those patients receiving total daily doses of 320 mg or less (0.3%), as summarized in Table 5 below. Both patients who had torsade de pointes in the group receiving >320 mg/day were receiving 640 mg/day. In the group receiving ≤320 mg daily, one case of TdP occurred at a daily dose of 320 mg on day 4 of treatment and one case occurred on a daily dose of 160 mg on day 1 of treatment.

[See table 5 above]

Prolongation of the QT interval is dose related, increasing from baseline an average of 25, 40, and 50 msec in the 80, 120, and 160 mg groups, respectively, in the clinical dose-response study. In this clinical trial BETAPACE AF™ treatment was not initiated if the QT interval was greater than 450 msec and during therapy the dose was reduced or discontinued if the QT interval was ≥520 msec.

Experience in patients with ventricular arrhythmias is also pertinent to the risk of torsade de pointes in patients with AFIB/AFL (see below).

Proarrhythmia in Ventricular Arrhythmia Patients: [see BETAPACE® (sotalol hydrochloride) Package Insert]. In patients with a history of sustained ventricular tachycardia, the incidence of torsade de pointes during sotalol treatment was 4% and worsened VT in about 1%; in patients with other less serious ventricular arrhythmias the incidence of torsade de pointes was 1% and new or worsened VT in about 0.7%. Additionally, in approximately 1% of patients, deaths were considered possibly drug related; such cases, although difficult to evaluate, may have been associated with proarrhythmic events.

Torsade de pointes arrhythmias in patients with VT/VF were dose related, as was the prolongation of QT (QT_c) interval, as shown in Table 6 below.

Continued on next page

Information on the Berlex products appearing here is based on the most current information available at the time of publication closing. Further information for these and other products may be obtained from the Medical Affairs Department, Berlex Laboratories, 300 Fairfield Road, Wayne, New Jersey 07470, 1-888-BERLEX-4. Information on Betaseron and Fludara may be obtained from Berlex Laboratories, 15049 San Pablo Avenue, Richmond, California 94804-0016, 1-800-888-4112.

Betapace AF—Cont.

Table 6
Percent Incidence of Torsade de Pointes and Mean QT_c Interval by Dose For Patients With Sustained VT/VF

Daily Dose (mg)	Incidence of Torsade de pointes	Mean QT_c*(msec)
80	0 (69)	463 (17)
160	0.5 (832)	467 (181)
320	1.6 (835)	473 (344)
480	4.4 (459)	483 (234)
640	3.7 (324)	490 (185)
>640	5.8 (103)	512 (62)

( ) Number of patients assessed
*highest on-therapy value

Table 7 below relates the incidence of torsade de pointes to on-therapy QTc and change in QTc from baseline. It should be noted, however, that the highest on-therapy QTc was in many cases the one obtained at the time of the torsade de pointes event, so that the table overstates the predictive value of a high QTc.
[See table 7 below]
In addition to dose and presence of sustained VT, other risk factors for torsade de pointes were gender (females had a higher incidence), excessive prolongation of the QTc interval and history of cardiomegaly or congestive heart failure. Patients with sustained ventricular tachycardia and a history of congestive heart failure appear to have the highest risk for serious proarrhythmia (7%). Of the ventricular arrhythmia patients experiencing torsade de pointes, approximately two-thirds spontaneously reverted to their baseline rhythm. The others were either converted electrically (D/C cardioversion or overdrive pacing) or treated with other drugs (see **OVERDOSAGE**). It is not possible to determine whether some sudden deaths represented episodes of torsade de pointes, but in some instances sudden death did follow a documented episode of torsade de pointes. Although sotalol therapy was discontinued in most patients experiencing torsade de pointes, 17% were continued on a lower dose.

Use with Drugs that Prolong QT Interval and Antiarrhythmic Agents:
The use of BETAPACE AF™ in conjunction with other drugs that prolong the QT interval has not been studied and is not recommended. Such drugs include many antiarrhythmics, some phenothiazines, cisapride, bepridil, tricyclic antidepressants, and certain oral macrolides. Class I or Class III antiarrhythmic agents should be withheld for at least three half-lives prior to dosing with BETAPACE AF.™ In clinical trials, BETAPACE AF™ was not administered to patients previously treated with oral amiodarone for >1 month in the previous three months. Class Ia antiarrhythmic drugs, such as disopyramide, quinidine and procainamide and other Class III drugs (e.g., amiodarone) are not recommended as concomitant therapy with BETAPACE AF,™ because of their potential to prolong refractoriness (**See WARNINGS**). There is only limited experience with the concomitant use of Class Ib or Ic antiarrhythmics.

Congestive Heart Failure: Sympathetic stimulation is necessary in supporting circulatory function in congestive heart failure, and beta-blockade carries the potential hazard of further depressing myocardial contractility and precipitating more severe failure. In patients who have heart failure controlled by digitalis and/or diuretics, BETAPACE AF™ should be administered cautiously. Both digitalis and sotalol slow AV conduction. As with all beta-blockers, caution is advised when initiating therapy in patients with any evidence of left ventricular dysfunction. In a pooled data base of four placebo-controlled AFIB/AFL and PSVT studies, new or worsening CHF occurred during therapy with BETAPACE AF™ in 5 (1.2%) of 415 patients. In these studies patients with uncontrolled heart failure were excluded (i.e. NYHA Functional Classes III or IV). In other premarketing sotalol studies, new or worsened congestive heart failure (CHF) occurred in 3.3% (n=3257) of patients and led to discontinuation in approximately 1% of patients receiving sotalol. The incidence was higher in patients presenting with sustained ventricular tachycardia/fibrillation (4.6%, n=1363), or a prior history of heart failure (7.3%, n=696). Based on a life-table analysis, the one-year incidence of new or worsened CHF was 3% in patients without a prior history and 10% in patients with a prior history of CHF. NYHA Classification was also closely associated to the incidence of new or worsened heart failure while receiving sotalol (1.8% in 1395 Class I patients, 4.9% in 1254 Class II patients and 6.1% in 278 Class III or IV patients).

Electrolyte Disturbances: BETAPACE AF™ should not be used in patients with hypokalemia or hypomagnesemia prior to correction of imbalance, as these conditions can exaggerate the degree of QT prolongation, and increase the potential for torsade de pointes. Special attention should be given to electrolyte and acid-base balance in patients experiencing severe or prolonged diarrhea or patients receiving concomitant diuretic drugs.

Bradycardia/Heart Block: The incidence of bradycardia (as determined by the investigators) in the supraventricular arrhythmia population treated with BETAPACE AF™ (N = 415) was 13%, and led to discontinuation in 2.4% of patients. Bradycardia itself increases the risk of torsade de pointes.

Recent Acute MI: Sotalol has been used in a controlled trial following an acute myocardial infarction without evidence of increased mortality (**See Safety in Patients with Structural Heart Disease**). Although specific studies of its use in treating atrial arrhythmias after infarction have not been conducted, the usual precautions regarding heart failure, avoidance of hypokalemia, bradycardia or prolonged QT interval apply.

The following warnings are related to the beta-blocking activity of BETAPACE AF.™

Abrupt Withdrawal: Hypersensitivity to catecholamines has been observed in patients withdrawn from beta-blocker therapy. Occasional cases of exacerbation of angina pectoris, arrhythmias and, in some cases, myocardial infarction have been reported after abrupt discontinuation of beta-blocker therapy. Therefore, it is prudent when discontinuing chronically administered BETAPACE AF,™ particularly in patients with ischemic heart disease, to carefully monitor the patient and consider the temporary use of an alternate beta-blocker if appropriate. If possible, the dosage of BETAPACE AF™ should be gradually reduced over a period of one to two weeks. If angina or acute coronary insufficiency develops, appropriate therapy should be instituted promptly. Patients should be warned against interruption or discontinuation of therapy without the physician's advice. Because coronary artery disease is common and may be unrecognized in patients receiving BETAPACE AF,™ abrupt discontinuation in patients with arrhythmias may unmask latent coronary insufficiency.

Non-Allergic Bronchospasm (e.g., chronic bronchitis and emphysema): **PATIENTS WITH BRONCHOSPASTIC DISEASES SHOULD IN GENERAL NOT RECEIVE BETA-BLOCKERS.** It is prudent, if BETAPACE AF™ (sotalol hydrochloride) is to be administered, to use the smallest effective dose, so that inhibition of bronchodilation produced by endogenous or exogenous catecholamine stimulation of $beta_2$ receptors may be minimized.

Anaphylaxis: While taking beta-blockers, patients with a history of anaphylactic reaction to a variety of allergens may have a more severe reaction on repeated challenge, either accidental, diagnostic or therapeutic. Such patients may be unresponsive to the usual doses of epinephrine used to treat the allergic reaction.

Anesthesia: The management of patients undergoing major surgery who are being treated with beta-blockers is controversial. Protracted severe hypotension and difficulty in restoring and maintaining normal cardiac rhythm after anesthesia have been reported in patients receiving beta-blockers.

Diabetes: In patients with diabetes (especially labile diabetes) or with a history of episodes of spontaneous hypoglycemia, BETAPACE AF™ should be given with caution since beta-blockade may mask some important premonitory signs of acute hypoglycemia; e.g., tachycardia.

Sick Sinus Syndrome: BETAPACE AF™ should be used only with extreme caution in patients with sick sinus syndrome associated with symptomatic arrhythmias, because it may cause sinus bradycardia, sinus pauses or sinus arrest. In patients with AFIB and sinus node dysfunction, the risk of torsade de pointes with BETAPACE AF™ therapy is increased, especially after cardioversion. Bradycardia following cardioversion in these patients is associated with QT_c interval prolongation which is augmented due to the reverse use dependence of the Class III effects of BETAPACE AF.™ Patients with AFIB/AFL associated with the sick sinus syndrome may be treated with BETAPACE AF™ if they have an implanted pacemaker for control of bradycardia symptoms.

Thyrotoxicosis: Beta-blockade may mask certain clinical signs (e.g., tachycardia) of hyperthyroidism. Patients suspected of developing thyrotoxicosis should be managed carefully to avoid abrupt withdrawal of beta-blockade which might be followed by an exacerbation of symptoms of hyperthyroidism, including thyroid storm. The beta-blocking effects of BETAPACE AF™ may be useful in controlling heart rate in AFIB associated with thyrotoxicosis but no study has been conducted to evaluate this.

PRECAUTIONS

RENAL IMPAIRMENT: BETAPACE AF™ (sotalol hydrochloride) is eliminated principally via the kidneys through glomerular filtration and to a small degree by tubular secretion. There is a direct relationship between renal function, as measured by serum creatinine or creatinine clearance, and the elimination rate of BETAPACE AF.™ Guidance for dosing in conditions of renal impairment can be found under "DOSAGE AND ADMINISTRATION".

Information for Patients:
Please refer to the patient package insert.
Prior to initiation of BETAPACE AF™ therapy, the patient should be advised to read the patient package insert and reread it each time therapy is renewed. The patient should be fully instructed on the need for compliance with the recommended dosing of BETAPACE AF,™ the potential interactions with drugs that prolong the QT interval and other antiarrhythmics, and the need for periodic monitoring of QT and renal function to minimize the risk of serious abnormal rhythms.

Medications and Supplements: Assessment of patients' medication history should include all over-counter, prescription and herbal/natural preparations with emphasis on preparations that may affect the pharmacodynamics of BETAPACE AF™ such as other cardiac antiarrhythmic drugs, some phenothiazines, cisapride, bepridil, tricyclic antidepressants and oral macrolides (See **WARNINGS and Use With Drugs That Prolong QT Interval and Antiarrhythmic Agents**). Patients should be instructed to notify their health care providers of any change in over-the-counter, prescription or supplement use. If a patient is hospitalized or is prescribed a new medication for any condition, the patient must inform the health care provider of ongoing BETAPACE AF™ therapy. Patients should also check with their health care provider and/or pharmacist prior to taking a new over-the-counter medicine.

Electrolyte Imbalance: If patients experience symptoms that may be associated with altered electrolyte balance, such as excessive or prolonged diarrhea, sweating, or vomiting, or loss of appetite or thirst, these conditions should be immediately reported to their health care provider.

Dosing Schedule: Patients should be instructed NOT to double the next dose if a dose is missed. The next dose should be taken at the usual time.

DRUG INTERACTIONS

Drugs undergoing CYP450 metabolism: Sotalol is primarily eliminated by renal excretion; therefore, drugs that are metabolized by CYP450 are not expected to alter the pharmacokinetics of sotalol.

Digoxin: Proarrhythmic events were more common in sotalol treated patients also receiving digoxin; it is not clear whether this represents an interaction or is related to the presence of CHF, a known risk factor for proarrhythmia, in the patients receiving digoxin.

Calcium blocking drugs: BETAPACE AF™ should be administered with caution in conjunction with calcium blocking drugs because of possible additive effects on atrioventricular conduction or ventricular function. Additionally, concomitant use of these drugs may have additive effects on blood pressure, possibly leading to hypotension.

Catecholamine-depleting agents: Concomitant use of catecholamine-depleting drugs, such as reserpine and guanethidine, with a beta-blocker may produce an excessive reduction of resting sympathetic nervous tone. Patients treated with BETAPACE AF™ plus a catecholamine depletor should therefore be closely monitored for evidence of hypotension and/or marked bradycardia which may produce syncope.

Insulin and oral antidiabetics: Hyperglycemia may occur, and the dosage of insulin or antidiabetic drugs may require adjustment. Symptoms of hypoglycemia may be masked.

Beta-2-receptor stimulants: Beta-agonists such as salbutamol, terbutaline and isoprenaline may have to be administered in increased dosages when used concomitantly with BETAPACE AF.™

Clonidine: Beta-blocking drugs may potentiate the rebound hypertension sometimes observed after discontinuation of clonidine; therefore, caution is advised when discontinuing clonidine in patients receiving BETAPACE AF.™

Other: No pharmacokinetic interactions were observed with hydrochloro-thiazide or warfarin.

Antacids: Administration of BETAPACE AF™ within 2 hours of antacids containing aluminum oxide and magne-

Table 7
Relationship Between QT_c Interval Prolongation and Torsade de Pointes

On-Therapy QT_c Interval (msec)	Incidence of Torsade de pointes	Change in QT_c Interval From Baseline (msec)	Incidence of Torsade de pointes
less than 500	1.3% (1787)	less than 65	1.6% (1516)
500–525	3.4% (236)	65–80	3.2% (158)
525–550	5.6% (125)	80–100	4.1% (146)
>550	10.8% (157)	100–130	5.2% (115)
		>130	7.1% (99)

( ) Number of patients assessed

sium hydroxide should be avoided because it may result in a reduction in Cmax and AUC of 26% and 20%, respectively and consequently in a 25% reduction in the bradycardic effect at rest. Administration of the antacid two hours after BETAPACE AF™ has no effect on the pharmacokinetics or pharmacodynamics of sotalol.

Drug/Laboratory Test Interactions

The presence of sotalol in the urine may result in falsely elevated levels of urinary metanephrine when measured by fluorimetric or photometric methods. In screening patients suspected of having a pheochromocytoma and being treated with sotalol, a specific method, such as a high performance liquid chromatographic assay with solid phase extraction (e.g., J. Chromatogr. 385:241, 1987) should be employed in determining levels of catecholamines.

Carcinogenesis, Mutagenesis, Impairment of Fertility: No evidence of carcinogenic potential was observed in rats during a 24-month study at 137–275 mg/kg/day (approximately 30 times the maximum recommended human oral dose (MRHD) as mg/kg or 5 times the MRHD as mg/m^2) or in mice, during a 24-month study at 4141–7122 mg/kg/ day (approximately 450–750 times the MRHD as mg/kg or 36–63 times the MRHD as mg/m^2).

Sotalol has not been evaluated in any specific assay of mutagenicity or clastogenicity.

No significant reduction in fertility occurred in rats at oral doses of 1000 mg/kg/day (approximately 100 times the MRHD as mg/kg or 9 times the MRHD as mg/m^2) prior to mating, except for a small reduction in the number of offspring per litter.

Pregnancy Category B: Reproduction studies in rats and rabbits during organo-genesis at 100 and 22 times the MRHD as mg/kg (9 and 7 times the MRHD as mg/m^2), respectively, did not reveal any teratogenic potential associated with sotalol HCl. In rabbits, a high dose of sotalol HCl (160 mg/kg/day) at 16 times the MRHD as mg/kg (6 times the MRHD as mg/m^2) produced a slight increase in fetal death likely due to maternal toxicity. Eight times the maximum dose (80 mg/kg/day or 3 times the MRHD as mg/m^2) did not result in an increased incidence of fetal deaths. In rats, 1000 mg/kg/day sotalol HCl, 100 times the MRHD (18 times the MRHD as mg/m^2), increased the number of early resorptions, while at 14 times the maximum dose (2.5 times the MRHD as mg/m^2), no increase in early resorptions was noted. However, animal reproduction studies are not always predictive of human response.

Although there are no adequate and well-controlled studies in pregnant women, sotalol HCl has been shown to cross the placenta, and is found in amniotic fluid. There has been a report of subnormal birth weight with sotalol. Therefore, BETAPACE AF™ should be used during pregnancy only if the potential benefit outweighs the potential risk.

Nursing Mothers: Sotalol is excreted in the milk of laboratory animals and has been reported to be present in human milk. Because of the potential for adverse reactions in nursing infants from BETAPACE AF,™ a decision should be made whether to discontinue nursing or to discontinue the drug, taking into account the importance of the drug to the mother.

Pediatric Use: The safety and effectiveness of BETAPACE AF™ in children have not been established.

ADVERSE REACTIONS

Adverse events that are clearly related to BETAPACE AF™ are those which are typical of its Class II (beta-blocking) and Class III (cardiac action potential duration prolongation) effects. The common documented beta-blocking adverse events (bradycardia, dyspnea, and fatigue) and Class III effects (QT interval prolongation) are dose related.

In a pooled clinical trial population consisting of four placebo-controlled studies with 275 patients with AFIB/AFL treated with 160–320 mg doses of BETAPACE AF,™ the following adverse events were reported at a rate of 2% or more in the 160–240 mg treated patients and greater than the rate in placebo patients (See Table 8). The data are presented by incidence of events in the BETAPACE AF™ and placebo groups by body system and daily dose. No significant irreversible non-cardiac end-organ toxicity was observed.

[See table 8 above]

Overall, discontinuation because of unacceptable adverse events was necessary in 17% of the patients, and occurred in 10% of patients less than two weeks after starting treatment. The most common adverse events leading to discontinuation of BETAPACE AF™ were: fatigue 4.6%, bradycardia 2.4%, proarrhythmia 2.2%, dyspnea 2%, and QT interval prolongation 1.4%.

In clinical trials involving 1292 patients with sustained VT/VF, the common adverse events (occurring in ≥ 2% of patients) were similar to those described for the AFIB/AFL population.

Occasional reports of elevated serum liver enzymes have occurred with sotalol therapy but no cause and effect relationship has been established. One case of peripheral neuropathy which resolved on discontinuation of sotalol and recurred when the patient was rechallenged with the drug was reported in an early dose tolerance study. Elevated blood glucose levels and increased insulin requirements can occur in diabetic patients.

Potential Adverse Effects

Foreign marketing experience with sotalol hydrochloride shows an adverse experience profile similar to that described above from clinical trials. Voluntary reports since introduction also include rare reports of: emotional lability, slightly clouded sensorium, incoordination, vertigo, paralysis, thrombocytopenia, eosinophilia, leukopenia, photosensitivity reaction, fever, pulmonary edema, hyperlipidemia, myalgia, pruritus, alopecia.

The oculomucocutaneous syndrome associated with the beta-blocker practolol has not been associated with BETAPACE AF™ during investigational use and foreign marketing experience.

Table 8
Incidence (%) of Common Adverse Events (≥2% in the 160–240 mg group and more frequent than on placebo) in Four Placebo-Controlled Studies of Patients with AFIB/AFL

Body System/ Adverse Event (Preferred Term)	Placebo N=282	Betapace AF™ Total Daily Dose 160–240 N=153	Betapace AF™ Total Daily Dose >240–320 N=122
CARDIOVASCULAR			
Abnormality ECG	0.4	3.3	2.5
Angina Pectoris	1.1	2.0	1.6
Bradycardia	2.5	13.1	12.3
Chest pain Cardiac/Non-Anginal	4.6	4.6	2.5
Disturbance Rhythm Atrial	2.1	2.0	1.6
Disturbance Rhythm Subjective	9.9	9.8	7.4
GASTROINTESTINAL			
Appetite Decreased	0.4	2.0	1.6
Diarrhea	2.1	5.2	5.7
Distention Abdomen	0.4	0.7	2.5
Dyspepsia/Heartburn	1.8	2.0	2.5
Nausea/Vomiting	5.3	7.8	5.7
Pain Abdomen	2.5	3.9	2.5
GENERAL			
Fatigue	8.5	19.6	18.9
Fever	0.7	0.7	3.3
Hyperhidrosis	3.2	5.2	4.9
Influenza	0.4	2.0	0.8
Sensation Cold	0.7	2.0	2.5
Weakness	3.2	5.2	4.9
MUSCULOSKELETAL/CONNECTIVE TISSUE			
Pain Chest Musculoskeletal	1.4	2.0	2.5
Pain Musculoskeletal	2.8	2.6	4.1
NERVOUS SYSTEM			
Dizziness	12.4	16.3	13.1
Headache	5.3	3.3	11.5
Insomnia	1.1	2.6	4.1
RESPIRATORY			
Cough	2.5	3.3	2.5
Dyspnea	7.4	9.2	9.8
Infection Upper Respiratory	1.1	2.6	3.3
Tracheobronchitis	0.7	0.7	3.3
SPECIAL SENSES			
Disturbance Vision	0.7	2.6	0.8

$$\text{creatinine clearance (male)} = \frac{(140\text{-age}) \times \text{body weight in kg}}{72 \times \text{serum creatinine (mg/dL)}}$$

$$\text{creatinine clearance (female)} = \frac{(140\text{-age}) \times \text{body weight in kg} \times 0.85}{72 \times \text{serum creatinine (mg/dL)}}$$

OVERDOSAGE

Intentional or accidental overdosage with sotalol has rarely resulted in death.

Symptoms and Treatment of Overdosage: The most common signs to be expected are bradycardia, congestive heart failure, hypotension, bronchospasm and hypoglycemia. In cases of massive intentional overdosage (2–16 grams) of sotalol the following clinical findings were seen: hypotension, bradycardia, cardiac asystole, prolongation of QT interval, torsade de pointes, ventricular tachycardia, and premature ventricular complexes. If overdosage occurs, therapy with BETAPACE AF™ should be discontinued and the patient observed closely. Because of the lack of protein binding, hemodialysis is useful for reducing sotalol plasma concentrations. Patients should be carefully observed until QT intervals are normalized and the heart rate returns to levels >50 bpm. The occurrence of hypotension following an overdose may be associated with an initial slow drug elimination phase (half life of 30 hours) thought to be due to a temporary reduction of renal function caused by the hypotension. In addition, if required, the following therapeutic measures are suggested:

Bradycardia or Cardiac Asystole:	Atropine, another anticholinergic drug, a beta-adrenergic agonist or transvenous cardiac pacing.
Heart Block:	(second and third degree) transvenous cardiac pacemaker.
Hypotension:	(depending on associated factors) epinephrine rather than isoproterenol or norepinephrine may be useful.
Bronchospasm:	Aminophylline or aerosol beta-2-receptor stimulant.
Torsade de pointes:	DC cardioversion, transvenous cardiac pacing, epinephrine, magnesium sulfate.

DOSAGE AND ADMINISTRATION

- Therapy with BETAPACE AF™ must be initiated (and, if necessary, titrated) in a setting that provides continuous electrocardiographic (ECG) monitoring and in the presence of personnel trained in the management of serious ventricular arrhythmias. Patients should continue to be monitored in this way for a minimum of 3 days on the maintenance dose. In addition, patients should not be discharged within 12 hours of electrical or pharmacological conversion to normal sinus rhythm.
- The QT interval is used to determine patient eligibility for BETAPACE AF™ treatment and for monitoring safety during treatment. The baseline QT interval must be ≤450 msec in order for a patient to be started on BETAPACE AF™ therapy. During initiation and titration, the QT interval should be monitored 2–4 hours after each dose. If the QT interval prolongs to 500 msec or greater, the dose must be reduced or the drug discontinued.
- **The dose of BETAPACE AF™ must be individualized according to calculated creatinine clearance.** In patients with a creatinine clearance >60 mL/min BETAPACE AF™ is administered twice daily (BID) while in those with a creatinine clearance between 40 and 60 mL/min, the dose is administered once daily (QD). In patients with a creatinine clearance less than 40 mL/min BETAPACE AF™ is contraindicated. The recommended initial dose of BETAPACE AF™ is 80 mg and is initiated as shown in the dosing algorithm described below. The 80 mg dose can be titrated upward to 120 mg during initial hospitalization or after discharge on 80 mg in the event of recurrence, by rehospitalization and repeating the same steps used during the initiation of therapy **(See Upward Titration of Dose)**.
- Patients with atrial fibrillation should be anticoagulated according to usual medical practice. Hypokalemia should be corrected before initiation of BETAPACE AF™ therapy **(See WARNINGS, Ventricular Arrhythmia)**.
- Patients to be discharged on BETAPACE AF™ therapy from an in-patient setting should have an adequate supply of BETAPACE AF,™ to allow uninterrupted therapy until the patient can fill a BETAPACE AF™ prescription.

Continued on next page

Information on the Berlex products appearing here is based on the most current information available at the time of publication closing. Further information for these and other products may be obtained from the Medical Affairs Department, Berlex Laboratories, 300 Fairfield Road, Wayne, New Jersey 07470, 1-888-BERLEX-4. Information on Betaseron and Fludara may be obtained from Berlex Laboratories, 15049 San Pablo Avenue, Richmond, California 94804-0016, 1-800-888-4112.

Betapace AF—Cont.

Initiation of BETAPACE AF™ Therapy

Step 1. Electrocardiographic assessment: Prior to administration of the first dose, the QT interval must be determined using an average of 5 beats. If the baseline QT is greater than 450 msec (JT ≥330 msec if QRS over 100 msec), BETAPACE AF™ is contraindicated.

Step 2: Calculation of creatinine clearance: Prior to the administration of the first dose, the patient's creatinine clearance should be calculated using the following formula: [See second table on previous page]

When serum creatinine is given in µmol/L, divide the value by 88.4 (1 mg/dL =88.4 µmol/L)

Step 3. Starting Dose: The starting dose of BETAPACE AF™ is 80 mg twice daily (BID) if the creatinine clearance is > 60 mL/min, and 80 mg once daily (QD) if the creatinine clearance is 40–60 mL/min. If the creatinine clearance is < 40 mL/min BETAPACE AF™ is contraindicated.

Step 4. Administer the appropriate daily dose of BETAPACE AF™ and begin continuous ECG monitoring with QT interval measurements 2–4 hours after each dose.

Step 5. If the 80 mg dose level is tolerated and the QT interval remains < 500 msec after at least 3 days (after 5 or 6 doses if patient receiving QD dosing), the patient can be discharged. Alternatively, during hospitalization, the dose can be increased to 120 mg bid and the patient followed for 3 days on this dose (followed for 5 or 6 doses if patient receiving QD doses).

The steps described above are summarized in the following diagram:

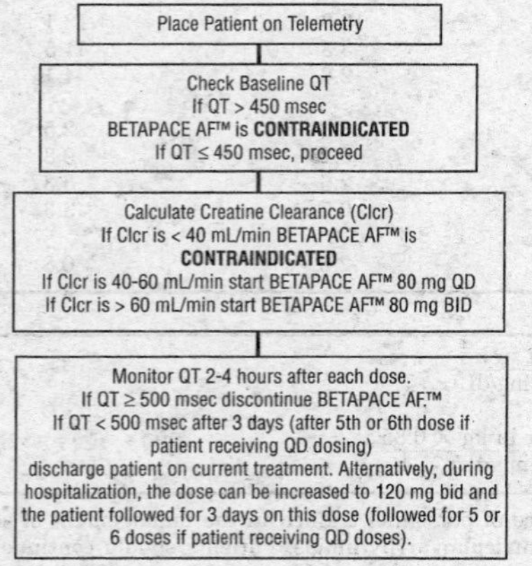

Place Patient on Telemetry
Check Baseline QT
If QT > 450 msec
BETAPACE AF™ is CONTRAINDICATED
If QT ≤ 450 msec, proceed
Calculate Creatine Clearance (Clcr)
If Clcr is < 40 mL/min BETAPACE AF™ is CONTRAINDICATED
If Clcr is 40-60 mL/min start BETAPACE AF™ 80 mg QD
If Clcr is > 60 mL/min start BETAPACE AF™ 80 mg BID
Monitor QT 2-4 hours after each dose.
If QT ≥ 500 msec discontinue BETAPACE AF™
If QT < 500 msec after 3 days (after 5th or 6th dose if patient receiving QD dosing)
discharge patient on current treatment. Alternatively, during hospitalization, the dose can be increased to 120 mg bid and the patient followed for 3 days on this dose (followed for 5 or 6 doses if patient receiving QD doses).

Upward Titration of Dose

If the 80 mg dose level (given BID or QD depending upon the creatinine clearance) does not reduce the frequency of relapses of AFIB/AFL and is tolerated without excessive QT interval prolongation (i.e. ≥ 520 msec), the dose level may be increased to 120 mg (BID or QD depending upon the creatinine clearance). As proarrhythmic events can occur not only at initiation of therapy, but also with each upward dosage adjustment, Steps 2 through 5 used during initiation of BETAPACE AF™ therapy should be followed when increasing the dose level. In the U.S. multicenter dose-response study, the 120 mg dose (BID or QD) was found to be the most effective in prolonging the time to ECG documented symptomatic recurrence of AFIB/AFL. If the 120 mg dose level does not reduce the frequency of early relapse of AFIB/AFL and is tolerated without excessive QT interval prolongation (≥520 msec), an increase to 160 mg (BID or QD depending upon the creatinine clearance), can be considered. Steps 2 through 5 used during the initiation of therapy should be used again to introduce such an increase.

Maintenance of BETAPACE AF™ Therapy

Renal function and QT should be re-evaluated regularly if medically warranted. If QT is 520 msec or greater (JT 430 msec or greater if QRS is > 100 msec), the dose of BETAPACE AF™ therapy should be reduced and patients should be carefully monitored until QT returns to less than 520 msec. If the QT interval is ≥ 520 msec while on the lowest maintenance dose level (80 mg) the drug should be discontinued. If renal function deteriorates, reduce the daily dose in half by administering the drug once daily as described in **Initiation of BETAPACE AF™ Therapy, Step 3.**

Special Considerations

The maximum recommended dose in patients with a calculated creatinine clearance greater than 60 mL/min is 160 mg BID, doses greater than 160mg BID have been associated with an increased incidence of torsades the pointes and are not recommended.

A patient who misses a dose should NOT double the next dose. The next dose should be taken at the usual time.

Transfer to BETAPACE AF™ from BETAPACE®

Patients with a history of symptomatic AFIB/AFL who are currently receiving BETAPACE® for the maintenance of normal sinus should be transferred to BETAPACE AF™ because of the significant differences in labeling (i.e., patient package insert, dosing administration, and safety information).

Transfer to BETAPACE AF™ from Other Antiarrhythmic Agents

Before starting BETAPACE AF,™ previous antiarrhythmic therapy should generally be withdrawn under careful monitoring for a minimum of 2–3 plasma half-lives if the patient's clinical condition permits (See **DRUG INTERACTIONS**). Treatment has been initiated in some patients receiving I.V. lidocaine without ill effect. After discontinuation of amiodarone, BETAPACE AF™ should not be initiated until the QT interval is normalized (See **WARNINGS**).

HOW SUPPLIED

BETAPACE AF™ (sotalol hydrochloride); capsule-shaped white scored tablets imprinted with the strength and "BERLEX" are available as follows:

NDC 50419-115-06 80 mg strength, bottle of 60 in unit use package
NDC 50419-115-11 80 mg strength, carton of 100 unit dose
NDC 50419-119-06 120 mg strength, bottle of 60 in unit use package
NDC 50419-119-11 120 mg strength, carton of 100 unit dose
NDC 50419-116-06 160 mg strength, bottle of 60 in unit use package
NDC 50419-116-11 160 mg strength, carton of 100 unit dose

Store at 25°C with excursions permitted between 15°–30°C.
Rx only

Manufactured by:
BERLEX® Laboratories, Wayne, NJ 07470
6072200 February 2000

Shown in Product Identification Guide, page 308

CLIMARA® ℞

[*clī-măr ′-a*]

estradiol transdermal system

Continuous Delivery for Once Weekly Application

PRESCRIBING INFORMATION

1. ESTROGENS HAVE BEEN REPORTED TO INCREASE THE RISK OF ENDOMETRIAL CARCINOMA IN POSTMENOPAUSAL WOMEN. Close clinical surveillance of all women taking estrogens is important. Adequate diagnostic measures, including endometrial sampling when indicated, should be undertaken to rule out malignancy in all cases of undiagnosed persistent or recurring abnormal vaginal bleeding. There is currently no evidence that "natural" estrogens are more or less hazardous than "synthetic" estrogens at equi-estrogenic doses.

2. ESTROGENS SHOULD NOT BE USED DURING PREGNANCY.

Estrogen therapy during pregnancy is associated with an increased risk of congenital defects in the reproductive organs of the fetus, and possibly other birth defects. Studies of women who received diethylstilbestrol (DES) during pregnancy have shown that female offspring have an increased risk of vaginal adenosis, squamous cell dysplasia of the uterine cervix, and clear cell vaginal cancer later in life; male offspring have an increased risk of urogenital abnormalities and possibly testicular cancer later in life. The 1985 DES Task Force concluded that use of DES during pregnancy is associated with a subsequent increased risk of breast cancer in the mothers, although a causal relationship remains unproven and the observed level of excess risk is similar to that for a number of other breast cancer risk factors.

There is no indication for estrogen therapy during pregnancy or during the immediate postpartum period. Estrogens are ineffective for the prevention or treatment of threatened or habitual abortion. Estrogens are not indicated for the prevention of postpartum breast engorgement.

DESCRIPTION

Climara®, estradiol transdermal system, is designed to release 17β-estradiol continuously upon application to intact skin. Four (6.5, 12.5, 18.75 and 25.0 cm²) systems are available to provide nominal *in vivo* delivery of 0.025, 0.05, 0.075 or 0.1 mg respectively of estradiol per day. The period of use is 7 days. Each system has a contact surface area of either 6.5, 12.5, 18.75 or 25.0 cm², and contains 2.0, 3.8, 5.7 or 7.6 mg of estradiol USP respectively. The composition of the systems per unit area is identical.

Estradiol USP (17β-estradiol) is a white, crystalline powder, chemically described as estra-1,3,5(10)-triene-3,17β-diol. It has an empirical formula of $C_{18}H_{24}O_2$ and molecular weight of 272.37. The structural formula is:

[Structural formula: H_3C, OH, H, H, H, HO]

The Climara® system comprises two layers. Proceeding from the visible surface toward the surface attached to the skin, these layers are (1) a translucent polyethylene film, and (2) an acrylate adhesive matrix containing estradiol USP. A protective liner (3) of siliconized or fluoropolymer-coated polyester film is attached to the adhesive surface and must be removed before the system can be used.

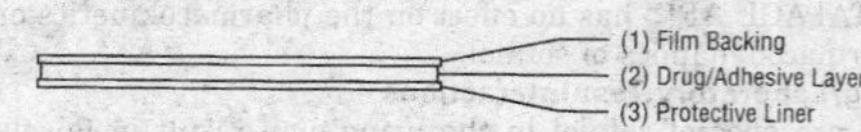

The active component of the system is 17β-estradiol. The remaining components of the system (acrylate copolymer adhesive, fatty acid esters, and polyethylene backing) are pharmacologically inactive.

CLINICAL PHARMACOLOGY

The Climara® system provides systemic estrogen replacement therapy by releasing 17β-estradiol, the major estrogenic hormone secreted by the human ovary.

Estrogens are largely responsible for the development and maintenance of the female reproductive system and secondary sexual characteristics. Although circulating estrogens exist in a dynamic equilibrium of metabolic interconversions, estradiol is the principal intracellular human estrogen and is substantially more potent than its metabolites, estrone and estriol, at the receptor level. The primary source of estrogen in normally cycling adult women is the ovarian follicle, which secretes 70 to 500 µg of estradiol daily, depending on the phase of the menstrual cycle. After menopause, most endogenous estrogen is produced by conversion of androstenedione, secreted by the adrenal cortex, to estrone by peripheral tissues. Thus, estrone and the sulfate conjugated form, estrone sulfate, are the most abundant circulating estrogens in postmenopausal women.

Circulating estrogens modulate the pituitary secretion of the gonadotropins. Luteinizing hormone (LH) and follicle stimulating hormone (FSH) through negative feedback mechanism and estrogen replacement therapy acts to reduce the elevated levels of these hormones seen in postmenopausal women.

A two-year clinical trial enrolled a total of 175 healthy, hysterectomized, postmenopausal, non-osteoporotic (i.e., lumbar spine bone mineral density > 0.9 gm/cm²) women at 10 study centers in the United States. 129 subjects were allocated to receive active treatment with 4 different doses of 17β-estradiol patches (6.5, 12.5, 15, 25 cm²) and 46 subjects were allocated to receive placebo patches. 77% of the randomized subjects (100 on active drug and 34 on placebo) contributed data to the analysis of percent change of A-P spine bone mineral density (BMD), the primary efficacy variable (see Figure 1). A statistically significant overall treatment effect at each timepoint was noted, implying bone preservation for all active treatment groups at all timepoints, as opposed to bone loss for placebo at all timepoints.

Figure 1
Mean Percent Change from Baseline in Lumbar Spine (A-P View) Bone Mineral Density by Treatment and Time last observation carried forward

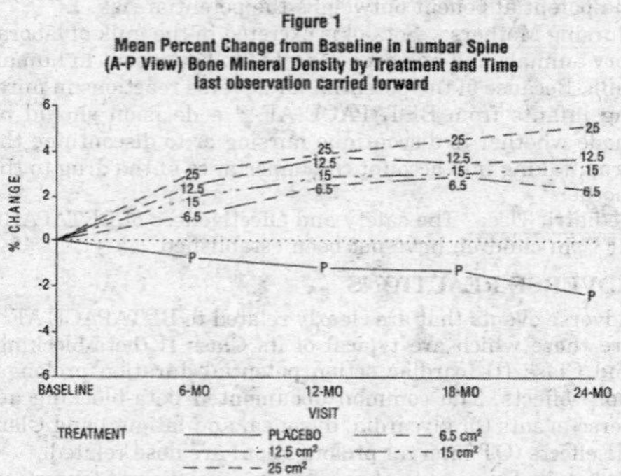

Percent change in BMD of the total hip (see Figure 2), was also statistically significantly different from placebo for all active treatment groups. The results of the measurements of biochemical markers supported the finding of efficacy for all doses of transdermal estradiol. Serum osteocalcin levels decreased, indicative of a decrease in bone formation, at all timepoints for all active treatment doses, statistically significantly different from placebo (which generally rose). Urinary deoxypyridinoline and pyridinoline changes also suggested a decrease in bone turnover for all active treatment groups.

Figure 2
Mean Percent Change from Baseline in Total Hip by Treatment and Time last observation carried forward

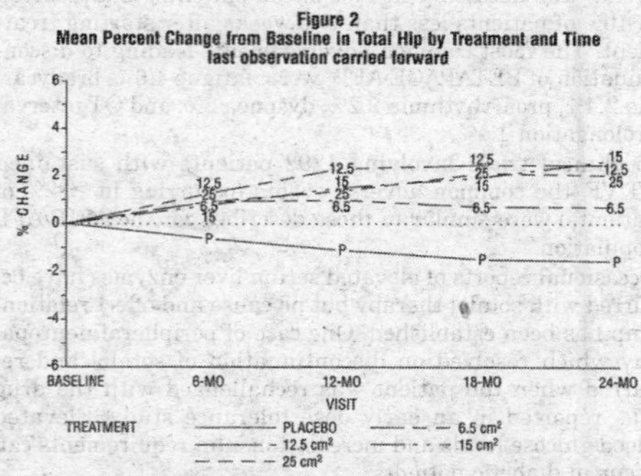

Footnote: This figure is based on 74% of the randomized subjects (95 on active drug and 34 on placebo).

PHARMACOKINETICS

Transdermal administration of Climara® produces mean serum concentrations of estradiol comparable to those produced by premenopausal women in the early follicular phase of the ovulatory cycle. The pharmacokinetics of estradiol following application of the Climara® system were investigated in 197 healthy postmenopausal women in six studies. In five of the studies Climara® system was applied to the abdomen and in a sixth study application to the buttocks and abdomen were compared.

Absorption: The Climara® transdermal delivery system continuously releases estradiol which is transported across intact skin leading to sustained circulating levels of estradiol during 7 day treatment period. The systemic availability of estradiol after transdermal administration is about 20 times higher than that after oral administration. This difference is due to the absence of first pass metabolism when estradiol is given by the transdermal route.

The bioavailability of Climara® was determined in two single dose studies after 1 week application of the Climara® system versus two consecutive 3 day and 4 day applications of the Estraderm® system. Mean estradiol serum concentrations observed during the treatment of the 25.0 and 12.5 cm^2 Climara® systems versus the 20 and 10 cm^2 Estraderm® systems are shown in Figures 3 and 4, respectively. Both sizes of Climara® maintained significantly lower peak and mean steady state estradiol levels than did the Estraderm® system; however, towards the end of each treatment period, the Climara® system maintained similar (day 6) or higher (day 7) serum estradiol levels than did the Estraderm® system. The fluctuation index with the Climara® system was 1/4 to 1/3 the fluctuation index observed with Estraderm.® However, this has not been shown to be clinically significant.

Figure 3

Observed Mean (± S.E.) Estradiol Serum Concentrations for a One Week Application of the Climara® system (25 cm²) and Consecutive Three Day and Four Day Application of the Estraderm® System (20 cm²) in 24 postmenopausal women

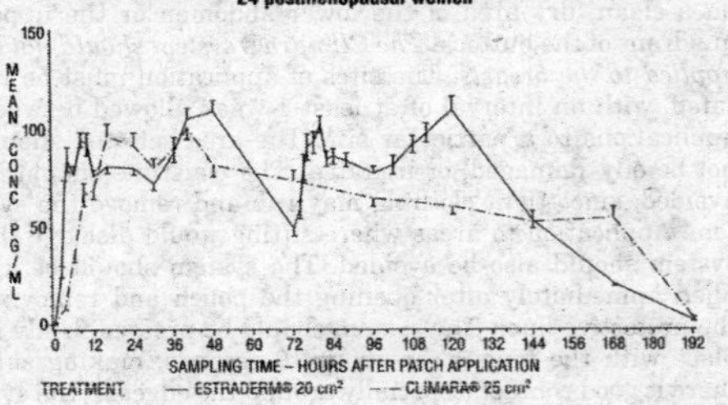

Figure 4

Observed Mean (± S.E.) Estradiol Serum Concentrations for a One Week Application of the Climara® system (12.5 cm²) and Consecutive Three Day and Four Day Application of the Estraderm® System (10 cm²) in 24 postmenopausal women

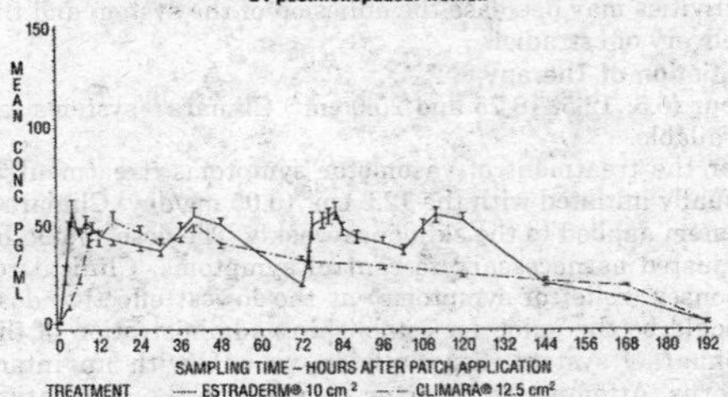

In a third bioavailability study, the Climara 6.5 cm^2 was studied with the Climara 12.5 cm^2 as reference. The mean estradiol levels in serum from the 2 sizes are shown in Figure 5.

Figure 5

Mean Serum 17β-Estradiol Concentrations vs. Time Profile following Application of a 6.5 cm² Transdermal Patch and Application of a 12.5 cm² Climara patch

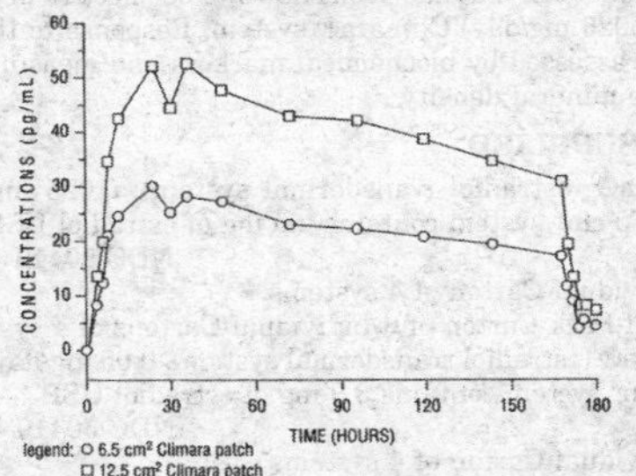

Dose proportionality was demonstrated for the Climara 6.5 cm^2 patch as compared to the Climara 12.5 cm^2 patch in a 2 week crossover study with a one week washout period between the two patches in 24 postmenopausal women.

Dose proportionality was also demonstrated for the Climara® system (12.5 cm^2 and 25 cm^2) in a 1 week study conducted in 54 postmenopausal women. The mean steady state levels (Cavg) of the estradiol during the application of Climara 25 cm^2 and 12.5 cm^2 on the abdomen were about 80 and 40 pg/mL, respectively.

In a 3 week multiple application study in 24 postmenopausal women, the 25.0 cm^2 Climara® system produced average peak estradiol concentrations (Cmax) of approximately 100 pg/mL. Trough values at the end of each wear interval (Cmin) were approximately 35 pg/mL. Nearly identical serum curves were seen each week, indicating little or no accumulation of estradiol in the body. Serum estrone peak and trough levels were 60 and 40 pg/mL, respectively.

Table 1
Pharmacokinetic Summary (Mean Estradiol Values)

Climara® Delivery Rate	Surface Area (cm^2)	Application Site	No. of Subjects	Dosing	Cmax (pg/mL)	Cmin (pg/mL)	Cavg (pg/mL)
0.025	6.5	Abdomen	24	Single	32	17	22
0.05	12.5	Abdomen	102	Single	71	29	41
0.1	25	Abdomen	139	Single	147	60	87
0.1	25	Buttock	38	Single	174	71	106

In a single dose randomized crossover study conducted to compare the effect of site of application, 38 postmenopausal women wore a single Climara® 25 cm^2 system for 1 week on the abdomen and buttocks. The estradiol serum concentration profiles are shown in Figure 6. Cmax and Cavg values were, respectively, 25% and 17% higher with the buttock application than with the abdomen application.

Figure 6

Observed Mean (± S.E.) Estradiol Serum Concentrations for a One Week Application of the Climara® system (25 cm²) to the abdomen and buttocks of 38 postmenopausal women

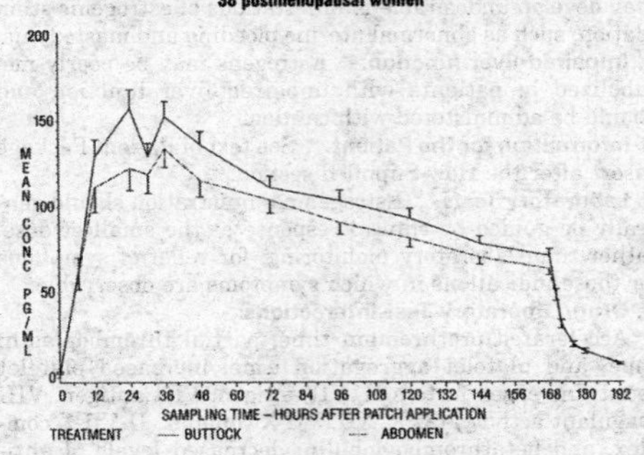

Table 1 provides a summary of estradiol pharmacokinetic parameters determined during evaluation of Climara®.

[See table 1 above]

The relative standard deviation of each pharmacokinetic parameter after application to the abdomen averaged 50%, which is indicative of the considerable intersubject variability associated with transdermal drug delivery. The relative standard deviation of each pharmacokinetic parameter after application to the buttock was lower than that after application to the abdomen (e.g., for Cmax 39% vs 62%, and for Cavg 35% vs 48%).

Distribution: The distribution of exogenous estrogens is similar to that of endogenous estrogens. Estrogens are widely distributed in the body and are generally found in higher concentrations in the sex hormone target organs. Estradiol and other naturally occurring estrogens are bound mainly to sex hormone binding globulin (SHBG), and to lesser degree to albumin.

Metabolism: Exogenous estrogens are metabolized in the same manner as endogenous estrogens. Circulating estrogens exist in a dynamic equilibrium of metabolic interconversions. These transformations take place mainly in the liver. Estradiol is converted reversibly to estrone, and both can be converted to estriol, which is the major urinary metabolite. Estrogens also undergo enterohepatic recirculation via sulfate and glucuronide conjugation in the liver, biliary secretion of conjugates into the intestine, and hydrolysis in the gut followed by reabsorption. In postmenopausal women a significant portion of the circulating estrogens exist as sulfate conjugates, especially estrone sulfate, which serves as a circulating reservoir for the formation of more active estrogens.

Excretion: Estradiol, estrone and estriol are excreted in the urine along with glucuronide and sulfate conjugates. After removal of the Climara® system, serum estradiol levels decline in about 12 hours to preapplication levels with an apparent half life of approximately 4 hours.

Special populations:

Race: There is no available information to establish the relevance of race for the absorption and pharmacokinetics of estradiol following transdermal application.

Patients with Renal Impairment: Total estradiol serum levels are higher in postmenopausal women with end stage renal disease (ESRD) receiving maintenance hemodialysis than in normal subjects at baseline and following oral doses of estradiol. Therefore, conventional transdermal estradiol doses used in individuals with normal renal function may be excessive for postmenopausal women with ESRD receiving maintenance hemodialysis.

Patients with Hepatic Impairment: Estrogens may be poorly metabolized in patients with impaired liver function and should be administered with caution.

INDICATIONS AND USAGE

Climara® is indicated in the:

1. Treatment of moderate to severe vasomotor symptoms associated with the menopause. There is no adequate evidence that estrogens are effective for nervous symptoms or depression which might occur during menopause and they should not be used to treat these conditions.
2. Treatment of vulval and vaginal atrophy.
3. Treatment of hypoestrogenism due to hypogonadism, castration or primary ovarian failure.
4. Treatment of abnormal uterine bleeding due to hormonal imbalance in the absence of organic pathology and only when associated with a hypoplastic or atrophic endometrium.
5. Prevention of Postmenopausal Osteoporosis (loss of bone mass). The mainstays of prevention of postmenopausal osteoporosis are estrogen, an adequate lifetime calcium and vitamin D intake, and exercise.

Estrogen replacement therapy reduces bone resorption and retards or halts postmenopausal bone loss. Case-controlled studies have shown an approximately 60% reduction in hip and wrist fractures in women whose estrogen replacement was begun within a few years of menopause. Studies also suggest that estrogen reduces the rate of vertebral fractures. Even when started as late as 6 years after menopause, estrogen prevents further loss of bone mass for as long as treatment is continued. When estrogen therapy is discontinued, bone mass declines at a rate comparable to the immediate postmenopausal period.

CONTRAINDICATIONS

Estrogens should not be used in individuals with any of the following conditions:

1. Known or suspected pregnancy (see Boxed Warning). Estrogens may cause fetal harm when administered to a pregnant woman.
2. Undiagnosed abnormal genital bleeding.
3. Known or suspected cancer of the breast except in appropriately selected patients being treated for metastatic disease.
4. Known or suspected estrogendependent neoplasia.
5. Active thrombophlebitis or thromboembolic disorders.

WARNINGS

1. Induction of malignant neoplasms.

Endometrial cancer. The reported endometrial cancer risk among unopposed estrogen users is about 2- to 12-fold greater than in nonusers, and appears dependent on duration of treatment and on estrogen dose. Most studies show no significant increased risk associated with use of estrogens for less than one year. The greatest risk appears associated with prolonged use—with increased risks of 15- to 24-fold for five to ten years or more. In three studies, persistence of risk was demonstrated for 8 to over 15 years after cessation of estrogen treatment. In one study a significant decrease in the incidence of endometrial cancer occurred six months after estrogen withdrawal. Concurrent progestin therapy may offset this risk but the overall health impact in postmenopausal women is not known (see Precautions).

Breast Cancer. While the majority of studies have not shown an increased risk of breast cancer in women who have ever used estrogen replacement therapy, some have reported a moderately increased risk (relative risks of 1.3–2.0) in those taking higher doses or those taking lower doses for prolonged periods of time, especially in excess of 10 years.

Congenital lesions with malignant potential. Estrogen therapy during pregnancy is associated with an increased risk of fetal congenital reproductive tract disorders, and possibly other birth defects. Studies of women who received DES during pregnancy have shown that female offspring have an increased risk of vaginal adenosis, squamous cell dysplasia of the uterine cervix, and clear cell vaginal cancer later in life; male offspring have an increased risk of urogenital abnormalities and possibly testicular cancer later in life. Although some of these changes are benign, others are precursors of malignancy.

2. Gallbladder disease. Two studies have reported a 2- to 4-fold increase in the risk of gallbladder disease requiring surgery in women receiving postmenopausal estrogens.

3. Cardiovascular disease. Large doses of estrogen (5 mg conjugated estrogens per day), comparable to those used to

Continued on next page

Information on the Berlex products appearing here is based on the most current information available at the time of publication closing. Further information for these and other products may be obtained from the Medical Affairs Department, Berlex Laboratories, 300 Fairfield Road, Wayne, New Jersey 07470, 1-888-BERLEX-4. Information on Betaseron and Fludara may be obtained from Berlex Laboratories, 15049 San Pablo Avenue, Richmond, California 94804-0016, 1-800-888-4112.

Climara—Cont.

treat cancer of the prostate and breast, have been shown in a large prospective clinical trial in men to increase the risks of nonfatal myocardial infarction, pulmonary embolism, and thrombophlebitis. These risks cannot necessarily be extrapolated from men to women. However, to avoid the theoretical cardiovascular risk to women caused by high estrogen doses, the dose for estrogen replacement therapy should not exceed the lowest effective dose.

4. **Elevated blood pressure.** Occasional blood pressure increases during estrogen replacement therapy have been attributed to idiosyncratic reactions to estrogens. More often, blood pressure has remained the same or has dropped. One study showed that postmenopausal estrogen users have higher blood pressure than nonusers. Two other studies showed slightly lower blood pressure among estrogen users compared to nonusers. Postmenopausal estrogen use does not increase the risk of stroke. Nonetheless, blood pressure should be monitored at regular intervals with estrogen use. Ethinyl estradiol and conjugated estrogens have been shown to increase renin substrate. In contrast to these oral estrogens, transdermally administered estradiol has been reported not to affect renin substrate.

5. **Hypercalcemia.** Administration of estrogens may lead to severe hypercalcemia in patients with breast cancer and bone metastases. If this occurs, the drug should be stopped and appropriate measures taken to reduce the serum calcium level.

PRECAUTIONS

A. General

1. Addition of a progestin. Studies of the addition of a progestin for 10 or more days of a cycle of estrogen administration have reported a lowered incidence of endometrial hyperplasia than would be induced by estrogen treatment alone. Morphological and biochemical studies of endometria suggest that 10 to 14 days of progestin are needed to provide maximal maturation of the endometrium and to reduce the likelihood of hyperplastic changes.

There are, however, possible risks that may be associated with the use of progestins in estrogen replacement regimens. These include: (1) adverse effects on lipoprotein metabolism (lowering HDL and raising LDL) which could diminish the purported cardioprotective effect of estrogen therapy (see Precautions D.4., below); (2) impairment of glucose tolerance; and (3) possible enhancement of mitotic activity in breast epithelial tissue, although few epidemiological data are available to address this point (see Precautions below). The choice of progestin, its dose, and its regimen may be important in minimizing these adverse effects, but these issues will require further study before they are clarified.

2. Cardiovascular risk. *A causal relationship between estrogen replacement therapy and reduction of cardiovascular disease in postmenopausal women has not been proven. Furthermore, the effect of added progestins on this putative benefit is not yet known.*

In recent years many published studies have suggested that there may be a cause-effect relationship between postmenopausal oral estrogen replacement therapy *without added progestins* and a decrease in cardiovascular disease in women. Although most of the observational studies that assessed this statistical association have reported a 20% to 50% reduction in coronary heart disease risk and associated mortality in estrogen takers, the following should be considered when interpreting these reports: (1) Because only one of these studies was randomized and it was too small to yield statistically significant results, all relevant studies were subject to selection bias. Thus, the apparently reduced risk of coronary artery disease cannot be attributed with certainty to estrogen replacement therapy. It may instead have been caused by lifestyle and medical characteristics of the women studied with the result that healthier women were selected for estrogen therapy. In general, treated women were of a higher socioeconomic and educational status, more slender, more physically active, more likely to have undergone surgical menopause, and less likely to have diabetes than the untreated women. Although some studies attempted to control for these selection factors, it is common for properly designed randomized trials to fail to confirm benefits suggested by less rigorous study designs. (2) Current medical practice often includes the use of concomitant progestin therapy with intact uteri (see PRECAUTIONS and WARNINGS). While the effects of added progestins on the risk of ischemic heart disease are not known, all available progestins reverse at least some of the favorable effects of estrogens on HDL and LDL levels. (3) While the effects of added progestins on the risk of breast cancer are also unknown, available epidemiological evidence suggests that progestins do not reduce, and may enhance, the moderately increased breast cancer incidence that has been reported with prolonged estrogen replacement therapy (see WARNINGS above).

Because relatively long-term use of estrogens by a woman with a uterus has been shown to induce endometrial cancer, physicians often recommend that women who are deemed candidates for hormone replacement should take progestins as well as estrogens. When considering prescribing concomitant estrogens and progestins for hormone replacement therapy, physicians and patients are advised to carefully weigh the potential benefits and risks of the added progestin. Large-scale randomized, placebo-controlled, prospective clinical trials are required to clarify these issues.

3. Physical examination. A complete medical and family history should be taken prior to the initiation of any estrogen therapy. The pretreatment and periodic physical examinations should include special reference to blood pressure, breasts, abdomen, and pelvic organs, and should include a Papanicolaou smear. As a general rule, estrogen should not be prescribed for longer than one year without reexamining the patient.

4. Hypercoagulability. Some studies have shown that women taking estrogen replacement therapy have hypercoagulability, primarily related to decreased anti-thrombin activity. This effect appears dose- and duration-dependent and is less pronounced than that associated with oral contraceptive use. Also, postmenopausal women tend to have increased coagulation parameters at baseline compared to premenopausal women. There is some suggestion that low dose postmenopausal mestranol may increase the risk of thromboembolism, although the majority of studies (of primarily conjugated estrogens users) report no such increase. There is insufficient information on hypercoagulability in women who have had previous thromboembolic disease.

5. Familial hyperlipoproteinemia. Estrogen therapy may be associated with massive elevations of plasma triglycerides leading to pancreatitis and other complications in patients with familial defects of lipoprotein metabolism.

6. Fluid retention. Because estrogens may cause some degree of fluid retention, conditions that might be exacerbated by this factor, such as asthma, epilepsy, migraine, and cardiac or renal dysfunction, require careful observation.

7. Uterine bleeding and mastodynia. Certain patients may develop undesirable manifestations of estrogenic stimulation, such as abnormal uterine bleeding and mastodynia.

8. Impaired liver function. Estrogens may be poorly metabolized in patients with impaired liver function and should be administered with caution.

B. Information for the Patient. See text of Patient Package Insert after the How Supplied section.

C. Laboratory Tests. Estrogen administration should generally be guided by clinical response at the smallest dose, rather than laboratory monitoring, for relief of symptoms for those indications in which symptoms are observable.

D. Drug/Laboratory Test Interactions.

1. Accelerated prothrombin time, partial thromboplastin time, and platelet aggregation time; increased platelet count; increased factors II, VII antigen, VIII antigen, VIII coagulant activity, IX, X, XII, VII-X complex, II-VII-X complex, and betathromboglobulin; decreased levels of antifactor Xa and antithrombin III, decreased antithrombin III activity; increased levels of fibrinogen and fibrinogen activity; increased plasminogen antigen and activity.
2. Increased thyroid-binding globulin (TBG) leading to increased circulating total thyroid hormone, as measured by protein-bound iodine (PBI), T4 levels (by column or by radioimmunoassay) or T3 levels by radioimmunoassay. T3 resin uptake is decreased, reflecting the elevated TBG. Free T4 and free T3 concentrations are unaltered.
3. Other binding proteins may be elevated in serum, i.e., corticosteroid binding globulin (CBG), sex hormone-binding globulin (SHBG), leading to increased circulating corticosteroids and sex steroids respectively. Free or biologically active hormone concentrations are unchanged. Other plasma proteins may be increased (angiotensinogen/renin substrate, alpha-1-antitrypsin, ceruloplasmin).
4. Increased plasma HDL and HDL-2 subfraction concentrations, reduced LDL cholesterol concentration, increased triglycerides levels.
5. Impaired glucose tolerance.
6. Reduced response to metyrapone test.
7. Reduced serum folate concentration.

E. Carcinogenesis, Mutagenesis, and Impairment of Fertility. See CONTRAINDICATIONS and WARNINGS. Long term continuous administration of natural and synthetic estrogens in certain animal species increases the frequency of carcinomas of the breast, uterus, cervix, vagina, testis, and liver.

F. Pregnancy Category X. See CONTRAINDICATIONS and BOXED WARNING. Estrogens should not be used during pregnancy.

G. Nursing Mothers. As a general principle, the administration of any drug to nursing mothers should be done only when clearly necessary since many drugs are excreted in human milk. In addition, estrogen administration to nursing mothers has been shown to decrease the quantity and quality of the milk.

ADVERSE REACTIONS

See WARNINGS and Boxed Warning regarding induction of neoplasia, adverse effects on the fetus, increased incidence of gallbladder disease, cardiovascular disease, elevated blood pressure, and hypercalcemia.

The most commonly reported adverse reaction to the Climara® system in clinical trials was skin irritation at the application site. In two well-controlled clinical studies, the overall rate of discontinuation due to skin irritation at the application site was 6.8%: 7.9% for the 12.5 cm^2 system and 5.3% for the 25.0 cm^2 system compared with 11.5% for the placebo system. Patients with known skin irritation to the patch were excluded from participation in the studies. In a 3-week comparative skin irritation study with the Estraderm® system, in 95 subjects, no statistically significant differences in irritation were observed. Some degree of irritation at the end of week three was seen in 25% of Estraderm® and 31% of Climara® subjects. Clinically significant irritation (mild erythema associated with symptoms or moderate to severe erythema) was evident at the end of week three in 11% of Estraderm® and 9% of Climara® subjects.

The following additional adverse reactions have been reported with estrogen therapy:

1. Genitourinary system.
Changes in vaginal bleeding pattern and abnormal withdrawal bleeding or flow, breakthrough bleeding, spotting. Increase in size of uterine leiomyomata. Vaginal candidiasis. Change in amount of cervical secretion.

2. Breasts.
Tenderness, enlargement.

3. Gastrointestinal.
Nausea, vomiting. Abdominal cramps, bloating. Cholestatic jaundice. Increased incidence of gallbladder disease.

4. Skin.
Chloasma or melasma that may persist when drug is discontinued. Erythema multiforme. Erythema nodosum. Hemorrhagic eruption. Loss of scalp hair. Hirsutism.

5. Eyes.
Steepening of corneal curvature. Intolerance to contact lenses.

6. Central Nervous System.
Headache, migraine, dizziness. Mental depression. Chorea.

7. Miscellaneous.
Increase or decrease in weight. Reduced carbohydrate tolerance. Aggravation of porphyria. Edema. Changes in libido.

OVERDOSAGE

Serious ill effects have not been reported following acute ingestion of large doses of estrogen-containing oral contraceptives by young children. Overdosage of estrogen may cause nausea and vomiting, and withdrawal bleeding may occur in females.

DOSAGE AND ADMINISTRATION

The adhesive side of the Climara® system should be placed on a clean, dry area of the lower abdomen or the upper quadrant of the buttock. *The Climara® system should not be applied to the breasts.* The sites of application must be rotated, with an interval of at least 1 week allowed between applications to a particular site. The area selected should not be oily, damaged, or irritated. The waistline should be avoided, since tight clothing may rub and remove the system. Application to areas where sitting would dislodge the system should also be avoided. The system should be applied immediately after opening the pouch and removing the protective liner. The system should be pressed firmly in place with the fingers for about 10 seconds, making sure there is good contact, especially around the edges. If the system lifts, apply pressure to maintain adhesion. In the event that a system should fall off, a new system should be applied for the remainder of the 7-day dosing interval. Only one system should be worn at any one time during the 7-day dosing interval. Swimming, bathing, or using a sauna while using the Climara® system has not been studied, and these activities may decrease the adhesion of the system and the delivery of estradiol.

Initiation of Therapy

Four (6.5, 12.5, 18.75 and 25.0 cm^2) Climara® systems are available.

For the treatment of vasomotor symptoms, treatment is usually initiated with the 12.5 cm^2 (0.05 mg/day) Climara® system applied to the skin once-weekly. The dose should be adjusted as necessary to control symptoms. Clinical responses (relief of symptoms) at the lowest effective dose should be the guide for establishing administration of the Climara® system, especially in women with an intact uterus. Attempts to taper or discontinue the medication should be made at 3- to 6-month intervals. In women who are not currently taking oral estrogens, treatment with the Climara® system can be initiated at once.

In women who are currently taking oral estrogen, treatment with the Climara® system can be initiated 1 week after withdrawal of oral therapy or sooner if symptoms reappear in less than 1 week.

For the prevention of postmenopausal osteoporosis, the minimum dose that has been shown to be effective is the 6.5 cm^2 (0.025 mg/day) Climara® system. Response to therapy can be assessed by biochemical markers and measurement of bone mineral density.

HOW SUPPLIED

Climara® (estradiol transdermal system), 0.025 mg/day–each 6.5 cm^2 system contains 2.0 mg of estradiol USP
NDC 50419-454-04
Individual Carton of 4 systems
Shelf Pack Carton of 6 Individual Cartons of 4 systems

Climara® (estradiol transdermal system), 0.05 mg/day–each 12.5 cm^2 system contains 3.9 mg of estradiol USP
NDC 50419-451-04
Individual Carton of 4 systems
Shelf Pack Carton of 6 Individual Cartons of 4 systems

Climara® (estradiol transdermal system), 0.075 mg/day–each 18.75 cm^2 system contains 5.7 mg of estradiol USP
NDC 50419-453-04
Individual Carton of 4 systems
Shelf Pack Carton of 6 Individual Cartons of 4 systems

Climara® (estradiol transdermal system), 0.1 mg/day–each 25.0 cm^2 system contains 7.6 mg of estradiol USP
NDC 50419-452-04
Individual Carton of 4 systems
Shelf Pack Carton of 6 Individual Cartons of 4 systems

Do not store above 86°F (30°C). Do not store unpouched. Apply immediately upon removal from the protective pouch.

Rx only

INFORMATION FOR THE PATIENT

INTRODUCTION

The Climara® system that your doctor has prescribed for you releases small amounts of estradiol through the skin in a continuous way. Estradiol is the same hormone that your ovaries produce abundantly before menopause. The dose of estradiol you require will depend upon your individual response. The dose is adjusted by the size of the Climara® system used; the systems are available in four sizes.

This leaflet describes when and how to use estrogens, and the risks and benefits of estrogen treatment.

Estrogens have important benefits but also some risks. You must decide, with your doctor, whether the risks to you of estrogen use are acceptable because of their benefits. If you use estrogens, check with your doctor to be sure you are using the lowest possible dose that works, and that you don't use them longer than necessary. How long you need to use estrogens will depend on the reason for use.

INFORMATION ABOUT CLIMARA®

How The Climara® System Works

The Climara® system contains 17β-estradiol. When applied to the skin as directed below, the Climara® system releases 17β-estradiol, which flows through the skin into the bloodstream.

How and Where to Apply the Climara® System

Each Climara® system is individually sealed in a protective pouch. To open the pouch, hold it vertically with the Climara® name facing you. Tear left to right using the top tear notch. Tear from bottom to top using the side tear notch. Pull the pouch open. The Climara® patch is the transparent plastic film attached to the clear thicker plastic backing. There is a silver-foil sticker securely attached to the inside of the pouch. This contains a moisture protectant (desiccant). **Do not remove it. Carefully remove the Climara® patch.** You'll notice that the patch is attached to a thicker, hard-plastic backing and that the patch itself is oval and transparent.

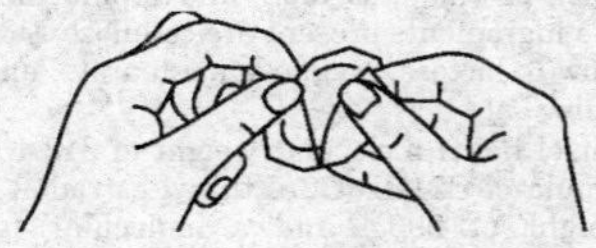

Apply the adhesive side of the Climara® system to a clean, dry area of the lower abdomen or the upper quadrant of the buttock. *Do not apply the Climara® system to your breasts.* The sites of application must be rotated, with an interval of at least 1 week allowed between applications to a particular site. The area selected should not be oily, damaged, or irritated. Avoid the waistline, since tight clothing may rub and remove the system. Application to areas where sitting would dislodge the system should also be avoided. Apply the system immediately after opening the pouch and removing the protective liner. Press the system firmly in place with the fingers for about 10 seconds, making sure there is good contact, especially around the edges.

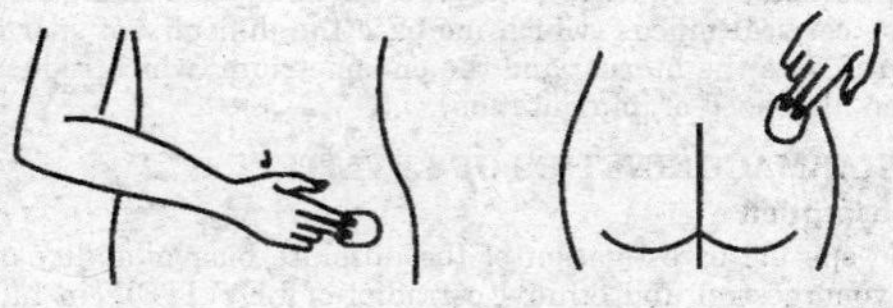

The Climara® system should be worn continuously for one week. You may wish to experiment with different locations when applying a new system, to find ones that are most comfortable for you and where clothing will not rub on the system.

When to Apply the Climara® System

The Climara® system should be changed once weekly.

When changing the system, remove the used Climara® system and discard it. Any adhesive that might remain on your skin can be easily rubbed off. Then place the new Climara® system on a different skin site. (The same skin site should not be used again for at least 1 week after removal of the system.)

Contact with water when you are bathing, swimming, or showering may affect the system. In the unlikely event that a system should fall off, a new system should be applied for the remainder of the 7-day dosing interval.

USES OF ESTROGEN

(Not every estrogen drug is approved for every use listed in this section. If you want to know which of these possible uses are approved for the medicine prescribed for you, ask your doctor or pharmacist to show you the professional labeling. You can also look up the specific estrogen product in a book called the "Physicians' Desk Reference", which is available in many book stores and public libraries. Generic drugs carry virtually the same labeling information as their brand name versions.)

- **To reduce moderate or severe menopausal symptoms.**
  Estrogens are hormones made by the ovaries of normal women. Between ages 45 and 55, the ovaries normally stop making estrogens. This leads to a drop in body estrogen levels which causes the "change of life" or menopause (the end of monthly menstrual periods). If both ovaries are removed during an operation before natural menopause takes place, the sudden drop in estrogen levels causes "surgical menopause".
  When the estrogen levels begin dropping, some women develop very uncomfortable symptoms, such as feelings of warmth in the face, neck, and chest, or sudden intense episodes of heat and sweating ("hot flashes" or "hot flushes"). Using estrogen drugs can help the body adjust to lower estrogen levels and reduce these symptoms. Most women have only mild menopausal symptoms or none at all and do not need to use estrogen drugs for these symptoms. Others may need to take estrogens for a few months while their bodies adjust to lower estrogen levels. The majority of women do not need estrogen replacement for longer than six months for these symptoms.
- **To treat vulval and vaginal atrophy** (itching, burning, dryness in or around the vagina, difficulty or burning on urination) associated with menopause.
- **To treat certain conditions in which a young woman's ovaries do not produce enough estrogen naturally.**
- **To treat certain types of abnormal vaginal bleeding due to hormonal imbalance when your doctor has found no serious cause of the bleeding.**
- **To treat certain cancers in special situations, in men and women.**
- **To prevent thinning of bones.**
  Osteoporosis is a thinning of the bones that makes them weaker and allows them to break more easily. The bones of the spine, wrists and hips break most often in osteoporosis. Both men and women start to lose bone mass after about age 40, but women lose bone mass faster after the menopause. Using estrogens after the menopause slows down bone thinning and may prevent bones from breaking. Lifelong adequate calcium intake, either in the diet (such as dairy products) or by calcium supplements (to reach a total daily intake of 1000 milligrams per day before menopause or 1500 milligrams per day after menopause), may help to prevent osteoporosis. Regular weight-bearing exercise (like walking and running for an hour, two or three times a week) may also help to prevent osteoporosis. Before you change your calcium intake or exercise habits, it is important to discuss these lifestyle changes with your doctor to find out if they are safe for you.
  Since estrogen use has some risks, only women who are likely to develop osteoporosis should use estrogens for prevention. Women who are likely to develop osteoporosis often have the following characteristics: white or Asian race, slim, cigarette smokers, and a family history of osteoporosis in a mother, sister, or aunt. Women who have relatively early menopause, often because their ovaries were removed during an operation ("surgical menopause"), are more likely to develop osteoporosis than women whose menopause happens at the average age.

WHO SHOULD NOT USE ESTROGENS

Estrogens should not be used:

- **During pregnancy (see Boxed Warning).**
  If you think you may be pregnant, do not use any form of estrogen-containing drug. Using estrogens while you are pregnant may cause your unborn child to have birth defects. Estrogens do not prevent miscarriage.
- **If you have unusual vaginal bleeding which has not been evaluated by your doctor (see Boxed Warning).**
  Unusual vaginal bleeding can be a warning sign of cancer of the uterus, especially if it happens after menopause. Your doctor must find out the cause of the bleeding so that he or she can recommend the proper treatment. Taking estrogens without visiting your doctor can cause you serious harm if your vaginal bleeding is caused by cancer of the uterus.
- **If you have had cancer.**
  Since estrogens increase the risk of certain types of cancer, you should not use estrogens if you have ever had cancer of the breast or uterus, unless your doctor recommends that the drug may help in the cancer treatment. (For certain patients with breast or prostate cancer, estrogens may help).
- **If you have any circulation problems.**
  Estrogen drugs should not be used except in unusually special situations in which your doctor judges that you need estrogen therapy so much that the risks are acceptable. Men and women with abnormal blood clotting conditions should avoid estrogen use (see Dangers of Estrogens, below).
- **When they do not work.**
  During menopause, some women develop nervous symptoms or depression. Estrogens do not relieve these symptoms. You may have heard that taking estrogens for years after menopause will keep your skin soft and supple and keep you feeling young. There is no evidence for these claims and such long-term estrogen use may have serious risks.
- **After childbirth or when breastfeeding a baby.**
  Estrogens should not be used to try to stop the breasts from filling with milk after a baby is born. Such treatment may increase the risk of developing blood clots (see Dangers of Estrogens, below).
  If you are breastfeeding, you should avoid using any drugs because many drugs pass through to the baby in the milk. While nursing a baby, you should take drugs only on the advice of your health care provider.

DANGERS OF ESTROGENS

- **Cancer of the uterus.**
  Your risk of developing cancer of the uterus gets higher the longer you use estrogens and the larger doses you use. One study showed that after women stop taking estrogens, this higher cancer risk quickly returns to the usual level of risk (as if you had never used estrogen therapy). Three other studies showed that the cancer risk stayed high for 8 to more than 15 years after stopping estrogen treatment. Because of this risk, **IT IS IMPORTANT TO TAKE THE LOWEST DOSE THAT WORKS AND TO TAKE IT ONLY AS LONG AS YOU NEED IT.**
  Using progestin therapy together with estrogen therapy may reduce the higher risk of uterine cancer related to estrogen use (but see Other Information, below).
  If you have had your uterus removed (total hysterectomy), there is no danger of developing cancer of the uterus.
- **Cancer of the breast.**
  Most studies have not shown a higher risk of breast cancer in women who have ever used estrogens. However, some studies have reported that breast cancer developed more often (up to twice the usual rate) in women who used estrogens for long periods of time (especially more than 10 years), or who used higher doses for shorter time periods.
  Regular breast examinations by a health professional and monthly self examination are recommended for all women.
- **Gallbladder disease.**
  Women who use estrogens after menopause are more likely to develop gallbladder disease needing surgery than women who do not use estrogens.
- **Abnormal blood clotting.**
  Taking estrogens may cause changes in your blood clotting system. These changes allow the blood to clot more easily, possibly allowing clots to form in your bloodstream. If blood clots do form in your bloodstream, they can cut off the blood supply to vital organs, causing serious problems. These problems may include a stroke (by cutting off blood to the brain), a heart attack (by cutting off blood to the heart), a pulmonary embolus (by cutting off blood to the lungs), or other problems. Any of these conditions may cause death or serious long term disability. However, most studies of low dose estrogen usage by women do not show an increased risk of these complications.

SIDE EFFECTS

In addition to the risks listed above, the following side effects have been reported with estrogen use:

— Nausea and vomiting.
— Breast tenderness or enlargement.
— Enlargement of benign tumors ("fibroids") of the uterus.
— Retention of excess fluid. This may make some conditions worsen, such as asthma, epilepsy, migraine, heart disease, or kidney disease.
— A spotty darkening of the skin, particularly on the face.

REDUCING RISK OF ESTROGEN USE

If you use estrogens, you can reduce your risks by doing these things:

- **See your doctor regularly.**
  While you are using estrogens, it is important to visit your doctor at least once a year for a check-up. If you develop vaginal bleeding while taking estrogens, you may need further evaluation. If members of your family have had breast cancer or if you have ever had breast lumps or an abnormal mammogram (breast x-ray), you may need to have more frequent breast examinations.
- **Reassess your need for estrogens.**
  You and your doctor should reevaluate whether or not you still need estrogens at least every six months.
- **Be alert for signs of trouble.**
  If any of these warning signals (or any other unusual symptoms) happen while you are using estrogens, call your doctor immediately:
  Abnormal bleeding from the vagina (possible uterine cancer)
  Pains in the calves or chest, sudden shortness of breath, or coughing blood (possible clot in the legs, heart, or lungs)
  Severe headache or vomiting, dizziness, faintness, changes in vision or speech, weakness or numbness of an arm or leg (possible clot in the brain or eye)

Continued on next page

Information on the Berlex products appearing here is based on the most current information available at the time of publication closing. Further information for these and other products may be obtained from the Medical Affairs Department, Berlex Laboratories, 300 Fairfield Road, Wayne, New Jersey 07470, 1-888-BERLEX-4. Information on Betaseron and Fludara may be obtained from Berlex Laboratories, 15049 San Pablo Avenue, Richmond, California 94804-0016, 1-800-888-4112.

Climara—Cont.

Breast lumps (possible breast cancer; ask your doctor or health professional to show you how to examine your breasts monthly)
Yellowing of the skin or eyes (possible liver problem)
Pain, swelling, or tenderness in the abdomen (possible gallbladder problem)

OTHER INFORMATION

1. Estrogens increase the risk of developing a condition (endometrial hyperplasia) that may lead to cancer of the lining of the uterus. Taking progestins, another hormone drug, with estrogens lowers the risk of developing this condition. Therefore, if your uterus has not been removed, your doctors may prescribe a progestin for you to take together with your estrogen.

You should know, however, that taking estrogens with progestins may have additional risks. These include:

— unhealthy effects on blood fats (especially a lowering of HDL blood cholesterol, the "good" blood fat which protects against heart disease);
— unhealthy effects on blood sugar (which might make a diabetic condition worse); and
— a possible further increase in breast cancer risk which may be associated with long-term estrogen use.

Some research has shown that estrogens taken *without* progestins may protect women against developing heart disease. However, this is not certain. The protection shown may have been caused by the characteristics of the estrogen-treated women, and not by the estrogen treatment itself. In general, treated women were slimmer, more physically active, and were less likely to have diabetes than the untreated women. These characteristics are known to protect against heart disease.

You are cautioned to discuss very carefully with your doctor or health care provider all the possible risks and benefits of long-term estrogen and progestin treatment as they affect you personally.

2. Your doctor has prescribed this drug for you and you alone. Do not give the drug to anyone else.

3. If you will be taking calcium supplements as part of the treatment to help prevent osteoporosis, check with your doctor about how much to take.

4. Keep this and all drugs out of the reach of children. In case of overdose, call your doctor, hospital or poison control center immediately.

5. This leaflet provides a summary of the most important information about estrogens. If you want more information, ask your doctor or pharmacist to show you the professional labeling. The professional labeling is also published in a book called the "Physicians' Desk Reference," which is available in book stores and public libraries. Generic drugs carry virtually the same labeling information as their brand name versions.

Do not store above 86° F(30° C). Do not store unpouched. Apply immediately upon removal from the protective pouch.

Rx only

Manufactured for Berlex Laboratories, Wayne, NJ 07470
Manufactured by 3M Pharmaceuticals, St. Paul, MN 55144
Berlex Component Code #6066300 (3M #621800)

May 1999

Shown in Product Identification Guide, page 308

LEVLITE™ 21 Tablets ℞
[lĕvlīt]
(levonorgestrel and ethinyl estradiol tablets, USP)
Rx only

LEVLITE™ 28 Tablets ℞
[lĕvlīt]
(levonorgestrel and ethinyl estradiol tablets, USP)
Rx only

TRI-LEVLEN® 21 ℞
[trī-lĕvlĕn]
Tablets
(levonorgestrel and ethinyl estradiol tablets—triphasic regimen)

TRI-LEVLEN® 28 ℞
[trī-lĕvlĕn]
Tablets
(levonorgestrel and ethinyl estradiol tablets—triphasic regimen)

LEVLEN® 21 ℞
[lĕvlĕn]
Tablets
(levonorgestrel and ethinyl estradiol tablets)

LEVLEN® 28 ℞
[lĕvlĕn]
Tablets
(levonorgestrel and ethinyl estradiol tablets)

Patients should be counseled that this product does not protect against HIV infection (AIDS) and other sexually transmitted diseases.

DESCRIPTION

LEVLITE™ 21 tablets

Each cycle of LEVLITE™ 21 (levonorgestrel and ethinyl estradiol tablets, USP) consists of 21 pink active tablets each containing 0.100 mg levonorgestrel and 0.020 mg ethinyl estradiol. The inactive ingredients are Calcium Carbonate USP, Corn Starch NF, Ferric Oxide/red/E 172 NF, Ferric Oxide/yellow/E 172 NF, Glycerin 85% Ph. Eur./ DAB, Lactose Monohydrate NF, Magnesium Stearate NF, Montanglycol Wax (Wax E) DAB, Polyethylene glycol 6,000 NF, Povidone 25,000 USP, Povidone 700,000 USP, Pregelatinized Starch NF (Modified Starch), Sucrose NF, Talc USP and Titanium Dioxide, E 171 USP.

LEVLITE™ 28 tablets

Each cycle of LEVLITE™ 28 (levonorgestrel and ethinyl estradiol tablets, USP) consists of 21 pink active tablets each containing 0.100 mg levonorgestrel and 0.020 mg ethinyl estradiol; and seven white tablets – inert. The inactive ingredients are Calcium Carbonate USP, Corn Starch NF, Ferric Oxide/red/E 172 NF, Ferric Oxide/yellow/E 172 NF, Glycerin 85% Ph. Eur./DAB, Lactose Monohydrate NF, Magnesium Stearate NF, Montanglycol Wax (Wax E) DAB, Polyethylene glycol 6,000 NF, Povidone 25,000 USP, Povidone 700,000 USP, Pregelatinized Starch NF (Modified Starch), Sucrose NF, Talc USP and Titanium Dioxide, E 171 USP.

TRI-LEVLEN® 21 tablets

Each cycle of TRI-LEVLEN® 21 (Levonorgestrel and Ethinyl Estradiol Tablets—Triphasic Regimen) tablets consists of three different drug phases as follows: Phase 1 comprised of 6 brown film-coated tablets, each containing 0.050 mg of levonorgestrel (d)(-)-13 beta-ethyl-17-alpha-ethinyl-17-beta-hydroxygon-4-en-3-one), a totally synthetic progestogen, and 0.030 mg of ethinyl estradiol (19-nor-17α-pregna-1,3,5(10)-trien-20-yne-3, 17-diol); phase 2 comprised of 5 white film-coated tablets, each containing 0.075 mg levonorgestrel and 0.040 mg ethinyl estradiol; and, phase 3 comprised of 10 light-yellow film-coated tablets, each containing 0.125 mg levonorgestrel and 0.030 mg ethinyl estradiol. The inactive ingredients present are cellulose, iron oxides, lactose, magnesium stearate, polacrilin potassium, polyethylene glycol, titanium dioxide, and hydroxypropyl methylcellulose.

TRI-LEVLEN® 28 tablets

Each cycle of TRI-LEVLEN® 28 (Levonorgestrel and Ethinyl Estradiol Tablets—Triphasic Regimen) tablets consists of three different drug phases as follows: Phase 1 comprised of 6 brown film-coated tablets, each containing 0.050 mg of levonorgestrel (d)(-)-13 beta-ethyl-17-alpha-ethinyl-17-beta-hydroxygon-4-en-3-one), a totally synthetic progestogen, and 0.030 mg of ethinyl estradiol (19-nor-17 α-pregna-1,3,5(10)-trien-20-yne-3, 17-diol); phase 2 comprised of 5 white film-coated tablets, each containing 0.075 mg levonorgestrel and 0.040 mg ethinyl estradiol; and phase 3 comprised of 10 light-yellow film-coated tablets, each containing 0.125 mg levonorgestrel and 0.030 mg ethinyl estradiol; then followed by 7 light-green film-coated inert tablets. The inactive ingredients present are cellulose, F D & C Blue 1, iron oxides, lactose, magnesium stearate, polacrilin potassium, polyethylene glycol, titanium dioxide, and hydroxypropyl methylcellulose.

LEVLEN® 21 tablets:

Each LEVLEN® 21 tablet (Levonorgestrel and Ethinyl Estradiol Tablets) contains 0.15 mg of levonorgestrel (d)(-)-13 beta-ethyl -17- alpha-ethinyl -17- beta-hydroxygon -4- en -3-one), a totally synthetic progestogen, and 0.03 mg of ethinyl estradiol (19-nor-17 α-pregna-1,3,5(10)-trien-20-yne-3, 17-diol). The inactive ingredients present are cellulose, FD&C Yellow 6, lactose, magnesium stearate, and polacrillin potassium.

LEVLEN® 28 tablets:

21 light-orange LEVLEN® tablets (Levonorgestrel and Ethinyl Estradiol Tablets), each containing 0.15 mg of levonorgestrel (d)(-)-13 beta-ethyl-17-alpha-ethinyl-17-beta-hydroxygon-4-en-3-one), a totally synthetic progestogen, and 0.03 mg of ethinyl estradiol (19-nor-17 α-pregna-1,3,5(10)-trien-20-yne-3, 17-diol), and 7 pink inert tablets. The inactive ingredients present are cellulose, D&C Red 30, FD&C Yellow 6, lactose, magnesium stearate, and polacrillin potassium.

Levonorgestrel has a molecular weight of 312.4 and a molecular formula of C21H28O2. Ethinyl estradiol has a molecular weight of 296.4 and a molecular formula of C20H24O2. The structural formulas are as follows:

Levonorgestrel   Ethinyl Estradiol

CLINICAL PHARMACOLOGY

Combination oral contraceptives act by suppression of gonadotropins. Although the primary mechanism of this action is inhibition of ovulation, other alterations include changes in the cervical mucus (which increase the difficulty of sperm entry into the uterus) and the endometrium (which reduce the likelihood of implantation).

PHARMACOKINETICS OF LEVLITE™

Absorption

No specific investigation of the absolute bioavailability of levonorgestrel and ethinyl estradiol of LEVLITE™ in humans has been conducted. However, literature indicates that levonorgestrel is rapidly and completely absorbed after oral administration and is not subject to first-pass metabolism. Ethinyl estradiol is rapidly and almost completely absorbed from the gastrointestinal tract but, due to first-pass metabolism in gut mucosa and liver, the absolute bioavailability of ethinyl estradiol is about 40%.

After a single dose of three LEVLITE™ Tablets to 17 women under fasting conditions, the extents of absorption of levonorgestrel and ethinyl estradiol were 98.6% and 99.0%, respectively, relative to the same dose of the 2 drugs when given as a microcrystalline suspension in water. The effect of food on the bioavailability of LEVLITE™ Tablets following oral administration has not been evaluated.

The pharmacokinetics of levonorgestrel and ethinyl estradiol following daily administration of LEVLITE™ Tablets for 21 days per cycle for three cycles, were determined in 18 women. Estimates of the pharmacokinetic parameters of levonorgestrel and ethinyl estradiol following single and multiple dose administration of LEVLITE™ Tablets are summarized in Table I. Mean levonorgestrel and ethinyl estradiol levels after a single dose and on day 21 at steady state are shown in Figure I.

The pharmacokinetics of total levonorgestrel are non-linear due to an increase in binding to SHBG, which is attributed to increased SHBG levels that are induced by the daily administration of ethinyl estradiol. Increased binding of levonorgestrel to SHBG leads to decreased clearance of levonorgestrel. Observed maximum levonorgestrel concen-

TABLE I MEAN (SD) PHARMACOKINETIC PARAMETERS OF LEVLITE™ AFTER SINGLE DOSE AND AFTER MULTIPLE DOSING FOR 3 CYCLES

Levonorgestrel

Day (cycle)	Cmax ng/mL	tmax h	AUC ng•h/mL	CL/F mL/min/kg	Vz L	SHBG nmol/L
1	2.36 (0.79)	1.3 (0.4)	29.2 (10.0)	1.0 (0.3)	129 (46)	64.5 (22.0)
			AUC (0–24h) ng•h/mL			
21 (1)	4.04 (2.08)	1.0 (0.3)	43.8 (22.4)	0.73 (0.34)	106 (42)	94.7 (37.4)
21 (3)	4.53 (1.94)	1.0 (0.3)	49.5 (24.5)	0.65 (0.33)	96 (35)	107.4 (45.8)

Ethinyl Estradiol

Day (cycle)	Cmax pg/mL	tmax h	AUC(0–24) pg•h/mL
1	49.5 (13.4)	1.5 (0.4)	298 (215)
21 (1)	66.2 (29.5)	1.4 (0.4)	596 (494)
21 (3)	58.1 (19.3)	1.4 (0.3)	417 (289)

Cmax = maximum concentration
tmax = time to maximum concentration
AUC = area under the drug concentration curve from time 0 to infinity
CL/f = oral clearance
Vz = volume of distribution
SHBG = sex hormone binding globulin
AUC (0–24) = area under the drug concentration time curve from time 0 to 24 hours; this represents the area for one dosing interval at steady state.

trations increased from day 1 to day 21 of the 1st and 3rd cycles by 66% and 83%, respectively.

FIGURE I

Mean Levonorgestrel Concentrations in Serum after single dose and on Day 21 of Cycles 1 and 3

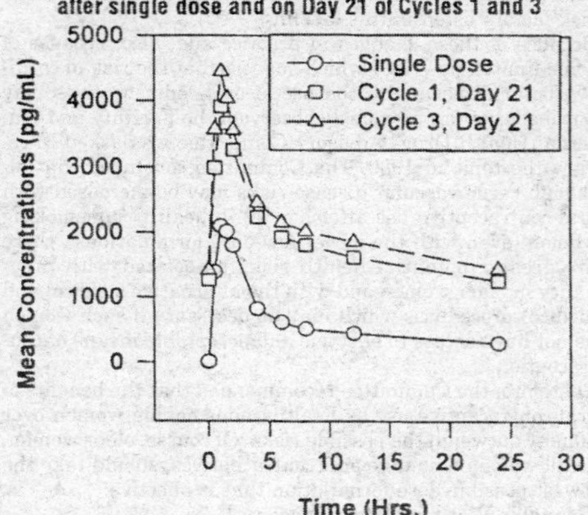

Mean Ethinyl Estradiol Concentrations in Serum after single dose and on Day 21 of Cycles 1 and 3

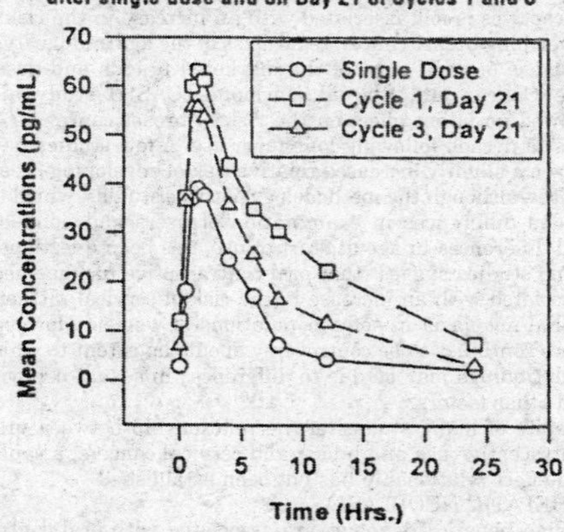

In calculating the mean concentration for ethinyl estradiol, any individual subject value below the quantifiable limit (i.e., 20 pg/mL) was converted to 0; and the 0 values were included for calculation of the mean concentration.

Table I provides a summary of levonorgestrel and ethinyl estradiol pharmacokinetic parameters.

[See table I at top of previous page]

Distribution

Levonorgestrel in serum is primarily bound to SHBG. Protein binding values for levonorgestrel are provided in Table II. Ethinyl estradiol is about 97% bound to plasma albumin. Ethinyl estradiol does not bind to SHBG, but induces SHBG synthesis.

[See table II above]

TABLE II. Protein binding (mean ± SD) of levonorgestrel in pools of serum samples collected from 18 women after a single dose of LEVLITE™, and following administration (once daily) over 3x21 days.

Parameter	Single Dose	Cycle 2	Cycle 4
% free	1.11 (0.27)	0.79 (0.22)	0.80 (0.23)
% SHBG-bound	64.5 (8.54)	75.6 (6.59)	74.7 (7.89)
% albumin-bound	34.4 (8.28)	23.6 (6.41)	24.5 (7.67)

Metabolism

Levonorgestrel: The most important metabolic pathway occurs in the reduction of the Δ4-3-oxo group and hydroxylation at positions 2α, 1β, and 16β, followed by conjugation. Most of the metabolites that circulate in the blood are sulfates of 3α, 5β-tetrahydro-levonorgestrel, while excretion occurs predominantly in the form of glucuronides. Some of the parent levonorgestrel also circulates as 17β-sulfate. Metabolic clearance rates may differ among individuals by several-fold, and this may account in part for the wide variation in levonorgestrel concentrations among users.

Ethinyl estradiol: Cytochrome P450 enzymes (CYP3A4) in the liver are responsible for the 2-hydroxylation that is the major oxidative reaction. The 2-hydroxy metabolite is further transformed by methylation and glucuronidation prior to urinary and fecal excretion. Levels of Cytochrome P450 (CYP3A) vary widely among individuals and can explain the variation in the rates of ethinyl estradiol 2-hydroxylation. Ethinyl estradiol is excreted in the urine and feces as glucuronide and sulfate conjugates and undergoes enterohepatic circulation.

Excretion

The elimination half-life for levonorgestrel after a single dose of LEVLITE™ is 25.4 ± 9.7 hours. Levonorgestrel and its metabolites are primarily excreted in the urine. The elimination half-life of ethinyl estradiol has been reported to be between 15 and 25 hours.

SPECIAL POPULATIONS for LEVLITE™

Hepatic Insufficiency

No formal studies have evaluated the effect of hepatic disease on the disposition of LEVLITE™. However, steroid hormones may be poorly metabolized in patients with impaired liver function.

Renal Insufficiency

No formal studies have evaluated the effect of renal disease on the disposition of LEVLITE™.

TABLE III. Percentage of women experiencing an unintended pregnancy during the first year of typical use and first year of perfect use of contraception and the percentage continuing use at the end of the first year. United States.

Method (1)	% of Women Experiencing an Accidental Pregnancy within the First Year of Use: Typical Use[1] (2)	Perfect Use[2] (3)	% of Women Continuing Use at One Year[3] (4)
Chance[4]	85	85	
Spermicides[5]	26	6	40
Periodic abstinence	25		63
Calendar		9	
Ovulation method		3	
Sympto-thermal[6]		2	
Post Ovulation		1	
Withdrawal	19	4	
Cap[7]			
Parous women	40	26	42
Nulliparous women	20	9	56
Sponge			
Parous women	40	20	42
Nulliparous women	20	9	56
Diaphragm[7]	20	6	56
Condom[8]			
Female (Reality)	21	5	56
Male	14	3	61
Pill	5		71
progestin only		0.5	
combined		0.1	
IUD			
Progesterone T	2	1.5	81
Copper T 380A	0.8	0.6	78
Lng 20	0.1	0.1	81
Depo Provera	0.3	0.3	70
Norplant and Norplant-2	0.05	0.05	88
Female sterilization	0.5	0.5	100
Male sterilization	0.15	0.10	100

Source: Trussell J, Contraceptive efficacy. In Hatcher RA, Trussell J, Stewart F, Cates W, Stewart GK, Kowal D, Guest F, *Contraceptive Technology:* Seventeenth Revised Edition. New York NY: Irvington Publishers, 1998, in press.

1 Among *typical* couples who initiate use of a method (not necessarily for the first time), the percentage who experience an accidental pregnancy during the first year if they do not stop use for any other reason.

2 Among couples who initiate use of a method (not necessarily for the first time) and who use it *perfectly* (both consistently and correctly), the percentage who experience an accidental pregnancy during the first year if they do not stop use for any other reason.

3 Among couples attempting to avoid pregnancy, the percentage who continue to use a method for one year.

4 The percentages becoming pregnant in columns (2) and (3) are based on data from populations where contraception is not used and from women who cease using contraception in order to become pregnant. Among such populations, about 89% become pregnant within one year. This estimate was lowered slightly (to 85%) to represent the percentage who would become pregnant within one year among women now relying on reversible methods of contraception if they abandoned contraception altogether.

5 Foams, creams, gels, vaginal suppositories, vaginal film.

6 Cervical mucus (ovulation) method supplemented by calendar in the pre-ovulatory and basal body temperature in the post-ovulatory phases.

7 With spermicidal cream or jelly.

8 Without spermicides.

Drug-Drug Interactions

Interactions between ethinyl estradiol and other drugs have been reported in the literature.

- *Interactions with Absorption.* Diarrhea may increase gastrointestinal motility and reduce hormone absorption. Similarly, any drug which reduces gut transit time may reduce hormone concentrations in the blood.
- *Interactions with Metabolism*
  Gastrointestinal Wall: Sulfation of ethinyl estradiol has been shown to occur in the gastrointestinal wall. Therefore, drugs which act as competitive inhibitors for sulfation in the gastrointestinal wall may increase ethinyl estradiol bioavailability.
- *Hepatic metabolism:* Interactions can occur with drugs that induce microsomal enzymes which can decrease ethinyl estradiol concentrations (e.g., rifampin, barbiturates, phenylbutazone, phenytoin, griseofulvin).
- *Interference with Enterohepatic Circulation:* Some clinical reports suggest that enterohepatic circulation of estrogens may decrease when certain antibiotic agents are given, which may reduce ethinyl estradiol concentrations (e.g., ampicillin, tetracycline).
- *Interference in the Metabolism of Other Drugs:* Ethinyl estradiol may interfere with the metabolism of other drugs by inhibiting hepatic microsomal enzymes or by inducing hepatic drug conjugation, particularly glucuronidation. Accordingly, plasma and tissue concentrations may either be increased or decreased, respectively (e.g., cyclosporin, theophylline).

INDICATIONS AND USAGE

Oral contraceptives are indicated for the prevention of pregnancy in women who elect to use this product as a method of contraception.

Oral contraceptives are highly effective. Table III lists the typical accidental pregnancy rates for users of combination oral contraceptives and other methods of contraception. The efficacy of these contraceptive methods, except sterilization, depends upon the reliability with which they are used. Correct and consistent use of methods can result in lower failure rates.

[See table III above]

CONTRAINDICATIONS

Oral contraceptives should not be used in women with any of the following conditions:

Thrombophlebitis or thromboembolic disorders.

A past history of deep-vein thrombophlebitis or thromboembolic disorders.

Cerebral-vascular or coronary-artery disease.

Known or suspected carcinoma of the breast.

Carcinoma of the endometrium or other known or suspected estrogen-dependent neoplasia.

Undiagnosed abnormal genital bleeding.

Continued on next page

Information on the Berlex products appearing here is based on the most current information available at the time of publication closing. Further information for these and other products may be obtained from the Medical Affairs Department, Berlex Laboratories, 300 Fairfield Road, Wayne, New Jersey 07470, 1-888-BERLEX-4. Information on Betaseron and Fludara may be obtained from Berlex Laboratories, 15049 San Pablo Avenue, Richmond, California 94804-0016, 1-800-888-4112.

Levlite/Tri-Levlen/Levlen—Cont.

Cholestatic jaundice of pregnancy or jaundice with prior pill use.
Hepatic adenomas or carcinomas.
Known or suspected pregnancy.

WARNINGS

> **Cigarette smoking increases the risk of serious cardiovascular side effects from oral-contraceptive use. This risk increases with age and with heavy smoking (15 or more cigarettes per day) and is quite marked in women over 35 years of age. Women who use oral contraceptives should be strongly advised not to smoke.**

The use of oral contraceptives is associated with increased risks of several serious conditions including myocardial infarction, thromboembolism, stroke, hepatic neoplasia, gallbladder disease, and hypertension, although the risk of serious morbidity or mortality is very small in healthy women without underlying risk factors. The risk of morbidity and mortality increases significantly in the presence of other underlying risk factors such as hypertension, hyperlipidemias, obesity and diabetes.

Practitioners prescribing oral contraceptives should be familiar with the following information relating to these risks. The information contained in this package insert is based principally on studies carried out in patients who used oral contraceptives with higher formulations of estrogens and progestogens than those in common use today. The effect of long-term use of the oral contraceptives with lower formulations of both estrogens and progestogens remains to be determined.

Throughout this labeling, epidemiologic studies reported are of two types: retrospective or case control studies and prospective or cohort studies. Case control studies provide a measure of the relative risk of a disease, namely, a ratio of the incidence of a disease among oral contraceptive users to that among nonusers. The relative risk does not provide information on the actual clinical occurrence of a disease. Cohort studies provide a measure of attributable risk, which is the difference in the incidence of disease between oral contraceptive users and nonusers. The attributable risk does provide information about the actual occurrence of a disease in the population. For further information, the reader is referred to a text on epidemiologic methods.

1. THROMBOEMBOLIC DISORDERS AND OTHER VASCULAR PROBLEMS

a. *Myocardial infarction*

An increased risk of myocardial infarction has been attributed to oral-contraceptive use. This risk is primarily in smokers or women with other underlying risk factors for coronary-artery disease such as hypertension, hypercholesterolemia, morbid obesity, and diabetes. The relative risk of heart attack for current oral contraceptive users has been estimated to be two to six. The risk is very low under the age of 30.

Smoking in combination with oral contraceptive use has been shown to contribute substantially to the incidence of myocardial infarctions in women in their mid-thirties or older with smoking accounting for the majority of excess cases. Mortality rates associated with circulatory disease have been shown to increase substantially in smokers over the age of 35 and nonsmokers over the age of 40 (Table IV) among women who use oral contraceptives.

[See table IV below]

Oral contraceptives may compound the effects of well-known risk factors, such as hypertension, diabetes, hyperlipidemias, age and obesity. In particular, some progestogens are known to decrease HDL cholesterol and cause glucose intolerance, while estrogens may create a state of hyperinsulinism. Oral contraceptives have been shown to increase blood pressure among users (see section 9 in "WARNINGS"). Similar effects on risk factors have been associated with an increased risk of heart disease. Oral contraceptives must be used with caution in women with cardiovascular disease risk factors.

b. *Thromboembolism*

An increased risk of thromboembolic and thrombotic disease associated with the use of oral contraceptives is well established. Case control studies have found the relative risk of users compared to nonusers to be 3 for the first episode of superficial venous thrombosis, 4 to 11 for deep vein thrombosis or pulmonary embolism, and 1.5 to 6 for women with predisposing conditions for venous thromboembolic disease. Cohort studies have shown the relative risk to be somewhat lower, about 3 for new cases and about 4.5 for new cases requiring hospitalization. The risk of thromboembolic disease due to oral contraceptives is not related to length of use and disappears after pill use is stopped.

A two- to four-fold increase in the relative risk of post-operative thromboembolic complications has been reported with the use of oral contraceptives. The relative risk of venous thrombosis in women who have predisposing conditions is twice that of women without such medical conditions. If feasible, oral contraceptives should be discontinued from at least four weeks prior to and for two weeks after elective surgery of a type associated with an increase in risk of thromboembolism and during and following prolonged immobilization. Since the immediate postpartum period is also associated with an increased risk of thromboembolism, oral contraceptives should be started no earlier than four to six weeks after delivery in women who elect not to breast-feed.

c. *Cerebrovascular diseases*

Oral contraceptives have been shown to increase both the relative and attributable risks of cerebrovascular events (thrombotic and hemorrhagic strokes), although, in general, the risk is greatest among older (>35 years), hypertensive women who also smoke. Hypertension was found to be a risk factor, for both users and nonusers, for both types of strokes, while smoking interacted to increase the risk for hemorrhagic strokes.

In a large study, the relative risk of thrombotic strokes has been shown to range from 3 for normotensive users to 14 for users with severe hypertension. The relative risk of hemorrhagic stroke is reported to be 1.2 for nonsmokers who used oral contraceptives, 2.6 for smokers who did not use oral contraceptives, 7.6 for smokers who used oral contraceptives, 1.8 for normotensive users and 25.7 for users with severe hypertension. The attributable risk is also greater in older women.

d. *Dose-related risk of vascular disease from oral contraceptives*

A positive association has been observed between the amount of estrogen and progestogen in oral contraceptives and the risk of vascular disease. A decline in serum high-density lipoproteins (HDL) has been reported with many progestational agents. A decline in serum high-density lipoproteins has been associated with an increased incidence of ischemic heart disease. Because estrogens increase HDL cholesterol, the net effect of an oral contraceptive depends on a balance achieved between doses of estrogen and progestogen and the nature and absolute amount of progestogen used in the contraceptive. The amount of both hormones should be considered in the choice of an oral contraceptive.

Minimizing exposure to estrogen and progestogen is in keeping with good principles of therapeutics. For any particular estrogen/progestogen combination, the dosage regimen prescribed should be one which contains the least amount of estrogen and progestogen that is compatible with a low failure rate and the needs of the individual patient. New acceptors of oral-contraceptive agents should be started on preparations containing the lowest estrogen content which provides satisfactory results in the individual.

e. *Persistence of risk of vascular disease*

There are two studies which have shown persistence of risk of vascular disease for ever-users of oral contraceptives. In a study in the United States, the risk of developing myocardial infarction after discontinuing oral contraceptives persists for at least 9 years for women aged 40–49 years who had used oral contraceptives for five or more years, but this increased risk was not demonstrated in other age groups. In another study in Great Britain, the risk of developing cerebrovascular disease persisted for at least 6 years after discontinuation of oral contraceptives, although excess risk was very small. However, both studies were performed with oral contraceptive formulations containing 50 micrograms or higher of estrogens.

2. ESTIMATES OF MORTALITY FROM CONTRACEPTIVE USE

One study gathered data from a variety of sources which have estimated the mortality rate associated with different methods of contraception at different ages (Table V). These estimates include the combined risk of death associated with contraceptive methods plus the risk attributable to pregnancy in the event of method failure. Each method of contraception has its specific benefits and risks. The study concluded that with the exception of oral contraceptive users 35 and older who smoke and 40 and older who do not smoke, mortality associated with all methods of birth control is less than that associated with childbirth.

The observation of a possible increase in risk of mortality with age for oral-contraceptive users is based on data gathered in the 1970's—but not reported until 1983. However, current clinical practice involves the use of lower estrogen dose formulations combined with careful restriction of oral-contraceptive use to women who do not have the various risk factors listed in this labeling.

Because of these changes in practice and, also, because of some limited new data which suggest that the risk of cardiovascular disease with the use of oral contraceptives may now be less than previously observed, the Fertility and Maternal Health Drugs Advisory Committee was asked to review the topic in 1989. The Committee concluded that although cardiovascular disease risks may be increased with oral-contraceptive use after age 40 in healthy nonsmoking women (even with the newer low-dose formulations), there are greater potential health risks associated with pregnancy in older women and with the alternative surgical and medical procedures which may be necessary if such women do not have access to effective and acceptable means of contraception.

Therefore, the Committee recommended that the benefits of oral-contraceptive use by healthy nonsmoking women over 40 may outweigh the possible risks. Of course, older women, as all women who take oral contraceptives, should take the lowest possible dose formulation that is effective.

[See table V at top of next page]

3. CARCINOMA OF THE REPRODUCTIVE ORGANS

Numerous epidemiological studies have been performed on the incidence of breast, endometrial, ovarian and cervical cancer in women using oral contraceptives. The overwhelming evidence in the literature suggests that use of oral contraceptives is not associated with an increase in the risk of developing breast cancer, regardless of the age and parity of first use or with most of the marketed brands and doses. The Cancer and Steroid Hormone (CASH) study also showed no latent effect on the risk of breast cancer for at least a decade following long-term use. A few studies have shown a slightly increased relative risk of developing breast cancer, although the methodology of these studies, which included differences in examination of users and nonusers and differences in age at start of use, has been questioned. Some studies suggest that oral-contraceptive use has been associated with an increase in the risk of cervical intraepithelial neoplasia in some populations of women. However, there continues to be controversy about the extent to which such findings may be due to differences in sexual behavior and other factors.

In spite of many studies of the relationship between oral-contraceptive use and breast and cervical cancers, a cause-and-effect relationship has not been established.

4. HEPATIC NEOPLASIA

Benign hepatic adenomas are associated with oral contraceptive use, although the incidence of benign tumors is rare in the United States. Indirect calculations have estimated the attributable risk to be in the range of 3.3 cases/100,000 for users, a risk that increases after four or more years of use. Rupture of rare, benign, hepatic adenomas may cause death through intra-abdominal hemorrhage.

Studies from Britain have shown an increased risk of developing hepatocellular carcinoma in long-term (>8 years) oral-contraceptive users. However, these cancers are extremely rare in the U.S. and the attributable risk (the excess incidence) of liver cancers in oral contraceptive users approaches less than one per million users.

5. OCULAR LESIONS

There have been clinical case reports of retinal thrombosis associated with the use of oral contraceptives. Oral contraceptives should be discontinued if there is unexplained partial or complete loss of vision; onset of proptosis or diplopia; papilledema; or retinal vascular lesions. Appropriate diagnostic and therapeutic measures should be undertaken immediately.

6. ORAL-CONTRACEPTIVE USE BEFORE OR DURING EARLY PREGNANCY

Extensive epidemiological studies have revealed no increased risk of birth defects in women who have used oral contraceptives prior to pregnancy. Studies also do not suggest a teratogenic effect, particularly insofar as cardiac anomalies and limb-reduction defects are concerned, when taken inadvertently during early pregnancy.

The administration of oral contraceptives to induce withdrawal bleeding should not be used as a test for pregnancy. Oral contraceptives should not be used during pregnancy to treat threatened or habitual abortion.

It is recommended that for any patient who has missed two consecutive periods, pregnancy should be ruled out before continuing oral-contraceptive use. If the patient has not adhered to the prescribed schedule, the possibility of pregnancy should be considered at the time of the first missed period. Oral contraceptive use should be discontinued if pregnancy is confirmed.

7. GALLBLADDER DISEASE

Earlier studies have reported an increased lifetime relative risk of gallbladder surgery in users of oral-contraceptives and estrogens. More recent studies, however, have shown that the relative risk of developing gallbladder disease among oral contraceptive users may be minimal. The recent findings of minimal risk may be related to the use of oral-contraceptive formulations containing lower hormonal doses of estrogens and progestogens.

8. CARBOHYDRATE AND LIPID METABOLIC EFFECTS

Oral contraceptives have been shown to cause glucose intolerance in a significant percentage of users. Oral contracep-

TABLE IV. (Adapted from P.M. Layde and V. Beral, Ref. #12.)

CIRCULATORY DISEASE MORTALITY RATES PER 100,000 WOMAN-YEARS BY AGE, SMOKING STATUS, AND ORAL CONTRACEPTIVE USE

AGE	EVER-USERS NON-SMOKING	EVER-USERS SMOKERS	CONTROLS NON-SMOKING	CONTROL SMOKERS
15–24	0.0	10.5	0.0	0.0
25–34	4.4	14.2	2.7	4.2
35–44	21.5	63.4	6.4	15.2
45+	52.4	206.7	11.4	27.9

tives containing greater than 75 micrograms of estrogens cause hyperinsulinism, while lower doses of estrogen cause less glucose intolerance. Progestogens increase insulin secretion and create insulin resistance, this effect varying with different progestational agents. However, in the nondiabetic woman, oral contraceptives appear to have no effect on fasting blood glucose. Because of these demonstrated effects, prediabetic and diabetic women should be carefully observed while taking oral-contraceptives.

A small proportion of women will have persistent hypertriglyceridemia while on the pill. As discussed earlier (see "WARNINGS" 1a. and 1d.), changes in serum triglycerides and lipoprotein levels have been reported in oral-contraceptive users.

9. ELEVATED BLOOD PRESSURE

An increase in blood pressure has been reported in women taking oral-contraceptives and this increase is more likely in older oral-contraceptive users and with continued use. Data from the Royal College of General Practitioners and subsequent randomized trials have shown that the incidence of hypertension increases with increasing quantities of progestogens.

Women with a history of hypertension or hypertension-related diseases, or renal disease should be encouraged to use another method of contraception. If women with hypertension elect to use oral contraceptives, they should be monitored closely, and if significant elevation of blood pressure occurs, oral contraceptives should be discontinued. For most women, elevated blood pressure will return to normal after stopping oral contraceptives, and there is no difference in the occurrence of hypertension among ever- and never-users.

10. HEADACHE

The onset or exacerbation of migraine or development of headache with a new pattern which is recurrent, persistent, or severe requires discontinuation of oral contraceptives and evaluation of the case.

11. BLEEDING IRREGULARITIES

Breakthrough bleeding and spotting are sometimes encountered in patients on oral contraceptives, especially during the first three months of use. The type and dose of progestogen may be important. Nonhormonal causes should be considered and adequate diagnostic measures taken to rule out malignancy or pregnancy in the event of breakthrough bleeding, as in the case of any abnormal vaginal bleeding. If pathology has been excluded, time or a change to another formulation may solve the problem. In the event of amenorrhea, pregnancy should be ruled out.

Some women may encounter post-pill amenorrhea or oligomenorrhea, especially when such a condition was preexistent.

PRECAUTIONS

1. GENERAL

Patients should be counseled that this product does not protect against HIV infection (AIDS) and other sexually transmitted diseases.

2. PHYSICAL EXAMINATION AND FOLLOW-UP

It is good medical practice for all women to have annual history and physical examinations, including women using oral contraceptives. The physical examination, however, may be deferred until after initiation of oral contraceptives if requested by the woman and judged appropriate by the clinician. The physical examination should include special reference to blood pressure, breasts, abdomen and pelvic organs, including cervical cytology and relevant laboratory tests. In case of undiagnosed, persistent, or recurrent abnormal vaginal bleeding, appropriate diagnostic measures should be conducted to rule out malignancy. Women with a strong family history of breast cancer or who have breast nodules should be monitored with particular care.

3. LIPID DISORDERS

Women who are being treated for hyperlipidemias should be followed closely if they elect to use oral contraceptives. Some progestogens may elevate LDL levels and may render the control of hyperlipidemias more difficult.

4. LIVER FUNCTION

If jaundice develops in any woman receiving such drugs, the medication should be discontinued. Steroid hormones may be poorly metabolized in patients with impaired liver function.

5. FLUID RETENTION

Oral contraceptives may cause some degree of fluid retention. They should be prescribed with caution, and only with careful monitoring, in patients with conditions which might be aggravated by fluid retention.

6. EMOTIONAL DISORDERS

Women with a history of depression should be carefully observed and the drug discontinued if depression recurs to a serious degree.

7. CONTACT LENSES

Contact-lens wearers who develop visual changes or changes in lens tolerance should be assessed by an ophthalmologist.

8. DRUG INTERACTIONS

Reduced efficacy and increased incidence of breakthrough bleeding and menstrual irregularities have been associated with concomitant use of rifampin. A similar association, though less marked, has been suggested with barbiturates, phenylbutazone, phenytoin sodium, and possibly with griseofulvin, ampicillin and tetracyclines.

9. INTERACTIONS WITH LABORATORY TESTS

Certain endocrine- and liver-function tests and blood components may be affected by oral contraceptives:

TABLE V—ANNUAL NUMBER OF BIRTH-RELATED OR METHOD-RELATED DEATHS ASSOCIATED WITH CONTROL OF FERTILITY PER 100,000 NONSTERILE WOMEN, BY FERTILITY-CONTROL METHOD ACCORDING TO AGE

Method of control and outcome	15–19	20–24	25–29	30–34	35–39	40–44
No fertility—control methods*	7.0	7.4	9.1	14.8	25.7	28.2
Oral contraceptives nonsmoker**	0.3	0.5	0.9	1.9	13.8	31.6
Oral contraceptives smoker**	2.2	3.4	6.6	13.5	51.1	117.2
IUD**	0.8	0.8	1.0	1.0	1.4	1.4
Condom*	1.1	1.6	0.7	0.2	0.3	0.4
Diaphragm/spermicide*	1.9	1.2	1.2	1.3	2.2	2.8
Periodic abstinence*	2.5	1.6	1.6	1.7	2.9	3.6

* Deaths are birth related
** Deaths are method related

Adapted from H.W. Ory, Family Planning Perspectives *15*:57–63, 1983.

a. Increased prothrombin and factors VII, VIII, IX and X; decreased antithrombin 3; increased norepinephrine-induced platelet aggregability.
b. Increased thyroid-binding globulin (TBG) leading to increased circulating total thyroid hormone, as measured by protein-bound iodine (PBI), T4 by column or by radioimmunoassay. Free T3 resin uptake is decreased, reflecting the elevated TBG, free T4 concentration is unaltered.
c. Other binding proteins may be elevated in serum.
d. Sex-binding globulins are increased and result in elevated levels of total circulating sex steroids and corticoids; however, free or biologically active levels remain unchanged.
e. Triglycerides may be increased.
f. Glucose tolerance may be decreased.
g. Serum folate levels may be depressed by oral-contraceptive therapy. This may be of clinical significance if a woman becomes pregnant shortly after discontinuing oral contraceptives.

10. CARCINOGENESIS

See "WARNINGS" section.

11. PREGNANCY

Pregnancy Category X. See "CONTRAINDICATIONS" and "WARNINGS" sections.

12. NURSING MOTHERS

Small amounts of oral-contraceptive steroids have been identified in the milk of nursing mothers, and a few adverse effects on the child have been reported, including jaundice and breast enlargement. In addition, oral contraceptives given in the postpartum period may interfere with lactation by decreasing the quantity and quality of breast milk. If possible, the nursing mother should be advised not to use oral contraceptives but to use other forms of contraception until she has completely weaned her child.

13. PEDIATRIC USE

Safety and efficacy of LEVLITE™ have been established in women of reproductive age. Safety and efficacy are expected to be the same for postpubertal adolescents under the age of 16 and for users 16 years and older. Use of this product before menarche is not indicated.

INFORMATION FOR THE PATIENT

See "Patient Labeling" printed below.

ADVERSE REACTIONS

An increased risk of the following serious adverse reactions has been associated with the use of oral contraceptives (see "WARNINGS" section).

- Thrombophlebitis
- Arterial thromboembolism
- Pulmonary embolism
- Myocardial infarction
- Cerebral hemorrhage
- Cerebral thrombosis
- Hypertension
- Gallbladder disease
- Hepatic adenomas or benign liver tumors

There is evidence of an association between the following conditions and the use of oral contraceptives, although additional confirmatory studies are needed:

- Mesenteric thrombosis
- Retinal thrombosis

The following adverse reactions have been reported in patients receiving oral contraceptives and are believed to be drug related:

- Nausea
- Vomiting
- Gastrointestinal symptoms, (such as abdominal cramps and bloating)
- Breakthrough bleeding
- Spotting
- Change in menstrual flow
- Amenorrhea
- Temporary infertility after discontinuation of treatment
- Edema
- Melasma which may persist
- Breast changes: tenderness, enlargement, secretion
- Change in weight (increase or decrease)
- Change in cervical erosion and secretion
- Diminution in lactation when given immediately postpartum
- Cholestatic jaundice
- Migraine
- Rash (allergic)
- Mental depression
- Reduced tolerance to carbohydrates
- Vaginal candidiasis
- Change in corneal curvature (steepening)
- Intolerance to contact lenses

The following adverse reactions have been reported in users of oral contraceptives and the association has been neither confirmed nor refuted:

- Premenstrual syndrome
- Cataracts
- Optic neuritis
- Changes in appetite
- Cystitis-like syndrome
- Headache
- Nervousness
- Dizziness
- Hirsutism
- Loss of scalp hair
- Erythema multiforme
- Erythema nodosum
- Hemorrhagic eruption
- Vaginitis
- Porphyria
- Impaired renal function
- Hemolytic uremic syndrome
- Budd-Chiari syndrome
- Acne
- Changes in libido
- Colitis

OVERDOSAGE

Serious ill effects have not been reported following acute ingestion of large doses of oral contraceptives by young children. Overdosage may cause nausea, and withdrawal bleeding may occur in females.

NON-CONTRACEPTIVE HEALTH BENEFITS

The following noncontraceptive health benefits related to the use of oral contraceptives are supported by epidemiological studies which largely utilized oral-contraceptive formulations containing doses exceeding 0.035 mg of ethinyl estradiol or 0.05 mg mestranol.

Effects on menses:
- increased menstrual cycle regularity
- decreased blood loss and decreased incidence of iron-deficiency anemia
- decreased incidence of dysmenorrhea

Effects related to inhibition of ovulation:
- decreased incidence of functional ovarian cysts
- decreased incidence of ectopic pregnancies

Effects from long-term use:
- decreased incidence of fibroadenomas and fibrocystic disease of the breast
- decreased incidence of acute pelvic inflammatory disease
- decreased incidence of endometrial cancer
- decreased incidence of ovarian cancer

DOSAGE AND ADMINISTRATION

LEVLITE™ 21 Tablets

To achieve maximum contraceptive effectiveness, LEVLITE™ 21 Tablets (levonorgestrel and ethinyl estradiol tablets, USP) must be taken exactly as directed at intervals not exceeding 24-hours.

LEVLITE™ 21 Tablets are a monophasic preparation. The dosage of LEVLITE™ 21 Tablets is one tablet daily for 21 consecutive days per menstrual cycle according to the prescribed schedule. Tablets are then discontinued for 7 days (three weeks on, one week off). It is recommended that LEVLITE™ 21 Tablets be taken at the same time each day, preferably after the evening meal or at bedtime. During the first cycle of medication, the patient should be instructed to take one pink LEVLITE™ 21 Tablet daily beginning on day one (1) of her menstrual cycle. (The first day of menstruation is day one.) The tablets are then discontinued for one week (7 days). Withdrawal bleeding usually occurs within 3 days following discontinuation of LEVLITE™ 21 Tablets. (If LEVLITE™ 21 Tablets are first taken later than the first day of the first menstrual cycle of medication or postpartum, contraceptive reliance should not be placed on LEVLITE™ 21

Continued on next page

Information on the Berlex products appearing here is based on the most current information available at the time of publication closing. Further information for these and other products may be obtained from the Medical Affairs Department, Berlex Laboratories, 300 Fairfield Road, Wayne, New Jersey 07470, 1-888-BERLEX-4. Information on Betaseron and Fludara may be obtained from Berlex Laboratories, 15049 San Pablo Avenue, Richmond, California 94804-0016, 1-800-888-4112.

Levlite/Tri-Levlen/Levlen—Cont.

Tablets until after the first 7 consecutive days of administration. The possibility of ovulation and conception prior to initiation of medication should be considered.)

When switching from another oral contraceptive, LEVLITE™ 21 Tablets should be started on the first day of bleeding following the last active tablet taken of the previous oral contraceptive.

The patient begins her next and all subsequent 21-day courses of LEVLITE™ 21 Tablets on the same day of the week that she began her first course, following the same schedule: 21 days on – 7 days off. She begins taking her pink tablets on the 8th day after discontinuance, regardless of whether or not a menstrual period has occurred or is still in progress. Any time the next cycle of LEVLITE™ 21 Tablets is started later than the 8th day, the patient should be protected by another means of contraception until she has taken a tablet daily for seven consecutive days.

If spotting or breakthrough bleeding occurs, the patient is instructed to continue on the same regimen. This type of bleeding is usually transient and without significance; however, if the bleeding is persistent or prolonged, the patient is advised to consult her physician. Although the occurrence of pregnancy is highly unlikely if LEVLITE™ 21 Tablets are taken according to directions, if withdrawal bleeding does not occur, the possibility of pregnancy must be considered. If the patient has not adhered to the prescribed schedule (missed one or more tablets or started taking them on a day later than she should have), the probability of pregnancy should be considered at the time of the first missed period and appropriate diagnostic measures taken before the medication is resumed. If the patient has adhered to the prescribed regimen and misses two consecutive periods, pregnancy should be ruled out before continuing the contraceptive regimen.

The risk of pregnancy increases with each tablet missed. For additional patient instructions regarding missed pills, see the "WHAT TO DO IF YOU MISS PILLS" section in the DETAILED PATIENT LABELING below. If breakthrough bleeding occurs following missed tablets, it will usually be transient and of no consequence.

In the nonlactating mother, LEVLITE™ 21 Tablets may be initiated postpartum, for contraception. When the tablets are administered in the postpartum period, the increased risk of thromboembolic disease associated with the postpartum period must be considered. (See "CONTRAINDICATIONS," "WARNINGS," and "PRECAUTIONS" concerning thromboembolic disease.) It is to be noted that early resumption of ovulation may occur if bromocriptine mesylate has been used for the prevention of lactation.

LEVLITE™ 28 Tablets

To achieve maximum contraceptive effectiveness, LEVLITE™ 28 Tablets (levonorgestrel and ethinyl estradiol tablets, USP) must be taken exactly as directed at intervals not exceeding 24-hours.

LEVLITE™ 28 Tablets are a monophasic preparation plus 7 inert tablets. The dosage of LEVLITE™ 28 Tablets is one tablet daily for 21 consecutive days per menstrual cycle plus 7 white inert tablets according to the prescribed schedule. It is recommended that LEVLITE™ 28 Tablets be taken at the same time each day, preferably after the evening meal or at bedtime. During the first cycle of medication, the patient should be instructed to take one pink LEVLITE™ 28 Tablet daily and then 7 white inert tablets for twenty-eight (28) consecutive days, beginning on day one (1) of her menstrual cycle. (The first day of menstruation is day one.) Withdrawal bleeding usually occurs within 3 days following the last pink tablet. (If LEVLITE™ 28 Tablets are first taken later than the first day of the first menstrual cycle of medication or postpartum, contraceptive reliance should not be placed on LEVLITE™ 28 Tablets until after the first 7 consecutive days of administration. The possibility of ovulation and conception prior to initiation of medication should be considered.)

When switching from another oral contraceptive, LEVLITE™ 28 Tablets should be started on the first day of bleeding following the last active tablet taken of the previous oral contraceptive.

The patient begins her next and all subsequent 28-day courses of LEVLITE™ 28 Tablets on the same day of the week that she began her first course, following the same schedule. She begins taking her pink tablets on the next day after ingestion of the last white tablet, regardless of whether or not a menstrual period has occurred or is still in progress. Anytime a subsequent cycle of LEVLITE™ 28 Tablets is started later than the next day, the patient should be protected by another means of contraception until she has taken a tablet daily for seven consecutive days.

If spotting or breakthrough bleeding occurs, the patient is instructed to continue on the same regimen. This type of bleeding is usually transient and without significance, however, if the bleeding is persistent or prolonged, the patient is advised to consult her physician. Although the occurrence of pregnancy is highly unlikely if LEVLITE™ 28 Tablets are taken according to directions, if withdrawal bleeding does not occur, the possibility of pregnancy must be considered. If the patient has not adhered to the prescribed schedule (missed one or more active tablets or started taking them on a day later than she should have), the probability of pregnancy should be considered at the time of the first missed period and appropriate diagnostic measures taken before the medication is resumed. If the patient has adhered to the prescribed regimen and misses two consecutive periods, pregnancy should be ruled out before continuing the contraceptive regimen.

The risk of pregnancy increases with each active (pink) tablet missed. For additional patient instructions regarding missed pills, see the "WHAT TO DO IF YOU MISS PILLS" section in the DETAILED PATIENT LABELING below. If breakthrough bleeding occurs following missed tablets, it will usually be transient and of no consequence. If the patient misses one or more white tablets, she is still protected against pregnancy provided she begins taking pink tablets again on the proper day.

In the nonlactating mother, LEVLITE™ 28 Tablets may be initiated postpartum, for contraception. When the tablets are administered in the postpartum period, the increased risk of thromboembolic disease associated with the postpartum period must be considered. (See "CONTRAINDICATIONS," "WARNINGS," and "PRECAUTIONS" concerning thromboembolic disease.) It is to be noted that early resumption of ovulation may occur if bromocriptine mesylate has been used for the prevention of lactation.

TRI-LEVLEN® 21 Tablets

To achieve maximum contraceptive effectiveness, TRI-LEVLEN® 21 Tablets (levonorgestrel and ethinyl estradiol tablets—triphasic regimen) should be taken exactly as directed and at intervals not exceeding 24-hours.

TRI-LEVLEN® 21 Tablets are a three-phase preparation. The dosage of TRI-LEVLEN® 21 Tablets is **one tablet** daily for 21 consecutive days per menstrual cycle in the following order: 6 brown tablets (phase 1), followed by 5 white tablets (phase 2), and then followed by the last 10 light-yellow tablets (phase 3), according to the prescribed schedule. Tablets are then discontinued for 7 days (three weeks on, one week off).

It is recommended that TRI-LEVLEN® 21 Tablets be taken at the same time each day. During the first cycle of medication, the patient should be instructed to take one TRI-LEVLEN® 21 Tablet daily in the order of 6 brown, 5 white and, finally, 10 light-yellow tablets for twenty-one (21) consecutive days, beginning on day one (1) of her menstrual cycle. (The first day of menstruation is day one.) The tablets are then discontinued for one week (7 days). Withdrawal bleeding usually occurs within 3 days following discontinuation of TRI-LEVLEN® 21 Tablets. (If an alternate starting regimen is used [Sunday Start or postpartum], contraceptive reliance should not be placed on TRI-LEVLEN® 21 Tablets until after the first 7 consecutive days of administration. The possibility of ovulation and conception prior to initiation of medication should be considered.)

The patient begins her next and all subsequent 21-day courses of TRI-LEVLEN® 21 Tablets on the same day of the week that she began her first course, following the same schedule: 21 days on—7 days off. She begins taking her brown tablets on the 8th day after discontinuance, regardless of whether or not a menstrual period has occurred or is still in progress. Any time the next cycle of TRI-LEVLEN® 21 Tablets is started later than the 8th day, the patient should be protected by another means of contraception until she has taken a tablet daily for seven consecutive days.

If spotting or breakthrough bleeding occurs, the patient is instructed to continue on the same regimen. This type of bleeding is usually transient and without significance; however, if the bleeding is persistent or prolonged, the patient is advised to consult her physician. Although the occurrence of pregnancy is highly unlikely if TRI-LEVLEN® 21 Tablets are taken according to directions, if withdrawal bleeding does not occur, the possibility of pregnancy must be considered. If the patient has not adhered to the prescribed schedule (missed one or more tablets or started taking them on a day later than she should have), the probability of pregnancy should be considered at the time of the first missed period and appropriate diagnostic measures taken before the medication is resumed. If the patient has adhered to the prescribed regimen and misses two consecutive periods, pregnancy should be ruled out before continuing the contraceptive regimen.

The risk of pregnancy increases with each active (brown, white, or light-yellow) tablet missed. For additional patient instructions regarding missed pills, see the "WHAT TO DO IF YOU MISS PILLS" section in the DETAILED PATIENT LABELING below. If breakthrough bleeding occurs following missed active tablets, it will usually be transient and of no consequence. If the patient misses one or more light-green tablets, she is still protected against pregnancy **provided** she begins taking brown tablets again on the proper day.

In the nonlactating mother, TRI-LEVLEN® 21 Tablets may be initiated postpartum, for contraception. When the tablets are administered in the postpartum period, the increased risk of thromboembolic disease associated with the postpartum period must be considered. (See "CONTRAINDICATIONS", "WARNINGS", and "PRECAUTIONS" concerning thromboembolic disease.) It is to be noted that early resumption of ovulation may occur if Parlodel® (bromocriptine mesylate) has been used for the prevention of lactation.

TRI-LEVLEN® 28 Tablets

To achieve maximum contraceptive effectiveness, TRI-LEVLEN® 28 Tablets (levonorgestrel and ethinyl estradiol tablets—triphasic regimen) should be taken exactly as directed and at intervals not exceeding 24-hours.

TRI-LEVLEN® 28 Tablets are a three-phase preparation plus 7 inert tablets. The dosage of TRI-LEVLEN® 28 Tablets is one tablet daily for 28 consecutive days per menstrual cycle in the following order: 6 brown tablets (phase 1), followed by 5 white tablets (phase 2), followed by 10 light-yellow tablets (phase 3), plus 7 light-green inert tablets according to the prescribed schedule.

It is recommended that TRI-LEVLEN® 28 Tablets be taken at the same time each day. During the first cycle of medication, the patient should be instructed to take one TRI-LEVLEN® 28 Tablet daily in the order of 6 brown, 5 white, 10 light-yellow tablets and then 7 light-green inert tablets for twenty-eight (28) consecutive days, beginning on day one (1) of her menstrual cycle. (The first day of menstruation is day one.) Withdrawal bleeding usually occurs within 3 days following the last light-yellow tablets. (If an alternate starting regimen is used [Sunday Start or postpartum], contraceptive reliance should not be placed on TRI-LEVLEN® 28 Tablets until after the first 7 consecutive days of administration. The possibility of ovulation and conception prior to initiation of medication should be considered.)

The patient begins her next and all subsequent 28-day courses of TRI-LEVLEN® 28 Tablets on the same day of the week that she began her first course, following the same schedule: She begins taking her brown tablets on the next day after ingestion of the last light-green tablet, regardless of whether or not a menstrual period has occurred or is still in progress. Any time a subsequent cycle of TRI-LEVLEN® 28 Tablets is started later than the next day, the patient should be protected by another means of contraception until she has taken a tablet daily for seven consecutive days.

If spotting or breakthrough bleeding occurs, the patient is instructed to continue on the same regimen. This type of bleeding is usually transient and without significance; however, if the bleeding is persistent or prolonged, the patient is advised to consult her physician. Although the occurrence of pregnancy is highly unlikely if TRI-LEVLEN® 28 Tablets are taken according to directions, if withdrawal bleeding does not occur, the possibility of pregnancy must be considered. If the patient has not adhered to the prescribed schedule (missed one or more active tablets or started taking them on a day later than she should have), the probability of pregnancy should be considered at the time of the first missed period and appropriate diagnostic measures taken before the medication is resumed. If the patient has adhered to the prescribed regimen and misses two consecutive periods, pregnancy should be ruled out before continuing the contraceptive regimen.

The risk of pregnancy increases with each active (brown, white, or light-yellow) tablet missed. For additional patient instructions regarding missed pills, see the "WHAT TO DO IF YOU MISS PILLS" section in the DETAILED PATIENT LABELING below. If breakthrough bleeding occurs following missed active tablets, it will usually be transient and of no consequence. If the patient misses one or more light-green tablets, she is still protected against pregnancy **provided** she begins taking brown tablets again on the proper day.

In the nonlactating mother, TRI-LEVLEN® 28 Tablets may be initiated postpartum, for contraception. When the tablets are administered in the postpartum period, the increased risk of thromboembolic disease associated with the postpartum period must be considered. (See "CONTRAINDICATIONS", "WARNINGS", and "PRECAUTIONS" concerning thromboembolic disease.) It is to be noted that early resumption of ovulation may occur if Parlodel® (bromocriptine mesylate) has been used for the prevention of lactation.

LEVLEN® 21 Tablets

To achieve maximum contraceptive effectiveness, LEVLEN® 21 Tablets (levonorgestrel and ethinyl estradiol tablets) should be taken exactly as directed and at intervals not exceeding 24-hours.

The dosage of LEVLEN® 21 Tablets is **one tablet** daily for 21 consecutive days per menstrual cycle according to the prescribed schedule. Tablets are then discontinued for 7 days (three weeks on, one week off).

It is recommended that LEVLEN® 21 Tablets be taken at the same time each day. During the first cycle of medication, the patient should be instructed to take one LEVLEN® 21 Tablet daily for twenty-one (21) consecutive days, beginning on day one (1) of her menstrual cycle. (The first day of menstruation is day one.) The tablets are then discontinued for one week (7 days). Withdrawal bleeding usually occurs within 3 days following discontinuation of LEVLEN® 21 Tablets. (If an alternate starting regimen is used [Sunday Start or postpartum], contraceptive reliance should not be placed on LEVLEN® 21 Tablets until after the first 7 consecutive days of administration. The possibility of ovulation and conception prior to initiation of medication should be considered.)

The patient begins her next and all subsequent 21-day courses of LEVLEN® 21 Tablets on the same day of the week that she began her first course, following the same schedule: 21 days on—7 days off. She begins taking her light-orange tablets on the 8th day after discontinuance, regardless of whether or not a menstrual period has occurred or is still in progress. Any time the next cycle of LEVLEN® 21 Tablets is started later than the 8th day, the patient should be protected by another means of contraception until she has taken a tablet daily for seven consecutive days.

If spotting or breakthrough bleeding occurs, the patient is instructed to continue on the same regimen. This type of bleeding is usually transient and without significance; however, if the bleeding is persistent or prolonged, the patient is advised to consult her physician. Although the occurrence of pregnancy is highly unlikely if LEVLEN® 21 Tablets are taken according to directions, if withdrawal bleeding does not occur, the possibility of pregnancy must be considered. If the patient has not adhered to the prescribed schedule (missed one or more tablets or started taking them on a day later than she should have), the probability of pregnancy should be considered at the time of the first missed period and appropriate diagnostic measures taken before the medication is resumed. If the patient has adhered to the prescribed regimen and misses two consecutive periods, pregnancy should be ruled out before continuing the contraceptive regimen.

In the nonlactating mother, LEVLEN® 21 Tablets may be initiated postpartum, for contraception. When the tablets are administered in the postpartum period, the increased risk of thromboembolic disease associated with the postpartum period must be considered. (See "CONTRAINDICATIONS", "WARNINGS", and "PRECAUTIONS" concerning thromboembolic disease.)

LEVLEN® 28 Tablets

To achieve maximum contraceptive effectiveness, LEVLEN® 28 Tablets (levonorgestrel and ethinyl estradiol tablets) should be taken exactly as directed at intervals not exceeding 24-hours.

The dosage of LEVLEN® 28 Tablets is one light-orange tablet daily for 21 consecutive days per menstrual cycle, followed by 7 pink insert tablets according to the prescribed schedule.

It is recommended that LEVLEN® 28 Tablets be taken at the same time each day. During the first cycle of medication, the patient should be instructed to take one TRI-LEVLEN® 28 Tablet daily in the order of 21 light orange and then 7 pink inert tablets for twenty-eight (28) consecutive days, beginning on day one (1) of her menstrual cycle. (The first day of menstruation is day one.) Withdrawal bleeding usually occurs within 3 days following the last light-orange tablet. (If an alternate starting regimen is used [Sunday Start or postpartum], contraceptive reliance should not be placed on LEVLEN® 28 Tablets until after the first 7 consecutive days of administration. The possibility of ovulation and conception prior to initiation of medication should be considered.)

The patient begins her next and all subsequent 28-day courses of LEVLEN® 28 Tablets on the same day of the week that she began her first course, following the same schedule. She begins taking her light-orange tablets on the next day after ingestion of the last pink tablet, regardless of whether or not a menstrual period has occurred or is still in progress. Any time a subsequent cycle of LEVLEN® 28 Tablets is started later than the next day, the patient should be protected by another means of contraception until she has taken a tablet daily for seven consecutive days.

If spotting or breakthrough bleeding occurs, the patient is instructed to continue on the same regimen. This type of bleeding is usually transient and without significance; however, if the bleeding is persistent or prolonged, the patient is advised to consult her physician. Although the occurrence of pregnancy is highly unlikely if LEVLEN® 28 Tablets are taken according to directions, if withdrawal bleeding does not occur, the possibility of pregnancy must be considered. If the patient has not adhered to the prescribed schedule (missed one or more active tablets or started taking them on a day later than she should have), the probability of pregnancy should be considered at the time of the first missed period and appropriate diagnostic measures taken before the medication is resumed. If the patient has adhered to the prescribed regimen and misses two consecutive periods, pregnancy should be ruled out before continuing the contraceptive regimen.

Any time the patient misses two or more tablets, she should also use another method of contraception until she has taken a tablet daily for seven consecutive days. If breakthrough bleeding occurs following missed active tablets, it usually will be transient and of no consequence. If the patient misses one or more pink tablets, she is still protected against pregnancy provided she begins taking the light-orange tablets again on the proper day.

In the nonlactating mother, LEVLEN® 28 Tablets may be initiated postpartum, for contraception. When the tablets are administered in the postpartum period, the increased risk of thromboembolic disease associated with the postpartum period must be considered. (See "CONTRAINDICATIONS", "WARNINGS", and "PRECAUTIONS" concerning thromboembolic disease.)

HOW SUPPLIED

LEVLITE™ 21 Tablets (levonorgestrel and ethinyl estradiol tablets, USP), are available in packages of 3 SLIDECASE® dispensers. Each cycle contains 21 round, unscored, coated tablets as follows:

In packages of 3 SLIDECASE® dispensers, NDC 50419-406-03

LEVLITE™ 28 Tablets (levonorgestrel and ethinyl estradiol tablets, USP), are available in packages of 3 SLIDECASE® dispensers. Each cycle contains 28 round, unscored coated tablets as follows:

In packages of 3 SLIDECASE® dispensers, NDC 50419-408-03

Keep at room temperature, approximately 25° C (77° F).

TRI-LEVLEN® 21 tablets (Levonorgestrel and Ethinyl Estradiol Tablets—Triphasic Regimen), are available in packages of 3 and 6 SLIDECASE® dispensers. Each cycle contains 21 round, film-coated tablets as follows:

NDC 50419-195, six brown tablets marked "B" on one side and "95" on the other side, each containing 0.050 mg levonorgestrel and 0.030 mg ethinyl estradiol;

NDC 50419-196, five white to off-white tablets marked "B" on one side and "96" on the other side, each containing 0.075 mg levonorgestrel and 0.040 mg ethinyl estradiol; and

NDC 50419-197, ten light-yellow tablets marked "B" on one side and "97" on the other side, each containing 0.125 mg levonorgestrel and 0.030 mg ethinyl estradiol.

In packages of:

3 SLIDECASE® dispensers .... NDC 50419-432-03

6 SLIDECASE® dispensers .... NDC 50419-432-06

TRI-LEVLEN® 28 tablets (Levonorgestrel and Ethinyl Estradiol Tablets—Triphasic Regimen), are available in packages of 3 and 6 SLIDECASE® dispensers. Each cycle contains 28 round, film-coated tablets as follows:

NDC 50419-195, six brown tablets marked "B" on one side and "95" on the other side, each containing 0.050 mg levonorgestrel and 0.030 mg ethinyl estradiol;

NDC 50419-196, five white to off-white tablets marked "B" on one side and "96" on the other side, each containing 0.075 mg levonorgestrel and 0.040 mg ethinyl estradiol;

NDC 50419-197, ten light-yellow tablets marked "B" on one side and "97" on the other side, each containing 0.125 mg levonorgestrel and 0.030 mg ethinyl estradiol; and

NDC 50419-111, seven light-green inert tablets marked "B" on one side and "11" on the other side.

In packages of:

3 SLIDECASE® dispensers .... NDC 50419-433-03

6 SLIDECASE® dispensers .... NDC 50419-433-06

LEVLEN® 21 tablets (Levonorgestrel and Ethinyl Estradiol Tablets), are available in packages of 3 SLIDECASE® dispensers. Each cycle contains 21 round, tablets as follows:

NDC 50419-021, 21 active light-orange tablets marked "B" on one side and "21" on the other side, each containing 0.15 mg levonorgestrel and 0.03 mg ethinyl estradiol;

In packages of:

3 SLIDECASE® dispensers .... NDC 50419-410-21

LEVLEN® 28 tablets (Levonorgestrel and Ethinyl Estradiol Tablets), are available in packages of 3 SLIDECASE® dispensers. Each cycle contains 28 round tablets as follows:

NDC 50419-021, 21 active, light-orange tablets marked "B" on one side and "21" on the other side, each containing 0.15 mg levonorgestrel and 0.03 mg ethinyl estradiol;

NDC 50419-028, 7 inert pink tablets marked "B" on one side and "28" on the other side.

In packages of:

3 SLIDECASE® dispensers .... NDC 50419-411-28

REFERENCES

References furnished upon request.

BRIEF SUMMARY PATIENT PACKAGE INSERT

This product (like all oral contraceptives) is intended to prevent pregnancy. It does not protect against HIV infection (AIDS) and other sexually transmitted diseases.

Oral contraceptives, also known as "birth-control pills" or "the pill", are taken to prevent pregnancy, and when taken correctly, have a failure rate of less than 1% per year when used without missing any pills. The typical failure rate of large numbers of pill users is less than 3% per year when women who miss pills are included. For most women oral contraceptives are also free of serious or unpleasant side effects. However, forgetting to take pills considerably increases the chances of pregnancy.

For the majority of women, oral contraceptives can be taken safely. But there are some women who are at high risk of developing certain serious diseases that can be life-threatening or may cause temporary or permanent disability or death. The risks associated with taking oral contraceptives increase significantly if you:

- smoke
- have high blood pressure, diabetes, high cholesterol
- have or have had clotting disorders, heart attack, stroke, angina pectoris, cancer of the breast or sex organs, jaundice, or malignant or benign liver tumors.

You should not take the pill if you suspect you are pregnant or have unexplained vaginal bleeding.

Cigarette smoking increases the risk of serious adverse effects on the heart and blood vessels from oral-contraceptive use. This risk increases with age and with heavy smoking (15 or more cigarettes per day) and is quite marked in women over 35 years of age. Women who use oral contraceptives should not smoke.

Most side effects of the pill are not serious. The most common such effects are nausea, vomiting, bleeding between menstrual periods, weight gain, breast tenderness, and difficulty wearing contact lenses. These side effects, especially nausea and vomiting may subside within the first three months of use.

The serious side effects of the pill occur very infrequently, especially if you are in good health and are young. However, you should know that the following medical conditions have been associated with or made worse by the pill:

1. Blood clots in the legs (thrombophlebitis), lungs (pulmonary embolism), stoppage or rupture of a blood vessel in the brain (stroke), blockage of blood vessels in the heart (heart attack and angina pectoris) or other organs of the body. As mentioned above, smoking increases the risk of heart attacks and strokes and subsequent serious medical consequences.

2. Liver tumors, which may rupture and cause severe bleeding. A possible but not definite association has been found with the pill and liver cancer. However, liver cancers are extremely rare. The chance of developing liver cancer from using the pill is thus even rarer.

3. High blood pressure, although blood pressure usually returns to normal when the pill is stopped.

The symptoms associated with these serious side effects are discussed in the detailed leaflet given to you with your supply of pills. Notify your doctor or healthcare provider if you notice any unusual physical disturbances while taking the pill. In addition, drugs such as rifampin, as well as some anticonvulsants and some antibiotics, may decrease oral contraceptive effectiveness.

Studies to date of women taking the pill have not shown an increase in the incidence of cancer of the breast or cervix. There is, however, insufficient evidence to rule out the possibility that pills may cause such cancers.

Taking the pill provides some important noncontraceptive benefits. These include less painful menstruation, less menstrual blood loss and anemia, fewer pelvic infections, and fewer cancers of the ovary and the lining of the uterus.

Be sure to discuss any medical condition you may have with your healthcare provider. Your healthcare provider will take a medical and family history before prescribing oral contraceptives and will examine you. The physicial examination may be delayed to another time if you request it and the healthcare provider believes that it is appropriate to postpone it.

You should be reexamined at least once a year while taking oral contraceptives. The detailed patient information booklet gives you further information which you should read and discuss with your healthcare provider.

DETAILED PATIENT PACKAGE INSERT

This product (like all oral contraceptives) is intended to prevent pregnancy. It does not protect against HIV infection (AIDS) and other sexually transmitted diseases.

INTRODUCTION

Any woman who considers using oral contraceptives (the "birth control pill" or the "pill") should understand the benefits and risks of using this form of birth control. This leaflet will give you much of the information you will need to make this decision and will also help you determine if you are at risk of developing any of the serious side effects of the pill. It will tell you how to use the pill properly so that it will be as effective as possible. However, this leaflet is not a replacement for a careful discussion between you and your healthcare provider. You should discuss the information provided in this leaflet with him or her, both when you first start taking the pill and during your revisits. You should also follow your healthcare provider's advice with regard to regular checks-ups while you are on the pill.

EFFECTIVENESS OF ORAL CONTRACEPTIVES

Oral contraceptives or "birth control pills" or "the pill" are used to prevent pregnancy and are more effective than other nonsurgical methods of birth control. When they are taken correctly, the chance of becoming pregnant is less than 1% when used perfectly, without missing pills. Typical failure rates are less than 3.0% per year. The chance of becoming pregnant increases with each missed pill during the menstrual cycle.

In comparison, typical failure rates for other nonsurgical methods of birth control during the first year of use are as follows:

[See first table at top of next page]

WHO SHOULD NOT TAKE ORAL CONTRACEPTIVES

Cigarette smoking increases the risk of serious adverse effects on the heart and blood vessels from oral-contraceptive use. This risk increases with age and with heavy smoking (15 or more cigarettes per day) and is quite marked in women over 35 years of age. Women who use oral contraceptives should not smoke.

Some women should not use the pill. For example, you should not take the pill if you are pregnant or think you may be pregnant. You should also not use the pill if you have had any of the following conditions:

- A history of heart attack or stroke
- Blood clots in the legs (thrombophlebitis), lungs (pulmonary embolism), or eyes
- A history of blood clots in the deep veins of your legs
- Chest pain (angina pectoris)
- Known or suspected breast cancer or cancer of the lining of the uterus, cervix or vagina
- Unexplained vaginal bleeding (until a diagnosis is reached by your doctor)
- Yellowing of the whites of the eyes or of the skin (jaundice) during pregnancy or during previous use of the pill
- Liver tumor (benign or cancerous)
- Known or suspected pregnancy

Tell your health-care provider if you have ever had any of these conditions. Your healthcare provider can recommend another method of birth control.

Continued on next page

Information on the Berlex products appearing here is based on the most current information available at the time of publication closing. Further information for these and other products may be obtained from the Medical Affairs Department, Berlex Laboratories, 300 Fairfield Road, Wayne, New Jersey 07470, 1-888-BERLEX-4. Information on Betaseron and Fludara may be obtained from Berlex Laboratories, 15049 San Pablo Avenue, Richmond, California 94804-0016, 1-800-888-4112.

Levlite/Tri-Levlen/Levlen—Cont.

OTHER CONSIDERATIONS BEFORE TAKING ORAL CONTRACEPTIVES

Tell your healthcare provider if you or any family member has ever had:

- Breast nodules, fibrocystic disease of the breast, an abnormal breast x-ray or mammogram
- Diabetes
- Elevated cholesterol or triglycerides
- High blood pressure
- Migraine or other headaches or epilepsy
- Mental depression
- Gallbladder, heart or kidney disease
- History of scanty or irregular menstrual periods

Women with any of these conditions should be checked often by their healthcare provider if they choose to use oral contraceptives. Also, be sure to inform your doctor or healthcare provider if you smoke or are on any medications.

RISKS OF TAKING ORAL CONTRACEPTIVES

1. RISK OF DEVELOPING BLOOD CLOTS

Blood clots and blockage of blood vessels are the most serious side effects of taking oral contraceptives and can be fatal. In particular, a clot in the legs can cause thrombophlebitis and a clot that travels to the lungs can cause a sudden blocking of the vessel carrying blood to the lungs. Rarely, clots occur in the blood vessels of the eye and may cause blindness, double vision, or impaired vision.

If you take oral contraceptives and need elective surgery, need to stay in bed for a prolonged illness or have recently delivered a baby, you may be at risk of developing blood clots. You should consult your doctor about stopping oral contraceptives three to four weeks before surgery and not taking oral contraceptives for 2 weeks after surgery or during bed rest. You should also not take oral contraceptives soon after delivery of a baby or a midtrimester pregnancy termination. It is advisable to wait for at least 4 weeks after delivery if you are not breast-feeding. If you are breast-feeding, you should wait until you have weaned your child before using the pill. (See also the section on Breast-Feeding in "GENERAL PRECAUTIONS".)

2. HEART ATTACKS AND STROKES

Oral contraceptives may increase the tendency to develop strokes (stoppage or rupture of blood vessels in the brain) and angina pectoris and heart attacks (blockage of blood vessels in the heart). Any of these conditions can cause death or serious disability.

Smoking greatly increases the possibility of suffering heart attacks and strokes. Furthermore, smoking and the use of oral contraceptives greatly increase the chances of developing and dying of heart disease.

3. GALLBLADDER DISEASE

Oral-contraceptive users probably have a greater risk than nonusers of having gallbladder disease, although this risk may be related to pills containing high doses of estrogens.

4. LIVER TUMORS

In rare cases, oral contraceptives can cause benign but dangerous liver tumors. These benign liver tumors can rupture and cause fatal internal bleeding. In addition, a possible but not definite association has been found with the pill and liver cancers in two studies, in which a few women who developed these very rare cancers were found to have used oral contraceptives for long periods. However, liver cancers are extremely rare. The chance of developing liver cancer from using the pill is thus even rarer.

5. CANCER OF THE REPRODUCTIVE ORGANS

There is, at present, no confirmed evidence that oral contraceptives increase the risk of cancer of the reproductive organs in human studies. Several studies have found no overall increase in the risk of developing breast cancer. However, women who use oral contraceptives and have a strong family history of breast cancer or who have breast nodules or abnormal mammograms should be closely followed by their doctors.

Some studies have found an increase in the incidence of cancer of the cervix in women who use oral contraceptives. However, this finding may be related to factors other than the use of oral contraceptives.

[See table V above]

In the above table, the risk of death from any birth-control method is less than the risk of childbirth, except for oral contraceptive users over the age of 35 who smoke and pill users over the age of 40 even if they do not smoke. It can be seen in the table that for women aged 15 to 39, the risk of death is highest with pregnancy (7 to 26 deaths per 100,000 women, depending on age). Among pill users who do not smoke, the risk of death was always lower than that associated with pregnancy for any age group, except for those women over the age of 40 when the risk increases to 32 deaths per 100,000 women, compared to 28 associated with pregnancy at that age. However, for pill users who smoke and are over the age of 35, the estimated number of deaths exceeds those for other methods of birth control. If a woman is over the age of 40 and smokes, her estimated risk of death is four times higher (117/100,000 women) than the estimated risk associated with pregnancy (28/100,000 women) in that age group.

The suggestion that women over 40 who don't smoke should not take oral contraceptives is based on information from older high-dose pills and on less-selective use of pills than is practiced today. An Advisory Committee of the FDA discussed this issue in 1989 and recommended that the ben-

Percentage of women experiencing an unintended pregnancy during the first year of typical use and first year of perfect use of contraception and the percentage continuing use at the end of the first year. United States.

Method (1)	% of Women Experiencing an Accidental Pregnancy within the First Year of Use: Typical Use[1] (2)	Perfect Use[2] (3)	% of Women Continuing Use at One Year[3] (4)
Chance[4]	85	85	
Spermicides[5]	26	6	40
Periodic abstinence	25		63
Calendar		9	
Ovulation method		3	
Sympto-thermal[6]		2	
Post Ovulation		1	
Withdrawal	19	4	
Cap[7]			
Parous women	40	26	42
Nulliparous women	20	9	56
Sponge			
Parous women	40	20	42
Nulliparous women	20	9	56
Diaphragm[7]	20	6	56
Condom[8]			
Female (Reality)	21	5	56
Male	14	3	61
Pill	5		71
progestin only		0.5	
combined		0.1	
IUD			
Progesterone T	2	1.5	81
Copper T 380A	0.8	0.6	78
Lng 20	0.1	0.1	81
Depo Provera	0.3	0.3	70
Norplant and Norplant-2	0.05	0.05	88
Female sterilization	0.5	0.5	100
Male sterilization	0.15	0.10	100

Source: Trussell J, Contraceptive efficacy. In Hatcher RA, Trussell J, Stewart F, Cates W, Stewart GK, Kowal D, Guest F, *Contraceptive Technology: Seventeenth Revised Edition.* New York NY: Irvington Publishers, 1998, in press.

1 Among *typical* couples who initiate use of a method (not necessarily for the first time), the percentage who experience an accidental pregnancy during the first year if they do not stop use for any other reason.

2 Among couples who initiate use of a method (not necessarily for the first time) and who use it *perfectly* (both consistently and correctly), the percentage who experience an accidental pregnancy during the first year if they do not stop use for any other reason.

3 Among couples attempting to avoid pregnancy, the percentage who continue to use a method for one year.

4 The percentages becoming pregnant in columns (2) and (3) are based on data from populations where contraception is not used and from women who cease using contraception in order to become pregnant. Among such populations, about 89% become pregnant within one year. This estimate was lowered slightly (to 85%) to represent the percentage who would become pregnant within one year among women now relying on reversible methods of contraception if they abandoned contraception altogether.

5 Foams, creams, gels, vaginal suppositories, vaginal film.

6 Cervical mucus (ovulation) method supplemented by calendar in the pre-ovulatory and basal body temperature in the post-ovulatory phases.

7 With spermicidal cream or jelly.

8 Without spermicides.

TABLE V. ANNUAL NUMBER OF BIRTH-RELATED OR METHOD-RELATED DEATHS ASSOCIATED WITH CONTROL OF FERTILITY PER 100,000 NONSTERILE WOMEN, BY FERTILITY-CONTROL METHOD ACCORDING TO AGE

Method of control and outcome	15–19	20–24	25–29	30–34	35–39	40–44
No fertility—control methods*	7.0	7.4	9.1	14.8	25.7	28.2
Oral contraceptives nonsmoker**	0.3	0.5	0.9	1.9	13.8	31.6
Oral contraceptives smoker**	2.2	3.4	6.6	13.5	51.1	117.2
IUD**	0.8	0.8	1.0	1.0	1.4	1.4
Condom*	1.1	1.6	0.7	0.2	0.3	0.4
Diaphragm/spermicide*	1.9	1.2	1.2	1.3	2.2	2.8
Periodic abstinence*	2.5	1.6	1.6	1.7	2.9	3.6

* Deaths are birth related

** Deaths are method related

Adapted from H.W. Ory, Family Planning Perspectives *15*:57–63, 1983.

efits of oral-contraceptive use by healthy, nonsmoking women over 40 years of age may outweigh the possible risks. However, all women, especially older women, are cautioned to use the lowest-dose pill that is effective.

WARNING SIGNALS

If any of these adverse effects occur while you are taking oral contraceptives, call your doctor immediately:

- Sharp chest pain, coughing of blood, or sudden shortness of breath (indicating a possible clot in the lung).
- Pain in the calf (indicating a possible clot in the leg).
- Crushing chest pain or heaviness in the chest (indicating a possible heart attack).
- Sudden severe headache or vomiting, dizziness or fainting, disturbances of vision or speech, weakness, or numbness in an arm or leg (indicating a possible stroke).
- Sudden partial or complete loss of vision (indicating a possible clot in the eye).
- Breast lumps (indicating possible breast cancer or fibrocystic disease of the breast; ask your doctor or healthcare provider to show you how to examine your breasts).
- Severe pain or tenderness in the stomach area (indicating a possibly ruptured liver tumor).
- Difficulty in sleeping, weakness, lack of energy, fatigue, or change in mood (possibly indicating severe depression).
- Jaundice or a yellowing of the skin or eyeballs, accompanied frequently by fever, fatigue, loss of appetite, dark-colored urine, or light-colored bowel movements (indicating possible liver problems).

SIDE EFFECTS OF ORAL CONTRACEPTIVES

1. VAGINAL BLEEDING

Irregular vaginal bleeding or spotting may occur while you are taking the pills. Irregular bleeding may vary from slight staining between menstrual periods to breakthrough bleeding which is a flow much like a regular period. Irregular bleeding occurs most often during the first few months of oral contraceptive use, but may also occur after you have been taking the pill for some time. Such bleeding may be temporary and usually does not indicate any serious problems. It is important to continue taking your pills on schedule. If the bleeding occurs in more than one cycle or lasts for more than a few days, talk to your doctor or healthcare provider.

2. CONTACT LENSES

If you wear contact lenses and notice a change in vision or an inability to wear your lenses, contact your doctor or healthcare provider.

3. FLUID RETENTION

Oral contraceptives may cause edema (fluid retention) with swelling of the fingers or ankles and may raise your blood pressure. If you experience fluid retention, contact your doctor or healthcare provider.

4. MELASMA

A spotty darkening of the skin is possible, particularly of the face.

5. OTHER SIDE EFFECTS

Other side effects may include change in appetite, headache, nervousness, depression, dizziness, loss of scalp hair, rash, and vaginal infections.

If any of these side effects bother you, call your doctor or healthcare provider.

GENERAL PRECAUTIONS

1. Missed periods and use of oral contraceptives before or during early pregnancy.

There may be times when you may not menstruate regularly after you have completed taking a cycle of pills. If you have taken your pills regularly and miss one menstrual period, continue taking your pills for the next cycle but be sure to inform your healthcare provider before doing so. If you have not taken the pills daily as instructed and missed a menstrual period, or if you missed two consecutive menstrual periods, you may be pregnant. Check with your healthcare provider immediately to determine whether you are pregnant. Do not continue to take oral contraceptives until you are sure you are not pregnant, but continue to use another method of contraception.

There is no conclusive evidence that oral contraceptive use is associated with an increase in birth defects when taken inadvertently during early pregnancy. Previously, a few studies had reported that oral contraceptives might be associated with birth defects, but these studies have not been confirmed. Nevertheless, oral contraceptives or any other drugs should not be used during pregnancy unless clearly necessary and prescribed by your doctor. You should check with your doctor about risks to your unborn child of any medication taken during pregnancy.

2. While breast-feeding

If you are breast-feeding, consult your doctor before starting oral contraceptives. Some of the drug will be passed on to the child in the milk. A few adverse effects on the child have been reported, including yellowing of the skin (jaundice) and breast enlargement. In addition, oral contraceptives may decrease the amount and quality of your milk. If possible, do not use oral contraceptives while breast-feeding. You should use another method of contraception since breast-feeding provides only partial protection from becoming pregnant and this partial protection decreases significantly as you breast-feed for longer periods of time. You should consider starting oral contraceptives only after you have weaned your child completely.

3. Laboratory tests

If you are scheduled for any laboratory tests, tell your doctor you are taking birth-control pills. Certain blood tests may be affected by birth-control pills.

4. Drug interactions

Certain drugs may interact with birth control pills to make them less effective in preventing pregnancy or cause an increase in breakthrough bleeding. Such drugs include rifampin, drugs used for epilepsy such as barbiturates (for example, phenobarbital) and phenytoin (Dilantin is one brand of this drug), phenylbutazone (Butazolidin is one brand) and possibly certain antibiotics. You may need to use an additional method of contraception during any cycle in which you take drugs that can make oral contraceptives less effective.

5. Sexually transmitted diseases

This product (like all oral contraceptives) is intended to prevent pregnancy. It does not protect against transmission of HIV (AIDS) and other sexually transmitted diseases such as chlamydia, genital herpes, genital warts, gonorrhea, hepatitis B, and syphilis.

HOW TO TAKE THE PILL

IMPORTANT POINTS TO REMEMBER

LEVLITE™, TRI-LEVLEN® and LEVLEN® Tablets

BEFORE YOU START TAKING YOUR PILLS:

1. BE SURE TO READ THESE DIRECTIONS:
   Before you start taking your pills.
   Anytime you are not sure what to do.
2. THE RIGHT WAY TO TAKE THE PILL IS TO TAKE ONE PILL EVERY DAY AT THE SAME TIME.
   If you miss pills you could get pregnant. This includes starting the pack late. The more pills you miss, the more likely you are to get pregnant.
3. MANY WOMEN HAVE SPOTTING OR LIGHT BLEEDING, OR MAY FEEL SICK TO THEIR STOMACH DURING THE FIRST 1–3 PACKS OF PILLS.
   If you do feel sick to your stomach, do not stop taking the pill. The problem will usually go away. If it doesn't go away, check with your doctor or clinic.
4. MISSING PILLS CAN ALSO CAUSE SPOTTING OR LIGHT BLEEDING, even when you make up these missed pills.
   On the days you take two pills, to make up for missed pills, you could also feel a little sick to your stomach.
5. IF YOU HAVE VOMITING OR DIARRHEA, for any reason, or IF YOU TAKE SOME MEDICINES, including some antibiotics, your pills may not work as well.
   Use a back-up method (such as condoms, foam, or sponge) until you check with your doctor or clinic.
6. IF YOU HAVE TROUBLE REMEMBERING TO TAKE THE PILL, talk to your doctor or clinic about how to make pill-taking easier or about using another method of birth control.
7. IF YOU HAVE ANY QUESTIONS OR ARE UNSURE ABOUT THE INFORMATION IN THIS LEAFLET, call your doctor or clinic.

BEFORE YOU START TAKING YOUR PILLS

LEVLITE™ Tablets

1. DECIDE WHAT TIME OF DAY YOU WANT TO TAKE YOUR PILL.
   It is important to take it at about the same time every day.
2. LOOK AT YOUR PILL PACK TO SEE IF IT HAS 21 OR 28 PILLS:
   The *21-pill* pack has 21 (pink) "active" pills (with hormones) to take for three weeks, followed by 1 week without pills.
   The *28-pill* pack has 21 (pink) "active" pills (with hormones) to take for three weeks, followed by 1 week of reminder pills (white) (without hormones).
3. ALSO FIND:
   1) where on the pack to start taking pills,
   2) in what order to take the pills (follow the arrows)

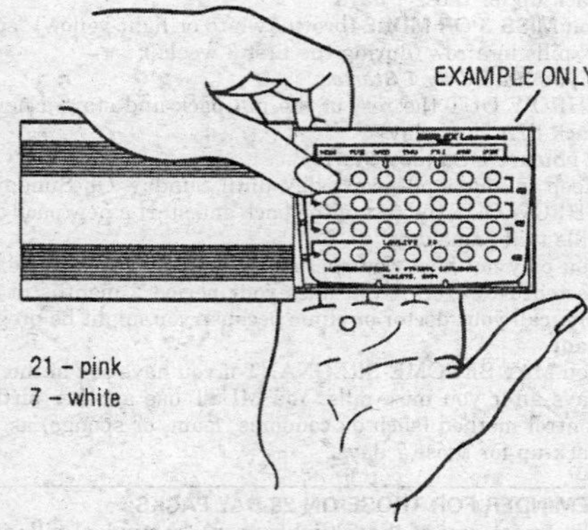

4. BE SURE YOU HAVE READY AT ALL TIMES:
   ANOTHER KIND OF BIRTH CONTROL (such as condoms, foam or sponge) to use as a back-up in case you miss pills.
   AN EXTRA, FULL PILL PACK.

TRI-LEVLEN® Tablets

1. DECIDE WHAT TIME OF DAY YOU WANT TO TAKE YOUR PILL.
   It is important to take it at about the same time every day.
2. LOOK AT YOUR PILL PACK TO SEE IF IT HAS 21 OR 28 PILLS:
   The 21-pill pack has 21 "active" (6 brown, 5 white and 10 light-yellow) pills (with hormones) to take for 3 weeks, followed by 1 week without pills.
   The 28-pill pack has 21 "active" (6 brown, 5 white and 10 light yellow) pills (with hormones) to take for 3 weeks, followed by 1 week of reminder (light-green) pills (without hormones).
3. ALSO FIND:
   1) where on the pack to start taking pills.
   2) in what order to take the pills (follow the arrows)

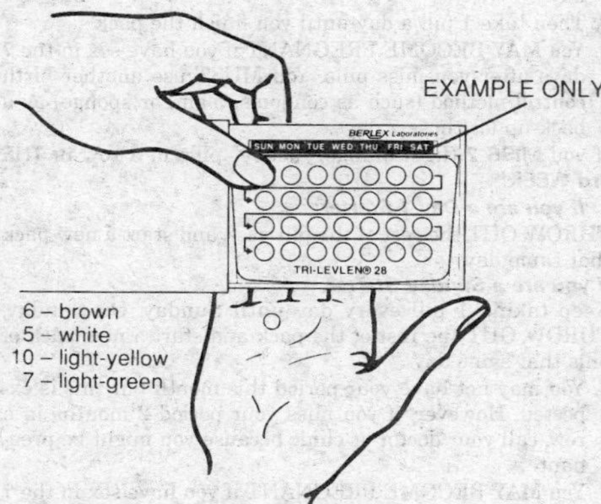

4. BE SURE YOU HAVE READY AT ALL TIMES:
   ANOTHER KIND OF BIRTH CONTROL (such as condoms, foam or sponge) to use as a back-up in case you miss pills.
   AN EXTRA, FULL PILL PACK.

LEVLEN® Tablets

1. DECIDE WHAT TIME OF DAY YOU WANT TO TAKE YOUR PILL.
   It is important to take it at about the same time every day.
2. LOOK AT YOUR PILL PACK TO SEE IF IT HAS 21 OR 28 PILLS:
   The 21-pill pack has 21 "active" (light-orange) pills (with hormones) to take for 3 weeks, followed by 1 week without pills.
   The 28-pill pack has 21 "active" (light-orange) pills (with hormones) to take for 3 weeks, followed by 1 week of reminder (pink) pills (without hormones).
3. ALSO FIND:
   1) where on the pack to start taking pills.
   2) in what order to take the pills (follow the arrows).

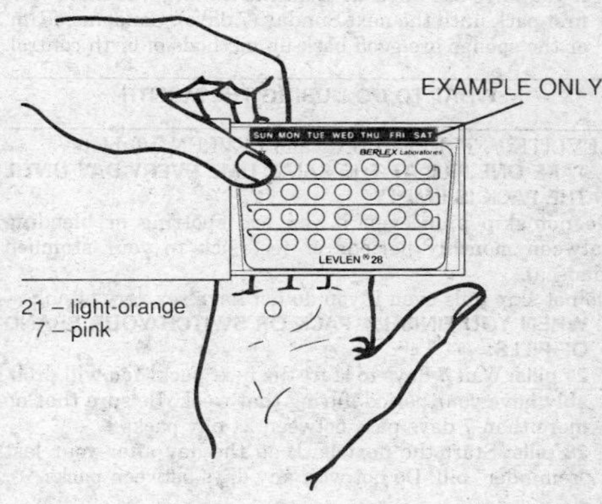

4. BE SURE YOU HAVE READY AT ALL TIMES:
   ANOTHER KIND OF BIRTH CONTROL (such as condoms, foam or sponge) to use as a back-up in case you miss pills.
   AN EXTRA, FULL PILL PACK.

WHEN TO START THE FIRST PACK OF PILLS

LEVLITE™ Tablets

You have a choice for which day to start taking your first pack of pills. Decide with your doctor or clinic which is the best day for you. Pick a time of day which will be easy to remember.

DAY 1 START:

1. Take the first (pink) "active" pill of the first pack during the *first 24 hours of your period.*
2. You will not need to use a back-up method of birth control, since you are starting the pill at the beginning of your period.

SUNDAY START:

1. Take the first (pink) "active" pill of the first pack on the *Sunday after your period starts,* even if you are still bleeding. If your period begins on Sunday, start the pack that same day.
2. *Use another method of birth control* as a back-up method if you have sex anytime from the Sunday you start your first pack until the next Sunday (7 days). Condoms, foam, or the sponge are good back-up methods of birth control.

TRI-LEVLEN® Tablets

You have a choice for which day to start taking your first pack of pills. Decide with your doctor or clinic which is the best day for you. Pick a time of day which will be easy to remember.

DAY 1 START:

1. Take the first "active" (brown) pill of the first pack during the first 24 hours of your period.
2. You will not need to use a back-up method of birth control, since you are starting the pill at the beginning of your period.

SUNDAY START:

1. Take the first "active" (brown) pill of the first pack on the Sunday after your period starts, even if you are still bleeding. If your period begins on Sunday, start the pack that same day.
2. Use another method of birth control as a back-up method if you have sex anytime from the Sunday you start your first pack until the next Sunday (7 days). Condoms, foam, or the sponge are good back-up methods of birth control.

LEVLEN® Tablets

You have a choice for which day to start taking your first pack of pills. Decide with your doctor or clinic which is the best day for you. Pick a time of day which will be easy to remember.

DAY 1 START:

1. Take the first "active" (light-orange) pill of the first pack during the first 24 hours of your period.

Continued on next page

Information on the Berlex products appearing here is based on the most current information available at the time of publication closing. Further information for these and other products may be obtained from the Medical Affairs Department, Berlex Laboratories, 300 Fairfield Road, Wayne, New Jersey 07470, 1-888-BERLEX-4. Information on Betaseron and Fludara may be obtained from Berlex Laboratories, 15049 San Pablo Avenue, Richmond, California 94804-0016, 1-800-888-4112.

Levlite/Tri-Levlen/Levlen—Cont.

2. You will not need to use a back-up method of birth control, since you are starting the pill at the beginning of your period.

SUNDAY START:

1. Take the first "active" (light-orange) pill of the first pack on the Sunday after your period starts, even if you are still bleeding. If your period begins on Sunday, start the pack that same day.
2. Use another method of birth control as a back-up method if you have sex anytime from the Sunday you start your first pack until the next Sunday (7 days). Condoms, foam, or the sponge are good back-up methods of birth control.

WHAT TO DO DURING THE MONTH

LEVLITE™, TRI-LEVLEN® and LEVLEN® Tablets

1. **TAKE ONE PILL AT THE SAME TIME EVERY DAY UNTIL THE PACK IS EMPTY**

Do not skip pills even if you are spotting or bleeding between monthly periods or feel sick to your stomach (nausea).

Do not skip pills even if you do not have sex very often.

2. **WHEN YOU FINISH A PACK OR SWITCH YOUR BRAND OF PILLS:**

21 pills: Wait 7 days to start the next pack. You will probably have your period during that week. Be sure that no more than 7 days pass between 21-day packs.

28 pills: Start the next pack on the day after your last "reminder" pill. Do not wait any days between packs.

WHAT TO DO IF YOU MISS PILLS

LEVLITE™ Tablets

If you **MISS 1** (pink) "active" pill:

1. Take it as soon as you remember. Take the next pill at your regular time. This means you may take two pills in one day.
2. You do not need to use a back-up birth control method if you have sex.

If you **MISS 2** (pink) "active" pills in a row in **WEEK 1 OR WEEK 2** of your pack:

1. Take two pills on the day you remember and two pills the next day.
2. Then take one pill a day until you finish the pack.
3. You MAY BECOME PREGNANT if you have sex in the 7 days after you miss pills. You MUST use another birth control method (such as condoms, foam, or sponge) as a back-up for those 7 days.

If you **MISS 2** (pink) "active" pills in a row in **THE 3rd WEEK:**

1. **If you are a Day 1 Starter:**

THROW OUT the rest of the pill pack and start a new pack that same day.

If you are a Sunday Starter:

Keep taking one pill every day until Sunday. On Sunday, THROW OUT the rest of the pack and start a new pack of pills that same day.

2. You may not have your period this month but this is expected. However, if you miss your period two months in a row, call your doctor or clinic because you might be pregnant.
3. You MAY BECOME PREGNANT if you have sex in the 7 days after you miss pills. You MUST use another birth control method (such as condoms, foam, or sponge) as a back-up for those 7 days.

If you **MISS 3 OR MORE** (pink) "active" pills in a row (during the first 3 weeks).

1. **If you are a Day 1 Starter:**
   THROW OUT the rest of the pill pack and start a new pack that same day.
   If you are a Sunday Starter:
   Keep taking 1 pill every day until Sunday. On Sunday, THROW OUT the rest of the pack and start a new pack of pills that same day.
2. You may not have your period this month but this is expected. However, if you miss your period two months in a row, call your doctor or clinic because you might be pregnant.
3. You MAY BECOME PREGNANT if you have sex in the 7 days after you miss pills. You MUST use another birth control method (such as condoms, foam, or sponge) as a back-up for those 7 days.

A REMINDER FOR THOSE ON 28-DAY PACKS:

If you forget any of the 7 (white) "reminder" pills in Week 4:
THROW AWAY the pills you missed.
Keep taking one pill each day until the pack is empty.
You do not need a back-up method.

FINALLY, IF YOU ARE STILL NOT SURE WHAT TO DO ABOUT THE PILLS YOU HAVE MISSED:

Use a BACK-UP METHOD anytime you have sex.

KEEP TAKING ONE ACTIVE PILL EACH DAY until you can reach your doctor or clinic.

TRI-LEVLEN® Tablets

If you **MISS 1** (brown, white or light yellow) "active" pill:

1. Take it as soon as you remember. Take the next pill at your regular time. This means you may take 2 pills in 1 day.
2. You do not need to use a back-up birth control method if you have sex.

If you **MISS 2** (brown or white) "active" pills in a row in **WEEK 1 OR WEEK 2** of your pack:

1. Take 2 pills on the day you remember and 2 pills the next day.
2. Then take 1 pill a day until you finish the pack.
3. YOU MAY BECOME PREGNANT if you have sex in the 7 days after you miss pills. You MUST use another birth control method (such as condoms, foam, or sponge) as a back-up for those 7 days.

If you **MISS 2** (light-yellow) "active" pills in a row in **THE 3rd WEEK:**

1. ***If you are a Day 1 Starter:***

THROW OUT the rest of the pill pack and start a new pack that same day.

If you are a Sunday Starter:

Keep taking 1 pill every day until Sunday. On Sunday, THROW OUT the rest of the pack and start a new pack of pills that same day.

2. You may not have your period this month but this is expected. However, if you miss your period 2 months in a row, call your doctor or clinic because you might be pregnant.
3. You MAY BECOME PREGNANT if you have sex in the 7 days after you miss pills. You MUST use another birth control method (such as condoms, foam, or sponge) as a back-up for those 7 days.

If you **MISS 3 OR MORE** (brown, white or light-yellow) "active" pills in a row (during the first 3 weeks).

1. ***If you are a Day 1 Starter:***
   THROW OUT the rest of the pill pack and start a new pack that same day.
   If you are a Sunday Starter:
   Keep taking 1 pill every day until Sunday. On Sunday, THROW OUT the rest of the pack and start a new pack of pills that same day.
2. You may not have your period this month but this is expected. However, if you miss your period 2 months in a row, call your doctor or clinic because you might be pregnant.
3. You MAY BECOME PREGNANT if you have sex in the 7 days after you miss pills. You MUST use another birth control method (such as condoms, foam, or sponge) as a back-up for those 7 days.

A REMINDER FOR THOSE ON 28-DAY PACKS:

If you forget any of the 7 (light-green) "reminder" pills in Week 4:
THROW AWAY the pills you missed.
Keep taking 1 pill each day until the pack is empty.
You do not need a back-up method if you start your next pack on time.

FINALLY, IF YOU ARE STILL NOT SURE WHAT TO DO ABOUT THE PILLS YOU HAVE MISSED:

Use a BACK-UP METHOD anytime you have sex.

KEEP TAKING ONE "ACTIVE" PILL EACH DAY until you can reach your doctor or clinic.

LEVLEN® Tablets

If you **MISS 1** (light-orange) "active" pill:

1. Take it as soon as you remember. Take the next pill at your regular time. This means you may take 2 pills in 1 day.
2. You do not need to use a back-up birth control method if you have sex.

If you **MISS 2** (light-orange) "active" pills in a row in **WEEK 1 OR WEEK 2** of your pack:

1. Take 2 pills on the day you remember and 2 pills the next day.
2. Then take 1 pill a day until you finish the pack.
3. You MAY BECOME PREGNANT if you have sex in the 7 days after you miss pills. You MUST use another birth control method (such as condoms, foam, or sponge) as a back-up for those 7 days.

If you **MISS 2** (light-orange) "active" pills in a row in **THE 3rd WEEK:**

1. ***If you are a Day 1 Starter:***

THROW OUT the rest of the pill pack and start a new pack that same day.

If you are a Sunday Starter:

Keep taking 1 pill every day until Sunday. On Sunday, THROW OUT the rest of the pack and start a new pack of pills that same day.

2. You may not have your period this month but this is expected. However, if you miss your period 2 months in a row, call your doctor or clinic because you might be pregnant.
3. You MAY BECOME PREGNANT if you have sex in the 7 days after you miss pills. You MUST use another birth control method (such as condoms, foam, or sponge) as a back-up for those 7 days.

If you **MISS 3 OR MORE** (light-orange) "active" pills in a row (during the first 3 weeks).

1. ***If you are a Day 1 Starter:***
   THROW OUT the rest of the pill pack and start a new pack that same day.
   If you are a Sunday Starter:
   Keep taking 1 pill every day until Sunday. On Sunday, THROW OUT the rest of the pack and start a new pack of pills that same day.
2. You may not have your period this month but this is expected. However, if you miss your period 2 months in a row, call your doctor or clinic because you might be pregnant.
3. You MAY BECOME PREGNANT if you have sex in the 7 days after you miss pills. You MUST use another birth control method (such as condoms, foam, or sponge) as a back-up for those 7 days.

A REMINDER FOR THOSE ON 28-DAY PACKS:

If you forget any of the 7 (pink) "reminder" pills in Week 4:
THROW AWAY the pills you missed.
Keep taking 1 pill each day until the pack is empty.
You do not need a back-up method if you start your next pack on time.

FINALLY, IF YOU ARE STILL NOT SURE WHAT TO DO ABOUT THE PILLS YOU HAVE MISSED:

Use a BACK-UP METHOD anytime you have sex.

KEEP TAKING ONE "ACTIVE" PILL EACH DAY until you can reach your doctor or clinic.

PREGNANCY DUE TO PILL FAILURE

The incidence of pill failure resulting in pregnancy is approximately less than 1.0% if taken every day as directed, but more typical failure rates are less than 3.0%. If failure does occur, the risk to the fetus is minimal.

RISKS TO THE FETUS

If you do become pregnant while using oral contraceptives, the risk to the fetus is small, on the order of no more than one per thousand. You should, however, discuss the risks to the developing child with your doctor.

PREGNANCY AFTER STOPPING THE PILL

There may be some delay in becoming pregnant after you stop using oral contraceptives, especially if you had irregular menstrual cycles before you used oral contraceptives. It may be advisable to postpone conception until you begin menstruating regularly once you have stopped taking the pill and desire pregnancy.

There does not appear to be any increase in birth defects in newborn babies when pregnancy occurs soon after stopping the pill.

OVERDOSAGE

Serious ill effects have not been reported following ingestion of large doses of oral contraceptives by young children. Overdosage may cause nausea and withdrawal bleeding in females. In case of overdosage, contact your healthcare provider or pharmacist.

OTHER INFORMATION

Your healthcare provider will take a medical and family history before prescribing oral contraceptives and will examine you. You should be re-examined at least once a year. Be sure to inform your healthcare provider if there is a family history of any of the conditions listed previously in this leaflet. Be sure to keep all appointments with your healthcare provider, because this is a time to determine if there are early signs of side effects of oral contraceptive use. Do not use the drug for any condition other than the one for which it was prescribed. This drug has been prescribed specifically for you; do not give it to others who may want birth-control pills.

HEALTH BENEFITS FROM ORAL CONTRACEPTIVES

In addition to preventing pregnancy, use of oral contraceptives may provide certain benefits. They are:

- Menstrual cycles may become more regular.
- Blood flow during menstruation may be lighter and less iron may be lost. Therefore, anemia due to iron deficiency is less likely to occur.
- Pain or other symptoms during menstruation may be encountered less frequently.
- Ovarian cysts may occur less frequently.
- Ectopic (tubal) pregnancy may occur less frequently.
- Noncancerous cysts or lumps in the breast may occur less frequently.
- Acute pelvic inflammatory disease may occur less frequently.
- Oral contraceptive use may provide some protection against developing two forms of cancer: cancer of the ovaries and cancer of the lining of the uterus.

If you want more information about birth-control pills, ask your doctor or pharmacist. They have a more technical leaflet called the Prescribing Information which you may wish to read.

Manufactured in Germany
Manufactured for:
BERLEX Laboratories, Wayne, NJ 07470

Revised Oct 1998 6071902
Revised July 1996 6070001
Revised Sept. 1996 6065802

Shown in Product Identification Guide, page 308

QUINAGLUTE ℞
DURA-TABS® TABLETS
[*kwĭn 'uh glōōt*]
(BRAND OF QUINIDINE GLUCONATE, EXTENDED-RELEASE TABLETS, USP)

DESCRIPTION

Quinidine is an antimalarial schizonticide and an antiarrhythmic agent with Class Ia activity; it is the d-isomer of quinine, and its molecular weight is 324.43. Quinidine gluconate is the gluconate salt of quinidine; its chemical name is cinchonan-9-ol, 6'-methoxy-, (9S)-, mono-D-gluconate; its structural formula is:

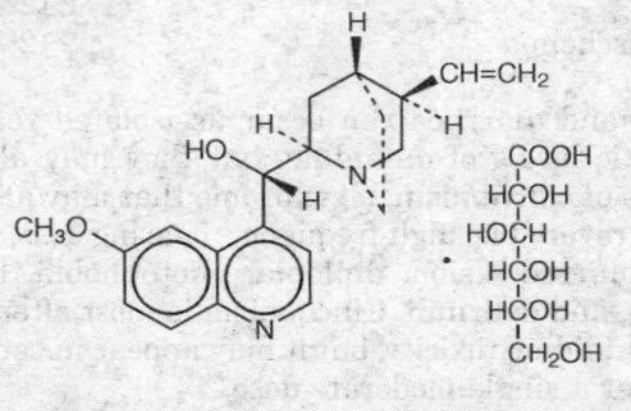

Its empirical formula is $C_{20}H_{24}N_2O_2 \cdot C_6H_{12}O_7$, and its molecular weight is 520.58, of which 62.3% is quinidine base. Each QUINAGLUTE DURA-TABS® tablet contains 324 mg of quinidine gluconate (202 mg of quinidine base) in a matrix to provide extended-release; the inactive ingredients include confectioner's sugar, magnesium stearate, corn starch and other ingredients. Meets USP Drug Release Test 4.

CLINICAL PHARMACOLOGY

Pharmacokinetics and Metabolism: The absolute **bioavailability** of quinidine from QUINAGLUTE® is 70–80%. Relative to a solution of quinidine sulfate, the bioavailability of quinidine from QUINAGLUTE® is reported to be 1.03. The less-than-complete bioavailability is thought to be due to first-pass elimination by the liver. Peak serum levels generally appear 3–5 hours after dosing; when the drug is taken with food, absorption is increased in both rate (27%) and extent (17%). The rate and extent of absorption of quinidine from QUINAGLUTE® are not significantly affected by the coadministration of an aluminum-hydroxide antacid. The rate of absorption of quinidine following the ingestion of grapefruit juice may be decreased.

The **volume of distribution** of quinidine is 2–3 L/kg in healthy young adults, but this may be reduced to as little as 0.5 L/kg in patients with congestive heart failure, or increased to 3–5 L/kg in patients with cirrhosis of the liver. At concentrations of 2–5 mg/L (6.5–16.2 µmol/L), the fraction of quinidine bound to plasma proteins (mainly to α_1-acid glycoprotein and to albumin) is 80–88% in adults and older children, but it is lower in pregnant women, and in infants and neonates it may be as low as 50–70%. Because α_1-acid glycoprotein levels are increased in response to stress, serum levels of total quinidine may be greatly increased in settings such as acute myocardial infarction, even though the serum content of unbound (active) drug may remain normal. Protein binding is also increased in chronic renal failure, but binding abruptly descends toward or below normal when heparin is administered for hemodialysis.

Quinidine **clearance** typically proceeds at 3–5 mL/min/kg in adults, but clearance in children may be twice or three times as rapid. The elimination half-life is 6–8 hours in adults and 3–4 hours in children. Quinidine clearance is unaffected by hepatic cirrhosis, so the increased volume of distribution seen in cirrhosis leads to a proportionate increase in the elimination half-life.

Most quinidine is eliminated hepatically via the action of cytochrome P450IIIA4; there are several different hydroxylated metabolites, and some of these have antiarrhythmic activity.

The most important of quinidine's metabolites is 3-hydroxyquinidine (3HQ), serum levels of which can approach those of quinidine in patients receiving conventional doses of QUINAGLUTE®. The volume of distribution of 3HQ appears to be larger than that of quinidine, and the elimination half-life of 3HQ is about 12 hours.

As measured by antiarrhythmic effects on animals, by QT_c prolongation in human volunteers, or by various *in vitro* techniques, 3HQ has at least half the antiarrhythmic activity of the parent compound, so it may be responsible for a substantial fraction of the effect of QUINAGLUTE® in chronic use.

When the urine pH is less than 7, about 20% of administered quinidine appears unchanged in the urine, but this fraction drops to as little as 5% when the urine is more alkaline. Renal clearance involves both glomerular filtration and active tubular secretion, moderated by (pH-dependent) tubular reabsorption. The net renal clearance is about 1 mL/min/kg in healthy adults.

When renal function is taken into account, quinidine clearance is apparently independent of patient age.

Assays of serum quinidine levels are widely available, but the results of modern assays may not be consistent with results cited in the older medical literature. The serum levels of quinidine cited in this package insert are those derived from specific assays, using either benzene extraction or (preferably) reverse-phase high-pressure liquid chromatography. In matched samples, older assays might unpredictably have given results that were as much as two or three times higher. A typical "therapeutic" concentration range is 2–6 mg/L (6.2–18.5 µmol/L).

Mechanisms of action

In patients with malaria, quinidine acts primarily as an intraerythrocytic schizonticide, with little effect upon sporozites or upon pre-erythrocytic parasites. Quinidine is gametocidal to *Plasmodium vivax* and *P. malariae*, but not to *P. falciparum*.

In cardiac muscle and in Purkinje fibers, quinidine depresses the rapid inward depolarizing sodium current, thereby slowing phase-0 depolarization and reducing the amplitude of the action potential without affecting the resting potential. In normal Purkinje fibers, it reduces the slope of phase-4 depolarization, shifting the threshold voltage upward toward zero. The result is slowed conduction and reduced automaticity in all parts of the heart, with increase of the effective refractory period relative to the duration of the action potential in the atria, ventricles, and Purkinje tissues. Quinidine also raises the fibrillation thresholds of the atria and ventricles, and it raises the ventricular *de*fibrillation threshold as well. Quinidine's actions fall into Class Ia in the Vaughn-Williams classification.

By slowing conduction and prolonging the effective refractory period, quinidine can interrupt or prevent reentrant arrhythmias and arrhythmias due to increased automaticity, including atrial flutter, atrial fibrillation, and paroxysmal supraventricular tachycardia.

In patients with sick sinus syndrome, quinidine can cause marked sinus node depression and bradycardia. In most patients, however, use of quinidine is associated with an increase in the sinus rate.

Like other antiarrhythmic drugs with Class Ia activity, quinidine prolongs the QT interval in a dose-related fashion. This may lead to increased ventricular automaticity and polymorphic ventricular tachycardias, including *torsades de pointes* (see **Warnings**).

In addition, quinidine has anticholinergic activity, it has negative inotropic activity, and it acts peripherally as an α-adrenergic antagonist (that is, as a vasodilator).

CLINICAL EFFECTS

Maintenance of sinus rhythm after conversion from atrial fibrillation: In six clinical trials (published between 1970 and 1984) with a total of 808 patients, quinidine (418 patients) was compared to nontreatment (258 patients) or placebo (132 patients) for the maintenance of sinus rhythm after cardioversion from chronic atrial fibrillation. Quinidine was consistently more efficacious in maintaining sinus rhythm, but a meta-analysis found that mortality in the quinidine-exposed patients (2.9%) was significantly greater than mortality in the patients who had not been treated with active drug (0.8%). Suppression of atrial fibrillation with quinidine has theoretical patient benefits (e.g., improved exercise tolerance; reduction in hospitalization for cardioversion; lack of arrhythmia-related palpitations, dyspnea and chest pain; reduced incidence of systemic embolism and/or stroke), but these benefits have never been demonstrated in clinical trials. Some of these benefits (e.g., reduction in stroke incidence) may be achievable by other means (anticoagulation).

By slowing the atrial rate in atrial flutter/fibrillation, quinidine can decrease the degree of atrioventricular block and cause an increase, sometimes marked, in the rate at which supraventricular impulses are successfully conducted by the atrioventricular node, with a resultant paradoxical increase in ventricular rate (see **Warnings**).

Non-life-threatening ventricular arrhythmias: In studies of patients with a variety of ventricular arrhythmias (mainly frequent ventricular premature beats and non-sustained ventricular tachycardia, quinidine (total n=502) has been compared with flecainide (n=141), mexiletine (n=246), propafenone (n=53), and tocainide (n=67). In each of these studies, the mortality in the quinidine group was numerically greater than the mortality in the comparator group. When the studies were combined in a meta-analysis, quinidine was associated with a statistically significant threefold relative risk of death.

At therapeutic doses, quinidine's only consistent effect upon the surface electrocardiogram is an increase in the QT interval. This prolongation can be monitored as a guide to safety, and it may provide better guidance than serum drug levels (see **Warnings**).

INDICATIONS AND USAGE

Conversion of atrial fibrillation/flutter: In patients with symptomatic atrial fibrillation/flutter whose symptoms are not adequately controlled by measures that reduce the rate of ventricular response, QUINAGLUTE® is indicated as a means of restoring normal sinus rhythm. If this use of QUINAGLUTE® does not restore sinus rhythm within a reasonable time (see **Dosage and Administration**), then QUINAGLUTE® should be discontinued.

Reduction of frequency of relapse into atrial fibrillation/flutter: Chronic therapy with QUINAGLUTE® is indicated for some patients at high risk of symptomatic atrial fibrillation/flutter, generally patients who have had previous episodes of atrial fibrillation/flutter that were so frequent and poorly tolerated as to outweigh, in the judgment of the physician and the patient, the risks of prophylactic therapy with QUINAGLUTE®. The increased risk of death should specifically be considered. QUINAGLUTE® should be used only after alternative measures (e.g., use of other drugs to control the ventricular rate) have been found to be inadequate.

In patients with histories of frequent symptomatic episodes of atrial fibrillation/flutter, the goal of therapy should be an increase in the average time between episodes. In most patients, the tachyarrhythmia *will recur* during therapy, and a single recurrence should not be interpreted as therapeutic failure.

Suppression of ventricular arrhythmias: QUINAGLUTE® is also indicated for the suppression of recurrent documented ventricular arrhythmias, such as sustained ventricular tachycardia, that in the judgment of the physician are life-threatening. Because of the proarryhthmic effects of quinidine, its use with ventricular arrhythmias of lesser severity is generally not recommended, and treatment of patients with asymptomatic ventricular premature contractions should be avoided. Where possible, therapy should be guided by the results of programmed electrical stimulation and/or Holter monitoring with exercise.

Antiarrhythmic drugs (including QUINAGLUTE®) have not been shown to enhance survival in patients with ventricular arrhythmias.

CONTRAINDICATIONS

Quinidine is contraindicated in patients who are known to be allergic to it, or who have developed thrombocytopenic purpura during prior therapy with quinidine or quinine.

In the absence of a functioning artificial pacemaker, quinidine is also contraindicated in any patient whose cardiac rhythm is dependent upon a junctional or idioventricular pacemaker, including patients in complete atrioventricular block.

Quinidine is also contraindicated in patients who, like those with myasthenia gravis, might be adversely affected by an anticholinergic agent.

WARNINGS

Mortality:

In many trials of antiarrhythmic therapy for non-life-threatening arrhythmias, active antiarrhythmic therapy has resulted in increased mortality; the risk of active therapy is probably greatest in patients with structural heart disease.

In the case of quinidine used to prevent or defer recurrence of atrial flutter/fibrillation, the best available data come from a meta-analysis described under *Clinical Pharmacology / Clinical Effects* **above. In the patients studied in the trials there analyzed, the mortality associated with the use of quinidine was more than three times as great as the mortality associated with the use of placebo.**

Another meta-analysis, also described under *Clinical Pharmacology / Clinical Effects,* **showed that in patients with various non-life-threatening ventricular arrhythmias, the mortality associated with the use of quinidine was consistently greater than that associated with the use of any of a variety of alternative antiarrhythmics.**

Proarrhythmic effects: Like many other drugs (including all other Class Ia antiarrhythmics), quinidine prolongs the QT_c interval, and this can lead to *torsades de pointes*, a life-threatening ventricular arrhythmia (see **Overdosage**). The risk of *torsades* is increased by bradycardia, hypokalemia, hypomagnesemia or high serum levels of quinidine, but it may appear in the absence of any of these risk factors. The best predictor of this arrhythmia appears to be the length of QT_c interval, and quinidine should be used with extreme care in patients who have preexisting long-QT syndromes, who have histories of *torsades de pointes* of any cause, or who have previously responded to quinidine (or other drugs that prolong ventricular repolarization) with marked lengthening of the QT_c interval. Estimation of the incidence of *torsades* in patients with therapeutic levels of quinidine is not possible from the available data.

Other ventricular arrhythmias that have been reported with quinidine include frequent extrasystoles, ventricular tachycardia, ventricular flutter, and ventricular fibrillation.

Paradoxical increase in ventricular rate in atrial flutter/fibrillation: When quinidine is administered to patients with atrial flutter/fibrillation, the desired pharmacologic reversion to sinus rhythm may (rarely) be preceded by a slowing of the atrial rate with a consequent increase in the rate of beats conducted to the ventricles. The resulting ventricular rate may be very high (greater than 200 beats per minute) and poorly tolerated. This hazard may be decreased if partial atrioventricular block is achieved prior to initiation of quinidine therapy, using conduction-reducing drugs such as digitalis, verapamil, diltiazem, or a β-receptor blocking agent.

Exacerbated bradycardia in sick sinus syndrome: In patients with the sick sinus syndrome, quinidine has been associated with marked sinus node depression and bradycardia.

Pharmacokinetic considerations: Renal or hepatic dysfunction causes the elimination of quinidine to be slowed, while congestive heart failure causes a reduction in quinidine's apparent volume of distribution. Any of these conditions can lead to quinidine toxicity if dosage is not appropriately reduced. In addition, interactions with coadministered drugs can alter the serum concentration and activity of quinidine, leading either to toxicity or to lack of efficacy if the dose of quinidine is not appropriately modified. (See **Precautions/Drug Interactions**.)

Vagolysis: Because quinidine opposes the atrial and A-V nodal effects of vagal stimulation, physical or pharmacological vagal maneuvers undertaken to terminate paroxysmal supraventricular tachycardia may be ineffective in patients receiving quinidine.

Continued on next page

Information on the Berlex products appearing here is based on the most current information available at the time of publication closing. Further information for these and other products may be obtained from the Medical Affairs Department, Berlex Laboratories, 300 Fairfield Road, Wayne, New Jersey 07470, 1-888-BERLEX-4. Information on Betaseron and Fludara may be obtained from Berlex Laboratories, 15049 San Pablo Avenue, Richmond, California 94804-0016, 1-800-888-4112.

Quinaglute—Cont.

PRECAUTIONS

Heart block

In patients without implanted pacemakers who are at high risk of complete atrioventricular block (e.g., those with digitalis intoxication, second degree atrioventricular block, or severe intraventricular conduction defects), quinidine should be used only with caution.

Drug and Diet Interactions

Altered pharmacokinetics of quinidine: Diltiazem significantly decreases the clearance and increases the $t_{1/2}$ of quinidine, but quinidine does not alter the kinetics of diltiazem.

Drugs that alkalinize the urine (**carbonic-anhydrase inhibitors, sodium bicarbonate, thiazide diuretics**) reduce renal elimination of quinidine.

By pharmacokinetic mechanisms that are not well understood, quinidine levels are increased by coadministration of **amiodarone** or **cimetidine**. Very rarely, and again by mechanisms not understood, quinidine levels are decreased by coadministration of **nifedipine**.

Hepatic elimination of quinidine may be accelerated by coadministration of drugs (**phenobarbital, phenytoin, rifampin**) that induce production of cytochrome P450IIIA4.

Perhaps because of competition for the P450IIIA4 metabolic pathway, quinidine levels rise when **ketaconazole** is coadministered.

Coadministration of **propranolol** usually does not affect quinidine pharmacokinetics, but in some studies the β-blocker appeared to cause increases in the peak serum levels of quinidine, decreases in quinidine's volume of distribution, and decreases in total quinidine clearance. The effects (if any) of coadministration of **other** β**-blockers** on quinidine pharmacokinetics have not been adequately studied.

Hepatic clearance of quinidine is significantly reduced during coadministration of **verapamil**, with corresponding increases in serum levels and half-life.

Grapefruit juice: Grapefruit juice inhibits P450 3A4-mediated metabolism of quinidine to 3-hydroxyquinidine. Although the clinical significance of this interaction is unknown, grapefruit juice should be avoided.

Dietary salt: The rate and extent of quinidine absorption may be affected by changes in dietary salt intake; a decrease in dietary salt intake may lead to an increase in plasma quinidine concentrations.

Altered pharmacokinetics of other drugs: Quinidine slows the elimination of **digoxin** and simultaneously reduces digoxin's apparent volume of distribution. As a result, serum digoxin levels may be as much as doubled. When quinidine and digoxin are coadministered, digoxin doses usually need to be reduced. Serum levels of **digitoxin** are also raised when quinidine is coadministered, although the effect appears to be smaller.

By a mechanism that is not understood, quinidine potentiates the anticoagulatory action of **warfarin**, and the anticoagulant dosage may need to be reduced.

Cytochrome P450IID6 is an enzyme critical to the metabolism of many drugs, notably including **mexiletine**, some **phenothiazines**, and most **polycyclic antidepressants**. Constitutional deficiency of cytochrome P450IID6 is found in less than 1% of Orientals, in about 2% of American blacks, and in about 8% of American whites. Testing with debrisoquine is sometimes used to distinguish the P450IID6-deficient "poor metabolizers" from the majority-phenotype "extensive metabolizers".

When drugs whose metabolism is P450IID6-dependent are given to poor metabolizers, the serum levels achieved are higher, sometimes much higher, than the serum levels achieved when identical doses are given to extensive metabolizers. To obtain similar clinical benefit without toxicity, doses given to poor metabolizers may need to be greatly reduced. In the case of prodrugs whose actions are actually mediated by P450IID6-produced metabolites (for example, **codeine** and **hydrocodone**, whose analgesic and antitussive effects appear to be mediated by morphine and hydromorphone, respectively), it may not be possible to achieve the desired clinical benefits in poor metabolizers.

Quinidine is not metabolized by cytochrome P450IID6, but therapeutic serum levels of quinidine inhibit the action of cytochrome P450IID6, effectively converting extensive metabolizers into poor metabolizers. Caution must be exercised whenever quinidine is prescribed together with drugs metabolized by cytochrome P450IID6.

Perhaps by competing for pathways of renal clearance, coadministration of quinidine causes an increase in serum levels of **procainamide**.

Serum levels of **haloperidol** are increased when quinidine is coadministered.

Presumably because both drugs are metabolized by cytochrome P450IIIA4, coadministration of quinidine causes variable slowing of the metabolism of **nifedipine**. Interactions with other dihydropyridine calcium channel blockers have not been reported, but these agents (including **felodipine, nicardipine,** and **nimodipine**) are all dependent upon P450IIIA4 for metabolism, so similar interactions with quinidine should be anticipated.

Altered pharmacodynamics of other drugs: Quinidine's anticholinergic, vasodilating, and negative inotropic actions may be additive to those of other drugs with these effects, and antagonistic to those of drugs with cholinergic, vasoconstricting, and positive inotropic effects. For example, when quinidine and **verapamil** are coadministered in doses that are each well tolerated as monotherapy, hypotension attributable to additive peripheral α-blockade is sometimes reported.

Quinidine potentiates the actions of depolarizing (succinylcholine, decamethonium) and nondepolarizing (*d*-tubocurarine, pancuronium) **neuromuscular blocking agents**. These phenomena are not well understood, but they are observed in animal models as well as in humans. In addition, *in vitro* addition of quinidine to the serum of pregnant women reduces the activity of pseudocholinesterase, an enzyme that is essential to the metabolism of succinylcholine.

Non-interactions of quinidine with other drugs: Quinidine has no clinically significant effect on the pharmacokinetics of **diltiazem, flecainide, mephenytoin, metoprolol, propafenone, propranolol, quinine, timolol,** or **tocainide.**

Conversely, the pharmacokinetics of quinidine are not significantly affected by **caffeine, ciprofloxacin, digoxin, felodipine, omeprazole,** or **quinine**. Quinidine's pharmacokinetics are also unaffected by cigarette smoking.

INFORMATION FOR PATIENTS

Before prescibing QUINAGLUTE® as prophylaxis against recurrence of atrial fibrillation, the physician should inform the patient of the risks and benefits to be expected (see **Clinical Pharmacology**). Discussion should include the facts

- that the goal of therapy will be a reduction (probably not to zero) in the frequency of episodes of atrial fibrillation; and
- that reduced frequency of fibrillatory episodes may be expected, if achieved, to bring symptomatic benefit; but
- that no data are available to show that reduced frequency of fibrillatory episodes will reduce the risks of irreversible harm through stroke or death; and in fact
- that such data as are available suggest that treatment with QUINAGLUTE® is likely to increase the patient's risk of death.

Carcinogenesis, mutagenesis, impairment of fertility

Animal studies to evaluate quinidine's carcinogenic or mutagenic potential have not been performed. Similarly, there are no animal data as to quinidine's potential to impair fertility.

Pregnancy

Pregnancy Category C. Animal reproductive studies have not been conducted with quinidine. There are no adequate and well-controlled studies in pregnant women. Quinidine should be given to a pregnant woman only if clearly needed. In one neonate whose mother had received quinidine throughout her pregnancy, the serum level of quinidine was equal to that of the mother, with no apparent ill effect. The level of quinidine in amniotic fluid was about three times higher than that found in serum.

Labor and Delivery

Quinine is said to be oxytocic in humans, but there are no adequate data as to quinidine's effects (if any) on human labor and delivery.

Nursing mothers

Quinidine is present in human milk at levels slightly lower than those in maternal serum; a human infant ingesting such milk should (scaling directly by weight) be expected to develop serum quinidine levels at least an order of magnitude lower than those of the mother. On the other hand, the pharmacokinetics and pharmacodynamics of quinidine in human infants have not been adequately studied, and neonates' reduced protein binding of quinidine may increase their risk of toxicity at low total serum levels. Administration of quinidine should (if possible) be avoided in lactating women who continue to nurse.

Geriatric use

Safety and efficacy of quinidine in elderly patients have not been systematically studied.

Pediatric use

In antimalarial trials, quinidine was as safe and effective in pediatric patients as in adults. Notwithstanding the known pharmacokinetic differences between children and adults (see **Pharmacokinetics and Metabolism**), children in these trials received the same doses (on a mg/kg basis) as adults. Safety and effectiveness of antiarrhythmic use in children have not been established.

ADVERSE REACTIONS

Quinidine preparations have been used for many years, but there are only sparse data from which to estimate the incidence of various adverse reactions. The adverse reactions most frequently reported have consistently been gastrointestinal, including diarrhea, nausea, vomiting, and heartburn/esophagitis.

In the reported study that was closest in character to the predominant approved use of QUINAGLUTE®, 86 adult outpatients with atrial fibrillation were followed for six months while they received slow-release quinidine bisulfate tablets, 600 mg (approximately 400 mg of quinidine base) twice daily. The incidences of adverse experiences reported more than once were as shown in the table below. The most serious quinidine-associated adverse reactions are described above under **Warnings.**

ADVERSE EXPERIENCES REPORTED MORE THAN ONCE IN 86 PATIENTS WITH ATRIAL FIBRILLATION

	Incidence (%)
diarrhea	21 (24%)
fever	5 (6%)
rash	5 (6%)
arrhythmia	3 (3%)
abnormal electrocardiogram	3 (3%)
nausea/vomiting	3 (3%)
dizziness	3 (3%)
headache	3 (3%)
asthenia	2 (2%)
cerebral ischemia	2 (2%)

Vomiting and diarrhea can occur as isolated reactions to therapeutic levels of quinidine, but they may also be the first signs of **cinchonism,** a syndrome that may also include tinnitus, reversible high-frequency hearing loss, deafness, vertigo, blurred vision, diplopia, photophobia, headache, confusion, and delirium. Cinchonism is most often a sign of chronic quinidine toxicity, but it may appear in sensitive patients after a single moderate dose.

A few cases of **hepatotoxicity,** including granulomatous hepatitis, have been reported in patients receiving quinidine. All of these have appeared during the first few weeks of therapy, and most (not all) have remitted once quinidine was withdrawn.

Autoimmune and inflammatory syndromes associated with quinidine therapy have included fever, urticaria, flushing, exfoliative rash, bronchospasm, psoriasiform rash, pruritus and lymphadenopathy, hemolytic anemia, vasculitis, thrombocytopenic purpura, uveitis, angioedema, agranulocytosis, the sicca syndrome, arthralgia, myalgia, elevation in serum levels of skeletal-muscle enzymes, a disorder resembling systemic lupus erythematosus, and pneumonitis.

Convulsions, apprehension, and ataxia have been reported, but it is not clear that these were not simply the results of hypotension and consequent cerebral hypoperfusion. There are many reports of syncope. Acute psychotic reactions have been reported to follow the first dose of quinidine, but these reactions appear to be extremely rare.

Other adverse reactions occasionally reported include depression, mydriasis, disturbed color perception, night blindness, scotomata, optic neuritis, visual field loss, photosensitivity, and abnormalities of pigmentation.

OVERDOSAGE

Overdoses with various oral formulations of quinidine have been well described. Death has been described after a 5-gram ingestion by a toddler, while an adolescent was reported to survive after ingesting 8 grams of quinidine.

The most important ill effects of acute quinidine overdoses are ventricular arrhythmias and hypotension. Other signs and symptoms of overdose may include vomiting, diarrhea, tinnitus, high-frequency hearing loss, vertigo, blurred vision, diplopia, photophobia, headache, confusion and delirium.

Arrhythmias: Serum quinidine levels can be conveniently assayed and monitored, but the electrocardiographic QT_c interval is a better predictor of quinidine-induced ventricular arrhythmias.

The necessary treatment of hemodynamically unstable polymorphic ventricular tachycardia (including *torsades de pointes*) is withdrawal of treatment with quinidine and either immediate cardioversion or, if a cardiac pacemaker is in place or immediately available, immediate overdrive pacing. After pacing or cardioversion, further management must be guided by the length of the QT_c interval.

Quinidine-associated ventricular tachyarrhythmias with normal underlying QT_c intervals have not been adequately studied. Because of the theoretical possibility of QT-prolonging effects that might be additive to those of quinidine, other antiarrhythmics with Class I (disopyramide, procainamide) or Class III activities should (if possible) be avoided. Similarly, although the use of bretylium in quinidine overdose has not been reported, it is reasonable to expect that the α-blocking properties of bretylium might be additive to those of quinidine, resulting in problematic hypotension.

If the postcardioversion QT_c interval is prolonged, then the precardioversion polymorphic ventricular tachycardia was (by definition) *torsades de pointes*. In this case, lidocaine and bretylium are unlikely to be of value, and other Class I antiarrhythmics (disopyramide, procainamide) are likely to exacerbate the situation. Factors contributing to QT_c prolongation (especially hypokalemia and hypomagnesemia) should be sought out and (if possible) aggressively corrected. Prevention of recurrent *torsades* may require sustained overdrive pacing or the cautious administration of isoproterenal (30–150 ng/kg/min).

Hypotension: Quinidine-induced hypotension that is not due to an arrhythmia is likely to be a consequence of quinidine-related α-blockade and vasorelaxation. Simple repletion of central volume (Trendelenburg positioning, saline infusion) may be sufficient therapy; other interventions reported to have been beneficial in this setting are those that increase peripheral vascular resistance, including α-agonist catecholamines (norepinephrine, metaraminol) and the Military Anti-Shock Trousers.

Treatment:

To obtain up-to-date information about the treatment of overdose, a good resource is your certified Regional Poison-Control Center. Telephone numbers of certified poison-control centers are listed in the Physicians' Desk Reference (PDR). In managing overdose, consider the possibilities of multiple-drug overdoses, drug-drug interactions, and unusual drug kinetics in your patient.

Accelerated removal: Adequate studies of orally-administered activated charcoal in human overdoses of quinidine have not been reported, but there are animal data showing significant enhancement of systemic elimination following this intervention, and there is at least one human case re-

port in which the elimination half-life of quinidine in the serum was apparently shortened by repeated gastric lavage. Activated charcoal should be avoided if an ileus is present; the conventional dose is 1 gram/kg, administered every 2–6 hours as a slurry with 8 mL/kg of tap water.
Although renal elimination of quinidine might theoretically be accelerated by maneuvers to acidify the urine, such maneuvers are potentially hazardous and of no demonstrated benefit.
Quinidine is not usefully removed from the circulation by dialysis.
Following quinidine overdose, drugs that delay elimination of quinidine (cimetidine, carbonic-anhydrase inhibitors, diltiazem, thiazide diuretics) should be withdrawn unless absolutely required.

DOSAGE AND ADMINISTRATION

The dose of quinidine delivered by QUINAGLUTE DURA-TABS® tablets may be titrated by breaking a tablet in half. If tablets are crushed or chewed, their extended-release properties will be lost.
The dosage of quinidine varies considerably depending upon the general condition and the cardiovascular state of the patient.

Conversion of atrial fibrillation/flutter to sinus rhythm
Especially in patients with known structural heart disease or other risk factors for toxicity, initiation or dose-adjustment of treatment with QUINAGLUTE® should generally be performed in a setting where facilities and personnel for monitoring and resuscitation are continuously available.
Patients with symptomatic atrial fibrillation/flutter should be treated with QUINAGLUTE® only after ventricular rate control (e.g., with digitalis or β-blockers) has failed to provide satisfactory control of symptoms.
Adequate trials have not identified an optimal regimen of QUINAGLUTE® for conversion of atrial fibrillation/flutter to sinus rhythm. In one reported regimen, the patient first receives two tablets (648 mg; 403 mg of quinidine base) of QUINAGLUTE® every eight hours. If this regimen has not resulted in conversion after 3 or 4 doses, then the dose is cautiously increased. If, at any point during administration, the QRS complex widens to 130% of its pre-treatment duration; the QT_c interval widens to 130% of its pre-treatment duration and is then longer than 500 ms; P waves disappear; or the patient develops significant tachycardia, symptomatic bradycardia, or hypotension, then QUINAGLUTE® is discontinued, and other means of conversion (e.g., direct-current cardioversion) are considered.
In another regimen sometimes used, the patient receives one tablet (324 mg; 202 mg of quinidine base) every eight hours for two days; then two tablets every twelve hours for two days; and finally two tablets every eight hours for up to four days. The four-day stretch may come at one of the lower doses if, in the judgment of the physician, the lower dose is the highest one that will be tolerated. The criteria for discontinuation of treatment with QUINAGLUTE ® are the same as in the other regimen.

Reduction in the frequency of relapse into atrial fibrillation/flutter
In a patient with a history of frequent symptomatic episodes of atrial fibrillation/flutter, the goal of therapy with QUINAGLUTE® should be an increase in the average time between episodes. In most patients, the tachyarrhythmia *will recur* during therapy with QUINAGLUTE®, and a single recurrence should not be interpreted as therapeutic failure.
Especially in patients with known structural heart disease or other risk factors for toxicity, initiation or dose adjustment of treatment with QUINAGLUTE® should generally be performed in a setting where facilities and personnel for monitoring and resuscitation are continuously available. Monitoring should be continued for two or three days after initiation of the regimen on which the patient will be discharged.
Therapy with QUINAGLUTE® should be begun with one tablet (324 mg; 202 mg of quinidine base) every eight or twelve hours. If this regimen is well tolerated, if the serum quinidine level is still well within the laboratory's therapeutic range, and if the average time between arrhythmic episodes has not been satisfactorily increased, then the dose may be cautiously raised. The total daily dosage should be reduced if the QRS complex widens to 130% of its pre-treatment duration; the QT_c interval widens to 130% of its pre-treatment duration and is then longer than 500 ms; P waves disappear; or the patient develops significant tachycardia, symptomatic bradycardia, or hypotension.

Suppression of life-threatening ventricular arrhythmias
Dosing regimens for the use of quinidine gluconate in suppressing life-threatening ventricular arrhythmias have not been adequately studied. Described regimens have generally been similar to the regimen described just above for the prophylaxis of symptomatic atrial fibrillation/flutter. Where possible, therapy should be guided by the results of programmed electrical stimulation and/or Holter monitoring with exercise.

HOW SUPPLIED

QUINAGLUTE DURA-TABS® tablets are 324 mg white to off-white, round tablets embossed with **C** in a flask design on one side and with a clock-like design on the other.

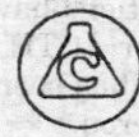 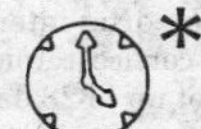 *

The tablets are available in bottles and unit-dose packages as follows:

bottle of 100	NDC 50419-101-10
bottle of 250	NDC 50419-101-25
bottle of 500	NDC 50419-101-50
unit-dose box of 100	NDC 50419-101-11

Store at 25° C (77° F); excursions permitted to 15–30° C (59–86°C).
[See USP Controlled Room Temperature]
*Tablet designs are registered trademarks of Berlex Laboratories

BERLEX® Laboratories, Wayne, NJ 07470
Rev. June 1999 6069504

Shown in Product Identification Guide, page 308

Berlex Laboratories
15049 SAN PABLO AVENUE, P.O. BOX 4099
RICHMOND, CA 94804-0099

Direct Inquiries to:
888-BERLEX-4

BETASERON® ℞
(Interferon beta-1b)

DESCRIPTION

Betaseron® (Interferon beta-1b) is a purified, sterile, lyophilized protein product produced by recombinant DNA techniques and formulated for use by injection. Interferon beta-1b is manufactured by bacterial fermentation of a strain of *Escherichia coli* that bears a genetically engineered plasmid containing the gene for human interferon $beta_{ser17}$. The native gene was obtained from human fibroblasts and altered in a way that substitutes serine for the cysteine residue found at position 17. Interferon beta-1b is a highly purified protein that has 165 amino acids and an approximate molecular weight of 18,500 daltons. It does not include the carbohydrate side chains found in the natural material.
The specific activity of Betaseron is approximately 32 million international units (IU)/mg Interferon beta-1b. Each vial contains 0.3 mg of Interferon beta-1b. The unit measurement is derived by comparing the antiviral activity of the product to the World Health Organization (WHO) reference standard of recombinant human interferon beta. Dextrose and Albumin Human, USP (15 mg each/vial) are added as stabilizers. Prior to 1993, a different analytical standard was used to determine potency. It assigned 54 million IU to 0.3 mg Interferon beta-1b.
Lyophilized Betaseron is a sterile, white to off-white powder intended for subcutaneous injection after reconstitution with the diluent supplied (Sodium Chloride, 0.54% Solution).

CLINICAL PHARMACOLOGY

General: Interferons are a family of naturally occurring proteins, which have molecular weights ranging from 15,000 to 21,000 daltons. Three major classes of interferons have been identified: alfa, beta, and gamma. Interferon beta-1b, interferon alfa, and interferon gamma have overlapping yet distinct biologic activities.[1–5] The activities of Interferon beta-1b are species-restricted and, therefore, the most pertinent pharmacologic information on Betaseron is derived from studies of human cells in culture and in humans.
Biologic Activities: Interferon beta-1b has been shown to possess both antiviral and immunoregulatory activities. The mechanisms by which Betaseron exerts its actions in multiple sclerosis (MS) are not clearly understood. However, it is known that the biologic response-modifying properties of Interferon beta-1b are mediated through its interactions with specific cell receptors found on the surface of human cells. The binding of Interferon beta-1b to these receptors induces the expression of a number of interferon-induced gene products (e.g., 2′, 5′-oligoadenylate synthetase, protein kinase, and indoleamine 2, 3-dioxygenase) that are believed to be the mediators of the biological actions of Interferon beta-1b.[1,3,6–10] A number of these interferon-induced products have been readily measured in the serum and cellular fractions of blood collected from patients treated with Interferon beta-1b.[11,12]
Pharmacokinetics: Because serum concentrations of Interferon beta-1b are low or not detectable following subcutaneous administration of 0.25 mg or less of Betaseron, pharmacokinetic information in patients with MS receiving the recommended dose of Betaseron is not available. Following single and multiple daily subcutaneous administrations of 0.5 mg Betaseron to healthy volunteers (N=12), serum Interferon beta-1b concentrations were generally below 100 IU/mL. Peak serum Interferon beta-1b concentrations occurred between 1 to 8 hours, with a mean peak serum interferon concentration of 40 IU/mL. Bioavailability, based on a total dose of 0.5 mg Betaseron given as two subcutaneous injections at different sites, was approximately 50%.
After intravenous administration of Betaseron (0.006 mg to 2.0 mg), similar pharmacokinetic profiles were obtained from healthy volunteers (N=12) and from patients with diseases other than MS (N=142). In patients receiving single intravenous doses up to 2.0 mg, increases in serum concentrations were dose proportional. Mean serum clearance values ranged from 9.4 $mL/min{\cdot}kg^{-1}$ to 28.9 $mL/min{\cdot}kg^{-1}$ and were independent of dose. Mean terminal elimination half-life values ranged from 8.0 minutes to 4.3 hours and mean steady-state volume of distribution values ranged from 0.25 L/kg to 2.88 L/kg. Three-times-a-week intravenous dosing for 2 weeks resulted in no accumulation of Interferon beta-1b in the serum of patients. Pharmacokinetic parameters after single and multiple intravenous doses of Betaseron were comparable.
Clinical Trials: The effectiveness of Betaseron in relapsing-remitting MS was evaluated in a double-blind, multiclinic (11 sites: 4 Canadian and 7 United States), randomized, parallel, placebo-controlled clinical investigation of 2 years duration. The study enrolled MS patients, aged 18 to 50, who were ambulatory (Kurtzke expanded disability status scale [EDSS] of ≤5.5), exhibited a relapsing-remitting clinical course, met Poser's criteria[13] for clinically definite and/or laboratory supported definite MS and had experienced at least two exacerbations over 2 years preceding the trial without exacerbation in the preceding month. Patients who had received prior immunosuppressant therapy were excluded.
An exacerbation was defined, per protocol, as the appearance of a new clinical sign/symptom or the clinical worsening of a previous sign/symptom (one that had been stable for at least 30 days) that persisted for a minimum of 24 hours.
Patients selected for study were randomized to treatment with either placebo (N=123), 0.05 mg of Betaseron (N=125), or 0.25 mg of Betaseron (N=124) self-administered subcutaneously every other day. Outcome based on the 372 randomized patients was evaluated after 2 years.
Patients who required more than three 28-day courses of corticosteroids were removed from the study. Minor analgesics (acetaminophen, codeine), antidepressants, and oral baclofen were allowed ad libitum but chronic nonsteroidal anti-inflammatory drug (NSAID) use was not allowed.
The primary, protocol defined, outcome assessment measures were 1) frequency of exacerbations per patient and 2) proportion of exacerbation free patients. A number of secondary outcome measures were also employed as described in Table 1.
In addition to clinical measures, annual magnetic resonance imaging (MRI) was performed and quantitated for extent of disease as determined by changes in total area of lesions. In a substudy of patients (N=52) at one site, MRIs were performed every 6 weeks and quantitated for disease activity as determined by changes in size and number of lesions.
Results at the protocol designated endpoint of 2 years (see TABLE 1): In the 2-year analysis, there was a 31% reduction in annual exacerbation rate, from 1.31 in the placebo group to 0.9 in the 0.25 mg group. The p-value for this difference was 0.0001. The proportion of patients free of exacerbations was 16% in the placebo group, compared with 25% in the Betaseron® (Interferon beta-1b) 0.25 mg group.
Of the 372 patients randomized, 72 (19%) failed to complete 2 full years on their assigned treatments. The reasons given for withdrawal varied with treatment assignment. Excessive use of steroids accounted for 11 of the 26 placebo withdrawals, but only 2 of the 21 withdrawals from the 0.05 mg assigned group and 1 of the 25 withdrawals from the 0.25 mg assigned group. Withdrawals for adverse events attributed to study article, however, were more common among Betaseron-treated patients: 1, 5, and 10 withdrew from the placebo, 0.05 mg, and 0.25 mg groups, respectively.
Over the 2-year period, there were 25 MS-related hospitalizations in the 0.25 mg Betaseron-treated group compared to 48 hospitalizations in the placebo group. In comparison, non-MS hospitalizations were evenly distributed among the groups, with 16 in the 0.25 mg Betaseron group and 15 in the placebo group. The average number of days of MS-related steroid use was 41 days in the 0.25 mg Betaseron group and 55 days in the placebo group (p=0.004).
MRI data were also analyzed for patients in this study. A frequency distribution of the observed percent changes in MRI area at the end of 2 years was obtained by grouping the percentages in successive intervals of equal width. Figure 1 displays a histogram of the proportions of patients who fell into each of these intervals. The median percent change in MRI area for the 0.25 mg group was −1.1% which was significantly smaller than the 16.5% observed for the placebo group (p=0.0001).
[See table 1 at top of next page]
[See figure 1 at top of next column]
In an evaluation of frequent MRI scans (every 6 weeks) on 52 patients at one site, the percent of scans with new or expanding lesions was 29% in the placebo group and 6% in the 0.25 mg treatment group (p=0.006).

Continued on next page

Information on the Berlex products appearing here is based on the most current information available at the time of publication closing. Further information for these and other products may be obtained from the Medical Affairs Department, Berlex Laboratories, 300 Fairfield Road, Wayne, New Jersey 07470, 1-888-BERLEX-4. Information on Betaseron and Fludara may be obtained from Berlex Laboratories, 15049 San Pablo Avenue, Richmond, California 94804-0016, 1-800-888-4112.

Betaseron—Cont.

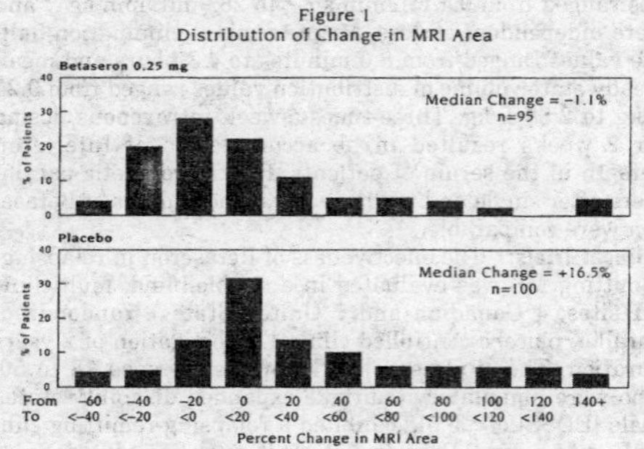

Figure 1
Distribution of Change in MRI Area

MRI scanning is viewed as a useful means to visualize changes in white matter that are believed to be a reflection of the pathologic changes that, appropriately located within the central nervous system (CNS), account for some of the signs and symptoms that typify relapsing-remitting MS. The exact relationship between MRI findings and the clinical status of patients is unknown. Changes in lesion area often do not correlate with clinical exacerbations probably because many of the lesions affect so-called "silent" regions of the CNS. Moreover, it is not clear what fraction of the lesions seen on MRI become foci of irreversible demyelinization (i.e., classic white matter plaques). The prognostic significance of the MRI findings in this study has not been evaluated.

At the end of 2 years on assigned treatment, patients in the study had the option of continuing on treatment under blinded conditions. Approximately 80% of patients under each treatment accepted. Although there was a trend toward patient benefit in the Betaseron® (Interferon beta-1b) groups during the third year, particularly in the 0.25 mg group, there was no statistically significant difference between the Betaseron-treated vs. placebo-treated patients in exacerbation rate, or in any of the secondary endpoints described in Table 1. As noted above, in the 2-year analysis, there was a 31% reduction in exacerbation rate in the 0.25 mg group, compared with placebo. The p-value for this difference was 0.0001. In the analysis of the third year alone, the difference between treatment groups was 28%. The p-value was 0.065. The lower number of patients may account for the loss of statistical significance, and lack of direct comparability among the patient groups in this extension study make the interpretation of these results difficult. The third year MRI data did not show a trend toward additional benefit in the Betaseron arm compared with the placebo arm.

Throughout the clinical trial, serum samples from patients were monitored for the development of antibodies to Interferon beta-1b. In patients receiving 0.25 mg of Betaseron (N=124) every other day in the clinical trial, 45% were found to have serum neutralizing activity at one or more of the time points tested. The relationship between antibody formation and clinical efficacy is not known.

TABLE 1
2 Year Study Results
Primary and Secondary Clinical Endpoints

Efficacy Parameters	Treatment Groups			Statistical Comparisons p-value		
Primary Endpoints	**Placebo (N=123)**	**0.05 mg (N=125)**	**0.25 mg (N=124)**	**Placebo vs 0.05 mg**	**0.05 mg vs 0.25 mg**	**Placebo vs 0.25 mg**
Annual exacerbation rate	1.31	1.14	0.90	0.005	0.113	**0.0001**
Proportion of exacerbation-free patients†	16%	18%	25%	0.609	0.288	**0.094**
Exacerbation frequency per patient 0†	20	22	29	0.151	0.077	**0.001**
1	32	31	39			
2	20	28	17			
3	15	15	14			
4	15	7	9			
≥5	21	16	8			
Secondary Endpoints††						
Median number of months to first on-study exacerbation	5	6	9	0.299	0.097	**0.010**
Rate of moderate or severe exacerbations per year	0.47	0.29	0.23	0.020	0.257	**0.001**
Mean number of moderate or severe exacerbation days per patient	44.1	33.2	19.5	0.229	0.064	**0.001**
Mean change in EDSS score‡ at endpoint	0.21	0.21	−0.07	0.995	0.108	**0.144**
Mean change in Scripps score‡‡ at endpoint	−0.53	−0.50	0.66	0.641	0.051	**0.126**
Median duration in days per exacerbation	36	33	35.5	ND	ND	**ND**
% change in mean MRI lesion area at endpoint	21.4%	9.8%	−0.9%	0.015	0.019	**0.0001**

ND -Not done
† 14 exacerbation-free patients (0 from placebo, 6 from 0.05 mg, and 8 from 0.25 mg) dropped out of the study before completing 6 months of therapy. These patients are excluded from this analysis.
†† Sequelae and Functional Neurologic Status, both required by protocol, were not analyzed individually but are included as a function of the EDSS.
‡ EDSS scores range from 0–10, with higher scores reflecting greater disability.
‡‡ Scripps neurologic rating scores range from 0–100, with smaller scores reflecting greater disability.

INDICATIONS AND USAGE

Betaseron is indicated for use in ambulatory patients with relapsing-remitting multiple sclerosis to reduce the frequency of clinical exacerbations. (See **CLINICAL PHARMACOLOGY, Clinical Trials** section.) Relapsing-remitting MS is characterized by recurrent attacks of neurologic dysfunction followed by complete or incomplete recovery. The safety and efficacy of Betaseron in chronic-progressive MS has not been evaluated.

CONTRAINDICATIONS

Betaseron is contraindicated in patients with a history of hypersensitivity to natural or recombinant interferon beta, Albumin Human USP, or any other component of the formulation.

WARNINGS

One suicide and 4 attempted suicides were observed among 372 study patients during a 3-year period. All five patients received Betaseron (three in the 0.05 mg group and two in the 0.25 mg). There were no attempted suicides in patients on study who did not receive Betaseron. Depression and suicide have been reported to occur in patients receiving interferon alfa, a related compound. Patients to be treated with Betaseron should be informed that depression and suicidal ideation may be a side effect of the treatment and should report these symptoms immediately to the prescribing physician. Patients exhibiting depression should be monitored closely and cessation of therapy should be considered.

Injection site necrosis (ISN) has been reported in 5% of patients in controlled clinical trials (see **ADVERSE REACTIONS** section). Typically, injection site necrosis occurs within the first 4 months of therapy, although post-marketing reports have been received of ISN occurring over 1 year after initiation of therapy. Necrosis may occur at single or multiple injection sites. The necrotic lesions are typically 3 cm or less in diameter, but larger areas have been reported. While necrosis has commonly extended only to subcutaneous fat, there are also reports of necrosis extending to and including fascia overlaying muscle. In some lesions where biopsy results are available, vasculitis has been reported. For some lesions debridement and, infrequently, skin grafting has been required.

As with any open lesion, it is important to avoid infection and, if it occurs, to treat the infection. Time to healing has varied depending on the severity of the necrosis at the time treatment was begun. In most cases healing was associated with scarring.

Some patients have experienced healing of necrotic skin lesions while Betaseron® (Interferon beta-1b) therapy continued, others have not. Whether to discontinue therapy following a single site of necrosis is dependent on the extent of necrosis. For patients who continue therapy with Betaseron® (Interferon beta-1b) after injection site necrosis has occurred, Betaseron should not be administered into the affected area until it is fully healed. If multiple lesions occur, therapy should be discontinued until healing occurs.

Patient understanding and use of aseptic self-injection techniques and procedures should be periodically reevaluated, particularly if injection site necrosis has occured.

PRECAUTIONS

General: Patients should be instructed in injection techniques to assure the safe self-administration of Betaseron. (See **PRECAUTIONS: Information to patients,** and **Betaseron Patient Information** sheet.)

Information to patients:

Instruction on self-injection technique and procedures. Patients should be instructed in the use of aseptic technique when administering Betaseron. Appropriate instruction for reconstitution of Betaseron and self-injection should be given including careful review of the **Betaseron Patient Information** sheet. If possible, the first injection should be performed under the supervision of an appropriately qualified health care professional.

Patients should be cautioned against the re-use of needles or syringes and instructed in safe disposal procedures. A puncture resistant container for disposal of used needles and syringes should be supplied to the patient along with instructions for safe disposal of full containers.

Patients should be advised of the importance of rotating areas of injection with each dose, to minimize the likelihood of severe injection site reactions or necrosis (see **Rotating Injection Sites** section of **Patient Information** sheet).

Patients should be cautioned not to change the dosage or the schedule of administration without medical consultation.

Awareness of adverse reactions. Serious adverse reactions associated with the use of Betaseron have been reported including depression and injection site necrosis (see **WARNINGS** section).

Patients should immediately report symptoms of depression or suicidal ideation to their physician. The symptoms of depression should be closely monitored by a physician.

Injection site necrosis was reported in 5% of patients in a controlled MS trial. If the patient experiences any break in the skin, which may be associated with blue-black discoloration, swelling, or drainage of fluid from the injection site, the patient should be advised to promptly contact their physician prior to continuing their Betaseron therapy.

Other injection site reactions occurred in eighty-five percent of patients in the controlled MS trial, at one or more times during therapy. There was redness, pain, swelling and discoloration. In general, these were transient and did not require discontinuation of therapy, but the nature and severity of all reported reactions should be carefully assessed (see **ADVERSE REACTIONS** section).

Flu-like symptoms are common following initiation of therapy with Betaseron. In the controlled MS clinical trial, acetaminophen was permitted for relief of fever or myalgia (see **ADVERSE REACTIONS** section).

Patients should be cautioned about the abortifacient potential of Betaseron (see **PRECAUTIONS, Pregnancy - Teratogenic effects**).

Laboratory tests: The following laboratory tests are recommended prior to initiating Betaseron therapy and at periodic intervals thereafter: hemoglobin, complete and differential white blood cell counts, platelet counts and blood chemistries including liver function tests. In the controlled MS trial, patients were monitored every 3 months. The study protocol stipulated that Betaseron therapy be discontinued in the event the absolute neutrophil count fell below 750/mm^3. When the absolute neutrophil count had returned to a value greater than 750/mm^3, therapy could be restarted at a 50% reduced dose. No patients were withdrawn or dose reduced for neutropenia or lymphopenia.

Similarly, if hepatic transaminase (SGOT/SGPT) levels exceeded 10 times the upper limit of normal, or if the serum bilirubin exceeded 5 times the upper limit of normal, therapy was discontinued. In each instance during the controlled MS trial, hepatic enzyme abnormalities returned to normal following discontinuation of therapy. When measurements had decreased to below these levels, therapy could be restarted at a 50% dose reduction, if clinically appropriate. Two patients were dose reduced for increased liver enzymes; one continued on treatment and one was ultimately withdrawn.

Drug interactions: Interactions between Betaseron and other drugs have not been fully evaluated. Although studies designed to examine drug interactions have not been done, it was noted that corticosteroid or ACTH treatment of relapses for periods of up to 28 days has been administered to patients (N=180) receiving Betaseron.

Betaseron administration to three cancer patients over a dose range of 0.025 mg to 2.2 mg led to a dose-dependent inhibition of antipyrine elimination.[14] The effect of alternate-day administration of 0.25 mg of Betaseron on drug metabolism in MS patients is unknown.

Carcinogenesis: The carcinogenic potential of Betaseron was evaluated by studying its effect on the morphological transformation of the mammalian cell line BALBc-3T3. No significant increases in transformation frequency were noted. No carcinogenicity data are available in animals or humans.

Betaseron® (Interferon beta-1b) was not mutagenic when assayed for genotoxicity in the Ames bacterial test in the presence or absence of metabolic activation.

Impairment of fertility: Studies in rhesus monkeys at doses up to 0.33 mg/kg/day (32 times the recommended human dose based on body surface area comparison*) in normally cycling rhesus female monkeys had no apparent adverse effects on the menstrual cycle or on associated hormonal profiles (progesterone and estradiol) when administered over 3 consecutive menstrual cycles. The extrapolability of animal doses to human doses is not known. Effects of Betaseron on normal cycling human females are not known.

*body surface dose based on 70 kg female

Pregnancy - Teratogenic effects: Pregnancy Category C: Betaseron was not teratogenic at doses up to 0.42 mg/kg/day in rhesus monkeys, but demonstrated a dose-related abortifacient activity when administered at doses ranging from 0.028 mg/kg/day (2.8 times the recommended human dose based on body surface area comparison) to 0.42 mg/kg/day (40 times the recommended human dose based on body surface area comparison). The extrapolability of animal doses to human doses is not known. Lower doses were not studied in monkeys. Spontaneous abortions while on treatment were reported in patients (N=4) who participated in the Betaseron MS clinical trial. Betaseron given to rhesus monkeys on gestation days 20 to 70 did not cause teratogenic effects, however, it is not known if teratogenic effects exist in humans. There are no adequate and well-controlled studies in pregnant women. If the patient becomes pregnant or plans to become pregnant while taking Betaseron, the patient should be apprised of the potential hazard to the fetus and it should be recommended that the patient discontinue therapy.

Nursing mothers: It is not known whether Betaseron is excreted in human milk. Because many drugs are excreted in human milk and because of the potential for serious adverse reactions in nursing infants from Betaseron, a decision should be made as to whether either to discontinue nursing or discontinue the drug, taking into account the importance of drug to the mother.

Pediatric use: Safety and efficacy in children under 18 years of age have not been established.

ADVERSE REACTIONS

Experience with Betaseron in patients with MS is limited to a total of 147 patients at the recommended dose of 0.25 mg every other day or more (see **CLINICAL PHARMACOLOGY, Clinical Trials** section). Consequently, adverse events that are associated with the use of Betaseron in MS patients at a low incidence may not have been observed in pre-marketing studies. Clinical experience with Betaseron in other populations (patients with cancer, HIV positive patients, etc.) provides additional data regarding adverse reactions; however, experience in non-MS populations may not be fully applicable to the MS population.

Injection site reactions (85%) and injection site necrosis (5%) occurred after administration of Betaseron. Inflammation, pain, hypersensitivity, necrosis, and non-specific reactions were significantly associated ($p<0.05$) with the 0.25 mg Betaseron-treated group. Only inflammation, pain, and necrosis were reported as severe events (see **WARNINGS** and **PRECAUTIONS** sections). The incidence rate for injection site reactions was calculated over the course of 3 years. This incidence rate decreased over time, with 79% of patients experiencing the event during the first 3 months of treatment compared to 47% during the last 6 months. The median time to the first occurrence of an injection site reaction was 7 days. Patients with injection site reactions reported these events 183.7 days per year. Three patients withdrew from the 0.25 mg Betaseron-treated group for injection site pain.

Flu-like symptom complex was reported in 76% of the patients treated with 0.25 mg Betaseron. A patient was defined as having a flu-like symptom complex if flu-like symptoms or at least two of the following symptoms were concurrently reported: fever, chills, myalgia, malaise, or sweating. Only myalgia, fever, and chills were reported as severe in more than 5% of the patients. The incidence rate for flu-like symptom complex was also calculated over the course of 3 years. The incidence rate of these events decreased over time, with 60% of patients experiencing the event during the first 3 months of treatment compared to 10% during the last 6 months. The median time to the first occurrence of flu-like symptom complex was 3.5 days and the median duration per patient was 7.5 days per year.

Laboratory abnormalities included absolute neutrophil count less than 1500/mm^3 (18%) (no patients had absolute neutrophil counts less than 500/mm^3), WBC less than 3000/mm^3 (16%), SGPT greater than 5 times baseline value (19%), and total bilirubin greater than 2.5 times baseline value (6%). Three patients were withdrawn from treatment with 0.25 mg Betaseron for abnormal liver enzymes including one following dose reduction (see **PRECAUTIONS, Laboratory Tests**).

Twenty-one (28%) of the 76 premenopausal females treated at 0.25 mg Betaseron and 10 (13%) of the 76 premenopausal females treated with placebo reported menstrual disorders. All of these reports were of mild to moderate severity and included: intermenstrual bleeding and spotting, early or delayed menses, decreased days of menstrual flow, and clotting and spotting during menstruation.

Mental disorders have been observed in patients in this study. Symptoms included depression, anxiety, emotional lability, depersonalization, suicide attempts, confusion, etc. In the treatment group, two patients withdrew for confusion. One suicide and four attempted suicides were also reported. It is not known whether these symptoms may be related to the underlying neurological basis of MS, to Betaseron treatment, or to a combination of both. Some similar symptoms have been noted in patients receiving interferon alfa and both interferons are thought to act through the same receptor. Patients who experience these symptoms should be closely monitored and cessation of therapy considered.

Additional common adverse clinical and laboratory events associated with the use of Betaseron® (Interferon beta-1b) are listed in the following paragraphs. These events occurred at an incidence of 5% or more in the 124 MS patients treated with 0.25 mg of Betaseron every other day for periods of up to 3 years in the controlled trial, and at an incidence that was at least twice that observed in the 123 placebo patients. Common adverse clinical and laboratory events associated with the use of Betaseron were: injection site reaction (85%), injection site necrosis (5%), palpitation (8%), hypertension (7%), tachycardia (6%), peripheral vascular disorders (5%), gastrointestinal disorders (6%), absolute neutrophil count <1500/mm^3 (18%), WBC <3000/mm^3 (16%), SGPT >5 times baseline value (19%), total bilirubin >2.5 times baseline value (6%), somnolence (6%), dyspnea (8%), laryngitis (6%), menstrual disorder (17%), cystitis (8%), breast pain (7%), pelvic pain (6%), and menorrhagia (6%).

TABLE 2
Adverse Reactions and Laboratory Abnormalities

Adverse Reaction	Placebo N=123	0.25 mg N=124
Body as a Whole		
Injection site reaction*	37%	85%
Headache	77%	84%
Fever*	41%	59%
Flu-like symptom complex*	56%	76%
Pain	48%	52%
Asthenia*	35%	49%
Chills*	19%	46%
Abdominal pain	24%	32%
Malaise*	3%	15%
Generalized edema	6%	8%
Pelvic pain	3%	6%
Injection site necrosis*	0%	5%
Cyst	2%	4%
Necrosis	0%	2%
Suicide attempt	0%	2%
Cardiovascular System		
Migraine	7%	12%
Palpitation*	2%	8%
Hypertension	2%	7%
Tachycardia	3%	6%
Peripheral vascular disorder	2%	5%
Hemorrhage	1%	3%
Digestive System		
Diarrhea	29%	35%
Constipation	18%	24%
Vomiting	19%	21%
Gastrointestinal disorder	3%	6%
Endocrine System		
Goiter	0%	2%
Hemic and Lymphatic System		
Lymphocytes less than 1500/mm^3	67%	82%
ANC < 1500/mm^{3*}	6%	18%
WBC < 3000/mm^{3*}	5%	16%
Lymphadenopathy	11%	14%
Metabolic and Nutritional Disorders		
SGPT > 5 times baseline*	6%	19%
Glucose < 55 mg/dL	13%	15%
Total bilirubin > 2.5 times baseline	2%	6%
Urine protein > 1+	3%	5%
SGOT > 5 times baseline*	0%	4%
Weight gain	0%	4%
Weight loss	2%	4%
Musculoskeletal System		
Myalgia*	28%	44%
Myasthenia	10%	13%
Nervous System		
Dizziness	28%	35%
Hypertonia	24%	26%
Anxiety	13%	15%
Nervousness	5%	8%
Somnolence	3%	6%
Confusion	2%	4%
Speech disorder	1%	3%
Convulsion	0%	2%
Hyperkinesia	0%	2%
Amnesia	0%	2%
Respiratory System		
Sinusitis	26%	36%
Dyspnea*	2%	8%
Laryngitis	2%	6%
Skin and Appendages		
Sweating*	11%	23%
Alopecia	2%	4%
Special Senses		
Conjunctivitis	10%	12%
Abnormal vision	4%	7%
Urogenital System		
Dysmenorrhea	11%	18%
Menstrual disorder*	8%	17%
Metrorrhagia	8%	15%
Cystitis	4%	8%
Breast pain	3%	7%
Menorrhagia	3%	6%
Urinary urgency	2%	4%
Fibrocystic breast	1%	3%
Breast neoplasm	0%	2%

* Significantly associated with Betaseron treatment.

A total of 277 MS patients have been treated with Betaseron® (Interferon beta-1b) in doses ranging from 0.025 mg to 0.5 mg. During the first 3 years of treatment, withdrawals due to clinical adverse events or laboratory abnormalities not mentioned above included: fatigue (2%, 6 patients), cardiac arrhythmia (<1%, 1 patient), allergic urticarial skin reaction to injections (<1%, 1 patient), headache (<1%, 1 patient), unspecified adverse events (<1%, 1 patient), and "felt sick" (<1%, 1 patient).

Table 2 enumerates adverse events and laboratory abnormalities that occurred at an incidence of 2% or more among the 124 MS patients treated with 0.25 mg Betaseron every other day for periods of up to 3 years in the controlled trial and at an incidence that was at least 2% more than that observed in the 123 placebo patients. Reported adverse events have been reclassified using the standard COSTART glossary to reduce the total number of terms employed in Table 2, terms so general as to be uninformative, and those events where a drug cause was remote have been excluded. It should be noted that the figures cited in the table cannot be used to predict the incidence of side effects in the course of usual medical practice where patient characteristics and other factors differ from those that prevailed in the clinical trials. The cited figures do provide the prescribing physician with some basis for estimating the relative contribution of drug and nondrug factors to the side effect incidence rate in the population studied.

Other events observed during premarketing evaluation of various doses of Betaseron in 1440 patients are listed in the paragraph that follows. Because most of the events were observed in open and uncontrolled studies, the role of Betaseron in their causation cannot be reliably determined. **Body as a Whole:** abscess, adenoma, anaphylactoid reaction, ascites, cellulitis, hernia, hydrocephalus, hypothermia, infection, peritonitis, photosensitivity, sarcoma, sepsis, and shock; **Cardiovascular System:** angina pectoris, arrhythmia, atrial fibrillation, cardiomegaly, cardiac arrest, cerebral hemorrhage, cerebral ischemia, endocarditis, heart failure, hypotension, myocardial infarct, pericardial effusion, postural hypotension, pulmonary embolus, spider angioma, subarachnoid hemorrhage, syncope, thrombophlebitis, thrombosis, varicose vein, vasospasm, venous pressure increased, ventricular extrasystoles, and ventricular fibrillation; **Digestive System:** aphthous stomatitis, cardiospasm, cheilitis, cholecystitis, cholelithiasis, duodenal ulcer, dry mouth, enteritis, esophagitis, fecal impaction, fecal incontinence, flatulence, gastritis, gastrointestinal hemorrhage, gingivitis, glossitis, hematemesis, hepatic neoplasia, hepatitis, hepatomegaly, ileus, increased salivation, intestinal obstruction, melena, nausea, oral leukoplakia, oral moniliasis, pancreatitis, periodontal abscess, proctitis, rectal hemor-

Continued on next page

Information on the Berlex products appearing here is based on the most current information available at the time of publication closing. Further information for these and other products may be obtained from the Medical Affairs Department, Berlex Laboratories, 300 Fairfield Road, Wayne, New Jersey 07470, 1-888-BERLEX-4. Information on Betaseron and Fludara may be obtained from Berlex Laboratories, 15049 San Pablo Avenue, Richmond, California 94804-0016, 1-800-888-4112.

Betaseron—Cont.

rhage, salivary gland enlargement, stomach ulcer, and tenesmus; **Endocrine System:** Cushing's Syndrome, diabetes insipidus, diabetes mellitus, hypothyroidism, and inappropriate ADH; **Hemic and Lymphatic System:** chronic lymphocytic leukemia, hemoglobin less than 9.4 g/100 mL, petechia, platelets less than 75,000/mm^3, and splenomegaly; **Metabolic and Nutritional Disorders:** alcohol intolerance, alkaline phosphatase greater than 5 times baseline value, BUN greater than 40 mg/dL, calcium greater than 11.5 mg/dL, cyanosis, edema, glucose greater than 160 mg/dL, glycosuria, hypoglycemic reaction, hypoxia, ketosis, and thirst; **Musculoskeletal System:** arthritis, arthrosis, bursitis, leg cramps, muscle atrophy, myopathy, myositis, ptosis, and tenosynovitis; **Nervous System:** abnormal gait, acute brain syndrome, agitation, apathy, aphasia, ataxia, brain edema, chronic brain syndrome, coma, delirium, delusions, dementia, depersonalization, diplopia, dystonia, encephalopathy, euphoria, facial paralysis, foot drop, hallucinations, hemiplegia, hypalgesia, hyperesthesia, incoordination, intracranial hypertension, libido decreased, manic reaction, meningitis, neuralgia, neuropathy, neurosis, nystagmus, oculogyric crisis, ophthalmoplegia, papilledema, paralysis, paranoid reaction, psychosis, reflexes decreased, stupor, subdural hematoma, torticollis, tremor, and urinary retention; **Respiratory System:** apnea, asthma, atelectasis, carcinoma of lung, hemoptysis, hiccup, hyperventilation, hypoventilation, interstitial pneumonia, lung edema, pleural effusion, pneumonia, and pneumothorax; **Skin and Appendages:** contact dermatitis, erythema nodosum, exfoliative dermatitis, furunculosis, hirsutism, leukoderma, lichenoid dermatitis, maculopapular rash, psoriasis, seborrhea, skin benign neoplasm, skin carcinoma, skin hypertrophy, skin necrosis, skin ulcer, urticaria, and vesiculobullous rash; **Special Senses:** blepharitis, blindness, deafness, dry eyes, ear pain, iritis, keratoconjunctivitis, mydriasis, otitis externa, otitis media, parosmia, photophobia, retinitis, taste loss, taste perversion, and visual field defect; **Urogenital System:** anuria, balanitis, breast engorgement, cervicitis, epididymitis, gynecomastia, hematuria, impotence, kidney calculus, kidney failure, kidney tubular disorder, leukorrhea, nephritis, nocturia, oliguria, polyuria, salpingitis, urethritis, urinary incontinence, uterine fibroids enlarged, uterine neoplasm, and vaginal hemorrhage.

DRUG ABUSE AND DEPENDENCE

No evidence or experience suggests that abuse or dependence occurs with Betaseron® (Interferon beta-1b) therapy; however, the risk of dependence has not been systematically evaluated.

DOSAGE AND ADMINISTRATION

The recommended dose of Betaseron for the treatment of ambulatory relapsing-remitting MS is 0.25 mg injected subcutaneously every other day. Limited data regarding the activity of a lower dose are presented above (see **CLINICAL PHARMACOLOGY, Clinical Trials**).

Evidence of efficacy beyond 2 years is not known since the primary evidence of efficacy derives from a 2-year, double-blind, placebo-controlled clinical trial (see **CLINICAL PHARMACOLOGY, Clinical Trials**). Safety data are not available beyond the third year. Patients were discontinued from this trial due to unremitting disease progression of 6 months or greater.

To reconstitute lyophilized Betaseron for injection, use a sterile syringe and needle to inject 1.2 mL of the diluent supplied, Sodium Chloride, 0.54% Solution, into the Betaseron vial. Gently swirl the vial of Betaseron to dissolve the drug completely; do not shake. Inspect the reconstituted product visually and discard the product before use if it contains particulate matter or is discolored. After reconstitution with accompanying diluent, Betaseron vials contain 0.25 mg Interferon beta-1b/mL of solution.

Withdraw 1 mL of reconstituted solution from the vial into a sterile syringe fitted with a 27-gauge needle and inject the solution subcutaneously. Sites for self-injection include arms, abdomen, hips, and thighs. A vial is suitable for single use only; unused portions should be discarded. (See **BETASERON PATIENT INFORMATION** sheet for **SELF-INJECTION PROCEDURE**.)

Stability:

The reconstituted product contains no preservative. Before reconstitution with diluent, store at 2° to 8°C (36° to 46°F). After reconstitution, if not used immediately, the product should be refrigerated and used within 3 hours. Avoid freezing.

If refrigeration is not possible, vials of Betaseron and diluent should be kept as cool as possible, below 30°C (86°F), away from heat and light, and used within 7 days.

HOW SUPPLIED

Betaseron is supplied as a lyophilized powder containing 0.3 mg of Interferon beta-1b, 15 mg Albumin Human USP, and 15 mg dextrose, USP. Drug is packaged in a clear glass, single-use vial (3 mL capacity); a separate vial containing 2 mL of diluent (Sodium Chloride, 0.54% solution) is included for each vial of drug. Store under refrigeration, between 2° to 8°C (36° to 46°F).

NDC 50419-521-03 0.3 mg/vial
NDC 50419-521-15 15 vials, 0.3 mg/vial

Caution: Federal law prohibits dispensing without prescription.

REFERENCES

1. Ruzicka FJ, et al. J Biol Chem, 1987; 262: 16142-16149. **2.** Uze G, et al. Cell, 1990; 60: 225-234. **3.** DeMaeyer E, et al. In: Interferons and other regulatory cytokines, NY, Wiley 1988. **4.** Colby CB, et al. J Immunol 1984; 133: 3091-3095. **5.** Pestka S, et al. Annu Rev Biochem 1987; 56: 727-777. **6.** Lengyel P, Annu Rev Biochem 1982; 51: 251-282. **7.** Witt PL, et al. J Interferon Res 1990; 10: 393-402. **8.** Schiller JH, et al. J Biol Resp Mod 1990; 9: 377-386. **9.** Rosenblum MG, et al. J Interferon Res 1990; 10: 141-151. **10.** Carlin JM, et al. J Immuno 1987; 130(7): 2414-2418. **11.** Witt PL, et al. J Immunotherapy 1993; 13: 191-200. **12.** Goldstein D, et al. J Natl Cancer Inst 1989; 81: 1061-1068. **13.** Poser CM, et al. Ann Neurol 1983; 13(3): 227-231. **14.** Blaschke TF, et al. Clinical Research 1985; 33(1): 19A.

Manufactured by:
CHIRON Corporation
Emeryville, CA 94608
U.S. License No. 1106
Distributed by:
BERLEX Laboratories
Richmond, CA 94804
U.S. Patent No. 4,588,585; 4,959,314; 4,737,462; 4,450,103

Part Number L -1172.2 Revision date 10/96
Printed in USA on Recycled Paper

BETASERON®
Interferon beta-1b

Read this patient information each time your prescription is filled because this information may have changed.

PATIENT INFORMATION

Betaseron® (Interferon beta-1b) is intended for use under the guidance and supervision of a physician. Your physician or his/her delegate should instruct you in the preparation of Betaseron for administration and in the technique of self injection. Do not attempt self-administration until you are sure that you understand the requirements for mixing the product and giving an injection to yourself.

Betaseron should be used as prescribed by your physician. However, if you miss a dose, take it as soon as you remember. Your next injection, however, should be scheduled about 48 hours later. While using Betaseron, please keep in mind the following facts:

- Betaseron must be kept cold. Be sure to store it in a refrigerator before and after reconstitution. Do not freeze.
- Keep syringes and needles away from children. Do not reuse needles or syringes. Discard used syringes and needles in a syringe disposal unit as instructed by your physician.
- Women: Betaseron should not be used during pregnancy or if you are trying to become pregnant. If you wish to become pregnant while using Betaseron, discuss the matter with your doctor. While using Betaseron, women of childbearing age should use birth control measures. If you do become pregnant you should discontinue treatment and contact your doctor immediately.
- Injection site reactions are common. They include redness, pain and swelling, and discoloration. Less frequently, injection site necrosis (skin breakdown and tissue destruction) has been observed. To minimize chances for a reaction, you should rotate injection sites as described on pages 3 and 4 or as recommended by your physician. Do not make an injection into skin that is tender, red, or hard. If you experience a break in the skin or drainage of fluid from the injection site, you should promptly contact your physician before continuing injections with Betaseron.
- Flu-like symptoms are also common. They include fever, chills, sweating, fatigue, and muscle aches. Taking Betaseron at night may help lessen the impact of flu-like symptoms.
- Depression, including suicide attempts, has been reported by patients. If you experience such symptoms, contact your physician promptly.
- As with any prescription medication, side effects related to therapy can occur. Consult with your physician if you have any problems, whether or not you think they may be related to Betaseron® (Interferon beta-1b).

SELF-INJECTION PROCEDURE

To mix the contents of one vial

Only the vial of diluent (liquid) that comes inside your prescription package should be used to dissolve the white cake of drug in the Betaseron vial.

1. Wash your hands thoroughly with soap and water.

2. Collect all your equipment before you begin the process. You'll need:

- vial of Diluent for Betaseron (Sodium Chloride 0.54%)
- vial of Betaseron
- 3-mL syringe with 21-gauge needle (1)
- 1-mL syringe with 27-gauge needle (1)
- alcohol wipes
- disposal unit (an opaque, puncture-resistant, sealable container for used syringes/needles)

NOTE: Be sure needle guards are on the needles tightly.

3. Remove the protective caps from both vials.

4. Use alcohol wipes to clean the tops of the vials—move in one direction and use one wipe per vial.

NOTE: Leave an alcohol wipe on top of each vial until you are ready to use it.

5. Resting your hands on a stable surface, remove the needle cover on the 3-mL syringe by pulling the cover straight off the needle.

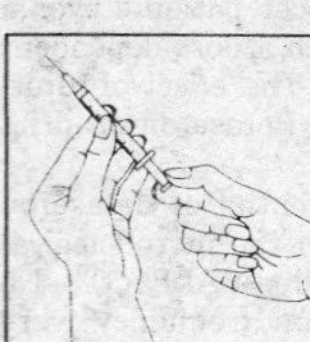

6. Pull back the plunger (on the 3-mL syringe) to the 1.2 mL mark.

NOTE: Read the labels on the vials—find the Diluent for Betaseron vial and throw away the alcohol wipe on top of it.

7. Holding the vial of Diluent for Betaseron® (Interferon beta-1b) on a stable surface, slowly insert the needle straight through the stopper, into the top of the vial.

NOTE: When inserting and removing needles from vials, be sure not to touch the needles or the rubber stoppers on the vials with your hands.

If you do touch a stopper, clean it with a fresh alcohol wipe. If you touch a needle, throw away the entire syringe into the disposal unit and start over with a new syringe.

If the needle touches any surface, throw away the entire syringe into the disposal unit and start over with a new syringe.

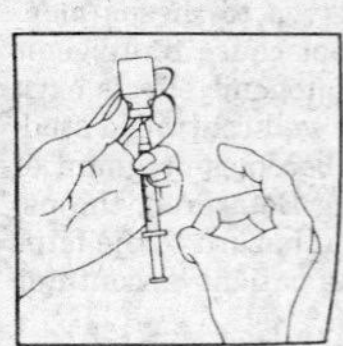

8. Push in the plunger all the way to gently inject air into the vial (leave the needle in the vial of Diluent for Betaseron).

9. Turn the vial of Diluent for Betaseron upside down.

NOTE: Keep the needle tip in the liquid.

10. Resting your hands on a stable surface, hold the vial and syringe in one hand and slowly pull back the plunger on the syringe to the 1.2 mL mark (to draw up that amount of liquid) with your other hand.

11. Keeping the vial upside down, gently tap the syringe until any air bubbles that formed rise to the top of the barrel of the syringe.

12. Carefully push in the plunger to eject ONLY THE AIR through the needle.

13. Remove the needle/syringe from the vial of Diluent for Betaseron.

NOTE: Find the Betaseron vial and throw away the alcohol wipe on top of it.

14. Holding the Betaseron vial on a stable surface, slowly insert the needle of the syringe (containing 1.2 mL of liquid) all the way through the stopper of the vial.

15. Push the plunger down slowly, directing the needle toward the side of the vial to allow the liquid to run down the inside wall (injecting Diluent for Betaseron directly onto the cake of drug will cause excess foaming).

16. Remove the needle/syringe from the Betaseron vial.

17. Throw away the 3 mL syringe into the disposal unit.

NOTE: Double-check that you are throwing away the correct syringe into the disposal unit.

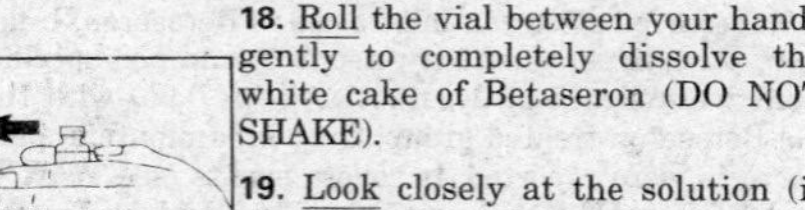

18. Roll the vial between your hands gently to completely dissolve the white cake of Betaseron (DO NOT SHAKE).

19. Look closely at the solution (it should be clear).

NOTE: If the mixture contains particles or is discolored, discard it and start again.

PREPARING THE INJECTION

1. Remove the needle guard of the 1 mL syringe and pull back the plunger to the 1 mL mark.

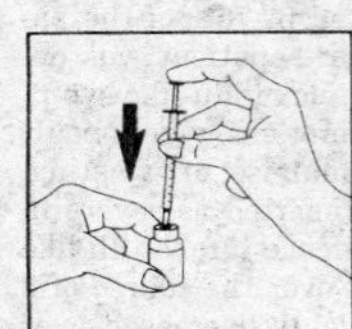

2. Insert the needle of the 1 mL syringe through the stopper of the vial of Betaseron solution.

3. Gently push the plunger all the way down to inject air into the vial (leave the needle in the vial).

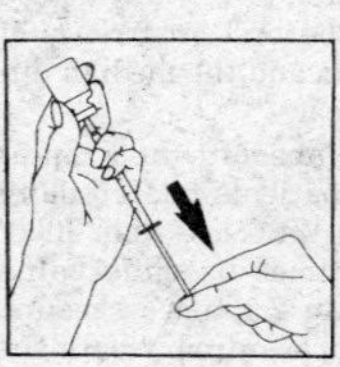

4. Turn the vial of Betaseron® (Interferon beta-1b) solution upside down.

NOTE: Keep the needle tip in the liquid.

5. Pull back the plunger to withdraw 1 mL of liquid into the syringe.

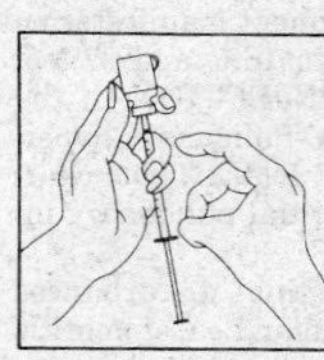

6. Hold the syringe with the needle pointing upward.

7. Tap the syringe gently until any air bubbles that formed rise to the top of the barrel of the syringe.

8. Carefully push in the plunger to eject ONLY THE AIR through the needle.

9. Remove the needle/syringe from the vial.
10. Recap the needle on the syringe.
NOTE: The injection should be administered immediately after mixing (if the injection is delayed, refrigerate the solution and inject it within 3 hours). Do not freeze.
11. Throw away unused portion of the solution remaining in the vial.

GIVING THE INJECTION

Subcutaneous (under the skin) self-administration

1. Choose an area for injection site (see diagrams for areas); use a different area each day.
- Abdomen—Areas 1 and 3
- Thighs— Areas 2 and 4
- Back of Arms—Areas 5 and 7
- Buttocks—Areas 6 and 8

NOTE: Do not use any areas in which you feel lumps, bumps, firm knots, or pain. Do not use any area in which the skin is discolored, depressed, scabbed, or has broken open. Talk to your doctor or healthcare professional about these or any other unusual conditions that you find.
Hold the syringe like a pencil or dart.
2. Use an alcohol wipe to clean the skin at the injection site; let it air dry.
3. Throw away the wipe.
4. Uncap the needle.

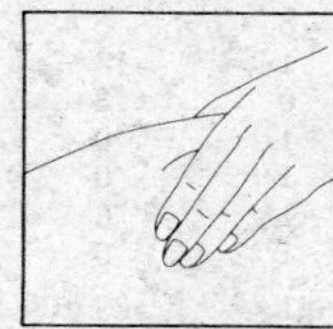

5. Gently pinch the skin together around the site (to lift it up a bit).

6. Resting your wrist on the skin near the site, stick the needle straight into the skin at a 90° angle with a quick, firm motion.

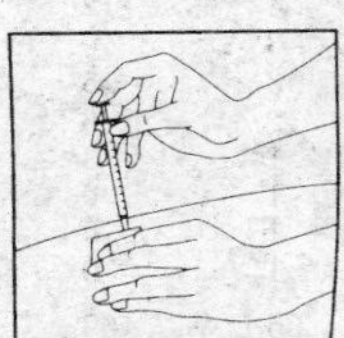

7. Inject the drug by using a slow, steady push (push the plunger all the way in until the syringe is empty).

8. Hold a swab on the injection site. Remove the needle from the skin.

9. Gently massage the injection site with a dry cotton ball or gauze.
10. Throw away the 1 mL syringe in the disposal unit.

INJECTION SITE

Picking an injection site

Betaseron® (Interferon beta-1b) should be injected into subcutaneous tissue (into the fat layer between the skin and the muscles beneath). The best areas for injection are where the skin is loose and soft (flabby), away from joints, nerves, bones, and other important structures.

Each day of injection you can choose an injection site from the upper, middle, or lower section of an area shown in the accompanying diagrams. It is a good idea to know where your injection will be given before you prepare your syringe. If there are any sites that are difficult for you to reach, you can ask your support person (or someone who has been trained to give injections) to help you.

Rotating injection sites

Each day of injection you can choose an injection site from the upper, middle, or lower section of an area shown in the accompanying diagrams.

To help prevent injection site reactions, you need to select a site in an area different from the area where you last injected yourself. You should not choose the same area for two injections in a row. Keeping a record of your injections will help make sure you rotate areas.

On the accompanying diagrams of the body, the areas of injection are numbered 1 through 8. Each area may be divided into three sections—upper, middle, and lower. If self-administering Betaseron, areas 1 through 4 may be the most convenient. Use the 8 areas in the following sequence:
- Your first 8 injections should be in a site in the upper section of each area (Rotation 1);
- The next 8 injections should be in a site in the middle section of each area (Rotation 2);
- And the next 8 should be in a site in the lower section of each area (Rotation 3).

By following this schedule, you will come back to your first injection site after 24 injections (48 days). If there are any sites that are difficult for you to reach, you can ask your support person, or someone who has been trained to give injections, to help you.
[See figure at top of next column]

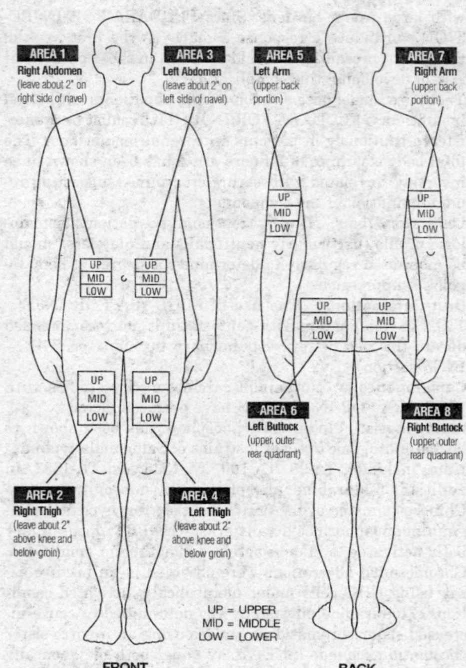

ROTATION 1	ROTATION 2	ROTATION 3
(Injections **1–8**)	(Injections **9–16**)	(Injections **17–24**)
Upper Area 1	Middle Area 1	Lower Area 1
Upper Area 2	Middle Area 2	Lower Area 2
Upper Area 3	Middle Area 3	Lower Area 3
Upper Area 4	Middle Area 4	Lower Area 4
Upper Area 5	Middle Area 5	Lower Area 5
Upper Area 6	Middle Area 6	Lower Area 6
Upper Area 7	Middle Area 7	Lower Area 7
Upper Area 8	Middle Area 8	Lower Area 8

Manufactured by:
CHIRON Corporation
Emeryville, CA 94608
U.S. License No. 1106
Distributed by:
BERLEX Laboratories
Richmond, CA 94804

Part Number L-1171.3 Revision date 12/97
Shown in Product Identification Guide, page 308

FLUDARA® ℞

(fludarabine phosphate)
FOR INJECTION
FOR INTRAVENOUS USE ONLY

> **WARNING:** FLUDARA FOR INJECTION should be administered under the supervision of a qualified physician experienced in the use of antineoplastic therapy. FLUDARA FOR INJECTION can severely suppress bone marrow function. When used at high doses in dose-ranging studies in patients with acute leukemia, FLUDARA FOR INJECTION was associated with severe neurologic effects, including blindness, coma, and death. This severe central nervous system toxicity occurred in 36% of patients treated with doses approximately four times greater (96 mg/m²/day for 5–7 days) than the recommended dose. Similar severe central nervous system toxicity has been rarely (≤0.2%) reported in patients treated at doses in the range of the dose recommended for chronic lymphocytic leukemia.
> Instances of life-threatening and sometimes fatal autoimmune hemolytic anemia have been reported to occur after one or more cycles of treatment with FLUDARA FOR INJECTION. Patients undergoing treatment with FLUDARA FOR INJECTION should be evaluated and closely monitored for hemolysis.
> In a clinical investigation using FLUDARA FOR INJECTION in combination with pentostatin (deoxycoformycin) for the treatment of refractory chronic lymphocytic leukemia (CLL), there was an unacceptably high incidence of fatal pulmonary toxicity. Therefore, the use of FLUDARA FOR INJECTION in combination with pentostatin is not recommended.

DESCRIPTION

FLUDARA FOR INJECTION contains fludarabine phosphate, a fluorinated nucleotide analog of the antiviral agent vidarabine, 9-β-D-arabinofuranosyladenine (ara-A) that is relatively resistant to deamination by adenosine deaminase. Each vial of sterile lyophilized solid cake contains 50 mg of the active ingredient fludarabine phosphate, 50 mg of mannitol, and sodium hydroxide to adjust pH to 7.7. The pH range for the final product is 7.2–8.2. Reconstitution with 2 mL of Sterile Water for Injection USP results in a solution containing 25 mg/mL of fludarabine phosphate intended for intravenous administration.

The chemical name for fludarabine phosphate is 9H-Purin-6-amine, 2-fluoro-9-(5-0-phosphono-β-D-arabinofuranosyl). The molecular formula of fludarabine phosphate is $C_{10}H_{13}FN_5O_7P$ (MW 365.2) and the structure is:

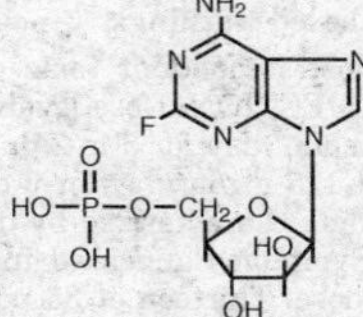

CLINICAL PHARMACOLOGY

Fludarabine phosphate is rapidly dephosphorylated to 2-fluoro-ara-A and then phosphorylated intracellularly by deoxycytidine kinase to the active triphosphate, 2-fluoro-ara-ATP. This metabolite appears to act by inhibiting DNA polymerase alpha, ribonucleotide reductase and DNA primase, thus inhibiting DNA synthesis. The mechanism of action of this antimetabolite is not completely characterized and may be multi-faceted.

Phase I studies in humans have demonstrated that fludarabine phosphate is rapidly converted to the active metabolite, 2-fluoro-ara-A, within minutes after intravenous infusion. Consequently, clinical pharmacology studies have focused on 2-fluoro-ara-A pharmacokinetics. In a study with 4 patients treated with 25 mg/m²/day for 5 days, the half-life of 2-fluoro-ara-A was approximately 10 hours. The mean total plasma clearance was 8.9 L/hr/m² and the mean volume of distribution was 98 L/m². Approximately 23% of the dose was excreted in the urine as unchanged 2-fluoro-ara-A. The mean C_{max} after the Day 1 dose was 0.57 mcg/mL and after the Day 5 dose was 0.54 mcg/mL. No information is available on pharmacokinetic parameters, other than C_{max}, following the Day 5 dose of 25 mg/m². Total body clearance of 2-fluoro-ara-A has been shown to be inversely correlated with serum creatinine, suggesting renal elimination of the compound.

A correlation was noted between the degree of absolute granulocyte count nadir and increased area under the concentration x time curve (AUC).

Two single-arm open-label studies of FLUDARA FOR INJECTION have been conducted in patients with CLL refractory to at least one prior standard alkylating-agent containing regimen. In a study conducted by M.D. Anderson Cancer Center (MDAH), 48 patients were treated with a dose of 22–40 mg/m² daily for 5 days every 28 days. Another study conducted by the Southwest Oncology Group (SWOG) involved 31 patients treated with a dose of 15–25 mg/m² daily for 5 days every 28 days. The overall objective response rates were 48% and 32% in the MDAH and SWOG studies, respectively. The complete response rate in both studies was 13%; the partial response rate was 35% in the MDAH study and 19% in the SWOG study. These response rates were obtained using standardized response criteria developed by the National Cancer Institute CLL Working Group[1] and were achieved in heavily pre-treated patients. The ability of FLUDARA FOR INJECTION to induce a significant rate of response in refractory patients suggests minimal cross-resistance with commonly used anti-CLL agents.

The median time to response in the MDAH and SWOG studies was 7 weeks (range of 1 to 68 weeks) and 21 weeks (range of 1 to 53 weeks) respectively. The median duration of disease control was 91 weeks (MDAH) and 65 weeks (SWOG). The median survival of all refractory CLL patients treated with FLUDARA FOR INJECTION was 43 weeks and 52 weeks in the MDAH and SWOG studies, respectively.

Rai stage improved to Stage II or better in 7 of 12 MDAH responders (58%) and in 5 of 7 SWOG responders (71%) who were Stage III or IV at baseline. In the combined studies, mean hemoglobin concentration improved from 9.0 g/dL at baseline to 11.8 g/dL at the time of response in a subgroup of anemic patients. Similarly, average platelet count improved from 63,500/mm³ to 103,300/mm³ at the time of response in a subgroup of patients who were thrombocytopenic at baseline.

INDICATIONS AND USAGE

FLUDARA FOR INJECTION is indicated for the treatment of patients with B-cell chronic lymphocytic leukemia (CLL)

Continued on next page

Information on the Berlex products appearing here is based on the most current information available at the time of publication closing. Further information for these and other products may be obtained from the Medical Affairs Department, Berlex Laboratories, 300 Fairfield Road, Wayne, New Jersey 07470, 1-888-BERLEX-4. Information on Betaseron and Fludara may be obtained from Berlex Laboratories, 15049 San Pablo Avenue, Richmond, California 94804-0016, 1-800-888-4112.

Fludara—Cont.

who have not responded to or whose disease has progressed during treatment with at least one standard alkylating-agent containing regimen. The safety and effectiveness of FLUDARA FOR INJECTION in previously untreated or nonrefractory patients with CLL have not been established.

CONTRAINDICATIONS

FLUDARA FOR INJECTION is contraindicated in those patients who are hypersensitive to this drug or its components.

WARNINGS (See boxed warning)

There are clear dose dependent toxic effects seen with FLUDARA FOR INJECTION. Dose levels approximately 4 times greater (96 mg/m^2/day for 5 to 7 days) than that recommended for CLL (25 mg/m^2/day for 5 days) were associated with a syndrome characterized by delayed blindness, coma and death. Symptoms appeared from 21 to 60 days following the last dose. Thirteen of 36 patients (36%) who received FLUDARA FOR INJECTION at high doses (96 mg/m^2/day for 5 to 7 days) developed this severe neurotoxicity. This syndrome has been reported rarely in patients treated with doses in the range of the recommended CLL dose of 25 mg/m^2/day for 5 days every 28 days. The effect of chronic administration of FLUDARA FOR INJECTION on the central nervous system is unknown, however, patients have received the recommended dose for up to 15 courses of therapy.

Severe bone marrow suppression, notably anemia, thrombocytopenia and neutropenia, has been reported in patients treated with FLUDARA FOR INJECTION. In a Phase I study in solid tumor patients, the median time to nadir counts was 13 days (range, 3–25 days) for granulocytes and 16 days (range, 2–32) for platelets. Most patients had hematologic impairment at baseline either as a result of disease or as a result of prior myelosuppressive therapy. Cumulative myelosuppression may be seen. While chemotherapy-induced myelosuppression is often reversible, administration of FLUDARA FOR INJECTION requires careful hematologic monitoring.

Instances of life-threatening and sometimes fatal autoimmune hemolytic anemia have been reported to occur after one or more cycles of treatment with FLUDARA FOR INJECTION in patients with or without a previous history of autoimmune hemolytic anemia or a positive Coombs' test and who may or may not be in remission from their disease. Steroids may or may not be effective in controlling these hemolytic episodes. The majority of patients rechallenged with FLUDARA FOR INJECTION developed a recurrence in the hemolytic process. The mechanism(s) which predispose patients to the development of this complication has not been identified. Patients undergoing treatment with FLUDARA FOR INJECTION should be evaluated and closely monitored for hemolysis.

Transfusion-associated graft-versus-host disease has been observed rarely after transfusion of non-irradiated blood in FLUDARA FOR INJECTION treated patients. Consideration should, therefore, be given to the use of irradiated blood products in those patients requiring transfusions while undergoing treatment with FLUDARA FOR INJECTION.

In a clinical investigation using FLUDARA FOR INJECTION in combination with pentostatin (deoxycoformycin) for the treatment of refractory chronic lymphocytic leukemia (CLL), there was an unacceptably high incidence of fatal pulmonary toxicity. Therefore, the use of FLUDARA FOR INJECTION in combination with pentostatin is not recommended.

Of the 133 CLL patients in the two trials, there were 29 fatalities during study. Approximately 50% of the fatalities were due to infection and 25% due to progressive disease.

Pregnancy Category D: FLUDARA FOR INJECTION may cause fetal harm when administered to a pregnant woman. Fludarabine phosphate was teratogenic in rats and in rabbits. Fludarabine phosphate was administered intravenously at doses of 0, 1, 10 or 30 mg/kg/day to pregnant rats on days 6 to 15 of gestation. At 10 and 30 mg/kg/day in rats, there was an increased incidence of various skeletal malformations. Fludarabine phosphate was administered intravenously at doses of 0, 1, 5 or 8 mg/kg/day to pregnant rabbits on days 6 to 15 of gestation. Dose-related teratogenic effects manifested by external deformities and skeletal malformations were observed in the rabbits at 5 and 8 mg/kg/day. Drug-related deaths or toxic effects on maternal and fetal weights were not observed. There are no adequate and well-controlled studies in pregnant women.

If FLUDARA FOR INJECTION is used during pregnancy, or if the patient becomes pregnant while taking this drug, the patient should be apprised of the potential hazard to the fetus. Women of childbearing potential should be advised to avoid becoming pregnant.

PRECAUTIONS

General: FLUDARA FOR INJECTION is a potent antineoplastic agent with potentially significant toxic side effects. Patients undergoing therapy should be closely observed for signs of hematologic and nonhematologic toxicity. Periodic assessment of peripheral blood counts is recommended to detect the development of anemia, neutropenia and thrombocytopenia.

Tumor lysis syndrome associated with FLUDARA FOR INJECTION treatment has been reported in CLL patients with large tumor burdens. Since FLUDARA FOR INJECTION can induce a response as early as the first week of treatment, precautions should be taken in those patients at risk of developing this complication.

There are inadequate data on dosing of patients with renal insufficiency. FLUDARA FOR INJECTION must be administered cautiously in patients with renal insufficiency. The total body clearance of 2-fluoro-ara-A has been shown to be inversely correlated with serum creatinine, suggesting renal elimination of the compound.

Laboratory Tests: During treatment, the patient's hematologic profile (particularly neutrophils and platelets) should be monitored regularly to determine the degree of hematopoietic suppression.

Drug Interactions: The use of FLUDARA FOR INJECTION in combination with pentostatin is not recommended due to the risk of severe pulmonary toxicity (see WARNINGS section).

Carcinogenesis: No animal carcinogenicity studies with FLUDARA FOR INJECTION have been conducted

Mutagenesis: Fludarabine phosphate has been shown to be non-mutagenic to several strains of Salmonella typhimurium, including TA-98, TA-100, TA-1535 and TA-1537. In addition, fludarabine phosphate was non-mutagenic to Chinese hamster ovary (CHO) cells at the hypoxanthine-guaninephosphoribosyltransferase (HGPRT) locus under both activated and non-activated metabolic conditions. Chromosomal aberrations were observed in an in vitro assay using CHO cells under metabolically activated conditions. Fludarabine phosphate was determined to cause increased sister chromatid exchanges using an in vitro sister chromatid exchange (SCE) assay under both metabolically activated and non-activated conditions. In addition, fludarabine phosphate has also been shown to be mutagenic as indicated by an increase in the number of micronucleated erythrocyte in the in vivo mouse micronucleus test at doses up to 1000 mg/kg.

Impairment of Fertility: Studies in mice, rats and dogs have demonstrated dose-related adverse effects on the male reproductive system. Observations consisted of a decrease in mean testicular weights in mice and rats with a trend toward decreased testicular weights in dogs and degeneration and necrosis of spermatogenic epithelium of the testes in mice, rats and dogs. The possible adverse effects on fertility in humans have not been adequately evaluated.

Pregnancy: Pregnancy Category D: (See WARNINGS section)

Nursing Mothers: It is not known whether this drug is excreted in human milk. Because many drugs are excreted in human milk and because of the potential for serious adverse reactions in nursing infants from FLUDARA FOR INJECTION, a decision should be made to discontinue nursing or discontinue the drug, taking into account the importance of the drug for the mother.

Pediatric Use: The safety and effectiveness of FLUDARA FOR INJECTION in children have not been established.

ADVERSE REACTIONS

The most common adverse events include myelosuppression (neutropenia, thrombocytopenia and anemia), fever and chills, infection, and nausea and vomiting. Other commonly reported events include malaise, fatigue, anorexia, and weakness. Serious opportunistic infections have occurred in CLL patients treated with FLUDARA FOR INJECTION. The most frequently reported adverse events and those reactions which are more clearly related to the drug are arranged below according to body system.

Hematopoietic Systems: Hematologic events (neutropenia, thrombocytopenia, and/or anemia) were reported in the majority of CLL patients treated with FLUDARA FOR INJECTION. During FLUDARA FOR INJECTION treatment of 133 patients with CLL, the absolute neutrophil count decreased to less than 500/mm^3 in 59% of patients, hemoglobin decreased from pretreatment values by at least 2 grams percent in 60%, and platelet count decreased from pretreatment values by at least 50% in 55%. Myelosuppression may be severe and cumulative. Bone marrow fibrosis occurred in one CLL patient treated with FLUDARA FOR INJECTION.

Life-threatening and sometimes fatal autoimmune hemolytic anemia have been reported to occur in patients receiving FLUDARA FOR INJECTION (see WARNINGS section). The majority of patients rechallenged with FLUDARA FOR INJECTION developed a recurrence in the hemolytic process.

Metabolic: Tumor lysis syndrome has been reported in CLL patients treated with FLUDARA FOR INJECTION. This complication may include hyperuricemia, hyperphosphatemia, hypocalcemia, metabolic acidosis, hyperkalemia, hematuria, urate crystalluria, and renal failure. The onset of this syndrome may be heralded by flank pain and hematuria.

Nervous System: (See WARNINGS section) Objective weakness, agitation, confusion, visual disturbances, and coma have occurred in CLL patients treated with FLUDARA FOR INJECTION at the recommended dose. Peripheral neuropathy has been observed in patients treated with FLUDARA FOR INJECTION and one case of wrist-drop was reported.

Pulmonary System: Pneumonia, a frequent manifestation of infection in CLL patients, occurred in 16%, and 22% of those treated with FLUDARA FOR INJECTION in the MDAH and SWOG studies, respectively. Pulmonary hypersensitivity reactions to FLUDARA FOR INJECTION characterized by dyspnea, cough and interstitial pulmonary infiltrate have been observed.

Gastrointestinal System: Gastrointestinal disturbances such as nausea and vomiting, anorexia, diarrhea, stomatitis and gastrointestinal bleeding have been reported in patients treated with FLUDARA FOR INJECTION.

Cardiovascular: Edema has been frequently reported. One patient developed a pericardial effusion possibly related to treatment with FLUDARA FOR INJECTION. No other severe cardiovascular events were considered to be drug related.

Genitourinary System: Rare cases of hemorrhagic cystitis have been reported in patients treated with FLUDARA FOR INJECTION.

Skin: Skin toxicity, consisting primarily of skin rashes, has been reported in patients treated with FLUDARA FOR INJECTION.

Data in the following table are derived from the 133 patients with CLL who received FLUDARA FOR INJECTION in the MDAH and SWOG studies.

PERCENT OF CLL PATIENTS REPORTING NON-HEMATOLOGIC ADVERSE EVENTS

ADVERSE EVENTS	MDAH (N=101)	SWOG (N=32)
ANY ADVERSE EVENT	88%	91%
BODY AS A WHOLE	72	84
FEVER	60	69
CHILLS	11	19
FATIGUE	10	38
INFECTION	33	44
PAIN	20	22
MALAISE	8	6
DIAPHORESIS	1	13
ALOPECIA	0	3
ANAPHYLAXIS	1	0
HEMORRHAGE	1	0
HYPERGLYCEMIA	1	6
DEHYDRATION	1	0
NEUROLOGICAL	21	69
WEAKNESS	9	65
PARESTHESIA	4	12
HEADACHE	3	0
VISUAL DISTURBANCE	3	15
HEARING LOSS	2	6
SLEEP DISORDER	1	3
DEPRESSION	1	0
CEREBELLAR SYNDROME	1	0
IMPAIRED MENTATION	1	0
PULMONARY	35	69
COUGH	10	44
PNEUMONIA	16	22
DYSPNEA	9	22
SINUSITIS	5	0
PHARYNGITIS	0	9
UPPER RESPIRATORY INFECTION	2	16
ALLERGIC PNEUMONITIS	0	6
EPISTAXIS	1	0
HEMOPTYSIS	1	6
BRONCHITIS	1	0
HYPOXIA	1	0
GASTROINTESTINAL	46	63
NAUSEA/VOMITING	36	31
DIARRHEA	15	13
ANOREXIA	7	34
STOMATITIS	9	0
GI BLEEDING	3	13
ESOPHAGITIS	3	0
MUCOSITIS	2	0
LIVER FAILURE	1	0
ABNORMAL LIVER FUNCTION TEST	1	3
CHOLELITHIASIS	0	3
CONSTIPATION	1	3
DYSPHAGIA	1	0
CUTANEOUS	17	18
RASH	15	15
PRURITUS	1	3
SEBORRHEA	1	0
GENITOURINARY	12	22
DYSURIA	4	3
URINARY INFECTION	2	15
HEMATURIA	2	3
RENAL FAILURE	1	0
ABNORMAL RENAL FUNCTION TEST	1	0
PROTEINURIA	1	0
HESITANCY	0	3
CARDIOVASCULAR	12	38
EDEMA	8	19
ANGINA	0	6
CONGESTIVE HEART FAILURE	0	3
ARRHYTHMIA	0	3
SUPRAVENTRICULAR TACHYCARDIA	0	3

MYOCARDIAL INFARCTION	0	3
DEEP VENOUS THROMBOSIS	1	3
PHLEBITIS	1	3
TRANSIENT ISCHEMIC ATTACK	1	0
ANEURYSM	1	0
CEREBROVASCULAR ACCIDENT	0	3
MUSCULOSKELETAL	7	16
MYALGIA	4	16
OSTEOPOROSIS	2	0
ARTHRALGIA	1	0
TUMOR LYSIS SYNDROME	1	0

More than 3000 patients received FLUDARA FOR INJECTION in studies of other leukemias, lymphomas, and other solid tumors. The spectrum of adverse effects reported in these studies was consistent with the data presented above.

OVERDOSAGE

High doses of FLUDARA FOR INJECTION (see Warnings) have been associated with an irreversible central nervous system toxicity characterized by delayed blindness, coma and death. High doses are also associated with severe thrombocytopenia and neutropenia due to bone marrow suppression. There is no known specific antidote for FLUDARA FOR INJECTION overdosage. Treatment consists of drug discontinuation and supportive therapy.

DOSAGE AND ADMINISTRATION

Usual Dose:

The recommended dose of FLUDARA FOR INJECTION is 25 mg/m^2 administered intravenously over a period of approximately 30 minutes daily for five consecutive days. Each 5 day course of treatment should commence every 28 days. Dosage may be decreased or delayed based on evidence of hematologic or nonhematologic toxicity. Physicians should consider delaying or discontinuing the drug if neurotoxicity occurs.

A number of clinical settings may predispose to increased toxicity from FLUDARA FOR INJECTION. These include advanced age, renal insufficiency, and bone marrow impairment. Such patients should be monitored closely for excessive toxicity and the dose modified accordingly.

The optimal duration of treatment has not been clearly established. It is recommended that three additional cycles of FLUDARA FOR INJECTION be administered following the achievement of a maximal response and then the drug should be discontinued.

Preparation of Solutions:

FLUDARA FOR INJECTION should be prepared for parenteral use by aseptically adding Sterile Water for Injection USP. When reconstituted with 2mL of Sterile Water for Injection, USP, the solid cake should fully dissolve in 15 seconds or less; each mL of the resulting solution will contain 25 mg of fludarabine phosphate, 25 mg of mannitol, and sodium hydroxide to adjust the pH to 7.7. The pH range for the final product is 7.2–8.2. In clinical studies, the product has been diluted in 100 cc or 125 cc of 5% Dextrose Injection USP or 0.9% Sodium Chloride USP.

Reconstituted FLUDARA FOR INJECTION contains no antimicrobial preservative and thus should be used within 8 hours of reconstitution. Care must be taken to assure the sterility of prepared solutions. Parenteral drug products should be inspected visually for particulate matter and discoloration prior to administration.

Handling and Disposal:

Procedures for proper handling and disposal should be considered. Consideration should be given to handling and disposal according to guidelines issued for cytotoxic drugs. Several guidelines on this subject have been published.[2–8] There is no general agreement that all of the procedures recommended in the guidelines are necessary or appropriate.

Caution should be exercised in the handling and preparation of FLUDARA FOR INJECTION solution. The use of latex gloves and safety glasses is recommended to avoid exposure in case of breakage of the vial or other accidental spillage. If the solution contacts the skin or mucous membranes, wash thoroughly with soap and water; rinse eyes thoroughly with plain water. Avoid exposure by inhalation or by direct contact of the skin or mucous membranes.

HOW SUPPLIED

FLUDARA FOR INJECTION is supplied as a white, lyophilized solid cake. Each vial contains 50 mg of fludarabine phosphate, 50 mg of mannitol and sodium hydroxide to adjust pH to 7.7. The pH range for the final product is 7.2–8.2. Store under refrigeration, between 2°–8°C (36°–46°F).

FLUDARA FOR INJECTION is supplied in a clear glass single dose vial (6mL capacity) and packaged in a single dose vial carton in a shelf pack of five.

CAUTION: Federal law prohibits dispensing without prescription.

NDC 50419-511-06

Manufactured by: Ben Venue Laboratories, Bedford, OH 44146

Manufactured for: Berlex Laboratories, Richmond, CA 94804

U. S. Patent Number: 4,357,324

REFERENCES

1. Cheson B.D., Bennett J.M., Rai K.R. et al. Guidelines for clinical protocols for chronic lymphocytic leukemia: Recommendations of the National Cancer Institute-Sponsored Working Group. Amer J Hematol 29:152–163, 1988.
2. Recommendations for the Safe Handling of Parenteral Antineoplastic Drugs. NIH Publication No. 83-2621. For sale by the Superintendent of Documents, U.S. Government Printing Office, Washington, D.C. 20402.
3. AMA Council Report. Guidelines for Handling Parenteral Antineoplastics, JAMA, 1985; March 15.
4. National Study Commission on Cytotoxic Exposure — Recommendations for Handling Cytotoxic Agents. Available from Louis P. Jeffrey, Sc.D., Chairman, National Study Commission on Cytotoxic Exposure, Massachusetts College of Pharmacy and Allied Health Sciences, 179 Longwood Avenue, Boston, Massachusetts 02115.
5. Clinical Oncological Society of Australia: Guidelines and Recommendations for Safe Handling of Antineoplastic Agents, Med. J. Australia 1983;1:426–428.
6. Jones, R.B. et al. Safe Handling of Chemotherapeutic Agents: A Report from the Mount Sinai Medical Center, Ca—A Cancer Journal for Clinicians 1983; Sept/Oct. 258–263.
7. American Society of Hospital Pharmacists Technical Assistance Bulletin on Handling Cytotoxic Drugs in Hospitals, Am. J. Hosp. Pharm. 1985; 42:131–137.
8. OSHA Work-Practice Guidelines for Personnel Dealing with Cytotoxic (antineoplastic) Drugs. Am. J. Hosp. Pharm. 1986; 43:1193–1204.

6063505 Rev. 1/96

Shown in Product Identification Guide, page 308

Berna Products, Corp.

4216 PONCE DE LEON BLVD.
CORAL GABLES, FL 33146

Direct Inquiries to:
Myrtha Entrialgo
(305) 443-2900
(800) 533-5899

For Medical Information Contact: Andres Murai, Jr
In Emergencies: Andres Murai, Jr.
(305) 443-2900
(800) 533-5899

Vivotif Berna® Vaccine

Typhoid Vaccine Live Oral Ty21a

DESCRIPTION

Vivotif Berna® (Typhoid Vaccine Live Oral Ty21a) is a live attenuated vaccine for oral administration only. The vaccine contains the attenuated strain *Salmonella typhi* Ty21a (1,2).

Vivotif Berna® Vaccine is manufactured by the Swiss Serum and Vaccine Institute. The vaccine strain is grown in fermentors under controlled conditions in medium containing a digest of yeast extract, an acid digest of casein, dextrose and galactose. The bacteria are collected by centrifugation, mixed with a stabilizer containing sucrose, ascorbic acid and amino acids, and lyophilized. The lyophilized bacteria are mixed with lactose and magnesium stearate and filled into gelatin capsules which are coated with an organic solution to render them resistant to dissolution in stomach acid. The enteric-coated, salmon/white capsules are then packaged in 4-capsule blisters for distribution. The contents of each enteric-coated capsule are shown in Table 1.

Table 1: Contents of one enteric-coated capsule of Vivotif Berna® Vaccine

Viable *S. typhi* Ty21a	2–6 $\times 10^9$ colony-forming units*
Non-viable *S. typhi* Ty21a	5–50 $\times 10^9$ bacterial cells
Sucrose	26–130 mg
Ascorbic acid	1–5 mg
Amino acid mixture	1.4–7 mg
Lactose	100–180 mg
Magnesium stearate	3.6–4.4 mg

* Vaccine potency (viable cell counts per capsule) is determined by inoculation of agar plates with appropriate dilutions of the vaccine suspended in physiological saline.

CLINICAL PHARMACOLOGY

Salmonella typhi is the etiological agent of typhoid fever, an acute, febrile enteric disease. Typhoid fever continues to be an important disease in many parts of the world. Travelers entering infected areas are at risk of contracting typhoid fever following the ingestion of contaminated food or water. Typhoid fever is considered to be endemic in most areas of Central and South America, the African continent, the Near East and the Middle East, Southeast Asia and the Indian subcontinent (3). There are approximately 500 cases of typhoid fever per year diagnosed in the United States (4). In 62% of these patients (data from 1975–1984) the disease was acquired outside of the United States while in 38% of the patients the disease was acquired within the United States (5). Of 340 cases acquired in the United States between 1977 and 1979, 23% of the cases were associated with typhoid carriers, 24% were due to food outbreaks, 23% were associated with the ingestion of contaminated food or water, 6% due to household contact with an infected person and 4% following exposure to *S. typhi* in a laboratory setting (6).

The majority of typhoid cases respond favorably to antibiotic therapy. However, the emergence of multi-drug resistant strains has greatly complicated therapy and cases of typhoid fever that are treated with ineffective drugs can be fatal (7). Approximately 2–4% of acute typhoid cases result in the development of a chronic carrier state (8). These nonsymptomatic carriers are the natural reservoir for *S. typhi* and can serve to maintain the disease in its endemic state or to directly infect individuals (3).

Virulent strains of *S. typhi* upon ingestion are able to pass through the stomach acid barrier, colonize the intestinal tract, penetrate the lumen and enter the lymphatic system and blood stream, thereby causing disease. One possible mechanism by which disease may be prevented is by evoking a local immune response in the intestinal tract. Such local immunity may be induced by oral ingestion of a live attenuated strain of *S. typhi* undergoing an aborted infection. The ability of *S. typhi* to cause disease and to induce a protective immune response is dependent upon the bacteria possessing a complete lipopolysaccharide (1). The *S. typhi* Ty21a vaccine strain, by virtue of a reduction in enzymes essential for lipopolysaccharide biosynthesis, is restricted in its ability to produce complete lipopolysaccharide (1,2). However, a sufficient quantity of complete lipopolysaccharide is synthesized to evoke a protective immune response. Despite low levels of lipopolysaccharide synthesis, the cells lyse before regaining a virulent phenotype due to the intracellular build-up of intermediates during lipopolysaccharide synthesis (1,2).

Results from clinical studies indicate that adults and children greater than 6 years of age may be protected against typhoid fever following the oral ingestion of 4 doses of Vivotif Berna® Vaccine (Typhoid Vaccine Live Oral Ty21a). The efficacy of the *S. typhi* Ty21a strain has been evaluated in a series of randomized, double-blind, controlled field trials. Suspected typhoid cases, detected by passive surveillance, were confirmed bacteriologically either by blood or bone marrow culture. The first trial was performed in Alexandria, Egypt with a study population of 32,388 children aged 6 to 7 years. Three doses of vaccine, in the form of a freshly reconstituted suspension administered after ingestion of 1 g of bicarbonate, were given on alternate days. Immunization resulted in a 95% decrease (95% confidence interval (CI) = 77%–99%) in the incidence of typhoid fever over a 3-year period of surveillance (9). A series of field trials were subsequently performed in Santiago, Chile to evaluate efficacy when the vaccine strain was administered in the form of an acid-resistant enteric-coated capsule. The initial trial involved 82,543 school-aged children, and compared 1 or 2 doses of vaccine given one week apart. After 24 months of surveillance vaccine efficacy was 29% (95% CI = 4%–47%) for the single dose schedule and 59% (95% CI = 41%–71%) for the 2-dose schedule (10). A further field trial was performed in Santiago, Chile involving 109,594 school-aged children (11). Three doses of enteric-coated capsules were administered either on alternate days (short immunization schedule) or 21 days apart (long immunization schedule). Following 36 months of surveillance vaccination resulted in a 67% (95% CI = 47%–79%) decrease in the incidence of typhoid fever in the short immunization schedule group and a 49% reduction (95% CI = 24%–66%) in the long immunization schedule group. After 48 months of surveillance the short immunization schedule resulted in a 69% (95% CI = 55%–80%) decrease in typhoid fever (12). An undiminished level of protection was observed during the fifth year of surveillance. A field trial was next conducted in Santiago, Chile to determine the relative efficacy of 2, 3 and 4 doses of enteric-coated vaccine administered on alternate days to school-aged children. Relative vaccine efficacy as determined by comparison of disease incidence within the three vaccinated groups was highest for the four dose regimen (13). The incidence of typhoid fever per 10^5 study subjects was 160.5 (95% CI = 130–191) for the three dose regimen versus 95.8 (95% CI = 71–121) for the four dose regimen ($p<0.004$). An additional field trial to determine vaccine efficacy was conducted in Plaju, Indonesia involving 20,543 individuals approximately 3 to 44 years of age (14). Due to logistical considerations three doses of enteric-coated capsules were administered at weekly intervals, a schedule known to provide suboptimal protection (11). After 30 months of surveillance vaccine efficacy for all age groups was 42% (95% CI = 23%–57%). Vaccine organisms can be shed transiently in the stool of vaccine recipients (16). However, secondary transmission of vaccine organisms has not been documented. Ty21a has not been isolated from blood cultures following immunization. At present, the precise mechanism(s) by which Vivotif Berna® Vaccine confers protection against typhoid fever is unknown. However, it is known that immunization of adult subjects can elicit a hu-

Continued on next page

Vivotif Berna—Cont.

moral anti-*S. typhi* LPS antibody response. Taking advantage of this fact, the seroconversion rate (defined as a Ú0.15 increase in optical density units over baseline determined in an ELISA) was compared in an open study between adults living in an endemic area (Chile) and non-endemic areas (United States and Switzerland) after the ingestion of 3 doses of vaccine. Comparable seroconversion rates were seen between these groups (15). *S. typhi* Ty21a cultured in medium not containing BHI induced an anti-*S. typhi* LPS antibody response comparable to that obtained with vaccine organisms cultured in medium containing BHI (15). Challenge studies in North American volunteers have shown that the Ty21a strain is capable of providing significant protection to an experimental challenge of *S. typhi* (16). Because of the very low incidence of typhoid fever in United States citizens, efficacy studies are not currently feasible in this population. However, the above observations support the expectation that Vivotif Berna® Vaccine will provide protection to recipients from non-typhoid endemic areas such as the United States.

INDICATIONS AND USAGE

Vivotif Berna® Vaccine (Typhoid Vaccine Live Oral Ty21a) is indicated for immunization of adults and children greater than 6 years of age against disease caused by *Salmonella typhi*. Routine typhoid vaccination is not recommended in the United States of America. Selective immunization against typhoid fever is recommended for the following groups: 1) travelers to areas in which there is a recognized risk of exposure to *S. typhi*, 2) persons with intimate exposure (e.g. household contact) to a *S. typhi* carrier, and 3) microbiology laboratorians who work frequently with *S. typhi*(7). There is no evidence to support the use of typhoid vaccine to control common source outbreaks, disease following natural disasters or in persons attending rural summer camps.

Not all recipients of Vivotif Berna® Vaccine will be fully protected against typhoid fever. Vaccinated individuals should continue to take personal precautions against exposure to typhoid organisms. The vaccine will not afford protection against species of *Salmonella* other than *Salmonella typhi* or other bacteria that cause enteric disease. The vaccine is not suitable for treatment of acute infections with *S. typhi*.

CONTRAINDICATIONS

Hypersensitivity to any component of the vaccine or the enteric-coated capsule. The vaccine should not be administered to persons during an acute febrile illness. Safety of the vaccine has not been demonstrated in persons deficient in their ability to mount a humoral or cell-mediated immune response, due to either a congenital or acquired immunodeficient state including treatment with immunosuppressive or antimitotic drugs. The vaccine should not be administered to these persons regardless of benefits.

WARNINGS

Vivotif Berna® (Typhoid Vaccine Live Oral Ty21a) is not to be taken during an acute gastrointestinal illness. The vaccine should not be administered to individuals receiving sulfonamides and antibiotics since these agents may be active against the vaccine strain and prevent a sufficient degree of multiplication to occur in order to induce a protective immune response. Postpone taking the vaccine if persistent diarrhea or vomiting is occurring. Unless a complete immunization schedule is followed, an optimum immune response may not be achieved. Not all recipients of Vivotif Berna® Vaccine will be fully protected against typhoid fever. Vaccinated individuals should continue to take personal precautions against exposure to typhoid organisms, i.e. travelers should take all necessary precautions to avoid contact or ingestion of potentially contaminated food or water.

Drug-Interactions

Several anti-malaria drugs, such as mefloquine, chloroquine and proguanil (not approved for use in US) possess antibacterial activity which may interfere with the immunogenicity of Vivotif Berna® Vaccine (17, 18). To determine the effect of these anti-malaria drugs on the humoral IgG or IgA anti-*S. typhi* immune response, healthy adult subjects were given mefloquine (250mg at weekly intervals; N=30) chloroquine (150mg at weekly intervals; N=30) or proguanil (200mg daily; N=30) together with the *S. typhi* Ty21a vaccine strain (19). Concomitant treatment with mefloquine or chloroquine did not result in a significant reduction in the serum anti-*S. typhi* immune response compared to subjects receiving vaccine strain only (N=45). The simultaneous administration of proguanil did effect a significant decrease in the immune response rate. These findings indicate that mefloquine and chloroquine can be administered together with Vivotif Berna® Vaccine. Proguanil should be administered only if 10 days or more have elapsed since the final dose of Vivotif Berna® Vaccine was ingested. The concomitant administration of oral polio vaccine or yellow fever vaccine does not suppress the immune response elicited by the Ty21a vaccine strain (19). There are no data regarding simultaneous administration of other parenteral vaccines or immunoglobulins with Vivotif Berna® Vaccine.

PRECAUTIONS

General

The health care provider should take all necessary precautions to ensure the safe and effective use of the vaccine. Patients should be questioned about previous reactions to this or similar products. The previous immunization history of the patient and current antibiotic usage should be obtained by the health care provider.

Information for Patients

It is essential that all 4 doses of vaccine be taken at the prescribed alternate day interval to obtain a maximal protective immune response. Vaccine potency is dependent upon storage under refrigeration [between 2°C and 8°C (35.6°F–46.4°F)]. The vaccine should be stored under refrigeration at all times. It is essential to replace unused vaccine in the refrigerator between doses. The vaccine capsule should be swallowed approximately 1 hour before a meal with a cold or luke-warm (temperature not to exceed body temperature, e.g., 37°C (98.6°F) drink. Care should be taken not to chew the vaccine capsule. The vaccine capsule should be swallowed as soon after placing in the mouth as possible. Not all recipients of Vivotif Berna® Vaccine (Typhoid Vaccine Live Oral Ty21a) will be fully protected against typhoid fever. Travelers should take all necessary precautions to avoid contact or ingestion of potentially contaminated food or water.

Several anti-malaria drugs, such as mefloquine, chloroquine and proguanil (not approved for use in US) possess antibacterial activity which may interfere with the immunogenicity of Vivotif Berna® Vaccine. Clinical results (see Warnings - Drug-Interactions) indicate that mefloquine and chloroquine can be administered together with Vivotif Berna® Vaccine. Proguanil should be administered only if 10 days or more have elapsed since the final dose of Vivotif Berna® Vaccine was ingested. Any serious adverse reactions related to the administration of the vaccine should be reported to your health care provider. You may also report an adverse reaction directly to the Vaccine Adverse Event Reporting System (1-800-822-7967) (20). Your health care provider should inform you of the benefits and risks of the vaccine, the importance of taking all 4 capsules in the correct schedule, and the importance of proper storage temperature of the capsules.

Carcinogenesis, Mutagenesis, Impairment of Fertility

Long-term studies in animals with Vivotif Berna® Vaccine have not been performed to evaluate carcinogenic potential, mutagenic potential or impairment of fertility.

Pregnancy

Category C

Animal reproduction studies have not been conducted with Vivotif Berna® Vaccine. It is not known whether Vivotif Berna® Vaccine can cause fetal harm when administered to pregnant woman or can affect reproduction capacity. Vivotif Berna® Vaccine should be given to a pregnant woman only if clearly needed.

Nursing Mothers

There is no data to warrant the use of this product in nursing mothers. It is not known if Vivotif Berna® Vaccine is excreted in human milk.

Pediatric Use

The safety and efficacy of Vivotif Berna® Vaccine has not been established in children under 6 years of age. This product is not indicated for use in children under 6 years of age.

ADVERSE REACTIONS

More than 1.4 million doses of Ty21a have been administered in controlled clinical trials and more than 150 million doses of Vivotif Berna® Vaccine (Typhoid Vaccine Live Oral Ty21a) have been marketed world-wide. Active surveillance for adverse reactions of enteric-coated capsules was performed in a pilot study (21) and in a subgroup of a large field trial (14) involving a total of 483 individuals receiving three vaccine doses. The overall symptom rates from both studies when vaccinated with capsules were combined and shown to be: abdominal pain (6.4%), nausea (5.8%), headache (4.8%), fever (3.3%), diarrhea (2.9%), vomiting (1.5%) and skin rash (1.0%). Only the incidence of nausea occured at a statistically higher frequency in the vaccinated group as compared to the placebo group (14). Administration of vaccine doses more than 5-fold higher than the currently recommended dose caused only mild reactions in an open study involving 155 healthy adult males (16).

Post-marketing surveillance has revealed that adverse reactions are infrequent and mild (17). Adverse reactions reported to the manufacturer during 1991-1995, during which time over 60 million doses (capsules) were administered, included: diarrhea (N=45), abdominal pain (N=42), nausea (N=35), fever (N=34), headache (N=26), skin rash (N=26), vomiting (N=18), or urticaria in the trunk and/or extremities (N=13). One isolated, non-fatal anaphylactic shock considered to be an allergic reaction to the vaccine was reported.

DOSAGE AND ADMINISTRATION

One capsule is to be swallowed approximately 1 hour before a meal with a cold or luke-warm [temperature not to exceed body temperature, e.g., 37 °C (98.6 °F)] drink on alternate days, e.g., days 1, 3, 5 and 7. Immunization (ingestion of all 4 doses of Vivotif Berna® Vaccine - Typhoid Vaccine Live Oral Ty21a) should be completed at least 1 week prior to potential exposure to *S. typhi*.

The blister containing the vaccine capsules should be inspected to ensure that the foil seal and capsules are intact. The vaccine capsule should not be chewed and should be swallowed as soon after placing in the mouth as possible. A complete immunization schedule is the ingestion of 4 vaccine capsules as described above.

Re-immunization

The optimum booster schedule for Vivotif Berna® Vaccine has not been determined. Efficacy has been shown to persist for at least 5 years. Further, there is no experience with Vivotif Berna® Vaccine as a booster in persons previously immunized with parenteral typhoid vaccine. It is recommended that a re-immunization dose consisting of four vaccine capsules taken on alternate days be given every 5 years under conditions of repeated or continued exposure to typhoid fever (7).

HOW SUPPLIED

A single foil blister contains 4 doses of vaccine in a single package. (NDC: 58337-0003-01)

STORAGE

Vivotif Berna® Vaccine (Typhoid Vaccine Live Oral Ty21a) is not stable when exposed to ambient temperatures. Vivotif Berna® Vaccine should therefore be shipped and stored between 2°C and 8°C (35.6–46.4°F). Each package of vaccine shows an expiration date. This expiration date is valid only if the product has been maintained at 2°C–8°C (35.6–46.4°F).

Vivotif Berna® Vaccine is manufactured by Swiss Serum and Vaccine Institute Berne, Switzerland, and distributed by Berna Products Corp., Coral Gables, FL 33146.

REFERENCES

1. Germanier R., E. Fürer. Isolation and characterisation of Gal E mutant Ty21a of *Salmonella typhi*: a candidate strain for a live, oral typhoid vaccine. J. Infect. Dis. 131: 553¤558, 1975.
2. Germanier R., E. Fürer. Characteristics of the attenuated oral vaccine strain *S. typhi* Ty21a. Develop. Biol. Standard 53: 3–7, 1983.
3. Miller S.I., E.L. Hohmann, D.A. Pegues. *Salmonella* (including *Salmonella typhi*). In: Principles and practice of infectious diseases. G.L. Mandell, J.E. Bennett, R. Dolin (ed.) fourth edition, Churchill Livingstone Inc. 2013-2033, 1995.
4. Centers for Disease Control. Summary of notifiable diseases, United States 1995. MMWR 44 (Supplement), 1996.
5. Ryan C.A., N.T. Hargrett-Bean, P.A. Blake. *Salmonella typhi* infections in the United States, 1975-1984: Increasing role of foreign travel. Rev. Infect. Dis. 11: 1 - 8, 1989.
6. Taylor D.N., R.A. Pollard, P.A. Blake. Typhoid in the United States and the Risk to the International Traveler. J. Infect. Dis. 148: 599–602, 1983.
7. Recommendations of the Advisory Committee on Immunization Practices (ACIP): Typhoid Immunization. MMWR 43 (RR-14), 1994
8. Ames, W.R., M. Robbins. Age and sex as factors in the development of the typhoid carrier state, and a model for estimating carrier prevalence. Am. J. Public Health 33: 221–230, 1943.
9. Wahdan M.H., C. Sérié, Y. Cerisier, S. Sallam, R. Germanier. A controlled field trial of live Salmonella typhi strain Ty21a oral vaccine against typhoid: three-year results. J. Infect. Dis. 145: 292–296, 1982.
10. Black R.E., M.M. Levine, C. Ferreccio, M.L. Clements, C. Lanata, J. Rooney, R. Germanier, Chilean Typhoid Committee. Efficacy of one or two doses of Ty21a *Salmonella typhi* vaccine in enteric-coated capsules in a controlled field trial. Vaccine 8: 81-84, 1990.
11. Levine M.M., C. Ferreccio, R.E. Black, R. Germanier, Chilean Typhoid Committee. Large-Scale Field Trial of Ty21a Live Oral Typhoid Vaccine in Enteric-Coated Capsule Formulation. Lancet 1: 1049–1052, 1987.
12. Levine M.M., C. Ferreccio, R.E. Black, C.O. Tacket, R. Germanier, Chilean Typhoid Committee. Progress in vaccines against typhoid fever. Rev. Inf. Dis. 11 (Supplement 3): S552-S567, 1989.
13. Ferreccio C., M.M. Levine, H. Rodriguez, R. Contreras, Chilean Typhoid Committee. Comparative efficacy of two, three, or four doses of Ty21a live oral typhoid vaccine in enteric-coated capsules: a field trial in endemic area. J. Inf. Dis. 159: 766-769, 1989.
14. Simanjuntak C.H., F.P. Paleologo, N.H. Punjabi, R. Darmowigoto, Soeprawoto, H. Totosudirjo, P. Haryanto, E. Suprijanto, N.D. Witham, S.L. Hoffman. Oral immunisation against typhoid fever in Indonesia with Ty21a vaccine. Lancet 338: 1055-1059, 1991.
15. Data on File, Swiss Serum and Vaccine Institute Berne, Switzerland.
16. Gilman R.H., R.B. Hornick, W.E. Woodward, H.L. DuPont, M.J. Snyder, M.M. Levine, J.P. Libonati. Evaluation of a UDP-glucose-4-epimeraseless mutant of *Salmonella typhi* as a live oral vaccine. J. Infect. Dis. 136: 717-723, 1977.
17. Cryz S.J. Jr., Post-marketing experience with live oral Ty21a Vaccine. Lancet; 341: 49-50, 1993. Data on File, Swiss Serum and Vaccine Institute Berne, Switzerland.
18. Horowitz H., CA. Carbonaro, Inhibition of the *Salmonella typhi* oral vaccine strain Ty21a, by mefloquine and chloroquine. J. Infect. Dis. 166: 1462-1464, 1992.
19. Kollaritsch H., J.U. Que, C. Kunz, G. Wiedermann, C. Herzog, S.J. Cryz Jr. Safety and immunogenicity of live oral cholera and typhoid vaccines administered alone or in combination with anti-malarial drugs, oral polio vaccine or yellow fever vaccine. J. Infect. Dis. (in press).
20. Vaccine Adverse Event Reporting System - United States. MMWR 39: 730–733, 1990.
21. Levine M.M., R.E. Black, C. Ferreccio, M.L. Clements, C. Lanata, J. Rooney, R. Gemanier. The efficacy of attenuated *Salmonella typhi* oral vaccine strain Ty21a evaluated in controlled field trials. In: Development of Vaccines and Drugs against Diarrhea. 11th Noble Confer-

ence, Stockholm, 1985, p. 90-101. J. Holmgren, A. Lindberg and R. Möllby (eds.). Studentlitteratur, Lund, Sweden, 1986.

Manufactured by:
Swiss Serum and Vaccine Institute Berne, Switzerland
US-Licence No. 21
Distributed by: Version:
Berna Products Corp., Coral Gables, FL 33146 April 1997
Shown in Product Identification Guide, page 308

Bertek Pharmaceuticals Inc.
781 CHESTNUT ROAD
MORGANTOWN, WV 26505

Direct Inquiries to:
(888) 823-7835
Fax: (304) 285-6453

Other Products Available:
NITREK® ℞

ACTICIN® ℞
[act' ĭ cĭn]
(permethrin) Cream 5%

DESCRIPTION
Acticin™ (permethrin) Cream 5% is a topical scabicidal agent for the treatment of infestation with *Sarcoptes scabiei* (scabies). It is available in an off-white, vanishing cream base. Acticin™ Cream is for topical use only.
Chemical Name: The permethrin used is an approximate 1:3 mixture of the cis and trans isomers of the pyrethroid (±)-3-phenoxybenzyl 3-(2,2-dichlorovinyl)-2,2-dimethylcyclopropanecarboxylate. Permethrin has a molecular formula of $C_{21}H_{20}Cl_2O_3$ and a molecular weight of 391.29. It is a yellow to light orange-brown, low melting solid or viscous liquid.

Each gram of Acticin™ Cream 5% contains permethrin 50 mg (5%) and the inactive ingredients butylated hydroxytoluene, carbomer 934P, coconut oil, glycerin, glyceryl stearate, isopropyl myristate, lanolin alcohols, light mineral oil, polyoxyethylene cetyl ethers, purified water, and sodium hydroxide. Formaldehyde 1 mg (0.1%) is added as a preservative.

CLINICAL PHARMACOLOGY
Permethrin, a pyrethroid, is active against a broad range of pests including lice, ticks, fleas, mites, and other arthropods. It acts on the nerve cell membrane to disrupt the sodium channel current by which the polarization of the membrane is regulated. Delayed repolarization and paralysis of the pests are the consequences of this disturbance.
Permethrin is rapidly metabolized by ester hydrolysis to inactive metabolites which are excreted primarily in the urine. Although the amount of permethrin absorbed after a single application of the 5% cream has not been determined precisely, data from studies with ^{14}C-labeled permethrin and absorption studies of the cream applied to patients with moderate to severe scabies indicate it is 2% or less of the amount applied.

INDICATIONS AND USAGE
Acticin™ Cream 5% is indicated for the treatment of infestation with *Sarcoptes scabiei* (scabies).

CONTRAINDICATIONS
Permethrin cream is contraindicated in patients with known hypersensitivity to any of its components, to any synthetic pyrethroid or pyrethrin.

WARNINGS
If hypersensitivity to permethrin cream occurs, discontinue use.

PRECAUTIONS
General: Scabies infestation is often accompanied by pruritis, edema and erythema. Treatment with permethrin cream may temporarily exacerbate these conditions.
Information for Patients: Patients with scabies should be advised that itching, mild burning and/or stinging may occur after application of permethrin cream. In clinical trials, approximately 75% of patients treated with permethrin cream who continued to manifest pruritis at 2 weeks had cessation by 4 weeks. If irritation persists, they should consult their physician. Permethrin cream may be very mildly irritating to the eyes. Patients should be advised to avoid contact with eyes during application and to flush with water immediately if permethrin cream gets in the eyes.
Carcinogenesis, Mutagenesis, Impairment of Fertility: Six carcinogenicity bioassays were evaluated with permethrin, three each in rats and mice. No tumorigenicity was seen in the rat studies. However, species-specific increases in pulmonary adenomas, a common benign tumor of mice of high spontaneous background incidence, were seen in the three mouse studies. In one of these studies there was an increased incidence of pulmonary alveolar-cell carcinomas and benign liver adenomas only in female mice when permethrin was given in their food at a concentration of 5000 ppm. Mutagenicity assays, which give useful correlative data for interpreting results from carcinogenicity bioassays in rodents, were negative. Permethrin showed no evidence of mutagenic potential in a battery of *in vitro* and *in vivo* genetic toxicity studies.
Permethrin did not have any adverse effect on reproductive function at a dose of 180 mg/kg/day orally in a three-generation rat study.
Pregnancy: *Teratogenic Effects:* Pregnancy Category B: Reproduction studies have been performed in mice, rats, and rabbits (200 to 400 mg/kg/day orally) and have revealed no evidence of impaired fertility or harm to the fetus due to permethrin. There are, however, no adequate and well-controlled studies in pregnant women. Because animal reproduction studies are not always predictive of human response, this drug should be used during pregnancy only if clearly needed.
Nursing Mothers: It is not known whether this drug is excreted in human milk. Because many drugs are excreted in human milk and because of the evidence for tumorigenic potential of permethrin in animal studies, consideration should be given to discontinuing nursing temporarily or withholding the drug while the mother is nursing.
Pediatric Use: Permethrin cream is safe and effective in pediatric patients two months of age and older. Safety and effectiveness in pediatric patients less than two months of age have not been established.

ADVERSE REACTIONS
In clinical trials, generally mild and transient burning and stinging followed application with permethrin cream in 10% of patients and was associated with the severity of infestation. Pruritis was reported in 7% of patients at various times post-application. Erythema, numbness, tingling, and rash were reported in 1 to 2% or less of patients (see PRECAUTIONS: General).

OVERDOSAGE
No instance of accidental ingestion of permethrin cream has been reported. If ingested, gastric lavage and general supportive measures should be employed.

DOSAGE AND ADMINISTRATION
Adults and children: Thoroughly massage Acticin™ (permethrin) Cream into the skin from the head to the soles of the feet. Scabies rarely infests the scalp of adults, although the hairline, neck, temple, and forehead may be infested in infants and geriatric patients. Usually 30 grams is sufficient for an average adult. The cream should be removed by washing (shower or bath) after 8 to 14 hours. Infants should be treated on the scalp, temple and forehead. ONE APPLICATION IS GENERALLY CURATIVE.
Patients may experience persistent pruritus after treatment. This is rarely a sign of treatment failure and is not an indication for retreatment. Demonstrable living mites after 14 days indicate that retreatment is necessary.

HOW SUPPLIED
Acticin™ (permethrin) Cream 5% (wt./wt.) is supplied in 60g tubes.

NDC Code	Strength	Quantity
62794-131-06	5%	60 g

Store at room temperature 15°–25°C (59°–77°F).
CAUTION: Federal (USA) law prohibits dispensing without prescription.
Distributed by: BERTEK PHARMACEUTICALS INC.
Morgantown WV. 26505

Manufactured by: Alpharma USPD Inc.
Baltimore, MD 21244

PN402.01C ACT-01
Rev. 02/00 VC1632
Shown in Product Identification Guide, page 308

AVITA® ℞
[ă vēt' ă]
(tretinoin cream)
CREAM, 0.025%
For Topical Use Only

DESCRIPTION
AVITA® Cream, a topical retinoid, contains tretinoin 0.025% by weight in a hydrophilic cream vehicle of stearic acid, polyolprepolymer-2, isopropyl myristate, polyoxyl 40 stearate, propylene glycol, stearyl alcohol, xanthan gum, sorbic acid, butylated hydroxytoluene, and purified water. Chemically, tretinoin is all-trans-retinoic acid (C20H2802; molecular weight 300.44 vitamin A acid) and has the following structural formula:
[See chemical structure at top of next column]

CLINICAL PHARMACOLOGY
Although the exact mode of action of tretinoin is unknown, current evidence suggests that topical tretinoin decreases cohesiveness of follicular epithelial cells with decreased microcomedo formation. Additionally, tretinoin stimulates mitotic activity and increased turnover of follicular epithelial cells causing extrusion of the comedones.
Pharmacokinetics:
In vitro and in vivo pharmacokinetic studies with AVITA® Cream indicate that less than 0.3% of the topically applied dose is bioavailable. Circulating plasma levels of both tretinoin and isotretinoin are only slightly elevated above those found in healthy normal controls.

CLINICAL STUDIES
In one vehicle-controlled clinical trial, AVITA® (tretinoin cream) Cream 0.025%, applied once daily was more effective than vehicle in the treatment of facial acne vulgaris of mild to moderate severity. Percent reductions in lesion count after treatment for 12 weeks in this study are shown in the following table:

	AVITA® Cream, 0.025%	Vehicle Cream
	N=75	N=58
Noninflammatory Lesions	45%	27%
Inflammatory Lesions	46%	32%
Total Lesions	46%	28%

N=Number of Subjects

INDICATIONS AND USAGE
AVITA® Cream is indicated for topical application in the treatment of acne vulgaris. The safety and efficacy of this product in the treatment of other disorders have not been established.

CONTRAINDICATIONS
The product should not be used if there is hypersensitivity to any of the ingredients.

PRECAUTIONS
General: If a reaction suggesting sensitivity or chemical irritation occurs, use of the medication should be discontinued. Exposure to sunlight, including sunlamps, should be minimized during the use of AVITA® Cream, and patients with sunburn should be advised not to use the product until fully recovered because of heightened susceptibility to sunlight as a result of the use of tretinoin. Patients who may be required to have considerable sun exposure due to occupation and those with inherent sensitivity to the sun should exercise particular caution. Use of sunscreen products and protective clothing over treated areas is recommended when exposure cannot be avoided. Whether extremes, such as wind or cold, also may be irritating to patients under treatment with tretinoin.
AVITA® Cream should be kept away from the eyes, the mouth, the paranasal creases, and mucous membranes. Topical use may induce severe local erythema and peeling at the site of application. If the degree of local irritation warrants, patients should be directed to temporarily use the medication less frequently, discontinue use temporarily, or discontinue use altogether. Efficacy at reduced frequencies of application has not been established. Tretinoin has been reported to cause severe irritation on eczematous skin and should be used with utmost caution in patients with this condition.
Information for Patients: See attached Patient Package Insert.
Drug Interactions: Concomitant topical medication, medicated or abrasive soaps and cleansers, soaps and cosmetics that have a strong drying effect, and products with high concentrations of alcohol, astringents, spices or lime should be used with caution because of possible interaction with tretinoin. Particular caution should be exercised in using preparations containing sulfur, resorcinol, or salicylic acid with AVITA® Cream. It also is advisable to "rest" a patient's skin until the effects of such preparations subside before use of AVITA® Cream is begun.
Carinogenesis Mutagenesis and Impairment of Fertility: In a life-time dermal study in CD-1 mice with another tretinoin cream, at 100 and 200 times the average recommended human topical clinical dose, and few skin tumors in the female mice and liver tumors in male mice were observed. The biological significance of these findings is not clear because they occurred at doses that exceeded the dermal maximally tolerated dose (MTD) of tretinoin and because they were within the background natural occurrence rate for these tumors in this strain of mice. There was no evidence of carcinogenic potential when tretinoin was administered topically at a dose five times the average recommended human topical clinical dose. For purposes of comparisons of the animal exposure to human exposure, the "recommended human topical clinical dose" is defined as 1.0 g of 0.025% AVITA® Cream applied daily to a 50 kg person. In a chronic, two-year bioassay of vitamin A acid in mice

Continued on next page

Avita Cream—Cont.

performed by Tsubura and Yamamoto, generalized amyloid deposition was reported in all vitamin A treated groups in the basal layer of the skin. In CD-1 mice, a similar study reported hyalinization at the treated skin sites and the incidence of this finding was 0/50, 3/50, 3/50, and 2/50 in male mice and 1/50, 0/50, 4/50, and 2/50 in female mice from the vehicle control, 0.25 mg/kg, 0.5 mg/kg, and 1 mg/kg groups, respectively.
Studies in hairless albino mice suggest that tretinoin may enhance the tumorigenic potential of carcinogenic doses of UVB and UVA light from a solar simulator. In other studies, when lightly pigmented hairless mice treated with tretinoin were exposed to carcinogenic doses of UVA/UVB light, the incidence and rate of development of skin tumors were either reduced or no effect was seen. Due to significantly different experimental conditions, no strict comparison of these disparate data is possible at this time. Although the significance of these studies to humans is not clear, patients should minimize exposure to sun.
The mutagenic potential of tretinoin was evaluated in the Ames assay and in the *in vivo* mouse micronucleus assay, both of which were negative.
Dermal Segment I and III studies with AVITA® Cream have not been performed in any species. In oral Segment I and Segment III studies in rats with tretinoin, decreased survival of neonates and growth retardation were observed at doses in excess of 2 mg/kg/day (> 400 times the average recommended human topical clinical dose).
Pregnancy: Pregnancy Category C.
Teratogenic Effects: Oral tretinoin has been shown to be teratogenic in rats, mice, rabbits, hamsters, and subhuman primates. It was teratogenic and fetotoxic in rats when given orally in doses 1000 times the average recommended human topical clinical dose. However, variations in teratogenic doses among various strains of rats have been reported. In the cynomolgus monkey, which metabolically is closer to humans for tretinoin than other species examined, fetal malformations were reported at oral doses of 10 mg/kg/day or greater, but none were observed at 5 mg/kg/day (1000 times the average recommended human topical clinical dose), although increased skeletal variations were observed at all doses. Dose-related increased embryolethality and abortion were reported. Similar results have also been reported in pigtail macaques.
Topical tretinoin in animal teratogenicity tests has generated equivocal results. There is evidence for teratogenicity (shortened or kinked tail) of topical tretinoin in Wistar rats at doses greater than 1 mg/kg/day (200 times the recommended human topical clinical dose) Anomalies (humerus: short 13%, bent 6%; os parietal incompletely ossified 14%) have also been reported in rats when 10 mg/kg/day was dermally applied.
Topical tretinoin (AVITA® Cream, 0.1%) has been shown to be teratogenic in rabbits when given in doses 91 times the topical human dose for cream (assuming a 50 mg adult applied 1.0 g of 0.1% cream topically). In this study, increased incidence of cleft palate and hydrocephaly was reported in the tretinoin-treated animals.
There are other reports, in New Zealand White rabbits with doses of approximately 80 times the recommended human topical clinical dose, of an increased incidence of domed head and hydrocephaly, typical of retinoid induced fetal malformations in this species.
When given subcutaneously to rabbits, tretinoin was teratogenic at 2 mg/kg/day but not at 1 mg/kg/day. These doses are approximately 400 and 200 times, respectively, the human topical dose of tretinoin cream, 0.025% (assuming a 50 kg adult applies 1.0 g of 0.025% cream topically).
In contrast, several well-controlled animal studies have shown that dermally applied tretinoin was not teratogenic at doses of 100 and 200 times the recommended human topical clinical dose, in rats and rabbits, respectively.
With widespread use of any drug, a small number of birth defect reports associated temporally with the administration of the drug would be expected by chance alone. Thirty cases of temporally associated congenital malformations have been reported during two decades of clinical use of another formulation of topical tretinoin (Retin-A). Although no definite pattern of teratogenicity and no causal association have been established from these cases, five of the reports describe the rare birth defect category, holoprosencephaly (defects associated with incomplete midline development of the forebrain). The significance of these spontaneous reports in terms of risk to the fetus is not known.
Nonteratogenic Effects: Dermal tretinoin has been shown to be fetotoxic in rabbits when administered in doses 100 times the recommended topical human clinical dose. Oral tretinoin has been shown to be fetotoxic in rats when administered in doses 500 times the recommended topical human clinical dose. There are, however, no adequate and well-controlled studies in pregnant women. AVITA® Cream should not be used during pregnancy.
Nursing Mothers: It is not known whether this drug is excreted in human milk. Because many drugs are excreted in human milk, caution should be exercised when AVITA® Cream is administered to a nursing woman.

ADVERSE REACTIONS

The skin of certain sensitive individuals may become excessively red, edematous, blistered, or crusted. If these effects occur, the medication should either be discontinued until the integrity of the skin is restored, or the medication dosing frequency should be adjusted temporarily to a level the patient can tolerate. However, efficacy has not been established for lower dosing frequencies. True contact allergy to topical tretinoin is rarely encountered. Temporary hyper- or hypopigmentation has been reported with repeated application of AVITA® Cream. Some individuals have been reported to have heightened susceptiblity to sunlight while under treatment with AVITA® Cream. Adverse effects of AVITA® Cream have been reversible upon discontinuation of therapy (see Dosage and Administration Section).

OVERDOSAGE

If medication is applied excessively, no more rapid or better results will be obtained and marked redness, peeling, or discomfort may occur. Oral ingestion of the drug may lead to the same side effects as those associated with excessive oral intake of vitamin A.

DOSAGE AND ADMINISTRATION

AVITA® Cream should be applied once a day, in the evening, to the skin where acne lesions appear, using enough to cover the entire affected area lightly. Application may cause a transient feeling of warmth or slight stinging. In cases where it has been necessary to temporarily discontinue therapy or reduce the frequency of applications, therapy may be resumed or frequency of application increased when the patients become able to tolerate the treatment. Alterations of dose frequency should be closely monitored by careful observation of the clinical therapeutic response and skin tolerance. Efficacy has not been established for less than once-daily dosing frequencies.
During the early weeks of therapy, an apparent increase in number and exacerbation of inflammatory acne lesions may occur. This is due, in part, to the action of the medication on deep, previously unseen lesions and should not be considered a reason to discontinue therapy. Therapeutic results should be noticed after two to three weeks but more than six weeks of therapy may be required before definite beneficial effects are seen. Patients treated with AVITA® Cream may use cosmetics, but the areas to be treated should be cleansed thoroughly before the medication is applied (see Precautions Section).

HOW SUPPLIED

AVITA® (tretinoin cream) Cream, 0.025% is supplied as:

NDC Code	Strength	Quantity
62794-141-02	0.025%	20 g
62794-141-03	0.025%	45 g

Storage Conditions: Store below 30°C (86°F); avoid freezing.
CAUTION: Rx only

Manufactured By:
DPT Laboratories
San Antonio, Texas 78215

Distributed By:
BERTEK PHARMACEUTICALS INC.
Morgantown WV, 26505
Revised February 1997 PN310.01C

Remove this portion before dispensing
AVITA®
(tretinoin cream)
CREAM, 0.025%

PATIENT INSTRUCTIONS
Acne Treatment
IMPORTANT
Read Directions Carefully Before Using
THIS LEAFLET TELLS YOU ABOUT AVITA® (TRETINOIN) CREAM ACNE TREATMENT AS PRESCRIBED BY YOUR PHYSICIAN. THIS PRODUCT IS TO BE USED ONLY ACCORDING TO YOUR DOCTOR'S INSTRUCTIONS, AND IT SHOULD NOT BE APPLIED TO OTHER AREAS OF THE BODY OR TO OTHER GROWTHS OR LESIONS. THE SAFETY AND EFFECTIVENESS OF THIS PRODUCT IN OTHER DISORDERS HAVE NOT BEEN EVALUATED. IF YOU HAVE ANY QUESTIONS, BE SURE TO ASK YOUR DOCTOR.

PRECAUTIONS

The effects of the sun on your skin. As you know, overexposure to natural sunlight or the artificial sunlight of a sunlamp can cause sunburn. Overexposure to the sun over many years may cause premature aging of the skin and even skin cancer. The chances of these effects occurring will vary depending on skin type, the climate and the care taken to avoid overexposure to the sun. Therapy with AVITA® Cream may make your skin more susceptible to sunburn and other adverse effects of the sun, so unprotected exposure to natural or artificial sunlight should be minimized.
Laboratory findings. *When laboratory mice are exposed to artificial sunlight, they often develop skin tumors. These sunlight-induced tumors may appear more quickly and in greater number if the mouse is also topically treated with the active ingredient in AVITA® Cream, tretinoin. In some studies, under different conditions, however, when mice treated with tretinoin were exposed to artificial sunlight, the incidence and rate of development of skin tumors was reduced. There is no evidence to date that tretinoin alone will cause the development of skin tumors in either laboratory animals or humans. However, investigations in this area are continuing.*
Use caution in the sun. When outside, even on hazy days, areas treated with AVITA® Cream should be protected. An effective sunscreen should be used any time you are outside (consult your physician for a recommendation of an SPF level which will provide you with the necessary high level of protection). For extended sun exposure, protective clothing, like a hat, should be worn. Do not use artificial sunlamps while you are using AVITA® Cream. If you do become sunburned, stop your therapy with AVITA® Cream until your skin has recovered.
Avoid excessive exposure to wind or cold. Extremes of climate tend to dry or burn normal skin treated with AVITA® Cream may be more vulnerable to these extremes. Your physician can recommend ways to manage your acne treatment under such conditions.
Possible problems. The skin of certain sensitive individuals may become excessively red, swollen, blistered, or crusted. If you are experiencing severe or persistent irritation, discontinue the use of AVITA® Cream and consult your physician.
There have been reports that, in some patients, areas treated with AVITA® Cream developed a temporary increase or decrease in the amount of skin pigment (color) present.
Use other medication only on your physician's advice. Only your physician knows which other medications may be helpful during treatment and will recommended them to you if necessary. Follow the physician's instructions carefully. In addition, you should avoid preparations that may dry or irritate your skin. These preparations may include certain astringents, toiletries containing alcohol, spices or lime, or certain medicated soaps, shampoos, and hair permanent solutions. Do not allow anyone else to use this medication.
Do not use other medications with AVITA® Cream which are not recommended by your doctor. The medications you have used in the past might cause unnecessary redness or peeling.
If you are pregnant, think you are pregnant, or are nursing an infant: No studies have been conducted in humans to establish the safety of AVITA® Cream in pregnant women. If you are pregnant, think you are pregnant, or are nursing a baby, consult your physician before using this medication.

AND WHILE YOU'RE ON AVITA® THERAPY

Use a mild non-medicated soap. avoid frequent washings and harsh scrubbing. Acne isn't caused by dirt, so no matter how hard you scrub, you can't wash it away. Washing too frequently or scrubbing too roughly may at times actually make your acne worse. Wash your skin gently with a mild, bland soap. Two or three times a day should be sufficient. Pat skin dry with a towel. Let the face dry 20 to 30 minutes before applying AVITA® Cream. Remember, excessive irritation such as rubbing, too much washing, use of other medications not suggested by your physician, etc., may worsen your acne.

HOW TO USE AVITA® (TRETINOIN) CREAM

To get the best results with AVITA® Cream therapy, it is necessary to use it properly. Forget about the instructions given for other products and the advice of friends. Just stick to the special plan your doctor has laid out for you and be patient. Remember, when AVITA® Cream is used properly, many users see improvement by 12 weeks. AGAIN FOLLOW INSTRUCTIONS – BE PATIENT – DON'T START AND STOP THERAPY ON YOUR OWN – IF YOU HAVE QUESTIONS, ASK YOUR DOCTOR.
To help you use the medication correctly, keep these simple instructions in mind.

- AVITA® Cream should be applied once a day, in the evening, or as directed by our physician, to the skin where acne lesions appear, using enough to cover the entire affected area lightly. First, wash with a mild soap and dry your skin gently. WAIT 20 to 30 MINUTES BEFORE APPLYING MEDICATION; it is important for skin to be completely dry in order to minimize possible irritation.
- It is better not to use more than the amount suggested by your physician or to apply more frequently than instructed. To much may irritate the skin, waste medication, and won't give faster or better results.
- Keep the medication away from the corners of the nose, mouth, eyes, and open wounds. *Spread away from these areas when applying.*
- *Cream:* Squeeze about a half inch or less of medications onto the fingertip. While that should be enough for your whole face, after you have had some experience with the medication you may find you need slightly more or less to do the job. The medications should become invisible almost immediately. If it is still visible, you are using too much. Cover the affected area lightly with AVITA® Cream by first dabbing it on your forehead, chin, and both cheeks, then spreading it over the entire affected area. Smooth gently into the skin.
- If needed, you may apply a moisturizer or a moisturizer with sunscreen that will not aggravate your acne (noncomedogenic) in the morning after you wash.

WHAT TO EXPECT WITH YOUR NEW TREATMENT

AVITA® Cream works deep inside your skin and this takes time. You cannot make AVITA® Cream work any faster by applying more than one dose each day, but an excess amount of AVITA® Cream may irritate your skin. Be patient.
There may be some discomfort or peeling during the early days of treatment. Some patients also notice that their skin begins to take on a blush.
These reactions do not happen to everyone. If they do, it is just skin adjusting to AVITA® Cream and this usually subsides within two to four weeks. These reactions can usually

be minimized by following instructions carefully. Should the effects become excessively troublesome, consult your doctor. BY THREE TO SIX WEEKS, some patients notice an appearance of new blemishes (papules and pustules). At this stage it is important to continue using AVITA® Cream.

If AVITA® Cream is going to have a beneficial effect for you, you should notice an improvement in your appearance by 6 to 12 weeks of therapy. Don't be discouraged if you see no immediate improvement. Don't stop treatment at the first signs of improvement.

Once your acne is under control you should continue regular application of AVITA® Cream until your physician instructs otherwise.

Manufactured By:
DPT Laboratories
San Antonio, Texas 78215

Distributed By:
BERTEK PHARMACEUTICALS INC.
Morgantown WV 26505
Revised February 1997

Shown in Product Identification Guide, page 308

AVITA® ℞
[*ă vēt' ă*]
(tretinoin gel)
GEL, 0.025%
For Topical Use Only

DESCRIPTION

AVITA® Gel, a topical retinoid, contains tretinoin 0.025% by weight in a gel vehicle of butylated hydroxytoluene, hydroxypropyl cellulose, polyolprepolymer-2, and ethanol (denatured with *tert*-butyl alcohol and brucine sulfate) 83% w/w. Chemically, tretinoin is all-*trans*-retinoic acid ($C_{20}H_{28}O_2$; molecular weight 300.44 vitamin A acid) and has the following structural formula:

CLINICAL PHARMACOLOGY

Although the exact mode of action of tretinoin is unknown, current evidence suggests that topical tretinoin decreases cohesiveness of follicular epithelial cells with decreased microcomedo formation. Additionally, tretinoin stimulates mitotic activity and increased turnover of follicular epithelial cells causing extrusion of the comedones.

Pharmacokinetics:

In vitro and in vivo pharmacokinetic studies with AVITA® Gel indicate that less than 0.3% of the topically applied dose is bioavailable. Circulating plasma levels of both tretinoin and isotretinoin are only slightly elevated above those found in healthy normal controls.

CLINICAL STUDIES

In two large vehicle-controlled clinical trials, AVITA® (tretinoin gel) Gel 0.025%, applied once daily was more effective than vehicle in the treatment of facial acne vulgaris of mild to moderate severity. Percent reductions in lesion counts after treatment for 12 weeks in these studies are shown in the following Tables:

Study 1	AVITA® Gel, 0.025%	Vehicle Gel
	N = 198	N= 204
Noninflammatory Lesions	-36%	-27%
Inflammatory Lesions	-35%	-25%
Total Lesions	-36%	-27%

Study 2	AVITA® Gel, 0.025%	Vehicle Gel
	N = 58	N= 58
Noninflammatory Lesions	-42%	-26%
Inflammatory Lesions	-38%	-23%
Total Lesions	-41%	-26%

N = Number of Subjects

INDICATIONS AND USAGE

AVITA® Gel is indicated for topical application in the treatment of acne vulgaris. The safety and efficacy of this product in the treatment of other disorders have not been established.

CONTRAINDICATIONS

The product should not be used if there is hypersensitivity to any of the ingredients.

WARNINGS

GELS ARE FLAMMABLE. Note: Keep away from heat and flame. Keep tube tightly closed.

PRECAUTIONS

General: If a reaction suggesting sensitivity or chemical irritation occurs, use of the medication should be discontinued. Exposure to sunlight, including sunlamps, should be minimized during the use of AVITA® Gel, and patients with sunburn should be advised not to use the product until fully recovered because of heightened susceptibility to sunlight as a result of the use of tretinoin. Patients who may be required to have considerable sun exposure due to occupation and those with inherent sensitivity to the sun should exercise particular caution. Use of sunscreen products and protective clothing over treated areas is recommended when exposure cannot be avoided. Weather extremes, such as wind or cold, also may be irritating to patients under treatment with tretinoin.

AVITA® Gel should be kept away from the eyes, the mouth, the paranasal creases, and mucous membranes. Topical use may induce severe local erythema and peeling at the site of application. If the degree of local irritation warrants, patients should be directed to temporarily use the medication less frequently, discontinue use temporarily, or discontinue use altogether. Efficacy at reduced frequencies of application has not been established. Tretinoin has been reported to cause severe irritation on eczematous skin and should be used with utmost caution in patients with this condition.

Information for Patients: See attached Patient Package Insert.

Drug Interactions: Concomitant topical medication, medicated or abrasive soaps and cleansers, soaps and cosmetics that have a strong drying effect, and products with high concentrations of alcohol, astringents, spices or lime should be used with caution because of possible interaction with tretinoin. Particular caution should be exercised in using preparations containing sulfur, resorcinol, or salicylic acid with AVITA® Gel. It also is advisable to "rest" a patient's skin until the effects of such preparations subside before use of AVITA® Gel is begun.

Carcinogenesis Mutagenesis and Impairment of Fertility: In a life-time dermal study in CD-1 mice with another tretinoin gel, at 100 and 200 times the average recommended human topical clinical dose, a few skin tumors in the female mice and liver tumors in male mice were observed. The biological significance of these findings is not clear because they occurred at doses that exceeded the dermal maximally tolerated dose (MTD) of tretinoin and because they were within the background natural occurrence rate for these tumors in this strain of mice. There was no evidence of carcinogenic potential when tretinoin was administered topically at a dose 5 times the average recommended human topical clinical dose. For purposes of comparisons of the animal exposure to human exposure, the "recommended human topical clinical dose" is defined as 1.0 g of 0.025% AVITA® Gel applied daily to a 50 kg person. In a chronic, two-year bioassay of Vitamin A acid in mice performed by Tsubura and Yamamoto, generalized amyloid deposition was reported in all Vitamin A treated groups in the basal layer of the skin. In CD-1 mice, a similar study reported hyalinization at the treated skin sites and the incidence of this finding was 0/50, 3/50, 3/50, and 2/50 in male mice and 1/50, 0/50, 4/50, and 2/50 in female mice from the vehicle control, 0.25 mg/kg, 0.5 mg/kg, and 1 mg/kg groups, respectively.

Studies in hairless albino mice suggest that tretinoin may enhance the tumorigenic potential of carcinogenic doses of UVB and UVA light from a solar simulator. In other studies, when lightly pigmented hairless mice treated with tretinoin were exposed to carcinogenic doses of UVA/UVB light, the incidence and rate of development of skin tumors were either reduced or no effect was seen. Due to significantly different experimental conditions, no strict comparison of these disparate data is possible at this time. Although the significance of these studies to humans is not clear, patients should minimize exposure to sun.

The mutagenic potential of tretinoin was evaluated in the Ames assay and in the *in vivo* mouse micronucleus assay, both of which were negative.

Dermal Segment I and III studies with AVITA® Gel have not been performed in any species. In oral Segment I and Segment III studies in rats with tretinoin, decreased survival of neonates and growth retardation were observed at doses in excess of 2 mg/kg/day (> 400 times the average recommended human topical clinical dose).

Pregnancy: Pregnancy Category C.

Teratogenic Effects: Oral tretinoin has been shown to be teratogenic in rats, mice, rabbits, hamsters, and subhuman primates. It was teratogenic and fetotoxic in rats when given orally in doses 1000 times the average recommended human topical clinical dose. However, variations in teratogenic doses among various strains of rats have been reported. In the cynomolgus monkey, which metabolically is closer to humans for tretinoin than other species examined, fetal malformations were reported at oral doses of 10 mg/kg/day or greater, but none were observed at 5 mg/kg/day (1000 times the average recommended human topical clinical dose), although increased skeletal variations were observed at all doses. Dose-related increased embryolethality and abortion were reported. Similar results have also been reported in pigtail macaques.

Topical tretinoin in animal teratogenicity tests has generated equivocal results. There is evidence for teratogenicity (shortened or kinked tail) of topical tretinoin in Wistar rats at doses greater than 1 mg/kg/day (200 times the recommended human topical clinical dose). Anomalies (humerus: short 13%, bent 6%; os parietal incompletely ossified 14%) have also been reported in rats when 10 mg/kg/day was dermally applied.

Topical tretinoin (AVITA® Gel, 0.025%) has been shown to be teratogenic in rabbits when given in doses 364 times the topical human dose for gel (assuming a 50 kg adult applies 1.0 g of 0.025% gel topically). In this study, increased incidence of cleft palate and hydrocephaly was reported in the tretinoin-treated animals.

There are other reports, in New Zealand White rabbits with doses of approximately 80 times the recommended human topical clinical dose, of an increased incidence of domed head and hydrocephaly, typical of retinoid-induced fetal malformations in this species.

When given subcutaneously to rabbits, tretinoin was teratogenic at 2 mg/kg/day but not at 1 mg/kg/day. These doses are approximately 400 and 200 times, respectively, the human topical dose of tretinoin gel, 0.025% (assuming a 50 kg adult applies 1.0 g of 0.025% gel topically).

In contrast, several well-controlled animal studies have shown that dermally applied tretinoin was not teratogenic at doses of 100 and 200 times the recommended human topical clinical dose, in rats and rabbits, respectively.

With widespread use of any drug, a small number of birth defect reports associated temporally with the administration of the drug would be expected by chance alone. Thirty cases of temporally associated congenital malformations have been reported during two decades of clinical use of another formulation of topical tretinoin (Retin A). Although no definite pattern of teratogenicity and no causal association have been established from these cases, 5 of the reports describe the rare birth defect category, holoprosencephaly (defects associated with incomplete midline development of the forebrain). The significance of these spontaneous reports in terms of risk to the fetus is not known.

Nonteratogenic Effects: Dermal tretinoin has been shown to be fetotoxic in rabbits when administered in doses 100 times the recommended topical human clinical dose. Oral tretinoin has been shown to be fetotoxic in rats when administered in doses 500 times the recommended topical human clinical dose. There are, however, no adequate and well-controlled studies in pregnant women. AVITA® Gel should not be used during pregnancy.

Nursing Mothers: It is not known whether this drug is excreted in human milk, caution should be exercised when AVITA® Gel is administered to a nursing woman.

ADVERSE REACTIONS

The skin of certain sensitive individuals may become excessively red, edematous, blistered, or crusted. If these effects occur, the medication should either be discontinued until the integrity of the skin is restored, or the medication dosing frequency should be adjusted temporarily to a level the patient can tolerate. However, efficacy has not been established for lower dosing frequencies. True contact allergy to topical tretinoin is rarely encountered. Temporary hyper- or hypopigmentation has been reported with repeated application of AVITA® Gel. Some individuals have been reported to have heightened susceptibility to sunlight while under treatment with AVITA® Gel. Adverse effects of AVITA® Gel have been reversible upon discontinuation of therapy (see Dosage and Administration Section).

OVERDOSAGE

If medication is applied excessively, no more rapid or better results will be obtained and marked redness, peeling, or discomfort may occur. Oral ingestion of the drug may lead to the same side effects as those associated with excessive oral intake of Vitamin A.

DOSAGE AND ADMINISTRATION

AVITA® Gel should be applied once a day, in the evening, to the skin where acne lesions appear, using enough to cover the entire affected area lightly. Application may cause a transient feeling of warmth or slight stinging. In cases where it has been necessary to temporarily discontinue therapy or reduce the frequency of application, therapy may be resumed or frequency of application increased when the patients become able to tolerate the treatment. Alterations of dose frequency should be closely monitored by careful observation of the clinical therapeutic response and skin tolerance. Efficacy has not been established for less than once-daily dosing frequencies.

During the early weeks of therapy, an *apparent* increase in number and exacerbation of inflammatory acne lesions may occur. This is due, in part, to the action of the medication on deep, previously unseen lesions and should not be considered a reason to discontinue therapy. Therapeutic results should be noticed after two to three weeks, but more than six weeks of therapy may be required before definite beneficial effects are seen. Patients treated with AVITA® Gel may use cosmetics, but the areas to be treated should be cleansed thoroughly before the medication is applied (see Precautions Section).

HOW SUPPLIED

AVITA® (tretinoin gel) Gel, 0.025% is supplied as:

NDC Code	Strength	Quantity
62794-140-02	0.025%	20 g
62794-140-03	0.025%	45 g

Storage Conditions: Store below 30°C (86°F); avoid freezing.

CAUTION: Federal (U.S.A.) law prohibits dispensing without prescription.

Continued on next page

Avita Gel—Cont.

Manufactured By:
DPT Laboratories
San Antonio, Texas 78215

Distributed by:
BERTEK PHARMACEUTICALS INC.
Morgantown WV 26505

December 1997 PN308.01C

Remove this portion before dispensing
AVITA®
(tretinoin gel)
GEL, 0.025%

PATIENT INSTRUCTIONS
Acne Treatment
IMPORTANT
Read Directions Carefully
Before Using

THIS LEAFLET TELLS YOU ABOUT AVITA® (TRETINOIN) ACNE TREATMENT AS PRESCRIBED BY YOUR PHYSICIAN. THIS PRODUCT IS TO BE USED ONLY ACCORDING TO YOUR DOCTOR'S INSTRUCTIONS, AND IT SHOULD NOT BE APPLIED TO OTHER AREAS OF THE BODY OR TO OTHER GROWTHS OR LESIONS. THE SAFETY AND EFFECTIVENESS OF THIS PRODUCT IN OTHER DISORDERS HAVE NOT BEEN EVALUATED. IF YOU HAVE ANY QUESTIONS, BE SURE TO ASK YOUR DOCTOR.

WARNINGS

GELS ARE FLAMMABLE. Note: Keep away from heat and flame. Keep tube tightly closed.

PRECAUTIONS

The effects of the sun on your skin. As you know, overexposure to natural sunlight or the artificial sunlight of a sunlamp can cause sunburn. Overexposure to the sun over many years may cause premature aging of the skin and even skin cancer. The chances of the these effects occurring will vary depending on skin type, the climate and the care taken to avoid overexposure to the sun. Therapy with AVITA® Gel may make your skin more susceptible to sunburn and other adverse effects of the sun, so unprotected exposure to natural or artificial sunlight should be minimized.

Laboratory findings. *When laboratory mice are exposed to artificial sunlight, they often develop skin tumors. These sunlight-induced tumors may appear more quickly and in greater number if the mouse is also topically treated with the active ingredient in AVITA® Gel, tretinoin. In some studies, under different conditions, however, when mice treated with tretinoin were exposed to artificial sunlight, the incidence and rate of development of skin tumors were reduced. There is no evidence to date that tretinoin alone will cause the development of skin tumors in either laboratory animals or humans. However, investigations in this area are continuing.*

Use caution in the sun. When outside, even on hazy days, areas treated with AVITA® Gel should be protected. An effective sunscreen should be used any time you are outside (consult your physician for a recommendation of an SPF level which will provide you with the necessary high level of protection). For extended sun exposure, protective clothing, like a hat, should be worn. Do not use artificial sunlamps while you are using AVITA® Gel. If you do become sunburned, stop your therapy with AVITA® Gel until your skin has recovered.

Avoid excessive exposure to wind or cold. Extremes of climate tend to dry or burn normal skin. Skin treated with AVITA® Gel may be more vulnerable to these extremes. Your physician can recommend ways to manage your acne treatment under such conditions.

Possible problems. The skin of certain sensitive individuals may become excessively red, swollen, blistered, or crusted. If you are experiencing severe or persistent irritation, discontinue the use of AVITA® Gel and consult your physician.

There have been reports that, in some patients, areas treated with AVITA® Gel developed a temporary increase or decrease in the amount of skin pigment (color) present.

Use other medication only on your physician's advice. Only your physician knows which other medications may be helpful during treatment and will recommend them to you if necessary. Follow the physician's instructions carefully. In addition, you should avoid preparations that may dry or irritate your skin. These preparations may include certain astringents, toiletries containing alcohol, spices or lime, or certain medicated soaps, shampoos, and hair permanent solutions. Do not allow anyone else to use this medication.

Do no use other medications with AVITA® Gel which are not recommended by your doctor. The medications you have used in the past might cause unnecessary redness or peeling.

If you are pregnant, think you are pregnant, or are nursing an infant: No studies have been conducted in humans to establish the safety of AVITA® Gel in pregnant women. If you are pregnant, think you are pregnant, or are nursing a baby, consult your physician before using this medication.

AND WHILE YOU'RE ON AVITA® THERAPY

Use a mild non-mediated soap. Avoid frequent washings and harsh scrubbing. Acne isn't caused by dirt, so no matter how hard you scrub, you can't wash it away. Washing too frequently or scrubbing too roughly may at times actually make your acne worse. Wash your skin gently with a mild, bland soap. Two or three times a day should be sufficient. Pat skin dry with a towel. Let the face dry 20 to 30 minutes before applying AVITA® Gel. Remember, excessive irritation such as rubbing, too much washing, use of other medications not suggested by your physician, etc., may worsen your acne.

HOW TO USE AVITA® (TRETINOIN) GEL

To get the best results with AVITA® Gel therapy, it is necessary to use it properly. Forget about the instructions given for other products and the advice of friends. Just stick to the special plan your doctor has laid out of you and be patient. Remember, when AVITA® Gel is *used properly,* many users see improvement by 12 weeks. AGAIN, FOLLOW INSTRUCTIONS – BE PATIENT – DON'T START AND STOP THERAPY ON YOUR OWN – IF YOU HAVE QUESTIONS, ASK YOUR DOCTOR.

To help you use the medication correctly, keep these simple instructions in mind.

- AVITA® Gel should be applied once a day, in the evening, or as directed by your physician, to the skin where acne lesions appear, using enough to cover the entire affected area lightly. First, wash with a mild soap and dry your skin gently. WAIT 20 to 30 MINUTES BEFORE APPLYING MEDICATION; it is important for skin to be completely dry in order to minimize possible irritation.
- It is better not to use more than the amount suggested by your physician or to apply more frequently than instructed. Too much may irritate the skin, waste medication, and won't give faster or better results.
- Keep the medication away from the corners of the nose, mouth, eyes, and open wounds. *Spread away from these areas when applying.*
- *Gel:* Squeeze about a half inch or less of medication onto the fingertip. While that should be enough for your whole face, after you have had some experience with the medication you may find you need slightly more or less to do the job. The medication should become invisible almost immediately. If it is still visible, or if dry flaking occurs from the gel *within a minute or so* you are using too much. Cover the affected area lightly with AVITA® Gel by first dabbing it on your forehead, chin, and both cheeks, then spreading it over the entire affected area. Smooth gently into the skin.
- If needed, you may apply a moisturizer or a moisturizer with sunscreen that will not aggravate your acne (noncomedogenic) in the morning after you wash.

WHAT TO EXPECT WITH YOUR NEW TREATMENT

AVITA® Gel works deep inside your skin and this takes time. You cannot make AVITA® Gel work any faster by applying more than one dose each day, but an excess amount of AVITA® Gel may irritate your skin. Be patient.

There may be some discomfort or peeling during the early days of treatment. Some patients also notice that their skin begins to take on a blush.

These reactions do not happen to everyone. If they do, it is just your skin adjusting to AVITA® Gel and this usually subsides within two to four weeks. These reactions can usually be minimized by following instructions carefully. Should the effects become excessively troublesome, consult your doctor.

BY THREE TO SIX WEEKS, some patients notice an appearance of new blemishes (papules and pustules). At this stage it is important to continue using AVITA® Gel.

If AVITA® Gel is going to have a beneficial effect for you, you should notice an improvement in your appearance by 6 to 12 weeks of therapy. Don't be discouraged if you see no immediate improvement. Don't stop treatment at the first signs of improvement.

Once your acne is under control you should continue regular application of AVITA® Gel until your physician instructs otherwise.

Manufactured By:
DPT Laboratories
San Antonio, Texas 78215

Distributed By:
BERTEK PHARMACEUTICALS INC
Morgantown WV 26505

December 1997

Shown in Product Identification Guide, page 308

CLORPRES™ ℞

[klōr prĕs]
(Clonidine Hydrochloride and Chlorthalidone)
TABLETS, USP
0.1 mg/15 mg, 0.2 mg/15 mg and 0.3 mg/15 mg

DESCRIPTION

CLORPRES™ is a combination of clonidine hydrochloride (a centrally acting antihypertensive agent) and chlorthalidone (a diuretic). CLORPRES™ is available as tablets for oral administration in three dosage strengths: 0.1 mg/15 mg, 0.2 mg/15 mg and 0.3 mg/15 mg of clonidine hydrochloride/chlorthalidone, respectively.

The inactive ingredients are ammonium chloride, colloidal silicon dioxide, croscarmellose sodium (Type A), magnesium stearate, microcrystalline cellulose, sodium lauryl sulfate, D&C yellow #10.

Clonidine Hydrochloride: Clonidine hydrochloride is an imidazoline derivative and exists as a mesomeric compound. The chemical name is 2-[(2,6-dichlorophenyl)imino]imidazoline monohydrochloride. The following are the structural formula, molecular formula and molecular weight:

$C_9H_9Cl_2N_3 \cdot HCl$
M.W. 266.56

Clonidine hydrochloride is an odorless, bitter, white crystalline substance soluble in water and alcohol.

Chlorthalidone: Chlorthalidone is a monosulfamyl diuretic that differs chemically from thiazide diuretics in that a double ring system is incorporated in its structure. It is 2-chloro-5-(1-hydroxy-3-oxo-1-isoindolinyl) benzenesulfonamide with the following structural formula, molecular formula and molecular weight:

$C_{14}H_{11}ClN_2O_4S$
M.W. 338.76

Chlorthalidone is practically insoluble in water, in ether and in chloroform; soluble in methanol; slightly soluble in alcohol.

CLINICAL PHARMACOLOGY

CLORPRES™: Clorpres produces a more pronounced antihypertensive response than occurs after either clonidine hydrochloride or chlorthalidone alone in equivalent doses.

Clonidine Hydrochloride: Clonidine hydrochloride acts relatively rapidly. The patient's blood pressure declines within 30 to 60 minutes after an oral dose, the maximum decrease occurring within 2 to 4 hours. The plasma level of clonidine hydrochloride peaks in approximately 3 to 5 hours and the plasma half-life ranges from 12 to 16 hours. The half-life increases up to 41 hours in patients with severe impairment of renal function. Following oral administration about 40 to 60% of the absorbed dose is recovered in the urine as unchanged drug in 24 hours. About 50% of the absorbed dose is metabolized in the liver.

Clonidine stimulates alpha-adrenoreceptors in the brain stem, resulting in reduced sympathetic outflow from the central nervous system and a decrease in peripheral resistance, renal vascular resistance, heart rate, and blood pressure. Renal blood flow and glomerular filtration rate remain essentially unchanged. Normal postural reflexes are intact and therefore orthostatic symptoms are mild and infrequent.

Acute studies with clonidine hydrochloride in humans have demonstrated a moderate reduction (15 to 20%) of cardiac output in the supine position with no change in the peripheral resistance; at a 45° tilt there is a smaller reduction in cardiac output and a decrease of peripheral resistance. During long-term therapy, cardiac output tends to return to control values, while peripheral resistance remains decreased. Slowing of the pulse rate has been observed in most patients given clonidine but the drug does not alter normal hemodynamic response to exercise.

Other studies in patients have provided evidence of a reduction in plasma renin activity and in the excretion of aldosterone and catecholamines, but the exact relationship of these pharmacologic actions to the antihypertensive effect has not been fully elucidated.

Clonidine acutely stimulates growth hormone release in both children and adults, but does not produce a chronic elevation of growth hormone with long-term use.

Tolerance may develop in some patients, necessitating a reevaluation of therapy.

Chlorthalidone: Chlorthalidone is a long-acting oral diuretic with antihypertensive activity. Its diuretic action commences a mean of 2.6 hours after dosing and continues for up to 72 hours. The drug produces diuresis with increased excretion of sodium and chloride. The diuretic effects of chlorthalidone and the benzothiadiazine (thiazide) diuretics appear to arise from similar mechanisms and the maximal effect of chlorthalidone and the thiazides appears to be similar. The site of action appears to be the distal convoluted tubule of the nephron. The diuretic effects of chlorthalidone lead to decreased extracellular fluid volume, plasma volume, cardiac output, total exchangeable sodium, glomerular filtration rate, and renal plasma flow. Although the mechanism of action of chlorthalidone and related drugs is not wholly clear, sodium and water depletion appear to provide a basis for its antihypertensive effect. Like the thiazide diuretics, chlorthalidone produces dose-related reductions in serum potassium levels, elevations in serum uric acid and blood glucose, and it can lead to decreased sodium and chloride levels.

The mean plasma half-life of chlorthalidone is about 40 to 60 hours. It is eliminated primarily as unchanged drug in the urine. Non-renal routes of elimination have yet to be clarified. In the blood, approximately 75% of the drug is bound to plasma proteins.

INDICATIONS AND USAGE

CLORPRES™ (clonidine hydrochloride USP/chlorthalidone USP) is indicated in the treatment of hypertension. **This fixed combination drug is not indicated for initial therapy**

of hypertension. Hypertension requires therapy titrated to the individual patient. If the fixed combination represents the dosage so determined, its use may be more convenient in patient management. The treatment of hypertension is not static, but must be reevaluated as conditions in each patient warrant.

CONTRAINDICATIONS

Anuria: CLORPRES™ is contraindicated in patients with known hypersensitivity to chlorthalidone or other sulfonamide-derived drugs.

WARNINGS

Chlorthalidone should be used with caution in severe renal disease. In patients with renal disease, chlorthalidone or related drugs may precipitate azotemia. Cumulative effects of the drug may develop in patients with impaired renal function. Chlorthalidone should be used with caution in patients with impaired hepatic function or progressive liver disease, because minor alterations of fluid and electrolyte balance may precipitate hepatic coma.

Sensitivity reactions may occur in patients with a history of allergy or bronchial asthma.

The possibility of exacerbation or activation of systemic lupus erythematosus has been reported with thiazide diuretics which are structurally related to chlorthalidone. However, systemic lupus erythematosus has not been reported following chlorthalidone administration.

PRECAUTIONS

Clonidine Hydrochloride: *General:* In patients who have developed localized contact sensitization to transdermal clonidine, substitution of oral clonidine hydrochloride therapy may be associated with the development of a generalized skin rash.

In patients who develop an allergic reaction from transdermal clonidine that extends beyond the local patch site (such as generalized skin rash, urticaria or angioedema), oral clonidine hydrochloride substitution may elicit a similar reaction.

As with all antihypertensive therapy, clonidine hydrochloride should be used with caution in patients with severe coronary insufficiency, recent myocardial infarction, cerebrovascular disease or chronic renal failure.

Withdrawal: Patients should be instructed not to discontinue therapy without consulting their physician. Sudden cessation of clonidine treatment has resulted in subjective symptoms such as nervousness, agitation and headache, accompanied or followed by a rapid rise in blood pressure and elevated catecholamine concentrations in the plasma, but such occurrences have usually been associated with previous administration of high oral doses (exceeding 1.2 mg/day) and/or with continuation of concomitant beta-blocker therapy. Rare instances of hypertensive encephalopathy and death have been reported. When discontinuing therapy with clonidine hydrochloride, the physician should reduce the dose gradually over 2 to 4 days to avoid withdrawl symptomatology.

An excessive rise in blood pressure following clonidine hydrochloride discontinuance can be reversed by administration of oral clonidine or by intravenous phentolamine. If therapy is to be discontinued in patients receiving beta-blockers and clonidine concurrently, beta-blockers should be discontinued several days before the gradual withdrawal of clonidine hydrochloride.

Perioperative Use: Administration of clonidine hydrochloride should be continued to within four hours of surgery and resumed as soon as possible thereafter. The blood pressure should be carefully monitored and appropriate measures instituted to control it as necessary.

Information for Patients: Patients who engage in potentially hazardous activities, such as operating machinery or driving, should be advised of a potential sedative effect of clonidine. Patients should be cautioned against interruption of clonidine hydrochloride therapy without a physician's advice.

Drug Interactions: If a patient receiving clonidine hydrochloride is also taking tricyclic antidepressants, the effect of clonidine may be reduced, thus necessitating an increase in dosage. Clonidine hydrochloride may enhance the CNS-depressive effects of alcohol, barbiturates or other sedatives. Amitriptyline in combination with clonidine enhances the manifestation of corneal lesions in rats (see Ocular Toxicity).

Ocular Toxicity: In several studies, oral clonidine hydrochloride produced a dose-dependent increase in the incidence and severity of spontaneously occurring retinal degeneration in albino rats treated for six months or longer. Tissue distribution studies in dogs and monkeys revealed that clonidine hydrochloride was concentrated in the choroid of the eye. In view of the retinal degeneration observed in rats, eye examinations were performed in 908 patients prior to the start of clonidine hydrochloride therapy, who were then examined periodically thereafter. In 353 of these 908 patients, examinations were performed for periods of 24 months or longer. Except for some dryness of the eyes, no drug-related abnormal ophthalmologic findings were recorded and clonidine hydrochloride did no alter retinal function as shown by specialized tests such as the electroretinogram and macular dazzle.

In rats, clonidine hydrochloride in combination with amitriptyline produced corneal lesions within 5 days.

Carcinogenesis, Mutagenesis, Impairment of Fertility: In a 132-week (fixed concentration) dietary administration study in rats, clonidine hydrochloride administered at 32 to 46 times the maximum recommended daily human oral dose was unassociated with evidence of carcinogenic potential.

Fertility of male or female rats was unaffected by clonidine hydrochloride doses as high as 150 mcg/kg or about 3 times the maximum recommended daily human oral dose (MRDHD). Fertility of female rats did, however, appear to be affected (in another experiment) at dose levels of 500 to 2000 mcg/kg or 10 to 40 times the MRDHD.

Usage in Pregnancy: *Teratogenic Effect. Pregnancy Category C:* Reproduction studies performed in rabbits at doses up to approximately 3 times the maximum recommended daily human dose (MRDHD) of clonidine hydrochloride have revealed no evidence of teratogenic or embryotoxic potential. In rats however, doses as low as 1/3 the MRDHD were associated with increased resorptions in a study in which dams were treated continuously from 2 months prior to mating. Increased resorptions were not associated with treatment at the same or at higher dose levels (up to 3 times the MRDHD) when dams were treated days 6 to 15 of gestation. Increased resorptions were observed at much higher levels (40 times the MRDHD) in rats and mice treated days 1 to 14 of gestation (lowest dose employed in that study was 500 mcg/kg). There are, however, no adequate and well-controlled studies in pregnant women. Because animal reproduction studies are not always predictive of human response, this drug should be used during pregnancy only if clearly needed.

Nursing Mothers: As clonidine hydrochloride is excreted in human milk, caution should be exercised when it is administered to a nursing woman.

Pediatric Use: Safety and effectiveness in the pediatric population have not been established.

Chlorthalidone: *General:* Hypokalemia and other electrolyte abnormalities, including hyponatremia and hypochloremic alkalosis, are common in patients receiving chlorthalidone. These abnormalities are dose-related but may occur even at the lowest marketed doses of chlorthalidone. Serum electrolytes should be determined before initiating therapy and at periodic intervals during therapy. Serum and urine electrolyte determinations are particularly important when the patient is vomiting excessively or receiving parenteral fluids. All patients taking chlorthalidone should be observed for clinical signs of electrolyte imbalance, including dryness of mouth, thirst, weakness, lethargy, drowsiness, muscle pains or cramps, muscular fatigue, hypotension, oliguria, tachycardia, palpitations and gastrointestinal disturbances, such as nausea and vomiting. Digitalis therapy may exaggerate metabolic effects of hypokalemia especially with reference to myocardial activity.

Any chloride deficit is generally mild and usually does not require specific treatment except under extraordinary circumstances (as in liver disease or renal disease). Dilutional hyponatremia may occur in edematous patients in hot weather: appropriate therapy is water restriction rather than administration of salt, except in rare instances when the hyponatremia is life-threatening. In cases of actual salt depletion, appropriate replacement is the therapy of choice.

Uric Acid: Hyperuricemia may occur or frank gout may be precipitated in certain patients receiving chlorthalidone.

Other: Increases in serum glucose may occur and latent diabetes mellitus may become manifest during chlorthalidone therapy (see PRECAUTIONS: Chlorthalidone: Drug Interactions). Chlorthalidone and related drugs may decrease serum PBI levels without signs of thyroid disturbance.

Information for Patients: Patients should inform their doctor if they have: 1) had an allergic reaction to chlorthalidone or other diuretics or have asthma 2) kidney disease 3) liver disease 4) gout 5) systemic lupus erythematosus, or 6) been taking other drugs such as cortisone, digitalis, lithium carbonate, or drugs for diabetes.

Patients should be cautioned to contact their physician if they experience any of the following symptoms of potassium loss: excess thirst, tiredness, drowsiness, restlessness, muscle pains or cramps, nausea, vomiting or increased heart rate or pulse.

Patients should also be cautioned that taking alcohol can increase the chance of dizziness occurring.

Laboratory Tests: Periodic determination of serum electrolytes to detect possible electrolyte imbalance should be performed at appropriate intervals.

All patients receiving chlorthalidone should be observed for clinical signs of fluid or electrolyte imbalance: namely, hyponatremia, hypochloremic alkalosis and hypokalemia. Serum and urine electrolyte determinations are particularly important when the patient is vomiting excessively or receiving parenteral fluids.

Drug Interactions: Chlorthalidone may add to or potentiate the action of other antihypertensive drugs. Insulin requirements in diabetic patients may be increased, decreased or unchanged. Higher dosage of oral hypoglycemic agents may be required. Chlorthalidone and related drugs may increase the responsiveness to tubocurarine. Clorthalidone and related drugs may decrease arterial responsiveness to norepinephrine. This diminution is not sufficient to preclude effectiveness of the pressor agent for therapeutic use. Lithium renal clearance is reduced by clorthalidone, increasing the risk of lithium toxicity.

Drug/Laboratory Test Interactions: Clorthalidone and related drugs may decrease serum PBI levels without signs of thyroid disturbance.

Carcinogenesis, Mutagenesis, Impairment of Fertility: No information is available.

Usage in Pregnancy: *Teratogenic Effects. Pregnancy Category B:* Reproduction studies have been performed in the rat and the rabbit at doses up to 420 times the human dose and have revealed no evidence of harm to the fetus due to clorthalidone. There are, however, no adequate and well-controlled studies in pregnant women. Because animal reproduction studies are not always predictive of human response, this drug should be used during pregnancy only if clearly needed.

Non-Teratogenic Effects: Thiazides cross the placental barrier and appear in cord blood. The use of clorthalidone and related drugs in pregnant women requires that the anticipated benefits of the drug be weighed against possible hazards to the fetus. These hazards include fetal or neonatal jaundice, thrombocytopenia, and possibly other adverse reactions that have occurred in the adult.

Nursing Mothers: Thiazides are excreted in human milk. Because of the potential for serious adverse reactions in nursing infants from clorthalidone, a decision should be made whether to discontinue nursing or to discontinue the drug, taking into account the importance of the drug to the mother.

Pediatric Use: Safety and effectiveness in the pediatric population have not been established.

ADVERSE REACTIONS

CLORPRES™ is generally well tolerated. Most adverse effects are mild and tend to diminish with continued therapy. The most frequent (which appears to be dose-related) are dry mouth, occurring in about 40 of 100 patients; drowsiness, about 33 in 100; dizziness, about 16 in 100; constipation and sedation, each about 10 in 100.

In addition to the reactions listed above, certain less frequent adverse experiences, which are shown below, have also been reported in patients receiving the component drugs of CLORPRES™ but in many cases patients were receiving concomitant medication and a causal relationship has not been established:

Clonidine Hydrochloride: *Gastrointestinal:* Nausea and vomiting, about 5 in 100 patients; anorexia and malaise, each about 1 in 100; mild transient abnormalities in liver function tests, about 1 in 100; rare reports of hepatitis; parotitis, rarely.

Metabolic: Weight gain, about 1 in 100 patients; gynecomastia, about 1 in 1000, transient elevation of blood glucose or serum creatinine phosphokinase, rarely.

Central Nervous System: Nervousness and agitation, about 3 in 100 patients; mental depression, about 1 in 100; headache, about 1 in 100; insomnia, about 5 in 1000. Vivid dreams or nightmares, other behavioral changes, restlessness, anxiety, visual and auditory hallucinations and delirium have been reported.

Cardiovascular: Orthostatic symptoms, about 3 in 100 patients; palpitations and tachycardia, and bradycardia, each about 5 in 1000. Raynaud's phenomenon, congestive heart failure, and electrocardiographic abnormalities, i.e., conduction disturbances and arrhythmias, have been reported rarely. Rare cases of sinus bradycardia and atrioventricular block have been reported, both with and without the use of concomitant digitalis.

Dermatological: Rash, about 1 in 100 patients; pruritus, about 7 in 1000; hives, angioneurotic edema and urticaria, about 5 in 1000, alopecia, about 2 in 1000.

Genitourinary: Decreased sexual activity, impotence and loss of libido, about 3 in 100 patients; nocturia, about 1 in 100; difficulty in micturition, about 2 in 1000; urinary retention, about 1 in 1000.

Other: Weakness, about 10 in 100 patients; fatigue, about 4 in 100; discontinuation syndrome, about 1 in 100; muscle or joint pain, about 6 in 1000 and cramps of the lower limbs, about 3 in 1000. Dryness, burning of the eyes, blurred vision, dryness of the nasal mucosa, pallor, weakly positive Coombs' test, increased sensitivity to alcohol and fever have been reported.

Chlorthalidone: *Gastrointestinal:* Anorexia, gastric irritation, nausea, vomiting, cramping, diarrhea, constipation, jaundice (intrahepatic cholestatic jaundice), pancreatitis.

Central Nervous System: Dizziness, vertigo, paresthesia, headache, xanthopsia.

Hematologic: Leukopenia, agranulocytosis, thrombocytopenia, aplastic anemia.

Dermatologic-Hypersensitivity: Purpura, photosensitivity, rash, urticaria, necrotizing angiitis (vasculitis) (cutaneous vasculitis), Lyell's syndrome (toxic epidermal necrolysis).

Cardiovascular: Orthostatic hypotension may occur and may be aggravated by alcohol, barbiturates or narcotics.

Other Adverse Reactions: Hyperglycemia, glycosuria, hyperuricemia, muscle spasm, weakness, restlessness, impotence.

Whenever adverse reactions are moderate or severe, chlorthalidone dosage should be reduced or therapy withdrawn.

OVERDOSAGE

Clonidine Hydrochloride: The signs and symptoms of clonidine hydrochloride ovedosage include hypotension, bradycardia, lethargy, irritability, weakness, somnolence, diminished or absent reflexes, miosis, vomiting and hypoventilation. With large overdoses, reversible cardiac conduction defects or arrhythmias, apnea, seizures and transient hypertension have been reported. The oral LD_{50} of clonidine in rats was 465 mg/kg, and in mice 206 mg/kg.

The general treatment of clonidine hydrochloride overdosage may include intravenous fluids as indicated. Bradycardia can be treated with intravenous atropine sulfate and hypotension with dopamine infusion in addition to intrave-

Continued on next page

Chlorpres—Cont.

nous fluids. Hypertension, associated with overdosage, has been treated with intravenous furosemide or diazoxide or alpha-blocking agents such as phentolamine. Tolazoline, an alpha-blocker, in intravenous doses of 10 mg at 30-minute intervals, may reverse clonidine's effects if other efforts fail. Routine hemodialysis is of limited benefit, since a maximum of 5% of circulating clonidine is removed.

In a patient who ingested 100 mg clonidine hydrochloride, plasma clonidine levels were 60 ng/mL (one hour), 190 ng/mL (1.5 hours), 370 ng/mL (two hours) and 120 ng/mL (5.5 and 6.5 hours). This patient developed hypertension followed by hypotension, bradycardia, apnea, hallucinations, semicoma, and premature ventricular contractions. The patient fully recovered after intensive treatment.

Chlorthalidone: Symptoms of acute overdosage include nausea, weakness, dizziness and disturbances of electrolyte balance. The oral LD_{50} of the drug in the mouse and the rat is more than 25,000 mg/kg body weight. The minimum lethal dose (MLD) in humans has not been established. There is no specific antidote but gastric lavage is recommended, followed by supportive treatment. Where necessary, this may include intravenous dextrose-saline with potassium, administered with caution.

DOSAGE AND ADMINISTRATION

The dosage must be determined by individual titration. (See INDICATIONS AND USAGE.)

Chlorthalidone is usually initiated at a dose of 25 mg once daily and may be increased to 50 mg if the response is insufficient after a suitable trial.

Clonidine hydrochloride is usually initiated at a dose of 0.1 mg twice daily. Elderly patients may benefit from a lower initial dose. Further increments of 0.1 mg/day may be made if necessary until the desired response is achieved. The therapeutic doses most commonly employed have ranged from 0.2 to 0.6 mg per day in divided doses.

One CLORPRES™ (clonidine hydrochloride/chlorthalidone) Tablet administered once or twice daily can be used to administer a minimum of 0.1 mg clonidine hydrochloride and 15 mg chlorthalidone to a maximum of 0.6 mg clonidine hydrochloride and 30 mg chlorthalidone.

HOW SUPPLIED

CLORPRES™ (clonidine hydrochloride and chlorthalidone) Tablets, USP are available containing:

0.1 mg clonidine hydrochloride, USP and 15 mg chlorthalidone, USP

or

0.2 mg clonidine hydrochloride, USP and 15 mg chlorthalidone, USP

or

0.3 mg clonidine hydrochloride, USP and 15 mg chlorthalidone, USP

The 0.1 mg/15 mg product is a yellow, round, scored tablet marked with M1. They are available as follows:

NDC 62794-001-01
bottles of 100 tablets

The 0.2 mg/15 mg product is a yellow, round, scored tablet marked with M27. They are available as follows:

NDC 62794-027-01
bottles of 100 tablets

The 0.3 mg/15 mg product is a yellow, round, scored tablet marked with M72. They are available as follows:

NDC 62794-072-01
bottles of 100 tablets

STORE AT CONTROLLED ROOM TEMPERATURE 15° to 30° C (59° to 86°F).

AVOID EXCESSIVE HUMIDITY.

Dispense in a tight, light-resistant container as defined in the USP using a child-resistant closure.

Rx only

BERTEK PHARMACEUTICALS INC.
Sugar Land, TX 77478

REVISED JUNE 1998
BKCLCH:R2

Shown in Product Identification Guide, page 308

DIGITEK® ℞

[dĭgĭ-tĕk]
(digoxin)
TABLETS, USP
℞ only

DESCRIPTION

DIGITEK (digoxin) is one of the cardiac (or digitalis) glycosides, a closely related group of drugs having in common specific effects on the myocardium. These drugs are found in a number of plants. Digoxin is extracted from the leaves of *Digitalis lanata.* The term "digitalis" is used to designate the whole group of glycosides. The glycosides are composed of two portions: a sugar and a cardenolide (hence "glycosides").

Digoxin is described chemically as (3 β, 5 β, 12 β)-3- [(*O*-2,6-dideoxy-β-*D*-*ribo*-hexopyranosyl-(1→4)-*O*-2,6-dideoxy-β-*D*-*ribo*-hexopyranosyl-(1→4)-2,6-dideoxy-β-*D*-*ribo*-hexopyranosyl)oxy]-12,14-dihydroxycard-20(22)-enolide. Its molecular formula is $C_{41}H_{64}O_{14}$, its molecular weight is 780.96, and the structural formula shown:

Digoxin exists as odorless white crystals that melt with decomposition above 230°C. The drug is practically insoluble in water and in ether; slightly soluble in diluted (50%) alcohol and in chloroform; and freely soluble in pyridine.

DIGITEK is supplied as 125-mcg (0.125-mg) or 250-mcg (0.25-mg) tablets for oral administration. Each tablet contains the labeled amount of digoxin USP and the following inactive ingredients: corn starch, croscarmellose sodium, microcrystalline cellulose, pregelatinized starch, lactose monohydrate and anhydrous lactose, silicon dioxide and stearic acid. In addition, the 0.125-mg tablet contains D&C Yellow No. 10 Aluminum Lake.

CLINICAL PHARMACOLOGY

Mechanism of Action: Digoxin inhibits sodium—potassium ATPase, an enzyme that regulates the quantity of sodium and potassium inside cells. Inhibition of the enzyme leads to an increase in the intracellular concentration of sodium and thus (by stimulation of sodium-calcium exchange) and increase in the intracellular concentration of calcium. The beneficial effects of digoxin result from direct actions on cardiac muscle, as well as indirect actions on the cardiovascular system mediated by effects on the autonomic nervous system. The autonomic effects include: (1) a vagomimetic action, which is responsible for the effects of digoxin on the sinoatrial and atrioventricular (AV) nodes; and (2) baroreceptor sensitization, which results in increased afferent inhibitory activity and reduced activity of the sympathetic nervous system and renin-angiotensin system for any given increment in mean arterial pressure. The pharmacologic consequences of these direct and indirect effects are: (1) an increase in the force and velocity of myocardial systolic contraction (positive inotropic action); (2) a decrease in the degree of activation of the sympathetic nervous system and renin-angiotensin system (neurohormonal deactivating effect); and (3) slowing of the heart rate and decreased conduction velocity through the AV node (vagomimetic effect). The effects of digoxin in heart failure are mediated by its positive inotropic and neurohormonal deactivating effects, whereas the effects of the drug in atrial arrhythmias are related to its vagomimetic actions. In high doses, digoxin increases sympathetic outflow from the central nervous system (CNS). This increase in sympathetic activity may be an important factor in digitalis toxicity.

Pharmacokinetics: ***Absorption:*** Following oral administration, peak serum concentrations of digoxin occur at 1 to 3 hours. Absorption of digoxin from digoxin tablets has been demonstrated to be 60% to 80% complete compared to an identical intravenous dose of digoxin (absolute bioavailability) or Digoxin Solution in Capsules (relative bioavailability). When digoxin tablets are taken after meals, the rate of absorption is slowed, but the total amount of digoxin absorbed is usually unchanged. When taken with meals high in bran fiber, however, the amount absorbed from an oral dose may be reduced. Comparisons of the systemic availability and equivalent doses for oral preparations of digoxin as shown in Table 1:

Table 1: Comparisons of the Systemic Availability and Equivalent Doses for Oral Preparations of Digoxin

Product	Absolute Bio-availability	Equivalent Doses(mcg)* Among Dosage Forms			
Digoxin Tablets	60–80%	62.5	125	250	500
Digoxin Pediatric Elixir	70–85%	62.5	125	250	500
Digoxin Solution In Capsules	90–100%	50	100	200	400
Digoxin Injection/IV	100%	50	100	200	400

* For example, 125-mcg Digoxin Tablets equivalent to 125 mcg Digoxin Pediatric Elixir equivalent to 100 mcg Digoxin Solution in Capsules equivalent to 100 mcg Digoxin Injection/IV.

In some patients, orally administered digoxin is converted to inactive reduction products (e.g., dihydrodigoxin) by colonic bacteria in the gut. Data suggest that one in ten patients treated with digoxin tablets will degrade 40% or more of the ingested dose. As a result, certain antibiotics may increase the absorption of digoxin in such patients. Although inactivation of these bacteria by antibiotics is rapid, the serum digoxin concentration will rise at a rate consistent with the elimination half-life of digoxin. The magnitude of rise in serum digoxin concentration relates to the extent of bacterial inactivation, and may be as must as two-fold in some cases.

Distribution: Following drug administration, a 6-to 8-hour tissue distribution phase is observed. This is followed by a much more gradual decline in the serum concentration of the drug, which is dependent on the elimination of digoxin from the body. The peak height and slope of the early portion (absorption/distribution phases) of the serum concentration-time curve are dependent upon the route of administration and the absorption characteristics of the formulation. Clinical evidence indicates that the early high serum concentrations do not reflect the concentration of digoxin at its site of action, but that with chronic use, the steady-state post-distribution serum concentrations are in equilibrium with tissue concentrations and correlate with pharmacologic effects. In individual patients, these post-distribution serum concentrations may be useful in evaluating therapeutic and toxic effects (see DOSAGE AND ADMINISTRATION: Serum Digoxin Concentrations).

Digoxin is concentrated in tissues and therefore has a large apparent volume of distribution. Digoxin crosses both the blood-brain barrier and the placenta. At delivery, the serum digoxin concentration in the newborn is similar to the serum concentration in the mother. Approximately 25% of digoxin in the plasma is bound to protein. Serum digoxin concentrations are not significantly altered by large changes in fat tissue weight, so that its distribution space correlates best with lean (i.e., ideal) body weight, not total body weight.

Metabolism: Only a small percentage (16%) of a dose of digoxin is metabolized. The end metabolites, which include 3 β-digoxigenin, 3-keto-digoxigenin, and their glucuronide and sulfate conjugates, are polar in nature and are postulated to be formed via hydrolysis, oxidation, and conjugation. The metabolism of digoxin is not dependent upon the cytochrome P-450 system, and digoxin is not known to induce or inhibit the cytochrome P-450 system.

Excretion: Elimination of digoxin follows first-order kinetics (that is, the quantity of digoxin eliminated at any time is proportional to the total body content). Following intravenous administration to healthy volunteers, 50% to 70% of a digoxin dose is excreted unchanged in the urine. Renal excretion of digoxin is proportional to glomerular filtration rate and is largely independent of urine flow. In healthy volunteers with normal renal function, digoxin has a half-life of 1.5 to 2 days. The half-life in anuric patients is prolonged to 3.5 to 5 days. Digoxin is not effectively removed from the body by dialysis, exchange transfusion or during cardiopulmonary bypass because most of the drug is bound to tissue and does not circulate in the blood.

Special Populations: Race differences in digoxin pharmacokinetics have not been formally studied. Because digoxin is primarily eliminated as unchanged drug via the kidney and because there are no important differences in creatinine clearance among races, pharmacokinetic differences due to race are not expected.

The clearance of digoxin can be primarily correlated with renal function as indicated by creatinine clearance. The Cockcroft and Gault formula for estimation of creatinine clearance includes age, body weight, and gender. A table that provides the usual daily maintenance dose requirements of DIGITEK Tablets based on creatinine clearance (per 70 kg) is presented in the DOSAGE AND ADMINISTRATION section.

Plasma digoxin profiles in patients with acute hepatitis generally fell within the range of profiles in a group of healthy subjects.

Pharmacodynamic and Clinical Effects: The times to onset of pharmacologic effect and to peak effect of preparations of digoxin are shown in Table 2:

Table 2: Times to Onset of Pharmacologic Effect and to Peak Effect of Preparations of Digoxin

Product	Time to Onset of Effect*	Time to Peak Effect*
Digoxin Tablets	0.5–2 hours	2–6 hours
Digoxin Pediatric Elixir	0.5–2 hours	2–6 hours
Digoxin Solution in Capsules	0.5–2 hours	2–6 hours
Digoxin Injection/IV	5—30 minutes†	1–4 hours

* Documented for ventricular response rate in atrial fibrillation, inotropic effects and electrocardiographic changes.
† Depending upon rate of infusion.

Chronic Atrial Fibrillation: In patients with chronic atrial fibrillation, digoxin slows rapid ventricular response in linear dose-response fashion from 0.25 to 0.75 mg/day. Digoxin should not be used for the treatment of multifocal atrial tachycardia.

INDICATIONS AND USAGE

Atrial Fibrillation: DIGITEK is indicated for the control of ventricular response rate in patients with chronic atrial fibrillation.

CONTRAINDICATIONS

Digitalis glycosides are contraindicated in patients with ventricular fibrillation or in patients with a known hypersensitivity to digoxin. A hypersensitivity reaction to other digitalis preparations usually constitutes a contraindication to digoxin.

WARNINGS

Sinus Node Disease and AV Block: Because digoxin slows sinoatrial and AV conduction, the drug commonly prolongs the PR interval. The drug may cause severe sinus bradycardia or sinoatrial block in patients with pre-existing sinus node disease and may cause advanced or complete heart block in patients with pre-existing incomplete AV block. In such patients consideration should be given to the insertion of a pacemaker before treatment with digoxin.

Accessory AV Pathway (Wolff-Parkinson-White Syndrome): After intravenous digoxin therapy, some patients with paroxysmal atrial fibrillation or flutter and a coexisting accessory AV pathway have developed increased antegrade conduction across the accessory pathway bypassing the AV node, leading to a very rapid ventricular response or ventricular fibrillation. Unless conduction down the accessory pathway has been blocked (either pharmacologically or by surgery), digoxin should not be used in such patients. The treatment of paroxysmal supraventricular tachycardia in such patients is usually direct-current cardioversion.

Use in Patients with Preserved Left Ventricular Systolic Function: Patients with certain disorders involving heart failure associated with preserved left ventricular ejection fraction may be particularly susceptible to toxicity of the drug. Such disorders include restrictive cardiomyopathy, constrictive pericarditis, amyloid heart disease, and acute cor pulmonale. Patients with idiopathic hypertrophic subaortic stenosis may have worsening of the outflow obstruction due to the inotropic effects of digoxin.

PRECAUTIONS

Use in Patients with Impaired Renal Function: Digoxin is primarily excreted by the kidneys; therefore, patients with impaired renal function require smaller than usual maintenance doses of digoxin (see DOSAGE AND ADMINISTRATION). Because of the prolonged elimination half-life, a longer period of time is required to achieve an initial or new steady-state serum concentration in patients with renal impairment than in patients with normal renal function. If appropriate care is not taken to reduce the dose of digoxin, such patients are at high risk for toxicity, and toxic effects will last longer in such patients than in patients with normal renal function.

Use in Patients with Electrolyte Disorders: In patients with hypokalemia or hypomagnesemia, toxicity may occur despite serum digoxin concentrations below 2 ng/mL, because potassium or magnesium depletion sensitizes the myocardium to digoxin. Therefore, it is desirable to maintain normal serum potassium and magnesium concentrations in patients being treated with digoxin. Deficiencies of these electrolytes may result from malnutrition, diarrhea, or prolonged vomiting, as well as the use of the following drugs or procedures: diuretics, amphotericin B, corticosteriods, antacids, dialysis, and mechanical suction of gastrointestinal secretions.

Hypercalcemia from any cause predisposes the patient to digitalis toxicity. Calcium, particularly when administered rapidly by the intravenous route, may produce serious arrhythmias in digitalized patients. On the other hand, hypocalcemia can nullify the effect of digoxin in humans; thus, digoxin may be ineffective until serum calcium is restored to normal. These interactions are related to the fact that digoxin affects contractility and excitability of the heart in a manner similar to that of calcium.

Use in Thyroid Disorders and Hypermetabolic States: Hypothyroidism may reduce the requirements for digoxin. Heart failure and/or atrial arrhythmias resulting from hypermetabolic or hyperdynamic states (e.g., hyperthyroidism, hypoxia, or arteriovenous shunt) are best treated by addressing the underlying condition. Atrial arrhythmias associated with hypermetabolic states are particularly resistant to digoxin treatment. Care must be taken to avoid toxicity if digoxin is used.

Use in Patients with Acute Myocardial Infarction: Digoxin should be used with caution in patients with acute myocardial infarction. The use of inotropic drugs in some patients in this setting may result in undesirable increases in myocardial oxygen demand and ischemia.

Use During Electrical Cardioversion: It may be desirable to reduce the dose of digoxin for 1 to 2 days prior to electrical cardioversion of atrial fibrillation to avoid the induction of ventricular arrhythmias, but physicians must consider the consequences of increasing the ventricular response if digoxin is withdrawn. If digitalis toxicity is suspected, elective cardioversion should be delayed. If it is not prudent to delay cardioversion, the lowest possible energy level should be selected to avoid provoking ventricular arrhythmias.

Laboratory Test Monitoring: Patients receiving digoxin should have their serum electrolytes and renal function (serum creatinine concentrations) assessed periodically; the frequency of assessments will depend on the clinical setting. For discussion of serum digoxin concentrations, see DOSAGE AND ADMINISTRATION section.

Drug Interactions: Potassium-depleting *diuretics* are a major contributing factor to digitalis toxicity. *Calcium*, particularly if administered rapidly by the intravenous route, may produce serious arrhythmias in digitalized patients. *Quinidine, verapamil, amiodarone, propafenone, indomethacin, itraconazole, alprazolam,* and *spironolactone* raise the serum digoxin concentration due to a reduction in clearance and/or in volume of distribution of the drug, with the implication that digitalis intoxication may result. *Erythromycin* and *clarithromycin* (and possibly other *macrolide antibiotics*) and *tetracycline* may increase digoxin absorption in patients who inactivate digoxin by bacterial metabolism in the lower intestine, so that digitalis intoxication may result (see CLINICAL PHARMACOLOGY: Absorption). *Propantheline* and *diphenoxylate*, by decreasing gut motility, may increase digoxin absorption. *Antacids, kaolin-pectin, sulfasalazine, neomycin, cholestyramine,* certain *anticancer drugs,* and *metoclopramide* may interfere with intestinal digoxin absorption, resulting in unexpectedly low serum concentrations. *Rifampin* may decrease serum digoxin concentration, especially in patients with renal dysfunction, by increasing the non-renal clearance of digoxin. There have been inconsistent reports regarding the effects of other drugs [e.g., *quinine, penicillamine*] on serum digoxin concentration. *Thyroid* administration to a digitalized, hypothyroid patient may increase the dose requirement of digoxin. Concomitant use of digoxin and *sympathomimetics* increases the risk of cardiac arrhythmias. *Succinylcholine* may cause a sudden extrusion of potassium from muscle cells, and may thereby cause arrhythmias in digitalized patients. Although beta-adrenergic blockers or calcium channel blockers and digoxin may be useful in combination to control atrial fibrillation, their additive effects on AV node conduction can result in advanced or complete heart block.

Due to the considerable variability of these interactions, the dosage of digoxin should be individualized when patients receive these medications concurrently. Furthermore, caution should be exercised when combining digoxin with any drug that may cause a significant deterioration in renal function, since a decline in glomerular filtration or tubular secretion may impair the excretion of digoxin.

Drug/Laboratory Test Interactions: The use of therapeutic doses of digoxin may cause prolongation of the PR interval and depression of the ST segment on the electrocardiogram. Digoxin may produce false positive ST-T changes on the electrocardiogram during exercise testing. These electrophysiologic effects reflect an expected effect of the drug and are not indicative of toxicity.

Carcinogenesis, Mutagenesis, Impairment of Fertility: There have been no long-term studies performed in animals to evaluate carcinogenic potential, nor have studies been conducted to assess the mutagenic potential of digoxin or its potential to affect fertility.

Pregnancy: ***Teratogenic Effects:*** Pregnancy Category C. Animal reproduction studies have not been conducted with digoxin. It is also not known whether digoxin can cause fetal harm when administered to a pregnant woman or can affect reproductive capacity. Digoxin should be given to a pregnant woman only if clearly needed.

Nursing Mothers: Studies have shown that digoxin concentrations in the mother's serum and milk are similar. However, the estimated exposure of a nursing infant to digoxin via breast feeding will be far below the usual infant maintenance dose. Therefore, this amount should have no pharmacologic effect upon the infant. Nevertheless, caution should be exercised when digoxin is administered to a nursing woman.

Pediatric Use: Newborn infants display considerable variability in their tolerance to digoxin. Premature and immature infants are particularly sensitive to the effects of digoxin, and the dosage of the drug must not only be reduced but must be individualized according to their degree of maturity. Digitalis glycosides can cause poisoning in children due to accidental ingestion.

Geriatric Use: The majority of clinical experience gained with digoxin has been in the elderly population. This experience has not identified differences in response or adverse effects between the elderly and younger patients. However, this drug is known to be substantially excreted by the kidney, and the risk of toxic reactions to this drug may be greater in patients with impaired renal function. Because elderly patients are more likely to have decreased renal function, care should be taken in dose selection, which should be based on renal function, and it may be useful to monitor renal function (see DOSAGE AND ADMINISTRATION).

ADVERSE REACTIONS

In general, the adverse reactions of digoxin are dose-dependent and occur at doses higher than those needed to achieve a therapeutic effect. Hence, adverse reactions are less common when digoxin is used within the recommended dose range or therapeutic serum concentration range and when there is careful attention to concurrent medications and conditions.

Because some patients may be particularly susceptible to side effects with digoxin, the dosage of the drug should always be selected carefully and adjusted as the clinical condition of the patient warrants. In the past, when high doses of digoxin were used and little attention was paid to clinical status or concurrent medications, adverse reactions to digoxin were more frequent and severe. Cardiac adverse reactions accounted for about one-half, gastrointestinal disturbances for about one-fourth, and CNS and other toxicity for about one-fourth of these adverse reactions. However, available evidence suggests that the incidence and severity of digoxin toxicity has decreased substantially in recent years. In recent controlled clinical trials, in patients with predominantly mild to moderate heart failure, the incidence of adverse experiences was comparable in patients taking digoxin and in those taking placebo. In a large mortality trial, the incidence of hospitalization for suspected digoxin toxicity was 2% in patients taking digoxin compared to 0.9% in patients taking placebo. In this trial, the most common manifestations of digoxin toxicity included gastrointestinal and cardiac disturbances; CNS manifestations were less common.

Adults: ***Cardiac:*** Therapeutic doses of digoxin may cause heart block in patients with pre-existing sinoatrial or AV conduction disorders; heart block can be avoided by adjusting the dose of digoxin. Prophylactic use of a cardiac pacemaker may be considered if the risk of heart block is considered unacceptable. High doses of digoxin may produce a variety of rhythm disturbances, such as first-degree, second-degree (Wenckebach), or third-degree heart block (including asystole); atrial tachycardia with block; AV dissociation; accelerated junctional (nodal) rhythm; unifocal or multiform ventricular premature contractions (especially bigeminy or trigeminy); ventricular tachycardia; and ventricular fibrillation. Digoxin produces PR prolongation and ST segment depression which should not by themselves be considered digoxin toxicity. Cardiac toxicity can also occur at therapeutic doses in patients who have conditions which may alter their sensitivity to digoxin (see WARNINGS and PRECAUTIONS).

Gastrointestinal: Digoxin may cause anorexia, nausea, vomiting and diarrhea. Rarely, the use of digoxin has been associated with abdominal pain, intestinal ischemia, and hemorrhagic necrosis of the intestines.

CNS: Digoxin can produce visual disturbances (blurred or yellow vision), headache, weakness, dizziness, apathy, confusion and mental disturbances (such as anxiety, depression, delirium, and hallucination).

Other: Gynecomastia has been occasionally observed following the prolonged use of digoxin. Thrombocytopenia and maculopapular rash and other skin reactions have been rarely observed.

The following table summarizes the incidence of those adverse experiences listed above for patients treated with digoxin tablets or placebo from two randomized, double-blind, placebo-controlled withdrawal trials. Patients in these trials were also receiving diuretics with or without angiotensin-converting enzyme inhibitors. These patients have been stable on digoxin, and were randomized to digoxin or placebo. The results shown in Table 3 reflect the experience in patients following dosage titration with the use of serum digoxin concentrations and careful follow-up. These adverse experiences are consistent with results from a large, placebo-controlled mortality trial (DIG trial) wherein over half the patients were not receiving digoxin prior to enrollment.

Table 3: Adverse Experiences in Two Parallel, Double-Blind, Placebo-Controlled Withdrawal Trials (Number of Patients Reporting)

Adverse Experience	Digoxin Patients (n=123)	Placebo Patients (n=125)
Cardiac		
Palpitation	1	4
Ventricular extrasystole	1	1
Tachycardia	2	1
Heart arrest	1	1
Gastrointestinal		
Anorexia	1	4
Nausea	4	2
Vomiting	2	1
Diarrhea	4	1
Abdonimal pain	0	6
CNS		
Headache	4	4
Dizziness	6	5
Mental disturbances	5	1
Other		
Rash	2	1
Death	4	3

Infants and Children: The side effects of digoxin in infants and children differ from those seen in adults in several respects. Although digoxin may produce anorexia, nausea, vomiting, diarrhea, and CNS disturbances in young patients, these are rarely the initial symptoms of overdosage. Rather, the earliest and most frequent manifestation of excessive dosing with digoxin in infants and children is the appearance of cardiac arrhythmias, including sinus bradycardia. In children, the use of digoxin may produce any arrhythmia. The most common are conduction disturbances or supraventricular tachyarrhythmias, such as atrial tachycardia (with or without block) and junctional (nodal) tachycardia. Ventricular arrhythmias are less common. Sinus bradycardia may be a sign of impending digoxin intoxication, especially in infants, even in the absence of first-degree heart block. Any arrhythmia or alteration in cardiac conduction that develops in a child taking digoxin should be assumed to be caused by digoxin, until further evaluation proves otherwise.

OVERDOSAGE

Treatment of Adverse Reactions Produced by Overdosage: Digoxin should be temporarily discontinued until the adverse reaction resolves. Every effort should also be made to correct factors that may contribute to the adverse reaction (such as electrolyte disturbances or concurrent medications). Once the adverse reaction has resolved, therapy with

Continued on next page

Digitek—Cont.

digoxin may be reinstituted, following a careful reassessment of dose.

Withdrawal of digoxin may be all that is required to treat the adverse reaction. However, when the primary manifestation of digoxin overdosage is a cardiac arrhythmia, additional therapy may be needed.

If the rhythm disturbance is a symptomatic bradyarrhythmia or heart block, consideration should be given to the reversal of toxicity with DIGIBIND® [Digoxin Immune Fab (Ovine)] (see below), the use of atropine, or the insertion of a temporary cardiac pacemaker. However, asymptomatic bradycardia or heart block related to digoxin may require only temporary withdrawal of the drug and cardiac monitoring of the patient.

If the rhythm disturbance is a ventricular arrhythmia, consideration should be given to the correction of electrolyte disorders, particularly if hypokalemia (see below) or hypomagnesemia is present. DIGIBIND® [Digoxin Immune Fab (Ovine)] is a specific antidote for digoxin and may be used to reverse potentially life-threatening ventricular arrhythmias due to digoxin overdosage.

Administration of Potassium: Every effort should be made to maintain the serum potassium concentration between 4 and 5.5 mmol/L. Potassium is usually administered orally, but when correction of the arrhythmia is urgent and the serum potassium concentration is low, potassium may be administered cautiously by intravenous route. The electrocardiogram should be monitored for any evidence of potassium toxicity (e.g., peaking of T waves) and to observe the effect on the arrhythmia. Potassium salts may be dangerous in patients who manifest bradycardia or heart block due to digoxin (unless primarily related to supraventricular tachycardia) and in the setting of massive digitalis overdosage (see Massive Digitalis Overdosage subsection).

Massive Digitalis Overdosage: Manifestations of life-threatening toxicity include ventricular tachycardia or ventricular fibrillation, or progressive bradyarrhythmias, or heart block. The administration of more than 10 mg of digoxin in a previously healthy adult or more than 4 mg in a previously healthy child, or a steady-state serum concentration greater than 10 ng/mL often results in cardiac arrest.

DIGIBIND® [Digoxin Immune Fab (Ovine)] should be used to reverse the toxic effects of ingestion of a massive overdose. The decision to administer DIGIBIND® [Digoxin Immune Fab (Ovine)] to a patient who has ingested a massive dose of digoxin but who has not yet manifested life-threatening toxicity should depend on the likelihood that life-threatening toxicity will occur (see above).

Patients with massive digitalis ingestion should receive large doses of activated charcoal to prevent absorption and bind digoxin in the gut during enteroenteric recirculation. Emesis or gastric lavage may be indicated especially if ingestion has occurred within 30 minutes of the patient's presentation at the hospital. Emesis should not be induced in patients who are obtunded. If a patient presents more than 2 hours after ingestion or already has toxic manifestations, it may be unsafe to induce vomiting or attempt passage of a gastric tube, because such maneuvers may induce an acute vagal episode that can worsen digitalis-related arrhythmias.

Severe digitalis intoxication can cause a massive shift of potassium from inside to outside the cell, leading to life-threatening hyperkalemia. The administration of potassium supplements in the setting of massive intoxication may be hazardous and should be avoided. Hyperkalemia caused by massive digitalis toxicity is best treated with DIGIBIND® [Digoxin Immune Fab (Ovine)]; initial treatment with glucose and insulin may also be required if hyperkalemia itself is acutely life-threatening.

DOSAGE AND ADMINISTRATION

General: Recommended dosages of digoxin may require considerable modification because of individual sensitivity of the patient to the drug, the presence of associated conditions, or the use of concurrent medications. In selecting a dose of digoxin, the following factors must be considered:

1. The body weight of the patient. Doses should be calculated based upon lean (i.e., ideal) body weight.
2. The patient's renal function, preferably evaluated on the basis of estimated creatinine clearance.
3. The patient's age. Infants and children require different doses of digoxin than adults. Also, advanced age may be indicative of diminished renal function even in patients with normal serum creatinine concentration (i.e., below 1.5 mg/dL)
4. Concomitant disease states, concurrent medications, or other factors likely to alter the pharmacokinetic or pharmacodynamic profile of digoxin (see PRECAUTIONS).

Serum Digoxin Concentrations: In general, the dose of digoxin used should be determined on clinical grounds. However, measurement of serum digoxin concentrations can be helpful to the clinician in determining the adequacy of digoxin therapy and in assigning certain probabilities to the likelihood of digoxin intoxication. About two-thirds of adults considered adequately digitalized (without evidence of toxicity) have serum digoxin concentrations ranging from 0.8 to 2 ng/mL. However, digoxin may produce clinical benefits even at serum concentrations below this range. About two-thirds of adult patients with clinical toxicity have serum digoxin concentrations greater than 2 ng/mL. However, since one third of patients with clinical toxicity have concentrations less than 2 ng/mL, values below 2 ng/mL do not rule out the possibility that a certain sign or symptom is related to digoxin therapy. Rarely, there are patients who are unable to tolerate digoxin at serum concentrations below 0.8 ng/mL. Consequently, the serum concentration of digoxin should always be interpreted in the overall clinical context, and an isolated measurement should not be used alone as the basis for increasing or decreasing the dose of the drug.

To allow adequate time for equilibration of digoxin between serum and tissue, sampling of serum concentrations should be done just before the next scheduled dose of the drug. If this is not possible, sampling should be done at least 6 to 8 hours after the last dose, regardless of the route of administration or the formulation used. On a once-daily dosing schedule, the concentration of digoxin will be 10% to 25% lower when sampled at 24 verses 8 hours, depending upon the patient's renal function. On a twice-daily dosing schedule, there will be only minor differences in serum digoxin concentrations whether sampling is done at 8 or 12 hour after a dose.

If a discrepancy exists between the reported serum concentration and the observed clinical response, the clinician should consider the following possibilities:

1. Analytical problems in the assay procedure.
2. Inappropriate serum sampling time.
3. Administration of a digitalis glycoside other than digoxin.
4. Conditions (described in WARNINGS and PRECAUTIONS) causing an alteration in the sensitivity of the patient to digoxin.
5. Serum digoxin concentration may decrease acutely during periods of exercise without any associated change in clinical efficacy due to increased binding of digoxin to skeletal muscle.

Atrial Fibrillation: For the treatment of chronic atrial fibrillation, digoxin should be titrated to the minimum dose which achieves the desired ventricular rate control without causing excessive adverse effects. Data are not available to establish the appropriate targets for resting or exercise rates. Peak digoxin body stores larger than 8 to 12 mcg/kg are often required.

Adults: Digitalization may be accomplished by either of two general approaches that vary in dosage and frequency of administration, but reach the same endpoint in terms of total amount of digoxin accumulated in the body.

1. If rapid digitalization is considered medically appropriate, it may be achieved by administering a loading dose based upon projected peak digoxin body stores. Maintenance dose can be calculated as a percentage of the loading dose.
2. More gradual digitalization may be obtained by beginning an appropriate maintenance dose, thus allowing digoxin body stores to accumulate slowly. Steady-state serum digoxin concentrations will be achieved in approximately five half-lives of the drug for the individual patient. Depending upon the patient's renal function, this will take between 1 and 3 weeks.

Rapid Digitalization with a Loading Dose: Because of altered digoxin distribution and elimination, projected peak body stores for patients with renal insufficiency should be conservative (i.e., 6 to 10 mcg/kg) [see PRECAUTIONS].

The loading dose should be administered in several portions, with roughly half the total given as the first dose. Additional fractions of this planned total dose may be given at 6- to 8-hour intervals, **with careful assessment of clinical response before each additional dose.**

If the patient's clinical response necessitates a change from the calculated loading dose of digoxin, then calculation of the maintenance dose should be based upon the amount actually given.

A single initial dose of 500 to 750 mcg (0.5 to 0.75 mg) of digoxin tablets usually produces a detectable effect in 0.5 to 2 hours that becomes maximal in 2 to 6 hours. Additional doses of 125 to 375 mcg (0.125 to 0.375 mg) may be given cautiously at 6- to 8-hour intervals until clinical evidence of an adequate effect is noted. The usual amount of digoxin tablets that a 70-kg patient requires to achieve 8 to 12 mcg/kg peak body stores is 750 to 1,250 mcg (0.75 to 1.25 mg).

Digoxin injection is frequently used to achieve rapid digitalization, with conversion to digoxin tablets or Digoxin Solution in Capsules for maintenance therapy. If patients are switched from intravenous to oral digoxin formulations, allowances must be made for differences in bioavailability when calculating maintenance dosages (see table, CLINICAL PHARMACOLOGY).

Maintenance Dosing: The doses of digoxin used in controlled trials have ranged from 125 to 500 mcg (0.125 to 0.5 mg) once daily. In these studies, the digoxin dose has been generally titrated according to the patient's age, lean body weight, and renal function. Therapy is generally initiated at a dose of 250 mcg (0.25 mg) once daily in patients under age 70 with good renal function, at a dose of 125 mcg (0.125 mg) once daily in patients over age 70 or with impaired renal function, and at a dose of 62.5 mcg (0.0625 mg) in patients with marked renal impairment. Doses may be increased every 2 weeks according to clinical response.

The maintenance dose should be based upon the percentage of the peak body stores lost each day through elimination. The following formula has had wide clinical use:

Maintenance Dose = Peak Body Stores (i.e., Loading Dose) × % Daily Loss/100

Where: % Daily Loss = 14 + Ccr/5

(Ccr is creatinine clearance, corrected to 70 kg body weight or 1.73 m^2 body surface area.)

Table 4 provides average daily maintenance dose requirements of digoxin tablets based upon lean body weight and renal function.

[See table 4 below]

Example: Based on the above table, a patient with an estimated lean body weight of 70 kg and a Ccr of 60mL/min, should be given a dose of 250 mcg (0.25 mg) daily of digoxin tablets, usually taken after the morning meal. If no loading dose is administered, steady-state serum concentrations in this patient should be anticipated at approximately 11 days.

Infants and Children: In general, divided daily dosing is recommended for infants and young children (under age 10). In the newborn period, renal clearance of digoxin is diminished and suitable dosage adjustments must be observed. This is especially pronounced in the premature infant. Beyond the immediate newborn period, children generally require proportionally larger doses than adults on the basis of body weight to surface area. Children over 10 years of age require adult dosages in proportion to their body weight. Some researchers have suggested that infants and young children tolerate slightly higher serum concentrations than do adults.

Daily maintenance doses for each group are given in Table 5 and should provide therapeutic effects with minimum risk of toxicity in most patients. These recommendations assume the presence of normal renal function:

Table 5: Daily Maintenance Doses in children with Normal Renal Function

Age	Daily Maintenance Dose (mcg/kg)
2 to 5 years	10 to 15
5 to 10 years	7 to 10
Over 10 years	3 to 5

In children with renal disease, digoxin must be carefully titrated based upon clinical response.

It cannot be overemphasized that both the adult and pediatric dosage guidelines provided are based upon average patient response and substantial individual variation can be expected. Accordingly, ultimate dosage selection must be based upon clinical assessment of the patient.

Dosage Adjustment when Changing Preparations: The difference in bioavailability between Digoxin Injection or Digoxin Solution in Capsules and Digoxin Pediatric Elixir or digoxin tablets must be considered when changing patients from one dosage form to another.

Table 4: Usual Daily Maintenance Dose Requirements (mcg) of DIGOXIN for Estimated Peak Body Stores of 10 mcg/kg

Corrected Ccr (mL/min per 70 kg)*	Lean Body Weight							Number of Days Before Steady-State Achieved†
	kg	50	60	70	80	90	100	
	lb	110	132	154	176	198	220	
0		62.5‡	125	125	125	187.5	187.5	22
10		125	125	125	187.5	187.5	187.5	19
20		125	125	187.5	187.5	187.5	250	16
30		125	187.5	187.5	187.5	250	250	14
40		125	187.5	187.5	250	250	250	13
50		187.5	187.5	250	250	250	250	12
60		187.5	187.5	250	250	250	375	11
70		187.5	250	250	250	250	375	10
80		187.5	250	250	250	375	375	9
90		187.5	250	250	250	375	500	8
100		250	250	250	375	375	500	7

*Ccr is creatinine clearance, corrected to 70 kg body weight or 1.73 m^2 body surface area.) *For adults*, if only serum creatinine concentrations (Scr) are available, a Ccr (corrected to 70 kg body weight) may be estimated in men as(140-age)/Scr. For women, this result should be multiplied by 0.85.

Note: This equation cannot be used for estimating creatinine clearance in infants or children.

†If no loading dose administered.

‡62.5 mcg = 0.0625 mg

Doses of 100 mcg (0.1 mg) and 200 mcg (0.2 mg) of Digoxin Solution in Capsules are approximately equivalent to 125-mcg (0.125-mg) and 250-mcg (0.25-mg) doses of digoxin tablets and Pediatric Elixir, respectively. (see table in CLINICAL PHARMACOLOGY: Pharmacokinetics).

HOW SUPPLIED

DIGITEK™ (digoxin) Tablets, USP 125 mcg (0.125 mg) are yellow, round tablets, and imprinted with **B 145** on the scored side of the tablets. They are available as follows:

NDC 62794-145-01
bottles of 100 tablets
NDC 62794-145-10
bottles of 1000 tablets
NDC 62794-145-56
bottles of 5000 tablets

DIGITEK™ (digoxin) Tablets, USP 250 mcg (0.25 mg) are white, round tablets, and imprinted with **B 146** on the scored side of the tablets. They are available as follows:

NDC 62794-146-01
bottles of 100 tablets
NDC 62794-146-10
bottles of 1000 tablets
NDC 62794-146-56
bottles of 5000 tablets

Store at 15° to 25°C (59° to 77°F) in a dry place and protect from light.
Dispense in a tight, light-resistant container as defined in the USP.

REVISED NOVEMBER 1999
BKDGTK:R2
8070-00

Distributed by
BERTEK PHARMACEUTICALS INC.
Morgantown, WV 26505
Manufactured by
AMIDE PHARMACEUTICAL, INC.,
101 East Main Street,
Little Falls, NJ 07424 USA

GRANULEX ℞

COMPOSITION

Each 0.82 cc. of medication delivered to the wound site contains Trypsin crystallized 0.1 mg., Balsam Peru 72.5 mg., Castor Oil 650.0 mg., and an emulsifier.

ACTION

Trypsin is intended for debridement of eschar and other necrotic tissue. It appears that in many instances removal of wound debris strengthens humoral defense mechanisms sufficiently to retard proliferation of local pathogens. Balsam Peru is an effective capillary bed stimulant used to increase circulation in the wound site area. Also, Balsam Peru has a mildly bactericidal action. Castor Oil is used to improve epithelialization by reducing premature epithelial desiccation and cornification. Also, it can act as a protective covering and aids in the reduction of pain.

INDICATIONS

For the treatment of decubitus ulcers, varicose ulcers, debridement of eschar, dehiscent wounds and sunburn.

USES

Granulex is in aerosol form which can be important to healing. It must be remembered, healing starts with a thin sheath of epithelium no more than a cell or two thick. Any rough movement or trauma can quickly destroy the healing tissue. Aerosols have the advantage of eliminating all extraneous physical contact with the wound. Granulex is easy to apply and quickly reduces odor frequently accompanying a decubitus ulcer. The wound may be left open or a wet bandage may be applied. As a suggestion; keep in mind wounds heal poorly in the presence of hemoglobin or zinc deficiency.

WARNING

Do not spray on fresh arterial clots. Avoid spraying in eyes. Flammable, do not expose to fire or open flame. Contents under pressure. Do not puncture or incinerate. Do not store at temperature above 120°F. Keep out of reach of children. Use only as directed. Intentional misuse by deliberately concentrating and inhaling the contents can be harmful or fatal.

DOSAGE

Apply a minimum of twice daily or as often as necessary. Shake well, press the aerosol valve and coat the wound rapidly but not excessively.

HOW SUPPLIED

2 oz. Aerosol NDC 62794-002-50
4 oz. Aerosol NDC 62794-002-51

KRISTALOSE™ ℞

[*krĭs' tă lōsĕ*]
(LACTULOSE)
For Oral Solution

DESCRIPTION

KRISTALOSE™ (Lactulose) is a synethetic disaccharide in the form of crystals for reconstitution prior to use for oral administration. Each 10 g of lactulose contains less than 0.3 g galactose and lactose as a total sum. The pH range is 3.0 to 7.0
Lactulose is a colonic acidifier which promotes laxation.
The chemical name for lactulose is 4-O-β-D-Galactopyranosyl-D-fructofuranose. It has the following structural formula:

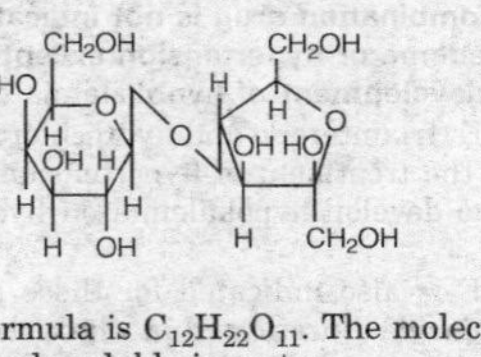

CH₂OH CH₂OH HO H O H OH H O OH HO H H H H OH H CH₂OH

The molecular formula is $C_{12}H_{22}O_{11}$. The molecular weight is 342.30. It is freely soluble in water.

CLINICAL PHARMACOLOGY

KRISTALOSE™ (Lactulose) is poorly absorbed from the gastrointestinal tract and no enzyme capable of hydrolysis of this disaccharide is present in human gastrointestinal tissue. As a result, oral doses of lactulose reach the colon virtually unchanged. In the colon, lactulose is broken down primarily to lactic acid, and also to small amounts of formic and acetic acids, by the action of colonic bacteria, which results in an increase in osmotic pressure and slight acidification of the colonic contents. This in turn causes an increase in stool water content and softens the stool.
Since lactulose does not exert its effect until it reaches the colon, and since transit time through the colon may be slow, 24 to 48 hours may be required to produce desired bowel movement.
Lactulose given orally to man and experimental animals resulted in only small amounts reaching the blood. Urinary excretion has been determined to be 3% or less and is essentially complete within 24 hours.

INDICATIONS AND USAGE

KRISTALOSE™ (Lactulose) for Oral Solution is indicated for the treatment of constipation. In patients with a history of chronic constipation, lactulose therapy increases the number of bowel movements per day and the number of days on which bowel movements occur.

CONTRAINDICATIONS

Since KRISTALOSE™ (Lactulose) for Oral Solution contains galactose (less than 0.3 g/10 g as a total sum with lactose), it is contraindicated in patients who require a low galactose diet.

WARNINGS

A theoretical hazard may exist for patients being treated with lactulose who may be required to undergo electrocautery procedures during proctoscopy or colonoscopy. Accumulation of H_2 gas in significant concentration in the presence of an electrical spark may result in an explosive reaction. Although this complication has not been reported with lactulose, patients on lactulose therapy undergoing such procedures should have a thorough bowel cleansing with a non-fermentable solution. Insufflation of CO_2 as an additional safeguard may be pursued but is considered to be a redundant measure.

PRECAUTIONS

General
Since KRISTALOSE™ (Lactulose) for Oral Solution contains galactose and lactose (less than 0.3 g/10 g as a total sum), it should be used with caution in diabetics.
Information for patients
In the event that an unusual diarrheal condition occurs, contact your physician.
Laboratory Tests
Elderly, debilitated patients who receive lactulose for more than six months should have serum electrolytes (potassium, chloride, carbon dioxide) measured periodically.
Drug Interactions
Results of preliminary studies in humans and rats suggest that nonabsorbable antacids given concurrently with lactulose may inhibit the desired lactulose-induced drop in colonic pH. Therefore, a possible lack of desired effect of treatment should be taken into consideration before such drugs are given concomitantly with lactulose.
Carcinogenesis, Mutagenesis, Impairment of Fertility
There are no known human data on long-term potential for carcinogenicity, mutagenicity, or impairment of fertility.
There are no known animal data on long-term potential for mutagenicity.
Administration of lactulose syrup in the diet of mice for 18 months in concentrations of 3 and 10 percent (v/w) did not produce any evidence of carcinogenicity.
In studies in mice, rats, and rabbits, doses of lactulose syrup up to 6 or 12 mL/kg/day produced no deleterious effects in breeding, conception, or parturition.
Pregnancy
Teratogenic Effects
Pregnancy Category B
Reproduction studies have been performed in mice, rats, and rabbits at doses up to 3 or 6 times the usual human oral dose and have revealed no evidence of impaired fertility or harm to the fetus due to lactulose. There are, however, no adequate and well-controlled studies in pregnant women. Because animal reproduction studies are not always predictive of human response, this drug should be used during pregnancy only if clearly needed.
Nursing Mothers
It is not known whether this drug is excreted in human milk. Because many drugs are excreted in human milk, caution should be exercised when lactulose is administered to a nursing woman.
Pediatric Use
Safety and effectiveness in pediatric patients have not been established.

ADVERSE REACTIONS

Precise frequency data are not available.
Initial dosing may produce flatulence and intestinal cramps, which are usually transient. Excessive dosage can lead to diarrhea with potential complications such as loss of fluids, hypokalemia, and hypernatremia.
Nausea and vomiting have been reported.

OVERDOSAGE

Signs and Symptoms
There have been no reports of accidental overdosage. In the event of overdosage, it is expected that diarrhea and abdominal cramps would be the major symptoms. Medication should be terminated.
Oral LD_{50}
The acute oral LD_{50} of the drug is 48.8 mL/kg in mice and greater than 30 mL/kg in rats.
Dialysis
Dialysis data are not available for lactulose. Its molecular similarity to sucrose, however, would suggest that it should be dialyzable.

DOSAGE AND ADMINISTRATION

The usual adult dosage is 10 g to 20 g of lactulose daily. The dose may be increased to 40 g daily if necessary. Twenty-four to forty-eight hours may be required to produce a normal bowel movement.
DIRECTIONS FOR PREPARATION
Dissolve contents of packet in half a glass (4 ounces) of water.
When Lactulose for Oral Solution is dissolved in water, the resulting solution may be colorless to a slightly pale yellow color.

HOW SUPPLIED

KRISTALOSE™ (Lactulose) for Oral Solution is available in 10 g and 20 g single dose packets in cartons of 30.

NDC 62794-501-17
Single dose packet of 10 g
NDC 62794-502-17
Single dose packet of 20 g

STORE AT ROOM TEMPERATURE, 15°–30°C (59°–86°F).
CAUTION: Federal law prohibits dispensing without prescription.
Distributed by
BERTEK PHARMACEUTICALS INC.
Sugar Land, TX 77478
Manufactured by
Inalco S.p.A.
Milan, Italy

BKKRST:R1
REVISED OCTOBER 1997

MAXZIDE® and MAXZIDE®-25 MG TABLETS ℞

[*măx 'zīde*]
BRAND OF (TRIAMTERENE AND HYDROCHLOROTHIAZIDE)

DESCRIPTION

MAXZIDE® (triamterene and hydrochlorothiazide) combines triamterene, a potassium-conserving diuretic, with the natriuretic agent, hydrochlorothiazide.
Each MAXZIDE® tablet contains:

Triamterene, USP .... 75 mg
Hydrochlorothiazide, USP .... 50 mg

Each MAXZIDE®-25 MG tablet contains:

Triamterene, USP .... 37.5 mg
Hydrochlorothiazide, USP .... 25 mg

MAXZIDE® and MAXZIDE®-25 MG tablets for oral administration contain the following inactive ingredients: Colloidal Silicon Dioxide, Croscarmellose Sodium, Magnesium Stearate, Microcrystalline Cellulose, Powdered Cellulose, Sodium Lauryl Sulfate and D&C Yellow #10. MAXZIDE®-25 MG tablets also contain FD&C Blue #1.
Triamterene is 2,4,7–triamino-6-phenylpteridine. Triamterene is practically insoluble in water, benzene, chloroform, ether and dilute alkali hydroxides. It is soluble in formic acid and sparingly soluble in methoxyethanol. Triamterene is very slightly soluble in acetic acid, alcohol and dilute mineral acids. Its molecular weight is 253.27. Its structural formula is:

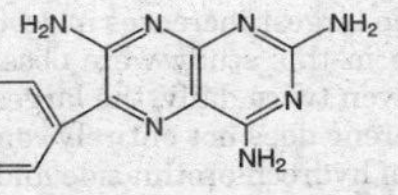

H_2N N N NH_2 N N NH_2

Continued on next page

Maxzide/Maxzide-25 —Cont.

Hydrochlorothiazide is 6-chloro-3,4-dihydro-2*H*-1,2,4, benzothiadiazine-7-sulfonamide 1,1–dioxide. Hydrochlorothiazide is slightly soluble in water and freely soluble in sodium hydroxide solution, n-butylamine and dimethylformamide. It is sparingly soluble in methanol and insoluble in ether, chloroform and dilute mineral acids. Its molecular weight is 297.73. Its structural formula is:

CLINICAL PHARMACOLOGY

MAXZIDE (triamterene and hydrochlorothiazide) is a diuretic, antihypertensive drug product, principally due to its hydrochlorothiazide component; the triamterene component of MAXZIDE reduces the excessive potassium loss which may occur with hydrochlorothiazide use.

Hydrochlorothiazide

Hydrochlorothiazide is a diuretic and antihypertensive agent. It blocks the renal tubular absorption of sodium and chloride ions. This natriuresis and diuresis is accomplished by a secondary loss of potassium and bicarbonate. Onset of hydrochlorothiazide's diuretic effect occurs within two hours and the peak action takes place in four hours. Diuretic activity persists for approximately six to twelve hours.

The exact mechanism of hydrochlorothiazide's antihypertensive action is not known although it may relate to the excretion and redistribution of body sodium. Hydrochlorothiazide does not affect normal blood pressure.

Following oral administration, peak hydrochlorothiazide plasma levels are attained in approximately two hours. It is excreted rapidly and unchanged in the urine.

Well-controlled studies have demonstrated that doses of hydrochlorothiazide as low as 25 mg given once daily are effective in treating hypertension, but the dose response has not been clearly established.

Triamterene

Triamterene is a potassium-conserving (antikaliuretic) diuretic with relatively weak natriuretic properties. It exerts its diuretic effect on the distal renal tubule to inhibit the reabsorption of sodium in exchange for potassium and hydrogen. With this action, triamterene increases sodium excretion and reduces the excessive loss of potassium and hydrogen associated with hydrochlorothiazide. Triamterene is not a competitive antagonist of the mineralocorticoids and its potassium-conserving effect is observed in patients with Addison's disease, ie, without aldosterone. Triamterene's onset and duration of activity is similar to hydrochlorothiazide. No predictable antihypertensive effect has been demonstrated with triamterene.

Triamterene is rapidly absorbed following oral administration. Peak plasma levels are achieved within one hour after dosing. Triamterene is primarily metabolized to the sulfate conjugate of hydroxytriamterene. Both the plasma and urine levels of this metabolite greatly exceed triamterene levels.

The amount of triamterene added to 50 mg of hydrochlorothiazide in MAXZIDE tablets was determined from steady-state dose response evaluations in which various doses of liquid preparations of triamterene were administered to hypertensive persons who developed hypokalemia with hydrochlorothiazide (50 mg given once daily). Single daily doses of 75 mg triamterene resulted in greater increases in serum potassium than lower doses (25 mg and 50 mg), while doses greater than 75 mg of triamterene resulted in no additional levels in serum potassium levels. The amount of triamterene added to the 25 mg of hydrochlorothiazide in MAXZIDE-25 MG tablets was also determined from steady-state dose response evaluations in which various doses of liquid preparations of triamterene were administered to hypertensive persons who developed hypokalemia with hydrochlorothiazide (25 mg given once daily). Single daily doses of 37.5 mg triamterene resulted in greater increases in serum potassium than a lower dose (25 mg), while doses greater than 37.5 mg of triamterene, ie, 75 and 100 mg, resulted in no additional elevations in serum potassium levels. The dose response relationship of triamterene was also evaluated in patients rendered hypokalemic by hydrochlorothiazide given 25 mg twice daily. Triamterene given twice daily increased serum potassium levels in a dose-related fashion. However, the combination of triamterene and hydrochlorothiazide given twice daily also appeared to produce an increased frequency of elevation in serum BUN and creatinine levels. The largest increases in serum potassium, BUN and creatinine in this study were observed with 50 mg of triamterene given twice daily, the largest dose tested. Ordinarily, triamterene does not entirely compensate for the kaliuretic effect of hydrochlorothiazide and some patients may remain hypokalemic while receiving triamterene and hydrochlorothiazide. In some individuals, however, it may induce hyperkalemia (see WARNINGS).

The triamterene and hydrochlorothiazide components of MAXZIDE and MAXZIDE-25 MG are well absorbed and are bioequivalent to liquid preparations of the individual components administered orally. Food does not influence the absorption of triamterene or hydrochlorothiazide from MAXZIDE or MAXZIDE-25 MG tablets. The hydrochlorothiazide components of MAXZIDE is bioequivalent to single entity hydrochlorothiazide tablet formulations.

INDICATIONS AND USAGE

This fixed combination drug is not indicated for the initial therapy of edema or hypertension except in individuals in whom the development of hypokalemia cannot be risked.

1. MAXZIDE (triamterene and hydrochlorothiazide) is indicated for the treatment of hypertension or edema in patients who develop hypokalemia on hydrochlorothiazide alone.
2. MAXZIDE is also indicated for those patients who require a thiazide diuretic and in whom the development of hypokalemia cannot be risked (eg, patients on concomitant digitalis preparations, or with a history of cardiac arryhthmias, etc.).

MAXZIDE may be used alone or in combination with other antihypertensive drugs, such as beta-blockers. Since MAXZIDE (triamterene and hydrochlorothiazide) may enhance the actions of these drugs, dosage adjustments may be necessary.

Usage in Pregnancy

The routine use of diuretics in an otherwise healthy woman is inappropriate and exposes mother and fetus to unnecessary hazard. Diuretics do not prevent development of toxemia of pregnancy, and there is no satisfactory evidence that they are useful in the treatment of developed toxemia. Edema during pregnancy may arise from pathological causes or from the physiologic and mechanical consequences of pregnancy. Thiazides are indicated in pregnancy when edema is due to pathologic causes, just as they are in absence of pregnancy. Dependent edema in pregnancy, resulting from restriction of venous return by the expanded uterus, is properly treated through elevation of the lower extremities and use of support hose; use of diuretics to lower intravascular volume in this case is illogical and unnecessary. There is hypervolemia during normal pregnancy which is harmful to neither the fetus nor the mother (in the absence of cardiovascular disease), but which is associated with edema, including generalized edema, in the majority of pregnant women. If this edema produces discomfort, increased recumbency will often provide relief. In rare instances, this edema may cause extreme discomfort which is not relieved by rest. In these cases, a short course of diuretics may provide relief and may be appropriate.

CONTRAINDICATIONS

Hyperkalemia

MAXZIDE (triamterene and hydrochlorothiazide) should not be used in the presence of elevated serum potassium levels (greater than or equal to 5.5 mEq/liter). If hyperkalemia develops, this drug should be discontinued and a thiazide alone should be substituted.

Antikaliuretic Therapy or Potassium Supplementation

MAXZIDE should not be given to patients receiving other potassium-conserving agents such as spironolactone, amiloride HCl or other formulations containing triamterene. Concomitant potassium supplementation in the form of medication, potassium-containing salt substitute or potassium-enriched diets should also not be used.

Impaired Renal Function

MAXZIDE is contraindicated in patients with anuria, acute and chronic renal insufficiency or significant renal impairment.

Hypersensitivity

MAXZIDE should not be used in patients who are hypersensitive to triamterene or hydrochlorothiazide or other sulfonamide-derived drugs.

WARNINGS

Hyperkalemia

Abnormal elevation of serum potassium levels (greater than or equal to 5.5 mEq/liter) can occur with all potassium-conserving diuretic combinations, including MAXZIDE. Hyperkalemia is more likely to occur in patients with renal impairment, diabetes (even without evidence of renal impairment), or elderly or severely ill patients. Since uncorrected hyperkalemia may be fatal, serum potassium levels must be monitored at frequent intervals especially in patients first receiving MAXZIDE, when dosages are changed or with any illness that may influence renal function.

If hyperkalemia is suspected, (warning signs include paresthesias, muscular weakness, fatigue, flaccid paralysis of the extremities, bradycardia and shock) an electrocardiogram (ECG) should be obtained. However, it is important to monitor serum potassium levels because mild hyperkalemia may not be associated with ECG changes.

If hyperkalemia is present, MAXZIDE (triamterene and hydrochlorothiazide) should be discontinued immediately and a thiazide alone should be substituted. If the serum potassium exceeds 6.5 mEq/liter, more vigorous therapy is required. The clinical situation dictates the procedures to be employed. These include the intravenous administration of calcium chloride solution, sodium bicarbonate solution and/or the oral or parenteral administration of glucose with a rapid-acting insulin preparation. Cationic exchange resins such as sodium polystyrene sulfonate may be orally or rectally administered. Persistent hyperkalemia may require dialysis.

The development of hyperkalemia associated with potassium-sparing diuretics is accentuated in the presence of renal impairment (see CONTRAINDICATIONS). Patients with mild renal functional impairment should not receive this drug without frequent and continuing monitoring of serum electrolytes. Cumulative drug effects may be observed in patients with impaired renal function. The renal clearances of hydrochlorothiazide and the pharmacologically active metabolite of triamterene, the sulfate ester of hydroxytriamterene, have been shown to be reduced and the plasma levels increased following MAXZIDE (triamterene and hydrochlorothiazide) administration to elderly patients and patients with impaired renal function.

Hyperkalemia has been reported in diabetic patients with the use of potassium-conserving agents even in the absence of apparent renal impairment. Accordingly, MAXZIDE (triamterene and hydrochlorothiazide) should be avoided in diabetic patients. If it is employed, serum electrolytes must be frequently monitored.

Because of the potassium-sparing properties of angiotensin-converting enzyme (ACE) inhibitors, MAXZIDE should be used cautiously, if at all, with these agents (see PRECAUTIONS, Drug Interactions).

Metabolic or Respiratory Acidosis

Potassium-conserving therapy should also be avoided in severely ill patients in whom respiratory or metabolic acidosis may occur. Acidosis may be associated with rapid elevations in serum potassium levels. If MAXZIDE is employed, frequent evaluations of acid/base balance and serum electrolytes are necessary.

PRECAUTIONS

General

Electrolyte Imbalance and BUN Increases

Patients receiving MAXZIDE (triamterene and hydrochlorothiazide) should be carefully monitored for fluid or electrolyte imbalances, ie, hyponatremia, hypochloremic alkalosis, hypokalemia and hypomagnesemia. Determination of serum electrolytes to detect possible electrolyte imbalance should be performed at appropriate intervals. Serum and urine electrolyte determinations are especially important and should be frequently performed when the patient is vomiting or receiving parenteral fluids. Warning signs or symptoms of fluid and electrolyte imbalance include: dryness of mouth, thirst, weakness, lethargy, drowsiness, restlessness, muscle pains or cramps, muscular fatigue, hypotension, oliguria, tachycardia and gastrointestinal disturbances such as nausea and vomiting.

Any chloride deficit during thiazide therapy is generally mild and usually does not require any specific treatment except under extraordinary circumstances (as in liver disease or renal disease). Dilutional hyponatremia may occur in edematous patients in hot weather; appropriate therapy is water restriction, rather than administration of salt, except in rare instances when the hyponatremia is life threatening. In actual salt depletion, appropriate replacement is the therapy of choice.

Hypokalemia may develop with thiazide therapy, especially with brisk diuresis, when severe cirrhosis is present, or during concomitant use of corticosteroids, ACTH, amphotericin B or after prolonged thiazide therapy. However, hypokalemia of this type is usually prevented by the triamterene component of MAXZIDE (triamterene and hydrochlorothiazide).

Interference with adequate oral electrolyte intake will also contribute to hypokalemia. Hypokalemia can sensitize or exaggerate the response of the heart to the toxic effects of digitalis (eg, increased ventricular irritability).

MAXZIDE (triamterene and hydrochlorothiazide) may produce an elevated blood urea nitrogen level (BUN), creatinine level or both. This is probably not the result of renal toxicity but is secondary to a reversible reduction of the glomerular filtration rate or a depletion of the intravascular fluid volume. Elevations in BUN and creatinine levels may be more frequent in patients receiving divided dose diuretic therapy. Periodic BUN and creatinine determinations should be made especially in elderly patients, patients with suspected or confirmed hepatic disease or renal insufficiencies. If azotemia increases, MAXZIDE (triamterene and hydrochlorothiazide) should be discontinued.

Hepatic Coma

MAXZIDE should be used with caution in patients with impaired hepatic function or progressive liver disease, since minor alterations of fluid and electrolyte balance may precipitate hepatic coma.

Renal Stones

Triamterene has been reported in renal stones in association with other calculus components. MAXZIDE should be used with caution in patients with histories of renal lithiasis.

Folic Acid Deficiency

Triamterene is a weak folic acid antagonist and may contribute to the appearance of megaloblastosis in instances where folic acid stores are decreased. In such patients, periodic blood elevations are recommended.

Hyperuricemia

Hyperuricemia may occur or acute gout may be precipitated in certain patients receiving thiazide therapy.

Metabolic and Endocrine Effects

The thiazides may decrease serum PBI levels without signs of thyroid disturbance.

Calcium excretion is decreased by thiazides. Pathological changes in the parathyroid gland with hypercalcemia and hypophosphatemia have been observed in a few patients on prolonged thiazide therapy. The common complications of hyperparathyroidism such as renal lithiasis, bone resorption, and peptic ulceration have not been seen. Thiazides should be discontinued before carrying out tests for parathyroid function.
Insulin requirements in diabetic patients may be increased, decreased or unchanged. Diabetes mellitus which has been latent may become manifest during thiazide administration.

Hypersensitivity
Sensitivity reactions to thiazides may occur in patients with or without a history of allergy or bronchial asthma.
Possible exacerbation or activation of systemic lupus erythematosus by thiazides has been reported.

Drug Interactions
Thiazides may add to or potentiate the action of other antihypertensive drugs.
The thiazides may decrease arterial responsiveness to norepinephrine. This diminution is not sufficient to preclude effectiveness of the pressor agent for therapeutic use. Thiazides have also been shown to increase the responsiveness to tubocurarine.
Lithium generally should not be given with diuretics because they reduce its renal clearance and add a high risk of lithium toxicity. Refer to the package insert on lithium before use of such concomitant therapy.
Acute renal failure has been reported in a few patients receiving indomethacin and formulations containing triamterene and hydrochlorothiazide. Caution is therefore advised when administering nonsteroidal anti-inflammatory agents with MAXZIDE (triamterene and hydrochlorothiazide).
Potassium-sparing agents should be used very cautiously, if at all, in conjunction with angiotensin-converting enzyme (ACE) inhibitors due to a greatly increased risk of hyperkalemia. Serum potassium should be monitored frequently.

Drug/Laboratory Test Interactions
Triamterene and quinidine have similar fluorescence spectra; thus MAXZIDE (triamterene and hydrochlorothiazide) may interfere with the measurement of quinidine.

Carcinogenesis, Mutagenesis, Impairment of Fertility
Studies have not been performed to evaluate the mutagenic or carcinogenic potential of MAXZIDE.

Hydrochlorothiazide
Two-year feeding studies in mice and rats conducted under the auspices of the National Toxicology Program (NTP) uncovered no evidence of a carcinogenic potential of hydrochlorothiazide in female mice (at doses of up to approximately 600 mg/kg/day) or in male and female rats (at doses of up to approximately 100 mg/kg/day). The NTP, however, found equivocal evidence for hepatocarcinogenicity in male mice.
Hydrochlorothiazide was not genotoxic in *in vitro* assays using strains TA 98, TA 100, TA 1535, TA 1537, and TA 1538 of *Salmonella typhimurium* (Ames assay) and in the Chinese Hamster Ovary (CHO) test for chromosomal aberrations, or in *in vivo* assays using mouse germinal cell chromosomes, Chinese hamster bone marrow chromosomes, and the *Drosophila* sex-linked recessive lethal trait gene. Positive test results were obtained only in the *in vitro* CHO Sister Chromatid Exchange (clastogenicity) and in the Mouse Lymphoma Cell (mutagenicity) assays, using concentrations of hydrochlorothiazide from 43 to 1300 μg/mL, and in the *Aspergillus nidulans* non-disjunction assay at an unspecified concentration.
Hydrochlorothiazide had no adverse effects on the fertility of mice and rats of either sex in studies wherein these species were exposed, via their diet, to doses of up to 100 and 4 mg/kg, respectively, prior to conception and throughout gestation.

Triamterene
Studies have not been performed to determine the carcinogenic or mutagenic potential of triamterene. Reproductive studies have been performed in rats at doses up to 30 times the human dose and have revealed no evidence of impaired fertility.

Pregnancy Category C
Teratogenic Effects—Animal reproduction studies have not been conducted with MAXZIDE. It is also not known if MAXZIDE can cause fetal harm when administered to a pregnant woman.

Hydrochlorothiazide
Studies in which hydrochlorothiazide was orally administered to pregnant mice and rats during their respective periods of major organogenesis at doses up to 3000 and 1000 mg hydrochlorothiazide/kg, respectively, provided no evidence of harm to the fetus. There are, however, no adequate and well-controlled studies in pregnant women.

Triamterene
Reproduction studies have been performed in rats at doses up to 30 times the human dose and have revealed no evidence of harm to the fetus due to triamterene. There are, however, no adequate and well-controlled studies in pregnant women.
Because animal reproduction studies are not always predictive of human response, MAXZIDE should be used during pregnancy only if clearly needed.

Nonteratogenic Effects
Thiazides and triamterene cross the placental barrier and appear in cord blood of animals. The use of MAXZIDE in pregnant women requires that the anticipated benefit be weighed against possible hazards to the fetus. These hazards include fetal or neonatal jaundice, thrombocytopenia following thiazides and possible other adverse reactions that have occurred in the adults.

Nursing Mothers
Thiazides appear and triamterene may appear in breast milk. If use of the drug product is deemed essential the patient should stop nursing.

Pediatric Use
The safety and effectiveness of MAXZIDE (triamterene and hydrochlorothiazide) in children has not been established.

ADVERSE REACTIONS

Side effects observed in association with the use of MAXZIDE, other combination products containing triamterene/hydrochlorothiazide, and products containing triamterene or hydrochlorothiazide include the following:
Gastrointestinal: jaundice (intrahepatic cholestatic jaundice), pancreatitis, nausea, appetite disturbance, taste alteration, vomiting, diarrhea, constipation, anorexia, gastric irritation, cramping.
Central Nervous System: drowsiness and fatigue, insomnia, headache, dizziness, dry mouth, depression, anxiety, vertigo, restlessness, paresthesias.
Cardiovascular: tachycardia, shortness of breath and chest pain, orthostatic hypotension (may be aggravated by alcohol, barbiturates or narcotics).
Renal: acute renal failure, acute interstitial nephritis, renal stones composed of triamterene in association with other calculus materials, urine discoloration.
Hematologic: leukopenia, agranulocytosis thrombocytopenia, aplastic anemia, hemolytic anemia and megaloblastosis.
Ophthalmic: xanthopsia, transient blurred vision.
Hypersensitivity: anaphylaxis, photosensitivity, rash, urticaria, purpura, necrotizing angiitis (vasculitis, cutaneous vasculitis), fever, respiratory distress including pneumonitis.
Other: muscle cramps and weakness, decreased sexual performance and sialadenitis.
Whenever adverse reactions are moderate to severe, therapy should be reduced or withdrawn.
Altered Laboratory Findings:
Serum Electrolytes: hyperkalemia, hypokalemia, hyponatremia, hypomagnesemia, hypochloremia (see WARNINGS, PRECAUTIONS).
Creatinine, Blood Urea Nitrogen: Reversible elevations in BUN and serum creatinine have been observed in hypertensive patients treated with MAXZIDE.
Glucose: hyperglycemia, glycosuria and diabetes mellitus (see PRECAUTIONS).
Serum Uric Acid, PBI and Calcium: (see PRECAUTIONS).
Other: Elevated liver enzymes have been reported in patients receiving MAXZIDE.

OVERDOSAGE

No specific data are available regarding MAXZIDE (triamterene and hydrochlorothiazide) overdosage in humans and no specific antidote is available.
Fluid and electrolyte imbalances are the most important concern. Excessive doses of the triamterene component may elicit hyperkalemia, dehydration, nausea, vomiting and weakness and possibly hypotension. Overdosing with hydrochlorothiazide has been associated with hypokalemia, hypochloremia, hyponatremia, dehydration, lethargy (may progress to coma) and gastrointestinal irritation. Treatment is symptomatic and supportive. Therapy with MAXZIDE (triamterene and hydrochlorothiazide) should be discontinued. Induce emesis or institute gastric lavage. Monitor serum electrolyte levels and fluid balance. Institute supportive measures as required to maintain hydration, electrolyte balance, respiratory, cardiovascular and renal functions.

DOSAGE AND ADMINISTRATION

The usual dose of MAXZIDE-25 MG is one or two tablets daily, given as a single dose, with appropriate monitoring of serum potassium (see WARNINGS). The usual dose of MAXZIDE is one tablet daily, with appropriate monitoring of serum potassium (see WARNINGS). There is no experience with the use of more than one MAXZIDE tablet daily or more than two MAXZIDE-25 MG tablets daily. Clinical experience with the administration of two MAXZIDE-25 MG tablets daily in divided doses (rather than as a single dose) suggests an increased risk of electrolyte imbalance and renal dysfunction.
Patients receiving 50 mg of hydrochlorothiazide who become hypokalemic may be transferred to MAXZIDE (triamterene and hydrochlorothiazide) directly. Patients receiving 25 mg hydrochlorothiazide who become hypokalemic may be transferred to MAXZIDE-25 MG (37.5 mg triamterene/25 mg hydrochlorothiazide) directly.
In patients requiring hydrochlorothiazide therapy and in whom hypokalemia cannot be risked therapy may be initiated with MAXZIDE-25 MG. If an optimal blood pressure response is not obtained with MAXZIDE-25 MG, the dose should be increased to two MAXZIDE-25 MG tablets daily as a single dose, or one MAXZIDE tablet daily. If blood pressure still is not controlled, another antihypertensive agent may be added (see PRECAUTIONS, Drug Interactions).
Clinical studies have shown that patients taking less bioavailable formulations of triamterene and hydrochlorothiazide in daily doses of 25–50 mg hydrochlorothiazide and 50–100 mg triamterene may be safely changed to one MAXZIDE-25 MG tablet daily. All patients changed from less bioavailable formulations to MAXZIDE should be monitored clinically for serum potassium after the transfer.

HOW SUPPLIED

MAXZIDE® (triamterene and hydrochlorothiazide) tablets are bowtie-shaped, flat-faced beveled, light yellow tablets, engraved with MAXZIDE on one side and scored on the other with B on the left and M8 on the right of the score. Each tablet contains 75 mg of triamterene, USP and 50 mg of hydrochlorothiazide, USP. They are supplied as follows:
NDC 62794-460-01—Bottle of 100 with CRC
NDC 62794-460-05—Bottle of 500
NDC 62794-460-88—Unit Dose 10 × 10s
MAXZIDE-25 MG (triamterene and hydrochlorothiazide) tablets are bowtie-shaped, flat-faced beveled, light green tablets, engraved with MAXZIDE on one side and scored on the other with B on the left and M9 on the right of the score. Each tablet contains 37.5 mg of triamterene, USP and 25 mg of hydrochlorothiazide, USP. They are supplied as follows:
NDC 62794-464-01—Bottle of 100 with CRC
NDC 62794-464-05—Bottle of 500
NDC 62794-464-88—Unit Dose 10 × 10s
Store at Controlled Room Temperature 15–30°C (59–86°F).
Protect from Light.
Dispense in a tight, light-resistant, child-resistant container.
BERTEK PHARMACEUTICALS INC.
Sugar Land, TX 77478
REVISED SEPTEMBER 1996 BKMAX:R3

Shown in Product Identification Guide, page 308

MENTAX® ℞

[mĕn-tax]
(butenafine HCl cream)
Cream, 1%
Rx only

CAUTION: Federal (USA) law prohibits dispensing without a prescription.

DESCRIPTION

Mentax® Cream, 1%, contains the synthetic antifungal agent, butenafine hydrochloride. Butenafine is a member of the class of antifungal compounds known as benzylamines which are structurally related to the allylamines.
Butenafine HCl is designated chemically as *N*-4-*tert*-butylbenzyl-*N*-methyl-1-naphthalenemethylamine hydrochloride. The compound has the empirical formula $C_{23}H_{27}N \bullet HCl$, a molecular weight of 353.93, and the following structural formula:

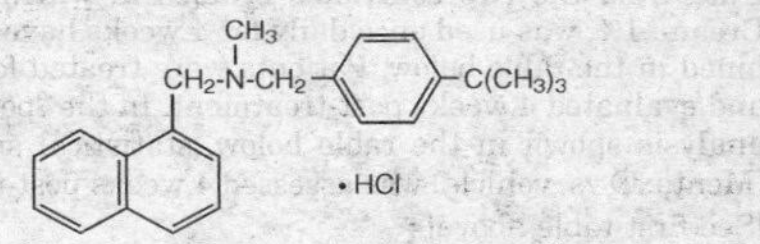

Butenafine HCl is a white, odorless, crystalline powder. It is freely soluble in methanol, ethanol, and chloroform, and slightly soluble in water. Each gram of Mentax® Cream, 1%, contains 10 mg of butenafine HCl in a white cream base of purified water USP, propylene glycol dicaprylate, glycerin USP, cetyl alcohol NF, glyceryl monostearate SE, white petrolatum USP, stearic acid NF, polyoxyethylene (23) cetyl ether, benzyl alcohol NF, diethanolamine NF, and sodium benzoate NF.

CLINICAL PHARMACOLOGY

Mechanism of Action
Butenafine HCl is a benzylamine derivative with a mode of action similar to that of the allylamine class of antifungal drugs. Butenafine HCl is hypothesized to act by inhibiting the epoxidation of squalene, thus blocking the biosynthesis of ergosterol, an essential component of fungal cell membranes. The benzylamine derivatives, like the allylamines, act at an earlier step in the ergosterol biosynthesis pathway than the azole class of antifungal drugs. Depending on the concentration of the drug and the fungal species tested, butenafine HCl may be fungicidal *in vitro*. However, the clinical significance of these *in vitro* data is unknown.

Pharmacokinetics
In one study conducted in healthy subjects for 14 days, 6 grams of Mentax® Cream, 1%, was applied once daily to the dorsal skin (3,000 cm^2) of 7 subjects, and 20 grams of the cream was applied once daily to the arms, trunk and groin areas (10,000 cm^2) of another 12 subjects. After 14 days of topical applications, the 6-gram dose group yielded a mean peak plasma butenafine HCl concentration, Cmax, of 1.4 ± 0.8 ng/mL, occurring at a mean time to the peak plasma concentration, Tmax, of 15 ± 8 hours, and a mean area under the plasma concentration-time curve, $AUC_{0-24\ hrs}$ of 23.9 ± 11.3 ng-hr/mL. For the 20-gram dose group, the mean Cmax was 5.0 ± 2.0 ng/mL, occurring at a mean Tmax of 6 ± 6 hours, and the mean $AUC_{0-24\ hrs}$ was 87.8 ± 45.3 ng-hr/mL. A biphasic decline of plasma butenafine HCl concentrations was observed with the half-lives estimated to be 35 hours and > 150 hours, respectively. At 72 hours after the last dose application, the mean plasma concentrations de-

Continued on next page

Mentax—Cont.

creased to 0.3 ± 0.2 ng/mL for the 6-gram dose group and 1.1 ± 0.9 ng/mL for the 20-gram dose group. Low levels of butenafine HCl remained in the plasma 7 days after the last dose application (mean: 0.1 ± 0.2 ng/mL for the 6-gram dose group, and 0.7 ± 0.5 ng/mL for the 20-gram dose group). The total amount (or % dose) of butenafine HCl absorbed through the skin into the systemic circulation has not been quantitated. It was determined that the primary metabolite in urine was formed through hydroxylation at the terminal *t*-butyl side-chain.

In 11 patients with tinea pedis, Mentax® Cream, 1%, was applied by the patients to cover the affected and immediately surrounding skin area once daily for 4 weeks, and a single blood sample was collected between 10 and 20 hours following dosing at 1, 2 and 4 weeks after treatment. The plasma butenafine HCl concentration ranged from undetectable to 0.3 ng/mL.

In 24 patients with tinea cruris, Mentax® Cream, 1 %, was applied by the patients to cover the affected and immediately surrounding skin area once daily for 2 weeks (mean average daily dose: 1.3 ± 0.2 g). A single blood sample was collected between 0.5 and 65 hours after the last dose, and the plasma butenafine HCl concentration ranged from undetectable to 2.52 ng/mL (mean ± SD: 0.91 ± 0.15 ng/mL). Four weeks after cessation of treatment, the plasma butenafine HCl concentration ranged from undetectable to 0.28 ng/mL.

Microbiology

Butenafine HCl has been shown to be active against most strains of the following microorganisms, both *in vitro* and in clinical infections as described in the INDICATIONS AND USAGE section:

Epidermophyton floccosum
Trichophyton mentagrophytes
Trichophyton rubrum
Trichophyton tonsurans

CLINICAL STUDIES

Interdigital Tinea Pedis

Once Daily Four Week Dosing

In the following data presentations, patients with interdigital tinea pedis in the absence of moccasin-type tinea pedis and onychomycosis were studied. The term **"Mycological Cure"** is defined as both negative KOH and culture. The term **"Effective Treatment"** refers to patients who had a "Mycological Cure" **and** an Investigator's Global of either "Excellent" (80% to 99% improvement) **or** "Cleared" (100% improvement). The term **"Overall Cure"** refers to patients who had both a "Mycological Cure" **and** an Investigator's Global Assessment of "Cleared" (100% improvement).

Data from the two controlled studies in which Mentax® Cream, 1%, was used once daily for 4 weeks have been combined in the table below. Patients were treated for 4 weeks and evaluated 4 weeks post-treatment. In the "per protocol" analysis shown in the table below, statistical significance (Mentax® vs. vehicle) was assessed 4 weeks post-treatment.

[See first table above]

Twice Daily One Week Dosing

In the following data presentations, patients with interdigital tinea pedis in the absence of moccasin-type tinea pedis were studied. Patients with concurrent onychomycosis were not excluded. The term **"Mycological Cure"** is defined as both negative KOH and culture. The term **"Effective Treatment"** refers to patients who had a "Mycological Cure" **and** an Investigator's Global of either "Excellent" (90% to 99% improvement) **or** "Cleared" (100% improvement). The term **"Overall Cure"** refers to patients who had both a "Mycological Cure" **and** an Investigator's Global Assessment of "Cleared" (100% improvement).

Data from the two controlled studies in which Mentax® Cream, 1%, was used twice daily for 1 week have been combined in the table below. Patients were treated for 1 week and evaluated 5 weeks post-treatment. In the "modified-intent-to-treat" analysis shown in the table below, statistical significance (Mentax® vs. vehicle) was assessed 5 weeks post-treatment.

[See second table above]

Tinea Corporis and Tinea Cruris

In the following data presentations, patients with tinea corporis or tinea cruris were studied. The term **"Mycological Cure"** is defined as both negative KOH and culture. The term **"Effective Treatment"** refers to patients who had a "Mycological Cure" **and** an Investigator's Global of either "Excellent" (90% to 99% improvement) **or** "Cleared" (100% improvement). The term **"Overall Cure"** refers to patients who had both a "Mycological Cure" **and** an Investigator's Global Assessment of "Cleared" (100% improvement).

Separate studies compared Mentax® Cream to vehicle applied once daily for 2 weeks in the treatment of tinea corporis and tinea cruris. Patients were treated for 2 weeks and evaluated 4 weeks post-treatment. All subjects with a positive baseline exam (including positive culture and KOH) and who were dispensed medication were included in the "modified intent-to-treat" analysis shown in the table below. Statistical significance (Mentax® vs. vehicle) was achieved for all patient outcome categories at Week 2 (end of treatment) and Week 6 (4 weeks post-treatment).

[See third table above]
[See fourth table above]

Interdigital Tinea Pedis: 4 Week Dosing Regimen

Patient Outcome Category	WEEK 4 (End of Treatment)		WEEK 8 (4 Weeks Post-Treatment)	
	Butenafine	Vehicle	Butenafine	Vehicle
Mycological Cure	89% (83/93)	57% (51/90)	90% (66/73)	38% (25/66)
Effective Treatment	57% (53/93)	28% (25/90)	74% (54/73)	26% (17/66)
Overall Cure	15% (14/93)	8% (7/90)	25% (18/73)	9% (6/66)

Interdigital Tinea Pedis: 1 Week Dosing Regimen

Patient Outcome Category	WEEK 1 (End of Treatment)		WEEK 6 (5 Weeks Post-Treatment)	
	Butenafine	Vehicle	Butenafine	Vehicle
Mycological Cure	44% (111/253)	28% (75/265)	79% (200/253)	20% (54/265)
Effective Treatment	5% (12/253)	3% (7/265)	38% (95/253)	7% (18/265)
Overall Cure	0.4% (1/253)	0.4% (1/265)	*15% (37/253)	0.7% (2/265)

*The Overall Cure rate of 15% is calculated from a 9% rate in one trial and a 20% rate in the second trial.

Tinea Corporis

Patient Outcome Category	WEEK 2 (End of Treatment)		WEEK 6 (4 Weeks Post-Treatment)	
	Butenafine	Vehicle	Butenafine	Vehicle
Mycological Cure	88% (37/42)	28% (10/36)	88% (37/42)	17% (6/36)
Effective Treatment	60% (25/42)	17% (6/36)	81% (34/42)	14% (5/36)
Overall Cure	31% (13/42)	3% (1/36)	67% (28/42)	14% (5/36)

Tinea Cruris

Patient Outcome Category	WEEK 2 (End of Treatment)		WEEK 6 (4 Weeks Post-Treatment)	
	Butenafine	Vehicle	Butenafine	Vehicle
Mycological Cure	78% (29/37)	11% (4/38)	81% (30/37)	13% (5/39)
Effective Treatment	57% (21/37)	8% (3/39)	73% (27/37)	5% (2/39)
Overall cure	32% (12/37)	8% (3/39)	62% (23/37)	3% (1/39)

INDICATIONS AND USAGE

Mentax® (butenafine HCl cream) Cream, 1%, is indicated for the topical treatment of the following superficial dermatophytoses: interdigital tinea pedis (athlete's foot), tinea corporis (ringworm) and tinea cruris (jock itch) due to *E. floccosum, T. mentagrophytes, T. rubrum,* and *T. tonsurans.* Butenafine HCl cream was not studied in immunocompromised patients. (See DOSAGE AND ADMINISTRATION).

CONTRAINDICATIONS

Mentax® (butenafine HCl cream) Cream, 1%, is contraindicated in individuals who have known or suspected sensitivity to Mentax® Cream, 1%, or any of its components.

WARNINGS

Mentax® (butenafine HCl cream) Cream, 1%, is not for ophthalmic, oral, or intravaginal use.

PRECAUTIONS

General

Mentax® Cream, 1%, is for external use only. If irritation or sensitivity develops with the use of Mentax® Cream, 1%, treatment should be discontinued and appropriate therapy instituted. Diagnosis of the disease should be confirmed either by direct microscopic examination of infected superficial epidermal tissue in a solution of potassium hydroxide or by culture on an appropriate medium.

Patients who are known to be sensitive to allylamine antifungals should use Mentax® (butenafine HCl cream) Cream, 1%, with caution, since cross-reactivity may occur. Use Mentax® Cream, 1%, as directed by the physician, and avoid contact with the eyes, nose, and mouth, and other mucous membranes.

Information for Patients

The patient should be instructed to:

1. Use Mentax® Cream, 1%, as directed by the physician. The hands should be washed after applying the medication to the affected area(s). Avoid contact with the eyes, nose, mouth, and other mucous membranes. Mentax® Cream, 1%, is for external use only.
2. Dry the affected area(s) thoroughly before application, if you wish to apply Mentax® Cream, 1%, after bathing.
3. Use the medication for the full treatment time recommended by the physician, even though symptoms may have improved. Notify the physician if there is no improvement after the end of the prescribed treatment period, or sooner, if the condition worsens (see below).
4. Inform the physician if the area of application shows signs of increased irritation, redness, itching, burning, blistering, swelling, or oozing.
5. Avoid the use of occlusive dressings unless otherwise directed by the physician.
6. Do not use this medication for any disorder other than that for which it was prescribed.

Drug Interactions

Potential drug interactions between Mentax® (butenafine HCl cream) Cream, 1%, and other drugs have not been systematically evaluated.

Carcinogenesis, Mutagenesis, Impairment of Fertility

Long-term studies to evaluate the carcinogenic potential of Mentax® Cream, 1%, have not been conducted. Two *in vitro* assays (bacterial reverse mutation test and chromosome aberration test in Chinese hamster lymphocytes) and one *in vivo* study (rat micronucleus bioassay) revealed no mutagenic or clastogenic potential for butenafine. Reproductive studies were conducted in which approximately 150 mg/m^2/day (25 mg/kg/day) of butenafine was administered subcutaneously, which is 5 times higher than the maximum recommended human topical dose (30 mg/m^2/day) for the treatment of tinea pedis, and six times higher than the anticipated maximum human topical dose (24 mg/m^2/day) for the treatment of tinea corporis or tinea cruris. At this dose in animals no adverse effects on male or female fertility were demonstrated.

Pregnancy

Teratogenic Effects: Pregnancy Category B

Subcutaneous or topical doses of butenafine at 150 to 300 mg/m^2/day (25 to 50 mg/kg/day) (equivalent to 5 to 10 times the maximum potential exposure at the recommended human topical dose for the treatment of tinea pedis, or 6 to 12 times the anticipated maximum exposure at the human topical dose for the treatment of tinea corporis or tinea cruris) during organogenesis in rats and rabbits were not teratogenic. There are, however, no adequate and well-controlled studies that have been conducted of topically-applied butenafine in pregnant women. Because animal reproduction studies are not always predictive of human response, this drug should be used during pregnancy only if clearly needed.

Nursing Mothers

It is not known if butenafine HCl is excreted in human milk. Because many drugs are excreted in human milk, caution should be exercised in prescribing Mentax® Cream, 1%, to a nursing women.

Pediatric Use

Safety and efficacy in pediatric patients below the age of 12 years have not been studied. Use of Mentax® Cream, 1%, in pediatric patients 12 to 16 years of age is supported by evidence from adequate and well-controlled studies of Mentax® Cream, 1%, in adults.

ADVERSE REACTIONS

In controlled clinical trials, 8 (approximately 1%) of 644 patients treated with Mentax® Cream, 1%, reported adverse events related to the skin. These included burning/stinging and worsening of the condition. No patient treated with Mentax® Cream, 1%, discontinued treatment due to an adverse event. In the vehicle-treated patients, two of 624 patients discontinued because of treatment site adverse events, one of which was severe burning/stinging and itching at the site of application.

In uncontrolled clinical trials, the most frequently reported adverse events in patients treated with Mentax® Cream, 1%, were: contact dermatitis, erythema, irritation, and itching, each occurring in less than 2% of patients.

OVERDOSAGE

Overdosage of butenafine HCl in humans has not been reported to date.

DOSAGE AND ADMINISTRATION

In the treatment of interdigital tinea pedis, Mentax® should be applied twice daily for 7 days OR once daily for 4 weeks (NOTE: in separate clinical trials, the 7 day dosing regimen was less efficacious than the 4 week regimen; see CLINICAL STUDIES. While the clinical significance of this difference is unknown, these data should be carefully considered before selecting the dosage regimen for patients at risk for the development of bacterial cellulitis of the lower extremity associated with interdigital cracking/fissuring).

Patients with tinea corporis or tinea cruris should apply Mentax® once daily for two weeks.

Sufficient Mentax® Cream should be applied to cover affected areas and immediately surrounding skin of patients with interdigital tinea pedis, tinea corporis, and tinea cruris. If a patient shows no clinical improvement after the treatment period, the diagnosis should be reviewed.

HOW SUPPLIED

Mentax® (butenafine HCl cream) Cream, 1%, is supplied in tubes in the following sizes:

15-gram tube (NDC 62794-151-02) 30-gram tube (NDC 62794-151-03)

STORE BETWEEN 5°C and 30°C (41° and 86°F).

Manufactured By: DPT Laboratories
San Antonio, Texas 78215

Distributed By: BERTEK PHARMACEUTICALS INC.
Morgantown WV 26505

July 1999
PN341.02H

Shown in Product Identification Guide, page 308

SULFAMYLON® CREAM ℞

Brand of MAFENIDE ACETATE CREAM, USP
Topical Antibacterial Agent for Adjunctive Therapy in Second- and Third-Degree Burns

DESCRIPTION

SULFAMYLON Cream is a soft, white, nonstaining, water-miscible, anti-infective cream for topical administration to burn wounds.

SULFAMYLON Cream spreads easily, and can be washed off readily with water. It has a slight acetic odor. Each gram of SULFAMYLON Cream contains mafenide acetate equivalent to 85 mg of the base. The cream vehicle consists of cetyl alcohol, stearyl alcohol, cetyl esters wax, polyoxyl 40 stearate, polyoxyl 8 stearate, glycerin, and water, with methylparaben, propylparaben, sodium metabisulfite, and edetate disodium as preservatives.

Chemically, mafenide acetate is α-Amino-ρ-toluenesulfonamide monoacetate and has the following structural formula:

$$H_2NO_2S-C_6H_4-CH_2NH_2 \cdot CH_3COOH$$

CLINICAL PHARMACOLOGY

SULFAMYLON Cream, applied topically, produces a marked reduction in the bacterial population present in the avascular tissues of second- and third-degree burns. Reduction in bacterial growth after application of SULFAMYLON Cream has also been reported to permit spontaneous healing of deep partial-thickness burns, and thus prevent conversion of burn wounds from partial thickness to full thickness. It should be noted, however, that delayed eschar separation has occurred in some cases.

Absorption and Metabolism. Applied topically, SULFAMYLON Cream diffuses through devascularized areas, is absorbed, and rapidly converted to a metabolite (ρ-carboxybenzenesulfonamide) which is cleared through the kidneys. SULFAMYLON is active in the presence of pus and serum, and its activity is not altered by changes in the acidity of the environment.

Antibacterial Activity. SULFAMYLON exerts bacteriostatic action against many gram-negative and gram-positive organisms, including *Pseudomonas aeruginosa* and certain strains of anaerobes.

INDICATIONS AND USAGE

SULFAMYLON Cream is a topical agent indicated for adjunctive therapy of patients with second- and third-degree burns.

CONTRAINDICATIONS

SULFAMYLON is contraindicated in patients who are hypersensitive to it. It is not known whether there is cross sensitivity to other sulfonamides.

WARNINGS

Fatal hemolytic anemia with disseminated intravascular coagulation, presumably related to a glucose-6-phosphate dehydrogenase deficiency, has been reported following therapy with SULFAMYLON Cream.

Contains sodium metabisulfite, a sulfite that may cause allergic-type reactions including anaphylactic symptoms and life-threatening or less severe asthmatic episodes in certain susceptible people. The overall prevalence of sulfite sensitivity in the general population is unknown and probably low. Sulfite sensitivity is seen more frequently in asthmatic than in nonasthmatic people.

PRECAUTIONS

SULFAMYLON and its metabolite, ρ-carboxybenzenesulfonamide, inhibit carbonic anhydrase, which may result in metabolic acidosis, usually compensated by hyperventilation. In the presence of impaired renal function, high blood levels of SULFAMYLON and its metabolite may exaggerate the carbonic anhydrase inhibition. Therefore, close monitoring of acid-base balance is necessary, particularly in patients with extensive second-degree or partial thickness burns and in those with pulmonary or renal dysfunction. Some burn patients treated with SULFAMYLON Cream have also been reported to manifest an unexplained syndrome of marked hyperventilation with resulting respiratory alkalosis (slightly alkaline blood pH, low arterial pCO_2, and decreased total CO_2); change in arterial pO_2 is variable. The etiology and significance of these findings are unknown.

Mafenide acetate cream should be used with caution in burn patients with acute renal failure.

SULFAMYLON Cream should be administered with caution to patients with history of hypersensitivity to mafenide. It is not known whether there is cross sensitivity to other sulfonamides.

Fungal colonization in and below the eschar may occur concomitantly with reduction of bacterial growth in the burn wound. However, fungal dissemination through the infected burn wound is rare.

Carcinogenesis, Mutagenesis, Impairment of Fertility. No long-term animal studies have been performed to evaluate the drug's potential in these areas.

Pregnancy Category C. Animal reproduction studies have not been conducted with SULFAMYLON. It is also not known whether SULFAMYLON can cause fetal harm when administered to a pregnant woman or can affect reproduction capacity. Therefore, the preparation is not recommended for the treatment of women of childbearing potential, unless the burned area covers more than 20% of the total body surface, or the need for the therapeutic benefit of SULFAMYLON Cream is, in the physician's judgment, greater than the possible risk to the fetus.

Nursing Mothers. It is not known whether mafenide acetate is excreted in human milk. Because many drugs are excreted in human milk and because of the potential for serious adverse reaction in nursing infants from SULFAMYLON, a decision should be made whether to discontinue nursing or to discontinue the drug, taking into account the importance of the drug to the mother.

Pediatric Use. Same as for adults. (See DOSAGE AND ADMINISTRATION.)

ADVERSE REACTIONS

It is frequently difficult to distinguish between an adverse reaction to SULFAMYLON Cream and the effect of a severe burn. A single case of bone marrow depression and a single case of an acute attack of porphyria have been reported following therapy with SULFAMYLON Cream. Fatal hemolytic anemia with disseminated intravascular coagulation, presumably related to a glucose-6-phosphate dehydrogenase deficiency, has been reported following therapy with SULFAMYLON Cream.

Dermatologic: The most frequently reported reaction was pain on application or a burning sensation. Rare occurrences are excoriation of new skin, and bleeding of skin.

Allergic: Rash, itching, facial edema, swelling, hives, blisters, erythema, and eosinophilia.

Respiratory: Tachypnea or hyperventilation, decrease in arterial pCO_2.

Metabolic: Acidosis, increase in serum chloride.

Accidental ingestion of SULFAMYLON Cream has been reported to cause diarrhea.

DOSAGE AND ADMINISTRATION

Prompt institution of appropriate measures for controlling shock and pain is of prime importance. The burn wounds are then cleansed and debrided, and SULFAMYLON Cream is applied with a sterile gloved hand. Satisfactory results can be achieved with application of the cream once or twice daily, to a thickness of approximately 1/16 inch; thicker application is not recommended. The burned areas should be covered with SULFAMYLON Cream at all times. Therefore, whenever necessary, the cream should be reapplied to any areas from which it has been removed (eg, by patient activity). The routine of administration can be accomplished in minimal time, since dressings usually are not required. If individual patient demands make them necessary, however, only a thin layer of dressing should be used.

When feasible, the patient should be bathed daily, to aid in debridement. A whirlpool bath is particularly helpful, but the patient may be bathed in bed or in a shower.

The duration of therapy with SULFAMYLON Cream depends on each patient's requirements. Treatment is usually continued until healing is progressing well or until the burn site is ready for grafting. *SULFAMYLON Cream should not be withdrawn from the therapeutic regimen while there is the possibility of infection.* However, if allergic manifestations occur during treatment with SULFAMYLON Cream, discontinuation of treatment should be considered.

If acidosis occurs and becomes difficult to control, particularly in patients with pulmonary dysfunction, discontinuing therapy with SULFAMYLON Cream for 24 to 48 hours while continuing fluid therapy may aid in restoring acid-base balance.

HOW SUPPLIED

16 ounce plastic jar (453.6 g)—NDC 0514-0101-54
Collapsible tubes of 4 ounces (113.4 g)—NDC 0514-0101-51
Collapsible tubes of 2 ounces (56.7 g)—NDC 0514-0101-50
Avoid exposure to excessive heat (temperatures above 104°F or 40°C).

Caution: U.S. Federal law prohibits dispensing without prescription.

DISTRIBUTED BY:
BERTEK PHARMACEUTICALS INC.
SUGAR LAND, TX 77478
1-888-823-7835

Revised May 1995

SULFAMYLON® ℞

[*sulfă ' mylŏn*]
(Mafenide Acetate, USP)
FOR 5% TOPICAL SOLUTION

DESCRIPTION

Mafenide acetate, USP is a synthetic antimicrobial agent designated chemically as α-amino-*p*-toluenesulfonamide monoacetate. It has the following structural formula:

$$H_2NO_2S-C_6H_4-CH_2NH_2 \cdot CH_3COOH$$

$$C_7H_{10}N_2O_2S \cdot C_2H_4O_2$$

M.W. 246.29

Mafenide acetate, USP is a white, crystalline powder which is freely soluble in water.

SULFAMYLON® For 5% Topical Solution is provided in packets containing 50 g of mafenide acetate to be reconstituted in 1000 mL of Sterile Water for Irrigation, USP or 0.9% Sodium Chloride Irrigation, USP. After mixing, the solution contains 5% w/v of mafenide acetate. The solution is an antimicrobial preparation suitable for topical administration. **The solution is not for injection.** The 5% topical solution is to be stored at room temperature, 25°–30°C (77°–86°F) and should be used within 48 hours after mixing.

CLINICAL PHARMACOLOGY

Mechanism of Action: The mechanism of action of mafenide is not known, but is different from that of the sulfonamides. Mafenide is not antagonized by pABA, serum, pus or tissue exudates, and there is no correlation between bacterial sensitivities to mafenide and to the sulfonamides. Its activity is not altered by changes in the acidity of the environment. The osmolality of the 5% topical solution is approximately 340 mOsm/kg.

Absorption and Metabolism: Applied topically, mafenide acetate diffuses through devascularized areas. Approximately 80% of a mafenide acetate dose is delivered to burned tissue over four hours following topical application of the 5% solution. Following application of mafenide acetate cream and solution, peak mafenide concentrations in human burned skin tissue occur at two and four hours, respectively. Peak tissue concentrations are similar following administration of the solution or cream. Once absorbed, mafenide is rapidly converted to an inactive metabolite (p-carboxybenzenesulfonamide) which is cleared through the kidneys. Clinical studies have shown that when applied topically to burns as an 11.2% mafenide acetate cream, blood levels of the parent drug peaked at 2-hours following application, ranging from 26 to 197 µg/mL for single doses of 14 to 77 g of mafenide acetate. Metabolite levels peaked at 3 hours, ranging from 10 to 340 µg/mL. Twenty-four hours after application, combined parent and metabolite blood levels had fallen to pretreatment levels.

Antimicrobial Activity: Mafenide acetate exerts broad bacteriostatic action against many gram-negative and gram-positive organisms, including *Pseudomonas aeruginosa* and certain strains of anaerobes.

***In Vitro* Cytotoxicity:** Data from *in vitro* studies on cell culture suggest that mafenide acetate may have a deleterious effect on human keratinocytes. The clinical significance of this information is unknown.

INDICATIONS AND USAGE

SULFAMYLON® For 5% Topical Solution is indicated for use as an adjunctive topical antimicrobial agent to control bacterial infection when used under moist dressings over meshed autografts on excised burn wounds.

Continued on next page

Sulfamylon Solution—Cont.

CONTRAINDICATIONS

SULFAMYLON® For 5% Topical Solution is contraindicated in patients who are hypersensitive to mafenide acetate. It is not known whether there is cross sensitivity to other sulfonamides.

WARNINGS

Fatal hemolytic anemia with disseminated intravascular coagulation, presumably related to a glucose-6-phosphate dehydrogenase deficiency, has been reported following therapy with mafenide acetate.

PRECAUTIONS

General: Mafenide acetate and its metabolite, p-carboxybenzenesulfonamide, inhibit carbonic anhydrase, which may result in metabolic acidosis, usually compensated by hyperventilation. In the presence of impaired renal function, high blood levels of mafenide acetate and its metabolite may exaggerate the carbonic anhydrase inhibition. Therefore, close monitoring of acid-base balance is necessary, particularly in patients with extensive second-degree or partial thickness burns and in those with pulmonary or renal dysfunction. Some burn patients treated with mafenide acetate have also been reported to manifest an unexplained syndrome of masked hyperventilation with resulting respiratory alkalosis (slightly alkaline blood pH, low arterial pCO_2, and decreased total CO_2); change in arterial pO_2 is variable. The etiology and significance of these findings are unknown.

Mafenide acetate should be used with caution in burn patients with acute renal failure.

Fungal colonization may occur concomitantly with reduction of bacterial growth in the burn wound. However, systemic fungal infection through the infected burn wound is rare.

Carcinogenesis, Mutagenesis, Impairment of Fertility: No long-term animal studies have been performed to evaluate the carcinogenic potential of mafenide acetate, however, the drug did not induce mutation in L5178Y mouse lymphoma cells at the TK locus.

Animal studies have not been performed to evaluate the potential effects of mafenide acetate on fertility.

Pregnancy: *Teratogenic Effects. Pregnancy Category C:* A teratology study performed in rats using oral doses of up to 600 mg/kg/day revealed no evidence of harm to the fetus due to mafenide acetate. There are no adequate data regarding the potential reproductive toxicity of mafenide acetate in a non-rodent species, nor are there adequate and well-controlled studies in pregnant women. Mafenide acetate should be used during pregnancy only if the potential benefit justifies the potential risk to the fetus.

Nursing Mothers: It is not known whether mafenide acetate is excreted in human milk. Because many drugs are excreted in human milk and because of the potential for serious adverse reactions in nursing infants from mafenide acetate, a decision should be made whether to discontinue nursing or to discontinue the drug, taking into account the importance of the drug to the mother.

Pediatric Use: The safety and effectiveness of SULFAMYLON® For 5% Topical Solution have been established in the age groups 3 months to 16 years.

Geriatric Use: No studies have been conducted to specifically examine the effects of mafenide acetate on burn wounds in geriatric patients.

ADVERSE REACTIONS

In the clinical setting of severe burns, it is often difficult to distinguish between an adverse reaction to mafenide acetate and burn sequelae. In a clinical study of pediatric patients with acute burns requiring autografts who received SULFAMYLON® 5% SOLUTION in addition to double antibiotic solution (DAB) wound therapy (neomycin sulfate 40 mg and polymyxin B 200,000 units/liter), the incidence of rash (4.6%) and itching (2.8%) in the group which received SULFAMYLON® 5% Solution was not different from that experienced with DAB dressings alone (5.7% and 1.3%, respectively).

From other clinical settings, a single case of bone marrow depression and a single case of an acute attack of porphyria have been reported following therapy with mafenide acetate. Fatal hemolytic anemia with disseminated intravascular coagulation, presumably related to a glucose-6-phosphate dehydrogenase deficiency, has been reported following therapy with mafenide acetate. The following adverse reactions have been reported with topical mafenide acetate therapy:

Dermatologic and Allergic: Pain or burning sensation, rash and pruritus (often localized to the area covered by the wound dressing), erythema, skin maceration from prolonged wet dressings, facial edema, swelling, hives, blisters, eosinophilia.

Respiratory or Metabolic: Tachypnea, hyperventilation, decrease in pCO_2, metabolic acidosis, increase in serum chloride.

OVERDOSAGE

Single oral doses of 2000 mg/kg of mafenide acetate as a 5% solution did not cause mortality or clinical symptoms of toxicity in rats.

DOSAGE AND ADMINISTRATION

SULFAMYLON® For 5% Topical Solution: *Directions for Preparation of the Solution:* SULFAMYLON® (Mafenide Acetate) For 5% Topical Solution is applied as a powder and is to be reconstituted with Sterile Water for Irrigation, USP or 0.9% Sodium Chloride Irrigation, USP. Aseptic techniques should be observed during preparation of the solution. Premeasured quantities of 50 g of mafenide acetate powder are provided in packets. The entire quantity of SULFAMYLON® should be emptied into a suitable container which contains 1000 mL of Sterile Water for Irrigation, USP or 0.9% Sodium Chloride Irrigation, USP and mixed until completely dissolved. **The resulting SULFAMYLON® (mafenide acetate, USP) 5% SOLUTION should be filtered through a 0.22 micron sterilizing grade filter prior to use.** The reconstituted/filtered solution should be stored at room temperature, 25°–30°C (77°–86°F), and should be used within 48 hours after preparation. **Not for Injection - For Topical Use Only.**

Directions for Use of the Solution: The grafted area should be covered with one layer of fine mesh gauze. An eight-ply burn dressing should be cut to the size of the graft and wetted with SULFAMYLON® 5% SOLUTION using an irrigation syringe and/or irrigation tubing until leaking is noticeable. If irrigation tubing is used, the tubing should be placed over the burn dressing in contact with the wound and covered with a second piece of eight-ply dressing. The irrigation dressing should be secured with a bolster dressing and wrapped as appropriate. The gauze dressing should be kept wet. In clinical studies, this has been accomplished by irrigating with a syringe or injecting the solution into the irrigation tubing every 4 hours or as necessary. If irrigation tubing is not used, the gauze dressing may be moistened every 6–8 hours or as necessary to keep wet.

Wound dressings may be left undisturbed, except for the irrigations, for up to five days. Additional soaks may be initiated until graft take is complete. Maceration of skin may result from wet dressings applied for intervals as short as 24 hours. Treatment is usually continued until autograft vascularization occurs and healing is progressing (typically occurring in about 5 days). Safety and effectiveness have not been established for longer than 5 days for an individual grafting procedure.

If allergic manifestations occur during treatment with SULFAMYLON® 5% SOLUTION, discontinuation of treatment should be considered. If acidosis occurs and becomes difficult to control, particularly in patients with pulmonary dysfunction, discontinuing the soaks with the mafenide acetate solution for 24 to 48 hours may aid in restoring acid-base balance (see PRECAUTIONS section). Dressing changes and monitoring the site for bacterial growth during this interruption should be adjusted accordingly.

HOW SUPPLIED

SULFAMYLON® (mafenide acetate, USP) For 5% Topical Solution is available in packets (NDC 62794-111-17) containing 50 g of mafenide acetate to be prepared using 1000 mL Sterile Water for Irrigation, USP or 0.9% Sodium Chloride Irrigation, USP. (See DOSAGE AND ADMINISTRATION: SULFAMYLON® For 5% Topical Solution: *Directions for Preparation of the Solution.*) The packets are supplied as follows:

Carton of five 50 g packets NDC 62794-111-98

Recommended Storage:

Packets – STORE PACKETS IN A DRY PLACE AT ROOM TEMPERATURE, 25°–30°C (77°–86°F)

Prepared Solution – STORE AT ROOM TEMPERATURE, 25°–30°C (77°–86°F).

USE WITHIN 48 HOURS OF PREPARATION.

Distributed by: Bertek Pharmaceuticals Inc.
Sugar Land, TX 77478
1-888-823-7835

Rx only

BKSFMN:R3
REVISED MARCH 1998

ZAGAM® ℞
(sparfloxacin) Tablets

DESCRIPTION

Zagam® (sparfloxacin) tablets contain sparfloxacin, a synthetic broad-spectrum antimicrobial agent for oral administration. Sparfloxacin, an aminodifluoroquinolone, is 5-Amino-1-cyclopropyl-7-(*cis*-3,5-dimethyl-1-piperazinyl)-6,8-difluoro-1,4-dihydro-4-oxo-3-quinolinecarboxylic acid. Its empirical formula is $C_{19}H_{22}F_2N_4O_3$ and it has the following chemical structure:

H, CH3, HN, H, CH3, F, N, H, F, COOH, NH2, O

Sparfloxacin has a molecular weight of 392.41. It occurs as a yellow crystalline powder. It is sparingly soluble in glacial acetic acid or chloroform, very slightly soluble in ethanol (95%), and practically insoluble in water and ether. It dissolves in dilute acetic acid or 0.1 N sodium hydroxide.

Zagam is available as a 200-mg round, white film-coated tablet. Each 200-mg tablet contains the following inactive ingredients: microcrystalline cellulose NF, corn starch NF, L-hydroxypropylcellulose NF, magnesium stearate NF, and colloidal silicone dioxide NF. The film coating contains: methylhydroxypropylcellulose USP, polyethylene glycol 6000, and titanium dioxide USP.

CLINICAL PHARMACOLOGY

Absorption: Sparfloxacin is well absorbed following oral administration with an absolute oral bioavailability of 92%. The mean maximum plasma sparfloxacin concentration following a single 400-mg oral dose was approximately 1.3 (±0.2) µg/mL. The area under the curve (mean $AUC_{0-\infty}$) following a single 400-mg oral dose was approximately 34 (±6.8) µg•hr/mL.

Steady-state plasma concentration was achieved on the first day by giving a loading dose that was double the daily dose. Mean (±SD) pharmacokinetic parameters observed for the 24-hour dosing interval with the recommended dosing regimen are shown below:

Dosing Regimen (mg/day)	Peak Cmax (µg/mL)	Trough C_{24} (µg/mL)	AUC $_{0\to24}$ hr. µg/mL
400 mg loading dose (day 1)	1.3 (±0.2)	0.5 (±0.1)	20.6 (±3.1)
200 mg q24 hours (steady-state)	1.1 (±0.1)	0.5 (±0.1)	18.7 (±2.6)

Maximum plasma concentrations for the initial oral 400-mg loading dose were typically achieved between 3 to 6 hours following administration with a mean value of approximately 4 hours. Maximum plasma concentrations for a 200-mg dose were also achieved between 3 to 6 hours after administration with a mean of about 4 hours.

Oral absorption of sparfloxacin is unaffected by administration with milk or food, including high fat meals. Concurrent administration of antacids containing magnesium hydroxide and aluminum hydroxide reduces the oral bioavailability of sparfloxacin by as much as 50%. (See **PRECAUTIONS, Information for Patients,** and **Drug Interactions.**)

Distribution: Upon reaching general circulation, sparfloxacin distributes well into the body, as reflected by the large mean steady-state volume of distribution (Vd_{ss}) of 3.9 (±0.8) L/kg. Sparfloxacin exhibits low plasma protein binding in serum at about 45%.

Sparfloxacin penetrates well into body fluids and tissues. Results of tissue and body fluid distribution studies demonstrated that oral administration of sparfloxacin produces sustained concentrations and that sparfloxacin concentrations in lower respiratory tract tissues and fluids generally exceed the corresponding plasma concentrations. The concentration of sparfloxacin in respiratory tissues (pulmonary parenchyma, bronchial wall, and bronchial mucosa) at 2 to 6 hours following standard oral dosing was approximately 3 to 6 times greater than the corresponding concentration in plasma. Concentrations in these respiratory tissues increase at up to 24 hours following dosing. Sparfloxacin is also highly concentrated into alveolar macrophages compared to plasma. Tissue or fluid to plasma sparfloxacin concentration ratios for respiratory tissues and fluids are:

[See table at top of next page]

Mean pleural effusion to plasma concentration ratios were 0.34 and 0.69 at 4 and 20 hours postdose, respectively.

Metabolism: Sparfloxacin is metabolized by the liver, primarily by phase II glucuronidation, to form a glucuronide conjugate. Its metabolism does not utilize or interfere with cytochrome-mediated oxidation, in particular cytochrome P450.

Excretion: The total body clearance and renal clearance of sparfloxacin were 11.4 (±3.5) and 1.5 (±0.5) L/hr, respectively. Sparfloxacin is excreted in both the feces (50%) and urine (50%). Approximately 10% of an orally administered dose is excreted in the urine as unchanged drug in patients with normal renal function. Following a 400-mg loading dose of sparfloxacin, the mean urine concentration 4 hours postdose was in excess of 12.0 µg/mL, and measurable concentrations of active drug persisted through six days for subjects with normal renal function.

The terminal elimination phase half-life ($t_{1/2}$) of sparfloxacin in plasma generally varies between 16 and 30 hours, with a mean $t_{1/2}$ of approximately 20 hours. The $t_{1/2}$ is independent of the administered dose, suggesting that sparfloxacin elimination kinetics are linear.

Special Populations

Geriatric: The pharmacokinetics of sparfloxacin are not altered in the elderly with normal renal function.

Pediatric: The pharmacokinetics of sparfloxacin in pediatric subjects have not been studied.

Gender: There are no gender differences in the pharmacokinetics of sparfloxacin.

Renal insufficiency: In patients with renal impairment (creatinine clearance <50 mL/min), the terminal elimination half-life of sparfloxacin is lengthened. Single or multiple doses of sparfloxacin in patients with varying degrees of renal impairment typically produce plasma concentrations that are twice those observed in subjects with normal renal function. (See **PRECAUTIONS: General** and **DOSAGE AND ADMINISTRATION.**)

Hepatic insufficiency: The pharmacokinetics of sparfloxacin are not altered in patients with mild or moderate hepatic impairment without cholestasis.

MICROBIOLOGY

Sparfloxacin has *in vitro* activity against a wide range of gram-negative and gram-positive microorganisms. Sparfloxacin exerts its antibacterial activity by inhibiting DNA gyrase, a bacterial topoisomerase. DNA gyrase is an essential enzyme which controls DNA topology and assists in DNA replication, repair, deactivation, and transcription. Quinolones differ in chemical structure and mode of action from β-lactam antibiotics. Quinolones may, therefore, be active against bacteria resistant to β-lactam antibiotics.
Although cross-resistance has been observed between sparfloxacin and other fluoroquinolones, some microorganisms resistant to other fluoroquinolones may be susceptible to sparfloxacin.
In vitro tests show that the combination of sparfloxacin and rifampin is antagonistic against *Staphylococcus aureus.*
Sparfloxacin has been shown to be active against most strains of the following microorganisms, both *in vitro* and in clinical infections as described in the **INDICATIONS AND USAGE** section:

Aerobic gram-positive microorganisms
Staphylococcus aureus
Streptococcus pneumoniae (penicillin-susceptible strains)
Aerobic gram-negative microorganisms
Enterobacter cloacae
Haemophilus influenzae
Haemophilus parainfluenzae
Klebsiella pneumoniae
Moraxella catarrhalis
Other microorganisms
Chlamydia pneumoniae
Mycoplasma pneumoniae

The following *in vitro* data are available, **but their clinical significance is unknown:**
Sparfloxacin exhibits *in vitro* minimal inhibitory concentrations (MIC's) of 1 μg/mL or less against most (≥90%) strains of the following microorganisms; however, the safety and effectiveness of sparfloxacin in treating clinical infections due to these microorganisms have not been established in adequate and well-controlled clinical trials.

Aerobic gram-positive microorganisms
Streptococcus agalactiae
Streptococcus pneumoniae (penicillin-resistant strains)
Streptococcus pyogenes
Viridans group streptococci
Aerobic gram-negative microorganisms
Acinetobacter anitratus
Acinetobacter lwoffi
Citrobacter diversus
Enterobacter aerogenes
Klebsiella oxytoca
Legionella pneumophila
Morganella morganii
Proteus mirabilis
Proteus vulgaris

SUSCEPTIBILITY TESTS

Dilution techniques: Quantitative methods are used to determine antimicrobial minimal inhibitory concentrations (MIC's). These MIC's provide estimates of the susceptibility of bacteria to antimicrobial compounds. The MIC's should be determined using a standardized procedure. Standardized procedures are based on a dilution method[1] (broth or agar) or equivalent with standardized inoculum concentrations and standardized concentrations of sparfloxacin powder. The MIC values should be interpreted according to the following criteria:
For testing aerobic microorganisms other than *Haemophilus influenzae, Haemophilus parainfluenzae,* and *Streptococcus pneumoniae:*

MIC (μg/mL)	Interpretation
≤1	Susceptible (S)
2	Intermediate (I)
≥4	Resistant (R)

For testing *Haemophilus influenzae* and *Haemophilus parainfluenzae:*[a]

MIC (μg/mL)	Interpretation
≤0.25	Susceptible (S)

[a] These interpretive standards are applicable only to broth microdilution susceptibility testing with *Haemophilus influenzae* and *Haemophilus parainfluenzae* using Haemophilus Test Medium[1].

The current absence of data on resistant strains precludes defining any categories other than "Susceptible." Strains yielding MIC results suggestive of a "nonsusceptible" category should be submitted to a reference laboratory for further testing.
For testing *Streptococcus pneumoniae:*[b]

MIC (μg/mL)	Interpretation
≤0.5	Susceptible (S)

[b] These interpretive standards are applicable only to broth microdilution susceptibility tests using cation-adjusted Mueller-Hinton broth with 2–5% lysed horse blood.

The current absence of data on resistant strains precludes defining any categories other than "Susceptible." Strains

Tissue to Plasma Sparfloxacin Concentration Mean Ratio (%CV)*

Respiratory tissues and fluids	n** value	Time of Collection Postdose: 2 to 6 hour	12 to 24 hour
alveolar macrophage	6/5	51.8 (88.7%)	68.1 (47.9%)
epithelial lining fluid	10/10	12.3 (26.7%)	17.6 (35.3%)
pulmonary parenchyma	8/7	5.9 (15.0%)	15.8 (32.0%)
bronchial wall	8/7	2.8 (16.0%)	5.7 (25.0%)
bronchial mucosa	6/5	2.7 (11.5%)	3.1 (11.6%)

* % CV (percent coefficient of variation)
** For tissues with two values, the first n is for 2 to 6 hours and the second n is for 12 to 24 hours.

yielding MIC results suggestive of a "nonsusceptible" category should be submitted to a reference laboratory for further testing.
A report of "Susceptible" indicates that the pathogen is likely to be inhibited if the antimicrobial compound in the blood reaches the concentration usually achievable. A report of "Intermediate" indicates that the result should be considered equivocal, and, if the microorganism is not fully susceptible to alternative, clinically feasible drugs, the test should be repeated. This category implies possible clinical applicability in body sites where the drug is physiologically concentrated or in situations where a high dosage of drug can be used. This category also provides a buffer zone which prevents small uncontrolled technical factors from causing major discrepancies in interpretation. A report of "Resistant" indicates that the pathogen is not likely to be inhibited if the antimicrobial compound in the blood reaches the concentration usually achievable; other therapy should be selected.
Standardized susceptibility test procedures require the use of laboratory control microorganisms to control the technical aspects of the laboratory procedures. Standard sparfloxacin powder should provide the following MIC values:

Microorganism	MIC Range (μg/mL)
Enterococcus faecalis ATCC 29212	0.12–0.5
Escherichia coli ATCC 25922	0.004–0.016
Haemophilus influenzae ATCC 49247[a]	0.004–0.016
Staphylococcus aureus ATCC 29213	0.03–0.12
Streptococcus pneumoniae ATCC 49619[b]	0.12–0.5

[a] This quality control range is applicable to only *H. influenzae* ATCC 49247 tested by a broth microdilution procedure using Haemophilus Test Medium (HTM)[1].
[b] This quality control range is applicable to only *S. pneumoniae* ATCC 49619 tested by a broth microdilution procedure using cation-adjusted Mueller-Hinton broth with 2–5% lysed horse blood.

Diffusion techniques: Quantitative methods that require measurement of zone diameters also provide reproducible estimates of the susceptibility of bacteria to antimicrobial compounds. One such standardized procedure[2] requires the use of standardized inoculum concentrations. This procedure uses paper disks impregnated with 5-μg sparfloxacin to test the susceptibility of microorganisms to sparfloxacin. Reports from the laboratory providing results of the standard single-disk susceptibility test with a 5-μg sparfloxacin disk should be interpreted according to the following criteria:
For aerobic microorganisms other than *Haemophilus influenzae, Haemophilus parainfluenzae,* and *Streptococcus pneumoniae:*

Zone Diameter (mm)	Interpretation
≥19	Susceptible (S)
16–18	Intermediate (I)
≤15	Resistant (R)

Haemophilus influenzae and *Haemophilus parainfluenzae* should not be tested by diffusion techniques. An MIC should be determined for these isolates.
For *Streptococcus pneumoniae:*[a]

Zone Diameter (mm)	Interpretation
≥19	Susceptible (S)

[a] These zone diameter standards for *Streptococcus pneumoniae* apply only to tests performed using Mueller-Hinton agar supplemented with 5% sheep blood and incubated in 5% CO_2.

The current absence of data on resistant strains precludes any category other than "Susceptible." Strains yielding zone diameter results suggestive of a "nonsusceptible" category should be submitted to a reference laboratory for further testing.
Interpretation should be as stated above for results using dilution techniques. Interpretation involves correlation of the diameter obtained in the disk test with the MIC for sparfloxacin.

As with standard dilution techniques, diffusion methods require the use of laboratory control microorganisms that are used to control the technical aspects of the laboratory procedures. For the diffusion technique, the 5-μg sparfloxacin disk should provide the following zone diameters in these laboratory quality control strains:

Microorganism	Zone Diameter (mm)
Escherichia coli ATCC 25922	30–38
Staphylococcus aureus ATCC 25923	27–33
Streptococcus pneumoniae ATCC 49619[a]	21–27

[a] These quality control limits apply to tests conducted with *S. pneumoniae* ATCC 49619 using Mueller-Hinton agar supplemented with 5% sheep blood incubated in 5% CO_2.

INDICATIONS AND USAGE

Zagam (sparfloxacin) is indicated for the treatment of adults (≥ 18 years of age) with the following infections caused by susceptible strains of the designated microorganisms:

Community-acquired pneumonia caused by *Chlamydia pneumoniae, Haemophilus influenzae, Haemophilus parainfluenzae, Moraxella catarrhalis, Mycoplasma pneumoniae,* or *Streptococcus pneumoniae*
Acute bacterial exacerbations of chronic bronchitis caused by *Chlamydia pneumoniae, Enterobacter cloacae, Haemophilus influenzae, Haemophilus parainfluenzae, Klebsiella pneumoniae, Moraxella catarrhalis, Staphylococcus aureus,* or *Streptococcus pneumoniae*

Appropriate culture and susceptibility tests should be performed before treatment in order to isolate and identify organisms causing the infection and to determine their susceptibility to sparfloxacin. Therapy with sparfloxacin may be initiated before results of these tests are known; once results become available, appropriate therapy should be selected. Culture and susceptibility testing performed periodically during therapy will provide information on the continued susceptibility of the pathogen to the antimicrobial agent and also on the possible emergence of bacterial resistance.

CONTRAINDICATIONS

Sparfloxacin is contraindicated for individuals with a history of hypersensitivity or photosensitivity reactions.
Torsade de pointes has been reported in patients receiving sparfloxacin concomitantly with disopyramide and amiodarone. Consequently, sparfloxacin is contraindicated for individuals receiving these drugs as well as other QT_c-prolonging antiarrhythmic drugs reported to cause torsade de pointes, such as class Ia antiarrhythmic agents (e.g., quinidine, procainamide), class III antiarrhythmic agents (e.g., sotalol), and bepridil. Sparfloxacin is contraindicated in patients with known QT_c prolongation or in patients being treated concomitantly with medications known to produce an increase in the QT_c interval and/or torsade de pointes (e.g., terfenadine). (See **WARNINGS** and **PRECAUTIONS.**)
It is essential to avoid exposure to the sun, bright natural light, and UV rays throughout the entire duration of treatment and for 5 days after treatment is stopped. Sparfloxacin is contraindicated in patients whose life-style or employment will not permit compliance with required safety precautions concerning phototoxicity. (See **WARNINGS** and **PRECAUTIONS.**)

WARNINGS

MODERATE TO SEVERE PHOTOTOXIC REACTIONS HAVE OCCURRED IN PATIENTS EXPOSED TO DIRECT OR INDIRECT SUNLIGHT OR TO ARTIFICIAL ULTRAVIOLET LIGHT (e.g., SUNLAMPS) DURING OR FOLLOWING TREATMENT. THESE REACTIONS HAVE ALSO OCCURRED IN PATIENTS EXPOSED TO SHADED OR DIFFUSE LIGHT, INCLUDING EXPOSURE THROUGH GLASS OR DURING CLOUDY WEATHER. PATIENTS SHOULD BE ADVISED TO DISCONTINUE SPARFLOXACIN THERAPY AT THE FIRST SIGNS OR SYMPTOMS OF A PHOTOTOXICITY REACTION SUCH AS A SENSATION OF SKIN BURNING, REDNESS, SWELLING, BLISTERS, RASH, ITCHING, OR DERMATITIS.
The overall incidence of drug related phototoxicity in the 1585 patients who received sparfloxacin during clinical tri-

Continued on next page

Zagam—Cont.

als with recommended dosage was 7.9% (n=126). Phototoxicity ranged from mild 4.1% (n=65) to moderate 3.3% (n=52) to severe 0.6% (n=9), with severe defined as involving at least significant curtailment of normal daily activity. The frequency of phototoxicity reactions characterized by blister formation was 0.8% (n=13) of which 3 were severe. The discontinuation rate due to phototoxicity independent of drug relationship was 1.1% (n=17).

As with some other types of phototoxicity, there is the potential for exacerbation of the reaction on re-exposure to sunlight or artificial ultraviolet light prior to complete recovery from the reaction. In a few cases, recovery from phototoxicity reactions was prolonged for several weeks. In rare cases, reactions have recurred up to several weeks after stopping sparfloxacin therapy.

EXPOSURE TO DIRECT AND INDIRECT SUNLIGHT (EVEN WHEN USING SUNSCREENS OR SUNBLOCKS) SHOULD BE AVOIDED WHILE TAKING SPARFLOXACIN AND FOR FIVE DAYS FOLLOWING THERAPY. SPARFLOXACIN THERAPY SHOULD BE DISCONTINUED IMMEDIATELY AT THE FIRST SIGNS OR SYMPTOMS OF PHOTOTOXICITY.

These phototoxic reactions have occurred with and without the use of sunscreens or sunblocks and have been associated with a single dose of sparfloxacin. However, a study in healthy volunteers has demonstrated that some sunscreen products, specifically those active in blocking UVA spectrum wavelengths (those containing the active ingredients octocrylene or Parsol® 1789), can moderate the photosensitizing effect of sparfloxacin. However, many over-the-counter sunscreens do not provide adequate UVA protection.

Increases in the QT_c interval have been observed in healthy volunteers treated with sparfloxacin. After a single loading dose of 400 mg, a mean increase in QT_c interval of 11 msec (2.9%) is seen; at steady-state the mean increase is 7 msec (1.9%). The magnitude of the QT_c effect does not increase with repeated administration, and the QT_c returns to baseline within 48 hours of the last dose. In clinical trials involving 1489 patients with a baseline QT_c measurement, the mean prolongation at steady-state was 10 msec (2.5%); 0.7% of patients had a QT_c interval greater than 500 msec; however, no arrhythmic effects were seen.

THE SAFETY AND EFFECTIVENESS OF SPARFLOXACIN IN CHILDREN, ADOLESCENTS (UNDER THE AGE OF 18 YEARS), PREGNANT WOMEN, AND LACTATING WOMEN HAVE NOT BEEN ESTABLISHED. (See **PRECAUTIONS—Pregnancy, Nursing Mothers;** and **Pediatric Use.**)

Sparfloxacin has been shown to cause arthropathy in immature dogs when given in oral doses of 25 mg/kg/day (approximately 1.9 times the highest human dose on a mg/m² basis) for seven consecutive days. Examination of the weight-bearing joints of the dogs revealed small erosive lesions of the cartilage. Other quinolones also produce erosions of cartilage of weight-bearing joints and other signs of arthropathy in immature animals of various species.

Convulsions and toxic psychoses have been reported in patients receiving quinolones, including sparfloxacin. Quinolones may also cause increased intracranial pressure and central nervous system stimulation which may lead to tremors, restlessness/agitation, anxiety/nervousness, lightheadedness, confusion, hallucinations, paranoia, depression, nightmares, insomnia, and, rarely, suicidal thoughts or acts. These reactions may occur following the first dose. If these reactions occur in patients receiving sparfloxacin, the drug should be discontinued and appropriate measures instituted. As with other quinolones, sparfloxacin should be used with caution in patients with a known or suspected CNS disorder that may predispose to seizures or lower the seizure threshold (e.g., severe cerebral arteriosclerosis, epilepsy) or in the presence of other risk factors that may predispose to seizures or lower the seizure threshold (e.g., certain drug therapy, renal dysfunction). Cases of seizure associated with hypoglycemia have been reported. (See **PRECAUTIONS: General Information for Patients, Drug Interactions** and **ADVERSE REACTIONS.**)

Serious and occasionally fatal hypersensitivity (including anaphylactoid or anaphylactic) reactions, some following the first dose, have been reported in patients receiving quinolones. Some reactions were accompanied by cardiovascular collapse, hypotension/shock, seizure, loss of consciousness, tingling, angioedema (including tongue, laryngeal, throat, or facial edema), airway obstruction (including bronchospasm, shortness of breath, and acute respiratory distress), dyspnea, urticaria, and/or itching. Only a few patients had a history of previous hypersensitivity reactions. If an allergic reaction to sparfloxacin occurs, the drug should be discontinued immediately. Serious acute hypersensitivity reactions may require immediate treatment with epinephrine, and other resuscitative measures including oxygen, intravenous fluids, antihistamines, corticosteroids, pressor amines, and airway management, including intubation, as clinically indicated.

Serious and sometimes fatal events, some due to hypersensitivity, and some due to uncertain etiology, have been reported rarely in patients receiving therapy with quinolones. These events may be severe and generally occur following the administration of multiple doses. Clinical manifestations may include one or more of the following: fever, rash or severe dermatologic reactions (e.g., toxic epidermal necrolysis, Stevens-Johnson Syndrome); vasculitis; arthralgia; myalgia; serum sickness; allergic pneumonitis; interstitial nephritis; acute renal insufficiency or failure; hepatitis; jaundice; acute hepatic necrosis or failure; anemia, including hemolytic and aplastic; thrombocytopenia, including thrombotic thrombocytopenic purpura; leukopenia; agranulocytosis; pancytopenia; and/or other hematologic abnormalities. The drug should be discontinued immediately at the first appearance of a skin rash or any other sign of hypersensitivity and supportive measures instituted. (See **PRECAUTIONS: Information for Patients** and **ADVERSE REACTIONS.**)

Pseudomembranous colitis has been reported with nearly all antibacterial agents, including sparfloxacin, and may range in severity from mild to life-threatening. Therefore, it is important to consider this diagnosis in patients who present with diarrhea subsequent to the administration of antibacterial agents.

Treatment with antibacterial agents alters the normal flora of the colon and may permit overgrowth of clostridia. Studies indicate that a toxin produced by *Clostridium difficile* is one primary cause of "antibiotic-associated colitis."

After the diagnosis of pseudomembranous colitis has been established, therapeutic measures should be initiated. Mild cases of pseudomembranous colitis usually respond to drug discontinuation alone. In moderate to severe cases, consideration should be given to management with fluids and electrolytes, protein supplementation, and treatment with an antibacterial drug clinically effective against *C. difficile* colitis.

Ruptures of the shoulder, hand, and Achilles tendons that required surgical repair or resulted in prolonged disability have been reported with sparfloxacin and other quinolones. Sparfloxacin should be discontinued if the patient experiences pain, inflammation, or rupture of a tendon. Patients should rest and refrain from exercise until the diagnosis of tendonitis or tendon rupture has been confidently excluded. Tendon rupture can occur at any time during or after therapy with sparfloxacin.

PRECAUTIONS

General: Adequate hydration of patients receiving sparfloxacin should be maintained to prevent the formation of a highly concentrated urine.

Administer sparfloxacin with caution in the presence of renal insufficiency. Careful clinical observation and appropriate laboratory studies should be performed prior to and during therapy since elimination of sparfloxacin may be reduced. Adjustment of the dosage regimen is necessary for patients with impaired renal function-creatinine clearance <50 mL/min. (See **CLINICAL PHARMACOLOGY** and **DOSAGE AND ADMINISTRATION.**)

Avoid the concomitant prescription of medications known to prolong the QT_c interval, e.g., erythromycin, terfenadine, astemizole, cisapride, pentamidine, tricyclic antidepressants, some antipsychotics including phenothiazines. (See **CONTRAINDICATIONS.**) Sparfloxacin is not recommended for use in patients with pro-arrhythmic conditions (e.g., hypokalemia, significant bradycardia, congestive heart failure, myocardial ischemia, and atrial fibrillation).

Moderate to severe phototoxicity reactions have been observed in patients exposed to direct sunlight while receiving drugs in this class. Excessive exposure to sunlight should be avoided. In clinical trials with sparfloxacin, phototoxicity was observed in approximately 7% of patients. Therapy should be discontinued if phototoxicity (e.g., a skin eruption) occurs.

As with other quinolones, sparfloxacin should be used with caution in any patient with a known or suspected CNS disorder that may predispose to seizures or lower the seizure threshold (e.g., severe cerebral arteriosclerosis, epilepsy) or in the presence of other risk factors that may predispose to seizures or lower the seizure threshold (e.g., certain drug therapy, renal dysfunction). (See **WARNINGS** and **Drug Interactions.**)

Information for Patients:

Patients should be advised:

- to avoid exposure to direct or indirect sunlight (including through glass, while using sunscreens and sunblocks, reflected sunlight, and cloudy weather) and exposure to artificial ultraviolet light (e.g., sunlamps) during treatment with sparfloxacin and for five days after therapy. If brief exposure to the sun cannot be avoided, patients should cover as much of their skin as possible with clothing;
- to discontinue sparfloxacin therapy at the first sign or symptom of phototoxicity reaction such as a sensation of skin burning, redness, swelling, blisters, rash, itching or dermatitis;
- that a patient who has experienced a phototoxic reaction with sparfloxacin should also be advised to avoid further exposure to sunlight and artificial ultraviolet light until the phototoxicity reaction has resolved and he or she has completely recovered from the reaction or for five days whichever is longer. In rare cases, reactions have recurred up to several weeks after stopping sparfloxacin therapy;
- that sparfloxacin may cause neurologic adverse effects (e.g., dizziness, lightheadedness) and that patients should know how they react to sparfloxacin before they operate an automobile or machinery or engage in other activities requiring mental alertness and coordination (see **WARNINGS** and **ADVERSE REACTIONS**);
- to discontinue treatment and inform their physician if they experience pain, inflammation, or rupture of a tendon, and to rest and refrain from exercise until the diagnosis of tendonitis or tendon rupture has been confidently excluded;
- that sparfloxacin can be taken with food or milk or caffeine-containing products;
- that mineral supplements or vitamins with iron, or zinc, or calcium may be taken 4 hours after sparfloxacin administration;
- that sucralfate or magnesium- and aluminum-containing antacids may be taken 4 hours after sparfloxacin administration (see **PRECAUTIONS—Drug Interactions**);
- that sparfloxacin may be associated with hypersensitivity reactions, even following the first dose, and to discontinue the drug at the first sign of a skin rash or other allergic reaction;
- to drink fluids liberally.

Drug Interactions:

Digoxin: Sparfloxacin has no effect on the pharmacokinetics of digoxin.

Methylxanthines: Sparfloxacin does not increase plasma theophylline concentrations. Since there is no interaction with theophylline, interaction with other methylxanthines such as caffeine is unlikely.

Warfarin: Sparfloxacin does not increase the anti-coagulant effect of warfarin.

Cimetidine: Cimetidine does not affect the pharmacokinetics of sparfloxacin.

Antacids and Sucralfate: Aluminum and magnesium cations in antacids and sucralfate form chelation complexes with sparfloxacin. The oral bioavailability of sparfloxacin is reduced when an aluminum-magnesium suspension is administered between 2 hours before and 2 hours after sparfloxacin administration. The oral bioavailability of sparfloxacin is not reduced when the aluminum-magnesium suspension is administered 4 hours following sparfloxacin administration.

Zinc/iron salts: Absorption of quinolones is reduced significantly by these preparations. These products may be taken 4 hours after sparfloxacin administration.

Probenecid: Probenecid does not alter the pharmacokinetics of sparfloxacin.

Drug/Laboratory Test Interactions:

Sparfloxacin therapy may produce false-negative culture results for *Mycobacterium tuberculosis* by suppression of mycobacterial growth.

Carcinogenesis, Mutagenesis, Impairment of Fertility:

Carcinogenesis: Sparfloxacin was not carcinogenic in mice or rats when administered for 104 weeks at daily oral doses 3.5–6.2 times greater than the maximum human dose (400 mg), respectively, based upon mg/m². These doses corresponded to plasma concentrations approximately equal to (mice) and 2.2 times greater than (rats) maximum human plasma concentrations.

Mutagenesis: Sparfloxacin was not mutagenic in *Salmonella typhimurium* TA98, TA100, TA1535, or TA1537, in *Escherichia coli* strain WP2 uvrA, nor in Chinese hamster lung cells. Sparfloxacin and other quinolones have been shown to be mutagenic in *Salmonella typhimurium* strain TA102 and to induce DNA repair in *Escherichia coli*, perhaps due to their inhibitory effect on bacterial DNA gyrase. Sparfloxacin induced chromosomal aberrations in Chinese hamster lung cells *in vitro* at cytotoxic concentrations; however, no increase in chromosomal aberrations or micronuclei in bone marrow cells was observed after sparfloxacin was administered orally to mice.

Impairment of Fertility: Sparfloxacin had no effect on the fertility or reproductive performance of male or female rats at oral doses up to 15.4 times the maximum human dose (400 mg) based upon mg/m² (equivalent to approximately 12 times the maximum human plasma concentration).

Pregnancy: Teratogenic effects: Pregnancy Category C Reproduction studies performed in rats, rabbits, and monkeys at oral doses 6.2, 4.4, and 2.6 times higher than the maximum human dose, respectively, based upon mg/m² (corresponding to plasma concentrations 4.5- and 6.5-fold higher than in humans in the monkey and rat, respectively) did not reveal any evidence of teratogenic effects. At these doses, sparfloxacin was clearly maternally toxic to the rabbit and monkey with evidence of slight maternal toxicity observed in the rat. When administered to pregnant rats at clearly maternally toxic doses (≥9.3 times the maximum human dose based upon mg/m²), sparfloxacin induced a dose-dependent increase in the incidence of fetuses with ventricular septal defects. Among the three species tested, this effect was specific to the rat. There are, however, no adequate and well-controlled studies in pregnant women. Sparfloxacin should be used during pregnancy only if the potential benefit justifies the potential risk to the fetus. (See **WARNINGS.**)

Nursing mothers: Sparfloxacin is excreted in human milk. Because of the potential for serious adverse reactions in infants nursing from mothers taking sparfloxacin, a decision should be made whether to discontinue nursing or to discontinue the drug, taking into account the importance of the drug to the mother. (See **WARNINGS.**)

Pediatric use: Safety and effectiveness have not been established in patients below the age of 18 years. Quinolones, including sparfloxacin, cause arthropathy and osteochondrosis in juvenile animals of several species. (See **WARNINGS.**)

ADVERSE REACTIONS

In clinical trials, most of the adverse events were mild to moderate in severity and transient in nature. During clinical investigations with the recommended dosage, 1585 patients received sparfloxacin and 1331 patients received a comparator. The discontinuation rate due to adverse events was 6.6% for sparfloxacin versus 5.6% for cefaclor, 14.8% for erythromycin, 8.9% for ciprofloxacin, 7.4% for ofloxacin, and 8.3% for clarithromycin.

The most frequently reported events (remotely, possibly, or probably drug related with an incidence of ≥1%) among sparfloxacin treated patients in the US phase 3 clinical trials with the recommended dosage were: photosensitivity reaction (7.9%), diarrhea (4.6%), nausea (4.3%), headache (4.2%), dyspepsia (2.3%), dizziness (2.0%), insomnia (1.9%), abdominal pain (1.8%), pruritus (1.8%), taste perversion (1.4%), and QT_c interval prolongation (1.3%), vomiting (1.3%), flatulence (1.1%) and vasodilatation (1.0%).

In US phase 3 clinical trials of shorter treatment duration than the recommended dosage, the most frequently reported events (incidence ≥1%, remotely, possibly, or probably drug related) were: headache (8.1%), nausea (7.6%), dizziness (3.8%), photosensitivity reaction (3.6%), pruritus (3.3%), diarrhea (3.2%), vaginal moniliasis (2.8%), abdominal pain (2.4%), asthenia (1.7%), dyspepsia (1.6%), somnolence (1.5%), dry mouth (1.4%), and rash (1.1%).

Additional possibly or probably related events that occurred in less than 1% of all patients enrolled in US phase 3 clinical trials are listed below:

BODY AS A WHOLE: fever, chest pain, generalized pain, allergic reaction, cellulitis, back pain, chills, face edema, malaise, accidental injury, anaphylactoid reaction, infection, mucous membrane disorder, neck pain, rheumatoid arthritis;

CARDIOVASCULAR: palpitation, electrocardiogram abnormal, hypertension, tachycardia, sinus bradycardia, PR interval shortened, angina pectoris, arrhythmia, atrial fibrillation, atrial flutter, complete AV block, first degree AV block, second degree AV block, cardiovascular disorder, hemorrhage, migraine, peripheral vascular disorder, supraventricular extrasystoles, ventricular extrasystoles, postural hypotension;

GASTROINTESTINAL: constipation, anorexia, gingivitis, oral moniliasis, stomatitis, tongue disorder, tooth disorder, gastroenteritis, increased appetite, mouth ulceration, flatulence, vomiting;

HEMATOLOGIC: cyanosis, ecchymosis, lymphadenopathy;

METABOLISM: gout, peripheral edema, thirst;

MUSCULOSKELETAL: arthralgia, arthritis, joint disorder, myalgia;

CENTRAL NERVOUS SYSTEM: paresthesia, hypesthesia, nervousness, somnolence, abnormal dreams, dry mouth, depression, tremor, anxiety, confusion, hallucinations, hyperesthesia, hyperkinesia, sleep disorder, hypokinesia, vertigo, abnormal gait, agitation, lightheadedness, emotional lability, euphoria, abnormal thinking, amnesia, twitching;

RESPIRATORY: asthma, epistaxis, pneumonia, rhinitis, pharyngitis, bronchitis, hemoptysis, sinusitis, cough increased, dyspnea, laryngismus, lung disorder, pleural disorder;

SKIN/HYPERSENSITIVITY: rash, maculopapular rash, dry skin, herpes simplex, sweating, urticaria, vesiculobullous rash, exfoliative dermatitis, acne, alopecia, angioedema, contact dermatitis, fungal dermatitis, furunculosis, pustular rash, skin discoloration, herpes zoster, petechial rash;

SPECIAL SENSES: ear pain, amblyopia, photophobia, tinnitus, conjunctivitis, diplopia, abnormality of accommodation, blepharitis, ear disorder, eye pain, lacrimation disorder, otitis media;

UROGENITAL: vaginitis, dysuria, breast pain, dysmenorrhea, hematuria, menorrhagia, nocturia, polyuria, urinary tract infection, kidney pain, leukorrhea, metrorrhagia, vulvovaginal disorder.

LABORATORY CHANGES: In the US phase 3 clinical trials, with the recommended dosage, the most frequently (incidence ≥1%) reported changes in laboratory parameters listed as adverse events, regardless of relationship to drug, were: elevated ALT (SGPT) (2.0%), AST (SGOT) (2.3%) and white blood cells (1.1%).

Increases for the following laboratory tests were reported in less than 1% of all patients enrolled in clinical trials: alkaline phosphatase, serum amylase, aPTT, blood urea nitrogen, calcium, creatinine, eosinophils, serum lipase, monocytes, neutrophils, total bilirubin, urine glucose, urine protein, urine red blood cells, and urine white blood cells.

Decreases for the following laboratory tests were reported in less than 1% of all patients enrolled in clinical trials: albumin, creatinine clearance, hematocrit, hemoglobin, lymphocytes, phosphorus, red blood cells, and sodium.

Increases and decreases for the following laboratory tests were reported in less than 1% of all patients in clinical trials: blood glucose, platelets, potassium, and white blood cells.

Postmarketing Adverse Events: The following are additional adverse events (regardless of relationship to drug) reported from worldwide postmarketing experience with sparfloxacin or other quinolones: acidosis, acute renal failure, agranulocytosis, albuminuria, anaphylactic shock, angioedema, anosmia, ataxia, bullous eruption, candiduria, cardiopulmonary arrest, cerebral thrombosis, convulsions, crystalluria, dysgeusia, dysphasia, ebrious feeling, embolism, erythema nodosum, exacerbation of myasthenia gravis, gastralgia, hemolytic anemia, hepatic necrosis, hepatitis, hiccough, hyperpigmentation, interstitial nephritis, interstitial pneumonia, intestinal perforation, jaundice, laryngeal or pulmonary edema, manic reaction, numbness, nystagmus, painful oral mucosa, pancreatitis, phobia, prolongation of prothrombin time, pseudomembranous colitis, Quincke's edema, renal calculi, rhabdomyolysis, sensory disturbance, Stevens-Johnson syndrome, squamous cell carcinoma, tendonitis, tendon rupture, tremor, thrombocytopenia, thrombocytopenia purpura, toxic epidermal necrolysis, toxic psychosis, urinary retention, uveitis, vaginal candidiasis, vasculitis.

Laboratory changes: elevation of serum triglycerides, serum cholesterol, blood glucose, serum potassium, decrease in WBC counts, RBC counts, hemoglobin level, hematocrit level, thrombocyte counts, elevation in GOT, GPT, ALP, LDH, γ-GTP, total bilirubin.

Organism	Sparfloxacin	Erythromycin*	Cefaclor
C. pneumoniae	19/22 (86.4%)	3/4 (75%)	5/5 (100%)
H. influenzae	20/24 (83.3%)	0	25/31 (80.6%)
H. parainfluenzae	61/63 (96.8%)	4/4 (100%)	31/41 (75.6%)
M. catarrhalis	7/8 (87.5%)	4/4 (100%)	5/6 (83.3%)
M. pneumoniae	36/39 (92.3%)	15/15 (100%)	20/24 (83.3%)
S. pneumoniae	39/41 (95.1%)	10/11 (90%)	16/17 (94.1%)

* Pathogen numbers were smaller since many of the strains were intrinsically resistant to erythromycin.

Event	Sparfloxacin n=387	Erythromycin n=209	Cefaclor n=162
Abdominal Pain	6 (1.6%)	18 (8.6%)	2 (1.2%)
Photosensitivity Reaction	16 (4.1%)	0	1 (0.6%)
QT Interval Prolonged	8 (2.1%)	2 (1.0%)	1 (0.6%)
Sinus Bradycardia	2 (0.5%)	6 (2.9%)	0
Diarrhea	15 (3.9%)	33 (15.8%)	7 (4.3%)
Flatulence	0	5 (2.4%)	0
Nausea	11 (2.8%)	32 (15.3%)	4 (2.5%)
Vomiting	10 (2.6%)	15 (7.2%)	1 (0.6%)
Insomnia	6 (1.6%)	5 (2.4%)	0

Organism	Sparfloxacin	Ofloxacin
H. parainfluenzae	104/109 (95.4%)	90/95 (94.7%)
H. influenzae	51/57 (89.5%)	61/65 (93.8%)
C. pneumoniae	37/45 (82.2%)	36/40 (90%)
M. catarrhalis	36/38 (94.7%)	33/34 (97.1%)
S. pneumoniae	30/34 (88.2%)	20/22 (90.9%)
S. aureus	16/19 (84.2%)	13/14 (92.9%)
K. pneumoniae	17/17 (100%)	15/17 (88.2%)
E. cloacae	12/13 (92.3%)	12/15 (80%)

OVERDOSAGE

In case of overdosage, the patient should be monitored in a suitably equipped medical facility and advised to avoid sun exposure for five days. ECG monitoring is recommended due to the possible prolongation of the QT_c interval. There is no known antidote for sparfloxacin overdosage.

It is not known whether sparfloxacin is dialyzable.

Single doses of sparfloxacin were relatively non-toxic via the oral route of administration in mice, rats, and dogs. No deaths occurred within a 14-day post-treatment observation period at the highest oral doses tested, up to 5000 mg/kg in either rodent species, or up to 600 mg/kg in the dog. Clinical signs observed included inactivity in mice and dogs, diarrhea in both rodent species, and vomiting, salivation, and tremors in dogs.

DOSAGE AND ADMINISTRATION

Zagam (sparfloxacin) can be taken with or without food.

The recommended daily dose of Zagam in patients with normal renal function is two 200-mg tablets taken on the first day as a loading dose. Thereafter, one 200-mg tablet should be taken every 24 hours for a total of 10 days of therapy (11 tablets).

The recommended daily dose of Zagam in patients with renal impairment (creatinine clearance <50 mL/min) is two 200-mg tablets taken on the first day as a loading dose. Thereafter, one 200-mg tablet should be taken every 48 hours for a total of 9 days of therapy (6 tablets).

CLINICAL STUDIES

Community-Acquired Pneumonia Studies

In two controlled clinical studies of community-acquired pneumonia conducted in the United States, sparfloxacin was compared to erythromycin and cefaclor. The patient clinical success and pathogen eradication rates for sparfloxacin were equivalent to those of the comparators. In these studies, the following pathogen eradication rates/presumed pathogen eradication rates were obtained:

[See first table above]

Safety

The following table lists possibly and probably drug-related adverse events that occurred in these studies at an incidence of ≥2%:

[See second table above]

Acute Bacterial Exacerbations of Chronic Bronchitis Study

In a controlled clinical study of acute bacterial exacerbations of chronic bronchitis conducted in the United States, sparfloxacin was compared to ofloxacin. In this study, the following pathogen eradication rates were obtained:

[See third table above]

Safety

The following table lists possibly and probably drug-related adverse events that occurred in the study at an incidence of ≥2% for either compound.

Event	Sparfloxacin (n=395)	Ofloxacin (n=403)
Headache	11 (2.8%)	6 (1.5%)
Photosensitivity Reaction	29 (7.3%)	3 (0.7%)
Diarrhea	6 (1.5%)	9 (2.2%)
Dyspepsia	8 (2.0%)	14 (3.5%)
Nausea	16 (4.1%)	29 (7.2%)
Dizziness	12 (3.0%)	10 (2.5%)
Insomnia	4 (1.0%)	46 (11.4%)
Taste Perversion	10 (2.5%)	10 (2.5%)

HOW SUPPLIED

Strength	Size		Description/Markings
200 mg	Blister Pack of 11 (RespiPac™)	NDC 62794-011-11	A white film coated, round bi convex tablet debossed with B over 11 one side of the tablet and blank on the other side
	Bottle of 55	011-55	

Store at Controlled Room Temperature 20 to 25°C (68 to 77°F) [see USP].

Caution: Federal law prohibits dispensing without a prescription.

Keep out of the reach of children.

ANIMAL PHARMACOLOGY

Sparfloxacin and other quinolones have been shown to cause arthropathy in juvenile animals of most species tested. (See **WARNINGS.**)

Sparfloxacin had no convulsive activity in mice when administered alone or in combination with the nonsteroidal anti-inflammatory agents ketoprofen, or naproxen.

References:

1. National Committee for Clinical Laboratory Standards. Methods for Dilution Antimicrobial Susceptibility Tests for Bacteria that Grow Aerobically—Third Edition. Approved Standard NCCLS Document M7-A3, Vol. 13, No. 25, NCCLS, Villanova, PA, December, 1993.

2. National Committee for Clinical Laboratory Standards. Performance Standards for Antimicrobial Disk Susceptibility Tests—Fifth Edition. Approved Standard NCCLS Document M2-A5, Vol. 13, No. 24, NCCLS, Villanova, PA, December 1993.

Distributed by Bertek Pharmaceuticals Inc.
Sugarland, TX 77478 USA
Manufactured by Rhone-Poulenc Rorer Pharmaceuticals
Collegeville, Pa 19426 USA
IN-0010A Bk2A6:R1
Rev 10/98

Shown in Product Identification Guide, page 308

Beutlich LP Pharmaceuticals

1541 SHIELDS DRIVE
WAUKEGAN, IL 60085-8304

Direct Inquiries to:
847-473-1100
800-238-8542
FAX 847–473-1122
E-mail fjb1541@worldnet.att.net
World Wide Web http://www.beutlich.com

CEO–TWO® EVACUANT SUPPOSITORY OTC

NDC #0283-0763-09

COMPOSITION

Each adult rectal suppository contains sodium bicarbonate and potassium bitartrate in a water soluble polyethylene glycol base.

HOW SUPPLIED

In packages of 10, white opaque suppositories. Keep in cool, dry place.
DO NOT REFRIGERATE
(See PDR For Nonprescription Drugs)

HURRICAINE® TOPICAL ANESTHETIC OTC

COMPOSITION

HURRICAINE contains 20% benzocaine in a flavored, water soluble polyethylene glycol base.

PACKAGING AVAILABLE

Gel
1 oz. Jar Wild Cherry NDC #0283-0871-31
1 oz. Jar Fresh Mint NDC #0283-0998-31
1 oz. Jar Pina Colada NDC #0283-0886-31
1 oz. Jar Watermelon NDC #0283-0293-31
1/6 oz. Tube Wild Cherry NDC #0283-0871-12
1/6 oz. Tube Watermelon NDC #0283-0293-12
Liquid
1 fl. oz. Jar Wild Cherry NDC #0283-0569-31
1 fl. oz. Jar Pina Colada NDC #0283-1886-31
1/6 oz. Tube Wild Cherry NDC #0283-0569-12
.25 ml Dry Handle Swab Wild Cherry NDC #0283-0693-01
Spray
2 oz. Aerosol Wild Cherry NDC #0283-0679-02
Spray Kit
2 oz. Aerosol Wild Cherry NDC #0283-0183-02 with 200 Disposable Extension Tubes
(See PDR For Nonprescription Drugs)

PERIDIN-C® OTC

Composition: Each orange colored tablet contains 2 popular antioxidants; Vitamin C and Bioflavonoids.
Ascorbic Acid 200 mg.
Hesperidin Complex 150 mg.
Hesperidin Methyl Chalcone 50 mg. F.D. & C. #6.

Dosage: 1 tablet daily or as directed.

How Supplied: In bottles of:
100 tablets NDC #0283-0597-01
500 tablets NDC #0283-0597-05

Biogen, Inc.

14 CAMBRIDGE CENTER
CAMBRIDGE, MA 02142

Direct Inquiries to:
Customer Service (800) 456-2255
Fax (617) 679-3100

AVONEX® ℞
[ăv ′-ə-nĕx]
INTERFERON BETA-1a

DESCRIPTION

AVONEX® (Interferon beta-1a) is produced by recombinant DNA technology. Interferon beta-1a is a 166 amino acid glycoprotein with a predicted molecular weight of approximately 22,500 daltons. It is produced by mammalian cells (Chinese Hamster Ovary cells) into which the human interferon beta gene has been introduced. The amino acid sequence of AVONEX® is identical to that of natural human interferon beta.

Using the World Health Organization (WHO) natural interferon beta standard, Second International Standard for Interferon, Human Fibroblast (Gb-23-902-531), AVONEX® has a specific activity of approximately 200 million international units (IU) of antiviral activity per mg; 30 mcg of AVONEX® contains 6 million IU of antiviral activity. The activity against other standards is not known.

AVONEX® is formulated as a sterile, white to off-white lyophilized powder for intramuscular injection after reconstitution with supplied diluent or Sterile Water for Injection, USP, preservative-free.

Each 1.0 mL (1.0 cc) of reconstituted AVONEX® contains 30 mcg of Interferon beta-1a, 15 mg Albumin Human, USP, 5.8 mg Sodium Chloride, USP, 5.7 mg Dibasic Sodium Phosphate, USP, and 1.2 mg Monobasic Sodium Phosphate, USP, at a pH of approximately 7.3.

CLINICAL PHARMACOLOGY

General

Interferons are a family of naturally occurring proteins and glycoproteins that are produced by eukaryotic cells in response to viral infection and other biological inducers. Interferon beta, one member of this family, is produced by various cell types including fibroblasts and macrophages. Natural interferon beta and Interferon beta-1a are glycosylated, with each containing a single N-linked complex carbohydrate moiety. Glycosylation of other proteins is known to affect their stability, activity, aggregation, biodistribution, and half-life in blood. However, the effects of glycosylation of interferon beta on these properties have not been fully defined.

Biologic Activities

Interferons are cytokines that mediate antiviral, antiproliferative and immunomodulatory activities in response to viral infection and other biological inducers. Three major interferons have been distinguished: alpha, beta, and gamma. Interferons alpha and beta form the Type I class of interferons, and interferon gamma is a Type II interferon. These interferons have overlapping but clearly distinct biological activities.

Interferon beta exerts its biological effects by binding to specific receptors on the surface of human cells. This binding initiates a complex cascade of intracellular events that leads to the expression of numerous interferon-induced gene products and markers. These include 2′, 5′-oligoadenylate synthetase, β_2-microglobulin, and neopterin. These products have been measured in the serum and cellular fractions of blood collected from patients treated with AVONEX® (Interferon beta-1a).

The specific interferon-induced proteins and mechanisms by which AVONEX® exerts its effects in multiple sclerosis have not been fully defined. Clinical studies conducted in MS patients showed that interleukin 10 (IL-10) levels in cerebrospinal fluid (CSF) were increased in patients treated with AVONEX® compared to placebo. However, no relationship has been established between absolute levels or changes in levels of IL-10 and clinical outcome in multiple sclerosis.

Pharmacokinetics

Pharmacokinetics of AVONEX® in multiple sclerosis patients have not been evaluated. The pharmacokinetic and pharmacodynamic profiles of AVONEX® in healthy subjects following doses of 30 mcg through 75 mcg have been investigated. Serum levels of Interferon beta-1a as measured by antiviral activity are slightly above detectable limits following a 30 mcg intramuscular (IM) dose, and increase with higher doses.

After an IM dose, serum levels of Interferon beta-1a typically peak between 3 and 15 hours and then decline at a rate consistent with a 10 hour elimination half-life. Serum levels of Interferon beta-1a may be sustained after IM administration due to prolonged absorption from the IM site. Systemic exposure, as determined by AUC and C_{max} values, is greater following IM than SC administration.

Subcutaneous administration of AVONEX® should not be substituted for intramuscular administration. Subcutaneous and intramuscular administration have been observed to have non-equivalent pharmacokinetic and pharmacodynamic parameters following administration to healthy volunteers.

Biological response markers (e.g., neopterin and β_2-microglobulin) are induced by Interferon beta-1a following parenteral doses of 15 mcg through 75 mcg in healthy subjects and treated patients. Biological response marker levels increase within 12 hours of dosing and remain elevated for at least 4 days. Peak biological response marker levels are typically observed 48 hours after dosing. The relationship of serum Interferon beta-1a levels or levels of these induced biological response markers to the mechanisms by which AVONEX® exerts its effects in multiple sclerosis is unknown.

Clinical Studies: Effects in Multiple Sclerosis

The clinical effects of AVONEX® (Interferon beta-1a) in multiple sclerosis were studied in a randomized, multicenter, double-blind, placebo-controlled study in patients with relapsing (stable or progressive) multiple sclerosis[1]. In this study, 301 patients received either 6 million IU (30 mcg) of AVONEX® (Interferon beta-1a) (n=158) or placebo (n=143) by IM injection once weekly. Patients were entered into the trial over a 2½ year period, received injections for up to 2 years, and continued to be followed until study completion. Two hundred eighty-two patients completed 1 year on study, and 172 patients completed 2 years on study. There were 144 patients treated with AVONEX® for more than 1 year, 115 patients for more than 18 months and 82 patients for 2 years.

All patients had a definite diagnosis of multiple sclerosis of at least 1 year duration and had at least 2 exacerbations in the 3 years prior to study entry (or 1 per year if the duration of disease was less than 3 years). At entry, study participants were without exacerbation during the prior 2 months and had Kurtzke Expanded Disability Status Scale (EDSS[2]) scores ranging from 1.0 to 3.5. Patients with chronic progressive multiple sclerosis were excluded from this study.

The primary outcome assessment was time to progression in disability, measured as an increase in the EDSS of at least 1.0 point that was sustained for at least 6 months. An increase in EDSS score reflects accumulation of disability. This endpoint was used to ensure that progression reflected permanent increase in disability rather than a transient effect due to an exacerbation.

Secondary outcomes included exacerbation frequency and results of magnetic resonance imaging (MRI) scans including gadolinium (Gd)-enhanced lesion number and volume and T2-weighted (proton density) lesion volume. Additional secondary endpoints included 2 upper limb (tested in both arms) and 3 lower limb function tests.

Twenty-three of the 301 patients (8%) discontinued treatment prematurely. Of these, 1 patient treated with placebo (1%) and 6 patients treated with AVONEX® (4%) discontinued treatment due to adverse events. Thirteen of these 23 patients remained on study and were evaluated for clinical endpoints.

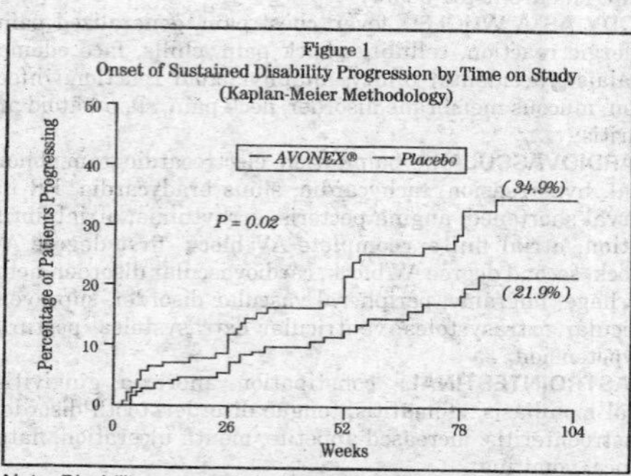

Note: Disability progression represents at least a 1.0 point increase in EDSS score sustained for at least 6 months.

Time to onset of sustained progression in disability was significantly longer in patients treated with AVONEX® than in patients receiving placebo (p=0.02). The Kaplan-Meier plots of these data are presented in Figure 1. The Kaplan-Meier estimate of the percentage of patients progressing by the end of 2 years was 34.9% for placebo-treated patients and 21.9% for AVONEX®-treated patients, indicating a slowing of the disease process. This represents a 37% reduction in the risk of accumulating disability in the AVONEX®-treated group compared to the placebo-treated group.

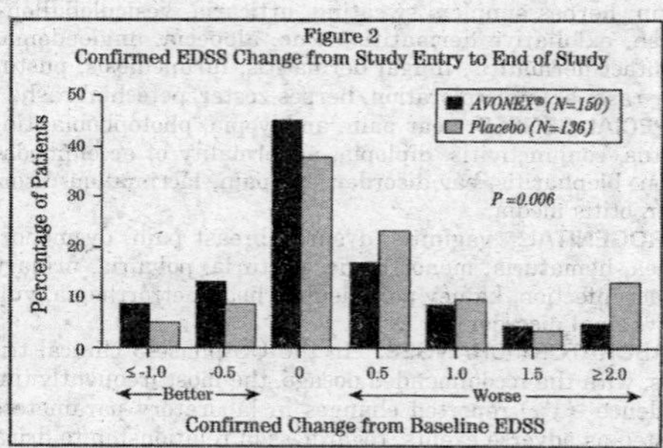

The distribution of confirmed EDSS change from study entry (baseline) to the end of the study is shown in Figure 2. There was a statistically significant difference between treatment groups in confirmed change for patients with at least 2 scheduled visits (136 placebo-treated and 150 AVONEX®-treated patients; p=0.006; see Table 1). Confirmed EDSS change was calculated as the difference between the EDSS score at study entry and 1 of the scores determined at the last 2 scheduled visits. If the EDSS score at either of the last 2 scheduled visits showed improvement (reduction in score), the higher score was used. Otherwise, the lower score was used. Nineteen patients had 1 score higher and 1 score lower than baseline; the higher score was used. The last 2 scheduled visits occurred at varying time points among patients.

The rate and frequency of exacerbations were determined as secondary outcomes. For all patients included in the study, irrespective of time on study, the annual exacerbation rate was 0.67 per year in the AVONEX®-treated group and 0.82 per year in the placebo-treated group (p=0.04).

AVONEX® (Interferon beta-1a) treatment significantly decreased the frequency of exacerbations in the subset of patients who were enrolled in the study for at least 2 years (87 placebo-treated patients and 85 AVONEX®-treated patients; p=0.03; see Table 1).

Gd-enhanced and T2-weighted (proton density) MRI scans of the brain were obtained in most patients at baseline and at the end of 1 and 2 years of treatment. Gd-enhancing lesions seen on brain MRI scans represent areas of breakdown of the blood brain barrier thought to be secondary to inflammation. Patients treated with AVONEX® demonstrated significantly lower Gd-enhanced lesion number after 1 and 2 years of treatment ($p \leq 0.05$; see Table 1). The volume of Gd-enhanced lesions was also analyzed, and showed similar treatment effects ($p \leq 0.03$). Percentage change in T2-weighted lesion volume from study entry to Year 1 was significantly lower in AVONEX®-treated than placebo-treated patients ($p=0.02$). A significant difference in T2-weighted lesion volume change was not seen between study entry and Year 2.

The exact relationship between MRI findings and the clinical status of patients is unknown. Changes in lesion area often do not correlate with changes in disability progression. The prognostic significance of the MRI findings in this study has not been evaluated.

Of the limb function tests, only 1 demonstrated a statistically significant difference between treatment groups (favoring AVONEX®).

A summary of the effects of AVONEX® on the primary and major secondary endpoints of this study is presented in Table 1.

Safety and efficacy of treatment with AVONEX® beyond 2 years are not known.

[See table 1 at right]

Table 1
Major Clinical Endpoints

Endpoint	Placebo	AVONEX®	P-Value
PRIMARY ENDPOINT:			
Time to sustained progression in disability (N: 143, 158)[1]	–See Figure 1–		0.02[2]
Percentage of patients progressing in disability at 2 years (Kaplan-Meier estimate)[1]	34.9%	21.9%	
SECONDARY ENDPOINTS:			
DISABILITY			
Mean confirmed change in EDSS from study entry to end of study (N: 136, 150)[1]	0.50	0.20	0.006[3]
EXACERBATIONS			
Number of exacerbations in subset completing 2 years (N: 87, 85)			
0	26%	38%	0.03[3]
1	30%	31%	
2	11%	18%	
3	14%	7%	
≥4	18%	7%	
Percentage of patients exacerbation-free in subset completing 2 years (N: 87, 85)	26%	38%	0.10[4]
Annual exacerbation rate (N: 143, 158)[1]	0.82	0.67	0.04[5]
MRI			
Number of Gd-enhanced lesions:			
At study entry (N: 132, 141)			
Mean (Median)	2.3 (1.0)	3.2 (1.0)	
Range	0-23	0-56	
Year 1 (N: 123, 134)			
Mean (Median)	1.6 (0)	1.0 (0)	0.02[3]
Range	0-22	0-28	
Year 2 (N: 82, 83)			
Mean (Median)	1.6 (0)	0.8 (0)	0.05[3]
Range	0-34	0-13	
T2 lesion volume:			
Percentage change from study entry to Year 1 (N: 116, 123)			
Median	-3.3%	-13.1%	0.02[3]
Percentage change from study entry to Year 2 (N: 83, 81)			
Median	-6.5%	-13.2%	0.36[3]

Note: (N: ,) denotes the number of evaluable placebo and AVONEX® (Interferon beta-1a) patients, respectively.
[1] *Patient data included in this analysis represent variable periods of time on study.*
[2] *Analyzed by Mantel-Cox (logrank) test.*
[3] *Analyzed by Mann-Whitney rank-sum test.*
[4] *Analyzed by Cochran-Mantel-Haenszel test.*
[5] *Analyzed by likelihood ratio test.*

INDICATIONS AND USAGE

AVONEX® (Interferon beta-1a) is indicated for the treatment of relapsing forms of multiple sclerosis to slow the accumulation of physical disability and decrease the frequency of clinical exacerbations. Safety and efficacy in patients with chronic progressive multiple sclerosis have not been evaluated.

CONTRAINDICATIONS

AVONEX® (Interferon beta-1a) is contraindicated in patients with a history of hypersensitivity to natural or recombinant interferon beta, human albumin, or any other component of the formulation.

WARNINGS

AVONEX® (Interferon beta-1a) should be used with caution in patients with depression. Depression and suicide have been reported to occur in patients receiving other interferon compounds. Depression and suicidal ideation are known to occur at an increased frequency in the multiple sclerosis population. A relationship between occurrence of depression and/or suicidal ideation and the use of AVONEX® has not been established. An equal incidence of depression was seen in the placebo-treated and AVONEX®-treated patients in the placebo-controlled multiple sclerosis study. Patients treated with AVONEX® should be advised to report immediately any symptoms of depression and/or suicidal ideation to their prescribing physicians. If a patient develops depression, cessation of AVONEX® therapy should be considered.

PRECAUTIONS

General

Caution should be exercised when administering AVONEX® (Interferon beta-1a) to patients with pre-existing seizure disorder. In the placebo-controlled study, 4 patients receiving AVONEX® experienced seizures, while no seizures occurred in the placebo group. Three of these 4 patients had no prior history of seizure. It is not known whether these events were related to the effects of multiple sclerosis alone, to AVONEX®, or to a combination of both. For patients with no prior history of seizure who develop seizures during therapy with AVONEX®, an etiologic basis should be established and appropriate anti-convulsant therapy instituted prior to considering resumption of AVONEX® treatment. The effect of AVONEX® administration on the medical management of patients with seizure disorder is unknown.

Patients with cardiac disease, such as angina, congestive heart failure, or arrhythmia, should be closely monitored for worsening of their clinical condition during initiation and continued treatment with AVONEX®. While AVONEX® does not have any known direct-acting cardiac toxicity, during the post-marketing period infrequent cases of congestive heart failure, cardiomyopathy, and cardiomyopathy with congestive heart failure have been reported in patients without known predisposition to these events or other known etiologies; in rare cases, these events have been temporally related to the administration of AVONEX®. In rare cases, these events have recurred upon rechallenge in patients with known predisposition.

Information to Patients

Patients should be informed of the most common adverse events associated with AVONEX® administration, including symptoms associated with flu syndrome (see Adverse Reactions section and precautions in Patient Information). Symptoms of flu syndrome are most prominent at the initiation of therapy and decrease in frequency with continued treatment. In the placebo-controlled study, patients were instructed to take 650 mg acetaminophen immediately prior to injection and for an additional 24 hours after each injection to modulate acute symptoms associated with AVONEX® administration.

Patients should be cautioned to report depression or suicidal ideation (see Warnings).

Patients should be advised about the abortifacient potential of interferon beta (see Pregnancy – Teratogenic Effects).

When a physician determines that AVONEX® can be used outside of the physician's office, persons who will be administering AVONEX® should receive instruction in reconstitution and injection, including the review of the injection procedures (see Dosage and Administration). If a patient is to self-administer, the physical ability of that patient to self-inject intramuscularly should be assessed. The first injection should be performed under the supervision of a qualified health care professional. A puncture-resistant container for disposal of needles and syringes should be used. Patients should be instructed in the technique and importance of proper syringe and needle disposal and be cautioned against reuse of these items.

Laboratory Tests

In addition to those laboratory tests normally required for monitoring patients with multiple sclerosis, complete blood and differential white blood cell counts, platelet counts, and blood chemistries, including liver function tests, are recommended during AVONEX® (Interferon beta-1a) therapy. During the placebo-controlled study, these tests were performed at least every 6 months. There were no significant differences between the placebo and AVONEX® groups in the incidence of liver enzyme elevation, leukopenia, or thrombocytopenia. However, these are known to be dose-related laboratory abnormalities associated with the use of interferons. Patients with myelosuppression may require more intensive monitoring of complete blood cell counts, with differential and platelet counts.

Drug Interactions

No formal drug interaction studies have been conducted with AVONEX® (Interferon beta-1a). In the placebo-controlled study, corticosteroids or ACTH were administered for treatment of exacerbations in some patients concurrently receiving AVONEX®. In addition, some patients receiving AVONEX® were also treated with anti-depressant therapy and/or oral contraceptive therapy. No unexpected adverse events were associated with these concomitant therapies.

Other interferons have been noted to reduce cytochrome P-450 oxidase-mediated drug metabolism. Formal hepatic drug metabolism studies with AVONEX® in humans have not been conducted. Hepatic microsomes isolated from AVONEX®-treated rhesus monkeys showed no influence of AVONEX® on hepatic P-450 enzyme metabolism activity.

As with all interferon products, proper monitoring of patients is required if AVONEX® is given in combination with myelosuppressive agents.

Carcinogenesis, Mutagenesis, and Impairment of Fertility

Carcinogenesis: No carcinogenicity data for Interferon beta-1a are available in animals or humans.

Mutagenesis: Interferon beta-1a was not mutagenic when tested in the Ames bacterial test and in an *in vitro* cytogenetic assay in human lymphocytes in the presence and absence of metabolic activation. These assays are designed to detect agents that interact directly with and cause damage to cellular DNA. Interferon beta-1a is a glycosylated protein that does not directly bind to DNA.

Impairment of Fertility: No studies were conducted to evaluate the effects of interferon beta on fertility in normal women or women with multiple sclerosis. It is not known whether Interferon beta-1a can affect human reproductive capacity.

Menstrual irregularities were observed in monkeys administered interferon beta at a dose 100 times the recommended weekly human dose (based upon a body surface area comparison). Anovulation and decreased serum progesterone levels were also noted transiently in some animals. These effects were reversible after discontinuation of drug. Treatment of monkeys with interferon beta at 2 times the recommended weekly human dose (based upon a body surface area comparison) had no effects on cycle duration or ovulation.

The accuracy of extrapolating animal doses to human doses is not known. In the placebo-controlled study, 6% of patients receiving placebo and 5% of patients receiving AVONEX® (Interferon beta-1a) experienced menstrual disorder. If menstrual irregularities occur in humans, it is not known how long they will persist following treatment.

Pregnancy - Teratogenic Effects

Pregnancy Category C: The reproductive toxicity of AVONEX® has not been studied in animals or humans. In pregnant monkeys given interferon beta at 100 times the recommended weekly human dose (based upon a body surface area comparison), no teratogenic or other adverse effects on fetal development were observed. Abortifacient activity was evident following 3 to 5 doses at this level. No abortifacient effects were observed in monkeys treated at 2 times the recommended weekly human dose (based upon a body surface area comparison). Although no teratogenic effects were seen in these studies, it is not known if teratogenic effects would be observed in humans. There are no adequate and well-controlled studies with interferons in pregnant women. If a woman becomes pregnant or plans to become pregnant while taking AVONEX®, she should be informed of the potential hazards to the fetus, and it should be recommended that the woman discontinue therapy.

Nursing Mothers

It is not known whether Interferon beta-1a is excreted in human milk. Because of the potential of serious adverse reactions in nursing infants, a decision should be made to either discontinue nursing or to discontinue AVONEX®.

Continued on next page

Avonex—Cont.

Pediatric Use
Safety and effectiveness in pediatric patients below the age of 18 years have not been established.

Geriatric Use
Safety and effectiveness in geriatric patients above the age of 65 years have not been established.

ADVERSE REACTIONS

The safety data describing the use of AVONEX® (Interferon beta-1a) in multiple sclerosis patients are based on the placebo-controlled trial in which 158 patients randomized to AVONEX® were treated for up to 2 years (see Clinical Studies).

The 5 most common adverse events associated (at $p \leq 0.075$) with AVONEX® treatment were flu-like symptoms (otherwise unspecified), muscle ache, fever, chills, and asthenia. The incidence of all 5 adverse events diminished with continued treatment.

One patient in the placebo group attempted suicide; no AVONEX®-treated patients attempted suicide. The incidence of depression was equal in the 2 treatment groups. However, since depression and suicide have been reported with other interferon products, AVONEX® (Interferon beta-1a) should be used with caution in patients with depression (see Warnings).

In the placebo-controlled study, 4 patients receiving AVONEX® experienced seizures, while no seizures occurred in the placebo group. Three of these 4 patients had no prior history of seizure. It is not known whether these events were related to the effects of multiple sclerosis alone, to AVONEX®, or to a combination of both (see Precautions).

Table 2 enumerates adverse events and selected laboratory abnormalities that occurred at an incidence of 2% or more among the 158 multiple sclerosis patients treated with 30 mcg of AVONEX® once weekly by IM injection. Reported adverse events have been classified using standard COSTART terms. Terms so general as to be uninformative and those events that were equal in incidence or more common in the placebo-treated patients have been excluded.

[See table 2 below]

AVONEX® (Interferon beta-1a) has also been evaluated in 290 patients with illnesses other than multiple sclerosis. The majority of these patients were enrolled in studies to evaluate AVONEX® treatment of chronic viral hepatitis B and C, in which the doses studied ranged from 15 mcg to 75 mcg, given SC, 3 times a week, for up to 6 months. The incidence of common adverse events in these studies was generally seen at a frequency similar to that seen in the placebo-controlled multiple sclerosis study. In these non-multiple sclerosis studies, inflammation at the site of the SC injection was seen in 52% of treated patients. In contrast, injection site inflammation was seen in 3% of multiple sclerosis patients receiving 30 mcg AVONEX® by IM injection. Subcutaneous injections were also associated with the following local reactions: injection site necrosis, injection site atrophy, injection site edema and injection site hemorrhage. None of the above was observed in the multiple sclerosis patients participating in the placebo-controlled study.

Other events observed during premarket and postmarket evaluation of AVONEX®, administered either SC or IM, are listed in the paragraph that follows. Because most of the events were observed in open and uncontrolled studies, or in marketed use, the role of AVONEX® (Interferon beta-1a) in their causation cannot be reliably determined. **Body as a Whole:** abscess, ascites, cellulitis, facial edema, hernia, injection site fibrosis, injection site hypersensitivity, injection site pain, lipoma, neoplasm, photosensitivity reaction, rigors, sepsis, sinus headache, toothache; **Cardiovascular System:** arrhythmia, arteritis, cardiomyopathy, congestive heart failure, heart arrest, hemorrhage, hypotension, palpitation, pericarditis, peripheral ischemia, peripheral vascular disorder, postural hypotension, pulmonary embolus, spider angioma, tachycardia, telangiectasia, vascular disorder; **Digestive System:** blood in stool, colitis, constipation, diverticulitis, dry mouth, gallbladder disorder, gastritis, gastrointestinal hemorrhage, gingivitis, gum hemorrhage, hepatitis, hepatoma, hepatomegaly, increased appetite, intestinal perforation, intestinal obstruction, liver function test abnormalities, periodontal abscess, periodontitis, proctitis, thirst, tongue disorder, vomiting; **Endocrine System:** hyperthyroidism, hypothyroidism; **Hemic and Lymphatic System:** coagulation time increased, ecchymosis, lymphadenopathy, petechia; **Metabolic and Nutritional Disorders:** abnormal healing, dehydration, hypoglycemia, hypomagnesemia, hypokalemia; **Musculoskeletal System:** arthritis, bone pain, myasthenia, osteonecrosis, synovitis; **Nervous System:** abnormal gait, amnesia, anxiety, Bell's Palsy, clumsiness, confusion, depersonalization, drug dependence, emotional lability, facial paralysis, hyperesthesia, hypertonia, increased libido, neurosis, paresthesia, psychosis, transient severe weakness; **Respiratory System:** bronchospasm, emphysema, hemoptysis, hiccup, hyperventilation, laryngitis, pharyngeal edema, pneumonia; **Skin and Appendages:** basal cell carcinoma, blisters, cold clammy skin, contact dermatitis, erythema, furunculosis, genital pruritus, nevus, pruritis, rash, seborrhea, skin ulcer, skin discoloration; **Special Senses:** abnormal vision, conjunctivitis, earache, eye pain, labyrinthitis, vitreous floaters; **Urogenital:** breast fibroadenosis, breast mass, dysuria, epididymitis, fibrocystic change of the breast, fibroids, gynecomastia, hematuria, kidney calculus, kidney pain, leukorrhea, menopause, nocturia, pelvic inflammatory disease, penis disorder, Peyronies Disease, polyuria, postmenopausal hemorrhage, prostatic disorder, pyelonephritis, testis disorder, urethral pain, urinary urgency, urinary retention, urinary incontinence, vaginal hemorrhage.

Table 2
Adverse Events and Selected Laboratory Abnormalities
in the Placebo-Controlled Study

Adverse Event	Placebo (N = 143)	AVONEX® (N = 158)
Body as a Whole		
Headache	57%	67%
Flu-like symptoms (otherwise unspecified)*	40%	61%
Pain	20%	24%
Fever*	13%	23%
Asthenia	13%	21%
Chills*	7%	21%
Infection	6%	11%
Abdominal pain	6%	9%
Chest pain	4%	6%
Injection site reaction	1%	4%
Malaise	3%	4%
Injection site inflammation	0%	3%
Hypersensitivity reaction	0%	3%
Ovarian cyst	0%	3%
Cardiovascular System		
Syncope	2%	4%
Vasodilation	1%	4%
Digestive System		
Nausea	23%	33%
Diarrhea	10%	16%
Dyspepsia	7%	11%
Anorexia	6%	7%
Hemic and Lymphatic System		
Anemia*	3%	8%
Eosinophils ≥ 10%	4%	5%
HCT (%) ≤ 32 (females) or ≤ 37 (males)	1%	3%
Ecchymosis injection site	1%	2%
Metabolic and Nutritional Disorders		
SGOT ≥ 3× ULN	1%	3%
Musculoskeletal System		
Muscle ache*	15%	34%
Arthralgia	5%	9%
Nervous System		
Sleep difficult	16%	19%
Dizziness	13%	15%
Muscle spasm	6%	7%
Suicidal tendency	1%	4%
Seizure	0%	3%
Speech disorder	0%	3%
Ataxia	0%	2%
Respiratory System		
Upper respiratory tract infection	28%	31%
Sinusitis	17%	18%
Dyspnea	3%	6%
Skin and Appendages		
Urticaria	2%	5%
Alopecia	1%	4%
Nevus	0%	3%
Herpes zoster	2%	3%
Herpes simplex	1%	2%
Special Senses		
Otitis media	5%	6%
Hearing decreased	0%	3%
Urogenital		
Vaginitis	2%	4%

Significantly associated with AVONEX® treatment ($p \leq 0.05$).

Serum Neutralizing Activity
Throughout the placebo-controlled multiple sclerosis study, serum samples from patients were monitored for the development of Interferon beta-1a neutralizing activity. During the study, 24% of AVONEX®-treated patients were found to have serum neutralizing activity at one or more time points tested. Fifteen percent of AVONEX®-treated patients tested positive for neutralizing activity at a level at which no placebo patient tested positive. The significance of the appearance of serum neutralizing activity is unknown.

DRUG ABUSE AND DEPENDENCE

There is no evidence that abuse or dependence occurs with AVONEX® (Interferon beta-1a) therapy. However, the risk of dependence has not been systematically evaluated.

DOSAGE AND ADMINISTRATION

The recommended dosage of AVONEX® (Interferon beta-1a) for the treatment of relapsing forms of multiple sclerosis is 30 mcg injected intramuscularly once a week (see Figure 3). AVONEX® is intended for use under the guidance and supervision of a physician. Patients may self-inject only if their physician determines that it is appropriate and with medical follow-up, as necessary, after proper training in intramuscular injection technique.

HOW SUPPLIED

AVONEX® (Interferon beta-1a) is supplied as a lyophilized powder in a single-use vial containing 33 mcg (6.6 million IU) of Interferon beta-1a, 16.5 mg Albumin Human, USP, 6.4 mg Sodium Chloride, USP, 6.3 mg Dibasic Sodium Phosphate, USP, and 1.3 mg Monobasic Sodium Phosphate, USP, and is preservative-free. Diluent is supplied in a single-use vial (Sterile Water for Injection, USP, preservative-free). Reconstitute AVONEX® with 1.1 mL (cc) of diluent and swirl gently to dissolve (approximate pH 7.3). Withdraw 1.0 mL (cc) for administration.

AVONEX® is available in the following package configuration (NDC 59627-001-03): Package (Administration Pack) containing four Administration Dose Packs (each containing one vial of AVONEX®, one 10 mL (10 cc) diluent vial, two alcohol wipes, one gauze pad, one 3 mL (cc) syringe, one Micro Pin®* vial access pin, one needle, and one adhesive bandage).

Stability and Storage
Vials of AVONEX® (Interferon beta-1a) must be stored in a 2–8°C (36–46°F) refrigerator. Should refrigeration be unavailable, AVONEX® can be stored at 25°C (77°F) for a period of up to 30 days. DO NOT EXPOSE TO HIGH TEMPERATURES. DO NOT FREEZE. Do not use beyond the expiration date stamped on the vial. Following reconstitution, it is recommended the product be used as soon as possible within 6 hours stored at 2–8°C (36–46°F). DO NOT FREEZE RECONSTITUTED AVONEX®.

REFERENCES

1. Jacobs LD, *et al.* Ann Neurol 1996; 39: 285-294.
2. Kurtzke JF. Neurol 1983; 33: 1444-1452.

AVONEX® (INTERFERON BETA-1a)
Manufactured by:
BIOGEN, INC.
14 Cambridge Center
Cambridge, MA 02142 USA

1-800-456-2255
U.S. Patent Pending
I63005-2 (4/00)
Rx only

**Micro Pin® is the trademark of B. Braun Medical Inc.*

Patient Information
AVONEX® (Interferon beta-1a) is intended for use under the guidance and supervision of a physician. If your physi-

cian recommends self-injection, you should be instructed in the preparation of AVONEX® for administration and in the technique of self-injection. Do not attempt self-administration until you are sure that you understand the requirements for preparing the product and giving an injection to yourself.

AVONEX® must be used as prescribed by your physician. However, if you miss a dose, take it as soon as you remember. You may resume your regular schedule, but 2 injections should not be administered within 2 days of each other. While using AVONEX®, please keep in mind the following facts:

- AVONEX® (Interferon beta-1a) must be kept cold. Be sure to store it in a refrigerator before and after reconstitution. Do not freeze. If refrigeration is not available, AVONEX® can be stored before reconstitution at 25°C (77°F) for up to 30 days. When storing outside of a refrigerator, do not allow AVONEX® to be exposed to high temperatures as may occur in a glove compartment or on a window sill.
- For treatment of multiple sclerosis, AVONEX® must be injected into the muscle (intramuscular injection).
- Keep syringes and needles away from children. Do not reuse needles or syringes. Discard used syringes and needles in a syringe disposal unit as instructed by your health care professional.
- Women: AVONEX® should not be used during pregnancy or if you are trying to become pregnant. If you wish to become pregnant while using AVONEX®, discuss the matter with your doctor. While using AVONEX®, women of childbearing age should use birth control measures. If you do become pregnant you should discontinue treatment and contact your doctor immediately.
- Flu-like symptoms are common. They include fever, chills, fatigue, and muscle ache. Your physician may recommend taking acetaminophen to help lessen the impact of flu-like symptoms.
- Depression has been reported by patients treated with interferon drugs. If you experience such symptoms, contact your physician promptly.
- As with any prescription medication, side effects related to therapy can occur. Consult with your physician if you have any problems, whether or not you think they may be related to AVONEX®.

FIGURE 3
RECONSTITUTION AND INJECTION

Read through entire instructions prior to starting procedure.

Wash hands prior to preparing medication and after the medication has been administered. Allow the AVONEX® (Interferon beta-1a) Administration Dose Pack to reach room temperature. Reconstitute AVONEX® using sterile technique, as discussed below.

The following supplies will be needed:

- vial of AVONEX® (white to off-white powder or cake)
- vial of diluent, single-use (Sterile Water for Injection, USP, preservative-free)
- syringe
- blue MICRO PIN® (vial access pin)
- sterile needle
- alcohol wipes
- gauze pad
- syringe disposal container
- adhesive bandage

Reconstitution with diluent vial

1. Remove the caps from the vial of AVONEX® and vial of diluent, and clean the rubber stopper of each vial with an alcohol wipe.

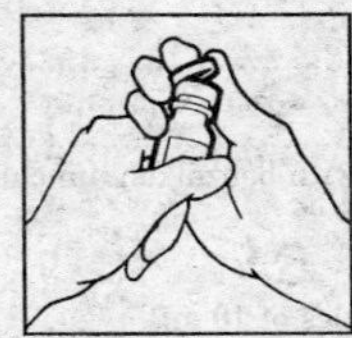

2. Remove the small protective cover from the syringe with a counter-clockwise turn.

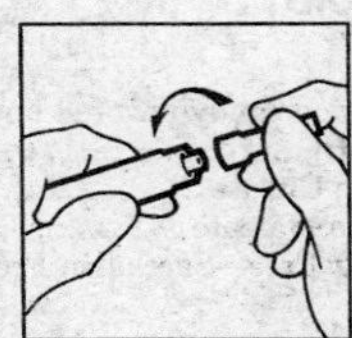

3. Attach the blue MICRO PIN® to the syringe with a **half turn** clockwise. ***CAUTION: Turning the MICRO PIN® more than half-way may make it difficult to remove.***

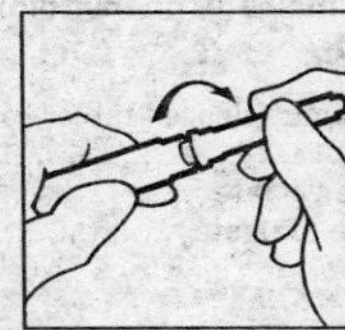

4. Pull the MICRO PIN® cover straight off; do not twist. Save for later use.

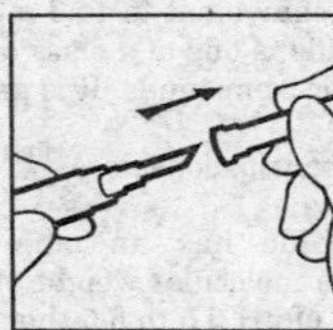

5. Pull back the syringe plunger to the 1.1 mL (cc) mark.

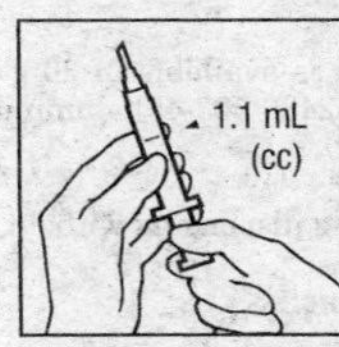

6. Firmly push the MICRO PIN® down through the center of the rubber stopper of the diluent vial.

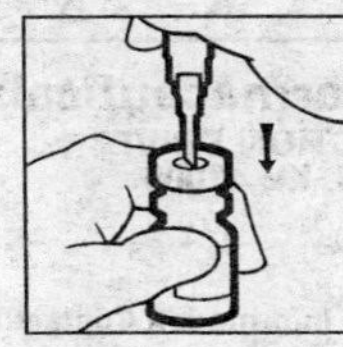

7. Inject air into the diluent vial by pushing down on the plunger until it cannot be pushed any further.
8. Turn the diluent vial and syringe upside down.
9. Keeping the MICRO PIN® in the fluid, withdraw 1.1 mL (cc) of diluent into the syringe by pulling back on the plunger.

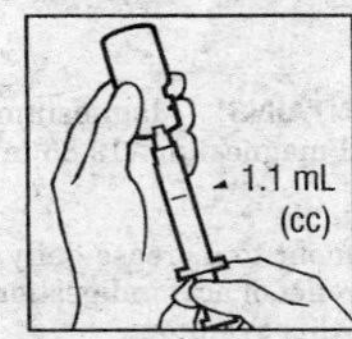

10. Tap the syringe gently to make any air bubbles rise to the top. If bubbles are present, press the plunger until the diluent is at the top of the syringe. Make sure there is still 1.1 mL (cc) of diluent in the syringe.

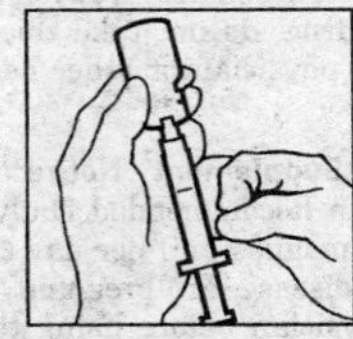

11. Pull the MICRO PIN® out of the diluent vial.
12. Firmly insert the MICRO PIN® through the center of the rubber stopper of the vial of AVONEX®.
13. ***Slowly*** inject the diluent. ***CAUTION: Rapid addition of the diluent may cause foaming, making it difficult to withdraw AVONEX®.***

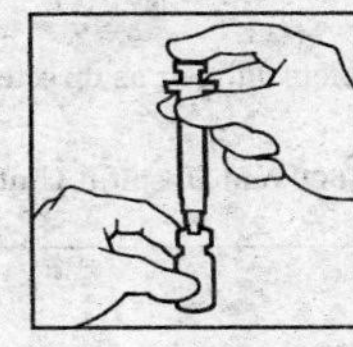

14. Without removing the syringe, ***gently*** swirl the vial until the AVONEX® is dissolved. ***CAUTION: DO NOT SHAKE.***

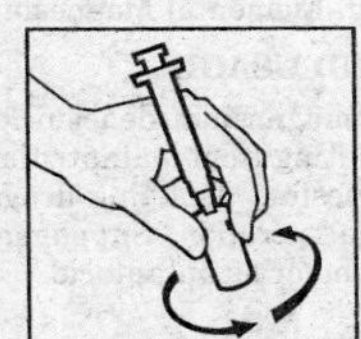

15. Check to see that all of the AVONEX® is dissolved.
16. Turn the vial and syringe upside down. Slowly withdraw 1.0 mL (cc) of AVONEX®. If bubbles appear, push solution ***slowly*** back into the vial and withdraw the solution again.

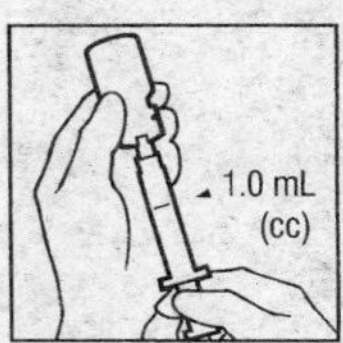

17. Check the contents of the syringe. Normal appearance is clear to slightly yellow solution. If appearance is not normal, do not use the syringe. Get a new set of materials, including syringe, and start again with Step 1.
18. With the vial still upside down, tap the syringe gently to make any air bubbles rise to the top. Then press the plunger until the AVONEX® is at the top of the syringe. Check the volume (should be 1.0 mL [cc]) and withdraw more medication if necessary. Withdraw the MICRO PIN® and syringe from the vial.
19. Replace the cover on the MICRO PIN® and remove from the syringe with a counterclockwise turn.
20. Attach a needle to the syringe with a half turn clockwise until the needle is secure.

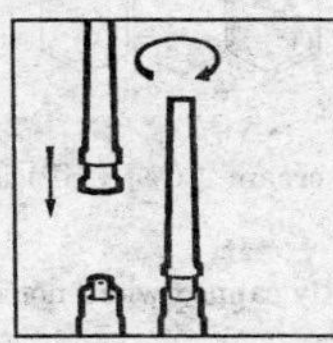

Injection

1. Use a new alcohol wipe to clean the skin at one of the recommended intramuscular injection sites. Pull the protective cover straight off the needle; do not twist.
2. With one hand, stretch the skin taut around the injection site. Hold the syringe with the other hand, making sure it is horizontal, until ready for injection. Insert the needle with a quick dart-like thrust at a 90° angle, through the skin and into the muscle. Expect to feel some resistance.

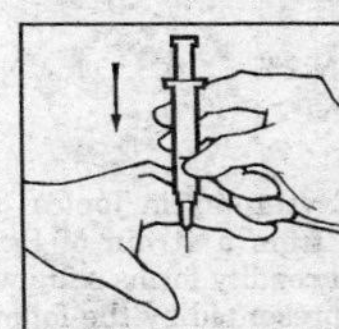

3. Once inserted, release the stretched skin and gently pull back slightly on the plunger and check for blood. If there is blood in the syringe, withdraw the needle from the injection site. Replace with a new needle and inject into a new site.
4. If you do not see blood, slowly push the plunger until the syringe is empty.

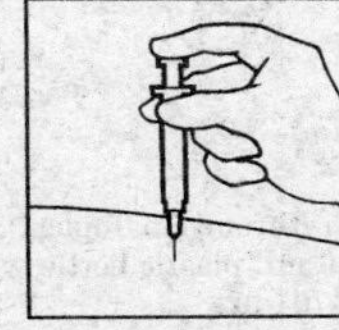

5. Hold a gauze pad near the needle at the injection site and pull the needle straight out. Use the pad to apply pressure to the site for a few seconds or rub gently in a circular motion.

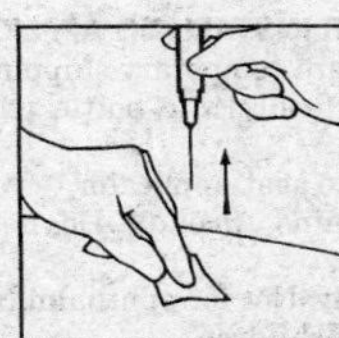

6. If there is bleeding at the site, wipe it off and, if necessary, apply an adhesive bandage.
7. Dispose of all supplies properly, including the diluent.

For information on over-the-counter drugs,
consult **PDR For Nonprescription Drugs**.

Bioglan Pharma, Inc.

**7 GREAT VALLEY PARKWAY, SUITE 301
MALVERN, PA 19355**

Direct Inquiries to:
Bioglan Pharma, Inc.
PHONE: 610-232-2000
FAX: 610-232-2020

MICANOL® ℞

(anthralin cream 1.0%, USP)
Topical treatment of psoriasis

DESCRIPTION

Micanol (anthralin cream 1.0%, USP) is a smooth, yellow cream containing 1% anthralin USP in an aqueous cream base of glyceryl monolaurate, glyceryl monomyristate, citric acid, sodium hydroxide and purified water.
The chemical name of anthralin is 1,8-dihydroxy-9-anthrone.
The structure is:

HOW SUPPLIED

Micanol (anthralin cream 1.0%, USP) is supplied in 50g tubes.
NDC 62436-401-01
Keep container tightly capped when not in use.
Avoid excessive heat.
Store at controlled room temperature 59°F–86°F (15°C–30°C).
Caution: Federal (U.S.A.) law prohibits dispensing without prescription.
Manufactured for Bioglan Pharma, Inc., Malvern, PA 19355 by Bioglan AB, Sweden
13212051

THERAMYCIN Z® ℞

ERYTHROMYCIN
TOPICAL SOLUTION 2%

DESCRIPTION

THERAMYCIN Z (Erythromycin Topical Solution 2%) is an antibiotic produced from a strain of *Streptomyces erythraeus.* It is basic and readily forms salts with acids. The active ingredient is represented by the following structure:

HOW SUPPLIED

THERAMYCIN Z (Erythromycin Topical Solution 2%), 2 fl oz (59.14 mL) in a 60 mL plastic bottle with applicator attached—NDC 62436-701-02.

STORAGE

THERAMYCIN Z (Erythromycin Topical Solution 2%) should be stored at Controlled Room Temperature 15°–30°C (59°–86°F). Preserve in a light-resistant container.

INSTRUCTIONS FOR INSTALLING APPLICATOR

1. Remove and discard temporary shipping cap.
2. Push applicator firmly into bottle using white cap as holder.
3. Screw cap down to seat applicator.

WARNINGS: Contains Alcohol—Do not use near open flame.
For external use only. Not for ophthalmic use.
Keep out of reach of children.
CAUTION: Federal law prohibits dispensing without prescription.
Manufactured specially for:
Bioglan Pharma, Inc.
Malvern, PA 19355

ZONALON® CREAM ℞

[*zŏn a lon*]
(doxepin hydrochloride cream), 5%
**FOR TOPICAL DERMATOLOGIC USE ONLY—
NOT FOR OPHTHALMIC, ORAL, OR INTRAVAGINAL USE.**

Prescribing information as of August 1998.

DESCRIPTION

ZONALON CREAM (doxepin hydrochloride cream) is a topical antipruritic cream. Each gram contains: 50 mg of doxepin hydrochloride (equivalent to 44.3 mg of doxepin).
Doxepin hydrochloride is one of a class of agents known as dibenzoxepin tricyclic compounds. It is an isomeric mixture of

N,N-Dimethyldibenz[*b,e*]oxepin-$\Delta^{11(6H),\gamma}$-propylamine hydrochloride

Doxepin hydrochloride has an empirical formula of $C_{19}H_{21}NO \cdot HCl$ and a molecular weight of 316.
The base is a cream of pH 3.5 to 5.5 that includes the inactive ingredients: sorbitol, cetyl alcohol, isopropyl myristate, glyceryl stearate, PEG-100 stearate, petrolatum, benzyl alcohol, titanium dioxide and purified water.

HOW SUPPLIED

ZONALON CREAM is available in 30 g (NDC 62436-523-30) and 45g (NDC 62436-523-45) aluminum tubes. Store at or below 27°C (80°F).

CAUTION

Federal law prohibits dispensing without prescription.
Manufactured for:
BIOGLAN PHARMA, Inc.
Malvern, PA 19355
by: DPT Laboratories, Inc.
San Antonio, TX 78215

Blaine Pharmaceuticals

**1515 PRODUCTION DRIVE
BURLINGTON, KY 41005**

Inquiries or Medical Information Contact:
(859) 283-9437
(800) 633-9353
FAX: (859) 283-9460
E-mail: blainepharma.com

MAG–OX 400™ OTC

DESCRIPTION

EACH TABLET CONTAINS: Magnesium Oxide, 400 mg [241.3 mg elemental magnesium (19.86 mEq)].

INDICATIONS

As a dietary supplement to increase daily intake of magnesium. Also used for relief of acid indigestion and upset stomach associated with this symptom.

DIRECTIONS

As an Adult Dietary Supplement - Take 1 to 2 tablets daily or as directed by a physician. **As an Adult Antacid** - Take 1 tablet 2 times a day or as directed by a physician.
DRUG INTERACTION PRECAUTION: Antacids may interact with certain prescription drugs. If you are presently taking a prescription drug, do not take this product without checking with your physician or other health professional.

WARNINGS

As an Adult Dietary Supplement - Not recommended for use in amounts over the Recommended Daily Intake (RDI) of 400 mg (elemental magnesium) per day (1 or 2 tablets). If you have a kidney disease, are pregnant, or are nursing a baby, consult a physician before using this product. May have a laxative effect. **As an Adult Antacid** - Do not take more than 2 tablets in a 24-hour period, or use this maximum dosage for more than 2 weeks, except under the advice and supervision of a physician. May have a laxative effect. As with any drug, if you are pregnant or nursing a baby, seek the advice of a health professional before using this product. Keep this and all drugs out of the reach of children. Store at controlled room temperature 15°–30°C (59°–86°F).

DOSAGE

Adult dose 1 to 2 tablets daily or as directed by a physician.

HOW SUPPLIED

Bottles of 120 and 1000 and Hospital Unit Dose (UD).

URO–MAG® OTC

DESCRIPTION

Each capsule contains Magnesium Oxide 140 mg. U.S.P. (Heavy), or 84.5 mg. Elemental Magnesium (6.93 mEq.)

INDICATIONS AND USAGE

Hypomagnesemia, magnesium deficiencies and/or magnesium depletion resulting from malnutrition, restricted diet, alcoholism or magnesium depleting drugs. For increasing urinary magnesium excretion. Supplemental magnesium during pregnancy and/or as an antacid.

WARNINGS

Do not take more than 4 capsules in a 24 hour period, or use this maximum dosage for more than 2 weeks, except under the advice and supervision of a physician. Do not use this product except under the advice and supervision of a physician if you have a kidney disease. May have laxative effect. As with any drug, if you are pregnant or nursing a baby, seek professional advice before using this product. Keep this and all medicines out of children's reach.

DOSAGE

Adult dose 4 to 5 capsules daily or as directed by a physician.

HOW SUPPLIED

Bottles of 100 and 1000 and Hospital Unit Dose (UD).

EDUCATIONAL MATERIAL

Samples available to physicians upon request.
(800)633-9353
E-mail: blainepharma.com

Blansett Pharmacal

**P.O. BOX 638
N. LITTLE ROCK, AR 72115**

Direct Inquiries to:
Customer Service
(501) 758-8635
FAX: (501) 758-5369

ANOLOR® 300 ℞

(butalbital, acetaminophen & caffeine)

Each opaque white capsule imprinted light green ANOLOR 300 and 51674-0009 contains:

Butalbital*	50 mg
*(WARNING: May be habit forming)	
Acetaminophen	325 mg
Caffeine	40 mg

HOW SUPPLIED

Bottles of 100

CORTANE-B™ *Aqueous* Ear Drops ℞

(chloroxylenol, pramoxine HCl, hydrocortisone)

Each 1 mL contains:

Chloroxylenol	1 mg
Pramoxine HCl	10 mg
Hydrocortisone	10 mg

In a bland *Aqueous* Vehicle

HOW SUPPLIED

Plastic dropper bottles of 10 mL.

CORTANE-B™ OTIC ℞

(chloroxylenol, hydrocortisone, pramoxine HCl)

Each 1 mL contains:

Chloroxylenol	1 mg
Pramoxine HCl	10 mg
Hydrocortisone	10 mg

In a bland vehicle with benzalkonium chloride as a preservative.

HOW SUPPLIED

Plastic dropper bottles of 10 mL.

NALEX®-A LIQUID ℞

[*nā-lĕx-ā*]

Each 5 mL pink cotton candy flavored liquid contains:

Phenylephrine HCl	5 mg
Phenyltoloxamine Citrate	7.5 mg
Chlorpheniramine Maleate	2.5 mg

Alcohol Free—Sugar Free—Saccharin Free

HOW SUPPLIED

Bottles of 16 oz.

NALEX®-A TABLETS (Dye Free) ℞

(chlorpheniramine maleate, phenyltoloxamine citrate, phenylephrine HCl)

Each white scored time released tablet contains:

Phenylephrine HCl	20 mg
Phenyltoloxamine Citrate	40 mg
Chlorpheniramine Maleate	4 mg

HOW SUPPLIED

Bottles of 100

Block Drug Company, Inc.

257 CORNELISON AVENUE
JERSEY CITY, NJ 07302

Direct Inquiries to:
Consumer Affairs
(201) 434-3000, Ext. 1308
FAX: (201) 432-6183

For Medical Information Contact:
Consumer Affairs
(800) 365-6500, Ext. 1308
FAX: (201) 432-6183

APHTHASOL® ℞

[*aph-thăsōl*]
(amlexanox oral paste), 5%
For Oral Cavity Use Only
Not for Ophthalmic Use

DESCRIPTION

Aphthasol contains 5% amlexanox in an adhesive oral paste. Chemically, amlexanox is 2-amino-7-isopropyl-5-oxo-5H-[1]benzopyrano[2,3-b] pyridine-3-carboxylic acid. It has a molecular formula of $C_{16}H_{14}N_2O_4$ and has a molecular weight of 298.30. Amlexanox is odorless, white to yellowish-white crystalline powder. The structural formula is:

Each gram of beige colored oral paste contains 50 mg of amlexanox in an adhesive oral paste base consisting of benzyl alcohol, gelatin, glyceryl monostearate, mineral oil, pectin, petrolatum, and sodium carboxymethylcellulose.

CLINICAL PHARMACOLOGY

The mechanism of action by which amlexanox accelerates healing of aphthous ulcers is unknown. *In vitro* studies have demonstrated amlexanox to be a potent inhibitor of the formation and/or release of inflammatory mediators (histamine and leukotrienes) from mast cells, neutrophils and mononuclear cells. Given orally to animals, amlexanox has demonstrated anti-allergic and anti-inflammatory activities and has been shown to suppress both immediate and delayed type hypersensitivity reactions. The relevance of these activities of amlexanox to its effects on aphthous ulcers has not been established.

Pharmacokinetics and Metabolism: After a single oral application of 100 mg of paste (5 mg amlexanox), maximal serum levels of approximately 120 ng/ml are observed at 2.4 hours. Most of the systemic absorption of amlexanox is via the gastrointestinal tract, and the amount absorbed directly through the active ulcer is not a significant portion of the applied dose. The half-life for elimination was 3.5 +/− 1.1 hours in healthy individuals. Approximately 17% of the dose is eliminated into the urine as unchanged amlexanox, a hydroxylated metabolite, and their conjugates. With multiple applications four times daily, steady state levels were reached within one week, and no accumulation was observed with up to four weeks of usage.

Clinical Studies: The safety of amlexanox oral paste, 5%, was established in a study in which 100 patients with aphthous ulcers applied the medication four times daily for 28 days with no significant topical or systemic adverse effects. The effectiveness was demonstrated in three controlled clinical studies of patients with mild to moderate aphthous ulcers which evaluated 464 patients receiving amlexanox oral paste, 5%, 465 patients receiving a placebo paste, and 195 patients receiving no treatment. Amlexanox oral paste, 5%, was shown to accelerate healing of aphthous ulcers in a statistically significant manner as compared to both vehicle and no treatment.

Amlexanox oral paste, 5%, versus no treatment: In the combined database of the two studies including a no treatment group, there was a significant difference in the rate of ulcer healing which translated to a reduction of 1.6 days in the median time to complete healing and a reduction of 1.3 days in the median time to complete pain relief. After 3 days of treatment there was a significant difference in both percent of patients with complete healing of ulcers (21% vs. 8%) and percent of patients with complete resolution of pain (44% vs. 20%).

Amlexanox oral paste, 5%, versus vehicle: In the combined database of the three studies, there was a significant difference in the rate of ulcer healing which translated into a reduction of 0.7 days in the median time to complete healing, and a reduction of 0.7 days in the median time to complete pain relief. After 4 days of treatment there was a significant difference in both percent of patients with complete healing of ulcers (37% vs. 27%) and percent of patients with complete resolution of pain (60% vs. 49%).

Pain relief occurred in conjunction with healing of the ulcers. Amlexanox oral paste, 5%, by itself, was not shown to be an analgesic medication. The safety and effectiveness of the product in immunocompromised individuals has not been assessed.

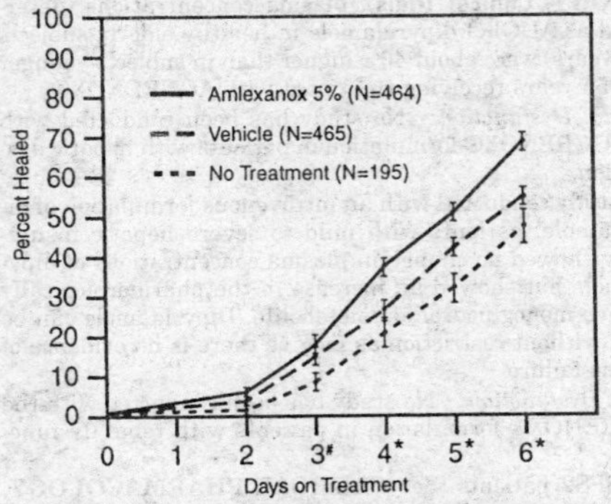

Results for amlexanox, 5%, vs. vehicle are based on three clinical trials. Results for amlexanox, 5%, vs. no treatment are based on two clinical trials.
* denotes statistically significant superiority of amlexanox, 5%, vs. vehicle and no treatment.
\# denotes statistically significant superiority of amlexanox, 5%, vs. no treatment.
Error bars represent Standard Error of the Mean.

INDICATIONS AND USAGE

Amlexanox oral paste, 5%, is indicated for the treatment of aphthous ulcers in people with normal immune systems.

CONTRAINDICATIONS

Amlexanox oral paste, 5%, is contraindicated in patients with known hypersensitivity to amlexanox or other ingredients in the formulation.

PRECAUTIONS

General: Wash hands immediately after applying amlexanox oral paste, 5%, directly to ulcers with the finger tips. In the event that a rash or contact mucositis occurs, discontinue use.

Information for Patients:

1. Apply the paste as soon as possible after noticing the symptoms of an aphthous ulcer. Continue to use the paste four times daily, preferably following oral hygiene after breakfast, lunch, dinner, and at bedtime.
2. Dry the ulcer(s) by gently patting it with a soft, clean cloth.
3. Wash your hands before applying the Aphthasol.
4. Moisten the tip of your index finger.
5. Squeeze a dab of paste approximately 1/4 inch (0.5 cm) onto a finger tip.
6. Gently dab the Aphthasol on to the ulcer. Repeat the process if you have more than one ulcer.
7. Wash your hands when you are done applying Aphthasol.
8. Wash eyes promptly if they should come in contact with the paste.
9. Use the paste until the ulcer heals. If significant healing or pain relief has not occurred in 10 days, consult your dentist or physician.
10. Keep out of the reach of children.

Carcinogenesis, Mutagenesis, Impairment of Fertility: Amlexanox was not carcinogenic when administered orally to rats for two years and to mice for 18 months. *In vitro* (Ames) and *in vivo* (mouse micronucleus) mutagenicity tests of amlexanox were negative. Amlexanox at doses up to two hundred times the projected human daily dose, on a mg/m^2 basis, did not significantly affect fertility or general reproductive performance in rats.

Pregnancy Category B: Teratology studies were performed with rats and rabbits at doses up to two hundred and six hundred times, respectively, the projected human daily dose, on a mg/m^2 basis. No adverse fetal effects were observed. At doses up to two hundred times the projected human daily dose, on a mg/m^2 basis, amlexanox did not have significant effect on peri- and postnatal development of rat fetuses. There are no adequate and well-controlled studies in pregnant women. Because animal reproduction studies are not always predictive of human response, this drug should be used during pregnancy only if clearly needed.

Nursing Mothers: Amlexanox was found in the milk of lactating rats; therefore, caution should be exercised when administering amlexanox oral paste, 5%, to a nursing woman.

Pediatric Use: Safety and effectiveness of amlexanox oral paste, 5%, in pediatric patients have not been established.

Geriatric Use: Clinical studies of Aphthasol did not include sufficient numbers of subjects aged 65 and over to determine whether they respond differently from younger subjects. Other reported clinical experience has not identified differences in responses between the elderly and younger patients. In general, dose selection for an elderly patient should be cautious, usually starting at the low end of the dosing range, reflecting the greater frequency of decreased hepatic, renal, or cardiac function, and of concomitant disease or other drug therapy.

ADVERSE REACTIONS

Adverse reactions considered related or possibly related to amlexanox oral paste, 5%, were not reported by more than 5% of patients. Adverse reactions reported by 1–2% of patients were transient pain, stinging and/or burning at the site of application. Infrequent (< 1%) adverse reactions in the clinical studies were contact mucositis, nausea, and diarrhea.

OVERDOSAGE

There are no reports of human ingestion overdosage. Ingestion of a full tube of 5 grams of paste would result in systemic exposure well below the maximum nontoxic dose of amlexanox in animals. Gastrointestinal upset such as diarrhea and vomiting could result from an overdose.

DOSAGE AND ADMINISTRATION

The paste should be applied as soon as possible after noticing the symptoms of an aphthous ulcer and should be used four times daily, preferably following oral hygiene after breakfast, lunch, dinner, and at bedtime. Squeeze a dab of paste approximately 1/4 inch (0.5 cm) onto a finger tip. With gentle pressure, dab the paste onto each ulcer in the mouth. Use of the medication should be continued until the ulcer heals. If significant healing or pain reduction has not occurred in 10 days, consult your dentist or physician.

HOW SUPPLIED

Amlexanox oral paste, 5%, is supplied in 5 gram tubes (NDC 10158-059-01). Amlexanox oral paste, 5%, should be stored at controlled room temperature, 15°–30°C (59°–86°F).

Manufactured for:

Oral Health Care Division
Block Drug Company, Inc.
Jersey City, NJ 07302

By Reedco, Inc.
Humacao, Puerto Rico 00791

Aphthasol® is a registered trademark of Block Drug Company, Inc.

March 1999 APH-PI-01

Boehringer Ingelheim Pharmaceuticals, Inc.

A subsidiary of Boehringer Ingelheim Corporation
900 RIDGEBURY ROAD
POST OFFICE BOX 368
RIDGEFIELD, CT 06877-0368

For Medical Information Contact:
1–800–542–6257
or email:
druginfo@rdg.boehringer-ingelheim.com

AGGRENOX® ℞

(aspirin/extended-release dipyridamole)
25 mg/200 mg capsules

PRESCRIBING INFORMATION

DESCRIPTION

AGGRENOX® is a combination antiplatelet agent intended for oral administration. Each hard gelatin capsule contains 200 mg dipyridamole in an extended-release form and 25 mg aspirin, as an immediate-release sugar-coated tablet. In addition, each capsule contains the following inactive ingredients: acacia, aluminum stearate, colloidal silicon dioxide, corn starch, dimethicone, hydroxypropyl methylcellulose, hydroxypropyl methylcellulose phthalate, lactose monohydrate, methacrylic acid copolymer, microcrystalline cellulose, povidone, stearic acid, sucrose, talc, tartaric acid, titanium dioxide, and triacetin.

Each capsule shell contains gelatin, red iron oxide and yellow iron oxide, titanium dioxide and water.

Dipyridamole

Dipyridamole is an antiplatelet agent chemically described as 2,6-bis(diethanolamino)-4,8-dipiperidino-pyrimido(5,4-d) pyrimidine (= dipyridamole). It has the following structural formula:

$C_{24}H_{40}N_8O_4$ Mol. Wt. 504.63

Dipyridamole is an odorless yellow crystalline substance, having a bitter taste. It is soluble in dilute acids, methanol and chloroform, and is practically insoluble in water.

Continued on next page

Aggrenox—Cont.

Aspirin

The antiplatelet agent aspirin (acetylsalicylic acid) is chemically known as benzoic acid, 2-(acetyloxy)-, and has the following structural formula:

OH
O
H_3C
O
$C_9H_8O_4$ Mol. Wt. 180.16

Aspirin is an odorless white needle-like crystalline or powdery substance. When exposed to moisture, aspirin hydrolyzes into salicylic and acetic acids, and gives off a vinegary odor. It is highly lipid soluble and slightly soluble in water.

CLINICAL PHARMACOLOGY

Mechanism of Action

The antithrombotic action of AGGRENOX® is the result of the additive antiplatelet effects of dipyridamole and aspirin.

Dipyridamole

Dipyridamole inhibits the uptake of adenosine into platelets, endothelial cells and erythrocytes *in vitro* and *in vivo;* the inhibition occurs in a dose-dependent manner at therapeutic concentrations (0.5–1.9 μg/mL). This inhibition results in an increase in local concentrations of adenosine which acts on the platelet A_2-receptor thereby stimulating platelet adenylate cyclase and increasing platelet cyclic-3′,5′-adenosine monophosphate (cAMP) levels. Via this mechanism, platelet aggregation is inhibited in response to various stimuli such as platelet activating factor (PAF), collagen and adenosine diphosphate (ADP).

Dipyridamole inhibits phosphodiesterase (PDE) in various tissues. While the inhibition of cAMP-PDE is weak, therapeutic levels of dipyridamole inhibit cyclic-3′,5′-guanosine monophosphate-PDE (cGMP-PDE), thereby augmenting the increase in cGMP produced by EDRF (endothelium-derived relaxing factor, now identified as nitric oxide).

Aspirin

Aspirin inhibits platelet aggregation by irreversible inhibition of platelet cyclo-oxygenase and thus inhibits the generation of thromboxane A_2, a powerful inducer of platelet aggregation and vasoconstriction.

Pharmacokinetics

There are no significant interactions between aspirin and dipyridamole. The kinetics of the components are unchanged by their coadministration as AGGRENOX®.

Dipyridamole

Absorption: Peak plasma levels of dipyridamole are achieved 2 hours (range 1–6 hours) after administration of a daily dose of 400 mg AGGRENOX® (given as 200 mg b.i.d.). The peak plasma concentration at steady-state is 1.98 μg/mL (1.01–3.99 μg/mL) and the steady-state trough concentration is 0.53 μg/mL (0.18–1.01 μg/mL).

Effect of Food: No food effect study has been conducted with the AGGRENOX® formulation.

Distribution: Dipyridamole is highly lipophilic (log P=3.71, pH=7); however, it has been shown that the drug does not cross the blood-brain barrier to any significant extent in animals. The steady-state volume of distribution of dipyridamole is about 92 L. Approximately 99% of dipyridamole is bound to plasma proteins, predominantly to alpha 1-acid glycoprotein and albumin.

Metabolism and Elimination: Dipyridamole is metabolized in the liver, primarily by conjugation with glucuronic acid, of which monoglucuronide which has low pharmacodynamic activity is the primary metabolite. In plasma, about 80% of the total amount is present as parent compound and 20% as monoglucuronide. Most of the glucuronide metabolite (about 95%) is excreted via bile into the feces, with some evidence of enterohepatic circulation. Renal excretion of parent compound is negligible and urinary excretion of the glucuronide metabolite is low (about 5%). With intravenous (i.v.) treatment of dipyridamole, a triphasic profile is obtained: a rapid alpha phase, with a half-life of about 3.4 minutes, a beta phase, with a half-life of about 39 minutes, (which, together with the alpha phase accounts for about 70% of the total area under the curve, AUC) and a prolonged elimination phase λ_z with a half-life of about 15.5 hours. Due to the extended absorption phase of the dipyridamole component, only the terminal phase is apparent from oral treatment with AGGRENOX® which, in trial 9.123 was 13.6 hours.

Special Populations:

Geriatric Patients: In ESPS2 (See **CLINICAL PHARMACOLOGY, Clinical Trials**), plasma concentrations (determined as AUC) of dipyridamole in healthy elderly subjects (>65 years) were about 40% higher than in subjects younger than 55 years receiving treatment with AGGRENOX®.

Hepatic Dysfunction: No study has been conducted with the AGGRENOX® formulation in patients with hepatic dysfunction.

In a study conducted with an intravenous formulation of dipyridamole, patients with mild to severe hepatic insufficiency showed no change in plasma concentrations of dipyridamole but showed an increase in the pharmacologically inactive monoglucuronide metabolite. Dipyridamole can be dosed without restriction as long as there is no evidence of hepatic failure.

Renal Dysfunction: No study has been conducted with the AGGRENOX® formulation in patients with renal dysfunction.

In ESPS2 patients (See **CLINICAL PHARMACOLOGY, Clinical Trials**), with creatinine clearances ranging from about 15 mL/min to >100 mL/min, no changes were observed in the pharmacokinetics of dipyridamole or its glucuronide metabolite if data were corrected for differences in age.

Aspirin

Absorption: Peak plasma levels of aspirin are achieved 0.63 hours (0.5–1 hour) after administration of a 50 mg aspirin daily dose from AGGRENOX® (given as 25 mg b.i.d.). The peak plasma concentration at steady-state is 319 ng/mL (175–463 ng/mL). Aspirin undergoes moderate hydrolysis to salicylic acid in the liver and the gastrointestinal wall, with 50%–75% of an administered dose reaching the systemic circulation as intact aspirin.

Distribution: Aspirin is poorly bound to plasma proteins and its apparent volume of distribution is low (10 L). Its metabolite, salicylic acid, is highly bound to plasma proteins, but its binding is concentration-dependent (nonlinear). At low concentrations (<100 μg/mL), approximately 90% of salicylic acid is bound to albumin. Salicylic acid is widely distributed to all tissues and fluids in the body, including the central nervous system, breast milk, and fetal tissues. Early signs of salicylate overdose (salicylism), including tinnitus (ringing in the ears), occur at plasma concentrations approximating 200 μg/mL (See **ADVERSE REACTIONS; OVERDOSAGE**).

Metabolism and Elimination: Aspirin is rapidly hydrolyzed in plasma to salicylic acid, with a half-life of 20 minutes. Plasma levels of aspirin are essentially undetectable 2–2.5 hours after dosing and peak salicylic acid concentrations occur 1 hour (range: 0.5–2 hours) after administration of aspirin. Salicylic acid is primarily conjugated in the liver to form salicyluric acid, a phenolic glucuronide, an acyl glucuronide, and a number of minor metabolites. Salicylate metabolism is saturable and total body clearance decreases at higher serum concentrations due to the limited ability of the liver to form both salicyluric acid and phenolic glucuronide. Following toxic doses (10–20 g), the plasma half-life may be increased to over 20 hours.

The elimination of acetylsalicylic acid follows first-order kinetics with AGGRENOX® and has a half-life of 0.33 hours. The half-life of salicylic acid is 1.71 hours. Both values correspond well with data from the literature at lower doses which state a resultant half-life of approximately 2–3 hours. At higher doses, the elimination of salicylic acid follows zero-order kinetics (i.e., the rate of elimination is constant in relation to plasma concentration), with an apparent half-life of 6 hours or higher. Renal excretion of unchanged drug depends upon urinary pH. As urinary pH rises above 6.5, the renal clearance of free salicylate increases from <5% to >80%. Alkalinization of the urine is a key concept in the management of salicylate overdose (See **OVERDOSAGE**). Following therapeutic doses, about 10% is excreted as salicylic acid and 75% as salicyluric acid, as the phenolic and acyl glucuronides, in urine.

Special Populations:

Hepatic Dysfunction: Aspirin is to be avoided in patients with severe hepatic insufficiency.

Renal Dysfunction: Aspirin is to be avoided in patients with severe renal failure (glomerular filtration rate less than 10 mL/min).

Clinical Trials

AGGRENOX® was studied in a double-blind, placebo-controlled, 24-month study (European Stroke Prevention Study 2, ESPS2) in which 6602 patients had an ischemic stroke (76%) or transient ischemic attack (TIA, 24%) within three months prior to entry. Patients were randomized to one of four treatment groups: AGGRENOX® (aspirin/extended-release dipyridamole) 25 mg/200 mg; extended-release dipyridamole (ER-DP) 200 mg alone; aspirin (ASA) 25 mg alone; or placebo. Patients received one capsule twice daily (morning and evening). Efficacy assessments included analyses of stroke (fatal or nonfatal) and death (from all causes) as confirmed by a blinded morbidity and mortality assessment group.

Stroke Endpoint:

AGGRENOX® reduced the risk of stroke by 22.1% compared to aspirin 50 mg/day alone (p =0.008) and reduced the risk of stroke by 24.4% compared to extended-release dipyridamole 400 mg/day alone (p = 0.002) (Table 1). AGGRENOX® reduced the risk of stroke by 36.8% compared to placebo (p < 0.001).

[See table 1 below]

ESPS2: Cumulative Stroke Rate (Fatal or Nonfatal) Over 24 Months Of Follow-Up

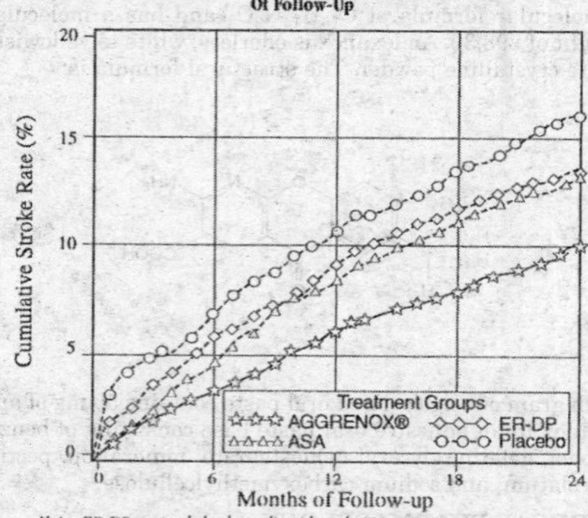

Note: ER-DP = extended-release dipyridamole 200 mg; ASA = aspirin 25 mg.
Note: The dosage regimen for all treatment groups is b.i.d.

Combined Stroke or Death Endpoint:

In ESPS2, AGGRENOX® reduced the risk of stroke or death by 12.1% compared to aspirin alone and by 10.3% compared to extended-release dipyridamole alone. These results were not statistically significant. AGGRENOX® reduced the risk of stroke or death by 24.2% compared to placebo.

Death Endpoint:

The incidence rate of all cause mortality was 11.3% for AGGRENOX®, 11.0% for aspirin alone, 11.4% for extended-release dipyridamole alone and 12.3% for placebo alone. The differences between the AGGRENOX®, aspirin alone and extended-release dipyridamole alone treatment groups were not statistically significant. These incidence rates for AGGRENOX® and aspirin alone are consistent with previous aspirin studies in stroke and TIA patients.

INDICATIONS AND USAGE

AGGRENOX® is indicated to reduce the risk of stroke in patients who have had transient ischemia of the brain or completed ischemic stroke due to thrombosis.

CONTRAINDICATIONS

AGGRENOX® is contraindicated in patients with hypersensitivity to dipyridamole, aspirin or any of the other product components.

Allergy: Aspirin is contraindicated in patients with known allergy to nonsteroidal anti-inflammatory drug products and in patients with the syndrome of asthma, rhinitis, and nasal polyps. Aspirin may cause severe urticaria, angioedema or bronchospasm (asthma).

Reye's Syndrome: Aspirin should not be used in children or teenagers for viral infections, with or without fever, because of the risk of Reye's syndrome with concomitant use of aspirin in certain viral illnesses.

Table 1: Summary of First Stroke (Fatal or Nonfatal) ESPS2: Intent-to-Treat Population

	Total Number of Patients n	Number of Patients With Stroke Within 2 Years n (%)	Kaplan-Meier Estimate of Survival at 2 Years (95% C.I.)	Gehan-Wilcoxon Test P-value	Risk Reduction at 2 Years	Odds Ratio (95% C.I.)
Individual Treatment Group						
AGGRENOX®	1650	157 (9.5%)	89.9% (88.4%, 91.4%)	—	—	—
ER-DP	1654	211 (12.8%)	86.7% (85.0%, 88.4%)	—	—	—
ASA	1649	206 (12.5%)	87.1% (85.4%, 88.7%)	—	—	—
Placebo	1649	250 (15.2%)	84.1% (82.2%, 85.9%)	—	—	—
Pairwise Treatment Group Comparisons						
AGGRENOX® vs. ER-DP	—	—	—	0.002**	24.4%	0.72 (0.58, 0.90)
AGGRENOX® vs. ASA	—	—	—	0.008**	22.1%	0.74 (0.59, 0.92)
AGGRENOX® vs. Placebo	—	—	—	<0.001**	36.8%	0.59 (0.48, 0.73)
ER-DP vs. Placebo	—	—	—	0.036*	16.5%	0.82 (0.67, 1.00)
ASA vs. Placebo	—	—	—	0.009**	18.9%	0.80 (0.66, 0.97)

*0.010 < p-value ≤0.050; **p-value ≤0.010.

Note: ER-DP = extended-release dipyridamole 200 mg; ASA = aspirin 25 mg. The dosage regimen for all treatment groups is b.i.d.

WARNINGS

Alcohol Warning: Patients who consume three or more alcoholic drinks every day should be counseled about the bleeding risks involved with chronic, heavy alcohol use while taking aspirin.

Coagulation Abnormalities: Even low doses of aspirin can inhibit platelet function leading to an increase in bleeding time. This can adversely affect patients with inherited or acquired (liver disease or vitamin K deficiency) bleeding disorders.

Gastrointestinal (GI) Side Effects: GI side effects include stomach pain, heartburn, nausea, vomiting, and gross GI bleeding. Although minor upper GI symptoms, such as dyspepsia, are common and can occur anytime during therapy, physicians should remain alert for signs of ulceration and bleeding, even in the absence of previous GI symptoms. Physicians should inform patients about the signs and symptoms of GI side effects and what steps to take if they occur.

Peptic Ulcer Disease: Patients with a history of active peptic ulcer disease should avoid using aspirin, which can cause gastric mucosal irritation and bleeding.

PRECAUTIONS

General

AGGRENOX® is not interchangeable with the individual components of aspirin and Persantine® Tablets.

Coronary Artery Disease: Dipyridamole has a vasodilatory effect and should be used with caution in patients with severe coronary artery disease (e.g., unstable angina or recently sustained myocardial infarction). Chest pain may be aggravated in patients with underlying coronary artery disease who are receiving dipyridamole.

For stroke or TIA patients for whom aspirin is indicated to prevent recurrent myocardial infarction (MI) or angina pectoris, the aspirin in this product may not provide adequate treatment for the cardiac indications.

Hepatic Insufficiency: Elevations of hepatic enzymes and hepatic failure have been reported in association with dipyridamole administration.

Hypotension: Dipyridamole should be used with caution in patients with hypotension since it can produce peripheral vasodilation.

Renal Failure: Avoid aspirin in patients with severe renal failure (glomerular filtration rate less than 10 mL/minute).

Risk of Bleeding: In ESPS2 the incidence of gastrointestinal bleeding was 68 patients (4.1%) in the AGGRENOX® group, 36 patients (2.2%) in the dipyridamole group, 52 patients (3.2%) in the aspirin group, and 34 patients (2.1%) in the placebo groups.

The incidence of intracranial hemorrhage was 9 patients (0.6%) in the AGGRENOX® group, 6 patients (0.5%) in the dipyridamole group, 6 patients (0.4%) in the aspirin group and 7 patients (0.4%) in the placebo groups.

Laboratory Tests

Aspirin has been associated with elevated hepatic enzymes, blood urea nitrogen and serum creatinine, hyperkalemia, proteinuria and prolonged bleeding time.

Dipyridamole has been associated with elevated hepatic enzymes.

Drug Interactions

No pharmacokinetic drug-drug interaction studies were conducted with the AGGRENOX® formulation. The following information was obtained from the literature.

Adenosine: Dipyridamole has been reported to increase the plasma levels and cardiovascular effects of adenosine. Adjustment of adenosine dosage may be necessary.

Angiotensin Converting Enzyme (ACE) Inhibitors: Due to the indirect effect of aspirin on the renin-angiotensin conversion pathway, the hyponatremic and hypotensive effects of ACE inhibitors may be diminished by concomitant administration of aspirin.

Acetazolamide: Concurrent use of aspirin and acetazolamide can lead to high serum concentrations of acetazolamide (and toxicity) due to competition at the renal tubule for secretion.

Anticoagulant Therapy (heparin and warfarin): Patients on anticoagulation therapy are at increased risk for bleeding because of drug-drug interactions and effects on platelets. Aspirin can displace warfarin from protein binding sites, leading to prolongation of both the prothrombin time and the bleeding time. Aspirin can increase the anticoagulant activity of heparin, increasing bleeding risk.

Anticonvulsants: Salicylic acid can displace protein-bound phenytoin and valproic acid, leading to a decrease in the total concentration of phenytoin and an increase in serum valproic acid levels.

Beta Blockers: The hypotensive effects of beta blockers may be diminished by the concomitant administration of aspirin due to inhibition of renal prostaglandins, leading to decreased renal blood flow and salt and fluid retention.

Cholinesterase Inhibitors: Dipyridamole may counteract the anticholinesterase effect of cholinesterase inhibitors, thereby potentially aggravating myasthenia gravis.

Diuretics: The effectiveness of diuretics in patients with underlying renal or cardiovascular disease may be diminished by the concomitant administration of aspirin due to inhibition of renal prostaglandins, leading to decreased renal blood flow and salt and fluid retention.

Methotrexate: Salicylate can inhibit renal clearance of methotrexate, leading to bone marrow toxicity, especially in the elderly or renal impaired.

Table 2: Incidence of Adverse Events in ESPS2*

Body System/Preferred Term	Indivdual Treatment Group							
	AGGRENOX®		ER-DP Alone		ASA Alone		Placebo	
Total Number Patients	1650		1654		1649		1649	
Total Number (%) of Patients With at Least One On-Treatment Adverse Event	1319	(79.9%)	1305	(78.9%)	1323	(80.2%)	1304	(79.1%)
Central & Peripheral Nervous System Disorders								
Headache	647	(39.2%)	634	(38.3%)	558	(33.8%)	543	(32.9%)
Convulsions	28	(1.7%)	15	(0.9%)	28	(1.7%)	26	(1.6%)
Gastro-Intestinal System Disorders								
Dyspepsia	303	(18.4%)	288	(17.4%)	299	(18.1%)	275	(16.7%)
Abdominal Pain	289	(17.5%)	255	(15.4%)	262	(15.9%)	239	(14.5%)
Nausea	264	(16.0%)	254	(15.4%)	210	(12.7%)	232	(14.1%)
Diarrhea	210	(12.7%)	257	(15.5%)	112	(6.8%)	161	(9.8%)
Vomiting	138	(8.4%)	129	(7.8%)	101	(6.1%)	118	(7.2%)
Hemorrhage Rectum	26	(1.6%)	22	(1.3%)	16	(1.0%)	13	(0.8%)
Melena	31	(1.9%)	10	(0.6%)	20	(1.2%)	13	(0.8%)
Hemorrhoids	16	(1.0%)	13	(0.8%)	10	(0.6%)	10	(0.6%)
GI Hemorrhage	20	(1.2%)	5	(0.3%)	15	(0.9%)	7	(0.4%)
Body as a Whole—General Disorders								
Pain	105	(6.4%)	88	(5.3%)	103	(6.2%)	99	(6.0%)
Fatigue	95	(5.8%)	93	(5.6%)	97	(5.9%)	90	(5.5%)
Back Pain	76	(4.6%)	77	(4.7%)	74	(4.5%)	65	(3.9%)
Accidental Injury	42	(2.5%)	24	(1.5%)	51	(3.1%)	37	(2.2%)
Malaise	27	(1.6%)	23	(1.4%)	26	(1.6%)	22	(1.3%)
Asthenia	29	(1.8%)	19	(1.1%)	17	(1.0%)	18	(1.1%)
Syncope	17	(1.0%)	13	(0.8%)	16	(1.0%)	8	(0.5%)
Psychiatric Disorders								
Amnesia	39	(2.4%)	40	(2.4%)	57	(3.5%)	34	(2.1%)
Confusion	18	(1.1%)	9	(0.5%)	22	(1.3%)	15	(0.9%)
Anorexia	19	(1.2%)	17	(1.0%)	10	(0.6%)	15	(0.9%)
Somnolence	20	(1.2%)	13	(0.8%)	18	(1.1%)	9	(0.5%)
Musculoskeletal System Disorders								
Arthralgia	91	(5.5%)	75	(4.5%)	91	(5.5%)	76	(4.6%)
Arthritis	34	(2.1%)	25	(1.5%)	17	(1.0%)	19	(1.2%)
Arthrosis	18	(1.1%)	22	(1.3%)	13	(0.8%)	14	(0.8%)
Myalgia	20	(1.2%)	16	(1.0%)	11	(0.7%)	11	(0.7%)
Respiratory System Disorders								
Coughing	25	(1.5%)	18	(1.1%)	32	(1.9%)	21	(1.3%)
Upper Respiratory Tract Infection	16	(1.0%)	9	(0.5%)	16	(1.0%)	14	(0.8%)
Cardiovascular Disorders, General								
Cardiac Failure	26	(1.6%)	17	(1.0%)	30	(1.8%)	25	(1.5%)
Platelet, Bleeding & Clotting Disorders								
Hemorrhage NOS	52	(3.2%)	24	(1.5%)	46	(2.8%)	24	(1.5%)
Epistaxis	39	(2.4%)	16	(1.0%)	45	(2.7%)	25	(1.5%)
Purpura	23	(1.4%)	8	(0.5%)	9	(0.5%)	7	(0.4%)
Neoplasm								
Neoplasma NOS	28	(1.7%)	16	(1.0%)	23	(1.4%)	20	(1.2%)
Red Blood Cell Disorders								
Anemia	27	(1.6%)	16	(1.0%)	19	(1.2%)	9	(0.5%)

*Reported by ≥1% of patients during AGGRENOX® treatment where the incidence was greater than in those treated with placebo.

Note: ER-DP = extended-release dipyridamole 200 mg; ASA = aspirin 25 mg.

Note: The dosage regimen for all treatment groups is b.i.d.

Note: NOS = not otherwise specified.

Table 3: Incidence of Adverse Events that Led to the Discontinuation of Treatment: Adverse Events with an Incidence of ≥1% in the AGGRENOX® group

	Treatment Groups							
	AGGRENOX®		ER-DP		ASA		Placebo	
Total Number of Patients	1650		1654		1649		1649	
Patients with at least one Adverse Event that led to treatment discontinuation	417	(25%)	419	(25%)	318	(19%)	352	(21%)
Headache	165	(10%)	166	(10%)	57	(3%)	69	(4%)
Dizziness	85	(5%)	97	(6%)	69	(4%)	68	(4%)
Nausea	91	(6%)	95	(6%)	51	(3%)	53	(3%)
Abdominal Pain	74	(4%)	64	(4%)	56	(3%)	52	(3%)
Dyspepsia	59	(4%)	61	(4%)	49	(3%)	46	(3%)
Vomiting	53	(3%)	52	(3%)	28	(2%)	24	(1%)
Diarrhea	35	(2%)	41	(2%)	9	(<1%)	16	(<1%)
Stroke	39	(2%)	48	(3%)	57	(3%)	73	(4%)
Transient Ischemic Attack	35	(2%)	40	(2%)	26	(2%)	48	(3%)
Angina Pectoris	23	(1%)	20	(1%)	16	(<1%)	26	(2%)

Note: ER-DP = extended-release dipyridamole 200 mg; ASA = aspirin 25 mg.
The dosage regimen for all treatment groups is b.i.d.

Nonsteroidal Anti-Inflammatory Drugs (NSAIDs): The concurrent use of aspirin with other NSAIDs may increase bleeding or lead to decreased renal function.

Oral Hypoglycemics: Moderate doses of aspirin may increase the effectiveness of oral hypoglycemic drugs, leading to hypoglycemia.

Uricosuric Agents (probenecid and sulfinpyrazone): Salicylates antagonize the uricosuric action of uricosuric agents.

Carcinogenesis, Mutagenesis, Impairment of Fertility:

Carcinogenesis: Dipyridamole: In a 111-week oral study in mice and in a 128–142-week oral study in rats, Persantine® (dipyridamole USP) produced no significant carcinogenic effects at doses of 8, 25 and 75 mg/kg. For a 50-kg person of average height (1.46 m^2 body surface area), the dose of dipyridamole at 75 mg/kg/day (225 mg/m^2/day in mice or 450 mg/m^2/day in rats) represents 0.76 or 1.5 times the recommended human dose (8 mg/kg/day or 296 mg/m^2/day) on a body surface area basis.

Mutagenicity: Combination of Dipyridamole and Aspirin: Mutagenicity testing with combination of dipyridamole and aspirin in a ratio of 1:5 revealed no mutagenic potential in the Ames test, *in vivo* chromosome aberration tests in mice and hamsters, oral micronucleus tests in mice and hamsters and dominant lethal test in mice. Aspirin induced chromosome aberrations in cultured human fibroblasts.

Fertility: Dipyridamole: Reproduction studies with Persantine® revealed no evidence of impaired fertility in rats at oral dosages of up to 500 mg/kg/day or 3000 mg/m^2/day (~10 times the recommended human dose on a body surface area basis). A significant reduction in number of corpora lutea with consequent reduction in implantations and live fetuses was, however, observed at dose of Persantine® of 1250 mg/kg/day or 7500 mg/m^2/day in rats (~25 times the recommended human dose on a body surface area basis).

Aspirin: Aspirin inhibits ovulation in rats.

Combination of Dipyridamole and Aspirin: Combination of dipyridamole and aspirin was not tested for effect on fertility and reproductive performance.

Continued on next page

Aggrenox—Cont.

Dipyridamole: Pregnancy Category B: Reproduction studies with dipyridamole have been performed in mice at doses up to 125 mg/kg (375 mg/m^2, ~1.3 times the recommended human dose), in rats at doses up to 1000 mg/kg (6000 mg/m^2, 20 times the recommended human dose) and in rabbits at doses up to 40 mg/kg (480 mg/m^2, ~1.6 times the recommended human dose) and have revealed no evidence of harm to the fetus.

Aspirin: Pregnancy Category D: Aspirin may produce adverse maternal effects: anemia, ante- or postpartum hemorrhage, prolonged gestation and labor. Maternal aspirin use during later stages of pregnancy may cause adverse fetal effects: low birth weight, increased incidence of intracranial hemorrhage in premature infants, stillbirths, neonatal death. Aspirin should be avoided 1 week prior to and during labor and delivery because it can result in excessive blood loss at delivery.

Reproduction studies have been performed with combination of dipyridamole and aspirin in a ratio of 1:4.4 in rats and rabbits and have revealed no teratogenic evidence at doses of up to 405 mg/kg/day in rats and 135 mg/kg/day in rabbits. However, treatment with combination of dipyridamole and aspirin at 405 mg/kg/day induced abortion in rats. The doses of dipyridamole at 75 mg/kg/day represent 1.5 times the recommended human dose on a body surface area basis. In these studies, aspirin itself was teratogenic at doses of 330 mg/kg/day (1980 mg/m^2/day) in rats (spina bifida, exencephaly, microphthalmia, and coelosomia) and 110 mg/kg/day (1320 mg/m^2/day) in rabbits (congested fetuses, agenesis of skull and upper jaw, generalized edema with malformation of the head, and diaphanous skin). The doses of aspirin at 330 mg/kg/day in rats and at 110 mg/kg/day in rabbits were ~54 and 36 times the recommended human dose, respectively, on a body surface area basis.

There were no adequate and well-controlled studies in pregnant women. AGGRENOX® should be used during pregnancy only if the potential benefit justifies the potential risk to the fetus. Due to the aspirin component, AGGRENOX® should be avoided in the third trimester of pregnancy.

Nursing Mothers

Dipyridamole (n=1) and aspirin are excreted in human breast milk in low concentrations. Therefore, caution should be exercised when AGGRENOX® is administered to a nursing woman.

Pediatric Use

Safety and effectiveness of AGGRENOX® in pediatric patients have not been studied. Due to the aspirin component, use of this product in the pediatric population is not recommended (See **CONTRAINDICATIONS**).

ADVERSE REACTIONS

A 24-month, multicenter, double-blind, randomized study (ESPS2) was conducted to compare the efficacy and safety of AGGRENOX® with placebo, extended-release dipyridamole alone and aspirin alone. The study was conducted in a total of 6602 male and female patients who had experienced a previous ischemic stroke or transient ischemia of the brain within three months prior to randomization.

Table 2 presents the incidence of adverse events that occurred in 1% or more of patients treated with AGGRENOX® where the incidence was also greater than in those patients treated with placebo. There is no clear benefit of the dipyridamole/aspirin combination over aspirin with respect to safety.

[See table 2 at top of previous page]

Discontinuation due to adverse events in ESPS2 was 25% for AGGRENOX®, 25% for extended-release dipyridamole, 19% for aspirin, and 21% for placebo (refer to Table 3).

[See table 3 on next page]

Other adverse events:

Adverse reactions that occurred in less than 1% of patients treated with AGGRENOX® in the ESPS2 study and that were medically judged to be possibly related to either dipyridamole or aspirin are listed below (See **WARNINGS**). *Body as a Whole:* Allergic reaction, fever. *Cardiovascular:* Hypotension. *Central Nervous System:* Coma, dizziness, paresthesia, cerebral hemorrhage, intracranial hemorrhage, subarachnoid hemorrhage. *Gastrointestinal:* Gastritis, ulceration and perforation. *Hearing & Vestibular Disorders:* Tinnitus, and deafness. Patients with high frequency hearing loss may have difficulty perceiving tinnitus. In these patients, tinnitus cannot be used as a clinical indicator of salicylism. *Heart Rate and Rhythm Disorders:* Tachycardia, palpitation, arrhythmia, supraventricular tachycardia. *Liver and Biliary System Disorders:* Cholelithiasis, jaundice, hepatic function abnormal. *Metabolic & Nutritional Disorders:* Hyperglycemia, thirst. *Platelet, Bleeding and Clotting Disorders:* Hematoma, gingival bleeding. *Psychiatric Disorders:* Agitation. *Reproductive:* Uterine hemorrhage. *Respiratory:* Hyperpnea, asthma, bronchospasm, hemoptysis, pulmonary edema. *Special Senses Other Disorders:* Taste loss. *Skin and Appendages Disorders:* Pruritus, urticaria. *Urogenital:* Renal insufficiency and failure, hematuria. *Vascular (Extracardiac) Disorders:* Flushing.

The following is a list of additional adverse reactions that have been reported either in the literature or are from postmarketing spontaneous reports for either dipyridamole or aspirin. *Body as a Whole:* Hypothermia, chest pain. *Cardiovascular:* Angina pectoris. *Central Nervous System:* Cerebral edema. *Fluid and Electrolyte:* Hyperkalemia, metabolic acidosis, respiratory alkalosis, hypokalemia. *Gastrointestinal:* Pancreatitis, Reye's syndrome, hematemesis. *Hearing and Vestibular Disorders:* Hearing loss. *Hypersensitivity:* Acute anaphylaxis, laryngeal edema. *Liver and Biliary System Disorders:* Hepatitis, hepatic failure. *Musculoskeletal:* Rhabdomyolysis. *Metabolic & Nutritional Disorders:* Hypoglycemia, dehydration. *Platelet, Bleeding and Clotting Disorders:* Prolongation of the prothrombin time, disseminated intravascular coagulation, coagulopathy, thrombocytopenia. *Reproductive:* Prolonged pregnancy and labor, stillbirths, lower birth weight infants, antepartum and postpartum bleeding. *Respiratory:* Tachypnea, dyspnea. *Skin and Appendages Disorders:* Rash, alopecia, angioedema, Stevens-Johnson syndrome. *Urogenital:* Interstitial nephritis, papillary necrosis, proteinuria. *Vascular (Extracardiac Disorders):* Allergic vasculitis.

The following is a list of additional adverse events that have been reported either in the literature or are from postmarketing spontaneous reports for either dipyridamole or aspirin. The causal relationship of these adverse events has not been established: anorexia, aplastic anemia, pancytopenia, thrombocytosis.

Laboratory Changes

Over the course of the 24-month study (ESPS2), patients treated with AGGRENOX® showed a decline (mean change from baseline) in hemoglobin of 0.25 g/dL, hematocrit of 0.75%, and erythrocyte count of $0.13 \times 10^6/mm^3$.

OVERDOSAGE

Because of the dose ratio of dipyridamole to aspirin, overdosage of AGGRENOX® is likely to be dominated by signs and symptoms of dipyridamole overdose. In case of real or suspected overdose, seek medical attention or contact a Poison Control Center immediately. Careful medical management is essential.

Dipyridamole

Based upon the known hemodynamic effects of dipyridamole, symptoms such as warm feeling, flushes, sweating, restlessness, feeling of weakness and dizziness may occur. A drop in blood pressure and tachycardia might also be observed.

Symptomatic treatment is recommended, possibly including a vasopressor drug. Gastric lavage should be considered. Since dipyridamole is highly protein bound, dialysis is not likely to be of benefit.

Aspirin

Salicylate toxicity may result from acute ingestion (overdose) or chronic intoxication. The early signs of salicylic overdose (salicylism), including tinnitus (ringing in the ears), occur at plasma concentrations approaching 200 µg/mL. Plasma concentrations of aspirin above 300 µg/mL are clearly toxic. Severe toxic effects are associated with levels above 400 µg/mL. A single lethal dose of aspirin in adults is not known with certainty but death may be expected at 30 g.

Treatment consists primarily of supporting vital functions, increasing salicylate elimination, and correcting the acid-base disturbance. Gastric emptying and/or lavage are recommended as soon as possible after ingestion, even if the patient has vomited spontaneously. After lavage and/or emesis, administration of activated charcoal, as a slurry, is beneficial, if less than 3 hours have passed since ingestion. Charcoal absorption should not be employed prior to emesis and lavage.

Severity of aspirin intoxication is determined by measuring the blood salicylate level. Acid-base status should be closely followed with serial blood gas and serum pH measurements. Fluid and electrolyte balance should also be maintained.

In severe cases, hyperthermia and hypovolemia are the major immediate threats to life. Children should be sponged with tepid water. Replacement fluid should be administered intravenously and augmented with correction of acidosis. Plasma electrolytes and pH should be monitored to promote alkaline diuresis of salicylate if renal function is normal. Infusion of glucose may be required to control hypoglycemia. Hemodialysis and peritoneal dialysis can be performed to reduce the body drug content. In patients with renal insufficiency or in cases of life-threatening intoxication, dialysis is usually required. Exchange transfusion may be indicated in infants and young children.

AGGRENOX®

A single oral dose of combination of dipyridamole and aspirin at doses of up to 6.75 g/kg in a ratio of 8:1 was non-lethal in rats. Decreased locomotor activity, prone position and piloerection were observed at doses of combination of dipyridamole and aspirin at 2.25 and 6.75 g/kg.

DOSAGE AND ADMINISTRATION

The recommended dose of AGGRENOX® is one capsule given orally twice daily, one in the morning and one in the evening. The capsules should be swallowed without chewing.

AGGRENOX® is not interchangeable with the individual components of aspirin and Persantine® Tablets.

HOW SUPPLIED

AGGRENOX® is available as a hard gelatin capsule, with a red cap and an ivory-colored body, 24.0 mm in length, containing yellow extended-release pellets incorporating dipyridamole and a round white tablet incorporating immediate-release aspirin. The capsule body is imprinted in red with the Boehringer Ingelheim logo and with "01A".

AGGRENOX® is supplied in bottles of 60 capsules (NDC 0597-0001-60).

Store at 25°C (77°F); excursions permitted to 15°–30°C (59°–86°F). Protect from excessive moisture.

Rx only AG-PI-4040830(11/11/99)

Manufactured by: Boehringer Ingelheim Pharma KG, Biberach, Germany

Distributed by: Boehringer Ingelheim Pharmaceuticals Inc., Ridgefield, CT 06877

Shown in Product Identification Guide, page 308

ALUPENT® ℞

[al 'u-pent]

(metaproterenol sulfate USP)

Bronchodilator

Tablets 10 mg		**BI-CODE 74**
Tablets 20 mg		**BI-CODE 72**
Inhalation Aerosol 10 ml		**BI-CODE 70**
Syrup 10 mg/5 ml		**BI-CODE 73**
Inhalation Solution 5%		**BI-CODE 71**
Inhalation Solution	**0.6%**	**BI-CODE 69**
Unit-dose Vials	**0.4%**	**BI-CODE 78**

Prescribing Information

DESCRIPTION

Alupent® (metaproterenol sulfate USP) Inhalation Aerosol is a bronchodilator administered by oral inhalation. The Alupent Inhalation Aerosol containing 150 mg of metaproterenol sulfate as micronized powder is sufficient medication for 200 inhalations. Each metered dose delivers through the mouthpiece 0.65 mg of metaproterenol sulfate (each ml contains 15 mg). The inert ingredients are dichlorodifluoromethane, dichlorotetrafluoroethane and trichloromonofluoromethane as propellants, and sorbitan trioleate.

Alupent Inhalation Solution is administered by oral inhalation with the aid of a nebulizer or an intermittent positive pressure breathing apparatus (IPPB). It contains Alupent 5% in a pH-adjusted aqueous solution containing benzalkonium chloride and edetate disodium as preservatives.

Alupent Inhalation Solution Unit-dose Vial is administered by oral inhalation with the aid of an IPPB. It contains Alupent 0.4% or 0.6% in a sterile pH-adjusted aqueous solution with edetate disodium and sodium chloride.

Alupent Syrup is an oral bronchodilator. Each teaspoonful (5 ml) of syrup contains 10 mg of metaproterenol sulfate. The inactive ingredients are edetate disodium, FD&C Red No. 40, hydroxyethylcellulose, imitation black cherry flavor, methylparaben, propylparaben, saccharin, sorbitol solution.

Alupent Tablets are administered orally. Each tablet contains metaproterenol sulfate 10 mg or 20 mg. The inactive ingredients are colloidal silicon dioxide, corn starch, dibasic calcium phosphate, lactose, magnesium stearate.

Chemically, Alupent is 1-(3,5 dihydroxyphenyl)-2-isopropylaminoethanol sulfate, a white crystalline, racemic mixture of two optically active isomers.

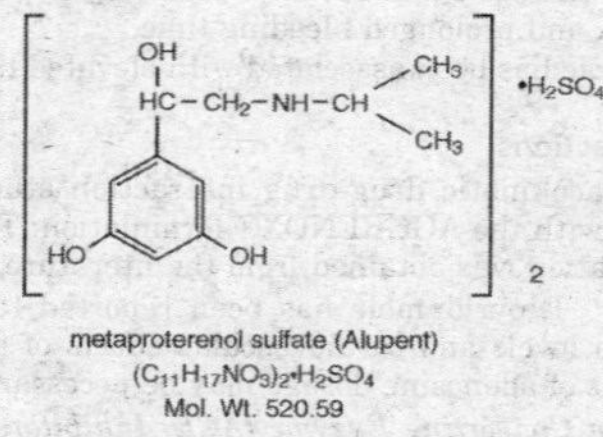

metaproterenol sulfate (Alupent)
$(C_{11}H_{17}NO_3)_2 \cdot H_2SO_4$
Mol. Wt. 520.59

CLINICAL PHARMACOLOGY

Alupent® (metaproterenol sulfate USP) is a potent beta-adrenergic stimulator. Alupent Inhalation Solutions have a rapid onset of action. It is postulated that beta-adrenergic stimulants produce many of their pharmacological effects by activation of adenyl cyclase, the enzyme which catalyzes the conversion of adenosine triphosphate to cyclic adenosine monophosphate.

In vitro studies and *in vivo* pharmacologic studies have demonstrated that Alupent® (metaproterenol sulfate USP) has a preferential effect on beta-2 adrenergic receptors compared with isoproterenol. While it is recognized that beta-2 adrenergic receptors are the predominant receptors in bronchial smooth muscle, recent data indicate that there is a population of beta-2 receptors in the human heart existing in a concentration between 10–50%. The precise function of these, however, is not yet established (see WARNINGS section).

The pharmacologic effects of beta adrenergic agonist drugs, including Alupent, are at least in part attributable to stimulation through beta adrenergic receptors of intracellular adenyl cyclase, the enzyme which catalyzes the conversion of adenosine triphosphate (ATP) to cyclic-3',5'-adenosine monophosphate (c-AMP). Increased c-AMP levels are associated with relaxation of bronchial smooth muscle and inhibition of release of mediators of immediate hypersensitivity from cells, especially from mast cells.

Pharmacokinetics: Absorption, biotransformation and excretion studies in humans following administration by inhalation have shown that approximately 3 percent of the actuated dose is absorbed intact through the lungs.

Absorption, biotransformation and excretion studies in humans following oral administration indicate that an average

of less than 10% of the drug is absorbed intact; it is not metabolized by catechol-O-methyl-transferase nor converted to glucuronide conjugates but is excreted primarily as the sulfate conjugate formed in the gut.
When administered orally or by inhalation, Alupent decreases reversible bronchospasm. Pulmonary function tests performed concomitantly usually show improvement following aerosol Alupent administration, e.g., an increase in the one-second forced expiratory volume (FEV_1), an increase in maximum expiratory flow rate, an increase in peak expiratory flow rate, an increase in forced vital capacity, and/or a decrease in airway resistance. The resultant decrease in airway obstruction may relieve the dyspnea associated with bronchospasm.
Controlled single- and multiple-dose studies have been performed with pulmonary function monitoring. The duration of effect of a single dose of Alupent Tablets 20 mg or Alupent Syrup (that is, the period of time during which there is a 15% or greater increase in FEV_1) was up to 4 hours.
Controlled single- and multiple-dose studies have been performed with pulmonary function monitoring. The duration of effect of a single dose of two to three inhalations of Alupent Inhalation Aerosol (that is, the period of time during which there is a 20% or greater increase in FEV_1) has varied from 1 to 5 hours.
In repetitive-dosing studies (up to q.i.d.) the duration of effect for a similar dose of Alupent Inhalation Aerosol has ranged from about 1 to 2.5 hours. Present studies are inadequate to explain the divergence in duration of the FEV_1 effect between single- and repetitive-dosing studies, respectively.
Following controlled single dose studies with Alupent Inhalation Solution by an intermittent positive pressure breathing apparatus (IPPB) and by hand-bulb nebulizers, significant improvement (15% or greater increase in FEV_1) occurred within 5 to 30 minutes and persisted for periods varying from 2 to 6 hours.
In these studies, the longer duration of effect occurred in the studies in which the drug was administered by IPPB, i.e., 6 hours, versus 2 to 3 hours when administered by hand-bulb nebulizer. In these studies, the doses used were 0.3 ml by IPPB and 10 inhalations by hand-bulb nebulizer.
In controlled repetitive-dosing studies with Alupent Inhalation Solution by IPPB and by hand-bulb nebulizer the onset of effect occurred within 5 to 30 minutes and duration ranged from 4 to 6 hours. In these studies, the doses used were 0.3 ml b.i.d. or t.i.d. when given by IPPB, and 10 inhalations q.i.d. (no more often than q4h) when given by hand-bulb nebulizer. As in the single dose studies, effectiveness was measured as a sustained increase in FEV_1 of 15% or greater. In these repetitive-dosing studies there was no apparent difference in duration between the two methods of delivery.
Clinical studies were conducted in which the effectiveness of Alupent® (metaproterenol sulfate USP) Inhalation Solution was evaluated by comparison with that of isoproterenol hydrochloride over periods of two to three months. Both drugs continued to produce significant improvement in pulmonary function throughout this period of treatment.
In two well-controlled studies in children 6 to 12 years of age with acute exacerbation of asthma, 70% of patients receiving Alupent Inhalation Solution (0.1 mL to 0.2 mL) showed improvement in pulmonary function as demonstrated by a 15% increase in FEV_1 above baseline.
Recent studies in laboratory animals (minipigs, rodents and dogs) recorded the occurrence of cardiac arrhythmias and sudden death (with histologic evidence of myocardial necrosis) when beta agonists and methylxanthines were administered concurrently. The significance of these findings when applied to humans is currently unknown.

INDICATIONS AND USAGE

Alupent® (metaproterenol sulfate USP) is indicated as a bronchodilator for bronchial asthma and for reversible bronchospasm which may occur in association with bronchitis and emphysema. Alupent Inhalation Solution 5% is additionally indicated for the treatment of acute asthmatic attacks in children age 6 years and older.

CONTRAINDICATIONS

Use in patients with cardiac arrhythmias associated with tachycardia is contraindicated.
Although rare, immediate hypersensitivity reactions and for Alupent Inhalation Solution 5% paradoxical bronchospasm can occur. Therefore, Alupent® (metaproterenol sulfate USP) is contraindicated in patients with a history of hypersensitivity to any of its components.

WARNINGS

Excessive use of adrenergic aerosols is potentially dangerous. Fatalities have been reported following excessive use of Alupent® (metaproterenol sulfate USP) as with other sympathomimetic inhalation preparations, and the exact cause is unknown. Cardiac arrest was noted in several cases.
Alupent, like other beta-adrenergic agonists, can produce a significant cardiovascular effect in some patients, as measured by pulse rate, blood pressure, symptoms and/or ECG changes. As with other beta-adrenergic aerosols, Alupent can produce paradoxical bronchospasm (which can be life threatening). If it occurs, the preparation should be discontinued immediately and alternative therapy instituted.
Alupent® (metaproterenol sulfate USP) should not be used more often than prescribed. Patients should be advised to contact their physician in the event that they do not respond to their usual dose of a sympathomimetic amine aerosol.

Population	Method of Administration	Usual Single Dose	Range	Dilution
Adult	Hand-bulb nebulizer	10 inhalations	5–15 inhalations	No dilution
12 years and older	IPPB or nebulizer	0.3 ml	0.2–0.3 ml	Diluted in approx. 2.5 ml saline solution or other diluent
Pediatric 6–12 years	Nebulizer	0.1 ml	0.1–0.2 ml	Diluted in saline solution to a total volume of 3 ml

PRECAUTIONS

General: Extreme care must be exercised with respect to the administration of additional sympathomimetic agents. Since metaproterenol is a sympathomimetic amine it should be used with caution in patients with cardiovascular disorders, including ischemic heart disease, hypertension or cardiac arrhythmias, in patients with hyperthyroidism or diabetes mellitus, and in patients who are unusually responsive to sympathomimetic amines or who have convulsive disorders. Significant changes in systolic and diastolic blood pressure could be expected to occur in some patients after use of any beta-adrenergic bronchodilator.
Physicians should recognize that a single dose of nebulized Alupent® (metaproterenol sulfate USP) in the treatment of acute asthma may alleviate symptoms and improve pulmonary function temporarily but fail to completely abort an attack.
Information for Patients: Extreme care must be exercised with respect to the administration of additional sympathomimetic agents. A sufficient interval of time should elapse prior to administration of another sympathomimetic agent.
Alupent Inhalation Solution 5% effects may last up to 6 hours or longer. It should not be used more often than recommended and the patient should not increase the number of inhalations or frequency of use without first consulting the physician. If symptoms of asthma get worse, adverse reactions occur, or the patient does not respond to the usual dose, the patient should be instructed to contact the physician immediately.
Alupent Tablets and Alupent Syrup should not be used more often than prescribed. If symptoms persist, patients should consult a physician promptly.
A single dose of nebulized Alupent in the treatment of an acute attack of asthma may not completely abort an attack.
Drug Interactions: Other beta-adrenergic aerosol bronchodilators should not be used concomitantly with Alupent® (metaproterenol sulfate USP) because they may have additive effects. Beta-adrenergic agonists should be administered with caution to patients being treated with monoamine oxidase inhibitors or tricyclic antidepressants, since the action of beta-adrenergic agonists on the vascular system may be potentiated.
Carcinogenesis/Mutagenesis/Impairment of Fertility: In an 18-month study in mice, Alupent produced a significant increase in benign hepatic adenomas in males and in benign ovarian tumors in females at doses corresponding to 31 and 62 times the maximum recommended dose (based on a 50 kg individual). In a 2-year study in rats, a nonsignificant incidence of benign leiomyomata of the mesovarium was noted at 62 times the maximum recommended dose. The relevance of these findings to man is not known. Mutagenic studies with Alupent have not been conducted. Reproduction studies in rats revealed no evidence of impaired fertility.
Pregnancy/Teratogenic Effects
PREGNANCY CATEGORY C: Alupent has been shown to be teratogenic and embryotoxic in rabbits when given orally in doses 620 times the human inhalation dose and 100 mg/kg or 62 times the maximum recommended human oral dose. These effects included skeletal abnormalities, hydrocephalus and skull bone separation.
Embryotoxicity has also been shown in mice when given orally at doses of 50 mg/kg or 31 times the maximum recommended human oral dose. Results of other oral reproduction studies in rats (40 mg/kg) and rabbits (50 mg/kg) have not revealed any teratogenic, embryotoxic or fetotoxic effects. There are no adequate and well-controlled studies in pregnant women. Alupent should be used during pregnancy only if the potential benefit justifies the potential risk to the fetus.
Nursing Mothers: It is not known whether Alupent is excreted in human milk; therefore, Alupent should be used during nursing only if the potential benefit justifies the possible risk to the newborn.
Pediatric Use: Safety and effectiveness in the pediatric population have not established under the age of 6 for Alupent Tablets, Syrup & Inhalation Solutions 5% and under the age of 12 for Inhalation Aerosol and Solution 0.4% & 0.6% UDV. See DOSAGE AND ADMINISTRATION.

ADVERSE REACTIONS

Adverse reactions are similar to those noted with other sympathomimetic agents. Adverse reactions such as tachycardia, hypertension, palpitations, nervousness, tremor, nausea and vomiting have been reported.
The most frequent adverse reaction to Alupent® (metaproterenol sulfate USP) administered by metered-dose inhaler among 251 patients in 90-day controlled clinical trials was nervousness. This was reported in 6.8% of patients. Less frequent adverse experiences, occurring in 1–4% of patients were headache, dizziness, palpitations, gastrointestinal distress, tremor, throat irritation, nausea, vomiting, cough and asthma exacerbation. Tachycardia occurred in less than 1% of patients.
Adverse experiences associated with Alupent Inhalation Solution 5% in at least 2% of 120 patients participating in multiple-dose clinical trial of 60 and 90-day (n=120) duration included nervousness (14.1%; n=17), cough (3.3%; n=4) headache (3.3%; n=4), tachycardia (2.5%; n=3) and tremor (2.5%; n=3).
Alupent Inhalation Solution 5% may be associated with a somewhat higher incidence of adverse reactions in children. In controlled clinical trials conducted in 160 pediatric patients the incidence of adverse reactions observed at the recommended doses was as follows: tachycardia, 16.6%; tremor, 33%; nausea, 14%; vomiting, 7.7%. The corresponding incidence in placebo-treated patients was: tachycardia, 7.6%; tremor, 20%; nausea, 7.7%; vomiting, 2.5%.
In two well-controlled studies in children 6 to 12 years of age with acute exacerbation of asthma, Alupent Inhalation Solution 5% was not efficacious in approximately 30% of patients, where efficacy was defined as a 15% increase in FEV_1 above baseline at two or more time points during the 1-hour testing period. In 8% of patients there was a decrease in FEV_1 of 10% or more from baseline at two or more time points during the testing period. Insufficient information exists to assess the relationship of drug administration to the decline in pulmonary function observed in these patients, but paradoxical bronchospasm is one possibility.
The most frequent adverse reactions to Alupent Inhalation Solution 0.4% and 0.6% are nervousness and tachycardia which occur in about 1 in 7 patients, tremor which occurs in about 1 in 20 patients and nausea which occurs in about 1 in 50 patients. Less frequent adverse reactions are hypertension, palpitations, vomiting and bad taste which occur in approximately 1 in 300 patients.
The following table of adverse experiences is derived from 26 controlled clinical trials with 496 patients treated with Alupent® (metaproterenol sulfate USP) Tablets:

ALUPENT® Tablets
Incidence of Adverse Events
Reported Among 496 Patients
Treated in 26 Controlled Clinical Trials

ADVERSE EXPERIENCE	Incidence Number of Patients	%
Cardiovascular		
Chest Pain	1	.2
Edema	1	.2
Hypertension	2	.4
Palpitations	19	3.8
Tachycardia	85	17.1
Central Nervous System		
Dizziness	12	2.4
Drowsiness	3	.6
Fatigue	7	1.4
Headache	35	7.0
Insomnia	9	1.8
Nervousness	100	20.2
Sensory disturbances	1	.2
Syncope	2	.4
Weakness	1	.2
Dermatological		
Diaphoresis	1	.2
Hives	1	.2
Pruritus	2	.4
Gastrointestinal		
Appetite changes	2	.4
Diarrhea	6	1.2
Gastrointestinal distress	15	3.0
Nausea	18	3.6
Vomiting	4	0.8
Musculoskeletal		
Pain	1	.2
Spasms	1	.2
Tremor	84	16.9
Ophthalmological		
Blurred vision	1	.2
Oro-Otolaryngeal		
Dry mouth/throat	2	.4
Laryngeal changes	1	.2
Bad taste	4	0.8
Respiratory		
Asthma exacerbation	10	2.0
Coughing	1	.2
Other		
Chatty	1	.2
Chills	1	.2

Continued on next page

Alupent—Cont.

Clonus noted on flexing foot	1	.2
Feverish	2	.4
Flu symptoms	1	.2
Facial and finger puffiness	1	.2

The incidence of adverse events occurring in at least 1% of the 1,120 patients treated with Alupent Syrup in 44 clinical trials are tachycardia (6.1%; n=68), nervousness (4.8%; n=54), tremor (1.6%; n=18), nausea (1.3%; n=15) and headache (1.1%; n=12).

It is important to recognize that adverse reactions from beta agonist bronchodilator solutions for nebulization may occur with the use of a new container of a product in patients who have previously tolerated that same product without adverse effect. There have been reports that indicate that such patients may subsequently tolerate replacement containers of the same product without adverse effect.

OVERDOSAGE

The expected symptoms with overdosage are those of excessive beta-adrenergic stimulation and/or any of the symptoms listed under adverse reactions, e.g. angina, hypertension or hypotension, arrhythmias, nervousness, headache, tremor, dry mouth, palpitation, nausea, dizziness, fatigue, malaise and insomnia.

Treatment consists of discontinuation of metaproterenol together with appropriate symptomatic therapy.

DOSAGE AND ADMINISTRATION

If Alupent® (metaproterenol sulfate USP) is administered before or after other sympathomimetic bronchodilators, caution should be exercised with respect to possible potentiation of adrenergic effects.

Inhalation Aerosol: The usual single dose is two to three inhalations. With repetitive dosing, inhalation should usually not be repeated more often than about every three to four hours. Total dosage per day should not exceed 12 inhalations. Alupent Inhalation Aerosol is not recommended for use in children under 12 years of age.

Usually, treatment need not be repeated more often than every four hours to relieve acute attacks of bronchospasm.

As with all medications, the physician should begin therapy with the lowest effective dose and then titrate the dosage according to the individual patient's requirements.

Alupent Inhalation Solution 5% is administered by oral inhalation with the aid of a nebulizer or an intermittent positive pressure breathing apparatus (IPPB).

Alupent Inhalation Solution 5% may be administered three to four times a day for the treatment of reversible airways disease in adults. A single dose of nebulized Alupent in the treatment of an acute attack of asthma may not completely abort an attack.

The dosage and administration are summarized in the table below:

[See table at top of previous page]

Inhalation Solution 0.4% and 0.6% Unit-dose Vials: Alupent Inhalation Solution Unit-dose Vial is administered by oral inhalation using an IPPB device. The usual adult dose is one vial per nebulization treatment. Each vial of Alupent Inhalation Solution 0.4% is equivalent to 0.2 ml Alupent Inhalation Solution 5% diluted to 2.5 ml with normal saline; each vial of Alupent Inhalation Solution 0.6% is equivalent to 0.3 ml Alupent Inhalation Solution 5% diluted to 2.5 ml with normal saline.

Usually, treatment need not be repeated more often than every 4 hours to relieve acute attacks of bronchospasm. As part of a total treatment program in chronic bronchospastic pulmonary diseases, Alupent Inhalation Solution Unit-dose vials may be administered three to four times a day.

As with all medications, the physician should begin therapy with the lowest effective dose and then titrate the dosage according to the individual patient's requirements.

Alupent Inhalation Solution Unit-dose Vial is not recommended for use in children under 12 years of age.

Syrup: *Children:* Aged six to nine years or weight under 60 lbs—one teaspoonful three or four times a day. Children over nine years or weight over 60 lbs—two teaspoonfuls three or four times a day. Clinical trial experience in children under the age of 6 is limited. Of 40 children treated with Alupent® (metaproterenol sulfate USP) Syrup for at least 1 month, daily doses of approximately 1.3 to 2.6 mg/kg were well tolerated. Adults—two teaspoonfuls three or four times a day.

It is recommended that the physician titrate the dosage according to each individual patient's response to therapy.

Tablets: *Adults:* The usual dose is 20 mg three or four times a day. *Children:* Aged six to nine years or weight under 60 lbs—10 mg three or four times a day. Over nine years or weight over 60 lbs—20 mg three or four times a day. Alupent tablets are not recommended for use in children under six years at this time. (Please refer to the CLINICAL PHARMACOLOGY section for further information on clinical experience with this product.) It is recommended that the physician titrate the dosage according to each individual patient's response to therapy.

HOW SUPPLIED

Inhalation Aerosol: Each 200 inhalations of Alupent® (metaproterenol sulfate USP) Inhalation Aerosol contains 150 mg of metaproterenol sulfate as a micronized powder in inert propellants. Each metered dose delivers through the mouthpiece 0.65 mg metaproterenol sulfate (each ml contains 15 mg). Alupent Inhalation Aerosol with Mouthpiece (NDC 0597-0070-17), net contents 14g (10 mL).The mouthpiece is white with a clear, colorless sleeve and a blue protective cap. Alupent Inhalation Aerosol Refill (NDC 0597-0070-18), net contents 14g (10 mL).

Note: The indented statement below is required by the Federal government's Clean Air Act for all products containing or manufactured with chlorofluorocarbons (CFCs).

> WARNING
>
> Contains trichloromonofluoromethane (CFC-11), dichlorodifluoromethane (CFC-12) and dichlorotetrafluoroethane (CFC-114), substances which harm public health and the environment by destroying ozone in the upper atmosphere.

A notice similar to the above WARNING has been placed in the "Instructions for Use" portion of the package insert pursuant to regulations of the United States Environmental Protection Agency.

Store between 59°F (15°C) and 77°F (25°C). Avoid excessive humidity.

Inhalation Solution: Alupent® (metaproterenol sulfate USP) Inhalation Solution is supplied as a 5% solution in bottles of 10 ml (NDC 0597-0071-75) or 30 ml (NDC 0597-0071-30) with accompanying calibrated dropper. Plastic cover on dropper should be discarded and not used to retain product. Store between 59°F (15°C) and 77°F (25°C). Protect from light. Do not use the solution if it is pinkish or darker than slightly yellow or contains a precipitate.

Alupent Inhalation Solution Unit-dose Vial is supplied as a 0.4% (NDC 0597-0078-62) or 0.6% (NDC 0597-0069-62) clear colorless or nearly colorless solution containing 2.5 ml with 25 vials per box. Each vial is made from a low-density polyethylene resin. Store below 77°F (25°C). Protect from light. Do not use the solution if it is pinkish or darker than slightly yellow or contains a precipitate.

Syrup: Alupent® (metaproterenol sulfate USP) is available as a cherry-flavored syrup, 10 mg per teaspoonful (5 ml) in 16 fl. oz. bottles (NDC 0597-0073-16). Store between 59°F (15°C) and 86°F (30°C). Protect from light.

Tablets: Alupent® (metaproterenol sulfate USP) is supplied in two dosage strengths as scored round white tablets in bottles of 100. Tablets of 10 mg coded BI/74 (NDC 0597-0074-01). Tablets of 20 mg coded BI/72 (NDC 0597-0072-01). *Storage for bottles:* Store between 59°F (15°C) and 86°F (30°C). Protect from light. Blisters no longer distributed.

Rx only.

AL-PI-7/95

Distributed by Boehringer Ingelheim Pharmaceuticals, Inc., Ridgefield, CT 06877

Licensed from Boehringer Ingelheim International GmbH

Shown in Product Identification Guide, page 308

ATROVENT® ℞

[*ă 'trō "vĕnt*]

(ipratropium bromide)
Inhalation Aerosol
Bronchodilator .... BI-CODE 82

Prescribing Information

DESCRIPTION

The active ingredient in Atrovent® (ipratropium bromide) Inhalation Aerosol is ipratropium bromide. It is an anticholinergic bronchodilator chemically described as 8-azoniabicyclo (3.2.1)-octane,3-(3-hydroxy-1-oxo-2-phenylpropoxy)-8-methyl-8-(1-methylethyl)-, bromide, monohydrate *(endo, syn)-*, (±)-: a synthetic quaternary ammonium compound, chemically related to atropine.

ipratropium bromide (Atrovent) — $C_{20}H_{30}BrNO_3 \cdot H_2O$ Mol. Wt. 430.4

Ipratropium bromide is a white crystalline substance, freely soluble in water and lower alcohols but insoluble in lipophilic solvents such as ether, chloroform, and fluorocarbons.

Atrovent Inhalation Aerosol is an inhalation aerosol for oral administration. The net weight is 14 grams; it yields 200 inhalations. Each actuation of the valve delivers 18 mcg of ipratropium bromide from the mouthpiece. The inert ingredients are dichlorodifluoromethane, dichlorotetrafluoroethane, and trichloromonofluoromethane as propellants and soya lecithin.

CLINICAL PHARMACOLOGY

Atrovent® (ipratropium bromide) is an anticholinergic (parasympatholytic) agent which, based on animal studies, appears to inhibit vagally mediated reflexes by antagonizing the action of acetylcholine, the transmitter agent released from the vagus nerve. Anticholinergics prevent the increases in intracellular concentration of cyclic guanosine monophosphate (cyclic GMP) which are caused by interaction of acetylcholine with the muscarinic receptor on bronchial smooth muscle.

The bronchodilation following inhalation of Atrovent is primarily a local, site-specific effect, not a systemic one. Much of an inhaled dose is swallowed as shown by fecal excretion studies. Atrovent is not readily absorbed into the systemic circulation either from the surface of the lung or from the gastrointestinal tract as confirmed by blood level and renal excretion studies.

The half-life of elimination is about 2 hours after inhalation or intravenous administration. Autoradiographic studies in rats have shown that Atrovent does not penetrate the blood-brain barrier.

In controlled 90 day studies in patients with bronchospasm associated with chronic obstructive pulmonary disease (chronic bronchitis and emphysema) significant improvements in pulmonary function (FEV_1 and $FEF_{25-75\%}$ increases of 15% or more) occurred within 15 minutes, reached a peak in 1–2 hours, and persisted for periods of 3 to 4 hours in the majority of patients and up to 6 hours in some patients. In addition, significant increases in Forced Vital Capacity (FVC) have been demonstrated.

Controlled clinical studies have demonstrated that Atrovent® (ipratropium bromide) does not alter either mucociliary clearance or the volume or viscosity of respiratory secretions. In studies without a positive control Atrovent did not alter pupil size, accommodation or visual acuity (See ADVERSE REACTIONS).

Ventilation/perfusion studies have shown no clinically significant effects on pulmonary gas exchange or arterial oxygen tension. Atrovent does not produce clinically significant changes in pulse rate or blood pressure.

INDICATIONS AND USAGE

Atrovent® (ipratropium bromide) Inhalation Aerosol is indicated as a bronchodilator for maintenance treatment of bronchospasm associated with chronic obstructive pulmonary disease, including chronic bronchitis and emphysema.

CONTRAINDICATIONS

Atrovent® (ipratropium bromide) Inhalation Aerosol is contraindicated in patients with a history of hypersensitivity to soya lecithin or related food products such as soybean and peanut. Atrovent should also not be taken by patients hypersensitive to any other components of the drug product or to atropine or its derivatives.

WARNINGS

Atrovent® (ipratropium bromide) is not indicated for the initial treatment of acute episodes of bronchospasm where rapid response is required. Immediate hypersensitivity reactions may occur after administration of ipratropium bromide, as demonstrated by rare cases of urticaria, angioedema, rash, bronchospasm and oropharyngeal edema.

PRECAUTIONS

General Atrovent® (ipratropium bromide) should be used with caution in patients with narrow-angle glaucoma, prostatic hypertrophy or bladder-neck obstruction.

Information for Patients Patients should be advised that temporary blurring of vision, precipitation or worsening of narrow-angle glaucoma or eye pain may result if the aerosol is sprayed into the eyes. If recommended dosage does not provide relief or symptoms become worse, patients should seek immediate medical attention. While taking Atrovent® Inhalation Aerosol, other inhaled drugs should not be used unless prescribed. (See illustrated Patient's Instructions for Use).

Drug Interactions Atrovent has been used concomitantly with other drugs, including sympathomimetic bronchodilators, methylxanthines, steroids and cromolyn sodium, commonly used in the treatment of chronic obstructive pulmonary disease, without adverse drug reactions. There are no formal studies fully evaluating the interaction effects of Atrovent and these drugs with respect to effectiveness.

Carcinogenesis, Mutagenesis, Impairment of Fertility Two-year oral carcinogenicity studies in rats and mice have revealed no carcinogenic potential at doses up to 1,250 times the maximum recommended human daily dose for Atrovent. Results of various mutagenicity studies were negative.

Fertility of male or female rats at oral doses up to approximately 10,000 times the maximum recommended human daily dose was unaffected by Atrovent administration. At doses above 18,000 times the maximum recommended human daily dose, increased resorption and decreased conception rates were observed.

Pregnancy *TERATOGENIC EFFECTS Pregnancy Category B:* Oral reproduction studies performed in mice, rats and rabbits (at doses approximately 2,000, 200,000 and 26,000 times the maximum recommended human daily dose, respectively) and inhalation reproduction studies in rats and rabbits (at doses approximately 312 and 375 times the maximum recommended human daily dose, respectively) have demonstrated no evidence of teratogenic effects as a result of Atrovent® (ipratropium bromide). However, no adequate or well controlled studies have been conducted in pregnant women. Because animal reproduction studies are not always predictive of human response, Atrovent® (ipratropium bromide) should be used during pregnancy only if clearly needed.

Nursing Mothers It is not known whether Atrovent is excreted in human milk. Although lipid-insoluble quaternary bases pass into breast milk, it is unlikely that Atrovent would reach the infant to an important extent, especially when taken by aerosol. However, because many drugs are excreted in human milk, caution should be exercised when Atrovent is administered to a nursing woman.

Pediatric Use Safety and effectiveness in the pediatric population below the age of 12 have not been established.

ADVERSE REACTIONS

Adverse reaction information concerning Atrovent® (ipratropium bromide) is derived from 90 day controlled clinical trials (N=254), other controlled clinical trials using recommended doses of Atrovent (N=377) and an uncontrolled study (N=1924). Additional information is derived from the foreign post-marketing experience and the published literature.

Adverse reactions occurring in greater than one percent of patients in the 90 day controlled clinical trials appear in the following table:

Reaction	Percent of Patients Ipratropium bromide N = 254	Metaproterenol sulfate N = 249
Cardiovascular		
Palpitations	1.8	1.6
Central Nervous System		
Nervousness	3.1	6.8
Dizziness	2.4	2.8
Headache	2.4	2.0
Dermatological		
Rash	1.2	0.4
Gastrointestinal		
Nausea	2.8	1.2
Gastrointestinal distress	2.4	2.8
Vomiting	0	1.2
Musculoskeletal		
Tremor	0	2.4
Ophthalmological		
Blurred vision	1.2	0.8
Oro-Otolaryngeal		
Dry mouth	2.4	0.8
Irritation from aerosol	1.6	1.6
Respiratory		
Cough	5.9	1.2
Exacerbation of symptoms	2.4	3.6

Additional adverse reactions reported in less than one percent of the patients considered possibly due to Atrovent include urinary difficulty, fatigue, insomnia and hoarseness. The large uncontrolled, open-label study included seriously ill patients. About 7% of patients treated discontinued the program because of adverse events.

Of the 2301 patients treated in the large uncontrolled study and in clinical trials other than the 90 day studies, the most common adverse reactions reported were: dryness of the oropharynx, about 5 in 100; cough, exacerbation of symptoms and irritation from aerosol, each about 3 in 100; headache, about 2 in 100; nausea, dizziness, blurred vision/difficulty in accommodation, and drying of secretions, each about 1 in 100. Less frequently reported adverse reactions that were possibly due to Atrovent® (ipratropium bromide) include tachycardia, paresthesias, drowsiness, coordination difficulty, itching, hives, flushing, alopecia, constipation, tremor, and mucosal ulcers.

Cases of precipitation or worsening of narrow-angle glaucoma, acute eye pain and hypotension have been reported. Allergic-type reactions such as skin rash, angioedema of tongue, lips and face, urticaria (including giant urticaria), laryngospasm and anaphylactic reaction have been reported, with positive rechallenge in some cases. Many of the patients had a history of allergies to other drugs and/or foods, including soybean. (See CONTRAINDICATIONS.)

OVERDOSAGE

Acute overdosage by inhalation is unlikely since Atrovent® (ipratropium bromide) is not well absorbed systemically after aerosol or oral administration. The oral LD_{50} of Atrovent ranged between 1001 and 2010 mg/kg in mice; between 1667 and more than 4000 mg/kg in rats; and between 400 and 1300 mg/kg in dogs.

DOSAGE AND ADMINISTRATION

The usual starting dose of Atrovent® (ipratropium bromide) is two inhalations (36 mcg) four times a day. Patients may take additional inhalations as required; however, the total number of inhalations should not exceed 12 in 24 hours.

HOW SUPPLIED

Atrovent® (ipratropium bromide) Inhalation Aerosol is supplied as a metered dose inhaler with a white mouthpiece which has a clear, colorless sleeve and a green protective cap.

Atrovent® Inhalation Aerosol with Mouthpiece (NDC 0597-0082-14), net contents 14 g. Atrovent® Inhalation Aerosol Refill (NDC 0597-0082-18), net contents 14 g. Each 14 gram vial provides sufficient medication for 200 inhalations. Each actuation delivers 18 mcg of ipratropium bromide from the mouthpiece.

Note: The indented statement below is required by the Federal government's Clean Air Act for all products containing or manufactured with chlorofluorocarbons (CFCs):

> **WARNING**
> Contains trichloromonofluoromethane (CFC-11), dichlorodifluoromethane (CFC-12) and dichlorotetrafluoroethane (CFC-114), substances which harm public health and the environment by destroying ozone in the upper atmosphere.

A notice similar to the above WARNING has been placed in the information for the patient of this product under the Environmental Protection Agency's (EPA's) regulations. The patient's warning states that the patient should consult his or her physician if there are questions or alternatives.

Store between 59°F (15°C) and 86°F (30°C). Avoid excessive humidity.

Keep out of children's reach. Shake well before using. Patients should be reminded to read and follow the accompanying "Instructions for Use," which should be dispensed with the product. As with most inhaled medications in aerosol canisters, the therapeutic effect of this medication may decrease when the canister is cold.

Warning: Discard the canister after you have used the labeled number of inhalations. The correct amount of medication in each inhalation cannot be assured after this point.

Rx only

AT-PI-4042170 039(3/99)

Manufactured by: 3M Pharmaceuticals, St. Paul, MN 55144
Pharmaceuticals, Inc., Ridgefield, CT 06877

Licensed from: Boehringer Ingelheim
International GmbH

Shown in Product Identification Guide, page 308

ATROVENT® ℞
[*ă 'trō "vĕnt*]
(ipratropium bromide)
Inhalation Solution .... BI-CODE 80

Prescribing Information

DESCRIPTION

The active ingredient in Atrovent® (ipratropium bromide) Inhalation Solution is ipratropium bromide monohydrate. It is an anticholinergic bronchodilator chemically described as 8-azoniabicyclo[3.2.1]-octane, 3-(3-hydroxy-1-oxo-2-phenylpropoxy)-8-methyl-8-(1-methylethyl)-, bromide, monohydrate *(endo, syn)*-, (±)-; a synthetic quaternary ammonium compound, chemically related to atropine.

H_3C $CH(CH_3)_2$ N^+ H H H O OC—CH— CH_2OH $Br^- \cdot H_2O$

ipratropium bromide monohydrate (Atrovent) $C_{20}H_{30}BrNO_3 \cdot H_2O$ Mol. Wt. 430.4

Ipratropium bromide is a white crystalline substance, freely soluble in water and lower alcohols. It is a quaternary ammonium compound and thus exists in an ionized state in aqueous solutions. It is relatively insoluble in non-polar media.

Atrovent Inhalation Solution is administered by oral inhalation with the aid of a nebulizer. It contains ipratropium bromide 0.02% (anhydrous basis) in a sterile, preservative-free, isotonic saline solution, pH-adjusted to 3.4 (3 to 4) with hydrochloric acid.

CLINICAL PHARMACOLOGY

Atrovent® (ipratropium bromide) is an anticholinergic (parasympatholytic) agent that, based on animal studies, appears to inhibit vagally-mediated reflexes by antagonizing the action of acetylcholine, the transmitter agent released from the vagus nerve.

Anticholinergics prevent the increases in intracellular concentration of cyclic guanosine monophosphate (cyclic GMP) that are caused by interaction of acetylcholine with the muscarinic receptor on bronchial smooth muscle.

The bronchodilation following inhalation of Atrovent is primarily a local, site-specific effect, not a systemic one. Much of an administered dose is swallowed but not absorbed, as shown by fecal excretion studies. Following nebulization of a 2 mg dose, a mean 7% of the dose was absorbed into the systemic circulation either from the surface of the lung or from the gastrointestinal tract. The half-life of elimination is about 1.6 hours after intravenous administration. Ipratropium bromide is minimally (0 to 9% in vitro) bound to plasma albumin and α_1-acid glycoproteins. It is partially metabolized. Autoradiographic studies in rats have shown that Atrovent does not penetrate the blood-brain barrier. Atrovent has not been studied in patients with hepatic or renal insufficiency. It should be used with caution in those patient populations.

In controlled 12-week studies in patients with bronchospasm associated with chronic obstructive pulmonary disease (chronic bronchitis and emphysema) significant improvements in pulmonary function (FEV_1 increases of 15% or more) occurred within 15 to 30 minutes, reached a peak in 1–2 hours, and persisted for periods of 4–5 hours in the majority of patients, with about 25–38% of the patients demonstrating increases of 15% or more for at least 7–8 hours. Continued effectiveness of Atrovent Inhalation Solution was demonstrated throughout the 12-week period. In addition, significant increases in forced vital capacity (FVC) have been demonstrated. However, Atrovent did not consistently produce significant improvement in subjective symptom scores nor in quality of life scores over the 12-week duration of study.

Additional controlled 12-week studies were conducted to evaluate the safety and effectiveness of Atrovent Inhalation Solution administered concomitantly with the beta adrenergic bronchodilator solutions metaproterenol and albuterol compared with the administration of each of the beta agonists alone. Combined therapy produced significant additional improvement in FEV_1 and FVC. On combined therapy, the median duration of 15% improvement in FEV_1 was 5–7 hours, compared with 3–4 hours in patients receiving a beta agonist alone.

INDICATIONS AND USAGE

Atrovent® (ipratropium bromide) Inhalation Solution administered either alone or with other bronchodilators, especially beta adrenergics, is indicated as a bronchodilator for maintenance treatment of bronchospasm associated with chronic obstructive pulmonary disease, including chronic bronchitis and emphysema.

CONTRAINDICATIONS

Atrovent® (ipratropium bromide) is contraindicated in known or suspected cases of hypersensitivity to ipratropium bromide, or to atropine and its derivatives.

WARNINGS

The use of Atrovent® (ipratropium bromide) Inhalation Solution as a single agent for the relief of bronchospasm in acute COPD exacerbation has not been adequately studied. Drugs with faster onset of action may be preferable as initial therapy in this sitsutation. Combination of Atrovent and beta agonists has not been shown to be more effective than either drug alone in reversing the bronchospasm associated with acute COPD exacerbation.

Immediate hypersensitivity reactions may occur after administration of ipratropium bromide, as demonstrated by rare cases of urticaria, angioedema, rash, bronchospasm and oropharyngeal edema.

PRECAUTIONS

General Atrovent® (ipratropium bromide) should be used with caution in patients with narrow-angle glaucoma, prostatic hypertrophy or bladder-neck obstruction.

Information for Patients Patients should be advised that temporary blurring of vision, precipitation or worsening of narrow-angle glaucoma or eye pain may result if the solution comes into direct contact with the eyes. Use of a nebulizer with mouthpiece rather than face mask may be preferable, to reduce the likelihood of the nebulizer solution reaching the eyes. Patients should be advised that Atrovent Inhalation Solution can be mixed in the nebulizer with albuterol or metaproterenol if used within one hour. Drug stability and safety of Atrovent Inhalation Solution when mixed with other drugs in a nebulizer have not been established. Patients should be reminded that Atrovent Inhalation Solution should be used consistently as prescribed throughout the course of therapy.

Drug Interactions Atrovent has been shown to be a safe and effective bronchodilator when used in conjuction with beta adrenergic bronchodilators. Atrovent has also been used with other pulmonary medications, including methylxanthines and corticosteroids, without adverse drug interactions.

Carcinogenesis, Mutagenesis, Impairment of Fertility: Two-year oral carcinogenicity studies in rats and mice have revealed no carcinogenic potential at dietary doses up to 6 mg/kg/day of Atrovent.

Results of various mutagenicity studies (Ames test, mouse dominant lethal test, mouse micronucleus test and chromosome aberration of bone marrow in Chinese hamsters) were negative.

Fertility of male or female rats at oral doses up to 50 mg/kg/day was unaffected by Atrovent administration. At doses above 90 mg/kg, increased resorption and decreased conception rates were observed.

Pregnancy *TERATOGENIC EFFECTS*

Pregnancy Category B. Oral reproduction studies performed in mice, rats and rabbits at doses of 10, 100, and 125 mg/kg respectively, and inhalation reproduction studies in rats and rabbits at doses of 1.5 and 1.8 mg/kg (or approximately 38 and 45 times the recommended human daily dose) respectively, have demonstrated no evidence of teratogenic effects as a result of Atrovent. However, no adequate or well-controlled studies have been conducted in pregnant women. Because animal reproduction studies are not always predictive of human response, Atrovent should be used during pregnancy only if clearly needed.

Nursing Mothers It is not known whether Atrovent is excreted in human milk. Although lipid-insoluble quaternary bases pass into breast milk, it is unlikely that Atrovent® (ipratropium bromide) would reach the infant to a signifi-

Continued on next page

Atrovent Solution—Cont.

cant extent, especially when taken by inhalation since Atrovent is not well absorbed systemically after inhalation or oral administration. However, because many drugs are excreted in human milk, caution should be exercised when Atrovent is administered to a nursing woman.

Pediatric Use: Safety and effectiveness in the pediatric population below the age of 12 have not been established.

ADVERSE REACTIONS

Adverse reaction information concerning Atrovent® (ipratropium bromide) Inhalation Solution is derived from 12-week active-controlled clinical trials. Additional information is derived from foreign post-marketing experience and the published literature.

All adverse events, regardless of drug relationship, reported by three percent or more patients in the 12-week controlled clinical trials appear in the table below:

[See table below]

Additional adverse reactions reported in less than three percent of the patients treated with Atrovent include tachycardia, palpitations, eye pain, urinary retention, urinary tract infection and urticaria. Cases of precipitation or worsening of narrow-angle glaucoma and acute eye pain have been reported.

Lower respiratory adverse reactions (bronchitis, dyspnea and bronchospasm) were the most common events leading to discontinuation of Atrovent therapy in the 12-week trials. Headache, mouth dryness and aggravation of COPD symptoms are more common when the total daily dose of Atrovent equals or exceeds 2,000 mcg.

Allergic-type reactions such a skin rash, angioedema of tongue, lips and face, urticaria, laryngospasm and anaphylactic reaction have been reported. Many of the patients had a history of allergies to other drugs and/or foods.

OVERDOSAGE

Acute systemic overdosage by inhalation is unlikely since Atrovent® (ipratropium bromide) is not well absorbed after inhalation at up to four-fold the recommended dose, or after oral administration at up to forty-fold the recommended dose. The oral LD_{50} of Atrovent ranged between 1001 and 2010 mg/kg in mice; between 1667 and more than 4000 mg/kg in rats; and between 400 and 1300 mg/kg in dogs.

DOSAGE AND ADMINISTRATION

The usual dosage of Atrovent® (ipratropium bromide) Inhalation Solution is 500 mcg (1 Unit-Dose Vial) administered three to four times a day by oral nebulization, with doses 6 to 8 hours apart. Atrovent Inhalation Solution Unit-Dose Vials contain 500 mcg ipratropium bromide anhydrous in 2.5 ml normal saline. Atrovent Inhalation Solution can be mixed in the nebulizer with albuterol or metaproterenol if used within one hour. Drug stability and safety of Atrovent Inhalation Solution when mixed with other drugs in a nebulizer have not been established.

HOW SUPPLIED

Atrovent® (ipratropium bromide) Inhalation Solution Unit Dose Vial is supplied as a 0.02% clear, colorless solution containing 2.5 ml with 25 vials per foil pouch (NDC 0597-0080-62).

Each vial is made from a low density polyethylene (LDPE) resin.

STORE BETWEEN 59°F (15°C) AND 86°F (30°C). PROTECT FROM LIGHT.

STORE UNUSED VIALS IN THE FOIL POUCH.

ATTENTION PHARMACIST: Detach "Patient's Instructions for Use" from Package Insert and dispense with solution.

Caution

Federal law prohibits dispensing without prescription.

AS-PI 6/96 Rev

Distributed by

Boehringer Ingelheim Pharmaceuticals, Inc. Ridgefield, CT 06877

Manufactured by Roxane Laboratories, Inc., Columbus, OH 43228

Licensed from Boehringer Ingelheim International GmbH

Shown in Product Identification Guide, page 309

ATROVENT® ℞
(ipratropium bromide)
Nasal Spray 0.03% (21 mcg/spray)

Prescribing Information

DESCRIPTION

The active ingredient in ATROVENT® Nasal Spray is ipratropium bromide monohydrate. It is an anticholinergic agent chemically described as 8-azoniabicyclo (3.2.1) octane,3-(3-hydroxy-1-oxo-2-phenylpropoxy)-8-methyl-8-(1-methylethyl)-, bromide, monohydrate *(endo,syn)*-, (±)- :a synthetic quaternary ammonium compound, chemically related to atropine. Its structural formula is:

[See chemical structure at top of next column]

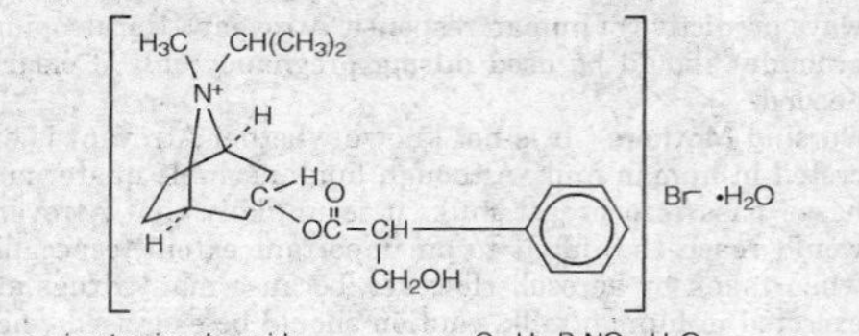

Ipratropium bromide is a white to off-white, crystalline substance. It is freely soluble in lower alcohols and water, existing in an ionized state in aqueous solutions, and relatively insoluble in non-polar media.

ATROVENT® (ipratropium bromide) Nasal Spray 0.03% is a metered-dose, manual pump spray unit which delivers

ipratropium bromide monohydrate $C_{20}H_{30}BrNO_3 \cdot H_2O$ Mol. Wt. 430.4

21 mcg (70μL) ipratropium bromide per spray on an anhydrous basis in an isotonic, aqueous solution with pH adjusted to 4.7. It also contains benzalkonium chloride, edetate disodium, sodium chloride, sodium hydroxide, hydrochloric acid, and purified water. Each bottle contains 345 sprays.

CLINICAL PHARMACOLOGY

Mechanism of Action

Ipratropium bromide is an anticholinergic agent that inhibits vagally-mediated reflexes by antagonizing the action of acetylcholine at the cholinergic receptor. In humans, ipratropium bromide has anti-secretory properties and, when applied locally, inhibits secretions from the serous and seromucous glands lining the nasal mucosa. Ipratropium bromide is a quaternary amine that minimally crosses the nasal and gastrointestinal membrane and the blood-brain barrier, resulting in a reduction of the systemic anticholinergic effects (e.g., neurologic, ophthalmic, cardiovascular, and gastrointestinal effects) that are seen with tertiary anticholinergic amines.

Pharmacokinetics

Absorption: Ipratropium bromide is poorly absorbed into the systemic circulation following oral administration (2–3%). Less than 20% of an 84 mcg per nostril dose was absorbed from the nasal mucosa of normal volunteers, induced-cold patients, or perennial rhinitis patients.

Distribution: Ipratropium bromide is minimally bound (0 to 9% *in vitro*) to plasma albumin and α1-acid glycoprotein. Its blood/plasma concentration ratio was estimated to be about 0.89. Studies in rats have shown that ipratropium bromide does not penetrate the blood-brain barrier.

Metabolism: Ipratropium bromide is partially metabolized to ester hydrolysis products, tropic acid and tropane. These metabolites appear to be inactive based on *in vitro* receptor affinity studies using rat brain tissue homogenates.

Elimination: After intravenous administration of 2 mg ipratropium bromide to 10 healthy volunteers, the terminal half-life of ipratropium was approximately 1.6 hours. The total body clearance and renal clearance were estimated to be 2,505 and 1,019 ml/min, respectively. The amount of the total dose excreted unchanged in the urine (Ae) within 24 hours was approximately one-half of the administered dose.

Pediatrics: Following administration of 42 mcg of ipratropium bromide per nostril two or three times a day in perennial rhinitis patients 6–18 years old, the mean amounts of the total dose excreted unchanged in the urine (8.6 to 11.1%) were higher than those reported in adult volunteers or adult perennial rhinitis patients (3.7 to 5.6%). Plasma ipratropium concentrations were relatively low (ranging from undetectable up to 0.49 ng/ml). No correlation of the amount of the total dose excreted unchanged in the urine (Ae) with age or gender was observed in the pediatric population.

Special Populations: Gender does not appear to influence the absorption or excretion of nasally administered ipratropium bromide. The pharmacokinetics of ipratropium bromide have not been studied in patients with hepatic or renal insufficiency or in the elderly.

Drug-Drug Interaction: No specific pharmacokinetic studies were conducted to evaluate potential drug-drug interactions.

Pharmacodynamics: In two single-dose trials (n=17), doses up to 336 mcg of ipratropium bromide did not significantly affect pupillary diameter, heart rate, or systolic/diastolic blood pressure. Similarly, in patients with induced-colds, ATROVENT (ipratropium bromide) Nasal Spray 0.06% (84 mcg/nostril four times a day), had no significant effects on pupillary diameter, heart rate or systolic/diastolic blood pressure.

Two nasal provocation trials in perennial rhinitis patients (n=44) using ipratropium bromide nasal spray showed a dose dependent increase in inhibition of methacholine induced nasal secretion with an onset of action within 15 minutes (time of first observation).

Controlled clinical trials demonstrated that intranasal fluorocarbon-propelled ipratropium bromide does not alter physiologic nasal functions (e.g., sense of smell, ciliary beat frequency, mucociliary clearance, or the air conditioning capacity of the nose).

Clinical Trials

The clinical trials for ATROVENT® (ipratropium bromide) Nasal Spray 0.03% were conducted in patients with nonallergic perennial rhinitis (NAPR) and in patients with allergic perennial rhinitis (APR). APR patients were those who experienced symptoms of nasal hypersecretion and nasal congestion or sneezing when exposed to specific perennial allergens (e.g., dust mites, molds) and were skin test positive to these allergens. NAPR patients were those who experienced symptoms of nasal hypersecretion and nasal congestion or sneezing throughout the year, but were skin test negative to common perennial allergens.

In four controlled, four- and eight-week comparisons of ATROVENT® (ipratropium bromide) Nasal Spray 0.03% (42 mcg per nostril, two or three times daily) with its vehi-

All Adverse Events, from a Double-blind, Parallel, 12-week Study of Patients with COPD*

PERCENT OF PATIENTS

	Atrovent® (500 mcg t.i.d) n=219	Alupent® 15 mg t.i.d) n=212	Atrovent®/Alupent® (500 mcg t.i.d/ 15 mg t.i.d) n=108	Albuterol(2.5 mg t.i.d) n=205	Atrovent®/ Albuterol (500 mcg t.i.d/ 2.5 mg t.i.d) n=100
Body as a Whole-General Disorders					
Headache	6.4	5.2	6.5	6.3	9.0
Pain	4.1	3.3	0.9	2.9	5.0
Influenza-like symptoms	3.7	4.7	6.5	0.5	1.0
Back pain	3.2	1.9	1.9	2.4	0.0
Chest pain	3.2	4.2	5.6	2.0	1.0
Cardiovascular Disorders					
Hypertension/Hypertension Aggravated	0.9	1.9	0.9	1.5	4.0
Central & Peripheral Nervous System					
Dizziness	2.3	3.3	1.9	3.9	4.0
Insomnia	0.9	0.5	4.6	1.0	1.0
Tremor	0.9	7.1	8.3	1.0	0.0
Nervousness	0.5	4.7	6.5	1.0	1.0
Gastrointestinal System Disorders					
Mouth Dryness	3.2	0.0	1.9	2.0	3.0
Nausea	4.1	3.8	1.9	2.9	2.0
Constipation	0.9	0.0	3.7	1.0	1.0
Musculo-Skeletal System Disorders					
Arthritis	0.9	1.4	0.9	0.5	3.0
Respiratory System Disorders (Lower)					
Coughing	4.6	8.0	6.5	5.4	6.0
Dyspnea	9.6	13.2	16.7	12.7	9.0
Bronchitis	14.6	24.5	15.7	16.6	20.0
Bronchospasm	2.3	2.8	4.6	5.4	5.0
Sputum Increased	1.4	1.4	4.6	3.4	0.0
Respiratory Disorder	0.0	6.1	6.5	2.0	4.0
Respiratory System Disorders (Upper)					
Upper Respiratory Tract Infection	13.2	11.3	9.3	12.2	16.0
Pharyngitis	3.7	4.2	5.6	2.9	4.0
Rhinitis	2.3	4.2	1.9	2.4	0.0
Sinusitis	2.3	2.8	0.9	5.4	4.0

* All adverse events, regardless of drug relationship, reported by three percent or more patients in the 12-week controlled clinical trials.

cle, in patients with allergic or nonallergic perennial rhinitis, there was a statistically significant decrease in the severity and duration of rhinorrhea in the ATROVENT® group throughout the entire study period. An effect was seen as early as the first day of therapy. There was no effect of ATROVENT® (ipratropium bromide) Nasal Spray 0.03% on degree of nasal congestion, sneezing, or postnasal drip. The response to ATROVENT® (ipratropium bromide) Nasal Spray 0.03% did not appear to be affected by the type of perennial rhinitis (NAPR or APR), age, or gender. No controlled clinical trials directly compared the efficacy of BID versus TID treatment.

INDICATIONS AND USAGE

ATROVENT® (ipratropium bromide) Nasal Spray 0.03% is indicated for the symptomatic relief of rhinorrhea associated with allergic and nonallergic perennial rhinitis in adults and children age 6 years and older. ATROVENT® (ipratropium bromide) Nasal Spray 0.03% does not relieve nasal congestion, sneezing, or postnasal drip associated with allergic or nonallergic perennial rhinitis.

CONTRAINDICATIONS

ATROVENT® (ipratropium bromide) Nasal Spray 0.03% is contraindicated in patients with a history of hypersensitivity to atropine or its derivatives, or to any of the other ingredients.

WARNINGS

Immediate hypersensitivity reactions may occur after administration of ipratropium bromide, as demonstrated by rare cases of urticaria, angioedema, rash, bronchospasm, and oropharyngeal edema.

PRECAUTIONS

General

ATROVENT® (ipratropium bromide) Nasal Spray 0.03% should be used with caution in patients with narrow-angle glaucoma, prostatic hypertrophy, or bladder-neck obstruction, particularly if they are receiving an anticholinergic by another route. Cases of precipitation or worsening of narrow-angle glaucoma and acute eye pain have been reported with direct eye contact of ipratropium bromide administered by oral inhalation.

Information for Patients

Patients should be advised that temporary blurring of vision, precipitation or worsening of narrow-angle glaucoma, or eye pain may result if ATROVENT® (ipratropium bromide) Nasal Spray 0.03% comes into direct contact with the eyes. Patients should be instructed to avoid spraying ATROVENT® (ipratropium bromide) Nasal Spray 0.03% in or around their eyes. Patients who experience eye pain, blurred vision, excessive nasal dryness, or episodes of nasal bleeding should be instructed to contact their doctor. Patients should be reminded to carefully read and follow the accompanying Patient's Instructions for Use.

Drug Interactions

No controlled clinical trials were conducted to investigate drug-drug interactions. ATROVENT® (ipratropium bromide) Nasal Spray 0.03% is minimally absorbed into the systemic circulation; nonetheless, there is some potential for an additive interaction with other concomitantly administered anticholinergic medications, including ATROVENT® for oral inhalation.

Carcinogenesis, Mutagenesis, Impairment of Fertility

In two-year carcinogenicity studies in rats and mice, ipratropium bromide at oral doses up to 6 mg/kg (approximately 190 and 95 times the maximum recommended daily intranasal dose in adults, respectively, and approximately 110 and 60 times the maximum recommended daily intranasal dose in children, respectively, on a mg/m^2 basis) showed no carcinogenic activity. Results of various mutagenicity studies (Ames test, mouse dominant lethal test, mouse micronucleus test, and chromosome aberration of bone marrow in Chinese hamsters) were negative.

Fertility of male or female rats was unaffected by ipratropium bromide at oral doses up to 50 mg/kg (approximately 1,600 times the maximum recommended daily intranasal dose in adults on a mg/m^2 basis). At an oral dose of 500 mg/kg (approximately 16,000 times the maximum recommended daily intranasal dose in adults on a mg/m^2 basis), ipratropium bromide produced a decrease in the conception rate.

Pregnancy

TERATOGENIC EFFECTS Pregnancy Category B. Oral reproduction studies were performed at doses of 10 mg/kg in mice, 1000 mg/kg in rats and 125 mg/kg in rabbits. These doses correspond, in each species respectively, to approximately 160, 32,000 and 8,000 times the maximum recommended daily intranasal dose in adults on a mg/m^2 basis. Inhalation reproduction studies were conducted in rats and rabbits at doses of 1.5 and 1.8 mg/kg respectively, (approximately 50 and 120 times, respectively, the maximum recommended daily intranasal dose in adults on a mg/m^2 basis). These studies demonstrated no evidence of teratogenic effects as a result of ipratropium bromide. At oral doses above 90 mg/kg in rats (approximately 2,900 times the maximum recommended daily intranasal dose in adults on a mg/m^2 basis) embryotoxicity was observed as increased resorption. This effect is not considered relevant to human use due to the large doses at which it was observed and the difference in route of administration. However, no adequate or well controlled studies have been conducted in pregnant women. Because animal reproduction studies are not always predictive of human response, ATROVENT® (ipratropium bromide) Nasal Spray 0.03% should be used during pregnancy only if clearly needed.

Nursing Mothers

It is known that some ipratropium bromide is systemically absorbed following nasal adminstration; however the portion which may be excreted in human milk is unknown. Although lipid-insoluble quaternary bases pass into breast milk, the minimal systemic absorption makes it unlikely that ipratropium bromide would reach the infant in an amount sufficient to cause a clinical effect. However, because many drugs are excreted in human milk, caution should be exercised when ATROVENT® (ipratropium bromide) Nasal Spray 0.03% is administered to a nursing woman.

Pediatric Use

The safety of ATROVENT® (ipratropium bromide) Nasal Spray 0.03% at a dose of two sprays (42 mcg) per nostril two or three times daily (total dose 168 to 252 mcg/day) has been demonstrated in 77 pediatric patients 6–12 years of age in placebo-controlled, 4-week trials and in 55 pediatric patients in active-controlled, 6 month trials. The effectiveness of ATROVENT® (ipratropium bromide) Nasal Spray 0.03% for the treatment of rhinorrhea associated with allergic and nonallergic perennial rhinitis in this pediatric age group is based on an extrapolation of the demonstrated efficacy of ATROVENT® (ipratropium bromide) Nasal Spray 0.03% in adults with these conditions and the likelihood that the disease course, pathophysiology, and the drug's effects are substantially similar to that of the adults. The recommended dose for the pediatric population is based on within and cross-study comparisons of the efficacy of ATROVENT® (ipratropium bromide) Nasal Spray 0.03% in adults and pediatric patients and on its safety profile in both adults and pediatric patients. The safety and effectiveness of ATROVENT® (ipratropium bromide) Nasal Spray 0.03% in patients under 6 years of age have not been established.

ADVERSE REACTIONS

Adverse reaction information on ATROVENT® (ipratropium bromide) Nasal Spray 0.03% in patients with perennial rhinitis was derived from four multicenter, vehicle-controlled clinical trials involving 703 patients (356 patients on ATROVENT® and 347 patients on vehicle), and a one-year, open-label, follow-up trial. In three of the trials, patients received ATROVENT® (ipratropium bromide) Nasal Spray 0.03% three times daily, for eight weeks. In the other trial, ATROVENT® (ipratropium bromide) Nasal Spray 0.03% was given to patients two times daily for four weeks. Of the 285 patients who entered the open-label, follow-up trial, 232 were treated for 3 months, 200 for 6 months, and 159 up to one year. The majority (>86%) of patients treated for one year were maintained on 42 mcg per nostril, two or three times daily, of ATROVENT® (ipratropium bromide) Nasal Spray 0.03%.

The following table shows adverse events, and the frequency that these adverse events led to the discontinuation of treatment, reported for patients who received ATROVENT® (ipratropium bromide) Nasal Spray 0.03% at the recommended dose of 42 mcg per nostril, or vehicle two or three times daily for four or eight weeks. Only adverse events reported with an incidence of at least 2.0% in the ATROVENT® group and higher in the ATROVENT® group than in the vehicle group are shown.

[See table above]

% of Patients Reporting Events+

	ATROVENT® Nasal Spray 0.03% (n=356)		Vehicle Control (n=347)	
	Incidence %	Discontinued %	Incidence %	Discontinued %
Headache	9.8	0.6	9.2	0
Upper respiratory tract infection	9.8	1.4	7.2	1.4
Epistaxis[1]	9.0	0.3	4.6	0.3
Rhinitis*				
Nasal dryness	5.1	0	0.9	0.3
Nasal irritation[2]	2.0	0	1.7	0.6
Other nasal symptoms[3]	3.1	1.1	1.7	0.3
Pharyngitis	8.1	0.3	4.6	0
Nausea	2.2	0.3	0.9	0

+ This table includes adverse events which occurred at an incidence rate of at least 2.0% in the ATROVENT® group and more frequently in the ATROVENT® group than in the vehicle group.

[1] Epistaxis reported by 7.0% of ATROVENT® patients and 2.3% of vehicle patients, blood-tinged mucus by 2.0% of ATROVENT® patients and 2.3% of vehicle patients.

[2] Nasal irritation includes reports of nasal itching, nasal burning, nasal irritation, and ulcerative rhinitis.

[3] Other nasal symptoms include reports of nasal congestion, increased rhinorrhea, increased rhinitis, posterior nasal drip, sneezing, nasal polyps and nasal edema.

* All events are listed by their WHO term; rhinitis has been presented by descriptive terms for clarification.

ATROVENT® (ipratropium bromide) Nasal Spray 0.03% was well tolerated by most patients. The most frequently reported nasal adverse events were transient episodes of nasal dryness or epistaxis. These adverse events were mild or moderate in nature, none was considered serious, none resulted in hospitalization and most resolved spontaneously or following a dose reduction. Treatment for nasal dryness and epistaxis was required infrequently (2% or less) and consisted of local application of pressure or a moisturizing agent (e.g., petroleum jelly or saline nasal spray). Patient discontinuation for epistaxis or nasal dryness was infrequent in both the controlled (0.3% or less) and one-year, open-label (2% or less) trials. There was no evidence of nasal rebound (i.e., a clinically significant increase in rhinorrhea, posterior nasal drip, sneezing or nasal congestion severity compared to baseline) upon discontinuation of double-blind therapy in these trials.

Adverse events reported by less than 2% of the patients receiving ATROVENT® (ipratropium bromide) Nasal Spray 0.03% during the controlled clinical trials or during the open-label follow-up trial, which are potentially related to ATROVENT®'s local effects or systemic anticholinergic effects include: dry mouth/throat, dizziness, ocular irritation, blurred vision, conjunctivitis, hoarseness, cough, and taste perversion. Additional anticholinergic effects noted with other ATROVENT® dosage forms (ATROVENT® Inhalation Solution, ATROVENT® Inhalation Aerosol, and ATROVENT® Nasal Spray 0.06%) include: precipitation or worsening of narrow angle glaucoma, urinary retention, prostatic disorders, tachycardia, constipation, and bowel obstruction.

There were infrequent reports of skin rash in both the controlled and uncontrolled clinical studies. Other allergic-type reactions such as angioedema of the throat, tongue, lips and face, urticaria, laryngospasm, and anaphylactic reactions have been reported with other ipratropium bromide products.

No controlled trial was conducted to address the relative incidence of adverse events of BID versus TID therapy.

OVERDOSAGE

Acute overdosage by intranasal administration is unlikely since ipratropium bromide is not well absorbed systemically after intranasal or oral administration. Following administration of a 20 mg oral dose (equivalent to ingesting more than four bottles of ATROVENT® Nasal Spray 0.03%) to 10 male volunteers, no change in heart rate or blood pressure was noted. Following a 2 mg intravenous infusion over 15 minutes to the same 10 male volunteers, plasma ipratropium concentrations of 22–45 ng/mL were observed (>100 times the concentrations observed following intranasal administration). Following intravenous infusion these 10 volunteers had a mean increase of heart rate of 50 bpm and less than 20 mmHg change in systolic or diastolic blood pressure at the time of peak ipratropium levels.

Oral median lethal doses of ipratropium bromide were greater than 1,000 mg/kg in mice (approximately 16,000 and 9,500 times the maximum recommended daily intranasal dose in adults and children, respectively, on a mg/m^2 basis), 1,700 mg/kg in rats (approximately 55,000 and 32,000 times the maximum recommended daily intranasal dose in adults and children, respectively, on a mg/m^2 basis), and 400 mg/kg in dogs (approximately 43,000 and 25,000 times the maximum recommended daily intranasal dose in adults and children, respectively, on a mg/m^2 basis).

DOSAGE AND ADMINISTRATION

The recommended dose of ATROVENT® (ipratropium bromide) Nasal Spray 0.03% is two sprays (42 mcg) per nostril two or three times daily (total dose 168 to 252 mcg/day) for the symptomatic relief of rhinorrhea associated with allergic and nonallergic perennial rhinitis in adults and children age 6 years and older. Optimum dosage varies with the response of the individual patient.

Initial pump priming requires seven sprays of the pump. If used regularly as recommended, no further priming is required. If not used for more than 24 hours, the pump will require two sprays, or if not used for more than seven days, the pump will require seven sprays to reprime.

HOW SUPPLIED

ATROVENT® (ipratropium bromide) Nasal Spray 0.03% is supplied in a white high density polyethylene (HDPE) bottle fitted with a white and clear metered nasal spray pump, a green safety clip to prevent accidental discharge of the spray, and a clear plastic dust cap. It contains 31.1 g of product formulation, 345 sprays, each delivering 21 mcg (70 µL)

Continued on next page

Atrovent Spray 0.03%—Cont.

of ipratropium per spray, or 28 days of therapy at the maximum recommended dose (two sprays per nostril three times a day).
Store tightly closed between 59°F (15°C) and 86°F (30°C). Avoid freezing. Keep out of reach of children.
Do not spray in the eyes.
Patients should be reminded to read and follow the accompanying Patient's Instructions for Use, which should be dispensed with the product.
Rx only.

AN.03-PI-11/98

Manufactured by: Boehringer Ingelheim Pharmaceuticals, Inc.
Ridgefield, CT 06877
Licensed from: Boehringer Ingelheim International GmbH

Shown in Product Identification Guide, page 308

ATROVENT® ℞
(ipratropium bromide)
Nasal Spray 0.06% (42 mcg/spray)

Prescribing Information

DESCRIPTION

The active ingredient in ATROVENT® Nasal Spray is ipratropium bromide monohydrate. It is an anticholinergic agent chemically described as 8-azoniabicyclo (3.2.1) octane,3-(3-hydroxy-1-oxo-2-phenylpropoxy)-8-methyl-8-(1-methylethyl)-, bromide, monohydrate (*endo, syn*)-, (±)- : a synthetic quaternary ammonium compound, chemically related to atropine. Its structural formula is:

ipratropium bromide monohydrate — $C_{20}H_{30}BrNO_3 \cdot H_2O$ Mol. Wt. 430.4

Ipratropium bromide is a white to off-white, crystalline substance. It is freely soluble in lower alcohols and water, existing in an ionized state in aqueous solutions, and relatively insoluble in non-polar media.
ATROVENT® (ipratropium bromide) Nasal Spray 0.06% is a metered-dose, manual pump spray unit which delivers 42 mcg ipratropium bromide (on an anhydrous basis) per spray (70µL) in an isotonic, aqueous solution with pH-adjusted to 4.7. It also contains benzalkonium chloride, edetate disodium, sodium chloride, sodium hydroxide, hydrochloric acid, and purified water. Each bottle contains 165 sprays.

CLINICAL PHARMACOLOGY

Mechanism of Action

Ipratropium bromide is an anticholinergic agent that inhibits vagally-mediated reflexes by antagonizing the action of acetylcholine at the cholinergic receptor. In humans, ipratropium bromide has anti-secretory properties and, when applied locally, inhibits secretions from the serous and seromucous glands lining the nasal mucosa. Ipratropium bromide is a quaternary amine that minimally crosses the nasal and gastrointestinal membrane and the blood-brain barrier, resulting in a reduction of the systemic anticholinergic effects (e.g., neurologic, ophthalmic, cardiovascular, and gastrointestinal effects) that are seen with tertiary anticholinergic amines.

Pharmacokinetics

Absorption: Ipratropium bromide is poorly absorbed into the systemic circulation following oral administration (2–3%). Less than 20% of an 84 mcg per nostril dose was absorbed from the nasal mucosa of normal volunteers, induced-cold adult volunteers, naturally-acquired common cold pediatric patients, or perennial rhinitis adult patients.
Distribution: Ipratropium bromide is minimally bound (0 to 9% *in vitro*) to plasma albumin and a_1-acid glycoprotein. Its blood/plasma concentration ratio was estimated to be about 0.89. Studies in rats have shown that ipratropium bromide does not penetrate the blood-brain barrier.
Metabolism: Ipratropium bromide is partially metabolized to ester hydrolysis products, tropic acid, and tropane. These metabolites appear to be inactive based on in vitro receptor affinity studies using rat brain tissue homogenates.
Elimination: After intravenous administration of 2 mg ipratropium bromide to 10 healthy volunteers, the terminal half-life of ipratropium bromide was approximately 1.6 hours. The total body clearance and renal clearance were estimated to be 2,505 and 1,019 ml/min respectively. The amount of the total dose excreted unchanged in the urine (Ae) within 24 hours was approximately one-half of the administered dose.
Pediatrics: Following administration of 84 mcg of ipratropium bromide per nostril three times a day in patients 5–18 years old (n=42) with a naturally-acquired common cold, the mean amount of the total dose excreted unchanged in the urine of 7.8% was comparable to 84 mcg per nostril four times a day in an adult induced common cold population (n=22) of 7.3 to 8.1%. Plasma ipratropium concentrations were relatively low (ranging from undetectable up to 0.62 ng/mL). No correlation of the amount of the total dose excreted unchanged in the urine (Ae) with age or gender was observed in the pediatric population.
Special Populations: Gender does not appear to influence the absorption or excretion of nasally administered ipratropium bromide. The pharmacokinetics of ipratropium bromide have not been studied in patients with hepatic or renal insufficiency or in the elderly.
Drug-Drug Interactions: No specific pharmacokinetic studies were conducted to evaluate potential drug-drug interactions.
Pharmacodynamics: In two single dose trials (n=17), doses up to 336 mcg of ipratropium bromide did not significantly affect pupillary diameter, heart rate, or systolic/diastolic blood pressure. Similarly, ATROVENT® Nasal Spray 0.06% in adult patients (n=22) with induced-colds, (84 mcg/nostril four times a day) and in pediatric patients (n=45) with naturally acquired common colds (84 mcg/nostril three times a day) had no significant effects on pupillary diameter, heart rate, or systolic/diastolic blood pressure.
Controlled clinical trials demonstrated that intranasal fluorocarbon-propelled ipratropium bromide does not alter physiologic nasal functions (e.g., sense of smell, ciliary beat frequency, mucociliary clearance, or the air conditioning capacity of the nose).

Clinical Trials

The clinical trials for ATROVENT® (ipratropium bromide) Nasal Spray 0.06% were conducted in patients with rhinorrhea associated with naturally occurring common colds. In two controlled four day comparisons of ATROVENT® (ipratropium bromide) Nasal Spray 0.06% (84 mcg per nostril, administered three or four times daily; n=352) with its vehicle (n=351), there was a statistically significant reduction of rhinorrhea, as measured by both nasal discharge weight and the patients' subjective assessment of severity of rhinorrhea using a visual analog scale. These significant differences were evident within one hour following dosing. There was no effect of ATROVENT® (ipratropium bromide) Nasal Spray 0.06% on degree of nasal congestion or sneezing. The response to ATROVENT® (ipratropium bromide) Nasal Spray 0.06% did not appear to be affected by age or gender. No controlled clinical trials directly compared the efficacy of three times daily versus four times daily treatment.

INDICATIONS AND USAGE

ATROVENT® (ipratropium bromide) Nasal Spray 0.06% is indicated for the symptomatic relief of rhinorrhea associated with the common cold for adults and children age 5 years and older. ATROVENT® (ipratropium bromide) Nasal Spray 0.06% does not relieve nasal congestion or sneezing associated with the common cold.
The safety and effectiveness of the use of ATROVENT® (ipratropium bromide) Nasal Spray 0.06% beyond four days in patients with the common cold has not been established.

CONTRAINDICATIONS

ATROVENT® (ipratropium bromide) Nasal Spray 0.06% is contraindicated in patients with a history of hypersensitivity to atropine or its derivatives, or to any of the other ingredients.

WARNINGS

Immediate hypersensitivity reactions may occur after administration of ipratropium bromide, as demonstrated by rare cases of urticaria, angioedema, rash, bronchospasm and oropharyngeal edema.

PRECAUTIONS

General

ATROVENT® (ipratropium bromide) Nasal Spray 0.06% should be used with caution in patients with narrow-angle glaucoma, prostatic hypertrophy or bladder neck obstruction, particularly if they are receiving an anticholinergic by another route. Cases of precipitation or worsening of narrow-angle glaucoma and acute eye pain have been reported with direct eye contact of ipratropium bromide administered by oral inhalation.

Information for Patients

Patients should be advised that temporary blurring of vision, precipitation or worsening of narrow-angle glaucoma or eye pain may result if ATROVENT® (ipratropium bromide) Nasal Spray 0.06% comes into direct contact with the eyes. Patients should be instructed to avoid spraying ATROVENT® (ipratropium bromide) Nasal Spray 0.06% in or around the eyes. Patients who experience eye pain, blurred vision, excessive nasal dryness or episodes of nasal bleeding should be instructed to contact their doctor. Patients should be reminded to carefully read and follow the accompanying Patient's Instructions for Use.

Drug Interactions

No controlled clinical trials were conducted to investigate potential drug-drug interactions. ATROVENT® (ipratropium bromide) Nasal Spray 0.06% is minimally absorbed into the systemic circulation; nonetheless, there is some potential for an additive interaction with other concomitantly administered anticholinergic medications, including ATROVENT® for oral inhalation.

Carcinogenesis, Mutagenesis, Impairment of Fertility

In two-year carcinogenicity studies in rats and mice, ipratropium bromide at oral doses up to 6 mg/kg (approximately 70 and 35 times the maximum recommended daily intranasal dose in adults, respectively, and approximately 45 and 25 times the maximum recommended daily intranasal dose in children, respectively, on a mg/m^2 basis) showed no carcinogenic activity. Results of various mutagenicity studies (Ames test, mouse dominant lethal test, mouse micronucleus test, and chromosome aberration of bone marrow in Chinese hamsters) were negative.
Fertility of male or female rats was unaffected by ipratropium bromide at oral doses up to 50 mg/kg (approximately 600 times the maximum recommended daily intranasal dose in adults on a mg/m^2 basis). At an oral dose of 500 mg/kg (approximately 16,000 times the maximum recommended daily intranasal dose in adults on a mg/ m^2 basis), ipratropium bromide produced a decrease in the conception rate.

Pregnancy

TERATOGENIC EFFECTS Pregnancy Category B. Oral reproduction studies were performed at doses of 10 mg/kg in mice, 1,000 mg/kg in rats and 125 mg/kg in rabbits. These doses correspond, in each species respectively, to approximately 60, 12,000, and 3,000 times the maximum recommended daily intranasal dose in adults on a mg/m^2 basis. Inhalation reproduction studies were conducted in rats and rabbits at doses of 1.5 and 1.8 mg/kg, respectively, (approximately 20 and 45 times, respectively, maximum recommended daily intranasal dose in adults on a mg/ m^2 basis). These studies demonstrated no evidence of teratogenic effects as a result of ipratropium bromide. At oral doses above 90 mg/kg in rats (approximately 1,100 times the maximum recommended daily intranasal dose in adults on a mg/ m^2 basis) embryotoxicity was observed as increased resorption. This effect is not considered relevant to human use due to the large doses at which it was observed and the difference in route of administration. However, no adequate or well controlled studies have been conducted in pregnant women. Because animal reproduction studies are not always predictive of human response, ipratropium bromide should be used during pregnancy only if clearly needed.

Nursing Mothers

It is known that some ipratropium bromide is systemically absorbed following nasal administration; however the portion which may be excreted in human milk is unknown. Although lipid-insoluble quaternary bases pass into breast milk, the minimal systemic absorption makes it unlikely that ipratropium bromide would reach the infant in an amount sufficient to cause a clinical effect. However, because many drugs are excreted in human milk, caution should be exercised when ATROVENT® (ipratropium bromide) Nasal Spray 0.06% is administered to a nursing woman.

Pediatric Use

The safety of ATROVENT (ipratropium bromide) Nasal Spray 0.06% at a dose of two sprays (84 mcg) per nostril three times a day (total dose 504 mcg/day) for two to four days has been demonstrated in two clinical trials involving 362 pediatric patients 5–11 years of age with naturally acquired common colds. In this pediatric population ATROVENT® (ipratropium bromide) Nasal Spray 0.06% had an adverse event profile similar to that observed in adolescent and adult patients. When ATROVENT® was concomitantly administered with an oral decongestant (pseudoephedrine HCl) in 122 children ages 5–12 years, and concomitantly administered with an oral decongestant/antihistamine combination (pseudoephedrine HCl/chlorpheniramine maleate) in 123 children ages 5–12 years, adverse event profiles were similar to ATROVENT® alone.
The effectiveness of ATROVENT® (ipratropium bromide) Nasal Spray 0.06% for the treatment of rhinorrhea associated with the common cold in this pediatric age group is based on extrapolation of the demonstrated efficacy of ATROVENT (ipratropium bromide) Nasal Spray 0.06% in adolescents and adults with this condition and the likelihood that the disease course, pathophysiology, and the drug's effects are substantially similar to that of adults. The recommended dose for the pediatric population is based on cross-study comparisons of the efficacy of ATROVENT (ipratropium bromide) Nasal Spray 0.06% in adults and pediatric patients and on its safety profile in both adults and pediatric patients. The safety and effectiveness of ATROVENT (ipratropium bromide) Nasal Spray 0.06% in pediatric patients under 5 years of age have not been established.

ADVERSE REACTIONS

Adverse reaction information on ATROVENT® (ipratropium bromide) Nasal Spray 0.06% in patients with the common cold was derived from two multicenter, vehicle-controlled clinical trials involving 1,276 patients (195 patients on ATROVENT® (ipratropium bromide) Nasal Spray 0.03%, 352 patients on ATROVENT® (ipratropium bromide) Nasal Spray 0.06%, 189 patients on ATROVENT® (ipratropium bromide) Nasal Spray 0.12%, 351 patients on vehicle and 189 patients receiving no treatment).
The following table shows adverse events reported for patients who received ATROVENT® (ipratropium bromide) Nasal Spray 0.06% at the recommended dose of 84 mcg per nostril, or vehicle, administered three or four times daily, where the incidence is 1% or greater in the ATROVENT® group and higher in the ATROVENT® group than in the vehicle group.

% of Patients Reporting Events[1] ATROVENT® Nasal Spray 0.06% (n = 352)	Vehicle Control (n = 351)	
Epistaxis[2]	8.2%	2.3%
Dry Mouth/Throat	1.4%	0.3%
Nasal Congestion	1.1%	0.0%
Nasal Dryness	4.8%	2.8%

[1] This table includes adverse events for which the incidence was 1% or greater in the ATROVENT® group and higher in the ATROVENT® group than in the vehicle group.

[2] Epistaxis reported by 5.4% of ATROVENT® patients and 1.4% of vehicle patients, blood tinged nasal mucus by 2.8% of ATROVENT® patients and 0.9% of vehicle patients.

ATROVENT® (ipratropium bromide) Nasal Spray 0.06% was well tolerated by most patients. The most frequently reported adverse events were transient episodes of nasal dryness or epistaxis. The majority of these adverse events (96%) were mild or moderate in nature, none was considered serious, and none resulted in hospitalization. No patient required treatment for nasal dryness, and only three patients (<1%) required treatment for epistaxis, which consisted of local application of pressure or a moisturizing agent (e.g., petroleum jelly). No patient receiving ATROVENT® (ipratropium bromide) Nasal Spray 0.06% was discontinued from the trial due to other nasal dryness or bleeding.

Adverse events reported by less than 1% of the patients receiving ATROVENT® (ipratropium bromide) Nasal Spray 0.06% during the controlled clinical trials which are potentially related to ATROVENT®'s local effects or systemic anticholinergic effects include: taste perversion, nasal burning, conjunctivitis, coughing, dizziness, hoarseness, palpitation, pharyngitis, tachycardia, thirst, tinnitus and blurred vision. Additional anticholinergic effects noted with other ATROVENT® dosage forms (ATROVENT® Inhalation Solution, ATROVENT® Inhalation Aerosol and ATROVENT® Nasal Spray 0.03%) include: precipitation or worsening of narrow-angle glaucoma, urinary retention, prostate disorders, constipation and bowel obstruction.

There were no reports of allergic-type reactions in the controlled clinical trials. Allergic-type reactions such as skin rash, angioedema of the tongue, lips and face, urticaria, laryngospasm and anaphylactic reactions have been reported with other ipratropium bromide products.

No controlled trial was conducted to address the relative incidence of adverse events for three times daily versus four times daily therapy.

OVERDOSAGE

Acute overdosage by intranasal administration is unlikely since ipratropium bromide is not well absorbed systemically after intranasal or oral administration. Following administration of a 20 mg oral dose (equivalent to ingesting more than two bottles of ATROVENT® Nasal Spray 0.06%) to 10 male volunteers, no change in heart rate or blood pressure was noted. Following a 2 mg intravenous infusion over 15 minutes to the same 10 male volunteers, plasma ipratropium concentrations of 22–45 ng/mL were observed (>100 times the concentrations observed following intranasal administration). Following intravenous infusion these 10 volunteers had a mean increase of heart rate of 50 bpm and less than 20 mm Hg change in systolic or diastolic blood pressure at the time of peak ipratropium levels.

Oral median lethal doses of ipratropium bromide were greater than: 1,000 mg/kg in mice (approximately 6,000 and 3,800 times the maximum recommended daily intranasal dose in adults and children, respectively, on a mg/m^2 basis) 1,700 mg/kg in rats (approximately 21,000 and 13,000 times the maximum recommended daily intranasal dose in adults and children, respectively, on a mg/m^2 basis) and 400 mg/kg in dogs (approximately 16,000 and 10,000 times the maximum recommended daily intranasal dose in adults and children, respectively, on a mg/m^2 basis).

DOSAGE AND ADMINISTRATION

The recommended dose of ATROVENT® (ipratropium bromide) Nasal Spray 0.06% is two sprays (84 mcg) per nostril three or four times daily (total dose 504 to 672 mcg/day) for symptomatic relief of rhinorrhea associated with the common cold in adults and children age 5 years and older. Optimum dosage varies with response of the individual patient. The recommended dose of ATROVENT® (ipratropium bromide) Nasal Spray 0.06% for children age 5–11 years is two sprays (84 mcg) per nostril three times daily (total dose of 504 mcg/day).

The safety and effectiveness of the use of ATROVENT® (ipratropium bromide) Nasal Spray 0.06% beyond four days in patients with the common cold have not been established.

Initial pump priming requires seven sprays of the pump. If used regularly as recommended, no further priming is required. If not used for more than 24 hours, the pump will require two sprays, or if not used for more than seven days, the pump will require seven sprays to reprime.

HOW SUPPLIED

ATROVENT® (ipratropium bromide) Nasal Spray 0.06% is supplied in a white high density polyethylene (HDPE) bottle fitted with a metered nasal spray pump, a green safety clip to prevent accidental discharge of the spray, and a clear plastic dust cap. It contains 16.6 g of product formulation, 165 sprays, each delivering 42 mcg of ipratropium bromide per spray (70 µL), or 10 days of therapy at the maximum recommended dose (two sprays per nostril four times a day).

Store tightly closed between 59°F (15°C) and 86°F (30°C). Avoid freezing. Keep out of reach of children. Do not spray in the eyes.

Patients should be reminded to read and follow the accompanying Patient's Instructions for Use, which should be dispensed with the product.

Rx only.

AN.06-PI-12/98

Manufactured by
Boehringer Ingelheim Pharmaceuticals, Inc.
Ridgefield, CT 06877

Licensed from
Boehringer Ingelheim International GmbH

Shown in Product Identification Guide, page 308

CATAPRES® ℞

[kah 'tah-pres]
(clonidine hydrochloride USP)
Oral Antihypertensive
Tablets of 0.1, 0.2 and 0.3 mg

Prescribing Information

DESCRIPTION

CATAPRES® (clonidine hydrochloride USP) is a centrally acting alpha-agonist hypotensive agent available as tablets for oral administration in three dosage strengths: 0.1 mg, 0.2 mg and 0.3 mg. The 0.1 mg tablet is equivalent to 0.087 mg of the free base.

The inactive ingredients are colloidal silicon dioxide, corn starch, dibasic calcium phosphate, FD&C Yellow No. 6, gelatin, glycerin, lactose, magnesium stearate, methylparaben, propylparaben. The CATAPRES 0.1 mg tablet also contains FD&C Blue No. 1 and FD&C Red No. 3.

Clonidine hydrochloride is an imidazoline derivative and exists as a mesomeric compound. The chemical name is 2-(2,6-dichlorophenylamino)-2-imidazoline hydrochloride. The following is the structural formula:

$C_9H_9Cl_2N_3 \cdot HCl$ Mol. Wt. 266.56

[See chemical structure at top of next column]

Clonidine hydrochloride is an odorless, bitter, white, crystalline substance soluble in water and alcohol.

CLINICAL PHARMACOLOGY

Clonidine stimulates alpha-adrenoreceptors in the brain stem. This action results in reduced sympathetic outflow from the central nervous system and in decreases in peripheral resistance, renal vascular resistance, heart rate, and blood pressure. CATAPRES (clonidine hydrochloride USP) acts relatively rapidly. The patient's blood pressure declines within 30 to 60 minutes after an oral dose, the maximum decrease occurring within 2 to 4 hours. Renal blood flow and glomerular filtration rate remain essentially unchanged. Normal postural reflexes are intact; therefore, orthostatic symptoms are mild and infrequent.

Acute studies with clonidine hydrochloride in humans have demonstrated a moderate reduction (15% to 20%) of cardiac output in the supine position with no change in the peripheral resistance: at a 45° tilt there is a smaller reduction in cardiac output and a decrease of peripheral resistance. During long-term therapy, cardiac output tends to return to control values, while peripheral resistance remains decreased. Slowing of the pulse rate has been observed in most patients given clonidine, but the drug does not alter normal hemodynamic response to exercise.

Tolerance to the antihypertensive effect may develop in some patients, necessitating a reevaluation of therapy.

Other studies in patients have provided evidence of a reduction in plasma renin activity and in the excretion of aldosterone and catecholamines. The exact relationship of these pharmacologic actions to the antihypertensive effect of clonidine has not been fully elucidated.

Clonidine acutely stimulates growth hormone release in both children and adults, but does not produce a chronic elevation of growth hormone with long-term use.

Pharmacokinetics: The plasma level of clonidine peaks in approximately 3 to 5 hours and the plasma half-life ranges from 12 to 16 hours. The half-life increases up to 41 hours in patients with severe impairment of renal function. Following oral administration, about 40–60% of the absorbed dose is recovered in the urine as unchanged drug in 24 hours. About 50% of the absorbed dose is metabolized in the liver.

INDICATIONS AND USAGE

CATAPRES® (clonidine hydrochloride USP) is indicated in the treatment of hypertension. CATAPRES may be employed alone or concomitantly with other antihypertensive agents.

CONTRAINDICATIONS

CATAPRES® (clonidine hydrochloride USP) Tablets should not be used in patients with known hypersensitivity to clonidine (see PRECAUTIONS).

WARNINGS

Withdrawal: Patients should be instructed not to discontinue therapy without consulting their physician. Sudden cessation of clonidine treatment has, in some cases, resulted in symptoms such as nervousness, agitation, headache, and tremor accompanied or followed by a rapid rise in blood pressure and elevated catecholamine concentrations in the plasma. The likelihood of such reactions to discontinuation of clonidine therapy appears to be greater after administration of higher doses or continuation of concomitant beta-blocker treatment and special caution is therefore advised in these situations. Rare instances of hypertensive encephalopathy, cerebrovascular accidents and death have been reported after clonidine withdrawal. When discontinuing therapy with CATAPRES®, the physician should reduce the dose gradually over 2 to 4 days to avoid withdrawal symptomatology.

An excessive rise in blood pressure following discontinuation of CATAPRES therapy can be reversed by administration of oral clonidine hydrochloride or by intravenous phentolamine. If therapy is to be discontinued in patients receiving a beta-blocker and clonidine concurrently, the beta-blocker should be withdrawn several days before the gradual discontinuation of CATAPRES.

Because children commonly have gastrointestinal illnesses that lead to vomiting, they may be particularly susceptible to hypertensive episodes resulting from abrupt inability to take medication.

PRECAUTIONS

General: In patients who have developed localized contact sensitization to CATAPRES-TTS® (clonidine), continuation of CATAPRES-TTS® or substitution of oral clonidine hydrochloride therapy may be associated with the development of a generalized skin rash.

In patients who develop an allergic reaction to CATAPRES-TTS, substitution of oral clonidine hydrochloride may also elicit an allergic reaction (including generalized rash, urticaria, or angioedema).

CATAPRES® (clonidine hydrochloride) should be used with caution in patients with severe coronary insufficiency, conduction disturbances, recent myocardial infarction, cerebrovascular disease or chronic renal failure.

Perioperative Use: Administration of CATAPRES should be continued to within four hours of surgery and resumed as soon as possible thereafter. Blood pressure should be carefully monitored during surgery and additional measures to control blood pressure should be available if required.

Information for Patients: Patients should be cautioned against interruption of CATAPRES therapy without their physician's advice.

Patients who engage in potentially hazardous activities, such as operating machinery or driving, should be advised of a possible sedative effect of clonidine. They should also be informed that this sedative effect may be increased by concomitant use of alcohol, barbiturates, or other sedating drugs.

Drug Interactions: Clonidine may potentiate the CNS-depressive effects of alcohol, barbiturates or other sedating drugs. If a patient receiving clonidine hydrochloride is also taking tricyclic antidepressants, the hypotensive effect of clonidine may be reduced, necessitating an increase in the clonidine dose.

Due to a potential for additive effects such as bradycardia and AV block, caution is warranted in patients receiving clonidine concomitantly with agents known to affect sinus node function or AV nodal conduction, e.g. digitalis, calcium channel blockers and beta-blockers.

Amitriptyline in combination with clonidine enhances the manifestation of corneal lesions in rats (See TOXICOLOGY).

Toxicology: In several studies with oral clonidine hydrochloride, a dose-dependent increase in the incidence and severity of spontaneous retinal degeneration was seen in albino rats treated for six months or longer. Tissue distribution studies in dogs and monkeys showed a concentration of clonidine in the choroid.

In view of the retinal degeneration seen in rats, eye examinations were performed during clinical trials in 908 patients before, and periodically after, the start of clonidine therapy. In 353 of these 908 patients, the eye examinations were carried out over periods of 24 months or longer. Except for some dryness of the eyes, no drug-related abnormal ophthalmological findings were recorded and, according to specialized tests such as electroretinography and macular dazzle, retinal function was unchanged.

In combination with amitriptyline, clonidine hydrochloride administration led to the development of corneal lesions in rats within five days.

Carcinogenesis, Mutagenesis, Impairment of Fertility: Chronic dietary administration of clonidine was not carcinogenic to rats (132 weeks) or mice (78 weeks) dosed, respectively, at up to 46 or 70 times the maximum recommended daily human dose as mg/kg (9 or 6 times the MRDHD on a mg/m^2 basis). There was no evidence of genotoxicity in the Ames test for mutagenicity or mouse micronucleus test for clastogenicity.

Continued on next page

Catapres—Cont.

Fertility of male or female rats was unaffected by clonidine doses as high as 150 mcg/kg (approximately 3 times the MRDHD). In a separate experiment, fertility of female rats appeared to be affected at dose levels of 500 to 2000 mcg/kg (10 to 40 times the oral MRDHD on a mg/kg basis; 2 to 8 times the MRDHD on a mg/m^2 basis).

Usage in Pregnancy: *TERATOGENIC EFFECTS Pregnancy Category C.* Reproduction studies performed in rabbits at doses up to approximately 3 times the oral maximum recommended daily human dose (MRDHD) of CATAPRES (clonidine hydrochloride) produced no evidence of a teratogenic or embryotoxic potential in rabbits. In rats, however, doses as low as $^1/_3$ the oral MRDHD ($^1/_{15}$ the MRDHD on a mg/m^2 basis) of clonidine were associated with increased resorptions in a study in which dams were treated continuously from two months prior to mating. Increased resorptions were not associated with treatment at the same time or at higher dose levels (up to 3 times the oral MRDHD) when the dams were treated on gestation days 6–15. Increases in resorption were observed at much higher dose levels (40 times the oral MRDHD on a mg/kg basis; 4 to 8 times the MRDHD on a mg/m^2 basis) in mice and rats treated on gestation days 1–14 (lowest dose employed in the study was 500 mcg/kg).

No adequate, well-controlled studies have been conducted in pregnant women. Because animal reproduction studies are not always predictive of human response, this drug should be used during pregnancy only if clearly needed.

Nursing Mothers: As clonidine hydrochloride is excreted in human milk, caution should be exercised when CATAPRES® (clonidine hydrochloride USP) is administered to a nursing woman.

Pediatric Use: Safety and effectiveness in pediatric patients below the age of twelve have not been established (See WARNINGS on Withdrawal).

ADVERSE REACTIONS

Most adverse effects are mild and tend to diminish with continued therapy. The most frequent (which appear to be dose-related) are dry mouth, occurring in about 40 of 100 patients; drowsiness, about 33 in 100; dizziness, about 16 in 100; constipation and sedation, each about 10 in 100.

The following less frequent adverse experiences have also been reported in patients receiving CATAPRES® (clonidine hydrochloride USP), but in many cases patients were receiving concomitant medication and a causal relationship has not been established.

Body as a Whole: Weakness, about 10 in 100 patients; fatigue, about 4 in 100; headache and withdrawal syndrome each about 1 in 100. Also reported were pallor; a weakly positive Coombs' test; increased sensitivity to alcohol; and fever.

Cardiovascular: Orthostatic symptoms, about 3 in 100 patients; palpitations and tachycardia, and bradycardia, each about 5 in 1000. Syncope, Raynaud's phenomenon, congestive heart failure, and electrocardiographic abnormalities (i.e., sinus node arrest, functional bradycardia, high degree AV block and arrhythmias) have been reported rarely. Rare cases of sinus bradycardia and atrioventricular block have been reported, both with and without the use of concomitant digitalis.

Central Nervous System: Nervousness and agitation, about 3 in 100 patients; mental depression, about 1 in 100 and insomnia, about 5 in 1000. Other behavioral changes, vivid dreams or nightmares, restlessness, anxiety, visual and auditory hallucinations and delirium have rarely been reported.

Dermatological: Rash, about 1 in 100 patients; pruritus, about 7 in 1000; hives, angioneurotic edema and urticaria, about 5 in 1000; alopecia, about 2 in 1000.

Gastrointestinal: Nausea and vomiting, about 5 in 100 patients; anorexia and malaise, each about 1 in 100; mild transient abnormalities in liver function tests, about 1 in 100; hepatitis, parotitis, constipation, pseudo-obstruction, and abdominal pain, rarely.

Genitourinary: Decreased sexual activity, impotence and loss of libido, about 3 in 100 patients; nocturia, about 1 in 100; difficulty in micturition, about 2 in 1000; urinary retention, about 1 in 1000.

Hematologic: Thrombocytopenia, rarely.

Metabolic: Weight gain, about 1 in 100 patients; gynecomastia, about 1 in 1000; transient elevation of blood glucose or serum creatine phosphokinase, rarely.

Musculoskeletal: Muscle or joint pain, about 6 in 1000 and leg cramps, about 3 in 1000.

Oro-otolaryngeal: Dryness of the nasal mucosa was rarely reported.

Ophthalmological: Dryness of the eyes, burning of the eyes and blurred vision were reported.

OVERDOSAGE

Hypertension may develop early and may be followed by hypotension, bradycardia, respiratory depression, hypothermia, drowsiness, decreased or absent reflexes, weakness, irritability and miosis. The frequency of CNS depression may be higher in children than adults. Large overdoses may result in reversible cardiac conduction defects or dysrhythmias, apnea, coma and seizures. Signs and symptoms of overdose generally occur within 30 minutes to two hours after exposure. As little as 0.1 mg of clonidine has produced signs of toxicity in children.

There is no specific antidote for clonidine overdose. Clonidine overdosage may result in the rapid development of CNS depression; therefore, induction of vomiting with ipecac syrup is not recommended. Gastric lavage may be indicated following recent and/or large ingestions. Administration of activated charcoal and/or a cathartic may be beneficial. Supportive care may include atropine sulfate for bradycardia, intravenous fluids and/or vasopressor agents for hypotension and vasodilators for hypertension. Naloxone may be a useful adjunct for the management of clonidine-induced respiratory depression, hypotension and/or coma; blood pressure should be monitored since the administration of naloxone has occasionally resulted in paradoxical hypertension. Tolazoline administration has yielded inconsistent results and is not recommended as first-line therapy. Dialysis is not likely to significantly enhance the elimination of clonidine.

The largest overdose reported to date involved a 28-year old male who ingested 100 mg of clonidine hydrochloride powder. This patient developed hypertension followed by hypotension, bradycardia, apnea, hallucinations, semicoma, and premature ventricular contractions. The patient fully recovered after intensive treatment. Plasma clonidine levels were 60 ng/ml after 1 hour, 190 ng/ml after 1.5 hours, 370 ng/ml after 2 hours, and 120 ng/ml after 5.5 and 6.5 hours. In mice and rats, the oral LD_{50} of clonidine is 206 and 465 mg/kg, respectively.

DOSAGE AND ADMINISTRATION

Adults: The dose of CATAPRES® (clonidine hydrochloride USP) must be adjusted according to the patient's individual blood pressure response. The following is a general guide to its administration.

Initial Dose: 0.1 mg tablet twice daily (morning and bedtime). Elderly patients may benefit from a lower initial dose.

Maintenance Dose: Further increments of 0.1 mg per day may be made at weekly intervals if necessary until the desired response is achieved. Taking the larger portion of the oral daily dose at bedtime may minimize transient adjustment effects of dry mouth and drowsiness. The therapeutic doses most commonly employed have ranged from 0.2 mg to 0.6 mg per day given in divided doses. Studies have indicated that 2.4 mg is the maximum effective daily dose, but doses as high as this have rarely been employed.

Renal Impairment: Dosage must be adjusted according to the degree of impairment, and patients should be carefully monitored. Since only a minimal amount of clonidine is removed during routine hemodialysis, there is no need to give supplemental clonidine following dialysis.

HOW SUPPLIED

CATAPRES® (clonidine hydrochloride USP) is supplied in scored oval tablets containing 0.1 mg, 0.2 mg or 0.3 mg of clonidine hydrochloride.

[See table below]

Store below 86°F (30°C).

Dispense in tight, light-resistant container.

Caution: Federal law prohibits dispensing without prescription.

CA-PI-8/96

Boehringer Ingelheim Pharmacueticals, Inc.
Ridgefield, CT 06877
Licensed from Boehringer Ingelheim International GmbH

Shown in Product Identification Guide, page 309

Dose (mg)	Color	Marking	Bottle of 100	Bottle of 1000	Unit Dose of 100
0.1	Tan	BI 6	NDC0597-0006-01	NDC0597-0006-10	NDC0597-0006-61
0.2	Orange	BI 7	NDC0597-0007-01	NDC0597-0007-10	NDC0597-0007-61
0.3	Peach	BI 11	NDC0597-0011-01		

CATAPRES-TTS® ℞

[*căt-a 'prĕss*]

(clonidine)

Transdermal Therapeutic System

Catapres-TTS® -1

Catapres-TTS® -2

Catapres-TTS® -3

Programmed delivery *in vivo* of 0.1, 0.2, or 0.3 mg clonidine per day, for one week.

Prescribing Information

DESCRIPTION

Catapres-TTS® (clonidine) is a transdermal system providing continuous systemic delivery of clonidine for 7 days at an approximately constant rate. Clonidine is a centrally acting alpha-agonist hypotensive agent. It is an imidazoline derivative with the chemical name 2, 6-dichloro-N-2-imidazolidinylidenebenzenamine and has the following chemical structure:

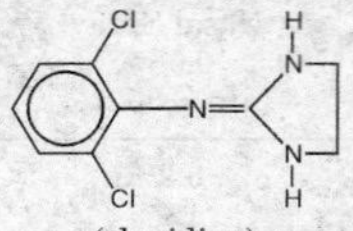

(clonidine)

System Structure and Components Catapres-TTS is a multilayered film, 0.2 mm thick, containing clonidine as the active agent. The system areas are 3.5 cm^2 (CATAPRES-TTS-1), 7.0 cm^2 (CATAPRES-TTS-2) and 10.5 cm^2 (CATAPRES-TTS-3) and the amount of drug released is directly proportional to the area (See Release Rate Concept). The composition per unit area is the same for all three doses.

Proceeding from the visible surface towards the surface attached to the skin, there are four consecutive layers: 1) a backing layer of pigmented polyester film; 2) a drug reservoir of clonidine, mineral oil, polyisobutylene, and colloidal silicon dioxide; 3) a microporous polypropylene membrane that controls the rate of delivery of clonidine from the system to the skin surface; 4) an adhesive formulation of clonidine, mineral oil, polyisobutylene, and colloidal silicon dioxide. Prior to use, a protective slit release liner of polyester that covers the adhesive layer is removed.

Cross section of the system:

Backing
Drug Reservoir
Control Membrane
Adhesive
Slit Release Liner

Release Rate Concept Catapres-TTS is programmed to release clonidine at an approximately constant rate for 7 days. The energy for drug release is derived from the concentration gradient existing between a saturated solution of drug in the system and the much lower concentration prevailing in the skin. Clonidine flows in the direction of the lower concentration at a constant rate, limited by the rate-controlling membrane, so long as a saturated solution is maintained in the drug reservoir.

Following system application to intact skin, clonidine in the adhesive layer saturates the skin site below the system. Clonidine from the drug reservoir then begins to flow through the rate-controlling membrane and the adhesive layer of the system into the systemic circulation via the capillaries beneath the skin. Therapeutic plasma clonidine levels are achieved 2 to 3 days after initial application of Catapres-TTS.

The 3.5, 7.0, and 10.5 cm^2 systems deliver 0.1, 0.2, and 0.3 mg of clonidine per day, respectively. To ensure constant release of drug for 7 days, the total drug content of the system is higher than the total amount of drug delivered. Application of a new system to a fresh skin site at weekly intervals continuously maintains therapeutic plasma concentrations of clonidine. If the Catapres-TTS is removed and not replaced with a new system, therapeutic plasma clonidine levels will persist for about 8 hours and then decline slowly over several days. Over this time period, blood pressure returns gradually to pretreatment levels.

CLINICAL PHARMACOLOGY

Clonidine stimulates alpha-adrenoreceptors in the brain stem. This action results in reduced sympathetic outflow from the central nervous system and in decreases in peripheral resistance, renal vascular resistance, heart rate, and blood pressure. Renal blood flow and glomerular filtration rate remain essentially unchanged. Normal postural reflexes are intact; therefore, orthostatic symptoms are mild and infrequent.

Acute studies with clonidine hydrochloride in humans have demonstrated a moderate reduction (15%–20%) of cardiac output in the supine position with no change in peripheral resistance; at a 45° tilt there is a smaller reduction in cardiac output and a decrease of peripheral resistance.

During long-term therapy, cardiac output tends to return to control values, while peripheral resistance remains decreased. Slowing of the pulse rate has been observed in most patients given clonidine, but the drug does not alter normal hemodynamic responses to exercise.

Tolerance to the antihypertensive effect may develop in some patients, necessitating a reevaluation of therapy.

Other studies in patients have provided evidence of a reduction in plasma renin activity and in the excretion of aldosterone and catecholamines. The exact relationship of these pharmacologic actions to the antihypertensive effect of clonidine has not been fully elucidated.

Clonidine acutely stimulates the release of growth hormone in children as well as adults but does not produce a chronic elevation of growth hormone with long-term use.

Pharmacokinetics The plasma half-life of clonidine is 12.7 ± 7 hours. Following oral administration, about 40–60% of the absorbed dose is recovered in the urine as unchanged drug within 24 hours. The remainder of the absorbed dose is metabolized in the liver.

INDICATIONS AND USAGE

Catapres-TTS® (clonidine) is indicated in the treatment of hypertension. It may be employed alone or concomitantly with other antihypertensive agents.

CONTRAINDICATIONS

Catapres-TTS® (clonidine) should not be used in patients with known hypersensitivity to clonidine or to any other component of the therapeutic system.

WARNINGS

Withdrawal Patients should be instructed not to discontinue therapy without consulting their physician. Sudden cessation of clonidine treatment has, in some cases, resulted in symptoms such as nervousness, agitation, headache, and confusion accompanied or followed by a rapid rise in blood pressure and elevated catecholamine concentrations in the plasma. The likelihood of such reactions to discontinuation of clonidine therapy appears to be greater after administration of higher doses or continuation of concomitant beta-blocker treatment and special caution is therefore advised in these situations. Rare instances of hypertensive encephalopathy, cerebrovascular accidents and death have been reported after clonidine withdrawal. When discontinuing therapy with Catapres, the physician should reduce the dose gradually over 2 to 4 days to avoid withdrawal symptomatology.

An excessive rise in blood pressure following discontinuation of Catapres-TTS® therapy can be reversed by administration of oral clonidine hydrochloride or by intravenous phentolamine. If therapy is to be discontinued in patients receiving a beta-blocker and clonidine concurrently, the beta-blocker should be withdrawn several days before the gradual discontinuation of Catapres-TTS®.

PRECAUTIONS

General In patients who have developed localized contact sensitization to Catapres-TTS® (clonidine) continuation of Catapres-TTS or substitution of oral clonidine hydrochloride therapy may be associated with development of a generalized skin rash.

In patients who develop an allergic reaction to Catapres-TTS, substitution of oral clonidine hydrochloride may also elicit an allergic reaction (including generalized rash, urticaria, or angioedema).

Catapres-TTS should be used with caution in patients with severe coronary insufficiency, conduction disturbances, recent myocardial infarction, cerebrovascular disease, or chronic renal failure.

In rare instances, loss of blood pressure control has been reported in patients using Catapres-TTS according to the instructions for use.

Perioperative Use Catapres-TTS therapy should not be interrupted during the surgical period. Blood pressure should be carefully monitored during surgery and additional measures to control blood pressure should be available if required. Physicians considering starting Catapres-TTS therapy during the perioperative period must be aware that therapeutic plasma clonidine levels are not achieved until 2 to 3 days after initial application of Catapres-TTS (see DOSAGE AND ADMINISTRATION).

Defibrillation or Cardioversion The transdermal clonidine systems should be removed before attempting defibrillation or cardioversion because of the potential for altered electrical conductivity which may increase the risk of arcing, a phenomenon associated with the use of defibrillators.

Information for Patients Patients should be cautioned against interruption of Catapres-TTS therapy without their physician's advice.

Patients who engage in potentially hazardous activities, such as operating machinery or driving, should be advised of a possible sedative effect of clonidine. They should also be informed that this sedative effect may be increased by concomitant use of alcohol, barbiturates, or other sedating drugs.

Patients should be instructed to consult their physicians promptly about the possible need to remove the patch if they observe moderate to severe localized erythema and/or vesicle formation at the site of application or generalized skin rash.

If a patient experiences isolated, mild localized skin irritation before completing 7 days of use, the system may be removed and replaced with a new system applied to a fresh skin site.

If the system should begin to loosen from the skin after application, the patient should be instructed to place the adhesive overlay directly over the system to ensure adhesion during its 7-day use.

Used Catapres-TTS patches contain a substantial amount of their initial drug content which may be harmful to infants and children if accidentally applied or ingested. THEREFORE, PATIENTS SHOULD BE CAUTIONED TO KEEP BOTH USED AND UNUSED CATAPRES-TTS PATCHES OUT OF THE REACH OF CHILDREN. After use, Catapres-TTS should be folded in half with the adhesive sides together and discarded away from children's reach.

Instructions for use, storage and disposal of the system are provided at the end of this monograph. These instructions also are included in each box of Catapres-TTS.

Drug Interactions Clonidine may potentiate the CNS-depressive effects of alcohol, barbiturates or other sedating drugs. If a patient receiving clonidine is also taking tricyclic antidepressants, the hypotensive effect of clonidine may be reduced, necessitating an increase in the clonidine dose.

Due to potential for additive effects such as bradycardia and AV block, caution is warranted in patients receiving clonidine concomitantly with agents known to affect sinus node function or AV nodal conduction e.g., digitalis, calcium channel blockers and beta-blockers.

	Programmed Delivery Clonidine *in vivo* Per Day Over 1 Week	Clonidine Content	Size	Code
Catapres-TTS®-1 (clonidine)	0.1 mg	2.5 mg	3.5 cm^2	BI-31
Catapres-TTS®-2 (clonidine)	0.2 mg	5.0 mg	7.0 cm^2	BI-32
Catapres-TTS®-3 (clonidine)	0.3 mg	7.5 mg	10.5 cm^2	BI-33

Amitriptyline in combination with clonidine enhances the manifestation of corneal lesions in rats (see TOXICOLOGY).

Toxicology In several studies with oral clonidine hydrochloride, a dose-dependent increase in the incidence and severity of spontaneous retinal degeneration was seen in albino rats treated for six months or longer. Tissue distribution studies in dogs and monkeys showed a concentration of clonidine in the choroid.

In view of the retinal degeneration seen in rats, eye examinations were performed during clinical trials in 908 patients before, and periodically after, the start of clonidine therapy. In 353 of these 908 patients, the eye examinations were carried out over periods of 24 months or longer. Except for some dryness of the eyes, no drug-related abnormal ophthalmological findings were recorded and, according to specialized tests such as electroretinography and macular dazzle, retinal function was unchanged.

In combination with amitriptyline, clonidine hydrochloride administration led to the development of corneal lesions in rats within 5 days.

Carcinogenesis, Mutagenesis, Impairment of Fertility Chronic dietary administration of clonidine was not carcinogenic to rats (132 weeks) or mice (78 weeks) dosed, respectively, at up to 46 to 70 times the maximum recommended daily human dose as mg/kg (9 or 6 times the MRDHD on a mg/m^2 basis). There was no evidence of genotoxicity in the Ames test for mutagenicity or mouse micronucleus test for clastogenicity.

Fertility of male and female rats was unaffected by clonidine doses as high as 150 mcg/kg (approximately 3 times the MRDHD). In a separate experiment, fertility of female rats appeared to be affected at dose levels of 500 to 2000 mcg/kg (10 to 40 times the oral MRDHD on a mg/kg basis; 2 to 8 times the MRDHD on a mg/m^2 basis).

Pregnancy *TERATOGENIC EFFECTS Pregnancy Category C.* Reproduction studies performed in rabbits at doses up to approximately 3 times the oral maximum recommended daily human dose (MRDHD) of Catapres (clonidine hydrochloride) produced no evidence of a teratogenic or embryotoxic potential in rabbits. In rats, however, doses as low as $1/3$ the oral MRDHD ($1/15$ the MRDHD on a mg/m^2 basis) of clonidine were associated with increased resorptions in a study in which dams were treated continuously from 2 months prior to mating. Increased resorptions were not associated with treatment at the same time or at higher dose levels (up to 3 times the oral MRDHD) when the dams were treated on gestation days 6–15. Increases in resorption were observed at much higher dose levels (40 times the oral MRDHD on a mg/kg basis; 4 to 8 times the MRDHD on a mg/m^2 basis) in mice and rats treated on gestation days 1–14 (lowest dose employed in the study was 500 mcg/kg). No adequate, well-controlled studies have been conducted in pregnant women. Because animal reproduction studies are not always predictive of human response, this drug should be used during pregnancy only if clearly needed.

Nursing Mothers As clonidine is excreted in human milk, caution should be exercised when Catapres-TTS is administered to a nursing woman.

Pediatric Use Safety and effectiveness in pediatric patients below the age of twelve have not been established (See Warnings on Withdrawal).

ADVERSE REACTIONS

Clinical trial experience with Catapres-TTS® Most systemic adverse effects during Catapres-TTS therapy have been mild and have tended to diminish with continued therapy. In a 3-month multiclinic trial of Catapres-TTS in 101 hypertensive patients, the systemic adverse reactions were, dry mouth (25 patients) and drowsiness (12) fatigue (6), headache (5), lethargy and sedation (3 each), insomnia, dizziness, impotence/sexual dysfunction, dry throat (2 each) and constipation, nausea, change in taste and nervousness (1 each).

In the above mentioned 3-month controlled clinical trial, as well as other uncontrolled clinical trials, the most frequent adverse reactions were dermatological and are described below.

In the 3-month trial, 51 of the 101 patients had localized skin reactions such as erythema (26 patients) and/or pruritus, particularly after using an adhesive overlay throughout the 7-day dosage interval. Allergic contact sensitization to Catapres-TTS was observed in 5 patients. Other skin reactions were localized vesiculation (7 patients), hyperpigmentation (5), edema (3), excoriation (3), burning (3), papules (1), throbbing (1), blanching (1), and a generalized macular rash (1).

In additional clinical experience, contact dermatitis resulting in treatment discontinuation was observed in 128 of 673 patients (about 19 in 100) after a mean duration of treatment of 37 weeks. The incidence of contact dermatitis was about 34 in 100 among white women, about 18 in 100 in white men, about 14 in 100 in black women, and approximately 8 in 100 in black men. Analysis of skin reaction data showed that the risk of having to discontinue Catapres-TTS treatment because of contact dermatitis was greatest between treatment weeks 6 and 26, although sensitivity may develop either earlier or later in treatment.

In a large-scale clinical acceptability and safety study by 451 physicians in a total of 3539 patients, other allergic reactions were recorded for which a causal relationship to Catapres-TTS was not established: maculopapular rash (10 cases); urticaria (2 cases); and angioedema of the face (2 cases), which also affected the tongue in one of the patients.

Marketing Experience with Catapres-TTS Other adverse effects reported since the drug has been marketed are listed below by body system. In this setting, an incidence or causal relationship cannot always be accurately determined. However, none of the events listed below occurred in a frequency greater than 0.5%.

Body as a Whole Fever, malaise, weakness and pallor, and withdrawal syndrome.

Cardiovascular Congestive heart failure; cerebrovascular accident; electrocardiographic abnormalities (i.e., bradycardia, sick sinus syndrome disturbances and arrhythmias); chest pain; orthostatic symptoms; syncope, increases in blood pressure; sinus bradycardia and atrioventricular block with and without the use of concomitant digitalis; Raynaud's phenomenon; tachycardia; bradycardia; and palpitations.

Central and Peripheral Nervous System/Psychiatric Delirium, mental depression, visual and auditory hallucinations, localized numbness, vivid dreams or nightmares, restlessness, anxiety, agitation, irritability, other behavioral changes, and drowsiness.

Dermatological Angioneurotic edema, localized or generalized rash, hives, urticaria, contact dermatitis, pruritus, alopecia, and localized hypo or hyperpigmentation.

Gastrointestinal Anorexia and vomiting.

Genitourinary Difficult micturition, loss of libido, and decreased sexual activity.

Metabolic Gynecomastia or breast enlargement and weight gain.

Musculoskeletal Muscle or joint pain, and leg cramps.

Ophthalmological Blurred vision, burning of the eyes and dryness of the eyes.

Adverse Events Associated with Oral Catapres Therapy Most adverse effects are mild and tend to diminish with continued therapy. The most frequent (which appear to be dose-related) are dry mouth, occurring in about 40 of 100 patients; drowsiness, about 33 in 100; dizziness, about 16 in 100; constipation and sedation, each about 10 in 100. The following less frequent adverse experiences have also been reported in patients receiving Catapres (clonidine hydrochloride USP), but in many cases patients were receiving concomitant medication and a causal relationship has not been established.

Body as A Whole Weakness, about 10 in 100 patients; fatigue, about 4 in 100; headache and withdrawal syndrome, each about 1 in 100. Also reported were pallor, a weakly positive Coombs' test, increased sensitivity to alcohol, and fever.

Cardiovascular Orthostatic symptoms, about 3 in 100 patients; palpitations and tachycardia, and bradycardia, each about 5 in 1000. Syncope, Raynaud's phenomenon, congestive heart failure, and electrocardiographic abnormalities (i.e., sinus node arrest, functional bradycardia, high degree AV block and arrhythmias) have been reported rarely. Rare cases of sinus bradycardia and AV block have been reported, both with and without the use of concomitant digitalis.

Central Nervous System Nervousness and agitation, about 3 in 100 patients; mental depression, about 1 in 100; and insomnia, about 5 in 1000. Other behavioral changes, vivid dreams or nightmares, restlessness, anxiety, visual and auditory hallucinations and delirium have rarely been reported.

Dermatological Rash, about 1 in 100 patients; pruritus, about 7 in 1000; hives, angioneurotic edema and urticaria, about 5 in 1000; alopecia, about 2 in 1000.

Gastrointestinal Nausea and vomiting, about 5 in 100 patients; anorexia and malaise, each about 1 in 100; mild transient abnormalities in liver function tests, about 1 in 100; hepatitis, parotitis, constipation, pseudo-obstruction, and abdominal pain, rarely.

Genitourinary Decreased sexual activity, impotence and loss of libido, about 3 in 100 patients; nocturia, about 1 in 100; difficulty in micturition, about 2 in 1000; urinary retention, about 1 in 1000.

Hematologic Thrombocytopenia, rarely.

Metabolic Weight gain, about 1 in 100 patients; gynecomastia, about 1 in 1000; transient elevation of blood glucose or serum creatine phosphokinase, rarely.

Musculoskeletal Muscle or joint pain, about 6 in 1000 and leg cramps, about 3 in 1000.

Oro-otolaryngeal Dryness of the nasal mucosa was rarely reported.

Ophthalmological Dryness of the eyes, burning of the eyes and blurred vision were reported.

Continued on next page

Catapres-TTS—Cont.

OVERDOSAGE

Hypertension may develop early and may be followed by hypotension, bradycardia, respiratory depression, hypothermia, drowsines, decreased or absent reflexes, weakness, irritability and miosis. The frequency of CNS depression may be higher in children than adults. Large overdoses may result in reversible cardiac conduction defects or dysrhythmias, apnea, coma and seizures. Signs and symptoms of overdose generally occur within 30 minutes to two hours after exposure. As little as 0.1 mg of clonidine has produced signs of toxicity in children.

If symptoms of poisoning occur following dermal exposure, remove all Catapres-TTS systems. After their removal, the plasma clonidine levels will persist for about 8 hours, then decline slowly over a period of several days. Rare cases of Catapres-TTS poisoning due to accidental or deliberate mouthing or ingestion of the patch have been reported, many of them involving children.

There is no specific antidote for clonidine overdosage. Ipecac syrup-induced vomiting and gastric lavage would not be expected to remove significant amounts of clonidine following dermal exposure. If the patch is ingested, whole bowel irrigation may be considered and the administration of activated charcoal and/or cathartic may be beneficial. Supportive care may include atropine sulfate for bradycardia, intravenous fluids and/or vasopressor agents for hypotension and vasodilators for hypertension. Naloxone may be a useful adjunct for the management of clonidine-induced respiratory depression, hypotension and/or coma; blood pressure should be monitored since the administration of naloxone has occasionally resulted in paradoxical hypertension. Tolazoline administration has yielded inconsistent results and is not recommended as first-line therapy. Dialysis is not likely to significantly enhance the elimination of clonidine.

The largest overdose reported to date, involved a 28-year-old male who ingested 100 mg of clonidine hydrochloride powder. This patient developed hypertension followed by hypotension, bradycardia, apnea, hallucinations, semicoma, and premature ventricular contractions. The patient fully recovered after intensive treatment. Plasma clonidine levels were 60 ng/mL after 1 hour, 190 ng/mL after 1.5 hours, 370 ng/mL after 2 hours, and 120 ng/mL after 5.5 and 6.5 hours. In mice and rats, the oral LD_{50} of clonidine is 206 and 465 mg/kg, respectively.

DOSAGE AND ADMINISTRATION

Apply Catapres-TTS® (clonidine) once every 7 days to a hairless area of intact skin on the upper outer arm or chest. Each new application of Catapres-TTS should be on a different skin site from the previous location. If the system loosens during 7-day wearing, the adhesive overlay should be applied directly over the system to ensure good adhesion. There have been rare reports of the need for patch changes prior to 7 days to maintain blood pressure control.

To initiate therapy, Catapres-TTS dosage should be titrated according to individual therapeutic requirements, starting with Catapres-TTS-1. If after one or two weeks the desired reduction in blood pressure is not achieved, increase the dosage by adding another Catapres-TTS-1 or changing to a larger system. An increase in dosage above two Catapres-TTS-3 is usually not associated with additional efficacy.

When substituting Catapres-TTS for oral clonidine or for other antihypertensive drugs, physicians should be aware that the antihypertensive effect of Catapres-TTS may not commence until 2–3 days after initial application. Therefore, gradual reduction of prior drug dosage is advised. Some or all previous antihypertensive treatment may have to be continued, particularly in patients with more severe forms of hypertension.

Renal Impairment Dosage must be adjusted according to the degree of impairment, and patients should be carefully monitored. Since only a minimal amount of clonidine is removed during routine hemodialysis, there is no need to give supplemental clonidine following dialysis.

HOW SUPPLIED

Catapres-TTS-1 (clonidine) and Catapres-TTS-2 are supplied as 4 pouched systems and 4 adhesive overlays per carton, 3 cartons per shipper (NDC 0597-0031-12 and 0597-0032-12, respectively). Catapres-TTS-3 is supplied as 4 pouched systems and 4 adhesive overlays per carton (NDC 0597-0033-34). See chart below.

[See table at top of previous page]

STORAGE AND HANDLING

Store below 86° F (30° C).

CAUTION Federal law prohibits dispensing without prescription.

CT-PI-830892(8/96)

Manufactured by
Alza Corporation, Palo Alto, California 94304
Distributed by
Boehringer Ingelheim Pharmaceuticals, Inc.
Ridgefield, CT 06877
Licensed from
Boehringer Ingelheim International GmbH

Shown in Product Identification Guide, page 309

COMBIPRES® ℞

[*kom 'be-pres*]

Each tablet contains: 0.1/15 mg, 0.2/15 mg, 0.3/15 mg of clonidine hydrochloride/chlorthalidone, respectively

Oral Antihypertensive

Tablets 0.1	**BI-CODE 08**
Tablets 0.2	**BI-CODE 09**
Tablets 0.3	**BI-CODE 10**

Prescribing Information

DESCRIPTION

Combipres® is a combination of clonidine hydrochloride (a centrally acting antihypertensive agent) and chlorthalidone (a diuretic). Combipres® is available as tablets for oral administration in three dosage strengths: 0.1/15 mg, 0.2/15 mg and 0.3/15 mg of clonidine hydrochloride/chlorthalidone, respectively.

The inactive ingredients are colloidal silicon dioxide, corn starch, dibasic calcium phosphate, gelatin, glycerin, lactose, magnesium stearate, methylparaben and propylparaben. The Combipres 0.1/15 mg tablet also contains FD&C Red No. 3. The Combipres 0.2/15 mg tablet also contains FD&C Blue No. 1.

Clonidine hydrochloride:

Clonidine hydrochloride is an imidazoline derivative and exists as a mesomeric compound. The chemical name is 2-(2,6-dichlorophenylamino)-2-imidazoline hydrochloride. The following is the structural formula:

$C_9H_9Cl_2N_3 \cdot HCl$
Mol. Wt. 266.56

Clonidine hydrochloride is an odorless, bitter, white, crystalline substance soluble in water and alcohol.

Chlorthalidone

Chlorthalidone is a monosulfamyl diuretic that differs chemically from thiazide diuretics in that a double ring system is incorporated in its structure. It is a racemic mixture of 2-chloro-5-(1-hydroxy-3-oxo-1-isoindolinyl) benzenesulfonamide with the following structural formula:

$C_{14}H_{11}Cl\ N_2O_4S$
Mol. Wt. 338.76

Chlorthalidone is practically insoluble in water, in ether and in chloroform; soluble in methanol; slightly soluble in alcohol.

CLINICAL PHARMACOLOGY

Combipres®:

Combipres produces a more pronounced antihypertensive response than occurs after either clonidine hydrochloride or chlorthalidone alone in equivalent doses.

Clonidine hydrochloride:

Clonidine hydrochloride acts relatively rapidly. The patient's blood pressure declines within 30 to 60 minutes after an oral dose, the maximum decrease occurring within 2 to 4 hours. The plasma level of clonidine hydrochloride peaks in approximately 3 to 5 hours and the plasma half-life ranges from 12 to 16 hours. The half-life increases up to 41 hours in patients with severe impairment of renal function. Following oral administration about 40–60% of the absorbed dose is recovered in the urine as unchanged drug in 24 hours. About 50% of the absorbed dose is metabolized in the liver. Clonidine stimulates alpha-adrenoreceptors in the brain stem, resulting in reduced sympathetic outflow from the central nervous system and a decrease in peripheral resistance, renal vascular resistance, heart rate, and blood pressure. Renal blood flow and glomerular filtration rate remain essentially unchanged. Normal postural reflexes are intact and therefore orthostatic symptoms are mild and infrequent.

Acute studies with clonidine hydrochloride in humans have demonstrated a moderate reduction (15 to 20%) of cardiac output in the supine position with no change in the peripheral resistance; at a 45° tilt there is a smaller reduction in cardiac output and a decrease of peripheral resistance. During long-term therapy, cardiac output tends to return to control values, while peripheral resistance remains decreased. Slowing of the pulse rate has been observed in most patients given clonidine but the drug does not alter normal hemodynamic response to exercise.

Other studies in patients have provided evidence of a reduction in plasma renin activity and in the excretion of aldosterone and catecholamines, but the exact relationship of these pharmacologic actions to the antihypertensive effect has not been fully elucidated.

Clonidine acutely stimulates growth hormone release in both children and adults, but does not produce a chronic elevation of growth hormone with long-term use.

Tolerance may develop in some patients, necessitating a reevaluation of therapy.

Chlorthalidone:

Chlorthalidone is a long-acting oral diuretic with antihypertensive activity. Its diuretic action commences a mean of 2.6 hours after dosing and continues for up to 72 hours. The drug produces diuresis with increased excretion of sodium and chloride. The diuretic effects of chlorthalidone and the benzothiadiazine (thiazide) diuretics appear to arise from similar mechanisms and the maximal effect of chlorthalidone and the thiazides appears to be similar. The site of action appears to be the distal convoluted tubule of the nephron. The diuretic effects of chlorthalidone lead to decreased extracellular fluid volume, plasma volume, cardiac output, total exchangeable sodium, glomerular filtration rate, and renal plasma flow. Although the mechanism of action of chlorthalidone and related drugs is not wholly clear, sodium and water depletion appear to provide a basis for its antihypertensive effect. Like the thiazide diuretics, chlorthalidone produces dose-related reductions in serum potassium levels, elevations in serum uric acid and blood glucose, and it can lead to decreased sodium and chloride levels.

The mean plasma half-life of chlorthalidone is about 40 to 60 hours. It is eliminated primarily as unchanged drug in the urine. Non-renal routes of elimination have yet to be clarified. In the blood, approximately 75% of the drug is bound to plasma proteins.

INDICATIONS AND USAGE

Combipres® (clonidine hydrochloride USP/chlorthalidone USP) is indicated in the treatment of hypertension. **This fixed combination drug is not indicated for initial therapy of hypertension. Hypertension requires therapy titrated to the individual patient. If the fixed combination represents the dosage so determined, its use may be more convenient in patient management. The treatment of hypertension is not static, but must be reevaluated as conditions in each patient warrant.**

CONTRAINDICATIONS

Anuria. Combipres® is contraindicated in patients with known hypersensitivity to chlorthalidone or other sulfonamide-derived drugs.

WARNINGS

Chlorthalidone should be used with caution in severe renal disease. In patients with renal disease, chlorthalidone or related drugs may precipitate azotemia. Cumulative effects of the drug may develop in patients with impaired renal function. Chlorthalidone should be used with caution in patients with impaired hepatic function or progressive liver disease, because minor alterations of fluid and electrolyte balance may precipitate hepatic coma.

Sensitivity reactions may occur in patients with a history of allergy or bronchial asthma. The possibility of exacerbation or activation of systemic lupus erythematosus has been reported with thiazide diuretics which are structurally related to chlorthalidone. However, systemic lupus erythematosus has not been reported following chlorthalidone administration.

PRECAUTIONS

Clonidine hydrochloride:

General: In patients who have developed localized contact sensitization to Catapres-TTS® (clonidine), substitution of oral clonidine hydrochloride therapy may be associated with the development of a generalized skin rash.

In patients who develop an allergic reaction from Catapres-TTS® (clonidine) that extends beyond the local patch site (such as generalized skin rash, urticaria, or angioedema), oral clonidine hydrochloride substitution may elicit a similar reaction.

As with all antihypertensive therapy, clonidine hydrochloride should be used with caution in patients with severe coronary insufficiency, recent myocardial infarction, cerebrovascular disease or chronic renal failure.

Withdrawal Patients should be instructed not to discontinue therapy without consulting their physician. Sudden cessation of clonidine treatment has resulted in subjective symptoms such as nervousness, agitation and headache, accompanied or followed by a rapid rise in blood pressure and elevated catecholamine concentrations in the plasma, but such occurrences have usually been associated with previous administration of high oral doses (exceeding 1.2 mg/day) and/or with continuation of concomitant beta-blocker therapy. Rare instances of hypertensive encephalopathy and death have been reported. When discontinuing therapy with clonidine hydrochloride, the physician should reduce the dose gradually over 2 to 4 days to avoid withdrawal symptomatology.

An excessive rise in blood pressure following clonidine hydrochloride discontinuance can be reversed by administration of oral clonidine or by intravenous phentolamine. If therapy is to be discontinued in patients receiving beta-blockers and clonidine concurrently, beta-blockers should be discontinued several days before the gradual withdrawal of clonidine hydrochloride.

Perioperative Use Administration of clonidine hydrochloride should be continued to within four hours of surgery and resumed as soon as possible thereafter. The blood pressure should be carefully monitored and appropriate measures instituted to control it as necessary.

Information for Patients Patients who engage in potentially hazardous activities, such as operating machinery or driving, should be advised of a potential sedative effect of clonidine. Patients should be cautioned against interruption of clonidine hydrochloride therapy without a physician's advice.

Drug Interactions If a patient receiving clonidine hydrochloride is also taking tricyclic antidepressants, the effect of clonidine may be reduced, thus necessitating an increase in dosage. Clonidine hydrochloride may enhance the CNS-depressive effects of alcohol, barbiturates or other sedatives. Amitriptyline in combination with clonidine enhances the manifestation of corneal lesions in rats (see OCULAR TOXICITY).

OCULAR TOXICITY

In several studies, oral clonidine hydrochloride produced a dose-dependent increase in the incidence and severity of spontaneously occurring retinal degeneration in albino rats treated for six months or longer. Tissue distribution studies in dogs and monkeys revealed that clonidine hydrochloride was concentrated in the choroid of the eye. In view of the retinal degeneration observed in rats, eye examinations were performed in 908 patients prior to the start of clonidine hydrochloride therapy, who were then examined periodically thereafter. In 353 of these 908 patients, examinations were performed for periods of 24 months or longer. Except for some dryness of the eyes, no drug-related abnormal ophthalmologic findings were recorded and clonidine hydrochloride did not alter retinal function as shown by specialized tests such as the electroretinogram and macular dazzle.

In rats, clonidine hydrochloride in combination with amitriptyline produced corneal lesions within 5 days.

Carcinogenesis, Mutagenesis, Impairment of Fertility In a 132-week (fixed concentration) dietary administration study in rats, clonidine hydrochloride administered at 32 to 46 times the maximum recommended daily human oral dose was unassociated with evidence of carcinogenic potential.

Fertility of male or female rats was unaffected by clonidine hydrochloride doses as high as 150 mcg/kg or about 3 times the maximum recommended daily human oral dose (MRDHD). Fertility of female rats did, however, appear to be affected (in another experiment) at dose levels of 500 to 2000 mcg/kg or 10 to 40 times the MRDHD.

Usage in Pregnancy

TERATOGENIC EFFECTS Pregnancy Category C. Reproduction studies performed in rabbits at doses up to approximately 3 times the maximum recommended daily human dose (MRDHD) of clonidine hydrochloride have revealed no evidence of teratogenic or embryotoxic potential. In rats however, doses as low as $^1/_3$ the MRDHD were associated with increased resorptions in a study in which dams were treated continuously from 2 months prior to mating. Increased resorptions were not associated with treatment at the same or at higher dose levels (up to 3 times the MRDHD) when dams were treated days 6–15 of gestation. Increased resorptions were observed at much higher levels (40 times the MRDHD) in rats and mice treated days 1–14 of gestation (lowest dose employed in that study was 500 mcg/kg). There are, however, no adequate and well-controlled studies in pregnant women. Because animal reproduction studies are not always predictive of human response, this drug should be used during pregnancy only if clearly needed.

Nursing Mothers As clonidine hydrochloride is excreted in human milk, caution should be exercised when it is administered to a nursing woman.

Pediatric Use Safety and effectiveness in the pediatric population have not been established.

Chlorthalidone: **General**

Hypokalemia and other electrolyte abnormalities, including hyponatremia and hypochloremic alkalosis, are common in patients receiving chlorthalidone. These abnormalities are dose-related but may occur even at the lowest marketed doses of chlorthalidone. Serum electrolytes should be determined before initiating therapy and at periodic intervals during therapy. Serum and urine electrolyte determinations are particularly important when the patient is vomiting excessively or receiving parenteral fluids. All patients taking chlorthalidone should be observed for clinical signs of electrolyte imbalance, including dryness of mouth, thirst, weakness, lethargy, drowsiness, restlessness, muscle pains or cramps, muscular fatigue, hypotension, oliguria, tachycardia, palpitations and gastrointestinal disturbances, such as nausea and vomiting. Digitalis therapy may exaggerate metabolic effects of hypokalemia especially with reference to myocardial activity.

Any chloride deficit is generally mild and usually does not require specific treatment except under extraordinary circumstances (as in liver disease or renal disease). Dilutional hyponatremia may occur in edematous patients in hot weather: appropriate therapy is water restriction, rather than administration of salt, except in rare instances when the hyponatremia is life-threatening. In cases of actual salt depletion, appropriate replacement is the therapy of choice.

Uric Acid Hyperuricemia may occur or frank gout may be precipitated in certain patients receiving chlorthalidone.

Other Increases in serum glucose may occur and latent diabetes mellitus may become manifest during chlorthalidone therapy (see PRECAUTIONS Drug Interactions). Chlorthalidone and related drugs may decrease serum PBI levels without signs of thyroid disturbance.

Information for Patients Patients should inform their doctor if they have: 1) had an allergic reaction to chlorthalidone or other diuretics or have asthma 2) kidney disease 3) liver disease 4) gout 5) systemic lupus erythematosus, or 6) been taking other drugs such as cortisone, digitalis, lithium carbonate, or drugs for diabetes.

Patients should be cautioned to contact their physician if they experience any of the following symptoms of potassium loss: excess thirst, tiredness, drowsiness, restlessness, muscle pains or cramps, nausea, vomiting or increased heart rate or pulse.

Patients should also be cautioned that taking alcohol can increase the chance of dizziness occurring.

Laboratory Tests Periodic determination of serum electrolytes to detect possible electrolyte imbalance should be performed at appropriate intervals.

All patients receiving chlorthalidone should be observed for clinical signs of fluid or electrolyte imbalance: namely, hyponatremia, hypochloremic alkalosis and hypokalemia. Serum and urine electrolyte determinations are particularly important when the patient is vomiting excessively or receiving parenteral fluids.

Drug Interactions Chlorthalidone may add to or potentiate the action of other antihypertensive drugs. Insulin requirements in diabetic patients may be increased, decreased or unchanged. Higher dosage of oral hypoglycemic agents may be required. Chlorthalidone and related drugs may increase the responsiveness to tubocurarine. Chlorthalidone and related drugs may decrease arterial responsiveness to norepinephrine. This diminution is not sufficient to preclude effectiveness of the pressor agent for therapeutic use. Lithium renal clearance is reduced by chlorthalidone, increasing the risk of lithium toxicity.

Drug/Laboratory Test Interactions Chlorthalidone and related drugs may decrease serum PBI levels without signs of thyroid disturbance.

Carcinogenesis, Mutagenesis, Impairment of Fertility No information is available.

Usage in Pregnancy

TERATOGENIC EFFECTS Pregnancy Category B. Reproduction studies have been performed in the rat and the rabbit at doses up to 420 times the human dose and have revealed no evidence of harm to the fetus due to chlorthalidone. There are, however, no adequate and well-controlled studies in pregnant women. Because animal reproduction studies are not always predictive of human response, this drug should be used during pregnancy only if clearly needed.

NON-TERATOGENIC EFFECTS Thiazides cross the placental barrier and appear in cord blood. The use of chlorthalidone and related drugs in pregnant women requires that the anticipated benefits of the drug be weighed against possible hazards to the fetus. These hazards include fetal or neonatal jaundice, thrombocytopenia, and possibly other adverse reactions that have occurred in the adult.

Nursing Mothers Thiazides are excreted in human milk. Because of the potential for serious adverse reactions in nursing infants from chlorthalidone, a decision should be made whether to discontinue nursing or to discontinue the drug, taking into account the importance of the drug to the mother.

Pediatric Use Safety and effectiveness in the pediatric population have not been established.

ADVERSE REACTIONS

Combipres® is generally well tolerated. Most adverse effects are mild and tend to diminish with continued therapy. The most frequent (which appear to be dose-related) are dry mouth, occurring in about 40 to 100 patients; drowsiness, about 33 in 100; dizziness, about 16 in 100; constipation and sedation, each about 10 in 100.

In addition to the reactions listed above, certain less frequent adverse experiences, which are shown below, have also been reported in patients receiving the component drugs of Combipres® but in many cases patients were receiving concomitant medication and a causal relationship has not been established:

Clonidine hydrochloride:

Gastrointestinal Nausea and vomiting, about 5 in 100 patients; anorexia and malaise, each about 1 in 100; mild transient abnormalities in liver function tests, about 1 in 100; rare reports of hepatitis; parotitis, rarely.

Metabolic Weight gain, about 1 in 100 patients; gynecomastia, about 1 in 1000, transient elevation of blood glucose or serum creatine phosphokinase, rarely.

Central Nervous System Nervousness and agitation, about 3 in 100 patients; mental depression, about 1 in 100; headache, about 1 in 100; insomnia, about 5 in 1000. Vivid dreams or nightmares, other behavioral changes, restlessness, anxiety, visual and auditory hallucinations and delirium have been reported.

Cardiovascular Orthostatic symptoms, about 3 in 100 patients; palpitations and tachycardia, and bradycardia, each about 5 in 1000. Raynaud's phenomenon, congestive heart failure, and electrocardiographic abnormalities i.e. conduction disturbances and arrhythmias have been reported rarely. Rare cases of sinus bradycardia and atrioventricular block have been reported, both with and without the use of concomitant digitalis.

Dermatological Rash, about 1 in 100 patients; pruritus, about 7 in 1000; hives, angioneurotic edema and urticaria, about 5 in 1000, alopecia, about 2 in 1000.

Genitourinary Decreased sexual activity, impotence and loss of libido, about 3 in 100 patients; nocturia, about 1 in 100; difficulty in micturition, about 2 in 1000; urinary retention, about 1 in 1000.

Other Weakness, about 10 in 100 patients; fatigue, about 4 in 100; discontinuation syndrome, about 1 in 100; muscle or joint pain, about 6 in 1000 and cramps of the lower limbs, about 3 in 1000. Dryness, burning of the eyes, blurred vision, dryness of the nasal mucosa, pallor, weakly positive Coombs' test, increased sensitivity to alcohol and fever have been reported.

Chlorthalidone:

Gastrointestinal: Anorexia, gastric irritation, nausea, vomiting, cramping, diarrhea, constipation, jaundice (intrahepatic cholestatic jaundice), pancreatitis.

Central Nervous System: Dizziness, vertigo, paresthesias, headache, xanthopsia.

Hematologic: Leukopenia, agranulocytosis, thrombocytopenia, aplastic anemia.

Dermatologic-Hypersensitivity: Purpura, photosensitivity, rash, urticaria, necrotizing angiitis (vasculitis) (cutaneous vasculitis), Lyell's syndrome (toxic epidermal necrolysis).

Cardiovascular: Orthostatic hypotension may occur and may be aggravated by alcohol, barbiturates or narcotics.

Other adverse reactions: Hyperglycemia, glycosuria, hyperuricemia, muscle spasm, weakness, restlessness, impotence. Whenever adverse reactions are moderate or severe, chlorthalidone dosage should be reduced or therapy withdrawn.

OVERDOSAGE

Clonidine hydrochloride:

The signs and symptoms of clonidine hydrochloride overdosage include hypotension, bradycardia, lethargy, irritability, weakness, somnolence, diminished or absent reflexes, miosis, vomiting and hypoventilation. With large overdoses, reversible cardiac conduction defects or arrhythmias, apnea, seizures and transient hypertension have been reported. The oral LD_{50} of clonidine in rats was 465 mg/kg, and in mice 206 mg/kg.

The general treatment of clonidine hydrochloride overdosage may include intravenous fluids as indicated. Bradycardia can be treated with intravenous atropine sulfate and hypotension with dopamine infusion in addition to intravenous fluids. Hypertension, associated with overdosage, has been treated with intravenous furosemide or diazoxide or alpha-blocking agents such as phentolamine. Tolazoline, an alpha-blocker, in intravenous doses of 10 mg at 30-minute intervals, may reverse clonidine's effects if other efforts fail. Routine hemodialysis is of limited benefit, since a maximum of 5% of circulating clonidine is removed.

In a patient who ingested 100 mg clonidine hydrochloride, plasma clonidine levels were 60 ng/ml (one hour), 190 ng/ml (1.5 hours), 370 ng/ml (two hours) and 120 ng/ml (5.5 and 6.5 hours). This patient developed hypertension followed by hypotension, bradycardia, apnea, hallucinations, semicoma, and premature ventricular contractions. The patient fully recovered after intensive treatment.

Chlorthalidone:

Symptoms of acute overdosage include nausea, weakness, dizziness and disturbances of electrolyte balance. The oral LD_{50} of the drug in the mouse and the rat is more than 25,000 mg/kg body weight. The minimum lethal dose (MLD) in humans has not been established. There is no specific antidote but gastric lavage is recommended, followed by supportive treatment. Where necessary, this may include intravenous dextrose-saline with potassium, administered with caution.

DOSAGE AND ADMINISTRATION

The dosage must be determined by individual titration. (See INDICATIONS AND USAGE.)

Chlorthalidone is usually initiated at a dose of 25 mg once daily and may be increased to 50 mg if the response is insufficient after a suitable trial.

Clonidine hydrochloride is usually initiated at a dose of 0.1 mg twice daily. Elderly patients may benefit from a lower initial dose. Further increments of 0.1 mg/day may be made if necessary until the desired response is achieved. The therapeutic doses most commonly employed have ranged from 0.2 to 0.6 mg per day in divided doses.

One Combipres® (clonidine hydrochloride/chlorthalidone) Tablet administered once or twice daily can be used to administer a minimum of 0.1 mg clonidine hydrochloride and 15 mg chlorthalidone to a maximum of 0.6 mg clonidine hydrochloride and 30 mg chlorthalidone.

HOW SUPPLIED

Combipres® 0.1/15 mg (each tablet contains clonidine hydrochloride USP, 0.1 mg + chlorthalidone USP, 15 mg) tablets are pink, oval shaped and single scored with the marking Bl 8. Available in bottles of 100 (NDC 0597-0008-01) and 1000 (NDC 0597-0008-10).

Combipres® 0.2/15 mg (each tablet contains clonidine hydrochloride USP 0.2 mg +chlorthalidone USP, 15 mg) tablets are blue, oval shaped and single scored with the marking Bl 9. Available in bottles of 100 (NDC 0597-0009-01) and 1000 (NDC 0597-0009-10).

Combipres® 0.3/15 mg (each tablet contains clonidine hydrochloride USP, 0.3 mg + chlorthalidone USP, 15 mg) tablets are white, oval shaped and single scored with the marking Bl 10. Available in bottles of 100 (NDC 0597-0010-01).

Store below 86°F (30°C). Avoid excessive humidity.

Dispense in tight, light-resistant container.

Caution: Federal law prohibits dispensing without prescription.

CM-PI-2/95 Rev.

Boehringer Ingelheim Pharmaceuticals, Inc.
Ridgefield, CT 06877
Licensed from Boehringer Ingelheim International GmbH

Shown in Product Identification Guide, page 309

Continued on next page

COMBIVENT® ℞

[*cŏmbĕvant*]
(ipratropium bromide and albuterol sulfate)
Inhalation Aerosol
Bronchodilator Aerosol
For Oral Inhalation Only
Prescribing Information

DESCRIPTION

Combivent® Inhalation Aerosol is a combination of ipratropium bromide and albuterol sulfate. Ipratropium bromide is an anticholinergic bronchodilator chemically described as 8-azoniabicyclo[3.2.1]octane, 3-(3-hydroxy-1-oxo-2-phenylpropoxy)-8-methyl- 8-(1-methylethyl)-, bromide, monohydrate *(endo,syn)*-,(±): a synthetic quaternary ammonium compound chemically related to atropine. Ipratropium bromide is a white to off-white crystalline substance, freely soluble in water and lower alcohols but insoluble in lipophilic solvents such as ether, chloroform and fluorocarbons. The structural formula is:

$C_{20}H_{30}BrNO_3 \cdot H_2O$ ipratropium bromide Mol. Wt. 430.4

Albuterol sulfate, chemically known as (1,3-benzenedimethanol, α'-[[(1,1-dimethylethyl) amino] methyl]-4-hydroxy, sulfate (2:1)(salt), (±)- is a relatively selective beta$_2$-adrenergic bronchodilator. Albuterol is the official generic name in the United States. The World Health Organization recommended name for the drug is salbutamol. Albuterol sulfate is a white to off-white crystalline powder, soluble in water and slightly soluble in ethanol. The structural formula is:

$(C_{13}H_{21}NO_3)_2 \cdot H_2SO_4$ albuterol sulfate Mol. Wt. 576.7

Combivent® Inhalation Aerosol contains a microcrystalline suspension of ipratropium bromide and albuterol sulfate in a pressurized metered-dose aerosol unit for oral inhalation administration. The 200 inhalation unit has a net weight of 14.7 grams. Each actuation meters 21 mcg of ipratropium bromide and 120 mcg of albuterol sulfate from the valve and delivers 18 mcg of ipratropium bromide and 103 mcg of albuterol sulfate (equivalent to 90 mcg albuterol base) from the mouthpiece. The excipients are dichlorodifluoromethane, dichlorotetrafluoroethane, and trichloromonofluoromethane as propellants and soya lecithin.

CLINICAL PHARMACOLOGY

Combivent® Inhalation Aerosol is a combination of the anticholinergic bronchodilator, ipratropium bromide, and the beta$_2$-adrenergic bronchodilator, albuterol sulfate.

Ipratropium Bromide:

Mechanism of Action

Ipratropium bromide is an anticholinergic (parasympatholytic) agent which, based on animal studies, appears to inhibit vagally mediated reflexes by antagonizing the action of acetylcholine, the transmitter agent released from the vagus nerve. Anticholinergics prevent the increases in intracellular concentration of cyclic guanosine monophosphate (cyclic GMP) which are caused by interaction of acetylcholine with the muscarinic receptor on bronchial smooth muscle.

Pharmacokinetics

The bronchodilation following inhalation of ipratropium bromide is primarily a local, site-specific effect, not a systemic one. Much of an administered dose is swallowed as shown by fecal excretion studies. Ipratropium bromide is a quaternary amine. It is not readily absorbed into the systemic circulation either from the surface of the lung or from the gastrointestinal tract as confirmed by blood level and renal excretion studies. Plasma levels of ipratropium bromide were below the assay sensitivity limit of 100 pg/mL.

The half-life of elimination is about 2 hours after inhalation or intravenous administration. Ipratropium bromide is minimally bound (0 to 9% *in vitro*) to plasma albumin and α$_1$-acid glycoprotein. It is partially metabolized to inactive ester hydrolysis products. Following intravenous administration, approximately one-half of the dose is excreted unchanged in the urine. Studies in rats have shown that ipratropium bromide does not penetrate the blood-brain barrier. The pharmacokinetics of Combivent® Inhalation Aerosol or ipratropium bromide have not been studied in patients with hepatic or renal insufficiency or in the elderly (See PRECAUTIONS).

Controlled clinical studies have demonstrated that ipratropium bromide does not alter either mucociliary clearance or the volume or viscosity of respiratory secretions. In studies without a positive control, ipratropium bromide did not alter pupil size, accommodation or visual acuity (See ADVERSE REACTIONS).

Ventilation/perfusion studies have shown no clinically significant effects on pulmonary gas exchange or arterial oxygen tension. At recommended doses, ipratropium bromide does not produce clinically significant changes in pulse rate or blood pressure.

Albuterol Sulfate:

Mechanism of Action

In-vitro studies and *in-vivo* pharmacologic studies have demonstrated that albuterol has a preferential effect on beta$_2$-adrenergic receptors compared with isoproterenol. While it is recognized that beta$_2$-adrenergic receptors are the predominant receptors on bronchial smooth muscle, recent data indicate that there is a population of beta$_2$-receptors in the human heart which comprise between 10% and 50% of cardiac beta-adrenergic receptors. The precise function of these receptors, however, is not yet established (See WARNINGS).

Activation of beta$_2$-adrenergic receptors on airway smooth muscle leads to the activation of adenylyl cyclase and to an increase in the intracellular concentration of cyclic-3',5'-adenosine monophosphate (cyclic AMP). This increase of cyclic AMP leads to the activation of protein kinase A, which inhibits the phosphorylation of myosin and lowers intracellular ionic calcium concentrations, resulting in relaxation. Albuterol relaxes the smooth muscles of all airways, from the trachea to the terminal bronchioles. Albuterol acts as a functional antagonist to relax the airway irrespective of the spasmogen involved, thus protecting against all bronchoconstrictor challenges. Increased cyclic AMP concentrations are also associated with the inhibition of release of mediators from mast cells in the airway.

Albuterol has been shown in most clinical trials to have more bronchial smooth muscle relaxation effect than isoproterenol at comparable doses while producing fewer cardiovascular effects. However, all beta-adrenergic drugs, including albuterol sulfate, can produce a significant cardiovascular effect in some patients (See PRECAUTIONS).

Pharmacokinetics

Albuterol is longer acting than isoproterenol in most patients because it is not a substrate for the cellular uptake processes for catecholamines nor for metabolism by catechol-O-methyl transferase. Instead, the drug is conjugatively metabolized to albuterol 4'-O-sulfate.

In a pharmacokinetic study in 12 healthy male volunteers of two inhalations of albuterol sulfate, 103 mcg dose/inhalation through the mouthpiece, peak plasma albuterol concentrations ranging from 419 to 802 pg/mL (mean 599 ± 122 pg/mL) were obtained within three hours post-administration. Following this single-dose administration, 30.8 ± 10.2% of the estimated mouthpiece dose was excreted unchanged in the 24 hour urine. Since albuterol sulfate is rapidly and completely absorbed, this study could not distinguish between pulmonary and gastrointestinal absorption. Intravenous pharmacokinetics of albuterol were studied in a comparable group of 16 healthy male volunteers; the mean terminal half-life following a 30-minute infusion of 1.5 mg was 3.9 hours with a mean clearance of 439 mL/min/1.73 m^2.

Intravenous albuterol studies in rats demonstrated that albuterol crossed the blood-brain barrier and reached brain concentrations amounting to about 5% of the plasma concentrations. In structures outside the blood-brain barrier (pineal and pituitary glands), the drug achieved concentrations more than 100 times those in whole brain.

Studies in pregnant rats with tritiated albuterol demonstrated that approximately 10% of the circulating maternal drug was transferred to the fetus. Disposition in fetal lungs was comparable to maternal lungs, but fetal liver disposition was 1% of maternal liver levels.

Studies in laboratory animals (minipigs, rodents, and dogs) have demonstrated the occurrence of cardiac arrhythmias and sudden death (with histologic evidence of myocardial necrosis) when beta-agonists and methylxanthines were administered concurrently. The significance of these findings when applied to humans is unknown.

Combivent® Inhalation Aerosol:

Mechanism of Action

Combivent® Inhalation Aerosol is expected to maximize the response to treatment in patients with chronic obstructive pulmonary disease (COPD) by reducing bronchospasm through two distinctly different mechanisms, anticholinergic (parasympatholytic) and sympathomimetic. Simultaneous administration of both an anticholinergic (ipratropium bromide) and a beta$_2$-sympathomimetic (albuterol sulfate) is designed to benefit the patient by producing a greater bronchodilator effect than when either drug is utilized alone at its recommended dosage.

Pharmacokinetics

In a crossover pharmacokinetic study in 12 healthy male volunteers comparing the pattern of absorption and excretion of two inhalations of Combivent® Inhalation Aerosol to the two active components individually, the co-administration of ipratropium bromide and albuterol sulfate from a single canister did not significantly alter the systemic absorption of either component. Ipratropium bromide levels remained below detectable limits (<100 pg/mL). Peak albuterol level obtained within 3 hours post-administration was 492 ± 132 pg/mL. Following this single administration, 27.1 ± 5.7% of the estimated mouthpiece dose was excreted unchanged in the 24 hour urine. From a pharmacokinetic perspective, the synergistic efficacy of Combivent® Inhalation Aerosol is likely to be due to a local effect on the muscarinic and beta$_2$-adrenergic receptors in the lung.

Clinical Trials

In two 12-week randomized, double-blind, active-controlled clinical trials, 1067 patients with chronic obstructive pulmonary disease (COPD) were evaluated for the bronchodilator efficacy of Combivent® Inhalation Aerosol (358 patients) in comparison to its components, ipratropium bromide (362 patients) and albuterol sulfate (347 patients).

Serial FEV$_1$ measurements (shown below as a percent change from test-day baseline) demonstrated that Combivent® Inhalation Aerosol produced significantly greater improvement in pulmonary function than either ipratropium bromide or albuterol sulfate when given separately.

The median time to onset of a 15% increase in FEV$_1$ was 15 minutes and the median time to peak FEV$_1$ was one hour for Combivent® Inhalation Aerosol and its components. The median duration of effect as measured by FEV$_1$ was 4–5 hours for Combivent® Inhalation Aerosol compared to 4 hours for ipratropium bromide and 3 hours for albuterol sulfate.

Percent Change in Adjusted Mean[a] FEV$_1$ From Test-Day Baseline–Endpoint Analysis of the Evaluable Data Set

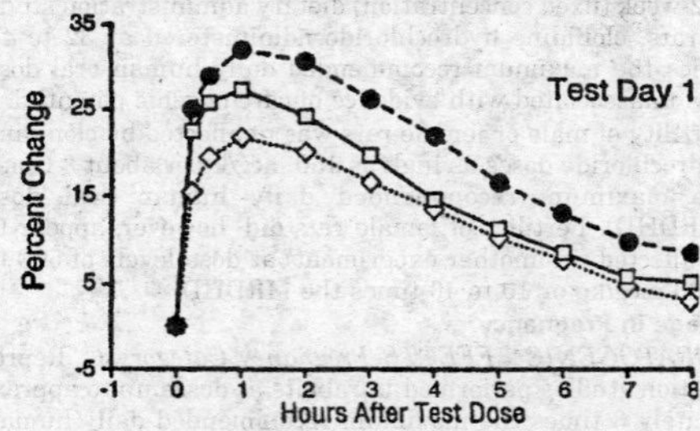

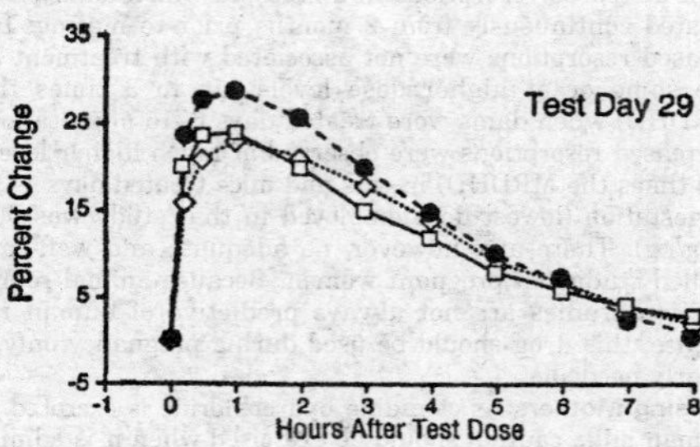

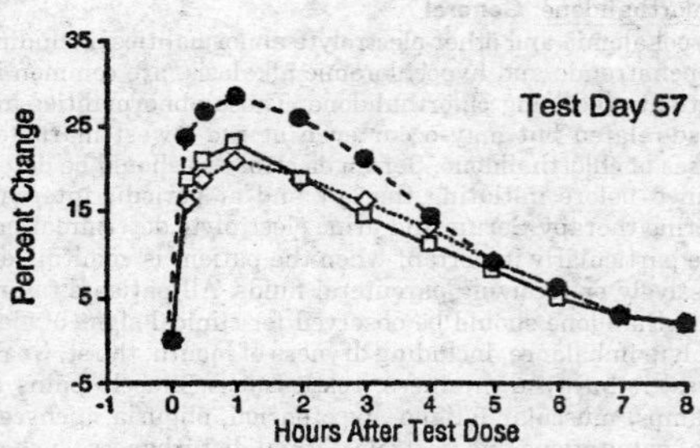

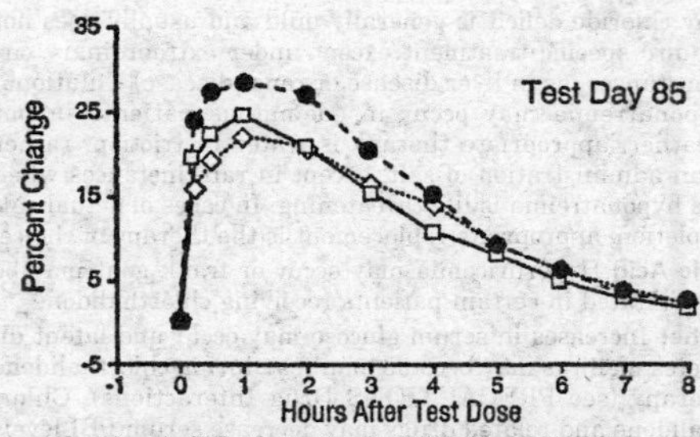

● Combivent (n=347) ◇ Ipratropium (n=355) □ Albuterol (n=331)
[a] Adjusted for test-day baseline FEV$_1$, center and treatment-by-center interaction

These studies demonstrated that each component of Combivent® Inhalation Aerosol contributed to the improvement in pulmonary function produced by the combination, especially during the first 4–5 hours after dosing, and that

Combivent® Inhalation Aerosol was significantly more effective than ipratropium bromide or albuterol sulfate administered alone.

In the two controlled twelve-week studies, Combivent® Inhalation Aerosol did not produce any change in the secondary efficacy parameters including symptom scores, physician global assessments and morning PEFR, all of which were monitored throughout the study period.

INDICATIONS AND USAGE

Combivent® Inhalation Aerosol is indicated for use in patients with chronic obstructive pulmonary disease (COPD) on a regular aerosol bronchodilator who continue to have evidence of bronchospasm and who require a second bronchodilator.

CONTRAINDICATIONS

Combivent® Inhalation Aerosol is contraindicated in patients with a history of hypersensitivity to soya lecithin or related food products such as soybean and peanut. Combivent® Inhalation Aerosol is also contraindicated in patients hypersensitive to any other components of the drug product or to atropine or its derivatives.

WARNINGS

1. Paradoxical Bronchospasm: Combivent® Inhalation Aerosol can produce paradoxical bronchospasm that can be life threatening. If it occurs, the preparation should be discontinued immediately and alternative therapy instituted. It should be recognized that paradoxical bronchospasm, when associated with inhaled formulations, frequently occurs with the first use of a new canister.

2. Cardiovascular Effect: The albuterol sulfate contained in Combivent® Inhalation Aerosol, like other beta-adrenergic agonists, can produce a clinically significant cardiovascular effect in some patients, as measured by pulse rate, blood pressure and/or symptoms. Although such effects are uncommon after administration of Combivent® Inhalation Aerosol at recommended doses, if they occur, discontinuation of the drug may be indicated. In addition, beta-adrenergic agents have been reported to produce ECG changes, such as flattening of the T wave, prolongation of the QTc interval, and ST segment depression. Therefore, Combivent® Inhalation Aerosol should be used with caution in patients with cardiovascular disorders, especially coronary insufficiency, cardiac arrhythmias and hypertension.

3. Do Not Exceed Recommended Dose: Fatalities have been reported in association with excessive use of inhaled sympathomimetic drugs, in patients with asthma. The exact cause of death is unknown, but cardiac arrest following an unexpected development of a severe acute asthmatic crisis and subsequent hypoxia is suspected.

4. Immediate Hypersensitivity Reactions: Immediate hypersensitivity reactions may occur after administration of ipratropium bromide or albuterol sulfate, as demonstrated by rare cases of urticaria, angioedema, rash, bronchospasm, anaphylaxis and oropharyngeal edema.

5. Storage Conditions: The contents of Combivent® Inhalation Aerosol are under pressure. Do not puncture. Do not use or store near heat or open flame. Exposure to temperatures above 120°F may cause bursting. Never throw the container into a fire or incinerator. Keep out of reach of children.

PRECAUTIONS

General

1. Effects Seen with Anticholinergic Drugs: Combivent® Inhalation Aerosol contains ipratropium bromide and, therefore, should be used with caution in patients with narrow-angle glaucoma, prostatic hypertrophy or bladder-neck obstruction.

2. Effects Seen with Sympathomimetic Drugs: Preparations containing sympathomimetic amines such as albuterol sulfate should be used with caution in patients with convulsive disorders, hyperthyroidism, or diabetes mellitus and in patients who are unusually responsive to sympathomimetic amines. Beta-adrenergic agents may also produce significant hypokalemia in some patients (possibly through intracellular shunting) which has the potential to produce adverse cardiovascular effects. The decrease in serum potassium is usually transient, not requiring supplementation.

3. Use in Hepatic or Renal Disease: Combivent® Inhalation Aerosol has not been studied in patients with hepatic or renal insufficiency. It should be used with caution in those patient populations.

Information for Patients

Patients should be cautioned to avoid spraying the aerosol into their eyes and be advised that this may result in precipitation or worsening of narrow-angle glaucoma, eye pain or discomfort, temporary blurring of vision, visual halos or colored images in association with red eyes from conjunctival and corneal congestion. Should any combination of these symptoms develop, consult your physician immediately.

The action of Combivent® Inhalation Aerosol should last 4–5 hours or longer. Combivent® Inhalation Aerosol should not be used more frequently than recommended. Do not increase the dose or frequency of Combivent® Inhalation Aerosol without consulting your physician. If you find that treatment with Combivent® Inhalation Aerosol becomes less effective for symptomatic relief, your symptoms become worse, and/or you need to use the product more frequently than usual, medical attention should be sought immediately. While you are taking Combivent® Inhalation Aerosol, other inhaled drugs should be taken only as directed by your physician. If you are pregnant or nursing, contact your physician about use of Combivent® Inhalation Aerosol. Appropriate use of Combivent® Inhalation Aerosol includes an understanding of the way it should be administered (See Patient's Instructions for Use).

Drug Interactions

Combivent® Inhalation Aerosol has been used concomitantly with other drugs, including sympathomimetic bronchodilators, methylxanthines and steroids, commonly used in the treatment of COPD, without adverse drug reactions. No formal drug interaction studies have been performed with Combivent® Inhalation Aerosol and these or other medications commonly used in the treatment of COPD.

Anticholinergic agents: Although ipratropium bromide is minimally absorbed into the systemic circulation, there is some potential for an additive interaction with concomitantly used anticholinergic medications. Caution is therefore advised in the co-administration of Combivent® Inhalation Aerosol with other anticholinergic-containing drugs.

Beta-adrenergic agents: Caution is advised in the co-administration of Combivent® Inhalation Aerosol and other sympathomimetic agents due to the increased risk of adverse cardiovascular effects.

Beta-receptor blocking agents and albuterol inhibit the effect of each other. Beta-receptor blocking agents should be used with caution in patients with hyperreactive airways.

Diuretics: The ECG changes and/or hypokalemia which may result from the administration of non-potassium sparing diuretics (such as loop or thiazide diuretics) can be acutely worsened by beta-agonists, especially when the recommended dose of the beta-agonist is exceeded. Although the clinical significance of these effects is not known, caution is advised in the co-administration of beta-agonist-containing drugs, such as Combivent® Inhalation Aerosol, with non-potassium sparing diuretics.

Monoamine oxidase inhibitors or tricyclic antidepressants: Combivent® Inhalation Aerosol should be administered with extreme caution to patients being treated with monoamine oxidase inhibitors or tricyclic antidepressants or within two weeks of discontinuation of such agents because the action of albuterol on the cardiovascular system may be potentiated.

Carcinogenesis, Mutagenesis, Impairment of Fertility

Ipratropium bromide: Two-year oral carcinogenicity studies in rats and mice have revealed no carcinogenic potential at doses up to 6 mg/kg/day. This dose corresponds to approximately 360 and 180 times the maximum recommended human daily inhalation dose in rats and mice respectively, on a mg/m^2 basis. Results of various mutagenicity studies (Ames test, mouse dominant lethal test, mouse micronucleus test and chromosome aberration of bone marrow in Chinese hamsters) were negative. Fertility of male or female rats at oral doses up to 50 mg/kg/day (approximately 3000 times the maximum recommended human daily inhalation dose on a mg/m^2 basis) was unaffected by ipratropium bromide administration. At doses above 90 mg/kg/day (approximately 5400 times the maximum recommended human daily inhalation dose on a mg/m^2 basis), increased resorption and decreased conception rates were observed.

Albuterol: Like other agents in its class, albuterol caused a significant dose-related increase in the incidence of benign leiomyomas of the mesovarium in a two-year study in the rat at dietary doses of 2, 10 and 50 mg/kg/day (approximately 20, 100 and 500 times the maximum recommended human daily inhalation dose on a mg/m^2 basis). In another study this effect was blocked by the co-administration of propranolol. The relevance of these findings to humans is not known. An 18-month study in mice at dietary doses up to 500 mg/kg/day (approximately 2500 times the maximum recommended human daily inhalation dose on a mg/m^2 basis) and a 99-week study in hamsters at oral doses up to 50 mg/kg/day (approximately 375 times the maximum recommended human daily inhalation dose on a mg/m^2 basis) revealed no evidence of tumorigenicity. Studies with albuterol revealed no evidence of mutagenesis. Reproduction studies in rats with albuterol sulfate revealed no evidence of impaired fertility.

Pregnancy

TERATOGENIC EFFECTS Pregnancy Category C.

Ipratropium bromide: *Pregnancy Category B.* Oral reproduction studies were performed at doses of 10 mg/kg in mice, 100 mg/kg in rats and 125 mg/kg in rabbits. These doses correspond, in each species, respectively, to approximately 300, 600 and 15,000 times the maximum recommended human daily inhalation dose on a mg/m^2 basis. Inhalation reproduction studies were conducted in rats and rabbits at doses of 1.5 and 1.8 mg/kg/day (approximately 90 and 210 times the maximum recommended human daily inhalation dose on a mg/m^2 basis). These studies have demonstrated no evidence of teratogenic effects as a result of ipratropium bromide.

Albuterol: *Pregnancy Category C.* Albuterol has been shown to be teratogenic in mice. A reproduction study in CD-1 mice given albuterol subcutaneously (0.025, 0.25 and 2.5 mg/kg) showed cleft palate formation in 5 of 111 (4.5%) fetuses at 0.25 mg/kg (equivalent to the maximum recommended human daily inhalation dose on a mg/m^2 basis) and in 10 of 108 (9.3%) fetuses at 2.5 mg/kg (approximately 10 times the maximum recommended human daily inhalation dose on a mg/m^2 basis). None was observed at 0.025 mg/kg (approximately one-tenth the maximum recommended human daily inhalation dose). Cleft palate also occurred in 22 of 72 (30.5%) fetuses treated with 2.5 mg/kg isoproterenol (positive control). A reproduction study with oral albuterol in Stride Dutch rabbits revealed cranioschisis in 7 of 19 (37%) fetuses at 50 mg/kg (approximately 1000 times the maximum recommended human daily inhalation dose on a mg/m^2 basis).

There are, however, no adequate and well-controlled studies of Combivent® Inhalation Aerosol, ipratropium bromide or albuterol sulfate, in pregnant women. Because animal reproduction studies are not always predictive of human response, Combivent® Inhalation Aerosol should be used during pregnancy only if the potential benefit justifies the potential risk to the fetus.

Labor and Delivery

Because of the potential for beta-agonist interference with uterine contractility, use of Combivent® Inhalation Aerosol for the treatment of COPD during labor should be restricted to those patients in whom the benefits clearly outweigh the risk.

Nursing Mothers

It is not known whether the components of Combivent® Inhalation Aerosol are excreted in human milk.

Ipratropium bromide: Although lipid-insoluble quaternary bases pass into breast milk, it is unlikely that the active component ipratropium bromide, would reach the infant to an important extent, especially when taken by aerosol. However, because many drugs are excreted in human milk, caution should be exercised when Combivent® Inhalation Aerosol is administered to a nursing mother.

Albuterol: Because of the potential for tumorigenicity shown for albuterol in animal studies, a decision should be made whether to discontinue nursing or to discontinue the drug, taking into account the importance of the drug to the mother.

Pediatric Use

Safety and effectiveness of Combivent® Inhalation Aerosol in pediatric patients have not been established.

ADVERSE REACTIONS

Adverse reaction information concerning Combivent® Inhalation Aerosol is derived from two 12-week controlled clinical trials (N=358 for Combivent® Inhalation Aerosol).

[See table above]

All Adverse Events (in percentages), from Two Large Double-Blind, Parallel, 12-Week Studies of Patients with COPD*

	Combivent® Ipratropium Bromide 36 mcg/Albuterol Sulfate 206 mcg q.i.d. N=358	Ipratropium Bromide 36 mcg q.i.d. N=362	Albuterol Sulfate 206 mcg q.i.d. N=347
Body as A Whole— General Disorders			
Headache	5.6	3.9	6.6
Pain	2.5	1.9	1.2
Influenza	1.4	2.2	2.9
Chest Pain	0.3	1.4	2.9
Gastrointestinal System Disorders			
Nausea	2.0	2.5	2.6
Respiratory System Disorders (Lower)			
Bronchitis	12.3	12.4	17.9
Dyspnea	4.5	3.9	4.0
Coughing	4.2	2.8	2.6
Respiratory Disorders	2.5	1.7	2.3
Pneumonia	1.4	2.5	0.6
Bronchospasm	0.3	3.9	1.7
Respiratory System Disorders (Upper)			
Upper Resp. Tract Infection	10.9	12.7	13.0
Pharyngitis	2.2	3.3	2.3
Sinusitis	2.3	1.9	0.9
Rhinitis	1.1	2.5	2.3

* All adverse events, regardless of drug relationship, reported by two percent or more patients in one or more treatment group in the 12-week controlled clinical trials.

Continued on next page

Combivent—Cont.

Additional adverse reactions, reported in less than two percent of the patients in the Combivent® Inhalation Aerosol treatment group include edema, fatigue, hypertension, dizziness, nervousness, paresthesia, tremor, dysphonia, insomnia, diarrhea, dry mouth, dyspepsia, vomiting, arrhythmia, palpitation, tachycardia, arthralgia, angina, increased sputum, taste perversion, and urinary tract infection/dysuria.
Allergic-type reactions such as skin rash, angioedema of tongue, lips and face, urticaria (including giant urticaria), laryngospasm and anaphylactic reaction have been reported, with positive rechallenge in some cases. Many of these patients had a history of allergies to other drugs and/or foods including soybean (See CONTRAINDICATIONS).
Additional information derived from the published literature and post-marketing surveillance on the use of ipratropium or albuterol inhalation aerosol singly or in combination that is not included in the lists above includes: cases of precipitation or worsening of narrow-angle glaucoma, acute eye pain, blurred vision, nasal congestion, drying of secretions, mucosal ulcers, irritation from aerosol, paradoxical bronchospasm, wheezing, exacerbation of COPD symptoms, heartburn, drowsiness, CNS stimulation, coordination difficulty, weakness, itching, flushing, alopecia, hypotension, gastrointestinal distress, constipation, and urinary difficulties.

OVERDOSAGE

The effects of overdosage are expected to be related primarily to albuterol sulfate. Acute overdosage with ipratropium bromide is unlikely since ipratropium bromide is not well absorbed systemically after aerosol or oral administration. The oral median lethal dose of ipratropium bromide ranged between 1001 and 2010 mg/kg in mice (approximately 30,000 and 60,000 times the maximum recommended human daily inhalation dose on a mg/m^2 basis, respectively); between 1667 and 4000 mg/kg in rats (approximately 100,000 and 240,000 times the maximum recommended human daily inhalation dose, respectively, on a mg/m^2 basis); and between 400 and 1300 mg/kg (approximately 80,000 and 260,000 times the maximum recommended human daily inhalation dose, respectively, on a mg/m^2 basis) in dogs. Whereas the oral median lethal dose of albuterol sulfate in mice and rats was greater than 2,000 mg/kg (approximately 10,000 and 20,000 times the maximum recommended human daily inhalation dose, respectively, on a mg/m^2 basis), the inhalational median lethal dose could not be determined. Manifestations of overdosage with albuterol may include anginal pain, hypertension, hypokalemia, tachycardia with rates up to 200 beats per minute and exaggeration of the pharmacologic effects listed in ADVERSE REACTIONS. As with all sympathomimetic aerosol medications, cardiac arrest and even death may be associated with abuse. Dialysis is not appropriate treatment for overdosage of albuterol as an inhalation aerosol; the judicious use of a cardiovascular beta-receptor blocker, such as metoprolol tartrate may be indicated.

DOSAGE AND ADMINISTRATION

The dose of Combivent® Inhalation Aerosol is two inhalations four times a day. Patients may take additional inhalations as required; however, the total number of inhalations should not exceed 12 in 24 hours. Safety and efficacy of additional doses of Combivent® Inhalation Aerosol beyond 12 puffs/24 hours have not been studied. Also, safety and efficacy of extra doses of ipratropium or albuterol in addition to the recommended doses of Combivent® Inhalation Aerosol have not been studied. It is recommended to "test-spray" three times before using for the first time and in cases where the aerosol has not been used for more than 24 hours.

HOW SUPPLIED

Combivent® Inhalation Aerosol is supplied as a metered-dose inhaler with a white mouthpiece which has a clear, colorless sleeve and an orange protective cap. The Combivent® Inhalation Aerosol canister should be used with the Combivent® Inhalation Aerosol actuator only. The actuator should not be used with other aerosol medications. Each actuation meters 21 mcg of ipratropium bromide and 120 mcg of albuterol sulfate from the valve and delivers 18 mcg of ipratropium bromide and 103 mcg of albuterol sulfate (equivalent to 90 mcg albuterol base) from the mouthpiece. Each 14.7 gram canister provides sufficient medication for 200 inhalations (NDC 0597-0013-14).
The canister should be discarded after the labeled number of actuations have been used. The amount of medication in each actuation cannot be assured after this point.
Store between 59° F (15° C) and 86° F (30° C). Avoid excessive humidity. For optimal results, the canister should be at room temperature before using. Shake well before using.
Note: The indented statement below is required by the Federal government's Clean Air Act for all products containing or manufactured with chlorofluorocarbons (CFCs):

> **Warning:** Contains trichloromonofluoromethane (CFC-11), dichlorodifluoromethane (CFC-12) and dichlorotetrafluoroethane (CFC-114), substances which harm public health and the environment by destroying ozone in the upper atmosphere.

A notice similar to the above **Warning** has been placed in the information for the patient of this product under the Environmental Protection Agency's (EPA's) regulations. The patient's warning states that the patient should consult his or her physician if there are any questions about alternatives.

Rx only.

CB-PI-4046880 029(2/99)

Manufactured by: 3M Pharmaceuticals, St. Paul, MN 55144
Ipratropium bromide licensed from: Boehringer Ingelheim International GmbH

Shown in Product Identification Guide, page 309

FLOMAX® ℞

[flō-măx]
(tamsulosin hydrochloride)
Capsules
Prescribing Information

DESCRIPTION

Tamsulosin hydrochloride is an antagonist of alpha$_{1A}$ adrenoceptors in the prostate.
Tamsulosin HCl is (-)-(*R*)-5-[2-[[2-(0-ethoxyphenoxy) ethyl]amino]propyl]-2-methoxybenzenesulfonamide, monohydrochloride. Tamsulosin HCl occurs as white crystals that melt with decomposition at approximately 230°C. It is sparingly soluble in water and in methanol, slightly soluble in glacial acetic acid and in ethanol, and practically insoluble in ether.
The empirical formula of tamsulosin HCl is $C_{20}H_{28}N_2O_5S \bullet HCl$. The molecular weight of tamsulosin HCl is 444.98. Its structural formula is:

Each FLOMAX capsule for oral administration contains tamsulosin HCl 0.4 mg, and the following inactive ingredients: methacrylic acid copolymer, microcrystalline cellulose, triacetin, polysorbate 80, sodium lauryl sulfate, calcium stearate, talc, FD&C blue No. 2, titanium dioxide, ferric oxide, gelatin, and trace amounts of shellac, industrial methylated spirit 74 OP, *n*-butyl alcohol, isopropyl alcohol, propylene glycol, dimethylpolysiloxane, and black iron oxide E172.

CLINICAL PHARMACOLOGY

The symptoms associated with benign prostatic hyperplasia (BPH) are related to bladder outlet obstruction, which is comprised of two underlying components: static and dynamic. The static component is related to an increase in prostate size caused, in part, by a proliferation of smooth muscle cells in the prostatic stroma. However, the severity of BPH symptoms and the degree of urethral obstruction do not correlate well with the size of the prostate. The dynamic component is a function of an increase in smooth muscle tone in the prostate and bladder neck leading to constriction of the bladder outlet. Smooth muscle tone is mediated by the sympathetic nervous stimulation of alpha$_1$ adrenoceptors, which are abundant in the prostate, prostatic capsule, prostatic urethra, and bladder neck. Blockade of these adrenoceptors can cause smooth muscles in the bladder neck and prostate to relax, resulting in an improvement in urine flow rate and a reduction in symptoms of BPH.
Tamsulosin, an alpha$_1$ adrenoceptor blocking agent, exhibits selectivity for alpha$_1$ receptors in the human prostate. At least three discrete alpha$_1$-adrenoceptor subtypes have been identified: alpha$_{1A}$, alpha$_{1B}$ and alpha$_{1D}$; their distribution differs between human organs and tissue. Approximately 70% of the alpha$_1$-receptors in human prostate are of the alpha$_{1A}$ subtype.
FLOMAX capsules are not intended for use as an antihypertensive drug.
Pharmacokinetics The pharmacokinetics of tamsulosin HCl have been evaluated in adult healthy volunteers and patients with BPH after single and/or multiple administration with doses ranging from 0.1 mg to 1 mg.
Absorption: Absorption of tamsulosin HCl from FLOMAX capsules 0.4 mg is essentially complete (>90%) following oral administration under fasting conditions. Tamsulosin HCl exhibits linear kinetics following single and multiple dosing, with achievement of steady-state concentrations by the fifth day of once-a-day dosing.
Effect of Food: The time to maximum concentration (T_{max}) is reached by four to five hours under fasting conditions and by six to seven hours when FLOMAX capsules are administered with food. Taking FLOMAX capsules under fasted conditions results in a 30% increase in bioavailability (AUC) and 40% to 70% increase in peak concentrations (C_{max}) compared to fed conditions (Figure 1).

Figure 1: Mean Plasma Tamsulosin HCl Concentrations Following Single-Dose Administration of FLOMAX capsules 0.4 mg Under Fasted and Fed Conditions (n=8).

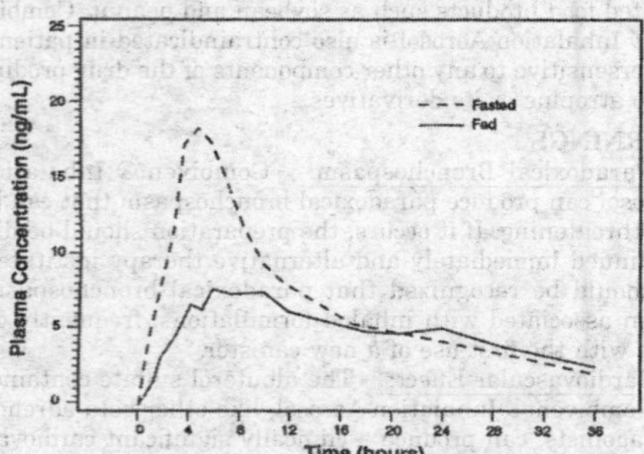

The effects of food on the pharmacokinetics of tamsulosin HCl are consistent regardless of whether a FLOMAX capsule is taken with a light breakfast or a high-fat breakfast (Table 1).
[See table 1 below]
Distribution: The mean steady-state apparent volume of distribution of tamsulosin HCl after intravenous administration to ten healthy male adults was 16L, which is suggestive of distribution into extracellular fluids in the body. Additionally, whole body autoradiographic studies in mice and rats and tissue distribution in rats and dogs indicate that tamsulosin HCl is widely distributed to most tissues including kidney, prostate, liver, gall bladder, heart, aorta, and brown fat, and minimally distributed to the brain, spinal cord, and testes. Tamsulosin HCl is extensively bound to human plasma proteins (94% to 99%), primarily alpha-1 acid glycoprotein (AAG), with linear binding over a wide concentration range (20 to 600 ng/mL). The results of two-way *in vitro* studies indicate that the binding of tamsulosin HCl to human plasma proteins is not affected by amitriptyline, diclofenac, glyburide, simvastatin plus simvastatin-hydroxy acid metabolite, warfarin, diazepam, propranolol, trichlormethiazide, or chlormadinone. Likewise, tamsulosin HCl had no effect on the extent of binding of these drugs.
Metabolism: There is no enantiomeric bioconversion from tamsulosin HCl [R(-) isomer] to the S(+) isomer in humans. Tamsulosin HCl is extensively metabolized by cytochrome P450 enzymes in the liver and less than 10% of the dose is excreted in urine unchanged. However, the pharmacokinetic profile of the metabolites in humans has not been established. Additionally, the cytochrome P450 enzymes that primarily catalyze the Phase I metabolism of tamsulosin HCl have not been conclusively identified. Therefore, possible interactions with other cytochrome P450 metabolized compounds cannot be discerned with current information. The metabolites of tamsulosin HCl undergo extensive conjugation to glucuronide or sulfate prior to renal excretion.
Incubations with human liver microsomes showed no evidence of clinically significant metabolic interactions between tamsulosin HCl and amitriptyline, albuterol (beta agonist), glyburide (glibenclamide) and finasteride (5alpha-

TABLE 1 Mean (± S.D.) Pharmacokinetic Parameters Following FLOMAX capsules 0.4 mg Once Daily or 0.8 mg Once Daily with a Light Breakfast, High-Fat Breakfast or Fasted

Pharmacokinetic Parameter	0.4 mg q.d. to healthy volunteers; n=23 (age range 18-32 years)		0.8 mg q.d. to healthy volunteers; n=22 (age range 55-75 years)		
	Light Breakfast	Fasted	Light Breakfast	High-Fat Breakfast	Fasted
Cmin (ng/mL)	4.0 ± 2.6	3.8 ± 2.5	12.3 ± 6.7	13.5 ± 7.6	13.3 ± 13.3
Cmax (ng/mL)	10.1 ± 4.8	17.1 ± 17.1	29.8 ± 10.3	29.1 ± 11.0	41.6 ± 15.6
Cmax/Cmin Ratio	3.1 ± 1.0	5.3 ± 2.2	2.7 ± 0.7	2.5 ± 0.8	3.6 ± 1.1
Tmax (hours)	6.0	4.0	7.0	6.6	5.0
T1/2 (hours)	–	–	–	–	14.9 ± 3.9
AUC$_\tau$ (ng•hr/mL)	151 ± 81.5	199 ± 94.1	440 ± 195	449 ± 217	557 ± 257

Cmin = observed minimum concentration
Cmax = observed maximum tamsulosin HCl plasma concentration
Tmax = median time-to-maximum concentration
T1/2 = observed half-life
AUC$_\tau$ = Area under the tamsulosin HCl plasma time curve over the dosing interval

reductase inhibitor for treatment of BPH). However, results of the *in vitro* testing of the tamsulosin HCl interaction with diclofenac and warfarin were equivocal.

Excretion: On administration of the radiolabeled dose of tamsulosin HCl to four healthy volunteers, 97% of the administered radioactivity was recovered, with urine (76%) representing the primary route of excretion compared to feces (21%) over 168 hours. Following intravenous or oral administration of an immediate-release formulation, the elimination half-life of tamsulosin HCl in plasma range from five to seven hours. Because of absorption rate-controlled pharmacokinetics with FLOMAX capsules, the apparent half-life of tamsulosin HCl is approximately 9 to 13 hours in healthy volunteers and 14 to 15 hours in the target population. Tamsulosin HCl undergoes restrictive clearance in humans, with a relatively low systemic clearance (2.88 L/h).

Special Populations: Geriatrics (Age): Cross-study comparison of FLOMAX capsules overall exposure (AUC) and half-life indicate that the pharmacokinetic disposition of tamsulosin HCl may be slightly prolonged in geriatric males compared to young, healthy male volunteers. Intrinsic clearance is independent of tamsulosin HCl binding to AAG, but diminishes with age, resulting in a 40% overall higher exposure (AUC) in subjects of age 55 to 75 years compared to subjects of age 20 to 32 years.

Renal Dysfunction: The pharmacokinetics of tamsulosin HCl have been compared in 6 subjects with mild – moderate ($30 \leq CL_{cr} < 70$ mL/min/1.73m^2) or moderate-severe ($10 \leq CL_{cr} < 30$ mL/min/1.73m^2) renal impairment and 6 normal subjects ($CL_{cr} < 90$ mL/min/1.73m^2). While a change in the overall plasma concentration of tamsulosin HCl was observed as the result of altered binding to AAG, the unbound (active) concentration of tamsulosin HCl, as well as the intrinsic clearance, remained relatively constant. Therefore, patients with renal impairment do not require an adjustment in FLOMAX capsules dosing. However, patients with endstage renal disease ($CL_{cr} < 10$ mL/min/1.73m^2) have not been studied.

Hepatic Dysfunction: The pharmacokinetics of tamsulosin HCl have been compared in 8 subjects with moderate hepatic dysfunction (Child-Pugh's classification: Grades A and B) and 8 normal subjects. While a change in the overall plasma concentration of tamsulosin HCl was observed as the result of altered binding to AAG, the unbound (active) concentration of tamsulosin HCl does not change significantly with only a modest (32%) change in intrinsic clearance of unbound tamsulosin HCl. Therefore, patients with moderate hepatic dysfunction do not require an adjustment in FLOMAX capsules dosage.

Drug-Drug Interactions: Nifedipine, Atenolol, Enalapril: In three studies in hypertensive subjects (age range 47–79 years) whose blood pressure was controlled with stable doses of Procardia XL®, atenolol, or enalapril for at least three months, FLOMAX capsules 0.4 mg for seven days followed by FLOMAX capsules 0.8 mg for another seven days (n=8 per study) resulted in no clinically significant effects on blood pressure and pulse rate compared to placebo (n=4 per study). Therefore, dosage adjustments are not necessary when FLOMAX capsules are administered concomitantly with Procardia XL®, atenolol, or enalapril.

Warfarin: A definitive drug-drug interaction study between tamsulosin HCl and warfarin was not conducted. Results from limited *in vitro* and *in vivo* studies are inconclusive. Therefore, caution should be exercised with concomitant administration of warfarin and FLOMAX capsules.

Digoxin and Theophylline: In two studies in healthy volunteers (n=10 per study; age range 19-39 years) receiving FLOMAX capsules 0.4 mg/day for two days, followed by FLOMAX capsules 0.8 mg/day for five to eight days, single intravenous doses of digoxin 0.5 mg or theophylline 5 mg/kg resulted in no change in the pharmacokinetics of digoxin or theophylline. Therefore, dosage adjustments are not necessary when a FLOMAX capsule is administered concomitantly with digoxin or theophylline.

Furosemide: The pharmacokinetic and pharmacodynamic interaction between FLOMAX capsules 0.8 mg/day (steady-state) and furosemide 20 mg intravenously (single dose) was evaluated in ten healthy volunteers (age range 21-40 years). FLOMAX capsules had no effect on the pharmacodynamics (excretion of electrolytes) of furosemide. While furosemide produced an 11% to 12% reduction in tamsulosin HCl Cmax and AUC, these changes are expected to be clinically insignificant and do not require adjustment of the FLOMAX capsules dosage.

Cimetidine: The effects of cimetidine at the highest recommended dose (400 mg every six hours for six days) on the pharmacokinetics of a single FLOMAX capsule 0.4 mg dose was investigated in ten healthy volunteers (age range 21-38 years). Treatment with cimetidine resulted in a significant decrease (26%) in the clearance of tamsulosin HCl which resulted in a moderate increase in tamsulosin HCl AUC (44%). Therefore, FLOMAX capsules should be used with caution in combination with cimetidine, particularly at doses higher than 0.4 mg.

Clinical Studies Four placebo-controlled clinical studies and one active-controlled clinical study enrolled a total of 2296 patients (1003 received FLOMAX capsules 0.4 mg once daily, 491 received FLOMAX capsules 0.8 mg once daily, and 802 were control patients) in the U.S. and Europe.

In the two U.S. placebo-controlled, double-blind, 13-week, multicenter studies [Study 1 (US92-03A) and Study 2 (US93-01)], 1486 men with the signs and symptoms of BPH were enrolled. In both studies, patients were randomized to either placebo, FLOMAX capsules 0.4 mg once daily, or FLOMAX capsules 0.8 mg once daily. Patients in FLOMAX capsules 0.8-mg once daily treatment groups received a dose of 0.4 mg once daily for one week before increasing to the 0.8-mg once daily dose. The primary efficacy assessments included: 1) total American Urological Association (AUA) Symptom Score questionnaire, which evaluated irritative (frequency, urgency, and nocturia), and obstructive (hesitancy, incomplete emptying, intermittency, and weak stream) symptoms, where a decrease in score is consistent with improvement in symptoms; and 2) peak urine flow rate, where an increased peak urine flow rate value over baseline is consistent with decreased urinary obstruction.

Mean changes from baseline to week 13 in total AUA Symptom Score were significantly greater for groups treated with FLOMAX capsules 0.4 mg and 0.8 mg once daily compared to placebo in both U.S. studies (Table 2, Figures 2A and 2B). The changes from baseline to week 13 in peak urine flow rate were also significantly greater for the FLOMAX capsules 0.4-mg and 0.8-mg once daily groups compared to placebo in Study 1, and for the FLOMAX capsules 0.8-mg once daily group in Study 2 (Table 2, Figures 3A and 3B). Overall there were no significant differences in improvement observed in total AUA Symptom Scores or peak urine flow rates between the 0.4-mg and the 0.8-mg dose groups with the exception that the 0.8-mg dose in Study 1 had a significantly greater improvement in total AUA Symptom Score compared to the 0.4-mg dose.

[See table 2 above]

TABLE 2 MEAN (± S.D.) CHANGES FROM BASELINE TO WEEK 13 IN TOTAL AUA SYMPTOM SCORE ** AND PEAK URINE FLOW RATE (ML/SEC)

	Total AUA Symptom Score		Peak Urine Flow Rate	
	Mean Baseline Value	Mean Change	Mean Baseline Value	Mean Change
Study 1 †				
FLOMAX capsules 0.8 mg once daily	19.9±4.9 n=247	−9.6*±6.7 n=237	9.57±2.51 n=247	1.78*±3.35 n=247
FLOMAX capsules 0.4 mg once daily	19.8±5.0 n=254	−8.3*±6.5 n=246	9.46±2.49 n=254	1.75*±3.57 n=254
Placebo	19.6±4.9 n=254	−5.5±6.6 n=246	9.75±2.54 n=254	0.52±3.39 n=253
Study 2 ‡				
FLOMAX capsules 0.8 mg once daily	18.2±5.6 n=244	−5.8*±6.4 n=238	9.96±3.16 n=244	1.79*±3.36 n=237
FLOMAX capsules 0.4 mg once daily	17.9±5.8 n=248	−5.1*±6.4 n=244	9.94±3.14 n=248	1.52±3.64 n=244
Placebo	19.2±6.0 n=239	−3.6±5.7 n=235	9.95±3.12 n=239	0.93±3.28 n=235

* Statistically significant difference from placebo (p-value ≤0.050; Bonferroni-Holm multiple test procedure);
**Total AUA Symptom Scores ranged from 0 to 35
† Peak urine flow rate measured 4 to 8 hours post dose at week 13
‡ Peak urine flow rate measured 24 to 27 hours post dose at week 13
Week 13: For patients not completing the 13 week study the last observation was carried forward.

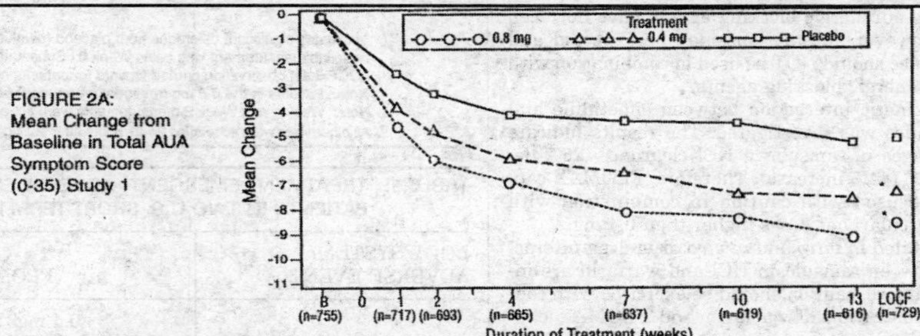

FIGURE 2A: Mean Change from Baseline in Total AUA Symptom Score (0-35) Study 1

* indicates significant difference from placebo (p-value ≤0.050).
B=Baseline determined approximately one week prior to the initial dose of double-blind medication at Week 0. Subsequent values are observed cases.
LOCF= Last observation carried forward for patients not completing the 13-week study.
Note: Patients in the 0.8 mg treatment group received 0.4 mg for the first week.
Note: Total AUA Symptom Scores range from 0 to 35.

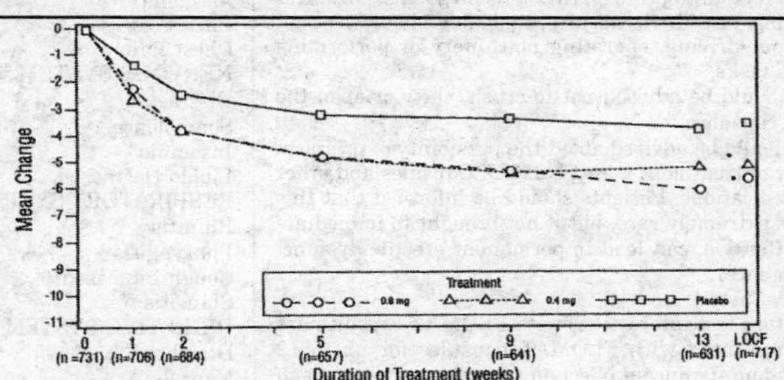

FIGURE 2B: Mean Change from Baseline in Total AUA Symptom Score (0-35) Study 2

* indicates significant difference from placebo (p-value ≤0.050).
Baseline measurement was taken Week 0. Subsequent values are observed cases.
LOCF= Last observation carried forward for patients not completing the 13-week study.
Note: Patients in the 0.8 mg treatment group received 0.4 mg for the first week.
Note: Total AUA Symptom Scores range from 0 to 35.

Mean total AUA Symptom Scores for both FLOMAX capsules 0.4-mg and 0.8-mg once daily groups showed a rapid decrease starting at one week after dosing and remained decreased through 13 weeks in both studies (Figures 2A and 2B).

In Study 1, 400 patients (53% of the originally randomized group) elected to continue in their originally assigned treatment groups in a double-blind, placebo controlled, 40 week extension trial (138 patients on 0.4 mg, 135 patients on 0.8 mg and 127 patients on placebo). Three hundred and twenty-three patients (43% of the originally randomized group) completed one year. Of these, 81% (97 patients) on 0.4 mg, 74% (75 patients) on 0.8 mg and 56% (57 patients) on placebo had a response ≥25% above baseline in total AUA Symptom Score at one year.

[See figures 2A & 2B above]

[See figures 3A & 3B at top of next page]

INDICATIONS AND USAGE

FLOMAX® (tamsulosin HCl) capsules are indicated for the treatment of the signs and symptoms of benign prostatic hyperplasia (BPH). FLOMAX capsules are not indicated for the treatment of hypertension.

Continued on next page

Flomax—Cont.

CONTRAINDICATIONS

FLOMAX capsules are contraindicated in patients known to be hypersensitive to tamsulosin HCl or any component of FLOMAX capsules.

WARNINGS

The signs and symptoms of orthostasis (postural hypotension, dizziness and vertigo) were detected more frequently in FLOMAX capsule treated patients than in placebo recipients. As with other alpha-adrenergic blocking agents there is a potential risk of syncope (see ADVERSE REACTIONS).

Patients beginning treatment with FLOMAX capsules should be cautioned to avoid situations where injury could result should syncope occur.

Rarely (probably less than one in fifty thousand patients), tamsulosin, like other alpha$_1$ antagonists, has been associated with priapism (persistent painful penile erection unrelated to sexual activity). Because this condition can lead to permanent impotence if not properly treated, patients must be advised about the seriousness of the condition (see Precautions: Information for Patients).

PRECAUTIONS

General

1) Carcinoma of the prostate: Carcinoma of the prostate and BPH cause many of the same symptoms. These two diseases frequently co-exist. Patients should be evaluated prior to the start of FLOMAX capsules therapy to rule out the presence of carcinoma of the prostate.

2) Drug-Drug Interactions: The pharmacokinetic and pharmacodynamic interactions between FLOMAX capsules and other alpha-adrenergic blocking agents have not been determined. However, interactions may be expected and FLOMAX capsules should NOT be used in combination with other alpha-adrenergic blocking agents.

The pharmacokinetic interaction between cimetidine and FLOMAX capsules was investigated. The results indicate significant changes in tamsulosin HCl clearance (26% decrease) and AUC (44% increase). Therefore, FLOMAX capsules should be used with caution in combination with cimetidine, particularly at doses higher than 0.4 mg.

Results from limited *in vitro* and *in vivo* drug-drug interaction studies between tamsulosin HCl and warfarin are inconclusive. Therefore, caution should be exercised with concomitant administration of warfarin and FLOMAX capsules.

(See also drug-drug interaction studies in CLINICAL PHARMACOLOGY, Pharmacokinetics subsection.)

Information for Patients (see Patient Package Insert)

Patients should be told about the possible occurrence of symptoms related to postural hypotension such as dizziness when taking FLOMAX capsules, and they should be cautioned about driving, operating machinery or performing hazardous tasks.

Patients should be advised not to crush, chew or open the FLOMAX capsules.

Patients should be advised about the possibility of priapism as a result of treatment with FLOMAX Capsules and other similar medications. Patients should be informed that this reaction is extremely rare, but if not brought to immediate medical attention, can lead to permanent erectile dysfunction (impotence).

Laboratory Tests

No laboratory test interactions with FLOMAX capsules are known. Treatment with FLOMAX capsules for up to 12 months had no significant effect on prostate-specific antigen (PSA).

Pregnancy Teratogenic Effects, Pregnancy Category B. Administration of tamsulosin HCl to pregnant female rats at dose levels up to 300 mg/kg/day (approximately 50 times the human therapeutic AUC exposure) revealed no evidence of harm to the fetus. Administration of tamsulosin HCl to pregnant rabbits at dose levels up to 50 mg/kg/day produced no evidence of fetal harm. FLOMAX capsules are not indicated for use in women.

Nursing Mothers FLOMAX capsules are not indicated for use in women.

Pediatric Use FLOMAX capsules are not indicated for use in pediatric populations.

Carcinogenesis, Mutagenesis, and Impairment of Fertility Rats administered doses up to 43 mg/kg/day in males and 52 mg/kg/day in females had no increases in tumor incidence with the exception of a modest increase in the frequency of mammary gland fibroadenomas in female rats receiving doses ≥ 5.4 mg/kg ($P < 0.015$). The highest doses of tamsulosin HCl evaluated in the rat carcinogenicity study produced systemic exposures (AUC) in rats 3 times the exposures in men receiving the maximum therapeutic dose of 0.8 mg/day.

Mice were administered doses up to 127 mg/kg/day in males and 158 mg/kg/day in females. There were no significant tumor findings in male mice. Female mice treated for 2 years with the two highest doses of 45 and 158 mg/kg/day had statistically significant increases in the incidence of mammary gland fibroadenomas ($P < 0.0001$) and adenocarcinomas ($P < 0.0075$). The highest dose levels of tamsulosin HCl evaluated in the mice carcinogenicity study produced systemic exposures (AUC) in mice 8 times the exposures in men receiving the maximum therapeutic dose of 0.8 mg/day.

The increased incidences of mammary gland neoplasms in female rats and mice were considered secondary to tamsulosin HCl-induced hyperprolactinemia. It is not known if FLOMAX capsules elevate prolactin in humans. The relevance for human risk of the findings of prolactin-mediated endocrine tumors in rodents is not known.

Tamsulosin HCl produced no evidence of mutagenic potential *in vitro* in the Ames reverse mutation test, mouse lymphoma thymidine kinase assay, unscheduled DNA repair synthesis assay, and chromosomal aberration assays in Chinese hamster ovary cells or human lymphocytes. There were no mutagenic effects in the *in vivo* sister chromatid exchange and mouse micronucleus assay.

Studies in rats revealed significantly reduced fertility in males dosed with single or multiple daily doses of 300 mg/kg/day of tamsulosin HCl (AUC exposure in rats about 50 times the human exposure with the maximum therapeutic dose). The mechanism of decreased fertility in male rats is considered to be an effect of the compound on the vaginal plug formation possibly due to changes of semen content or impairment of ejaculation. The effects on fertility were reversible showing improvement by 3 days after a single dose and 4 weeks after multiple dosing. Effects on fertility in males were completely reversed within nine weeks of discontinuation of multiple dosing. Multiple doses of 10 and 100 mg/kg/day tamsulosin HCl (1/5 and 16 times the anticipated human AUC exposure) did not significantly alter fertility in male rats. Effects of tamsulosin HCl on sperm counts or sperm function have not been evaluated. Studies in females rats revealed significant reductions in fertility after single or multiple dosing with 300 mg/kg/day of the R-isomer or racemic mixture of tamsulosin HCl, respectively. In female rats, the reductions in fertility after single doses were considered to be associated with impairments in fertilization. Multiple dosing with 10 or 100 mg/kg/day of the racemic mixture did not significantly alter fertility in female rats.

ADVERSE REACTIONS

The incidence of treatment-emergent adverse events has been ascertained from six short-term U.S. and European placebo-controlled clinical trials in which daily doses of 0.1 to 0.8 mg FLOMAX capsules were used. These studies evaluated safety in 1783 patients treated with FLOMAX capsules and 798 patients administered placebo. Table 3 sum-

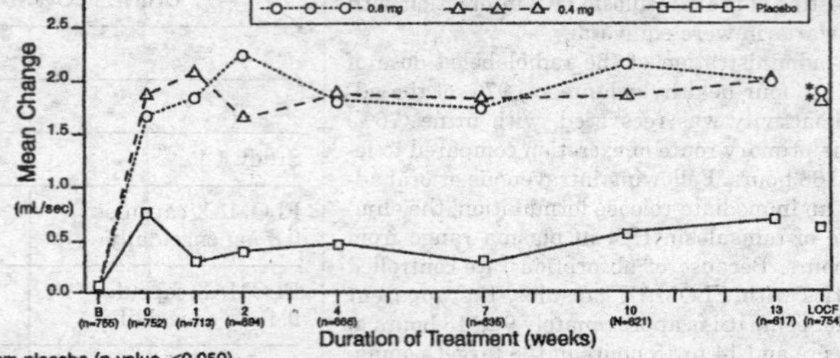

* indicates significant difference from placebo (p-value ≤0.050).
B=Baseline determined approximately one week prior to the initial dose of double-blind medication at Week 0. Subsequent values are observed cases.
LOCF= Last observation carried forward for patients not completing the 13-week study.
Note: The uroflowmetry assessments at week 0 were recorded 4-8 hours after patients received the first dose of double-blind medication. Measurements at each visit were scheduled 4-8 hours after dosing (approximately peak plasma tamsulosin concentration).
Note: Patients in the 0.8 mg treatment groups received 0.4 for the first week.

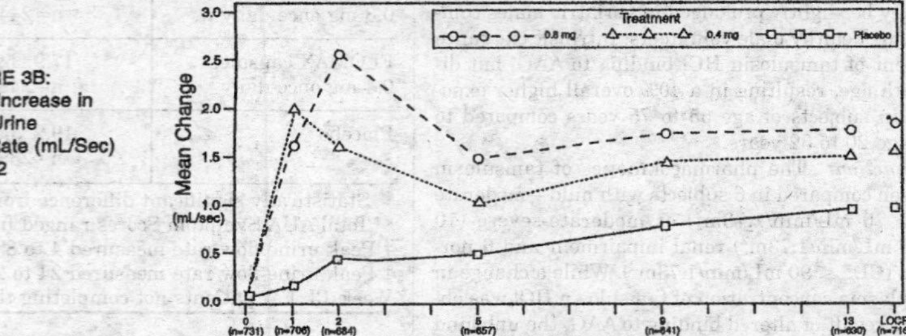

* indicates significant difference from placebo (p-value ≤0.050).
Baseline measurement was taken Week 0. Subsequent values are observed cases.
LOCF=Last observation carried forward for patients not completing the 13-week study.
Note: Patients in the 0.8 mg treatment group received 0.4 mg for the first week.
Note: Week 1 and Week 2 measurements were scheduled 4-8 hours after dosing (approximate peak plasma tamsulosin concentration).
All other visits were scheduled 24-27 hours after dosing (approximate trough tamsulosin concentration).

TABLE 3. TREATMENT EMERGENT[1] ADVERSE EVENTS OCCURRING IN ≥2% OF FLOMAX CAPSULES OR PLACEBO PATIENTS IN TWO U.S. SHORT-TERM PLACEBO-CONTROLLED CLINICAL STUDIES

BODY SYSTEM/ ADVERSE EVENT	FLOMAX CAPSULES GROUPS		PLACEBO
	0.4 mg n=502	0.8 mg n=492	n=493
BODY AS WHOLE			
Headache	97 (19.3%)	104 (21.1%)	99 (20.1%)
Infection	45 (9.0%)	53 (10.8%)	37 (7.5%)
Asthenia	39 (7.8%)	42 (8.5%)	27 (5.5%)
Back Pain	35 (7.0%)	41 (8.3%)	27 (5.5%)
Chest Pain	20 (4.0%)	20 (4.1%)	18 (3.7%)
NERVOUS SYSTEM			
Dizziness	75 (14.9%)	84 (17.1%)	50 (10.1%)
Somnolence	15 (3.0%)	21 (4.3%)	8 (1.6%)
Insomnia	12 (2.4%)	7 (1.4%)	3 (0.6%)
Libido Decreased	5 (1.0%)	10 (2.0%)	6 (1.2%)
RESPIRATORY SYSTEM			
Rhinitis	66 (13.1%)	88 (17.9%)	41 (8.3%)
Pharyngitis	29 (5.8%)	25 (5.1%)	23 (4.7%)
Cough Increased	17 (3.4%)	22 (4.5%)	12 (2.4%)
Sinusitis	11 (2.2%)	18 (3.7%)	8 (1.6%)
DIGESTIVE SYSTEM			
Diarrhea	31 (6.2%)	21 (4.3%)	22 (4.5%)
Nausea	13 (2.6%)	19 (3.9%)	16 (3.2%)
Tooth Disorder	6 (1.2%)	10 (2.0%)	7 (1.4%)
UROGENITAL SYSTEM			
Abnormal Ejaculation	42 (8.4%)	89 (18.1%)	1 (0.2%)
SPECIAL SENSES			
Amblyopia	1 (0.2%)	10 (2.0%)	2 (0.4%)

[1]A treatment-emergent adverse event was defined as any event satisfying one of the following criteria:
- The adverse event occurred for the first time after initial dosing with double-blind study medication.
- The adverse event was present prior to or at the time of initial dosing with double-blind study medication and subsequently increased in severity during double-blind treatment;

or
- The adverse event was present prior to or at the time of initial dosing with double-blind study medication, disappeared completely, and then reappeared during double-blind treatment.

marizes the treatment-emergent adverse events that occurred in ≥ 2% of patients receiving either FLOMAX capsules 0.4 mg, or 0.8 mg and at an incidence numerically higher than that in the placebo group during two 13-week U.S. trials (US92-03A and US93-01) conducted in 1487 men.

[See table 3 on previous page]

Signs and Symptoms of Orthostasis In the two U.S. studies, symptomatic postural hypotension was reported by 0.2% of patients (1 of 502) in the 0.4-mg group, 0.4% of patients (2 of 492) in the 0.8-mg group, and by no patients in the placebo group. Syncope was reported by 0.2% of patients (1 of 502) in the 0.4-mg group, 0.4% of patients (2 of 492) in the 0.8-mg group and 0.6% of patients (3 of 493) in the placebo group. Dizziness was reported by 15% of patients (75 of 502) in the 0.4-mg group, 17% of patients (84 of 492) in the 0.8-mg group, and 10% of patients (50 of 493) in the placebo group. Vertigo was reported by 0.6% of patients (3 of 502) in the 0.4-mg group, 1% of patients (5 of 492) in the 0.8 mg group and by 0.6% of patients (3 of 493) in the placebo group.

Multiple testing for orthostatic hypotension was conducted in a number of studies. Such a test was considered positive if it met one or more of the following criteria: (1) a decrease in systolic blood pressure of ≥20 mmHg upon standing from the supine position during the orthostatic tests; (2) a decrease in diastolic blood pressure ≥10mmHg upon standing, with the standing diastolic blood pressure <65 mmHg during the orthostatic test; (3) an increase in pulse rate of ≥20 bpm upon standing with a standing pulse rate ≥100 bpm during the orthostatic test; and (4) the presence of clinical symptoms (faintness, lightheadedness/lightheaded, dizziness, spinning sensation, vertigo, or postural hypotension) upon standing during the orthostatic test.

Following the first dose of double-blind medication in Study 1, a positive orthostatic test result at 4 hours post-dose was observed in 7% of patients (37 of 498) who received FLOMAX capsules 0.4 mg once daily and in 3% of the patients (8 of 253) who received placebo. At 8 hours post-dose, a positive orthostatic test result was observed for 6% of the patients (31 of 498) who received FLOMAX capsules 0.4 mg once daily and 4% (9 of 250) who received placebo (Note: patients in the 0.8-mg group received 0.4 mg once daily for the first week of Study 1).

In Studies 1 and 2, at least one positive orthostatic test result was observed during the course of these studies for 81 of the 502 patients (16%) in the FLOMAX capsules 0.4-mg once daily group, 92 of the 491 patients (19%) in the FLOMAX capsules 0.8-mg once daily group and 54 of the 493 patients (11%) in the placebo group.

Because orthostasis was detected more frequently in FLOMAX capsule-treated patients than in placebo recipients, there is a potential risk of syncope (see WARNINGS).

Abnormal Ejaculation Abnormal ejaculation includes ejaculation failure, ejaculation disorder, retrograde ejaculation and ejaculation decrease. As shown in Table 3, abnormal ejaculation was associated with FLOMAX capsules administration and was dose-related in the U.S. studies. Withdrawal from these clinical studies of FLOMAX capsules because of abnormal ejaculation was also dose-dependent with 8 of 492 patients (1.6%) in the 0.8-mg group, and no patients in the 0.4-mg or placebo groups discontinuing treatment due to abnormal ejaculation.

Post-Marketing Experience Allergic-type reactions such as skin rash, pruritus, angioedema of tongue, lips and face and urticaria have been reported with positive rechallenge in some cases. Priapism has been reported rarely. Infrequent reports of palpitations, constipation and vomiting have been received during the post-marketing period.

OVERDOSAGE

Should overdosage of FLOMAX capsules lead to hypotension (See WARNINGS and ADVERSE REACTIONS), support of the cardiovascular system is of first importance. Restoration of blood pressure and normalization of heart rate may be accomplished by keeping the patient in the supine position. If this measure is inadequate, then administration of intravenous fluids should be considered. If necessary, vasopressors should then be used and renal function should be monitored and supported as needed. Laboratory data indicate that tamsulosin HCl is 94% to 99% protein bound; therefore, dialysis is unlikely to be of benefit.

One patient reported an overdose of thirty 0.4-mg FLOMAX capsules. Following the ingestion of the capsules, the patient reported a severe headache.

DOSAGE AND ADMINISTRATION

FLOMAX capsules 0.4 mg once daily is recommended as the dose for the treatment of the signs and symptoms of BPH. It should be administered approximately one-half hour following the same meal each day.

For those patients who fail to respond to the 0.4-mg dose after two to four weeks of dosing, the dose of FLOMAX capsules can be increased to 0.8 mg once daily. If FLOMAX capsules administration is discontinued or interrupted for several days at either the 0.4-mg or 0.8-mg dose, therapy should be started again with the 0.4-mg once daily dose.

HOW SUPPLIED

FLOMAX capsules 0.4 mg are supplied in high density polyethylene bottles containing 100 or 1000 hard gelatin capsules with olive green opaque cap and orange opaque body. The capsules are imprinted on one side with "Flomax 0.4 mg" and on the other side with "BI 58."

NDC 0597-0058-01
FLOMAX Capsules
0.4 mg, 100 capsules
NDC 0597-0058-10
FLOMAX Capsules
0.4 mg, 1000 capsules

℞ only.

Store at controlled room temperature 20°-25° C (68°-77° F). Keep FLOMAX capsules and all medicines out of reach of children FL-PI-SRT10(11/99)

Marketed by:
Boehringer Ingelheim Pharmaceuticals, Inc.
Ridgefield, CT 06877
and
Abbott Laboratories Inc.
North Chicago, IL 60064
Licensed from and Manufactured by:
Yamanouchi Pharmaceutical Co., Ltd.
3–11 Nihonbashi-Honcho 2-Chome
Chuo-ku, Tokyo 103-8411, Japan

Shown in Product Identification Guide, page 309

MEXITIL® ℞

[mex ' ĭ-til]
(mexiletine hydrochloride, USP)
Oral Antiarrhythmic
Capsules of

150 mg	**BI-CODE 66**
200 mg	**BI-CODE 67**
250 mg	**BI-CODE 68**

Prescribing Information

DESCRIPTION

Mexitil® (mexiletine hydrochloride, USP) is an orally active antiarrhythmic agent available as 150 mg, 200 mg and 250 mg capsules. 100 mg of mexiletine hydrochloride is equivalent to 83.31 mg of mexiletine base. It is a white to off-white crystalline powder with slightly bitter taste, freely soluble in water and in alcohol. Mexitil® has a pKa of 9.2.

Chemically, Mexitil® is 1-methyl-2-(2, 6-xylyloxy) ethylamine hydrochloride and has the following structural formula:

$C_{11}H_{17}NO{\cdot}HCl$ mexiletine hydrochloride, USP
Mol. Wt. 215.73 (Mexitil)

Mexitil® Capsules contain the following inactive ingredients: colloidal silicon dioxide, corn starch, magnesium stearate, titanium dioxide, gelatin, FD&C Red No. 40, D&C Red No. 28 and FD&C Blue No. 1; the Mexitil® 150 mg and 250 mg capsules also contain FD&C Yellow No. 10. Mexitil® capsules may contain one or more of the following components: sodium lauryl sulfate, sodium proprionate, edetate calcium disodium, benzyl alcohol, carboxymethylcellulose sodium, glycerin, butylparaben, propylparaben, methylparaben, pharmaceutical glaze, ethylene glycol monoethylether, soya lecithin, dimethylpolysiloxane, refined shellac (food grade) and other inactive ingredients.

CLINICAL PHARMACOLOGY

Mechanism of Action

Mexitil® (mexiletine hydrochloride, USP) is a local anesthetic, antiarrhythmic agent, structurally similar to lidocaine, but orally active. In animal studies, Mexitil® has been shown to be effective in the suppression of induced ventricular arrhythmias, including those induced by glycoside toxicity and coronary artery ligation. Mexitil®, like lidocaine, inhibits the inward sodium current, thus reducing the rate of rise of the action potential, Phase 0. Mexitil® decreased the effective refractory period (ERP) in Purkinje fibers. The decrease in ERP was of lesser magnitude than the decrease in action potential duration (APD), with a resulting increase in the ERP/APD ratio.

Electrophysiology in Man Mexiletine is a Class 1B antiarrhythmic compound with electrophysiologic properties in man similar to lidocaine, but dissimilar from quinidine, procainamide, and disopyramide.

In patients with normal conduction systems, Mexitil® has a minimal effect on cardiac impulse generation and propagation. In clinical trials, no development of second-degree or third-degree AV block was observed. Mexitil® did not prolong ventricular depolarization (QRS duration) or repolarization (QT intervals) as measured by electrocardiography. Theoretically, therefore, Mexitil® may be useful in the treatment of ventricular arrhythmias associated with a prolonged QT interval.

In patients with pre-existing conduction defects, depression of the sinus rate, prolongation of sinus node recovery time, decreased conduction velocity and increased effective refractory period of the intraventricular conduction system have occasionally been observed.

The antiarrhythmic effect of Mexitil® has been established in controlled comparative trials against placebo, quinidine, procainamide and disopyramide. Mexitil®, at doses of 200–400 mg q8h, produced a significant reduction of ventricular premature beats, paired beats, and episodes of non-sustained ventricular tachycardia compared to placebo and was similar in effectiveness to the active agents. Among all patients entered into the studies, about 30% in each treatment group had a 70% or greater reduction in PVC count and about 40% failed to complete the 3 month studies because of adverse effects. Follow-up of patients from the controlled trials has demonstrated continued effectiveness of Mexitil® in long-term use.

Hemodynamics Hemodynamic studies in a limited number of patients, with normal or abnormal myocardial function, following oral administration of Mexitil®, have shown small, usually not statistically significant, decreases in cardiac output and increases in systemic vascular resistance, but no significant negative inotropic effect. Blood pressure and pulse rate remain essentially unchanged. Mild depression of myocardial function, similar to that produced by lidocaine, has occasionally been observed following intravenous Mexitil® therapy in patients with cardiac disease.

Pharmacokinetics Mexitil® is well absorbed (~90%) from the gastrointestinal tract. Unlike lidocaine, its first-pass metabolism is low. Peak blood levels are reached in two to three hours. In normal subjects, the plasma elimination half-life of Mexitil® is approximately 10–12 hours. It is 50–60% bound to plasma protein, with a volume of distribution of 5–7 liters/kg. Mexitil® is metabolized in the liver. Approximately 10% is excreted unchanged by the kidney. While urinary pH does not normally have much influence on elimination, marked changes in urinary pH influence the rate of excretion: acidification accelerates excretion, while alkalinization retards it.

Several metabolites of mexiletine have shown minimal antiarrhythmic activity in animal models. The most active is the minor metabolite N-methylmexiletine, which is less than 20% as potent as mexiletine. The urinary excretion of N-methylmexiletine in man is less than 0.5%. Thus the therapeutic activity of Mexitil® is due to the parent compound.

Hepatic impairment prolongs the elimination half-life of Mexitil®. In eight patients with moderate to severe liver disease, the mean half-life was approximately 25 hours.

Consistent with the limited renal elimination of Mexitil®, little change in the half-life has been detected in patients with reduced renal function. In eight patients with creatinine clearance less than 10 ml/min, the mean plasma elimination half-life was 15.7 hours; in seven patients with creatinine clearance between 11–40 ml/min, the mean half-life was 13.4 hours.

The absorption rate of Mexitil® is reduced in clinical situations such as acute myocardial infarction in which gastric emptying time is increased. Narcotics, atropine and magnesium-aluminum hydroxide have also been reported to slow the absorption of Mexitil®. Metoclopramide has been reported to accelerate absorption.

Mexiletine plasma levels of at least 0.5 mcg/ml are generally required for therapeutic response. An increase in the frequency of central nervous system adverse effects has been observed when plasma levels exceed 2.0 mcg/ml. Thus the therapeutic range is approximately 0.5 to 2.0 mcg/ml. Plasma levels within the therapeutic range can be attained with either three times daily or twice daily dosing but peak to trough differences are greater with the latter regimen, creating the possibility of adverse effects at peak and arrhythmic escape at trough. Nevertheless, some patients may be transferred successfully to the twice daily regimen (See DOSAGE AND ADMINISTRATION).

INDICATIONS AND USAGE

Mexitil® is indicated for the treatment of documented ventricular arrhythmias, such as sustained ventricular tachycardia, that, in the judgement of the physician, are life-threatening. Because of the proarrhythmic effects of Mexitil®, its use with lesser arrhythmias is generally not recommended. Treatment of patients with asymptomatic ventricular premature contractions should be avoided.

Initiation of Mexitil® treatment, as with other antiarrhythmic agents used to treat life-threatening arrhythmias, should be carried out in the hospital.

Antiarrhythmic drugs have not been shown to enhance survival in patients with ventricular arrhythmias.

CONTRAINDICATIONS

Mexitil® (mexiletine hydrochloride, USP) is contraindicated in the presence of cardiogenic shock or pre-existing second- or third-degree AV block (if no pacemaker is present).

WARNINGS: Mortality: In the National Heart, Lung and Blood Institute's Cardiac Arrhythmia Suppression Trial (CAST), a long-term, multicentered, randomized, double-blind study in patients with asymptomatic non-life-threatening ventricular arrhythmias who had a myocardial infarction more than six days but less than two years previously, an excessive mortality or non-fatal cardiac arrest rate (7.7%) was seen in patients treated with encainide or flecainide compared with that seen in patients assigned to carefully matched placebo-treated groups (3.0%). The average duration of treatment with encainide or flecainide in this study was ten months.

The applicability of the CAST results to other populations (e.g., those without recent myocardial infarction) is uncertain. Considering the known proarrhythmic properties of Mexitil® and the lack of evidence of improved survival for any antiarrhythmic drug in patients without life-threatening arrhythmias, the use of

Continued on next page

Mexitil—Cont.

Mexitil® as well as other antiarrhythmic agents should be reserved for patients with life-threatening ventricular antiarrhythmia.

Acute Liver Injury In postmarketing experience abnormal liver function tests have been reported, some in the first few weeks of therapy with Mexitil® (mexiletine hydrochloride, USP). Most of these have been observed in the setting of congestive heart failure or ischemia and their relationship to Mexitil® has not been established.

PRECAUTIONS

General If a ventricular pacemaker is operative, patients with second or third degree heart block may be treated with Mexitil® (mexiletine hydrochloride, USP) if continuously monitored. A limited number of patients (45 of 475 in controlled clinical trials) with pre-existing first degree AV block were treated with Mexitil®; none of these patients developed second or third degree AV block. Caution should be exercised when it is used in such patients or in patients with pre-existing sinus node dysfunction or intraventricular conduction abnormalities.

Like other antiarrhythmics Mexitil® (mexiletine hydrochloride, USP) can cause worsening of arrhythmias. This has been uncommon in patients with less serious arrhythmias (frequent premature beats or non-sustained ventricular tachycardia: see ADVERSE REACTIONS), but is of greater concern in patients with life-threatening arrhythmias such as sustained ventricular tachycardia. In patients with such arrhythmias subjected to programmed electrical stimulation or to exercise provocation, 10–15% of patients had exacerbation of the arrhythmia, a rate not greater than that of other agents.

Mexitil® should be used with caution in patients with hypotension and severe congestive heart failure because of the potential for aggravating these conditions.

Since Mexitil® is metabolized in the liver, and hepatic impairment has been reported to prolong the elimination half-life of Mexitil®, patients with liver disease should be followed carefully while receiving Mexitil®. The same caution should be observed in patients with hepatic dysfunction secondary to congestive heart failure.

Concurrent drug therapy or dietary regimens which may markedly alter urinary pH should be avoided during Mexitil® therapy. The minor fluctuations in urinary pH associated with normal diet do not affect the excretion of Mexitil®.

SGOT Elevation and Liver Injury: In three-month controlled trials, elevations of SGOT greater than three times the upper limit of normal occurred in about 1% of both mexiletine-treated and control patients. Approximately 2% of patients in the mexiletine compassionate use program had elevations of SGOT greater than or equal to three times the upper limit of normal. These elevations frequently occurred in association with identifiable clinical events and therapeutic measures such as congestive heart failure, acute myocardial infarction, blood transfusions and other medications. These elevations were often asymptomatic and transient, usually not associated with elevated bilirubin levels and usually did not require discontinuation of therapy. Marked elevations of SGOT (>1000 U/L) were seen before death in four patients with end-stage cardiac disease (severe congestive heart failure, cardiogenic shock).

Rare instances of severe liver injury, including hepatic necrosis, have been reported in association with Mexitil® treatment. It is recommended that patients in whom an abnormal liver test has occurred, or who have signs or symptoms suggesting liver dysfunction, be carefully evaluated. If persistent or worsening elevation of hepatic enzymes is detected, consideration should be given to discontinuing therapy.

Blood Dyscrasias: Among 10,867 patients treated with mexiletine in the compassionate use program, marked leukopenia (neutrophils less than 1000/mm^3) or agranulocytosis were seen in 0.06% and milder depressions of leukocytes were seen in 0.08%, and thrombocytopenia was observed in 0.16%. Many of these patients were seriously ill and receiving concomitant medications with known hematologic adverse effects. Rechallenge with mexiletine in several cases was negative. Marked leukopenia or agranulocytosis did not occur in any patient receiving Mexitil® alone; five of the six cases of agranulocytosis were associated with procainamide (sustained release preparations in four) and one with vinblastine. If significant hematologic changes are observed, the patient should be carefully evaluated, and, if warranted, Mexitil® should be discontinued. Blood counts usually return to normal within one month of discontinuation. (See ADVERSE REACTIONS.)

Convulsions (seizures) did not occur in Mexitil® controlled clinical trials. In the compassionate use program, convulsions were reported in about 2 of 1000 patients. Twenty-eight percent of these patients discontinued therapy. Convulsions were reported in patients with and without a prior history of seizures. Mexiletine should be used with caution in patients with known seizure disorder.

Drug Interactions In a large compassionate use program Mexitil® has been used concurrently with commonly employed antianginal, antihypertensive, and anticoagulant drugs without observed interactions. A variety of antiarrhythmics such as quinidine or propranolol were also added, sometimes with improved control of ventricular ectopy. When phenytoin or other hepatic enzyme inducers such as rifampin and phenobarbital have been taken concurrently with Mexitil®, lowered Mexitil® plasma levels have been reported. Monitoring of Mexitil® plasma levels is recommended during such concurrent use to avoid ineffective therapy.

In a formal study, benzodiazepines were shown not to affect Mexitil® plasma concentrations. ECG intervals (PR, QRS and QT) were not affected by concurrent Mexitil® and digoxin, diuretics, or propranolol.

Concurrent administration of cimetidine and Mexitil® has been reported to increase, decrease, or leave unchanged Mexitil® plasma levels; therefore patients should be followed carefully during concurrent therapy.

Mexitil® does not alter serum digoxin levels but magnesium-aluminum hydroxide, when used to treat gastrointestinal symptoms due to Mexitil®, has been reported to lower serum digoxin levels.

Concurrent use of Mexitil® and theophylline may lead to increased plasma theophylline levels. One controlled study in eight normal subjects showed a 72% mean increase (range 35–136%) in plasma theophylline levels. This increase was observed at the first test point which was the second day after starting Mexitil®. Theophylline plasma levels returned to pre-Mexitil® values within 48 hours after discontinuing Mexitil®. If Mexitil® and theophylline are to be used concurrently, theophylline blood levels should be monitored, particularly when the Mexitil® dose is changed. An appropriate adjustment in theophylline dose should be considered.

Additionally, in one controlled study in five normal subjects and seven patients, the clearance of caffeine was decreased 50% following the administration of Mexitil®.

Carcinogenesis, Mutagenesis and Impairment of Fertility Studies of carcinogenesis in rats (24 months) and mice (18 months) did not demonstrate any tumorigenic potential. Mexitil® was found to be non-mutagenic in the Ames test. Mexitil® did not impair fertility in the rat.

Pregnancy/Teratogenic Effects *PREGNANCY CATEGORY C:* Reproduction studies performed with Mexitil® (mexiletine hydrochloride, USP) in rats, mice and rabbits at doses up to four times the maximum human oral dose (24 mg/kg in a 50 kg patient) revealed no evidence of teratogenicity or impaired fertility but did show an increase in fetal resorption. There are no adequate and well-controlled studies in pregnant women; this drug should be used in pregnancy only if the potential benefit justifies the potential risk to the fetus.

Nursing Mothers Mexitil® appears in human milk in concentrations similar to those observed in plasma. Therefore, if the use of Mexitil® is deemed essential, an alternative method of infant feeding should be considered.

Pediatric Use Safety and effectiveness in the pediatric population have not been established.

COMPARATIVE INCIDENCE (%) OF ADVERSE EVENTS AMONG PATIENTS TREATED WITH MEXILETINE OR CONTROL DRUGS IN THE 12-WEEK, DOUBLE-BLIND TRIALS

	Mexiletine N = 430	Quinidine N = 262	Procainamide N = 78	Disopyramide N = 69
Cardiovascular				
Palpitations	4.3	4.6	1.3	5.8
Chest Pain	2.6	3.4	1.3	2.9
Angina/Angina-like Pain	1.7	1.9	2.6	2.9
Increased Ventricular Arrhythmias/PVC's	1.0	2.7	2.6	—
Digestive				
Nausea/Vomiting/Heartburn	39.3	21.4	33.3	14.5
Diarrhea	5.2	33.2	2.6	8.7
Constipation	4.0	—	6.4	11.6
Changes in Appetite	2.6	1.9	—	—
Abdominal Pain/Cramps/Discomfort	1.2	1.5	—	1.4
Central Nervous System				
Dizziness/Lightheadedness	18.9	14.1	14.1	2.9
Tremor	13.2	2.3	3.8	1.4
Coordination Difficulties	9.7	1.1	1.3	—
Changes in Sleep Habits	7.1	2.7	11.5	8.7
Weakness	5.0	5.3	7.7	2.9
Nervousness	5.0	1.9	6.4	5.8
Fatigue	3.8	5.7	5.1	1.4
Speech Difficulties	2.6	0.4	—	—
Confusion/Clouded Sensorium	2.6	—	3.8	—
Paresthesias/Numbness	2.4	2.3	2.6	—
Tinnitus	2.4	1.5	—	—
Depression	2.4	1.1	1.3	1.4
Other				
Blurred Vision/Visual Disturbances	5.7	3.1	5.1	7.2
Headache	5.7	6.9	7.7	4.3
Rash	4.2	3.8	10.3	1.4
Dyspnea/Respiratory	3.3	3.1	5.1	2.9
Dry Mouth	2.8	1.9	5.1	14.5
Arthralgia	1.7	2.3	5.1	1.4
Fever	1.2	3.1	2.6	—

ADVERSE REACTIONS

Mexitil® (mexiletine hydrochloride, USP) commonly produces reversible gastrointestinal and nervous system adverse reactions but is otherwise well tolerated. Mexitil® has been evaluated in 483 patients in one-month and three-month controlled studies and in over 10,000 patients in a large compassionate use program. Dosages in the controlled studies ranged from 600–1200 mg/day; some patients (8%) in the compassionate use program were treated with higher daily doses (1600–3200 mg/day). In the three-month controlled trials comparing Mexitil® to quinidine, procainamide and disopyramide, the most frequent adverse reactions were upper gastrointestinal distress (41%), lightheadedness (10.5%), tremor (12.6%) and coordination difficulties (10.2%). Similar frequency and incidence were observed in the one-month placebo-controlled trial. Although these reactions were generally not serious, and were dose-related and reversible with a reduction in dosage, by taking the drug with food or antacid or by therapy discontinuation, they led to therapy discontinuation in 40% of patients in the controlled trials. A tabulation of the adverse events reported in the one-month placebo-controlled trial follows:

COMPARATIVE INCIDENCE (%) OF ADVERSE EVENTS AMONG PATIENTS TREATED WITH MEXILETINE AND PLACEBO IN THE 4-WEEK, DOUBLE-BLIND CROSSOVER TRIAL

	Mexiletine N = 53	Placebo N = 49
Cardiovascular		
Palpitations	7.5	10.2
Chest Pain	7.5	4.1
Increased Ventricular Arrhythmias/PVC's	1.9	—
Digestive		
Nausea/Vomiting/Heartburn	39.6	6.1
Central Nervous System		
Dizziness/Lightheadedness	26.4	14.3
Tremor	13.2	—
Nervousness	11.3	6.1
Coordination Difficulties	9.4	—
Changes in Sleep Habits	7.5	16.3
Paresthesias/Numbness	3.8	2.0
Weakness	1.9	4.1
Fatigue	1.9	2.0
Tinnitus	1.9	4.1
Confusion/Clouded Sensorium	1.9	2.0
Other		
Headache	7.5	6.1
Blurred Vision/Visual Disturbances	7.5	2.0
Dyspnea/Respiratory	5.7	10.2
Rash	3.8	2.0
Non-specific Edema	3.8	—

A tabulation of adverse reactions occurring in one percent or more of patients in the three-month controlled studies follows:
[See table at top of previous page]
Less than 1%: Syncope, edema, hot flashes, hypertension, short-term memory loss, loss of consciousness, other psychological changes, diaphoresis, urinary hesitancy/retention, malaise, impotence/decreased libido, pharyngitis, congestive heart failure.
An additional group of over 10,000 patients has been treated in a program allowing administration of Mexitil® (mexiletine hydrochloride, USP) under compassionate use circumstances. These patients were seriously ill with the large majority on multiple drug therapy. Twenty-four percent of the patients continued in the program for one year or longer. Adverse reactions leading to therapy discontinuation occurred in 15 percent of patients (usually upper gastrointestinal system or nervous system effects). In general, the more common adverse reactions were similar to those in the controlled trials. Less common adverse events possibly related to Mexitil® use include:
Cardiovascular System: Syncope and hypotension, each about 6 in 1000; bradycardia, about 4 in 1000; angina/angina-like pain, about 3 in 1000; edema, atrioventricular block/conduction disturbances and hot flashes, each about 2 in 1000; atrial arrhythmias, hypertension and cardiogenic shock, each about 1 in 1000.
Central Nervous System: Short-term memory loss, about 9 in 1000 patients; hallucinations and other psychological changes, each about 3 in 1000; psychosis and convulsions/seizures, each about 2 in 1000; loss of consciousness, about 6 in 10,000.
Digestive: Dysphagia, about 2 in 1000; peptic ulcer, about 8 in 10,000; upper gastrointestinal bleeding, about 7 in 10,000; esophageal ulceration, about 1 in 10,000. Rare cases of severe hepatitis/acute hepatic necrosis.
Skin: Rare cases of exfoliative dermatitis and Stevens-Johnson Syndrome with Mexitil® (mexiletine hydrochloride, USP) treatment have been reported.
Laboratory: Abnormal liver function tests, about 5 in 1000 patients; positive ANA and thrombocytopenia, each about 2 in 1000; leukopenia (including neutropenia and agranulocytosis), about 1 in 1000; myelofibrosis, about 2 in 10,000 patients.
Other: Diaphoresis, about 6 in 1000; altered taste, about 5 in 1000; salivary changes, hair loss and impotence/decreased libido, each about 4 in 1000; malaise, about 3 in 1000; urinary hesitancy/retention, each about 2 in 1000; hiccups, dry skin, laryngeal and pharyngeal changes and changes in oral mucous membranes, each about 1 in 1000; SLE syndrome, about 4 in 10,000.
Hematology: Blood dyscrasias were not seen in the controlled trials but did occur among the 10,867 patients treated with mexiletine in the compassionate use program (see PRECAUTIONS).
Myelofibrosis was reported in two patients in the compassionate use program: one was receiving long-term thiotepa therapy and the other had pretreatment myeloid abnormalities.
In postmarketing experience, there have been isolated, spontaneous reports of pulmonary changes including pulmonary fibrosis during Mexitil® therapy with or without other drugs or diseases that are known to produce pulmonary toxicity. A causal relationship to Mexitil® therapy has not been established. In addition, there have been isolated reports of exacerbation of congestive heart failure in patients with pre-existing compromised ventricular function. There have been rare reports of pancreatitis associated with Mexitil® treatment.

OVERDOSAGE

Clinical findings associated with Mexitil® overdosage have included nausea, hypotension, sinus bradycardia, paresthesia, seizures, bundle branch block, AV heart block, asystole, ventricular tachyarrhythmia, including ventricular fibrillation, cardiovascular collapse and coma. The lowest known dose in a fatality case was 4.4g with postmortem serum mexiletine level of 34–37 mcg/ml (Jequier P. et al. Lancet 1976: 1 (7956): 429). Patients have recovered from ingestion of 4g to 18g of mexiletine (Frank S.E. et al. *Am J Emerg Med* 1991: 9:43–48).
There is no specific antidote for Mexitil®. Management of Mexitil® overdosage includes general supportive measures, close observation and monitoring of vital signs. In addition, the use of pharmacologic interventions (e.g., pressor agents, atropine or anticonvulsants) or transvenous cardiac pacing is suggested, depending on the patient's clinical condition.

DOSAGE AND ADMINISTRATION

The dosage of Mexitil® (mexiletine hydrochloride, USP) must be individualized on the basis of response and tolerance, both of which are dose-related. Administration with food or antacid is recommended. Initiate Mexitil® therapy with 200 mg every eight hours when rapid control of arrhythmia is not essential. A minimum of two to three days between dose adjustments is recommended. Dose may be adjusted in 50 or 100 mg increments up or down.
As with any antiarrhythmic drug, clinical and electrocardiographic evaluation (including Holter monitoring if necessary for evaluation) are needed to determine whether the desired antiarrhythmic effect has been obtained and to guide titration and dose adjustment.
Satisfactory control can be achieved in most patients by 200 to 300 mg given every eight hours with food or antacid. If satisfactory response has not been achieved at 300 mg q8h, and the patient tolerates Mexitil® well, a dose of 400 mg q8h may be tried. As the severity of CNS side effects increases with total daily dose, the dose should not exceed 1200 mg/day.
In general, patients with renal failure will require the usual doses of Mexitil®. Patients with severe liver disease, however, may require lower doses and must be monitored closely. Similarly, marked right-sided congestive heart failure can reduce hepatic metabolism and reduce the needed dose. Plasma level may also be affected by certain concomitant drugs (see PRECAUTIONS: Drug Interactions).
Loading Dose: When rapid control of ventricular arrhythmia is essential, an initial loading dose of 400 mg of Mexitil® may be administered, followed by a 200 mg dose in eight hours. Onset of therapeutic effect is usually observed within 30 minutes to two hours.
Q12H Dosage Schedule: Some patients responding to Mexitil® may be transferred to a 12-hour dosage schedule to improve convenience and compliance. If adequate suppression is achieved on a Mexitil® dose of 300 mg or less every eight hours, the same total daily dose may be given in divided doses every 12 hours while carefully monitoring the degree of suppression of ventricular ectopy. This dose may be adjusted up to a maximum of 450 mg every 12 hours to achieve the desired response.
Transferring to Mexitil: The following dosage schedule, based on theoretical considerations rather than experimental data, is suggested for transferring patients from other Class I oral antiarrhythmic agents to Mexitil®: Mexitil® treatment may be initiated with a 200 mg dose, and titrated to response as described above, 6–12 hours after the last dose of quinidine sulfate, 3–6 hours after the last dose of procainamide, 6–12 hours after the last dose of disopyramide or 8–12 hours after the last dose of tocainide.
In patients in whom withdrawal of the previous antiarrhythmic agent is likely to produce life-threatening arrhythmias, hospitalization of the patient is recommended.
When transferring from lidocaine to Mexitil®, the lidocaine infusion should be stopped when the first oral dose of Mexitil® is administered. The infusion line should be left open until suppression of the arrhythmia appears to be satisfactorily maintained. Consideration should be given to the similarity of the adverse effects of lidocaine and Mexitil® and the possibility that they may be additive.

HOW SUPPLIED

Mexitil® (mexiletine hydrochloride, USP) is supplied in hard gelatin capsules containing 150 mg, 200 mg or 250 mg of mexiletine hydrochloride:
Mexitil® 150 mg capsules are red and caramel with the marking BI 66. Available in bottles of 100 (NDC 0597-0066-01) and individually blister-sealed unit-dose cartons of 100 (NDC 0597-0066-61).
Mexitil® 200 mg capsules are red with the marking BI 67. Available in bottles of 100 (NDC 0597-0067-01) and individually blister-sealed unit-dose cartons of 100 (NDC 0597-0067-61).
Mexitil® 250 mg capsules are red and aqua green with the marking BI 68. Available in bottles of 100 (NDC 0597-0068-01) and individually blister-sealed unit-dose cartons of 100 (NDC 0597-0068-61).
Store at room temperature 20–25°C (68–77°F).
Caution: Federal law prohibits dispensing without prescription.

ME-PI-7/96 Rev.

Boehringer Ingelheim
Pharmaceuticals, Inc.
Ridgefield, Connecticut 06877
Licensed from
Boehringer Ingelheim
International GmbH

Shown in Product Identification Guide, page 309

MICARDIS® ℞

(telmisartan)
Tablets 40 mg and 80 mg
Prescribing Information

USE IN PREGNANCY

When used in pregnancy during the second and third trimesters, drugs that act directly on the renin-angiotensin system can cause injury and even death to the developing fetus. When pregnancy is detected, MICARDIS® tablets should be discontinued as soon as possible. **See WARNINGS: Fetal/Neonatal Morbidity and Mortality**

DESCRIPTION

MICARDIS® (telmisartan) is a nonpeptide angiotensin II receptor (type AT_1) antagonist.
Telmisartan is chemically described as 4'-[(1,4'-dimethyl-2'-propyl[2,6'-bi-1H-benzimidazol]-1'-yl)methyl]-[1,1'-biphenyl]-2-carboxylic acid. Its empirical formula is $C_{33}H_{30}N_4O_2$, its molecular weight is 514.63, and its structural formula is:

Telmisartan is a white to off-white, odorless crystalline powder. It is practically insoluble in water and in the pH range of 3 to 9, sparingly soluble in strong acid (except insoluble in hydrochloric acid), and soluble in strong base.
MICARDIS® is available as tablets for oral administration, containing either 40 mg or 80 mg of telmisartan. The tablets contain the following inactive ingredients: sodium hydroxide, meglumine, povidone, sorbitol, and magnesium stearate. MICARDIS® tablets are hygroscopic and require protection from moisture.

CLINICAL PHARMACOLOGY

Mechanism of Action

Angiotensin II is formed from angiotensin I in a reaction catalyzed by angiotensin-converting enzyme (ACE, kininase II). Angiotensin II is the principal pressor agent of the renin-angiotensin system, with effects that include vasoconstriction, stimulation of synthesis and release of aldosterone, cardiac stimulation, and renal reabsorption of sodium. Telmisartan blocks the vasoconstrictor and aldosterone-secreting effects of angiotensin II by selectively blocking the binding of angiotensin II to the AT_1 receptor in many tissues, such as vascular smooth muscle and the adrenal gland. Its action is therefore independent of the pathways for angiotensin II synthesis.
There is also an AT_2 receptor found in many tissues, but AT_2 is not known to be associated with cardiovascular homeostasis. Telmisartan has much greater affinity (>3,000 fold) for the AT_1 receptor than for the AT_2 receptor.
Blockade of the renin-angiotensin system with ACE inhibitors, which inhibit the biosynthesis of angiotensin II from angiotensin I, is widely used in the treatment of hypertension. ACE inhibitors also inhibit the degradation of bradykinin, a reaction also catalyzed by ACE. Because telmisartan does not inhibit ACE (kininase II), it does not affect the response to bradykinin. Whether this difference has clinical relevance is not yet known. Telmisartan does not bind to or block other hormone receptors or ion channels known to be important in cardiovascular regulation.
Blockade of the angiotensin II receptor inhibits the negative regulatory feedback of angiotensin II on renin secretion, but the resulting increased plasma renin activity and angiotensin II circulating levels do not overcome the effect of telmisartan on blood pressure.

Pharmacokinetics

General
Following oral administration, peak concentrations (C_{max}) of telmisartan are reached in 0.5–1 hour after dosing. Food slightly reduces the bioavailability of telmisartan, with a reduction in the area under the plasma concentration-time curve (AUC) of about 6% with the 40 mg tablet and about 20% after a 160 mg dose. The absolute bioavailability of telmisartan is dose dependent. At 40 and 160 mg the bioavailability was 42% and 58%, respectively. The pharmacokinetics of orally administered telmisartan are nonlinear over the dose range 20–160 mg, with greater than proportional increases of plasma concentrations (C_{max} and AUC) with increasing doses. Telmisartan shows bi-exponential decay kinetics with a terminal elimination half-life of approximately 24 hours. Trough plasma concentrations of telmisartan with once daily dosing are about 10–25% of peak plasma concentrations. Telmisartan has an accumulation index in plasma of 1.5 to 2.0 upon repeated once daily dosing.
Metabolism and Elimination
Following either intravenous or oral administration of ^{14}C-labeled telmisartan, most of the administered dose (>97%) was eliminated unchanged in feces via biliary excretion; only minute amounts were found in the urine (0.91% and 0.49% of total radioactivity, respectively).
Telmisartan is metabolized by conjugation to form a pharmacologically inactive acylglucuronide; the glucuronide of the parent compound is the only metabolite that has been identified in human plasma and urine. After a single dose, the glucuronide represents approximately 11% of the measured radioactivity in plasma. The cytochrome P450 isoenzymes are not involved in the metabolism of telmisartan.
Total plasma clearance of telmisartan is >800 mL/min. Terminal half-life and total clearance appear to be independent of dose.
Distribution
Telmisartan is highly bound to plasma proteins (>99.5%), mainly albumin and α_1-acid glycoprotein. Plasma protein binding is constant over the concentration range achieved with recommended doses. The volume of distribution for telmisartan is approximately 500 liters, indicating additional tissue binding.

Special Populations

Pediatric: Telmisartan pharmacokinetics have not been investigated in patients <18 years of age.
Geriatric: The pharmacokinetics of telmisartan do not differ between the elderly and those younger than 65 years (see DOSAGE AND ADMINISTRATION).
Gender: Plasma concentrations of telmisartan are generally 2–3 times higher in females than in males. In clinical trials, however, no significant increases in blood pressure response or in the incidence of orthostatic hypotension were found in women. No dosage adjustment is necessary.
Renal Insufficiency: Renal excretion does not contribute to the clearance of telmisartan. Based on modest experience in patients with mild-to-moderate renal impairment (creatinine clearance of 30–80 mL/min, mean clearance approximately 50 mL/min), no dosage adjustment is necessary in

Continued on next page

Micardis—Cont.

patients with decreased renal function. Telmisartan is not removed from blood by hemofiltration (see PRECAUTIONS, and DOSAGE AND ADMINISTRATION).

Hepatic Insufficiency: In patients with hepatic insufficiency, plasma concentrations of telmisartan are increased, and absolute bioavailability approaches 100% (see PRECAUTIONS, and DOSAGE AND ADMINISTRATION).

Drug Interactions: See PRECAUTIONS, Drug Interactions.

Pharmacodynamics

In normal volunteers, a dose of telmisartan 80 mg inhibited the pressor response to an intravenous infusion of angiotensin II by about 90% at peak plasma concentrations with approximately 40% inhibition persisting for 24 hours.

Plasma concentration of angiotensin II and plasma renin activity (PRA) increased in a dose-dependent manner after single administration of telmisartan to healthy subjects and repeated administration to hypertensive patients. The once-daily administration of up to 80 mg telmisartan to healthy subjects did not influence plasma aldosterone concentrations. In multiple dose studies with hypertensive patients, there were no clinically significant changes in electrolytes (serum potassium or sodium), or in metabolic function (including serum levels of cholesterol, triglycerides, HDL, LDL, glucose, or uric acid).

In 30 hypertensive patients with normal renal function treated for 8 weeks with telmisartan 80 mg or telmisartan 80 mg in combination with hydrochlorothiazide 12.5 mg, there were no clinically significant changes from baseline in renal blood flow, glomerular filtration rate, filtration fraction, renovascular resistance, or creatinine clearance.

Clinical Trials

The antihypertensive effects of MICARDIS® (telmisartan) have been demonstrated in six principal placebo-controlled clinical trials, studying a range of 20–160 mg; one of these examined the antihypertensive effects of telmisartan and hydrochlorothiazide in combination. The studies involved a total of 1773 patients with mild-to-moderate hypertension (diastolic blood pressure of 95–114 mmHg), 1031 of whom were treated with telmisartan. Following once daily administration of telmisartan, the magnitude of blood pressure reduction from baseline after placebo subtraction was approximately (SBP/DBP) 6–8 / 6 mmHg for 20 mg, 9–13 / 6–8 mmHg for 40 mg, and 12–13 / 7–8 mmHg for 80 mg. Larger doses (up to 160 mg) did not appear to cause a further decrease in blood pressure.

Upon initiation of antihypertensive treatment with telmisartan, blood pressure was reduced after the first dose, with a maximal reduction by about 4 weeks. With cessation of treatment with MICARDIS® tablets, blood pressure gradually returned to baseline values over a period of several days to one week. During long term studies (without placebo control) the effect of telmisartan appeared to be maintained for up to at least one year. The antihypertensive effect of telmisartan is not influenced by patient age, gender, weight or body mass index. Blood pressure response in black patients (usually a low-renin population) is noticeably less than that in Caucasian patients. This has been true for most, but not all, angiotensin II antagonists and ACE inhibitors.

In a controlled study, the addition of telmisartan to hydrochlorothiazide produced an additional dose-related reduction in blood pressure that was similar in magnitude to the reduction achieved with telmisartan monotherapy. Hydrochlorothiazide also had an added blood pressure effect when added to telmisartan.

The onset of antihypertensive activity occurs within 3 hours after administration of a single oral dose. At doses of 20, 40, and 80 mg, the antihypertensive effect of once daily administration of telmisartan is maintained for the full 24-hour dose interval. With automated ambulatory blood pressure monitoring and conventional blood pressure measurements, the 24-hour trough-to-peak ratio for 40–80 mg doses of telmisartan was 70–100% for both systolic and diastolic blood pressure. The incidence of symptomatic orthostasis after the first dose in all controlled trials was low (0.04%).

There were no changes in the heart rate of patients treated with telmisartan in controlled trials.

INDICATIONS AND USAGE

MICARDIS® (telmisartan) is indicated for the treatment of hypertension. It may be used alone or in combination with other antihypertensive agents.

CONTRAINDICATIONS

MICARDIS® is contraindicated in patients who are hypersensitive to any component of this product.

WARNINGS

Fetal/Neonatal Morbidity and Mortality

Drugs that act directly on the renin-angiotensin system can cause fetal and neonatal morbidity and death when administered to pregnant women. Several dozen cases have been reported in the world literature in patients who were taking angiotensin converting enzyme inhibitors. When pregnancy is detected, MICARDIS® tablets should be discontinued as soon as possible.

The use of drugs that act directly on the renin-angiotensin system during the second and third trimesters of pregnancy has been associated with fetal and neonatal injury, including hypotension, neonatal skull hypoplasia, anuria, reversible or irreversible renal failure, and death. Oligohydramnios has also been reported, presumably resulting from decreased fetal renal function; oligohydramnios in this setting has been associated with fetal limb contractures, craniofacial deformation, and hypoplastic lung development. Prematurity, intrauterine growth retardation, and patent ductus arteriosus have also been reported, although it is not clear whether these occurrences were due to exposure to the drug.

These adverse effects do not appear to have resulted from intrauterine drug exposure that has been limited to the first trimester. Mothers whose embryos and fetuses are exposed to an angiotensin II receptor antagonist only during the first trimester should be so informed. Nonetheless, when patients become pregnant, physicians should have the patient discontinue the use of MICARDIS® tablets as soon as possible.

Rarely (probably less often than once in every thousand pregnancies), no alternative to an angiotensin II receptor antagonist will be found. In these rare cases, the mothers should be apprised of the potential hazards to their fetuses, and serial ultrasound examinations should be performed to assess the intra-amniotic environment.

If oligohydramnios is observed, MICARDIS® tablets should be discontinued unless it is considered life-saving for the mother. Contraction stress testing (CST), a non-stress test (NST), or biophysical profiling (BPP) may be appropriate, depending upon the week of pregnancy. Patients and physicians should be aware, however, that oligohydramnios may not appear until after the fetus has sustained irreversible injury.

Infants with histories of *in utero* exposure to an angiotensin II receptor antagonist should be closely observed for hypotension, oliguria, and hyperkalemia. If oliguria occurs, attention should be directed toward support of blood pressure and renal perfusion. Exchange transfusion or dialysis may be required as a means of reversing hypotension and/or substituting for disordered renal function.

There is no clinical experience with the use of MICARDIS® tablets in pregnant women. No teratogenic effects were observed when telmisartan was administered to pregnant rats at oral doses of up to 50 mg/kg/day and to pregnant rabbits at oral doses up to 45 mg/kg/day. In rabbits, embryolethality associated with maternal toxicity (reduced body weight gain and food consumption) was observed at 45 mg/kg/day [about 6.4 times the maximum recommended human dose (MRHD) of 80 mg on a mg/m^2 basis]. In rats, maternally toxic (reduction in body weight gain and food consumption) telmisartan doses of 15 mg/kg/day (about 1.9 times the MRHD on a mg/m^2 basis), administered during late gestation and lactation, were observed to produce adverse effects in neonates, including reduced viability, low birth weight, delayed maturation, and decreased weight gain. Telmisartan has been shown to be present in rat fetuses during late gestation and in rat milk. The no observed effect doses for developmental toxicity in rats and rabbits, 5 and 15 mg/kg/day, respectively, are about 0.64 and 3.7 times, on a mg/m^2 basis, the maximum recommended human dose of telmisartan (80 mg/day).

Hypotension in Volume-Depleted Patients

In patients with an activated renin-angiotensin system, such as volume- and/or salt-depleted patients (e.g., those being treated with high doses of diuretics), symptomatic hypotension may occur after initiation of therapy with MICARDIS® tablets. This condition should be corrected prior to administration of MICARDIS® tablets, or treatment should either start under close medical supervision or with a reduced dose of an AII antagonist (this may require use of a drug other than MICARDIS® as it is not possible to give less than 40 mg at present).

If hypotension does occur, the patient should be placed in the supine position and, if necessary, given an intravenous infusion of normal saline. A transient hypotensive response is not a contraindication to further treatment, which usually can be continued without difficulty once the blood pressure has stabilized.

PRECAUTIONS

General

Impaired Hepatic Function: As the majority of telmisartan is eliminated by biliary excretion, patients with biliary obstructive disorders or hepatic insufficiency can be expected to have reduced clearance. MICARDIS® tablets should be used with caution in these patients, but there is no way to reduce the dose below 40 mg; an alternative treatment can be considered.

Impaired Renal Function: As a consequence of inhibiting the renin-angiotensin-aldosterone system, changes in renal function may be anticipated in susceptible individuals. In patients whose renal function may depend on the activity of the renin-angiotensin-aldosterone system (e.g., patients with severe congestive heart failure), treatment with angiotensin-converting enzyme inhibitors and angiotensin receptor antagonists has been associated with oliguria and/or progressive azotemia and (rarely) with acute renal failure and/or death. Similar results may be anticipated in patients treated with MICARDIS® tablets.

In studies of ACE inhibitors in patients with unilateral or bilateral renal artery stenosis, increases in serum creatinine or blood urea nitrogen were observed. There has been no long term use of MICARDIS® tablets in patients with unilateral or bilateral renal artery stenosis but an effect similar to that seen with ACE inhibitors should be anticipated.

Information for Patients

Pregnancy: Female patients of childbearing age should be told about the consequences of second- and third-trimester exposure to drugs that act on the renin-angiotensin system, and they should also be told that these consequences do not appear to have resulted from intrauterine drug exposure that has been limited to the first trimester. These patients should be asked to report pregnancies to their physicians as soon as possible.

Drug Interactions

Digoxin: When telmisartan was coadministered with digoxin, median increases in digoxin peak plasma concentration (49%) and in trough concentration (20%) were observed. It is, therefore, recommended that digoxin levels be monitored when initiating, adjusting, and discontinuing telmisartan to avoid possible over- or under-digitalization.

Warfarin: Telmisartan administered for 10 days slightly decreased the mean warfarin trough plasma concentration; this decrease did not result in a change in International Normalized Ratio (INR).

Other Drugs: Coadministration of telmisartan did not result in a clinically significant interaction with acetaminophen, amlodipine, glibenclamide, hydrochlorothiazide or ibuprofen. Telmisartan is not metabolized by the cytochrome P450 system and had no effects *in vitro* on cytochrome P450 enzymes, except for some inhibition of CYP2C19. Telmisartan is not expected to interact with drugs that inhibit cytochrome P450 enzymes; it is also not expected to interact with drugs metabolized by cytochrome P450 enzymes, except for possible inhibition of the metabolism of drugs metabolized by CYP2C19.

Carcinogenesis, Mutagenesis, Impairment of Fertility

There was no evidence of carcinogenicity when telmisartan was administered in the diet to mice and rats for up to 2 years. The highest doses administered to mice (1000 mg/kg/day) and rats (100 mg/kg/day) are, on a mg/m^2 basis, about 59 and 13 times, respectively, the maximum recommended human dose (MRHD) of telmisartan. These same doses have been shown to provide average systemic exposures to telmisartan >100 times and >25 times, respectively, the systemic exposure in humans receiving the MRHD (80 mg/day).

Genotoxicity assays did not reveal any telmisartan-related effects at either the gene or chromosome level. These assays included bacterial mutagenicity tests with Salmonella and *E coli* (Ames), a gene mutation test with Chinese hamster V79 cells, a cytogenetic test with human lymphocytes, and a mouse micronucleus test.

No drug-related effects on the reproductive performance of male and female rats were noted at 100 mg/kg/day (the highest dose administered), about 13 times, on a mg/m^2 basis, the MRHD of telmisartan. This dose in the rat resulted in an average systemic exposure (telmisartan AUC as determined on day 6 of pregnancy) at least 50 times the average systemic exposure in humans at the MRHD (80 mg/day).

Pregnancy

Pregnancy Categories C (first trimester) and D (second and third trimesters). See WARNINGS: Fetal/Neonatal Morbidity and Mortality.

Nursing Mothers

It is not known whether telmisartan is excreted in human milk, but telmisartan was shown to be present in the milk of lactating rats. Because of the potential for adverse effects on the nursing infant, a decision should be made whether to discontinue nursing or discontinue the drug, taking into account the importance of the drug to the mother.

Pediatric Use

Safety and effectiveness in pediatric patients have not been established.

Geriatric Use

Of the total number of patients receiving MICARDIS® in clinical studies, 551 (18.6%) were 65 to 74 years of age and 130 (4.4%) were 75 years or older. No overall differences in effectiveness and safety were observed in these patients compared to younger patients and other reported clinical experience has not identified differences in responses between the elderly and younger patients, but greater sensitivity of some older individuals cannot be ruled out.

ADVERSE REACTIONS

MICARDIS® has been evaluated for safety in more than 3700 patients, including 1900 treated for over six months and more than 1300 for over one year. Adverse experiences have generally been mild and transient in nature and have only infrequently required discontinuation of therapy.

In placebo-controlled trials involving 1041 patients treated with various doses of telmisartan (20–160 mg) monotherapy for up to 12 weeks, an overall incidence of adverse events similar to that of placebo was observed.

Adverse events occurring at an incidence of 1% or more in patients treated with telmisartan and at a greater rate than in patients treated with placebo, irrespective of their causal association, are presented in the following table.

	Telmisartan n = 1455 %	Placebo n = 380 %
Upper respiratory tract infection	7	6
Back pain	3	1
Sinusitis	3	2
Diarrhea	3	2
Pharyngitis	1	0

In addition to the adverse events in the table, the following events occurred at a rate of 1% but were at least as frequent

in the placebo group: influenza-like symptoms, dyspepsia, myalgia, urinary tract infection, abdominal pain, headache, dizziness, pain, fatigue, coughing, hypertension, chest pain, nausea and peripheral edema.
Discontinuation of therapy due to adverse events was required in 2.8% of 1455 patients treated with MICARDIS® tablets and 6.1% of 380 placebo patients in placebo-controlled clinical trials.
The incidence of adverse events was not dose-related and did not correlate with gender, age, or race of patients.
The incidence of cough occurring with telmisartan in six placebo-controlled trials was identical to that noted for placebo-treated patients (1.6%).
In addition to those listed above, adverse events that occurred in more than 0.3% of 3500 patients treated with MICARDIS® monotherapy in controlled or open trials are listed below. It cannot be determined whether these events were causally related to MICARDIS® tablets:
Autonomic Nervous System: impotence, increased sweating, flushing; *Body as a Whole:* allergy, fever, leg pain, malaise; *Cardiovascular:* palpitation, dependent edema, angina pectoris, tachycardia, leg edema, abnormal ECG; *CNS:* insomnia, somnolence, migraine, vertigo, paresthesia, involuntary muscle contractions, hypoaesthesia; *Gastrointestinal:* flatulence, constipation, gastritis, vomiting, dry mouth, hemorrhoids, gastroenteritis, enteritis, gastroesophageal reflux, toothache, non-specific gastrointestinal disorders; *Metabolic:* gout, hypercholesterolemia, diabetes mellitus; *Musculoskeletal:* arthritis, arthralgia, leg cramps; *Psychiatric:* anxiety, depression, nervousness; *Resistance Mechanism:* infection, fungal infection, abscess, otitis media; *Respiratory:* asthma, bronchitis, rhinitis, dyspnea, epistaxis; *Skin:* dermatitis, rash, eczema, pruritus; *Urinary:* micturition frequency, cystitis; *Vascular:* cerebrovascular disorder; and *Special Senses:* abnormal vision, conjunctivitis, tinnitus, earache.
A single case of angioedema was reported (among a total of 3781 patients treated with telmisartan).

Clinical Laboratory Findings

In placebo-controlled clinical trials, clinically relevant changes in standard laboratory test parameters were rarely associated with administration of MICARDIS® tablets.
Hemoglobin: A greater than 2 g/dL decrease in hemoglobin was observed in 0.8% telmisartan patients compared with 0.3% placebo patients. No patients discontinued therapy due to anemia.
Creatinine: A 0.5 mg/dL rise or greater in creatinine was observed in 0.4% telmisartan patients compared with 0.3% placebo patients. One telmisartan-treated patient discontinued therapy due to increases in creatinine and blood urea nitrogen.
Liver enzymes: Occasional elevations of liver chemistries occurred in patients treated with telmisartan; all marked elevations occurred at a higher frequency with placebo. No telmisartan-treated patients discontinued therapy due to abnormal hepatic function.

OVERDOSAGE

Limited data are available with regard to overdosage in humans. The most likely manifestation of overdosage with MICARDIS® tablets would be hypotension, dizziness and tachycardia; bradycardia could occur from parasympathetic (vagal) stimulation. If symptomatic hypotension should occur, supportive treatment should be instituted. Telmisartan is not removed by hemodialysis.

DOSAGE AND ADMINISTRATION

Dosage must be individualized. The usual starting dose of MICARDIS® tablets is 40 mg once a day. Blood pressure response is dose related over the range of 20–80 mg (see CLINICAL PHARMACOLOGY: Clinical Trials).

Special Populations: Patients with depletion of intravascular volume should have the condition corrected or MICARDIS® tablets should be initiated under close medical supervision (see WARNINGS: Hypotension in Volume-Depleted Patients).

Patients with biliary obstructive disorders or hepatic insufficiency should have treatment started under close medical supervision (see PRECAUTIONS: General, *Impaired Hepatic Function*, and *Impaired Renal Function*).

Most of the antihypertensive effect is apparent within two weeks and maximal reduction is generally attained after four weeks. When additional blood pressure reduction beyond that achieved with 80 mg MICARDIS® is required, a diuretic may be added.
No initial dosing adjustment is necessary for elderly patients or patients with mild-to-moderate renal impairment. Patients on dialysis may develop orthostatic hypotension; their blood pressure should be closely monitored.
MICARDIS® tablets may be administered with other antihypertensive agents.
MICARDIS® tablets may be administered with or without food.

HOW SUPPLIED

MICARDIS® is available as white, oblong-shaped, uncoated tablets containing telmisartan 40 mg or 80 mg. Tablets are marked with the BOEHRINGER INGELHEIM logo on one side, and on the other side, with a decorative score and either 51H or 52H for the 40 mg and 80 mg strengths, respectively. Tablets are provided as follows:
MICARDIS® (telmisartan) tablets 40 mg are individually blister-sealed in cartons of 28 tablets as 4 × 7 cards (NDC 0597-0040-28).
MICARDIS® (telmisartan) tablets 80 mg are individually blister-sealed in cartons of 28 tablets as 4 × 7 cards (NDC 0597-0041-28).

Storage

Store at 25°C (77°F); excursions permitted to 15–30°C (59–86°F) (see USP Controlled Room Temperature). Tablets should not be removed from blisters until immediately before administration.

Rx only.

MC-PI-862080 (11/98)

Manufactured by: Boehringer Ingelheim Pharma KG, Ingelheim, Germany
Distributed by: Boehringer Ingelheim Pharmaceuticals, Inc., Ridgefield, CT
Licensed from: Boehringer Ingelheim International GmbH, Ingelheim, Germany

Shown in Product Identification Guide, page 309

MOBIC® ℞
(meloxicam) Tablets 7.5 mg
Prescribing Information

DESCRIPTION

MOBIC® (meloxicam), an oxicam derivative, is a member of the enolic acid group of nonsteroidal anti-inflammatory drugs (NSAIDs). Each yellow tablet contains meloxicam 7.5 mg for oral administration. It is chemically designated as 4-hydroxy-2-methyl-*N*-(5-methyl-2-thiazolyl)-2*H*-1,2-benzothiazine-3-carboxamide 1, 1-dioxide. The molecular weight is 351.4. Its empirical formula is $C_{14}H_{13}N_3O_4S_2$ and it has the following structural formula.

Meloxicam is a yellow solid, practically insoluble in water, with higher solubility observed in strong acids and bases. It is very slightly soluble in methanol. Meloxicam has an apparent partition coefficient $(\log P)_{app} = 0.1$ in *n*-octanol/buffer pH 7.4. Meloxicam has pKa values of 1.1 and 4.2.
MOBIC is available as a tablet for oral administration containing 7.5 mg meloxicam.
The inactive ingredients in MOBIC include colloidal silicon dioxide, crospovidone, lactose monohydrate, magnesium stearate, microcrystalline cellulose, povidone and sodium citrate dihydrate.

CLINICAL PHARMACOLOGY

Mechanism of Action

Meloxicam is a nonsteroidal anti-inflammatory drug (NSAID) that exhibits anti-inflammatory, analgesic, and antipyretic activities in animal models. The mechanism of action of meloxicam, like that of other NSAIDs, may be related to prostaglandin synthetase (cyclooxygenase) inhibition.

Pharmacokinetics

Absorption The absolute bioavailability of meloxicam capsules was 89% following a single oral dose of 30 mg compared with 30 mg IV bolus injection. Meloxicam capsules have been shown to be bioequivalent to MOBIC tablets. Following single intravenous doses, dose-proportional pharmacokinetics were shown in the range of 5 mg to 60 mg. After multiple oral doses the pharmacokinetics of meloxicam capsules were dose-proportional over the range of 7.5 mg to 15 mg. Mean C_{max} was achieved within four to five hours after a 7.5 mg meloxicam tablet was taken under fasted conditions, indicating a prolonged drug absorption. The rate or extent of absorption was not affected by multiple dose administration, suggesting linear pharmacokinetics. With multiple dosing, steady state conditions were reached by day 5. A second meloxicam concentration peak occurs around 12 to 14 hours post-dose suggesting gastrointestinal recirculation.
[See table 1 at top of next page]
Food and Antacid Effects Drug intake after a high fat breakfast (75 g of fat) did not affect extent of absorption of meloxicam capsules, but led to 22% higher C_{max} values. Mean C_{max} values were achieved between five and six hours. No pharmacokinetic interaction was detected with concomitant administration of antacids. MOBIC tablets can be administered without regard to timing of meals and antacids.
Distribution The mean volume of distribution (Vss) of meloxicam is approximately 10 L. Meloxicam is ~ 99.4% bound to human plasma proteins (primarily albumin) within the therapeutic dose range. The fraction of protein binding is independent of drug concentration, over the clinically relevant concentration range, but decreases to ~99% in patients with renal disease. Meloxicam penetration into human red blood cells, after oral dosing, is less than 10%. Following a radiolabeled dose, over 90% of the radioactivity detected in the plasma was present as unchanged meloxicam.
Meloxicam concentrations in synovial fluid, after a single oral dose, range from 40% to 50% of those in plasma. The free fraction in synovial fluid is 2.5 times higher than in plasma, due to the lower albumin content in synovial fluid as compared to plasma. The significance of this penetration is unknown.
Metabolism Meloxicam is almost completely metabolized to four pharmacologically inactive metabolites. The major metabolite, 5′-carboxy meloxicam (60% of dose), from P-450 mediated metabolism was formed by oxidation of an intermediate metabolite 5′-hydroxymethyl meloxicam which is also excreted to a lesser extent (9% of dose). *In vitro* studies indicate that cytochrome P-450 2C9 plays an important role in this metabolic pathway with a minor contribution of the CYP 3A4 isozyme. Patients' peroxidase activity is probably responsible for the other two metabolites which account for 16% and 4% of the administered dose, respectively.
Excretion Meloxicam excretion is predominantly in the form of metabolites, and occurs to equal extents in the urine and feces. Only traces of the unchanged parent compound are excreted in the urine (0.2%) and feces (1.6%). The extent of the urinary excretion was confirmed for unlabeled multiple 7.5 mg doses: 0.5%, 6% and 13% of the dose were found in urine in the form of meloxicam, and the 5′-hydroxymethyl and 5′-carboxy metabolites, respectively. There is significant biliary and/or enteral secretion of the drug. This was demonstrated when oral administration of cholestyramine following a single IV dose of meloxicam decreased the AUC of meloxicam by 50%.
The mean elimination half-life ($t_{1/2}$) ranges from 15 hours to 20 hours. The elimination half-life is constant across dose levels indicating linear metabolism within the therapeutic dose range. Plasma clearance ranges from 7 to 9 mL/min.

Special Populations

Pediatric The pharmacokinetics of MOBIC in pediatric patients under 18 years of age have not been investigated.
Geriatric Elderly males (≥ 65 years of age) exhibited meloxicam plasma concentrations and steady state pharmacokinetics similar to young males. Elderly females (≥ 65 years of age) had a 47% higher AUC_{ss} and 32% higher $C_{max\ ss}$ as compared to younger females (≤ 55 years of age) after body weight normalization. Despite the increased total concentrations in the elderly females, the adverse event profile was comparable for both elderly patient populations. A smaller free fraction was found in elderly female patients in comparison to elderly male patients.
Gender Young females exhibited slightly lower plasma concentrations relative to young males. After single doses of 7.5 mg MOBIC, the mean elimination half-life was 19.5 hours for the female group as compared to 23.4 hours for the male group. At steady state, the data were similar (17.9 hours vs. 21.4 hours). This pharmacokinetic difference due to gender is likely to be of little clinical importance. There was linearity of pharmacokinetics and no appreciable difference in the C_{max} or T_{max} across genders.
Hepatic Insufficiency Following a single 15 mg dose of meloxicam there was no marked difference in plasma concentrations in subjects with mild (Child-Pugh Class I) and moderate (Child-Pugh Class II) hepatic impairment compared to healthy volunteers. Protein binding of meloxicam was not affected by hepatic insufficiency. No dose adjustment is necessary in mild to moderate hepatic insufficiency. Patients with severe hepatic impairment (Child-Pugh Class III) have not been adequately studied.
Renal Insufficiency Meloxicam pharmacokinetics have been investigated in subjects with different degrees of renal insufficiency. Total drug plasma concentrations decreased with the degree of renal impairment while free AUC values were similar. Total clearance of meloxicam increased in these patients probably due to the increase in free fraction leading to an increased metabolic clearance. There is no need for dose adjustment in patients with mild to moderate renal failure (CrCL >15 mL/min). Patients with severe renal insufficiency have not been adequately studied. The use of MOBIC in subjects with severe renal impairment is not recommended (see WARNINGS, Advanced Renal Disease).
Hemodialysis Following a single dose of meloxicam, the free C_{max} plasma concentrations were higher in patients with renal failure on chronic hemodialysis (1% free fraction) in comparison to healthy volunteers (0.3% free fraction). Hemodialysis did not lower the total drug concentration in plasma; therefore, additional doses are not necessary after hemodialysis. Meloxicam is not dialyzable.

CLINICAL TRIALS

The use of MOBIC for the treatment of the signs and symptoms of osteoarthritis of the knee and hip was evaluated in a double-blind controlled trial in the U.S. involving 464 patients treated with MOBIC for 12 weeks. MOBIC (3.75 mg, 7.5 mg and 15 mg daily) was compared to placebo. The four primary endpoints were investigator's global assessment, patient global assessment, patient pain assessment, and total WOMAC score (a self-administered questionnaire addressing pain, function and stiffness). Patients on MOBIC 7.5 mg daily and MOBIC 15 mg daily showed significant improvement in each of these endpoints compared with placebo.
The use of MOBIC for the management of signs and symptoms of osteoarthritis was evaluated in six double-blind, active-controlled trials outside the U.S. in which a total of 9589 patients were treated for 4 weeks to 6 months. In these trials, the efficacy of MOBIC, in doses of 7.5 and 15 mg/day, was comparable to piroxicam 20 mg/day and diclofenac SR 100 mg/day and consistent with the efficacy seen in the U.S. trial.

INDICATIONS AND USAGE

MOBIC is indicated for relief of the signs and symptoms of osteoarthritis.

Continued on next page

Mobic—Cont.

CONTRAINDICATIONS

MOBIC is contraindicated in patients with known hypersensitivity to meloxicam. It should not be given to patients who have experienced asthma, urticaria, or allergic-type reactions after taking aspirin or other NSAIDs. Severe, rarely fatal, anaphylactic-like reactions to NSAIDs have been reported in such patients (see WARNINGS, Anaphylactoid Reactions, and PRECAUTIONS, Pre-existing Asthma).

WARNINGS

Gastrointestinal (GI) Effects–Risk of GI Ulceration, Bleeding, and Perforation:

Serious gastrointestinal toxicity, such as inflammation, bleeding, ulceration, and perforation of the stomach, small intestine or large intestine, can occur at any time, with or without warning symptoms, in patients treated with nonsteroidal anti-inflammatory drugs (NSAIDs). Minor upper gastrointestinal problems, such as dyspepsia, are common and may also occur at any time during NSAID therapy. Therefore, physicians and patients should remain alert for ulceration and bleeding, even in the absence of previous GI symptoms. Patients should be informed about the signs and/or symptoms of serious GI toxicity and the steps to take if they occur. The utility of periodic laboratory monitoring has not been demonstrated, nor has it been adequately assessed. Only one in five patients who develop a serious upper GI adverse event on NSAID therapy is symptomatic. It has been demonstrated that upper GI ulcers, gross bleeding or perforation, caused by NSAIDs, appear to occur in approximately 1% of the patients treated for 3–6 months, and in about 2–4% of patients treated for one year. These trends continue thus, increasing the likelihood of developing a serious GI event at some time during the course of therapy. However, even short-term therapy is not without risk.

NSAIDs should be prescribed with extreme caution in those with a prior history of ulcer disease or gastrointestinal bleeding. Most spontaneous reports of fatal GI events are in elderly or debilitated patients and therefore special care should be taken in treating this population. **To minimize the potential risk for an adverse GI event, the lowest effective dose should be used for the shortest possible duration.** For high-risk patients, alternate therapies that do not involve NSAIDs should be considered.

Studies have shown that patients with a *prior history of peptic ulcer disease and/or gastrointestinal bleeding* and who use NSAIDs, have a greater than 10-fold risk for developing a GI bleed than patients with neither of these risk factors. In addition to a past history of ulcer disease, pharmacoepidemiological studies have identified several other co-therapies or co-morbid conditions that may increase the risk for GI bleeding such as: treatment with oral corticosteroids, treatment with anticoagulants, longer duration of NSAID therapy, smoking, alcoholism, older age, and poor general health status.

Anaphylactoid Reactions

As with other NSAIDs, anaphylactoid reactions have occurred in patients without known prior exposure to MOBIC. MOBIC should not be given to patients with the aspirin triad. This symptom complex typically occurs in asthmatic patients who experience rhinitis with or without nasal polyps, or who exhibit severe, potentially fatal bronchospasm after taking aspirin or other NSAIDs (see CONTRAINDICATIONS and PRECAUTIONS, Pre-existing Asthma). Emergency help should be sought in cases where an anaphylactoid reaction occurs.

Advanced Renal Disease

In cases with advanced kidney disease, treatment with MOBIC is not recommended. If NSAID therapy must be initiated, close monitoring of the patient's kidney function is advisable (see PRECAUTIONS, Renal Effects).

Pregnancy

In late pregnancy, as with other NSAIDs, MOBIC should be avoided because it may cause premature closure of the ductus arteriosus.

PRECAUTIONS

General

MOBIC cannot be expected to substitute for corticosteroids or to treat corticosteroid insufficiency. Abrupt discontinuation of corticosteroids may lead to disease exacerbation. Patients on prolonged corticosteroid therapy should have their therapy tapered slowly if a decision is made to discontinue corticosteroids.

The pharmacological activity of MOBIC in reducing inflammation and possibly fever may diminish the utility of these diagnostic signs in detecting complications of presumed noninfectious, painful conditions.

Hepatic Effects

Borderline elevations of one or more liver tests may occur in up to 15% of patients taking NSAIDs, including MOBIC. These laboratory abnormalities may progress, may remain unchanged, or may be transient with continuing therapy. Notable elevations of ALT or AST (approximately three or more times the upper limit of normal) have been reported in approximately 1% of patients in clinical trials with NSAIDs. In addition, rare cases of severe hepatic reactions, including jaundice and fatal fulminant hepatitis, liver necrosis and hepatic failure, some of them with fatal outcomes, have been reported with NSAIDs.

Patients with signs and/or symptoms suggesting liver dysfunction, or in whom an abnormal liver test has occurred, should be evaluated for evidence of the development of a more severe hepatic reaction while on therapy with MOBIC. If clinical signs and symptoms consistent with liver disease develop, or if systemic manifestations occur (e.g., eosinophilia, rash, etc.), MOBIC should be discontinued.

Table 1 Single Dose and Steady State Pharmacokinetic Parameters for Oral 7.5 and 15 mg Meloxicam (Mean and % CV)[1]

	Steady State			Single Dose	
Pharmacokinetic Parameters (% CV)	**Healthy male adults (Fed)[2]**	**Elderly males (Fed)[2]**	**Elderly females (Fed)[2]**	**Renal failure (Fasted)**	**Hepatic insufficiency (Fasted)**
	7.5 mg[3] tablets	**15 mg capsules**	**15 mg capsules**	**15 mg capsules**	**15 mg capsules**
N	**18**	**5**	**8**	**12**	**12**
C_{max} [μg/mL]	1.05 (20)	2.3 (59)	3.2 (24)	0.59 (36)	0.84 (29)
t_{max} [h]	4.9 (8)	5 (12)	6 (27)	4 (65)	10 (87)
$t_{1/2}$ [h]	20.1 (29)	21 (34)	24 (34)	18 (46)	16 (29)
CL/f [mL/min]	8.8 (29)	9.9 (76)	5.1 (22)	19 (43)	11 (44)
V_Z/f^4 [L]	14.7 (32)	15 (42)	10 (30)	26 (44)	14 (29)

[1]The parameter values in the Table are from various studies;
[2]not under high fat conditions;
[3]MOBIC tablets;
[4]$V_Z/f = Dose/(AUC \bullet K_{el})$

Table 2 Adverse Events (%) Occurring in ≥ 2% of MOBIC Patients in a 12-Week Osteoarthritis Placebo and Active-Controlled Trial

	Placebo	MOBIC 7.5 mg daily	MOBIC 15 mg daily	Diclofenac 100 mg daily
No. of Patients	**157**	**154**	**156**	**153**
Gastrointestinal	17.2	20.1	17.3	28.1
Abdominal Pain	2.5	1.9	2.6	1.3
Diarrhea	3.8	7.8	3.2	9.2
Dyspepsia	4.5	4.5	4.5	6.5
Flatulence	4.5	3.2	3.2	3.9
Nausea	3.2	3.9	3.8	7.2
Body as a Whole				
Accident Household	1.9	4.5	3.2	2.6
Edema[1]	2.5	1.9	4.5	3.3
Fall	0.6	2.6	0.0	1.3
Influenza-Like Symptoms	5.1	4.5	5.8	2.6
Central and Peripheral Nervous System				
Dizziness	3.2	2.6	3.8	2.0
Headache	10.2	7.8	8.3	5.9
Respiratory				
Pharyngitis	1.3	0.6	3.2	1.3
Upper Respiratory Tract Infection	1.9	3.2	1.9	3.3
Skin				
Rash[2]	2.5	2.6	0.6	2.0

[1]WHO preferred terms edema, edema dependent, edema peripheral and edema legs combined
[2]WHO preferred terms rash, rash erythematous and rash maculo-papular combined

Renal Effects

Caution should be used when initiating treatment with MOBIC in patients with considerable dehydration. It is advisable to rehydrate patients first and then start therapy with MOBIC. Caution is also recommended in patients with pre-existing kidney disease (see WARNINGS, Advanced Renal Disease).

Long-term administration of NSAIDs has resulted in renal papillary necrosis and other renal medullary changes. Renal toxicity has also been seen in patients in whom renal prostaglandins have a compensatory role in the maintenance of renal perfusion. In these patients, administration of NSAIDs may cause dose-dependent reduction in prostaglandin formation and, secondarily, in renal blood flow, which may precipitate overt renal decompensation. Patients at greatest risk of this reaction are those with impaired renal function, heart failure, liver dysfunction, those taking diuretics and ACE inhibitors, and the elderly. Discontinuation of NSAID therapy is usually followed by recovery to the pretreatment state.

The extent to which metabolites may accumulate in patients with renal failure has not been studied with MOBIC. Because some MOBIC metabolites are excreted by the kidney, patients with significantly impaired renal function should be more closely monitored.

Hematological Effects

Anemia is sometimes seen in patients receiving NSAIDs, including MOBIC. This may be due to fluid retention, GI blood loss, or an incompletely described effect upon erythropoiesis. Patients on long-term treatment with NSAIDs, including MOBIC, should have their hemoglobin or hematocrit checked if they exhibit any signs or symptoms of anemia.

Drugs which inhibit the biosynthesis of prostaglandins may interfere to some extent with platelet function and vascular responses to bleeding.

NSAIDs inhibit platelet aggregation and have been shown to prolong bleeding time in some patients. Unlike aspirin their effect on platelet function is quantitatively less, or of shorter duration, and reversible. MOBIC does not generally affect platelet counts, prothrombin time (PT), or partial thromboplastin time (PTT). Patients receiving MOBIC who may be adversely affected by alterations in platelet function, such as those with coagulation disorders or patients receiving anticoagulants, should be carefully monitored.

Fluid Retention and Edema

Fluid retention and edema have been observed in some patients taking NSAIDs, including MOBIC. Therefore, as with other NSAIDs, MOBIC should be used with caution in patients with fluid retention, hypertension, or heart failure.

Pre-existing Asthma

Patients with asthma may have aspirin-sensitive asthma. The use of aspirin in patients with aspirin-sensitive asthma has been associated with severe bronchospasm which can be fatal. Since cross reactivity, including bronchospasm, between aspirin and other nonsteroidal anti-inflammatory drugs has been reported in such aspirin-sensitive patients, MOBIC should not be administered to patients with this form of aspirin sensitivity and should be used with caution in patients with pre-existing asthma.

Information for Patients

MOBIC, like other drugs of its class, can cause discomfort and, rarely, more serious side effects, such as gastrointestinal bleeding, which may result in hospitalization and even fatal outcomes. Although serious GI tract ulcerations and bleeding can occur without warning symptoms, patients should be alert for the signs and symptoms of ulcerations and bleeding, and should ask for medical advice when observing any indicative signs or symptoms. Patients should be made aware of the importance of this follow-up (see WARNINGS, Gastrointestinal (GI) Effects—Risk of GI Ulceration, Bleeding and Perforation).

Patients should report to their physicians signs or symptoms of gastrointestinal ulceration or bleeding, skin rash, weight gain, or edema.

Patients should be informed of the warning signs and symptoms of hepatotoxicity (e.g., nausea, fatigue, lethargy, pruritus, jaundice, right upper quadrant tenderness, and "flu-like" symptoms). If these occur, patients should be instructed to stop therapy and seek immediate medical therapy.

Patients should also be instructed to seek immediate emergency help in the case of an anaphylactoid reaction (see WARNINGS, Anaphylactoid Reactions).

In late pregnancy, as with other NSAIDs, MOBIC should be avoided because it may cause premature closure of the ductus arteriosus.

Laboratory Tests

Patients on long-term treatment with NSAIDs should have their CBC and a chemistry profile checked periodically. If clinical signs and symptoms consistent with liver or renal disease develop, systemic manifestations occur (e.g., eosinophilia, rash, etc.) or if abnormal liver tests persist or worsen, MOBIC should be discontinued.

Drug Interactions

ACE inhibitors Reports suggest that NSAIDs may diminish the antihypertensive effect of angiotensin-converting enzyme (ACE) inhibitors. This interaction should be given consideration in patients taking NSAIDs concomitantly with ACE inhibitors.

Aspirin Concomitant administration of aspirin (1000 mg TID) to healthy volunteers tended to increase the AUC (10%) and C_{max} (24%) of meloxicam. The clinical significance of this interaction is not known; however, as with other NSAIDs, concomitant administration of meloxicam and aspirin is not generally recommended because of the potential for increased adverse effects. Concomitant administration of low-dose aspirin with MOBIC may result in an increased rate of GI ulceration or other complications, compared to use of MOBIC alone. MOBIC is not a substitute for aspirin for cardiovascular prophylaxis.

Cholestyramine Pretreatment for four days with cholestyramine significantly increased the clearance of meloxicam by 50%. This resulted in a decrease in $t_{1/2}$, from 19.2 hours to 12.5 hours, and a 35% reduction in AUC. This suggests the existence of a recirculation pathway for meloxicam in the gastrointestinal tract. The clinical relevance of this interaction has not been established.

Cimetidine Concomitant administration of 200 mg cimetidine QID did not alter the single-dose pharmacokinetics of 30 mg meloxicam.

Digoxin Meloxicam 15 mg once daily for 7 days did not alter the plasma concentration profile of digoxin after β-acetyldigoxin administration for 7 days at clinical doses. *In vitro* testing found no protein binding drug interaction between digoxin and meloxicam.

Furosemide Clinical studies, as well as post-marketing observations, have shown that NSAIDs can reduce the natriuretic effect of furosemide and thiazide diuretics in some patients. This effect has been attributed to inhibition of renal prostaglandin synthesis. Studies with furosemide agents and meloxicam have not demonstrated a reduction in natriuretic effect. Furosemide single and multiple dose pharmacodynamics and pharmacokinetics are not affected by multiple doses of meloxicam. Nevertheless, during concomitant therapy with furosemide and MOBIC, patients should be observed closely for signs of declining renal function (see PRECAUTIONS, Renal Effects), as well as to assure diuretic efficacy.

Lithium In clinical trials, NSAIDs have produced an elevation of plasma lithium levels and a reduction in renal lithium clearance. In a study conducted in healthy subjects, mean pre-dose lithium concentration and AUC were increased by 21% in subjects receiving lithium doses ranging from 804 to 1072 mg BID with meloxicam 15 mg QD as compared to subjects receiving lithium alone. These effects have been attributed to inhibition of renal prostaglandin synthesis by MOBIC. Patients on lithium treatment should be closely monitored when MOBIC is introduced or withdrawn.

Methotrexate A study in 13 rheumatoid arthritis (RA) patients evaluated the effects of multiple doses of meloxicam on the pharmacokinetics of methotrexate taken once weekly. Meloxicam did not have a significant effect on the pharmacokinetics of single doses of methotrexate. *In vitro*, methotrexate did not displace meloxicam from its human serum binding sites.

Warfarin Anticoagulant activity should be monitored, particularly in the first few days after initiating or changing MOBIC therapy in patients receiving warfarin or similar agents, since these patients are at an increased risk of bleeding. The effect of meloxicam on the anticoagulant effect of warfarin was studied in a group of healthy subjects receiving daily doses of warfarin that produced an INR (International Normalized Ratio) between 1.2 and 1.8. In these subjects, meloxicam did not alter warfarin pharmacokinetics and the average anticoagulant effect of warfarin as determined by prothrombin time. However, one subject showed an increase in INR from 1.5 to 2.1. Caution should be used when administering MOBIC with warfarin since patients on warfarin may experience changes in INR and an increased risk of bleeding complications when a new medication is introduced.

Carcinogenesis, Mutagenesis, Impairment of Fertility

No carcinogenic effect of meloxicam was observed in rats given oral doses up to 0.8 mg/kg/day (approximately 0.4-fold the human dose at 15 mg/day for a 50 kg adult based on body surface area conversion) for 104 weeks or in mice given oral doses up to 8.0 mg/kg/day (approximately 2.2-fold the human dose, as noted above) for 99 weeks.

Meloxicam was not mutagenic in an Ames assay, or clastogenic in a chromosome aberration assay with human lymphocytes and an *in vivo* micronucleus test in mouse bone marrow.

Meloxicam did not impair male and female fertility in rats at oral doses up to 9 and 5 mg/kg/day, respectively (4.9-fold and 2.5-fold the human dose, as noted above). However, an increased incidence of embryolethality at oral doses ≥ 1 mg/kg/day (0.5-fold the human dose, as noted above) was observed in rats when dams were given meloxicam 2 weeks prior to mating and during early embryonic development.

Table 3 Adverse Events (%) Occurring in ≥ 2% of MOBIC Patients in 4 to 6 Weeks and 6 Month Active-Controlled Osteoarthritis Trials

	4–6 Weeks Controlled Trials		6 Month Controlled Trials	
	MOBIC 7.5 mg daily	MOBIC 15 mg daily	MOBIC 7.5 mg daily	MOBIC 15 mg daily
No. of Patients	**8955**	**256**	**169**	**306**
Gastrointestinal	11.8	18.0	26.6	24.2
Abdominal Pain	2.7	2.3	4.7	2.9
Constipation	0.8	1.2	1.8	2.6
Diarrhea	1.9	2.7	5.9	2.6
Dyspepsia	3.8	7.4	8.9	9.5
Flatulence	0.5	0.4	3.0	2.6
Nausea	2.4	4.7	4.7	7.2
Vomiting	0.6	0.8	1.8	2.6
Body as a Whole				
Edema[1]	0.6	2.0	2.4	1.6
Pain	0.9	2.0	3.6	5.2
Central and Peripheral Nervous System				
Dizziness	1.1	1.6	2.4	2.6
Headache	2.4	2.7	3.6	2.6
Hematologic				
Anemia	0.1	0.0	4.1	2.9
Musculo-Skeletal				
Arthralgia	0.5	0.0	5.3	1.3
Back Pain	0.5	0.4	3.0	0.7
Psychiatric				
Insomnia	0.4	0.0	3.6	1.6
Respiratory				
Coughing	0.2	0.8	2.4	1.0
Upper Respiratory Tract Infection	0.2	0.0	8.3	7.5
Skin				
Pruritus	0.4	1.2	2.4	0.0
Rash[2]	0.3	1.2	3.0	1.3
Urinary				
Micturition Frequency	0.1	0.4	2.4	1.3
Urinary Tract Infection	0.3	0.4	4.7	6.9

[1]WHO preferred terms edema, edema dependent, edema peripheral and edema legs combined
[2]WHO preferred terms rash, rash erythematous and rash maculo-papular combined

Pregnancy

Teratogenic Effects: Pregnancy Category C.

Meloxicam caused an increased incidence of septal defect of the heart, a rare event, at an oral dose of 60 mg/kg/day (64.5-fold the human dose at 15 mg/day for a 50 kg adult based on body surface area conversion) and embryolethality at oral doses ≥ 5 mg/kg/day (5.4-fold the human dose, as noted above) when rabbits were treated throughout organogenesis. Meloxicam was not teratogenic in rats up to an oral dose of 4 mg/kg/day (approximately 2.2-fold the human dose, as noted above) throughout organogenesis. An increased incidence of stillbirths was observed when rats were given oral doses ≥ 1 mg/kg/day throughout organogenesis. Meloxicam crosses the placental barrier. There are no adequate and well-controlled studies in pregnant women. MOBIC should be used during pregnancy only if the potential benefit justifies the potential risk to the fetus.

Nonteratogenic Effects: Meloxicam caused a reduction in birth index, live births, and neonatal survival at oral doses ≥ 0.125 mg/kg/day (approximately 0.07-fold the human dose at 15 mg/day for a 50 kg adult based on body surface area conversion) when rats were treated during the late gestation and lactation period. No studies have been conducted to evaluate the effect of meloxicam on the closure of the ductus arteriosus in humans; use of meloxicam during the third trimester of pregnancy should be avoided.

Labor and Delivery

Studies in rats with meloxicam, as with other drugs known to inhibit prostaglandin synthesis, showed an increased incidence of stillbirths, increased length of delivery time, and delayed parturition at oral dosages ≥ 1 mg/kg/day (approximately 0.5-fold the human dose at 15 mg/day for a 50 kg adult based on body surface area conversion), and decreased pup survival at an oral dose of 4 mg/kg/day (approximately 2.1-fold the human dose, as noted above) throughout organogenesis. Similar findings were observed in rats receiving oral dosages ≥ 0.125 mg/kg/day (approximately 0.07-fold the human dose, as noted above) during late gestation and the lactation period.

Nursing Mothers

Studies of meloxicam excretion in human milk have not been conducted; however, meloxicam was excreted in the milk of lactating rats at concentrations higher than those in plasma. Because of the potential for serious adverse reactions in nursing infants from MOBIC, a decision should be made whether to discontinue nursing or to discontinue the drug, taking into account the importance of the drug to the mother.

Pediatric Use

Safety and effectiveness in pediatric patients under 18 years of age have not been established.

Geriatric Use

As with any NSAID, caution should be exercised in treating the elderly (65 years and older).

ADVERSE REACTIONS

The MOBIC phase 2/3 clinical trial database includes 10,122 patients treated with MOBIC 7.5 mg/day and 3,505 patients treated with MOBIC 15 mg/day. MOBIC at these doses was administered to 661 patients for at least 6 months and to 312 patients for at least one year. Approximately 10,500 of these patients were treated in ten placebo and/or active-controlled osteoarthritis trials. Gastrointestinal (GI) adverse events were the most frequently reported adverse events in all treatment groups across MOBIC trials.

A 12-week multicenter, double-blind, randomized trial was conducted in patients with osteoarthritis of the knee or hip to compare the efficacy and safety of MOBIC with placebo and with an active control. Table 2 depicts adverse events that occurred in ≥ 2% of the MOBIC treatment groups.

[See table 2 on previous page]

The adverse events that occurred with MOBIC in ≥ 2% of patients treated short-term (4–6 weeks) and long-term (6 months) in active-controlled osteoarthritis trials are presented in Table 3.

[See table 3 above]

As with other NSAIDs, higher doses of MOBIC (e.g., chronic daily 30 mg dose) were associated with an increased risk of serious GI events, therefore the daily dose of MOBIC should not exceed 15 mg.

The following is a list of adverse drug reactions occurring in < 2% of patients receiving MOBIC in clinical trials involving approximately 15,400 patients. Adverse reactions reported only in worldwide post-marketing experience or the literature are shown in italics and are considered rare (< 0.1%).

Body as a Whole: allergic reaction, *anaphylactoid reactions including shock,* face edema, fatigue, fever, hot flushes, malaise, syncope, weight decrease, weight increase **Cardiovascular:** angina pectoris, cardiac failure, hypertension, hypotension, myocardial infarction, vasculitis **Central and Peripheral Nervous System:** convulsions, paresthesia, tremor, vertigo **Gastrointestinal:** colitis, dry mouth, duodenal ulcer, eructation, esophagitis, gastric ulcer, gastritis, gastroesophageal reflux, gastrointestinal hemorrhage, hematemesis, hemorrhagic duodenal ulcer, hemorrhagic gastric ulcer, intestinal perforation, melena, pancreatitis, perforated duodenal ulcer, perforated gastric ulcer, stomatitis ulcerative **Heart Rate and Rhythm:** arrhythmia, palpitation, tachycar-

Continued on next page

Mobic—Cont.

dia **Hematologic:** *agranulocytosis,* leukopenia, purpura, thrombocytopenia **Liver and Biliary System:** ALT increased, AST increased, bilirubinemia, GGT increased, hepatitis, *jaundice, liver failure* **Metabolic and Nutritional:** dehydration **Psychiatric Disorders:** abnormal dreaming, anxiety, appetite increased, confusion, depression, nervousness, somnolence **Respiratory:** asthma, bronchospasm, dyspnea **Skin and Appendages:** alopecia, angioedema, bullous eruption, *erythema multiforme,* photosensitivity reaction, pruritus, *Stevens-Johnson syndrome,* sweating increased, *toxic epidermal necrolysis,* urticaria **Special Senses:** abnormal vision, conjunctivitis, taste perversion, tinnitus **Urinary System:** albuminuria, BUN increased, creatinine increased, hematuria, *interstitial nephritis,* renal failure.

OVERDOSAGE

There is limited experience with meloxicam overdose. Four cases have taken 6 to 11 times the highest recommended dose; all recovered. Cholestyramine is known to accelerate the clearance of meloxicam.

Symptoms following acute NSAID overdose are usually limited to lethargy, drowsiness, nausea, vomiting, and epigastric pain, which are generally reversible with supportive care. Gastrointestinal bleeding can occur. Severe poisoning may result in hypertension, acute renal failure, hepatic dysfunction, respiratory depression, coma, convulsions, cardiovascular collapse, and cardiac arrest. Anaphylactoid reactions have been reported with therapeutic ingestion of NSAIDs, and may occur following an overdose.

Patients should be managed with symptomatic and supportive care following an NSAID overdose. In cases of acute overdose, gastric lavage followed by activated charcoal is recommended. Gastric lavage performed more than one hour after overdose has little benefit in the treatment of overdose. Administration of activated charcoal is recommended for patients who present 1–2 hours after overdose. For substantial overdose or severely symptomatic patients, activated charcoal may be administered repeatedly. Accelerated removal of meloxicam by 4 gm oral doses of cholestyramine given three times a day was demonstrated in a clinical trial. Administration of cholestyramine may be useful following an overdose. Forced diuresis, alkalinization of urine, hemodialysis, or hemoperfusion may not be useful due to high protein binding.

DOSAGE AND ADMINISTRATION

The lowest dose of MOBIC should be sought for each patient. For the treatment of osteoarthritis the recommended starting and maintenance dose of MOBIC is 7.5 mg once daily. Some patients may receive additional benefit by increasing the dose to 15 mg once daily. The maximum recommended daily dose of MOBIC is 15 mg.

MOBIC may be taken without regard to timing of meals.

HOW SUPPLIED

MOBIC is available as a yellow, round, biconvex, uncoated tablet containing meloxicam 7.5 mg. The tablet is impressed with the Boehringer Ingelheim logo on one side, and on the other side, the letter "M". MOBIC is available as follows:

NDC 0597-0029-30; Bottles of 30
NDC 0597-0029-01; Bottles of 100
NDC 0597-0029-61; Unit dose packages of 100 (10 blister cards of 10 tablets each)

Store at 25°C (77°F); excursions permitted to 15°C–30°C (59°F–86°F). Keep in a dry place.

Dispense in a tight container.

Rx only MB-PI-4058550/US/4

Manufactured by:
Boehringer Ingelheim Pharma KG
Ingelheim, Germany

Marketed by:
Boehringer Ingelheim Pharmaceuticals, Inc.
Ridgefield, CT 06877, USA
and
Abbott Laboratories
North Chicago, IL 60064, USA

Licensed from:
Boehringer Ingelheim International GmbH

Shown in Product Identification Guide, page 309

PERSANTINE® Tablets ℞

[per-san 'tēn]
(dipyridamole USP)

Tablets of 25 mg .... BI-CODE 17
Tablets of 50 mg .... BI-CODE 18
Tablets of 75 mg .... BI-CODE 19

Prescribing Information

DESCRIPTION Dipyridamole USP is a platelet inhibitor chemically described as 2,6-bis-(diethanolamino)-4,8-dipiperidino-pyrimido-(5,4-d) pyrimidine. It has the following structural formula:

[See chemical structure at top of next column]

Dipyridamole is an odorless yellow crystalline powder, having a bitter taste. It is soluble in dilute acids, methanol and chloroform, and practically insoluble in water.

PERSANTINE tablets for oral administration contain:

Active Ingredient *TABLETS 25, 50, and 75 mg:* dipyridamole USP 25, 50, and 75 mg respectively.

$C_{24}H_{40}N_8O_4$ Mol. Wt. 504.63

Inactive Ingredients *TABLETS 25, 50, and 75 mg:* acacia, carnauba wax, corn starch, FD&C blue No. 1 aluminum lake, D&C yellow No. 10 aluminum lake, D&C red No. 30 aluminum lake, lactose, magnesium stearate, polyethylene glycol, povidone, shellac, sodium benzoate, sucrose, talc, titanium dioxide, white wax.

CLINICAL PHARMACOLOGY It is believed that platelet reactivity and interaction with prosthetic cardiac valve surfaces, resulting in abnormally shortened platelet survival time, is a significant factor in thromboembolic complications occurring in connection with prosthetic heart valve replacement.

PERSANTINE tablets have been found to lengthen abnormally shortened platelet survival time in a dose-dependent manner.

In three randomized controlled clinical trials involving 854 patients who had undergone surgical placement of a prosthetic heart valve, PERSANTINE tablets, in combination with warfarin, decreased the incidence of postoperative thromboembolic events by 62 to 91% compared to warfarin treatment alone. The incidence of thromboembolic events in patients receiving the combination of PERSANTINE tablets and warfarin ranged from 1.2 to 1.8%. In three additional studies involving 392 patients taking PERSANTINE tablets and coumarin-like anticoagulants, the incidence of thromboembolic events ranged from 2.3 to 6.9%.

In these trials, the coumarin anticoagulant was begun between 24 hours and 4 days postoperatively, and the PERSANTINE tablets were begun between 24 hours and 10 days postoperatively. The length of follow-up in these trials varied from 1 to 2 years.

PERSANTINE tablets do not influence prothrombin time or activity measurements when administered with warfarin.

Mechanism of Action Dipyridamole is a platelet adhesion inhibitor, although the mechanism of action has not been fully elucidated. The mechanism may relate to inhibition of red blood cell uptake of adenosine, itself an inhibitor of platelet reactivity, phosphodiesterase inhibition leading to increased cyclic-3', 5'-adenosine monophosphate within platelets, and inhibition of thromboxane A_2 formation which is a potent stimulator of platelet activation.

Hemodynamics In dogs intraduodenal doses of dipyridamole of 0.5 to 4.0 mg/kg produced dose-related decreases in systemic and coronary vascular resistance leading to decreases in systemic blood pressure and increases in coronary blood flow. Onset of action was in about 24 minutes and effects persisted for about 3 hours.

Similar effects were observed following IV PERSANTINE in doses ranging from 0.025 to 2.0 mg/kg.

In man the same qualitative hemodynamic effects have been observed. However, acute intravenous administration of PERSANTINE may worsen regional myocardial perfusion distal to partial occlusion of coronary arteries.

Pharmacokinetics and Metabolism Following an oral dose of PERSANTINE tablets, the average time to peak concentration is about 75 minutes. The decline in plasma concentration following a dose of PERSANTINE tablets fits a two-compartment model. The alpha half-life (the initial decline following peak concentration) is approximately 40 minutes. The beta half-life (the terminal decline in plasma concentration) is approximately 10 hours. Dipyridamole is highly bound to plasma proteins. It is metabolized in the liver where it is conjugated as a glucuronide and excreted with the bile.

INDICATIONS AND USAGE PERSANTINE tablets are indicated as an adjunct to coumarin anticoagulants in the prevention of postoperative thromboembolic complications of cardiac valve replacement.

CONTRAINDICATIONS None known.

PRECAUTIONS General PERSANTINE tables should be used with caution in patients with hypotension since it can produce peripheral vasodilation.

Carcinogenesis, Mutagenesis, Impairment of Fertility In a 111 week oral study in mice and in a 128-142 week oral study in rats, dipyridamole USP produced no significant carcinogenic effects at doses of 8, 25 and 75 mg/kg (1, 3.1 and 9.4 times the maximum recommended daily human dose). Mutagenicity testing with dipyridamole was negative. Reproduction studies with dipyridamole revealed no evidence of impaired fertility in rats at dosages up to 60 times the maximum recommended human dose. A significant reduction in number of corpora lutea with consequent reduction in implantations and live fetuses was, however, observed at 155 times the maximum recommended human dose.

Teratogenic Effects *PREGNANCY CATEGORY B* Reproduction studies have been performed in mice at doses up to 125 mg/kg (15.6 times the maximum recommended daily human dose), rats at doses up to 1000 mg/kg (125 times the maximum recommended daily human dose) and rabbits at doses up to 40 mg/kg (5 times the maximum recommended daily human dose) and have revealed no evidence of harm to the fetus due to dipyridamole. There are, however, no adequate and well-controlled studies in pregnant women. Because animal reproduction studies are not always predictive of human response, this drug should be used during pregnancy only if clearly needed.

Nursing Mothers As dipyridamole is excreted in human milk, caution should be exercised when PERSANTINE® (dipyridamole USP) tablets are administered to a nursing woman.

Pediatric Use Safety and effectiveness in the pediatric population below the age of 12 years has not been established.

ADVERSE REACTIONS Adverse reactions at therapeutic doses are usually minimal and transient. On long-term use of PERSANTINE tablets initial side effects usually disappear. The following reactions were reported in two heart valve replacement trials comparing PERSANTINE tablets and warfarin therapy to either warfarin alone or warfarin and placebo:

	Persantine tablets/ Warfarin (N=147)	Placebo/ Warfarin (N=170)
Dizziness	13.6%	8.2%
Abdominal distress	6.1%	3.5%
Headache	2.3%	0.0
Rash	2.3%	1.1%

Other reactions from uncontrolled studies include diarrhea, vomiting, flushing and pruritus. In addition, angina pectoris has been reported rarely and there have been rare reports of liver dysfunction. On those uncommon occasions when adverse reactions have been persistent or intolerable, they have ceased on withdrawal of the medication.

When PERSANTINE tablets were administered concomitantly with warfarin, bleeding was no greater in frequency or severity than that observed when warfarin was administered alone.

In postmarketing reporting experience, there have been rare reports of larynx edema, fatigue, malaise, myalgia, arthritis, nausea, dyspepsia, paresthesia, hepatitis, alopecia, cholelithiasis, palpitation, and tachycardia.

OVERDOSAGE Hypotension, if it occurs, is likely to be of short duration, but a vasopressor drug may be used if necessary. The oral LD_{50} in mice is 2,150 mg/kg. Single oral doses of 6,000 mg/kg in rats and 350 mg/kg in dogs were lethal. Symptoms of acute toxicity included ataxia, decreased locomotion and diarrhea in rodents and emesis, ataxia and depression in dogs. Since PERSANTINE tablets are highly protein bound, dialysis is not likely to be of benefit.

DOSAGE AND ADMINISTRATION *Adjunctive Use in Prophylaxis of Thromboembolism after Cardiac Valve Replacement.* The recommended dose is 75-100 mg four times daily as an adjunct to the usual warfarin therapy. Please note that aspirin is not to be administered concomitantly with coumarin anticoagulants.

HOW SUPPLIED PERSANTINE tablets are available as round, orange, sugar-coated tablets of 25 mg, 50 mg and 75 mg coded BI/17, BI/18 and BI/19 respectively.

They are available in the following package sizes:

25 mg Tablets
Bottles of 100 (NDC 0597-0017-01)
Bottles of 1000 (NDC 0597-0017-10)
Unit Dose Packages of 100 (NDC 0597-0017-61)
50 mg Tablets
Bottles of 100 (NDC 0597-0018-01)
Bottles of 1000 (NDC 0597-0018-10)
Unit Dose Packages of 100 (NDC 0597-0018-61)
75 mg Tablets
Bottles of 100 (NDC 0597-0019-01)
Bottles of 500 (NDC 0597-0019-05)
Unit Dose Packages of 100 (NDC 0597-0019-61)

Store below 86°F (30°C).

Caution: Federal law prohibits dispensing without prescription.

PE-PI-10/97 Rev

Boehringer Ingelheim
Pharmaceuticals, Inc.
Ridgefield, CT 06877

Licensed from
Boehringer Ingelheim
International GmbH

Shown in Product Identification Guide, page 309

SERENTIL® ℞

[seh-ren 'til]
(mesoridazine besylate) USP

Tablets, 10 mg .... BI-CODE 20
Tablets, 25 mg .... BI-CODE 21
Tablets, 50 mg .... BI-CODE 22
Tablets, 100 mg .... BI-CODE 23
Concentrate of 25 mg/ml .... BI-CODE 25
Ampuls of 1 ml (25 mg) .... BI-CODE 27
Rx only

Prescribing Information
CAUTION:
Federal law prohibits dispensing without prescription.

DESCRIPTION

Serentil® (mesoridazine besylate), the besylate salt of a metabolite of thioridazine, is a phenothiazine tranquilizer which is effective in the treatment of schizophrenia, organic brain disorders, alcoholism and psychoneuroses. Serentil® (mesoridazine besylate) is 10-[2(1-methyl-2-piperidyl) ethyl]-2-(methyl-sulfinyl)-phenothiazine [as the besylate].

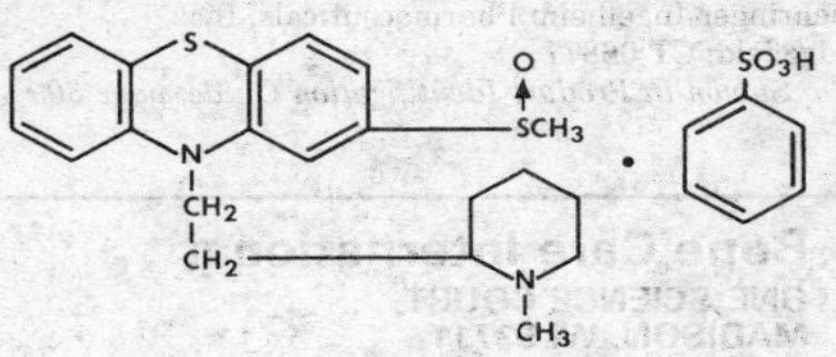

Tablet, 10 mg, for oral administration
ACTIVE INGREDIENT: mesoridazine (as the besylate), 10 mg. *INACTIVE INGREDIENTS*: acacia, carnauba wax, colloidal silicon dioxide, FD&C Red No. 40 aluminum lake, lactose, microcrystalline cellulose, povidone, sodium benzoate, starch, stearic acid, sucrose, synthetic black iron oxide, talc, titanium dioxide and other ingredients.

Tablet, 25 mg, for oral administration
ACTIVE INGREDIENT: mesoridazine (as the besylate), 25 mg. *INACTIVE INGREDIENTS*: acacia, carnauba wax, colloidal silicon dioxide, FD&C Red No. 40 aluminum lake, lactose, microcrystalline cellulose, povidone, sodium benzoate, stearic acid, sucrose, synthetic black iron oxide, talc, titanium dioxide and other ingredients.

Tablet, 50 mg, for oral administration
ACTIVE INGREDIENT: mesoridazine (as the besylate), 50 mg. *INACTIVE INGREDIENTS*: acacia, carnauba wax, colloidal silicon dioxide, FD&C Red No. 40 aluminum lake, gelatin, lactose, microcrystalline cellulose, povidone, sodium benzoate, starch, stearic acid, sucrose, synthetic black iron oxide, talc, titanium dioxide and other ingredients.

Tablet, 100 mg, for oral administration
ACTIVE INGREDIENT: mesoridazine (as the besylate), 100 mg. *INACTIVE INGREDIENTS*: acacia, carnauba wax, colloidal silicon dioxide, FD&C Red No. 40 aluminum lake, gelatin, lactose, microcrystalline cellulose, povidone, sodium benzoate, starch, stearic acid, sucrose, synthetic black iron oxide, talc, titanium dioxide and other ingredients.

Ampuls, 1 mL, for intramuscular administration
ACTIVE INGREDIENT: mesoridazine (as the besylate), 25 mg. *INACTIVE INGREDIENTS*: edetate disodium USP, 0.5 mg; sodium chloride USP, 7.2 mg; carbon dioxide gas (bone dry) q.s., water for injection USP, q.s. to 1 ml.

Concentrate, for oral administration
ACTIVE INGREDIENT: mesoridazine (as the besylate), 25 mg per mL. *INACTIVE INGREDIENTS*: alcohol, 0.61% by volume; citric acid; FD&C Red No. 40; flavors; methylparaben; propylparaben; purified water; sodium citrate, sorbitol.

ACTIONS

Based upon animal studies, Serentil® (mesoridazine besylate), as with other phenothiazines, acts indirectly on reticular formation, whereby neuronal activity into reticular formation is reduced without affecting its intrinsic ability to activate the cerebral cortex. In addition, the phenothiazines exhibit at least part of their activities through depression of hypothalamic centers. Neurochemically, the phenothiazines are thought to exert their effects by a central adrenergic blocking action.

INDICATIONS

In clinical studies Serentil® (mesoridazine besylate) has been found useful in the following disease states:

Schizophrenia Serentil® (mesoridazine besylate) is effective in the treatment of schizophrenia. It substantially reduces the severity of emotional withdrawal, conceptual disorganization, anxiety, tension, hallucinatory behavior, suspiciousness and blunted affect in schizophrenic patients. As with other phenothiazines, patients refractory to previous medication may respond to Serentil® (mesoridazine besylate).

Behavioral Problems in Mental Deficiency and Chronic Brain Syndrome The effect of Serentil® (mesoridazine besylate) was found to be excellent or good in the management of hyperactivity and uncooperativeness associated with mental deficiency and chronic brain syndrome.

Alcoholism—Acute and Chronic Serentil® (mesoridazine besylate) ameliorates anxiety, tension, depression, nausea and vomiting in both acute and chronic alcoholics without producing hepatic dysfunction or hindering the functional recovery of the impaired liver.

Psychoneurotic Manifestations Serentil® (mesoridazine besylate) reduces the symptoms of anxiety and tension, prevalent symptoms often associated with neurotic components of many disorders, and benefits personality disorders in general.

CONTRAINDICATIONS

As with other phenothiazines, Serentil® (mesoridazine besylate) is contraindicated in severe central nervous system depression or comatose states from any cause including drug induced central nervous system depression (see WARNINGS).

Serentil® (mesoridazine besylate) is contraindicated in individuals who have previously shown hypersensitivity to the drug.

WARNINGS

Tardive Dyskinesia Tardive dyskinesia, a syndrome consisting of potentially irreversible, involuntary, dyskinetic movements may develop in patients treated with neuroleptic (antipsychotic) drugs. Although the prevalence of the syndrome appears to be highest among the elderly, especially elderly women, it is impossible to rely upon prevalence estimates to predict, at the inception of neuroleptic treatment, which patients are likely to develop the syndrome. Whether neuroleptic drug products differ in their potential to cause tardive dyskinesia is unknown.

Both the risk of developing the syndrome and the likelihood that it will become irreversible are believed to increase as the duration of treatment and the total cumulative dose of neuroleptic drugs administered to the patient increase. However, the syndrome can develop, although much less commonly, after relatively brief treatment periods at low doses.

There is no known treatment for established cases of tardive dyskinesia, although the syndrome may remit, partially or completely, if neuroleptic treatment is withdrawn. Neuroleptic treatment itself, however, may suppress (or partially suppress) the signs and symptoms of the syndrome and thereby may possibly mask the underlying disease process. The effect that symptomatic suppression has upon the long-term course of the syndrome is unknown.

Given these considerations, neuroleptics should be prescribed in a manner that is most likely to minimize the occurrence of tardive dyskinesia. Chronic neuroleptic treatment should generally be reserved for patients who suffer from a chronic illness 1) that is known to respond to neuroleptic drugs, and 2) for which alternative, equally effective but potentially less harmful treatments are *not* available or appropriate. In patients who do require chronic treatment, the smallest dose and the shortest duration of treatment producing a satisfactory clinical response should be sought. The need for continued treatment should be reassessed periodically.

If signs and symptoms of tardive dyskinesia appear in a patient on neuroleptics, drug discontinuation should be considered. However, some patients may require treatment despite the presence of the syndrome.

(For further information about the description of tardive dyskinesia and its clinical detection, please refer to the sections on Information for Patients and Adverse Reactions).

Neuroleptic Malignant Syndrome (NMS) A potentially fatal symptom complex sometimes referred to as Neuroleptic Malignant Syndrome (NMS) has been reported in association with antipsychotic drugs. Clinical manifestations of NMS are hyperpyrexia, muscle rigidity, altered mental status and evidence of autonomic instability (irregular pulse or blood pressure, tachycardia, diaphoresis, and cardiac dysrhythmias).

The diagnostic evaluation of patients with this syndrome is complicated. In arriving at a diagnosis, it is important to identify cases where the clinical presentation includes both serious medical illness (e.g., pneumonia, systemic infection, etc.) and untreated or inadequately treated extrapyramidal signs and symptoms (EPS). Other important considerations in the differential diagnosis include central anticholinergic toxicity, heat stroke, drug fever and primary central nervous system (CNS) pathology.

The management of NMS should include 1) immediate discontinuation of antipsychotic drugs and other drugs not essential to concurrent therapy, 2) intensive symptomatic treatment and medical monitoring, and 3) treatment of any concomitant serious medical problems for which specific treatments are available. There is no general agreement about specific pharmacological treatment regimens for uncomplicated NMS.

If a patient requires antipsychotic drug treatment after recovery from NMS, the potential reintroduction of drug therapy should be carefully considered. The patient should be carefully monitored, since recurrences of NMS have been reported.

Where patients are participating in activities requiring complete mental alertness, (e.g., driving) it is advisable to administer the phenothiazines cautiously and to increase the dosage gradually.

Central Nervous System Depressants As in the case of other phenothiazines, Serentil® (mesoridazine besylate) is capable of potentiating central nervous system depressants (e.g., alcohol, anesthetics, barbiturates, narcotics, opiates, other psychoactive drugs, etc.) as well as atropine and phosphorus insecticides. Severe respiratory depression and respiratory arrest have been reported when a patient was given Serentil® (mesoridazine besylate) and a concomitant high dose of a barbiturate.

Usage in Pregnancy The safety of this drug in pregnancy has not been established; hence, it should be given only when the anticipated benefits to be derived from treatment exceed the possible risks to mother and fetus.

Usage in Children The use of Serentil® (mesoridazinebesylate) in children under 12 years of age is not recommended, because safe conditions for its use have not been established.

PRECAUTIONS

While ocular changes have not to date been related to Serentil® (mesoridazine besylate), one should be aware that such changes have been seen with other drugs of this class. Because of possible hypotensive effects, reserve parenteral administration for bedfast patients or for acute ambulatory cases, and keep patient lying down for at least one-half hour after injection.

Leukopenia and/or agranulocytosis have been attributed to phenothiazine therapy. A single case of transient granulocytopenia has been associated with Serentil® (mesoridazine besylate). Since convulsive seizures have been reported, patients receiving anticonvulsant medication should be maintained on that regimen while receiving Serentil® (mesoridazine besylate).

Neuroleptic drugs elevate prolactin levels; the elevation persists during chronic administration. Tissue culture experiments indicate that approximately one-third of human breast cancers are prolactin dependent in vitro, a factor of potential importance if the prescription of these drugs is contemplated in a patient with a previously detected breast cancer. Although disturbances such as galactorrhea, amenorrhea, gynecomastia, and impotence have been reported, the clinical significance of elevated serum prolactin levels is unknown for most patients. An increase in mammary neoplasms has been found in rodents after chronic administration of neuroleptic drugs. Neither clinical studies nor epidemiologic studies conducted to date, however, have shown an association between chronic administration of these drugs and mammary tumorigenesis; the available evidence is considered too limited to be conclusive at this time.

INFORMATION FOR PATIENTS Given the likelihood that some patients exposed chronically to neuroleptics will develop tardive dyskinesia, it is advised that all patients in whom chronic use is contemplated be given, if possible, full information about this risk.

ADVERSE REACTIONS

Drowsiness and hypotension were the most prevalent side effects encountered. Side effects tended to reach their maximum level of severity early with the exception of a few (rigidity and motoric effects) which occurred later in therapy. With the exceptions of tremor and rigidity, adverse reactions were generally found among those patients who received relatively high doses early in treatment. Clinical data showed no tendency for the investigators to terminate treatment because of side effects.

Serentil® (mesoridazine besylate) has demonstrated a remarkably low incidence of adverse reactions when compared with other phenothiazine compounds.

Central Nervous System Drowsiness, Parkinson's syndrome, dizziness, weakness, tremor, restlessness, ataxia, dystonia, rigidity, slurring, akathisia, motoric reactions (opisthotonos) have been reported.

Autonomic Nervous System Dry mouth, nausea and vomiting, fainting, stuffy nose, photophobia, constipation and blurred vision have occurred in some instances.

Genitourinary System Inhibition of ejaculation, impotence, enuresis, incontinence, and priapism have been reported.

Skin Itching, rash, hypertrophic papillae of the tongue and angioneurotic edema have been reported.

Cardiovascular System Hypotension and tachycardia have been reported. EKG changes have occurred in some instances (see PHENOTHIAZINE DERIVATIVES: Cardiovascular Effects).

PHENOTHIAZINE DERIVATIVES It should be noted that efficacy, indications and untoward effects have varied with the different phenothiazines. The physician should be aware that the following have occurred with one or more phenothiazines and should be considered whenever one of these drugs is used.

Autonomic Reactions Miosis, obstipation, anorexia, paralytic ileus.

Cutaneous Reactions Erythema, exfoliative dermatitis, contact dermatitis.

Blood Dyscrasias Agranulocytosis, leukopenia, eosinophilia, thrombocytopenia, anemia, aplastic anemia, pancytopenia.

Allergic Reactions Fever, laryngeal edema, angioneurotic edema, asthma.

Hepatotoxicity Jaundice, biliary stasis.

Cardiovascular Effects Changes in the terminal portion of the electrocardiogram, including prolongation of the Q-T interval, lowering and inversion of the T wave and appearance of a wave tentatively identified as a bifid T or a U wave have been observed in some patients receiving the phenothiazine tranquilizers, including Serentil® (mesoridazine besylate). To date, these appear to be due to altered repolarization and not related to myocardial damage. They appear to be reversible. While there is no evidence at present that these changes are in any way precursors of any significant disturbance of cardiac rhythm, it should be noted that sudden and unexpected deaths apparently due to cardiac arrest have occurred in patients previously showing characteristic electrocardiographic changes while taking the drug. The use of periodic electrocardiograms has been proposed but would appear to be of questionable value as a predictive device. Hypotension, rarely resulting in cardiac arrest, has been noted.

Extrapyramidal Symptoms Akathisia, agitation, motor restlessness, dystonic reactions, trismus, torticollis, opisthotonos, oculogyric crises, tremor, muscular rigidity, akinesia.

Tardive Dyskinesia Chronic use of neuroleptics may be associated with the development of tardive dyskinesia. The salient features of this syndrome are described in the WARNINGS section and below.

The syndrome is characterized by involuntary choreoathetoid movements which variously involve the tongue, face,

Continued on next page

Serentil—Cont.

mouth, lips, or jaw (e.g., protrusion of the tongue, puffing of cheeks, puckering of the mouth, chewing movements), trunk and extremities. The severity of the syndrome and the degree of impairment produced vary widely.
The syndrome may become clinically recognizable either during treatment, upon dosage reduction, or upon withdrawal of treatment. Movements may decrease in intensity and may disappear altogether if further treatment with neuroleptics is withheld. It is generally believed that reversibility is more likely after short rather than long-term neuroleptic exposure. Consequently, early detection of tardive dyskinesia is important. To increase the likelihood of detecting the syndrome at the earliest possible time, the dosage of neuroleptic drug should be reduced periodically (if clinically possible) and the patient observed for signs of the disorder. This maneuver is critical, for neuroleptic drugs may mask the signs of the syndrome.
Endocrine Disturbances Menstrual irregularities, altered libido, gynecomastia, lactation, weight gain, edema. False positive pregnancy tests have been reported.
Urinary Disturbances Retention, incontinence.
Others Hyperpyrexia. Behavioral effects suggestive of a paradoxical reaction have been reported. These include excitement, bizarre dreams, aggravation of psychoses and toxic confusional states. More recently, a peculiar skin-eye syndrome has been recognized as a side effect following long-term treatment with phenothiazines. This reaction is marked by progressive pigmentation of areas of the skin or conjunctiva and/or accompanied by discoloration of the exposed sclera and cornea. Opacities of the anterior lens and cornea described as irregular or stellate in shape have also been reported. Systemic lupus erythematosus-like syndrome.

OVERDOSAGE

Symptoms of Acute Overdosage

— Drowsiness, confusion, disorientation, agitation, coma, death.
— Dryness of mouth, edema of glottis, laryngeal spasms, nasal congestion, blurred vision, vomiting.
— Hyperpyrexia, dilated pupils, muscle rigidity, hyperactive reflexes, areflexia.
— Stupor, and CNS depression or stimulation with convulsions followed by respiratory depression.
— Cardiac abnormalities, including Q.R.S. changes, tachycardia, hypotension, bilateral bundle branch block, ventricular fibrillation, shock, cardiac arrest and congestive heart failure. (See case descriptions below).

Treatment of Acute Overdosage No specific antidote is known. The drug is not dialyzable. Treatment should include:

— *General supportive* measures with *emesis* and *gastric lavage*.
— *Respiratory assistance* is apparently the most effective measure when indicated.
— The *administration of barbiturates* for control of convulsions alleviates an increase in the cardiac work load, but should be undertaken with caution to avoid potentiation of respiratory depression.
— *Intramuscular paraldehyde* or *diazepam* provides anticonvulsant activity with less respiratory depression than do the barbiturates; diazepam seems to be preferred.
— The use of *digitalis and/or physostigmine* may be considered in case of serious cardiovascular abnormalities or cardiac failure.
— Due to several cases of severe cardiotoxicity following Serentil® (mesoridazine besylate) overdose, *continuous ECG monitoring* of these patients is recommended. Two cases are described below:

Marrs-Simon P.A. et al. ("Cardiotoxic Manifestations of Mesoridazine Overdose", *Ann Emerg Med.* 1988;17:1074-1078) describes the management of a 20 year old female who experienced severe cardiotoxicity following an overdose of mesoridazine. The paper also describes similar cases from the published literature.
The serum mesoridazine level in a 115 lb. patient following ingestion of 4.5 to 6.0 grams of Serentil® (mesoridazine besylate) was 2.5 mcg/mL. She was comatose, hypotensive, convulsing, and had ECG changes. Twenty-four hours later, after hemoperfusion with activated charcoal, the mesoridazine blood levels fell to 1.3 mcg/mL and the patient was normotensive and responsive.

DOSAGE AND ADMINISTRATION

The dosage of Serentil® (mesoridazine besylate) as in most medications, should be adjusted to the needs of the individual. The lowest effective dosage should always be used. When maximum response is achieved, dosage may be reduced gradually to a maintenance level.
Schizophrenia For most patients, regardless of severity, a starting dose of 50 mg t.i.d. is recommended. The usual optimum total daily dose range is 100-400 mg per day.
Behavioral Problems in Mental Deficiency and Chronic Brain Syndrome For most patients a starting dose of 25 mg t.i.d. is recommended. The usual optimum total daily dose range is 75-300 mg per day.
Alcoholism For most patients the usual starting dose is 25 mg b.i.d. The usual optimum total daily dose range is 50-200 mg per day.
Psychoneurotic Manifestations For most patients the usual starting dose is 10 mg t.i.d. The usual optimum total daily dose range is 30-150 mg per day.
Injectable Form In those situations in which an intramuscular form of medication is indicated, Serentil® (mesoridazine besylate) injectable is available. For most patients a starting dose of 25 mg is recommended. The dose may be repeated in 30 to 60 minutes, if necessary. The usual optimum total daily dose range is 25-200 mg per day.

HOW SUPPLIED

Tablets 10 mg (NDC 0597-0020-01), 25 mg (NDC 0597-0021-01), 50 mg (NDC 0597-0022-01), and 100 mg (NDC 0597-0023-01) mesoridazine (as the besylate). Bottles of 100.
Ampuls 1 mL [25 mg mesoridazine (as the besylate)]. Boxes of 20 (NDC 0597-0027-02).
Concentrate Contains 25 mg mesoridazine (as the besylate) per mL, alcohol, USP, 0.61% by volume. Immediate containers: Amber glass bottles of 4 fl oz (118 mL) packaged in cartons of 12 bottles, with an accompanying dropper graduated to deliver 10 mg, 25 mg, and 50 mg of mesoridazine (as the besylate) (NDC 0597-0025-04).

STORAGE

Tablets: Below 86°F (30°C). Injection: Below 86°F (30°C); protect from light. Oral solution: Below 77°F (25°C); protect from light; dispense in amber glass bottles only.
The concentrate may be diluted with distilled water, acidified tap water, orange juice or grape juice.
Each dose should be diluted just prior to administration. Preparation and storage of bulk dilutions is not recommended.
Additional information available to physicians.

PHARMACOLOGY

Pharmacological studies in laboratory animals have established that Serentil® (mesoridazine besylate) has a spectrum of pharmacodynamic actions typical of a major tranquilizer. In common with other tranquilizers it inhibits spontaneous motor activity in mice, prolongs thiopental and hexobarbital sleeping time in mice and produces spindles and block of arousal reaction in the EEG of rabbits. It is effective in blocking spinal reflexes in the cat and antagonizes d-amphetamine excitation and toxicity in grouped mice. It shows a moderate adrenergic blocking activity in vitro and in vivo and antagonizes 5-hydroxytryptamine in vivo. Intravenously administered, it lowers the blood pressure of anesthetized dogs. It has a weak antiacetylcholine effect in vitro.
The most outstanding activity of Serentil® (mesoridazine besylate) is seen in tests developed to investigate antiemotive activity of drugs. Such tests are those in which the rat reacts to acute or chronic stress by increased defecation (emotogenic defecation) or tests in which "emotional mydriasis" is elicited in the mouse by an electric shock. In both of these tests Serentil® (mesoridazine besylate) is effective in reducing emotive reactions. Its ED_{50} in inhibiting emotogenic defecation in the rat is 0.053 mg/kg (subcutaneous administration). Serentil® (mesoridazine besylate) has a potent antiemetic action. The intravenous ED_{50} against apomorphine-induced emesis in the dog is 0.64 mg/kg. Serentil® (mesoridazine besylate), in common with other phenothiazines, demonstrates antiarrhythmic activity in anesthetized dogs.
Metabolic studies in the dog and rabbit with tritium labeled mesoridazine demonstrate that the compound is well absorbed from the gastrointestinal tract. The biological half-life of Serentil® (mesoridazine besylate) in these studies appears to be somewhere between 24 and 48 hours. Although significant urinary excretion was observed following the administration of Serentil® (mesoridazine besylate), these studies also suggest that biliary excretion is an important excretion route for mesoridazine and/or its metabolites.

Toxicity Studies
Acute LD_{50} (mg/kg):

Route	Mouse	Rat	Rabbit	Dog
Oral	560±62.5	644±48	MLD=800	MLD=800
I.M.	—	509M 584 F	405	—
I.V.	26±0.08	—	—	—

Chronic toxicity studies were conducted in rats and dogs. Rats were administered Serentil® (mesoridazine besylate) orally seven days per week for a period of seventeen months in doses up to 160 mg/kg per day. Dogs were administered Serentil® (mesoridazine besylate) orally seven days per week for a period of thirteen months. The daily dosage of the drug was increased during the period of this test such that the "top-dose" group received a daily dose of 120 mg/kg of mesoridazine for the last month of the study.
Untoward effects that occurred upon chronic administration of high dose levels included:
Rats Reduction of food intake, slowed weight gain, morphological changes in pituitary-supported endocrine organs, and melanin-like pigment deposition in renal tissues.
Dogs Emesis, muscle tremors, decreased food intake and death associated with aspiration of oral-gastric contents into the respiratory system.
Increased intrauterine resorptions were seen with Serentil® (mesoridazine besylate) in rats at 70 mg/kg and in rabbits at 125 mg/kg but not at 60 and 100 mg/kg, respectively. No drug related teratology was suggested by these reproductive studies.

Local irritation from the intramuscular injection of Serentil® (mesoridazine besylate) was of the same order of magnitude as with other phenothiazines.

SE-PI-7/96 Rev

Manufactured by:
Sandoz Pharmaceuticals Corporation,
East Hanover, NJ 07936
Distributed by:
Boehringer Ingelheim Pharmaceuticals, Inc.
Ridgefield, CT 06877

Shown in Product Identification Guide, page 309

Bone Care International

ONE SCIENCE COURT
MADISON, WI 53711

Direct Inquiries to:
Professional Services Department
TELEPHONE: (888)-389-4242 extension 554
FAX: (608)-236-0313

HECTOROL® CAPSULES ℞

[*heck'-tōrōl*]
(Doxercalciferol)

DESCRIPTION

Doxercalciferol, the active ingredient in Hectorol, is a synthetic vitamin D analog that undergoes metabolic activation *in vivo* to form 1α,25-dihydroxyvitamin D_2 (1α,25-$(OH)_2D_2$), a naturally occurring, biologically active form of Vitamin D_2. Hectorol is available as soft gelatin capsules containing 2.5 mcg doxercalciferol. Each capsule also contains butylated hydroxyanisole (BHA), ethanol, and fractionated triglyceride of coconut oil. Gelatin capsule shells contain glycerin, D&C Yellow No. 10, and titanium dioxide.
Doxercalciferol is a colorless crystalline compound with a calculated molecular weight of 412.66 and a molecular formula of $C_{28}H_{44}O_2$. It is soluble in oils and organic solvents, but is relatively insoluble in water. Chemically, doxercalciferol is (1α,3β,5Z,7E,22E)-9,10-secoergosta-5,7, 10(19)22-tetraene-1,3-diol and has the following structural formula:

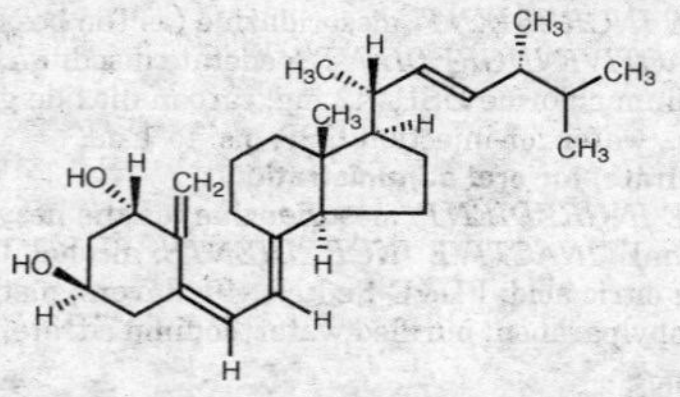

Other names frequently used for doxercalciferol are 1α-OH-D_2, 1α-hydroxyvitamin D_2, and 1α-hydroxyergocalciferol.

CLINICAL PHARMACOLOGY

Vitamin D levels in humans depend on two sources: (1) exposure to the ultraviolet rays of the sun for conversion of 7-dehydrocholesterol in the skin to vitamin D_3 (cholecalciferol) and (2) dietary intake of either vitamin D_2 (ergocalciferol) or vitamin D_3. Vitamin D_2 and vitamin D_3 must be metabolically activated in the liver and the kidney before becoming fully active on target tissues. The initial step in the activation process is the introduction of a hydroxyl group in the side chain at C-25 by the hepatic enzyme, CYP 27 (a vitamin D-25-hydroxylase). The products of this reaction are 25-$(OH)D_2$ and 25-$(OH)D_3$, respectively. Further hydroxylation of these metabolites occurs in the mitochondria of kidney tissue, catalyzed by renal 25-hydroxyvitamin D-1-α-hydroxylase to produce 1α,25-$(OH)_2D_2$, the primary biologically active form of vitamin D_2, and 1α,25-$(OH)_2D_3$ (calcitriol), the biologically active form of vitamin D_3.
Mechanism of action
Calcitriol (1α,25-$(OH)_2D_3$) and 1α,25-$(OH)_2D_2$ regulate blood calcium at levels required for essential body functions. Specifically, the biologically active vitamin D metabolites control the intestinal absorption of dietary calcium, the tubular reabsorption of calcium by the kidney and, in conjunction with parathyroid hormone (PTH), the mobilization of calcium from the skeleton. They act directly on bone cells (osteoblasts) to stimulate skeletal growth, and on the parathyroid glands to suppress PTH synthesis and secretion. These functions are mediated by the interaction of these biologically active metabolites with specific receptor proteins in the various target tissues. In uremic patients, deficient production of biologically active vitamin D metabolites leads to secondary hyperparathyroidism, which contributes to the development of metabolic bone disease in patients with renal failure.
Pharmacokinetics and Metabolism
Doxercalciferol is absorbed from the gastrointestinal tract and activated by CYP 27 in the liver to form 1α,25-$(OH)_2D_2$ (major metabolite) and 1α,24-dihydroxyvitamin D_2 (minor metabolite). Activation of doxercalciferol does not require the involvement of the kidneys.
In healthy volunteers, peak blood levels of 1α,25-$(OH)_2D_2$, the major metabolite of doxercalciferol, are attained at 11–12 hours after repeated oral doses of 5 to 15 mcg of Hec-

torol and the mean half-life of $1\alpha,25\text{-(OH)}_2D_2$ elimination is approximately 32 to 37 hours with a range of up to 96 hours. The half-life in patients with end-stage renal disease (ESRD) on dialysis appears to be similar. Hemodialysis causes a temporary increase in $1\alpha,25\text{-(OH)}_2D_2$ mean concentrations, presumably due to volume contraction. $1\alpha,25\text{-(OH)}_2D_2$ is not removed from blood during hemodialysis.

Clinical Studies

The safety and effectiveness of Hectorol were evaluated in two clinical studies in patients with chronic renal disease on hemodialysis. After randomization to two groups, eligible patients underwent an 8-week washout period during which no vitamin D derivatives were administered to either group. Subsequently, all patients received Hectorol in an open-label fashion for 16 weeks followed by a double-blind period of 8 weeks during which patients received either Hectorol or placebo. The initial dose of Hectorol during the open-label phase was 10 micrograms after each dialysis session (3 times weekly) for a total of 30 mcg per week. The dosage of Hectorol was adjusted as necessary by the investigator in order to achieve intact parathyroid hormone (iPTH) levels within a targeted range of 150 to 300 pg/mL. The maximum dosage was limited to 20 mcg after each dialysis (60 mcg/week). If at any time during the trial iPTH fell below 150 pg/mL, Hectorol was immediately suspended and restarted at a lower dosage the following week.

Results:

Decreases in plasma iPTH from baseline values were calculated, using, as baseline, the average of the last 3 values obtained during the 8-week washout phase and are displayed in the table below.

[See first table at right]

In both studies, Hectorol treatment resulted in a statistically significant reduction from baseline in mean iPTH levels during the open-label period. During the double-blind period (weeks 17 to 24), the reduction in mean iPTH levels was maintained in the Hectorol treatment group compared to a return to near baseline in the placebo group.

In the clinical trials, the values for iPTH varied widely from patient to patient and from week to week for individual patients. The following table shows the numbers of patients within each group who achieved and maintained iPTH levels below 300 pg/mL during the open-label and double-blind phases.

[See second table at right]

During the 8-week double-blind phase, more patients achieved and maintained the target range of values for iPTH with Hectorol than with placebo.

		iPTH means ± s.d. (n*) p Value v. Baseline p Value v. Placebo	
		Hectorol	Placebo
Study A	Baseline	797.2 ± 443.8 (30) n.a. 0.97	847.1 ± 765.5 (32)
	Week 16 (open-label)	384.3 ± 397.8 (24) <.001 0.72	526.5 ± 872.2 (29) <.001
	Week 24 (double-blind)	404.4 ± 262.9 (21) <.001 0.008	672.6 ± 356.9 (24) 0.70
Study B	Baseline	973.9 ± 567.0 (41) n.a. 0.81	990.4 ± 488.3 (35)
	Week 16 (open label)	476.1 ± 444.5 (37) <.001 0.91	485.9 ± 443.4 (32) <.001
	Week 24 (double-blind)	459.8 ± 443.0 (35) <.001 <.001	871.9 ± 623.6 (30) <0.65

* all subjects; last value carried to discontinuation

		Number of times iPTH ≤300 pg/mL					
		Only 1		Only 2		≥ 3	
		Hectorol	Placebo	Hectorol	Placebo	Hectorol	Placebo
Study A	Weeks 1–16 (open-label)	2/30	2/32	0/30	0/32	22/30	23/32
	Weeks 17–24 (double-blind)	0/24	9/29	3/24	1/29	17/24	5/29
Study B	Weeks 1–16 (open-label)	2/41	4/35	1/41	0/35	29/41	21/35
	Weeks 17–24 (double-blind)	2/37	6/32	1/37	4/32	26/37	4/32

INDICATIONS AND USAGE

Hectorol is indicated for the reduction of elevated iPTH levels in the management of secondary hyperparathyroidism in patients undergoing chronic renal dialysis.

CONTRAINDICATIONS

Hectorol should not be given to patients with a tendency towards hypercalcemia or evidence of vitamin D toxicity.

WARNINGS

Overdosage of any form of vitamin D is dangerous (see **OVERDOSAGE**). Progressive hypercalcemia due to overdosage of vitamin D and its metabolites may be so severe as to require emergency attention. Acute hypercalcemia may exacerbate tendencies to cardiac arrhythmias and seizures and will affect the action of digitalis drugs. Chronic hypercalcemia can lead to generalized vascular calcification and other soft-tissue calcification. The serum calcium times serum phosphorus (Ca X P) product should not be allowed to exceed 70. Radiographic evaluation of suspect anatomical regions may be useful in the early detection of this condition.

Since doxercalciferol is a precursor for $1\alpha,25\text{-(OH)}_2D_2$, a potent metabolite of vitamin D, pharmacologic doses of vitamin D and its derivatives should be withheld during doxercalciferol treatment to avoid possible additive effects and hypercalcemia.

Oral calcium-based or other non-aluminum containing phosphate binders and a low phosphate diet should be used to control serum phosphorus levels in patients undergoing dialysis. Uncontrolled serum phosphorus exacerbates secondary hyperparathyroidism and can lessen the effectiveness of doxercalciferol in reducing blood PTH levels. After initiating doxercalciferol therapy, the dose of phosphate binders should be decreased to correct persistent mild hypercalcemia (10.6 to 11.2 mg/dL for 3 consecutive determinations) or increased to correct persistent mild hyperphosphatemia (7.0 to 8.0 mg/dL for 3 consecutive determinations).

Magnesium containing antacids and Hectorol should not be used concomitantly in patients on chronic renal dialysis because such use may lead to the development of hypermagnesemia.

PRECAUTIONS

General

The principal adverse effects of treatment with Hectorol are hypercalcemia, hyperphosphatemia, and oversuppression of PTH. Prolonged hypercalcemia can lead to calcification of soft tissues, including the heart and arteries, and hyperphosphatemia can exacerbate hyperparathyroidism. Oversuppression of PTH may lead to adynamic bone syndrome. All of these potential adverse effects should be managed by regular patient monitoring and appropriate dosage adjustments. During treatment with Hectorol, patients usually require dose titration, as well as adjustment in co-therapy (i.e., dietary phosphate binders) in order to effect and sustain PTH suppression while maintaining serum calcium and phosphorus within prescribed ranges.

In four adequate and well-controlled studies, the incidence of hypercalcemia and hyperphosphatemia increased during therapy with Hectorol. The observed increases during Hectorol treatment, although occurring at a low rate, underscore the importance of regular safety monitoring of serum calcium and phosphorus levels throughout treatment. Patients with higher pre-treatment serum levels of calcium or phosphorus were more likely to experience hypercalcemia or hyperphosphatemia. Therefore, Hectorol should not be given to patients with a recent history of hypercalcemia or hyperphosphatemia, or evidence of vitamin D toxicity.

Information for the Patient

The patient, spouse, or guardian should be informed about compliance with dosage instructions, adherence to instructions about diet, calcium supplementation, and avoidance of the use of nonprescription drugs without prior approval from their physician. Patients should also be carefully informed about the symptoms of hypercalcemia (see **ADVERSE REACTIONS** section).

Laboratory Tests

For dialysis patients, serum or plasma iPTH and serum calcium, phosphorus, and alkaline phosphatase should be determined periodically. In the early phase of treatment, iPTH, serum calcium, and serum phosphorus should be determined prior to initiation of Hectorol treatment and weekly thereafter.

Drug Interactions

Cholestyramine has been reported to reduce intestinal absorption of fat-soluble vitamins; therefore, it may impair intestinal absorption of doxercalciferol. Magnesium-containing antacids and Hectorol should not be used concomitantly, because such use may lead to the development of hypermagnesemia. (see **WARNINGS**) The use of mineral oil or other substances that may affect absorption of fat may influence the absorption and availability of Hectorol. Although not examined specifically, both enzyme inducers (such as glutethimide and phenobarbital) and enzyme inhibitors (such as phenytoin) may affect the 25-hydroxylation of Hectorol and may necessitate dose adjustments.

Carcinogenesis, Mutagenesis, Impairment of Fertility

Long-term studies in animals to evaluate the carcinogenic potential of Hectorol have not been conducted. No evidence of genetic toxicity was observed in an *in vitro* bacterial mutagenicity assay (Ames test) or a mouse lymphoma gene mutation assay. Hectorol caused structural chromatid and chromosome aberrations in an *in vitro* human lymphocyte clastogenicity assay with metabolic activation. However, Hectorol was negative in an *in vivo* mouse micronucleus clastogenicity assay. Hectorol had no effect on male or female fertility in rats at oral doses up to 2.5 mcg/kg/day (approximately 3 times the maximum recommended human dose of 60 mcg/week based on mcg/m^2 body surface area).

Use in Pregnancy

Pregnancy Category B

Reproduction studies in rats and rabbits, at doses up to 20 mcg/kg/day and 0.1 mcg/kg/day (approximately 25 times and less than the maximum recommended human dose of 60 mcg/week based on mcg/m^2 body surface area, respectively) have revealed no teratogenic or fetotoxic effects due to Hectorol. There are, however, no adequate and well-controlled studies in pregnant women. Because animal reproduction studies are not always predictive of human response, this drug should be used during pregnancy only if clearly needed.

Nursing Mothers

It is not known whether this drug is excreted in human milk. Because other vitamin D derivatives are excreted in human milk and because of the potential for serious adverse reactions in nursing infants from doxercalciferol, a decision should be made whether to discontinue nursing or to discontinue the drug, taking into account the importance of the drug to the mother.

Pediatric Use

Safety and efficacy of Hectorol in pediatric patients have not been established.

Hepatic Insufficiency

Since patients with hepatic insufficiency may not metabolize Hectorol appropriately, the drug should be used with caution in patients with impaired hepatic function. More frequent monitoring of iPTH, calcium, and phosphorus levels should be done in such individuals.

ADVERSE REACTIONS

Hectorol has been evaluated for safety in clinical studies in 165 patients with chronic renal disease on hemodialysis. In two placebo-controlled, double-blind, multicenter studies, discontinuation of therapy due to any adverse event occurred in 2.9% of 138 patients treated with Hectorol for four to six months (dosage titrated to achieve target iPTH levels, see **CLINICAL PHARMACOLOGY/Clinical Studies**) and in 3.3% of 61 patients treated with placebo for two months. Adverse events occurring in the Hectorol group at a frequency of 2% or greater and more frequently than in the placebo group are presented in the following table:

[See first table at bottom of next page]

Potential adverse effects of Hectorol are, in general, similar to those encountered with excessive vitamin D intake. The early and late signs and symptoms of vitamin D intoxication associated with hypercalcemia include:

Early

Weakness, headache, somnolence, nausea, vomiting, dry mouth, constipation, muscle pain, bone pain, and metallic taste.

Continued on next page

Hectorol—Cont.

Late
Polyuria, polydipsia, anorexia, weight loss, nocturia, conjunctivitis (calcific), pancreatitis, photophobia, rhinorrhea, pruritus, hyperthermia, decreased libido, elevated blood urea nitrogen (BUN), albuminuria, hypercholesterolemia, elevated serum aspartate transaminase (AST) and alanine transaminase (ALT), ectopic calcification, hypertension, cardiac arrhythmias, and, rarely, overt psychosis.

OVERDOSAGE

Administration of Hectorol to patients in excess doses can cause hypercalcemia, hypercalciuria, hyperphosphatemia, and over-suppression of PTH secretion leading in certain cases to adynamic bone disease. High intake of calcium and phosphate concomitant with Hectorol may lead to similar abnormalities. High levels of calcium in the dialysate bath may contribute to hypercalcemia.

Treatment of Hypercalcemia and Overdosage
General treatment of hypercalcemia (greater than 1 mg/dL above the upper limit of the normal range) consists of immediate suspension of Hectorol therapy, institution of a low calcium diet, and withdrawal of calcium supplements. Serum calcium levels should be determined at least weekly until normocalcemia ensues. Hypercalcemia usually resolves in 2 to 7 days. When serum calcium levels have returned to within normal limits, Hectorol therapy may be reinstituted at a dose that is at least 2.5 mcg lower than prior therapy. Serum calcium levels should be obtained weekly after all dosage changes and during subsequent dosage titration. Persistent or markedly elevated serum calcium levels may be corrected by dialysis against a reduced calcium or calcium-free dialysate.

Treatment of Accidental Overdosage of Doxercalciferol
The treatment of acute accidental overdosage of Hectorol should consist of general supportive measures. If drug ingestion is discovered within a relatively short time (10 minutes), induction of emesis or gastric lavage may be of benefit in preventing further absorption. If drug ingestion is discovered later than 10 minutes post-ingestion, the administration of mineral oil may promote its fecal elimination. Serial serum electrolyte determinations (especially calcium), rate of urinary calcium excretion, and assessment of electrocardiographic abnormalities due to hypercalcemia should be obtained. Such monitoring is critical in patients receiving digitalis. Discontinuation of supplemental calcium and institution of a low calcium diet are also indicated in accidental overdosage. If persistent and markedly elevated serum calcium levels occur, there are a variety of therapeutic alternatives which may be considered. These include the use of drugs such as phosphates and corticosteroids as well as measures to induce diuresis. Also, one may consider dialysis against a calcium-free dialysate.

DOSAGE AND ADMINISTRATION

The optimal dose of Hectorol must be carefully determined for each patient.
The recommended initial dose of Hectorol is 10.0 mcg administered three times weekly at dialysis (approximately every other day). The initial dose should be adjusted, as needed, in order to lower blood iPTH into the range of 150 to 300 pg/mL. The dose may be increased at 8-week intervals by 2.5 mcg if iPTH is not lowered by 50% and fails to reach the target range. The maximum recommended dose of Hectorol is 20 mcg administered three times a week at dialysis for a total of 60 mcg per week. Drug administration should be suspended if iPTH falls below 100 pg/mL and restarted one week later at a dose that is at least 2.5 mcg lower than the last administered dose. During titration, iPTH, serum calcium, and serum phosphorus levels should be obtained weekly. If hypercalcemia, hyperphosphatemia, or a serum calcium times serum phosphorus product greater than 70 is noted, the drug should be immediately suspended until these parameters are appropriately lowered. Then, the drug should be restarted at a dose that is at least 2.5 mcg lower. Dosing must be individualized and based on iPTH levels with monitoring of serum calcium and serum phosphorus levels. The following is a suggested approach in dose titration:
[See second table below]

HOW SUPPLIED

NDC 64894-825-50
2.5 mcg doxercalciferol in soft gelatin, sunshine yellow, oval capsules, imprinted **BCI**; bottles of 50.
Store at controlled room temperature 20° to 25°C (68° to 77°F) [see USP].

HECTOROL® INJECTION ℞

[heck'-tŏrōl]
(Doxercalciferol)

DESCRIPTION

Doxercalciferol, the active ingredient in Hectorol, is a synthetic vitamin D analog that undergoes metabolic activation *in vivo* to form 1α,25-dihydroxyvitamin D_2 (1α,25-$(OH)_2D_2$), a naturally occurring, biologically active form of vitamin D_2. Hectorol is available as a sterile, clear, colorless, aqueous solution for intravenous injection. Each milliliter (mL) of solution contains doxercalciferol, 2 mcg; TWEEN® Polysorbate 20, 4 mg; sodium chloride, 1.5 mg; sodium ascorbate, 10 mg, sodium phosphate, dibasic 7.6 mg; sodium phosphate, monobasic 1.8 mg; and disodium edetate, 1.1 mg.
Doxercalciferol is a colorless crystalline compound with a calculated molecular weight of 412.66 and a molecular formula of $C_{28}H_{44}O_2$. It is soluble in oils and organic solvents, but is relatively insoluble in water. Chemically, doxercalciferol is (1α,3β,5Z,7E,22E)-9,10-secoergosta-5,7,10(19) 22-tetraen-1,3-diol and has the following structural formula:

Other names frequently used for doxercalciferol are 1α-hydroxyvitamin D_2, 1α-OH-D_2, and 1α-hydroxyergocalciferol.

CLINICAL PHARMACOLOGY

Vitamin D levels in humans depend on two sources: (1) exposure to the ultraviolet rays of the sun for conversion of 7-dehydrocholesterol in the skin to vitamin D_3 (cholecalciferol) and (2) dietary intake of either vitamin D_2 (ergocalciferol) or vitamin D_3. Vitamin D_2 and vitamin D_3 must be metabolically activated in the liver and kidney before becoming fully active on target tissues. The initial step in the activation process is the introduction of an hydroxyl group in the side chain at C-25 by an hepatic enzyme, CYP 27 (a vitamin D-25-hydroxylase). The products of this reaction are 25-$(OH)D_2$ and 25-$(OH)D_3$, respectively. Further hydroxylation of these metabolites occurs in the mitochondria of kidney tissue, catalyzed by renal 25-hydroxyvitamin D-1-α-hydroxylase to produce 1α,25-$(OH)_2D_2$, the primary biologically active form of vitamin D_2, and 1α,25-$(OH)_2D_3$ (calcitriol), the biologically active form of vitamin D_3.

Mechanism of Action
Calcitriol (1α,25-$(OH)_2D_3$) and 1α,25-$(OH)_2D_2$ regulate blood calcium at levels required for essential body functions. Specifically, the biologically active vitamin D metabolites control the intestinal absorption of dietary calcium, the tubular reabsorption of calcium by the kidney and, in conjunction with parathyroid hormone (PTH), the mobilization of calcium from the skeleton. They act directly on bone cells (osteoblasts) to stimulate skeletal growth, and on the parathyroid glands to suppress PTH synthesis and secretion. These functions are mediated by the interaction of these biologically active metabolites with specific receptor proteins in the various target tissues. In uremic patients, deficient production of biologically active vitamin D metabolites (due to lack of or insufficient 25-hydroxyvitamin D-1-alpha-hydroxylase activity) leads to secondary hyperparathyroidism, which contributes to the development of metabolic bone disease in patients with renal failure.

Pharmacokinetics and Metabolism
After intravenous administration, doxercalciferol is activated by CYP 27 in the liver to form 1α,25-$(OH)_2D_2$ (major metabolite) and 1α,24-dihydroxyvitamin D_2 (minor metabolite). Activation of doxercalciferol does not require the involvement of the kidneys.
Peak blood levels of 1α,25-$(OH)_2D_2$ are reached at 8+/−5.9 hours (mean +/−SD) after a single intravenous dose of 5 µg of doxercalciferol. The mean elimination half-life of 1α,25-$(OH)_2D_2$ after an oral dose is approximately 32 to 37 hours with a range of up to 96 hours. The mean elimination half-life in patients with end stage renal disease (ESRD) and in healthy volunteers appears to be similar following an oral dose. Hemodialysis causes a temporary increase in 1α,25-$(OH)_2D_2$ mean concentrations presumably due to volume contraction. 1α,25-$(OH)_2D_2$ is not removed from blood during hemodialysis.

Clinical Studies
The safety and effectiveness of Hectorol Injection were evaluated in two open-label, single-arm, multi-centered clinical studies (Study C and Study D) in a total of 70 patients with chronic renal disease on hemodialysis. Patients in Study C were an average age of 54 years (range: 23–73), were 50% male, and were 61% Black, 25% Caucasian, and 14% Hispanic, and had been on hemodialysis for an average of 65 months. Patients in Study D were an average age of 51 years (range: 28–76), were 48% male, and 100% Black and had been on hemodialysis for an average of 61 months. This group of 70 of the 138 patients who had been treated with Hectorol Capsules in prior clinical studies (Study A and Study B) received Hectorol Injection in an open-label fashion for 12 weeks following an 8-week washout (control) period. Dosing of Hectorol Injection was initiated at the rate of 4.0 mcg administered at the end of each dialysis session (3 times weekly) for a total of 12.0 mcg per week. The dosage of Hectorol was adjusted in an attempt to achieve iPTH levels within a targeted range of 150 to 300 pg/mL. The dosage was increased by 2.0 mcg per dialysis session after 8 weeks of treatment if the iPTH levels remained above 300 pg/mL

Adverse Events Reported by ≥2% of Hectorol treated patients and more frequently than placebo during the double-blind phase of two Clinical Studies

Adverse Event	Hectorol® (n=61) %	Placebo (n=61) %
Body as a Whole		
Abscess	3.3	0.0
Headache	27.9	18.0
Malaise	27.9	19.7
Cardiovascular System		
Bradycardia	6.6	4.9
Digestive System		
Anorexia	4.9	3.3
Constipation	3.3	3.3
Dyspepsia	4.9	1.6
Nausea/Vomiting	21.3	19.7
Musculo-Skeletal System		
Arthralgia	4.9	0.0
Metabolic and Nutritional		
Edema	34.4	21.3
Weight increase	4.9	0.0
Nervous System		
Dizziness	11.5	9.8
Sleep disorder	3.3	0.0
Respiratory System		
Dyspnea	11.5	6.6
Skin		
Pruritis	8.2	6.6

A patient who reported the same medical term more than once was counted only once for that medical term.

Initial Dosing

iPTH Level	Hectoral Dose
>400 pg/mL	10.0 mcg three times per week at dialysis.

Dose Titration

iPTH Level	Hectoral Dose
Decreased by <50% and above 300 pg/mL	Increase by 2.5 mcg at eight-week intervals as necessary
150–300 pg/mL	Maintain
<100 pg/mL	Suspend for one week, then resume at a dose that is at least 2.5 mcg lower

and were greater than 50% of baseline levels. The maximum dosage was limited to 18.0 mcg per week. If at any time during the trial iPTH fell below 150 pg/mL, Hectorol Injection was immediately suspended and restarted at a lower dosage the following week.

Results:
Fifty-two of the 70 patients who were treated with Hectorol Injection achieved iPTH levels ≤ 300 pg/mL. Forty-one of these patients exhibited plasma iPTH levels ≤ 300 pg/mL on at least 3 occasions. Thirty-six patients had plasma iPTH levels < 150 pg/mL on at least one occasion during study participation.
Mean weekly doses in Study C ranged from 8.9 mcg to 12.5 mcg. In Study D, the mean weekly doses ranged from 9.1 mcg to 11.6 mcg.
Decreases in plasma iPTH from baseline values were calculated, using, as baseline, the average of the last 3 values obtained during the 8-week washout period and are displayed in the table below. Plasma iPTH levels were measured weekly during the 12-week study.
[See first table above]
In both studies, iPTH levels increased progressively and significantly in 62.9% of patients during the 8-week washout (control) period during which no vitamin D derivatives were administered. In contrast, Hectorol Injection treatment resulted in a clinically significant reduction (at least 30%) from baseline in mean iPTH levels during the 12-week open-label treatment period in more than 92% of the 70 treated patients.
The following table shows the numbers of patients who achieved iPTH levels below 300 pg/mL on one, two, or three or more non-consecutive occasions during the 12-week treatment period. Thirty-seven of 70 patients (53%) had plasma iPTH levels within the targeted range (150–300 pg/mL) during Weeks 10–12.

	Number of times iPTH ≤ 300 pg/mL		
	1	2	≥ 3
Study C	3/28	0/28	16/28
Study D	4/42	4/42	25/42

INDICATIONS AND USAGE

Hectorol is indicated for the reduction of elevated iPTH levels in the management of secondary hyperparathyroidism in patients undergoing chronic renal dialysis.

CONTRAINDICATIONS

Hectorol should not be given to patients with a tendency towards hypercalcemia or current evidence of vitamin D toxicity.

WARNINGS

Overdosage of any form of vitamin D, including Hectorol, is dangerous (see **OVERDOSAGE**). Progressive hypercalcemia due to overdosage of vitamin D and its metabolites may be so severe as to require emergency attention. Acute hypercalcemia may exacerbate tendencies for cardiac arrhythmias and seizures and may potentiate the action of digitalis drugs. Chronic hypercalcemia can lead to generalized vascular calcification and other soft-tissue calcification. The serum calcium times serum phosphorus (Ca X P) product should not be allowed to exceed 70. Radiographic evaluation of suspect anatomical regions may be useful in the early detection of this condition.
Since doxercalciferol is a precursor for 1α,25-$(OH)_2D_2$, a potent metabolite of vitamin D, pharmacologic doses of vitamin D and its derivatives should be withheld during doxercalciferol treatment to avoid possible additive effects and hypercalcemia.
Oral calcium-based or other non aluminum-containing phosphate binders and a low phosphate diet should be used to control serum phosphorus levels in patients undergoing dialysis. Uncontrolled serum phosphorus exacerbates secondary hyperparathyroidism and can lessen the effectiveness of doxercalciferol in reducing blood PTH levels. After initiating doxercalciferol therapy, the dose of phosphate binders should be decreased to correct persistent mild hypercalcemia (10.6 to 11.2 mg/dL for 3 consecutive determinations), or increased to correct persistent mild hyperphosphatemia (7.0 to 8.0 mg/dL for 3 consecutive determinations).
Magnesium-containing antacids and Hectorol should not be used concomitantly in patients on chronic renal dialysis because such use may lead to the development of hypermagnesemia.

PRECAUTIONS

General
The principal adverse effects of treatment with Hectorol Injection are hypercalcemia, hyperphosphatemia, and oversuppression of iPTH (less than 150 pg/mL). Prolonged hypercalcemia can lead to calcification of soft tissues, including the heart and arteries, and hyperphosphatemia can exacerbate hyperparathyroidism. Oversuppression of iPTH may lead to adynamic bone syndrome. All of these potential adverse effects should be managed by regular patient monitoring and appropriate dosage adjustments. During treatment with Hectorol, patients usually require dose titration, as well as adjustment in co-therapy (i.e., dietary phosphate binders) in order to maximize iPTH suppression while maintaining serum calcium and phosphorus levels within prescribed ranges.
In two open-label, single-arm, multi-centered studies, the incidence of hypercalcemia and hyperphosphatemia increased during therapy with Hectorol Injection (see **ADVERSE REACTIONS** section). The observed increases during Hectorol treatment underscore the importance of regular safety monitoring of serum calcium and phosphorus levels throughout treatment. Patients with higher pretreatment serum levels of calcium (> 10.5 mg/dL) or phosphorus (> 6.9 mg/dL) were more likely to experience hypercalcemia or hyperphosphatemia. Therefore, Hectorol should not be given to patients with a recent history of hypercalcemia or hyperphosphatemia, or evidence of vitamin D toxicity.
[See second table above]

iPTH summary data for patients receiving Hectorol Injection

iPTH Level	Study C (n=28)	Study D (n=42)	Combined protocols (n=70)
Baseline (Mean of Weeks –2, –1 and 0)			
Mean (SE)	698 (60)	762 (65)	736 (46)
Median	562	648	634
On-treatment (Week 12[1])			
Mean (SE)	406 (63)	426 (60)	418 (43)
Median	311	292	292
Change from Baseline[2]			
Mean (SE)	–292 (55)	–336 (41)	–318 (33)
Median	–274	–315	–304
P-value[3]	.004	.001	<.001

[1] Values were carried forward for the two patients on study for 10 weeks
[2] Treatment iPTH minus baseline iPTH
[3] Wilcoxon one-sample test

Incidence Rates of Hypercalcemia and Hyperphosphatemia in Two Phase 3 Studies with Hectorol Injection

Study	Hypercalcemia (per 100 patient weeks)		Hyperphosphatemia (per 100 patient weeks)	
	Washout (Off Treatment)	Open-Label (Treatment)	Washout (Off Treatment)	Open-Label (Treatment)
Study C	0.9	0.9	0.9	2.4
Study D	0.3	1.0	1.2	3.7

Information for the Patient
The patient, spouse, or guardian should be informed about compliance with instructions about diet and calcium supplementation and avoidance of the use of nonprescription drugs without prior approval from their physician. Patients should also be carefully informed about the symptoms of hypercalcemia (see **ADVERSE REACTIONS** section).
Laboratory Tests
Serum levels of iPTH, calcium, and phosphorus should be determined prior to initiation of Hectorol treatment. During the early phase of treatment (i.e., first 12 weeks), serum iPTH, calcium, and phosphorus levels should be determined weekly. For dialysis patients in general, serum or plasma iPTH and serum calcium, phosphorus, and alkaline phosphatase should be determined periodically.
Drug Interactions
Specific drug interaction studies have not been conducted. Magnesium-containing antacids and Hectorol should not be used concomitantly, because such use may lead to the development of hypermagnesemia. (See **WARNINGS**.) Although not examined specifically, enzyme inducers (such as glutethimide and phenobarbitol) may affect the 25-hydroxylation of Hectorol and may necessitate dosage adjustments.
Carcinogenesis, Mutagenesis, Impairment of Fertility
Long-term studies in animals to evaluate the carcinogenic potential of doxercalciferol have not been conducted. No evidence of genetic toxicity was observed in an *in vitro* bacterial mutagenicity assay (Ames test) or a mouse lymphoma gene mutation assay. Doxercalciferol caused structural chromatid and chromosome aberrations in an *in vitro* human lymphocyte clastogenicity assay with metabolic activation. However, doxercalciferol was negative in an *in vivo* mouse micronucleus clastogenicity assay. Doxercalciferol had no effect on male or female fertility in rats at oral doses up to 2.5 mcg/kg/day (approximately 3 times the maximum recommended human oral dose of 60 mcg/wk based on mcg/m^2 body surface area).
Use in Pregnancy
Pregnancy Category B
Reproduction studies in rats and rabbits, at doses up to 20 mcg/kg/day and 0.1 mcg/kg/day (approximately 25 times and less than the maximum recommended human oral dose of 60 mcg/week based on mcg/m^2 body surface area, respectively) have revealed no teratogenic or fetotoxic effects due to doxercalciferol. There are, however, no adequate and well-controlled studies in pregnant women. Because animal reproduction studies are not always predictive of human response, this drug should be used during pregnancy only if clearly needed.
Nursing Mothers
It is not known whether doxercalciferol is excreted in human milk. Because other vitamin D derivatives are excreted in human milk and because of the potential for serious adverse reactions in nursing infants from doxercalciferol, a decision should be made whether to discontinue nursing or to discontinue the drug, taking into account the importance of the drug to the mother.
Pediatric Use
Safety and efficacy of Hectorol in pediatric patients have not been established.
Geriatric Use
Of the 70 patients treated with Hectorol Injection in the two Phase 3 clinical studies, 12 patients were 65 years or over. In these studies, no overall differences in efficacy or safety were observed between patients 65 years or older and younger patients.
Hepatic Insufficiency
Studies examining the influence of hepatic insufficiency on the metabolism of Hectorol were inconclusive. Since patients with hepatic insufficiency may not metabolize doxercalciferol appropriately, the drug should be used with caution in patients with impaired hepatic function. More frequent monitoring of iPTH, calcium, and phosphorus levels should be done in such individuals.

ADVERSE REACTIONS

Hectorol Injection has been evaluated for safety in 70 patients with chronic renal disease on hemodialysis (who had been previously treated with oral Hectorol) from two 12-week, open-label, single-arm, multi-centered studies. (Dosage titrated to achieve target plasma iPTH levels, see **CLINICAL PHARMACOLOGY/Clinical Studies).**
Because there was no placebo group included in the studies of Hectorol Injection, the table below provides the adverse event incidence rates from placebo-controlled studies of oral Hectorol.

Adverse Events Reported by ≥2% of Hectorol Treated Patients and More Frequently Than Placebo During the Double-blind Phase of Two Clinical Studies

Adverse Event	Hectorol (n=61) %	Placebo (n=61) %
Body as a Whole		
Abscess	3.3	0.0
Headache	27.9	18.0
Malaise	27.9	19.7
Cardiovascular System		
Bradycardia	6.6	4.9
Digestive System		
Anorexia	4.9	3.3
Constipation	3.3	3.3
Dyspepsia	4.9	1.6
Nausea/Vomiting	21.3	19.7

Continued on next page

Hectorol—Cont.

Musculo-Skeletal System		
Arthralgia	4.9	0.0
Metabolic and Nutritional		
Edema	34.4	21.3
Weight increase	4.9	0.0
Nervous System		
Dizziness	11.5	9.8
Sleep disorder	3.3	0.0
Respiratory System		
Dyspnea	11.5	6.6
Skin		
Pruritis	8.2	6.6

A patient who reported the same medical term more than once was counted only once for that medical term.

Potential adverse effects of Hectorol are, in general, similar to those encountered with excessive vitamin D intake. The early and late signs and symptoms of vitamin D intoxication associated with hypercalcemia include:

Early

Weakness, headache, somnolence, nausea, vomiting, dry mouth, constipation, muscle pain, bone pain, and metallic taste.

Late

Polyuria, polydipsia, anorexia, weight loss, nocturia, conjunctivitis (calcific), pancreatitis, photophobia, rhinorrhea, pruritus, hyperthermia, decreased libido, elevated blood urea nitrogen (BUN), albuminuria, hypercholesterolemia, elevated serum aspartate transaminase (AST) and alanine transaminase (ALT), ectopic calcification, hypertension, cardiac arrhythmias and, rarely, overt psychosis.

OVERDOSAGE

Administration of Hectorol to patients in excess doses can cause hypercalcemia, hypercalciuria, hyperphosphatemia, and over-suppression of PTH secretion leading in certain cases to adynamic bone disease. High intake of calcium and phosphate concomitant with Hectorol may lead to similar abnormalities. High levels of calcium in the dialysate bath may contribute to hypercalcemia.

Treatment of Hypercalcemia and Overdosage

General treatment of hypercalcemia (greater than 1 mg/dL above the upper limit of the normal range) consists of immediate suspension of Hectorol therapy, institution of a low calcium diet, and withdrawal of calcium supplements. Serum calcium levels should be determined at least weekly until normocalcemia ensues. Hypercalcemia usually resolves in 2 to 7 days. When serum calcium levels have returned to within normal limits, Hectorol therapy may be reinstituted at a dose that is at least 1.0 mcg lower than prior therapy. Serum calcium levels should be obtained weekly after all dosage changes and during subsequent dosage titration. Persistent or markedly elevated serum calcium levels may be corrected by dialysis against a reduced calcium or calcium-free dialysate.

Treatment of Accidental Overdosage of Hectorol

The treatment of acute accidental overdosage of Hectorol should consist of general supportive measures. Serial serum electrolyte determinations (especially calcium), rate of urinary calcium excretion, and assessment of electrocardiographic abnormalities due to hypercalcemia should be obtained. Such monitoring is critical in patients receiving digitalis. Discontinuation of supplemental calcium and a low calcium diet are also indicated in accidental overdosage. If persistent and markedly elevated serum calcium levels occur, there are a variety of therapeutic alternatives which may be considered. These include the use of drugs such as phosphates and corticosteroids as well as measures to induce diuresis. Also, one may consider dialysis against a calcium-free dialysate.

DOSAGE AND ADMINISTRATION

Adult Administration:

The optimal dose of Hectorol must be carefully determined for each patient.

The recommended initial dose of Hectorol is 4.0 mcg administered as a bolus dose three times weekly at the end of dialysis (approximately every other day). The initial dose should be adjusted, as needed, in order to lower blood iPTH into the range of 150 to 300 pg/mL. The dose may be increased at 8-week intervals by 1.0 – 2.0 mcg if iPTH is not lowered by 50% and fails to reach the target range. Dosages higher than 18 mcg weekly have not been studied. Drug administration should be suspended if iPTH falls below 100 pg/mL and restarted one week later at a dose which is at least 1.0 mcg lower than the last administered dose. During titration, iPTH, serum calcium, and serum phosphorus levels should be obtained weekly. If hypercalcemia, hyperphosphatemia, or a serum calcium times phosphorus product greater than 70 is noted, the drug should be immediately suspended until these parameters are appropriately lowered. Then, the drug should be restarted at a dose which is 1.0 mcg lower.

Dosing must be individualized and based on iPTH levels with monitoring of serum calcium and serum phosphorus levels. The following is a suggested approach in dose titration:

Initial Dosing

PTH Level	Hectorol Dose
> 400 pg/mL	4.0 mcg three times per week at the end of dialysis, or approximately every other day

Dose Titration

Decreased by < 50% and above 300 pg/mL	Increase by 1.0 to 2.0 mcg at eight-week intervals as necessary
150–300 pg/mL	Maintain
< 100 pg/mL	Suspend for one week, then resume at a dose that is at least 1.0 mcg lower

Discard unused portion.

HOW SUPPLIED

Hectorol (doxercalciferol) Injection is supplied in pre-scored 1 mL and 2 mL amber glass ampules containing 2.0 mcg and 4.0 mcg.

Store at 15° to 25°C (59° to 77°F). Protect from light.

888-389-4242
P-0002 4/00

Braintree Laboratories, Inc.

P.O. BOX 850929
BRAINTREE, MA 02185-0929

Direct Inquiries to:
Harry P. Keegan, President
(781) 843-2202

For Medical Information Contact:
In Emergencies:
Jack DiPalma, M.D.
(800) 874-6756

GoLYTELY® ℞
[go-lit 'lē]
(PEG-3350 and Electrolytes For Oral Solution)

NuLYTELY® ℞
[new-lit 'lē]
(PEG-3350, Sodium Chloride, Sodium Bicarbonate and Potassium Chloride for Oral Solution)

DESCRIPTION

GoLYTELY®

A white powder in a 4 liter jug for reconstitution, containing 236 g polyethylene glycol 3350, 22.74 g sodium sulfate (anhydrous), 6.74 g sodium bicarbonate, 5.86 g sodium chloride, 2.97 g potassium chloride. When dissolved in water to a volume of 4 liters, GoLYTELY (PEG-3350 and electrolytes for oral solution) is an isosmotic solution having a mildly salty taste. GoLYTELY is administered orally or via nasogastric tube as a gastrointestinal lavage.

NuLYTELY®

A white powder for reconstitution containing 420 g polyethylene glycol 3350, 5.72 g sodium bicarbonate, 11.2 g sodium chloride, 1.48 g potassium chloride. When dissolved in water to a volume of 4 liters, NuLYTELY (PEG-3350, sodium chloride, sodium bicarbonate and potassium chloride for oral solution) is an isosmotic solution having a pleasant mineral water taste. NuLYTELY is administered orally or via nasogastric tube as a gastrointestinal lavage.

CLINICAL PHARMACOLOGY

GoLYTELY and NuLYTELY induce a diarrhea which rapidly cleanses the bowel, usually within four hours. The osmotic activity of polyethylene glycol 3350 and the electrolyte concentration result in virtually no net absorption or excretion of ions or water. Accordingly, large volumes may be administered without significant changes in fluid or electrolyte balance.

INDICATIONS AND USAGE

GoLYTELY®

GoLYTELY is indicated for bowel cleansing prior to colonoscopy and barium enema X-ray examination.

NuLYTELY®

NuLYTELY is indicated for bowel cleansing prior to colonoscopy.

CONTRAINDICATIONS

GoLYTELY and NuLYTELY are contraindicated in patients known to be hypersensitive to any of the components. GoLYTELY and NuLYTELY are contraindicated in patients with gastrointestinal obstruction, gastric retention, bowel perforation, toxic colitis, toxic megacolon or ileus.

WARNINGS

GoLYTELY®

No additional ingredients, e.g. flavorings, should be added to the solution. GoLYTELY should be used with caution in patients with severe ulcerative colitis.

NuLYTELY®

No additional ingredients, e.g. flavorings, should be added to the solution. NuLYTELY should be used with caution in patients with severe ulcerative colitis. Use of NuLYTELY in children younger than 2 years of age should be carefully monitored for occurrence of possible hypoglycemia, as this solution has no caloric substrate. Dehydration has been reported in 1 child and hypokalemia has been reported in 3 children.

PRECAUTIONS

General: Patients with impaired gag reflex, unconscious, or semiconscious patients, and patients prone to regurgitation or aspiration should be observed during the administration of GoLYTELY or NuLYTELY, especially if it is administered via nasogastric tube. If a patient experiences severe bloating, distention or abdominal pain, administration should be slowed or temporarily discontinued until the symptoms abate. If gastrointestinal obstruction or perforation is suspected, appropriate studies should be performed to rule out these conditions before administration of GoLYTELY or NuLYTELY.

Information for Patients: GoLYTELY and NuLYTELY produce a watery stool which cleanses the bowel before examination. Prepare the solution according to the instructions on the bottle. It is more palatable if chilled. For best results, no solid food should be consumed during the 3 to 4 hour period before drinking the solution, but in no case should solid foods be eaten within 2 hours of taking GoLYTELY or NuLYTELY.

GoLYTELY®: Drink 240 mL (8 oz.) every 10 minutes. Rapid drinking of each portion is better than drinking small amounts continuously.

NuLYTELY®: Adults drink 240 mL (8 oz.) every 10 minutes. Continue drinking until the watery stool is clear and free of solid matter. This usually requires at least 3 liters and it is best to drink all of the solution. Any unused portion should be discarded. Pediatric patients (aged 6 months or greater) drink 25 mL/kg/hour. Continue drinking until the watery stool is clear and free of solid matter. Any unused portion should be discarded. Use of NuLYTELY in children younger than 2 years of age should be carefully monitored for occurrence of possible hypoglycemia, as this solution has no caloric substrate. Dehydration has been reported in 1 child and hypokalemia has been reported in 3 children.

The first bowel movement should occur approximately one hour after the start of GoLYTELY or NuLYTELY administration. You may experience some abdominal bloating and distention before the bowels start to move. If severe discomfort or distention occur, stop drinking temporarily or drink each portion at longer intervals until these symptoms disappear.

Drug Interactions: Oral medication administered within one hour of the start of administration of GoLYTELY or NuLYTELY may be flushed from the gastrointestinal tract and not absorbed.

Carcinogenesis, Mutagenesis, Impairment of Fertility: Carcinogenic and reproductive studies with animals have not been performed.

Pregnancy: Category C. Animal reproduction studies have not been conducted with GoLYTELY and NuLYTELY. It is also not known whether GoLYTELY and NuLYTELY can cause fetal harm when administered to a pregnant woman or can affect reproductive capacity. GoLYTELY and NuLYTELY should be given to a pregnant woman only if clearly needed.

Pediatric Use:

GoLYTELY®

Safety and effectiveness in children have not been established.

NuLYTELY®

Safety and effectiveness of NuLYTELY in pediatric patients aged 6 months and older is supported by evidence from adequate and well-controlled clinical trials of NuLYTELY in adults with additional safety and efficacy data from published studies of similar formulations.

ADVERSE REACTIONS

Nausea, abdominal fullness and bloating are the most common adverse reactions (occurring in up to 50% of patients) to administration of GoLYTELY or NuLYTELY. Abdominal cramps, vomiting and anal irritation occur less frequently. These adverse reactions are transient and subside rapidly. Isolated cases of urticaria, rhinorrhea, dermatitis and (rarely) anaphylactic reaction have been reported which may represent allergic reactions.

Published literature contains isolated reports of serious adverse reactions following the administration of PEG-ELS products in patients over 60 years of age. These adverse events include upper GI bleeding from Mallory-Weiss Tear, esophageal perforation, asystole, sudden dyspnea with pulmonary edema, and "butterfly-like" infiltrate on chest X-ray after vomiting and aspirating PEG.

DOSAGE AND ADMINISTRATION

GoLYTELY®

The recommended dose for adults is 4 liters of GoLYTELY solution prior to gastrointestinal examination, as ingestion of this dose produces a satisfactory preparation in over 95% of patients. Ideally, the patient should fast for approximately three or four hours prior to GoLYTELY administration, but in no case should solid food be given for at least two hours before the solution is given.

GoLYTELY is usually administered orally, but may be given via nasogastric tube to patients who are unwilling or unable to drink the solution. **Oral administration** is at a rate of 240 mL (8 oz.) every 10 minutes, until 4 liters are consumed or the rectal effluent is clear. Rapid drinking of each portion is preferred to drinking small amounts continuously. **Nasogastric tube administration** is at the rate of 20–30 mL per minute (1.2–1.8 liters per hour). The first bowel movement should occur approximately one hour after the start of GoLYTELY administration.

Various regimens have been used. One method is to schedule patients for examination in midmorning or later, allowing the patients three hours for drinking and an additional one hour period for complete bowel evacuation. Another method is to administer GoLYTELY on the evening before the examination, particularly if the patient is to have a barium enema.

NuLYTELY®

NuLYTELY is usually administered orally, but may be given via nasogastric tube to patients who are unwilling or unable to drink the solution. Ideally, the patient should fast for approximately three or four hours prior to NuLYTELY administration, but in no case should solid food be given for at least two hours before the solution is given.

Oral administration:

Adults: At a rate of 240 mL (8 oz.) every 10 minutes, until the rectal effluent is clear or 4 liters are consumed.

Pediatric Patients (aged 6 months or greater): At a rate of 25 mL/kg/hour, until the rectal effluent is clear.

Rapid drinking of each portion is preferred to drinking small amounts continuously.

Nasogastric tube administration:

Adults: At a rate of 20–30 mL per minute (1.2–1.8 liters per hour).

Pediatric Patients (aged 6 months or greater): At a rate of 25 mL/kg/hour, until the rectal effluent is clear.

The first bowel movement should occur approximately one hour after the start of NuLYTELY administration. Ingestion of 4 liters of NuLYTELY solution prior to gastrointestinal examination produces satisfactory preparation in over 95% of patients.

Various regimens have been used. One method is to schedule patients for examination in midmorning or later, allowing the patients three hours for drinking and an additional one hour period for complete bowel evacuation. Another method is to administer NuLYTELY on the evening before the examination.

Preparation of the solution:

GoLYTELY® solution is prepared by filling the container to the 4 liter mark with water and shaking vigorously several times to insure that the ingredients are dissolved. Dissolution is facilitated by using lukewarm water. The solution is more palatable if chilled before administration. The reconstituted solution should be refrigerated and used within 48 hours. Discard any unused portion.

NuLYTELY® solution is prepared by filling the container to the 4 liter mark with water and shaking vigorously several times to insure that the ingredients are dissolved. Dissolution is facilitated by using lukewarm water. The solution is more palatable if chilled before administration. However, chilled solution is not recommended for infants. The reconstituted solution should be refrigerated and used within 48 hours. Discard any unused portion.

HOW SUPPLIED

GoLYTELY®

In powdered form, for oral administration as a solution following reconstitution.

GoLYTELY® is available in a disposable jug and a packet in powdered form containing: **Disposable Jug:** polyethylene glycol 3350 236 g, sodium sulfate (anhydrous) 22.74 g, sodium bicarbonate 6.74 g, sodium chloride 5.86 g, potassium chloride 2.97 g. When made up to 4 liters volume with water, the solution contains PEG-3350 17.6 mmol/L, sodium 125 mmol/L, sulfate 40 mmol/L, chloride 35 mmol/L, bicarbonate 20 mmol/L and potassium 10 mmol/L. **Packet:** polyethylene glycol 3350 227.1 g, anhydrous sodium sulfate 21.5 g, sodium bicarbonate 6.36 g, sodium chloride 5.53 g, potassium chloride 2.82 g. When made up to 1 gallon volume with water, the solution contains PEG-3350 60g/L, sodium sulfate 5.68 g/L, sodium bicarbonate 1.68 g/L, sodium chloride 1.46 g/L and potassium chloride 0.745 g/L.

Pineapple Flavor GoLYTELY is available in a disposable jug in powdered form containing: polyethylene glycol 3350 236 g, sodium sulfate (anhydrous) 22.74 g, sodium bicarbonate 6.74 g, sodium chloride 5.86 g, potassium chloride 2.97 g, flavoring ingredients 3.0 g. When made up to 4 liters volume with water, the solution contains PEG-3350 17.6 mmol/L, sodium 125 mmol/L, sulfate 40 mmol/L, chloride 35 mmol/L, bicarbonate 20 mmol/L and potassium 10 mmol/L.

NuLYTELY®

NuLYTELY, Cherry NuLYTELY, Lemon-Lime NuLYTELY and Orange NuLYTELY are available in a disposable jug, in powdered form, for oral administration as a solution following reconstitution.

Each jug contains:

NuLYTELY: polyethylene glycol 3350 420 g, sodium bicarbonate 5.72 g, sodium chloride 11.2 g, potassium chloride 1.48 g. When made up to 4 liters volume with water, the solution contains PEG-3350 31.3 mmol/L, sodium 65 mmol/L, chloride 53 mmol/L, bicarbonate 17 mmol/L and potassium 5 mmol/L.

Cherry NuLYTELY: polyethylene glycol 3350 420 g, sodium bicarbonate 5.72 g, sodium chloride 11.2 g, potassium chloride 1.48 g and flavoring ingredients 2.0 g. When made up to 4 liters volume with water, the solution contains PEG-3350 31.3 mmol/L, sodium 65 mmol/L, chloride 53 mmol/L, bicarbonate 17 mmol/L and potassium 5 mmol/L.

Lemon-Lime NuLYTELY: polyethylene glycol 3350 420 g, sodium bicarbonate 5.72 g, sodium chloride 11.2 g, potassium chloride 1.48 g and flavoring ingredients 2.0 g. When made up to 4 liters volume with water, the solution contains PEG-3350 31.3 mmol/L, sodium 65 mmol/L, chloride 53 mmol/L, bicarbonate 17 mmol/L and potassium 5 mmol/L.

Orange NuLYTELY: polyethylene glycol 3350 420 g, sodium bicarbonate 5.72 g, sodium chloride 11.2 g, potassium chloride 1.48 g and flavoring ingredients 2.0 g. When made up to 4 liters volume with water, the solution contains PEG-3350 31.3 mmol/L, sodium 65 mmol/L, chloride 53 mmol/L, bicarbonate 17 mmol/L and potassium 5 mmol/L.

STORAGE: Store in sealed container at 25°C. When reconstituted, keep solution refrigerated. Use within 48 hours. Discard unused portion.

GoLYTELY	NDC 52268-100-01
GoLYTELY 1 Gallon Packet	NDC 52268-700-01
Pineapple Flavor GoLYTELY	NDC 52268-101-01
NuLYTELY	NDC 52268-300-01
Cherry Flavor NuLYTELY	NDC 52268-301-01
Lemon-Lime Flavor NuLYTELY	NDC 52268-302-01
Orange Flavor NuLYTELY	NDC 52268-303-01

Rx only

Distributed by Braintree Laboratories, Inc., Braintree, MA 02185

Shown in Product Identification Guide, page 309

MIRALAX™ ℞

[*mīra 'lăx*]

Polyethylene Glycol 3350, NF Powder

Full Prescribing Information

DESCRIPTION

A white powder for reconstitution. MiraLax (polyethylene glycol 3350, NF) is a synthetic polyglycol having an average molecular weight of 3350. The actual molecular weight is not less than 90.0 percent and not greater than 110.0 percent of the nominal value. The chemical formula is $HO(C_2H_4O)_nH$ in which n represents the average number of oxyethylene groups. Below 55°C it is a free flowing white powder freely soluble in water.

MiraLax is an osmotic agent for the treatment of constipation.

CLINICAL PHARMACOLOGY

Pharmacology: MiraLax is an osmotic agent which causes water to be retained with the stool.

Essentially, complete recovery of MiraLax was shown in normal subjects without constipation. Attempts at recovery of MiraLax in constipated patients resulted in incomplete and highly variable recovery. In vitro study showed indirectly that MiraLax was not fermented into hydrogen or methane by the colonic microflora in human feces. MiraLax appears to have no effect on the active absorption or secretion of glucose or electrolytes. There is no evidence of tachyphylaxis.

CLINICAL TRIALS

In one study, patients with less than 3 bowel movements per week were randomized to MiraLax, 17 grams, or placebo for 14 days. An increase in bowel movement frequency was observed for both treatment groups during the first week of treatment. MiraLax was statistically superior to placebo during the second week of treatment.

In another study, patients with 3 bowel movements or less per week and/or less than 300 grams of stool per week were randomized to 2 dose levels of MiraLax or placebo for 10 days each. Success was defined by an increase in both bowel movement frequency and daily stool weight. For both parameters, superiority of the 17 gram dose of MiraLax over placebo was demonstrated.

INDICATIONS AND USAGE

For the treatment of occasional constipation. This product should be used for 2 weeks or less or as directed by a physician.

CONTRAINDICATIONS

MiraLax is contraindicated in patients with known or suspected bowel obstruction and patients known to be allergic to polyethylene glycol.

WARNINGS

Patients with symptoms suggestive of bowel obstruction (nausea, vomiting, abdominal pain or distention) should be evaluated to rule out this condition before initiating MiraLax therapy.

PRECAUTIONS

General: Patients presenting with complaints of constipation should have a thorough medical history and physical examination to detect associated metabolic, endocrine and neurogenic conditions, and medications. A diagnostic evaluation should include a structural examination of the colon. Patients should be educated about good defecatory and eating habits (such as high fiber diets) and lifestyle changes (adequate dietary fiber and fluid intake, regular exercise) which may produce more regular bowel habits.

MiraLax should be administered dissolved in approximately 8 ounces of water.

Information for Patients: MiraLax softens the stool and increases the frequency of bowel movements by retaining water in the stool. It should always be taken by mouth after being dissolved in 8 ounces of water. Should unusual cramps, bloating, or diarrhea occur, consult your physician. Two to 4 days may be required to produce a bowel movement. This product should be used for 2 weeks or less or as directed by a physician. Prolonged, frequent or excessive use of MiraLax may result in electrolyte imbalance and dependence on laxatives.

Laboratory Tests: No clinically significant effects on laboratory tests have been demonstrated.

Drug Interactions: No specific drug interactions have been demonstrated.

Carcinogenesis, Mutagenesis, Impairment of Fertility: Long term carcinogenicity studies, genetic toxicity studies and reproductive toxicity studies in animals have not been performed with MiraLax.

Pregnancy: Category C. Animal reproductive studies have not been performed with MiraLax. It is also not known whether MiraLax can cause fetal harm when administered to a pregnant woman, or can effect reproductive capacity. MiraLax should only be administered to a pregnant woman if clearly needed.

Pediatric Use: Safety and effectiveness in pediatric patients has not been established.

Geriatric Use: There is no evidence for special considerations when MiraLax is administered to elderly patients. In geriatric nursing home patients a higher incidence of diarrhea occurred at the recommended 17 gram dose. If diarrhea occurs MiraLax should be discontinued.

ADVERSE REACTIONS

Nausea, abdominal bloating, cramping and flatulence may occur. High doses may produce diarrhea and excessive stool frequency, particularly in elderly nursing home patients.

Patients taking other medications containing polyethylene glycol have occasionally developed urticaria suggestive of an allergic reaction.

OVERDOSAGE

There have been no reports of accidental overdosage. In the event of overdosage diarrhea would be the expected major event. If an overdose of drug occurred without concomitant ingestion of fluid, dehydration due to diarrhea may result. Medication should be terminated and free water administered. The oral LD_{50} is >50 gm/Kg in mice, rats and rabbits.

DOSAGE AND ADMINISTRATION

The usual dose is 17 grams (about 1 heaping tablespoon) of powder per day (or as directed by physician) in 8 ounces of water. Each bottle of MiraLax is supplied with a measuring cap marked to contain 17 grams of laxative powder when filled to the indicated line.

Two to 4 days (48 to 96 hours) may be required to produce a bowel movement.

HOW SUPPLIED

In powdered form, for oral administration after dissolution in water. MiraLax is available in two package sizes; a 14 oz. container of 255 grams of laxative powder and a 26 oz. container of 527 grams of laxative powder.

The cap on each bottle is marked with a measuring line and may be used to measure a single MiraLax dose of 17 grams (about 1 heaping tablespoon).

Rx only

STORAGE

Store at 25 degrees C (77 degrees F); excursions permitted to 15–30 degrees C (59–86 degrees F). See USP "Controlled Room Temperature."

Distributed by Braintree Laboratories, Inc., Braintree, MA 02185

D 4/00

Shown in Product Identification Guide, page 309

PhosLo® ℞

[*phos "lō '*]

Calcium Acetate Tablets

DESCRIPTION

Each white round tablet (stamped "BRA 200") contains 667 mg of calcium acetate, USP (anhydrous; $Ca(CH_3COO)_2$; MW=158.17 grams) equal to 169 mg (8.45 mEq) calcium, and 10 mg of the inert binder, polyethylene glycol 8000 NF.

CLINICAL PHARMACOLOGY

Patients with advanced renal insufficiency (creatinine clearance less than 30 ml/min) exhibit phosphate retention and some degree of hyperphosphatemia. The retention of phosphate plays a pivotal role in causing secondary hyperparathyroidism associated with osteodystrophy, and soft-tissue calcification. The mechanism by which phosphate retention

Continued on next page

Phoslo—Cont.

leads to hyperparathyroidism is not clearly delineated. Therapeutic efforts directed toward the control of hyperphosphatemia include reduction in the dietary intake of phosphate, inhibition of absorption of phosphate in the intestine with phosphate binders, and removal of phosphate from the body by more efficient methods of dialysis. The rate of removal of phosphate by dietary manipulation or by dialysis is insufficient. Dialysis patients absorb 40% to 80% of dietary phosphorus. Therefore, the fraction of dietary phosphate absorbed from the diet needs to be reduced by using phosphate binders in most renal failure patients on maintenance dialysis. Calcium acetate (PhosLo) when taken with meals, combines with dietary phosphate to form insoluble calcium phosphate which is excreted in the feces. Maintenance of serum phosphorus below 6.0 mg/dl is generally considered as a clinically acceptable outcome of treatment with phosphate binders. PhosLo is highly soluble at neutral pH, making the calcium readily available for binding to phosphate in the proximal small intestine.
Orally administered calcium acetate from pharmaceutical dosage forms has been demonstrated to be systemically absorbed up to approximately 40% under fasting conditions and up to approximately 30% under nonfasting conditions. This range represents data from both healthy subjects and renal dialysis patients under various conditions.

INDICATIONS AND USAGE

PhosLo is indicated for the control of hyperphosphatemia in end stage renal failure and does not promote aluminum absorption.

CONTRAINDICATIONS

Patients with hypercalcemia.

WARNINGS

Patients with end stage renal failure may develop hypercalcemia when given calcium with meals. No other calcium supplements should be given concurrently with PhosLo. Progressive hypercalcemia due to overdose of PhosLo may be severe as to require emergency measures. Chronic hypercalcemia may lead to vascular calcification, and other soft-tissue calcification. The serum calcium level should be monitored twice weekly during the early dose adjustment period. **The serum calcium times phosphate (CaXP) product should not be allowed to exceed 66.** Radiographic evaluation of suspect anatomical region may be helpful in early detection of soft-tissue calcification.

PRECAUTIONS

General: Excessive dosage of PhosLo induces hypercalcemia; therefore, early in the treatment during dosage adjustment serum calcium should be determined twice weekly. Should hypercalcemia develop, the dosage should be reduced or the treatment discontinued immediately depending on the severity of hypercalcemia. PhosLo should not be given to patients on digitalis, because hypercalcemia may precipitate cardiac arrhythmias. PhosLo therapy should always be started at low dose and should not be increased without careful monitoring of serum calcium. An estimate of daily dietary calcium intake should be made initially and the intake adjusted as needed. Serum phosphorus should also be determined periodically.
Information for the Patient: The patient should be informed about compliance with dosage instructions, adherence to instructions about diet and avoidance of the use of nonprescription antacids. Patients should be informed about the symptoms of hypercalcemia (see ADVERSE REACTIONS section).
Drug Interactions: PhosLo may decrease the bioavailability of tetracyclines.
Carcinogenesis, Mutagenesis, Impairment of Fertility: Long term animal studies have not been performed to evaluate the carcinogenic potential or effect on fertility of PhosLo.
Pregnancy: Teratogenic Effects: Category C. Animal reproduction studies have not been conducted with PhosLo. It is also not known whether PhosLo can cause fetal harm when administered to a pregnant woman or can effect reproduction capacity. PhosLo should be given to a pregnant woman only if clearly needed.
Pediatric Use: Safety and efficacy of PhosLo have not been established.

ADVERSE REACTIONS

In clinical studies, patients have occasionally experienced nausea during PhosLo therapy. Hypercalcemia may occur during treatment with PhosLo. Mild hypercalcemia (Ca>10.5 mg/dl) may be asymptomatic or manifest itself as constipation, anorexia, nausea and vomiting. More severe hypercalcemia (Ca>12 mg/dl) is associated with confusion, delerium, stupor and coma. Mild hypercalcemia is easily controlled by reducing the PhosLo dose or temporarily discontinuing therapy. Severe hypercalcemia can be treated by acute hemodialysis and discontinuing PhosLo therapy.
Decreasing dialysate calcium concentration could reduce the incidence and severity of PhosLo induced hypercalcemia. The long-term effect of PhosLo on the progression of vascular or soft-tissue calcification has not been determined. Isolated cases of pruritus have been reported which may represent allergic reactions.

OVERDOSAGE

Administration of PhosLo in excess of the appropriate daily dosage can cause severe hypercalcemia (See Adverse Reactions).

DOSAGE AND ADMINISTRATION

The recommended initial dose of PhosLo for the adult dialysis patient is 2 tablets with each meal. The dosage may be increased gradually to bring the serum phosphate value below 6 mg/dl, as long as hypercalcemia does not develop. Most patients require 3–4 tablets with each meal.
Store at controlled room temperature, 15°–30°C.

HOW SUPPLIED

In tablet form for oral administration. Each white round tablet contains 667 mg of calcium acetate (anhydrous $Ca(CH_3COO)_2$; MW=158.17 grams) equal to 169 mg (8.45 mEq) calcium, and 10 mg of the inert binder, polyethylene glycol 8000.
NDC 52268-200-01 P 5/99
Rx only
Manufactured for Braintree Laboratories, Inc.,
Braintree, MA 02185-0929
Shown in Product Identification Guide, page 309

Bristol-Myers Products

(A Bristol-Myers Squibb Company)
345 PARK AVENUE
NEW YORK, NY 10154

Direct Inquiries to:
Products Division
Consumer Affairs Department
1350 Liberty Avenue
Hillside, NJ 07207
(800) 468-7746

EXCEDRIN® MIGRAINE OTC

Pain Reliever/Pain Reliever Aid

ACTIVE INGREDIENTS

Each tablet, caplet or geltab contains Acetaminophen 250mg, Aspirin 250mg and Caffeine 65mg.

INACTIVE INGREDIENTS

(tablet and caplet) benzoic acid, carnauba wax, hydroxypropylcellulose, hydroxypropyl methylcellulose, microcrystalline cellulose, mineral oil, polysorbate 20, povidone, propylene glycol, simethicone emulsion, sorbitan monolaurate, stearic acid, may also contain: FD&C blue no. 1, titanium dioxide.

INACTIVE INGREDIENTS

(geltab) benzoic acid, D&C yellow #10 lake, disodium EDTA, FD&C blue #1 lake, FD&C red #40 lake, ferric oxide, gelatin, glycerin, hydroxypropylcellulose, hydroxypropyl methylcellulose, maltitol solution, microcrystalline cellulose, mineral oil, pepsin, polysorbate 20, povidone, propylene glycol, propyl gallate, simethicone emulsion, sorbitan monolaurate, stearic acid, titanium dioxide.

USE

Treats migraine.

WARNINGS

Reye's syndrome: Children and teenagers should not use this drug for chicken pox, or flu symptoms before a doctor is consulted about Reye's syndrome, a rare but serious illness reported to be associated with aspirin.
Allergy alert: aspirin may cause a severe allergic reaction which may include: • hives • facial swelling • asthma (wheezing) • shock
Alcohol warning: If you consume 3 or more alcoholic drinks every day, ask your doctor whether you should take acetaminophen and aspirin or other pain relievers/fever reducers. Acetaminophen and aspirin may cause liver damage and stomach bleeding.
Caffeine warning: The recommended dose of this product contains about as much caffeine as a cup of coffee. Limit the use of caffeine-containing medications, foods, or beverages while taking this product because too much caffeine may cause nervousness, irritability, sleeplessness, and, occasionally, rapid heart beat.
Do not use • if you have ever had an allergic reaction to any other pain reliever/fever reducer
Ask a doctor before use if you have
• never had migraines diagnosed by a health professional • a headache that is different from your usual migraines • the worst headache of your life • fever and stiff neck • headaches beginning after or caused by head injury, exertion, coughing or bending • experienced your first headache after the age of 50 • daily headaches • asthma • bleeding problems • ulcers • stomach problems such as heartburn, upset stomach, or stomach pain that do not go away or recur • a migraine so severe as to require bed rest • problems or serious side effects from taking pain relievers or fever reducers
Ask a doctor or pharmacist before use if you are taking a prescription drug for: • anticoagulation (thinning of the blood) • diabetes • gout • arthritis
Stop use and ask a doctor if
- an allergic reaction occurs. Seek medical help right away.
- your migraine is not relieved or worsens after first dose
- new or unexpected symptoms occur
- ringing in the ears or loss of hearing occurs

If pregnant or breast-feeding, ask a health professional before use. It is especially important not to use aspirin during the last 3 months of pregnancy unless definitely directed to do so by a doctor because it may cause problems in the unborn child or complications during delivery.
Keep out of reach of children. In case of overdose, get medical help or contact a Poison Control Center right away. Quick medical attention is critical for adults as well as for children even if you do not notice any signs or symptoms.

DIRECTIONS

- adults: take 2 (tablets, caplets or geltabs) with a glass of water
- if symptoms persist or worsen, ask your doctor
- do not take more than 2 tablets in 24 hours, unless directed by a doctor
- under 18 years of age: ask a doctor.

OVERDOSE

Acetylcysteine As An Antidote For Acetaminophen Overdose
Acetaminophen is rapidly absorbed from the upper gastrointestinal tract with peak plasma levels occurring between 30 and 60 minutes after therapeutic doses and usually within 4 hours following an overdose. The parent compound, which is nontoxic, is extensively metabolized in the liver to form principally the sulfate and glucuronide conjugates which are also nontoxic and are rapidly excreted in the urine. A small fraction of an ingested dose is metabolized in the liver by the cytochrome P-450 mixed function oxidase enzyme system to form a reactive, potentially toxic, intermediate metabolite which preferentially conjugates with hepatic glutathione to form the nontoxic cysteine and mercapturic acid derivatives which are then excreted by the kidney. Therapeutic doses of acetaminophen do not saturate the glucuronide and sulfate conjugation pathways and do not result in the formation of sufficient reactive metabolite to deplete glutathione stores. However, following ingestion of a large overdose (150 mg/kg or greater) the glucuronide and sulfate conjugation pathways are saturated resulting in a larger fraction of the drug being metabolized via the P-450 pathway. The increased formation of reactive metabolite may deplete the hepatic stores of glutathione with subsequent binding of the metabolite to protein molecules within the hepatocyte resulting in cellular necrosis. Acetylcysteine has been shown to reduce the extent of liver injury following acetaminophen overdose. Early symptoms following a potentially hepatotoxic overdose may include: nausea, vomiting, diaphoresis and general malaise. Clinical and laboratory evidence of hepatic toxicity may not be apparent until 48 to 72 hours postingestion. In most adults and adolescents, regardless of the quantity of acetaminophen reported to have been ingested, administer acetylcysteine immediately. Acetylcysteine therapy should be initiated and continued for a full course of therapy. Its effectiveness depends on early administration, with benefit seen principally in patients treated within 16 hours of the overdose. If acetaminophen plasma assay capability is not available, and the estimated acetaminophen ingestion exceeds 150 mg/kg., acetylcysteine therapy should be initiated and continued for a full course of therapy.
For full prescription information, refer to the acetylcysteine package insert. Do not await the results of assays for acetaminophen level before initiating treatment with acetylcysteine. The following additional procedures are recommended: The stomach should be emptied promptly by lavage or by induction of emesis with syrup of ipecac. A serum acetaminophen assay should be obtained as early as possible, but no sooner than four hours following ingestion. Liver function studies should be obtained initially and repeated at 24-hour intervals. For additional emergency information call your regional poison center or toll-free (1-800-525-6115) to the Rocky Mountain Poison Center for assistance in diagnosis and for directions in the use of acetylcysteine as an antidote.

HOW SUPPLIED

EXCEDRIN® MIGRAINE is supplied as:
Coated white circular tablets or coated white caplets with letter "E" debossed on one side. Supplied in bottles of 24's, 50's, 100's, 175's, 275's (tablets) are available in club store packages. Coated round geltabs–green on one side, white on the other, printed with black "E" on one side. Supplied in bottles of 24's, 50's and 100's (2 bottles of 50 each).
Store at 20–25°C (68–77°F).
For use under U.S. Patent No. 5972916
Shown in Product Identification Guide, page 309

For information on over-the-counter drugs, consult **PDR For Nonprescription Drugs.**

Bristol-Myers Squibb Company

P.O. BOX 4500
PRINCETON, NJ 08543-4500

For Medical Information Contact:
Generally:
Bristol-Myers Squibb Drug Information Department
P.O. Box 4500
Princeton, NJ 08543-4500
(800) 321–1335

Adverse Drug Experiences
and Product Defects Reporting call
between 8:30 AM–4:30 PM EST:
(609) 818-3737

Sales and Ordering:
Orders may be placed by:
1. Calling your purchase orders toll-free between 8:30 AM–5:00 PM EST:
(800) 631-5244
2. Mailing your purchase orders to:
Bristol-Myers Squibb U.S. Pharmaceuticals
Attn: Customer Service
P.O. Box 5250
Princeton, NJ 08543-5250
3. Faxing your purchase orders to:
(800) 523-2965
4. Transmitting computer-to-computer on the NWDA and UCS formats through Ordernet Services use: DEA# PE0048579

AVALIDE® ℞

[avă-līde]
(irbesartan-hydrochlorothiazide)
Tablets
Rx only

USE IN PREGNANCY
When used in pregnancy during the second and third trimesters, drugs that act directly on the renin-angio tensin system can cause injury and even death to the developing fetus. When pregnancy is detected, AVALIDE should be discontinued as soon as possible. (See **WARNINGS: Fetal/Neonatal Morbidity and Mortality**.)

DESCRIPTION

AVALIDE®* (irbesartan-hydrochlorothiazide) Tablets is a combination of an angiotensin II receptor antagonist (AT1 subtype), irbesartan, and a thiazide diuretic, hydrochlorothiazide (HCTZ).

Irbesartan is a non-peptide compound, chemically described as a 2-butyl-3-[[2′-(1*H*-tetrazol-5-yl) [1, 1′-biphenyl]-4-yl]-methyl]-1,3-diazaspiro [4,4] non-1-en-4-one. Its empirical formula is $C_{25}H_{28}N_6O$, and its structural formula is:

[structural formula: O, N, N, $(CH_2)_3CH_3$, N, N, N, N, H]

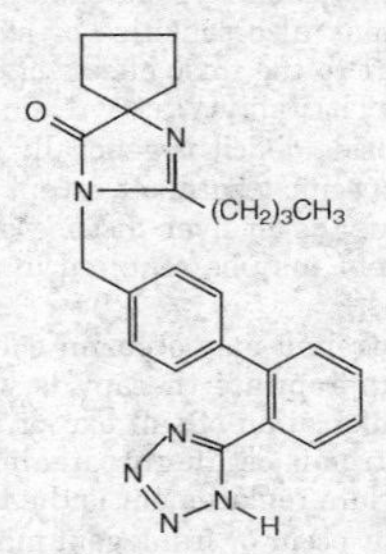

Irbesartan is a white to off-white crystalline powder with a molecular weight of 428.5. It is a nonpolar compound with a partition coefficient (octanol/water) of 10.1 at pH of 7.4. Irbesartan is slightly soluble in alcohol and methylene chloride and practically insoluble in water.

Hydrochlorothiazide is 6-chloro-3,4-dihydro- 2*H*-1,2,4-benzo - thiadiazine - 7 - sulfonamide 1,1 - dioxide. Its empirical formula is $C_7H_8ClN_3O_4S_2$ and its structural formula is:

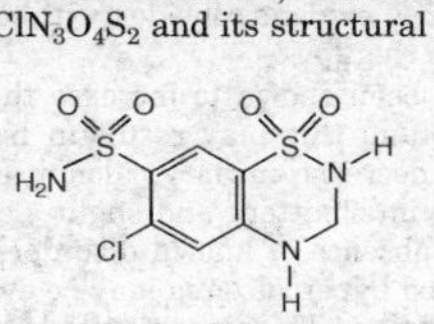

[structural formula: O O, S, H_2N, O O, S, N, H, Cl, N, H]

Hydrochlorothiazide is a white, or practically white, crystalline powder with a molecular weight of 297.7. Hydrochlorothiazide is slightly soluble in water and freely soluble in sodium hydroxide solution.

AVALIDE is available for oral administration in tablets containing 150 mg or 300 mg of irbesartan combined with 12.5 mg of hydrochlorothiazide. Inactive ingredients include: lactose monohydrate, microcrystalline cellulose, pregelatinized starch, croscarmellose sodium, ferric oxide red, ferric oxide yellow, silicon dioxide, and magnesium stearate.

CLINICAL PHARMACOLOGY

Mechanism Of Action

Irbesartan

Angiotensin II is a potent vasoconstrictor formed from angiotensin I in a reaction catalyzed by angiotensin-converting enzyme (ACE, kininase II). Angiotensin II is the principal pressor agent of the renin-angiotensin system (RAS) and also stimulates aldosterone synthesis and secretion by adrenal cortex, cardiac contraction, renal resorption of sodium, activity of the sympathetic nervous system, and smooth muscle cell growth. Irbesartan blocks the vasoconstrictor and aldosterone-secreting effects of angiotensin II by selectively binding to the AT_1 angiotensin II receptor. There is also an AT_2 receptor in many tissues, but it is not involved in cardiovascular homeostasis.

Irbesartan is a specific competitive antagonist of AT_1 receptors with a much greater affinity (more than 8500-fold) for the AT_1 receptor than for the AT_2 receptor, and no agonist activity.

Blockade of the AT_1 receptor removes the negative feedback of angiotensin II on renin secretion, but the resulting increased plasma renin activity and circulating angiotensin II do not overcome the effects of irbesartan on blood pressure.

Irbesartan does not inhibit ACE or renin or affect other hormone receptors or ion channels known to be involved in the cardiovascular regulation of blood pressure and sodium homeostasis. Because irbesartan does not inhibit ACE, it does not affect the response to bradykinin; whether this has clinical relevance is not known.

Hydrochlorothiazide

Hydrochlorothiazide is a thiazide diuretic. Thiazides affect the renal tubular mechanisms of electrolyte reabsorption, directly increasing excretion of sodium and chloride in approximately equivalent amounts. Indirectly, the diuretic action of hydrochlorothiazide reduces plasma volume, with consequent increases in plasma renin activity, increases in aldosterone secretion, increases in urinary potassium loss, and decreases in serum potassium. The renin-aldosterone link is mediated by angiotensin II, so coadministration of an angiotensin II receptor antagonist tends to reverse the potassium loss associated with these diuretics.

The mechanism of the antihypertensive effect of thiazides is not fully understood.

*Registered trademark of Sanofi-Synthelabo, Inc.

Pharmacokinetics

Irbesartan

Irbesartan is an orally active agent that does not require biotransformation into an active form. The oral absorption of irbesartan is rapid and complete with an average absolute bioavailability of 60–80%. Following oral administration of irbesartan, peak plasma concentrations of irbesartan are attained at 1.5–2 hours after dosing. Food does not affect the bioavailability of irbesartan.

Irbesartan exhibits linear pharmacokinetics over the therapeutic dose range.

The terminal elimination half-life of irbesartan averaged 11–15 hours. Steady-state concentrations are achieved within 3 days. Limited accumulation of irbesartan (<20%) is observed in plasma upon repeated once-daily dosing.

Hydrochlorothiazide

When plasma levels have been followed for at least 24 hours, the plasma half-life has been observed to vary between 5.6 and 14.8 hours.

Metabolism and Elimination

Irbesartan

Irbesartan is metabolized via glucuronide conjugation and oxidation. Following oral or intravenous administration of ^{14}C-labeled irbesartan, more than 80% of the circulating plasma radioactivity is attributable to unchanged irbesartan. The primary circulating metabolite is the inactive irbesartan glucuronide conjugate (approximately 6%). The remaining oxidative metabolites do not add appreciably to irbesartan's pharmacologic activity.

Irbesartan and its metabolites are excreted by both biliary and renal routes. Following either oral or intravenous administration of ^{14}C-labeled irbesartan, about 20% of radioactivity is recovered in the urine and the remainder in the feces, as irbesartan or irbesartan glucuronide.

In vitro studies of irbesartan oxidation by cytochrome P450 isoenzymes indicated irbesartan was oxidized primarily by 2C9; metabolism by 3A4 was negligible. Irbesartan was neither metabolized by, nor did it substantially induce or inhibit, isoenzymes commonly associated with drug metabolism (1A1, 1A2, 2A6, 2B6, 2D6, 2E1). There was no induction or inhibition of 3A4.

Hydrochlorothiazide

Hydrochlorothiazide is not metabolized but is eliminated rapidly by the kidney. At least 61 percent of the oral dose is eliminated unchanged within 24 hours.

Distribution

Irbesartan

Irbesartan is 90% bound to serum proteins (primarily albumin and α_1-acid glycoprotein) with negligible binding to cellular components of blood. The average volume of distribution is 53–93 liters. Total plasma and renal clearances are in the range of 157–176 and 3.0–3.5 mL/min, respectively. With repetitive dosing, irbesartan accumulates to no clinically relevant extent.

Studies in animals indicate that radiolabeled irbesartan weakly crosses the blood brain barrier and placenta. Irbesartan is excreted in the milk of lactating rats.

Hydrochlorothiazide

Hydrochlorothiazide crosses the placental but not the blood-brain barrier and is excreted in breast milk.

Special Populations

Pediatric: Irbesartan pharmacokinetics have not been investigated in patients <18 years of age.

Gender: No gender related differences in pharmacokinetics were observed in healthy elderly (age 65–80 years) or in healthy young (age 18–40 years) subjects. In studies of hypertensive patients, there was no gender difference in half-life or accumulation, but somewhat higher plasma concentrations of irbesartan were observed in females (11–44%). No gender-related dosage adjustment is necessary.

Geriatric: In elderly subjects (age 65–80 years), irbesartan elimination half-life was not significantly altered, but AUC and C_{max} values were about 20–50% greater than those of young subjects (age 18–40 years). No dosage adjustment is necessary in the elderly.

Race: In healthy black subjects, irbesartan AUC values were approximately 25% greater than whites; there were no differences in C_{max} values.

Renal Insufficiency: The pharmacokinetics of irbesartan were not altered in patients with renal impairment or in patients on hemodialysis. Irbesartan is not removed by hemodialysis. No dosage adjustment is necessary in patients with mild to severe renal impairment unless a patient with renal impairment is also volume depleted. (See **WARNINGS: Hypotension in Volume- or Salt-depleted Patients** and **DOSAGE AND ADMINISTRATION**.)

Hepatic Insufficiency: The pharmacokinetics of irbesartan following repeated oral administration were not significantly affected in patients with mild to moderate cirrhosis of the liver. No dosage adjustment is necessary in patients with hepatic insufficiency.

Drug Interactions: (See **PRECAUTIONS: Drug Interactions**.)

Pharmacodynamics

Irbesartan

In healthy subjects, single oral irbesartan doses of up to 300 mg produced dose-dependent inhibition of the pressor effect of angiotensin II infusions. Inhibition was complete (100%) 4 hours following oral doses of 150 mg or 300 mg and partial inhibition was sustained for 24 hours (60% and 40% at 300 mg and 150 mg, respectively).

In hypertensive patients, angiotensin II receptor inhibition following chronic administration of irbesartan causes a 1.5–2 fold rise in angiotensin II plasma concentration and a 2–3 fold increase in plasma renin levels. Aldosterone plasma concentrations generally decline following irbesartan administration, but serum potassium levels are not significantly affected at recommended doses.

In hypertensive patients, chronic oral doses of irbesartan (up to 300 mg) had no effect on glomerular filtration rate, renal plasma flow or filtration fraction. In multiple dose studies in hypertensive patients, there were no clinically important effects on fasting triglycerides, total cholesterol, HDL-cholesterol, or fasting glucose concentrations. There was no effect on serum uric acid during chronic oral administration and no uricosuric effect.

Hydrochlorothiazide

After oral administration of hydrochlorothiazide, diuresis begins within 2 hours, peaks in about 4 hours and lasts about 6 to 12 hours.

Clinical Studies

Irbesartan

The antihypertensive effects of irbesartan were examined in seven (7) major placebo-controlled 8–12 week trials in patients with baseline diastolic blood pressures of 95–110 mmHg. Doses of 1–900 mg were included in these trials in order to fully explore the dose-range of irbesartan. These studies allowed a comparison of once- or twice-daily regimens at 150 mg/day, comparisons of peak and trough effects, and comparisons of response by gender, age, and race. Two of the seven placebo-controlled trials identified above and two additional placebo-controlled studies examined the antihypertensive effects of irbesartan and hydrochlorothiazide in combination.

The seven (7) studies of irbesartan monotherapy included a total of 1915 patients randomized to irbesartan (1–900 mg) and 611 patients randomized to placebo. Once-daily doses of 150 to 300 mg provided statistically and clinically significant decreases in systolic and diastolic blood pressure with trough (24 hour post-dose) effects after 6–12 weeks of treatment compared to placebo, of about 8–10/5–6 and 8–12/5–8 mmHg, respectively. No further increase in effect was seen at dosages greater than 300 mg. The dose-response relationships for effects on systolic and diastolic pressure are shown in Figures 1 and 2.

[See figures at top of next column]

Once-daily administration of therapeutic doses of irbesartan gave peak effects at around 3–6 hours and, in one continuous ambulatory blood pressure monitoring study, and again around 14 hours. This was seen with both once-daily and twice-daily dosing. Trough-to-peak ratios for systolic and diastolic response were generally between 60–70%. In a continuous ambulatory blood pressure monitoring study, once-daily dosing with 150 mg gave trough and mean 24-hour responses similar to those observed in patients receiving twice-daily dosing at the same total daily dose.

Continued on next page

Avalide—Cont.

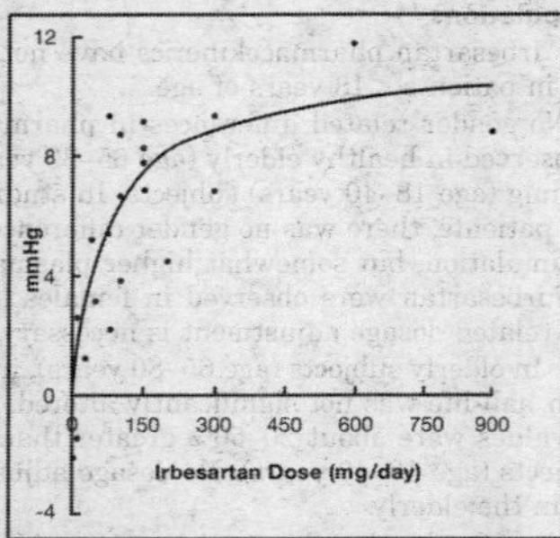

Figure 1. Placebo-subtracted reduction in trough SeSBP; integrated analysis

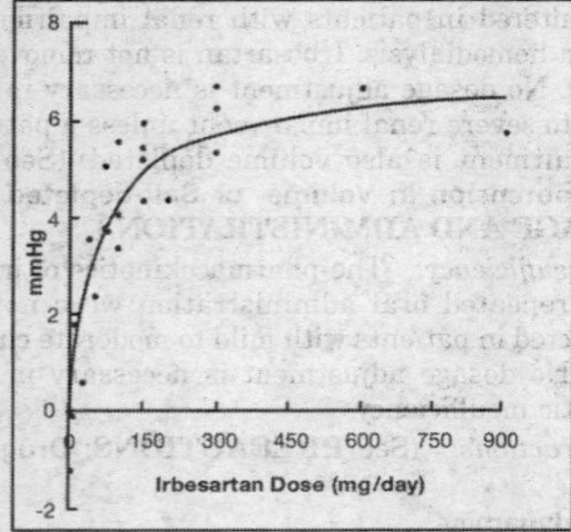

Figure 2. Placebo-subtracted reduction in trough SeDBP; integrated analysis

Analysis of age, gender, and race subgroups of patients showed that men and women, and patients over and under 65 years of age, had generally similar responses. Irbesartan was effective in reducing blood pressure regardless of race, although the effect was somewhat less in blacks (usually a low-renin population). Black patients typically show an improved response with the addition of a low dose diuretic (e.g., 12.5 mg hydrochlorothiazide).

The effect of irbesartan is apparent after the first dose and is close to the full observed effect at 2 weeks. At the end of the 8-week exposure, about 2/3 of the antihypertensive effect was still present 1 week after the last dose. Rebound hypertension was not observed. There was essentially no change in average heart rate in irbesartan-treated patients in controlled trials.

Irbesartan-Hydrochlorothiazide

The antihypertensive effects of AVALIDE (irbesartan-hydrochlorothiazide) Tablets were examined in 4 placebo-controlled studies of 8–12 weeks in patients with mild-moderate hypertension. These trials included 1914 patients randomized to fixed doses of irbesartan (37.5 to 300 mg) and concomitant hydrochlorothiazide (6.25 to 25 mg). One factorial study compared all combinations of irbesartan (37.5, 100 and 300 mg or placebo) and hydrochlorothiazide (6.25, 12.5, and 25 mg or placebo). The irbesartan-hydrochlorothiazide combinations of 75/12.5 mg and 150/12.5 mg were compared to their individual components and placebo in a separate study. A third study investigated the ambulatory blood pressure responses to irbesartan-hydrochlorothiazide (75/12.5 mg and 150/12.5 mg) and placebo after 8 weeks of dosing. Another trial investigated the effects of the addition of irbesartan (75 mg) in patients not controlled on hydrochlorothiazide (25 mg) alone.

In controlled trials, the addition of irbesartan 150–300 mg to hydrochlorothiazide doses of 6.25, 12.5 or 25 mg produced further dose-related reductions in blood pressure of 8–10/3–6 mmHg, comparable to those achieved with the same monotherapy dose of irbesartan. The addition of hydrochlorothiazide to irbesartan produced further dose-related reductions in blood pressure at trough (24 hours post-dose) of 5–6/2–3 mmHg (12.5 mg) and 7–11/4–5 mmHg (25 mg), also comparable to effects achieved with hydrochlorothiazide alone. Once-daily dosing with 150 mg irbesartan and 12.5 mg hydrochlorothiazide, 300 mg irbesartan and 12.5 mg hydrochlorothiazide, or 300 mg irbesartan and 25 mg hydrochlorothiazide produced mean placebo-adjusted blood pressure reductions at trough (24 hours post-dosing) of about 13–15/7–9, 14/9–12, and 19–21/11–12 mmHg, respectively. Peak effects occurred at 3–6 hours, with the trough-to-peak ratios >65%.

In another study, irbesartan (75–150 mg) or placebo was added on a background of 25 mg hydrochlorothiazide in patients not adequately controlled (SeDBP 93–120 mmHg) on hydrochlorothiazide (25 mg) alone. The addition of irbesartan (75–150 mg) gave an additive effect (systolic/diastolic) at trough (24 hours post-dosing) of 11/7 mmHg.

There was no difference in response for men and women or in patients over or under 65 years of age. Black patients had a larger response to hydrochlorothiazide than non-black patients and a smaller response to irbesartan. The overall response to the combination was similar for black and non-black patients.

INDICATIONS AND USAGE

AVALIDE (irbesartan-hydrochlorothiazide) Tablets is indicated for the treatment of hypertension. This fixed dose combination is not indicated for initial therapy (see **DOSAGE AND ADMINISTRATION**).

CONTRAINDICATIONS

AVALIDE is contraindicated in patients who are hypersensitive to any component of this product.

Because of the hydrochlorothiazide component, this product is contraindicated in patients with anuria or hypersensitivity to other sulfonamide-derived drugs.

WARNINGS

Fetal/Neonatal Morbidity and Mortality

Drugs that act directly on the renin-angiotensin system can cause fetal and neonatal morbidity and death when administered to pregnant women. Several dozen cases have been reported in the world literature in patients who were taking angiotensin converting enzyme inhibitors. When pregnancy is detected, AVALIDE (irbesartan-hydrochlorothiazide) Tablets should be discontinued as soon as possible.

The use of drugs that act directly on the renin-angiotensin system during the second and third trimesters of pregnancy has been associated with fetal and neonatal injury, including hypotension, neonatal skull hypoplasia, anuria, reversible or irreversible renal failure, and death. Oligohydramnios has also been reported, presumably resulting from decreased fetal renal function; oligohydramnios in this setting has been associated with fetal limb contractures, craniofacial deformation, and hypoplastic lung development. Prematurity, intrauterine growth retardation, and patent ductus arteriosus have also been reported, although it is not clear whether these occurrences were due to exposure to the drug.

These adverse effects do not appear to have resulted from intrauterine drug exposure that has been limited to the first trimester.

Mothers whose embryos and fetuses are exposed to an angiotensin II receptor antagonist only during the first trimester should be so informed. Nonetheless, when patients become pregnant, physicians should have the patient discontinue the use of AVALIDE as soon as possible.

Rarely (probably less often than once in every thousand pregnancies), no alternative to a drug acting on the renin-angiotensin system will be found. In these rare cases, the mothers should be apprised of the potential hazards to their fetuses, and serial ultrasound examinations should be performed to assess the intraamniotic environment.

If oligohydramnios is observed, AVALIDE (irbesartan-hydrochlorothiazide) Tablets should be discontinued unless it is considered life-saving for the mother. Contraction stress testing (CST), a non-stress test (NST), or biophysical profiling (BPP) may be appropriate depending upon the week of pregnancy. Patients and physicians should be aware, however, that oligohydramnios may not appear until after the fetus has sustained irreversible injury.

Infants with histories of *in utero* exposure to an angiotensin II receptor antagonist should be closely observed for hypotension, oliguria, and hyperkalemia. If oliguria occurs, attention should be directed toward support of blood pressure and renal perfusion. Exchange transfusion or dialysis may be required as a means of reversing hypotension and/or substituting for disordered renal function.

When pregnant rats were treated with irbesartan from day 0 to day 20 of gestation (oral doses of 50, 180, and 650 mg/kg/day), increased incidences of renal pelvic cavitation, hydroureter and/or absence of renal papilla were observed in fetuses at doses ≥50 mg/kg/day [approximately equivalent to the maximum recommended human dose (MRHD), 300 mg/day, on a body surface area basis]. Subcutaneous edema was observed in fetuses at doses ≥180 mg/kg/day (about 4 times the MRHD on a body surface area basis). As these anomalies were not observed in rats in which irbesartan exposure (oral doses of 50, 150 and 450 mg/kg/day) was limited to gestation days 6–15, they appear to reflect late gestational effects of the drug. In pregnant rabbits, oral doses of 30 mg irbesartan/kg/day were associated with maternal mortality and abortion. Surviving females receiving this dose (about 1.5 times the MRHD on a body surface area basis) had a slight increase in early resorptions and a corresponding decrease in live fetuses. Irbesartan was found to cross the placental barrier in rats and rabbits.

Radioactivity was present in the rat and rabbit fetus during late gestation and in rat milk following oral doses of radiolabeled irbesartan.

Studies in which hydrochlorothiazide was administered to pregnant mice and rats during their respective periods of major organogenesis at doses up to 3000 and 1000 mg/kg/day, respectively, provided no evidence of harm to the fetus.

A development toxicity study was performed in rats with doses of 50/50 and 150/150 mg/kg/day irbesartan-hydrochlorothiazide. Although the high dose combination appeared to be more toxic to the dams than either drug alone, there did not appear to be an increase in toxicity to the developing embryos.

Thiazides cross the placental barrier and appear in cord blood. There is a risk of fetal or neonatal jaundice, thrombocytopenia, and possibly other adverse reactions that have occurred in adults.

Hypotension in Volume- or Salt-depleted Patients

Excessive reduction of blood pressure was rarely seen in patients with uncomplicated hypertension treated with irbesartan alone (<0.1%) or with irbesartan-hydrochlorothiazide (approximately 1%). Initiation of antihypertensive therapy may cause symptomatic hypotension in patients with intravascular volume- or sodium-depletion, e.g., in patients treated vigorously with diuretics or in patients on dialysis. Such volume depletion should be corrected prior to administration of antihypertensive therapy.

If hypotension occurs, the patient should be placed in the supine position and, if necessary, given an intravenous infusion of normal saline. A transient hypotensive response is not a contraindication to further treatment, which usually can be continued without difficulty once the blood pressure has stabilized.

Hydrochlorothiazide

Hepatic Impairment

Thiazides should be used with caution in patients with impaired hepatic function or progressive liver disease, since minor alterations of fluid and electrolyte balance may precipitate hepatic coma.

Hypersensitivity Reaction

Hypersensitivity reactions to hydrochlorothiazide may occur in patients with or without a history of allergy or bronchial asthma, but are more likely in patients with such a history.

Systemic Lupus Erythematosus

Thiazide diuretics have been reported to cause exacerbation or activation of systemic lupus erythematosus.

Lithium Interaction

Lithium generally should not be given with thiazides (see **PRECAUTIONS**: **Drug Interactions**; *Hydrochlorothiazide, Lithium*).

PRECAUTIONS

General

Irbesartan-Hydrochlorothiazide

In double-blind clinical trials of various doses of irbesartan and hydrochlorothiazide, the incidence of hypertensive patients who developed hypokalemia (serum potassium <3.5 mEq/L) was 7.5% versus 6.0% for placebo; the incidence of hyperkalemia (serum potassium >5.7 mEq/L) was <1.0% versus 1.7% for placebo. No patient discontinued due to increases or decreases in serum potassium. Overall, the combination of irbesartan and hydrochlorothiazide had no effect on serum potassium. Higher doses of irbesartan ameliorated the hypokalemic response to hydrochlorothiazide.

Hydrochlorothiazide

Periodic determination of serum electrolytes to detect possible electrolyte imbalance should be performed at appropriate intervals. All patients receiving thiazide therapy should be observed for clinical signs of fluid or electrolyte imbalance: hyponatremia, hypochloremic alkalosis, and hypokalemia. Serum and urine electrolyte determinations are particularly important when the patient is vomiting excessively or receiving parenteral fluids. Warning signs or symptoms of fluid and electrolyte imbalance, irrespective of cause, include dryness of mouth, thirst, weakness, lethargy, drowsiness, restlessness, confusion, seizures, muscle pains or cramps, muscular fatigue, hypotension, oliguria, tachycardia, and gastrointestinal disturbances such as nausea and vomiting.

Hypokalemia may develop, especially with brisk diuresis, when severe cirrhosis is present, or after prolonged therapy. Interference with adequate oral electrolyte intake will also contribute to hypokalemia. Hypokalemia may cause cardiac arrhythmia and may also sensitize or exaggerate the response of the heart to the toxic effects of digitalis (e.g., increased ventricular irritability).

Although any chloride deficit is generally mild and usually does not require specific treatment except under extraordinary circumstances (as in liver disease or renal disease), chloride replacement may be required in the treatment of metabolic alkalosis.

Dilutional hyponatremia may occur in edematous patients in hot weather; appropriate therapy is water restriction, rather than administration of salt except in rare instances when the hyponatremia is life-threatening. In actual salt depletion, appropriate replacement is the therapy of choice.

Hyperuricemia may occur or frank gout may be precipitated in certain patients receiving thiazide therapy.

In diabetic patients dosage adjustments of insulin or oral hypoglycemic agents may be required. Hyperglycemia may occur with thiazide diuretics. Thus latent diabetes mellitus may become manifest during thiazide therapy.

The antihypertensive effects of the drug may be enhanced in the post sympathectomy patient. If progressive renal impairment becomes evident consider withholding or discontinuing diuretic therapy.

Thiazides have been shown to increase the urinary excretion of magnesium; this may result in hypomagnesemia.

Thiazides may decrease urinary calcium excretion. Thiazides may cause intermittent and slight elevation of serum calcium in the absence of known disorders of calcium metabolism. Marked hypercalcemia may be evidence of hidden hyperparathyroidism. Thiazides should be discontinued before carrying out tests for parathyroid function.

Increases in cholesterol and triglyceride levels may be associated with thiazide diuretic therapy.

Impaired Renal Function

As a consequence of inhibiting the renin-angiotensin-aldosterone system, changes in renal function may be anticipated in susceptible individuals. In patients whose renal function may depend on the activity of the renin-angiotensin-aldosterone system (e.g., patients with severe congestive heart failure), treatment with angiotensin converting enzyme inhibitors has been associated with oliguria and/or progressive azotemia and (rarely) with acute renal failure and/or death. Irbesartan would be expected to behave similarly. In studies of ACE inhibitors in patients with unilateral or bilateral renal artery stenosis, increases in serum creatinine or BUN have been reported. There has been no known use of irbesartan in patients with unilateral or bilateral renal artery stenosis, but a similar effect should be anticipated.

Thiazides should be used with caution in severe renal disease. In patients with renal disease, thiazides may precipitate azotemia. Cumulative effects of the drug may develop in patients with impaired renal function.

Information For Patients

Pregnancy: Female patients of childbearing age should be told about the consequences of second- and third-trimester exposure to drugs that act on the renin-angiotensin system, and they should also be told that these consequences do not appear to have resulted from intrauterine drug exposure that has been limited to the first trimester. These patients should be asked to report pregnancies to their physicians as soon as possible.

Symptomatic Hypotension: A patient receiving AVALIDE (irbesartan-hydrochlorothiazide) Tablets should be cautioned that lightheadedness can occur, especially during the first days of therapy, and that it should be reported to the prescribing physician. The patients should be told that if syncope occurs, AVALIDE should be discontinued until the physician has been consulted.

All patients should be cautioned that inadequate fluid intake, excessive perspiration, diarrhea, or vomiting can lead to an excessive fall in blood pressure, with the same consequences of lightheadedness and possible syncope.

Drug Interactions

Irbesartan

No significant drug-drug pharmacokinetic (or pharmacodynamic) interactions have been found in interaction studies with hydrochlorothiazide, digoxin, warfarin, and nifedipine. *In vitro* studies show significant inhibition of the formation of oxidized irbesartan metabolites with the known cytochrome CYP 2C9 substrates/inhibitors sulphenazole, tolbutamide and nifedipine. However, in clinical studies the consequences of concomitant irbesartan on the pharmacodynamics of warfarin were negligible. Concomitant nifedipine or hydrochlorothiazide had no effect on irbesartan pharmacokinetics. Based on *in vitro* data, no interaction would be expected with drugs whose metabolism is dependent upon cytochrome P450 isozymes 1A1, 1A2, 2A6, 2B6, 2D6, 2E1, or 3A4.

In separate studies of patients receiving maintenance doses of warfarin, hydrochlorothiazide, or digoxin, irbesartan administration for 7 days had no effect on the pharmacodynamics of warfarin (prothrombin time) or the pharmacokinetics of digoxin. The pharmacokinetics of irbesartan were not affected by coadministration of nifedipine or hydrochlorothiazide.

Hydrochlorothiazide

When administered concurrently the following drugs may interact with thiazide diuretics:

Alcohol, Barbiturates, Or Narcotics — potentiation of orthostatic hypotension may occur.

Antidiabetic Drugs (oral agents and insulin) — dosage adjustment of the antidiabetic drug may be required.

Other Antihypertensive Drugs — additive effect or potentiation.

Cholestyramine And Colestipol Resins — absorption of hydrochlorothiazide is impaired in the presence of anionic exchange resins. Single doses of either cholestyramine or colestipol resins bind the hydrochlorothiazide and reduce its absorption from the gastrointestinal tract by up to 85 and 43 percent, respectively.

Corticosteroids, ACTH — intensified electrolyte depletion, particularly hypokalemia.

Pressor Amines (e.g., Norepinephrine) — possible decreased response to pressor amines but not sufficient to preclude their use.

Skeletal Muscle Relaxants, Nondepolarizing (e.g., Tubocurarine) — possible increased responsiveness to the muscle relaxant.

Lithium — should not generally be given with diuretics. Diuretic agents reduce the renal clearance of lithium and add a high risk of lithium toxicity. Refer to the package insert for lithium preparations before use of such preparations with AVALIDE.

Non-steroidal Anti-inflammatory Drugs — in some patients, the administration of a non-steroidal anti-inflammatory agent can reduce the diuretic, natriuretic, and antihypertensive effects of loop, potassium-sparing and thiazide diuretics. Therefore, when AVALIDE (irbesartan-hydrochlorothiazide) Tablets and non-steroidal anti-inflammatory agents are used concomitantly, the patient should be observed closely to determine if the desired effect of the diuretic is obtained.

Carcinogenesis, Mutagenesis, Impairment Of Fertility

Irbesartan-Hydrochlorothiazide

No carcinogenicity studies have been conducted with the irbesartan-hydrochlorothiazide combination.

Irbesartan-hydrochlorothiazide was not mutagenic in standard *in vitro* tests (Ames microbial test and Chinese hamster mammalian-cell forward gene-mutation assay). Irbesartan-hydrochlorothiazide was negative in tests for induction of chromosomal aberrations (*in vitro* — human lymphocyte assay; *in vivo* — mouse micronucleus study). The combination of irbesartan and hydrochlorothiazide has not been evaluated in definitive studies of fertility.

	Irbesartan/HCTZ (n=898) (%)	Placebo (n=236) (%)	Irbesartan (n=400) (%)	HCTZ (n=380) (%)
Body as a Whole				
Chest Pain	2	1	2	2
Fatigue	7	3	4	3
Influenza	3	1	2	2
Cardiovascular				
Edema	3	3	2	2
Tachycardia	1	0	1	1
Gastrointestinal				
Abdominal Pain	2	1	2	2
Dyspepsia/heartburn	2	1	0	2
Nausea/vomiting	3	0	2	0
Immunology				
Allergy	1	0	1	1
Musculoskeletal				
Musculoskeletal Pain	7	5	6	10
Nervous System				
Dizziness	8	4	6	5
Dizziness Orthostatic	1	0	1	1
Renal/Genitourinary				
Abnormality Urination	2	1	1	2

Irbesartan (mg)	HCTZ (mg)	NDC 0087-xxxx-xx for unit of use			
		Bottle of			Blister of
		30	90	500	100
150	12.5	2775–31	2775–32	2775–15	2775–35
300	12.5	2776–31	2776–32	2776–15	2776–35

Irbesartan

No evidence of carcinogenicity was observed when irbesartan was administered at doses of up to 500/1000 mg/kg/day (males/females, respectively) in rats and 1000 mg/kg/day in mice for up to two years. For male and female rats, 500 mg/kg/day provided an average systemic exposure to irbesartan ($AUC_{0\text{-}24hours}$, bound plus unbound) about 3 and 11 times, respectively, the average systemic exposure in humans receiving the maximum recommended dose (MRD) of 300 mg irbesartan/day, whereas 1000 mg/kg/day (administered to females only) provided an average systemic exposure about 21 times that reported for humans at the MRD. For male and female mice, 1000 mg/kg/day provided an exposure to irbesartan about 3 and 5 times, respectively, the human exposure at 300 mg/day.

Irbesartan was not mutagenic in a battery of *in vitro* tests (Ames microbial test, rat hepatocyte DNA repair test, V79 mammalian-cell forward gene-mutation assay). Irbesartan was negative in several tests for induction of chromosomal aberrations (*in vitro*-human lymphocyte assay; *in vivo*-mouse micronucleus study).

Irbesartan had no adverse effects on fertility or mating of male or female rats at oral doses ≤650 mg/kg/day, the highest dose providing a systemic exposure to irbesartan ($AUC_{0\text{-}24hours}$, bound plus unbound) about 5 times that found in humans receiving the maximum recommended dose of 300 mg/day.

Hydrochlorothiazide

Two-year feeding studies in mice and rats conducted under the auspices of the National Toxicology Program (NTP) uncovered no evidence of a carcinogenic potential of hydrochlorothiazide in female mice (at doses of up to approximately 600 mg/kg/day) or in male and female rats (at doses of up to approximately 100 mg/kg/day). The NTP, however, found equivocal evidence for hepatocarcinogenicity in male mice. Hydrochlorothiazide was not genotoxic *in vitro* in the Ames mutagenicity assay of *Salmonella typhimurium* strains TA 98, TA 100, TA 1535, TA 1537, and TA 1538 and in the Chinese Hamster Ovary (CHO) test for chromosomal aberrations, or in vivo in assays using mouse germinal cell chromosomes, Chinese hamster bone marrow chromosomes, and the *Drosophila* sex-linked recessive lethal trait gene. Positive test results were obtained only in the *in vitro* CHO Sister Chromatid Exchange (clastogenicity) and in the Mouse Lymphoma Cell (mutagenicity) assays, using concentrations of hydrochlorothiazide from 43 to 1300 mg/mL, and in the *Aspergillus nidulans* non-disjunction assay at an unspecified concentration.

Hydrochlorothiazide had no adverse effects on the fertility of mice and rats of either sex in studies wherein these species were exposed, via their diet, to doses of up to 100 and 4 mg/kg, respectively, prior to mating and throughout gestation.

Pregnancy

Pregnancy Categories C (first trimester) and D (second and third trimesters)

(See **WARNINGS: Fetal/Neonatal Morbidity and Mortality.**)

Nursing Mothers

It is not known whether irbesartan is excreted in human milk, but irbesartan or some metabolite of irbesartan is secreted at low concentration in the milk of lactating rats. Because of the potential for adverse effects on the nursing infant, a decision should be made whether to discontinue nursing or discontinue the drug, taking into account the importance of the drug to the mother.

Thiazides appear in human milk. Because of the potential for adverse effects on the nursing infant, a decision should be made whether to discontinue nursing or discontinue the drug, taking into account the importance of the drug to the mother.

Pediatric Use

Safety and effectiveness in pediatric patients have not been established.

Geriatric Use

Of the total number of patients in controlled clinical studies of hypertension with AVALIDE, 143 patients (16.0%) were 65 years and over, while 21 (2.3%) were 75 years and over. No overall differences in effectiveness or safety were observed between these patients and younger patients, but greater sensitivity of some older individuals cannot be ruled out.

ADVERSE REACTIONS

Irbesartan-hydrochlorothiazide

AVALIDE (irbesartan-hydrochlorothiazide) Tablets has been evaluated for safety in 898 patients treated for essential hypertension. In clinical trials with AVALIDE, no adverse experiences peculiar to this combination drug product have been observed. Adverse experiences have been limited to those that were reported previously with irbesartan and/or hydrochlorothiazide (HCTZ). The overall incidence of adverse experiences reported with the combination was comparable to placebo. In general, treatment with AVALIDE was well tolerated. For the most part, adverse experiences have been mild and transient in nature and have not required discontinuation of therapy. In controlled clinical trials, discontinuation of AVALIDE therapy due to clinical adverse experiences was required in only 3.6%. This incidence was significantly less (p=0.023) than the 6.8% of patients treated with placebo who discontinued therapy.

In these double-blind controlled clinical trials, the following adverse experiences reported with AVALIDE occurred in ò1% of patients, and more often on the irbesartan-hydrochlorothiazide combination then on placebo, regardless of drug relationship:

[See first table above]

The following adverse events were also reported at a rate of 1% or greater, but were as, or more, common in the placebo group: headache, sinus abnormality, cough, URI, pharyngitis, diarrhea, rhinitis, urinary tract infection, rash, anxiety/nervousness, and muscle cramp.

Adverse events occurred at about the same rates in men and women, older and younger patients, and black and non-black patients.

Irbesartan

Other adverse experiences that have been reported with irbesartan, without regard to causality are listed below:

Body as a Whole: fever, chills, orthostatic effects, facial edema, upper extremity edema

Cardiovascular: flushing, hypertension, cardiac murmur, myocardial infarction, angina pectoris, hypotension, syncope, arrhythmic/conduction disorder, cardio-respiratory arrest, heart failure, hypertensive crisis

Dermatologic: pruritus, dermatitis, ecchymosis, erythema face, urticaria

Endocrine/Metabolic/Electrolyte Imbalances: sexual dysfunction, libido change, gout

Gastrointestinal: diarrhea, constipation, gastroenteritis, flatulence, abdominal distention

Continued on next page

Avalide—Cont.

Musculoskeletal/Connective Tissue: musculoskeletal trauma, extremity swelling, muscle cramp, arthritis, muscle ache, musculoskeletal chest pain, joint stiffness, bursitis, muscle weakness
Nervous System: anxiety/nervousness, sleep disturbance, numbness, somnolence, vertigo, emotional disturbance, depression, paresthesia, tremor, transient ischemic attack, cerebrovascular accident
Renal/Genitourinary: prostate disorder
Respiratory: cough, upper respiratory infection, epistaxis, tracheobronchitis, congestion, pulmonary congestion, dyspnea, wheezing
Special Senses: vision disturbance, hearing abnormality, ear infection, ear pain, conjunctivitis.
Hydrochlorothiazide
Other adverse experiences that have been reported with hydrochlorothiazide, without regard to causality, are listed below:
Body As A Whole: weakness
Digestive: pancreatitis, jaundice (intrahepatic cholestatic jaundice), sialadenitis, cramping, gastric irritation
Hematologic: aplastic anemia, agranulocytosis, leukopenia, hemolytic anemia, thrombocytopenia
Hypersensitivity: purpura, photosensitivity, urticaria, necrotizing angiitis (vasculitis and cutaneous vasculitis), fever, respiratory distress including pneumonitis and pulmonary edema, anaphylactic reactions
Metabolic: hyperglycemia, glycosuria, hyperuricemia
Musculoskeletal: muscle spasm
Nervous System/Psychiatric: restlessness
Renal: renal failure, renal dysfunction, interstitial nephritis
Skin: erythema multiforme including Stevens-Johnson syndrome, exfoliative dermatitis including toxic epidermal necrolysis
Special Senses: transient blurred vision, xanthopsia.
Post-Marketing Experience
The following adverse reactions have been reported in post-marketing experience: Rare cases of urticaria and angioedema (involving swelling of the face, lips, pharynx, and/or tongue); hyperkalemia.

Laboratory Test Findings
In controlled clinical trials, clinically important changes in standard laboratory parameters were rarely associated with administration of AVALIDE (irbesartan-hydrochlorothiazide) Tablets.
Creatinine, Blood Urea Nitrogen: Minor increases in blood urea nitrogen (BUN) or serum creatinine were observed in 2.3 and 1.1 percent, respectively, of patients with essential hypertension treated with AVALIDE alone. No patient discontinued taking AVALIDE due to increased BUN. One patient discontinued taking AVALIDE due to a minor increase in serum creatinine.
Hemoglobin: Mean decreases of approximately 0.2 g/dL occurred in patients treated with AVALIDE alone, but were rarely of clinical importance. This compared to a mean of 0.4 g/dL in patients receiving placebo. No patients were discontinued due to anemia.
Liver Function Tests: Occasional elevations of liver enzymes and/or serum bilirubin have occurred. In patients with essential hypertension treated with AVALIDE alone, one patient was discontinued due to elevated liver enzymes.
Serum Electrolytes: (See **PRECAUTIONS**.)

OVERDOSAGE
Irbesartan
No data are available in regard to overdosage in humans. However, daily doses of 900 mg for 8 weeks were well-tolerated. The most likely manifestations of overdosage are expected to be hypotension and tachycardia; bradycardia might also occur from overdose. Irbesartan is not removed by hemodialysis.
To obtain up-to-date information about the treatment of overdosage, a good resource is a certified Regional Poison-Control Center. Telephone numbers of certified poison-control centers are listed in the *Physicians' Desk Reference* (PDR). In managing overdose, consider the possibilities of multiple-drug interactions, drug-drug interactions, and un usual drug kinetics in the patient.
Laboratory determinations of serum levels of irbesartan are not widely available, and such determinations have, in any event, no established role in the management of irbesartan overdose.
Acute oral toxicity studies with irbesartan in mice and rats indicated acute lethal doses were in excess of 2000 mg/kg, about 25- and 50-fold the maximum recommended human dose (300 mg) on a mg/m^2 basis, respectively.
Hydrochlorothiazide
The most common signs and symptoms of overdose observed in humans are those caused by electrolyte depletion (hypokalemia, hypochloremia, hyponatremia) and dehydration resulting from excessive diuresis. If digitalis has also been administered, hypokalemia may accentuate cardiac arrhythmias. The degree to which hydrochlorothiazide is removed by hemodialysis has not been established. The oral LD_{50} of hydrochlorothiazide is greater than 10 g/kg in both mice and rats.

DOSAGE AND ADMINISTRATION
The recommended initial dose of irbesartan is 150 mg once daily. Patients requiring further reduction in blood pressure should be titrated to 300 mg once daily.
A lower initial dose of irbesartan (75 mg) is recommended in patients with depletion of intravascular volume (e.g., patients treated vigorously with diuretics or on hemodialysis) (see **WARNING: Hypotension in Volume- or Salt-depleted Patients**). Patients not adequately treated by the maximum dose of 300 mg once daily are unlikely to derive additional benefit from a higher dose or twice-daily dosing.
Hydrochlorothiazide is effective in doses of 12.5 to 50 mg once daily.
To minimize dose-independent side effects, it is usually appropriate to begin combination therapy only after a patient has failed to achieve the desired effect with monotherapy.
The side effects (see **WARNINGS**) of irbesartan are generally rare and apparently independent of dose; those of hydrochlorothiazide are a mixture of dose-dependent (primarily hypokalemia) and dose-independent phenomena (e.g., pancreatitis), the former much more common than the latter. Therapy with any combination of irbesartan and hydrochlorothiazide will be associated with both sets of dose-independent side effects.
AVALIDE may be administered with other antihypertensive agents.
AVALIDE may be administered with or without food.

Replacement Therapy
The combination may be substituted for the titrated components.

Dose Titration by Clinical Effect
A patient whose blood pressure is inadequately controlled by irbesartan or hydrochlorothiazide alone may be switched to once daily AVALIDE. Recommended doses of AVALIDE, in order of increasing mean effect, are (irbesartan-hydrochlorothiazide) 150/12.5 mg, 300/12.5 mg, and 300/25 mg (two 150/12.5 mg tablets). The largest incremental effect will likely be in the transition from monotherapy to 150/12.5 mg. (See **CLINICAL PHARMACOLOGY: Clinical Studies**). It takes 2–4 weeks for the blood pressure to stabilize after a change in the dose of AVALIDE.
The usual dose of AVALIDE is one tablet once daily. More than two tablets once daily is not recommended. The maximal antihypertensive effect is attained about 2–4 weeks after initiation of therapy.

Use in Patients with Renal Impairment
The usual regimens of therapy with AVALIDE may be followed as long as the patient's creatinine clearance is >30 mL/min. In patients with more severe renal impairment, loop diuretics are preferred to thiazides, so AVALIDE is not recommended.

Patients with Hepatic Impairment
No dosage adjustment is necessary in patients with hepatic impairment.

HOW SUPPLIED
AVALIDE® (irbesartan-hydrochlorothiazide) Tablets are peach, biconvex, and oval with a heart debossed on one side and 2775 or 2776 on the reverse, supplied as follows:
[See second table on previous page]

Storage
Store at a temperature between 15°C and 30°C (59°F and 86° F) [See USP].
Manufactured and Distributed by:
Bristol-Myers Squibb Company
Princeton, NJ 08543-4500
Comarketed by:
Sanofi-Synthelabo, Inc.
New York, NY 10016
1030329A1 Revised November 1999
N1401-01
B4-B001-11-99
Shown in Product Identification Guide, page 309

AVAPRO® ℞
[*avă-prō*]
(irbesartan)
Tablets

> **USE IN PREGNANCY**
> **When used in pregnancy during the second and third trimesters, drugs that act directly on the renin-angiotensin system can cause injury and even death to the developing fetus.** When pregnancy is detected, AVAPRO should be discontinued as soon as possible. See **WARNINGS: Fetal/Neonatal Morbidity and Mortality.**

DESCRIPTION
AVAPRO* (irbesartan) is an angiotensin II receptor (AT_1 subtype) antagonist.
Irbesartan is a non-peptide compound, chemically described as a 2-butyl-3-[[2′-(1*H*-tetrazol-5-yl) [1, 1′-biphenyl]-4-yl]methyl]-1,3-diazaspiro [4,4] non-1-en-4-one.
Its empirical formula is $C_{25}H_{28}N_6O$, and the structural formula:
[See chemical structure at top of next column]
Irbesartan is a white to off-white crystalline powder with a molecular weight of 428.5. It is a nonpolar compound with a partition coefficient (octanol/water) of 10.1 at pH of 7.4. Irbesartan is slightly soluble in alcohol and methylene chloride and practically insoluble in water.
AVAPRO is available for oral administration in unscored tablets containing 75 mg, 150 mg, or 300 mg of irbesartan.

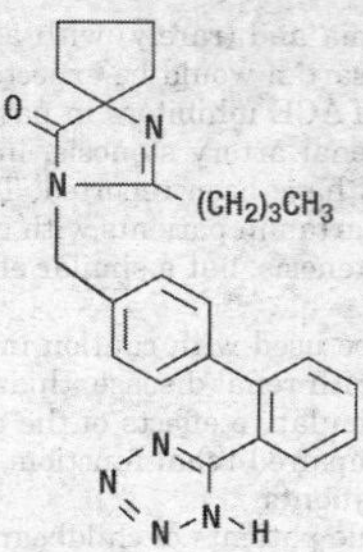

Inactive ingredients include: lactose, microcrystalline cellulose, pregelatinized starch, croscarmellose sodium, poloxamer 188, silicon dioxide and magnesium stearate.

CLINICAL PHARMACOLOGY
Mechanism of Action
Angiotensin II is a potent vasoconstrictor formed from angiotensin I in a reaction catalyzed by angiotensin-converting enzyme (ACE, kininase II). Angiotensin II is the principal pressor agent of the renin-angiotensin system (RAS) and also stimulates aldosterone synthesis and secretion by adrenal cortex, cardiac contraction, renal resorption of sodium, activity of the sympathetic nervous system, and smooth muscle cell growth. Irbesartan blocks the vasoconstrictor and aldosterone-secreting effects of angiotensin II by selectively binding to the AT_1 angiotensin II receptor. There is also an AT_2 receptor in many tissues, but it is not involved in cardiovascular homeostasis.
Irbesartan is a specific competitive antagonist of AT_1 receptors with a much greater affinity (more than 8500-fold) for the AT_1 receptor than for the AT_2 receptor and no agonist activity.
Blockade of the AT_1 receptor removes the negative feedback of angiotensin II on renin secretion, but the resulting increased plasma renin activity and circulating angiotensin II do not overcome the effects of irbesartan on blood pressure.
Irbesartan does not inhibit ACE or renin or affect other hormone receptors or ion channels known to be involved in the cardiovascular regulation of blood pressure and sodium homeostasis. Because irbesartan does not inhibit ACE, it does not affect the response to bradykinin; whether this has clinical relevance is not known.

*Registered trademark of Sanofi-Synthelabo, Inc.

Pharmacokinetics
Irbesartan is an orally active agent that does not require biotransformation into an active form. The oral absorption of irbesartan is rapid and complete with an average absolute bioavailability of 60–80%. Following oral administration of AVAPRO (irbesartan), peak plasma concentrations of irbesartan are attained at 1.5–2 hours after dosing. Food does not affect the bioavailability of AVAPRO.
Irbesartan exhibits linear pharmacokinetics over the therapeutic dose range.
The terminal elimination half-life of irbesartan averaged 11–15 hours. Steady-state concentrations are achieved within 3 days. Limited accumulation of irbesartan (<20%) is observed in plasma upon repeated once-daily dosing.

Metabolism and Elimination
Irbesartan is metabolized via glucuronide conjugation and oxidation. Following oral or intravenous administration of ^{14}C-labeled irbesartan, more than 80% of the circulating plasma radioactivity is attributable to unchanged irbesartan. The primary circulating metabolite is the inactive irbesartan glucuronide conjugate (approximately 6%). The remaining oxidative metabolites do not add appreciably to irbesartan's pharmacologic activity.
Irbesartan and its metabolites are excreted by both biliary and renal routes. Following either oral or intravenous administration of ^{14}C-labeled irbesartan, about 20% of radioactivity is recovered in the urine and the remainder in the feces, as irbesartan or irbesartan glucuronide.
In vitro studies of irbesartan oxidation by cytochrome P450 isoenzymes indicated irbesartan was oxidized primarily by 2C9; metabolism by 3A4 was negligible. Irbesartan was neither metabolized by, nor did it substantially induce or inhibit, isoenzymes commonly associated with drug metabolism (1A1, 1A2, 2A6, 2B6, 2D6, 2E1). There was no induction or inhibition of 3A4.

Distribution
Irbesartan is 90% bound to serum proteins (primarily albumin and α_1-acid glycoprotein) with negligible binding to cellular components of blood. The average volume of distribution is 53–93 liters. Total plasma and renal clearances are in the range of 157–176 and 3.0–3.5 mL/min, respectively. With repetitive dosing, irbesartan accumulates to no clinically relevant extent.
Studies in animals indicate that radiolabeled irbesartan weakly crosses the blood brain barrier and placenta. Irbesartan is excreted in the milk of lactating rats.

Special Populations
Pediatric: Irbesartan pharmacokinetics have not been investigated in patients <18 years of age.
Gender: No gender related differences in pharmacokinetics were observed in healthy elderly (age 65–80 years) or in healthy young (age 18–40 years) subjects. In studies of hypertensive patients, there was no gender difference in half-life or accumulation, but somewhat higher plasma concentrations of irbesartan were observed in females (11–44%). No gender-related dosage adjustment is necessary.

Geriatric: In elderly subjects (age 65–80 years), irbesartan elimination half-life was not significantly altered, but AUC and C_{max} values were about 20–50% greater than those of young subjects (age 18–40 years). No dosage adjustment is necessary in the elderly.
Race: In healthy black subjects, irbesartan AUC values were approximately 25% greater than whites; there were no differences in C_{max} values.
Renal Insufficiency: The pharmacokinetics of irbesartan were not altered in patients with renal impairment or in patients on hemodialysis. Irbesartan is not removed by hemodialysis. No dosage adjustment is necessary in patients with mild to severe renal impairment unless a patient with renal impairment is also volume depleted. (See **WARNINGS: Hypotension in Volume- or Salt-depleted Patients** and **DOSAGE AND ADMINISTRATION.**)
Hepatic Insufficiency: The pharmacokinetics of irbesartan following repeated oral administration were not significantly affected in patients with mild to moderate cirrhosis of the liver. No dosage adjustment is necessary in patients with hepatic insufficiency.
Drug Interactions: (See **PRECAUTIONS: Drug Interactions.**)

Pharmacodynamics

In healthy subjects, single oral irbesartan doses of up to 300 mg produced dose-dependent inhibition of the pressor effect of angiotensin II infusions. Inhibition was complete (100%) 4 hours following oral doses of 150 mg or 300 mg and partial inhibition was sustained for 24 hours (60% and 40% at 300 mg and 150 mg, respectively).

In hypertensive patients, angiotensin II receptor inhibition following chronic administration of irbesartan causes a 1.5–2 fold rise in angiotensin II plasma concentration and a 2–3 fold increase in plasma renin levels. Aldosterone plasma concentrations generally decline following irbesartan administration, but serum potassium levels are not significantly affected at recommended doses.

In hypertensive patients, chronic oral doses of irbesartan (up to 300 mg) had no effect on glomerular filtration rate, renal plasma flow or filtration fraction. In multiple dose studies in hypertensive patients, there were no clinically important effects on fasting triglycerides, total cholesterol, HDL-cholesterol, or fasting glucose concentrations. There was no effect on serum uric acid during chronic oral administration, and no uricosuric effect.

Clinical Studies

The antihypertensive effects of AVAPRO (irbesartan) were examined in seven (7) major placebo-controlled 8–12 week trials in patients with baseline diastolic blood pressures of 95–110 mmHg. Doses of 1–900 mg were included in these trials in order to fully explore the dose-range of irbesartan. These studies allowed comparison of once- or twice-daily regimens at 150 mg/day, comparisons of peak and trough effects, and comparisons of response by gender, age, and race. Two of the seven placebo-controlled trials identified above examined the antihypertensive effects of irbesartan and hydrochlorothiazide in combination.

The seven (7) studies of irbesartan monotherapy included a total of 1915 patients randomized to irbesartan (1–900 mg) and 611 patients randomized to placebo. Once-daily doses of 150 and 300 mg provided statistically and clinically significant decreases in systolic and diastolic blood pressure with trough (24 hours post-dose) effects after 6–12 weeks of treatment compared to placebo, of about 8–10/5–6 and 8–12/5–8 mmHg, respectively. No further increase in effect was seen at dosages greater than 300 mg. The dose-response relationships for effects on systolic and diastolic pressure are shown in Figures 1 and 2.

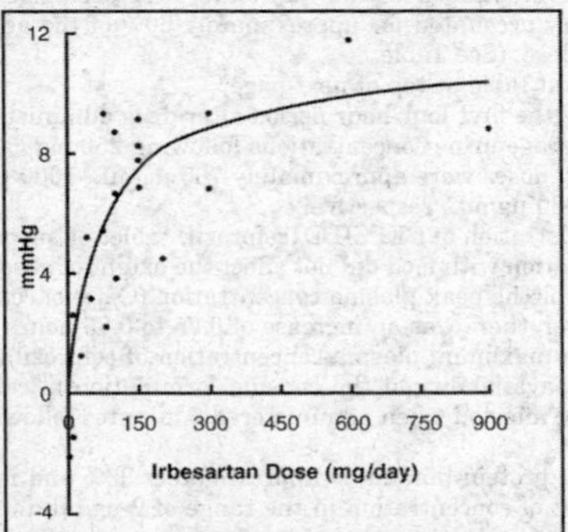

Figure 1. Placebo-subtracted reduction in trough SeSBP; integrated analysis

[See figure 2 at top of next column]

Once-daily administration of therapeutic doses of irbesartan gave peak effects at around 3–6 hours and, in one ambulatory blood pressure monitoring study, again around 14 hours. This was seen with both once-daily and twice-daily dosing. Trough-to-peak ratios for systolic and diastolic response were generally between 60–70%. In a continuous ambulatory blood pressure monitoring study, once-daily dosing with 150 mg gave trough and mean 24-hour responses similar to those observed in patients receiving twice-daily dosing at the same total daily dose.

In controlled trials, the addition of irbesartan to hydrochlorothiazide doses of 6.25, 12.5, or 25 mg produced further

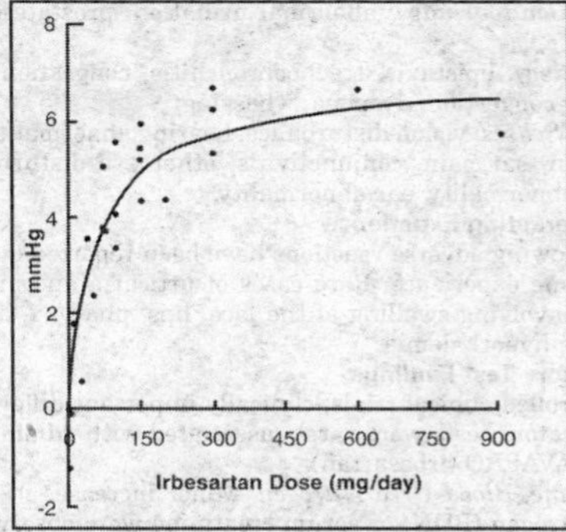

Figure 2. Placebo-subtracted reduction in trough SeDBP; integrated analysis

dose-related reductions in blood pressure similar to those achieved with the same monotherapy dose of irbesartan. HCTZ also had an approximately additive effect.

Analysis of age, gender, and race subgroups of patients showed that men and women, and patients over and under 65 years of age, had generally similar responses. Irbesartan was effective in reducing blood pressure regardless of race, although the effect was somewhat less in blacks (usually a low-renin population).

The effect of irbesartan is apparent after the first dose and it is close to its full observed effect at 2 weeks. At the end of an 8-week exposure, about 2/3 of the antihypertensive effect was still present one week after the last dose. Rebound hypertension was not observed. There was essentially no change in average heart rate in irbesartan-treated patients in controlled trials.

INDICATIONS AND USAGE

AVAPRO (irbesartan) is indicated for the treatment of hypertension. It may be used alone or in combination with other antihypertensive agents.

CONTRAINDICATIONS

AVAPRO is contraindicated in patients who are hypersensitive to any component of this product.

WARNINGS

Fetal/Neonatal Morbidity and Mortality

Drugs that act directly on the renin-angiotensin system can cause fetal and neonatal morbidity and death when administered to pregnant women. Several dozen cases have been reported in the world literature in patients who were taking angiotensin-converting-enzyme inhibitors. When pregnancy is detected, AVAPRO should be discontinued as soon as possible.

The use of drugs that act directly on the renin-angiotensin system during the second and third trimesters of pregnancy has been associated with fetal and neonatal injury, including hypotension, neonatal skull hypoplasia, anuria, reversible or irreversible renal failure, and death. Oligohydramnios has also been reported, presumably resulting from decreased fetal renal function; oligohydramnios in this setting has been associated with fetal limb contractures, craniofacial deformation, and hypoplastic lung development. Prematurity, intrauterine growth retardation, and patent ductus arteriosus have also been reported, although it is not clear whether these occurrences were due to exposure to the drug.

These adverse effects do not appear to have resulted from intrauterine drug exposure that has been limited to the first trimester.

Mothers whose embryos and fetuses are exposed to an angiotensin II receptor antagonist only during the first trimester should be so informed. Nonetheless, when patients become pregnant, physicians should have the patient discontinue the use of AVAPRO as soon as possible.

Rarely (probably less often than once in every thousand pregnancies), no alternative to a drug acting on the renin-angiotensin system will be found. In these rare cases, the mothers should be apprised of the potential hazards to their fetuses, and serial ultrasound examinations should be performed to assess the intraamniotic environment.

If oligohydramnios is observed, AVAPRO should be discontinued unless it is considered life-saving for the mother. Contraction stress testing (CST), a non-stress test (NST), or biophysical profiling (BPP) may be appropriate depending upon the week of pregnancy. Patients and physicians should be aware, however, that oligohydramnios may not appear until after the fetus has sustained irreversible injury.

Infants with histories of *in utero* exposure to an angiotensin II receptor antagonist should be closely observed for hypotension, oliguria, and hyperkalemia. If oliguria occurs, attention should be directed toward support of blood pressure and renal perfusion. Exchange transfusion or dialysis may be required as means of reversing hypotension and/or substituting for disordered renal function.

When pregnant rats were treated with irbesartan from day 0 to day 20 of gestation (oral doses of 50, 180, and 650 mg/kg/day), increased incidences of renal pelvic cavitation, hydroureter and/or absence of renal papilla were observed in fetuses at doses ≥50 mg/kg/day [approximately equivalent to the maximum recom mended human dose (MRHD), 300 mg/day, on a body surface area basis]. Subcutaneous edema was observed in fetuses at doses ≥180 mg/kg/day (about 4 times the MRHD on a body surface area basis). As these anomalies were not observed in rats in which irbesartan exposure (oral doses of 50, 150 and 450 mg/kg/day) was limited to gestation days 6–15, they appear to reflect late gestational effects of the drug. In pregnant rabbits, oral doses of 30 mg irbesartan/kg/day were associated with maternal mortality and abortion. Surviving females receiving this dose (about 1.5 times the MRHD on a body surface area basis) had a slight increase in early resorptions and a corresponding decrease in live fetuses. Irbesartan was found to cross the placental barrier in rats and rabbits.

Radioactivity was present in the rat and rabbit fetus during late gestation and in rat milk following oral doses of radiolabeled irbesartan.

Hypotension in Volume- or Salt-depleted Patients

Excessive reduction of blood pressure was rarely seen (<0.1%) in patients with uncomplicated hypertension. Initiation of antihypertensive therapy may cause symptomatic hypotension in patients with intravascular volume- or sodium-depletion, e.g., in patients treated vigorously with diuretics or in patients on dialysis. Such volume depletion should be corrected prior to administration of AVAPRO (irbesartan), or a low starting dose should be used (see **DOSAGE AND ADMINISTRATION**).

If hypotension occurs, the patient should be placed in the supine position and, if necessary, given an intravenous infusion of normal saline. A transient hypotensive response is not a contraindication to further treatment, which usually can be continued without difficulty once the blood pressure has stabilized.

PRECAUTIONS

Impaired Renal Function

As a consequence of inhibiting the renin-angiotensin-aldosterone system, changes in renal function may be anticipated in susceptible individuals. In patients whose renal function may depend on the activity of the renin-angiotensin-aldosterone system (e.g., patients with severe congestive heart failure), treatment with angiotensin-converting-enzyme inhibitors has been associated with oliguria and/or progressive azotemia and (rarely) with acute renal failure and/or death. AVAPRO would be expected to behave similarly. In studies of ACE inhibitors in patients with unilateral or bilateral renal artery stenosis, increases in serum creatinine or BUN have been reported. There has been no known use of AVAPRO in patients with unilateral or bilateral renal artery stenosis, but a similar effect should be anticipated.

Information for Patients

Pregnancy: Female patients of childbearing age should be told about the consequences of second- and third-trimester exposure to drugs that act on the renin-angiotensin system, and they should also be told that these consequences do not appear to have resulted from intrauterine drug exposure that has been limited to the first trimester. These patients should be asked to report pregnancies to their physicians as soon as possible.

Drug Interactions

No significant drug-drug pharmacokinetic (or pharmacodynamic) interactions have been found in interaction studies with hydrochlorothiazide, digoxin, warfarin, and nifedipine. *In vitro* studies show significant inhibition of the formation of oxidized irbesartan metabolites with the known cytochrome CYP 2C9 substrates/inhibitors sulphenazole, tolbutamide and nifedipine. However, in clinical studies the consequences of concomitant irbesartan on the pharmacodynamics of warfarin were negligible. Based on *in vitro* data, no interaction would be expected with drugs whose metabolism is dependent upon cytochrome P450 isozymes 1A1, 1A2, 2A6, 2B6, 2D6, 2E1, or 3A4.

In separate studies of patients receiving maintenance doses of warfarin, hydrochlorothiazide, or digoxin, irbesartan administration for 7 days had no effect on the pharmacodynamics of warfarin (prothrombin time) or pharmacokinetics of digoxin. The pharmacokinetics of irbesartan were not affected by coadministration of nifedipine or hydrochlorothiazide.

Carcinogenesis, Mutagenesis, Impairment of Fertility

No evidence of carcinogenicity was observed when irbesartan was administered at doses of up to 500/1000 mg/kg/day (males/females, respectively) in rats and 1000 mg/kg/day in mice for up to two years. For male and female rats, 500 mg/kg/day provided an average systemic exposure to irbesartan (AUC_{0-24h}, bound plus unbound) about 3 and 11 times, respectively, the average systemic exposure in humans receiving the maximum recommended dose (MRD) of 300 mg irbesartan/day, whereas 1000 mg/kg/day (administered to females only) provided an average systemic exposure about 21 times that reported for humans at the MRD. For male and female mice, 1000 mg/kg/day provided an exposure to irbesartan about 3 and 5 times, respectively, the human exposure at 300 mg/day.

Irbesartan was not mutagenic in a battery of *in vitro* tests (Ames microbial test, rat hepatocyte DNA repair test, V79 mammalian-cell forward gene-mutation assay). Irbesartan was negative in several tests for induction of chromosomal aberrations (*in vitro*-human lymphocyte assay; *in vivo*-mouse micronucleus study).

Irbesartan had no adverse effects on fertility or mating of male or female rats at oral doses ≤650 mg/kg/day, the high-

Continued on next page

Avapro—Cont.

est dose providing a systemic exposure to irbesartan (AUC_{0-24h}, bound plus unbound) about 5 times that found in humans receiving the maximum recommended dose of 300 mg/day.

Pregnancy

Pregnancy Categories C (first trimester) and D (second and third trimester). See **WARNINGS: Fetal/Neonatal Morbidity and Mortality.**

Nursing Mothers

It is not known whether irbesartan is excreted in human milk, but irbesartan or some metabolite of irbesartan is secreted at low concentration in the milk of lactating rats. Because of the potential for adverse effects on the nursing infant, a decision should be made whether to discontinue nursing or discontinue the drug, taking into account the importance of the drug to the mother.

Pediatric Use

Safety and effectiveness in pediatric patients have not been established.

Geriatric Use

Of the total number of patients receiving AVAPRO (irbesartan) in controlled clinical studies, 911 patients (18.5%) were 65 years and over, while 150 patients (3.0%) were 75 years and over. No overall differences in effectiveness or safety were observed between these patients and younger patients, but greater sensitivity of some older individuals cannot be ruled out.

ADVERSE REACTIONS

AVAPRO has been evaluated for safety in more than 4300 patients with hypertension and about 5000 subjects overall. This experience includes 1303 patients treated for over 6 months and 407 patients for 1 year or more. Treatment with AVAPRO was well-tolerated, with an incidence of adverse events similar to placebo. These events generally were mild and transient with no relationship to the dose of AVAPRO.

In placebo-controlled clinical trials, discontinuation of therapy due to a clinical adverse event was required in 3.3 percent of patients treated with AVAPRO, versus 4.5 percent of patients given placebo.

In placebo-controlled clinical trials, the adverse event experiences that occurred in at least 1% of patients treated with AVAPRO (n=1965) and at a higher incidence versus placebo (n=641) included diarrhea (3% vs. 2%), dyspepsia/heartburn (2% vs. 1%), musculoskeletal trauma (2% vs. 1%), fatigue (4% vs. 3%), and upper respiratory infection (9% vs. 6%). None of these differences were significant.

The following adverse events occurred at an incidence of 1% or greater in patients treated with irbesartan, but were at least as frequent or more frequent in patients receiving placebo: abdominal pain, anxiety/nervousness, chest pain, dizziness, edema, headache, influenza, musculoskeletal pain, pharyngitis, nausea/ vomiting, rash, rhinitis, sinus abnormality, tachycardia and urinary tract infection.

Irbesartan use was not associated with an increased incidence of dry cough, as is typically associated with ACE inhibitor use. In placebo controlled studies, the incidence of cough in irbesartan treated patients was 2.8% versus 2.7% in patients receiving placebo.

The incidence of hypotension or orthostatic hypotension was low in irbesartan treated patients (0.4%), unrelated to dosage, and similar to the incidence among placebo treated patients (0.2%). Dizziness, syncope, and vertigo were reported with equal or less frequency in patients receiving irbesartan compared with placebo.

In addition, the following potentially important events occurred in less than 1% of the 1965 patients and at least 5 patients (0.3%) receiving irbesartan in clinical studies, and those less frequent, clinically significant events (listed by body system). It cannot be determined whether these events were causally related to irbesartan:

Body as a Whole: fever, chills, facial edema, upper extremity edema;

Cardiovascular: flushing, hypertension, cardiac murmur, myocardial infarction, angina pectoris, arrhythmic/conduction disorder, cardio-respiratory arrest, heart failure, hypertensive crisis;

Dermatologic: pruritus, dermatitis, ecchymosis, erythema face, urticaria;

Endocrine/Metabolic/Electrolyte Imbalances: sexual dysfunction, libido change, gout;

Gastrointestinal: constipation, oral lesion, gastroenteritis, flatulence, abdominal distention;

Musculoskeletal/Connective Tissue: extremity swelling, muscle cramp, arthritis, muscle ache, musculoskeletal chest pain, joint stiffness, bursitis, muscle weakness;

Nervous System: sleep disturbance, numbness, somnolence, emotional disturbance, depression, paresthesia, tremor, transient ischemic attack, cerebrovascular accident;

Renal/Genitourinary: abnormal urination, prostate disorder;

Respiratory: epistaxis, tracheobronchitis, congestion, pulmonary congestion, dyspnea, wheezing;

Special Senses: vision disturbance, hearing abnormality, ear infection, ear pain, conjunctivitis, other eye disturbance, eyelid abnormality, ear abnormality.

Post-Marketing Experience

The following adverse reactions have been reported in post-marketing experience: Rare cases of urticaria and angioedema (involving swelling of the face, lips, pharynx, and/or tongue); hyperkalemia.

Laboratory Test Findings

In controlled clinical trials, clinically important differences in laboratory tests were rarely associated with administration of AVAPRO (irbesartan).

Creatinine, Blood Urea Nitrogen: Minor increases in blood urea nitrogen (BUN) or serum creatinine were observed in less than 0.7% of patients with essential hypertension treated with AVAPRO alone versus 0.9% on placebo. (See **PRECAUTIONS: Impaired Renal Function.**)

Hematologic: Mean decreases in hemoglobin of 0.2 g/dL were observed in 0.2% of patients receiving AVAPRO compared to 0.3% of placebo treated patients. Neutropenia (<1000 cells/mm^3) occurred at similar frequencies among patients receiving AVAPRO (0.3%) and placebo treated patients (0.5%).

OVERDOSAGE

No data are available in regard to overdosage in humans. However, daily doses of 900 mg for 8 weeks were well-tolerated. The most likely manifestations of overdosage are expected to be hypotension and tachycardia; bradycardia might also occur from overdose. Irbesartan is not removed by hemodialysis.

To obtain up-to-date information about the treatment of overdosage, a good resource is a certified Regional Poison-Control Center. Telephone numbers of certified poison-control centers are listed in the *Physicians' Desk Reference* (PDR). In managing overdose, consider the possibilities of multiple-drug interactions, drug-drug interactions, and unusual drug kinetics in the patient.

Laboratory determinations of serum levels of irbesartan are not widely available, and such determinations have, in any event, no known established role in the management of irbesartan overdose.

Acute oral toxicity studies with irbesartan in mice and rats indicated acute lethal doses were in excess of 2000 mg/kg, about 25- and 50-fold the maximum recommended human dose (300 mg) on a mg/m^2 basis, respectively.

DOSAGE AND ADMINISTRATION

The recommended initial dose of AVAPRO is 150 mg once daily. Patients requiring further reduction in blood pressure should be titrated to 300 mg once daily.

A low dose of a diuretic may be added, if blood pressure is not controlled by AVAPRO alone. Hydrochlorothiazide has been shown to have an additive effect (see **CLINICAL PHARMACOLOGY: Clinical Studies**). Patients not adequately treated by the maximum dose of 300 mg once daily are unlikely to derive additional benefit from a higher dose or twice-daily dosing.

No dosage adjustment is necessary in elderly patients, or in patients with hepatic impairment or mild to severe renal impairment.

AVAPRO may be administered with other antihypertensive agents.

AVAPRO may be administered with or without food.

Volume- and Salt-depleted Patients

A lower initial dose of AVAPRO (75 mg) is recommended in patients with depletion of intravascular volume or salt (e.g., patients treated vigorously with diuretics or on hemodialysis) (see **WARNINGS: Hypotension in Volume- or Salt-depleted Patients**).

HOW SUPPLIED

AVAPRO® (irbesartan) is available as white to off-white biconvex oval tablets, debossed with a heart shape on one side and a portion of the NDC code on the other. Unit-of-use bottles contain 30, 90, or 500 tablets and blister packs contain 100 tablets, as follows:

[See table below]

Storage

Store at a temperature between 15° C and 30° C (59° F and 86° F) [USP].

Manufactured and Distributed by:
Bristol-Myers Squibb Co:
Princeton, NJ 08543-4500
Comarketed by:
sanofi~synthelabo
New York, NY 10016

	75 mg	150 mg	300 mg
Debossing	2771	2772	2773
Bottle of 30	0087-2771-31	0087-2772-31	0087-2773-31
Bottle of 90	0087-2771-32	0087-2772-32	0087-2773-32
Bottle of 500	0087-2771-15	0087-2772-15	0087-2773-15
Blister of 100	0087-2771-35	0087-2772-35	0087-2773-35

Revised November 1999 1017108A2
P0617-02

Shown in Product Identification Guide, page 309

CEFZIL® ℞
[*sĕf -zil*]
(CEFPROZIL) Tablets
250 mg and 500 mg

CEFZIL® ℞
(CEFPROZIL)
for Oral Suspension
125 mg/5 mL and 250 mg/5 mL

Rx only

DESCRIPTION

CEFZIL® (cefprozil) is a semi-synthetic broad-spectrum cephalosporin antibiotic.

Cefprozil is a cis and trans isomeric mixture (≥ 90% cis). The chemical name for the monohydrate is (6R, 7R)-7-[(R)-2-amino-2-(p-hydroxyphenyl)acetamido]-8-oxo-3-propenyl-5-thia-1-azabicyclo[4.2.0]oct-2-ene-2-carboxylic acid monohydrate, and the structural formula is:

Cefprozil is a white to yellowish powder with a molecular formula for the monohydrate of $C_{18}H_{19}N_3O_5S \cdot H_2O$ and a molecular weight of 407.45.

CEFZIL (cefprozil) tablets and CEFZIL for oral suspension are intended for oral administration.

CEFZIL tablets contain cefprozil equivalent to 250 mg or 500 mg of anhydrous cefprozil. In addition, each tablet contains the following inactive ingredients: cellulose, hydroxypropylmethylcellulose, magnesium stearate, methylcellulose, simethicone, sodium starch glycolate, polyethylene glycol, polysorbate 80, sorbic acid and titanium dioxide. The 250 mg tablets also contain FD&C Yellow No. 6.

CEFZIL for oral suspension contains cefprozil equivalent to 125 mg or 250 mg anhydrous cefprozil per 5 mL constituted suspension. In addition, the oral suspension contains the following inactive ingredients: aspartame, cellulose, citric acid, colloidal silicone dioxide, FD&C Red No. 3, flavors (natural and artificial), glycine, polysorbate 80, simethicone, sodium benzoate, sodium carboxymethylcellulose, sodium chloride, and sucrose.

CLINICAL PHARMACOLOGY

The pharmacokinetic data were derived from the capsule formulation; however, bioequivalence has been demonstrated for the oral solution, capsule, tablet and suspension formulations under fasting conditions.

Following oral administration of cefprozil to fasting subjects, approximately 95% of the dose was absorbed. The average plasma half-life in normal subjects was 1.3 hours, while the steady state volume of distribution was estimated to be 0.23 L/kg. The total body clearance and renal clearance rates were approximately 3 mL/min/kg and 2.3 mL/min/kg, respectively.

Average peak plasma concentrations after administration of 250 mg, 500 mg, or 1 g doses of cefprozil to fasting subjects were approximately 6.1, 10.5, and 18.3 µg/mL, respectively, and were obtained within 1.5 hours after dosing. Urinary recovery accounted for approximately 60% of the administered dose. (See Table.)

[See first table at top of next page]

During the first four-hour period after drug administration, the average urine concentrations following 250 mg, 500 mg, and 1 g doses were approximately 700 µg/mL, 1000 µg/mL, and 2900 µg/mL, respectively.

Administration of CEFZIL® (cefprozil) tablet or suspension formulation with food did not affect the extent of absorption (AUC) or the peak plasma concentration (C_{max}) of cefprozil. However, there was an increase of 0.25 to 0.75 hours in the time to maximum plasma concentration of cefprozil (T_{max}). The bioavailability of the capsule formulation of cefprozil was not affected when administered 5 minutes following an antacid.

Plasma protein binding is approximately 36% and is independent of concentration in the range of 2 µg/mL to 20 µg/mL.

There was no evidence of accumulation of cefprozil in the plasma in individuals with normal renal function following multiple oral doses of up to 1000 mg every 8 hours for 10 days.

In patients with reduced renal function, the plasma half-life may be prolonged up to 5.2 hours depending on the degree of the renal dysfunction. In patients with complete absence of renal function, the plasma half-life of cefprozil has been shown to be as long as 5.9 hours. The half-life is shortened during hemodialysis. Excretion pathways in patients with markedly impaired renal function have not been determined. (See **PRECAUTIONS** and **DOSAGE AND ADMINISTRATION.**)

In patients with impaired hepatic function, the half-life increases to approximately 2 hours. The magnitude of the changes does not warrant a dosage adjustment for patients with impaired hepatic function.

The average AUC observed in elderly subjects (≥ 65 years of age) is approximately 35–60% higher relative to young adults, and the average AUC in females is approximately 15–20% higher than in males. The magnitude of these age- and gender-related changes in the pharmacokinetics of cefprozil is not sufficient to necessitate dosage adjustments.
Adequate data on CSF levels of cefprozil are not available.
Comparable pharmacokinetic parameters of cefprozil are observed between pediatric patients (6 months–12 years) and adults following oral administration of selected matched doses. The maximum concentrations are achieved at 1–2 hours after dosing. The plasma elimination half-life is approximately 1.5 hours. In general, the observed plasma concentrations of cefprozil in pediatric patients at the 7.5, 15, and 30 mg/kg doses are similar to those observed within the same time frame in normal adult subjects at the 250, 500 and 1000 mg doses, respectively. The comparative plasma concentrations of cefprozil in pediatric patients and adult subjects at the equivalent dose level are presented in the table below.
[See second table at right]

Dosage (mg)	Mean Plasma Cefprozil* Concentration (μg/mL)			8-hour Urinary Excretion (%)
	Peak appx. 1.5 hr	4 hr	8 hr	
250 mg	6.1	1.7	0.2	60%
500 mg	10.5	3.2	0.4	62%
1000 mg	18.3	8.4	1.0	54%

* Data represent mean values of 12 healthy volunteers.

Population	Dose	Mean (SD) Plasma Cefprozil Concentrations (μg/mL)				$T_{1/2}$ (hr)
		1 hr	2 hr	4 hr	6 hr	
children (n = 18)	7.5 mg/kg	4.70 (1.57)	3.99 (1.24)	0.91 (0.30)	0.23[a] (0.13)	0.94 (0.32)
adults (n =12)	250 mg	4.82 (2.13)	4.92 (1.13)	1.70[b] (0.53)	0.53 (0.17)	1.28 (0.34)
children (n = 19)	15 mg/kg	10.86 (2.55)	8.47 (2.03)	2.75 (1.07)	0.61[c] (0.27)	1.24 (0.43)
adults (n = 12)	500 mg	8.39 (1.95)	9.42 (0.98)	3.18[d] (0.76)	1.00[d] (0.24)	1.29 (0.14)
children (n = 10)	30 mg/kg	6.69 (4.26)	17.61 (6.39)	8.66 (2.70)	–	2.06 (0.21)
adults (n = 12)	1000 mg	11.99 (4.67)	16.95 (4.07)	8.36 (4.13)	2.79 (1.77)	1.27 (0.12)

[a]n = 11; [b]n = 5; [c]n = 9; [d]n = 11.

Microbiology
Cefprozil has *in vitro* activity against a broad range of gram-positive and gram-negative bacteria. The bactericidal action of cefprozil results from inhibition of cell-wall synthesis. Cefprozil has been shown to be active against most strains of the following microorganisms both *in vitro* and in clinical infections as described in the **INDICATIONS AND USAGE** section.

Aerobic gram-positive microorganisms:
Staphylococcus aureus (including β-lactamase-producing strains)
NOTE: Cefprozil is inactive against methicillin-resistant staphylococci.
Streptococcus pneumoniae
Streptococcus pyogenes

Aerobic gram-negative microorganisms:
Haemophilus influenzae (including β-lactamase-producing strains)
Moraxella (Branhamella) catarrhalis (including β-lactamase-producing strains)
The following *in vitro* data are available; however, their clinical significance is unknown. Cefprozil exhibits *in vitro* minimum inhibitory concentrations (MIC's) of 8 μg/mL or less against most (≥90%) strains of the following microorganisms; however, the safety and effectiveness of cefprozil in treating clinical infections due to these microorganisms have not been established in adequate and well-controlled clinical trials.

Aerobic gram-positive microorganisms:
Enterococcus durans
Enterococcus faecalis
Listeria monocytogenes
Staphylococcus epidermidis
Staphylococcus saprophyticus
Staphylococcus warneri
Streptococcus agalactiae
Streptococci (Groups C, D, F, and G)
viridans group Streptococci
NOTE: Cefprozil is inactive against *Enterococcus faecium.*

Aerobic gram-negative microorganisms:
Citrobacter diversus
Escherichia coli
Klebsiella pneumoniae
Neisseria gonorrhoeae (including β-lactamase-producing strains)
Proteus mirabilis
Salmonella spp.
Shigella spp.
Vibrio spp.
NOTE: Cefprozil is inactive against most strains of *Acinetobacter, Enterobacter, Morganella morganii, Proteus vulgaris, Providencia, Pseudomonas,* and *Serratia.*

Anaerobic microorganisms:
Prevotella (Bacteroides) melaninogenicus
Clostridium difficile
Clostridium perfringens
Fusobacterium spp.
Peptostreptococcus spp.
Propionibacterium acnes
NOTE: Most strains of the *Bacteroides fragilis* group are resistant to cefprozil.
Susceptibility Tests
Dilution Techniques: Quantitative methods are used to determine antimicrobial minimal inhibitory concentrations (MIC's). These MIC's provide estimates of the susceptibility of bacteria to antimicrobial compounds. The MIC's should be determined using a standardized procedure. Standardized procedures are based on a dilution method[1,2] (broth or agar) or equivalent with standardized inoculum concentrations and standardized concentrations of cefprozil powder. The MIC values should be interpreted according to the following criteria:

MIC (μg/mL)	Interpretation
≤ 8	Susceptible (S)
16	Intermediate (I)
≥ 32	Resistant (R)

A report of "Susceptible" indicates that the pathogen is likely to be inhibited if the antimicrobial compound in the blood reaches the concentrations usually achievable. A report of "Intermediate" indicates that the result should be considered equivocal, and, if the microorganism is not fully susceptible to alternative, clinically feasible drugs, the test should be repeated. This category implies possible clinical applicability in body sites where the drug is physiologically concentrated or in situations where high dosage of drug can be used. This category also provides a buffer zone which prevents small uncontrolled technical factors from causing major discrepancies in interpretation. A report of "Resistant" indicates that the pathogen is not likely to be inhibited if the antimicrobial compound in the blood reaches the concentrations usually achievable; other therapy should be selected.
Standardized susceptibility test procedures require the use of laboratory control microorganisms to control the technical aspects of the laboratory procedures. Standard cefprozil powder should provide the following MIC values:

Microorganism	MIC (μg/mL)
Enterococcus faecalis ATCC 29212	4–16
Escherichia coli ATCC 25922	1–4
Haemophilus influenzae ATCC 49766	1–4
Staphylococcus aureus ATCC 29213	0.25–1
Streptococcus pneumoniae ATCC 49619	0.25–1

Diffusion Techniques: Quantitative methods that require measurement of zone diameters also provide reproducible estimates of the susceptibility of bacteria to antimicrobial compounds. One such standardized procedure[3] requires the use of standardized inoculum concentrations. This procedure uses paper disks impregnated with 30 μg cefprozil to test the susceptibility of microorganisms to cefprozil.
Reports from the laboratory providing results of the standard single-disk susceptibility test with a 30 μg cefprozil disk should be interpreted according to the following criteria:

Zone diameter (mm)	Interpretation
≥ 18	Susceptible (S)
15–17	Intermediate (I)
≤ 14	Resistant (R)

Interpretation should be as stated above for results using dilution techniques. Interpretation involves correlation of the diameter obtained in the disk test with the MIC for cefprozil.
As with standardized dilution techniques, diffusion methods require the use of laboratory control microorganisms that are used to control the technical aspects of the laboratory procedures. For the diffusion technique, the 30 μg cefprozil disk should provide the following zone diameters in these laboratory test quality control strains.

Microorganism	Zone diameter (mm)
Escherichia coli ATCC 25922	21–27
Haemophilus influenzae ATCC 49766	20–27
Staphylococcus aureus ATCC 25923	27–33
Streptococcus pneumoniae ATCC 49619	25–32

INDICATIONS AND USAGE

CEFZIL (cefprozil) is indicated for the treatment of patients with mild to moderate infections caused by susceptible strains of the designated microorganisms in the conditions listed below:
UPPER RESPIRATORY TRACT
Pharyngitis/tonsillitis caused by *Streptococcus pyogenes.*
NOTE: The usual drug of choice in the treatment and prevention of streptococcal infections, including the prophylaxis of rheumatic fever, is penicillin given by the intramuscular route. Cefprozil is generally effective in the eradication of *Streptococcus pyogenes* from the nasopharynx; however, substantial data establishing the efficacy of cefprozil in the subsequent prevention of rheumatic fever are not available at present.
Otitis Media caused by *Streptococcus pneumoniae, Haemophilus influenzae* (including β-lactamase-producing strains) and *Moraxella (Branhamella) catarrhalis* (including β-lactamase-producing strains). (See **CLINICAL STUDIES** section.)
NOTE: In the treatment of otitis media due to β-lactamase producing organisms, cefprozil had bacteriologic eradication rates somewhat lower than those observed with a product containing a specific β-lactamase inhibitor. In considering the use of cefprozil, lower overall eradication rates should be balanced against the susceptibility patterns of the common microbes in a given geographic area and the increased potential for toxicity with products containing β-lactamase inhibitors.
Acute Sinusitis caused by *Streptococcus pneumoniae, Haemophilus influenzae* (including β-lactamase-producing strains) and *Moraxella (Branhamella) catarrhalis* (including β-lactamase-producing strains).
LOWER RESPIRATORY TRACT
Secondary Bacterial Infection of Acute Bronchitis and Acute Bacterial Exacerbation of Chronic Bronchitis caused by *Streptococcus pneumoniae, Haemophilus influenzae* (including β-lactamase-producing strains), and *Moraxella (Branhamella) catarrhalis* (including β-lactamase-producing strains).
SKIN AND SKIN STRUCTURE
Uncomplicated Skin and Skin-Structure Infections caused by *Staphylococcus aureus* (including penicillinase-producing strains), and *Streptococcus pyogenes.* Abscesses usually require surgical drainage.
Culture and susceptiblity testing should be performed when appropriate to determine susceptibility of the causative organism to cefprozil.

CONTRAINDICATIONS

CEFZIL (cefprozil) is contraindicated in patients with known allergy to the cephalosporin class of antibiotics.

WARNINGS

BEFORE THERAPY WITH CEFZIL IS INSTITUTED, CAREFUL INQUIRY SHOULD BE MADE TO DETERMINE WHETHER THE PATIENT HAS HAD PREVIOUS HYPERSENSITIVITY REACTIONS TO CEFZIL, CEPHALOSPORINS, PENICILLINS, OR OTHER DRUGS. IF THIS PRODUCT IS TO BE GIVEN TO PENICILLIN-SENSITIVE PATIENTS, CAUTION SHOULD BE EXERCISED BECAUSE CROSS-SENSITIVITY AMONG β-LACTAM ANTIBIOTICS HAS BEEN CLEARLY DOCUMENTED AND MAY OCCUR IN UP TO 10% OF PATIENTS WITH A HISTORY OF PENICILLIN ALLERGY. IF AN ALLERGIC REACTION TO CEFZIL OCCURS, DISCONTINUE THE DRUG. SERIOUS ACUTE HYPERSENSITIVITY REACTIONS MAY REQUIRE TREATMENT WITH EPINEPHRINE AND OTHER EMERGENCY MEASURES, INCLUDING OXYGEN, INTRAVENOUS FLUIDS, INTRAVENOUS ANTIHISTAMINES, CORTICOSTEROIDS, PRESSOR AMINES, AND AIRWAY MANAGEMENT, AS CLINICALLY INDICATED.
Pseudomembranous colitis has been reported with nearly all antibacterial agents, including cefprozil, and may range in severity from mild to life threatening. Therefore, it is important to consider this diagnosis in patients who present with diarrhea subsequent to the administration of antibacterial agents.
Treatment with antibacterial agents alters the normal flora of the colon and may permit overgrowth of clostridia. Studies indicate that a toxin produced by *Clostridium difficile* is one primary cause of "antibiotic-associated" colitis.
After the diagnosis of pseudomembranous colitis has been established, appropriate therapeutic measures should be initiated. Mild cases of pseudomembranous colitis usually respond to drug discontinuation alone. In moderate to severe cases, consideration should be given to management with fluids and electrolytes, protein supplementation, and treatment with an antibacterial drug clinically effective against *Clostridium difficile* colitis.

Continued on next page

Cefzil—Cont.

Population/Infection	Dosage (mg)	Duration (days)
ADULTS (13 years and older)		
UPPER RESPIRATORY TRACT		
Pharyngitis/Tonsillitis	500 q 24h	10*
Acute Sinusitis (For moderate to severe infections, the higher dose should be used)	250 q 12h or 500 q 12h	10
LOWER RESPIRATORY TRACT		
Secondary Bacterial Infection of Acute Bronchitis and Acute Bacterial Exacerbation of Chronic Bronchitis	500 q 12h	10
SKIN AND SKIN STRUCTURE		
Uncomplicated Skin and Skin Structure Infections	250 q 12h or 500 q 24h or 500 q 12h	10
CHILDREN (2 years – 12 years)		
UPPER RESPIRATORY TRACT†		
Pharyngitis/Tonsillitis	7.5 mg/kg q 12h	10*
SKIN AND SKIN STRUCTURE†		
Uncomplicated Skin and Skin Structure Infections	20 mg/kg q 24h	10
INFANTS & CHILDREN (6 months – 12 years)		
UPPER RESPIRATORY TRACT†		
Otitis Media (See **INDICATIONS AND USAGE** and **CLINICAL STUDIES**sections)	15 mg/kg q 12h	10
Acute Sinusitis (For moderate to severe infections, the higher dose should be used	7.5 mg/kg q 12h 15 mg/kg	10

* In the treatment of infections due to *Streptococcus pyogenes*, CEFZIL should be administered for at least 10 days.
† Not to exceed recommended adult doses.

U.S. Acute Otitis Media Study
Cefprozil vs β-lactamase inhibitor-containing control drug

EFFICACY:

Pathogen	% of Cases with Pathogen (n = 155)	Outcome
S. pneumoniae	48.4%	cefprozil success rate 5% better than control
H. influenzae	35.5%	cefprozil success rate 17% less than control
M. catarrhalis	13.5%	cefprozil success rate 12% less than control
S. pyogenes	2.6%	cefprozil equivalent to control
Overall	100.0%	cefprozil success rate 5% less than control

SAFETY:
The incidence of adverse events, primarily diarrhea and rash*, were clinically and statistically significantly higher in the control arm versus the cefprozil arm.

PRECAUTIONS

General
In patients with known or suspected renal impairment (see **DOSAGE AND ADMINISTRATION**), careful clinical observation and appropriate laboratory studies should be done prior to and during therapy. The total daily dose of CEFZIL (cefprozil) should be reduced in these patients because high and/or prolonged plasma antibiotic concentrations can occur in such individuals from usual doses. Cephalosporins, including CEFZIL, should be given with caution to patients receiving concurrent treatment with potent diuretics since these agents are suspected of adversely affecting renal function.
Prolonged use of CEFZIL may result in the overgrowth of nonsusceptible organisms. Careful observation of the patient is essential.
If superinfection occurs during therapy, appropriate measures should be taken.
Cefprozil should be prescribed with caution in individuals with a history of gastrointestinal disease particularly colitis.
Positive direct Coombs' tests have been reported during treatment with cephalosporin antibiotics.

Information for Patients
Phenylketonurics: CEFZIL (cefprozil) for oral suspension contains phenylalanine 28 mg per 5 mL (1 teaspoonful) constituted suspension for both the 125 mg/5 mL and 250 mg/5 mL dosage forms.

Drug Interactions
Nephrotoxicity has been reported following concomitant administration of aminoglycoside antibiotics and cephalosporin antibiotics. Concomitant administration of probenecid doubled the AUC for cefprozil.
The bioavailability of the capsule formulation of cefprozil was not affected when administered 5 minutes following an antacid.

Drug/Laboratory Test Interactions
Cephalosporin antibiotics may produce a false positive reaction for glucose in the urine with copper reduction tests (Benedict's or Fehling's solution or with Clinitest®[4] tablets), but not with enzyme-based tests for glycosuria (e.g., Tes-Tape®[5]). A false negative reaction may occur in the ferricyanide test for blood glucose. The presence of cefprozil in the blood does not interfere with the assay of plasma or urine creatinine by the alkaline picrate method.

Carcinogenesis, Mutagenesis, and Impairment of Fertility
Long term *in vivo* studies have not been performed to evaluate the carcinogenic potential of cefprozil.
Cefprozil was not found to be mutagenic in either the Ames *Salmonella* or *E. coli* WP2 urvA reversion assays or the Chinese hamster ovary cell HGPRT forward gene mutation assay and it did not induce chromosomal abnormalities in Chinese hamster ovary cells or unscheduled DNA synthesis in rat hepatocytes *in vitro*. Chromosomal aberrations were not observed in bone marrow cells from rats dosed orally with over 30 times the highest recommended human dose based upon mg/m^2.
Impairment of fertility was not observed in male or female rats given oral doses of cefprozil up to 18.5 times the highest recommended human dose based upon mg/m^2.

Pregnancy: Teratogenic Effects. Pregnancy Category B
Reproduction studies have been performed in rabbits, mice and rats using oral doses of cefprozil of 0.8, 8.5 and 18.5 times the maximum daily human dose (1000 mg) based upon mg/m^2, and have revealed no harm to the fetus. There are, however, no adequate and well-controlled studies in pregnant women. Because animal reproduction studies are not always predictive of human response, this drug should be used during pregnancy only if clearly needed.

Labor and Delivery
Cefprozil has not been studied for use during labor and delivery. Treatment should only be given if clearly needed.

Nursing Mothers
Small amounts of cefprozil (< 0.3% of dose) have been detected in human milk following administration of a single 1 gram dose to lactating women. The average levels over 24 hours ranged from 0.25 to 3.3 µg/mL. Caution should be exercised when CEFZIL is administered to a nursing woman, since the effect of cefprozil on nursing infants is unknown.

Pediatric Use: (See **INDICATIONS AND USAGE** and **DOSAGE AND ADMINISTRATION**.)
The safety and effectiveness of cefprozil in the treatment of otitis media have been established in the age groups 6 months to 12 years. Use of CEFZIL for the treatment of otitis media is supported by evidence from adequate and well-controlled studies of cefprozil in pediatric patients. (See **CLINICAL STUDIES** section.)
The safety and effectiveness of cefprozil in the treatment of pharyngitis/ tonsillitis or uncomplicated skin and skin structure infections have been established in the age groups 2 to 12 years. Use of CEFZIL for the treatment of these infections is supported by evidence from adequate and well-controlled studies of cefprozil in pediatric patients.
The safety and effectiveness of cefprozil in the treatment of acute sinusitis have been established in the age groups 6 months to 12 years. Use of CEFZIL in these age groups is supported by evidence from adequate and well-controlled studies of cefprozil in adults.
Safety and effectiveness in pediatric patients below the age of 6 months have not been established for the treatment of otitis media or acute sinusitis or below the age of 2 years for the treatment of pharyngitis/tonsillitis or uncomplicated skin and skin structure infections. However, accumulation of other cephalosporin antibiotics in newborn infants (resulting from prolonged drug half-life in this age group) has been reported.

Geriatric Use
Healthy geriatric volunteers (≥ 65 years old) who received a single 1 g dose of cefprozil had 35%–60% higher AUC and 40% lower renal clearance values when compared to healthy adult volunteers 20–40 years of age. In clinical studies, when geriatric patients received the usual recommended adult doses, clinical efficacy and safety were acceptable and comparable to results in non-geriatric adult patients.

ADVERSE REACTIONS

The adverse reactions to cefprozil are similar to those observed with other orally administered cephalosporins. Cefprozil was usually well tolerated in controlled clinical trials. Approximately 2% of patients discontinued cefprozil therapy due to adverse events.
The most common adverse effects observed in patients treated with cefprozil are:
Gastrointestinal: Diarrhea (2.9%), nausea (3.5%), vomiting (1%) and abdominal pain (1%).
Hepatobiliary: Elevations of AST (SGOT) (2%), ALT (SGPT) (2%), alkaline phosphatase (0.2%), and bilirubin values (<0.1%). As with some penicillins and some other cephalosporin antibiotics, cholestatic jaundice has been reported rarely.
Hypersensitivity: Rash (0.9%), urticaria (0.1%). Such reactions have been reported more frequently in children than in adults. Signs and symptoms usually occur a few days after initiation of therapy and subside within a few days after cessation of therapy.
CNS: Dizziness (1%). Hyperactivity, headache, nervousness, insomnia, confusion, and somnolence have been reported rarely (<1%). All were reversible.
Hematopoietic: Decreased leukocyte count (0.2%), eosinophilia (2.3%).
Renal: Elevated BUN (0.1%), serum creatinine (0.1%).
Other: Diaper rash and superinfection (1.5%), genital pruritus and vaginitis (1.6%).
The following adverse events, regardless of established causal relationship to CEFZIL, have been rarely reported during post-marketing surveillance: anaphylaxis, angioedema, colitis (including pseudomembranous colitis), erythema multiforme, fever, serum-sickness like reactions, Stevens-Johnson Syndrome and thrombocytopenia.

Cephalosporin class paragraph
In addition to the adverse reactions listed above which have been observed in patients treated with cefprozil, the following adverse reactions and altered laboratory tests have been reported for cephalosporin-class antibiotics:
Aplastic anemia, hemolytic anemia, hemorrhage, renal dysfunction, toxic epidermal necrolysis, toxic nephropathy, prolonged prothrombin time, positive Coombs' test, elevated LDH, pancytopenia, neutropenia, agranulocytosis. Several cephalosporins have been implicated in triggering seizures, particularly in patients with renal impairment, when the dosage was not reduced. (See **DOSAGE AND ADMINISTRATION** and **OVERDOSAGE**.)
If seizures associated with drug therapy occur, the drug should be discontinued. Anticonvulsant therapy can be given if clinically indicated.

OVERDOSAGE

Single 5000 mg/kg oral doses of cefprozil caused no mortality or signs of toxicity in adult, weanling, or neonatal rats, or adult mice. A single oral dose of 3000 mg/kg caused diarrhea and loss of appetite in cynomolgus monkeys, but no mortality.
Cefprozil is eliminated primarily by the kidneys. In case of severe overdosage, especially in patients with compromised renal function, hemodialysis will aid in the removal of cefprozil from the body.

DOSAGE AND ADMINISTRATION

CEFZIL (cefprozil) is administered orally.
[See first table above]

Renal Impairment
Cefprozil may be administered to patients with impaired renal function. The following dosage schedule should be used.

Creatinine Clearance (mL/min)	Dosage (mg)	Dosing Interval
30–120	standard	standard
0–29*	50% of standard	standard

* Cefprozil is in part removed by hemodialysis; therefore, cefprozil should be administered after the completion of hemodialysis.

European Acute Otitis Media Study
Cefprozil vs β-lactamase inhibitor-containing control drug

EFFICACY:

Pathogen	% of Cases with Pathogen (n = 47)	Outcome
S. pneumoniae	51.0%	cefprozil equivalent to control
H. influenzae	29.8%	cefprozil equivalent to control
M. catarrhalis	6.4%	cefprozil equivalent to control
S. pyogenes	12.8%	cefprozil equivalent to control
Overall	100.0%	cefprozil equivalent to control

SAFETY:
The incidence of adverse events in the cefprozil arm was comparable to the incidence of adverse events in the control arm (agent that contained a specific β-lactamase inhibitor).

Hepatic Impairment
No dosage adjustment is necessary for patients with impaired hepatic function.

HOW SUPPLIED

CEFZIL® (Cefprozil) Tablets
Each light orange film-coated tablet, imprinted with "7720" on one side and "250" on the other, contains the equivalent of 250 mg anhydrous cefprozil.

Bottles of 100 Tablets	**NDC** 0087-7720-60
Cartons of 100 Tablets	**NDC** 0087-7720-66

(10 strips containing 10 tablets on each strip)

Each white film-coated tablet, imprinted with "7721" on one side and "500" on the other, contains the equivalent of 500 mg anhydrous cefprozil.

Bottles of 50 Tablets	**NDC** 0087-7721-50
Bottles of 100 Tablets	**NDC** 0087-7721-60
Cartons of 100 Tablets	**NDC** 0087-7721-66

(10 strips containing 10 tablets on each strip)

Store at controlled room temperature, 59° to 86° F (15° to 30° C).

CEFZIL® (Cefprozil) For Oral Suspension
Each 5 mL of constituted suspension contains the equivalent of 125 mg anhydrous cefprozil.

50 mL Bottle	**NDC** 0087-7718-40
75 mL Bottle	**NDC** 0087-7718-62
100 mL Bottle	**NDC** 0087-7718-64

Each 5 mL of constituted suspension contains the equivalent of 250 mg anhydrous cefprozil.

50 mL Bottle	**NDC** 0087-7719-40
75 mL Bottle	**NDC** 0087-7719-62
100 mL Bottle	**NDC** 0087-7719-64

All powder formulations for oral suspension contain cefprozil in a bubble-gum flavored mixture.

Reconstitution Directions for Oral Suspension
Prepare the suspension at the time of dispensing; for ease in preparation, add water in two portions and shake well after each aliquot.

Total Amount of Water Required for Reconstitution

Bottle Size	Final Concentration 125 mg/ 5 mL	Final Concentration 250 mg/5 mL
50 mL	36 mL	36 mL
75 mL	54 mL	54 mL
100 mL	72 mL	72 mL

After mixing, store in a refrigerator and discard unused portion after 14 days.
Store at 59° to 77° F (15° to 25° C) prior to constitution.
U.S. Patent No. 4,520,022

CLINICAL STUDIES

Study One:
In a controlled clinical study of **acute otitis media** performed in the United States where significant rates of β-lactamase producing organisms were found, cefprozil was compared to an oral antimicrobial agent that contained a specific β-lactamase inhibitor. In this study, using very strict evaluability criteria and microbiologic and clinical response criteria at the 10-16 days post-therapy follow-up, the following presumptive bacterial eradication/clinical cure outcomes (i.e. clinical success) and safety results were obtained:
[See second table on previous page]

Age Group	Cefprozil	Control
6 months-2 years	21%	41%
3–12 years	10%	19%

*The majority of these involved the diaper area in young children.

Study Two:
In a controlled clinical study of **acute otitis media** performed in Europe, cefprozil was compared to an oral antimicrobial agent that contained a specific β-lactamase inhibitor. As expected in a European population, this study population had a lower incidence of β-lactamase-producing organisms than usually seen in U.S. trials. In this study, using very strict evaluability criteria and microbiologic and clinical response criteria at the 10–16 days post-therapy follow-up, the following presumptive bacterial eradication/clinical cure outcomes (i.e. clinical success) were obtained:
[See table at top of page]

REFERENCES

1. National Committee for Clinical Laboratory Standards. *Methods for Dilution Antimicrobial Susceptibility Tests for Bacteria that Grow Aerobically*—Third Edition. Approved Standard NCCLS Document M7-A3, Vol. 13, No. 25, NCCLS, Villanova, PA, December, 1993.
2. National Committee for Clinical Laboratory Standards. *Methods for Antimicrobial Susceptibility Testing of Anaerobic Bacteria*—Third Edition. Approved Standard NCCLS Document M11-A3, Vol. 13, No. 26, NCCLS, Villanova, PA, December, 1993.
3. National Committee for Clinical Laboratory Standards. *Performance Standards for Antimicrobial Disk Susceptibility Tests*—Fifth Edition. Approved Standard NCCLS Document M2-A5, Vol. 13, No. 24, NCCLS, Villanova, PA, December, 1993.
4. Clinitest® is a registered trademark of the Bayer Corporation.
5. Tes-Tape® is a registered trademark of Eli Lilly and Company.

7718DIM-12
51-004077-03
Revised March 1998

Bristol-Myers Squibb Company
Princeton, New Jersey 08543
USA

Shown in Product Identification Guide, page 309

CORZIDE® 40/5 ℞
[cŏr-zīde]
CORZIDE® 80/5
Nadolol and Bendroflumethiazide Tablets

Rx only

DESCRIPTION

CORZIDE (Nadolol and Bendroflumethiazide Tablets) for oral administration combines two antihypertensive agents: CORGARD® (nadolol), a nonselective beta-adrenergic blocking agent, and NATURETIN® (bendroflumethiazide), a thiazide diuretic-antihypertensive. Formulations: 40 mg and 80 mg nadolol per tablet combined with 5 mg bendroflumethiazide. Inactive ingredients: cellulose, colorant (FD&C Blue No. 2), lactose, magnesium stearate, povidone, sodium starch glycolate, and starch.

Nadolol
Nadolol is a white crystalline powder. It is freely soluble in ethanol, soluble in hydrochloric acid, slightly soluble in water and in chloroform, and very slightly soluble in sodium hydroxide.
Nadolol is designated chemically as 1-(*tert*-butylamino)-3-[(5,6,7,8-tetrahydro-*cis*-6,7-dihydroxy-1-naphthyl)oxy]-2-propanol. Structural formula:

OH, H, H, OH, $OCH_2CHCH_2NHC(CH_3)_3$, OH

$C_{17}H_{27}NO_4$ MW 309.40

Bendroflumethiazide
Bendroflumethiazide is a white crystalline powder. It is soluble in alcohol and in sodium hydroxide, and insoluble in hydrochloric acid, water, and chloroform.
Bendroflumethiazide is designated chemically as 3-benzyl-3,4-dihydro-6-(trifluoromethyl)-2*H*-1,2,4-benzothiadiazine-7-sulfonamide 1,1-dioxide. Structural formula:

NH_2SO_2, O, O, S, NH, CF_3, N, H, CH_2

$C_{15}H_{14}F_3N_3O_4S_2$ MW 421.41

CLINICAL PHARMACOLOGY

Nadolol
Nadolol is a nonselective beta-adrenergic receptor blocking agent. Clinical pharmacology studies have demonstrated beta-blocking activity by showing (1) reduction in heart rate and cardiac output at rest and on exercise, (2) reduction of systolic and diastolic blood pressure at rest and on exercise, (3) inhibition of isoproterenol-induced tachycardia, and (4) reduction of reflex orthostatic tachycardia.
Nadolol specifically competes with beta-adrenergic receptor agonists for available beta receptor sites; it inhibits both the $beta_1$ receptors located chiefly in cardiac muscle and the $beta_2$ receptors located chiefly in the bronchial and vascular musculature, inhibiting the chronotropic, inotropic, and vasodilator responses to beta-adrenergic stimulation proportionately. Nadolol has no intrinsic sympathomimetic activity and, unlike some other beta-adrenergic blocking agents, nadolol has little direct myocardial depressant activity and does not have an anesthetic-like membrane-stabilizing action. Animal and human studies show that nadolol slows the sinus rate and depresses AV conduction. In dogs, only minimal amounts of nadolol were detected in the brain relative to amounts in blood and other organs and tissues. Nadolol has low lipophilicity as determined by octanol/water partition coefficient, a characteristic of certain beta-blocking agents that has been correlated with the limited extent to which these agents cross the blood-brain barrier, their low concentration in the brain, and low incidence of CNS-related side effects.
In controlled clinical studies, nadolol at doses of 40 to 320 mg/day has been shown to decrease both standing and supine blood pressure, the effect persisting for approximately 24 hours after dosing.
The mechanism of the antihypertensive effects of beta-adrenergic receptor blocking agents has not been established; however, factors that may be involved include (1) competitive antagonism of catecholamines at peripheral (non-CNS) adrenergic neuron sites (especially cardiac) leading to decreased cardiac output, (2) a central effect leading to reduced tonic-sympathetic nerve outflow to the periphery, and (3) suppression of renin secretion by blockade of the beta-adrenergic receptors responsible for renin release from the kidneys.
While cardiac output and arterial pressure are reduced by nadolol therapy, renal hemodynamics are stable, with preservation of renal blood flow and glomerular filtration rate.
By blocking catecholamine-induced increases in heart rate, velocity and extent of myocardial contraction, and blood pressure, nadolol generally reduces the oxygen requirements of the heart at any given level of effort, making it useful for many patients in the long-term management of angina pectoris. On the other hand, nadolol can increase oxygen requirements by increasing left ventricular fiber length and end diastolic pressure, particularly in patients with heart failure.
Although beta-adrenergic receptor blockade is useful in treatment of angina and hypertension, there are also situations in which sympathetic stimulation is vital. For example, in patients with severely damaged hearts, adequate ventricular function may depend on sympathetic drive. Beta-adrenergic blockade may worsen AV block by preventing the necessary facilitating effects of sympathetic activity on conduction. $Beta_2$-adrenergic blockade results in passive bronchial constriction by interfering with endogenous adrenergic bronchodilator activity in patients subject to bronchospasm and may also interfere with exogenous bronchodilators in such patients.
Absorption of nadolol after oral dosing is variable, averaging about 30 percent. Peak serum concentrations of nadolol usually occur in three to four hours after oral administration and the presence of food in the gastrointestinal tract does not affect the rate or extent of nadolol absorption. Approximately 30 percent of the nadolol present in serum is reversibly bound to plasma protein.
Unlike many other beta-adrenergic blocking agents, nadolol is not metabolized by the liver and is excreted unchanged, principally by the kidneys.
The half-life of therapeutic doses of nadolol is about 20 to 24 hours, permitting once-daily dosage. Because nadolol is excreted predominantly in the urine, its half-life increases in renal failure (see **PRECAUTIONS, General,** and **DOSAGE AND ADMINISTRATION**). Steady state serum concentrations of nadolol are attained in six to nine days with once-daily dosage in persons with normal renal function. Because of variable absorption and different individual responsiveness, the proper dosage must be determined by titration.
Exacerbation of angina and, in some cases, myocardial infarction and ventricular dysrhythmias have been reported after abrupt discontinuation of therapy with beta-adrenergic blocking agents in patients with coronary artery disease. Abrupt withdrawal of these agents in patients without coronary artery disease has resulted in transient symptoms, including tremulousness, sweating, palpitation, headache, and malaise. Several mechanisms have been proposed to explain these phenomena, among them increased sensitivity to catecholamines because of increased numbers of beta receptors.

Bendroflumethiazide
The mechanism of action of bendroflumethiazide results in an interference with the renal tubular mechanism of electrolyte reabsorption. At maximal therapeutic dosage all thiazides are approximately equal in their diuretic potency.
Thiazides increase excretion of sodium and chloride in approximately equivalent amounts. Natriuresis causes a secondary loss of potassium and bicarbonate.
The mechanism of the antihypertensive effect of thiazides is unknown. Thiazides do not affect normal blood pressure.
Onset of action of thiazides occurs in two hours and the peak effect at about four hours. Duration of action persists for approximately six to 12 hours. Thiazides are eliminated rapidly by the kidney.

INDICATIONS

CORZIDE (Nadolol and Bendroflumethiazide Tablets) is indicated in the management of hypertension.
This fixed combination drug is not indicated for initial therapy of hypertension. If the fixed combination represents the dose titrated to the individual patient's needs, it may be more convenient than the separate components.

Continued on next page

Corzide—Cont.

CONTRAINDICATIONS

Nadolol

Nadolol is contraindicated in bronchial asthma, sinus bradycardia and greater than first degree conduction block, cardiogenic shock, and overt cardiac failure (see **WARNINGS**).

Bendroflumethiazide

Bendroflumethiazide is contraindicated in anuria. It is also contraindicated in patients who have previously demonstrated hypersensitivity to bendroflumethiazide or other sulfonamide-derived drugs.

WARNINGS

Nadolol

Cardiac Failure—Sympathetic stimulation may be a vital component supporting circulatory function in patients with congestive heart failure, and its inhibition by beta-blockade may precipitate more severe failure. Although beta-blockers should be avoided in overt congestive heart failure, if necessary, they can be used with caution in patients with a history of failure who are well compensated, usually with digitalis and diuretics. Beta-adrenergic blocking agents do not abolish the inotropic action of digitalis on heart muscle.

IN PATIENTS WITHOUT A HISTORY OF HEART FAILURE, continued use of beta-blockers can, in some cases, lead to cardiac failure. Therefore, at the first sign or symptom of heart failure, the patient should be digitalized and/or treated with diuretics, and the response observed closely, or nadolol should be discontinued (gradually, if possible).

Exacerbation of Ischemic Heart Disease Following Abrupt Withdrawal—Hypersensitivity to catecholamines has been observed in patients withdrawn from beta-blocker therapy; exacerbation of angina and, in some cases, myocardial infarction have occurred after *abrupt* discontinuation of such therapy. When discontinuing chronically administered nadolol, particularly in patients with ischemic heart disease, the dosage should be gradually reduced over a period of one to two weeks and the patient should be carefully monitored. If angina markedly worsens or acute coronary insufficiency develops, nadolol administration should be reinstituted promptly, at least temporarily, and other measures appropriate for the management of unstable angina should be taken. Patients should be warned against interruption or discontinuation of therapy without the physician's advice. Because coronary artery disease is common and may be unrecognized, it may be prudent not to discontinue nadolol therapy abruptly even in patients treated only for hypertension.

Nonallergic Bronchospasm (e.g., chronic bronchitis, emphysema)—PATIENTS WITH BRONCHOSPASTIC DISEASES SHOULD IN GENERAL NOT RECEIVE BETA-BLOCKERS. Nadolol should be administered with caution since it may block bronchodilation produced by endogenous or exogenous catecholamine stimulation of beta$_2$ receptors.

Major Surgery—Because beta-blockade impairs the ability of the heart to respond to reflex stimuli and may increase the risks of general anesthesia and surgical procedures, resulting in protracted hypotension or low cardiac output, it has generally been suggested that such therapy should be withdrawn several days prior to surgery. Recognition of the increased sensitivity to catecholamines of patients recently withdrawn from beta-blocker therapy, however, has made this recommendation controversial. If possible, beta-blockers should be withdrawn well before surgery takes place. In the event of emergency surgery, the anesthesiologist should be informed that the patient is on beta-blocker therapy. The effects of nadolol can be reversed by administration of beta-receptor agonists such as isoproterenol, dopamine, dobutamine, or levarterenol. Difficulty in restarting and maintaining the heart beat has also been reported with beta-adrenergic receptor blocking agents.

Diabetes and Hypoglycemia—Beta-adrenergic blockade may prevent the appearance of permonitory signs and symptoms (e.g., tachycardia and blood pressure changes) of acute hypoglycemia. This is especially important with labile diabetics. Beta-blockade also reduces the release of insulin in response to hyperglycemia; therefore, it may be necessary to adjust the dose of antidiabetic drugs.

Thyrotoxicosis—Beta-adrenergic blockade may mask certain clinical signs (e.g., tachycardia) of hyperthyroidism. Patients suspected of developing thyrotoxicosis should be managed carefully to avoid abrupt withdrawal of beta-adrenergic blockade which might precipitate a thyroid storm.

Bendroflumethiazide

Thiazides should be used with caution in severe renal disease. In patients with renal disease, thiazides may precipitate azotemia. Cumulative effects of the drug may develop in patients with impaired renal function.

Thiazides should be used with caution in patients with impaired hepatic function or progressive liver disease, since minor alterations of fluid and electrolyte balance may precipitate hepatic coma.

Sensitivity reactions may occur in patients with or without a history of allergy or bronchial asthma.

The possibility of exacerbation or activation of systemic lupus erythematosus has been reported.

Lithium generally should not be given with diuretics; diuretic agents reduce the renal clearance of lithium and add a high risk of lithium toxicity. Refer to the package insert for lithium preparations before use of such concomitant therapy.

PRECAUTIONS

General

Nadolol

Nadolol should be used with caution in patients with impaired renal function (see **DOSAGE AND ADMINISTRATION**).

Bendroflumethiazide

Periodic determination of serum electrolytes to detect possible electrolyte imbalance should be performed at appropriate intervals.

All patients receiving thiazide therapy should be observed for clinical signs of fluid or electrolyte imbalance, namely: hyponatremia, hypochloremic alkalosis, and hypokalemia. Serum and urine electrolyte determinations are particularly important when the patient is vomiting excessively or receiving parenteral fluids. Warning signs or symptoms of fluid and electrolyte imbalance may include: dryness of the mouth, thirst, weakness, lethargy, drowsiness, restlessness, muscle pains or cramps, muscular fatigue, hypotension, oliguria, tachycardia, and gastrointestinal disturbances, such as nausea or vomiting.

Hypokalemia may develop, especially with brisk diuresis or when severe cirrhosis is present.

Interference with adequate oral electrolyte intake will also contribute to hypokalemia. Hypokalemia can sensitize or exaggerate the response of the heart to the toxic effects of digitalis (e.g., increased ventricular irritability). Concurrent administration of a potassium-sparing diuretic or potassium supplements may be indicated in these patients.

Any chloride deficit is generally mild and usually does not require specific treatment except under extraordinary circumstances (as in liver disease or renal disease). Dilutional hyponatremia may occur in edematous patients in hot weather; appropriate therapy is water restriction, rather than administration of salt, except in rare instances when the hyponatremia is life-threatening. In actual salt depletion, appropriate replacement is the therapy of choice.

Hyperuricemia may occur or frank gout may be precipitated in certain patients receiving thiazide therapy.

Latent diabetes mellitus may become manifest during thiazide administration.

The antihypertensive effect of thiazide diuretics may be enhanced in the postsympathectomy patient.

If progressive renal impairment becomes evident, as indicated by a rising nonprotein nitrogen or blood urea nitrogen (BUN), a careful reappraisal of therapy is necessary with consideration given to withholding or discontinuing diuretic therapy.

Thiazides may decrease serum PBI levels without signs of thyroid disturbance.

Calcium excretion is decreased by thiazides. Pathological changes in the parathyroid gland with hypercalcemia and hypophosphatemia have been observed in a few patients on prolonged thiazide therapy. The common complications of hyperparathyroidism such as renal lithiasis, bone resorption, and peptic ulceration have not been seen. Thiazides should be discontinued before carrying out tests for parathyroid function.

Thiazides have been shown to increase the urinary excretion of magnesium; this may result in hypomagnesemia.

Information for Patients

Patients, especially those with evidence of coronary artery insufficiency, should be warned against interruption or discontinuation of therapy without the physician's advice. Although cardiac failure rarely occurs in properly selected patients, patients being treated with beta-adrenergic blocking agents should be advised to consult the physician at the first sign or symptom of impending failure.

The patient should also be advised of a proper course in the event of an inadvertently missed dose.

The patient should be informed of symptoms that would suggest potential adverse effects and told to report them promptly.

Laboratory Tests

Serum electrolyte levels should be regularly monitored (see **WARNINGS, Bendroflumethiazide**, also **PRECAUTIONS, General, Bendroflumethiazide**).

Drug Interactions

Nadolol

When administered concurrently the following drugs may interact with beta-adrenergic receptor blocking agents:

Anesthetics, general—exaggeration of the hypotension induced by general anesthetics (see **WARNINGS, Nadolol, Major Surgery**).

Antidiabetic drugs (oral agents and insulin)—hypoglycemia or hyperglycemia; adjust dosage of antidiabetic drug accordingly (see **WARNINGS, Nadolol, Diabetes and Hypoglycemia**).

Catecholamine-depleting drugs (e.g., reserpine)—additive effect; monitor closely for evidence of hypotension and/or excessive bradycardia (e.g., vertigo, syncope, postural hypotension).

Response to Treatment for Anaphylactic Reaction—While taking beta-blockers, patients with a history of severe anaphylactic reaction to a variety of allergens may be more reactive to repeated challenge, either accidental, diagnostic, or therapeutic. Such patients may be unresponsive to the usual doses of epinephrine used to treat allergic reaction.

Bendroflumethiazide

When administered concurrently the following drugs may interact with thiazide diuretics:

Alcohol, barbiturates, or narcotics—potentiation of orthostatic hypotension may occur.

Amphotericin B, corticosteroids, or corticotropin (ACTH)—may intensify electrolyte imbalance, particularly hypokalemia. Monitor potassium levels; use potassium replacements if necessary.

Anticoagulants (oral)—dosage adjustments of anticoagulant medication may be necessary since bendroflumethiazide may decrease their effects.

Antigout medications—dosage adjustments of antigout medication may be necessary since bendroflumethiazide may raise the level of blood uric acid.

Other antihypertensive medications (e.g., ganglionic or peripheral adrenergic blocking agents)—dosage adjustments may be necessary since bendroflumethiazide may potentiate their effects.

Antidiabetic drugs (oral agents and insulin)—since thiazides may elevate blood glucose levels, dosage adjustments of antidiabetic agents may be necessary.

Calcium salts—increased serum calcium levels due to decreased excretion may occur. If calcium must be prescribed monitor serum calcium levels and adjust calcium dosage accordingly.

Cardiac glycosides—enhanced possibility of digitalis toxicity associated with hypokalemia. Monitor potassium levels; use potassium replacement if necessary.

Cholestyramine resin and colestipol HCL—may delay or decrease absorption of bendroflumethiazide. Sulfonamide diuretics should be taken at least one hour before or four to six hours after these medications.

Diazoxide—enhanced hyperglycemic, hyperuricemic, and antihypertensive effects. Be cognizant of possible interaction; monitor blood glucose and serum uric acid levels.

Lithium salts—may enhance lithium toxicity due to reduced renal clearance. Avoid concurrent use; if lithium must be prescribed monitor serum lithium levels and adjust lithium dosage accordingly. (See **WARNINGS**)

MAO inhibitors—dosage adjustments of one or both agents may be necessary since hypotensive effects are enhanced.

Nondepolarizing muscle relaxants, preanesthetics and anesthetics used in surgery (e.g., tubocurarine chloride and gallamine triethiodide)—effects of these agents may be potentiated; dosage adjustments may be required. Monitor and correct any fluid and electrolyte imbalances prior to surgery if feasible.

Nonsteroidal anti-inflammatory agents—in some patients, the administration of a nonsteroidal anti-inflammatory agent can reduce the diuretic, natriuretic, and antihypertensive effect of loop, potassium-sparing or thiazide diuretics. Therefore, when bendroflumethiazide and nonsteroidal anti-inflammatory agents are used concomitantly, the patient should be observed closely to determine if the desired effect of the diuretic is obtained.

Methenamine—possible decreased effectiveness due to alkalinization of the urine.

Pressor amines (e.g., norepinephrine)—decreased arterial responsiveness, but not sufficient to preclude effectiveness of the pressor agent for therapeutic use. Use caution in patients taking both medications who undergo surgery. Administer preanesthetic and anesthetic agents in reduced dosage, and if possible, discontinue bendroflumethiazide one week prior to surgery.

Probenecid or sulfinpyrazone—increased dosage of these agents may be necessary since bendroflumethiazide may have hyperuricemic effects.

Drug/Laboratory Test Interactions

Bendroflumethiazide may produce false-negative results with the phentolamine and tyramine tests; may interfere with the phenosulfonphthalein test due to decrease excretion; and it may cause diagnostic interference of serum electrolyte levels, blood and urine glucose levels, and a decrease in serum PBI levels without signs of thyroid disturbance.

Carcinogenesis, Mutagenesis, Impairment of Fertility

Nadolol

In chronic oral toxicologic studies (one to two years) in mice, rats, and dogs, nadolol did not produce any significant toxic effects. In two-year oral carcinogenicity studies in rats and mice, nadolol did not produce any neoplastic, preneoplastic, or nonneoplastic pathologic lesions. In fertility and general reproductive performance studies in rats, nadolol caused no adverse effect.

Bendroflumethiazide

Studies have not been performed to evaluate carcinogenic potential, mutagenesis, or whether this drug adversely affects fertility in males or females.

Pregnancy—Teratogenic Effects

Nadolol

Category C. In animal reproduction studies with nadolol, evidence of embryo- and fetotoxicity was found in rabbits, but not in rats or hamsters, at doses 5 to 10 times greater (on a mg/kg basis) than the maximum indicated human dose. No teratogenic potential was observed in any of these species.

There are no adequate and well-controlled studies in pregnant women. Nadolol should be used during pregnancy only if the potential benefit justifies the potential risk to the fetus. Neonates whose mothers are receiving nadolol at parturition have exhibited bradycardia, hypoglycemia, and associated symptoms.

Bendroflumethiazide

Category C. Animal reproduction studies have not been conducted with bendroflumethiazide. It is also not known whether this drug can cause fetal harm when administered to a pregnant woman or can affect reproduction capacity. Bendroflumethiazide should be given to a pregnant woman only if clearly needed.

Pregnancy—Nonteratogenic Effects

Thiazides cross the placental barrier and appear in cord blood. The use of thiazides in pregnant women requires that the anticipated benefit be weighed against possible hazards to the fetus. These hazards include fetal or neonatal jaundice, thrombocytopenia, and possibly other adverse reactions which have occurred in the adult.

Nursing Mothers

Both nadolol and bendroflumethiazide are excreted in human milk. Because of the potential for serious adverse reactions in nursing infants from both drugs, a decision should be made whether to discontinue nursing or to discontinue therapy taking into account the importance of CORZIDE (Nadolol and Bendroflumethiazide Tablets) to the mother.

Pediatric Use

Safety and effectiveness in pediatric patients have not been established.

ADVERSE REACTIONS

Nadolol

Most adverse effects have been mild and transient and have rarely required withdrawal of therapy.

Cardiovascular—Bradycardia with heart rates of less than 60 beats per minute occurs commonly, and heart rates below 40 beats per minute and/or symptomatic bradycardia were seen in about 2 of 100 patients. Symptoms of peripheral vascular insufficiency, usually of the Raynaud type, have occurred in approximately 2 of 100 patients. Cardiac failure, hypotension, and rhythm/conduction disturbances have each occurred in about 1 of 100 patients. Single instances of first degree and third degree heart block have been reported; intensification of AV block is a known effect of beta-blockers (see also **CONTRAINDICATIONS**, **WARNINGS**, and **PRECAUTIONS**).

Central Nervous System—Dizziness or fatigue has been reported in approximately 2 of 100 patients; paresthesias, sedation, and change in behavior have each been reported in approximately 6 of 1000 patients.

Respiratory—Bronchospasm has been reported in approximately 1 of 1000 patients (see **CONTRAINDICATIONS** and **WARNINGS**).

Gastrointestinal—Nausea, diarrhea, abdominal discomfort, constipation, vomiting, indigestion, anorexia, bloating, and flatulence have been reported in 1 to 5 of 1000 patients.

Miscellaneous—Each of the following has been reported in 1 to 5 of 1000 patients: rash; pruritus; headache; dry mouth, eyes, or skin; impotence or decreased libido; facial swelling; weight gain; slurred speech; cough; nasal stuffiness; sweating; tinnitus; blurred vision. Reversible alopecia has been reported infrequently.

The following adverse reactions have been reported in patients taking nadolol and/or other beta-adrenergic blocking agents, but no causal relationship to nadolol has been established.

Central Nervous System—Reversible mental depression progressing to catatonia; visual disturbances; hallucinations; an acute reversible syndrome characterized by disorientation for time and place, short-term memory loss, emotional lability with slightly clouded sensorium, and decreased performance on neuropsychometrics.

Gastrointestinal—Mesenteric arterial thrombosis; ischemic colitis; elevated liver enzymes.

Hematologic—Agranulocytosis; thrombocytopenic or nonthrombocytopenic purpura.

Allergic—Fever combined with aching and sore throat; laryngospasm; respiratory distress.

Miscellaneous—Pemphigoid rash; hypertensive reaction in patients with pheochromocytoma; sleep disturbances; Peyronie's disease.

The oculomucocutaneous syndrome associated with the beta-blocker practolol has not been reported with nadolol.

Bendroflumethiazide

Gastrointestinal—Nausea, vomiting, cramping and anorexia are not uncommon; diarrhea, constipation, gastric irritation, abdominal bleeding, jaundice (intrahepatic cholestatic jaundice), hepatitis, and sialadenitis occasionally occur; and pancreatitis has been reported.

Central Nervous System—Dizziness, vertigo, paresthesia, headache, and xanthopsia occasionally occur.

Hematologic—Leukopenia, agranulocytosis, thrombocytopenia, hemolytic anemia, and aplastic anemia have been reported.

Dermatologic-Hypersensitivity—Purpura, exfoliative dermatitis, pruritus, ecchymosis, urticaria, necrotizing angiitis (vasculitis, cutaneous vasculitis), respiratory distress including penumonitis, fever, and anaphylactic reactions occasionally occur; photosensitivity and rash have been reported.

Cardiovascular—Orthostatic hypotension may occur and may be potentiated by coadministration with certain other drugs (e.g., alcohol, barbiturates, narcotics, other antihypertensive medications, etc.; see **PRECAUTIONS, Drug Interactions**).

Other—Muscle spasm, weakness, or restlessness is not uncommon; hyperglycemia, glycosuria, metabolic acidosis in diabetic patients, hyperuricemia, allergic glomerulonephritis, and transient blurred vision occassionally occur.

Whenever adverse reactions are moderate or severe, thiazide dosage should be reduced or therapy withdrawn.

OVERDOSAGE

In the event of overdosage, nadolol may cause excessive bradycardia, cardiac failure, hypotension, or bronchospasm. In addition to the expected diuresis, overdosage of bendroflumethiazide may produce varying degrees of lethargy which may progress to coma with minimal depression of respiration and cardiovascular function and without significant serum elecrolyte changes or dehydration. The mechanism of thiazide-induced CNS depression is unknown. Gastrointestinal irritation may occur. Transitory increase in BUN has been reported, and serum electrolyte changes may occur, especially in patients with impaired renal function.

Treatment

Nadolol can be removed from the general circulation by hemodialysis. In determining the duration of corrective therapy, note must be taken of the long duration of the effect of nadolol. In addition to gastric lavage, the following measures should be employed, as appropriate.

Excessive Bradycardia—Administer atropine (0.25 to 1.0 mg). If there is no response to vagal blockade, administer isoproterenol cautiously.

Cardiac Failure—Administer a digitalis glycoside and diuretic. It has been reported that glucagon may also be useful in this situation.

Hypotension—Administer vasopressors, e.g., epinephrine or levarterenol. (There is evidence that epinephrine may be the drug of choice.)

Bronchospasm—Administer a beta$_2$-stimulating agent and/or a theophylline derivative.

Stupor or Coma—Supportive therapy as warranted.

Gastrointestinal Effects—Syptomatic treatment as needed.

BUN and/or Serum Electrolyte Abnormalities—Institute supportive measures as required to maintain hydration, electrolyte balance, respiration, and cardiovascular and renal function.

DOSAGE AND ADMINISTRATION

DOSAGE MUST BE INDIVIDUALIZED (SEE **INDICATIONS**). CORZIDE MAY BE ADMINISTERED WITHOUT REGARD TO MEALS.

Bendroflumethiazide is usually given at a dose of 5 mg daily. The usual initial dose of nadolol is 40 mg once daily whether used alone or in combination with a diuretic. Bendroflumethiazide in CORZIDE is 30 percent more bioavailable than that of 5 mg Naturetin tablets. Conversion from 5 mg NATURETIN to CORZIDE represents a 30 percent increase in dose of bendroflumethiazide.

The initial dose of CORZIDE (Nadolol and Bendroflumethiazide Tablets) may therefore be the 40 mg/5 mg tablet once daily. When the antihypertensive response is not satisfactory, the dose may be increased by administering the 80 mg/5 mg tablet once daily.

When necessary, another hypertensive agent may be added gradually beginning with 50 percent of the usual recommended starting dose to avoid an excessive fall in blood pressure.

Dosage Adjustment in Renal Failure—Absorbed nadolol is excreted principally by the kidneys and, although nonrenal elimination does occur, dosage adjustments are necessary in patients with renal impairment. The following dose intervals are recommended:

Creatinine Clearance (mL/min/1.73m^2)	Dosage Interval (hours)
>50	24
31–50	24–36
10–30	24–48
<10	40–60

HOW SUPPLIED

CORZIDE (Nadolol and Bendroflumethiazide Tablets)

- **40 mg nadolol combined with 5 mg bendroflumethiazide** in bottles of 100 tablets (NDC 0003-0283-50).
- **80 mg nadolol combined with 5 mg bendroflumethiazide** in bottles of 100 tablets (NDC 0003-0284-50).

Round, biconvex tablets are white to bluish white with dark blue specks. Each tablet has a full bisect bar. Tablet identification numbers: 40 mg/5 mg combination, **283**; 80 mg/5 mg combination, **284**.

Storage

Keep bottle tightly closed. Store at room temperature; avoid excessive heat.

A Bristol-Myers Squibb Company
Princeton, NJ 08543 USA

Revised May 2000

DURICEF® ℞

[dur 'ĭ-sef]

(cefadroxil monohydrate, USP)

Rx only

DESCRIPTION

DURICEF® (cefadroxil monohydrate, USP) is a semisynthetic cephalosporin antibiotic intended for oral administration. It is a white to yellowish-white crystalline powder. It is soluble in water and it is acid-stable. It is chemically designated as 5-Thia-1-azabicyclo[4.2.0]oct-2-ene-2-carboxylic acid, 7-[[amino(4-hydroxy-phenyl)acetyl] amino]-3-methyl-8-oxo-, monohydrate, [6R-[6α,7β(R*)]]-. It has the formula $C_{16}H_{17}N_3O_5S \bullet H_2O$ and the molecular weight of 381.40. It has the following structural formula:

DURICEF film-coated tablets, 1 g, contain the following inactive ingredients: microcrystalline cellulose, hydroxypropyl methylcellulose, magnesium stearate, polyethylene glycol, polysorbate 80, simethicone emulsion, and titanium dioxide.

DURICEF for Oral Suspension contains the following inactive ingredients: FD&C Yellow No. 6, flavors (natural and artificial), polysorbate 80, sodium benzoate, sucrose, and xanthan gum.

DURICEF capsules contain the following inactive ingredients: D&C Red No. 28, FD&C Blue No. 1, FD&C Red No. 40, gelatin, magnesium stearate, and titanium dioxide.

CLINICAL PHARMACOLOGY

DURICEF is rapidly absorbed after oral administration. Following single doses of 500 and 1000 mg, average peak serum concentrations were approximately 16 and 28 µg/mL, respectively. Measurable levels were present 12 hours after administration. Over 90% of the drug is excreted unchanged in the urine within 24 hours. Peak urine concentrations are approximately 1800 µg/mL during the period following a single 500-mg oral dose. Increases in dosage generally produce a proportionate increase in DURICEF urinary concentration. The urine antibiotic concentration, following a 1-g dose, was maintained well above the MIC of susceptible urinary pathogens for 20 to 22 hours.

Microbiology

In vitro tests demonstrate that the cephalosporins are bactericidal because of their inhibition of cell-wall synthesis. Cefadroxil has been shown to be active against the following organisms both *in vitro* and in clinical infections (see INDICATIONS AND USAGE):

Beta-hemolytic streptococci
Staphylococci, including penicillinase-producing strains
Streptococcus (Diplococcus) pneumoniae
Escherichia coli
Proteus mirabilis
Klebsiella species
Moraxella (Branhamella) catarrhalis

Note: Most strains of *Enterococcus faecalis* (formerly *Streptococcus faecalis*) and *Enterococcus faecium* (formerly *Streptococcus faecium*) are resistant to DURICEF (cefadroxil monohydrate, USP). It is not active against most strains of *Enterobacter* species, *Morganella morganii* (formerly *Proteus morganii*), and *P. vulgaris*. It has no activity against *Pseudomonas* species and *Acinetobacter calcoaceticus* (formerly *Mima* and *Herellea* species).

Susceptibility tests: Diffusion techniques

The use of antibiotic disk susceptibility test methods which measure zone diameter give an accurate estimation of antibiotic susceptibility. One such standard procedure[1] which has been recommended for use with disks to test susceptibility of organisms to cefadroxil uses the cephalosporin class (cephalothin) disk. Interpretation involves the correlation of the diameters obtained in the disk test with the minimum inhibitory concentration (MIC) for cefadroxil.

Reports from the laboratory giving results of the standard single-disk susceptibility test with a 30 µg cephalothin disk should be interpreted according to the following criteria:

Zone Diameter (mm)	Interpretation
≥ 18	(S) Susceptible
15–17	(I) Intermediate
≤ 14	(R) Resistant

A report of "Susceptible" indicates that the pathogen is likely to be inhibited by generally achievable blood levels. A report of "Intermediate susceptibility" suggests that the organism would be susceptible if high dosage is used or if the infection is confined to tissue and fluids (eg, urine) in which high antibiotic levels are attained. A report of "Resistant" indicates that achievable concentrations of the antibiotic are unlikely to be inhibitory and other therapy should be selected.

Standardized procedures require the use of laboratory control organisms. The 30 µg cephalothin disk should give the following zone diameters:

Organism	Zone Diameter (mm)
Staphylococcus aureus ATCC 25923	29–37
Escherichia coli ATCC 25922	17–22

Dilution Techniques

When using the NCCLS agar dilution or broth dilution (including microdilution) method[2] or equivalent, a bacterial isolate may be considered susceptible if the MIC (minimum

Continued on next page

Duricef—Cont.

inhibitory concentration) value for cephalothin is 8 µg/mL or less. Organisms are considered resistant if the MIC is 32 µg/mL or greater. Organisms with an MIC value of less than 32 µg/mL but greater than 8 µg/mL are intermediate.
As with standard diffusion methods, dilution procedures require the use of laboratory control organisms. Standard cephalothin powder should give MIC values in the range of 0.12 µg/mL and 0.5 µg/mL for *Staphylococcus aureus* ATCC 29213. For *Escherichia coli* ATCC 25922, the MIC range should be between 4.0 µg/mL and 16.0 µg/mL. For *Streptococcus faecalis* ATCC 29212, the MIC range should be between 8.0 and 32.0 µg/mL.

INDICATIONS AND USAGE

DURICEF (cefadroxil monohydrate, USP) is indicated for the treatment of patients with infection caused by susceptible strains of the designated organisms in the following diseases:
Urinary tract infections caused by *E. coli, P. mirabilis,* and *Klebsiella* species.
Skin and skin structure infections caused by staphylococci and/or streptococci.
Pharyngitis and/or tonsillitis caused by *Streptococcus pyogenes* (Group A beta-hemolytic streptococci).
Note: Only penicillin by the intramuscular route of administration has been shown to be effective in the prophylaxis of rheumatic fever. DURICEF is generally effective in the eradication of streptococci from the oropharynx. However, data establishing the efficacy of DURICEF for the prophylaxis of subsequent rheumatic fever are not available.
Note: Culture and susceptibility tests should be initiated prior to and during therapy. Renal function studies should be performed when indicated.

CONTRAINDICATIONS

DURICEF (cefadroxil monohydrate, USP) is contraindicated in patients with known allergy to the cephalosporin group of antibiotics.

WARNINGS

BEFORE THERAPY WITH DURICEF IS INSTITUTED, CAREFUL INQUIRY SHOULD BE MADE TO DETERMINE WHETHER THE PATIENT HAS HAD PREVIOUS HYPERSENSITIVITY REACTIONS TO CEFADROXIL, CEPHALOSPORINS, PENICILLINS, OR OTHER DRUGS. IF THIS PRODUCT IS TO BE GIVEN TO PENICILLIN-SENSITIVE PATIENTS, CAUTION SHOULD BE EXERCISED BECAUSE CROSS-SENSITIVITY AMONG BETA-LACTAM ANTIBIOTICS HAS BEEN CLEARLY DOCUMENTED AND MAY OCCUR IN UP TO 10% OF PATIENTS WITH A HISTORY OF PENICILLIN ALLERGY.
IF AN ALLERGIC REACTION TO DURICEF OCCURS, DISCONTINUE THE DRUG. SERIOUS ACUTE HYPERSENSITIVITY REACTIONS MAY REQUIRE TREATMENT WITH EPINEPHRINE AND OTHER EMERGENCY MEASURES, INCLUDING OXYGEN, INTRAVENOUS FLUIDS, INTRAVENOUS ANTIHISTAMINES, CORTICOSTEROIDS, PRESSOR AMINES, AND AIRWAY MANAGEMENT, AS CLINICALLY INDICATED.
Pseudomembranous colitis has been reported with nearly all antibacterial agents, including cefadroxil, and may range from mild to life-threatening. Therefore, it is important to consider this diagnosis in patients who present with diarrhea subsequent to the administration of antibacterial agents.
Treatment with antibacterial agents alters the normal flora of the colon and may permit overgrowth of clostridia. Studies indicate that a toxin produced by *Clostridium difficile* is a primary cause of "antibiotic-associated colitis."
After the diagnosis of pseudomembranous colitis has been established, therapeutic measures should be initiated. Mild cases of pseudomembranous colitis usually respond to discontinuation of the drug alone. In moderate to severe cases, consideration should be given to management with fluids and electrolytes, protein supplementation and treatment with an antibacterial drug effective against *Clostridium difficile.*

PRECAUTIONS

General
DURICEF should be used with caution in the presence of markedly impaired renal function (creatinine clearance rate of less than 50 mL/min/1.73 M^2). (See DOSAGE AND ADMINISTRATION.) In patients with known or suspected renal impairment, careful clinical observation and appropriate laboratory studies should be made prior to and during therapy.
Prolonged use of DURICEF may result in the overgrowth of nonsusceptible organisms. Careful observation of the patient is essential. If superinfection occurs during therapy, appropriate measures should be taken.
DURICEF® (cefadroxil monohydrate, USP) should be prescribed with caution in individuals with history of gastrointestinal disease, particularly colitis.
Drug/Laboratory Test Interactions
Positive direct Coombs' tests have been reported during treatment with the cephalosporin antibiotics. In hematologic studies or in transfusion cross-matching procedures when antiglobulin tests are performed on the minor side or in Coombs' testing of newborns whose mothers have received cephalosporin antibiotics before parturition, it should be recognized that a positive Coombs' test may be due to the drug.

DAILY DOSAGE OF DURICEF® SUSPENSION

Child's Weight				
lbs	kg	125 mg/5 mL	250 mg/5 mL	500 mg/5 mL
10	4.5	1 tsp	—	
20	9.1	2 tsp	1 tsp	
30	13.6	3 tsp	$1\frac{1}{2}$ tsp	
40	18.2	4 tsp	2 tsp	1 tsp
50	22.7	5 tsp	$2\frac{1}{2}$ tsp	$1\frac{1}{4}$ tsp
60	27.3	6 tsp	3 tsp	$1\frac{1}{2}$tsp
70 & above	31.8+	—	—	2 tsp

Reconstitution Directions for Oral Suspension

Bottle Size	Reconstitution Directions
100 mL	Suspend in a total of 67 mL water. Method: Tap bottle lightly to loosen powder. Add 67 mL of water in two portions. Shake well after each addition.
75 mL	Suspend in a total of 51 mL water. Method: Tap bottle lightly to loosen powder. Add 51 mL of water in two portions. Shake well after each addition.
50 mL	Suspend in a total of 34 mL water. Method: Tap bottle lightly to loosen powder. Add 34 mL of water in two portions. Shake well after each addition.

After reconstitution, store in refrigerator. Shake well before using. Keep container tightly closed. Discard unused portion after 14 days.

Creatinine Clearance	Dosage Interval
0–10 mL/min	36 hours
10–25 mL/min	24 hours
25–50 mL/min	12 hours

Carcinogenesis, Mutagenesis, and Impairment of Fertility: No long-term studies have been performed to determine carcinogenic potential. No genetic toxicity tests have been performed.
Pregnancy: Pregnancy Category B: Reproduction studies have been performed in mice and rats at doses up to 11 times the human dose and have revealed no evidence of impaired fertility or harm to the fetus due to cefadroxil monohydrate. There are, however, no adequate and well controlled studies in pregnant women. Because animal reproduction studies are not always predictive of human response, this drug should be used during pregnancy only if clearly needed.
Labor and Delivery: DURICEF (cefadroxil monohydrate, USP) has not been studied for use during labor and delivery. Treatment should only be given if clearly needed.
Nursing Mothers: Caution should be exercised when cefadroxil monohydrate is administered to a nursing mother.
Pediatric Use: (See DOSAGE AND ADMINISTRATION.)

ADVERSE REACTIONS

Gastrointestinal
Onset of pseudomembranous colitis symptoms may occur during or after antibiotic treatment (see WARNINGS). Dyspepsia, nausea and vomiting have been reported rarely. Diarrhea has also occurred.
Hypersensitivity
Allergies (in the form of rash, urticaria, angioedema, and pruritis) have been observed. These reactions usually subsided upon discontinuation of the drug. Anaphylaxis has also been reported.
Other
Other reactions have included hepatic dysfunction including cholestasis and elevations in serum transaminase, genital pruritus, genital moniliasis, vaginitis, moderate transient neutropenia, fever. Agranulocytosis, thrombocytopenia, idiosyncratic hepatic failure, erythema multiforme, Stevens-Johnson syndrome, serum sickness, and arthralgia have been rarely reported.
In addition to the adverse reactions listed above which have been observed in patients treated with cefadroxil, the following adverse reactions and altered laboratory tests have been reported for cephalosporin-class antibiotics:
Toxic epidermal necrolysis, abdominal pain, superinfection, renal dysfunction, toxic nephropathy, aplastic anemia, hemolytic anemia, hemorrhage, prolonged prothrombin time, positive Coombs' test, increased BUN, increased creatinine, elevated alkaline phosphatase, elevated aspartate aminotransferase (AST), elevated alanine aminotransferase (ALT), elevated bilirubin, elevated LDH, eosinophilia, pancytopenia, neutropenia.
Several cephalosporins have been implicated in triggering seizures, particularly in patients with renal impairment, when the dosage was not reduced (see DOSAGE AND ADMINISTRATION and OVERDOSAGE). If seizures associated with drug therapy occur, the drug should be discontinued. Anticonvulsant therapy can be given if clinically indicated.

OVERDOSAGE

A study of children under six years of age suggested that ingestion of less than 250 mg/kg of cephalosporins is not associated with significant outcomes. No action is required other than general support and observation. For amounts greater than 250 mg/kg, induce gastric emptying.
In five anuric patients, it was demonstrated that an average of 63% of a 1 g oral dose is extracted from the body during a 6-8 hour hemodialysis session.

DOSAGE AND ADMINISTRATION

DURICEF is acid-stable and may be administered orally without regard to meals. Administration with food may be helpful in diminishing potential gastrointestinal complaints occasionally associated with oral cephalosporin therapy.
Adults
Urinary Tract Infections: For uncomplicated lower urinary tract infections (i.e., cystitis) the usual dosage is 1 or 2 g per day in single (q.d.) or divided doses (b.i.d.).
For all other urinary tract infections the usual dosage is 2 g per day in divided doses (b.i.d.).
Skin and Skin Structure Infections: For skin and skin structure infections the usual dosage is 1 g per day in single (q.d.) or divided doses (b.i.d.).
Pharyngitis and Tonsillitis: Treatment of group A beta-hemolytic streptococcal pharyngitis and tonsillitis—1 g per day in single (q.d.) or divided doses (b.i.d.) for 10 days.
Children
For urinary tract infections, the recommended daily dosage for children is 30 mg/kg/day in divided doses every 12 hours. For pharyngitis, tonsillitis, and impetigo, the recommended daily dosage for children is 30 mg/kg/day in a single dose or in equally divided doses every 12 hours. For other skin and skin structure infections, the recommended daily dosage is 30 mg/kg/day in equally divided doses every 12 hours. In the treatment of beta-hemolytic streptococcal infections, a therapeutic dosage of DURICEF should be administered for at least 10 days.
See chart for total daily dosage for children.
[See first table above]
In patients with renal impairment, the dosage of cefadroxil monohydrate should be adjusted according to creatinine clearance rates to prevent drug accumulation. The following schedule is suggested. In adults, the initial dose is 1000 mg of DURICEF (cefadroxil monohydrate, USP) and the maintenance dose (based on the creatinine clearance rate [mL/min/1.73 M^2]) is 500 mg at the time intervals listed below.
[See second table above]
Patients with creatinine clearance rates over 50 mL/min may be treated as if they were patients having normal renal function.
[See third table above]

HOW SUPPLIED

DURICEF® (cefadroxil monohydrate, USP) 500 mg Capsules: opaque, maroon and white hard gelatin capsules, imprinted with "PPP" and "784" on one end and with "DURICEF" and "500 mg" on the other end. Capsules are supplied as follows:
NDC 0087-0784-46 Bottle of 50
Store at controlled room temperature (15°-30°C).
DURICEF® 1 gram Tablets: white to off white, top bisected, oval shaped, imprinted with "PPP" on one side of the bisect and "785" on the other side of the bisect. Tablets are supplied as follows:
NDC 0087-0785-43 Bottle of 50
NDC 0087-0785-45 4 packs of 10 individually labeled blisters with 1 tablet per blister
Store at controlled room temperature (15°-30°C).

DURICEF® for Oral Suspension is orange-pineapple flavored, and is supplied as follows:

125 mg/5 mL	**NDC** 0087-0786-41	100 mL Bottle
250 mg/5 mL	**NDC** 0087-0782-41	100 mL Bottle
500 mg/5 mL	**NDC** 0087-0783-05	75 mL Bottle
	NDC 0087-0783-41	100 mL Bottle

Prior to reconstitution: Store at controlled room temperature (15°-30°C).

REFERENCES

1. National Committee for Clinical Laboratory Standards, Approved Standard, *Performance Standards for Antimicrobial Disk Susceptibility Test*, 4th Edition, Vol. 10 (7): M2-A4, Villanova, PA, April, 1990. **2.** National Committee for Clinical Laboratory Standards, Approved Standard: *Methods for Dilution Antimicrobial Susceptibility Tests for Bacteria that Grow Aerobically*, 2nd Edition, Vol. 10 (8): M7-A2, Villanova, PA, April, 1990.

0782DIM-08 Revised February 2000
E3-B001-02-00

Bristol-Myers Squibb Co
Princeton, NJ 08543
USA

Shown in Product Identification Guide, page 309

GLUCOPHAGE® ℞

[*GLUE-coe-fahj*]
(metformin hydrochloride tablets)
500 mg, 850 mg, and 1000 mg
Rx only

DESCRIPTION

GLUCOPHAGE (metformin hydrochloride tablets) is an oral antihyperglycemic drug used in the management of non-insulin-dependent diabetes mellitus (type 2 diabetes). Metformin hydrochloride (N,N-dimethylimidodicarbonimidic diamide hydrochloride) is not chemically or pharmacologically related to the oral sulfonylureas. The structural formula is as shown:

$$\begin{array}{l} H_3C \\ \quad N - C - NH - C - NH_2 \bullet HCl \\ H_3C \quad \| \qquad\quad \| \\ \qquad NH \qquad NH \end{array}$$

Metformin hydrochloride is a white to off-white crystalline compound with a molecular formula of $C_4H_{11}N_5 \bullet HCl$ and a molecular weight of 165.63. Metformin hydrochloride is freely soluble in water and is practically insoluble in acetone, ether and chloroform. The pK_a of metformin is 12.4. The pH of a 1% aqueous solution of metformin hydrochloride is 6.68.

GLUCOPHAGE tablets contain 500 mg, 850 mg, and 1000 mg of metformin hydrochloride. Each tablet contains the active ingredients povidone and magnesium stearate. In addition, the coating for the 500 mg and 850 mg contains hydroxypropyl methylcellulose (hypromellose) and the coating for the 1000 mg contains hydroxypropyl methylcellulose and polyethylene glycol.

CLINICAL PHARMACOLOGY

Antidiabetic Activity

GLUCOPHAGE is an antihyperglycemic agent which improves glucose tolerance in type 2 diabetes subjects, lowering both basal and postprandial plasma glucose. Its pharmacologic mechanisms of action are different from those of sulfonylureas. GLUCOPHAGE decreases hepatic glucose production, decreases intestinal absorption of glucose and improves insulin sensitivity (increases peripheral glucose uptake and utilization). Unlike sulfonylureas, GLUCOPHAGE does not produce hypoglycemia in either diabetic or nondiabetic subjects (except in special circumstances, see PRECAUTIONS) and does not cause hyperinsulinemia. With metformin therapy, insulin secretion remains unchanged while fasting insulin levels and day-long plasma insulin response may actually decrease.

In a double-blind, placebo-controlled, multicenter U.S. clinical trial involving obese type 2 diabetes patients whose hyperglycemia was not adequately controlled with dietary management alone (baseline fasting plasma glucose [FPG] of approximately 240 mg/dL), treatment with GLUCOPHAGE (up to 2.55 g/day) for 29 weeks resulted in significant mean net reductions in fasting and postprandial plasma glucose (PPG) and HbA_{1c} of 59 mg/dL, 83 mg/dL, and 1.8%, respectively, compared to placebo group (see Table 1).

[See table 1 above]

Table 1. GLUCOPHAGE vs Placebo
Summary of Mean Changes from Baseline* in Plasma Glucose HbA_{1c} and Body Weight, at Final Visit (29-week study)

	GLUCOPHAGE (n = 141)	Placebo (n = 145)	P-Value
FPG (mg/dL)			
Baseline	241.5	237.7	NS
Change at FINAL VISIT	–53.0	6.3	0.001**
Hemoglobin A_{1c} (%)			
Baseline	8.4	8.2	NS
Change at FINAL VISIT	–1.4	0.4	0.001**
Body Weight (lbs)			
Baseline	201.0	206.0	NS
Change at FINAL VISIT	–1.4	–2.4	NS

* All patients on diet therapy at Baseline
** Statistically significant

Monotherapy with GLUCOPHAGE may be effective in patients who have not responded to sulfonylureas or who have only a partial response to sulfonylureas or who have ceased to respond to sulfonylureas. In such patients, if adequate glycemic control is not attained with GLUCOPHAGE monotherapy, the combination of GLUCOPHAGE and a sulfonylurea may have a synergistic effect, since both agents act to improve glucose tolerance by different but complementary mechanisms.

A 29-week, double-blind, placebo-controlled study of GLUCOPHAGE and glyburide, alone and in combination, was conducted in obese type 2 diabetes patients who had failed to achieve adequate glycemic control while on maximum doses of glyburide (baseline FPG of approximately 250 mg/dL) (see Table 2). Patients randomized to continue on glyburide experienced worsening of glycemic control, with mean increases in FPG, PPG and HbA_{1c} of 14 mg/dL, 3 mg/dL and 0.2%, respectively. In contrast, those randomized to GLUCOPHAGE (metformin hydrochloride tablets) (up to 2.5 g/day) did not experience a deterioration in glycemic control, but rather a slight improvement, with mean reductions in FPG, PPG and HbA_{1c} of 1 mg/dL, 6 mg/dL and 0.4%, respectively. The combination of GLUCOPHAGE and glyburide was synergistic in reducing FPG, PPG and HbA_{1c} levels by 63 mg/dL, 65 mg/dL, and 1.7%, respectively. Compared to results of glyburide treatment alone, the net differences with combination treatment were –77 mg/dL, –68 mg/dL and –1.9%, respectively (see Table 2).

[See table 2 above]

Table 2. Combined GLUCOPHAGE/Glyburide (Comb) vs Glyburide (Glyb) or Glucophage (GLU) Monotherapy: Summary of Mean Changes from Baseline* in Plasma Glucose, HbA_{1c} and Body Weight, at Final Visit (29-week study)

	Comb (n = 213)	Glyb (n = 209)	GLU (n = 210)	P-values Glyb vs Comb	GLU vs Comb	GLU vs Glyb
Fasting Plasma Glucose (mg/dL)						
Baseline	250.5	247.5	253.9	NS	NS	NS
Change at FINAL VISIT	–63.5	13.7	–0.9	0.001**	0.001**	0.025**
Hemoglobin A_{1c} (%)						
Baseline	8.8	8.5	8.9	NS	NS	0.007**
Change at FINAL VISIT	–1.7	0.2	–0.4	0.001**	0.001**	0.001**
Body Weight (lbs)						
Baseline	202.2	203.0	204.0	NS	NS	NS
Change at FINAL VISIT	0.9	–0.7	–8.4	0.011**	0.001**	0.001**

* All patients on glyburide, 20 mg/day, at Baseline
** Statistically significant

The magnitude of the decline in fasting blood glucose concentration following the institution of GLUCOPHAGE (metformin hydrochloride tablets) therapy is proportional to the level of fasting hyperglycemia. Non-insulin-dependent diabetics with higher fasting glucose concentrations will experience greater declines in plasma glucose and glycosylated hemoglobin.

GLUCOPHAGE has a modest favorable effect on serum lipids, which are often abnormal in type 2 diabetes patients. In clinical studies, particularly when baseline levels were abnormally elevated, GLUCOPHAGE, alone or in combination with a sulfonylurea, lowered mean fasting serum triglycerides, total cholesterol and LDL cholesterol levels and had no adverse effects on other lipid levels (see Table 3).

[See table 3 above]

Table 3. Summary of Mean Percent Reduction of Major Serum Lipid Variables at Final Visit (29-week study)

	Glucophage vs. Placebo (% Change from Baseline)		Combined Glucophage/Glyburide vs. Monotherapy (% Change from Baseline)		
	Glucophage (n = 141)	Placebo (n = 145)	Glucophage (n = 210)	Glucophage/ Glyburide (n = 213)	Glyburide (n = 209)
Total Cholesterol	–5%*	1%	–2%	–4%**	1%
Total Triglycerides	–16%	1%	–3%**	–8%**	4%
LDL-Cholesterol	–8%*	1%	–4%**	–6%**	3%
HDL-Cholesterol	2%	–1%	5%	3%	1%

* $P < 0.05$ vs. Placebo
** $P < 0.05$ vs. Glyburide

In contrast to sulfonylureas, body weight of individuals on GLUCOPHAGE tends to remain stable or may even decrease somewhat (see Tables 1 and 2).

A 24 week, double-blind, placebo-controlled study of GLUCOPHAGE and insulin vs insulin plus placebo was conducted in type 2 diabetic patients who failed to achieve adequate glycemic control on insulin alone (see Table 4). Patients randomized to receive GLUCOPHAGE and insulin achieved a reduction in the HbA_{1c} of 2.10%, compared to a 1.56% reduction in HbA_{1c} achieved by insulin and placebo. The improvement in glycemic control was achieved at the final study visit with 16% less insulin, 93.0 U/day vs 110.6 U/day, GLUCOPHAGE and insulin vs insulin and placebo, respectively, p=0.04. Eighty-one percent of patients had an HbA_{1c} value below 8% with GLUCOPHAGE compared with 50% in the placebo group.

[See table 4 on next page]

A second double-blind placebo-controlled study (n=51), with 16 weeks of randomized treatment, demonstrated that in type 2 diabetic patients controlled on insulin for 8 weeks with an average HbA_{1c} of 7.46 ± 0.97%, the addition of metformin maintained equivalent glycemic control (HbA_{1c} 7.15 ± 0.61 vs 6.97 ± 0.62 for metformin and placebo, respectively) with 19% less insulin vs baseline (reduction of 23.68 ± 30.22 vs an increase of 0.43 ± 25.20 units for metformin and placebo, p<0.01). In addition, this study demonstrated that the combination of metformin and insulin resulted in a reduction in body weight of 3.11 ± 4.30 lbs, compared to an increase of 1.30 ± 6.08 lbs for placebo, p=0.01.

In summary, metformin-treated patients showed significant improvement in all parameters of glycemic control (FPG, PPG and HbA_{1c}), stabilization or decrease in body weight, and a tendency to improvement in the lipid profile, particularly when baseline values are abnormally elevated.

Pharmacokinetics

Absorption and Bioavailability

The absolute bioavailability of a 500 mg metformin hydrochloride tablet given under fasting conditions is approximately 50–60%. Studies using single oral doses of metformin tablets of 500 mg and 1500 mg, and 850 mg to 2550 mg, indicate that there is a lack of dose proportionality with increasing doses, which is due to decreased absorption rather than an alteration in elimination. Food decreases the extent and slightly delays the absorption of metformin, as

Continued on next page

Glucophage—Cont.

shown by approximately a 40% lower peak concentration and 25% lower AUC in plasma and a 35 minute prolongation of time to peak plasma concentration following administration of a single 850 mg tablet of metformin with food, compared to the same tablet strength administered fasting. The clinical relevance of these decreases is unknown.

Distribution

The apparent volume of distribution (V/F) of metformin following single oral doses of 850 mg averaged 654 ± 358 L. Metformin is negligibly bound to plasma proteins in contrast to sulfonylureas which are more than 90% protein bound. Metformin partitions into erythrocytes, most likely as a function of time. At usual clinical doses and dosing schedules of GLUCOPHAGE (metformin hydrochloride tablets), steady state plasma concentrations of metformin are reached within 24–48 hours and are generally < 1 µg/mL. During controlled clinical trials, maximum metformin plasma levels did not exceed 5 µg/mL, even at maximum doses.

Metabolism and Elimination

Intravenous single-dose studies in normal subjects demonstrate that metformin is excreted unchanged in the urine and does not undergo hepatic metabolism (no metabolites have been identified in humans) nor biliary excretion. Renal clearance (see Table 5) is approximately 3.5 times greater than creatinine clearance which indicates that tubular secretion is the major route of metformin elimination. Following oral administration, approximately 90% of the absorbed drug is eliminated via the renal route within the first 24 hours, with a plasma elimination half-life of approximately 6.2 hours. In blood, the elimination half-life is approximately 17.6 hours, suggesting that the erythrocyte mass may be a compartment of distribution.

Special Populations

Type 2 Diabetes Subjects

In the presence of normal renal function, there are no differences between single or multiple dose pharmacokinetics of metformin between diabetics and nondiabetics (see Table 5), nor is there any accumulation of metformin in either group at usual clinical doses.

Renal Insufficiency

In subjects with decreased renal function (based on measured creatinine clearance), the plasma and blood half-life of metformin is prolonged and the renal clearance is decreased in proportion to the decrease in creatinine clearance (see Table 5).

Hepatic Insufficiency

No pharmacokinetic studies have been conducted in subjects with hepatic insufficiency.

Geriatrics

Limited data from controlled pharmacokinetic studies of metformin in healthy elderly subjects suggest that total plasma clearance is decreased, the half-life is prolonged and C_{max} is increased, compared to healthy young subjects. From these data, it appears that the change in metformin pharmacokinetics with aging is primarily accounted for by a change in renal function (see Table 5).

[See table 5 below]

Pediatrics

No pharmacokinetic studies have been conducted in pediatric subjects.

Gender

Metformin pharmacokinetic parameters did not differ significantly in diabetic and nondiabetic subjects when analyzed according to gender (males = 19, females = 16). Similarly, in controlled clinical studies in patients with type 2 diabetes, the antihyperglycemic effect of GLUCOPHAGE (metformin hydrochloride tablets) was comparable in males and females.

Race

No studies of metformin pharmacokinetic parameters according to race have been performed. In controlled clinical studies of GLUCOPHAGE in patients with type 2 diabetes, the antihyperglycemic effect was comparable in whites (n = 249), blacks (n = 51) and hispanics (n = 24).

INDICATIONS AND USE

GLUCOPHAGE (metformin hydrochloride tablets), as monotherapy, is indicated as an adjunct to diet to lower blood glucose in patients with type 2 diabetes whose hyperglycemia cannot be satisfactorily managed on diet alone.

GLUCOPHAGE may be used concomitantly with a sulfonylurea or insulin to improve glycemic control.

In initiating treatment for type 2 diabetes, diet should be emphasized as the primary form of treatment.

Caloric restriction and weight loss are essential in the obese diabetic patient. Proper dietary management alone may be effective in controlling the blood glucose and symptoms of hyperglycemia. Loss of blood glucose control in diet-managed patients may be transient, thus requiring only short-term pharmacologic therapy. The importance of regular physical activity should also be stressed, and cardiovascular risk factors should be identified and corrective measures taken where possible. If this treatment program fails to reduce symptoms and/or blood glucose, the use of GLUCOPHAGE alone or GLUCOPHAGE plus a sulfonylurea should be considered.

If, after a suitable trial of such treatments, glucose control still has not been achieved, consideration should be given to the use of insulin. Judgments should be based on regular clinical and laboratory evaluations.

Table 4. Combined GLUCOPHAGE/Insulin vs Insulin Summary of Mean Changes from Baseline in HbA_{1c} and Daily Insulin Dose

	GLUCOPHAGE	Placebo	Treatment difference Mean ± SE
N	26	28	
Hemoglobin A_{1c} (%)			
Baseline	8.95	9.32	
Change at FINAL VISIT	−2.10	−1.56	0.54 ± 0.43[a]
Insulin Dose (U/day)			
Baseline	93.12	94.64	
Change at FINAL VISIT	−0.15	+15.93	−16.08 ± 7.77[b]

[a] Statistically significant using analysis of covariance with baseline as covariate (P=0.04)
Not significant using analysis of variance (values shown in table)
[b] Statistically significant for insulin (P=0.04)

Table 5. Select Mean (± S.D.) Metformin Pharmacokinetic Parameters Following Single or Multiple Oral Doses of GLUCOPHAGE

Subject Groups: GLUCOPHAGE dose[a] (number of subjects)	C_{max}[b] (µg/mL)	t_{max}[c] (hrs)	Renal Clearance (mL/min)
Healthy, nondiabetic adults:			
500 mg SD[d] (24)	1.03 (± 0.33)	2.75 (± 0.81)	600 (± 132)
850 mg SD (74)[e]	1.60 (± 0.38)	2.64 (± 0.82)	552 (± 139)
850 mg t.i.d. for 19 doses[f] (9)	2.01 (± 0.42)	1.79 (± 0.94)	642 (± 173)
Adults with type 2 diabetes:			
850 mg SD (23)	1.48 (± 0.5)	3.32 (±1.08)	491 (± 138)
850 mg t.i.d. for 19 doses[f] (9)	1.90 (±0.62)	2.01 (± 1.22)	550 (± 160)
Elderly[g], healthy nondiabetic adults:			
850 mg SD (12)	2.45 (± 0.70)	2.71 (± 1.05)	412 (± 98)
Renal-impaired adults: 850 mg SD			
Mild (CL_{cr}[h] 61–90 mL/min) (5)	1.86 (± 0.52)	3.20 (± 0.45)	384 (± 122)
Moderate (CL_{cr} 31–60 mL/min) (4)	4.12 (± 1.83)	3.75 (± 0.50)	108 (± 57)
Severe (CL_{cr} 10–30 mL/min) (6)	3.93 (± 0.92)	4.01 (± 1.10)	130 (± 90)

[a]–All doses given fasting except the first 18 doses of the multiple dose studies;
[b]–Peak plasma concentration;
[c]–Time to peak plasma concentration;
[d]–SD = single dose;
[e]–Combined results (average means) of five studies: mean age 32 years (range 23–59 yrs).
[f]–Kinetic study done following dose 19, given fasting.
[g]–Elderly subjects, mean age 71 years (range 65–81 years).
[h]–CL_{cr} = creatinine clearance normalized to body surface area of 1.73 m^2.

CONTRAINDICATIONS

GLUCOPHAGE is contraindicated in patients with:

1. Renal disease or renal dysfunction (e.g., as suggested by serum creatinine levels ≥ 1.5 mg/dL [males], ≥ 1.4 mg/dL [females] or abnormal creatinine clearance) which may also result from conditions such as cardiovascular collapse (shock), acute myocardial infarction, and septicemia (see WARNINGS and PRECAUTIONS).
2. Congestive heart failure requiring pharmacologic treatment.
3. GLUCOPHAGE should be temporarily discontinued in patients undergoing radiologic studies involving intravascular administration of iodinated contrast materials, because use of such products may result in acute alteration of renal function. (See also PRECAUTIONS).
4. Known hypersensitivity to metformin hydrochloride.
5. Acute or chronic metabolic acidosis, including diabetic ketoacidosis, with or without coma. Diabetic ketoacidosis should be treated with insulin.

WARNINGS

Lactic acidosis:

Lactic acidosis is a rare, but serious, metabolic complication that can occur due to metformin accumulation during treatment with GLUCOPHAGE; when it occurs, it is fatal in approximately 50% of cases. Lactic acidosis may also occur in association with a number of pathophysiologic conditions, including diabetes mellitus, and whenever there is significant tissue hypoperfusion and hypoxemia. Lactic acidosis is characterized by elevated blood lactate levels (>5 mmol/L), decreased blood pH, electrolyte disturbances with an increased anion gap, and an increased lactate/pyruvate ratio. When metformin is implicated as the cause of lactic acidosis, metformin plasma levels > 5 µg/mL are generally found.

The reported incidence of lactic acidosis in patients receiving metformin hydrochloride is very low (approximately 0.03 cases/1000 patient-years, with approximately 0.015 fatal cases/1000 patient-years). Reported cases have occurred primarily in diabetic patients with significant renal insufficiency, including both intrinsic renal disease and renal hypoperfusion, often in the setting of multiple concomitant medical/surgical problems and multiple concomitant medications. Patients with congestive heart failure requiring pharmacologic management, in particular those with unstable or acute congestive heart failure who are at risk of hypoperfusion and hypoxemia are at increased risk of lactic acidosis. The risk of lactic acidosis increases with the degree of renal dysfunction and the patient's age. The risk of lactic acidosis may, therefore, be significantly decreased by regular monitoring of renal function in patients taking GLUCOPHAGE and by use of the minimum effective dose of GLUCOPHAGE. In particular, treatment of the elderly should be accompanied by careful monitoring of renal function. GLUCOPHAGE treatment should not be initiated in patients ≥ 80 years of age unless measurement of creatinine clearance demonstrates that renal function is not reduced, as these patients are more susceptible to developing lactic acidosis. In addition, GLUCOPHAGE should be promptly withheld in the presence of any condition associated with hypoxemia, dehydration or sepsis. Because impaired hepatic function may significantly limit the ability to clear lactate, GLUCOPHAGE should generally be avoided in patients with clinical or laboratory evidence of hepatic disease. Patients should be cautioned against excessive alcohol intake, either acute or chronic, when taking GLUCOPHAGE (metformin hydrochloride tablets), since alcohol potentiates the effects of metformin hydrochloride on lactate metabolism. In addition, GLUCOPHAGE should be temporarily discontinued prior to any intravascular radiocontrast study and for any surgical procedure (see also PRECAUTIONS).

The onset of lactic acidosis often is subtle, and accompanied only by nonspecific symptoms such as malaise, myalgias, respiratory distress, increasing somnolence and nonspecific abdominal distress. There may be associated hypothermia, hypotension and resistant bradyarrhythmias with more marked acidosis. The patient and the patient's physician must be aware of the possible importance of such symptoms and the patient should be instructed to notify the physician immediately if they occur (see also PRECAUTIONS). GLUCOPHAGE (metformin hydrochloride tablets) should be withdrawn until the situation is clarified. Serum electrolytes, ketones, blood glucose and, if indicated, blood pH, lactate levels and even blood metformin levels may be useful. Once a patient is stabilized on any dose level of GLUCOPHAGE, gastrointestinal symptoms, which are common during initiation of therapy, are unlikely to be drug related. Later occurrence of gastrointestinal symptoms could be due to lactic acidosis or other serious disease.

Levels of fasting venous plasma lactate above the upper limit of normal but less than 5 mmol/L in patients taking GLUCOPHAGE do not necessarily indicate impending lactic acidosis and may be explainable by other mechanisms, such as poorly controlled diabetes or obesity, vigorous physical activity or technical problems in sample handling. (See also PRECAUTIONS.)

Lactic acidosis should be suspected in any diabetic patient with metabolic acidosis lacking evidence of ketoacidosis (ketonuria and ketonemia).
Lactic acidosis is a medical emergency that must be treated in a hospital setting. In a patient with lactic acidosis who is taking GLUCOPHAGE, the drug should be discontinued immediately and general supportive measures promptly instituted. Because metformin hydrochloride is dialyzable (with a clearance of up to 170 mL/min under good hemodynamic conditions), prompt hemodialysis is recommended to correct the acidosis and remove the accumulated metformin. Such management often results in prompt reversal of symptoms and recovery. (See also CONTRAINDICATIONS and PRECAUTIONS).

PRECAUTIONS

General

Monitoring of renal function—GLUCOPHAGE is known to be substantially excreted by the kidney, and the risk of metformin accumulation and lactic acidosis increases with the degree of impairment of renal function. Thus, patients with serum creatinine levels above the upper limit of normal for their age should not receive GLUCOPHAGE. In patients with advanced age, GLUCOPHAGE should be carefully titrated to establish the minimum dose for adequate glycemic effect, because aging is associated with reduced renal function. In elderly patients, renal function should be monitored regularly and, generally, GLUCOPHAGE should not be titrated to the maximum dose (see DOSAGE AND ADMINISTRATION). For patients ≥ 80 years of age, see WARNINGS. Before initiation of GLUCOPHAGE therapy and at least annually thereafter, renal function should be assessed and verified as normal. In patients in whom development of renal dysfunction is anticipated, renal function should be assessed more frequently and GLUCOPHAGE discontinued if evidence of renal impairment is present.

Use of concomitant medications that may affect renal function or metformin disposition—Concomitant medication(s) that may affect renal function or result in significant hemodynamic change or may interfere with the disposition of GLUCOPHAGE, such as cationic drugs that are eliminated by renal tubular secretion (See Drug Interactions), should be used with caution.

Radiologic studies involving the use of intravascular iodinated contrast materials (for example, intravenous urogram, intravenous cholangiography, angiography, and computed tomography (CT) scans with contrast materials)—Intravascular contrast studies with iodinated materials can lead to acute alteration of renal function and have been associated with lactic acidosis in patients receiving GLUCOPHAGE (see CONTRAINDICATIONS). Therefore, in patients in whom any such study is planned, GLUCOPHAGE should be discontinued at the time of or prior to the procedure, and withheld for 48 hours subsequent to the procedure and reinstituted only after renal function has been re-evaluated and found to be normal.

Hypoxic states—Cardiovascular collapse (shock) from whatever cause, acute congestive heart failure, acute myocardial infarction and other conditions characterized by hypoxemia have been associated with lactic acidosis and may also cause prerenal azotemia. When such events occur in patients on GLUCOPHAGE therapy, the drug should be promptly discontinued.

Surgical procedures—GLUCOPHAGE therapy should be temporarily suspended for any surgical procedure (except minor procedures not associated with restricted intake of food and fluids) and should not be restarted until the patient's oral intake has resumed and renal function has been evaluated as normal.

Alcohol intake—Alcohol is known to potentiate the effect of metformin on lactate metabolism. Patients, therefore, should be warned against excessive alcohol intake, acute or chronic, while recieving GLUCOPHAGE.

Impaired hepatic function—Since impaired hepatic function has been associated with some cases of lactic acidosis, GLUCOPHAGE should generally be avoided in patients with clinical or laboratory evidence of hepatic disease.

Vitamin B_{12} levels—A decrease to subnormal levels of previously normal serum vitamin B_{12} levels, without clinical manifestations, is observed in approximately 7% of patients receiving GLUCOPHAGE in controlled clinical trials of 29 weeks duration. Such decrease, possibly due to interference with B_{12} absorption from the B_{12}-intrinsic factor complex, is, however, very rarely associated with anemia and appears to be rapidly reversible with discontinuation of GLUCOPHAGE (metformin hydrochloride tablets) or vitamin B_{12} supplementation. Measurement of hematologic parameters on an annual basis is advised in patients on GLUCOPHAGE and any apparent abnormalities should be appropriately investigated and managed (see Laboratory Tests).

Certain individuals (those with inadequate vitamin B_{12} or calcium intake or absorption) appear to be predisposed to developing subnormal vitamin B_{12} levels. In these patients, routine serum vitamin B_{12} measurements at two- to three-year intervals may be useful.

Change in clinical status of previously controlled diabetic—A diabetic patient previously well controlled on GLUCOPHAGE (metformin hydrochloride tablets) who develops laboratory abnormalities or clinical illness (especially vague and poorly defined illness) should be evaluated promptly for evidence of ketoacidosis or lactic acidosis. Evaluation should include serum electrolytes and ketones, blood glucose and, if indicated, blood pH, lactate, pyruvate and metformin levels. If acidosis of either form occurs, GLUCOPHAGE must be stopped immediately and other appropriate corrective measures initiated (see also WARNINGS).

Hypoglycemia—Hypoglycemia does not occur in patients receiving GLUCOPHAGE alone under usual circumstances of use, but could occur when caloric intake is deficient, when strenuous exercise is not compensated by caloric supplementation, or during concomitant use with other glucose-lowering agents (such as sulfonylureas or insulin) or ethanol.

Elderly, debilitated or malnourished patients, and those with adrenal or pituitary insufficiency or alcohol intoxication are particularly susceptible to hypoglycemic effects. Hypoglycemia may be difficult to recognize in the elderly, and in people who are taking beta-adrenergic blocking drugs.

Loss of control of blood glucose—When a patient stabilized on any diabetic regimen is exposed to stress such as fever, trauma, infection, or surgery, a temporary loss of glycemic control may occur. At such times, it may be necessary to withhold GLUCOPHAGE and temporarily administer insulin. GLUCOPHAGE may be reinstituted after the acute episode is resolved.

The effectiveness of oral antidiabetic drugs in lowering blood glucose to a targeted level decreases in many patients over a period of time. This phenomenon, which may be due to progression of the underlying disease or to diminished responsiveness to the drug, is known as secondary failure, to distinguish it from primary failure in which the drug is ineffective during initial therapy. Should secondary failure occur with GLUCOPHAGE or sulfonylurea monotherapy, combined therapy with GLUCOPHAGE and sulfonylurea may result in a response. Should secondary failure occur with combined GLUCOPHAGE/sulfonylurea therapy, it may be necessary to initiate insulin therapy.

Information for Patients

Patients should be informed of the potential risks and advantages of GLUCOPHAGE and of alternative modes of therapy. They should also be informed about the importance of adherence to dietary instructions, of a regular exercise program, and of regular testing of blood glucose, glycosylated hemoglobin, renal function and hematologic parameters.

The risks of lactic acidosis, its symptoms, and conditions that predispose to its development, as noted in the WARNINGS and PRECAUTIONS sections should be explained to patients. Patients should be advised to discontinue GLUCOPHAGE immediately and to promptly notify their health practitioner if unexplained hyperventilation, myalgia, malaise, unusual somnolence or other nonspecific symptoms occur. Once a patient is stabilized on any dose level of GLUCOPHAGE, gastrointestinal symptoms, which are common during initiation of therapy, are unlikely to be drug related. Later occurrence of gastrointestinal symptoms could be due to lactic acidosis or other serious disease.

Patients should be counselled against excessive alcohol intake, either acute or chronic, while receiving GLUCOPHAGE.

GLUCOPHAGE alone does not usually cause hypoglycemia, although it may occur when GLUCOPHAGE is used in conjunction with oral sulfonylureas and insulin. When initiating combination therapy, the risks of hypoglycemia, its symptoms and treatment, and conditions that predispose to its development should be explained to patients.

(See Patient Labeling Printed Below)

Laboratory Tests

Response to all diabetic therapies should be monitored by periodic measurements of fasting blood glucose and glycosylated hemoglobin levels, with a goal of decreasing these levels toward the normal range. During initial dose titration, fasting glucose can be used to determine the therapeutic response. Thereafter, both glucose and glycosylated hemoglobin should be monitored. Measurements of glycosylated hemoglobin may be especially useful for evaluating long-term control (see also DOSAGE AND ADMINISTRATION).

Initial and periodic monitoring of hematologic parameters (e.g., hemoglobin/hematocrit and red blood cell indices) and renal function (serum creatinine) should be performed, at least on an annual basis. While megaloblastic anemia has rarely been seen with GLUCOPHAGE therapy, if this is suspected, vitamin B_{12} deficiency should be excluded.

Drug Interactions

Glyburide: In a single-dose interaction study in type 2 diabetes subjects, co-administration of metformin and glyburide did not result in any changes in either metformin pharmacokinetics or pharmacodynamics. Decreases in glyburide AUC and C_{max} were observed, but were highly variable. The single-dose nature of this study and the lack of correlation between glyburide blood levels and pharmacodynamic effects, makes the clinical significance of this interaction uncertain (see DOSAGE AND ADMINISTRATION: Concomitant GLUCOPHAGE and Oral Sulfonylurea Therapy).

Furosemide: A single-dose, metformin-furosemide drug interaction study in healthy subjects demonstrated that pharmacokinetic parameters of both compounds were affected by co-administration. Furosemide increased the metformin plasma and blood C_{max} by 22% and blood AUC by 15%, without any significant change in metformin renal clearance. When administered with metformin, the C_{max} and AUC of furosemide were 31% and 12% smaller, respectively, than when administered alone, and the terminal half-life was decreased by 32%, without any significant change in furosemide renal clearance. No information is available about the interaction of metformin and furosemide when co-administered chronically.

Nifedipine: A single-dose, metformin-nifedipine drug interaction study in normal healthy volunteers demonstrated that co-administration of nifedipine increased plasma metformin C_{max} and AUC by 20% and 9%, respectively, and increased the amount excreted in the urine. T_{max} and half-life were unaffected. Nifedipine appears to enhance the absorption of metformin. Metformin had minimal effects on nifedipine.

Cationic Drugs: Cationic drugs (e.g., amiloride, digoxin, morphine, procainamide, quinidine, quinine, ranitidine, triamterene, trimethoprim, and vancomycin) that are eliminated by renal tubular secretion theoretically have the potential for interaction with metformin by competing for common renal tubular transport systems. Such interaction between metformin and oral cimetidine has been observed in normal healthy volunteers in both single- and multiple-dose, metformin-cimetidine drug interaction studies, with a 60% increase in peak metformin plasma and whole blood concentrations and a 40% increase in plasma and whole blood metformin AUC. There was no change in elimination half-life in the single-dose study. Metformin had no effect on cimetidine pharmacokinetics. Although such interactions remain theoretical (except for cimetidine), careful patient monitoring and dose adjustment of GLUCOPHAGE and/or the interfering drug is recommended in patients who are taking cationic medications that are excreted via the proximal renal tubular secretory system.

Other: Certain drugs tend to produce hyperglycemia and may lead to loss of glycemic control. These drugs include thiazide and other diuretics, corticosteroids, phenothiazines, thyroid products, estrogens, oral contraceptives, phenytoin, nicotinic acid, sympathomimetics, calcium channel blocking drugs, and isoniazid. When such drugs are administered to a patient receiving GLUCOPHAGE, the patient should be closely observed to maintain adequate glycemic control.

In healthy volunteers, the pharmacokinetics of metformin and propranolol and metformin and Ibuprofen were not affected when co-administered in single-dose interaction studies.

Metformin is negligibly bound to plasma proteins and is, therefore, less likely to interact with highly protein-bound drugs such as salicylates, sulfonamides, chloramphenicol, and probenecid, as compared to the sulfonylureas, which are extensively bound to serum proteins.

Carcinogenesis, Mutagenesis, Impairment of Fertility

Long-term carcinogenicity studies have been performed in rats (dosing duration of 104 weeks) and mice (dosing duration of 91 weeks) at doses up to and including 900 mg/kg/day and 1500 mg/kg/day, respectively. These doses are both approximately three times the maximum recommended human daily dose on a body surface area basis. No evidence of carcinogenicity with metformin was found in either male or female mice. Similarly, there was no tumorigenic potential observed with metformin in male rats. However, an increased incidence of benign stromal uterine polyps was seen in female rats treated with 900 mg/kg/day.

No evidence of a mutagenic potential of metformin was found in the Ames test (*S. typhimurium*), gene mutation test (mouse lymphoma cells), chromosomal aberrations test (human lymphocytes), or *in vivo* micronuclei formation test (mouse bone marrow).

Fertility of male or female rats was unaffected by metformin administration at doses as high as 600 mg/kg/day, or approximately two times the maximum recommended human daily dose on a body surface area basis.

Pregnancy

Teratogenic Effects

Pregnancy Category B. Safety in pregnant women has not been established. Metformin was not teratogenic in rats and rabbits at doses up to 600 mg/kg/day, or about two times the maximum recommended human daily dose on a body surface area basis. Determination of fetal concentrations demonstrated a partial placental barrier to metformin. Because animal reproduction studies are not always predictive of human response, any decision to use this drug should be balanced against the benefits and risks.

Because recent information suggests that abnormal blood glucose levels during pregnancy are associated with a higher incidence of congenital abnormalities, there is a consensus among experts that insulin be used during pregnancy to maintain blood glucose levels as close to normal as possible.

Nursing Mothers

Studies in lactating rats show that metformin is excreted into milk and reaches levels comparable to those in plasma. Similar studies have not been conducted in nursing mothers, but caution should be exercised in such patients, and a decision should be made whether to discontinue nursing or to discontinue the drug, taking into account the importance of the drug to the mother.

Pediatric Use

Safety and effectiveness in pediatric patients have not been established. Studies in maturity-onset diabetes of the young (MODY) have not been conducted.

Geriatric Use

Controlled clinical studies of GLUCOPHAGE (metformin hydrochloride tablets) did not include sufficient numbers of

Continued on next page

Glucophage—Cont.

elderly patients to determine whether they respond differently from younger patients, although other reported clinical experience has not identified differences in responses between the elderly and younger patients. GLUCOPHAGE is known to be substantially excreted by the kidney and because the risk of serious adverse reactions to the drug is greater in patients with impaired renal function, it should only be used in patients with normal renal function (see CONTRAINDICATIONS, CLINICAL PHARMACOLOGY: Pharmacokinetics). Because aging is associated with reduced renal function, GLUCOPHAGE should be used with caution as age increases. Care should be taken in dose selection and should be based on careful and regular monitoring of renal function. Generally, elderly patients should not be titrated to the maximum dose of GLUCOPHAGE (see also WARNINGS and DOSAGE AND ADMINISTRATION).

ADVERSE REACTIONS

Lactic Acidosis: See WARNINGS, PRECAUTIONS and OVERDOSAGE Sections.

Gastrointestinal Reactions: Gastrointestinal symptoms (diarrhea, nausea, vomiting, abdominal bloating, flatulence, and anorexia) are the most common reactions to GLUCOPHAGE and are approximately 30% more frequent in patients on monotherapy than in placebo-treated patients, particularly during initiation of GLUCOPHAGE therapy. These symptoms are generally transient and resolve spontaneously during continued treatment. Occasionally, temporary dose reduction may be useful. In controlled trials, GLUCOPHAGE was discontinued due to gastrointestinal reactions in approximately 4% of patients.

Because gastrointestinal symptoms during therapy initiation appear to be dose-related, they may be decreased by gradual dose escalation and by having patients take GLUCOPHAGE with meals (see DOSAGE AND ADMINISTRATION).

Because significant diarrhea and/or vomiting may cause dehydration and prerenal azotemia, under such circumstances, GLUCOPHAGE should be temporarily discontinued.

For patients who have been stabilized on GLUCOPHAGE, nonspecific gastrointestinal symptoms should not be attributed to therapy unless intercurrent illness or lactic acidosis have been excluded.

Special Senses: During initiation of GLUCOPHAGE therapy, approximately 3% of patients may complain of an unpleasant or metallic taste, which usually resolves spontaneously.

Dermatologic Reactions: The incidence of rash/dermatitis in controlled clinical trials was comparable to placebo for GLUCOPHAGE monotherapy and to sulfonylurea for GLUCOPHAGE/sulfonylurea therapy.

Hematologic: (See also PRECAUTIONS). During controlled clinical trials of 29 weeks duration, approximately 9% of patients on GLUCOPHAGE monotherapy and 6% of patients on GLUCOPHAGE/sulfonylurea therapy developed asymptomatic subnormal serum vitamin B_{12} levels; serum folic acid levels did not decrease significantly. However, only five cases of megaloblastic anemia have been reported with metformin administration (none during U.S. clinical studies) and no increased incidence of neuropathy has been observed. Therefore, serum B_{12} levels should be appropriately monitored or periodic parenteral B_{12} supplementation considered.

DRUG ABUSE AND DEPENDENCE

GLUCOPHAGE possesses no pharmacodynamic properties, either primary or secondary, which could be expected to result in abuse as a recreational drug or addiction.

OVERDOSAGE

Hypoglycemia has not been seen with ingestion of up to 85 grams of GLUCOPHAGE, although lactic acidosis has occurred in such circumstances (see WARNINGS). Metformin is dialyzable with a clearance of up to 170 mL/min under good hemodynamic conditions. Therefore, hemodialysis may be useful for removal of accumulated drug from patients in whom metformin overdosage is suspected.

DOSAGE AND ADMINISTRATION

There is no fixed dosage regimen for the management of hyperglycemia in diabetes mellitus with GLUCOPHAGE or any other pharmacologic agent. Dosage of GLUCOPHAGE must be individualized on the basis of both effectiveness and tolerance, while not exceeding the maximum recommended daily dose of 2550 mg. GLUCOPHAGE should be given in divided doses with meals and should be started at a low dose, with gradual dose escalation, as described below, both to reduce gastrointestinal side effects and to permit identification of the minimum dose required for adequate glycemic control of the patient.

During treatment initiation and dose titration (see Recommended Dosing Schedule), fasting plasma glucose should be used to determine the therapeutic response to GLUCOPHAGE and identify the minimum effective dose for the patient. Thereafter, glycosylated hemoglobin should be measured at intervals of approximately three months. **The therapeutic goal should be to decrease both fasting plasma glucose and glycosylated hemoglobin levels to normal or near normal by using the lowest effective dose of GLUCOPHAGE (metformin hydrochloride tablets), either when used as monotherapy or in combination with sulfonylurea or insulin.**

Monitoring of blood glucose and glycosylated hemoglobin will also permit detection of primary failure, i.e., inadequate lowering of blood glucose at the maximum recommended dose of medication, and secondary failure, i.e., loss of an adequate blood glucose lowering response after an initial period of effectiveness.

Short-term administration of GLUCOPHAGE may be sufficient during periods of transient loss of control in patients usually well-controlled on diet alone.

Recommended Dosing Schedule

In general, clinically significant responses are not seen at doses below 1500 mg per day. However, a lower recommended starting dose and gradually increased dosage is advised to minimize gastrointestinal symptoms.

The usual starting dose of GLUCOPHAGE is 500 mg twice a day or 850 mg once a day, given with meals. Dosage increases should be made in increments of 500 mg weekly or 850 mg every 2 weeks, up to a total of 2000 mg per day, given in divided doses. Patients can also be titrated from 500 mg twice a day to 850 mg twice a day after 2 weeks. For those patients requiring additional glycemic control, GLUCOPHAGE may be given to a maximum daily dose of 2550 mg per day. Doses above 2000 mg may be better tolerated given three times a day with meals.

Transfer from Other Antidiabetic Therapy

When transferring patients from standard oral hypoglycemic agents other than chlorpropamide to GLUCOPHAGE, no transition period generally is necessary. When transferring patients from chlorpropamide, care should be exercised during the first two weeks because of the prolonged retention of chlorpropamide in the body, leading to overlapping drug effects and possible hypoglycemia.

Concomitant GLUCOPHAGE and Oral Sulfonylurea Therapy

If patients have not responded to four weeks of the maximum dose of GLUCOPHAGE monotherapy, consideration should be given to gradual addition of an oral sulfonylurea while continuing GLUCOPHAGE at the maximum dose, even if prior primary or secondary failure to a sulfonylurea has occurred. Clinical and pharmacokinetic drug-drug interaction data are currently available only for metformin plus glyburide (glibenclamide). Published clinical information exists for the use of metformin with either chlorpropamide, tolbutamide or glipizide. No published clinical information exists regarding concomitant use of metformin with acetohexamide or tolazamide.

With concomitant GLUCOPHAGE and sulfonylurea therapy, the desired control of blood glucose may be obtained by adjusting the dose of each drug. However, attempts should be made to identify the minimum effective dose of each drug to achieve this goal. With concomitant GLUCOPHAGE and sulfonylurea therapy, the risk of hypoglycemia associated with sulfonylurea therapy continues and may be increased. Appropriate precautions should be taken. (See Package Insert of the respective sulfonylurea).

If patients have not satisfactorily responded to one to three months of concomitant therapy with the maximum dose of GLUCOPHAGE and the maximum dose of an oral sulfonylurea, institution of insulin therapy and discontinuation of these oral agents should be considered.

Concomitant GLUCOPHAGE and Insulin Therapy

The current insulin dose should be continued upon initiation of GLUCOPHAGE therapy. GLUCOPHAGE therapy should be initiated at 500 mg once daily in patients on insulin therapy. For patients not responding adequately, the dose of GLUCOPHAGE should be increased by 500 mg after approximately 1 week and by 500 mg every week thereafter until adequate glycemic control is achieved. The maximum recommended daily dose is 2500 mg. (See Recommended Dosing Schedule; GLUCOPHAGE 500 mg Tablets.) It is recommended that the insulin dose be decreased by 10% to 25% when fasting plasma glucose concentrations decrease to less than 120 mg/dL in patients receiving concomitant insulin and GLUCOPHAGE. Further adjustment should be individualized based on glucose-lowering response.

Specific Patient Populations

GLUCOPHAGE is not recommended for use in pregnancy or for use in pediatric patients.

The initial and maintenance dosing of GLUCOPHAGE should be conservative in patients with advanced age, due to the potential for decreased renal function in this population. Any dosage adjustment should be based on a careful assessment of renal function. Generally, elderly patients should not be titrated to the maximum dose of GLUCOPHAGE.

Monitoring of renal function is necessary to aid in prevention of lactic acidosis, particularly in the elderly. (see WARNINGS.)

In debilitated or malnourished patients, the dosing should also be conservative and based on a careful assessment of renal function.

HOW SUPPLIED

GLUCOPHAGE® (metformin hydrochloride tablets)
[See table below]

GLUCOPHAGE 500 mg tablets are round, white to off-white, film coated tablets debossed with BMS 6060 around the periphery of the tablet on one side and 500 debossed across the face of the other side.

GLUCOPHAGE 850 mg tablets are round, white to off-white, film coated tablets debossed with BMS 6070 around the periphery of the tablet on one side and 850 debossed across the face of the other side.

GLUCOPHAGE 1000 mg tablets are white, oval, biconvex, film coated tablets with BMS 6071 debossed on one side and 1000 debossed on the opposite side and with a bisect line on both sides.

Storage

Store between 15°–30° C (59°–86° F).
Dispense in light resistant container.

PATIENT INFORMATION ABOUT GLUCOPHAGE® (metformin hydrochloride tablets)

WARNING: A small number of people who have taken Glucophage have developed a serious condition called lactic acidosis. Properly functioning kidneys are needed to help prevent lactic acidosis. Most people with kidney problems should not take Glucophage. (See Question Nos. 10–14).

Q1. Why do I need to take GLUCOPHAGE?

Your doctor has prescribed GLUCOPHAGE (GLUE-coe-fahj) to treat your type 2 diabetes. This is also known as non-insulin-dependent diabetes mellitus.

Q2. What is type 2 diabetes?

People with diabetes are not able to make enough insulin and/or respond normally to the insulin their body does make. When this happens, sugar (glucose) builds up in the blood. This can lead to serious medical problems including kidney damage, amputations and blindness. Diabetes is also closely linked to heart disease. The main goal of treating diabetes is to lower your blood sugar to a normal level.

Q3. Why is it important to control type 2 diabetes?

Studies have shown that good control of blood sugar can prevent or delay complications such as blindness.

Q4. How is type 2 diabetes usually controlled?

High blood sugar can be lowered by diet and exercise, by a number of oral medications and by insulin injections. Before taking GLUCOPHAGE you should first try to control your diabetes by exercise and weight loss. Even if you are taking GLUCOPHAGE, you should still exercise and follow the diet recommended for your diabetes.

Q5. Does GLUCOPHAGE work differently from other glucose-control medications?

Yes it does. Until GLUCOPHAGE (metformin hydrochloride tablets) was introduced, all the available oral glucose-control medications were from the same chemical group called sulfonylureas. These drugs lower blood sugar primarily by causing more of the body's own insulin to be released. GLUCOPHAGE lowers the amount of sugar in your blood by helping your body respond better to its own insulin. GLUCOPHAGE (metformin hydrochloride tablets) does not cause your body to produce more insulin. Therefore, GLUCOPHAGE rarely causes hypoglycemia (low blood sugar) and it doesn't usually cause weight gain.

Q6. What happens if my blood sugar is still too high?

When blood sugar cannot be lowered enough by either GLUCOPHAGE (metformin hydrochloride tablets) or a sulfonylurea, the two medications may be effective taken together. However, if you are unable to maintain your blood sugar with diet, exercise and glucose-control medication taken orally, then your doctor may prescribe injectable insulin to control your diabetes.

Q7. Why would I take GLUCOPHAGE if I am already on insulin?

Because adding GLUCOPHAGE to insulin can help you better control your blood sugar while reducing the insulin dose and possibly reducing your weight.

Q8. Can GLUCOPHAGE cause side effects?

GLUCOPHAGE, like all blood-sugar lowering medications, can cause side effects in some patients. Most of these side effects are minor and will go away after you've taken GLUCOPHAGE for a while. However, there are also serious, but rare side effects related to GLUCOPHAGE (see below).

Q9. What kind of side effects can GLUCOPHAGE cause?

If side effects occur, they usually occur during the first few weeks of therapy. They are normally minor ones such as diarrhea, nausea and upset stomach. Taking your GLUCOPHAGE with meals can help reduce these side effects. Although these side effects are likely to go away, call your doctor if you have severe discomfort or if these effects last for more than a few weeks. Some patients may need to have their dose lowered or stop taking GLUCOPHAGE, either temporarily or permanently. Although these problems occur in up to one-third of patients when they first start taking GLUCOPHAGE, you should tell your doctor if the problems come back or start later on during the therapy.

About three out of one hundred people report having a temporary unpleasant or metallic taste when they start taking GLUCOPHAGE.

500 mg	Bottles of 100	NDC 0087-6060-05
500 mg	Bottles of 500	NDC 0087-6060-10
850 mg	Bottles of 100	NDC 0087-6070-05
850 mg	Bottles of 300	NDC 0087-6070-10
1000 mg	Bottles of 100	NDC 0087-6071-11
1000 mg	Bottles of 500	NDC 0087-6071-12

Q10. Are there any serious side effects that GLUCOPHAGE can cause?
GLUCOPHAGE rarely causes serious side effects. The most serious side effect that GLUCOPHAGE can cause is called lactic acidosis.
Q11. What is lactic acidosis and can it happen to me?
Lactic acidosis is caused by a buildup of lactic acid in the blood. Lactic acidosis associated with GLUCOPHAGE is rare and has occurred mostly in people whose kidneys were not working normally. Lactic acidosis has been reported in about one in 33,000 patients taking GLUCOPHAGE over the course of a year. Although rare, if lactic acidosis does occur, it can be fatal in up to half the cases.
It's also important for your liver to be working normally when you take GLUCOPHAGE. Your liver helps remove lactic acid from your bloodstream.
Your doctor will monitor your diabetes and may perform blood tests on you from time to time to make sure your kidneys and your liver are functioning normally.
There is no evidence that GLUCOPHAGE causes harm to the kidneys or liver.
Q12. Are there other risk factors for lactic acidosis?
Your risk of developing lactic acidosis from taking GLUCOPHAGE is very low as long as your kidneys and liver are healthy. However, some factors can increase your risk because they can affect kidney and liver function. You should discuss your risk with your physician. You should not take GLUCOPHAGE if:
- You have chronic kidney or liver problems
- You have congestive heart failure which is treated with medications, e.g., digoxin (Lanoxin®) or furosemide (Lasix®)
- You drink alcohol excessively (all the time or short-term "binge" drinking)
- You are seriously dehydrated (have lost a large amount of body fluids)
- You are going to have certain x-ray procedures with injectable contrast agents
- You are going to have surgery
- You develop a serious condition such as a heart attack, severe infection, or a stroke
- You are ≥ 80 years of age and have NOT had your kidney function tested.

Q13. What are the symptoms of lactic acidosis?
Some of the symptoms include: feeling very weak, tired or uncomfortable; unusual muscle pain, trouble breathing, unusual or unexpected stomach discomfort, feeling cold, feeling dizzy or lightheaded, or suddenly developing a slow or irregular heartbeat.
If you notice these symptoms, or if your medical condition has suddenly changed, stop taking GLUCOPHAGE and call your doctor right away. Lactic acidosis is a medical emergency that must be treated in a hospital.
Q14. What does my doctor need to know to decrease my risk of lactic acidosis?
Tell your doctor if you have an illness that results in severe vomiting, diarrhea and/or fever, or if your intake of fluids is generally reduced. These situations can lead to severe dehydration, and it may be necessary to stop taking GLUCOPHAGE temporarily.
You should let your doctor know if you are going to have any surgery or specialized x-ray procedures that require injection of contrast agents. GLUCOPHAGE therapy will need to be stopped temporarily in such instances.
Q15. Can I take GLUCOPHAGE with other medications?
Remind your doctor that you are taking GLUCOPHAGE when any new drug is prescribed or a change is made in how you take a drug already prescribed. GLUCOPHAGE may interfere with the way some drugs work and some drugs may interfere with the action of GLUCOPHAGE.
Q16. What if I become pregnant while taking GLUCOPHAGE?
Tell your doctor if you plan to become pregnant or have become pregnant. As with other oral glucose-control medications, you should not take GLUCOPHAGE during pregnancy.
Usually your doctor will prescribe insulin while you are pregnant. As with all medications, you and your doctor should discuss the use of GLUCOPHAGE if you are nursing a child.
Q17. How do I take GLUCOPHAGE?
Your doctor will tell you how many GLUCOPHAGE tablets to take and how often. This should also be printed on the label of your prescription. You will probably be started on a low dose of GLUCOPHAGE and your dosage will be increased gradually until your blood sugar is controlled.
Q18. Where can I get more information about GLUCOPHAGE?
This leaflet is a summary of the most important information about GLUCOPHAGE. If you have any questions or problems, you should talk to your doctor or other healthcare provider about type 2 diabetes as well as GLUCOPHAGE and its side effects. There is also a leaflet (package insert) written for health professionals that your pharmacist can let you read.
GLUCOPHAGE® is a registered trademark of LIPHA s.a. Licensed to Bristol-Myers Squibb Company.
Revised December 1999 6060DIM-08
F5-B001R-12-99

Bristol-Myers Squibb Co
Distributed by:
Bristol-Myers Squibb Company
Princeton, NJ 08543 USA
Shown in Product Identification Guide, page 309

GLUCOVANCE™
(Glyburide and Metformin HCl Tablets)

(Please consult the MANUFACTURERS' INDEX or the BRAND AND GENERIC NAME INDEX for product page number)

MONOPRIL® ℞
[mŏnō-prĭll]
Fosinopril Sodium
Tablets
Rx only

USE IN PREGNANCY
When used in pregnancy during the second and third trimesters, ACE inhibitors can cause injury and even death to the developing fetus. When pregnancy is detected, MONOPRIL should be discontinued as soon as possible. **See WARNINGS: Fetal/Neonatal Morbidity and Mortality.**

DESCRIPTION
MONOPRIL (fosinopril sodium tablets) is the sodium salt of fosinopril, the ester prodrug of an angiotensin converting enzyme (ACE) inhibitor, fosinoprilat. It contains a phosphinate group capable of specific binding to the active site of angiotensin converting enzyme. Fosinopril sodium is designated chemically as: L-proline, 4-cyclohexyl-1-[[[2-methyl-1-(1-oxopropoxy) propoxy] (4-phenylbutyl) phosphinyl] acetyl]-, sodium salt, *trans*-.
Fosinopril sodium is a white to off-white crystalline powder. It is soluble in water (100 mg/mL), methanol, and ethanol and slightly soluble in hexane.
Its empirical formula is $C_{30}H_{45}NNaO_7P$, and its molecular weight is 585.65.
MONOPRIL is available for oral administration as 10 mg, 20 mg, and 40 mg tablets. Inactive ingredients include: lactose, microcrystalline cellulose, crospovidone, povidone, and sodium stearyl fumarate.

CLINICAL PHARMACOLOGY
Mechanism of Action
In animals and humans, fosinopril sodium is hydrolyzed by esterases to the pharmacologically active form, fosinoprilat, a specific competitive inhibitor of angiotensin converting enzyme (ACE).
ACE is a peptidyl dipeptidase that catalyzes the conversion of angiotensin I to the vasoconstrictor substance, angiotensin II. Angiotensin II also stimulates aldosterone secretion by the adrenal cortex. Inhibition of ACE results in decreased plasma angiotensin II, which leads to decreased vasopressor activity and to decreased aldosterone secretion. The latter decrease may result in a small increase of serum potassium.
In 647 hypertensive patients treated with fosinopril alone for an average of 29 weeks, mean increases in serum potassium of 0.1 mEq/L were observed. Similar increases were observed among all patients treated with fosinopril, including those receiving concomitant diuretic therapy. Removal of angiotensin II negative feedback on renin secretion leads to increased plasma renin activity.
ACE is identical to kininase, an enzyme that degrades bradykinin. Whether increased levels of bradykinin, a potent vasodepressor peptide, play a role in the therapeutic effects of MONOPRIL remains to be elucidated.
While the mechanism through which MONOPRIL lowers blood pressure is believed to be primarily suppression of the renin-angiotensin-aldosterone system, MONOPRIL has an antihypertensive effect even in patients with low-renin hypertension. Although MONOPRIL was antihypertensive in all races studied, black hypertensive patients (usually a low-renin hypertensive population) had a smaller average response to ACE inhibitor monotherapy than non-black patients.
In patients with heart failure, the beneficial effects of MONOPRIL are thought to result primarily from suppression of the renin-angiotensin-aldosterone system; inhibition of the angiotensin converting enzyme produces decreases in both preload and afterload.
Pharmacokinetics and Metabolism
Following oral administration, fosinopril (the prodrug) is absorbed slowly. The absolute absorption of fosinopril averaged 36% of an oral dose. The primary site of absorption is the proximal small intestine (duodenum/jejunum). While the rate of absorption may be slowed by the presence of food in the gastrointestinal tract, the extent of absorption of fosinopril is essentially unaffected.
Fosinoprilat is highly protein-bound (approximately 99.4%), has a relatively small volume of distribution, and has negligible binding to cellular components in blood. After single and multiple oral doses, plasma levels, areas under plasma concentration-time curves (AUCs) and peak concentrations (Cmaxs) are directly proportional to the dose of fosinopril. Times to peak concentrations are independent of dose and are achieved in approximately 3 hours.
After an oral dose of radiolabeled fosinopril, 75% of radioactivity in plasma was present as active fosinoprilat, 20–30% as a glucuronide conjugate of fosinoprilat, and 1–5% as a *p*-hydroxy metabolite of fosinoprilat. Since fosinoprilat is not biotransformed after intravenous administration, fosinopril, not fosinoprilat, appears to be the precursor for the glucuronide and *p*-hydroxy metabolites. In rats, the p-hydroxy metabolite of fosinoprilat is as potent an inhibitor of ACE as fosinoprilat; the glucuronide conjugate is devoid of ACE inhibitory activity.
After intravenous administration, fosinoprilat was eliminated approximately equally by the liver and kidney. After oral administration of radiolabeled fosinopril, approximately half of the absorbed dose is excreted in the urine and the remainder is excreted in the feces. In two studies involving healthy subjects, the mean body clearance of intravenous fosinoprilat was between 26 and 39 mL/min.
In healthy subjects, the terminal elimination half-life (t1/2) of an intravenous dose of radiolabeled fosinoprilat is approximately 12 hours. In hypertensive patients with normal renal and hepatic function, who received repeated doses of fosinopril, the effective t1/2 for accumulation of fosinoprilat averaged 11.5 hours. In patients with heart failure, the effective t1/2 was 14 hours.
In patients with mild-to-severe renal insufficiency (creatinine clearance 10–80 mL/min/1.73m^2), the clearance of fosinoprilat does not differ appreciably from normal, because of the large contribution of hepatobiliary elimination. In patients with end-stage renal disease (creatinine clearance < 10 mL/min/1.73m^2), the total body clearance of fosinoprilat is approximately one-half of that in patients with normal renal function. (See **DOSAGE AND ADMINISTRATION**.)
Fosinopril is not well dialyzed. Clearance of fosinoprilat by hemodialysis and peritoneal dialysis averages 2% and 7%, respectively, of urea clearances.
In patients with hepatic insufficiency (alcoholic or biliary cirrhosis), the extent of hydrolysis of fosinopril is not appreciably reduced, although the rate of hydrolysis may be slowed; the apparent total body clearance of fosinoprilat is approximately one-half of that in patients with normal hepatic function.
In elderly (male) subjects (65–74 years old) with clinically normal renal and hepatic function, there appear to be no significant differences in pharmacokinetic parameters for fosinoprilat compared to those of younger subjects (20–35 years old).
Fosinoprilat was found to cross the placenta of pregnant animals.
Studies in animals indicate that fosinopril and fosinoprilat do not cross the blood-brain barrier.
Pharmacodynamics and Clinical Effects
Serum ACE activity was inhibited by ≥90% at 2 to 12 hours after single doses of 10 to 40 mg of fosinopril. At 24 hours, serum ACE activity remained suppressed by 85%, 93%, and 93% in the 10, 20, and 40 mg dose groups, respectively.
Hypertension
Administration of MONOPRIL (fosinopril sodium tablets) to patients with mild-to-moderate hypertension results in a reduction of both supine and standing blood pressure to about the same extent with no compensatory tachycardia. Symptomatic postural hypotension is infrequent, although it can occur in patients who are salt- and/or volume-depleted (see **WARNINGS**). Use of MONOPRIL in combination with thiazide diuretics gives a blood pressure-lowering effect greater than that seen with either agent alone.
Following oral administration of single doses of 10–40 mg, MONOPRIL lowered blood pressure within one hour, with peak reductions achieved 2–6 hours after dosing. The antihypertensive effect of a single dose persisted for 24 hours. Following four weeks of monotherapy in placebo-controlled trials in patients with mild-to-moderate hypertension, once-daily doses of 20–80 mg lowered supine or seated systolic and diastolic blood pressures 24 hours after dosing by an average of 8–9/6–7 mmHg more than placebo. The trough effect was about 50–60% of the peak diastolic response and about 80% of the peak systolic response.
In most trials, the antihypertensive effect of MONOPRIL increased during the first several weeks of repeated measurements. The antihypertensive effect of MONOPRIL has been shown to continue during long-term therapy for at least 2 years. Abrupt withdrawal of MONOPRIL has not resulted in a rapid increase in blood pressure.
Limited experience in controlled and uncontrolled trials combining fosinopril with a calcium channel blocker or a loop diuretic has indicated no unusual drug-drug interactions. Other ACE inhibitors have had less than additive effects with beta-adrenergic blockers, presumably because both drugs lower blood pressure by inhibiting parts of the renin-angiotensin system.
ACE inhibitors are generally less effective in blacks than in non-blacks. The effectiveness of MONOPRIL was not influenced by age, sex, or weight.
In hemodynamic studies in hypertensive patients, after three months of therapy, responses (changes in BP, heart rate, cardiac index, and PVR) to various stimuli (e.g., isometric exercise, 45° head-up tilt, and mental challenge) were unchanged compared to baseline, suggesting that MONOPRIL does not affect the activity of the sympathetic nervous system. Reduction in systemic blood pressure appears to have been mediated by a decrease in peripheral vascular resistance without reflex cardiac effects. Similarly, renal, splanchnic, cerebral, and skeletal muscle blood flow were unchanged compared to baseline, as was glomerular filtration rate.
Heart Failure
In a randomized, double-blind, placebo-controlled trial, 179 patients with heart failure, all receiving diuretics and some

Continued on next page

Monopril—Cont.

receiving digoxin, were administered single doses of 1, 20, or 40 mg of MONOPRIL or placebo. Doses of 20 and 40 mg of MONOPRIL resulted in acute decreases in pulmonary capillary wedge pressure (preload) and mean arterial blood pressure and systemic vascular resistance (afterload). One hundred fifty-five of these patients were re-randomized to once-daily therapy with MONOPRIL (1, 20, or 40 mg) for an additional 10 weeks. Hemodynamic measurements made 24 hours after dosing showed (relative to baseline) continued reduction in pulmonary capillary wedge pressure, mean arterial blood pressure, right atrial pressure and an increase in cardiac index and stroke volume for the 20 and 40 mg dose groups. No tachyphylaxis was seen.

MONOPRIL was studied in 3 double-blind, placebo-controlled, 12–24 week trials including a total of 734 patients with heart failure, with MONOPRIL doses from 10 to 40 mg daily. Concomitant therapy in 2 of these 3 trials included diuretics and digitalis; in the third trial patients were receiving only diuretics. All 3 trials showed statistically significant benefits of MONOPRIL therapy, compared to placebo, in one or more of the following: exercise tolerance (one study), symptoms of dyspnea, orthopnea and paroxysmal nocturnal dyspnea (2 studies), NYHA classification (2 studies), hospitalization for heart failure (2 studies), study withdrawals for worsening heart failure (2 studies), and/or need for supplemental diuretics (2 studies). Favorable effects were maintained for up to two years. Effects of MONOPRIL on long-term mortality in heart failure have not been evaluated. The once-daily dosage for the treatment of congestive heart failure was the only dosage regimen used during clinical trial development and was determined by the measurement of hemodynamic responses.

INDICATIONS AND USAGE

MONOPRIL is indicated for the treatment of hypertension. It may be used alone or in combination with thiazide diuretics.

MONOPRIL is indicated in the management of heart failure as adjunctive therapy when added to conventional therapy including diuretics with or without digitalis (see **DOSAGE AND ADMINISTRATION**).

In using MONOPRIL (consideration should be given to the fact that another angiotensin converting enzyme inhibitor, captopril, has caused agranulocytosis, particularly in patients with renal impairment or collagen-vascular disease. Available data are insufficient to show that MONOPRIL (fosinopril sodium tablets) does not have a similar risk (see **WARNINGS**).

In considering use of MONOPRIL, it should be noted that in controlled trials ACE inhibitors have an effect on blood pressure that is less in black patients than in non-blacks. In addition, ACE inhibitors (for which adequate data are available) cause a higher rate of angioedema in black than in non-black patients (see **WARNINGS: Angioedema**).

CONTRAINDICATIONS

MONOPRIL (fosinopril sodium tablets) is contraindicated in patients who are hypersensitive to this product or to any other angiotensin converting enzyme inhibitor (e.g., a patient who has experienced angioedema with any other ACE inhibitor therapy).

WARNINGS

Anaphylactoid and Possibly Related Reactions

Presumably because angiotensin-converting enzyme inhibitors affect the metabolism of eicosanoids and polypeptides, including endogenous bradykinin, patients receiving ACE inhibitors (including MONOPRIL) may be subject to a variety of adverse reactions, some of them serious.

Angioedema: Angioedema involving the extremities, face, lips, mucous membranes, tongue, glottis or larynx has been reported in patients treated with ACE inhibitors. If angioedema involves the tongue, glottis or larynx, airway obstruction may occur and be fatal. If laryngeal stridor or angioedema of the face, lips, mucous membranes, tongue, glottis or extremities occurs, treatment with MONOPRIL should be discontinued and appropriate therapy instituted immediately. **Where there is involvement of the tongue, glottis, or larynx, likely to cause airway obstruction, appropriate therapy, e.g., subcutaneous epinephrine solution 1:1000 (0.3 mL to 0.5 mL) should be promptly administered** (see **PRECAUTIONS: Information for Patients** and **ADVERSE REACTIONS**).

Anaphylactoid reactions during desensitization: Two patients undergoing desensitizing treatment with hymenoptera venom while receiving ACE inhibitors sustained life-threatening anaphylactoid reactions. In the same patients, these reactions were avoided when ACE inhibitors were temporarily withheld, but they reappeared upon inadvertent rechallenge.

Anaphylactoid reactions during membrane exposure: Anaphylactoid reactions have been reported in patients dialyzed with high-flux membranes and treated concomitantly with an ACE inhibitor. Anaphylactoid reactions have also been reported in patients undergoing low-density lipoprotein apheresis with dextran sulfate absorption.

Hypotension

MONOPRIL can cause symptomatic hypotension. Like other ACE inhibitors, fosinopril has been only rarely associated with hypotension in uncomplicated hypertensive patients. Symptomatic hypotension is most likely to occur in patients who have been volume- and/or salt-depleted as a result of prolonged diuretic therapy, dietary salt restriction, dialysis, diarrhea, or vomiting. Volume and/or salt depletion should be corrected before initiating therapy with MONOPRIL.

In patients with heart failure, with or without associated renal insufficiency, ACE inhibitor therapy may cause excessive hypotension, which may be associated with oliguria or azotemia and, rarely, with acute renal failure and death. In such patients, MONOPRIL therapy should be started under close medical supervision; they should be followed closely for the first 2 weeks of treatment and whenever the dose of fosinopril or diuretic is increased. Consideration should be given to reducing the diuretic dose in patients with normal or low blood pressure who have been treated vigorously with diuretics or who are hyponatremic.

If hypotension occurs, the patient should be placed in a supine position, and, if necessary, treated with intravenous infusion of physiological saline. MONOPRIL treatment usually can be continued following restoration of blood pressure and volume.

Neutropenia/Agranulocytosis

Another angiotensin converting enzyme inhibitor, captopril, has been shown to cause agranulocytosis and bone marrow depression, rarely in uncomplicated patients, but more frequently in patients with renal impairment, especially if they also have a collagen-vascular disease such as systemic lupus erythematosus or scleroderma. Available data from clinical trials of fosinopril are insufficient to show that fosinopril does not cause agranulocytosis at similar rates. Monitoring of white blood cell counts should be considered in patients with collagen-vascular disease, especially if the disease is associated with impaired renal function.

Fetal/Neonatal Morbidity and Mortality

ACE inhibitors can cause fetal and neonatal morbidity and death when administered to pregnant women. Several dozen cases have been reported in the world literature. When pregnancy is detected, ACE inhibitors should be discontinued as soon as possible.

The use of ACE inhibitors during the second and third trimesters of pregnancy has been associated with fetal and neonatal injury, including hypotension, neonatal skull hypoplasia, anuria, reversible or irreversible renal failure, and death. Oligohydramnios has also been reported, presumably resulting from decreased fetal renal function; oligohydramnios in this setting has been associated with fetal limb contractures, craniofacial deformation, and hypoplastic lung development. Prematurity, intrauterine growth retardation, and patent ductus arteriosus have also been reported, although it is not clear whether these occurrences were due to the ACE-inhibitor exposure.

These adverse effects do not appear to have resulted from intrauterine ACE-inhibitor exposure that has been limited to the first trimester. Mothers whose embryos and fetuses are exposed to ACE inhibitors only during the first trimester should be so informed. Nonetheless, when patients become pregnant, physicians should make every effort to discontinue the use of fosinopril as soon as possible.

Rarely (probably less often than once in every thousand pregnancies), no alternative to ACE inhibitors will be found. In these rare cases, the mothers should be apprised of the potential hazards to their fetuses, and serial ultrasound examinations should be performed to assess the intraamniotic environment.

If oligohydramnios is observed, fosinopril should be discontinued unless it is considered life-saving for the mother. Contraction stress testing (CST), a non-stress test (NST), or biophysical profiling (BPP) may be appropriate, depending upon the week of pregnancy. Patients and physicians should be aware, however, that oligohydramnios may not appear until after the fetus has sustained irreversible injury.

Infants with histories of *in utero* exposure to ACE inhibitors should be closely observed for hypotension, oliguria, and hyperkalemia. If oliguria occurs, attention should be directed toward support of blood pressure and renal perfusion. Exchange transfusion or dialysis may be required as a means of reversing hypotension and/or substituting for disordered renal function. Fosinopril is poorly dialyzed from the circulation of adults by hemodialysis and peritoneal dialysis. There is no experience with any procedure for removing fosinopril from the neonatal circulation.

When fosinopril was given to pregnant rats at doses about 80 to 250 times (on a mg/kg basis) the maximum recommended human dose, three similar orofacial malformations and one fetus with *situs inversus* were observed among the offspring. No teratogenic effects of fosinopril were seen in studies in pregnant rabbits at doses up to 25 times (on a mg/kg basis) the maximum recommended human dose.

Hepatic Failure

Rarely, ACE Inhibitors have been associated with a syndrome that starts with cholestatic jaundice and progresses to fulminant hepatic necrosis and (sometimes) death. The mechanism of this syndrome is not understood. Patients receiving ACE inhibitors who develop jaundice or marked elevations of hepatic enzymes should discontinue the ACE inhibitor and receive appropriate medical follow-up.

PRECAUTIONS

General

Impaired Renal Function: As a consequence of inhibiting the renin-angiotensin-aldosterone system, changes in renal function may be anticipated in susceptible individuals. In patients with severe congestive heart failure whose renal function may depend on the activity of the renin-angiotensin-aldosterone system, treatment with angiotensin converting enzyme inhibitors, including MONOPRIL (fosinopril sodium tablets), may be associated with oliguria and/or progressive azotemia and (rarely) with acute renal failure and/or death.

In hypertensive patients with renal artery stenosis in a solitary kidney or bilateral renal artery stenosis, increases in blood urea nitrogen and serum creatinine may occur. Experience with another angiotensin converting enzyme inhibitor suggests that these increases are usually reversible upon discontinuation of ACE inhibitor and/or diuretic therapy. In such patients, renal function should be monitored during the first few weeks of therapy. Some hypertensive patients with no apparent pre-existing renal vascular disease have developed increases in blood urea nitrogen and serum creatinine, usually minor and transient, especially when MONOPRIL has been given concomitantly with a diuretic. This is more likely to occur in patients with pre-existing renal impairment. Dosage reduction of MONOPRIL and/or discontinuation of the diuretic may be required.

Evaluation of patients with hypertension or heart failure should always include assessment of renal function (see DOSAGE AND ADMINISTRATION).

Impaired renal function decreases total clearance of fosinoprilat and approximately doubles AUC. In general, no adjustment of dosing is needed. However, patients with heart failure and severely reduced renal function may be more sensitive to the hemodynamic effects (e.g. hypotension) of ACE inhibition (see **CLINICAL PHARMACOLOGY**).

Hyperkalemia: In clinical trials, hyperkalemia (serum potassium greater than 10% above the upper limit of normal) has occurred in approximately 2.6% of hypertensive patients receiving MONOPRIL (fosinopril sodium tablets). In most cases, these were isolated values which resolved despite continued therapy. In clinical trials, 0.1% of patients (two patients) were discontinued from therapy due to an elevated serum potassium. Risk factors for the development of hyperkalemia include renal insufficiency, diabetes mellitus, and the concomitant use of potassium-sparing diuretics, potassium supplements, and/or potassium-containing salt substitutes, which should be used cautiously, if at all, with MONOPRIL (see **PRECAUTIONS: Drug Interactions**).

Cough: Presumably due to the inhibition of the degradation of endogenous bradykinin, persistent nonproductive cough has been reported with all ACE inhibitors, always resolving after discontinuation of therapy. ACE inhibitor-induced cough should be considered in the differential diagnosis of cough.

Impaired Liver Function: Since fosinopril is primarily metabolized by hepatic and gut wall esterases to its active moiety, fosinoprilat, patients with impaired liver function could develop elevated plasma levels of unchanged fosinopril. In a study in patients with alcoholic or biliary cirrhosis, the extent of hydrolysis was unaffected, although the rate was slowed. In these patients, the apparent total body clearance of fosinoprilat was decreased and the plasma AUC approximately doubled.

Surgery/Anesthesia: In patients undergoing surgery or during anesthesia with agents that produce hypotension, fosinopril will block the angiotensin II formation that could otherwise occur secondary to compensatory renin release. Hypotension that occurs as a result of this mechanism can be corrected by volume expansion.

Hemodialysis

Recent clinical observations have shown an association of hypersensitivity-like (anaphylactoid) reactions during hemodialysis with high-flux dialysis membranes (e.g., AN69) in patients receiving ACE inhibitors as medication. In these patients, consideration should be given to using a different type of dialysis membrane or a different class of medication. (See **WARNINGS: Anaphylactoid reactions during membrane exposure.**)

Information for Patients

Angioedema: Angioedema, including laryngeal edema, can occur with treatment with ACE inhibitors, especially following the first dose. Patients should be advised to immediately report to their physician any signs or symptoms suggesting angioedema (e.g., swelling of face, eyes, lips, tongue, larynx, mucous membranes, and extremities; difficulty in swallowing or breathing; hoarseness) and to discontinue therapy. (See **WARNINGS: Angioedema** and **ADVERSE REACTIONS**.)

Symptomatic Hypotension: Patients should be cautioned that lightheadedness can occur, especially during the first days of therapy, and it should be reported to a physician. Patients should be told that if syncope occurs, MONOPRIL (fosinopril sodium tablets) should be discontinued until the physician has been consulted.

All patients should be cautioned that inadequate fluid intake or excessive perspiration, diarrhea, or vomiting can lead to an excessive fall in blood pressure, with the same consequences of lightheadedness and possible syncope.

Hyperkalemia: Patients should be told not to use potassium supplements or salt substitutes containing potassium without consulting the physician.

Neutropenia: Patients should be told to promptly report any indication of infection (e.g., sore throat, fever), which could be a sign of neutropenia.

Pregnancy: Female patients of childbearing age should be told about the consequences of second- and third-trimester exposure to ACE inhibitors, and they should also be told that these consequences do not appear to have resulted from intrauterine ACE-inhibitor exposure that has been limited to the first trimester. These patients should be asked to report pregnancies to their physicians as soon as possible.

Drug Interactions

With diuretics: Patients on diuretics, especially those with intravascular volume depletion, may occasionally experience an excessive reduction of blood pressure after initiation of therapy with MONOPRIL (fosinopril sodium tablets). The possibility of hypotensive effects with MONOPRIL can be minimized by either discontinuing the diuretic or increasing salt intake prior to initiation of treatment with MONOPRIL. If this is not possible, the starting dose should be reduced and the patient should be observed closely for several hours following an initial dose and until blood pressure has stabilized (see **DOSAGE AND ADMINISTRATION**).

With potassium supplements and potassium-sparing diuretics: MONOPRIL can attenuate potassium loss caused by thiazide diuretics. Potassium-sparing diuretics (spironolactone, amiloride, triamterene, and others) or potassium supplements can increase the risk of hyperkalemia. Therefore, if concomitant use of such agents is indicated, they should be given with caution, and the patient's serum potassium should be monitored frequently.

With lithium: Increased serum lithium levels and symptoms of lithium toxicity have been reported in patients receiving ACE inhibitors during therapy with lithium. These drugs should be coadministered with caution, and frequent monitoring of serum lithium levels is recommended. If a diuretic is also used, the risk of lithium toxicity may be increased.

With antacids: In a clinical pharmacology study, coadministration of an antacid (aluminum hydroxide, magnesium hydroxide, and simethicone) with fosinopril reduced serum levels and urinary excretion of fosinoprilat as compared with fosinopril administrated alone, suggesting that antacids may impair absorption of fosinopril. Therefore, if concomitant administration of these agents is indicated, dosing should be separated by 2 hours.

Other: Neither MONOPRIL nor its metabolites have been found to interact with food. In separate single or multiple dose pharmacokinetic interaction studies with chlorthalidone, nifedipine, propranolol, hydrochlorothiazide, cimetidine, metoclopramide, propantheline, digoxin, and warfarin, the bioavailability of fosinoprilat was not altered by coadministration of fosinopril with any one of these drugs. In a study with concomitant administration of aspirin and MONOPRIL, the bioavailability of unbound fosinoprilat was not altered.

In a pharmacokinetic interaction study with warfarin, bioavailability parameters, the degree of protein binding, and the anticoagulant effect (measured by prothrombin time) of warfarin were not significantly changed.

Drug/Laboratory Test Interaction

Fosinopril may cause a false low measurement of serum digoxin levels with the Digi-Tab® RIA Kit for Digoxin. Other kits, such as the Coat-A-Count® RIA Kit, may be used.

Carcinogenesis, Mutagenesis, and Impairment of Fertility

No evidence of a carcinogenic effect was found when fosinopril was given in the diet to mice and rats for up to 24 months at doses up to 400 mg/kg/day. On a body weight basis, the highest dose in mice and rats is about 250 times the maximum human dose of 80 mg, assuming a 50 kg subject. On a body surface area basis, in mice, this dose is 20 times the maximum human dose; in rats, this dose is 40 times the maximum human dose. Male rats given the highest dose level had a slightly higher incidence of mesentery/omentum lipomas.

Neither fosinopril nor the active fosinoprilat was mutagenic in the Ames microbial mutagen test, the mouse lymphoma forward mutation assay, or a mitotic gene conversion assay. Fosinopril was also not genotoxic in a mouse micronucleus test *in vivo* and a mouse bone marrow cytogenetic assay *in vivo*.

In the Chinese hamster ovary cell cytogenetic assay, fosinopril increased the frequency of chromosomal aberrations when tested without metabolic activation at a concentration that was toxic to the cells. However, there was no increase in chromosomal aberrations at lower drug concentrations without metabolic activation or at any concentration with metabolic activation.

There were no adverse reproductive effects in male and female rats treated with 15 or 60 mg/kg daily. On a body weight basis, the high dose of 60 mg/kg is about 38 times the maximum recommended human dose. On a body surface area basis, this dose is 6 times the maximum recommended human dose. There was no effect on pairing time prior to mating in rats until a daily dose of 240 mg/kg, a toxic dose, was given; at this dose, a slight increase in pairing time was observed. On a body weight basis, this dose is 150 times the maximum recommended human dose. On a body surface area basis, this dose is 24 times the maximum recommended human dose.

Pregnancy Categories C (first trimester) and D (second and third trimesters)

See WARNINGS: Fetal/Neonatal Morbidity and Mortality.

Nursing Mothers

Ingestion of 20 mg daily for three days resulted in detectable levels of fosinoprilat in breast milk. MONOPRIL (fosinopril sodium tablets) should not be administered to nursing mothers.

Geriatric Use

Of the total number of patients who received fosinopril in US clinical studies of MONOPRIL, 13% were 65 and older while 1.3% were 75 and older. No overall differences in effectiveness or safety were observed between these patients and younger patients, and other reported clinical experience has not identified differences in response between the elderly and younger patients, but greater sensitivity of some older individuals cannot be ruled out.

In a pharmacokinetic study comparing elderly (65–74 years old) and non-elderly (20–35 years old) healthy volunteers, there were no differences between the groups in peak fosinoprilat levels or area under the plasma concentration time curve (AUC).

Pediatric Use

Safety and effectiveness in pediatric patients have not been established.

Clinical Adverse Events in Placebo-Controlled Trials (Hypertension)

	MONOPRIL (N=688) Incidence (Discontinuation)	Placebo (N=184) Incidence (Discontinuation)
Cough	2.2 (0.4)	0.0 (0.0)
Dizziness	1.6 (0.0)	0.0 (0.0)
Nausea/Vomiting	1.2 (0.4)	0.5 (0.0)

Clinical Adverse Events in Placebo-Controlled Trials (Heart Failure)

	MONOPRIL (N = 361) Incidence (Discontinuation)	**Placebo (N = 373) Incidence (Discontinuation)**
Dizziness	11.9 (0.6)	5.4 (0.3)
Cough	9.7 (0.8)	5.1 (0.0)
Hypotension	4.4 (0.8)	0.8 (0.0)
Musculoskeletal Pain	3.3 (0.0)	2.7 (0.0)
Nausea/Vomiting	2.2 (0.6)	1.6 (0.3)
Diarrhea	2.2 (0.0)	1.3 (0.0)
Chest Pain (non-cardiac)	2.2 (0.0)	1.6 (0.0)
Upper Respiratory Infection	2.2 (0.0)	1.3 (0.0)
Orthostatic Hypotension	1.9 (0.0)	0.8 (0.0)
Subjective Cardiac Rhythm Disturbance	1.4 (0.6)	0.8 (0.3)
Weakness	1.4 (0.3)	0.5 (0.0)

ADVERSE REACTIONS

MONOPRIL (fosinopril sodium tablets) has been evaluated for safety in more than 2100 individuals in hypertension and heart failure trials, including approximately 530 patients treated for a year or more. Generally adverse events were mild and transient, and their frequency was not prominently related to dose within the recommended daily dosage range.

Hypertension

In placebo-controlled clinical trials (688 MONOPRIL-treated patients), the usual duration of therapy was two to three months. Discontinuations due to any clinical or laboratory adverse event were 4.1 and 1.1 percent in MONOPRIL-treated and placebo-treated patients, respectively. The most frequent reasons (0.4 to 0.9%) were headache, elevated transaminases, fatigue, cough (see **PRECAUTIONS: General,** *Cough*), diarrhea, and nausea and vomiting.

During clinical trials with any MONOPRIL (fosinopril sodium tablets) regimen, the incidence of adverse events in the elderly (≥ 65 years old) was similar to that seen in younger patients.

Clinical adverse events probably or possibly related or of uncertain relationship to therapy, occurring in at least 1% of patients treated with MONOPRIL alone and at least as frequent on MONOPRIL as on placebo in placebo-controlled clinical trials are shown in the table below.

[See first table above]

The following events were also seen at >1% on MONOPRIL but occurred in the placebo group at a greater rate: headache, diarrhea, fatigue, and sexual dysfunction. Other clinical events probably or possibly related, or of uncertain relationship to therapy occurring in 0.2 to 1.0% of patients (except as noted) treated with MONOPRIL in controlled or uncontrolled clinical trials (N = 1479) and less frequent, clinically significant events include (listed by body system):

General: Chest pain, edema, weakness, excessive sweating.

Cardiovascular: Angina/myocardial infarction, cerebrovascular accident, hypertensive crisis, rhythm disturbances, palpitations, hypotension, syncope, flushing, claudication.

Orthostatic hypotension occurred in 1.4% of patients treated with fosinopril monotherapy. Hypotension or orthostatic hypotension was a cause for discontinuation of therapy in 0.1% of patients.

Dermatologic: Urticaria, rash, photosensitivity, pruritus.

Endocrine/Metabolic: Gout, decreased libido.

Gastrointestinal: Pancreatitis, hepatitis, dysphagia, abdominal distention, abdominal pain, flatulence, constipation, heartburn, appetite/weight change, dry mouth.

Hematologic: Lymphadenopathy.

Immunologic: Angioedema. (See **WARNINGS: Angioedema**).

Musculoskeletal: Arthralgia, musculoskeletal pain, myalgia/muscle cramp.

Nervous/Psychiatric: Memory disturbance, tremor, confusion, mood change, paresthesia, sleep disturbance, drowsiness, vertigo.

Respiratory: Bronchospasm, pharyngitis, sinusitis/rhinitis, laryngitis/hoarseness, epistaxis. A symptom-complex of cough, bronchospasm, and eosinophilia has been observed in two patients treated with fosinopril.

Special Senses: Tinnitus, vision disturbance, taste disturbance, eye irritation.

Urogenital: Renal insufficiency, urinary frequency.

Heart Failure

In placebo-controlled clinical trials (361 MONOPRIL-treated patients), the usual duration of therapy was 3–6 months. Discontinuations due to any clinical or laboratory adverse event, except for heart failure, were 8.0% and 7.5% in MONOPRIL-treated and placebo-treated patients, respectively. The most frequent reason for discontinuation of MONOPRIL was angina pectoris (1.1%). Significant hypotension after the first dose of MONOPRIL occurred in 14/590 (2.4%) of patients; 5/590 (0.8%) patients discontinued due to first dose hypotension.

Clinical adverse events probably or possibly related or of uncertain relationship to therapy, occurring in at least 1% of patients treated with MONOPRIL and at least as common as the placebo group, in placebo-controlled trials are shown in the table below.

[See second table above]

The following events also occurred at a rate of 1% or more on MONOPRIL (fosinopril sodium tablets) but occurred on placebo more often: fatigue, dyspnea, headache, rash, abdominal pain, muscle cramp, angina pectoris, edema, and insomnia.

The incidence of adverse events in the elderly (≥65 years old) was similar to that seen in younger patients.

Other clinical events probably or possibly related, or of uncertain relationship to therapy occurring in 0.4 to 1.0% of patients (except as noted) treated with MONOPRIL (fosinopril sodium tablets) in controlled clinical trials (N = 516) and less frequent, clinically significant events include (listed by body system):

General: Fever, influenza, weight gain, hyperhidrosis, sensation of cold, fall, pain.

Cardiovascular: Sudden death, cardiorespiratory arrest, shock (0.2%), atrial rhythm disturbance, cardiac rhythm disturbances, non anginal chest pain, edema lower extremity, hypertension, syncope, conduction disorder, bradycardia, tachycardia.

Dermatologic: pruritus.

Endocrine/Metabolic: Gout, sexual dysfunction.

Gastrointestinal: Hepatomegaly, abdominal distension, decreased appetite, dry mouth, constipation, flatulence.

Immunologic: Angioedema (0.2%).

Musculoskeletal: Muscle ache, swelling of an extremity, weakness of an extremity.

Nervous/Psychiatric: Cerebral infarction, TIA, depression, numbness, paresthesia, vertigo, behavior change, tremor.

Respiratory: Abnormal vocalization, rhinitis, sinus abnormality, tracheobronchitis, abnormal breathing, pleuritic chest pain.

Special Senses: Vision disturbance, taste disturbance.

Urogenital: Abnormal urination, kidney pain.

Fetal/Neonatal Morbidity and Mortality

See WARNINGS: Fetal/Neonatal Morbidity and Mortality.

Potential Adverse Effects Reported with ACE Inhibitors

Body as a whole: Anaphylactoid reactions (see **WARNINGS: Anaphylactoid and possible related reactions** and **PRECAUTIONS: Hemodialysis**).

Other medically important adverse effects reported with ACE inhibitors include: Cardiac arrest; eosinophilic pneumonitis; neutropenia/agranulocytosis, pancytopenia, anemia (including hemolytic and aplastic), thrombocytopenia; acute renal failure; hepatic failure, jaundice (hepatocellular or cholestatic); symptomatic hyponatremia; bullous pemphigus, exfoliative dermatitis; a syndrome which may include:

Continued on next page

Monopril—Cont.

arthralgia/arthritis, vasculitis, serositis, myalgia, fever, rash or other dermatologic manifestations, a positive ANA, leukocytosis, eosinophilia, or an elevated ESR.

Laboratory Test Abnormalities

Serum Electrolytes: Hyperkalemia, (see **PRECAUTIONS**); hyponatremia, (see **PRECAUTIONS: Drug Interactions,** *With diuretics*).

BUN/Serum Creatinine: Elevations, usually transient and minor, of BUN or serum creatinine have been observed. In placebo-controlled clinical trials, there were no significant differences in the number of patients experiencing increases in serum creatinine (outside the normal range or 1.33 times the pre-treatment value) between the fosinopril and placebo treatment groups. Rapid reduction of longstanding or markedly elevated blood pressure by any antihypertensive therapy can result in decreases in the glomerular filtration rate and, in turn, lead to increases in BUN or serum creatinine. (See **PRECAUTIONS: General.**)

Hematology: In controlled trials, a mean hemoglobin decrease of 0.1 g/dL was observed in fosinopril-treated patients. In individual patients decreases in hemoglobin or hematocrit were usually transient, small, and not associated with symptoms. No patient was discontinued from therapy due to the development of anemia. *Other:* Neutropenia (see **WARNINGS**), leukopenia and eosinophilia.

Liver Function Tests: Elevations of transaminases, LDH, alkaline phosphatase and serum bilirubin have been reported. Fosinopril therapy was discontinued because of serum transaminase elevations in 0.7% of patients. In the majority of cases, the abnormalities were either present at baseline or were associated with other etiologic factors. In those cases which were possibly related to fosinopril therapy, the elevations were generally mild and transient and resolved after discontinuation of therapy.

OVERDOSAGE

Oral doses of fosinopril at 2600 mg/kg in rats were associated with significant lethality. Human overdoses of fosinopril have not been reported, but the most common manifestation of human fosinopril overdosage is likely to be hypotension.

Laboratory determinations of serum levels of fosinoprilat and its metabolites are not widely available, and such determinations have, in any event, no established role in the management of fosinopril overdose. No data are available to suggest physiological maneuvers (e.g., maneuvers to change the pH of the urine) that might accelerate elimination of fosinopril and its metabolites. Fosinoprilat is poorly removed from the body by both hemodialysis and peritoneal dialysis.

Angiotensin II could presumably serve as a specific antagonist-antidote in the setting of fosinopril overdose, but angiotensin II is essentially unavailable outside of scattered research facilities. Because the hypotensive effect of fosinopril is achieved through vasodilation and effective hypovolemia, it is reasonable to treat fosinopril overdose by infusion of normal saline solution.

DOSAGE AND ADMINISTRATION

Hypertension

The recommended initial dose of MONOPRIL (is 10 mg once a day, both as monotherapy and when the drug is added to a diuretic. Dosage should then be adjusted according to blood pressure response at peak (2–6 hours) and trough (about 24 hours after dosing) blood levels. The usual dosage range needed to maintain a response at trough is 20–40 mg but some patients appear to have a further response to 80 mg. In some patients treated with once daily dosing, the antihypertensive effect may diminish toward the end of the dosing interval. If trough response is inadequate, dividing the daily dose should be considered. If blood pressure is not adequately controlled with MONOPRIL alone, a diuretic may be added.

Concomitant administration of MONOPRIL with potassium supplements, potassium salt substitutes, or potassium-sparing diuretics can lead to increases of serum potassium (see **PRECAUTIONS**).

In patients who are currently being treated with a diuretic, symptomatic hypotension occasionally can occur following the initial dose of MONOPRIL. To reduce the likelihood of hypotension, the diuretic should, if possible, be discontinued two to three days prior to beginning therapy with MONOPRIL (see **WARNINGS**). Then, if blood pressure is not controlled with MONOPRIL alone, diuretic therapy should be resumed. If diuretic therapy cannot be discontinued, an initial dose of 10 mg of MONOPRIL should be used with careful medical supervision for several hours and until blood pressure has stabilized. (See **WARNINGS; PRECAUTIONS: Information for Patients and Drug Interactions.**)

Since concomitant administration of MONOPRIL with potassium supplements, or potassium-containing salt substitutes or potassium-sparing diuretics may lead to increases in serum potassium, they should be used with caution (see **PRECAUTIONS**).

Heart Failure

Digitalis is not required for MONOPRIL to manifest improvements in exercise tolerance and symptoms. Most placebo-controlled clinical trial experience has been with both digitalis and diuretics present as background therapy.

The usual starting dose of MONOPRIL should be 10 mg once daily. Following the initial dose of MONOPRIL, the patient should be observed under medical supervision for at least two hours for the presence of hypotension or orthostasis and, if present, until blood pressure stabilizes. An initial dose of 5 mg is preferred in heart failure patients with moderate to severe renal failure or those who have been vigorously diuresed.

Dosage should be increased, over a several week period, to a dose that is maximal and tolerated but not exceeding 40 mg once daily. The usual effective dosage range is 20 to 40 mg once daily.

The appearance of hypotension, orthostasis, or azotemia early in dose titration should not preclude further careful dose titration. Consideration should be given to reducing the dose of concomitant diuretic.

For Hypertensive or Heart Failure Patients With Renal Impairment: In patients with impaired renal function, the total body clearance of fosinoprilat is approximately 50% slower than in patients with normal renal function. Since hepatobiliary elimination partially compensates for diminished renal elimination, the total body clearance of fosinoprilat does not differ appreciably with any degree of renal insufficiency (creatinine clearances <80 mL/min/1.73m^2), including end-stage renal failure (creatinine clearance <10 mL/min/1.73m^2). This relative constancy of body clearance of active fosinoprilat, resulting from the dual route of elimination, permits use of the usual dose in patients with any degree of renal impairment. (See **WARNINGS: Anaphylactoid reactions during membrane exposure** and **PRECAUTIONS: Hemodialysis.**)

Shown in Product Identification Guide, page 309

HOW SUPPLIED

Monopril (fosinopril sodium tablets)

10 mg tablets: White to off-white, biconvex flat-end diamond shaped, compressed partially scored tablets with **BMS** on one side and **Monopril 10** on the other. They are supplied in bottles of 30 (NDC 0087-0158-22), bottles of 90 (NDC 0087-0158-46), and 1000 (NDC 0087-0158-85). Bottles contain a desiccant canister.

20 mg tablets: White to off-white, oval shaped, compressed tablets with **BMS** on one side and **Monopril 20** on the other. They are supplied in bottles of 30 (NDC 0087-0609-41), bottles of 90 (NDC 0087-0609-42), and 1000 (NDC 0087-0609-85). Bottles contain a desiccant canister.

40 mg tablets: White to off-white, biconvex hexagonal shaped, compressed tablets with **BMS** on one side and **Monopril 40** on the other. They are supplied in bottles of 30 (NDC 0087-1202-12) and bottles of 90 (NDC 0087-1202-13). Bottles contain a desiccant canister.

UNIMATIC® unit-dose packs containing 100 tablets are also available for each potency: **10 mg** (NDC 0087-0158-45) and **20 mg** (NDC 0087-0609-45).

STORAGE

Store between 15° C (59° F) and 30° C (86° F). Avoid prolonged exposure to temperatures above 30° C (86° F). Keep bottles tightly closed (protect from moisture).

J4-502K
F4-B001-08-99 1081010A2
0158DIM-08 51-006144-02
Revised: August 1999

Bristol-Myers Squibb Company
Princeton, NJ 08543 USA

Shown in Product Identification Guide, page 309

PLAVIX® ℞

[*plă vĭks*]
clopidogrel bisulfate
tablets
Rx only

DESCRIPTION

PLAVIX* (clopidogrel bisulfate) is an inhibitor of ADP-induced platelet aggregation acting by direct inhibition of adenosine diphosphate (ADP) binding to its receptor and of the subsequent ADP-mediated activation of the glycoprotein GPIIb/IIIa complex. Chemically it is methyl (+)-(*S*)-α-(2-chlorophenyl)-6,7-dihydrothieno[3,2-c]pyridine-5(4*H*)-acetate sulfate (1:1). The empirical formula of clopidogrel bisulfate is $C_{16}H_{16}Cl\ NO_2S \bullet H_2SO_4$ and its molecular weight is 419.9.

The structural formula is as follows:

Clopidogrel bisulfate is a white to off-white powder. It is practically insoluble in water at neutral pH but freely soluble at pH 1. It also dissolves freely in methanol, dissolves sparingly in methylene chloride, and is practically insoluble in ethyl ether. It has a specific optical rotation of about +56°.

PLAVIX for oral administration is provided as pink, round, biconvex, debossed film-coated tablets containing 97.875 mg of clopidogrel bisulfate which is the molar equivalent of 75 mg of clopidogrel base.

Each tablet contains anhydrous lactose, hydrogenated castor oil, microcrystalline cellulose, polyethylene glycol 6000 and pregelatinized starch as inactive ingredients. The pink film coating contains ferric oxide (red), hydroxypropyl methylcellulose 2910, polyethylene glycol 6000 and titanium dioxide. The tablets are polished with Carnauba wax.

---

*Registered trademark of Sanofi-Synthelabo, Inc.

CLINICAL PHARMACOLOGY

Mechanism of Action

Clopidogrel is an inhibitor of platelet aggregation. A variety of drugs that inhibit platelet function have been shown to decrease morbid events in people with established atherosclerotic cardiovascular disease as evidenced by stroke or transient ischemic attacks, myocardial infarction, or need for bypass or angioplasty. This indicates that platelets participate in the initiation and/or evolution of these events and that inhibiting them can reduce the event rate.

Pharmacodynamic Properties

Clopidogrel selectively inhibits the binding of adenosine diphosphate (ADP) to its platelet receptor and the subsequent ADP-mediated activation of the glycoprotein GPIIb/IIIa complex, thereby inhibiting platelet aggregation. Biotransformation of clopidogrel is necessary to produce inhibition of platelet aggregation, but an active metabolite responsible for the activity of the drug has not been isolated. Clopidogrel also inhibits platelet aggregation induced by agonists other than ADP by blocking the amplification of platelet activation by released ADP. Clopidogrel does not inhibit phosphodiesterase activity.

Clopidogrel acts by irreversibly modifying the platelet ADP receptor. Consequently, platelets exposed to clopidogrel are affected for the remainder of their lifespan.

Dose dependent inhibition of platelet aggregation can be seen 2 hours after single oral doses of PLAVIX. Repeated doses of 75 mg PLAVIX per day inhibit ADP-induced platelet aggregation on the first day, and inhibition reaches steady state between Day 3 and Day 7. At steady state, the average inhibition level observed with a dose of 75 mg PLAVIX per day was between 40% and 60%. Platelet aggregation and bleeding time gradually return to baseline values after treatment is discontinued, generally in about 5 days.

Pharmacokinetics and Metabolism

After repeated 75-mg oral doses of clopidogrel (base), plasma concentrations of the parent compound, which has no platelet inhibiting effect, are very low and are generally below the quantification limit (0.00025 mg/L) beyond 2 hours after dosing. Clopidogrel is extensively metabolized by the liver. The main circulating metabolite is the carboxylic acid derivative, and it too has no effect on platelet aggregation. It represents about 85% of the circulating drug-related compounds in plasma.

Following an oral dose of ^{14}C-labeled clopidogrel in humans, approximately 50% was excreted in the urine and approximately 46% in the feces in the 5 days after dosing. The elimination half-life of the main circulating metabolite was 8 hours after single and repeated administration. Covalent binding to platelets accounted for 2% of radiolabel with a half-life of 11 days.

Effect of Food: Administration of PLAVIX (clopidogrel bisulfate) with meals did not significantly modify the bioavailability of clopidogrel as assessed by the pharmacokinetics of the main circulating metabolite.

Absorption and Distribution: Clopidogrel is rapidly absorbed after oral administration of repeated doses of 75 mg clopidogrel (base), with peak plasma levels (≅3 mg/L) of the main circulating metabolite occurring approximately 1 hour after dosing. The pharmacokinetics of the main circulating metabolite are linear (plasma concentrations increased in proportion to dose) in the dose range of 50 to 150 mg of clopidogrel. Absorption is at least 50% based on urinary excretion of clopidogrel-related metabolites.

Clopidogrel and the main circulating metabolite bind reversibly *in vitro* to human plasma proteins (98% and 94%, respectively). The binding is nonsaturable *in vitro* up to a concentration of 100 µg/mL.

Metabolism and Elimination: *In vitro* and *in vivo*, clopidogrel undergoes rapid hydrolysis into its carboxylic acid derivative. In plasma and urine, the glucuronide of the carboxylic acid derivative is also observed.

Special Populations

Geriatric Patients: Plasma concentrations of the main circulating metabolite are significantly higher in elderly (≥75 years) compared to young healthy volunteers but these higher plasma levels were not associated with differences in platelet aggregation and bleeding time. No dosage adjustment is needed for the elderly.

Renally Impaired Patients: After repeated doses of 75 mg PLAVIX per day, plasma levels of the main circulating metabolite were lower in patients with severe renal impairment (creatinine clearance from 5 to 15 mL/min) compared to subjects with moderate renal impairment (creatinine clearance 30 to 60 mL/min) or healthy subjects. Although inhibition of ADP-induced platelet aggregation was lower (25%) than that observed in healthy volunteers, the prolongation of bleeding time was similar to healthy volunteers receiving 75 mg of PLAVIX per day. No dosage adjustment is needed in renally impaired patients.

Gender: No significant difference was observed in the plasma levels of the main circulating metabolite between males and females. In a small study comparing men and women, less inhibition of ADP-induced platelet aggregation was observed in women, but there was no difference in prolongation of bleeding time. In the large, controlled clinical study (Clopidogrel vs. Aspirin in Patients at Risk of Ischemic Events; CAPRIE), the incidence of clinical outcome events, other adverse clinical events, and abnormal clinical laboratory parameters was similar in men and women.

Race: Pharmacokinetic differences due to race have not been studied.

CLINICAL STUDIES

The clinical evidence for the efficacy of PLAVIX is derived from the CAPRIE (Clopidogrel vs. Aspirin in Patients at Risk of Ischemic Events) trial. This was a 19,185-patient, 304-center, international, randomized, double-blind, parallel-group study comparing PLAVIX (75 mg daily) to aspirin (325 mg daily). The patients randomized had: 1) recent histories of myocardial infarction (within 35 days); 2) recent histories of ischemic stroke (within 6 months) with at least a week of residual neurological signs; or 3) objectively established peripheral arterial disease. Patients received randomized treatment for an average of 1.6 years (maximum of 3 years).

The trial's primary outcome was the time to first occurrence of new ischemic stroke (fatal or not), new myocardial infarction (fatal or not), or other vascular death. Deaths not easily attributable to nonvascular causes were all classified as vascular.

Outcome Events of the Primary Analysis

Patients	PLAVIX 9599	aspirin 9586
IS (fatal or not)	438 (4.56%)	461 (4.81%)
MI (fatal or not)	275 (2.86%)	333 (3.47%)
Other vascular death	226 (2.35%)	226 (2.36%)
Total	939 (9.78%)	1020 (10.64%)

As shown in the table, PLAVIX (clopidogrel bisulfate) was associated with a lower incidence of outcome events of every kind. The overall risk reduction (9.78% vs. 10.64%) was 8.7%, P=0.045. Similar results were obtained when all-cause mortality and all-cause strokes were counted instead of vascular mortality and ischemic strokes (risk reduction 6.9%). In patients who survived an on-study stroke or myocardial infarction, the incidence of subsequent events was again lower in the PLAVIX group.

The curves showing the overall event rate are shown in the figure. The event curves separated early and continued to diverge over the 3-year follow-up period.

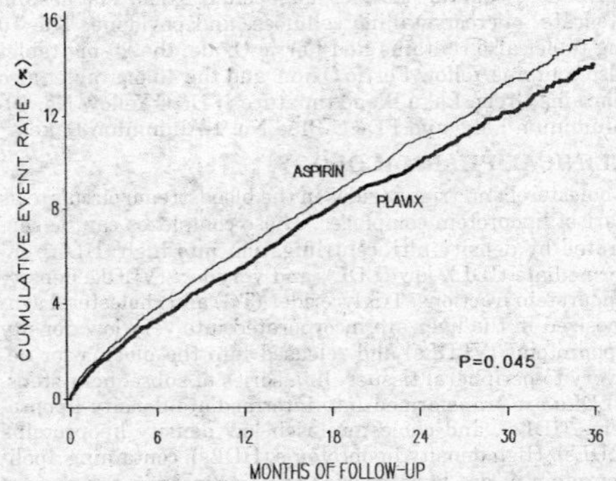

Although the statistical significance favoring PLAVIX over aspirin was marginal (P=0.045), and represents the result of a single trial that has not been replicated, the comparator drug, aspirin, is itself effective (vs. placebo) in reducing cardiovascular events in patients with recent myocardial infarction or stroke. Thus, the difference between PLAVIX and placebo, although not measured directly, is substantial. The CAPRIE trial included a population that was randomized on the basis of 3 entry criteria. The efficacy of PLAVIX relative to aspirin was heterogeneous across these randomized subgroups (P=0.043). It is not clear whether this difference is real or a chance occurrence. Although the CAPRIE trial was not designed to evaluate the relative benefit of PLAVIX over aspirin in the individual patient subgroups, the benefit appeared to be strongest in patients who were enrolled because of peripheral vascular disease (especially those who also had a history of myocardial infarction) and weaker in stroke patients. In patients who were enrolled in the trial on the sole basis of a recent myocardial infarction, PLAVIX (clopidogrel bisulfate) was not numerically superior to aspirin.

In the meta-analyses of studies of aspirin vs. placebo in patients similar to those in CAPRIE, aspirin was associated with a reduced incidence of atherothrombotic events. There was a suggestion of heterogeneity in these studies too, with the effect strongest in patients with a history of myocardial infarction, weaker in patients with a history of stroke, and not discernible in patients with a history of peripheral vascular disease. With respect to the inferred comparison of PLAVIX to placebo, there is no indication of heterogeneity.

INDICATIONS AND USAGE

PLAVIX (clopidogrel bisulfate) is indicated for the reduction of atherosclerotic events (myocardial infarction, stroke, and vascular death) in patients with atherosclerosis documented by recent stroke, recent myocardial infarction, or established peripheral arterial disease.

Adverse Events Occurring in ≥2.5% of PLAVIX Patients

Body System Event	PLAVIX [n=9599] % Incidence (% Discontinuation)	Aspirin [n=9586] % Incidence (% Discontinuation)
Body as a Whole—general disorders		
Chest Pain	8.3 (0.2)	8.3 (0.3)
Accidental Injury	7.9 (0.1)	7.3 (0.1)
Influenza-like symptoms	7.5 (<0.1)	7.0 (<0.1)
Pain	6.4 (0.1)	6.3 (0.1)
Fatigue	3.3 (0.1)	3.4 (0.1)
Cardiovascular disorders, general		
Edema	4.1 (<0.1)	4.5 (<0.1)
Hypertension	4.3 (<0.1)	5.1 (<0.1)
Central & peripheral nervous system disorders		
Headache	7.6 (0.3)	7.2 (0.2)
Dizziness	6.2 (0.2)	6.7 (0.3)
Gastrointestinal system disorders		
Abdominal pain	5.6 (0.7)	7.1 (1.0)
Dyspepsia	5.2 (0.6)	6.1 (0.7)
Diarrhea	4.5 (0.4)	3.4 (0.3)
Nausea	3.4 (0.5)	3.8 (0.4)
Metabolic & nutritional disorders		
Hypercholesterolemia	4.0 (0)	4.4 (<0.1)
Musculo-skeletal system disorders		
Arthralgia	6.3 (0.1)	6.2 (0.1)
Back Pain	5.8 (0.1)	5.3 (<0.1)
Platelet, bleeding, & clotting disorders		
Purpura	5.3 (0.3)	3.7 (0.1)
Epistaxis	2.9 (0.2)	2.5 (0.1)
Psychiatric disorders		
Depression	3.6 (0.1)	3.9 (0.2)
Respiratory system disorders		
Upper resp tract infection	8.7 (<0.1)	8.3 (<0.1)
Dyspnea	4.5 (0.1)	4.7 (0.1)
Rhinitis	4.2 (0.1)	4.2 (<0.1)
Bronchitis	3.7 (0.1)	3.7 (0)
Coughing	3.1 (<0.1)	2.7 (<0.1)
Skin & appendage disorders		
Rash	4.2 (0.5)	3.5 (0.2)
Pruritus	3.3 (0.3)	1.6 (0.1)
Urinary system disorders		
Urinary tract infection	3.1 (0)	3.5 (0.1)

CONTRAINDICATIONS

The use of PLAVIX is contraindicated in the following conditions:

- Hypersensitivity to the drug substance or any component of the product.
- Active pathological bleeding such as peptic ulcer or intracranial hemorrhage.

WARNINGS

Thrombotic thrombocytopenic purpura (TTP): TTP has been reported rarely following use of PLAVIX, sometimes after a short exposure (<2weeks). TTP is a serious condition requiring prompt treatment. It is characterized by thrombocytopenia, microangiopathic hemolytic anemia (schistocytes [fragmented RBCs] seen on peripheral smear), neurological findings, renal dysfunction, and fever. TTP was not seen during clopidogrel's clinical trials, which included over 11,300 clopidogrel-treated patients. In world-wide postmarketing experience, however, TTP has been reported at a rate of about four cases per million patients exposed, or about 11 cases per million patient-years. The background rate is thought to be about four cases per million person-years.

PRECAUTIONS

General

As with other anti-platelet agents, PLAVIX should be used with caution in patients who may be at risk of increased bleeding from trauma, surgery, or other pathological conditions. If a patient is to undergo elective surgery and an antiplatelet effect is not desired, PLAVIX should be discontinued 7 days prior to surgery.

GI Bleeding: PLAVIX prolongs the bleeding time. In CAPRIE, PLAVIX was associated with a rate of gastrointestinal bleeding of 2.0%, vs. 2.7% on aspirin. PLAVIX should be used with caution in patients who have lesions with a propensity to bleed (such as ulcers). Drugs that might induce such lesions (such as aspirin and other nonsteroidal anti-inflammatory drugs [NSAIDs]) should be used with caution in patients taking PLAVIX.

Use in Hepatically Impaired Patients: Experience is limited in patients with severe hepatic disease, who may have bleeding diatheses. PLAVIX should be used with caution in this population.

Information for Patients

Patients should be told that it may take them longer than usual to stop bleeding when they take PLAVIX, and that they should report any unusual bleeding to their physician. Patients should inform physicians and dentists that they are taking PLAVIX before any surgery is scheduled and before any new drug is taken.

Drug Interactions

Study of specific drug interactions yielded the following results:

Aspirin: Aspirin did not modify the clopidogrel-mediated inhibition of ADP-induced platelet aggregation. Concomitant administration of 500 mg of aspirin twice a day for 1 day did not significantly increase the prolongation of bleeding time induced by PLAVIX. PLAVIX potentiated the effect of aspirin on collagen-induced platelet aggregation. The safety of chronic concomitant administration of aspirin and PLAVIX has not been established.

Heparin: In a study in healthy volunteers, PLAVIX did not necessitate modification of the heparin dose or alter the effect of heparin on coagulation. Coadministration of heparin had no effect on inhibition of platelet aggregation induced by PLAVIX. The safety of this combination has not been established, however, and concomitant use should be undertaken with caution.

Nonsteroidal Anti-Inflammatory Drugs (NSAIDs): In healthy volunteers receiving naproxen, concomitant administration of PLAVIX was associated with increased occult gastrointestinal blood loss. NSAIDs and PLAVIX should be coadministered with caution.

Warfarin: The safety of the coadministration of PLAVIX (clopidogrel bisulfate) with warfarin has not been established. Consequently, concomitant administration of these two agents should be undertaken with caution. (See **Precautions-General**).

Other Concomitant Therapy: No clinically significant pharmacodynamic interactions were observed when PLAVIX was coadministered with **atenolol, nifedipine,** or both atenolol and nifedipine. The pharmacodynamic activity of PLAVIX was also not significantly influenced by the coadministration of **phenobarbital, cimetidine** or **estrogen**.

The pharmacokinetics of **digoxin** or **theophylline** were not modified by the coadministration of PLAVIX (clopidogrel bisulfate).

At high concentrations *in vitro*, clopidogrel inhibits P_{450} (2C9). Accordingly, PLAVIX may interfere with the metabolism of **phenytoin, tamoxifen, tolbutamide, warfarin, torsemide, fluvastatin,** and many **non-steroidal anti-inflammatory agents,** but there are no data with which to predict the magnitude of these interactions. Caution should be used when any of these drugs is coadministered with PLAVIX.

In addition to the above specific interaction studies, patients entered into CAPRIE received a variety of concomitant medications **including diuretics, beta-blocking agents,**

Continued on next page

Plavix—Cont.

angiotensin converting enzyme inhibitors, calcium antagonists, cholesterol lowering agents, coronary vasodilators, antidiabetic agents, antiepileptic agents and **hormone replacement therapy** without evidence of clinically significant adverse interactions.

Drug/Laboratory Test Interactions

None known.

Carcinogenesis, Mutagenesis, Impairment of Fertility

There was no evidence of tumorigenicity when clopidogrel was administered for 78 weeks to mice and 104 weeks to rats at dosages up to 77 mg/kg per day, which afforded plasma exposures >25 times that in humans at the recommended daily dose of 75 mg.

Clopidogrel was not genotoxic in four *in vitro* tests (Ames test, DNA-repair test in rat hepatocytes, gene mutation assay in Chinese hamster fibroblasts, and metaphase chromosome analysis of human lymphocytes) and in one *in vivo* test (micronucleus test by oral route in mice).

Clopidogrel was found to have no effect on fertility of male and female rats at oral doses up to 400 mg/kg per day (52 times the recommended human dose on a mg/m^2 basis).

Pregnancy

Pregnancy Category B. Reproduction studies performed in rats and rabbits at doses up to 500 and 300 mg/kg/day (respectively, 65 and 78 times the recommended daily human dose on a mg/m^2 basis), revealed no evidence of impaired fertility or fetotoxicity due to clopidogrel. There are, however, no adequate and well-controlled studies in pregnant women. Because animal reproduction studies are not always predictive of a human response, PLAVIX should be used during pregnancy only if clearly needed.

Nursing Mothers

Studies in rats have shown that clopidogrel and/or its metabolites are excreted in the milk. It is not known whether this drug is excreted in human milk. Because many drugs are excreted in human milk and because of the potential for serious adverse reactions in nursing infants, a decision should be made whether to discontinue nursing or to discontinue the drug, taking into account the importance of the drug to the nursing woman.

Pediatric Use

Safety and effectiveness in the pediatric population have not been established.

ADVERSE REACTIONS

PLAVIX has been evaluated for safety in more than 11,300 patients, including over 7,000 patients treated for 1 year or more. The overall tolerability of PLAVIX was similar to that of aspirin regardless of age, gender and race, with an approximately equal incidence (13%) of patients withdrawing from treatment because of adverse reactions. The clinically important adverse events observed in CAPRIE are discussed below.

Hemorrhagic: In patients receiving PLAVIX in CAPRIE, gastrointestinal hemorrhage occurred at a rate of 2.0%, and required hospitalization in 0.7%. In patients receiving aspirin, the corresponding rates were 2.7% and 1.1%, respectively. The incidence of intracranial hemorrhage was 0.4% for PLAVIX compared to 0.5% for aspirin.

Neutropenia/agranulocytosis: Ticlopidine, a drug chemically similar to PLAVIX, is associated with a 0.8% rate of severe neutropenia (less than 450 neutrophils/μL). Patients in CAPRIE (see Clinical Trials) were intensively monitored for neutropenia. Severe neutropenia was observed in six patients, four on PLAVIX and two on aspirin. Two of the 9599 patients who received PLAVIX (clopidogrel bisulfate) and none of the 9586 patients who received aspirin had neutrophil counts of zero.

One of the four PLAVIX patients was receiving cytotoxic chemotherapy, and another recovered and returned to the trial after only temporarily interrupting treatment with PLAVIX.

Although the risk of myelotoxicity with PLAVIX thus appears to be quite low, this possibility should be considered when a patient receiving PLAVIX demonstrates fever or other sign of infection.

Gastrointestinal: Overall, the incidence of gastrointestinal events (e.g. abdominal pain, dyspepsia, gastritis and constipation) in patients receiving PLAVIX (clopidogrel bisulfate) was 27.1%, compared to 29.8% in those receiving aspirin.

The incidence of peptic, gastric or duodenal ulcers was 0.7% for PLAVIX and 1.2% for aspirin.

Cases of diarrhea were reported in 4.5% of patients in the PLAVIX group compared to 3.4% in the aspirin group. However, these were rarely severe (PLAVIX=0.2% and aspirin=0.1%).

The incidence of patients withdrawing from treatment because of gastrointestinal adverse reactions was 3.2% for PLAVIX and 4.0% for aspirin.

Rash and Other Skin Disorders: The incidence of skin and appendage disorders in patients receiving PLAVIX was 15.8% (0.7% serious); the corresponding rate in aspirin patients was 13.1% (0.5% serious).

The overall incidence of patients withdrawing from treatment because of skin and appendage disorders adverse reactions was 1.5% for PLAVIX and 0.8% for aspirin.

Adverse events occurring in ≥2.5% of patients on PLAVIX in the CAPRIE controlled clinical trial are shown below regardless of relationship to PLAVIX. The median duration of therapy was 20 months, with a maximum of 3 years.

[See table at top of previous page]

Incidence of discontinuation, regardless of relationship to therapy, is shown in parentheses.

Other adverse experiences of potential importance occurring in 1% to 2.5% of patients receiving PLAVIX (clopidogrel bisulfate) in the CAPRIE controlled clinical trial are listed below regardless of relationship to PLAVIX. In general, the incidence of these events was similar in the aspirin-treated group.

Autonomic Nervous System Disorders: Syncope, Palpitation. *Body as a Whole - general disorders:* Asthenia, Hernia. *Cardiovascular disorders:* Cardiac failure. *Central and peripheral nervous system disorders:* Cramps legs, Hypoaesthesia, Neuralgia, Paresthesia, Vertigo. *Gastrointestinal system disorders:* Constipation, Vomiting. *Heart rate and rhythm disorders:* Fibrillation atrial. *Liver and biliary system disorders:* Hepatic enzymes increased. *Metabolic and nutritional disorders:* Gout, hyperuricemia, non-protein nitrogen (NPN) increased. *Musculo-skeletal system disorders:* Arthritis, Arthrosis. *Platelet, bleeding & clotting disorders:* GI hemorrhage, hematoma, platelets decreased. *Psychiatric disorders:* Anxiety, Insomnia. *Red blood cell disorders:* Anemia. *Respiratory system disorders:* Pneumonia, Sinusitis. *Skin and appendage disorders:* Eczema, Skin ulceration. *Urinary system disorders:* Cystitis. *Vision disorders:* Cataract, Conjunctivitis.

Other potentially serious adverse events which may be of clinical interest but were rarely reported (<1%) in patients who received PLAVIX are listed below regardless of relationship to PLAVIX. In general, the incidence of these events was similar in the aspirin group.

Body as a whole: Allergic reaction, necrosis ischemic. *Cardiovascular disorders:* Edema generalized. *Gastrointestinal system disorders:* Gastric ulcer perforated, gastritis hemorrhagic, upper GI ulcer hemorrhagic. *Liver and Biliary system disorders:* Bilirubinemia, hepatitis infectious, liver fatty. *Platelet, bleeding and clotting disorders:* hemarthrosis, hematuria, hemoptysis, hemorrhage intracranial, hemorrhage retroperitoneal, hemorrhage of operative wound, ocular hemorrhage, pulmonary hemorrhage, purpura allergic, thrombocytopenia. *Red blood cell disorders:* Anemia aplastic, anemia hypochromic. *Reproductive disorders, female:* Menorrhagia. *Respiratory system disorders:* Hemothorax. *Skin and appendage disorders:* Bullous eruption, rash erythematous, rash maculopapular, urticaria. *White cell and reticuloendothelial system disorders:* Agranulocytosis, granulocytopenia, leukemia, leukopenia, neutrophils decreased.

Postmarketing Experience

The following events have been reported spontaneously from worldwide postmarketing experience; very rare cases of hypersensitivity reactions including angioedema, bronchospasms, and anaphylactoid reactions. Suspected thrombotic thrombocytopenic purpura (TTP) has been reported as part of the world-wide postmarketing experience, see **WARNINGS**.

OVERDOSAGE

One case of deliberate overdosage with PLAVIX was reported in the large, controlled clinical study. A 34-year-old woman took a single 1,050-mg dose of PLAVIX (equivalent to 14 standard 75-mg tablets). There were no associated adverse events. No special therapy was instituted, and she recovered without sequelae.

No adverse events were reported after single oral administration of 600 mg (equivalent to 8 standard 75-mg tablets) of PLAVIX in healthy volunteers. The bleeding time was prolonged by a factor of 1.7, which is similar to that typically observed with the therapeutic dose of 75 mg of PLAVIX per day.

A single oral dose of clopidogrel at 1500 or 2000 mg/kg was lethal to mice and to rats and at 3000 mg/kg to baboons. Symptoms of acute toxicity were vomiting (in baboons), prostration, difficult breathing, and gastrointestinal hemorrhage in all species.

Recommendations About Specific Treatment:

Based on biological plausibility, platelet transfusion may be appropriate to reverse the pharmacological effects of PLAVIX if quick reversal is required.

DOSAGE AND ADMINISTRATION

The recommended dose of PLAVIX is 75 mg once daily with or without food.

No dosage adjustment is necessary for elderly patients or patients with renal disease. (See **Clinical Pharmacology: Special Populations**.)

HOW SUPPLIED

PLAVIX (clopidogrel bisulfate) is available as a pink, round, biconvex, film-coated tablet debossed with "75" on one side and "1171" on the other. Tablets are provided as follows:

NDC 63653-1171-6 bottles of 30
NDC 63653-1171-1 bottles of 90
NDC 63653-1171-5 bottles of 500
NDC 63653-1171-3 blisters of 100

Storage

Store at 25° C (77° F); excursions permitted to 15°–30° C (59°–86° F) [See USP Controlled Room Temperature]

Manufactured by:
Sanofi-Synthelabo, Inc.
New York, NY 10016

Distributed by:
Bristol-Myers Squibb/Sanofi Pharmaceuticals Partnership
New York, NY 10016

Sanofi-Synthelabo/Bristol-Myers Squibb Company

PLAVIX® is a registered trademark of Sanofi-Synthelabo

Revised: April 2000 J4-643F 1171DIM-07
B1-B001-05-00 1077549A4 1081251A5

Shown in Product Identification Guide, page 309

PRAVACHOL® ℞

[pră-vă-chol]

(pravastatin sodium)

Tablets

Rx only

DESCRIPTION

PRAVACHOL® (pravastatin sodium) is one of a new class of lipid-lowering compounds, the HMG-CoA reductase inhibitors, which reduce cholesterol biosynthesis. These agents are competitive inhibitors of 3-hydroxy-3-methylglutaryl-coenzyme A (HMG-CoA) reductase, the enzyme catalyzing the early rate-limiting step in cholesterol biosynthesis, conversion of HMG-CoA to mevalonate.

Pravastatin sodium is designated chemically as 1-Naphthalene-heptanoic acid, 1,2,6,7,8,8a-hexahydro-β,δ,6-trihydroxy-2-methyl-8-(2-methyl-1-oxobutoxy)-, monosodium salt, [1S-[1α(βS*,δS*),2α,6α,8β(R*),8aα]]-. Structural formula:

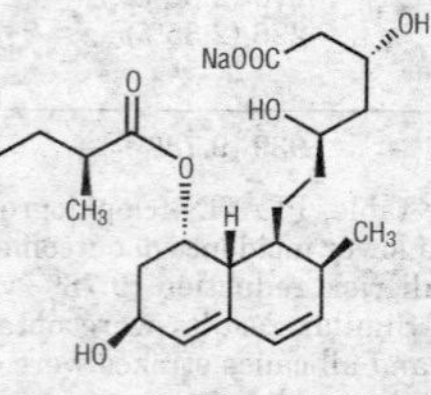

Pravastatin sodium is an odorless, white to off-white, fine or crystalline powder. It is a relatively polar hydrophilic compound with a partition coefficient (octanol/water) of 0.59 at a pH of 7.0. It is soluble in methanol and water (>300 mg/mL), slightly soluble in isopropanol, and practically insoluble in acetone, acetonitrile, chloroform, and ether.

PRAVACHOL is available for oral administration as 10 mg, 20 mg and 40 mg tablets. Inactive ingredients include: croscarmellose sodium, lactose, magnesium oxide, magnesium stearate, microcrystalline cellulose, and povidone. The 10 mg tablet also contains Red Ferric Oxide, the 20 mg tablet also contains Yellow Ferric Oxide, and the 40 mg tablet also contains Green Lake Blend (mixture of D&C Yellow No. 10-Aluminum Lake and FD&C Blue No. 1-Aluminum Lake).

CLINICAL PHARMACOLOGY

Cholesterol and triglycerides in the bloodstream circulate as part of lipoprotein complexes. These complexes can be separated by density ultracentrifugation into high (HDL), intermediate (IDL), low (LDL), and very low (VLDL) density lipoprotein fractions. Triglycerides (TG) and cholesterol synthesized in the liver are incorporated into very low density lipoproteins (VLDLs) and released into the plasma for delivery to peripheral tissues. In a series of subsequent steps, VLDLs are transformed into intermediate density lipoproteins (IDLs), and cholesterol-rich low density lipoproteins (LDLs). High density lipoproteins (HDLs), containing apolipoprotein A, are hypothesized to participate in the reverse transport of cholesterol from tissues back to the liver.

PRAVACHOL produces its lipid-lowering effect in two ways. First, as a consequence of its reversible inhibition of HMG-CoA reductase activity, it effects modest reductions in intracellular pools of cholesterol. This results in an increase in the number of LDL-receptors on cell surfaces and enhanced receptor-mediated catabolism and clearance of circulating LDL. Second, pravastatin inhibits LDL production by inhibiting hepatic synthesis of VLDL, the LDL precursor.

Clinical and pathologic studies have shown that elevated levels of total cholesterol (Total-C), low density lipoprotein cholesterol (LDL-C), and apolipoprotein B (Apo B – a membrane transport complex for LDL) promote human atherosclerosis. Similarly, decreased levels of HDL-cholesterol (HDL-C) and its transport complex, apolipoprotein A, are associated with the development of atherosclerosis. Epidemiologic investigations have established that cardiovascular morbidity and mortality vary directly with the level of Total-C and LDL-C and inversely with the level of HDL-C. Like LDL, cholesterol-enriched triglyceride-rich lipoproteins, including VLDL, IDL, and remnants, can also promote atherosclerosis. Elevated plasma TG are frequently found in a triad with low HDL-C levels and small LDL particles, as well as in association with non-lipid metabolic risk factors for coronary heart disease. As such, total plasma TG has not consistently been shown to be an independent risk factor for CHD. Furthermore, the independent effect of raising HDL or lowering TG on the risk of coronary and cardiovascular morbidity and mortality has not been determined.

In both normal volunteers and patients with hypercholesterolemia, treatment with PRAVACHOL reduced Total-C, LDL-C, and apolipoprotein B. PRAVACHOL also reduced VLDL-C and TG and produced increases in HDL-C and apolipoprotein A. The effects of pravastatin on Lp (a), fibrinogen, and certain other independent biochemical risk markers for coronary heart disease are unknown. Although pravastatin is relatively more hydrophilic than other HMG-CoA reductase inhibitors, the effect of relative hydrophilicity, if any, on either efficacy or safety has not been established.

In one primary (West of Scotland Coronary Prevention Study – WOS)[1] and two secondary (Long-term Intervention with Pravastatin in Ischemic Disease – LIPID[2] and the Cholesterol and Recurrent Events – CARE[3]) prevention studies, PRAVACHOL has been shown to reduce cardiovascular morbidity and mortality across a wide range of cholesterol levels (see **Clinical Studies**).

Pharmacokinetics/Metabolism

PRAVACHOL (pravastatin sodium) is administered orally in the active form. In clinical pharmacology studies in man, pravastatin is rapidly absorbed, with peak plasma levels of parent compound attained 1 to 1.5 hours following ingestion. Based on urinary recovery of radiolabeled drug, the average oral absorption of pravastatin is 34% and absolute bioavailability is 17%. While the presence of food in the gastrointestinal tract reduces systemic bioavailability, the lipid-lowering effects of the drug are similar whether taken with, or 1 hour prior, to meals.

Pravastatin undergoes extensive first-pass extraction in the liver (extraction ratio 0.66), which is its primary site of action, and the primary site of cholesterol synthesis and of LDL-C clearance. *In vitro* studies demonstrated that pravastatin is transported into hepatocytes with substantially less uptake into other cells. In view of pravastatin's apparently extensive first-pass hepatic metabolism, plasma levels may not necessarily correlate perfectly with lipid-lowering efficacy. Pravastatin plasma concentrations [including: area under the concentration-time curve (AUC), peak (C_{max}), and steady-state minimum (C_{min})] are directly proportional to administered dose. Systemic bioavailability of pravastatin administered following a bedtime dose was decreased 60% compared to that following an AM dose. Despite this decrease in systemic bioavailability, the efficacy of pravastatin administered once daily in the evening, although not statistically significant, was marginally more effective than that after a morning dose. This finding of lower systemic bioavailability suggests greater hepatic extraction of the drug following the evening dose. Steady-state AUCs, C_{max} and C_{min} plasma concentrations showed no evidence of pravastatin accumulation following once or twice daily administration of PRAVACHOL (pravastatin sodium) tablets. Approximately 50% of the circulating drug is bound to plasma proteins. Following single dose administration of ^{14}C-pravastatin, the elimination half-life ($t_{1/2}$) for total radioactivity (pravastatin plus metabolites) in humans is 77 hours.

Pravastatin, like other HMG-CoA reductase inhibitors, has variable bioavailability. The coefficient of variation, based on between-subject variability, was 50% to 60% for AUC.

Approximately 20% of a radiolabeled oral dose is excreted in urine and 70% in the feces. After intravenous administration of radiolabeled pravastatin to normal volunteers, approximately 47% of total body clearance was via renal excretion and 53% by non-renal routes (i.e., biliary excretion and biotransformation). Since there are dual routes of elimination, the potential exists both for compensatory excretion by the alternate route as well as for accumulation of drug and/or metabolites in patients with renal or hepatic insufficiency.

In a study comparing the kinetics of pravastatin in patients with biopsy confirmed cirrhosis (N=7) and normal subjects (N=7), the mean AUC varied 18-fold in cirrhotic patients and 5-fold in healthy subjects. Similarly, the peak pravastatin values varied 47-fold for cirrhotic patients compared to 6-fold for healthy subjects.

Biotransformation pathways elucidated for pravastatin include: (a) isomerization to 6-epi pravastatin and the 3α-hydroxyisomer of pravastatin (SQ 31,906), (b) enzymatic ring hydroxylation to SQ 31,945, (c) ω-1 oxidation of the ester side chain, (d) β-oxidation of the carboxy side chain, (e) ring oxidation followed by aromatization, (f) oxidation of a hydroxyl group to a keto group, and (g) conjugation. The major degradation product is the 3α-hydroxy isomeric metabolite, which has one-tenth to one-fortieth the HMG-CoA reductase inhibitory activity of the parent compound.

In a single oral dose study using pravastatin 20 mg, the mean AUC for pravastatin was approximately 27% greater and the mean cumulative urinary excretion (CUE) approximately 19% lower in elderly men (65 to 75 years old) compared with younger men (19 to 31 years old). In a similar study conducted in women, the mean AUC for pravastatin was approximately 46% higher and the mean CUE approximately 18% lower in elderly women (65 to 78 years old) compared with younger women (18 to 38 years old). In both studies, C_{max}, T_{max} and $t^{1/2}$ values were similar in older and younger subjects.

Clinical Studies

Prevention of Coronary Heart Disease

In the Pravastatin Primary Prevention Study (West of Scotland Coronary Prevention Study – WOS),[1] the effect of PRAVACHOL (pravastatin sodium) on fatal and nonfatal coronary heart disease (CHD) was assessed in 6595 men 45–64 years of age, without a previous myocardial infarction (MI), and with LDL-C levels between 156–254 mg/dL (4–6.7 mmol/L). In this randomized, double-blind, placebo-controlled study, patients were treated with standard care, including dietary advice, and either PRAVACHOL 40 mg daily (N=3302) or placebo (N=3293) and followed for a median duration of 4.8 years. Median (25th, 75th percentile) percent changes from baseline after 6 months of pravastatin treatment in Total C, LDL-C, TG, and HDL were -20.3 (-26.9, -11.7), -27.7 (-36.0, -16.9), -9.1 (-27.6, 12.5), and 6.7 (-2.1, 15.6), respectively.

Table 1 LIPID—Primary and Secondary Endpoints

Event	Pravastatin (N = 4512)	Placebo (N = 4502)	Risk Reduction	*P*-value
	Number (%) of Subjects			
Primary Endpoint				
CHD mortality	287 (6.4)	373 (8.3)	24%	0.0004
Secondary Endpoints				
Total mortality	498 (11.0)	633 (14.1)	23%	<0.0001
CHD mortality or non-fatal MI	557 (12.3)	715 (15.9)	24%	<0.0001
Myocardial revascularization procedures (CABG or PTCA)	584 (12.9)	706 (15.7)	20%	<0.0001
Stroke				
All-cause	169 (3.7)	204 (4.5)	19%	0.0477
Non-hemorrhagic	154 (3.4)	196 (4.4)	23%	0.0154
Cardiovasacular mortality	331 (7.3)	433 (9.6)	25%	<0.0001

Table 2 CARE—Primary and Secondary Endpoints

Event	Pravastatin (N = 2081)	Placebo (N = 2078)	Risk Reduction	*P*-value
	Number (%) of Subjects			
Primary Endpoint				
CHD mortality or nonfatal MI*	212 (10.2)	274 (13.2)	24%	0.003
Secondary Endpoints				
Myocardial revascularization procedures (CABG or PTCA)	294 (14.1)	391 (18.8)	27%	<0.001
Stroke or TIA	93 (4.5)	124 (6.0)	26%	0.029

* The risk reduction due to treatment with PRAVACHOL was consistent in both sexes.

PRAVACHOL significantly reduced the rate of first coronary events (either coronary heart disease (CHD) death or nonfatal MI) by 31% [248 events in the placebo group (CHD death=44, nonfatal MI=204) vs 174 events in the PRAVACHOL group (CHD death=31, nonfatal MI=143), p=0.0001 (see figure below)]. The risk reduction with PRAVACHOL was similar and significant throughout the entire range of baseline LDL cholesterol levels. This reduction was also similar and significant across the age range studied with a 40% risk reduction for patients younger than 55 years and a 27% risk reduction for patients 55 years and older. The Pravastatin Primary Prevention Study included only men and therefore it is not clear to what extent these data can be extrapolated to a similar population of female patients.

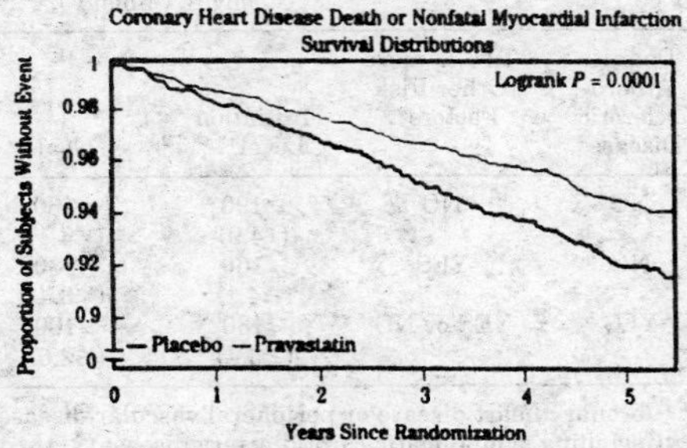

PRAVACHOL also significantly decreased the risk for undergoing myocardial revascularization procedures (coronary artery bypass graft [CABG] surgery or percutaneous transluminal coronary angioplasty [PTCA]) by 37% (80 vs 51 patients, p=0.009) and coronary angiography by 31% (128 vs 90, p=0.007). Cardiovascular deaths were decreased by 32% (73 vs 50, p=0.03) and there was no increase in death from non-cardiovascular causes.

Secondary Prevention of Cardiovascular Events

In the Long-term Intervention with Pravastatin in Ischemic Disease (LIPID)[2] study, the effect of PRAVACHOL, 40 mg daily, was assessed in 9014 patients (7498 men; 1516 women; 3514 elderly patients [age ≥65 years]; 782 diabetic patients) who had experienced either an MI (5754 patients) or had been hospitalized for unstable angina pectoris (3260 patients) in the preceding 3–36 months. Patients in this multicenter, double-blind, placebo-controlled study participated for an average of 5.6 years (median of 5.9 years) and at randomization had total cholesterol between 114 and 563 mg/dL (mean 219 mg/dL), LDL-C between 46 and 274 mg/dL (mean 150 mg/dL), triglycerides between 35 and 2710 mg/dL (mean 160 mg/dL), and HDL-C between 1 and 103 mg/dL (mean 37 mg/dL). At baseline, 82% of patients were receiving aspirin and 76% were receiving antihypertensive medication. Treatment with PRAVACHOL significantly reduced the risk for total mortality by reducing coronary death (see Table 1). The risk reduction due to treatment with PRAVACHOL on CHD mortality was consistent regardless of age. PRAVACHOL significantly reduced the risk for total mortality (by reducing CHD death) and CHD events (CHD mortality or nonfatal MI) in patients who qualified with a history of either MI or hospitalization for unstable angina pectoris.

[See table 1 above]

In the Cholesterol and Recurrent Events (CARE)[3] study the effect of PRAVACHOL, 40 mg daily, on coronary heart disease death and nonfatal MI was assessed in 4159 patients (3583 men and 576 women) who had experienced a myocardial infarction in the preceding 3–20 months and who had normal (below the 75th percentile of the general population) plasma total cholesterol levels. Patients in this double-blind, placebo controlled study participated for an average of 4.9 years and had a mean baseline total cholesterol of 209 mg/dL. LDL cholesterol levels in this patient population ranged from 101 mg/dL–180 mg/dL (mean = 139 mg/dL). At baseline, 84% of patients were receiving aspirin and 82% were taking antihypertensive medications. Median (25th, 75th percentile) percent changes from baseline after 6 months of pravastatin treatment in Total C, LDL-C, TG, and HDL were -22.0 (-28.4, -14.9), -32.4 (-39.9, -23.7), -11.0 (-26.5, 8.6), and 5.1 (-2.9, 12.7), respectively. Treatment with PRAVACHOL significantly reduced the rate of first recurrent coronary events (either CHD death or nonfatal MI), the risk of undergoing revascularization procedures (PTCA, CABG), and the risk for stroke or transient ischemic attack (TIA) (see Table 2).

[See table 2 above]

In the Pravastatin Limitation of Atherosclerosis in the Coronary Arteries (PLAC I)[4] study, the effect of pravastatin therapy on coronary atherosclerosis was assessed by coronary angiography in patients with coronary disease and moderate hypercholesterolemia (baseline LDL-C range = 130–190 mg/dL). In this double-blind, multicenter, controlled clinical trial angiograms were evaluated at baseline and at three years in 264 patients. Although the difference between pravastatin and placebo for the primary endpoint (per-patient change in mean coronary artery diameter) and one of two secondary endpoints (change in percent lumen diameter stenosis) did not reach statistical significance, for the secondary endpoint of change in minimum lumen diameter, statistically significant slowing of disease was seen in the pravastatin treatment group (p=0.02).

In the Regression Growth Evaluation Statin Study (REGRESS)[5], the effect of pravastatin on coronary atherosclerosis was assessed by coronary angiography in 885 patients with angina pectoris, angiographically documented coronary artery disease and hypercholesterolemia (baseline total cholesterol range = 160–310 mg/dL). In this double-blind, multicenter, controlled clinical trial, angiograms were evaluated at baseline and at two years in 653 patients (323 treated with pravastatin). Progression of coronary atherosclerosis was significantly slowed in the pravastatin group as assessed by changes in mean segment diameter (p=0.037) and minimum obstruction diameter (p=0.001).

Analysis of pooled events from PLAC I, the Pravastatin, Lipids and Atherosclerosis in the Carotids Study (PLAC II)[6], REGRESS, and the Kuopio Atherosclerosis Prevention Study (KAPS)[7] (combined N=1891) showed that treatment with pravastatin was associated with a statistically significant reduction in the composite event rate of fatal and nonfatal myocardial infarction (46 events or 6.4% for placebo versus 21 events or 2.4% for pravastatin, p=0.001). The predominant effect of pravastatin was to reduce the rate of nonfatal myocardial infarction.

Primary Hypercholesterolemia (Fredrickson Type IIa and IIb)

PRAVACHOL (pravastatin sodium) is highly effective in reducing Total-C, LDL-C and Triglycerides (TG) in patients with heterozygous familial, presumed familial combined and non-familial (non-FH) forms of primary hypercholesterolemia, and mixed dyslipidemia. A therapeutic response is seen within 1 week, and the maximum response usually is achieved within 4 weeks. This response is maintained during extended periods of therapy. In addition, PRAVACHOL

Continued on next page

Pravachol—Cont.

is effective in reducing the risk of acute coronary events in hypercholesterolemic patients with and without previous myocardial infarction.

A single daily dose is as effective as the same total daily dose given twice a day. In multicenter, double-blind, placebo-controlled studies of patients with primary hypercholesterolemia, treatment with pravastatin in daily doses ranging from 10 mg to 40 mg consistently and significantly decreased Total-C, LDL-C, TG, and Total-C/HDL-C and LDL-C/HDL-C ratios; modestly decreased VLDL-C and produced variable increases in HDL-C.

Primary Hypercholesterolemia Study
Dose Response of PRAVACHOL*
Once Daily Administration At Bedtime

Dose	Total-C	LDL-C	HDL-C	TG
10 mg	−16%	−22%	+ 7%	−15%
20 mg	−24%	−32%	+ 2%	−11%
40 mg	−25%	−34%	+12%	−24%

*Mean percent change from baseline after 8 weeks

In another clinical trial, patients treated with pravastatin in combination with cholestyramine (70% of patients were taking cholestyramine 20 or 24 g per day) had reductions equal to or greater than 50% in LDL-C. Furthermore, pravastatin attenuated cholestyramine-induced increases in TG levels (which are themselves of uncertain clinical significance).

Hypertriglyceridemia (Fredrickson Type IV)

The response to pravastatin in patients with Type IV hyperlipidemia (baseline TG > 200 mg/dL and LDL-C < 160 mg/dL) was evaluated in a subset of 429 patients from the Cholesterol and Recurrent Events (CARE) study. For pravastatin-treated subjects, the median (min, max) baseline triglyceride level was 246.0 (200.5, 349.5) mg/dL. [See first table above]

Dysbetalipoproteinemia (Fredrickson Type III)

The response to pravastatin in two double-blind crossover studies of 46 patients with genotype E2/E2 and Fredrickson Type III dysbetalipoproteinemia is shown in the table below. [See second table above]

Patients With Fredrickson Type IV Hyperlipidemia
Median (25th,75th percentile) Percent Change From Baseline

	Pravastatin 40 mg (N=429)	Placebo (N=430)
Triglycerides	−21.1 (−34.8, 1.3)	−6.3 (−23.1, 18.3)
Total-C	−22.1 (−27.1, −14.8)	0.2 (−6.9, 6.8)
LDL-C	−31.7 (−39.6, −21.5)	0.7 (−9.0, 10.0)
HDL-C	7.4 (−1.2, 17.7)	2.8 (−5.7, 11.7)
Non-HDL-C	−27.2 (−34.0, −18.5)	−0.8 (−8.2, 7.0)

Patients With Fredrickson Type III Dysbetalipoproteinemia
Median (min, max) Percent Change From Baseline

	Median (min, max) at Baseline (mg/dL)	Median % Change (min, max) Pravastatin 40 mg (N=20)
Study 1		
Total-C	386.5 (245.0, 672.0)	−32.7 (−58.5, 4.6)
Triglycerides	443.0 (275.0, 1299.0)	−23.7 (−68.5, 44.7)
VLDL-C*	206.5 (110.0, 379.0)	−43.8 (−73.1, −14.3)
LDL-C*	117.5 (80.0, 170.0)	−40.8 (−63.7, 4.6)
HDL-C	30.0 (18.0, 88.0)	6.4 (−45.0, 105.6)
Non-HDL-C	344.5 (215.0, 646.0)	−36.7 (−66.3, 5.8)
*N=14		
	Median (min, max) at Baseline (mg/dL)	**Median % Change (min, max) Pravastatin 40 mg (N=26)**
Study 2		
Total-C	340.3 (230.1, 448.6)	−31.4 (−54.5, −13.0)
Triglycerides	343.2 (212.6, 845.9)	−11.9 (−56.5, 44.8)
VLDL-C	145.0 (71.5, 309.4)	−35.7 (−74.7, 19.1)
LDL-C	128.6 (63.8, 177.9)	−30.3 (−52.2, 13.5)
HDL-C	38.7 (27.1, 58.0)	5.0 (−17.7, 66.7)
Non-HDL-C	295.8 (195.3, 421.5)	−35.5 (−81.0, −13.5)

INDICATIONS AND USAGE

Therapy with PRAVACHOL (pravastatin sodium) should be considered in those individuals at increased risk for atherosclerosis-related clinical events as a function of cholesterol level, the presence or absence of coronary heart disease, and other risk factors.

Primary Prevention of Coronary Events

In hypercholesterolemic patients without clinically evident coronary heart disease, PRAVACHOL (pravastatin sodium) is indicated to:

- Reduce the risk of myocardial infarction
- Reduce the risk of undergoing myocardial revascularization procedures
- Reduce the risk of cardiovascular mortality with no increase in death from non-cardiovascular causes

Secondary Prevention of Cardiovascular Events

In patients with clinically evident coronary heart disease, PRAVACHOL is indicated to:

- Reduce the risk of total mortality by reducing coronary death
- Reduce the risk of myocardial infarction
- Reduce the risk of undergoing myocardial revascularization procedures
- Reduce the risk of stroke and stroke/transient ischemic attack (TIA)
- Slow the progression of coronary atherosclerosis

Hyperlipidemia

PRAVACHOL is indicated as an adjunct to diet to reduce elevated Total-C, LDL-C, Apo B, and TG levels and to increase HDL-C in patients with primary hypercholesterolemia and mixed dyslipidemia (Fredrickson Type IIa and IIb).[8]

PRAVACHOL is indicated as adjunctive therapy to diet for the treatment of patients with elevated serum triglyceride levels (Fredrickson Type IV).

PRAVACHOL is indicated for the treatment of patients with primary dysbetalipoproteinemia (Fredrickson Type III) who do not respond adequately to diet.

Lipid-altering agents should be used in addition to a diet restricted in saturated fat and cholesterol when the response to diet and other nonpharmacological measures alone has been inadequate (see NCEP Guidelines below).

Prior to initiating therapy with pravastatin, secondary causes for hypercholesterolemia (e.g., poorly controlled diabetes mellitus, hypothyroidism, nephrotic syndrome, dysproteinemias, obstructive liver disease, other drug therapy, alcoholism) should be excluded, and a lipid profile performed to measure Total-C, HDL-C, and TG. For patients with triglycerides (TG) <400 mg/dL (<4.5 mmol/L), LDL-C can be estimated using the following equation:

$$\text{LDL-C} = \text{Total-C} - \text{HDL-C} - \tfrac{1}{5}\,\text{TG}$$

For TG levels >400 mg/dL (>4.5 mmol/L), this equation is less accurate and LDL-C concentrations should be determined by ultracentrifugation. In many hypertriglyceridemic patients, LDL-C may be low or normal despite elevated Total-C. In such cases, HMG-CoA reductase inhibitors are not indicated.

Lipid determinations should be performed at intervals of no less than four weeks and dosage adjusted according to the patient's response to therapy.

The National Cholesterol Education Program's Treatment Guidelines are summarized below:

Definite Athero-sclerotic Disease*	Two or more Other Risk Factors**	LDL Cholesterol mg/dL (mmol/L) Initiation Level***	Goal
NO	NO	≥190 (>4.9)	<160 (<4.1)
NO	YES	≥160 (≥4.1)	<130 (<3.4)
YES	YES or NO	≥130 (≥3.4)	≤100 (≤2.6)

* Coronary heart disease or peripheral vascular disease (including symptomatic carotid artery disease).

** Other risk factors for coronary heart disease (CHD) include: age (males: ≥45 years; females: ≥55 years or premature menopause without estrogen replacement therapy); family history of premature CHD; current cigarette smoking; hypertension; confirmed HDL-C <35 mg/dL (<0.91 mmol/L); and diabetes mellitus. Subtract one risk factor if HDL-C is ≥60 mg/dL (≥1.6 mmol/L).

*** In CHD patients with LDL-C levels 100–129 mg/dL, the physician should exercise clinical judgement in deciding whether to initiate drug treatment.

At the time of hospitalization for an acute coronary event, consideration can be given to initiating drug therapy at discharge if the LDL-C is ≥130 mg/dL (see NCEP Guidelines, above).

Since the goal of treatment is to lower LDL-C, the NCEP recommends that LDL-C levels be used to initiate and assess treatment response. Only if LDL-C levels are not available, should the Total-C be used to monitor therapy.

As with other lipid-lowering therapy, PRAVACHOL (pravastatin sodium) is not indicated when hypercholesterolemia is due to hyperalphalipoproteinemia (elevated HDL-C).

CONTRAINDICATIONS

Hypersensitivity to any component of this medication.

Active liver disease or unexplained, persistent elevations in liver function tests (see **WARNINGS**).

Pregnancy and lactation. Atherosclerosis is a chronic process and discontinuation of lipid-lowering drugs during pregnancy should have little impact on the outcome of long-term therapy of primary hypercholesterolemia. Cholesterol and other products of cholesterol biosynthesis are essential components for fetal development (including synthesis of steroids and cell membranes). Since HMG-CoA reductase inhibitors decrease cholesterol synthesis and possibly the synthesis of other biologically active substances derived from cholesterol, they are contraindicated during pregnancy and in nursing mothers. **Pravastatin should be administered to women of childbearing age only when such patients are highly unlikely to conceive and have been informed of the potential hazards.** If the patient becomes pregnant while taking this class of drug, therapy should be discontinued immediately and the patient apprised of the potential hazard to the fetus (see **PRECAUTIONS: Pregnancy**).

WARNINGS

Liver Enzymes

HMG-CoA reductase inhibitors, like some other lipid-lowering therapies, have been associated with biochemical abnormalities of liver function. Increases of serum transaminase (ALT, AST) values to more than 3 times the upper limit of normal occurring on 2 or more (not necessarily sequential) occasions have been reported in 1.3% of patients treated with pravastatin in the US over an average period of 18 months. These abnormalities were not associated with cholestasis and did not appear to be related to treatment duration. In those patients in whom these abnormalities were believed to be related to pravastatin and who were discontinued from therapy, the transaminase levels usually fell slowly to pretreatment levels. These biochemical findings are usually asymptomatic although worldwide experience indicates that anorexia, weakness, and/or abdominal pain may also be present in rare patients.

In the largest long-term placebo-controlled clinical trial with pravastatin (Pravastatin Primary Prevention Study; see **CLINICAL PHARMACOLOGY**), the overall incidence of AST and/or ALT elevations to greater than three times the upper limit of normal was 1.05% in the pravastatin group as compared to 0.75% in the placebo group. One (0.03%) pravastatin-treated patient and 2 (0.06%) placebo-treated patients were discontinued because of transaminase elevations. Of the patients with normal liver function at week 12, three of 2875 treated with pravastatin (0.10%) and one of the 2919 placebo patients (0.03%) had elevations of AST greater than three times the upper limit of normal on two consecutive measurements and/or discontinued due to elevations in transaminase levels during the 4.8 years (median treatment) of the study.

It is recommended that liver function tests be performed prior to and at 12 weeks following initiation of therapy or the elevation of dose. Patients who develop increased transaminase levels or signs and symptoms of liver disease should be monitored with a second liver function evaluation to confirm the finding and be followed thereafter with frequent liver function tests until the abnormality(ies) return to normal. Should an increase in AST or ALT of three times the upper limit of normal or greater persist, withdrawal of pravastatin therapy is recommended.

Active liver disease or unexplained transaminase elevations are contraindications to the use of pravastatin (see **CONTRAINDICATIONS**). Caution should be exercised when pravastatin is administered to patients with a history of liver disease or heavy alcohol ingestion (see **CLINICAL PHARMACOLOGY: Pharmacokinetics/Metabolism**). Such patients should be closely monitored, started at the lower end of the recommended dosing range, and titrated to the desired therapeutic effect.

Skeletal Muscle

Rare cases of rhabdomyolysis with acute renal failure secondary to myoglobinuria have been reported with pravastatin and other drugs in this class. Uncomplicated myalgia has also been reported in pravastatin-treated patients (see **ADVERSE REACTIONS**). Myopathy, defined as muscle aching or muscle weakness in conjunction with increases in creatine phosphokinase (CPK) values to greater than 10 times the upper normal limit, was rare (<0.1%) in pravastatin clinical trials. Myopathy should be considered in any patient with diffuse myalgias, muscle tenderness or weakness, and/or marked elevation of CPK. Patients should be advised to report promptly unexplained muscle pain, tenderness or weakness, particularly if accompanied by malaise or fever. **Pravastatin therapy should be discontinued if markedly elevated CPK levels occur or myopathy is diagnosed or suspected. Pravastatin therapy should also be temporarily withheld in any patient experiencing an acute or serious condition predisposing to the development of renal failure secondary to rhabdomyolysis, e.g., sepsis; hypotension; major surgery; trauma; severe metabolic, endocrine, or electrolyte disorders; or uncontrolled epilepsy.**

The risk of myopathy during treatment with another HMG-CoA reductase inhibitor is increased with concurrent therapy with either erythromycin, cyclosporine, niacin, or fibrates. However, neither myopathy nor significant increases in CPK levels have been observed in three reports involving a total of 100 post-transplant patients (24 renal and 76 cardiac) treated for up to two years concurrently with pravastatin 10–40 mg and cyclosporine. Some of these patients also received other concomitant immunosuppressive therapies. Further, in clinical trials involving small numbers of patients who were treated concurrently with pravastatin and niacin, there were no reports of myopathy. Also, myopathy was not reported in a trial of combination pravastatin (40 mg/day) and gemfibrozil (1200 mg/day), although 4 of 75 patients on the combination showed marked CPK elevations versus one of 73 patients receiving placebo. There was a trend toward more frequent CPK elevations and patient withdrawals due to musculoskeletal symptoms in the group receiving combined treatment as compared with the groups receiving placebo, gemfibrozil, or pravastatin monotherapy (see **PRECAUTIONS: Drug Interactions**). **The use of fibrates alone may occasionally be associated with myopathy. The combined use of pravastatin and fibrates should be avoided unless the benefit of further alterations in lipid levels is likely to outweigh the increased risk of this drug combination.**

PRECAUTIONS

General

PRAVACHOL (pravastatin sodium) may elevate creatine phosphokinase and transaminase levels (see **ADVERSE REACTIONS**). This should be considered in the differential diagnosis of chest pain in a patient on therapy with pravastatin.

Homozygous Familial Hypercholesterolemia. Pravastatin has not been evaluated in patients with rare homozygous familial hypercholesterolemia. In this group of patients, it has been reported that HMG-CoA reductase inhibitors are less effective because the patients lack functional LDL receptors.

Renal Insufficiency. A single 20 mg oral dose of pravastatin was administered to 24 patients with varying degrees of renal impairment (as determined by creatinine clearance). No effect was observed on the pharmacokinetics of pravastatin or its 3α-hydroxy isomeric metabolite (SQ 31,906). A small increase was seen in mean AUC values and half-life (t½) for the inactive enzymatic ring hydroxylation metabolite (SQ 31,945). Given this small sample size, the dosage administered, and the degree of individual variability, patients with renal impairment who are receiving pravastatin should be closely monitored.

Information for Patients

Patients should be advised to report promptly unexplained muscle pain, tenderness or weakness, particularly if accompanied by malaise or fever (see **WARNINGS: Skeletal Muscle**).

Drug Interactions

Immunosuppressive Drugs, Gemfibrozil, Niacin (Nicotinic Acid), Erythromycin: See **WARNINGS: Skeletal Muscle.**

Cytochrome P450 3A4 Inhibitors: In vitro and *in vivo* data indicate that pravastatin is not metabolized by cytochrome P450 3A4 to a clinically significant extent. This has been shown in studies with known cytochrome P450 3A4 inhibitors (see diltiazem and itraconazole below). Other examples of cytochrome P450 3A4 inhibitors include ketoconazole, mibefradil, and erythromycin.

Diltiazem—Steady-state levels of diltiazem (a known, weak inhibitor of P450 3A4) had no effect on the pharmacokinetics of pravastatin. In this study, the AUC and C_{max} of another HMG-CoA reductase inhibitor which is known to be metabolized by cytochrome P450 3A4 increased by factors of 3.6 and 4.3, respectively.

Itraconazole—The mean AUC and C_{max} for pravastatin were increased by factors of 1.7 and 2.5, respectively, when given with itraconazole (a potent P450 3A4 inhibitor which also inhibits p-glycoprotein transport) as compared to placebo. The mean t½ was not affected by itraconazole, suggesting that the relatively small increases in C_{max} and AUC were due solely to increased bioavailability rather than a decrease in clearance, consistent with inhibition of p-glycoprotein transport by itraconazole. This drug transport system is thought to affect bioavailability and excretion of HMG-CoA reductase inhibitors, including pravastatin. The AUC and C_{max} of another HMG-CoA reductase inhibitor which is known to be metabolized by cytochrome P450 3A4 increased by factors of 19 and 17, respectively, when given with itraconazole.

Antipyrine: Since concomitant administration of pravastatin had no effect on the clearance of antipyrine, interactions with other drugs metabolized via the same hepatic cytochrome isozymes are not expected.

Cholestyramine/Colestipol: Concomitant administration resulted in an approximately 40 to 50% decrease in the mean AUC of pravastatin. However, when pravastatin was administered 1 hour before or 4 hours after cholestyramine or 1 hour before colestipol and a standard meal, there was no clinically significant decrease in bioavailability or therapeutic effect. (See **DOSAGE AND ADMINISTRATION: Concomitant Therapy.**)

Warfarin: Pravastatin had no clinically significant effect on prothrombin time when administered in a study to normal elderly subjects who were stabilized on warfarin.

Cimetidine: The $AUC_{0-12\ hr}$ for pravastatin when given with cimetidine was not significantly different from the AUC for pravastatin when given alone. A significant difference was observed between the AUC's for pravastatin when given with cimetidine compared to when administered with antacid.

Digoxin: In a crossover trial involving 18 healthy male subjects given pravastatin and digoxin concurrently for 9 days, the bioavailability parameters of digoxin were not affected. The AUC of pravastatin tended to increase, but the overall bioavailability of pravastatin plus its metabolites SQ 31,906 and SQ 31,945 was not altered.

Cyclosporine: Some investigators have measured cyclosporine levels in patients on pravastatin, and to date, these results indicate no clinically meaningful elevations in cyclosporine levels. In one single-dose study, pravastatin levels were found to be increased in cardiac transplant patients receiving cyclosporine.

Gemfibrozil: In a crossover study in 20 healthy male volunteers given concomitant single doses of pravastatin and gemfibrozil, there was a significant decrease in urinary excretion and protein binding of pravastatin. In addition, there was a significant increase in AUC, C_{max}, and T_{max} for the pravastatin metabolite SQ 31,906. Combination therapy with pravastatin and gemfibrozil is generally not recommended.

In interaction studies with *aspirin, antacids* (1 hour prior to PRAVACHOL), *cimetidine, nicotinic acid*, or *probucol*, no statistically significant differences in bioavailability were seen when PRAVACHOL (pravastatin sodium) was administered.

Endocrine Function

HMG-CoA reductase inhibitors interfere with cholesterol synthesis and lower circulating cholesterol levels and, as such, might theoretically blunt adrenal or gonadal steroid hormone production. Results of clinical trials with pravastatin in males and post-menopausal females were inconsistent with regard to possible effects of the drug on basal steroid hormone levels. In a study of 21 males, the mean testosterone response to human chorionic gonadotropin was significantly reduced ($p<0.004$) after 16 weeks of treatment with 40 mg of pravastatin. However, the percentage of patients showing a ≥50% rise in plasma testosterone after human chorionic gonadotropin stimulation did not change significantly after therapy in these patients. The effects of HMG-CoA reductase inhibitors on spermatogenesis and fertility have not been studied in adequate numbers of patients. The effects, if any, of pravastatin on the pituitary-gonadal axis in pre-menopausal females are unknown. Patients treated with pravastatin who display clinical evidence of endocrine dysfunction should be evaluated appropriately. Caution should also be exercised if an HMG-CoA reductase inhibitor or other agent used to lower cholesterol levels is administered to patients also receiving other drugs (e.g., ketoconazole, spironolactone, cimetidine) that may diminish the levels or activity of steroid hormones.

CNS Toxicity

CNS vascular lesions, characterized by perivascular hemorrhage and edema and mononuclear cell infiltration of perivascular spaces, were seen in dogs treated with pravastatin at a dose of 25 mg/kg/day, a dose that produced a plasma drug level about 50 times higher than the mean drug level in humans taking 40 mg/day. Similar CNS vascular lesions have been observed with several other drugs in this class.

A chemically similar drug in this class produced optic nerve degeneration (Wallerian degeneration of retinogeniculate fibers) in clinically normal dogs in a dose-dependent fashion starting at 60 mg/kg/day, a dose that produced mean plasma drug levels about 30 times higher than the mean drug level in humans taking the highest recommended dose (as measured by total enzyme inhibitory activity). This same drug also produced vestibulocochlear Wallerian-like degeneration and retinal ganglion cell chromatolysis in dogs treated for 14 weeks at 180 mg/kg/day, a dose which resulted in a mean plasma drug level similar to that seen with the 60 mg/kg/day dose.

Carcinogenesis, Mutagenesis, Impairment of Fertility

In a 2-year study in rats fed pravastatin at doses of 10, 30, or 100 mg/kg body weight, there was an increased incidence of hepatocellular carcinomas in males at the highest dose ($p<0.01$). Although rats were given up to 125 times the human dose (HD) on a mg/kg body weight basis, serum drug levels were only 6 to 10 times higher than those measured in humans given 40 mg pravastatin as measured by AUC. In a 2-year study in mice fed pravastatin at doses of 250 and 500 mg/kg/day, there was an increased incidence of hepatocellular carcinomas in males and females at both 250 and 500 mg/kg/day ($p<0.0001$). At these doses, lung adenomas in females were increased ($p=0.013$). Serum drug levels were 30 to 40 times (250 mg/kg/day) and 50 times (500 mg/kg/day) that of humans given 40 mg pravastatin, as measured by AUC. In another 2-year study in mice with doses at up to 100 mg/kg/day (producing plasma drug levels up to 5 times human drug levels at 40 mg), there were no drug-induced tumors.

No evidence of mutagenicity was observed *in vitro*, with or without rat-liver metabolic activation, in the following studies: microbial mutagen tests, using mutant strains of *Salmonella typhimurium* or *Escherichia coli*; a forward mutation assay in L5178Y TK +/− mouse lymphoma cells; a chromosomal aberration test in hamster cells; and a gene conversion assay using *Saccharomyces cerevisiae*. In addition, there was no evidence of mutagenicity in either a dominant lethal test in mice or a micronucleus test in mice.

In a study in rats, with daily doses up to 500 mg/kg, pravastatin did not produce any adverse effects on fertility or general reproductive performance. However, in a study with another HMG-CoA reductase inhibitor, there was decreased fertility in male rats treated for 34 weeks at 25 mg/kg body weight, although this effect was not observed in a subsequent fertility study when this same dose was administered for 11 weeks (the entire cycle of spermatogenesis, including epididymal maturation). In rats treated with this same reductase inhibitor at 180 mg/kg/day, seminiferous tubule degeneration (necrosis and loss of spermatogenic epithelium) was observed. Although not seen with pravastatin, two similar drugs in this class caused drug-related testicular atrophy, decreased spermatogenesis, spermatocytic degeneration, and giant cell formation in dogs. The clinical significance of these findings is unclear.

Pregnancy

Pregnancy Category X.

See **CONTRAINDICATIONS**.

Safety in pregnant women has not been established. Pravastatin was not teratogenic in rats at doses up to 1000 mg/kg daily or in rabbits at doses of up to 50 mg/kg daily. These doses resulted in 20x (rabbit) or 240x (rat) the human exposure based on surface area (mg/meter^2). Rare reports of congenital anomalies have been received following intrauterine exposure to other HMG-CoA reductase inhibitors. In a review[9] of approximately 100 prospectively followed pregnancies in women exposed to simvastatin or lovastatin, the incidences of congenital anomalies, spontaneous abortions and fetal deaths/stillbirths did not exceed what would be expected in the general population. The number of cases is adequate only to exclude a three-to-four-fold increase in congenital anomalies over the background incidence. In 89% of the prospectively followed pregnancies, drug treatment was initiated prior to pregnancy and was discontinued at some point in the first trimester when pregnancy was identified. As safety in pregnant women has not been established and there is no apparent benefit to therapy with PRAVACHOL during pregnancy (see **CONTRAINDICATIONS**), treatment should be immediately discontinued as soon as pregnancy is recognized. PRAVACHOL (pravastatin sodium) should be administered to women of child-bearing potential only when such patients are highly unlikely to conceive and have been informed of the potential hazards.

Nursing Mothers

A small amount of pravastatin is excreted in human breast milk. Because of the potential for serious adverse reactions in nursing infants, women taking PRAVACHOL should not nurse (see **CONTRAINDICATIONS**).

Pediatric Use

Safety and effectiveness in individuals less than 18 years old have not been established. Hence, treatment in patients less than 18 years old is not recommended at this time.

Geriatric Use

Two secondary prevention trials with pravastatin (CARE and LIPID) included a total of 6,593 subjects treated with pravastatin 40 mg for periods ranging up to 6 years. Across these two studies, 36.1% of pravastatin subjects were aged 65 and older and 0.8% were aged 75 and older. The beneficial effect of pravastatin in elderly subjects in reducing cardiovascular events and in modifying lipid profiles was similar to that seen in younger subjects. The adverse event profile in the elderly was similar to that in the overall population. Other reported clinical experience has not identified differences in responses to pravastatin between elderly and younger patients.

Mean pravastatin AUCs are slightly (25–50%) higher in elderly subjects than in healthy young subjects, but mean C_{max}, T_{max} and $t^{1/2}$ values are similar in both age groups and substantial accumulation of pravastatin would not be expected in the elderly (see **CLINICAL PHARMACOLOGY: Pharmacokinetics/Metabolism**).

ADVERSE REACTIONS

Pravastatin is generally well tolerated; adverse reactions have usually been mild and transient. In 4-month long placebo-controlled trials, 1.7% of pravastatin-treated patients and 1.2% of placebo-treated patients were discontinued from treatment because of adverse experiences attributed to study drug therapy; this difference was not statistically significant. In long-term studies, the most common reasons for discontinuation were asymptomatic serum transaminase increases and mild, non-specific gastrointestinal complaints. (See also **PRECAUTIONS: Geriatric Use** section).

Continued on next page

Pravachol—Cont.

Adverse Clinical Events
All adverse clinical events (regardless of attribution) reported in more than 2% of pravastatin-treated patients in the placebo-controlled trials are identified in the table below; also shown are the percentages of patients in whom these medical events were believed to be related or possibly related to the drug:
[See table below]
In three large, placebo-controlled trials (West of Scotland Coronary Prevention study [WOS], Cholesterol and Recurrent Events study [CARE], and Long-term Intervention with Pravastatin in Ischemic Disease study [LIPID]) involving a total of 19,768 patients treated with PRAVACHOL (N=9895) or placebo (N=9873), the safety and tolerability profile in the pravastatin group was comparable to that of the placebo group over the median 4.8 to 5.9 years of follow-up.
The following effects have been reported with drugs in this class; not all the effects listed below have necessarily been associated with pravastatin therapy:
Skeletal: myopathy, rhabdomyolysis, arthralgia.
Neurological: dysfunction of certain cranial nerves (including alteration of taste, impairment of extra-ocular movement, facial paresis), tremor, vertigo, memory loss, paresthesia, peripheral neuropathy, peripheral nerve palsy, anxiety, insomnia, depression.
Hypersensitivity Reactions: An apparent hypersensitivity syndrome has been reported rarely which has included one or more of the following features: anaphylaxis, angioedema, lupus erythematous-like syndrome, polymyalgia rheumatica, dermatomyositis, vasculitis, purpura, thrombocytopenia, leukopenia, hemolytic anemia, positive ANA, ESR increase, eosinophilia, arthritis, arthralgia, urticaria, asthenia, photosensitivity, fever, chills, flushing, malaise, dyspnea, toxic epidermal necrolysis, erythema multiforme, including Stevens-Johnson syndrome.
Gastrointestinal: pancreatitis, hepatitis, including chronic active hepatitis, cholestatic jaundice, fatty change in liver, and, rarely, cirrhosis, fulminant hepatic necrosis, and hepatoma; anorexia, vomiting.
Skin: alopecia, pruritus. A variety of skin changes (e.g., nodules, discoloration, dryness of skin/mucous membranes, changes to hair/nails) have been reported.
Reproductive: gynecomastia, loss of libido, erectile dysfunction.
Eye: progression of cataracts (lens opacities), ophthalmoplegia.
Laboratory Abnormalities: elevated transaminases, alkaline phosphatase, and bilirubin; thyroid function abnormalities.

Laboratory Test Abnormalities
Increases in serum transaminase (ALT, AST) values and CPK have been observed (see **WARNINGS**).
Transient, asymptomatic eosinophilia has been reported. Eosinophil counts usually returned to normal despite continued therapy. Anemia, thrombocytopenia, and leukopenia have been reported with HMG-CoA reductase inhibitors.

Concomitant Therapy
Pravastatin has been administered concurrently with cholestyramine, colestipol, nicotinic acid, probucol and gemfibrozil. Preliminary data suggest that the addition of either probucol or gemfibrozil to therapy with lovastatin or pravastatin is not associated with greater reduction in LDL-cholesterol than that achieved with lovastatin or pravastatin alone. No adverse reactions unique to the combination or in addition to those previously reported for each drug alone have been reported. Myopathy and rhabdomyolysis (with or without acute renal failure) have been reported when another HMG-CoA reductase inhibitor was used in combination with immunosuppressive drugs, gemfibrozil, erythromycin, or lipid-lowering doses of nicotinic acid. Concomitant therapy with HMG-CoA reductase inhibitors and these agents is generally not recommended. (See **WARNINGS: Skeletal Muscle** and **PRECAUTIONS: Drug Interactions.**)

OVERDOSAGE
To date, there are two reported cases of overdosage with pravastatin, both of which were asymptomatic and not associated with clinical laboratory abnormalities. If an overdose occurs, it should be treated symptomatically and supportive measures should be instituted as required.

DOSAGE AND ADMINISTRATION
The patient should be placed on a standard cholesterol-lowering diet before receiving PRAVACHOL (pravastatin sodium) and should continue on this diet during treatment with PRAVACHOL (see NCEP Treatment Guidelines for details on dietary therapy).
The recommended starting dose is 10, 20 or 40 mg once daily. PRAVACHOL can be administered as a single dose at any time of the day, with or without food. In patients with a history of significant renal or hepatic dysfunction, a starting dose of 10 mg daily is recommended.
Since the maximal effect of a given dose is seen within 4 weeks, periodic lipid determinations should be performed at this time and dosage adjusted according to the patient's response to therapy and established treatment guidelines.
In patients taking immunosuppressive drugs such as cyclosporine (see **WARNINGS: Skeletal Muscle**) concomitantly with pravastatin, therapy should begin with 10 mg of pravastatin once-a-day at bedtime and titration to higher doses should be done with caution. Most patients treated with this combination received a maximum pravastatin dose of 20 mg/day.

Concomitant Therapy
The lipid-lowering effects of PRAVACHOL on total and LDL cholesterol are enhanced when combined with a bile-acid-binding resin. When administering a bile-acid-binding resin (e.g., cholestyramine, colestipol) and pravastatin, PRAVACHOL should be given either 1 hour or more before or at least 4 hours following the resin. See also **ADVERSE REACTIONS: Concomitant Therapy.**

HOW SUPPLIED
PRAVACHOL® (pravastatin sodium) Tablets are supplied as:
10 mg tablets: Pink to peach, rounded, rectangular-shaped, biconvex with a P embossed on one side and PRAVACHOL 10 engraved on the opposite side. They are supplied in bottles of 90 (NDC 0003-5154-05). Bottles contain a desiccant canister.
20 mg tablets: Yellow, rounded, rectangular-shaped, biconvex with a P embossed on one side and PRAVACHOL 20 engraved on the opposite side. They are supplied in bottles of 90 (NDC 0003-5178-05) and bottles of 1000 (NDC 0003-5178-75). Bottles contain a desiccant canister.
40 mg tablets: Green, rounded, rectangular-shaped, biconvex with a P embossed on one side and PRAVACHOL 40 engraved on the opposite side. They are supplied in bottles of 90 (NDC 0003-5194-10). Bottles contain a desiccant canister.
Unimatic® unit-dose packs containing 100 tablets are also available for the **20 mg** (NDC 0003-5178-06) potency.

Storage
Do not store above 86° F (30° C). Keep tightly closed (protect from moisture). Protect from light.

REFERENCES
1. Shepherd J, et al. Prevention of coronary heart disease with pravastatin in men with hypercholesterolemia (WOS). *N Engl J Med* 1995;333:1301–7.
2. The Long-term Intervention with Pravastatin in Ischemic Disease Group. Prevention of cardiovascular events and death with pravastatin in patients with coronary heart disease and a broad range of initial cholesterol levels (LIPID). *N Engl J Med* 1998;339:1349–1357.
3. Sacks FM, et al. The effect of pravastatin on coronary events after myocardial infarction in patients with average cholesterol levels (CARE). *N Engl J Med.* 1996;335:1001–9.
4. Pitt B, et al. Pravastatin Limitation of Atherosclerosis in the Coronary Arteries (PLAC I): Reduction in Atherosclerosis Progression and Clinical Events. *J Am Coll Cardiol* 1995;26:1133–9.
5. Jukema JW, et al. Effects of Lipid Lowering by Pravastatin on Progression and Regression of Coronary Artery Disease in Symptomatic Man With Normal to Moderately Elevated Serum Cholesterol Levels. The Regression Growth Evaluation Statin Study (REGRESS). *Circulation* 1995;91:2528–2540.
6. Crouse JR, et al. Pravastatin, lipids, and atherosclerosis in the carotid arteries: design features of a clinical trial with carotid atherosclerosis outcome (PLAC II). *Controlled Clinical Trials* 13:495, 1992.
7. Salonen R, et al. Kuopio Atherosclerosis Prevention Study (KAPS). A population-based primary preventive trial of the effect of LDL lowering on atherosclerotic progression in carotid and femoral arteries. Research Institute of Public Health, University of Kuopio, Finland. *Circulation* 92:1758, 1995.
8. Fredrickson DS, et, al. Fat transport in lipoproteins–an integrated approach to mechanisms and disorders. *N Engl J Med* 1967; 276:34–42, 94–102, 148–156, 215–224, 273–281.
9. Manson JM, Freyssinges C, Ducrocq MB, Stephenson WP. Postmarketing Surveillance of Lovastatin and Simvastatin Exposure During Pregnancy. *Reproductive Toxicology* 10(6):439–446, 1996.

Bristol-Myers Squibb Co.
Princeton, NJ 08543
D3-B001-07-00 5154DIM-15
Revised July 2000
Shown in Product Identification Guide, page 309

	All Events		Events Attributed to Study Drug	
Body System/Event	**Pravastatin (N = 900) %**	**Placebo (N = 411) %**	**Pravastatin (N = 900) %**	**Placebo (N = 411) %**
Cardiovascular				
Cardiac Chest Pain	4.0	3.4	0.1	0.0
Dermatologic Rash	4.0*	1.1	1.3	0.9
Gastrointestinal				
Nausea/Vomiting	7.3	7.1	2.9	3.4
Diarrhea	6.2	5.6	2.0	1.9
Abdominal Pain	5.4	6.9	2.0	3.9
Constipation	4.0	7.1	2.4	5.1
Flatulence	3.3	3.6	2.7	3.4
Heartburn	2.9	1.9	2.0	0.7
General				
Fatigue	3.8	3.4	1.9	1.0
Chest Pain	3.7	1.9	0.3	0.2
Influenza	2.4*	0.7	0.0	0.0
Musculoskeletal				
Localized Pain	10.0	9.0	1.4	1.5
Myalgia	2.7	1.0	0.6	0.0
Nervous System				
Headache	6.2	3.9	1.7*	0.2
Dizziness	3.3	3.2	1.0	0.5
Renal/Genitourinary				
Urinary Abnormality	2.4	2.9	0.7	1.2
Respiratory				
Common Cold	7.0	6.3	0.0	0.0
Rhinitis	4.0	4.1	0.1	0.0
Cough	2.6	1.7	0.1	0.0

*Statistically significantly different from placebo.

SERZONE® ℞
[sĕr-zonĕ]
(nefazodone hydrochloride) Tablets
Rx only

DESCRIPTION
SERZONE® (nefazodone hydrochloride) is an antidepressant for oral administration with a chemical structure unrelated to selective serotonin reuptake inhibitors, tricyclics, tetracyclics, or monoamine oxidase inhibitors (MAOI).
Nefazodone hydrochloride is a synthetically derived phenylpiperazine antidepressant. The chemical name for nefazodone hydrochloride is 2-[3-[4-(3-chlorophenyl)-1-piperazinyl]propyl]-5-ethyl-2,4-dihydro-4-(2-phenoxyethyl)-3H-1,2,4-triazol-3-one monohydrochloride. The molecular formula is $C_{25}H_{32}ClN_5O_2 \cdot HCl$, which corresponds to a molecular weight of 506.5. The structural formula is:

Nefazodone hydrochloride is a nonhygroscopic, white crystalline solid. It is freely soluble in chloroform, soluble in propylene glycol, and slightly soluble in polyethylene glycol and water.
SERZONE is supplied as hexagonal tablets containing 50 mg, 100 mg, 150 mg, 200 mg, or 250 mg of nefazodone hydrochloride and the following inactive ingredients: microcrystalline cellulose, povidone, sodium starch glycolate, colloidal silicon dioxide, magnesium stearate, and iron oxides (red and/or yellow) as colorants.

CLINICAL PHARMACOLOGY
Pharmacodynamics
The mechanism of action of nefazodone, as with other antidepressants, is unknown.
Preclinical studies have shown that nefazodone inhibits neuronal uptake of serotonin and norepinephrine.
Nefazodone occupies central 5-HT_2 receptors at nanomolar concentrations, and acts as an antagonist at this receptor. Nefazodone was shown to antagonize alpha$_1$-adrenergic receptors, a property which may be associated with postural hypotension. *In vitro* binding studies showed that nefazodone had no significant affinity for the following receptors: alpha$_2$ and beta adrenergic, 5-HT_{1A}, cholinergic, dopaminergic, or benzodiazepine.

Pharmacokinetics
Nefazodone hydrochloride is rapidly and completely absorbed but is subject to extensive metabolism, so that its

absolute bioavailability is low, about 20%, and variable. Peak plasma concentrations occur at about one hour and the half-life of nefazodone is 2–4 hours.
Both nefazodone and its pharmacologically similar metabolite, hydroxynefazodone, exhibit nonlinear kinetics for both dose and time, with AUC and C_{max} increasing more than proportionally with dose increases and more than expected upon multiple dosing over time, compared to single dosing. For example, in a multiple-dose study involving BID dosing with 50, 100, and 200 mg, the AUC for nefazodone and hydroxynefazodone increased by about 4-fold with an increase in dose from 200 to 400 mg per day; C_{max} increased by about 3-fold with the same dose increase. In a multiple-dose study involving BID dosing with 25, 50, 100, and 150 mg, the accumulation ratios for nefazodone and hydroxynefazodone AUC, after 5 days of BID dosing relative to the first dose, ranged from approximately 3 to 4 at the lower doses (50–100 mg/day) and from 5 to 7 at the higher doses (200–300 mg/day); there were also approximately 2- to 4-fold increases in C_{max} after 5 days of BID dosing relative to the first dose, suggesting extensive and greater than predicted accumulation of nefazodone and its hydroxy metabolite with multiple dosing. Steady-state plasma nefazodone and metabolite concentrations are attained within 4 to 5 days of initiation of BID dosing or upon dose increase or decrease.
Nefazodone is extensively metabolized after oral administration by n-dealkylation and aliphatic and aromatic hydroxylation, and less than 1% of administered nefazodone is excreted unchanged in urine. Attempts to characterize three metabolites identified in plasma, hydroxynefazodone (HO-NEF), meta-chlorophenylpiperazine (mCPP), and a triazole-dione metabolite, have been carried out. The AUC (expressed as a multiple of the AUC for nefazodone dosed at 100 mg BID) and elimination half-lives for these three metabolites were as follows:

AUC Multiples and $T_{1/2}$ for
Three Metabolites of Nefazodone (100 mg BID)

Metabolite	AUC Multiple	$T_{1/2}$
HO-NEF	0.4	1.5 – 4 h
mCPP	0.07	4 – 8 h
Triazole-dione	4.0	18 h

HO-NEF possesses a pharmacological profile qualitatively and quantitatively similar to that of nefazodone. mCPP has some similarities to nefazodone, but also has agonist activity at some serotonergic receptor subtypes. The pharmacological profile of the triazole-dione metabolite has not yet been well characterized. In addition to the above compounds, several other metabolites were present in plasma but have not been tested for pharmacological activity.
After oral administration of radiolabeled nefazodone, the mean half-life of total label ranged between 11 and 24 hours. Approximately 55% of the administered radioactivity was detected in urine and about 20–30% in feces.
Distribution—Nefazodone is widely distributed in body tissues, including the central nervous system (CNS). In humans the volume of distribution of nefazodone ranges from 0.22 to 0.87 L/kg.
Protein Binding—At concentrations of 25–2500 ng/mL nefazodone is extensively (>99%) bound to human plasma proteins *in vitro*. The administration of 200 mg BID of nefazodone for 1 week did not increase the fraction of unbound warfarin in subjects whose prothrombin times had been prolonged by warfarin therapy to 120–150% of the laboratory control (see **PRECAUTIONS** section, **Drug Interactions** subsection). While nefazodone did not alter the *in vitro* protein binding of chlorpromazine, desipramine, diazepam, diphenylhydantoin, lidocaine, prazosin, propranolol, or verapamil, it is unknown whether or not displacement of either nefazodone or these drugs occurs *in vivo*. There was a 5% decrease in the protein binding of haloperidol; this is probably of no clinical significance.
Effect of Food—Food delays the absorption of nefazodone and decreases the bioavailability of nefazodone by approximately 20%.
Renal Disease—In studies involving 29 renally impaired patients, renal impairment (creatinine clearances ranging from 7 to 60 mL/min/1.73m²) had no effect on steady-state nefazodone plasma concentrations.
Liver Disease—In a multiple-dose study of patients with liver cirrhosis, the AUC values for nefazodone and HO-NEF at steady state were approximately 25% greater than those observed in normal volunteers.
Age/Gender Effects—After single doses of 300 mg to younger and older patients, C_{max} and AUC for nefazodone and hydroxynefazodone were up to twice as high in the older patients. With multiple doses, however, differences were much smaller, 10–20%. A similar result was seen for gender, with a higher C_{max} and AUC in women after single doses but no difference after multiple doses.
Treatment with SERZONE should be initiated at half the usual dose in elderly patients, especially women (see **DOSAGE AND ADMINISTRATION** section), but the therapeutic dose range is similar in younger and older patients.

Clinical Efficacy Trial Results

Studies in Outpatients with Depression

During its premarketing development, the efficacy of SERZONE was evaluated at doses within the therapeutic range in five well-controlled, short-term (6–8 weeks) clinical investigations. These trials enrolled outpatients meeting DSM-III or DSM-IIIR criteria for major depression. Among these trials, two demonstrated the effectiveness of SERZONE, and two provided additional support for that conclusion.
One trial was a 6-week dose-titration study comparing SERZONE in two dose ranges (up to 300 mg/day and up to 600 mg/day [mean modal dose for this group was about 400 mg/day], on a BID schedule) and placebo. The second trial was an 8-week dose-titration study comparing SERZONE (up to 600 mg/day; mean modal dose was 375 mg/day), imipramine (up to 300 mg/day), and placebo, all on a BID schedule. Both studies demonstrated SERZONE, at doses titrated between 300 mg to 600 mg/day (therapeutic dose range), to be superior to placebo on at least three of the following four measures: 17-Item Hamilton Depression Rating Scale or HDRS (total score), Hamilton Depressed Mood item, Clinical Global Impressions (CGI) Severity score, and CGI Improvement score. Significant differences were also found for certain factors of the HDRS (e.g., anxiety factor, sleep disturbance factor, and retardation factor). In the two supportive studies, SERZONE was titrated up to 500 or 600 mg/day (mean modal doses of 462 mg/day and 363 mg/day). In the fifth study, the differentiation in response rates between SERZONE and placebo was not statistically significant. Three additional trials were conducted using subtherapeutic doses of SERZONE.
There were no efficacy studies focusing specifically on the elderly or on men and women separately. Overall, approximately two thirds of patients in these trials were women, and an analysis of the effects of gender on outcome did not suggest any differential responsiveness on the basis of sex. There were too few elderly patients in these trials to reveal possible age-related differences in response.
Since its initial marketing as an antidepressant drug product, additional clinical investigations of SERZONE have been conducted. These studies explored SERZONE's use under conditions not evaluated fully at the time initial marketing approval was granted.

Studies in "Inpatients"

Two studies were conducted to evaluate SERZONE's effectiveness in hospitalized depressed patients. These were 6-week, dose-titration trials comparing SERZONE (up to 600 mg/day) and placebo, on a BID schedule. In one study, SERZONE was superior to placebo. In this study, the mean modal dose of SERZONE was 503 mg/day, and 85% of these inpatients were melancholic; at baseline, patients were distributed at the higher end of the 7-point CGI Severity scale, as follows: 4=moderately ill (17%); 5=markedly ill (48%); 6=severely ill (32%). In the other study, the differentiation in response rates between SERZONE and placebo was not statistically significant. This result may be explained by the "high" rate of spontaneous improvement among the patients randomized to placebo.

Studies of "Relapse Prevention in Patients Recently Recovered (Clinically) from Depression"

Two studies were conducted to assess SERZONE's capacity to maintain a clinical remission in acutely depressed patients who were judged to have responded adequately (HDRS total score ≤10) after a 16-week period of open treatment with SERZONE (titration up to 600 mg/day). In one study, SERZONE was superior to placebo. In this study, patients (n=131) were randomized to continuation on SERZONE or placebo for an additional 36 weeks (1 year total). This study demonstrated a significantly lower relapse rate (HDRS total score ≥18) for patients taking SERZONE compared to those on placebo. The second study was of appropriate design and power, but the sample of patients admitted for evaluation did not suffer relapses at a high enough incidence to provide a meaningful test of SERZONE's efficacy for this use.

Comparisons of Clinical Trial Results

Highly variable results have been seen in the clinical development of all antidepressant drugs. Furthermore, in those circumstances when the drugs have not been studied in the same controlled clinical trial(s), comparisons among the findings of studies evaluating the effectiveness of different antidepressant drug products are inherently unreliable. Because conditions of testing (e.g., patient samples, investigators, doses of the treatments administered and compared, outcome measures, etc.) vary among trials, it is virtually impossible to distinguish a difference in drug effect from a difference due to one or more of the confounding factors just enumerated.

INDICATIONS AND USAGE

SERZONE (nefazodone hydrochloride) is indicated for the treatment of depression.
The efficacy of SERZONE in the treatment of depression was established in 6–8 week controlled trials of outpatients and in a 6-week controlled trial of depressed inpatients whose diagnoses corresponded most closely to the DSM-III or DSM-IIIR category of major depressive disorder (see **CLINICAL PHARMACOLOGY** section).
A major depressive episode implies a prominent and relatively persistent depressed or dysphoric mood that usually interferes with daily functioning (nearly every day for at least 2 weeks). It must include either depressed mood or loss of interest or pleasure and at least five of the following nine symptoms: depressed mood, loss of interest in usual activities, significant change in weight and/or appetite, insomnia or hypersomnia, psychomotor agitation or retardation, increased fatigue, feelings of guilt or worthlessness, slowed thinking or impaired concentration, a suicide attempt or suicidal ideation.
The efficacy of SERZONE in reducing relapse in patients with major depression who were judged to have had a satisfactory clinical response to 16 weeks of open-label SERZONE treatment for an acute depressive episode has been demonstrated in a randomized placebo-controlled trial (see **CLINICAL PHARMACOLOGY** section). Although remitted patients were followed for as long as 36 weeks in the study cited (i.e., 52 weeks total), the physician who elects to use SERZONE for extended periods should periodically reevaluate the long-term usefulness of the drug for the individual patient.

CONTRAINDICATIONS

Coadministration of terfenadine, astemizole, cisapride, pimozide, or carbamazepine with SERZONE (nefazodone hydrochloride) is contraindicated (see **WARNINGS** and **PRECAUTIONS** sections).
SERZONE is contraindicated in patients with known hypersensitivity to nefazodone or other phenylpiperazine antidepressants.
The coadministration of triazolam and nefazodone causes a significant increase in the plasma level of triazolam (see **WARNINGS** and **PRECAUTIONS** sections), and a 75% reduction in the initial triazolam dosage is recommended if the two drugs are to be given together. Because not all commercially available dosage forms of triazolam permit a sufficient dosage reduction, the coadministration of triazolam and SERZONE should be avoided for most patients, including the elderly.

WARNINGS

Potential for Interaction with Monoamine Oxidase Inhibitors

In patients receiving antidepressants with pharmacological properties similar to nefazodone in combination with a monoamine oxidase inhibitor (MAOI), there have been reports of serious, sometimes fatal, reactions. For a selective serotonin reuptake inhibitor (SSRI), these reactions have included hyperthermia, rigidity, myoclonus, autonomic instability with possible rapid fluctuations of vital signs, and mental status changes that include extreme agitation progressing to delirium and coma. These reactions have also been reported in patients who have recently discontinued that drug and have been started on an MAOI. Some cases presented with features resembling neuroleptic malignant syndrome. Severe hyperthermia and seizures, sometimes fatal, have been reported in association with the combined use of tricyclic antidepressants and MAOIs. These reactions have also been reported in patients who have recently discontinued these drugs and have been started on an MAOI.
Although the effects of combined use of nefazodone and MAOI have not been evaluated in humans or animals, because nefazodone is an inhibitor of both serotonin and norepinephrine reuptake, it is recommended that nefazodone not be used in combination with an MAOI, or within 14 days of discontinuing treatment with an MAOI. At least 1 week should be allowed after stopping nefazodone before starting an MAOI.

Interaction with Triazolobenzodiazepines

Interaction studies of nefazodone with two triazolobenzodiazepines, i.e., triazolam and alprazolam, metabolized by cytochrome P450 3A4, have revealed substantial and clinically important increases in plasma concentrations of these compounds when administered concomitantly with nefazodone.

Triazolam

When a single oral 0.25-mg dose of triazolam was coadministered with nefazodone (200 mg BID) at steady state, triazolam half-life and AUC increased 4-fold and peak concentrations increased 1.7-fold. Nefazodone plasma concentrations were unaffected by triazolam. ***Coadministration of nefazodone potentiated the effects of triazolam on psychomotor performance tests.*** If triazolam is coadministered with SERZONE, a 75% reduction in the initial triazolam dosage is recommended. Because not all commercially available dosage forms of triazolam permit sufficient dosage reduction, coadministration of triazolam with SERZONE should be avoided for most patients, including the elderly. In the exceptional case where coadministration of triazolam with SERZONE may be considered appropriate, only the lowest possible dose of triazolam should be used (see **CONTRAINDICATIONS** and **PRECAUTIONS** sections).

Alprazolam

When alprazolam (1 mg BID) and nefazodone (200 mg BID) were coadministered, steady-state peak concentrations, AUC and half-life values for alprazolam increased by approximately 2-fold. Nefazodone plasma concentrations were unaffected by alprazolam. If alprazolam is coadministered with SERZONE, a 50% reduction in the initial alprazolam dosage is recommended. No dosage adjustment is required for SERZONE.

Potential Terfenadine, Astemizole, Cisapride, and Pimozide Interactions

Terfenadine, astemizole, cisapride, and pimozide are all metabolized by the cytochrome P450 3A4 (CYP3A4) isozyme, and it has been demonstrated that ketoconazole, erythromycin, and other inhibitors of CYP3A4 can block the metabolism of these drugs, which can result in increased plasma concentrations of parent drug. Increased plasma

Continued on next page

Serzone—Cont.

concentrations of terfenadine, astemizole, cisapride, and pimozide are associated with QT prolongation and with rare cases of serious cardiovascular adverse events, including death, due principally to ventricular tachycardia of the torsades de pointes type. Nefazodone has been shown *in vitro* to be an inhibitor of CYP3A4. Consequently, it is recommended that nefazodone not be used in combination with either terfenadine, astemizole, cisapride, or pimozide (see **CONTRAINDICATIONS** and **PRECAUTIONS** sections).

Interaction with Carbamazepine

The coadministration of carbamazepine 200 mg BID with nefazodone 200 mg BID, at steady state for both drugs, resulted in almost 95% reductions in AUCs for nefazodone and hydroxynefazodone, likely resulting in insufficient plasma nefazodone and hydroxynefazodone concentrations for achieving an antidepressant effect for SERZONE. Consequently, it is recommended that SERZONE not be used in combination with carbamazepine (see **CONTRAINDICATIONS** and **PRECAUTIONS** sections).

PRECAUTIONS

General

Postural Hypotension

A pooled analysis of the vital signs monitored during placebo-controlled premarketing studies revealed that 5.1% of nefazodone patients compared to 2.5% of placebo patients ($p \leq 0.01$) met criteria for a potentially important decrease in blood pressure at some time during treatment (systolic blood pressure ≤90 mmHg *and* a change from baseline of ≥20 mmHg). While there was no difference in the proportion of nefazodone and placebo patients having adverse events characterized as 'syncope' (nefazodone, 0.2%; placebo, 0.3%), the rates for adverse events characterized as 'postural hypotension' were as follows: nefazodone (2.8%), tricyclic antidepressants (10.9%), SSRI (1.1%), and placebo (0.8%). Thus, the prescriber should be aware that there is some risk of postural hypotension in association with nefazodone use. SERZONE should be used with caution in patients with known cardiovascular or cerebrovascular disease that could be exacerbated by hypotension (history of myocardial infarction, angina, or ischemic stroke) and conditions that would predispose patients to hypotension (dehydration, hypovolemia, and treatment with antihypertensive medication).

Activation of Mania/Hypomania

During premarketing testing, hypomania or mania occurred in 0.3% of nefazodone-treated unipolar patients, compared to 0.3% of tricyclic- and 0.4% of placebo-treated patients. In patients classified as bipolar the rate of manic episodes was 1.6% for nefazodone, 5.1% for the combined tricyclic-treated groups, and 0% for placebo-treated patients. Activation of mania/hypomania is a known risk in a small proportion of patients with major affective disorder treated with other marketed antidepressants. As with all antidepressants, SERZONE (nefazodone hydrochloride) should be used cautiously in patients with a history of mania.

Suicide

The possibility of a suicide attempt is inherent in depression and may persist until significant remission occurs. Close supervision of high-risk patients should accompany initial drug therapy. Prescriptions for SERZONE should be written for the smallest quantity of tablets consistent with good patient management in order to reduce the risk of overdose.

Seizures

During premarketing testing, a recurrence of a petit mal seizure was observed in a patient receiving nefazodone who had a history of such seizures. In addition, one nonstudy participant reportedly experienced a convulsion (type not documented) following a multiple-drug overdose (see **OVERDOSAGE** section). Rare occurrences of convulsions (including grand mal seizures) following nefazodone administration have been reported since market introduction. A causal relationship to nefazodone has not been established (see **ADVERSE REACTIONS** section).

Priapism

While priapism did not occur during premarketing experience with nefazodone, rare reports of priapism have been received since market introduction. A causal relationship to nefazodone has not been established (see **ADVERSE REACTIONS** section). If patients present with prolonged or inappropriate erections, they should discontinue therapy immediately and consult their physicians. If the condition persists for more than 24 hours, a urologist should be consulted to determine appropriate management.

Use in Patients with Concomitant Illness

SERZONE has not been evaluated or used to any appreciable extent in patients with a recent history of myocardial infarction or unstable heart disease. Patients with these diagnoses were systematically excluded from clinical studies during the product's premarketing testing. Evaluation of electrocardiograms of 1153 patients who received nefazodone in 6- to 8-week, double-blind, placebo-controlled trials did not indicate that nefazodone is associated with the development of clinically important ECG abnormalities. However, sinus bradycardia, defined as heart rate ≤50 bpm and a decrease of at least 15 bpm from baseline, was observed in 1.5% of nefazodone-treated patients compared to 0.4% of placebo-treated patients ($p \leq 0.05$). Because patients with a recent history of myocardial infarction or unstable heart disease were excluded from clinical trials, such patients should be treated with caution.

In patients with cirrhosis of the liver, the AUC values of nefazodone and HO-NEF were increased by approximately 25%.

Information for Patients

Physicians are advised to discuss the following issues with patients for whom they prescribe SERZONE:

Time to Response/Continuation

As with all antidepressants, several weeks on treatment may be required to obtain the full antidepressant effect. Once improvement is noted, it is important for patients to continue drug treatment as directed by their physician.

Interference With Cognitive and Motor Performance

Since any psychoactive drug may impair judgment, thinking, or motor skills, patients should be cautioned about operating hazardous machinery, including automobiles, until they are reasonably certain that SERZONE therapy does not adversely affect their ability to engage in such activities.

Pregnancy

Patients should be advised to notify their physician if they become pregnant or intend to become pregnant during therapy.

Nursing

Patients should be advised to notify their physician if they are breast-feeding an infant (see **PRECAUTIONS** section, **Nursing Mothers** subsection).

Concomitant Medication

Patients should be advised to inform their physicians if they are taking, or plan to take, any prescription or over-the-counter drugs, since there is a potential for interactions. Significant caution is indicated if SERZONE is to be used in combination with XANAX®[1], concomitant use with HALCION®[1] should be avoided for most patients including the elderly, and concomitant use with SELDANE®[2], HISMANAL®[3], PROPULSID®[3], or ORAP®[4] is contraindicated (see **CONTRAINDICATIONS** and **WARNINGS** sections).

Alcohol

Patients should be advised to avoid alcohol while taking SERZONE.

Allergic Reactions

Patients should be advised to notify their physician if they develop a rash, hives, or a related allergic phenomenon.

Laboratory Tests

There are no specific laboratory tests recommended.

Drug Interactions

Drugs Highly Bound to Plasma Protein

Because nefazodone is highly bound to plasma protein (see **CLINICAL PHARMACOLOGY** section, **Pharmacokinetics** subsection), administration of SERZONE to a patient taking another drug that is highly protein bound may cause increased free concentrations of the other drug, potentially resulting in adverse events. Conversely, adverse effects could result from displacement of nefazodone by other highly bound drugs.

Warfarin—There were no effects on the prothrombin or bleeding times or upon the pharmacokinetics of R-warfarin when nefazodone (200 mg BID) was administered for 1 week to subjects who had been pretreated for 2 weeks with warfarin. Although the coadministration of nefazodone did decrease the subjects' exposure to S-warfarin by 12%, the lack of effects on the prothrombin and bleeding times indicates this modest change is not clinically significant. Although these results suggest no adjustments in warfarin dosage are required when nefazodone is administered to patients stabilized on warfarin, such patients should be monitored as required by standard medical practices.

CNS-Active Drugs

Monoamine Oxidase Inhibitors—See **WARNINGS** section.

Haloperidol—When a single oral 5-mg dose of haloperidol was coadministered with nefazodone (200 mg BID) at steady state, haloperidol apparent clearance decreased by 35% with no significant increase in peak haloperidol plasma concentrations or time of peak. This change is of unknown clinical significance. Pharmacodynamic effects of haloperidol were generally not altered significantly. There were no changes in the pharmacokinetic parameters for nefazodone. Dosage adjustment of haloperidol may be necessary when coadministered with nefazodone.

Lorazepam—When lorazepam (2 mg BID) and nefazodone (200 mg BID) were coadministered to steady state, there was no change in any pharmacokinetic parameter for either drug compared to each drug administered alone. Therefore, dosage adjustment is not necessary for either drug when coadministered.

Triazolam/Alprazolam-See **CONTRAINDICATIONS** and **WARNINGS** sections.

Alcohol—Although nefazodone did not potentiate the cognitive and psychomotor effects of alcohol in experiments with normal subjects, the concomitant use of SERZONE and alcohol in depressed patients is not advised.

Buspirone—In a study of steady-state pharmacokinetics in healthy volunteers, coadministration of buspirone (2.5 or 5 mg BID) with nefazodone (250 mg BID) resulted in marked increases in plasma buspirone concentrations (increases up to 20-fold in C_{max} and up to 50-fold in AUC) and statistically significant decreases (about 50%) in plasma concentrations of the buspirone metabolite 1-pyrimidinylpiperazine. With 5-mg BID doses of buspirone, slight increases in AUC were observed for nefazodone (23%) and its metabolites hydroxynefazodone (17%) and mCPP (9%). The side effect profile for subjects receiving buspirone 2.5 mg BID and nefazodone 250 mg BID was similar to that for subjects receiving either drug alone. Subjects receiving buspirone 5 mg BID and nefazodone 250 mg BID experienced side effects such as lightheadedness, asthenia, dizziness, and somnolence. If the two drugs are to be used in combination, a low dose of buspirone (e.g., 2.5 mg BID) is recommended. Subsequent dose adjustment of either drug should be based on clinical assessment.

Pimozide—See **CONTRAINDICATIONS**, **WARNINGS**, and **PRECAUTIONS:** *Pharmacokinetics of Nefazodone in 'Poor Metabolizers' and Potential Interaction with Drugs that Inhibit and/or Are Metabolized by Cytochrome P450 Isozymes.*

Fluoxetine—When fluoxetine (20 mg QD) and nefazodone (200 mg BID) were administered at steady state there were no changes in the pharmacokinetic parameters for fluoxetine or its metabolite, norfluoxetine. Similarly, there were no changes in the pharmacokinetic parameters of nefazodone or HO-NEF; however, the mean AUC levels of the nefazodone metabolites mCPP and triazole-dione increased by 3- to 6-fold and 1.3-fold, respectively. When a 200-mg dose of nefazodone was administered to subjects who had been receiving fluoxetine for 1 week, there was an increased incidence of transient adverse events such as headache, lightheadedness, nausea, or paresthesia, possibly due to the elevated mCPP levels. Patients who are switched from fluoxetine to nefazodone without an adequate washout period may experience similar transient adverse events. The possibility of this happening can be minimized by allowing a washout period before initiating nefazodone therapy and by reducing the initial dose of nefazodone. Because of the long half-life of fluoxetine and its metabolites, this washout period may range from one to several weeks depending on the dose of fluoxetine and other individual patient variables.

Phenytoin—Pretreatment for 7 days with 200 mg BID of nefazodone had no effect on the pharmacokinetics of a single 300-mg oral dose of phenytoin. However, due to the nonlinear pharmacokinetics of phenytoin, the failure to observe a significant effect on the single-dose pharmacokinetics of phenytoin does not preclude the possibility of a clinically significant interaction with nefazodone when phenytoin is dosed chronically. However, no change in the initial dosage of phenytoin is considered necessary and any subsequent adjustment of phenytoin dosage should be guided by usual clinical practices.

Desipramine—When nefazodone (150 mg BID) and desipramine (75 mg QD) were administered together there were no changes in the pharmacokinetics of desipramine or its metabolite, 2-hydroxy desipramine. There were also no changes in the pharmacokinetics of nefazodone or its triazole-dione metabolite, but the AUC and C_{max} of mCPP increased by 44% and 48%, respectively, while the AUC of HO-NEF decreased by 19%. No changes in doses of either nefazodone or desipramine are necessary when the two drugs are given concomitantly. Subsequent dose adjustments should be made on the basis of clinical response.

Lithium—In 13 healthy subjects the coadministration of nefazodone (200 mg BID) with lithium (500 mg BID) for 5 days (steady-state conditions) was found to be well tolerated. When the two drugs were coadministered, there were no changes in the steady-state pharmacokinetics of either lithium, nefazodone, or its metabolite HO-NEF; however, there were small decreases in the steady-state plasma concentrations of two nefazodone metabolites, mCPP and triazole-dione, which are considered not to be of clinical significance. Therefore, no dosage adjustment of either lithium or nefazodone is required when they are coadministered.

Carbamazepine—The coadministration of nefazodone (200 mg BID) for 5 days to 12 healthy subjects on carbamazepine who had achieved steady state (200 mg BID) was found to be well tolerated. Steady-state conditions for carbamazepine, nefazodone, and several of their metabolites were achieved by day 5 of coadministration. With coadministration of the two drugs there were significant increases in the steady-state C_{max} and AUC of carbamazepine (23% and 23%, respectively), while the steady-state C_{max} and the AUC of the carbamazepine metabolite, 10,11 epoxycarbamazepine, decreased by 21% and 20%, respectively. The coadministration of the two drugs significantly reduced the steady-state C_{max} and AUC of nefazodone by 86% and 93%, respectively. Similar reductions in the C_{max} and AUC of HO-NEF were also observed (85% and 94%), while the reductions in C_{max} and AUC of mCPP and triazole-dione were more modest (13% and 44% for the former and 28% and 57% for the latter). Due to the potential for coadministration of carbamazepine to result in insufficient plasma nefazodone and hydroxynefazodone concentrations for achieving an antidepressant effect for SERZONE, it is recommended that SERZONE not be used in combination with carbamazepine (see **CONTRAINDICATIONS** and **WARNINGS** sections).

General Anesthetics—Little is known about the potential for interaction between nefazodone and general anesthetics; therefore, prior to elective surgery, SERZONE should be discontinued for as long as clinically feasible.

Other CNS-Active Drugs—The use of nefazodone in combination with other CNS-active drugs has not been systematically evaluated. Consequently, caution is advised if concomitant administration of SERZONE (nefazodone hydrochloride) and such drugs is required.

Cimetidine

When nefazodone (200 mg BID) and cimetidine (300 mg QID) were coadministered for one week, no change in the steady-state pharmacokinetics of either nefazodone or cimetidine was observed compared to each dosed alone. Therefore, dosage adjustment is not necessary for either drug when coadministered.

Theophylline
When nefazodone (200 mg BID) was given to patients being treated with theophylline (600–1200 mg/day) for chronic obstructive pulmonary disease, there was no change in the steady-state pharmacokinetics of either nefazodone or theophylline. FEV_1 measurements taken when theophylline and nefazodone were coadministered did not differ from baseline dosage (i.e., when theophylline was administered alone). Therefore, dosage adjustment is not necessary for either drug when coadministered.
Cardiovascular-Active Drugs
Digoxin—When nefazodone (200 mg BID) and digoxin (0.2 mg QD) were coadministered for 9 days to healthy male volunteers (n=18) who were phenotyped as CYP2D6 extensive metabolizers, C_{max}, C_{min}, and AUC of digoxin were increased by 29%, 27%, and 15%, respectively. Digoxin had no effects on the pharmacokinetics of nefazodone and its active metabolites. Because of the narrow therapeutic index of digoxin, caution should be exercised when nefazodone and digoxin are coadministered; plasma level monitoring for digoxin is recommended.
Propranolol—The coadministration of nefazodone (200 mg BID) and propranolol (40 mg BID) for 5.5 days to healthy male volunteers (n=18), including 3 poor and 15 extensive CYP2D6 metabolizers, resulted in 30% and 14% reductions in C_{max} and AUC of propranolol, respectively, and a 14% reduction in C_{max} for the metabolite, 4-hydroxypropranolol. The kinetics of nefazodone, hydroxynefazodone, and triazole-dione were not affected by coadministration of propranolol. However, C_{max}, C_{min}, and AUC of m-chlorophenylpiperazine were increased by 23%, 54%, and 28%, respectively. No change in initial dose of either drug is necessary and dose adjustments should be made on the basis of clinical response.
HMG-CoA Reductase Inhibitors—When single 40-mg doses of simvastatin or atorvastatin, both substrates of CYP3A4, were given to healthy adult volunteers who had received SERZONE 200 mg BID for 6 days, approximately 20-fold increases in plasma concentrations of simvastatin and simvastatin acid and 3- to 4-fold increases in plasma concentrations of atorvastatin and atorvastatin lactone were seen. These effects appear to be due to the inhibition of CYP3A4 by SERZONE because, in the same study, SERZONE had no significant effect on the plasma concentrations of pravastatin, which is not metabolized by CYP3A4 to a clinically significant extent.
There have been rare reports of rhabdomyolysis involving patients receiving the combination of SERZONE and either simvastatin or lovastatin, also a substrate of CYP3A4 (see **ADVERSE REACTIONS: Postintroduction Clinical Experience** section). Rhabdomyolysis has been observed in patients receiving HMG-CoA reductase inhibitors administered alone (at recommended dosages) and in particular, for certain drugs in this class, when given in combination with inhibitors of the CYP3A4 isozyme.
Caution should be used if SERZONE is administered in combination with HMG-CoA reductase inhibitors that are metabolized by CYP3A4, such as simvastatin, atorvastatin, and lovastatin, and dosage adjustments of these HMG-CoA reductase inhibitors are recommended. Since metabolic interactions are unlikely between SERZONE and HMG-CoA reductase inhibitors that undergo little or no metabolism by the CYP3A4 isozyme, such as pravastatin or fluvastatin, dosage adjustments should not be necessary.
Immunosuppressive Agents
There have been rare reports of increased blood concentrations of cyclosporine and tacrolimus into toxic ranges when patients received these drugs concomitantly with SERZONE. Both cyclosporine and tacrolimus are substrates of CYP3A4, and nefazodone is known to inhibit this enzyme. If either cyclosporine or tacrolimus is administered with SERZONE, blood concentrations of the immunosuppressive agent should be monitored and dosage adjusted accordingly.
Pharmacokinetics of Nefazodone in 'Poor Metabolizers' and Potential Interaction with Drugs that Inhibit and/or Are Metabolized by Cytochrome P450 Isozymes
CYP3A4 Isozyme—Nefazodone has been shown *in vitro* to be an inhibitor of CYP3A4. This is consistent with the interactions observed between nefazodone and triazolam, alprazolam, buspirone, atorvastatin, and simvastatin, drugs metabolized by this isozyme. Consequently, caution is indicated in the combined use of nefazodone with any drugs known to be metabolized by CYP3A4. In particular, the combined use of nefazodone with triazolam should be avoided for most patients, including the elderly. The combined use of nefazodone with terfenadine, astemizole, cisapride, or pimozide is contraindicated (see **CONTRAINDICATIONS** and **WARNINGS** sections).
CYP2D6 Isozyme—A subset (3% to 10%) of the population has reduced activity of the drug-metabolizing enzyme CYP2D6. Such individuals are referred to commonly as "poor metabolizers" of drugs such as debrisoquin, dextromethorphan, and the tricyclic antidepressants. The pharmacokinetics of nefazodone and its major metabolites are not altered in these "poor metabolizers." Plasma concentrations of one minor metabolite (mCPP) are increased in this population; the adjustment of SERZONE dosage is not required when administered to "poor metabolizers." Nefazodone and its metabolites have been shown *in vitro* to be extremely weak inhibitors of CYP2D6. Thus, it is not likely that nefazodone will decrease the metabolic clearance of drugs metabolized by this isozyme.
CYP1A2 Isozyme—Nefazodone and its metabolites have been shown *in vitro* not to inhibit CYP1A2. Thus, metabolic interactions between nefazodone and drugs metabolized by this isozyme are unlikely.

Electroconvulsive Therapy (ECT)
There are no clinical studies of the combined use of ECT and nefazodone.

Carcinogenesis, Mutagenesis, Impairment of Fertility
Carcinogenesis
There is no evidence of carcinogenicity with nefazodone. The dietary administration of nefazodone to rats and mice for 2 years at daily doses of up to 200 mg/kg and 800 mg/kg, respectively, which are approximately 3 and 6 times, respectively, the maximum human daily dose on a mg/m^2 basis, produced no increase in tumors.
Mutagenesis
Nefazodone has been shown to have no genotoxic effects based on the following assays: bacterial mutation assays, a DNA repair assay in cultured rat hepatocytes, a mammalian mutation assay in Chinese hamster ovary cells, an *in vivo* cytogenetics assay in rat bone marrow cells, and a rat dominant lethal study.
Impairment of Fertility
A fertility study in rats showed a slight decrease in fertility at 200 mg/kg/day (approximately three times the maximum human daily dose on a mg/m^2 basis) but not at 100 mg/kg/day (approximately 1.5 times the maximum human daily dose on a mg/m^2 basis).

Pregnancy
Teratogenic Effects—Pregnancy Category C
Reproduction studies have been performed in pregnant rabbits and rats at daily doses up to 200 and 300 mg/kg, respectively (approximately 6 and 5 times, respectively, the maximum human daily dose on a mg/m^2 basis). No malformations were observed in the offspring as a result of nefazodone treatment. However, increased early pup mortality was seen in rats at a dose approximately five times the maximum human dose, and decreased pup weights were seen at this and lower doses, when dosing began during pregnancy and continued until weaning. The cause of these deaths is not known. The no-effect dose for rat pup mortality was 1.3 times the human dose on a mg/m^2 basis. There are no adequate and well-controlled studies in pregnant women. Nefazodone should be used during pregnancy only if the potential benefit justifies the potential risk to the fetus.

Labor and Delivery
The effect of SERZONE (nefazodone hydrochloride) on labor and delivery in humans is unknown.

Nursing Mothers
It is not known whether SERZONE or its metabolites are excreted in human milk. Because many drugs are excreted in human milk, caution should be exercised when SERZONE is administered to a nursing woman.

Pediatric Use
Safety and effectiveness in individuals below 18 years of age have not been established.

Geriatric Use
Over 500 elderly (≥65 years) individuals participated in clinical studies with nefazodone. No unusual adverse age-related phenomena were identified in this cohort of elderly patients treated with nefazodone. Due to the increased systemic exposure to nefazodone seen in single-dose studies in elderly patients (see **CLINICAL PHARMACOLOGY** section, **Pharmacokinetics** subsection), treatment should be initiated at half the usual dose, but titration upward should take place over the same range as in younger patients (see **DOSAGE AND ADMINISTRATION** section). The usual precautions should be observed in elderly patients who have concomitant medical illnesses or who are receiving concomitant drugs.

ADVERSE REACTIONS

Associated with Discontinuation of Treatment
Approximately 16% of the 3496 patients who received SERZONE (nefazodone hydrochloride) in worldwide premarketing clinical trials discontinued treatment due to an adverse experience. The more common (≥1%) events in clinical trials associated with discontinuation and considered to be drug related (i.e., those events associated with dropout at a rate approximately twice or greater for SERZONE compared to placebo) included: nausea (3.5%), dizziness (1.9%), insomnia (1.5%), asthenia (1.3%), and agitation (1.2%).

Incidence in Controlled Trials
Commonly Observed Adverse Events in Controlled Clinical Trials
The most commonly observed adverse events associated with the use of SERZONE (incidence of 5% or greater) and not seen at an equivalent incidence among placebo-treated patients (i.e., significantly higher incidence for SERZONE compared to placebo, $p \leq 0.05$), derived from the table below, were: somnolence, dry mouth, nausea, dizziness, constipation, asthenia, lightheadedness, blurred vision, confusion, and abnormal vision.
Adverse Events Occurring at an Incidence of 1% or More Among SERZONE-Treated Patients
The table that follows enumerates adverse events that occurred at an incidence of 1% or more, and were more frequent than in the placebo group, among SERZONE-treated patients who participated in short-term (6- to 8-week) placebo-controlled trials in which patients were dosed with SERZONE (nefazodone hydrochloride) to ranges of 300 to 600 mg/day. This table shows the percentage of patients in each group who had at least one episode of an event at some time during their treatment. Reported adverse events were classified using standard COSTART-based Dictionary terminology.
The prescriber should be aware that these figures cannot be used to predict the incidence of side effects in the course of usual medical practice where patient characteristics and other factors differ from those which prevailed in the clinical trials. Similarly, the cited frequencies cannot be compared with figures obtained from other clinical investigations involving different treatments, uses, and investigators. The cited figures, however, do provide the prescribing physician with some basis for estimating the relative contribution of drug and nondrug factors to the side-effect incidence rate in the population studied.

Treatment-Emergent Adverse Experience Incidence in 6- to 8-Week Placebo-Controlled Clinical Trials[1], SERZONE 300 to 600 mg/day Dose Range

		Percent of Patients	
Body System	Preferred Term	SERZONE (n=393)	Placebo (n=394)
Body as a Whole	Headache	36	33
	Asthenia	11	5
	Infection	8	6
	Flu syndrome	3	2
	Chills	2	1
	Fever	2	1
	Neck rigidity	1	0
Cardiovascular	Postural hypotension	4	1
	Hypotension	2	1
Dermatological	Pruritus	2	1
	Rash	2	1
Gastrointestinal	Dry mouth	25	13
	Nausea	22	12
	Constipation	14	8
	Dyspepsia	9	7
	Diarrhea	8	7
	Increased appetite	5	3
	Nausea & vomiting	2	1
Metabolic	Peripheral edema	3	2
	Thirst	1	<1
Musculoskeletal	Arthralgia	1	<1
Nervous	Somnolence	25	14
	Dizziness	17	5
	Insomnia	11	9
	Lightheadedness	10	3
	Confusion	7	2
	Memory impairment	4	2
	Paresthesia	4	2
	Vasodilatation[2]	4	2
	Abnormal dreams	3	2
	Concentration decreased	3	1
	Ataxia	2	0
	Incoordination	2	1
	Psychomotor retardation	2	1
	Tremor	2	1
	Hypertonia	1	0
	Libido decreased	1	<1
Respiratory	Pharyngitis	6	5
	Cough increased	3	1
Special Senses	Blurred vision	9	3
	Abnormal vision[3]	7	1
	Tinnitus	2	1
	Taste perversion	2	1
	Visual field defect	2	0
Urogenital	Urinary frequency	2	1
	Urinary tract infection	2	1
	Urinary retention	2	1
	Vaginitis[4]	2	1
	Breast pain[4]	1	<1

[1] Events reported by at least 1% of patients treated with SERZONE and more frequent than the placebo group are included; incidence is rounded to the nearest 1% (<1% indicates an incidence less than 0.5%). Events for which the SERZONE incidence was equal to or less than placebo are not listed in the table, but included the following: abdominal pain, pain, back pain, accidental injury, chest pain, neck pain, palpitation, migraine, sweating, flatulence, vomiting, anorexia, tooth disorder, weight gain, edema, myalgia, cramp, agitation, anxiety, depression, hypesthesia, CNS stimulation, dysphoria, emotional lability, sinusitis, rhinitis, dysmenorrhea[4], dysuria.
[2] Vasodilatation—flushing, feeling warm.
[3] Abnormal vision—scotoma, visual trails.
[4] Incidence adjusted for gender.

Continued on next page

Serzone—Cont.

Dose Dependency of Adverse Events
The table that follows enumerates adverse events that were more frequent in the SERZONE (nefazodone hydrochloride) dose range of 300 to 600 mg/day than in the SERZONE dose range of up to 300 mg/day. This table shows only those adverse events for which there was a statistically significant difference (p≤0.05) in incidence between the SERZONE dose ranges as well as a difference between the high dose range and placebo.
[See table below]
Vital Sign Changes
(See **PRECAUTIONS** section, *Postural Hypotension* subsection.)
Weight Changes
In a pooled analysis of placebo-controlled premarketing studies, there were no differences between nefazodone and placebo groups in the proportions of patients meeting criteria for potentially important increases or decreases in body weight (a change of ≥7%).
Laboratory Changes
Of the serum chemistry, serum hematology, and urinalysis parameters monitored during placebo-controlled premarketing studies with nefazodone, a pooled analysis revealed a statistical trend between nefazodone and placebo for hematocrit, i.e., 2.8% of nefazodone patients met criteria for a potentially important decrease in hematocrit (≤37% male or ≤32% female) compared to 1.5% of placebo patients (0.05≤0.10). Decreases in hematocrit, presumably dilutional, have been reported with many other drugs that block alpha$_1$-adrenergic receptors. There was no apparent clinical significance of the observed changes in the few patients meeting these criteria.
ECG Changes
Of the ECG parameters monitored during placebo-controlled premarketing studies with nefazodone, a pooled analysis revealed a statistically significant difference between nefazodone and placebo for sinus bradycardia, i.e., 1.5% of nefazodone patients met criteria for a potentially important decrease in heart rate (≤50 bpm and a decrease of ≥15 bpm) compared to 0.4% of placebo patients (p<0.05). There was no obvious clinical significance of the observed changes in the few patients meeting these criteria.

Other Events Observed During the Premarketing Evaluation of SERZONE
During its premarketing assessment, multiple doses of SERZONE (nefazodone hydrochloride) were administered to 3496 patients in clinical studies, including more than 250 patients treated for at least one year. The conditions and duration of exposure to SERZONE varied greatly, and included (in overlapping categories) open and double-blind studies, uncontrolled and controlled studies, inpatient and outpatient studies, fixed-dose and titration studies. Untoward events associated with this exposure were recorded by clinical investigators using terminology of their own choosing. Consequently, it is not possible to provide a meaningful estimate of the proportion of individuals experiencing adverse events without first grouping similar types of untoward events into a smaller number of standardized event categories.
In the tabulations that follow, reported adverse events were classified using standard COSTART-based Dictionary terminology. The frequencies presented, therefore, represent the proportion of the 3496 patients exposed to multiple doses of SERZONE who experienced an event of the type cited on at least one occasion while receiving SERZONE. All reported events are included except those already listed in the Treatment-Emergent Adverse Experience Incidence table, those events listed in other safety-related sections of this insert, those adverse experiences subsumed under COSTART terms that are either overly general or excessively specific so as to be uninformative, those events for which a drug cause was very remote, and those events which were not serious and occurred in fewer than two patients.
It is important to emphasize that, although the events reported occurred during treatment with SERZONE, they were not necessarily caused by it.
Events are further categorized by body system and listed in order of decreasing frequency according to the following definitions: frequent adverse events are those occurring on one or more occasions in at least 1/100 patients (only those not already listed in the tabulated results from placebo-controlled trials appear in this listing); infrequent adverse events are those occurring in 1/100 to 1/1000 patients; rare events are those occurring in fewer than 1/1000 patients.
Body as a whole—Infrequent: allergic reaction, malaise, photosensitivity reaction, face edema, hangover effect, abdomen enlarged, hernia, pelvic pain, and halitosis. *Rare:* cellulitis.
Cardiovascular system—Infrequent: tachycardia, hypertension, syncope, ventricular extrasystoles, and angina pectoris. *Rare:* AV block, congestive heart failure, hemorrhage, pallor, and varicose vein.
Dermatological system—Infrequent: dry skin, acne, alopecia, urticaria, maculopapular rash, vesiculobullous rash, and eczema.
Gastrointestinal system—Frequent: gastroenteritis. *Infrequent:* eructation, periodontal abscess, abnormal liver function tests, gingivitis, colitis, gastritis, mouth ulceration, stomatitis, esophagitis, peptic ulcer, and rectal hemorrhage. *Rare:* glossitis, hepatitis, dysphagia, gastrointestinal hemorrhage, oral moniliasis, and ulcerative colitis.
Hemic and lymphatic system—Infrequent: ecchymosis, anemia, leukopenia, and lymphadenopathy.
Metabolic and nutritional system—Infrequent: weight loss, gout, dehydration, lactic dehydrogenase increased, SGOT increased, and SGPT increased. *Rare:* hypercholesteremia and hypoglycemia.
Musculoskeletal system—Infrequent: arthritis, tenosynovitis, muscle stiffness, and bursitis. *Rare:* tendinous contracture.
Nervous system—Infrequent: vertigo, twitching, depersonalization, hallucinations, suicide attempt, apathy, euphoria, hostility, suicidal thoughts, abnormal gait, thinking abnormal, attention decreased, derealization, neuralgia, paranoid reaction, dysarthria, increased libido, suicide, and myoclonus. *Rare:* hyperkinesia, increased salivation, cerebrovascular accident, hyperesthesia, hypotonia, ptosis, and neuroleptic malignant syndrome.
Respiratory system—Frequent: dyspnea and bronchitis. *Infrequent:* asthma, pneumonia, laryngitis, voice alteration, epistaxis, hiccup. *Rare:* hyperventilation and yawn.
Special senses—Frequent: eye pain. *Infrequent:* dry eye, ear pain, abnormality of accommodation, diplopia, conjunctivitis, mydriasis, keratoconjunctivitis, hyperacusis, and photophobia. *Rare:* deafness, glaucoma, night blindness, and taste loss.
Urogenital system—Frequent: impotence[a]. *Infrequent:* cystitis, urinary urgency, metrorrhagia[a], amenorrhea[a], polyuria, vaginal hemorrhage[a], breast enlargement[a], menorrhagia[a], urinary incontinence, abnormal ejaculation[a], hematuria, nocturia, and kidney calculus. *Rare:* uterine fibroids enlarged[a], uterine hemorrhage[a], anorgasmia, and oliguria.

[a]Adjusted for gender.

Postintroduction Clinical Experience
Postmarketing experience with SERZONE has shown an adverse experience profile similar to that seen during the premarketing evaluation of nefazodone. Voluntary reports of adverse events temporally associated with SERZONE have been received since market introduction that are not listed above and for which a causal relationship has not been established. These include:
Rare occurrences of convulsions (including grand mal seizures) and priapism (see **PRECAUTIONS** section);
Rare reports of rhabdomyolysis involving patients receiving the combination of SERZONE and lovastatin or simvastatin (see **PRECAUTIONS** section);
Rare reports of liver necrosis and liver failure, in some cases leading to liver transplantation and/or death.

DRUG ABUSE AND DEPENDENCE
Controlled Substance Class
SERZONE (nefazodone hydrochloride) is not a controlled substance.
Physical and Psychological Dependence
In animal studies, nefazodone did not act as a reinforcer for intravenous self-administration in monkeys trained to self-administer cocaine, suggesting no abuse liability. In a controlled study of abuse liability in human subjects, nefazodone showed no potential for abuse.
Nefazodone has not been systematically studied in humans for its potential for tolerance, physical dependence, or withdrawal. While the premarketing clinical experience with nefazodone did not reveal any tendency for a withdrawal syndrome or any drug-seeking behavior, it is not possible to predict on the basis of this limited experience the extent to which a CNS-active drug will be misused, diverted, and/or abused once marketed. Consequently, physicians should carefully evaluate patients for a history of drug abuse and follow such patients closely, observing them for signs of misuse or abuse of SERZONE (e.g., development of tolerance, dose escalation, drug-seeking behavior).

OVERDOSAGE
Human Experience
In premarketing clinical studies, there were seven reports of nefazodone overdose alone or in combination with other pharmacological agents. The amount of nefazodone ingested ranged from 1000 mg to 11,200 mg. Commonly reported symptoms from overdose of nefazodone included nausea, vomiting, and somnolence. One nonstudy participant took 2000–3000 mg of nefazodone with methocarbamol and alcohol; this person reportedly experienced a convulsion (type not documented). None of these patients died.
In postmarketing experience, overdose with SERZONE alone and in combination with alcohol and/or other substances has been reported. Commonly reported symptoms were similar to those reported from overdose in premarketing experience. While there have been rare reports of fatalities in patients taking overdoses of nefazodone, predominantly in combination with alcohol and/or other substances, no causal relationship to nefazodone has been established.
Overdosage Management
Treatment should consist of those general measures employed in the management of overdosage with any antidepressant.
Ensure an adequate airway, oxygenation, and ventilation. Monitor cardiac rhythm and vital signs. General supportive and symptomatic measures are also recommended. Induction of emesis is not recommended. Gastric lavage with a large-bore orogastric tube with appropriate airway protection, if needed, may be indicated if performed soon after ingestion, or in symptomatic patients.
Activated charcoal should be administered. Due to the wide distribution of nefazodone in body tissues, forced diuresis, dialysis, hemoperfusion, and exchange transfusion are unlikely to be of benefit. No specific antidotes for nefazodone are known.
In managing overdosage, consider the possibility of multiple drug involvement. The physician should consider contacting a poison control center for additional information on the treatment of any overdose. Telephone numbers for certified poison control centers are listed in the *Physicians' Desk Reference* (PDR).

DOSAGE AND ADMINISTRATION
Initial Treatment
The recommended starting dose for SERZONE (nefazodone hydrochloride) is 200 mg/day, administered in two divided doses (BID). In the controlled clinical trials establishing the antidepressant efficacy of SERZONE, the effective dose range was generally 300 to 600 mg/day. Consequently, most patients, depending on tolerability and the need for further clinical effect, should have their dose increased. Dose increases should occur in increments of 100 mg/day to 200 mg/day, again on a BID schedule, at intervals of no less than 1 week. As with all antidepressants, several weeks on treatment may be required to obtain a full antidepressant response.
Dosage for Elderly or Debilitated Patients
The recommended initial dose for elderly or debilitated patients is 100 mg/day on a BID schedule. These patients often have reduced nefazodone clearance and/or increased sensitivity to the side effects of CNS-active drugs. It may also be appropriate to modify the rate of subsequent dose titration. As steady-state plasma levels do not change with age, the final target dose based on a careful assessment of the patient's clinical response may be similar in healthy younger and older patients.
Maintenance/Continuation/Extended Treatment
There is no body of evidence available from controlled trials to indicate how long the depressed patient should be treated with SERZONE. It is generally agreed, however, that pharmacological treatment for acute episodes of depression should continue for up to 6 months or longer. Whether the dose of antidepressant needed to induce remission is identical to the dose needed to maintain euthymia is unknown. Systematic evaluation of the efficacy of SERZONE has shown that efficacy is maintained for periods of up to 36 weeks following 16 weeks of open-label acute treatment (treated for 52 weeks total) at dosages that averaged 438 mg/day. For most patients, their maintenance dose was that associated with response during acute treatment. (See **CLINICAL PHARMACOLOGY** section.) The safety of SERZONE in long-term use is supported by data from both double-blind and open-label trials involving more than 250 patients treated for at least one year.
Switching Patients to or from a Monoamine Oxidase Inhibitor
At least 14 days should elapse between discontinuation of an MAOI and initiation of therapy with SERZONE. In addition, at least 7 days should be allowed after stopping SERZONE before starting an MAOI.

HOW SUPPLIED
SERZONE® (nefazodone hydrochloride) tablets are hexagonal tablets imprinted with BMS and the strength (i.e., 100 mg) on one side and the identification code number on the other. The 100 mg and 150 mg tablets are bisect scored on both tablet faces. The 50 mg, 200 mg, and 250 mg tablets are unscored.

Dose Dependency of Adverse Events in Placebo-Controlled Trials[1]
Percent of Patients

Body System	Preferred Term	SERZONE 300–600 mg/day (n = 209)	SERZONE ≤ 300 mg/day (n = 211)	Placebo (n = 212)
Gastrointestinal	Nausea	23	14	12
	Constipation	17	10	9
Nervous	Somnolence	28	16	13
	Dizziness	22	11	4
	Confusion	8	2	1
Special Senses	Abnormal vision	10	0	2
	Blurred vision	9	3	2
	Tinnitus	3	0	1

[1] Events for which there was a statistically significant difference (p≤0.05) between the nefazodone dose groups.

NDC CODE	*DESCRIPTION*
NDC 0087-0031-47	50 mg light pink tablet, bottle of 60
NDC 0087-0032-31	100 mg white tablet, bottle of 60
NDC 0087-0032-44	100 mg white tablet, blister pack of 100
NDC 0087-0039-31	150 mg peach tablet, bottle of 60
NDC 0087-0039-01	150 mg peach tablet, blister pack of 100
NDC 0087-0033-31	200 mg light yellow tablet, bottle of 60
NDC 0087-0033-44	200 mg light yellow tablet, blister pack of 100
NDC 0087-0041-31	250 mg white tablet, bottle of 60

U.S. Patent No. 4,338,317

Store at room temperature, below 40° C (104° F) and dispense in a tight container.

REFERENCES

1. HALCION® and XANAX® are registered trademarks of the Upjohn Company.
2. SELDANE® is a registered trademark of Merrell Pharmaceuticals, Incorporated, a subsidiary of Hoechst Marion Roussel.
3. HISMANAL® and PROPULSID® are registered trademarks of Janssen Pharmaceutica, Incorporated.
4. ORAP® is a registered trademark of Gate Pharmaceuticals, a division of Teva Pharmaceuticals USA.

Bristol-Myers Squibb Co.
Princeton, NJ 08543
Revised April 2000 Printed in USA
0032DIM-14 P4460-13
D5-B001-04-00

Shown in Product Identification Guide, page 309

STADOL NS® Ⓒ ℞

[stā ′-dŏl]
(butorphanol tartrate)
Nasal Spray
Rx only

DESCRIPTION

Butorphanol tartrate is a synthetically derived opioid agonist-antagonist analgesic of the phenanthrene series. The chemical name is (-)-17-(cyclobutylmethyl) morphinan-3, 14-diol [S-(R*,R*)] - 2,3 - dihydroxybutanedioate (1:1) (salt). The molecular formula is $C_{21}H_{29}NO_2{,}C_4H_6O_6$, which corresponds to a molecular weight of 477.55. Butorphanol tartrate is a white crystalline substance. The dose is expressed as the tartrate salt. One milligram of the salt is equivalent to 0.68 mg of the free base. The n-octanol/aqueous buffer partition coefficient of butorphanol is 180:1 at pH 7.5. STADOL NS (butorphanol tartrate) is an aqueous solution of butorphanol tartrate for administration as a metered spray to the nasal mucosa. Each bottle of STADOL NS contains 2.5 mL of a 10 mg/mL solution of butorphanol tartrate with sodium chloride, citric acid, and benzethonium chloride in purified water with sodium hydroxide and/or hydrochloric acid added to adjust the pH to 5.0. The pump reservoir must be fully primed (see **PATIENT INSTRUCTIONS**) prior to initial use. After initial priming each metered spray delivers an average of 1.0 mg of butorphanol tartrate and the 2.5 mL bottle will deliver an average of 14–15 doses of STADOL NS. If not used for 48 hours or longer, the unit must be reprimed (see **PATIENT INSTRUCTIONS**). With intermittent use requiring repriming before each dose, the 2.5 mL bottle will deliver an average of 8–10 doses of STADOL NS depending on how much repriming is necessary.

CLINICAL PHARMACOLOGY

General Pharmacology and Mechanism of Action: Butorphanol is a mixed agonist-antagonist with low intrinsic activity at receptors of the μ-opioid type (morphine-like). It is also an agonist at κ-opioid receptors. Its interactions with these receptors in the central nervous system apparently mediate most of its pharmacologic effects, including analgesia. In addition to analgesia, CNS effects include depression of spontaneous respiratory activity and cough, stimulation of the emetic center, miosis and sedation. Effects possibly mediated by non-CNS mechanisms include alteration in cardiovascular resistance and capacitance, bronchomotor tone, gastrointestinal secretory and motor activity and bladder sphincter activity. In an animal model, the dose of butorphanol tartrate required to antagonize morphine analgesia by 50% was similar to that for nalorphine, less than that for pentazocine and more than that for naloxone. The pharmacological activity of butorphanol metabolites has not been studied in humans; in animal studies, butorphanol metabolites have demonstrated some analgesic activity. In human studies of butorphanol (see **Clinical Trials**), sedation is commonly noted at doses of 0.5 mg or more. Narcosis is produced by 10–12 mg doses of butorphanol administered over 10–15 minutes intravenously. Butorphanol, like other mixed agonist-antagonists with a high affinity for the κ-receptor, may produce unpleasant psychotomimetic effects in some individuals. Nausea and/or vomiting may be produced by doses of 1 mg or more administered by any route. In human studies involving individuals without significant respiratory dysfunction, 2 mg of butorphanol IV and 10 mg of morphine sulfate IV depressed respiration to a comparable degree. At higher doses, the magnitude of respiratory depression with butorphanol is not appreciably increased; however, the duration of respiratory depression is longer. Respiratory depression noted after administration of butorphanol to humans by any route is reversed by treatment with naloxone, a specific opioid antagonist (see **OVERDOSAGE: Treatment** section). Butorphanol tartrate demonstrates antitussive effects in animals at doses less than those required for analgesia. Hemodynamic changes noted during cardiac catheterization in patients receiving single 0.025 mg/kg intravenous doses of butorphanol have included increases in pulmonary artery pressure, wedge pressure and vascular resistance, increases in left ventricular end diastolic pressure and in systemic arterial pressure.

Table 1
Mean Pharmacokinetic Parameters of Butorphanol in Young and Elderly Subjects[a]

	Intravenous		Nasal	
Parameters	Young	Elderly	Young	Elderly
T_{max}[b] (hr)			0.62 (0.32)[e] (0.15–1.50)[g]	1.03 (0.74) (0.25–3.00)
C_{max}[c] (ng/mL)			1.04 (0.40) (0.35–1.97)	0.90 (0.57) (0.10–2.68)
AUC (inf)[d] (hr•ng/mL)	7.24 (1.57) (4.40–9.77)	8.71 (2.02) (4.76–13.03)	4.93 (1.24) (2.16–7.27)	5.24 (2.27) (0.30–10.34)
Half-life (hr)	4.56 (1.67) (2.06–8.70)	5.61 (1.36) (3.25–8.79)	4.74 (1.57) (2.89–8.79)	6.56 (1.51) (3.75–9.17)
Absolute Bioavailability (%)			69 (16) (44–113)	61 (25) (3–121)
Volume of Distribution[f] (L)	487 (155) (305–901)	552 (124) (305–737)		
Total Body Clearance (L/hr)	99 (23) (70–154)	82 (21) (52–143)		

(a) Young subjects (n = 24) are from 20 to 40 years old and elderly (n = 24) are greater than 65 years of age.
(b) Time to peak plasma concentration.
(c) Peak plasma concentration normalized to 1 mg dose.
(d) Area under the plasma concentration-time curve after a 1 mg dose.
(e) Mean (1 S.D.)
(f) Derived from IV data.
(g) (range of observed values)

Pharmacodynamics The analgesic effect of butorphanol is influenced by the route of administration. Onset of analgesia is within a few minutes for intravenous administration, within 15 minutes for intramuscular injection, and within 15 minutes for the nasal spray doses. Peak analgesic activity occurs within 30–60 minutes following intravenous and intramuscular administration and within 1–2 hours following the nasal spray administration. The duration of analgesia varies depending on the pain model as well as the route of administration, but is generally 3–4 hours with IM and IV doses as defined by the time 50% of patients required remedication. In postoperative studies, the duration of analgesia with IV or IM butorphanol was similar to morphine, meperidine, and pentazocine when administered in the same fashion at equipotent doses (see **Clinical Trials**). Compared to the injectable form and other drugs in this class, STADOL NS (butorphanol tartrate) has a longer duration of action (4–5 hours) (see **Clinical Trials**).

Pharmacokinetics: STADOL (butorphanol tartrate) Injection is rapidly absorbed after IM injection and peak plasma levels are reached in 20–40 minutes. After nasal administration, mean peak blood levels of 0.9–1.04 ng/mL occur at 30–60 minutes after a 1 mg dose (see Table 1). The absolute bioavailability of STADOL NS is 60–70% and is unchanged in patients with allergic rhinitis. In patients using a nasal vasoconstrictor (oxymetazoline) the fraction of the dose absorbed was unchanged, but the rate of absorption was slowed. The peak plasma concentrations were approximately half those achieved in the absence of the vasoconstrictor. Following its initial absorption/distribution phase, the single dose pharmacokinetics of butorphanol by the intravenous, intramuscular, and nasal routes of administration are similar (see Figure 1).

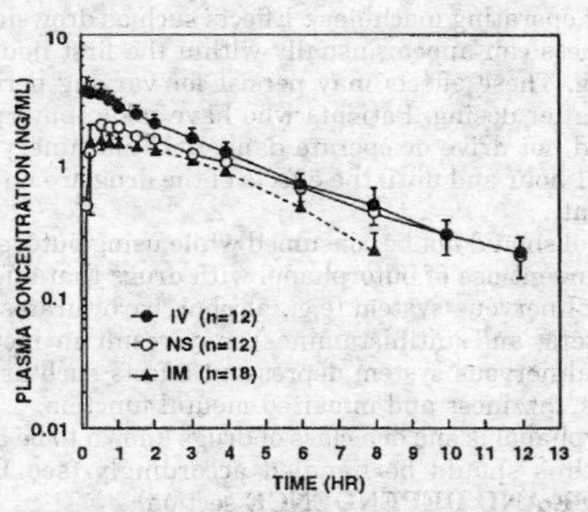

Figure 1—Butorphanol Plasma Levels After IV, IM and Nasal Spray Administration of 2 mg Dose

Serum protein binding is independent of concentration over the range achieved in clinical practice (up to 7 ng/mL) with a bound fraction of approximately 80%.

The volume of distribution of butorphanol varies from 305–901 liters and total body clearance from 52–154 liters/hr (see Table 1).

[See table 1 above]

Dose proportionality for STADOL NS has been determined at steady state in doses up to 4 mg at 6 hour intervals. Steady state is achieved within 2 days. The mean peak plasma concentration at steady state was 1.8-fold (maximal 3-fold) following a single dose. The drug is transported across the blood-brain and placental barriers and into human milk (see **PRECAUTIONS: Labor and Delivery** and **Nursing Mothers** sections). Butorphanol is extensively metabolized in the liver. Metabolism is qualitatively and quantitatively similar following intravenous, intramuscular, or nasal administration. Oral bioavailability is only 5–17% because of extensive first-pass metabolism of butorphanol. The major metabolite of butorphanol is hydroxybutorphanol, while norbutorphanol is produced in small amounts. Both have been detected in plasma following administration of butorphanol, with norbutorphanol present at trace levels at most time points. The elimination half-life of hydroxybutorphanol is about 18 hours and, as a consequence, considerable accumulation (~ 5-fold) occurs when butorphanol is dosed to steady state (1 mg transnasally q6h for 5 days). Elimination occurs by urine and fecal excretion. When ^3H labelled butorphanol is administered to normal subjects, most (70–80%) of the dose is recovered in the urine, while approximately 15% is recovered in the feces. About 5% of the dose is recovered in the urine as butorphanol. Forty-nine percent is eliminated in the urine as hydroxybutorphanol. Less than 5% is excreted in the urine as norbutorphanol. Butorphanol pharmacokinetics in the elderly differ from younger patients (see Table 1). The mean absolute bioavailability of STADOL NS (butorphanol tartrate) in elderly women (48%) was less than that in elderly men (75%), young men (68%) or young women (70%). Elimination half-life is increased in the elderly (6.6 hours as opposed to 4.7 hours in younger subjects). In renally impaired patients with creatinine clearances < 30 mL/min the elimination half-life is approximately doubled and the total body clearance is approximately one half (10.5 hours [clearance 150 L/h] as compared to 5.8 hours [clearance 260 L/h] in normals). No effect was observed on C_{max} or T_{max} after a single dose. For further recommendations refer to **PRECAUTIONS: Hepatic and Renal Disease, Drug Interactions,** and **Geriatric Use** sections and to the **CLINICAL PHARMACOLOGY: Individualization of Dosage** section below.

Clinical Trials: The effectiveness of opioid analgesics varies in different pain syndromes. Studies with STADOL Injection have been performed in postoperative (primarily abdominal and orthopedic) pain and pain during labor and delivery, as preoperative and preanesthetic medication, and as a supplement to balanced anesthesia (see below). Studies with STADOL NS have been performed in postoperative (general, orthopedic, oral, cesarean section) pain, in postepisiotomy pain, in pain of musculoskeletal origin, and in migraine headache pain (see below).

Use in the Management of Pain: *Postoperative Pain:* The analgesic efficacy of STADOL (butorphanol tartrate) Injection in postoperative pain was investigated in several double-blind active-controlled studies involving 958 butorphanol-treated patients. The following doses were found to have approximately equivalent analgesic effect: 2 mg butorphanol, 10 mg morphine, 40 mg pentazocine and 80 mg meperidine. After intravenous administration of STADOL Injection, onset and peak analgesic effect occurred by the time of first observation (30 minutes). After intramuscular administration, pain relief onset occurred at 30 minutes or less,

Continued on next page

Stadol NS—Cont.

and peak effect occurred between 30 minutes and 1 hour. The duration of action of STADOL Injection was 3–4 hours when defined as the time necessary for pain intensity to return to pretreatment level or the time to retreatment. The analgesic efficacy of STADOL NS was evaluated (approximately 35 patients per treatment group) in a general and orthopedic surgery trial. Single doses of STADOL NS (1 or 2 mg) and IM meperidine (37.5 or 75 mg) were compared. Analgesia provided by 1 and 2 mg doses of STADOL NS was similar to 37.5 and 75 mg meperidine, respectively, with onset of analgesia within 15 minutes and peak analgesic effect within 1 hour. The median duration of pain relief was 2.5 hours with 1 mg STADOL NS, 3.5 hours with 2 mg STADOL NS, and 3.3 hours with either dose of meperidine. In a postcesarean section trial, STADOL NS administered to 35 patients as two 1 mg doses 60 minutes apart was compared with a single 2 mg dose of STADOL NS or a single 2 mg IV dose of STADOL Injection (37 patients each). Onset of analgesia was within 15 minutes for all STADOL regimens. Peak analgesic effects of 2 mg intravenous STADOL Injection and STADOL NS were similar in magnitude. The duration of pain relief provided by both 2 mg STADOL NS regimens was approximately 4.5 hours and was greater than intravenous STADOL Injection (2.6 hours).

Migraine Headache Pain: The analgesic efficacy of two 1 mg doses 1 hour apart of STADOL NS in migraine headache pain was compared with a single dose of 10 mg IM methadone (31 and 32 patients, respectively). Significant onset of analgesia occurred within 15 minutes for both STADOL NS and IM methadone. Peak analgesic effect occurred at 2 hours for STADOL NS and 1.5 hours for methadone. The median duration of pain relief was 6 hours with STADOL NS and 4 hours with methadone as judged by the time when approximately half of the patients remedicated. In two other trials in patients with migraine headache pain, a 2 mg initial dose of STADOL NS followed by an additional 1 mg dose 1 hour later (76 patients) was compared with either 75 mg IM meperidine (24 patients) or placebo (72 patients). Onset, peak activity and duration were similar with both active treatments; however, the incidence of adverse experiences (nausea, vomiting, dizziness) was higher in these two trials with the 2 mg initial dose of STADOL NS than in the trial with the 1 mg initial dose.

Preanesthetic Medication: STADOL Injection (2 mg and 4 mg) and meperidine (80 mg) were studied for use as preanesthetic medication in hospitalized surgical patients. Patients received a single intramuscular dose of either STADOL Injection or meperidine approximately 90 minutes prior to anesthesia. The anesthesia regimen included barbiturate induction, followed by nitrous oxide and oxygen with halothane or enflurane, with or without a muscle relaxant. Anesthetic preparation was rated as satisfactory in all 42 STADOL Injection patients regardless of the type of surgery.

Balanced Anesthesia: STADOL Injection administered intravenously (mean dose 2 mg) was compared to intravenous morphine sulfate (mean dose 10 mg) as premedication shortly before thiopental induction, followed by balanced anesthesia in 50 ASA Class 1 and 2 patients. Anesthesia was then maintained by repeated intravenous doses, averaging 4.6 mg STADOL Injection and 22.8 mg morphine per patient. Anesthetic induction and maintenance were generally rated as satisfactory with both STADOL Injection (25 patients) and morphine (25 patients) regardless of the type of surgery performed. Emergence from anesthesia was comparable with both agents.

Labor (see **PRECAUTIONS**): The analgesic efficacy of intravenous STADOL Injection was studied in pain during labor. In a total of 145 patients STADOL Injection (1 mg and 2 mg) was as effective as 40 mg and 80 mg of meperidine (144 patients) in the relief of pain in labor with no effect on the duration or progress of labor. Both drugs readily crossed the placenta and entered fetal circulation. The condition of the infants in these studies, determined by Apgar scores at 1 and 5 minutes (8 or above) and time to sustained respiration, showed that STADOL Injection had the same effects on the infants as meperidine. In these studies neurobehavioral testing in infants exposed to STADOL Injection at a mean of 18.6 hours after delivery, showed no significant differences between treatment groups.

Individualization of Dosage: Use of butorphanol in geriatric patients, patients with renal impairment, patients with hepatic impairment, and during labor requires extra caution (see below and the appropriate sections in **PRECAUTIONS**). The usual recommended dose for initial nasal administration is 1 mg (1 spray in **one** nostril). If adequate pain relief is not achieved within 60–90 minutes, an additional 1 mg dose may be given. The initial dose sequence outlined above may be repeated in 3–4 hours as required after the second dose of the sequence. For the management of severe pain, an initial dose of 2 mg (1 spray in **each** nostril) may be used in patients who will be able to remain recumbent in the event drowsiness or dizziness occurs. In such patients additional doses should not be given for 3–4 hours. The incidence of adverse events is higher with an initial 2 mg dose (see **Clinical Trials**). The initial dose sequence in elderly patients and patients with renal or hepatic impairment should be limited to 1 mg followed by 1 mg in 90–120 minutes. The repeat dose sequence in these patients should be determined by the patient's response rather than at fixed times but will generally be no less than at 6 hour intervals (see **PRECAUTIONS**).

INDICATIONS AND USAGE

STADOL NS (butorphanol tartrate) is indicated for the management of pain when the use of an opioid analgesic is appropriate.

CONTRAINDICATIONS

STADOL NS is contraindicated in patients hypersensitive to butorphanol tartrate or the preservative benzethonium chloride in STADOL NS or STADOL Injection in the multidose vial.

WARNINGS

Patients Dependent on Narcotics: Because of its opioid antagonist properties, butorphanol is not recommended for use in patients dependent on narcotics. Such patients should have an adequate period of withdrawal from opioid drugs prior to beginning butorphanol therapy. In patients taking opioid analgesics chronically, butorphanol has precipitated withdrawal symptoms such as anxiety, agitation, mood changes, hallucinations, dysphoria, weakness and diarrhea. Because of the difficulty in assessing opioid tolerance in patients who have recently received repeated doses of narcotic analgesic medication, caution should be used in the administration of butorphanol to such patients.

Drug Abuse and Dependence

Drug Abuse—Butorphanol tartrate, by all routes of administration, has been associated with episodes of abuse.

Of the cases received, there were more reports of abuse with the nasal spray formulation than with the injectable formulation.

Physical Dependence, Tolerance, and Withdrawal—Prolonged, continuous use of butorphanol tartrate may result in physical dependence or tolerance (a decrease in response to a given dose). Abrupt cessation of use by patients with physical dependence may result in symptoms of withdrawal.

Note—Proper patient selection, dose and prescribing limitations, appropriate directions for use, and frequent monitoring are important to minimize the risk of abuse and physical dependence. (See **DRUG ABUSE AND DEPENDENCE** section below.)

PRECAUTIONS

General: Hypotension associated with syncope during the first hour of dosing with STADOL NS (butorphanol tartrate) has been reported rarely, particularly in patients with past history of similar reactions to opioid analgesics. Therefore, patients should be advised to avoid activities with potential risks. **Head Injury and Increased Intracranial Pressure:** As with other opioids, the use of butorphanol in patients with head injury may be associated with carbon dioxide retention and secondary elevation of cerebrospinal fluid pressure, drug-induced miosis, and alterations in mental state that would obscure the interpretation of the clinical course of patients with head injuries. In such patients, butorphanol should be used only if the benefits of use outweigh the potential risks.

Disorders of Respiratory Function or Control: Butorphanol may produce respiratory depression, especially in patients receiving other CNS active agents, or patients suffering from CNS diseases or respiratory impairment.

Hepatic and Renal Disease: In patients with severe hepatic or renal disease the initial dosage interval for STADOL NS (butorphanol tartrate) should be increased to 6–8 hours until the response has been well characterized. Subsequent doses should be determined by patient response rather than being scheduled at fixed intervals (see **CLINICAL PHARMACOLOGY: Individualization of Dosage** section). **Cardiovascular Effects:** Because butorphanol may increase the work of the heart, especially the pulmonary circuit, the use of butorphanol in patients with acute myocardial infarction, ventricular dysfunction, or coronary insufficiency should be limited to those situations where the benefits clearly outweigh the risk (see **CLINICAL PHARMACOLOGY**). Severe hypertension has been reported rarely during butorphanol therapy. In such cases, butorphanol should be discontinued and the hypertension treated with antihypertensive drugs. In patients who are not opioid dependent, naloxone has also been reported to be effective.

Use in Ambulatory Patients

1. Opioid analgesics, including butorphanol, impair the mental and physical abilities required for the performance of potentially dangerous tasks such as driving a car or operating machinery. Effects such as drowsiness or dizziness can appear, usually within the first hour after dosing. These effects may persist for varying periods of time after dosing. Patients who have taken butorphanol should not drive or operate dangerous machinery for at least 1 hour and until the effects of the drug are no longer present.
2. Alcohol should not be consumed while using butorphanol. Concurrent use of butorphanol with drugs that affect the central nervous system (e.g., alcohol, barbiturates, tranquilizers, and antihistamines) may result in increased central nervous system depressant effects such as drowsiness, dizziness and impaired mental function.
3. Butorphanol is one of a class of drugs known to be abused and thus should be handled accordingly (see **DRUG ABUSE AND DEPENDENCE** section).
4. Patients should be instructed on the proper use of STADOL NS (see **PATIENT INSTRUCTIONS**).

Drug Interactions: Concurrent use of butorphanol with central nervous system depressants (e.g., alcohol, barbiturates, tranquilizers, and antihistamines) may result in increased central nervous system depressant effects. When used concurrently with such drugs, the dose of butorphanol should be the smallest effective dose and the frequency of dosing reduced as much as possible when administered concomitantly with drugs that potentiate the action of opioids. In healthy volunteers, the pharmacokinetics of a 1-mg dose of butorphanol administered as STADOL NS were not affected by the coadministration of a single 6-mg subcutaneous dose of sumatriptan. The pharmacokinetics of a 1-mg dose of butorphanol administered as STADOL NS were not affected by the coadministration of cimetidine (300 mg QID). Conversely, the administration of STADOL NS (1 mg butorphanol QID) did not alter the pharmacokinetics of a 300-mg dose of cimetidine. It is not known if the effects of butorphanol are altered by concomitant medications that affect hepatic metabolism of drugs (erythromycin, theophylline, etc.), but physicians should be alert to the possibility that a smaller initial dose and longer intervals between doses may be needed. The fraction of STADOL NS absorbed is unaffected by the concomitant administration of a nasal vasoconstrictor (oxymetazoline), but the rate of absorption is decreased. Therefore, a slower onset can be anticipated if STADOL NS is administered concomitantly with, or immediately following, a nasal vasoconstrictor. No information is available about the use of butorphanol concurrently with MAO inhibitors.

Information for Patients (see **PRECAUTIONS: Use in Ambulatory Patients**).

Carcinogenesis, Mutagenesis, Impairment of Fertility: Two-year carcinogenicity studies were conducted in mice and rats given butorphanol tartrate in the diet up to 60 mg/kg/day (180 mg/m^2 for mice and 354 mg/m^2 for rats). There was no evidence of carcinogenicity in either species in these studies. Butorphanol was not genotoxic in *S. typhimurium* or *E. coli* assays or in unscheduled DNA synthesis and repair assays conducted in cultured human fibroblast cells. Rats treated orally with 160 mg/kg/day (944 mg/m^2) had a reduced pregnancy rate. However, a similar effect was not observed with a 2.5 mg/kg/day (14.75 mg/m^2) subcutaneous dose.

Pregnancy: Pregnancy Category C: Reproduction studies in mice, rats and rabbits during organogenesis did not reveal any teratogenic potential to butorphanol. However, pregnant rats treated subcutaneously with butorphanol at 1 mg/kg (5.9 mg/m^2) had a higher frequency of stillbirths than controls. Butorphanol at 30 mg/kg/oral (360 mg/m^2) and 60 mg/kg/oral (720 mg/m^2) also showed higher incidences of post-implantation loss in rabbits. There are no adequate and well-controlled studies of STADOL in pregnant women before 37 weeks of gestation. STADOL should be used during pregnancy only if the potential benefit justifies the potential risk to the infant.

Labor and Delivery: There have been rare reports of infant respiratory distress/apnea following the administration of STADOL Injection during labor. The reports of respiratory distress/apnea have been associated with administration of a dose within 2 hours of delivery, use of multiple doses, use with additional analgesic or sedative drugs, or use in preterm pregnancies (see **OVERDOSAGE: Treatment**). In a study of 119 patients, the administration of 1 mg of IV STADOL Injection during labor was associated with transient (10–90 minutes) sinusoidal fetal heart rate patterns, but was not associated with adverse neonatal outcomes. In the presence of an abnormal fetal heart rate pattern, STADOL Injection should be used with caution. STADOL NS is not recommended during labor or delivery because there is no clinical experience with its use in this setting.

Nursing Mothers: Butorphanol has been detected in milk following administration of STADOL (butorphanol tartrate) Injection to nursing mothers. The amount an infant would receive is probably clinically insignificant (estimated 4 µg/L of milk in a mother receiving 2 mg IM four times a day). Although there is no clinical experience with the use of STADOL NS in nursing mothers, it should be assumed that butorphanol will appear in the milk in similar amounts following the nasal route of administration.

Pediatric Use: Butorphanol is not recommended for use in patients below 18 years of age because safety and efficacy have not been established in this population.

Geriatric Use: The initial dose of STADOL Injection recommended for elderly patients is half the usual dose at twice the usual interval. Subsequent doses and intervals should be based on the patient response (see **CLINICAL PHARMACOLOGY: Individualization of Dosage** section). Initially a 1 mg dose of STADOL NS should generally be used in geriatric patients and 90–120 minutes should elapse before deciding whether a second 1 mg dose is needed (see **CLINICAL PHARMACOLOGY: Individualization of Dosage** section). Due to changes in clearance, the mean half-life of butorphanol is increased by 25% (to over 6 hours) in patients over the age of 65 years. Elderly patients may be more sensitive to its side effects. Results from a long-term clinical safety trial suggest that elderly patients may be less tolerant of dizziness due to STADOL NS than younger patients.

ADVERSE REACTIONS

Clinical Trial Experience: A total of 2446 patients were studied in butorphanol clinical trials. Approximately half received STADOL Injection with the remainder receiving STADOL NS. In nearly all cases the type and incidence of side effects with butorphanol by any route were those commonly observed with opioid analgesics. The adverse experiences described below are based on data from short-term and long-term clinical trials in patients receiving butorphanol by any route. There has been no attempt to correct for placebo effect or to subtract the frequencies reported by placebo-treated patients in controlled trials. The most frequently reported adverse experiences across all clinical trials with STADOL Injection and STADOL NS were somnolence (43%), dizziness (19%), nausea and/or vomiting (13%). In long-term trials with STADOL NS only, nasal congestion (13%) and insomnia (11%) were frequently reported.

The following adverse experiences were reported at a frequency of 1% or greater in clinical trials and were considered to be probably related to the use of butorphanol. **Body as a Whole:** asthenia/lethargy, headache, sensation of heat. **Cardiovascular:** vasodilation, palpitations. **Digestive:** anorexia, constipation, dry mouth, nausea and/or vomiting, stomach pain. **Nervous:** anxiety, confusion, dizziness, euphoria, floating feeling, insomnia, nervousness, paresthesia, somnolence, tremor. **Respiratory:** bronchitis, cough, dyspnea, epistaxis, nasal congestion, nasal irritation, pharyngitis, rhinitis, sinus congestion, sinusitis, upper respiratory infection. **Skin and Appendages:** sweating/clammy, pruritis. **Special Senses:** blurred vision, ear pain, tinnitus, unpleasant taste.

The following adverse experiences were reported with a frequency of less than 1% in clinical trials and were considered to be probably related to the use of butorphanol. **Cardiovascular:** hypotension, syncope. **Nervous:** abnormal dreams, agitation, dysphoria, hallucinations, hostility, withdrawal symptoms. **Skin and Appendages:** rash/hives. **Urogenital:** impaired urination.

The following infrequent additional adverse experiences were reported in a frequency of less than 1% of the patients studied in short-term STADOL NS trials and under circumstances where the association between these events and butorphanol administration is unknown. They are being listed as alerting information for the physician. **Body as a Whole:** edema. **Cardiovascular:** chest pain, hypertension, tachycardia. **Nervous:** depression. **Respiratory:** shallow breathing.

Postmarketing Experience: Postmarketing experience with STADOL NS and STADOL Injection has shown an adverse event profile similar to that seen during the premarketing evaluation of butorphanol by all routes of administration. Adverse experiences that were associated with the use of STADOL NS or STADOL Injection and that are not listed above have been chosen for inclusion below because of their seriousness, frequency of reporting, or probable relationship to butorphanol. Because they are reported voluntarily from a population of unknown size, estimates of frequency cannot be made. These adverse experiences include apnea, convulsion, delusion, drug dependence, excessive drug effect associated with transient difficulty speaking and/or executing purposeful movements, overdose, and vertigo. Reports of butorphanol overdose with a fatal outcome have usually but not always been associated with ingestion of multiple drugs.

DRUG ABUSE AND DEPENDENCE

STADOL (butorphanol tartrate) Injection, and STADOL NS (butorphanol tartrate) Nasal Spray are listed in Schedule IV of the Controlled Substances Act (CSA). Proper patient selection, dose and prescribing limitations, appropriate directions for use, and frequent monitoring are important to minimize the risk of abuse and physical dependence with butorphanol tartrate. Special care should be exercised in administering butorphanol to patients with a history of drug abuse or to patients receiving the drug on a continuous basis for an extended period.

Clinical Trial Experience: In all clinical trials, less than 1% of patients using STADOL NS had experiences that suggested the development of physical dependence or tolerance. Much of this information is based on experience with patients who did not have prolonged continuous exposure to STADOL NS. However, in one controlled clinical trial where patients with chronic pain from nonmalignant disease were treated with STADOL NS (n=303) or placebo (n=99) for up to 6 months, overuse (which may suggest the development of tolerance) was reported in nine (2.9%) patients receiving STADOL NS and no patients receiving placebo. Probable withdrawal symptoms were reported in eight (2.6%) patients using STADOL NS and no patients receiving placebo in the chronic nonmalignant pain study. Most of these patients abruptly discontinued STADOL NS after extended use or high doses. Symptoms suggestive of withdrawal included anxiety, agitation, tremulousness, diarrhea, chills, sweats insomnia, confusion, incoordination, and hallucinations.

Postmarketing Experience: Butorphanol tartrate has been associated with episodes of abuse and dependence. Of the cases received, there were more reports of abuse with the nasal spray formulation than with the injectable formulation.

OVERDOSAGE

Clinical Manifestations: The clinical manifestations of butorphanol overdose are those of opioid drugs in general. Consequences of overdose vary with the amount of butorphanol ingested and individual response to the effects of opiates. The most serious symptoms are hypoventilation, cardiovascular insufficiency, coma, and death. Butorphanol overdose may be associated with ingestion of multiple drugs (see **ADVERSE REACTIONS: Postmarketing Experience** section). Overdose can occur due to accidental or intentional misuse of butorphanol, especially in young children who may gain access to the drug in the home.

Treatment: The management of suspected butorphanol overdosage includes maintenance of adequate ventilation, peripheral perfusion, normal body temperature, and protection of the airway. Patients should be under continuous observation with adequate serial measures of mental state, responsiveness and vital signs. Oxygen and ventilatory assistance should be available with continual monitoring by pulse oximetry if indicated. In the presence of coma, placement of an artificial airway may be required. An adequate intravenous portal should be maintained to facilitate treatment of hypotension associated with vasodilation. The use of a specific opioid antagonist such as naloxone should be considered. As the duration of butorphanol action usually exceeds the duration of action of naloxone, repeated dosing with naloxone may be required. In managing cases of suspected butorphanol overdose, the possibility of multiple drug ingestion should always be considered.

DOSAGE AND ADMINISTRATION

Factors to be considered in determining the dose are age, body weight, physical status, underlying pathological condition, use of other drugs, type of anesthesia to be used, and surgical procedure involved. Use in the elderly, in patients with hepatic or renal disease, or in labor requires extra caution (see **PRECAUTIONS** section and **CLINICAL PHARMACOLOGY: Individualization of Dosage** section). The following doses are for patients who do not have impaired hepatic or renal function and who are not on CNS active agents.

Use for Pain: The usual recommended dose for initial nasal administration is 1 mg (1 spray in **one** nostril). Adherence to this dose reduces the incidence of drowsiness and dizziness. If adequate pain relief is not achieved within 60–90 minutes, an additional 1 mg dose may be given. The initial dose sequence outlined above may be repeated in 3–4 hours as required after the second dose of the sequence. Depending on the severity of the pain, an initial dose of 2 mg (1 spray in **each** nostril) may be used in patients who will be able to remain recumbent in the event drowsiness or dizziness occurs. In such patients single additional 2 mg doses should not be given for 3–4 hours. **Use in Balanced Anesthesia:** The use of STADOL NS is not recommended because it has not been studied in induction or maintenance of anesthesia. **Labor:** The use of STADOL NS (butorphanol tartrate) is not recommended as it has not been studied in labor.

Safety and Handling: STADOL NS is an open delivery system with increased risk of exposure to health care workers. In the priming process, a certain amount of butorphanol may be aerosolized; therefore, the pump sprayer should be aimed away from the patient or other people or animals. The disposal of Schedule IV controlled substances must be consistent with State and Federal Regulations. The unit should be disposed of by unscrewing the cap, rinsing the bottle, and placing the parts in a waste container.

HOW SUPPLIED

STADOL NS® (butorphanol tartrate) Nasal Spray is supplied in a child-resistant prescription vial containing a metered-dose spray pump with protective clip and dust cover, a bottle of nasal spray solution, and a patient instruction leaflet. On average, one bottle will deliver 14–15 doses if no repriming is necessary. NDC 0087-5650-41 - 10 mg per mL, 2.5 mL bottle

PHARMACIST ASSEMBLY INSTRUCTIONS FOR STADOL NS NASAL SPRAY: The pharmacist will assemble STADOL NS prior to dispensing to the patient, according to the following instructions: 1. Open the child-resistant prescription vial and remove the spray pump and solution bottle. 2. Assemble STADOL NS by first unscrewing the white cap from the solution bottle and screwing the pump unit tightly onto the bottle. Make sure the clear cover is on the pump unit. 3. Return the STADOL NS bottle to the child-resistant prescription vial for dispensing to the patient.

Storage Conditions: Store at 25° C (77° F) controlled room temperature. See USP. Parenteral drug products should be inspected visually for particulate matter and discoloration prior to administration, whenever solution and container permit.

Revised May 1999 565001DIL-5
1081557A1

STADOL NS also promoted by:
Cephalon, Inc.

Bristol-Myers Squibb Company
Princeton, New Jersey 08543-4500
USA

A4-B001-05-99

Shown in Product Identification Guide, page 309

TEQUIN™ ℞
(gatifloxacin)
Tablets
TEQUIN™ ℞
(gatifloxacin)
Injection
Rx only
(Patient Information Included)

TEQUIN™ is available as TEQUIN (gatifloxacin) Tablets for oral administration and as TEQUIN (gatifloxacin) Injection for intravenous administration.

DESCRIPTION

TEQUIN contains gatifloxacin, a synthetic broad-spectrum 8-methoxyfluoroquinolone antibacterial agent for oral or intravenous administration. Chemically, gatifloxacin is (±)-1-cyclopropyl-6-fluoro-1, 4-dihydro-8-methoxy-7-(3-methyl-1-piperazinyl)-4-oxo-3-quinolinecarboxylic acid sesquihydrate.

The chemical structure is:

Its empirical formula is $C_{19}H_{22}FN_3O_4 \bullet 1.5\ H_2O$ and its molecular weight is 402.42. Gatifloxacin is a sesquihydrate crystalline powder and is white to pale yellow in color. It exists as a racemate, with no net optical rotation. The solubility of the compound is pH dependent. The maximum aqueous solubility (40–60 mg/mL) occurs at a pH range of 2 to 5.

TEQUIN Tablets

TEQUIN Tablets are available as 200 mg and 400 mg white, film-coated tablets and contain the following inactive ingredients: hydroxypropyl methylcellulose, magnesium stearate, methylcellulose, microcrystalline cellulose, polyethylene glycol, polysorbate 80, simethicone, sodium starch glycolate, sorbic acid, and titanium dioxide.

TEQUIN Injection

TEQUIN Injection is available in 20 mL (200 mg) and 40 mL (400 mg) single-use vials as a sterile, preservative-free aqueous solution of gatifloxacin with pH ranging from 3.5 to 5.5. TEQUIN Injection is also available in ready-to-use 100 mL (200 mg) and 200 mL (400 mg) flexible bags as a sterile, preservative-free aqueous solution of gatifloxacin with pH ranging from 3.5 to 5.5. The appearance of the intravenous solution may range from light yellow to greenish-yellow in color. The color does not affect nor is it indicative of product stability.

The intravenous formulation contains dextrose, anhydrous, USP or dextrose, monohydrate, USP and Water for Injection, USP, and may contain hydrochloric acid and/or sodium hydroxide for pH adjustment.

CLINICAL PHARMACOLOGY

Gatifloxacin is administered as a racemate, with the disposition and antibacterial activity of the R- and S-enantiomers virtually identical.

Absorption

Gatifloxacin is well absorbed from the gastrointestinal tract after oral administration and can be given without regard to food. The absolute bioavailability of gatifloxacin is 96%. Peak plasma concentrations of gatifloxacin usually occur 1–2 hours after oral dosing.

The oral and intravenous routes of administration for TEQUIN (gatifloxacin) can be considered interchangeable, since the pharmacokinetics of gatifloxacin after 1-hour intravenous administration are similar to those observed for orally administered gatifloxacin when equal doses are administered (Figure 1) (see **DOSAGE AND ADMINISTRATION**).

FIGURE 1.
Mean Plasma Concentration-Time Profiles of Gatifloxacin Following Intravenous (IV) and Oral (PO) Administration of a Single 400 mg Dose to Healthy Subjects.

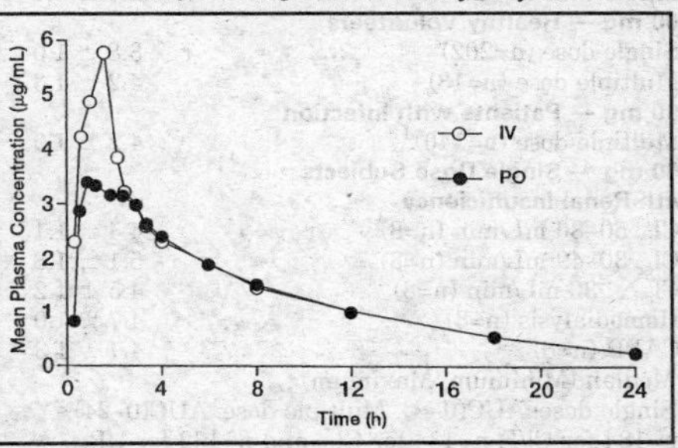

Pharmacokinetics

The mean (SD) pharmacokinetic parameters of gatifloxacin following oral administration to healthy subjects with bacterial infections and subjects with renal insufficiency are listed in Table 1. The mean (SD) pharmacokinetic parameters of gatifloxacin following intravenous administration to healthy subjects are listed in Table 2.

[See table 1 at bottom of next page]
[See table 2 at bottom of next page]

Gatifloxacin pharmacokinetics are linear and time-independent at doses ranging from 200 to 800 mg administered over a period of up to 14 days. Steady-state concentrations are achieved by the third daily oral or intravenous dose of gatifloxacin. The mean steady-state peak and trough plasma concentrations attained following a dosing regimen of 400 mg once daily are approximately 4.2 µg/mL and 0.4 µg/mL, respectively, for oral administration and 4.6 µg/mL and 0.4 µg/mL, respectively, for intravenous administration.

Distribution

Serum protein binding of gatifloxacin is approximately 20% in volunteers and is concentration independent. Consistent

Continued on next page

Tequin—Cont.

with the low protein binding, concentrations of gatifloxacin in saliva were approximately equal to those in plasma (mean [range] saliva:plasma ratio was 0.88 [0.46–1.57]). The mean volume of distribution of gatifloxacin at steady-state (Vd_{ss}) ranged from 1.5 to 2.0 L/kg. Gatifloxacin is widely distributed throughout the body into many body tissues and fluids. Rapid distribution of gatifloxacin into tissues results in higher gatifloxacin concentrations in most target tissues than in serum (Table 3).

[See table 3 at top of next page]

Metabolism

Gatifloxacin undergoes limited biotransformation in humans with less than 1% of the dose excreted in the urine as ethylenediamine and methylethylenediamine metabolites.

In vitro studies with cytochrome P450 isoenzymes (CYP) indicate that gatifloxacin does not inhibit CYP3A4, CYP2D6, CYP2C9, CYP2C19, or CYP1A2, suggesting that gatifloxacin is unlikely to alter the pharmacokinetics of drugs metabolized by these enzymes (e.g., midazolam, cyclosporine, warfarin, theophylline).

In vivo studies in animals and humans indicate that gatifloxacin is not an enzyme inducer; therefore, gatifloxacin is unlikely to alter the metabolic elimination of itself or other co-administered drugs.

Excretion

Gatifloxacin is excreted as unchanged drug primarily by the kidney. More than 70% of an administered TEQUIN (gatifloxacin) dose was recovered as unchanged drug in the urine within 48 hours following oral and intravenous administration, and 5% was recovered in the feces. Less than 1% of the dose is recovered in the urine as two metabolites. Crystals of gatifloxacin have not been observed in the urine of normal, healthy human subjects following administration of intravenous or oral doses up to 800 mg.

The mean elimination half-life of gatifloxacin ranges from 7 to 14 hours and is independent of dose and route of administration. Renal clearance is independent of dose with mean value ranging from 124 to 161 mL/min. The magnitude of this value, coupled with the significant decrease in the elimination of gatifloxacin seen with concomitant probenecid administration, indicates that gatifloxacin undergoes both glomerular filtration and tubular secretion. Gatifloxacin may also undergo minimal biliary and/or intestinal elimination, since 5% of dose was recovered in the feces as unchanged drug. This finding is supported by the 5-fold higher concentration of gatifloxacin in the bile compared to the plasma (mean bile:plasma ratio [range] 5.34 [0.33–14.0]).

Special Populations

Patients with Bacterial Infections

The pharmacokinetics of gatifloxacin were similar between healthy volunteers and patients with infection, when underlying renal function was taken into account (see Table 1).

Geriatric

Following a single oral 400 mg dose of gatifloxacin in young (18–40 years) and elderly (≥ 65 years) male and female subjects, there were only modest differences in the pharmacokinetics of gatifloxacin noted in female subjects; elderly females had a 21% increase in C_{max} and a 32% increase in $AUC_{(0-\infty)}$ compared to young females. These differences were mainly due to decreasing renal function with increasing age and are not thought to be clinically important. No dosage adjustment based on age alone is necessary for elderly subjects when administering TEQUIN (gatifloxacin).

Pediatric

The pharmacokinetics of gatifloxacin in pediatric populations (< 18 years of age) have not been established.

Gender

Following a single oral 400 mg dose of gatifloxacin in male and female subjects, there were only modest differences in the pharmacokinetics of gatifloxacin, mainly confined to elderly subjects. Elderly females had a 21% increase in C_{max} and a 33% increase in $AUC_{(0-\infty)}$ compared to elderly males. Both results were accounted for by gender-related differences in body weight and are not thought to be clinically important. Dosage adjustment of TEQUIN is not necessary based on gender.

Chronic Hepatic Disease

Following a single oral 400 mg dose of gatifloxacin in healthy subjects and in subjects with moderate hepatic impairment (Child-Pugh B classification of cirrhosis), C_{max} and $AUC_{(0-\infty)}$ values for gatifloxacin were modestly higher (32% and 23% respectively). Due to the concentration-dependent antimicrobial activity associated with quinolones, the modestly higher C_{max} values in the subjects with moderate hepatic impairment are not expected to negatively impact the outcome of TEQUIN therapy in this population. Dosage adjustment of TEQUIN is not necessary in patients with moderate hepatic impairment. The effect of severe hepatic impairment on the pharmacokinetics of TEQUIN is unknown.

Renal Insufficiency

Following administration of a single oral 400 mg dose of gatifloxacin to subjects with varying degrees of renal impairment, apparent total clearance of gatifloxacin (Cl/F) was reduced and systemic exposure (AUC) was increased commensurate with the decrease in renal function (see Table 1). Total gatifloxacin clearance was reduced 57% in moderate renal insufficiency (Cl_{cr} 30–49 mL/min) and 77% in severe renal insufficiency ($Cl_{cr} < 30$ mL/min). Systemic exposure to gatifloxacin was approximately 2 times higher in moderate renal insufficiency and approximately 4 times higher in severe renal insufficiency, compared to subjects with normal renal function. Mean C_{max} values were modestly increased. A reduced dosage of TEQUIN is recommended in patients with creatinine clearance < 40 mL/min, including patients requiring hemodialysis or continuous ambulatory peritoneal dialysis (CAPD). (See **PRECAUTIONS: General** and **DOSAGE AND ADMINISTRATION: Impaired Renal Function**.)

Diabetes Mellitus

The pharmacokinetics of gatifloxacin in patients with type 2 diabetes (non-insulin-dependent diabetes mellitus), following TEQUIN 400 mg orally for 10 days, were comparable to those in healthy subjects.

Glucose Homeostasis

No clinically significant changes in glucose tolerance (via measurement of oral glucose challenge) and glucose homeostasis (via measurement of fasting serum glucose, serum insulin and c-peptide) were observed following single or multiple intravenous infusion doses of 200 to 800 mg TEQUIN (gatifloxacin) in healthy volunteers, or 400 mg oral doses of TEQUIN for 10 days in patients with type 2 diabetes (non-insulin-dependent diabetes mellitus). Transient modest increases in serum insulin and decreases in glucose concentrations were noted with the first dose of intravenous or oral gatifloxacin. Following multiple oral doses of TEQUIN in patients with type 2 non-insulin-dependent diabetes mellitus controlled with glyburide, decreases in serum insulin concentrations were noted following oral glucose challenge; however, these decreases were not accompanied by changes in serum glucose levels. (See **PRECAUTIONS: General.**)

Photosensitivity Potential

In a study of the skin response to ultraviolet and visible radiation conducted in 48 healthy, male Caucasian volunteers (12 per group), the minimum erythematous dose was measured for ciprofloxacin (500 mg BID), lomefloxacin (400 mg QD), gatifloxacin (400 mg QD), and placebo before and after drug administration for 7 days. In this study, gatifloxacin was comparable to placebo at all wavelengths tested and had a lower potential for producing delayed photosensitivity skin reactions than ciprofloxacin or lomefloxacin.

Electrocardiogram

In volunteer studies assessing oral and IV doses ranging from 200 to 800 mg, 55 subjects had 76 paired valid ECGs. There were no subjects with abnormal QTc intervals (> 450 msec); the mean ± SD change in QTc interval was 2.9 ± 16.5 msec.

There is limited information available on the potential for a pharmacodynamic interaction in humans between gatifloxacin and drugs that prolong the QTc interval of an electrocardiogram. Therefore, gatifloxacin should not be used with Class IA and Class III antiarrhythmics. (See **WARNINGS** and **PRECAUTIONS**.)

Spirometry

No clinically significant changes in spirometry were observed following single or multiple 200 mg, 400 mg, 600 mg, and 800 mg intravenous infusion doses of TEQUIN in healthy volunteers.

Drug-Drug Interactions

Systemic exposure to TEQUIN is increased following concomitant administration of TEQUIN and probenecid, and is reduced by concomitant administration of TEQUIN and ferrous sulfate or antacids containing aluminum or magnesium salts. TEQUIN can be administered 4 hours before the administration of dietary supplements containing zinc, magnesium, or iron (such as multivitamins).

Probenecid: Concomitant administration of TEQUIN (single oral 200 mg dose) with probenecid (500 mg BID × 1 day) resulted in a 42% increase in AUC and a 44% longer half-life of gatifloxacin.

Iron: When TEQUIN (single oral 400 mg dose) was administered concomitantly with ferrous sulfate (single oral

Table 1: Gatifloxacin Pharmacokinetic Parameters — Oral Administration

	C_{max} (μg/mL)	T_{max}[a] (h)	AUC[b] (μg·h/mL)	$T_{1/2}$ (h)	Cl/F (mL/min)	Cl_R (mL/min)	UR (%)
200 mg — Healthy Volunteers							
Single dose (n=12)	2.0 ± 0.4	1.00 (0.50, 2.50)	14.2 ± 0.4	—	241 ± 40	—	73.8 ± 10.9
400 mg — Healthy Volunteers							
Single dose (n=202)[c]	3.8 ± 1.0	1.00 (0.50, 6.00)	33.0 ± 6.2	7.8 ± 1.3	210 ± 44	151 ± 46	72.4 ± 18.1
Multiple dose (n=18)	4.2 ± 1.3	1.00 (0.50, 4.00)	34.4 ± 5.7	7.1 ± 0.6	199 ± 31	159 ± 34	80.2 ± 12.1
400 mg — Patients with Infection							
Multiple dose (n=140)[d]	4.2 ± 1.9	—	51.3 ± 20.4	—	147 ± 48	—	—
400 mg — Single Dose Subjects with Renal Insufficiency							
Cl_{cr} 50–80 mL/min (n=8)	4.4 ± 1.1	1.13 (0.75, 2.00)	48.0 ± 12.7	11.2 ± 2.8	148 ± 41	124 ± 38	83.7 ± 7.8
Cl_{cr} 30–49 mL/min (n=8)	5.1 ± 1.8	0.75 (0.50, 6.00)	74.9 ± 12.6	17.2 ± 8.5	92 ± 17	67 ± 24	71.1 ± 17.4
Cl_{cr} < 30 mL/min (n=8)	4.5 ± 1.2	1.50 (0.50, 6.00)	149.3 ± 35.6	30.7 ± 8.4	48 ± 16	23 ± 13	44.7 ± 13.0
Hemodialysis (n=8)	4.7 ± 1.0	1.50 (1.00, 3.00)	180.3 ± 34.4	35.7 ± 7.0	38 ± 8	—	—
CAPD (n=8)	4.7 ± 1.3	1.75 (0.50, 3.00)	227.0 ± 60.0	40.3 ± 8.3	31 ± 8	—	—

[a] Median (Minimum, Maximum)
[b] Single dose: AUC(0–∞), Multiple dose: AUC(0–24)
[c] n=184 for Cl/F, n=134 for Cl_R, and n=132 for UR;
[d] Based on the patient population pharmacokinetic modeling, n=103 for C_{max}

C_{max}: Maximum serum concentration; T_{max}: Time to C_{max}; AUC: Area under concentration versus time curve; $T_{1/2}$: Serum half-life; Cl/F: Apparent total clearance; Cl_R: Renal clearance; UR: Urinary recovery.

Table 2: Gatifloxacin Pharmacokinetic Parameters — Intravenous Administration

	C_{max} (μg/mL)	T_{max}[a] (h)	AUC[b] (μg·h/mL)	$T_{1/2}$ (h)	Vd_{ss} (L/kg)	Cl (mL/min)	Cl_R (mL/min)	UR (%)
200 mg — Healthy Volunteers								
Single dose (n=12)	2.2 ± 0.3	1.00 (0.67, 1.50)	15.9 ± 2.6	11.1 ± 4.1	1.9 ± 0.1	214 ± 36	155 ± 32	71.7 ± 6.8
Multiple dose (n=8)[c]	2.4 ± 0.4	1.00 (0.67, 1.00)	16.8 ± 3.6	12.3 ± 4.6	2.0 ± 0.3	207 ± 44	155 ± 55	72.4 ± 16.4
400 mg — Healthy Volunteers								
Single dose (n=30)	5.5 ± 1.0	1.00 (0.50, 1.00)	35.1 ± 6.7	7.4 ± 1.6	1.5 ± 0.2	196 ± 33	124 ± 41	62.3 ± 16.7
Multiple dose (n=5)	4.6 ± 0.6	1.00 (1.00, 1.00)	35.4 ± 4.6	13.9 ± 3.9	1.6 ± 0.5	190 ± 24	161 ± 43	83.5 ± 13.8

[a] Median (Minimum, Maximum)
[b] Single dose: AUC(0–∞), Multiple dose: AUC(0–24)
[c] n=7 for Cl_R and UR

C_{max}: Maximum serum concentration; T_{max}: Time to C_{max}; AUC: Area under concentration versus time curve; $T_{1/2}$: Serum half-life; Vd_{ss}: Volume of distribution; Cl: Total clearance; Cl_R: Renal clearance; UR: Urinary recovery.

Table 3: Gatifloxacin Tissue — Fluid/Serum Ratio (Range)[a]

Fluid or Tissue	Tissue-Fluid/Serum Ratio (Range)[a]
Respiratory	
Alveolar macrophages	26.5 (10.9–61.1)
Bronchial mucosa	1.65 (1.12–2.22)
Lung epithelial lining fluid	1.67 (0.81–4.46)
Lung parenchyma	4.09 (0.50–9.22)
Sinus mucosa	1.78 (1.17–2.49)
Sputum (Multiple dose)	1.28 (0.49–2.38)
Reproductive	
Ejaculate	1.07 (0.86–1.32)
Seminal fluid	1.01 (0.81–1.21)
Vagina	1.22 (0.57–1.63)
Cervix	1.45 (0.56–2.64)

[a]Mean of individual ratios collected over 24 hours following single (100, 150, 200, 300, or 400 mg) or multiple (150 or 200 mg BID) doses of gatifloxacin.

325 mg dose), bioavailability of gatifloxacin was reduced (54% reduction in mean C_{max} and 35% reduction in mean AUC). Administration of TEQUIN (single oral 400 mg dose) 2 hours after or 2 hours before ferrous sulfate (single oral 325 mg dose) did not significantly alter the oral bioavailability of gatifloxacin. (See **DOSAGE AND ADMINISTRATION**.)

Antacids: When TEQUIN (gatifloxacin) (single oral 400 mg dose) was administered 2 hours before, concomitantly, or 2 hours after an aluminum/magnesium-containing antacid (1800 mg of aluminum oxide and 1200 mg of magnesium hydroxide single oral dose), there was a 15%, 69%, and 47% reduction in C_{max} and a 17%, 64%, and 40% reduction in AUC of gatifloxacin, respectively. An aluminum/magnesium-containing antacid did not have a clinically significant effect on the pharmacokinetics of gatifloxacin when administered 4 hours after gatifloxacin administration (single oral 400 mg dose). (See **DOSAGE AND ADMINISTRATION**.)

Milk, Calcium, and Calcium-containing Antacids: No significant pharmacokinetic interactions occur when milk or calcium carbonate is administered concomitantly with TEQUIN (gatifloxacin). Concomitant administration of 200 mL of milk or 1000 mg of calcium carbonate with TEQUIN (200 mg gatifloxacin dose for the milk study and 400 mg gatifloxacin dose for the calcium carbonate study) had no significant effect on the pharmacokinetics of gatifloxacin. TEQUIN can be administered 4 hours before the administration of dietary supplements containing zinc, magnesium, or iron (such as multivitamins).

Minor pharmacokinetic interactions occur following concomitant administration of gatifloxacin and digoxin; a priori dosage adjustments of either drug are not warranted.

Digoxin: Overall, only modest increases in C_{max} and AUC of digoxin were noted (12% and 19% respectively) in 8 of 11 healthy volunteers who received concomitant administration of TEQUIN (400 mg oral tablet, once daily for 7 days) and digoxin (0.25 mg orally, once daily for 7 days). In 3 of 11 subjects, however, a significant increase in digoxin concentrations was observed. In these 3 subjects, digoxin C_{max} increased by 18%, 29%, and 58% while digoxin AUC increased by 66%, 104%, and 79%, and digoxin clearance decreased by 40%, 51%, and 45%. Although dose adjustments for digoxin are not warranted with initiation of gatifloxacin treatment, patients taking digoxin should be monitored for signs and/or symptoms of toxicity. In patients who display signs and/or symptoms of digoxin intoxication, serum digoxin concentrations should be determined, and digoxin dosage should be adjusted as appropriate. The pharmacokinetics of gatifloxacin was not altered by digoxin.

No significant pharmacokinetic interactions occur when cimetidine, midazolam, theophylline, warfarin, or glyburide is administered concomitantly with TEQUIN. These results and the data from *in vitro* studies suggest that gatifloxacin is unlikely to significantly alter the metabolic clearance of drugs metabolized by CYP3A, CYP1A2, CYP2C9, CYP2C19, and CYP2D6 isoenzymes.

Cimetidine: Administration of TEQUIN (single oral dose of 200 mg) 1 hour after cimetidine (single oral dose of 200 mg) had no significant effect on the pharmacokinetics of gatifloxacin. These results suggest that absorption of gatifloxacin is expected to be unaffected by H_2-receptor antagonists like cimetidine.

Midazolam: TEQUIN administration had no significant effect on the systemic clearance of intravenous midazolam. A single intravenous dose of midazolam (0.0145 mg/kg) had no effect on the steady-state pharmacokinetics of gatifloxacin (once daily oral doses of 400 mg for 5 days). These results are consistent with the lack of effect of TEQUIN (gatifloxacin) *in vitro* studies with the human CYP3A4 isoenzyme.

Theophylline: Concomitant administration of TEQUIN (once daily oral doses of 400 mg for 5 days) and theophylline (300 mg BID oral dose for 10 days) had no significant effect on the pharmacokinetics of either drug. These results are consistent with the lack of effect of TEQUIN in *in vitro* studies with the human CYP1A2 isoenzyme.

Warfarin: Concomitant administration of TEQUIN (once daily oral doses of 400 mg for 11 days) and warfarin (single oral dose of 25 mg) had no significant effect on the pharmacokinetics of either drug nor was the prothrombin time significantly altered. These results are consistent with the lack of effect of TEQUIN in *in vitro* studies with the human CYP2C9, CYP1A2, CYP3A4 and CYP2C19 isoenzymes. (See **PRECAUTIONS: Drug Interactions**.)

Glyburide: Concomitant administration of TEQUIN (once daily oral doses of 400 mg for 10 days) and glyburide (steady-state once daily regimen) in patients with type 2 diabetes mellitus had no significant effects on the disposition of either drug, nor were the fasting glucose levels significantly changed. These results are consistent with the lack of effect of TEQUIN in *in vitro* studies with the human CYP3A4 isoenzyme.

Microbiology

Gatifloxacin is an 8-methoxyfluoroquinolone with *in vitro* activity against a wide range of gram-negative and gram-positive microorganisms. The antibacterial action of gatifloxacin results from inhibition of DNA gyrase and topoisomerase IV. DNA gyrase is an essential enzyme that is involved in the replication, transcription and repair of bacterial DNA. Topoisomerase IV is an enzyme known to play a key role in the partitioning of the chromosomal DNA during bacterial cell division. It appears that the C-8-methoxy moiety contributes to enhanced activity and lower selection of resistant mutants of gram-positive bacteria compared to the non-methoxy C-8 moiety.

The mechanism of action of fluoroquinolones including gatifloxacin is different from that of penicillins, cephalosporins, aminoglycosides, macrolides, and tetracyclines. Therefore, fluoroquinolones may be active against pathogens that are resistant to these antibiotics. There is no cross-resistance between gatifloxacin and the mentioned classes of antibiotics.

From *in vitro* synergy tests, gatifloxacin, as with other fluoroquinolones, is antagonistic with rifampin against enterococci.

Resistance to gatifloxacin *in vitro* develops slowly via multiple-step mutations. Resistance to gatifloxacin *in vitro* occurs at a general frequency of between 1×10^{-7} to 10^{-10}. Although cross-resistance has been observed between gatifloxacin and some other fluoroquinolones, some microorganisms resistant to other fluoroquinolones may be susceptible to gatifloxacin.

Gatifloxacin has been shown to be active against most strains of the following microorganisms, both *in vitro* and in clinical infections as described in the **INDICATIONS AND USAGE** section:

Aerobic gram-positive microorganisms
- *Staphylococcus aureus* (methicillin-susceptible strains only)
- *Streptococcus pneumoniae* (penicillin-susceptible strains)

Aerobic gram-negative microorganisms
- *Escherichia coli*
- *Haemophilus influenzae*
- *Haemophilus parainfluenzae*
- *Klebsiella pneumoniae*
- *Moraxella catarrhalis*
- *Neisseria gonorrhoeae*
- *Proteus mirabilis*

Other microorganisms
- *Chlamydia pneumoniae*
- *Legionella pneumophila*
- *Mycoplasma pneumoniae*

The following *in vitro* data are available, **but their clinical significance is unknown.**

Gatifloxacin exhibits *in vitro* minimum inhibitory concentrations (MICs) of ≤ 2 μg/mL (≤ 1 μg/mL for *Streptococcus pneumoniae*) against most (90%) strains of the following microorganisms; however, the safety and effectiveness of gatifloxacin in treating clinical infections due to these microorganisms have not been established in adequate and well-controlled clinical trials.

Aerobic gram-positive microorganisms
- *Staphylococcus saprophyticus*
- *Streptococcus pneumoniae* (penicillin-resistant strains)
- *Streptococcus pyogenes*

Aerobic gram-negative microorganisms
- *Acinetobacter lwoffii*
- *Citrobacter koseri*
- *Citrobacter freundii*
- *Enterobacter aerogenes*
- *Enterobacter cloacae*
- *Klebsiella oxytoca*
- *Morganella morganii*
- *Proteus vulgaris*

Anaerobic microorganisms
- *Peptostreptococcus* spp

NOTE: The activity of gatifloxacin against *Treponema pallidum* has not been evaluated; however, other quinolones are not active against *Treponema pallidum* (see **WARNINGS**).

NOTE: Extended-spectrum β-lactamase producing gram-negative microorganisms may have reduced susceptibility to quinolones.

Susceptibility Tests

Dilution techniques: Quantitative methods are used to determine antimicrobial minimum inhibitory concentrations (MICs). These MICs provide estimates of the susceptibility of bacteria to antimicrobial compounds. The MICs should be determined using a standardized procedure. Standardized procedures are based on a dilution method[1] (broth or agar) or equivalent with standardized inoculum concentrations and standardized concentrations of gatifloxacin powder. The MIC values should be interpreted according to the following criteria:

For testing *Enterobacteriaceae* and *Staphylococcus* species:

MIC (μg/mL)	Interpretation
≤2.0	Susceptible (S)
4.0	Intermediate (I)
≥8.0	Resistant (R)

For testing *Haemophilus influenzae* and *Haemophilus parainfluenzae*[a]:

MIC (μg/mL)	Interpretation
≤0.5	Susceptible (S)

[a] This interpretive standard is applicable only to broth microdilution susceptibility tests with *Haemophilus influenzae* and *Haemophilus parainfluenzae* using *Haemophilus* Test Medium (HTM).

The current absence of data on resistant strains precludes defining any results other than "Susceptible". Strains yielding MIC results suggestive of a "nonsusceptible" category should be submitted to a reference laboratory for further testing.

For testing *Streptococccus pneumoniae*[b]:

MIC (μg/mL)	Interpretation
≤1.0	Susceptible (S)
2.0	Intermediate (I)
≥4.0	Resistant (R)

[b] These interpretive standards are applicable only to broth microdilution susceptibility tests using cation-adjusted Mueller-Hinton broth with 2–5% lysed horse blood.

For testing *Neisseria gonorrhoeae*[c]:

MIC (μg/mL)	Interpretation
≤0.125	Susceptible (S)
0.25	Intermediate (I)
≥0.5	Resistant (R)

[c] These interpretive standards are applicable to agar dilution tests with GC agar base and 1% defined growth supplement.

A report of "Susceptible" indicates that the pathogen is likely to be inhibited if the antimicrobial compound in the blood reaches the concentration usually achievable. A report of "Intermediate" indicates that the result should be considered equivocal, and if the microorganism is not fully susceptible to alternative, clinically feasible drugs, the test should be repeated. This category implies possible clinical applicability in body sites where the drug is physiologically concentrated or in situations where high dosage of drug can be used. This category also provides a buffer zone which prevents small uncontrolled technical factors from causing major discrepancies in interpretation. A report of "Resistant" indicates that the pathogen is not likely to be inhibited if the antimicrobial compound in the blood reaches the concentration usually achievable; other therapy should be selected.

Standardized susceptibility test procedures require the use of laboratory control microorganisms to control the technical aspects of the laboratory procedures. Standard gatifloxacin powder should provide the following MIC values:

Microorganism	MIC Range (μg/mL)
Enterococcus faecalis ATCC 29212	0.12 – 1.0
Escherichia coli ATCC 25922	0.008 – 0.03
Haemophilus influenzae ATCC 49247[d]	0.004 – 0.03
Neisseria gonorrhoeae ATCC 49226[e]	0.002 – 0.016
Pseudomonas aeruginosa ATCC 27853	0.5 – 2.0
Staphylococcus aureus ATCC 29213	0.03 – 0.12
Streptococcus pneumoniae ATCC 49619[f]	0.12 – 0.5

[d] This quality control range is applicable to only *H. influenzae* ATCC 49247 tested by a broth microdilution procedure using HTM.[1]

Continued on next page

Tequin—Cont.

[e] This quality control range is applicable to only *N. gonorrhoeae* ATCC 49226 tested by an agar dilution procedure using GC agar base with 1% defined growth supplement.[1]
[f] This quality control range is applicable to only *S. pneumoniae* ATCC 49619 tested by a microdilution procedure using cation-adjusted Mueller-Hinton broth with 2–5% lysed horse blood.[1]

Diffusion techniques: Quantitative methods that require measurement of zone diameters also provide reproducible estimates of the susceptibility of bacteria to antimicrobial compounds. One such standardized procedure[2] requires the use of standardized inoculum concentrations. This procedure uses paper disks impregnated with 5 µg gatifloxacin to test the susceptibility of microorganisms to gatifloxacin.
Reports from the laboratory providing results of the standard single-disk susceptibility test with a 5 µg gatifloxacin disk should be interpreted according to the following criteria:
The following zone diameter interpretive criteria should be used for testing *Enterobacteriaceae* and *Staphylococcus* species:

Zone Diameter (mm)	Interpretation
≥18	Susceptible (S)
15 – 17	Intermediate (I)
≤14	Resistant (R)

For testing *Haemophilus influenzae* and *Haemophilus parainfluenzae* [g]:

Zone Diameter (mm)	Interpretation
≥18	Susceptible (S)

[g] This zone diameter standards is applicable only to tests with *Haemophilus influenzae* and *Haemophilus parainfluenzae* using *Haemophilus* Test Medium (HTM).[2]

The current absence of data on resistant strains precludes defining any results other than "Susceptible". Strains yielding MIC results suggestive of a "nonsusceptible" category should be submitted to a reference laboratory for further testing.

For testing *Streptococcus pneumoniae* [h]:

Zone Diameter (mm)	Interpretation
≥18	Susceptible (S)
15 – 17	Intermediate (I)
≤14	Resistant (R)

[h] These zone diameter standards only apply to tests performed using Mueller-Hinton agar supplemented with 5% sheep blood incubated in 5% CO_2.[2]

For testing *Neisseria gonorrhoeae* [i]:

Zone Diameter (mm)	Interpretation
≥38	Susceptible (S)
34 – 37	Intermediate (I)
≤33	Resistant (R)

[i] These interpretive standards are applicable to disk diffusion tests with GC agar base and 1% defined growth supplement incubated in 5% CO_2.

Interpretation should be as stated above for results using dilution techniques. Interpretation involves correlation of the diameter obtained in the disk test with the MIC for gatifloxacin.[2]
As with standardized dilution techniques, methods require the use of laboratory control microorganisms that are used to control the technical aspects of the laboratory procedures. For the diffusion technique, the 5 µg gatifloxacin disk should provide the following zone diameters in these laboratory quality control strains:

Microorganism	Zone Diameter Range (mm)
Escherichia coli ATCC 25922	30–37
Haemophilus influenzae ATCC 49247[j]	33–41
Neisseria gonorrhoeae ATCC 49226[k]	45–56
Pseudomonas aeruginosa ATCC 27853	20–28
Staphylococcus aureus ATCC 25923	27–33
Streptococcus pneumoniae ATCC 49619[l]	24–31

[j] This quality control range applies to tests conducted with *Haemophilus influenzae* ATCC 49247 using *Haemophilus* Test Medium (HTM)[2].
[k] This quality control range is only applicable to tests conducted with *N. gonorrhoeae* ATCC 49226 performed by disk diffusion using GC agar base and 1% defined growth supplement.[2]
[l] This quality control range is applicable only to tests conducted with *S. pneumoniae* ATCC 49619 performed by disk diffusion using Mueller-Hinton agar supplemented with 5% defibrinated sheep blood.

INDICATIONS AND USAGE

TEQUIN (gatifloxacin) is indicated for the treatment of infections due to susceptible strains of the designated microorganisms in the conditions listed below. (See **DOSAGE AND ADMINISTRATION.**)

Acute bacterial exacerbation of chronic bronchitis due to *Streptococcus pneumoniae, Haemophilus influenzae, Haemophilus parainfluenzae, Moraxella catarrhalis, or Staphylococcus aureus.*

Acute sinusitis due to *Streptococcus pneumoniae* or *Haemophilus influenzae.*

Community-acquired pneumonia due to *Streptococcus pneumoniae, Haemophilus influenzae, Haemophilus parainfluenzae, Moraxella catarrhalis, Staphylococcus aureus, Mycoplasma pneumoniae, Chlamydia pneumoniae,* or *Legionella pneumophila.*

Uncomplicated urinary tract infections (cystitis) due to *Escherichia coli, Klebsiella pneumoniae,* or *Proteus mirabilis.*

Complicated urinary tract infections due to *Escherichia coli, Klebsiella pneumoniae,* or *Proteus mirabilis.*

Pyelonephritis due to *Escherichia coli.*

Uncomplicated urethral and cervical gonorrhea due to *Neisseria gonorrhoeae.* **Acute, uncomplicated rectal infections in women** due to *Neisseria gonorrhoeae.* (See **WARNINGS.**)

Appropriate culture and susceptibility tests should be performed before treatment in order to isolate and identify organisms causing infection and to determine their susceptibility to gatifloxacin. Therapy with TEQUIN (gatifloxacin) may be initiated before results of these tests are known; once results become available, appropriate therapy should be continued.

CONTRAINDICATIONS

TEQUIN is contraindicated in persons with a history of hypersensitivity to gatifloxacin or any member of the quinolone class of antimicrobial agents.

WARNINGS

THE SAFETY AND EFFECTIVENESS OF GATIFLOXACIN IN PEDIATRIC PATIENTS, ADOLESCENTS (LESS THAN 18 YEARS OF AGE), PREGNANT WOMEN, AND LACTATING WOMEN HAVE NOT BEEN ESTABLISHED. (See **PRECAUTIONS: Pediatric Use, Pregnancy,** and **Nursing Mothers** subsections.)

GATIFLOXACIN MAY HAVE THE POTENTIAL TO PROLONG THE QTc INTERVAL OF THE ELECTROCARDIOGRAM IN SOME PATIENTS. DUE TO THE LACK OF CLINICAL EXPERIENCE, GATIFLOXACIN SHOULD BE AVOIDED IN PATIENTS WITH KNOWN PROLONGATION OF THE QTc INTERVAL, PATIENTS WITH UNCORRECTED HYPOKALEMIA, AND PATIENTS RECEIVING CLASS IA (E.G., QUINIDINE, PROCAINAMIDE) OR CLASS III (E.G., AMIODARONE, SOTALOL) ANTIARRHYTHMIC AGENTS.

Pharmacokinetic studies between gatifloxacin and drugs that prolong the QTc interval such as cisapride, erythromycin, antipsychotics, and tricyclic antidepressants have not been performed. Gatifloxacin should be used with caution when given concurrently with these drugs, as well as in patients with ongoing proarrhythmic conditions, such as clinically significant bradycardia or acute myocardial ischemia. No cardiovascular morbidity or mortality attributable to QTc prolongation occurred with gatifloxacin treatment in over 4000 patients, including 118 patients concurrently receiving drugs known to prolong the QTc interval and 139 patients with uncorrected hypokalemia (ECG monitoring was not performed).

The likelihood of QTc prolongation may increase with increasing concentrations of the drug; therefore, the recommended dose should not be exceeded. QTc prolongation may lead to an increased risk for ventricular arrhythmias including torsades de pointes.

As with other members of the quinolone class, gatifloxacin has caused arthropathy and/or chondrodysplasia in immature dogs. The relevance of these findings to the clinical use of gatifloxacin is unknown. (See **ANIMAL PHARMACOLOGY.**)

Convulsions, increased intracranial pressure, and psychosis have been reported in patients receiving quinolones. Quinolones may also cause central nervous system (CNS) stimulation, which may lead to tremors, restlessness, lightheadedness, confusion, hallucinations, paranoia, depression, nightmares and insomnia. These reactions may occur following the first dose. If these reactions occur in patients receiving gatifloxacin, the drug should be discontinued and appropriate measures instituted. (See **ADVERSE REACTIONS.**)

As with other quinolones, TEQUIN (gatifloxacin) should be used with caution in patients with known or suspected CNS disorders, such as severe cerebral atherosclerosis, epilepsy, and other factors that predispose to seizures.

Serious and occasionally fatal hypersensitivity and/or anaphylactic reactions have been reported in patients receiving therapy with quinolones. These reactions may occur following the first dose. Some reactions have been accompanied by cardiovascular collapse, hypotension/shock, seizure, loss of consciousness, tingling, angioedema (including tongue, laryngeal, throat or facial edema/swelling), airway obstruction (including bronchospasm, shortness of breath, and acute respiratory distress), dyspnea, urticaria, itching and other serious skin reactions.

TEQUIN should be discontinued at the first appearance of a skin rash or any other sign of hypersensitivity. Serious acute hypersensitivity reactions may require treatment with epinephrine and other resuscitative measures, including oxygen, intravenous fluids, antihistamines, corticosteroids, pressor amines, and airway management, as clinically indicated. (See **PRECAUTIONS.**)

Serious and sometimes fatal events, some due to hypersensitivity and some due to uncertain etiology, have been reported in patients receiving antibacterial therapy. These events may be severe and generally occur following the administration of multiple doses. Clinical manifestations may include one or more of the following: fever, rash or severe dermatologic reactions (e.g., toxic epidermal necrolysis, Stevens-Johnson syndrome); vasculitis, arthralgia, myalgia, serum sickness; allergic pneumonitis, interstitial nephritis; acute renal insufficiency or failure; hepatitis, jaundice, acute hepatic necrosis or failure; anemia, including hemolytic and aplastic; thrombocytopenia, including thrombotic thrombocytopenic purpura; leukopenia; agranulocytosis; pancytopenia; and/or other hematologic abnormalities.

Pseudomembranous colitis has been reported with nearly all antibacterial agents, including TEQUIN (gatifloxacin), and may range in severity from mild to life-threatening. It is important, therefore, to consider this diagnosis in patients who present with diarrhea subsequent to the administration of any antibacterial agent.

Treatment with antibacterial agents alters the flora of the colon and may permit overgrowth of clostridia. Studies indicate that a toxin produced by *Clostridium difficile* is the primary cause of "antibiotic-associated colitis."

After the diagnosis of pseudomembranous colitis has been established, therapeutic measures should be initiated. Mild cases of pseudomembranous colitis usually respond to drug discontinuation alone. In moderate to severe cases, consideration should be given to management with fluids and electrolytes, protein supplementation, and treatment with an antibacterial drug clinically effective against *C. difficile* colitis.

Although not seen in clinical trials of TEQUIN, ruptures of the shoulder, hand, and Achilles tendons that required surgical repair or resulted in prolonged disability have been reported in patients receiving quinolones. TEQUIN should be discontinued if the patient experiences pain, inflammation or rupture of a tendon. Patients should rest and refrain from exercise until the diagnosis of tendonitis or tendon rupture has been confidently excluded. Tendon rupture can occur during or after therapy with quinolones.

Gatifloxacin has not been shown to be effective in the treatment of syphilis. Antimicrobial agents used in high doses for short periods of time to treat gonorrhea may mask or delay the symptoms of incubating syphilis. All patients with gonorrhea should have a serologic test for syphilis at the time of diagnosis.

PRECAUTIONS

General

Quinolones may cause central nervous system (CNS) events including nervousness, agitation, insomnia, anxiety, nightmares, or paranoia. (See **WARNINGS** and **PRECAUTIONS: Information for Patients.**)

Administer gatifloxacin with caution in the presence of renal insufficiency. Careful clinical observation and appropriate laboratory studies should be performed prior to and during therapy since elimination of gatifloxacin may be reduced. In patients with impaired renal function (creatinine clearance < 40 mL/min), adjustment of the dosage regimen is necessary to avoid the accumulation of gatifloxacin due to decreased clearance. (See **CLINICAL PHARMACOLOGY** and **DOSAGE AND ADMINISTRATION.**)

As with other quinolones, disturbances of blood glucose, including symptomatic hyper- and hypoglycemia, have been reported, usually in diabetic patients receiving concomitant treatment with an oral hypoglycemic (e.g., glyburide) or with insulin. In these patients, the monitoring of blood glucose is recommended. (See **CLINICAL PHARMACOLOGY** and **ADVERSE REACTIONS.**)

Information for Patients (See **Patient Information** Section)

To assure safe and effective use of TEQUIN, the following information and instructions should be communicated to the patient when appropriate.

Patients should be advised:

- that TEQUIN may produce changes in the electrocardiogram (QTc interval prolongation);
- that TEQUIN should be avoided in patients receiving Class IA (e.g., quinidine, procainimide) or Class III (e.g., amiodarone, sotalol) antiarrhythmic agents;
- that TEQUIN should be used with caution in patients receiving drugs that may effect the QTc interval such as cisapride, erythromycin, antipsychotics, and tricyclic antidepressants;
- to inform their physician of any personal or family history of QTc prolongation or proarrhythmic conditions such as recent hypokalemia, significant bradycardia, or recent myocardial ischemia;
- to inform their physician of any other medications when taken concurrently with TEQUIN, including over-the-counter medications;
- to contact their physician if they experience palpitations or fainting spells while taking TEQUIN (gatifloxacin);
- that TEQUIN Tablets may be taken with or without meals;

- that TEQUIN Tablets should be taken 4 hours before any aluminum- or magnesium-based antacids (see **PRECAUTIONS: Drug Interactions**);
- that TEQUIN Tablets should be taken at least 4 hours before the administration of ferrous sulfate or dietary supplements containing zinc, magnesium, or iron (such as multivitamins) (see **PRECAUTIONS: Drug Interactions**);
- that TEQUIN should be taken 4 hours before VIDEX® (didanosine) buffered tablets, buffered solution, or buffered powder for oral suspension;
- that TEQUIN may be associated with hypersensitivity reactions, even following the first dose, and to discontinue the drug at the first sign of a skin rash, hives or other skin reactions, difficulty in swallowing or breathing, any swelling suggesting angioedema (e.g., swelling of the lips, tongue, face, tightness of the throat, hoarseness), or other symptoms of an allergic reaction (see **WARNINGS** and **ADVERSE REACTIONS**);
- that if they are diabetic and are being treated with insulin or an oral hypoglycemic agent and a hypoglycemic reaction occurs, they should discontinue gatifloxacin and consult a physician (see **PRECAUTIONS: General**);
- to discontinue treatment; rest and refrain from exercise; and inform their physician if they experience pain, inflammation, or rupture of a tendon;
- that TEQUIN may cause dizziness and lightheadedness; therefore, patients should know how they react to this drug before they operate an automobile or machinery or engage in activities requiring mental alertness or coordination;
- that phototoxicity has been reported in patients receiving certain quinolones. There was no phototoxicity seen with gatifloxacin at the recommended dose. In keeping with good medical practice, avoid excessive sunlight or artificial ultraviolet light (e.g. tanning beds). If sunburn-like reaction or skin eruptions occur, contact their physician. (See **CLINICAL PHARMACOLOGY: Photosensitivity Potential**);
- that convulsions have been reported in patients receiving quinolones, and they should notify their physician before taking this drug if there is a history of this condition.

Drug Interactions

TEQUIN (gatifloxacin) can be taken 4 hours before ferrous sulfate, dietary supplements containing zinc, magnesium, or iron (such as multivitamins), or aluminum/magnesium-containing antacids without any significant pharmacokinetic interactions. (See **CLINICAL PHARMACOLOGY**.)

Milk, calcium carbonate, cimetidine, theophylline, warfarin glyburide, or midazolam: No significant interactions have been observed when administered concomitantly with TEQUIN. No dosage adjustments are necessary when these drugs are administered concomitantly with TEQUIN. (See **CLINICAL PHARMACOLOGY**.)

Digoxin: Concomitant administration of TEQUIN and digoxin did not produce significant alteration of the pharmacokinetics of gatifloxacin; however, an increase in digoxin concentrations was observed for 3 of 11 subjects. Patients taking digoxin should therefore be monitored for signs and/or symptoms of toxicity. In patients who display signs and/or symptoms of digoxin intoxication, serum digoxin concentrations should be determined, and digoxin dosage should be adjusted as appropriate. (See **CLINICAL PHARMACOLOGY**.)

Probenecid: The systemic exposure of TEQUIN is significantly increased following the concomitant administration of TEQUIN and probenecid. (See **CLINICAL PHARMACOLOGY**.)

Warfarin: In subjects receiving warfarin, no significant change in clotting time was observed when gatifloxacin was coadministered. However, because some quinolones have been reported to enhance the effects of warfarin or its derivatives, prothrombin time or other suitable anticoagulation test should be monitored closely if a quinolone antimicrobial is administered with warfarin or its derivatives.

Nonsteroidal anti-inflammatory drugs (NSAIDS): Although not observed with gatifloxacin in preclinical and clinical trials, the concomitant administration of nonsteroidal anti-inflammatory drugs with a quinolone may increase the risks of CNS stimulation and convulsions (see **WARNINGS**).

Laboratory Test Interactions

There are no reported laboratory test interactions.

Carcinogenesis, Mutagenesis, Impairment of Fertility

B6C3F1 mice given gatifloxacin in the diet for 18 months at doses with an average intake up to 81 mg/kg/day in males and 90 mg/kg/day in females showed no increases in neoplasms. These doses are approximately 0.13 and 0.18 times the maximum recommended human dose based upon daily systemic exposure (AUC).

In a 2-year dietary carcinogenicity study in Fischer 344 rats, no increases in neoplasms were seen in males given doses up to 47 mg/kg/day and females given up to 139 mg/kg/day. These doses are approximately 0.36 (males) and 0.81 (females) times the maximum recommended human dose based upon daily systemic exposure. A statistically significant increase in the incidence of large granular lymphocyte (LGL) leukemia was seen in males treated with a high dose of 100 mg/kg/day (approximately 0.74 times the maximum recommended human dose based upon daily systemic exposure) versus controls. Although Fischer 344 rats have a high spontaneous background rate of LGL leukemia, the incidence in high-dose males slightly exceeded the historical control range established for this strain. The findings in high-dose males are not considered a concern with regard to the safe use of gatifloxacin in humans.

In genetic toxicity tests, gatifloxacin was not mutagenic in several strains of bacteria used in the Ames test; however, it was mutagenic to *Salmonella* strain TA102. Gatifloxacin was negative in four *in vivo* assays that included oral and intravenous micronucleus tests in mice, an oral cytogenetics test in rats, and an oral DNA repair test in rats. Gatifloxacin was positive in *in vitro* gene-mutation assays in Chinese hamster V-79 cells and *in vitro* cytogenetics assays in Chinese hamster CHL/IU cells. These findings were not unexpected; similar findings have been seen with other quinolones and may be due to the inhibitory effects of high concentrations on eukaryotic type II DNA topoisomerase.

There were no adverse effects on fertility or reproduction in rats given gatifloxacin orally at doses up to 200 mg/kg/day (approximately equivalent to the maximum human dose based on systemic exposure [AUC]).

Pregnancy: Category C

There were no teratogenic effects observed in rats or rabbits at oral gatifloxacin doses up to 150 or 50 mg/kg, respectively (approximately 0.7 and 1.9 times the maximum human dose based on systemic exposure). However, skeletal malformations were observed in fetuses from rats given 200 mg/kg/day orally or 60 mg/kg/day intravenously during organogenesis. Developmental delays in skeletal ossification, including wavy ribs, were observed in fetuses from rats given oral doses of ≥ 150 mg/kg or intravenous doses of ≥ 30 mg/kg daily during organogenesis, suggesting that gatifloxacin is slightly fetotoxic at these doses. Similar findings have been seen with other quinolones. These changes were not seen in rats or rabbits given oral doses of gatifloxacin up to 50 mg/kg (approximately 0.2 and 1.9 times the maximum human dose, respectively, based on systemic exposure).

When rats were given oral doses of 200 mg/kg of gatifloxacin beginning in late pregnancy and continuing throughout lactation, late postimplantation loss increased, as did neonatal and perinatal mortalities. These observations also suggest fetotoxicity. Similar findings have been seen with other quinolones.

Because there are no adequate and well-controlled studies in pregnant women, TEQUIN (gatifloxacin) should be used during pregnancy only if the potential benefit outweighs the potential risk to the fetus.

Nursing Mothers

Gatifloxacin is excreted in the breast milk of rats. It is not known whether this drug is excreted in human milk. Because many drugs are excreted in human milk, caution should be exercised when gatifloxacin is administered to a nursing woman.

Pediatric Use

The safety and effectiveness of gatifloxacin in pediatric populations (< 18 years of age) have not been established. Quinolones, including gatifloxacin, cause arthropathy and osteochondrotoxicity in juvenile animals (rats and dogs).

Geriatric Use

In multiple-dose clinical trials of gatifloxacin (N = 2891), 22% of patients were ≥65 years of age and 10% were ≥75 years of age. No overall differences in safety or efficacy were observed between these subjects and younger subjects, and other reported clinical experience has not identified differences in responses between the elderly and younger patients, but greater sensitivity of some older individuals cannot be ruled out.

This drug is known to be substantially excreted by the kidney, and the risk of toxic reactions to this drug may be greater in patients with impaired renal function. Because elderly patients are more likely to have decreased renal function, care should be taken in dose selection, and it may be useful to monitor renal function. (See **DOSAGE AND ADMINISTRATION**.)

ADVERSE REACTIONS

Over 4000 patients have been treated with gatifloxacin in single- and multiple-dose clinical efficacy trials worldwide. In gatifloxacin studies, the majority of adverse reactions were described as mild in nature. Gatifloxacin was discontinued for adverse events thought related to drug in 2.9% of patients.

Drug-related adverse events classified as possibly, probably, or definitely related with a frequency of ≥3% in patients receiving gatifloxacin in single- and multiple-dose clinical trials are as follows: nausea 8%, vaginitis 6%, diarrhea 4%, headache 3%, dizziness 3%.

In patients who were treated with either intravenous gatifloxacin or with intravenous followed by oral therapy, the incidence of adverse events was similar to those who received oral therapy alone. Local injection site reactions (redness at injection site) were noted in 5% of patients.

Additional drug-related adverse events (possibly, probably, or definitely related) considered clinically relevant that occurred in ≥0.1% to <3% of patients receiving gatifloxacin in single- and multiple-dose clinical trials are as follows:

Body as a Whole: allergic reaction, chills, fever, back pain, chest pain

Cardiovascular System: palpitation

Digestive System: abdominal pain, constipation, dyspepsia, glossitis, oral moniliasis, stomatitis, mouth ulcer, vomiting

Metabolic/Nutritional System: peripheral edema

Nervous System: abnormal dream, insomnia, paresthesia, tremor, vasodilatation, vertigo

Respiratory System: dyspnea, pharyngitis

Skin/Appendages: rash, sweating

Special Senses: abnormal vision, taste perversion, tinnitus

Urogenital System: dysuria, hematuria

Additional drug-related adverse events considered clinically relevant that occurred in <0.1% (rare adverse events) of patients receiving gatifloxacin in single- and multiple-dose clinical trials are as follows: abnormal thinking, agitation, alcohol intolerance, anorexia, anxiety, arthalgia, arthritis, asthenia, asthma (bronchospasm), ataxia, bone pain, bradycardia, breast pain, cheilitis, colitis, confusion, convulsion, cyanosis, depersonalization, depression, diabetes mellitus, dry skin, dysphagia, ear pain, ecchymosis, edema, epistaxis, euphoria, eye pain, face edema, flatulence, gastritis, gastrointestional hemorrhage, gingivitis, halitosis, hallucination, hematemesis, hostility, hyperesthesia, hyperglycemia, hypertension, hypertonia, hyperventilation, hypoglycemia, leg cramp, lymphadenopathy, maculopapular rash, metrorrhagia, migraine, mouth edema, myalgia, myasthenia, neck pain, nervousness, panic attack, paranoia, parosmia, pruritus, pseudomembranous colitis, psychosis, ptosis, rectal hemorrhage, somnolence, stress, substernal chest pain, tachycardia, taste loss, thirst, tongue edema, vesiculobullous rash.

Laboratory Changes

Clinically relevant changes in laboratory parameters, without regard to drug relationship, occurred in fewer than 1% of TEQUIN-treated patients. These included the following: neutropenia, increased ALT or AST levels, alkaline phosphatase, bilirubin, serum amylase, and electrolytes abnormalities. It is not known whether these abnormalities were caused by the drug or the underlying condition being treated.

OVERDOSAGE

Gatifloxacin exhibits a low potential for acute toxicity in animal studies. The minimum lethal oral doses in rats and dogs were greater than 2000 mg/kg and 1000 mg/kg, respectively. The minimum lethal intravenous dose was 144 mg/kg in rats and greater than 45 mg/kg in dogs. Clinical signs observed included decreased activity and respiratory rate, vomiting, tremors, and convulsions.

In the event of acute oral overdose, the stomach should be emptied by inducing vomiting or by gastric lavage. The patient should be carefully observed (including ECG monitoring) and given symptomatic and supportive treatment. Adequate hydration should be maintained. Gatifloxacin is not efficiently removed from the body by hemodialysis (approximately 14% recovered over 4 hours) or by chronic ambulatory peritoneal dialysis (CAPD) (approximately 11% recovered over 8 days).

DOSAGE AND ADMINISTRATION

The recommended dosage for TEQUIN (gatifloxacin) Tablets or TEQUIN Injection is described in Table 4. Doses of TEQUIN are administered once every 24 hours. These recommendations apply to all patients with a creatinine clearance ≥40 mL/min. For patients with a creatinine clearance <40 mL/min, see the **Impaired Renal Function** subsection.

TEQUIN can be administered without regard to food, including milk and dietary supplements containing calcium. Oral doses of TEQUIN should be administered at least 4 hours before the administration of ferrous sulfate, dietary supplements containing zinc, magnesium, or iron (such as multivitamins), aluminum/magnesium-containing antacids, or VIDEX® (didanosine) buffered tablets, buffered solution, or buffered powder for oral suspension.

TEQUIN can be administered without regard to age (≥18 years), or gender.

When switching from intravenous to oral dosage administration, no dosage adjustment is necessary. Patients whose therapy is started with TEQUIN Injection may be switched to TEQUIN Tablets when clinically indicated at the discretion of the physician.

TEQUIN (gatifloxacin) Injection should be administered by INTRAVENOUS infusion only. It is not intended for intramuscular, intrathecal, intraperitoneal, or subcutaneous administration.

Single-use vials require dilution prior to administration. (See *Preparation of Gatifloxacin for Intravenous Administration.*)

TEQUIN Injection should be administered by intravenous infusion over a period of 60 minutes. CAUTION: RAPID OR BOLUS INTRAVENOUS INFUSION SHOULD BE AVOIDED.

[See table 4 at top of next page]

Impaired Renal Function

Since gatifloxacin is eliminated primarily by renal excretion, a dosage modification of TEQUIN (gatifloxacin) is recommended for patients with creatinine clearance < 40 mL/min, including patients on hemodialysis and on CAPD. The recommended dosage of TEQUIN is:

[See table 5 on next page]

Administer TEQUIN (gatifloxacin) after a dialysis session for patients on hemodialysis.

Single 400 mg dose TEQUIN regimen (for the treatment of uncomplicated urinary tract infections and gonorrhea) and 200 mg once daily for 3 days TEQUIN regimen (for the treatment of uncomplicated urinary tract infections) require no dosage adjustment in patients with impaired renal function.

The following formula may be used to estimate creatinine clearance:

[See third table from top on next page]

Continued on next page

Tequin—Cont.

Chronic Hepatic Disease
No adjustment in the dosage of TEQUIN is necessary in patients with moderate hepatic impairment (Child-Pugh Class B). There are no data in patients with severe hepatic impairment (Child-Pugh Class C). (See **CLINICAL PHARMACOLOGY**.)

Intravenous Administration
Preparation of Gatifloxacin for Intravenous Administration TEQUIN solution in single-use vials: TEQUIN Injection is supplied in single-use 20 or 40 mL vials (10 mg/mL) containing a concentrated solution of gatifloxacin in 5% dextrose (200 or 400 mg of gatifloxacin, respectively). (See **HOW SUPPLIED**.) THESE TEQUIN INJECTION SINGLE-USE VIALS MUST BE FURTHER DILUTED WITH AN APPROPRIATE SOLUTION PRIOR TO INTRAVENOUS ADMINISTRATION. The concentration of the resulting diluted solution should be 2 mg/mL prior to administration.
Compatible intravenous solutions: Any of the following intravenous solutions may be used to prepare a 2 mg/mL gatifloxacin solution:

- 5% Dextrose Injection, USP
- 0.9% Sodium Chloride Injection, USP
- 5% Dextrose and 0.9% Sodium Chloride Injection, USP
- Lactated Ringer's and 5% Dextrose Injection, USP
- 5% Sodium Bicarbonate Injection, USP
- Plasma-Lyte® 56 and 5% Dextrose Injection (Multiple Electrolytes and Dextrose Injection, Type 1, USP)
- M/6 Sodium Lactate Injection, USP
- Water for Injection, USP

Gatifloxacin solutions at 2 mg/mL also have been shown to be compatible with 20 mEq/L Potassium Chloride in 5% Dextrose and 0.45% Sodium Chloride Injection, USP.
This intravenous drug product should be inspected visually for particulate matter prior to dilution and administration. Samples containing visible particles should be discarded. Since no preservative or bacteriostatic agent is present in this product, aseptic technique must be used in preparation of the final intravenous solution. Since the vials are for single-use only, any unused portion remaining in the vial should be discarded.
Since only limited data are available on the compatibility of gatifloxacin intravenous injection with other intravenous substances, additives or other medications should not be added to TEQUIN (gatifloxacin) Injection in single-use vials or infused simultaneously through the same intravenous line.
If the same intravenous line is used for sequential infusion of different drugs, the line should be flushed before and after infusion of TEQUIN Injection with an infusion solution compatible with TEQUIN Injection and with any other drug(s) administered via this common line.
If TEQUIN Injection is to be given concomitantly with another drug, each drug should be given separately in accordance with the recommended dosage and route of administration for each drug.
TEQUIN Injection premix in single-use flexible containers: TEQUIN Injection is also available in ready-to-use 100 and 200 mL flexible bags containing a dilute solution of 200 or 400 mg gatifloxacin in 5% dextrose. NO FURTHER DILUTION OF THIS PREPARATION IS NECESSARY.
This intravenous drug product should be inspected visually for particulate matter prior to administration. Samples containing visible particles should be discarded.
Since the premix flexible bags are for single use only, any unused portion should be discarded.
Since only limited data are available on the compatibility of gatifloxacin intravenous injection with other intravenous substances, additives or other medications should not be added to TEQUIN (gatifloxacin) Injection in flexible containers or infused simultaneously through the same intravenous line. If the same intravenous line is used for sequential infusion of different drugs, the line should be flushed before and after infusion of TEQUIN Injection with an infusion solution compatible with TEQUIN Injection and with any other drug(s) administered via this common line.
Instructions for the use of TEQUIN Injection premix in flexible containers:
To open:

1. Tear outer wrap at the notch and remove solution container.
2. Check the container for minute leaks by squeezing the inner bag firmly. If leaks are found, or if the seal is not intact, discard the solution, as the sterility may be compromised.
3. Use only if solution is clear and light yellow to greenish-yellow in color.
4. Use sterile equipment.
5. **WARNING: Do not use flexible containers in series connections.** Such use could result in air embolism due to residual air being drawn from the primary container before administration of the fluid from the secondary container is complete.

Preparation for administration:

1. Close flow control clamp of administration set.
2. Remove cover from port at bottom of container.
3. Insert piercing pin of administration set into port with a twisting motion until the pin is firmly seated. **NOTE: See full directions on administration set carton.**
4. Suspend container from hanger.
5. Squeeze and release drip chamber to establish proper fluid level in chamber during infusion of TEQUIN Injection premix in flexible containers.
6. Open flow control clamp to expel air from set. Close clamp.
7. Regulate rate of administration with flow control clamp.

Table 4: Gatifloxacin — Dosage Guidelines

INFECTION[a]	DAILY DOSE[b]	DURATION
Acute Bacterial Exacerbation of Chronic Bronchitis	400 mg	7–10 days
Acute Sinusitis	400 mg	10 days
Community-acquired Pneumonia	400 mg	7–14 days
Uncomplicated Urinary Tract Infections (cystitis)	400 mg or 200 mg	Single dose 3 days
Complicated Urinary Tract Infections	400 mg	7–10 days
Acute Pyelonephritis	400 mg	7–10 days
Uncomplicated Urethal Gonorrhea in Men; Endocervical and Rectal Gonorrhea in Women	400 mg	Single dose

[a] due to the designated pathogens (see **INDICATIONS AND USAGE**).
[b] for either the oral or intravenous routes of administration for TEQUIN (see **CLINICAL PHARMACOLOGY**).

Table 5: Recommended Dosage of TEQUIN in Adult Patients with Renal Impairment

Creatinine Clearance	Initial Dose	Subsequent Dose[a]
≥ 40 mL/min	400 mg	400 mg every day
< 40 mL/min	400 mg	200 mg every day
Hemodialysis	400 mg	200 mg every day
Continuous peritoneal dialysis	400 mg	200 mg every day

[a] Start subsequent dose on Day 2 of dosing.

$$\text{Men: Creatinine Clearance (mL/min)} = \frac{\text{Weight (kg)} \times (140\text{-age})}{72 \times \text{serum creatinine (mg/dL)}}$$

Women: 0.85 × the value calculated for men.

Stability of TEQUIN Injection as Supplied
When stored under recommended conditions, TEQUIN Injection, as supplied in 20 mL and 40 mL vials and in 100 mL and 200 mL flexible containers, is stable through the expiration date printed on the label.
Stability of TEQUIN Injection Following Dilution
TEQUIN Injection, when diluted in a compatible intravenous fluid to a concentration of 2 mg/mL, is stable for 14 days when stored between 20°C–26°C or when stored under refrigeration between 2°C–8°C.
TEQUIN Injection, when diluted to a concentration of 2 mg/mL in a compatible intravenous fluid EXCEPT FOR 5% SODIUM BICARBONATE INJECTION, USP, may be stored for up to 6 months at -25°C–10°C (-13°F–14°F). Frozen solutions may be thawed at controlled room temperature. Solutions that have been thawed are stable for 14 days after removal from the freezer when stored between 20°C–25°C or when stored under refrigeration between 2°C–8°C. Solutions should not be refrozen

Plasma-Lyte® is a registered trademark of Baxter International, Inc.

HOW SUPPLIED

Tablets
TEQUIN™ (gatifloxacin) Tablets are available as 200 mg and 400 mg white, film-coated tablets. The tablets are almond shaped and biconvex and contain gatifloxacin sesquihydrate equivalent to either 200 mg or 400 mg gatifloxacin.
TEQUIN Tablets are packaged in bottles, unit dose blister strips, and blister packs of 7 tablets (TEQUIN Teq-Paq™) in the following configurations:
200 mg tablets—color: white; shape: biconvex; debossing: "BMS" on one side and "TEQUIN" and "200" on the other.
Bottles of 30 (NDC 0015-1117-50)
Blister pack of 100 (NDC 0015-1117-80)
400 mg tablets—color: white; shape: biconvex; debossing: "BMS" on one side and "TEQUIN" and "400" on the other.
Bottles of 50 (NDC 0015-1177-60)
Blister pack of 100 (NDC 0015-1177-80)
Carton of 2 TEQUIN Teq-Paqs (7 tablets each) (NDC 0015-1177-19)
Storage
Store at 25°C (77°F); excursions permitted to 15–30°C (59–86°F) [see USP Controlled Room Temperature].

Intravenous Solution — Single-Use Vials
TEQUIN™ (gatifloxacin) Injection is available for intravenous administration in the following configurations:
Single-use vials containing a clear, light yellow to greenish-yellow solution at a concentration of 10 mg/mL gatifloxacin.
10 mg/mL (200 mg), 20 mL vials (NDC 0015-1178-80)
10 mg/mL (400 mg), 40 mL vials (NDC 0015-1179-80)
Storage
Store at 25°C (77°F); excursions permitted to 15–30°C (59–86°F) [see USP Controlled Room Temperature].

Intravenous Solution — Premix Bags
TEQUIN Injection is also available in ready-to-use flexible bags containing a dilute solution of 200 mg or 400 mg of gatifloxacin in 5% dextrose. Premix bags are manufactured by Abbott Laboratories in North Chicago, IL.
2 mg/mL (200 mg), 100 mL flexible container (NDC 0015-1180-80)
2 mg/mL (400 mg), 200 mL flexible container (NDC 0015-1181-80)
Storage
Store at 25°C (77°F); excursions permitted to 15–30°C (59–86°F) [see USP Controlled Room Temperature].
Do not freeze.

ANIMAL PHARMACOLOGY

In contrast to some other quinolone antibacterials, there was no evidence of phototoxicity when gatifloxacin was evaluated in the hairless mouse or guinea pig models using simulated sunlight or UVA radiation, respectively.
Unlike some other members of the quinolone class, crystalluria, ocular toxicity, and testicular degeneration were not observed in 6-month repeat dose studies with rats or dogs given gatifloxacin.
While some quinolone antibacterials have proconvulsant activity that is exacerbated with concomitant use of nonsteroidal antiinflammatory drugs (NSAID), gatifloxacin did not produce an increase in seizure activity when administered intravenously to mice at doses up to 100 mg/kg in combination with the NSAID fenbufen.
Quinolone antibacterials have been shown to cause arthropathy in immature animals. There is no evidence of arthropathy in fully mature rats and dogs given gatifloxacin for 6 months at doses of 240 or 24 mg/kg, respectively (approximately 1.5 times the maximum human dose in both species based on systemic exposure). Arthropathy and chondrodysplasia were observed in immature dogs given 10 mg/kg gatifloxacin orally for 7 days (approximately equal to the maximum human dose based upon systemic exposure) [see **WARNINGS**]. The relevance of these findings to the clinical use of gatifloxacin is unknown.
Some other members of the quinolone class have been shown to cause prolongation of the QT interval in dogs. Intravenous 10 mg/kg bolus doses of gatifloxacin had no effect on QT interval in anesthetized dogs.

REFERENCES

1. National Committee for Clinical Laboratory Standards. *Methods for Dilution Antimicrobial Susceptibility Tests for Bacteria That Grows Aerobically* – Fourth Edition; Approved Standard, NCCLS, Wayne, PA, Document M7-A4, Vol. 17, No. 2, NCCLS, January 1997.
2. National Committee for Clinical Laboratory Standards. *Performance Standards for Antimicrobial Disk Susceptibility Tests* – Sixth Edition; Approved Standard, NCCLS, Wayne, PA, Document M2-A6, Vol. 17, No. 1, NCCLS, January 1997.

Patient Information About:
TEQUIN™ (gatifloxacin)
200 mg and 400 mg Tablets
This section contains important information about TEQUIN (gatifloxacin) that you should read before you begin treatment. This section does not list all the benefits and risks of TEQUIN and does not take the place of discussions with your doctor or healthcare professional about your medical condition or your treatment. If you have questions, talk with your healthcare professional. The medicine described here can only be prescribed by a licensed healthcare professional. Only your healthcare professional can determine if TEQUIN is right for you.

What is TEQUIN?
TEQUIN (*pronounced TEK win*) is an antibiotic used to treat lung, sinus, or urinary tract infections, and also to

treat certain sexually transmitted diseases caused by germs called bacteria. TEQUIN kills many of the kinds of bacteria that can infect the lungs, sinus, and urinary tract and that cause certain sexually transmitted diseases. TEQUIN has been shown in a large number of clinical trials to be safe and effective for the treatment of bacterial infections.
Sometimes viruses, rather than bacteria, may infect the lungs and sinuses (for example, the common cold). TEQUIN, like all other antibiotics, does not kill viruses.
The sexually transmitted disease called gonorrhea is treated by TEQUIN. Other diseases called syphilis or non-gonococcal disease are not treated by TEQUIN.
You should contact your doctor if you think your condition is not improving while taking TEQUIN. TEQUIN Tablets are white and contain either 200 mg or 400 mg of active drug.

How and when should I take TEQUIN?
TEQUIN should be taken once a day for 1 to 14 days depending on your prescription. It should be swallowed whole and may be taken with or without food. Try to take the tablet at the same time each day.
You may begin to feel better quickly; however, in order to make sure that all bacteria are killed, you should complete the full course of medication. Do not take more than the prescribed dose of TEQUIN. Try not to miss a dose, but if you do, take it as soon as possible. If it is almost time for the next dose, skip the missed dose and continue your regular dose.

Who should not take TEQUIN?
You should avoid TEQUIN (gatifloxacin) if you have ever had a severe allergic reaction to any medicine in the group of antibiotics known as "quinolones" such as CIPRO® (ciprofloxacin) or LEVAQUIN® (levofloxacin).
You should avoid TEQUIN if you have a rare condition known as congenital prolongation of the QTc interval. If any of your family members have this condition, you should inform your healthcare professional.
You should avoid TEQUIN if you are being treated for heart rhythm disturbances with certain medicines such as quinidine, procainamide, amiodarone, or sotalol. Inform your healthcare professional if you are taking a heart rhythm drug.
TEQUIN should be avoided in patients with a condition known as hypokalemia (low blood potassium). Hypokalemia may be caused by medicines called diuretics such as furosemide and hydrochlorothiazide. If you are taking a diuretic you should speak with your healthcare professional.
If you are pregnant or planning to become pregnant while taking TEQUIN, talk to your doctor before taking this medication. TEQUIN is not recommended for use during pregnancy or nursing, as the effects on the unborn child or nursing infant are unknown
TEQUIN is not recommended for children.

What about other medications I am taking?
It is important to let your healthcare provider know all of the medicines that you are using.

- It is important to let your healthcare provider know if you are taking certain medicines that can have an effect on an electrocardiogram test, such as cisapride, erythromycin, some antidepressants, and some antipsychotic drugs.
- You should tell your healthcare professional if you are taking medicines called diuretics (also sometimes called water pills) such as furosemide and hydrochlorothiazide, because diuretics can sometimes cause low potassium.
- Many antacids and multivitamins may interfere with the absorption of TEQUIN (gatifloxacin) and may prevent it from working properly. You should take TEQUIN 4 hours before taking these products.

What are the possible side effects of TEQUIN?
TEQUIN is generally well tolerated. The most common side effects that can occur while taking TEQUIN are usually mild and include nausea, vomiting, stomach pain, diarrhea, dizziness, and headache. You should be careful about driving or operating machinery until you are sure TEQUIN does not cause dizziness. If you notice any side effects not mentioned in this section or if you have any questions or concerns about the side effects you are experiencing, please discuss them with your healthcare professional.
In a few people, TEQUIN, like some other antibiotics, may produce a small effect on the heart that is seen on an electrocardiogram test. Although this has not caused any problems in more than 4000 patients who have taken TEQUIN in clinical trials, in theory, it could result in extremely rare cases of abnormal heartbeat, which may be dangerous. Contact your healthcare professional if you develop heart palpitations (fast beating) or have fainting spells.

Where can I get more information about TEQUIN?
This section is a summary of the most important information about TEQUIN. It does not include everything there is to know about TEQUIN. If you have any questions or problems, you should talk to your doctor or healthcare provider. There is also a leaflet (Package Insert) written for healthcare professionals that your pharmacist can let you read. You may want to read this information and discuss it with your doctor or healthcare professional. Remember, no written information can replace careful discussion with your doctor.

Remember

- Take your dose of TEQUIN once a day.
- Complete the course of medication (take all of the pills) even if you are feeling better.
- Do not use TEQUIN for another condition or give it to others.
- Store TEQUIN tablets at room temperature in a tightly sealed container.
- Throw away TEQUIN when it is outdated or no longer needed by flushing it down the toilet.
- Keep this and all medications out of reach of children.

CIPRO® (ciprofloxacin) is a registered trademark of the Bayer Corporation.
LEVAQUIN® (levofloxacin) is a registered trademark of Ortho-McNeil Pharmaceutical, Inc.
Bristol-Myers Squibb Company
Princeton, NJ 08543 U.S.A.
Also marketed by:
Schering Corporation
Kenilworth, NJ 07033
E5-B001-04-00 Revised April 2000
J4-677B
Licensed from Kyorin Pharmaceutical Company, Limited
Tokyo, Japan

Shown in Product Identification Guide, page 309

Bristol-Myers Squibb Dermatology® A Bristol-Myers Squibb Company

P.O. BOX 4500
PRINCETON, NJ 08543-4500

For Medical Information Contact:
Generally:
Bristol-Myers Squibb Drug Information Department
P.O. Box 4500
Princeton, NJ 08543-4500
(800) 321-1335
Adverse Drug Experiences
and Product Defects Reporting call
between 8:30 AM–4:30 PM EST:
(609) 818-3737
Sales and Ordering:
Orders may be placed by:
1. Calling your purchase orders toll-free between 8:30 AM–5:00 PM EST:
(800) 531-5244
2. Mailing your purchase orders to:
Bristol-Myers Squibb U.S. Pharmaceuticals
Attn: Customer Service
P.O. Box 5250
Princeton, NJ 08543-5250
3. Faxing your purchase orders to:
(800) 523–2965
4. Transmitting computer-to-computer on the NWDA and UCS formats through Ordernet Services use: DEA# PE0048579

VANIQA™ ℞

(eflornithine hydrochloride)
Cream, 13.9%
For topical dermatological use only. Not for ophthalmic, oral or intravaginal use.
Rx only

DESCRIPTION

VANIQA™ is a cream containing 13.9% (139 mg/g) of anhydrous eflornithine hydrochloride as eflornithine hydrochloride monohydrate (150 mg/g).
Chemically, eflornithine hydrochloride is (±) -2-(difluoromethyl) ornithine monohydrochloride monohydrate, with the empirical formula $C_6H_{12}F_2N_2O_2$•HCl• H_2O, a molecular weight of 236.65 and the following structural formula:

[Structural formula: F, F, OH, H_2N, H_2N, O, • HCl, • H_2O]

Anhydrous eflornithine hydrochloride has an empirical formula $C_6H_{12}F_2N_2O_2$• HCl and a molecular weight of 218.65.
Other ingredients include: ceteareth-20, cetearyl alcohol, dimethicone, glyceryl stearate, methylparaben, mineral oil, PEG-100 stearate, phenoxyethanol, propylparaben, stearyl alcohol and water.

CLINICAL PHARMACOLOGY

Pharmacodynamics
There are no studies examining the inhibition of the enzyme ornithine decarboxylase (ODC) in human skin following the application of topical eflornithine. However, there are studies in the literature that report the inhibition of ODC activity in skin following oral eflornithine. It is postulated that topical eflornithine hydrochloride irreversibly inhibits skin ODC activity. This enzyme is necessary in the synthesis of polyamines. Animal data indicate that inhibition of ornithine decarboxylase inhibits cell division and synthetic functions, which affect the rate of hair growth. VANIQA has been shown to retard the rate of hair growth in non-clinical and clinical studies.

Pharmacokinetics
The mean percutaneous absorption of eflornithine in women with unwanted facial hair, from a 13.9% w/w cream formulation, is < 1% of the radioactive dose, following either single or multiple doses under conditions of clinical use, that included shaving within 2 hours before radiolabeled dose application in addition to other forms of cutting or plucking and tweezing to remove facial hair. Steady-state was reached within four days of twice-daily application. The apparent steady-state plasma $t_{1/2}$ of eflornithine was approximately 8 hours. Following twice-daily application of 0.5 g of the cream (total dose 1.0 g/day; 139 mg as anhydrous eflornithine hydrochloride), under conditions of clinical use in women with unwanted facial hair (n=10), the steady-state C_{max}, C_{trough} and AUC_{12hr} were approximately 10 ng/mL, 5 ng/mL, and 92 ng•hr/mL, respectively, expressed in terms of the anhydrous free base of eflornithine hydrochloride. At steady-state, the dose-normalized peak concentrations (C_{max}) and the extent of daily systemic exposure (AUC) of eflornithine following twice-daily application of 0.5 g of the cream (total dose 1.0 g/day) is estimated to be approximately 100- and 60-fold lower, respectively, when compared to 370 mg/day once-daily oral doses. This compound is not known to be metabolized and is primarily excreted unchanged in the urine.

INDICATIONS AND USAGE

VANIQA (eflornithine hydrochloride) Cream, 13.9% is indicated for the reduction of unwanted facial hair in women. VANIQA has only been studied on the face and adjacent involved areas under the chin of affected individuals. Usage should be limited to these areas of involvement.

CLINICAL TRIALS

Results of topical dermal studies for contact sensitization, photocontact sensitization, and photocontact irritation reveal that under conditions of clinical use, VANIQA is not expected to cause contact sensitization, phototoxic, or photosensitization reactions. Results of the topical dermal study for contact irritation did reveal that VANIQA could cause irritation reactions in clinical use in susceptible individuals or under conditions of exaggerated use.
Two randomized double-blind studies involving 594 female patients (393 treated with VANIQA, 201 with vehicle) treated twice daily for up to 24 weeks evaluated the efficacy of VANIQA in the reduction of unwanted facial hair in women. Women in the trial had a customary frequency of removal of facial hair two or more times per week. Women with facial conditions such as severe inflammatory acne, women who were pregnant, and nursing mothers were excluded from the studies. Physicians assessed the improvement or worsening from the baseline condition (Physician's Global Assessment [PGA]), 48 hours after shaving, of all treated areas. Statistically significant improvement for VANIQA versus vehicle was seen in each of these studies for "marked improvement" or greater response (24-week time point; p≤0.001). Marked improvement was seen consistently at 8 weeks after initiation of treatment and continued throughout the 24 weeks of treatment. Hair growth approached pretreatment levels within 8 weeks of treatment withdrawal. The success rate over time is graphically presented below for each pivotal trial.

[See graphic at top of next page]

Approximately 32% of patients showed marked improvement or greater (protocol definition of clinical success) after 24 weeks of treatment with VANIQA, compared to 8% with the vehicle. Combined results of these two trials through 24 weeks are presented below.

PGA Outcome	VANIQA	Vehicle
Clear/almost clear	5%	0%
Marked improvement	27%	8%
Improved	26%	26%
No improvement/worse/missing	42%	66%

Subgroup analyses appeared to suggest greater benefit for Whites than non-Whites (37% vs. 22% success, respectively; p=0.017). However, non-Whites, mostly Black subjects, did have significant treatment benefit with 22% graded as success on VANIQA compared to 5% on vehicle.
About 12% of women in the clinical trials were postmenopausal. Significant improvement in PGA outcome versus vehicle was seen in postmenopausal women (38% compared to 0%, p≤0.001).
VANIQA statistically significantly reduced how bothered patients felt by their facial hair and by the time spent removing, treating, or concealing facial hair. These patient-observable differences were seen as early as 8 weeks after initiating treatment. Hair growth approached pretreatment levels within 8 weeks of treatment withdrawal.
Clinical trials with VANIQA involved over 1370 women with unwanted facial hair of skin types I-VI, of whom 68% were White, 17% Black, 11% Hispanic-Latino, 2% Asian-Pacific Islander, 0.6% American Native, and 1.3% other.

CONTRAINDICATIONS

VANIQA is contraindicated in patients with a history of sensitivity to any components of the preparation.

WARNINGS

Discontinue use if hypersensitivity occurs.

PRECAUTIONS

General
For external use only.

Continued on next page

Vaniqa—Cont.

Transient stinging or burning may occur when applied to abraded or broken skin.

Information For Patients

Patients using VANIQA (eflornithine hydrochloride) Cream, 13.9% should receive the following information and instructions:

1. This medication is not a depilatory, but rather appears to retard hair growth to improve the condition and the patient's appearance. Patients will likely need to continue using a hair removal method (e.g., shaving, plucking, etc.) in conjunction with VANIQA.
2. Onset of improvement was seen after as little as 4–8 weeks of treatment in the 24-week clinical trials. The condition may return to pretreatment levels 8 weeks after discontinuing treatment.
3. If skin irritation or intolerance develops, direct the patient to temporarily reduce the frequency of application (e.g., once a day). If irritation continues, the patient should discontinue use of the product.

Refer to the Patient Information Leaflet for additional important information and instructions.

Drug Interactions

It is not known if VANIQA has any interaction with other topically applied drug products.

Carcinogenesis, Mutagenesis and Impairment of Fertility

In a 12-month photocarcinogenicity study in hairless albino mice, animals treated with the vehicle alone showed an increased incidence of skin tumors induced by exposure to ultraviolet (UVA/UVB) light, whereas mice treated topically with VANIQA at doses up to 600 mg/kg [19X the Maximum Recommended Human Dose (MRHD) based on body surface area (BSA)] showed an incidence of skin tumors equivalent to untreated-control animals.

A two-year dermal carcinogenicity study in CD- 1 mice treated with VANIQA revealed no evidence of carcinogenicity at daily doses up to 600 mg/kg (950X the MRHD based on AUC comparisons).

Eflornithine did not elicit mutagenic effects in an Ames reverse-mutation assay or clastogenicity in primary human lymphocytes, with and without metabolic activation. In a dermal micronucleus assay, eflornithine hydrochloride cream, 13.9% at doses up to 900 mg/kg (58X the MRHD based on BSA) in rats yielded no evidence of genotoxicity.

In a dermal fertility and early embryonic development study in rats treated with VANIQA there were no adverse reproductive effects at doses up to 450 mg/kg (29X the MRHD based on BSA). In a peri- and postnatal study in rats, eflornithine administered in the drinking water was associated with maternal toxicity and reduced pup weights at doses of at least 625 mg/kg (40X the MRHD based on BSA) and a slightly reduced fertility index, which was considered to be of questionable biological significance, at 1698 mg/kg (110X the MRHD based on BSA). No effects were seen with an oral dose of 223 mg/kg (14X the MRHD based on BSA). In the latter study, the multiples of the human exposure are likely much higher, since eflornithine is well absorbed orally in rats, whereas minimal absorption occurs in humans treated topically.

Pregnancy

Teratogenic Effects: Pregnancy Category C

In the first dermal embryo-fetal development study in rats treated with eflornithine hydrochloride cream, 13.9%, (in which no precautions were taken to prevent ingestion of drug from application sites), maternal toxicity and fetal effects including reduced numbers of live fetuses, decreased fetal weights, and delayed ossification and development of the viscera were observed at doses of 225 and 450 mg/kg (15X and 29X the MRHD based on BSA, respectively). When the study was repeated under conditions that avoided ingestion from application sites, no maternal, fetal or teratogenic effects were observed at doses up to 450 mg/kg (29X the MRHD based on BSA). In the first study in which no precautions were taken to prevent ingestion, circulating plasma levels were 11- to 14-fold higher than in the second study in which ingestion was prevented. In a dermal embryo-fetal development study in rabbits treated with VANIQA (eflornithine hydrochloride) Cream, 13.9% no adverse maternal or fetal effects occurred at doses up to 90 mg/kg (11X the MRHD based on BSA). Significant dermal irritation, as well as possible ingestion of VANIQA occurred at 300 mg/kg/day (36X the MRHD based on BSA) and was associated with maternal deaths, abortions, increased fetal resorptions, and reduced fetal weights. Fetotoxicity in the absence of maternal toxicity has been reported in oral studies with eflornithine with fetal no-effect doses of 80 mg/kg in rats and 45 mg/kg in rabbits. In these studies, no evidence of teratogenicity was observed in rats given up to 200 mg/kg or in rabbits given up to 135 mg/kg.

Although VANIQA was not formally studied in pregnant patients, 22 pregnancies occurred during the trials. Nineteen of these pregnancies occurred while patients were using VANIQA. Of the 19 pregnancies, there were 9 healthy infants, 4 spontaneous abortions, 5 induced/elective abortions, and 1 birth defect (Down's Syndrome to a 35-year-old). Because there are no adequate and well-controlled studies in pregnant women, the risk/benefit ratio of using VANIQA in women with unwanted facial hair who are pregnant should be weighed carefully with serious consideration for either not implementing or discontinuing use of VANIQA

Nursing Mothers

It is not known whether or not eflornithine hydrochloride is excreted in human milk. Caution should be exercised when VANIQA is administered to a nursing woman.

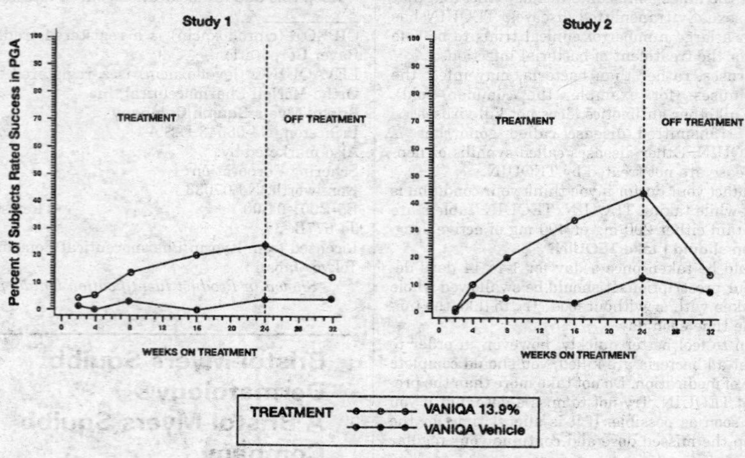

Adverse Event Term	Vehicle-Controlled Studies		Vehicle-Controlled and Open-Label Studies
	VANIQA (n=393)	*Vehicle (n=201)*	*VANIQA (n=1373)*
Acne	21.3	21.4	10.8
Pseudofolliculitis Barbae	16.3	15.4	4.9
Stinging Skin	7.9	2.5	4.1
Headache	3.8	5.0	4.0
Burning Skin	4.3	2.0	3.5
Dry Skin	1.8	3.0	3.3
Pruritus (itching)	3.8	4.0	3.1
Erythema (redness)	1.3	0.0	2.5
Tingling Skin	3.6	1.5	2.2
Dyspepsia	2.5	2.0	1.9
Skin Irritation	1.0	1.0	1.8
Rash	2.8	0.0	1.5
Alopecia	1.5	2.5	1.3
Dizziness	1.5	1.5	1.3
Folliculitis	0.5	0.0	1.0
Hair Ingrown	0.3	2.0	0.9
Facial Edema	0.3	3.0	0.7
Anorexia	1.0	2.0	0.7
Nausea	0.5	1.0	0.7
Asthenia	0.0	1.0	0.3
Vertigo	0.3	1.0	0.1

Pediatric Use

The safety and effectiveness of this product have not been established in pediatric patients less than 12 years of age.

Geriatric Use

Of the 1373 patients on active treatment in clinical studies of VANIQA, approximately 7% were 65 years or older and approximately 1% were 75 or older. No apparent differences in safety were observed between older patients and younger patients.

ADVERSE REACTIONS

Adverse events reported for most body systems occurred at similar frequencies in VANIQA and vehicle control groups. The most frequent adverse events related to treatment with VANIQA were skin-related. The following table notes the percentage of adverse events associated with the use of VANIQA or its vehicle that occurred at greater than 1% in both the vehicle-controlled studies and the open-label safety studies up to 1 year of continuous use.

[See second table above]

Treatment related skin adverse events that occurred in less than 1% of the subjects treated with VANIQA are: bleeding skin, cheilitis, contact dermatitis, swelling of lips, herpes simplex, numbness and rosacea.

Adverse events were primarily mild in intensity and generally resolved without medical treatment or discontinuation of VANIQA. Only 2% of subjects discontinued studies due to an adverse event related to use of VANIQA (eflornithine hydrochloride) Cream, 13.9%.

Laboratory Test Abnormalities

No laboratory test abnormalities have been consistently found to be associated with VANIQA. In an open labeled study, some patients showed an increase in their transaminases; however, the clinical significance of these findings is not known.

OVERDOSAGE

Overdosage information with VANIQA is unavailable. Given the low percutaneous penetration of this drug, overdosage via the topical route is not expected (see **CLINICAL PHARMACOLOGY**). However, should very high topical doses (e.g., multiple tubes per day) or oral ingestion be encountered (a 30 g tube contains 4.2 g of eflornithine hydrochloride), the patient should be monitored, and appropriate supportive measures administered as necessary.

(Note: Use of an intravenous formulation of eflornithine hydrochloride at high doses (400 mg/kg/day or approximately 24 g/day) for the treatment of *Trypanosoma brucei gambiense* infection (African sleeping sickness) has been associated with adverse events and laboratory abnormalities. Adverse events in this setting have included hair loss, facial swelling, seizures, hearing impairment, stomach upset, loss of appetite, headache, weakness and dizziness. A variety of hematological toxicities, including anemia, thrombocytopenia and leukopenia have also been observed, but these were usually reversible upon discontinuation of treatment.)

DOSAGE AND ADMINISTRATION

Apply a thin layer of VANIQA to affected areas of the face and adjacent involved areas under the chin and rub in thoroughly. Do not wash treated area for at least 4 hours. Use twice daily at least 8 hours apart or as directed by a physician. The patient should continue to use hair removal techniques as needed in conjunction with VANIQA. (VANIQA should be applied at least 5 minutes after hair removal.) Cosmetics or sunscreens may be applied over treated areas after cream has dried.

HOW SUPPLIED

VANIQA TM (eflornithine hydrochloride) Cream, 13.9% is available as:

30 gram tube NDC 0072-1500-30
Net wt. 60 gram (2-30 gram tubes) NDC 0072-1500-65

STORAGE

Store at 25°C (77°F); excursions permitted to 15°C-30°C (59°F-86°F) [See USP Controlled Room Temperature]. Do not freeze. See tube crimp and carton end for expiration date and lot number.

Patient Information Leaflet for VANIQA™

(eflornithine hydrochloride) Cream, 13.9%

INFORMATION FOR PATIENTS

This section contains important information about VANIQA that you should read before you begin treatment. This section does not list all the benefits and risks of VANIQA and does not take the place of discussions with your doctor or healthcare professional about your condition or your treatment. If you have questions, talk with your healthcare professional. The medicine described here can only be prescribed by a licensed healthcare professional. Only your healthcare professional can determine if VANIQA is right for you.

What is VANIQA?

VANIQA (pronounced "VAN-i-ka") is a prescription medication applied to the skin for the reduction of unwanted facial hair in women.

The active ingredient in VANIQA is eflornithine hydrochloride. VANIQA also contains ceteareth-20, cetearyl alcohol, dimethicone, glyceryl stearate, methylparaben, mineral oil, PEG-100 stearate, phenoxyethanol, propylparaben, stearyl alcohol and water.

How does VANIQA work?

VANIQA interferes with an enzyme found in the hair follicle of the skin needed for hair growth. This results in slower hair growth and improved appearance where VANIQA is applied.

VANIQA does not permanently remove hair or "cure" unwanted facial hair. It is not a depilatory. Your treatment program should include continuation of any hair removal technique you are currently using. VANIQA will help you manage your condition and improve your appearance.

Improvement in the condition occurs gradually. Don't be discouraged if you see no immediate improvement. Be patient. Improvement may be seen as early as 4 to 8 weeks of treatment. Improvement may take longer in some individuals. If no improvement is seen after 6 months of use, discontinue use. Clinical studies show that in about 8 weeks after stopping treatment with VANIQA, the hair will return to the same condition as before beginning treatment.

Who should not use VANIQA?

You should not use VANIQA if you are allergic to any of the ingredients in the cream. All ingredients are listed on the tube and at the beginning of this leaflet.

You should not use VANIQA if you are less than 12 years of age.

What should you tell your doctor before using VANIQA?

If you are allergic to any of the ingredients, tell your doctor.

If you are pregnant or plan to become pregnant, discuss with your doctor whether you should use VANIQA during pregnancy. No clinical studies have been performed in pregnant women.

If you are breast feeding, consult your doctor before using VANIQA. It is not known if VANIQA is passed to infants through breast milk.

If you are taking any prescription medicines, non-prescription medicines or using any facial or skin creams, check with your physician before use of VANIQA.

How should I use VANIQA?

Use VANIQA only for the condition for which it was prescribed by your doctor. Do not give it to other people or allow other people to use it.

You will need to continue your normal procedures for hair removal until desired results have been achieved. You may then be less bothered by the time spent in removing hair or the frequency of hair removal. VANIQA is to be used twice daily, at least eight hours apart, or as directed by your doctor. VANIQA is for external use only.

Follow the instructions for application of VANIQA carefully. Apply a thin layer of VANIQA to the affected areas of the face and adjacent involved areas under the chin and rub in thoroughly. You should not wash the treatment areas for at least 4 hours after application of VANIQA (eflornithine hydrochloride) Cream, 13.9%.

VANIQA may cause temporary redness, rash, burning, stinging or tingling, especially when the skin is damaged. If irritation continues, stop use of VANIQA and contact your doctor. Avoid getting the medication in your eyes or inside your nose or mouth. If the product gets in your eyes, rinse thoroughly with water and contact your doctor.

If you forget or miss a dose of VANIQA do not try to "make it up". Return to your normal application schedule as soon as you can.

You may use your normal cosmetics or sunscreen after applying VANIQA, but you should wait a few minutes to allow the treatment to be absorbed before applying them.

If your condition gets worse with treatment, stop use of VANIQA and contact your doctor.

What are the possible side effects of VANIQA?

VANIQA may cause temporary redness, stinging, burning, tingling or rash on areas of the skin where it is applied. Folliculitis (hair bumps) may also occur. If these persist, consult your doctor.

How should VANIQA be stored?

VANIQA (eflornithine hydrochloride) Cream, 13.9%, should be stored at 15°C-30°C (59°F-86°F). Do not freeze.

Keep this and all medicines out of the reach of children.

This medicine was prescribed for your particular condition. Do not use it for another condition or give it to anyone else. This summary does not include everything there is to know about VANIQA. If you have questions or concerns, or want more information about VANIQA, your doctor or pharmacist has the complete prescribing information upon which this leaflet is based. You may want to read it and discuss it with your doctor or health care professional. Remember, no written summary can replace careful discussion with your doctor.

Westwood-Squibb Colton Holdings Partnership
Plainsboro, NJ USA 08536
Manufactured by Bristol-Myers Squibb Company,
Buffalo, NY USA 14213
U.S.Patent Nos.: 5,648,394 and 4,720,489
Under license from Westwood-Squibb Colton Holdings Partnership
Bristol-Myers Squibb Company
Princeton, NJ 08543 U.S.A.
A2-B001-07-00 Issue date: July 2000
03-6049-0 03-6054-0

For information on the following products, see listing under WESTWOOD-SQUIBB PHARMACEUTICALS, INC.:

Dovonex Cream
Dovonex Ointment
Dovonex Scalp Solution
Lac-Hydrin Cream
Lac-Hydrin Lotion
Ultravate Cream
Ultravate Ointment

Bristol-Myers Squibb Oncology/ Immunology Division

A Bristol-Myers Squibb Company
P.O. BOX 4500
PRINCETON, NJ 08543-4500

For Medical Information Contact:

Generally:

Bristol-Myers Squibb Drug Information Department
P.O. Box 4500
Princeton, NJ 08543-4500
(800) 426-7644

Adverse Drug Experiences

and Product Defects Reporting call
between 8:30 AM–4:30 PM EST:
(609) 818-3737

Sales and Ordering:

Orders may be placed by:

1. Calling the following toll-free number between 8:30 AM–5:00 PM EST:
   Continental U.S.: (800) 631-5244
   Alaska-Hawaii: (800) 631-5244
2. Mail orders and all inquiries should be sent to:
   Bristol-Myers Squibb Oncology Division
   Attn: Customer Service
   P.O. Box 5250
   Princeton, NJ 08543-5250
3. Faxing your purchase orders to:
   (800) 523-2965
4. Transmitting computer-to-computer on the NWDA and UCS formats through Ordernet Services use: DEA #PE0048579

BiCNU® ℞

(carmustine for injection)
℞ ONLY

WARNINGS

BiCNU® (carmustine for injection) should be administered under the supervision of a qualified physician experienced in the use of cancer chemotherapeutic agents. Bone marrow suppression, notably thrombocytopenia and leukopenia, which may contribute to bleeding and overwhelming infections in an already compromised patient, is the most common and severe of the toxic effects of BiCNU (see **WARNINGS** and **ADVERSE REACTIONS**).

Since the major toxicity is delayed bone marrow suppression, blood counts should be monitored weekly for at least 6 weeks after a dose (see **ADVERSE REACTIONS**). At the recommended dosage, courses of BiCNU should not be given more frequently than every 6 weeks.

The bone marrow toxicity of BiCNU is cumulative and therefore dosage adjustment must be considered on the basis of nadir blood counts from prior dose (see **Dosage Adjustment Table** under **DOSAGE AND ADMINISTRATION**).

Pulmonary toxicity from BiCNU appears to be dose related. Patients receiving greater than 1400 mg/m^2 cumulative dose are at significantly higher risk than those receiving less.

Delayed pulmonary toxicity can occur years after treatment, and can result in death, particularly in patients treated in childhood (see **ADVERSE REACTIONS**, and **PRECAUTIONS**: **Pediatric Use**).

DESCRIPTION

BiCNU® (carmustine for injection) is one of the nitrosoureas used in the treatment of certain neoplastic diseases. It is 1,3-bis (2-chloroethyl)-1-nitrosourea. It is lyophilized pale yellow flakes or congealed mass with a molecular weight of 214.06. It is highly soluble in alcohol and lipids, and poorly soluble in water. BiCNU is administered by intravenous infusion after reconstitution as recommended.

The structural formula is:

$$Cl\text{-}CH_2\text{-}CH_2\text{-}\underset{NO}{N}\text{-}\overset{O}{\overset{\|}{C}}\text{-}NH\text{-}CH_2\text{-}CH_2\text{-}Cl$$

Sterile BiCNU is available in 100 mg single dose vials of lyophilized material.

CLINICAL PHARMACOLOGY

Although it is generally agreed that carmustine alkylates DNA and RNA, it is not cross resistant with other alkylators. As with other nitrosoureas, it may also inhibit several key enzymatic processes by carbamoylation of amino acids in proteins.

Intravenously administered carmustine is rapidly degraded, with no intact drug detectable after 15 minutes. However, in studies with C^{14}-labeled drug, prolonged levels of the isotope were detected in the plasma and tissue, probably representing radioactive fragments of the parent compound.

It is thought that the antineoplastic and toxic activities of carmustine may be due to metabolites. Approximately 60% to 70% of a total dose is excreted in the urine in 96 hours and about 10% as respiratory CO_2. The fate of the remainder is undetermined.

Because of the high lipid solubility and the relative lack of ionization at physiological pH, carmustine crosses the blood-brain barrier quite effectively. Levels of radioactivity in the CSF are ≥ 50% of those measured concurrently in plasma.

INDICATIONS AND USAGE

BiCNU is indicated as palliative therapy as a single agent or in established combination therapy with other approved chemotherapeutic agents in the following:

1. Brain tumors–glioblastoma, brainstem glioma, medulloblastoma, astrocytoma, ependymoma, and metastatic brain tumors.
2. Multiple myeloma–in combination with prednisone.
3. Hodgkin's Disease–as secondary therapy in combination with other approved drugs in patients who relapse while being treated with primary therapy, or who fail to respond to primary therapy.
4. Non-Hodgkin's lymphomas–as secondary therapy in combination with other approved drugs for patients who relapse while being treated with primary therapy, or who fail to respond to primary therapy.

CONTRAINDICATIONS

BiCNU should not be given to individuals who have demonstrated a previous hypersensitivity to it.

WARNINGS

Since the major toxicity is delayed bone marrow suppression, blood counts should be monitored weekly for at least 6 weeks after a dose (see **ADVERSE REACTIONS**). At the recommended dosage, courses of BiCNU should not be given more frequently than every 6 weeks.

The bone marrow toxicity of BiCNU is cumulative and therefore dosage adjustment must be considered on the basis of nadir blood counts from prior dose (see **Dosage Adjustment Table** under **DOSAGE AND ADMINISTRATION**).

Pulmonary toxicity from BiCNU appears to be dose related. Patients receiving greater than 1400 mg/m^2 cumulative dose are at significantly higher risk than those receiving less. Additionally delayed onset pulmonary fibrosis occurring up to 17 years after treatment has been reported in patients who receive BiCNU in childhood and early adolescence (see **ADVERSE REACTIONS**).

Long-term use of nitrosoureas has been reported to be associated with the development of secondary malignancies.

Liver and renal function tests should be monitored periodically (see **ADVERSE REACTIONS**).

Continued on next page

BiCNU—Cont.

BiCNU may cause fetal harm when administered to a pregnant woman. BiCNU has been shown to be embryotoxic in rats and rabbits and teratogenic in rats when given in doses equivalent to the human dose. There are no adequate and well-controlled studies in pregnant women. If this drug is used during pregnancy, or if the patient becomes pregnant while taking (receiving) this drug, the patient should be apprised of the potential hazard to the fetus. Women of childbearing potential should be advised to avoid becoming pregnant.

BiCNU has been administered through an intraarterial intracarotid route; this procedure is investigational and has been associated with ocular toxicity.

PRECAUTIONS

General: In all instances where the use of BiCNU (carmustine for injection) is considered for chemotherapy, the physician must evaluate the need and usefulness of the drug against the risks of toxic effects or adverse reactions. Most such adverse reactions are reversible if detected early. When such effects or reactions do occur, the drug should be reduced in dosage or discontinued and appropriate corrective measures should be taken according to the clinical judgment of the physician. Reinstitution of BiCNU therapy should be carried out with caution, and with adequate consideration of the further need for the drug and alertness as to possible recurrence of toxicity.

Laboratory Tests: Due to delayed bone marrow suppression, blood counts should be monitored weekly for at least 6 weeks after a dose.

Baseline pulmonary function studies should be conducted along with frequent pulmonary function tests during treatment. Patients with a baseline below 70% of the predicted Forced Vital Capacity (FVC) or Carbon Monoxide Diffusing Capacity (DL_{CO}) are particularly at risk.

Since BiCNU may cause liver dysfunction, it is recommended that liver function tests be monitored.

Renal function tests should also be monitored periodically.

Carcinogenesis, Mutagenesis, Impairment of Fertility: BiCNU is carcinogenic in rats and mice, producing a marked increase in tumor incidence in doses approximating those employed clinically. Nitrosourea therapy does have carcinogenic potential in humans (see **ADVERSE REACTIONS**). BiCNU also affects fertility in male rats at doses somewhat higher than the human dose.

Pregnancy: Pregnancy "Category D". (See **WARNINGS** section.)

Nursing Mothers: It is not known whether this drug is excreted in human milk. Because of the potential for serious adverse events in nursing infants, nursing should be discontinued while taking BiCNU.

Pediatric Use: Safety and effectiveness in children have not been established. Delayed onset pulmonary fibrosis occurring up to 17 years after treatment, has been reported in a long-term study of patients who received BiCNU in childhood and early adolescence (1–16 years). Eight out of the 17 patients (47%) who survived childhood brain tumors, including all the five patients initially treated at less than five years of age, died of pulmonary fibrosis. Therefore, the risks and benefits of BiCNU therapy must be carefully considered, due to the extremely high risk of pulmonary toxicity. (See **ADVERSE REACTIONS: Pulmonary Toxicity.**)

ADVERSE REACTIONS

Pulmonary Toxicity: Pulmonary toxicity characterized by pulmonary infiltrates and/or fibrosis has been reported to occur from 9 days to 43 months after treatment with BiCNU and related nitrosoureas. Most of these patients were receiving prolonged therapy with total doses of BiCNU greater than 1400 mg/m^2. However, there have been reports of pulmonary fibrosis in patients receiving lower total doses. Other risk factors include past history of lung disease and duration of treatment. Cases of fatal pulmonary toxicity with BiCNU have been reported.

Additionally, delayed onset pulmonary fibrosis occurring up to 17 years after treatment has been reported in a long-term study with 17 patients who received BiCNU in childhood and early adolescence (1–16 years) in cumulative doses ranging from 770 to 1800 mg/m^2 combined with cranial radiotherapy for intracranial tumors. Chest x-rays demonstrated pulmonary hypoplasia with upper zone contraction. Gallium scans were normal in all cases. Thoracic CT scans have demonstrated an unusual pattern of upper zone fibrosis. There was some late reduction of pulmonary function in all long-term survivors. This form of lung fibrosis may be slowly progressive and has resulted in death in some cases. In this long-term study, 8 of 17 died of delayed pulmonary lung fibrosis, including all those initially treated (5 of 17) at less than 5 years of age.

Hematologic Toxicity: A frequent and serious toxicity of BiCNU is delayed myelosuppression. It usually occurs 4 to 6 weeks after drug administration and is dose related. Thrombocytopenia occurs at about 4 weeks postadministration and persists for 1 to 2 weeks. Leukopenia occurs at 5 to 6 weeks after a dose of BiCNU and persists for 1 to 2 weeks. Thrombocytopenia is generally more severe than leukopenia. However, both may be dose-limiting toxicities.

BiCNU may produce cumulative myelosuppression, manifested by more depressed indices or longer duration of suppression after repeated doses.

The occurrence of acute leukemia and bone marrow dysplasias have been reported in patients following long-term nitrosourea therapy.

Anemia also occurs, but is less frequent and less severe than thrombocytopenia or leukopenia.

Gastrointestinal Toxicity: Nausea and vomiting after I.V. administration of BiCNU are noted frequently. This toxicity appears within 2 hours of dosing, usually lasting 4 to 6 hours, and is dose related. Prior administration of antiemetics is effective in diminishing and sometimes preventing this side effect.

Hepatotoxicity: A reversible type of hepatic toxicity, manifested by increased transaminase, alkaline phosphatase, and bilirubin levels, has been reported in a small percentage of patients receiving BiCNU.

Nephrotoxicity: Renal abnormalities consisting of progressive azotemia, decrease in kidney size and renal failure have been reported in patients who received large cumulative doses after prolonged therapy with BiCNU and related nitrosoureas. Kidney damage has also been reported occasionally in patients receiving lower total doses.

Other Toxicities: Accidental contact of reconstituted BiCNU with skin has caused burning and hyperpigmentation of the affected areas.

Rapid I.V. infusion of BiCNU may produce intensive flushing of the skin and suffusion of the conjunctiva within 2 hours, lasting about 4 hours. It is also associated with burning at the site of injection although true thrombosis is rare.

Neuroretinitis, chest pain, headache, allergic reaction, hypotension and tachycardia have been reported as part of ongoing surveillance.

OVERDOSAGE

No proven antidotes have been established for BiCNU overdosage.

DOSAGE AND ADMINISTRATION

The recommended dose of BiCNU as a single agent in previously untreated patients is 150 to 200 mg/m^2 intravenously every 6 weeks. This may be given as a single dose or divided into daily injections such as 75 to 100 mg/m^2 on 2 successive days. When BiCNU is used in combination with other myelosuppressive drugs or in patients in whom bone marrow reserve is depleted, the doses should be adjusted accordingly.

Doses subsequent to the initial dose should be adjusted according to the hematologic response of the patient to the preceding dose. The following schedule is suggested as a guide to dosage adjustment:

Nadir After Prior Dose		Percentages of Prior Dose to be Given
Leukocytes/mm^3	Platelets/mm^3	
>4000	>100,000	100%
3000–3999	75,000–99,999	100%
2000–2999	25,000–74,999	70%
<2000	<25,000	50%

A repeat course of BiCNU (carmustine for injection) should not be given until circulating blood elements have returned to acceptable levels (platelets above 100,000/mm^3, leukocytes above 4,000/mm^3), and this is usually in 6 weeks. Adequate number of neutrophils should be present on a peripheral blood smear. Blood counts should be monitored weekly and repeat courses should not be given before 6 weeks because the hematologic toxicity is delayed and cumulative.

Administration Precautions: As with other potentially toxic compounds, caution should be exercised in handling BiCNU and preparing the solution of BiCNU. Accidental contact of reconstituted BiCNU with the skin has caused transient hyperpigmentation of the affected areas. The use of gloves is recommended. If BiCNU lyophilized material or solution contacts the skin or mucosa, immediately wash the skin or mucosa thoroughly with soap and water.

The reconstituted solution should be used intravenously only and should be administered by I.V. drip. Injection of BiCNU over shorter periods of time than 1 to 2 hours may produce intense pain and burning at the site of injection.

Preparation of Intravenous Solutions: First, dissolve BiCNU with 3 mL of the supplied sterile diluent (Dehydrated Alcohol Injection, USP). Second, aseptically add 27 mL Sterile Water for Injection, USP. Each mL of resulting solution contains 3.3 mg of BiCNU in 10% ethanol. Such solutions should be protected from light.

Reconstitution as recommended results in a clear, colorless to yellowish solution which may be further diluted with 5% Dextrose Injection, USP. Parenteral drug products should be inspected visually for particulate matter and discoloration prior to administration, whenever solution and container permit.

Important Note: The lyophilized dosage formulation contains no preservatives and is not intended for use as a multiple dose vial.

Stability: Unopened vials of the dry drug must be stored in a refrigerator (2°C to 8°C, 36°F to 46°F). The recommended storage of unopened vials provides a stable product for 2 years. After reconstitution as recommended, BiCNU is stable for 8 hours at room temperature (25°C, 77°F), protected from light.

Vials reconstituted as directed and further diluted to a concentration of 0.2 mg/mL in 5% Dextrose Injection, USP, should be stored at room temperature, protected from light and utilized within 8 hours.

Glass containers were used for the stability data provided in this section. Only use glass containers for BiCNU administration.

Important Note: BiCNU has a low melting point (30.5°C to 32.0°C or 86.9°F to 89.6°F). Exposure of the drug to this temperature or above will cause the drug to liquefy and appear as an oil film on the vials. This is a sign of decomposition and vials should be discarded. If there is a question of adequate refrigeration upon receipt of this product, immediately inspect the larger vial in each individual carton. Hold the vial to the bright light for inspection. The BiCNU will appear as a very small amount of dry flakes or dry congealed mass. If this is evident, the BiCNU is suitable for use and should be refrigerated immediately.

Procedures for proper handling and disposal of anticancer drugs should be considered. Several guidelines on this subject have been published.[1–7] There is no general agreement that all of the procedures recommended in the guidelines are necessary or appropriate.

HOW SUPPLIED

BiCNU® (carmustine for injection). Each package includes a vial containing 100 mg carmustine and a vial containing 3 mL sterile diluent.

NDC 0015-3012-38

Store dry powder in refrigerator (2°C to 8°C, 36°F to 46°F). For information on package sizes available refer to the current price schedule.

REFERENCES

1. Recommendations for the Safe Handling of Parenteral Antineoplastic Drugs. NIH Publication No. 83-2621. For sale by the Superintendent of Documents, US Government Printing Office, Washington, DC 20402.
2. AMA Council Report. Guidelines for Handling Parenteral Antineoplastics. *JAMA* 1985; 253(11):1590–1592.
3. National Study Commission on Cytotoxic Exposure-Recommendations for Handling Cytotoxic Agents. Available from Louis P. Jeffrey, ScD, Chairman, National Study Commission on Cytotoxic Exposure, Massachusetts College of Pharmacy and Allied Health Sciences, 179 Longwood Avenue, Boston, Massachusetts 02115.
4. Clinical Oncological Society of Australia. Guidelines and Recommendations for Safe Handling of Antineoplastic Agents. *Med J Australia* 1983; 1:426–428.
5. Jones, RB, et al: Safe Handling of Chemotherapeutic Agents. A Report from the Mount Sinai Medical Center. *CA–A Cancer Journal for Clinicians* 1983; (Sept/Oct)258–263.
6. American Society of Hospital Pharmacists Technical Assistance Bulletin on Handling Cytotoxic and Hazardous Drugs. *Am J Hosp Pharm* 1990; 47:1033–1049.
7. Controlling Occupational Exposure to Hazardous Drugs. (OSHA WORK PRACTICE GUIDELINES). *Am J Health-Syst Pharm* 1996; 53:1669–1685.

Manufactured by:
Ben Venue Laboratories, Inc., Bedford, Ohio 44146
Distributed by:
BRISTOL LABORATORIES®
ONCOLOGY PRODUCTS
A Bristol-Myers Squibb Company
Princeton, NJ 08543
U.S.A.
H1-B001-12-98 P7980-06
Revised: June 1998

BLENOXANE® ℞

[blĕn-ŏx-ānĕ]
(bleomycin sulfate for injection, USP)
Rx ONLY

WARNING

It is recommended that BLENOXANE® (bleomycin sulfate for injection, USP) be administered under the supervision of a qualified physician experienced in the use of cancer chemotherapeutic agents. Appropriate management of therapy and complications is possible only when adequate diagnostic and treatment facilities are readily available.

Pulmonary fibrosis is the most severe toxicity associated with BLENOXANE. The most frequent presentation is pneumonitis occasionally progressing to pulmonary fibrosis. Its occurrence is higher in elderly patients and in those receiving greater than 400 units total dose, but pulmonary toxicity has been observed in young patients and those treated with low doses.

A severe idiosyncratic reaction consisting of hypotension, mental confusion, fever, chills, and wheezing has been reported in approximately 1% of lymphoma patients treated with BLENOXANE.

DESCRIPTION

BLENOXANE® (bleomycin sulfate for injection, USP) is a mixture of cytotoxic glycopeptide antibiotics isolated from a strain of *Streptomyces verticillus*. It is freely soluble in water.

Note: A unit of bleomycin is equal to the formerly used milligram activity. The term milligram activity is a misnomer and was changed to units to be more precise.

CLINICAL PHARMACOLOGY

Although the exact mechanism of action of BLENOXANE is unknown, available evidence would seem to indicate that the main mode of action is the inhibition of DNA synthesis with some evidence of lesser inhibition of RNA and protein synthesis.

In mice, high concentrations of BLENOXANE are found in the skin, lungs, kidneys, peritoneum, and lymphatics. Tumor cells of the skin and lungs have been found to have high concentrations of BLENOXANE in contrast to the low concentrations found in hematopoietic tissue. The low concentrations of BLENOXANE found in bone marrow may be related to high levels of BLENOXANE degradative enzymes found in that tissue.

In patients with normal renal function, 60% to 70% of an administered dose is recovered in the urine as active bleomycin. In patients with a creatinine clearance of > 35 mL per minute, the serum or plasma terminal elimination half-life of bleomycin is approximately 115 minutes. In patients with a creatinine clearance of < 35 mL per minute, the plasma or serum terminal elimination half-life increases exponentially as the creatinine clearance decreases. It was reported that patients with moderately severe renal failure excreted less than 20% of the dose in the urine. This result would suggest that severe renal impairment could lead to accumulation of the drug in blood.

Information on the dose proportionality of bleomycin is not available.

When administered intrapleurally for the treatment of malignant pleural effusion, BLENOXANE acts as a sclerosing agent.

Following intrapleural administration to a limited number of patients (n=4), the resultant bleomycin plasma concentrations suggest a systemic absorption of approximately 45%.

The safety and efficacy of BLENOXANE 60 units and tetracycline (1 gm) as treatment for malignant pleural effusion were evaluated in a multicenter, randomized trial. Patients were required to have cytologically positive pleural effusion, good performance status (0,1,2), lung re-expansion following tube thoracostomy with drainage rates of 100 mL/24 hr. or less, no prior intrapleural therapy, no prior systemic BLENOXANE therapy, no chest irradiation and no recent change in systemic therapy. Overall survival did not differ between the BLENOXANE 60 units (n=44) and tetracycline (n=41) groups. Of patients evaluated within 30 days of instillation, the recurrence rate was 36% (10/28) with BLENOXANE and 67% (18/27) with tetracycline (p=0.023). Toxicity was similar between groups.

INDICATIONS AND USAGE

BLENOXANE should be considered a palliative treatment. It has been shown to be useful in the management of the following neoplasms either as a single agent or in proven combinations with other approved chemotherapeutic agents:

Squamous Cell Carcinoma: Head and neck (including mouth, tongue, tonsil, nasopharynx, oropharynx, sinus, palate, lip, buccal mucosa, gingivae, epiglottis, skin, larynx), penis, cervix, and vulva. The response to BLENOXANE is poorer in patients with previously irradiated head and neck cancer.

Lymphomas: Hodgkin's Disease, non-Hodgkin's lymphoma.

Testicular Carcinoma: Embryonal cell, choriocarcinoma, and teratocarcinoma.

BLENOXANE has also been shown to be useful in the management of:

Malignant Pleural Effusion: BLENOXANE is effective as a sclerosing agent for the treatment of malignant pleural effusion and prevention of recurrent pleural effusions.

CONTRAINDICATIONS

BLENOXANE is contraindicated in patients who have demonstrated a hypersensitive or an idiosyncratic reaction to it.

WARNINGS

Patients receiving BLENOXANE must be observed carefully and frequently during and after therapy. It should be used with extreme caution in patients with significant impairment of renal function or compromised pulmonary function.

Pulmonary toxicities occur in 10% of treated patients. In approximately 1%, the nonspecific pneumonitis induced by BLENOXANE progresses to pulmonary fibrosis, and death. Although this is age and dose related, the toxicity is unpredictable. Frequent roentgenograms are recommended (see **ADVERSE REACTIONS: Pulmonary** section).

A severe idiosyncratic reaction (similar to anaphylaxis) consisting of hypotension, mental confusion, fever, chills, and wheezing has been reported in approximately 1% of lymphoma patients treated with BLENOXANE. Since these reactions usually occur after the first or second dose, careful monitoring is essential after these doses (see **ADVERSE REACTIONS: Idiosyncratic Reactions** section).

Renal or hepatic toxicity, beginning as a deterioration in renal or liver function tests, have been reported, infrequently. These toxicities may occur, however, at any time after initiation of therapy.

Usage in Pregnancy:

Pregnancy "Category D"—BLENOXANE can cause fetal harm when administered to a pregnant woman. It has been shown to be teratogenic in rats. Administration of intraperitoneal doses of 1.5 mg/kg/day to rats (about 1.6 times the recommended human dose on a unit/m^2 basis) on days 6–15 of gestation caused skeletal malformations, shortened innominate artery and hydroureter. BLENOXANE is abortifacient but not teratogenic in rabbits, at I.V. doses of 1.2 mg/kg/day (about 2.4 times the recommended human dose on a unit/m^2 basis) given on gestation days 6–18.

There have been no studies in pregnant women. If BLENOXANE is used during pregnancy, or if the patient becomes pregnant while receiving this drug, the patient should be apprised of the potential hazard to the fetus. Women of childbearing potential should be advised to avoid becoming pregnant during therapy with BLENOXANE.

PRECAUTIONS

General: Bleomycin clearance may be reduced in patients with impaired renal function. No guidelines have been established for dose adjustments, but bleomycin should be used with extreme caution in patients with significant renal impairment.

Carcinogenesis, Mutagenesis, and Impairment of Fertility: The carcinogenic potential of BLENOXANE (bleomycin sulfate for injection, USP) in humans is unknown. A study in F344-type male rats demonstrated an increased incidence of nodular hyperplasia after induced lung carcinogenesis by nitrosamines, followed by treatment with bleomycin. In another study where the drug was administered to rats by subcutaneous injection at 0.35 mg/kg weekly (3.82 units/m^2 weekly or about 30% at the recommended human dose), necropsy findings included dose related injection site fibrosarcomas as well as various renal tumors. Bleomycin has been shown to be mutagenic both *in vitro* and *in vivo*. The effects of bleomycin on fertility have not been studied.

Pregnancy: Pregnancy "Category D". (See **WARNINGS** section.)

Nursing Mothers: It is not known whether the drug is excreted in human milk. Because many drugs are excreted in human milk and because of the potential for serious adverse reactions in nursing infants, it is recommended that nursing be discontinued by women receiving BLENOXANE therapy.

Pediatric Use: Safety and effectiveness of BLENOXANE in pediatric patients have not been established.

ADVERSE REACTIONS

Pulmonary: This is potentially the most serious side effect, occurring in approximately 10% of treated patients. The most frequent presentation is pneumonitis occasionally progressing to pulmonary fibrosis. Approximately 1% of patients treated have died of pulmonary fibrosis. Pulmonary toxicity is both dose and age related, being more common in patients over 70 years of age and in those receiving over 400 units total dose. This toxicity, however, is unpredictable and has been seen occasionally in young patients receiving low doses. Some published reports have suggested that the risk of pulmonary toxicity may be increased when bleomycin is used in combination with G-CSF (filgrastim) or other cytokines. However, randomized clinical studies completed to date have not demonstrated an increased risk of pulmonary complications in patients treated with bleomycin and G-CSF.

Because of lack of specificity of the clinical syndrome, the identification of patients with pulmonary toxicity due to BLENOXANE has been extremely difficult. The earliest symptom associated with BLENOXANE pulmonary toxicity is dyspnea. The earliest sign is fine rales.

Radiographically, BLENOXANE-induced pneumonitis produces nonspecific patchy opacities, usually of the lower lung fields. The most common changes in pulmonary function tests are a decrease in total lung volume and a decrease in vital capacity. However, these changes are not predictive of the development of pulmonary fibrosis.

The microscopic tissue changes due to BLENOXANE toxicity include bronchiolar squamous metaplasia, reactive macrophages, atypical alveolar epithelial cells, fibrinous edema, and interstitial fibrosis. The acute stage may involve capillary changes and subsequent fibrinous exudation into alveoli producing a change similar to hyaline membrane formation and progressing to a diffuse interstitial fibrosis resembling the Hamman-Rich syndrome. These microscopic findings are nonspecific; e.g., similar changes are seen in radiation pneumonitis and pneumocystic pneumonitis.

To monitor the onset of pulmonary toxicity, roentgenograms of the chest should be taken every 1 to 2 weeks (see **WARNINGS** section). If pulmonary changes are noted, treatment should be discontinued until it can be determined if they are drug related. Recent studies have suggested that sequential measurement of the pulmonary diffusion capacity for carbon monoxide (DL_{CO}) during treatment with BLENOXANE may be an indicator of subclinical pulmonary toxicity. It is recommended that the DL_{CO} be monitored monthly if it is to be employed to detect pulmonary toxicities, and thus the drug should be discontinued when the DL_{CO} falls below 30% to 35% of the pretreatment value.

Because of bleomycin's sensitization of lung tissue, patients who have received bleomycin are at greater risk of developing pulmonary toxicity when oxygen is administered in surgery. While long exposure to very high oxygen concentrations is a known cause of lung damage, after bleomycin administration, lung damage can occur at lower concentrations that are usually considered safe. Suggested preventive measures are:

1. Maintain Fl O_2 at concentrations approximating that of room air (25%) during surgery and the postoperative period.
2. Monitor carefully fluid replacement, focusing more on colloid administration rather than crystalloid.

Sudden onset of an acute chest pain syndrome suggestive of pleuropericarditis has been rarely reported during BLENOXANE infusions. Although each patient must be individually evaluated, further courses of BLENOXANE do not appear to be contraindicated.

Pulmonary adverse events which may be related to the intrapleural administration of BLENOXANE have been reported only rarely.

Idiosyncratic Reactions: In approximately 1% of the lymphoma patients treated with BLENOXANE, an idiosyncratic reaction, similar to anaphylaxis clinically, has been reported. The reaction may be immediate or delayed for several hours, and usually occurs after the first or second dose (see **WARNINGS** section). It consists of hypotension, mental confusion, fever, chills, and wheezing. Treatment is symptomatic including volume expansion, pressor agents, antihistamines, and corticosteroids.

Integument and Mucous Membranes: These are the most frequent side effects, being reported in approximately 50% of treated patients. These consist of erythema, rash, striae, vesiculation, hyperpigmentation, and tenderness of the skin. Hyperkeratosis, nail changes, alopecia, pruritus, and stomatitis have also been reported. It was necessary to discontinue BLENOXANE therapy in 2% of treated patients because of these toxicities.

Scleroderma-like skin changes have also been reported as part of postmarketing surveillance.

Skin toxicity is a relatively late manifestation usually developing in the 2nd and 3rd week of treatment after 150 to 200 units of BLENOXANE have been administered and appears to be related to the cumulative dose.

Intrapleural administration of BLENOXANE has occasionally been associated with local pain. Hypotension possibly requiring symptomatic treatment has been reported infrequently. Death has been very rarely reported in association with BLENOXANE pleurodesis in these very seriously ill patients.

Other: Vascular toxicities coincident with the use of BLENOXANE in combination with other antineoplastic agents have been reported rarely. The events are clinically heterogeneous and may include myocardial infarction, cerebrovascular accident, thrombotic microangiopathy (HUS) or cerebral arteritis. Various mechanisms have been proposed for these vascular complications. There are also reports of Raynaud's phenomenon occurring in patients treated with BLENOXANE in combination with vinblastine with or without cisplatin or, in a few cases, with BLENOXANE as a single agent. It is currently unknown if the cause of Raynaud's phenomenon in these cases is the disease, underlying vascular compromise, BLENOXANE, vinblastine, hypomagnesemia, or a combination of any of these factors.

Fever, chills, and vomiting were frequently reported side effects. Anorexia and weight loss are common and may persist long after termination of this medication. Pain at tumor site, phlebitis, and other local reactions were reported infrequently.

Malaise was also reported as part of postmarketing surveillance.

DOSAGE AND ADMINISTRATION

Because of the possibility of an anaphylactoid reaction, lymphoma patients should be treated with 2 units or less for the first two doses. If no acute reaction occurs, then the regular dosage schedule may be followed.

The following dose schedule is recommended: **Squamous cell carcinoma, non-Hodgkin's lymphoma, testicular carcinoma**—0.25 to 0.50 units/kg (10 to 20 units/m^2) given intravenously, intramuscularly, or subcutaneously weekly or twice weekly.

Hodgkin's Disease: 0.25 to 0.50 units/kg (10 to 20 units/m^2) given intravenously, intramuscularly, or subcutaneously weekly or twice weekly. After a 50% response, a maintenance dose of 1 unit daily or 5 units weekly intravenously or intramuscularly should be given.

Pulmonary toxicity of BLENOXANE (bleomycin sulfate for injection, USP) appears to be dose related with a striking increase when the total dose is over 400 units. Total doses over 400 units should be given with great caution.

Note: When BLENOXANE is used in combination with other antineoplastic agents, pulmonary toxicities may occur at lower doses.

Improvement of Hodgkin's Disease and testicular tumors is prompt and noted within 2 weeks. If no improvement is seen by this time, improvement is unlikely. Squamous cell cancers respond more slowly, sometimes requiring as long as 3 weeks before any improvement is noted.

Malignant Pleural Effusion: 60 units administered as a single dose bolus intrapleural injection (see **ADMINISTRATION: Intrapleural** section).

ADMINISTRATION

BLENOXANE may be given by the intramuscular, intravenous, subcutaneous or intrapleural routes.

Continued on next page

Blenoxane—Cont.

Intramuscular or Subcutaneous: The BLENOXANE 15 units vial should be reconstituted with 1 to 5 mL of Sterile Water for Injection, USP; Sodium Chloride for Injection, 0.9%, USP; or Sterile Bacteriostatic Water for Injection, USP. The BLENOXANE 30 units vial should be reconstituted with 2 to 10 mL of the above diluents.

Intravenous: The contents of the 15 units or 30 units vial should be dissolved in 5 mL or 10 mL, respectively of Sodium Chloride for Injection, 0.9%, USP and administered slowly over a period of 10 minutes.

Intrapleural: 60 units of BLENOXANE is dissolved in 50–100 mL sodium chloride injection 0.9%, and administered through a thoracostomy tube following drainage of excess pleural fluid and confirmation of complete lung expansion. The literature suggests that successful pleurodesis is, in part, dependent upon complete drainage of the pleural fluid and reestablishment of negative intrapleural pressure prior to instillation of a sclerosing agent. Therefore, the amount of drainage from the chest tube should be as minimal as possible prior to instillation of BLENOXANE. Although there is no conclusive evidence to support this contention, it is generally accepted that chest tube drainage should be less than 100 mL in a 24 hour period prior to sclerosis. However, BLENOXANE instillation may be appropriate when drainage is between 100–300 mL under clinical conditions that necessitate sclerosis therapy. The thoracostomy tube is clamped after BLENOXANE instillation. The patient is moved from the supine to the left and right lateral positions several times during the next four hours. The clamp is then removed and suction reestablished. The amount of time the chest tube remains in place following sclerosis is dictated by the clinical situation.

The intrapleural injection of topical anesthetics or systemic narcotic analgesia is generally not required.

Parenteral drug products should be inspected visually for particulate matter and discoloration prior to administration, whenever solution and container permit.

HOW SUPPLIED

BLENOXANE® (bleomycin sulfate for injection, USP) is available as follows:

NDC 0015-3010-20, 15 units per vial as bleomycin sulfate for injection, USP.

NDC 0015-3063-01, 30 units per vial as bleomycin sulfate for injection, USP.

Stability: The sterile powder is stable under refrigeration 2°C (36°F) to 8°C (46°F) and should not be used after the expiration date is reached.

BLENOXANE should not be reconstituted or diluted with D_5W or other dextrose containing diluents. When reconstituted in D_5W and analyzed by HPLC, BLENOXANE demonstrates a loss of A_2 and B_2 potency that does not occur when BLENOXANE is reconstituted in 0.9% sodium chloride.

BLENOXANE is stable for 24 hours at room temperature in Sodium Chloride.

Procedures for proper handling and disposal of anticancer drugs should be considered. Several guidelines on this subject have been published.[1–7] There is no general agreement that all of the procedures recommended in the guidelines are necessary or appropriate.

REFERENCES

1. Recommendations for the Safe Handling of Parenteral Antineoplastic Drugs. NIH Publication No. 83-2621. For sale by the Superintendent of Documents, US Government Printing Office, Washington, DC 20402.
2. AMA Council Report. Guidelines for Handling Parenteral Antineoplastics. *JAMA* 1985; 253(11):1590–1592.
3. National Study Commission on Cytotoxic Exposure—Recommendations for Handling Cytotoxic Agents. Available from Louis P. Jeffrey, ScD, Chairman, National Study Commission on Cytotoxic Exposure, Massachusetts College of Pharmacy and Allied Health Sciences, 179 Longwood Avenue, Boston, Massachusetts 02115.
4. Clinical Oncological Society of Australia: Guidelines and Recommendations for Safe Handling of Antineoplastic Agents. *Med J Australia* 1983; 1:426–428.
5. Jones RB, et al: Safe Handling of Chemotherapeutic Agents: A Report from the Mount Sinai Medical Center. *CA–A Cancer Journal for Clinicians* 1983; (Sept/Oct) 258–263.
6. American Society of Hospital Pharmacists Technical Assistance Bulletin on Handling Cytotoxic and Hazardous Drugs. *Am J Hosp Pharm* 1990; 47:1033–1049.
7. Controlled Occupational Exposure to Hazardous Drugs (OSHA WORK PRACTICE GUIDELINES) *Am J Health-Syst Pharm* 1996; 53:1669–1685.

Manufactured by: **Nippon Kayaku Co., Ltd.**
Tokyo, Japan

Distributed by:
Mead Johnson
ONCOLOGY PRODUCTS
A Bristol-Myers Squibb Company
Princton, NJ 08543
U.S.A.

H2-B001-9-99 1018230A2
Revised: April 1999

Shown in Product Identification Guide, page 310

CeeNU® ℞

[*cē 'nū*]
(lomustine)
Capsules
Rx ONLY

> **WARNINGS**
>
> CeeNU® (lomustine) should be administered under the supervision of a qualified physician experienced in the use of cancer chemotherapeutic agents.
>
> Bone marrow suppression, notably thrombocytopenia and leukopenia, which may contribute to bleeding and overwhelming infections in an already compromised patient, is the most common and severe of the toxic effects of CeeNU (see **WARNINGS** and **ADVERSE REACTIONS**).
>
> Since the major toxicity is delayed bone marrow suppression, blood counts should be monitored weekly for at least 6 weeks after a dose (see **ADVERSE REACTIONS**). At the recommended dosage, courses of CeeNU should not be given more frequently than every 6 weeks.
>
> The bone marrow toxicity of CeeNU is cumulative and therefore dosage adjustment must be considered on the basis of nadir blood counts from prior dose (see **Dosage Adjustment Table** under **DOSAGE AND ADMINISTRATION**).

DESCRIPTION

CeeNU® (lomustine [CCNU]) Capsules is one of the nitrosoureas used in the treatment of certain neoplastic diseases. It is 1-(2-chloro-ethyl)-3-cyclohexyl-1-nitrosourea. It is a yellow powder with the empirical formula of $C_9H_{16}ClN_3O_2$ and a molecular weight of 233.71. CeeNU is soluble in 10% ethanol (0.05 mg per mL) and in absolute alcohol (70 mg per mL). CeeNU is relatively insoluble in water (<0.05 mg per mL).

It is relatively unionized at a physiological pH.

Inactive ingredients in CeeNU capsules are: magnesium stearate and mannitol.

The structural formula is:

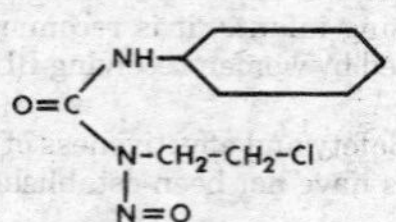

CeeNU is available in 10 mg, 40 mg, and 100 mg capsules for oral administration.

CLINICAL PHARMACOLOGY

Although it is generally agreed that CeeNU alkylates DNA and RNA, it is not cross resistant with other alkylators. As with other nitrosoureas, it may also inhibit several key enzymatic processes by carbamoylation of amino acids in proteins.

CeeNU may be given orally. Following oral administration of radioactive CeeNU at doses ranging from 30 mg/m^2 to 100 mg/m^2, about half of the radioactivity given was excreted in the form of degradation products within 24 hours. The serum half-life of the metabolites ranges from 16 hours to 2 days. Tissue levels are comparable to plasma levels at 15 minutes after intravenous administration.

Because of the high lipid solubility and the relative lack of ionization at physiological pH, CeeNU crosses the blood-brain barrier quite effectively. Levels of radioactivity in the CSF are 50% or greater than those measured concurrently in plasma.

INDICATIONS AND USAGE

CeeNU has been shown to be useful as a single agent in addition to other treatment modalities, or in established combination therapy with other approved chemotherapeutic agents in the following:

Brain tumors: both primary and metastatic, in patients who have already received appropriate surgical and/or radiotherapeutic procedures.

Hodgkin's Disease: secondary therapy in combination with other approved drugs in patients who relapse while being treated with primary therapy, or who fail to respond to primary therapy.

CONTRAINDICATIONS

CeeNU should not be given to individuals who have demonstrated a previous hypersensitivity to it.

WARNINGS

Since the major toxicity is delayed bone marrow suppression, blood counts should be monitored weekly for at least 6 weeks after a dose (see **ADVERSE REACTIONS**). At the recommended dosage, courses of CeeNU should not be given more frequently than every 6 weeks.

The bone marrow toxicity of CeeNU is cumulative and therefore dosage adjustment must be considered on the basis of nadir blood counts from prior dose (see **Dosage Adjustment Table** under **DOSAGE AND ADMINISTRATION**).

Pulmonary toxicity from CeeNU appears to be dose related (see **ADVERSE REACTIONS**).

Long-term use of nitrosoureas has been reported to be possibly associated with the development of secondary malignancies.

Liver and renal function tests should be monitored periodically (see **ADVERSE REACTIONS**).

Pregnancy: Pregnancy "Category D". CeeNU can cause fetal harm when administered to a pregnant woman. CeeNU is embryotoxic and teratogenic in rats and embryotoxic in rabbits at dose levels equivalent to the human dose. There are no adequate and well controlled studies in pregnant women. If this drug is used during pregnancy, or if the patient becomes pregnant while taking (receiving) this drug, the patient should be apprised of the potential hazard to the fetus. Women of childbearing potential should be advised to avoid becoming pregnant.

PRECAUTIONS

General: In all instances where the use of CeeNU is considered for chemotherapy, the physician must evaluate the need and usefulness of the drug against the risks of toxic effects or adverse reactions. Most such adverse reactions are reversible if detected early. When such effects or reactions do occur, the drug should be reduced in dosage or discontinued and appropriate corrective measures should be taken according to the clinical judgment of the physician. Reinstitution of CeeNU therapy should be carried out with caution and with adequate consideration of the further need for the drug and alertness as to possible recurrence of toxicity.

Laboratory Tests: Due to delayed bone marrow suppression, blood counts should be monitored weekly for at least 6 weeks after a dose.

Baseline pulmonary function studies should be conducted along with frequent pulmonary function tests during treatment. Patients with a baseline below 70% of the predicted Forced Vital Capacity (FVC) or Carbon Monoxide Diffusing Capacity (DL_{co}) are particularly at risk.

Since CeeNU (lomustine) Capsules may cause liver dysfunction, it is recommended that liver function tests be monitored periodically.

Renal function tests should also be monitored periodically.

Carcinogenesis, Mutagenesis, Impairment of Fertility: CeeNU is carcinogenic in rats and mice, producing a marked increase in tumor incidence in doses approximating those employed clinically. Nitrosourea therapy does have carcinogenic potential in humans (see **ADVERSE REACTIONS**). CeeNU also affects fertility in male rats at doses somewhat higher than the human dose.

Pregnancy: Pregnancy "Category D". (See **WARNINGS**.)

Nursing Mothers: It is not known whether this drug is excreted in human milk. Because many drugs are excreted in human milk and because of the potential for serious adverse reactions in nursing infants from CeeNU, a decision should be made whether to discontinue nursing or to discontinue the drug, taking into account the importance of the drug to the mother.

Pediatric Use: See **ADVERSE REACTIONS, Pulmonary Toxicity,** and **DOSAGE AND ADMINISTRATION.**

Information for the Patient: Patients receiving CeeNU should be given the following information and instructions by the physician:

1. Patients should be told that CeeNU is an anticancer drug and belongs to the group of medicines known as alkylating agents.
2. In order to provide the proper dose of CeeNU, patients should be aware that there may be two or more different types and colors of capsules in the container dispensed by the pharmacist.
3. Patients should be told that CeeNU is given as a single oral dose and will not be repeated for at least 6 weeks.
4. Patients should be told that nausea and vomiting usually last less than 24 hours, although loss of appetite may last for several days.
5. If any of the following reactions occur, notify the physician: fever, chills, sore throat, unusual bleeding or bruising, shortness of breath, dry cough, swelling of feet or lower legs, mental confusion, or yellowing of eyes and skin.

ADVERSE REACTIONS

Hematologic Toxicity: The most frequent and most serious toxicity of CeeNU is delayed myelosuppression. It usually occurs 4 to 6 weeks after drug administration and is dose related. Thrombocytopenia occurs at about 4 weeks postadministration and persists for 1 to 2 weeks. Leukopenia occurs at 5 to 6 weeks after a dose of CeeNU and persists for 1 to 2 weeks. Approximately 65% of patients receiving 130 mg/m^2 develop white blood counts below 5000 wbc/mm^3. Thirty-six percent developed white blood counts below 3000 wbc/mm^3. Thrombocytopenia is generally more severe than leukopenia. However, both may be dose-limiting toxicities. **CeeNU may produce cumulative myelosuppression, manifested by more depressed indices or longer duration of suppression after repeated doses.**

The occurrence of acute leukemia and bone marrow dysplasias have been reported in patients following long-term nitrosourea therapy.

Anemia also occurs, but is less frequent and less severe than thrombocytopenia or leukopenia.

Pulmonary Toxicity: Pulmonary toxicity characterized by pulmonary infiltrates and/or fibrosis has been reported rarely with CeeNU. Onset of toxicity has occurred after an interval of 6 months or longer from the start of therapy with cumulative doses of CeeNU usually greater than 1100 mg/m^2. There is one report of pulmonary toxicity at a cumulative dose of only 600 mg.

Delayed onset pulmonary fibrosis occurring up to 17 years after treatment has been reported in patients who received related nitrosoureas in childhood and early adolescence

(1–16 years) combined with cranial radiotherapy for intracranial tumors. There appeared to be some late reduction of pulmonary function of all long-term survivors. This form of lung fibrosis may be slowly progressive and has resulted in death in some cases. In this long-term study of carmustine, all those initially treated at less than five years of age died of delayed pulmonary fibrosis.

Gastrointestinal Toxicity: Nausea and vomiting may occur 3 to 6 hours after an oral dose and usually lasts less than 24 hours. Prior administration of antiemetics is effective in diminishing and sometimes preventing this side effect. Nausea and vomiting can also be reduced if CeeNU is administered to fasting patients.

Hepatotoxicity: A reversible type of hepatic toxicity, manifested by increased transaminase, alkaline phosphatase and bilirubin levels, has been reported in a small percentage of patients receiving CeeNU.

Nephrotoxicity: Renal abnormalities consisting of progressive azotemia, decrease in kidney size and renal failure have been reported in patients who received large cumulative doses after prolonged therapy with CeeNU. Kidney damage has also been reported occasionally in patients receiving lower total doses.

Other Toxicities: Stomatitis, alopecia, optic atrophy, and visual disturbances such as blindness have been reported infrequently.

Neurological reactions such as disorientation, lethargy, ataxia, and dysarthria have been noted in some patients receiving CeeNU. However, the relationship to medication in these patients is unclear.

OVERDOSAGE

No proven antidotes have been established for CeeNU overdosage.

DOSAGE AND ADMINISTRATION

The recommended dose of CeeNU in adult and pediatric patients as a single agent in previously untreated patients is 130 mg/m^2 as a single oral dose every 6 weeks. In individuals with compromised bone marrow function, the dose should be reduced to 100 mg/m^2 every 6 weeks. When CeeNU is used in combination with other myelosuppressive drugs, the doses should be adjusted accordingly.

Doses subsequent to the initial dose should be adjusted according to the hematologic response of the patient to the preceding dose. The following schedule is suggested as a guide to dosage adjustment:

Nadir After Prior Dose		Percentage of Prior Dose to be Given
Leukocytes	Platelets	
> 4000	> 100,000	100%
3000–3999	75,000–99,999	100%
2000–2999	25,000–74,999	70%
< 2000	< 25,000	50%

A repeat course of CeeNU should not be given until circulating blood elements have returned to acceptable levels (platelets above 100,000/ mm^3; leukocytes above 4000/mm^3) and this is usually in 6 weeks. Adequate number of neutrophils should be present on a peripheral blood smear. Blood counts should be monitored weekly and repeat courses should not be given before 6 weeks because the hematologic toxicity is delayed and cumulative.

HOW SUPPLIED

The dose pack of CeeNU® (lomustine)
NDC 0015-3034-10 Capsules contains:
2–100 mg capsules (Green/Green)
2–40 mg capsules (White/Green)
2–10 mg capsules (White/White)

Stability: CeeNU Capsules are stable for the lot life indicated on package labeling when stored at room temperature in well closed containers. Avoid excessive heat (over 40°C, 104°F).

Directions to the Pharmacist: The dose pack contains a total of 300 mg and will provide enough medication for titration of a single dose. The total dose prescribed by the physician can be obtained (to within 10 mg) by determining the appropriate combination of the enclosed capsule strengths. The appropriate number of capsules of each size should be placed in a single vial to which the patient information label (gummed label provided) explaining the differences in the appearance of the capsules is affixed. Each color-coded capsule is imprinted with the dose in milligrams.

A patient information sticker, to be placed on dispensing container, is enclosed.

Also available: Individual bottles of 20 capsules each.
NDC 0015-3032-20—100 mg capsules (Green/Green)
NDC 0015-3031-20—40 mg capsules (White/Green)
NDC 0015-3030-20—10 mg capsules (White/White)

Procedures for proper handling and disposal of anticancer drugs should be considered. Several guidelines on this subject have been published.[1–7] There is no general agreement that all of the procedures recommended in the guidelines are necessary or appropriate.

REFERENCES

1. Recommendations for the Safe Handling of Parenteral Antineoplastic Drugs. NIH Publication No. 83-2621. For sale by the Superintendent of Documents, US Government Printing Office, Washington, DC 20402.
2. AMA Council Report. Guidelines for Handling Parenteral Antineoplastics. *JAMA* 1985; 253 (11):1590–1592.
3. National Study Commission on Cytotoxic Exposure—Recommendations for Handling Cytotoxic Agents. Available from Louis P. Jeffrey, ScD, Chairman, National Study Commission on Cytotoxic Exposure, Massachusetts College of Pharmacy and Allied Health Sciences, 179 Longwood Avenue, Boston, Massachusetts 02115.
4. Clinical Oncological Society of Australia. Guidelines and Recommendations for Safe Handling of Antineoplastic Agents. *Med J Australia* 1983; 1:426–428.
5. Jones RB, et al: Safe Handling of Chemotherapeutic Agents: A Report from the Mount Sinai Medical Center. *CA-A Cancer Journal for Clinicians* 1983; (Sept/Oct)258–263.
6. American Society of Hospital Pharmacists Technical Assistance Bulletin on Handling Cytotoxic and Hazardous Drugs. *Am J Hosp Pharm* 1990; 47:1033–1049.
7. Controlling Occupational Exposure to Hazardous Drugs. (OSHA WORK PRACTICE GUIDELINES). *Am J Health-Syst Pharm* 1996; 53:1669–1685.

BRISTOL LABORATORIES®
ONCOLOGY PRODUCTS
A Bristol-Myers Squibb Company
Princeton, NJ 08543
U.S.A.
Made in Italy
H3-B001-1-00 1050973
Revised June 1998

Lyophilized *CYTOXAN*® ℞

[*sī-taks 'an*]
(cyclophosphamide for injection, USP)

***CYTOXAN*® Tablets**
(cyclophosphamide tablets, USP)
℞ ONLY

DESCRIPTION

Lyophilized CYTOXAN® (cyclophosphamide for injection, USP) is a sterile white lyophilized cake, or partially broken cake, containing 75 mg mannitol per 100 mg cyclophosphamide (anhydrous). CYTOXAN® Tablets (cyclophosphamide tablets, USP) are for oral use and contain 25 mg or 50 mg cyclophosphamide (anhydrous). Inactive ingredients in CYTOXAN tablets are: acacia, FD&C Blue No. 1, D&C Yellow No. 10 Aluminum Lake, lactose, magnesium stearate, starch, stearic acid, and talc. Cyclophosphamide is a synthetic antineoplastic drug chemically related to the nitrogen mustards. Cyclophosphamide is a white crystalline powder with the molecular formula $C_7H_{15}Cl_2N_2O_2P \bullet H_2O$ and a molecular weight of 279.1. The chemical name for cyclophosphamide is 2-[bis(2-chloroethyl)amino]tetrahydro-2H-1,3,2-oxazaphosphorine 2-oxide monohydrate. Cyclophosphamide is soluble in water, saline, or ethanol and has the following structural formula:

O, P, O, NH, $N(CH_2CH_2Cl)_2 \bullet H_2O$

CLINICAL PHARMACOLOGY

CYTOXAN (cyclophosphamide) is biotransformed principally in the liver to active alkylating metabolites by a mixed function microsomal oxidase system. These metabolites interfere with the growth of susceptible rapidly proliferating malignant cells. The mechanism of action is thought to involve cross-linking of tumor cell DNA.

CYTOXAN is well absorbed after oral administration with a bioavailability greater than 75%. The unchanged drug has an elimination half-life of 3 to 12 hours. It is eliminated primarily in the form of metabolites, but from 5% to 25% of the dose is excreted in urine as unchanged drug. Several cytotoxic and noncytotoxic metabolites have been identified in urine and in plasma. Concentrations of metabolites reach a maximum in plasma 2 to 3 hours after an intravenous dose. Plasma protein binding of unchanged drug is low but some metabolites are bound to an extent greater than 60%. It has not been demonstrated that any single metabolite is responsible for either the therapeutic or toxic effects of cyclophosphamide. Although elevated levels of metabolites of cyclophosphamide have been observed in patients with renal failure, increased clinical toxicity in such patients has not been demonstrated.

INDICATIONS AND USAGE

Malignant Diseases: CYTOXAN, although effective alone in susceptible malignancies, is more frequently used concurrently or sequentially with other antineoplastic drugs. The following malignancies are often susceptible to CYTOXAN treatment:

1. Malignant lymphomas (Stages III and IV of the Ann Arbor staging system), Hodgkin's disease, lymphocytic lymphoma (nodular or diffuse), mixed-cell type lymphoma, histiocytic lymphoma, Burkitt's lymphoma. **2.** Multiple myeloma. **3.** Leukemias: Chronic lymphocytic leukemia, chronic granulocytic leukemia (it is usually ineffective in acute blastic crisis), acute myelogenous and monocytic leukemia, acute lymphoblastic (stem-cell) leukemia in children (CYTOXAN given during remission is effective in prolonging its duration). **4.** Mycosis fungoides (advanced disease). **5.** Neuroblastoma (disseminated disease). **6.** Adenocarcinoma of the ovary. **7.** Retinoblastoma. **8.** Carcinoma of the breast.

Nonmalignant Disease—Biopsy Proven "Minimal Change" Nephrotic Syndrome in Children: CYTOXAN is useful in carefully selected cases of biopsy proven "minimal change" nephrotic syndrome in children but should not be used as primary therapy. In children whose disease fails to respond adequately to appropriate adrenocorticosteroid therapy or in whom the adrenocorticosteroid therapy produces or threatens to produce intolerable side effects, CYTOXAN may induce a remission. CYTOXAN is not indicated for the nephrotic syndrome in adults or for any other renal disease.

CONTRAINDICATIONS

Continued use of cyclophosphamide is contraindicated in patients with severely depressed bone marrow function. Cyclophosphamide is contraindicated in patients who have demonstrated a previous hypersensitivity to it. (See **WARNINGS** and **PRECAUTIONS**.)

WARNINGS

Carcinogenesis, Mutagenesis, Impairment of Fertility: Second malignancies have developed in some patients treated with cyclophosphamide used alone or in association with other antineoplastic drugs and/or modalities. Most frequently, they have been urinary bladder, myeloproliferative, or lymphoproliferative malignancies. Second malignancies most frequently were detected in patients treated for primary myeloproliferative or lymphoproliferative malignancies or nonmalignant disease in which immune processes are believed to be involved pathologically.

In some cases, the second malignancy developed several years after cyclophosphamide treat ment had been discontinued. In a single breast cancer trial utilizing two to four times the standard dose of cyclophosphamide in conjunction with doxorubicin a small number of cases of secondary acute myeloid leukemia occurred within two years of treatment initiation. Urinary bladder malignancies generally have occurred in patients who previously had hemorrhagic cystitis. In patients treated with cyclophosphamide-containing regimens for a variety of solid tumors, isolated case reports of secondary malignancies have been published. One case of carcinoma of the renal pelvis was reported in a patient receiving long-term cyclophosphamide therapy for cerebral vasculitis. The possibility of cyclophosphamide-induced malignancy should be considered in any benefit-to-risk assessment for use of the drug.

Cyclophosphamide can cause fetal harm when administered to a pregnant woman and such abnormalities have been reported following cyclophosphamide therapy in pregnant women. Abnormalities were found in two infants and a six-month-old fetus born to women treated with cyclophosphamide. Ectrodactylia was found in two of the three cases. Normal infants have also been born to women treated with cyclophosphamide during pregnancy, including the first trimester. If this drug is used during pregnancy, or if the patient becomes pregnant while taking (receiving) this drug, the patient should be apprised of the potential hazard to the fetus. Women of childbearing potential should be advised to avoid becoming pregnant.

Cyclophosphamide interferes with oogenesis and spermatogenesis. It may cause sterility in both sexes. Development of sterility appears to depend on the dose of cyclophosphamide, duration of therapy, and the state of gonadal function at the time of treatment. Cyclophosphamide-induced sterility may be irreversible in some patients.

Amenorrhea associated with decreased estrogen and increased gonadotropin secretion develops in a significant proportion of women treated with cyclophosphamide. Affected patients generally resume regular menses within a few months after cessation of therapy. Girls treated with cyclophosphamide during prepubescence generally develop secondary sexual characteristics normally and have regular menses. Ovarian fibrosis with apparently complete loss of germ cells after prolonged cyclophosphamide treatment in late prepubescence has been reported. Girls treated with cyclophosphamide during prepubescence subsequently have conceived.

Men treated with cyclophosphamide may develop oligospermia or azoospermia associated with increased gonadotropin but normal testosterone secretion. Sexual potency and libido are unimpaired in these patients. Boys treated with cyclophosphamide during prepubescence develop secondary sexual characteristics normally, but may have oligospermia or azoospermia and increased gonadotropin secretion. Some degree of testicular atrophy may occur. Cyclophosphamide-induced azoospermia is reversible in some patients, though the reversibility may not occur for several years after cessation of therapy. Men temporarily rendered sterile by cyclophosphamide have subsequently fathered normal children.

Urinary System: Hemorrhagic cystitis may develop in patients treated with cyclophosphamide. Rarely, this condition can be severe and even fatal. Fibrosis of the urinary bladder, sometimes extensive, also may develop with or without accompanying cystitis. Atypical urinary bladder epithelial cells may appear in the urine. These adverse effects appear to depend on the dose of cyclophosphamide and the duration of therapy. Such bladder injury is thought to be due to cyclophosphamide metabolites excreted in the urine. Forced fluid intake helps to assure an ample output of urine, necessitates frequent voiding, and reduces the time the drug remains in the bladder. This helps to prevent cystitis. Hematuria usually resolves in a few days after cyclophosphamide treatment is stopped, but it may persist. Medical and/or surgical supportive treatment may be required, rarely, to treat protracted cases of severe hemorrhagic cystitis. It is usually

Continued on next page

Cytoxan—Cont.

necessary to discontinue cyclophosphamide therapy in instances of severe hemorrhagic cystitis.

Cardiac Toxicity: Although a few instances of cardiac dysfunction have been reported following use of recommended doses of cyclophosphamide, no causal relationship has been established. Acute cardiac toxicity has been reported with doses as low as 2.4 g/m² to as high as 26 g/m², usually as a portion of an intensive antineoplastic multidrug regimen or in conjunction with transplantation procedures. In a few instances with high doses of cyclophosphamide, severe, and sometimes fatal, congestive heart failure has occurred after the first cyclophosphamide dose. Histopathologic examination has primarily shown hemorrhagic myocarditis. Hemopericardium has occurred secondary to hemorrhagic myocarditis and myocardial necrosis. Pericarditis has been reported independent of any hemopericardium.

No residual cardiac abnormalities, as evidenced by electrocardiogram or echocardiogram appear to be present in patients surviving episodes of apparent cardiac toxicity associated with high doses of cyclophosphamide.

Cyclophosphamide has been reported to potentiate doxorubicin-induced cardiotoxicity.

Infections: Treatment with cyclophosphamide may cause significant suppression of immune responses. Serious, sometimes fatal, infections may develop in severely immunosuppressed patients. Cyclophosphamide treatment may not be indicated or should be interrupted or the dose reduced in patients who have or who develop viral, bacterial, fungal, protozoan, or helminthic infections.

Other: Anaphylactic reactions have been reported; death has also been reported in association with this event. Possible cross-sensitivity with other alkylating agents has been reported.

PRECAUTIONS

General: Special attention to the possible development of toxicity should be exercised in patients being treated with cyclophosphamide if any of the following conditions are present.

1. Leukopenia **2.** Thrombocytopenia **3.** Tumor cell infiltration of bone marrow **4.** Previous X-ray therapy **5.** Previous therapy with other cytotoxic agents **6.** Impaired hepatic function **7.** Impaired renal function

Laboratory Tests: During treatment, the patient's hematologic profile (particularly neutrophils and platelets) should be monitored regularly to determine the degree of hematopoietic suppression. Urine should also be examined regularly for red cells which may precede hemorrhagic cystitis.

Drug Interactions: The rate of metabolism and the leukopenic activity of cyclophosphamide reportedly are increased by chronic administration of high doses of phenobarbital.

The physician should be alert for possible combined drug actions, desirable or undesirable, involving cyclophosphamide even though cyclophosphamide has been used successfully concurrently with other drugs, including other cytotoxic drugs.

Cyclophosphamide treatment, which causes a marked and persistent inhibition of cholinesterase activity, potentiates the effect of succinylcholine chloride.

If a patient has been treated with cyclophosphamide within 10 days of general anesthesia, the anesthesiologist should be alerted.

Adrenalectomy: Since cyclophosphamide has been reported to be more toxic in adrenalectomized dogs, adjustment of the doses of both replacement steroids and cyclophosphamide may be necessary for the adrenalectomized patient.

Wound Healing: Cyclophosphamide may interfere with normal wound healing.

Carcinogenesis, Mutagenesis, Impairment of Fertility: See **WARNINGS** section for information on carcinogenesis, mutagenesis, and impairment of fertility.

Pregnancy: Pregnancy "Category D". (See **WARNINGS**.)

Nursing Mothers: Cyclophosphamide is excreted in breast milk. Because of the potential for serious adverse reactions and the potential for tumorigenicity shown for cyclophosphamide in humans, a decision should be made whether to discontinue nursing or to discontinue the drug, taking into account the importance of the drug to the mother.

ADVERSE REACTIONS

Information on adverse reactions associated with the use of CYTOXAN (cyclophosphamide) is arranged according to body system affected or type of reaction. The adverse reactions are listed in order of decreasing incidence. The most serious adverse reactions are described in the **WARNINGS** section.

Reproductive System: See **WARNINGS** section for information on impairment of fertility.

Digestive System: Nausea and vomiting commonly occur with cyclophosphamide therapy. Anorexia and, less frequently, abdominal discomfort or pain and diarrhea may occur. There are isolated reports of hemorrhagic colitis, oral mucosal ulceration and jaundice occurring during therapy. These adverse drug effects generally remit when cyclophosphamide treatment is stopped.

Skin and Its Structures: Alopecia occurs commonly in patients treated with cyclophosphamide. The hair can be expected to grow back after treatment with the drug or even during continued drug treatment, though it may be different in texture or color. Skin rash occurs occasionally in patients receiving the drug. Pigmentation of the skin and changes in nails can occur. Very rare reports of Stevens-Johnson syndrome and toxic epidermal necrolysis have been received during postmarketing surveillance; due to the nature of spontaneous adverse event reporting, a definitive causal relationship to cyclophosphamide has not been established.

Hematopoietic System: Leukopenia occurs in patients treated with cyclophosphamide, is related to the dose of drug, and can be used as a dosage guide. Leukopenia of less than 2000 cells/mm³ develops commonly in patients treated with an initial loading dose of the drug, and less frequently in patients maintained on smaller doses. The degree of neutropenia is particularly important because it correlates with a reduction in resistance to infections. Fever without documented infection has been reported in neutropenic patients. Thrombocytopenia or anemia develop occasionally in patients treated with CYTOXAN (cyclophosphamide). These hematologic effects usually can be reversed by reducing the drug dose or by interrupting treatment. Recovery from leukopenia usually begins in 7 to 10 days after cessation of therapy.

Urinary System: See **WARNINGS** section for information on cystitis and urinary bladder fibrosis.

Hemorrhagic ureteritis and renal tubular necrosis have been reported to occur in patients treated with cyclophosphamide. Such lesions usually resolve following cessation of therapy.

Infections: See **WARNINGS** section for information on reduced host resistance to infections.

Carcinogenesis: See **WARNINGS** section for information on carcinogenesis.

Respiratory System: Interstitial pneumonitis has been reported as part of the postmarketing experience. Interstitial pulmonary fibrosis has been reported in patients receiving high doses of cyclophosphamide over a prolonged period.

Other: Anaphylactic reactions have been reported; death has also been reported in association with this event. Possible cross-sensitivity with other alkylating agents has been reported. SIADH (syndrome of inappropriate ADH secretion) has been reported with the use of cyclophosphamide. Malaise and asthenia have been reported as part of the postmarketing experience.

OVERDOSAGE

No specific antidote for cyclophosphamide is known. Overdosage should be managed with supportive measures, including appropriate treatment for any concurrent infection, myelosuppression, or cardiac toxicity should it occur.

DOSAGE AND ADMINISTRATION

Treatment of Malignant Diseases—Adults and Children: When used as the only oncolytic drug therapy, the initial course of CYTOXAN for patients with no hematologic deficiency usually consists of 40 to 50 mg/kg given intravenously in divided doses over a period of 2 to 5 days. Other intravenous regimens include 10 to 15 mg/kg given every 7 to 10 days or 3 to 5 mg/kg twice weekly.

Oral CYTOXAN dosing is usually in the range of 1 to 5 mg/kg/day for both initial and maintenance dosing.

Many other regimens of intravenous and oral CYTOXAN have been reported. Dosages must be adjusted in accord with evidence of antitumor activity and/or leukopenia. The total leukocyte count is a good, objective guide for regulating dosage. Transient decreases in the total white blood cell count to 2000 cells/mm³ (following short courses) or more persistent reduction to 3000 cells/mm³ (with continuing therapy) are tolerated without serious risk of infection if there is no marked granulocytopenia.

When CYTOXAN is included in combined cytotoxic regimens, it may be necessary to reduce the dose of CYTOXAN as well as that of the other drugs.

CYTOXAN and its metabolites are dialyzable although there are probably quantitative differences depending upon the dialysis system being used. Patients with compromised renal function may show some measurable changes in pharmacokinetic parameters of CYTOXAN metabolism, but there is no consistent evidence indicating a need for CYTOXAN dosage modification in patients with renal function impairment.

Treatment of Nonmalignant Diseases—Biopsy Proven "Minimal Change" Nephrotic Syndrome In Children: An oral dose of 2.5 to 3 mg/kg daily for a period of 60 to 90 days is recommended. In males, the incidence of oligospermia and azoospermia increases if the duration of CYTOXAN treatment exceeds 60 days. Treatment beyond 90 days increases the probability of sterility. Adrenocorticosteroid therapy may be tapered and discontinued during the course of CYTOXAN therapy. See **PRECAUTIONS** section concerning hematologic monitoring.

Preparation and Handling of Solutions: Parenteral drug products should be inspected visually for particulate matter and discoloration prior to administration, whenever solution and container permit.

Lyophilized CYTOXAN should be prepared for parenteral use by adding Sterile Water for Injection, USP, to the vial and shaking to dissolve. Use the quantity of diluent shown below to reconstitute the product.

Dosage Strength	Lyophilized CYTOXAN Quantity of Diluent
100 mg	5 mL
200 mg	10 mL
500 mg	20–25 mL
1 g	50 mL
2 g	80–100 mL

Solutions of Lyophilized CYTOXAN may be injected intravenously, intramuscularly, intraperitoneally, or intrapleurally or they may be infused intravenously in the following:

- Dextrose Injection, USP (5% dextrose)
- Dextrose and Sodium Chloride Injection, USP (5% dextrose and 0.9% sodium chloride)
- 5% Dextrose and Ringer's Injection
- Lactated Ringer's Injection, USP
- Sodium Chloride Injection, USP (0.45% sodium chloride)
- Sodium Lactate Injection, USP (1/6 molar sodium lactate)

Reconstituted Lyophilized CYTOXAN is chemically and physically stable for 24 hours at room temperature or for six days in the refrigerator; it does not contain any antimicrobial preservative and thus care must be taken to assure the sterility of prepared solutions.

The osmolarities of solutions of Lyophilized CYTOXAN, and normal saline are found in the following table:

Lyophilized CYTOXAN	mOsm/L
4 mL diluent per 100 mg cyclophosphamide	219
5 mL diluent per 100 mg cyclophosphamide	172

Lyophilized CYTOXAN is slightly hypotonic.

Extemporaneous liquid preparations of CYTOXAN for oral administration may be prepared by dissolving Lyophilized CYTOXAN in Aromatic Elixir, N.F. Such preparations should be stored under refrigeration in glass containers and used within 14 days.

HOW SUPPLIED

Lyophilized CYTOXAN® (cyclophosphamide for injection, USP) contains 75 mg of mannitol per 100 mg of cyclophosphamide (anhydrous) and is supplied in vials for single-dose use.

Lyophilized CYTOXAN® (cyclophosphamide for injection, USP). U.S. Patent No. 4,537,883

[See first table above]

NDC 0015-0539-41	100 mg vials, carton of 12, case of 1 carton
NDC 0015-0546-41	200 mg vials, carton of 12, case of 1 carton
NDC 0015-0547-41	500 mg vials, carton of 12, case of 1 carton
NDC 0015-0548-41	1.0 g vials, carton of 6
NDC 0015-0549-41	2.0 g vials, carton of 6

CYTOXAN® Tablets (cyclophosphamide tablets, USP), 25 mg, and CYTOXAN® Tablets, 50 mg, are white tablets with blue flecks containing 25 mg and 50 mg cyclophosphamide (anhydrous), respectively.

[See second table above]

CYTOXAN® Tablets (cyclophosphamide tablets, USP).

NDC 0015-0503-01	50 mg, bottles of 100
NDC 0015-0503-02	50 mg, bottles of 1000
NDC 0015-0504-01	25 mg, bottles of 100

Storage at or below 77°F (25°C) is recommended; this product will withstand brief exposure to temperatures up to 86°F (30°C) but should be protected from temperatures above 86°F (30°C).

Procedures for proper handling and disposal of anticancer drugs should be considered. Several guidelines on this subject have been published.[1–7] There is no general agreement that all of the procedures recommended in the guidelines are necessary or appropriate.

REFERENCES

1. Recommendations for the Safe Handling of Parenteral Antineoplastic Drugs. NIH Publication No. 83-2621. For sale by the Superintendent of Documents, US Government Printing Office, Washington, DC 20402.
2. AMA Council Report. Guidelines for Handling Parenteral Antineoplastics. *JAMA* 1985; 253(11):1590–1592.
3. National Study Commission on Cytotoxic Exposure—Recommendations for Handling Cytotoxic Agents. Available from Louis P. Jeffrey, ScD, Chairman, National Study Commission on Cytotoxic Exposure, Massachusetts College of Pharmacy and Allied Health Sciences, 179 Longwood Avenue, Boston, Massachusetts 02115.
4. Clinical Oncological Society of Australia. Guidelines and Recommendations for Safe Handling of Antineoplastic Agents. *Med J Australia* 1983; 1:426–428.
5. Jones RB, et al: Safe Handling of Chemotherapeutic Agents: A Report from the Mount Sinai Medical Center. CA—*A Cancer Journal for Clinicians* 1983; (Sept/Oct)258–263.
6. American Society of Hospital Pharmacists Technical Assistance Bulletin on Handling Cytotoxic and Hazardous Drugs. *Am J Hosp Pharm* 1990; 47:1033–1049.
7. Controlling Occupational Exposure to Hazardous Drugs. (OSHA Work Practice Guidelines). *Am J Health-Syst Pharm* 1996; 53:1669–1685.

Mead Johnson
ONCOLOGY PRODUCTS
A Bristol-Myers Squibb Company
Princeton, NJ 08543
U.S.A.

H4-B001-5-00 0539DIM-08
1079968A1 Revised January 2000

Shown in Product Identification Guide, page 310

DROXIA™ ℞

[*drŏx-ē-ă*]
(hydroxyurea capsules, USP)
℞ ONLY

> **WARNING**
> Treatment of patients with DROXIA™ (hydroxyurea capsules, USP) may be complicated by severe, sometimes life-threatening, adverse effects. DROXIA should be administered under the supervision of a physician experienced in the use of this medication for the treatment of sickle cell anemia.
> Hydroxyurea is mutagenic and clastogenic, and causes cellular transformation to a tumorigenic phenotype. Hydroxyurea is thus unequivocally genotoxic and a presumed transspecies carcinogen which implies a carcinogenic risk to humans. In patients receiving long-term hydroxyurea for myeloproliferative disorders, such as polycythemia vera and thrombocythemia, secondary leukemias have been reported. It is unknown whether this leukemogenic effect is secondary to hydroxyurea or is associated with the patients' underlying disease. The physician and patient must very carefully consider the potential benefits of DROXIA relative to the undefined risk of developing secondary malignancies.

DESCRIPTION

DROXIA™ (hydroxyurea capsules, USP) is available for oral use as capsules providing 200 mg, 300 mg and 400 mg hydroxyurea. Inactive ingredients: citric acid, gelatin, lactose, magnesium stearate, sodium phosphate, titanium dioxide and capsule colorants: FD&C Blue #1 and FD&C Green #3 (200 mg capsules); D&C Red #28, D&C Red #33 and FD&C Blue #1 (300 mg capsules); D&C Red #28, D&C Red #33 and D&C Yellow #10 (400 mg capsules).
Hydroxyurea is an essentially tasteless, white crystalline powder. Its structural formula is:

$$H_2N-\overset{\displaystyle O}{\overset{\|}{C}}-NH-OH$$

CLINICAL PHARMACOLOGY

Mechanism of Action: The precise mechanism by which hydroxyurea produces its cytotoxic and cytoreductive effects is not known. However, various studies support the hypothesis that hydroxyurea causes an immediate inhibition of DNA synthesis by acting as a ribonucleotide reductase inhibitor, without interfering with the synthesis of ribonucleic acid or of protein.
The mechanisms by which DROXIA produces its beneficial effects in patients with sickle cell anemia (SCA) are uncertain. Known pharmacologic effects of DROXIA that may contribute to its beneficial effects include increasing hemoglobin F levels in RBCs, decreasing neutrophils, increasing the water content of RBCs, increasing deformability of sickled cells, and altering the adhesion of RBCs to endothelium.
Pharmacokinetics:
Absorption—Hydroxyurea is readily absorbed after oral administration. Peak plasma levels are reached in 1 to 4 hours after an oral dose. With increasing doses, disproportionately greater mean peak plasma concentrations and AUCs are observed.
There are no data on the effect of food on the absorption of hydroxyurea.
Distribution—Hydroxyurea distributes rapidly and widely in the body with an estimated volume of distribution approximating total body water.
Plasma to ascites fluid ratios range from 2:1 to 7.5:1. Hydroxyurea concentrates in leukocytes and erythrocytes.
Metabolism—Up to 50% of an oral dose undergoes conversion through metabolic pathways that are not fully characterized. In one minor pathway, hydroxyurea may be degraded by urease found in intestinal bacteria. Acetohydroxamic acid was found in the serum of three leukemic patients receiving hydroxyurea and may be formed from hydroxylamine resulting from action of urease on hydroxyurea.
Excretion—Excretion of hydroxyurea in humans is a nonlinear process occurring through two pathways. One is saturable, probably hepatic metabolism; the other is first-order renal excretion. In adults with SCA, mean cumulative urinary hydroxyurea excretion was 62% of the administered dose at 8-hours.
Special Populations:
Geriatric, Gender, Race—No information is available regarding pharmacokinetic differences due to age, gender or race.
Pediatric—No pharmacokinetic data are available in pediatric patients treated with hydroxyurea for SCA.
Renal Insufficiency—There are no data that support specific guidance for dosage adjustment in patients with renal impairment. As renal excretion is a pathway of elimination, consideration should be given to decreasing the dosage of hydroxyurea in patients with renal impairment. Close monitoring of hematologic parameters is advised in these patients.
Hepatic Insufficiency—There are no data that support specific guidance for dosage adjustment in patients with hepatic impairment. Close monitoring of hematologic parameters is advised in these patients.
Drug Interactions—There are no data on concomitant use of hydroxyurea with other drugs in humans.

Event	Hydroxyurea (N=152)	Placebo (N=147)	Percent Change vs Placebo	P Value
Median yearly rate of painful crises*	2.5	4.6	−46	=0.001
Median yearly rate of painful crises requiring hospitalization	1.0	2.5	−60	=0.0027
Median time to first painful crisis (months)	2.76	1.35	+104	=0.014
Median time to second painful crisis (months)	6.58	4.13	+59	=0.0024
Incidence of chest syndrome (# episodes)	56	101	−45	=0.003
Number of patients transfused	55	79	−30	=0.002
Number of units of blood transfused	423	670	−37	=0.003

* A painful crisis was defined in the study as acute sickling-related pain that resulted in a visit to a medical facility, that lasted more than 4 hours, and that required treatment with a parenteral narcotic or NSAID. Chest syndrome, priapism, and hepatic sequestration were included in this definition.

CLINICAL STUDIES

The efficacy of hydroxyurea in sickle cell anemia was assessed in a large clinical study (Multicenter Study of Hydroxyurea in Sickle Cell Anemia)[1].
The study was a randomized, double-blind, placebo-controlled trial that evaluated 299 adult patients (≥ 18 years) with moderate to severe disease (≥ 3 painful crises yearly). The trial was stopped by the Data Safety Monitoring Committee, after accrual was completed but before the scheduled 24 months of follow-up was completed in all patients, based on observations of fewer painful crises among patients receiving hydroxyurea.
Compared to placebo treatment, treatment with hydroxyurea resulted in a significant decrease in the yearly rate of painful crises, the yearly rate of painful crises requiring hospitalization, the incidence of chest syndrome, the number of patients transfused, and units of blood transfused. Hydroxyurea treatment significantly increased the median time to both first and second painful crises.
Although patients with 3 or more painful crises during the preceding 12 months were eligible for the study, most of the benefit in crisis reduction was seen in the patients with 6 or more painful crises during the preceding 12 months.
[See table above]
No deaths were attributed to treatment with hydroxyurea, and none of the patients developed neoplastic disorders during the study. Treatment was permanently stopped for medical reasons in 14 hydroxyurea-treated (2 patients with myelotoxicity) and 6 placebo-treated patients. (See **ADVERSE REACTIONS** section.)
Fetal Hemoglobin: In patients with SCA treated with hydroxyurea, fetal hemoglobin (HbF) increases 4 to 12 weeks after initiation of treatment. In general, average HbF levels correlate with dose and plasma level with possible plateauing at higher dosages.
A clear relation between reduction in crisis frequency and increased HbF or F-cell levels has not been demonstrated. The dose-related cytoreductive effects of hydroxyurea, particularly on neutrophils, was the factor most strongly correlated with reduced crisis frequency.

INDICATIONS AND USAGE

DROXIA (hydroxyurea capsules, USP) is indicated to reduce the frequency of painful crises and to reduce the need for blood transfusions in adult patients with sickle cell anemia with recurrent moderate to severe painful crises (generally at least 3 during the preceding 12 months).

CONTRAINDICATIONS

DROXIA is contraindicated in patients who have demonstrated a previous hypersensitivity to hydroxyurea or any other component of its formulation.

WARNINGS

DROXIA is a cytotoxic and myelosuppressive agent. DROXIA should not be given if bone marrow function is markedly depressed, as indicated by neutrophils below 2000 cells/mm^3; a platelet count below 80,000/mm^3; a hemoglobin level below 4.5 g/dL; or reticulocytes below 80,000/mm^3 when the hemoglobin concentration is below 9 g/dL. Neutropenia is generally the first and most common manifestation of hematologic suppression. (See **DOSAGE AND ADMINISTRATION** section.) Thrombocytopenia and anemia occur less often, and are seldom seen without a preceding leukopenia. Recovery from myelosuppression is usually rapid when therapy is interrupted. DROXIA causes macrocytosis, which may mask the incidental development of folic acid deficiency. Prophylactic administration of folic acid is recommended.
Hydroxyurea should be used with caution in patients with renal dysfunction. (See **DOSAGE AND ADMINISTRATION** section.)
Carcinogenesis and Mutagenesis: (See **Boxed WARNING** section.) Hydroxyurea is genotoxic in a wide range of test systems and is thus presumed to be a human carcinogen. In patients receiving long-term hydroxyurea for myeloproliferative disorders, such as polycythemia vera and thrombocythemia, secondary leukemia has been reported. It is unknown whether this leukemogenic effect is secondary to hydroxyurea or is associated with the patients' underlying disease. Skin cancer has also been reported in patients receiving long-term hydroxyurea.
Conventional long-term studies to evaluate the carcinogenic potential of DROXIA have not been performed. However, intraperitoneal administration of 125–250 mg/kg hydroxyurea (about 0.6–1.2 times the maximum recommended human oral daily dose on a mg/m^2 basis) thrice weekly for 6 months to female rats increased the incidence of mammary tumors in rats surviving to 18 months compared to control. Hydroxyurea is mutagenic *in vitro* to bacteria, fungi, protozoa, and mammalian cells. Hydroxyurea is clastogenic *in vitro* (hamster cells, human lymphoblasts) and *in vivo* (SCE assay in rodents, mouse micronucleus assay). Hydroxyurea causes the transformation of rodent embryo cells to a tumorigenic phenotype.
Pregnancy: DROXIA can cause fetal harm when administered to a pregnant woman. Hydroxyurea is embryotoxic and causes fetal malformations (partially ossified cranial bones, absence of eye sockets, hydrocephaly, bipartite sternebrae, missing lumbar vertebrae) at 180 mg/kg/day (about 0.8 times the maximum recommended human daily dose on a mg/m^2 basis) in rats and at 30 mg/kg/day (about 0.3 times the maximum recommended human daily dose on a mg/m^2 basis) in rabbits. Embryotoxicity was characterized by decreased fetal viability, reduced live litter sizes, and developmental delays. Hydroxyurea crosses the placenta. Single doses of ≥ 375 mg/kg (about 1.7 times the maximum recommended human daily dose on a mg/m^2 basis) to rats caused growth retardation and impaired learning ability. There are no adequate and well-controlled studies in pregnant women. If this drug is used during pregnancy or if the patient becomes pregnant while taking this drug, the patient should be apprised of the potential harm to the fetus. Women of childbearing potential should be advised to avoid becoming pregnant.

PRECAUTIONS

Therapy with DROXIA requires close supervision. Some patients treated at the recommended initial dose of 15 mg/kg/day have experienced severe or life-threatening myelosuppression, requiring interruption of treatment and dose reduction. The hematologic status of the patient, as well as kidney and liver function should be determined prior to, and repeatedly during treatment. Treatment should be interrupted if neutrophil levels fall to < 2000/mm^3; platelets fall to < 80,000/mm^3; hemoglobin declines to less than 4.5 g/dL; or if reticulocytes fall below 80,000/mm^2 when the hemoglobin concentration is below 9 g/dL. Following recovery, treatment may be resumed at lower doses (see **DOSAGE AND ADMINISTRATION** section).
Patients must be able to follow directions regarding drug administration and their monitoring and care.
Carcinogenesis, Mutagenesis, and Impairment of Fertility: See **WARNINGS** and **Boxed WARNING** sections for Carcinogenesis and Mutagenesis information.
Impairment of Fertility—Hydroxyurea administered to male rats at 60 mg/kg/day (about 0.3 times the maximum recommended human daily dose on a mg/m^2 basis) produced testicular atrophy, decreased spermatogenesis, and significantly reduced their ability to impregnate females.
Pregnancy: Pregnancy "Category D". (See **WARNINGS** section.)
Nursing Mothers: Hydroxyurea is excreted in human milk. Because of the potential for serious adverse reactions with hydroxyurea, a decision should be made either to discontinue nursing or to discontinue the drug, taking into account the importance of the drug to the mother.
Pediatric Use: Safety and effectiveness in pediatric patients have not been established.
Drug Interactions: Prospective studies on the potential for hydroxyurea to interact with other drugs have not been performed.
Information for Patients: (See **Patient Information** at end of labeling.) Patients should be reminded that this medication must be handled with care. People who are not taking DROXIA (hydroxyurea capsules, USP) should not be exposed to it. If the powder from the capsule is spilled, it should be wiped up immediately with a damp disposable towel and discarded in a closed container, such as a plastic bag. The medication should be kept away from children and pets.
The necessity of monitoring blood counts every two weeks, throughout the duration of therapy, should be emphasized. For additional information, see the accompanying **Patient Information** leaflet.

Continued on next page

Droxia—Cont.

ADVERSE REACTIONS

Sickle Cell Anemia: In patients treated for sickle cell anemia in the Multicenter Study of Hydroxyurea in Sickle Cell Anemia[1], the most common adverse reactions were hematologic, with neutropenia, and low reticulocyte and platelet levels necessitating temporary cessation in almost all patients. Hematologic recovery usually occurred in two weeks.

Non-hematologic events that possibly were associated with treatment include hair loss, skin rash, fever, gastrointestinal disturbances, weight gain, bleeding and parvovirus B-19 infection; however, these non-hematologic events occurred with similar frequencies in the hydroxyurea and placebo treatment groups. Melanonychia has also been reported in patients receiving DROXIA for SCA.

Other: Adverse events associated with the use of hydroxyurea in the treatment of neoplastic diseases, in addition to hematologic effects include: gastrointestinal symptoms (stomatitis, anorexia, nausea, vomiting, diarrhea, and constipation), and dermatological reactions such as maculopapular rash, skin ulceration, dermatomyositis-like skin changes, peripheral erythema and facial erythema. Hyperpigmentation, atrophy of skin and nails, scaling and violet papules have been observed in some patients after several years of long-term daily maintenance therapy with hydroxyurea. Skin cancer has been reported. Dysuria and alopecia occur very rarely. Large doses may produce moderate drowsiness. Neurological disturbances have occurred extremely rarely and were limited to headache, dizziness, disorientation, hallucinations, and convulsions. Hydroxyurea occasionally may cause temporary impairment of renal tubular function accompanied by elevations in serum uric acid, BUN, and creatinine levels. Abnormal BSP retention has been reported. Fever, chills, malaise, edema, asthenia, and elevation of hepatic enzymes have also been reported.

The association of hydroxyurea with the development of acute pulmonary reactions consisting of diffuse pulmonary infiltrates, fever and dyspnea has been rarely reported. Pulmonary fibrosis also has been reported rarely.

OVERDOSAGE

Acute mucocutaneous toxicity has been reported in patients receiving hydroxyurea at dosages several times the therapeutic dose. Soreness, violet erythema, edema on palms and soles followed by scaling of hands and feet, severe generalized hyperpigmentation of the skin, and stomatitis have been observed.

DOSAGE AND ADMINISTRATION

Dosage should be based on the patient's actual or ideal weight, whichever is less. The initial dose of DROXIA is 15 mg/kg/day as a single dose. The patient's blood count must be monitored every two weeks. (See **WARNINGS** section.)

If blood counts are in an **acceptable range***, the dose may be increased by 5 mg/kg/day every 12 weeks until a maximum tolerated dose (the highest dose that does not produce **toxic**** blood counts over 24 consecutive weeks), or 35 mg/kg/day, is reached.

If blood counts are between the **acceptable range*** and **toxic****, the dose is not increased.

If blood counts are considered **toxic****, DROXIA should be discontinued until hematologic recovery. Treatment may then be resumed after reducing the dose by 2.5 mg/kg/day from the dose associated with hematologic toxicity. DROXIA may then be titrated up or down, every 12 weeks in 2.5 mg/kg/day increments, until the patient is at a stable dose that does not result in hematologic toxicity for 24 weeks. Any dosage on which a patient develops hematologic toxicity twice should not be tried again.

***acceptable range =**
neutrophils $\geq$ 2500 cells/mm^3,
platelets $\geq$ 95,000/mm^3,
hemoglobin > 5.3 g/dL and
reticulocytes $\geq$ 95,000/mm^3 if the hemoglobin concentration < 9 g/dL.

****toxic =**
neutrophils < 2000 cells/mm^3,
platelets < 80,000/mm^3,
hemoglobin < 4.5 g/dL and
reticulocytes < 80,000/mm^3 if the hemoglobin concentration < 9 g/dL.

Renal Insufficiency: There are no data that support specific guidance for dosage adjustment in patients with renal impairment. As renal excretion is a pathway of elimination, consideration should be given to decreasing the dosage of DROXIA in patients with renal impairment. Close monitoring of hematologic parameters is advised in these patients.

Hepatic Insufficiency: There are no data that support specific guidance for dosage adjustment in patients with hepatic impairment. Close monitoring of hematologic parameters is advised in these patients.

Procedures for proper handling and disposal of cytotoxic drugs should be considered. Several guidelines on this subject have been published.[2–8] There is no general agreement that all of the procedures recommended in the guidelines are necessary or appropriate.

HOW SUPPLIED

DROXIA™ (hydroxyurea capsules, USP).

200 mg capsules packaged in HDPE bottles of 60 with a plastic safety screw cap. (**NDC** 0003-6335-17). The cap and body are opaque blue-green. The capsule is marked in black ink on both the cap and body with **DROXIA** and **6335**.

300 mg capsules packaged in HDPE bottles of 60 with a plastic safety screw cap. (**NDC** 0003-6336-17). The cap and body are opaque purple. The capsule is marked in black ink on both the cap and body with **DROXIA** and **6336**.

400 mg capsules packaged in HDPE bottles of 60 with a plastic safety screw cap. (**NDC** 0003-6337-17). The cap and body are opaque reddish-orange. The capsule is marked in black ink on both the cap and body with **DROXIA** and **6337**.

Storage: Store at 25° C (77° F); excursions permitted to 15–30° C (59–86° F). Keep tightly closed.

REFERENCES

1. Charache, S, et al: Hydroxyurea and Sickle Cell Anemia: Clinical Utility of a Myelosuppressive "Switching" Agent. *Medicine* 1996; 75:300–326.
2. Recommendations for the Safe Handling of Parenteral Antineoplastic Drugs. NIH Publications. No. 83-2621. For sale by the Superintendent of Documents, US Government Printing Office, Washington, DC 20402.
3. AMA Council Report: Guidelines for Handling Parenteral Antineoplastics. *JAMA* 1985; 253(11):1590–1592.
4. National Study Commission on Cytotoxic Exposure-Recommendations for Handling Cytotoxic Agents. Available from Louis P. Jeffrey, ScD, Chairman, National Study Commission on Cytotoxic Exposure, Massachusetts College of Pharmacy and Allied Health Sciences, 179 Longwood Avenue, Boston, MA 02115.
5. Clinical Oncological Society of Australia: Guidelines and Recommendations for Safe Handling of Antineoplastic Agents. *Med J Australia* 1983; 1:426–428.
6. Jones RB, et al: Safe Handling of Chemotherapeutic Agents: A Report from the Mount Sinai Medical Center, *CA—A Cancer Journal for Clinicians*. 1983; (Sept./Oct.)258–263.
7. American Society of Hospital Pharmacists Technical Assistance Bulletin on Handling Cytotoxic and Hazardous Drugs. *Am J Hosp Pharm* 1990; 47:1033–1049.
8. Controlling Occupational Exposure to Hazardous Drugs. (OSHA Work—Practice Guidelines). *Am J Health—Syst Pharm* 1996; 53:1669–1685.

Patient Information About
***DROXIA*™ Capsules**
(generic name = hydroxyurea)

WHAT IS THE MOST IMPORTANT INFORMATION I SHOULD KNOW ABOUT DROXIA?

DROXIA (pronounced drock-SEE-yuh) capsules are used to treat sickle cell anemia in adults. DROXIA reduces the frequency of painful crises and reduces the need for blood transfusions.

- It is VERY IMPORTANT that you have regular blood counts so that your doctor can decrease or increase the DROXIA dose as needed to avoid serious complications.
- The most serious side effects of DROXIA involve the blood and may include severely low white blood cell counts (leukopenia, neutrophenia), which can decrease your resistance to infections; severely low red blood cell counts (anemia); or severely low platelet counts (thrombocytopenia), which can cause bleeding. Almost all patients who received DROXIA in clinical studies needed to have their medication stopped for a time to allow their low blood counts to return to acceptable levels.
- If you get pregnant, DROXIA may harm or cause death to your unborn child. You should not become pregnant while taking DROXIA. Make sure you use a contraceptive method. *Tell your doctor if you become pregnant or plan to become pregnant while taking DROXIA.*
- DROXIA may decrease the ability of men to father children and women to have children.
- Laboratory tests and reports in humans suggest DROXIA may increase your risk of developing cancer, especially if it is taken for a long time. However, it is still uncertain whether DROXIA causes cancer.

WHAT IS DROXIA?

DROXIA is a prescription medicine that is used to reduce the frequency of painful crises and reduce the need for blood transfusions in adults with sickle cell anemia. How DROXIA works is not certain but it may work by reducing the number of white blood cells and/or increasing red blood cells that carry fetal hemoglobin (HbF). Fetal hemoglobin may prevent sickling.

WHAT IS SICKLE CELL ANEMIA?

Sickle cell anemia is an inherited disorder of the red blood cells. Red blood cells carry oxygen to all parts of the body by using a protein called hemoglobin. Normal red blood cells contain only normal hemoglobin and are shaped like indented disks. These cells are very flexible and move easily through small blood vessels.

In sickle cell anemia, the red blood cells contain sickle hemoglobin, which causes them to change to a rigid, spiked shape (sickle shape) after oxygen is released. Sickled cells get stuck and form plugs in small blood vessels. These plugs restrict blood flow, causing damage to surrounding tissues resulting in a painful crisis.

Because there are blood vessels in all parts of the body, painful crises can occur anywhere in your body. In addition, sickle cells are trapped and destroyed in the liver and spleen. This results in a shortage of red blood cells (anemia).

WILL DROXIA CURE MY SICKLE CELL ANEMIA?

No. However, DROXIA may help you better control your sickle cell anemia, but it is important to follow your doctor's instructions carefully.

In a study of adults taking recommended doses, daily treatment with DROXIA resulted in fewer painful crises, fewer patients with "acute chest syndrome" (a pneumonia-like condition that leads to difficulty in breathing) and less need for blood transfusions.

WHO SHOULD NOT TAKE DROXIA CAPSULES?

Do not take DROXIA capsules if you are allergic to any of the ingredients. Besides the active ingredient hydroxyurea, DROXIA capsules contain the following inactive ingredients: citric acid, gelatin, lactose, magnesium stearate, sodium phosphate, titanium dioxide and capsule colorants. Tell your doctor if you think you have ever had an allergic reaction.

If you get pregnant, DROXIA (hydroxyurea capsules, USP) may harm or cause death to your unborn child. You should not become pregnant while taking DROXIA. Make sure you use a contraceptive method. *Tell your doctor if you become pregnant or plan to become pregnant while taking DROXIA.*

HOW DO I TAKE DROXIA CAPSULES?

Always follow your doctor's instructions carefully when taking DROXIA capsules or *any* prescription medication. The usual dose of DROXIA may range from as few as one to several capsules per day. DROXIA is usually taken once a day. You should try to take it at the same time each day. Your doctor will determine the proper starting dose of DROXIA for you based on your weight and blood count. The dose will then be increased slowly to your maximum tolerated dose (maximum dose that does NOT produce severely low blood counts). **Your doctor should measure your blood counts every two weeks after you begin treatment with DROXIA.** Depending on the results, your dosage may be adjusted or the drug may be stopped for a while.

DROXIA is a medication that *must* be handled with care. People who are not taking DROXIA should not be exposed to it. If the powder from the capsule is spilled, it should be wiped up *immediately* with a damp disposable towel and discarded in a closed container, such as a plastic bag.

If you accidentally take an overdose of DROXIA capsules, seek medical attention immediately. Contact your doctor, local poison control center, or emergency room.

WHAT IF I MISS A DOSE OF DROXIA CAPSULES?

Try not to miss your dose of DROXIA, but if you do, take it as soon as possible. If it is almost time for your next dose, skip the missed dose and resume your regular dosing schedule. *Do not take two doses during the same day.* If you miss more than one dose, call your doctor for instructions.

WHAT SHOULD I AVOID WHILE TAKING DROXIA CAPSULES?

Some other medications can increase your risk of experiencing serious side effects from DROXIA. While you are taking DROXIA capsules, you should inform your doctor of all prescription and over-the-counter medicines that you are taking.

In nursing mothers, DROXIA is present in breast milk. Because of the potential for side effects in the newborn, you should discontinue nursing your baby while taking DROXIA.

WHAT ARE THE POSSIBLE SIDE EFFECTS OF DROXIA CAPSULES?

As with other medicines, DROXIA may cause unwanted effects, although it is not always possible to tell whether such effects are caused by DROXIA, another medication you may be taking, or your sickle cell anemia. *Any* side effects or unusual symptoms that you experience should be reported to your doctor, particularly if they persist or are troublesome.

The most serious side effects of DROXIA involve the blood, and may include severely low white blood cell counts (leukopenia, neutropenia), which can decrease your resistance to infections; severely low red blood cell counts (anemia); or severely low platelet counts (thrombocytopenia), which can cause bleeding. Almost all patients who received DROXIA in clinical studies needed to have their medication stopped for a time to allow their low blood counts to return to acceptable levels.

The side effects reported most often by adults with sickle cell anemia participating in studies of DROXIA included hair loss, skin rash, fever, stomach and/or bowel disturbances, weight gain, bleeding, virus infection, and discolored nails (melanonychia), but these were equally common in people getting a placebo (sugar pill).

Skin cancer and leukemia, which can be fatal, have been reported in patients receiving long-term hydroxyurea for conditions other than sickle cell anemia. In laboratory tests DROXIA causes changes in chromosomes and DNA (genetic material) that strongly suggest it can cause cancer in people, especially if it is taken for a long time.

ARE REGULAR BLOOD COUNTS NECESSARY WHILE TAKING DROXIA CAPSULES?

Yes. Your doctor should measure your blood counts every two weeks while you are taking DROXIA. Your DROXIA dose will require adjustment based on these regular blood counts. Serious problems can occur if the DROXIA dose is not adjusted on time.

WHAT ELSE SHOULD I KNOW ABOUT DROXIA CAPSULES?

If you have kidney or liver disease, close monitoring of your blood count, kidney and liver function will be required.

Because it may not be possible to detect a deficiency of folic acid in patients taking DROXIA, your doctor may prescribe a folic acid supplement for you.

WHAT ELSE SHOULD I DO TO CONTROL MY SICKLE CELL CRISES?

Because painful crises can be brought on by factors such as infection, dehydration, worsening anemia, emotional stress, extreme temperature exposure, or ingestion of substances such as alcohol or other recreational drugs, you should be aware of the following general guidelines that will help keep you pain-free:

- Seek immediate medical attention when a fever develops or signs of infection appear.
- Avoid smoking and drinking more than 1–2 alcoholic beverages a day.
- Drink 8 to 10 glasses of water or other fluid each day.
- Avoid any types of physical exertion that seem to bring on painful crises or other discomfort.
- Avoid extreme temperature changes and dress appropriately in hot and cold weather.

This medicine was prescribed for your particular condition. Do not use DROXIA Capsules for another condition or give it to others. Keep DROXIA Capsules and all medicines out of the reach of children. Discard DROXIA Capsules when they are outdated or no longer needed by flushing the contents of your bottle down the toilet.

The summary does not include everything there is to know about DROXIA Capsules. Medicines are sometimes prescribed for purposes other than those listed in a **Patient Information** leaflet. If you have questions or concerns, or want more information about DROXIA Capsules, your physician and pharmacist have the complete prescribing information upon which this leaflet is based. You may want to read it and discuss it with your doctor. Remember, no written summary can replace careful discussion with your doctor.

This **Patient Information** leaflet has been approved by the U.S. Food and Drug Administration.

BRISTOL LABORATORIES
ONCOLOGY PRODUCTS
A Bristol-Myers Squibb Company
Princeton, NJ 08543
U.S.A.
Made in Italy
U4-B001-7-99 1053547
Issued: April 1999

Shown in Product Identification Guide, page 310

ETOPOPHOS® ℞

[*ē-top-ō-phos*]
(etoposide phosphate) for Injection
Rx ONLY

WARNINGS

ETOPOPHOS® (etoposide phosphate) for Injection should be administered under the supervision of a qualified physician experienced in the use of cancer chemotherapeutic agents. Severe myelosuppression with resulting infection or bleeding may occur.

DESCRIPTION

ETOPOPHOS® (etoposide phosphate) for Injection is an antineoplastic agent which is available for intravenous infusion as a sterile lyophile in single-dose vials containing etoposide phosphate equivalent to 100 mg etoposide, 32.7 mg sodium citrate, USP and 300 mg dextran 40.

Etoposide phosphate is a water soluble ester of etoposide (commonly known as VP-16), a semi-synthetic derivative of podophyllotoxin. The water solubility of etoposide phosphate lessens the potential for precipitation following dilution and during intravenous administration.

The chemical name for etoposide phosphate is: 4′-Demethylepipodophyllotoxin 9-[4,6-O-(R)-ethylidene-β-D-glucopyranoside], 4′-(dihydrogen phosphate).

Etoposide phosphate has the following structure:

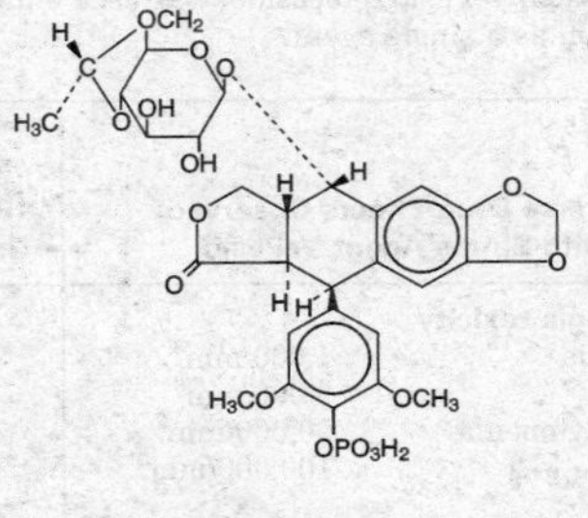

CLINICAL PHARMACOLOGY

The *in vitro* cytotoxicity observed for etoposide phosphate is significantly less than that seen with etoposide which is believed due to the necessity for conversion *in vivo* to the active moiety, etoposide, by dephosphorylation. The mechanism of action is believed to be the same as that of etoposide. Etoposide has been shown to cause metaphase arrest in chick fibroblasts. Its main effect, however, appears to be at the G_2 portion of the cell cycle in mammalian cells. Two different dose-dependent responses are seen. At high concentrations (10 µg/mL or more), lysis of cells entering mitosis is observed. At low concentrations (0.3 to 10 µg/mL), cells are inhibited from entering prophase. It does not interfere with microtubular assembly. The predominant macromolecular effect of etoposide appears to be the induction of DNA strand breaks by an interaction with DNA-topoisomerase II or the formation of free radicals.

ETOPOPHOS Bioequivalence: Following intravenous administration of ETOPOPHOS, etoposide phosphate is rapidly and completely converted to etoposide in plasma. A direct comparison of the pharmacokinetic parameters [area under the concentration time curve (AUC) and the maximum plasma concentration (C_{max})] of etoposide following intravenous administration of molar equivalent doses of ETOPOPHOS and VePesid® (etoposide) was made in two randomized cross-over studies in patients with a variety of malignancies. In the first study of 41 evaluable patients, the etoposide mean ± S.D. AUC values were 168.3 ± 48.2 µg•hr/mL and 156.7 ± 43.4 µg•hr/mL following administration of molar equivalent doses of 150 mg/m^2 ETOPOPHOS or VePesid with a 3.5 hour infusion time; the corresponding mean ± S.D. C_{max} values were 20.0 ± 3.7 µg/mL and 19.6 ± 4.2 µg/mL, respectively. The point estimate (90% confidence interval) for the bioavailability of etoposide from ETOPOPHOS, relative to VePesid, was 107% (105%, 110%) for AUC and 103% (99%, 106%) for C_{max}. In the second study of 29 evaluable patients following intravenous administration of 90, 100 and 110 mg/m^2 molar equivalents of ETOPOPHOS or VePesid with a 60 minute infusion time, the etoposide mean ± S.D. AUC values (normalized to the 100 mg/m^2 dose) were 96.1 ± 22.6 µg•hr/mL and 86.5 ± 25.8 µg•hr/mL, respectively; the corresponding mean ± S.D. C_{max} values (normalized to the 100 mg/m^2 dose) were 20.1 ± 4.1 µg/mL and 19.0 ± 5.1 µg/mL, respectively. The point estimate (90% confidence interval) for the bioavailability of etoposide from ETOPOPHOS, relative to VePesid, was 113% (107%, 119%) for AUC and 107% (101%, 113%) for C_{max} indicating bioequivalence. Results from both studies demonstrated no statistically significant differences in the AUC and C_{max} parameters for etoposide when administered as ETOPOPHOS or VePesid. In addition, in the latter study, there were no statistically significant differences in the pharmacodynamic parameters (hematologic toxicity) after administration of ETOPOPHOS or VePesid. Following VePesid administration, the mean nadir values (expressed as percent decrease from baseline) for leukocytes, granulocytes, hemoglobin and thrombocytes were 67.2 ± 17.0%, 84.1 ± 14.6%, 22.6 ± 9.8% and 46.4 ± 21.9%, respectively; the corresponding values after administration of ETOPOPHOS were 67.3 ± 14.2%, 81.0 ± 16.5%, 21.4 ± 9.9% and 44.1 ± 20.7%, respectively.

Because of the similarity of pharmacokinetics and pharmacodynamics of etoposide after administration of either ETOPOPHOS or VePesid, the following information on VePesid should be considered:

VePesid Pharmacokinetics: On intravenous administration, the disposition of etoposide is best described as a biphasic process with a distribution half-life of about 1.5 hours and terminal elimination half-life ranging from 4 to 11 hours. Total body clearance values range from 33 to 48 mL/min or 16 to 36 mL/min/m^2 and, like the terminal elimination half-life, are independent of dose over a range 100-600 mg/m^2. Over the same dose range, the AUC and the C_{max} values increase linearly with dose. Etoposide does not accumulate in the plasma following daily administration of 100 mg/m^2 for 4 to 5 days. After intravenous infusion the C_{max} and AUC values exhibit marked intra- and inter-subject variability.

The mean volumes of distribution at steady state fall in the range of 18 to 29 liters or 7 to 17 L/m^2. Etoposide enters the CSF poorly. Although it is detectable in CSF and intracerebral tumors, the concentrations are lower than in extracerebral tumors and in plasma. Etoposide concentrations are higher in normal lung than in lung metastases and are similar in primary tumors and normal tissues of the myometrium. *In vitro*, etoposide is highly protein bound (97%) to human plasma proteins. An inverse relationship between plasma albumin levels and etoposide renal clearance is found in children. In a study determining the effect of other therapeutic agents on the *in vitro* binding of carbon-14 labeled etoposide to human serum proteins, only phenylbutazone, sodium salicylate, and aspirin displaced protein-bound etoposide at concentrations achieved *in vivo*.

Etoposide binding ratio correlates directly with serum albumin in patients with cancer and in normal volunteers. The unbound fraction of etoposide significantly correlated with bilirubin in a population of cancer patients. Data have suggested a significant inverse correlation between serum albumin concentration and free fraction of etoposide (see **PRECAUTIONS** section).

After intravenous administration of ^{3}H-etoposide (70–290 mg/m^2), mean recoveries of radioactivity in the urine range from 42% to 67%, and fecal recoveries range from 0 to 16% of the dose. Less than 50% of an intravenous dose is excreted in the urine as etoposide with mean recoveries of 8% to 35% within 24 hours.

In children, approximately 55% of the dose of VePesid (etoposide) is excreted in the urine as etoposide in 24 hours. The mean renal clearance of etoposide is 7 to 10 mL/min/m^2 or 35% of the total body clearance over a dose of 80 to 600 mg/m^2. Etoposide, therefore, is cleared by both renal and nonrenal processes, i.e., metabolism and biliary excretion. The effect of renal disease on plasma etoposide clearance is not known in children.

Biliary excretion appears to be a minor route of etoposide elimination. Only 6% or less of an intravenous dose is recovered in the bile as etoposide. Metabolism accounts for most of the nonrenal clearance of etoposide. The major urinary metabolite of etoposide in adults and children is the hydroxy acid [4′-demethylepipodophyllic acid-9-(4,6-0-(R)-ethylidene-β-D-glucopyranoside)], formed by opening of the lactone ring. It is also present in human plasma, presumably as the **trans** isomer. Glucuronide and/or sulfate conjugates of etoposide are excreted in human urine and represent 5% to 22% of the dose. In addition, O-demethylation of the dimethoxyphenol ring occurs through the CYP450 3A4 isoenzyme pathway to produce the corresponding catechol.

In adults, the total body clearance of etoposide is correlated with creatinine clearance, serum albumin concentration, and nonrenal clearance. Patients with impaired renal function receiving etoposide have exhibited reduced total body clearance, increased AUC and a lower volume of distribution at steady state (see **PRECAUTIONS** section). Use of cisplatin therapy is associated with reduced total body clearance. In children, elevated serum SGPT levels are associated with reduced drug total body clearance. Prior use of cisplatin may also result in a decrease of etoposide total body clearance in children.

Although some minor differences in pharmacokinetic parameters between age and gender have been observed, these differences were not considered clinically significant.

Clinical Studies: A total of 7 clinical trials with 365 patients treated (368 entered) provide the data base for the human experience summarized in this insert. Five phase I trials evaluated etoposide phosphate given on a days 1, 3 and 5 or days 1 through 5 schedule. In two trials the drug was given over 5 minutes and in three over 30 minutes. The following table summarizes the doses, schedules, infusion times and numbers of patients entered in the phase I experience.

Dose Escalation (Phase I) Trials of Etoposide Phosphate

Study	Schedule Q 21 days	Infusion Time	Dose Range (mg/m^2)	Number of Patients Entered
002	Days 1–5	30 minutes	25–110	68
005	Days 1, 3, 5	30 minutes	50–175	39
006	Days 1–5	30 minutes	50–125	28
008	Days 1, 3, 5	5 minutes	50–200	36
009	Days 1–5	5 minutes	50–125	27

Two trials evaluated the pharmacokinetic equivalence of etoposide and etoposide phosphate. A phase I study (002) was expanded at the higher doses to compare the pharmacokinetic profile of etoposide following administration of etoposide or etoposide phosphate. Another, multi-institutional trial (012), was conducted at a dose of 150 mg/m^2 using a days 1, 3 and 5 schedule and a crossover design.

The seventh trial (011) was a randomized study in which patients with limited or extensive small cell lung cancer and no prior therapy were treated with either cisplatin plus etoposide or cisplatin plus etoposide phosphate. Patients received 20 mg/m^2/day of cisplatin for 5 days and 80 mg/m^2/day of etoposide or etoposide phosphate. A total of 121 patients were randomized and 120 treated (60 per group). Response rates, time to response, duration of response, time to progression, time to worsening performance status and survival were similar in the two groups whether the analysis was done for patients with limited or extensive disease or for the entire population. The following table summarizes the results regardless of disease extent.

[See table at top of next page]

The most prominent side effects were myelosuppression and GI toxicity. Sixty-eight percent of patients treated with etoposide phosphate plus cisplatin had neutrophils less than 500/mm^3 at some time during treatment as did 88% of those getting etoposide and cisplatin. Over 85% in each group had nausea and/or vomiting. No differences in the pattern or severity of side effects were observed.

INDICATION AND USAGE

ETOPOPHOS (etoposide phosphate) for Injection is indicated in the management of the following neoplasms:

Refractory Testicular Tumors: ETOPOPHOS for Injection in combination therapy with other approved chemotherapeutic agents in patients with refractory testicular tumors who have already received appropriate surgical, chemotherapeutic, and radiotherapeutic therapy.

Small Cell Lung Cancer: ETOPOPHOS for Injection in combination with other approved chemotherapeutic agents as first line treatment in patients with small cell lung cancer.

CONTRAINDICATIONS

ETOPOPHOS (etoposide phosphate) for Injection is contraindicated in patients who have demonstrated a previous hypersensitivity to etoposide, etoposide phosphate, or any other component of the formulations.

WARNINGS

Patients being treated with ETOPOPHOS must be frequently observed for myelosuppression both during and after therapy. Myelosuppression resulting in death has been reported following etoposide administration. Dose-limiting

Continued on next page

Etopophos—Cont.

bone marrow suppression is the most significant toxicity associated with ETOPOPHOS therapy. Therefore, the following studies should be obtained at the start of therapy and prior to each subsequent cycle of ETOPOPHOS: platelet count, hemoglobin, white blood cell count, and differential. The occurrence of a platelet count below 50,000/mm^3 or an absolute neutrophil count below 500/mm^3 is an indication to withhold further therapy until the blood counts have sufficiently recovered. The toxicity of rapidly infused ETOPOPHOS in patients with impaired renal or hepatic function has not been adequately evaluated. The toxicity profile of ETOPOPHOS when infused at doses >175 mg/m^2 has not been delineated.

Physicians should be aware of the possible occurrence of an anaphylactic reaction manifested by chills, fever, tachycardia, bronchospasm, dyspnea and hypotension. Higher rates of anaphylactic-like reactions have been reported in children who received infusions of etoposide at concentrations higher than those recommended. The role that concentration of infusion (or rate of infusion) plays in the development of anaphylactic-like reactions is uncertain. (See **ADVERSE REACTIONS** section.) Treatment is symptomatic. The infusion should be terminated immediately, followed by the administration of pressor agents, corticosteroids, antihistamines, or volume expanders at the discretion of the physician.

ETOPOPHOS can cause fetal harm when administered to a pregnant woman. Etoposide has been shown to be teratogenic in mice and rats, and it is therefore likely that ETOPOPHOS is also teratogenic.

In rats, an intravenous etoposide dose of 0.4 mg/kg/day (about 1/20th of the human dose on a mg/m^2 basis) during organogenesis caused maternal toxicity, embryotoxicity, and teratogenicity (skeletal abnormalities, exencephaly, encephalocele, and anophthalmia); higher doses of 1.2 and 3.6 mg/kg/day (about 1/7th and 1/2 of the human dose on a mg/m^2 basis) resulted in 90% and 100% embryonic resorptions. In mice, a single 1.0 mg/kg (1/16th of the human dose on a mg/m^2 basis) dose of etoposide administered intraperitoneally on days 6, 7, or 8 of gestation caused embryotoxicity, cranial abnormalities, and major skeletal malformations. An i.p. dose of 1.5 mg/kg (about 1/10th of the human dose on a mg/m^2 basis) on day 7 of gestation caused an increase in the incidence of intrauterine death and fetal malformations and a significant decrease in the average fetal body weight.

If this drug is used during pregnancy, or if the patient becomes pregnant while receiving this drug, the patient should be warned of the potential hazard to the fetus. Women of childbearing potential should be advised to avoid becoming pregnant.

ETOPOPHOS should be considered a potential carcinogen in humans. The occurrence of acute leukemia with or without a preleukemic phase has been reported in rare instances in patients treated with etoposide alone or in association with other neoplastic agents. The risk of development of a preleukemic or leukemic syndrome is unclear. Carcinogenicity tests with ETOPOPHOS have not been conducted in laboratory animals.

PRECAUTIONS

General: In all instances where the use of ETOPOPHOS is considered for chemotherapy, the physician must evaluate the need and usefulness of the drug against the risk of adverse reactions. Most such adverse reactions are reversible if detected early. If severe reactions occur, the drug should be reduced in dosage or discontinued and appropriate corrective measures should be taken according to the clinical judgement of the physician. Reinstitution of ETOPOPHOS therapy should be carried out with caution, and with adequate consideration of the further need for the drug and alertness as to possible recurrence of toxicity.

Patients with low serum albumin may be at an increased risk for etoposide associated toxicities.

Laboratory Tests: Periodic complete blood counts should be done during the course of ETOPOPHOS treatment. They should be performed prior to each cycle of therapy and at appropriate intervals during and after therapy.

Carcinogenesis (see WARNINGS section), Mutagenesis, Impairment of Fertility: ETOPOPHOS was non-mutagenic in *in vitro* Ames microbial mutagenicity assay and the *E. coli* WP2 uvrA reverse mutation assay. Since ETOPOPHOS is rapidly and completely converted to etoposide *in vivo* and etoposide has been shown to be mutagenic in Ames assay, ETOPOPHOS should be considered as a potential mutagen *in vivo*.

In rats, an oral dose of ETOPOPHOS at 86.0 mg/kg/day (about 10 times the human dose on a mg/m^2 basis) or above administered for 5 consecutive days resulted in irreversible testicular atrophy. Irreversible testicular atrophy was also present in rats treated with ETOPOPHOS intravenously for 30 days at 5.11 mg/kg/day (about 1/2 of the human dose on a mg/m^2 basis).

Pregnancy: Pregnancy "Category D". (See **WARNINGS** section.)

Nursing Mothers: It is not known whether this drug is excreted in human milk. Because many drugs are excreted in human milk and because of the potential for serious adverse reactions in nursing infants from ETOPOPHOS, a decision should be made whether to discontinue nursing or to discontinue the drug, taking into account the importance of the drug to the mother.

Response to Treatment for All Patients

	Etoposide Phosphate plus Cisplatin	Etoposide plus Cisplatin	P-value
Complete Responses:	15%	15%	1.000*
Partial Responses:	46%	43%	0.855*
Overall Response Rate:	61%	58%	0.854*
Median Time to Response:	48 days	46 days	0.596**
Median Response Duration:	273 days	241 days	0.141***
Median Time to Progression:	211 days	213 days	0.500***
Median Time to Worsening Performance Status:	210 days	149 days	0.472***
Median Survival:	348 days	318 days	0.780***

* Fisher's Exact Test
** Wilcoxon Rank Sum test
*** Logrank test

Pediatric Use: Safety and effectiveness in pediatric patients have not been established. Anaphylactic reactions have been reported in pediatric patients who received etoposide (see **WARNINGS** section).

Drug Interactions: Caution should be exercised when administering ETOPOPHOS with drugs that are known to inhibit phosphatase activities (e.g., levamisole hydrochloride). High-dose cyclosporin A resulting in concentrations above 2000 ng/mL administered with oral etoposide has led to an 80% increase in etoposide exposure with a 38% decrease in total body clearance of etoposide compared to etoposide alone.

Renal Impairment: In patients with impaired renal function, the following initial dose modification should be considered based on measured creatinine clearance:

Measured Creatinine Clearance	>50 mL/min	15–50 mL/min
etoposide	100% of dose	75% of dose

Subsequent etoposide dosing should be based on patient tolerance and clinical effect. Equivalent dose adjustments of ETOPOPHOS should be used.

Data are not available in patients with creatinine clearances <15 mL/min and further dose reduction should be considered in these patients.

ADVERSE REACTIONS

ETOPOPHOS has been found to be well tolerated as a single agent in clinical studies involving 206 patients with a wide variety of malignancies, and in combination with cisplatin in 60 patients with small cell lung cancer. The most frequent clinically significant adverse experiences were leukopenia and neutropenia.

The incidences of adverse experiences in the table that follows are derived from studies in which ETOPOPHOS (etoposide phosphate) for Injection was administered as a single agent. A total of 98 patients received total doses at or above 450 mg/m^2 on a 5 consecutive days or days 1, 3 and 5 schedule during the first course of therapy.

Summary of Adverse Events Reported with Single Agent ETOPOPHOS Following Course 1 at Total Five Day Doses of ≥450 mg/m^2

		Percent of Patients
Hematologic toxicity		
Leukopenia	< 4000/mm^3	91
	< 1000/mm^3	17
Neutropenia	< 2000/mm^3	88
	< 500/mm^3	37
Thrombocytopenia	< 100,000/mm^3	23
	< 50,000/mm^3	9
Anemia	< 11 g/dL	72
	< 8 g/dL	19
Gastrointestinal toxicity		
Nausea and/or Vomiting		37
Anorexia		16
Muscositis		11
Constipation		8
Abdominal Pain		7
Diarrhea		6
Taste Alteration		6
Asthenia/Malaise		39
Alopecia		33
Chills and/or Fever		24
Dizziness		5
Extravasation/Phlebitis		5

Since etoposide phosphate is converted to etoposide, those adverse experiences that are associated with VePesid (etoposide) can be expected to occur with ETOPOPHOS.

Hematologic Toxicity: Myelosuppression after ETOPOPHOS administration is dose related and dose limiting with the leukocyte nadir counts occurring from day 15 to day 22 after initiation of drug therapy, granulocyte nadir counts occurring day 12–19 after initiation of drug therapy, and platelet nadirs occurring from day 10–15. Bone marrow recovery usually occurs by day 21 but may be delayed, and no cumulative toxicity has been reported. Fever and infection have also been reported in patients with neutropenia. Death associated with myelosuppression has been reported following etoposide administration.

Gastrointestinal Toxicity: Nausea and vomiting are the major gastrointestinal toxicities. The severity of such nausea and vomiting is generally mild to moderate with treatment discontinuation required in 1% of patients. Nausea and vomiting can usually be controlled with standard antiemetic therapy.

Blood Pressure Changes: In clinical studies, one hundred fifty-one patients were treated with ETOPOPHOS with infusion times ranging from thirty minutes to three and one-half hours. Sixty-three patients received ETOPOPHOS as a five minute bolus infusion. Four patients experienced one or more episodes of hypertension and eight patients experienced one or more episodes of hypotension, which may or may not be drug related. One episode of hypotension was reported among those patients who received a five minute bolus infusion. If clinically significant hypotension or hypertension occurs with ETOPOPHOS, appropriate supportive therapy should be initiated.

Allergic Reactions: Anaphylactic type reactions characterized by chills, rigors, tachycardia, bronchospasm, dyspnea, diaphoresis, fever, pruritus, hypertension or hypotension, loss of consciousness, nausea, and vomiting have been reported to occur in 3% (7/245) of all patients treated with ETOPOPHOS. Facial flushing was reported in 2% and skin rashes in 3% of patients receiving ETOPOPHOS. These reactions have usually responded promptly to the cessation of the infusion and administration of pressor agents, corticosteroids, antihistamines, or volume expanders as appropriate; however, the reactions can be fatal. Hypertension and/or flushing have also been reported. Blood pressure usually normalizes within a few hours after cessation of the initial infusion.

Anaphylactic-like reactions have occurred during the initial infusion of ETOPOPHOS (see **WARNINGS** section). Facial/tongue swelling, coughing, diaphoresis, cyanosis, tightness in throat, laryngospasm, back pain, and/or loss of consciousness have sometimes occurred in association with the above reactions. In addition, an apparent hypersensitivity-associated apnea has been reported rarely.

Rash, urticaria, and/or pruritus have infrequently been reported at recommended doses. At investigational doses, a generalized pruritic erythematous maculopapular rash, consistent with perivasculitis, has been reported.

Alopecia: Reversible alopecia, sometimes progressing to total baldness, was observed in up to 44% of patients.

Other Toxicities: The following adverse reactions have been infrequently reported: abdominal pain, aftertaste, constipation, dysphagia, fever, transient cortical blindness, interstitial pneumonitis/pulmonary fibrosis, optic neuritis, pigmentation, seizure (occasionally associated with allergic reactions), Stevens-Johnson Syndrome, toxic epidermal necrolysis, and a single report of radiation recall dermatitis. Rarely, hepatic toxicity may be seen.

The incidences of adverse reactions in the table that follows are derived from multiple data bases from studies in 2,081 patients when VePesid (etoposide) was used either orally or by injection as a single agent.

Adverse Drug Effects Observed with Single Agent VePesid		Percent Range of Reported Incidence
Hematologic toxicity		
Leukopenia	< 1,000/mm^3	3–17
	< 4,000/mm^3	60–91
Thrombocytopenia	< 50,000/mm^3	1–20
	< 100,000/mm^3	22–41
Anemia		0–33
Gastrointestinal toxicity		
Nausea and Vomiting		31–43
Abdominal Pain		0–2
Anorexia		10–13
Diarrhea		1–13
Stomatitis		1–6
Hepatic		0–3

Alopecia	8–66
Peripheral Neurotoxicity	1–2
Hypotension	1–2
Allergic Reaction	1–2

OVERDOSAGE

No proven antidotes have been established for ETOPOPHOS (etoposide phosphate) for Injection overdosage in humans. In mice, a single intravenous dose of rapidly administered ETOPOPHOS was lethal at or above 120 mg/kg (about 7 times human dose on a mg/m^2 basis) and was associated with clinical signs of neurotoxicity.

DOSAGE AND ADMINISTRATION

The usual dose of VePesid for Injection in testicular cancer in combination with other approved chemotherapeutic agents ranges from 50 to 100 mg/m^2/day on days 1 through 5 to 100 mg/m^2/day on days 1, 3, and 5. Equivalent doses of ETOPOPHOS should be used.

In small cell lung cancer, the VePesid for Injection dose in combination with other approved chemotherapeutic drugs ranges from 35 mg/m^2/day for 4 days to 50 mg/m^2/day for 5 days. Equivalent doses of ETOPOPHOS should be used.

For recommended dosing adjustments in patients with renal impairment, see **PRECAUTIONS** section.

ETOPOPHOS solutions may be administered at infusion rates from 5 to 210 minutes. Chemotherapy courses are repeated at 3- to 4-week intervals after adequate recovery from any toxicity.

The dosage should be modified to take into account the myelosuppressive effect of other drugs in the combination or the effects of prior x-ray therapy or chemotherapy which may have compromised bone marrow reserve.

Administration Precautions: As with other potentially toxic compounds, caution should be exercised in handling and preparing the solution of ETOPOPHOS. Skin reactions associated with accidental exposure to ETOPOPHOS may occur. The use of gloves is recommended. If ETOPOPHOS solution contacts the skin or mucosa, immediately and thoroughly wash the skin with soap and water and flush the mucosa with water.

Preparation for Intravenous Administration: Prior to use, the content of each vial must be reconstituted with either 5 mL or 10 mL Sterile Water for Injection, USP; 5% Dextrose Injection, USP; 0.9% Sodium Chloride Injection, USP; Sterile Bacteriostatic Water for Injection with Benzyl Alcohol; or Bacteriostatic Sodium Chloride for Injection with Benzyl Alcohol to a concentration equivalent to 20 mg/mL or 10 mg/mL etoposide (22.7 mg/mL or 11.4 mg/mL etoposide phosphate), respectively. Following reconstitution the solution may be administered without further dilution or it can be further diluted to concentrations as low as 0.1 mg/mL etoposide with either 5% Dextrose Injection, USP or 0.9% Sodium Chloride Injection, USP.

Solutions of ETOPOPHOS should be prepared in an aseptic manner. Parenteral drug products should be inspected visually for particulate matter and discoloration prior to administration whenever solution and container permit.

STABILITY

Unopened vials of ETOPOPHOS (etoposide phosphate) for Injection are stable until the date indicated on the package when stored under refrigeration 2°–8°C (36°–46°F) in the original package. When reconstituted and/or diluted as directed, ETOPOPHOS solutions can be stored in glass or plastic containers at controlled room temperature 20°–25°C (68°–77°F) or under refrigeration 2°–8°C (36° to 46° F) for 24 hours. Refrigerated solutions of ETOPOPHOS should be used immediately upon return to room temperature.

HOW SUPPLIED

NDC 0015-3404-20

Individually cartoned single-dose vials with white flip-off seals containing etoposide phosphate equivalent to 100 mg etoposide.

STORAGE

Store the unopened vials under refrigeration 2°–8° C (36°–46° F). Retain in original package to protect from light.

HANDLING AND DISPOSAL

Procedures for proper handling and disposal of anticancer drugs should be considered. Several guidelines on this subject have been published.[1–7] There is no general agreement that all of the procedures recommended in the guidelines are necessary or appropriate.

REFERENCES

1. Recommendations for the Safe Handling of Parenteral Antineoplastic Drugs. NIH Publication No. 83-2621. For sale by the Superintendent of Documents, US Government Printing Office, Washington, DC 20402.
2. AMA Council Report. Guidelines for Handling Parenteral Antineoplastics. *JAMA* 1985; 253(11):1590–1592.
3. National Study Commission on Cytotoxic Exposure—Recommendations for Handling Cytotoxic Agents. Available from Louis P. Jeffrey, ScD, Chairman, National Study Commission on Cytotoxic Exposure, Massachusetts College of Pharmacy and Allied Health Sciences, 179 Longwood Avenue, Boston, Massachusetts 02115.
4. Clinical Oncological Society of Australia. Guidelines and Recommendations for Safe Handling of Antineoplastic Agents. *Med J Australia* 1983; 1:426–428.
5. Jones RB, et al: Safe Handling of Chemotherapeutic Agents: A Report from the Mount Sinai Medical Center. *CA-A Cancer Journal for Clinicians* 1983; (Sept/Oct)258–263.
6. American Society of Hospital Pharmacists Technical Assistance Bulletin on Handling Cytotoxic and Hazardous Drugs. *Am J Hosp Pharm* 1990; 47:1033–1049.
7. OSHA Work-Practice Guidelines for Personnel Dealing with Cytotoxic (Antineoplastic) Drugs. *Am J Hosp Pharm* 1986; 43:1193-1204.

BRISTOL LABORATORIES®
ONCOLOGY PRODUCTS
A Bristol-Myers Squibb Company
Princeton, NJ 08543
U.S.A.

U2-B001-3-99 3404DIM-04
51-004164-03 Revised: December 1997

Shown in Product Identification Guide, page 310

HYDREA® ℞
[*hī-drea*]
(hydroxyurea capsules, USP)
℞ ONLY

DESCRIPTION

HYDREA® (hydroxyurea capsules, USP) is an antineoplastic agent, available for oral use as capsules providing 500 mg hydroxyurea. Inactive ingredients: citric acid, colorants (D&C Yellow No. 10, FD&C Blue No. 1, FD&C Red 40 and D&C Red 28), gelatin, lactose, magnesium stearate, sodium phosphate, and titanium dioxide.

Hydroxyurea occurs as an essentially tasteless, white crystalline powder. Its structural formula is:

$$H_2N-\overset{\displaystyle O}{\overset{\|}{C}}-NH-OH$$

CLINICAL PHARMACOLOGY

Mechanism of Action: The precise mechanism by which hydroxyurea produces its antineoplastic effects cannot, at present, be described. However, the reports of various studies in tissue culture in rats and humans lend support to the hypothesis that hydroxyurea causes an immediate inhibition of DNA synthesis by acting as a ribonucleotide reductase inhibitor, without interfering with the synthesis of ribonucleic acid or of protein. This hypothesis explains why, under certain conditions, hydroxyurea may induce teratogenic effects.

Three mechanisms of action have been postulated for the increased effectiveness of concomitant use of hydroxyurea therapy with irradiation on squamous cell (epidermoid) carcinomas of the head and neck. *In vitro* studies utilizing Chinese hamster cells suggest that hydroxyurea (1) is lethal to normally radioresistant S-stage cells, and (2) holds other cells of the cell cycle in the G1 or pre-DNA synthesis stage where they are most susceptible to the effects of irradiation. The third mechanism of action has been theorized on the basis of *in vitro* studies of HeLa cells: it appears that hydroxyurea, by inhibition of DNA synthesis, hinders the normal repair process of cells damaged but not killed by irradiation, thereby decreasing their survival rate; RNA and protein syntheses have shown no alteration.

Pharmacokinetics:

Absorption—Hydroxyurea is readily absorbed after oral administration. Peak plasma levels are reached in 1 to 4 hours after an oral dose. With increasing doses, disproportionately greater mean peak plasma concentrations and AUCs are observed.

There are no data on the effect of food on the absorption of hydroxyurea.

Distribution—Hydroxyurea distributes rapidly and widely in the body with an estimated volume of distribution approximating total body water.

Plasma to ascites fluid ratios range from 2:1 to 7.5:1. Hydroxyurea concentrates in leukocytes and erythrocytes.

Metabolism—Up to 50% of an oral dose undergoes conversion through metabolic pathways that are not fully characterized. In one minor pathway, hydroxyurea may be degraded by urease found in intestinal bacteria. Acetohydroxamic acid was found in the serum of three leukemic patients receiving hydroxyurea and may be formed from hydroxylamine resulting from action of urease on hydroxyurea.

Excretion—Excretion of hydroxyurea in humans is a nonlinear process occurring through two pathways. One is saturable, probably hepatic metabolism; the other is first-order renal excretion.

Special Populations:

Geriatric, Gender, Race—No information is available regarding pharmacokinetic differences due to age, gender or race.

Pediatric—No pharmacokinetic data are available in pediatric patients treated with hydroxyurea.

Renal Insufficiency—There are no data that support specific guidance for dosage adjustment in patients with renal impairment. As renal excretion is a pathway of elimination, consideration should be given to decreasing the dosage of hydroxyurea in patients with renal impairment. Close monitoring of hematologic parameters is advised in these patients.

Hepatic Insufficiency—There are no data that support specific guidance for dosage adjustment in patients with hepatic impairment. Close monitoring of hematologic parameters is advised in these patients.

Drug Interactions—There are no data on concomitant use of hydroxyurea with other drugs in humans.

Animal Pharmacology and Toxicology:

The oral LD_{50} of hydroxyurea is 7330 mg/kg in mice and 5780 mg/kg in rats, given as a single dose.

In subacute and chronic toxicity studies in the rat, the most consistent pathological findings were an apparent dose-related mild to moderate bone marrow hypoplasia as well as pulmonary congestion and mottling of the lungs. At the highest dosage levels (1260 mg/kg/day for 37 days then 2520 mg/kg/day for 40 days), testicular atrophy with absence of spermatogenesis occurred; in several animals, hepatic cell damage with fatty metamorphosis was noted. In the dog, mild to marked bone marrow depression was a consistent finding except at the lower dosage levels. Additionally, at the higher dose levels (140 to 420 mg or 140 to 1260 mg/kg/week given 3 or 7 days weekly for 12 weeks), growth retardation, slightly increased blood glucose values, and hemosiderosis of the liver or spleen were found; reversible spermatogenic arrest was noted. In the monkey, bone marrow depression, lymphoid atrophy of the spleen, and degenerative changes in the epithelium of the small and large intestines were found. At the higher, often lethal, doses (400 to 800 mg/kg/day for 7 to 15 days), hemorrhage and congestion were found in the lungs, brain, and urinary tract. Cardiovascular effects (changes in heart rate, blood pressure, orthostatic hypotension, EKG changes) and hematological changes (slight hemolysis, slight methemoglobinemia) were observed in some species of laboratory animals at doses exceeding clinical levels.

INDICATIONS AND USAGE

Significant tumor response to HYDREA (hydroxyurea capsules, USP) has been demonstrated in melanoma, resistant chronic myelocytic leukemia, and recurrent, metastatic, or inoperable carcinoma of the ovary.

Hydroxyurea used concomitantly with irradiation therapy is intended for use in the local control of primary squamous cell (epidermoid) carcinomas of the head and neck, excluding the lip.

CONTRAINDICATIONS

Hydroxyurea is contraindicated in patients with marked bone marrow depression, i.e., leukopenia (<2500 WBC) or thrombocytopenia (<100,000), or severe anemia.

HYDREA is contraindicated in patients who have demonstrated a previous hypersensitivity to hydroxyurea or any other component of its formulation.

WARNINGS

Treatment with hydroxyurea should not be initiated if bone marrow function is markedly depressed (see **CONTRAINDICATIONS**). Bone marrow suppression may occur, and leukopenia is generally its first and most common manifestation. Thrombocytopenia and anemia occur less often, and are seldom seen without a preceding leukopenia. However, the recovery from myelosuppression is rapid when therapy is interrupted. It should be borne in mind that bone marrow depression is more likely in patients who have previously received radiotherapy or cytotoxic cancer chemotherapeutic agents; hydroxyurea should be used cautiously in such patients.

Patients who have received irradiation therapy in the past may have an exacerbation of postirradiation erythema.

Severe anemia must be corrected before initiating therapy with hydroxyurea.

Erythrocytic abnormalities: megaloblastic erythropoiesis, which is self-limiting, is often seen early in the course of hydroxyurea therapy. The morphologic change resembles pernicious anemia, but is not related to vitamin B_{12} or folic acid deficiency. Hydroxyurea may also delay plasma iron clearance and reduce the rate of iron utilization by erythrocytes, but it does not appear to alter the red blood cell survival time.

Hydroxyurea should be used with caution in patients with marked renal dysfunction.

Elderly patients may be more sensitive to the effects of hydroxyurea, and may require a lower dose regimen.

In patients receiving long-term hydroxyurea for myeloproliferative disorders, such as polycythemia vera and thrombocythemia, secondary leukemia has been reported. It is unknown whether this leukemogenic effect is secondary to hydroxyurea or associated with the patients' underlying disease.

Carcinogenesis and Mutagenesis: Hydroxyurea is genotoxic in a wide range of test systems and is thus presumed to be a human carcinogen. In patients receiving long-term hydroxyurea for myeloproliferative disorders, such as polycythemia vera and and thrombocythemia, secondary leukemia has been reported. It is unknown whether this leukemogenic effect is secondary to hydroxyurea or is associated with the patients' underlying disease. Skin cancer has also been reported in patients receiving long-term hydroxyurea.

Conventional long-term studies to evaluate the carcinogenic potential of hydroxyurea have not been performed. However, intraperitoneal administration of 125–250 mg/kg hydroxyurea (about 0.6–1.2 times the maximum recommended human oral daily dose on a mg/m^2 basis) thrice weekly for 6 months to female rats increased the incidence of mammary tumors in rats surviving to 18 months compared to control.

Hydroxyurea is mutagenic *in vitro* to bacteria, fungi, protozoa, and mammalian cells. Hydroxyurea is clastogenic *in vitro* (hamster cells, human lymphoblasts) and *in vivo* (SCE

Continued on next page

Hydrea—Cont.

assay in rodents, mouse micronucleus assay). Hydroxyurea causes the transformation of rodent embryo cells to a tumorigenic phenotype.

Pregnancy: Drugs which affect DNA synthesis, such as hydroxyurea, may be potential mutagenic agents. The physician should carefully consider this possibility before administering this drug to male or female patients who may contemplate conception.

HYDREA (hydroxyurea capsules, USP) can cause fetal harm when administered to a pregnant woman. Hydroxyurea is embryotoxic and causes fetal malformations (partially ossified cranial bones, absence of eye sockets, hydrocephaly, bipartite sternebrae, missing lumbar vertebrae) at 180 mg/kg/day (about 0.8 times the maximum recommended human daily dose on a mg/m^2 basis) in rats and at 30 mg/kg/day (about 0.3 times the maximum recommended human daily dose on a mg/m^2 basis) in rabbits. Embryotoxicity was characterized by decreased fetal viability, reduced live litter sizes, and developmental delays. Hydroxyurea crosses the placenta. Single doses of ≥375 mg/kg (about 1.7 times the maximum recommended human daily dose on a mg/m^2 basis) to rats caused growth retardation and impaired learning ability. There are no adequate and well-controlled studies in pregnant women. If this drug is used during pregnancy or if the patient becomes pregnant while taking this drug, the patient should be apprised of the potential harm to the fetus. Women of childbearing potential should be advised to avoid becoming pregnant.

PRECAUTIONS

Therapy with hydroxyurea requires close supervision. The complete status of the blood, including bone marrow examination, if indicated, as well as kidney function and liver function should be determined prior to, and repeatedly during, treatment. The determination of the hemoglobin level, total leukocyte counts, and platelet counts should be performed at least once a week throughout the course of hydroxyurea therapy. If the white blood cell count decreases to less than 2500/mm^3, or the platelet count to less than 100,000/mm^3, therapy should be interrupted until the values rise significantly toward normal levels. Severe anemia, if it occurs, should be managed without interrupting hydroxyurea therapy.

Carcinogenesis, Mutagenesis, and Impairment of Fertility: See **WARNINGS** for Carcinogenesis and Mutagenesis information.

Impairment of Fertility—Hydroxyurea administered to male rats at 60 mg/kg/day (about 0.3 times the maximum recommended human daily dose on a mg/m^2 basis) produced testicular atrophy, decreased spermatogenesis, and significantly reduced their ability to impregnate females.

Pregnancy: Pregnancy Category D. (See **WARNINGS.**)

Nursing Mothers: Hydroxyurea is excreted in human milk.

Because of the potential for serious adverse reactions with hydroxyurea, a decision should be made whether to discontinue nursing or to discontinue the drug, taking into account the importance of the drug to the mother.

Pediatric Use: Safety and effectiveness in pediatric patients have not been established.

Drug Interactions: Prospective studies on the potential for hydroxyurea to interact with other drugs have not been performed.

Concurrent use of hydroxyurea and other myelosuppressive agents or radiation therapy may increase the likelihood of bone marrow depression or other adverse events. (See **WARNINGS** and **ADVERSE REACTIONS**).

Since hydroxyurea may raise the serum uric acid level, dosage adjustment of uricosuric medication may be necessary.

Information for Patients: HYDREA is a medication that must be handled with care. People who are not taking HYDREA should not be exposed to it. If the powder from the capsule is spilled, it should be wiped up immediately with a damp disposable towel and discarded in a closed container, such as a plastic bag. The medication should be kept away from children and pets.

ADVERSE REACTIONS

Adverse reactions have been primarily bone marrow depression (leukopenia, anemia, and occasionally thrombocytopenia), and less frequently gastrointestinal symptoms (stomatitis, anorexia, nausea, vomiting, diarrhea, and constipation), and dermatological reactions such as maculopapular rash, skin ulceration, dermatomyositis-like skin changes, peripheral, and facial erythema. Hyperpigmentation, atrophy of skin and nails, scaling and violet papules have been observed in some patients after several years of long-term daily maintenance therapy with HYDREA. Skin cancer has been reported. Dysuria and alopecia occur very rarely. Large doses may produce moderate drowsiness. Neurological disturbances have occurred extremely rarely and were limited to headache, dizziness, disorientation, hallucinations, and convulsions. HYDREA occasionally may cause temporary impairment of renal tubular function accompanied by elevations in serum uric acid, BUN, and creatinine levels. Abnormal BSP retention has been reported. Fever, chills, malaise, edema, asthenia, and elevation of hepatic enzymes have also been reported.

Adverse reactions observed with combined hydroxyurea and irradiation therapy are similar to those reported with the use of hydroxyurea or radiation treatment alone. These effects primarily include bone marrow depression (anemia and leukopenia), gastric irritation, and mucositis. Almost all patients receiving an adequate course of combined hydroxyurea and irradiation therapy will demonstrate concurrent leukopenia. Platelet depression (<100,000 cells/mm^3) has occurred rarely and only in the presence of marked leukopenia. HYDREA may potentiate some adverse reactions usually seen with irradiation alone, such as gastric distress and mucositis.

The association of hydroxyurea with the development of acute pulmonary reactions consisting of diffuse pulmonary infiltrates, fever and dyspnea has been rarely reported. Pulmonary fibrosis also has been reported rarely.

OVERDOSAGE

Acute mucocutaneous toxicity has been reported in patients receiving hydroxyurea at dosages several times the therapeutic dose. Soreness, violet erythema, edema on palms and soles followed by scaling of hands and feet, severe generalized hyperpigmentation of the skin, and stomatitis have also been observed.

DOSAGE AND ADMINISTRATION

Procedures for proper handling and disposal of antineoplastic drugs should be considered. Several guidelines on this subject have been published.[1–7] There is no general agreement that all of the procedures recommended in the guidelines are necessary or appropriate.

Because of the rarity of melanoma, resistant chronic myelocytic leukemia, carcinoma of the ovary, and carcinomas of the head and neck in pediatric patients, dosage regimens have not been established.

All dosage should be based on the patient's actual or ideal weight, whichever is less. Concurrent use of HYDREA (hydroxyurea capsules, USP) with other myelosuppressive agents may require adjustment of dosages.

SOLID TUMORS

Intermittent Therapy: 80 mg/kg administered orally as a *single* dose every *third* day.

Continuous Therapy: 20 to 30 mg/kg administered orally as a *single* dose *daily*.

Concomitant Therapy with Irradiation: *Carcinoma of the head and neck*—80 mg/kg administered orally as a *single* dose every *third* day.

Administration of hydroxyurea should begin at least seven days before initiation of irradiation and continued during radiotherapy as well as indefinitely afterwards provided that the patient may be kept under adequate observation and evidences no unusual or severe reactions.

RESISTANT CHRONIC MYELOCYTIC LEUKEMIA

Until the intermittent therapy regimen has been evaluated, CONTINUOUS therapy (20 to 30 mg/kg administered orally as a *single* dose *daily*) is recommended.

An adequate trial period for determining the antineoplastic effectiveness of hydroxyurea is six weeks of therapy. When there is regression in tumor size or arrest in tumor growth, therapy should be continued indefinitely. Therapy should be interrupted if the white blood cell count drops below 2500/mm^3, or the platelet count below 100,000/mm^3. In these cases, the counts should be re-evaluated after three days, and therapy resumed when the counts return to acceptable levels. Since the hematopoietic rebound is prompt, it is usually necessary to omit only a few doses. If prompt rebound has not occurred during combined HYDREA and irradiation therapy, irradiation may also be interrupted. However, the need for postponement of irradiation has been rare; radiotherapy has usually been continued using the recommended dosage and technique. Severe anemia, if it occurs, should be corrected without interrupting hydroxyurea therapy. Because hematopoiesis may be compromised by extensive irradiation or by other antineoplastic agents, it is recommended that hydroxyurea be administered cautiously to patients who have recently received extensive radiation therapy or chemotherapy with other cytotoxic drugs.

Pain or discomfort from inflammation of the mucous membranes at the irradiated site (mucositis) is usually controlled by measures such as topical anesthetics and orally administered analgesics. If the reaction is severe, hydroxyurea therapy may be temporarily interrupted; if it is extremely severe, irradiation dosage may, in addition, be temporarily postponed. However, it has rarely been necessary to terminate these therapies.

Severe gastric distress, such as nausea, vomiting, and anorexia, resulting from combined therapy may usually be controlled by temporary interruption of hydroxyurea administration.

Renal Insufficiency: There are no data that support specific guidance for dosage adjustments in patients with renal impairment. As renal excretion is a pathway of elimination, consideration should be given to decreasing the dosage of HYDREA in patients with renal impairment. Close monitoring of hematologic parameters is advised in these patients.

Hepatic Insufficiency: There are no data that support specific guidance for dosage adjustment in patients with hepatic impairment. Close monitoring of hematologic parameters is advised in these patients.

HOW SUPPLIED

Hydrea® (hydroxyurea capsules, USP)

500 mg capsules in bottles of 100 (**NDC** 0003-0830-50).

Capsule identification number: 830. The cap is opaque green and the body is opaque pink. They are imprinted on both sections in black ink with "HYDREA" and "830".

Storage: Store at 25°C (77°F); excursions permitted to 15–30°C (59–86°F). Keep tightly closed.

REFERENCES

1. Recommendations for the Safe Handling of Parenteral Antineoplastic Drugs. *NIH Publications* No. 83-2621. For sale by the Superintendent of Documents, US Government Printing Office, Washington, DC 20402.
2. AMA Council Report. Guidelines for Handling Parenteral Antineoplastics. *JAMA* 1985; 253(11):1590–1592.
3. *National Study Commission on Cytotoxic Exposure*—Recommendations for Handling Cytotoxic Agents. Available from Louis P. Jeffrey, ScD, Chairman, National Study Commission on Cytotoxic Exposure, *Massachusetts College of Pharmacy and Allied Health Sciences,* 179 Longwood Avenue, Boston, MA 02115.
4. Clinical Oncological Society of Australia. Guidelines and Recommendations for Safe Handling of Antineoplastic Agents. *Med J Australia* 1983; 1:426–428.
5. Jones RB, et al. Safe Handling of Chemotherapeutic Agents: A Report from the Mount Sinai Medical Center, *CA-A Cancer Journal for Clinicians* 1983; (Sept/Oct)258–263.
6. American Society of Hospital Pharmacists Technical Assistance Bulletin on Handling Cytotoxic and Hazardous Drugs. *Am J Hosp Pharm* 1990; 47:1033–1049.
7. Controlling Occupational Exposure to Hazardous Drugs. (OSHA WORK PRACTICE GUIDELINES). *Am J Health-Syst Pharm* 1996;53:1669–1685.

BRISTOL-MYERS SQUIBB
ONCOLOGY
Bristol-Myers Squibb Company
Princeton, NJ 08543
U.S.A.

Made in Italy

K8-B001-6-00 1053327A1

Revised: January 2000

IFEX® ℞

[ī-fĕx]

(ifosfamide for injection)

Rx ONLY

> **WARNING**
>
> IFEX® should be administered under the supervision of a qualified physician experienced in the use of cancer chemotherapeutic agents. Urotoxic side effects, especially hemorrhagic cystitis, as well as CNS toxicities such as confusion and coma have been associated with the use of IFEX. When they occur, they may require cessation of IFEX therapy. Severe myelosuppression has been reported. (See **ADVERSE REACTIONS** section.)

DESCRIPTION

IFEX® (ifosfamide for injection) single-dose vials for constitution and administration by intravenous infusion each contain 1 gram or 3 grams of sterile ifosfamide. Ifosfamide is a chemotherapeutic agent chemically related to the nitrogen mustards and a synthetic analog of cyclophosphamide. Ifosfamide is 3-(2-chloroethyl)-2-[(2-chloroethyl)amino]tetrahydro-2H-1,3,2-oxazaphosphorine 2-oxide. The molecular formula is $C_7H_{15}Cl_2N_2O_2P$ and its molecular weight is 261.1. Its structural formula is:

Ifosfamide is a white crystalline powder that is soluble in water.

CLINICAL PHARMACOLOGY

Ifosfamide has been shown to require metabolic activation by microsomal liver enzymes to produce biologically active metabolites. Activation occurs by hydroxylation at the ring carbon atom 4 to form the unstable intermediate 4-hydroxyifosfamide. This metabolite rapidly degrades to the stable urinary metabolite 4-ketoifosfamide. Opening of the ring results in formation of the stable urinary metabolite, 4-carboxyifosfamide. These urinary metabolites have not been found to be cytotoxic. N, N-*bis* (2-chloroethyl)-phosphoric acid diamide (ifosphoramide) and acrolein are also found. Enzymatic oxidation of the chloroethyl side chains and subsequent dealkylation produces the major urinary metabolites, dechloroethyl ifosfamide and dechloroethyl cyclophosphamide. The alkylated metabolites of ifosfamide have been shown to interact with DNA.

In vitro incubation of DNA with activated ifosfamide has produced phosphotriesters. The treatment of intact cell nuclei may also result in the formation of DNA-DNA cross-links. DNA repair most likely occurs in G-1 and G-2 stage cells.

Pharmacokinetics: Ifosfamide exhibits dose-dependent pharmacokinetics in humans. At single doses of 3.8–5.0 g/m^2, the plasma concentrations decay biphasically and the mean terminal elimination half-life is about 15 hours. At doses of 1.6–2.4 g/m^2/day, the plasma decay is monoexponential and the terminal elimination half-life is about 7 hours. Ifosfamide is extensively metabolized in humans and the metabolic pathways appear to be saturated at high doses.

After administration of doses of 5 g/m² of ^{14}C-labeled ifosfamide, from 70% to 86% of the dosed radioactivity was recovered in the urine, with about 61% of the dose excreted as parent compound. At doses of 1.6–2.4 g/m² only 12% to 18% of the dose was excreted in the urine as unchanged drug within 72 hours.

Two different dechloroethylated derivatives of ifosfamide, 4-carboxyifosfamide, thiodiacetic acid and cysteine conjugates of chloroacetic acid have been identified as the major urinary metabolites of ifosfamide in humans and only small amounts of 4-hydroxyifosfamide and acrolein are present. Small quantities (nmole/mL) of ifosfamide mustard and 4-hydroxyifosfamide are detectable in human plasma. Metabolism of ifosfamide is required for the generation of the biologically active species and while metabolism is extensive, it is also quite variable among patients.

In a study at Indiana University, 50 fully evaluable patients with germ cell testicular cancer were treated with IFEX in combination with cisplatin and either vinblastine or etoposide after failing (47 of 50 patients) at least two prior chemotherapy regimens consisting of cisplatin/vinblastine/bleomycin, (PVB), cisplatin/vinblastine/actinomycin D/bleomycin/cyclophosphamide, (VAB6), or the combination of cisplatin and etoposide. Patients were selected for remaining cisplatin sensitivity because they had previously responded to a cisplatin containing regimen and had not progressed while on the cisplatin containing regimen or within 3 weeks of stopping it. Patients served as their own control based on the premise that long term complete responses could not be achieved by retreatment with a reg imen to which they had previously responded and subsequently relapsed.

Ten of 50 fully evaluable patients were still alive 2 to 5 years after treatment. Four of the 10 long term survivors were rendered free of cancer by surgical resection after treatment with the ifosfamide regimen; median survival for the entire group of 50 fully evaluable patients was 53 weeks.

INDICATION AND USAGE

IFEX, used in combination with certain other approved antineoplastic agents, is indicated for third line chemotherapy of germ cell testicular cancer. It should ordinarily be used in combination with a prophylactic agent for hemorrhagic cystitis, such as mesna.

CONTRAINDICATIONS

Continued use of IFEX is contraindicated in patients with severely depressed bone marrow function (See **WARNINGS** and **PRECAUTIONS** sections). IFEX is also contraindicated in patients who have demonstrated a previous hypersensitivity to it.

WARNINGS

Urinary System: Urotoxic side effects, especially hemorrhagic cystitis, have been frequently associated with the use of IFEX. It is recommended that a urinalysis should be obtained prior to each dose of IFEX. If microscopic hematuria (greater than 10 RBCs per high power field), is present, then subsequent administration should be withheld until complete resolution.

Further administration of IFEX should be given with vigorous oral or parenteral hydration.

Hematopoietic System: When IFEX is given in combination with other chemotherapeutic agents, severe myelosuppression is frequently observed. Close hematologic monitoring is recommended. White blood cell (WBC) count, platelet count and hemoglobin should be obtained prior to each administration and at appropriate intervals. Unless clinically essential, IFEX should not be given to patients with a WBC count below 2000/µL and/or a platelet count below 50,000/µL.

Central Nervous System: Neurologic manifestations consisting of somnolence, confusion, hallucinations and in some instances, coma, have been reported following IFEX therapy. The occurrence of these symptoms requires discontinuing IFEX therapy. The symptoms have usually been reversible and supportive therapy should be maintained until their complete resolution.

Pregnancy: Animal studies indicate that the drug is capable of causing gene mutations and chromosomal damage *in vivo*. Embryotoxic and teratogenic effects have been observed in mice, rats and rabbits at doses 0.05 to 0.075 times the human dose. Ifosfamide can cause fetal damage when administered to a pregnant woman. If IFEX (ifosfamide for injection) is used during pregnancy, or if the patient becomes pregnant while taking this drug, the patient should be apprised of the potential hazard to the fetus.

PRECAUTIONS

General: IFEX should be given cautiously to patients with impaired renal function as well as to those with compromised bone marrow reserve, as indicated by: leukopenia, granulocytopenia, extensive bone marrow metastases, prior radiation therapy, or prior therapy with other cytotoxic agents.

Laboratory Tests: During treatment, the patient's hematologic profile (particularly neutrophils and platelets) should be monitored regularly to determine the degree of hematopoietic suppression. Urine should also be examined regularly for red cells which may precede hemorrhagic cystitis.

Drug Interactions: The physician should be alert for possible combined drug actions, desirable or undesirable, involving ifosfamide even though ifosfamide has been used successfully concurrently with other drugs, including other cytotoxic drugs.

Adverse Reaction	* Incidence (%)	Adverse Reaction	* Incidence (%)
Alopecia	83	Coagulopathy	< 1
Nausea-Vomiting	58	Constipation	< 1
Hematuria	46	Dermatitis	< 1
Gross Hematuria	12	Diarrhea	< 1
CNS Toxicity	12	Fatigue	< 1
Infection	8	Hypertension	< 1
Renal Impairment	6	Hypotension	< 1
Liver Dysfunction	3	Malaise	< 1
Phlebitis	2	Polyneuropathy	< 1
Fever	1	Pulmonary Symptoms	< 1
Allergic Reaction	< 1	Salivation	< 1
Anorexia	< 1	Stomatitis	< 1
Cardiotoxicity	< 1		

*Based upon 2,070 patients from the published literature in 30 single agent studies.

Wound Healing: Ifosfamide may interfere with normal wound healing.

Pregnancy: Pregnancy "Category D". (See **WARNINGS** section.)

Nursing Mothers: Ifosfamide is excreted in breast milk. Because of the potential for serious adverse events and the tumorigenicity shown for ifosfamide in animal studies, a decision should be made whether to discontinue nursing or to discontinue the drug, taking into account the importance of the drug to the mother.

Carcinogenesis, Mutagenesis, Impairment of Fertility: Ifosfamide has been shown to be carcinogenic in rats, with female rats showing a significant incidence of leiomyosarcomas and mammary fibroadenomas.

The mutagenic potential of ifosfamide has been documented in bacterial systems *in vitro* and mammalian cells *in vivo*. *In vivo*, ifosfamide has induced mutagenic effects in mice and *Drosophila melanogaster* germ cells, and has induced a significant increase in dominant lethal mutations in male mice as well as recessive sex-linked lethal mutations in *Drosophila*.

In pregnant mice, resorptions increased and anomalies were present at day 19 after a 30 mg/m² dose of ifosfamide was administered on day 11 of gestation. Embryolethal effects were observed in rats following the administration of 54 mg/m² doses of ifosfamide from the 6th through the 15th day of gestation and embryotoxic effects were apparent after dams received 18 mg/m² doses over the same dosing period. Ifosfamide is embryotoxic to rabbits receiving 88 mg/m²/day doses from the 6th through the 18th day after mating. The number of anomalies was also significantly increased over the control group.

Pediatric Use: Safety and effectiveness in pediatric patients have not been established.

ADVERSE REACTIONS

In patients receiving IFEX as a single agent, the dose-limiting toxicities are myelosuppression and urotoxicity. Dose fractionation, vigorous hydration, and a protector such as mesna can significantly reduce the incidence of hematuria, especially gross hematuria, associated with hemorrhagic cystitis. At a dose of 1.2 g/m² daily for 5 consecutive days, leukopenia, when it occurs, is usually mild to moderate. Other significant side effects include alopecia, nausea, vomiting, and central nervous system toxicities.

[See table above]

Hematologic Toxicity: Myelosuppression was dose related and dose limiting. It consisted mainly of leukopenia and, to a lesser extent, thrombocytopenia. A WBC count < 3000/µL is expected in 50% of the patients treated with IFEX single agent at doses of 1.2 g/m² per day for 5 consecutive days. At this dose level, thrombocytopenia (platelets < 100,000/µL) occurred in about 20% of the patients. At higher dosages, leukopenia was almost universal, and at total dosages of 10–12 g/m²/cycle, one half of the patients had a WBC count below 1000/µL and 8% of patients had platelet counts less than 50,000/µL. Myelosuppression was usually reversible and treatment can be given every 3 to 4 weeks. When IFEX is used in combination with other myelosuppressive agents, adjustments in dosing may be necessary. Patients who experience severe myelosuppression are potentially at increased risk for infection. Anemia has been reported as part of postmarketing surveillance.

Digestive System: Nausea and vomiting occurred in 58% of the patients who received IFEX. They were usually controlled by standard antiemetic therapy. Other gastrointestinal side effects include anorexia, diarrhea, and in some cases, constipation.

Urinary System: Urotoxicity consisted of hemorrhagic cystitis, dysuria, urinary frequency and other symptoms of bladder irritation. Hematuria occurred in 6% to 92% of patients treated with IFEX. The incidence and severity of hematuria can be significantly reduced by using vigorous hydration, a fractionated dose schedule and a protector such as mesna. At daily doses of 1.2 g/m² for 5 consecutive days without a protector, microscopic hematuria is expected in about one half of the patients and gross hematuria in about 8% of patients.

Renal toxicity occurred in 6% of the patients treated with ifosfamide as a single agent. Clinical signs, such as elevation in BUN or serum creatinine or decrease in creatinine clearance, were usually transient. They were most likely to be related to tubular damage. One episode of renal tubular acidosis which progressed into chronic renal failure was reported. Proteinuria and acidosis also occurred in rare instances. Metabolic acidosis was reported in 31% of patients in one study when IFEX was administered at doses of 2.0 to 2.5 g/m²/day for 4 days. Renal tubular acidosis, Fanconi syndrome, renal rickets and acute renal failure have been reported. Close clinical monitoring of serum and urine chemistries including phosphorus, potassium, alkaline phosphatase and other appropriate laboratory studies is recommended. Appropriate replacement therapy should be administered as indicated.

Central Nervous System: CNS side effects were observed in 12% of patients treated with IFEX. Those most commonly seen were somnolence, confusion, depressive psychosis, and hallucinations. Other less frequent symptoms include dizziness, disorientation, and cranial nerve dysfunction. Seizures and coma with death were occasionally reported. The incidence of CNS toxicity may be higher in patients with altered renal function.

Other: Alopecia occurred in approximately 83% of the patients treated with IFEX as a single agent. In combination, this incidence may be as high as 100%, depending on the other agents included in the chemotherapy regimen.

Increases in liver enzymes and/or bilirubin were noted in 3% of the patients. Other less frequent side effects included phlebitis, pulmonary symptoms, fever of unknown origin, allergic reactions, stomatitis, cardiotoxicity, and polyneuropathy.

OVERDOSAGE

No specific antidote for IFEX (ifosfamide for injection) is known. Management of overdosage would include general supportive measures to sustain the patient through any period of toxicity that might occur.

DOSAGE AND ADMINISTRATION

IFEX should be administered intravenously at a dose of 1.2 g/m² per day for 5 consecutive days. Treatment is repeated every 3 weeks or after recovery from hematologic toxicity (Platelets ≥ 100,000/µL, WBC ≥ 4,000/µL). In order to prevent bladder toxicity, IFEX should be given with extensive hydration consisting of at least 2 liters of oral or intravenous fluid per day. A protector, such as mesna, should also be used to prevent hemorrhagic cystitis. IFEX should be administered as a slow intravenous infusion lasting a minimum of 30 minutes. Although IFEX has been administered to a small number of patients with compromised hepatic and/or renal function, studies to establish optimal dose schedules of IFEX in such patients have not been conducted.

Preparation for Intravenous Administration/Stability: Injections are prepared for parenteral use by adding *Sterile Water for Injection, USP*, or *Sterile Bacteriostatic Water for Injection, USP* (benzyl alcohol or parabens preserved), to the vial and shaking to dissolve. Use the quantity of diluent shown below to constitute the product:

Dosage Strength	Quantity of Diluent	Final Concentration
1 gram	20 mL	50 mg/mL
3 grams	60 mL	50 mg/mL

Solutions of ifosfamide may be diluted further to achieve concentrations of 0.6 to 20 mg/mL in the following fluids:

5% Dextrose Injection, USP
0.9% Sodium Chloride Injection, USP
Lactated Ringer's Injection, USP
Sterile Water for Injection, USP

Because essentially identical stability results were obtained for Sterile Water admixtures as for the other admixtures (5% Dextrose Injection, 0.9% Sodium Chloride Injection, and Lactated Ringer's Injection), the use of large volume parenteral glass bottles, Viaflex bags or PAB™ bags that contain intermediate concentrations or mixtures of excipients (e.g., 2.5% Dextrose Injection, 0.45% Sodium Chloride Injection, or 5% Dextrose and 0.9% Sodium Chloride Injection) is also acceptable.

Constituted or constituted and further diluted solutions of IFEX should be refrigerated and used within 24 hours.

Parenteral drug products should be inspected visually for particulate matter and discoloration prior to administration.

HOW SUPPLIED

IFEX® (ifosfamide for injection) is only available in combination packages with the uroprotective agent MESNEX® (mesna) Injection.

Continued on next page

Ifex—Cont.

IFEX (ifosfamide for injection)/MESNEX® (mesna) Injection.

NDC 0015-3556-26 — 5 × 1-gram Single Dose Vial of IFEX
— 3 × 1-gram Multidose Vial of of MESNEX

NDC 0015-3554-27 — 10 × 1-gram Single Dose Vial of IFEX
— 10 × 1-gram Multidose Vial of MESNEX

NDC 0015-3564-15 — 2 × 3-gram Single Dose Vial of IFEX
— 6 × 1-gram Multidose Vial of MESNEX

Store at controlled room temperature 20°C to 25°C (68°F to 77°F). Protect from temperatures above 30°C (86°F).

Procedures for proper handling and disposal of anticancer drugs should be considered. Skin reactions associated with accidental exposure to IFEX may occur. The use of gloves is recommended. If IFEX solution contacts the skin or mucosa, immediately wash the skin thoroughly with soap and water or rinse the mucosa with copious amounts of water. Several guidelines on this subject have been published.[1–7] There is no general agreement that all of the procedures recommended in the guidelines are necessary or appropriate.

REFERENCES

1. Recommendations for the Safe Handling of Parenteral Antineoplastic Drugs. NIH Publication No. 83-2621. For sale by the Superintendent of Documents, US Government Printing Office, Washington, DC 20402.
2. AMA Council Report. Guidelines for Handling Parenteral Antineoplastics. *JAMA* 1985; 253(11):1590–1592.
3. National Study Commission on Cytotoxic Exposure—Recommendations for Handling Cytotoxic Agents. Available from Louis P. Jeffrey, ScD, Chairman, National Study Commission on Cytotoxic Exposure, Massachusetts College of Pharmacy and Allied Health Sciences, 179 Longwood Avenue, Boston, Massachusetts 02115.
4. Clinical Oncological Society of Australia. Guidelines and Recommendations for Safe Handling of Antineoplastic Agents. *Med J Australia* 1983; 1:426–428.
5. Jones, RB, et al: Safe Handling of Chemotherapeutic Agents: A Report from the Mount Sinai Medical Center. *CA—A Cancer Journal for Clinicians* 1983; (Sept/Oct)258–263.
6. American Society of Hospital Pharmacists Technical Assistance Bulletin on Handling Cytotoxic and Hazardous Drugs. *Am J Hosp Pharm* 1990; 47:1033–1049.
7. Controlling Occupational Exposure to Hazardous Drugs. (OSHA WORK PRACTICE GUIDELINES.) *Am J Health Syst-Pharm* 1996; 53:1669–1685.

Distributed by:
Mead Johnson
ONCOLOGY PRODUCTS
A Bristol-Myers Squibb Company
Princeton, NJ 08543
U.S.A.
Manufactured by:
ASTA MEDICA
A Degussa Company
Frankfurt am Mein
Germany
H5-B001-12-98 N0054-01
Revised: June 1998

Shown in Product Identification Guide, page 310

LYSODREN® ℞

[līso 'dren]
(mitotane tablets, USP)
Rx Only

> **WARNINGS**
> LYSODREN® (mitotane tablets, USP) should be administered under the supervision of a qualified physician experienced in the uses of cancer chemotherapeutic agents. LYSODREN should be temporarily discontinued immediately following shock or severe trauma since adrenal suppression is its prime action. Exogenous steroids should be administered in such circumstances, since the depressed adrenal may not immediately start to secrete steroids.

DESCRIPTION

LYSODREN® (mitotane tablets, USP) is an oral chemotherapeutic agent. It is best known by its trivial name, o,p'-DDD, and is chemically, 1,1-dichloro-2-(o-chlorophenyl)-2-(p-chlorophenyl) ethane. The chemical structure is shown below.

CHCl2 CH Cl Cl

LYSODREN is a white granular solid composed of clear colorless crystals. It is tasteless and has a slight pleasant aromatic odor. It is soluble in ethanol, isooctane and carbon tetrachloride. It has a molecular weight of 320.05.

Inactive ingredients in LYSODREN tablets are: avicel, Polyethylene Glycol 3350, silicon dioxide, and starch.

LYSODREN is available as 500 mg scored tablets for oral administration.

CLINICAL PHARMACOLOGY

LYSODREN can best be described as an adrenal cytotoxic agent, although it can cause adrenal inhibition, apparently without cellular destruction. Its biochemical mechanism of action is unknown. Data are available to suggest that the drug modifies the peripheral metabolism of steroids as well as directly suppressing the adrenal cortex. The administration of LYSODREN alters the extra-adrenal metabolism of cortisol in man; leading to a reduction in measurable 17-hydroxy corticosteroids, even though plasma levels of corticosteroids do not fall. The drug apparently causes increased formation of 6-B-hydroxyl cortisol.

Data in adrenal carcinoma patients indicate that about 40% of oral LYSODREN is absorbed and approximately 10% of administered dose is recovered in the urine as a water-soluble metabolite. A variable amount of metabolite (1% to 17%) is excreted in the bile and the balance is apparently stored in the tissues.

Following discontinuation of LYSODREN, the plasma terminal half-life has ranged from 18 to 159 days. In most patients blood levels become undetectable after 6 to 9 weeks. Autopsy data have provided evidence that LYSODREN is found in most tissues of the body; however, fat tissues are the primary site of storage. LYSODREN is converted to a water-soluble metabolite.

No unchanged LYSODREN has been found in urine or bile.

INDICATIONS AND USAGE

LYSODREN is indicated in the treatment of inoperable adrenal cortical carcinoma of both functional and nonfunctional types.

CONTRAINDICATIONS

LYSODREN should not be given to individuals who have demonstrated a previous hypersensitivity to it.

WARNINGS

LYSODREN should be temporarily discontinued immediately following shock or severe trauma, since adrenal suppression is its prime action. Exogenous steroids should be administered in such circumstances, since the depressed adrenal may not immediately start to secrete steroids.

LYSODREN should be administered with care to patients with liver disease other than metastatic lesions from the adrenal cortex, since the metabolism of LYSODREN may be interfered with and the drug may accumulate.

All possible tumor tissues should be surgically removed from large metastatic masses before LYSODREN administration is instituted. This is necessary to minimize the possibility of infarction and hemorrhage in the tumor due to a rapid cytotoxic effect of the drug.

Long-term continuous administration of high doses of LYSODREN may lead to brain damage and impairment of function. Behavioral and neurological assessments should be made at regular intervals when continuous LYSODREN treatment exceeds 2 years.

A substantial percentage of the patients treated show signs of adrenal insufficiency. It therefore appears necessary to watch for and institute steroid replacement in those patients. However, some investigators have recommended that steroid replacement therapy be administered concomitantly with LYSODREN. It has been shown that the metabolism of exogenous steroids is modified and consequently somewhat higher doses than normal replacement therapy may be required.

PRECAUTIONS

General: Adrenal insufficiency may develop in patients treated with LYSODREN (mitotane tablets, USP), and adrenal steroid replacement should be considered for these patients.

Since sedation, lethargy, vertigo, and other CNS side effects can occur, ambulatory patients should be cautioned about driving, operating machinery, and other hazardous pursuits requiring mental and physical alertness.

Drug Interactions: LYSODREN has been reported to accelerate the metabolism of warfarin by the mechanism of hepatic microsomal enzyme induction, leading to an increase in dosage requirements for warfarin. Therefore, physicians should closely monitor patients for a change in anticoagulant dosage requirements when administering LYSODREN to patients on coumarin-type anticoagulants. In addition, LYSODREN should be given with caution to patients receiving other drugs susceptible to the influence of hepatic enzyme induction.

Carcinogenesis, Mutagenesis, Impairment of Fertility: The carcinogenic and mutagenic potentials of LYSODREN are unknown. However, the mechanism of action of this compound suggests that it probably has less carcinogenic potential than other cytotoxic chemotherapeutic drugs.

Pregnancy: Pregnancy "Category C". Animal reproduction studies have not been conducted with LYSODREN. It is also not known whether LYSODREN can cause fetal harm when administered to a pregnant woman or can affect reproduction capacity. LYSODREN should be given to a pregnant woman only if clearly needed.

Nursing Mothers: It is not known whether this drug is excreted in human milk. Because many drugs are excreted in human milk and because of the potential for adverse reactions in nursing infants from mitotane, a decision should be made whether to discontinue nursing or to discontinue the drug, taking into account the importance of the drug to the mother.

Pediatric Use: Safety and effectiveness in pediatric patients have not been established.

ADVERSE REACTIONS

A very high percentage of patients treated with LYSODREN have shown at least one type of side effect. The main types of adverse reactions consist of the following:

1. Gastrointestinal disturbances, which consist of anorexia, nausea or vomiting, and in some cases diarrhea, occur in about 80% of the patients.
2. Central nervous system side effects occur in 40% of the patients. These consist primarily of depression as manifested by lethargy and somnolence (25%), and dizziness or vertigo (15%).
3. Skin toxicity has been observed in about 15% of the cases. These skin changes consist primarily of transient skin rashes which do not seem to be dose related. In some instances, this side effect subsided while the patients were maintained on the drug without a change of dose. Infrequently occurring side effects involve the eye (visual blurring, diplopia, lens opacity, toxic retinopathy); the genitourinary system (hematuria, hemorrhagic cystitis, and albuminuria); cardiovascular system (hypertension, orthostatic hypotension, and flushing); and some miscellaneous effects including generalized aching, hyperpyrexia, and lowered protein bound iodine (PBI).

OVERDOSAGE

No proven antidotes have been established for LYSODREN overdosage.

DOSAGE AND ADMINISTRATION

The recommended treatment schedule is to start the patient at 2 to 6 g of LYSODREN per day in divided doses, either three or four times a day. Doses are usually increased incrementally to 9 to 10 g per day. If severe side effects appear, the dose should be reduced until the maximum tolerated dose is achieved. If the patient can tolerate higher doses and improved clinical response appears possible, the dose should be increased until adverse reactions interfere. Experience has shown that the maximum tolerated dose (MTD) will vary from 2 to 16 g per day, but has usually been 9 to 10 g per day. The highest doses used in the studies to date were 18 to 19 g per day.

Treatment should be instituted in the hospital until a stable dosage regimen is achieved.

Treatment should be continued as long as clinical benefits are observed. Maintenance of clinical status or slowing of growth of metastatic lesions can be considered clinical benefits if they can clearly be shown to have occurred.

If no clinical benefits are observed after 3 months at the maximum tolerated dose, the case would generally be considered a clinical failure. However, 10% of the patients who showed a measurable response required more than 3 months at the MTD. Early diagnosis and prompt institution of treatment improve the probability of a positive clinical response. Clinical effectiveness can be shown by reduction in tumor mass; reduction in pain, weakness or anorexia; and reduction of symptoms and signs due to excessive steroid production.

A number of patients have been treated intermittently with treatment being restarted when severe symptoms have reappeared. Patients often do not respond after the third or fourth such course. Experience accumulated to date suggests that continuous treatment with the maximum possible dosage of LYSODREN is the best approach.

Procedures for proper handling and disposal of anticancer drugs should be considered. Several guidelines on this subject have been published.[1–7] There is no general agreement that all of the procedures recommended in the guidelines are necessary or appropriate.

HOW SUPPLIED

LYSODREN® (mitotane tablets, USP)
NDC 0015-3080-60 – 500 mg Tablets, bottle of 100
STORAGE
Tablets may be stored at room temperature.

REFERENCES

1. Recommendations for the Safe Handling of Parenteral Antineoplastic Drugs. NIH Publication No. 83-2621. For sale by the Superintendent of Documents, US Government Printing Office, Washington, DC 20402.
2. AMA Council Report. Guidelines for Handling Parenteral Antineoplastics. *JAMA* 1985; 253(11)1590–1592.
3. National Study Commission on Cytotoxic Exposure—Recommendations for Handling Cytotoxic Agents. Available from Louis P. Jeffrey, ScD, Chairman, National Study Commission on Cytotoxic Exposure, Massachusetts College of Pharmacy and Allied Health Sciences, 179 Longwood Avenue, Boston, Massachusetts 02115.
4. Clinical Oncological Society of Australia: Guidelines and Recommendations for Safe Handling of Antineoplastic Agents. *Med J Australia* 1983; 1:426–428.
5. Jones, RB, et al: Safe Handling of Chemotherapeutic Agents: A Report from the Mount Sinai Medical Center. *CA—A Cancer Journal for Clinicians* 1983; (Sept/Oct) 258–263.
6. American Society of Hospital Pharmacists Technical Assistance Bulletin on Handling Cytotoxic Drugs in Hospitals. *Am J Hosp Pharm* 1990; 47:1033–1049.
7. Controlling Occupational Exposure to Hazardous Drugs. (OSHA Work-Practice Guidelines). *Am J Health-Syst Pharm* 1996;53:1669–1685.

Distributed by:
BRISTOL LABORATORIES®
ONCOLOGY PRODUCTS
A Bristol-Myers Squibb Company
Princeton, NJ 08543
U.S.A.
Made in Italy
H6-B001-7-99 1050972
Revised April 1999

MEGACE® ORAL SUSPENSION ℞

[*mĕg 'ace*]
(megestrol acetate)
Rx ONLY

DESCRIPTION

MEGACE® (megestrol acetate) Oral Suspension contains megestrol acetate, a synthetic derivative of the naturally occurring steroid hormone, progesterone. Megestrol acetate is a white, crystalline solid chemically designated as 17α-(acetyloxy)-6-methylpregna-4,6-diene-3,20-dione. Solubility at 37°C in water is 2 µg per mL, solubility in plasma is 24 µg per mL. Its molecular weight is 384.51.

The empirical formula is $C_{24}H_{32}O_4$ and the structural formula is represented as follows:

MEGACE Oral Suspension is supplied as an oral suspension containing 40 mg of micronized megestrol acetate per mL.

MEGACE Oral Suspension contains the following inactive ingredients: alcohol (max. 0.06% v/v from flavor), citric acid, lemon-lime flavor, polyethylene glycol, polysorbate 80, purified water, sodium benzoate, sodium citrate, sucrose and xanthan gum.

CLINICAL PHARMACOLOGY

Several investigators have reported on the appetite enhancing property of megestrol acetate and its possible use in cachexia. The precise mechanism by which megestrol acetate produces effects in anorexia and cachexia is unknown at the present time.

There are several analytical methods used to estimate megestrol acetate plasma concentrations, including gas chromatography-mass fragmentography (GC-MF), high pressure liquid chromatography (HPLC) and radioimmunoassay (RIA). The GC-MF and HPLC methods are specific for megestrol acetate and yield equivalent concentrations. The RIA method reacts to megestrol acetate metabolites and is, therefore, non-specific and indicates higher concentrations than the GC-MF and HPLC methods. Plasma concentrations are dependent, not only on the method used, but also on intestinal and hepatic inactivation of the drug, which may be affected by factors such as intestinal tract motility, intestinal bacteria, antibiotics administered, body weight, diet and liver function.

The major route of drug elimination in humans is urine. When radiolabeled megestrol acetate was administered to humans in doses of 4 to 90 mg, the urinary excretion within 10 days ranged from 56.5% to 78.4% (mean 66.4%) and fecal excretion ranged from 7.7% to 30.3% (mean 19.8%). The total recovered radioactivity varied between 83.1% and 94.7% (mean 86.2%). Megestrol acetate metabolites which were identified in urine constituted 5% to 8% of the dose administered. Respiratory excretion as labeled carbon dioxide and fat storage may have accounted for at least part of the radioactivity not found in urine and feces.

Plasma steady state pharmacokinetics of megestrol acetate were evaluated in 10 adult, cachectic male patients with acquired immunodeficiency syndrome (AIDS) and an involuntary weight loss greater than 10% of baseline. Patients received single oral doses of 800 mg/day of MEGACE Oral Suspension for 21 days. Plasma concentration data obtained on day 21 were evaluated for up to 48 hours past the last dose.

Mean (±1SD) peak plasma concentration (C_{max}) of megestrol acetate was 753 (±539) ng/mL. Mean area under the concentration time-curve (AUC) was 10476 (±7788) ng × hr/mL. Median T_{max} value was five hours. Seven of 10 patients gained weight in three weeks.

Additionally, 24 adult, asymptomatic HIV seropositive male subjects were dosed once daily with 750 mg of MEGACE Oral Suspension. The treatment was administered for 14 days. Mean C_{max} and AUC values 490 (±238) ng/mL and 6779 (±3048) hr × ng/mL, respectively. The median T_{max} value was three hours. The mean C_{min} value was 202 (±101) ng/mL. The mean % of fluctuation value was 107 (±40).

The relative bioavailability of MEGACE 40 mg tablets and MEGACE Oral Suspension has not been evaluated. The effect of food on the bioavailability of MEGACE Oral Suspension has not been evaluated.

MEGACE (megestrol acetate) Oral Suspension Clinical Efficacy Trials

	Trial 1 Study Accrual Dates 11/88 to 12/90				Trial 2 Study Accrual Dates 5/89 to 4/91	
Megestrol Acetate, mg/day	0	100	400	800	0	800
Entered Patients	38	82	75	75	48	52
Evaluable Patients	28	61	53	53	29	36
Mean Change in Weight (lb.) Baseline to 12 Weeks	0.0	2.9	9.3	10.7	-2.1	11.2
% Patients ≥5 Pound Gain at Last Evaluation in 12 Weeks	21	44	57	64	28	47
Mean Changes in Body Composition*:						
Fat Body Mass (lb.)	0.0	2.2	2.9	5.5	1.5	5.7
Lean Body Mass (lb.)	-1.7	-0.3	1.5	2.5	-1.6	-0.6
Water (liters)	-1.3	-0.3	0.0	0.0	-0.1	-0.1
% Patients With Improved Appetite:						
At time of Max. Wt. Change	50	72	72	93	48	69
At Last Evaluation in 12 Wks.	50	72	68	89	38	67
Mean Change in Daily Caloric Intake: Baseline to Time of Maximum Weight Change	-107	326	308	646	30	464

*Based on bioelectrical impedence analysis determinations at last evaluation in 12 weeks.

DESCRIPTION OF CLINICAL STUDIES

The clinical efficacy of MEGACE Oral Suspension was assessed in two clinical trials. One was a multicenter, randomized, double-blind, placebo-controlled study comparing megestrol acetate (MA) at doses of 100 mg, 400 mg, and 800 mg per day versus placebo in AIDS patients with anorexia/cachexia and significant weight loss. Of the 270 patients entered on study, 195 met all inclusion/exclusion criteria, had at least two additional post baseline weight measurements over a 12 week period or had one post baseline weight measurement but dropped out for therapeutic failure. The percent of patients gaining five or more pounds at maximum weight gain in 12 study weeks was statistically significantly greater for the 800 mg (64%) and 400 mg (57%) MA-treated groups than for the placebo group (24%). Mean weight increased from baseline to last evaluation in 12 study weeks in the 800 mg MA-treated group by 7.8 pounds, the 400 mg MA group by 4.2 pounds, the 100 mg MA group by 1.9 pounds, and decreased in the placebo group by 1.6 pounds. Mean weight changes at 4, 8 and 12 weeks for patients evaluable for efficacy in the two clinical trials are shown graphically. Changes in body composition during the 12 study weeks as measured by bioelectrical impedance analysis showed increases in non-water body weight in the MA-treated groups (see **Clinical Studies Table**). In addition, edema developed or worsened in only 3 patients.

Greater percentages of MA-treated patients in the 800 mg group (89%), the 400 mg group (68%) and the 100 mg group (72%), than in the placebo group (50%), showed an improvement in appetite at last evaluation during the 12 study weeks. A statistically significant difference was observed between the 800 mg MA-treated group and the placebo group in the change in caloric intake from baseline to time of maximum weight change. Patients were asked to assess weight change, appetite, appearance, and overall perception of well-being in a 9 question survey. At maximum weight change only the 800 mg MA-treated group gave responses that were statistically significantly more favorable to all questions when compared to the placebo-treated group. A dose response was noted in the survey with positive responses correlating with higher dose for all questions.

The second trial was a multicenter, randomized, double-blind, placebo-controlled study comparing megestrol acetate 800 mg/day versus placebo in AIDS patients with anorexia/cachexia and significant weight loss. Of the 100 patients entered on study, 65 met all inclusion/exclusion criteria, had at least two additional post baseline weight measurements over a 12 week period or had one post baseline weight measurement but dropped out for therapeutic failure. Patients in the 800 mg MA-treated group had a statistically significantly larger increase in mean maximum weight change than patients in the placebo group. From baseline to study week 12, mean weight increased by 11.2 pounds in the MA-treated group and decreased 2.1 pounds in the placebo group. Changes in body composition as measured by bioelectrical impedance analysis showed increases in non-water weight in the MA-treated group (see **Clinical Studies Table**). No edema was reported in the MA-treated group. A greater percentage of MA-treated patients (67%) than placebo-treated patients (38%) showed an improvement in appetite at last evaluation during the 12 study weeks; this difference was statistically significant. There were no statistically significant differences between treatment groups in mean caloric change or in daily caloric intake at time to maximum weight change. In the same 9 question survey referenced in the first trial, patients' assessments of weight change, appetite, appearance, and overall perception of well-being showed increases in mean scores in MA-treated patients as compared to the placebo group.

In both trials, patients tolerated the drug well and no statistically significant differences were seen between the treatment groups with regard to laboratory abnormalities, new opportunistic infections, lymphocyte counts, T_4 counts, T_8 counts, or skin reactivity tests (see **ADVERSE REACTIONS**).

[See table above]

The following figures are the results of mean weight changes for patients evaluable for efficacy in trials 1 and 2.

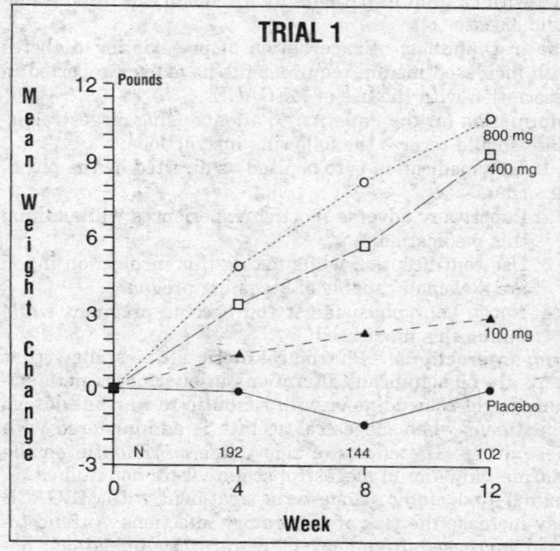

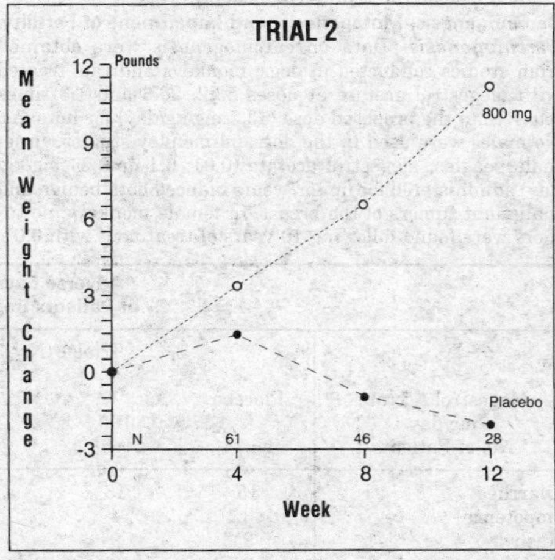

INDICATIONS AND USAGE

MEGACE (megestrol acetate) Oral Suspension is indicated for the treatment of anorexia, cachexia, or an unexplained, significant weight loss in patients with a diagnosis of acquired immunodeficiency syndrome (AIDS).

CONTRAINDICATIONS

History of hypersensitivity to megestrol acetate or any component of the formulation. Known or suspected pregnancy.

WARNINGS

Megestrol acetate may cause fetal harm when administered to a pregnant woman. For animal data on fetal effects (see

Continued on next page

Megace O.S.—Cont.

PRECAUTIONS: Impairment of Fertility). There are no adequate and well-controlled studies in pregnant women. If this drug is used during pregnancy, or if the patient becomes pregnant while taking (receiving) this drug, the patient should be apprised of the potential hazard to the fetus. Women of childbearing potential should be advised to avoid becoming pregnant.

Megestrol acetate is not intended for prophylactic use to avoid weight loss.

(See also **PRECAUTIONS: Carcinogenesis, Mutagenesis, and Impairment of Fertility**.)

Although the glucocorticoid activity of MEGACE Oral Suspension has not been fully evaluated, evidence of adrenal suppression has been observed. Clinical cases of new onset diabetes, exacerbation of pre-existing diabetes, and Cushing's syndrome have been reported in association with the use of MEGACE. Cases of clinically apparent adrenal insufficiency have also been reported in association with MEGACE. The possibility of adrenal suppression should be considered in any patient taking or withdrawing from chronic MEGACE therapy who presents with symptoms of adrenal insufficiency such as hypotension, nausea, vomiting, dizziness, or weakness. Laboratory evaluation for adrenal insufficiency and replacement stress doses of a rapidly acting glucocorticoid may be indicated for such patients. Failure to recognize inhibition of the hypothalmic-pituitary-adrenal axis may result in death.

PRECAUTIONS

General: Therapy with MEGACE Oral Suspension for weight loss should only be instituted after treatable causes of weight loss are sought and addressed. These treatable causes include possible malignancies, systemic infections, gastrointestinal disorders affecting absorption, endocrine disease and renal or psychiatric diseases.

Effects on HIV viral replication have not been determined. Use with caution in patients with a history of thromboembolic disease.

Use in Diabetics: Exacerbation of pre-existing diabetes with increased insulin requirements have been reported in association with the use of MEGACE.

Information for the Patients: Patients using megestrol acetate should receive the following instructions:

1. This medication is to be used as directed by the physician.
2. Report any adverse reaction experiences while taking this medication.
3. Use contraception while taking this medication if you are a woman capable of becoming pregnant.
4. Notify your physician if you become pregnant while taking this medication.

Drug Interactions: Pharmacokinetic studies show that there are no significant alterations in pharmacokinetic parameters of zidovudine or with rifabutin to warrant dosage adjustment when megestrol acetate is administered with these drugs. The effects of zidovudine or rifabutin on the pharmacokinetics of megestrol acetate were not studied.

Animal Toxicology: Long-term treatment with MEGACE may increase the risk of respiratory infections. A trend toward increased frequency of respiratory infections, decreased lymphocyte counts and increased neutrophil counts was observed in a two-year chronic toxicity/carcinogenicity study of megestrol acetate conducted in rats.

Carcinogenesis, Mutagenesis, and Impairment of Fertility:
Carcinogenesis—Data on carcinogenesis were obtained from studies conducted in dogs, monkeys and rats treated with megestrol acetate at doses 53.2, 26.6 and 1.3 times *lower* than the proposed dose (13.3 mg/kg/day) for humans. No males were used in the dog and monkey studies. In female beagles, megestrol acetate (0.01, 0.1 or 0.25 mg/kg/day) administered for up to 7 years induced both benign and malignant tumors of the breast. In female monkeys, no tumors were found following 10 years of treatment with 0.01, 0.1 or 0.5 mg/kg/day megestrol acetate. Pituitary tumors were observed in female rats treated with 3.9 or 10 mg/kg/day of megestrol acetate for 2 years. The relationship of these tumors in rats and dogs to humans is unknown but should be considered in assessing the risk-to-benefit ratio when prescribing MEGACE Oral Suspension and in surveillance of patients on therapy. (See **WARNINGS**.)

Mutagenesis—No mutagenesis data are currently available.

Impairment of Fertility—Perinatal/postnatal (segment III) toxicity studies were performed in rats at doses (0.05–12.5 mg/kg) *less* than that indicated for humans (13.3 mg/kg); in these low dose studies, the reproductive capability of male offspring of megestrol acetate-treated females was impaired. Similar results were obtained in dogs. Pregnant rats treated with megestrol acetate showed a reduction in fetal weight and number of live births, and feminization of male fetuses. No toxicity data are currently available on male reproduction (spermatogenesis).

Pregnancy: Pregnancy "Category X". (See **WARNINGS** and **PRECAUTIONS: Impairment of Fertility**.) No adequate animal teratology information is available at clinically relevant doses.

Nursing Mothers: Because of the potential for adverse effects on the newborn, nursing should be discontinued if MEGACE Oral Suspension is required.

Use in HIV-Infected Women: Although megestrol acetate has been used extensively in women for the treatment of endometrial and breast cancers, its use in HIV-infected women has been limited.

All 10 women in the clinical trials reported breakthrough bleeding.

Pediatric Use: Safety and effectiveness in pediatric patients have not been established.

ADVERSE REACTIONS

Clinical Adverse Events: Adverse events which occurred in at least 5% of patients in any arm of the two clinical efficacy trials and the open trial are listed below by treatment group. All patients listed had at least one post baseline visit during the 12 study weeks. These adverse events should be considered by the physician when prescribing MEGACE Oral Suspension.

[See table below]

Adverse events which occurred in 1% to 3% of all patients enrolled in the two clinical efficacy trials with at least one follow-up visit during the first 12 weeks of the study are listed below by body system. Adverse events occurring less than 1% are not included. There were no significant differences between incidence of these events in patients treated with megestrol acetate and patients treated with placebo.

Body as a Whole—abdominal pain, chest pain, infection, moniliasis and sarcoma

Cardiovascular System—cardiomyopathy and palpitation

Digestive System—constipation, dry mouth, hepatomegaly, increased salivation and oral moniliasis

Hemic and Lymphatic System—leukopenia

Metabolic and Nutritional—LDH increased, edema and peripheral edema

Nervous System—paresthesia, confusion, convulsion, depression, neuropathy, hypesthesia and abnormal thinking

Respiratory System—dyspnea, cough, pharyngitis and lung disorder

Skin and Appendages—alopecia, herpes, pruritus, vesiculobullous rash, sweating and skin disorder

Special Senses—amblyopia

Urogenital System—albuminuria, urinary incontinence, urinary tract infection and gynecomastia

Postmarketing—Postmarketing reports associated with MEGACE (megestrol acetate) Oral Suspension include thromboembolic phenomena including thrombophlebitis, pulmonary embolism and glucose intolerance (see **WARNINGS** and **PRECAUTIONS**).

OVERDOSAGE

No serious unexpected side effects have resulted from studies involving MEGACE Oral Suspension administered in dosages as high as 1200 mg/day. Megestrol acetate has not been tested for dialyzability; however, due to its low solubility it is postulated that dialysis would not be an effective means of treating overdose.

Adverse Events
% of Patients Reporting

	Trial 1 (N=236)				Trial 2 (N=87)		Open Label Trial
Megestrol Acetate mg/day No. of Patients	Placebo 0 N=34	100 N=68	400 N=69	800 N=65	Placebo 0 N=38	800 N=49	1200 N=176
Diarrhea	15	13	8	15	8	6	10
Impotence	3	4	6	14	0	4	7
Rash	9	9	4	12	3	2	6
Flatulence	9	0	1	9	3	10	6
Hypertension	0	0	0	8	0	0	4
Asthenia	3	2	3	6	8	4	5
Insomnia	0	3	4	6	0	0	1
Nausea	9	4	0	5	3	4	5
Anemia	6	3	3	5	0	0	0
Fever	3	6	4	5	3	2	1
Libido Decreased	3	4	0	5	0	2	1
Dyspepsia	0	0	3	3	5	4	2
Hyperglycemia	3	0	6	3	0	0	3
Headache	6	10	1	3	3	0	3
Pain	6	0	0	2	5	6	4
Vomiting	9	3	0	2	3	6	4
Pneumonia	6	2	0	2	3	0	1
Urinary Freq.	0	0	1	2	5	2	1

DOSAGE AND ADMINISTRATION

The recommended adult initial dosage of MEGACE Oral Suspension is 800 mg/day (20 mL/day). Shake container well before using.

In clinical trials evaluating different dose schedules, daily doses of 400 and 800 mg/day were found to be clinically effective.

A plastic dosage cup with 10 mL and 20 mL markings is provided for convenience.

HOW SUPPLIED

MEGACE® (megestrol acetate) Oral Suspension is available as a lemon-lime flavored oral suspension containing 40 mg of micronized megestrol acetate per mL.

NDC 0015-0508-42 Bottles of 240 mL (8 fl. oz.)

STORAGE

Store MEGACE Oral Suspension between 15°–25°C (59°–77°F) and dispense in a tight container. Protect from heat.

SPECIAL HANDLING

Health Hazard Data: There is no threshold limit value established by OSHA, NIOSH, or ACGIH.

Exposure or "overdose" at levels approaching recommended dosing levels could result in side effects described above (see **WARNINGS** and **ADVERSE REACTIONS**). Women at risk of pregnancy should avoid such exposure.

Mead Johnson
ONCOLOGY PRODUCTS
A Bristol-Myers Squibb Company
Princeton, NJ 08543
U.S.A.

H7-B001A-3-00 J4-651A

Revised: February 2000

Shown in Product Identification Guide, page 310

MEGACE® ℞

[mĕg 'ace]

(megestrol acetate tablets, USP)

℞ ONLY

DESCRIPTION

MEGACE® (megestrol acetate tablets, USP) is a synthetic, antineoplastic and progestational drug. Megestrol acetate is a white, crystalline solid chemically designated as 17α-acetyloxy-6-methylpregna-4,6-diene-3, 20-dione. Solubility at 37°C in water is 2 mcg per mL, solubility in plasma is 24 mcg per mL. Its molecular weight is 384.51. The empirical formula is $C_{24}H_{32}O_4$ and the structural formula is represented as follows:

megestrol acetate tablets, USP

MEGACE is supplied as tablets for oral administration containing 20 mg and 40 mg megestrol acetate.

MEGACE tablets contain the following inactive ingredients: acacia, calcium phosphate, FD&C Blue No. 1 Aluminum Lake, lactose, magnesium stearate, silicon dioxide colloidal, and starch.

CLINICAL PHARMACOLOGY

While the precise mechanism by which MEGACE produces its antineoplastic effects against endometrial carcinoma is unknown at the present time, inhibition of pituitary gonadotrophin production and resultant decrease in estrogen secretion may be factors. There is evidence to suggest a local effect as a result of the marked changes brought about by the direct instillation of progestational agents into the endometrial cavity. The antineoplastic action of megestrol acetate on carcinoma of the breast is effected by modifying the action of other steroid hormones and by exerting a direct cytotoxic effect on tumor cells.[1] In metastatic cancer, hormone receptors may be present in some tissues but not others. The receptor mechanism is a cyclic process whereby estrogen produced by the ovaries enters the target cell, forms a complex with cytoplasmic receptor and is transported into the cell nucleus. There it induces gene transcription and leads to the alteration of normal cell functions. Pharmacologic doses of megestrol acetate not only decrease the number of hormone-dependent human breast cancer cells but also is capable of modifying and abolishing the stimulatory effects of estrogen on these cells. It has been suggested[2] that progestins may inhibit in one of two ways: by interfering with either the stability, availability, or turnover of the estrogen receptor complex in its interaction with genes or in conjunction with the progestin receptor complex, by interacting directly with the genome to turn off specific estrogen-responsive genes.

There are several analytical methods used to estimate MEGACE plasma levels, including mass fragmentography, gas chromatography (GC), high pressure liquid chromatography (HPLC), and radioimmunoassay. The plasma levels by HPLC assay or radioimmunoassay methods are about one-sixth those obtained by the GC method. The plasma levels are dependent not only on the method used, but also on intestinal and hepatic inactivation of the drug, which may be affected by factors such as intestinal tract motility, intestinal bacteria, antibiotics administered, body weight, diet, and liver function.[3,4]

Metabolites account for only 5% to 8% of the administered dose and are considered negligible.[5] The major route of drug elimination in humans is the urine. When radio-labeled megestrol acetate was administered to humans in doses of 4 to 90 mg, the urinary excretion within 10 days ranged from 56.5% to 78.4% (mean 66.4%) and fecal excretion ranged from 7.7% to 30.3% (mean 19.8%). The total recovered radioactivity varied between 83.1% and 94.7% (mean 86.2%). Respiratory excretion as labeled carbon dioxide and fat storage may have accounted for at least part of the radioactivity not found in the urine and feces.

In normal male volunteers (n=23) who received 160 mg of megestrol acetate given as a 40 mg qid regimen, the oral absorption of MEGACE appeared to be variable. Plasma levels were assayed by a high pressure liquid chromatographic (HPLC) procedure. Peak drug levels for the first 40 mg dose ranged from 10 to 56 ng/mL (mean 27.6 ng/mL) and the times to peak concentrations ranged from 1.0 to 3.0 hours (mean 2.2 hours). Plasma elimination half-life ranged from 13.0 to 104.9 hours (mean 34.2 hours). The steady state plasma concentrations for a 40 mg qid regimen have not been established.

INDICATION AND USAGE

MEGACE is indicated for the palliative treatment of advanced carcinoma of the breast or endometrium (i.e., recurrent, inoperable, or metastatic disease). It should not be used in lieu of currently accepted procedures such as surgery, radiation, or chemotherapy.

CONTRAINDICATIONS

History of hypersensitivity to megestrol acetate or any component of the formulation.

WARNINGS

Megestrol acetate may cause fetal harm when administered to a pregnant woman. Fertility and reproduction studies with high doses of megestrol acetate have shown a reversible feminizing effect on some male rat fetuses.[6] There are no adequate and well-controlled studies in pregnant women. If this drug is used during pregnancy, or if the patient becomes pregnant while taking (receiving) this drug, the patient should be apprised of the potential hazard to the fetus. Women of childbearing potential should be advised to avoid becoming pregnant.

The use of MEGACE (megestrol acetate tablets, USP) in other types of neoplastic disease is not recommended.

(See also **PRECAUTIONS: Carcinogenesis, Mutagenesis, and Impairment of Fertility.**)

Although the glucocorticoid activity of MEGACE tablets has not been fully evaluated, evidence of adrenal suppression has been observed. Clinical cases of new onset diabetes, exacerbation of pre-existing diabetes, and Cushing's syndrome have been reported in association with the use of MEGACE. Cases of clinically apparent adrenal insufficiency have also been reported in association with MEGACE. The possibility of adrenal suppression should be considered in any patient taking or withdrawing from chronic MEGACE therapy who presents with symptoms of adrenal insufficiency such as hypotension, nausea, vomiting, dizziness, or weakness. Laboratory evaluation for adrenal insufficiency and replacement stress doses of a rapidly acting glucocorticoid may be indicated for such patients. Failure to recognize inhibition of the hypothalmic-pituitary-adrenal axis may result in death.

PRECAUTIONS

General: Close surveillance is indicated for any patient treated for recurrent or metastatic cancer. Use with caution in patients with a history of thromboembolic disease.

Use in Diabetics: Exacerbation of pre-existing diabetes with increased insulin requirements has been reported in association with the use of MEGACE.

Information for the Patients: Patients using megestrol acetate should receive the following instructions:

1. This medication is to be used as directed by the physician.
2. Report any adverse reaction experiences while taking this medication.

Laboratory Tests: Breast malignancies in which estrogen and/or progesterone receptors are positive are more likely to respond to MEGACE.[7, 8, 9]

Carcinogenesis, Mutagenesis, and Impairment of Fertility: Administration of megestrol acetate to female dogs for up to 7 years is associated with an increased incidence of both benign and malignant tumors of the breast.[10] Comparable studies in rats and studies in monkeys are not associated with an increased incidence of tumors. The relationship of the dog tumors to humans is unknown but should be considered in assessing the benefit-to-risk ratio when prescribing MEGACE and in surveillance of patients on therapy.[10,11] (See **WARNINGS**.)

Pregnancy: Pregnancy "Category D". (See **WARNINGS**.)

Nursing Mothers: Because of the potential for adverse effects on the newborn, nursing should be discontinued if MEGACE is required for treatment of cancer.

Pediatric Use: Safety and effectiveness in pediatric patients have not been established.

ADVERSE REACTIONS

Weight Gain: Weight gain is a frequent side effect of MEGACE.[12,13] This gain has been associated with increased appetite and is not necessarily associated with fluid retention.

Thromboembolic Phenomena: Thromboembolic phenomena including thrombophlebitis and pulmonary embolism (in some cases fatal) have been reported.

Glucocorticoid Effects: (See **WARNINGS**.)

Other Adverse Reactions: Heart failure, nausea and vomiting, edema, breakthrough menstrual bleeding, dyspnea, tumor flare (with or without hypercalcemia), hyperglycemia, glucose intolerance, alopecia, hypertension, carpal tunnel syndrome, mood changes, hot flashes, malaise, asthenia, lethargy, sweating and rash.

OVERDOSAGE

No serious unexpected side effects have resulted from studies involving MEGACE administered in dosages as high as 1600 mg/day. Oral administration of large, single doses of megestrol acetate (5 g/kg) did not produce toxic effects in mice.[6] Megestrol acetate has not been tested for dialyzability; however, due to its low solubility it is postulated that this would not be an effective means of treating overdose.

DOSAGE AND ADMINISTRATION

Breast Cancer: 160 mg/day (40 mg q.i.d.).

Endometrial Carcinoma: 40–320 mg/day in divided doses.

At least 2 months of continuous treatment is considered an adequate period for determining the efficacy of MEGACE.

HOW SUPPLIED

MEGACE® (megestrol acetate tablets, USP) is available as light blue, scored tablets containing 20 mg or 40 mg megestrol acetate, USP.

NDC 0015-0595-01	20 mg tablet, bottles of 100
NDC 0015-0596-41	40 mg tablet, bottles of 100
NDC 0015-0596-45	40 mg tablet, bottles of 500
NDC 0015-0596-46	40 mg tablet, bottles of 250

STORAGE

Store MEGACE at room temperature; protect from temperatures above 40°C (104°F).

SPECIAL HANDLING

Health Hazard Data: There is no threshold limit value established by OSHA, NIOSH, or ACGIH.

Exposure or "overdose" at levels approaching recommended dosing levels could result in side effects described above (see **WARNINGS** and **ADVERSE REACTIONS**). Women at risk of pregnancy should avoid such exposure.

REFERENCES

1. Allegra JC, Kiefer SM: Mechanisms of Action of Progestational Agents. *Semin Oncol* 1985; 12(Suppl 1):3.
2. DeSombre ER, Kuivanen PC: Progestin Modulation of Estrogen-Dependent Marker Protein Synthesis in the Endometrium. *Semin Oncol* 1985; 12(Suppl 1):6.
3. Alexieva-Figusch J, Blankenstein MA, Hop WCJ, et al: Treatment of Metastatic Breast Cancer Patients with Different Dosages of Megestrol Acetate: Dose Relations, Metabolic and Endocrine Effects. *Eur J Cancer Clin Oncol* 1984; 20:33-40.
4. Gaver RC, Movahhed HS, Farmen RH, Pittman KA: Liquid Chromatographic Procedure for the Quantitative Analysis of Megestrol Acetate in Human Plasma. *J Pharm Sci* 1985; 74:664.
5. Cooper JM, Kellie AE: The Metabolism of Megestrol Acetate (17-alpha-acetoxy-6-methylpregna-4,6-diene-3, 20-dione) in Women. *Steroids* 1968;11:133.
6. David A, Edwards K, Fellowes KP, Plummer JM: Anti-Ovulatory and Other Biological Properties of Megestrol Acetate. *J Reprod Fertil* 1963; 5:331.
7. McGuire WL, Clark GM: The Prognostic Role of Progesterone Receptors in Human Breast Cancer. *Semin Oncol* 1983; 10(suppl 4):2.
8. Horwitz KB: The Central Role of Progesterone Receptors and Progestational Agents in the Management and Treatment of Breast Cancer. *Semin Oncol* 1988; 15(Suppl 1):14.
9. Bonomi P, Johnson P, Anderson K, Wolter J, Bunting N, Strauss A, Roseman D, Shorey W, Econonou S: Primary Hormonal Therapy of Advanced Breast Cancer with Megestrol Acetate: Predictive Value of Estrogen Receptor and Progesterone Receptor Levels. *Semin Oncol* 1985; 12(Suppl 1):48-54.
10. Nelson LW, Weikel JH Jr., Reno FE: Mammary Nodules in Dogs During Four Years' Treatment with Megestrol Acetate or Chlormadinone Acetate. *J Natl Cancer Inst* 1973; 51:1303.
11. Owen LN, Briggs MH: Contraceptive Steroid Toxicology in the Beagle Dog and its Relevance to Human Carcinogenicity. *Curr Med Res Opin* 1976; 4:309.
12. Ansfield FJ, Kallas GJ, Singson JP: Clinical Results with Megestrol Acetate in Patients with Advanced Carcinoma of the Breast. *Surg Gynecol Obstet* 1982; 155: 888.
13. Alexieva-Figusch J, van Gilse HA, Hop WCJ, et al: Progestin Therapy in Advanced Breast Cancer: Megestrol Acetate—An Evaluation of 160 Treated Cases. *Cancer* 1980; 46:2369.

Mead Johnson
ONCOLOGY PRODUCTS
A Bristol-Myers Squibb Company
Princeton, NJ 08543
U.S.A.

H7-B001-3-00 595DIM-08
Revised: February 2000

Shown in Product Identification Guide, page 310

MESNEX® Rx ONLY

[*mĕs-nĕx*]
(Mesna) Injection

DESCRIPTION

MESNEX® (mesna) Injection is a detoxifying agent to inhibit the hemorrhagic cystitis induced by ifosfamide (IFEX®). The active ingredient mesna is a synthetic sulfhydryl compound designated as sodium 2-mercaptoethane sulfonate with a molecular formula of $C_2H_5NaO_3S_2$ and a molecular weight of 164.18. Its structural formula is as follows:

$HS\text{-}CH_2\text{-}CH_2SO_3\text{-}Na^+$

MESNEX Injection is a sterile, nonpyrogenic, aqueous solution of clear and colorless appearance in clear glass single dose ampules or multidose vials for intravenous administration. MESNEX Injection contains 100 mg/mL mesna, 0.25 mg/mL edetate disodium and sodium hydroxide for pH adjustment. MESNEX Injection multidose vials also contain 10.4 mg of benzyl alcohol as a preservative. The solution has a pH range of 6.5–8.5.

CLINICAL PHARMACOLOGY

MESNEX was developed as a prophylactic agent to prevent the hemorrhagic cystitis induced by ifosfamide.

Analogous to the physiological cysteine-cystine system, following intravenous administration, mesna is rapidly oxidized to its only metabolite, mesna disulfide (dimesna). Mesna disulfide remains in the intravascular compartment and is rapidly eliminated by the kidneys.

In the kidney, the mesna disulfide is reduced to the free thiol compound, mesna, which reacts chemically with the urotoxic ifosfamide metabolites (acrolein and 4-hydroxy-ifosfamide) resulting in their detoxification. The first step in the detoxification process is the binding of mesna to 4-hydroxy-ifosfamide forming a nonurotoxic 4-sulfoethylthioifosfamide. Mesna also binds to the double bonds of acrolein and other urotoxic metabolites.

After administration of an 800 mg dose the half-lives of mesna and dimesna in the blood are 0.36 hours and 1.17 hours respectively. Approximately 32% and 33% of the administered dose was eliminated in the urine in 24 hours as mesna and dimesna respectively. The majority of the dose recovered was eliminated within 4 hours. Mesna has a volume of distribution of 0.652 L/kg and a plasma clearance of 1.23 L/kg/hour.

Ifosfamide has been shown to have dose dependent pharmacokinetics in humans. At doses of 2–4 g, its terminal elimination half-life is about 7 hours. As a result, in order to maintain adequate levels of mesna in the urinary bladder during the course of elimination of the urotoxic ifosfamide metabolites, repeated doses of MESNEX are required.

Based on the pharmacokinetic profiles of mesna and ifosfamide as discussed above, MESNEX was given as bolus doses prior to ifosfamide and at 4 and 8 hours after ifosfamide administration. The hemorrhagic cystitis produced by ifosfamide is dose dependent. At a dose of 1.2 g/m² ifosfamide administered daily for 5 days, 16–26% of the patients who received conventional uroprophylaxis (high fluid intake, alkalinization of the urine and the administration of diuretics) developed hematuria > 50 rbc/hpf or macrohematuria). In contrast, none of the patients who received MESNEX together with this dose of ifosfamide developed hematuria. Higher doses of ifosfamide from 2 to 4 g/m² administered for three to five days, produced hematuria in 31 to 100% of the patients. When MESNEX was administered together with these doses of ifosfamide the incidence of hematuria was less than 7%.

INDICATIONS AND USAGE

MESNEX has been shown to be effective as a prophylactic agent in reducing the incidence of ifosfamide-induced hemorrhagic cystitis.

CONTRAINDICATIONS

MESNEX is contraindicated in patients known to be hypersensitive to mesna or other thiol compounds.

WARNINGS

Allergic reactions to mesna were reported in patients with autoimmune disorders. The majority of the patients received high doses of mesna orally. The symptoms ranged from mild hypersensitivity to systemic anaphylactic reactions.

MESNEX has been developed as an agent to prevent ifosfamide-induced hemorrhagic cystitis. It will not prevent or alleviate any of the other adverse reactions or toxicities associated with ifosfamide therapy.

MESNEX does not prevent hemorrhagic cystitis in all patients. Up to 6% of patients treated with mesna have developed hematuria (> 50 rbc/hpf or WHO grade 2 and above). As a result, a morning specimen of urine should be examined for the presence of hematuria (red blood cells) each day prior to ifosfamide therapy. If hematuria develops when MESNEX is given with ifosfamide according to the recommended dosage schedule, depending on the severity of the hematuria, dosage reductions or discontinuation of ifosfamide therapy may be initiated.

Continued on next page

Mesnex—Cont.

In order to obtain adequate protection, MESNEX must be administered with each dose of ifosfamide as outlined in the **"DOSAGE AND ADMINISTRATION"** section. MESNEX is not effective in preventing hematuria due to other pathological conditions such as thrombocytopenia.
Because of the benzyl alcohol content, the multidose vial should not be used in neonates or infants and should be used with caution in older pediatric patients.

PRECAUTIONS

Laboratory Tests: A false positive test for urinary ketones may arise in patients treated with MESNEX (mesna) Injection. In this test, a red-violet color develops which, with the addition of glacial acetic acid, will return to violet.
Pediatrics: Because of the benzyl alcohol content, the multidose vial should not be used in neonates or infants and should be used with caution in older pediatric patients.
Drug Interactions: *In vitro* and *in vivo* animal tumor models have shown that mesna does not have any effect on the antitumor efficacy of concomitantly administered cytotoxic agents.
Carcinogenesis, Mutagenesis and Impairment of Fertility: No long term animal studies have been performed to evaluate the carcinogenic potential of mesna. The Ames Salmonella typhimurium test, mouse micronucleus assay and frequency of sister chromatid exchange and chromosomal aberrations in PHA-stimulated lymphocytes *in vitro* assays revealed no mutagenic activity.
Pregnancy: Pregnancy "Category B". Reproduction studies in rats and rabbits with oral doses up to 1000 mg/kg have revealed no harm to the fetus due to mesna. It is not known whether MESNEX can cause fetal harm when administered to a pregnant woman or can affect reproductive capacity. MESNEX should be given to a pregnant woman only if the benefits clearly outweigh any possible risks.
Teratology studies in rats and rabbits have shown no effects.
Nursing Mothers: It is not known whether mesna or dimesna is excreted in human milk. Because many drugs are excreted in human milk and because of the potential for adverse reactions in nursing infants from mesna, a decision should be made whether to discontinue nursing or discontinue the drug, taking into account the importance of the drug to the mother.

ADVERSE REACTIONS

Because mesna is used in combination with ifosfamide and other chemotherapeutic agents with documented toxicities, it is difficult to distinguish the adverse reactions which may be due to MESNEX from those caused by the concomitantly administered cytostatic agents. As a result, the adverse reaction profile of MESNEX was determined in three Phase I studies (16 subjects) utilizing intravenous and oral administration and two controlled studies in which ifosfamide and mesna were compared to ifosfamide and standard prophylaxis.
In Phase I studies in which I.V. bolus doses of 0.8 to 1.6 g/m^2 MESNEX were administered as single or three repeated doses to a total of 10 patients, a bad taste in the mouth (100%) and soft stools (70%) were reported. At intravenous and oral bolus doses of 2.4 g/m^2 which are approximately 10 times the recommended clinical doses (0.24 g/m^2) headache (50%), fatigue (33%), nausea (33%), diarrhea (83%), limb pain (50%), hypotension (17%) and allergy (17%) have also been reported in the 6 patients who participated in this study.
In controlled clinical studies, adverse reactions which can be reasonably associated with mesna were vomiting, diarrhea and nausea.

OVERDOSAGE

There is no known antidote for MESNEX.

DOSAGE AND ADMINISTRATION

For the prophylaxis of ifosfamide-induced hemorrhagic cystitis, MESNEX may be given on a fractionated dosing schedule of bolus intravenous injections as outlined below.
MESNEX is given as intravenous bolus injections in a dosage equal to 20% of the ifosfamide dosage (w/w) at the time of ifosfamide administration and 4 and 8 hours after each dose of ifosfamide. The total daily dose of mesna is 60% of the ifosfamide dose.
The recommended dosing schedule is outlined below:

	0 hours	4 hours	8 hours
Ifosfamide	1.2 g/m^2	–	–
MESNEX	240 mg/m^2	240 mg/m^2	240 mg/m^2

In order to maintain adequate protection, this dosing schedule should be repeated on each day that ifosfamide is administered. When the dosage of ifosfamide is adjusted (either increased or decreased), the dose of MESNEX should be modified accordingly. When exposed to oxygen, mesna is oxidized to the disulfide, dimesna. As a result, if the ampules are used, any unused mesna remaining in the ampules after dosing should be discarded and new ampules used for each administration.
The MESNEX multidose vials may be stored and used for up to 8 days.

PREPARATION OF INTRAVENOUS SOLUTIONS/STABILITY
For I.V. administration the drug can be diluted by adding the MESNEX Injection solution to any of the following fluids obtaining final concentrations of 20 mg mesna/mL fluid:

- 5% Dextrose Injection, USP
- 5% Dextrose and 0.2% Sodium Chloride Injection, USP
- 5% Dextrose and 0.33% Sodium Chloride Injection, USP
- 5% Dextrose and 0.45% Sodium Chloride Injection, USP
- 0.92% Sodium Chloride Injection, USP
- Lactated Ringer's Injection, USP

For example:
One mL of MESNEX (mesna) Injection multidose vial 100 mg/mL may be added to 4 mL, or one ampule of MESNEX Injection 200 mg/2 mL may be added to 8 mL of any of the solutions listed above to create a final concentration of 20 mg mesna/mL fluid.
Diluted solutions are chemically and physically stable for 24 hours at 25°C (77°F).
Mesna is not compatible with cisplatin.
Parenteral drug products should be inspected visually for particulate matter and discoloration prior to administration.

HOW SUPPLIED

MESNEX® (mesna) Injection 100 mg/mL
NDC 0015-3560-41
200 mg Single Dose Ampule, Box of 15 Ampules of 2-mL (color-ring coding: turquoise/yellow)
NDC 0015-3563-02
1 g Multidose Vial,
Box of 1 vial of 10 mL
NDC 0015-3563-03
1 g Multidose Vial,
Box of 10 vials of 10 mL
Store at controlled room temperature 15–30°C (59°–86°F).
U.S. Patent No.: 4,220,660
Distributed by:
Mead Johnson
ONCOLOGY PRODUCTS
A Bristol-Myers Squibb Company
Princeton, NJ 08543
U.S.A.
Manufactured by:
ASTA MEDICA
A Degussa Company
Frankfurt am Mein
Germany
H8-B001-5-98 N1217-00
Revised: March 1998

Shown in Product Identification Guide, page 310

MUTAMYCIN® ℞

[*mū″-tĕ-mī′-sĭn*]
(mitomycin for injection, USP)
Rx ONLY

> **WARNING**
> MUTAMYCIN® (mitomycin for injection, USP) should be administered under the supervision of a qualified physician experienced in the use of cancer chemotherapeutic agents. Appropriate management of therapy and complications is possible only when adequate diagnostic and treatment facilities are readily available.
> Bone marrow suppression, notably thrombocytopenia and leukopenia, which may contribute to overwhelming infections in an already compromised patient, is the most common and severe of the toxic effects of MUTAMYCIN (see **WARNINGS** and **ADVERSE REACTIONS** sections).
> Hemolytic Uremic Syndrome (HUS) a serious complication of chemotherapy, consisting primarily of microangiopathic hemolytic anemia, thrombocytopenia, and irreversible renal failure has been reported in patients receiving systemic MUTAMYCIN. The syndrome may occur at any time during systemic therapy with MUTAMYCIN as a single agent or in combination with other cytotoxic drugs, however, most cases occur at doses ≥ 60 mg of MUTAMYCIN. Blood product transfusion may exacerbate the symptoms associated with this syndrome.
> The incidence of the syndrome has not been defined.

DESCRIPTION

MUTAMYCIN® (mitomycin for injection, USP) (also known as mitomycin and/or mitomycin-C) is an antibiotic isolated from the broth of *Streptomyces caespitosus* which has been shown to have antitumor activity. The compound is heat stable, has a high melting point, and is freely soluble in organic solvents.

ACTION

MUTAMYCIN selectively inhibits the synthesis of deoxyribonucleic acid (DNA). The guanine and cytosine content correlates with the degree of MUTAMYCIN-induced cross-linking. At high concentrations of the drug, cellular RNA and protein synthesis are also suppressed.
In humans, MUTAMYCIN is rapidly cleared from the serum after intravenous administration. Time required to reduce the serum concentration by 50% after a 30 mg bolus injection is 17 minutes. After injection of 30 mg, 20 mg, or 10 mg I.V., the maximal serum concentrations were 2.4 µg/mL, 1.7 µg/mL, and 0.52 µg/mL, respectively. Clearance is effected primarily by metabolism in the liver, but metabolism occurs in other tissues as well. The rate of clearance is inversely proportional to the maximal serum concentration because, it is thought, of saturation of the degradative pathways.
Approximately 10% of a dose of MUTAMYCIN is excreted unchanged in the urine. Since metabolic pathways are saturated at relatively low doses, the percent of a dose excreted in urine increases with increasing dose. In children, excretion of intravenously administered MUTAMYCIN is similar.
Animal Toxicology: MUTAMYCIN has been found to be carcinogenic in rats and mice. At doses approximating the recommended clinical dose in man, it produces a greater than 100% increase in tumor incidence in male Sprague-Dawley rats, and a greater than 50% increase in tumor incidence in female Swiss mice.

INDICATIONS

MUTAMYCIN is not recommended as single-agent, primary therapy. It has been shown to be useful in the therapy of disseminated adenocarcinoma of the stomach or pancreas in proven combinations with other approved chemotherapeutic agents and as palliative treatment when other modalities have failed. MUTAMYCIN is not recommended to replace appropriate surgery and/or radiotherapy.

CONTRAINDICATIONS

MUTAMYCIN is contraindicated in patients who have demonstrated a hypersensitive or idiosyncratic reaction to it in the past.
MUTAMYCIN is contraindicated in patients with thrombocytopenia, coagulation disorder, or an increase in bleeding tendency due to other causes.

WARNINGS

Patients being treated with MUTAMYCIN must be observed carefully and frequently during and after therapy.
The use of MUTAMYCIN results in a high incidence of bone marrow suppression, particularly thrombocytopenia and leukopenia. Therefore, the following studies should be obtained repeatedly during therapy and for at least eight weeks following therapy: platelet count, white blood cell count, differential, and hemoglobin. The occurrence of a platelet count below 100,000/mm^3 or a WBC below 4,000/mm^3 or a progressive decline in either is an indication to withhold further therapy until blood counts have recovered above these levels.
Patients should be advised of the potential toxicity of this drug, particularly bone marrow suppression. Deaths have been reported due to septicemia as a result of leukopenia due to the drug.
Patients receiving MUTAMYCIN should be observed for evidence of renal toxicity. MUTAMYCIN should not be given to patients with a serum creatinine greater than 1.7 mg percent.
Usage in Pregnancy: Safe use of MUTAMYCIN in pregnant women has not been established. Teratological changes have been noted in animal studies. The effect of MUTAMYCIN on fertility is unknown.

PRECAUTIONS

Acute shortness of breath and severe bronchospasm have been reported following the administration of vinca alkaloids in patients who had previously or simultaneously received MUTAMYCIN. The onset of this acute respiratory distress occurred within minutes to hours after the vinca alkaloid injection. The total number of doses for each drug has varied considerably. Bronchodilators, steroids and/or oxygen have produced symptomatic relief.
A few cases of adult respiratory distress syndrome have been reported in patients receiving MUTAMYCIN in combination with other chemotherapy and maintained at FIO_2 concentrations greater than 50% perioperatively. Therefore, caution should be exercised using only enough oxygen to provide adequate arterial saturation since oxygen itself is toxic to the lungs. Careful attention should be paid to fluid balance and overhydration should be avoided.
Bladder fibrosis/contraction has been reported with intravesical administration (not an approved route of administration), which in rare cases has required cystectomy.
Nursing Mothers: It is not known if mitomycin is excreted in human milk. Because many drugs are excreted in human milk and because of the potential for serious adverse reactions in nursing infants from mitomycin, it is recommended that nursing be discontinued when receiving mitomycin therapy.
Pediatric Use: Safety and effectiveness in pediatric patients have not been established.

ADVERSE REACTIONS

Bone Marrow Toxicity: This was the most common and most serious toxicity, occurring in 605 of 937 patients (64.4%). Thrombocytopenia and/or leukopenia may occur anytime within 8 weeks after onset of therapy with an average time of 4 weeks. Recovery after cessation of therapy was within 10 weeks. About 25% of the leukopenic or thrombocytopenic episodes did not recover. MUTAMYCIN produces cumulative myelosuppression.
Integument and Mucous Membrane Toxicity: This has occurred in approximately 4% of patients treated with MUTAMYCIN (mitomycin for injection, USP). Cellulitis at the injection site has been reported and is occasionally severe. Stomatitis and alopecia also occur frequently. Rashes are rarely reported. The most important dermatological problem with this drug, however, is the necrosis and consequent sloughing of tissue which results if the drug is extravasated during injection. Extravasation may occur with or without an accompanying stinging or burning sensation and

even if there is adequate blood return when the injection needle is aspirated. There have been reports of delayed erythema and/or ulceration occurring either at or distant from the injection site, weeks to months after MUTAMYCIN, even when no obvious evidence of extravasation was observed during administration. Skin grafting has been required in some of the cases.

Renal Toxicity: 2% of 1,281 patients demonstrated a statistically significant rise in creatinine. There appeared to be no correlation between total dose administered or duration of therapy and the degree of renal impairment.

Pulmonary Toxicity: This has occurred infrequently but can be severe and may be life threatening. Dyspnea with a nonproductive cough and radiographic evidence of pulmonary infiltrates may be indicative of MUTAMYCIN-induced pulmonary toxicity. If other etiologies are eliminated, MUTAMYCIN therapy should be discontinued. Steroids have been employed as treatment of this toxicity, but the therapeutic value has not been determined. A few cases of adult respiratory distress syndrome have been reported in patients receiving MUTAMYCIN in combination with other chemotherapy and maintained at FIO_2 concentrations greater than 50% perioperatively.

Hemolytic Uremic Syndrome (HUS): This serious complication of chemotherapy, consisting primarily of microangiopathic hemolytic anemia (hematocrit ≤ 25%), thrombocytopenia (≤ 100,000/mm^3), and irreversible renal failure (serum creatinine ≥ 1.6 mg/dL) has been reported in patients receiving systemic MUTAMYCIN. Microangiopathic hemolysis with fragmented red blood cells on peripheral blood smears has occurred in 98% of patients with the syndrome. Other less frequent complications of the syndrome may include pulmonary edema (65%), neurologic abnormalities (16%), and hypertension. Exacerbation of the symptoms associated with HUS has been reported in some patients receiving blood product transfusions. A high mortality rate (52%) has been associated with this syndrome.

The syndrome may occur at any time during systemic therapy with MUTAMYCIN as a single agent or in combination with other cytotoxic drugs. Less frequently, HUS has also been reported in patients receiving combinations of cytotoxic drugs not including MUTAMYCIN. Of 83 patients studied, 72 developed the syndrome at total doses exceeding 60 mg of MUTAMYCIN. Consequently, patients receiving ≥ 60 mg of MUTAMYCIN should be monitored closely for unexplained anemia with fragmented cells on peripheral blood smear, thrombocytopenia, and decreased renal function.

The incidence of the syndrome has not been defined.

Therapy for the syndrome is investigational.

Cardiac Toxicity: Congestive heart failure, often treated effectively with diuretics and cardiac glycosides, has rarely been reported. Almost all patients who experienced this side effect had received prior doxorubicin therapy.

Acute Side Effects Due to MUTAMYCIN were fever, anorexia, nausea, and vomiting. They occurred in about 14% of 1,281 patients.

Other: Headache, blurring of vision, confusion, drowsiness, syncope, fatigue, edema, thrombophlebitis, hematemesis, diarrhea, and pain. These did not appear to be dose related and were not unequivocally drug related. They may have been due to the primary or metastatic disease processes. Malaise and asthenia have been reported as part of postmarketing surveillance. Bladder fibrosis/contraction has been reported with intravesical administration (see **PRECAUTIONS**).

DOSAGE AND ADMINISTRATION

MUTAMYCIN should be given intravenously only, using care to avoid extravasation of the compound. If extravasation occurs, cellulitis, ulceration, and slough may result.

Each vial contains either mitomycin 5 mg and mannitol 10 mg, mitomycin 20 mg and mannitol 40 mg, or mitomycin 40 mg and mannitol 80 mg. To administer, add Sterile Water for Injection, 10 mL, 40 mL, or 80 mL respectively. Shake to dissolve. If product does not dissolve immediately, allow to stand at room temperature until solution is obtained.

After full hematological recovery (see guide to dosage adjustment) from any previous chemotherapy, the following dosage schedule may be used at 6 to 8 week intervals:

20 mg/m^2 intravenously as a single dose via a functioning intravenous catheter.

Because of cumulative myelosuppression, patients should be fully reevaluated after each course of MUTAMYCIN, and the dose reduced if the patient has experienced any toxicities. Doses greater than 20 mg/m^2 have not been shown to be more effective, and are more toxic than lower doses.

The following schedule is suggested as a guide to dosage adjustment:

Nadir After Prior Dose		
Leukocytes/mm^3	Platelets/mm^3	Percentage of Prior Dose to be Given
> 4000	> 100,000	100%
3000–3999	75,000–99,999	100%
2000–2999	25,000–74,999	70%
< 2000	< 25,000	50%

No repeat dosage should be given until leukocyte count has returned to 4000/mm^3 and platelet count to 100,000/mm^3. When MUTAMYCIN is used in combination with other myelosuppressive agents, the doses should be adjusted accordingly. If the disease continues to progress after two courses of MUTAMYCIN, the drug should be stopped since chances of response are minimal.

STABILITY

1. **Unreconstituted** MUTAMYCIN stored at room temperature is stable for the lot life indicated on the package. Avoid excessive heat (over 40°C, 104°F).
2. **Reconstituted** with Sterile Water for Injection to a concentration of 0.5 mg per mL, MUTAMYCIN is stable for 14 days refrigerated or 7 days at room temperature.
3. **Diluted** in various I.V. fluids at room temperature, to a concentration of 20 to 40 micrograms per mL:

I.V. Fluid	Stability
5% Dextrose Injection	3 hours
0.9% Sodium Chloride Injection	12 hours
Sodium Lactate Injection	24 hours

4. The combination of MUTAMYCIN (5 mg to 15 mg) and heparin (1,000 units to 10,000 units) in 30 mL of 0.9% Sodium Chloride Injection is stable for 48 hours at room temperature.

Procedures for proper handling and disposal of anticancer drugs should be considered. Several guidelines on this subject have been published.[1–7] There is no general agreement that all of the procedures recommended in the guidelines are necessary or appropriate.

HOW SUPPLIED

MUTAMYCIN® (mitomycin for injection, USP)

NDC 0015-3001-20 —Each vial contains 5 mg mitomycin.
NDC 0015-3002-20—Each vial contains 20 mg mitomycin.
NDC 0015-3059-20—Each vial contains 40 mg mitomycin.

For information on package sizes available, refer to the current price schedule.

REFERENCES

1. Recommendations for the Safe Handling of Parenteral Antineoplastic Drugs. NIH Publication No. 83–2621. For sale by the Superintendent of Documents, US Government Printing Office, Washington, DC 20402.
2. AMA Council Report. Guidelines for Handling Parenteral Antineoplastics. *JAMA* 1985; 253 (11):1590–1592.
3. National Study Commission on Cytotoxic Exposure—Recommendations for Handling Cytotoxic Agents. Available from Louis P. Jeffrey, ScD, Chairman, National Study Commission on Cytotoxic Exposure, Massachusetts College of Pharmacy and Allied Health Sciences, 179 Longwood Avenue, Boston, Massachusetts 02115.
4. Clinical Oncological Society of Australia. Guidelines and Recommendations for Safe Handling of Antineoplastic Agents. *Med J Australia* 1983; 1:426–428.
5. Jones RB, et al: Safe Handling of Chemotherapeutic Agents: A Report from the Mount Sinai Medical Center. *CA–A Cancer Journal for Clinicians* 1983; (Sept/Oct) 258–263.
6. American Society of Hospital Pharmacists Technical Assistance Bulletin on Handling Cytotoxic and Hazardous Drugs. *Am J Hosp Pharm* 1990; 47:1033–1049.
7. Controlling Occupational Exposure to Hazardous Drugs (OSHA WORK PRACTICE GUIDELINES). *Am J Health-Syst Pharm* 1996; 53:1669–1685.

BRISTOL-MYERS SQUIBB
ONCOLOGY
Bristol-Myers Squibb Company
Princeton, NJ 08543
U.S.A.

H9-B001-6-00 3001DIM-31
1080027A1 Revised January 2000

Shown in Product Identification Guide, page 310

MYCOSTATIN® ℞

[*mīk 'ō-stat "in*]
(nystatin lozenges, USP)
PASTILLES
℞ ONLY

DESCRIPTION

Nystatin is a polyene antifungal antibiotic obtained from *Streptomyces noursei*. Structural formula:

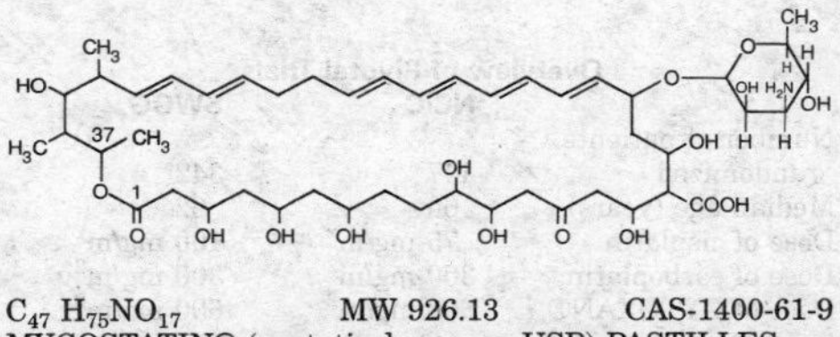

$C_{47}H_{75}NO_{17}$ MW 926.13 CAS-1400-61-9

MYCOSTATIN® (nystatin lozenges, USP) PASTILLES are round, light to dark gold-colored troches designed to dissolve slowly in the mouth. Each MYCOSTATIN PASTILLE provides 200,000 units nystatin. Inactive ingredients: anise oil, cinnamon oil, gelatin, sucrose, and other ingredients.

CLINICAL PHARMACOLOGY

Nystatin is both fungistatic and fungicidal *in vitro* against a wide variety of yeasts and yeast-like fungi. *Candida albicans* demonstrates no significant resistance to nystatin *in vitro* on repeated subculture in increasing levels of nystatin; other *Candida* species become quite resistant. Generally, resistance does not develop *in vivo*. Nystatin acts by binding to sterols in the cell membrane of susceptible fungi with a resultant change in membrane permeability allowing leakage of intracellular components. Nystatin exhibits no activity against bacteria, protozoa, trichomonads, or viruses.

Pharmacokinetics: Gastrointestinal absorption of nystatin is insignificant. Most orally administered nystatin is passed unchanged in the stool. Significant concentrations of nystatin may appear occasionally in the plasma of patients with renal insufficiency during oral therapy with conventional dosage forms.

Mean nystatin concentrations in excess of those required *in vitro* to inhibit growth of clinically significant *Candida* persisted in saliva for approximately two hours after the start of oral dissolution of two MYCOSTATIN PASTILLES (400,000 units nystatin) administered simultaneously to 12 healthy volunteers.

INDICATIONS AND USAGE

MYCOSTATIN PASTILLES are indicated for the treatment of candidiasis in the oral cavity.

CONTRAINDICATIONS

MYCOSTATIN PASTILLES are contraindicated in those patients with a history of hypersensitivity to any of the components.

PRECAUTIONS

General: This medication is not to be used for the treatment of systemic mycoses.

In order to achieve maximum effect from the medication, MYCOSTATIN (nystatin lozenges, USP) PASTILLES must be allowed to dissolve slowly in the mouth; therefore, patients for whom the MYCOSTATIN PASTILLE is prescribed, including pediatric patients and the elderly, must be competent to utilize the dosage form as intended.

If irritation or hypersensitivity develops with MYCOSTATIN PASTILLES, treatment should be discontinued and appropriate therapy instituted.

Information for the Patient: Patients taking this medication should receive the following information and instructions:

1. Use as directed; the medication is not for any disorder other than for which it was prescribed.
2. Allow the MYCOSTATIN PASTILLE to dissolve slowly in the mouth; **do not chew or swallow the PASTILLE.**
3. The patient should be advised regarding replacement of any missed doses.
4. There should be no interruption or discontinuation of medication until the prescribed course of treatment is completed even though symptomatic relief may occur within a few days.
5. If symptoms of local irritation develop, the physician should be notified promptly.
6. Good oral hygiene, including proper care of dentures, is particularly important for denture wearers.

Laboratory Tests: If there is a lack of therapeutic response, appropriate microbiological studies (e.g., KOH smears and/or cultures) should be repeated to confirm the diagnosis of candidiasis and rule out other pathogens before instituting another course of therapy.

Carcinogenesis, Mutagenesis, Impairment of Fertility: Studies have not been performed to evaluate carcinogenic or mutagenic potential, or possible impairment of fertility in males or females.

Pregnancy: Teratogenic Effects: "Category C". Animal reproduction studies have not been conducted with nystatin. It is also not known whether nystatin can cause fetal harm when administered to a pregnant woman or can affect reproduction capacity. MYCOSTATIN PASTILLES should be dispensed to a pregnant woman only if clearly needed.

Nursing Mothers: It is not known whether nystatin is excreted in human milk. Although gastrointestinal absorbtion is insignificant, caution should be exercised when nystatin is prescribed for a nursing woman.

Pediatric Use: The use of MYCOSTATIN PASTILLES has not been systematically studied in pediatric patients.

ADVERSE REACTIONS

MYCOSTATIN PASTILLES are generally well tolerated by all age groups, even during prolonged use. Rarely, oral irritation or sensitization may occur. Nausea has been reported occasionally during therapy.

Large oral doses of nystatin have occasionally produced diarrhea, gastrointestinal distress, nausea and vomiting. Rash, including urticaria has been reported rarely. Stevens-Johnson syndrome has been reported very rarely.

OVERDOSAGE

Oral doses of nystatin in excess of five million units daily have caused nausea and gastrointestinal upset. There have been no reports of serious toxic effects or superinfections (See **CLINICAL PHARMACOLOGY, Pharmacokinetics**).

DOSAGE AND ADMINISTRATION

Pediatric Patients and Adults: The recommended dose is one or two MYCOSTATIN (nystatin lozenges, USP) PASTILLES (200,000 or 400,000 units nystatin) four or five times daily for as long as 14 days if necessary. The dosage regimen should be continued for at least 48 hours after disappearance of oral symptoms.

Continued on next page

Mycostatin—Cont.

Dosage should be discontinued if symptoms persist after the initial 14 day period of treatment (see **PRECAUTIONS, Laboratory Tests**).

Administration: MYCOSTATIN PASTILLES must be allowed to dissolve slowly in the mouth, and should not be chewed or swallowed whole.

HOW SUPPLIED

MYCOSTATIN® (nystatin lozenges, USP) PASTILLES, 200,000 units nystatin each, in packages containing 30 pleasant-tasting PASTILLES (**NDC** 0003-0543-20).

ALSO AVAILABLE

MYCOSTATIN® (nystatin, USP) is also available as a ready-to-use oral suspension, oral tablets, vaginal tablets, and topical powder, cream, and ointment (see package inserts accompanying those products for complete information).

Storage: Refrigerate between 2° and 8°C (36° and 46°F).

Manufactured by:

Ernest Jackson & Co., Ltd., Crediton, Devon, England

Distributed by:

Mead Johnson
ONCOLOGY PRODUCTS
A Bristol-Myers Squibb Company
Princeton, NJ 08543
U.S.A.

1099698

K1-B001-12-99 Revised August 1999

PARAPLATIN® ℞

[păr-a-plătin]
(carboplatin for injection)
Rx ONLY

> **WARNING**
> PARAPLATIN® (carboplatin for injection) should be administered under the supervision of a qualified physician experienced in the use of cancer chemotherapeutic agents. Appropriate management of therapy and complications is possible only when adequate treatment facilities are readily available.
> Bone marrow suppression is dose related and may be severe, resulting in infection and/or bleeding. Anemia may be cumulative and may require transfusion support. Vomiting is another frequent drug-related side effect.
> Anaphylactic-like reactions to PARAPLATIN have been reported and may occur within minutes of PARAPLATIN administration. Epinephrine, corticosteroids, and antihistamines have been employed to alleviate symptoms.

DESCRIPTION

PARAPLATIN® (carboplatin for injection) is supplied as a sterile, lyophilized white powder available in single-dose vials containing 50 mg, 150 mg, and 450 mg of carboplatin for administration by intravenous infusion. Each vial contains equal parts by weight of carboplatin and mannitol.

Carboplatin is a platinum coordination compound that is used as a cancer chemotherapeutic agent. The chemical name for carboplatin is platinum, diammine [1,1-cyclobutane-dicarboxylato(2-)-0,0′]-, (SP-4-2), and has the following structural formula:

[structural formula: H_3N, H_3N, Pt, O, O]

Carboplatin is a crystalline powder with the molecular formula of $C_6H_{12}N_2O_4Pt$ and a molecular weight of 371.25. It is soluble in water at a rate of approximately 14 mg/mL, and the pH of a 1% solution is 5–7. It is virtually insoluble in ethanol, acetone, and dimethylacetamide.

CLINICAL PHARMACOLOGY

Carboplatin, like cisplatin, produces predominantly interstrand DNA cross-links rather than DNA-protein cross-links. This effect is apparently cell-cycle nonspecific. The aquation of carboplatin, which is thought to produce the active species, occurs at a slower rate than in the case of cisplatin. Despite this difference, it appears that both carboplatin and cisplatin induce equal numbers of drug-DNA cross-links, causing equivalent lesions and biological effects. The differences in potencies for carboplatin and cisplatin appear to be directly related to the difference in aquation rates.

In patients with creatinine clearances of about 60 mL/min or greater, plasma levels of intact carboplatin decay in a biphasic manner after a 30-minute intravenous infusion of 300 to 500 mg/m² of Paraplatin. The initial plasma half-life (alpha) was found to be 1.1 to 2 hours (N = 6), and the post-distribution plasma half-life (beta) was found to be 2.6 to 5.9 hours (N = 6). The total body clearance, apparent volume of distribution and mean residence time for carboplatin are 4.4 L/hour, 16 L and 3.5 hours, respectively. The C_{max} values and areas under the plasma concentration vs. time curves from 0 to infinity (AUC inf) increase linearly with dose, although the increase was slightly more than dose proportional. Carboplatin, therefore, exhibits linear pharmacokinetics over the dosing range studied (300–500 mg/m²).

Carboplatin is not bound to plasma proteins. No significant quantities of protein-free, ultrafilterable platinum-containing species other than carboplatin are present in plasma. However, platinum from carboplatin becomes irreversibly bound to plasma proteins and is slowly eliminated with a minimum half-life of 5 days.

The major route of elimination of carboplatin is renal excretion. Patients with creatinine clearances of approximately 60 mL/min or greater excrete 65% of the dose in the urine within 12 hours and 71% of the dose within 24 hours. All of the platinum in the 24-hour urine is present as carboplatin. Only 3% to 5% of the administered platinum is excreted in the urine between 24 and 96 hours. There are insufficient data to determine whether biliary excretion occurs.

In patients with creatinine clearances below 60 mL/min the total body and renal clearances of carboplatin decrease as the creatinine clearance decreases. PARAPLATIN dosages should therefore be reduced in these patients (see **DOSAGE AND ADMINISTRATION**).

ADVERSE EXPERIENCES IN PATIENTS WITH OVARIAN CANCER NCIC STUDY

		PARAPLATIN Arm Percent*	Cisplatin Arm Percent*	P-Values**
Bone Marrow				
Thrombocytopenia	< 100,000/mm³	70	29	< 0.001
	< 50,000/mm³	41	6	< 0.001
Neutropenia	< 2,000 cells/mm³	97	96	n.s.
	< 1,000 cells/mm³	81	79	n.s.
Leukopenia	< 4,000 cells/mm³	98	97	n.s.
	< 2,000 cells/mm³	68	52	0.001
Anemia	< 11 g/dL	91	91	n.s.
	< 8 g/dL	18	12	n.s.
Infections		14	12	n.s.
Bleeding		10	4	n.s.
Transfusions		42	31	0.018
Gastrointestinal				
Nausea and vomiting		93	98	0.010
Vomiting		84	97	< 0.001
Other GI side effects		50	62	0.013
Neurologic				
Peripheral neuropathies		16	42	< 0.001
Ototoxicity		13	33	< 0.001
Other sensory side effects		6	10	n.s.
Central neurotoxicity		28	40	0.009
Renal				
Serum creatinine elevations		5	13	0.006
Blood urea elevations		17	31	< 0.001
Hepatic				
Bilirubin elevations		5	3	n.s.
SGOT elevations		17	13	n.s.
Alkaline phosphatase elevations		–	–	–
Electrolytes loss				
Sodium		10	20	0.005
Potassium		16	22	n.s.
Calcium		16	19	n.s.
Magnesium		63	88	< 0.001
Other side effects				
Pain		36	37	n.s.
Asthenia		40	33	n.s.
Cardiovascular		15	19	n.s.
Respiratory		8	9	n.s.
Allergic		12	9	n.s.
Genitourinary		10	10	n.s.
Alopecia+		50	62	0.017
Mucositis		10	9	n.s.

* Values are in percent of evaluable patients
* * n.s. = not significant, p > 0.05
\+ May have been affected by cyclophosphamide dosage delivered

CLINICAL STUDIES

Use with Cyclophosphamide for Initial Treatment of Ovarian Cancer: In two prospectively randomized, controlled studies conducted by the National Cancer Institute of Canada, Clinical Trials Group (NCIC) and the Southwest Oncology Group (SWOG), 789 chemotherapy naive patients with advanced ovarian cancer were treated with PARAPLATIN or cisplatin, both in combination with cyclophosphamide, every 28 days for six courses before surgical reevaluation. The following results were obtained from both studies:

COMPARATIVE EFFICACY

Overview of Pivotal Trials

	NCIC	SWOG
Number of patients randomized	447	342
Median age (years)	60	62
Dose of cisplatin	75 mg/m²	100 mg/m²
Dose of carboplatin	300 mg/m²	300 mg/m²
Dose of CYTOXAN® (cyclophosphamide, USP)	600 mg/m²	600 mg/m²
Residual tumor <2 cm (number of patients)	39% (174/447)	14% (49/342)

Clinical Response in Measurable Disease Patients

	NCIC	SWOG
Carboplatin (number of patients)	60% (48/80)	58% (48/83)
Cisplatin (number of patients)	58% (49/85)	43% (33/76)
95% C.I. of difference (Carboplatin - Cisplatin)	(-13.9%, 18.6%)	(-2.3%, 31.1%)

Pathologic Complete Response*

	NCIC	SWOG
Carboplatin (number of patients)	11% (24/224)	10% (17/171)
Cisplatin (number of patients)	15% (33/223)	10% (17/171)
95% C.I. of difference (Carboplatin - Cisplatin)	(-10.7%, 2.5%)	(-6.9%, 6.9%)

* 114 PARAPLATIN and 109 Cisplatin patients did not undergo second look surgery in NCIC study. 90 PARAPLATIN and 106 Cisplatin patients did not undergo second look surgery in SWOG study.

Progression-Free Survival (PFS)

	NCIC	SWOG
Median		
Carboplatin	59 weeks	49 weeks
Cisplatin	61 weeks	47 weeks
2-year PFS*		
Carboplatin	31%	21%
Cisplatin	31%	21%
95% C.I. of difference (Carboplatin - Cisplatin)	(-9.3, 8.7)	(-9.0, 9.4)
3-year PFS*		
Carboplatin	19%	8%
Cisplatin	23%	14%
95% C.I. of difference (Carboplatin - Cisplatin)	(-11.5, 4.5)	(-14.1, 0.3)
Hazard Ratio**	1.10	1.02
95% C.I. (Carboplatin - Cisplatin)	(0.89, 1.35)	(0.81, 1.29)

* Kaplan-Meier Estimates
Unrelated deaths occurring in the absence of progression were counted as events (progression) in this analysis.
** Analysis adjusted for factors found to be of prognostic significance were consistent with unadjusted analysis.

	Survival	
	NCIC	**SWOG**
Median		
Carboplatin	110 weeks	86 weeks
Cisplatin	99 weeks	79 weeks
2-year Survival*		
Carboplatin	51.9%	40.2%
Cisplatin	48.4%	39.0%
95% C.I. of difference (Carboplatin - Cisplatin)	(-6.2, 13.2)	(-9.8, 12.2)
3-year Survival*		
Carboplatin	34.6%	18.3%
Cisplatin	33.1%	24.9%
95% C.I. of difference (Carboplatin - Cisplatin)	(-7.7, 10.7)	(-15.9, 2.7)
Hazard Ratio**	0.98	1.01
95% C.I. (Carboplatin - Cisplatin)	(0.78, 1.23)	(0.78, 1.30)

* Kaplan-Meier Estimates
** Analysis adjusted for factors found to be of prognostic significance were consistent with unadjusted analysis.

COMPARATIVE TOXICITY

The pattern of toxicity exerted by the PARAPLATIN (carboplatin for injection)-containing regimen was significantly different from that of the cisplatin-containing combinations. Differences between the two studies may be explained by different cisplatin dosages and by different supportive care. The PARAPLATIN-containing regimen induced significantly more thrombocytopenia and, in one study, significantly more leukopenia and more need for transfusional support. The cisplatin-containing regimen produced significantly more anemia in one study. However, no significant differences occurred in incidences of infections and hemorrhagic episodes.

Non-hematologic toxicities (emesis, neurotoxicity, ototoxicity, renal toxicity, hypomagnesemia, and alopecia) were significantly more frequent in the cisplatin-containing arms.

[See table at top of previous page]
[See table at top right of page]

Use as a Single Agent for Secondary Treatment of Advanced Ovarian Cancer: In two prospective, randomized controlled studies in patients with advanced ovarian cancer previously treated with chemotherapy, PARAPLATIN (carboplatin for injection) achieved six clinical complete responses in 47 patients. The duration of these responses ranged from 45 to 71+ weeks.

ADVERSE EXPERIENCES IN PATIENTS WITH OVARIAN CANCER SWOG STUDY

		PARAPLATIN Arm Percent*	Cisplatin Arm Percent*	P-Values**
Bone Marrow				
Thrombocytopenia	< 100,000/mm^3	59	35	< 0.001
	< 50,000/mm^3	22	11	0.006
Neutropenia	< 2,000 cells/mm^3	95	97	n.s.
	< 1,000 cells/mm^3	84	78	n.s.
Leukopenia	< 4,000 cells/mm^3	97	97	n.s.
	< 2,000 cells/mm^3	76	67	n.s.
Anemia	< 11 g/dL	88	87	n.s.
	< 8 g/dL	8	24	< 0.001
Infections		18	21	n.s.
Bleeding		6	4	n.s.
Transfusions		25	33	n.s.
Gastrointestinal				
Nausea and vomiting		94	96	n.s.
Vomiting		82	91	0.007
Other GI side effects		40	48	n.s.
Neurologic				
Peripheral neuropathies		13	28	0.001
Ototoxicity		12	30	< 0.001
Other sensory side effects		4	6	n.s.
Central neurotoxicity		23	29	n.s.
Renal				
Serum creatinine elevations		7	38	< 0.001
Blood urea elevations		–	–	–
Hepatic				
Bilirubin elevations		5	3	n.s.
SGOT elevations		23	16	n.s.
Alkaline phosphatase elevations		29	20	n.s.
Electrolytes loss				
Sodium		–	–	–
Potassium		–	–	–
Calcium		–	–	–
Magnesium		58	77	< 0.001
Other side effects				
Pain		54	52	n.s.
Asthenia		43	46	n.s.
Cardiovascular		23	30	n.s.
Respiratory		12	11	n.s.
Allergic		10	11	n.s.
Genitourinary		11	13	n.s.
Alopecia+		43	57	0.009
Mucositis		6	11	n.s.

* Values are in percent of evaluable patients
** n.s. = not significant, $p > 0.05$
\+ May have been affected by cyclophosphamide dosage delivered

INDICATIONS

Initial Treatment of Advanced Ovarian Carcinoma: PARAPLATIN is indicated for the initial treatment of advanced ovarian carcinoma in established combination with other approved chemotherapeutic agents. One established combination regimen consists of PARAPLATIN and cyclophosphamide (CYTOXAN®). Two randomized controlled studies conducted by the NCIC and SWOG with PARAPLATIN vs. cisplatin, both in combination with cyclophosphamide, have demonstrated equivalent overall survival between the two groups (see **CLINICAL STUDIES**).

There is limited statistical power to demonstrate equivalence in overall pathologic complete response rates and long term survival (≥ 3 years) because of the small number of patients with these outcomes: the small number of patients with residual tumor < 2 cm after initial surgery also limits the statistical power to demonstrate equivalence in this subgroup.

Secondary Treatment of Advanced Ovarian Carcinoma: PARAPLATIN is indicated for the palliative treatment of patients with ovarian carcinoma recurrent after prior chemotherapy, including patients who have been previously treated with cisplatin.

Within the group of patients previously treated with cisplatin, those who have developed progressive disease while receiving cisplatin therapy may have a decreased response rate.

CONTRAINDICATIONS

PARAPLATIN is contraindicated in patients with a history of severe allergic reactions to cisplatin or other platinum-containing compounds, or mannitol.

PARAPLATIN should not be employed in patients with severe bone marrow depression or significant bleeding.

WARNINGS

Bone marrow suppression (leukopenia, neutropenia, and thrombocytopenia) is dose-dependent and is also the dose-limiting toxicity. Peripheral blood counts should be frequently monitored during PARAPLATIN treatment and, when appropriate, until recovery is achieved. Median nadir occurs at day 21 in patients receiving single-agent PARAPLATIN. In general, single intermittent courses of PARAPLATIN should not be repeated until leukocyte, neutrophil, and platelet counts have recovered.

Since anemia is cumulative, transfusions may be needed during treatment with PARAPLATIN, particularly in patients receiving prolonged therapy.

Bone marrow suppression is increased in patients who have received prior therapy, especially regimens including cisplatin. Marrow suppression is also increased in patients with impaired kidney function. Initial PARAPLATIN dosages in these patients should be appropriately reduced (see **DOSAGE AND ADMINISTRATION**) and blood counts should be carefully monitored between courses. The use of PARAPLATIN in combination with other bone marrow suppressing therapies must be carefully managed with respect to dosage and timing in order to minimize additive effects.

PARAPLATIN has limited nephrotoxic potential, but concomitant treatment with aminoglycosides has resulted in increased renal and/or audiologic toxicity, and caution must be exercised when a patient receives both drugs. Clinically significant hearing loss has been reported to occur in pediatric patients when PARAPLATIN was administered at higher than recommended doses in combination with other ototoxic agents.

PARAPLATIN can induce emesis, which can be more severe in patients previously receiving emetogenic therapy. The incidence and intensity of emesis have been reduced by using premedication with antiemetics. Although no conclusive efficacy data exist with the following schedules of PARAPLATIN, lengthening the duration of single intravenous administration to 24 hours or dividing the total dose over five consecutive daily pulse doses has resulted in reduced emesis.

Although peripheral neurotoxicity is infrequent, its incidence is increased in patients older than 65 years and in patients previously treated with cisplatin. Pre-existing cisplatin-induced neurotoxicity does not worsen in about 70% of the patients receiving PARAPLATIN (carboplatin for injection) as secondary treatment.

Loss of vision, which can be complete for light and colors, has been reported after the use of PARAPLATIN with doses higher than those recommended in the package insert. Vision appears to recover totally or to a significant extent within weeks of stopping these high doses.

As in the case of other platinum coordination compounds, allergic reactions to PARAPLATIN have been reported. These may occur within minutes of administration and should be managed with appropriate supportive therapy. There is increased risk of allergic reactions including anaphylaxis in patients previously exposed to platinum therapy. (See **CONTRAINDICATIONS** and **ADVERSE REACTIONS: Allergic Reactions.**)

High dosages of PARAPLATIN (more than four times the recommended dose) have resulted in severe abnormalities of liver function tests.

PARAPLATIN may cause fetal harm when administered to a pregnant woman. PARAPLATIN has been shown to be embryotoxic and teratogenic in rats. There are no adequate and well-controlled studies in pregnant women. If this drug is used during pregnancy, or if the patient becomes pregnant while receiving this drug, the patient should be apprised of the potential hazard to the fetus. Women of childbearing potential should be advised to avoid becoming pregnant.

PRECAUTIONS

General: Needles or intravenous administration sets containing aluminum parts that may come in contact with PARAPLATIN should not be used for the preparation or administration of the drug. Aluminum can react with carboplatin causing precipitate formation and loss of potency.

Drug Interactions: The renal effects of nephrotoxic compounds may be potentiated by PARAPLATIN.

Carcinogenesis, Mutagenesis, Impairment of Fertility: The carcinogenic potential of carboplatin has not been studied, but compounds with similar mechanisms of action and mutagenicity profiles have been reported to be carcinogenic. Carboplatin has been shown to be mutagenic both *in vitro* and *in vivo*. It has also been shown to be embryotoxic and teratogenic in rats receiving the drug during organogenesis. Secondary malignancies have been reported in association with multi-drug therapy.

Pregnancy: Pregnancy "Category D". (See **WARNINGS.**)

Nursing Mothers: It is not known whether carboplatin is excreted in human milk. Because there is a possibility of toxicity in nursing infants secondary to PARAPLATIN treatment of the mother, it is recommended that breast feeding be discontinued if the mother is treated with PARAPLATIN.

Pediatric Use: Safety and effectiveness in pediatric patients have not been established (see **WARNINGS, Audiologic Toxicity**).

ADVERSE REACTIONS

For a comparison of toxicities when carboplatin or cisplatin was given in combination with cyclophosphamide, see the COMPARATIVE TOXICITY subsection of the **CLINICAL STUDIES** section.

[See table at top of next page]

In the narrative section that follows, the incidences of adverse events are based on data from 1,893 patients with various types of tumors who received PARAPLATIN (carboplatin for injection) as single-agent therapy.

Hematologic Toxicity: Bone marrow suppression is the dose-limiting toxicity of PARAPLATIN. Thrombocytopenia with platelet counts below 50,000/mm^3 occurs in 25% of the

Continued on next page

Paraplatin—Cont.

patients (35% of pretreated ovarian cancer patients); neutropenia with granulocyte counts below 1,000/mm^3 occurs in 16% of the patients (21% of pretreated ovarian cancer patients); leukopenia with WBC counts below 2,000/mm^3 occurs in 15% of the patients (26% of pretreated ovarian cancer patients). The nadir usually occurs about day 21 in patients receiving single-agent therapy. By day 28, 90% of patients have platelet counts above 100,000/mm^3; 74% have neutrophil counts above 2,000/mm^3; 67% have leukocyte counts above 4,000/mm^3.

Marrow suppression is usually more severe in patients with impaired kidney function. Patients with poor performance status have also experienced a higher incidence of severe leukopenia and thrombocytopenia.

The hematologic effects, although usually reversible, have resulted in infectious or hemorrhagic complications in 5% of the patients treated with PARAPLATIN, with drug related death occurring in less than 1% of the patients. Fever has also been reported in patients with neutropenia.

Anemia with hemoglobin less than 11 g/dL has been observed in 71% of the patients who started therapy with a baseline above that value. The incidence of anemia increases with increasing exposure to PARAPLATIN. Transfusions have been administered to 26% of the patients treated with PARAPLATIN (44% of previously treated ovarian cancer patients).

Bone marrow depression may be more severe when PARAPLATIN is combined with other bone marrow suppressing drugs or with radiotherapy.

Gastrointestinal Toxicity: Vomiting occurs in 65% of the patients (81% of previously treated ovarian cancer patients) and in about one-third of these patients it is severe. Carboplatin, as a single agent or in combination, is significantly less emetogenic than cisplatin; however, patients previously treated with emetogenic agents, especially cisplatin, appear to be more prone to vomiting. Nausea alone occurs in an additional 10% to 15% of patients. Both nausea and vomiting usually cease within 24 hours of treatment and are often responsive to antiemetic measures. Although no conclusive efficacy data exist with the following schedules, prolonged administration of PARAPLATIN, either by continuous 24-hour infusion or by daily pulse doses given for five consecutive days, was associated with less severe vomiting than the single dose intermittent schedule. Emesis was increased when PARAPLATIN was used in combination with other emetogenic compounds. Other gastrointestinal effects observed frequently were pain, in 17% of the patients; diarrhea, in 6%; and constipation, also in 6%.

Neurologic Toxicity: Peripheral neuropathies have been observed in 4% of the patients receiving PARAPLATIN (6% of pretreated ovarian cancer patients) with mild paresthesias occurring most frequently. Carboplatin therapy produces significantly fewer and less severe neurologic side effects than does therapy with cisplatin. However, patients older than 65 years and/or previously treated with cisplatin appear to have an increased risk (10%) for peripheral neuropathies. In 70% of the patients with pre-existing cisplatin-induced peripheral neurotoxicity, there was no worsening of symptoms during therapy with PARAPLATIN. Clinical ototoxicity and other sensory abnormalities such as visual disturbances and change in taste have been reported in only 1% of the patients. Central nervous system symptoms have been reported in 5% of the patients and appear to be most often related to the use of antiemetics.

Although the overall incidence of peripheral neurologic side effects induced by PARAPLATIN is low, prolonged treatment, particularly in cisplatin pretreated patients, may result in cumulative neurotoxicity.

Nephrotoxicity: Development of abnormal renal function test results is uncommon, despite the fact that carboplatin, unlike cisplatin, has usually been administered without high-volume fluid hydration and/or forced diuresis. The incidences of abnormal renal function tests reported are 6% for serum creatinine and 14% for blood urea nitrogen (10% and 22%, respectively, in pretreated ovarian cancer patients). Most of these reported abnormalities have been mild and about one-half of them were reversible.

Creatinine clearance has proven to be the most sensitive measure of kidney function in patients receiving PARAPLATIN, and it appears to be the most useful test for correlating drug clearance and bone marrow suppression. Twenty-seven percent of the patients who had a baseline value of 60 mL/min or more demonstrated a reduction below this value during PARAPLATIN therapy.

Hepatic Toxicity: The incidences of abnormal liver function tests in patients with normal baseline values were reported as follows: total bilirubin, 5%; SGOT, 15%; and alkaline phosphatase, 24%; (5%, 19%, and 37%, respectively, in pretreated ovarian cancer patients). These abnormalities have generally been mild and reversible in about one-half of the cases, although the role of metastatic tumor in the liver may complicate the assessment in many patients. In a limited series of patients receiving very high dosages of PARAPLATIN and autologous bone marrow transplantation, severe abnormalities of liver function tests were reported.

Electrolyte Changes: The incidences of abnormally decreased serum electrolyte values reported were as follows: sodium, 29%; potassium, 20%; calcium, 22%; and magnesium, 29%; (47%, 28%, 31%, and 43%, respectively, in pretreated ovarian cancer patients). Electrolyte supplementation was not routinely administered concomitantly with

ADVERSE EXPERIENCES IN PATIENTS WITH OVARIAN CANCER

		First Line Combination Therapy* Percent	Second Line Single Agent Therapy** Percent
Bone Marrow			
Thrombocytopenia	< 100,000/mm^3	66	62
	< 50,000/mm^3	33	35
Neutropenia	< 2,000 cells/mm^3	96	67
	< 1,000 cells/mm^3	82	21
Leukopenia	< 4,000 cells/mm^3	97	85
	< 2,000 cells/mm^3	71	26
Anemia	< 11 g/dL	90	90
	< 8 g/dL	14	21
Infections		16	5
Bleeding		8	5
Transfusions		35	44
Gastrointestinal			
Nausea and vomiting		93	92
Vomiting		83	81
Other GI side effects		46	21
Neurologic			
Peripheral neuropathies		15	6
Ototoxicity		12	1
Other sensory side effects		5	1
Central neurotoxicity		26	5
Renal			
Serum creatinine elevations		6	10
Blood urea elevations		17	22
Hepatic			
Bilirubin elevations		5	5
SGOT elevations		20	19
Alkaline phosphatase elevations		29	37
Electrolytes loss			
Sodium		10	47
Potassium		16	28
Calcium		16	31
Magnesium		61	43
Other side effects			
Pain		44	23
Asthenia		41	11
Cardiovascular		19	6
Respiratory		10	6
Allergic		11	2
Genitourinary		10	2
Alopecia+		49	2
Mucositis		8	1

***Use with Cyclophosphamide for Initial Treatment of Ovarian Cancer:** Data are based on the experience of 393 patients with ovarian cancer (regardless of baseline status) who received initial combination therapy with PARAPLATIN and cyclophosphamide in two randomized controlled studies conducted by SWOG and NCIC (see **CLINICAL STUDIES**).

Combination with cyclophosphamide as well as duration of treatment may be responsible for the differences that can be noted in the adverse experience table.

* ***Single Agent Use for the Secondary Treatment of Ovarian Cancer:** Data are based on the experience of 553 patients with previously treated ovarian carcinoma (regardless of baseline status) who received single-agent PARAPLATIN.

PARAPLATIN, and these electrolyte abnormalities were rarely associated with symptoms.

Allergic Reactions: Hypersensitivity to PARAPLATIN has been reported in 2% of the patients. These allergic reactions have been similar in nature and severity to those reported with other platinum-containing compounds, i.e., rash, urticaria, erythema, pruritus, and rarely bronchospasm and hypotension. Anaphylactic reactions have been reported as part of postmarketing surveillance (see **WARNINGS**). These reactions have been successfully managed with standard epinephrine, corticosteroid, and antihistamine therapy.

Injection Site Reactions: Injection site reactions, including redness, swelling, and pain, have been reported during postmarketing surveillance. Necrosis associated with extravasation has also been reported.

Other Events: Pain and asthenia were the most frequently reported miscellaneous adverse effects; their relationship to the tumor and to anemia was likely. Alopecia was reported (3%). Cardiovascular, respiratory, genitourinary, and mucosal side effects have occurred in 6% or less of the patients. Cardiovascular events (cardiac failure, embolism, cerebrovascular accidents) were fatal in less than 1% of the patients and did not appear to be related to chemotherapy. Cancer-associated hemolytic uremic syndrome has been reported rarely.

Malaise, anorexia and hypertension have been reported as part of postmarketing surveillance.

OVERDOSAGE

There is no known antidote for PARAPLATIN overdosage. The anticipated complications of overdosage would be secondary to bone marrow suppression and/or hepatic toxicity.

DOSAGE AND ADMINISTRATION

NOTE: Aluminum reacts with carboplatin causing precipitate formation and loss of potency, therefore, needles or intravenous sets containing aluminum parts that may come in contact with the drug must not be used for the preparation or administration of PARAPLATIN.

Single Agent Therapy: PARAPLATIN (carboplatin for injection), as a single agent, has been shown to be effective in patients with recurrent ovarian carcinoma at a dosage of 360 mg/m^2 I.V. on day 1 every 4 weeks (alternatively see **Formula Dosing**). In general, however, single intermittent courses of PARAPLATIN should not be repeated until the neutrophil count is at least 2,000 and the platelet count is at least 100,000.

Combination Therapy with Cyclophosphamide: In the chemotherapy of advanced ovarian cancer, an effective combination for previously untreated patients consists of:

PARAPLATIN—300 mg/m^2 I.V. on day 1 every four weeks for six cycles (alternatively see **Formula Dosing**).

Cyclophosphamide (CYTOXAN®)—600 mg/m^2 I.V. on day 1 every 4 weeks for six cycles. For directions regarding the use and administration of cyclophosphamide (CYTOXAN®), please refer to its package insert. (See **CLINICAL STUDIES**.)

Intermittent courses of PARAPLATIN in combination with cyclophosphamide should not be repeated until the neutrophil count is at least 2,000 and the platelet count is at least 100,000.

Dose Adjustment Recommendations: Pretreatment platelet count and performance status are important prognostic factors for severity of myelosuppression in previously treated patients.

The suggested dose adjustments for single agent or combination therapy shown in the table below are modified from controlled trials in previously treated and untreated patients with ovarian carcinoma. Blood counts were done weekly, and the recommendations are based on the lowest post-treatment platelet or neutrophil value.

Platelets	Neutrophils	Adjusted Dose* (From Prior Course)
> 100,000	> 2,000	125%
50–100,000	500–2,000	No Adjustment
< 50,000	< 500	75%

*Percentages apply to PARAPLATIN as a single agent or to both PARAPLATIN and cyclophosphamide in combination. In the controlled studies, dosages were also adjusted at a lower level (50% to 60%) for severe myelosuppression. Escalations above 125% were not recommended for these studies.

PARAPLATIN is usually administered by an infusion lasting 15 minutes or longer. No pre- or post-treatment hydration or forced diuresis is required.

Patients with Impaired Kidney Function: Patients with creatinine clearance values below 60 mL/min are at increased risk of severe bone marrow suppression. In renally-impaired patients who received single agent PARAPLATIN therapy, the incidence of severe leukopenia, neutropenia, or thrombocytopenia has been about 25% when the dosage modifications in the table below have been used.

Baseline Creatinine Clearance	Recommended Dose on Day 1
41–59 mL/min	250 mg/m^2
16–40 mL/min	200 mg/m^2

The data available for patients with severely impaired kidney function (creatinine clearance below 15 mL/min) are too limited to permit a recommendation for treatment.

These dosing recommendations apply to the initial course of treatment. Subsequent dosages should be adjusted according to the patient's tolerance based on the degree of bone marrow suppression.

Formula Dosing: Another approach for determining the initial dose of PARAPLATIN is the use of mathematical formulae, which are based on a patient's pre-existing renal function or renal function and desired platelet nadir. Renal excretion is the major route of elimination for carboplatin. (See **CLINICAL PHARMACOLOGY**.) The use of dosing formulae, as compared to empirical dose calculation based on body surface area, allows compensation for patient variations in pretreatment renal function that might otherwise result in either underdosing (in patients with above average renal function) or overdosing (in patients with impaired renal function).

A simple formula for calculating dosage, based upon a patient's glomerular filtration rate (GFR in mL/min) and PARAPLATIN target area under the concentration versus time curve (AUC in mg/mL• min), has been proposed by Calvert. In these studies, GFR was measured by ^{51}Cr-EDTA clearance.

CALVERT FORMULA FOR CARBOPLATIN DOSING

Total Dose (mg)=(target AUC) × (GFR + 25)

Note: With the Calvert formula, the total dose of PARAPLATIN is calculated in mg, not mg/m^2.

The target AUC of 4-6 mg/mL• min using single agent PARAPLATIN appears to provide the most appropriate dose range in previously treated patients. This study also showed a trend between the AUC of single agent PARAPLATIN administered to previously treated patients and the likelihood of developing toxicity.

% Actual Toxicity in Previously Treated Patients		
AUC (mg/mL•min)	Gr 3 or Gr 4 Thrombocytopenia	Gr 3 or Gr 4 Leukopenia
4 to 5	16%	13%
6 to 7	33%	34%

PREPARATION OF INTRAVENOUS SOLUTIONS

Immediately before use, the content of each vial must be reconstituted with either Sterile Water for Injection, USP, 5% Dextrose in Water (D_5W), or 0.9% Sodium Chloride Injection, USP, according to the following schedule:

Vial Strength	Diluent Volume
50 mg	5 mL
150 mg	15 mL
450 mg	45 mL

These dilutions all produce a carboplatin concentration of 10 mg/mL.

PARAPLATIN can be further diluted to concentrations as low as 0.5 mg/mL with 5% Dextrose in Water (D_5W) or 0.9% Sodium Chloride Injection, USP.

STABILITY

Unopened vials of PARAPLATIN are stable for the life indicated on the package when stored at controlled room temperature 15°–30°C (59°–86°F), and protected from light.

When prepared as directed, PARAPLATIN solutions are stable for 8 hours at room temperature (25°C). Since no antibacterial preservative is contained in the formulation, it is recommended that PARAPLATIN solutions be discarded 8 hours after dilution.

Parenteral drug products should be inspected visually for particulate matter and discoloration prior to administration.

HOW SUPPLIED

PARAPLATIN® (carboplatin for injection)

NDC 0015-3213-30 **50 mg** vials, individually cartoned, shelf packs of 10 cartons, 10 shelf packs per case. (Yellow flip-off seals)

NDC 0015-3214-30 **150 mg** vials, individually cartoned, shelf packs of 10 cartons, 10 shelf packs per case. (Violet flip-off seals)

NDC 0015-3215-30 **450 mg** vials, individually cartoned, shelf packs of 6 cartons, 10 shelf packs per case. (Blue flip-off seals)

STORAGE

Store the unopened vials at controlled room temperature 15°–30°C (59°–86°F). Protect unopened vials from light. Solutions for infusion should be discarded 8 hours after preparation.

HANDLING AND DISPOSAL

Procedures for proper handling and disposal of anti-cancer drugs should be considered. Several guidelines on this subject have been published.[1–7] There is no general agreement that all of the procedures recommended in the guidelines are necessary or appropriate.

REFERENCES

1. Recommendations for the Safe Handling of Parenteral Antineoplastic Drugs. NIH Publication No. 83-2621. For sale by the Superintendent of Documents, US Government Printing Office, Washington, DC 20402.
2. AMA Council Report. Guidelines for Handling Parenteral Antineoplastics. *JAMA* 1985; 253(11):1590–1592.
3. National Study Commission on Cytotoxic Exposure—Recommendations for Handling Cytotoxic Agents. Available from Louis P. Jeffrey, ScD, Chairman, National Study Commission on Cytotoxic Exposure, Massachusetts College of Pharmacy and Allied Health Sciences, 179 Longwood Avenue, Boston, Massachusetts 02115.
4. Clinical Oncological Society of Australia. Guidelines and Recommendations for Safe Handling of Antineoplastic Agents. *Med J Australia* 1983; 1:426–428.
5. Jones RB, et al: Safe Handling of Chemotherapeutic Agents: A Report from the Mount Sinai Medical Center. *CA–A Cancer Journal for Clinicians* 1983; (Sept/Oct)258–263.
6. American Society of Hospital Pharmacists Technical Assistance Bulletin on Handling Cytotoxic and Hazardous Drugs. *Am J Hosp Pharm* 1990; 47:1033–1049.
7. Controlling Occupational Exposure to Hazardous Drugs. (OSHA WORK PRACTICE GUIDELINES). *Am J Health-Syst Pharm* 1996; 53:1669–1685.

U.S. Patent Nos. 4,140,707
4,657,927

BRISTOL LABORATORIES®
ONCOLOGY PRODUCTS
A Bristol-Myers Squibb Company
Princeton, NJ 08543
U.S.A.

K2-B001-5-00 3213DIM-12
1080187A2 Revised February 2000

Shown in Product Identification Guide, page 310

PLATINOL®-AQ ℞

[*plă-tin-ŏl*]
(cisplatin injection)
Rx ONLY

WARNING

PLATINOL®-AQ (cisplatin injection) should be administered under the supervision of a qualified physician experienced in the use of cancer chemotherapeutic agents. Appropriate management of therapy and complications is possible only when adequate diagnostic and treatment facilities are readily available.

Cumulative renal toxicity associated with PLATINOL-AQ is severe. Other major dose-related toxicities are myelosuppression, nausea, and vomiting.

Ototoxicity, which may be more pronounced in children, and is manifested by tinnitus, and/or loss of high frequency hearing and occasionally deafness, is significant.

Anaphylactic-like reactions to PLATINOL-AQ have been reported. Facial edema, bronchoconstriction, tachycardia, and hypotension may occur within minutes of PLATINOL-AQ administration. Epinephrine, corticosteroids, and antihistamines have been effectively employed to alleviate symptoms (see **WARNINGS** and **ADVERSE REACTIONS**).

Exercise caution to prevent inadvertent PLATINOL-AQ overdose. Doses greater than 100 mg/m^2/cycle once every 3 to 4 weeks are rarely used. Care must be taken to avoid inadvertent PLATINOL-AQ overdose due to confusion with PARAPLATIN® (carboplatin) or prescribing practices that fail to differentiate daily doses from total dose per cycle.

DESCRIPTION

PLATINOL®-AQ (cisplatin injection) is a clear, colorless, sterile aqueous solution, each mL containing 1 mg cisplatin and 9 mg Sodium Chloride, USP. HCl and/or Sodium Hydroxide is added to adjust pH of the solution.

The active ingredient, cisplatin, is a yellow to orange crystalline powder with the molecular formula $PtCl_2H_6N_2$, and a molecular weight of 300.1. Cisplatin is a heavy metal complex containing a central atom of platinum surrounded by two chloride atoms and two ammonia molecules in the cis position. It is soluble in water or saline at 1 mg/mL and in dimethylformamide at 24 mg/mL. It has a melting point of 207°C.

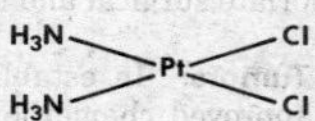

CLINICAL PHARMACOLOGY

Plasma concentrations of the parent compound, cisplatin, decay monoexponentially with a half-life of about 20 to 30 minutes following bolus administrations of 50 or 100 mg/m^2 doses. Monoexponential decay and plasma half-lives of about 0.5 hour are also seen following two hour or seven hour infusions of 100 mg/m^2. After the latter, the total-body clearances and volumes of distribution at steady-state for cisplatin are about 15 to 16 L/h/m^2 and 11 to 12 L/m^2.

Due to its unique chemical structure, the chlorine atoms of cisplatin are more subject to chemical displacement reactions by nucleophiles, such as water or sulfhydryl groups, than to enzyme-catalyzed metabolism. At physiological pH in the presence of 0.1M NaCl, the predominant molecular species are cisplatin and monohydroxymonochloro *cis*-diammine platinum (II) in nearly equal concentrations. The latter, combined with the possible direct displacement of the chlorine atoms by sulfhydryl groups of amino acids or proteins, accounts for the instability of cisplatin in biological matrices. The ratios of cisplatin to total free (ultrafilterable) platinum in the plasma vary considerably between patients and range from 0.5 to 1.1 after a dose of 100 mg/m^2.

Cisplatin does not undergo the instantaneous and reversible binding to plasma proteins that is characteristic of normal drug-protein binding. However, the platinum from cisplatin, but not cisplatin itself, becomes bound to several plasma proteins including albumin, transferrin, and gamma globulin. Three hours after a bolus injection and two hours after the end of a three-hour infusion, 90% of the plasma platinum is protein bound. The complexes between albumin and the platinum from cisplatin do not dissociate to a significant extent and are slowly eliminated with a minimum half-life of five days or more.

Following cisplatin doses of 20 to 120 mg/m^2, the concentrations of platinum are highest in liver, prostate, and kidney, somewhat lower in bladder, muscle, testicle, pancreas, and spleen and lowest in bowel, adrenal, heart, lung, cerebrum, and cerebellum. Platinum is present in tissues for as long as 180 days after the last administration. With the exception of intracerebral tumors, platinum concentrations in tumors are generally somewhat lower than the concentrations in the organ where the tumor is located. Different metastatic sites in the same patient may have different platinum concentrations. Hepatic metastases have the highest platinum concentrations, but these are similar to the platinum concentrations in normal liver. Maximum red blood cell concentrations of platinum are reached within 90 to 150 minutes after a 100 mg/m^2 dose of cisplatin and decline in a biphasic manner with a terminal half-life of 36 to 47 days.

Over a dose range of 40 to 140 mg cisplatin/m^2 given as a bolus injection or as infusions varying in length from 1 hour to 24 hours, from 10% to about 40% of the administered platinum is excreted in the urine in 24 hours. Over five days following administration of 40 to 100 mg/m^2 doses given as rapid, 2 to 3 hour, or 6 to 8 hour infusions, a mean of 35% to 51% of the dosed platinum is excreted in the urine. Similar mean urinary recoveries of platinum of about 14% to 30% of the dose are found following five daily administrations of 20, 30, or 40 mg/m^2/day. Only a small percentage of the administered platinum is excreted beyond 24 hours post-infusion and most of the platinum excreted in the urine in 24 hours is excreted within the first few hours. Platinum-containing species excreted in the urine are the same as those found following the incubation of cisplatin with urine from healthy subjects, except that the proportions are different.

The parent compound, cisplatin, is excreted in the urine and accounts for 13% to 17% of the dose excreted within one hour after administration of 50 mg/m^2. The mean renal clearance of cisplatin exceeds creatinine clearance and is 62 and 50 mL/min/m^2 following administration of 100 mg/m^2 as 2 hour or 6 to 7 hour infusions, respectively.

The renal clearance of free (ultrafilterable) platinum also exceeds the glomerular filtration rate indicating that cisplatin or other platinum-containing molecules are actively secreted by the kidneys. The renal clearance of free platinum is nonlinear and variable and is dependent on dose, urine flow rate, and individual variability in the extent of active secretion and possible tubular reabsorption.

There is a potential for accumulation of ultrafilterable platinum plasma concentrations whenever cisplatin is administered on a daily basis but not when dosed on an intermittent basis.

No significant relationships exist between the renal clearance of either free platinum or cisplatin and creatinine clearance.

Although small amounts of platinum are present in the bile and large intestine after administration of cisplatin, the fecal excretion of platinum appears to be insignificant.

INDICATIONS

PLATINOL-AQ (cisplatin injection) is indicated as therapy to be employed as follows:

Metastatic Testicular Tumors: In established combination therapy with other approved chemotherapeutic agents in patients with metastatic testicular tumors who have al-

Continued on next page

Platinol-AQ—Cont.

ready received appropriate surgical and/or radiotherapeutic procedures.

Metastatic Ovarian Tumors: In established combination therapy with other approved chemotherapeutic agents in patients with metastatic ovarian tumors who have already received appropriate surgical and/or radiotherapeutic procedures. An established combination consists of PLATINOL-AQ and CYTOXAN® (cyclophosphamide). PLATINOL-AQ, as a single agent, is indicated as secondary therapy in patients with metastatic ovarian tumors refractory to standard chemotherapy who have not previously received PLATINOL-AQ therapy.

Advanced Bladder Cancer: PLATINOL-AQ is indicated as a single agent for patients with transitional cell bladder cancer which is no longer amenable to local treatments such as surgery and/or radiotherapy.

CONTRAINDICATIONS

PLATINOL-AQ is contraindicated in patients with preexisting renal impairment. PLATINOL-AQ should not be employed in myelosuppressed patients, or patients with hearing impairment.

PLATINOL-AQ is contraindicated in patients with a history of allergic reactions to PLATINOL-AQ or other platinum-containing compounds.

WARNINGS

PLATINOL-AQ produces cumulative nephrotoxicity which is potentiated by aminoglycoside antibiotics. The serum creatinine, BUN, creatinine clearance, and magnesium, sodium, potassium, and calcium levels should be measured prior to initiating therapy, and prior to each subsequent course. At the recommended dosage, PLATINOL-AQ should not be given more frequently than once every 3 to 4 weeks (see **ADVERSE REACTIONS**).

There are reports of severe neuropathies in patients in whom regimens are employed using higher doses of PLATINOL-AQ or greater dose frequencies than those recommended. These neuropathies may be irreversible and are seen as paresthesias in a stocking-glove distribution, areflexia, and loss of proprioception and vibratory sensation.

Loss of motor function has also been reported.

Anaphylactic-like reactions to PLATINOL-AQ have been reported. These reactions have occurred within minutes of administration to patients with prior exposure to PLATINOL-AQ, and have been alleviated by administration of epinephrine, corticosteroids, and antihistamines.

Since ototoxicity of PLATINOL-AQ is cumulative, audiometric testing should be performed prior to initiating therapy and prior to each subsequent dose of drug (see **ADVERSE REACTIONS**).

PLATINOL-AQ can cause fetal harm when administered to a pregnant woman. PLATINOL-AQ is mutagenic in bacteria and produces chromosome aberrations in animal cells in tissue culture. In mice PLATINOL-AQ is teratogenic and embryotoxic. If this drug is used during pregnancy or if the patient becomes pregnant while taking this drug, the patient should be apprised of the potential hazard to the fetus. Patients should be advised to avoid becoming pregnant.

The carcinogenic effect of PLATINOL-AQ was studied in BD IX rats. PLATINOL-AQ was administered i.p. to 50 BD IX rats for 3 weeks, 3×1 mg/kg body weight per week. Four hundred and fifty-five days after the first application, 33 animals died, 13 of them related to malignancies: 12 leukemias and 1 renal fibrosarcoma.

The development of acute leukemia coincident with the use of PLATINOL-AQ has rarely been reported in humans. In these reports, PLATINOL-AQ was generally given in combination with other leukemogenic agents.

PRECAUTIONS

Peripheral blood counts should be monitored weekly. Liver function should be monitored periodically. Neurologic examination should also be performed regularly (see **ADVERSE REACTIONS**).

Drug Interactions: Plasma levels of anticonvulsant agents may become subtherapeutic during cisplatin therapy.

In a randomized trial in advanced ovarian cancer, response duration was adversely affected when pyridoxine was used in combination with altretamine (hexamethylmelamine) and PLATINOL-AQ.

Carcinogenesis, Mutagenesis, Impairment of Fertility: See **WARNINGS**.

Pregnancy: Pregnancy "Category D". (See **WARNINGS**.)

Nursing Mothers: Cisplatin has been reported to be found in human milk; patients receiving PLATINOL-AQ should not breast feed.

Pediatric Use: Safety and effectiveness in pediatric patients have not been established.

ADVERSE REACTIONS

Nephrotoxicity: Dose-related and cumulative renal insufficiency is the major dose-limiting toxicity of PLATINOL-AQ. Renal toxicity has been noted in 28% to 36% of patients treated with a single dose of 50 mg/m^2. It is first noted during the second week after a dose and is manifested by elevations in BUN and creatinine, serum uric acid and/or a decrease in creatinine clearance. **Renal toxicity becomes more prolonged and severe with repeated courses of the drug. Renal function must return to normal before another dose of PLATINOL-AQ can be given.**

Impairment of renal function has been associated with renal tubular damage. The administration of PLATINOL-AQ using a 6- to 8-hour infusion with intravenous hydration, and mannitol has been used to reduce nephrotoxicity. However, renal toxicity still can occur after utilization of these procedures.

Ototoxicity: Ototoxicity has been observed in up to 31% of patients treated with a single dose of PLATINOL-AQ 50 mg/m^2, and is manifested by tinnitus and/or hearing loss in the high frequency range (4,000 to 8,000 Hz). Decreased ability to hear normal conversational tones may occur occasionally. Deafness after the initial dose of PLATINOL-AQ has been reported rarely. Ototoxic effects may be more severe in children receiving PLATINOL-AQ. Hearing loss can be unilateral or bilateral and tends to become more frequent and severe with repeated doses. Ototoxicity may be enhanced with prior or simultaneous cranial irradiation. It is unclear whether PLATINOL-AQ induced ototoxicity is reversible. Ototoxic effects may be related to the peak plasma concentration of PLATINOL-AQ. Careful monitoring of audiometry should be performed prior to initiation of therapy and prior to subsequent doses of PLATINOL-AQ.

Vestibular toxicity has also been reported.

Ototoxicity may become more severe in patients being treated with other drugs with nephrotoxic potential.

Hematologic: Myelosuppression occurs in 25% to 30% of patients treated with PLATINOL-AQ. The nadirs in circulating platelets and leukocytes occur between days 18 to 23 (range 7.5 to 45) with most patients recovering by day 39 (range 13 to 62). Leukopenia and thrombocytopenia are more pronounced at higher doses (>50 mg/m^2). Anemia (decrease of 2 g hemoglobin/100 mL) occurs at approximately the same frequency and with the same timing as leukopenia and thrombocytopenia. Fever and infection have also been reported in patients with neutropenia.

In addition to anemia secondary to myelosuppression, a Coombs' positive hemolytic anemia has been reported. In the presence of cisplatin hemolytic anemia, a further course of treatment may be accompanied by increased hemolysis and this risk should be weighed by the treating physician.

The development of acute leukemia coincident with the use of PLATINOL-AQ has rarely been reported in humans. In these reports, PLATINOL-AQ (cisplatin injection) was generally given in combination with other leukemogenic agents.

Gastrointestinal: Marked nausea and vomiting occur in almost all patients treated with PLATINOL-AQ, and are occasionally so severe that the drug must be discontinued. Nausea and vomiting usually begin within 1 to 4 hours after treatment and last up to 24 hours. Various degrees of vomiting, nausea and/or anorexia may persist for up to 1 week after treatment.

Delayed nausea and vomiting (begins or persists 24 hours or more after chemotherapy) has occurred in patients attaining complete emetic control on the day of PLATINOL-AQ therapy.

Diarrhea has also been reported.

OTHER TOXICITIES

Vascular toxicities coincident with the use of PLATINOL-AQ in combination with other antineoplastic agents have been reported rarely. The events are clinically heterogeneous and may include myocardial infarction, cerebrovascular accident, thrombotic microangiopathy (HUS), or cerebral arteritis. Various mechanisms have been proposed for these vascular complications. There are also reports of Raynaud's phenomenon occurring in patients treated with the combination of bleomycin, vinblastine with or without PLATINOL-AQ. It has been suggested that hypomagnesemia developing coincident with the use of PLATINOL-AQ may be an added, although not essential, factor associated with this event. However, it is currently unknown if the cause of Raynaud's phenomenon in these cases is the disease, underlying vascular compromise, bleomycin, vinblastine, hypomagnesemia, or a combination of any of these factors.

Serum Electrolyte Disturbances: Hypomagnesemia, hypocalcemia, hyponatremia, hypokalemia, and hypophosphatemia have been reported to occur in patients treated with PLATINOL-AQ and are probably related to renal tubular damage. Tetany has occasionally been reported in those patients with hypocalcemia and hypomagnesemia. Generally, normal serum electrolyte levels are restored by administering supplemental electrolytes and discontinuing PLATINOL-AQ.

Inappropriate antidiuretic hormone syndrome has also been reported.

Hyperuricemia: Hyperuricemia has been reported to occur at approximately the same frequency as the increases in BUN and serum creatinine. It is more pronounced after doses greater than 50 mg/m^2, and peak levels of uric acid generally occur between 3 to 5 days after the dose. Allopurinol therapy for hyperuricemia effectively reduces uric acid levels.

Neurotoxicity (see **WARNINGS**): Neurotoxicity, usually characterized by peripheral neuropathies, has been reported. The neuropathies usually occur after prolonged therapy (4 to 7 months); however, neurologic symptoms have been reported to occur after a single dose. Although symptoms and signs of PLATINOL-AQ neuropathy usually develop during treatment, symptoms of neuropathy may begin 3 to 8 weeks after the last dose of PLATINOL-AQ, although this is rare. PLATINOL-AQ therapy should be discontinued when the symptoms are first observed. The neuropathy, however, may progress further even after stopping treatment. Preliminary evidence suggests peripheral neuropathy may be irreversible in some patients.

Lhermitte's sign, dorsal column myelopathy, and autonomic neuropathy have also been reported.

Loss of taste and seizures have also been reported.

Muscle cramps, defined as localized, painful, involuntary skeletal muscle contractions of sudden onset and short duration, have been reported and were usually associated in patients receiving a relatively high cumulative dose of PLATINOL-AQ and with a relatively advanced symptomatic stage of peripheral neuropathy.

Ocular Toxicity: Optic neuritis, papilledema, and cerebral blindness have been reported infrequently in patients receiving standard recommended doses of PLATINOL-AQ. Improvement and/or total recovery usually occurs after discontinuing PLATINOL-AQ. Steroids with or without mannitol have been used; however, efficacy has not been established.

Blurred vision and altered color perception have been reported after the use of regimens with higher doses of PLATINOL-AQ or greater dose frequencies than those recommended in the package insert. The altered color perception manifests as a loss of color discrimination, particularly in the blue-yellow axis. The only finding on funduscopic exam is irregular retinal pigmentation of the macular area.

Anaphylactic-like Reactions: Anaphylactic-like reactions have been occasionally reported in patients previously exposed to PLATINOL-AQ. The reactions consist of facial edema, wheezing, tachycardia, and hypotension within a few minutes of drug administration. Reactions may be controlled by intravenous epinephrine with corticosteroids and/or antihistamines as indicated. Patients receiving PLATINOL-AQ should be observed carefully for possible anaphylactic-like reactions and supportive equipment and medication should be available to treat such a complication.

Hepatotoxicity: Transient elevations of liver enzymes, especially SGOT, as well as bilirubin, have been reported to be associated with PLATINOL-AQ administration at the recommended doses.

Other Events: Other toxicities reported to occur infrequently are cardiac abnormalities, hiccups, elevated serum amylase, and rash. Alopecia, malaise, and asthenia have been reported as part of postmarketing surveillance.

Local soft tissue toxicity has rarely been reported following extravasation of PLATINOL-AQ. Severity of the local tissue toxicity appears to be related to the concentration of the PLATINOL-AQ solution. Infusion of solutions with a PLATINOL-AQ concentration greater than 0.5 mg/mL may result in tissue cellulitis, fibrosis, and necrosis.

OVERDOSAGE

Caution should be exercised to prevent inadvertent overdosage with PLATINOL-AQ. Acute overdosage with this drug may result in kidney failure, liver failure, deafness, ocular toxicity (including detachment of the retina), significant myelosuppression, intractable nausea and vomiting and/or neuritis. In addition, death can occur following overdosage.

No proven antidotes have been established for PLATINOL-AQ overdosage. Hemodialysis, even when initiated four hours after the overdosage, appears to have little effect on removing platinum from the body because of PLATINOL-AQ's rapid and high degree of protein binding. Management of overdosage should include general supportive measures to sustain the patient through any period of toxicity that may occur.

DOSAGE AND ADMINISTRATION

Note: Needles or intravenous sets containing aluminum parts that may come in contact with PLATINOL-AQ should not be used for preparation or administration. Aluminum reacts with PLATINOL-AQ, causing precipitate formation and a loss of potency.

Metastatic Testicular Tumors: The usual PLATINOL-AQ dose for the treatment of testicular cancer in combination with other approved chemotherapeutic agents is 20 mg/m^2 I.V. daily for 5 days per cycle.

Metastatic Ovarian Tumors: The usual PLATINOL-AQ dose for the treatment of metastatic ovarian tumors in combination with CYTOXAN (cyclophosphamide) is 75–100 mg/m^2 I.V. per cycle once every 4 weeks, (Day 1).

The dose of CYTOXAN when used in combination with PLATINOL-AQ is 600 mg/m^2 I.V. once every 4 weeks, (Day 1).

For directions for the administration of CYTOXAN, refer to the CYTOXAN package insert.

In combination therapy, PLATINOL-AQ and CYTOXAN are administered sequentially.

As a single agent, PLATINOL-AQ should be administered at a dose of 100 mg/m^2 I.V. per cycle once every 4 weeks.

Advanced Bladder Cancer: PLATINOL-AQ (cisplatin injection) should be administered as a single agent at a dose of 50–70 mg/m^2 I.V. per cycle once every 3 to 4 weeks depending on the extent of prior exposure to radiation therapy and/or prior chemotherapy. For heavily pretreated patients an initial dose of 50 mg/m^2 per cycle repeated every four weeks is recommended.

Pretreatment hydration with 1 to 2 liters of fluid infused for 8 to 12 hours prior to a PLATINOL-AQ dose is recommended. The drug is then diluted in 2 liters of 5% Dextrose in 1/2 or 1/3 normal saline containing 37.5 g of mannitol, and infused over a 6- to 8-hour period. If diluted solution is not to be used within 6 hours, protect solution from light. Do not dilute PLATINOL-AQ in just 5% Dextrose Injection. Adequate hydration and urinary output must be maintained during the following 24 hours.

A repeat course of PLATINOL-AQ should not be given until the serum creatinine is below 1.5 mg/100 mL, and/or the BUN is below 25 mg/100 mL. A repeat course should not be given until circulating blood elements are at an acceptable level (platelets ≥100,000/mm^3, WBC ≥4,000/mm^3). Subsequent doses of PLATINOL-AQ should not be given until an audiometric analysis indicates that auditory acuity is within normal limits.

As with other potentially toxic compounds, caution should be exercised in handling the aqueous solution. Skin reactions associated with accidental exposure to cisplatin may occur. The use of gloves is recommended. If PLATINOL-AQ contacts the skin or mucosa, immediately and thoroughly wash the skin with soap and water and flush the mucosa with water.

The aqueous solution should be used intravenously only and should be administered by I.V. infusion over a 6- to 8-hour period.

NOTE TO PHARMACIST: Exercise caution to prevent inadvertent PLATINOL-AQ overdosage. Please call prescriber if dose greater than 100 mg/m^2 per cycle. Aluminum and flip-off seal of vial have been imprinted with the following statement: **CALL DR. IF DOSE>100 MG/M^2/CYCLE.**

STABILITY

PLATINOL-AQ is a sterile, multidose vial without preservatives.

Store at 15°C–25°C. Do not refrigerate. Protect unopened container from light.

The cisplatin remaining in the amber vial following initial entry is stable for 28 days protected from light or for 7 days under fluorescent room light.

Procedures for proper handling and disposal of anticancer drugs should be considered. Several guidelines on this subject have been published.[1–7] There is no general agreement that all of the procedures recommended in the guidelines are necessary or appropriate.

HOW SUPPLIED

PLATINOL®-AQ (cisplatin injection)

NDC 0015-3220-22—Each multidose vial contains 50 mg of cisplatin

NDC 0015-3221-22—Each multidose vial contains 100 mg of cisplatin

REFERENCES

1. Recommendations for the Safe Handling of Parenteral Antineoplastic Drugs. NIH Publication No. 83-2621. For sale by the Superintendent of Documents, US Government Printing Office, Washington, DC 20402.
2. AMA Council Report. Guidelines for Handling Parenteral Antineoplastics. *JAMA* 1985; 253(11):1590–1592.
3. National Study Commission on Cytotoxic Exposure—Recommendations for Handling Cytotoxic Agents. Available from Louis P. Jeffrey, ScD, Chairman, National Study Commission on Cytotoxic Exposure, Massachusetts College of Pharmacy and Allied Health Sciences, 179 Longwood Avenue, Boston, Massachusetts 02115.
4. Clinical Oncological Society of Australia. Guidelines and Recommendations for Safe Handling of Antineoplastic Agents. *Med J Australia* 1983; 1:426–428.
5. Jones RB, et al: Safe Handling of Chemotherapeutic Agents: A Report from the Mount Sinai Medical Center. *CA–A Cancer Journal for Clinicians* 1983; (Sept/Oct)258–263.
6. American Society of Hospital Pharmacists Technical Assistance Bulletin on Handling Cytotoxic and Hazardous Drugs. *Am J Hosp Pharm* 1990; 47:1033–1049.
7. Controlling Occupational Exposure to Hazardous Drugs. (OSHA WORK PRACTICE GUIDELINES). *Am J Health-Syst Pharm* 1996; 53:1669–1685.

BRISTOL-MYERS SQUIBB ONCOLOGY

Bristol-Myers Squibb Company
Princeton, NJ 08543
U.S.A.

K3-B002-5-00 3220DIM-19
1080225A2 Revised October 1999

Shown in Product Identification Guide, page 310

RUBEX® ℞

[*rŭ-bex*]

(doxorubicin hydrochloride for injection, USP)

FOR INTRAVENOUS USE ONLY

℞ ONLY

WARNINGS

1. Severe local tissue necrosis will occur if there is extravasation during administration (see **DOSAGE AND ADMINISTRATION** section). Doxorubicin must not be given by the intramuscular or subcutaneous route.
2. Myocardial toxicity manifested in its most severe form by potentially fatal congestive heart failure may occur either during therapy or months to years after termination of therapy. The probability of developing impaired myocardial function based on a combined index of signs, symptoms and decline in left ventricular ejection fraction (LVEF) is estimated to be 1% to 2% at a total cumulative dose of 300 mg/m^2 of doxorubicin, 3% to 5% at a dose of 400 mg/m^2, 5% to 8% at 450 mg/m^2 and 6% to 20% at 500 mg/m^2.* The risk of developing CHF increases rapidly with increasing total cumulative doses of doxorubicin in excess of 450 mg/m^2. This toxicity may occur at lower cumulative doses in patients with prior mediastinal irradiation or on concurrent cyclophosphamide therapy or with pre-existing heart disease.
3. Dosage should be reduced in patients with impaired hepatic function.
4. Severe myelosuppression may occur.
5. Doxorubicin should be administered only under the supervision of a physician who is experienced in the use of cancer chemotherapeutic agents.

*Data on file at Pharmacia & Upjohn.

DESCRIPTION

Doxorubicin is a cytotoxic anthracycline antibiotic isolated from cultures of *Streptomyces peucetius* var. *caesius*. Doxorubicin consists of a naphthacenequinone nucleus linked through a glycosidic bond at ring atom 7 to an amino sugar, daunosamine.

Chemically, doxorubicin hydrochloride is: (8*S*,10*S*)-10-[(3-Amino-2,3,6-trideoxy-α-L-*lyxo*-hexopyranosyl)-oxy]-8-glycoloyl-7,8,9,10-tetrahydro-6,8,11-trihydroxy-1-methoxy-5,12-naphthacenedione hydrochloride [*25316-40-9*].

The structural formula is as follows:

$C_{27}H_{29}NO_{11}$ •HCl Molecular Weight — 579.99

Doxorubicin binds to nucleic acids, presumably by specific intercalation of the planar anthracycline nucleus with the DNA double helix. The anthracycline ring is lipophilic but the saturated end of the ring system contains abundant hydroxyl groups adjacent to the amino sugar, producing a hydrophilic center. The molecule is amphoteric, containing acidic functions in the ring phenolic groups and a basic function in the sugar amino group. It binds to cell membranes as well as plasma proteins. RUBEX® (doxorubicin hydrochloride for injection, USP) is for intravenous use only. It is available in 50 mg and 100 mg single dose vials as a lyophilized, sterile powder with added lactose (anhydrous), 250 mg and 500 mg, respectively.

CLINICAL PHARMACOLOGY

The cytotoxic effect of doxorubicin on malignant cells and its toxic effects on various organs are thought to be related to nucleotide base intercalation and cell membrane lipid binding activities of doxorubicin. Intercalation inhibits nucleotide replication and action of DNA and RNA polymerases. The interaction of doxorubicin with topoisomerase II to form DNA-cleavable complexes appears to be an important mechanism of doxorubicin cytocidal activity. Doxorubicin cellular membrane binding may effect a variety of cellular functions. Enzymatic electron reduction of doxorubicin by a variety of oxidases, reductases and dehydrogenases generate highly reactive species including the hydroxyl free radical OH^-. Free radical formation has been implicated in doxorubicin cardiotoxicity by means of Cu (II) and Fe (III) reduction at the cellular level.

Animal studies have shown activity in a spectrum of experimental tumors, immunosuppression, carcinogenic properties in rodents, induction of a variety of toxic effects, including delayed and progressive cardiac toxicity, myelosuppression in all species and atrophy to testes in rats and dogs.

Pharmacokinetic studies, determined in patients with various types of tumors undergoing either single or multi-agent therapy have shown that doxorubicin follows a multiphasic disposition after intravenous injection. The initial distributive half-life of approximately 5.0 minutes suggests rapid tissue uptake of doxorubicin, while its slow elimination from tissues is reflected by a terminal half-life of 20 to 48 hours. Steady-state distribution volumes exceed 20 to 30 L/kg and are indicative of extensive drug uptake into tissues. Plasma clearance is in the range of 8 to 20 mL/min/kg and is predominately by metabolism and biliary excretion. Approximately 40% of the dose appears in the bile in 5 days while only 5% to 12% of the drug and its metabolites appear in the urine during the same time period. Binding of doxorubicin and its major metabolite, doxorubicinol to plasma proteins is about 74% to 76% and is independent of plasma concentration of doxorubicin up to 2 μM. Enzymatic reduction at the 7 position and cleavage of the daunosamine sugar yields aglycones which are accompanied by free radical formation, the local production of which may contribute to the cardiotoxic activity of doxorubicin. Disposition of doxorubicinol (DOX-OL) in patients is formation rate limited. The terminal half-life of DOX-OL is similar to doxorubicin. The relative exposure of DOX-OL, compared to doxorubicin ranges between 0.4 to 0.6. In urine, <3% of the dose was recovered as DOX-OL over 7 days. A published clinical study involving 6 men and 21 women with no prior anthracycline therapy reported a significantly higher median doxorubicin clearance in the men compared to the women (113 versus 44 L/hr). However, the terminal half-life of doxorubicin was longer in men compared to the women (54 versus 35 hrs).

In four patients dose-independent pharmacokinetics have been shown for doxorubicin in the dose range of 30 to 70 mg/m^2. Systemic clearance of doxorubicin is significantly reduced in obese women with ideal body weight greater than 130%. There was a significant reduction in clearance without any change in volume of distribution in obese patients when compared with normal patients with less than 115% ideal body weight. The clearance of doxorubicin and doxorubicinol was also reduced in patients with impaired hepatic function. Doxorubicin was excreted in the milk of one lactating patient, with peak milk concentration at 24 hours after treatment being approximately 4.4-fold greater than the corresponding plasma concentration. Doxorubicin was detectable in the milk up to 72 hours after therapy with 70 mg/m^2 of doxorubicin given as a 15 minute intravenous infusion and 100 mg/m^2 of cisplatin as a 26 hour intravenous infusion. The peak concentration of doxorubicinol in milk at 24 hours was 0.2 μM and AUC up to 24 hours was 16.5 μM.hr while the AUC for doxorubicin was 9.9 μM.hr. Doxorubicin does not cross the blood brain barrier.

INDICATIONS AND USAGE

RUBEX (doxorubicin hydrochloride for injection, USP) has been used successfully to produce regression in disseminated neoplastic conditions such as acute lymphoblastic leukemia, acute myeloblastic leukemia, Wilms' tumor, neuroblastoma, soft tissue and bone sarcomas, breast carcinoma, ovarian carcinoma, transitional cell bladder carcinoma, thyroid carcinoma, gastric carcinoma, Hodgkin's disease, malignant lymphoma and bronchogenic carcinoma in which the small cell histologic type is the most responsive compared to other cell types.

CONTRAINDICATIONS

Doxorubicin therapy should not be started in patients who have marked myelosuppression induced by previous treatment with other antitumor agents or by radiotherapy. Doxorubicin treatment is contraindicated in patients who received previous treatment with complete cumulative doses of doxorubicin, daunorubicin, idarubicin and/or other anthracyclines and anthracenes.

WARNINGS

Special attention must be given to the cardiotoxicity induced by doxorubicin. Irreversible myocardial toxicity, manifested in its most severe form by life-threatening and potentially fatal congestive heart failure, may occur either during therapy or months to years after termination of therapy. The probability of developing impaired myocardial function, based on a combined index of signs, symptoms and decline in left ventricular ejection fraction (LVEF) is estimated to be 1% to 2% at a total cumulative dose of 300 mg/m^2 of doxorubicin, 3% to 5% at a dose of 400 mg/m^2, 5% to 8% at a dose of 450 mg/m^2 and 6% to 20% at a dose of 500 mg/m^2 given in a schedule of a bolus injection once every 3 weeks (data on file at Pharmacia & Upjohn). In a retrospective review by Von Hoff *et al*, the probability of developing congestive heart failure was reported to be 5/168 (3%) at a cumulative dose of 430 mg/m^2 of doxorubicin, 8/110 (7%) at 575 mg/m^2 and 3/14 (21%) at 728 mg/m^2. The cumulative incidence of CHF was 2.2%. In a prospective study of doxorubicin in combination with cyclophosphamide, fluorouracil and/or vincristine in patients with breast cancer or small cell lung cancer, the cumulative incidence of congestive heart failure was 5% to 6%. The probability of CHF at various cumulative doses of doxorubicin was 1.5% at 300 mg/m^2, 4.9% at 400 mg/m^2, 7.7% at 450 mg/m^2 and 20.5% at 500 mg/m^2.

Cardiotoxicity may occur at lower doses in patients with prior mediastinal irradiation, concurrent cyclophosphamide therapy and advanced age. Data also suggest that pre-existing heart disease is a co-factor for increased risk of doxorubicin cardiotoxicity. In such cases, cardiac toxicity may occur at doses lower than the respective recommended cumulative dose of doxorubicin. Studies have suggested that concomitant administration of doxorubicin and calcium channel entry blockers may increase the risk of doxorubicin cardiotoxicity. The total dose of doxorubicin administered to the individual patient should also take into account previous or concomitant therapy with related compounds such as daunorubicin, idarubicin and mitoxantrone. Cardiomyopathy and/or congestive heart failure may be encountered several months or years after discontinuation of doxorubicin therapy.

The risk of congestive heart failure and other acute manifestations of doxorubicin cardiotoxicity in children may be as much or lower than in adults. Children appear to be at particular risk for developing delayed cardiac toxicity in that doxorubicin induced cardiomyopathy impairs myocardial growth as children mature, subsequently leading to possible development of congestive heart failure during early adulthood. As many as 40% of children may have subclinical cardiac dysfunction and 5% to 10% of children may develop congestive heart failure on long term follow-up. This late cardiac toxicity may be related to the dose of doxorubicin. The longer the length of follow-up the greater the increase in the detection rate.

Treatment of doxorubicin induced congestive heart failure includes the use of digitalis, diuretics, after load reducers such as angiotensin I converting enzyme (ACE) inhibitors, low salt diet, and bed rest. Such intervention may relieve symptoms and improve the functional status of the patient.

Monitoring Cardiac Function: In adult patients severe cardiac toxicity may occur precipitously without antecedent

Continued on next page

Rubex—Cont.

ECG changes. Cardiomyopathy induced by anthracyclines is usually associated with very characteristic histopathologic changes on an endomyocardial biopsy (EM biopsy), and a decrease of left ventricular ejection fraction (LVEF), as measured by multi-gated radionuclide angiography (MUGA scans) and/or echocardiogram (ECHO), from pretreatment baseline values. However, it has not been demonstrated that monitoring of the ejection fraction will predict when individual patients are approaching their maximally tolerated cumulative dose of doxorubicin. Cardiac function should be carefully monitored during treatment to minimize the risk of cardiac toxicity. A baseline cardiac evaluation with an ECG, LVEF, and /or an echocardiogram (ECHO) is recommended especially in patients with risk factors for increased cardiac toxicity (pre-existing heart disease, mediastinal irradiation, or concurrent cyclophosphamide therapy). Subsequent evaluations should be obtained at a cumulative dose of doxorubicin of at least 400 mg/m^2 and periodically thereafter during the course of therapy. Children are at increased risk for developing delayed cardiotoxicity following doxorubicin administration and therefore a follow-up cardiac evaluation is recommended periodically to monitor for this delayed cardiotoxicity.

In adults, a 10% decline in LVEF to below the lower limit of normal or an absolute LVEF of 45%, or a 20% decline in LVEF at any level is indicative of deterioration in cardiac function. In children, deterioration in cardiac function during or after the completion of therapy with doxorubicin is indicated by a drop in fractional shortening (FS) by an absolute value of ≥ 10 percentile units or below 29%, and a decline in LVEF of 10 percentile units or an LVEF below 55%. In general, if test results indicate deterioration in cardiac function associated with doxorubicin, the benefit of continued therapy should be carefully evaluated against the risk of producing irreversible cardiac damage.

Acute life-threatening arrhythmias have been reported to occur during or within a few hours after doxorubicin administration.

There is a high incidence of bone marrow depression, primarily of leukocytes, requiring careful hematologic monitoring. With the recommended dose schedule, leukopenia is usually transient, reaching its nadir 10 to 14 days after treatment with recovery usually occurring by the 21st day. White blood counts as low as 1000/mm^3 are to be expected during treatment with appropriate doses of doxorubicin. Red blood cell and platelet levels should also be monitored since they may also be depressed. Hematologic toxicity may require dose reduction or suspension or delay of doxorubicin therapy. Persistent severe myelosuppression may result in superinfection or hemorrhage.

Doxorubicin may potentiate the toxicity of other anticancer therapies. Exacerbation of cyclophosphamide induced hemorrhagic cystitis and enhancement of the hepatotoxicity of 6-mercaptopurine have been reported. Radiation induced toxicity to the myocardium, mucosae, skin and liver have been reported to be increased by the administration of doxorubicin.

Since metabolism and excretion of doxorubicin occurs predominantly by the hepatobiliary route, toxicity to recommended doses of doxorubicin can be enhanced by hepatic impairment, therefore, prior to the individual dosing, evaluation of hepatic function is recommended using conventional laboratory tests such as SGOT, SGPT, alkaline phosphatase and bilirubin (see **DOSAGE AND ADMINISTRATION** section).

Necrotizing colitis manifested by typhlitis (cecal inflammation), bloody stools and severe and sometimes fatal infections have been associated with a combination of doxorubicin given by I.V. push daily for 3 days and cytarabine given by continuous infusion daily for 7 or more days.

On intravenous administration of doxorubicin, extravasation may occur with or without an accompanying stinging or burning sensation, even if blood returns well on aspiration of the infusion needle (see **DOSAGE AND ADMINISTRATION** section). If any signs or symptoms of extravasation have occurred, the injection or infusion should be immediately terminated and restarted in another vein.

Pregnancy "Category D"—Safe use of doxorubicin in pregnancy has not been established. Doxorubicin is embryotoxic and teratogenic in rats and embryotoxic and abortifacient in rabbits. There are no adequate and well-controlled studies in pregnant women. If doxorubicin is to be used during pregnancy, or if the patient becomes pregnant during therapy, the patient should be apprised of the potential hazard to the fetus. Women of childbearing age should be advised to avoid becoming pregnant.

PRECAUTIONS

General: Doxorubicin is not an anti-microbial agent.

Information for Patients: RUBEX (doxorubicin hydrochloride for injection, USP) imparts a red coloration to the urine for 1 to 2 days after administration, and patients should be advised to expect this during active therapy.

Drug Interactions:

Paclitaxel—Two published studies report that initial administration of paclitaxel infused over 24 hours followed by doxorubicin administered over 48 hours resulted in a significant decrease in doxorubicin clearance with more profound neutropenic and stomatitis episodes than the reverse sequence of administration.

Progesterone—In a published study, progesterone was given intravenously to patients with advanced malignancies (ECOG PS <2) at high doses (up to 10 g over 24 hours) concomitantly with a fixed doxorubicin dose (60 mg/m^2) via bolus. Enhanced doxorubicin-induced neutropenia and thrombocytopenia were observed.

Verapamil—A study of the effects of verapamil on the acute toxicity of doxorubicin in mice revealed higher initial peak concentrations of doxorubicin in the heart with a higher incidence and severity of degenerative changes in cardiac tissue resulting in a shorter survival.

Cyclosporine—The addition of cyclosporine to doxorubicin may result in increases in AUC for both doxorubicin and doxorubicinol possibly due to a decrease in clearance of parent drug and a decrease in metabolism of doxorubicinol. Literature reports suggest that adding cyclosporine to doxorubicin results in more profound and prolonged hematologic toxicity than doxorubicin alone. Coma and/or seizures have also been described.

Literature reports have also described the following drug interactions: phenobarbital increases the elimination of doxorubicin, phenytoin levels may be decreased by doxorubicin, streptozocin (Zanosar®) may inhibit hepatic metabolism of doxorubicin, and administration of live vaccines to immunosuppressed patients including those undergoing cytotoxic chemotherapy may be hazardous.

Laboratory Tests: Initial treatment with doxorubicin requires observation of the patient and periodic monitoring of complete blood counts, hepatic function tests, and radionuclide left ventricular ejection fraction (See **WARNINGS** section).

Like other cytotoxic drugs, doxorubicin may induce "tumor lysis syndrome" and hyperuricemia in patients with rapidly growing tumors. Appropriate supportive and pharmacologic measures may prevent or alleviate this complication.

Carcinogenesis, Mutagenesis, Impairment of Fertility: Formal long-term carcinogenicity studies have not been conducted with doxorubicin. Doxorubicin and related compounds have been shown to have mutagenic and carcinogenic properties when tested in experimental models (including bacterial systems, mammalian cells in culture, and female Sprague-Dawley rats).

The possible adverse effect on fertility in males and females in humans or experimental animals have not been adequately evaluated. Testicular atrophy was observed in rats and dogs.

A variant of chemotherapy-related acute non-lymphocytic leukemia has been reported to occur infrequently a few years after multiple drug treatment of some neoplasms, which sometimes included doxorubicin. The exact role of doxorubicin has not been elucidated.

Pregnancy "Category D". (See **WARNINGS** section.)

Nursing Mothers: Because of the potential for serious adverse reactions in nursing infants from doxorubicin, mothers should be advised to discontinue nursing during doxorubicin therapy.

ADVERSE REACTIONS

Dose-limiting toxicities of therapy are myelosuppression and cardiotoxicity. Other reactions reported are:

Cardiotoxicity: (See **WARNINGS** section.)

Cutaneous: Reversible complete alopecia occurs in most cases. Hyperpigmentation of nailbeds and dermal creases, primarily in children, and onycholysis have been reported in a few cases. Recall of skin reaction due to prior radiotherapy has occurred with doxorubicin administration.

Gastrointestinal: Acute nausea and vomiting occurs frequently and may be severe. This may be alleviated by antiemetic therapy. Mucositis (stomatitis and esophagitis) may occur 5 to 10 days after administration. The effect may be severe leading to ulceration and represents a site of origin for severe infections. The dosage regimen consisting of administration of doxorubicin on three successive days results in greater incidence and severity of mucositis. Ulceration and necrosis of the colon, especially the cecum, may occur leading to bleeding or severe infections which can be fatal. This reaction has been reported in patients with acute nonlymphocytic leukemia treated with a 3-day course of doxorubicin combined with cytarabine. Anorexia and diarrhea have been occasionally reported.

Vascular: Phlebosclerosis has been reported especially when small veins are used or a single vein is used for repeated administration. Facial flushing may occur if the injection is given too rapidly.

Local: Severe cellulitis, vesication and tissue necrosis will occur if extravasation of doxorubicin occurs during administration. Erythematous streaking along the vein proximal to the site of the injection has been reported (see **DOSAGE AND ADMINISTRATION** section).

Hematologic: The occurrence of secondary acute myeloid leukemia with or without a preleukemic phase has been reported rarely in patients concurrently treated with doxorubicin in association with DNA-damaging antineoplastic agents. Such cases could have a short (1–3 years) latency period.

Hypersensitivity: Fever, chills and urticaria have been reported occasionally. Anaphylaxis may occur. A case of apparent cross sensitivity to lincomycin has been reported.

Other: Conjunctivitis and lacrimation occur rarely.

OVERDOSAGE

Acute overdosage with doxorubicin enhances the toxic effects of mucositis, leukopenia and thrombocytopenia. Treatment of acute overdosage consists of treatment of the severely myelosuppressed patient with hospitalization, antimicrobials, platelet transfusions and symptomatic treatment of mucositis. Use of hemopoietic growth factor (G-CSF, GM-CSF) may be considered.

Cumulative dosage with doxorubicin increases the risk of cardiomyopathy and resultant congestive heart failure (See **WARNINGS** section). Treatment consists of vigorous management of congestive heart failure with digitalis preparations, diuretics, and after load reducers such as ACE inhibitors.

DOSAGE AND ADMINISTRATION

Care in the administration of doxorubicin hydrochloride will reduce the chance of perivenous infiltration (See **WARNINGS** section). It may also decrease the chance of local reactions such as urticaria and erythematous streaking. On intravenous administration of doxorubicin, extravasation may occur with or without an accompanying burning or stinging sensation, even if blood returns well on aspiration of the infusion needle. If any signs or symptoms of extravasation have occurred, the injection or infusion should be immediately terminated and restarted in another vein. If extravasation is suspected, intermittent application of ice to the site for 15 min., q.i.d. × 3 days may be useful. The benefit of local administration of drugs has not been clearly established. Because of the progressive nature of extravasation reactions, close observation and plastic surgery consultation is recommended. Blistering, ulceration and/or persistent pain are indications for wide excision surgery, followed by split-thickness skin grafting.

The most commonly used dose schedule when used as a single agent is 60 to 75 mg/m^2 as a single intravenous injection administered at 21-day intervals. The lower dosage should be given to patients with inadequate marrow reserves due to old age, or prior therapy, or neoplastic marrow infiltration. RUBEX (doxorubicin hydrochloride for injection, USP) has been used concurrently with other approved chemotherapeutic agents. Evidence is available that in some types of neoplastic disease combination chemotherapy is superior to single agents. The benefits and risks of such therapy continue to be elucidated. When used in combination with other chemotherapy drugs, the most commonly used dosage of doxorubicin is 40 to 50 mg/m^2 given as a single intravenous injection every 21 to 28 days. Doxorubicin dosage must be reduced in case of hyperbilirubinemia as follows:

Plasma bilirubin concentration (mg/dL)	Dosage reduction (%)
1.2–3.0	50
3.1–5.0	75

Reconstitution Directions: RUBEX 50 mg and 100 mg vials should be reconstituted with 25 mL and 50 mL, respectively, of Sodium Chloride Injection, USP (0.9%) to give a final concentration of 2 mg/mL of doxorubicin hydrochloride. An appropriate volume of air should be withdrawn from the vial during reconstitution to avoid excessive pressure buildup. Bacteriostatic diluents are not recommended.

After adding the diluent, the vial should be shaken and the contents allowed to dissolve. The reconstituted solution is stable for 7 days at room temperature and 15 days under refrigeration 2°–8°C (36°–46°F). It should be protected from exposure to sunlight and any unused solution should be discarded.

It is recommended that doxorubicin be slowly administered into the tubing of a freely running intravenous infusion of Sodium Chloride Injection, USP or 5% Dextrose Injection, USP. The tubing should be attached to a Butterfly® needle inserted preferably into a large vein. If possible, avoid veins over joints or in extremities with compromised venous or lymphatic drainage. The rate of administration is dependent on the size of the vein and the dosage. However, the dose should be administered in not less than 3 to 5 minutes. Local erythematous streaking along the vein as well as facial flushing may be indicative of too rapid an administration. A burning or stinging sensation may be indicative of perivenous infiltration and the infusion should be immediately terminated and restarted in another vein. Perivenous infiltration may occur painlessly.

Doxorubicin should not be mixed with heparin or fluorouracil since it has been reported that these drugs are incompatible to the extent that a precipitate may form. Until specific compatibility data are available, it is not recommended that doxorubicin be mixed with other drugs.

Parenteral drug products should be inspected visually for particulate matter and discoloration prior to administration, whenever solution and container permit.

Handling and Disposal: Skin reactions associated with doxorubicin have been reported. Skin accidently exposed to doxorubicin should be rinsed copiously with soap and warm water, and if the eyes are involved, standard irrigation techniques should be used immediately. The use of goggles, gloves, and protective gowns is recommended during preparation and administration of the drug.

Procedures for proper handling and disposal of anticancer drugs should be considered. Several guidelines on this subject have been published.[1–7] There is no general agreement that all of the procedures recommended in the guidelines are necessary or appropriate.

HOW SUPPLIED

RUBEX® (doxorubicin hydrochloride for injection, USP) is available as follows:

50 mg— Each single-dose vial contains 50 mg of doxorubicin HCI, USP as a sterile red-orange lyophilized powder, **NDC** 0015-3352-22. Available as one individually cartoned vial.

100 mg— Each single-dose vial contains 100 mg of doxorubicin HCl, USP as a sterile red-orange lyophilized powder, **NDC** 0015-3353-22. Available as one individually cartoned vial.

Storage: Store dry powder at controlled room temperature 15°–30°C (59°–86°F).

The reconstituted solution is stable for 7 days at room temperature or 15 days under refrigeration 2°–8°C (36°–46°F). Protect from exposure to sunlight. Retain in carton until time of use.

Discard unused portion.

REFERENCES

1. Recommendations for the Safe Handling of Parenteral Antineoplastic Drugs. NIH Publication No. 83-2621. For sale by the Superintendent of Documents, US Government Printing Office, Washington, DC 20402.
2. AMA Council Report. Guidelines for Handling Parenteral Antineoplastics. *JAMA* 1985; 253 (11):1590–1592.
3. National Study Commission on Cytotoxic Exposure—Recommendations for Handling Cytotoxic Agents. Available from Louis P. Jeffrey, ScD, Chairman, National Study Commission on Cytotoxic Exposure, Massachusetts College of Pharmacy and Allied Health Sciences, 179 Longwood Avenue, Boston, Massachusetts 02115.
4. Clinical Oncological Society of Australia. Guidelines and Recommendations for Safe Handling of Antineoplastic Agents. *Med J Australia* 1983; 1:426–428.
5. Jones RB, et al: Safe Handling of Chemotherapeutic Agents: A Report from the Mount Sinai Medical Center. *CA-A Cancer Journal for Clinicians* 1983; (Sept/Oct) 258–263.
6. American Society of Hospital Pharmacists Technical Assistance Bulletin on Handling Cytotoxic and Hazardous Drugs. *Am J Hosp Pharm* 1990; 47:1033–1049.
7. Controlling Occupational Exposure to Hazardous Drugs. (OSHA WORK PRACTICE GUIDELINES). *Am J Health—Syst Pharm* 1996;53:1669–1685.

Mead Johnson
ONCOLOGY PRODUCTS
A Bristol-Myers Squibb Company
Princeton, NJ 08543
U.S.A.
K9-B001-6-99 3351DIM-07
51-004726-03 Revised: March 1999

TAXOL® ℞

[tăx-al]

(paclitaxel) Injection

(Patient Information Included)

℞ ONLY

WARNING

TAXOL® (paclitaxel) Injection should be administered under the supervision of a physician experienced in the use of cancer chemotherapeutic agents. Appropriate management of complications is possible only when adequate diagnostic and treatment facilities are readily available.

Anaphylaxis and severe hypersensitivity reactions characterized by dyspnea and hypotension requiring treatment, angioedema, and generalized urticaria have occurred in 2%–4% of patients receiving TAXOL in clinical trials. Fatal reactions have occurred in patients despite premedication. All patients should be pretreated with corticosteroids, diphenhydramine, and H_2 antagonists. (See **DOSAGE AND ADMINISTRATION**.) Patients who experience severe hypersensitivity reactions to TAXOL should not be rechallenged with the drug.

TAXOL therapy should not be given to patients with solid tumors who have baseline neutrophil counts of less than 1,500 cells/mm^3 and should not be given to patients with AIDS-related Kaposi's sarcoma if the baseline neutrophil count is less than 1000 cells/mm^3. In order to monitor the occurrence of bone marrow suppression, primarily neutropenia, which may be severe and result in infection, it is recommended that frequent peripheral blood cell counts be performed on all patients receiving TAXOL.

DESCRIPTION

TAXOL® (paclitaxel) Injection is a clear colorless to slightly yellow viscous solution. It is supplied as a nonaqueous solution intended for dilution with a suitable parenteral fluid prior to intravenous infusion. TAXOL is available in 30 mg (5 mL), 100 mg (16.7 mL), and 300 mg (50 mL) multidose vials. Each mL of sterile nonpyrogenic solution contains 6 mg paclitaxel, 527 mg of purified Cremophor® EL* (polyoxyethylated castor oil) and 49.7% (v/v) dehydrated alcohol, USP.

Paclitaxel is a natural product with antitumor activity. TAXOL is obtained via a semi-synthetic process from *Taxus baccata*. The chemical name for paclitaxel is 5β,20-Epoxy-1,2α,4,7β,10β,13α-hexahydroxytax-11-en-9-one 4,10-diacetate 2-benzoate 13-ester with (2*R*,3*S*)-*N*-benzoyl-3-phenylisoserine.

Paclitaxel has the following structural formula:

[See chemical structure at top of next column]

Table 1: Summary of Pharmacokinetic Parameters – Mean Values

Dose (mg/m²)	Infusion Duration (h)	N (patients)	C_{max} (ng/mL)	AUC (0–∞) (ng·h/mL)	T-HALF (h)	CL_T (L/h/m²)
135	24	2	195	6300	52.7	21.7
175	24	4	365	7993	15.7	23.8
135	3	7	2170	7952	13.1	17.7
175	3	5	3650	15007	20.2	12.2

C_{max} = Maximum plasma concentration
AUC (0–∞) = Area under the plasma concentration-time curve from time 0 to infinity
CL_T = Total body clearance

Paclitaxel is a white to off-white crystalline powder with the empirical formula $C_{47}H_{51}NO_{14}$ and a molecular weight of 853.9. It is highly lipophilic, insoluble in water, and melts at around 216–217°C.

CLINICAL PHARMACOLOGY

Paclitaxel is a novel antimicrotubule agent that promotes the assembly of microtubules from tubulin dimers and stabilizes microtubules by preventing depolymerization. This stability results in the inhibition of the normal dynamic reorganization of the microtubule network that is essential for vital interphase and mitotic cellular functions. In addition, paclitaxel induces abnormal arrays or "bundles" of microtubules throughout the cell cycle and multiple asters of microtubules during mitosis.

Following intravenous administration of TAXOL, paclitaxel plasma concentrations declined in a biphasic manner. The initial rapid decline represents distribution to the peripheral compartment and elimination of the drug. The later phase is due, in part, to a relatively slow efflux of paclitaxel from the peripheral compartment.

Pharmacokinetic parameters of paclitaxel following 3- and 24-hour infusions of TAXOL at dose levels of 135 and 175 mg/m^2 were determined in a Phase 3 randomized study in ovarian cancer patients and are summarized in the following table:

[See table 1 above]

It appeared that with the 24-hour infusion of TAXOL, a 30% increase in dose (135 mg/m^2 versus 175 mg/m^2) increased the C_{max} by 87%, whereas the AUC (0-∞) remained proportional. However, with a 3-hour infusion, for a 30% increase in dose, the C_{max} and AUC (0-∞) were increased by 68% and 89%, respectively. The mean apparent volume of distribution at steady state, with the 24-hour infusion of TAXOL, ranged from 227 to 688 L/m^2, indicating extensive extravascular distribution and/or tissue binding of paclitaxel.

The pharmacokinetics of paclitaxel were also evaluated in adult cancer patients who received single doses of 15–135 mg/m^2 given by 1-hour infusions (n=15), 30–275 mg/m^2 given by 6-hour infusions (n=36), and 200–275 mg/m^2 given by 24-hour infusions (n=54) in Phase 1 & 2 studies. Values for CL_T and volume of distribution were consistent with the findings in the Phase 3 study. The pharmacokinetics of TAXOL in patients with AIDS-related Kaposi's sarcoma have not been studied.

* Cremophor® EL is the registered trademark of BASF Aktiengesellschaft. Cremophor® EL is further purified by a Bristol-Myers Squibb Company proprietary process before use.

In vitro studies of binding to human serum proteins, using paclitaxel concentrations ranging from 0.1 to 50 µg/mL, indicate that between 89%–98% of drug is bound; the presence of cimetidine, ranitidine, dexamethasone, or diphenhydramine did not affect protein binding of paclitaxel.

After intravenous administration of 15–275 mg/m^2 doses of TAXOL (paclitaxel) Injection as 1-, 6-, or 24-hour infusions, mean values for cumulative urinary recovery of unchanged drug ranged from 1.3% to 12.6% of the dose, indicating extensive non-renal clearance. In five patients administered a 225 or 250 mg/m^2 dose of radiolabeled TAXOL as a 3-hour infusion, a mean of 71% of the radioactivity was excreted in the feces in 120 hours, and 14% was recovered in the urine. Total recovery of radioactivity ranged from 56% to 101% of the dose. Paclitaxel represented a mean of 5% of the administered radioactivity recovered in the feces, while metabolites, primarily 6α-hydroxypaclitaxel, accounted for the balance. *In vitro* studies with human liver microsomes and tissue slices showed that paclitaxel was metabolized primarily to 6α-hydroxypaclitaxel by the cytochrome P450 isozyme CYP2C8; and to two minor metabolites, 3'-*p*-hydroxypaclitaxel and 6α, 3'-*p*-dihydroxypaclitaxel, by CYP3A4. *In vitro*, the metabolism of paclitaxel to 6α-hydroxypaclitaxel was inhibited by a number of agents (ketoconazole, verapamil, diazepam, quinidine, dexamethasone, cyclosporin, teniposide, etoposide, and vincristine), but the concentrations used exceeded those found *in vivo* following normal therapeutic doses. Testosterone, 17α-ethinyl estradiol, retinoic acid, and quercetin, a specific inhibitor of CYP2C8, also inhibited the formation of 6α-hydroxypaclitaxel *in vitro*. The pharmacokinetics of paclitaxel may also be altered *in vivo* as a result of interactions with compounds that are substrates, inducers, or inhibitors of CYP2C8 and/or CYP3A4. (See **PRECAUTIONS: Drug Interactions**.) The effect of renal or hepatic dysfunction on the disposition of paclitaxel has not been investigated.

Possible interactions of paclitaxel with concomitantly administered medications have not been formally investigated.

CLINICAL STUDIES

Ovarian Carcinoma:

First-Line Data—The safety and efficacy of TAXOL followed by cisplatin in patients with advanced ovarian cancer and no prior chemotherapy were evaluated in two Phase 3 multicenter, randomized, controlled trials. In an Intergroup study led by the European Organization for Research and Treatment of Cancer involving the Scandinavian Group NOCOVA, the National Cancer Institute of Canada, and the Scottish Group, 680 patients with Stage II_{B-C}, III, or IV disease (optimally or non-optimally debulked) received either TAXOL 175 mg/m^2 infused over 3 hours followed by cisplatin 75 mg/m^2 (Tc) or cyclophosphamide 750 mg/m^2 followed by cisplatin 75 mg/m^2 (Cc) for a median of six courses. Although the protocol allowed further therapy, only 15% received both drugs for nine or more courses. In a study conducted by the Gynecological Oncology Group (GOG), 410 patients with Stage III or IV disease (>1 cm residual disease after staging laparotomy or distant metastases) received either TAXOL 135 mg/m^2 infused over 24 hours followed by cisplatin 75 mg/m^2 or cyclophosphamide 750 mg/m^2 followed by cisplatin 75 mg/m^2 for six courses.

In both studies, patients treated with TAXOL in combination with cisplatin had significantly higher response rate, longer time to progression, and longer survival time compared with standard therapy. These differences were also significant for the subset of patients in the Intergroup study with non-optimally debulked disease, although the study was not fully powered for subset analyses (Tables 2A and 2B). Kaplan-Meier survival curves for each study are shown in Figures 1 and 2.

[See table 2A at top of next page]
[See table 2B on next page]

Figure 1. Survival: Cc Versus Tc (Intergroup)

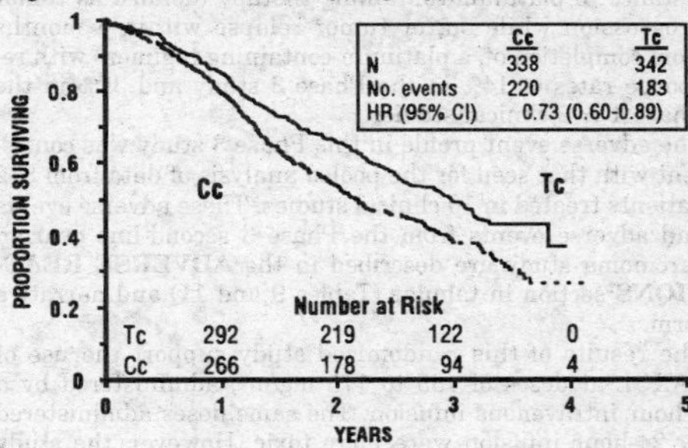

Figure 2. Survival: Cc Versus Tc (GOG-111)

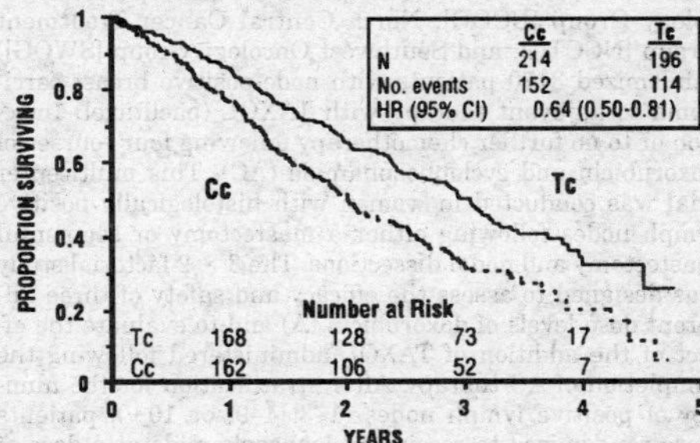

The adverse event profile for patients receiving TAXOL (paclitaxel) Injection in combination with cisplatin in these studies was qualitatively consistent with that seen for the pooled analysis of data from 812 patients treated with sin-

Continued on next page

Taxol—Cont.

gle-agent TAXOL in 10 clinical studies. These adverse events and adverse events from the Phase 3 first-line ovarian carcinoma studies are described in the **ADVERSE REACTIONS** section in tabular (Tables 9 and 10) and narrative form.

Second-Line Data—Data from five Phase 1 & 2 clinical studies (189 patients), a multicenter randomized Phase 3 study (407 patients), as well as an interim analysis of data from more than 300 patients enrolled in a treatment referral center program were used in support of the use of TAXOL in patients who have failed initial or subsequent chemotherapy for metastatic carcinoma of the ovary. Two of the Phase 2 studies (92 patients) utilized an initial dose of 135 to 170 mg/m^2 in most patients (>90%) administered over 24 hours by continuous infusion. Response rates in these two studies were 22% (95% Cl: 11% to 37%) and 30% (95% Cl: 18% to 46%) with a total of 6 complete and 18 partial responses in 92 patients. The median duration of overall response in these two studies measured from the first day of treatment was 7.2 months (range: 3.5–15.8 months) and 7.5 months (range: 5.3–17.4 months), respectively. The median survival was 8.1 months (range: 0.2–36.7 months) and 15.9 months (range: 1.8–34.5+ months).

The Phase 3 study had a bifactorial design and compared the efficacy and safety of TAXOL, administered at two different doses (135 or 175 mg/m^2) and schedules (3- or 24-hour infusion). The overall response rate for the 407 patients was 16.2% (95% Cl: 12.8% to 20.2%), with 6 complete and 60 partial responses. Duration of response, measured from the first day of treatment was 8.3 months (range: 3.2–21.6 months). Median time to progression was 3.7 months (range: 0.1+ – 25.1+ months). Median survival was 11.5 months (range: 0.2–26.3+ months).

Response rates, median survival, and median time to progression for the 4 arms are given in the following table.

[See table 3 at right]

Analyses were performed as planned by the bifactorial study design described in the protocol, by comparing the two doses (135 or 175 mg/m^2) irrespective of the schedule (3 or 24 hours) and the two schedules irrespective of dose. Patients receiving the 175 mg/m^2 dose had a response rate similar to that for those receiving the 135 mg/m^2 dose: 18% vs. 14% (p=0.28). No difference in response rate was detected when comparing the 3-hour with the 24-hour infusion: 15% vs. 17% (p=0.50). Patients receiving the 175 mg/m^2 dose of TAXOL had a longer time to progression than those receiving the 135 mg/m^2 dose: median 4.2 vs. 3.1 months (p=0.03). The median time to progression for patients receiving the 3-hour vs. the 24-hour infusion was 4.0 months vs. 3.7 months, respectively. Median survival was 11.6 months in patients receiving the 175 mg/m^2 dose of TAXOL and 11.0 months in patients receiving the 135 mg/m^2 dose (p=0.92). Median survival was 11.7 months for patients receiving the 3-hour infusion of TAXOL and 11.2 months for patients receiving the 24-hour infusion (p=0.91). These statistical analyses should be viewed with caution because of the multiple comparisons made.

TAXOL remained active in patients who had developed resistance to platinum-containing therapy (defined as tumor progression while on, or tumor relapse within 6 months from completion of, a platinum-containing regimen) with response rates of 14% in the Phase 3 study and 31% in the Phase 1 & 2 clinical studies.

The adverse event profile in this Phase 3 study was consistent with that seen for the pooled analysis of data from 812 patients treated in 10 clinical studies. These adverse events and adverse events from the Phase 3 second-line ovarian carcinoma study are described in the **ADVERSE REACTIONS** section in tabular (Tables 9 and 11) and narrative form.

The results of this randomized study support the use of TAXOL at doses of 135 to 175 mg/m^2, administered by a 3-hour intravenous infusion. The same doses administered by 24-hour infusion were more toxic. However, the study had insufficient power to determine whether a particular dose and schedule produced superior efficacy.

Breast Carcinoma:

Adjuvant Therapy—A Phase 3 intergroup study (Cancer and Leukemia Group B [CALGB], Eastern Cooperative Oncology Group [ECOG], North Central Cancer Treatment Group [NCCTG], and Southwest Oncology Group [SWOG]) randomized 3170 patients with node-positive breast carcinoma to adjuvant therapy with TAXOL (paclitaxel) Injection or to no further chemotherapy following four courses of doxorubicin and cyclophosphamide (AC). This multicenter trial was conducted in women with histologically positive lymph nodes following either a mastectomy or segmental mastectomy and nodal dissections. The 3 × 2 factorial study was designed to assess the efficacy and safety of three different dose levels of doxorubicin (A) and to evaluate the effect of the addition of TAXOL administered following the completion of AC therapy. After stratification for the number of positive lymph nodes (1–3, 4–9, or 10+), patients were randomized to receive cyclophosphamide at a dose of 600 mg/m^2 and doxorubicin at doses of either 60 mg/m^2 (on day 1), 75 mg/m^2 (in two divided doses on days 1 and 2), or 90 mg/m^2 (in two divided doses on days 1 and 2 with prophylactic G-CSF support and ciprofloxacin) every 3 weeks for four courses and either TAXOL 175 mg/m^2 as a 3-hour infusion every 3 weeks for four additional courses or no additional chemotherapy. Patients whose tumors were positive were to receive subsequent tamoxifen treatment (20 mg daily for 5 years); patients who received segmental mastectomies prior to study were to receive breast irradiation after recovery from treatment-related toxicities.

At the time of the current analysis, median follow-up was 30.1 months. Of the 2066 patients who were hormone receptor positive, 93% received tamoxifen. The primary analyses of disease-free survival and overall survival used multivariate Cox models, which included TAXOL administration, doxorubicin dose, number of positive lymph nodes, tumor size, menopausal status, and estrogen receptor status as factors. Based on the model for disease-free survival, patients receiving AC followed by TAXOL had a 22% reduction in the risk of disease recurrence compared to patients randomized to AC alone (Hazard Ratio [HR] = 0.78, 95% CI 0.67–0.91, p=0.0022). They also had a 26% reduction in the risk of death (HR = 0.74, 95% CI 0.60–0.92, p=0.0065). For disease-free survival and overall survival, p values were not adjusted for interim analyses. Kaplan-Meier curves are shown in Figures 3 and 4. Increasing the dose of doxorubicin higher than 60 mg/m^2 had no effect on either disease-free survival or overall survival.

[See figures 3 & 4 in next column]

Subset analyses— Subsets defined by variables of known prognostic importance in adjuvant breast carcinoma were examined, including number of positive lymph nodes, tumor size, hormone receptor status, and menopausal status. Such analyses must be interpreted with care, as the most secure finding is the overall study result. In general, a reduction in hazard similar to the overall reduction was seen with TAXOL for both disease-free and overall survival in all of the larger subsets with one exception; patients with receptor-positive tumors had a smaller reduction in hazard (HR = 0.92) for disease-free survival with TAXOL than other groups. Results of subset analyses are shown in Table 4.

Table 2A: Efficacy in the Phase 3 First-Line Ovarian Carcinoma Studies

	Intergroup (non-optimally debulked subset) T175/3[a] c75 (n=218)		C750[a] c75 (n=227)	GOG-111 T135/24[a] c75 (n=196)		C750[a] c75 (n=214)
• Clinical Response[b]	(n=153)		(n=153)	(n=113)		(n=127)
- rate (percent)	58		43	62		48
- p-value[c]		0.016			0.04	
• Time to Progression						
- median (months)	13.2		9.9	16.6		13.0
- p-value[c]		0.0060			0.0008	
- hazzard ratio (HR)[c]		0.76			0.70	
- 95% Cl[c]		0.62–0.92			0.56–0.86	
• Survival						
- median (months)	29.5		21.9	35.5		24.2
- p-value[c]		0.0057			0.0002	
- hazard ratio[c]		0.73			0.64	
- 95% Cl[c]		0.58–0.91			0.50–0.81	

[a] TAXOL dose in mg/m^2/infusion duration in hours; cyclophosphamide and cisplatin doses in mg/m^2.
[b] Among patients with measurable disease only.
[c] Unstratified for the Intergroup Study, Stratified for Study GOG-111.

Table 2B: Efficacy in the Phase 3 First-Line Ovarian Carcinoma Intergroup Study

	T175/3[a] c75 (n=342)		C750[a] c75 (n=338)
• Clinical Response[b]	(n=162)		(n=161)
- rate (percent)	59		45
- p-value[c]		0.014	
• Time to Progression			
- median (months)	15.3		11.5
- p-value[c]		0.0005	
- hazard ratio[c]		0.74	
- 95% Cl[c]		0.63–0.88	
• Survival			
- median (months)	35.6		25.9
- p-value[c]		0.0016	
- hazard ratio[c]		0.73	
- 95% Cl[c]		0.60–0.89	

[a] TAXOL dose in mg/m^2/infusion duration in hours; cyclophosphamide and cisplatin doses in mg/m^2.
[b] Among patients with measurable disease only.
[c] Unstratified.

Table 3: Efficacy in the Phase 3 Second-Line Ovarian Carcinoma Study

	175/3 (n=96)	175/24 (n=106)	135/3 (n=99)	135/24 (n=106)
• Response				
- rate (percent)	14.6	21.7	15.2	13.2
- 95% Confidence Interval	(8.5–23.6)	(14.5–31.0)	(9.0–24.1)	(7.7–21.5)
• Time to Progression				
- median (months)	4.4	4.2	3.4	2.8
- 95% Confidence Interval	(3.0–5.6)	(3.5–5.1)	(2.8–4.2)	(1.9–4.0)
• Survival				
- median (months)	11.5	11.8	13.1	10.7
- 95% Confidence Interval	(8.4–14.4)	(8.9–14.6)	(9.1–14.6)	(8.1–13.6)

Figure 3. Disease-Free Survival: AC Versus AC+T

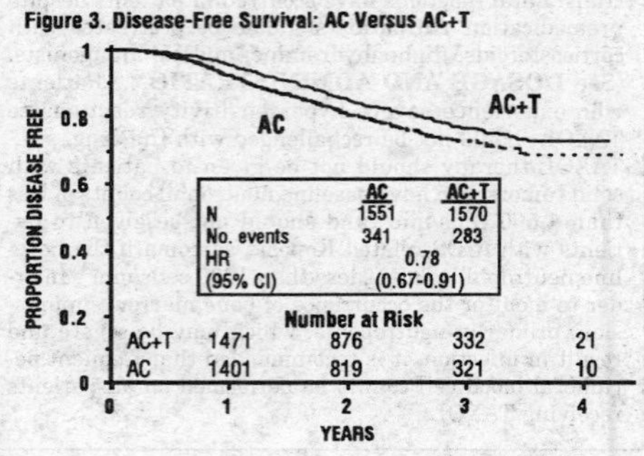

Figure 4. Survival: AC Versus AC+T

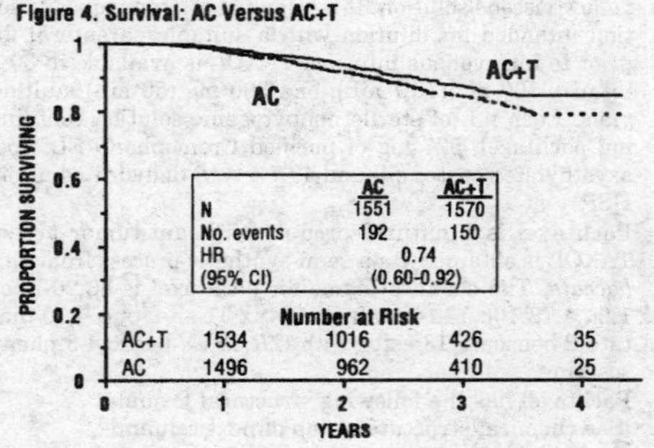

[See table 4 at right]
These retrospective subgroup analyses suggest that the beneficial effect of TAXOL (paclitaxel) Injection is clearly established in the receptor-negative subgroup, but the benefit in receptor-positive patients is not yet clear. With respect to menopausal status, the benefit of TAXOL is consistent (see Table 4 and Figures 5–8).

Figure 5. Disease-Free Survival - Receptor Status Negative/Unknown AC Versus AC+T

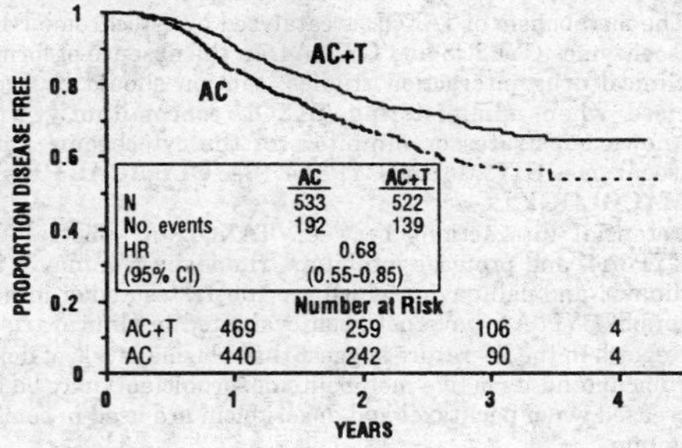

Figure 6. Disease-Free Survival - Receptor Status Positive AC Versus AC+T

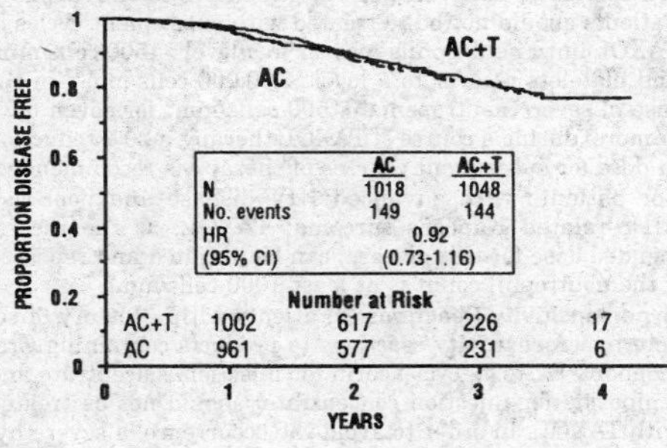

Figure 7. Disease-Free Survival - Premenopausal AC Versus AC+T

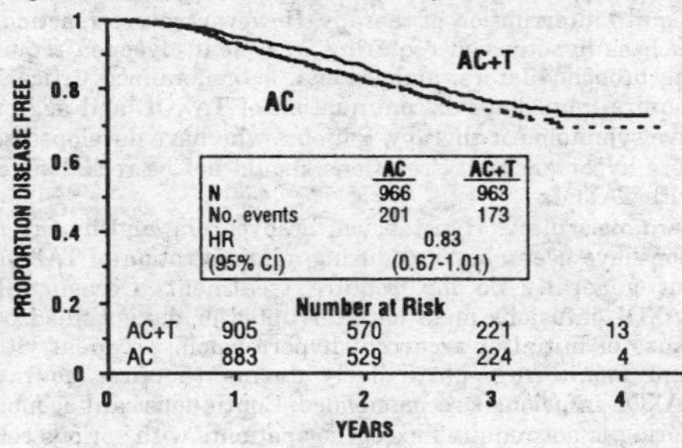

Figure 8. Disease-Free Survival - Postmenopausal AC Versus AC+T

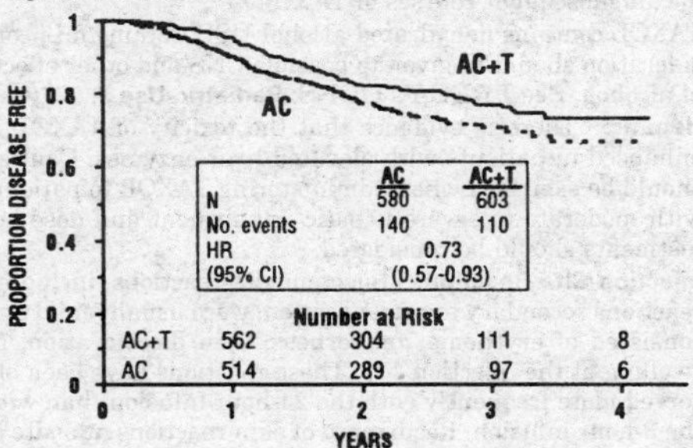

The adverse event profile for the patients who received TAXOL subsequent to AC was consistent with that seen in the pooled analysis of data from 812 patients (Table 9) treated with single-agent TAXOL in 10 clinical studies. These adverse events are described in the **ADVERSE REACTIONS** section in tabular (Tables 9 and 12) and narrative form.

After Failure of Initial Chemotherapy—Data from 83 patients accrued in three Phase 2 open label studies and from 471 patients enrolled in a Phase 3 randomized study were available to support the use of TAXOL in patients with metastatic breast carcinoma.

Phase 2 open label studies—Two studies were conducted in 53 patients previously treated with a maximum of one prior chemotherapeutic regimen. TAXOL was administered in these two trials as a 24-hour infusion at initial doses of 250 mg/m^2 (with G-CSF support) or 200 mg/m^2. The response rates were 57% (95% CI: 37% to 75%) and 52% (95% CI: 32% to 72%), respectively. The third Phase 2 study was conducted in extensively pretreated patients who had failed anthracycline therapy and who had received a minimum of two chemotherapy regimens for the treatment of metastatic disease. The dose of TAXOL was 200 mg/m^2 as a 24-hour infusion with G-CSF support. Nine of 30 patients achieved a partial response, for a response rate of 30% (95% CI: 15% to 50%).

Phase 3 randomized study—This multicenter trial was conducted in patients previously treated with one or two regimens of chemotherapy. Patients were randomized to receive TAXOL at a dose of either 175 mg/m^2 or 135 mg/m^2 given as a 3-hour infusion. In the 471 patients enrolled, 60% had symptomatic disease with impaired performance status at study entry, and 73% had visceral metastases. These patients had failed prior chemotherapy either in the adjuvant setting (30%), the metastatic setting (39%), or both (31%). Sixty-seven percent of the patients had been previously exposed to anthracyclines and 23% of them had disease considered resistant to this class of agents.

The overall response rate for the 454 evaluable patients was 26% (95% CI: 22% to 30%), with 17 complete and 99 partial responses. The median duration of response, measured from the first day of treatment, was 8.1 months (range: 3.4–18.1+ months). Overall for the 471 patients, the median time to progression was 3.5 months (range: 0.03–17.1 months). Median survival was 11.7 months (range: 0–18.9 months).

Response rates, median survival and median time to progression for the 2 arms are given in the following table.

Table 5: Efficacy in Breast Cancer after Failure of Initial Chemotherapy or Within 6 Months of Adjuvant Chemotherapy

	175/3 (n=235)		135/3 (n=236)
· Response			
- rate (percent)	28		22
- p-value		0.135	
· Time to Progression			
- median (months)	4.2		3.0
- p-value		0.027	
· Survival			
- median (months)	11.7		10.5
- p-value		0.321	

The adverse event profile of the patients who received single-agent TAXOL (paclitaxel) Injection in the Phase 3 study was consistent with that seen for the pooled analysis of data from 812 patients treated in 10 clinical studies. These adverse events and adverse events from the Phase 3 breast carcinoma study are described in the **ADVERSE REACTIONS** section in tabular (Tables 9 and 13) and narrative form.

Non-Small Cell Lung Carcinoma (NSCLC)—In a Phase 3 open label randomized study conducted by the ECOG, 599 patients were randomized to either TAXOL (T) 135 mg/m^2 as a 24-hour infusion in combination with cisplatin (c) 75 mg/m^2, TAXOL (T) 250 mg/m^2 as a 24-hour infusion in combination with cisplatin (c) 75 mg/m^2 with G-CSF support, or cisplatin (c) 75 mg/m^2 on day 1, followed by etoposide (VP) 100 mg/m^2 on days 1, 2, and 3 (control).

Response rates, median time to progression, median survival, and one-year survival rates are given in the following table. The reported p-values have not been adjusted for multiple comparisons. There were statistically significant differences favoring each of the TAXOL plus cisplatin arms for response rate and time to tumor progression. There was no statistically significant difference in survival between either TAXOL plus cisplatin arm and the cisplatin plus etoposide arm.

[See table 6 above]

In the ECOG study, the Functional Assessment of Cancer Therapy-Lung (FACT-L) questionnaire had seven subscales that measured subjective assessment of treatment. Of the seven, the Lung Cancer Specific Symptoms subscale favored the TAXOL 135 mg/m^2/24 hour plus cisplatin arm compared to the cisplatin/etoposide arm. For all other factors, there was no difference in the treatment groups.

The adverse event profile for patients who received TAXOL in combination with cisplatin in this study was generally consistent with that seen for the pooled analysis of data from 812 patients treated with single-agent TAXOL in 10 clinical studies. These adverse events and adverse events from the Phase 3 first-line NSCLC study are described in the **ADVERSE REACTIONS** section in tabular (Tables 9 and 14) and narrative form.

AIDS-Related Kaposi's Sarcoma—Data from two Phase 2 open label studies support the use of TAXOL as second-line therapy in patients with AIDS-related Kaposi's sarcoma. Fifty-nine of the 85 patients enrolled in these studies had previously received systemic therapy, including interferon alpha (32%), DaunoXome® (31%), DOXIL® (2%), and doxorubicin containing chemotherapy (42%), with 64% having received prior anthracyclines. Eighty-five percent of the pretreated patients had progressed on, or could not tolerate, prior systemic therapy.

Continued on next page

Table 4: Subset Analyses—Adjuvant Breast Carcinoma Study

Patient Subset	No. of Patients	Disease-Free Survival: No. of Recurrences	Disease-Free Survival: Hazard Ratio (95% CI)	Overall Survival: No. of Deaths	Overall Survival: Hazard Ratio (95% CI)
· No. of Positive Nodes					
1–3	1449	221	0.72 (0.55–0.94)	107	0.76 (0.52–1.12)
4–9	1310	274	0.78 (0.61–0.99)	148	0.66 (0.47–0.91)
10+	360	129	0.93 (0.66–1.31)	87	0.90 (0.59–1.36)
· Tumor Size (cm)					
≤ 2	1096	153	0.79 (0.57–1.08)	67	0.73 (0.45–1.18)
> 2 and ≤ 5	1611	358	0.79 (0.64–0.97)	201	0.74 (0.56–0.98)
>5	397	111	0.75 (0.51–1.08)	72	0.73 (0.46–1.16)
· Menuopausal Status					
Pre	1929	374	0.83 (0.67–1.01)	187	0.72 (0.54–0.97)
Post	1183	250	0.73 (0.57–0.93)	155	0.77 (0.56–1.06)
· Receptor Status					
Positive[a]	2066	293	0.92 (0.73–1.16)	126	0.83 (0.59–1.18)
Negative/Unknown[b]	1055	331	0.68 (0.55–0.85)	216	0.71 (0.54–0.93)

[a]Positive for either estrogen or progesterone receptors.
[b]Negative or missing for both estrogen and progesterone receptors (both missing: n=15).

Table 6: Efficacy Parameters in the Phase 3 First-Line NSCLC Study

	T135/24 c75 (n=198)	T250/24 c75 (n=201)	VP100[a] c75 (n=200)
· Response			
- rate (percent)	25	23	12
- p-value[b]	0.001	<0.001	
· Time to Progression			
- median (months)	4.3	4.9	2.7
- p-value[b]	0.05	0.004	
· Survival			
- median (months)	9.3	10.0	7.4
- p-value[b]	0.12	0.08	
· One-Year Survival			
- percent of patients	36	40	32

[a] Etoposide (VP) 100 mg/m^2 was administered I.V. on days 1, 2 and 3.
[b] Compared to cisplatin/etoposide.

Taxol—Cont.

In Study CA139–174 patients received TAXOL at 135 mg/m^2 as a 3-hour infusion every 3 weeks (intended dose intensity 45 mg/m^2/week). If no dose-limiting toxicity was observed, patients were to receive 155 mg/m^2 and 175 mg/m^2 in subsequent courses. Hematopoietic growth factors were not to be used initially. In Study CA139–281 patients received TAXOL at 100 mg/m^2 as a 3-hour infusion every 2 weeks (intended dose intensity 50 mg/m^2/week). In this study patients could be receiving hematopoietic growth factors before the start of TAXOL therapy, or this support was to be initiated as indicated; the dose of TAXOL was not increased. The dose intensity of TAXOL used in this patient population was lower than the dose intensity recommended for other solid tumors.

All patients had widespread and poor-risk disease. Applying the ACTG staging criteria to patients with prior systemic therapy, 93% were poor risk for extent of disease (T_1), 88% had a CD4 count <200 cells/mm^3 (I_1), and 97% had poor risk considering their systemic illness (S_1).

All patients in Study CA139–174 had a Karnofsky performance status of 80 or 90 at baseline; in Study CA139–281, there were 26 (46%) patients with a Karnofsky performance status of 70 or worse at baseline.

Table 7: Extent of Disease at Study Entry

	Percent of Patients Prior Systemic Therapy (n=59)
Visceral ± edema ± oral ± cutaneous	42
Edema or lymph nodes ± oral ± cutaneous	41
Oral ± cutaneous	10
Cutaneous only	7

Although the planned dose intensity in the two studies was slightly different (45 mg/m^2/week in Study CA139–174 and 50 mg/m^2/week in Study CA139–281), delivered dose intensity was 38–39 mg/m^2/week in both studies, with a similar range (20–24 to 51–61).

DaunoXome® is a registered trademark of NeXstar Pharmaceuticals, Inc.

DOXIL® is a registered trademark of Sequus Pharmaceuticals, Inc.

Efficacy—The efficacy of TAXOL (paclitaxel) Injection was evaluated by assessing cutaneous tumor response according to the amended ACTG criteria and by seeking evidence of clinical benefit in patients in six domains of symptoms and/or conditions that are commonly related to AIDS-related Kaposi's sarcoma.

Cutaneous Tumor Response (Amended ACTG Criteria)—The objective response rate was 59% (95% CI: 46% to 72%)(35 of 59 patients) in patients with prior systemic therapy. Cutaneous responses were primarily defined as flattening of more than 50% of previously raised lesions.

Table 8: Overall Best Response (Amended ACTG Criteria)

	Percent of Patients Prior Systemic Therapy (n=59)
Complete response	3
Partial response	56
Stable disease	29
Progression	8
Early death/toxicity	3

The median time to response was 8.1 weeks and the median duration of response measured from the first day of treatment was 10.4 months (95% CI: 7.0 to 11.0 months) for the patients who had previously received systemic therapy. The median time to progression was 6.2 months (95% CI: 4.6 to 8.7 months).

Additional Clinical Benefit—Most data on patient benefit were assessed retrospectively (plans for such analyses were not included in the study protocols). Nonetheless, clinical descriptions and photographs indicated clear benefit in some patients, including instances of improved pulmonary function in patients with pulmonary involvement, improved ambulation, resolution of ulcers, and decreased analgesic requirements in patients with KS involving the feet and resolution of facial lesions and edema in patients with KS involving the face, extremities, and genitalia.

Safety—The adverse event profile of TAXOL administered to patients with advanced HIV disease and poor-risk AIDS-related Kaposi's sarcoma was generally similar to that seen in a pooled analysis of data from 812 patients with solid tumors. These adverse events and adverse events from the Phase 2 second-line Kaposi's sarcoma studies are described in the **ADVERSE REACTIONS** section in tabular (Tables 9 and 15) and narrative form. In this immunosuppressed patient population, however, a lower dose intensity of TAXOL and supportive therapy including hematopoietic growth factors in patients with severe neutropenia are recommended. Patients with AIDS-related Kaposi's sarcoma may have more severe hematologic toxicities than patients with solid tumors.

INDICATIONS

TAXOL is indicated as first-line and subsequent therapy for the treatment of advanced carcinoma of the ovary. As first-line therapy, TAXOL is indicated in combination with cisplatin.

TAXOL is indicated for the adjuvant treatment of node-positive breast cancer administered sequentially to standard doxorubicin-containing combination chemotherapy. In the clinical trial, there was an overall favorable effect on disease-free and overall survival in the total population of patients with receptor-positive and receptor-negative tumors, but the benefit has been specifically demonstrated by available data (median follow-up 30 months) only in the patients with estrogen and progesterone receptor-negative tumors. (See **CLINICAL STUDIES: Breast Carcinoma.**)

TAXOL is indicated for the treatment of breast cancer after failure of combination chemotherapy for metastatic disease or relapse within 6 months of adjuvant chemotherapy. Prior therapy should have included an anthracycline unless clinically contraindicated.

TAXOL, in combination with cisplatin, is indicated for the first-line treatment of non-small cell lung cancer in patients who are not candidates for potentially curative surgery and/or radiation therapy.

TAXOL is indicated for the second-line treatment of AIDS-related Kaposi's sarcoma.

CONTRAINDICATIONS

TAXOL is contraindicated in patients who have a history of hypersensitivity reactions to TAXOL or other drugs formulated in Cremophor® EL (polyoxyethylated castor oil).

TAXOL should not be used in patients with solid tumors who have baseline neutrophil counts of <1500 cells/mm^3 or in patients with AIDS-related Kaposi's sarcoma with baseline neutrophil counts of <1000 cells/mm^3.

WARNINGS

Anaphylaxis and severe hypersensitivity reactions characterized by dyspnea and hypotension requiring treatment, angioedema, and generalized urticaria have occurred in 2%–4% of patients receiving TAXOL in clinical trials. Fatal reactions have occurred in patients despite premedication. All patients should be pretreated with corticosteroids, diphenhydramine, and H_2 antagonists. (See **DOSAGE AND ADMINISTRATION**.) Patients who experience severe hypersensitivity reactions to TAXOL should not be rechallenged with the drug.

Bone marrow suppression (primarily neutropenia) is dose-dependent and is the dose-limiting toxicity. Neutrophil nadirs occurred at a median of 11 days. TAXOL should not be administered to patients with baseline neutrophil counts of less than 1500 cells/mm^3 (<1000 cells/mm^3 for patients with KS). Frequent monitoring of blood counts should be instituted during TAXOL treatment. Patients should not be retreated with subsequent cycles of TAXOL until neutrophils recover to a level >1500 cells/mm^3 (>1000 cells/mm^3 for patients with KS) and platelets recover to a level >100,000 cells/mm^3.

Severe conduction abnormalities have been documented in <1% of patients during TAXOL therapy and in some cases requiring pacemaker placement. If patients develop significant conduction abnormalities during TAXOL infusion, appropriate therapy should be administered and continuous cardiac monitoring should be performed during subsequent therapy with TAXOL.

Pregnancy: TAXOL can cause fetal harm when administered to a pregnant woman. Administration of paclitaxel during the period of organogenesis to rabbits at doses of 3.0 mg/kg/day (about 0.2 the daily maximum recommended human dose on a mg/m^2 basis) caused embryo- and fetotoxicity, as indicated by intrauterine mortality, increased resorptions, and increased fetal deaths. Maternal toxicity was also observed at this dose. No teratogenic effects were observed at 1.0 mg/kg/day (about 1/15 the daily maximum recommended human dose on a mg/m^2 basis); teratogenic potential could not be assessed at higher doses due to extensive fetal mortality.

There are no adequate and well-controlled studies in pregnant women. If TAXOL is used during pregnancy, or if the patient becomes pregnant while receiving this drug, the patient should be apprised of the potential hazard to the fetus. Women of childbearing potential should be advised to avoid becoming pregnant.

IVEX-2® is a registered trademark of the Millipore Corporation.

PRECAUTIONS

Contact of the undiluted concentrate with plasticized polyvinyl chloride (PVC) equipment or devices used to prepare solutions for infusion is not recommended. In order to minimize patient exposure to the plasticizer DEHP [di-(2-ethylhexyl)phthalate], which may be leached from PVC infusion bags or sets, diluted TAXOL (paclitaxel) Injection solutions should preferably be stored in bottles (glass, polypropylene) or plastic bags (polypropylene, polyolefin) and administered through polyethylene-lined administration sets.

TAXOL should be administered through an in-line filter with a microporous membrane not greater than 0.22 microns. Use of filter devices such as IVEX-2® filters which incorporate short inlet and outlet PVC-coated tubing has not resulted in significant leaching of DEHP.

Drug Interactions: In a Phase I trial using escalating doses of TAXOL (110–200 mg/m^2) and cisplatin (50 or 75 mg/m^2) given as sequential infusions, myelosuppression was more profound when TAXOL was given after cisplatin than with the alternate sequence (i.e., TAXOL before cisplatin). Pharmacokinetic data from these patients demonstrated a decrease in paclitaxel clearance of approximately 33% when TAXOL was administered following cisplatin.

The metabolism of TAXOL is catalyzed by cytochrome P450 isoenzymes CYP2C8 and CYP3A4. In the absence of formal clinical drug interaction studies, caution should be exercised when administering TAXOL concomitantly with known substrates or inhibitors of the cytochrome P450 isoenzymes CYP2C8 and CYP3A4. (See **CLINICAL PHARMACOLOGY**.)

Potential interactions between TAXOL, a substrate of CYP3A4, and protease inhibitors (ritonavir, saquinavir, indinavir, and nelfinavir), which are substrates and/or inhibitors of CYP3A4, have not been evaluated in clinical trials.

Reports in the literature suggest that plasma levels of doxorubicin (and its active metabolite doxorubicinol) may be increased when paclitaxel and doxorubicin are used in combination.

Hematology: TAXOL therapy should not be administered to patients with baseline neutrophil counts of less than 1,500 cells/mm^3. In order to monitor the occurrence of myelotoxicity, it is recommended that frequent peripheral blood cell counts be performed on all patients receiving TAXOL. Patients should not be re-treated with subsequent cycles of TAXOL until neutrophils recover to a level >1500 cells/mm^3 and platelets recover to a level >100,000 cells/mm^3. In the case of severe neutropenia (<500 cells/mm^3 for seven days or more) during a course of TAXOL therapy, a 20% reduction in dose for subsequent courses of therapy is recommended. For patients with advanced HIV disease and poor-risk AIDS-related Kaposi's sarcoma, TAXOL, at the recommended dose for this disease, can be initiated and repeated if the neutrophil count is at least 1000 cells/mm^3.

Hypersensitivity Reactions: Patients with a history of severe hypersensitivity reactions to products containing Cremophor® EL (e.g., cyclosporin for injection concentrate and teniposide for injection concentrate) should not be treated with TAXOL. In order to avoid the occurrence of severe hypersensitivity reactions, all patients treated with TAXOL should be premedicated with corticosteroids (such as dexamethasone), diphenhydramine and H_2 antagonists (such as cimetidine or ranitidine). Minor symptoms such as flushing, skin reactions, dyspnea, hypotension, or tachycardia do not require interruption of therapy. However, severe reactions, such as hypotension requiring treatment, dyspnea requiring bronchodilators, angioedema, or generalized urticaria require immediate discontinuation of TAXOL and aggressive symptomatic therapy. Patients who have developed severe hypersensitivity reactions should not be rechallenged with TAXOL.

Cardiovascular: Hypotension, bradycardia, and hypertension have been observed during administration of TAXOL, but generally do not require treatment. Occasionally TAXOL infusions must be interrupted or discontinued because of initial or recurrent hypertension. Frequent vital sign monitoring, particularly during the first hour of TAXOL infusion, is recommended. Continuous cardiac monitoring is not required except for patients with serious conduction abnormalities. (See **WARNINGS**.)

Nervous System: Although, the occurrence of peripheral neuropathy is frequent, the development of severe symptomatology is unusual and requires a dose reduction of 20% for all subsequent courses of TAXOL.

TAXOL contains dehydrated alcohol USP, 396 mg/mL; consideration should be given to possible CNS and other effects of alcohol. (See **PRECAUTIONS: Pediatric Use.**)

Hepatic: There is evidence that the toxicity of TAXOL is enhanced in patients with elevated liver enzymes. Caution should be exercised when administering TAXOL to patients with moderate to severe hepatic impairment and dose adjustments should be considered.

Injection Site Reaction: Injection site reactions, including reactions secondary to extravasation, were usually mild and consisted of erythema, tenderness, skin discoloration, or swelling at the injection site. These reactions have been observed more frequently with the 24-hour infusion than with the 3-hour infusion. Recurrence of skin reactions at a site of previous extravasation following administration of TAXOL at a different site, i.e., "recall", has been reported rarely.

Rare reports of more severe events such as phlebitis, cellulitis, induration, skin exfoliation, necrosis, and fibrosis have been received as part of the continuing surveillance of TAXOL safety. In some cases the onset of the injection site reaction either occurred during a prolonged infusion or was delayed by a week to ten days.

A specific treatment for extravasation reactions is unknown at this time. Given the possibility of extravasation, it is advisable to closely monitor the infusion site for possible infiltration during drug administration.

Carcinogenesis, Mutagenesis, Impairment of Fertility: The carcinogenic potential of TAXOL has not been studied. Paclitaxel has been shown to be clastogenic *in vitro* (chromosome aberrations in human lymphocytes) and *in vivo* (micronucleus test in mice). Paclitaxel was not mutagenic in the Ames test or the CHO/HGPRT gene mutation assay.

Administration of paclitaxel prior to and during mating produced impairment of fertility in male and female rats at doses equal to or greater than 1 mg/kg/day (about 0.04 the daily maximum recommended human dose on a mg/m^2 basis). At this dose, paclitaxel caused reduced fertility and reproductive indices, and increased embryo- and fetotoxicity. (See WARNINGS.)

Pregnancy: Pregnancy "Category D". (See **WARNINGS**.)

Nursing Mothers: It is not known whether the drug is excreted in human milk. Following intravenous administration of carbon-14 labeled TAXOL to rats on days 9 to 10 postpartum, concentrations of radioactivity in milk were higher than in plasma and declined in parallel with the plasma concentrations. Because many drugs are excreted in human milk and because of the potential for serious adverse reactions in nursing infants, it is recommended that nursing be discontinued when receiving TAXOL therapy.

Pediatric Use: The safety and effectiveness of TAXOL in pediatric patients have not been established.

There have been reports of central nervous system (CNS) toxicity (rarely associated with death) in a clinical trial in pediatric patients in which TAXOL was infused intravenously over 3 hours at doses ranging from 350 mg/m^2 to 420 mg/m^2. The toxicity is most likely attributable to the high dose of the ethanol component of the TAXOL (paclitaxel) Injection vehicle given over a short infusion time. The use of concomitant antihistamines may intensify this effect. Although a direct effect of the paclitaxel itself cannot be discounted, the high doses used in this study (over twice the recommended adult dosage) must be considered in assessing the safety of TAXOL for use in this population.

ADVERSE REACTIONS

Pooled Analysis of Adverse Event Experiences from Single-Agent Studies: Data in the following table are based on the experience of 812 patients (493 with ovarian carcinoma and 319 with breast carcinoma) enrolled in 10 studies who received single-agent TAXOL. Two hundred and seventy-five patients were treated in eight Phase 2 studies with TAXOL doses ranging from 135 to 300 mg/m^2 administered over 24 hours (in four of these studies, G-CSF was administered as hematopoietic support). Three hundred and one patients were treated in the randomized Phase 3 ovarian carcinoma study which compared two doses (135 or 175 mg/m^2) and two schedules (3 or 24 hours) of TAXOL. Two hundred and thirty-six patients with breast carcinoma received TAXOL (135 or 175 mg/m^2) administered over 3 hours in a controlled study.

[See table 9 above]

None of the observed toxicities were clearly influenced by age.

Table 9: Summary[a] of Adverse Events in Patients With Solid Tumors Receiving Single-Agent TAXOL

		Percent of Patients (n=812)
• Bone Marrow[b]		
- Neutropenia	< 2,000/mm^3	90
	< 500/mm^3	52
- Leukopenia	< 4,000/mm^3	90
	< 1,000/mm^3	17
- Thrombocytopenia	< 100,000/mm^3	20
	< 50,000/mm^3	7
- Anemia	< 11 g/dL	78
	< 8 g/dL	16
- Infections		30
- Bleeding		14
- Red Cell Transfusions		25
- Platelet Transfusions		2
• Hypersensitivity Reactions[b]		
- All		41
- Severe[†]		2
• Cardiovascular		
- Vital Sign Changes[c]		
- Bradycardia (n=537)		3
- Hypotension (n=532)		12
- Significant Cardiovascular Events		1
• Abnormal ECG		
- All PTS		23
- Pts with normal baseline (n=559)		14
• Peripheral Neuropathy		
- Any symptoms		60
- Severe symptoms[†]		3
• Myalgia/Arthralgia		
- Any symptoms		60
- Severe symptoms[†]		8
• Gastrointestinal		
- Nausea and vomiting		52
- Diarrhea		38
- Mucositis		31
• Alopecia		87
• Hepatic(Pts with normal baseline and on study data)		
- Bilirubin elevations (N=765)		7
- Alkaline phosphatase elevations (N=575)		22
- AST (SGOT) elevations (N=591)		19
• Injection Site Reaction		13

[a] Based on worst course analysis.
[b] All patients received premedication.
[c] During the first 3 hours of infusion.
[†] Severe events are defined as at least Grade III toxicity.

Disease-Specific Adverse Event Experiences First-Line Ovary in Combination: For the 1084 patients who were evaluable for safety in the Phase 3 first-line ovary combination therapy studies, Table 10 shows the incidence of important adverse events. For both studies, the analysis of safety was based on all courses of therapy (six courses for the GOG-111 study and up to nine courses for the Intergroup study).

[See table 10 at top of next page]

Second-Line Ovary: For the 403 patients who received single-agent TAXOL (paclitaxel) Injection in the Phase 3 second-line ovarian carcinoma study, the following table shows the incidence of important adverse events.

[See table 11 on next page]

Myelosuppression was dose and schedule related, with the schedule effect being more prominent. The development of severe hypersensitivity reactions (HSRs) was rare; 1% of the patients and 0.2% of the courses overall. There was no apparent dose or schedule effect seen for the HSRs. Peripheral neuropathy was clearly dose-related, but schedule did not appear to affect the incidence.

Adjuvant Breast: For the Phase 3 adjuvant breast carcinoma study, the following table shows the incidence of important severe adverse events for the 3121 patients (total population) who were evaluable for safety as well as for a group of 325 patients (early population) who, per the study protocol, were monitored more intensively than other patients.

[See table 12 on page 1065]

The incidence of an adverse event for the total population likely represents an underestimation of the actual incidence given that safety data were collected differently based on enrollment cohort. However, since safety data were collected consistently across regimens, the safety of the sequential addition of TAXOL (paclitaxel) Injection following AC therapy may be compared with AC therapy alone. Compared to patients who received AC alone, patients who received AC followed by TAXOL experienced more Grade III/IV neurosensory toxicity, more Grade III/IV myalgia/arthralgia, more Grade III/IV neurologic pain (5% vs 1%), more Grade III/IV flu-like symptoms (5% vs 3%), and more Grade III/IV hyperglycemia (3% vs 1%). During the additional four courses of treatment with TAXOL, two deaths (0.1%) were attributed to treatment. During TAXOL treatment, Grade IV neutropenia was reported for 15% of patients, Grade II/III neurosensory toxicity for 15%, Grade II/III myalgias for 23%, and alopecia for 46%.

The incidences of severe hematologic toxicities, infections, mucositis, and cardiovascular events increased with higher doses of doxorubicin.

Breast Cancer After Failure of Initial Chemotherapy: For the 458 patients who received single-agent TAXOL in the Phase 3 breast carcinoma study, the following table shows the incidence of important adverse events by treatment arm (each arm was administered by a 3-hour infusion).

[See table 13 on page 1065]

Myelosuppression and peripheral neuropathy were dose related. There was one severe hypersensitivity reaction (HSR) observed at the dose of 135 mg/m^2.

First-Line NSCLC in Combination: In the study conducted by the Eastern Cooperative Oncology Group (ECOG), patients were randomized to either TAXOL (T) 135 mg/m^2 as a 24-hour infusion in combination with cisplatin (c) 75 mg/m^2, TAXOL (T) 250 mg/m^2 as a 24-hour infusion in combination with cisplatin (c) 75 mg/m^2 with G-CSF support, or cisplatin (c) 75 mg/m^2 on day 1, followed by etoposide (VP) 100 mg/m^2 on days 1, 2 and 3 (control).

The following table shows the incidence of important adverse events.

[See table 14 on page 1066]

Toxicity was generally more severe in the high-dose TAXOL (paclitaxel) Injection treatment arm (T250/c75) than in the low-dose TAXOL arm (T135/c75). Compared to the cisplatin/etoposide arm, patients in the low-dose TAXOL arm experienced more arthralgia/myalgia of any grade and more severe neutropenia. The incidence of febrile neutropenia was not reported in this study.

Kaposi's Sarcoma: The following table shows the frequency of important adverse events in the 85 patients with KS treated with two different single-agent TAXOL regimens.

[See table 15 on page 1066]

As demonstrated in this table, toxicity was more pronounced in the study utilizing TAXOL at a dose of 135 mg/m^2 every 3 weeks than in the study utilizing TAXOL at a dose of 100 mg/m^2 every 2 weeks. Notably, severe neutropenia (76% versus 35%), febrile neutropenia (55% versus 9%), and opportunistic infections (76% versus 54%) were more common with the former dose and schedule. The differences between the two studies with respect to dose escalation and use of hematopoietic growth factors, as described above, should be taken into account. (See **CLINICAL STUDIES: Aids-Related Kaposi's Sarcoma.**) Note also that only 26% of the 85 patients in these studies received concomitant treatment with protease inhibitors, whose effect on paclitaxel metabolism has not yet been studied.

Adverse Event Experiences by Body System: Unless otherwise noted, the following discussion refers to the overall safety database of 812 patients with solid tumors treated with single-agent TAXOL in clinical studies. Toxicities that occurred with greater severity or frequency in previously untreated patients with ovarian carcinoma or NSCLC who received TAXOL in combination with cisplatin or in patients with breast cancer who received TAXOL after doxorubicin/cyclophosphamide in the adjuvant setting and that occurred with a difference that was clinically significant in these populations are also described. The frequency and severity of important adverse events for the Phase 3 ovarian carcinoma, breast carcinoma, NSCLC, and the Phase 2 Kaposi's sarcoma studies are presented above in tabular form by treatment arm. In addition, rare events have been reported from postmarketing experience or from other clinical studies. The frequency and severity of adverse events have been generally similar for patients receiving TAXOL for the treatment of ovarian, breast, or lung carcinoma or Kaposi's sarcoma, but patients with AIDS-related Kaposi's sarcoma may have more frequent and severe hematologic toxicity, infections, and febrile neutropenia. These patients require a lower dose intensity and supportive care. (See **CLINICAL STUDIES: Aids-Related Kaposi's Sarcoma.**) Toxicities that were observed only in or were noted to have occurred with greater severity in the population with Kaposi's sarcoma and that occurred with a difference that was clinically significant in this population are described.

Hematologic: Bone marrow suppression was the major dose-limiting toxicity of TAXOL. Neutropenia, the most important hematologic toxicity, was dose and schedule dependent and was generally rapidly reversible. Among patients treated in the Phase 3 second-line ovarian study with a 3-hour infusion, neutrophil counts declined below 500 cells/mm^3 in 14% of the patients treated with a dose of 135 mg/m^2 compared to 27% at a dose of 175 mg/m^2 ($p=0.05$). In the same study, severe neutropenia (<500 cells/mm^3) was more frequent with the 24-hour than with the 3-hour infusion; infusion duration had a greater impact on myelosuppression than dose. Neutropenia did not appear to increase with cumulative exposure and did not appear to be more frequent nor more severe for patients previously treated with radiation therapy.

In the study where TAXOL was administered to patients with ovarian carcinoma at a dose of 135 mg/m^2/24 hours in combination with cisplatin versus the control arm of cyclophosphamide plus cisplatin, the incidences of grade IV neutropenia and of febrile neutropenia were significantly greater in the TAXOL plus cisplatin arm than in the control arm. Grade IV neutropenia occurred in 81% on the TAXOL (paclitaxel) Injection plus cisplatin arm versus 58% on the cyclophosphamide plus cisplatin arm, and febrile neutropenia occurred in 15% and 4% respectively. On the TAXOL/cisplatin arm, there were 35/1074 (3%) courses with fever in which Grade IV neutropenia was reported at some time during the course. When TAXOL followed by cisplatin was administered to patients with advanced NSCLC in the ECOG study, the incidences of Grade IV neutropenia were 74% (TAXOL 135 mg/m^2/24 hours followed by cisplatin) and 65% (TAXOL 250 mg/m^2/24 hours followed by cisplatin and G-CSF) compared with 55% in patients who received cisplatin/etoposide.

Continued on next page

Taxol—Cont.

Fever was frequent (12% of all treatment courses). Infectious episodes occurred in 30% of all patients and 9% of all courses; these episodes were fatal in 1% of all patients, and included sepsis, pneumonia and peritonitis. In the Phase 3 second-line ovarian study, infectious episodes were reported in 20% and 26% of the patients treated with a dose of 135 mg/m^2 or 175 mg/m^2 given as 3-hour infusions, respectively. Urinary tract infections and upper respiratory tract infections were the most frequently reported infectious complications. In the immunosuppressed patient population with advanced HIV disease and poor-risk AIDS-related Kaposi's sarcoma, 61% of the patients reported at least one opportunistic infection. (See **CLINICAL STUDIES: AIDS-Related Kaposi's Sarcoma**.) The use of supportive therapy, including G-CSF, is recommended for patients who have experienced severe neutropenia. (See **DOSAGE AND ADMINISTRATION**.)

Thrombocytopenia was uncommon, and almost never severe (<50,000 cells/mm^3). Twenty percent of the patients experienced a drop in their platelet count below 100,000 cells/mm^3 at least once while on treatment; 7% had a platelet count <50,000 cells/mm^3 at the time of their worst nadir. Bleeding episodes were reported in 4% of all courses and by 14% of all patients but most of the hemorrhagic episodes were localized and the frequency of these events was unrelated to the TAXOL dose and schedule. In the Phase 3 second-line ovarian study, bleeding episodes were reported in 10% of the patients; no patients treated with the 3-hour infusion received platelet transfusions. In the adjuvant breast carcinoma trial, the incidence of severe thrombocytopenia and platelet transfusions increased with higher doses of doxorubicin.

Anemia (Hb <11 g/dL) was observed in 78% of all patients and was severe (Hb <8 g/dL) in 16% of the cases. No consistent relationship between dose or schedule and the frequency of anemia was observed. Among all patients with normal baseline hemoglobin, 69% became anemic on study but only 7% had severe anemia. Red cell transfusions were required in 25% of all patients and in 12% of those with normal baseline hemoglobin levels.

Hypersensitivity Reactions (HSRs): All patients received premedication prior to TAXOL (see **WARNINGS** and **PRECAUTIONS: Hypersensitivity Reactions**). The frequency and severity of HSRs were not affected by the dose or schedule of TAXOL administration. In the Phase 3 second-line ovarian study, the 3-hour infusion was not associated with a greater increase in HSRs when compared to the 24-hour infusion. Hypersensitivity reactions were observed in 20% of all courses and in 41% of all patients. These reactions were severe in less than 2% of the patients and 1% of the courses. No severe reactions were observed after course 3 and severe symptoms occurred generally within the first hour of TAXOL infusion. The most frequent symptoms observed during these severe reactions were dyspnea, flushing, chest pain, and tachycardia.

The minor hypersensitivity reactions consisted mostly of flushing (28%), rash (12%), hypotension (4%), dyspnea (2%), tachycardia (2%), and hypertension (1%). The frequency of hypersensitivity reactions remained relatively stable during the entire treatment period.

Rare reports of chills and reports of back pain in association with hypersensitivity reactions have been received as part of the continuing surveillance of TAXOL safety.

Cardiovascular: Hypotension, during the first 3 hours of infusion, occurred in 12% of all patients and 3% of all courses administered. Bradycardia, during the first 3 hours of infusion, occurred in 3% of all patients and 1% of all courses. In the Phase 3 second-line ovarian study, neither dose nor schedule had an effect on the frequency of hypotension and bradycardia. These vital sign changes most often caused no symptoms and required neither specific therapy nor treatment discontinuation. The frequency of hypotension and bradycardia were not influenced by prior anthracycline therapy.

Significant cardiovascular events possibly related to single-agent TAXOL occurred in approximately 1% of all patients. These events included syncope, rhythm abnormalities, hypertension and venous thrombosis. One of the patients with syncope treated with TAXOL at 175 mg/m^2 over 24 hours had progressive hypotension and died. The arrhythmias included asymptomatic ventricular tachycardia, bigeminy and complete AV block requiring pacemaker placement. Among patients with NSCLC treated with TAXOL in combination with cisplatin in the Phase 3 study, significant cardiovascular events occurred in 12%–13%. This apparent increase in cardiovascular events is possibly due to an increase in cardiovascular risk factors in patients with lung cancer.

Electrocardiogram (ECG) abnormalities were common among patients at baseline. ECG abnormalities on study did not usually result in symptoms, were not dose-limiting, and required no intervention. ECG abnormalities were noted in 23% of all patients. Among patients with a normal ECG prior to study entry, 14% of all patients developed an abnormal tracing while on study. The most frequently reported ECG modifications were non-specific repolarization abnormalities, sinus bradycardia, sinus tachycardia, and premature beats. Among patients with normal ECGs at baseline, prior therapy with anthracyclines did not influence the frequency of ECG abnormalities.

Cases of myocardial infarction have been reported rarely. Congestive heart failure has been reported typically in patients who have received other chemotherapy, notably anthracyclines. (See **PRECAUTIONS: Drug Interactions**.)

Table 10: Frequency[a] of Important Adverse Events in the Phase 3 for First-Line Ovarian Carcinoma Studies

	Percent of Patients			
	Intergroup		GOG-111	
	T175/3[b] c75[c] (n=339)	C750[c] c75[c] (n=336)	T135/24[b] c75[c] (n=196)	C750[c] c75[c] (n=213)
• Bone Marrow				
- Neutropenia				
< 2,000/mm^3	91[d]	95[d]	96	92
< 500/mm^3	33[d]	43[d]	81[d]	58[d]
- Thrombocytopenia				
< 100,000/mm^3[e]	21[d]	33[d]	26	30
< 50,000/mm^3	3[d]	7[d]	10	9
- Anemia				
< 11 g/dL[f]	96	97	88	86
< 8 g/dL	3[d]	8[d]	13	9
- Infections	25	27	21	15
- Febrile Neutropenia	4	7	15[d]	4[d]
• Hypersensitivity Reactions				
- All	11[d]	6[d]	8[d,g]	1[d,g]
- Severe[†]	1	1	3[d,g]	—[d,g]
• Neurotoxicity[h]				
- Any symptoms	87[d]	52[d]	25	20
- Severe symptoms[†]	21[d]	2[d]	3[d]	—[d]
• Nausea/Vomiting				
- Any symptoms	88	93	65	69
- Severe symptoms[†]	18	24	10	11
• Myalgia/Arthralgia				
- Any symptoms	60[d]	27[d]	9[d]	2[d]
- Severe symptoms[†]	6[d]	1[d]	1	—
• Diarrhea				
- Any symptoms	37[d]	29[d]	16[d]	8[d]
- Severe symptoms[†]	2	3	4	1
• Asthenia				
- Any symptoms	NC	NC	17[d]	10[d]
- Severe symptoms[†]	NC	NC	1	1
• Alopecia				
- Any symptoms	96[d]	89[d]	55[d]	37[d]
- Severe symptoms[†]	51[d]	21[d]	6	8

[a] Based on worst course analysis.
[b] TAXOL (T) dose in mg/m^2/infusion duration in hours.
[c] Cyclophosphamide (C) or cisplatin (c) dose in mg/m^2.
[d] $p<0.05$ by Fisher exact test.
[e] <130,000/mm^3 in the Intergroup study.
[f] <12 g/dL in the Intergroup study.
[g] All patients received premedication.
[h] In the GOG-111 study, neurotoxicity was collected as peripheral neuropathy and the Intergroup study, neurotoxicity was collected as either neuromotor or neurosensory symptoms.
[†] Severe events are defined as at least Grade III toxicity.
NC Not Collected.

Table 11: Frequency[a] of Important Adverse Events in the Phase 3 Second-Line Ovarian Carcinoma Study

		Percent of Patients (n=812)			
		175/3[b] (n=95)	175/24[b] (n=105)	135/3[b] (n=98)	135/24[b] (n=105)
• Bone Marrow					
- Neutropenia	< 2,000/mm^3	78	98	78	98
	< 500/mm^3	27	75	14	67
- Thrombocytopenia	< 100,000/mm^3	4	18	8	6
	< 50,000/mm^3	1	7	2	1
- Anemia	< 11 g/dL	84	90	68	88
	< 8 g/dL	11	12	6	10
- Infections		26	29	20	18
• Hypersensitivity Reactions[c]					
- All		41	45	38	45
- Severe[†]		2	0	2	1
• Peripheral Neuropathy					
- Any symptoms		63	60	55	42
- Severe symptoms[†]		1	2	0	0
• Mucositis					
- Any symptoms		17	35	21	25
- Severe symptoms[†]		0	3	0	2

[a] Based on worst course analysis.
[b] TAXOL dose in mg/m^2/infusion duration in hours.
[c] All patients received premedication.
[†] Severe events are defined as at least Grade III toxicity.

Rare reports of atrial fibrillation and supraventricular tachycardia have been received as part of the continuing surveillance of TAXOL safety.

Respiratory: Rare reports of interstitial pneumonia, lung fibrosis, and pulmonary embolism have been received as part of the continuing surveillance of TAXOL safety. Rare reports of radiation pneumonitis have been received in patients receiving concurrent radiotherapy.

Neurologic: The assessment of neurologic toxicity was conducted differently among the studies as evident from the data reported in each individual study (see Tables 9-15). Moreover, the frequency and severity of neurologic manifestations were influenced by prior and/or concomitant therapy with neurotoxic agents.

In general, the frequency and severity of neurologic manifestations were dose-dependent in patients receiving single-agent TAXOL (paclitaxel) Injection. Peripheral neuropathy was observed in 60% of all patients (3% severe) and in 52% (2% severe) of the patients without pre-existing neuropathy. The frequency of peripheral neuropathy increased with cumulative dose. Neurologic symptoms were observed in 27% of the patients after the first course of treatment and in 34%–51% from course 2 to 10. Peripheral neuropathy was the cause of TAXOL discontinuation in 1% of all patients. Sensory symptoms have usually improved or resolved within several months of TAXOL discontinuation. Pre-existing neuropathies resulting from prior therapies are not a contraindication for TAXOL therapy.

In the Intergroup first-line ovarian carcinoma study (see Table 10), neurotoxicity included reports of neuromotor and neurosensory events. The regimen with TAXOL 175 mg/m^2 given by 3-hour infusion plus cisplatin 75 mg/m^2 resulted in a greater incidence and severity of neurotoxicity than the regimen containing cyclophosphamide and cisplatin, 87% (21% severe) versus 52% (2% severe), respectively. The duration of grade III or IV neurotoxicity cannot be determined with precision for the Intergroup study since the resolution dates of adverse events were not collected in the case report forms for this trial and complete follow-up documentation was available only in a minority of these patients. In the GOG first-line ovarian carcinoma study, neurotoxicity was reported as peripheral neuropathy. The regimen with TAXOL 135 mg/m^2 given by 24-hour infusion plus cisplatin 75 mg/m^2 resulted in an incidence of neurotoxicity that was similar to the regimen containing cyclophosphamide plus cisplatin, 25% (3% severe) versus 20% (0% severe), respectively. Cross-study comparison of neurotoxicity in the Intergroup and GOG trials suggests that when TAXOL is given in combination with cisplatin 75 mg/m^2, the incidence of severe neurotoxicity is more common at a TAXOL dose of 175 mg/m^2 given by 3-hour infusion (21%) than at a dose of 135 mg/m^2 given by 24-hour infusion (3%).

In patients with NSCLC, administration of TAXOL followed by cisplatin resulted in a greater incidence of severe neurotoxicity compared to the incidence in patients with ovarian or breast cancer treated with single-agent TAXOL. Severe neurosensory symptoms were noted in 13% of NSCLC patients receiving TAXOL 135 mg/m^2 by 24-hour infusion followed by cisplatin 75 mg/m^2 and 8% of NSCLC patients receiving cisplatin/etoposide (see Table 14).

Other than peripheral neuropathy, serious neurologic events following TAXOL administration have been rare (<1%) and have included grand mal seizures, syncope, ataxia, and neuroencephalopathy.

Rare reports of autonomic neuropathy resulting in paralytic ileus have been received as part of the continuing surveillance of TAXOL safety. Optic nerve and/or visual disturbances (scintillating scotomata) have also been reported, particularly in patients who have received higher doses than those recommended. These effects generally have been reversible. However, rare reports in the literature of abnormal visual evoked potentials in patients have suggested persistent optic nerve damage. Postmarketing reports of ototoxicity (hearing loss and tinnitus) have also been received.

Arthralgia/Myalgia: There was no consistent relationship between dose or schedule of TAXOL and the frequency or severity of arthralgia/myalgia. Sixty percent of all patients treated experienced arthralgia/myalgia; 8% experienced severe symptoms. The symptoms were usually transient, occurred two or three days after TAXOL administration, and resolved within a few days. The frequency and severity of musculoskeletal symptoms remained unchanged throughout the treatment period.

Hepatic: No relationship was observed between liver function abnormalities and either dose or schedule of TAXOL administration. Among patients with normal baseline liver function 7%, 22%, and 19% had elevations in bilirubin, alkaline phosphatase, and AST (SGOT), respectively. Prolonged exposure to TAXOL was not associated with cumulative hepatic toxicity.

Rare reports of hepatic necrosis and hepatic encephalopathy leading to death have been received as part of the continuing surveillance of TAXOL safety.

Renal: Among the patients treated for Kaposi's sarcoma with TAXOL, five patients had renal toxicity of grade III or IV severity. One patient with suspected HIV nephropathy of grade IV severity had to discontinue therapy. The other four patients had renal insufficiency with reversible elevations of serum creatinine.

Gastrointestinal (GI): Nausea/vomiting, diarrhea, and mucositis were reported by 52%, 38%, and 31% of all patients, respectively. These manifestations were usually mild to moderate. Mucositis was schedule dependent and occurred more frequently with the 24-hour than with the 3-hour infusion.

In patients with poor-risk AIDS-related Kaposi's sarcoma, nausea/ vomiting, diarrhea, and mucositis were reported by 69%, 79%, and 28% of patients, respectively. One third of patients with Kaposi's sarcoma complained of diarrhea prior to study start. (See **CLINICAL STUDIES: AIDS-Related Kaposi's Sarcoma.**)

In the first-line Phase 3 ovarian carcinoma studies, the incidence of nausea and vomiting when TAXOL was administered in combination with cisplatin appeared to be greater compared with the database for single-agent TAXOL in ovarian and breast carcinoma. In addition, diarrhea of any grade was reported more frequently compared to the control arm, but there was no difference for severe diarrhea in these studies.

Rare reports of intestinal obstruction, intestinal perforation, pancreatitis, ischemic colitis, and dehydration have been received as part of the continuing surveillance of TAXOL safety. Rare reports of neutropenic enterocolitis (typhlitis), despite the coadministration of G-CSF, were observed in patients treated with TAXOL alone and in combination with other chemotherapeutic agents.

Injection Site Reaction: Injection site reactions, including reactions secondary to extravasation, were usually mild and consisted of erythema, tenderness, skin discoloration, or swelling at the injection site. These reactions have been observed more frequently with the 24-hour infusion than with the 3-hour infusion. Recurrence of skin reactions at a site of previous extravasation following administration of TAXOL at a different site, i.e., "recall", has been reported rarely.

Rare reports of more severe events such as phlebitis, cellulitis, induration, skin exfoliation, necrosis, and fibrosis have been received as part of the continuing surveillance of TAXOL safety. In some cases the onset of the injection site reaction either occurred during a prolonged infusion or was delayed by a week to ten days.

A specific treatment for extravasation reactions is unknown at this time. Given the possibility of extravasation, it is advisable to closely monitor the infusion site for possible infiltration during drug administration.

Other Clinical Events: Alopecia was observed in almost all (87%) of the patients. Transient skin changes due to TAXOL (paclitaxel) Injection-related hypersensitivity reactions have been observed, but no other skin toxicities were significantly associated with TAXOL administration. Nail changes (changes in pigmentation or discoloration of nail bed) were uncommon (2%). Edema was reported in 21% of all patients (17% of those without baseline edema); only 1% had severe edema and none of these patients required treatment discontinuation. Edema was most commonly focal and disease-related. Edema was observed in 5% of all courses for patients with normal baseline and did not increase with time on study.

Rare reports of skin abnormalities related to radiation recall as well as reports of maculopapular rash and pruritus have been received as part of the continuing surveillance of TAXOL safety.

Reports of asthenia and malaise have been received as part of the continuing surveillance of TAXOL safety. In the Phase 3 trial of TAXOL 135 mg/m^2 over 24 hours in combination with cisplatin as first-line therapy of ovarian cancer, asthenia was reported in 17% of the patients, significantly greater than the 10% incidence observed in the control arm of cyclophosphamide/cisplatin.

Accidental Exposure: Upon inhalation, dyspnea, chest pain, burning eyes, sore throat, and nausea have been reported. Following topical exposure, events have included tingling, burning, and redness.

Table 12: Frequency[a] of Important Severe[b] Adverse Events in the Phase 3 Adjuvant Breast Carcinoma Study

	Percent of Patients			
	Early Population		Total Population	
	AC[c] (n=166)	AC[c] followed by T[d] (n=159)	AC[c] (n=1551)	AC[c] followed by T[d] (n=1570)
• Bone Marrow[e]				
- Neutropenia < 500/mm^3	79	76	48	50
- Thrombocytopenia < 50,000/mm^3	27	25	11	11
- Anemia < 8 g/dL	17	21	8	8
- Infections	6	14	5	6
- Fever without infection	—	3	<1	1
• Hypersensitivity Reactions[f]	1	4	1	2
• Cardiovascular Events	1	2	1	2
• Neuromotor Toxicity	1	1	<1	1
• Neurosensory Toxicity	—	3	<1	3
• Myalgia/Arthralgia	—	2	<1	2
• Nausea/Vomiting	13	18	8	9
• Mucositis	13	4	6	5

[a] Based on worst course analysis.
[b] Severe events are defined as at least Grade III toxicity.
[c] Patients received 600 mg/m^2 cyclophosphamide and doxorubicin (AC) at doses of either 60 mg/m^2, 75 mg/m^2, or 90 mg/m^2 (with prophylactic G-CSF support and ciprofloxacin), every 3 weeks for four courses.
[d] TAXOL (T) following four courses of AC at a dose of 175 mg/m^2/3 hours every 3 weeks for four courses.
[e] The incidence of febrile neutropenia was not reported in this study.
[f] All patients were to receive premedication.

Table 13: Frequency[a] of Important Adverse Events in the Phase 3 of Breast Cancer After Failure of Initial Chemotherapy of Within 6 Months of Adjuvant Chemotherapy

		Percent of Patients	
		175/3[b] (n=229)	135/3[b] (n=229)
• Bone Marrow			
- Neutropenia	< 2,000/mm^3	90	81
	< 500/mm^3	28	19
- Thrombocytopenia	< 100,000/mm^3	11	7
	< 50,000/mm^3	3	2
- Anemia	< 11 g/dL	55	47
	< 8 g/dL	4	2
- Infections		23	15
- Febrile Neutropenia		2	2
• Hypersensitivity Reactions[c]			
- All		36	31
- Severe[†]		0	<1
• Peripheral Neuropathy			
- Any symptoms		70	46
- Severe symptoms[†]		7	3
• Mucositis			
- Any symptoms		23	17
- Severe symptoms[†]		3	<1

[a] Based on worst course analysis.
[b] TAXOL dose in mg/m^2/infusion duration in hours.
[c] All patients received premedication.
[†] Severe events are defined as at least Grade III toxicity.

OVERDOSAGE

There is no known antidote for TAXOL overdosage. The primary anticipated complications of overdosage would consist of bone marrow suppression, peripheral neurotoxicity, and mucositis. Overdoses in pediatric patients may be associated with acute ethanol toxicity (see **PRECAUTIONS: Pediatric Use**).

DOSAGE AND ADMINISTRATION

Note: Contact of the undiluted concentrate with plasticized PVC equipment or devices used to prepare solutions for infusion is not recommended. In order to minimize patient exposure to the plasticizer DEHP [di-(2-ethylhexyl)phthalate], which may be leached from PVC infusion bags or sets, diluted TAXOL solutions should be stored in bottles (glass, polypropylene) or plastic bags (polypropylene, polyolefin) and administered through polyethylene-lined administration sets.

All patients should be premedicated prior to TAXOL administration in order to prevent severe hypersensitivity reactions. Such premedication may consist of dexamethasone 20 mg PO administered approximately 12 and 6 hours before TAXOL, diphenhydramine (or its equivalent) 50 mg I.V. 30 to 60 minutes prior to TAXOL, and cimetidine (300 mg) or ranitidine (50 mg) I.V. 30 to 60 minutes before TAXOL.

For patients with **carcinoma of the ovary,** the following regimens are recommended (see **CLINICAL STUDIES: Ovarian Carcinoma**):

1) For previously untreated patients with carcinoma of the ovary, one of the following recommended regimens may be given every 3 weeks. In selecting the appropriate regimen, differences in toxicities should be considered (see Table 10 in **ADVERSE REACTIONS: Disease-Specific Adverse Event Experiences**).

Continued on next page

Taxol—Cont.

a. TAXOL administered intravenously over 3 hours at a dose of 175 mg/m^2 followed by cisplatin at a dose of 75 mg/m^2; or
b. TAXOL administered intravenously over 24 hours at a dose of 135 mg/m^2 followed by cisplatin at a dose of 75 mg/m^2.

2) In patients previously treated with chemotherapy for carcinoma of the ovary, TAXOL has been used at several doses and schedules; however, the optimal regimen is not yet clear. The recommended regimen is TAXOL 135 mg/m^2 or 175 mg/m^2 administered intravenously over 3 hours every 3 weeks.

For patients with **carcinoma of the breast**, the following regimens are recommended (see **CLINICAL STUDIES: Breast Carcinoma**):

1) For the adjuvant treatment of node-positive breast cancer, the recommended regimen is TAXOL, at a dose of 175 mg/m^2 intravenously over 3 hours every 3 weeks for four courses administered sequentially to doxorubicin-containing combination chemotherapy. The clinical trial used four courses of doxorubicin and cyclophosphamide (See **CLINICAL STUDIES: Breast Carcinoma**).
2) After failure of initial chemotherapy for metastatic disease or relapse within 6 months of adjuvant chemotherapy, TAXOL at a dose of 175 mg/m^2 administered intravenously over 3 hours every 3 weeks has been shown to be effective.

For patients with **non-small cell lung carcinoma**, the recommended regimen, given every 3 weeks, is TAXOL administered intravenously over 24 hours at a dose of 135 mg/m^2 followed by cisplatin, 75 mg/m^2.

For patients with **AIDS-related Kaposi's sarcoma,** TAXOL admini-stered at a dose of 135 mg/m^2 given intravenously over 3 hours every 3 weeks or at a dose of 100 mg/m^2 given intravenously over 3 hours every 2 weeks is recommended (dose intensity 45–50 mg/m^2/week). In the two clinical trials evaluating these schedules (see **CLINICAL STUDIES: AIDS-Related Kaposi's Sarcoma**), the former schedule (135 mg/m^2 every 3 weeks) was more toxic than the latter. In addition, all patients with low performance status were treated with the latter schedule (100 mg/m^2 every 2 weeks).

Based upon the immunosuppression in patients with advanced HIV disease, the following modifications are recommended in these patients:

1) Reduce the dose of dexamethasone as one of the three premedication drugs to 10 mg PO (instead of 20 mg PO);
2) Initiate or repeat treatment with TAXOL only if the neutrophil count is at least 1000 cells/mm^3;
3) Reduce the dose of subsequent courses of TAXOL by 20% for patients who experience severe neutropenia (neutrophil <500 cells/mm^3 for a week or longer); and
4) Initiate concomitant hematopoietic growth factor (G-CSF) as clinically indicated.

For the therapy of patients with solid tumors (ovary, breast, and NSCLC), courses of TAXOL should not be repeated until the neutrophil count is at least 1,500 cells/mm^3 and the platelet count is at least 100,000 cells/mm^3. TAXOL should not be given to patients with AIDS-related Kaposi's sarcoma if the baseline or subsequent neutrophil count is less than 1000 cells/mm^3. Patients who experience severe neutropenia (neutrophil <500 cells/mm^3 for a week or longer) or severe peripheral neuropathy during TAXOL (paclitaxel) Injection therapy should have dosage reduced by 20% for subsequent courses of TAXOL. The incidence of neurotoxicity and the severity of neutropenia increase with dose.

Preparation and Administration Precautions: TAXOL is a cytotoxic anticancer drug and, as with other potentially toxic compounds, caution should be exercised in handling TAXOL. The use of gloves is recommended. If TAXOL solution contacts the skin, wash the skin immediately and thoroughly with soap and water. Following topical exposure, events have included tingling, burning, and redness. If TAXOL contacts mucous membranes, the membranes should be flushed thoroughly with water. Upon inhalation, dyspnea, chest pain, burning eyes, sore throat, and nausea have been reported.

Given the possibility of extravasation, it is advisable to closely monitor the infusion site for possible infiltration during drug administration. (See **PRECAUTIONS: Injection Site Reaction.**)

Preparation for Intravenous Administration: TAXOL must be diluted prior to infusion. TAXOL should be diluted in 0.9% Sodium Chloride Injection, USP; 5% Dextrose Injection, USP; 5% Dextrose and 0.9% Sodium Chloride Injection, USP, or 5% Dextrose in Ringer's Injection to a final concentration of 0.3 to 1.2 mg/mL. The solutions are physically and chemically stable for up to 27 hours at ambient temperature (approximately 25¡C) and room lighting conditions. Parenteral drug products should be inspected visually for particulate matter and discoloration prior to administration whenever solution and container permit.

Upon preparation, solutions may show haziness, which is attributed to the formulation vehicle. No significant losses in potency have been noted following simulated delivery of the solution through i.v. tubing containing an in-line (0.22 micron) filter.

Data collected for the presence of the extractable plasticizer DEHP [di-(2-ethylhexyl)phthalate] show that levels increase with time and concentration when dilutions are prepared in PVC containers. Consequently, the use of plasticized PVC containers and administration sets is not recommended. TAXOL solutions should be prepared and stored in glass, polypropylene, or polyolefin containers. Non-PVC containing administration sets, such as those which are polyethylene-lined, should be used.

TAXOL should be administered through an in-line filter with a microporous membrane not greater than 0.22 microns. Use of filter devices such as IVEX-2® filters which incorporate short inlet and outlet PVC-coated tubing has not resulted in significant leaching of DEHP.

Table 14: Frequency[a] of Important Adverse Events in the Phase 3 for First-Line NSCLC

		Percent of Patients		
		T135/24[b] c75 (n=195)	T250/24[c] c75 (n=197)	VP100[d] c75 (n=196)
• Bone Marrow				
- Neutropenia	< 2,000/mm^3	89	86	84
	< 500/mm^3	74[e]	65	55
- Thrombocytopenia	< normal	48	68	62
	< 50,000/mm^3	6	12	16
- Anemia	< normal	94	96	95
	< 8 g/dL	22	19	28
- Infections		38	31	35
• Hypersensitivity Reactions[f]				
- All		16	27	13
- Severe[†]		1	4[e]	1
• Arthralgia/Myalgia				
- Any symptoms		21[e]	2[e]	9
- Severe symptoms[†]		3	11	1
• Nausea/Vomiting				
- Any symptoms		85	87	81
- Severe symptoms[†]		27	29	22
• Mucositis				
- Any symptoms		18	28	16
- Severe symptoms[†]		1	4	2
• Neuromotor Toxicity				
- Any symptoms		37	47	44
- Severe symptoms[†]		6	12	7
• Neurosenory Toxicity				
- Any symptoms		48	61	25
- Severe symptoms[†]		13	28[e]	8
• Cardiovascular Events				
- Any symptoms		33	39	24
- Severe symptoms[†]		13	12	8

[a] Based on worst course analysis.
[b] TAXOL (T) dose in mg/m^2/infusion duration in hours; cisplatin (c) dose in mg/m^2.
[c] TAXOL dose in mg/m^2/infusions duration in hours with G-CSF support; cisplatin dose in mg/m^2.
[d] Etoposide (VP) dose in mg/m^2 was administered I.V. on days 1, 2 and 3; cisplatin dose in mg/m^2.
[e] $p<0.05$
[f] All patients received premedication.
[†] Severe events are defined as at least Grade III toxicity.

Table 15: Frequency[a] of Important Adverse Events in the AIDS-Related Kaposi's Sarcoma Studies

		Percent of Patients	
		Study CA139-174 TAXOL 135/3[b] q 3wk (n=29)	Study CA139-281 TAXOL 100/3[b] q 2wk (n=56)
• Bone Marrow			
- Neutropenia	< 2,000/mm^3	100	95
	< 500/mm^3	76	35
- Thrombocytopenia	< 100,000/mm^3	52	27
	< 50,000/mm^3	17	5
- Anemia	< 11 g/dL	86	73
	< 8 g/dL	34	25
- Febrile Neutropenia		55	9
• Opportunistic Infection			
- Any		76	54
- Cytomegalovirus		45	27
- Herpes Simplex		38	11
- *Pnemocystis carinii*		14	21
- *M. avium-intracellulare*		24	4
- Candidiasis, esophageal		7	9
- Cryptospridiosis		7	7
- Cryptococcal meningitis		3	2
- Leukoencephalopathy		—	2
• Hypersensitivity Reaction[c]			
- All		14	9
• Cardiovascular			
- Hypotension		17	9
- Bradycardia		3	—
• Peripheral Neuropathy			
- Any		79	46
- Severe [†]		10	2
• Myalgia/Arthralgia			
- Any		93	48
- Severe[†]		14	16
• Gastrointestinal			
- Nausea and Vomiting		69	70
- Diarrhea		90	73
- Mucositis		45	20
• Renal (creatinine elevation)			
- Any		34	18
- Severe[†]		7	5
• Discontinuation for drug toxicity		7	16

[a] Based on worst course analysis.
[b] TAXOL dose in mg/m^2/infusion duration in hours.
[c] All patients received premedication.
[†] Severe events are defined as at least Grade III toxicity.

The Chemo Dispensing Pin™ device or similar devices with spikes should not be used with vials of TAXOL since they can cause the stopper to collapse resulting in loss of sterile integrity of the TAXOL solution.

Stability: Unopened vials of TAXOL Injection are stable until the date indicated on the package when stored between 20°–25°C (68°–77°F), in the original package. Neither freezing nor refrigeration adversely affects the stability of the product. Upon refrigeration components in the TAXOL vial may precipitate, but will redissolve upon reaching room temperature with little or no agitation. There is no impact on product quality under these circumstances. If the solution remains cloudy or if an insoluble precipitate is noted, the vial should be discarded. Solutions for infusion prepared as recommended are stable at ambient temperature (approximately 25°C) and lighting conditions for up to 27 hours.

HOW SUPPLIED

NDC 0015-3475-30 30 mg/5 mL multidose vial individually packaged in a carton.

NDC 0015-3476-30 100 mg/16.7 mL multidose vial individually packaged in a carton.

NDC 0015-3479-11 300 mg/50 mL multidose vial individually packaged in a carton.

Storage: Store the vials in original cartons between 20°–25°C (68°–77°F). Retain in the original package to protect from light.

Handling and Disposal: Procedures for proper handling and disposal of anticancer drugs should be considered. Several guidelines on this subject have been published.[1–7] There is no general agreement that all of the procedures recommended in the guidelines are necessary or appropriate.

REFERENCES

1. Recommendations for the Safe Handling of Parenteral Antineoplastic Drugs. NIH Publication No. 83–2621. For sale by the Superintendent of Documents, US Government Printing Office, Washington, DC 20402.
2. AMA Council Report. Guidelines for Handling Parenteral Antineoplastics. *JAMA* 1985; 253(11):1590–1592.
3. National Study Commission on Cytotoxic Exposure-Recommendations for Handling Cytotoxic Agents. Available from Louis P. Jeffrey, Chairman, National Study Commission on Cytotoxic Exposure, Massachusetts College of Pharmacy and Allied Health Sciences, 179 Longwood Avenue, Boston, Massachusetts, 02115.
4. Clinical Oncological Society of Australia. Guidelines and Recommendations for Safe Handling of Antineoplastic Agents. *Med J Australia* 1983; 1:426–428.
5. Jones RB, et al: Safe Handling of Chemotherapeutic Agents: A Report from the Mount Sinai Medical Center. *CA-A Cancer Journal for Clinicians* 1983; (Sept/Oct) 258–263.
6. American Society of Hospital Pharmacists Technical Assistance Bulletin on Handling Cytotoxic and Hazardous Drugs. *Am J Hosp Pharm* 1990; 47:1033–1049.
7. Controlling Occupational Exposure to Hazardous Drugs. (OSHA WORK-PRACTICE GUIDELINES.) *Am J Health-Syst Pharm* 1996; 53:1669–1685.

Chemo Dispensing Pin™ is a trademark of B. Braun Medical Incorporated.

PATIENT INFORMATION

***TAXOL*® Injection**

(generic name = paclitaxel)

WHAT IS TAXOL?

TAXOL is a prescription cancer medicine. It is injected into a vein and it is used to treat different types of tumors. The tumors include advanced ovary and breast cancer. The tumors also include certain lung cancers (non-small cell) in people who cannot have surgery or radiation therapy. TAXOL may also be used to treat AIDS-related Kaposi's sarcoma.

WHAT IS CANCER?

Under normal conditions, the cells in your body divide and grow in an orderly, controlled way. Cell division and growth are necessary for the human body to perform its functions and to repair itself, when necessary. Cancer cells are different from normal cells because they are not able to control their own growth. The reasons for this abnormal growth are not yet fully understood.

A tumor is a mass of unhealthy cells that are dividing and growing fast and in an uncontrolled way. When a tumor invades surrounding healthy body tissue it is known as a malignant tumor. A malignant tumor can spread (metastasize) from its original site to other parts of the body if not found and treated early.

HOW DOES TAXOL WORK?

TAXOL is a type of medical treatment called chemotherapy. The purpose of chemotherapy is to kill cancer cells or prevent their growth.

All cells, whether they are healthy cells or cancer cells, go through several stages of growth. During one of the stages, the cell starts to divide. TAXOL may stop the cells from dividing and growing, so they eventually die. In addition, normal cells may also be affected by TAXOL causing some of the side effects. (See **WHAT ARE THE POSSIBLE SIDE EFFECTS OF TAXOL?** below.)

WHO SHOULD NOT TAKE TAXOL?

Patients who have a history of hypersensitivity (allergic reactions) to TAXOL or other drugs containing Cremophor® EL* (polyoxyethylated castor oil), like cyclosporine or teniposide, should not be given TAXOL. In addition, TAXOL should not be given to patients with dangerously low white blood cell counts.

HOW IS TAXOL GIVEN?

TAXOL is injected into a vein [intravenous (I.V.) infusion]. Before you are given TAXOL, you will have to take certain medicines (premedications) to prevent or reduce the chance you will have a serious allergic reaction. Such reactions have occurred in a small number of patients while receiving TAXOL and have been rarely fatal. (See **WHAT ARE THE POSSIBLE SIDE EFFECTS OF TAXOL?** below).

WHAT ARE THE POSSIBLE SIDE EFFECTS OF TAXOL?

Most patients taking TAXOL will experience side effects, although it is not always possible to tell whether such effects are caused by TAXOL, another medicine they may be taking, or the cancer itself. Important side effects are described below; however, some patients may experience other side effects that are less common. *Report any unusual symptoms to your doctor.*

Important side effects observed in studies of patients taking TAXOL were as follows:

— *Allergic reactions.* Allergic reactions can vary in degrees of severity. They may cause death in rare cases. When a severe allergic reaction develops, it usually occurs at the time the medicine is entering the body (during TAXOL infusion). Allergic reactions may cause trouble breathing, very low blood pressure, sudden swelling, and/or hives or rash. The likelihood of a serious allergic reaction is lowered by the use of several kinds of medicines that are given to you before the TAXOL infusion.

— *Heart and blood vessel (cardiovascular) effects.* TAXOL may cause a drop in heart rate (bradycardia) and low blood pressure (hypotension). The patient usually does not notice these changes. These changes usually do not require treatment. Your heart function, including blood pressure and pulse, will be monitored while you are receiving the medicine. You should notify your doctor if you have a history of heart disease.

— *Infections due to low white blood cell count.* Among the body's defenses against bacterial infections are white blood cells. Between your TAXOL treatment cycles, you will often have blood tests to check your white blood cell counts. TAXOL usually causes a brief drop in white blood cells. *If you have a fever (temperature above 100.4°F) or other sign of infection, tell your doctor right away. Sometimes serious infections develop that require treatment in the hospital with antibiotics. Serious illness or death could result if such infections are not treated when white blood cell counts are low.*

— *Hair loss.* Complete hair loss, or alopecia, almost always occurs with TAXOL. This usually involves the loss of eyebrows, eyelashes, and pubic hair, as well as scalp hair. It can occur suddenly after treatment has begun, but usually happens 14 to 21 days after treatment. *Hair generally grows back after you've finished your TAXOL treatment.*

— *Joint and muscle pain.* You may get joint and muscle pain a few days after your TAXOL (paclitaxel) Injection treatment. These symptoms usually disappear in a few days. Although pain medicine may not be necessary, tell your doctor if you are uncomfortable.

— *Irritation at the injection site.* TAXOL sometimes causes irritation at the site where it enters the vein. Reactions may include discomfort, redness, swelling, inflammation (of the surrounding skin or of the vein itself), and ulceration (open sores). These reactions are usually caused by the I.V. (intravenous) fluid leaking into the surrounding area. *If you notice anything unusual at the site of the injection (needle), either during or after treatment, tell your doctor right away.*

— *Low red blood cell count.* Red blood cells deliver oxygen to tissues throughout all parts of the body and take carbon dioxide from the tissues by using a protein called hemoglobin. A lowering of the volume of red blood cells may occur following TAXOL treatment causing anemia. Some patients may need a blood transfusion to treat the anemia.

Patients can feel tired, tire easily, appear pale, and become short of breath. Contact your doctor if you experience any of these symptoms following TAXOL treatment.

— *Mouth or lip sores (mucositis).* Some patients develop redness and/or sores in the mouth or on the lips. These symptoms might occur a few days after the TAXOL treatment and usually decrease or disappear within one week. Talk with your doctor about proper mouth care and other ways to prevent or reduce your chances of developing mucositis.

— *Numbness, tingling, or burning in the hands and/or feet (neuropathy).* These symptoms occur often with TAXOL and usually get better or go away without medication within several months of completing treatment. However, if you are uncomfortable, tell your doctor so that he/she can decide the best approach for relief of your symptoms.

— *Stomach upset and diarrhea.* Some patients experience nausea, vomiting, and/or diarrhea following TAXOL use. If you experience nausea or stomach upset, tell your doctor. Diarrhea will usually disappear without treatment; however, *if you experience severe abdominal or stomach area pain and/or severe diarrhea, tell your doctor right away.*

Talk with your doctor or other healthcare professional to discuss ways to prevent or reduce some of these side effects.

Because this leaflet does not include all possible side effects that can occur with TAXOL, it is important to talk with your doctor about other possible side effects.

CAN I TAKE TAXOL IF I AM PREGNANT OR NURSING A BABY?

TAXOL could harm the fetus when given to a pregnant woman. Women should avoid becoming pregnant while they are undergoing treatment with TAXOL. *Tell your doctor if you become pregnant or plan to become pregnant while taking TAXOL.*

Because studies have shown TAXOL to be present in the breast milk of animals receiving the drug, it may be present in human breast milk as well. Therefore, nursing a baby while taking TAXOL is NOT recommended.

This medicine was prescribed for your particular condition. This summary does not include everything there is to know about TAXOL. Medicines are sometimes prescribed for purposes other than those listed in a Patient Information Leaflet. If you have questions or concerns, or want more information about TAXOL, your doctor and pharmacist have the complete prescribing information upon which this guide is based. You may want to read it and discuss it with your doctor. Remember, no written summary can replace careful discussion with your doctor.

* Cremophor® EL is the registered trademark of BASF Aktiengesellschaft. Cremophor® is further purified by a Bristol-Myers Squibb Company proprietary process before use.

This Patient Information Leaflet has been approved by the U.S. Food and Drug Administration.

MeadJohnson
ONCOLOGY PROUCTS
A Britol-Myers Squibb Company
Princeton, NJ 08543
U.S.A.

K4-B001-7-00 Based on: 1109663A5
347630DIM-11 (4/00) Revised January 2000

Shown in Product Identification Guide, page 310

TESLAC® Ⓒ℞

[*tĕs-lăc*]

(testolactone tablets, USP)

Rx ONLY

DESCRIPTION

TESLAC® (testolactone tablets, USP) is available for oral administration as tablets providing 50 mg testolactone per tablet. Testolactone is a synthetic anti-neoplastic agent that is structurally distinct from the androgen steroid nucleus in possessing a six-membered lactone ring in place of the usual five-membered carbocyclic D-ring. Testolactone is chemically designated as 13-hydroxy-3-oxo-13,17-secoandrosta-1,4-dien-17-oic acid δ-lactone. Graphic formula:

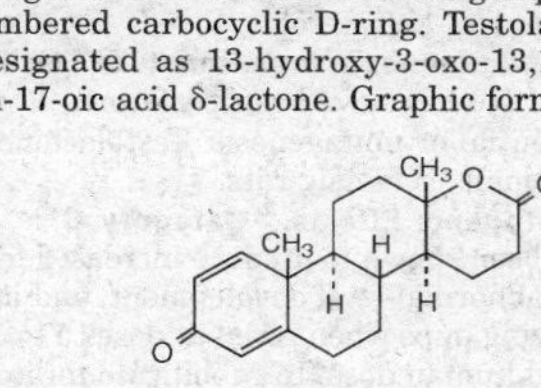

$C_{19}H_{24}O_3$ MW 300.40 CAS-968-93-4

Inactive ingredients: calcium stearate, cornstarch, gelatin, and lactose.

Testolactone is a white, odorless, crystalline solid, soluble in ethanol and slightly soluble in water.

CLINICAL PHARMACOLOGY

Although the precise mechanism by which testolactone produces its clinical antineoplastic effects has not been established, its principal action is reported to be inhibition of steroid aromatase activity and consequent reduction in estrone synthesis from adrenal androstenedione, the major source of estrogen in postmenopausal women. Based on *in vitro* studies, the aromatase inhibition may be noncompetitive and irreversible. This phenomenon may account for the persistence of testolactone's effect on estrogen synthesis after drug withdrawal.

Despite some similarity to testosterone, testolactone has no *in vivo* androgenic effect. No other hormonal effects have been reported in clinical studies in patients receiving testolactone. In one study, testolactone administered orally (1000 mg/day) was reported to increase renal tubular reabsorption of calcium but to have no effect on serum calcium concentration. The mechanism of the hypocalciuric effect is unknown. No clinical effects in humans of testolactone on adrenal function have been reported; however, one study noted an increase in urinary excretion of 17-ketosteroids in most of the patients treated with 150 mg/day orally.

Testolactone is well absorbed from the gastrointestinal tract. It is metabolized to several derivatives in the liver, all of which preserve the lactone D-ring. These metabolites, as well as some unmetabolized drug, are excreted in the urine. Additional pharmacokinetic data in humans are unavailable.

For information concerning carcinogenesis, mutagenesis, pregnancy, and lactation, see the corresponding **PRECAUTIONS** sections.

Continued on next page

Teslac—Cont.

In animals, parenteral but not oral testolactone reduced cortisone acetate induced hepatic glycogen deposits. In animal tests conducted to detect any hormonal activity for testolactone, some evidence of antiandrogenic and antiglucocorticoid activity was seen; increased growth rate in the newborn was suggested. However there was no clear manifestation of androgenic, estrogenic or antiestrogenic, progestational or antiprogestational, gonadotropin-like or antigonadotropic effects. Testolactone did not demonstrate anti-inflammatory, mineralocorticoid-like, or glucocorticoid-like properties.

INDICATIONS AND USAGE

TESLAC (testolactone tablets, USP) is recommended as adjunctive therapy in the palliative treatment of advanced or disseminated breast cancer in postmenopausal women when hormonal therapy is indicated. It may also be used in women who were diagnosed as having had disseminated breast carcinoma when premenopausal, in whom ovarian function has been subsequently terminated.

TESLAC was found to be effective in approximately 15 percent of patients with advanced or disseminated mammary cancer evaluated according to the following criteria: 1) those with a measurable decrease in size of all demonstrable tumor masses; 2) those in whom more than 50 percent of nonosseous lesions decreased in size although all bone lesions remained static; and 3) those in whom more than 50 percent of total lesions improved while the remainder were static.

CONTRAINDICATIONS

Testolactone is contraindicated in the treatment of breast cancer in men and in patients with a history of hypersensitivity to the drug.

PRECAUTIONS

Information for Patients: The physician should be consulted regarding missed doses. Notify the physician if adverse reactions occur or become more pronounced.

Laboratory Tests: Plasma calcium levels should be routinely determined in any patient receiving therapy for mammary cancer, particularly during periods of active remission of bony metastases. If hypercalcemia occurs, appropriate measures should be instituted.

Drug Interactions: When administered concurrently, testolactone may increase the effects of oral anticoagulants; monitor and adjust anticoagulant dosage accordingly.

Drug/Laboratory Test Interactions: Physiologic effects of testolactone may result in decreased estradiol concentrations with radioimmunoassays for estradiol, increased plasma calcium concentrations (see **PRECAUTIONS, Laboratory Tests** section), and increased 24-hour urinary excretion of creatine and 17-ketosteroids.

Carcinogenesis, Mutagenesis, Impairment of Fertility: No long-term animal studies have been performed to evaluate carcinogenic potential or mutagenesis. Testolactone did not affect fertility in male or female rats.

Pregnancy: Teratogenic Effects, "Category C": In rats, testolactone has been shown to produce increased fetal mortality, increased abnormal fetal development, and increased mortality in growing pups when given at doses 5 to 15 times the recommended human dose. In rabbits, no teratologic effects were observed at doses 2.5 to 7.5 times the recommended human dose. There are no adequate and well controlled studies in pregnant women. Testolactone is intended for use only in postmenopausal women and should not be used during pregnancy.

Nursing Mothers: It is not known whether this drug is excreted in human milk. Because many drugs are excreted in human milk, a decision should be made whether or not to discontinue nursing.

Pediatric Use: Safety and effectiveness in children have not been established.

ADVERSE REACTIONS

Certain signs and symptoms have been reported in association with the use of this drug but, in these instances, it is often impossible to determine the relationship of the underlying disease and drug administration to the reported reaction. Such reactions include maculopapular erythema, increase in blood pressure, paresthesia, malaise, aches and edema of the extremities, glossitis, anorexia and nausea and vomiting. Alopecia alone and with associated nail growth disturbance have been reported rarely; these side effects subsided without interruption of treatment.

DRUG ABUSE AND DEPENDENCE

TESLAC is classified as a controlled substance under the Anabolic Steroids Control Act of 1990 and has been assigned to Schedule III.

OVERDOSAGE

There have been no reports of acute overdosage with testolactone tablets.

DOSAGE AND ADMINISTRATION

The recommended oral dose is 250 mg qid.

In order to evaluate the response, therapy with testolactone should be continued for a minimum of three months unless there is active progression of the disease.

HOW SUPPLIED

TESLAC® (testolactone tablets, USP)

50 mg/tablet: bottles of 100 (**NDC** 0003-0690-50). Each round, white, biconvex tablet is imprinted with the identification number 690.

Storage

Store at controlled room temperature 25°C (77°F).

Mead Johnson
ONCOLOGY PRODUCTS
A Bristol-Myers Squibb Company
Princeton, NJ 08543
U.S.A.
Made in Australia

K5-B001-7-99 J4-666

Revised December 1998

VePesid® ℞

[*vĕ-pesid*]
(etoposide)
For Injection and Capsules
Rx ONLY

> **WARNINGS**
> VePesid® should be administered under the supervision of a qualified physician experienced in the use of cancer chemotherapeutic agents. Severe myelosuppression with resulting infection or bleeding may occur.

DESCRIPTION

VePesid® (etoposide) (also commonly known as VP-16) is a semisynthetic derivative of podophyllotoxin used in the treatment of certain neoplastic diseases. It is 4'-demethylepipodophyllotoxin 9-[4,6-0-(R)-ethylidene-β-D-glucopyranoside]. It is very soluble in methanol and chloroform, slightly soluble in ethanol, and sparingly soluble in water and ether. It is made more miscible with water by means of organic solvents. It has a molecular weight of 588.58 and a molecular formula of $C_{29}H_{32}O_{13}$.

VePesid may be administered either intravenously or orally. VePesid For Injection is available in 100 mg (5 mL), 150 mg (7.5 mL), 500 mg (25 mL), or 1 gram (50 mL), sterile, multiple dose vials. The pH of the clear, nearly colorless to yellow liquid is 3 to 4. Each mL contains 20 mg etoposide, 2 mg citric acid, 30 mg benzyl alcohol, 80 mg modified polysorbate 80/tween 80, 650 mg polyethylene glycol 300, and 30.5 percent (v/v) alcohol. Vial headspace contains nitrogen.

VePesid is also available as 50 mg pink capsules. Each liquid filled, soft gelatin capsule contains 50 mg of etoposide in a vehicle consisting of citric acid, glycerin, purified water, and polyethylene glycol 400. The soft gelatin capsules contain gelatin, glycerin, sorbitol, purified water, and parabens (ethyl and propyl) with the following dye system: iron oxide (red) and titanium dioxide; the capsules are printed with edible ink.

The structural formula is:

CLINICAL PHARMACOLOGY

VePesid has been shown to cause metaphase arrest in chick fibroblasts. Its main effect, however, appears to be at the G_2 portion of the cell cycle in mammalian cells. Two different dose-dependent responses are seen. At high concentrations (10 µg/mL or more), lysis of cells entering mitosis is observed. At low concentrations (0.3 to 10 µg/mL), cells are inhibited from entering prophase. It does not interfere with microtubular assembly. The predominant macromolecular effect of etoposide appears to be the induction of DNA strand breaks by an interaction with DNA topoisomerase II or the formation of free radicals.

Pharmacokinetics: On intravenous administration, the disposition of etoposide is best described as a biphasic process with a distribution half-life of about 1.5 hours and terminal elimination half-life ranging from 4 to 11 hours. Total body clearance values range from 33 to 48 mL/min or 16 to 36 mL/min/m^2 and, like the terminal elimination half-life, are independent of dose over a range 100–600 mg/m^2. Over the same dose range, the areas under the plasma concentration vs. time curves (AUC) and the maximum plasma concentration (Cmax) values increase linearly with dose. Etoposide does not accumulate in the plasma following daily administration of 100 mg/m^2 for 4 to 5 days.

The mean volumes of distribution at steady state fall in the range of 18 to 29 liters or 7 to 17 L/m^2. Etoposide enters the CSF poorly. Although it is detectable in CSF and intracerebral tumors, the concentrations are lower than in extracerebral tumors and in plasma. Etoposide concentrations are higher in normal lung than in lung metastases and are similar in primary tumors and normal tissues of the myometrium. *In vitro*, etoposide is highly protein bound (97%) to human plasma proteins. An inverse relationship between plasma albumin levels and etoposide renal clearance is found in children. In a study determining the effect of other therapeutic agents on the *in vitro* binding of carbon-14 labeled etoposide to human serum proteins, only phenylbutazone, sodium salicylate, and aspirin displaced protein-bound etoposide at concentrations achieved *in vivo*.[1]

Etoposide binding ratio correlates directly with serum albumin in patients with cancer and in normal volunteers. The unbound fraction of etoposide significantly correlated with bilirubin in a population of cancer patients.[2,3] Data have suggested a significant inverse correlation between serum albumin concentration and free fraction of etoposide (see **PRECAUTIONS** section).

After intravenous administration of ^{3}H-etoposide (70–290 mg/m^2), mean recoveries of radioactivity in the urine range from 42 to 67%, and fecal recoveries range from 0 to 16% of the dose. Less than 50% of an intravenous dose is excreted in the urine as etoposide with mean recoveries of 8 to 35% within 24 hours.

In children, approximately 55% of the dose is excreted in the urine as etoposide in 24 hours. The mean renal clearance of etoposide is 7 to 10 mL/min/m^2 or about 35% of the total body clearance over a dose range of 80 to 600 mg/m^2. Etoposide, therefore, is cleared by both renal and nonrenal processes, i.e., metabolism and biliary excretion. The effect of renal disease on plasma etoposide clearance is not known. Biliary excretion appears to be a minor route of etoposide elimination. Only 6% or less of an intravenous dose is recovered in the bile as etoposide. Metabolism accounts for most of the nonrenal clearance of etoposide. The major urinary metabolite of etoposide in adults and children is the hydroxy acid [4'-demethylepipodophyllic acid-9-(4,6-0-(R)-ethylidene-β-D-glucopyranoside)], formed by opening of the lactone ring. It is also present in human plasma, presumably as the **trans** isomer. Glucuronide and/or sulfate conjugates of etoposide are excreted in human urine and represent 5 to 22% of the dose. In addition, O-demethylation of the dimethoxyphenol ring occurs through the CYP450 3A4 isoenzyme pathway to produce the corresponding catechol.

After either intravenous infusion or oral capsule administration, the Cmax and AUC values exhibit marked intra- and inter-subject variability. This results in variability in the estimates of the absolute oral bioavailability of etoposide oral capsules.

Cmax and AUC values for orally administered etoposide capsules consistently fall in the same range as the Cmax and AUC values for an intravenous dose of one-half the size of the oral dose. The overall mean value of oral capsule bioavailability is approximately 50% (range 25–75%). The bioavailability of etoposide capsules appears to be linear up to a dose of at least 250 mg/m^2.

There is no evidence of a first-pass effect for etoposide. For example, no correlation exists between the absolute oral bioavailability of etoposide capsules and nonrenal clearance. No evidence exists for any other differences in etoposide metabolism and excretion after administration of oral capsules as compared to intravenous infusion.

In adults, the total body clearance of etoposide is correlated with creatinine clearance, serum albumin concentration, and nonrenal clearance. Patients with impaired renal function receiving etoposide have exhibited reduced total body clearance, increased AUC and a lower volume of distribution at steady state (see **PRECAUTIONS** section). Use of cisplatin therapy is associated with reduced total body clearance. In children, elevated serum SGPT levels are associated with reduced drug total body clearance. Prior use of cisplatin may also result in a decrease of etoposide total body clearance in children.

Although some minor differences in pharmacokinetic parameters between age and gender have been observed, these differences were not considered clinically significant.

INDICATIONS AND USAGE

VePesid (etoposide) is indicated in the management of the following neoplasms:

Refractory Testicular Tumors: VePesid For Injection in combination therapy with other approved chemotherapeutic agents in patients with refractory testicular tumors who have already received appropriate surgical, chemotherapeutic, and radiotherapeutic therapy.

Adequate data on the use of VePesid Capsules in the treatment of testicular cancer are not available.

Small Cell Lung Cancer: VePesid For Injection and/or Capsules in combination with other approved chemotherapeutic agents as first line treatment in patients with small cell lung cancer.

CONTRAINDICATIONS

VePesid is contraindicated in patients who have demonstrated a previous hypersensitivity to etoposide or any component of the formulation.

WARNINGS

Patients being treated with VePesid must be frequently observed for myelosuppression both during and after therapy. Myelosuppression resulting in death has been reported. Dose-limiting bone marrow suppression is the most significant toxicity associated with VePesid therapy. Therefore, the following studies should be obtained at the start of therapy and prior to each subsequent cycle of VePesid: platelet count, hemoglobin, white blood cell count, and differential.

The occurrence of a platelet count below 50,000/mm^3 or an absolute neutrophil count below 500/mm^3 is an indication to withhold further therapy until the blood counts have sufficiently recovered.

Physicians should be aware of the possible occurrence of an anaphylactic reaction manifested by chills, fever, tachycardia, bronchospasm, dyspnea, and hypotension. Higher rates of anaphylactic-like reactions have been reported in children who received infusions at concentrations higher than those recommended. The role that concentration of infusion (or rate of infusion) plays in the development of anaphylactic-like reactions is uncertain. (See **ADVERSE REACTIONS** section.) Treatment is symptomatic. The infusion should be terminated immediately, followed by the administration of pressor agents, corticosteroids, antihistamines, or volume expanders at the discretion of the physician.

For parenteral administration, VePesid should be given only by slow intravenous infusion (usually over a 30 to 60 minute period) since hypotension has been reported as a possible side effect of rapid intravenous injection.

Pregnancy: VePesid can cause fetal harm when administered to a pregnant woman. Etoposide has been shown to be teratogenic in mice and rats.

In rats, an intravenous etoposide dose of 0.4 mg/kg/day (about 1/20th of the human dose on a mg/m^2 basis) during organogenesis caused maternal toxicity, embryotoxicity, and teratogenicity (skeletal abnormalities, exencephaly, encephalocele, and anophthalmia); higher doses of 1.2 and 3.6 mg/kg/day (about 1/7th and 1/2 of human dose on a mg/m^2 basis) resulted in 90 and 100% embryonic resorptions. In mice, a single 1.0 mg/kg (1/16th of human dose on a mg/m^2 basis) dose of etoposide administered intraperitoneally on days 6, 7, 8 of gestation caused embryotoxicity, cranial abnormalities, and major skeletal malformations. An I.P. dose of 1.5 mg/kg (about 1/10th of human dose on a mg/m^2 basis) on day 7 of gestation caused an increase in the incidence of intrauterine death and fetal malformations and a significant decrease in the average fetal body weight.

Women of childbearing potential should be advised to avoid becoming pregnant. If this drug is used during pregnancy, or if the patient becomes pregnant while receiving this drug, the patient should be warned of the potential hazard to the fetus.

VePesid should be considered a potential carcinogen in humans. The occurrence of acute leukemia with or without a preleukemic phase has been reported in rare instances in patients treated with etoposide alone or in association with other neoplastic agents. The risk of development of a preleukemic or leukemic syndrome is unclear. Carcinogenicity tests with VePesid have not been conducted in laboratory animals.

PRECAUTIONS

General: In all instances where the use of VePesid is considered for chemotherapy, the physician must evaluate the need and usefulness of the drug against the risk of adverse reactions. Most such adverse reactions are reversible if detected early. If severe reactions occur, the drug should be reduced in dosage or discontinued and appropriate corrective measures should be taken according to the clinical judgment of the physician. Reinstitution of VePesid therapy should be carried out with caution, and with adequate consideration of the further need for the drug and alertness as to possible recurrence of toxicity.

Patients with low serum albumin may be at an increased risk for etoposide associated toxicities.

Laboratory Tests: Periodic complete blood counts should be done during the course of VePesid treatment. They should be performed prior to each cycle of therapy and at appropriate intervals during and after therapy. At least one determination should be done prior to each dose of VePesid.

Renal Impairment: In patients with impaired renal function, the following initial dose modification should be considered based on measured creatinine clearance:

Measured Creatinine Clearance	> 50 mL/min	15–50 mL/min
etoposide	100% of dose	75% of dose

Subsequent VePesid dosing should be based on patient tolerance and clinical effect.

Data are not available in patients with creatinine clearances <15 mL/min and further dose reduction should be considered in these patients.

Carcinogenesis, (see **WARNINGS** section) **Mutagenesis, Impairment of Fertility:** Etoposide has been shown to be mutagenic in Ames assay.

Treatment of Swiss-Albino mice with 1.5 mg/kg I.P. of VePesid on day 7 of gestation increased the incidence of intrauterine death and fetal malformations as well as significantly decreased the average fetal body weight. Maternal weight gain was not affected.

Irreversible testicular atrophy was present in rats treated with etoposide intravenously for 30 days at 0.5 mg/kg/day (about 1/16th of the human dose on a mg/m^2 basis).

Pregnancy: Pregnancy "Category D". (See **WARNINGS** section.)

Nursing Mothers: It is not known whether this drug is excreted in human milk. Because many drugs are excreted in human milk and because of the potential for serious adverse reactions in nursing infants from VePesid (etoposide), a decision should be made whether to discontinue nursing or to discontinue the drug, taking into account the importance of the drug to the mother.

Pediatric Use: Safety and effectiveness in pediatric patients have not been established.

VePesid For Injection contains polysorbate 80. In premature infants, a life-threatening syndrome consisting of liver and renal failure, pulmonary deterioration, thrombocytopenia, and ascites has been associated with an injectable vitamin E product containing polysorbate 80. Anaphylactic reactions have been reported in pediatric patients. (See **WARNINGS** section.)

Drug Interactions: High-dose cyclosporine resulting in concentrations above 2000 ng/mL administered with oral etoposide has led to an 80% increase in etoposide exposure with a 38% decrease in total body clearance of etoposide compared to etoposide alone.

ADVERSE REACTIONS

The following data on adverse reactions are based on both oral and intravenous administration of VePesid as a single agent, using several different dose schedules for treatment of a wide variety of malignancies.

Hematologic Toxicity: Myelosuppression is dose related and dose limiting, with granulocyte nadirs occurring 7 to 14 days after drug administration and platelet nadirs occurring 9 to 16 days after drug administration. Bone marrow recovery is usually complete by day 20, and no cumulative toxicity has been reported. Fever and infection have also been reported in patients with neutropenia. Death associated with myelosuppression has been reported.

The occurrence of acute leukemia with or without a preleukemic phase has been reported rarely in patients treated with VePesid in association with other antineoplastic agents. (See **WARNINGS** section.)

Gastrointestinal Toxicity: Nausea and vomiting are the major gastrointestinal toxicities. The severity of such nausea and vomiting is generally mild to moderate with treatment discontinuation required in 1% of patients. Nausea and vomiting can usually be controlled with standard antiemetic therapy. Mild to severe mucositis/esophagitis may occur. Gastrointestinal toxicities are slightly more frequent after oral administration than after intravenous infusion.

Hypotension: Transient hypotension following rapid intravenous administration has been reported in 1% to 2% of patients. It has not been associated with cardiac toxicity or electrocardiographic changes. No delayed hypotension has been noted. To prevent this rare occurrence, it is recommended that VePesid be administered by slow intravenous infusion over a 30- to 60-minute period. If hypotension occurs, it usually responds to cessation of the infusion and administration of fluids or other supportive therapy as appropriate. When restarting the infusion, a slower administration rate should be used.

Allergic Reactions: Anaphylactic-like reactions characterized by chills, fever, tachycardia, bronchospasm, dyspnea, and/or hypotension have been reported to occur in 0.7% to 2% of patients receiving intravenous VePesid and in less than 1% of the patients treated with the oral capsules. These reactions have usually responded promptly to the cessation of the infusion and administration of pressor agents, corticosteroids, antihistamines, or volume expanders as appropriate; however, the reactions can be fatal. Hypertension and/or flushing have also been reported. Blood pressure usually normalizes within a few hours after cessation of the infusion. Anaphylactic-like reactions have occurred during the initial infusion of VePesid.

Facial/tongue swelling, coughing, diaphoresis, cyanosis, tightness in throat, laryngospasm, back pain, and/or loss of consciousness have sometimes occurred in association with the above reactions. In addition, an apparent hypersensitivity-associated apnea has been reported rarely.

Rash, urticaria, and/or pruritus have infrequently been reported at recommended doses. At investigational doses, a generalized pruritic erythematous maculopapular rash, consistent with perivasculitis, has been reported.

Alopecia: Reversible alopecia, sometimes progressing to total baldness, was observed in up to 66% of patients.

Other Toxicities: The following adverse reactions have been infrequently reported: abdominal pain, aftertaste, constipation, dysphagia, asthenia, fatigue, malaise, somnolence, transient cortical blindness, optic neuritis, interstitial pneumonitis/pulmonary fibrosis, fever, seizure (occasionally associated with allergic reactions), Stevens-Johnson syndrome, and toxic epidermal necrolysis, pigmentation, and a single report of radiation recall dermatitis.

Hepatic toxicity, generally in patients receiving higher doses of the drug than those recommended, has been reported with VePesid. Metabolic acidosis has also been reported in patients receiving higher doses.

Reports of extravasation with swelling have been received postmarketing. Rarely extravasation has been associated with necrosis and venous induration.

The incidences of adverse reactions in the table that follows are derived from multiple data bases from studies in 2,081 patients when VePesid was used either orally or by injection as a single agent.

[See table above]

ADVERSE DRUG EFFECT	PERCENT RANGE OF REPORTED INCIDENCE
Hematologic toxicity	
Leukopenia (less than 1,000 WBC/mm^3)	3–17
Leukopenia (less than 4,000 WBC/mm^3)	60–91
Thrombocytopenia (less than 50,000 platelets/mm^3)	1–20
Thrombocytopenia (less than 100,000 platelets/mm^3)	22–41
Anemia	0–33
Gastrointestinal toxicity	
Nausea and vomiting	31–43
Abdominal pain	0–2
Anorexia	10–13
Diarrhea	1–13
Stomatitis	1–6
Hepatic	0–3
Alopecia	8–66
Peripheral neurotoxicity	1–2
Hypotension	1–2
Allergic Reaction	1–2

OVERDOSAGE

No proven antidotes have been established for VePesid overdosage.

DOSAGE AND ADMINISTRATION

Note: Plastic devices made of acrylic or ABS (a polymer composed of acrylonitrile, butadiene, and styrene) have been reported to crack and leak when used with *undiluted* VePesid For Injection.

VePesid For Injection: The usual dose of VePesid For Injection in testicular cancer in combination with other approved chemotherapeutic agents ranges from 50 to 100 mg/m^2/day on days 1 through 5 to 100 mg/m^2/day on days 1, 3, and 5.

In small cell lung cancer, the VePesid For Injection dose in combination with other approved chemotherapeutic drugs ranges from 35 mg/m^2/day for 4 days to 50 mg/m^2/day for 5 days.

For recommended dosing adjustments in patients with renal impairment, see **PRECAUTIONS** section.

Chemotherapy courses are repeated at 3- to 4-week intervals after adequate recovery from any toxicity.

VePesid (etoposide) Capsules: In small cell lung cancer, the recommended dose of VePesid Capsules is two times the I.V. dose rounded to the nearest 50 mg.

The dosage, by either route, should be modified to take into account the myelosuppressive effects of other drugs in the combination or the effects of prior x-ray therapy or chemotherapy which may have compromised bone marrow reserve.

Administration Precautions: As with other potentially toxic compounds, caution should be exercised in handling and preparing the solution of VePesid. Skin reactions associated with accidental exposure to VePesid may occur. The use of gloves is recommended. If VePesid solution contacts the skin or mucosa, immediately and thoroughly wash the skin with soap and water and flush the mucosa with water.

Preparation for Intravenous Administration: VePesid For Injection must be diluted prior to use with either 5% Dextrose Injection, USP, or 0.9% Sodium Chloride Injection, USP, to give a final concentration of 0.2 to 0.4 mg/mL. If solutions are prepared at concentrations above 0.4 mg/mL, precipitation may occur. Hypotension following rapid intravenous administration has been reported, hence, it is recommended that the VePesid solution be administered over a 30- to 60-minute period. A longer duration of administration may be used if the volume of fluid to be infused is a concern. **VePesid should not be given by rapid intravenous injection.**

Parenteral drug products should be inspected visually for particulate matter and discoloration (see **DESCRIPTION** section) prior to administration whenever solution and container permit.

Stability: Unopened vials of VePesid For Injection are stable for 24 months at room temperature (25°C). Vials diluted

Continued on next page

Vepesid—Cont.

as recommended to a concentration of 0.2 or 0.4 mg/mL are stable for 96 and 24 hours, respectively, at room temperature (25°C) under normal room fluorescent light in both glass and plastic containers.
VePesid Capsules must be stored under refrigeration 2°–8°C (36°– 46°F). The capsules are stable for 24 months under such refrigeration conditions.
Procedures for proper handling and disposal of anticancer drugs should be considered. Several guidelines on this subject have been published.[4–10] There is no general agreement that all of the procedures recommended in the guidelines are necessary or appropriate.

HOW SUPPLIED

VePesid® (etoposide) For Injection
NDC 0015-3095-20 – 100 mg/5 mL Sterile, Multiple Dose Vial, 10's
NDC 0015-3084-20 – 150 mg/7.5 mL Sterile, Multiple Dose Vial
NDC 0015-3061-20 – 500 mg/25 mL Sterile, Multiple Dose Vial
NDC 0015-3062-20 – 1 gram/50 mL Sterile, Multiple Dose Vial
VePesid® (etoposide) Capsules
NDC 0015-3091-45 – 50 mg pink capsules with "BRISTOL 3091" printed in black in blisterpacks of 20 individually labeled blisters, each containing one capsule.
Capsules are to be stored under refrigeration 2°–8°C (36°–46°F).
DO NOT FREEZE.
Dispense in child-resistant containers.
For information on package sizes available, refer to the current price schedule.

REFERENCES

1. Gaver RC, Deeb G: The Effect of Other Drugs on the *in vitro* Binding of 14C-Etoposide to Human Serum Proteins. *Proc Am Assoc Cancer Res* 1989; 30:A2132.
2. Stewart CF, et al: Altered Protein Binding of Etoposide in Patients with Cancer. *Clin Pharmacol Ther* 1989; 45: 49–55.
3. Stewart CF, et al: Prospective Evaluation of a Model for Predicting Etoposide Plasma Protein Binding in Cancer Patients. *Proc Am Assoc Cancer Res* 1989; 30:A958.
4. Recommendations for the Safe Handling of Parenteral Antineoplastic Drugs. NIH Publication No. 83-2621. For sale by the Superintendent of Documents, US Government Printing Office, Washington, DC 20402.
5. AMA Council Report. Guidelines for Handling Parenteral Antineoplastics. *JAMA* 1985; 253(11):1590–1592.
6. National Study Commission on Cytotoxic Exposure—Recommendations for Handling Cytotoxic Agents. Available from Louis P. Jeffrey, ScD, Chairman, National Study Commission on Cytotoxic Exposure, Massachusetts College of Pharmacy and Allied Health Sciences, 179 Longwood Avenue, Boston, Massachusetts 02115.
7. Clinical Oncological Society of Australia. Guidelines and Recommendations for Safe Handling of Antineoplastic Agents. *Med J Australia* 1983; 1:426–428.
8. Jones RB, et al: Handling of Chemotherapeutic Agents: A Report from the Mount Sinai Medical Center. *CA-A Cancer Journal for Clinicians* 1983; (Sept/Oct)258–263.
9. American Society of Hospital Pharmacists Technical Assistance Bulletin on Handling Cytotoxic and Hazardous Drugs. *Am J Hosp Pharm* 1990; 47:1033–1049.
10. Controlling Occupational Exposure to Hazardous Drugs. (OSHA WORK PRACTICE GUIDELINES). *Am J Health-Syst Pharm* 1996; 53:1669–1685.

Capsules:
Manufactured by:
R.P. Scherer GmbH
Eberback/Baden, Germany
Injection:
BRISTOL LABORATORIES
Oncology Products
A Bristol-Myers Squibb Co.
Princeton, New Jersey 08543 U.S.A.
Distributed by:
BRISTOL LABORATORIES®
ONCOLOGY PRODUCTS
A Bristol-Myers Squibb Company
Princeton, NJ 08543
U.S.A.
K6-B001-12-98 1047844
Revised September 1998

Shown in Product Identification Guide, page 310

VIDEX® ℞

[*vī-dex*]
(didanosine)

VIDEX® (didanosine) Chewable/Dispersible Buffered Tablets

VIDEX® (didanosine) Buffered Powder for Oral Solution

VIDEX® (didanosine) Pediatric Powder for Oral Solution
Rx ONLY

(Please consult the MANUFACTURERS' INDEX or the BRAND AND GENERIC NAME INDEX for product page number)

Shown in Product Identification Guide, page 310

VUMON® ℞

[*vū 'mŏn*]
(teniposide injection)
℞ ONLY

WARNING
VUMON® (teniposide injection) is a cytotoxic drug, which should be administered under the supervision of a qualified physician experienced in the use of cancer chemotherapeutic agents. Appropriate management of therapy and complications is possible only when adequate treatment facilities are readily available.
Severe myelosuppression with resulting infection or bleeding may occur. Hypersensitivity reactions, including anaphylaxis-like symptoms, may occur with initial dosing or at repeated exposure to VUMON. Epinephrine, with or without corticosteroids and antihistamines has been employed to alleviate hypersensitivity reaction symptoms.

DESCRIPTION

VUMON® (teniposide injection) (also commonly known as VM-26), is supplied as a sterile nonpyrogenic solution in a nonaqueous medium intended for dilution with a suitable parenteral vehicle prior to intravenous infusion. VUMON is available in 50 mg (5 mL) ampules. Each mL contains 10 mg teniposide, 30 mg benzyl alcohol, 60 mg N,N-dimethylacetamide, 500 mg purified Cremophor® EL (polyoxyethylated castor oil)* and 42.7 percent (V/V) dehydrated alcohol. The pH of the clear solution is adjusted to approximately 5 with maleic acid.
Teniposide is a semisynthetic derivative of podophyllotoxin. The chemical name for teniposide is 4′-demethylepipodophyllotoxin 9-[4,6-0-(R)-2- thenylidene-β-D-glucopyranoside]. Teniposide differs from etoposide, another podophyllotoxin derivative, by the substitution of a thenylidene group on the glucopyranoside ring.
Teniposide has the following structural formula:

Teniposide is a white to off-white crystalline powder with the empirical formula $C_{32}H_{32}O_{13}S$ and a molecular weight of 656.66. It is a lipophilic compound with a partition coefficient value (octanol/water) of approximately 100. Teniposide is insoluble in water and ether. It is slightly soluble in methanol and very soluble in acetone and dimethylformamide.

CLINICAL PHARMACOLOGY

Teniposide is a phase-specific cytotoxic drug, acting in the late S or early G_2 phase of the cell cycle, thus preventing cells from entering mitosis.
Teniposide causes dose-dependent single- and double-stranded breaks in DNA and DNA: protein cross-links. The mechanism of action appears to be related to the inhibition of type II topoisomerase activity since teniposide does not intercalate into DNA or bind strongly to DNA. The cytotoxic effects of teniposide are related to the relative number of double-stranded DNA breaks produced in cells, which are a reflection of the stabilization of a topoisomerase II-DNA intermediate.
Teniposide has a broad spectrum of *in vivo* antitumor activity against murine tumors, including hematologic malignancies and various solid tumors. Notably, teniposide is active against sublines of certain murine leukemias with acquired resistance to cisplatin, doxorubicin, amsacrine, daunorubicin, mitoxantrone or vincristine.
Plasma drug levels declined biexponentially following intravenous infusion (155 mg/m² over 1 to 2.5 hours) of VUMON given to eight children (4–11 years old) with newly diagnosed acute lymphoblastic leukemia (ALL). The observed average pharmacokinetic parameters and associated coefficients of variation (CV%) based on a two-compartmental model analysis of the data are as follows:
[See table below]
There appears to be some association between an increase in serum alkaline phosphatase or gamma glutamyl-transpeptidase and a decrease in plasma clearance of teniposide. Therefore, caution should be exercised if VUMON is to be administered to patients with hepatic dysfunction.
In adults, at doses of 100 to 333 mg/m²/day, plasma levels increased linearly with dose. Drug accumulation in adult patients did not occur after daily administration of VUMON for 3 days. In pediatric patients, maximum plasma concentrations (C_{max}) after infusions of 137 to 203 mg/m² over a period of one to two hours exceeded 40 µg/mL; by 20 to 24 hours after infusion plasma levels were generally < 2µg/mL.
Renal clearance of parent teniposide accounts for about 10 percent of total body clearance. In adults, after intravenous administration of 10 mg/kg or 67 mg/m² of tritium-labeled teniposide, 44 percent of the radiolabel was recovered in urine (parent drug and metabolites) within 120 hours after dosing. From 4 to 12 percent of a dose is excreted in urine as parent drug. Fecal excretion of radioactivity within 72 hours after dosing accounted for 0 to 10 percent of the dose. Mean steady-state volumes of distribution range from 8 to 44 L/m² for adults and 3 to 11 L/m² for children. The blood-brain barrier appears to limit diffusion of teniposide into the brain, although in a study in patients with brain tumors, CSF levels of teniposide were higher than CSF levels reported in other studies of patients who did not have brain tumors.
Teniposide is highly protein bound. *In vitro* plasma protein binding of teniposide is >99 percent. The high affinity of teniposide for plasma proteins may be an important factor in limiting distribution of drug within the body. Steady state volume of distribution of the drug increases with a decrease in plasma albumin levels. Therefore, careful monitoring of children with hypoalbuminemia is indicated during therapy. Levels of teniposide in saliva, CSF and malignant ascites fluid are low relative to simultaneously measured plasma levels.

* Cremophor® EL is the registered trademark of BASF Aktiengesellschaft. Cremophor® EL is further purified by a Bristol-Myers Squibb Company proprietary process before use.

The pharmacokinetic characteristics of teniposide differ from those of etoposide, another podophyllotoxin. Teniposide is more extensively bound to plasma proteins, and its cellular uptake is greater. Teniposide also has a lower systemic clearance, a longer elimination half-life, and is excreted in the urine as parent drug to a lesser extent than etoposide.
In a study at St. Jude Children's Research Hospital (SJCRH), 9 children with acute lymphocytic leukemia (ALL) failing induction therapy with a cytarabine-containing regimen, were treated with VUMON (teniposide injection) plus cytarabine. Three of these patients were induced into complete remission with durations of remission of 30 weeks, 59 weeks, and 13 years. In another study at SJCRH, 16 children with ALL refractory to vincristine/prednisone-containing regimens were treated with VUMON plus vincristine and prednisone. Three of these patients were induced into complete remission with durations of remission of 5.5, 37, and 73 weeks. In these two studies patients served as their own control based on the premise that long-term complete remissions could not be achieved by re-treatment with drugs to which they had previously failed to respond.

INDICATION AND USAGE

VUMON, in combination with other approved anticancer agents, is indicated for induction therapy in patients with refractory childhood acute lymphoblastic leukemia.

CONTRAINDICATIONS

VUMON is generally contraindicated in patients who have demonstrated a previous hypersensitivity to teniposide and/or Cremophor® EL (polyoxyethylated castor oil).

WARNINGS

VUMON is a potent drug and should be used only by physicians experienced in the administration of cancer chemotherapeutic drugs. Blood counts as well as renal and hepatic function tests should be carefully monitored prior to and during therapy.
Patients being treated with VUMON should be observed frequently for myelosuppression both during and after therapy. Dose-limiting bone marrow suppression is the most significant toxicity associated with VUMON therapy. Therefore, the following studies should be obtained at the start of therapy and prior to each subsequent dose of VUMON: hemoglobin, white blood cell count and differential and platelet count. If necessary, repeat bone marrow examination should be performed prior to the decision to continue therapy in the setting of severe myelosuppression.
Physicians should be aware of the possible occurrence of a hypersensitivity reaction variably manifested by chills, fever, urticaria, tachycardia, bronchospasm, dyspnea, hypertension or hypotension and facial flushing. This reaction may occur with the first dose of VUMON and may be life

Parameter	Mean	CV%
Total body clearance (mL/min/m²)	10.3	25
Volume at steady-state (L/m²)	3.1	30
Terminal half-life (hours)	5.0	44
Volume of central compartment (L/m²)	1.5	36
Rate constant, central to peripheral (1/hours)	0.47	62
Rate constant, peripheral to central (1/hours)	0.42	37

threatening if not treated promptly with antihistamines, corticosteroids, epinephrine, intravenous fluids and other supportive measures as clinically indicated. The exact cause of these reactions is unknown. They may be due to the Cremophor® EL (polyoxyethylated castor oil) component of the vehicle or to teniposide itself.[1] Patients who have experienced prior hypersensitivity reactions to VUMON are at risk for recurrence of symptoms and should only be re-treated with VUMON if the antileukemic benefit already demonstrated clearly outweighs the risk of a probable hypersensitivity reaction for that patient. When a decision is made to re-treat a patient with VUMON in spite of an earlier hypersensitivity reaction, the patient should be pretreated with corticosteroids and antihistamines and receive careful clinical observation during and after VUMON infusion. In the clinical experience with VUMON at SJCRH and the National Cancer Institute (NCI), re-treatment of patients with prior hypersensitivity reactions has been accomplished using measures described above. To date, there is no evidence to suggest cross-sensitization between VUMON and VePesid® (etoposide).

One episode of sudden death, attributed to probable arrhythmia and intractable hypotension has been reported in an elderly patient receiving VUMON combination therapy for a non-leukemic malignancy. (See ADVERSE REACTIONS.) Patients receiving VUMON treatment should be under continuous observation for at least the first 60 minutes following the start of the infusion and at frequent intervals thereafter. If symptoms or signs of anaphylaxis occur, the infusion should be stopped immediately, followed by the administration of epinephrine, corticosteroids, antihistamines, pressor agents, or volume expanders at the discretion of the physician. An aqueous solution of epinephrine 1:1000 and a source of oxygen should be available at the bedside.

For parenteral administration, VUMON should be given only by slow intravenous infusion (lasting at least 30- to 60-minutes) since hypotension has been reported as a possible side effect of rapid intravenous injection, perhaps due to a direct effect of Cremophor® EL.[2,3] If clinically significant hypotension develops, the VUMON infusion should be discontinued. The blood pressure usually normalizes within hours in response to cessation of the infusion and administration of fluids or other supportive therapy as appropriate. If the infusion is restarted, a slower administration rate should be used and the patient should be carefully monitored.

Acute central nervous system depression and hypotension have been observed in patients receiving investigational infusions of high-dose VUMON who were pretreated with antiemetic drugs. The depressant effects of the antiemetic agents and the alcohol content of the VUMON formulation may place patients receiving higher than recommended doses of VUMON at risk for central nervous system depression.

Pregnancy: Pregnancy "Category D".

VUMON may cause fetal harm when administered to a pregnant woman. VUMON has been shown to be teratogenic and embryotoxic in laboratory animals. In pregnant rats intravenous administration of VUMON, 0.1–3 mg/kg (0.6–18 mg/m^2), every second day from day 6 to day 16 post coitum caused dose-related embryotoxicity and teratogenicity. Major anomalies included spinal and rib defects, deformed extremities, anophthalmia and celosomia.

There are no adequate and well-controlled studies in pregnant women. If VUMON is used during pregnancy, or if the patient becomes pregnant while receiving this drug, the patient should be apprised of the potential hazard to the fetus. Women of childbearing potential should be advised to avoid becoming pregnant during therapy with VUMON.

PRECAUTIONS

General: In all instances where the use of VUMON is considered for chemotherapy, the physician must evaluate the need and usefulness of the drug against the risk of adverse reactions. Most such adverse reactions are reversible if detected early. If severe reactions occur, the drug should be reduced in dosage or discontinued and appropriate corrective measures should be taken according to the clinical judgment of the physician. Reinstitution of VUMON therapy should be carried out with caution, and with adequate consideration of the further need for the drug and alertness as to possible recurrence of toxicity.

VUMON must be administered as an intravenous infusion. Care should be taken to ensure that the intravenous catheter or needle is in the proper position and functional prior to infusion. Improper administration of VUMON may result in extravasation causing local tissue necrosis and/or thrombophlebitis. In some instances, occlusion of central venous access devices has occurred during 24-hour infusion of VUMON at a concentration of 0.1 to 0.2 mg/mL. Frequent observation during these infusions is necessary to minimize this risk.[4,5]

Laboratory Tests: Periodic complete blood counts and assessments of renal and hepatic function should be done during the course of VUMON treatment. They should be performed prior to therapy and at clinically appropriate intervals during and after therapy. There should be at least one determination of hematologic status prior to therapy with VUMON.

Drug Interactions: In a study in which 34 different drugs were tested, therapeutically relevant concentrations of tolbutamide, sodium salicylate and sulfamethizole displaced protein-bound teniposide in fresh human serum to a small but significant extent. Because of the extremely high binding of teniposide to plasma proteins, these small decreases in binding could cause substantial increases in free drug levels in plasma which could result in potentiation of drug toxicity. Therefore, caution should be used in administering VUMON (teniposide injection) to patients receiving these other agents. There was no change in the plasma kinetics of teniposide when coadministered with methotrexate. However, the plasma clearance of methotrexate was slightly increased. An increase in intracellular levels of methotrexate was observed *in vitro* in the presence of teniposide.

Carcinogenesis, Mutagenesis, Impairment of Fertility: Children at SJCRH with ALL in remission who received maintenance therapy with VUMON at weekly or twice weekly doses (plus other chemotherapeutic agents), had a relative risk of developing secondary acute nonlymphocytic leukemia (ANLL) approximately 12 times that of patients treated according to other less intensive schedules.[6]

A short course of VUMON for remission-induction and/or consolidation therapy was not associated with an increased risk of secondary ANLL, but the number of patients assessed was small. The potential benefit from VUMON must be weighed on a case by case basis against the potential risk of the induction of a secondary leukemia. The carcinogenicity of teniposide has not been studied in laboratory animals. Compounds with similar mechanisms of action and mutagenicity profiles have been reported to be carcinogenic and teniposide should be considered a potential carcinogen in humans. Teniposide has been shown to be mutagenic in various bacterial and mammalian genetic toxicity tests. These include positive mutagenic effects in the Ames/Salmonella and *B. subtilis* bacterial mutagenicity assays. Teniposide caused gene mutations in both Chinese hamster ovary cells and mouse lymphoma cells and DNA damage as measured by alkaline elution in human lung carcinoma derived cell lines. In addition, teniposide induced aberrations in chromosome structure in primary cultures of human lymphocytes *in vitro* and in L5178y/TK +/− mouse lymphoma cells *in vitro*. Chromosome aberrations were observed *in vivo* in the embryonic tissue of pregnant Swiss albino mice treated with teniposide. Teniposide also caused a dose-related increase in sister chromatid exchanges in Chinese hamster ovary cells and it has been shown to be embryotoxic and teratogenic in rats receiving teniposide during organogenesis. Treatment of pregnant rats I.V. with doses between 1.0 and 3.0 mg/kg/day on alternate days from day 6 to 16 post coitum caused retardation of embryonic development, prenatal mortality and fetal abnormalities.

Pregnancy: Pregnancy "Category D". (See **WARNINGS.**)

Nursing Mothers: It is not known whether this drug is excreted in human milk. Because many drugs are excreted in human milk and because of the potential for serious adverse reactions in nursing infants, a decision should be made whether to discontinue nursing or to discontinue the drug, taking into account the importance of VUMON therapy to the mother.

Patients with Down's Syndrome: Patients with both Down's Syndrome and leukemia may be especially sensitive to myelosuppressive chemotherapy, therefore, initial dosing with VUMON should be reduced in these patients. It is suggested that the first course of VUMON should be given at half the usual dose. Subsequent courses may be administered at higher dosages depending on the degree of myelosuppression and mucositis encountered in earlier courses in an individual patient.

ADVERSE REACTIONS

The table below presents the incidences of adverse reactions derived from an analysis of data contained within literature reports of 7 studies involving 303 pediatric patients in which VUMON was administered by injection as a single agent in a variety of doses and schedules for a variety of hematologic malignancies and solid tumors. The total number of patients evaluable for a given event was not 303 since the individual studies did not address the occurrence of each event listed. Five of these seven studies assessed VUMON activity in hematologic malignancies, such as leukemia. Thus, many of these patients had abnormal hematologic status at start of therapy with VUMON and were expected to develop significant myelosuppression as an endpoint of treatment.

[See table above]

Single-Agent VUMON
Summary of Toxicity for All Evaluable Pediatric Patients

Toxicity	Incidence in Evaluable Patients (%)
Hematologic Toxicity	
Myelosuppression, nonspecified	75
Leukopenia (< 3,000 WBC/µL)	89
Neutropenia (<2,000 ANC/µL)	95
Thrombocytopenia (< 100,000 plt/µL)	85
Anemia	88
Non-Hematologic Toxicity	
Mucositis	76
Diarrhea	33
Nausea/vomiting	29
Infection	12
Alopecia	9
Bleeding	5
Hypersensitivity reactions	5
Rash	3
Fever	3
Hypotension/Cardiovascular	2
Neurotoxicity	<1
Hepatic dysfunction	<1
Renal dysfunciton	<1
Metabolic abnormalities	<1

Hematologic Toxicity: VUMON, when used with other chemotherapeutic agents for the treatment of ALL, results in severe myelosuppression. Early onset of profound myelosuppression with delayed recovery can be expected when using the doses and schedules of VUMON necessary for treatment of refractory ALL, since bone marrow hypoplasia is a desired endpoint of therapy. The occurrence of acute nonlymphocytic leukemia (ANLL), with or without a preleukemic phase, has been reported in patients treated with VUMON in combination with other antineoplastic agents. See **PRECAUTIONS, Carcinogenesis, Mutagenesis, Impairment of Fertility.**

Gastrointestinal Toxicity: Nausea and vomiting are the most common gastrointestinal toxicities, having occurred in 29 percent of evaluable pediatric patients. The severity of this nausea and vomiting is generally mild to moderate.

Hypotension: Transient hypotension following rapid intravenous administration has been reported in 2 percent of evaluable pediatric patients. One episode of sudden death, attributed to probable arrhythmia and intractable hypotension, has been reported in an elderly patient receiving VUMON combination therapy for a non-leukemic malignancy. No other cardiac toxicity or electrocardiographic changes have been documented. No delayed hypotension has been noted.

Allergic Reactions: Hypersensitivity reactions characterized by chills, fever, tachycardia, flushing, bronchospasm, dyspnea, and blood pressure changes (hypertension or hypotension) have been reported to occur in approximately 5 percent of evaluable pediatric patients receiving intravenous VUMON. The incidence of hypersensitivity reactions to VUMON appears to be increased in patients with brain tumors, and in patients with neuroblastoma.[1]

Central Nervous System: Acute central nervous system depression and hypotension have been observed in patients receiving investigational infusions of high-dose VUMON (teniposide injection) who were pretreated with antiemetic drugs. The depressant effects of the antiemetic agents and the alcohol content of the VUMON formulation may place patients receiving higher than recommended doses of VUMON at risk for central nervous system depression.

Alopecia: Alopecia, sometimes progressing to total baldness, was observed in 9 percent of evaluable pediatric patients who received VUMON as single agent therapy. It was usually reversible.

OVERDOSAGE

There is no known antidote for VUMON overdosage. The anticipated complications of overdosage are secondary to bone marrow suppression. Treatment should consist of supportive care including blood products and antibiotics as indicated.

DOSAGE AND ADMINISTRATION

NOTE: Contact of undiluted VUMON with plastic equipment or devices used to prepare solutions for infusion may result in softening or cracking and possible drug product leakage. This effect has *not* been reported with *diluted solutions* of VUMON.

In order to prevent extraction of the plasticizer DEHP [di(2-ethylhexyl)phtalate], solutions of VUMON should be prepared in non-DEHP containing LVP containers such as glass or polyolefin plastic bags or containers.

Continued on next page

Vumon—Cont.

VUMON solutions should be administered with non-DEHP containing I.V. administration sets.
In one study, childhood ALL patients failing induction therapy with a cytarabine-containing regimen were treated with the combination of VUMON 165 mg/m^2 and cytarabine 300 mg/m^2 intravenously, twice weekly for 8–9 doses. In another study, patients with childhood ALL refractory to vincristine/prednisone-containing regimens were treated with the combination of VUMON 250 mg/m^2 and vincristine 1.5 mg/m^2 intravenously, weekly for 4–8 weeks and prednisone 40 mg/m^2 orally × 28 days.
Adequate data in patients with hepatic insufficiency and/or renal insufficiency are lacking, but dose adjustments may be necessary for patients with significant renal or hepatic impairment.

Preparation and Administration Precautions: VUMON is a cytotoxic anticancer drug and as with other potentially toxic compounds, caution should be exercised in handling and preparing the solution of VUMON. Skin reactions associated with accidental exposure to VUMON may occur. The use of gloves is recommended. If VUMON solution contacts the skin, immediately wash the skin thoroughly with soap and water. If VUMON contacts mucous membranes, the membranes should be flushed thoroughly with water.

Preparation for Intravenous Administration: VUMON must be diluted with either 5 percent Dextrose Injection, USP or 0.9 percent Sodium Chloride Injection, USP, to give final teniposide concentrations of 0.1 mg/mL, 0.2 mg/mL, 0.4 mg/mL or 1.0 mg/mL. Solutions prepared in 5 percent Dextrose Injection, USP or 0.9 percent Sodium Chloride Injection, USP at teniposide concentrations of 0.1 mg/mL, 0.2 mg/mL or 0.4 mg/mL are stable at room temperature for up to 24 hours after preparation. VUMON solutions prepared at a final teniposide concentration of 1.0 mg/mL should be administered within 4 hours of preparation to reduce the potential for precipitation. **Refrigeration of VUMON solutions is not recommended.** Stability and use times are identical in glass and plastic parenteral solution containers.
Although solutions are chemically stable under the conditions indicated, precipitation of teniposide may occur at the recommended concentrations, especially if the diluted solution is subjected to more agitation than is recommended to prepare the drug solution for parenteral administration.[7] In addition, storage time prior to administration should be minimized and care should be taken to avoid contact of the diluted solution with other drugs or fluids. Parenteral drug products should be inspected visually for particulate matter and discoloration prior to administration whenever solution and container permit. **Precipitation has been reported during 24-hour infusions of VUMON diluted to teniposide concentrations of 0.1 to 0.2 mg/mL, resulting in occlusion of central venous access catheters in several patients.[4,5] Heparin solution can cause precipitation of teniposide, therefore, the administration apparatus should be flushed thoroughly with 5 percent Dextrose Injection or 0.9 percent Sodium Chloride Injection, USP before and after administration of VUMON.[5]**
Hypotension has been reported following rapid intravenous administration; it is recommended that the VUMON solution be administered over at least a 30 to 60-minute period. **VUMON should not be given by rapid intravenous injection.**
In a 24-hour study under simulated conditions of actual use of the product relative to dilution strength, diluent and administration rates, dilutions at 0.1 to 1.0 mg/mL were chemically stable for at least 24 hours. Data collected for the presence of the extractable DEHP [di(2-ethylhexyl)phtalate] from PVC containers show that levels increased with time and concentration of the solutions. The data appeared similar for 0.9 percent Sodium Chloride Injection, USP, and 5 percent Dextrose Injection, USP. Consequently, the use of PVC containers is not recommended.
Similarly, the use of non-DEHP I.V. administration sets is recommended. Lipid administration sets or low DEHP containing nitroglycerin sets will keep patients' exposure to DEHP at low levels and are suitable for use. The diluted solutions are chemically and physically compatible with the recommended I.V. administration sets and LVP containers for up to 24 hours at ambient room temperature and lighting conditions. **Because of the potential for precipitation, compatibility with other drugs, infusion materials or I.V. pumps cannot be assured.**

Stability: Unopened ampules of VUMON are stable until the date indicated on the package when stored under refrigeration (2°–8°C) in the original package. Freezing does not adversely affect the product.

HOW SUPPLIED

VUMON® (teniposide injection)

NDC 0015-3075-19
50 mg/5 mL sterile clear, colorless glass ampules individually packaged in a carton.

NDC 0015-3075-97
50 mg/5 mL sterile clear, colorless glass ampules individually nested in a carton tray of 10 ampules per tray.

Storage: Store the unopened ampules under refrigeration (2°–8°C). Retain in original package to protect from light.

Handling and Disposal: Procedures for proper handling and disposal of anticancer drugs should be considered. Several guidelines on this subject have been published.[8–14] There is no general agreement that all of the procedures recommended in the guidelines are necessary or appropriate.

REFERENCES

1. O'Dwyer PJ, et al: Hypersensitivity Reactions to Teniposide (VM-26): An Analysis. *J Clin Oncol* 1986; 4(8):1262–1269.
2. Lorenz W, et al: Histamine Release in Dogs by Cremophor® EL and Its Derivatives. *Agents and Actions* 1977; 7(1):63–67.
3. Lassus M, et al: Allergic Reactions Associated with Cremophor Containing Antineoplastics. *Proc Am Soc Clin Oncol* 1985; 4:268 (Abstract C-1042).
4. Strong D, Morris L: Precipitation of Teniposide During Infusion. *Am J Hosp Pharm*; Mar 1990; Letter, 47:512,518.
5. Bogardus J, et al: Precipitation of Teniposide During Infusion. *Am J Hosp Pharm*; Mar 1990; Letter, 47:518–519.
6. Pui C-H, et al: Acute Myeloid Leukemia in Children Treated with Epipodophyllotoxins for Acute Lymphoblastic Leukemia. *N Engl J Med* 1991; 325: 1682–1687.
7. Deardoff D, Schmidt C: Mixing Additives in Plastic LVPs. *Am J Hosp Pharm*; Dec 1980; Letter, 37:1610,1613.
8. Recommendations for the Safe Handling of Parenteral Antineoplastic Drugs. NIH Publication No. 83–2621. For sale by the Superintendent of Documents, US Government Printing Office, Washington, DC 20402.
9. AMA Council Report. Guidelines for Handling Parenteral Antineoplastics. *JAMA* 1985; 253(11):1590–1592.
10. National Study Commission on Cytotoxic Exposure—Recommendations for Handling Cytotoxic Agents. Available from Louis P. Jeffrey, Chairman, National Study Commission on Cytotoxic Exposure, Massachusetts College of Pharmacy and Allied Health Sciences, 179 Longwood Avenue, Boston, Massachusetts 02115.
11. Clinical Oncological Society of Australia. Guidelines and Recommendations for Safe Handling of Antineoplastic Agents. *Med J Australia* 1983; 1:426–428.
12. Jones RB, et al: Safe Handling of Chemotherapeutic Agents: A Report from the Mount Sinai Medical Center. *CA-A Cancer Journal for Clinicians* 1983; (Sept/Oct) 258–263.
13. American Society of Hospital Pharmacists Technical Assistance Bulletin on Handling Cytotoxic Drugs in Hospitals. *Am J Hosp Pharm* 1990; 47:1033–1049.
14. Controlling Occupational Exposure to Hazardous Drugs (OSHA WORK PRACTICE GUIDELINES). *Am J Health-Syst Pharm* 1996;53:1669–1685.

U.S. Patent No. 3,524,844

BRISTOL LABORATORIES®
ONCOLOGY PRODUCTS
A Bristol-Myers Squibb Company
Princeton, NJ 08543
U.S.A.
Made in Italy

K7-B001-2-00 1050966A1
Issued October 1998

ZERIT® ℞
(stavudine)
[*zə 'rĭt*]

ZERIT® Capsules
(stavudine)

ZERIT® for Oral Solution
(stavudine)
Rx ONLY

> WARNING
> **LACTIC ACIDOSIS AND SEVERE HEPATOMEGALY WITH STEATOSIS, INCLUDING FATAL CASES, HAVE BEEN REPORTED WITH THE USE OF NUCLEOSIDE ANALOGUES ALONE OR IN COMBINATION, INCLUDING STAVUDINE AND OTHER ANTIRETROVIRALS (SEE WARNINGS).**

DESCRIPTION

ZERIT® is the brand name for stavudine (d4T), a synthetic thymidine nucleoside analogue, active against the Human Immunodeficiency Virus (HIV).
ZERIT (stavudine) Capsules are supplied for oral administration in strengths of 15, 20, 30, and 40 mg of stavudine. Each capsule also contains inactive ingredients microcrystalline cellulose, sodium starch glycolate, lactose, and magnesium stearate. The hard gelatin shell consists of gelatin, silicon dioxide, sodium lauryl sulfate, titanium dioxide, and iron oxides.
ZERIT (stavudine) for Oral Solution is supplied as a dye-free, fruit-flavored powder in bottles with child-resistant closures providing 200 mL of a 1 mg/mL stavudine solution upon constitution with water per label instructions. The powder for oral solution contains the following inactive ingredients: methylparaben, propylparaben, sodium carboxymethylcellulose, sucrose, and antifoaming and flavoring agents.
The chemical name for stavudine is 2′,3′-didehydro-3′-deoxythymidine. Stavudine has the following structural formula:

Stavudine is a white to off-white crystalline solid with the molecular formula $C_{10}H_{12}N_2O_4$ and a molecular weight of 224.2. The solubility of stavudine at 23°C is approximately 83 mg/mL in water and 30 mg/mL in propylene glycol. The n-octanol/water partition coefficient of stavudine at 23°C is 0.144.

MICROBIOLOGY

Mechanism of Action: Stavudine, a nucleoside analogue of thymidine, inhibits the replication of HIV in human cells *in vitro*. Stavudine is phosphorylated by cellular kinases to the active metabolite stavudine triphosphate. Stavudine triphosphate inhibits the activity of HIV reverse transcriptase both by competing with the natural substrate deoxythymidine triphosphate (K_i=0.0083 to 0.032 μM), and by its incorporation into viral DNA causing a termination of DNA chain elongation because stavudine lacks the essential 3′-OH group. Stavudine triphosphate inhibits cellular DNA polymerase beta and gamma, and markedly reduces the synthesis of mitochondrial DNA.

***In Vitro* HIV Susceptibility:** The *in vitro* antiviral activity of stavudine was measured in peripheral blood mononuclear cells, monocytic cells, and lymphoblastoid cell lines. The concentration of drug necessary to inhibit viral replication by 50% (ED_{50}) ranged from 0.009 to 4 mM against laboratory and clinical isolates of HIV-1. Stavudine had additive and synergistic activity in combination with didanosine and zalcitabine, respectively, *in vitro*. Stavudine combined with zidovudine had additive or antagonistic activity *in vitro* depending upon the molar ratios of the agents tested. The relationship between *in vitro* susceptibility of HIV to stavudine and the inhibition of HIV replication in humans has not been established.

Drug Resistance: HIV isolates with reduced susceptibility to stavudine have been selected *in vitro* and were also obtained from patients treated with stavudine. Phenotypic analysis of HIV isolates from stavudine-treated patients revealed, in 3 of 20 paired isolates, a 4- to 12-fold decrease in susceptibility to stavudine *in vitro*. The genetic basis for these susceptibility changes has not been identified. The clinical relevance of changes in stavudine suceptibility has not been established.

Cross-resistance: Five of 11 stavudine post-treatment isolates developed moderate resistance to zidovudine (9- to 176-fold) and 3 of those 11 isolates developed moderate resistance to didanosine (7- to 29-fold). The clinical relevance of these findings is unknown.

CLINICAL PHARMACOLOGY

Pharmacokinetics in Adults: The pharmacokinetics of stavudine have been evaluated in HIV-infected adult and pediatric patients (Table 1). Peak plasma concentrations (C_{max}) and area under the plasma concentration-time curve (AUC) increased in proportion to dose after both single and multiple doses ranging from 0.03 to 4 mg/kg. There was no significant accumulation of stavudine with repeated administration every 6, 8, or 12 hours.

Absorption—Following oral administration, stavudine is rapidly absorbed, with peak plasma concentrations occurring within 1 hour after dosing. The systemic exposure to stavudine is the same following administration as capsules or solution.

Distribution—Binding of stavudine to serum proteins was negligible over the concentration range of 0.01 to 11.4 μg/mL. Stavudine distributes equally between red blood cells and plasma.

Metabolism—The metabolic fate of stavudine has not been elucidated in humans.

Excretion—Renal elimination accounted for about 40% of the overall clearance regardless of the route of administration. The mean renal clearance was about twice the average endogenous creatinine clearance, indicating active tubular secretion in addition to glomerular filtration.

[See table 1 at top of next page]

Special Populations:

Pediatric—For pharmacokinetic properties of stavudine in pediatric patients, see Table 1.

Renal Insufficiency—Data from two studies indicated that the apparent oral clearance of stavudine decreased and the terminal elimination half-life increased as creatinine clearance decreased (see Table 2). C_{max} and T_{max} were not significantly altered by renal insufficiency. The mean ± SD hemodialysis clearance value of stavudine was 120 ± 18 mL/min (n=12); the mean ± SD percentage of the stavudine dose recovered in the dailysate, timed to occur between 2–6 hours post-dose, was 31 ± 5%. Based on these observations, it is recommended that ZERIT (stavudine) dosage be modified in patients with reduced creatinine clearance and in patients receiving maintenance hemodialysis (see **DOSAGE AND ADMINISTRATION** section).

[See table 2 at top of next page]

Hepatic Insufficiency—Stavudine pharmacokinetics were not altered in 5 non-HIV-infected patients with hepatic impairment secondary to cirrhosis (Child-Pugh classification B or C) following the administration of a single 40 mg dose.

Geriatric—Stavudine pharmacokinetics have not been studied in patients >65 years of age.
Gender—A population pharmacokinetic analysis of stavudine concentrations collected during a controlled clinical study in HIV-infected patients showed no clinically important differences between males (n=291) and females (n=27).
Race—A population pharmacokinetic analysis of stavudine concentrations collected during a controlled clinical study in HIV-infected patients (233 Caucasian, 39 African American, 41 Hispanic, 1 Asian, and 4 Other). The results of this analysis showed no clinically important differences associated with race.
Drug Interactions—Drug interaction studies have demonstrated that there are no clinically significant interactions between stavudine and the following: didanosine, lamivudine, or nelfinavir.
Zidovudine may competitively inhibit the intracellular phosphorylation of stavudine. Therefore, use of zidovudine in combination with ZERIT is not recommended.

INDICATIONS AND USAGE

ZERIT, in combination with other antiretroviral agents, is indicated for the treatment of HIV-1 infection (see CLINICAL STUDIES).

CLINICAL STUDIES

Combination Therapy: The combination use of ZERIT is based on the results of clinical studies in HIV-infected patients in double- and triple-combination regimens with other antiretroviral agents.
One of these studies (START 1) was a multicenter, randomized, open-label study comparing ZERIT (40 mg BID) plus lamivudine plus indinavir to zidovudine plus lamivudine plus indinavir in 202 treatment-naive patients. Both regimens resulted in a similar magnitude or inhibition of HIV RNA levels and increases in CD4 cell counts through 48 weeks.
Monotherapy: The efficacy of ZERIT was demonstrated in a randomized, double-blind study (AI455–019, conducted 1992-1994) comparing ZERIT with zidovudine in 822 patients with a spectrum of HIV-related symptoms. The outcome in terms of progression of HIV disease and death was similar for both drugs.

CONTRAINDICATIONS

ZERIT is contraindicated in patients with clinically significant hypersensitivity to stavudine or to any of the components contained in the formulation.

WARNINGS

1. Lactic Acidosis/Severe Hepatomegaly with Steatosis: Lactic acidosis and severe hepatomegaly with steatosis, including fatal cases, have been reported with the use of nucleoside analogues alone or in combination, including stavudine and other antiretrovirals. A majority of these cases have been in women. Obesity and prolonged nucleoside exposure may be risk factors. Particular caution should be exercised when administering ZERIT to any patient with known risk factors for liver disease; however, cases have also been reported in patients with no known risk factors. Treatment with ZERIT should be suspended in any patient who develops clinical or laboratory findings suggestive of lactic acidosis or pronounced hepatotoxicity (which may include hepatomegaly and steatosis even in the absence of marked transaminase elevations).
2. Peripheral Neuropathy: Peripheral neuropathy, manifested by numbness, tingling, or pain in the hands or feet, has been reported in patients receiving ZERIT (stavudine) therapy. Peripheral neuropathy has occurred more frequently in patients with advanced HIV disease, a history of neuropathy, or concurrent neurotoxic drug therapy, including didanosine (see **ADVERSE REACTIONS**).

PRECAUTIONS

Information for Patients: Patients should be informed that an important toxicity of ZERIT is peripheral neuropathy. Patients should be aware that peripheral neuropathy is manifested by numbness, tingling, or pain in hands or feet, and that these symptoms should be reported to their physicians. Patients should be counseled that peripheral neuropathy occurs with greatest frequency in patients who have advanced HIV disease or a history of peripheral neuropathy, and that dose modification and/or discontinuation of ZERIT may be required if toxicity develops.
Caregivers of young children receiving ZERIT therapy should be instructed regarding detection and reporting of peripheral neuropathy.
Patients should be informed that when ZERIT is used in combination with other agents with similar toxicities, the incidence of adverse events may be higher than when ZERIT is used alone. These patients should be followed closely.
Patients should be informed that ZERIT is not a cure for HIV infection, and that they may continue to acquire illnesses associated with HIV infection, including opportunistic infections. Patients should be advised to remain under the care of a physician when using ZERIT. They should be advised that ZERIT therapy has not been shown to reduce the risk of transmission of HIV to others through sexual contact or blood contamination. Patients should be informed that the long-term effects of ZERIT are unknown at this time.
Patients should be informed that the Centers for Disease Control and Prevention (CDC) recommend that HIV-infected mothers not nurse newborn infants to reduce the risk of postnatal transmission of HIV infection.
Drug Interactions: Zidovudine may competitively inhibit the intracellular phosphorylation of stavudine. Therefore, use of zidovudine in combination with ZERIT is not recommended. (See **CLINICAL PHARMACOLOGY**.)

Table 1
Mean ±SD Pharmacokinetic Parameters of Stavudine in Adult and Pediatric HIV-infected Patients

Parameter	Adult Patients	n	Pediatric Patients	n
Oral bioavailability (F)	86.4 ± 18.2%	25	76.9 ± 31.7%	20
Volume of distribution[a] (VD)	58 ± 21 L	44	18.5 ± 9.2 L/m^2	21
Apparent oral volume of distribution[b] (VD/F)	66 ± 22 L	71	not determined	—
Ratio of CSF: plasma concentrations (as %)[c]	not determined	—	59 ± 35%	8
Total body clearance[a] (CL)	8.3 ± 2.3 mL/min/kg	44	247 ± 94 mL/min/m^2	21
Apparent oral clearance[b] (CL/F)	8.0 ± 2.6 mL/min/kg	113	333 ± 87 mL/min/m^2	20
Elimination half-life ($T_{1/2}$), I.V. dose[a]	1.15 ± 0.35 hr	44	1.11 ± 0.28 hr	21
Elimination half-life ($T_{1/2}$) oral dose[b]	1.44 ± 0.30 hr	115	0.96 ± 0.26 hr	20
Urinary recovery of stavudine (% of dose)	39 ± 23%	88	34 ± 16%	19

[a] following 1 hour I.V. infusion
[b] following single oral dose
[c] following multiple oral doses

Table 2
Mean ± SD Pharmacokinetic Parameter Values Single 40-mg Oral Dose of ZERIT

	Creatinine Clearance			
	>50 mL/min (n=10)	26–50 mL/min (n=5)	9–25 mL/min (n=5)	Hemodialysis Patients* (n=11)
CL_{cr}(mL/min)	104 ± 28	41 ± 5	17 ± 3	NA
CL/F (mL/min)	335 ± 57	191 ± 39	116 ± 25	105 ± 17
CL_R(mL/min)	167 ± 65	73 ± 18	17 ± 3	NA
$T_{1/2}$ (h)	1.7 ± 0.4	3.5 ± 2.5	4.6 ± 0.9	5.4 ± 1.4

CL_{cr} = creatinine clearance
CL/F = apparent oral clearance
CL_R = renal clearance
$T_{1/2}$ = terminal elimination half-life
NA = not applicable
*Determined while patients were off dialysis.

Carcinogenesis, Mutagenesis, Impairment of Fertility: In 2-year carcinogenicity studies in mice and rats, stavudine was noncarcinogenic at doses which produced exposures (AUC) 39 and 168 times, respectively, human exposure at the recommended clinical dose. Benign and malignant liver tumors in mice and rats and malignant urinary bladder tumors in male rats occurred at levels of exposure 250 (mice) and 732 (rats) times human exposure at the recommended clinical dose.
Stavudine was not mutagenic in the Ames, *E. coli* reverse mutation, or the CHO/HGPRT mammalian cell forward gene mutation assays, with and without metabolic activation. Stavudine produced positive results in the *in vitro* human lymphocyte clastogenesis and mouse fibroblast assays, and in the *in vivo* mouse micronucleus test. In the *in vitro* assays, stavudine elevated the frequency of chromosome aberrations in human lymphocytes (concentrations of 25 to 250 µg/mL, without metabolic activation) and increased the frequency of transformed foci in mouse fibroblast cells (concentrations of 25 to 2500 µg/mL, with and without metabolic activation). In the *in vivo* micronucleus assay, stavudine was clastogenic in bone marrow cells following oral stavudine administration to mice at dosages of 600 to 2000 mg/kg/day for 3 days.
No evidence of impaired fertility was seen in rats with exposures (based on C_{max}) up to 216 times that observed following a clinical dosage of 1 mg/kg/day.
Pregnancy: Pregnancy "Category C". Reproduction studies have been performed in rats and rabbits with exposures (based on C_{max}) up to 399 and 183 times, respectively, of that seen at a clinical dosage of 1 mg/kg/day and have revealed no evidence of teratogenicity. The incidence in fetuses of a common skeletal variation, unossified or incomplete ossification of sternebra, was increased in rats at 399 times human exposure, while no effect was observed at 216 times human exposure. A slight post-implantation loss was noted at 216 times the human exposure with no effect noted at approximately 135 times the human exposure. An increase in early rat neonatal mortality (birth to 4 days of age) occurred at 399 times the human exposure, while survival of neonates was unaffected at approximately 135 times the human exposure. A study in rats showed that stavudine is transferred to the fetus through the placenta. The concentration in fetal tissue was approximately one-half the concentration in maternal plasma. There are no adequate and well-controlled studies in pregnant women. Because animal reproduction studies are not always predictive of human response, stavudine should be used during pregnancy only if clearly needed.
Antiretrovial Pregnancy Registry: To monitor maternal-fetal outcomes of pregnant women exposed to stavudine and other antiretroviral agents, an Antiretroviral Pregnancy Registry has been established. Physicians are encouraged to register patients by calling (800) 258-4263.
Nursing Mothers: Studies in lactating rats demonstrated that stavudine is excreted in milk. Although it is not known whether stavudine is excreted in human milk, there exists the potential for adverse effects from stavudine in nursing infants. Mothers should be instructed to discontinue nursing if they are receiving stavudine. This instruction is consistent with the Centers for Disease Control recommendation that HIV-infected mothers not breast-feed their infants to avoid risking postnatal transmission of HIV infection.
Pediatric Use: Use of stavudine in pediatric patients is supported by evidence from adequate and well-controlled studies of stavudine in adults with additional pharmacokinetic and safety data in pediatric patients.
Adverse events that were reported to occur in 105 pediatric patients receiving ZERIT 2 mg/kg/day for a median of 6.4 months in study ACTG 240 were generally similar to those reported in adults.
Stavudine pharmacokinetics have been evaluated in 25 HIV-infected pediatric patients ranging in age from 5 weeks to 15 years and in weight from 2 to 43 kg after I.V. or oral administration of single doses and BID regimens (see **CLINICAL PHARMACOLOGY**, Table 1).

ADVERSE REACTIONS

Adults: ZERIT therapy has been associated with peripheral neuropathy, which can be severe, is dose related, and occurs more frequently in patients being treated with neurotoxic drug therapy, including didanosine, in patients with advanced HIV infection, or in patients who have previously experienced peripheral neuropathy.
Patients should be monitored for the development of neuropathy, which is usually manifested by numbness, tingling, or pain in the feet or hands. Stavudine-related peripheral neuropathy may resolve if therapy is withdrawn promptly. In some cases, symptoms may worsen temporarily following discontinuation of therapy. If symptoms resolve completely, patients may tolerate resumption of treatment at one-half the dose (see **DOSAGE AND ADMINISTRATION**). If neuropathy recurs after resumption of ZERIT, permanent discontinuation of ZERIT should be considered.
When ZERIT is used in combination with other agents with similar toxicities, the incidence of adverse events may be higher than when ZERIT is used alone. Patients treated with ZERIT in combination with didanosine may be at increased risk for adverse events such as pancreatitis, peripheral neuropathy, and liver function abnormalities. (See **WARNINGS** and **PRECAUTIONS**).

Continued on next page

Zerit—Cont.

Selected clinical adverse events that occurred in adult patients receiving ZERIT (stavudine) in a controlled monotherapy trial (Study AI455-019) are provided in Table 3.

Table 3
Selected Clinical Adverse Events in Study AI455-019[a] (Monotherapy)

Adverse Events	Percent (%)	
	ZERIT (40 mg BID) (n=412)	zidovudine (200 mg TID) (n=402)
Headache	54	49
Diarrhea	50	44
Peripheral Neurologic Symptoms/Neuropathy	52	39
Rash	40	35
Nausea and Vomiting	39	44

[a] Median duration of stavudine therapy = 79 weeks; median duration of zidovudine therapy = 53 weeks.

Pancreatitis was observed in three of the 412 adult patients who received ZERIT in a controlled monotherapy study.
Selected clinical adverse events that occurred in antiretroviral naive adult patients receiving ZERIT from two controlled combination studies are provided in Table 4.
[See table 4 above]
Pancreatitis resulting in death was observed in one patient who received ZERIT plus didanosine plus indinavir in the START 2 study.
Selected laboratory abnormalities reported in a controlled monotherapy study (Study AI455-019) are provided in Table 5.

Table 5
Selected Adult Laboratory Abnormalities in Study AI455-019[a,b]

Parameter	Percent (%)	
	ZERIT (40 mg BID) (n=412)	zidovudine (200 mg TID) (n=402)
AST (SGOT) (>5.0 × ULN)	11	10
ALT (SGPT) (>5.0 × ULN)	13	11
Amylase (≥1.4 × ULN)	14	13

[a] Data presented for patients for whom laboratory evaluations were performed.
[b] Median duration of stavudine therapy = 79 weeks; median duration of zidovudine therapy = 53 weeks.
ULN = upper limit of normal.

Selected laboratory abnormalities reported in two controlled combination studies are provided in Tables 6 and 7.
[See table 6 above]
[See table 7 above]

Observed During Clinical Practice: The following events have been identified during post-approval use of ZERIT (stavudine). Because they are reported voluntarily from a population of unknown size, estimates of frequency cannot be made. These events have been chosen for inclusion due to their seriousness, frequency of reporting, causal connection to ZERIT, or a combination of these factors.
Body as a Whole—abdominal pain, allergic reaction, and chills/fever.
Digestive Disorders—anorexia.
Hematologic Disorders—anemia, leukopenia, and thrombocytopenia.
Liver—lactic acidosis and hepatic steatosis (see **WARNINGS**), hepatitis and liver failure.
Musculoskeletal—myalgia.
Nervous—insomnia.
Pediatric Patients: Adverse reactions and serious laboratory abnormalities in pediatric patients were similar in type and frequency to those seen in adult patients.

OVERDOSAGE

Experience with adults treated with 12 to 24 times the recommended daily dosage revealed no acute toxicity. Complications of chronic overdosage include peripheral neuropathy and hepatic toxicity. Stavudine can be removed by hemodialysis; the mean ± SD hemodialysis clearance of stavudine is 120 ± 18 mL/min. Whether stavudine is eliminated by peritoneal dialysis has not been studied.

DOSAGE AND ADMINISTRATION

The interval between doses of ZERIT should be 12 hours. ZERIT may be taken without regard to meals.
Adults: The recommended dose based on body weight is as follows:

40 mg twice daily for patients ≥60 kg.
30 mg twice daily for patients <60 kg.

Table 4
Selected Clinical Adverse Events in START 1 and START 2[a] Studies (Combination Therapy)

Adverse Events	Percent (%)			
	START 1		START 2	
	ZERIT+ lamivudine+ indinavir (n=100[b])	zidovudine+ lamivudine+ indinavir (n=102)	ZERIT+ didanosine+ indinavir (n=102[b])	zidovudine+ lamivudine+ indinavir (n=103)
Nausea	43	63	53	67
Diarrhea	34	16	45	39
Headache	25	26	46	37
Rash	18	13	30	18
Vomiting	18	33	30	35
Peripheral Neurologic Symptoms/Neuropathy	8	7	21	10

[a] START 2 compared two triple-combination regimens in 205 treatment-naive patients. Patients received either ZERIT (40 mg BID) plus didanosine plus indinavir or zidovudine plus lamivudine plus indinavir.
[b] Duration of stavudine therapy = 48 weeks.

Table 6
Selected Laboratory Abnormalities in START 1 and START 2 Studies (Grades 3–4)

Parameter	Percent of Patients			
	START 1		START 2	
	ZERIT+ lamivudine+ indinavir (n=100)	zidovudine+ lamivudine+ indinavir (n=102)	ZERIT+ didanosine+ indinavir (n=102)	zidovudine+ lamivudine+ indinavir (n=103)
Bilirubin (> 2.6 × ULN)	7	6	16	8
SGOT (AST) (>5 × ULN)	5	2	7	7
SGPT (ALT) (>5 × ULN)	6	2	8	5
GGT (>5 × ULN)	2	2	5	2
Lipase (>2 × ULN)	6	3	5	5
Amylase (>2 × ULN)	4	<1	8	2

ULN = upper limit of normal.

Table 7
Selected Laboratory Abnormalities in START 1 and START 2 Studies (All Grades)

Parameter	Percent (%)			
	START 1		START 2	
	ZERIT+ lamivudine+ indinavir (n=100)	zidovudine+ lamivudine+ indinavir (n=102)	ZERIT+ didanosine+ indinavir (n=102)	zidovudine+ lamivudine+ indinavir (n=103)
Total Bilirubin	65	60	68	55
SGOT (AST)	42	20	53	20
SGPT (ALT)	40	20	50	18
GGT	15	8	28	12
Lipase	27	12	26	19
Amylase	21	19	31	17

Table 9

Product Strength	Capsule Shell Color	Markings on Capsule (in Black Ink)	Capsules per Bottle	NDC No.
15 mg	Light yellow & dark red	BMS 1964 15	60	0003-1964-01
20 mg	Light brown	BMS 1965 20	60	0003-1965-01
30 mg	Light orange & dark orange	BMS 1966 30	60	0003-1966-01
40 mg	Dark orange	BMS 1967 40	60	0003-1967-01

Pediatrics: The recommended dose for pediatric patients weighing less than 30 kg is 1 mg/kg/dose, given every 12 hours. Pediatric patients weighing 30 kg or greater should receive the recommended adult dosage.
Dosage Adjustment: Patients should be monitored for the development of peripheral neuropathy, which is usually manifested by numbness, tingling, or pain in the feet or hands. These symptoms may be difficult to detect in young children (see **WARNINGS**). If these symptoms develop during treatment, stavudine therapy should be interrupted. Symptoms may resolve if therapy is withdrawn promptly. In some cases, symptoms may worsen temporarily following discontinuation of therapy. If symptoms resolve completely, patients may tolerate resumption of treatment at one-half the recommended dose.

20 mg twice daily for patients ≥60 kg.
15 mg twice daily for patients <60 kg.

If neuropathy recurs after resumption of ZERIT, permanent discontinuation of ZERIT should be considered.
Renal Impairment—ZERIT may be administered to adult patients with impaired renal function with adjustment in dose as shown in Table 8.

Table 8
Recommended Dosage Adjustment for Renal Impairment

Creatinine Clearance (mL/min)	Recommended ZERIT Dose by Patient Weight	
	≥60 kg	<60 kg
>50	40 mg every 12 hours	30 mg every 12 hours
26–50	20 mg every 12 hours	15 mg every 12 hours
10–25	20 mg every 24 hours	15 mg every 24 hours

Since urinary excretion is also a major route of elimination of stavudine in pediatric patients, the clearance of stavudine may be altered in children with renal impairment. Although there are insufficient data to recommend a specific dose adjustment of ZERIT in this patient population, a reduction in the dose and/or an increase in the interval between doses should be considered.

Hemodialysis Patients—The recommended dose is 20 mg every 24 hours (≥60 kg) or 15 mg every 24 hours (<60 kg), administered after the completion of hemodialysis and at the same time of day on non-dialysis days.

Method of Preparation:

ZERIT (stavudine) for Oral Solution

Prior to dispensing, the pharmacist must constitute the dry powder with purified water to a concentration of 1 mg stavudine per mL of solution, as follows:

1. Add 202 mL of purified water to the container.
2. Shake container vigorously until the powder dissolves completely. Constitution in this way produces 200 mL (deliverable volume) of 1 mg/mL stavudine solution. The solution may appear slightly hazy.
3. Dispense solution in original container with measuring cup provided. Instruct patient to shake the container vigorously prior to measuring each dose and to store the tightly closed container in a refrigerator, 36° to 46°F (2° to 8°C). Discard any unused portion after 30 days.

HOW SUPPLIED

ZERIT® (stavudine) Capsules are available in the following strengths and configurations of plastic bottles with child-resistant closures:

[See table 9 on previous page]

ZERIT® (stavudine) for Oral Solution is a dye-free, fruit-flavored powder that provides 1 mg of stavudine per mL of solution upon constitution with water. Directions for solution preparation are included on the product label and in the **DOSAGE AND ADMINISTRATION** section of this insert. ZERIT for Oral Solution (NDC No. 0003-1968-01) is available in child-resistant containers that provide 200 mL of solution after constitution with water.

US Patent No.: 4,978,655

Storage: ZERIT Capsules should be stored in tightly closed containers at controlled room temperature, 59° to 86°F (15° to 30°C).

ZERIT (stavudine) for Oral Solution should be protected from excessive moisture and stored in tightly closed containers at controlled room temperature, 59° to 86°F (15° to 30°C). After constitution, store tightly closed containers of ZERIT for Oral Solution in a refrigerator, 36° to 46°F (2° to 8°C). Discard any unused portion after 30 days.

BRISTOL-MYERS SQUIBB
IMMUNOLOGY
Bristol-Myers Squibb Company
Princeton, NJ 08543
U.S.A.

F9-B001-8-99 1017718A4

Revised August 1999

Shown in Product Identification Guide, page 310

BTG Pharmaceuticals

70 WOOD AVENUE SOUTH
ISELIN, NJ 08830

For Medical Information or Emergencies Contact:
(800) 741-2698

For Customer Service and Ordering:
(800) 741-2698
FAX: (800) 741-2696

DELATESTRYL® Ⓒℝ

Testosterone Enanthate
Injection USP
in UNIMATIC® Single Dose Syringes
and Multiple Dose Vials

CAUTION: Federal law prohibits dispensing without prescription.

DESCRIPTION

DELATESTRYL (Testosterone Enanthate Injection) provides testosterone enanthate, a derivative of the primary endogenous androgen testosterone, for intramuscular administration. In their active form, androgens have a 17-beta-hydroxy group. Esterification of the 17-beta-hyroxy group increases the duration of action of testosterone; hydrolysis to free testosterone occurs *in vivo.* Each mL of sterile, colorless to pale yellow solution provides 200 mg testosterone enanthate in sesame oil with 5 mg chlorobutanol (chloral derivative) as a preservative.

Testosterone enanthate is designated chemically as androst-4-en-3-one, 17-[(1-oxoheptyl)-oxy]-, (17β)-. Structural formula:

$OCO(CH_2)_5CH_3$ CH_3 H CH_3 H H O

$C_{26}H_{40}O_3$ MW 400.60

CLINICAL PHARMACOLOGY

Endogenous androgens are responsible for the normal growth and development of the male sex organs and for maintenance of secondary sex characteristics. These effects include growth and maturation of prostate, seminal vesicles, penis, and scrotum; development of male hair distribution, such as beard, pubic, chest, and axillary hair; laryngeal enlargement; vocal chord thickening; alterations in body musculature; and fat distribution.

Androgens also cause retention of nitrogen, sodium, potassium, and phosphorus, and decreased urinary excretion of calcium. Androgens have been reported to increase protein anabolism and decrease protein catabolism. Nitrogen balance is improved only when there is sufficient intake of calories and protein.

Androgens are responsible for the growth spurt of adolescence and for the eventual termination of linear growth which is brought about by fusion of the epiphyseal growth centers. In children, exogenous androgens accelerate linear growth rates but may cause a disproportionate advancement in bone maturation. Use over long periods may result in fusion of the epiphyseal growth centers and termination of growth process. Androgens have been reported to stimulate the production of red blood cells by enhancing the production of erythropoietic stimulating factor.

During exogenous administration of androgens, endogenous testosterone release is inhibited through feedback inhibition of pituitary luteinizing hormone (LH). At large doses of exogenous androgens, spermatogenesis may also be suppressed through feedback inhibition of pituitary follicle stimulating hormone (FSH).

There is a lack of substantial evidence that androgens are effective in fractures, surgery, convalescence, and functional uterine bleeding.

Pharmacokinetics

Testosterone esters are less polar than free testosterone. Testosterone esters in oil injected intramuscularly are absorbed slowly from the lipid phase; thus testosterone enanthate can be given at intervals of two to four weeks.

Testosterone in plasma is 98 percent bound to a specific testosterone-estradiol binding globulin, and about two percent is free. Generally, the amount of this sex-hormone binding globulin in the plasma will determine the distribution of testosterone between free and bound forms, and the free testosterone concentration will determine its half-life.

About 90 percent of a dose of testosterone is excreted in the urine as glucuronic and sulfuric acid conjugates of testosterone and its metabolites; about six percent of a dose is excreted in the feces, mostly in the unconjugated form. Inactivation of testosterone occurs primarily in the liver. Testosterone is metabolized to various 17-keto steroids through two different pathways. There are considerable variations of the half-life of testosterone as reported in the literature, ranging from 10 to 100 minutes.

In responsive tissues, the activity of testosterone appears to depend on reduction to dihydrotestosterone, which binds to cytosol receptor proteins. The steroid-receptor complex is transported to the nucleus where it initiates transcription events and cellular changes related to androgen action.

INDICATIONS AND USAGE

Males

DELATESTRYL (Testosterone Enanthate Injection) is indicated for replacement therapy in conditions associated with a deficiency or absence of endogenous testosterone.

Primary hypogonadism (congenital or acquired)—Testicular failure due to cryptorchidism, bilateral torsion, orchitis, vanishing testis syndrome, or orchidectomy.

Hypogonadotropic hypogonadism (congenital or acquired)—Idiopathic gonadotropin or luteinizing hormone-releasing hormone (LHRH) deficiency, or pituitary-hypothalamic injury from tumors, trauma, or radiation. (Appropriate adrenal cortical and thyroid hormone replacement therapy are still necessary, however, and are actually of primary importance.)

If the above conditions occur prior to puberty, androgen replacement therapy will be needed during the adolescent years for development of secondary sexual characteristics. Prolonged androgen treatment will be required to maintain sexual characteristics in these and other males who develop testosterone deficiency after puberty.

Delayed puberty—DELATESTRYL (Testosterone Enanthate Injection) may be used to stimulate puberty in carefully selected males with clearly delayed puberty. These patients usually have a familial pattern of delayed puberty that is not secondary to a pathological disorder; puberty is expected to occur spontaneously at a relatively late date. Brief treatment with conservative doses may occasionally be justified in these patients if they do not respond to psychological support. The potential adverse effect on bone maturation should be discussed with the patient and parents prior to androgen administration. An x-ray of the hand and wrist to determine bone age should be obtained every six months to assess the effect of treatment on the epiphyseal centers (see WARNINGS).

Females

Metastatic mammary cancer—DELATESTRYL (Testosterone Enanthate Injection) may be used secondarily in women with advancing inoperable metastatic (skeletal) mammary cancer who are one to five years postmenopausal. Primary goals of therapy in these women include ablation of the ovaries. Other methods of counteracting estrogen activity are adrenalectomy, hypophysectoy, and/or antiestrogen therapy. This treatment has also been used in premenopausal women with breast cancer who have benefited from oophorectomy and are considered to have a hormone-responsive tumor. Judgment concerning androgen therapy should be made by an oncologist with expertise in this field.

CONTRAINDICATIONS

Androgens are contraindicated in men with carcinomas of the breast or with known or suspected carcinomas of the prostate and in women who are or may become pregnant. When administered to pregnant women, androgens cause virilization of the external genitalia of the female fetus. This virilization includes clitoromegaly, abnormal vaginal development, and fusion of genital folds to form a scrotal-like structure. The degree of masculinization is related to the amount of drug given and the age of the fetus and is most likely to occur in the female fetus when the drugs are given in the first trimester. If the patient becomes pregnant while taking androgens, she should be apprised of the potential hazard to the fetus.

This preparation is also contraindicated in patients with a history of hypersensitivity to any of its components.

WARNINGS

In patients with breast cancer and in immobilized patients, androgen therapy may cause hypercalcemia by stimulating osteolysis. In patients with cancer, hypercalcemia may indicate progression of bony metastasis. If hypercalcemia occurs, the drug should be discontinued and appropriate measures instituted.

Prolonged use of high doses of androgens has been associated with the development of peliosis hepatis and hepatic neoplasms including hepatocellular carcinoma (see PRECAUTIONS, Carcinogenesis). Peliosis hepatis can be a life-threatening or fatal complication.

If cholestatic hepatitis with jaundice appears or if liver function tests become abnormal, the androgen should be discontinued and the etiology should be determined. Drug-induced jaundice is reversible when the medication is discontinued.

Geriatric patients treated with androgens may be at an increased risk for the development of prostatic hypertrophy and prostatic carcinoma.

Due to sodium and water retention, edema with or without congestive heart failure may be a serious complication in patients with preexisting cardiac, renal, or hepatic disease. In addition to discontinuation of the drug, diuretic therapy may be required. If the administration of testosterone enanthate is restarted, a lower dose should be used.

Gynecomastia frequently develops and occasionally persists in patients being treated for hypogonadism.

Androgen therapy should be used cautiously in healthy males with delayed puberty. The effect on bone maturation should be monitored by assessing bone age of the wrist and hand every six months. In children, androgen treatment may accelerate bone maturation without producing compensatory gain in linear growth. This adverse effect may result in compromised adult stature. The younger the child the greater the risk of compromising final mature height.

PRECAUTIONS

General

Women should be observed for signs of virilization (deepening of the voice, hirsutism, acne, clitoromegaly, and menstrual irregularities). Discontinuation of drug therapy at the time of evidence of mild virilism is necessary to prevent irreversible virilization. Such virilization is usual following androgen use at high doses and is not prevented by concomitant use of estrogens. A decision may be made by the patient and the physician that some virilization will be tolerated during treatment for breast carcinoma.

Because androgens may alter serum cholesterol concentration, caution should be used when administering these drugs to patients with a history of myocardial infarction or coronary artery disease. Serial determinations of serum cholesterol should be made and therapy adjusted accordingly. A causal relationship between myocardial infarction and hypercholesterolemia has not been established.

Information for Patients

Male adolescent patients receiving androgens for delayed puberty should have bone development checked every six months.

The physician should instruct patients to report any of the following side effects of androgens:

Adult or adolescent males—too frequent or persistent erections of the penis.

Women—hoarseness, acne, changes in menstrual periods, or more facial hair.

All patients—Any nausea, vomiting, changes in skin color, or ankle swelling.

Laboratory Tests

Women with disseminated breast carcinoma should have frequent determination of urine and serum calcium levels during the course of androgen therapy (see WARNINGS).

Periodic (every six months) X-ray examinations of bone age should be made during treatment of pre-pubertal males to determine the rate of bone maturation and the effects of androgen therapy on the epiphyseal centers.

Hemoglobin and hematocrit should be checked periodically for polycythemia in patients who are receiving high doses of androgens.

Continued on next page

Delatestryl—Cont.

Drug Interactions

When administering concurrently, the following drugs may interact with androgens:

Anticoagulants, oral—C-17 substituted derivatives of testosterone, such as methandrostenolone, have been reported to decrease the anticoagulant requirement. Patients receiving oral anticoagulant therapy require close monitoring especially when androgens are started or stopped.

Antidiabetic drugs and insulin—In diabetic patients, the metabolic effects of androgens may decrease blood glucose and insulin requirements.

ACTH and corticosteroids—Enhanced tendency toward edema. Use caution when giving these drugs together, especially in patients with hepatic or cardiac disease.

Oxyphenbutazone—Elevated serum levels of oxyphenbutazone may result.

Drug/Laboratory Test Interferences

Androgens may decrease levels of thyroxine-binding globulin, resulting in decreased total T_4 serum levels and increased resin uptake of T_3 and T_4. Free thyroid hormone levels remain unchanged, however, and there is no clinical evidence of thyroid dysfunction.

Carcinogenesis

Testosterone has been tested by subcutaneous injection and implantation in mice and rats. The implant induced cervical-uterine tumors in mice, which metastasized in some cases. There is suggestive evidence that injection of testosterone into some strains of female mice increases their susceptibility to hepatoma. Testosterone is also known to increase the number of tumors and decrease the degree of differentiation of chemically induced carcinomas of the liver in rats.

There are rare reports of hepatocellular carcinoma in patients receiving long-term therapy with androgens in high doses. Withdrawal of the drugs did not lead to regression of the tumors in all cases.

Geriatric patients treated with androgens may be at an increased risk for the development of prostatic hypertrophy and prostatic carcinoma.

Pregnancy: Teratogenic Effects

Category X (see CONTRAINDICATIONS).

Nursing Mothers

It is not known whether androgens are excreted in human milk. Because many drugs are excreted in human milk and because of the potential for serious adverse reactions in nursing infants from androgens, a decision should be made whether to discontinue nursing or to discontinue the drug, taking into account the importance of the drug to the mother.

Pediatric Use

Androgen therapy should be used very cautiously in pediatric patients and only by specialists who are aware of the adverse effects on bone maturation. Skeletal maturation must be monitored every six months by an X-ray of the hand and wrist (see INDICATIONS AND USAGE, and WARNINGS).

ADVERSE REACTIONS

Endocrine and Urogenital, Female—The most common side effects of androgen therapy are amenorrhea and other menstrual irregularities, inhibition of gonadotropin secretion, and virilization, including deepening of the voice and clitoral enlargement. The latter usually is not reversible after androgens are discontinued. When administered to a pregnant woman, androgens cause virilization of the external genitalia of the female fetus. *Male*—Gynecomastia, and excessive frequency and duration of penile erections. Oligospermia may occur at high dosages (see CLINICAL PHARMACOLOGY).

Skin and Appendages—Hirsutism, male pattern baldness, and acne.

Fluid and Electrolyte Disturbances—Retention of sodium, chloride, water, potassium, calcium (see WARNINGS), and inorganic phosphates.

Gastrointestinal—Nausea, cholestatic jaundice, alterations in liver function tests; rarely, hepatocellular neoplasms, peliosis hepatis (see WARNINGS).

Hematologic—Suppression of clotting factors II, V, VII, and X; bleeding in patients on concomitant anticoagulant therapy; polycythemia.

Nervous System—Increased or decreased libido, headache, anxiety, depression, and generalized paresthesia.

Metabolic—Increased serum cholesterol.

Miscellaneous—Rarely, anaphylactoid reactions; inflammation and pain at injection site.

DRUG ABUSE AND DEPENDENCE

DELATESTRYL is classified as a controlled substance under the Anabolic Steroids Control Act of 1990 and has been assigned to Schedule III.

OVERDOSAGE

There have been no reports of acute overdosage with androgens.

DOSAGE AND ADMINISTRATOIN

Dosage and duration of therapy with DELATESTRYL (Testosterone Enanthate Injection) will depend on age, sex, diagnosis, patient's response to treatment, and appearance of adverse effects. When properly given, injections of DELATESTRYL are well tolerated. Care should be taken to inject the preparation deeply into the gluteal muscle following the usual precautions for intramuscular administration. In general, total doses above 400 mg per month are not required because of the prolonged action of the preparation. Injections more frequently than every two weeks are rarely indicated. NOTE: Use of a wet needle or wet syringe may cause the solution to become cloudy; however, this does not affect the potency of the material. Parenteral drug products should be inspected visually for particulate matter and discoloration prior to administration, whenever solution and container permit. DELATESTRYL is a clear, colorless to pale yellow solution.

Male hypogonadism: As replacement therapy, i.e., for eunuchism, the suggested dosage is 50 to 400 mg every 2 to 4 weeks.

In males with delayed puberty: Various dosage regimens have been used; some call for lower dosages initially with gradual increases as puberty progresses, with or without a decrease in maintenance levels. Other regimens call for higher dosage to induce pubertal changes and lower dosage for maintenance after puberty. The chronological and skeletal ages must be taken into consideration, both in determining the initial dose and in adjusting the dose. Dosage is within the range of 50 to 200 mg every 2 to 4 weeks for a limited duration, for example, 4 to 6 months. X-rays should be taken at appropriate intervals to determine the amount of bone maturation and skeletal development (see INDICATIONS AND USAGE, and WARNINGS).

Palliation of inoperable mammary cancer in women: A dosage of 200 to 400 mg every 2 to 4 weeks is recommended. Women with metastatic breast carcinoma must be followed closely because androgen therapy occasionally appears to accelerate the disease.

HOW SUPPLIED

DELATESTRYL (Testosterone Enanthate Injection USP) is available in 1 mL (200 mg/mL) Unimatic single dose syringes (NDC 54396-328-16). Each syringe is supplied with a sterile disposable 20-gauge, $1^1/_2$-inch needle.

DELATESTRYL is also available in 5 mL (200 mg/mL) multiple dose vials (NDC 54396-328-40).

Storage

DELATESTRYL (Testosterone Enanthate Injection USP) should be stored at room temperature. Warming and rotating the syringe unit or vial between the palms of the hands will redissolve any crystals that may have formed during storage at low temperatures.

Directions for Use of **UNIMATIC®** *single dose syringe*

1) Screw the threaded tip of the plunger rod clockwise into the cartridge plunger and push forward a few millimeters to break any friction between the cartridge plunger and syringe barrel.

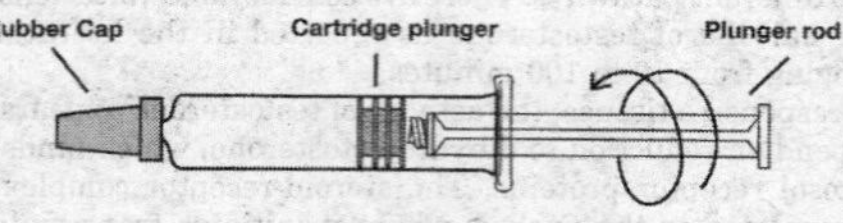

2) Holding syringe erect, aseptically remove the rubber cap from the tip of the syringe and attach the sterile, disposable needle using a push-twist action.

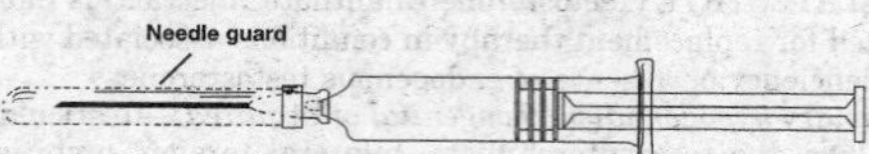

3) Remove the needle guard, hold the syringe erect, and push plunger forward until a drop appears at tip of needle and all of the air is evacuated. Following the usual aspiration procedure, complete the injection.

4) Destroy the needle and syringe immediately after use.

UNIMATIC is a registered trademark of E. R. Squibb & Sons, Inc.

Mfd. for: BTG Pharmaceuticals Corp., Iselin, NJ 08830
by: Bristol-Myers Squibb, Princeton, NJ 08543
Revised October 1995 J4-484D

Shown in Product Identification Guide, page 310

OXANDRIN® Ⓒ℞

(oxandrolone tablets, USP)

DESCRIPTION

Oxandrin® oral tablets contain 2.5 mg of the anabolic steroid oxandrolone. Oxandrolone is 17β-hydroxy-17α-methyl-2-oxa-5α-androstan-3-one with the following structural formula:

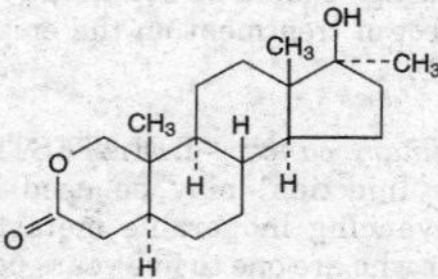

Inactive ingredients include cornstarch, lactose, magnesium stearate, and hydroxypropyl methylcellulose.

CLINICAL PHARMACOLOGY

Anabolic steroids are synthetic derivatives of testosterone. Certain clinical effects and adverse reactions demonstrate the androgenic properties of this class of drugs. Complete dissociation of anabolic and androgenic effects has not been achieved. The actions of anabolic steroids are therefore similar to those of male sex hormones with the possibility of causing serious disturbances of growth and sexual development if given to young children. Anabolic steroids suppress the gonadotropic functions of the pituitary and may exert a direct effect upon the testes.

During exogenous administration of anabolic androgens, endogenous testosterone release is inhibited through inhibition of pituitary luteinizing hormone (LH). At large doses, spermatogenesis may be suppressed through feedback inhibition of pituitary follicle-stimulating hormone (FSH).

Anabolic steroids have been reported to increase low-density lipoproteins and decrease high-density lipoproteins. These levels revert to normal on discontinuation of treatment.

INDICATIONS AND USAGE

Oxandrin is indicated as adjunctive therapy to promote weight gain after weight loss following extensive surgery, chronic infections, or severe trauma, and in some patients who without definite pathophysiologic reasons fail to gain or to maintain normal weight, to offset the protein catabolism associated with prolonged administration of corticosteroids, and for the relief of the bone pain frequently accompanying osteoporosis (See **DOSAGE AND ADMINISTRATION**).

DRUG ABUSE AND DEPENDENCE

Oxandrolone is classified as a controlled substance under the Anabolic Steroids Control Act of 1990 and has been assigned to Schedule III (non-narcotic).

CONTRAINDICATIONS

1. Known or suspected carcinoma of the prostate or the male breast.
2. Carcinoma of the breast in females with hypercalcemia (androgenic anabolic steroids may stimulate osteolytic bone resorption).
3. Pregnancy, because of possible masculinization of the fetus. Oxandrin has been shown to cause embryotoxicity, fetotoxicity, infertility, and masculinization of female animal offspring when given in doses 9 times the human dose.
4. Nephrosis, the nephrotic phase of nephritis.
5. Hypercalcemia.

WARNINGS

PELIOSIS HEPATIS, A CONDITION IN WHICH LIVER AND SOMETIMES SPLENIC TISSUE IS REPLACED WITH BLOOD-FILLED CYSTS, HAS BEEN REPORTED IN PATIENTS RECEIVING ANDROGENIC ANABOLIC STEROID THERAPY. THESE CYSTS ARE SOMETIMES PRESENT WITH MINIMAL HEPATIC DYSFUNCTION, BUT AT OTHER TIMES THEY HAVE BEEN ASSOCIATED WITH LIVER FAILURE. THEY ARE OFTEN NOT RECOGNIZED UNTIL LIFE-THREATENING LIVER FAILURE OR INTRA-ABDOMINAL HEMORRHAGE DEVELOPS. WITHDRAWAL OF DRUG USUALLY RESULTS IN COMPLETE DISAPPEARANCE OF LESIONS.

LIVER CELL TUMORS ARE ALSO REPORTED. MOST OFTEN THESE TUMORS ARE BENIGN AND ANDROGEN-DEPENDENT, BUT FATAL MALIGNANT TUMORS HAVE BEEN REPORTED. WITHDRAWAL OF DRUG OFTEN RESULTS IN REGRESSION OR CESSATION OF PROGRESSION OF THE TUMOR. HOWEVER, HEPATIC TUMORS ASSOCIATED WITH ANDROGENS OR ANABOLIC STEROIDS ARE MUCH MORE VASCULAR THAN OTHER HEPATIC TUMORS AND MAY BE SILENT UNTIL LIFE-THREATENING INTRA-ABDOMINAL HEMORRHAGE DEVELOPS. BLOOD LIPID CHANGES THAT ARE KNOWN TO BE ASSOCIATED WITH INCREASED RISK OF ATHEROSCLEROSIS ARE SEEN IN PATIENTS TREATED WITH ANDROGENS OR ANABOLIC STEROIDS. THESE CHANGES INCLUDE DECREASED HIGH-DENSITY LIPOPROTEINS AND SOMETIMES INCREASED LOW-DENSITY LIPOPROTEINS. THE CHANGES MAY BE VERY MARKED AND COULD HAVE A SERIOUS IMPACT ON THE RISK OF ATHEROSCLEROSIS AND CORONARY ARTERY DISEASE.

Cholestatic hepatitis and jaundice may occur with 17-alpha-alkylated androgens at a relatively low dose. If cholestatic hepatitis with jaundice appears or if liver function tests become abnormal, oxandrolone should be discontinued and the etiology should be determined. Drug-induced jaundice is reversible when the medication is discontinued.

In patients with breast cancer, anabolic steroid therapy may cause hypercalcemia by stimulating osteolysis. Oxandrolone therapy should be discontinued if hypercalcemia occurs.

Edema with or without congestive heart failure may be a serious complication in patients with pre-existing cardiac, renal, or hepatic disease. Concomitant administration of adrenal cortical steroid or ACTH may increase the edema.

In children, androgen therapy may accelerate bone maturation without producing compensatory gain in linear growth. This adverse effect results in compromised adult height. The younger the child, the greater the risk of compromising final mature height. The effect on bone maturation should be monitored by assessing bone age of the left wrist and hand every 6 months (See **PRECAUTIONS**: **Laboratory tests**).

Geriatric patients treated with androgenic anabolic steroids may be at an increased risk for the development of prostatic hypertrophy and prostatic carcinoma.

ANABOLIC STEROIDS HAVE NOT BEEN SHOWN TO ENHANCE ATHLETIC ABILITY.

PRECAUTIONS

General:

Women should be observed for signs of virilization (deepening of the voice, hirsutism, acne, clitoromegaly). Discontinuation of drug therapy at the time of evidence of mild virilism is necessary to prevent irreversible virilization. Some virilizing changes in women are irreversible even after prompt discontinuance of therapy and are not prevented by concomitant use of estrogens. Menstrual irregularities may also occur.

Anabolic steroids may cause suppression of clotting factors II, V, VII, and X, and an increase in prothrombin time.

Information for patients:

The physician should instruct patients to report any of the following side effects of androgens:

Males: Too frequent or persistent erections of the penis, appearance or aggravation of acne.

Females: Hoarseness, acne, changes in menstrual periods, or more facial hair.

All patients: Nausea, vomiting, changes in skin color, or ankle swelling.

Laboratory tests:

Women with disseminated breast carcinoma should have frequent determination of urine and serum calcium levels during the course of therapy (See **WARNINGS**).

Because of the hepatotoxicity associated with the use of 17-alpha-alkylated androgens, liver function tests should be obtained periodically.

Periodic (every 6 months) x-ray examinations of bone age should be made during treatment of children to determine the rate of bone maturation and the effects of androgen therapy on the epiphyseal centers.

Serum lipids and high-density lipoprotein cholesterol determinations should be done periodically as androgenic anabolic steroids have been reported to increase low-density lipoproteins. Serum cholesterol levels may increase during therapy. Therefore, caution is required when administering these agents to patients with a history of myocardial infarction or coronary artery disease. Serial determinations of serum cholesterol should be made and therapy adjusted accordingly.

Hemoglobin and hematocrit should be checked periodically for polycythemia in patients who are receiving high doses of anabolic steroids.

Drug interactions

Anticoagulants:

Anabolic steroids may increase sensitivity to oral anticoagulants. Dosage of the anticoagulant may have to be decreased in order to maintain desired prothrombin time. Patients receiving oral anticoagulant therapy require close monitoring, especially when anabolic steroids are started or stopped.

Oral hypoglycemic agents:

Oxandrolone may inhibit the metabolism of oral hypoglycemic agents.

Adrenal steroids or ACTH:

In patients with edema, concomitant administration with adrenal cortical steroids or ACTH may increase the edema.

Drug/Laboratory test interactions:

Anabolic steroids may decrease levels of thyroxine-binding globulin, resulting in decreased total T_4 serum levels and increased resin uptake of T_3 and T_4. Free thyroid hormone levels remain unchanged. In addition, a decrease in PBI and radioactive iodine uptake may occur.

Carcinogenesis, mutagenesis, impairment of fertility

Animal data:

Oxandrolone has not been tested in laboratory animals for carcinogenic or mutagenic effects. In 2-year chronic oral rat studies, a dose-related reduction of spermatogenesis and decreased organ weights (testes, prostate, seminal vesicles, ovaries, uterus, adrenals, and pituitary) were shown.

Human data:

Liver cell tumors have been reported in patients receiving long-term therapy with androgenic anabolic steroids in high doses (See **WARNINGS**). Withdrawal of the drugs did not lead to regression of the tumors in all cases.

Geriatric patients treated with androgenic anabolic steroids may be at an increased risk for the development of prostatic hypertrophy and prostatic carcinoma.

Pregnancy:

Teratogenic effects—Pregnancy Category X (See **CONTRAINDICATIONS**).

Nursing mothers:

It is not known whether anabolic steroids are excreted in human milk. Because of the potential of serious adverse reactions in nursing infants from oxandrolone, a decision should be made whether to discontinue nursing or to discontinue the drug, taking into account the importance of the drug to the mother.

Pediatric use:

Anabolic agents may accelerate epiphyseal maturation more rapidly than linear growth in children and the effect may continue for 6 months after the drug has been stopped. Therefore, therapy should be monitored by x-ray studies at 6-month intervals in order to avoid the risk of compromising adult height. Androgenic anabolic steroid therapy should be used very cautiously in children and only by specialists who are aware of the effects on bone maturation (See **WARNINGS**).

ADVERSE REACTIONS

The following adverse reactions have been associated with use of anabolic steroids:

Hepatic: Cholestatic jaundice with, rarely, hepatic necrosis and death. Hepatocellular neoplasms and peliosis hepatis with long-term therapy (See **WARNINGS**). Reversible changes in liver function tests also occur including increased bromsulfophthalein (BSP) retention, and increases in serum bilirubin, aspartate aminotransferase (AST, SGOT) and alkaline phosphatase.

In *males:*

Prepubertal: Phallic enlargement and increased frequency or persistence of erections.

Postpubertal: Inhibition of testicular function, testicular atrophy and oligospermia, impotence, chronic priapism, epididymitis, and bladder irritability.

In *females:*

Clitoral enlargement, menstrual irregularities.

CNS: Habituation, excitation, insomnia, depression, and changes in libido.

Hematologic: Bleeding in patients on concomitant anticoagulant therapy.

Breast: Gynecomastia.

Larynx: Deepening of the voice in females.

Hair: Hirsutism and male pattern baldness in females.

Skin: Acne (especially in females and prepubertal males).

Skeletal: Premature closure of epiphyses in children (See **PRECAUTIONS**: **Pediatric use**).

Fluid and electrolytes: Edema, retention of serum electrolytes (sodium chloride, potassium, phosphate, calcium).

Metabolic/Endocrine: Decreased glucose tolerance (See **PRECAUTIONS**: **Laboratory tests**), increased creatinine excretion, increased serum levels of creatinine phosphokinase (CPK). Masculinization of the fetus. Inhibition of gonadotropin secretion.

OVERDOSAGE

No symptoms or signs associated with overdosage have been reported. It is possible that sodium and water retention may occur.

The oral LD_{50} of oxandrolone in mice and dogs is greater than 5,000 mg/kg. No specific antidote is known, but gastric lavage may be used.

DOSAGE AND ADMINISTRATION

Therapy with anabolic steroids is adjunctive to and not a replacement for conventional therapy. The duration of therapy with Oxandrin (oxandrolone) will depend on the response of the patient and the possible appearance of adverse reactions. Therapy should be intermittent.

Adults: The *usual adult* dosage of Oxandrin is one 2.5-mg tablet 2 to 4 times daily. However, the response of individuals to anabolic steroids varies, and a daily dosage of as little as 2.5 mg or as much as 20 mg may be required to achieve the desired response. A course of therapy of 2 to 4 weeks is usually adequate. This may be repeated intermittently as indicated.

Children: For children the total daily dosage of Oxandrin is ≤ 0.1 mg per kilogram body weight or ≤ 0.045 mg per pound of body weight. This may be repeated intermittently as indicated.

HOW SUPPLIED

Oxandrin 2.5-mg tablets are oval, white, and scored with BTG on one side and "11" on each side of the scoreline on the other side; bottles of 100 (NDC 54396-111-11).

Rx only

Revised: Apr. 17, 1998

Manufactured for
BTG Pharmaceuticals by:
G.D. Searle & Co.
Chicago, IL 60680
Address medical inquires to:
BTG Pharmaceuticals
Medical Affairs
70 Wood Avenue South
Iselin, NJ 08830
BTG PHARMACEUTICALS

BTG PHARMACEUTICALS
OXANDRIN® CIII
(oxandrolone tablets, USP)

A05268-1

Shown in Product Identification Guide, page 310

For information on over-the-counter drugs, consult **PDR For Nonprescription Drugs**.

J.R. Carlson Laboratories, Inc.

15 COLLEGE DR.
ARLINGTON HEIGHTS, IL 60004-1985

Direct Inquiries to:
Customer Service
(847) 255-1600
FAX: (847) 255-1605

For Medical Information Contact:
In Emergencies:
Customer Service
(847) 255-1600
FAX: (847) 255-1605

ACES® OTC

DESCRIPTION

ACES provides four natural antioxidant nutrients.

Two Soft Gels Contain:		% U.S. RDA
Beta-Carotene (Pro-Vitamin A)	10,000 IU	200%
Vitamin C (Calcium Ascorbate)	1000 mg	1667%
Vitamin E (d-Alpha Tocopherol)	400 IU	1333%
Selenium (L-selenomethionine)	100 mcg	*

RDA: Recommended Daily Allowance—Adults
*U.S. RDA not determined

The nutrients in ACES are: Beta Carotene—(Pro-vitamin A) derived from tiny sea plants or algae (*D. salina*) grown in the fresh ocean waters off southern Australia; Vitamin C provided as the gentle, buffered calcium ascorbate; Vitamin E 100% natural-source from soy, the most biologically active form; And Selenium—organically bound with the essential nutrient methionine to promote assimilation.

Suggested Use: For dietary supplementation, take two soft gels daily, preferably at mealtime.

Corn-free. Wheat-free. Milk-free. Sugar-free. Yeast-free. Preservative-free. Soft Gel Contents: Nutrients listed above, soybean oil, vegetable stearin, lecithin, beeswax. Soft Gel Shell: Beef gelatin, glycerin, water, carob.

HOW SUPPLIED

In bottles of 50, 90, 200, and 360.
Also available as *ACES ® plus ZINC.*

E-GEMS® OTC

DESCRIPTION

100% natural-source vitamin E (d-alpha tocopheryl acetate) soft gels. Available in 8 strengths: 30 IU, 100 IU, 200 IU, 400 IU, 600 IU, 800 IU, 1000 IU, 1200 IU.

HOW SUPPLIED

Supplied in a variety of bottle sizes.

Carnrick Laboratories A Business Unit of Elan Pharmaceuticals

45 HORSE HILL ROAD
CEDAR KNOLLS, NJ 07927

Direct Inquiries to:
For Medical Information Contact:
(888) NEURO-05
(888) 638-7605

To Report Adverse Events Contact:
(877) ELAN GSS
(877) 352-6477

MIDRIN® ℞
[*mid 'rin*]

CAUTION

Federal law prohibits dispensing without prescription.

DESCRIPTION

Each red capsule with pink band contains Isometheptene Mucate 65 mg., Dichloralphenazone 100 mg., and Acetaminophen 325 mg.

Isometheptene Mucate is a white crystalline powder having a characteristic aromatic odor and bitter taste. It is an unsaturated aliphatic amine with sympathomimetic properties.

Dichloralphenazone is a white, microcrystalline powder, with slight odor and tastes saline at first, becoming acrid. It is a mild sedative.

Acetaminophen, a non-salicylate, occurs as a white, odorless, crystalline powder possessing a slightly bitter taste.

Continued on next page

Midrin—Cont.

Midrin® capsules contain FD&C Yellow No. 6 as a color additive.

ACTIONS

Isometheptene Mucate, a sympathomimetic amine, acts by constricting dilated cranial and cerebral arterioles, thus reducing the stimuli that lead to vascular headaches. Dichloralphenazone, a mild sedative, reduces the patient's emotional reaction to the pain of both vascular and tension headaches. Acetaminophen raises the threshold to painful stimuli, thus exerting an analgesic effect against all types of headaches.

INDICATIONS

For relief of tension and vascular headaches.*

> * Based on a review of this drug (isometheptene mucate) by the National Academy of Sciences-National Research Council and/or other information, FDA has classified the other indication as "possibly" effective in the treatment of migraine headache.
> Final classification of the less-than-effective indication requires further investigation.

CONTRAINDICATIONS

Midrin® is contraindicated in glaucoma and/or severe cases of renal disease, hypertension, organic heart disease, hepatic disease and in those patients who are on monoamine-oxidase (MAO) inhibitor therapy.

PRECAUTIONS

Caution should be observed in hypertension, peripheral vascular disease and after recent cardiovascular attacks.

ADVERSE REACTIONS

Transient dizziness and skin rash may appear in hypersensitive patients. This can usually be eliminated by reducing the dose.

DOSAGE AND ADMINISTRATION

FOR RELIEF OF MIGRAINE HEADACHE: The usual adult dosage is two capsules at once, followed by one capsule every hour until relieved, up to 5 capsules within a twelve hour period.

FOR RELIEF OF TENSION HEADACHE: The usual adult dosage is one or two capsules every four hours up to 8 capsules a day.

HOW SUPPLIED

Red capsules imprinted with pink band, the letter "C" and 86120. Bottles of 50 capsules, NDC 0086-0120-05. Bottles of 100 capsules, NDC 0086-0120-10. Bottles of 250 capsules, NDC 0086-0120-25. Store at controlled room temperature 15°–30°C (59°–86°F) in a dry place.

The most recent revision of this labeling is July 1997.

Manufactured for Carnrick Laboratories

Shown in Product Identification Guide, page 310

NAPRELAN® ℞

[nă' prĕ-lăn]

(naproxen sodium)

CONTROLLED-RELEASE TABLETS

Equivalent to 375 mg and 500 mg naproxen

DESCRIPTION

NAPRELAN®* contains naproxen sodium, a member of the arylacetic acid group of nonsteroidal anti-inflammatory drugs (NSAIDs). Naprelan® uses the proprietary IPDAS™ (Intestinal Protective Drug Absorption System) technology. It is a rapidly disintegrating tablet system combining an immediate release component and a sustained release component of microparticles that are widely dispersed, allowing absorption of the active ingredient throughout the gastrointestinal (GI) tract, maintaining blood levels over 24 hours. The chemical name for naproxen sodium is 2-naphthaleneacetic acid, 6-methoxy-α-methyl-sodium salt, (S)- with the following structural formula:

CH_3 | CHCOONa ; CH_3O

Naproxen sodium

Molecular Formula: $C_{14}H_{13}NaO_3$ Molecular Weight: 252.24

Naproxen sodium is an odorless crystalline powder, white to creamy in color. It is soluble in methanol and water.

Naprelan® contains 412.5 mg or 550 mg of naproxen sodium, equivalent to 375 mg and 500 mg of naproxen and 37.5 mg and 50 mg sodium respectively. Each Naprelan® tablet also contains the following inactive ingredients: ammonio methacrylate copolymer Type A, ammonio methacrylate copolymer Type B, citric acid, crospovidone, magnesium stearate, methacrylic acid copolymer Type A, microcrystalline cellulose, povidone, and talc. The tablet coating contains hydroxypropyl methylcellulose, polyethylene glycol, and titanium dioxide.

*Registered trademark of Élan Corporation, plc

Pharmacokinetic Parameters at Steady State Day 5 (Mean of 24 Subjects)

Parameter (units)	naproxen 500 mg Q12h/5 days (1000 mg)			Naprelan® 2 × 500 mg tablets (1000 mg) Q24h/5 days		
	Mean	SD	Range	Mean	SD	Range
AUC 0-24 (mcgxh/mL)	1446	168	1167–1858	1448	145	1173–1774
C_{max} (mcg/mL)	95	13	71–117	94	13	74–127
C_{avg} (mcg/mL)	60	7	49–77	60	6	49–74
C_{min} (mcg/mL)	36	9	13–51	33	7	23–48
T_{max} (hrs)	3	1	1–4	5	2	2–10

CLINICAL PHARMACOLOGY

Naproxen is a nonsteroidal anti-inflammatory drug (NSAID), with analgesic and antipyretic properties. As with other NSAIDs, its mode of action is not fully understood; however, its ability to inhibit prostaglandin synthesis may be involved in the anti-inflammatory effect.

PHARMACOKINETICS

Although naproxen itself is well absorbed, the sodium salt form is more rapidly absorbed resulting in higher peak plasma levels for a given dose. Approximately 30% of the total naproxen sodium dose in Naprelan® is present in the dosage form as an immediate release component. The remaining naproxen sodium is coated as microparticles to provide sustained release properties. After oral administration, plasma levels of naproxen are detected within 30 minutes of dosing, with peak plasma levels occurring approximately 5 hours after dosing. The observed terminal elimination half-life of naproxen from both immediate release naproxen sodium and Naprelan® is approximately 15 hours. Steady state levels of naproxen are achieved in 3 days and the degree of naproxen accumulation in the blood is consistent with this.

Plasma Naproxen Concentrations
Mean of 24 Subjects (+/-2SD)
(Steady State, Day 5)

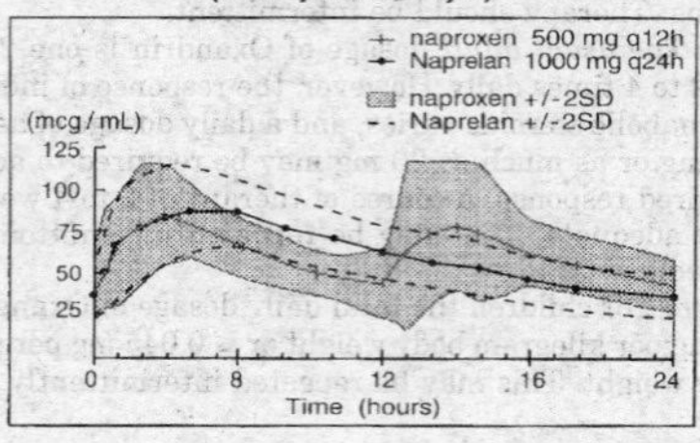

[See table above]

Absorption

Naproxen itself is rapidly and completely absorbed from the GI tract with an *in vivo* bioavailability of 95%. Based on the pharmacokinetic profile, the absorption phase of Naprelan® occurs in the first 4–6 hours after administration. This coincides with disintegration of the tablet in the stomach, the transit of the sustained release microparticles through the small intestine and into the proximal large intestine. An *in vivo* imaging study has been performed in healthy volunteers which confirms rapid disintegration of the tablet matrix and dispersion of the microparticles.

The absorption rate from the sustained release particulate component of Naprelan® is slower than that for conventional naproxen sodium tablets. It is this prolongation of drug absorption processes which maintains plasma levels and allows for once daily dosing.

Food Effects

No significant food effects were observed when twenty-four subjects were given a single dose of Naprelan® 500 mg either after an overnight fast or 30 minutes after a meal. In common with conventional naproxen and naproxen sodium formulations, food causes a slight decrease in the rate of naproxen absorption following Naprelan® administration.

Distribution

Naproxen has a volume of distribution of 0.16 L/kg. At therapeutic levels naproxen is greater than 99% albumin-bound. At doses of naproxen greater than 500 mg/day there is a less than proportional increase in plasma levels due to an increase in clearance caused by saturation of plasma protein binding at higher doses. However the concentration of unbound naproxen continues to increase proportionally to dose. Naprelan® exhibits similar dose proportional characteristics.

Metabolism

Naproxen is extensively metabolized to 6-0-desmethyl naproxen and both parent and metabolites do not induce metabolizing enzymes.

Elimination

The elimination half-life of Naprelan® and conventional naproxen is approximately 15 hours. Steady state conditions are attained after 2–3 doses of Naprelan®. Most of the drug is excreted in the urine, primarily as unchanged naproxen (less than 1%), 6-0-desmethyl naproxen (less than 1%) and their glucuronide or other conjugates (66–92%). A small amount (<5%) of the drug is excreted in the feces. The rate of excretion has been found to coincide closely with the rate of clearance from the plasma. In patients with renal failure metabolites may accumulate.

Special Populations

Pediatric Use

No pediatric studies have been performed with Naprelan®, thus safety of Naprelan in pediatric populations has not been established.

Renal Insufficiency

Naproxen pharmacokinetics have not been determined in subjects with renal insufficiency. Given that naproxen is metabolized and conjugates are primarily excreted by the kidneys, the potential exists for naproxen metabolites to accumulate in the presence of renal insufficiency.

CLINICAL STUDIES

RHEUMATOID ARTHRITIS

The use of Naprelan for the management of the signs and symptoms of rheumatoid arthritis was assessed in a 12 week double-blind, randomized, placebo and active-controlled study in 348 patients. Two Naprelan 500 mg tablets (1000 mg) once daily and naproxen 500 mg tablets twice daily (1000 mg) were more effective than placebo. Clinical effectiveness was demonstrated at one week and continued for the duration of the study.

OSTEOARTHRITIS

The use of Naprelan® for the management of the signs and symptoms of osteoarthritis of the knee was assessed in a 12 week double-blind, placebo and active-controlled study in 347 patients. Two Naprelan® 500 mg tablets (1000 mg) once daily and naproxen 500 mg tablets twice daily (1000 mg) were more effective than placebo. Clinical effectiveness was demonstrated at one week and continued for the duration of the study.

ANALGESIA

The onset of the analgesic effect of Naprelan® was seen within 30 minutes in a pharmacokinetic/pharmacodynamic study of patients with pain following oral surgery. In controlled clinical trials, naproxen has been used in combination with gold, D-penicillamine, methotrexate and corticosteroids. Its use in combination with salicylate is not recommended because there is evidence that aspirin increases the rate of excretion of naproxen and data are inadequate to demonstrate that naproxen and aspirin produce greater improvement over that achieved with aspirin alone. In addition, as with other NSAIDs the combination may result in higher frequency of adverse events than demonstrated for either product alone.

SPECIAL STUDIES

In a double-blind randomized, parallel group study, 19 subjects received either two Naprelan® 500 mg tablets (1000 mg) once daily or naproxen 500 mg tablets (1000 mg) twice daily for 7 days. Mucosal biopsy scores and endoscopic scores were lower in the subjects who received Naprelan®. In another double-blind, randomized, crossover study, 23 subjects received two Naprelan® 500 mg tablets (1000 mg) once daily, naproxen 500 mg tablets (1000 mg) twice daily and aspirin 650 mg four times daily (2600 mg) for 7 days each. There were significantly fewer duodenal erosions seen with Naprelan® than with either naproxen or aspirin. There were significantly fewer gastric erosions with both Naprelan® and naproxen than with aspirin.

The clinical significance of these findings is unknown.

Individualization of Dosage

RHEUMATOID ARTHRITIS, OSTEOARTHRITIS, AND ANKYLOSING SPONDYLITIS

Naprelan® like other NSAIDs shows considerable variation in response. The recommended starting dose of Naprelan® in adults is two Naprelan® 375 mg tablets (750 mg) once daily, or two Naprelan® 500 mg tablets (1000 mg) once daily. Patients already taking naproxen 250 mg, 375 mg or 500 mg twice daily (morning and evening) may have their total daily dose replaced with Naprelan® as a single daily dose.

During long-term administration, the dose of Naprelan® may be adjusted up or down depending on the clinical response of the patient.

In patients who tolerate lower doses of Naprelan® well, the dose may be increased to three Naprelan® 500 mg tablets (1500 mg) once daily for limited periods when a higher level of anti-inflammatory/analgesic activity is required. When treating patients, especially at the higher dose levels, the physician should observe sufficient increased clinical benefit to offset the potential increased risk. (See **Clinical Pharmacology**). The lowest effective dose should be sought and used in every patient.

Symptomatic improvement in arthritis usually begins within one week; however, treatment for two weeks may be required to achieve a therapeutic benefit. A lower dose should be considered in patients with renal or hepatic impairment or in elderly patients (see **Precautions**). Studies indicate that although total plasma concentration of naproxen is unchanged, the unbound plasma fraction of naproxen is increased in the elderly. Caution is advised when high doses are required and some adjustment of dosage may be required in elderly patients. As with other drugs used in the elderly it is prudent to use the lowest effective dose.

ANALGESIA, DYSMENORRHEA, BURSITIS, AND TENDINITIS

The recommended starting dose is two Naprelan® 500 mg tablets (1000 mg) once daily. For patients requiring greater analgesic benefit, three Naprelan® 500 mg tablets (1500 mg) may be used for a limited period. Thereafter, the total daily dose should not exceed two Naprelan® 500 mg tablets (1000 mg).

ACUTE GOUT

The recommended dose on the first day is two or three Naprelan® 500 mg tablets (1000–1500 mg) once daily, followed by two Naprelan® 500 mg tablets (1000 mg) once daily, until the attack has subsided.

INDICATIONS AND USAGE

Naprelan® is indicated for the treatment of rheumatoid arthritis, osteoarthritis, ankylosing spondylitis, tendinitis, bursitis and acute gout. It is also indicated in the relief of mild to moderate pain and the treatment of primary dysmenorrhea.

CONTRAINDICATIONS

All naproxen products are contraindicated in patients who have had allergic reactions to prescription as well as to over-the-counter products containing naproxen. Anaphylactoid reactions may occur in patients without previous known exposure or hypersensitivity to aspirin, naproxen, or other NSAIDs, or in individuals with a history of angioedema, urticaria, bronchospastic reactivity (e.g. asthma), and nasal polyps. Anaphylactoid reactions, like anaphylaxis, may have a fatal outcome. Therefore, careful questioning of patients for such things as asthma, nasal polyps, urticaria, and hypotension associated with NSAIDs before starting therapy is important. In addition, if such symptoms occur during therapy, treatment with Naprelan® should be discontinued.

WARNINGS

RISK OF GI ULCERATION, BLEEDING AND PERFORATION WITH NSAID THERAPY

Serious GI toxicity such as bleeding, ulceration and perforation, can occur at any time, with or without warning symptoms, in patients treated chronically with NSAID therapy. Although minor upper GI problems, such as dyspepsia, are common, usually developing early in therapy, physicians should remain alert for ulcerations and bleeding in patients treated chronically with NSAIDs even in the absence of previous GI tract symptoms. In patients observed in clinical trials with naproxen of several months to two years duration, symptomatic upper GI ulcers, gross bleeding or perforation appear to occur in approximately 1% of patients treated for 3–6 months, and in about 2–4% of patients treated for one year. Physicians should inform patients about the signs and/or symptoms of serious GI toxicity and what steps to take if they occur.

Studies to date with all naproxen products have not identified any subset of patients not at risk of developing peptic ulceration and bleeding or any differences between different naproxen products in their propensity to cause peptic ulceration and bleeding. Except for a prior history of serious GI events and other risk factors known to be associated with peptic ulcer disease, such as alcoholism, smoking etc., no risk factors (e.g., age, sex) have been associated with increased risk. Elderly or debilitated patients seem to tolerate ulceration or bleeding less well than other individuals and most spontaneous reports of fatal GI events are in this population. Studies to date are inconclusive concerning the relative risk of various NSAIDs in causing such reactions. High doses of any NSAID probably carry a greater risk of these reactions, although controlled clinical trials showing this do not exist in most cases. In considering the use of relatively large doses (within the recommended dosage range), sufficient benefit should be anticipated to offset the potential increased risk of GI toxicity.

PRECAUTIONS

GENERAL

NAPRELAN® SHOULD NOT BE USED CONCOMITANTLY WITH OTHER NAPROXEN PRODUCTS SINCE THEY ALL CIRCULATE IN THE PLASMA AS THE NAPROXEN ANION.

The antipyretic and anti-inflammatory activities of the drug may reduce fever and inflammation, thus diminishing their utility as diagnostic signs.

Because of adverse eye findings in animal studies with drugs of this class, it is recommended that ophthalmic studies be carried out if any change or disturbance in vision occurs.

Renal Effects

As with other NSAIDs, long term administration of naproxen to animals has resulted in renal papillary necrosis and other abnormal renal pathology. In humans, there have been reports of acute interstitial nephritis, hematuria, proteinuria, and occasionally nephrotic syndrome associated with naproxen-containing products and other NSAIDs since they have been marketed.

A second form of renal toxicity has been seen in patients taking naproxen as well as other NSAIDs. In patients with prerenal conditions with reduction in renal blood flow or blood volume, renal prostaglandins have a supportive role in the maintenance of renal perfusion. Administration of a NSAID may cause a dose-dependent reduction in prostaglandin formation and may precipitate overt renal decompensation. Patients at greatest risk of this reaction are those with impaired renal function, heart failure, liver dysfunction, diuretic use, and the elderly. Discontinuation of NSAID therapy is typically followed by recovery to the pretreatment state.

Naproxen and its metabolites are eliminated primarily by the kidneys, therefore the drug should be used with great caution in patients with significantly impaired renal function and the monitoring of serum creatinine and/or creatinine clearance is advised in these patients. Caution should be used if the drug is given to patients with creatinine clearance of less than 20 mL/minute because accumulation of naproxen has been seen in such patients.

Hepatic Effects

As with other NSAIDs, borderline elevations of one or more liver tests may occur in up to 15% of patients. These abnormalities may progress, may remain essentially unchanged, or may resolve with continued therapy. The ALT (SGPT) is probably the most sensitive indicator of liver dysfunction. Meaningful (3 times the upper limit of normal) elevations of ALT (SGPT) or AST (SGOT) occurred in controlled clinical trials in less than 1% of patients. A patient with symptoms and/or signs suggesting liver dysfunction, or in whom an abnormal liver test has occurred, should be evaluated for evidence of the development of more severe hepatic reaction while on therapy with naproxen. Severe hepatic reactions, including jaundice and cases of fatal hepatitis have been reported with naproxen as with other NSAIDs. Although such reactions are rare, if abnormal liver tests persist or worsen, if clinical signs and symptoms consistent with liver disease develop, or if systemic manifestations occur (e.g. eosinophilia, rash, fever, etc.), naproxen should be discontinued. Chronic alcoholic liver disease and probably other diseases with decreased or abnormal plasma proteins (albumin) reduce the total plasma concentration of naproxen, but the plasma concentration of unbound naproxen is increased. Caution is advised when high doses are required and some adjustment of dosage may be required in these patients. It is prudent to use the lowest effective dose.

Fluid Retention and Edema

Peripheral edema has been observed in some patients receiving naproxen. Naprelan® (naproxen sodium) tablets contain 37.5 mg or 50 mg of sodium (1.5 mEq or 2.0 mEq respectively). This should be considered in patients whose overall intake of sodium must be severely restricted. For these reasons, Naprelan® should be used with caution in patients with fluid retention, hypertension or heart failure.

INFORMATION FOR PATIENTS

Naprelan®, like other drugs of its class, is not free of side effects. This formulation of naproxen can cause discomfort and, rarely, there are more serious side effects, such as GI bleeding, which may result in hospitalization and even fatal outcomes. NSAIDs are often essential agents in the management of arthritis and have a major role in the treatment of pain but they also may be commonly employed for conditions which are less serious. Physicians may wish to discuss with their patients the potential risks (see **Warnings**, **Precautions**, and **Adverse Reactions**) and likely benefits of Naprelan® treatment.

Caution should be exercised by patients whose activities require alertness if they experience drowsiness, dizziness, vertigo or depression during therapy with naproxen.

LABORATORY TESTS

Because serious GI tract ulceration and bleeding can occur without warning symptoms, physicians should follow patients chronically treated with Naprelan® for the signs and symptoms of ulceration and bleeding, and should inform them of the importance of this follow-up and what they should do if certain signs and symptoms do appear. Patients with initial hemoglobin values of 10 grams or less who are to receive long-term therapy should have hemoglobin values determined periodically. (See **Warnings**—RISK OF GI ULCERATION, BLEEDING AND PERFORATION WITH NSAID THERAPY).

Drug Interactions

The use of NSAIDs in patients who are receiving ACE inhibitors may potentiate renal disease states (See **Precautions**—*Renal Effects*). *In vitro* studies have shown that naproxen anion, because of its affinity for protein, may displace from their binding sites other drugs which are also albumin-bound (see **Clinical Pharmacology**—PHARMACOKINETICS).

Theoretically, the naproxen anion itself could likewise be displaced. Short-term controlled studies failed to show that taking the drug significantly affects prothrombin times when administered to individuals on coumarin-type anticoagulants. Caution is advised nonetheless, since interactions have been seen with other non steroidal agents of this class. Similarly, patients receiving the drug and a hydantoin, sulfonamide or sulfonylurea should be observed for signs of toxicity to these drugs.

Concomitant administration of naproxen and aspirin is not recommended because naproxen is displaced from its binding sites during the concomitant administration of aspirin, resulting in lower plasma concentrations and peak plasma levels.

The natriuretic effect of furosemide has been reported to be inhibited by some drugs of this class. Inhibition of renal lithium clearance leading to increases in plasma lithium concentrations has also been reported. Naproxen and other NSAIDs can reduce the antihypertensive effect of propranolol and other beta-blockers.

Probenecid given concurrently increases naproxen anion plasma levels and extends its plasma half-life significantly. Caution should be used if naproxen is administered concomitantly with methotrexate. Naproxen, naproxen sodium and other NSAIDs have been reported to reduce the tubular secretion of methotrexate in an animal model, possibly increasing the toxicity of methotrexate.

DRUG/LABORATORY TEST INTERACTIONS

Naproxen may decrease platelet aggregation and prolong bleeding time. This effect should be kept in mind when bleeding times are determined. The administration of naproxen may result in increased urinary values for 17-ketogenic steroids because of an interaction between the drug and/or its metabolites with m-dinitrobenzene used in this assay. Although 17-hydroxy-corticosteroid measurements (Porter-Silber test) do not appear to be artifactually altered, it is suggested that therapy with naproxen be temporarily discontinued 72 hours before adrenal function tests are performed if the Porter-Silber test is to be used.

Naproxen may interfere with some urinary assays of 5-hydroxy indoleacetic acid (5HIAA).

CARCINOGENESIS

A two year study was performed in rats to evaluate the carcinogenic potential of naproxen at doses of 8 mg/kg/day, 16 mg/kg/day, and 24 mg/kg/day (50 mg/m^2, 100 mg/m^2, and 150 mg/m^2). The maximum dose used was 0.28 times the systemic exposure to humans at the recommended dose. No evidence of tumorigenicity was found.

PREGNANCY

Teratogenic Effects: Pregnancy Category B

Reproduction studies have been performed in rats at 20 mg/kg/day (125 mg/m^2/day, 0.23 times the human systemic exposure) rabbits at 20 mg/kg/day (220 mg/m^2/day, 0.27 times the human systemic exposure) and mice at 170 mg/kg/day (510 mg/m^2/day, 0.28 times the human systemic exposure) with no evidence of impaired fertility or harm to the fetus due to the drug. There are no adequate and well-controlled studies in pregnant women. Because animal reproduction studies are not always predictive of human response, Naprelan® should be used during pregnancy only if the potential benefits justify the potential risks to the fetus.

Nonteratogenic Effects

There is some evidence to suggest that when inhibitors of prostaglandin synthesis are used to delay preterm labor there is an increased risk of neonatal complications such as necrotizing enterocolitis, patent ductus arteriosus, and intracranial hemorrhage. Naproxen treatment given in the late pregnancy to delay parturition has been associated with persistent pulmonary hypertension, renal dysfunction, and abnormal prostaglandin E levels in preterm infants. Because of the known effect of drugs of this class on the human fetal cardiovascular system (closure of ductus arteriosus), use during third trimester should be avoided.

NURSING MOTHERS

The naproxen anion has been found in the milk of lactating women at a concentration of approximately 1% of that found in the plasma. Because of the possible adverse effects of prostaglandin-inhibiting drugs on neonates, use in nursing mothers should be avoided.

PEDIATRIC USE

No pediatric studies have been performed with Naprelan®, thus safety of Naprelan® in pediatric populations has not been established.

ADVERSE REACTIONS

As with all drugs in this class, the frequency and severity of adverse events depends on several factors: the dose of the drug and duration of treatment; the age, the sex, physical condition of the patient; any concurrent medical diagnoses or individual risk factors.

The following adverse reactions are divided into three parts based on frequency and whether or not the possibility exists of a causal relationship between drug usage and these adverse events. In those reactions listed as "Probable Causal Relationship" there is at least one case for each adverse reaction where there is evidence to suggest that there is a causal relationship between drug usage and the reported event. The adverse reactions reported were based on the results from two double-blind controlled clinical trials of three months duration with an additional nine month open-label extension. A total of 542 patients received Naprelan® either in the double-blind period or in the nine month open-label

Continued on next page

Naprelan—Cont.

extension. Of these 542 patients, 232 received Naprelan®, 167 were initially treated with Naprosyn and 143 were initially treated with placebo. Adverse reactions reported by patients who received Naprelan® are shown by body system. Those adverse reactions observed with naproxen but not reported in controlled trials with Naprelan® are italicized.

The most frequent adverse events from the double-blind and open-label clinical trials were headache (15%), followed by dyspepsia (14%), and flu syndrome (10%). The incidence of other adverse events occurring in 3%–9% of the patients are marked with an asterisk.

Those reactions occurring in less than 3% of the patients are unmarked.

INCIDENCE GREATER THAN 1% (PROBABLE CAUSAL RELATIONSHIP)

Body as a Whole—Pain (back)*, pain*, infection*, fever, injury (accident), asthenia, pain chest, headache (15%), flu syndrome (10%). Gastrointestinal—Nausea*, diarrhea*, constipation*, abdominal pain*, flatulence, gastritis, vomiting, dysphagia, dyspepsia (14%), *heartburn**, *stomatitis*.

Hematologic—Anemia, ecchymosis.

Respiratory—Pharyngitis*, rhinitis*, sinusitis*, bronchitis, cough increased.

Renal—Urinary tract infection*, cystitis.

Dermatologic—Skin rash*, *skin eruptions**, *ecchymoses**, *purpura*.

Metabolic and Nutrition—Peripheral edema, hyperglycemia.

Central Nervous System—Dizziness, paresthesia, insomnia, *drowsiness**, *lightheadedness*.

Cardiovascular—Hypertension, *edema**, *dyspnea**, *palpitations*.

Musculoskeletal—Cramps (leg), myalgia, arthralgia, joint disorder, tendon disorder.

Special Senses—*Tinnitus**, *hearing disturbances, visual disturbances*.

General—*Thirst*.

INCIDENCE LESS THAN 1% (PROBABLE CAUSAL RELATIONSHIP)

Body as a Whole—Abscess, monilia, neck rigid, pain neck, abdomen enlarged, carcinoma, cellulitis, edema general, LE syndrome, malaise, mucous membrane disorder, allergic reaction, pain pelvic.

Gastrointestinal—Anorexia, cholecystitis, cholelithiasis, eructation, GI hemorrhage, rectal hemorrhage, stomatitis aphthous, stomatitis ulcer, ulcer mouth, ulcer stomach, periodontal abscess, cardiospasm, colitis, esophagitis, gastroenteritis, GI disorder, rectal disorder, tooth disorder, hepatosplenomegaly, liver function abnormality, melena, ulcer esophagus, *hematemesis, jaundice, pancreatitis, necrosis*.

Renal—Dysmenorrhea, dysuria, kidney function abnormality, nocturia, prostate disorder, pyelonephritis, carcinoma breast, urinary incontinence, kidney calculus, kidney failure, menorrhagia, metrorrhagia, neoplasm breast, nephrosclerosis, hematuria, pain kidney, pyuria, urine abnormal, urinary frequency, urinary retention, uterine spasm, vaginitis, *glomerular nephritis, hyperkalemia, interstitial nephritis, nephrotic syndrome, renal disease, renal failure, renal papillary necrosis*.

Hematologic—Leukopenia, bleeding time increased, eosinophilia, abnormal RBC, abnormal WBC, thrombocytopenia, *agranulocytosis, granulocytopenia*.

Central Nervous System—Depression, anxiety, hypertonia, nervousness, neuralgia, neuritis, vertigo, amnesia, confusion, co-ordination, abnormal diplopia, emotional lability, hematoma subdural, paralysis, *dream abnormalities, inability to concentrate, muscle weakness*.

Dermatologic: Angiodermatitis, herpes simplex, dry skin, sweating, ulcer skin, acne, alopecia, dermatitis contact, eczema, herpes zoster, nail disorder, skin necrosis, subcutaneous nodule, pruritus, urticaria, neoplasm skin, *photosensitive dermatitis, photosensitivity reactions resembling porphyria cutaneous tarda, epidermolysis bullosa*.

Special Senses—Amblyopia, scleritis, cataract, conjunctivitis, deaf, ear disorder, keratoconjunctivitis, lacrimation disorder, otitis media, pain eye.

Cardiovascular—Angina pectoris, coronary artery disease, myocardial infarction, deep thrombophlebitis, vasodilation, vascular anomaly, arrhythmia, bundle branch block, abnormal ECG, heart failure right, hemorrhage, migraine, aortic stenosis, syncope, tachycardia, *congestive heart failure*.

Respiratory—Asthma, dyspnea, lung edema, laryngitis, lung disorder, epistaxis, pneumonia, respiratory distress, respiratory disorder, *eosinophilic pneumonitis*.

Musculoskeletal—Myasthenia, bone disorder, spontaneous bone fracture, fibrotendinitis, bone pain, ptosis, spasm general, bursitis.

Metabolic and Nutrition—Creatinine increase, glucosuria, hypercholesteremia, albuminuria, alkalosis, BUN increased, dehydration, edema, glucose tolerance decrease, hyperuricemia, hypokalemia, SGOT increase, SGPT increase, weight decrease.

General—*Anaphylactoid reactions, angioneurotic edema, menstrual disorders, hypoglycemia, pyrexia (chills and fevers)*.

INCIDENCE LESS THAN 1% (CAUSAL RELATIONSHIP UNKNOWN)

Other adverse reactions listed in the naproxen package label, but not reported by those who received Naprelan® are shown in italics. These observations are being listed as alerting information to the physician.

Hematologic—*Aplastic anemia, hemolytic anemia*.

Central Nervous System: *Aseptic meningitis, cognitive dysfunction*.

Dermatologic—*Epidermal necrolysis, erythema multiforme, Stevens-Johnson syndrome*.

Gastrointestinal—*Non-peptic GI ulceration, ulcerative stomatitis*.

Cardiovascular—*Vasculitis*.

OVERDOSAGE

Significant naproxen overdosage may be characterized by drowsiness, heartburn, indigestion, nausea or vomiting. Because naproxen sodium may be rapidly absorbed, high and early blood levels should be anticipated. A few patients have experienced seizures, but it is not clear whether or not these were drug-related. It is not known what dose of the drug would be life threatening. The oral LD_{50} of the drug is 500 mg/kg in rats, 1200 mg/kg in mice, 4000 mg/kg in hamsters and greater than 1000 mg/kg in dogs.

Should a patient ingest a large number of tablets, accidentally or purposefully, the stomach may be emptied and usual supportive measures employed. In animals 0.5 g/kg of activated charcoal was effective in reducing plasma levels of naproxen. Hemodialysis does not decrease the plasma concentration of naproxen because of the high degree of its protein binding.

DOSAGE AND ADMINISTRATION

RHEUMATOID ARTHRITIS, OSTEOARTHRITIS, AND ANKYLOSING SPONDYLITIS

The usual daily dose of Naprelan® is two Naprelan® 375 mg tablets (750 mg) once daily, or two Naprelan® 500 mg tablets (1000 mg) once a day. Both larger and smaller doses may be required in individual patients (see **Individualization of Dosage**). Regardless of indication, the dosage should be individualized to achieve effective dose and minimize adverse events, however the maximum daily dose is three Naprelan® 500 mg once daily.

MANAGEMENT OF PAIN, PRIMARY DYSMENORRHEA, AND ACUTE TENDINITIS AND BURSITIS

The recommended starting dose is two Naprelan® 500 mg tablets (1000 mg) once daily. For patients requiring greater analgesic benefit, three Naprelan® 500 mg tablets (1500 mg) may be used for a limited period. Thereafter, the total daily dose should not exceed two Naprelan® 500 mg tablets (1000 mg).

ACUTE GOUT

The recommended dose on the first day is two to three Naprelan® 500 mg tablets (1000–1500 mg) once daily, followed by two Naprelan® 500 mg tablets (1000 mg) once daily, until the attack has subsided.

HOW SUPPLIED

Naprelan® (naproxen sodium) Controlled-Release Tablets are available as follows:

Naprelan® 375: white, capsule-shaped tablet with "N" on one side and "901" on the reverse; in bottles of 100; NDC 0086-0090-10. Each tablet contains 412.5 mg naproxen sodium equivalent to 375 mg naproxen.

Naprelan® 500: white, capsule-shaped tablet with "N" on one side and "902" on the reverse; in bottles of 75; NDC 0086-0091-75. Each tablet contains 550 mg naproxen sodium equivalent to 500 mg naproxen.

Rx Only

US Patent 5,637,320

Store at controlled room temperature, 20°–25° C (68°–77° F).

Dispense in a well-closed container.

Manufactured for:
Carnick Laboratories
Division of Elan Pharmaceuticals
Cedar Knolls, NJ 07927
by élan pharma ltd.
Athlone, Ireland
700920 Revised January 7, 1999

Shown in Product Identification Guide, page 310

SKELAXIN® ℞

brand of metaxalone

CAUTION

Federal law prohibits dispensing without prescription.

DESCRIPTION

Each pale rose, scored tablet contains: metaxalone, 400 mg. Skelaxin® (metaxalone) has the following chemical structure and name:

5-[(3,4-dimethylphenoxy)methyl]-2 oxazolidinone

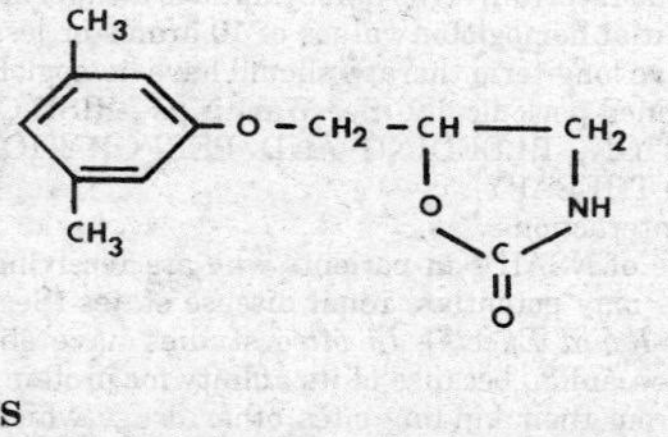

ACTIONS

The mechanism of action of metaxalone in humans has not been established, but may be due to general central nervous system depression. It has no direct action on the contractile mechanism of striated muscle, the motor end plate or the nerve fiber.

INDICATIONS

Skelaxin® (metaxalone) is indicated as an adjunct to rest, physical therapy, and other measures for the relief of discomforts associated with acute, painful musculoskeletal conditions. The mode of action of this drug has not been clearly identified, but may be related to its sedative properties. Metaxalone does not directly relax tense skeletal muscles in man.

CONTRAINDICATIONS

Metaxalone is contraindicated in individuals who have shown hypersensitivity to the drug. Metaxalone should not be administered to patients with a known tendency to drug-induced, hemolytic, or other anemias. It is contraindicated in patients with significantly impaired renal or hepatic function.

PRECAUTIONS

Elevation in cephalin flocculation tests without concurrent changes in other liver function parameters have been noted. Hence, it is recommended that metaxalone be administered with great care to patients with pre-existing liver damage and that serial liver function studies be performed as required.

False-positive Benedict's tests, due to an unknown reducing substance, have been noted. A glucose-specific test will differentiate findings.

Pregnancy: Reproduction studies have been performed in rats and have revealed no evidence of impaired fertility or harm to the fetus due to metaxalone. Reactions reports from marketing experience have not revealed evidence of fetal injury, but such experience cannot exclude the possibility of infrequent or subtle damage to the human fetus. Safe use of metaxalone has not been established with regard to possible adverse effects upon fetal development. Therefore, metaxalone tablets should not be used in women who are or may become pregnant and particularly during early pregnancy unless in the judgment of the physician the potential benefits outweigh the possbile hazards.

Nursing Mothers: It is not known whether this drug is secreted in human milk. As a general rule, nursing should not be undertaken while a patient is on a drug since many drugs are excreted in human milk.

Pediatric Use: Safety and effectiveness in children 12 years of age and below have not been established.

ADVERSE REACTIONS

The most frequent reactions to metaxalone include nausea, vomiting, gastrointestinal upset, drowsiness, dizziness, headache, and nervousness or "irritability." Other adverse reactions are: hypersensitivity reaction, characterized by a light rash with or without pruritus; leukopenia; hemolytic anemia; jaundice.

DOSAGE

The recommended dose for adults and children over 12 years of age is two tablets (800 mg) three to four times a day.

MANAGEMENT OF OVERDOSAGE

Gastric lavage and supportive therapy as indicated. (When determining the LD_{50} in rats and mice, progressive sedation, hypnosis and finally respiratory failure were noted as the dosage increased. In dogs, no LD_{50} could be determined as the higher doses produced an emetic action in 15 to 30 minutes). No documented case of major toxicity has been reported.

HOW SUPPLIED

Skelaxin® (metaxalone) is available as a 400 mg. pale rose tablet, inscribed with 8662 on the scored side and "C" on the other. Available in bottles of 100 (NDC 0086-0062-10) and in bottles of 500 (NDC 0086-0062-50).

Store at Controlled Room Temperature, between 15°C and 30°C (59°F and 86°F).

1/98

Manufactured for Carnrick Laboratories

Shown in Product Identification Guide, page 310

IDENTIFICATION PROBLEM?
Turn to the **Product Identification Guide,** where you'll find more than 1600 products pictured in actual size and full color.

Celgene Corporation

7 POWDER HORN DRIVE
WARREN, NJ 07059

Direct Inquiries to:
(732) 271-1001
(800) 890-4619
Customer Service
888-4-CELGENE
888-423-5436
Medical Services
732-805-3905
732-805-3667 fax
Drug Safety
732-805-3667
732-271-4115 fax

THALOMID® Capsules ℞

[*thălō-mĭd*]
(thalidomide)

WARNING: SEVERE, LIFE-THREATENING HUMAN BIRTH DEFECTS
IF THALIDOMIDE IS TAKEN DURING PREGNANCY, IT CAN CAUSE SEVERE BIRTH DEFECTS OR DEATH TO AN UNBORN BABY. THALIDOMIDE SHOULD NEVER BE USED BY WOMEN WHO ARE PREGNANT OR WHO COULD BECOME PREGNANT WHILE TAKING THE DRUG. EVEN A SINGLE DOSE [1 CAPSULE (50 mg)] TAKEN BY A PREGNANT WOMAN DURING HER PREGNANCY CAN CAUSE SEVERE BIRTH DEFECTS.
BECAUSE OF THIS TOXICITY AND IN AN EFFORT TO MAKE THE CHANCE OF FETAL EXPOSURE TO THALOMID® (thalidomide) AS NEGLIGIBLE AS POSSIBLE, THALOMID® (thalidomide) IS APPROVED FOR MARKETING ONLY UNDER A SPECIAL RESTRICTED DISTRIBUTION PROGRAM APPROVED BY THE FOOD AND DRUG ADMINISTRATION. THIS PROGRAM IS CALLED THE "SYSTEM FOR THALIDOMIDE EDUCATION AND PRESCRIBING SAFETY *S.T.E.P.™)*".
UNDER THIS RESTRICTED DISTRIBUTION PROGRAM, ONLY PRESCRIBERS AND PHARMACISTS REGISTERED WITH THE PROGRAM ARE ALLOWED TO PRESCRIBE AND DISPENSE THE PRODUCT. IN ADDITION, PATIENTS MUST BE ADVISED OF, AGREE TO, AND COMPLY WITH THE REQUIREMENTS OF THE *S.T.E.P.S.™* PROGRAM IN ORDER TO RECEIVE PRODUCT.
PLEASE SEE THE FOLLOWING BOXED WARNINGS CONTAINING SPECIAL INFORMATION FOR PRESCRIBERS, FEMALE PATIENTS, AND MALE PATIENTS ABOUT THIS RESTRICTED DISTRIBUTION PROGRAM.

PRESCRIBERS

THALOMID® (thalidomide) may be prescribed only by licensed prescribers who are registered in the *S.T.E.P.S.*™ program and understand the risk of teratogenicity if thalidomide is used during pregnancy.

Major human fetal abnormalities related to thalidomide administration during pregnancy have been documented: amelia (absence of limbs), phocomelia (short limbs), hypoplasticity of the bones, absence of bones, external ear abnormalities (including anotia, micro pinna, small or absent external auditory canals), facial palsy, eye abnormalities (anophathalmos, microphthalmos), and congenital heart defects. Alimentary tract, urinary tract, and genital malformations have also been documented.[1] Mortality at or shortly after birth has been reported at about 40%.[2]

Effective contraception (see **CONTRAINDICATIONS**) must be used for at least 1 month before beginning thalidomide therapy, during thalidomide therapy, and for 1 month following discontinuation of thalidomide therapy. Reliable contraception is indicated even where there has been a history of infertility, unless due to hysterectomy or because the patient has been post-menopausal for at least 24 months. Two reliable forms of contraception must be used simultaneously unless continuous abstinence from reproductive heterosexual sexual intercourse is the chosen method. Women of childbearing potential should be referred to a qualified provider of contraceptive methods, if needed. Sexually mature women who have not undergone a hysterectomy or who have not been post-menopausal for at least 24 consecutive months (i.e., who have had menses at some time in the preceding 24 consecutive months) are considered to be women of child-bearing potential.

Before starting treatment, women of childbearing potential should have a pregnancy test (sensitivity of at least 50 mIU/mL). The test should be performed within the 24 hours prior to beginning therapy. A prescription for thalidomide for a woman of childbearing potential must not be issued by the prescriber until a written report of a negative pregnancy test has been obtained by the prescriber.

Once treatment has started, pregnancy testing should occur weekly during the first month of use, then monthly thereafter in women with regular menstrual cycles. If menstrual cycles are irregular, the pregnancy testing should occur every 2 weeks. Pregnancy testing and counseling should be performed if a patient misses her period or if there is any abnormality in menstrual bleeding.

If pregnancy does occur during thalidomide treatment, thalidomide must be discontinued immediately.

Any suspected fetal exposure to THALOMID® (thalidomide) must be reported immediately to the FDA *via* the MedWATCH number at 1-800-FDA-1088 and also to Celgene Corporation. The patient should be referred to an obstetrician/gynecologist experienced in reproductive toxicity for further evaluation and counseling.

FEMALE PATIENTS

Thalidomide is contraindicated in WOMEN of childbearing potential unless alternative therapies are considered inappropriate AND the patient MEETS ALL OF THE FOLLOWING CONDITIONS (i.e., she is essentially unable to become pregnant while on thalidomide therapy):

- she understands and can reliably carry out instructions.
- she is capable of complying with the mandatory contraceptive measures, pregnancy testing, patient registration, and patient survey as described in the System for Thalidomide Education and Prescribing Safety (*S.T.E.P.S.*™) program.
- she has received both oral and written warnings of the hazards of taking thalidomide during pregnancy and of exposing a fetus to the drug.
- she has received both oral and written warnings of the risk of possible contraception failure and of the need to use two reliable forms of contraception simultaneously (see **CONTRAINDICATIONS**), unless continuous abstinence from reproductive heterosexual intercourse is the chosen method. (Sexually mature women who have not undergone a hysterectomy or who have not been post-menopausal for at least 24 consecutive months (i.e., who have had menses at some time in the preceding 24 consecutive months) are considered to be women of childbearing potential.).
- she acknowledges, in writing, her understanding of these warnings and of the need for using two reliable methods of contraception for one month prior to starting thalidomide therapy, during thalidomide therapy, and for one month after stopping thalidomide therapy.
- she has had a negative pregnancy test with a sensitivity of at least 50 mIU/mL, within the 24 hours prior to beginning therapy. (See **PRECAUTIONS, CONTRAINDICATIONS.**)
- if the patient is between 12 and 18 years of age, her parent or legal guardian must have read this material and agreed to ensure compliance with the above.

MALE PATIENTS

Thalidomide is contraindicated in sexually mature MALES unless the PATIENT MEETS ALL OF THE FOLLOWING CONDITIONS:

- he understands and can reliably carry out instructions.
- he is capable of complying with the mandatory contraceptive measures that are appropriate for men, patient registration, and patient survey as described in the *S.T.E.P.S.*™ program.
- he has received both oral and written warnings of the hazards of taking thalidomide and exposing a fetus to the drug.
- he has received both oral and written warnings of the risk of possible contraception failure and of the need to use barrier contraception when having sexual intercourse with women of childbearing potential, even if he has undergone successful vasectomy.
- he acknowledges, in writing, his understanding of these warnings and of the need for using barrier contraception (latex condom), even if he has undergone successful vasectomy, when having sexual intercourse with women of childbearing potential. Sexually mature women who have not undergone a hysterectomy or who have not been post-menopausal for at least 24 consecutive months (i.e., who have had menses at some time in the preceding 24 consecutive months) are considered to be women of child-bearing potential.
- if the patient is between 12 and 18 years of age, his parent or legal guardian must have read this material and agreed to ensure compliance with the above.

DESCRIPTION

THALOMID® (thalidomide), α-(N-phthalimido)glutarimide, is an immunomodulatory agent. The empirical formula for thalidomide is $C_{13}H_{10}N_2O_4$ and the gram molecular weight is 258.2. The CAS number of thalidomide is 50-35-1.

Note: • asymmetric carbon atom

Thalidomide is an off-white to white, nearly odorless, crystalline powder that is soluble at 25°C in dimethyl sulfoxide and sparingly soluble in water and ethanol. The glutarimide moiety contains a single asymmetric center and, therefore, may exist in either of two optically active forms designated S-(-) or R-(+). THALOMID® (thalidomide) is an equal mixture of the S-(-) and R-(+) forms and, therefore, has a net optical rotation of zero.

THALOMID® (thalidomide) is available in 50 mg capsules for oral administration. Active ingredient: thalidomide. Inactive ingredients: anhydrous lactose, microcrystalline cellulose, polyvinylpyrrolidone, stearic acid, colloidal anhydrous silica, and gelatin.

CLINICAL PHARMACOLOGY

Mechanism of Action

Thalidomide is an immunomodulatory agent with a spectrum of activity that is not fully characterized. In patients with erythema nodosum leprosum (ENL) the mechanism of action is not fully understood.

Available data from *in vitro* studies and preliminary clinical trials suggest that the immunologic effects of this compound can vary substantially under different conditions, but, may be related to suppression of excessive tumor necrosis factor-alpha (TNF-α) production and down-modulation of selected cell surface adhesion molecules involved in leukocyte migration[3,4,5,6]. For example, administration of thalidomide has been reported to decrease circulating levels of TNF-α in patients with ENL[3], however, it has also been shown to increase plasma TNF-α levels in HIV-seropositive patients[7].

Pharmacokinetics and Drug Metabolism

Absorption

The absolute bioavailability of thalidomide from THALOMID® (thalidomide) capsules has not yet been characterized in human subjects due to its poor aqueous solubility. In studies of both healthy volunteers and subjects with Hansen's disease, the mean time to peak plasma concentrations (T_{max}) of THALOMID® (thalidomide) ranged from 2.9 to 5.7 hours indicating that THALOMID® (thalidomide) is slowly absorbed from the gastrointestinal tract. While the extent of absorption (as measured by area under the curve [AUC]) is proportional to dose in healthy subjects, the observed peak concentration (C_{max}) increased in a less than proportional manner (see Table 1 below). This lack of C_{max} dose proportionality, coupled with the observed increase in T_{max} values, suggests that the poor solubility of thalidomide in aqueous media may be hindering the rate of absorption.

[See table 1 at top of next page]

Co-administration of THALOMID® (thalidomide) with a high fat meal causes minor (<10%) changes in the observed AUC and C_{max} values: however, it causes an increase in T_{max} to approximately 6 hours.

Distribution

It is not known whether thalidomide is present in the ejaculate of males.

The extent of plasma protein binding of thalidomide is unknown.

Metabolism

At the present time, the exact metabolic route and fate of thalidomide is not known in humans. Thalidomide itself does not appear to be hepatically metabolized to any large extent, but appears to undergo non-enzymatic hydrolysis in plasma to multiple metabolites. In a repeat dose study in which THALOMID® (thalidomide) 200 mg was administered to 10 healthy females for 18 days, thalidomide displayed similar pharmacokinetic profiles on the first and last day of dosing. This suggests that thalidomide does not induce or inhibit its own metabolism.

Elimination

As indicated in Table 1 (above) the mean half-life of elimination ranges from approximately 5 to 7 hours following a single dose and is not altered upon multiple dosing. As noted in the metabolism subsection, the precise metabolic fate and route of elimination of thalidomide in humans is not known at this time. Thalidomide itself has a renal clearance of 1.15 mL/minute with less than 0.7% of the dose excreted in the urine as unchanged drug. Following a single dose, urinary levels of thalidomide were undetectable 48 hrs after dosing. Although thalidomide is thought to be hydrolyzed to a number of metabolites[8], only a very small amount (0.02% of the administered dose) of 4-OH-thalidomide was identified in the urine of subjects 12 to 24 hours after dosing.

Pharmacokinetic Data in Special Populations

HIV-seropositive Subjects: There is no apparent significant difference in measured pharmacokinetic parameter values between healthy human subjects and HIV-seropositive subjects following single dose administration of THALOMID® (thalidomide) capsules.

Patients with Hansen's Disease: Analysis of data from a small study in Hansen's patients suggests that these patients, relative to healthy subjects, may have an increased bioavailability of THALOMID® (thalidomide). The increase is reflected both in an increased area under the curve and in increased peak plasma levels. The clinical significance of this increase is unknown.

Patients with Renal Insufficiency: The pharmacokinetics of thalidomide in patients with renal dysfunction have not been determined.

Patients with Hepatic Disease: The pharmacokinetics of thalidomide in patients with hepatic impairment have not been determined.

Continued on next page

Thalomid—Cont.

Age: Analysis of the data from pharmacokinetic studies in healthy volunteers and patients with Hansen's disease ranging in age from 20 to 69 years does not reveal any age-related changes.

Pediatric: No pharmacokinetic data are available in subjects below the age of 18 years.

Gender: While a comparative trial of the effects of gender on thalidomide pharmacokinetic has not been conducted, examination of the data for thalidomide does not reveal any significant gender differences in pharmacokinetic parameter values.

Race: Pharmacokinetic differences due to race have not been studied.

Clinical Studies

The primary data demonstrating the efficacy of thalidomide in the treatment of the cutaneous manifestations of moderate to severe ENL are derived from the published medical literature and from a retrospective study of 102 patients treated by the U.S. Public Health Service.

Two double blind, randomized, controlled trials reported the dermatologic response to a 7 day course of 100 mg thalidomide (four times daily) or control. Dosage was lower for patients under 50 kg in weight.

[See table 2 at right]

Waters[11] reported the results of two studies, both double blind, randomized, placebo controlled, crossover trials in a total of 10 hospitalized, steroid-dependent patients with chronic ENL treated with 100 mg thalidomide or placebo (three times daily). All patients also received dapsone. The primary endpoint was reduction in weekly steroid dosage.

[See table 3 at right]

Data on the efficacy of thalidomide in prevention of ENL relapse were derived from a retrospective evaluation of 102 patients treated with the auspices of the U.S. Public Health Service. A subset of patients with ENL controlled on thalidomide demonstrated repeated relapse upon drug withdrawal and remission with reinstitution of therapy.

Twenty U.S. patients between the ages of 11 and 17 years were treated with thalidomide, generally at 100 mg daily. Response rates and safety profiles were similar to that observed in the adult population.

Thirty-two other published studies containing over 1600 patients consistently report generally successful treatment of the cutaneous manifestations of moderate to severe ENL with thalidomide.

INDICATIONS AND USAGE

THALOMID® (thalidomide) is indicated for the acute treatment of the cutaneous manifestations of moderate to severe erythema nodosum leprosum (ENL). THALOMID® (thalidomide) is not indicated as monotherapy for such ENL treatment in the presence of moderate to severe neuritis.

THALOMID® (thalidomide) is also indicated as maintenance therapy for prevention and suppression of the cutaneous manifestations of ENL recurrence.

CONTRAINDICATIONS (See BOXED WARNINGS.)

Pregnancy: Category X

Due to its known human teratogenicity, even following a single dose, thalidomide is contraindicated in pregnant women and women capable of becoming pregnant. (See **BOXED WARNINGS.**) When there is no alternative treatment, women of childbearing potential may be treated with thalidomide provided adequate precautions are taken to avoid pregnancy. Women must commit either to abstain continuously from heterosexual sexual intercourse or to use two methods of reliable birth control, including at least one highly effective method (*e.g.,* IUD, hormonal contraception, tubal ligation, or partner's vasectomy) and one additional effective method (*e.g.,* latex condom, diaphragm, or cervical cap), beginning 4 weeks prior to initiating treatment with thalidomide, during therapy with thalidomide, and continuing for 4 weeks following discontinuation of thalidomide therapy. If hormonal or IUD contraception is medically contraindicated (see also **PRECAUTIONS: Drug Interactions**), two other effective or highly effective methods may be used. Women of childbearing potential being treated with thalidomide should have pregnancy testing (sensitivity of at least 50 mIU/mL). The test should be performed within the 24 hours before beginning thalidomide therapy and then weekly during the first month of thalidomide therapy, then monthly thereafter in women with regular menstrual cycles or every 2 weeks in women with irregular menstrual cycles. Pregnancy testing and counseling should be performed if a patient misses her period or if there is any abnormality in menstrual bleeding. If pregnancy occurs during thalidomide treatment, thalidomide must be immediately discontinued. Under these conditions, the patient should be referred to an obstetrician/gynecologist experienced in reproductive toxicity for further evaluation and counseling.

THALOMID® (thalidomide) is contraindicated in patients who have demonstrated hypersensitivity to the drug and its components.

WARNINGS (See BOXED WARNINGS.)

Birth defects:

Thalidomide can cause severe birth defects in humans, (See **BOXED WARNINGS** and **CONTRAINDICATIONS.**) Patients should be instructed to take thalidomide only as prescribed and not to share their thalidomide with anyone else. Because it is not known whether or not thalidomide is present in the ejaculate of males receiving the drug, males receiving thalidomide must always use a latex condom when engaging in sexual activity with women of childbearing potential.

Table 1
Pharmacokinetic Parameter Values for THALOMID® (thalidomide) Mean (%CV)

Population/ Single Dose	$AUC_{0-\infty}$ (μg-hr/mL)	C_{max} (μg/mL)	T_{max} (hrs)	Half-life (hrs)
Healthy Subjects (n=14)				
50 mg	4.9 (16%)	0.62 (52%)	2.9 (66%)	5.52 (37%)
200 mg	18.9 (17%)	1.76 (30%)	3.5 (57%)	5.53 (25%)
400 mg	36.4 (26%)	2.82 (28%)	4.3 (37%)	7.29 (36%)
Patients with Hansen's Disease (n=6)				
400 mg	46.4 (44.1%)	3.44 (52.6%)	5.7 (27%)	6.86 (17%)

Table 2
Double Blind, Controlled Clinical Trials of Thalidomide in Patients with ENL: Cutaneous Response

Reference	No. of Patients	No. Treatment Courses*	Percent Responding**	
Iyer *et al.*[9] Bull World Health Organization 1971; 45:719	92	204	Thalidomide 75%	Aspirin 25%
Sheskin *et al.*[10] Int J Lep 1969; 37:135	52	173	Thalidomide 66%	Placebo 10%

*In patients with cutaneous lesions
**Iyer: Complete response or lesions absent
**Sheskin: Complete Improvement + "striking" improvement (i.e., >50% improvement)

Table 3
Double Blind, Controlled Trial of Thalidomide in Patients with ENL: Reduction in Steroid Dosage

Reference	Duration of Treatment	No. of Patients	Number Responding Thalidomide	Placebo
Waters[11]	4 weeks	9	4/5	0/4
Lep Rev 1971; 42:26	6 weeks (crossover)	8	8/8	1/8

Drowsiness and somnolence:

Thalidomide frequently causes drowsiness and somnolence. Patients should be instructed to avoid situations where drowsiness may be a problem and not to take other medications that may cause drowsiness without adequate medical advice. Patients should be advised as to the possible impairment of mental and/or physical abilities required for the performance of hazardous tasks, such as driving a car or operating other complex or dangerous machinery.

Peripheral neuropathy:

Thalidomide is known to cause nerve damage that may be permanent. Peripheral neuropathy is a common, potentially severe, side effect of treatment with thalidomide that may be irreversible. Peripheral neuropathy generally occurs following chronic use over a period of months, however, reports following relatively short term use also exist. The correlation with cumulative dose is unclear. Symptoms may occur some time after thalidomide treatment has been stopped and may resolve slowly or not at all. Few reports of neuropathy have arisen in the treatment of ENL despite long-term thalidomide treatment. However, the inability clinically to differentiate thalidomide neuropathy from the neuropathy often seen in Hansen's disease makes it difficult to determine accurately the incidence of thalidomide-related neuropathy in ENL patients treated with thalidomide.

Patients should be examined at monthly intervals for the first 3 months of thalidomide therapy to enable the clinician to detect early signs of neuropathy, which include numbness, tingling or pain in the hands and feet. Patients should be evaluated periodically thereafter during treatment. Patients should be regularly counseled, questioned, and evaluated for signs or symptoms of peripheral neuropathy. Consideration should be given to electrophysiological testing, consisting of measurement of sensory nerve action potential (SNAP) amplitudes at baseline and thereafter every 6 months in an effort to detect asymptomatic neuropathy. If symptoms of drug-induced neuropathy develop, thalidomide should be discontinued immediately to limit further damage, if clinically appropriate. Usually, treatment with thalidomide should only be reinitiated if the neuropathy returns to baseline status. Medications known to be associated with neuropathy should be used with caution in patients receiving thalidomide.

Dizziness and orthostatic hypotension:

Patients should also be advised that thalidomide may cause dizziness and orthostatic hypotension and that, therefore, they should sit upright for a few minutes prior to standing up from a recumbent position.

Neutropenia:

Decreased white blood cell counts, including neutropenia, have been reported in association with the clinical use of thalidomide. Treatment should not be initiated with an absolute neutrophil count (ANC) of $<750/mm^3$. White blood cell count and differential should be monitored on an ongoing basis, especially in patients who may be more prone to neutropenia, such as patients who are HIV-seropositive. If ANC decreases to below $750/mm^3$ while on treatment, the patient's medication regimen should be re-evaluated and, if the neutropenia persists, consideration should be given to withholding thalidomide if clinically appropriate.

Increased HIV-Viral Load:

If a randomized, placebo controlled trial of thalidomide in an HIV-seropositive patient population, plasma HIV RNA levels were found to increase (median change = 0.42 $\log_{10}$ copies HIV RNA/mL, p = 0.04 compared to placebo)[7]. A similar trend was observed in a second, unpublished study conducted in patients who were HIV-seropositive[12]. The clinical significance of this increase is unknown. Both studies were conducted prior to availability of highly active antiretroviral therapy. Until the clinical significance of this finding is further understood, in HIV-seropositive patients, viral load should be measured after the first and third months of treatment and every 3 months thereafter.

PRECAUTIONS

Hypersensitivity:

Hypersensitivity to THALOMID® (thalidomide) has been reported. Signs and symptoms have included the occurrence of erythematous macular rash, possibly associated with fever, tachycardia, and hypotension, and if severe, may necessitate interruption of therapy. If the reaction recurs when dosing is resumed, THALOMID® (thalidomide) should be discontinued.

Bradycardia:

Bradycardia in association with thalidomide use has been reported. At present there have been no reports of bradycardia requiring medical or other intervention. The clinical significance and underlying etiology of the bradycardia noted in some thalidomide-treated patients are presently unknown.

Stevens-Johnson Syndrome:

Serious dermatologic reactions including Stevens-Johnson syndrome, which may be fatal, have been reported. THALOMID® should be discontinued if a skin rash occurs and only resumed following appropriate clinical evaluation. If the rash is exfoliative, purpuric, or bullous or if Stevens-Johnson syndrome or toxic epidermal necrolysis is suspected, use of THALOMID® should not be resumed.

Information for Patients (See BOXED WARNINGS.)

Patients should be instructed about the potential teratogenicity of thalidomide and the precautions that must be taken to preclude fetal exposure as per the *S.T.E.P.S.*™ program and boxed warnings in this package insert. Patients should be instructed to take thalidomide only as prescribed in compliance with all of the provisions of the *S.T.E.P.S.*™ Restricted Distribution Program.

Patients should be instructed not to share medication with anyone else.

Patients should be instructed that thalidomide frequently causes drowsiness and somnolence. Patients should be instructed to avoid situations where drowsiness may be a problem and not to take other medications that may cause drowsiness without adequate medical advice. Patients should be advised as to the possible impairment of mental and/or physical abilities required for the performance of hazardous tasks, such as driving a car or operating other complex machinery. Patients should be instructed that thalidomide may potentiate the somnolence caused by alcohol.

Patients should be instructed that thalidomide can cause peripheral neuropathies that may be initially signaled by numbness, tingling, or pain or a burning sensation in the feet or hands. Patients should be instructed to report such occurrences to their prescriber immediately.

Patients should also be instructed that thalidomide may cause dizziness and orthostatic hypotension and that, therefore, they should sit upright for a few minutes prior to standing up from a recumbent position.
Patients should be instructed that they are not permitted to donate blood while taking thalidomide. In addition, male patients should be instructed that are not permitted to donate sperm while taking thalidomide.

Laboratory Tests

Pregnancy Testing: **(See BOXED WARNINGS.)** Women of childbearing potential should have pregnancy testing performed (sensitivity of at least 50 mIU/mL). The test should be performed within the 24 hours prior to beginning thalidomide therapy and then weekly during the first month of use, then monthly thereafter in women with regular menstrual cycles or every 2 weeks in women with irregular menstrual cycles. Pregnancy testing should also be performed if a patient misses her period or if there is any abnormality in menstrual bleeding.
Neutropenia: **(See WARNINGS.)**
HIV Viral Load: **(See WARNINGS.)**

Drug Interactions

Thalidomide has been reported to enhance the sedative activity of barbiturates, alcohol, chlorpromazine, and reserpine.
Peripheral Neuropathy: Medications known to be associated with peripheral neuropathy should be used with caution in patients receiving thalidomide.
Oral Contraceptives: In 10 healthy women, the pharmacokinetic profiles of norethindrone and ethinyl estradiol following administration of a single dose containing 1.0 mg of norethindrone acetate and 75 µg of ethinyl estradiol were studied. The results were similar with and without coadministration of thalidomide 200 mg/day to steady-state levels.

Important Non-Thalidomide Drug Interactions

Drugs That Interfere with Hormonal Contraceptives: Concomitant use of HIV-protease inhibitors, griseofulvin, rifampin, rifabutin, phenytoin, or carbamazepine with hormonal contraceptive agents, may reduce the effectiveness of the contraception. Therefore, women requiring treatment with one or more of these drugs must use two OTHER effective or highly effective methods of contraception or abstain from reproductive heterosexual sexual intercourse.

Carcinogenesis, Mutagenesis, Impairment of Fertility

Long-term carcinogenicity tests have not been conducted using thalidomide. Thalidomide gave no evidence of mutagenic effects when assayed in *in vitro* bacterial (*Salmonella typhimurium* and *Escherichia coli*; Ames mutagenicity test), *in vitro* mammalian (AS52 Chinese hampster ovary cells; AS52/XPRT mammalian cell forward gene mutation assay) and *in vivo* mammalian (CD-1 mice; *in vivo* micronucleus test) test systems.
Animal studies to characterize the effects of thalidomide on fertility have not been conducted.

Pregnancy

Pregnancy Category X: **See BOXED WARNINGS and CONTRAINDICATIONS.**
Because of the known human teratogenicity of thalidomide, thalidomide is contraindicated in women who are or may become pregnant and who are not using the two required types of birth control or who are not continually abstaining from reproductive heterosexual sexual intercourse. If thalidomide is taken during pregnancy, it can cause severe birth defects or death to an unborn baby. Thalidomide should never be used by women who are pregnant or who could become pregnant while taking the drug. Even a single dose [1 capsule (50 mg)] taken by a pregnant women can cause birth defects. If pregnancy does occur during treatment, the drug should be immediately discontinued. Under these conditions, the patient should be referred to an obstetrician/gynecologist experienced in reproductive toxicity for further evaluation and counselling. Any suspected fetal exposure to THALOMID® (thalidomide) must be reported to the FDA *via* the MedWatch program at 1-800-FDA-1088 and also to Celgene Corporation.
Animal studies to characterize the effects of thalidomide on late stage pregnancy have not been conducted.

Use in Nursing Mothers

It is not known whether thalidomide is excreted in human milk. Because many drugs are excreted in human milk and because of the potential for serious adverse reactions in nursing infants from thalidomide, a decision should be made whether to discontinue nursing or to discontinue the drug, taking into account the importance of the drug to the mother.

Pediatric Use

Safety and effectiveness in pediatric patients below the age of 12 years have not been established.

Geriatric Use

No systemic studies in geriatric patients have been conducted. Thalidomide has been used in clinical trials in patients up to 90 years of age. Adverse events in patients over the age of 65 years did not appear to differ in kind from those reported in younger individuals

ADVERSE REACTIONS

The most serious toxicity associated with thalidomide is its documented human teratogenicity. (See **BOXED WARNINGS** and **CONTRAINDICATIONS**). The risk of severe birth defects, primarily phocomelia or death to the fetus, is extremely high during the critical period of pregnancy. The critical period is estimated, depending on the source of information, to range from 35 to 50 days after the last menstrual period. The risk of other potentially severe birth defects outside this critical period is unknown, but may be significant. Based on present knowledge, thalidomide must not be used at any time during pregnancy.

Table 4
Summary of Adverse Events (AEs)
Reported in Celgene-sponsored Controlled Clinical Trials

Body System/Adverse Event	All AEs Reported in ENL Patients	AEs Reported in ≥3 HIV-seropositive Patients Thalidomide		Placebo
	50 to 300 mg/day (N=24)	100 mg/day (N=36)	200 mg/day (N=32)	(N=35)
Body as a Whole	**16 (66.7%)**	**18 (50.0%)**	**19 (59.4%)**	**13 (37.1%)**
Abdominal pain	1 (4.2%)	1 (2.8%)	1 (3.1%)	4 (11.4%)
Accidental injury	1 (4.2%)	2 (5.6%)	0	1 (2.9%)
Asthenia	2 (8.3%)	2 (5.6%)	7 (21.9%)	1 (2.9%)
Back pain	1 (4.2%)	2 (5.6%)	0	0
Chills	1 (4.2%)	0	3 (9.4%)	4 (11.4%)
Facial edema	1 (4.2%)	0	0	0
Fever	0	7 (19.4%)	7 (21.9%)	6 (17.1%)
Headache	3 (12.5%)	6 (16.7%)	6 (18.7%)	4 (11.4%)
Infection	0	3 (8.3%)	2 (6.3%)	1 (2.9%)
Malaise	2 (8.3%)	0	0	0
Neck pain	1 (4.2%)	0	0	0
Neck rigidity	1 (4.2%)	0	0	0
Pain	2 (8.3%)	0	1 (3.1%)	2 (5.7%)
Digestive System	**5 (20.8%)**	**16 (44.4%)**	**16 (50.0%)**	**15 (42.9%)**
Anorexia	0	1 (2.8%)	3 (9.4%)	2 (5.7%)
Constipation	1 (4.2%)	1 (2.8%)	3 (9.4%)	0
Diarrhea	1 (4.2%)	4 (11.1%)	6 (18.7%)	6 (17.1%)
Dry mouth	0	3 (8.3%)	3 (9.4%)	2 (5.7%)
Flatulence	0	3 (8.3%)	0	2 (5.7%)
Liver function tests multiple abnormalities	0	0	3 (9.4%)	0
Nausea	1 (4.2%)	0	4 (12.5%)	1 (2.9%)
Oral moniliasis	1 (4.2%)	4 (11.1%)	2 (6.3%)	0
Tooth pain	1 (4.2%)	0	0	0
Hemic and Lymphatic	**0**	**8 (22.2%)**	**13 (40.6%)**	**10 (28.6%)**
Anemia	0	2 (5.6%)	4 (12.5%)	3 (8.6%)
Leukopenia	0	6 (16.7%)	8 (25.0%)	3 (8.6%)
Lymphadenopathy	0	2 (5.6%)	4 (12.5%)	3 (8.6%)
Metabolic and Endocrine Disorders	**1 (4.2%)**	**8 (22.2%)**	**12 (37.5%)**	**8 (22.9%)**
Edema peripheral	1 (4.2%)	3 (8.3%)	1 (3.1%)	0
Hyperlipemia	0	2 (5.6%)	3 (9.4%)	1 (2.9%)
SGOT increased	0	1 (2.8%)	4 (12.5%)	2 (5.7%)
Nervous System	**13 (54.2%)**	**19 (52.8%)**	**18 (56.3%)**	**12 (34.3%)**
Agitation	0	0	3 (9.4%)	0
Dizziness	1 (4.2%)	7 (19.4%)	6 (18.7%)	0
Insomnia	0	0	3 (9.4%)	2 (5.7%)
Nervousness	0	1 (2.8%)	3 (9.4%)	0
Neuropathy	0	3 (8.3%)	0	0
Paresthesia	0	2 (5.6%)	5 (15.6%)	4 (11.4%)
Somnolence	9 (37.5%)	13 (36.1%)	12 (37.5%)	4 (11.4%)
Tremor	1 (4.2%)	0	0	0
Vertigo	2 (8.3%)	0	0	0
Respiratory System	**3 (12.5%)**	**9 (25.0%)**	**6 (18.7%)**	**9 (25.7%)**
Pharyngitis	1 (4.2%)	3 (8.3%)	2 (6.3%)	2 (5.7%)
Rhinitis	1 (4.2%)	0	0	4 (11.4%)
Sinusitis	1 (4.2%)	3 (8.3%)	1 (3.1%)	2 (5.7%)
Skin and Appendages	**10 (41.7%)**	**17 (47.2%)**	**18 (56.3%)**	**19 (54.3%)**
Acne	0	4 (11.1%)	1 (3.1%)	0
Dermatitis fungal	1 (4.2%)	2 (5.6%)	3 (9.4%)	0
Nail disorder	1 (4.2%)	0	1 (3.1%)	0
Pruritus	2 (8.3%)	1 (2.8%)	2 (6.3%)	2 (5.7%)
Rash	5 (20.8%)	9 (25.0%)	8 (25.0%)	11 (31.4%)
Rash maculo-papular	1 (4.2%)	6 (16.7%)	6 (18.7%)	2 (5.7%)
Sweating	0	0	4 (12.5%)	4 (11.4%)
Urogenital System	**2 (8.3%)**	**6 (16.7%)**	**2 (6.3%)**	**4 (11.4%)**
Albuminuria	0	3 (8.3%)	1 (3.1%)	2 (5.7%)
Hematuria	0	4 (11.1%)	0	1 (2.9%)
Impotence	2 (8.3%)	1 (2.8%)	0	0

Thalidomide is associated with drowsiness/somnolence, peripheral neuropathy, dizziness/orthostatic hypotension, neutropenia, and HIV viral load increase. **(See WARNINGS.)**
Hypersensitivity to THALOMID® (thalidomide) and bradycardia in patients treated with thalidomide have been reported. **(See PRECAUTIONS.)**
Somnolence, dizziness, and rash are the most commonly observed adverse events associated with the use of thalidomide. Thalidomide has been studied in controlled and uncontrolled clinical trials in patients with ENL and in people who are HIV-seropositive. In addition, thalidomide has been administered investigationally for more than 20 years in numerous indications. Adverse event profiles from these uses are summarized in the sections that follow.

Other Adverse Events:

Due to the nature of the longitudinal data that form the basis of this product's safety evaluation, no determination has been made of the causal relationship between the reported adverse events listed below and thalidomide. These lists are of various adverse events noted by investigators in patients to whom they had administered thalidomide under various conditions.

Incidence in Controlled Clinical Trials

Table 4 lists treatment-emergent signs and symptoms that occurred in THALOMID® (thalidomide)-treated patients in controlled clinical trials in ENL. Doses ranged from 50 to 300 mg/day. All adverse events were mild to moderate in severity, and none resulted in discontinuation. Table 4 also lists treatment-emegent adverse events that occurred in at least 3 of the THALOMID® (thalidomide)-treated HIV-seropositive patients who participated in an 8-week, placebo controlled clinical trial. Events that were more frequent in the placebo-treated group are not included. (**See WARNINGS, PRECAUTIONS**, and **DRUG INTERACTIONS**.)
[See table 4 above]

Other Adverse Events Observed in ENL Patients

Thalidomide in doses up to 400 mg/day has been administered investigationally in the United States over a 19-year period in 1465 patients with ENL. The published literature describes the treatment of an additional 1678 patients. To provide a meaningful estimate of the proportion of the individuals having adverse events, similar types of events were grouped into a smaller number of standardized categories using a modified COSTART dictionary/terminology. These categories are used in the listing below. All reported events are included except those already listed in the previous table. Due to the fact that these data were collected from uncontrolled studies, the incidence rate cannot be determined. As mentioned previously, **no causal relationship between thalidomide and these events can be conclusively determined at this time.**
These are reports of all adverse events noted by investigators in patients to whom they had administered thalidomide.
Body as a Whole: Abdomen enlarged, fever, photosensitivity, upper extremity pain.
Cardiovascular System: Bradycardia, hypertension, hypotension, peripheral vascular disorder, tachycardia.
Digestive System: Anorexia, appetite increase/weight gain, dry mouth, dyspepsia, enlarged liver, eructation, flatulence, increased liver function tests, intestinal obstruction, vomiting.
Hemic and Lymphatic: ESR decrease, eosinophilia, granulocytopenia, hypochromic anemia, leukemia, leukocytosis, leukopenia, MCV elevated, RBC abnormal, spleen palpable, thrombocytopenia.

Continued on next page

Thalomid—Cont.

Metabolic and Endocrine: ADH inappropriate, alkaline phosphatase, amyloidosis, bilirubinemia, BUN increased, creatinine increased, cyanosis, diabetes, edema, electrolyte abnormalities, hyperglycemia, hyperkalemia, hyperuricemia, hypocalcemia, hypoproteinemia, LDH increased, phosphorus decreased, SGPT increased.
Muscular Skeletal: Arthritis, bone tenderness, hypertonia, joint disorder, leg cramps, myalgia, myasthenia, periosteal disorder.
Nervous System: Abnormal thinking, agitation, amnesia, anxiety, causalgia, circumoral paresthesia, confusion, depression, euphoria, hyperesthesia, insomnia, nervousness, neuralgia, neuritis, neuropathy, paresthesia, peripheral neuritis, psychosis, vasodilation.
Respiratory System: Cough, emphysema, epistaxis, pulmonary embolus, rales, upper respiratory infection, voice alteration.
Skin and Appendages: Acne, alopecia, dry skin, eczematous rash, exfoliative dermatitis, ichtyosis, perifollicular thickening, skin necrosis, seborrhea, sweating, urticaria, vesiculobullous rash.
Special Senses: Amblyopia, deafness, dry eye, eye pain, tinnitus.
Urogenital: Decreased creatinine clearance, hematuria, orchitis, proteinuria, pyuria, urinary frequency.

Other Adverse Events Observed in HIV-seropositive Patients

In addition to controlled clinical trials, THALOMID® (thalidomide) has been used in uncontrolled studies in 145 patients. Less frequent adverse events that have been reported in these HIV-seropositive patients treated with THALOMID® (thalidomide) were grouped into a smaller number of standardized categories using modified COSTART dictionary/terminology and these categories are used in the listing below. Adverse events that have already been included in the tables and narrative above, or that are too general to be informative are not listed.
Body as a Whole Ascites, AIDS, allergic reaction, cellulitis, chest pain, chills and fever, cyst, decreased CD4 count, facial edema, flu syndrome, hernia, hormone level altered, moniliasis, photosensitivity reaction, sarcoma, sepsis, viral infection.
Cardiovascular System: Angina pectoris, arrhythmia, atrial fibrillation, bradycardia, cerebral ischemia, cerebrovascular accident, congestive heart failure, deep thrombophlebitis, heart arrest, heart failure, hypertension, hypotension, murmur, myocardial infarct, palpitation, pericarditis, peripheral vascular disorder, postural hypotension, syncope, tachycardia, thrombophlebitis, thrombosis.
Digestive System: Cholangitis, cholestatic jaundice, colitis, dyspepsia, dysphagia, esophagitis, gastroenteritis, gastrointestinal disorder, gastrointestinal hemorrhage, gum disorder, hepatitis, pancreatitis, parotid gland enlargement, periodontitis, stomatitis, tongue discoloration, tooth disorder.
Hemic and Lymphatic: Aplastic anemia, macrocytic anemia, megaloblastic anemia, microcytic anemia.
Metabolic and Endocrine: Avitaminosis, bilirubinemia, dehydration, hypercholesteremia, hypoglycemia, increased alkaline phosphatase, increased lipase, increased serum creatinine, peripheral edema.
Muscular Skeletal: Myalgia, myasthenia.
Nervous System: Abnormal gait, ataxia, decreased libido, decreased reflexes, dementia, dysesthesia, dyskinesia, emotional lability, hostility, hypalgesia, hyperkinesia, incoordination, meningitis, neurologic disorder, tremor, vertigo.
Respiratory System: Apnea, bronchitis, lung disorder, lung edema, pneumonia (including *Pneumocystis carinii* pneumonia), rhinitis.

Skin and Appendages: Angioedema, benign skin neoplasm, eczema, herpes simplex, incomplete Stevens-Johnson syndrome, nail disorder, pruritus, psoriasis, skin discoloration, skin disorder.
Special Senses: Conjunctivitis, eye disorder, lacrimination disorder, retinitis, taste perversion.

Other Adverse Events in the Published Literature or Reported from Other Sources

The following additional events have been identified either in the published literature or from spontaneous reports from other sources: acute renal failure, amenorrhea, aphthous stomatitis, bile duct obstruction, carpal tunnel, chronic myelogenous leukemia, diplopia, dysesthesia, dyspnea, enuresis, erythema nodosum, erythroleukemia, foot drop, galactorrhea, gynecomastia, hangover effect, hypomagnesemia, hypothroidism, lymphedema, lymphopenia, metrorrhagia, migraine, myxedema, nodular sclerosing Hodgkin's disease, nystagmus, oliguria, pancytopenia, petechiae, purpura, Raynaud's syndrome, stomach ulcer, and suicide attempt.

DRUG ABUSE AND DEPENDENCE

Physical and psychological dependence has not been reported in patients taking thalidomide. However, as with other tranquilizers/hypnotics, thalidomide too has been reported to create in patients habituation to its soporific effects.

OVERDOSAGE

There have been three cases of overdose reported, all attempted suicides. There have been no reported fatalities in doses up to 14.4 grams, and all patients recovered without reported squelae.

DOSAGE AND ADMINISTRATION

THALOMID® (thalidomide) MUST ONLY BE ADMINISTERED IN COMPLIANCE WITH ALL OF THE TERMS OUTLINED IN THE *S.T.E.P.S.*™ PROGRAM. THALOMID® (thalidomide) MAY ONLY BE PRESCRIBED BY PRESCRIBERS REGISTERED WITH THE *S.T.E.P.S.*™ PROGRAM AND MAY ONLY BE DISPENSED BY PHARMACISTS REGISTERED WITH THE *S.T.E.P.S.*™ PROGRAM.

Drug prescribing to women of childbearing potential should be contingent upon initial and continued confirmed negative results of pregnancy testing.

For an episode of cutaneous ENL, THALOMID® (thalidomide) dosing should be initiated at 100 to 300 mg/day, administered once daily with water, preferably at bedtime and at least 1 hour after the evening meal. Patients weighing less than 50 kilograms should be started at the low end of the dose range.

In patients with a severe cutaneous ENL reaction, or in those who have previously required higher doses to control the reaction, THALOMID® (thalidomide) dosing may be initiated at higher doses up to 400 mg/day once daily at bedtime or in divided doses with water, at least 1 hour after meals.

In patients with moderate to severe neuritis associated with a severe ENL reaction, corticosteroids may be started concomitantly with THALOMID® (thalidomide). Steroid usage can be tapered and discontinued when the neuritis has ameliorated.

Dosing with THALOMID® (thalidomide) should usually continue until signs and symptoms of active reaction have subsided, usually a period of at least 2 weeks. Patients may then be tapered off medication in 50 mg decrements every 2 to 4 weeks.

Patients who have a documented history of requiring prolonged maintenance to prevent the recurrence of cutaneous ENL or who flare during tapering, should be maintained on the minimum dose necessary to control the reaction. Tapering off medication should be attempted every 3 to 6 months, in decrements of 50 mg every 2 to 4 weeks.

HOW SUPPLIED

(THIS PRODUCT IS ONLY SUPPLIED TO PHARMACISTS REGISTERED WITH THE *S.T.E.P.S.*™ PROGRAM—See BOXED WARNINGS.)

THALOMID® (thalidomide) is supplied in hard gelatin, 50 mg capsules [white opaque], imprinted "Celgene" with a "do not get pregnant" logo.

Boxes of 140 containing 10 prescription packs of 14 capsules each (NDC 59572-105-92).

Boxes of 280 containing 10 prescription packs of 28 capsules each (NDC 59572-105-93).

STORAGE AND DISPENSING

PHARMACISTS NOTE:

DRUG MUST ONLY BE DISPENSED IN NO MORE THAN A 1-MONTH SUPPLY AND ONLY ON PRESENTATION OF A NEW PRESCRIPTION WRITTEN WITHIN THE PREVIOUS 7 DAYS. SPECIFIC INFORMED CONSENT (copy attached as part of this package insert) AND COMPLIANCE WITH THE MANDATORY PATIENT REGISTRY AND SURVEY ARE REQUIRED FOR ALL PATIENTS (MALE AND FEMALE) PRIOR TO DISPENSING BY THE PHARMACIST.

This drug must not be packaged.

Store at 59 to 86°F; 15 to 30°C. Protect from light.

Rx only and only able to be prescribed and dispensed under the terms of the *S.T.E.P.*™ Restricted Distribution Program

Manufactured for Celgene Corporation
7 Powder Horn Drive
Warren, New Jersey 07059

Important Information and Warnings For All Patients Taking THALOMID® (thalidomide)

WARNING: SERIOUS HUMAN BIRTH DEFECTS
IF THALIDOMIDE IS TAKEN DURING PREGNANCY, IT CAN CAUSE SEVERE BIRTH DEFECTS OR DEATH TO AN UNBORN BABY. THALIDOMIDE SHOULD NEVER BE USED BY WOMEN WHO ARE PREGNANT OR WHO COULD BECOME PREGNANT WHILE TAKING THE DRUG. EVEN A SINGLE DOSE [1 CAPSULE (50 mg)] TAKEN BY A PREGNANT WOMAN CAN CAUSE SEVERE BIRTH DEFECTS.

CONSENT FOR WOMEN:

INIT:____ 1. I understand that I must not take THALOMID® (thalidomide) if I am pregnant, breast-feeding a baby, or able to get pregnant and not using the required two methods of birth control.

INIT:____ 2. I understand that severe birth defects can occur with the use of THALOMID® (thalidomide). I have been warned by my doctor that my unborn baby will almost certainly have serious birth defects or may even die if I am pregnant or become pregnant while taking THALOMID® (thalidomide).

INIT:____ 3. I understand that if I am able to become pregnant, I must use at least one highly effective method and one additional effective method of birth control (contraception) AT THE SAME TIME:

At least one highly effective method		One additional effective method
IUD	AND	Latex condom
Hormonal (birth control pills, injections, or implants)		Diaphragm
Tubal ligation		Cervical cap
Partner's vasectomy		

These birth control methods must be used for at least 4 weeks before starting THALOMID® (thalidomide) therapy, all during THALOMID® (thalidomide) therapy, and for at least 4 weeks after THALOMID® (thalidomide) therapy has stopped. I must use these methods even if I am infertile, unless I have had a hysterectomy or because I have been post-menopausal for at least 24 months (been through the changes of life). The only exception is if I completely avoid heterosexual sexual intercourse. If a hormonal (birth control pills, injections, or implants) or IUD method is not medically possible for me, I may use another highly effective method or two barrier methods AT THE SAME TIME.

INIT:____ 4. I know that I must have a pregnancy test done by my doctor within the 24 hours prior to starting THALOMID® (thalidomide) therapy, then every week during the first 4 weeks of THALOMID® (thalidomide) therapy. I will then have a pregnancy test every 4 weeks if I have regular menstrual cycles, or every 2 weeks if my cycles are irregular while I am taking THALOMID® (thalidomide).

INIT:____ 5. I know that I must immediately stop taking THALOMID® (thalidomide) and inform my doctor if I become pregnant while taking the drug; if I miss my menstrual period, or experience unusual menstrual bleeding; stop using birth control; or think, FOR ANY REASON, that I may be pregnant. If my doctor is not available, I can call 1-888-668-2528 for information on emergency contraception.

INIT:____ 6. I am not now pregnant, nor will I try to become pregnant for at least 4 weeks after I have completely finished taking THALOMID® (thalidomide).

INIT:____ 7. I understand that THALOMID® (thalidomide) will be prescribed ONLY for me. I must NOT share it with ANYONE, even someone who has symptoms similar to mine. It must be kept out of the reach of children and should never be given to women who are able to have children.

INIT:____ 8. I have read the THALOMID® (thalidomide) patient brochure and/or viewed the videotape, "Important Information for Men and Women Taking THALOMID® (thalidomide)". I understand the contents, including other possible health problems from THALOMID® (thalidomide), so-called "side effects". I know that I cannot donate blood while taking THALOMID® (thalidomide).

INIT:____ 9. My doctor has answered any questions I have asked.

INIT:____ 10. I understand that I must participate in a survey and patient registry while I am on THALOMID® (thalidomide), which will require completing additional forms.

CONSENT FOR MEN:

INIT:____ 1. I understand that I must not take THALOMID® (thalidomide) if I cannot avoid unprotected sex with a woman, even if I have had a successful vasectomy.

INIT:____ 2. I understand that severe birth defects or death to an unborn baby have occurred when women took thalidomide during pregnancy.

INIT:____ 3. I have been told by my doctor that I must NEVER have unprotected sex with a woman because it is not known if the drug is present in semen or sperm. My doctor has explained that I must either completely avoid heterosexual sexual intercourse or I must use a latex condom EVERY TIME I have sexual intercourse with a female partner while I am taking THALOMID® (thalidomide) – and for 4 weeks after I stop taking the drug, even if I have had a successful vasectomy.

INIT:____ 4. I also know that I must inform my doctor if I have had unprotected sex with a woman; or if I think, FOR ANY REASON, that my sexual partner may be pregnant. If my doctor is not available, I can call 1-888-668-2528 for information on emergency contraception.

INIT:____5. I understand that THALOMID® (thalidomide) will be prescribed ONLY for me. I must NOT share it with ANYONE, even someone who has symptoms similar to mine. It must be kept out of the reach of children and should never be given to women who are able to have children.

INIT:____6. I have read the THALOMID® (thalidomide) patient brochure and/or viewed the videotape, "Important Information for Men and Women Taking THALOMID® (thalidomide)". I understand the contents, including other possible health problems from THALOMID® (thalidomide), so-called "side effects". I know that I cannot donate blood or semen while taking THALOMID® (thalidomide).

INIT:____7. My doctor has answered any questions I have asked.

INIT:____8. I understand that I must participate in a survey and patient registry while I am on THALOMID® (thalidomide), which will require completing additional forms.

Authorization:

This information has been read aloud to me in the language of my choice. I understand that if I do not follow all of my doctor's instructions, I will not be able to receive THALOMID® (thalidomide). I now authorize my doctor to begin my treatment with THALOMID® (thalidomide).

Patient Name (please print)	Social Security No. (Only last six digits required)	Date of Birth (mo./day/yr.)

Patient, Parent/ Guardian Signature	Date (mo./day/yr.)

I have fully explained to the patient the nature, purpose, and risks of the treatment described above, especially the risks to women of childbearing potential. I have asked the patient if she/he has any questions regarding her/his treatment with THALOMID® (thalidomide) and have answered those questions to the best of my ability. I will ensure that the appropriate components of the patient consent form are completed. In addition, I will comply with all of my obligations and responsibilities as a prescriber registered under the *S.T.E.P.S.*™ restricted distribution program.

Physician Name (please print)	DEA No.

Physician Signature	Date (mo./day/yr.)

REFERENCES

1. Manson JM. 1986. Teratogenicity. Cassarett and Doull's Toxicology: The Basic Science of Poisons. Third Edition. Pages 195–220. New York: MacMillan Publishing Co.
2. Smithels RW and Newman CG. 1992. J. Med. Genet. 29(10):716–723.
3. Sampaio EP, Kaplan G, Miranda A, *et al.* 1993. J. Infect. Dis. 168(2):408–414.
4. Sarno EN, Grau GE, Vieira LM, *et al.* 1991. Clin. Exp. Immunol. 84:103–108.
5. Sampaio EP, Moreira AL, Sarno EN, *et al.* 1992. J. Exp. Med. 175:1729–1737.
6. Nogueira AC, Neubert R, Helge H, *et al.* 1994. Life Sciences. 55(2):77–92.
7. Jacobson JM, Greenspan JS, Spritzler J, *et al.* 1997. New Eng. J. Med. 336(21):1487–1493.
8. Schumaker H, Smith RL, and Williams RT. 1965. Br. J. Pharmacol. 25:324–337.
9. Iyer CGS, Languillon J, Ramanujam K, *et al.* 1971. Bull. WHO. 45:719–732.
10. Sheskin J and Convit J. 1969. Intl. J. Leprosy. 37:135–146.
11. Waters MFR. 1971. Lepr. Rev. 42:26–42.
12. Unpublished data, on file at Celgene.

THALPI.003 11/99 CG

Shown in Product Identification Guide, page 310

For EMERGENCY telephone numbers, consult the **Manufacturers' Index**.

Centocor, Inc.

200 GREAT VALLEY PARKWAY
MALVERN, PA 19355

Direct General Inquiries to:
Ph: (610) 651-6000
(888) 874-3083
Fax: (610) 651-6100

Medical Emergency Contact:
Ph: 1-800-457-6399

For Medical Information/Adverse Experience Reporting Contact:
Medical Information & Product Surveillance
Ph: (800) 457-6399
Fax: (610) 651-6197

REMICADE® ℞
INFLIXIMAB
recombinant
For IV Injection

DESCRIPTION

REMICADE® (infliximab) is a chimeric $IgG1_{\kappa}$ monoclonal antibody with an approximate molecular weight of 149,100 daltons. It is composed of human constant and murine variable regions. Infliximab binds specifically to human tumor necrosis factor alpha (TNFα) with an association constant of 10^{10} M^{-1}. Infliximab is produced by a recombinant cell line cultured by continuous perfusion and is purified by a series of steps that includes measures to inactivate and remove viruses.

REMICADE is supplied as a sterile, white, lyophilized powder for intravenous infusion. Following reconstitution with 10 mL of Sterile Water for Injection, USP, the resulting pH is approximately 7.2. Each single-use vial contains 100 mg infliximab, 500 mg sucrose, 0.5 mg polysorbate 80, 2.2 mg monobasic sodium phosphate and 6.1 mg dibasic sodium phosphate. No preservatives are present.

CLINICAL PHARMACOLOGY

General

Infliximab neutralizes the biological activity of TNFα by binding with high affinity to the soluble and transmembrane forms of TNFα and inhibits binding of TNFα with its receptors.[1–4] Infliximab does not neutralize TNFβ (lymphotoxin α), a related cytokine that utilizes the same receptors as TNFα. Biological activities attributed to TNFα include: induction of pro-inflammatory cytokines such as IL-1 and IL-6, enhancement of leukocyte migration by increasing endothelial layer permeability and expression of adhesion molecules by endothelial cells and leukocytes, activation of neutrophil and eosinophil functional activity, induction of acute phase reactants and other liver proteins, as well as tissue degrading enzymes produced by synoviocytes and/or chondrocytes. Cells expressing transmembrane TNFα bound by infliximab can be lysed *in vitro* by complement or effector cells.[2] Infliximab inhibits the functional activity of TNFα in a wide variety of *in vitro* bioassays utilizing human fibroblasts, endothelial cells, neutrophils,[3] B and T lymphocytes and epithelial cells. Anti-TNFα antibodies reduce disease activity in the cotton-top tamarin colitis model, and decrease synovitis and joint erosions in a murine model of collagen-induced arthritis. Infliximab prevents disease in transgenic mice that develop polyarthritis as a result of constitutive expression of human TNFα, and, when administered after disease onset, allows eroded joints to heal.

Pharmacodynamics

Elevated concentrations of TNFα have been found in the joints of rheumatoid arthritis patients[5] and the stools of Crohn's disease patients[6] and correlate with elevated disease activity. In Crohn's disease, treatment with REMICADE reduced infiltration of inflammatory cells and TNFα production in inflamed areas of the intestine, and reduced the proportion of mononuclear cells from the lamina propria able to express TNFα and interferon γ.[4] In rheumatoid arthritis, treatment with REMICADE reduced infiltration of inflammatory cells into inflamed areas of the joint as well as expression of molecules mediating cellular adhesion [E-selectin, intercellular adhesion molecule-1 (ICAM-1) and vascular cell adhesion molecule-1 (VCAM-1)], chemoattraction [interleukin 8 (IL-8) and monocyte chemotactic protein (MCP-1)] and tissue degradation [matrix metalloproteinase (MMP) 1 and 3].[4] After treatment with REMICADE, patients with Crohn's disease or rheumatoid arthritis exhibited decreased levels of serum interleukin 6 (IL-6) and C-reactive protein (CRP) compared to baseline. Peripheral blood lymphocytes from REMICADE-treated patients showed no significant decrease in number or in proliferative responses to *in vitro* mitogenic stimulation when compared to cells from untreated patients.

Pharmacokinetics

Single intravenous infusions of 1 to 20 mg/kg showed a predictable and linear relationship between the dose administered and the maximum serum concentration and area under the concentration-time curve. The volume of distribution at steady state was independent of dose and indicated that infliximab was distributed primarily within the vascular compartment. Median pharmacokinetic results for the recommended doses of 3 mg/kg in rheumatoid arthritis and 5 mg/kg in Crohn's disease indicate that the terminal half-life of infliximab is 8.0 to 9.5 days.

Following an initial dose of REMICADE, repeated infusions at 2 and 6 weeks in fistulizing Crohn's disease and rheumatoid arthritis patients resulted in predictable concentration-time profiles following each treatment. No systemic accumulation of infliximab occurred upon continued repeated treatment with 3 mg/kg or 10 mg/kg at 4- or 8-week intervals in rheumatoid arthritis patients or patients with moderate or severe Crohn's disease retreated with 4 infusions of 10 mg/kg REMICADE at 8-week intervals. No major differences in clearance or volume of distribution were observed in patient subgroups defined by age or weight. It is not known if there are differences in clearance or volume of distribution between gender subgroups or in patients with marked impairment of hepatic or renal function.

CLINICAL STUDIES

Rheumatoid Arthritis

The safety and efficacy of REMICADE when given in conjunction with methotrexate (MTX) were assessed in a multicenter, randomized, double-blind, placebo-controlled study of 428 patients with active rheumatoid arthritis despite treatment with MTX (the Anti-TNF Trial in Rheumatoid Arthritis with Concomitant Therapy or ATTRACT). The median age of patients enrolled was 54 years, with a median duration of disease of 8.4 years and a median number of swollen and tender joints of 20 and 31 respectively. All patients were to have received MTX for ≥ 6 months and be on a stable dose ≥ 12.5 mg/week for 4 weeks prior to study. All REMICADE and placebo groups continued their stable dose of MTX and folic acid.

In addition to MTX, patients received placebo, 3 mg/kg or 10 mg/kg of REMICADE by intravenous infusion at weeks 0, 2 and 6 followed by additional infusions every four or eight weeks thereafter. Concurrent use of stable doses of oral corticosteroids (10 mg/day) and/or nonsteroidal anti-inflammatory drugs was also permitted. The primary endpoint was the proportion of patients at week 30 who attained an improvement in signs and symptoms as measured by the American College of Rheumatology criteria, (ACR 20). An ACR 20 response is defined as at least a 20% improvement in both tender and swollen joint counts and in 3 of the following 5 criteria: physician global assessment, patient global assessment, functional/disability measure, visual analog pain scale and erythrocyte sedimentation rate (ESR) or CRP.

At week 30, 43/86 (50%) of patients treated every 8 weeks with 3 mg/kg of REMICADE plus MTX attained an ACR 20 compared with 18/88 (20%) of patients treated with placebo plus MTX (p<0.001). Higher doses and/or more frequent administrations did not result in higher response rates. Results are shown in Figure 1.

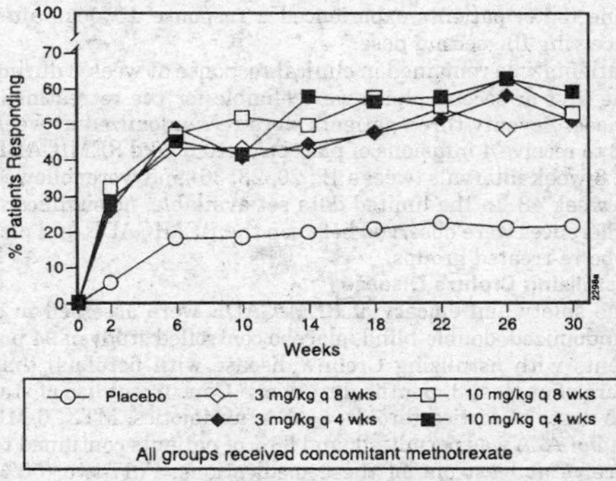

Figure 1. Percentage of Patients who Achieved an ACR 20.

At week 30, the ACR 50 response was 27% for patients treated with 3 mg/kg REMICADE (infliximab) every 8 weeks plus MTX, compared to 5% for patients treated with placebo plus MTX (p<0.001). The ACR 70 response was 8% for patients treated with 3 mg/kg REMICADE every 8 weeks plus MTX and 0% for patients treated with placebo plus MTX. Patients receiving 3 mg/kg REMICADE every 8 weeks demonstrated superior improvement in all ACR response components except HAQ compared to patients treated with placebo plus MTX (Table 1). Data on use of REMICADE without concurrent MTX are limited (see *PRECAUTIONS, Immunogenicity*).[7,8]

[See table 1 at top of next page]

Active Crohn's Disease

The safety and efficacy of REMICADE were assessed in a randomized, double-blind, placebo-controlled dose ranging study of 108 patients with moderate to severe active Crohn's disease[9] [Crohn's Disease Activity Index (CDAI) ≥220≤400]. All patients had experienced an inadequate response to prior conventional therapies, including corticosteroids (60% of patients), 5-aminosalicylates (5-ASA) (60%) and/or 6-mercaptopurine/azathioprine (6-MP/AZA) (37%). Concurrent use of stable dose regimens of corticosteroids, 5-ASA, 6-MP and/or AZA was permitted and 92% of patients continued to receive at least one of these medications.

The study was divided into three phases. In the first phase, patients were randomized to receive a single intravenous

Continued on next page

Remicade—Cont.

(IV) dose of placebo, 5, 10 or 20 mg/kg of REMICADE. The primary endpoint was the proportion of patients who experienced a clinical response, defined as a decrease in CDAI by ≥70 points from baseline at the 4-week evaluation and without an increase in Crohn's disease medications or surgery for Crohn's disease. Patients who responded at week 4 were followed to week 12. Secondary endpoints included the proportion of patients who were in clinical remission at week 4 (CDAI <150), and clinical response over time.

At week 4, four of twenty-five (16%) of the placebo patients achieved a clinical response vs. twenty-two of twenty-seven (82%) of the patients receiving 5 mg/kg REMICADE ($p < 0.001$, two-sided, Fisher's Exact test). One of twenty-five (4%) placebo patients and thirteen of twenty-seven (48%) patients receiving 5 mg/kg REMICADE achieved a CDAI <150 at week 4. The maximum response to any dose of REMICADE was observed within 2 to 4 weeks. The proportion of patients responding gradually diminished over the 12 weeks of the evaluation period. There was no evidence of a dose response; doses higher than 5 mg/kg did not result in a greater proportion of responders. Results are shown in Figure 2.

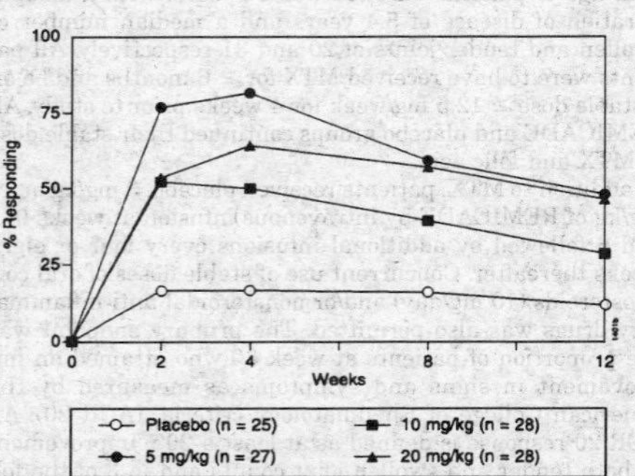

Figure 2. Response (≥70 point decrease in CDAI) to a Single IV REMICADE or Placebo Dose.

During the 12-week period following infusion, patients treated with REMICADE compared to placebo demonstrated improvement in outcomes measured by the Inflammatory Bowel Disease Questionnaire.

In the second phase, 29 patients who did not respond to the single dose of 5, 10 or 20 mg/kg of REMICADE entered the open label phase and received a single 10 mg/kg dose of REMICADE 4 weeks after the initial dose. Ten of twenty-nine (34%) patients experienced a response 4 weeks after receiving the second dose.

Patients who remained in clinical response at week 8 during the first or second phase were eligible for the retreatment phase. Seventy-three patients were re-randomized at week 12 to receive 4 infusions of placebo or 10 mg/kg REMICADE at 8-week intervals (weeks 12, 20, 28, 36) and were followed to week 48. In the limited data set available, no significant differences were observed between the REMICADE and placebo re-treated groups.

Fistulizing Crohn's Disease

The safety and efficacy of REMICADE were assessed in a randomized, double-blind, placebo controlled study of 94 patients with fistulizing Crohn's disease with fistula(s) that were of at least 3 months duration.[10] Concurrent use of stable doses of corticosteroids, 5-ASA, antibiotics, MTX, 6-MP and/or AZA was permitted, and 83% of patients continued to receive at least one of these medications. Fifty-two (55%) had multiple cutaneously draining fistulas, 90% of patients had fistula(s) in the perianal area and 10% had abdominal fistula(s).

Patients received 3 doses of placebo, 5 or 10 mg/kg REMICADE at weeks 0, 2 and 6 and were followed up to 26 weeks. The primary endpoint was the proportion of patients who experienced a clinical response, defined as ≥50% reduction from baseline in the number of fistula(s) draining upon gentle compression, on at least two consecutive visits, without an increase in medication or surgery for Crohn's disease.

Eight of thirty-one (26%) patients in the placebo arm achieved a clinical response vs. twenty-one of the thirty-one (68%) patients in the 5 mg/kg REMICADE arm ($p = 0.002$, two-sided, Fisher's Exact test). Eighteen of thirty-two (56%) patients in the 10 mg/kg arm achieved a clinical response. The median time to onset of response in the REMICADE-treated group was 2 weeks. The median duration of response was 12 weeks; after 22 weeks there was no difference between either dose of REMICADE and placebo in the proportion of patients in response (Figure 3). New fistula(s) developed in approximately 15% of both REMICADE and placebo-treated patients.

[See figure 3 in next column]

Seven of sixty (12%) evaluable REMICADE-treated patients, compared to one of thirty-one (3.5%) placebo-treated patients, developed an abscess in the area of fistulas between 8 and 16 weeks after the last infusion of REMICADE. Six of the REMICADE patients who developed an abscess had experienced a clinical response (see *ADVERSE REACTIONS, Infections*).

Table 1

MEDIAN VALUES AT BASELINE & WEEK 30 FOR ACR COMPONENTS

Parameter	Placebo + MTX Baseline	Placebo + MTX 30 weeks	3 mg/kg q 8 wks REMICADE + MTX Baseline	3 mg/kg q 8 wks REMICADE + MTX 30 weeks
No. of Tender Joints	24	16	32	12
No. of Swollen Joints	19	13	19	9
Pain[a]	6.7	5.9	7.0	3.8
Physician's Global Assessment[a]	6.5	5.0	6.1	2.6
Patient's Global Assessment[a]	6.2	5.5	6.6	3.6
Disability Index (HAQ)[b]	1.8	1.5	1.8	1.5
CRP (mg/dL)	3.0	2.3	3.1	0.8
ESR (mm/hr)	39	35	40	24

[a] Visual Analog Scale (0=best, 10=worst)

[b] Health Assessment Questionnaire, measurement of 8 categories: dressing and grooming, arising, eating, walking, hygiene, reach, grip, and activities

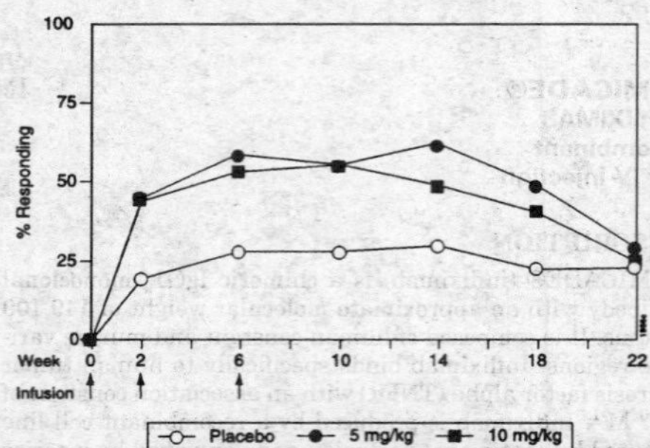

Figure 3. Response [fistula(s) closure] with Three Doses of REMICADE (infliximab) or Placebo.

Dose regimens other than dosing at weeks 0, 2 and 6 have not been studied. Studies have not been done to assess the effects of REMICADE on healing of the internal fistular canal, on closure of non-cutaneously draining fistulas (e.g., entero-entero), or on cutaneously draining fistulas in locations other than perianal and periabdominal.

INDICATIONS AND USAGE

Rheumatoid Arthritis

REMICADE, in combination with methotrexate, is indicated for the reduction in signs and symptoms of rheumatoid arthritis in patients who have had an inadequate response to methotrexate.

Crohn's Disease

REMICADE is indicated for the reduction in signs and symptoms of Crohn's disease in patients with moderately to severely active Crohn's disease who have had an inadequate response to conventional therapy.

The safety and efficacy of therapy continued beyond a single dose have not been established (see *DOSAGE AND ADMINISTRATION*).

REMICADE is indicated for the reduction in the number of draining enterocutaneous fistulae in patients with fistulizing Crohn's disease.

The safety and efficacy of therapy continued beyond three doses have not been studied (see *DOSAGE AND ADMINISTRATION*).

CONTRAINDICATIONS

REMICADE should not be administered to patients with known hypersensitivity to any murine proteins or other component of the product.

WARNINGS

RISK OF INFECTIONS

SERIOUS INFECTIONS, INCLUDING SEPSIS AND FATAL INFECTIONS, HAVE BEEN REPORTED IN PATIENTS RECEIVING TNF-BLOCKING AGENTS. MANY OF THE SERIOUS INFECTIONS IN PATIENTS TREATED WITH REMICADE HAVE OCCURRED IN PATIENTS ON CONCOMITANT IMMUNOSUPPRESSIVE THERAPY THAT, IN ADDITION TO THEIR CROHN'S DISEASE OR RHEUMATOID ARTHRITIS, COULD PREDISPOSE THEM TO INFECTIONS. CAUTION SHOULD BE EXERCISED WHEN CONSIDERING THE USE OF REMICADE IN PATIENTS WITH A CHRONIC INFECTION OR A HISTORY OF RECURRENT INFECTION. REMICADE SHOULD NOT BE GIVEN TO PATIENTS WITH A CLINICALLY IMPORTANT, ACTIVE INFECTION. PATIENTS WHO DEVELOP A NEW INFECTION WHILE UNDERGOING TREATMENT WITH REMICADE SHOULD BE MONITORED CLOSELY. IF A PATIENT DEVELOPS A SERIOUS INFECTION OR SEPSIS, REMICADE THERAPY SHOULD BE DISCONTINUED (see *ADVERSE REACTIONS, Infections*).

Hypersensitivity

REMICADE has been associated with hypersensitivity reactions that vary in their time of onset. Most hypersensitivity reactions, which include urticaria, dyspnea, and/or hypotension, have occurred during or within 2 hours of infliximab infusion. However, in some cases, serum sickness-like reactions have been observed in Crohn's disease patients 3 to 12 days after REMICADE therapy was reinstituted following an extended period without REMICADE treatment. Symptoms associated with these reactions include fever, rash, headache, sore throat, myalgias, polyarthralgias, hand and facial edema and/or dysphagia. These reactions were associated with marked increase in antibodies to infliximab, loss of detectable serum concentrations of REMICADE, and possible loss of drug efficacy. REMICADE should be discontinued for severe reactions. Medications for the treatment of hypersensitivity reactions (e.g., acetaminophen, antihistamines, corticosteroids and/or epinephrine) should be available for immediate use in the event of a reaction (see *ADVERSE REACTIONS, Infusion-related Reactions*).

PRECAUTIONS

Autoimmunity

Treatment with REMICADE may result in the formation of autoantibodies and, rarely, in the development of a lupus-like syndrome. If a patient develops symptoms suggestive of a lupus-like syndrome following treatment with REMICADE, treatment should be discontinued (see *ADVERSE REACTIONS, Autoantibodies/Lupus-like Syndrome*).

Malignancy

Patients with long duration of Crohn's disease or rheumatoid arthritis and chronic exposure to immunosuppressant therapies are more prone to develop lymphomas (see *ADVERSE REACTIONS, Malignancies/Lymphoproliferative Disease*). The impact of treatment with REMICADE on these phenomena is unknown.

Immunogenicity

Treatment with REMICADE can be associated with the development of antibodies to infliximab (also referred to as human antichimeric antibodies, HACA). One hundred thirty-four of the 199 Crohn's disease patients treated with REMICADE were evaluated for the development of infliximab-specific antibodies; 18 (13%) were antibody-positive (the majority at low titer, <1:20). Patients who were antibody-positive were more likely to experience an infusion reaction (see *ADVERSE REACTIONS, Infusion-related Reactions*). Antibody development was lower among rheumatoid arthritis and Crohn's disease patients receiving immunosuppressant therapies such as 6-MP, AZA or MTX. With repeated dosing of REMICADE, serum concentrations of infliximab were higher in rheumatoid arthritis patients who received concomitant MTX. There are limited data available on the development of antibodies to infliximab in patients receiving long-term treatment with REMICADE. Because immunogenicity analyses are product-specific, comparison of antibody rates to those from other products is not appropriate.

Vaccinations

No data are available on the response to vaccination or on the secondary transmission of infection by live vaccines in patients receiving anti-TNF therapy. It is recommended that live vaccines not be given concurrently.

Drug Interactions

Specific drug interaction studies, including interactions with MTX, have not been conducted. The majority of patients in rheumatoid arthritis or Crohn's disease clinical trials received one or more concomitant medications. In rheumatoid arthritis, concomitant medications besides MTX were nonsteroidal anti-inflammatory agents, folic acid, corticosteroids and/or narcotics. Concomitant Crohn's disease medications were antibiotics, antivirals, corticosteroids, 6-MP/AZA and aminosalicylates. Patients with Crohn's disease who received immunosuppressants tended to experience fewer infusion reactions compared to patients on no immunosuppressants (see *PRECAUTIONS, Immunogenicity* and *ADVERSE REACTIONS, Infusion-related Reactions*).

Carcinogenesis, Mutagenesis and Impairment of Fertility

Long-term studies in animals have not been performed to evaluate the carcinogenic potential. No clastogenic or mutagenic effects of infliximab were observed in the *in vivo* mouse micronucleus test or the *Salmonella-Escherichia coli* (Ames) assay, respectively. Chromosomal aberrations were not observed in an assay performed using human lymphocytes. It is not known whether infliximab can impair fertility in humans. No impairment of fertility was observed in a fertility and general reproduction toxicity study conducted in mice using an analogous antibody that selectively inhibits the functional activity of mouse TNFα.

Pregnancy Category C

Since infliximab does not cross-react with TNFα in species other than humans and chimpanzees, animal reproduction studies have not been conducted with REMICADE (infliximab). It is not known whether REMICADE can cause fetal harm when administered to a pregnant woman or can affect reproduction capacity while infliximab is present in the serum (see *CLINICAL PHARMACOLOGY, Pharmacokinetics*). REMICADE should be given to a pregnant woman only if clearly needed. No evidence of maternal toxicity, embryotoxicity or teratogenicity was observed in a developmental toxicity study conducted in mice using an analogous antibody that selectively inhibits the functional activity of mouse TNFα.

Nursing Mothers

It is not known whether infliximab is excreted in human milk or absorbed systemically after ingestion. Because many drugs and immunoglobulins are excreted in human milk, and because of the potential for adverse reactions in nursing infants from REMICADE, a decision should be made whether to discontinue nursing or to discontinue the drug, taking into account the importance of the drug to the mother.

Pediatric Use

Safety and effectiveness of REMICADE in patients with juvenile rheumatoid arthritis and in pediatric patients with Crohn's disease have not been established.

Geriatric Use

In the ATTRACT study, no overall differences were observed in effectiveness or safety in the 72 patients aged 65 or older compared to younger patients. In Crohn's disease studies, there were insufficient numbers of patients aged 65 or older to determine whether they respond differently from patients aged 18 to 65. Because there is a higher incidence of infections in the elderly population in general, caution should be used in treating the elderly (see *ADVERSE REACTIONS, Infections*).

ADVERSE REACTIONS

A total of 771 patients were treated with REMICADE in clinical trials. In both rheumatoid arthritis and Crohn's disease trials, approximately 5% of patients discontinued REMICADE because of adverse experiences. The most common reasons for discontinuation of treatment were dyspnea, urticaria and headache.

Infusion-related Reactions

Acute infusion reactions

An infusion reaction was defined as any adverse event occurring during the infusion or within 1 to 2 hours after the infusion. Seventeen percent of REMICADE-treated patients in all clinical trials experienced an infusion reaction compared to 7% of placebo-treated patients. Among the 3284 REMICADE infusions, 4% were accompanied by nonspecific symptoms such as fever or chills, 1% were accompanied by pruritus or urticaria, 1% were accompanied by cardiopulmonary reactions (primarily chest pain, hypotension, hypertension or dyspnea), and 0.1% were accompanied by combined symptoms of pruritus/urticaria and cardiopulmonary reactions. Less than 2% of patients discontinued REMICADE because of infusion reactions, and all patients recovered with treatment and/or discontinuation of infusion. REMICADE infusions beyond the initial infusion in rheumatoid arthritis patients were not associated with a higher incidence of reactions.

Patients with Crohn's disease who became positive for antibodies to infliximab were more likely to develop infusion reactions than were those who were negative (36% vs. 11% respectively). Use of concomitant immunosuppressant agents appeared to reduce the frequency of antibodies to infliximab and infusion reactions (see *PRECAUTIONS, Immunogenicity* and *Drug Interactions*).

Reactions following readministration

In a clinical trial of forty patients with Crohn's disease retreated with infliximab following a 2 to 4 year period without infliximab treatment, 10 patients experienced adverse events manifesting 3 to 12 days following infusion of which 6 were considered serious. Signs and symptoms included myalgia and/or arthralgia with fever and/or rash, with some patients also experiencing pruritus, facial, hand or lip edema, dysphagia, urticaria, sore throat, and headache. Patients experiencing these adverse events had not experienced infusion-related adverse events associated with their initial infliximab therapy. Of the 40 patients enrolled, these adverse events occurred in 9 of 23 (39%) who had received liquid formulation which is no longer in use and 1 of 17 (6%) who received lyophilized formulation. The clinical data are not adequate to determine if occurrence of these reactions is due to differences in formulation. Patients' signs and symptoms improved substantially or resolved with treatment in all cases. There are insufficient data on the incidence of these events after drug-free intervals of less than 2 years. However, these events have been observed infrequently in clinical trials and post-marketing surveillance at intervals of less than 1 year.

Infections

In REMICADE clinical trials, infections were reported by 26% of REMICADE-treated patients (average of 27 weeks of follow-up) and by 16% of placebo-treated patients (average of 20 weeks of follow-up). The infections most frequently reported were upper respiratory tract infections (including, sinusitis, pharyngitis, and bronchitis) and urinary tract infections. No increased risk of serious infections or sepsis has been observed with Remicade compared to placebo. Among REMICADE-treated patients, these serious infections included pneumonia, cellulitis, pyelonephritis and sepsis. In the ATTRACT study, one patient died with disseminated tuberculosis and one died with disseminated coccidioidomycosis. The relationship to REMICADE is unknown (see *WARNINGS, Risk of Infections*). Twelve percent of patients with fistulizing Crohn's disease developed a new abscess 8 to 16 weeks after the last infusion of REMICADE (see *CLINICAL STUDIES, Fistulizing Crohn's Disease*).

Autoantibodies/Lupus-like Syndrome

Patients were tested for autoantibodies at multiple time points. In the rheumatoid arthritis ATTRACT study, 23% of REMICADE-treated patients developed antinuclear antibodies (ANA) between screening and last evaluation, compared to 6% of placebo-treated patients. Anti-dsDNA antibodies developed in approximately 4% of REMICADE-treated patients, compared to none of the placebo-treated patients. No association was seen between REMICADE dose/schedule and development of ANA or anti-dsDNA.

Table 2

ADVERSE EVENTS IN RHEUMATOID ARTHRITIS AND CROHN'S DISEASE TRIALS

	RHEUMATOID ARTHRITIS		CROHN'S DISEASE	
	Placebo (n=133)	REMICADE (infliximab) (n=555)	Placebo (n=56)	REMICADE (n=199)
Avg. weeks of follow-up	22.3	26.9	14.7	27.0
Respiratory				
Upper respiratory infection	13%	20%	9%	16%
Coughing	5%	10%	0%	5%
Sinusitis	3%	9%	2%	5%
Rhinitis	4%	8%	4%	6%
Pharyngitis	5%	8%	5%	9%
Bronchitis	2%	4%	2%	7%
Gastrointestinal				
Nausea	17%	14%	4%	17%
Abdominal Pain	7%	8%	4%	12%
Vomiting	10%	5%	0%	9%
Other				
Headache	10%	20%	21%	23%
Rash	4%	9%	5%	6%
Fatigue	5%	6%	5%	11%
Fever	4%	6%	7%	10%
Back pain	2%	6%	4%	5%
Pain	4%	6%	5%	9%
Urinary tract infection	3%	6%	4%	3%
Pruritus	0%	5%	2%	5%
Moniliasis	2%	3%	0%	5%

Of Crohn's disease patients treated with REMICADE who were evaluated for antinuclear antibodies (ANA), 34% developed ANA between screening and last evaluation. Anti-dsDNA antibodies developed in approximately 9% of Crohn's disease patients treated with REMICADE. The development of anti-dsDNA antibodies was not related to either the dose or duration of REMICADE treatment. However, baseline therapy with an immunosuppressant in Crohn's disease patients was associated with reduced development of anti-dsDNA antibodies (3% compared to 21% in patients not receiving any immunosuppressant). Crohn's disease patients were approximately 2 times more likely to develop anti-dsDNA antibodies if they were ANA-positive at study entry.

Three patients developed clinical symptoms consistent with a lupus-like syndrome, two with rheumatoid arthritis and one with Crohn's disease. All three patients improved following discontinuation of therapy and appropriate medical treatment (see *PRECAUTIONS, Autoimmunity*).

Malignancies/Lymphoproliferative Disease

Five new and 2 recurrent malignancies were observed in 6 of 771 patients treated with REMICADE for up to 36 weeks in clinical trials. These were non-Hodgkin's B-cell lymphoma, breast cancer, melanoma, squamous cell cancer of the skin, and basal cell cancer. There are insufficient data to determine whether Remicade contributed to the development of these malignancies. The observed rates and incidences were similar to those expected for the populations studied [11,12] (see *PRECAUTIONS, Malignancy*).

Other Adverse Reactions

Adverse events occurring at a frequency of at least 5% in trials in patients with rheumatoid arthritis or Crohn's disease are shown in Table 2. Patients with Crohn's disease who were treated with REMICADE were more likely than patients with rheumatoid arthritis to experience adverse events associated with gastrointestinal symptoms.

[See table 2 above]

Serious adverse events by body system that occurred in all patients treated with REMICADE at frequencies <2% are as follows:

Body as a whole: abdominal hernia, chest pain, fall, pain

Blood: splenic infarction, splenomegaly

Cardiovascular: hypertension, hypotension, syncope

Central & Peripheral Nervous: dizziness, headache, upper motor neuron lesion

Collagen: lupus erythematosus syndrome, rheumatoid nodules

Ear and Hearing: ceruminosis

Gastrointestinal: abdominal pain, Crohn's disease, diarrhea, gastric ulcer, intestinal obstruction, intestinal perforation, intestinal stenosis, nausea, pancreatitis, proctalgia, vomiting

Heart Rate and Rhythm: palpitation, tachycardia

Liver and Biliary: cholecystitis

Metabolic and Nutritional: dehydration, pancreatic insufficiency, weight decrease

Musculoskeletal: arthropathy, back pain, bone fracture, myalgia, tendon disorder, tendon injury

Myo-, Endo-, Pericardial and Coronary Valve: cardiac failure, myocardial ischemia

Neoplasms: lymphoma

Platelet, Bleeding and Clotting: thrombocytopenia

Psychiatric: anxiety, confusion, delirium, depression, somnolence, suicide attempt

Red Blood Cell: anemia

Resistance Mechanism: abscess, cellulitis, fever, infection bacterial, sepsis

Respiratory: adult respiratory distress syndrome, bronchitis, coughing, dyspnea, pleurisy, pneumonia, pulmonary infiltration, respiratory insufficiency

Skin and Appendages: furunculosis, rash, increased sweating

Urinary: azotemia, dysuria, hydronephrosis, kidney infarction, renal failure, ureteral obstruction

Vascular (Extracardiac): brain infarction, pulmonary embolism, thrombophlebitis deep

White cell and Reticuloendothelial: leukopenia, lymphadenopathy

A greater proportion of patients enrolled into the ATTRACT trial who received REMICADE plus MTX experienced mild, transient elevations (<2 times the upper limit of normal) in AST or ALT (37% each) compared to patients treated with placebo plus MTX (AST: 24%, ALT: 29%). Five (1.5%) patients treated with REMICADE and MTX experienced more prolonged elevations in their ALT.

OVERDOSAGE

Single doses up to 20 mg/kg have been administered without any direct toxic effect. In case of overdosage, it is recommended that the patient be monitored for any signs or symptoms of adverse reactions or effects and appropriate symptomatic treatment instituted immediately.

DOSAGE AND ADMINISTRATION

Rheumatoid Arthritis

The recommended dose of REMICADE is 3 mg/kg given as an intravenous infusion followed with additional 3 mg/kg doses at 2 and 6 weeks after the first infusion then every 8 weeks thereafter. Remicade should be given in combination with methotrexate.

Crohn's Disease

The recommended dose of REMICADE is 5 mg/kg given as a single intravenous infusion for treatment of moderately to severely active Crohn's disease. In patients with fistulizing disease, an initial 5 mg/kg dose should be followed with additional 5 mg/kg doses at 2 and 6 weeks after the first infusion.

There are insufficient safety and efficacy data for the use of REMICADE in Crohn's disease beyond the recommended duration (see *WARNINGS, Hypersensitivity; ADVERSE REACTIONS, Infusion-related Reactions;* and *INDICATIONS AND USAGE*).

Preparation and administration instructions: Use aseptic technique.

REMICADE vials do not contain antibacterial preservatives. Therefore, the vials after reconstitution should be used immediately, not re-entered or stored. The diluent to be used for reconstitution is 10 mL of Sterile Water for Injection, USP. The total dose of the reconstituted product must be further diluted to 250 mL with 0.9% Sodium Chloride Injection, USP. The infusion concentration should range between 0.4 mg/mL and 4 mg/mL. The REMICADE infusion should begin within 3 hours of preparation.

1. Calculate the dose and the number of REMICADE vials needed. Each REMICADE vial contains 100 mg of infliximab. Calculate the total volume of reconstituted REMICADE solution required.
2. Reconstitute each REMICADE vial with 10 mL of Sterile Water for Injection, USP, using a syringe equipped with a 21-gauge or smaller needle. Remove the flip-top from the vial and wipe the top with an alcohol swab. Insert the syringe needle into the vial through the center of the rubber stopper and direct the stream of Sterile Water for Injection, USP, to the glass wall of the vial. Do not use the vial if the vacuum is not present. Gently swirl the solution by rotating the vial to dissolve the lyophilized powder. Avoid prolonged or vigorous agitation. DO NOT SHAKE. Foaming of the solution on reconstitution is not unusual. Allow the reconstituted solution to stand for 5 minutes. The solution should be colorless to light yellow

Continued on next page

Remicade—Cont.

and opalescent, and the solution may develop a few translucent particles as infliximab is a protein. Do not use if opaque particles, discoloration, or other foreign particles are present.

3. Dilute the total volume of the reconstituted REMICADE solution dose to 250 mL with 0.9% Sodium Chloride Injection, USP, by withdrawing a volume of 0.9% Sodium Chloride Injection, USP, equal to the volume of reconstituted REMICADE from the 0.9% Sodium Chloride Injection, USP, 250 mL bottle or bag. Slowly add the total volume of reconstituted REMICADE solution to the 250 mL infusion bottle or bag. Gently mix.
4. The infusion solution must be administered over a period of not less than 2 hours and must use an infusion set with an in-line, sterile, non-pyrogenic, low-protein-binding filter (pore size of 1.2-μm or less). Any unused portion of the infusion solution should not be stored for reuse.
5. No physical biochemical compatibility studies have been conducted to evaluate the co-administration of REMICADE with other agents. REMICADE should not be infused concomitantly in the same intravenous line with other agents.
6. Parenteral drug products should be inspected visually for particulate matter and discoloration prior to administration, whenever solution and container permit. If visibly opaque particles, discoloration or other foreign particulates are observed, the solution should not be used.

Storage

Store the lyophilized product under refrigeration at 2°C to 8°C (36°F to 46°F). Do not freeze. Do not use beyond the expiration date. This product contains no preservative.

HOW SUPPLIED

REMICADE (infliximab) lyophilized concentrate for IV injection is supplied in individually-boxed single-use vials in the following strength:

NDC 57894-030-01 100 mg infliximab in a 20-mL vial

REFERENCES

1. Knight DM, Trinh H, Le J, Siegel S, Shealy D, McConough M, Scallon B, Moore MA, Vilcek J, Daddona P, Ghrayeb J. Construction and initial characterization of a mouse-human chimeric anti-TNF antibody. *Molec Immunol* 1993;30:1443–1453.
2. Scallon BJ, Moore MA, Trinh H, Knight DM, Ghrayeb J. Chimeric anti-TNFα monoclonal antibody cA2 binds recombinant transmembrane TNFα and activates immune effector functions. *Cytokine* 1995;7:251–259.
3. Siegel SA, Shealy DJ, Nakada MT, Le J, Woulfe DS, Probert L, Kollias G, Ghrayeb J, Vilcek J, Daddona PE. The mouse/human chimeric monoclonal antibody cA2 neutralizes TNF *in vitro* and protects transgenic mice from cachexia and TNF lethality *in vivo*. *Cytokine* 1995;7:15–25.
4. Data on file.
5. Chu CQ, Field M, Feldmann M and Maini RN. Localization of tumor necrosis factor alpha in synovial tissues and at the cartilage-pannus junction in patients with rheumatoid arthritis. *Arthritis and Rheum* 1991;34:1125–1132.
6. Braegger CP, Nicholls S, Murch SH, Stephens S, MacDonald TT. Tumour necrosis factor alpha in stool as a marker of intestinal inflammation. *Lancet* 1992;339:89–91.
7. Maini RN, Breedveld FC, Kalden JR, Smolen JS, Davis D, Macfarlane JD, Antoni C, Leeb B, Elliott MJ, Woody JN, Schaible TF, Feldmann M. Therapeutic efficacy of multiple intravenous infusions of anti-tumor necrosis factor α monoclonal antibody combined with low-dose weekly methotrexate in rheumatoid arthritis. *Arthritis Rheum* 1998;41(9);1552–1563.
8. Elliott MJ, Maini RN, Feldmann M, et al. Randomised double-blind comparison of chimeric monoclonal antibody to tumour necrosis factor alpha (cA2) versus placebo in rheumatoid arthritis. *Lancet* 1994 Oct 22;344(8930):1105–1110.
9. Targan SR, Hanauer SR, van Deventer SJH, Mayer L, Present D, Braakman T, DeWoody K, Schaible TF, Rutgeerts PJ. A short-term study of chimeric monoclonal antibody cA2 to tumor necrosis factor α for Crohn's disease. *N Engl J Med* 1997;337(15):1029–1035.
10. Present DH, Rutgeerts P, Targan S, Hanauer SB, Mayer L, van Hogezand RA, Podolsky DK, Sands B, Braakman T, DeWoody KL, Schaible TF, van Deventer SJH: Infliximab for the treatment of fistulas in patients with Crohn's disease. *N Engl J Med* 1999;340:1398–1405.
11. Greenstein AJ, Mullin GE, Strauchen JA, Heimann T, et al. Lymphoma in inflammatory bowel disease. *Cancer* 1992;69:1119–21.
12. Jones M, Symmons D, Finn J, Wolfe F. Does exposure to immunosuppressive therapy increase the 10 year malignancy and mortality risks in rheumatoid arthritis? A matched cohort study. *Br J Rheum* 1996;35:738–45.

Centocor, Inc., Malvern, PA 19355, USA License #1242
1-800-457-6399 9 November 1999

Shown in Product Identification Guide, page 310

RETAVASE® ℞

Reteplase,
recombinant

DESCRIPTION

Retavase® (Reteplase) is a non-glycosylated deletion mutein of tissue plasminogen activator (tPA), containing the kringle 2 and the protease domains of human tPA. Retavase® contains 355 of the 527 amino acids of native tPA (amino acids 1–3 and 176–527). Retavase® is produced by recombinant DNA technology in E. coli. The protein is isolated as inactive inclusion bodies from E. coli, converted into its active form by an in vitro folding process and purified by chromatographic separation. The molecular weight of Reteplase is 39,571 daltons.

Potency is expressed in units (U) using a reference standard which is specific for Retavase® and is not comparable with units used for other thrombolytic agents.

Retavase® is a sterile, white, lyophilized powder for intravenous bolus injection after reconstitution with Sterile Water for Injection, USP (without preservatives). Following reconstitution, the pH is 6.0 ± 0.3. Retavase® is supplied as a 10.4 U vial to ensure sufficient drug for administration of each 10 U dose. Each single-use vial contains:

10.4 U (18.1 mg) Vial	
Reteplase	18.1 mg
Tranexamic Acid	8.32 mg
Dipotassium Hydrogen Phosphate	136.24 mg
Phosphoric Acid	51.27 mg
Sucrose	364.0 mg
Polysorbate 80	5.20 mg

CLINICAL PHARMACOLOGY

General

Retavase® is a recombinant plasminogen activator which catalyzes the cleavage of endogenous plasminogen to generate plasmin. Plasmin in turn degrades the fibrin matrix of the thrombus, thereby exerting its thrombolytic action.[1,2] In a controlled trial, 36 of 56 patients treated for an acute myocardial infarction (AMI) had a decrease in fibrinogen levels to below 100 mg/dL by 2 hours following the administration of Retavase® as a double-bolus intravenous injection (10 + 10 U) in which 10 U (17.4 mg) was followed 30 minutes later by a second bolus of 10 U (17.4 mg).[3] The mean fibrinogen level returned to the baseline value by 48 hours.

Pharmacokinetics

Based on the measurement of thrombolytic activity, Retavase® is cleared from plasma at a rate of 250–450 mL/min, with an effective half-life of 13–16 minutes. Retavase® is cleared primarily by the liver and kidney.

Clinical Studies

The safety and efficacy of Retavase® were evaluated in three controlled clinical trials in which Retavase® was compared to other thrombolytic agents. The INJECT study was designed to assess the relative effects of Retavase® or the Streptase® brand of Streptokinase upon mortality rates at 35 days following an AMI. The other studies (RAPID 1 and RAPID 2) were arteriographic studies which compared the effect on coronary patency of Retavase® to two regimens of Alteplase (a tissue plasminogen activator; Activase® in the USA and Actilyse® in Europe) in patients with an AMI. In all three studies, patients were treated with aspirin (initial doses of 160 mg to 350 mg and subsequent doses of 75 mg to 350 mg) and heparin (a 5,000 U IV bolus prior to the administration of Retavase®, followed by a 1000 U/hour continuous IV infusion for at least 24 hours).[3,4,5] The safety and efficacy of Retavase® have not been evaluated using antithrombotic or antiplatelet regimens other than those described above.

Retavase® (10 + 10 U) was compared to Streptokinase (1.5 million units over 60 minutes) in a double-blind, randomized, European study (INJECT), which studied 6,010 patients treated within 12 hours of the onset of symptoms of AMI. To be eligible for enrollment, patients had to have chest pain consistent with coronary ischemia and ST segment elevation, or a bundle branch block pattern on the EKG. Patients with known cerebrovascular or other bleeding risks or those with a systolic blood pressure >200 mm Hg or a diastolic blood pressure >100 mm Hg were excluded from enrollment. The results of the primary endpoint (mortality at 35 days), six month mortality and selected other 35 day endpoints are shown in Table 1 for patients receiving study medications.

[See table 1 below]

For morality, stroke and the combined outcome of mortality or stroke, the 95% confidence intervals in Table 1 reflect the range within which the true difference in outcomes probably lies and includes the possibility of no difference. The incidences of congestive heart failure and of cardiogenic shock were significantly lower among patients treated with Retavase®.

The total incidence of stroke was similar between the groups. However, more patients treated with Retavase® experienced hemorrhagic strokes than patients treated with Streptokinase. An exploratory analysis indicated that the incidence of intracranial hemorrhage was higher among older patients or those with elevated blood pressure. The incidence of intracranial hemorrhage among the 698 patients treated with Retavase® who were older than 70 years was 2.2%. Intracranial hemorrhage occurred in 8 of the 332 (2.4%) patients treated with Retavase® who had an initial systolic blood pressure >160 mm Hg and in 15 of the 2,629 (0.6%) Retavase® patients who had an initial systolic blood pressure <160 mm Hg.

Two arteriographic studies (RAPID 1 and RAPID 2) were performed utilizing open-label administration of the study agents and a blinded review of the arteriograms. In RAPID 1, patients were treated within 6 hours of the onset of symptoms, and in RAPID 2, patients were treated within 12 hours of the onset of symptoms. Both studies evaluated coronary artery perfusion through the infarct-related artery 90 minutes after the initiation of therapy as the primary endpoint. Some patients in each study also had perfusion through the infarct-related artery evaluated at 60 minutes after the initiation of therapy. In RAPID 1, Retavase® (in doses of 10 + 10 U, 15 U, or 10 + 5 U) was compared to a 3 hour regimen of Alteplase (100 mg administered over 3 hrs). In RAPID 2, Retavase® (10 + 10 U) was compared to an accelerated regimen of Alteplase (100 mg administered over 1.5 hrs). The percentages of patients with partial or complete flow (TIMI grades 2 or 3) and complete flow (TIMI grade 3), are shown along with ventricular function assessments in Table 2. The follow-up arteriogram was performed at a median of 8 (RAPID 1) and 5 (RAPID 2) days following the administration of the thrombolytics. In RAPID 1 the best patency results were obtained with the 10 + 10 U dose. In RAPID 2, the percentage of patients with partial or complete flow and the percentage of patients with complete flow was significantly higher with Retavase® than with Alteplase at 90 minutes after the initiation of therapy. In both clinical trials the reocclusion rates were similar for Retavase® and Alteplase. The relationship between coronary artery patency and clinical efficacy has not been established.

[See table 2 at bottom of next page]

Approximately 70% (RAPID 1) and 78% (RAPID 2) of the patients in the arteriographic studies underwent optional arteriography at 60 minutes following the administration of the study agents. In both trials the percentage of patients with complete flow at 60 minutes was significantly higher with Retavase® than with Alteplase. Neither RAPID clinical trial was designed nor powered to compare the efficacy or safety of Retavase® and Alteplase with respect to the outcomes of mortality and stroke.

INDICATIONS AND USAGE

Retavase® (Reteplase) is indicated for use in the management of acute myocardial infarction (AMI) in adults for the improvement of ventricular function following AMI, the reduction of the incidence of congestive heart failure and the reduction of mortality associated with AMI. Treatment should be initiated as soon as possible after the onset of AMI symptoms (see **CLINICAL PHARMACOLOGY**).

CONTRAINDICATIONS

Because thrombolytic therapy increases the risk of bleeding, Retavase® is contraindicated in the following situations:

- **Active internal bleeding**
- **History of cerebrovascular accident**
- **Recent intracranial or intraspinal surgery or trauma (see WARNINGS)**

Table 1
INJECT TRIAL
Incidence of Selected Outcomes

Enpoint	Retavase® n = 2,965	Streptokinase n = 2,971	Retavase®-Streptokinase difference (95% CI)	P Value
35 Day mortality	8.9%	9.4%	-0.5 (-2.0, 0.9)	0.49*
6 Month mortality†	11.0%	12.1%	-1.1 (-2.7, 0.6)	0.22
Combined outcome of 35 day mortality or nonfatal stroke within 35 days	9.6%	10.2%	-0.6 (-2.1, 1.0)	0.47
Heart failure	24.8%	28.1%	-3.3 (-5.6, -1.1)	0.004
Cardiogenic shock	4.6%	5.8%	-1.2 (-2.4, -0.1)	0.03
Any stroke	1.4%	1.1%	0.3 (-0.3, 0.8)	0.34
Intrancranial hemorrhage	0.8%	0.4%	0.4 (0.0, 0.8)	0.04

*p value for the exploratory analysis comparing Retavase® versus Streptokinase.
†Kaplan-Meier estimates.

- **Intracranial neoplasm, arteriovenous malformation, or aneurysm**
- **Known bleeding diathesis**
- **Severe uncontrolled hypertension**

WARNINGS

Bleeding

The most common complication encountered during Retavase® therapy is bleeding. The sites of bleeding include both internal bleeding sites (intracranial, retroperitoneal, gastrointestinal, genitourinary, or respiratory) and superficial bleeding sites (venous cutdowns, arterial punctures, sites of recent surgical intervention). The concomitant use of heparin anticoagulation may contribute to bleeding. In clinical trials some of the hemorrhage episodes occurred one or more days after the effects of Retavase® had dissipated, but while heparin therapy was continuing.

As fibrin is lysed during Retavase® therapy, bleeding from recent puncture sites may occur. Therefore, thrombolytic therapy requires careful attention to all potential bleeding sites (including catheter insertion sites, arterial and venous puncture sites, cutdown sites, and needle puncture sites). Noncompressible arterial puncture must be avoided and internal jugular and subclavian venous punctures should be avoided to minimize bleeding from noncompressible sites.

Should an arterial puncture be necessary during the administration of Retavase®, it is preferable to use an upper extremity vessel that is accessible to manual compression. Pressure should be applied for at least 30 minutes, a pressure dressing applied, and the puncture site checked frequently for evidence of bleeding.

Intramuscular injections and nonessential handling of the patient should be avoided during treatment with Retavase®. Venipunctures should be performed carefully and only as required.

Should serious bleeding (not controllable by local pressure) occur, concomitant anticoagulant therapy should be terminated immediately. In addition, the second bolus of Retavase® should not be given if serious bleeding occurs before it is administered.

Each patient being considered for therapy with Retavase® should be carefully evaluated and anticipated benefits weighed against the potential risks associated with therapy.

In the following conditions, the risks of Retavase® therapy may be increased and should be weighed against the anticipated benefits:

- Recent major surgery, e.g., coronary artery bypass graft, obstetrical delivery, organ biopsy
- Previous puncture of noncompressible vessels
- Cerebrovascular disease
- Recent gastrointestinal or genitourinary bleeding
- Recent trauma
- Hypertension: systolic BP ≥180 mm Hg and/or diastolic BP ≥110 mm Hg
- High likelihood of left heart thrombus, e.g., mitral stenosis with atrial fibrillation
- Acute pericarditis
- Subacute bacterial endocarditis
- Hemostatic defects including those secondary to severe hepatic or renal disease
- Severe hepatic or renal dysfunction
- Pregnancy
- Diabetic hemorrhagic retinopathy or other hemorrhagic ophthalmic conditions
- Septic thrombophlebitis or occluded AV cannula at a seriously infected site
- Advanced age
- Patients currently receiving oral anticoagulants, e.g., warfarin sodium
- Any other condition in which bleeding constitutes a significant hazard or would be particularly difficult to manage because of its location

Cholesterol Embolization

Cholesterol embolism has been reported rarely in patients treated with thrombolytic agents; the true incidence is unknown. This serious condition, which can be lethal, is also associated with invasive vascular procedures (e.g., cardiac catheterization, angiography, vascular surgery) and/or anticoagulant therapy. Clinical features of cholesterol embolism may include livedo reticularis, "purple toe" syndrome, acute renal failure, gangrenous digits, hypertension, pancreatitis, myocardial infarction, cerebral infarction, spinal cord infarction, retinal artery occlusion, bowel infarction, and rhabdomyolysis.

Arrhythmias

Coronary thrombolysis may result in arrhythmias associated with reperfusion. These arrhythmias (such as sinus bradycardia, accelerated idioventricular rhythm, ventricular premature depolarizations, ventricular tachycardia) are not different from those often seen in the ordinary course of acute myocardial infarction and should be managed with standard antiarrhythmic measures. It is recommended that antiarrhythmic therapy for bradycardia and/or ventricular irritability be available when Retavase® is administered.

PRECAUTIONS

General

Standard management of myocardial infarction should be implemented concomitantly with Retavase® treatment. Arterial and venous punctures should be minimized (see **WARNINGS**). In addition, the second bolus of Retavase® should not be given if the serious bleeding occurs before it is administered. In the event of serious bleeding, any concomitant heparin should be terminated immediately. Heparin effects can be reversed by protamine.

Readministration

There is no experience with patients receiving repeat courses of therapy with Retavase®. Retavase® did not induce the formation of Retavase® specific antibodies in any of the approximately 2,400 patients who were tested for antibody formation in clinical trials. If an anaphylactoid reaction occurs, the second bolus of Retavase® should not be given, and appropriate therapy should be initiated.

Drug Interactions

The interaction of Retavase® with other cardioactive drugs has not been studied. In addition to bleeding associated with heparin and vitamin K antagonists, drugs that alter platelet function (such as aspirin, dipyridamole, and abciximab) may increase the risk of bleeding if administered prior to or after Retavase® therapy.

Drug/Laboratory Test Interactions

Administration of Retavase® may cause decreases in plasminogen and fibrinogen. During Retavase® therapy, if coagulation tests and/or measurements of fibrinolytic activity are performed, the results may be unreliable unless specific precautions are taken to prevent in vitro artifacts. Retavase® is an enzyme that when present in blood in pharmacologic concentrations remains active under in vitro conditions. This can lead to degradation of fibrinogen in blood samples removed for analysis. Collection of blood samples in the presence of PPACK (chloromethylketone) at 2 μM concentrations was used in clinical trials of prevent in vitro fibrinolytic artifacts.[6]

Use of Antithrombotics

Heparin and aspirin have been administered concomitantly with and following the administration of Retavase® in the management of acute myocardial infarction. Because heparin, aspirin, or Retavase® may cause bleeding complications, careful monitoring for bleeding is advised, especially at arterial puncture sites.

Carcinogenesis, Mutagenesis, Impairment of Fertility

Long-term studies in animals have not been performed to evaluate the carcinogenic potential of Retavase®. Studies to determine mutagenicity, chromosomal aberrations, gene mutations, and micronuclei induction were negative at all concentrations tested. Reproductive toxicity studies in rats revealed no effects on fertility at doses up to 15 times the human dose (4.31 U/kg).

Pregnancy Category C

Reteplase has been shown to have an abortifacient effect in rabbits when given in doses 3 times the human dose (0.86 U/kg). Reproduction studies performed in rats at doses up to 15 times the human dose (4.31 U/kg) revealed no evidence of fetal anomalies; however, Reteplase administered to pregnant rabbits resulted in hemorrhaging in the genital tract, leading to abortions in mid-gestation. There are no adequate and well-controlled studies in pregnant women. The most common complication of thrombolytic therapy is bleeding and certain conditions, including pregnancy, can increase this risk. Reteplase should be used during pregnancy only if the potential benefit justifies the potential risk to the fetus.

Nursing Mothers

It is not known whether Retavase® is excreted in human milk. Because many drugs are excreted in human milk, caution should be exercised when Retavase® is administered to a nursing woman.

Pediatric Use

Safety and effectiveness of Retavase® in pediatric patients have not been established.

ADVERSE REACTIONS

Bleeding

The most frequent adverse reaction associated with Retavase® is bleeding (see **WARNINGS**). The types of bleeding events associated with thrombolytic therapy may be broadly categorized as either intracranial hemorrhage or other types of hemorrhage.

- Intracranial hemorrhage (see **CLINICAL PHARMACOLOGY**)
  In the INJECT clinical trial the rate of in-hospital, intracranial hemorrhage among all patients treated with Retavase® was 0.8% (23 of 2,965 patients). As seen with Retavase® and other thrombolytic agents, the risk for intracranial hemorrhage is increased in patients with advanced age or with elevated blood pressure.
- Other types of hemorrhage
  The incidence of other types of bleeding events in clinical studies of Retavase® varied depending upon the use of arterial catheterization of other invasive procedures and whether the study was performed in Europe or the USA. The overall incidence of any bleeding event in patients treated with Retavase® in clinical studies (n = 3,805) was 21.1%. The rates for bleeding events, regardless of severity, for the 10 + 10 U Retavase® regimen from controlled clinical studies are summarized in Table 3.

Table 3
Retavase® Hemorrhage Rates

Bleeding Site	INJECT	RAPID 1 and RAPID 2	
	Europe n = 2,965	USA n = 210	Europe n = 113
Injection Site*	4.6%	48.6%	19.5%
Gastrointestinal	2.5%	9.0%	1.8%
Genitourinary	1.6%	9.5%	0.9%
Anemia, site unknown	2.6%	1.4%	0.9%

*includes the arterial catheterization site (all patients in the RAPID studies underwent arterial catheterization).

In these studies the severity and sites of bleeding events were comparable for Retavase® and the comparison thrombolytic agents.

Should serious bleeding in a critical location (intracranial, gastrointestinal, retroperitoneal, pericardial) occur, any concomitant heparin should be terminated immediately. In addition, the second bolus of Retavase® should not be given if the serious bleeding occurs before it is administered. Death and permanent disability are not uncommonly reported in patients who have experienced stroke (including intracranial bleeding) and other serious bleeding episodes.

Fibrin which is part of the hemostatic plug formed at needle puncture sites will be lysed during Retavase® therapy. Therefore, Retavase® therapy requires careful attention to potential bleeding sites (e.g., catheter insertion sites, arterial puncture sites).

Allergic Reactions

Among the 2,965 patients receiving Retavase® in the INJECT trial, serious allergic reactions were noted in 3 patients, with one patient experiencing dyspnea and hypotension. No anaphylactoid reactions were observed among the 3,856 patients treated with Retavase® in initial clinical trials. In an ongoing clinical trial two anaphylactoid reactions have been reported among approximately 2,500 patients receiving Retavase®.

Other Adverse Reactions

Patients administered Retavase® as treatment for myocardial infarction have experienced many events which are frequent sequelae of myocardial infarction and may or may not

Continued on next page

Table 2
RAPID 1 and RAPID 2 TRIALS
Arteriographic Results

Outcome	RAPID 2			RAPID 1*		
	Retavase® (10 +10 U)	Alteplase (Accelerated regimen)	p	Retavase® (10 +10 U)	Alteplase (Standard regimen)	p
90 minute patency rates	n = 157	n = 146		n = 142	n = 145	
TIMI 2 or 3 TIMI 3	83% 60%	73% 45%	0.03 0.01	85% 63%	77% 49%	0.08 0.02
Follow-up patency rates	n = 128	n = 113		n = 123	n = 123	
TIMI 2 or 3 TIMI 3	89% 75%	90% 77%	0.76 0.72	95% 88%	88% 71%	0.04 0.001
Follow-up ejection fraction mean %	n = 89	n = 77		n = 91	n = 84	
	52%	54%	0.25	53%	49%	0.03
Follow-up regional wall motion	n = 87	n = 72		n = 84	n = 80	
Standard deviation from mean normal value	-2.3	-2.3	0.96	-2.2	-2.6	0.02

*p values represent one of multiple dose comparisons.

Retavase—Cont.

be attributable to Retavase® therapy. These events include cardiogenic shock, arrhythmias (e.g., sinus bradycardia, accelerated idioventricular rhythm, ventricular premature depolarizations, supraventricular tachycardia, ventricular tachycardia, ventricular fibrillation), AV block, pulmonary edema, heart failure, cardiac arrest, recurrent ischemia, reinfarction, myocardial rupture, mitral regurgitation, pericardial effusion, pericarditis, cardiac tamponade, venous thrombosis and embolism, and electromechanical dissociation. These events can be life-threatening and may lead to death. Other adverse events have been reported, including nausea and/or vomiting, hypotension, and fever.

DOSAGE AND ADMINISTRATION

Retavase® (Reteplase) is for intravenous administration only. Retavase® is administered as a 10 + 10 U double-bolus injection. Each bolus is administered as an intravenous injection over 2 minutes. The second bolus is given 30 minutes after initiation of the first bolus injection. Each bolus injection should be given via an intravenous line in which no other medication is being simultaneously injected or infused. No other medication should be added to the injection solution containing Retavase®. There is no experience with patients receiving repeat courses of therapy with Retavase®.

Heparin and Retavase® are incompatible when combined in solution. Do not administer heparin and Retavase® simultaneously in the same intravenous line. If Retavase® is to be injected through an intravenous line containing heparin, a normal saline or 5% dextrose (D5W) solution should be flushed through the line prior to and following the Retavase® injection.

Although the value of anticoagulants and antiplatelet drugs during and following administration of Retavase® has not been studied, heparin has been administered concomitantly in more than 99% of patients. Aspirin has been given either during and/or following heparin treatment. Studies assessing the safety and efficacy of Retavase® without adjunctive therapy with heparin and aspirin have not been performed.

Reconstitution—Retavase® Kit and Retavase® Half-Kit: Reconstitution should be carried out using the diluent and dispensing pin provided with Retavase®. It is important that Retavase® be reconstituted only with the supplied Sterile Water for Injection, USP (without preservatives). The reconstituted preparation results in a colorless solution containing Retavase® 1 unit/mL. Slight foaming upon reconstitution is not unusual; allowing the vial to stand undisturbed for several minutes is usually sufficient to allow dissipation of any large bubbles.

Because Retavase® contains no antibacterial preservatives, it should be reconstituted immediately before use. When reconstituted as directed, the solution may be used within 4 hours when stored at 2–30°C (36–86°F). Prior to administration, the product should be visually inspected for particulate matter and discoloration.

Reconstitution Instructions—Retavase® Kit and Retavase® Half-Kit: Use aseptic technique throughout.

Step 1: Withdraw 10 mL of Sterile Water for Injection, USP (SWFI) from the supplied vial into a sterile 10 mL syringe.

Step 2: Open the package containing the dispensing pin. Remove the protective cap from the luer lock port of the dispensing pin and connect the sterile 10mL syringe to the dispensing pin.
Remove the protective flip-cap from one vial of Retavase®.

Step 3: Remove the protective cap from the spike end of the dispensing pin, and insert the spike into the vial of Retavase® until the security clips lock onto the vial.
Transfer the 10 mL of SWFI through the dispensing pin into the vial of Retavase®.

Step 4: With the dispensing pin and syringe still attached to the vial, swirl the vial gently to dissolve the Retavase®. **DO NOT SHAKE.**

Step 5: Withdraw 10 mL of Retavase® reconstituted solution back into the syringe. A small amount of solution will remain in the vial due to overfill.

Step 6: Detach the syringe from the dispensing pin, and attach a sterile needle.

Step 7: The 10 mL bolus dose is now ready for administration.

Safely discard all used reconstitution components and the empty Retavase® vial according to institutional procedures.

HOW SUPPLIED

Retavase® Kit	NDC 57894-040-01
Retavase® Half-Kit	NDC 57894-040-02

Retavase®, is supplied as a sterile, preservative-free, lyophilized powder in 10.4 unit (equivalent to 18.1 mg Retavase®) vials without a vacuum, in the following packaging configurations:

Retavase® Kit: 2 single-use Retavase® vials 10.4 units (18.1 mg), 2 single-use diluent vials for reconstitution (10 mL Sterile Water for Injection, USP), 2 sterile 10 mL syringes, 2 sterile dispensing pins, 4 sterile needles, 2 alcohol swabs and a package insert:

Retavase® Half-Kit: 1 single-use Retavase® vial 10.4 units (18.1 mg), 1 single-use diluent vial for reconstitution (10 mL Sterile Water for Injection, USP), a sterile dispensing pin and a package insert.

Storage: Store Retavase® at 2–25°C (36–77°F). The box should remain sealed until use to protect the lyophilisate from exposure to light. Do not use beyond the expiration date printed on the box.

References

1. Martin U, Sponer G, Strein K. Evaluation of thrombolytic and systemic effects of the novel recombinant plasminogen activator BM 06.022 compared with alteplase, anistreplase, streptokinase and urokinase in a canine model of coronary artery thrombosis. *JACC.* 1992;19:433–440.
2. Kohnert U, Rudolph R, Verheijen JH. Biochemical properties of the kringle 2 and protease domains are maintained in the refolded t-PA deletion variant BM 06.022. *Protein Engineering.* 1992; 5:93–100.
3. Smalling R, Bode C, Kalbfleisch J, et al. More rapid, complete, and stable coronary thrombolysis with bolus administration of reteplase compared with alteplase infusion in acute myocardial infarction. *Circulation.* 1995;91: 2725–2732.
4. Bode C, Smalling R, Gunther B, et al. Randomized comparison of coronary thrombolysis achieved with double bolus reteplase (recombinant plasminogen activator) and front-loaded, accelerated alteplase (recombinant tissue plasminogen activator) in patients with acute myocardial infarction. *Circulation.* 1996;94:891–898.
5. INJECT Study Group. Randomised, double-blind comparison of reteplase double-bolus administration with streptokinase in acute myocardial infarction (INJECT): trial to investigate equivalence. *Lancet.* 1995;346:329–336.
6. Martin U, Gärtner D, Markl HJ, et al. D-PHE-PRO-ARGCHLOROMETHYLKETONE prevents in vitro fibrinogen reduction by the novel recombinant plasminogen activator BM 06.022. *Ann Hematol.* 1992;64(suppl)A47.

Retavase®,
Reteplase, recombinant
Manufactured by:
Centocor, Inc.
Malvern, PA 19355
U.S. License Number 1242

0711001

Shown in Product Identification Guide, page 310

Cephalon, Inc.

145 BRANDYWINE PARKWAY
WEST CHESTER, PA 19380

For Medical Information Contact:
(800) 896-5855
Adverse Drug Experiences:
(800) 896-5855
Customer Service:
(888) 535-2374

PROVIGIL® Ⓒ Ɽ
(MODAFINIL)
Tablets

DESCRIPTION

PROVIGIL (modafinil) is a wakefulness-promoting agent for oral administration. Modafinil is a racemic compound. The chemical name for modafinil is 2-[(diphenylmethyl) sulfinyl]acetamide. The molecular formula is $C_{15}H_{15}NO_2S$ and the molecular weight is 273.36.

The chemical structure is:

Modafinil is a white to off-white, crystalline powder that is practically insoluble in water and cyclohexane. It is sparingly to slightly soluble in methanol and acetone. PROVIGIL tablets contain 100 mg or 200 mg of modafinil and the following inactive ingredients: lactose, corn starch, magnesium silicate, croscarmellose sodium, povidone, magnesium stearate, and talc.

CLINICAL PHARMACOLOGY

Mechanism of Action and Pharmacology

The precise mechanism(s) through which modafinil promotes wakefulness is unknown. Modafinil has wake-promoting actions like sympathomimetic agents including amphetamine and methylphenidate, although the pharmacologic profile is not identical to that of sympathomimetic amines.

At pharmacologically relevant concentrations, modafinil does not bind to most potentially relevant receptors for sleep/wake regulation, including those for norepinephrine, serotonin, dopamine, GABA, adenosine, histamine-3, melatonin, or benzodiazepines. Modafinil also does not inhibit the activities of MAO-B or phosphodiesterases II-V.

Modafinil is not a direct- or indirect-acting dopamine receptor agonist and is inactive in several *in vivo* preclinical models capable of detecting enhanced dopaminergic activity. *In vitro*, modafinil binds to the dopamine reuptake site and causes an increase in extracellular dopamine, but no increase in dopamine release. In a preclinical model, the wakefulness induced by amphetamine, but not modafinil, is antagonized by the dopamine receptor antagonist haloperidol.

Modafinil does not appear to be a direct or indirect α_1-adrenergic agonist. Although modafinil-induced wakefulness can be attenuated by the α_1-adrenergic receptor antagonist, prazosin, in assay systems known to be responsive to α-adrenergic agonists, modafinil has no activity. Modafinil does not display sympathomimetic activity in the rat vas deferens preparations (agonist-stimulated or electrically stimulated) nor does it increase the formation of the adrenergic receptor-mediated second messenger phosphatidyl inositol in *in vitro* models. Unlike sympathomimetic agents, modafinil does not reduce cataplexy in narcoleptic canines and has minimal effects on cardiovascular and hemodynamic parameters.

In the cat, equal wakefulness-promoting doses of methylphenidate and amphetamine increased neuronal activation throughout the brain. Modafinil at an equivalent wakefulness-promoting dose selectively and prominently increased neuronal activation in more discrete regions of the brain. The relationship of this finding in cats to the effects of modafinil in humans is unknown.

In addition to its wakefulness-promoting effects and increased locomotor activity in animals, in humans, PROVIGIL produces psychoactive and euphoric effects, alterations in mood, perception, thinking, and feelings typical of other CNS stimulants. Modafinil is reinforcing, as evidenced by its self-administration in monkeys previously trained to self-administer cocaine; modafinil was also partially discriminated as stimulant-like.

The optical enantiomers of modafinil have similar pharmacological actions in animals. The enantiomers have not been individually studied in humans. Two major metabolites of modafinil, modafinil acid and modafinil sulfone, do not appear to contribute to the CNS-activating properties of modafinil.

Pharmacokinetics

Modafinil is a racemic compound, whose enantiomers have different pharmacokinetics (e.g., the half-life of the *l*-isomer is approximately three times that of the *d*-isomer in humans). The enantiomers do not interconvert. At steady state, total exposure to the *l*-isomer is approximately three times that for the *d*-isomer. The trough concentration (C_{minss}) of circulating modafinil after once daily dosing consists of 90% of the *l*-isomer and 10% of the *d*-isomer. The effective elimination half-life of modafinil after multiple doses is about 15 hours. The enantiomers of modafinil exhibit linear kinetics upon multiple dosing of 200–600 mg/day once daily in healthy volunteers. Apparent steady states of total modafinil and *l*-(-)-modafinil are reached after 2–4 days of dosing.

Absorption and Distribution

Absorption of PROVIGIL tablets is rapid, with peak plasma concentrations occurring at 2–4 hours. The bioavailability of PROVIGIL tablets is approximately equal to that of an aqueous suspension. The absolute oral bioavailability was not determined due to the aqueous insolubility (<1 mg/mL) of modafinil, which precluded intravenous administration. Food has no effect on overall PROVIGIL bioavailability; however, its absorption (t_{max}) may be delayed by approximately one hour if taken with food.

Modafinil is well distributed in body tissue with an apparent volume of distribution (~0.9 L/kg) larger than the volume of total body water (0.6 L/kg). In human plasma, *in vitro*, modafinil is moderately bound to plasma protein (~60%, mainly to albumin). At serum concentrations obtained at steady state after doses of 200 mg/day, modafinil exhibits no displacement of protein binding of warfarin, diazepam, or propranolol. Even at much larger concentrations (1000 μM; >25 times the C_{max} of 40 μM at steady state at 400 mg/day), modafinil has no effect on warfarin binding. Modafinil acid at concentrations >500 μM decreases the extent of warfarin binding, but these concentrations are >35 times those achieved therapeutically.

Metabolism and Elimination

The major route of elimination (~90%) is metabolism, primarily by the liver, with subsequent renal elimination of the metabolites. Urine alkalinization has no effect on the elimination of modafinil.

Metabolism occurs through hydrolytic deamidation, S-oxidation, aromatic ring hydroxylation, and glucuronide conjugation. Less than 10% of an administered dose is excreted as the parent compound. In a clinical study using radiolabeled modafinil, a total of 81% of the administered radioactivity was recovered in 11 days post-dose, predominantly in the urine (80% vs. 1.0% in the feces). The largest fraction of the drug in urine was modafinil acid, but at least six other metabolites were present in lower concentrations. Only two metabolites reach appreciable concentrations in plasma, i.e., modafinil acid and modafinil sulfone. In preclinical models, modafinil acid, modafinil sulfone, 2-[(diphenylmethyl)sulfonyl]acetic acid and 4-hydroxy modafinil, were inactive or did not appear to mediate the arousal effects of modafinil.

In humans, modafinil shows a possible induction effect on its own metabolism after chronic administration of doses ≥400 mg/day. Induction of hepatic metabolizing enzymes, most importantly cytochrome P-450 (CYP) 3A4, has also been observed *in vitro* after incubation of primary cultures of human hepatocytes with modafinil. (For further discussion of the effects of modafinil on CYP enzyme activities see **PRECAUTIONS, Drug Interactions**).

Drug-Drug Interactions: Because modafinil is a reversible inhibitor of the drug-metabolizing enzyme CYP2C19, coadministration of modafinil with drugs such as diazepam, phenytoin and propranolol, which are largely eliminated via that pathway, may increase the circulating levels of those compounds. In addition, in individuals deficient in the enzyme CYP2D6 (i.e., 7–10% of the Caucasian population; similar or lower in other populations), the levels of CYP2D6 substrates such as tricyclic antidepressants and selective serotonin reuptake inhibitors, which have ancillary routes of elimination through CYP2C19, may be increased by coadministration of modafinil. Dose adjustments may be necessary for patients being treated with these and similar medications (See **PRECAUTIONS, Drug Interactions**).

Chronic administration of modafinil may also cause modest induction of the metabolizing enzyme CYP3A4, thus reducing the levels of co-administered substrates for that enzyme system, such as steroidal contraceptives, cyclosporine and, to a lesser degree, theophylline. Dose adjustments may be necessary for patients being treated with these and similar medications (See **PRECAUTIONS, Drug Interactions**).

An apparent concentration-related suppression of CYP2C9 activity was observed in human hepatocytes after exposure to modafinil *in vitro*. Although no other indication of CYP2C9 suppression has been observed, the *in vitro* results suggest that there is potential for metabolic interaction between PROVIGIL and CYP2C9 substrates, such as warfarin or phenytoin (See **PRECAUTIONS, Drug Interactions**).

Special Populations

Gender Effect: The pharmacokinetics of modafinil are not affected by gender.

Age Effect: A slight decrease (~20%) in the oral clearance (CL/F) of modafinil was observed in a single dose study at 200 mg in 12 subjects with a mean age of 63 years (range 53–72 years), but the change was considered unlikely to be clinically significant. In a multiple dose study (300 mg/day) in 12 patients with a mean age of 82 years (range 67–87 years), the mean levels of modafinil in plasma were approximately two times those historically obtained in matched younger subjects. Due to potential effects from the multiple concomitant medications with which most of the patients were being treated, the apparent difference in modafinil pharmacokinetics may not be attributable solely to the effects of aging. However, the results suggest that the clearance of modafinil may be reduced in the elderly (See **DOSAGE AND ADMINISTRATION**).

Race Effect: The influence of race on the pharmacokinetics of modafinil has not been studied.

Renal Impairment: In a single dose 200 mg modafinil study, severe chronic renal failure (creatinine clearance ≤20 mL/min) did not significantly influence the pharmacokinetics of modafinil, but exposure to modafinil acid (an inactive metabolite) was increased 9 fold (See **PRECAUTIONS**).

Hepatic Impairment: Pharmacokinetics and metabolism were examined in patients with cirrhosis of the liver (6 M and 3 F). Three patients had stage B or B+ cirrhosis (per the Child criteria) and 6 patients had stage C or C+ cirrhosis. Clinically 8 of 9 patients were icteric and all had ascites. In these patients, the oral clearance of modafinil was decreased by about 60% and the steady state concentration was doubled compared to normal patients. The dose of PROVIGIL should be reduced in patients with severe hepatic impairment (See **PRECAUTIONS** and **DOSAGE AND ADMINISTRATION**).

CLINICAL TRIALS

The effectiveness of PROVIGIL in reducing the excessive daytime sleepiness (EDS) associated with narcolepsy was established in two US 9-week, multicenter, placebo-controlled, two-dose (200 mg per day and 400 mg per day) parallel-group, double-blind studies of outpatients who met the ICD-9 and American Sleep Disorders Association criteria for narcolepsy (which are also consistent with the American Psychiatric Association DSM-IV criteria). These criteria include either 1) recurrent daytime naps or lapses into sleep that occur almost daily for at least three months, plus sudden bilateral loss of postural muscle tone in association with intense emotion (cataplexy) or 2) a complaint of excessive sleepiness or sudden muscle weakness with associated features: sleep paralysis, hypnagogic hallucinations, automatic behaviors, disrupted major sleep episode; and polysomnography demonstrating one of the following: sleep latency less than 10 minutes or rapid eye movement (REM) sleep latency less than 20 minutes. In addition, for entry into these studies, all patients were required to have objectively documented excessive daytime sleepiness, a Multiple Sleep Latency Test (MSLT) with two or more sleep onset REM periods, and the absence of any other clinically significant active medical or psychiatric disorder. The MSLT, an objective daytime polysomnographic assessment of the patient's ability to fall asleep in an unstimulating environment, measures latency (in minutes) to sleep onset averaged over 4 test sessions at 2-hour intervals following nocturnal polysomnography. For each test session, the subject was told to lie quietly and attempt to sleep. Each test session was terminated after 20 minutes if no sleep occurred or 15 minutes after sleep onset.

In both studies, the primary measures of effectiveness were 1) sleep latency, as assessed by the Maintenance of Wakefulness Test (MWT) and 2) the change in the patient's overall disease status, as measured by the Clinical Global Impression of Change (CGI-C). For a successful trial, both measures had to show significant improvement.

The MWT measures latency (in minutes) to sleep onset averaged over 4 test sessions at 2 hour intervals following nocturnal polysomnography. For each test session, the subject was asked to attempt to remain awake without using extraordinary measures. Each test session was terminated after 20 minutes if no sleep occurred or 10 minutes after sleep onset. The CGI-C is a 7-point scale, centered at *No Change*, and ranging from *Very Much Worse* to *Very Much Improved*. Patients were rated by evaluators who had no access to any data about the patients other than a measure of their baseline severity. Evaluators were not given any specific guidance about the criteria they were to apply when rating patients.

Other assessments of effect included the Multiple Sleep Latency Test (MSLT), Epworth Sleepiness Scale (ESS; a series of questions designed to assess the degree of sleepiness in everyday situations) the Steer Clear Performance Test (SCPT; a computer-based evaluation of a patient's ability to avoid hitting obstacles in a simulated driving situation), standard nocturnal polysomnography, and patient's daily sleep log. Patients were also assessed with the Quality of Life in Narcolepsy (QOLIN) scale, which contains the validated SF-36 health questionnaire.

Both studies demonstrated improvement in objective and subjective measures of excessive daytime sleepiness for both the 200 mg and 400 mg doses compared to placebo. Patients treated with either dose of PROVIGIL showed a statistically significantly enhanced ability to remain awake on the MWT (all p values <0.001) at weeks 3, 6, 9, and endpoint compared to placebo and a statistically significantly greater global improvement, as rated on the CGI-C scale (all p values <0.05).

The average sleep latencies (in minutes) on the MWT at endpoint in the 2 controlled trials are shown in the table below:

Table 1. MWT Average Sleep Latency at Endpoint
Average Sleep Latency at Endpoint

		PROVIGIL	
	Placebo	200 mg*	400 mg*
Trial 1	5.07	8.18	8.90
Trial 2	5.35	8.28	7.86

*significantly different from placebo for both trials ($p<0.001$)

The percentages of patients who showed any degree of improvement on the CGI-C in the two clinical trials are shown in the table below:

Table 2. Clinical Global Impression of Change (CGI-C)
Percent of Patients Who Improved at Endpoint

		PROVIGIL	
	Placebo	200 mg*	400 mg*
Trial 1	37%	64%	72%
Trial 2	38%	58%	60%

*significantly different from placebo for both trials (Trial 1: $p<0.001$; Trial 2: $p<0.01$)

Similar statistically significant treatment-related improvements were seen on other measures of impairment in narcolepsy, including a decrease in the propensity to fall asleep on the MSLT ($p<0.001$ for each dose in comparison to placebo) and a statistically significant lessening of patient-assessed level of daytime sleepiness on the ESS ($p<0.001$ for each dose in comparison to placebo).

Although PROVIGIL tended to be numerically superior to placebo on several of the other outcome measures, there were no consistent statistically significant differences between drug and placebo on these measures.

Nighttime sleep measured with nocturnal polysomnography was not affected by the use of PROVIGIL.

The effectiveness of modafinil in long-term use (greater than 9 weeks) has not been systematically evaluated in placebo-controlled trials. The physician who elects to prescribe PROVIGIL tablets for an extended time should periodically re-evaluate long-term usefulness for the individual patient.

INDICATIONS AND USAGE

PROVIGIL is indicated to improve wakefulness in patients with excessive daytime sleepiness associated with narcolepsy.

CONTRAINDICATIONS

PROVIGIL is contraindicated in patients with known hypersensitivity to modafinil.

PRECAUTIONS

General

Although modafinil has not been shown to produce functional impairment, any drug affecting the CNS may alter judgment, thinking or motor skills. Patients should be cautioned about operating an automobile or other hazardous machinery until they are reasonably certain that PROVIGIL therapy will not adversely affect their ability to engage in such activities.

Cardiovascular System

In clinical studies of PROVIGIL, signs and symptoms including chest pain, palpitations, dyspnea and transient ischemic T-wave changes on ECG were observed in three subjects in association with mitral valve prolapse or left ventricular hypertrophy. It is recommended that PROVIGIL tablets not be used in patients with a history of left ventricular hypertrophy or ischemic ECG changes, chest pain, arrhythmia or other clinically significant manifestations of mitral valve prolapse in association with CNS stimulant use.

Modafinil has not been evaluated or used to any appreciable extent in patients with a recent history of myocardial infarction or unstable angina, and such patients should be treated with caution.

Modafinil has not been systematically evaluated in patients with hypertension. Periodic monitoring of hypertensive patients may be appropriate.

Central Nervous System

One healthy male volunteer developed ideas of reference, paranoid delusions, and auditory hallucinations in association with multiple daily 600 mg doses of PROVIGIL and sleep deprivation. There was no evidence of psychosis 36 hours after drug discontinuation. Caution should be exercised when PROVIGIL is given to patients with a history of psychosis.

Patients with Severe Renal Impairment

In patients with severe renal impairment (mean creatinine clearance = 16.6 mL/min), a 200 mg single dose of modafinil did not lead to increased exposure to modafinil but resulted in much higher exposure to the inactive metabolite, modafinil acid, than is seen in subjects with normal renal function. There is little information available about the safety of such levels of this metabolite (See **CLINICAL PHARMACOLOGY**).

Patients with Severe Hepatic Impairment

In patients with severe hepatic impairment, with or without cirrhosis (See **CLINICAL PHARMACOLOGY**), PROVIGIL should be administered at a reduced dose as the clearance of modafinil was decreased compared to that in normal subjects (See **DOSAGE AND ADMINISTRATION**).

Elderly Patients

To the extent that elderly patients may have diminished renal and/or hepatic function, dosage reductions should be considered (See **DOSAGE AND ADMINISTRATION**).

Patients Using Contraceptives

The effectiveness of steroidal contraceptives may be reduced when used with PROVIGIL tablets and for one month after discontinuation of therapy (See *Potential Interactions with Drugs That Inhibit, Induce, or are Metabolized by Cytochrome P-450 Isoenzymes and Other Hepatic Enzymes*). Alternative or concomitant methods of contraception are recommended for patients treated with PROVIGIL tablets, and for one month after discontinuation of PROVIGIL.

Information for Patients

Physicians are advised to discuss the following issues with patients for whom they prescribe PROVIGIL tablets.

Pregnancy

Animal studies to assess the effects of modafinil on reproduction and the developing fetus were not conducted at adequately high doses or according to guidelines which would ensure a comprehensive evaluation of the potential of modafinil to adversely affect fertility, or cause embryolethality or teratogenicity (See *Impairment of Fertility* and **Pregnancy**).

Patients should be advised to notify their physician if they become pregnant or intend to become pregnant during therapy. Patients should be cautioned regarding the potential increased risk of pregnancy when using steroidal contraceptives (including depot or implantable contraceptives) with PROVIGIL tablets and for one month after discontinuation of therapy.

Nursing

Patients should be advised to notify their physician if they are breast feeding an infant.

Concomitant Medication

Patients should be advised to inform their physician if they are taking, or plan to take, any prescription or over-the-counter drugs, because of the potential for interactions between PROVIGIL tablets and other drugs.

Alcohol

Patients should be advised that the use of PROVIGIL in combination with alcohol has not been studied. Patients should be advised that it is prudent to avoid alcohol while taking PROVIGIL tablets.

Allergic Reactions

Patients should be advised to notify their physician if they develop a rash, hives, or a related allergic phenomenon.

Drug Interactions

CNS Active Drugs

Methylphenidate—In a single-dose study in healthy volunteers, coadministration of modafinil (200 mg) with methylphenidate (40 mg) did not cause any significant alterations in the pharmacokinetics of either drug. However, the absorption of PROVIGIL may be delayed by approximately one hour when coadministered with methylphenidate.

Clomipramine—The coadministration of a single dose of clomipramine (50 mg) on the first of three days of treatment with modafinil (200 mg/day) in healthy volunteers did not show an effect on the pharmacokinetics of either drug. However, one incident of increased levels of clomipramine and its active metabolite desmethylclomipramine has been reported in a patient with narcolepsy during treatment with modafinil (See *Potential Interactions with Drugs That In-*

Continued on next page

Provigil—Cont.

hibit, Induce, or are Metabolized by Cytochrome P-450 Isoenzymes and Other Hepatic Enzymes).

Triazolam—In a single-dose pharmacodynamic study with PROVIGIL in healthy volunteers (50, 100 or 200 mg) and triazolam (0.25 mg), no clinically important alterations in the safety profile of modafinil or triazolam were noted.

Monoamine Oxidase (MAO) Inhibitors—Interaction studies with monoamine oxidase inhibitors have not been performed. Therefore, caution should be used when concomitantly administering MAO inhibitors and modafinil.

Potential Interactions with Drugs That Inhibit, Induce, or are Metabolized by Cytochrome P-450 Isoenzymes and Other Hepatic Enzymes

In a controlled study in patients with narcolepsy, chronic dosing of PROVIGIL at 400 mg/day once daily resulted in a ~20% mean decrease in modafinil plasma trough concentrations by week 9, relative to those at week 3, suggesting that chronic administration of PROVIGIL might have caused induction of its metabolism. In addition, coadministration of potent inducers of CYP3A4 (e.g., carbamazepine, phenobarbital, rifampin) or inhibitors of CYP3A4 (e.g., ketoconazole, itraconazole) could alter the levels of modafinil due to the partial involvement of that enzyme in the metabolic elimination of the compound.

In *in vitro* studies using primary human hepatocyte cultures, modafinil was shown to slightly induce CYP1A2, CYP2B6 and CYP3A4 in a concentration-dependent manner. Although induction results based on *in vitro* experiments are not necessarily predictive of response *in vivo*, caution needs to be exercised when PROVIGIL is coadministered with drugs that depend on these three enzymes for their clearance. Specifically, lower blood levels of such drugs could result. In the case of CYP1A2 and CYP2B6, no other evidence of enzyme induction has been observed. A modest induction of CYP3A4 by modafinil has been indicated by other results, hence the clearance of CYP3A4 substrates such as cyclosporine, steroidal contraceptives and, to a lesser degree, theophylline, may be increased.

One case of an interaction between modafinil and cyclosporine has been reported in a 41 year old woman who had undergone an organ transplant. After one month of administration of 200 mg/day of modafinil, cyclosporine blood levels were decreased by 50%. The interaction was postulated to be due to the increased metabolism of cyclosporine, since no other factor expected to affect the disposition of the drug had changed.

The exposure of human hepatocytes to modafinil *in vitro* produced an apparent concentration-related suppression of expression of CYP2C9 activity. The clinical relevance of this finding is unclear, since no other indication of CYP2C9 suppression has been observed. However, monitoring of prothrombin times is suggested as a precaution for the first several months of coadministration of PROVIGIL and warfarin, a CYP2C9 substrate, and thereafter whenever PROVIGIL dosing is changed. In addition, patients receiving PROVIGIL and phenytoin, a CYP2C9 substrate, concomitantly should be monitored for signs of phenytoin toxicity.

In vitro studies using human liver microsomes showed that modafinil has little or no capacity to inhibit the major CYP enzymes except for CYP2C19, which is reversibly inhibited at pharmacologically relevant concentrations of modafinil. Drugs that are largely eliminated via CYP2C19 metabolism, such as diazepam, propranolol, phenytoin or S-mephenytoin may have prolonged elimination upon coadministration with PROVIGIL and may require dosage reduction.

In addition, CYP2C19 provides an ancillary pathway for the metabolism of certain tricyclic antidepressants (e.g., clomipramine and desipramine) that are primarily metabolized by CYP2D6. In tricyclic-treated patients deficient in CYP2D6 (i.e., those who are poor metabolizers of debrisoquine; 7–10% of the Caucasian population; similar or lower in other populations), the amount of metabolism by CYP2C19 may be substantially increased. PROVIGIL may cause elevation of the levels of the tricyclics in this subset of patients. Physicians should be aware that a reduction in the dose of tricyclic agents might be needed in these patients.

Carcinogenesis, Mutagenesis, Impairment of Fertility

Carcinogenesis

Carcinogenicity studies were conducted in which modafinil was administered in the diet to mice for 78 weeks and to rats for 104 weeks at doses of 6, 30 and 60 mg/kg/day. The highest dose studied represents 1.5 times (mouse) or 3 times (rat) greater than the maximum recommended human daily dose of 200 mg on a mg/m^2 basis. There was no evidence of tumorigenesis associated with modafinil administration in these studies, but because the mouse study used an inadequate high dose that was not representative of a maximum tolerated dose, the carcinogenic potential of modafinil has not been fully evaluated.

Mutagenesis

There was no evidence of mutagenic or clastogenic potential of modafinil in a series of assays. It was not mutagenic in the *in vitro* Ames bacterial reverse mutation test, the *in vitro* mouse lymphoma/TK locus assay in the presence or absence of metabolic activation; and it was not clastogenic in the *in vitro* human lymphocyte chromosomal aberration assay in the presence or absence of metabolic activation, or in two *in vivo* mouse bone marrow micronucleus assays. Modafinil did not increase unscheduled DNA synthesis in rat hepatocytes. In a cell transformation assay in BALB/3T3 mouse embryo cells, modafinil did not cause an increase in the frequency of transformed foci in the presence or absence of metabolic activation.

Table 3. Incidence of Treatment-Emergent Adverse Experiences in US 9-Week Placebo-Controlled Clinical Trials[1] with PROVIGIL (200 mg and 400 mg) Daily

Body System	Preferred Term	Modafinil (n = 369)	Placebo (n = 185)
Body as a Whole	Headache	50%	40%
	Chest pain	2%	1%
	Neck pain	2%	1%
	Chills	2%	0%
	Rigid Neck	1%	0%
	Fever/Chills	1%	0%
Digestive	Nausea	13%	4%
	Diarrhea	8%	4%
	Dry mouth	5%	1%
	Anorexia	5%	1%
	Abnormal liver function[2]	3%	2%
	Vomiting	2%	1%
	Mouth ulcer	1%	0%
	Gingivitis	1%	0%
	Thirst	1%	0%
Respiratory System	Rhinitis	11%	8%
	Pharyngitis	6%	3%
	Lung disorder	4%	2%
	Dyspnea	2%	1%
	Asthma	1%	0%
	Epistaxis	1%	0%
Nervous System	Nervousness	8%	6%
	Dizziness	5%	4%
	Depression	4%	3%
	Anxiety	4%	1%
	Cataplexy	3%	2%
	Insomnia	3%	1%
	Paresthesia	3%	1%
	Dyskinesia[3]	2%	0%
	Hypertonia	2%	0%
	Confusion	1%	0%
	Amnesia	1%	0%
	Emotional lability	1%	0%
	Ataxia	1%	0%
	Tremor	1%	0%
Cardiovascular	Hypotension	2%	1%
	Hypertension	2%	0%
	Vasodilation	1%	0%
	Arrhythmia	1%	0%
	Syncope	1%	0%
Hemic/Lymphatic	Eosinophilia	2%	0%
Special Senses	Amblyopia	2%	1%
	Abnormal vision	2%	0%
Metabolic/Nutritional	Hyperglycemia	1%	0%
	Albuminuria	1%	0%
Musculco-skeletal	Joint disorder	1%	0%
Skin/Appendages	Herpes simplex	1%	0%
	Dry skin	1%	0%
Urgoenital	Abnormal urine	1%	0%
	Urinary retention	1%	0%
	Abnormal ejaculation[4]	1%	0%

[1] Events reported by at least 1% of patients treated with PROVIGIL that were more frequent than in the placebo group are included; incidence is rounded to the nearest 1%. The adverse experience terminology is coded using a standard modified COSTART Dictionary.
Events for which the PROVIGIL incidence was at least 1%, but equal to or less than placebo are not listed in the table. These events included the following: infection, back pain, pain, hypothermia, abdominal pain, flu syndrome, allergic reaction, fever, asthenia, accidental injury, general edema, tachycardia, palpitations, migraine, ventricular extrasystole, bradycardia, dyspepsia, tooth disorder, constipation, flatulence, increased appetite, gastroenteritis, GI disorder, ecchymosis, anemia, leukocytosis, peripheral edema, increased weight, increased SGOT, myalgia, arthritis, arthralgia, somnolence, thinking abnormality, leg cramps, sleep disorder, hallucinations, hyperkinesia, decreased libido, increased cough, sinusitis, bronchitis, pneumonia, rash, sweating, pruritus, skin disorder, psoriasis, ear pain, eye pain, ear disorder, taste perversion, dysmenorrhea[4], urinary tract infection, pyuria, hematuria, cystitis, and disturbed menses[4].

[2] Elevated liver enzymes.

[3] Oro-facial dyskinesias.

[4] Incidence adjusted for gender.

Impairment of Fertility

When modafinil was administered orally to male and female rats prior to and throughout mating and gestation at doses up to 100 mg/kg/day (4.8 times the maximum recommended daily dose of 200 mg on a mg/m^2 basis) no effects on fertility were seen. The study to evaluate these effects, however, did not use sufficiently high doses or large enough sample size to adequately assess effects on fertility.

Pregnancy

Pregnancy Category C: Embryotoxicity was observed in the absence of maternal toxicity when rats received oral modafinil throughout the period of organogenesis. At a dose of 200 mg/kg/day (10 times the maximum recommended daily human dose of 200 mg on a mg/m^2 basis) there was an increase in resorption, hydronephrosis, and skeletal variations. The no-effect dose for these effects was 100 mg/kg/day (5 times the maximum recommended daily human dose on a mg/m^2 basis). When rabbits received oral modafinil throughout organogenesis at doses up to 100 mg/kg/day (10 times the maximum recommended daily human dose on a mg/m^2 basis), no embryotoxicity was seen. Neither of these studies, however, used optimal doses for the evaluation of embryotoxicity. Although a threshold dose for embryotoxicity has been identified, the full spectrum of potential toxic effects on the fetus has not been characterized. When rats were dosed throughout gestation and lactation at doses up to 200 mg/kg/day, no developmental toxicity was noted postnatally in the offspring. There are no adequate and well-controlled trials with modafinil in pregnant women and this drug should be used during pregnancy only if the potential benefit outweighs the potential risk.

Labor and Delivery

The effect of modafinil on labor and delivery in humans has not been systematically investigated. Seven normal births occurred in patients who had received modafinil during pregnancy. One patient gave birth 3 weeks earlier than the expected range of delivery dates (estimated using ultrasound) to a healthy male infant. One woman with a history of spontaneous abortions suffered a spontaneous abortion while being treated with modafinil.

Nursing Mothers

It is not known whether modafinil or its metabolites are excreted in human milk. Because many drugs are excreted in human milk, caution should be exercised when PROVIGIL tablets are administered to a nursing woman.

PEDIATRIC USE
Safety and effectiveness in individuals below 16 years of age have not been established.
GERIATRIC USE
Safety and effectiveness in individuals above 65 years of age have not been established. Experience in a limited number of patients (15) who were greater than 65 years of age in US clinical trials showed an incidence of adverse experiences similar to other age groups.

ADVERSE REACTIONS
Modafinil has been evaluated for safety in over 2200 subjects, of whom more than 900 subjects with narcolepsy or narcolepsy/hypersomnia were given at least one dose of modafinil. Modafinil has been found to be generally well-tolerated. In controlled clinical trials, most adverse experiences were mild to moderate.
The most commonly observed adverse events (≥5%) associated with the use of modafinil more frequently than placebo-treated patients in controlled US and foreign studies were headache, infection, nausea, nervousness, anxiety, and insomnia.
In US placebo-controlled Phase 3 clinical trials, 5% of the 369 patients who received PROVIGIL discontinued due to an adverse experience. The most frequent (≥1%) reasons for discontinuation that occurred at a higher rate for PROVIGIL than placebo patients were headache (1%), nausea (1%), depression (1%) and nervousness (1%). In foreign, controlled clinical trials, reasons for discontinuation were similar to those in US trials. In a Canadian clinical trial, a 35 year old obese narcoleptic male with a prior history of syncopal episodes experienced a 9-second episode of asystole while sleeping after 27 days of modafinil treatment (300 mg/day in divided doses).
Incidence in Controlled Trials
The following table presents the adverse experiences that occurred in narcolepsy patients at a rate of 1% or more and were more frequent in patients treated with PROVIGIL than in placebo patients in US placebo-controlled clinical trials.
The prescriber should be aware that the figures provided below cannot be used to predict the frequency of adverse experiences in the course of usual medical practice, where patient characteristics and other factors may differ from those occurring during clinical studies. Similarly, the cited frequencies cannot be directly compared with figures obtained from other clinical investigations involving different treatments, uses, or investigators. Review of these frequencies, however, provides prescribers with a basis to estimate the relative contribution of drug and non-drug factors to the incidence of adverse events in the population studied.
[See table 3 at top of previous page]
Dose Dependency of Adverse Events
In the US Phase 3 clinical trials, the only adverse experience that was more frequent (≥5% difference) in the PROVIGIL dose group of 400 mg/day than in the PROVIGIL dose group of 200 mg/day and placebo was headache.
Vital Sign Changes
There were no consistent effects or patterns of change in vital signs for patients treated with PROVIGIL enrolled in the US Phase 3 clinical trials.
Weight Changes
There were no clinically significant differences in body weight change in patients treated with PROVIGIL compared to placebo-treated patients.
Laboratory Changes
Clinical chemistry, hematology, and urinalysis parameters were monitored in US Phase 1, 2 and 3 studies. In these studies, mean plasma levels of gamma-glutamyl transferase (GGT) were found to be higher following administration of PROVIGIL, but not placebo. Few subjects (1%), however, had GGT elevations outside of the normal range. Shift to higher, but not clinically significantly abnormal, GGT values appeared to increase with time in the population treated with PROVIGIL in the 9-week US phase 3 clinical trials. No differences were apparent in alkaline phosphatase, alanine aminotransferase, aspartate aminotransferase, total protein, albumin, or total bilirubin.
Although there were more abnormal eosinophil counts following PROVIGIL administration than placebo in US Phase 1 and 2 studies, the difference does not appear to be clinically significant. Observed shifts were from normal to high.
ECG Changes
No treatment-emergent pattern of ECG abnormalities was found in US Phase 1, 2, and 3 studies following administration of PROVIGIL.

DRUG ABUSE AND DEPENDENCE
Controlled Substance Class
Modafinil (PROVIGIL) is listed in Schedule IV of the Controlled Substances Act.
Abuse Potential and Dependence
In addition to its wakefulness-promoting effect and increased locomotor activity in animals, in humans, PROVIGIL produces psychoactive and euphoric effects, alterations in mood, perception, thinking and feelings typical of other CNS stimulants. In *in vitro* binding studies, modafinil binds to the dopamine reuptake site and causes an increase in extracellular dopamine, but no increase in dopamine release. Modafinil is reinforcing, as evidenced by its self-administration in monkeys previously trained to self-administer cocaine. In some studies, modafinil was also partially discriminated as stimulant-like. Physicians should follow patients closely, especially those with a history of drug and/or stimulant (e.g., methylphenidate, amphetamine, or cocaine) abuse. Patients should be observed for signs of misuse or abuse (e.g., incrementation of doses or drug-seeking behavior).
The abuse potential of modafinil (200, 400, and 800 mg) was assessed relative to methylphenidate (45 and 90 mg) in an inpatient study in individuals experienced with drugs of abuse. Results from this clinical study demonstrated that modafinil produced psychoactive and euphoric effects and feelings consistent with other scheduled CNS stimulants (methylphenidate).
Withdrawal
The effects of modafinil withdrawal were monitored following 9 weeks of modafinil use in one US Phase 3 controlled clinical trial. No specific symptoms of withdrawal were observed during 14 days of observation, although sleepiness returned in narcoleptic patients.

OVERDOSAGE
Human Experience
A total of 151 doses of 1000 mg/day (5 times the maximum recommended daily dose of 200 mg) or more, have been recorded for 32 individuals. Doses of 4500 mg and 4000 mg were taken intentionally by two patients participating in foreign depression studies. In both cases, the adverse experiences observed were limited, expected, and not life-threatening, and the patients recovered fully by the following day. The adverse experiences included excitation or agitation, insomnia, and slight or moderate elevations in hemodynamic parameters. In neither of these cases nor in other instances of doses of more than 1000 mg/day, including experience with up to 21 consecutive days of dosing at 1200 mg/day, were any unexpected effects or specific organ toxicities observed. Other observed high dose effects in clinical studies have included anxiety, irritability, aggressiveness, confusion, nervousness, tremor, palpitations, sleep disturbances, nausea, diarrhea and decreased prothrombin time.
Overdose Management
No specific antidote to the toxic effects of modafinil overdose has been identified to date. Such overdoses should be managed with primarily supportive care, including cardiovascular monitoring. If there are no contraindications, induced emesis or gastric lavage should be considered. There are no data to suggest the utility of dialysis or urinary acidification or alkalinization in enhancing drug elimination. The physician should consider contacting a poison-control center on the treatment of any overdose.

DOSAGE AND ADMINISTRATION
The dose of PROVIGIL is 200 mg/day, given as a single dose in the morning.
Doses of 400 mg/day, given as a single dose, have been well tolerated, but there is no consistent evidence that this dose confers additional benefit beyond that of the 200 mg dose (See **CLINICAL PHARMACOLOGY, CLINICAL TRIALS**).
In patients with severe hepatic impairment, the dose of PROVIGIL should be reduced to one-half of that recommended for patients with normal hepatic function (See **CLINICAL PHARMACOLOGY** and **PRECAUTIONS**).
There is inadequate information to determine safety and efficacy of dosing in patients with severe renal impairment (See **CLINICAL PHARMACOLOGY** and **PRECAUTIONS**).
In elderly patients, elimination of PROVIGIL and its metabolites may be reduced as a consequence of aging. Therefore, consideration should be given to the use of lower doses in this population (See **CLINICAL PHARMACOLOGY** and **PRECAUTIONS**).

HOW SUPPLIED: PROVIGIL® (MODAFINIL) TABLETS
100 mg Each capsule-shaped, white, uncoated tablet is debossed with "PROVIGIL" on one side and "100 MG" on the other.
NDC 63459-100-01—Bottles of 100
200 mg Each capsule-shaped, white, scored, uncoated tablet is debossed with "PROVIGIL" on one side and "200 MG" on the other.
NDC 63459-200-01—Bottles of 100
Store at 20°–25° C (68°–77° F).
Caution: Federal law prohibits dispensing without prescription.
Manufactured for:
Cephalon, Inc.
West Chester, PA 19380

13360-2
R2 12/99
Shown in Product Identification Guide, page 310

For EMERGENCY telephone numbers, consult the **Manufacturers' Index**.

Cetylite Industries, Inc.
9051 RIVER ROAD
P.O. BOX 90006
PENNSAUKEN, NJ 08110-0700

Direct Inquiries to:
Mr. Stanley L. Wachman, President
(856) 665-6111
(800) 257-7740
FAX: (856) 665-5408

CETACAINE® ℞
[*set'a-cane"*]
TOPICAL ANESTHETIC

ACTIVE INGREDIENTS

Benzocaine	14.0%
Butyl Aminobenzoate	2.0%
Tetracaine Hydrochloride	2.0%

CONTAINS

Benzalkonium Chloride	0.5%
Cetyl Dimethyl Ethyl Ammonium Bromide	0.005%

In bland, water-soluble base.

ACTION
The onset of Cetacaine produced anesthesia is rapid (approximately 30 seconds) and the duration of anesthesia is typically 30–60 minutes, when used as directed. This effect is due to the rapid onset, but short duration of action of Benzocaine coupled with the slow onset, but extended duration of Tetracaine HCl and bridged by the intermediate action of Butamben.
It is believed that all of these agents act by reversibly blocking nerve conduction. Speed and duration of action is determined by the ability of the agent to be absorbed by the mucous membrane and nerve sheath and then to diffuse out, and ultimately be metabolized (primarily by plasma cholinesterases) to inert metabolites which are excreted in the urine.

INDICATIONS
Cetacaine is a topical anesthetic indicated for the production of anesthesia of all accessible mucous membrane except the eyes. Cetacaine Spray is indicated for use to control pain or gagging. Cetacaine in all forms is indicated to control pain and for use for surgical or endoscopic or other procedures in the ear, nose, mouth, pharynx, larynx, trachea, bronchi, and esophagus. It may also be used for vaginal or rectal procedures when feasible.

DOSAGE AND ADMINISTRATION
Cetacaine Spray should be applied for approximately one second or less for normal anesthesia. Only a limited quantity of Cetacaine is required for anesthesia. Spray in excess of two seconds is contraindicated. Average expulsion rate of residue from spray, at normal temperatures, is 200 mg per second.
Tissue need not be dried prior to application of Cetacaine. Cetacaine should be applied directly to the site where pain control is required. Cetacaine Liquid may be applied with a cotton applicator or directly to tissue. The cotton applicator should not be held in position for extended periods of time, since local reactions to benzoate topical anesthetics are related to the length of time of application.

ADVERSE REACTIONS
Hypersensitivity Reactions: Unpredictable adverse reactions (ie, hypersensitivity, including anaphylaxis) are extremely rare.
Localized allergic reactions may occur after prolonged or repeated use of any aminobenzoate anesthetic. The most common adverse reaction caused by local anesthetics is contact dermatitis charaterized by erythema and pruritus that may progress to vesiculation and oozing. This occurs most commonly in patients following prolonged self-medication, which is contraindicated. If rash, urticaria, edema, or other manifestations of allergy develop during use, the drug should be discontinued. To minimize the possibility of a serious allergic reaction, Cetacaine preparations should not be applied for prolonged periods except under continual supervision. Dehydration of the epithelium or an escharotic effect may also result from prolonged contact.

PRECAUTION
On rare occasions, methemoglobinemia has been reported in connection with the use of benzocaine-containing products. Care should be used not to exceed a two second spray. If a patient becomes cyanotic, treat appropriately to counteract (such as with methylene blue, if medically indicated).
USE IN PREGNANCY
Safe use of Cetacaine has not been established with respect to possible adverse effects upon fetal development. Therefore, Cetacaine should not be used during early pregnancy, unless in the judgement of a physician, the potential ben-

Continued on next page

Cetacaine—Cont.

efits outweigh the unknown hazards. Routine precaution for the use of any topical anesthetic should be observed when Cetacaine is used.

Appropriate pediatric dosage has not been established for this product.

CONTRAINDICATIONS

Cetacaine is not suitable and should never be used for injection. Do not use on the eyes. To avoid excessive systemic absorption, Cetacaine should not be applied to large areas of denuded or inflamed tissue. Cetacaine should not be administered to patients who are hypersensitive to any of its ingredients or to patients known to have cholinesterase deficiencies. Tolerance may vary with the status of the patient. Dosage should be reduced in the debilitated elderly, acutely ill, and very young patients.

Individual dosage of tetracaine hydrochloride in excess of 20 mg is contraindicated. Cetacaine should not be used under dentures or cotton rolls, as retention of the active ingredients under a denture or cotton roll could possibly cause an escharotic effect. Routine precaution for the use of any topical anesthetic should be observed when using Cetacaine.

Jetco® Cannula for Cetacaine Spray

- The supplied 4" stainless steel Jetco® cannula (J-4) for Cetacaine Spray is especially designed for accessibility and application of Cetacaine, at the required site of pain control.
- The Jetco cannula is also available in 6", (J-6) and 8" curved configuration, (J-8).
- Replacement Jetco cannulas are available.
- The Jetco cannula is inserted firmly into the protruding plastic stem on each bottle of Cetacaine Spray.
- The Jetco cannula may be removed and reinserted as many times as required for cleansing or sterilization, and is autoclavable.

PACKAGING AVAILABLE

Cetacaine Spray 56 g. including propellant.
Cetacaine Liquid 56 g.
Cetacaine Hospital Gel 29 g. Tube.

CAUTION

Federal law prohibits dispensing Cetacaine without prescription.

CETYLITE
INDUSTRIES, INC.
9051 River Road
Pennsauken, NJ 08110-3293
1-800-257-7740
www.cetylite.com
Made in U.S.A. Rev. 11/99

Shown in Product Identification Guide, page 310

Chiron Corporation

4560 HORTON STREET
EMERYVILLE, CA 94608-2916

For Medical Information Contact:
Generally:
Professional Services (7:00 AM to 5:00 PM PST):
(800) CHIRON-8 selection #2
(800) 244-7668 selection #2
FAX: (510) 923-3435
e-mail: drug__info@cc.chiron.com
In Emergencies:
(7:00 AM to 5:00 PM PST):
(800) CHIRON-8 selection #3
(800) 244-7668 selection #3
After Hours and Weekend Emergencies:
(415) 487-8335
Sales and Ordering:
(800) CHIRON-8 selection #1
(800) 244-7668 selection #1
FAX: (510) 923-3434

DEPOCYT™ ℞

(cytarabine liposome injection)
For Intrathecal Use Only
50 mg vial
Rx only

WARNING

DepoCyt™ (cytarabine liposome injection) should be administered only under the supervision of a qualified physician experienced in the use of intrathecal cancer chemotherapeutic agents. Appropriate management of complications is possible only when adequate diagnostic and treatment facilities are readily available. In all clinical studies, chemical arachnoiditis, a syndrome manifested primarily by nausea, vomiting, headache and fever, was a common adverse event. If left untreated, chemical arachnoiditis may be fatal. The incidence and severity of chemical arachnoiditis can be reduced by coadministration of dexamethasone (see WARNINGS). Patients receiving DepoCyt should be treated concurrently with dexamethasone to mitigate the symptoms of chemical arachnoiditis (see DOSAGE AND ADMINISTRATION).

DESCRIPTION

DepoCyt™ (cytarabine liposome injection) is a sterile, injectable suspension of the antimetabolite cytarabine, encapsulated into multivesicular lipid-based particles. Chemically, cytarabine is 4-amino-1-β-D-arabinofuranosyl-2(1H)-pyrimidinone, also known as cytosine arabinoside ($C_9H_{13}N_3O_5$, molecular weight 243.22).

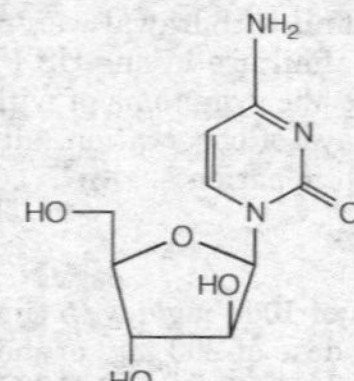

The following is an artist's rendition of a DepoCyt particle:

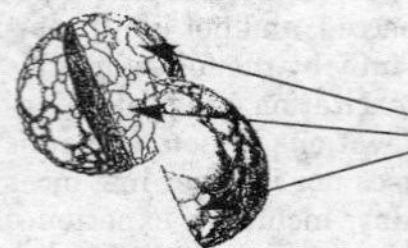

Nonconcentric vesicles, each with an internal, aqueous chamber containing encapsulated cytarabine solution, surrounded by a bilayer lipid membrane.

DepoCyt is available in 5 mL, ready-to-use, single-use vials containing 50 mg of cytarabine. DepoCyt is formulated as a sterile, nonpyrogenic, white to off-white suspension of cytarabine in Sodium Chloride 0.9% w/v in Water for Injection. DepoCyt is preservative-free. Cytarabine, the active ingredient, is present at a concentration of 10 mg/mL and is encapsulated in the particles. Inactive ingredients at their respective approximate concentrations are cholesterol, 4.1 mg/mL; triolein, 1.2 mg/mL; dioleoylphosphatidylcholine (DOPC), 5.7 mg/mL; and dipalmitoylphosphatidylglycerol (DPPG), 1.0 mg/mL. The pH of the product falls within the range from 5.5 to 8.5.

CLINICAL PHARMACOLOGY

Mechanism of Action

DepoCyt™ (cytarabine liposome injection) is a sustained-release formulation of the active ingredient cytarabine designed for direct administration into the cerebrospinal fluid (CSF). Cytarabine is a cell cycle phase-specific antineoplastic agent, affecting cells only during the S-phase of cell division. Intracellularly, cytarabine is converted into cytarabine-5'-triphosphate (ara-CTP), which is the active metabolite. The mechanism of action is not completely understood, but it appears that ara-CTP acts primarily through inhibition of DNA polymerase. Incorporation into DNA and RNA may also contribute to cytarabine cytotoxicity. Cytarabine is cytotoxic to a wide variety of proliferating mammalian cells in culture.

Pharmacokinetics

The pharmacokinetics of DepoCyt administered intrathecally to patients at a 50 mg dose every 2 weeks is currently under investigation. However, preliminary analysis of the pharmacokinetic data show that following DepoCyt intrathecal administration in patients, in either the lumbar sac or by intraventricular reservoir, peak levels of free cytarabine were observed within 5 hours in both the ventricle and lumbar sac. These peak levels were followed by a biphasic elimination profile with a terminal phase half-life of 100 to 263 hours over a dose range of 12.5 mg to 75 mg. In contrast, intrathecal administration of 30 mg of free cytarabine showed a biphasic CSF concentration profile with a terminal phase half-life of 3.4 hours. Since the transfer rate of cytarabine from the CSF to plasma is slow and the conversion of cytarabine to ara-U in the plasma is fast, systemic exposure to cytarabine was negligible following intrathecal administration of DepoCyt, 50 mg or 75 mg.

Metabolism and Elimination

The primary route of elimination of cytarabine is metabolism to the inactive compound ara-U (1-β-D-arabinofuranosyluracil or uracilarabinoside), followed by urinary excretion of ara-U. In contrast to systemically administered cytarabine, which is rapidly metabolized to ara-U, conversion to ara-U in the CSF is negligible after intrathecal administration because of the significantly lower cytidine deaminase activity in the CNS tissues and CSF. The CSF clearance rate of cytarabine is similar to the CSF bulk flow rate of 0.24 mL/min.

Drug Interactions

No formal assessments of pharmacokinetic drug-drug interactions between DepoCyt and other agents have been conducted.

Special Populations

The effects of gender or race on the pharmacokinetics of DepoCyt have not been studied, nor has the effect of renal or hepatic impairment.

CLINICAL STUDIES

DepoCyt™ (cytarabine liposome injection) was studied in clinical trials that enrolled patients with neoplastic meningitis due to solid tumors, lymphoma, or leukemia. A randomized multicenter, multi-arm study involving a total of 99 patients compared 50 mg of DepoCyt administered every 2 weeks to standard intrathecal chemotherapy administered twice a week to patients with either solid tumors, lymphoma, or leukemia. For patients with lymphoma, standard therapy consisted of 50 mg of unencapsulated cytarabine given twice a week. Thirty-three lymphoma patients (17 DepoCyt, 16 cytarabine) were enrolled. Patients went off study if they had not achieved a complete response defined as clearing of the CSF from all previously positive sites in the absence of progression of neurological symptoms, after 4 weeks of treatment with study drug. Patients were to receive concurrent treatment with dexamethasone to minimize symptoms associated with chemical arachnoiditis, a known toxicity of intrathecal cytarabine and methotrexate (see WARNINGS and DOSAGE AND ADMINISTRATION).

Lymphoma

Approval of DepoCyt for lymphomatous meningitis is based on an increased complete response with DepoCyt compared to control unencapsulated cytarabine. There has been no demonstration of an improved clinical outcome as a result of the increased response rate. In the controlled trial, complete response was prospectively defined as (a) conversion, confirmed by a blinded central pathologist, from a positive examination of the CSF for malignant cells to a negative examination on two separate occasions (at least 3 days apart, on day 29 and later) at all intitially positive sites, together with (b) an absence of neurologic progression during the treatment period.

The complete response rates in the controlled study of lymphoma are shown in Table 1, giving results for all of the 33 lymphoma patients randomized. Although there was a plan for central pathology review of the data, in 4 of the 7 responding patients on the DepoCyt arm this was not accomplished and these cases were considered to have had a complete response based on the reading of an unblinded pathologist. The median overall survival of all treated patients was 99.5 days on the DepoCyt arm and 63 days on the cytarabine arm. In both arms the majority of patients died from progressive systemic disease, not the neoplastic meningitis.

Table 1: Complete Responses in Patients with Lymphomatous Meningitis in the Controlled Study

Intent-to-treat	
DepoCyt™	**Cytarabine**
7/17 (41%)	1/16 (6%)

INDICATIONS

DepoCyt™ (cytarabine liposome injection) is indicated for the intrathecal treatment of lymphomatous meningitis. This indication is based on demonstration of increased complete response rate compared to unencapsulated cytarabine. There are no controlled trials that demonstrate a clinical benefit resulting from this treatment, such as improvement in disease-related symptoms, or increased time to disease progression, or increased survival.

CONTRAINDICATIONS

DepoCyt™ (cytarabine liposome injection) is contraindicated in patients who are hypersensitive to cytarabine or any component of the formulation, and in patients with active meningeal infection.

WARNINGS (see boxed WARNING)

DepoCyt™ (cytarabine liposome injection) should be administered only under the supervision of a qualified physician experienced in the use of cancer chemotherapeutic agents. Appropriate management of complications is possible only when adequate diagnostic and treatment facilities are readily available. Chemical arachnoiditis, a syndrome manifested primarily by nausea, vomiting, headache, and fever has been a common adverse event in all studies. If left untreated, chemical arachnoiditis may be fatal. The incidence and severity of chemical arachnoiditis can be reduced by coadministration of dexamethasone. Patients receiving DepoCyt should be treated concurrently with dexamethasone to mitigate the symptoms of chemical arachnoiditis (see DOSAGE AND ADMINISTRATION).

During the clinical studies, 2 deaths related to DepoCyt were reported. One patient died after developing encephalopathy 36 hours after an intraventricular dose of DepoCyt, 125 mg. This patient was receiving concurrent whole-brain irradiation and had previously received systemic chemotherapy with cyclophosphamide, doxorubicin, and fluorouracil, as well as intraventricular methotrexate. The other patient received DepoCyt, 50 mg by the intraventricular route and developed focal seizures progressing to status epilepticus. This patient died approximately 8 weeks after the last dose of study medication. The death of 1 additional patient was considered "possibly" related to DepoCyt. He was a 63-year-old with extensive lymphoma involving the nasopharynx, brain, and meninges with multiple neurologic deficits who died of apparent disease progression 4 days after his second dose of DepoCyt.

After intrathecal administration of free cytarabine the most frequently reported reactions are nausea, vomiting and fever. Intrathecal administration of free cytarabine may cause myelopathy and other neurologic toxicity and can rarely lead to a permanent neurologic deficit. Administration of intrathecal cytarabine in combination with other chemotherapeutic agents or with cranial/spinal irradiation may increase this risk of neurotoxicity.

Blockage to CSF flow may result in increased free cytarabine concentrations in the CSF and an increased risk of neurotoxicity.

Pregnancy Category D

There are no studies assessing the reproductive toxicity of DepoCyt. Cytarabine, the active component of DepoCyt, can cause fetal harm if a pregnant woman is exposed to the drug systemically. Three anecdotal cases of major limb malformations have been reported in infants after their mothers received intravenous cytarabine, alone or in combination with other agents, during the first trimester. The concern for fetal harm following intrathecal DepoCyt administration is low, however, because systemic exposure to cytarabine is negligible. Cytarabine was teratogenic in mice (cleft palate, phocomelia, deformed appendages, skeletal abnormalities) when doses ≥ 2 mg/kg/day were administered IP during the period of organogenesis (about 0.2 times the recommended human dose on mg/m^2 basis), and in rats (deformed appendages) when 20 mg/kg was administered as a single IP dose on day 12 of gestation (about 4 times the recommended human dose on mg/m^2 basis). Single IP doses of 50 mg/kg in rats (about 10 times the recommended human dose on mg/m^2 basis) on day 14 of gestation also caused reduced prenatal and postnatal brain size and permanent impairment of learning ability. Cytarabine was embryotoxic in mice when administered during the period of organogenesis. Embryotoxicity was characterized by decreased fetal weight at 0.5 mg/kg/day (about 0.05 times the recommended human dose on mg/m^2 basis), and increased early and late resorptions and decreased live litter sizes at 8 mg/kg/day (approximately equal to the recommended human dose on mg/m^2 basis). There are no adequate and well-controlled studies in pregnant women. If this drug is used during pregnancy or if the patient becomes pregnant while taking this drug, the patient should be apprised of the potential harm to the fetus. Despite the low apparent risk for fetal harm, women of childbearing potential should be advised to avoid becoming pregnant.

PRECAUTIONS

General Precautions

DepoCyt™ (cytarabine liposome injection) has the potential of producing serious toxicity (see boxed WARNING). All patients receiving DepCyt should be treated concurrently with dexamethasone to mitigate the symptoms of chemical arachnoiditis (see DOSAGE AND ADMINISTRATION). Toxic effects may be related to a single dose or to cumulative administration. Because toxic effects can occur at any time during therapy (although they are most likely within 5 days of drug administration), patients receiving intrathecal therapy with DepoCyt should be monitored continuously for the development of neurotoxicity. If patients develop neurotoxicity, subsequent doses of DepoCyt should be reduced, and DepoCyt should be discontinued if toxicity persists.

Some patients with neoplastic meningitis receiving treatment with DepoCyt may require concurrent radiation or systemic therapy with other chemotherapeutic agents; this may increase the rate of adverse events.

Anaphylactic reactions following intravenous administration of free cytarabine have been reported.

Although significant systemic exposure to free cytarabine following intrathecal treatment is not expected, some effect on bone marrow function cannot be excluded. Systemic toxicity due to intravenous administration of cytarabine consists primarily of bone marrow suppression with leukopenia, thrombocytopenia, and anemia. Accordingly, careful monitoring of the hematopoietic system is advised.

Transient elevations in CSF protein and white blood cells have been observed in patients following DepoCyt administration and have also been noted after intrathecal treatment with methotrexate or cytarabine.

Information for the Patient

Patients should be informed about the expected adverse events of headache, nausea, vomiting, and fever, and about the early signs and symptoms of neurotoxicity. The importance of concurrent dexamethasone administration should be emphasized at the initiation of each cycle of DepoCyt treatment. Patients should be instructed to seek medical attention if signs or symptoms of neurotoxicity develop, or if oral dexamethasone is not well tolerated (see DOSAGE AND ADMINISTRATION).

Drug Interactions

No formal drug interaction studies of DepoCyt and other drugs were conducted. Concomitant administration of DepoCyt with other antineoplastic agents administered by the intrathecal route has not been studied. With intrathecal cytarabine and other cytotoxic agents administered intrathecally, enhanced neurotoxicity has been associated with coadministration of drugs.

Laboratory Test Interactions

Since DepoCyt particles are similar in size and appearance to white blood cells, care must be taken in interpreting CSF examinations following DepoCyt administration.

Carcinogenesis, Mutagenesis, Impairment of Fertility

No carcinogenicity, mutagenicity, or impairment of fertility studies have been conducted with DepoCyt. The active ingredient of DepoCyt, cytarabine, was mutagenic in *in vitro* tests and was clastogenic *in vitro* (chromosome aberrations and SCE in human leukocytes) and *in vivo* (chromosome aberrations and SCE assay in rodent bone marrow, mouse micronucleus assay). Cytarabine caused the transformation of hamster embryo cells and rat H43 cells *in vitro*. Cytarabine was clastogenic to meiotic cells; a dose-dependent increase in sperm-head abnormalities and chromosomal aberrations

Figure 1: Incidence and Severity of Chemical Arachnoiditis by Cycle in Patients with Lymphomatous Meningitis in the Randomized Study

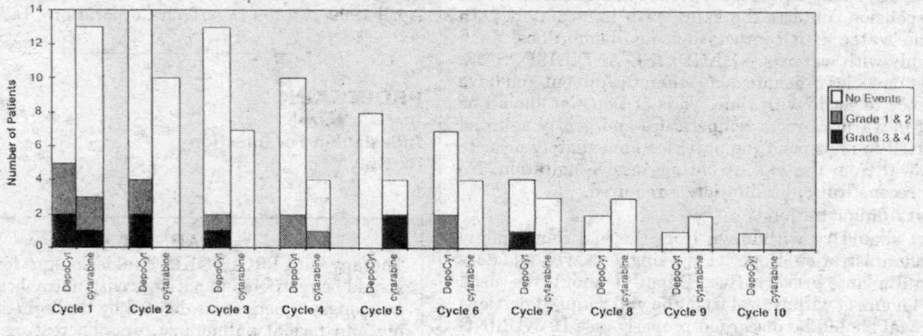

Table 2: Comparison of Adverse Events Occurring in ≥ 10% of Patients, by Cycle. Patients with Lymphomatous Meningitis Receiving DepoCyt™ or Cytarabine (ara-C) in the Randomized Study

	All Adverse Events %		Grade 3 or 4 Adverse Events %	
Number of Cycles	**n = 74**	**n = 45**	**n = 74**	**n = 45**
Body System/Adverse Event	**DepoCyt™**	**ara-C**	**DepoCyt™**	**ara-C**
Body as a Whole	53	60	18	22
Headache*	28	9	5	2
Asthenia	19	33	5	9
Fever*	11	24	4	0
Back pain*	7	11	0	2
Pain	11	20	3	0
Nervous System	45	53	18	18
Confusion	14	7	4	2
Somnolence	12	11	4	2
Abnormal gait	4	11	1	2
Digestive System	27	44	7	9
Nausea*	11	16	0	4
Vomiting*	12	18	3	2
Constipation	7	11	0	0
Metabolic and Nutritional Disorders	16	24	0	0
Peripheral edema	7	11	0	0
Hemic and Lymphatic System	19	22	11	13
Neutropenia	9	11	8	11
Thrombocytopenia	8	16	5	11
Anemia	1	13	1	4
Urogenital System	11	20	3	2
Urinary incontinence	3	11	0	0
Special Senses	16	18	1	2

*Components of chemical arachnoiditis.

occurred in mice given IP cytarabine. Impairment of Fertility: No studies assessing the impact of cytarabine on fertility are available in the literature. Because the systemic exposure to free cytarabine following intrathecal treatment with DepoCyt was negligible, the risk of impaired fertility after intrathecal DepoCyt is likely to be low.

Pregnancy

Pregnancy Category D (see WARNINGS).

Nursing Mothers

It is not known whether cytarabine is excreted in human milk following intrathecal DepoCyt administration. The systemic exposure to free cytarabine following intrathecal treatment with DepoCyt was negligible. Despite the low apparent risk, because many drugs are excreted in human milk and because of the potential for serious adverse reactions in nursing infants, the use of DepoCyt is not recommended in nursing women.

Pediatric Use

The safety and efficacy of DepoCyt in pediatric patients has not been established.

ADVERSE REACTIONS

The toxicity database consists of the observations made during an early uncontrolled study and the controlled multi-arm study described above. In the early study, patients received DepoCyt™ (cytarabine liposome injection) at doses ranging from 12.5 mg to 125 mg. In the randomized multi-arm study, DepoCyt was administered at a dose of 50 mg every 2 weeks and was compared to standard intrathecal chemotherapy (cytarabine or methotrexate) in patients with lymphoma, leukemia, and solid tumors; 28 lymphoma patients, 5 leukemia patients, and 59 solid tumor patients received study drug.

Arachnoiditis is an expected and well-documented side effect of both neoplastic meningitis and of intrathecal chemotherapy. For clinical studies of DepoCyt, chemical arachnoiditis was defined as the occurrence of any one of the symptoms of neck rigidity, neck pain, meningism or any two of the symptoms of nausea, vomiting, headache, fever, back pain, or CSF pleocytosis; the grade assigned to an episode of chemical arachnoiditis was the highest severity grade of its component symptoms. Since most of the adverse events reported in the trials were transient episodes associated with drug exposure, the incidence of these events is best expressed by drug cycle. A cycle of treatment for all treatment groups was defined as the 14-day period between DepoCyt doses. The duration of reported symptoms was from 1 to 5 days. Although it was sometimes difficult to distinguish between drug-related chemical arachnoiditis, infectious meningitis, or disease progression, >90% of the chemical arachnoiditis cases reported occurred within 48 hours of the administration of intrathecal drug, indicating a drug etiology. The incidence and severity of chemical arachnoiditis by cycle in patients with lymphomatous meningitis in the controlled study are shown in Figure 1.

In the early study, chemical arachnoiditis was observed in 100% of cycles without dexamethasone prophylaxis; with concurrent administration of dexamethasone, chemical arachnoiditis was observed in 33% of cycles. Patients receiving DepoCyt should be treated concurrently with dexamethasone to mitigate the symptoms of chemical arachnoiditis (see DOSAGE AND ADMINISTRATION).

[See figure 1 above]

Table 2 shows the rate of all adverse events occurring in ≥10 % of patients, as a rate per cycle in the lymphoma randomized study.

[See table 2 above]

OVERDOSAGE

No overdosages with DepoCyt™ (cytarabine liposome injection) have been reported. An overdose with DepoCyt may be associated with severe chemical arachnoiditis including encephalopathy.

In an early uncontrolled study without dexamethasone prophylaxis, single doses up to 125 mg were administered. One patient at the 125 mg dose level died of encephalopathy 36 hours after receiving an intraventricular dose of DepoCyt (see WARNINGS). This patient, however, was also receiving concomitant whole brain irradiation and had previously received intraventricular methotrexate.

There is no antidote for overdose of intrathecal DepoCyt or unencapsulated cytarabine released from DepoCyt. Exchange of CSF with isotonic saline has been carried out in a case of intrathecal overdose of free cytarabine, and such a procedure may be considered in the case of DepoCyt overdose. Management of overdose should be directed at maintaining vital functions.

DOSAGE AND ADMINISTRATION

Preparation of DepoCyt™ (cytarabine liposome injection)

DepoCyt is a cytotoxic anticancer drug and, as with other potentially toxic compounds, caution should be used in han-

Continued on next page

DepoCyt—Cont.

dling DepoCyt. The use of gloves is recommended. If DepoCyt suspension contacts the skin, wash immediately with soap and water. If it contacts mucous membranes, flush thoroughly with water (see HANDLING AND DISPOSAL). DepoCyt particles are more dense than the diluent and have a tendency to settle with time. Vials of DepoCyt should be allowed to warm to room temperature and gently agitated or inverted to resuspend the particles immediately prior to withdrawal from the vial. Avoid aggressive agitation. No further reconstitution or dilution is required.

DepoCyt Administration

DepoCyt should be withdrawn from the vial immediately before administration. DepoCyt is a single-use vial and does not contain any preservative; DepoCyt should be used within 4 hours of withdrawal from the vial. Unused portions of each vial should be discarded properly (see HANDLING AND DISPOSAL). Do not save any unused portions for later administration. Do not mix DepoCyt with any other medications.

In-line filters must not be used when administering DepoCyt. DepoCyt is administered directly into the CSF via an intraventricular reservoir or by direct injection into the lumbar sac. DepoCyt should be injected slowly over a period of 1–5 minutes. Following drug administration by lumbar puncture, the patient should be instructed to lie flat for 1 hour. Patients should be observed by the physician for immediate toxic reactions.

Patients should be started on dexamethasone 4 mg bid either PO or IV for 5 days beginning on the day of DepoCyt injection.

DepoCyt must only be administered by the intrathecal route.

Further dilution of DepoCyt is not recommended.

Dosing Regimen

For the treatment of lymphomatous meningitis, DepoCyt 50 mg (one vial of DepoCyt) is recommended to be given according to the following schedule:

Induction therapy: DepoCyt, 50 mg, administered intrathecally (intraventricular or lumbar puncture) every 14 days for 2 doses (weeks 1 and 3).

Consolidation therapy: DepoCyt, 50 mg, administered intrathecally (intraventricular or lumbar puncture) every 14 days for 3 doses (weeks 5, 7 and 9) followed by 1 additional dose at week 13.

Maintenance: DepoCyt, 50 mg, administered intrathecally (intraventricular or lumbar puncture) every 28 days for 4 doses (weeks 17, 21, 25 and 29).

If drug-related neurotoxicity develops, the dose should be reduced to 25 mg. If toxicity persists, treatment with DepoCyt should be discontinued.

HANDLING AND DISPOSAL

Procedures for proper handling and disposal of anticancer drugs should be considered. Several guidelines on this subject have been published.[1–7] There is no general agreement that all of the procedures recommended in the guidelines are necessary or appropriate.

HOW SUPPLIED

DepoCyt™ (cytarabine liposome injection) is supplied as a sterile, white to off-white suspension in 5 mL glass, single use vials.

Refrigerate at 2° to 8°C (36° to 46°F). Protect from freezing and avoid aggressive agitation.

Available as individual carton containing one ready to use vial. **NDC 53905-331-01.**

Do not use beyond expiration date printed on the label.

REFERENCES

1. *Recommendations for the Safe Handling of Parenteral Antineoplastic Drugs.* Publication NIH 83-2621. For sale by the Superintendent of Documents, U.S. Government Printing Office, Washington, DC 20402.
2. Council on Scientific Affairs. Guidelines for handling parenteral antineoplastics. *JAMA.* 1985; 253:1590–1592.
3. National Study Commission on Cytotoxic Exposure. *Recommendations for handling cytotoxic agents.* Available from Louis P. Jeffrey, ScD, Chairman, National Study Commission on Cytotoxic Exposure, Massachusetts College of Pharmacy and Allied Health Sciences, 179 Longwood Avenue, Boston, Massachusetts 02115.
4. Clinical Oncological Society of Australia. Guidelines and recommendations for safe handling of antineoplastic agents. *Med J Australia.* 1983;1:426–428.
5. Jones RB, et al. Safe handling of chemotherapeutic agents: a report from the Mount Sinai Medical Center. *CA J Clin.* 1983;33:258–263.
6. American Society of Hospital Pharmacists Technical Assistance Bulletin on Handling Cytotoxic and Hazardous Drugs. *Am J Hosp Pharm.* 1990; 47:1033–1049.
7. Controlling Occupational Exposure to Hazardous Drugs (OSHA Work-Practice Guidelines). *Am J Health-Syst Pharm.* 1996;53:1669–1685.

Rx only

For additional information, contact Chiron Corporation Professional Services at (800) 244-7668, Selection 2.

Manufactured by:
Skyepharma Inc.
San Diego, CA 92121

Distributed by:
Chiron Corporation
Emeryville, CA 94608
U.S. Patent Nos. 5,807,572; 5,723,147
April 1999 ©1999 DepoTech Corporation L-7125

PROLEUKIN® ℞

[*prō-lū ʹ-kin*]
Aldesleukin For Injection
Rx Only

> **WARNINGS**
>
> Therapy with PROLEUKIN® (aldesleukin) for injection should be restricted to patients with normal cardiac and pulmonary functions as defined by thallium stress testing and formal pulmonary function testing. Extreme caution should be used in patients with a normal thallium stress test and a normal pulmonary function test who have a history of cardiac or pulmonary disease.
>
> PROLEUKIN should be administered in a hospital setting under the supervision of a qualified physician experienced in the use of anti cancer agents. An intensive care facility and specialists skilled in cardiopulmonary or intensive care medicine must be available.
>
> PROLEUKIN administration has been associated with capillary leak syndrome (CLS) which is characterized by a loss of vascular tone and extravasation of plasma proteins and fluid into the extravascular space. CLS results in hypotension and reduced organ perfusion which may be severe and can result in death. CLS may be associated with cardiac arrhythmias (supraventricular and ventricular), angina, myocardial infarction, respiratory insufficiency requiring intubation, gastrointestinal bleeding or infarction, renal insufficiency, edema, and mental status changes.
>
> PROLEUKIN treatment is associated with impaired neutrophil function (reduced chemotaxis) and with an increased risk of disseminated infection, including sepsis and bacterial endocarditis. Consequently, preexisting bacterial infections should be adequately treated prior to initiation of PROLEUKIN therapy. Patients with indwelling central lines are particularly at risk for infection with gram positive microorganisms. Antibiotic prophylaxis with oxacillin, nafcillin, ciprofloxacin, or vancomycin has been associated with a reduced incidence of staphylococcal infections.
>
> PROLEUKIN administration should be withheld in patients developing moderate to severe lethargy or somnolence; continued administration may result in coma.

DESCRIPTION

PROLEUKIN® (aldesleukin) for injection, a human recombinant interleukin-2 product, is a highly purified protein with a molecular weight of approximately 15,300 daltons. The chemical name is des-alanyl-1, serine-125 human interleukin-2. PROLEUKIN, a lymphokine, is produced by recombinant DNA technology using a genetically engineered *E. coli* strain containing an analog of the human interleukin-2 gene. Genetic engineering techniques were used to modify the human IL-2 gene, and the resulting expression clone encodes a modified human interleukin-2. This recombinant form differs from native interleukin-2 in the following ways: a) PROLEUKIN is not glycosylated because it is derived from *E. coli*; b) the molecule has no N-terminal alanine; the codon for this amino acid was deleted during the genetic engineering procedure; c) the molecule has serine substituted for cysteine at amino acid position 125; this was accomplished by site specific manipulation during the genetic engineering procedure; and d) the aggregation state of PROLEUKIN is likely to be different from that of native interleukin-2.

The *in vitro* biological activities of the native nonrecombinant molecule have been reproduced with PROLEUKIN.[1,2]

PROLEUKIN is supplied as a sterile, white to off-white, lyophilized cake in single-use vials intended for intravenous (IV) administration. When reconstituted with 1.2 mL Sterile Water for Injection, USP, each mL contains 18 million IU (1.1 mg) PROLEUKIN, 50 mg mannitol, and 0.18 mg sodium dodecyl sulfate, buffered with approximately 0.17 mg monobasic and 0.89 mg dibasic sodium phosphate to a pH of 7.5 (range 7.2 to 7.8). The manufacturing process for PROLEUKIN involves fermentation in a defined medium containing tetracycline hydrochloride. The presence of the antibiotic is not detectable in the final product. PROLEUKIN contains no preservatives in the final product.

PROLEUKIN biological potency is determined by a lymphocyte proliferation bioassay and is expressed in International Units (IU) as established by the World Health Organization 1st International Standard for Interleukin-2 (human). The relationship between potency and protein mass is as follows:

18 million (18×10^6) IU PROLEUKIN = 1.1 mg protein

CLINICAL PHARMACOLOGY

PROLEUKIN® (aldesleukin) has been shown to possess the biological activities of human native interleukin-2.[1,2]

In vitro studies performed on human cell lines demonstrate the immunoregulatory properties of PROLEUKIN, including: a) enhancement of lymphocyte mitogenesis and stimulation of long-term growth of human interleukin-2 dependent cell lines; b) enhancement of lymphocyte cytotoxicity; c) induction of killer cell (lymphokine-activated (LAK) and natural (NK)) activity; and d) induction of interferon-gamma production.

The *in vivo* administration of PROLEUKIN in animals and humans produces multiple immunological effects in a dose dependent manner. These effects include activation of cellular immunity with profound lymphocytosis, eosinophilia, and thrombocytopenia, and the production of cytokines including tumor necrosis factor, IL-1 and gamma interferon.[3]

In vivo experiments in murine tumor models have shown inhibition of tumor growth.[4] The exact mechanism by which PROLEUKIN mediates its antitumor activity in animals and humans is unknown.

Pharmacokinetics: PROLEUKIN exists as biologically active, non-covalently bound microaggregates with an average size of 27 recombinant interleukin-2 molecules. The solubilizing agent, sodium dodecyl sulfate, may have an effect on the kinetic properties of this product.

The pharmacokinetic profile of PROLEUKIN is characterized by high plasma concentrations following a short IV infusion, rapid distribution into the extravascular space and elimination from the body by metabolism in the kidneys with little or no bioactive protein excreted in the urine. Studies of IV PROLEUKIN in sheep and humans indicate that upon completion of infusion, approximately 30% of the administered dose is detectable in plasma. This finding is consistent with studies in rats using radiolabeled PROLEUKIN, which demonstrate a rapid (<1 min) uptake of the majority of the label into the lungs, liver, kidney, and spleen.

The serum half-life (T 1/2) curves of PROLEUKIN remaining in the plasma are derived from studies done in 52 cancer patients following a 5-minute IV infusion. These patients were shown to have a distribution and elimination T 1/2 of 13 and 85 minutes, respectively.

Following the initial rapid organ distribution, the primary route of clearance of circulating PROLEUKIN is the kidney. In humans and animals, PROLEUKIN is cleared from the circulation by both glomerular filtration and peritubular extraction in the kidney.[5–8] This dual mechanism for delivery of PROLEUKIN to the proximal tubule may account for the preservation of clearance in patients with rising serum creatinine values. Greater than 80% of the amount of PROLEUKIN distributed to plasma, cleared from the circulation and presented to the kidney is metabolized to amino acids in the cells lining the proximal convoluted tubules. In humans, the mean clearance rate in cancer patients is 268 mL/min.

The relatively rapid clearance of PROLEUKIN has led to dosage schedules characterized by frequent, short infusions. Observed serum levels are proportional to the dose of PROLEUKIN.

Immunogenicity: Fifty-seven of 77 (74%) metastatic renal cell carcinoma patients treated with an every 8-hour PROLEUKIN regimen and 33 of 50 (66%) metastatic melanoma patients treated with a variety of IV regimens developed low titers of non-neutralizing anti-PROLEUKIN antibodies. Neutralizing antibodies were not detected in this group of patients, but have been detected in 1/106 (<1%) patients treated with IV PROLEUKIN using a wide variety of schedules and doses. The clinical significance of anti-PROLEUKIN antibodies is unknown.

Clinical Experience: Two hundred fifty-five patients with metastatic renal cell cancer (metastatic RCC) were treated with single agent PROLEUKIN in 7 clinical studies conducted at 21 institutions. Two hundred seventy patients with metastatic melanoma were treated with single agent PROLEUKIN in 8 clinical studies conducted at 22 institutions. Patients enrolled in trials of single agent PROLEUKIN were required to have an Eastern Cooperative Oncology Group (ECOG) Performance Status (PS) of 0 or 1 and normal organ function as determined by cardiac stress test, pulmonary function tests, and creatinine ≤1.5 mg/dL. Patients with brain metastases, active infections, organ allografts and diseases requiring steroid treatment were excluded.

PROLEUKIN was given by 15 min IV infusion every 8 hours for up to 5 days (maximum of 14 doses). No treatment was given on days 6 to 14 and then dosing was repeated for up to 5 days on days 15 to 19 (maximum of 14 doses). These 2 cycles constituted 1 course of therapy. Patients could receive a maximum of 28 doses during a course of therapy. In practice >90% of patients had doses withheld. Metastatic RCC patients received a median of 20 of 28 scheduled doses of PROLEUKIN. Metastatic melanoma patients received a median of 18 of 28 scheduled doses of PROLEUKIN during the first course of therapy. Doses were withheld for specific toxicities (See **"DOSAGE AND ADMINISTRATION"** section, **"Dose Modifications"** subsection and **"ADVERSE REACTIONS"** section).

In the renal cell cancer studies (n=255), objective response was seen in 37 (15%) patients, with 17 (7%) complete and 20 (8%) partial responders (See Table I). The 95% confidence interval for objective response was 11% to 20%. Onset of tumor regression was observed as early as 4 weeks after completion of the first course of treatment, and in some cases, tumor regression continued for up to 12 months after the start of treatment. Responses were observed in both lung and non-lung sites (e.g., liver, lymph node, renal bed occurrences, soft tissue). Responses were also observed in patients with individual bulky lesions and high tumor burden.

In the metastatic melanoma studies (n=270), objective response was seen in 43 (16%) patients, with 17 (6%) complete and 26 (10%) partial responders (See Table I). The 95% confidence interval for objective response was 12% to 21%. Responses in metastatic melanoma patients were observed in both visceral and non-visceral sites (e.g., lung, liver, lymph node, soft tissue, adrenal, subcutaneous). Responses were also observed in patients with individual bulky lesions and large cumulative tumor burden.

[See table I at right]

An analysis of prognostic factors showed that a better ECOG performance status (see Table II) was significantly associated with response.

[See table II at right]

TABLE I
PROLEUKIN CLINICAL RESPONSE DATA

	METASTATIC RCC		METASTATIC MELANOMA	
	Number of Responding Patients (response rate)	Median Response Duration in Months (range)	Number of Responding Patients (response rate)	Median Response Duration in Months (range)
CR's	17 (7%)	80+* (7 to 131+)	17 (6%)	59+* (3 to 122+)
PR's	20 (8%)	20 (3 to 126+)	26 (10%)	6 (1 to 111+)
PR's + CR's	37 (15%)	54 (3 to 131+)	43 (16%)	9 (1 to 122+)

(+) sign means ongoing

* Median duration not yet observed; a conservative value is presented which represents the minimum median duration of response.

TABLE II
PROLEUKIN CLINICAL RESPONSE BY ECOG PERFORMANCE STATUS (PS)

Pre Treatment ECOG PS	METASTATIC RCC CR	PR	METASTATIC MELANOMA CR	PR
0	14/166 (8%)	16/166 (10%)	14/191 (7%)	22/191 (12%)
≥1	3/89 (3%)	4/89 (4%)	3/79 (4%)	4/79 (5%)

INDICATIONS AND USAGE

PROLEUKIN® (aldesleukin) is indicated for the treatment of adults with metastatic renal cell carcinoma (metastatic RCC).

PROLEUKIN is indicated for the treatment of adults with metastatic melanoma.

Careful patient selection is mandatory prior to the administration of PROLEUKIN. See "**CONTRAINDICATIONS**", "**WARNINGS**" and "**PRECAUTIONS**" sections regarding patient screening, including recommended cardiac and pulmonary function tests and laboratory tests.

Evaluation of clinical studies to date reveals that patients with more favorable ECOG performance status (ECOG PS O) at treatment initiation respond better to PROLEUKIN, with a higher response rate and lower toxicity (See "**CLINICAL PHARMACOLOGY**" section, "**Clinical Experience**" subsection and "**ADVERSE REACTIONS**" section). Therefore, selection of patients for treatment should include assessment of performance status.

Experience in patients with ECOG PS >1 is extremely limited.

CONTRAINDICATIONS

PROLEUKIN® (aldesleukin) is contraindicated in patients with a known history of hypersensitivity to interleukin-2 or any component of the PROLEUKIN formulation.

PROLEUKIN is contraindicated in patients with an abnormal thallium stress test or abnormal pulmonary function tests and those with organ allografts. Retreatment with PROLEUKIN is contraindicated in patients who have experienced the following drug-related toxicities while receiving an earlier course of therapy:

- Sustained ventricular tachycardia (≥5 beats)
- Cardiac arrhythmias not controlled or unresponsive to management
- Chest pain with ECG changes, consistent with angina or myocardial infarction
- Cardiac tamponade
- Intubation for >72 hours
- Renal failure requiring dialysis >72 hours
- Coma or toxic psychosis lasting >48 hours
- Repetitive or difficult to control seizures
- Bowel ischemia/perforation
- GI bleeding requiring surgery

WARNINGS

See boxed "**WARNINGS**"

Because of the severe adverse events which generally accompany PROLEUKIN® (aldesleukin) therapy at the recommended dosages, thorough clinical evaluation should be performed to identify patients with significant cardiac, pulmonary, renal, hepatic, or CNS impairment in whom PROLEUKIN is contraindicated. Patients with normal cardiovascular, pulmonary, hepatic, and CNS function may experience serious, life threatening or fatal adverse events. Adverse events are frequent, often serious, and sometimes fatal.

Should adverse events, which require dose modification occur, dosage should be withheld rather than reduced (See "**DOSAGE AND ADMINISTRATION**" section, "**Dose Modifications**" subsection).

PROLEUKIN has been associated with exacerbation of preexisting or initial presentation of autoimmune disease and inflammatory disorders. Exacerbation of Crohn's disease, scleroderma, thyroiditis, inflammatory arthritis, diabetes mellitus, oculo-bulbar myasthenia gravis, crescentic IgA glomerulonephritis, cholecystitis, cerebral vasculitis, Stevens-Johnson syndrome and bullous pemphigoid, has been reported following treatment with IL-2.

All patients should have thorough evaluation and treatment of CNS metastases and have a negative scan prior to receiving PROLEUKIN therapy. New neurologic signs, symptoms, and anatomic lesions following PROLEUKIN therapy have been reported in patients without evidence of CNS metastases. Clinical manifestations included changes in mental status, speech difficulties, cortical blindness, limb or gait ataxia, hallucinations, agitation, obtundation, and coma. Radiological findings included multiple and, less commonly, single cortical lesions on MRI and evidence of demyelination. Neurologic signs and symptoms associated with PROLEUKIN therapy usually improve after discontinuation of PROLEUKIN therapy; however, there are reports of permanent neurologic defects. One case of possible cerebral vasculitis, responsive to dexamethasone, has been reported. In patients with known seizure disorders, extreme caution should be exercised as PROLEUKIN may cause seizures.

PRECAUTIONS

General: Patients should have normal cardiac, pulmonary, hepatic, and CNS function at the start of therapy. (See "**PRECAUTIONS**" section, "**Laboratory Tests**" subsection).

Capillary leak syndrome (CLS) begins immediately after PROLEUKIN® (aldesleukin) treatment starts and is marked by increased capillary permeability to protein and fluids and reduced vascular tone. In most patients, this results in a concomitant drop in mean arterial blood pressure within 2 to 12 hours after the start of treatment. With continued therapy, clinically significant hypotension (defined as systolic blood pressure below 90 mm Hg or a 20 mm Hg drop from baseline systolic pressure) and hypoperfusion will occur. In addition, extravasation of protein and fluids into the extravascular space will lead to the formation of edema and creation of new effusions.

Medical management of CLS begins with careful monitoring of the patient's fluid and organ perfusion status. This is achieved by frequent determination of blood pressure and pulse, and by monitoring organ function, which includes assessment of mental status and urine output. Hypovolemia is assessed by catheterization and central pressure monitoring.

Flexibility in fluid and pressor management is essential for maintaining organ perfusion and blood pressure. Consequently, extreme caution should be used in treating patients with fixed requirements for large volumes of fluid (e.g., patients with hypercalcemia). Administration of IV fluids, either colloids or crystalloids is recommended for treatment of hypovolemia. Correction of hypovolemia may require large volumes of IV fluids but caution is required because unrestrained fluid administration may exacerbate problems associated with edema formation or effusions. With extravascular fluid accumulation, edema is common and ascites, pleural or pericardial effusions may develop. Management of these events depends on a careful balancing of the effects of fluid shifts so that neither the consequences of hypovolemia (e.g., impaired organ perfusion) nor the consequences of fluid accumulations (e.g., pulmonary edema) exceed the patient's tolerance.

Clinical experience has shown that early administration of dopamine (1 to 5 μg/kg/min) to patients manifesting capillary leak syndrome, before the onset of hypotension, can help to maintain organ perfusion particularly to the kidney and thus preserve urine output. Weight and urine output should be carefully monitored. If organ perfusion and blood pressure are not sustained by dopamine therapy, clinical investigators have increased the dose of dopamine to 6 to 10 μg/kg/min or have added phenylephrine hydrochloride (1 to 5 μg/kg/min) to low dose dopamine (See "**ADVERSE REACTIONS**" section). Prolonged use of pressors, either in combination or as individual agents, at relatively high doses, may be associated with cardiac rhythm disturbances. If there has been excessive weight gain or edema formation, particularly if associated with shortness of breath from pulmonary congestion, use of diuretics, once blood pressure has normalized, has been shown to hasten recovery. **NOTE: Prior to the use of any product mentioned, the physician should refer to the package insert for the respective product.**

PROLEUKIN® (aldesleukin) treatment should be withheld for failure to maintain organ perfusion as demonstrated by altered mental status, reduced urine output, a fall in the systolic blood pressure below 90 mm Hg or onset of cardiac arrhythmias (See "**DOSAGE AND ADMINISTRATION**" section, "**Dose Modifications**" subsection). Recovery from CLS begins soon after cessation of PROLEUKIN therapy. Usually, within a few hours, the blood pressure rises, organ perfusion is restored and reabsorption of extravasated fluid and protein begins.

Kidney and liver function are impaired during PROLEUKIN treatment. Use of concomitant nephrotoxic or hepatotoxic medications may further increase toxicity to the kidney or liver.

Mental status changes including irritability, confusion, or depression which occur while receiving PROLEUKIN may be indicators of bacteremia or early bacterial sepsis, hypoperfusion, occult CNS malignancy, or direct PROLEUKIN-induced CNS toxicity. Alterations in mental status due solely to PROLEUKIN therapy may progress for several days before recovery begins. Rarely, patients have sustained permanent neurologic deficits (See "**PRECAUTIONS**" section "**Drug Interactions**" subsection).

Exacerbation of preexisting autoimmune disease or initial presentation of autoimmune and inflammatory disorders has been reported following PROLEUKIN alone or in combination with interferon (See "**PRECAUTIONS**" section "**Drug Interactions**" subsection and "**ADVERSE REACTIONS**" section). Hypothyroidism, sometimes preceded by hyperthyroidism, has been reported following PROLEUKIN treatment. Some of these patients required thyroid replacement therapy. Changes in thyroid function may be a manifestation of autoimmunity. Onset of symptomatic hyperglycemia and/or diabetes mellitus has been reported during PROLEUKIN therapy.

PROLEUKIN enhancement of cellular immune function may increase the risk of allograft rejection in transplant patients.

Laboratory Tests: The following clinical evaluations are recommended for all patients, prior to beginning treatment and then daily during drug administration.

- Standard hematologic tests-including CBC, differential and platelet counts
- Blood chemistries-including electrolytes, renal and hepatic function tests
- Chest x-rays

Serum creatinine should be ≤1.5 mg/dL prior to initiation of PROLEUKIN treatment.

All patients should have baseline pulmonary function tests with arterial blood gases. Adequate pulmonary function should be documented (FEV_1 >2 liters or ≥75% of predicted for height and age) prior to initiating therapy.

All patients should be screened with a stress thallium study. Normal ejection fraction and unimpaired wall motion should be documented. If a thallium stress test suggests minor wall motion abnormalities further testing is suggested to exclude significant coronary artery disease.

Daily monitoring during therapy with PROLEUKIN should include vital signs (temperature, pulse, blood pressure, and respiration rate), weight, and fluid intake and output. In a patient with a decreased systolic blood pressure, especially less than 90 mm Hg, constant cardiac rhythm monitoring should be conducted. If an abnormal complex or rhythm is seen, an ECG should be performed. Vital signs in these hypotensive patients should be taken hourly.

During treatment, pulmonary function should be monitored on a regular basis by clinical examination, assessment of vital signs and pulse oximetry. Patients with dyspnea or clinical signs of respiratory impairment (tachypnea or rales) should be further assessed with arterial blood gas determination. These tests are to be repeated as often as clinically indicated.

Cardiac function should be assessed daily by clinical examination and assessment of vital signs. Patients with signs or symptoms of chest pain, murmurs, gallops, irregular rhythm or palpitations should be further assessed with an ECG examination and cardiac enzyme evaluation. Evidence of myocardial injury, including findings compatible with myocardial infarction or myocarditis, has been reported. Ventricular hypokinesia due to myocarditis may be persistent for several months. If there is evidence of cardiac ischemia or congestive heart failure, PROLEUKIN therapy should be held, and a repeat thallium study should be done.

Drug Interactions: PROLEUKIN may affect central nervous function. Therefore, interactions could occur following concomitant administration of psychotropic drugs (e.g., narcotics, analgesics, antiemetics, sedatives, tranquilizers).

Concurrent administration of drugs possessing nephrotoxic (e.g., aminoglycosides, indomethacin), myelotoxic (e.g., cytotoxic chemotherapy), cardiotoxic (e.g., doxorubicin) or hepatotoxic (e.g., methotrexate, asparaginase) effects with PROLEUKIN may increase toxicity in these organ systems. The safety and efficacy of PROLEUKIN in combination with any antineoplastic agents have not been established.

In addition, reduced kidney and liver function secondary to PROLEUKIN treatment may delay elimination of concomitant medications and increase the risk of adverse events from those drugs.

Hypersensitivity reactions have been reported in patients receiving combination regimens containing sequential high dose PROLEUKIN and antineoplastic agents, specifically, dacarbazine, cis-platinum, tamoxifen and interferon-alfa.

Continued on next page

Proleukin—Cont.

These reactions consisted of erythema, pruritus, and hypotension and occurred within hours of administration of chemotherapy. These events required medical intervention in some patients.
Myocardial injury, including myocardial infarction, myocarditis, ventricular hypokinesia, and severe rhabdomyolysis appear to be increased in patients receiving PROLEUKIN and interferon-alfa concurrently.
Exacerbation or the initial presentation of a number of autoimmune and inflammatory disorders has been observed following concurrent use of interferon-alfa and PROLEUKIN, including crescentic IgA glomerulonephritis, oculobulbar myasthenia gravis, inflammatory arthritis, thyroiditis, bullous pemphigoid, and Stevens-Johnson syndrome.
Although glucocorticoids have been shown to reduce PROLEUKIN-induced side effects including fever, renal insufficiency, hyperbilirubinemia, confusion, and dyspnea, concomitant administration of these agents with PROLEUKIN may reduce the antitumor effectiveness of PROLEUKIN and thus should be avoided.[12]
Beta-blockers and other antihypertensives may potentiate the hypotension seen with PROLEUKIN.
Delayed Adverse Reactions to Iodinated Contrast Media: A review of the literature revealed that 12.6% (range 11–28%) of 501 patients treated with various interleukin-2 containing regimens who were subsequently administered radiographic iodinated contrast media experienced acute, atypical adverse reactions. The onset of symptoms usually occurred within hours (most commonly 1 to 4 hours) following the administration of contrast media. These reactions include fever, chills, nausea, vomiting, pruritus, rash, diarrhea, hypotension, edema, and oliguria. Some clinicians have noted that these reactions resemble the immediate side effects caused by interleukin-2 administration, however the cause of contrast reactions after interleukin-2 therapy is unknown. Most events were reported to occur when contrast media was given within 4 weeks after the last dose of interleukin-2. These events were also reported to occur when contrast media was given several months after interleukin-2 treatment.[13]
Carcinogenesis, Mutagenesis, Impairment of Fertility: There have been no studies conducted assessing the carcinogenic or mutagenic potential of PROLEUKIN.
There have been no studies conducted assessing the effect of PROLEUKIN on fertility. It is recommended that this drug not be administered to fertile persons of either gender not practicing effective contraception.
Pregnancy: *Pregnancy Category C.* PROLEUKIN has been shown to have embryolethal effects in rats when given in doses at 27 to 36 times the human dose (scaled by body weight). Significant maternal toxicities were observed in pregnant rats administered PROLEUKIN by IV injection at doses 2.1 to 36 times higher than the human dose during critical period of organogenesis. No evidence of teratogenicity was observed other than that attributed to maternal toxicity. There are no adequate well-controlled studies of PROLEUKIN in pregnant women. PROLEUKIN should be used during pregnancy only if the potential benefit justifies the potential risk to the fetus.
Nursing Mothers: It is not known whether this drug is excreted in human milk. Because many drugs are excreted in human milk and because of the potential for serious adverse reactions in nursing infants from PROLEUKIN, a decision should be made whether to discontinue nursing or to discontinue the drug, taking into account the importance of the drug to the mother.
Pediatric Use: Safety and effectiveness in children under 18 years of age have not been established.
Geriatric Use: There were a small number of patients aged 65 and over in clinical trials of PROLEUKIN; experience is limited to 27 patients, eight with metastatic melanoma and nineteen with metastatic renal cell carcinoma. The response rates were similar in patients 65 years and over as compared to those less than 65 years of age. The median number of courses and the median number of doses per course were similar between older and younger patients.
PROLEUKIN is known to be substantially excreted by the kidney, and the risk of toxic reactions to this drug may be greater in patients with impaired renal function. The pattern of organ system toxicity and the proportion of patients with severe toxicities by organ system were generally similar in patients 65 and older and younger patients. There was a trend, however, towards an increased incidence of severe urogenital toxicities and dyspnea in the older patients.

ADVERSE REACTIONS

The rate of drug-related deaths in the 255 metastatic RCC patients who received single-agent PROLEUKIN® (aldesleukin) was 4% (11/255); the rate of drug-related deaths in the 270 metastatic melanoma patients who received single-agent PROLEUKIN was 2% (6/270).
The following data on common adverse events (reported in greater than 10% of patients, any grade), presented by body system, decreasing frequency and by preferred term (COSTART) are based on 525 patients (255 with renal cell cancer and 270 with metastatic melanoma) treated with the recommended infusion dosing regimen.
[See table III above]
The following data on life-threatening adverse events (reported in greater than 1% of patients, grade 4), presented by body system, and by preferred term (COSTART) are based on 525 patients (255 with renal cell cancer and 270 with metastatic melanoma) treated with the recommended infusion dosing regimen.
[See table IV above]

TABLE III
ADVERSE EVENTS OCCURRING IN ≥10% OF PATIENTS
(n=525)

Body System	% Patients	Body System	% Patients
Body as a Whole		Metabolic and Nutritional Disorders	
Chills	52	Bilirubinemia	40
Fever	29	Creatinine increase	33
Malaise	27	Peripheral edema	28
Asthenia	23	SGOT increase	23
Infection	13	Weight gain	16
Pain	12	Edema	15
Abdominal pain	11	Acidosis	12
Abdomen enlarged	10	Hypomagnesium	12
Cardiovascular		Hypocalcemia	11
Hypotension	71	Alkaline phosphatase increase	10
Tachycardia	23	Nervous	
Vasodilation	13	Confusion	34
Supraventricular tachycardia	12	Somnolence	22
Cardiovascular disorder[a]	11	Anxiety	12
Arrhythmia	10	Dizziness	11
Digestive		Respiratory	
Diarrhea	67	Dyspnea	43
Vomiting	50	Lung disorder[b]	24
Nausea	35	Respiratory disorder[c]	11
Stomatitis	22	Cough increase	11
Anorexia	20	Rhinitis	10
Nausea and vomiting	19	Skin and Appendages	
Hemic and Lymphatic		Rash	42
Thrombocytopenia	37	Pruritus	24
Anemia	29	Exfoliative dermatitis	18
Leukopenia	16	Urogenital	
		Oliguria	63

[a] Cardiovascular disorder: fluctuations in blood pressure, asymptomatic ECG changes, CHF.
[b] Lung disorder: physical findings associated with pulmonary congestion, rales, rhonchi.
[c] Respiratory disorder: ARDS, CXR infiltrates, unspecified pulmonary changes.

TABLE IV
LIFE-THREATENING (GRADE 4) ADVERSE EVENTS
(n=525)

Body System	# (%) Patients	Body System	# (%) Patients
Body as a Whole		Metabolic and Nutritional Disorders	
Fever	5 (1%)	Bilirubinemia	13 (2%)
Infection	7 (1%)	Creatinine increase	5 (1%)
Sepsis	6 (1%)	SGOT increase	3 (1%)
Cardiovascular		Acidosis	4 (1%)
Hypotension	15 (3%)	Nervous	
Supraventricular tachycardia	3 (1%)	Confusion	5 (1%)
Cardiovascular disorder[a]	7 (1%)	Stupor	3 (1%)
Myocardial infarct	7 (1%)	Coma	8 (2%)
Ventricular tachycardia	5 (1%)	Psychosis	7 (1%)
Heart arrest	4 (1%)	Respiratory	
Digestive		Dyspnea	5 (1%)
Diarrhea	10 (2%)	Respiratory disorder[c]	14 (3%)
Vomiting	7 (1%)	Apnea	5 (1%)
Hemic and Lymphatic		Urogenital	
Thrombocytopenia	5 (1%)	Oliguria	33 (6%)
Coagulation disorder[b]	4 (1%)	Anuria	25 (5%)
		Acute kidney failure	3 (1%)

[a] Cardiovascular disorder: fluctuations in blood pressure.
[b] Coagulation disorder: intravascular coagulopathy.
[c] Respiratory disorder: ARDS, respiratory failure, intubation.

The following life-threatening (grade 4) events were reported by <1% of the 525 patients: hypothermia; shock; bradycardia; ventricular extrasystoles; myocardial ischemia; syncope; hemorrhage; atrial arrhythmia; phlebitis; AV block second degree; endocarditis; pericardial effusion; peripheral gangrene; thrombosis; coronary artery disorder; stomatitis; nausea and vomiting; liver function tests abnormal; gastrointestinal hemorrhage; hematemesis; bloody diarrhea; gastrointestinal disorder; intestinal perforation; pancreatitis; anemia; leukopenia; leukocytosis; hypocalcemia; alkaline phosphatase increase; BUN increase; hyperuricemia; NPN increase; respiratory acidosis; somnolence; agitation; neuropathy; paranoid reaction; convulsion; grand mal convulsion; delirium; asthma, lung edema; hyperventilation; hypoxia; hemoptysis; hypoventilation; pneumothorax; mydriasis; pupillary disorder; kidney function abnormal; kidney failure; acute tubular necrosis.
In an additional population of greater than 1,800 patients treated with PROLEUKIN-based regimens using a variety of doses and schedules (e.g., subcutaneous, continuous infusion, administration with LAK cells) the following serious adverse events were reported: duodenal ulceration; bowel necrosis; myocarditis; supraventricular tachycardia; permanent or transient blindness secondary to optic neuritis; transient ischemic attacks; meningitis; cerebral edema; pericarditis; allergic interstitial nephritis; tracheo-esophageal fistula.
In the same clinical population, the following fatal events each occurred with a frequency of <1%: malignant hyperthermia; cardiac arrest; myocardial infarction; pulmonary emboli; stroke; intestinal perforation; liver or renal failure; severe depression leading to suicide; pulmonary edema; respiratory arrest; respiratory failure.
In patients with both metastatic RCC and metastatic melanoma, those with ECOG PS of 1 or higher had a higher treatment-related mortality, and serious adverse events.
Most adverse reactions are self-limiting and, usually, but not invariably, reverse or improve within 2 or 3 days of discontinuation of therapy. Examples of adverse reactions with permanent sequelae include: myocardial infarction, bowel perforation/infarction, and gangrene.
In post marketing experience, the following serious adverse events have been reported in a variety of treatment regimens that include interleukin-2: anaphylaxis; cellulitis; injection site necrosis; retroperitoneal hemorrhage; cardiomyopathy; cerebral hemorrhage; fatal endocarditis; hypertension; cholecystitis; colitis; gastritis; hepatitis; hepatosplenomegaly; intestinal obstruction; hyperthyroidism, neutropenia; myopathy; myositis; rhabdomyolysis; cerebral lesions; encephalopathy; extrapyramidal syndrome; insomnia; neuralgia; neuritis; neuropathy (demyelination); urticaria; pneumonia (bacterial, fungal, viral).
Exacerbation or initial presentation of a number of autoimmune and inflammatory disorders have been reported (See "**WARNINGS**" section, "**PRECAUTIONS**" section, "**Drug Interactions**" subsection). Persistent but nonprogressive vitiligo has been observed in malignant melanoma patients treated with interleukin-2. Synergistic, additive and novel toxicities have been reported with PROLEUKIN used in combination with other drugs. Novel toxicities include delayed adverse reactions to iodinated contrast media and hypersensitivity reactions to antineoplastic agents (See "**PRECAUTIONS**" section, "**Drug Interactions**" subsection).
Experience has shown the following concomitant medications to be useful in the management of patients on PRO-

LEUKIN therapy: a) standard antipyretic therapy, including nonsteroidal anti-inflammatories (NSAIDs), started immediately prior to PROLEUKIN to reduce fever. Renal function should be monitored as some NSAIDs may cause synergistic nephrotoxicity; b) meperidine used to control the rigors associated with fever; c) H_2 antagonists given for prophylaxis of gastrointestinal irritation and bleeding; d) antiemetics and antidiarrheals used as needed to treat other gastrointestinal side effects. Generally these medications were discontinued 12 hours after the last dose of PROLEUKIN.

Patients with indwelling central lines have a higher risk of infection with gram positive organisms.[9–11] A reduced incidence of staphylococcal infections in PROLEUKIN studies has been associated with the use of antibiotic prophylaxis which includes the use of oxacillin, nafcillin, ciprofloxacin, or vancomycin. Hydroxyzine or diphenhydramine has been used to control symptoms from pruritic rashes and continued until resolution of pruritus. Topical creams and ointments should be applied as needed for skin manifestations. Preparations containing a steroid (e.g., hydrocortisone) should be avoided. **NOTE: Prior to the use of any product mentioned, the physician should refer to the package insert for the respective product.**

OVERDOSAGE

Side effects following the use of PROLEUKIN® (aldesleukin) appear to be dose-related. Exceeding the recommended dose has been associated with a more rapid onset of expected dose-limiting toxicities. Symptoms which persist after cessation of PROLEUKIN should be monitored and treated supportively. Life-threatening toxicities may be ameliorated by the intravenous administration of dexamethasone, which may also result in loss of the therapeutic effects of PROLEUKIN.[12] **NOTE: Prior to the use of dexamethasone, the physician should refer to the package insert for this product.**

DOSAGE AND ADMINISTRATION

The recommended PROLEUKIN® (aldesleukin) for injection treatment regimen is administered by a 15-minute IV infusion every 8 hours. Before initiating treatment, carefully review the "**INDICATIONS AND USAGE**", "**CONTRAINDICATIONS**", "**WARNINGS**", "**PRECAUTIONS**", and "**ADVERSE REACTIONS**" sections, particularly regarding patient selection, possible serious adverse events, patient monitoring and withholding dosage. The following schedule has been used to treat adult patients with metastatic renal cell carcinoma (metastatic RCC) or metastatic melanoma. Each course of treatment consists of two 5-day treatment cycles separated by a rest period.

600,000 IU/kg (0.037 mg/kg) dose administered every 8 hours by a 15-minute IV infusion for a maximum of 14 doses. Following 9 days of rest, the schedule is repeated for another 14 doses, for a maximum of 28 doses per course, as tolerated. During clinical trials, doses were frequently withheld for toxicity (See "**Clinical Experience**" and "**Dose Modifications**" subsections). Metastatic RCC patients treated with this schedule received a median of 20 of the 28 doses during the first course of therapy. Metastatic melanoma patients received a median of 18 doses during the first course of therapy.

Retreatment: Patients should be evaluated for response approximately 4 weeks after completion of a course of therapy and again immediately prior to the scheduled start of the next treatment course. Additional courses of treatment should be given to patients only if there is some tumor shrinkage following the last course and retreatment is not contraindicated (See "**CONTRAINDICATIONS**" section). Each treatment course should be separated by a rest period of at least 7 weeks from the date of hospital discharge.

Dose Modifications: Dose modification for toxicity should be accomplished by withholding or interrupting a dose rather than reducing the dose to be given. Decisions to stop, hold, or restart PROLEUKIN therapy must be made after a global assessment of the patient. With this in mind, the following guidelines should be used:

[See first table above]

[See second table above]

Retreatment with PROLEUKIN is contraindicated in patients who have experienced the following toxicities:

Body System	
Cardiovascular	Sustained ventricular tachycardia (≥5 beats)
	Cardiac rhythm disturbances not controlled or unresponsive to management
	Chest pain with ECG changes, consistent with angina or myocardial infarction
	Cardiac tamponade
Respiratory	Intubation for >72 hours
Urogenital	Renal failure requiring dialysis >72 hours
Nervous	Coma or toxic psychosis lasting >48 hours
	Repetitive or difficult to control seizures
Digestive	Bowel ischemia/perforation
	GI bleeding requiring surgery

Doses should be held and restarted according to the following:

Body System	Hold dose for	Subsequent doses may be given if
Cardiovascular	Atrial fibrillation, supraventricular tachycardia, or bradycardia that requires treatment or is recurrent or persistent	Patient is asymptomatic with full recovery to normal sinus rhythm
	Systolic bp <90 mm Hg with increasing requirements for pressors	Systolic bp ≥90 mmHg and stable or improving requirements for pressors
	Any ECG change consistent with MI, ischemia or myocarditis with or without chest pain; suspicion of cardiac ischemia	Patient is asymptomatic, MI and myocarditis have been ruled out, clinical suspicion of angina is low; there is no evidence of ventricular hypokinesia
Respiratory	O_2 saturation <90%	O_2 saturation >90%
Nervous	Mental status changes, including moderate confusion or agitation	Mental status changes completely resolved
Body as a Whole	Sepsis syndrome, patient is clinically unstable	Sepsis syndrome has resolved, patient is clinically stable, infection is under treatment
Urogenital	Serum creatinine > 4.5 mg/dL or a serum creatinine of ≥4 mg/dL in the presence of severe volume overload, acidosis, or hyperkalemia	Serum creatinine <4 mg/dL and fluid and electrolyte status is stable
	Persistent oliguria, urine output of <10 mL/hour for 16 to 24 hours with rising serum creatinine	Urine output >10 mL/hour with a decrease of serum creatinine >1.5 mg/dL or normalization of serum creatinine
Digestive	Signs of hepatic failure including encephalopathy, increasing ascites, liver pain, hypoglycemia	All signs of hepatic failure have resolved*
	Stool guaiac repeatedly >3-4+	Stool guaiac negative
Skin	Bullous dermatitis or marked worsening of preexisting skin condition, avoid topical steroid therapy	Resolution of all signs of bullous dermatitis

* Discontinue all further treatment for that course. A new course of treatment, if warranted, should be initiated no sooner than 7 weeks after cessation of adverse event and hospital discharge.

Reconstitution and Dilution Directions: Reconstitution and dilution procedures other than those recommended may alter the delivery and/or pharmacology of PROLEUKIN and thus should be avoided.

1. PROLEUKIN® (aldesleukin) is a sterile, white to off-white, preservative-free, lyophilized powder suitable for IV infusion upon reconstitution and dilution. **EACH VIAL CONTAINS 22 MILLION IU (1.3 MG) OF PROLEUKIN AND SHOULD BE RECONSTITUTED ASEPTICALLY WITH 1.2 ML OF STERILE WATER FOR INJECTION, USP. WHEN RECONSTITUTED AS DIRECTED, EACH ML CONTAINS 18 MILLION IU (1.1 MG) PROLEUKIN.** The resulting solution should be a clear, colorless to slightly yellow liquid. The vial is for single-use only and any unused portion should be discarded.
2. During reconstitution, the Sterile Water for Injection, USP should be directed at the side of the vial and the contents gently swirled to avoid excess foaming. DO NOT SHAKE.
3. The dose of PROLEUKIN, reconstituted with Sterile Water for Injection, USP (without preservative) should be diluted aseptically in 50 mL of 5% Dextrose Injection, USP (D5W) and infused over a 15-minute period.
   In cases where the total dose of PROLEUKIN is 1.5 mg or less (e.g., a patient with a body weight of less than 40 kilograms), the dose of PROLEUKIN should be diluted in a smaller volume of D5W. Concentrations of PROLEUKIN below 30 µg/mL and above 70 µg/mL have shown increased variability in drug delivery. Dilution and delivery of PROLEUKIN outside of this concentration range should be avoided.
4. Glass bottles and plastic (polyvinyl chloride) bags have been used in clinical trials with comparable results. It is recommended that plastic bags be used as the dilution container since experimental studies suggest that use of plastic containers results in more consistent drug delivery. **In-line filters should not be used when administering PROLEUKIN.**
5. Before and after reconstitution and dilution, store in a refrigerator at 2° to 8°C (36° to 46°F). Do not freeze. Administer PROLEUKIN within 48 hours of reconstitution. The solution should be brought to room temperature prior to infusion in the patient.
6. Reconstitution or dilution with Bacteriostatic Water for Injection, USP, or 0.9% Sodium Chloride Injection, USP should be avoided because of increased aggregation. PROLEUKIN should not be coadministered with other drugs in the same container.
7. Parenteral drug products should be inspected visually for particulate matter and discoloration prior to administration, whenever solution and container permit.

HOW SUPPLIED

PROLEUKIN® (aldesleukin) for injection is supplied in individually boxed single-use vials. Each vial contains 22 × 10^6 IU of PROLEUKIN. Discard unused portion.

NDC 53905-991-01 Individually boxed single-use vial

Store vials of lyophilized PROLEUKIN in a refrigerator at 2° to 8°C (36° to 46°F). PROTECT FROM LIGHT. Store in carton until time of use.

Reconstituted or diluted PROLEUKIN is stable for up to 48 hours at refrigerated and room temperatures, 2° to 25°C (36° to 77°F). However, since this product contains no preservative, the reconstituted and diluted solutions should be stored in the refrigerator.

Do not use beyond the expiration date printed on the vial.

NOTE: This product contains no preservative.

Rx Only

REFERENCES

1. Doyle MV, Lee MT, Fong S. Comparison of the biological activities of human recombinant interleukin-2[125] and native interleukin-2. *J Biol Response Mod* 1985; **4**:96-109.
2. Ralph P, Nakoinz I, Doyle M, et al. Human B and T lymphocyte stimulating properties of interleukin-2 (IL-2) muteins. In: *Immune Regulation by Characterized Polypeptides*. Alan R. Liss, Inc. 1987; 453-62.
3. Winkelhake JL and Gauny SS. Human recombinant interleukin-2 as an experimental therapeutic. *Pharmacol Rev* 1990; **42**:1-28.
4. Rosenberg SA, Mule JJ, Spiess PJ, et al. Regression of established pulmonary metastases and subcutaneous tumor mediated by the systemic administration of high-dose recombinant interleukin-2. *J Exp Med* 1985; **161**: 1169-88.
5. Konrad MW, Hemstreet G, Hersh EM, et al. Pharmacokinetics of recombinant interleukin-2 in humans. *Cancer Res* 1990; **50**:2009-17.
6. Donohue JH and Rosenberg SA. The fate of interleukin-2 after *in vivo* administration. *J Immunol* 1983; **130**: 2203-8.
7. Koths K, Halenbeck R. Pharmacokinetic studies on ^{35}S-labeled recombinant interleukin-2 in mice. In: Sorg C and Schimpl A, eds. *Cellular And Molecular Biology Of Lymphokines*. Academic Press: Orlando, FL, 1985;779.
8. Gibbons JA, Luo ZP, Hansen ER et al. Quantitation of the renal clearance of interleukin-2 using nephrectomized and ureter ligated rats. *J Pharmacol Exp Ther* 1995; **272**: 119-125.
9. Bock SN, Lee RE, Fisher B, et al. A prospective randomized trial evaluating prophylactic antibiotics to prevent triple-lumen catheter-related sepsis in patients treated with immunotherapy. *J Clin Oncol* 1990; **8**:161-69.
10. Hartman LC, Urba WJ, Steis RG, et al. Use of prophylactic antibiotics for prevention of intravascular catheter-related infections in interleukin-2-treated patients. *J Natl Cancer Inst* 1989; **81**:1190-93.

Continued on next page

Proleukin—Cont.

11. Snydman DR, Sullivan B, Gill M, et al. Nosocomial sepsis associated with interleukin-2. *Ann Intern Med* 1990; **112**:102-07.
12. Mier JW, Vachino G, Klempner MS, et al. Inhibition of interleukin-2-induced tumor necrosis factor release by dexamethasone: Prevention of an acquired neutrophil chemotaxis defect and differential suppression of interleukin-2 associated side effects. *Blood* 1990; **76**:1933-40.
13. Choyke PL, Miller DL, Lotze MT, et al. Delayed reactions to contrast media after interleukin-2-immunotherapy. *Radiology* 1992; **183**:111-114.

Manufactured by:
Chiron Corporation
Emeryville, CA 94608
U.S. License No. 1106
Distributed by:
Chiron Corporation
Emeryville, CA 94608
For additional information, contact Chiron Corporations Professional Services 1-800-244-7668, selection 2.
U.S. Patent Nos. RE 33653; 4,530,787; 4,569,790; 4,604,377; 4,748,234; 4,572,798; 4,853,332; 4,959,314; 5,464,939

10000340 Revised June 2000

Rabies Vaccine
RABAVERT®
Rabies Vaccine for Human Use ℞

DESCRIPTION

RabAvert, rabies vaccine, produced by Chiron Behring GmbH & Co is a sterile freeze-dried vaccine obtained by growing the fixed-virus strain Flury LEP in primary cultures of chicken fibroblasts. The strain Flury LEP was obtained from American Type Culture Collection as the 59th egg passage. The growth medium for propagation of the virus is a synthetic cell culture medium with the addition of human albumin, polygeline (processed bovine gelatin) and antibiotics. The virus is inactivated with β-propiolactone, and further processed by zonal centrifugation in a sucrose density-gradient. The vaccine is lyophilized after addition of a stabilizer solution which consists of buffered polygeline and potassium glutamate. One dose of reconstituted vaccine contains less than 12 mg polygeline (processed bovine gelatin), 1 mg potassium glutamate and 0.3 mg sodium EDTA. Small quantities of bovine serum are used in the cell culture process. Testing of the product components and excipients using currently available methods has not detected any adventitious agents. Further, bovine components originate only from source countries known to be free of bovine spongioform encephalopathy. Minimal amounts of chicken protein may be present in the final product; ovalbumin content is less than 3 ng/dose (1 mL), based on ELISA. Antibiotics (neomycin, chlortetracycline, amphotericin B) added during cell and virus propagation are largely removed during subsequent steps in the manufacturing process. In the final vaccine, neomycin is present at <1 μg, chlortetracycline at < 20 ng, and amphotericin B at < 2 ng per dose. RabAvert is intended for intramuscular (IM) injection. The vaccine contains no preservative and should be used immediately after reconstitution with the supplied diluent (Water For Injection, USP). The potency of the final product is determined by the NIH mouse potency test using the US reference standard. The potency of one dose (1.0 mL) RabAvert is at least 2.5 IU of rabies antigen. RabAvert is a white, freeze-dried vaccine for reconstitution with the diluent prior to use; the reconstituted vaccine is a clear to slightly opaque, colorless suspension.

CLINICAL PHARMACOLOGY

Rabies in the United States

Over the last 100 years, the epidemiology of rabies in animals in the United States has changed dramatically. More than 90% of all animal rabies cases reported annually to the Centers for Disease Control and Prevention (CDC) now occur in wildlife, whereas before 1960 the majority were in domestic animals. The principal rabies hosts today are wild carnivores and bats. Annual human deaths have fallen from more than a hundred at the turn of the century to one to two per year despite major outbreaks of animal rabies in several geographic areas. Within the United States, only Hawaii has remained rabies free. Although rabies among humans is rare in the United States, every year tens of thousands of people receive rabies vaccine for post-exposure prophylaxis. Rabies is almost invariably fatal due to encephalomyelitis. Modern day prophylaxis has proven nearly 100% successful; most human fatalities now occur in people who fail to seek medical treatment, usually because they do not recognize a risk in the animal contact leading to the infection. Inappropriate post-exposure prophylaxis may also result in clinical rabies. Survival after clinical rabies is extremely rare, and is associated with severe brain damage and permanent disability.

RabAvert (in combination with passive immunization with Human Rabies Immune Globulin (HRIG) and local wound treatment) in post-exposure immunization against rabies has been shown to protect, patients of all age groups from rabies, when the vaccine was administered according to the World Health Organization (WHO) guidelines and as soon as possible after rabid animal contact. Anti-rabies antibody titers after immunization have been shown to reach levels well above the minimal protective level of 0.5 IU/mL within 14 days after initiating the immunization series. The minimal antibody titer accepted as seroconversion is 0.5 IU, measured by the rapid fluorescent inhibition test (RFFIT) as specified by the WHO (1, 2) or a 1:5 titer (complete inhibition in RFFIT at 1:5 dilution) as specified by the CDC. Vaccine failure has only been reported when key elements of rabies post-exposure regimens were omitted or when the vaccine has been incorrectly administered.

Pre-exposure Immunization

The immunogenicity of RabAvert has been demonstrated in clinical trials conducted in different countries such as the USA (3, 4), UK (5), Croatia (6), and Thailand (7, 8, 9). When administered according to the recommended immunization schedule (days 0, 7, 21), 100% of subjects attained a protective titer. Two studies carried out in the USA in 101 subjects antibody titers > 0.5 IU/mL were obtained by day 28 in all subjects. In studies carried out in Thailand in 22 subjects, and in Croatia in 25 subjects, antibody titers of > 0.5 IU/mL were obtained by day 14 (injections on days 0, 7, 21) in all subjects.

The ability of RabAvert to boost previously immunized subjects was evaluated in three clinical trials. In the Thailand study, pre-exposure booster doses were administered to 10 individuals. Antibody titers of > 0.5 IU/mL were present at baseline on day 0 in all subjects (8). Titers after a booster dose were enhanced from geometric mean titers (GMT) of 1.91 IU/mL to 23.66 IU/mL on day 30. In an additional booster study, individuals known to have been immunized with Human Diploid Cell Vaccine (HDCV) were boosted with RabAvert. In this study, a booster response was observed on day 14 for all (22/22) individuals (10). In a trial carried out in the USA (3), a RabAvert IM booster dose resulted in a significant increase in titers in all (35/35) subjects, regardless of whether they had received RabAvert or HDCV as the primary vaccine.

Persistence of antibody after immunization with RabAvert has been evaluated. In a trial performed in the UK, neutralizing antibody titers > 0.5 IU/mL were present 2 years after immunization in all sera (6/6) tested.

Post-exposure Immunization

RabAvert, when used in the recommended post-exposure WHO program of 5 to 6 IM injections of 1 mL (days 0, 3, 7, 14, 30, and one optionally on day 90) provided protective titers of neutralizing antibody (> 0.5 IU/mL) in 158/160 patients (7, 8, 11–14) within 14 days and in 215/216 patients by day 28–38.

Of these, 203 were followed for at least 10 months. No case of rabies was observed (7, 8, 11–18). Some patients received HRIG, 20–30 IU per kg body weight, or Equine Rabies Immune Globulin (ERIG), 40 IU per kg body weight, at the time of the first dose. In most studies (7, 8, 11, 15), the addition of either HRIG or ERIG caused a slight decrease in GMTs which was neither clinically relevant nor statistically significant. In one study (14), patients receiving HRIG had significantly lower ($p < 0.05$) GMTs on day 14; however, again this was not clinically relevant. After day 14 there was no statistical significance.

The results of several studies of normal volunteers who have been given the WHO regimen of vaccine for post-exposure use (10, 19–22) i.e., "simulated" post-exposure use, show that with sampling by day 28–30, 205/208 vaccinees had protective titers > 0.5 IU/mL.

Over a 10 year (7/85 – 6/95) period, 46 reports of suspected post-exposure vaccine failure have been evaluated (11.8 million doses distributed). In each case, post-exposure treatment had not been in compliance with WHO recommendations.

INDICATIONS AND USAGE

RabAvert is indicated for pre-exposure immunization, in both primary series and booster dose, and for post-exposure prophylaxis against rabies.

There are no data on the interchangeable use of different rabies vaccines in a single pre- or post-exposure series. Therefore the vaccine from a single manufacturer should be used for the complete series whenever possible. If vaccines from other manufacturers are administered during the immunization series, an adequate antibody response should be confirmed by appropriate serologic tests. However, for booster immunization, RabAvert was shown to elicit satisfactory antibody level responses in 41 persons who received a primary series with HDCV (3, 10).

A. Pre-exposure Immunization—See Table 1

Pre-exposure Immunization Schedule

Pre-exposure immunization consists of three doses of RabAvert 1.0 mL, intramuscularly (deltoid region), one each on days 0, 7, and 21 or 28 ([23] see also Table 1 for criteria for pre-exposure immunization).

Pre-exposure immunization should be offered to persons in high-risk groups, such as veterinarians, animal handlers, wildlife officers, certain laboratory workers, and persons spending time in foreign countries where rabies is endemic. Persons whose activities bring them into contact with potentially rabid dogs, cats, foxes, skunks, bats, or other species at risk of having rabies should also be considered for pre-exposure prophylaxis.

Pre-exposure immunization is given for several reasons. First, it may provide protection to persons with inapparent exposure to rabies. Second, it may protect persons whose post-exposure therapy might be expected to be delayed. Finally, although it does not eliminate the need for prompt therapy after a rabies exposure, it simplifies therapy by eliminating the need for globulin and decreasing the number of doses of vaccine needed. This is of particular importance for persons at high risk of being exposed in countries where the available rabies immunizing products may carry a higher risk of adverse reactions.

In some instances, pre-exposure immunization should be boosted periodically in an effort to provide continuous protection (see Table 1); each booster immunization consists of a single dose. See **Clinical Pharmacology**. Serum antibody determinations before and after booster immunization may be helpful in determining both the need for a booster dose and the timing of such a dose.

[See table 1 at left]

B. Post-exposure Immunization—See Table 2

The following recommendations are only a guide. In applying them, take into account the animal species involved, the circumstances of the bite or other exposure, the immunization status of the animal, and presence of rabies in the region (as outlined below). Local or state public health officials should be consulted if questions arise about the need for rabies prophylaxis (23).

[See table 2 at bottom of next page]

In the United States, the following factors should be considered before antirabies treatment is initiated.

Species of Biting Animal

Carnivorous wild animals (especially skunks, raccoons, foxes and coyotes) and bats are the animals most commonly infected with rabies and have caused most of the indigenous cases of human rabies in the United States since 1960. Unless an animal is tested and shown not to be rabid, post-exposure prophylaxis should be initiated upon bite or nonbite exposure to the animals. (See definition in "Type of Exposure" below). If treatment has been initiated and subsequent testing in a qualified laboratory shows the exposing animal is not rabid, treatment can be discontinued (23).

The likelihood that a domestic dog or cat is infected with rabies varies from region to region; hence the need for post-exposure prophylaxis also varies (23).

Rodents (such as squirrels, hamsters, guinea pigs, gerbils, chipmunks, rats, and mice) and lagomorphs (including rab-

Table 1: Criteria for Pre-exposure immunization

Risk Category and Nature of Risk	Typical Populations	Pre-exposure regimen
Continuous. Virus present continuously, often in high concentrations. Aerosol, mucous membrane, bite, or nonbite exposures may go unrecognized.	Rabies research lab workers,* rabies biologics production workers.	Primary course. Serologic testing every 6 months; booster vaccination when antibody level falls below acceptable level.*
Frequent. Exposure usually episodic, with source recognized, but exposure may also be unrecognized. Aerosol, mucous membrane, bite or nonbite exposure.	Rabies, diagnostic lab workers,* spelunkers, veterinarians and staff, and animal-control and wildlife workers in rabies enzootic areas. Travelers visiting foreign areas of enzootic rabies for more than 30 days.	Primary course. Booster vaccination or serologic testing every 2 years.**
Infrequent (greater than population-at large). Exposure nearly always episodic with source recognized. Mucous membrane, bite, or nonbite exposure.	Veterinarians and animal-control and wildlife workers in areas of low rabies enzooticity. Veterinary students.	Primary course. No routine booster vaccination or serologic testing.**
Rare (population-at-large). Exposures always episodic. Mucous membrane, or bite with source unrecognized.	US population-at-large, including individuals in rabies epizootic areas.	No vaccination necessary.

Adapted from the recommendations of the Immunization Practices Advisory Committee (ACIP) on rabies prevention. MMWR, 1991; 40 (Suppl. RR-3): 1–19.

* Judgment of relative risk and extra monitoring of vaccination status of laboratory workers is the responsibility of the laboratory supervisor (see US Department of Health and Human Service's Biosafety in Microbiological and Biomedical Laboratories, 1984).

** Minimal acceptable antibody level is complete virus neutralization at a 1:5 serum dilution by RFFIT. Booster dose should be administered if the titer falls below this level.

bits and hares) are rarely found to be infected with rabies and have not been known to cause human rabies in the United States. In these cases, the state or local health department should be consulted before a decision is made to initiate post-exposure antirabies prophylaxis (23).

Circumstances of Biting Incident

An UNPROVOKED attack is more likely than a provoked attack to indicate the animal is rabid. Bites inflicted on a person attempting to feed or handle an apparently healthy animal should generally be regarded as PROVOKED.

Type of Exposure

Rabies is transmitted by introducing the virus into open cuts or wounds in skin or via mucous membranes. The likelihood of rabies infection varies with the nature and extent of exposure. Two categories of exposure should be considered:

Bite: Any penetration of the skin by teeth. Bites to the face and hands carry the highest risk, but the site of the bite should not influence the decision to begin treatment (23).

Nonbite: Scratches, abrasions, open wounds, or mucous membranes contaminated with saliva or other potentially infectious material, such as brain tissue, from a rabid animal. Casual contact, such as petting a rabid animal (without a bite or nonbite exposure as described above), does not constitute an exposure and is not an indication for prophylaxis. There have been two instances of airborne rabies acquire in laboratories and two probable airborne rabies cases acquired in a bat-infested cave in Texas (23).

The only documented cases for rabies from human-to-human transmission occurred in four patients in the United States and overseas who received corneas transplanted from persons who died of rabies undiagnosed at the time of death (2). Stringent guidelines for acceptance of donor corneas should reduce this risk.

Bite and nonbite exposure from humans with rabies theoretically could transmit rabies, although no cases of rabies acquired this way have been documented. Each potential exposure to human rabies should be carefully evaluated to minimize unnecessary rabies prophylaxis (23).

Post-exposure Immunization Schedule

The essential components of rabies post-exposure prophylaxis are prompt local treatment of wounds and immunization, including administration, in most instances of both globulin and vaccine (Table 2).

A complete course of post-exposure immunization for previously unvaccinated adults and children consists of a total of 5 doses, each 1.0 mL: one IM injection on each of days 0, 3, 7, 14 and 28.

1. Local Treatment of Wounds

Immediate and thorough washing of all bite wounds and scratches with soap and water is an important measure for preventing rabies. In animal studies, simple local wound cleansing has been shown to reduce markedly the likelihood of rabies. Whenever possible, bite injuries should not be sutured to avoid further and/or deeper contamination. Tetanus prophylaxis and measures to control bacterial infection should be given as indicated (23).

2. Specific Treatment of Rabies

The injection schedule for post-exposure prophylaxis depends on whether the patient has had or has not had previous immunization against rabies. For persons who have not previously been immunized against rabies, the schedule consists of an initial injection IM of HRIG exactly 20 IU per kilogram body weight in total. If anatomically feasible, up to half of the dose of HRIG should be thoroughly infiltrated in and around the wound(s) and the remainder should be administered IM in the gluteal region. HRIG is administered only once (for specific instructions for HRIG use, see the product package insert). The HRIG injection is followed by a series of 5 individual injections of RabAvert (1.0 mL each) given IM on days 0, 3,7, 14 and 28. Administration of HRIG and RabAvert should be given at separate sites using separate syringes. Post-exposure rabies prophylaxis should begin the same day exposure occurred or as soon after exposure as possible. The combined use of HRIG and RabAvert is recommended for both bite and non-bite exposures, regardless of the interval between exposure and initiation of treatment.

In the event that HRIG is not readily available for the initiation of treatment, it can be given through the seventh day after administration of the first dose of vaccine. HRIG is not indicated beyond the seventh day because an antibody response to RabAvert is presumed to have begun by that time (23).

The sooner treatment is begun after exposure, the better. However, there have been instances in which the decision to begin treatment was made as late as 6 months or longer after exposure due to delay in recognition that an exposure has occurred. Post-exposure antirabies immunization should always include administration of both passive antibody and immunization with the exception of persons who have previously received complete immunization regimens (pre-exposure or post-exposure) with a cell culture vaccine, or persons who have been immunized with other types of vaccines and have had documented rabies antibody titers. Persons who have previously received rabies immunization should receive 2 IM doses of RabAvert: 1 on day 0 and another on day 3. They should not be given HRIG.

3. Treatment Outside the United States

If post-exposure immunization is begun outside the United States with regimens or products that are not used in the United States, it may be desirable to provide additional treatment when the patient reaches the USA. State or local health departments should be contacted for specific advice in such cases (23).

CONTRAINDICATIONS

In view of the almost invariably fatal outcome of rabies, there is no contraindication to post-exposure immunization. However, if an alternative product (e.g. HDCV or Rabies Vaccine Adsorbed [RVA]) is not available, care should be taken if the vaccine is to be administered to persons known to be sensitive to processed bovine gelatin, chicken protein, neomycin, chlortetracycline and amphotericin B in trace amounts, which may be present in the vaccine and may cause an allergic reaction in such individuals.

WARNINGS

Serious systemic anaphylactic reactions have been reported and neuroparalytic events have been reported in temporal association with RabAvert, rabies vaccine, administration. Against the background of 11.8 million doses distributed worldwide as of June 30, 1995, 10 cases of encephalitis (1 death) or meningitis, 7 cases of transient paralysis (including 2 cases of Guillain-Barré Syndrome), 1 case of myelitis, 1 case of retrobulbar neuritis, and 2 cases of suspected multiple sclerosis have been temporally associated with the use of RabAvert. Also 2 cases of anaphylactic shock have been reported. Such events pose a dilemma for the attending physician. A patient's risk of developing rabies must be carefully considered, however, before deciding to discontinue immunization.

RABAVERT MUST NOT BE USED SUBCUTANEOUSLY OR INTRADERMALLY!

RabAvert must be injected intramuscularly. For adults, the deltoid area is the preferred site of immunization; for small children, administration into the anterolateral zone of the thigh is preferred. The use of the gluteal region should be avoided, since administration in this area may result in lower neutralizing antibody titers (2).

DO NOT INJECT INTRAVASCULARLY!

Unintentional intravascular injection may result in systemic reactions, including shock. Immediate measures include catecholamines, volume replacement, high doses of corticosteroids, and oxygen.

Development of active immunity after vaccination may be impaired in immune-compromised individuals. Please refer to *Drug Interactions*, under **Precautions.**

PRECAUTIONS

General

Care is to be taken by the heath care provider for the safe and effective use of the product. The health care provider should also question the patient, parent or guardian about 1) the current health status of the vaccinee; and 2) reactions to a previous dose of RabAvert, or a similar product. Pre-exposure vaccination should be postponed in the case of sick and convalescent persons, and those considered to be in the incubation stage of an infectious disease. A separate, sterile syringe and needle or a sterile disposable unit should be used for each patient to prevent transmission of hepatitis and other infectious agents from person to person. Needles should not be recapped and should be properly disposed of. As with any vaccine, vaccination with RabAvert may not protect 100% of susceptible individuals.

Hypersensitivity

RabAvert is produced in chick embryo cell culture. Persons with a history of anaphylactic, anaphylactoid, or other immediate reactions (e.g. hives, swelling of the mouth and throat, difficulty breathing, hypotension, or shock) subsequent to egg ingestion should not be immunized with this vaccine. At present there is no evidence that persons are at increased risk if they have egg hypersensitivities that are not anaphylactic or anaphylactoid in nature; however, in this case, HDCV rabies vaccines or RVA should be administered. There is no evidence to indicate that persons with allergies to chickens or feathers are at increased risk of reaction to vaccines produced in chick embryo cell culture.

Since reconstituted RabAvert contains traces of processed bovine gelatin, chicken protein, neomycin, chlortetracycline and amphotericin B, the possibility of allergic reactions in individuals sensitive to these substances should be considered when administering the vaccine.

Epinephrine injection (1:1000) must be immediately available should anaphylactic or other allergic reactions occur.

When a person with a history of hypersensitivity must be given RabAvert, antihistamines may be given; epinephrine (1:1000), volume replacement, corticosteroids and oxygen should be readily available to counteract anaphylactic reactions.

Drug Interactions

Corticosteroids, other immunosuppressive agents, antimalarials and immunosuppressive illnesses can interfere with the development of active immunity after vaccination, and may diminish the protective efficacy of the vaccine. Pre-exposure prophylaxis should be administered to such persons with the awareness that the immune response may be inadequate. Immunosuppressive agents should not be administered during post-exposure therapy unless essential for the treatment of other conditions. When rabies post-exposure prophylaxis is administered to persons receiving corticosteroids or other immunosuppressive therapy, or who are immunosuppressed, it is important that a serum sample be tested for rabies antibody to ensure that an acceptable antibody response has been induced (23).

Rabies Immune Globulin must not be administered at more than the recommended dose, since response to active immunization may be impaired.

Use in Pregnancy

Category C. Animal reproduction studies have not been conducted with RabAvert. It is also not known whether RabAvert can cause fetal harm when administered to a pregnant woman or can affect reproduction capacity. RabAvert should be given to a pregnant woman only if clearly needed. However, because of the potential consequences of inadequately treated rabies exposure, and limited data which indicate that fetal abnormalities have not been associated with rabies vaccination, pregnancy is not considered a contraindication to post-exposure prophylaxis. If there is substantial risk of exposure to rabies, pre-exposure prophylaxis may also be indicated during pregnancy. However, in such instances, consideration should be given to removing the pregnant woman from the high risk environment.

Carcinogenesis, Mutagenesis, Impairment of Fertility

Long-term studies with RabAvert have not been conducted to assess the potential for carcinogenesis, mutagenesis, or impairment of fertility.

ADVERSE REACTIONS

SEE ALSO **WARNINGS** AND **CONTRAINDICATIONS** SECTIONS FOR ADDITIONAL STATEMENTS

Local reactions such as induration, swelling and reddening have been reported more often than systemic reactions. In a comparative trial in normal volunteers, Dreesen *et al.* (3, 24) described their experience with RabAvert compared to a HDCV rabies vaccine. Nineteen subjects received RabAvert and 20 received HDCV. The most commonly reported adverse reaction was pain at the injection site, reported in 45% of the HDCV group, and 34% of the RabAvert group. Localized lymphadenopathy was reported in about 15% of each group. The most common systemic reactions were malaise (15% RabAvert group vs. 25% HDCV group), headache (10% RabAvert group vs. 20% HDCV group), and dizziness (15% RabAvert group vs. 10% HDCV group). In a recent study in the USA (4), 83 subjects received RabAvert and 82 received HDCV. Again the most common adverse reaction was pain at the injection site in 80% in the HDCV group and 84% in the RabAvert group. The most common systemic reactions were headache (52% RabAvert group vs. 45% HDCV group), myalgia (53% RabAvert group vs. 38% HDCV group) and malaise (20% RabAvert group vs. 17% HDCV group). None of the adverse events was serious, almost all adverse events were of mild or moderate intensity. Statistically significant differences between vaccination groups were not found. Both vaccines were generally well tolerated.

Table 2: Rabies Post-exposure Prophylaxis Guide (Advisory Committee on Immunization Practices [ACIP]) (23)

Animal type	Evaluation and disposition of animal	Post-exposure prophylaxis recommendations
Dogs and cats	Healthy and available for 10 days observation	Should not begin prophylaxis unless animal develops symptoms of rabies*
	Rabid or suspected rabid	Immediate immunization
	Unknown (escaped)	Consult public health officials
Skunks, raccoons, bats, foxes, and most other carnivores; woodchucks	Regarded as rabid unless geographic area is known to be free of rabies or until animal proven negative by laboratory tests**	Immediate immunization
Livestock, rodents, and lagomorphs (rabbits and hares)	Consider individually	Consult public health officials. Bites of squirrels, hamsters, guinea pigs, gerbils, chipmunks, rats, mice, other rodents, rabbits, and hares almost never require antirabies treatment

* During the 10-day holding period, begin treatment with HRIG and RabAvert rabies vaccine at first sign of rabies in a dog or cat that has bitten someone. The symptomatic animal should be killed immediately and tested.

**The animal should be killed and tested as soon as possible. Holding for observation is not recommended. Discontinue vaccine if immunofluorescence test results of the animal are negative.

Continued on next page

RabAvert—Cont.

Uncommonly observed adverse events include temperatures above 38°C (100°F), swollen lymph nodes, and gastrointestinal complaints. In rare cases, patients have experienced severe headache, fatigue, circulatory reactions, sweating, chills, monoarthritis and allergic reactions; transient paresthesias and one case of suspected urticaria pigmentosa have also been reported.

Type III hypersensitivity reactions in pre-exposure booster immunizations have been reported with one HDCV rabies vaccine (25–27). These reactions are thought to be due to small amounts of human serum albumin (HSA) rendered allergenic by β-propiolactone (23, 28, 29). Human serum albumin (HSA) is present in RabAvert at concentrations less than 0.3μg/dose. No type III hypersensitivity reactions have been observed with RabAvert (30).

Serious systemic anaphylactic reactions or neuroparalytic events have been reported in association with RabAvert administration. Against a background of 11.8 million doses distributed world-wide 10 cases of encephalitis (1 death) or meningitis, 7 cases of transient paralysis including 2 cases of Guillain-Barré Syndrome, 1 case of myelitis, 1 case of retrobulbar neuritis, and 2 cases of suspected multiple sclerosis have been temporally associated with the use of RabAvert. Also, 2 cases of anaphylactic shock have been reported. A patient's risk of developing rabies must be carefully considered, however, before deciding to discontinue immunization (see **Warnings**).

The use of corticosteroids to treat life-threatening neuroparalytic reactions may inhibit the development of immunity to rabies (see **Precautions,** Drug Interactions).

Once initiated, rabies prophylaxis should not be interrupted or discontinued because of local or mild systemic adverse reactions to rabies vaccine. Usually such reactions can be successfully managed with anti-inflammatory and antipyretic agents.

Reporting of Adverse Events

Adverse events should be reported by the health care provider or patient to the US Department of Health and Human Services (DHHS) Vaccine Adverse Event Reporting System (VAERS). Report forms and information about reporting requirements or completion of the form can be obtained from VAERS by calling the toll-free number 1-800-822-7967 (26). In the USA, such events can be reported to the Professional Services Department, Chiron Corporation: phone: 1-888-CHIRON7.

DOSAGE AND ADMINISTRATION

The individual dose is 1 mL, given intramuscularly.

Administer in adults by IM injection into the deltoid muscle or, in the case of small children, into the anterolateral zone of the thigh. The gluteal area should be avoided for vaccine injections, since administration in this area may result in lower neutralizing antibody titers. Care should be taken to avoid injection into or near blood vessels and nerves. After aspiration, if blood or any suspicious discoloration appears in the syringe, do not inject but discard contents and repeat procedure using a new dose of vaccine, at a different site.

Instructions for Reconstituting RabAvert

Using the longer of the 2 needles supplied, transfer the entire contents of the diluent vial into the vaccine vial. Mix gently to avoid foaming. The white, freeze-dried vaccine dissolves to give a clear or slightly opaque suspension. Withdraw the total amount of dissolved vaccine into the syringe and replace the long needle with the smaller needle for IM injection. The reconstituted vaccine should be used immediately.

Parenteral drug products should be inspected visually for particulate matter and discoloration prior to administration. If either of these conditions exists, the vaccine should not be administered. A separate, sterile syringe and needle or a sterile disposable unit should be used for each patient to prevent transmission of hepatitis and other infectious agents from person to person. Needles should not be recapped and should be properly disposed of. No data are available regarding the concurrent administration of RabAvert rabies vaccine with other vaccines.

Pediatric Use

Children and adults receive the same dose of 1 mL, given IM.

Only limited data on the safety and efficacy of RabAvert in the pediatric age group are available. However, in four studies some pre-exposure and post-exposure experience has been gained (17, 31, 32, 33).

Pre-exposure:

Pre-exposure administration of RabAvert in 11 Thai children from the age of 2 years and older resulted in antibody levels higher than 0.5 IU/mL on day 14 in all children (32). In another study in Mexico, 15/21 children aged 7–18 years had antibody titers of ≥ 0.5 IU/mL on day 14, and all 21 children had antibody titers of ≥ 0.5 IU/mL on day 30. Only mild local pain was noted in approximately one quarter of the children (33).

Post-exposure:

In a 10-year serosurveillance study, RabAvert has been administered to 91 children aged 1 to 5 years and 436 children and adolescents aged 6 to 20 years (17). The vaccine was effective in both age groups. None of these patients developed rabies.

One newborn has received RabAvert on an immunization schedule of days 0, 3, 7, 14 and 30; the antibody concentration on day 37 was 2.34 IU/mL. There were no clinically significant adverse events (31).

A. Pre-exposure Dosage

1. Primary Immunization

In the United States, the Advisory Committee on Immunization Practices (ACIP) recommends three injections of 1.0 mL each: one injection on day 0 and one on day 7, and one either on day 21 or 28 (for criteria for pre-exposure immunization, see Table 1).

2. Booster Immunization

The individual booster dose is 1 mL, given intramuscularly. Booster immunization is given to persons who have received previous rabies immunization and remain at increased risk of rabies exposure by reasons of occupation.

Persons who work with live rabies virus in research laboratories or vaccine production facilities (continuous-risk category: see Table 1) should have a serum sample tested for rabies antibodies every 6 months. Booster doses of vaccine should be given to maintain a serum titer > 1:5 serum dilution by the RFFIT.

The frequent-risk category includes other laboratory workers such as those doing rabies diagnostic testing, spelunkers, veterinarians and staff, animal-control and wildlife officers in areas where rabies is epizootic, and international travelers living or visiting (for > 30 days) in areas where canine rabies is endemic. Persons among this group should have a serum sample tested for rabies antibodies every 2 years and, if the titer is less than complete neutralization at a 1:5 serum dilution by RFFIT, should have a booster dose of vaccine. Alternatively, a booster can be administered in the absence of a titer determination.

Veterinarians and animal-control and wildlife officers working in areas of low rabies enzooticity (infrequent-exposure group) do not require routine pre-exposure booster doses of RabAvert after completion of a full primary pre-exposure immunization scheme (Table 1).

B. Post-exposure Dosage

Immunization should begin as soon as possible after exposure. A complete course of immunization consists of a total of 5 injections of 1 mL each: one injection on each of days 0, 3, 7, 14 and 28 in conjunction with the administration of HRIG on day 0. For children, see *Pediatric Use* section, above.

Begin with the administration of HRIG. Give 20 IU/kg body weight.

This formula is applicable to all age groups, including children. The recommended dosage of HRIG should not exceed 20 IU/kg body weight because it may otherwise interfere with active antibody production. Since vaccine-induced antibody appears within 1 week, HRIG is not indicated more than 7 days after initiating post-exposure immunization with RabAvert. If possible, up to one-half the dose of HRIG should be thoroughly infiltrated in the area around the wound and the rest should be administered IM, in a different site from the rabies vaccine, preferably in the gluteal area.

Because the antibody response following the recommended immunization regimen with RabAvert has been satisfactory, routine post-immunization serologic testing is not recommended. Serologic testing is indicated in unusual circumstances, as when the patient is known to be immunosuppressed. Contact state health department or CDC for recommendations.

C. Post-exposure Therapy of Previously Immunized Persons

When rabies exposure occurs in an immunized person who was vaccinated according to the recommended regimen with RabAvert or other tissue culture vaccines or who had previously demonstrated rabies antibody, that person should receive two IM doses (1.0 mL each) of RabAvert: one immediately and one 3 days later. HRIG should not be given in these cases. Persons should be considered to have been immunized previously if they received pre- or post-exposure prophylaxis with RabAvert or other tissue culture vaccines or have been documented to have had an adequate antibody response to duck embryo rabies vaccine. If the immune status of a previously vaccinated person is not known, full primary post-exposure antirabies treatment (HRIG plus 5 doses of vaccine) may be necessary. In such cases, if antibodies can be demonstrated in a serum sample collected before vaccine is given, treatment can be discontinued after at least two doses of vaccine.

HOW SUPPLIED

Package with:

1 vial of freeze-dried vaccine containing a single dose

1 disposable syringe

1 longer needle for reconstitution, 21 gauge × 1.5″

1 vial of sterile Water For Injection, USP (1 mL)

1 smaller needle for injection, 25 gauge × 1″

N.D.C.# 53905-501-01 CAUTION: Federal law prohibits dispensing without a prescription

Storage

RabAvert should be stored protected from light at 2°C to 8°C (36°F to 46°F). After reconstitution the vaccine is to be used immediately. The vaccine may not be used after the expiration date given on package and container.

REFERENCES

1. Smith JS, Yager, PA & Baer, GM. A rapid reproducible test for determining rabies neutralisation antibody. Bull WHO. 1973; 48: 535–541.
2. Eighth Report of the WHO Expert Committee on Rabies. WHO Technical Report Series, no. 824; 1992.
3. Dreesen DW, et al. Two-year comparative trial on the immunogenicity and adverse effects of purified chick embryo cell rabies vaccine for pre-exposure immunization. Vaccine. 1989; 7: 397–400.
4. Dreesen DW. Investigation of antibody response to purified chick embryo cell tissue culture vaccine (PCECV) or human diploid cell culture vaccine (HDCV) in health volunteers. Study synopsis 7USA401RA, September 1996–December 1996 (unpublished).
5. Nicholson KG, et al. Pre-exposure studies with purified chick embryo cell culture rabies vaccine and human diploid cell vaccine: serological and clinical responses in man. Vaccine. 1987; 5: 208–210.
6. Vodopija I, et al. An evaluation of second generation tissue culture rabies vaccines for use in man: a four-vaccine comparative immunogenicity study using a pre-exposure vaccination schedule and an abbreviated 2-1-1 post-exposure schedule. Vaccine. 1986; 4: 245–248.
7. Wasi C, et al. Purified chick embryo cell rabies vaccine (letter). Lancet. 1986; 1: 40.
8. Wasi C. Rabies prophylaxis with purified chick embryo (PCEC) rabies vaccine. Protocol 8T—201RA, 1983–1984 (unpublished).
9. Wasi C. Personal communication to Behringwerke AG, 1990.
10. Bijok U, et al. Clinical trials in healthy volunteers with the new purified chick embryo cell rabies vaccine for man. J Commun Dis. 1984; 16: 61–69.
11. Vodopija I. Post-exposure rabies prophylaxis with purified chick embryo cell (PCEC) rabies vaccine. Protocol 7YU-201RA, 1983–1985 (unpublished).
12. John J. Evaluation of purified chick embryo cell culture (PCEC) rabies vaccine, 1987 (unpublished).
13. Tanphaichitra D, Siristonpun Y. Study of the efficacy of a purified chick embryo cell vaccine in patients bitten by rabid animals. Intern Med. 1987; 3: 158–160.
14. Thongcharoen P, et al. Effectiveness of new economical schedule of rabies postexposure prophylaxis using purified chick embryo cell tissue culture rabies vaccine. Protocol 7T—301lP, 1993 (unpublished).
15. Ljubicic M, et al. Efficacy of PCEC vaccines in post-exposure rabies prophylaxis. In: Vodopija, Nicholson, Smerdel & Bijok (eds.): Improvements in rabies post-exposure treatment (Proceedings of a meeting in Dubrovnik, Yugoslavia). Zagreb Institute of Public Health 1985.
16. Madhusudana SN, Tripathi KK. Post exposure studies with human diploid cell rabies vaccine and purified chick embryo cell vaccine: Comparative Serological Responses in Man. Int. Med Microbiol. 1989; 271: 345–350.
17. Sehgal S, et al. Ten year longitudinal study of efficacy and safety of purified chick embryo cell vaccine for pre- and post-exposure prophylaxis of rabies in Indian population. J Commun Dis. 1995; 27: 36–43.
18. Sehgal S, et al. Cinical evaluation of purified chick embryo cell antirabies vaccine for post-exposure treatment. J Commun Dis. 1988; 20: 293–300.
19. Suntharasamai P, et al.: Purified chick embryo cell rabies vaccine: economical multisite intradermal regimen for post-exposure prophylaxis. Epidemiol Infect. 1987; 99 (3): 755–765.
20. Meesomboon V, et al. Antibody response to PCEC-rabies vaccine. J. Commun.Dis. 1987; 13: 130–136.
21. Sehgal S. Report of the trials of PCEC (Purified Chick Embryo Cell) rabies vaccine in India. In: Vodopija, Nicholson, Smerdel & Bijok (eds.): Improvements in rabies post-exposure treatment (Proceedings of a meeting in Dubrovnik, Yugoslavia). Zagreb Institute of Public Heath 1985 pp. 71–75.
22. Lesic L, Petrovic M. Study Report: Findings of Clinical Trials on Rabipur PCEC, Rabies Vaccine. National Reference Laboratory for Rabies, Novi Sad, Yugoslavia, 1988 (unpublished).
23. Centers for Disease Control. Rabies Prevention – United States, 1991. Recommendations of the Immunization Practices Advisory Committee (ACIP). MMWR. 1991; 40 (RR-3): 1–19.
24. Dreesen D. et al.: A comparative study of cell culture rabies vaccine: Immunogenicity and safety. Protocol 8USA301RA, 1985–1986 (unpublished).
25. Centers for Disease Control. Systemic allergic reactions following immunization with HDC rabies vaccine. MMWR. 1984; 33: 185–187.
26. Centers for Disease Control. Rabies Prevention - United States. MMWR. 1984; 33: 393–402.
27. Dreesen DW, et al. Immune complex-like disease in 23 persons following a booster dose of rabies HDC vaccine. Vaccine. 1986; 4: 45–49.
28. Anderson, MC, et al. The role of specific IgE and beta-propiolactone in reactions resulting from booster dose of human diploid rabies cell vaccine. J Allergy Clin. Immunol. 1987; 80: 861–868.
29. Swanson MC, et al. IgE and IgG antibodies to beta-propiolactone and human serum albumin associated with urticarial reactions to rabies vaccine. J Infect Dis. 1987; 155: 909–913.
30. Marwick C. Changes recommended in use of human diploid cell rabies vaccine (news). JAMA. 1985; 245: 14–15.
31. Lumbiganon P, Wasi C. Survival after rabies immunisation in newborn infant of affected mother. Lancet. 1990; 336: 319–332.
32. Lumbiganon P, et al. Pre-exposure vaccination with purified chick embryo cell rabies vaccines in children. Asian Pacific J Allergy Immunol, 1989; 7: 99–101.
33. Gonzales de Ciso. Comparative evaluation of PCEC and Fluenzalida vaccines. Protocol 8Mex201RA, 1983–1984 (unpublished).

Manufactured by:
Chiron Behring GmbH & Co,
D-35006 Marburg, Germany
Distributed by:
Chiron Corporation
Emeryville, CA 94608, USA

Rev. 10/97

Shown in Product Identification Guide, page 311

CibaGeneva Pharmaceuticals

Ciba-Geigy Corporation

Geneva Pharmaceuticals, Inc.

PLEASE NOTE:

Due to the merger of CibaGeneva Pharmaceuticals and Sandoz Pharmaceuticals Corporation, please refer to **Novartis Pharmaceuticals Corporation** for branded product information and **Geneva Pharmaceuticals, Inc.** for branded generic product information.

Colgate Oral Pharmaceuticals, Inc.

a subsidiary of Colgate-Palmolive Company
ONE COLGATE WAY
CANTON, MA 02021 U.S.A.

Direct Inquiries to:
Professional Services Department
(800) 226-5428

For Medical Information Contact:
In Emergencies:
Pittsburgh Poison Control
(412) 692-5596

LURIDE® DROPS ℞
brand of sodium fluoride
oral solution

1.69 fl oz (50 mL) bottles, calibrated dropper

LURIDE® LOZI-TABS® ℞
brand of sodium fluoride

120 tablet bottles 0.25 mg F vanilla
120 tablet bottles 0.5 mg F grape
120 tablet bottles 1 mg F cherry

PERIOGARD® ℞
(chlorhexidine gluconate
oral rinse, 0.12%)

16 fl oz bottles

PREVIDENT 5000 PLUS® ℞
brand of 1.1% Sodium Fluoride
prescription dental cream

1.8 oz. (51g) net wt. tubes Spearmint or Fruitastic™ Twin Pack (two 1.8 oz (51g) net wt. tubes) Spearmint

CollaGenex Pharmaceuticals, Inc.

41 UNIVERSITY DRIVE
NEWTOWN, PA 18940

Direct inquiries to:
888-339-5678

PERIOSTAT® ℞
[*pĕrĭo-stat*]
(doxycycline hyclate capsules)

DESCRIPTION

Periostat® is available as a 20 mg capsule formulation of doxycycline hyclate for oral administration.
Doxycycline is synthetically derived from oxytetracycline.

Pharmacokinetic Parameters for Periostat®

	n	Cmax (ng/mL)	Tmax (hr)	Cl/F (L/hr)	$t_{1/2}$ (hr)
Single dose 20 mg	42	400 ± 142	1.5 (0.5–4.0)	3.80 ± 0.85	18.4 ± 5.38
Steady-State 20 mg BID	30	790 ± 285	2 (0.98–12.0)	3.76 ± 1.06	Not Determined

Clinical Results at Nine Months as an Adjunct to SRP

Parameter	Baseline Pocket Depth 0–3 mm	4–6 mm	≥ 7 mm
Number of Patients	90	90	79
Mean Gain in ALv			
Periostat® 20 mg BID	0.25 mm	1.03 mm*	1.55 mm*
Placebo	0.20 mm	0.86 mm	1.17 mm
Mean Decrease in PD			
Periostat® 20 mg BID	0.16 mm**	0.95 mm**	1.68 mm**
Placebo	0.05 mm	0.69 mm	1.20 mm
% of Sites with loss of ALv ≥2 mm			
Periostat® 20 mg BID	1.9%	1.3%	0.3%*
Placebo	2.2%	2.4%	3.6%
% of Sites with BOP			
Periostat® 20 mg BID	39%**	64%*	75%
Placebo	46%	70%	80%

*$p<0.050$ vs. the placebo control group.
**$p<0.010$ vs. the placebo control group.

The structural formula of doxycycline hyclate is:

with an empirical formula of $(C_{22}H_{24}N_2O_8 \cdot HCl)_2 \cdot C_2H_6O \cdot H_2O$ and a molecular weight of 1025.89. The chemical designation for doxycycline is 4-(dimethylamino)-1,4,4a,5,5a,6,11,12a-octahydro-3,5,10,12,12a-pentahydroxy-6-methyl-1,11-dioxo-2-naphthacenecarboxamide monohydrochloride, compound with ethyl alcohol (2:1), monohydrate.
Doxycycline hyclate is a light-yellow crystalline powder which is soluble in water.
Inert ingredients in the formulation are: hard gelatin capsules; magnesium stearate; and microcrystalline cellulose. Each capsule contains doxycycline hyclate equivalent to 20 mg of doxycycline.

CLINICAL PHARMACOLOGY

After oral administration, doxycycline hyclate is rapidly and nearly completely absorbed from the gastrointestinal tract. Doxycycline is eliminated with a half-life of approximately 18 hours by renal and fecal excretion of unchanged drug.
Mechanism of Action: Doxycycline has been shown to inhibit collagenase activity in vitro.[1] Additional studies have shown that doxycycline reduces the elevated collagenase activity in the gingival crevicular fluid of patients with adult periodontitis.[2,3] The clinical significance of these findings is not known.
Microbiology: Doxycycline is a member of the tetracycline class of antibiotics. The dosage of doxycycline achieved with this product during administration is well below the concentration required to inhibit microorganisms commonly associated with adult periodontitis. Clinical studies with this product demonstrated no effect on total anaerobic and facultative bacteria in plaque samples from patients administered this dose regimen for 9 to 18 months. This product **should not** be used for reducing the numbers of or eliminating those microorganisms associated with periodontitis.
Pharmacokinetics
The pharmacokinetics of doxycycline following oral administration of Periostat® were investigated in 3 volunteer studies involving 87 adults. Additionally, doxycycline pharmacokinetics have been characterized in numerous scientific publications.[4] Pharmacokinetic parameters for Periostat® following single oral doses and at steady-state in healthy subjects are presented as follows:
[See first table above]
Absorption: Doxycycline is virtually completely absorbed after oral administration. Following 20 mg doxycycline, twice a day, in healthy volunteers, the mean peak concentration in plasma was 790 ng/mL and the average steady-state concentration was 482 ng/mL. The effect of food on the absorption of doxycycline from Periostat® has not been studied.
Distribution: Doxycycline is greater than 90% bound to plasma proteins. Its apparent volume of distribution is variously reported as between 52.6 and 134 L.[4,6]
Metabolism: Major metabolites of doxycycline have not been identified. However, enzyme inducers such as barbiturates, carbamazepine, and phenytoin decrease the half-life of doxycycline.
Excretion: Doxycycline is excreted in the urine and feces as unchanged drug. It is variously reported that between 29% and 55.4% of an administered dose can be accounted for in the urine by 72 hours.[5,6] Half-life averaged 18 hours in subjects receiving a single 20 mg doxycycline dose.
Special Populations
Geriatric: Doxycycline pharmacokinetics have not been evaluated in geriatric patients.
Pediatric: Doxycycline pharmacokinetics have not been evaluated in pediatric patients. (See **WARNINGS**.)
Gender: A study was conducted in 42 subjects where doxycycline pharmacokinetics were compared in men and women. It was observed that C_{max} was approximately 1.7-fold higher in women than in men. There were no apparent differences in other pharmacokinetic parameters.
Race: Differences in doxycycline pharmacokinetics among racial groups have not been evaluated.
Renal Insufficiency: Studies have shown no significant difference in serum half-life of doxycycline in patients with normal and severely impaired renal function. Hemodialysis does not alter the half-life of doxycycline.
Hepatic Insufficiency: Doxycycline pharmacokinetics have not been evaluated in patients with hepatic insufficiency.
Drug Interactions: See "Precautions"

Clinical Study

In a randomized, multi-centered, double-blind, 9-month Phase 3 study involving 190 adult patients with periodontal disease [at least two probing sites per quadrant of between 5 and 9 mm pocket depth (PD) and attachment level (ALv)], the effects of oral administration of 20 mg twice a day of doxycycline hyclate plus scaling and root planing (SRP) were compared to placebo control plus SRP. Both treatment groups were administered a course of scaling and root planing in 2 quadrants at Baseline. Measurements of ALv, PD and bleeding-on-probing (BOP) were obtained at Baseline, 3, 6, and 9 months from each site about each tooth in the two quadrants that received SRP using the UNC-15 manual probe. Each tooth site was categorized into one of three strata based on Baseline PD: 0–3 mm (no disease), 4–6 mm (mild/moderate disease), ≥ 7 mm (severe disease). For each stratum and treatment group, the following were calculated at month 3, 6, and 9: mean change in ALv from baseline, mean change in PD from baseline, mean percentage of tooth sites per patient exhibiting attachment loss of ≥ 2 mm from baseline, and percentage of tooth sites with bleeding on probing. The results are summarized in the following table. [See second table above]

INDICATIONS AND USAGE

Periostat® is indicated for use as an adjunct to scaling and root planing to promote attachment level gain and to reduce pocket depth in patients with adult periodontitis.

CONTRAINDICATIONS

This drug is contraindicated in persons who have shown hypersensitivity to any of the tetracyclines.

WARNINGS

THE USE OF DRUGS OF THE TETRACYCLINE CLASS DURING TOOTH DEVELOPMENT (LAST HALF OF PREGNANCY, INFANCY AND CHILDHOOD TO THE AGE OF 8 YEARS) MAY CAUSE PERMANENT DISCOLORATION OF THE TEETH (YELLOW-GRAY-BROWN). This adverse reaction is more common during long-term use of the drugs but has been observed following repeated short-term courses. Enamel hypoplasia has also been reported.

Continued on next page

Periostat—Cont.

TETRACYCLINE DRUGS, THEREFORE, SHOULD NOT BE USED IN THIS AGE GROUP AND IN PREGNANT OR NURSING MOTHERS UNLESS THE POTENTIAL BENEFITS MAY BE ACCEPTABLE DESPITE THE POTENTIAL RISKS.

All tetracyclines form a stable calcium complex in any bone forming tissue. A decrease in fibula growth rate has been observed in premature infants given oral tetracyclines in doses of 25 mg/kg every 6 hours. This reaction was shown to be reversible when the drug was discontinued.

Doxycycline can cause fetal harm when administered to a pregnant woman. Results of animal studies indicate that tetracyclines cross the placenta, are found in fetal tissues, and can have toxic effects on the developing fetus (often related to retardation of skeletal development). Evidence of embryotoxicity has also been noted in animals treated early in pregnancy. If any tetracyclines are used during pregnancy, or if the patient becomes pregnant while taking this drug, the patient should be apprised of the potential hazard to the fetus.

The catabolic action of the tetracyclines may cause an increase in BUN. Studies to date indicate that this does not occur with the use of doxycycline in patients with impaired renal function.

Photosensitivity manifested by an exaggerated sunburn reaction has been observed in some individuals taking tetracyclines. Patients apt to be exposed to direct sunlight or ultraviolet light should be advised that this reaction can occur with tetracycline drugs, and treatment should be discontinued at the first evidence of skin erythema.

PRECAUTIONS

While no overgrowth by opportunistic microorganisms such as yeast were noted during clinical studies, as with other antimicrobials, Periostat® therapy may result in overgrowth of nonsusceptible microorganisms including fungi.

The use of tetracyclines may increase the incidence of vaginal candidiasis.

Periostat® should be used with caution in patients with a history or predisposition to oral candidiasis. The safety and effectiveness of Periostat® has not been established for the treatment of periodontitis in patients with coexistant oral candidiasis.

If superinfection is suspected, appropriate measures should be taken.

Laboratory Tests: In long term therapy, periodic laboratory evaluations of organ systems, including hematopoietic, renal, and hepatic studies should be performed.

Drug Interactions: Because tetracyclines have been shown to depress plasma prothrombin activity, patients who are on anticoagulant therapy may require downward adjustment of their anticoagulant dosage.

Since bacteriostatic antibiotics, such as the tetracycline class of antibiotics, may interfere with the bactericidal action of members of the b-lactam (e.g. penicillin) class of antibiotics, it is not advisable to administer these antibiotics concomitantly.

Absorption of tetracyclines is impaired by antacids containing aluminum, calcium, or magnesium, and by iron-containing preparations. Absorption is also impaired by bismuth subsalicylate.

Barbiturates, carbamazepine, and phenytoin decrease the half-life of doxycycline.

The concurrent use of tetracycline and Penthrane (methoxyfluorane) has been reported to result in fatal renal toxicity. Concurrent use of tetracycline may render oral contraceptives less effective.

Drug/Laboratory Test Interactions: False elevations of urinary catecholamine levels may occur due to interference with the fluorescence test.

Carcinogenesis, Mutagenesis, Impairment of Fertility: Doxycycline hyclate has not been evaluated for carcinogenic potential in long-term animal studies. Evidence of oncogenic activity was obtained in studies with related compounds, i.e., oxytetracycline (adrenal and pituitary tumors), and minocycline (thyroid tumors).

Doxycycline hyclate demonstrated no potential to cause genetic toxicity in an *in vitro* point mutation study with mammalian cells (CHO/HGPRT forward mutation assay) or in an *in vivo* micronucleus assay conducted in CD-1 mice. However, data from an *in vitro* assay with CHO cells for potential to cause chromosomal aberrations suggest that doxycycline hyclate is a weak clastogen.

Oral administration of doxycycline hyclate to male and female Sprague-Dawley rats adversely affected fertility and reproductive performance, as evidenced by increased time for mating to occur, reduced sperm motility, velocity, and concentration, abnormal sperm morphology, and increased pre- and post-implantation losses. Doxycycline hyclate induced reproductive toxicity at all dosages that were examined in this study, as even the lowest dosage tested (50 mg/kg/day) induced a statistically significant reduction in sperm velocity. Note that 50 mg/kg/day is approximately 10 times the amount of doxycycline hyclate contained in the recommended daily dose of Periostat® for a 60 kg human when compared on the basis of body surface area estimates (mg/m^2). Although doxycycline impairs the fertility of rats when administered at sufficient dosage, the effect of Periostat® on human fertility is unknown.

Pregnancy: ***Teratogenic Effects:*** Pregnancy Category D. (See WARNINGS.) Results from animal studies indicate that doxycycline crosses the placenta and is found in fetal tissues.

Nonteratogenic effects: (See WARNINGS.)

Labor and Delivery: The effect of tetracyclines on labor and delivery is unknown.

Nursing Mothers: Tetracyclines are excreted in human milk. Because of the potential for serious adverse reactions in nursing infants from doxycycline, the use of Periostat® in nursing mothers is contraindicated. (See WARNINGS.)

Pediatric Use: The use of Periostat® in infancy and childhood is contraindicated. (See WARNINGS.)

ADVERSE REACTIONS

Adverse Reactions in Clinical Trials of Periostat®: In clinical trials of adult patients with periodontal disease 213 patients received Periostat® 20 mg BID over a 9–12 month period. The most frequent adverse reactions occurring in studies involving treatment with Periostat® or placebo are listed below:

Incidence (%) of Adverse Reactions in Periostat Clinical Trials

Adverse Reaction	Periostat 20 mg BID (n=213)	Placebo (n=215)
Headache	55 (26%)	56 (26%)
Common Cold	47 (22%)	46 (21%)
Flu Symptoms	24 (11%)	40 (19%)
Tooth Ache	14 (7%)	28 (13%)
Periodontal Abscess	8 (4%)	21 (10%)
Tooth Disorder	13 (6%)	19 (9%)
Nausea	17 (8%)	12 (6%)
Sinusitis	7 (3%)	18 (8%)
Injury	11 (5%)	18 (8%)
Dyspepsia	13 (6%)	5 (2%)
Sore Throat	11 (5%)	13 (6%)
Joint Pain	12 (6%)	8 (4%)
Diarrhea	12 (6%)	8 (4%)
Sinus Congestion	11 (5%)	11 (5%)
Coughing	9 (4%)	11 (5%)
Sinus Headache	8 (4%)	8 (4%)
Rash	8 (4%)	6 (3%)
Back Pain	7 (3%)	8 (4%)
Back Ache	4 (2%)	9 (4%)
Menstrual Cramp	9 (4%)	5 (2%)
Acid Indigestion	8 (4%)	7 (3%)
Pain	8 (4%)	5 (2%)
Infection	4 (2%)	6 (3%)
Gum Pain	1 (%)	6 (3%)
Bronchitis	7 (3%)	5 (2%)
Muscle Pain	2 (1%)	6 (3%)

Note: Percentages are based on total number of study participants in each treatment group.

Adverse Reactions for Tetracyclines: The following adverse reactions have been observed in patients receiving tetracyclines:

Gastrointestinal: anorexia, nausea, vomiting, diarrhea, glossitis, dysphagia, enterocolitis, and inflammatory lesions (with vaginal candidiasis) in the anogenital region. Hepatotoxicity has been reported rarely. Rare instances of esophagitis and esophageal ulcerations have been reported in patients receiving the capsule forms of the drugs in the tetracycline class. Most of these patients took medications immediately before going to bed. (SEE DOSAGE AND ADMINISTRATION.)

Skin: maculopapular and erythematous rashes. Exfoliative dermatitis has been reported but is uncommon. Photosensitivity is discussed above. (See WARNINGS.)

Renal toxicity: Rise in BUN has been reported and is apparently dose related. (See WARNINGS.)

Hypersensitivity reactions: urticaria, angioneurotic edema, anaphylaxis, anaphylactoid purpura, serum sickness, pericarditis, and exacerbation of systemic lupus erythematosus.

Blood: Hemolytic anemia, thrombocytopenia, neutropenia, and eosinophilia have been reported.

OVERDOSAGE

In case of overdosage, discontinue medication, treat symptomatically and institute supportive measures. Dialysis does not alter serum half-life and thus would not be of benefit in treating cases of overdose.

DOSAGE AND ADMINISTRATION

THE DOSAGE OF PERIOSTAT® DIFFERS FROM THAT OF DOXYCYCLINE USED TO TREAT INFECTIONS. EXCEEDING THE RECOMMENDED DOSAGE MAY RESULT IN AN INCREASED INCIDENCE OF SIDE EFFECTS INCLUDING THE DEVELOPMENT OF RESISTANT MICROORGANISMS.

Periostat® 20 mg twice daily as an adjunct following scaling and root planing may be administered for up to 9 months. Safety beyond 12 months and efficacy beyond 9 months have not been established.

Periostat® should be administered at least one hour prior to morning and evening meals.

Administration of adequate amounts of fluid along with the capsules is recommended to wash down the drug and reduce the risk of esophageal irritation and ulceration. (SEE ADVERSE REACTIONS.)

HOW SUPPLIED

Periostat® (white capsule imprinted with "Periostat™") containing doxycycline hyclate equivalent to 20 mg doxycycline. Bottle of 100 (NDC 27280-007-01).

Storage: All products are to be stored at controlled room temperatures of 59 °F–86 °F (15 °C–30 °C) and dispensed in tight, light-resistant containers (USP).

Rx Only

PERIOSTAT® is a trademark of CollaGenex Pharmaceuticals, Inc., Newtown, PA 18940.

Manufactured by
Applied Analytical Inc.
Wilmington, NC 28403
Marketed by
CollaGenex Pharmaceuticals, Inc.
Newtown, PA 18940
U.S. Patents 4,666,897
and RE 34,656

REFERENCES

1. Golub L.M., Sorsa T., Lee H-M, Ciancio S., Sorbi D., Ramamurthy N.S., Gruber B., Salo T., Konttinen Y.T.: Doxycycline Inhibits Neutrophil (PMN)-type Matrix Metalloproteinases in Human Adult Periodontitis Gingiva. J. Clin. Periodontol 1995; 22: 100–109.
2. Golub L.M., Ciancio S., Ramamurthy N.S., Leung M., McNamara T.F.: Low-dose Doxycycline Therapy: Effect on Gingival and Crevicular Fluid Collagenase Activity in Humans. J. Periodont Res 1990; 25: 321–330.
3. Golub L.M., Lee H.M., Greenwald R.A., Ryan M.E., Salo T., Giannobile W.V.: A Matrix Metalloproteinase Inhibitor Reduces Bone-type Collagen Degradation Fragments and Specific Collagenases in Gingival Crevicular Fluid During Adult Periodontitis. Inflammation Research 1997; 46: 310–319.
4. Saivain S., Houin G.: Clinical Pharmacokinetics of Doxycycline and Minocycline. Clin. Pharmacokinetics 1988; 15: 355–366.
5. Schach von Wittenau M., Twomey T.: The Disposition of Doxycycline by Man and Dog. Chemotherapy 1971; 16: 217–228.
6. Campistron G., Coulais Y., Caillard C., Mosser J., Pontagnier H., Houin G.: Pharmacokinetics and Bioavailability of Doxycycline in Humans. Arzneimittel Forschung 1986; 36: 1705–1707.

Connetics Corporation

3400 WEST BAYSHORE ROAD
PALO ALTO, CA 94303

Direct Inquiries to:
(650) 843-2800
FAX: (650) 843-2899
www.connetics.com

For Medical Information Contact:
Medical Information Department
(650) 843-2800
FAX: (650) 843-2898
E-mail: medicalaffairs@connetics.com

LUXIQ™ ℞

[lux-ĭk]
(betamethasone valerate) Foam, 0.12%

For Dermatologic Use Only
Not for Ophthalmic Use

DESCRIPTION

Luxíq contains betamethasone valerate, USP, a synthetic corticosteroid, for topical dermatologic use. The corticosteroids constitute a class of primarily synthetic steroids used topically as anti-inflammatory agents.

Chemically, betamethasone valerate is 9-fluoro-11β,17,21-trihydroxy-16β-methylpregna-1,4-diene-3, 20-dione 17-valerate, with the empirical formula $C_{27}H_{37}FO_6$, a molecular weight of 476.58 (CAS Registry Number 2152-44-5) and the following structural formula:

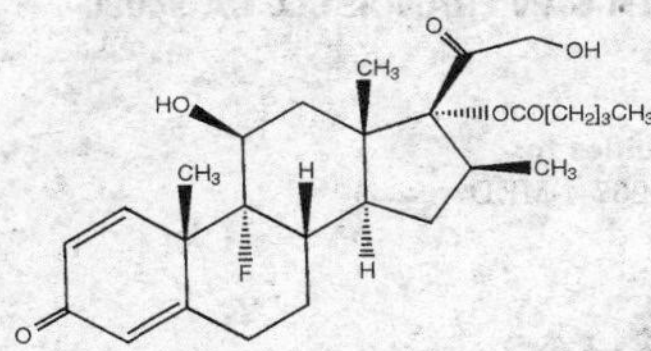

Betamethasone 17-valerate

Betamethasone valerate is a white to practically white, odorless crystalline powder, and is practically insoluble in water, freely soluble in acetone and in chloroform, soluble in alcohol, and slightly soluble in benzene and in ether.
Each gram of Luxíq contains 1.2 mg betamethasone valerate, USP, in a hydroalcoholic, thermolabile foam. The foam also contains ethanol (60.4%), purified water, propylene glycol, cetyl alcohol, stearyl alcohol, polysorbate 60, citric acid, and potassium citrate, and is dispensed from an aluminum can pressurized with a hydrocarbon propellant (propane/butane).

CLINICAL PHARMACOLOGY

Like other topical corticosteroids, betamethasone valerate foam has anti-inflammatory, anti-pruritic, and vasoconstrictive properties. The mechanism of the anti-inflammatory activity of the topical steroids, in general, is unclear. However, corticosteroids are thought to act by the induction of phospholipase A_2 inhibitory proteins, collectively called lipocortins. It is postulated that these proteins control the biosynthesis of potent mediators of inflammation such as prostaglandins and leukotrienes by inhibiting the release of their common precursor arachidonic acid. Arachidonic acid is released from membrane phospholipids by phospholipase A_2.

Pharmacokinetics:
Topical corticosteroids can be absorbed from intact healthy skin. The extent of percutaneous absorption of topical corticosteroids is determined by many factors, including the vehicle and the integrity of the epidermal barrier. Occlusion, inflammation and/or other disease processes in the skin may also increase percutaneous absorption.
The use of pharmacodynamic endpoints for assessing the systemic exposure of topical corticosteroids is necessary due to the fact that circulating levels are well below the level of detection. Once absorbed through the skin, topical corticosteroids are handled through pharmacokinetic pathways similar to systemically administered corticosteroids. They are metabolized, primarily in the liver, and are then excreted by the kidneys. In addition, some corticosteroids and their metabolites are also excreted in the bile.

CLINICAL STUDIES

The safety and efficacy of Luxíq has been demonstrated in a four-week trial. An adequate and well-controlled clinical trial was conducted in 190 patients with moderate to severe scalp psoriasis. Patients were treated twice daily for four weeks with Luxíq Foam, Placebo foam, a commercially available betamethasone valerate lotion 0.12% (formerly expressed as 0.1% betamethasone), or Placebo lotion. At four weeks of treatment, study results of 159 patients demonstrated that the efficacy of Luxíq Foam in treating scalp psoriasis is superior to that of Placebo foam, and is comparable to that of a currently marketed BMV lotion (see Table below).
[See first table above]

Subjects with Target Lesion Parameter Clear at Endpoint	Luxíq Foam n (%)	BMV Lotion n (%)	Placebo foam n (%)
Scaling	30 (47%)	22 (35%)	2 (6%)
Erythema	26 (41%)	16 (25%)	2 (6%)
Plaque Thickness	42 (66%)	25 (40%)	5 (16%)
Investigator's Global: Subjects Completely Clear or Almost Clear at Endpoint	43 (67%)	29 (46%)	6 (19%)

INDICATIONS AND USAGE

Luxíq is a medium potency of topical corticosteroid indicated for relief of the inflammatory and pruritic manifestations of corticosteroid-responsive dermatoses of the scalp.

CONTRAINDICATIONS

Luxíq is contraindicated in patients who are hypersensitive to betamethasone valerate, to other corticosteroids, or to any ingredient in this preparation.

PRECAUTIONS

General: Systemic absorption of topical corticosteroids has caused reversible hypothalamic-pituitary-adrenal (HPA) axis suppression with the potential for glucocorticosteroid insufficiency after withdrawal of treatment. Manifestations of Cushing's syndrome, hyperglycemia, and glucosuria can also be produced in some patients by systemic absorption of topical corticosteroids while on treatment.
Conditions which augment systemic absorption include the application of the more potent steroids, use over large surface areas, prolonged use, and the addition of occlusive dressings.
Therefore, patients applying a topical steroid to a large surface area or to areas under occlusion should be evaluated periodically for evidence of HPA axis suppression. If HPA axis suppression is noted, an attempt should be made to withdraw the drug, to reduce the frequency of application, or to substitute a less potent steroid.
Recovery of HPA axis function is generally prompt upon discontinuation of topical corticosteroids. Infrequently, signs and symptoms of glucocorticosteroid insufficiency may occur requiring supplemental systemic corticosteroids. For information on systemic supplementation, see prescribing information for those products.
Pediatric patients may be more susceptible to systemic toxicity from equivalent doses due to their larger skin surface to body mass ratios. (See **PRECAUTIONS—Pediatric Use.**)
If irritation develops, Luxíq should be discontinued and appropriate therapy instituted. Allergic contact dermatitis with corticosteroids is usually diagnosed by observing a failure to heal rather than noting a clinical exacerbation, as with most topical products not containing corticosteroids. Such an observation should be corroborated with appropriate diagnostic patch testing.
In the presence of dermatological infections, the use of an appropriate antifungal or antibacterial agent should be instituted. If a favorable response does not occur promptly, use of Luxíq should be discontinued until the infection has been adequately controlled.

Information for Patients: Patients using topical corticosteroids should receive the following information and instructions:

1. This medication is to be used as directed by the physician. It is for external use only. Avoid contact with the eyes.
2. This medication should not be used for any disorder other than for which it was prescribed.
3. The treated scalp area should not be bandaged or otherwise covered or wrapped so as to be occlusive unless directed by the physician.
4. Patients should report to their physician any signs of local adverse reactions.
5. As with other corticosteroids, therapy should be discontinued when control is achieved. If no improvement is seen within 2 weeks, contact the physician.

Laboratory Tests: The following tests may be helpful in evaluating patients for HPA axis suppression:
ACTH stimulation test
A.M. plasma cortisol test
Urinary free cortisol test

Carcinogenesis, Mutagenesis, and Impairment of Fertility: Long-term animal studies have not been performed to evaluate the carcinogenic potential or the effect on fertility of betamethasone valerate.
Betamethasone was genotoxic in the *in vitro* human peripheral blood lymphocyte chromosome aberration assay with metabolic activation and in the *in vivo* mouse bone marrow micronucleus assay.

Pregnancy Category C: Corticosteroids have been shown to be teratogenic in laboratory animals when administered systemically at relatively low dosage levels. Some corticosteroids have been shown to be teratogenic after dermal application in laboratory animals. There are no adequate and well-controlled studies in pregnant women. Therefore, Luxíq should be used during pregnancy only if the potential benefit justifies the potential risk to the fetus.
Drugs of this class should not be used extensively on pregnant patients, in large amounts, or for prolonged period of time.

Nursing Mothers: Systemically administered corticosteroids appear in human milk and could suppress growth, interfere with endogenous corticosteroid production, or cause other untoward effects. It is not known whether topical administration of corticosteroids could result in sufficient systemic absorption to produce detectable quantities in breast milk. Because many drugs are excreted in human milk, caution should be exercised when Luxíq is administered to a nursing woman.

Pediatric Use: Safety and effectiveness in pediatric patients have not been established. Because of a higher ratio of skin surface area to body mass, pediatric patients are at a greater risk than adults of HPA axis suppression and Cushing's syndrome when they are treated with topical corticosteroids. They are therefore also at greater risk of adrenal insufficiency during and/or after withdrawal of treatment. Adverse effects including striae have been reported with inappropriate use of topical corticosteroids in infants and children.
Hypothalamic-pituitary-adrenal (HPA) axis suppression, Cushing's syndrome, linear growth retardation, delayed weight gain, and intracranial hypertension have been reported in children receiving topical corticosteroids. Manifestations of adrenal suppression in children include low plasma cortisol levels and an absence of response to ACTH stimulation. Manifestations of intracranial hypertension include bulging fontanelles, headaches, and bilateral papilledema.
Administration of topical corticosteroids to children should be limited to the least amount compatible with an effective therapeutic regimen. Chronic corticosteroid therapy may interfere with the growth and development of children.

ADVERSE REACTIONS

The most frequent adverse event was burning/itching/stinging at the application site; the incidence and severity of this event were as follows:
[See second table above]

Incidence and severity of burning/itching/stinging

Product	Total incidence	Maximum severity		
		Mild	Moderate	Severe
Luxíq Foam n=63	34 (54%)	28 (44%)	5 (8%)	1 (2%)
Betamesthasone valerate lotion n=63	33 (52%)	26 (41%)	6 (10%)	1 (2%)
Placebo Foam n=32	24 (75%)	13 (41%)	7 (22%)	4 (12%)
Placebo Lotion n=30	20 (67%)	12 (40%)	5 (17%)	3 (10%)

Other adverse events which were considered to be possibly, probably, or definitely related to Luxíq occurred in 1 patient each; these were paresthesia, pruritus, acne, alopecia, and conjunctivitis.
The following additional local adverse reactions have been reported with topical corticosteroids, and they may occur more frequently with the use of occlusive dressings. These reactions are listed in an approximately decreasing order of occurrence: irritation; dryness; folliculitis; acneiform eruptions; hypopigmentation; perioral dermatitis; allergic contact dermatitis; secondary infection; skin atrophy; striae; and miliaria.
Systemic absorption of topical corticosteroids has produced reversible hypothalamic-pituitary-adrenal (HPA) axis suppression, manifestations of Cushing's syndrome, hyperglycemia, and glucosuria in some patients.

OVERDOSAGE

Topically applied Luxíq can be absorbed in sufficient amounts to produce systemic effects. (See **PRECAUTIONS**)

DOSAGE AND ADMINISTRATION

Note: For proper dispensing of foam, can must be inverted. For application to the scalp invert can and dispense a small amount of Luxíq onto a saucer or other cool surface. Do not dispense directly onto hands as foam will begin to melt immediately upon contact with warm skin. Pick up small amounts of foam with fingers and gently massage into affected area until foam disappears. Repeat until entire affected scalp area is treated. Apply twice daily, once in the morning and once at night.
As with other corticosteroids, therapy should be discontinued when control is achieved. If no improvement is seen within 2 weeks, reassessment of the diagnosis may be necessary.
Luxíq should not be used with occlusive dressings until directed by a physician.

HOW SUPPLIED

Luxíq is supplied in a 100-gram aluminum can; box of one: NDC 63032-21-00
Store at controlled room temperature 68–77°F (20–25°C).
WARNING
FLAMMABLE. AVOID FIRE, FLAME OR SMOKING DURING USE. Keep out of reach of children. Contents under pressure. Do not puncture or incinerate container. Do not expose to heat or store at temperatures above 120°F (49°C).
Manufactured for:
Connetics Corporation
Palo Alto, CA 94303 USA

Continued on next page

Luxiq—Cont.

By:
CCL Pharmaceuticals, Inc.
Runcorn WA7 1NU UK
M-(LB-0156) February 1999
Shown in Product Identification Guide, page 311

Cooke Pharma

1404 OLD COUNTY ROAD
BELMONT, CA 94002

Direct Inquiries to:
Customer Service Dept.
(888) 808-6838

HEARTBAR® OTC

L-arginine-enriched
Medical Food

DESCRIPTION

The HeartBar® is a medical food for the dietary management of cardiovascular disease. These ingredients are placed in a convenient and pleasant-tasting nutrition bar. The major active ingredient in the HeartBar is L-arginine, which is an amino acid required for the production of nitric oxide (NO). Each 50g bar contains L-arginine (3 g) and other amino acids, folate (200 µcg) and other B-complex vitamins, antioxidant vitamins E (200 IU) and C (250 mg), niacin (25 mg) and phytoestrogens. These nutrients are combined in a fruit, fiber, and soy protein-based nutrition bar. One HeartBar contains 13 g of protein (10g of soy protein), 27 g of carbohydrate (20 g of sugars, 3 g of fiber), 2.5 g of fat (no saturated fat, 0 mg of cholesterol), and 190 calories. HeartBar does not require a prescription but is to be used under the supervision of a health care professional.

COMPOSITION (original flavor)

High fructose corn syrup, soy protein isolate, fructose, toasted soy pieces, raisins, vanilla cookie pieces (including wheat flour), L-arginine HCl, natural and artificial flavors, oat fiber, D-alpha-tocopherol acetate, sodium ascorbate, dipotassium phosphate, niacinamide, pyridoxine hydrochloride, folic acid, cyanocobalamin.

CLINICAL BACKGROUND

The major active ingredient of the HeartBar, L-arginine, is a semi-essential amino acid, and is the precursor for endothelium-derived nitric oxide (NO). NO is a potent vasodilator, and a major regulator of vasomotion and blood pressure. In addition, NO inhibits platelet aggregation, vascular smooth muscle proliferation and adherence of leukocytes to the vessel wall, key processes in atherosclerosis and restenosis.

Endothelium-derived NO activity is reduced in patients with cardiovascular disease; this abnormality contributes to insufficient blood flow, elevated blood pressure, as well as progression of disease. L-arginine has been shown to enhance the synthesis of NO. In humans, L-arginine improves vasodilation, enhances coronary and peripheral blood flow, and inhibits platelet aggregation.

The usual dietary intake of L-arginine is about 3 to 5 g/day, which in some cardiovascular conditions, may not be sufficient intake to maintain healthy NO levels. Two HeartBars/day provides an additional 6 g of L-arginine. The other active ingredients of the HeartBar contribute to the production of, or help prevent the breakdown of NO further augmenting the activity of NO.

The HeartBar has been tested clinically in several patient populations and shown to be effective in improving blood flow. In two separate studies of individuals with total cholesterol over 230 mg/dl (n=41 & n=39), two HeartBars/day restored flow-mediated vasodilation to normal within one and two weeks respectively (compared to no change with placebo).

In patients with peripheral arterial disease secondary to atherosclerosis (n=39), 2 HeartBars/day for 2 weeks improved pain-free walking distances by 66% (compared to placebo of 18%). In addition to this improvement in physical function, these patients experienced an improvement in quality of life scores as measured by the SF-36 Medical Outcomes Survey.

In patients with stable angina (n=36), 2 HeartBars/day for 2 weeks improved flow-mediated vasodilation. This was associated with a 22% increase in exercise time, 43% increase in work performance and a significant improvement in quality of life as measured by SF-36 and Seattle Angina Questionnaire scores.

In a study of diabetic patients (n=10), there was no change in pre- and post-prandial serum glucose measures or glycosylated hemoglobin during 3 months of HeartBar use at 2 bars/day.

PHARMACOKINETICS

Following the administration of 1 HeartBar, plasma arginine levels rise from 68±27 µM/L to a peak of 119±48 µM/L within one hour of ingestion. Arginine levels are maintained above those of individuals on an arginine-free diet for at least 8 hours after ingestion. A similar pattern of arginine levels is observed following the ingestion of a single HeartBar after a week of b.i.d. use. After 2 weeks, trough L-arginine levels are 42% higher than levels before HeartBar use. These arginine levels compare favorably with L-arginine administration by capsular form.

PRECAUTIONS

Diabetics

Each HeartBar is equal to 2 carbohydrate exchanges. Although in a randomized study, there was no effect of regular use on daily fasting and post-prandial serum glucose or glycosylated hemoglobin measures, diabetics should monitor their blood glucose carefully while initiating regular use of the HeartBar. The effect of L-arginine on retinopathy is not known, therefore, those with diabetic retinopathy should not use HeartBar.

Renal Failure Patients

The HeartBar contains 13 g of protein. This amount of protein should be considered when determining total daily protein load.

Allergies

The base of the bar is of soy protein, which is generally considered hypoallergenic. The original flavor also contains a small amount of wheat flour, is low in gluten but not gluten-free. Therefore, individuals with allergies to wheat products or gluten intolerance should be cautious.

Sepsis

The hypotension associated with sepsis is, in part, mediated by excessive NO production. Such patients should not be given HeartBar.

ADVERSE REACTIONS

No serious adverse reactions have been demonstrated or reported in clinical trials or in the HeartBar Safety-In-Use study of over 2 years duration.

Minor adverse reactions are infrequent, generally related to gastrointestinal disturbances and appear unrelated to the L-arginine in the bar (Adverse events were just as common in the group given placebo bar). In a two-week study of the HeartBar, 4 of 41 individuals reported increased flatulence that resolved after several days of bar use. One of 41 individuals complained of increased frequency of bowel movements and soft stools. In a 10-week study of the HeartBar, 2 of 41 individuals reported dry mouth. A change in bowel habits was reported by 1 individual in each of the placebo and HeartBar groups. Use of HeartBar has not been associated with increased incidence of herpes cold sore formation.

The HeartBar is not indicated for individuals with co-existing conditions of diabetic retinopathy or neoplastic disease because the effect of L-arginine on the progression of these disorders is unknown.

ADMINISTRATION

Symptomatic or high-risk population
One HeartBar twice daily
At-risk population
One HeartBar daily

HOW SUPPLIED

Individually wrapped bars, cartons of 16 and cases of 64. Also available in 20g trial size.

<u>Original Flavor</u>	
Individual Bars	NDC 63535-10102
By Carton	NDC 63535-10103
By Case	NDC 63535-10104
<u>Cranberry Flavor</u>	
Individual Bars	NDC 63535-10302
By Carton	NDC 63535-10303
By Case	NDC 63535-10304
<u>Peanut Butter Flavor</u>	
Individual Bars	NDC 63535-10502
By Carton	NDC 63535-10503
By Case	NDC 63535-10504

REFERENCES

J. P. Cooke, V. J. Dzau, *Annu. Rev. Med.* **48**, 489–509 (1997).
A. J. Maxwell, J. P. Cooke, *Curr Opin Nephrol Hypertens* **7**, 63–70 (1998).
A. J. Maxwell, B. A. Anderson, M. P. Zapien, J. P. Cooke, *CV Drugs & Therapy* **14**, 357–364 (2000).
A. J. Maxwell, B. A. Anderson, J. P. Cooke, *Vascular Med* **5**, 11–19 (2000).
A. J. Maxwell, *Nutrition & MD* **25**, 1–4 (1999).
A. J. Maxwell, M. P. Zapien, B. A. Anderson, P. H. Stone, *J Am Coll Cardiol* **35**, 408A (2000).

Shown in Product Identification Guide, page 311

For information on over-the-counter drugs, consult **PDR For Nonprescription Drugs**.

COR Therapeutics, Inc.

256 EAST GRAND AVENUE
SOUTH SAN FRANCISCO, CA 94080

Direct Inquiries to:
Ph: 1-888-267-4-MED

INTEGRILIN® ℞

[In-tĕg-rĭl-in]
(eptifibatide)
Injection
For Intravenous Administration

DESCRIPTION

Eptifibatide is a cyclic heptapeptide containing six amino acids and one mercaptopropionyl (des-amino cysteinyl) residue. An interchain disulfide bridge is formed between the cysteine amide and the mercaptopropionyl moieties. Chemically it is N^6-(aminoiminomethyl)-N^2-(3-mercapto-1-oxopropyl-L-lysylglycyl-L-α-aspartyl-L-tryptophyl-L-prolyl-L-cysteinamide, cyclic (1→6)-disulfide. Eptifibatide binds to the platelet receptor glycoprotein (GP) IIb/IIIa of human platelets and inhibits platelet aggregation.

The eptifibatide peptide is produced by solution-phase peptide synthesis, and is purified by preparative reverse-phase liquid chromatography and lyophilized. The structural formula is:

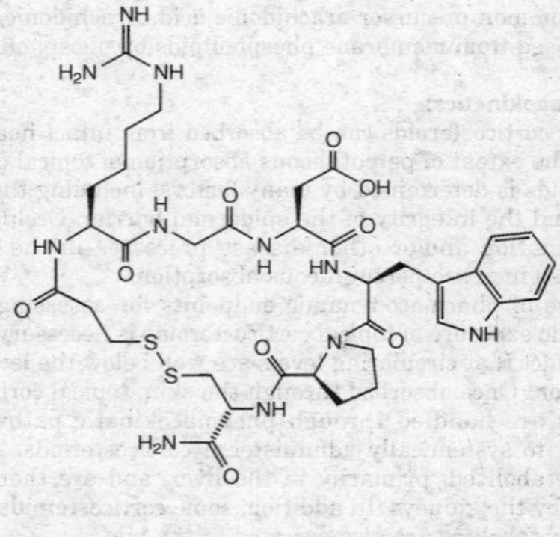

INTEGRILIN (eptifibatide) Injection is a clear, colorless, sterile, non-pyrogenic solution for intravenous (IV) use. Each 10-mL vial contains 2 mg/mL of eptifibatide and each 100-mL vial contains 0.75 mg/mL of eptifibatide. Each vial of either size also contains 5.25 mg/mL citric acid and sodium hydroxide to adjust the pH to 5.25.

CLINICAL PHARMACOLOGY

Mechanism of Action. Eptifibatide reversibly inhibits platelet aggregation by preventing the binding of fibrinogen, von Willebrand factor, and other adhesive ligands to GP IIb/IIIa. When administered intravenously, eptifibatide inhibits *ex vivo* platelet aggregation in a dose- and concentration-dependent manner. Platelet aggregation inhibition is reversible following cessation of the eptifibatide infusion; this is thought to result from dissociation of eptifibatide from the platelet.

Pharmacodynamics. Infusion of eptifibatide into baboons caused a dose-dependent inhibition of *ex vivo* platelet aggregation, with complete inhibition of aggregation achieved at infusion rates greater than 5.0 µg/kg/min. In a baboon model that is refractory to aspirin and heparin, doses of eptifibatide that inhibit aggregation prevented acute thrombosis with only a modest prolongation (2- to 3-fold) of the bleeding time. Platelet aggregation in dogs was also inhibited by infusions of eptifibatide, with complete inhibition at 2.0 µg/kg/min. This infusion dose completely inhibited canine coronary thrombosis induced by coronary artery injury (Folts model).

Human pharmacodynamic data were obtained in healthy subjects and in patients presenting with unstable angina (UA) or non-Q-wave myocardial infarction (NQMI) and/or undergoing percutaneous coronary interventions. Studies in healthy subjects enrolled only males; patient studies enrolled approximately one third women. In these studies, eptifibatide inhibited *ex vivo* platelet aggregation induced by adenosine diphosphate (ADP) and other agonists in a dose- and concentration-dependent manner. The effect of eptifibatide was observed immediately after administration of a 180 µg/kg intravenous bolus. Table 1 shows the effects of the two doses of eptifibatide used in the two principal clinical studies on *ex vivo* platelet aggregation induced by 20 µM ADP in PPACK-anticoagulated platelet-rich plasma and on bleeding time.

Table 1
Platelet Inhibition and Bleeding Time

	IMPACT II 135/0.5*	PURSUIT 180/ 2.0**
Inhibition of platelet aggregation 15 min. after bolus	69%	84%
Inhibition of platelet aggregation at steady state	40–50%	>90%
Bleeding-time prolongation at steady state	<5×	<5×
Inhibition of platelet aggregation 4h after infusion discontinuation	<30%	<50%
Bleeding-time prolongation 6h after infusion discontinuation	1×	1.4×

*135 µg/kg bolus followed by a continuous infusion of 0.5 µg/kg/min
**180 µg/kg bolus followed by a continuous infusion of 2.0 µg/kg/min

When administered alone, eptifibatide has no measurable effect on prothrombin time (PT) or activated partial thromboplastin time (aPTT). (See also PRECAUTIONS: Drug Interactions.)
There were no important differences between men and women or between age groups in the pharmacodynamic properties of eptifibatide. Differences among ethnic groups have not been assessed.
Pharmacokinetics. The pharmacokinetics of eptifibatide are linear and dose-proportional for bolus doses ranging from 90 to 250 µg/kg and infusion rates from 0.5 to 3.0 µg/kg/min. Plasma elimination half-life is approximately 2.5 hours. The recommended regimens of a bolus followed by an infusion produce an early peak level, followed by a small decline with attainment of steady state within 4–6 hours. The extent of eptifibatide binding to human plasma protein is about 25%.
Excretion and Metabolism. Clearance in patients with coronary artery disease is 55–58 mL/kg/h. In healthy subjects, renal clearance accounts for approximately 50% of total body clearance, with the majority of the drug excreted in the urine as eptifibatide, deamidated eptifibatide, and other, more polar metabolites. No major metabolites have been detected in human plasma. Clinical studies have included 2418 patients with serum creatinine between 1.0 and 2.0 mg/dL (for the 180 µg/kg bolus and the 2.0 µg/kg/min infusion) and 7 patients with serum creatinine between 2.0 and 4.0 mg/dL (for the 135 µg/kg bolus and the 0.5 µg/kg/min infusion), without dose adjustment. No data are available in patients with more severe degrees of renal impairment, but plasma eptifibatide levels are expected to be higher in such patients (see CONTRAINDICATIONS).
Special Populations. Patients in clinical studies were older than the subjects in clinical pharmacology studies, and they had lower total body eptifibatide clearance and higher eptifibatide plasma levels. Clinical studies were conducted in patients aged 20 to 94 years with coronary artery disease without dose adjustment for age. Because patients over 75 years of age were enrolled into the PURSUIT clinical study only if their body weight exceeded 50 kg, minimal data are available on lighter-weight patients over 75 years of age. Men and women showed no important differences in the pharmacokinetics of eptifibatide.

CLINICAL STUDIES

Eptifibatide was studied in two placebo-controlled, randomized studies, one (PURSUIT) in patients with acute coronary syndrome (unstable angina (UA) or non-Q-wave myocardial infarction (NQMI)), the other (IMPACT II) in patients about to undergo a percutaneous cardiovascular intervention (PCI; balloon angioplasty in most cases, but sometimes directional atherectomy, transluminal extraction catheter atherectomy, rotational ablation atherectomy, or excimer-laser angioplasty).
Acute coronary syndrome is defined as prolonged (≥10 minutes) symptoms of cardiac ischemia within the previous 24 hours associated with either ST-segment changes (elevation between 0.6 mm and 1 mm or depression >0.5 mm), T-wave inversion (>1 mm), or positive CK-MB. This definition includes "unstable angina" and "non-Q-wave myocardial infarction" but excludes myocardial infarction that is associated with Q waves or greater degrees of ST-segment elevation.
PURSUIT was a 726-center, 27-country, double-blind, randomized, placebo-controlled study in 10,948 patients presenting with UA or NQMI. Patients could be enrolled only if they had experienced cardiac ischemia at rest (≥10 minutes) within the previous 24 hours and had either ST-segment changes (elevations between 0.6 mm and 1 mm or depression >0.5 mm), T-wave inversion (>1 mm), or increased CK-MB. Important exclusion criteria included a history of bleeding diathesis, evidence of abnormal bleeding within the previous 30 days, uncontrolled hypertension, major surgery within the previous 6 weeks, stroke within the previous 30 days, any history of hemorrhagic stroke, serum creatinine >2.0 mg/dL, dependency on renal dialysis, or platelet count <100,000/mm^3.
Patients were randomized to either placebo, eptifibatide 180 µg/kg bolus followed by a 2.0 µg/kg/min infusion (180/2.0), or eptifibatide 180 µg/kg bolus followed by a 1.3 µg/kg/min infusion (180/1.3). The infusion was continued for 72 hours, until hospital discharge, or until the time of coronary artery bypass grafting (CABG), whichever occurred first, except that if PCI was performed, the eptifibatide infusion was continued for 24 hours after the procedure, allowing for a duration of infusion up to 96 hours.
The lower-infusion-rate arm was stopped after the first interim analysis when the two active-treatment arms appeared to have the same incidence of bleeding.
Patient age ranged from 20 to 94 (mean 63) years, and 65% were male. The patients were 89% Caucasian, 6% Hispanic, and 5% Black, recruited in the United States and Canada (40%), Western Europe (39%), Eastern Europe (16%), and Latin America (5%).
This was a "real world" study; each patient was managed according to the usual standards of the investigational site; frequencies of angiography, PCI, and CABG therefore differed widely from site to site and from country to country. Of the patients in PURSUIT, 13% were managed with PCI during drug infusion, of whom 50% received intracoronary stents; 87% were managed medically (without PCI during drug infusion).
The majority of patients received aspirin (75–325 mg once daily). Heparin was administered intravenously or subcutaneously, at the physician's discretion, most commonly as an intravenous bolus of 5000 U followed by a continuous infusion of 1000 U/h. For patients weighing less than 70 kg, the recommended heparin bolus dose was 60 U/kg followed by a continuous infusion of 12 U/kg/h. A target aPTT of 50–70 seconds was recommended. A total of 1250 patients underwent PCI within 72 hours after randomization, in which case they received intravenous heparin to maintain an activated clotting time (ACT) of 300–350 seconds.
The primary endpoint of the study was the occurrence of death from any cause or new myocardial infarction (MI) (evaluated by a blinded Clinical Endpoints Committee) within 30 days of randomization.
Compared to placebo, eptifibatide administered as a 180 µg/kg bolus followed by a 2.0 µg/kg/min infusion significantly (p=0.042) reduced the incidence of endpoint events (see Table 2). The reduction in the incidence of endpoint events in patients receiving eptifibatide was evident early during treatment, and this reduction was maintained through at least 30 days (see Figure 1). Table 2 also shows the incidence of the components of the primary endpoint, death (whether or not preceded by an MI) and new MI in surviving patients at 30 days.
[See table 2 above]

Table 2
Clinical Events in The PURSUIT Study

Death or MI	Placebo (n = 4739) n (%)	Eptifibatide (180/2.0) (n = 4722) n (%)	p-value
3 days	359 (7.6%)	279 (5.9%)	0.001
7 days	552 (11.6%)	477 (10.1%)	0.016
30 days			
Death or MI (Primary Endpoint)	745 (15.7%)	672 (14.2%)	0.042
Death	177 (3.7%)	165 (3.5%)	
Nonfatal MI	568 (12.0%)	507 (10.7%)	

Figure 1
Kaplan-Meier Plot of Time to Death or Myocardial Infarction Within 30 Days of Randomization

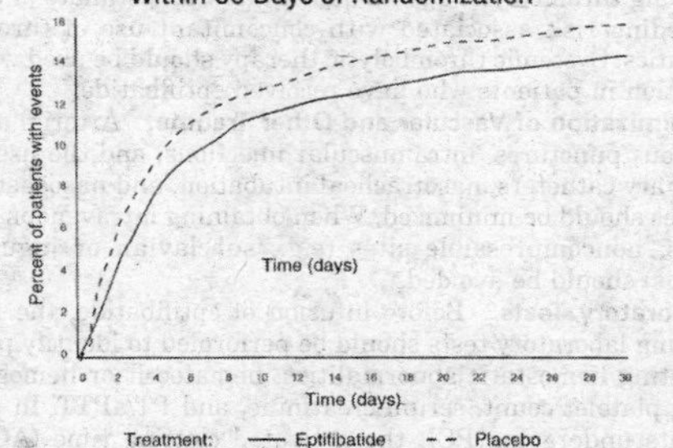

The effect of eptifibatide in PURSUIT did not appear to vary with patients' age. There were too few non-Caucasian patients to reach any conclusion as to possible differences related to race. Analysis of the PURSUIT results reveals a complex interaction of treatment, gender, and region. Throughout the world, eptifibatide was significantly less beneficial in women than in men, and in the overall study eptifibatide in women was nonsignificantly worse than placebo. These results were, however, strikingly heterogeneous across the several regions; eptifibatide appeared much worse than placebo in women in Latin America, while effects in men and women were scarcely distinguishable (relative risk reductions of 23% and 18%, respectively) in the U.S. and Canada. These results may reflect (a) genuine biological interactions between eptifibatide and gender, (b) interactions between eptifibatide and unknown international differences in concomitant therapy delivered to men and women, and (c) the play of chance, but the relative contributions of these possible factors are unknown.
Treatment with eptifibatide prior to determination of patient management strategy reduced clinical events regardless of whether patients ultimately underwent diagnostic catheterization, revascularization (i.e., PCI or CABG surgery) or continued to receive medical management alone. Table 3 shows the incidence of death or MI within 72 hours.

Table 3
Clinical Events (Death or MI) in the PURSUIT Study Within 72 Hours of Randomization

	Placebo	Eptifibatide 180/2.0
Overall Patient Population	n=4739	n=4722
- At 72 hours	7.6%	5.9%
Patients undergoing early PCI	n=631	n=619
- Pre-procedure (nonfatal MI only)	5.5%	1.8%
- At 72 hours	14.4%	9.0%
Patients not undergoing early PCI	n=4108	n=4103
- At 72 hours	6.5%	5.4%

All of the effect of eptifibatide was established within 72 hours (during the period of drug infusion), regardless of management strategy. Moreover, for patients undergoing early PCI, a reduction in events was evident prior to the procedure.
Follow-up data were available through 165 days for 10,611 patients enrolled in the PURSUIT trial (96.9 percent of the initial enrollment). This follow-up included 4,566 patients who received eptifibatide at the 180/2.0 dose. As reported by the investigators, the occurrence of death from any cause or new myocardial infarction for patients followed for at least 165 days was reduced from 13.6 percent with placebo to 12.1 percent with eptifibatide 180/2.0.
IMPACT II was a multi-center, double-blind, randomized, placebo-controlled study conducted in the United States in 4010 patients undergoing PCI. Major exclusion criteria included a history of bleeding diathesis, major surgery within 6 weeks of treatment, gastrointestinal bleeding within 30 days, any stroke or structural CNS abnormality, uncontrolled hypertension, PT >1.2 times control, hematocrit <30%, platelet count <100,000/mm^3, and pregnancy.
Patient age ranged from 24 to 89 (mean 60) years, and 75% were male. The patients were 92% Caucasian, 5% Black, and 3% Hispanic. Patients were randomly assigned to one of three treatment regimens, each incorporating a bolus dose initiated immediately prior to PCI followed by a continuous infusion lasting 20–24 hours: 1) 135 µg/kg bolus followed by a continuous infusion of 0.5 µg/kg/min of eptifibatide (135/0.5); 2) 135 µg/kg bolus followed by a continuous infusion of 0.75 µg/kg/min of eptifibatide (135/0.75); or 3) a matching placebo bolus followed by a matching placebo continuous infusion. Each patient received aspirin and an intravenous heparin bolus of 100 U/kg, with additional bolus infusions of up to 2000 additional units of heparin every 15 minutes to maintain an activated clotting time (ACT) of 300–350 seconds.
The primary endpoint was the composite of death, MI, or urgent revascularization, analyzed at 30 days after randomization in all patients who received at least one dose of study drug.
As shown in Table 4, each eptifibatide regimen reduced the rate of death, MI, or urgent intervention, although at 30 days, this finding was statistically significant only in the lower-dose eptifibatide group. As in the PURSUIT study, the effects of eptifibatide were seen early and persisted throughout the 30-day period.
[See table 4 at top of next page]
At the time of randomization, approximately 25% of the IMPACT II patients suffered from only chronic stable angina, or had had no angina at all since a remote (more than 14 days prior) myocardial infarction. At the other extreme, approximately 40% of the IMPACT II patients had ongoing acute coronary syndromes, including patients with rest angina, others with refractory recurrent angina, others with early post-infarction angina, and others about to receive percutaneous interventions during or immediately following acute myocardial infarction. The remaining patients had various histories of recent and remote acute coronary syndromes; data are not available to describe what fraction of these underwent PCI within only a day or two of an acute episode. The IMPACT II study was not powered to obtain stable estimates of efficacy in subpopulations defined by degree of acuity, but (as shown in Table 5) the data suggest that the benefit of eptifibatide was not limited to patients with ongoing acute coronary syndromes.

Continued on next page

Integrilin—Cont.

[See table 5 at right]

INDICATIONS AND USAGE

INTEGRILIN is indicated:

- For the treatment of patients with acute coronary syndrome (UA/NQMI), including patients who are to be managed medically and those undergoing percutaneous coronary intervention (PCI). In this setting, INTEGRILIN has been shown to decrease the rate of a combined endpoint of death or new myocardial infarction.
- For the treatment of patients undergoing PCI. In this setting, INTEGRILIN has been shown to decrease the rate of a combined endpoint of death, new myocardial infarction, or need for urgent intervention.

In the clinical studies of eptifibatide, most patients received heparin and aspirin, as described in CLINICAL TRIALS.

CONTRAINDICATIONS

Treatment with eptifibatide is contraindicated in patients with:

- A history of bleeding diathesis, or evidence of active abnormal bleeding within the previous 30 days.
- Severe hypertension (systolic blood pressure >200 mm Hg or diastolic blood pressure >110 mm Hg) not adequately controlled on antihypertensive therapy.
- Major surgery within the preceding 6 weeks.
- History of stroke within 30 days or any history of hemorrhagic stroke.
- Current or planned administration of another parenteral GP IIb/IIIa inhibitor.
- Platelet count <100,000/mm^3.
- Serum creatinine ≥4.0 mg/dL. In patients with serum creatinine levels between 2.0 mg/dL and 4.0 mg/dL, the 135μg/kg bolus and 0.5 μg/kg/min infusion should be administered.
- Dependency on renal dialysis.
- Known hypersensitivity to any component of the product.

WARNINGS

Bleeding. Bleeding is the most common complication encountered during eptifibatide therapy. Administration of eptifibatide is associated with an increase in major and minor bleeding, as classified by the criteria of the Thrombolysis in Myocardial Infarction Study group (TIMI), (see ADVERSE REACTIONS). Most major bleeding associated with eptifibatide has been at the arterial access site for cardiac catheterization or from the gastrointestinal or genitourinary tract.

In patients undergoing percutaneous coronary interventions, patients receiving eptifibatide experience an increased incidence of major bleeding compared to those receiving placebo. Special care should be employed to minimize the risk of bleeding among these patients (see PRECAUTIONS).

If bleeding cannot be controlled with pressure, infusion of eptifibatide and concomitant heparin should be stopped immediately.

PRECAUTIONS

Bleeding Precautions

Care of the Femoral Artery Access Site in Patients Undergoing Percutaneous Coronary Intervention (PCI). In patients undergoing PCI, treatment with eptifibatide is associated with an increase in major and minor bleeding at the site of arterial sheath placement. After PCI, eptifibatide infusion should be continued for 20–24 hours. The femoral artery sheath may be removed during treatment with eptifibatide, but only after heparin has been discontinued and its effects largely reversed. In the IMPACT II study, heparin use was discouraged after the PCI procedure if the coronary lesion appeared angiographically stable. Early sheath removal was encouraged in both the IMPACT II and the PURSUIT studies while study drug was being infused. Prior to removing the sheath, it was recommended that heparin be discontinued for 3–4 hours and that an aPTT of <45 seconds be documented. In any case, both heparin and eptifibatide should be discontinued and sheath hemostasis should be achieved by standard compressive techniques at least 4 hours before hospital discharge.

Use of Thrombolytics, Anticoagulants, and Other Antiplatelet Agents. In the IMPACT II and PURSUIT studies, eptifibatide was used concomitantly with heparin and aspirin (see CLINICAL STUDIES). Because eptifibatide inhibits platelet aggregation, caution should be employed when it is used with other drugs that affect hemostasis, including **thrombolytics, oral anticoagulants, non-steroidal anti-inflammatory drugs, dipyridamole, ticlopidine, and clopidogrel.** To avoid potentially additive pharmacologic effects, concomitant treatment with **other inhibitors of platelet receptor GP IIb/IIIa** should be avoided.

There is only a small experience with concomitant use of eptifibatide and **thrombolytics.** In a study of 180 patients with acute myocardial infarction (AMI), eptifibatide (in regimens up to a bolus of 180 μg/kg followed by a continuous infusion of 0.75 μg/kg/min for 24 hours) was administered concomitantly with the approved "accelerated" regimen of alteplase, a thrombolytic agent. The studied regimens of eptifibatide did not increase the incidence of major bleeding or transfusion compared to the incidence seen when alteplase was given alone.

In the IMPACT II study, 15 patients received a thrombolytic agent in conjunction with the 135/0.5 dosing regimen, 2 of whom experienced a major bleed. In the PURSUIT study, 40

Table 4
Clinical Events in the IMPACT II Study

	Placebo n (%)	Eptifibatide (135/0.5) n (%)	Eptifibatide (135/0.75) n (%)
Patients	1285	1300	1286
Abrupt Closure	65 (5.1%)	36 (2.8%)	43 (3.3%)
p-value vs. placebo		0.003	0.030
Death, MI, or Urgent Intervention			
24 hours	123 (9.6%)	86 (6.6%)	89 (6.9%)
p-value vs. placebo		0.006	0.014
48 hours	131 (10.2%)	99 (7.6%)	102 (7.9%)
p-value vs. placebo		0.021	0.045
30 days (primary endpoint)	149 (11.6%)	118 (9.1%)	128 (10.0%)
p-value vs. placebo		0.035	0.179
Death or MI			
30 days	110 (8.6%)	89 (6.8%)	95 (7.4%)
p-value vs. placebo		0.102	0.272
6 months	151 (11.9%)*	136 (10.6%)*	130 (10.3%)*
p-value vs. placebo		0.297	0.182

*Kaplan-Meier estimate of event rate

Table 5
Clinical Events at 30 Days in the IMPACT II Study, Stratified by Acuity at Time of Randomization

Classification of Patients (%)	Placebo n (%)	Eptifibatide 135/0.5 n (%)	Eptifibatide 135/0.75 n (%)
Ongoing ACS, MI ongoing or within past 24h (41.3%)	538 (11.5%)	532 (10.0%)	527 (10.6%)
Others (58.7%)	747 (11.6%)	768 (8.5%)	759 (9.5%)

Table 6
Major Bleeding by Maximal aPTT Within 72 Hours in the PURSUIT Study

	Placebo n (%)	Eptifibatide 180/1.3* n (%)	Eptifibatide 180/2.0 n (%)
Maximum aPTT (seconds)			
<50	44/721(6.1%)	21/244(8.6%)	44/743(5.9%)
50-70 (recommended)	92/908(10.1%)	28/259(10.8%)	99/883(11.2%)
>70	281/2786(10.1%)	99/891(11.1%)	345/2811(12.3%)

*Administered only until the first interim analysis

patients who received eptifibatide at the 180/2.0 dosing regimen received a thrombolytic agent, 10 of whom experienced a major bleed.

In another AMI study involving 181 patients, eptifibatide (in regimens up to a bolus of 180 μg/kg followed by a continuous infusion of up to 2.0 μg/kg/min for up to 72 hours) was administered concomitantly with streptokinase (1.5 million units over 60 minutes), another thrombolytic agent. At the highest studied infusion rates (1.3 μg/kg/min and 2.0 μg/kg/min), eptifibatide was associated with an increase in the incidence of bleeding and transfusions compared to the incidence seen when streptokinase was given alone.

These limited data on the use of eptifibatide in patients receiving thrombolytic agents do not allow an estimate of the bleeding risk associated with concomitant use of thrombolytics. Systemic thrombolytic therapy should be used with caution in patients who have received eptifibatide.

Minimization of Vascular and Other Trauma. Arterial and venous punctures, intramuscular injections, and the use of urinary catheters, nasotracheal intubation, and nasogastric tubes should be minimized. When obtaining intravenous access, noncompressible sites (e.g., subclavian or jugular veins) should be avoided.

Laboratory Tests. Before infusion of eptifibatide, the following laboratory tests should be performed to identify preexisting hemostatic abnormalities: hematocrit or hemoglobin, platelet count, serum creatinine, and PT/aPTT. In patients undergoing PCI, the activated clotting time (ACT) should also be measured.

Maintaining Target aPTT and ACT. The aPTT should be maintained between 50 and 70 seconds unless PCI is to be performed. In patients treated with heparin, bleeding can be minimized by close monitoring of the aPTT. Table 6 displays the risk of major bleeding according to the maximum aPTT attained within 72 hours in the PURSUIT study.

[See table 6 above]

During PCI, the PURSUIT study stipulated a target ACT of between 300 and 350 seconds. Patients receiving an eptifibatide 180 μg/kg bolus followed by a 2 μg/kg/min infusion experienced an increased incidence of bleeding relative to placebo, primarily at the femoral artery access site.

The aPTT or ACT should be checked prior to arterial sheath removal. The sheath should not be removed unless the aPTT is <45 seconds or the ACT is <150 seconds.

Thrombocytopenia. If the patient experiences a confirmed platelet decrease to <100,000/mm^3, INTEGRILIN and heparin should be discontinued and the condition appropriately monitored and treated.

Renal Insufficiency. Based on results of clinical studies with eptifibatide (which did not adjust dose for renal function) and the fact that the drug is cleared equally by renal and nonrenal mechanisms, dose adjustment is unnecessary for patients with mild to moderate renal impairment (serum creatinine <2.0 mg/dL for the 180 μg/kg bolus and the 2.0 μg/kg/min infusion and <4.0 mg/dL for the 135 μg/kg bolus and the 0.5 μg/kg/min infusion). For patients with serum creatinine >2.0 mg/dL and <4.0 mg/dL, eptifibatide should be administered as a 135 μg/kg bolus followed by a 0.5 μg/kg/min infusion. Plasma eptifibatide levels are expected to be higher in patients with more severe renal impairment, but no data are available for such patients or for patients on renal dialysis. *In vitro* studies have indicated that eptifibatide may be cleared from plasma by dialysis.

Geriatric Use. The PURSUIT and IMPACT II clinical studies enrolled patients up to the age of 94 years (45% were age 65 and over; 12% were age 75 and older). There was no apparent difference in efficacy between older and younger patients treated with eptifibatide. The incidence of bleeding complications was higher in the elderly in both placebo and eptifibatide groups, and the incremental risk of eptifibatide-associated bleeding was greater in the older patients. No dose adjustment was made for elderly patients, but patients over 75 years of age had to weigh at least 50 kg to be enrolled in the PURSUIT study because of concern about an increased risk of bleeding in this subgroup (see also ADVERSE REACTIONS).

Carcinogenesis, Mutagenesis, Impairment of Fertility. No long-term studies in animals have been performed to evaluate the carcinogenic potential of eptifibatide. Eptifibatide was not genotoxic in the Ames test, the mouse lymphoma cell (L 5178Y, TK$^{+/-}$) forward mutation test, the human lymphocyte chromosome aberration test, or the mouse micronucleus test. Administered by continuous intravenous infusion at total daily doses up to 72 mg/kg/day (about 4 times the recommended maximum daily human dose on a body surface area basis), eptifibatide had no effect on fertility and reproductive performance of male and female rats.

Pregnancy. Pregnancy Category B. Teratology studies have been performed by continuous intravenous infusion of eptifibatide in pregnant rats at total daily doses of up to 72 mg/kg/day (about 4 times the recommended maximum daily human dose on a body surface area basis) and in pregnant rabbits at total daily doses of up to 36 mg/kg/day (also about 4 times the recommended maximum daily human dose on a body surface area basis). These studies revealed no evidence of harm to the fetus due to eptifibatide. There are, however, no adequate and well-controlled studies in pregnant women with eptifibatide. Because animal reproduction studies are not always predictive of human response, eptifibatide should be used during pregnancy only if clearly needed.

Pediatric Use. Safety and effectiveness of eptifibatide in pediatric patients have not been studied.

Nursing Mothers. It is not known whether eptifibatide is excreted in human milk. Because many drugs are excreted in human milk, caution should be exercised when eptifibatide is administered to a nursing mother.

ADVERSE REACTIONS

A total of 14,718 patients were treated in the two Phase III clinical trials (PURSUIT and IMPACT II). Of these, 8737 received eptifibatide: 1300 at 135/0.5 for up to 24 hours, 1286 at 135/0.75 for up to 24 hours, 1472 at 180/1.3 for up to 72 hours, and 4679 at 180/2.0 for up to 72 hours. The other 5981 patients received placebo. These 14,718 patients had a mean age of 62 years (range 20 to 94 years). Eighty-nine percent of the patients were Caucasian, with the remainder being predominantly Black (5%) and Hispanic (5%). Sixty-seven percent were men.

Because of the different regimens used in PURSUIT and IMPACT II, data from the two studies were not pooled.

Bleeding. The incidences of bleeding events and transfusions in the PURSUIT and IMPACT II studies are shown in Table 7. Bleeding was classified as major or minor by the criteria of the TIMI study group. Major bleeding events consisted of intracranial hemorrhage and other bleeding that led to decreases in hemoglobin greater than 5 g/dL. Minor bleeding events included spontaneous gross hematuria, spontaneous hematemesis, other observed blood loss with a hemoglobin decrease of more than 3 g/dL, and other hemoglobin decreases that were greater than 4 g/dL but less than 5 g/dL. In patients who received transfusions, the corresponding loss in hemoglobin was estimated through an adaptation period of the method of Landefeld *et al.*

[See table 7 at right]

Table 7
Bleeding Events and Transfusions in the PURSUIT and IMPACT II Studies

PURSUIT	Placebo n (%)	Eptifibatide 180/1.3* n (%)	Eptifibatide 180/2.0 n (%)
Patients	4696	1472	4679
Major bleeding[a]	425 (9.3%)	152 (10.5%)	498 (10.8%)
Minor bleeding[a]	347 (7.6%)	152 (10.5%)	604 (13.1%)
Requiring Transfusions[b]	490 (10.4%)	188 (12.8%)	601 (12.8%)

IMPACT II	Placebo n (%)	Eptifibatide 135/0.5 n (%)	Eptifibatide 135/0.75 n (%)
Patients	1285	1300	1286
Major bleeding[a]	55 (4.5%)	55 (4.4%)	58 (4.7%)
Minor bleeding[a]	115 (9.3%)	146 (11.7%)	177 (14.2%)
Requiring Transfusions[b]	66 (5.1%)	71 (5.5%)	74 (5.8%)

Note: denominator is based on patients for whom data are available
*Administered only until the first interim analysis
[a] For major and minor bleeding, patients are counted only once according to the most severe classification.
[b] Includes transfusions of whole blood, packed red blood cells, fresh frozen plasma, cryoprecipitate, platelets, and autotransfusion during the initial hospitalization.

As shown in Tables 8 and 9, the overall incidence of major bleeding in these studies was strongly related to the incidence of coronary artery bypass graft (CABG) surgery; the excess bleeding seen with eptifibatide, however, was seen only among the patients who did not undergo CABG.

In the PURSUIT study, the greatest increase in major bleeding in eptifibatide-treated patients compared to placebo was associated with bleeding at the femoral artery access site (2.8% versus 1.3%). Oropharyngeal (primarily gingival), genito-urinary, gastrointestinal, and retroperitoneal bleeding were also seen more commonly in eptifibatide-treated patients compared to placebo. Among patients experiencing a major bleed in the IMPACT II study, an increase in bleeding on eptifibatide versus placebo was observed only for the femoral artery access site (3.2% versus 2.8%).

Tables 8 and 9 display the incidence of TIMI major bleeding according to the cardiac procedures carried out in the PURSUIT and IMPACT II studies, respectively. The most common bleeding complications were related to cardiac revascularization (CABG-related or femoral artery access site bleeding).

[See table 8 at right]
[See table 9 at right]

Table 8
Major Bleeding by Procedures in the PURSUIT Study

	Placebo n (%)	Eptifibatide 180/1.3* n (%)	Eptifibatide 180/2.0 n (%)
Patients	4577	1451	4604
Overall Incidence of Major Bleeding	425 (9.3%)	152 (10.5%)	498 (10.8%)
Breakdown by Procedure:			
CABG	375 (8.2%)	123 (8.5%)	377 (8.2%)
Angioplasty without CABG	27 (0.6%)	16 (1.1%)	64 (1.4%)
Angiography without angioplasty or CABG	11 (0.2%)	7 (0.5%)	29 (0.6%)
Medical Therapy Only	12 (0.3%)	6 (0.4%)	28 (0.6%)

Denominators are based on the total number of patients whose TIMI classification was resolved.
*Administered only until the first interim analysis

Table 9
Major Bleeding by Procedures in the IMPACT II Study

	Placebo n (%)	Eptifibatide 135/0.5 n (%)	Eptifibatide 135/0.75 n (%)
Patients	1230	1249	1245
Overall Incidence of Major Bleeding	55 (4.5%)	55 (4.4%)	58 (4.7%)
Breakdown of Bleeding by Procedure:			
CABG	35 (2.8%)	23 (1.8%)	26 (2.1%)
Angioplasty without CABG	20 (1.6%)	32 (2.6%)	32 (2.7%)

Denominators are based on the total number of patients whose TIMI classification was resolved.

In the PURSUIT study, the risk of major bleeding with eptifibatide increased inversely with patient weight. This relationship was most apparent for patients weighing less than 70 kg. These trends were not apparent in the IMPACT II study.

Bleeding adverse events resulting in discontinuation of study drug were more frequent among patients receiving eptifibatide than placebo (8% versus 1% in PURSUIT, 3.5% versus 1.9% in IMPACT II).

Intracranial Hemorrhage and Stroke. Intracranial hemorrhage was rare in the PURSUIT clinical study, with only 3 patients in the placebo group, 1 patient in the group treated with eptifibatide 180/1.3 and 5 patients in the group treated with eptifibatide 180/2.0 experiencing a hemorrhagic stroke within 30 days of randomization. The overall incidence of stroke was 0.5% in patients receiving eptifibatide 180/1.3, 0.7% in patients receiving eptifibatide 180/2.0, and 0.8% in placebo patients within 30 days of randomization.

In the IMPACT II study, intracranial hemorrhage was experienced by 1 patient treated with eptifibatide 135/0.5, 2 patients treated with eptifibatide 135/0.75 and 2 patients in the placebo group. The overall incidence of stroke was 0.5% in patients receiving 135/0.5 eptifibatide, 0.7% in patients receiving eptifibatide 135/0.75 and 0.7% in the placebo group.

Thrombocytopenia. In the PURSUIT and IMPACT II studies, the incidence of thrombocytopenia (<100,000/mm^3 or ≥50% reduction from baseline) and the incidence of platelet transfusions were similar between patients treated with eptifibatide and placebo.

Allergic Reactions. In the IMPACT II study, anaphylaxis was reported in 1 patient (0.08%) on placebo and in no patients on eptifibatide. In the PURSUIT study, anaphylaxis was reported in 7 patients receiving placebo (0.15%) and 7 patients receiving eptifibatide 180/2.0 (0.16%). In the IMPACT II study, 2 patients (1 patient (0.04%) receiving eptifibatide and 1 patient (0.08%) receiving placebo) discontinued study drug because of allergic reactions. In the PURSUIT study, anaphylaxis was given as a reason for drug discontinuation in 3 patients (0.05%) who received eptifibatide and in none of the patients who received placebo.

The potential for development of antibodies to eptifibatide has been studied in 433 subjects. Eptifibatide was nonantigenic in 412 patients receiving a single administration of eptifibatide (135 µg/kg bolus followed by a continuous infusion of either 0.5 µg/kg/min or 0.75 µg/kg/min), and in 21 subjects to whom eptifibatide (135 µg/kg bolus followed by a continuous infusion of 0.75 µg/kg/min) was administered twice, 28 days apart. In both cases, plasma for antibody detection was collected approximately 30 days after each dose. The development of antibodies to eptifibatide at higher doses has not been evaluated.

Other Adverse Reactions. Serious non-bleeding events occurred in 19% of the eptifibatide and 19% of the placebo patients in the PURSUIT study. The only serious non-bleeding adverse event that occurred at a rate of at least 1% and was more common with eptifibatide than placebo (7% versus 6%) was hypotension. Most of the serious non-bleeding events consisted of cardiovascular events typical of an unstable angina population. In the IMPACT II study, serious non-bleeding events that occurred in greater than 1% of patients were uncommon and similar in incidence between placebo- and eptifibatide-treated patients.

Discontinuation of study drug due to adverse events other than bleeding was uncommon in both the PURSUIT and IMPACT II studies, with no single event occurring in >0.5% of the study population. In the PURSUIT study, non-bleeding adverse events leading to discontinuation occurred in the eptifibatide and placebo groups in the following body systems with an incidence of ≥0.1%: cardiovascular system (0.3% and 0.3%), digestive system (0.1% and 0.1%), hemic/lymphatic system (0.1% and 0.1%), nervous system (0.3% and 0.4%), urogenital system (0.1% and 0.1%), and whole body system (0.2% and 0.2%). In the IMPACT II study, non-bleeding adverse events leading to discontinuation occurred in the 135/0.5 eptifibatide and placebo groups in the following body systems with an incidence of ≥0.1%: whole body (0.3% and 0.1%), cardiovascular system (1.4% and 1.4%), digestive system (0.2% and 0%), hemic/lymphatic system (0.2% and 0%), nervous system (0.3% and 0.2%), and respiratory system (0.1% and 0.1%).

OVERDOSAGE

There has been only limited experience with overdosage of eptifibatide. There were 8 patients in the IMPACT II study and 9 patients in the PURSUIT study who received bolus doses and/or infusion doses more than double those called for in the protocols, or who were identified by the investigator as having received an overdose. None of these patients experienced an intracranial bleed or other major bleeding.

Eptifibatide was not lethal to rats, rabbits, or monkeys when administered by continuous intravenous infusion for 90 minutes at a total dose of 45 mg/kg (about 2 to 5 times the recommended maximum daily human dose on a body surface area basis). Symptoms of acute toxicity were loss of righting reflex, dyspnea, ptosis, and decreased muscle tone in rabbits and petechial hemorrhages in the femoral and abdominal areas of monkeys.

DOSAGE AND ADMINISTRATION

The safety and efficacy of eptifibatide has been established in clinical studies that employed concomitant use of heparin and aspirin. Different dose regimens of eptifibatide were used in the major clinical studies. (See CLINICAL STUDIES.)

Acute Coronary Syndrome. The recommended adult dosage of eptifibatide in patients with acute coronary syndrome is an intravenous bolus of 180 µg/kg as soon as possible following diagnosis, followed by a continuous infusion of 2.0 µg/kg/min until hospital discharge or initiation of CABG surgery, up to 72 hours. If a patient is to undergo a percutaneous coronary intervention (PCI) while receiving eptifibatide, consideration can be given to decreasing the infusion

Continued on next page

Integrilin—Cont.

rate to 0.5 μg/kg/min (the infusion rate in IMPACT II) at the time of the procedure. Infusion should be continued for an additional 20–24 hours after the procedure, allowing for up to 96 hours of therapy. In the PURSUIT study, patients weighing more than 121 kg received a maximum bolus of 22.6 mg (11.3 mL of the 2 mg/mL injection) followed by a maximum infusion of 15 mg (20 mL of the 0.75 mg/mL injection) per hour.

Percutaneous Coronary Intervention (PCI) in patients not presenting with an acute coronary syndrome. The recommended adult dosage of eptifibatide in patients undergoing PCI and not presenting with an acute coronary syndrome is an intravenous bolus of 135 μg/kg administered immediately before the initiation of PCI followed by a continuous infusion of 0.5 μg/kg/min for 20–24 hours. In the IMPACT II study, there was little experience in patients weighing more than 143 kg.

In patients who undergo coronary artery bypass graft surgery, eptifibatide infusion should be discontinued prior to surgery.

In the clinical trials that showed eptifibatide to be effective, most patients received concomitant aspirin and heparin. The aspirin doses used in the clinical studies were as follows:

Acute Coronary Syndrome (PURSUIT Study)	Angioplasty (IMPACT II Study)
160 mg initially, then 75–325 mg daily	75–325 mg 1–24 hours prior to intervention

The initial target aPTT in the PURSUIT study was 50–70 seconds, and the recommended heparin dosing was:

- if weight ≥70 kg, 5000 U bolus followed by infusion of 1000 U/hr
- if weight <70 kg, 60 U/kg bolus followed by infusion of 12 U/kg/hr

When these patients were to undergo PCI, the target ACT was 300–350 seconds, and the recommended heparin doses were:

Initial Heparin Bolus

ACT (seconds)	Heparin Bolus
<150	100 U/kg (10,000 U maximum)
151–225	75 U/kg
226–299	50 U/kg
≥300	none

Repeat Heparin Bolus*

ACT (seconds)	Heparin Bolus
<275	50 U/kg
275–299	25 U/kg
≥300	none

*based on hourly ACT determinations

In the IMPACT II study, the target ACT was 300–350 seconds before the procedure and ≤ 350 seconds thereafter. The recommended heparin doses were:

- prior to intervention: 100 U/kg bolus
- during intervention: up to 2000 U bolus q15min
- after intervention: infusion at physician's discretion

Patients requiring thrombolytic therapy had eptifibatide infusions stopped and were discontinued from the studies.

Instructions for Administration

1. Like other parenteral drug products, INTEGRILIN solutions should be inspected visually for particulate matter and discoloration prior to administration, whenever solution and container permit.
2. INTEGRILIN may be administered in the same intravenous line as alteplase, atropine, dobutamine, heparin, lidocaine, meperidine, metoprolol, midazolam, morphine, nitroglycerin, or verapamil. INTEGRILIN should not be administered through the same intravenous line as furosemide.
3. INTEGRILIN may be administered in the same IV line with 0.9% NaCl or 0.9% NaCl/5% dextrose. With either vehicle, the infusion may also contain up to 60 mEq/L of potassium chloride. No incompatibilities have been observed with intravenous administration sets. No compatibility studies have been performed with PVC bags.
4. The bolus dose of INTEGRILIN should be withdrawn from the 10-mL vial into a syringe. The bolus dose should be administered by IV push over 1–2 minutes.
5. Immediately following the bolus dose administration, a continuous infusion of INTEGRILIN should be initiated. When using an intravenous infusion pump, INTEGRILIN should be administered undiluted directly from the 100-mL vial. The 100-mL vial should be spiked with a vented infusion set. Care should be taken to center the spike within the circle on the stopper top.

INTEGRILIN is to be administered by volume according to patient weight. Patients should receive study drug according to the following table:

[See table 1 below]
[See table 2 below]

HOW SUPPLIED

INTEGRILIN (eptifibatide) Injection is supplied as a sterile solution in 10-mL vials containing 20 mg of eptifibatide (NDC 0085-1177-01) and 100-mL vials containing either 75 mg of eptifibatide (NDC 0085-1136-01) or 200 mg of eptifibatide (NDC 0085-1177-02).

Vials should be stored refrigerated at 2–8°C (36–46°F). Vials may be transferred to room temperature storage* for a period not to exceed 2 months. Upon transfer, vial cartons must be marked by the dispensing pharmacist with a "DISCARD BY" date (2 months from the transfer date or the labeled expiration date, whichever comes first).

Do not use beyond the labeled expiration date. Protect from light until administration. Discard any unused portion left in the vial.

* USP controlled Room Temperature: 25°C (77°F) with excursions permitted between 15–30°C (59–86°F).

Rx only

Marketed By:
COR Therapeutics, Inc.
South San Francisco, CA 94080
and
Key Pharmaceuticals, Inc.
Kenilworth, NJ 07033

Distributed By:
Key Pharmaceuticals, Inc.
Kenilworth, NJ 07033

1. INTEGRILIN Dosing Chart by Weight for Patients With Acute Coronary Syndrome (180 μg/kg Bolus and 2μg/kg/min Infusion)

Patient Weight (kg)	Patient Weight (lb)	180μg/kg Bolus Volume (from 2 mg/mL vial)	2.0 μg/kg/min Infusion Volume (from 2 mg/mL 100-mL vial)	2.0 μg/kg/min Infusion Volume (from 0.75 mg/mL 100-mL vial)
37–41	81–91	3.4 mL	2.0 mL/h	6.0 mL/h
42–46	92–102	4.0 mL	2.5 mL/h	7.0 mL/h
47–53	103–117	4.5 mL	3.0 mL/h	8.0 mL/h
54–59	118–130	5.0 mL	3.5 mL/h	9.0 mL/h
60–65	131–143	5.6 mL	3.8 mL/h	10.0 mL/h
66–71	144–157	6.2 mL	4.0 mL/h	11.0 mL/h
72–78	158–172	6.8 mL	4.5 mL/h	12.0 mL/h
79–84	173–185	7.3 mL	5.0 mL/h	13.0 mL/h
85–90	186–198	7.9 mL	5.3 mL/h	14.0 mL/h
91–96	199–212	8.5 mL	5.6 mL/h	15.0 mL/h
97–103	213–227	9.0 mL	6.0 mL/h	16.0 mL/h
104–109	228–240	9.5 mL	6.4 mL/h	17.0 mL/h
110–115	241–253	10.2 mL	6.8 mL/h	18.0 mL/h
116–121	254–267	10.7 mL	7.0 mL/h	19.0 mL/h
>121	>267	11.3 mL	7.5 mL/h	20.0 mL/h

2. INTEGRILIN Dosing Chart by Weight for Patients Without Acute Coronary Syndromes Undergoing PCI (135 μg/kg Bolus and 0.5 μg/kg/min Infusion)

Patient Weight (kg)	Patient Weight (lb)	135 μg/kg Bolus Volume (from 2 mg/mL vial)	0.5 μg/kg/min Infusion Volume (from 2 mg/mL 100-mL vial)	0.5 μg/kg/min Infusion Volume (from 0.75 mg/mL 100-mL vial)
40–55	88–121	3.4 mL	0.7 mL/h	2.0 mL/h
56–68	122–150	4.2 mL	0.9 mL/h	2.5 mL/h
69–80	151–176	5.1 mL	1.1 mL/h	3.0 mL/h
81–93	177–205	5.9 mL	1.3 mL/h	3.5 mL/h
94–105	206–231	6.8 mL	1.5 mL/h	4.0 mL/h
106–118	232–260	7.6 mL	1.7 mL/h	4.5 mL/h
119–131	261–288	8.4 mL	1.9 mL/h	5.0 mL/h
132–143	289–315	9.2 mL	2.1 mL/h	5.5 mL/h

Issued December 1999
Rev 6
Shown in Product Identification Guide, page 311

Cypros Pharmaceutical Corporation

(For product information, see QUESTCOR PHARMACEUTICALS, INC.)

Daiichi Pharmaceutical Corp.

**11 PHILIPS PARKWAY
MONTVALE, NJ 07645**

Direct Inquiries to:
Medical Services Department
Ph: (877) 324-4244 (877-DAIICHI)
Fax: (888) 727-5666
For Medical Emergencies and Product Information Contact:
Medical Services Department
Ph: (888) 727-2500
Fax: (888) 272-7979

EVOXAC™ Capsules ℞
(cevimeline hydrochloride)

DESCRIPTION

Cevimeline is cis-2'-methylspiro (1-azabicyclo [2.2.2] octane-3, 5' -[1,3] oxathiolane) hydrochloride, hydrate (2:1). Its empirical formula is $C_{10}H_{17}NOS.HCl.1/2H_2O$, and its structural formula is:

Cevimeline has a molecular weight of 244.79. It is a white to off white crystalline powder with a melting point range of 201 to 203°C. It is freely soluble in alcohol and chloroform, very soluble in water, and virtually insoluble in ether. The pH of a 1% solution ranges from 4.6 to 5.6. Inactive ingredients include lactose monohydrate, hydroxypropyl cellulose, and magnesium stearate.

CLINICAL PHARMACOLOGY

Pharmacodynamics

Cevimeline is a cholinergic agonist which binds to muscarinic receptors. Muscarinic agonists in sufficient dosage can increase secretion of exocrine glands, such as salivary and sweat glands and increase tone of the smooth muscle in the gastrointestinal and urinary tracts.

Pharmacokinetics

Absorption: After administration of a single 30 mg capsule, cevimeline was rapidly absorbed with a mean time to peak concentration of 1.5 to 2 hours. No accumulation of active drug or its metabolites was observed following multiple dose administration. When administered with food, there is a decrease in the rate of absorption, with a fasting T_{MAX} of 1.53 hours and a T_{MAX} of 2.86 hours after a meal; the peak concentration is reduced by 17.3%. Single oral doses across the clinical dose range are dose proportional.

Distribution: Cevimeline has a volume of distribution of approximately 6L/kg and is <20% bound to human plasma proteins. This suggests that cevimeline is extensively bound to tissues; however, the specific binding sites are unknown.

Metabolism: Isozymes CYP2D6 and CYP3A3/4 are responsible for the metabolism of cevimeline. After 24 hours, 86.7% of the dose was recovered (16.0% unchanged, 44.5% as cis and trans-sulfoxide, 22.3% of the dose as glucuronic acid conjugate and 4% of the dose as N-oxide of cevimeline). Approximately 8% of the trans-sulfoxide metabolite is then converted into the corresponding glucuronic acid conjugate and eliminated. Cevimeline did not inhibit cytochrome P450 isozymes 1A2, 2A6, 2C9, 2C19, 2D6, 2E1, and 3A4.

Excretion: The mean half-life of cevimeline is 5+/−1 hours. After 24 hours, 84% of a 30 mg dose of cevimeline was excreted in urine. After seven days, 97% of the dose was recovered in the urine and 0.5% was recovered in the feces.

Special Populations: The effects of renal impairment, hepatic impairment, or ethnicity on the pharmacokinetics of cevimeline have not been investigated.

Clinical Studies

Cevimeline has been shown to improve the symptoms of dry mouth in patients with Sjögren's Syndrome.

A 6-week, randomized, double blind, placebo-controlled study was conducted in 75 patients (10 men, 65 women) with a mean age of 53.6 years (range 33–75). The racial distribution was Caucasian 92%, Black 1% and other 7%. The effects of cevimeline at 30 mg tid (90 mg/day) and 60 mg tid (180 mg/day) were compared to those of placebo. Patients were evaluated by a measure called global improvement, which is defined as a response of "better" to the question, "Please rate the overall condition of your dry mouth now compared with how you felt before starting treatment in this study." Patients also had the option of selecting "worse" or "no change" as answers. Seventy-six percent of the patients in the 30 mg tid group reported a global improvement in their dry mouth symptoms compared to 35% of the patients in the placebo group. This difference was statistically significant at p=0.0043. There was no evidence that patients in the 60 mg tid group had better global evaluation scores than the patients in the 30 mg tid group.

A 12-week, randomized, double-blind, placebo-controlled study was conducted in 197 patients (10 men, 187 women) with a mean age of 54.5 years (range 23–74). The racial distribution was Caucasian 91.4%, Black 3% and other 5.6%. The effects of cevimeline at 15 mg tid (45 mg/day) and 30 mg tid (90 mg/day) were compared to those of placebo. Statistically significant global improvement in the symptoms of dry mouth (p=0.0004) was seen for the 30 mg tid group compared to placebo, but not for the 15 mg group compared to placebo. Salivary flow showed statistically significant increases at both doses of cevimeline during the study compared to placebo.

A second 12-week, randomized, double-blind, placebo-controlled study was conducted in 212 patients (11 men, 201 women) with a mean age of 55.3 years (range 24–75). The racial distribution was Caucasian 88.7%, Black 1.9% and other 9.4%. The effects of cevimeline at 15 mg tid (45 mg/day) and 30 mg tid (90 mg/day) were compared to those of placebo. No statistically significant differences were noted in the patient global evaluations. However, there was a higher placebo response rate in this study compared to the aforementioned studies. The 30 mg tid group showed a statistically significant increase in salivary flow from pre-dose to post-dose compared to placebo (p=0.0017).

INDICATIONS AND USAGE

Cevimeline is indicated for the treatment of symptoms of dry mouth in patients with Sjögren's Syndrome.

CONTRAINDICATIONS

Cevimeline is contraindicated in patients with uncontrolled asthma, known hypersensitivity to cevimeline, and when miosis is undesirable, e.g., in acute iritis and in narrow-angle (angle-closure) glaucoma.

WARNINGS

Cardiovascular Disease:

Cevimeline can potentially alter cardiac conduction and/or heart rate. Patients with significant cardiovascular disease may potentially be unable to compensate for transient changes in hemodynamics or rhythm induced by EVOXAC™. EVOXAC™ should be used with caution and under close medical supervision in patients with a history of cardiovascular disease evidenced by angina pectoris or myocardial infarction.

Pulmonary Disease:

Cevimeline can potentially increase airway resistance, bronchial smooth muscle tone, and bronchial secretions. Cevimeline should be administered with caution and with close medical supervision to patients with controlled asthma, chronic bronchitis, or chronic obstructive pulmonary disease.

Ocular:

Ophthalmic formulations of muscarinic agonists have been reported to cause visual blurring which may result in decreased visual acuity, especially at night and in patients with central lens changes, and to cause impairment of depth perception. Caution should be advised while driving at night or performing hazardous activities in reduced lighting.

PRECAUTIONS

General:

Cevimeline toxicity is characterized by an exaggeration of its parasympathomimetic effects. These may include: headache, visual disturbance, lacrimation, sweating, respiratory distress, gastrointestinal spasm, nausea, vomiting, diarrhea, atrioventricular block, tachycardia, bradycardia, hypotension, hypertension, shock, mental confusion, cardiac arrhythmia, and tremors.

Cevimeline should be administered with caution to patients with a history of nephrolithiasis or cholelithiasis. Contractions of the gallbladder or biliary smooth muscle could precipitate complications such as cholecystitis, cholangitis and biliary obstruction. An increase in the ureteral smooth muscle tone could theoretically precipitate renal colic or ureteral reflux in patients with nephrolithiasis.

Information for Patients: Patients should be informed that cevimeline may cause visual disturbances, especially at night, that could impair their ability to drive safely.

If a patient sweats excessively while taking cevimeline, dehydration may develop. The patient should drink extra water and consult a health care provider.

Drug Interactions:

Cevimeline should be administered with caution to patients taking beta adrenergic antagonists, because of the possibility of conduction disturbances. Drugs with parasympathomimetic effects administered concurrently with cevimeline can be expected to have additive effects. Cevimeline might interfere with desirable antimuscarinic effects of drugs used concomitantly.

Drugs which inhibit CYP2D6 and CYP3A3/4 also inhibit the metabolism of cevimeline. Cevimeline should be used with caution in individuals known or suspected to be deficient in CYP2D6 activity, based on previous experience, as they may be at a higher risk of adverse events. In an *in vitro* study, cytochrome P450 isozymes 1A2, 2A6, 2C9, 2C19, 2D6, 2E1, and 3A4 were not inhibited by exposure to cevimeline.

Carcinogenesis, Mutagenesis and Impairment of Fertility:

Lifetime carcinogenicity studies were conducted in CD-1 mice and F-344 rats. A statistically significant increase in the incidence of adenocarcinomas of the uterus was observed in female rats that received cevimeline at a dosage of 100 mg/kg/day (approximately 8 times the maximum human exposure based on comparison of AUC data). No other significant differences in tumor incidence were observed in either mice or rats.

Cevimeline exhibited no evidence of mutagenicity or clastogenicity in a battery of assays that included an Ames test, an *in vitro* chromosomal aberration study in mammalian cells, a mouse lymphoma study in L5178Y cells, or a micronucleus assay conducted *in vivo* in ICR mice.

Cevimeline did not adversely affect the reproductive performance or fertility of male Sprague-Dawley rats when administered for 63 days prior to mating and throughout the period of mating at dosages up to 45 mg/kg/day (approximately 5 times the maximum recommended dose for a 60 kg human following normalization of the data on the basis of body surface area estimates). Females that were treated with cevimeline at dosages up to 45 mg/kg/day from 14 days prior to mating through day seven of gestation exhibited a statistically significantly smaller number of implantations than did control animals.

Pregnancy:

Pregnancy Category C.

Cevimeline was associated with a reduction in the mean number of implantations when given to pregnant Sprague-Dawley rats from 14 days prior to mating through day seven of gestation at a dosage of 45 mg/kg/day (approximately 5 times the maximum recommended dose for a 60 kg human when compared on the basis of body surface area estimates). This effect may have been secondary to maternal toxicity. There are no adequate and well-controlled studies in pregnant women. Cevimeline should be used during pregnancy only if the potential benefit justifies the potential risk to the fetus.

Nursing Mothers:

It is not known whether this drug is secreted in human milk. Because many drugs are excreted in human milk, and because of the potential for serious adverse reactions in nursing infants from EVOXAC™, a decision should be made whether to discontinue nursing or discontinue the drug, taking into account the importance of the drug to the mother.

Pediatric Use:

Safety and effectiveness in pediatric patients have not been established.

Geriatric Use:

Although clinical studies of cevimeline included subjects over the age of 65, the numbers were not sufficient to determine whether they respond differently from younger subjects. Special care should be exercised when cevimeline treatment is initiated in an elderly patient, considering the greater frequency of decreased hepatic, renal, or cardiac function, and of concomitant disease or other drug therapy in the elderly.

ADVERSE REACTIONS

Cevimeline was administered to 1777 patients during clinical trials worldwide, including Sjögren's patients and patients with other conditions. In placebo-controlled Sjögren's studies in the U.S., 320 patients received cevimeline doses ranging from 15 mg tid to 60 mg tid, of whom 93% were women and 7% were men. Demographic distribution was 90% Caucasian, 5% Hispanic, 3% Black and 2% of other origin. In these studies, 14.6% of patients discontinued treatment with cevimeline due to adverse events.

The following adverse events associated with muscarinic agonism were observed in the clinical trials of cevimeline in Sjögren's syndrome patients:

Adverse Event	Cevimeline 30 mg (tid) n*=533	Placebo (tid) n=164
Excessive Sweating	18.7%	2.4%
Nausea	13.8%	7.9%
Rhinitis	11.2%	5.4%
Diarrhea	10.3%	10.3%
Excessive Salivation	2.2%	0.6%
Urinary Frequency	0.9%	1.8%
Asthenia	0.5%	0.0%
Flushing	0.3%	0.6%
Polyuria	0.1%	0.6%

*n is the total number of patients exposed to the dose at any time during the study.

In addition, the following adverse events (≥3% incidence) were reported in the Sjögren's clinical trials:

Adverse Event	Cevimeline 30 mg (tid) n*=533	Placebo (tid) n=164
Headache	14.4%	20.1%
Sinusitis	12.3%	10.9%
Upper Respiratory Tract Infection	11.4%	9.1%
Dyspepsia	7.8%	8.5%
Abdominal Pain	7.6%	6.7%
Urinary Tract Infection	6.1%	3.0%
Coughing	6.1%	3.0%
Pharyngitis	5.2%	5.4%
Vomiting	4.6%	2.4%
Injury	4.5%	2.4%
Back Pain	4.5%	4.2%
Rash	4.3%	6.0%
Conjunctivitis	4.3%	3.6%
Dizziness	4.1%	7.3%
Bronchitis	4.1%	1.2%
Arthralgia	3.7%	1.8%
Surgical Intervention	3.3%	3.0%
Fatigue	3.3%	1.2%
Pain	3.3%	3.0%
Skeletal Pain	2.8%	1.8%
Insomnia	2.4%	1.2%
Hot Flushes	2.4%	0.0%
Rigors	1.3%	1.2%
Anxiety	1.3%	1.2%

*n is the total number of patients exposed to the dose at any time during the study.

The following events were reported in Sjögren's patients at incidences of <3% and ≥1%: constipation, tremor, abnormal vision, hypertonia, peripheral edema, chest pain, myalgia, fever, anorexia, eye pain, earache, dry mouth, vertigo, salivary gland pain, pruritus, influenza-like symptoms, eye infection, post-operative pain, vaginitis, skin disorder, depression, hiccup, hyporeflexia, infection, fungal infection, sialoadenitis, otitis media, erythematous rash, pneumonia, edema, salivary gland enlargement, allergy, gastroesophageal reflux, eye abnormality, migraine, tooth disorder, epistaxis, flatulence, toothache, ulcerative stomatitis, anemia, hypoesthesia, cystitis, leg cramps, abscess, eructation, moniliasis, palpitation, increased amylase, xerophthalmia, allergic reaction.

The following events were reported rarely in treated Sjögren's patients (<1%): Causal relation is unknown:

Body as a Whole Disorders: aggravated allergy, precordial chest pain, abnormal crying, hematoma, leg pain, edema, periorbital edema, activated pain trauma, pallor, changed sensation temperature, weight decrease, weight increase, chocking, mouth edema, syncope, malaise, face edema, substernal chest pain

Cardiovascular Disorders: abnormal ECG, heart disorder, heart murmur, aggravated hypertension, hypotension, arrhythmia, extrasystoles, t wave inversion, tachycardia, supraventricular tachycardia, angina pectoris, myocardial infarction, pericarditis, pulmonary embolism, peripheral ischemia, superficial phlebitis, purpura, deep thrombophlebitis, vascular disorder, vasculitis, hypertension

Digestive Disorders: appendicitis, increased appetite, ulcerative colitis, diverticulitis, duodenitis, dysphagia, enterocolitis, gastric ulcer, gastritis, gastroenteritis, gastrointestinal hemorrhage, gingivitis, glossitis, rectum hemorrhage, hemorrhoids, ileus, irritable bowel syndrome, melena, mucositis, esophageal stricture, esophagitis, oral hemorrhage, peptic ulcer, periodontal destruction, rectal disorder, stomatitis, tenesmus, tongue discoloration, tongue disorder, geographic tongue, tongue ulceration, dental caries

Endocrine Disorders: increased glucocorticoids, goiter, hypothyroidism

Hematologic Disorders: thrombocytopenic purpura, thrombocythemia, thrombocytopenia, hypochromic anemia, eosinophilia, granulocytopenia, leucopenia, leukocytosis, cervical lymphadenopathy, lymphadenopathy

Liver and Biliary System Disorders: cholelithiasis, increased gamma-glutamyl transferase, increased hepatic enzymes, abnormal hepatic function, viral hepatitis, increased serum glutamate exaloacetic transaminase (SGOT)(also called AST-aspartate aminotransferase), increased serum glutamate pyruvate transaminase (SGPT)(also called ALT-alanine aminotransferase)

Metabolic and Nutritional Disorders: dehydration, diabetes mellitus, hypercalcemia, hypercholesterolemia, hyperglycemia, hyperlipemia, hypertriglyceridemia, hyperuricemia, hypoglycemia, hypokalemia, hyponatremia, thirst

Musculoskeletal Disorders: arthritis, aggravated arthritis, arthropathy, femoral head avascular necrosis, bone disorder, bursitis, costochondritis, plantar fasciitis, muscle weakness, osteomyelitis, osteoporosis, synovitis, tendinitis, tenosynovitis

Neoplasms: basal cell carcinoma, squamous carcinoma

Nervous Disorders: carpal tunnel syndrome, coma, abnormal coordination, dysesthesia, dyskinesia, dysphonia, aggravated multiple sclerosis, involuntary muscle contractions, neuralgia, neuropathy, paresthesia, speech disorder, agitation, confusion, depersonalization, aggravated depression, abnormal dreaming, emotional lability, manic reaction, paroniria, somnolence, abnormal thinking, hyperkinesia, hallucination

Miscellaneous Disorders: fall, food poisoning, heat stroke, joint dislocation, post-operative hemorrhage

Resistance Mechanism Disorders: cellulitis, herpes simplex, herpes zoster, bacterial infection, viral infection, genital moniliasis, sepsis

Respiratory Disorders: asthma, bronchospasm, chronic obstructive airway disease, dyspnea, hemoptysis, laryngitis,

Continued on next page

Evoxac—Cont.

nasal ulcer, pleural effusion, pleurisy, pulmonary congestion, pulmonary fibrosis, respiratory disorder
Rheumatologic Disorders: aggravated rheumatoid arthritis, lupus erythematosus rash, lupus erythematosus syndrome
Skin and Appendages Disorders: acne, alopecia, burn, dermatitis, contact dermatitis, lichenoid dermatitis, eczema, furunculosis, hyperkeratosis, lichen planus, nail discoloration, nail disorder, onychia, onychomycosis, paronychia, photosensitivity reaction, rosacea, scleroderma, seborrhea, skin discoloration, dry skin, skin exfoliation, skin hypertrophy, skin ulceration, urticaria, verruca, bullous eruption, cold clammy skin
Special Senses Disorders: deafness, decreased hearing, motion sickness, parosmia, taste perversion, blepharitis, cataract, corneal opacity, corneal ulceration, diplopia, glaucoma, anterior chamber eye hemorrhage, keratitis, keratoconjunctivitis, mydriasis, myopia, photopsia, retinal deposits, retinal disorder, scleritis, vitreous detachment, tinnitus
Urogenital Disorders: epididymitis, prostatic disorder, abnormal sexual function, amenorrhea, female breast neoplasm, malignant female breast neoplasm, female breast pain, positive cervical smear test, dysmenorrhea, endometrial disorder, intermenstrual bleeding, leukorrhea, menorrhagia, menstrual disorder, ovarian cyst, ovarian disorder, genital pruritus, uterine hemorrhage, vaginal hemorrhage, atrophic vaginitis, albuminuria, bladder discomfort, increased blood urea nitrogen, dysuria, hematuria, micturition disorder, nephrosis, nocturia, increased nonprotein nitrogen, pyelonephritis, renal calculus, abnormal renal function, renal pain, strangury, urethral disorder, abnormal urine, urinary incontinence, decreased urine flow, pyuria

In one subject with lupus erythematosus receiving concomitant multiple drug therapy, a highly elevated ALT level was noted after the fourth week of cevimeline therapy. In two other subjects receiving cevimeline in the clinical trials, very high AST levels were noted. The significance of these findings is unknown.

Additional adverse events (relationship unknown) which occurred in other clinical studies (patient population different from Sjögren's patients) are as follows:
cholinergic syndrome, blood pressure fluctuation, cardiomegaly, postural hypotension, aphasia, convulsions, abnormal gait, hyperesthesia, paralysis, abnormal sexual function, enlarged abdomen, change in bowel habits, gum hyperplasia, intestinal obstruction, bundle branch block, increased creatine phosphokinase, electrolyte abnormality, glycosuria, gout, hyperkalemia, hyperproteinemia, increased lactic dehydrogenase (LDH), increased alkaline phosphatase, failure to thrive, abnormal platelets, aggressive reaction, amnesia, apathy, delirium, delusion, dementia, illusion, impotence, neurosis, paranoid reaction, personality disorder, hyperhemoglobinemia, apnea, atelectasis, yawning, oliguria, urinary retention, distended vein, lymphocytosis

MANAGEMENT OF OVERDOSE

Management of the signs and symptoms of acute overdosage should be handled in a manner consistent with that indicated for other muscarinic agonists: general supportive measures should be instituted. If medically indicated, atropine, an anti-cholinergic agent, may be of value as an antidote for emergency use in patients who have had an overdose of cevimeline. If medically indicated, epinephrine may also be of value in the presence of severe cardiovascular depression or bronchoconstriction. It is not known if cevimeline is dialyzable.

DOSAGE AND ADMINISTRATION

The recommended dose of cevimeline is 30 mg taken three times a day. There is insufficient safety information to support doses greater than 30 mg tid. There is also insufficient evidence for additional efficacy of cevimeline at doses greater than 30 mg tid.

HOW SUPPLIED

EVOXAC™ is available as white, hard gelatin capsules of cevimeline hydrochloride containing 30 mg of cevimeline imprinted with "EVOXAC™", "30 mg", and a black bar above "30 mg". It is supplied in child resistant bottles of 100 capsules (NDC 63395-201-13).

Store at 25°C (77°F) excursion permitted to 15°–30°C (59°–86°F)

Rx Only

Manufactured by:
YAMANOUCHI PHARMA TECHNOLOGIES, INC.
Palo Alto, CA 94304
for:
SnowBrand Pharmaceuticals, Inc.
Rockville, MD 20850
Distributed and Marketed by:
Daiichi Pharmaceutical Corporation,
Montvale, NJ 07645
SRT11 02/2000

Shown in Product Identification Guide, page 311

FLOXIN® Otic ℞

[flox-in]
(ofloxacin otic solution) 0.3%

DESCRIPTION

FLOXIN® Otic (ofloxacin otic solution) 0.3% is a sterile aqueous anti-infective (anti-bacterial) solution for otic use. Chemically, ofloxacin has three condensed 6-membered rings made up of a fluorinated carboxyquinolone with a benzoxazine ring. The chemical name of ofloxacin is: (±)-9-fluoro-2,3-dihydro-3-methyl-10-(4-methyl-1-piperazinyl)-7-oxo-7*H*-pyrido [1,2,3-*de*]-1,4-benzoxazine- 6-carboxylic acid. The empirical formula of ofloxacin is $C_{18}H_{20}FN_3O_4$ and its molecular weight is 361.38. The structural formula is:

FLOXIN® Otic contains 0.3% (3mg/mL) ofloxacin with benzalkonium chloride (0.0025%), sodium chloride (0.9%), and water for injection. Hydrochloric acid and sodium hydroxide are added to adjust the pH to 6.5 ± 0.5.

CLINICAL PHARMACOLOGY

Pharmacokinetics: Drug concentrations in serum (in subjects with tympanostomy tubes and perforated tympanic membranes), in otorrhea, and in mucosa of the middle ear (in subjects with perforated tympanic membranes) were determined following otic administration of ofloxacin solution. In two single-dose studies, mean ofloxacin serum concentrations were low in adult patients with tympanostomy tubes, with and without otorrhea, after otic administration of a 0.3% solution (4.1 ng/mL (n=3) and 5.4 ng/mL (n=5), respectively). In adults with perforated tympanic membranes, the maximum serum drug level of ofloxacin detected was 10 ng/mL after administration of a 0.3% solution. Ofloxacin was detectable in the middle ear mucosa of some adult subjects with perforated tympanic membranes (11 of 16 subjects). The variability of ofloxacin concentration in middle ear mucosa was high. The concentrations ranged from 1.2 to 602 µg/g after otic administration of a 0.3% solution. Ofloxacin was present in high concentrations in otorrhea (389–2850 µg/g, n=13) 30 minutes after otic administration of a 0.3% solution in subjects with chronic suppurative otitis media and perforated tympanic membranes. However, the measurement of ofloxacin in the otorrhea does not necessarily reflect the exposure of the middle ear to ofloxacin.

Microbiology: Ofloxacin has *in vitro* activity against a wide range of gram-negative and gram-positive microorganisms. Ofloxacin exerts its antibacterial activity by inhibiting DNA gyrase, a bacterial topoisomerase. DNA gyrase is an essential enzyme which controls DNA topology and assists in DNA replication, repair, deactivation, and transcription. Cross-resistance has been observed between ofloxacin and other fluoroquinolones. There is generally no cross-resistance between ofloxacin and other classes of antibacterial agents such as beta-lactams or aminoglycosides.

Ofloxacin has been shown to be active against most strains of the following microorganisms, both *in vitro* and clinically in otic infections as described in the **INDICATIONS AND USAGE** section.

AEROBES, GRAM-POSITIVE:
Staphylococcus aureus
Streptococcus pneumoniae

AEROBES, GRAM-NEGATIVE:
Haemophilus influenzae
Moraxella catarrhalis
Proteus mirabilis
Pseudomonas aeruginosa

INDICATIONS AND USAGE

FLOXIN® Otic (ofloxacin otic solution) 0.3% is indicated for the treatment of infections caused by susceptible strains of the designated microorganisms in the specific conditions listed below:

Otitis Externa in adults and pediatric patients, one year and older, due to *Staphylococcus aureus* and *Pseudomonas aeruginosa.*

Chronic Suppurative Otitis Media in patients 12 years and older with perforated tympanic membranes due to *Staphylococcus aureus, Proteus mirabilis, and Pseudomonas aeruginosa.*

Acute Otitis Media in pediatric patients one year and older with tympanostomy tubes due to *Staphylococcus aureus, Streptococcus pneumoniae, Haemophilus influenzae, Moraxella catarrhalis,* and *Pseudomonas aeruginosa.*

CONTRAINDICATIONS

FLOXIN® Otic (ofloxacin otic solution) 0.3% is contraindicated in patients with a history of hypersensitivity to ofloxacin, to other quinolones, or to any of the components in this medication.

WARNINGS

NOT FOR OPHTHALMIC USE.
NOT FOR INJECTION.

Serious and occasionally fatal hypersensitivity (anaphylactic) reactions, some following the first dose, have been reported in patients receiving systemic quinolones, including ofloxacin. Some reactions were accompanied by cardiovascular collapse, loss of consciousness, angioedema (including laryngeal, pharyngeal or facial edema), airway obstruction, dyspnea, urticaria, and itching. If an allergic reaction to ofloxacin is suspected, stop the drug. Serious acute hypersensitivity reactions may require immediate emergency treatment. Oxygen and airway management, including intubation, should be administered as clinically indicated.

PRECAUTIONS

General: As with other anti-infective preparations, prolonged use may result in over-growth of nonsusceptible organisms, including fungi. If the infection is not improved after one week, cultures should be obtained to guide further treatment. If otorrhea persists after a full course of therapy, or if two or more episodes of otorrhea occur within six months, further evaluation is recommended to exclude an underlying condition such as cholesteatoma, foreign body, or a tumor.

The systemic administration of quinolones, including ofloxacin at doses much higher than given or absorbed by the otic route, has led to lesions or erosions of the cartilage in weight-bearing joints and other signs of arthropathy in immature animals of various species.

Young growing guinea pigs dosed in the middle ear with 0.3% ofloxacin otic solution showed no systemic effects, lesions or erosions of the cartilage in weight-bearing joints, or other signs of arthropathy. No drug-related structural or functional changes of the cochlea and no lesions in the ossicles were noted in the guinea pig following otic administration of 0.3% ofloxacin for one month.

No signs of local irritation were found when 0.3% ofloxacin was applied topically in the rabbit eye. Ofloxacin was also shown to lack dermal sensitizing potential in the guinea pig maximization study.

Information for Patients: Avoid contaminating the applicator tip with material from the fingers or other sources. This precaution is necessary if the sterility of the drops is to be preserved. Systemic quinolones, including ofloxacin, have been associated with hypersensitivity reactions, even following a single dose. Discontinue use immediately and contact your physician at the first sign of a rash or allergic reaction.

Otitis Externa

Prior to administration of FLOXIN® Otic in patients with otitis externa, the solution should be warmed by holding the bottle in the hand for one or two minutes to avoid dizziness which may result from the instillation of a cold solution. The patient should lie with the affected ear upward, and then the drops should be instilled. This position should be maintained for five minutes to facilitate penetration of the drops into the ear canal. Repeat, if necessary, for the opposite ear (see **DOSAGE AND ADMINISTRATION**).

Acute Otitis Media and Chronic Suppurative Otitis Media

In pediatric patients (from 1 to 12 years old) with acute otitis media with tympanostomy tubes and in patients with chronic suppurative otitis media with perforated tympanic membranes, prior to administration, the solution should be warmed by holding the bottle in the hand for one or two minutes to avoid dizziness which may result from the instillation of a cold solution. The patient should lie with the affected ear upward, and then the drops should be instilled. The tragus should then be pumped 4 times by pushing inward to facilitate penetration of the drops into the middle ear. This position should be maintained for five minutes. Repeat, if necessary, for the opposite ear (see **DOSAGE AND ADMINISTRATION**).

Drug Interactions: Specific drug interactions studies have not been conducted with FLOXIN® Otic.

Carcinogenesis, Mutagenesis, Impairment of Fertility

Long-term studies to determine the carcinogenic potential of ofloxacin have not been conducted. Ofloxacin was not mutagenic in the Ames test, the sister chromatid exchange assay (Chinese hamster and human cell lines), the unscheduled DNA synthesis (UDS) assay using human fibroblasts, the dominant lethal assay, or the mouse micronucleus assay. Ofloxacin was positive in the rat hepatocyte UDS assay, and in the mouse lymphoma assay. In rats, ofloxacin did not affect male or female reproductive performance at oral doses up to 360 mg/kg/day. This would be over 1000 times the maximum recommended clinical dose, based upon body surface area, assuming total absorption of ofloxacin from the ear of a patient treated with FLOXIN® Otic twice per day.

Pregnancy

Teratogenic Effects: Pregnancy Category C. Ofloxacin has been shown to have an embryocidal effect in rats at a dose of 810 mg/kg/day and in rabbits at 160 mg/kg/day.

These dosages resulted in decreased fetal body weights and increased fetal mortality in rats and rabbits, respectively. Minor fetal skeletal variations were reported in rats receiving doses of 810 mg/kg/day. Ofloxacin has not been shown to be teratogenic at doses as high as 810 mg/kg/day and 160 mg/kg/day when administered to pregnant rats and rabbits, respectively.

Ofloxacin has not been shown to have any adverse effects on the developing embryo or fetus at doses relevant to the amount of ofloxacin that will be delivered ototopically at the recommended clinical doses.

Nonteratogenic Effects: Additional studies in the rat demonstrated that doses up to 360 mg/kg/day during late gestation had no adverse effects on late fetal development, labor, delivery, lactation, neonatal viability, or growth of the newborn. There are, however, no adequate and well-controlled studies in pregnant women. FLOXIN® Otic should be used during pregnancy only if the potential benefit justifies the potential risk to the fetus.

Nursing Mothers: In nursing women, a single 200 mg oral dose resulted in concentrations of ofloxacin in milk which were similar to those found in plasma. It is not known whether ofloxacin is excreted in human milk following topical otic administration. Because of the potential for serious adverse reactions from ofloxacin in nursing infants, a decision should be made whether to discontinue nursing or to discontinue the drug, taking into account the importance of the drug to the mother.

Pediatric Use: No changes in hearing function occurred in 30 pediatric subjects treated with ofloxacin otic and tested for audiometric parameters. Although safety and efficacy have been demonstrated in pediatric patients one year and older, safety and effectiveness in infants below the age of one year have not been established. Although quinolones, including ofloxacin, have been shown to cause arthropathy in immature animals after systemic administration, young growing guinea pigs dosed in the middle ear with 0.3% ofloxacin otic solution for one month showed no systemic effects, quinolone-induced lesions, erosions of the cartilage in weight-bearing joints, or other signs of arthropathy.

ADVERSE REACTIONS

In the Phase III registration trials, a total of 885 subjects were treated with ofloxacin otic solution. This included 229 subjects with otitis externa (with intact tympanic membranes) and 656 subjects with acute otitis media with tympanostomy tubes or chronic suppurative otitis media with perforated tympanic membranes. The reported treatment-related adverse events are listed below:

Subjects with Otitis Externa

The following treatment-related adverse events occurred in 1% or more of the subjects with intact tympanic membranes.

Adverse Event	Frequency (n=229)
Pruritus	4%
Application Site Reaction	3%
Dizziness	1%
Earache	1%
Vertigo	1%

The following treament-related adverse events were each reported in a single subject: dermatitis, eczema, erythematous rash, follicular rash, rash, hypoaesthesia, tinnitus, dyspepsia, hot flushes, flushing, and otorrhagia.

Subjects with Acute Otitis Media with Tympanostomy Tubes and Subjects with Chronic Suppurative Otitis Media with Perforated Tympanic Membranes

The following treatment-related adverse events occurred in 1% or more of the subjects with non-intact tympanic membranes.

Adverse Event	Frequency (n=656)
Taste Perversion	7%
Earache	1%
Pruritus	1%
Paraesthesia	1%
Rash	1%
Dizziness	1%

Other treatment-related adverse reactions reported in subjects with non-intact tympanic membranes included: diarrhea (0.6%), nausea (0.3%), vomiting (0.3%), dry mouth (0.5%), headache (0.3%), vertigo (0.5%), otorrhagia (0.6%), tinnitus (0.3%), fever (0.3%). The following treatment-related adverse events were each reported in a single subject: application site reaction, otitis externa, urticaria, abdominal pain, dysaesthesia, hyperkinesia, halitosis, inflammation, pain, insomnia, coughing, pharyngitis, rhinitis, sinusitis, and tachycardia.

DOSAGE AND ADMINISTRATION

Otitis Externa: The recommended dosage regimen for the treatment of otitis externa is:

For pediatric patients (from 1 to 12 years old): Five drops (0.25 mL, 0.75 mg ofloxacin) instilled into the affected ear twice daily for ten days.

For patients 12 years and older: Ten drops (0.5 mL, 1.5 mg ofloxacin) instilled into the affected ear twice daily for ten days. The solution should be warmed by holding the bottle in the hand for one or two minutes to avoid dizziness which may result from the instillation of a cold solution. The patient should lie with the affected ear upward, and then the drops should be instilled. This position should be maintained for five minutes to facilitate penetration of the drops into the ear canal. Repeat, if necessary, for the opposite ear.

Acute Otitis Media in Pediatric Patients with Tympanostomy Tubes: The recommended dosage regimen for the treatment of acute otitis media in pediatric patients (from one to 12 years old) with tympanostomy tubes is:

Five drops (0.25 mL, 0.75 mg ofloxacin) instilled into the affected ear twice daily for ten days. The solution should be warmed by holding the bottle in the hand for one or two minutes to avoid dizziness which may result from the instillation of a cold solution. The patient should lie with the affected ear upward, and then the drops should be instilled. The tragus should then be pumped 4 times by pushing inward to facilitate penetration of the drops into the middle ear. This position should be maintained for five minutes. Repeat, if necessary, for the opposite ear.

Chronic Suppurative Otitis Media with Perforated Tympanic Membranes: The recommended dosage regimen for the treatment of chronic suppurative otitis media with perforated tympanic membranes in patients 12 years and older is:

Ten drops (0.5 mL, 1.5 mg ofloxacin) instilled into the affected ear twice daily for fourteen days. The solution should be warmed by holding the bottle in the hand for one or two minutes to avoid dizziness which may result from the instillation of a cold solution. The patient should lie with the affected ear upward, before instilling the drops. The tragus should then be pumped 4 times by pushing inward to facilitate penetration into the middle ear. This position should be maintained for five minutes. Repeat, if necessary, for the opposite ear.

HOW SUPPLIED

FLOXIN® Otic (ofloxacin otic solution) 0.3% is supplied in plastic dropper bottles containing 5 mL and 10 mL. The NDC codes are: 63395-101-05 FLOXIN® Otic 5 mL 63395-101-10 FLOXIN® Otic 10 mL

Note: Store at 15–25°C (59–77°F).

Caution: Federal (U.S.A.) law prohibits dispensing without prescription.

DAIICHI PHARMACEUTICAL CORPORATION
Montvale, NJ 07645
October 15, 1999

Medication Guide

FLOXIN® (FLOX-IN) **Otic**
(ofloxacin otic solution) 0.3%

IMPORTANT PATIENT INFORMATION AND INSTRUCTIONS. READ BEFORE USE.

What is FLOXIN Otic?

FLOXIN Otic is an antibiotic in a sterile solution used to treat ear infections caused by certain bacteria found in:

- patients (12 years and older) who have a middle ear infection and have a hole in the eardrum
- pediatric patients (between 1 and 12) who have a middle ear infection and have a tube in the eardrum
- patients (1 year and older) who have an infection in the ear canal

Middle Ear Infection: A middle ear infection is a bacterial infection behind the eardrum. People with a hole or a tube in the eardrum may notice a discharge (fluid draining) in the ear canal.

Ear Canal Infection: An ear canal infection (also known as "Swimmer's Ear") is a bacterial infection of the ear canal. The ear canal and the outer part of the ear may swell, turn red, and be painful. Also, a fluid discharge may appear in the ear canal.

Who should NOT use FLOXIN Otic?

- Do not use this product if allergic to ofloxacin or to other quinolone antibiotics.
- Do not give this product to pediatric patients who are less than one year old.

How should FLOXIN Otic be given?

1. Wash hands

The person giving FLOXIN Otic should wash his/her hands with soap and water.

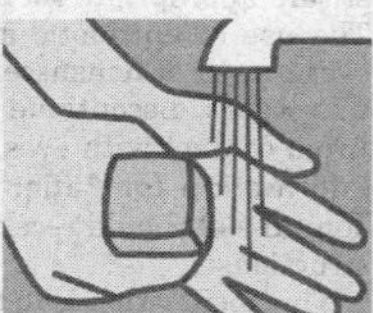

2. Clean ear & warm bottle

Gently clean any discharge that can be removed easily from the outer ear. DO NOT INSERT ANY OBJECT OR SWAB INTO THE EAR CANAL.

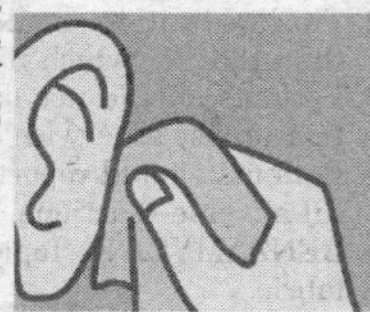

Hold the bottle of FLOXIN Otic in the hand for one or two minutes to warm the solution.

3. Add drops

The person receiving FLOXIN Otic should lie on his/her side with the infected ear up. Patients (12 and older) should have **10 drops** of FLOXIN Otic put into the infected ear. Pediatric patients under 12 should have **5 drops** put into the infected ear. The tip of the bottle should not touch the fingers or the ear or any other surfaces.

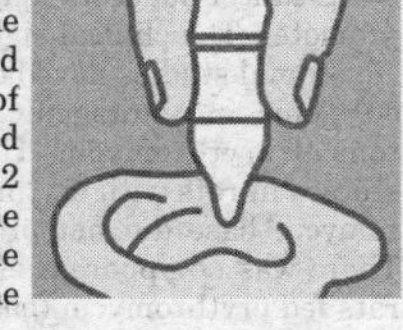

BE SURE TO FOLLOW INSTRUCTIONS BELOW FOR THE PATIENT'S SPECIFIC EAR INFECTION.

4. Press ear or pull ear

For a **Middle Ear Infection**: While the person receiving FLOXIN Otic lies on his/her side, the person giving the drops should gently press the

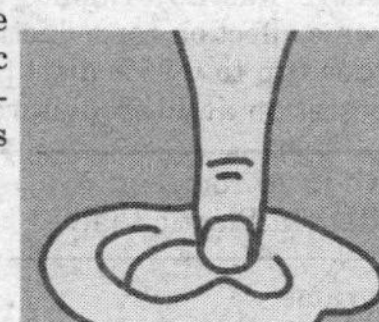

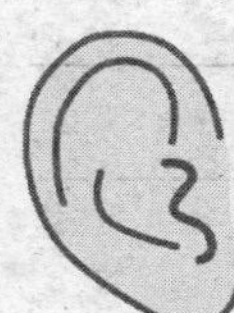

TRAGUS (see diagram) 4 times in a pumping motion. This will allow the drops to pass through the hole or tube in the eardrum and into the middle ear.

For an **Ear Canal Infection ("Swimmer's Ear")**: While the person receiving the drops lies on his/her side, the person giving the drops should gently pull the outer ear upward and backward. This will allow the ear drops to flow down into the ear canal.

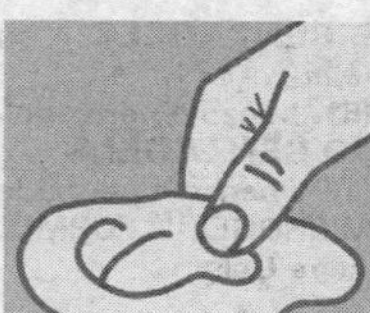

5. Stay on side

The person who received the ear drops should remain on his/her side for at least 5 minutes.

Repeat Steps 2–5 for the other ear if both ears are infected.

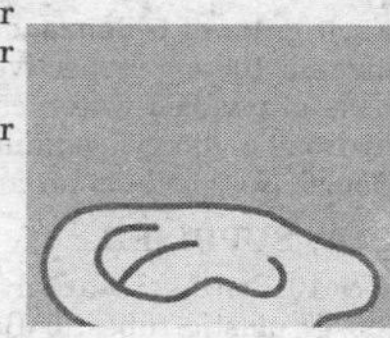

How often should FLOXIN® Otic be given?

FLOXIN Otic ear drops should be given 2 times each day (about 12 hours apart, for example, 8 AM and 8 PM) in each infected ear unless the doctor has instructed otherwise. The best times to use the ear drops are in the morning and at night. It is very important to use the ear drops for as long as the doctor has instructed, **even if the symptoms improve**. If FLOXIN Otic ear drops are not used for as long as the doctor has instructed, the infection may return.

What if a dose is missed?

If a dose of FLOXIN Otic is missed, it should be given as soon as possible. If it is almost time for the next dose, skip the missed dose and go back to the regular dosing schedule. Do not use a double dose unless the doctor has instructed you to do so. If the infection is not improved after one week, you should consult your doctor. If you have two or more episodes of drainage within six months, it is recommended you see your doctor for further evaluation.

What activities should be avoided while using FLOXIN Otic?

It is important that the infected ear(s) remain clean and dry. When bathing, avoid getting the infected ear(s) wet. Avoid swimming unless the doctor has instructed otherwise.

What are the possible side effects of FLOXIN Otic?

During the testing of FLOXIN Otic, the most common side effect was a bitter taste which happened in 7% of patients with a middle ear infection. This may occur when some of the drops pass from the middle ear to the back of the mouth. This side effect is not serious and there is no need to stop the medicine if this should happen. Other side effects were:

For Middle Ear Infections: Earache (1%), itching (1%), abnormal sensation (1%), rash (1%) and dizziness (1%).

For Ear Canal Infections: Itching (4%), discomfort upon application (3%), dizziness (1%), earache (1%) and light headedness (1%).

If any of these side effects occur, call the doctor.

If an allergic reaction to FLOXIN Otic occurs, stop using the product and contact your doctor.

DO NOT TAKE FLOXIN Otic BY MOUTH.

If FLOXIN Otic is accidentally swallowed or overdose occurs, call the doctor immediately. This medicine is available only with a doctor's prescription. Use only as directed. Do not use this medicine if outdated. If you wish to learn more about FLOXIN Otic ask the doctor or pharmacist.

HOW SUPPLIED

Plastic dropper bottles containing 5 mL and 10 mL
Store at 15° to 25° C (59°–77° F)

FLOXIN Otic is manufactured for:
Daiichi Pharmaceutical Corp.
Montvale, NJ 07645

By:
Parkedale Pharmaceuticals Inc.
Rochester, MI 48307

This Medication Guide has been approved by the U.S. Food and Drug Administration.
Revised: (11/22/99)

Shown in Product Identification Guide, page 311

Dermik Laboratories, Inc.

1050 WESTLAKES DRIVE
BERWYN, PA 19312

Direct Inquiries to:
QUALITY ASSURANCE QUESTIONS:
John Chiles
Sr QA Specialist
(610) 454-2432
REGULATORY AFFAIRS QUESTIONS:
Ron Panner
Sr Director, WW Reg Affairs
(610) 454-3026

For Medical Information Contact:
PRODUCT INFORMATION/ADVERSE DRUG EXPERIENCES/EMERGENCIES
Medical Information and Education
(800) 340-7502
(610) 454-8110

Continued on next page

5 BENZAGEL® ℞
[*ben-za-jel*]
(5% benzoyl peroxide) and
10 BENZAGEL® ℞
(10% benzoyl peroxide)
MICROGEL™ FORMULA
Acne Gels

DESCRIPTION

Each gram of **5 Benzagel®** and **10 Benzagel®** contains 50 mg and 100 mg respectively, of benzoyl peroxide in a gel vehicle of purified water, carbomer 940, 14% alcohol, sodium hydroxide, dioctyl sodium sulfosuccinate and fragrances.
Benzoyl peroxide is an antibacterial and keratolytic agent.

HOW SUPPLIED

5 & 10 Benzagel® are available in 1.5 oz (42.5 g) and 3 oz (85 g) plastic tubes; 5 Benzagel® contains 50 mg benzoyl peroxide per gram and 10 Benzagel® contains 100 mg benzoyl peroxide per gram.
Store at room temperature.
5-Benzagel 1.5 oz NDC 0066-0430-15
5-Benzagel 3.0 oz NDC 0066-0430-30
10-Benzagel 1.5 oz NDC 0066-0431-15
10 Benzagel 3.0 oz NDC 0066-0431-30
CR-5733N Rev. 12/96

BENZAMYCIN® ℞
[*ben 'za-mi "sin*]
(erythromycin-benzoyl peroxide topical gel)
Topical gel: erythromycin (3%), benzoyl peroxide (5%)
For Dermatological Use Only - Not for Ophthalmic Use
Reconstitute Before Dispensing

DESCRIPTION

BENZAMYCIN® Topical Gel contains erythromycin [(3R*, 4S*, 5S*, 6R*, 7R*, 9R*, 11R*, 12R*, 13S*, 14R*)-4-[(2,6-Dideoxy-3-*C*-methyl-3-*O*-methyl-α-L-*ribo*-hexopyranosyl)-oxy]-14-ethyl-7,12,13-trihydroxy-3,5,7,9,11,13-hexamethyl-6-[[3,4,6-trideoxy-3-(dimethylamino)-β-D-*xylo*-hexopyranosyl]oxy]oxacyclotetradecane-2,10-dione]. Erythromycin is a macrolide antibiotic produced from a strain of *Saccharopolyspora erythraea* (formerly *Streptomyces erythreus*). It is a base and readily forms salts with acids.
Chemically, erythromycin is ($C_{37}H_{67}NO_{13}$). It has the following structural formula:

Erythromycin has the molecular weight of 733.94. It is a white crystalline powder and has a solubility of approximately 1 mg/mL in water and is soluble in alcohol at 25°C. BENZAMYCIN Topical Gel also contains benzoyl peroxide for topical use. Benzoyl peroxide is an antibacterial and keratolytic agent.
Chemically, benzoyl peroxide is ($C_{14}H_{10}O_4$). It has the following structural formula:

Benzoyl peroxide has the molecular weight of 242.23. It is a white granular powder and is sparingly soluble in water and alcohol and soluble in acetone, chloroform and ether.
Each gram of BENZAMYCIN Topical Gel contains, as dispensed, 30 mg (3%) of erythromycin and 50 mg (5%) of benzoyl peroxide in a base of purified water USP, carbomer 940 NF, alcohol 20%, sodium hydroxide NF, docusate sodium and fragrance.

CLINICAL PHARMACOLOGY

The exact mechanism by which erythromycin reduces lesions of acne vulgaris is not fully known; however, the effect appears to be due in part to the antibacterial activity of the drug.
Benzoyl peroxide has a keratolytic and desquamative effect which may also contribute to its efficacy. Benzoyl peroxide has been shown to be absorbed by the skin where it is converted to benzoic acid.

MICROBIOLOGY

Erythromycin acts by inhibition of protein synthesis in susceptible organisms by reversibly binding to 50 **S** ribosomal subunits, thereby inhibiting translocation of aminoacyl transfer-RNA and inhibiting polypeptide synthesis. Antagonism has been demonstrated *in vitro* between erythromycin, lincomycin, chloramphenicol and clindamycin.
Benzoyl peroxide is an antibacterial agent which has been shown to be effective against *Propionibacterium acnes*, an anaerobe found in sebaceous follicles and comedones. The antibacterial action of benzoyl peroxide is believed to be due to the release of active oxygen.

INDICATIONS AND USAGE

BENZAMYCIN Topical Gel is indicated for the topical treatment of acne vulgaris.

CONTRAINDICATIONS

BENZAMYCIN Topical Gel is contraindicated in those individuals who have shown hypersensitivity to any of its components.

WARNINGS

Pseudomembranous colitis has been reported with nearly all antibacterial agents, including erythromycin, and may range in severity from mild to life-threatening. Therefore, it is important to consider this diagnosis in patients who present with diarrhea subsequent to the administration of antibacterial agents.
Treatment with antibacterial agents alters the normal flora of the colon and may permit overgrowth of clostridia. Studies indicate that a toxin produced by *Clostridium difficile* is one primary cause of "antibiotic-associated colitis."
After the diagnosis of pseudomembranous colitis has been established, therapeutic measures should be initiated. Mild cases of pseudomembranous colitis usually respond to drug discontinuation alone. In moderate to severe cases, consideration should be given to management with fluids and electrolytes, protein supplementation and treatment with an antibacterial drug clinically effective against *C. difficile* colitis.

PRECAUTIONS

General: For topical use only; not for ophthalmic use. Concomitant topical acne therapy should be used with caution because a possible cumulative irritancy effect may occur, especially with the use of peeling, desquamating or abrasive agents. If severe irritation develops, discontinue use and institute appropriate therapy.
The use of antibiotic agents may be associated with the overgrowth of nonsusceptible organisms including fungi. If this occurs, discontinue use and take appropriate measures.
Avoid contact with eyes and all mucous membranes.
Information for Patients: Patients using BENZAMYCIN Topical Gel should receive the following information and instructions:

1. This medication is to be used as directed by the physician. It is for external use only. Avoid contact with the eyes, nose, mouth, and all mucous membranes.
2. This medication should not be used for any disorder other than that for which it was prescribed.
3. Patients should not use any other topical acne preparation unless otherwise directed by physician.
4. Patients should report to their physician any signs of local adverse reactions.
5. BENZAMYCIN® Topical Gel may bleach hair or colored fabric.
6. Keep product refrigerated and discard after 3 months.

CARCINOGENESIS, MUTAGENESIS AND IMPAIRMENT OF FERTILITY
Data from a study using mice known to be highly susceptible to cancer suggests that benzoyl peroxide acts as a tumor promoter. The clinical significance of this is unknown.
No animal studies have been performed to evaluate the carcinogenic and mutagenic potential or effects on fertility of topical erythromycin. However, long-term (2-year) oral studies in rats with erythromycin ethylsuccinate and erythromycin base did not provide evidence of tumorigenicity. There was no apparent effect on male or female fertility in rats fed erythromycin (base) at levels up to 0.25% of diet.
Pregnancy: Teratogenic Effects: Pregnancy CATEGORY C: Animal reproduction studies have not been conducted with BENZAMYCIN Topical Gel or benzoyl peroxide.
There was no evidence of teratogenicity or any other adverse effect on reproduction in female rats fed erythromycin base (up to 0.25% diet) prior to and during mating, during gestation and through weaning of two successive litters.
There are no well-controlled trials in pregnant women with BENZAMYCIN Topical Gel. It also is not known whether BENZAMYCIN Topical Gel can cause fetal harm when administered to a pregnant woman or can affect reproductive capacity. BENZAMYCIN Topical Gel should be given to a pregnant woman only if clearly needed.
Nursing Women: It is not known whether BENZAMYCIN Topical Gel is excreted in human milk after topical application. However, erythromycin is excreted in human milk following oral and parenteral erythromycin administration. Therefore, caution should be exercised when erythromycin is administered to a nursing woman.
Pediatric Use: Safety and effectiveness of this product in pediatric patients below the age of 12 have not been established.

ADVERSE REACTIONS

In controlled clinical trials, the total incidence of adverse reactions associated with the use of BENZAMYCIN Topical Gel was approximately 3%. These were dryness and urticarial reaction.
The following additional local adverse reactions have been reported occasionally: irritation of the skin including peeling, itching, burning sensation, erythema, inflammation of the face, eyes and nose, and irritation of the eyes. Skin discoloration, oiliness and tenderness of the skin have also been reported.

DOSAGE AND ADMINISTRATION

BENZAMYCIN Topical Gel should be applied twice daily, morning and evening, or as directed by a physician, to affected areas after the skin is thoroughly washed, rinsed with warm water and gently patted dry.

How Supplied and Compounding Directions:
[See table below]
Prior to dispensing, tap vial until powder flows freely. Add indicated amount of ethyl alcohol (70%) to vial (to the mark) and immediately shake to completely dissolve erythromycin. Add this solution to gel and stir until homogeneous in appearance (1 to 1 ½ minutes). BENZAMYCIN Topical Gel should then be stored under refrigeration. Do not freeze. Place a 3-month expiration date on the label.
NOTE: ***Prior to reconstitution,* store at room temperature between 15° and 30°C (59°–86°F).**
***After reconstitution,* store under refrigeration between 2° and 8°C (36°–46°F).**
Do not freeze. Keep tightly closed. Keep out of the reach of children.
Caution: Federal (U.S.A.) law prohibits dispensing without prescription.
U.S. Patent Nos. 4,387,107 and 4,497,794.
Manufactured by Rhône-Poulenc Rorer Puerto Rico Inc.
Manati, Puerto Rico
For **Dermik Laboratories, Inc.**
A Rhône-Poulenc Rorer Company
Collegeville, PA 19426
Rev. 2/96 IN-7121P
BENZAMYCIN®
(erythromycin-benzoyl
peroxide topical gel)

PLEASE READ COMPLETE COMPOUNDING DIRECTIONS

NOTE: TAP VIAL UNTIL ALL POWDER FLOWS FREELY. ADD ETHYL ALCOHOL (70%) TO VIAL (TO THE MARK) AND **IMMEDIATELY** SHAKE/DISSOLVE **COMPLETELY.**

Size (Net Weight)	NDC 0066-	Benzoyl Peroxide Gel	Active Erythromycin Powder (In Plastic Vial)	Ethyl Alcohol (70%) To Be Added
11.65 grams (as dispensed) SAMPLE	0510-05	10 grams	0.4 grams	1.5 mL
23.3 grams (as dispensed)	0510-23	20 grams	0.8 grams	3 mL
46.6 grams (as dispensed)	0510-46	40 grams	1.6 grams	6 mL

DRITHOCREME® ℞
[*drĭth'ocrēm*]
(anthralin) 0.1%, 0.25%, 0.5%, 1.0% (HP)

DESCRIPTION

Drithocreme® is a pale yellow topical cream containing 0.1%, 0.25%, 0.5% or 1.0% (HP) anthralin USP in a base of white petrolatum, sodium lauryl sulfate, cetostearyl alcohol, ascorbic acid, salicylic acid, chlorocresol and purified water. The chemical name of anthralin is 1,8-dihydroxy-9-anthrone.

HOW SUPPLIED

50g tubes
Drithocreme 0.1% NDC 0066-7200-50
Drithocreme 0.25% NDC 0066-7201-50
Drithocreme 0.5% NDC 0066-7202-50
Drithocreme HP 1% NDC 0066-7203-50
Caution: Federal law prohibits dispensing without prescription.
Distributed by
DERMIK LABORATORIES, INC.
A RHÔNE-POULENC RORER COMPANY
COLLEGEVILLE, PA 19426
Made in UK. Rev. 1/97 IN-1660B (LTF 089)

DRITHO-SCALP® ℞
(anthralin) 0.25%, 0.5%

HYTONE® ℞
[*hī-tōne*]
(hydrocortisone)
Cream, Lotion

HYTONE® ℞
[*hī-tōne*]
(hydrocortisone)
Ointment

KLARON® ℞
[*klă - rŏn*]
(sodium sulfacetamide lotion)
Lotion, 10%

DESCRIPTION

Each mL of **Klaron®** (sodium sulfacetamide lotion) **Lotion, 10%** contains 100 mg of sodium sulfacetamide in a vehicle consisting of purified water; propylene glycol; lauramide DEA (and) diethanolamine; polyethylene glycol 400, monolaurate; hydroxyethyl cellulose; sodium chloride; sodium metabisulfite; methylparaben; xanthan gum; EDTA and simethicone.

Sodium sulfacetamide is a sulfonamide with antibacterial activity. Chemically, sodium sulfacetamide is N′ -[(4-aminophenyl) sulfonyl] - acetamide, monosodium salt, monohydrate. The structural formula is:

$NH_2-C_6H_4-SO_2N(Na)COCH_3 \cdot H_2O$

CLINICAL PHARMACOLOGY

The most widely accepted mechanism of action of sulfonamides is the Woods-Fildes theory, based on sulfonamides acting as a competitive inhibitor of para-aminobenzoic acid (PABA) utilization, an essential component for bacterial growth. While absorption through intact skin in humans has not been determined, *in vitro* studies with human cadaver skin indicated a percutaneous absorption of about 4%. Sodium sulfacetamide is readily absorbed from the gastrointestinal tract when taken orally and excreted in the urine largely unchanged. The biological half-life has been reported to be between 7 to 13 hours.

INDICATIONS

Klaron Lotion is indicated in the topical treatment of *acne vulgaris*.

CONTRAINDICATIONS

Klaron Lotion is contraindicated for use by patients having known hypersensitivity to sulfonamides or any other component of this preparation (see **WARNINGS** section).

WARNINGS

Fatalities have occurred, although rarely, due to severe reactions to sulfonamides including Stevens-Johnson syndrome, toxic epidermal necrolysis, fulminant hepatic necrosis, agranulocytosis, aplastic anemia, and other blood dyscrasias. Hypersensitivity reactions may occur when a sulfonamide is readministered, irrespective of the route of administration. Sensitivity reactions have been reported in individuals with no prior history of sulfonamide hypersensitivity. At the first sign of hypersensitivity, skin rash or other reactions, discontinue use of this preparation (see **ADVERSE REACTIONS** section).

Klaron Lotion contains sodium metabisulfite, a sulfite that may cause allergic-type reactions including anaphylactic symptoms and life-threatening or less severe asthmatic episodes in certain susceptible people. The overall prevalence of sulfite sensitivity in the general population is unknown and probably low. Sulfite sensitivity is seen more frequently in asthmatic than in non-asthmatic people (see **CONTRAINDICATIONS** section).

PRECAUTIONS

General: For external use only. Keep away from eyes. If irritation develops, use of the product should be discontinued and appropriate therapy instituted. Patients should be carefully observed for possible local irritation or sensitization during long-term therapy. Hypersensitivity reactions may occur when a sulfonamide is readministered irrespective of the route of administration, and cross-sensitivity between different sulfonamides may occur. Sodium sulfacetamide can cause reddening and scaling of the skin. Particular caution should be employed if areas of involved skin to be treated are denuded or abraded.

Keep out of reach of children.

Carcinogenesis, Mutagenesis and Impairment of Fertility: Long-term studies in animals have not been performed to evaluate carcinogenic potential.

Pregnancy - Category C: Animal reproduction studies have not been conducted with **Klaron® Lotion**. It is also not known whether **Klaron Lotion** can cause fetal harm when administered to a pregnant woman or can affect reproduction capacity. **Klaron Lotion** should be given to a pregnant woman only if clearly needed.

Kernicterus may occur in the newborn as a result of treatment of a pregnant woman at term with orally administered sulfonamide. There are no adequate and well controlled studies of **Klaron Lotion** in pregnant women, and it is not known whether topically applied sulfonamides can cause fetal harm when administered to a pregnant woman.

Nursing Mothers: It is not known whether sodium sulfacetamide is excreted in the human milk following topical use of **Klaron Lotion**. Systemically administered sulfonamides are capable of producing kernicterus in the infants of lactating women. Small amounts of orally administered sulfonamides have been reported to be eliminated in human milk. Because many drugs are excreted in human milk, caution should be exercised in prescribing for nursing women.

Pediatric Use: Safety and effectiveness in pediatric patients under the age of 12 have not been established.

ADVERSE REACTIONS

In controlled clinical trials for the management of *acne vulgaris*, the occurrence of adverse reactions associated with the use of **Klaron Lotion** was infrequent and restricted to local events. The total incidence of adverse reactions reported in these studies was less than 2%. Only one of 105 patients treated with **Klaron Lotion** had adverse reactions of erythema, itching and edema. It has been reported that sodium sulfacetamide may cause local irritation, stinging and burning. While the irritation may be transient, occasionally, the use of medication has to be discontinued.

DOSAGE AND ADMINISTRATION

Apply a thin film to affected areas twice daily.

HOW SUPPLIED

2 FL OZ (59 mL) bottles (**NDC** 0066-7500-02).
Store at room temperature.
Caution: Federal law prohibits dispensing without prescription.
Marketed by
Dermik Laboratories, Inc.
A Rhône-Poulenc Rorer Company
Collegeville, PA, USA 19426
Rev. 12/96 IN-5178C

NORITATE™ ℞
(metronidazole cream)
Cream, 1%
FOR TOPICAL USE ONLY
(NOT FOR OPHTHALMIC USE)

DESCRIPTION

NORITATE™ (metronidazole cream) **Cream, 1%**, contains metronidazole, USP. Chemically, metronidazole is 2-methyl-5-nitro-1*H*-imidazole-1-ethanol. The molecular formula for metronidazole is $C_6H_9N_3O_3$. It has the following structural formula:

[Structural formula: imidazole ring with O_2N, CH_3 and CH_2CH_2OH substituents]

Metronidazole has a molecular weight of 171.16. It is a white to pale yellow crystalline powder. It is slightly soluble in alcohol and has a solubility in water of 10 mg/mL at 20°C. Metronidazole is a member of the imidazole class of antibacterial agents and is classified as an antiprotozoal and anti-bacterial agent.

NORITATE is an emollient cream; each gram contains 10 mg micronized metronidazole USP, in a base of purified water USP, stearic acid NF, glyceryl monostearate NF, glycerin USP, methylparaben NF, triethanolamine NF and propylparaben NF.

CLINICAL PHARMACOLOGY

Pharmacokinetics: When one gram dose of NORITATE cream, 1%, was applied in a single application to the face of 16 healthy volunteers, low concentrations of metronidazole were detected in the plasma of 7 of the volunteers. The mean ± SD C_{max} of metronidazole was 27.6 ± 7.3 ng/mL, which is about 1% of the value reported for a single 250 mg oral dose of metronidazole. The time to maximum plasma concentration (T_{max}) in the volunteers with detectable metronidazole was 8–12 hours after topical application.

Pharmacodynamics: The mechanisms by which metronidazole acts in reducing inflammatory lesions of rosacea are unknown.

Clinical Studies: Safety and efficacy of NORITATE were evaluated in two randomized vehicle-controlled clinical studies for the treatment of rosacea, which excluded patients who had nodules, moderate or severe rhinophyma, dense telangiectases, plaque-like facial edema or ocular involvement and those who had a history of not responding to metronidazole therapy for rosacea. Of the patients included in the efficacy database (n=416), there were 142 men and 274 women. Endpoint efficacy data comparisons for patients treated with daily NORITATE or vehicle applications are listed below.

[See table above]

Inflammatory Lesion Counts and Erythema Severity Scores in Two Clinical Trials for Rosacea

	Noritate				Vehicle			
	Study 1		Study 2		Study 1		Study 2	
	N	Result	N	Result	N	Result	N	Result
Papules + Pustules Count								
Baseline	89	15	92	19	50	18	49	17
Week-10	80	7*	82	8	45	15	41	12
Reduction		49%*		58%*		17%		30%
Papules Count								
Baseline	89	13	92	17	50	15	49	15
Week-10	80	7*	82	7	45	12	41	11
Reduction		41%*		55%*		14%		28%
Erythema Score								
Baseline	89	2.2	92	2.3	50	2.2	49	2.2
Week-10	80	1.3*	82	1.4*	45	1.7	40	1.8
Reduction		42%*		40%*		25%		19%

* Statistically significant differences between NORITATE and vehicle groups with p≤0.05. Erythema scores: 0=none, 1=mild, 2=moderate and 3=severe.

Safety Studies: Studies of contact sensitization (n=258), phototoxicity (n=21), and photocontact sensitization (n=29) of NORITATE were conducted. No evidence of sensitization or phototoxicity was seen in these studies.

INDICATIONS AND USAGE

NORITATE is indicated for the topical treatment of inflammatory lesions and erythema of rosacea.

CONTRAINDICATIONS

NORITATE is contraindicated in those patients with a history of hypersensitivity to metronidazole or to any other ingredient in this formulation.

PRECAUTIONS

General: If a reaction suggesting local skin irritation occurs, patients should be directed to discontinue use of the medication. Conjunctivitis associated with topical use of metronidazole on the face has been reported. Contact with the eyes should be avoided. Metronidazole is a nitroimidazole and should be used with care in patients with evidence of, or history of, blood dyscrasia.

Information for Patients: Patients using NORITATE™ should receive the following information and instructions:

1. This medication is to be used as directed.
2. It is for external use only.
3. Avoid contact with the eyes.
4. Cleanse affected area(s) before applying NORITATE.
5. This medication should not be used for any disorder other than that for which it is prescribed.
6. Patients should report any adverse reaction to their physician.

Drug Interactions: Oral metronidazole has been reported to potentiate the anticoagulant effect of coumarin and warfarin resulting in a prolongation of prothrombin time. Drug interactions should be kept in mind when NORITATE is prescribed for patients who are receiving anticoagulant treatment, although they are less likely to occur with topical metronidazole administration because of low absorption. (See **CLINICAL PHARMACOLOGY, Pharmacokinetics** section)

Carcinogenesis, Mutagenesis and Impairment of Fertility: Metronidazole has shown evidence of carcinogenic activity in a number of studies involving chronic, oral administration in mice and rats but not in studies involving hamsters. In several long term studies in mice, oral doses of approximately 225 mg/m^2/day or greater (approximately 37 times the human topical dose on a mg/m^2 basis) were associated with an increase in pulmonary tumors and lymphomas. Several long term oral studies in the rat have shown statistically significant increases in mammary and hepatic tumors at doses >885 mg/m^2/day (144 times the topical human dose).

Metronidazole has shown evidence of mutagenic activity in several *in vitro* bacterial assay systems. In addition, a dose-related increase in the frequency of micronuclei was observed in mice after intraperitoneal injections. An increase in chromosomal aberrations in peripheral blood lymphocytes was reported in patients with Crohn's disease who were treated with 200 to 1200 mg/day of metronidazole for 1 to 24 months. However, in another study, no increase in chromosomal aberrations in circulating lymphocytes was observed in patients with Crohn's disease treated with the drug for 8 months.

In one published study, using albino hairless mice, intraperitoneal administration of metronidazole at a dose of 45 mg/m^2/day (approximately 7 times the human topical dose on a mg/m^2 basis) was associated with an increase in ultraviolet

Continued on next page

Noritate—Cont.

radiation-induced skin carcinogenesis. Neither dermal carcinogenicity nor photocarcinogenicity studies have been performed with NORITATE or any marketed metronidazole formulations.

Pregnancy: *Teratogenic Effects*: Pregnancy Category B. There are no adequate and well controlled studies with the use of NORITATE in pregnant women.

Metronidazole crosses the placental barrier and enters the fetal circulation rapidly. No fetotoxicity was observed after oral administration of metronidazole to rats or mice at 200 and 20 times, respectively, the expected clinical dose. However, oral metronidazole has shown carcinogenic activity in rodents. Because animal reproduction studies are not always predictive of human response, NORITATE should be used during pregnancy only if clearly needed.

Nursing Mothers: After oral administration, metronidazole is secreted in breast milk in concentrations similar to those found in the plasma. Even though blood levels taken after topical metronidazole application are significantly lower than those achieved after oral metronidazole, a decision should be made whether to discontinue nursing or to discontinue the drug, taking into account the importance of the drug to the mother and the risk to the infant.

Pediatric Use: Safety and effectiveness in pediatric patients have not been established.

ADVERSE REACTIONS

Safety data from 302 patients who used NORITATE (n=200) or vehicle control (n=102) once daily in clinical trials and experienced an adverse event considered to be treatment-related include: application site reaction (NORITATE 1, vehicle 1), condition aggravated (NORITATE 1, vehicle 0), paresthesia (NORITATE 0, vehicle 1), acne (NORITATE 1, vehicle 0), dry skin (NORITATE 0, vehicle 2). The majority of adverse reactions were mild to moderate in severity.

Two patients treated with NORITATE once daily discontinued treatment because of adverse events: one for a severe flare of comedonal acne and one for rosacea aggravated.

DOSAGE AND ADMINISTRATION

Areas to be treated should be cleansed before application of NORITATE. Apply and rub in a thin film of NORITATE once daily to entire affected area(s). Patients may use cosmetics after application of NORITATE.

HOW SUPPLIED

Cream—30 gram aluminum tube NDC 0066-9850-30.

Caution: Federal law prohibits dispensing without a prescription. Keep out of the reach of children.

Storage Conditions: Store at controlled room temperature: 20 to 25°C (68 to 77°F).

Marketed by:
Dermik Laboratories, Inc.
A Rhône-Poulenc Rorer Company
Collegeville, PA 19426 Rev. 09/97
Made in Canada IN-0040
688097-20-0

PENLAC™ Nail Lacquer ℞

[pĕn-lack]
(ciclopirox) Topical Solution, 8%

Full Prescribing Information
FOR USE ON FINGERNAILS AND TOENAILS AND IMMEDIATELY ADJACENT SKIN ONLY
NOT FOR USE IN EYES
CAUTION
Federal Law Prohibits Dispensing Without Prescription

DESCRIPTION

PENLAC™ NAIL LACQUER (ciclopirox) Topical Solution, 8%, contains a synthetic antifungal agent, ciclopirox. It is intended for topical use on fingernails and toenails and immediately adjacent skin.

Each gram of PENLAC™ NAIL LACQUER (ciclopirox) Topical Solution, 8%, contains 80 mg ciclopirox in a solution base consisting of ethyl acetate, NF; isopropyl alcohol, USP; and butyl monoester of poly[methylvinyl ether/maleic acid] in isopropyl alcohol. Ethyl acetate and isopropyl alcohol are solvents that vaporize after application.

PENLAC™ NAIL LACQUER (ciclopirox) Topical Solution, 8%, is a clear, colorless to slightly yellowish solution.

The chemical name for ciclopirox is 6-cyclohexyl-1-hydroxy-4-methyl-2(1H)-pyridone, with the empirical formula $C_{12}H_{17}NO_2$ and a molecular weight of 207.27. The CAS Registry Number is [29342-05-0]. The chemical structure is:

OH
N O
CH_3

CLINICAL PHARMACOLOGY

Microbiology

Mechanism of Action

The mechanism of action of ciclopirox has been investigated using various *in vitro* and *in vivo* infection models. One *in vitro* study suggested that ciclopirox acts by chelation of polyvalent cations (Fe^{+3} or Al^{+3}) resulting in the inhibition of the metal-dependent enzymes that are responsible for the degradation of peroxides within the fungal cell. The clinical significance of this observation is not known.

Activity *in vitro* and *ex vivo*

In vitro methodologies employing various broth or solid media with and without additional nutrients have been utilized to determine ciclopirox minimum inhibitory concentration (MIC) values for the dermatophytic molds.[1, 2] As a consequence, a broad range of MIC values, 1–20 μg/mL, were obtained for *Trichophyton rubrum* and *Trichophyton mentagrophytes* species. Correlation between *in vitro* MIC results and clinical outcome has yet to be established for ciclopirox.

One *ex vivo* study was conducted evaluating 8% ciclopirox against new and established *Trichophyton rubrum* and *Trichophyton mentagrophytes* infections in ovine hoof material.[3] After 10 days of treatment the growth of *T. rubrum* and *T. mentagrophytes* in the established infection model was very minimally affected. Elimination of the molds from hoof material was not achieved in either the new or established infection models.

Susceptibility testing for *Trichophyton rubrum* species

In vitro susceptibility testing methods for determining ciclopirox MIC values against the dermatophytic molds, including *Trichophyton rubrum* species, have not been standardized or validated. Ciclopirox MIC values will vary depending on the susceptibility testing method employed, composition and pH of media and the utilization of nutritional supplements. Breakpoints to determine whether clinical isolates of *Trichophyton rubrum* are susceptible or resistant to ciclopirox have not been established.

Resistance

Studies have not been conducted to evaluate drug resistance development in *T. rubrum* species exposed to 8% ciclopirox topical solution. Studies assessing cross-resistance to ciclopirox and other known antifungal agents have not been performed.

Antifungal Drug Interactions

No studies have been conducted to determine whether ciclopirox might reduce the effectiveness of systemic antifungal agents for onychomycosis. Therefore, the concomitant use of 8% ciclopirox topical solution and systemic antifungal agents for onychomycosis, is not recommended.

Pharmacokinetics

As demonstrated in pharmacokinetic studies in animals and man, ciclopirox olamine is rapidly absorbed after oral administration and completely eliminated in all species via feces and urine. Most of the compound is excreted either unchanged or as glucuronide. After oral administration of 10 mg of radiolabeled drug (14C-ciclopirox) to healthy volunteers, approximately 96% of the radioactivity was excreted renally within 12 hours of administration. Ninety-four percent of the renally excreted radioactivity was in the form of glucuronides. Thus, glucuronidation is the main metabolic pathway of this compound.

Systemic absorption of ciclopirox was determined in 5 patients with dermatophytic onychomycoses, after application of PENLAC™ NAIL LACQUER Topical Solution, 8%, to all 20 digits and adjacent 5 mm of skin once daily for six months. Random serum concentrations and 24 hour urinary excretion of ciclopirox were determined at two weeks and at 1, 2, 4 and 6 months after initiation of treatment and 4 weeks post-treatment. In this study, ciclopirox serum levels ranged from 12–80 ng/mL. Based on urinary data, mean absorption of ciclopirox from the dosage form was <5% of the applied dose. One month after cessation of treatment, serum and urine levels of ciclopirox were below the limit of detection.

In two vehicle-controlled trials, patients applied PENLAC™ NAIL LACQUER Topical Solution, 8%, to all toenails and affected fingernails. Out of a total of 66 randomly selected patients on active treatment, 24 had detectable serum ciclopirox concentrations at some point during the dosing interval (range 10.0–24.6 ng/mL). It should be noted that eleven of these 24 patients took concomitant medication containing ciclopirox as ciclopirox olamine (Loprox® Cream, 0.77%).

The penetration of the PENLAC™ NAIL LACQUER Topical Solution, 8%, was evaluated in an *in vitro* investigation. Radiolabeled ciclopirox applied once to onychomycotic toenails that were avulsed demonstrated penetration up to a depth of approximately 0.4 mm. As expected, nail plate concentrations decreased as a function of nail depth. The clinical significance of these findings in nail plates is unknown. Nail bed concentrations were not determined.

INDICATIONS AND USAGE

(To understand fully the indication for this product, please read the entire INDICATION AND USAGE section of the labeling.)

PENLAC™ NAIL LACQUER Topical Solution, 8%, as a component of a comprehensive management program, is indicated as topical treatment in immunocompetent patients with mild to moderate onychomycosis of fingernails and toenails without lunula involvement, due to *Trichophyton rubrum*. The comprehensive management program includes removal of the unattached, infected nails as frequently as monthly, by a health care professional who has special competence in the diagnosis and treatment of nail disorders, including minor nail procedures.

- No studies have been conducted to determine whether ciclopirox might reduce the effectiveness of systemic antifungal agents for onychomycosis. Therefore, the concomitant use of 8% ciclopirox topical solution and systemic antifungal agents for onychomycosis, is not recommended.
- PENLAC™ NAIL LACQUER Topical Solution, 8%, should be used only under medical supervision as described above.
- The effectiveness and safety of PENLAC™ NAIL LACQUER Topical Solution, 8%, in the following populations has not been studied. The clinical trials with use of PENLAC™ NAIL LACQUER Topical Solution, 8%, excluded patients who: were pregnant or nursing, planned to become pregnant, had a history of immunosuppression (e.g., extensive, persistent, or unusual distribution of dermatomycoses, extensive seborrheic dermatitis, recent or recurring herpes zoster, or persistent herpes simplex), were HIV seropositive, received organ transplant, required medication to control epilepsy, were insulin dependent diabetics or had diabetic neuropathy. Patients with severe plantar (moccasin) tinea pedis were also excluded.
- The safety and efficacy of using PENLAC™ NAIL LACQUER Topical Solution, 8%, daily for greater than 48 weeks have not been established.

Clinical Trials Data

The results of use of PENLAC™ NAIL LACQUER Topical Solution, 8%, in treatment of onychomycosis of the toenail without lunula involvement were obtained from two double-blind, placebo-controlled studies conducted in the US. In these studies, patients with onychomycosis of the great toenails without lunula involvement were treated with ciclopirox topical solution, 8%, in conjunction with monthly removal of the unattached, infected toenail by the investigator. PENLAC™ NAIL LACQUER Topical Solution, 8%, was applied for 48 weeks. At baseline, patients had 20–65% involvement of the target great toenail plate. Statistical significance was demonstrated in one of two studies for the endpoint "complete cure" (clear nail and negative mycology), and in two studies for the endpoint "almost clear" (≤10% nail involvement and negative mycology) at the end of study. These results are presented below.

[See table above]

At Week 48 (plus Last Observation Carried Forward) for the Intent-to-Treat (ITT) Population

	Study 312		Study 313	
	Active	Vehicle	Active	Vehicle
Complete Cure*	6/110 (5.5%)	1/109 (0.9%)	10/118 (8.5%)	0/117 (0%)
Almost Clear**	7/107 (6.5%)	1/108 (0.9%)	14/116 (12%)	1/115 (0.9%)
Negative Mycology Alone***	30/105 (29%)	12/106 (11%)	41/115 (36%)	10/114 (9%)

*Clear nail and negative mycology
**≤10% nail involvement and negative mycology
***Negative KOH and negative culture

The summary of reported patient outcomes for the ITT population at 12 weeks following the end of treatment are presented below. Note that post-treatment efficacy assessments were scheduled only for patients who achieved a complete cure.

[See table at bottom of next page]

CONTRAINDICATIONS

PENLAC™ NAIL LACQUER Topical Solution, 8%, is contraindicated in individuals who have shown hypersensitivity to any of its components.

WARNINGS

PENLAC™ NAIL LACQUER Topical Solution, 8%, is not for ophthalmic, oral, or intravaginal use. For use on nails and immediately adjacent skin only.

PRECAUTIONS

If a reaction suggesting sensitivity or chemical irritation should occur with the use of PENLAC™ NAIL LACQUER Topical Solution, 8%, treatment should be discontinued and appropriate therapy instituted.

So far there is no relevant clinical experience with patients with insulin dependent diabetes or who have diabetic neuropathy. The risk of removal of the unattached, infected nail, by the health care professional and trimming by the patient, should be carefully considered before prescribing to patients with a history of insulin dependent diabetes mellitus or diabetic neuropathy.

Information for Patients

Patients should have detailed instructions regarding the use of PENLAC™ NAIL LACQUER Topical Solution, 8%, as a component of a comprehensive management program for onychomycosis in order to achieve maximum benefit with the use of this product.

The patient should be told to:

1. Use PENLAC™ NAIL LACQUER Topical Solution, 8%, as directed by a health care professional. Avoid contact with the eyes and mucous membranes. Contact with skin other than skin immediately surrounding the treated nail(s) should be avoided. PENLAC™ NAIL LACQUER Topical Solution, 8%, is for external use only.
2. PENLAC™ NAIL LACQUER Topical Solution, 8%, should be applied evenly over the entire nail plate and 5 mm of surrounding skin. If possible, PENLAC™ NAIL LACQUER Topical Solution, 8%, should be applied to the nail bed, hyponychium, and the under surface of the nail plate when it is free of the nail bed (e.g., onycholysis). Contact with the surrounding skin may produce mild, transient irritation (redness).
3. Removal of the unattached, infected nail, as frequently as monthly, by a health care professional is needed with use of this medication.
4. Inform a health care professional if the area of application shows signs of increased irritation (redness, itching, burning, blistering, swelling, oozing).
5. Up to 48 weeks of daily applications with PENLAC™ NAIL LACQUER Topical Solution, 8%, and professional removal of the unattached, infected nail, as frequently as monthly, are considered the full treatment needed to achieve a clear or almost clear nail (defined as 10% or less residual nail involvement).
6. Six months of therapy with professional removal of the unattached, infected nail may be required before initial improvement of symptoms is noticed.
7. A completely clear nail may not be achieved with use of this medication. In clinical studies less than 12% of patients were able to achieve either a completely clear or almost clear toenail.
8. Do not use the medication for any disorder other than that for which it is prescribed.
9. Do not use nail polish or other nail cosmetic products on the treated nails.
10. Avoid use near heat or open flame, because product is flammable.

Carcinogenesis, Mutagenesis, Impairment of Fertility:

No carcinogenicity study was conducted with PENLAC™ NAIL LACQUER Topical Solution, 8%, formulation. A carcinogenicity study of ciclopirox (1% and 5% solutions in polyethylene glycol 400) in female mice dosed topically twice per week for 50 weeks followed by a 6-month drug-free observation period prior to necropsy revealed no evidence of tumors at the application sites.

In human systemic tolerability studies following daily application (~340 mg of PENLAC™ NAIL LACQUER Topical Solution, 8%) in subjects with distal subungual onychomycosis, the average maximal serum level of ciclopirox was 31±28 ng/mL after two months of once daily applications. This level was 159 times lower than the lowest toxic dose and 115 times lower than the highest nontoxic dose in rats and dogs fed 7.7 and 23.1 mg ciclopirox (as ciclopirox olamine)/kg/day.

The following *in vitro* genotoxicity tests have been conducted with ciclopirox: evaluation of gene mutation in Ames *Salmonella* and *E. coli* assays (negative); chromosome aberration assays in V79 Chinese hamster lung fibroblasts, with and without metabolic activation (positive); gene mutation assay in the HGPRT-test with V79 Chinese hamster lung fibroblasts (negative); unscheduled DNA synthesis in human A549 cells (negative); and BALB/c3T3 cell transformation assay (negative). In an *in vivo* Chinese hamster bone marrow cytogenetic assay, ciclopirox was negative for chromosome aberrations at 5,000 mg/kg.

The following *in vitro* genotoxicity tests were conducted with PENLAC™ NAIL LACQUER Topical Solution, 8%: Ames *Salmonella* test (negative); unscheduled DNA synthesis in the rat hepatocytes (negative); cell transformation assay in BALB/c3T3 cell assay (positive). The positive response of the lacquer formulation in the BALB/c3T3 test was attributed to its butyl monoester of poly[methylvinyl ether/maleic acid] resin component (Gantrez® ES-435), which also tested positive in this test. The cell transformation assay may have been confounded because of the film-forming nature of the resin. Gantrez® ES-435 tested nonmutagenic in both the *in vitro* mouse lymphoma forward mutation assay with or without activation and unscheduled DNA synthesis assay in rat hepatocytes.

Oral reproduction studies in rats at doses up to 3.85 mg ciclopirox (as ciclopirox olamine)/kg/day [equivalent to approximately 1.4 times the potential exposure at the maximum recommended human topical dose (MRHTD)] did not reveal any specific effects on fertility or other reproductive parameters. MRHTD (mg/m^2) is based on the assumption of 100% systemic absorption of 27.12 mg ciclopirox (~340 mg PENLAC™ NAIL LACQUER Topical Solution, 8%) that will cover all the fingernails and toenails including 5 mm proximal and lateral fold area plus onycholysis to a maximal extent of 50%.

Pregnancy

Teratogenic effects: Pregnancy Category B

Teratology studies in mice, rats, rabbits, and monkeys at oral doses of up to 77, 23, 23, or 38.5 mg, respectively, of ciclopirox as ciclopirox olamine/kg/day (14, 8, 17, and 28 times MRHTD), or in rats and rabbits receiving topical doses of up to 92.4 and 77 mg/kg/day, respectively (33 and 55 times MRHTD), did not indicate any significant fetal malformations.

There are no adequate or well-controlled studies of topically applied ciclopirox in pregnant women. PENLAC™ NAIL LACQUER Topical Solution, 8%, should be used during pregnancy only if the potential benefit justifies the potential risk to the fetus.

Nursing Mothers

It is not known whether this drug is excreted in human milk. Since many drugs are excreted in human milk, caution should be exercised when PENLAC™ NAIL LACQUER Topical Solution, 8%, is administered to a nursing woman.

Pediatric Use

Safety and effectiveness in pediatric patients have not been established.

Geriatric Use

Clinical studies of PENLAC™ NAIL LACQUER Topical Solution, 8%, did not include sufficient numbers of subjects aged 65 and over to determine whether they respond differently from younger subjects. Other reported clinical experience has not identified differences in responses between elderly and younger patients.

ADVERSE REACTIONS

In the vehicle-controlled clinical trials conducted in the US, 9% (30/327) of patients treated with PENLAC™ NAIL LACQUER Topical Solution and 7% (23/328) of patients treated with vehicle reported treatment-emergent adverse events (TEAE) considered by the investigator to be causally related to the test material.

The incidence of these adverse events, within each body system, was similar between the treatment groups except for Skin and Appendages: 8% (27/327) and 4% (14/328) of subjects in the ciclopirox and vehicle groups reported at least one adverse event, respectively. The most common were rash-related adverse events: periungual erythema and erythema of the proximal nail fold were reported more frequently in patients treated with PENLAC™ NAIL LACQUER Topical Solution (5% [16/327]) than in patients treated with vehicle (1% [3/328]). Other TEAEs thought to be causally related included nail disorders such as shape change, irritation, ingrown toenail, and discoloration.

The incidence of nail disorders was similar between the treatment groups (2% [6/327] in the PENLAC™ NAIL LACQUER Topical Solution group and 2% [7/328] in the vehicle group). Moreover, application site reactions and/or burning of the skin occurred in 1% of patients treated with PENLAC™ NAIL LACQUER Topical Solution (3/327) and vehicle (4/328).

A 21-Day Cumulative Irritancy study was conducted under conditions of semi-occlusion. Mild reactions were seen in 46% of patients with the PENLAC™ NAIL LACQUER Topical Solution, 32% with the vehicle and 2% with the negative control, but all were reactions of mild transient erythema. There was no evidence of allergic contact sensitization for either the PENLAC™ NAIL LACQUER Topical Solution, 8%, or the vehicle base. In the vehicle-controlled studies, one patient treated with PENLAC™ NAIL LACQUER Topical Solution, 8%, discontinued treatment due to a rash, localized to the palm (causal relation to test material undetermined).

Use of PENLAC™ NAIL LACQUER Topical Solution, 8%, for 48 additional weeks was evaluated in an open-label extension study conducted in patients previously treated in the vehicle-controlled studies. Three percent (9/281) of subjects treated with PENLAC™ NAIL LACQUER Topical Solution, 8%, experienced at least one TEAE that the investigator thought was causally related to the test material. Mild rash in the form of periungual erythema (1% [2/281]) and nail disorders (1% [4/281]) were the most frequently reported. Four patients discontinued because of TEAEs. Two of the four had events considered to be related to test material: one patient's great toenail "broke away" and another had an elevated creatine phosphokinase level on Day 1 (after 48 weeks of treatment with vehicle in the previous vehicle-controlled study).

DOSAGE AND ADMINISTRATION

PENLAC™ NAIL LACQUER Topical Solution, 8%, should be used as a component of a comprehensive management program for onychomycosis. Removal of the unattached, infected nail, as frequently as monthly, by a health care professional, weekly trimming by the patient, and daily application of the medication are all integral parts of this therapy.

Nail Care By Health Care Professionals

Removal of the unattached, infected nail, as frequently as monthly, trimming of onycholytic nail, and filing of excess horny material should be performed by professionals trained in treatment of nail disorders.

Nail Care By Patient

Patients should file away (with emery board) loose nail material and trim nails, as required, every seven days after PENLAC™ NAIL LACQUER Topical Solution, 8%, is removed with alcohol.

PENLAC™ NAIL LACQUER Topical Solution, 8%, should be applied once daily (preferably at bedtime or eight hours before washing) to all affected nails with the applicator brush provided. The PENLAC™ NAIL LACQUER Topical Solution, 8%, should be applied evenly over the entire nail plate.

If possible, PENLAC™ NAIL LACQUER Topical Solution, 8%, should be applied to the nail bed, hyponychium, and the under surface of the nail plate when it is free of the nail bed (e.g., onycholysis).

The PENLAC™ NAIL LACQUER Topical Solution, 8%, should not be removed on a daily basis. Daily applications should be made over the previous coat and removed with alcohol every seven days. This cycle should be repeated throughout the duration of therapy.

HOW SUPPLIED

PENLAC™ NAIL LACQUER (ciclopirox) Topical Solution, 8%, is supplied in 3.3 mL (NDC 0066-8008-01) glass bottles with screw caps which are fitted with brushes.

Protect from light (e.g., store bottle in the carton after every use).

PENLAC™ NAIL LACQUER (ciclopirox) Topical Solution, 8%, should be stored at room temperature between 59° and 86°F (15° and 30°C).

CAUTION: Flammable. Keep away from heat and flame.
Rx ONLY.

REFERENCES:

1. Dittmar W., Lohaus G. 1973. HOE296, A new antimycotic compound with a broad antimicrobial spectrum. *Arzneim-Forsch./Drug Res.* 23:670–674.
2. Niewerth et. al., 1998. Antimicrobial susceptibility testing of dermatophytes: Comparison of the agar macrodilution and broth micro dilution tests. *Chemotherapy.* 44:31–35.
3. Yang et. al. 1997. A new simulation model for studying in vitro topical penetration of antifungal drugs into hard keratin. *J. Mycol. Med.* 7:195–98.

Gantrez is a registered trademark of GAF Corporation

PENLAC™ NAIL LACQUER (ciclopirox) Topical Solution, 8%

Patient Information and Instructions

Patients should have detailed instructions regarding the use of PENLAC™ NAIL LACQUER Topical Solution, 8%, as a component of a comprehensive management program for onychomycosis in order to achieve maximum benefit with the use of this product. Discuss your treatment plan with your health care professional for regular removal of the unattached, infected nail.

Before using this medication, tell your doctor if you:

- Are pregnant or nursing
- Are an insulin dependent diabetic or have diabetic neuropathy
- Have a history of immunosuppression
- Are immunocompromised (e.g., received an organ transplant, etc.)
- Require medication to control epilepsy
- Use or require topical corticosteroids on a repeated monthly basis
- Use steroid inhalers on a regular basis

Patient Information:

- Use PENLAC™ NAIL LACQUER Topical Solution, 8%, as directed by your health care professional.
- PENLAC™ NAIL LACQUER Topical Solution, 8%, is for external use only.
- Contact with skin other than skin immediately surrounding the treated nail(s) should be avoided.
- Avoid contact with the eyes and mucous membranes.
- Removal of the unattached, infected nail, as frequently as monthly, by your health care professional is needed with use of this medication to obtain maximal benefit with use of this product.
- Inform your health care professional if the area of application shows signs of increased irritation (redness, itching, burning, blistering, swelling, oozing).

Continued on next page

Post-treatment Week 12 Data for Patients Who Achieved Complete Cure at Week 48

	Study 312		Study 313	
	Active	Vehicle	Active	Vehicle
Number of Treated Patients	112	111	119	118
Complete Cure at Week 48	6	1	10	0
Post-treatment Week 12 Outcomes:				
Patients Missing All Week 12 Assessments	2	0	2	0
Patients with Week 12 Assessments	4	1	8	0
Complete Cure	3	1	4	0
Almost Clear	2*	1	1*	0
Negative Mycology	3	1	5	0

*Four patients (from studies 312 and 313) who were completely cured did not have post-treatment Week 12 planimetry data.

Penlac—Cont.

- Up to 48 weeks of daily applications with PENLAC™ NAIL LACQUER Topical Solution, 8%, and professional removal, as frequently as monthly, of the unattached, infected nail are considered the full treatment time to achieve a clear or almost clear nail (defined as 10% or less residual nail involvement). Six months of therapy with professional removal of the unattached infected nail may be required before initial improvement of symptoms is noticed.
- A completely clear nail may not be achieved with use of this medication. In clinical studies less than 12% of patients were able to achieve either a clear or almost clear toenail.
- Do not use nail polish or other nail cosmetic products on the treated nails.
- Avoid use near heat or open flame, because product is flammable.

Patient Instructions

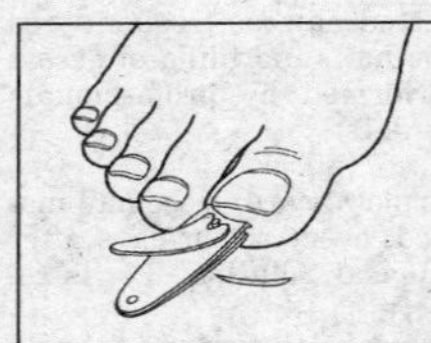

1. Before starting treatment, remove any loose nail or nail material using nail clippers or nail files.

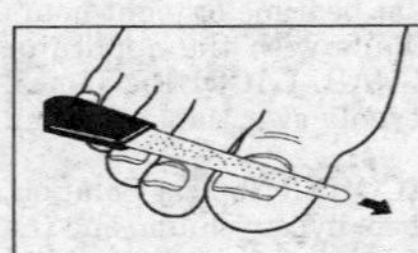

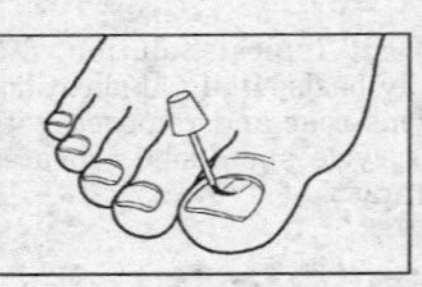

2. Apply PENLAC™ NAIL LACQUER Topical Solution, 8%, once daily (preferably at bedtime) to all affected nails with the applicator brush provided. Apply the lacquer evenly over the entire nail. Where possible, nail lacquer should also be applied to the underside of the nail and to the skin beneath it. Allow lacquer to dry (approximately 30 seconds) before putting on socks or stockings. After applying medication, wait 8 hours before taking a bath or shower.
3. Apply PENLAC™ NAIL LACQUER Topical Solution, 8%, daily over the previous coat.
4. Once a week, remove the PENLAC™ NAIL LACQUER Topical Solution, 8%, with alcohol. Remove as much as possible of the damaged nail using scissors, nail clippers, or nail files.

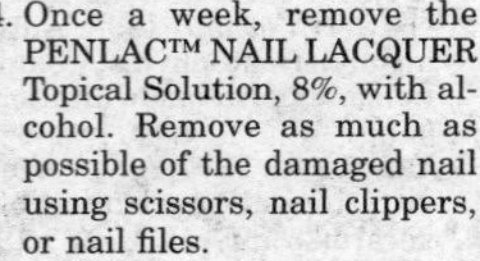

5. Repeat process (steps 2 through 4).

Please Note:

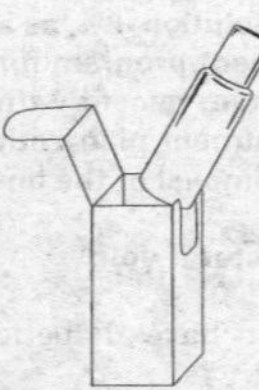

1. To prevent screw cap from sticking to the bottle, do not allow solution to get into the bottle threads.
2. To prevent the solution from drying out, bottle should be closed tightly after every use.
3. To protect from light, replace bottle into carton after each use.

Prescribing Information as of January 2000
Mfd. by: Aventis Pharma Deutschland GmbH
D-65926 Frankfurt am Main
Germany
Made in Germany
Marketed by: DERMIK LABORATORIES, INC.
Collegeville, PA 19426

PSORCON® CREAM ℞
[*sŏr-kon*]
(diflorasone diacetate cream) 0.05%

PSORCON® OINTMENT ℞
[*sŏr-kon*]
(diflorasone diacetate ointment) 0.05%
Not for Ophthalmic Use

DESCRIPTION

Each gram of **psorcon** Ointment contains 0.5 mg diflorasone diacetate in an ointment base.

Chemically, diflorasone diacetate is 6α, 9-difluoro-11β,17,21-trihydroxy-16β-methylpregna-1,4-diene-3,20-dione 17,21-diacetate. The structural formula is represented below:

Each gram of **psorcon** Ointment contains 0.5 mg diflorasone diacetate in an ointment base of propylene glycol, glyceryl monostearate and white petrolatum.

HOW SUPPLIED

psorcon Ointment 0.05% is available in the following size tubes:

15 gram	NDC 0066-0071-17
30 gram	NDC 0066-0071-31
60 gram	NDC 0066-0071-60

Store at controlled room temperature 20° to 25°C (68° to 77°F) [see USP].

Caution: Federal law prohibits dispensing without prescription.

Manufactured by
Pharmacia & Upjohn Company
Kalamazoo, MI, USA 49001
For
Dermik Laboratories, Inc.
A Rhône-Poulenc Rorer Company
Collegeville, PA, USA 19426
Revised October 1996 813 377 208α
IN-7191J 691694

PSORCON® E™ emollient cream ℞
(diflorasone diacetate cream) 0.05%
Not For Ophthalmic Use

DESCRIPTION

Each gram of **Psorcon E** Emollient Cream contains 0.5 mg diflorasone diacetate in a cream base.

Chemically, diflorasone diacetate is: 6α,9-difluoro - 11β,17,21 - trihydroxy - 16β - methyl-pregna - 1,4 - diene - 3,20 - dione 17,21 - diacetate. The structural formula is represented below:

Each gram of **Psorcon E** Emollient Cream contains 0.5 mg diflorasone diacetate in a hydrophilic vanishing cream base of propylene glycol, stearyl alcohol, cetyl alcohol, sorbitan monostearate, polysorbate 60, mineral oil and purified water.

CLINICAL PHARMACOLOGY

Topical corticosteroids share anti-inflammatory, antipruritic and vasoconstrictive actions.

The mechanism of anti-inflammatory activity of the topical corticosteroids is unclear. Various laboratory methods, including vasoconstrictor assays, are used to compare and predict potencies and/or clinical efficacies of the topical corticosteroids. There is some evidence to suggest that a recognizable correlation exists between vasoconstrictor potency and therapeutic efficacy in man.

Pharmacokinetics: The extent of percutaneous absorption of topical corticosteroids is determined by many factors including the vehicle, the integrity of the epidermal barrier, and the use of occlusive dressings.

Topical corticosteroids can be absorbed from normal intact skin. Inflammation and/or other disease processes in the skin increase percutaneous absorption. Occlusive dressings substantially increase the percutaneous absorption of topical corticosteroids. Thus, occlusive dressings may be a valuable therapeutic adjunct for treatment of resistant dermatoses. (See **DOSAGE AND ADMINISTRATION**.)

Once absorbed through the skin, topical corticosteroids are handled through pharmacokinetic pathways similar to systemically administered corticosteroids. Corticosteroids are bound to plasma proteins in varying degrees. They are metabolized primarily in the liver and are then excreted by the kidneys. Some of the topical corticosteroids and their metabolites are also excreted into the bile.

INDICATIONS AND USAGE

Topical corticosteroids are indicated for relief of the inflammatory and pruritic manifestations of corticosteroid responsive dermatoses.

CONTRAINDICATIONS

Topical steroids are contraindicated in those patients with a history of hypersensitivity of any of the components of the preparation.

PRECAUTIONS

General: Systemic absorption of topical corticosteroids has produced reversible hypothalamic-pituitary-adrenal (HPA) axis suppression, manifestations of Cushings's syndrome, hyperglycemia, and glucosuria in some patients.

Conditions which augment systemic absorption include the application of the more potent steroids, use over large surface areas, prolonged use, and the addition of occlusive dressings.

Therefore, patients receiving a large dose of a potent topical steroid applied to a large surface area or under an occlusive dressing should be evaluated periodically for evidence of HPA axis suppression by using the urinary free cortisol and ACTH stimulation tests. If HPA axis suppression is noted, an attempt should be made to withdraw the drug, to reduce the frequency of application, or to substitute a less potent steroid.

Recovery of HPA axis function is generally prompt and complete upon discontinuation of the drug. Infrequently, signs and symptoms of steroid withdrawal may occur, requiring supplemental systemic corticosteroids.

Pediatric patients may absorb proportionally larger amounts of topical corticosteroids and thus be more susceptible to systemic toxicity. (See **PRECAUTIONS: Pediatric Use.**)

If irritation develops, topical corticosteroids should be discontinued and appropriate therapy instituted.

In the presence of dermatological infections, the use of an appropriate antifungal or antibacterial agent should be instituted. If a favorable response does not occur promptly, the corticosteroid should be discontinued until the infection has been adequately controlled.

Information for the Patient: Patients using topical corticosteroids should receive the following information and instructions:

1. This medication is to be used as directed by the physician. It is for external use only. Avoid contact with the eyes.
2. Patients should be advised not to use this medication for any disorder other than for which it was prescribed.
3. The treated skin area should not be bandaged or otherwise covered or wrapped as to be occlusive unless directed by the physician.
4. Patients should report any signs of local adverse reactions especially under occlusive dressing.
5. Parents of pediatric patients should be advised not to use tight-fitting diapers or plastic pants on an infant or child being treated in the diaper area, as these garments may constitute occlusive dressings.

Laboratory Tests: The following tests may be helpful in evaluating the HPA axis suppression:

Urinary free cortisol test
ACTH stimulation test

Carcinogenesis, Mutagenesis, and Impairment of Fertility: Long-term animal studies have not been performed to evaluate the carcinogenic potential or the effect on fertility of topical corticosteroids.

Studies to determine mutagenicity with prednisolone and hydrocortisone have revealed negative results.

Pregnancy Category C: Corticosteroids are generally teratogenic in laboratory animals when administered systemically at relatively low dosage levels. The more potent corticosteroids have been shown to be teratogenic after dermal application in laboratory animals. There are no adequate and well-controlled studies in pregnant women on teratogenic effects from topically applied corticosteroids. Therefore, topical corticosteroids should be used during pregnancy only if the potential benefit justifies the potential risk to the fetus. Drugs of this class should not be used extensively on pregnant patients, in large amounts, or for prolonged periods of time.

Nursing Mothers: It is not known whether topical administration of corticosteroids could result in sufficient systemic absorption to produce detectable quantities in breast milk. Systemically administered corticosteroids are secreted into breast milk in quantities **not** likely to have a deleterious effect on the infant. Nevertheless, caution should be exercised when topical corticosteroids are administered to a nursing woman.

Pediatric Use: Safety and effectiveness of **Psorcon E** (diflorasone diacetate cream) in pediatric patients have not been established. Because of a higher ratio of skin surface area to body mass, pediatric patients are at a greater risk than adults of HPA-axis suppression when they are treated with topical corticosteroids. They are, therefore, also at greater risk of glucocorticosteroid insufficiency after withdrawal of treatment and of Cushing's syndrome while on treatment. Adverse effects including striae have been reported with inappropriate use of topical corticosteroids in pediatric patients.

HPA axis suppression, Cushing's syndrome, and intracranial hypertension have been reported in pediatric patients receiving topical corticosteroids. Manifestations of adrenal suppression in pediatric patients include linear growth retardation, delayed weight gain, low plasma cortisol levels, and absence of response to ACTH stimulation. Manifestations of intracranial hypertension include bulging fontanelles, headaches, and bilateral papilledema.

Administration of topical corticosteroids to pediatric patients should be limited to the least amount compatible with an effective therapeutic regimen. Chronic corticosteroid therapy may interfere with the growth and development of pediatric patients.

ADVERSE REACTIONS

The following local adverse reactions have been reported with topical corticosteroids, but may occur more frequently with the use of occlusive dressings. These reactions are listed in an approximate decreasing order of occurrence:

1. Burning
2. Itching
3. Irritation
4. Dryness
5. Folliculitis
6. Hypertrichosis
7. Acneiform eruptions
8. Hypopigmentation
9. Perioral dermatitis
10. Allergic contact dermatitis
11. Maceration of the skin
12. Secondary infection
13. Skin atrophy
14. Striae
15. Miliaria

OVERDOSAGE

Topically applied corticosteroids can be absorbed in sufficient amounts to produce systemic effects. (See **PRECAUTIONS**.)

DOSAGE AND ADMINISTRATION

Psorcon E Emollient Cream should be applied to the affected areas as a thin film from one to three times daily depending on the severity or resistant nature of the condition.

Occlusive dressings may be used for the management of psoriasis or recalcitrant conditions.

If an infection develops, the use of occlusive dressings should be discontinued and appropriate antimicrobial therapy initiated.

HOW SUPPLIED

Psorcon E Emollient Cream is available in the following size tubes:

15 gram	NDC 0066-0272-17
30 gram	NDC 0066-0272-31
60 gram	NDC 0066-0272-60

Store at controlled room temperature, 20° to 25° C (68° to 77°F) [see USP].

Rx only

Manufactured for

Dermik Laboratories, Inc.

A Rhône-Poulenc Rorer Company

Collegeville, PA, USA 19426

By Pharmacia & Upjohn Company

Kalamazoo, MI, USA 49001

Revised June 1998

IN-7154J 817 504 002A

691694

PSORCON® E™ emollient ointment ℞

(diflorasone diacetate ointment) 0.05%

Not For Ophthalmic Use

DESCRIPTION

Each gram of **Psorcon E** Emollient Ointment contains 0.5 mg diflorasone diacetate in an ointment base.

Chemically, diflorasone diacetate is: 6α,9-difluoro - 11β, 17,21 - trihydroxy - 16β - methyl-pregna - 1,4-diene - 3,20 - dione 17,21 - diacetate. The structural formula is represented below:

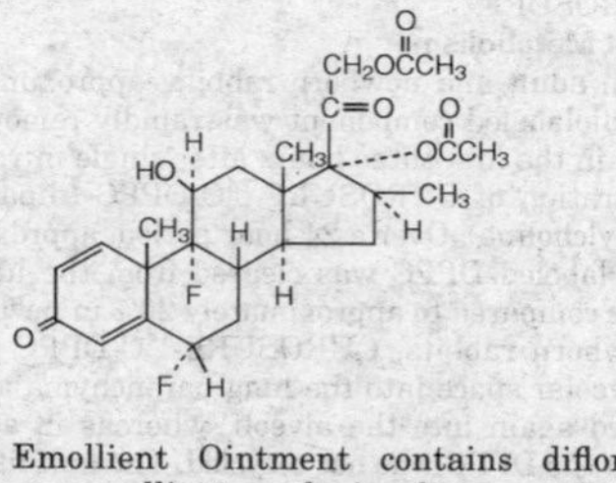

Psorcon E Emollient Ointment contains diflorasone diacetate in an emollient, occlusive base consisting of polyoxypropylene 15-stearyl ether, stearic acid, lanolin alcohol and white petrolatum.

CLINICAL PHARMACOLOGY

Topical corticosteroids share anti-inflammatory, antipruritic and vasoconstrictive actions.

The mechanism of anti-inflammatory activity of the topical corticosteroids is unclear. Various laboratory methods, including vasoconstrictor assays, are used to compare and predict potencies and/or clinical efficacies of the topical corticosteroids. There is some evidence to suggest that a recognizable correlation exists between vasoconstrictor potency and therapeutic efficacy in man.

Pharmacokinetics: The extent of percutaneous absorption of topical corticosteroids is determined by many factors including the vehicle, the integrity of the epidermal barrier, and the use of occlusive dressings.

Topical corticosteroids can be absorbed from normal intact skin. Inflammation and/or other disease processes in the skin increase percutaneous absorption. Occlusive dressings substantially increase the percutaneous absorption of topical corticosteroids. Thus, occlusive dressings may be a valuable therapeutic adjunct for treatment of resistant dermatoses. (See **DOSAGE AND ADMINISTRATION**.)

Once absorbed through the skin, topical corticosteroids are handled through pharmacokinetic pathways similar to systemically administered corticosteroids. Corticosteroids are bound to plasma proteins in varying degrees. They are metabolized primarily in the liver and are then excreted by the kidneys. Some of the topical corticosteroids and their metabolites are also excreted into the bile.

INDICATIONS AND USAGE

Topical corticosteroids are indicated for relief of the inflammatory and pruritic manifestations of corticosteroid responsive dermatoses.

CONTRAINDICATIONS

Topical steroids are contraindicated in those patients with a history of hypersensitivity to any of the components of the preparation.

PRECAUTIONS

General: Systemic absorption of topical corticosteroids has produced reversible hypothalamic-pituitary-adrenal (HPA) axis suppression, manifestations of Cushing's syndrome, hyperglycemia, and glucosuria in some patients.

Conditions which augment systemic absorption include the application of the more potent steroids, use over large surface areas, prolonged use, and the addition of occlusive dressings.

Therefore, patients receiving a large dose of a potent topical steroid applied to a large surface area or under an occlusive dressing should be evaluated periodically for evidence of HPA axis suppression by using the urinary free cortisol and ACTH stimulation tests. If HPA axis suppression is noted, an attempt should be made to withdraw the drug, to reduce the frequency of application, or to substitute a less potent steroid.

Recovery of HPA axis function is generally prompt and complete upon discontinuation of the drug. Infrequently, signs and symptoms of steroid withdrawal may occur, requiring supplemental systemic corticosteroids.

Pediatric patients may absorb proportionally larger amounts of topical corticosteroids and thus be more susceptible to systemic toxicity. (See **PRECAUTIONS: Pediatric Use**.)

If irritation develops, topical corticosteroids should be discontinued and appropriate therapy instituted.

In the presence of dermatological infections, the use of an appropriate antifungal or antibacterial agent should be instituted. If a favorable response does not occur promptly, the corticosteroid should be discontinued until the infection has been adequately controlled.

Information for the Patient: Patients using topical corticosteroids should receive the following information and instructions:

1. This medication is to be used as directed by the physician. It is for external use only. Avoid contact with the eyes.
2. Patients should be advised not to use this medication for any disorder other than for which it was prescribed.
3. The treated skin area should not be bandaged or otherwise covered or wrapped as to be occlusive unless directed by the physician.
4. Patients should report any signs of local adverse reactions especially under occlusive dressing.
5. Parents of pediatric patients should be advised not to use tight-fitting diapers or plastic pants on an infant or child being treated in the diaper area, as these garments may constitute occlusive dressings.

Laboratory Tests: The following tests may be helpful in evaluating the HPA axis suppression:

Urinary free cortisol test

ACTH stimulation test

Carcinogenesis, Mutagenesis, and Impairment of Fertility: Long-term animal studies have not been performed to evaluate the carcinogenic potential or the effect on fertility of topical corticosteroids.

Studies to determine mutagenicity with prednisolone and hydrocortisone have revealed negative results.

Pregnancy Category C: Corticosteroids are generally teratogenic in laboratory animals when administered systemically at relatively low dosage levels. The more potent corticosteroids have been shown to be teratogenic after dermal application in laboratory animals. There are no adequate and well-controlled studies in pregnant women on teratogenic effects from topically applied corticosteroids. Therefore, topical corticosteroids should be used during pregnancy only if the potential benefit justifies the potential risk to the fetus. Drugs of this class should not be used extensively on pregnant patients, in large amounts, or for prolonged periods of time.

Nursing Mothers: It is not known whether topical administration of corticosteroids could result in sufficient systemic absorption to produce detectable quantities in breast milk. Systemically administered corticosteroids are secreted into breast milk in quantities **not** likely to have a deleterious effect on the infant. Nevertheless, caution should be exercised when topical corticosteroids are administered to a nursing woman.

Pediatric Use: Safety and effectiveness of **Psorcon E** (diflorasone diacetate ointment) in pediatric patients have not been estblished. Because of a higher ratio of skin surface area to body mass, pediatric patients are at a greater risk than adults of HPA-axis suppression when they are treated with topical corticosteroids. They are, therefore, also at greater risk of glucocorticosteroid insufficiency after withdrawal of treatment and of Cushing's syndrome while on treatment. Adverse effects including striae have been reported with inappropriate use of topical corticosteroids in pediatric patients.

HPA axis suppression, Cushing's syndrome, and intracranial hypertension have been reported in pediatric patients receiving topical corticosteroids. Manifestations of adrenal suppression in pediatric patients include linear growth retardation, delayed weight gain, low plasma cortisol levels, and absence of response to ACTH stimulation. Manifestations of intracranial hypertension include bulging fontanelles, headaches, and bilateral papilledema.

Administration of topical corticosteroids to pediatric patients should be limited to the least amount compatible with an effective therapeutic regimen. Chronic corticosteroid therapy may interfere with the growth and development of pediatric patients.

ADVERSE REACTIONS

The following local adverse reactions have been reported with topical corticosteroids, but may occur more frequently with the use of occlusive dressings. These reactions are listed in an approximate decreasing order of occurrence:

1. Burning
2. Itching
3. Irritation
4. Dryness
5. Folliculitis
6. Hypertrichosis
7. Acneiform eruptions
8. Hypopigmentation
9. Perioral dermatitis
10. Allergic contact dermatitis
11. Maceration of the skin
12. Secondary infection
13. Skin atrophy
14. Striae
15. Miliaria

OVERDOSAGE

Topically applied corticosteroids can be absorbed in sufficient amounts to produce systemic effects. (See **PRECAUTIONS**.)

DOSAGE AND ADMINISTRATION

Topical cortisteroids should be applied to the affected area as a thin film from one to four times daily depending on the severity of the condition.

Occlusive dressings may be used for the management of psoriasis or recalcitrant conditions.

If an infection develops, the use of occlusive dressings should be discontinued and appropriate antimicrobial therapy initiated.

HOW SUPPLIED

Psorcon E Emollient Ointment is available as follows:

15 gram tube	NDC 0066-0275-17
30 gram tube	NDC 0066-0275-31
60 gram tube	NDC 0066-0275-60

Store at controlled room temperature, 20° to 25° C (68° to 77° F) [see USP].

Rx only

Manufactured for

Dermik Laboratories, Inc.

A Rhône-Poulenc Rorer Company

Collegeville, PA, USA 19426

By Pharmacia & Upjohn Company

Kalamazoo, MI, USA 49001

Revised June 1998

IN-7119J 817 503 002A

691694

SULFACET-R® Lotion ℞

[sul-fa-set]

(Sodium Sulfacetamide 10% and Sulfur 5%)

DESCRIPTION

Each mL of **Sulfacet-R® Lotion** (sodium sulfacetamide 10% and sulfur 5%) as dispensed contains 100 mg of sodium sulfacetamide and 50 mg of sulfur in a tinted lotion of 2-bromo-2-nitropropane-1, 3 diol, attapulgite, butylparaben, hydroxyethyl cellulose, iron oxides, lauramide DEA (and) diethanolamine, methylparaben, polyethylene glycol 400 monolaurate, propylene glycol, purified water, silicone emulsion, sodium chloride, sodium metabisulfite, sodium polynaphthalenesulfonate, talc, titanium dioxide, xanthan gum, and zinc oxide. Color Blender contains an additional inactive ingredient, polyethylene glycol 400, NF.

Sodium sulfacetamide is a sulfonamide with antibacterial activity while sulfur acts as a keratolytic agent. Chemically sodium sulfacetamide is N'-[(4-aminophenyl) sulfonyl]-acetamide, monosodium salt, monohydrate.

The structural formula is:

Sulfacetamide Sodium

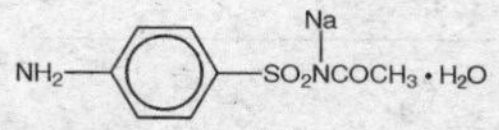

CLINICAL PHARMACOLOGY

The most widely accepted mechanism of action of sulfonamides is the Woods-Fildes theory which is based on the fact that sulfonamides act as competitive antagonists to para-aminobenzoic acid (PABA), an essential component for bacterial growth. While absorption through intact skin has not been determined, sodium sulfacetamide is readily absorbed

Continued on next page

Sulfacet-R—Cont.

from the gastrointestinal tract when taken orally and excreted in the urine, largely unchanged. The biological half-life has variously been reported as 7 to 12.8 hours.
The exact mode of action of sulfur in the treatment of acne is unknown, but it has been reported that it inhibits the growth of *p. acnes* and the formation of free fatty acids.

INDICATIONS

Sulfacet-R® Lotion is indicated in the topical control of acne vulgaris, acne rosacea and seborrheic dermatitis.

CONTRAINDICATIONS

Sulfacet-R Lotion is contraindicated for use by patients having known hypersensitivity to sulfonamides, sulfur, or any other component of this preparation. **Sulfacet-R Lotion** is not to be used by patients with kidney disease.

WARNINGS

Although rare, sensitivity to sodium sulfacetamide may occur. Therefore, caution and careful supervision should be observed when prescribing this drug for patients who may be prone to hypersensitivity to topical sulfonamides. Systemic toxic reactions such as agranulocytosis, acute hemolytic anemia, purpura hemorrhagica, drug fever, jaundice, and contact dermatitis indicate hypersensitivity to sulfonamides. Particular caution should be employed if areas of denuded or abraded skin are involved.
Contains sodium metabisulfite, a sulfite that may cause allergic-type reactions including anaphylactic symptoms and life-threatening or less severe asthmatic episodes in certain susceptible people. The overall prevalence of sulfite sensitivity in the general population is unknown and probably low. Sulfite sensitivity is seen more frequently in asthmatic than in nonasthmatic people.

PRECAUTIONS

General: If irritation develops, use of the product should be discontinued and appropriate therapy instituted. For external use only. Keep away from eyes. Patients should be carefully observed for possible local irritation or sensitization during long-term therapy. The object of this therapy is to achieve desquamation without irritation, but sodium sulfacetamide and sulfur can cause reddening and scaling of epidermis. These side effects are not unusual in the treatment of acne vulgaris, but patients should be cautioned about the possibility. Keep out of the reach of children.
Carcinogenesis, Mutagenesis and Impairment of Fertility: Long-term studies in animals have not been performed to evaluate carcinogenic potential.
Pregnancy: Category C. Animal reproduction studies have not been conducted with Sulfacet-R Lotion. It is also not known whether Sulfacet-R Lotion can cause fetal harm when administered to a pregnant woman or can affect reproduction capacity. Sulfacet-R Lotion should be given to a pregnant woman only if clearly needed.
Nursing Mothers: It is not known whether sodium sulfacetamide is excreted in the human milk following topical use of Sulfacet-R Lotion. However, small amounts of orally administered sulfonamides have been reported to be eliminated in human milk. In view of this and because many drugs are excreted in human milk, caution should be exercised when Sulfacet-R Lotion is administered to a nursing woman.
Pediatric Use: Safety and effectiveness in pediatric patients under the age of 12 have not been established.

ADVERSE REACTIONS

Although rare, sodium sulfacetamide may cause local irritation.

DOSAGE AND ADMINISTRATION

Shake well before using. Apply a thin film to affected areas with light massaging to blend in each application 1 to 3 times daily. Each package contains a Dermik Color Blender-trademark which enables the patient to alter the basic shade of the lotion so that it matches the skin color exactly.
(Important to the Pharmacist: At the time of dispensing, add contents of Sulfa-Pak™ vial* to the bottle. Shake well and/or stir with a glass rod to insure uniform dispersion. Place expiration date of four (4) months on bottle label.)
*Sulfa-Pak™ vial contains 2.1 g of sodium sulfacetamide.

HOW SUPPLIED

25 g bottles (NDC 0066-0028-25).
CAUTION: Federal law prohibits dispensing without prescription.
Dermik Laboratories, Inc.
A Rhône-Poulenc Rorer Company Rev. 11/96
Collegeville, PA, USA 19426 CR-5055R

SULFACET-R® TINT FREE LOTION ℞
[sul-fă-set]
(Sodium Sulfacetamide 10% and Sulfur 5%)

VANOXIDE®-HC LOTION ℞
[vă-noxīde]
(benzoyl peroxide 50 mg, hydrocortisone 5 mg)

VYTONE® CREAM 1% ℞
[vī-tōne]
(hydrocortisone-iodoquinol)

ZETAR® EMULSION (Coal Tar) ℞
[zē-tar]

DEY

**2751 NAPA VALLEY CORPORATE DRIVE
NAPA, CA 94558**

Direct Inquiries to:
Alan Witten
(800) 755-5560
FAX: (707) 224-8918
www.deyinc.com

For Medical Information Contact:
In Emergencies:
Mary Lou Freathy
(707) 224-3200
FAX: (707) 224-1415

Brand Name or Generic Name	Concentration Or Size	NDC or Product #
Acetylcysteine Solution USP (Mucosil™) (℞)	Acetylcysteine Solution 10%	
	Twelve 4 mL Vials	49502-181-04
	Three 30 mL Vials	49502-181-30
Acetylcysteine Solution USP (Mucosil™) (℞)	Acetylcysteine Solution 20%	
	Twelve 4 mL Vials	49502-182-04
	Three 30 mL Vials	49502-182-30
Albuterol Inhalation Aerosol (℞)	One 17 g Inhaler 200 Metered Inhalations	49502-333-17
	One 17g Refill	49502-333-27
Shown in Product Identification Guide, page 311		
Albuterol Sulfate Inhalation Solution (℞)	Twenty-Five 3 mL Vials 0.083% (expressed as Albuterol)	49502-697-03
	Thirty 3 mL Vials 0.083% (expressed as Albuterol)	49502-697-33
	Sixty 3 mL Vials 0.083% (expressed as Albuterol)	49502-697-60
Shown in Product Identification Guide, page 311		
Albuterol Sulfate Inhalation Solution 0.5% (℞)	One 20 mL Concentrate	49502-105-01
Shown in Product Identification Guide, page 311		
Curosurf® (℞) (poractant alfa) Intratracheal Suspension	One 1.5 mL Vial (120 mg)	49502-180-01
	One 3 mL Vial (240 mg)	49502-180-03
Shown in Product Identification Guide, page 311		
EasiVent™ Valved Holding Chamber (℞)		49502-207-01
Shown in Product Identification Guide, page 311		
EpiPen® Epinephrine Auto-Injector (℞)	0.3 mg	49502-500-01
EpiPen® Jr. Epinephrine Auto-Injector (℞)	0.15 mg	49502-501-01
Shown in Product Identification Guide, page 311		
Cromolyn Sodium Inhalation Solution USP (℞)	Sixty 2 mL Vials 20 mg/2mL	49502-689-02
	One Hundred Twenty 2 mL Vials 20 mg/2mL	49502-689-12
Shown in Product Identification Guide, page 311		
Ipratropium Bromide Inhalation Solution (℞)	Twenty-five 2.5 mL Vials (0.5 mg/2.5 mL)	49502-685-03
	Thirty 2.5 ml vials (0.5/2.5 mL)	49502-685-33
	Sixty 2.5 mL Vials (0.5/2.5 mL)	49502-685-60
Shown in Product Identification Guide, page 311		
Metaproterenol Sulfate Inhalation Solution USP (℞)	Twenty-five 2.5 mL Vials 0.4%	49502-678-03
	Twenty-five 2.5 mL Vials 0.6%	49502-676-03
Sodium Chloride Inhalation Solution USP (OTC)	One Hundred 3 mL Vials 0.45%	49502-820-03
	One Hundred 5 mL Vials 0.45%	49502-820-05
	One Hundred 3 mL Vials 0.9%	49502-830-03
	One Hundred 5 mL Vials 0.9%	49502-830-05
	Fifty 15 mL Vials 0.9%	49502-830-50
Sodium Chloride Solution (℞)	Fifty 15 mL Vials 3%	49502-640-15
	Fifty 15 mL Vials 10%	49502-641-15

CUROSURF® ℞
(poractant alfa)
INTRATRACHEAL SUSPENSION

DESCRIPTION

CUROSURF® (poractant alfa) Intratracheal Suspension is a sterile, non-pyrogenic pulmonary surfactant intended for intratracheal use only. It is an extract of natural porcine lung surfactant consisting of 99% polar lipids (mainly phospholipids) and 1% hydrophobic low molecular weight proteins (surfactant associated proteins SP-B and SP-C). It is suspended in 0.9% sodium chloride solution. The pH is adjusted as required with sodium bicarbonate to a pH of 6.2 (5.5–6.5). CUROSURF contains no preservatives.
CUROSURF is a white to creamy white suspension of poractant alfa. Each milliliter of surfactant mixture contains 80 mg of surfactant (including 74 mg of total phospholipids, 54 mg of phosphatidylcholine of which 30.5 mg is dipalmitoyl phosphatidylcholine) and 1 mg of protein including 0.3 mg of SP-B.

CLINICAL PHARMACOLOGY

Mechanism of Action
Endogenous pulmonary surfactant reduces surface tension at the air-liquid interface of the alveoli during ventilation and stabilizes the alveoli against collapse at resting transpulmonary pressures. A deficiency of pulmonary surfactant in preterm infants results in Respiratory Distress Syndrome (RDS) characterized by poor lung expansion, inadequate gas exchange, and a gradual collapse of the lungs (atelectasis). CUROSURF compensates for the deficiency of surfactant and restores surface activity to the lungs of these infants.
Activity
In vitro—CUROSURF lowers minimum surface tension to ≤4mN/m as measured by the Wilhelmy Balance System.
In vivo—In several pharmacodynamic studies, CUROSURF improved lung compliance, pulmonary gas exchange, or survival in premature rabbits.
Pharmacokinetics
CUROSURF is administered directly to the target organ, the lung, where biophysical effects occur at the alveolar surface. No human pharmacokinetic studies to characterize the absorption, biotransformation, or excretion of CUROSURF have been performed. Non-clinical studies have been performed to evaluate the disposition of phospholipids present in CUROSURF.
Animal Metabolism
In both adult and newborn rabbits, approximately 50% of the radiolabeled component was rapidly removed from the alveoli in the first three hours after single intratracheal administration of CUROSURF-^{14}C-DPPC (dipalmitoylphosphatidylcholine). Over a 24-hour period, approximately 45% of the labeled DPPC was cleared from the lungs of adult rabbits compared to approximately 20% in newborn rabbits. In newborn rabbits, CUROSURF-^{14}C-DPPC passed from the alveolar space into the lung parenchyma and then was secreted again into the alveoli, whereas in adult rabbits, most of the DPPC was not recycled. The half-life in the lung appeared to be about 25 hours in adult rabbits and 67 hours in newborn rabbits.
The concentration of ^{14}C-DPPC in alveolar macrophages was ≤2% of that in the lung in newborn and adult rabbits. Of the total ^{14}C-DPPC recovered in newborn rabbits, $<0.6\%$ was found in the serum, liver, kidneys, and brain, respectively, at 48 hours.
No information is available about the metabolic rate of the surfactant-associated proteins in CUROSURF.

CLINICAL STUDIES

The clinical efficacy of CUROSURF was demonstrated in one single-dose study (Study 1) and one multiple-dose study (Study 2) in the treatment of established neonatal RDS involving approximately 500 infants. Each study was randomized, multicenter, and controlled.
In Study 1, infants 700–2000g birth weight with RDS requiring mechanical ventilation and a $FiO_2 \geq 0.60$ were enrolled. CUROSURF 2.5 mL/kg single dose (200 mg/kg) or control (disconnection from the ventilator and manual ventilation for 2 minutes) was administered after RDS developed and before 15 hours of age. The results from Study 1 are shown below in Table 1.

[See table 1 at right]
In Study 2, infants 700–2000g birth weight with RDS requiring mechanical ventilation and a $FiO_2 \geq 0.60$ were enrolled. In this two-arm trial, CUROSURF was administered after RDS developed and before 15 hours of age, as a single-dose or as multiple doses. In the single-dose arm, infants received CUROSURF 2.5mL/kg (200mg/kg). In the multiple-dose arm, the initial dose of CUROSURF was 2.5mL/kg (200mg/kg) and subsequent doses of CUROSURF were 1.25mL/kg (100mg/kg). The results from Study 2 are shown below in Table 2.
[See table 2 at right]

ACUTE CLINICAL EFFECTS
As with other surfactants, marked improvements in oxygenation may occur within minutes of the administration of CUROSURF.

INDICATION AND USAGE

CUROSURF is indicated for the treatment (rescue) of Respiratory Distress Syndrome (RDS) in premature infants. CUROSURF reduces mortality and pneumothoraces associated with RDS.

WARNINGS

CUROSURF is intended for intratracheal use only.
THE ADMINISTRATION OF EXOGENOUS SURFACTANTS, INCLUDING CUROSURF, CAN RAPIDLY AFFECT OXYGENATION AND LUNG COMPLIANCE. Therefore, infants receiving CUROSURF should receive frequent clinical and laboratory assessments so that oxygen and ventilatory support can be modified to respond to respiratory changes. CUROSURF should only be administered by those trained and experienced in the care, resuscitation, and stabilization of pre-term infants.
TRANSIENT ADVERSE EFFECTS SEEN WITH THE ADMINISTRATION OF CUROSURF INCLUDE BRADYCARDIA, HYPOTENSION, ENDOTRACHEAL TUBE BLOCKAGE, AND OXYGEN DESATURATION. These events require stopping Curosurf administration and taking appropriate measures to alleviate the condition. After the patient is stable, dosing may proceed with appropriate monitoring.

PRECAUTIONS

General
Correction of acidosis, hypotension, anemia, hypoglycemia, and hypothermia is recommended prior to CUROSURF administration.
Surfactant administration can be expected to reduce the severity of RDS but will not eliminate the mortality and morbidity associated with other complications of prematurity.
Sufficient information is not available on the effects of administering initial doses of CUROSURF other than 2.5 mL/kg (200 mg/kg), subsequent doses other than 1.25 mL/kg (100 mg/kg), administration of more than three total doses, dosing more frequently than every 12 hours, or initiating therapy with CUROSURF more than 15 hours after diagnosing RDS. Adequate data are not available on the use of CUROSURF in conjunction with experimental therapies of RDS, e.g., high-frequency ventilation.

Carcinogenesis, Mutagenesis, Impairment of Fertility
Studies to assess potential carcinogenic and reproductive effects of CUROSURF, or other surfactants, have not been conducted.
Mutagenicity studies of CUROSURF, which included the Ames test, gene mutation assay in Chinese hamster V79 cells, chromosomal aberration assay in Chinese hamster ovarian cells, unscheduled DNA synthesis in HELA S3 cells, and *in vivo* mouse nuclear test, were negative.

ADVERSE REACTIONS

Transient adverse effects seen with the administration of CUROSURF include bradycardia, hypotension, endotracheal tube blockage, and oxygen desaturation.
The rates of common complications of prematurity observed in Study 1 are shown below in Table 3.
[See table 3 above]
Immunological studies have not demonstrated differences in levels of surfactant-antisurfactant immune complexes and anti-CUROSURF antibodies between patients treated with CUROSURF and patients who received control treatment.

FOLLOW-UP EVALUATIONS
Seventy-six infants (45 treated with CUROSURF) were evaluated at 1 year of age and 73 infants (44 treated with CUROSURF) at 2 years of age. Data from follow-up evaluations for weight and length, persistent respiratory symptoms, incidence of cerebral palsy, visual impairment, or auditory impairment was similar between treatment groups. In 16 patients (10 treated with CUROSURF and 6 controls) evaluated at 5.5 years of age, the developmental quotient, derived using the Griffiths Mental Developmental Scales, was similar between groups.

OVERDOSAGE

There have been no reports of overdosage following the administration of CUROSURF.
In the event of accidental overdosage, and only if there are clear clinical effects on the infant's respiration, ventilation, or oxygenation, as much of the suspension as possible should be aspirated and the infant should be managed with supportive treatment, with particular attention to fluid and electrolyte balance.

DOSAGE AND ADMINISTRATION

FOR INTRATRACHEAL ADMINISTRATION ONLY.
CUROSURF should be administered by, or under the supervision of, clinicians experienced in intubation, ventilatory management, and general care of premature infants.

TABLE 1

EFFICACY PARAMETER	SINGLE DOSE CUROSURF n=78	CONTROL n=67	P-VALUE
	%	%	
MORTALITY at 28 DAYS (ALL CAUSES)	31	48	≤0.05
BRONCHOPULMONARY DYSPLASIA#	18	22	N.S.
PNEUMOTHORAX	21	36	≤0.05
PULMONARY INTERSTITIAL EMPHYSEMA	21	38	≤0.05

#Bronchopulmonary dysplasia (BPD) diagnosed by positive x-ray and supplemental oxygen dependence at 28 days of life.
N.S.: not statistically significant

TABLE 2

EFFICACY PARAMETER	SINGLE-DOSE CUROSURF n=184	MULTIPLE-DOSE CUROSURF n=173	P-VALUE
	%	%	
MORTALITY at 28 DAYS (ALL CAUSES)	21	13	0.048
BPD	18	18	N.S.
PNEUMOTHORAX	17	9	0.03
PULMONARY INTERSTITIAL EMPHYSEMA	27	22	N.S.

N.S.: not statistically significant

TABLE 3
COMPLICATIONS OF PREMATURITY

	CUROSURF 2.5 mL/kg (200 mg/kg) n=78	CONTROL* n=66
	%	%
Acquired Pneumonia	17	21
Acquired Septicemia	14	18
Bronchopulmonary Dysplasia	18	22
Intracranial Hemorrhage	51	64
Patent Ductus Arteriosus	60	48
Pneumothorax	21	36
Pulmonary Interstitial Emphysema	21	38

*Control patients were disconnected from the ventilator and manually ventilated for 2 minutes. No surfactant was instilled.

TABLE 4

WEIGHT (grams)	INITIAL DOSE 2.5 mL/kg	REPEAT DOSE 1.25 mL/kg	WEIGHT (grams)	INITIAL DOSE 2.5 mL/kg	REPEAT DOSE 1.25 mL/kg
	EACH DOSE (mL)			EACH DOSE (mL)	
600–650	1.60	0.80	1301–1350	3.30	1.65
651–700	1.70	0.85	1351–1400	3.50	1.75
701–750	1.80	0.90	1401–1450	3.60	1.80
751–800	2.00	1.00	1451–1500	3.70	1.85
801–850	2.10	1.05	1501–1550	3.80	1.90
851–900	2.20	1.10	1551–1600	4.00	2.00
901–950	2.30	1.15	1601–1650	4.10	2.05
951–1000	2.50	1.25	1651–1700	4.20	2.10
1001–1050	2.60	1.30	1701–1750	4.30	2.15
1051–1100	2.70	1.35	1751–1800	4.50	2.25
1101–1150	2.80	1.40	1801–1850	4.60	2.30
1151–1200	3.00	1.50	1851–1900	4.70	2.35
1201–1250	3.10	1.55	1901–1950	4.80	2.40
1251–1300	3.20	1.60	1951–2000	5.00	2.50

Marked improvements in oxygenation and lung compliance may occur within minutes of administration of CUROSURF. Therefore, the infant should receive frequent clinical and laboratory assessments such that oxygen and ventilator support can be modified to respond to respiratory status changes.

Dosage
The initial dose of CUROSURF is 2.5 mL per kg birth weight. Up to 2 subsequent doses of 1.25 mL/kg birth weight can be administered at 12-hour intervals if needed (i.e., in infants who remain intubated and require mechanical ventilation and supplemental oxygen). Dosages may be determined from the following CUROSURF dosing chart for a range of birth weights.
[See table 4 above]

Directions for Use
CUROSURF should be inspected visually for discoloration prior to administration. The color of CUROSURF is white to creamy white. CUROSURF should be stored in a refrigerator at +2 to +8°C (36–46°F). Before use, the vial should be slowly warmed to room temperature and gently turned upside-down, in order to obtain a uniform suspension. DO NOT SHAKE.
Unopened, unused vials of CUROSURF that have warmed to room temperature can be returned to refrigerated storage within 24 hours for future use. Do not warm to room temperature and return to refrigerated storage more than once. Protect from light. Each single-use vial should be entered only once and the vial with any unused material should be discarded after the initial entry.

General
CUROSURF is administered intratracheally by instillation through a 5-French end-hole catheter (cut to a standard length of 8 cm) inserted into the infant's endotracheal tube, with the tip positioned distally in the endotracheal tube. The catheter tip should not extend beyond the distal tip of the endotracheal tube. Each dose of CUROSURF should be administered as two aliquots, with each aliquot administered into one of the two main bronchi by positioning the infant with either the right or left side dependent.
Before administering CUROSURF, assure proper placement and patency of the endotracheal tube. At the discretion of the clinician, the endotracheal tube may be suctioned before administering CUROSURF. The infant should be allowed to stabilize before proceeding with dosing.

Initial Dose
The initial recommended dose of CUROSURF is 2.5 mL/kg birth weight. This dose may be determined from the CUROSURF dosing chart (see Table 4).
Slowly withdraw the entire contents of the vial of CUROSURF into a 3 or 5mL plastic syringe through a large-gauge needle (e.g., at least 20 gauge). Attach the pre-cut 8 cm 5 French catheter to the syringe. Fill the catheter with CUROSURF. Discard excess CUROSURF through the catheter so that only the total dose to be given remains in the syringe.
Immediately before CUROSURF administration, the infant's ventilator settings should be changed to a rate of 40–60 breaths/minute, inspiratory time 0.5 second, and supplemental oxygen sufficient to maintain $SaO_2 > 92\%$. Keep the infant in a neutral position (head and body in alignment without inclination). Briefly disconnect the endotracheal tube from the ventilator. Insert the pre-cut 5 French catheter into the endotracheal tube and instill the first aliquot (1.25 mL/kg birth weight) of CUROSURF. The infant should be positioned such that either the right or left side is dependent for this aliquot. After the first aliquot of the surfactant is instilled, remove the catheter from the endotracheal tube and manually ventilate the infant with 100% oxygen at a rate of 40–60 breaths/minute for one minute. When the infant is stable, reposition the infant such that the other side is dependent and administer the remaining aliquot using the same procedures. After instillation of the second aliquot, remove the catheter without flushing. Do not suction airways for 1 hour after surfactant instillation unless signs of significant airway obstruction occur.
After completion of the dosing procedure, resume usual ventilator management and clinical care. In the clinical trials, ventilator management was modified to maintain a PaO_2 of about 55mmHg, $PaCO_2$ of 35–45, and pH >7.3.

Continued on next page

Curosurf—Cont.

Repeat doses
Up to two repeat doses of 1.25 mL/kg birth weight each may be administered, using the same technique described for the initial dose. Repeat doses should be administered, at approximately 12-hour intervals, in infants who remain intubated and in whom RDS is considered responsible for their persisting or deteriorating respiratory status. The maximum recommended total dose (sum of the initial and up to two repeat doses) is 5 mL/kg.

Dosing Precautions
Transient episodes of bradycardia, decreased oxygen saturation, reflux of the surfactant into the endotracheal tube, and airway obstruction have occurred during the dosing procedure of CUROSURF. These events require interrupting the administration of CUROSURF and taking the appropriate measures to alleviate the condition. After stabilization, dosing may resume with appropriate monitoring.

HOW SUPPLIED
CUROSURF® (poractant alfa) Intratracheal Suspension (NDC Numbers: 49502-180-01 [1.5 mL]; 49502-180-03 [3 mL]) is available in sterile, ready-to-use rubber-stoppered clear glass vials containing 1.5 mL (120 mg phospholipids) or 3 mL (240 mg phospholipids) of suspension. One vial per carton.
Store CUROSURF Intratracheal Suspension in a refrigerator at +2 to +8°C (36–46°F). Unopened vials of CUROSURF may be warmed to room temperature for up to 24 hours prior to use. CUROSURF should not be warmed to room temperature and returned to the refrigerator more than once. PROTECT FROM LIGHT. Do not shake. Vials are for single use only. After opening the vial discard the unused portion of the drug.
Rx only.
Manufactured for:
DEY
2751 Napa Valley Corporate Drive
Napa, CA 94558
Manufactured by and licensed from:
Chiesi Farmaceutici, S.p.A.
Parma, Italy 43100
03-572-02 A
6/00

Shown in Product Identification Guide, page 311

EASIVENT™ ℞

Valved Holding Chamber For Use With Metered Dose Inhalers

Instructions For Use With Metered-Dose Inhalers
Read complete instructions carefully before use.

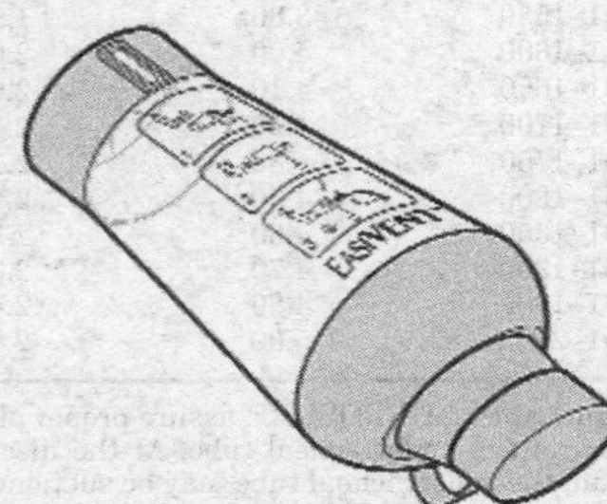

Retail Product No: 49502-207-01
EasiVent™ Valved Holding Chamber is designed to assist with metered dose inhaler (MDI) aerosol medication delivery. Using your inhaler with EasiVent™ Valved Holding Chamber is easier than using your MDI alone. It helps deliver medication from your MDI to your lungs by selectively removing most large particles that normally stay in the mouth and throat, thus allowing the smaller particles to enter and be deposited in the lungs.
Please read all instructions for your EasiVent™ Valved Holding Chamber before your first use. Always remember your MDI canister contains the medicine your doctor has prescribed for you. When using EasiVent™ Valved Holding Chamber, only use as many doses (puffs) as directed by your doctor.

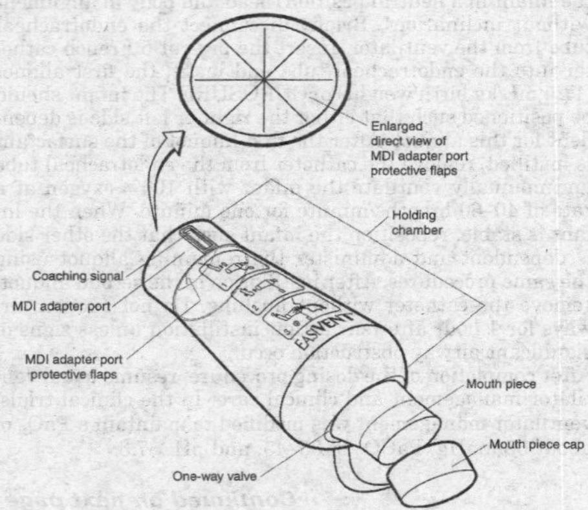

1 Remove both your inhaler and the EasiVent™ Valved Holding Chamber from their boxes.

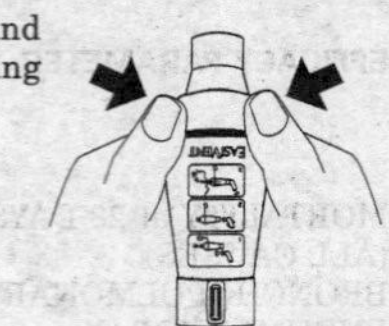

2 To open the EasiVent™ Valved Holding Chamber remove the mouthpiece cap from the EasiVent Valved Holding Chamber and hold the unit in both hands with the mouthpiece facing away from your body. Press down on the mouthpiece with both thumbs.

3 Remove the mouthpiece cap from your MDI.

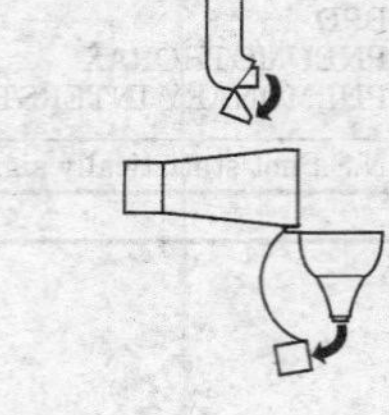

4 Visually inspect the EasiVent™ Valved Holding Chamber for any objects that do not belong there before each use.
5 Close the EasiVent™ Valved Holding Chamber and confirm that it is closed. Confirm that all parts are secure.

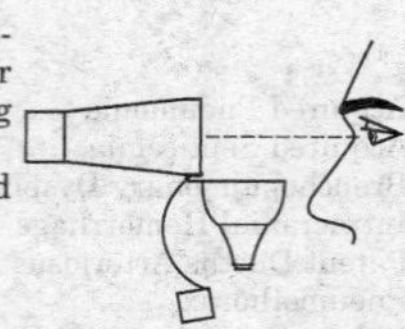

6 Vigorously shake the MDI 4 or 5 times. Place the MDI mouthpiece into the MDI adapter port at the end of the EasiVent™ Valved Holding Chamber (see illustration). Be sure the MDI is completely inserted into the adapter port of the EasiVent™ Valved Holding Chamber.
7 Place the mouthpiece of the EasiVent™ Valved Holding Chamber in your mouth, closing your lips tightly around the mouthpiece.

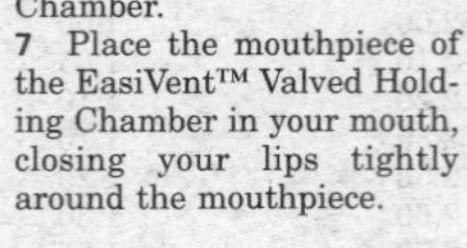

8 Exhale normally and press down firmly on the MDI one time to release one puff of medication. Immediately begin inhaling slowly and deeply THROUGH THE MOUTH until a full breath is taken. If you hear a whistle from the coaching signal, inhale more slowly.

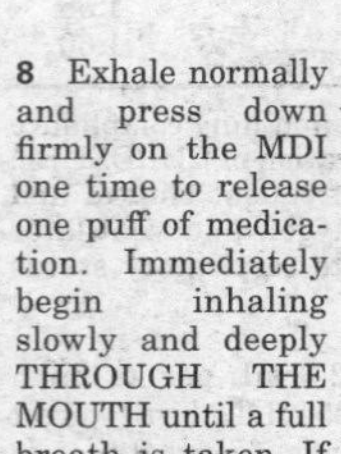

9 Remove the EasiVent™ Valved Holding Chamber from your mouth; hold your breath for 5 to 10 seconds (to improve medicine delivery) before exhaling normally.
10 If your doctor has prescribed more than one dose (puff) of medication, you should wait at least one minute between puffs, and repeat steps 6 through 8 as necessary.
11 After use, remove the MDI from the adapter port and replace the mouthpiece cap on your MDI. Open the EasiVent™ Valved Holding Chamber (see item 2) and store your MDI inside. Close the lid (ensuring that it closes easily) and replace the mouthpiece cap.

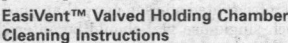

EasiVent™ Valved Holding Chamber Cleaning Instructions
The EasiVent™ Valved Holding Chamber is manufactured from high quality, durable plastic and latex free materials. It is recomended you clean the device once a week to prevent medication build-up inside the unit.

1 Separate the lid and body of the EasiVent™ Valved Holding Chamber at the midpoint as shown.

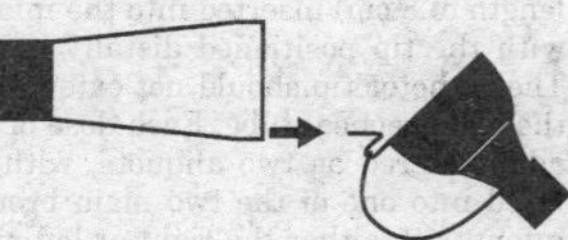

2 Remove the mouthpiece cover. Wash the EasiVent™ Valved Holding Chamber BY HAND in warm water with a mild soap. Rinse all parts with clean water, shake out any excess water, and allow to air dry or use a soft cloth.

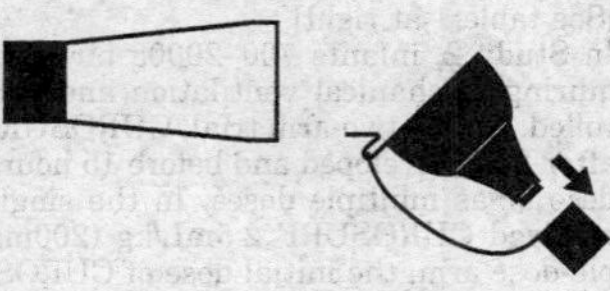

3 Be sure that all parts are dry before reassembling your EasiVent™ Valved Holding Chamber. Insert the tab of the lid into the slot on the chamber as shown, replace the mouthpiece cap, and close the lid (ensuring that it closes easily).

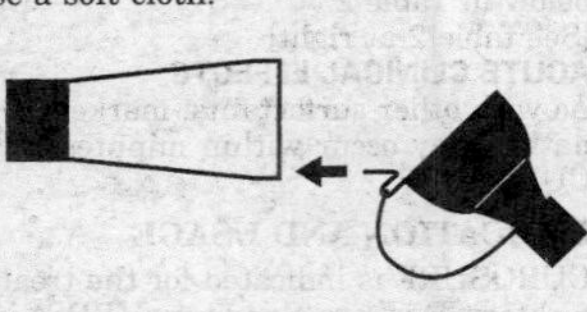

Masks
Masks are available for the EasiVent™ Valved Holding Chamber in small, medium and large sizes.
CAUTION: Federal (USA) law restricts this device to sale by or on the order of a physician.
Manufactured for
Dey
Napa, CA 94558, U.S.A.
by DHD Healthcare
Canastota, NY 13032, U.S.A.
Pat. Pending
For information call:
1-800-527-4278
1/99
03-552-00

Shown in Product Identification Guide, page 311

EPIPEN® 0.3 mg brand of ℞

EPINEPHRINE AUTO-INJECTOR
Auto-Injector for Intramuscular Injection of Epinephrine For the Emergency Treatment of Allergic Reactions (Anaphylaxis)
Delivers 0.3 mg intramuscular dose of epinephrine from epinephrine injection, USP, 1:1000 (0.3 mL).

EPIPEN® JR. 0.15 mg ℞

EPINEPHRINE AUTO-INJECTOR
Auto-Injector for Intramuscular Injection of Epinephrine For the Emergency Treatment of Allergic Reactions (Anaphylaxis)
Delivers 0.15 mg intramuscular dose of epinephrine from epinephrine injection, USP, 1:2000 (0.3 mL).

IMPORTANT INFORMATION

- **DO NOT REMOVE SAFETY CAP UNTIL READY FOR USE.**
- **ONLY 0.3 ML OF SOLUTION IS DISPENSED. THE MAJORITY OF THE DRUG PRODUCT, 1.7 ML, REMAINS IN THE AUTO-INJECTOR AFTER ACTIVATION.**
- **THE UNIT CONTAINS NO LATEX.**

DESCRIPTION
The EpiPen and EpiPen Jr. auto-injectors contain 2 mL epinephrine injection for emergency intramuscular use. Each EpiPen auto-injector delivers a single dose of 0.3 mg epinephrine from epinephrine injection, USP, 1:1000 (0.3 mL) in a sterile solution.
Each EpiPen Jr. auto-injector delivers a single dose of 0.15 mg epinephrine from epinephrine injection, USP, 1:2000 (0.3 mL) in a sterile solution.
For stability purposes, approximately 1.7 mL remains in the auto-injector after activation.
Each 0.3 mL in EpiPen contains 0.3 mg epinephrine, 1.8 mg sodium chloride, 0.5 mg sodium metabisulfite, hydrochloric acid to adjust pH, and Water for Injection. The pH range is 2.2–5.0.
Each 0.3 mL in EpiPen Jr. contains 0.15 mg epinephrine, 1.8 mg sodium chloride, 0.5 mg sodium metabisulfite, hydrochloric acid to adjust pH, and Water for Injection. The pH range is 2.2–5.0.
Epinephrine is a sympathomimetic catecholamine. Chemically, epinephrine is B-(3, 4-dihydroxyphenyl)-a-methylaminoethanol, with the following structure:

OH
HO — C — CH_2NHCH_3
HO H

It deteriorates rapidly on exposure to air or light, turning pink from oxidation to adrenochrome and brown from the formation of melanin. Epinephrine solutions which show evidence of discoloration should be replaced.

CLINICAL PHARMACOLOGY
Epinephrine is a sympathomimetic drug, acting on both alpha and beta receptors. It is the drug of choice for the emergency treatment of severe allergic reactions (Type I) to insect stings or bites, foods, drugs, and other allergens. It can also be used in the treatment of idiopathic or exercise-induced anaphylaxis. Epinephrine when given subcutaneously or intramuscularly has a rapid onset and short duration of action. The strong vasoconstrictor action of epinephrine through its effect on alpha adrenergic receptors acts

quickly to counter vasodilation and increased vascular permeability which can lead to loss of intravascular fluid volume and hypotension during anaphylactic reactions. Epinephrine through its action on beta receptors on bronchial smooth muscle causes bronchial smooth muscle relaxation which alleviates wheezing and dyspnea. Epinephrine also alleviates pruritis, urticaria, and angioedema and may be effective in relieving gastrointestinal and genitourinary symptoms associated with anaphylaxis.

INDICATIONS AND USAGE

Epinephrine is indicated in the emergency treatment of allergic reactions (anaphylaxis) to insect stings or bites, foods, drugs and other allergens as well as idiopathic or exercise-induced anaphylaxis. The EpiPen and EpiPen Jr. auto-injectors are intended for immediate self-administration by a person with a history of an anaphylactic reaction. Such reactions may occur within minutes after exposure and consist of flushing, apprehension, syncope, tachycardia, thready or unobtainable pulse associated with a fall in blood pressure, convulsions, vomiting, diarrhea and abdominal cramps, involuntary voiding, wheezing, dyspnea due to laryngeal spasm, pruritis, rashes, uticaria or angioedema. The EpiPen and EpiPen Jr. are designed as emergency supportive therapy only and are not a replacement or substitute for immediate medical or hospital care.

CONTRAINDICATIONS

There are no absolute contraindications to the use of epinephrine in a life-threatening situation.

WARNINGS

Epinephrine is light sensitive and should be stored in the tube provided. Store at room temperature (15°–30°C/59°–86°F). Do not refrigerate. Before using, check to make sure solution in auto-injector is not discolored. Replace the auto-injector if the solution is discolored or contains a precipitate. Avoid possible inadvertent intravascular administration. EpiPen and EpiPen Jr. should **only** be injected into the anterolateral aspect of the thigh. DO NOT INJECT INTO BUTTOCK.

Large doses or accidental intravenous injection of epinephrine may result in cerebral hemorrhage due to sharp rise in blood pressure. DO NOT INJECT INTRAVENOUSLY. Rapidly acting vasodilators can counteract the marked pressor effects of epinehrine.

Epinephrine is the preferred treatment for serious allergic or other emergency situations even through this product contains sodium metabisulfite, a sulfite that may in other products cause allergic-type reactions including anaphylactic symptoms or life-threatening or less severe asthmatic episodes in certain susceptible persons. The alternatives to using epinephrine in a life-threatening situation may not be satisfactory. The presence of a sulfite in this product should not deter administration of the drug for treatment of serious allergic or other emergency situations.

Accidental injection into the hands or feet may result in loss of blood flow to the affected area and should be avoided. If there is an accidental injection into these areas, advise the patient to go immediately to the nearest emergency room for treatment. EpiPen and EpiPen Jr. should **only** be injected into the anterolateral aspect of the thigh.

PRECAUTIONS

Epinephrine is essential for the treatment of anaphylaxis. Patients with a history of severe allergic reactions (anaphylaxis) to insect stings or bites, foods, drugs, and other allergens as well as idiopathic and exercise-induced anaphylaxis should be carefully instructed about the circumstances under which this life-saving medication should be used. It must be clearly determined that the patient is at risk of future anaphylaxis, since the following risks may be associated with epinephrine administration (see Dosage and Administration).

Epinephrine is ordinarily administered with extreme caution to patients who have heart disease. Use of epinephrine with drugs that may sensitize the heart to arrhythmias, e.g., digitalis, mercurial diurectics, or quinidine, ordinarily is not recommended. Anginal pain may be induced by epinephrine in patients with coronary insufficiency.

The effects of epinephrine may be potentiated by tricyclic antidepressants and monoamine oxidase inhibitors.

Some patients may be at greater risk of developing adverse reactions after epinephrine administration. These include: hyperthyroid individuals, individuals with cardiovascular disease, hypertension, or diabetes, elderly individuals, pregnant women, pediatric patients under 30 kg (66 lbs.) body weight using EpiPen, and pediatric patients under 15 kg (33 lbs.) body weight using EpiPen Jr.

Despite these concerns, epinephrine is essential for the treatment of anaphylaxis. Therefore, patients with these conditions, and/or any other person who might be in a position to administer EpiPen or EpiPen Jr. to a patient experiencing anaphylaxis should be carefully instructed in regard to the circumstances under which this life-saving medication should be used.

CARCINOGENESIS, MUTAGENESIS, IMPAIRMENT OF FERTILITY

Studies of epinephrine in animals to evaluate the carcinogenic and mutagenic potential or the effect on fertility have not been conducted. This should not prevent the use of this life-saving medication under the conditions noted under INDICATIONS AND USAGE and as indicated under PRECAUTIONS above.

USAGE IN PREGNANCY

Pregnancy Category C: Epinephrine has been shown to be teratogenic in rats when given in doses about 25 times the human dose. There are no adequate and well-controlled studies in pregnant women. Epinephrine should be used during pregnancy only if the potential benefit justifies the potential risk to the fetus.

PEDIATRIC USE

Epinephrine may be given safely to pediatric patients at a dosage appropriate to body weight (see Dosage and Administration).

ADVERSE REACTIONS

Side effects of epinephrine may include palpitations, tachycardia, sweating, nausea and vomiting, respiratory difficulty, pallor, dizziness, weakness, tremor, headache, apprehension, nervousness and anxiety.

Cardiac arrhythmias may follow administration of epinephrine.

OVERDOSAGE

Overdosage or inadvertent intravascular injection of epinephrine may cause cerebral hemorrhage resulting from a sharp rise in blood pressure. Fatalities may also result from pulmonary edema because of peripheral vascular constriction together with cardiac stimulation.

DOSAGE AND ADMINISTRATION

A physician who prescribes EpiPen or EpiPen Jr. should take appropriate steps to insure that the patient (or parent) understands the indications and use of this device thoroughly. The physician should review with the patient or any other person who might be in a position to administer EpiPen or EpiPen Jr. to a patient experiencing anaphylaxis, in detail, the patient instructions and operation of the EpiPen or EpiPen Jr. auto-injector. Inject the delivered dose of the EpiPen auto-injector (0.3 mL epinephrine injection, USP, 1:1000) or the EpiPen Jr. auto-injector (0.3 mL epinephrine injection, USP, 1:2000) intramuscularly into the anterolateral aspect of the thigh, through clothing if necessary. See detailed Directions for Use on the accompanying Patient Instructions.

Usual epinephrine adult dose for allergic emergencies is 0.3 mg. For pediatric use, the appropriate dosage may be 0.15 or 0.30 mg depending upon the body weight of the patient. A dosage of 0.01 mg/kg body weight is recommended. EpiPen Jr., which provides a dosage of 0.15 mg, may be more appropriate for patients weighing less than 30 kg. However, the prescribing physician has the option of prescribing more or less than these amounts, based on careful assessment of each individual patient and recognizing the life-threatening nature of the reactions for which this drug is being prescribed. The physician should consider using other forms of injectable epinephrine if doses lower than 0.15 mg are felt to be necessary.

With severe persistent anaphylaxis, repeat injections with an additional EpiPen may be necessary.

Parenteral drug products should be periodically inspected visually by the patient for particulate matter or discoloration and should be replaced if these are present.

HOW SUPPLIED

EpiPen auto-injectors (epinephrine injection, USP, 1:1000, 0.3 mL) are available in individual cartons, NDC 49502-500-01.

EpiPen Jr. auto-injectors (epinephrine injection, USP, 1:2000, 0.3 mL) are available in individual cartons, NDC 49502-501-01.

Store in a dark place at room temperature (15°–30°C/59°–86°F). Do not refrigerate. Contains no latex.

Rx only.

DEY

Manufactured for Dey, Napa, California, 94558, U.S.A
by Meridian Medical Technologies, Inc.,
Columbia, MD 21046, U.S.A.

Shown in Product Identification Guide, page 311

Dista Products Company

Division of Eli Lilly and Company
General Offices
LILLY CORPORATE CENTER
INDIANAPOLIS, INDIANA 46285

Direct Inquiries to:
Dista Products and Eli Lilly and Company
Lilly Corporate Center
Indianapolis, IN 46285
(317) 276-2000
www.dista.com

For Medical Information Contact:
Lilly Research Laboratories
Lilly Corporate Center
Indianapolis, IN 46285
(800) 545-5979

LEGEND

Identi-Code®—*Formula Identification Code, Dista*
Identi-Dose®—*Unit Dose Medication, Dista*
Pulvules®—*Filled Gelatin Capsules, Dista*
℞Pak—*Prescription Package, Dista*

IDENTI-CODE® Index
(formula identification code, Dista)
Provides Positive Product Identification

A letter-number symbol, a 4-digit number, the name of the product, the strength of the product, or a combination of these appears on each Dista capsule and tablet and on each label of pediatric liquids and powders for oral suspension. The letter/number or 4-digit number identifies the product.

Identi-
Code® Product Name

Coated **Tablets**

Pulvules®

3104 Prozac®
Composition (Each Pulvule®): fluoxetine hydrochloride, 10 mg (equiv. to fluoxetine)

3105 Prozac®
Composition (Each Pulvule®): fluoxetine hydrochloride, 20 mg (equiv. to fluoxetine)

3107 Prozac®
Composition (Each Pulvule®): fluoxetine hydrochloride, 40 mg (equiv. to fluoxetine)

402 Keflex®
Composition (Each Pulvule®): Cephalexin, USP, 250 mg

403 Keflex®
Composition (Each Pulvule®): Cephalexin, USP, 500 mg

UNIT-DOSE PACKAGING

Identi-Dose® (unit dose medication, Dista) Closed-circuit control of medication from pharmacy to nurse to patient and return. Simplifies counting and dispensing whether in single-unit or prescription-size quantities. Fits into any dispensing system for ready identification and legibility, better inventory control, protection from contamination, easier handling and recording under Medicare, prevention of drug loss through pilferage or spilling, better control of Federal Controlled Substances, and less chance of medication errors.

The following products are available through normal channels of supply:

Identi-Dose®
Pulvules®
No.
3104 Prozac®, 10 mg
3105 Prozac®, 20 mg
3107 Prozac®, 40 mg

ILOTYCIN® ℞

[*ī-lō-tĭ ′-sĭn*]
(erythromycin)
Ophthalmic Ointment, USP, 0.5%
(Sterile)

DESCRIPTION

Ilotycin® (Erythromycin Ophthalmic Ointment, USP) belongs to the macrolide group of antibiotics. It is basic and readily forms a salt when combined with an acid. The base, as crystals or powder, is slightly soluble in water, moderately soluble in ether, and readily soluble in alcohol or chloroform. Erythromycin is an antibiotic produced from a strain of *Streptomyces erythraeus*. The special sterile ophthalmic ointment base flows freely over the conjunctiva. It has the following structural formula:

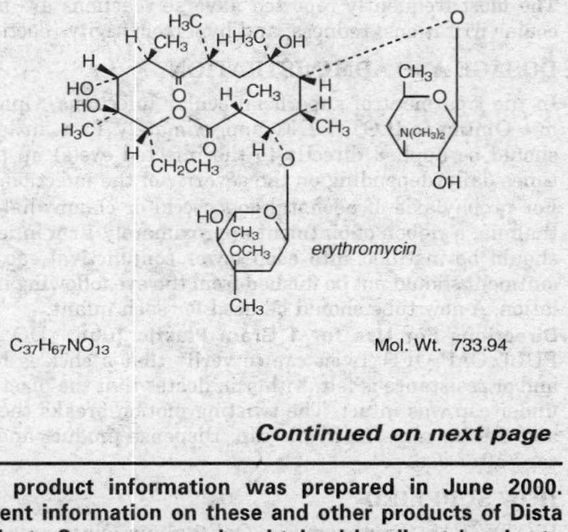

erythromycin

$C_{37}H_{67}NO_{13}$ Mol. Wt. 733.94

Continued on next page

This product information was prepared in June 2000. Current information on these and other products of Dista Products Company may be obtained by direct inquiry to Lilly Research Laboratories, Lilly Corporate Center, Indianapolis, Indiana 46285, (800) 545-5979.

Ilotycin—Cont.

Chemical Name: (3R*, 4S*, 5S*, 6R*, 7R*, 9R*, 11R*, 12R*, 13S*, 14R*)-4-[(2,6-Dideoxy-3-C-methyl-3-*O*-methyl-α-L-*ribo*-hexopyranosyl)oxy]-14-ethyl-7, 12, 13-trihydroxy-3, 5, 7, 9, 11, 13-hexamethyl-6-[[3, 4, 6-trideoxy-3-(dimethylamino)-β-D-*xylo*-hexopyranosyl]oxy]oxacyclotetradecane-2,10-dione.

Each Gram Contains: ACTIVE: Erythromycin, USP, 5 mg (0.5%); INACTIVES: White Petrolatum, Mineral Oil.

CLINICAL PHARMACOLOGY

Microbiology—Erythromycin inhibits protein synthesis without affecting nucleic acid synthesis. Erythromycin is usually active against the following organisms *in vitro* and in clinical infections:

Streptococcus pyogenes (group A β-hemolytic)
Alpha-hemolytic streptococci (viridans group)
Staphylococcus aureus, including penicillinase-producing strains (methicillin-resistant staphylococci are uniformly resistant to erythromycin)
Streptococcus pneumoniae
Mycoplasma pneumoniae (Eaton Agent, PPLO)
Haemophilus influenzae (not all strains of this organism are susceptible at the erythromycin concentrations ordinarily achieved)
Treponema pallidum
Corynebacterium diphtheriae
Neisseria gonorrhoeae
Chlamydia trachomatis

INDICATIONS AND USAGE

For the treatment of superficial ocular infections involving the conjunctiva and/or cornea caused by organisms susceptible to Ilotycin®.

For prophylaxis of ophthalmia neonatorum due to *N. gonorrhoeae* or *C. trachomatis.*

The effectiveness of erythromycin in the prevention of ophthalmia caused by penicillinase-producing *N. gonorrhoeae* is not established.

For infants born to mothers with clinically apparent gonorrhea, intravenous or intramuscular injections of aqueous crystalline penicillin G should be given; a single dose of 50,000 units for term infants or 20,000 units for infants of low birth weight. Topical prophylaxis alone is inadequate for these infants.

CONTRAINDICATIONS

This drug is contraindicated in patients with a history of hypersensitivity to erythromycin.

PRECAUTIONS

General—The use of antimicrobial agents may be associated with the overgrowth of nonsusceptible organisms including fungi; in such a case, antibiotic administration should be stopped and appropriate measures taken.

Information for Patients—Avoid contaminating the tip of container with material from the eye, fingers, or other source.

Carcinogenesis, Mutagenesis, Impairment of Fertility —Two year oral studies conducted in rats with erythromycin did not provide evidence of tumorigenicity. Mutagenicity studies have not been conducted. No evidence of impaired fertility or harm to the fetus that appeared related to erythromycin was reported in these studies.

Pregnancy—Pregnancy Category B—Reproduction studies have been performed in rats, mice, and rabbits using erythromycin and its various salts and esters, at doses that were several multiples of the usual human dose. There are, however, no adequate and well-controlled studies in pregnant women. Because animal reproductive studies are not always predictive of human response, the erythromycins should be used during pregnancy only if clearly needed.

Nursing Mothers—Caution should be exercised when erythromycin is administered to a nursing woman.

Pediatric Use—See INDICATIONS AND USAGE and DOSAGE AND ADMINISTRATION.

ADVERSE REACTIONS

The most frequently reported adverse reactions are minor ocular irritations, redness, and hypersensitivity reactions.

DOSAGE AND ADMINISTRATION

In the treatment of superficial ocular infections, Ophthalmic Ointment ILOTYCIN® approximately 1 cm in length should be applied directly to the infected eye(s) up to six times daily, depending on the severity of the infection.

For prophylaxis of neonatal gonococcal or chlamydial ophthalmia, a ribbon of ointment approximately 1 cm in length should be instilled into each lower conjunctival sac. The ointment should not be flushed from the eye following instillation. A new tube should be used for each infant.

Directions For Use for 1 Gram Plastic Tube: DO NOT PULL CAP OFF. Twist cap to verify that a click is heard and/or resistance is felt. Either indicates that the plastic tip under cap was intact. The twisting motion breaks the seal and the tip remains in the cap. Dispense product and discard after use.

HOW SUPPLIED

ILOTYCIN® (Erythromycin Ophthalmic Ointment, USP, 0.5%) No. 52 is available in the following sizes:

1/8 oz. (3.5 g) tamper-resistant tube—(NDC 0777-1863-17-Prod. No. FL09234

DO NOT USE IF BOTTOM RIDGE OF TUBE CAP IS EXPOSED.

1 g plastic container (in cartons of 50)—(NDC 0777-1863-55)-Prod. No. FL09232

DO NOT USE IF CLICK IS NOT HEARD AND/OR RESISTANCE IS NOT FELT.

Storage: Store between 15°–30°C (59°–86°F).
KEEP OUT OF REACH OF CHILDREN.

Caution: Federal law prohibits dispensing without prescription.

KEFLEX® ℞

[*kĕf 'lĕks*]
(cephalexin)
USP

DESCRIPTION

Keflex® (Cephalexin, USP) is a semisynthetic cephalosporin antibiotic intended for oral administration. It is 7-(D-α-Amino-α-phenylacetamido)-3-methyl-3-cephem-4-carboxylic acid monohydrate. Cephalexin has the molecular formula $C_{16}H_{17}N_3O_4S \cdot H_2O$ and the molecular weight is 365.41.

Cephalexin has the following structural formula:

HO O CH3 • H2O N— H H2N H S H H

The nucleus of cephalexin is related to that of other cephalosporin antibiotics. The compound is a zwitterion; ie, the molecule contains both a basic and an acidic group. The isoelectric point of cephalexin in water is approximately 4.5 to 5.

The crystalline form of cephalexin which is available is a monohydrate. It is a white crystalline solid having a bitter taste. Solubility in water is low at room temperature; 1 or 2 mg/mL may be dissolved readily, but higher concentrations are obtained with increasing difficulty.

The cephalosporins differ from penicillins in the structure of the bicyclic ring system. Cephalexin has a *D*-phenylglycyl group as substituent at the 7-amino position and an unsubstituted methyl group at the 3-position.

Each Pulvule® contains cephalexin monohydrate equivalent to 250 mg (720 µmol) or 500 mg (1,439 µmol) of cephalexin. The Pulvules also contain cellulose, D & C Yellow No. 10, F D & C Blue No. 1, F D & C Yellow No. 6, gelatin, magnesium stearate, silicone, titanium dioxide, and other inactive ingredients.

After mixing, each 5 mL of Keflex, for Oral Suspension, will contain cephalexin monohydrate equivalent to 125 mg (360 µmol) or 250 mg (720 µmol) of cephalexin. The suspensions also contain flavors, methylcellulose, silicone, sodium lauryl sulfate, and sucrose. The 125-mg suspension contains F D & C Red No. 40, and the 250-mg suspension contains F D & C Yellow No. 6.

CLINICAL PHARMACOLOGY

Human Pharmacology —Keflex is acid stable and may be given without regard to meals. It is rapidly absorbed after oral administration. Following doses of 250 mg, 500 mg, and 1 g, average peak serum levels of approximately 9, 18, and 32 µg/mL respectively were obtained at 1 hour. Measurable levels were present 6 hours after administration. Cephalexin is excreted in the urine by glomerular filtration and tubular secretion. Studies showed that over 90% of the drug was excreted unchanged in the urine within 8 hours. During this period, peak urine concentrations following the 250-mg, 500-mg, and 1-g doses were approximately 1,000, 2,200, and 5,000 µg/mL respectively.

Microbiology—In vitro tests demonstrate that the cephalosporins are bactericidal because of their inhibition of cell-wall synthesis. Cephalexin has been shown to be active against most strains of the following microorganisms both *in vitro* and in clinical infections as described in the INDICATIONS AND USAGE section.

Aerobes, Gram-positive:
Staphylococcus aureus (including penicillinase-producing strains)
Staphylococcus epidermidis (penicillin-susceptible strains)
Streptococcus pneumoniae
Streptococcus pyogenes

Aerobes, Gram-negative:
Escherichia coli
Haemophilus influenzae
Klebsiella pneumoniae
Moraxella (Branhamella) catarrhalis
Proteus mirabilis

Note—Methicillin-resistant staphylococci and most strains of enterococci (*Enterococcus faecalis* [formerly *Streptococcus faecalis*]) are resistant to cephalosporins, including cephalexin. It is not active against most strains of *Enterobacter* spp, *Morganella morganii* and *Proteus vulgaris.* It has no activity against *Pseudomonas* spp or *Acinetobacter calcoaceticus.*

Susceptibility Tests —**Diffusion techniques**: Quantitative methods that require measurement of zone diameters provide reproducible estimates of the susceptibility of bacteria to antimicrobial compounds. One such standardized procedure[1] that has been recommended for use with disks to test the susceptibility of microorganisms to cephalexin uses the 30-µg cephalothin disk. Interpretation involves correlation of the diameter obtained in the disk test with the minimal inhibitory concentration (MIC) for cephalexin.

Reports from the laboratory providing results of the standard single-disk susceptibility test with a 30-µg cephalothin disk should be interpreted according to the following criteria:

Zone Diameter (mm)	Interpretation
≥18	(S) Susceptible
15–17	(I) Intermediate
≤14	(R) Resistant

A report of "Susceptible" indicates that the pathogen is likely to be inhibited by usually achievable concentrations of the antimicrobial compound in blood. A report of "Intermediate" indicates that the result should be considered equivocal, and, if the microorganism is not fully susceptible to alternative, clinically feasible drugs, the test should be repeated. This category implies possible clinical applicability in body sites where the drug is physiologically concentrated or in situations where high dosage of drug can be used. This category also provides a buffer zone that prevents small uncontrolled technical factors from causing major discrepancies in interpretation. A report of "Resistant" indicates that usually achievable concentrations of the antimicrobial compound in the blood are unlikely to be inhibitory and that other therapy should be selected.

Measurement of MIC or MBC and achieved antimicrobial compound concentrations may be appropriate to guide therapy in some infections. (See CLINICAL PHARMACOLOGY section for information on drug concentrations achieved in infected body sites and other pharmacokinetic properties of this antimicrobial drug product.)

Standardized susceptibility test procedures require the use of laboratory control microorganisms. The 30-µg cephalothin disk should provide the following zone diameters in these laboratory test quality control strains:

Microorganism	Zone Diameter (mm)
E. coli ATCC 25922	15–21
S. aureus ATCC 25923	29–37

Dilution techniques:
Quantitative methods that are used to determine MICs provide reproducible estimates of the susceptibility of bacteria to antimicrobial compounds. One such standardized procedure uses a standardized dilution method[2] (broth, agar, microdilution) or equivalent with cephalothin powder. The MIC values obtained should be interpreted according to the following criteria:

MIC (µg/mL)	Interpretation
≤8	(S) Susceptible
16	(I) Intermediate
≥32	(R) Resistant

Interpretation should be as stated above for results using diffusion techniques.

As with standard diffusion techniques, dilution methods require the use of laboratory control microorganisms. Standard cephalothin powder should provide the following MIC values:

Microorganism	MIC (µg/mL)
E. coli ATCC 25922	4–16
S. aureus ATCC 29213	0.12–0.5

INDICATIONS AND USAGE

Keflex is indicated for the treatment of the following infections when caused by susceptible strains of the designated microorganisms:

Respiratory tract infections caused by *S. pneumoniae* and *S. pyogenes* (Penicillin is the usual drug of choice in the treatment and prevention of streptococcal infections, including the prophylaxis of rheumatic fever. Keflex is generally effective in the eradication of streptococci from the nasopharynx; however, substantial data establishing the efficacy of Keflex in the subsequent prevention of rheumatic fever are not available at present.)

Otitis media due to *S. pneumoniae, H. influenzae,* staphylococci, streptococci, and *M. catarrhalis*

Skin and skin structure infections caused by staphylococci and/or streptococci

Bone infections caused by staphylococci and/or *P. mirabilis*

Genitourinary tract infections, including acute prostatitis, caused by *E. coli, P. mirabilis,* and *K. pneumoniae*

Note —Culture and susceptibility tests should be initiated prior to and during therapy. Renal function studies should be performed when indicated.

CONTRAINDICATIONS

Keflex is contraindicated in patients with known allergy to the cephalosporin group of antibiotics.

WARNINGS

BEFORE CEPHALEXIN THERAPY IS INSTITUTED, CAREFUL INQUIRY SHOULD BE MADE CONCERNING PREVIOUS HYPERSENSITIVITY REACTIONS TO CEPHALOSPORINS AND PENICILLIN. CEPHALOSPORIN C DERIVATIVES SHOULD BE GIVEN CAUTIOUSLY TO PENICILLIN-SENSITIVE PATIENTS.

SERIOUS ACUTE HYPERSENSITIVITY REACTIONS MAY REQUIRE EPINEPHRINE AND OTHER EMERGENCY MEASURES.

There is some clinical and laboratory evidence of partial cross-allergenicity of the penicillins and the cephalosporins. Patients have been reported to have had severe reactions (including anaphylaxis) to both drugs.

Any patient who has demonstrated some form of allergy, particularly to drugs, should receive antibiotics cautiously. No exception should be made with regard to Keflex.

Pseudomembranous colitis has been reported with nearly all antibacterial agents, including cephalexin, and may range from mild to life threatening. Therefore, it is important to consider this diagnosis in patients with diarrhea subsequent to the administration of antibacterial agents.

Treatment with antibacterial agents alters the normal flora of the colon and may permit overgrowth of clostridia. Studies indicate that a toxin produced by *Clostridium difficile* is one primary cause of antibiotic-associated colitis.

After the diagnosis of pseudomembranous colitis has been established, appropriate therapeutic measures should be initiated. Mild cases of pseudomembranous colitis usually respond to drug discontinuation alone. In moderate to severe cases, consideration should be given to management with fluids and electrolytes, protein supplementation, and treatment with an antibacterial drug clinically effective against *Clostridium difficile* colitis.

Usage in Pregnancy —Safety of this product for use during pregnancy has not been established.

PRECAUTIONS

General —Patients should be followed carefully so that any side effects or unusual manifestations of drug idiosyncrasy may be detected. If an allergic reaction to Keflex occurs, the drug should be discontinued and the patient treated with the usual agents (eg, epinephrine or other pressor amines, antihistamines, or corticosteroids).

Prolonged use of Keflex may result in the overgrowth of nonsusceptible organisms. Careful observation of the patient is essential. If superinfection occurs during therapy, appropriate measures should be taken.

Positive direct Coombs' tests have been reported during treatment with the cephalosporin antibiotics. In hematologic studies or in transfusion cross-matching procedures when antiglobulin tests are performed on the minor side or in Coombs' testing of newborns whose mothers have received cephalosporin antibiotics before parturition, it should be recognized that a positive Coombs' test may be due to the drug.

Keflex should be administered with caution in the presence of markedly impaired renal function. Under such conditions, careful clinical observation and laboratory studies should be made because safe dosage may be lower than that usually recommended.

Indicated surgical procedures should be performed in conjunction with antibiotic therapy.

As a result of administration of Keflex, a false-positive reaction for glucose in the urine may occur. This has been observed with Benedict's and Fehling's solutions and also with Clinitest® tablets.

As with other β-lactams, the renal excretion of cephalexin is inhibited by probenecid.

Broad-spectrum antibiotics should be prescribed with caution in individuals with a history of gastrointestinal disease, particularly colitis.

Usage in Pregnancy —Pregnancy Category B —The daily oral administration of cephalexin to rats in doses of 250 or 500 mg/kg prior to and during pregnancy, or to rats and mice during the period of organogenesis only, had no adverse effect on fertility, fetal viability, fetal weight, or litter size. Note that the safety of cephalexin during pregnancy in humans has not been established.

Cephalexin showed no enhanced toxicity in weanling and newborn rats as compared with adult animals. Nevertheless, because the studies in humans cannot rule out the possibility of harm, Keflex should be used during pregnancy only if clearly needed.

Nursing Mothers —The excretion of cephalexin in the milk increased up to 4 hours after a 500-mg dose; the drug reached a maximum level of 4 μg/mL, then decreased gradually, and had disappeared 8 hours after administration. Caution should be exercised when Keflex is administered to a nursing woman.

ADVERSE REACTIONS

Gastrointestinal —Symptoms of pseudomembranous colitis may appear either during or after antibiotic treatment. Nausea and vomiting have been reported rarely. The most frequent side effect has been diarrhea. It was very rarely severe enough to warrant cessation of therapy. Dyspepsia, gastritis, and abdominal pain have also occurred. As with some penicillins and some other cephalosporins, transient hepatitis and cholestatic jaundice have been reported rarely.

Hypersensitivity —Allergic reactions in the form of rash, urticaria, angioedema, and, rarely, erythema multiforme, Stevens-Johnson syndrome, or toxic epidermal necrolysis have been observed. These reactions usually subsided upon discontinuation of the drug. In some of these reactions, supportive therapy may be necessary. Anaphylaxis has also been reported.

Other reactions have included genital and anal pruritus, genital moniliasis, vaginitis and vaginal discharge, dizziness, fatigue, headache, agitation, confusion, hallucinations, arthralgia, arthritis, and joint disorder. Reversible interstitial nephritis has been reported rarely. Eosinophilia, neutropenia, thrombocytopenia, and slight elevations in AST and ALT have been reported.

OVERDOSAGE

Signs and Symptoms —Symptoms of oral overdose may include nausea, vomiting, epigastric distress, diarrhea, and hematuria. If other symptoms are present, it is probably secondary to an underlying disease state, an allergic reaction, or toxicity due to ingestion of a second medication.

Treatment —To obtain up-to-date information about the treatment of overdose, a good resource is your certified Regional Poison Control Center. Telephone numbers of certified poison control centers are listed in the *Physicians' Desk Reference (PDR)*. In managing overdosage, consider the possibility of multiple drug overdoses, interaction among drugs, and unusual drug kinetics in your patient.

Unless 5 to 10 times the normal dose of cephalexin has been ingested, gastrointestinal decontamination should not be necessary.

Protect the patient's airway and support ventilation and perfusion. Meticulously monitor and maintain, within acceptable limits, the patient's vital signs, blood gases, serum electrolytes, etc. Absorption of drugs from the gastrointestinal tract may be decreased by giving activated charcoal, which, in many cases, is more effective than emesis or lavage; consider charcoal instead of or in addition to gastric emptying. Repeated doses of charcoal over time may hasten elimination of some drugs that have been absorbed. Safeguard the patient's airway when employing gastric emptying or charcoal.

Forced diuresis, peritoneal dialysis, hemodialysis, or charcoal hemoperfusion have not been established as beneficial for an overdose of cephalexin; however, it would be extremely unlikely that one of these procedures would be indicated.

The oral median lethal dose of cephalexin in rats is >5,000 mg/kg.

DOSAGE AND ADMINISTRATION

Keflex is administered orally.

Adults —The adult dosage ranges from 1 to 4 g daily in divided doses. The usual adult dose is 250 mg every 6 hours. For the following infections, a dosage of 500 mg may be administered every 12 hours: streptococcal pharyngitis, skin and skin structure infections, and uncomplicated cystitis in patients over 15 years of age. Cystitis therapy should be continued for 7 to 14 days. For more severe infections or those caused by less susceptible organisms, larger doses may be needed. If daily doses of Keflex greater than 4 g are required, parenteral cephalosporins, in appropriate doses, should be considered.

Pediatric Patients —The usual recommended daily dosage for pediatric patients is 25 to 50 mg/kg in divided doses. For streptococcal pharyngitis in patients over 1 year of age and for skin and skin structure infections, the total daily dose may be divided and administered every 12 hours.

Keflex Suspension

Weight	125 mg/5 mL
10 kg (22 lb)	1/2 to 1 tsp q.i.d.
20 kg (44 lb)	1 to 2 tsp q.i.d.
40 kg (88 lb)	2 to 4 tsp q.i.d
Weight	**250 mg/5 mL**
10 kg (22 lb)	1/4 to 1/2 tsp q.i.d.
20 kg (44 lb)	1/2 to 1 tsp q.i.d.
40 kg (88 lb)	1 to 2 tsp q.i.d.
or	
Weight	**125 mg/5 mL**
10 kg (22 lb)	1 to 2 tsp b.i.d.
20 kg (44 lb)	2 to 4 tsp b.i.d.
40 kg (88 lb)	4 to 8 tsp b.i.d.
Weight	**250 mg/5 mL**
10 kg (22 lb)	1/2 to 1 tsp b.i.d.
20 kg (44 lb)	1 to 2 tsp b.i.d.
40 kg (88 lb)	2 to 4 tsp b.i.d.

In severe infections, the dosage may be doubled.

In the therapy of otitis media, clinical studies have shown that a dosage of 75 to 100 mg/kg/day in 4 divided doses is required.

In the treatment of β-hemolytic streptococcal infections, a therapeutic dosage of Keflex should be administered for at least 10 days.

HOW SUPPLIED

Keflex® For Oral Suspension, (or cephalexin, USP), is available in:

The 125 mg per 5 mL oral suspension* is available as follows:

100-mL Bottles	NDC 0777-2321-48 (M-201)
200-mL Bottles	NDC 0777-2321-89 (M-201)

The 250 mg per 5 mL oral suspension* is available as follows:

100-mL Bottles	NDC 0777-2368-48 (M-202)
200-mL Bottles	NDC 0777-2368-89 (M-202)
ID†100	NDC 0777-2368-33 (M-202)

Keflex® Pulvules®, (or cephalexin, USP), are available in:

The 250 mg Pulvules are a white powder filled into size 2 Para-Posilok® Caps (opaque white and opaque dark green) that are imprinted with "Dista" and identity code "H69" on the green cap, and Keflex 250 on the white body in edible black ink. They are available as follows:

Bottles of 20	NDC 0777-0869-20 (PU402)
Bottles of 100	NDC 0777-0869-02 (PU402)

The 500 mg Pulvules are a white powder filled into an elongated, size 0 Para-Posilok Caps (opaque light green and opaque dark green) that are imprinted with "Dista" and identity code "H71" on the dark green cap, and Keflex 500 on the light green body in edible black ink. They are available as follows:

Bottles of 20	NDC 0777-0871-20 (PU403)
Bottles of 100	NDC 0777-0871-02 (PU403)

* After mixing, store in a refrigerator. May be kept for 14 days without significant loss of potency. Shake well before using. Keep tightly closed.

† Identi-Dose® (unit dose medication, Dista).

Store at controlled room temperature, 15° to 30°C (59° to 86°F).

REFERENCES

1. National Committee for Clinical Laboratory Standards: Performance standards for antimicrobial disk susceptibility tests—5th ed. Approved Standard NCCLS Document M2-A5, Vol 13, No 24, NCCLS, Villanova, PA, 1993.
2. National Committee for Clinical Laboratory Standards: Methods for dilution antimicrobial susceptibility tests for bacteria that grow aerobically—3rd ed. Approved Standard NCCLS Document M7-A3, Vol 13, No 25, NCCLS, Villanova, PA, 1993.

Literature revised December 15, 1998.

PV 0360 DPP [121598]

NALFON® ℞

[*năl 'fŏn*]

(fenoprofen calcium)

USP

Capsules

DESCRIPTION

Nalfon® (Fenoprofen Calcium Capsules, USP) is a nonsteroidal, anti-inflammatory, antiarthritic drug. Nalfon capsules contain fenoprofen calcium as the dihydrate in an amount equivalent to 200 mg (0.826 mmol) or 300 mg (1.24 mmol) of fenoprofen. The capsules also contain cellulose, gelatin, iron oxides, silicone, titanium dioxide, and other inactive ingredients. The 300-mg capsules also contain D & C Yellow No. 10 and F D & C Yellow No. 6.

Chemically, Nalfon is an arylacetic acid derivative.

The structural formula is as follows:

CH_3CHCOO^- $Ca \cdot 2H_2O$ $[\ ]_2$

Benzeneacetic acid, α-methyl-3-phenoxy-, calcium salt dihydrate, (±)-

Nalfon is a white crystalline powder that has the empirical formula $C_{30}H_{26}CaO_6 \cdot 2H_2O$ representing a molecular weight of 558.65. At 25°C, it dissolves to a 15 mg/mL solution in alcohol (95%). It is slightly soluble in water and insoluble in benzene.

The *p*Ka of Nalfon is 4.5 at 25°C.

CLINICAL PHARMACOLOGY

Nalfon is a nonsteroidal, anti-inflammatory, antiarthritic drug that also possesses analgesic and antipyretic activities. Its exact mode of action is unknown, but it is thought that prostaglandin synthetase inhibition is involved. Nalfon has been shown to inhibit prostaglandin synthetase isolated from bovine seminal vesicles. Reproduction studies in rats have shown Nalfon to be associated with prolonged labor and difficult parturition when given during late pregnancy. Evidence suggests that this may be due to decreased uterine contractility resulting from the inhibition of prostaglandin synthesis. Its action is not mediated through the adrenal gland.

Fenoprofen shows anti-inflammatory effects in rodents by inhibiting the development of redness and edema in acute inflammatory conditions and by reducing soft-tissue swelling and bone damage associated with chronic inflammation. It exhibits analgesic activity in rodents by inhibiting the writhing response caused by the introduction of an irritant into the peritoneal cavities of mice and by elevating pain thresholds that are related to pressure in edematous hindpaws of rats. In rats made febrile by the subcutaneous administration of brewer's yeast, fenoprofen produces antipyretic action. These effects are characteristic of nonsteroidal, anti-inflammatory, antipyretic, analgesic drugs.

The results in humans confirmed the anti-inflammatory and analgesic actions found in animals. The emergence and

Continued on next page

This product information was prepared in June 2000. Current information on these and other products of Dista Products Company may be obtained by direct inquiry to Lilly Research Laboratories, Lilly Corporate Center, Indianapolis, Indiana 46285, (800) 545-5979.

Nalfon—Cont.

degree of erythemic response were measured in adult male volunteers exposed to ultraviolet irradiation. The effects of Nalfon, aspirin, and indomethacin were each compared with those of a placebo. All 3 drugs demonstrated anti-erythemic activity.

In patients with rheumatoid arthritis, the anti-inflammatory action of Nalfon has been evidenced by relief of pain, increase in grip strength, and reductions in joint swelling, duration of morning stiffness, and disease activity (as assessed by both the investigator and the patient). The anti-inflammatory action of Nalfon has also been evidenced by increased mobility (ie, a decrease in the number of joints having limited motion).

The use of Nalfon in combination with gold salts or corticosteroids has been studied in patients with rheumatoid arthritis. The studies, however, were inadequate in demonstrating whether further improvement is obtained by adding Nalfon to maintenance therapy with gold salts or steroids. Whether or not Nalfon used in conjunction with partially effective doses of a corticosteroid has a "steroid-sparing" effect is unknown.

In patients with osteoarthritis, the anti-inflammatory and analgesic effects of Nalfon have been demonstrated by reduction in tenderness as a response to pressure and reductions in night pain, stiffness, swelling, and overall disease activity (as assessed by both the patient and the investigator). These effects have also been demonstrated by relief of pain with motion and at rest and increased range of motion in involved joints.

In patients with rheumatoid arthritis and osteoarthritis, clinical studies have shown Nalfon to be comparable to aspirin in controlling the aforementioned measures of disease activity, but mild gastrointestinal reactions (nausea, dyspepsia) and tinnitus occurred less frequently in patients treated with Nalfon than in aspirin-treated patients. It is not known whether Nalfon causes less peptic ulceration than does aspirin.

In patients with pain, the analgesic action of Nalfon has produced a reduction in pain intensity, an increase in pain relief, improvement in total analgesia scores, and a sustained analgesic effect.

Under fasting conditions, Nalfon is rapidly absorbed, and peak plasma levels of 50 µg/mL are achieved within 2 hours after oral administration of 600-mg doses. Good dose proportionality was observed between 200-mg and 600-mg doses in fasting male volunteers. The plasma half-life is approximately 3 hours. About 90% of a single oral dose is eliminated within 24 hours as fenoprofen glucuronide and 4'-hydroxyfenoprofen glucuronide, the major urinary metabolites of fenoprofen. Fenoprofen is highly bound (99%) to albumin.

The concomitant administration of antacid (containing both aluminum and magnesium hydroxide) does not interfere with absorption of Nalfon.

There is less suppression of collagen-induced platelet aggregation with single doses of Nalfon than there is with aspirin.

INDICATIONS AND USAGE

Nalfon is indicated for relief of the signs and symptoms of rheumatoid arthritis and osteoarthritis. It is recommended for the treatment of acute flare-ups and exacerbations and for the long-term management of these diseases.

Nalfon is also indicated for the relief of mild to moderate pain.

CONTRAINDICATIONS

Nalfon is contraindicated in patients who have shown hypersensitivity to it.

The drug should not be administered to patients with a history of significantly impaired renal function.

Nalfon should not be given to patients in whom aspirin and other nonsteroidal anti-inflammatory drugs induce the symptoms of asthma, rhinitis, or urticaria, because cross-sensitivity to these drugs occurs in a high proportion of such patients.

WARNINGS

Risk of GI Ulceration, Bleeding, and Perforation with NSAID Therapy —Serious gastrointestinal toxicity, such as bleeding, ulceration, and perforation, can occur at any time, with or without warning symptoms, in patients treated chronically with NSAID therapy. Although minor upper gastrointestinal problems, such as dyspepsia, are common, usually developing early in therapy, physicians should remain alert for ulceration and bleeding in patients treated chronically with NSAIDs, even in the absence of previous GI tract symptoms. In patients observed in clinical trials of several months to 2 years duration, symptomatic upper GI ulcers, gross bleeding, or perforation appear to occur in approximately 1% of patients treated for 3 to 6 months, and in about 2% to 4% of patients treated for 1 year. Physicians should inform patients about the signs and/or symptoms of serious GI toxicity and what steps to take if they occur.

Studies to date have not identified any subset of patients not at risk of developing peptic ulceration and bleeding. Except for a prior history of serious GI events and other risk factors known to be associated with peptic ulcer disease, such as alcoholism, smoking, etc, no risk factors (eg, age, sex) have been associated with increased risk. Elderly or debilitated patients seem to tolerate ulceration or bleeding less well than other individuals and most spontaneous reports of fatal GI events are in this population. Studies to date are inconclusive concerning the relative risk of various NSAIDs in causing such reactions. High doses of any NSAID probably carry a greater risk of these reactions, although controlled clinical trials showing this do not exist in most cases. In considering the use of relatively large doses (within the recommended dosage range), sufficient benefit should be anticipated to offset the potential increased risk of GI toxicity.

Since Nalfon has been marketed, there have been reports of genitourinary tract problems in patients taking it. The most frequently reported problems have been episodes of dysuria, cystitis, hematuria, interstitial nephritis, and nephrotic syndrome. This syndrome may be preceded by the appearance of fever, rash, arthralgia, oliguria, and azotemia and may progress to anuria. There may also be substantial proteinuria, and, on renal biopsy, electron microscopy has shown foot process fusion and T-lymphocyte infiltration in the renal interstitium. Early recognition of the syndrome and withdrawal of the drug have been followed by rapid recovery. Administration of steroids and the use of dialysis have also been included in the treatment. Because a syndrome with some of these characteristics has also been reported with other nonsteroidal anti-inflammatory drugs, it is recommended that patients who have had these reactions with other such drugs not be treated with Nalfon. In patients with possibly compromised renal function, periodic renal function examinations should be done.

PRECAUTIONS

General —Renal Effects —There have been reports of acute interstitial nephritis and nephrotic syndrome (*see* Contraindications *and* Warnings).

A second form of renal toxicity has been seen in patients with prerenal conditions leading to a reduction in renal blood flow or blood volume, in which renal prostaglandins play a supportive role in the maintenance of renal perfusion. In these patients, administration of an NSAID may cause a dose-dependent reduction in prostaglandin formation and may precipitate overt renal decompensation at any time. Patients at greatest risk for this reaction are those with impaired renal function, heart failure, liver dysfunction, those taking diuretics, and the elderly. Discontinuation of NSAID therapy is typically followed by recovery to the pretreatment state.

Since Nalfon is primarily eliminated by the kidneys, patients with possibly compromised renal function (such as the elderly) should be monitored periodically, especially during long-term therapy. For such patients, it may be anticipated that a lower daily dosage will avoid excessive drug accumulation.

Miscellaneous —Peripheral edema has been observed in some patients taking Nalfon; therefore, Nalfon should be used with caution in patients with compromised cardiac function or hypertension. The possibility of renal involvement should be considered.

Studies to date have not shown changes in the eyes attributable to the administration of Nalfon. However, adverse ocular effects have been observed with other anti-inflammatory drugs. Eye examinations, therefore, should be performed if visual disturbances occur in patients taking Nalfon.

Caution should be exercised by patients whose activities require alertness if they experience CNS side effects while taking Nalfon.

Since the safety of Nalfon has not been established in patients with impaired hearing, these patients should have periodic tests of auditory function during prolonged therapy with Nalfon.

Information for Patients —Nalfon, like other drugs of its class, is not free of side effects. The side effects of these drugs can cause discomfort and, rarely, there are more serious side effects, such as gastrointestinal bleeding, which may result in hospitalization and even fatal outcomes.

NSAIDs (Nonsteroidal Anti-Inflammatory Drugs) are often essential agents in the management of arthritis and have a major role in the treatment of pain, but they also may be commonly employed for conditions which are less serious.

Physicians may wish to discuss with their patients the potential risks (*see* Warnings, Precautions, *and* Adverse Reactions sections) and likely benefits of NSAID treatment, particularly when the drugs are used for less serious conditions where treatment without NSAIDs may represent an acceptable alternative to both the patient and physician.

Laboratory Tests —In chronic studies in rats, high doses of Nalfon caused elevation of serum transaminase and hepatocellular hypertrophy. In clinical trials, some patients developed elevation of serum transaminase, LDH, and alkaline phosphatase that persisted for some months and usually, but not always, declined despite continuation of the drug. The significance of this is unknown. It is recommended, therefore, that Nalfon be discontinued if any significant liver abnormality occurs.

As with other nonsteroidal anti-inflammatory drugs, borderline elevations in 1 or more liver tests may occur in up to 15% of patients. These abnormalities may progress, may remain essentially unchanged, or may be transient with continued therapy. The SGPT (ALT) test is probably the most sensitive indicator of liver dysfunction. Meaningful (ie, 3 times the upper limit of normal) elevations of SGPT or SGOT (AST) occurred in controlled clinical trials in less than 1% of patients. A patient with symptoms and/or signs suggesting liver dysfunction, or in whom an abnormal liver test has occurred, should be evaluated for evidence of the development of more severe hepatic reactions while using Nalfon.

Severe hepatic reactions, including jaundice and cases of fatal hepatitis, have been reported with Nalfon, as with other nonsteroidal anti-inflammatory drugs. As a result, during long-term therapy, liver function tests should be monitored periodically. Although such reactions are rare, if liver tests continue to be abnormal or worsen, if clinical signs and symptoms consistent with liver disease develop, or if systemic manifestations occur (eg, eosinophilia and rash), Nalfon should be discontinued. If this drug is to be used in the presence of impaired liver function, it must be done under strict observation.

Patients with initial low hemoglobin values who are receiving long-term therapy with Nalfon should have a hemoglobin determination made at reasonable intervals.

Nalfon decreases platelet aggregation and may prolong bleeding time. Patients who may be adversely affected by prolongation of the bleeding time should be carefully observed when Nalfon is administered.

Because serious GI tract ulceration and bleeding can occur without warning symptoms, physicians should follow chronically treated patients for the signs and symptoms of ulceration and bleeding and should inform them of the importance of this follow-up (*see* Risk of GI Ulcerations, Bleeding and Perforation with NSAID Therapy *under* Warnings).

Laboratory Test Interactions —Amerlex-M kit assay values of total and free triiodothyronine in patients receiving Nalfon have been reported as falsely elevated on the basis of a chemical cross-reaction that directly interferes with the assay. Thyroid-stimulating hormone, total thyroxine, and thyrotropin-releasing hormone response are not affected.

Drug Interactions —The coadministration of aspirin decreases the biologic half-life of fenoprofen because of an increase in metabolic clearance that results in a greater amount of hydroxylated fenoprofen in the urine. Although the mechanism of interaction between fenoprofen and aspirin is not totally known, enzyme induction and displacement of fenoprofen from plasma albumin binding sites are possibilities. Because Nalfon has not been shown to produce any additional effect beyond that obtained with aspirin alone and because aspirin increases the rate of excretion of Nalfon, the concomitant use of Nalfon and salicylates is not recommended.

Chronic administration of phenobarbital, a known enzyme inducer, may be associated with a decrease in the plasma half-life of fenoprofen. When phenobarbital is added to or withdrawn from treatment, dosage adjustment of Nalfon may be required.

In vitro studies have shown that fenoprofen, because of its affinity for albumin, may displace from their binding sites other drugs that are also albumin bound, and this may lead to drug interaction. Theoretically, fenoprofen could likewise be displaced. Patients receiving hydantoins, sulfonamides, or sulfonylureas should be observed for increased activity of these drugs and, therefore, signs of toxicity from these drugs. In patients receiving coumarin-type anticoagulants, the addition of Nalfon to therapy could prolong the prothrombin time. Patients receiving both drugs should be under careful observation. Patients treated with Nalfon may be resistant to the effects of loop diuretics.

In patients receiving Nalfon and a steroid concomitantly, any reduction in steroid dosage should be gradual in order to avoid the possible complications of sudden steroid withdrawal.

Usage in Pregnancy —Safe use of Nalfon during pregnancy and lactation has not been established; therefore, administration to pregnant patients and nursing mothers is not recommended. Reproduction studies have been performed in rats and rabbits. When fenoprofen was given to rats during pregnancy and continued until the time of labor, parturition was prolonged. Similar results have been found with other nonsteroidal anti-inflammatory drugs that inhibit prostaglandin synthetase.

Usage in Pediatric Patients —Safety and effectiveness in pediatric patients have not been established.

ADVERSE REACTIONS

During clinical studies for rheumatoid arthritis, osteoarthritis, or mild to moderate pain and studies of pharmacokinetics, complaints were compiled from a checklist of potential adverse reactions, and the following data emerged. These encompass observations in 6,786 patients, including 188 observed for at least 52 weeks. For comparison, data are also presented from complaints received from the 266 patients who received placebo in these same trials. During short-term studies for analgesia, the incidence of adverse reactions was markedly lower than that seen in longer-term studies.

INCIDENCE GREATER THAN 1%

Probable Causal Relationship

Digestive System —During clinical trials with Nalfon, the most common adverse reactions were gastrointestinal in nature and occurred in 20.8% of patients receiving Nalfon as compared to 16.9% of patients receiving placebo. In descending order of frequency, these reactions included dyspepsia (10.3%, Nalfon, vs 2.3%, placebo), nausea (7.7% vs 7.1%), constipation (7% vs 1.5%), vomiting (2.6% vs 1.9%), abdominal pain (2% vs 1.1%), and diarrhea (1.8% vs 4.1%).

The drug was discontinued because of adverse gastrointestinal reactions in less than 2% of patients during premarketing studies.

Nervous System —The most frequent adverse neurologic reactions were headache (8.7% treated vs 7.5% placebo) and somnolence (8.5% vs 6.4%). Dizziness (6.5% vs 5.6%), tremor (2.2% vs 0.4%), and confusion (1.4% vs none) were noted less frequently.

Nalfon was discontinued in less than 0.5% of patients because of these side effects during premarketing studies.

Skin and Appendages —Increased sweating (4.6% vs 0.4%), pruritus (4.2% vs 0.8%), and rash (3.7% vs 0.4%) were reported.

Nalfon was discontinued in about 1% of patients because of an adverse effect related to the skin during premarketing studies.

Special Senses —Tinnitus (4.5% vs 0.4%), blurred vision (2.2% vs none), and decreased hearing (1.6% vs none) were reported.

Nalfon was discontinued in less than 0.5% of patients because of adverse effects related to the special senses during premarketing studies.

Cardiovascular —Palpitations (2.5% vs 0.4%).

Nalfon was discontinued in about 0.5% of patients because of adverse cardiovascular reactions during premarketing studies.

Miscellaneous —Nervousness (5.7% vs 1.5%), asthenia (5.4% vs 0.4%), peripheral edema (5.0% vs 0.4%), dyspnea (2.8% vs none), fatigue (1.7% vs 1.5%), upper respiratory infection (1.5% vs 5.6%), and nasopharyngitis (1.2% vs none).

INCIDENCE LESS THAN 1%

Probable Causal Relationship

The following adverse reactions, occurring in less than 1% of patients, were reported in controlled clinical trials and voluntary reports made since Nalfon was initially marketed. The probability of a causal relationship exists between Nalfon and these adverse reactions:

Digestive System —Gastritis, peptic ulcer with/without perforation, gastrointestinal hemorrhage, anorexia, flatulence, dry mouth, and blood in the stool. Increases in alkaline phosphatase, LDH, and SGOT, jaundice, and cholestatic hepatitis were observed (*see* Precautions).

Genitourinary Tract —Renal failure, dysuria, cystitis, hematuria, oliguria, azotemia, anuria, interstitial nephritis, nephrosis, and papillary necrosis (*see* Warnings).

Hypersensitivity —Angioedema (angioneurotic edema).

Hematologic —Purpura, bruising, hemorrhage, thrombocytopenia, hemolytic anemia, aplastic anemia, agranulocytosis, and pancytopenia.

Miscellaneous —Anaphylaxis, urticaria, malaise, insomnia, and tachycardia.

INCIDENCE LESS THAN 1%

Causal Relationship Unknown

Other reactions reported either in clinical trials or spontaneously, occurred in circumstances in which a causal relationship could not be established. However, with these rarely reported reactions, the possibility of such a relationship cannot be excluded. Therefore, these observations are listed to alert the physician.

Skin and Appendages —Exfoliative dermatitis, toxic epidermal necrolysis, Stevens-Johnson syndrome, and alopecia.

Digestive System —Aphthous ulcerations of the buccal mucosa, metallic taste, and pancreatitis.

Cardiovascular —Atrial fibrillation, pulmonary edema, electrocardiographic changes, and supraventricular tachycardia.

Nervous System —Depression, disorientation, seizures, and trigeminal neuralgia.

Special Senses —Burning tongue, diplopia, and optic neuritis.

Miscellaneous —Personality change, lymphadenopathy, mastodynia, and fever.

OVERDOSAGE

Signs and Symptoms —Symptoms of overdose appear within several hours and generally involve the gastrointestinal and central nervous systems. They include dyspepsia, nausea, vomiting, abdominal pain, dizziness, headache, ataxia, tinnitus, tremor, drowsiness, and confusion. Hyperpyrexia, tachycardia, hypotension, and acute renal failure may occur rarely following overdose. Respiratory depression and metabolic acidosis have also been reported following overdose with certain NSAIDs.

Treatment —To obtain up-to-date information about the treatment of overdose, a good resource is your certified Regional Poison Control Center. Telephone numbers of certified poison control centers are listed in the *Physicians' Desk Reference (PDR)*. In managing overdosage, consider the possibility of multiple drug overdoses, interaction among drugs, and unusual drug kinetics in your patient.

Protect the patient's airway and support ventilation and perfusion. Meticulously monitor and maintain, within acceptable limits, the patient's vital signs, blood gases, serum electrolytes, etc. Absorption of drugs from the gastrointestinal tract may be decreased by giving activated charcoal, which, in many cases, is more effective than emesis or lavage; consider charcoal instead of or in addition to gastric emptying. Repeated doses of charcoal over time may hasten elimination of some drugs that have been absorbed. Safeguard the patient's airway when employing gastric emptying or charcoal.

Alkalinization of the urine, forced diuresis, peritoneal dialysis, hemodialysis, and charcoal hemoperfusion do not enhance systemic drug elimination.

DOSAGE AND ADMINISTRATION

Analgesia —For the treatment of mild to moderate pain, the recommended dosage is 200 mg every 4 to 6 hours, as needed.

Rheumatoid Arthritis and Osteoarthritis —The suggested dosage is 300 to 600 mg, 3 or 4 times a day. The dose should be tailored to the needs of the patient and may be increased or decreased depending on the severity of the symptoms. Dosage adjustments may be made after initiation of drug therapy or during exacerbations of the disease. Total daily dosage should not exceed 3,200 mg.

If gastrointestinal complaints occur, Nalfon may be administered with meals or with milk. Although the total amount absorbed is not affected, peak blood levels are delayed and diminished.

Patients with rheumatoid arthritis generally seem to require larger doses of Nalfon than do those with osteoarthritis. The smallest dose that yields acceptable control should be employed.

Although improvement may be seen in a few days in many patients, an additional 2 to 3 weeks may be required to gauge the full benefits of therapy.

HOW SUPPLIED

Capsules:

200 mg* (white and ocher) (UC5966)—(RX681) (100's) NDC 63304-681-01

300 mg* (yellow and ocher) (UC5967)—(RX682) (100's) NDC 63304-682-01

* Equivalent to fenoprofen.

Store at controlled room temperature, 59° to 86°F (15° to 30°C).

Rx only

Literature revised May 24, 1999

PV 1021 UFP [052499]

PROZAC® ℞

[*prō 'zăk*]

(fluoxetine hydrochloride)

DESCRIPTION

Prozac® (Fluoxetine Hydrochloride) is an antidepressant for oral administration; it is chemically unrelated to tricyclic, tetracyclic, or other available antidepressant agents. It is designated (±)-N-methyl-3-phenyl-3-[(α,α,α-trifluoro-*p*-tolyl)oxy]propylamine hydrochloride and has the empirical formula of $C_{17}H_{18}F_3NO \cdot HCl$. Its molecular weight is 345.79. The structural formula is:

$F_3C-C_6H_4-O-CH(C_6H_5)CH_2CH_2NHCH_3 \cdot HCl$

Fluoxetine hydrochloride is a white to off-white crystalline solid with a solubility of 14 mg/mL in water.

Each Pulvule® contains fluoxetine hydrochloride equivalent to 10 mg (32.3 μmol), 20 mg (64.7 μmol), or 40 mg (129.3 μmol) of fluoxetine. The Pulvules also contain starch, gelatin, silicone, titanium dioxide, iron oxide, and other inactive ingredients. The 10 mg and 20 mg Pulvules also contain F D & C Blue No. 1, and the 40 mg Pulvule also contains F D & C Blue No. 1 and F D & C Yellow No. 6.

Each tablet contains fluoxetine hydrochloride equivalent to 10 mg (32.3 μmol) of fluoxetine. The tablets also contain microcrystalline cellulose, magnesium stearate, crospovidone, hydroxypropyl methylcellulose, titanium dioxide, polyethylene glycol, and yellow iron oxide. In addition to the above ingredients, the 10 mg tablet contains F D & C Blue No. 1 aluminum lake, and polysorbate 80.

The oral solution contains fluoxetine hydrochloride equivalent to 20 mg/5 mL (64.7 μmol) of fluoxetine. It also contains alcohol 0.23%, benzoic acid, flavoring agent, glycerin, purified water, and sucrose.

CLINICAL PHARMACOLOGY

Pharmacodynamics:

The antidepressant, antiobsessive-compulsive, and antibulimic actions of fluoxetine are presumed to be linked to its inhibition of CNS neuronal uptake of serotonin. Studies at clinically relevant doses in man have demonstrated that fluoxetine blocks the uptake of serotonin into human platelets. Studies in animals also suggest that fluoxetine is a much more potent uptake inhibitor of serotonin than of norepinephrine.

Antagonism of muscarinic, histaminergic, and α_1-adrenergic receptors has been hypothesized to be associated with various anticholinergic, sedative, and cardiovascular effects of classical tricyclic antidepressant drugs. Fluoxetine binds to these and other membrane receptors from brain tissue much less potently in vitro than do the tricyclic drugs.

Absorption, Distribution, Metabolism, and Excretion:

Systemic Bioavailability—In man, following a single oral 40 mg dose, peak plasma concentrations of fluoxetine from 15 to 55 ng/mL are observed after 6 to 8 hours.

The Pulvule, tablet, and oral solution dosage forms of fluoxetine are bioequivalent. Food does not appear to affect the systemic bioavailability of fluoxetine, although it may delay its absorption inconsequentially. Thus, fluoxetine may be administered with or without food.

Protein Binding—Over the concentration range from 200 to 1,000 ng/mL, approximately 94.5% of fluoxetine is bound in vitro to human serum proteins, including albumin and α_1-glycoprotein. The interaction between fluoxetine and other highly protein-bound drugs has not been fully evaluated, but may be important (*see* Precautions).

Enantiomers—Fluoxetine is a racemic mixture (50/50) of *R*-fluoxetine and *S*-fluoxetine enantiomers. In animal models, both enantiomers are specific and potent serotonin uptake inhibitors with essentially equivalent pharmacologic activity. The *S*-fluoxetine enantiomer is eliminated more slowly and is the predominant enantiomer present in plasma at steady state.

Metabolism—Fluoxetine is extensively metabolized in the liver to norfluoxetine and a number of other, unidentified metabolites. The only identified active metabolite, norfluoxetine, is formed by demethylation of fluoxetine. In animal models, *S*-norfluoxetine is a potent and selective inhibitor of serotonin uptake and has activity essentially equivalent to *R*- or *S*-fluoxetine. *R*-norfluoxetine is significantly less potent than the parent drug in the inhibition of serotonin uptake. The primary route of elimination appears to be hepatic metabolism to inactive metabolites excreted by the kidney.

Clinical Issues Related to Metabolism/Elimination—The complexity of the metabolism of fluoxetine has several consequences that may potentially affect fluoxetine's clinical use.

Variability in Metabolism—A subset (about 7%) of the population has reduced activity of the drug metabolizing enzyme cytochrome P450IID6. Such individuals are referred to as "poor metabolizers" of drugs such as debrisoquin, dextromethorphan, and the tricyclic antidepressants. In a study involving labeled and unlabeled enantiomers administered as a racemate, these individuals metabolized *S*-fluoxetine at a slower rate and thus achieved higher concentrations of *S*-fluoxetine. Consequently, concentrations of *S*-norfluoxetine at steady state were lower. The metabolism of *R*-fluoxetine in these poor metabolizers appears normal. When compared with normal metabolizers, the total sum at steady state of the plasma concentrations of the 4 active enantiomers was not significantly greater among poor metabolizers. Thus, the net pharmacodynamic activities were essentially the same. Alternative, nonsaturable pathways (non-IID6) also contribute to the metabolism of fluoxetine. This explains how fluoxetine achieves a steady-state concentration rather than increasing without limit.

Because fluoxetine's metabolism, like that of a number of other compounds including tricyclic and other selective serotonin antidepressants, involves the P450IID6 system, concomitant therapy with drugs also metabolized by this enzyme system (such as the tricyclic antidepressants) may lead to drug interactions (*see* Drug Interactions *under* Precautions).

Accumulation and Slow Elimination—The relatively slow elimination of fluoxetine (elimination half-life of 1 to 3 days after acute administration and 4 to 6 days after chronic administration) and its active metabolite, norfluoxetine (elimination half-life of 4 to 16 days after acute and chronic administration), leads to significant accumulation of these active species in chronic use and delayed attainment of steady state, even when a fixed dose is used. After 30 days of dosing at 40 mg/day, plasma concentrations of fluoxetine in the range of 91 to 302 ng/mL and norfluoxetine in the range of 72 to 258 ng/mL have been observed. Plasma concentrations of fluoxetine were higher than those predicted by single-dose studies, because fluoxetine's metabolism is not proportional to dose. Norfluoxetine, however, appears to have linear pharmacokinetics. Its mean terminal half-life after a single dose was 8.6 days and after multiple dosing was 9.3 days. Steady state levels after prolonged dosing are similar to levels seen at 4–5 weeks.

The long elimination half-lives of fluoxetine and norfluoxetine assure that, even when dosing is stopped, active drug substance will persist in the body for weeks (primarily depending on individual patient characteristics, previous dosing regimen, and length of previous therapy at discontinuation). This is of potential consequence when drug discontinuation is required or when drugs are prescribed that might interact with fluoxetine and norfluoxetine following the discontinuation of Prozac.

Liver Disease—As might be predicted from its primary site of metabolism, liver impairment can affect the elimination of fluoxetine. The elimination half-life of fluoxetine was prolonged in a study of cirrhotic patients, with a mean of 7.6 days compared to the range of 2 to 3 days seen in subjects without liver disease; norfluoxetine elimination was also delayed, with a mean duration of 12 days for cirrhotic patients compared to the range of 7 to 9 days in normal subjects. This suggests that the use of fluoxetine in patients with liver disease must be approached with caution. If fluoxetine is administered to patients with liver disease, a lower or less frequent dose should be used (*see* Precautions *and* Dosage and Administration).

Continued on next page

This product information was prepared in June 2000. Current information on these and other products of Dista Products Company may be obtained by direct inquiry to Lilly Research Laboratories, Lilly Corporate Center, Indianapolis, Indiana 46285, (800) 545-5979.

Prozac—Cont.

Renal Disease—In depressed patients on dialysis (N=12), fluoxetine administered as 20 mg once daily for two months produced steady-state fluoxetine and norfluoxetine plasma concentrations comparable to those seen in patients with normal renal function. While the possibility exists that renally excreted metabolites of fluoxetine may accumulate to higher levels in patients with severe renal dysfunction, use of a lower or less frequent dose is not routinely necessary in renally impaired patients (*see* Use in Patients With Concomitant Illness *under* Precautions *and* Dosage and Administration).

Age—The disposition of single doses of fluoxetine in healthy elderly subjects (greater than 65 years of age) did not differ significantly from that in younger normal subjects. However, given the long half-life and nonlinear disposition of the drug, a single-dose study is not adequate to rule out the possibility of altered pharmacokinetics in the elderly, particularly if they have systemic illness or are receiving multiple drugs for concomitant diseases. The effects of age upon the metabolism of fluoxetine have been investigated in 260 elderly but otherwise healthy depressed patients (≥60 years of age) who received 20 mg fluoxetine for 6 weeks. Combined fluoxetine plus norfluoxetine plasma concentrations were 209.3 ± 85.7 ng/mL at the end of 6 weeks. No unusual age-associated pattern of adverse events was observed in those elderly patients.

Clinical Trials:

Depression—The efficacy of Prozac for the treatment of patients with depression (≥18 years of age) has been studied in 5- and 6-week placebo-controlled trials. Prozac was shown to be significantly more effective than placebo as measured by the Hamilton Depression Rating Scale (HAM-D). Prozac was also significantly more effective than placebo on the HAM-D subscores for depressed mood, sleep disturbance, and the anxiety subfactor.

Two 6-week controlled studies comparing Prozac, 20mg, and placebo have shown Prozac, 20 mg daily, to be effective in the treatment of elderly patients (≥60 years of age) with depression. In these studies, Prozac produced a significantly higher rate of response and remission as defined respectively by a 50% decrease in the HAM-D score and a total endpoint HAM-D score of ≤8. Prozac was well tolerated and the rate of treatment discontinuations due to adverse events did not differ between Prozac (12%) and placebo (9%).

A study was conducted involving depressed outpatients who had responded (modified HAMD-17 score of ≤ 7 during each of the last 3 weeks of open-label treatment and absence of major depression by DSM-III-R criteria) by the end of an initial 12–week open treatment phase on Prozac 20 mg/day. These patients (N=298) were randomized to continuation on double-blind Prozac 20 mg/day or placebo. At 38 weeks (50 weeks total), a statistically significantly lower relapse rate (defined as symptoms sufficient to meet a diagnosis of major depression for 2 weeks or a modified HAMD-17 score of ≥ 14 for 3 weeks) was observed for patients taking Prozac compared to those on placebo.

Obsessive-Compulsive Disorder—The effectiveness of Prozac for the treatment for obsessive-compulsive disorder (OCD) was demonstrated in two 13-week, multicenter, parallel group studies (Studies 1 and 2) of adult outpatients who received fixed Prozac doses of 20, 40, or 60 mg/day (on a once a day schedule, in the morning) or placebo. Patients in both studies had moderate to severe OCD (DSM-III-R), with mean baseline ratings on the Yale-Brown Obsessive Compulsive Scale (YBOCS, total score) ranging from 22 to 26. In Study 1, patients receiving Prozac experienced mean reductions of approximately 4 to 6 units on the YBOCS total score, compared to a 1-unit reduction for placebo patients. In Study 2, patients receiving Prozac experienced mean reductions of approximately 4 to 9 units on the YBOCS total score, compared to a 1-unit reduction for placebo patients. While there was no indication of a dose response relationship for effectiveness in Study 1, a dose response relationship was observed in Study 2, with numerically better responses in the 2 higher dose groups. The following table provides the outcome classification by treatment group on the Clinical Global Impression (CGI) improvement scale for studies 1 and 2 combined:

Outcome Classification (%) on CGI Improvement Scale for Completers in Pool of Two OCD Studies

Outcome Classification	Placebo	Prozac 20 mg	40 mg	60 mg
Worse	8%	0%	0%	0%
No Change	64%	41%	33%	29%
Minimally Improved	17%	23%	28%	24%
Much Improved	8%	28%	27%	28%
Very Much Improved	3%	8%	12%	19%

Exploratory analyses for age and gender effects on outcome did not suggest any differential responsiveness on the basis of age or sex.

Bulimia Nervosa—The effectiveness of Prozac for the treatment of bulimia was demonstrated in two 8-week and one 16-week, multicenter, parallel group studies of adult outpatients meeting DSM-III-R criteria for bulimia. Patients in the 8-week studies received either 20 mg/day or 60 mg/day of Prozac or placebo in the morning. Patients in the 16-week study received a fixed Prozac dose of 60 mg/day (once a day) or placebo. Patients in these 3 studies had moderate to severe bulimia with median binge-eating and vomiting frequencies ranging from 7 to 10 per week and 5 to 9 per week, respectively. In these 3 studies, Prozac, 60 mg, but not 20 mg, was statistically significantly superior to placebo in reducing the number of binge-eating and vomiting episodes per week. The statistically significantly superior effect of 60 mg vs placebo was present as early as week 1 and persisted throughout each study. The Prozac related reduction in bulimic episodes appeared to be independent of baseline depression as assessed by the Hamilton Depression Rating Scale. In each of these 3 studies, the treatment effect, as measured by differences between Prozac, 60 mg, and placebo on median reduction from baseline in frequency of bulimic behaviors at endpoint, ranged from 1 to 2 episodes per week for binge-eating and 2 to 4 episodes per week for vomiting. The size of the effect was related to baseline frequency, with greater reductions seen in patients with higher baseline frequencies. Although some patients achieved freedom from binge-eating and purging as a result of treatment, for the majority, the benefit was a partial reduction in the frequency of binge-eating and purging.

INDICATIONS AND USAGE

Depression—Prozac is indicated for the treatment of depression. The efficacy of Prozac was established in 5- and 6-week trials with depressed adult and geriatric outpatients (≥18 years of age) whose diagnoses corresponded most closely to the DSM-III (currently DSM-IV) category of major depressive disorder (*see* Clinical Trials *under* Clinical Pharmacology).

A major depressive episode (DSM-IV) implies a prominent and relatively persistent (nearly every day for at least 2 weeks) depressed or dysphoric mood that usually interferes with daily functioning, and includes at least 5 of the following 9 symptoms: depressed mood; loss of interest in usual activities; significant change in weight and/or appetite; insomnia or hypersomnia; psychomotor agitation or retardation; increased fatigue; feelings of guilt or worthlessness; slowed thinking or impaired concentration; a suicide attempt or suicidal ideation.

The antidepressant action of Prozac in hospitalized depressed patients has not been adequately studied.

The efficacy of Prozac in maintaining an antidepressant response for up to 38 weeks following 12 weeks of open-label acute treatment (50 weeks total) was demonstrated in a placebo-controlled trial. The usefulness of the drug in patients receiving Prozac for extended periods should be reevaluated periodically (*see* Clinical Trials *under* Clinical Pharmacology).

Obsessive-Compulsive Disorder—Prozac is indicated for the treatment of obsessions and compulsions in patients with obsessive-compulsive disorder (OCD), as defined in the DSM-III-R; ie, the obsessions or compulsions cause marked distress, are time-consuming, or significantly interfere with social or occupational functioning.

The efficacy of Prozac was established in 13-week trials with obsessive-compulsive outpatients whose diagnoses corresponded most closely to the DSM-III-R category of obsessive-compulsive disorder (*see* Clinical Trials *under* Clinical Pharmacology).

Obsessive-compulsive disorder is characterized by recurrent and persistent ideas, thoughts, impulses, or images (obsessions) that are ego-dystonic and/or repetitive, purposeful, and intentional behaviors (compulsions) that are recognized by the person as excessive or unreasonable.

The effectiveness of Prozac in long-term use, ie, for more than 13 weeks, has not been systematically evaluated in placebo-controlled trials. Therefore, the physician who elects to use Prozac for extended periods should periodically reevaluate the long-term usefulness of the drug for the individual patient (*see* Dosage and Administration).

Bulimia Nervosa—Prozac is indicated for the treatment of binge-eating and vomiting behaviors in patients with moderate to severe bulimia nervosa.

The efficacy of Prozac was established in 8 to 16 week trials for adult outpatients with moderate to severe bulimia nervosa, ie, at least 3 bulimic episodes per week for 6 months (*see* Clinical Trials *under* Clinical Pharmacology).

The effectiveness of Prozac in long-term use, ie, for more than 16 weeks, has not been systematically evaluated in placebo-controlled trials. Therefore, the physician who elects to use Prozac for extended periods should periodically reevaluate the long-term usefulness of the drug for the individual patient (*see* Dosage and Administration).

CONTRAINDICATIONS

Prozac is contraindicated in patients known to be hypersensitive to it.

Monoamine Oxidase Inhibitors—There have been reports of serious, sometimes fatal, reactions (including hyperthermia, rigidity, myoclonus, autonomic instability with possible rapid fluctuations of vital signs, and mental status changes that include extreme agitation progressing to delirium and coma) in patients receiving fluoxetine in combination with a monoamine oxidase inhibitor (MAOI), and in patients who have recently discontinued fluoxetine and are then started on an MAOI. Some cases presented with features resembling neuroleptic malignant syndrome. Therefore, Prozac should not be used in combination with an MAOI, or within a minimum of 14 days of discontinuing therapy with an MAOI. Since fluoxetine and its major metabolite have very long elimination half-lives, at least 5 weeks (perhaps longer, especially if fluoxetine has been prescribed chronically and/or at higher doses [*see* Accumulation and Slow Elimination *under* Clinical Pharmacology]) should be allowed after stopping Prozac before starting an MAOI.

WARNINGS

Rash and Possibly Allergic Events—In US fluoxetine clinical trials, 7% of 10,782 patients developed various types of rashes and/or urticaria. Among the cases of rash and/or urticaria reported in premarketing clinical trials, almost a third were withdrawn from treatment because of the rash and/or systemic signs or symptoms associated with the rash. Clinical findings reported in association with rash include fever, leukocytosis, arthralgias, edema, carpal tunnel syndrome, respiratory distress, lymphadenopathy, proteinuria, and mild transaminase elevation. Most patients improved promptly with discontinuation of fluoxetine and/or adjunctive treatment with antihistamines or steroids, and all patients experiencing these events were reported to recover completely.

In premarketing clinical trials, 2 patients are known to have developed a serious cutaneous systemic illness. In neither patient was there an unequivocal diagnosis, but 1 was considered to have a leukocytoclastic vasculitis, and the other, a severe disquamating syndrome that was considered variously to be a vasculitis or erythema multiforme. Other patients have had systemic syndromes suggestive of serum sickness.

Since the introduction of Prozac, systemic events, possibly related to vasculitis, have developed in patients with rash. Although these events are rare, they may be serious, involving the lung, kidney, or liver. Death has been reported to occur in association with these systemic events.

Anaphylactoid events, including bronchospasm, angioedema, and urticaria alone and in combination, have been reported.

Pulmonary events, including inflammatory processes of varying histopathology and/or fibrosis, have been reported rarely. These events have occurred with dyspnea as the only preceding symptom.

Whether these systemic events and rash have a common underlying cause or are due to different etiologies or pathogenic processes is not known. Furthermore, a specific underlying immunologic basis for these events has not been identified. Upon the appearance of rash or of other possibly allergic phenomena for which an alternative etiology cannot be identified, Prozac should be discontinued.

PRECAUTIONS

General

Anxiety and Insomnia—In US placebo-controlled clinical trials for depression, 12% to 16% of patients treated with Prozac and 7% to 9% of patients treated with placebo reported anxiety, nervousness, or insomnia.

In US placebo-controlled clinical trials for obsessive-compulsive disorder, insomnia was reported in 28% of patients treated with Prozac and in 22% of patients treated with placebo. Anxiety was reported in 14% of patients treated with Prozac and in 7% of patients treated with placebo.

In US placebo-controlled clinical trials for bulimia nervosa, insomnia was reported in 33% of patients treated with Prozac, 60 mg, and 13% of patients treated with placebo. Anxiety and nervousness were reported respectively in 15% and 11% of patients treated with Prozac, 60 mg, and in 9% and 5% of patients treated with placebo.

Among the most common adverse events associated with discontinuation (incidence at least twice that for placebo and at least 1% for Prozac in clinical trials collecting only a primary event associated with discontinuation) in US placebo-controlled fluoxetine clinical trials were anxiety (2% in OCD), insomnia (1% in combined indications and 2% in bulimia), and nervousness (1% in depression) (see Table 3, below).

Altered Appetite and Weight—Significant weight loss, especially in underweight depressed or bulimic patients, may be an undersirable result of treatment with Prozac.

In US placebo-controlled clinical trials for depression, 11% of patients treated with Prozac and 2% of patients treated with placebo reported anorexia (decreased appetite). Weight loss was reported in 1.4% of patients treated with Prozac and in 0.5% of patients treated with placebo. However, only rarely have patients discontinued treatment with Prozac because of anorexia or weight loss.

In US placebo-controlled clinical trials for OCD, 17% of patients treated with Prozac and 10% of patients treated with placebo reported anorexia (decreased appetite). One patient discontinued treatment with Prozac because of anorexia.

In US placebo-controlled clinical trials for bulimia nervosa, 8% of patients treated with Prozac, 60 mg, and 4% of patients treated with placebo reported anorexia (decreased appetite). Patients treated with Prozac, 60 mg, on average lost 0.45 kg compared with a gain of 0.16 kg by patients treated with placebo in the 16-week double-blind trial. Weight change should be monitored during therapy.

Activation of Mania/Hypomania—In US placebo-controlled clinical trials for depression, mania/hypomania was reported in 0.1% of patients treated with Prozac and 0.1% of patients treated with placebo. Activation of mania/hypomania has also been reported in a small proportion of patients with Major Affective Disorder treated with marketed antidepressants.

In US placebo-controlled clinical trials for OCD, mania/hypomania was reported in 0.8% of patients treated with Prozac and no patients treated with placebo. No patients reported mania/hypomania in US placebo-controlled clinical trials for bulimia. In all US Prozac clinical trials, 0.7% of 10,782 patients reported mania/hypomania.

Seizures—In US placebo-controlled clinical trials for depression, convulsions (or events described as possibly having been seizures) were reported in 0.1% of patients treated with Prozac and 0.2% of patients treated with placebo. No patients reported convulsions in US placebo-controlled clinical trials for either OCD or bulimia. In all US Prozac clinical trials, 0.2% of 10,782 patients reported convulsions. The percentage appears to be similar to that associated with other marketed antidepressants. Prozac should be introduced with care in patients with a history of seizures.

Suicide—The possibility of a suicide attempt is inherent in depression and may persist until significant remission occurs. Close supervision of high risk patients should accompany initial drug therapy. Prescriptions for Prozac should be written for the smallest quantity of capsules consistent with good patient management, in order to reduce the risk of overdose.

Because of well-established comorbidiy between OCD and depression and bulimia and depression, the same precautions observed when treating patients with depression should be observed when treating patients with OCD or bulimia.

The Long Elimination Half-Lives of Fluoxetine and Its Metabolites—Because of the long elimination half-lives of the parent drug and its major active metabolite, changes in dose will not be fully reflected in plasma for several weeks, affecting both strategies for titration to final dose and withdrawal from treatment (*see* Clinical Pharmacology *and* Dosage and Administration).

Use in Patients With Concomitant Illness—Clinical experience with Prozac in patients with concomitant systemic illness is limited. Caution is advisable in using Prozac in patients with diseases or conditions that could affect metabolism or hemodynamic responses.

Fluoxetine has not been evaluated or used to any appreciable extent in patients with a recent history of myocardial infarction or unstable heart disease. Patients with these diagnoses were systematically excluded from clinical studies during the product's premarket testing. However, the electrocardiograms of 312 patients who received Prozac in double-blind trials were retrospectively evaluated; no conduction abnormalities that resulted in heart block were observed. The mean heart rate was reduced by approximately 3 beats/min.

In subjects with cirrhosis of the liver, the clearances of fluoxetine and its active metabolite, norfluoxetine, were decreased, thus increasing the elimination half-lives of these substances. A lower or less frequent dose should be used in patients with cirrhosis.

Studies in depressed patients on dialysis did not reveal excessive accumulation of fluoxetine or norfluoxetine in plasma (*see* Renal Disease *under* Clinical Pharmacology). Use of a lower or less frequent dose for renally impaired patients is not routinely necessary (*see* Dosage and Administration).

In patients with diabetes, Prozac may alter glycemic control. Hypoglycemia has occurred during therapy with Prozac, and hyperglycemia has developed following discontinuation of the drug. As is true with many other types of medication when taken concurrently by patients with diabetes, insulin and/or oral hypoglycemic dosage may need to be adjusted when therapy with Prozac is instituted or discontinued.

Interference With Cognitive and Motor Performance—Any psychoactive drug may impair judgment, thinking, or motor skills, and patients should be cautioned about operating hazardous machinery, including automobiles, until they are reasonably certain that the drug treatment does not affect them adversely.

Information for Patients—Physicians are advised to discuss the following issues with patients for whom they prescribe Prozac:

Because Prozac may impair judgment, thinking, or motor skills, patients should be advised to avoid driving a car or operating hazardous machinery until they are reasonably certain that their performance is not affected.

Patients should be advised to inform their physician if they are taking or plan to take any prescription or over-the-counter drugs or alcohol.

Patients should be advised to notify their physician if they become pregnant or intend to become pregnant during therapy.

Patients should be advised to notify their physician if they are breast feeding an infant.

Patients should be advised to notify their physician if they develop a rash or hives.

Laboratory Tests—There are no specific laboratory tests recommended.

Drug Interactions—As with all drugs, the potential for interaction by a variety of mechanisms (eg, pharmacodynamic, pharmacokinetic drug inhibition or enhancement, etc) is a possibility (*see* Accumulation and Slow Elimination *under* Clinical Pharmacology).

Drugs Metabolized by P450IID6—Approximately 7% of the normal population has a genetic defect that leads to reduced levels of activity of the cytochrome P450 isoenzyme P450IID6. Such individuals have been referred to as "poor metabolizers" of drugs such as debrisoquin, dextromethorphan, and tricyclic antidepressants. Many drugs, such as most antidepressants, including fluoxetine and other selective uptake inhibitors of serotonin, are metabolized by this isoenzyme; thus, both the pharmacokinetic properties and relative proportion of metabolites are altered in poor metabolizers. However, for fluoxetine and its metabolite the sum of the plasma concentrations of the 4 active enantiomers is comparable between poor and extensive metabolizers (*see* Variability in Metabolism *under* Clinical Pharmacology).

Fluoxetine, like other agents that are metabolized by P450IID6, inhibits the activity of this isoenzyme, and thus may make normal metabolizers resemble "poor metabolizers." Therapy with medications that are predominantly metabolized by the P450IID6 system and that have a relatively narrow therapeutic index (*see* list below), should be initiated at the low end of the dose range if a patient is receiving fluoxetine concurrently or has taken it in the previous 5 weeks. Thus, his/her dosing requirements resemble those of "poor metabolizers." If fluoxetine is added to the treatment regimen of a patient already receiving a drug metabolized by P450IID6, the need for decreased dose of the original medication should be considered. Drugs with a narrow therapeutic index represent the greatest concern (eg, flecainide, vinblastine, and tricyclic antidepressants).

Drugs Metabolized by Cytochrome P450IIIA4—In an in vivo interaction study involving co-administration of fluoxetine with single doses of terfenadine (a cytochrome P450IIIA4 substrate), no increase in plasma terfenadine concentrations occurred with concomitant fluoxetine. In addition, in vitro studies have shown ketoconazole, a potent inhibitor of P450IIIA4 activity, to be at least 100 times more potent than fluoxetine or norfluoxetine as an inhibitor of the metabolism of several substrates for this enzyme, including astemizole, cisapride, and midazolam. These data indicate that fluoxetine's extent of inhibition of cytochrome P450IIIA4 activity is not likely to be of clinical significance.

CNS Active Drugs—The risk of using Prozac in combination with other CNS active drugs has not been systematically evaluated. Nonetheless, caution is advised if the concomitant administration of Prozac and such drugs is required. In evaluating individual cases, consideration should be given to using lower initial doses of the concomitantly administered drugs, using conservative titration schedules, and monitoring of clinical status (*see* Accumulation and Slow Elimination *under* Clinical Pharmacology).

Anticonvulsants—Patients on stable doses of phenytoin and carbamazepine have developed elevated plasma anticonvulsant concentrations and clinical anticonvulsant toxicity following initiation of concomitant fluoxetine treatment.

Antipsychotics—Some clinical data suggests a possible pharmacodynamic and/or pharmacokinetic interaction between serotonin specific reuptake inhibitors (SSRIs) and antipsychotics. Elevation of blood levels of haloperidol and clozapine has been observed in patients receiving concomitant fluoxetine. A single case report has suggested possible additive effects of primozide and fluoxetine leading to bradycardia.

Benzodiazepines—The half-life of concurrently administered diazepam may be prolonged in some patients (*see* Accumulation and Slow Elimination *under* Clinical Pharmacology). Coadministration of alprazolam and fluoxetine has resulted in increased alprazolam plasma concentrations and in further psychomotor performance decrement due to increased alprazolam levels.

Lithium—There have been reports of both increased and decreased lithium levels when lithium was used concomitantly with fluoxetine. Cases of lithium toxicity and increased serotonergic effects have been reported. Lithium levels should be monitored when these drugs are administered concomitantly.

Tryptophan—Five patients receiving Prozac in combination with tryptophan experienced adverse reactions, including agitation, restlessness, and gastrointestinal distress.

Monoamine Oxidase Inhibitors—*See* Contraindications.

Other Antidepressants—In two studies, previously stable plasma levels of imipramine and desipramine have increased greater than 2 to 10-fold when fluoxetine has been administered in combination. This influence may persist for three weeks or longer after fluoxetine is discontinued. Thus, the dose of tricyclic antidepressant (TCA) may need to be reduced and plasma TCA concentrations may need to be monitored temporarily when fluoxetine is coadministered or has been recently discontinued (*see* Accumulation and Slow Elimination *under* Clinical Pharmacology, and Drugs Metabolized by P450IID6 *under* Drug Interactions).

Potential Effects of Coadministration of Drugs Tightly Bound to Plasma Proteins—Because fluoxetine is tightly bound to plasma protein, the administration of fluoxetine to a patient taking another drug that is tightly bound to protein (eg, Coumadin, digitoxin) may cause a shift in plasma concentrations potentially resulting in an adverse effect. Conversely, adverse effects may result from displacement of protein bound fluoxetine by other tightly bound drugs (*see* Accumulation and Slow Elimination *under* Clinical Pharmacology).

Warfarin—Altered anti-coagulant effects, including increased bleeding, have been reported when fluoxetine is coadministered with warfarin. Patients receiving warfarin therapy should receive careful coagulation monitoring when fluoxetine is initiated or stopped.

Electroconvulsive Therapy—There are no clinical studies establishing the benefit of the combined use of ECT and fluoxetine. There have been rare reports of prolonged seizures in patients on fluoxetine receiving ECT treatment.

Carcinogenesis, Mutagenesis, Impairment of Fertility—There is no evidence of carcinogenicity, mutagenicity, or impairment of fertility with Prozac.

Carcinogenicity—The dietary administration of fluoxetine to rats and mice for 2 years at doses of up to 10 and 12 mg/kg/day, respectively (approximately 1.2 and 0.7 times, respectively, the maximum recommended human dose [MRHD] of 80 mg on a mg/m^2 basis), produced no evidence of carcinogenicity.

Mutagenicity—Fluoxetine and norfluoxetine have been shown to have no genotoxic effects based on the following assays: bacterial mutation assay, DNA repair assay in cultured rat hepatocytes, mouse lymphoma assay, and in vivo sister chromatid exchange assay in Chinese hamster bone marrow cells.

Impairment of Fertility—Two fertility studies conducted in rats at doses of up to 7.5 and 12.5 mg/kg/day (approximately 0.9 and 1.5 times the MRHD on a mg/m^2 basis), indicated that fluoxetine had no adverse effects on fertility.

Pregnancy—Pregnancy Category C: In embryo-fetal development studies in rats and rabbits, there was no evidence of teratogenicity following administration of up to 12.5 and 15 mg/kg/day, respectively (1.5 and 3.6 times, respectively, the maximum recommended human dose [MRHD] of 80 mg on a mg/m^2 basis) throughout organogenesis. However, in rat reproduction studies, an increase in stillborn pups, a decrease in pup weight, and an increase in pup deaths during the first 7 days postpartum occurred following maternal exposure to 12 mg/kg/day (1.5 times the MRHD on a mg/m^2 basis) during gestation or 7.5 mg/kg/day (0.9 times the MRHD on a mg/m^2 basis) during gestation and lactation. There was no evidence of developmental neurotoxicity in the surviving offspring of rats treated with 12 mg/kg/day during gestation. The no-effect dose for rat pup mortality was 5 mg/kg/day (0.6 times the MRHD on a mg/m^2 basis). Prozac should be used during pregnancy only if the potential benefit justifies the potential risk to the fetus.

Labor and Delivery—The effect of Prozac on labor and delivery in humans is unknown. However, because fluoxetine crosses the placenta and because of the possibility that fluoxetine may have adverse effects on the newborn, fluoxetine should be used during labor and delivery only if the potential benefit justifies the potential risk to the fetus.

Nursing Mothers—Because Prozac is excreted in human milk, nursing while on Prozac is not recommended. In 1 breast milk sample, the concentration of fluoxetine plus norfluoxetine was 70.4 ng/mL. The concentration in the mother's plasma was 295.0 ng/mL. No adverse effects on the infant were reported. In another case, an infant nursed by a mother on Prozac developed crying, sleep disturbance, vomiting, and watery stools. The infant's plasma drug levels were 340 ng/mL of fluoxetine and 208 ng/mL of norfluoxetine on the second day of feeding.

Pediatric Use—Safety and effectiveness in pediatric patients have not been established.

Geriatric Use—U.S. fluoxetine clinical trials (10,782 patients) included 687 patients ≥ 65 years of age and 93 patients ≥ 75 years of age. The efficacy in geriatric patients has been established (*see* Clinical Trials *under* Clinical Pharmacology). For pharmacokinetic information in geriatric patients see Age under Clinical Pharmacology. No overall differences in safety or effectiveness were observed between these subjects and younger subjects, and other reported clinical experience has not identified differences in responses between the elderly and younger patients, but greater sensitivity of some older individuals cannot be ruled out. As with other SSRIs, fluoxetine has been associated with cases of clinically significant hyponatremia in elderly patients (*see* Hyponatremia *under* Precautions).

Hyponatremia—Cases of hyponatremia (some with serum sodium lower than 110 mmol/L) have been reported. The hyponatremia appeared to be reversible when Prozac was discontinued. Although these cases were complex with varying possible etiologies, some were possibly due to the syndrome of inappropriate antidiuretic hormone secretion (SIADH). The majority of these occurrences have been in older patients and in patients taking diuretics or who were otherwise volume depleted. In two 6-week controlled studies in patients ≥ 60 years of age, 10 of 323 fluoxetine patients and 6 of 327 placebo recipients had a lowering of serum sodium below the reference range; this difference was not statistically significant. The lowest observed concentration was 129 mmol/L. The observed decreases were not clinically significant.

Platelet Function—There have been rare reports of altered platelet function and/or abnormal results from laboratory studies in patients taking fluoxetine. While there have been reports of abnormal bleeding in several patients taking fluoxetine, it is unclear whether fluoxetine had a causative role.

ADVERSE REACTIONS

Multiple doses of Prozac had been administered to 10,782 patients with various diagnoses in US clinical trials as of May 8, 1995. Adverse events were recorded by clinical in-

Continued on next page

This product information was prepared in June 2000. Current information on these and other products of Dista Products Company may be obtained by direct inquiry to Lilly Research Laboratories, Lilly Corporate Center, Indianapolis, Indiana 46285, (800) 545-5979.

Prozac—Cont.

vestigators using descriptive terminology of their own choosing. Consequently, it is not possible to provide a meaningful estimate of the proportion of individuals experiencing adverse events without first grouping similar types of events into a limited (ie, reduced) number of standardized event categories.

In the tables and tabulations that follow, COSTART Dictionary terminology has been used to classify reported adverse events. The stated frequencies represent the proportion of individuals who experienced, at least once, a treatment-emergent adverse event of the type listed. An event was considered treatment-emergent if it occurred for the first time or worsened while receiving therapy following baseline evaluation. It is important to emphasize that events reported during therapy were not necessarily caused by it.

The prescriber should be aware that the figures in the tables and tabulations cannot be used to predict the incidence of side effects in the course of usual medical practice where patient characteristics and other factors differ from those that prevailed in the clinical trials. Similarly, the cited frequencies cannot be compared with figures obtained from other clinical investigations involving different treatments, uses, and investigators. The cited figures, however, do provide the prescribing physician with some basis for estimating the relative contribution of drug and nondrug factors to the side effect incidence rate in the population studied.

Incidence in US Placebo-Controlled Clinical Trials (excluding data from extensions of trials)—Table 1 enumerates the most common treatment-emergent adverse events associated with the use of Prozac (incidence of at least 5% for Prozac and at least twice that for placebo within at least one of the indications) for the treatment of depression, OCD, and bulimia in US controlled clinical trials. Table 2 enumerates treatment-emergent adverse events that occurred in 2% or more patients treated with Prozac and with incidence greater than placebo who participated in US controlled clinical trials comparing Prozac with placebo in the treatment of depression, OCD, or bulimia. Table 2 provides combined data for the pool of studies that are provided separately by indication in Table 1.

[See table 1 above]

TABLE 2.
TREATMENT-EMERGENT ADVERSE EVENTS: INCIDENCE IN US DEPRESSION, OCD, AND BULIMIA PLACEBO-CONTROLLED CLINICAL TRIALS

	Percentage of Patients Reporting Event	
	Depression, OCD, and bulimia combined	
Body System/ Adverse Event*	Prozac (N=2444)	Placebo (N=1331)
Body as a Whole		
Headache	21	20
Asthenia	12	6
Flu Syndrome	5	4
Fever	2	1
Cardiovascular System		
Vasodilatation	3	1
Palpitation	2	1
Digestive System		
Nausea	23	10
Diarrhea	12	8
Anorexia	11	3
Dry mouth	10	7
Dyspepsia	8	5
Flatulence	3	2
Vomiting	3	2
Metabolic and Nutritional Disorders		
Weight loss	2	1
Nervous System		
Insomnia	20	11
Anxiety	13	8
Nervousness	13	9
Somnolence	13	6
Dizziness	10	7
Tremor	10	3
Libido decreased	4	—
Respiratory System		
Pharyngitis	5	4
Yawn	3	—
Skin and Appendages		
Sweating	8	3
Rash	4	3
Pruritus	3	2
Special Senses		
Abnormal vision	3	1

*Included are events reported by at least 2% of patients taking Prozac, except the following events, which had an incidence on placebo ≥Prozac (depression, OCD, and bulimia combined): abdominal pain, abnormal dreams, accidental injury, back pain, chest pain, constipation, cough increased, depression (includes suicidal thoughts), dysmenorrhea, gastrointestinal disorder, infection, myalgia, pain, paresthesia, rhinitis, sinusitis, thinking abnormal.
—Incidence less than 1%.

TABLE 1—MOST COMMON TREATMENT-EMERGENT ADVERSE EVENTS: INCIDENCE IN US DEPRESSION, OCD, AND BULIMIA PLACEBO-CONTROLLED CLINICAL TRIALS

	Percentage of patients reporting event					
	Depression		OCD		Bulimia	
Body System/ Adverse Event	Prozac (N=1728)	Placebo (N=975)	Prozac (N=266)	Placebo (N=89)	Prozac (N=450)	Placebo (N=267)
Body as a Whole						
Asthenia	9	5	15	11	21	9
Flu syndrome	3	4	10	7	8	3
Cardiovascular System						
Vasodilatation	3	2	5	—	2	1
Digestive System						
Nausea	21	9	26	13	29	11
Anorexia	11	2	17	10	8	4
Dry mouth	10	7	12	3	9	6
Dyspepsia	7	5	10	4	10	6
Nervous System						
Insomnia	16	9	28	22	33	13
Anxiety	12	7	14	7	15	9
Nervousness	14	9	14	15	11	5
Somnolence	13	6	17	7	13	5
Tremor	10	3	9	1	13	1
Libido decreased	3	—	11	2	5	1
Abnormal dreams	1	1	5	2	5	3
Respiratory System						
Pharyngitis	3	3	11	9	10	5
Sinusitis	1	4	5	2	6	4
Yawn	—	—	7	—	11	—
Skin and Appendages						
Sweating	8	3	7	—	8	3
Rash	4	3	6	3	4	4
Urogenital System						
Impotence†	2	—	—	—	7	—
Abnormal ejaculation†	—	—	7	—	7	—

†Denominator used was for males only (N=690 Prozac depression; N=410 placebo depression; N=116 Prozac OCD; N=43 placebo OCD; N=14 Prozac bulimia; N=1 placebo bulimia).
—Incidence less than 1%.

TABLE 3—MOST COMMON ADVERSE EVENTS ASSOCIATED WITH DISCONTINUATION IN US DEPRESSION, OCD, AND BULIMIA PLACEBO-CONTROLLED CLINICAL TRIALS

Depression, OCD, and bulimia combined (N=1108)	Depression (N=392)	OCD (N=266)	Bulimia (N=450)
—	—	Anxiety (2%)	—
Insomnia (1%)	—	—	Insomnia (2%)
—	Nervousness (1%)	—	—
—	—	Rash (1%)	—

Associated with Discontinuation in US Placebo-Controlled Clinical Trials (excluding data from extensions of trials)—Table 3 lists the adverse events associated with discontinuation of Prozac treatment (incidence at least twice that for placebo and at least 1% for Prozac in clinical trials collecting only a primary event associated with discontinuation) in depression, OCD, and bulimia.

[See table 3 above]

Other Events Observed In All US Clinical Trials—Following is a list of all treatment-emergent adverse events reported at anytime by individuals taking fluoxetine in US clinical trials (10,782 patients) except (1) those listed in the body or footnotes of Table 1 or 2 above or elsewhere in labeling; (2) those for which the COSTART terms were uninformative or misleading; (3) those events for which a causal relationship to Prozac use was considered remote; and (4) events occurring in only 1 patient treated with Prozac and which did not have a substantial probability of being acutely life-threatening.

Events are classified within body system categories using the following definitions: frequent adverse events are defined as those occurring on 1 or more occasions in at least 1/100 patients; infrequent adverse events are those occurring in 1/100 to 1/1,000 patients; rare events are those occurring in less than 1/1,000 patients.

Body as a Whole—*Frequent:* chills; *Infrequent:* chills and fever, face edema, intentional overdose, malaise, pelvic pain, suicide attempt; *Rare:* abdominal syndrome acute, hypothermia, intentional injury, neuroleptic malignant syndrome, photosensitivity reaction.

Cardiovascular System—*Frequent:* hemorrhage, hypertension; *Infrequent:* angina pectoris, arrhythmia, congestive heart failure, hypotension, migraine, myocardial infarct, postural hypotension, syncope, tachycardia, vascular headache; *Rare:* atrial fibrillation, bradycardia, cerebral embolism, cerebral ischemia, cerebrovascular accident, extrasystoles, heart arrest, heart block, pallor, peripheral vascular disorder, phlebitis, shock, thrombophlebitis, thrombosis, vasospasm, ventricular arrhythmia, ventricular extrasystoles, ventricular fibrillation.

Digestive System—*Frequent:* increased appetite, nausea and vomiting; *Infrequent:* aphthous stomatitis, cholelithiasis, colitis, dysphagia, eructation, esophagitis, gastritis, gastroenteritis, glossitis, gum hemmorhage, hyperchlorhydria, increased salivation, liver function tests abnormal, melena, mouth ulceration, nausea/vomiting/diarrhea, stomach ulcer, stomatitis, thirst; *Rare:* biliary pain, bloody diarrhea, cholecystitis, duodenal ulcer, enteritis, esophageal ulcer, fecal incontinence, gastrointestinal hemorrhage, hematemesis, hemorrhage of colon, hepatitis, intestinal obstruction, liver fatty deposit, pancreatitis, peptic ulcer, rectal hemorrhage, salivary gland enlargement, stomach ulcer hemorrhage, tongue edema.

Endocrine System—*Infrequent:* hypothyroidism: *Rare:* diabetic acidosis, diabetes mellitus.

Hemic and Lymphatic System—*Infrequent:* anemia, ecchymosis; *Rare:* blood dyscrasia, hypochromic anemia, leukopenia, lymphedema, lymphocytosis, petechia, purpura, thrombocythemia, thrombocytopenia.

Metabolic and Nutritional—*Frequent:* weight gain; *Infrequent:* dehydration, generalized edema, gout, hypercholesteremia, hyperlipemia, hypokalemia, preipheral edema, *Rare:* alcohol intolerance, alkaline phosphatase increased, BUN increased, creatine phosphokinase increased, hyperkalemia, hyperuricemia, hypocalcemia, iron deficiency anemia, SGPT increased.

Musculoskeletal System—*Infrequent:* arthritis, bone pain, bursitis, leg cramps, tenosynovitis; *Rare:* arthrosis, chondrodystrophy, myasthenia, myopathy, myositis, osteomyelitis, osteoporosis, rheumatoid arthritis.

Nervous System—*Frequent:* agitation, amnesia, confusion, emotional lability, sleep disorder; *Infrequent:* abnormal gait, acute brain syndrome, akathisia, apathy, ataxia, buccoglossal syndrome, CNS depression, CNS stimulation, depersonalization, euphoria, hallucinations, hostility, hyperkinesia, hypertonia, hypesthesia, incoordination, libido increased, myoclonus, nueralgia, neuropathy, neurosis, paranoid reaction, personality disorder†, psychosis, vertigo; *Rare:* abnormal electroencephalogram, antisocial reaction, circumoral paresthesia, coma, delusions, dysarthria, dystonia, extrapyramidal syndrome, foot drop, hyperesthesia, neuritis, paralysis, reflexes decreased, reflexes increased, stupor.

Respiratory System—*Infrequent:* asthma, epistaxis, hiccup, hyperventilation; *Rare:* apnea, atelectasis, cough decreased, emphysema, hemoptysis, hypoventilation, hypoxia, larynx edema, lung edema, pneumothorax, stridor.

Skin and Appendages—*Infrequent:* acne, alopecia, contact dermatitis, eczema, maculopapular rash, skin discoloration, skin ulcer, vesiculobullous rash; *Rare:* furunculosis, herpes zoster, hirsutism, petechial rash, psoriasis, purpuric rash, pustular rash, seborrhea.

Special Senses—*Frequent:* ear pain, taste perversion, tinnitus; *Infrequent:* conjunctivitis, dry eyes, mydriasis, photophobia; *Rare:* blepharitis, deafness, diplopia, exophthalmos, eye hemorrhage, glaucoma, hyperacusis, iritis, parosmia, scleritis, strabismus, taste loss, visual field defect.

Urogenital System—*Frequent:* urinary frequency; *Infrequent:* abortion*, albuminuria, amenorrhea*, anorgasmia, breast enlargement, breast pain, cystitis, dysuria, female lactation*, fibrocystic breast*, hematuria, leukorrhea*, menorrhagia*, metrorrhagia*, nocturia, polyuria, urinary incontinence, urinary retention, urinary urgency, vaginal hemorrhage*; *Rare:* breast engorgement, glycosuria, hypomenorrhea*, kidney pain, oliguria, priapism*, uterine hemorrhage*, uterine fibroids enlarged*.

† Personality disorder is the COSTART term for designating non-aggressive objectionable behavior.

* Adjusted for gender

Postintroduction Reports—Voluntary reports of adverse events temporally associated with Prozac that have been received since market introduction and that may have no causal relationship with the drug include the following: aplastic anemia, atrial fibrillation, cerebral vascular accident, cholestatic jaundice, confusion, dyskinesia (including, for example, a case of buccal-lingual-masticatory syndrome with involuntary tongue protrusion reported to develop in a 77-year-old female after 5 weeks of fluoxetine therapy and which completely resolved over the next few months following drug discontinuation), eosinophilic pneumonia, epidermal necrolysis, erythema nodosum, exfoliative dermatitis, gynecomastia, heart arrest, hepatic failure/necrosis, hyperprolactinemia, immune-related hemolytic anemia, kidney failure, misuse/abuse, movement disorders developing in patients with risk factors including drugs associated with such events and worsening of preexisting movement disorders, neuroleptic malignant syndrome-like events, pancreatitis, pancytopenia, priapism, pulmonary embolism, QT prolongation, Stevens-Johnson syndrome, sudden unexpected death, suicidal ideation, thrombocytopenia, thrombocytopenic purpura, vaginal bleeding after drug withdrawal, and violent behaviors.

DRUG ABUSE AND DEPENDENCE

Controlled Substance Class—Prozac is not a controlled substance.

Physical and Psychological Dependence—Prozac has not been systematically studied, in animals or humans, for its potential for abuse, tolerance or physical dependence. While the premarketing clinical experience with Prozac did not reveal any tendency for a withdrawal syndrome or any drug-seeking behavior, these observations were not systematic and it is not possible to predict on the basis of this limited experience the extent to which a CNS-active drug will be misused, diverted, and/or abused once marketed. Consequently, physicians should carefully evaluate patients for history of drug abuse and follow such patients closely, observing them for signs of misuse or abuse of Prozac (eg, development of tolerance, incrementation of dose, drug-seeking behavior).

OVERDOSAGE

Human Experience—As of December 1987, there were 2 deaths among approximately 38 reports of acute overdose with fluoxetine, either alone or in combination with other drugs and/or alcohol. One death involved a combined overdose with approximately 1,800 mg of fluoxetine and an undetermined amount of maprotiline. Plasma concentrations of fluoxetine and maprotiline were 4.57 mg/L and 4.18 mg/L, respectively. A second death involved 3 drugs yielding plasma concentrations as follows: fluoxetine, 1.93 mg/L; norfluoxetine, 1.10 mg/L; codeine, 1.80 mg/L; temazepam, 3.80 mg/L.

One other patient who reportedly took 3,000 mg of fluoxetine experienced 2 grand mal seizures that remitted spontaneously without specific anticonvulsant treatment (*see* Management of Overdose). The actual amount of drug absorbed may have been less due to vomiting.

Nausea and vomiting were prominent in overdoses involving higher fluoxetine doses. Other prominent symptoms of overdose included agitation, restlessness, hypomania, and other signs of CNS excitation. Except for the 2 deaths noted above, all other overdose cases recovered without residua.

Since introduction, reports of death attributed to overdosage of fluoxetine alone have been extremely rare.

Animal Experience—Studies in animals do not provide precise or necessarily valid information about the treatment of human overdose. However, animal experiments can provide useful insights into possible treatment strategies.

The oral median lethal dose in rats and mice was found to be 452 and 248 mg/kg respectively. Acute high oral doses produced hyperirritability and convulsions in several animal species.

Among 6 dogs purposely overdosed with oral fluoxetine, 5 experienced grand mal seizures. Seizures stopped immediately upon the bolus intravenous administration of a standard veterinary dose of diazepam. In this short-term study, the lowest plasma concentration at which a seizure occurred was only twice the maximum plasma concentration seen in humans taking 80 mg/day, chronically.

In a separate single-dose study, the ECG in dogs given high doses did not reveal prolongation of the PR, QRS, or QT intervals. Tachycardia and an increase in blood pressure were observed. Consequently, the value of the ECG in predicting cardiac toxicity is unknown. Nonetheless, the ECG should ordinarily be monitored in cases of human overdose (*see* Management of Overdose).

Management of Overdose—Treatment should consist of those general measures employed in the management of overdosage with any antidepressant.

Ensure an adequate airway, oxygenation, and ventilation. Monitor cardiac rhythm and vital signs. General supportive and symptomatic measures are also recommended. Induction of emesis is not recommended. Gastric lavage with a large-bore orogastric tube with appropriate airway protection, if needed, may be indicated if performed soon after ingestion, or in symptomatic patients.

Activated charcoal should be administered. Due to the large volume of distribution of this drug, forced diuresis, dialysis, hemoperfusion and exchange transfusion are unlikely to be of benefit. No specific antidotes for fluoxetine are known.

A specific caution involves patients who are taking or have recently taken fluoxetine and might ingest excessive quantities of a tricyclic antidepressant. In such a case, accumulation of the parent tricyclic and/or an active metabolite may increase the possibility of clinically significant sequelae and extend the time needed for close medical observation (*see* Other Antidepressants *under* Precautions).

Based on experience in animals, which may not be relevant to humans, fluoxetine-induced seizures that fail to remit spontaneously may respond to diazepam.

In managing overdosage, consider the possibility of multiple drug involvement. The physician should consider contacting a poison control center for additional information on the treatment of any overdose. Telephone numbers for certified poison control centers are listed in the *Physicians' Desk Reference (PDR)*.

DOSAGE AND ADMINISTRATION

Depression—

Initial Treatment—In controlled trials used to support the efficacy of fluoxetine, patients were administered morning doses ranging from 20 mg to 80 mg/day. Studies comparing fluoxetine 20, 40, and 60 mg/day to placebo indicate that 20 mg/day is sufficient to obtain a satisfactory antidepressant response in most cases. Consequently, a dose of 20 mg/day, administered in the morning, is recommended as the initial dose.

A dose increase may be considered after several weeks if no clinical improvement is observed. Doses above 20 mg/day may be administered on a once a day (morning) or b.i.d. schedule (ie, morning and noon) and should not exceed a maximum dose of 80 mg/day.

As with other antidepressants, the full antidepressant effect may be delayed until 4 weeks of treatment or longer.

As with many other medications, a lower or less frequent dosage should be used in patients with hepatic impairment. A lower or less frequent dosage should also be considered for the elderly (*see* Geriatric Use *under* Precautions), and for patients with concurrent disease or on multiple concomitant medications. Dosage adjustments for renal impairment are not routinely necessary (*see* Liver Disease and Renal Disease *under* Clinical Pharmacology, *and* Use in Patients with Concomitant Illness *under* Precautions).

Maintenance/Continuation/Extended Treatment—It is generally agreed that acute episodes of depression require several months or longer of sustained pharmacologic therapy. Whether the dose of antidepressant needed to induce remission is identical to the dose needed to maintain and/or sustain euthymia is unknown.

Systematic evaluation of Prozac has shown that its antidepressant efficacy is maintained for periods of up to 38 weeks following 12 weeks of open-label acute treatment (50 weeks total) at a dose of 20 mg/day (*see* Clinical Trials *under* Clinical Pharmacology).

Obsessive-Compulsive Disorder—

Initial Treatment—In the controlled clinical trials of fluoxetine supporting its effectiveness in the treatment of obsessive-compulsive disorder, patients were administered fixed daily doses of 20, 40, or 60 mg of fluoxetine or placebo (*see* Clinical Trials *under* Clinical Pharmacology). In one of these studies, no dose response relationship for effectiveness was demonstrated. Consequently, a dose of 20 mg/day, administered in the morning, is recommended as the initial dose. Since there was a suggestion of a possible dose response relationship for effectiveness in the second study, a dose increase may be considered after several weeks if insufficient clinical improvement is observed. The full therapeutic effect may be delayed until 5 weeks of treatment or longer.

Doses above 20 mg/day may be administered on a once a day (ie, morning) or b.i.d. schedule (ie, morning and noon). A dose range of 20 to 60 mg/day is recommended, however, doses of up to 80 mg/day have been well tolerated in open studies of OCD. The maximum fluoxetine dose should not exceed 80 mg/day.

As with the use of Prozac in depression, a lower or less frequent dosage should be used in patients with hepatic impairment. A lower or less frequent dosage should also be considered for the elderly (*see* Geriatric Use *under* Precautions), and for patients with concurrent disease or on multiple concomitant medications. Dosage adjustments for renal impairment are not routinely necessary (*see* Liver Disease and Renal Disease *under* Clinical Pharmacology, *and* Use in Patients with Concomitant Illness *under* Precautions).

Maintenance/Continuation Treatment—While there are no systematic studies that answer the question of how long to continue Prozac, OCD is a chronic condition and it is reasonable to consider continuation for a responding patient. Although the efficacy of Prozac after 13 weeks has not been documented in controlled trials, patients have been continued in therapy under double-blind conditions for up to an additional 6 months without loss of benefit. However, dosage adjustments should be made to maintain the patient on the lowest effective dosage, and patients should be periodically reassessed to determine the need for treatment.

Bulimia Nervosa—

Initial Treatment—In the controlled clinical trials of fluoxetine supporting its effectiveness in the treatment of bulimia nervosa, patients were administered fixed daily fluoxetine doses of 20 or 60 mg, or placebo (*see* Clinical Trials *under* Clinical Pharmacology). Only the 60 mg dose was statistically significantly superior to placebo in reducing the frequency of binge-eating and vomiting. Consequently, the recommended dose is 60 mg/day, administered in the morning. For some patients it may be advisable to titrate up to this target dose over several days. Fluoxetine doses above 60 mg/day have not been systematically studied in patients with bulimia.

As with the use of Prozac in depression and OCD, a lower or less frequent dosage should be used in patients with hepatic impairment. A lower or less frequent dosage should also be considered for the elderly (*see* Geriatric Use *under* Precautions), and for patients with concurrent disease or on multiple concomitant medications. Dosage adjustments for renal impairment are not routinely necessary (*see* Liver Disease and Renal Disease *under* Clinical Pharmacology, *and* Use in Patients with Concomitant Illness *under* Precautions).

Maintenance/Continuation Treatment—While there are no systematic studies that answer the question of how long to continue Prozac, bulimia is a chronic condition and it is reasonable to consider continuation for a responding patient. Although the efficacy of Prozac after 16 weeks has not been documented in controlled trials, some patients have been continued in therapy under double-blind conditions for up to an additional 6 months without loss of benefit. However, patients should be periodically reassessed to determine the need for continued treatment.

Switching Patients to a Tricyclic Antidepressant (TCA): Dosage of a TCA may need to be reduced, and plasma TCA concentrations may need to be monitored temporarily when fluoxetine is coadministered or has been recently discontinued (*see* Other Antidepressants *under* Drug Interactions).

Switching Patients to or from a Monoamine Oxidase Inhibitor:

At least 14 days should elapse between discontinuation of an MAOI and initiation of therapy with Prozac. In addition, at least 5 weeks, perhaps longer, should be allowed after stopping Prozac before starting an MAOI (*see* Contraindications and Precautions).

HOW SUPPLIED

The following products are manufactured by Eli Lilly and Company for Dista Products Company.

Prozac® Pulvules®, USP, are available in:

The 10 mg* Pulvule is opaque green and green, imprinted with DISTA 3104 on the cap and Prozac 10 mg on the body:

NDC 0777-3104-02 (PU3104) - Bottles of 100
NDC 0777-3104-07 (PU3104) - Bottles of 2000
NDC 0777-3104-82 (PU3104) - 20 FlexPak™§ blister cards of 31

The 20 mg* Pulvule is an opaque green cap and off-white body, imprinted with DISTA 3105 on the cap and Prozac 20 mg on the body:

NDC 0777-3105-30 (PU3105) - Bottles of 30
NDC 0777-3105-02 (PU3105) - Bottles of 100
NDC 0777-3105-07 (PU3105) - Bottles of 2000
NDC 0777-3105-33 (PU3105) - (ID†100) Blisters
NDC 0777-3105-82 (PU3105) - 20 FlexPak™§ blister cards of 31

The 40 mg* Pulvule is an opaque green cap and opaque orange body, imprinted with DISTA 3107 on the cap and Prozac 40 mg on the body:

NDC 0777-3107-30 (PU3107) - Bottles of 30

Liquid, Oral Solution is available in:
20 mg* per 5 mL with mint flavor:

NDC 0777-5120-58 (MS-5120‡) - Bottles of 120 mL

The following products are manufactured and distributed by Eli Lilly and Company.

Prozac® Tablets are available in:

The 10 mg* tablet is green, elliptical shaped, and scored, with PROZAC 10 depossed on opposite side of score.

Continued on next page

This product information was prepared in June 2000. Current information on these and other products of Dista Products Company may be obtained by direct inquiry to Lilly Research Laboratories, Lilly Corporate Center, Indianapolis, Indiana 46285, (800) 545-5979.

Prozac—Cont.

NDC 0002-4006-30 (TA4006) - Bottles of 30
NDC 0002-4006-02 (TA4006) - Bottles of 100

*Fluoxetine base equivalent.
†Identi-Dose® (unit dose medication, Lilly).
‡Dispense in a tight, light-resistant container.
§FlexPak™ (flexible blister card, Lilly).
Store at controlled room temperature, 59° to 86°F (15° to 30°C).

ANIMAL TOXICOLOGY

Phospholipids are increased in some tissues of mice, rats, and dogs given fluoxetine chronically. This effect is reversible after cessation of fluoxetine treatment. Phospholipid accumulation in animals has been observed with many cationic amphiphilic drugs, including fenfluramine, imipramine, and rantidine. The significance of this effect to humans is unknown.

Rx only

Literature revised August 11, 1999
PV 3312 DPP [081199]

Shown in Product Identification Guide, page 311

DJ Pharma Inc.

12730 HIGH BLUFF BLVD
SUITE 160
SAN DIEGO, CA 92130

For Direct Inquiries:
1-877-DJ Pharm
1-877-357-4276

CEDAX® ℞

(ceftibuten capsules)
and
(ceftibuten for oral suspension)
FOR ORAL USE ONLY

DESCRIPTION

CEDAX (ceftibuten capsules) and (ceftibuten for oral suspension) contain the active ingredient ceftibuten as ceftibuten dihydrate. Ceftibuten dihydrate is a semisynthetic cephalosporin antibiotic for oral administration. Chemically, it is (+)-(6R,7R)-7-[(Z)-2-(2-Amino-4-thiazolyl)-4-carboxycrotonamido]-8-oxo-5-thia-1-azabicyclo[4.2.0]oct-2-ene-2-carboxylic acid, dihydrate. Its molecular formula is $C_{15}H_{14}N_4O_6S_2 \cdot 2H_2O$. Its molecular weight is 446.43 as the dihydrate.

Ceftibuten dihydrate has the following structural formula:

CEDAX Capsules contain ceftibuten dihydrate equivalent to 400 mg of ceftibuten. Inactive ingredients contained in the capsule formulation include: magnesium stearate, microcrystalline cellulose, and sodium starch glycolate. The capsule shell and/or band contains gelatin, sodium lauryl sulfate, titanium dioxide, and polysorbate 80. The capsule shell may also contain benzyl alcohol, sodium propionate, edetate calcium disodium, butylparaben, propylparaben, and methylparaben.

CEDAX Oral Suspension after reconstitution contains ceftibuten dihydrate equivalent to 90 mg of ceftibuten per 5 mL. CEDAX Oral Suspension is cherry flavored and contains the inactive ingredients: cherry flavoring, polysorbate 80, silicon dioxide, simethicone, sodium benzoate, sucrose (approximately 1 g/5 mL), titanium dioxide, and xanthan gum.

CLINICAL PHARMACOLOGY

PHARMACOKINETICS

Absorption:

CEDAX CAPSULES

Ceftibuten is rapidly absorbed after oral administration of CEDAX Capsules. The plasma concentrations and pharmacokinetic parameters of ceftibuten after a single 400-mg dose of CEDAX Capsules to 12 healthy adult male volunteers (20 to 39 years of age) are displayed in the table below. When CEDAX Capsules were administered once daily for 7 days, the average C_{max} was 17.9 µg/mL on day 7. Therefore, ceftibuten accumulation in plasma is about 20% at steady state.

CEDAX ORAL SUSPENSION

Ceftibuten is rapidly absorbed after oral administration of CEDAX Oral Suspension. The plasma concentrations and pharmacokinetic parameters of ceftibuten after a single 9-mg/kg dose of CEDAX Oral Suspension to 32 fasting pediatric patients (6 months to 12 years of age) are displayed in the following table:

[See table below]

The absolute bioavailability of CEDAX Oral Suspension has not been determined. The plasma concentrations of ceftibuten in pediatric patients are dose proportional following single doses of CEDAX Capsules of 200 mg and 400 mg and of CEDAX Oral Suspension between 4.5 mg/kg and 9 mg/kg.

Distribution:

CEDAX CAPSULES

The average apparent volume of distribution (V/F) of ceftibuten in 6 adult subjects is 0.21 L/kg (± 1 SD = 0.03 L/kg).

CEDAX ORAL SUSPENSION

The average apparent volume of distribution (V/F) of ceftibuten in 32 fasting pediatric patients is 0.5 L/kg (± 1 SD = 0.02 L/kg).

Protein Binding:

Ceftibuten is 65% bound to plasma proteins. The protein binding is independent of plasma ceftibuten concentration.

Tissue Penetration:

Bronchial secretions: In a study of 15 adults administered a single 400-mg dose of ceftibuten and scheduled to undergo bronchoscopy, the mean concentrations in epithelial lining fluid and bronchial mucosa were 15% and 37%, respectively, of the plasma concentrations.

Sputum: Ceftibuten sputum levels average approximately 7% of the concomitant plasma ceftibuten level. In a study of 24 adults administered ceftibuten 200 mg bid or 400 mg qd, the average C_{max} in sputum (1.5 µg/mL) occurred at 2 hours postdose and the average C_{max} in plasma (17 µg/mL) occurred at 2 hours postdose.

Middle-ear fluid (MEF): In a study of 12 pediatric patients administered 9 mg/kg, ceftibuten MEF area under the curve (AUC) averaged approximately 70% of the plasma AUC. In the same study, C_{max} values were 14.3 ± 2.7 µg/mL in MEF at 4 hours postdose and 14.5 ± 3.7 µg/mL in plasma at 2 hours postdose.

Parameter	Average Plasma Concentration (in µg/mL of ceftibuten after a single 400-mg dose) and Derived Pharmacokinetic Parameters (± 1 SD) (n = 12 healthy adult males)	Average Plasma Concentration (in µg/mL of ceftibuten after a single 9-mg/kg dose) and Derived Pharmacokinetic Parameters (± 1 SD) (n = 32 pediatric patients)
1.0 h	6.1 (5.1)	9.3 (6.3)
1.5 h	9.9 (5.9)	8.6 (4.4)
2.0 h	11.3 (5.2)	11.2 (4.6)
3.0 h	13.3 (3.0)	9.0 (3.4)
4.0 h	11.2 (2.9)	6.6 (3.1)
6.0 h	5.8 (1.6)	3.8 (2.5)
8.0 h	3.2 (1.0)	1.6 (1.3)
12.0 h	1.1 (0.4)	0.5 (0.4)
C_{max}, µg/mL	15.0 (3.3)	13.4 (4.9)
T_{max}, h	2.6 (0.9)	2.0 (1.0)
AUC, µg•h/mL	73.7 (16.0)	56.0 (16.9)
T½, h	2.4 (0.2)	2.0 (0.6)
Total body clearance (Cl/F) mL/min/kg	1.3 (0.3)	2.9 (0.7)

Tonsillar tissue: Data on ceftibuten penetration into tonsillar tissue are not available.

Cerebrospinal fluid: Data on ceftibuten penetration into cerebrospinal fluid are not available.

Metabolism and Excretion:

A study with radiolabeled ceftibuten administered to 6 healthy adult male volunteers demonstrated that *cis*-ceftibuten is the predominant component in both plasma and urine. About 10% of ceftibuten is converted to the *trans*-isomer. The *trans*-isomer is approximately $^1/_8$ as antimicrobially potent as the *cis*-isomer.

Ceftibuten is excreted in the urine; 95% of the administered radioactivity was recovered either in urine or feces. In 6 healthy adult male volunteers, approximately 56% of the administered dose of ceftibuten was recovered from urine and 39% from the feces within 24 hours. Because renal excretion is a significant pathway of elimination, patients with renal dysfunction and patients undergoing hemodialysis require dosage adjustment (see **DOSAGE AND ADMINISTRATION**).

Food Effect on Absorption:

Food affects the bioavailability of ceftibuten from CEDAX Capsules and CEDAX Oral Suspension.

The effect of food on the bioavailability of CEDAX Capsules was evaluated in 26 healthy male volunteers who ingested 400 mg of CEDAX Capsules after an overnight fast or immediately after a standardized breakfast. Results showed that food delays the time of C_{max} by 1.75 hours, decreases the C_{max} by 18%, and decreases the extent of absorption (AUC) by 8%.

The effect of food on the bioavailability of CEDAX Oral Suspension was evaluated in 18 healthy adult male volunteers who ingested 400 mg of CEDAX Oral Suspension after an overnight fast or immediately after a standardized breakfast. Results obtained demonstrated a decrease in C_{max} of 26% and an AUC of 17% when CEDAX Oral Suspension was administered with a high-fat breakfast, and a decrease in C_{max} of 17% and in AUC of 12% when CEDAX Oral Suspension was administered with a low-calorie nonfat breakfast (see **PRECAUTIONS**).

Bioequivalence of Dosage Formulations:

A study in 18 healthy adult male volunteers demonstrated that a 400-mg dose of CEDAX Capsules produced equivalent concentrations to a 400-mg dose of CEDAX Oral Suspension. Average C_{max} values were 15.6 (3.1) µg/mL for the capsule and 17.0 (3.2) µg/mL for the suspension. Average AUC values were 80.1 (14.4) µg•hr/mL for the capsule and 87.0 (12.2) µg•hr/mL for the suspension.

Special Populations:

Geriatric patients: Ceftibuten pharmacokinetics have been investigated in elderly (65 years of age and older) men (n = 8) and women (n = 4). Each volunteer received ceftibuten 200-mg capsules twice daily for 3½ days. The average C_{max} was 17.5 (3.7) µg/mL after 3½ days of dosing compared to 12.9 (2.1) µg/mL after the first dose; ceftibuten accumulation in plasma was 40% at steady state. Information regarding the renal function of these volunteers was not available; therefore, the significance of this finding for clinical use of CEDAX Capsules in elderly patients is not clear. Ceftibuten dosage adjustment in elderly patients may be necessary (see **DOSAGE AND ADMINISTRATION**).

Patients with renal insufficiency: Ceftibuten pharmacokinetics have been investigated in adult patients with renal dysfunction. The ceftibuten plasma half-life increased and apparent total clearance (Cl/F) decreased proportionately with increasing degree of renal dysfunction. In 6 patients with moderate renal dysfunction (creatinine clearance 30 to 49 mL/min). The plasma half-life of ceftibuten increased to 7.1 hours and Cl/F decreased to 30 mL/min. In 6 patients with severe renal dysfunction (creatinine clearance 5 to 29 mL/min), the half-life increased to 13.4 hours and Cl/F decreased to 16 mL/min. In 6 functionally anephric patients (creatinine clearance <5 mL/min), the half-life increased to 22.3 hours and Cl/F decreased to 11 mL/min (a 7- to 8-fold change compared to healthy volunteers). Hemodialysis removed 65% of the drug from the blood in 2 to 4 hours. These changes serve as the basis for dosage adjustment recommendations in adult patients with mild to severe renal dysfunction (see **DOSAGE AND ADMINISTRATION**).

Microbiology:

Ceftibuten exerts its bactericidal action by binding to essential target proteins of the bacterial cell wall. This binding leads to inhibition of cell-wall synthesis.

Ceftibuten is stable in the presence of most plasmid-mediated beta-lactamases, but it is not stable in the presence of chromosomally-mediated cephalosporinases produced in organisms such as *Bacteroides, Citrobacter, Enterobacter, Morganella,* and *Serratia*. Like other beta-lactam agents, ceftibuten should not be used against strains resistant to beta-lactams due to general mechanisms such as permeability or penicillin-binding protein changes like penicillin-resistant *S. pneumoniae*.

Ceftibuten has been shown to be active against most strains of the following organisms both *in vitro* and in clinical infections (see **INDICATIONS AND USAGE**):

Gram-positive aerobes:

Streptococcus pneumoniae (penicillin-susceptible strains only)
Streptococcus pyogenes

Gram-negative aerobes:

Haemophilus influenzae (including β-lactamase-producing strains)

Moraxella catarrhalis (including β-lactamase-producing strains)

There are no known organisms which are potential pathogens in the indications approved for ceftibuten for which ceftibuten exhibits *in vitro* activity but for which the safety and efficacy of ceftibuten in treating clinical infections due to these organisms, have not been established in adequate and well-controlled trials.

NOTE: Ceftibuten is INACTIVE *in vitro* against *Acinetobacter, Bordetella, Campylobacter, Enterobacter, Enterococcus, Flavobacterium, Hafnia, Listeria, Pseudomonas, Staphylococcus,* and *Streptococcus* (except *pneumoniae* and *pyogenes*) species. In addition, it shows little *in vitro* activity against most anaerobes, including most species of *Bacteroides.*

Susceptibility testing:

Dilution Techniques: Quantitative methods are used to determine antimicrobial minimal inhibitory concentrations (MICs). These MICs provide estimates of the susceptibility of bacteria to antimicrobial compounds. The MICs should be determined using a standardized procedure. Standardized procedures are based on a dilution method (broth, agar, or microdilution) or equivalent with standardized inoculum concentrations and standardized concentrations of ceftibuten powder. The MIC values should be interpreted according to the following criteria when testing *Haemophilus* species using Haemophilus Test Media (HTM):

MIC (μg/mL)	Interpretation
≤2	(S) Susceptible

The current absence of resistant strains precludes defining any categories other than "Susceptible". Strains yielding results suggestive of a "Nonsusceptible" category should be submitted to a reference laboratory for further testing.

A report of "Susceptible" implies that an infection due to the strain may be appropriately treated with the dosage of antimicrobial agent recommended for that type of infection and infecting species, unless otherwise contraindicated.

Ceftibuten is indicated for penicillin-susceptible only strains of *Streptococcus pneumoniae.* A pneumococcal isolate that is susceptible to penicillin (MIC ≤0.06 μg/mL) can be considered susceptible to ceftibuten for approved indications. Testing of ceftibuten against penicillin-intermediate or penicillin-resistant isolates is not recommended. Reliable interpretive criteria for ceftibuten are not currently available. Physicians should be informed that clinical response rates with ceftibuten may be lower in strains that are not penicillin-susceptible.

Standardized susceptibility test procedures require the use of laboratory control microorganisms to control the technical aspect of laboratory procedures. Standard ceftibuten powder should provide the following MIC values:

Organism	MIC range (μg/mL)
Haemophilus influenzae ATCC 49247	0.25–1.0

Diffusion Techniques: Quantitative methods that require measurement of zone diameters also provide estimates of the susceptibility of bacteria to antimicrobial compounds. One such standardized procedure requires the use of standardized inoculum concentrations. This procedure uses paper disks impregnated with 30 μg of ceftibuten to test the susceptibility of microorganisms to ceftibuten.

Reports from the laboratory providing results of the standard single-disk susceptibility test with a 30-μg ceftibuten disk should be interpreted according to the following criteria when testing *Haemophilus* species using Haemophilus Test Media (HTM):

Zone Diameter (mm)	Interpretation
≥28	(S) Susceptible

The current absence of resistant strains precludes defining any categories other than "Susceptible". Strains yielding results suggestive of a "Nonsusceptible" category should be submitted to a reference laboratory for further testing.

Interpretation should be as stated above for results using dilution techniques.

Ceftibuten is indicated for penicillin-susceptible only strains of *Streptococcus pneumoniae*. Pneumococcal isolates with oxacillin zone sizes of ≥20 mm are susceptible to penicillin and can be considered susceptible for approved indications. Reliable disk diffusion tests for ceftibuten do not yet exist.

As with standardized dilution techniques, diffusion methods require the use of laboratory control microorganisms that are used to control the technical aspects of the laboratory procedures. For the diffusion technique, the 30-μg ceftibuten disk should provide the following zone diameters in these laboratory test quality control strains:

Organism	Zone diameter (mm)
Haemophilus influenzae ATCC 49247	29–35

Cephalosporin-class disks should not be used to test for susceptibility to ceftibuten.

INDICATIONS AND USAGE

CEDAX (ceftibuten) is indicated for the treatment of individuals with mild-to-moderate infections caused by susceptible strains of the designated microorganisms in the specific conditions listed below (see **DOSAGE AND ADMINISTRATION** and **CLINICAL STUDIES** section).

ADVERSE REACTIONS
CEFTIBUTEN CAPSULES
US CLINICAL TRIALS IN ADULT PATIENTS
(n = 1092)

Incidence equal to or greater than 1%	Nausea Headache Diarrhea Dyspepsia Dizziness Abdominal pain Vomiting	4% 3% 3% 2% 1% 1% 1%
Incidence less than 1% but greater than 0.1%	Anorexia, Constipation, Dry mouth, Dyspnea, Dysuria, Eructation, Fatigue, Flatulence, Loose stools, Moniliasis, Nasal congestion, Paresthesia, Pruritus, Rash, Somnolence, Taste perversion, Urticaria, Vaginitis	

LABORATORY VALUE CHANGES*
CEFTIBUTEN CAPSULES
US CLINICAL TRIALS IN ADULT PATIENTS

Incidence equal to or greater than 1%	↑ BUN ↑ Eosinophils ↓ Hemoglobin ↑ ALT (SGPT) ↑ Bilirubin	4% 3% 2% 1% 1%
Incidence less than 1% but greater than 0.1%	↑ Alk phosphatase ↑ Creatinine ↑ Platelets ↓ Platelets ↓ Leukocytes ↑ AST (SGOT)	

*Changes in laboratory values with possible clinical significance regardless of whether or not the investigator thought that the change was due to drug toxicity.

Acute Bacterial Exacerbations of Chronic Bronchitis due to *Haemophilus influenzae* (including β-lactamase-producing strains), *Moraxella catarrhalis* (including β-lactamase-producing strains), or *Streptococcus pneumoniae* (penicillin-susceptible strains only).

NOTE: In acute bacterial exacerbations of chronic bronchitis clinical trials where *Moraxella catarrhalis* was isolated from infected sputum at baseline, ceftibuten clinical efficacy was 22% less than control.

Acute Bacterial Otitis Media due to *Haemophilus influenzae* (including β-lactamase-producing strains), *Moraxella catarrhalis* (including β-lactamase-producing strains), or *Streptococcus pyogenes.*

NOTE: Although ceftibuten used empirically was equivalent to comparators in the treatment of clinically and/or microbiologically documented acute otitis media, the efficacy against *Streptococcus pneumoniae* was 23% less than control. Therefore, ceftibuten should be given empirically **only** when adequate antimicrobial coverage against *Streptococcus pneumoniae* has been previously administered.

Pharyngitis and Tonsillitis due to *Streptococcus pyogenes.*

NOTE: Only penicillin by the intramuscular route of administration has been shown to be effective in the prophylaxis of rheumatic fever. Ceftibuten is generally effective in the eradication of *Streptococcus pyogenes* from the oropharynx; however, data establishing the efficacy of the CEDAX product for the prophylaxis is of subsequent rheumatic fever are not available.

CONTRAINDICATIONS

CEDAX (ceftibuten) is contraindicated in patients with known allergy to the cephalosporin group of antibiotics.

WARNINGS

BEFORE THERAPY WITH THE CEDAX PRODUCT IS INSTITUTED, CAREFUL INQUIRY SHOULD BE MADE TO DETERMINE WHETHER THE PATIENT HAS HAD PREVIOUS HYPERSENSITIVITY REACTIONS TO CEFTIBUTEN, OTHER CEPHALOSPORINS, PENICILLINS, OR OTHER DRUGS. IF THIS PRODUCT IS TO BE GIVEN TO PENICILLIN-SENSITIVE PATIENTS, CAUTION SHOULD BE EXERCISED BECAUSE CROSS HYPERSENSITIVITY AMONG BETA-LACTAM ANTIBIOTICS HAS BEEN CLEARLY DOCUMENTED AND MAY OCCUR IN UP TO 10% OF PATIENTS WITH A HISTORY OF PENICILLIN ALLERGY. IF AN ALLERGIC REACTION TO THE CEDAX PRODUCT OCCURS, DISCONTINUE THE DRUG. SERIOUS ACUTE HYPERSENSITIVITY REACTIONS MAY REQUIRE TREATMENT WITH EPINEPHRINE AND OTHER EMERGENCY MEASURES, INCLUDING OXYGEN, INTRAVENOUS FLUIDS, INTRAVENOUS ANTIHISTAMINES, CORTICOSTEROIDS, PRESSOR AMINES, AND AIRWAY MANAGEMENT, AS CLINICALLY INDICATED.

Psudomembranous colitis has been reported with nearly all antibacterial agents, including ceftibuten, and may range in severity from mild to life threatening. Therefore, it is important to consider this diagnosis in patients who present with diarrhea subsequent to the administration of antibacterial agents.

Treatment with antibacterial agents alters normal flora of the colon and may permit overgrowth of clostridia. Studies indicate that a toxin produced by *Clostridium difficile* is one primary cause of "antibiotic-associated colitis".

After the diagnosis of pseudomembranous colitis has been established, appropriate therapeutic measures should be initiated. Mild cases of pseudomembranous colitis usually respond to drug discontinuation alone. In moderate to severe cases, consideration should be given to management with fluids and electrolytes, protein supplementation, and treatment with an antibacterial drug clinically effective against *Clostridium difficile.*

PRECAUTIONS

General:

As with other broad-spectrum antibiotics, prolonged treatment may result in the possible emergence and overgrowth of resistant organisms. Careful observation of the patient is essential. If superinfection occurs during therapy, appropriate measures should be taken.

The dose of ceftibuten may require adjustment in patients with varying degrees of renal insufficiency, particularly in patients with creatinine clearance less than 50 mL/min or undergoing hemodialysis (see **DOSAGE AND ADMINISTRATION**). Ceftibuten is readily dialyzable. Dialysis patients should be monitored carefully, and administration of ceftibuten should occur immediately following dialysis.

Ceftibuten should be prescribed with caution to individuals with a history of gastrointestinal disease, particularly colitis.

Information to Patients:

Patients should be informed that:

- If the patient is diabetic, he/she should be informed that CEDAX Oral Suspension contains 1 gram sucrose per teaspoon of suspension.
- CEDAX Oral Suspension should be taken at least 2 hours before a meal or at least 1 hour after a meal (see **CLINICAL PHARMACOLOGY, Food Effect on Absorption**).

Drug Interactions:

Theophylline: Twelve healthy male volunteers were administered one 200-mg ceftibuten capsule twice daily for 6 days. With the morning dose of ceftibuten on day 6, each volunteer received a single intravenous infusion of theophylline (4 mg/kg). The pharmacokinetics of theophylline were not altered. The effect of ceftibuten on the pharmacokinetics of theophylline administered orally has not been investigated.

Antacids or H_2-receptor antagonists: The effect of increased gastric pH on the bioavailability of ceftibuten was evaluated in 18 healthy adult volunteers. Each volunteer was administered one 400-mg ceftibuten capsule. A single dose of liquid antacid did not affect the C_{max} or AUC of ceftibuten; however, 150 mg of ranitidine q12h for 3 days increased the ceftibuten C_{max} by 23% and ceftibuten AUC by 16%. The clinical relevance of these increases is not known.

Drug/Laboratory Test Interactions:

There have been no chemical or laboratory test interactions with ceftibuten noted to date. False-positive direct Coombs' tests have been reported during treatment with other cephalosporins. Therefore, it should be recognized that a positive Coombs' test could be due to the drug. The results of assays using red cells from healthy subjects to determine whether ceftibuten would cause direct Coombs' reactions *in vitro* showed no positive reaction at ceftibuten concentrations as high as 40 μg/mL.

Carcinogenesis, Mutagenesis, Impairment of Fertility:

Long-term animal studies have not been performed to evaluate the carcinogenic potential of ceftibuten. No mutagenic

Continued on next page

Cedax—Cont.

effects were seen in the following studies: *in vitro* chromosome assay in human lymphocytes, *in vivo* chromosome assay in mouse bone marrow cells. Chinese Hamster Ovary (CHO) cell point mutation assay at the hypoxanthine-guanine phosphoribosyl transferase (HGPRT) locus, and in a bacterial reversion point mutation test (Ames). No impairment of fertility occurred when rats were administered ceftibuten orally up to 2000 mg/kg/day (approximately 43 times the human dose based on mg/m^2/day).

Pregnancy: Teratogenic effects: Pregnancy Category B:
Ceftibuten was not teratogenic in the pregnant rat at oral doses up to 400 mg/kg/day (approximately 8.6 times the human dose based on mg/m^2/day). Ceftibuten was not teratogenic in the pregnant rabbit at oral doses up to 40 mg/kg/day (approximately 1.5 times the human dose based on mg/m^2/day) and has revealed no evidence of harm to the fetus. There are no adequate and well-controlled studies in pregnant women. Because animal reproduction studies are not always predictive of human response, this drug should be used during pregnancy only if clearly needed.

Labor and Delivery:
Ceftibuten has not been studied for use during labor and delivery. Its use during such clinical situations should be weighed in terms of potential risk and benefit to both mother and fetus.

Nursing Mothers:
It is not known whether ceftibuten (at recommended dosages) is excreted in human milk. Because many drugs are excreted in human milk, caution should be exercised when ceftibuten is administered to a nursing woman.

Pediatric Use:
The safety and efficacy of ceftibuten in infants less than 6 months of age has not been established.

Geriatric Patients:
The usual adult dosage recommendation may be followed for patients in this age group. However, these patients should be monitored closely, particularly their renal function, as dosage adjustment may be required.

ADVERSE EVENTS

Clinical Trials:
CEDAX CAPSULES (adult patients)
In clinical trials, 1728 adult patients (1092 US and 636 international) were treated with the recommended dose of ceftibuten capsules (400 mg per day). There were no deaths or permanent disabilities thought due to drug toxicity in any of the patients in these studies. Thirty-six of 1728 (2%) patients discontinued medication due to adverse events thought by the investigators to be possibly, probably, or almost certainly related to drug toxicity. The discontinuations were primarily for gastrointestinal disturbances, usually diarrhea, vomiting, or nausea. Six of 1728 (0.3%) patients were discontinued due to rash or pruritus thought related to ceftibuten administration.
In the US trials, the following adverse events were thought by the investigators to be possibly, probably, or almost certainly related to ceftibuten capsules in multiple-dose clinical trials (n = 1092 ceftibuten-treated patients).
[See table at top of previous page]
CEDAX ORAL SUSPENSION (pediatric patients)
In clinical trials, 1152 pediatric patients (772 US and 380 international), 97% of whom were younger than 12 years of age, were treated with the recommended dose of ceftibuten (9 mg/kg once daily up to a maximum dose of 400 mg per day) for 10 days. There were no deaths, life-threatening adverse events, or permanent disabilities in any of the patients in these studies. Eight of 1152 (<1%) patients discontinued medication due to adverse events thought by the investigators to be possibly, probably, or almost certainly related to drug toxicity. The discontinuations were primarily (7 out of 8) for gastrointestinal disturbances, usually diarrhea or vomiting. One patient was discontinued due to a cutaneous rash thought possibly related to ceftibuten administration.
In the US trials, the following adverse events were thought by the investigators to be possibly, probably, or almost certainly related to ceftibuten oral suspension in multiple-dose clinical trials (n = 722 ceftibuten-treated patients).
[See first table above]
[See second table above]

In Post-marketing Experience:
The following adverse experiences have been reported during worldwide post-marketing surveillance: aphasia, jaundice, melena, psychosis, serum sickness-like reactions, stridor, and toxic epidermal necrolysis.

Cephalosporin-class Adverse Reactions:
In addition to the adverse reactions listed above that have been observed in patients treated with ceftibuten capsules, the following adverse events and altered laboratory tests have been reported for cephalosporin-class antibiotics:

allergic reactions, anaphylaxis, drug fever, Stevens-Johnson syndrome, renal dysfunction, toxic nephropathy, hepatic cholestasis, aplastic anemia, hemolytic anemia, hemorrhage, false-positive test for urinary glucose, neutropenia, pancytopenia, and agranulocytosis. Pseudomembranous colitis; onset of symptoms may occur during or after antibiotic treatment (see **WARNINGS**).

Several cephalosporins have been implicated in triggering seizures, particularly in patients with renal impairment when the dosage was not reduced (see **DOSAGE AND ADMINISTRATION** and **OVERDOSAGE**). If seizures associated with drug therapy occur, the drug should be discontinued. Anticonvulsant therapy can be given if clinically indicated.

ADVERSE REACTIONS
CEFTIBUTEN ORAL SUSPENSION
US CLINICAL TRIALS IN PEDIATRIC PATIENTS
(n = 772)

Incidence equal to or greater than 1%	Diarrhea* Vomiting Abdominal pain Loose stools	4% 2% 2% 2%
Incidence less than 1% but greater than 0.1%	Agitation, Anorexia, Dehydration, Diaper dermatitis, Dizziness, Dyspepsia, Fever, Headache, Hematuria, Hyperkinesia, Insomnia, Irritability, Nausea, Pruritus, Rash, Rigors, Urticaria	

*NOTE: The incidence of diarrhea in pediatric patients ≤2 years old was 8% (23/301) compared with 2% (9/471) in pediatric patients >2 years old.

LABORATORY VALUE CHANGES*
CEFTIBUTEN ORAL SUSPENSION
US CLINICAL TRIALS IN PEDIATRIC PATIENTS

Incidence equal to or greater than 1%	↑ Eosinophils ↑ BUN ↓ Hemoglobin ↑ Platelets	3% 2% 1% 1%
Incidence less than 1% but greater than 0.1%	↑ ALT (SGPT) ↑ AST (SGOT) ↑ Alk phosphatase ↑ Bilirubin ↑ Creatinine	

*Changes in laboratory values with possible clinical significance regardless of whether or not the investigator thought that the change was due to drug toxicity.

Type of infection (as qualified in the **INDICATIONS AND USAGE** section of this labeling)	Daily Maximum Dose	Dose and Frequency	Duration
ADULTS (12 years of age and older): Acute Bacterial Exacerbations of Chronic Bronchitis due to *H. influenzae* (including β-lactamase-producing strains), *M. catarrhalis* (including β-lactamase-producing strains), or *Streptococcus pneumoniae*(penicillin-susceptible strains only). (See **INDICATIONS AND USAGE—NOTE.**) Pharyngitis and tonsillitus due to *S. pyogenes.* Acute Bacterial Otitis Media due to *H. influenzae* (including β-lactamase-producing strains), *M. catarrhalis* (including β-lactamase-producing strains), or *S. pyogenes.* (See **INDICATIONS AND USAGE—NOTE.**)	400 mg	400 mg QD	10 days
PEDIATRIC PATIENTS: Pharyngitis and tonsillitis due to *S. pyogenes* Acute Bacterial Otitis Media due to *H. influenzae* (including β-lactamase-producing strains), and *M. Catarrhalis* (including β-lactamase-producing strains), or *S. pyogenes.* See **INDICATIONS AND USAGE—NOTE.**)	400 mg	9 mg/kg QD	10 days

OVERDOSAGE

Overdosage of cephalosporins can cause cerebral irritation leading to convulsions. Ceftibuten is readily dialyzable and significant quantities (65% of plasma concentrations) can be removed from the circulation by a single hemodialysis session. Information does not exist with regard to removal of ceftibuten by peritoneal dialysis.

DOSAGE AND ADMINISTRATION

The recommended doses of CEDAX Oral Suspension are presented in the table below. **CEDAX Oral Suspension must be administered at least 2 hours before or 1 hour after a meal.**
[See third table above]

CEFTIBUTEN ORAL SUSPENSION
PEDIATRIC DOSAGE CHART

CHILD'S WEIGHT	90 mg/5 mL
10 kg 22 lbs	1 tsp QD
20 kg 44 lbs	2 tsp QD
40 kg 88 lbs	4 tsp QD

Pediatric patients weighing more than 45 kg should receive the maximum daily dose of 400 mg.

Renal Impairment:
CEDAX Capsules and CEDAX Oral Suspension may be administered at normal doses in the presence of impaired renal function with creatinine clearance of 50 mL/min or greater. The recommendations for dosing in patients with varying degrees of renal insufficiency are presented in the following table.

Creatinine Clearance (mL/min)	Recommended Dosing Schedules
>50	9 mg/kg or 400 mg Q24h (normal dosing schedule)
30–49	4.5 mg/kg or 200 mg Q24h
5–29	2.25 mg/kg or 100 mg Q24h

Hemodialysis Patients:
In patients undergoing hemodialysis two or three times weekly, a single 400-mg dose of ceftibuten capsules or a single dose of 9 mg/kg (maximum of 400 mg of ceftibuten) oral suspension may be administered at the end of each hemodialysis session.

Directions for Mixing CEDAX Oral Suspension:
[See first table at top of next page]
After mixing, the suspension may be kept for 14 days and must be stored in the refrigerator. Keep tightly closed. Shake well before each use. Discard any unused portion after 14 days.

DIRECTIONS FOR MIXING CEDAX ORAL SUSPENSION

Final Concentration	Bottle Size	Amount of Water	Directions
90 mg per 5 mL	30 mL	Suspend in 28 mL of water	First tap the bottle to loosen powder. Then add water in two portions, shaking well after each aliquot.
	60 mL	Suspend in 53 mL of water	
	90 mL	Suspend in 78 mL of water	
	120 mL	Suspend in 103 mL of water	

BACTERIOLOGICAL OUTCOME
ACUTE BACTERIAL EXACERBATIONS OF CHRONIC BRONCHITIS

	Ceftibuten (400 mg QD)	Control
Bacteriological Eradication Rates		
Haemophilus influenzae	45/62 (73%)	26/36 (72%)
H. parainfluenzae	10/10	4/6
Moraxella catarrhalis	33/46 (72%)	32/34 (94%)
Streptococcus pneumoniae	23/35 (66%)	14/20 (70%)

BACTERIOLOGICAL OUTCOME
ACUTE BACTERIAL OTITIS MEDIA

	Ceftibuten 9 mg/kg QD	Control
Bacteriological Eradication Rates		
Haemophilus influenzae	56/67 (81%)	29/38 (76%)
Moraxella catarrhalis	20/26 (77%)	13/17 (77%)
Streptococcus pneumoniae	68/105 (65%)	35/40 (88%)
Streptococcus pyogenes	13/15 (87%)	5/5

HOW SUPPLIED

CEDAX Capsules, containing 400 mg of ceftibuten (as ceftibuten dihydrate) are white, opaque capsules imprinted with the product name and strength, are available as follows:

20 Capsules/Bottle (NDC 64455-0691-01)
100 Capsules/Bottle (NDC 64455-0691-02)
Unit-dose dispensing (10 strips of 4 capsules each) (NDC 64455-0691-03)

Store the capsules between 2° and 25°C (36° and 77°F). Replace cap securely after each opening.

CEDAX Oral Suspension is an off-white to cream-colored powder that, when reconstituted as directed, contains ceftibuten equivalent to 90 mg/5mL, supplied as follows:

90 mg/5 mL

18 mg/mL	30-mL Bottle	(NDC 64455-0777-03)
18 mg/mL	60-mL Bottle	(NDC 64455-0777-01)
18 mg/mL	90-mL Bottle	(NDC 64455-0777-04)
18 mg/mL	120-mL Bottle	(NDC 64455-0777-02)

Prior to reconstitution, the powder must be stored between 2° and 25°C (36° and 77°F). Once it is reconstituted, the oral suspension is stable for 14 days when stored in the refrigerator between 2° and 8°C (36° and 46°F).

CLINICAL STUDIES

Acute Bacterial Exacerbations of Chronic Bronchitis:
Three clinical trials (two domestic, the third abroad) have been conducted testing ceftibuten in the treatment of acute exacerbations of chronic bronchitis (AECB). Overall, the clinical outcome among patients who had signs and symptoms of AECB, who had a gram stain showing a predominance of PMNs and few epithelial cells, and who were evaluated at approximately 1 to 2 weeks after completing therapy were equivalent to comparators. The bacterial eradication rates of specific pathogens are presented below. [See second table above]

Acute Bacterial Otitis Media:
Four clinical trials (three domestic, the fourth abroad) have been conducted testing ceftibuten in the treatment of acute bacterial otitis media. Overall, the clinical outcome among patients who had signs and symptoms of acute bacterial otitis media and who were evaluated at approximately 1 to 2 weeks after completing therapy were equivalent to comparators. Tympanocentesis was performed on patients in three of the above-mentioned studies; the bacterial eradication rates of specific pathogens are presented below. [See third table above]

REFERENCES

1. National Committee for Clinical Laboratory Standards. Method for Dilution Antimicrobial Susceptibility Tests for Bacteria that Grow Aerobically—Third Edition. Approved Standard NCCLS Document M7-A3, Vol. 13, No. 25, NCCLS, Villanova, PA. December, 1993.
2. National Committee for Clinical Laboratory Standards. Performance Standards for Antimicrobial Disk Susceptibility Tests—Fifth Edition. Approved Standard NCCLS Document M2-A5, Vol. 13, No. 24, NCCLS, Villanova, PA. December, 1993.

DJ Pharma Inc.
San Diego, CA 92130 USA
Licensed by Shionogi and Co., Ltd., Japan
Manufactured by Schering Corporation B-23926903
Distributed by DJ Pharma Inc. **24111105T**
Rev. 4/00

D.A. CHEWABLE™ Tablets ℞

DESCRIPTION

Each D.A. CHEWABLE TABLET for oral administration contains:

chlorpheniramine maleate	2 mg
phenylephrine HCl	10 mg
methscopolamine nitrate	1.25 mg

in an orange-flavored and orange-colored chewable tablet.
Chlorpheniramine maleate is an antihistamine having the chemical name: 2-Pyridinepropanamine, γ-(4chlorophenyl)-*N,N*-dimethyl-,(Z)-2-butenedioate(1:1)
Phenylephrine HCl is a decongestant having the chemical name:
Benzenemethanol, 3-hydroxy-α[(methylamino) methyl]-,hydrochloride.
Methscopolamine nitrate is an anticholinergic having the chemical name: 3-Oxa-9-azoniatricyclo$[3.3.1.0^{2,4}]$ nonane, 7-(3-hydroxy-1-oxo-2-phenylpropoxy)-9,9-dimethyl-, nitrate, [7(*S*)-(1 α, 2 β, 4 β, 5 α, 7 β)]-
Inactive ingredients: artificial orange flavor, aspartame, colloidal silicon dioxide, croscarmellose sodium, FD&C yellow #6 (aluminum lake), magnesium stearate, malic acid, mannitol, microcrystalline cellulose, vanillin.

HOW SUPPLIED

D.A. CHEWABLE Tablets are available as orange flavored and orange colored scored tablets imprinted with *DURA* on one side and *CHEW* on the other.
Bottles of 100 (NDC 64455-013-01).
Store at room temperature, 15°–25°C (59°–77°F).
Dispense in a tight, light-resistant container (USP/NF) with a child-resistant closure.
Rx only
Manufactured for:
DJ Pharma, Inc.
San Diego, CA 92130
Manufactured by
Anabolic, Inc.
Irvine, CA 92614
Revised October 1998
DACT005K98

DURA-VENT® ℞
DECONGESTANT/EXPECTORANT TABLET

DESCRIPTION

Each DURA-VENT white, scored tablet for oral administration contains:

Phenylpropanolamine hydrochloride	75 mg
Guaifenesin	600 mg

in a special base to provide a prolonged therapeutic effect.
Phenylpropanolamine hydrochloride is a decongestant having the chemical name:
Benzenemethanol, α-(1-aminoethyl)-, hydrochloride, (*R**, *S**)-,(±).
Guaifenesin is an expectorant having the chemical name: 1,2-Propanediol, 3-(2-methoxyphenoxy)-.
Inactive ingredients: dicalcium phosphate, hydrogenated cottonseed oil, magnesium stearate, methylcellulose, microcrystalline cellulose, silicon dioxide, stearic acid, tricalcium phosphate.

HOW SUPPLIED

DURA-VENT is available as a white, scored tablet imprinted with 7.5/7.5 on one side and *DURA* on the other.
Bottles of 100 (NDC 64455-006-01).
Bottles of 600 (NDC 64455-006-06).
Store at room temperature, 15°–25°C (59°–77°F).
Dispense in a tight, light-resistant container (USP/NF) with a child-resistant closure.
Rx only.
Manufactured for DJ Pharma, Inc. San Diego, CA 92130
Manufactured by Anabolic, Inc., Irvine CA 92614
DV001l98

D.A. II® Tablet ℞
Dura-Vent®/DA Tablet

DESCRIPTION

Antihistamine/decongestant/anticholinergic combination tablets for oral use.

D.A. II™ Tablet

Each white, capsule-shaped tablet contains:

chlorpheniramine maleate	4 mg
phenylephrine HCl	10 mg
methscopolamine nitrate	1.25 mg

In a specially prepared base to provide a prolonged therapeutic effect.
Inactive ingredients: dicalcium phosphate, hydrogenated cottonseed oil, magnesium stearate, methylcellulose, stearic acid, microcrystalline cellulose, and silicon dioxide.

Dura-Vent®/DA Tablet

Each light brown, scored tablet contains:

chlorpheniramine maleate	8 mg
phenylephrine HCl	20 mg
methscopolamine nitrate	2.5 mg

In a specially prepared base to provide a prolonged therapeutic effect.
Inactive ingredients: D&C yellow #10 (aluminum lake), dicalcium phosphate, FD&C blue #1 (aluminum lake), FD&C red #40 (aluminum lake), hydrogenated cottonseed oil, magnesium stearate, methylcellulose, silica gel, and stearic acid.
Chlorpheniramine maleate is an antihistamine having the chemical name: 2-Pyridinepropanamine, γ-(4-chlorophenyl)-*N,N*-dimethyl-, (Z)-2-butenedioate(1:1).
Phenylephrine HCl is a decongestant having the chemical name: Benzenemethanol, 3-hydroxy-α-[(methylamino) methyl]-, hydrochloride.
Methscopolamine nitrate is an anticholinergic having the chemical name: 3-Oxa-9-azonlatricyclo $[3.3.1.0^{2\ 4}]$ nonane, 7-(3-hydroxy-1-oxo-2-phenylpropoxy)-9,9-dimethyl-,nitrate, [7(S)-(1α, 2β, 4β, 5α, 7β)]-.

HOW SUPPLIED

D.A. II is available as a white, capsule-shaped tablet imprinted with *DURA* on one side and *DA II* on the other.
Bottles of 100 (NDC 64455-028-01).
Dura-Vent/DA is available as a light brown, scored tablet imprinted with *DURA* on one side and *DA* on the other.
Bottles of 100 (NDC 64455-008-01).
Store at room temperature 15°–25°C (59°–77°F). Dispense in a tight, light-resistant container (USP/NF) with a child-resistant closure.
Rx only.
Manufactured for
DJ Pharma, Inc.
San Diego, CA 92130
Manufactured by
Anabolic, Inc.
Irvine, CA 92614
Revised October 1998 DURA197D98

FENESIN™ ℞
ORAL EXPECTORANT TABLET

DESCRIPTION

Each light blue, scored, sustained-release tablet provides 600 mg guaifenesin in a specially-prepared base to provide a prolonged therapeutic effect. Guaifenesin is an expectorant having the chemical name: 1,2-Propanediol, 3-(2-methoxy phenoxy)-.
Inactive Ingredients: colloidal silicon dioxide, FD&C Blue #1, partially hydrogenated cottonseed oil, dicalcium phosphate, hydroxypropyl methylcellulose, magnesium stearate, stearic acid.

HOW SUPPLIED

Fenesin is available as a light blue, scored tablet embossed with DURA on one side and 009 on the other.
Bottles of 100 (NDC 64455-009-01)
Bottles of 600 (NDC 64455-009-06)
Store at room temperature, 15°–25°C (59°–77°F).
Dispense in a tight, light-resistant container (USP/NF) with a child-resistant closure.

Continued on next page

Fenesin—Cont.

Rx only
Manufactured for DJ Pharma, Inc., San Diego, CA 92130
Manufactured by Anabolic, Inc., Irvine, CA 92614
Revised October 1998 F001J98

FENESIN™ DM ℞
ANTITUSSIVE/EXPECTORANT TABLET

DESCRIPTION

Each dark blue, scored tablet for oral administration contains:
dextromethorphan
hydrobromide .... 30 mg
guaifenesin .... 600 mg
in a special base to provide a prolonged therapeutic effect.

HOW SUPPLIED

Fenesin DM is available as a dark blue, scored tablet embossed with *Dura* on one side and *FDM 014* on the other.
Bottles of 100 (NDC 64455-014-01).
Store at controlled room temperature 15°–25°C (59°–77°F).
Dispense in a tight, light-resistant container (USP/NF) with a child-resistant closure.
Rx only
Manufactured for DJ Pharma, Inc., San Diego, CA 92130
Manufactured by Anabolic, Inc., Irvine, CA 92614
Revised October 1998 FDM003F98

GUAI-VENT™ /PSE ℞
DECONGESTANT/EXPECTORANT

DESCRIPTION

Each Guai-Vent/PSE white, uncoated, scored, sustained-release tablet for oral administration contains:
pseudoephedrine hydrochloride .... 120 mg
guaifenesin .... 600 mg
in a special base to provide a prolonged therapeutic effect.

HOW SUPPLIED

Guai-Vent/PSE tablets are white, uncoated, scored and coated with *"015"* on one side and *"DURA"* on the scored side.
Bottles of 100 (NDC 64455-015-01).
Store at controlled room temperature (59°–77°F or 15°–25°C). Dispense in a tight, light-resistant container as defined in USP/NF with a child-resistant closure.
Rx only.
Manufactured for DJ Pharma, Inc. San Diego, CA 92130
Manufactured by Anabolic, Inc., Irvine, CA 92614
Revised October 1998 GPSE001E98

KEFTAB® ℞
[kĕf 'tăb]
cephalexin hydrochloride, USP

DESCRIPTION

Keftab is a semisynthetic cephalosporin antibiotic intended for oral administration. Chemically, it is designated 7-(D-2-Amino-2-phenylacetamido)-3-methyl-3-cephem-4-carboxylic acid hydrochloride monohydrate, and the chemical formula is $C_{16}H_{17}N_3O_4S \cdot HCl \cdot H_2O$. The molecular weight is 401.87, and it has the following structural formula:

The nucleus of cephalexin hydrochloride is related to that of other cephalosporin antibiotics. The compound is the hydrochloride salt of cephalexin. The isoelectric point of cephalexin in water is approximately 4.5 to 5.
Cephalexin hydrochloride is in crystalline form and is a monohydrate. It is a white crystalline solid having a bitter taste. Solubility in water is high at room temperature; greater than 10 mg/mL may be dissolved readily.
The cephalosporins differ from penicillins in the structure of the bicyclic ring system. Cephalexin has a *D*-phenylglycyl group as substituent at the 7-amino position and an unsubstituted methyl group at the 3-position.
Each tablet contains cephalexin hydrochloride equivalent to 500 mg (1.439 µmol) cephalexin. The tablets also contain D & C Yellow No. 10, F D & C Blue No. 1, F D & C Red No. 40, magnesium stearate, silicon dioxide, stearic acid, sucrose, titanium dioxide, and other inactive ingredients.

CLINICAL PHARMACOLOGY

Human Pharmacology—Keftab is acid stable and may be given without regard to meals. It is rapidly absorbed after oral administration. Following doses of 250 mg and 500 mg, average peak serum levels of approximately 9 and 18 µg/mL respectively were obtained at 1 hour and declined to 1.6 and 3.4 µg/mL respectively at 3 hours. Measurable levels were present 6 hours after administration. Cephalexin is excreted in the urine by glomerular filtration and tubular secretion. Studies showed that approximately 70% of the drug was excreted unchanged in the urine within 12 hours. During the first 6 hours, average urine concentrations following the 250-mg and 500-mg doses were approximately 200 µg/mL (range, 54 to 663) and 500 µg/mL (range, 137 to 1,306) respectively. The average serum half-life is 1.1 hours.
Microbiology—In vitro tests demonstrate that the cephalosporins are bactericidal because of their inhibition of cell-wall synthesis. Keftab is active against the following organisms in vitro:
β-hemolytic streptococci
Staphylococcus aureus, including penicillinase-producing strains
Streptococcus pneumoniae
Escherichia coli
Proteus mirabilis
Klebsiella spp.
Haemophilus influenzae
Moraxella (Branhamella) catarrhalis
Note—Most strains of enterococci (*Enterococcus faecalis* [formerly *Streptococcus faecalis*]) and a few strains of staphylococci are resistant to Keftab. When tested by in vitro methods, staphylococci exhibit cross-resistance between Keftab and methicillin-type antibiotics. Keftab is not active against most strains of *Enterobacter* spp., *Morganella morganii* (formerly *Proteus morganii*), *Serratia* spp., and *Proteus vulgaris*. It has no activity against *Pseudomonas* or *Acinetobacter* spp.
Disk Susceptibility Tests—Quantitative methods that require measurement of zone diameters give the most precise estimates of antibiotic susceptibility. One such procedure[1] has been recommended for use with cephalosporin class (cephalothin) disks for testing susceptibility to cephalexin. The currently accepted zone diameter interpretation for the cephalothin disks' is appropriate for determining susceptibility to cephalexin. Interpretations correlate zone diameters of the disk test with MIC values for cephalexin. With this procedure, a report from the laboratory of "resistant" indicates a zone diameter of 14 mm or less and suggests that the infecting organism is not likely to respond to therapy. A report of "susceptibility" indicates a zone diameter of 18 mm or greater. A report of "intermediate susceptibility" indicates zone diameters between 15 and 17 mm and suggests that the organism would be susceptible if the infection is confined to the urine, in which high antibiotic levels can be obtained, or if high dosage is used in other types of infection.
Standardized procedures require use of control organisms.[1] The 30-µg cephalothin disk should give zone diameters between 18 and 23 mm and 25 and 37 mm for the reference strains *E. coli* ATCC 25922 and *S. aureus* ATCC 25923 respectively.

INDICATIONS AND USAGE

Keftab is indicated for the treatment of the following infections when caused by susceptible strains of the designated microorganisms:
Respiratory tract infections caused by *S. pneumoniae* and group A β-hemolytic streptococci (Penicillin is the usual drug of choice in the treatment and prevention of streptococcal infections, including the prophylaxis of rheumatic fever. Keftab is generally effective in the eradication of streptococci from the nasopharynx; however, substantial data establishing the efficacy of Keftab in the subsequent prevention of rheumatic fever are not available at present.)
Skin and skin structure infections caused by *S. aureus* and/or β-hemolytic streptococci.
Bone infections caused by *S. aureus* and/or *P. mirabilis*.
Genitourinary tract infections, including acute prostatitis, caused by *E. coli, P. mirabilis*, and *Klebsiella* spp.
Note—Culture and susceptibility tests should be initiated prior to and during therapy. Renal function studies should be performed when indicated.

CONTRAINDICATIONS

Keftab is contraindicated in patients with known allergy to the cephalosporin group of antibiotics.

WARNINGS

BEFORE CEPHALEXIN THERAPY IS INSTITUTED, CAREFUL INQUIRY SHOULD BE MADE CONCERNING PREVIOUS HYPERSENSITIVITY REACTIONS TO CEPHALOSPORINS AND PENICILLIN.
CEPHALOSPORIN C DERIVATIVES SHOULD BE GIVEN CAUTIOUSLY TO PENICILLIN-SENSITIVE PATIENTS.
SERIOUS ACUTE HYPERSENSITIVITY REACTIONS MAY REQUIRE EPINEPHRINE AND OTHER EMERGENCY MEASURES.
There is some clinical and laboratory evidence of partial cross-allergenicity of the penicillins and the cephalosporins. Patients have been reported to have had severe reactions (including anaphylaxis) to both drugs.
Any patient who has demonstrated some form of allergy, particularly to drugs, should receive antibiotics cautiously. No exception should be made with regard to Keftab.
Pseudomembranous colitis has been reported with virtually all broad-spectrum antibiotics (including macrolides, semisynthetic penicillins, and cephalosporins); therefore, it is important to consider its diagnosis in patients who develop diarrhea in association with the use of antibiotics. Such colitis may range in severity from mild to life threatening.
Treatment with broad-spectrum antibiotics alters the normal flora of the colon and may permit overgrowth of clostridia. Studies indicate that a toxin produced by *Clostridium difficile* is a primary cause of antibiotic-associated colitis.
Mild cases of pseudomembranous colitis usually respond to drug discontinuance alone. In moderate to severe cases, management should include sigmoidoscopy, appropriate bacteriologic studies, and fluid, electrolyte, and protein supplementation. When the colitis does not improve after the drug has been discontinued or when it is severe, treatment with an oral antibacterial drug effective against *C. difficile* is recommended. Other causes of colitis should be ruled out.

PRECAUTIONS

General—Patients should be followed carefully so that any side effects or unusual manifestations of drug idiosyncrasy may be detected. If an allergic reaction to Keftab occurs, the drug should be discontinued and the patient treated with the usual agents (eg, epinephrine or other pressor amines, antihistamines, or corticosteroids).
Prolonged use of Keftab may result in the overgrowth of nonsusceptible organisms. Careful observation of the patient is essential. If superinfection occurs during therapy, appropriate measures should be taken.
Positive direct Coombs' tests have been reported during treatment with the cephalosporin antibiotics. In hematologic studies or in transfusion cross-matching procedures when antiglobulin tests are performed on the minor side or in Coombs' testing of newborns whose mothers have received cephalosporin antibiotics before parturition, it should be recognized that a positive Coombs' test may be due to the drug.
Keftab should be administered with caution in the presence of markedly impaired renal function. Under such conditions, careful clinical observation and laboratory studies should be made because safe dosage may be lower than that usually recommended.
As a result of administration of Keftab, a false-positive reaction for glucose in the urine may occur. This has been observed with Benedict's and Fehling's solutions and also with Clinitest® tablets.
Broad-spectrum antibiotics should be prescribed with caution in individuals with a history of gastrointestinal disease, particularly colitis.
Pregnancy—Pregnancy Category B—Reproduction studies have been performed on rats in doses of 250 or 500 mg/kg/day and have revealed no evidence of impaired fertility or harm to the fetus due to cephalexin. There are, however, no adequate and well-controlled studies in pregnant women. Because animal reproduction studies are not always predictive of human response, this drug should be used during pregnancy only if clearly needed.
Nursing Mothers—The excretion of cephalexin in the milk increased up to 4 hours after a 500-mg dose; the drug reached a maximum level of 4 µg/mL, then decreased gradually, and had disappeared 8 hours after administration. A decision should be considered to discontinue nursing temporarily during therapy with Keftab.
Pediatric Use—Safety and effectiveness in pediatric patients have not been established.

ADVERSE REACTIONS

Gastrointestinal—Symptoms of pseudomembranous colitis may appear either during or after antibiotic treatment. Nausea and vomiting have been reported rarely. The most frequent side effect has been diarrhea. It was very rarely severe enough to warrant cessation of therapy. Abdominal pain, gastritis, and dyspepsia have also occurred. As with some penicillins and some other cephalosporins, transient hepatitis and cholestatic jaundice have been reported rarely.
Hypersensitivity—Allergic reactions in the form of rash, urticaria, angioedema, and, rarely, erythema multiforme, Stevens-Johnson syndrome, or toxic epidermal necrolysis have been observed. These reactions usually subsided upon discontinuation of the drug. In some of these reactions, supportive therapy may be necessary. Anaphylaxis has also been reported.
Other reactions have included genital and anal pruritus, genital moniliasis, vaginitis and vaginal discharge, dizziness, fatigue, headache, agitation, confusion, hallucinations, arthralgia, arthritis, and joint disorder. Reversible interstitial nephritis has been reported rarely. Eosinophilia, neutropenia, thrombocytopenia, slight elevations in aspartate aminotransferase (AST) and alanine aminotransferase (ALT), and elevated creatinine and BUN have been reported.
In addition to the adverse reactions listed above that have been observed in patients treated with Keftab, the following adverse reactions and altered laboratory tests have been reported for cephalosporin class antibiotics:
Adverse Reactions—Allergic reactions, including fever, colitis, renal dysfunction, toxic nephropathy, and hepatic dysfunction, including cholestasis.
Several cephalosporins have been implicated in triggering seizures, particularly in patients with renal impairment when the dosage was not reduced (*see* Indications and Usage *and* Precautions, General). If seizures associated with drug therapy should occur, the drug should be discontinued. Anticonvulsant therapy can be given if clinically indicated.
Altered Laboratory Tests—Increased prothrombin time, increased alkaline phosphatase, and leukopenia.

OVERDOSAGE

Signs and Symptoms—Symptoms of oral overdose may include nausea, vomiting, epigastric distress, diarrhea, and hematuria. If other symptoms are present, it is probably

secondary to an underlying disease state, an allergic reaction, or toxicity due to ingestion of a second medication.
Treatment—To obtain up-to-date information about the treatment of overdose, a good resource is your certified Regional Poison Control Center. Telephone numbers of certified poison control centers are listed in the *Physicians' Desk Reference (PDR)*. In managing overdosage, consider the possibility of multiple drug overdoses, interaction among drugs, and unusual drug kinetics in your patient.
Unless 5 to 10 times the normal dose of cephalexin has been ingested, gastrointestinal decontamination should not be necessary.
Protect the patient's airway and support ventilation and perfusion. Meticulously monitor and maintain, within acceptable limits, the patient's vital signs, blood gases, serum electrolytes, etc. Absorption of drugs from the gastrointestinal tract may be decreased by giving activated charcoal, which, in many cases, is more effective than emesis or lavage; consider charcoal instead of or in addition to gastric emptying. Repeated doses of charcoal over time may hasten elimination of some drugs that have been absorbed. Safeguard the patient's airway when employing gastric emptying or charcoal.
Forced diuresis, peritoneal dialysis, hemodialysis, or charcoal hemoperfusion have not been established as beneficial for an overdose of cephalexin; however, it should be extremely unlikely that one of these procedures would be indicated.
The oral median lethal dose of cephalexin in rats is 5,000 mg/kg.

DOSAGE AND ADMINISTRATION

Keftab is administered orally.
The adult dosage ranges from 1 to 4 g daily in divided doses. For the following infections, a dosage of 500 mg may be administered every 12 hours: streptococcal pharyngitis, skin and skin structure infections, and uncomplicated cystitis. Cystitis therapy should be continued for 7 to 14 days. For other infections, the usual dosing is every 6 hours. For more severe infections or those caused by less susceptible organisms, larger doses may be needed. If daily doses of Keftab greater than 4 g are required, parenteral cephalosporins, in appropriate doses, should be considered.

HOW SUPPLIED

Tablets (elliptical-shaped):
500 mg* (dark-green) (UC5395)—(100s) NDC 64455-034-01
Store at controlled room temperature, 59° to 86°F (15° to 30°C).
*Equivalent to cephalexin
CAUTION—Federal (USA) law prohibits dispensing without prescription.
Literature revised Oct. 1, 1997
PV 2061 UCP
KEF010B0997
1. 21 CFR 460.1 *Federal Register* 1987; 838-842.
DJ Pharma, Inc.
Manufactured by
Eli Lilly and Company
Indianapolis, IN, USA 46285
DJ Pharma Inc.
San Diego, CA 92130

RONDEC® Oral Drops ℞
RONDEC® Syrup ℞
RONDEC® Tablet ℞
RONDEC-TR® Tablet ℞

DESCRIPTION

Antihistamine/Decongestant for oral use

For infants (1–18 months)
RONDEC® Oral Drops ℞
Each dropperful (1 mL) contains carbinoxamine maleate, 2 mg; pseudoephedrine hydrochloride, 25 mg.
Inactive Ingredients: Citric acid, DC Red No. 33, FDC Yellow No. 6, glycerin, methylparaben, propylparaben, purified water, sodium benzoate, sodium citrate, sorbitol and artificial flavoring.

For pediatric patients (over 18 months)
RONDEC® Syrup ℞
Each teaspoonful (5 mL) contains carbinoxamine maleate, 4 mg; pseudoephedrine hydrochloride, 60 mg.
Inactive Ingredients: Citric acid, DC Red No. 33, FDC Yellow No. 6, glycerin, methylparaben, propylparaben, purified water, sodium benzoate, sodium citrate, sorbitol and artificial flavoring.

For adults and pediatric patients (6 yrs. and over)
RONDEC® Tablet ℞
Each tablet contains carbinoxamine maleate, 4 mg; pseudoephedrine hydrochloride, 60 mg.
Inactive Ingredients: Cellulosic polymers, FDC Yellow No. 6, hydrogenated vegetable oil wax, lactose, magnesium stearate, microcrystalline cellulose, polyethylene glycol, povidone, propylene glycol, silicon dioxide, sodium starch glycolate, sorbitan monooleate, titanium dioxide and vanillin.

For adults and adolescents (12 yrs. and over)
RONDEC-TR® Tablet ℞
Each timed-release tablet contains carbinoxamine maleate, 8 mg; pseudoephedrine hydrochloride, 120 mg.
Inactive Ingredients: Castor oil, cellulosic polymers, confectioner's sugar, cornstarch, FDC Blue No. 1, lactose, magnesium stearate, methyl acrylate-methyl methacrylate copolymer, microcrystalline cellulose, povidone, propylene glycol, sorbitan monooleate and titanium dioxide.

HOW SUPPLIED

Rondec Oral Drops, berry-flavored, in 30-mL bottles for dropper dosage, **NDC** 64455-020-03. Calibrated shatterproof dropper enclosed in each carton. Container meets safety closure requirements.
Rondec Syrup, berry-flavored, in 16-fl-oz (1-pint) bottles, **NDC** 64455-021-48; and 4-fl-oz bottles, **NDC** 64455-021-12. Dispense in USP tight glass container.
Rondec Tablet, in bottles of 100, **NDC** 64455-022-01; and bottles of 500, **NDC** 64455-022-05. Each orange-colored tablet marked with ⊓ and the number 5726 for professional identification. Dispense in USP tight container.
Rondec-TR Tablet, in bottles of 100, **NDC** 64455-025-01. Each blue-colored tablet marked with ⊓ and the number 6240 for professional identification. Dispense in USP tight container.
Recommended storage: Store below 86°F (30°C).
Rx only
Revised: June, 1998
Manufactured by: Abbott Laboratories
North Chicago, IL 60064 U.S.A.
Manufactured for: DJ Pharma, Inc.
San Diego, C.A. 92130
R002D98

RONDEC®-DM Syrup ℞
RONDEC®-DM Oral Drops ℞

DESCRIPTION

Antihistamine/Decongestant/ Antitussive for oral use

for adults and pediatric patients (18 months and over)
RONDEC®-DM Syrup ℞
Each teaspoonful (5 mL) contains:

carbinoxamine maleate	4 mg
pseudoephedrine hydrochloride	60 mg
dextromethorphan hydrobromide	15 mg

Inactive Ingredients: Citric acid, DC Red No. 33, FDC Blue No. 1, glycerin, menthol, purified water, sodium benzoate, sodium citrate, sorbitol, natural and artificial flavoring and other ingredients.

for infants (1–18 months)
RONDEC®-DM Oral Drops ℞
Each dropperful (1 mL) contains:

carbinoxamine maleate	2 mg
pseudoephedrine hydrochloride	25 mg
dextromethorphan hydrobromide	4 mg

Inactive Ingredients: Citric acid, DC Red No. 33, FDC Blue No. 1, glycerin, menthol, purified water, sodium benzoate, sodium citrate, sorbitol, natural and artificial flavoring and other ingredients.

HOW SUPPLIED

Rondec-DM Syrup, grape-flavored, in 16-fl-oz (1-pint) bottles, **NDC** 64455-024-48; and 4-fl-oz bottles, **NDC** 64455-024-12. Dispense in USP tight, light-resistant, glass container. Avoid exposure to excessive heat.
Rondec-DM Oral Drops, grape-flavored, in 30-mL bottles for dropper dosage. Calibrated, shatterproof dropper enclosed in each carton. Container meets safety closure requirements **NDC** 64455-020-03. Avoid exposure to excessive heat.
Rx only
Revised June, 1998
Manufactured by: Abbott Laboratories
North Chicago, IL 60064 U.S.A.
Manufactured for: DJ Pharma, Inc.
San Diego, CA 92130
RDM001C98

IDENTIFICATION PROBLEM?
Turn to the **Product Identification Guide,** where you'll find more than 1600 products pictured in actual size and full color.

Dow Hickam Pharmaceuticals

for product information see Bertek Pharmaceuticals Inc.

DuPont Pharma

WILMINGTON, DE 19880

DUPONT PHARMA
Chestnut Run Plaza, Hickory Run
P.O. Box 80723
Wilmington, DE 19880-0723
(302) 992-5000

Address all product-related inquiries to:
Medical Affairs Department

For Product Information/Adverse Drug Experience Reporting, call
Product Information
(302) 992-4240 or 1-800-474-2762

COUMADIN® TABLETS ℞
(Warfarin Sodium Tablets, USP) Crystalline
Anticoagulant
COUMADIN® FOR INJECTION ℞
(Warfarin Sodium for Injection, USP)
Rx only

DESCRIPTION

COUMADIN (crystalline warfarin sodium), is an anticoagulant which acts by inhibiting vitamin K-dependent coagulation factors. Chemically, it is 3-(α-acetonylbenzyl)-4-hydroxycoumarin and is a racemic mixture of the R- and S-enantiomers. Crystalline warfarin sodium is an ispropanol clathrate. The crystallization of warfarin sodium virtually eliminates trace impurities present in amorphous warfarin. Its empirical formula is $C_{19}H_{15}NaO_4$ and its structural formula may be represented by the following:

ONa CH₂COCH₃

Crystalline warfarin sodium occurs as a white, odorless, crystalline powder, is discolored by light and is very soluble in water; freely soluble in alcohol; very slightly soluble in chloroform and in ether.
COUMADIN Tablets for oral use also contain:

All strengths:	Lactose, starch and magnesium stearate
1 mg:	D&C Red No. 6 Barium Lake
2 mg:	FD&C Blue No. 2 Aluminum Lake and FD&C Red No. 40 Aluminum Lake
2-1/2 mg:	D&C Yellow No. 10 Aluminum Lake and FD&C Blue No. 1 Aluminum Lake
3 mg:	FD&C Yellow No. 6 Aluminum Lake, FD&C Blue No. 2 Aluminum Lake and FD&C Red No. 40 Aluminum Lake
4 mg:	FD&C Blue No. 1 Aluminum Lake
5 mg:	FD&C Yellow No. 6 Aluminum Lake
6 mg:	FD&C Yellow No. 6 Aluminum Lake and FD&C Blue No. 1 Aluminum Lake
7-1/2 mg:	D&C Yellow No. 10 Aluminum Lake and FD&C Yellow No. 6 Aluminum Lake
10 mg:	Dye Free

COUMADIN for Injection is supplied as a sterile, lyophilized powder, which, after reconstitution with 2.7 mL sterile Water for Injection, contains:

Warfarin Sodium	2 mg/mL
Sodium Phosphate, Dibasic, Heptahydrate	4.98 mg/mL
Sodium Phosphate, Monobasic, Monohydrate	0.194 mg/mL
Sodium Chloride	0.1 mg/mL
Mannitol	38.0 mg/mL
Sodium Hydroxide, as needed for pH adjustment to	8.1 to 8.3

CLINICAL PHARMACOLOGY

COUMADIN and other coumarin anticoagulants act by inhibiting the synthesis of vitamin K dependent clotting factors, which include Factors II, VII, IX, and X, and the anticoagulant proteins C and S. Half-lives of these clotting factors are as follows: Factor II—60 hours, VII—4–6 hours, IX—24 hours, and X—48–72 hours. The half-lives of proteins C and S are approximately 8 hours and 30 hours, respectively. The resultant *in vivo* effect is a sequential depression of Factors VII, IX, X and II activities. Vitamin K is an essential cofactor for the post ribosomal synthesis of the

Continued on next page

Coumadin—Cont.

TABLE 1
CLINICAL STUDIES OF WARFARIN IN NON-RHEUMATIC AF PATIENTS*

Study	N		PT Ratio	INR	Thromboembolism		% Major Bleeding	
	Warfarin-Treated Patients	Control Patients			% Risk Reduction	*p*-value	Warfarin-Treated Patients	Control Patients
AFASAK	335	336	1.5-2.0	2.8-4.2	60	0.027	0.6	0.0
SPAF	210	211	1.3-1.8	2.0-4.5	67	0.01	1.9	1.9
BAATAF	212	208	1.2-1.5	1.5-2.7	86	<0.05	0.9	0.5
CAFA	187	191	1.3-1.6	2.0-3.0	45	0.25	2.7	0.5
SPINAF	260	265	1.2-1.5	1.4-2.8	79	0.001	2.3	1.5

* All study results of warfarin vs. control are based on intention-to-treat analysis and include ischemic stroke and systemic thromboembolism, excluding hemorrhage and transient ischemic attacks.

TABLE 2

Event	Warfarin (N=607)	Placebo (N=607)	RR (95%CI)	% Risk Reduction (p-value)
Total Patient Years of Follow-up	2018	1944		
Total Mortality	94 (4.7/100 py)	123 (6.3/100 py)	0.76 (0.60, 0.97)	24 (p=0.030)
Vascular Death	82 (4.1/100 py)	105 (5.4/100 py)	0.78 (0.60, 1.02)	22 (p=0.068)
Recurrent MI	82 (4.1/100 py)	124 (6.4/100 py)	0.66 (0.51, 0.85)	34 (p=0.001)
Cerebrovascular Event	20 (1.0/100 py)	44 (2.3/100 py)	0.46 (0.28, 0.75)	54 (p=0.002)

RR=Relative risk; Risk reduction=(I - RR); CI=Confidence interval; MI=Myocardial infarction; py=patient years

vitamin K dependent clotting factors. The vitamin promotes the biosynthesis of γ-carboxyglutamic acid residues in the proteins which are essential for biological activity. Warfarin is thought to interfere with clotting factor synthesis by inhibition of the regeneration of vitamin K_1 epoxide. The degree of depression is dependent upon the dosage administered. Therapeutic doses of warfarin decrease the total amount of the active form of each vitamin K dependent clotting factor made by the liver by approximately 30% to 50%. An anticoagulation effect generally occurs within 24 hours after drug administration. However, peak anticoagulant effect may be delayed 72 to 96 hours. The duration of action of a single dose of racemic warfarin is 2 to 5 days. The effects of COUMADIN may become more pronounced as effects of daily maintenance doses overlap. Anticoagulants have no direct effect on an established thrombus, nor do they reverse ischemic tissue damage. However, once a thrombus has occurred, the goal of anticoagulant treatment is to prevent further extension of the formed clot and prevent secondary thromboembolic complications which may result in serious and possibly fatal sequelae.

Pharmacokinetics: COUMADIN is a racemic mixture of the R- and S-enantiomers. The S-enantiomer exhibits 2–5 times more anticoagulant activity than the R-enantiomer in humans, but generally has a more rapid clearance.

Absorption: COUMADIN is essentially completely absorbed after oral administration with peak concentration generally attained within the first 4 hours.

Distribution: There are no differences in the apparent volumes of distribution after intravenous and oral administration of single doses of warfarin solution. Warfarin distributes into a relatively small apparent volume of distribution of about 0.14 liter/kg. A distribution phase lasting 6 to 12 hours is distinguishable after rapid intravenous or oral administration of an aqueous solution. Using a one compartment model, and assuming complete bioavailability, estimates of the volumes of distribution of R- and S-warfarin are similar to each other and to that of the racemate. Concentrations in fetal plasma approach the maternal values, but warfarin has not been found in human milk (see WARNINGS—Lactation). Approximately 99% of the drug is bound to plasma proteins.

Metabolism: The elimination of warfarin is almost entirely by metabolism. COUMADIN is stereoselectively metabolized by hepatic microsomal enzymes (cytochrome P-450) to inactive hydroxylated metabolites (predominant route) and by reductases to reduced metabolites (warfarin alcohols). The warfain alcohols have minimal anticoagulant activity. The metabolites are principally excreted into the urine; and to a lesser extent into the bile. The metabolites of warfarin that have been identified include dehydrowarfarin, two diastereoisomer alcohols, 4′-, 6-, 7-, 8- and 10-hydroxywarfarin. The Cytochrome P-450 isozymes involved in the metabolism of warfarin include 2C9, 2C19, 2C8, 2C18, 1A2, and 3A4. 2C9 is likely to be the principal form of human liver P-450 which modulates the *in vivo* anticoagulant activity of warfarin.

Excretion: The terminal half-life of warfarin after a single dose is approximately one week; however, the effective half-life ranges from 20 to 60 hours, with a mean of about 40 hours. The clearance of R-warfarin is generally half that of S-warfarin, thus as the volumes of distribution are similar, the half-life of R-warfarin is longer than that of S-warfarin. The half-life of R-warfarin ranges from 37 to 89 hours, while that of S-warfarin ranges from 21 to 43 hours. Studies with radiolabeled drug have demonstrated that up to 92% of the orally administered dose is recovered in urine. Very little warfarin is excreted unchanged in urine. Urinary excretion is in the form of metabolites.

Elderly: Patients 60 years or older appear to exhibit greater than expected PT/INR response to the anticoagulant effects of warfarin. The cause of the increased sensitivity to the anticoagulant effects of warfarin in this age group is unknown. This increased anticoagulant effect from warfarin may be due to a combination of pharmacokinetic and pharmacodynamic factors. Racemic warfarin clearance may be unchanged or reduced with increasing age. Limited information suggests there is no difference in the clearance of S-warfarin in the elderly versus young subjects. However, there may be a slight decrease in the clearance of R-warfarin in the elderly as compared to the young. Therefore, as patient age increases, a lower dose of warfarin is usually required to produce a therapeutic level of anticoagulation.

Renal Dysfunction: Renal clearance is considered to be a minor determinant of anticoagulant response to warfarin. No dosage adjustment is necessary for patients with renal failure.

Hepatic Dysfunction: Hepatic dysfunction can potentiate the response to warfarin through impaired synthesis of clotting factors and decreased metabolism of warfarin.

The administration of COUMADIN via the intravenous (IV) route should provide the patient with the same concentration of an equal oral dose, but maximum plasma concentration will be reached earlier. However, the full anticoagulant effect of a dose of warfarin may not be achieved until 72–96 hours after dosing, indicating that the administration of IV COUMADIN should not provide any increased biological effect or earlier onset of action.

Clinical Trials

Atrial Fibrillation (AF): In five prospective randomized controlled clinical trials involving 3711 patients with non-rheumatic AF, warfarin significantly reduced the risk of systemic thromboembolism including stroke (See Table 1). The risk reduction ranged from 60% to 86% in all except one trial (CAFA: 45%) which stopped early due to published positive results from two of these trials. The incidence of major bleeding in these trials ranged from 0.6 to 2.7% (See Table 1). Meta-analysis findings of these studies revealed that the effects of warfarin in reducing thromboembolic events including stroke were similar at either moderately high INR (2.0–4.5) or low INR (1.4–3.0). There was a significant reduction in minor bleeds at the low INR. Similar data from clinical studies in valvular atrial fibrillation patients are not available.

[See table 1 above]

Myocardial Infarction: WARIS (The Warfarin Re-Infarction Study) was a double-blind, randomized study of 1214 patients 2 to 4 weeks post-infarction treated with warfarin to a target INR of 2.8 to 4.8. [But note that a lower INR was achieved and increased bleeding was associated with INR's above 4.0; (see DOSAGE AND ADMINISTRATION)]. The primary endpoint was a combination of total mortality and recurrent infarction. A secondary endpoint of cerebrovascular events was assessed. Mean follow-up of the patients was 37 months. The results for each endpoint separately, including an analysis of vascular death, are provided in the following table:

[See table 2 above]

Mechanical and Bioprosthetic Heart Valves: In a prospective, randomized, open label, positive-controlled study (Mok et al, 1985) in 254 patients, the thromboembolic-free interval was found to be significantly greater in patients with mechanical prosthetic heart valves treated with warfarin alone compared with dipyridamole-aspirin (p<0.005) and pentoxifylline-aspirin (p<0.05) treated patients. Rates of thromboembolic events in these groups were 2.2, 8.6, and 7.9/100 patient years, respectively. Major bleeding rates were 2.5, 0.0, and 0.9/100 patient years, respectively.

In a prospective, open label, clinical trial (Saour et al, 1990) comparing moderate (INR 2.65) vs. high intensity (INR 9.0) warfarin therapies in 258 patients with mechanical prosthetic heart valves, thromboembolism occurred with similar frequency in the two groups (4.0 and 3.7 events/100 patient years, respectively). Major bleeding was more common in the high intensity group (2.1 events/100 patient years) vs. 0.95 events/100 patient years in the moderate intensity group.

In a randomized trial (Turpie et al, 1988) in 210 patients comparing two intensities of warfarin therapy (INR 2.0–2.25 vs. INR 2.5–4.0) for a three-month period following tissue heart valve replacement, thromboembolism occurred with similar frequency in the two groups (major embolic events 2.0% vs. 1.9%, respectively and minor embolic events 10.8% vs. 10.2%, respectively). Major bleeding complications were more frequent with the higher intensity (major hemorrhages 4.6%) vs. none in the lower intensity.

INDICATIONS AND USAGE

COUMADIN (Warfarin Sodium) is indicated for the prophylaxis and/or treatment of venous thrombosis and its extension, and pulmonary embolism.

COUMADIN is indicated for the prophylaxis and/or treatment of the thromboembolic complications associated with atrial fibrillation and/or cardiac valve replacement.

COUMADIN is indicated to reduce the risk of death, recurrent myocardial infarction, and thromboembolic events such as stroke or systemic embolization after myocardial infarction.

CONTRAINDICATIONS

Anticoagulation is contraindicated in any localized or general physical condition or personal circumstance in which the hazard of hemorrhage might be greater than the potential clinical benefits of anticoagulation, such as:

Pregnancy: COUMADIN is contraindicated in women who are or may become pregnant because the drug passes through the placental barrier and may cause fatal hemorrhage to the fetus *in utero*. Furthermore, there have been reports of birth malformations in children born to mothers who have been treated with warfarin during pregnancy.

Embryopathy characterized by nasal hypoplasia with or without stippled epiphyses (chondrodysplasia punctata) has been reported in pregnant women exposed to warfarin during the first trimester. Central nervous system abnormalities also have been reported, including dorsal midline dysplasia characterized by agenesis of the corpus callosum, Dandy-Walker malformation, and midline cerebellar atrophy. Ventral midline dysplasia, characterized by optic atrophy, and eye abnormalities have been observed. Mental retardation, blindness, and other central nervous system abnormalities have been reported in association with second and third trimester exposure. Although rare, teratogenic reports following *in utero* exposure to warfarin include urinary tract anomalies such as single kidney, asplenia, anencephaly, spina bifida, cranial nerve palsy, hydrocephalus, cardiac defects and congenital heart disease, polydactyly, deformities of toes, diaphragmatic hernia, corneal leukoma, cleft palate, cleft lip, schizencephaly, and microcephaly.

Spontaneous abortion and still birth are known to occur and a higher risk of fetal mortality is associated with the use of warfarin. Low birth weight and growth retardation have also been reported.

Women of childbearing potential who are candidates for anticoagulant therapy should be carefully evaluated and the indications critically reviewed with the patient. If the patient becomes pregnant while taking this drug, she should be apprised of the potential risks to the fetus, and the possibility of termination of the pregnancy should be discussed in light of those risks.

Hemorrhagic tendencies or blood dyscrasias.

Recent or contemplated surgery of: (1) central nervous system; (2) eye; (3) traumatic surgery resulting in large open surfaces.

Bleeding tendencies associated with active ulceration or overt bleeding of: (1) gastrointestinal, genitourinary or respiratory tracts; (2) cerebrovascular hemorrhage; (3) aneurysms-cerebral, dissecting aorta; (4) pericarditis and pericardial effusions; (5) bacterial endocarditis.

Threatened abortion, eclampsia and preeclampsia.

Inadequate laboratory facilities.

Unsupervised patients with senility, alcoholism, or psychosis or other lack of patient cooperation.

Spinal puncture and other diagnostic or therapeutic procedures with potential for uncontrollable bleeding.

Miscellaneous: major regional, lumbar block anesthesia, malignant hypertension and known hypersensitivity to warfarin or to any other components of this product.

WARNINGS

The most serious risks associated with anticoagulant therapy with warfarin sodium are hemorrhage in any tissue or organ and, less frequently (<0.1%), necrosis and/or gangrene of skin and other tissues. The risk of hemorrhage is related to the level of intensity and the duration of anticoagulant therapy. Hemorrhage and necrosis have in some cases been reported to result in death or permanent disability. Necrosis appears to be associated with local thrombosis and usually appears within a few days of the start of anticoagulant therapy. In severe cases of necrosis, treatment through debridement or amputation of the affected tissue, limb, breast or penis has been reported. Careful diagnosis is required to determine whether necrosis is caused by an underlying disease. Warfarin therapy should be discontinued when warfarin is suspected to be the cause of developing necrosis and heparin therapy may be considered for anticoagulation. Although various treatments have been attempted, no treatment for necrosis has been considered uniformly effective. See below for information on predisposing conditions. These and other risks associated with anticoagulant therapy must be weighed against the risk of thrombosis or embolization in untreated cases.

It cannot be emphasized too strongly that treatment of each patient is a highly individualized matter. COUMADIN, a narrow therapeutic range (index) drug, may be affected by factors such as other drugs and dietary Vitamin K. Dosage should be controlled by periodic determinations of prothrombin time (PT)/International Normalized Ratio (INR) or other suitable coagulation tests. Determinations of whole blood clotting and bleeding times are not effective measures for control of therapy. Heparin prolongs the one-stage PT. When heparin and COUMADIN are administered concomitantly, refer below to CONVERSION FROM HEPARIN THERAPY for recommendations.

Caution should be observed when COUMADIN is administered in any situation or in the presence of any predisposing condition where added risk of hemorrhage, necrosis, and/or gangrene is present.

Anticoagulation therapy with COUMADIN may enhance the release of atheromatous plaque emboli, thereby increasing the risk of complications from systemic cholesterol microembolization, including the "purple toes syndrome." Discontinuation of COUMADIN therapy is recommended when such phenomena are observed.

Systemic atheroemboli and cholesterol microemboli can present with a variety of signs and symptoms including purple toes syndrome, livedo reticularis, rash, gangrene, abrupt and intense pain in the leg, foot, or toes, foot ulcers, myalgia, penile gangrene, abdominal pain, flank or back pain, hematuria, renal insufficiency, hypertension, cerebral ischemia, spinal cord infarction, pancreatitis, symptoms simulating polyarteritis, or any other sequelae of vascular compromise due to embolic occlusion. The most commonly involved visceral organs are the kidneys followed by the pancreas, spleen, and liver. Some cases have progressed to necrosis or death.

Purple toes syndrome is a complication of oral anticoagulation characterized by a dark, purplish or mottled color of the toes, usually occurring between 3–10 weeks, or later, after the initiation of therapy with warfarin or related compounds. Major features of this syndrome include purple color of plantar surfaces and sides of the toes that blanches on moderate pressure and fades with elevation of the legs; pain and tenderness of the toes; waxing and waning of the color over time. While the purple toes syndrome is reported to be reversible, some cases progress to gangrene or necrosis which may require debridement of the affected area, or may lead to amputation.

Heparin-induced thrombocytopenia: COUMADIN should be used with caution in patients with heparin-induced thrombocytopenia and deep venous thrombosis. Cases of venous limb ischemia, necrosis, and gangrene have occurred in patients with heparin-induced thrombocytopenia and deep venous thrombosis when heparin treatment was discontinued and warfarin therapy was started or continued. In some patients sequelae have included amputation of the involved area and/or death (Warkentin et al, 1997).

A severe elevation (>50 seconds) in activated partial thromboplastin time (aPTT) with a PT/INR in the desired range has been identified as an indication of increased risk of postoperative hemorrhage.

The decision to administer anticoagulants in the following conditions must be based upon the clinical judgment in which the risks of anticoagulant therapy are weighed against the benefits:

Lactation: COUMADIN appears in the milk of nursing mothers in an inactive form. Infants nursed by mothers treated with COUMADIN had no change in prothrombin time (PTs). Effects in premature infants have not been evaluated.

Severe to moderate hepatic or renal insufficiency.

Infectious diseases or disturbances of intestinal flora: sprue, antibiotic therapy.

Trauma which may result in internal bleeding.

Surgery or trauma resulting in large exposed raw surfaces.

Indwelling catheters.

Severe to moderate hypertension.

Known or suspected deficiency in protein C mediated anticoagulant response: Hereditary or acquired deficiencies of protein C or its cofactor, protein S, have been associated with tissue necrosis following warfarin administration. Not all patients with these conditions develop necrosis, and tissue necrosis occurs in patients without these deficiencies. Inherited resistance to activated protein C has been described in many patients with venous thromboembolic disorders but has not yet been evaluated as a risk factor for tissue necrosis. The risk associated with these conditions, both for recurrent thrombosis and for adverse reactions, is difficult to evaluate since it does not appear to be the same for everyone. Decisions about testing and therapy must be made on an individual basis. It has been reported that concomitant anticoagulation therapy with heparin for 5 to 7 days during initiation of therapy with COUMADIN may minimize the incidence of tissue necrosis. Warfarin therapy should be discontinued when warfarin is suspected to be the cause of developing necrosis and heparin therapy may be considered for anticoagulation.

Miscellaneous: polycythemia vera, vasculitis, and severe diabetes.

Minor and severe allergic/hypersensitivity reactions and anaphylactic reactions have been reported.

Classes of Drugs

5-lipoxygenase Inhibitor	Antineoplastics†	Hypnotics†
Adrenergic Stimulants, Central	Antiparasitic/Antimicrobials	Hypolipidemics†
Alcohol Abuse Reduction Preparations	Antiplatelet Drugs/Effects	Leukotriene Receptor Antagonist
Analgesics	Antithyroid Drugs†	Monoamine Oxidase Inhibitors
Anesthetics, Inhalation	Beta-Adrenergic Blockers	Narcotics, prolonged
Antiandrogen	Bromelains	Nonsteroidal Anti-Inflammatory Agents
Antiarrhythmics†	Cholelitholytic Agents	Psychostimulants
Antibiotics†	Diabetes Agents, Oral	Pyrazolones
Aminoglycosides (oral)	Diuretics†	Salicylates
Cephalosporins, parenteral	Fungal Medications, Systemic†	Selective Serotonin Reuptake Inhibitors
Macrolides	Gastric Acidity and Peptic Ulcer Agents†	Steroids, Adrenocortical†
Miscellaneous	Gastrointestinal	Steroids, Anabolic (17-Alkyl Testosterone Derivatives)
Penicillins, intravenous, high dose	Prokinetic Agents	Thrombolytics
Quinolones (fluoroquinolones)	Ulcerative Colitis Agents	Thyroid Drugs
Sulfonamides, long acting	Gout Treatment Agents	Tuberculosis Agents†
Tetracyclines	Hemorrheologic Agents	Uricosuric Agents
Anticoagulants	Hepatotoxic Drugs	Vaccines
Anticonvulsants†	Herbal Medicines	Vitamins†
Antidepressants†	Hyperglycemic Agents	
Antimalarial Agents	Hypertensive Emergency Agents	

Specific Drugs Reported

acetaminophen	fenoprofen	penicillin G, intravenous
alcohol†	fluconazole	pentoxifylline
allopurinol	fluorouracil	phenylbutazone
aminosalicylic acid	fluoxetine	phenytoin†
amiodarone HCl	flutamide	piperacillin
aspirin	fluvastatin	piroxicam
azithromycin	fluvoxamine	prednisone†
capecitabine	glucagon	propafenone
cefamandole	halothane	propoxyphene
cefazolin	heparin	propranolol
cefoperazone	ibuprofen	propylthiouracil†
cefotetan	ifosfamide	quinidine
cefoxitin	indomethacin	quinine
ceftriaxone	influenza virus vaccine	ranitidine†
celecoxib	itraconazole	rofecoxib
chenodiol	ketoprofen	sertraline
chloramphenicol	ketorolac	simvastatin
chloral hydrate†	levamisole	stanozolol
chlorpropamide	levothyroxine	streptokinase
cholestyramine†	liothyronine	sulfamethizole
cimetidine	lovastatin	sulfamethoxazole
ciprofloxacin	mefenamic acid	sulfinpyrazone
cisapride	methimazole†	sulfisoxazole
clarithromycin	methyldopa	sulindac
clofibrate	methylphenidate	tamoxifen
COUMADIN overdose	methylsalicylate ointment (topical)	tetracycline
cyclophosphamide†	metronidazole	thyroid
danazol	miconazole	ticarcillin
danshen (Chinese herb)	moricizine hydrochloride†	ticlopidine
dextran	nalidixic acid	tissue plasminogen activator (t-PA)
dextrothyroxine	naproxen	tolbutamide
diazoxide	neomycin	tramadol
diclofenac	norfloxacin	trimethoprim/sulfamethoxazole
dicumarol	ofloxacin	urokinase
diflunisal	olsalazine	valproate
disulfiram	omeprazole	vitamin E
doxycycline	oxaprozin	zafirlukast
erythromycin	oxymetholone	zileuton
ethacrynic acid	paroxetine	
fenofibrate		

also: other medications affecting blood elements which may modify hemostasis
dietary deficiencies
prolonged hot weather
unreliable PT/INR determinations

†Increased and decreased PT/INR responses have been reported.

In patients with acquired or inherited warfarin resistance, decreased therapeutic responses to COUMADIN have been reported. Exaggerated therapeutic responses have been reported in other patients.

Patients with congestive heart failure may exhibit greater than expected PT/INR response to COUMADIN, thereby requiring more frequent laboratory monitoring, and reduced doses of COUMADIN.

Concomitant use of anticoagulants with streptokinase or urokinase is not recommended and may be hazardous. (Please note recommendations accompanying these preparations.)

PRECAUTIONS

Periodic determination of PT/INR or other suitable coagulation test is essential.

Numerous factors, alone or in combination, including travel, changes in diet, environment, physical state and medication may influence response of the patient to anticoagulants. It is generally good practice to monitor the patient's response with additional PT/INR determinations in the period immediately after discharge from the hospital, and whenever other medications are initiated, discontinued or taken irregularly. The following factors are listed for reference; however, other factors may also affect the anticoagulant response.

Drugs may interact with COUMADIN through pharmacodynamic or pharmacokinetic mechanisms. Pharmacodynamic mechanisms for drug interactions with COUMADIN are synergism (impaired hemostasis, reduced clotting factor synthesis), competitive antagonism (vitamin K), and altered physiologic control loop for vitamin K metabolism (hereditary resistance). Pharmacokinetic mechanisms for drug interactions with COUMADIN are mainly enzyme induction, enzyme inhibition, and reduced plasma protein binding. It is important to note that some drugs may interact by more than one mechanism.

The following factors, alone or in combination, may be responsible for INCREASED PT/INR response:

ENDOGENEOUS FACTORS:

blood dyscrasia - see CONTRAINDICATIONS	hepatic disorders
cancer	infectious hepatitis
collagen vascular disease	jaundice
congestive heart failure	hyperthyroidism
diarrhea	poor nutritional state
elevated temperature	steatorrhea
	vitamin K deficiency

EXOGENOUS FACTORS:

Potential drug interactions with COUMADIN are listed below by drug class and by specific drugs.

[See table at top of page]

The following factors, alone or in combination, may be responsible for DECREASED PT/INR response:

Continued on next page

Coumadin—Cont.

ENDOGENOUS FACTORS:

edema hereditary coumarin resistance hyperlipemia	hypothyroidism nephrotic syndrome

EXOGENOUS FACTORS:

Potential drug interactions with COUMADIN (Warfarin Sodium) are listed below by drug class and by specific drugs.
[See first table at right]

Classes of Drugs

Adrenal Corticol Steroid Inhibitors Antacids Antianxiety Agents Antiarrhythmics† Antibiotics† Anticonvulsants† Antidepressants† Antihistamines Antineoplastics†	Antipsychotic Medications Antithyroid Drugs† Barbiturates Diuretics† Enteral Nutritional Supplements Fungal Medications, Systemic† Gastric Acidity and Peptic Ulcer Agents†	Hypnotics† Hypolipidemics† Immunosuppressives Oral Contraceptives, Estrogen Containing Steroids, Adrenocortical† Tuberculosis Agents† Vitamins†

Specific Drugs Reported

alcohol† aminoglutethimide amobarbital atorvastatin azathioprine butabarbital butalbital carbamazepine chloral hydrate† chlordiazepoxide chlorthalidone cholestyramine† corticotropin cortisone	COUMADIN underdosage cyclophosphamide† dicloxacillin ethchlorvynol glutethimide griseofulvin haloperidol meprobamate 6-mercaptopurine methiamazole† moricizine hydrochloride† nafcillin paraldehyde pentobarbital	phenobarbital phenytoin† prednisone† primidone propylthiouracil† ranitidine† rifampin secobarbital spironolactone sucralfate trazodone vitamin C (high dose) vitamin K

also: diet high in vitamin K
unreliable PT/INR determinations

†Increased and decreased PT/INR responses have been reported.

Because a patient may be exposed to a combination of the above factors, the net effect of COUMADIN on PT/INR response may be unpredictable. More frequent PT/INR monitoring is therefore advisable. Medications of unknown interaction with coumarins are best regarded with caution. When these medications are started or stopped, more frequent PT/INR monitoring is advisable.

It has been reported that concomitant administration of warfarin and ticlopidine may be associated with cholestatic hepatitis.

Effect on Other Drugs: Coumarins may also affect the action of other drugs. Hypoglycemic agents (chlorpropamide and tolbutamide) and anticonvulsants (phenytoin and phenobarbital) may accumulate in the body as a result of interference with either their metabolism or excretion.

Special Risk Patients: COUMADIN is a narrow therapeutic range (index) drug, and caution should be observed when warfarin sodium is administered to certain patients such as the elderly or debilitated or when administered in any situation or physical condition where added risk of hemorrhage is present.

Intramuscular (I.M.) injections of concomitant medications should be confined to the upper extremities which permits easy access for manual compression, inspections for bleeding and use of pressure bandages.

Caution should be observed when COUMADIN (or warfarin) is administered concomitantly with nonsteroidal anti-inflammatory drugs (NSAIDs), including aspirin, to be certain that no change in anticoagulation dosage is required. In addition to specific drug interactions that might affect PT/INR, NSAIDs, including aspirin, can inhibit platelet aggregation, and can cause gastrointestinal bleeding, peptic ulceration and/or perforation.

Acquired or inherited warfarin resistance should be suspected if large daily doses of COUMADIN are required to maintain a patient's PT/INR within a normal therapeutic range.

Information for Patients: The objective of anticoagulant therapy is to decrease the clotting ability of the blood so that thrombosis is prevented, while avoiding spontaneous bleeding. Effective therapeutic levels with minimal complications are in part dependent upon cooperative and well-instructed patients who communicate effectively with their physician. Patients should be advised: Strict adherence to prescribed dosage schedule is necessary. Do not take or discontinue any other medication, including salicylates (e.g., aspirin and topical analgesics) and other over-the-counter medications except on advice of the physician. Avoid alcohol consumption. Do not take COUMADIN during pregnancy and do not become pregnant while taking it (see CONTRAINDICATIONS). Avoid any activity or sport that may result in traumatic injury. Prothrombin time tests and regular visits to physician or clinic are needed to monitor therapy. Carry identification stating that COUMADIN is being taken. If the prescribed dose of COUMADIN is forgotten, notify the physician immediately. Take the dose as soon as possible on the same day but do not take a double dose of COUMADIN the next day to make up for missed doses. The amount of vitamin K in food may affect therapy with COUMADIN. Eat a normal, balanced diet maintaining a consistent amount of vitamin K. Avoid drastic changes in dietary habits, such as eating large amounts of green leafy vegetables. Contact physician to report any illness, such as diarrhea, infection or fever. Notify physician immediately if any unusual bleeding or symptoms occur. Signs and symptoms of bleeding include: pain, swelling or discomfort, prolonged bleeding from cuts, increased menstrual flow or vaginal bleeding, nosebleeds, bleeding of gums from brushing, unusual bleeding or bruising, red or dark brown urine, red or tar black stools, headache, dizziness, or weakness. If therapy with COUMADIN is discontinued, patients should be cautioned that the anticoagulant effects of COUMADIN may persist for about 2 to 5 days. **Patients should be informed that all warfarin sodium, USP, products represent the same medication, and should not be taken concomitantly, as overdosage may result.**

Carcinogenesis, Mutagenesis, Impairment of Fertility: Carcinogenicity and mutagenicity studies have not been performed with COUMADIN. The reproductive effects of COUMADIN have not been evaluated.

Use in Pregnancy: Pregnancy Category X—See CONTRAINDICATIONS.

Pediatric Use: Safety and effectiveness in pediatric patients below the age of 18 have not been established, in randomized, controlled clinical trials. However, the use of COUMADIN in pediatric patients is well-documented for the prevention and treatment of thromboembolic events. Difficulty achieving and maintaining therapeutic PT/INR ranges in the pediatric patient has been reported. More frequent PT/INR determinations are recommended because of possible changing warfarin requirements.

TABLE 3
Relationship Between INR and PT Ratios
For Thromboplastins With Different ISI Values (Sensitivities)

	PT RATIOS				
	ISI 1.0	**ISI 1.4**	**ISI 1.8**	**ISI 2.3**	**ISI 2.8**
INR = 2.0–3.0	2.0–3.0	1.6–2.2	1.5–1.8	1.4–1.6	1.3–1.5
INR = 2.5–3.5	2.5–3.5	1.9–2.4	1.7–2.0	1.5–1.7	1.4–1.6

Geriatric Use: Patients 60 years or older appear to exhibit greater than expected PT/INR response to the anticoagulant effects of warfarin (see CLINICAL PHARMACOLOGY). COUMADIN is contraindicated in any unsupervised patient with senility. Caution should be observed with administration of warfarin sodium to elderly patients in any situation or physical condition where added risk of hemorrhage is present. Low initiation doses of warfarin are recommended for elderly patients (see DOSAGE AND ADMINISTRATION).

ADVERSE REACTIONS

Potential adverse reactions to COUMADIN may include:

- Fatal or nonfatal hemorrhage from any tissue or organ. This is a consequence of the anticoagulant effect. The signs, symptoms, and severity will vary according to the location and degree or extent of the bleeding. Hemorrhagic complications may present as paralysis; paresthesia; headache, chest, abdomen, joint, muscle or other pain; dizziness; shortness of breath, difficult breathing or swallowing; unexplained swelling; weakness; hypotension; or unexplained shock. Therefore, the possibility of hemorrhage should be considered in evaluating the condition of any anticoagulated patient with complaints which do not indicate an obvious diagnosis. Bleeding during anticoagulant therapy does not always correlate with PT/INR. (See OVERDOSAGE—Treatment.)
- Bleeding which occurs when the PT/INR is within the therapeutic range warrants diagnostic investigation since it may unmask a previously unsuspected lesion, e.g., tumor, ulcer, etc.
- Necrosis of skin and other tissues. (See WARNINGS.)
- Adverse reactions reported infrequently include: hypersensitivity/allergic reactions, systemic cholesterol microembolization, purple toes syndrome, hepatitis, cholestatic hepatic injury, jaundice, elevated liver enzymes, vasculitis, edema, fever, rash, dermatitis, including bullous eruptions, urticaria, abdominal pain including cramping, flatulence/bloating, fatigue, lethargy, malaise, asthenia, nausea, vomiting, diarrhea, pain, headache, dizziness, taste perversion, pruritus, alopecia, cold intolerance, and paresthesia including feeling cold and chills.

Rare events of tracheal or tracheobronchial calcification have been reported in association with long-term warfarin therapy. The clinical significance of this event is unknown.

Priapism has been associated with anticoagulant administration, however, a causal relationship has not been established.

OVERDOSAGE

Signs and Symptoms: Suspected or over abnormal bleeding (e.g., appearance of blood in stools or urine, hematuria, excessive menstrual bleeding, melena, petechiae, excessive bruising or persistent oozing from superficial injuries) are early manifestations of anticoagulation beyond a safe and satisfactory level.

Treatment: Excessive anticoagulation, with or without bleeding, may be controlled by discontinuing COUMADIN therapy and if necessary, by administration of oral or parenteral vitamin K_1. (Please see recommendations accompanying vitamin K_1 preparations prior to use.)

Such use of vitamin K_1 reduces response to subsequent COUMADIN therapy. Patients may return to a pretreatment thrombotic status following the rapid reversal of a prolonged PT/INR. Resumption of COUMADIN administration reverses the effect of vitamin K, and a therapeutic PT/INR can again be obtained by careful dosage adjustment. If rapid anticoagulation is indicated, heparin may be preferable for initial therapy.

If minor bleeding progresses to major bleeding, give 5 to 25 mg (rarely up to 50 mg) parenteral vitamin K_1. In emergency situations of severe hemorrhage, clotting factors can be returned to normal by administering 200 to 500 mL of fresh whole blood or fresh frozen plasma, or by giving commercial Factor IX complex.

A risk of hepatitis and other viral diseases is associated with the use of these blood products; Factor IX complex is also associated with an increased risk of thrombosis. Therefore, these preparations should be used only in exceptional or life-threatening bleeding episodes secondary to COUMADIN (Warfarin Sodium) overdosage.

Purified Factor IX preparations should not be used because they cannot increase the levels of prothrombin, Factor VII and Factor X which are also depressed along with the levels of Factor IX as a result of COUMADIN treatment. Packed red blood cells may also be given if significant blood loss has occurred. Infusions of blood or plasma should be monitored carefully to avoid precipitating pulmonary edema in elderly patients or patients with heart disease.

DOSAGE AND ADMINISTRATION

The dosage and administration of COUMADIN must be individualized for each patient according to the particular patient's PT/INR response to the drug. The dosage should be adjusted based upon the patient's PT/INR. (See LABORATORY CONTROL below for full discussion on INR.)

Venous Thromboembolism (including pulmonary embolism): Available clinical evidence indicates that an INR of 2.0–3.0 is sufficient for prophylaxis and treatment of venous thromboembolism and minimizes the risk of hemorrhage associated with higher INRs. In patients with risk factors for recurrent venous thromboembolism including venous insufficiency, inherited thrombophilia, idiopathic venous thromboembolism, and a history of thrombotic events, consideration should be given to longer term therapy (Schulman et al, 1995 and Schulman et al, 1997).

Atrial Fibrillation: Five recent clinical trials evaluated the effects of warfarin in patients with non-valvular atrial fibrillation (AF). Meta-analysis findings of these studies revealed that the effects of warfarin in reducing thromboembolic events including stroke were similar at either moderately high INR (2.0–4.5) or low INR (1.4–3.0). There was a significant reduction in minor bleeds at the low INR. Similar data from clinical studies in valvular atrial fibrillation patients are not available. The trials in non-valvular atrial fibrillation support the American College of Chest Physicians' (ACCP) recommendation that an INR of 2.0–3.0 be used for long term warfarin therapy in appropriate AF patients.

Post-Myocardial Infarction: In post-myocardial infarction patients, COUMADIN therapy should be initiated early

(2–4 weeks post-infarction) and dosage should be adjusted to maintain an INR of 2.5–3.5 long-term. The recommendation is based on the results of the WARIS study in which treatment was initiated 2 to 4 weeks after the infarction. In patients thought to be at an increased risk of bleeding complications or on aspirin therapy, maintenance of COUMADIN therapy at the lower end of this INR range is recommended.

Mechanical and Bioprosthetic Heart Valves: In patients with mechanical heart valve(s), long term prophylaxis with warfarin to an INR of 2.5–3.5 is recommended. In patients with bioprosthetic heart valve(s), based on limited data, the American College of Chest Physicians recommends warfarin therapy to an INR of 2.0–3.0 for 12 weeks after valve insertion. In patients with additional risk factors such as atrial fibrillation or prior thromboembolism, consideration should be given for longer term therapy.

Recurrent Systemic Embolism: In cases where the risk of thromboembolism is great, such as in patients with recurrent systemic emboli, a higher INR may be required.

An INR of greater than 4.0 appears to provide no additional therapeutic benefit in most patients and is associated with a higher risk of bleeding.

Initial Dosage: The dosing of COUMADIN must be individualized according to patient's sensitivity to the drug as indicated by the PT/INR. Use of a large loading dose may increase the incidence of hemorrhagic and other complications, does not offer more rapid protection against thrombi formation, and is not recommended. Low initiation doses are recommended for elderly and/or debilitated patients and patients with potential to exhibit greater than expected PT/INR response to COUMADIN (see PRECAUTIONS). It is recommended that COUMADIN therapy be initiated with a dose of 2 to 5 mg per day with dosage adjustments based on the results of PT/INR determinations.

Maintenance: Most patients are satisfactorily maintained at a dose of 2 to 10 mg daily. Flexibility of dosage is provided by breaking scored tablets in half. The individual dose and interval should be gauged by the patient's prothrombin response.

Duration of Therapy: The duration of therapy in each patient should be individualized. In general, anticoagulant therapy should be continued until the danger of thrombosis and embolism has passed.

Missed Dose: The anticoagulant effect of COUMADIN persists beyond 24 hours. If the patient forgets to take the prescribed dose of COUMADIN at the scheduled time, the dose should be taken as soon as possible on the same day. The patients should not take the missed dose by doubling the daily dose to make up for missed doses, but should refer back to his or her physician.

Intravenous Route of Administration: COUMADIN for Injection provides an alternate administration route for patients who cannot receive oral drugs. The IV dosages would be the same as those that would be used orally if the patient could take the drug by the oral route. COUMADIN for Injection should be administered as a slow bolus injection over 1 to 2 minutes into a peripheral vein. It is not recommended for intramuscular administration. The vial should be reconstituted with 2.7 mL of sterile Water for Injection and inspected for particulate matter and discoloration immediately prior to use. Do not use if either particulate matter and/or discoloration is noted. After reconstitution, COUMADIN for Injection is chemically and physically stable for 4 hours at room temperature. It does not contain any antimicrobial preservative and, thus, care must be taken to assure the sterility of the prepared solution. The vial is not recommended for multiple use and unused solutions should be discarded.

LABORATORY CONTROL The PT reflects the depression of vitamin K dependent Factors VII, X and II. There are several modifications of the one-stage PT and the physician should become familiar with the specific method used in his laboratory. The degree of anticoagulation indicated by any range of PTs may be altered by the type of thromboplastin used; the appropriate therapeutic range must be based on the experience of each laboratory. The PT should be determined daily after the administration of the initial dose until PT/INR results stabilize in the therapeutic range. Intervals between subsequent PT/INR determinations should be based upon the physician's judgment of the patient's reliability and response to COUMADIN in order to maintain the individual within the therapeutic range. Acceptable intervals for PT/INR determinations are normally within the range of one to four weeks after a stable dosage has been determined. To ensure adequate control, it is recommended that additional PT tests are done when other warfarin products are interchanged with warfarin sodium tablets, USP, as well as whenever other medications are initiated, discontinued, or taken irregularly (see PRECAUTIONS).

Different thromboplastin reagents vary substantially in their sensitivity to sodium warfarin-induced effects on PT. To define the appropriate therapeutic regimen it is important to be familiar with the sensitivity of the thromboplastin reagent used in the laboratory and its relationship to the International Reference Preparation (IRP), a sensitive thromboplastin reagent prepared from human brain.

A system of standardizing the PT in oral anticoagulant control was introduced by the World Health Organization in 1983. It is based upon the determination of an International Normalized Ratio (INR) which provides a common basis for communication of PT results and interpretations of therapeutic ranges. The INR system of reporting is based on a logarithmic relationship between the PT ratios of the test and reference preparation. The INR is the PT ratio that would be obtained if the International Reference Preparation (IRP), which has an ISI of 1.0, were used to perform the test. Early clinical studies of oral anticoagulants, which formed the basis for recommended therapeutic ranges of 1.5 to 2.5 times control mean normal PT, used sensitive human brain thromboplastin. When using the less sensitive rabbit brain thromboplastins commonly employed in PT assays today, adjustments must be made to the targeted PT range that reflect this decrease in sensitivity.

The INR can be calculated as: INR = (observed PT ratio)^{ISI} where the ISI (International Sensitivity Index) is the correction factor in the equation that relates the PT ratio of the local reagent to the reference preparation and is a measure of the sensitivity of a given thromboplastin to reduction of vitamin K-dependent coagulation factors; the lower the ISI, the more "sensitive" the reagent and the closer the derived INR will be to the observed PT ratio.[1]

The proceedings and recommendations of the 1992 National Conference on Antithrombotic Therapy[2–4] review and evaluate issues related to oral anticoagulant therapy and the sensitivity of thromboplastin reagents and provide additional guidelines for defining the appropriate therapeutic regimen.

The conversion of the INR to PT ratios for the less-intense (INR 2.0–3.0) and more intense (INR 2.5–3.5) therapeutic range recommended by the ACCP for thromboplastins over a range of ISI values is shown in Table 3.[5]

[See table 3 on previous page]

TREATMENT DURING DENTISTRY AND SURGERY The management of patients who undergo dental and surgical procedures requires close liaison between attending physicians, surgeons and dentists. PT/INR determination is recommended just prior to any dental or surgical procedure. In patients undergoing minimal invasive procedures who must be anticoagulated prior to, during, or immediately following these procedures, adjusting the dosage of COUMADIN to maintain the PT/INR at the low end of the therapeutic range may safely allow for continued anticoagulation. The operative site should be sufficiently limited and accessible to permit the effective use of local procedures for hemostasis. Under these conditions, dental and minor surgical procedures may be performed without undue risk of hemorrhage. Some dental or surgical procedures may necessitate the interruption of COUMADIN therapy. When discontinuing COUMADIN even for a short period of time, the benefits and risks should be strongly considered.

CONVERSION FROM HEPARIN THERAPY Since the anticoagulant effect of COUMADIN is delayed, heparin is preferred initially for rapid anticoagulation. Conversion to COUMADIN may begin concomitantly with heparin therapy or may be delayed 3 to 6 days. To ensure continuous anticoagulation, it is advisable to continue full dose heparin therapy and that COUMADIN therapy be overlapped with heparin for 4 to 5 days, until COUMADIN has produced the desired therapeutic response as determined by PT/INR. When COUMADIN has produced the desired PT/INR or prothrombin activity, heparin may be discontinued.

COUMADIN may increase the aPTT test, even in the absence of heparin. During initial therapy with COUMADIN, the interference with heparin anticoagulation is of minimal clinical significance.

As heparin may affect the PT/INR, patients receiving both heparin and COUMADIN should have blood for PT/INR determination drawn at least:

- 5 hours after the last IV bolus dose of heparin, or
- 4 hours after cessation of a continuous IV infusion of heparin, or
- 24 hours after the last subcutaneous heparin injection.

HOW SUPPLIED

Tablets: For oral use, single scored with one face imprinted numerically with 1, 2, 2–1/2, 3, 4, 5, 6, 7–1/2 or 10 superimposed and inscribed with "COUMADIN" and with the opposite face inscribed with "DuPont." COUMADIN is available in bottles and Hospital Unit-Dose Blister Packages with potencies and colors as follows:

[See table above]

	100's	1000's	Hospital Unit-Dose Blister Package of 100
1 mg pink	NDC 0056-0169-70	NDC 0056-0169-90	NDC 0056-0169-75
2 mg lavender	NDC 0056-0170-70	NDC 0056-0170-90	NDC 0056-0170-75
2-1/2 mg green	NDC 0056-0176-70	NDC 0056-0176-90	NDC 0056-0176-75
3 mg tan	NDC 0056-0188-70	NDC 0056-0188-90	NDC 0056-0188-75
4 mg blue	NDC 0056-0168-70	NDC 0056-0168-90	NDC 0056-0168-75
5 mg peach	NDC 0056-0172-70	NDC 0056-0172-90	NDC 0056-0172-75
6 mg teal	NDC 0056-0189-70	NDC 0056-0189-90	NDC 0056-0189-75
7-1/2 mg yellow	NDC 0056-0173-70		NDC 0056-0173-75
10 mg white (Dye Free)	NDC 0056-0174-70		NDC 0056-0174-75

Protect from light. Store at controlled room temperature (59°–86°F, 15°–30°C). Dispense in a tight, light-resistant container as defined in the USP.

Hospital Unit-Dose Blister Packages are to be stored in carton until contents have been used.

Injection: Available for intravenous use only. Not recommended for intramuscular administration. Reconstitute with 2.7 mL of sterile Water for Injection to yield 2 mg/mL. Net contents 5.4 mg lyophilized powder. Maximum yield 2.5 mL.

5 mg vial (box of 6) NDC 0590-0324-35

Protect from light. Keep vial in box until used. Store at controlled room temperature (59°–86°F, 15°–30°C).

After reconstitution, store at controlled room temperature (59°–86°F, 15°–30°C) and use within 4 hours.

Do not refrigerate. Discard any unused solution.

REFERENCES

1. Poller, L.: Laboratory Control of Anticoagulant Therapy. Seminars in Thrombosis and Hemostasis, Vol. 12, No. 1, pp. 13–19, 1986.
2. Hirsh, J.: Is the Dose of Warfarin Prescribed by American Physicians Unnecessarily High? *Arch Int Med*, Vol. 147, pp. 769–771, 1987.
3. Cook, D.J., Guyatt, H.G., Laupacis, A., Sackett, D.L.: Rules of Evidence and Clinical Recommendations on the Use of Antithrombotic Agents. Chest ACCP Consensus Conference on Antithrombotic Therapy. *Chest*, Vol. 102(Suppl), pp. 305S–311S, 1992.
4. Hirsh, J., Dalen, J., Deykin, D., Poller, L.: Oral Anticoagulants Mechanism of Action, Clinical Effectiveness, and Optimal Therapeutic Range. Chest ACCP Consensus Conference on Antithrombotic Therapy. *Chest*, Vol. 102(Suppl), pp. 312S–326S, 1992.
5. Hirsh, J., M.D., F.C.C.P.: Hamilton Civic Hospitals Research Center, Hamilton, Ontario, Personal Communication.

Distributed by:
DuPont Pharma
Wilmington, Delaware 19880

6466-04/Rev. November, 1999

Shown in Product Identification Guide, page 311

INNOHEP® ℞

[in-ō-hep]

(tinzaparin sodium injection)
For Subcutaneous Use Only
Rx Only

SPINAL/EPIDURAL HEMATOMAS

When neuraxial anesthesia (epidural/spinal anesthesia) or spinal puncture is employed, patients anticoagulated or scheduled to be anticoagulated with low molecular weight heparins or heparinoids for prevention of thromboembolic complications are at risk of developing an epidural or spinal hematoma which can result in long-term or permanent paralysis.

The risk of these events is increased by the use of indwelling epidural catheters for administration of analgesia or by the concomitant use of drugs affecting hemostasis such as non-steroidal anti-inflammatory drugs (NSAIDs), platelet inhibitors, or other anticoagulants. The risk also appears to be increased by traumatic or repeated epidural or spinal puncture.

Patients should be frequently monitored for signs and symptoms of neurological impairment. If neurological compromise is noted, urgent treatment is necessary.

The physician should consider the potential benefit versus risk before neuraxial intervention in patients anticoagulated or to be anticoagulated for thromboprophylaxis (see also WARNINGS, Hemorrhage, and PRECAUTIONS, Drug Interactions).

DESCRIPTION

INNOHEP is a sterile solution, containing tinzaparin sodium, a low molecular weight heparin. It is available in a multiple dose 2 mL vial.

Each 2 mL vial contains 20,000 anti-Factor Xa IU (anti-Xa) of tinzaparin sodium per mL, for a total of 40,000 IU, and 3.1 mg/mL sodium metabisulfite as a stabilizer. The vial contains 10 mg/mL benzyl alcohol as a preservative. Sodium hydroxide may be added to achieve a pH range of 5.0 to 7.5.

Table 1
Composition of 20,000 anti-Xa IU/mL INNOHEP (tinzaparin sodium injection)

Component	Quantity per mL
Tinzaparin sodium	20,000 anti-Xa IU
Benzyl alcohol, USP	10 mg
Sodium metabisulfite, USP	3.106 mg[1]
Sodium hydroxide, USP	as necessary
Water for Injection, USP	q.s. to 1 mL

[1]Corresponding to 3.4 mg/mL sodium bisulfite

Tinzaparin sodium is the sodium salt of a low molecular weight heparin obtained by controlled enzymatic depoly-

Continued on next page

Innohep—Cont.

merization of heparin from porcine intestinal mucosa using heparinase from *Flavobacterium heparinum*. The majority of the components have a 2-O-sulpho-4-enepyranosuronic acid structure at the non-reducing end and a 2-N,6-O-disulpho-D-glucosamine structure at the reducing end of the chain.

Potency is determined by means of a biological assay and interpreted by the first International Low Molecular Weight Heparin Standard as units of anti-factor Xa (anti-Xa) activity per milligram. The mean tinzaparin sodium anti-factor Xa activity is approximately 100 IU per milligram. The average molecular weight ranges between 5,500 and 7,500 daltons. The molecular weight distribution is:

<2,000	Daltons	<10%
2,000 to 8,000	Daltons	60% to 72%
>8,000	Daltons	22% to 36%

Structural Formula:

n= 1 to 25, R = H or SO_3Na, R' = H or SO_3Na or $COCH_3$
R_2 = H and R_3 = COONa or R_2 = COONa and R_3= H

CLINICAL PHARMACOLOGY

Tinzaparin sodium is a low molecular weight heparin with antithrombotic properties. Tinzaparin sodium inhibits reactions that lead to the clotting of blood including the formation of fibrin clots, both *in vitro* and *in vivo*. It acts as a potent co-inhibitor of several activated coagulation factors, especially Factors Xa and IIa (thrombin). The primary inhibitory activity is mediated through the plasma protease inhibitor, antithrombin.

Bleeding time is usually unaffected by tinzaparin sodium. Activated partial thromboplastin time (aPTT) is prolonged by therapeutic doses of tinzaparin sodium used in the treatment of deep vein thrombosis (DVT). Prothrombin time (PT) may be slightly prolonged with tinzaparin sodium treatment but usually remains within the normal range. Neither aPTT nor PT can be used for therapeutic monitoring of tinzaparin sodium.

Neither unfractionated heparin nor tinzaparin sodium have intrinsic fibrinolytic activity; therefore, they do not lyse existing clots. Tinzaparin sodium induces release of tissue factor pathway inhibitor, which may contribute to the antithrombotic effect. Heparin is also known to have a variety of actions that are independent of its anticoagulant effects. These include interactions with endothelial cell growth factors, inhibition of smooth muscle cell proliferation, activation of lipoprotein lipase, suppression of aldosterone secretion, and induction of platelet aggregation.

Pharmacokinetics/Pharmacodynamics

Anti-Xa and anti-IIa activities are the primary biomarkers for assessing tinzaparin sodium exposure because plasma concentrations of low molecular weight heparins cannot be measured directly. Because of analytical assay limitations, anti-Xa activity is the more widely used biomarker. The measurements of anti-Xa and anti-IIa activities in plasma serve as surrogates for the concentrations of molecules which contain the high-affinity binding site for antithrombin (anti-Xa and anti-IIa activities). Monitoring patients based on anti-Xa activity is generally not advised. The data are provided in Figure 1 and Table 2 below.

Studies with tinzaparin sodium in healthy volunteers and patients have been conducted with both fixed- and weight-adjusted dose administration. Recommended therapy with tinzaparin sodium is based on weight-adjusted dosing (see **DOSAGE AND ADMINISTRATION**).

Figure 1
Mean and Standard Deviation of Anti-Xa Activity Following a Single SC Administration of 175 IU/kg and 4,500 IU* Tinzaparin Sodium to Healthy Volunteers

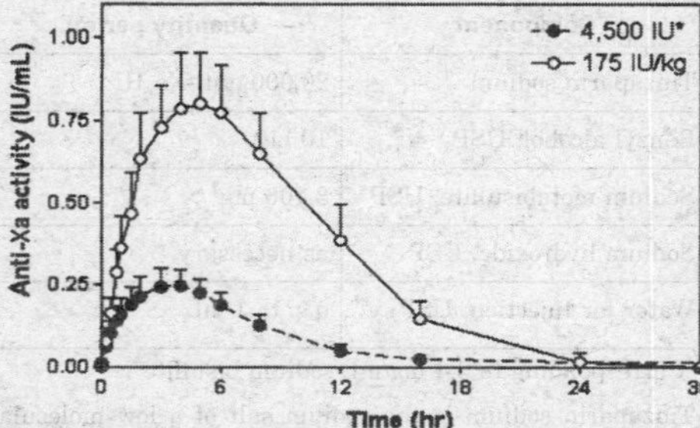

*Dosing based on fixed dose of 4,500 IU. Mean dose administered was 64.3 IU/kg.

Table 2
Summary of Pharmacokinetic Parameters (Mean and Standard Deviation) Based on Anti-Xa Activity Following a Single SC Administration of Tinzaparin Sodium to Healthy Volunteers

Parameter	Dose	
	4,500 IU*	175 IU/kg
C_{max} (IU/mL)	0.25 (0.05)	0.87 (0.24)
T_{max} (hr)	3.7 (0.9)	4.7 (1.1)
$AUC_{0-\infty}$ (IU*hr/mL)	2.0 (0.5)	9.6 (1.6)
Half-life (hr)	3.4 (1.7)	3.9 (0.9)

*Dosing based on fixed dose of 4,500 IU. Mean dose administered was 64.3 IU/kg.

Absorption

Plasma levels of anti-Xa activity increase in the first 2 to 3 hours following SC injection of tinzaparin sodium and reach a maximum within 4 to 5 hours. Maximum concentrations (C_{max}) of 0.25 and 0.87 IU/mL are achieved following a single SC fixed dose of 4,500 IU (approximately 64.3 IU/kg) and weight-adjusted dose of 175 IU/kg of tinzaparin sodium, respectively. Following a single SC injection of tinzaparin sodium, the mean anti-Xa to anti-IIa activity ratio, based on the area under the anti-Xa and anti-IIa time profiles, is 2.8 and is higher than that of unfractionated heparin (approximately 1.2). The absolute bioavailability (following 4,500 IU SC and intravenous [IV] administrations) is 86.7% based on anti-Xa activity. Based on the extent of absorption ($AUC_{0-\infty}$), a comparison of 4,500 IU and 12,250 IU doses indicates that increases in anti-Xa activity are greater than dose proportional relative to the increase in dose.

Distribution

The volume of distribution of tinzaparin sodium ranges from 3.1 L to 5.0 L. These values are similar in magnitude to blood volume, suggesting that the distribution of anti-Xa activity is limited to the central compartment.

Metabolism

Low molecular weight heparins are partially metabolized by desulphation and depolymerization.

Elimination

In healthy volunteers, the elimination half-life following SC administration of 4,500 IU or 175 IU/kg tinzaparin sodium is approximately 3–4 hours based on anti-Xa activity. Clearance following IV administration of 4,500 IU tinzaparin sodium is approximately 1.7 L/hr. The primary route of elimination is renal.

Special Populations

Population Pharmacokinetics

Anti-Xa concentrations from approximately 180 patients receiving SC tinzaparin sodium once daily (175 IU/kg body weight) as the treatment of proximal DVT and approximately 240 patients undergoing elective hip replacement surgery receiving SC tinzaparin sodium once daily (~65 IU/kg body weight) were analyzed by population pharmacokinetic methods. The results indicate that neither age nor gender significantly alter tinzaparin sodium clearance based on anti-Xa activity (see **PRECAUTIONS, General**). However, a reduction in tinzaparin sodium clearance was observed in patients with impaired renal function (reduced calculated creatinine clearance). Weight is also an important factor for the prediction of tinzaparin sodium clearance, consistent with the recommendation that INNOHEP therapy be based on weight-adjusted dosing (see **DOSAGE AND ADMINISTRATION**).

Renal Impairment

In 6 patients undergoing hemodialysis for chronic renal failure, the half-life of anti-Xa activity following a single IV dose of 75 IU/kg of tinzaparin sodium was prolonged compared to that for healthy volunteers (5.2 versus 1.6 hours). In patients being treated with tinzaparin sodium (175 IU/kg) for DVT, a population pharmacokinetic (PK) analysis determined that tinzaparin sodium clearance based on anti-Xa activity was related to creatinine clearance calculated by the Cockroft Gault equation. In this PK analysis, a reduction in tinzaparin sodium clearance in moderate (30–50 mL/min) and severe (<30 mL/min) renal impairment was observed. Patients with severe renal impairment exhibited a 24% reduction in tinzaparin sodium clearance relative to the remainder of the patients in the study. Patients with severe renal impairment should be dosed with caution (see **PRECAUTIONS**).

Hepatic Impairment

No prospective studies have assessed tinzaparin sodium pharmacokinetics or pharmacodynamics in hepatically-impaired patients. However, the hepatic route is not a major route of elimination of low molecular weight heparins (see **WARNINGS, Hemorrhage**).

Elderly

No prospective studies have assessed tinzaparin sodium pharmacokinetics or pharmacodynamics in healthy elderly volunteers. Since renal function is known to decline with age, elderly patients may show reduced elimination of tinzaparin sodium.

Obesity

No prospective studies have assessed tinzaparin sodium pharmacokinetics or pharmacodynamics in obese subjects. Based on the results of the population PK analysis, dosing should be based on body weight; body weight adjusted exposure is sufficient to explain tinzaparin sodium clearance differences observed in patients of different body mass index (BMI). Clinical trial experience is limited in patients with a BMI >40 kg/m².

CLINICAL STUDIES

Treatment of Acute Deep Vein Thrombosis (DVT) With or Without Pulmonary Embolism (PE)

In a randomized, multicenter, double-blind trial, INNOHEP (tinzaparin sodium injection) was compared to unfractionated heparin in 435 hospitalized patients with symptomatic, proximal DVT. Six percent of the enrolled patients had symptomatic pulmonary embolism confirmed by segmental or greater lung scan defect. The study patients ranged in age from 19 to 92 years (mean 61 ± 17 years), 55% were male, 88% were white and 8% black. Patients received either INNOHEP SC once daily according to body weight (175 IU/kg) and a placebo IV bolus followed by continuous placebo IV infusion, or unfractionated heparin as an initial IV bolus dose (5,000 IU) followed by continuous IV infusion of unfractionated heparin with the rate adjusted according to the aPTT (1.5 to 2.5 times control value) and a once daily SC placebo injection. Treatment continued for approximately 6 days, and both treatment groups also received oral warfarin sodium starting on Day 2 which continued to Day 90 with doses titrated to a target INR of 2.0 to 3.0.

The 90-day cumulative thromboembolic (TE) rate [recurrent DVT or PE] with INNOHEP was not significantly different than the rate with unfractionated heparin. The data are provided in Table 3.

Table 3
Efficacy of Once Daily INNOHEP in the Treatment of Acute Deep Vein Thrombosis

Indication Treatment of Acute DVT	Dosing Regimen INNOHEP[1] 175 IU/kg Once Daily SC n (%)	Heparin[1] 5,000 IU Bolus then aPTT Adjusted Continuous Infusion IV n (%)
Intent to Treat Population[2]	216 (100%)	219 (100%)
Patient Outcome at 90 Days		
Total TE[3] Events	6 (2.8%)[4]	15 (6.8%)[4]
DVTs	3 (1.4%)	9 (4.1%)
PEs	3 (1.4%)	6 (2.7%)

[1] Patients were also treated with warfarin sodium commencing within 24-48 hours of tinzaparin sodium or standard heparin therapy.
[2] All randomized patients who received at least one dose of active study drug
[3] TE = thromboembolic events (DVT and/or PE)
[4] The 95% Confidence Interval (CI) for the total TE event rate difference (4.0%) was 0.07%, 8.07%.

Mortality with INNOHEP was 4.6% (10 patients) and with heparin 9.6% (21 patients). The 95% confidence interval (CI) for the mortality difference was 0.16%, 9.76%.

In a multicenter, open-label, randomized clinical trial, INNOHEP was compared to unfractionated heparin as initial treatment for hospitalized patients with symptomatic PE not requiring thrombolytic therapy, embolectomy, or vena cava interruption. Patients were excluded if they carried an unusually high risk for thromboembolic and/or bleeding events or other complications. Of the 608 patients treated, 422 had documented DVT. Prior to determination of study eligibility and randomization, patients were allowed to receive unfractionated heparin; 78% of the patients received unfractionated heparin at therapeutic doses for up to 24 hours, and an additional 4% received heparin at therapeutic doses for greater than 24 hours. After randomization, INNOHEP was administered SC once daily, 175 IU/kg body weight; heparin as an initial IV bolus (50 IU/kg) followed by continuous IV infusion with the rate adjusted according to the aPTT (2 to 3 times control value). For both groups, treatment continued for approximately 8 days. All patients also received oral anticoagulant treatment starting in the first 3 days which continued to Day 90.

Thromboembolic events were infrequent for both treatment groups. No difference was observed between the two treatment groups for incidence of recurrence of thromboembolic events.

INDICATIONS AND USAGE

INNOHEP is indicated for the treatment of acute symptomatic deep vein thrombosis with or without pulmonary embolism when administered in conjunction with warfarin sodium. The safety and effectiveness of INNOHEP were established in hospitalized patients.

CONTRAINDICATIONS

INNOHEP is contraindicated in patients with active major bleeding, in patients with (or history of) heparin-induced thrombocytopenia, or in patients with hypersensitivity to tinzaparin sodium.

Patients with known hypersensitivity to heparin, sulfites, benzyl alcohol, or pork products should not be treated with INNOHEP.

WARNINGS

INNOHEP is not intended for intramuscular or intravenous administration.

INNOHEP cannot be used interchangeably (unit for unit) with heparin or other low molecular weight heparins as they differ in manufacturing process, molecular weight distribution, anti-Xa and anti-IIa activities, units, and dosage. Each of these medications has its own instructions for use.

INNOHEP should not be used in patients with a history of heparin-induced thrombocytopenia (see CONTRAINDICATIONS).

Hemorrhage: INNOHEP, like other anticoagulants, should be used with extreme caution in conditions with increased risk of hemorrhage, such as bacterial endocarditis; severe uncontrolled hypertension; congenital or acquired bleeding disorders including hepatic failure and amyloidosis; active ulcerative and angiodysplastic gastrointestinal disease; hemorrhagic stroke; shortly after brain, spinal or ophthalmological surgery, or in patients treated concomitantly with platelet inhibitors. Bleeding can occur at any site during therapy with INNOHEP. An unexplained fall in hematocrit, hemoglobin, or blood pressure should lead to serious consideration of a hemorrhagic event. If severe hemorrhage occurs, INNOHEP should be discontinued.

Spinal or epidural hematomas can occur with the associated use of low molecular weight heparins or heparinoids and spinal/epidural anesthesia or spinal puncture which can result in long-term or permanent paralysis. The risk of these events is higher with the use of post-operative indwelling epidural catheters or with the concomitant use of additional drugs affecting hemostasis such as NSAIDs (see boxed WARNING and PRECAUTIONS, Drug Interactions).

Thrombocytopenia: Thrombocytopenia can occur with the administration of INNOHEP.

In clinical studies, thrombocytopenia (platelet count <100,000/mm^3 if baseline value ≥150,000/mm^3, ≥50% decline if baseline <150,000/mm^3) was identified in 1% of patients given INNOHEP; severe thrombocytopenia (platelet count less than 50,000/mm^3) occurred in 0.13%.

Thrombocytopenia of any degree should be monitored closely. If the platelet count falls below 100,000/mm^3, INNOHEP should be discontinued. Cases of thrombocytopenia with disseminated thrombosis have also been observed in clinical practice with heparins, and low molecular weight heparins, including tinzaparin sodium. Some of these cases were complicated by organ infarction or limb ischemia.

Hypersensitivity: INNOHEP contains sodium metabisulfite, a sulfite that may cause allergic-type reactions including anaphylactic symptoms and life-threatening asthmatic episodes in certain susceptible people. The overall prevalence of sulfite sensitivity in the general population is unknown, but is probably low. Sulfite sensitivity is more frequent in asthmatic people than in non-asthmatic people.

Priapism: Priapism has been reported from post-marketing surveillance as a rare occurrence. In some cases surgical intervention was required.

Miscellaneous: INNOHEP multiple dose vial contains benzyl alcohol as a preservative. The administration of medications containing benzyl alcohol as a preservative to premature neonates has been associated with a fatal "Gasping Syndrome". Because benzyl alcohol may cross the placenta, INNOHEP preserved with benzyl alcohol should be used with caution in pregnant women only if clearly needed (see **PRECAUTIONS, Pregnancy**).

PRECAUTIONS

General: INNOHEP should not be mixed with other injections or infusions.

INNOHEP should be used with care in patients with a bleeding diathesis, uncontrolled arterial hypertension, or a history of recent gastrointestinal ulceration, diabetic retinopathy, and hemorrhage.

Consistent with expected age-related changes in renal function, elderly patients and patients with renal insufficiency may show reduced elimination of tinzaparin sodium. INNOHEP should be used with care in these patients (see **CLINICAL PHARMACOLOGY, *Special Populations***).

Laboratory Tests: Periodic complete blood counts including platelet count and hematocrit or hemoglobin, and stool tests for occult blood are recommended during treatment with INNOHEP. When administered at the recommended doses, routine anticoagulation tests such as prothrombin time (PT) and activated partial thromboplastin time (aPTT) are relatively insensitive measures of INNOHEP activity and, therefore, are unsuitable for monitoring.

Drug Interactions: Because of increased risk of bleeding, INNOHEP should be used with caution in patients receiving oral anticoagulants, platelet inhibitors (e.g., salicylates, dipyridamole, sulfinpyrazone, dextran, and NSAIDs including ketorolac tromethamine), and thrombolytics. If co-administration is essential, close clinical and laboratory monitoring of these patients is advised (see **PRECAUTIONS, Laboratory Tests**).

Laboratory Test Interactions

Elevation of Serum Transaminases: Asymptomatic reversible increases in aspartate (AST [SGOT]) and alanine (ALT [SGPT] aminotransferase levels have occurred in patients during treatment with INNOHEP (see **ADVERSE REACTIONS, Elevations of Serum Aminotransferases**). Similar increases in transaminase levels have also been observed in patients and volunteers treated with heparin and other low molecular weight heparins.

Since aminotransferase determinations are important in the differential diagnosis of myocardial infarction, liver disease, and pulmonary emboli, elevations that might be caused by drugs like INNOHEP should be interpreted with caution.

Carcinogenesis, Mutagenesis, Impairment of Fertility: No long-term studies in animals have been performed to evaluate the carcinogenic potential of tinzaparin sodium.

Tinzaparin sodium displayed no genotoxic potential in an *in vitro* bacterial cell mutation assay (AMES test), *in vitro* Chinese hamster ovary cell forward gene mutation test, *in vitro* human lymphocyte chromosomal aberration assay, and *in vivo* mouse micronucleus assay. Tinzaparin sodium at subcutaneous doses up to 1800 IU/kg/day in rats (about 2 times the maximum recommended human dose based on body surface area) was found to have no effect on fertility and reproductive performance.

Pregnancy

Teratogenic Effects: *Pregnancy Category B:* Teratogenicity studies have been performed in rats at subcutaneous doses up to 1800 IU/kg/day (about 2 times the maximum recommended human dose based on body surface area) and in rabbits at subcutaneous doses up to 1900 IU/kg/day (about 4 times the maximum recommended human dose based on body surface area) and have revealed no evidence of impaired fertility or harm to the fetus due to tinzaparin sodium. There are, however, no adequate and well-controlled studies in pregnant women. Because animal reproduction studies are not always predictive of human response, this drug should be used during pregnancy only if clearly needed.

There has been one case each reported of cleft palate, optic nerve hypoplasia, and trisomy 21 (Down's) syndrome in infants of women who received INNOHEP during pregnancy. A cause and effect relationship has not been established.

Non-teratogenic Effects: There have been four reports of fetal death/miscarriage in pregnant women receiving INNOHEP who had high risk pregnancies and/or a prior history of spontaneous abortion. Approximately 6% of pregnancies were complicated by fetal distress. There have been spontaneous reports of one case each of pulmonary hypoplasia or muscular hypotonia in infants of women receiving INNOHEP during pregnancy. A cause and effect relationship for the above observations has not been established.

Approximately 10% of pregnant women receiving INNOHEP experienced significant vaginal bleeding. A cause and effect relationship has not been established.

If INNOHEP is used during pregnancy, or if the patient becomes pregnant while taking this drug, the patient should be apprised of potential hazards to the fetus.

Cases of "Gasping Syndrome" have occurred in premature infants when large amounts of benzyl alcohol have been administered (99–404 mg/kg/day). The 2 mL vial of INNOHEP contains 20 mg of benzyl alcohol (10 mg of benzyl alcohol per mL) (see **WARNINGS, Miscellaneous**).

Nursing Mothers: In studies where tinzaparin sodium was administered subcutaneously to lactating rats, very low levels of tinzaparin sodium were found in breast milk. It is not know whether tinzaparin sodium is excreted in human milk. Because many drugs are excreted in human milk, caution should be exercised when INNOHEP is administered to nursing women.

Pediatric Use: Safety and effectiveness of tinzaparin sodium in pediatric patients have not been established.

Geriatric Use: In clinical studies for the treatment of DVT, 58% of patients were 65 or older and 29% were 75 and over. No significant overall differences in safety or effectiveness were observed between these subjects and younger subjects, and other reported clinical experience has not identified differences in responses between the elderly and younger patients, but greater sensitivity to tinzaparin sodium of some older individuals cannot be ruled out.

ADVERSE REACTIONS

Bleeding: Bleeding is the most common adverse event associated with INNOHEP (tinzaparin sodium injection); however, the incidence of major bleeding is low. In clinical trials, the definition of major bleeding included bleeding accompanied by ≥2 gram/dL decrease in hemoglobin, requiring transfusion of 2 or more units of blood products, or bleeding which was intracranial, retroperitoneal, or into a major prosthetic joint. The data are provided in Table 4.

Table 4
Major Bleeding Events[1] in Treatment of Acute Deep Vein Thrombosis With or Without Pulmonary Embolism

Indication	Treatment Group[1]	
Treatment of Acute DVT With or Without PE	INNOHEP (N=519) %	Heparin (N=524) %
Major Bleeding Events[2]	0.8[3]	2.7[3]

[1] INNOHEP 175 IU/kg once daily SC. Unfractionated heparin initial IV bolus of 5,000 IU followed by continuous IV infusion adjusted to an aPTT of 1.5 to 2.5 or initial IV bolus of 50 IU/kg followed by continuous IV infusion adjusted to an aPTT of 2.0 to 3.0. In all groups treatment continued for approximately 6 to 8 days, and all patients received oral anticoagulant treatment commencing in the first 2 to 3 days.

[2] Bleeding accompanied by ≥2 gram/dL decline in hemoglobin, requiring transfusion of 2 or more units of blood products, or bleeding which was intracranial, retroperitoneal, or into a major prosthetic joint

[3] The 95% CI on the difference in major bleeding event rates (1.9%) was 0.33%, 3.47%.

Thrombocytopenia: In clinical studies thrombocytopenia was identified in 1% of patients treated with INNOHEP. Severe thrombocytopenia (platelet count <50,000/mm^3) occurred in 0.13% (see **WARNINGS, Thrombocytopenia**).

Elevations of Serum Aminotransferases: Asymptomatic increases in aspartate (AST [SGOT]) and/or alanine (ALT [SGPT]) aminotransferase levels greater than 3 times the upper limit of normal of the laboratory reference range have been reported in up to 8.8% and 13% for AST and ALT, respectively, of patients receiving tinzaparin sodium for the treatment of DVT. Similar increases in aminotransferase levels have also been observed in patients and healthy volunteers treated with heparin and other low molecular weight heparins. Such elevations are reversible and are rarely associated with increases in bilirubin (see **PRECAUTIONS, Laboratory Tests**).

Local Reactions: Mild local irritation, pain, hematoma, and ecchymosis may follow SC injection of INNOHEP. Injection site hematoma has been reported in approximately 16% of INNOHEP treated patients.

Hypersensitivity: Anaphylactic/anaphylactoid reactions may occur in association with INNOHEP use (see CONTRAINDICATIONS and WARNINGS).

Adverse Events: Adverse events with INNOHEP or heparin reported at a frequency of ≥1% in clinical trials with patients undergoing treatment for proximal DVT with or without PE, are provided in Table 5.

Table 5
Adverse Events Occurring in ≥1% in Treatment of Acute Deep Vein Thrombosis With or Without Pulmonary Embolism Studies

Adverse Event	Treatment Group[1] INNOHEP (N=519) n (%)	Heparin (N=524) n (%)
Urinary Tract Infection	19 (3.7%)	18 (3.4%)
Pulmonary Embolism	12 (2.3%)	12 (2.3%)
Chest Pain	12 (2.3%)	8 (1.5%)
Epistaxis	10 (1.9%)	7 (1.3%)
Headache	9 (1.7%)	9 (1.7%)
Nausea	9 (1.7%)	10 (1.9%)
Hemorrhage NOS	8 (1.5%)	23 (4.4%)
Back Pain	8 (1.5%)	2 (0.4%)
Fever	8 (1.5%)	11 (2.1%)
Pain	8 (1.5%)	7 (1.3%)
Constipation	7 (1.3%)	9 (1.7%)
Rash	6 (1.2%)	8 (1.5%)
Dyspnea	6 (1.2%)	9 (1.7%)
Vomiting	5 (1.0%)	8 (1.5%)
Hematuria	5 (1.0%)	6 (1.1%)
Abdominal Pain	4 (0.8%)	6 (1.1%)
Diarrhea	3 (0.6%)	7 (1.3%)
Anemia	0	7 (1.3%)

NOS = not otherwise specified

[1] INNOHEP 175 IU/kg once daily SC. Unfractionated heparin initial IV bolus of 5,000 IU followed by continuous IV infusion adjusted to an aPTT of 1.5 to 2.5 or initial IV bolus of 50 IU/kg followed by continuous IV infusion adjusted to an aPTT of 2.0 to 3.0. In all groups treatment continued for approximately 6 to 8 days, and all patients received oral anticoagulant treatment commencing in the first 2 to 3 days.

Other Adverse Events in Completed or Ongoing Trials: Other adverse events reported at a frequency of ≥1% in 4,000 patients who received INNOHEP in completed or ongoing clinical trials are listed by body system:

Body as a Whole: injection site hematoma, reaction unclassified.

Cardiovascular Disorders, General: hypotension, hypertension.

Central and Peripheral Nervous System Disorders: dizziness.

Continued on next page

Innohep—Cont.

Gastrointestinal System Disorders: flatulence, gastrointestinal disorder (not otherwise specified), dyspepsia.
Heart Rate and Rhythm Disorders: tachycardia.
Myo-, Endo-, Pericardial and Valve Disorders: angina pectoris.
Platelet, Bleeding and Clotting Disorders: hematoma, thrombocytopenia.
Psychiatric Disorders: insomnia, confusion.
Red Blood Cell Disorders: anemia.
Resistance Mechanism Disorders: healing impaired, infection.
Respiratory System Disorders: pneumonia, respiratory disorder.
Skin and Appendages Disorders: rash erythematous, pruritus, bullous eruption, skin disorder.
Urinary System Disorders: urinary retention, dysuria.
Vascular (Extracardiac) Disorders: thrombophlebitis deep, thrombophlebitis leg deep.
Serious adverse events reported in clinical trials or from post-marketing experience are included in Table 6 and 7, respectively.

Table 6
Serious Adverse Events Associated with INNOHEP in Clinical Trials

Category	Serious Adverse Event
Bleeding-related	Anorectal bleeding Cerebral/intracranial bleeding Epistaxis Gastrointestinal hemorrhage Hemarthrosis Hematemesis Hematuria Hemorrhage NOS Injection site bleeding Melena Purpura Retroperitoneal/intra-abdominal bleeding Vaginal hemorrhage Wound hematoma
Organ dysfunction	Angina pectoris Cardiac arrhythmia Dependent edema Myocardial infarction/coronary thrombosis Thromboembolism
Fetal/neonatal	Congenital anomaly Fetal death Fetal distress
Cutaneous	Bullous eruption Erythematous rash Skin necrosis
Hematologic	Granulocytopenia Thrombocytopenia
Allergic reactions	Allergic reaction
Injection site reaction	Cellulitis
Neoplastic	Neoplasm

Table 7
Other Serious Adverse Events Associated with INNOHEP from Post-Marketing Surveillance

Category	Serious Adverse Event
Organ dysfunction	Cholestatic hepatitis Increase in hepatic enzymes Peripheral ischemia Priapism
Bleeding-related	Hemoptysis Ocular hemorrhage Rectal bleeding
Cutaneous reactions	Epidermal necrolysis Ischemic necrosis Urticaria
Hematologic	Agranulocytosis Pancytopenia Thrombocythemia
Injection site reactions	Abscess Necrosis
Allergic reactions	Angioedema
Fetal/neonatal	Neonatal hypotonia
General	Acute febrile reaction

Ongoing Safety Surveillance: When neuraxial anesthesia (epidural/spinal anesthesia) or spinal puncture is employed, patients anticoagulated or scheduled to be anticoagulated with low molecular weight heparins or heparinoids for prevention of thromboembolic complications are at risk of developing an epidural or spinal hematoma which can result in long-term or permanent paralysis (see **boxed WARNING**).
INNOHEP was first introduced in foreign markets in 1991. There have been no reports of spinal epidural hematoma in association with neuraxial anesthesia or spinal puncture with INNOHEP in clinical trials or in post-marketing surveillance.
There has been one case of spinal epidural hematoma with INNOHEP administered at a therapeutic dose in a patient who had not received neuraxial anesthesia or spinal puncture.

Table 8
INNOHEP Weight-based Dosing for Treatment of Deep Vein Thrombosis With or Without Symptomatic Pulmonary Embolism

Patient Body Weight in Pounds	DVT Treatment 175 IU/kg SC Once Daily 20,000 IU per mL: Dose (IU)	Amount (mL)	Patient Body Weight in Kilograms
68–80	6,000	0.3	31–36
81–94	7,000	0.35	37–42
95–107	8,000	0.4	43–48
108–118	9,000	0.45	49–53
119–131	10,000	0.5	54–59
132–144	11,000	0.55	60–65
145–155	12,000	0.6	66–70
156–168	13,000	0.65	71–76
169–182	14,000	0.7	77–82
183–195	15,000	0.75	83–88
196–206	16,000	0.8	89–93
207–219	17,000	0.85	94–99
220–232	18,000	0.9	100–105
233–243	19,000	0.95	106–110
244–256	20,000	1	111–116
257–270	21,000	1.05	117–122

OVERDOSAGE

Symptoms/Treatment: Accidental overdosage of INNOHEP may lead to bleeding complications. Nosebleeds, blood in urine or tarry stools may be noted as the first signs of bleeding. Easy bruising or petechial hemorrhages may precede frank bleeding. In case of minor bleeding, the patient should be monitored for signs of more severe bleeding. Of patients known to have received an overdose of tinzaparin sodium in clinical trials, defined as one or more doses >200 IU/kg for the treatment of DVT or >100 IU/kg for the prevention of DVT, approximately 16% experienced a bleeding complication.
Of spontaneous reports of probable overdosing with tinzaparin sodium, approximately 81% were accompanied by bleeding, usually hematoma. Most patients who have bleeding complications while receiving INNOHEP can be controlled by discontinuing INNOHEP, applying pressure to the site, if possible, and replacing volume and hemostatic blood elements (e.g., red blood cells, fresh frozen plasma, platelets) as required. In the event that this is ineffective, protamine sulfate can be administered.
In cases of serious bleeding or large overdose, protamine sulfate (1% solution) can be given by slow IV infusion at a dose of 1 mg protamine for every 100 anti-Xa IU of INNOHEP (tinzaparin sodium injection) given. A second infusion of 0.5 mg protamine sulfate per 100 anti-Xa IU of INNOHEP may be administered if the aPTT measured 2 to 4 hours after the first infusion remains prolonged. Even with the additional dose of protamine, the aPTT may remain more prolonged than would usually be found following administration of protamine to reverse unfractionated heparin. Protamine does not completely neutralize tinzaparin sodium anti-Xa activity (maximum about 60%).
Particular care should be taken to avoid overdosage with protamine sulfate. Administration of protamine sulfate can cause severe hypotensive and anaphylactoid reactions. Because fatal reactions have been reported with protamine sulfate, it should be given only when resuscitation facilities are readily available. For additional information consult the labeling of Protamine Sulfate Injection, USP, products.
Single subcutaneous doses of tinzaparin sodium at 22,000 and 7,700 IU/kg (about 10 and 7 times the maximum recommended human dose, respectively, based upon body surface area) were lethal to mice and rats, respectively. Symptoms of acute toxicity included hematoma formation and bleeding at the injection site, anemia, decreased motor activity, unsteady gait, piloerection, and ptosis.

DOSAGE AND ADMINISTRATION

All patients should be evaluated for bleeding disorders before administration of INNOHEP. Since coagulation parameters are unsuitable for monitoring INNOHEP activity, routine monitoring of coagulation parameters is not required (see **PRECAUTIONS, Laboratory Tests**).

Adult Dosage
The recommended dose of INNOHEP for the treatment of DVT with or without PE is 175 anti-Xa IU/kg of body weight, administered SC once daily for at least 6 days and until the patient is adequately anticoagulated with warfarin (INR at least 2.0 for two consecutive days). Warfarin sodium therapy should be initiated when appropriate (usually within 1–3 days of INNOHEP initiation).
As INNOHEP may theoretically affect the PT/INR, patients receiving both INNOHEP and warfarin should have blood for PT/INR determination drawn just prior to the next scheduled dose of INNOHEP.
Table 8 provides INNOHEP doses for the treatment of DVT with or without PE. It is necessary to calculate the appropriate INNOHEP dose for patient weights not displayed in Table 8.
An appropriately calibrated syringe should be used to assure withdrawal of the correct volume of drug from INNOHEP vials.
[See table 8 above]
To calculate the volume (mL) of an INNOHEP 175 anti-Xa IU per kg subcutaneous dose for treatment of deep vein thrombosis:

Patient weight (kg) × 0.00875 mL/kg = volume to be administered (mL) subcutaneously

Administration
INNOHEP is a clear, colorless to slightly yellow solution, and as with other parenteral drug products should be inspected visually for particulate matter and discoloration prior to administration.
INNOHEP is administered by SC injection. It must not be administered by intramuscular or intravenous injection.
Subcutaneous Injection Technique: Patients should be lying down (supine) or sitting and INNOHEP administered by deep SC injection. Administration should be alternated between the left and right anterolateral and left and right posterolateral abdominal wall. The injection site should be varied daily. The whole length of the needle should be introduced into a skin fold held between the thumb and forefinger; the skin fold should be held throughout the injection. To minimize bruising, do not rub the injection site after completion of the injection.

HOW SUPPLIED

INNOHEP is available in a multiple dose 2 mL vial in the following packages:

Box of 1	2 mL vial (20,000 anti-Xa IU per mL) NDC 0056-0342-08
Box of 10	2 mL vials (20,000 anti-Xa IU per mL) NDC 0056-0342-53

Store at 25°C (77°F); excursions permitted to 15°–30°C (59°–86°F) [See USP Controlled Room Temperature].
Keep out of the reach of children.

Manufactured for:
DuPont Pharma
Wilmington, DE 19880 USA
By:
Leo Pharmaceutical Products
Ballerup, Denmark
Innohep® is a registered trademark of Leo Pharmaceutical Products.

6536-00/July, 2000

LODOSYN® ℞
(CARBIDOPA)
TABLETS

When LODOSYN® (Carbidopa) is to be given to carbidopa-naive patients who are being treated with levodopa, the two drugs should be given at the same time, starting with no more than 20 to 25 percent of the previous daily dosage of levodopa when given without LODOSYN (Carbidopa). At least twelve hours should elapse between the last dose of levodopa and initiation of therapy with LODOSYN (Carbidopa) and levodopa. See the WARNINGS and DOSAGE AND ADMINISTRATION sections before initiating therapy.

DESCRIPTION

Carbidopa, an inhibitor of aromatic amino acid decarboxylation, is a white, crystalline compound, slightly soluble in water, with a molecular weight of 244.3. It is designated chemically as (−)-L-α-hydrazino-α-methyl-β-(3,4-dihydroxybenzene) propanoic acid monohydrate. Its empirical formula is $C_{10}H_{14}N_2O_4 \bullet H_2O$, and its structural formula is:

[Structural formula: OH; HO; CH_3; $-CH_2CCOOH \bullet H_2O$; $NHNH_2$]

LODOSYN (Carbidopa) tablets contain 25 mg of carbidopa. Inactive ingredients are cellulose, FD&C Yellow 6, magnesium stearate and starch.
Tablet content is expressed in terms of anhydrous carbidopa which has a molecular weight of 226.3.

CLINICAL PHARMACOLOGY

Parkinson's disease is a progressive, neurodegenerative disorder of the extrapyramidal nervous system affecting the mobility and control of the skeletal muscular system. Its characteristic features include resting tremor, rigidity, and bradykinetic movements. Symptomatic treatments, such as levodopa therapies, may permit the patient better mobility.

Mechanism of Action

Current evidence indicates that symptoms of Parkinson's disease are related to depletion of dopamine in the corpus striatum. Administration of dopamine is ineffective in the treatment of Parkinson's disease apparently because it does not cross the blood-brain barrier. However, levodopa, the metabolic precursor of dopamine, does cross the blood-brain barrier, and presumably is converted to dopamine in the brain. This is thought to be the mechanism whereby levodopa relieves symptoms of Parkinson's disease.

Pharmacodynamics

When levodopa is administered orally it is rapidly decarboxylated to dopamine in extracerebral tissues so that only a small portion of a given dose is transported unchanged to the central nervous system. For this reason, large doses of levodopa are required for adequate therapeutic effect and these may often be accompanied by nausea and other adverse reactions, some of which are attributable to dopamine formed in extracerebral tissues.

The incidence of levodopa-induced nausea and vomiting is less when LODOSYN is used with levodopa than when levodopa is used without LODOSYN. In many patients this reduction in nausea and vomiting will permit more rapid dosage titration.

Carbidopa inhibits decarboxylation of peripheral levodopa. Carbidopa has not been demonstrated to have any overt pharmacodynamic actions in the recommended doses. It does not appear to cross the blood-brain barrier readily and does not affect the metabolism of levodopa within the central nervous system at doses of carbidopa that are recommended for maximum effective inhibition of peripheral decarboxylation of levodopa.

Since its decarboxylase-inhibiting activity is limited primarily to extracerebral tissues, administration of carbidopa with levodopa makes more levodopa available for transport to the brain. However, since levodopa and carbidopa compete with certain amino acids for transport across the gut wall, the absorption of levodopa and carbidopa may be impaired in some patients on a high protein diet.

Pharmacokinetics

Carbidopa reduces the amount of levodopa required to produce a given response by about 75 percent and, when administered with levodopa, increases both plasma levels and the plasma half-life of levodopa, and decreases plasma and urinary dopamine and homovanillic acid.

In clinical pharmacologic studies, simultaneous administration of separate tablets of carbidopa and levodopa produced greater urinary excretion of levodopa in proportion to the excretion of dopamine when compared to the two drugs administered at separate times.

Supplemental pyridoxine (vitamin B_6) can be given to patients when they are receiving carbidopa and levodopa concomitantly or as SINEMET* CR (Carbidopa-Levodopa) Sustained-Release or SINEMET* (Carbidopa-Levodopa). Previous reports in the medical literature cautioned that high doses of vitamin B_6 should not be taken by patients on levodopa therapy alone because exogenously administered pyridoxine would enhance the metabolism of levodopa to dopamine. The introduction of carbidopa to levodopa therapy, which inhibits the peripheral decarboxylation of levodopa to dopamine, counteracts the metabolic-enhancing effect of pyridoxine.

Carbidopa is combined with levodopa in SINEMET (Carbidopa-Levodopa) and SINEMET CR (Carbidopa-Levodopa) Sustained-Release tablets. These combination tablets are available in three strengths for SINEMET: SINEMET 10-100 (Carbidopa-Levodopa), SINEMET 25-250 (Carbidopa-Levodopa) (1:10 ratio of carbidopa to levodopa) and SINEMET 25-100 (Carbidopa-Levodopa) (1:4 ratio of carbidopa to levodopa), and in two strengths for SINEMET CR: SINEMET CR 50-200 (Carbidopa-Levodopa) Sustained-Release and SINEMET CR 25-100 (Carbidopa-Levodopa) Sustained-Release (1:4 ratio of carbidopa to levodopa). Clinical trials show that these ratios of carbidopa and levodopa provide useful therapeutic effects in most patients.

INDICATIONS AND USAGE

LODOSYN is indicated for use with SINEMET (Carbidopa-Levodopa) or with levodopa in the treatment of the symptoms of idiopathic Parkinson's disease (paralysis agitans), postencephalitic parkinsonism, and symptomatic parkinsonism which may follow injury to the nervous system by carbon monoxide intoxication and/or manganese intoxication.

LODOSYN is for use with SINEMET (Carbidopa-Levodopa) in patients for whom the dosage of SINEMET (Carbidopa-Levodopa) provides less than adequate daily dosage (usually 70 mg daily) of carbidopa.

LODOSYN is for use with levodopa in the occasional patient whose dosage requirement of carbidopa and levodopa necessitates separate titration of each entity.

LODOSYN is used with SINEMET (Carbidopa-Levodopa) or with levodopa to permit the administration of lower doses of levodopa with reduced nausea and vomiting, more rapid dosage titration, and with a somewhat smoother response. However, patients with markedly irregular ("on-off") responses to levodopa have not been shown to benefit from the addition of carbidopa.

Since carbidopa prevents the reversal of levodopa effects caused by pyridoxine, supplemental pyridoxine (vitamin B_6), can be given to patients when they are receiving carbidopa and levodopa concomitantly or as SINEMET (Carbidopa-Levodopa).

Although the administration of LODOSYN permits control of parkinsonism and Parkinson's disease with much lower doses of levodopa, there is no conclusive evidence at present that this is beneficial other than in reducing nausea and vomiting, permitting more rapid titration, and providing a somewhat smoother response to levodopa.

Certain patients who responded poorly to levodopa alone have improved when carbidopa and levodopa were given concurrently. This was most likely due to decreased peripheral decarboxylation of levodopa rather than to a primary effect of carbidopa on the peripheral nervous system. Carbidopa has not been shown to enhance the intrinsic efficacy of levodopa.

In considering whether to give LODOSYN with SINEMET (Carbidopa-Levodopa) or with levodopa to patients who have nausea and/or vomiting, the physician should be aware that, while many patients may be expected to improve, some may not. Since one cannot predict which patients are likely to improve, this can only be determined by a trial of therapy. It should be further noted that in controlled trials comparing carbidopa and levodopa with levodopa alone, about half the patients with nausea and/or vomiting on levodopa alone improved spontaneously despite being retained on the same dose of levodopa during the controlled portion of the trial.

CONTRAINDICATIONS

LODOSYN is contraindicated in patients with known hypersensitivity to any component of this drug.

Nonselective monoamine oxidase (MAO) inhibitors are contraindicated for use with levodopa or carbidopa-levodopa combination products with or without LODOSYN. These inhibitors must be discontinued at least two weeks prior to initiating therapy with levodopa. SINEMET (Carbidopa-Levodopa), or levodopa may be administered concomitantly with the manufacturer's recommended dose of an MAO inhibitor with selectivity for MAO type B (e.g., selegiline HCl) (see PRECAUTIONS, *Drug Interactions*).

Levodopa or carbidopa-levodopa products, with or without LODOSYN, are contraindicated in patients with narrow-angle glaucoma.

Because levodopa or carbidopa-levodopa products, with or without LODOSYN, may activate a malignant melanoma, they should not be used in patients with suspicious, undiagnosed skin lesions or a history of melanoma.

WARNINGS

LODOSYN (Carbidopa) has no antiparkinsonian effect when given alone. It is indicated for use with SINEMET (Carbidopa-Levodopa) or levodopa. LODOSYN (Carbidopa) does not decrease adverse reactions due to central effects of levodopa.

When LODOSYN (Carbidopa) is to be given to carbidopa-naive patients who are being treated with levodopa alone, the two drugs should be given at the same time. At least twelve hours should elapse between the last dose of levodopa and initiation of therapy with LODOSYN (Carbidopa) and levodopa in combination. Start with no more than one-fifth (20%) to one-fourth (25%) of the previous daily dosage of levodopa when given without LODOSYN (Carbidopa). See the DOSAGE AND ADMINISTRATION section before initiation therapy.

As with levodopa, concomitant administration of LODOSYN and levodopa may cause involuntary movements and mental disturbances. These reactions are thought to be due to increased brain dopamine following administration of levodopa. All patients should be observed carefully for the development of depression with concomitant suicidal tendencies. Patients with past or current psychoses should be treated with caution. *Because* LODOSYN (Carbidopa) *permits more levodopa to reach the brain and, thus, more dopamine to be formed, dyskinesias may occur at lower levodopa dosages and sooner with concomitant use of* LODOSYN (Carbidopa) *and levodopa or carbidopa-levodopa combination products than with levodopa alone.* The occurrence of dyskinesias may require levodopa dosage reduction.

Levodopa, with or without LODOSYN, should be administered cautiously to patients with severe cardiovascular or pulmonary disease, bronchial asthma, renal, hepatic, or endocrine disease.

Care should be exercised in administering levodopa, with or without LODOSYN, to patients with a history of myocardial infarction who have residual atrial, nodal, or ventricular arrhythmias. In such patients, cardiac function should be monitored with particular care during the period of initial dosage adjustment, in a facility with provisions for intensive cardiac care.

As with levodopa alone there is a possibility of upper gastrointestinal hemorrhage in patients with a history of peptic ulcer.

Neuroleptic Malignant Syndrome (NMS): Sporadic cases of a symptom complex resembling NMS have been reported in association with dose reductions or withdrawal of certain antiparkinsonian agents such as levodopa, SINEMET (Carbidopa-Levodopa), or SINEMET CR (Carbidopa-Levodopa) Sustained-Release. Therefore, patients should be observed carefully when the dosage of levodopa is reduced abruptly or discontinued, especially if the patient is receiving neuroleptics.

NMS is an uncommon but life-threatening syndrome characterized by fever or hyperthermia. Neurological findings, including muscle rigidity, involuntary movements, altered consciousness, mental status changes; other disturbances such as autonomic dysfunction, tachycardia, tachypnea, sweating, hyper- or hypotension; laboratory findings, such as creatine phosphokinase elevation, leukocytosis, myoglobinuria, and increased serum myoglobin, have been reported.

The early diagnosis of this condition is important for the appropriate management of these patients. Considering NMS as a possible diagnosis and ruling out other acute illnesses (e.g., pneumonia, systemic infection, etc.) is essential. This may be especially complex if the clinical presentation includes both serious medical illness and untreated or inadequately treated extrapyramidal signs and symptoms (EPS). Other important considerations in the differential diagnosis include central anticholinergic toxicity, heat stroke, drug fever, and primary central nervous system (CNS) pathology.

The management of NMS should include: 1) intensive symptomatic treatment and medical monitoring and 2) treatment of any concomitant serious medical problems for which specific treatments are available. Dopamine agonists, such as bromocriptine, and muscle relaxants, such as dantrolene, are often used in the treatment of NMS; however, their effectiveness has not been demonstrated in controlled studies.

PRECAUTIONS

General

As with levodopa alone, periodic evaluations of hepatic, hematopoietic, cardiovascular, and renal function are recommended during extended concomitant therapy with LODOSYN and levodopa, or with LODOSYN and SINEMET (Carbidopa-Levodopa), or any combination of these drugs.

Patients with chronic wide-angle glaucoma may be treated cautiously with LODOSYN and levodopa or SINEMET, or any combination of these drugs, just as with levodopa alone, provided the intraocular pressure is well controlled and the patient is monitored carefully for changes in intraocular pressure during therapy.

Laboratory Tests

Abnormalities in laboratory tests may include elevations of liver function tests such as alkaline phosphatase, SGOT (AST), SGPT (ALT), lactic dehydrogenase, and bilirubin. Abnormalities in blood urea nitrogen and positive Coombs test have also been reported. Commonly, levels of blood urea nitrogen, creatinine, and uric acid are lower during concomitant administration of carbidopa and levodopa than with levodopa alone.

Levodopa and carbidopa-levodopa combination products may cause a false-positive reaction for urinary ketone bodies when a test tape is used for determination of ketonuria.

Continued on next page

Lodosyn—Cont.

This reaction will not be altered by boiling the urine specimen. False-negative tests may result with the use of glucose-oxidase methods of testing for glucosuria.

Drug Interactions

Caution should be exercised when the following drugs are administered concomitantly with LODOSYN (Carbidopa) given with levodopa or carbidopa-levodopa combination products.

Symptomatic postural hypotension has occurred when LODOSYN, given with levodopa or carbidopa-levodopa combination products, was added to the treatment of a patient receiving antihypertensive drugs. Therefore, when therapy with LODOSYN, given with or without levodopa or carbidopa-levodopa combination products, is started, dosage adjustment of the antihypertensive drug may be required.

For patients receiving monoamine oxidase inhibitors, see CONTRAINDICATIONS. Concomitant therapy with selegiline and carbidopa-levodopa may be associated with severe orthostatic hypotension not attributable to carbidopa-levodopa alone (see CONTRAINDICATIONS.

There have been rare reports of adverse reactions, including hypertension and dyskinesia, resulting from the concomitant use of tricyclic antidepressants and carbidopa-levodopa preparations.

Dopamine D_2 receptor antagonists (e.g., phenothiazines, butyrophenones, risperidone) and isoniazid may reduce the therapeutic effects of levodopa. In addition, the beneficial effects of levodopa in Parkinson's disease have been reported to be reversed by phenytoin and papaverine. Patients taking these drugs with LODOSYN and levodopa or carbidopa-levodopa combination products should be carefully observed for loss of therapeutic response.

Iron salts may reduce the bioavailability of carbidopa and levodopa.The clinical relevance is unclear.

Although metoclopramide may increase the bioavailability of levodopa by increasing gastric emptying, metoclopramide may also adversely affect disease control by its dopamine receptor antagonist properties.

Carcinogenesis, Mutagenesis, Impairment of Fertility

Carcinogenesis

There were no significant differences between treated and control rats with respect to mortality or neoplasia in a 96-week study of carbidopa at oral doses of 25, 45, or 135 mg/kg/day.

Combination of carbidopa and levodopa (10–20, 10–50, 10–100 mg/kg/day) were given orally to rats for 106 weeks. No effect on mortality or incidence and type of neoplasia was seen when compared to concurrent controls.

Mutagenesis

Mutagenicity studies have not been performed with either carbidopa or the combination of carbidopa and levodopa.

Fertility

Carbidopa had no effect on the mating performance, fertility, or survival of the young when administered orally to rats at doses of 30, 60, or 120 mg/kg/day. The highest dose caused a moderate decrease in body weight gain in males. The administration of carbidopa-levodopa at dose levels of 10–20, 10–50, or 10–100 mg/kg/day did not adversely affect the fertility of male or female rats, their reproductive performance, or the growth and survival of the young.

Pregnancy

Pregnancy Category C: There are no adequate and well-controlled studies with LODOSYN in pregnant women. It has been reported from individual cases that levodopa crosses the human placental barrier, enters the fetus, and is metabolized. Carbidopa concentrations in fetal tissue appeared to be minimal. LODOSYN should be used during pregnancy only if the potential benefit justifies the potential risk to the fetus.

Carbidopa, at doses as high as 120 mg/kg/day, was without teratogenic effects in the mouse or rabbit. In the rabbit, but not in the mouse, carbidopa-levodopa produced visceral anomalies, similar to those seen with levodopa alone, at approximately 7 times the maximum recommended human dose. The teratogenic effect of levodopa in rabbits was unchanges by the concomitant administration of carbidopa.

Nursing Mothers

It is not known whether carbidopa or levodopa is excreted in human milk. Because many drugs are excreted in human milk, and because of their potential for serious adverse reactions in nursing infants, a decision should be made whether to discontinue nursing or to discontinue the drug, taking into account the importance of the drug to the nursing woman.

Pediatric Use

Safety and effectiveness in pediatric patients have not been established, and use of the drug in patients below the age of 18 is not recommended.

ADVERSE REACTIONS

Carbidopa has not been demonstrated to have any overt pharmacodynamic actions in the recommended doses. The only adverse reactions that have been observed have been with concomitant use of carbidopa with other drugs such as levodopa, and with carbidopa-levodopa combination products.

When LODOSYN is administered concomitantly with levodopa or carbidopa-levodopa combination products, the most common adverse reactions have included dyskinesias such as choreiform, dystonic, and other involuntary movements, and nausea. Other adverse reactions reported with LODOSYN when administered concomitantly with levodopa alone or carbidopa-levodopa combination products were psychotic episodes including delusions, hallucinations, and paranoid ideation, depression with or without development of suicidal tendencies, and dementia. Convulsions also have occurred; however, a causal relationship with concomitant use of LODOSYN and levodopa has not been established.

The following other adverse reactions have been reported with levodopa and carbidopa-levodopa combination products. These same adverse reactions may also occur when LODOSYN is administered with these products.

Body as a Whole: abdominal pain and distress, asthenia, chest pain, fatigue.

Cardiovascular: cardiac irregularities, hypertension, myocardial infarction, hypotension including orthostatic hypotension, palpitation, phlebitis, syncope.

Gastrointestinal: anorexia, bruxism, burning sensation of the tongue, constipation, dark saliva, development of duodenal ulcer, diarrhea, dry mouth, dyspepsia, dysphagia, flatulence, gastrointestinal bleeding, gastrointestinal pain, heartburn, hiccups, sialorrhea, taste alterations, vomiting.

Hematologic: hemolytic and non-hemolytic anemia, leukopenia, thrombocytopenia, agranulocytosis.

Hypersensitivity: angioedema, urticaria, pruritus, Henoch-Schonlein purpura, bullous lesions (including pemphigus-like reactions).

Metabolic: edema, weight gain, weight loss.

Musculoskeltetal: back pain, leg pain, muscle cramps, shoulder pain.

Nervous System/Psychiatric: agitation, anxiety, ataxia, blepharospasm (which may be taken as an early sign of excess dosage; consideration of dosage reduction may be made at this time); bradykinetic episodes ("on-off" phenomenon), confusion, decreased mental acuity, disorientation, euphoria, dizziness, dream abnormalities including nightmares, extrapyramidal disorder, falling, gait abnormalities, headache, increased tremor, insomnia, memory impairment, muscle twitching, nervousness, numbness, paresthesia, peripheral neuropathy, somnolence, trismus, activation of latent Horner's syndrome, increased libido.

Respiratory: upper respiratory infection, dyspnea, pharyngeal pain, cough.

Skin: flushing, increased sweating, malignant melanoma (see also CONTRAINDICATIONS), rash, alopecia, dark sweat.

Special Senses: oculogyric crises, diplopia, blurred vision, dilated pupils.

Urogenital: dark urine, priapism, urinary frequency, urinary incontinence, urinary retention, urinary tract infection.

Laboratory Tests: abnormalities in alkaline phosphatase, SGOT (AST), SGPT (ALT), lactic dehydrogenase, bilirubin, blood urea nitrogen (BUN), Coombs test; elevated serum glucose; decreased hemoglobin and hematocrit; decreased white blood cell count and serum potassium; increased serum creatinine and uric acid; white blood cells, bacteria and blood in the urine; protein and glucose in the urine.

Miscellaneous: bizarre breathing patterns, faintness, hoarseness, hot flashes, malaise, neuroleptic malignant syndrome, sense of stimulation.

OVERDOSAGE

No reports of overdose with LODOSYN have been received. Management of overdosage with carbidopa is the same as that with levodopa or carbidopa-levodopa preparations.

In the event of overdosage, general supportive measures should be employed, along with immediate gastric lavage. Intravenous fluids should be administered judiciously, and an adequate airway maintained. Electrocardiographic monitoring should be instituted and the patient carefully observed for the development or arrhythmias; if required, appropriate antiarrhythmic therapy should be given. The possibility that the patient may have taken other drugs as well as LODOSYN should be taken into consideration. To date, no experience has been reported with dialysis; hence, its value in overdosage is not known. Pyridoxine is not effective in reversing the actions of LODOSYN.

Based on studies in which high doses of levodopa and/or carbidopa were administered, a significant proportion of rats and mice given single oral doses of levodopa of approximately 1500–2000 mg/kg are expected to die. A significant proportion of infant rats of both sexes are expected to die at a dose of 800 mg/kg. A significant proportion of rats are expected to die after treatment with similar doses of carbidopa. The addition of carbidopa in a 1:10 ratio with levodopa increases the dose at which a significant proportion of mice are expected to die to 3360 mg/kg.

DOSAGE AND ADMINISTRATION

Whether given with SINEMET (Carbidopa-Levodopa) or with levodopa, the optimal daily dosage of LODOSYN must be determined by careful titration. Most patients respond to a 1:10 proportion of carbidopa and levodopa, provided the daily dosage of carbidopa is 70 mg or more a day. The maximum daily dosage of carbidopa should not exceed 200 mg, since clinical experience with larger dosages is limited. If the patient is taking SINEMET (Carbidopa-Levodopa), the amount of carbidopa in SINEMET (Carbidopa-Levodopa) should be considered when calculating the total amount of LODOSYN to be administered each day.

Patients Receiving SINEMET (Carbidopa-Levodopa) *Who Require Additional Carbidopa*

Some patients taking SINEMET (Carbidopa-Levodopa) may not have adequate reduction in nausea and vomiting when the dosage of carbidopa is less than 70 mg a day, and the doage of levodopa is less than 700 mg a day. When these patients are taking SINEMET 10-100** (Carbidopa-Levodopa), 25 mg of LODOSYN may be given with the first dose of SINEMET (Carbidopa-Levodopa) each day. Additional doses of 12.5 mg or 25 mg may be given during the day with each dose of SINEMET (Carbidopa-Levodopa). When patients are taking SINEMET 25–250*** (Carbidopa-Levodopa) or SINEMET 25–100† (Carbidopa-Levodopa), 25 mg of LODOSYN may be given with any dose of SINEMET (Carbidopa-Levodopa) as required for optimum therapeutic response. The maximum daily dosage of carbidopa, given as LODOSYN and as SINEMET (Carbidopa-Levodopa), should not exceed 200 mg.

Patients Requiring Individual Titration of Carbidopa and Levodopa Dosage

Although SINEMET (Carbidopa-Levodopa) is the preferred method of carbidopa and levodopa administration, there may be an occasional patient who requires individually titrated doses of these two drugs. **In these patients, LODOSYN (Carbidopa) should be initiated at a dosage of 25 mg three or four times a day. The two drugs should be given at the same time, starting with no more than one-fifth (20%) to one-fourth (25%) of the previous or recommended daily dosage of levodopa when given without LODOSYN (Carbidopa). In patients already receiving levodopa therapy, at least twelve hours should elapse between the last dose of levodopa and initiation of therapy with LODOSYN (Carbidopa) and levodopa. A convenient way to initiate therapy in these patients is in the morning following a night when the patient has not taken levodopa for at least twelve hours.** Physicians who prescribe separate doses of LODOSYN and levodopa should be thoroughly familiar with the directions for use of each drug.

Dosage Adjustment

Dosage of LODOSYN may be adjusted by adding or omitting one-half or one tablet a day. Because both therapeutic and adverse responses occur more rapidly with combined therapy than when only levodopa is given, patients should be monitored closely during the dose adjustment period. Specifically, involuntary movements will occur more rapidly when LODOSYN and levodopa are given concomitantly than when levodopa is given without LODOSYN. The occurrence of involuntary movements may require dosage reduction. Blepharospasm may be a useful early sign of excess dosage in some patients.

Current evidence indicates other standard antiparkinsonian drugs may be continued while carbidopa and levodopa are being administered. However, the dosage of such other standard antiparkinsonian drugs may require adjustment.

Interruption of Therapy

Sporadic cases of a symptom complex resembling the Neuroleptic Malignant Syndrome (NMS) have been associated with dose reductions and withdrawal of SINEMET (Carbidopa-Levodopa) or SINEMET CR (Carbidopa-Levodopa) Sustained-Release. Patients should be observed carfully if abrupt reduction or discontinuation of SINEMET (Carbidopa-Levodopa) or SINEMET CR (Carbidopa-Levodopa) Sustained-Release is required, especially if the patient is receiving neuroleptics. (See WARNINGS.)

If general anesthesia is required, therapy may be continued as long as the patient is permitted to take fluids and medication by mouth. When therapy is interrupted temporarily, the patient should be observed for symptoms resembling NMS, and the usual daily dosage may be resumed as soon as the patient is able to take medication orally.

HOW SUPPLIED

Tablets LODOSYN, 25 mg, are orange, round, compressed tablets, that are scored and coded 511 on one side and LODOSYN on the other.

They are supplied as follows:

NDC 0056-0511-68 bottles of 100.

** SINEMET 10-100 (Carbidopa-Levodopa) contains 10 mg of carbidopa and 100 mg of levodopa.

*** SINEMET 25-250 (Carbidopa-Levodopa) contains 25 mg of carbidopa and 250 mg of levodopa.

† SINEMET 25-100 (Carbidopa-Levodopa) contains 25 mg of carbidopa and 100 mg of levodopa.

Manufactured by:
MERCK & CO., INC.
West Point, PA 19486, USA
For:
DuPont Pharma
Wilmington, Delaware 19880
Issued June 1999

6298-04

REVIA® ℞

(naltrexone hydrochloride tablets)
Rx only

DESCRIPTION:

REVIA (naltrexone hydrochloride), an opioid antagonist, is a synthetic congener of oxymorphone with no opioid agonist properties. Naltrexone differs in structure from oxymorphone in that the methyl group on the nitrogen atom is replaced by a cyclopropylmethyl group. REVIA is also related to the potent opioid antagonist, naloxone, or n-allylnoroxymorphone.

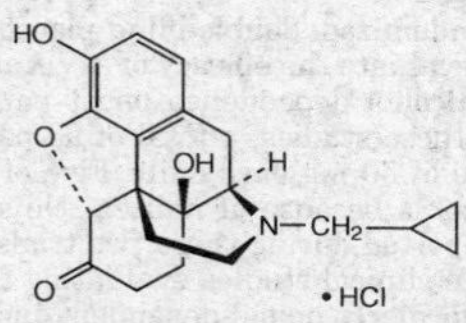

naltrexone hydrochloride

REVIA is a white, crystalline compound. The hydrochloride salt is soluble in water to the extent of about 100 mg/mL. REVIA is available in scored film-coated tablets containing 50 mg of naltrexone hydrochloride.
REVIA Tablets also contain: lactose, microcrystalline cellulose, crospovidone, colloidal silicon dioxide, magnesium stearate, hydroxypropyl methylcellulose, titanium dioxide, polyethylene glycol, polysorbate 80, yellow iron oxide and red iron oxide.

CLINICAL PHARMACOLOGY:

Pharmacodynamic Actions: REVIA is a pure opioid antagonist. It markedly attenuates or completely blocks, reversibly, the subjective effects of intravenously administered opioids.
When co-administered with morphine, on a chronic basis, REVIA blocks the physical dependence to morphine, heroin and other opioids.
REVIA has few, if any, intrinsic actions besides its opioid blocking properties. However, it does produce some pupillary constriction, by an unknown mechanism.
The administration of REVIA is not associated with the development of tolerance or dependence. In subjects physically dependent on opioids, REVIA will precipitate withdrawal symptomatology.
Clinical studies indicate that 50 mg of REVIA will block the pharmacologic effects of 25 mg of intravenously administered heroin for periods as long as 24 hours. Other data suggest that doubling the dose of REVIA provides blockade for 48 hours, and tripling the dose of REVIA provides blockade for about 72 hours.
REVIA blocks the effects of opioids by competitive binding (i.e., analogous to competitive inhibition of enzymes) at opioid receptors. This makes the blockade produced potentially surmountable, but overcoming full naltrexone blockade by administration of very high doses of opiates has resulted in excessive symptoms of histamine release in experimental subjects.
The mechanism of action of REVIA in alcoholism is not understood; however, involvement of the endogenous opioid system is suggested by preclinical data. REVIA, an opioid receptor antagonist, competitively binds to such receptors and may block the effects of endogenous opioids. Opioid antagonists have been shown to reduce alcohol consumption by animals, and REVIA has been shown to reduce alcohol consumption in clinical studies.
REVIA is not aversive therapy and does not cause a disulfiram-like reaction either as a result of opiate use or ethanol ingestion.

Pharmacokinetics:
REVIA is a pure opioid receptor antagonist. Although well absorbed orally, naltrexone is subject to significant first pass metabolism with oral bioavailability estimates ranging from 5 to 40%. The activity of naltrexone is believed to be due to both parent and the 6-β-naltrexol metabolite. Both parent drug and metabolites are excreted primarily by the kidney (53% to 79% of the dose), however, urinary excretion of unchanged naltrexone accounts for less than 2% of an oral dose and fecal excretion is a minor elimination pathway. The mean elimination half-life (T-1/2) values for naltrexone and 6-β-naltrexol are 4 hours and 13 hours, respectively. Naltrexone and 6-β-naltrexol are dose proportional in terms of AUC and C_{max} over the range of 50 to 200 mg and do not accumulate after 100 mg daily doses.

Absorption:
Following oral administration, naltrexone undergoes rapid and nearly complete absorption with approximately 96% of the dose absorbed from the gastrointestinal tract. Peak plasma levels of both naltrexone and 6-β-naltrexol occur within one hour of dosing.

Distribution:
The volume of distribution for naltrexone following intravenous administration is estimated to be 1350 liters. *In vitro* tests with human plasma show naltrexone to be 21% bound to plasma proteins over the therapeutic dose range.

Metabolism:
The systemic clearance (after intravenous administration) of naltrexone is ~3.5 L/min, which exceeds liver blood flow (~1.2 L/min). This suggests both that naltrexone is a highly extracted drug (>98% metabolized) and that extra-hepatic sites of drug metabolism exist. The major metabolite of naltrexone is 6-β-naltrexol. Two other minor metabolites are 2-hydroxy-3-methoxy-6-β-naltrexol and 2-hydroxy-3-methyl-naltrexone. Naltrexone and its metabolites are also conjugated to form additional metabolic products.

Elimination:
The renal clearance for naltrexone ranges from 30-127 mL/min and suggests that renal elimination is primarily by glomerular filtration. In comparison, the renal clearance for 6-β-naltrexol ranges from 230-369 mL/min, suggesting an additional renal tubular secretory mechanism. The urinary excretion of unchanged naltrexone accounts for less than 2% of an oral dose; urinary excretion of unchanged and conjugated 6-β-naltrexol accounts for 43% of an oral dose. The pharmacokinetic profile of naltrexone suggests that naltrexone and its metabolites may undergo enterohepatic recycling.

Hepatic and Renal Impairment:
Naltrexone appears to have extra-hepatic sites of drug metabolism and its major metabolite undergoes active tubular secretion (see **Metabolism** above). Adequate studies of naltrexone in patients with severe hepatic or renal impairment have not been conducted (see **PRECAUTIONS: Special Risk Patients**).

Clinical Trials:
Alcoholism:
The efficacy of REVIA as an aid to the treatment of alcoholism was tested in placebo-controlled, outpatient, double blind trials. These studies used a dose of REVIA 50 mg once daily for 12 weeks as an adjunct to social and psychotherapeutic methods when given under conditions that enhanced patient compliance. Patients with psychosis, dementia, and secondary psychiatric diagnoses were excluded from these studies.
In one of these studies, 104 alcohol-dependent patients were randomized to receive either REVIA 50 mg once daily or placebo. In this study, REVIA proved superior to placebo in measures of drinking including abstention rates (51% vs. 23%), number of drinking days, and relapse (31% vs. 60%). In a second study with 82 alcohol-dependent patients, the group of patients receiving REVIA were shown to have lower relapse rates (21% vs. 41%), less alcohol craving, and fewer drinking days compared with patients who received placebo, but these results depended on the specific analysis used.
The clinical use of REVIA as adjunctive pharmacotherapy for the treatment of alcoholism was also evaluated in a multicenter safety study. This study of 865 individuals with alcoholism included patients with comorbid psychiatric conditions, concomitant medications, polysubstance abuse and HIV disease. Results of this study demonstrated that the side effect profile of REVIA appears to be similar in both alcoholic and opioid dependent populations, and that serious side effects are uncommon.
In the clinical studies, treatment with REVIA supported abstinence, prevented relapse and decreased alcohol consumption. In the uncontrolled study, the patterns of abstinence and relapse were similar to those observed in the controlled studies. REVIA was not uniformly helpful to all patients, and the expected effect of the drug is a modest improvement in the outcome of conventional treatment.

Treatment of Opioid Addiction:
REVIA has been shown to produce complete blockade of the euphoric effects of opioids in both volunteer and addict populations. When administered by means that enforce compliance, it will produce an effective opioid blockade, but has not been shown to affect the use of cocaine or other non-opioid drugs of abuse.
There are no data that demonstrate an unequivocally beneficial effect of REVIA on rates of recidivism among detoxified, formerly opioid-dependent individuals who self-administer the drug. The failure of the drug in this setting appears to be due to poor medication compliance.
The drug is reported to be of greatest use in good prognosis opioid addicts who take the drug as part of a comprehensive occupational rehabilitative program, behavioral contract, or other compliance-enhancing protocol. REVIA, unlike methadone or LAAM (levo-alpha-acetylmethadol), does not reinforce medication compliance and is expected to have a therapeutic effect only when given under external conditions that support continued use of the medication.

Individualization of Dosage:
DO NOT ATTEMPT TREATMENT WITH REVIA UNLESS, IN THE MEDICAL JUDGEMENT OF THE PRESCRIBING PHYSICIAN, THERE IS NO REASONABLE POSSIBILITY OF OPIOID USE WITHIN THE PAST 7-10 DAYS. IF THERE IS ANY QUESTION OF OCCULT OPIOID DEPENDENCE, PERFORM A NALOXONE CHALLENGE TEST.

Treatment of Alcoholism:
The placebo-controlled studies that demonstrated the efficacy of REVIA as an adjunctive treatment of alcoholism used a dose regimen of REVIA 50 mg once daily for up to 12 weeks. Other dose regimens or durations of therapy were not studied in these trials.
Physicians are advised that 5-15% of patients taking REVIA for alcoholism will complain of non-specific side effects, chiefly gastrointestinal upset. Prescribing physicians have tried using an initial 25 mg dose, splitting the daily dose, and adjusting the time of dosing with limited success. No dose or pattern of dosing has been shown to be more effective than any other in reducing these complaints for all patients.

Treatment of Opioid Dependence:
Once the patient has been started on REVIA, 50 mg once a day will produce adequate clinical blockade of the actions of parenterally administered opioids. As with many non-agonist treatments for addiction, REVIA is of proven value only when given as part of a comprehensive plan of management that includes some measure to ensure the patient takes the medication.
A flexible approach to a dosing regimen may be employed to enhance compliance. Thus, patients may receive 50 mg of REVIA (naltrexone hydrochloride) every weekday with a 100 mg dose on Saturday or patients may receive 100 mg every other day, or 150 mg every third day. Several of the clinical studies reported in the literature have employed the following dosing regimen: 100 mg on Monday, 100 mg on Wednesday, and 150 mg on Friday. This dosing schedule appeared to be acceptable to many REVIA patients successfully maintaining their opioid-free state.
Experience with the supervised administration of a number of potentially hepatotoxic agents suggests that supervised administration and single doses of REVIA higher than 50 mg may have an associated increased risk of hepatocellular injury, even though three-times a week dosing has been well tolerated in the addict population and in initial clinical trials in alcoholism. Clinics using this approach should balance the possible risks against the probable benefits and may wish to maintain a higher index of suspicion for drug-associated hepatitis and ensure patients are advised of the need to report non-specific abdominal complaints (see **Information for Patients**).

INDICATIONS AND USAGE:

REVIA is indicated:
In the treatment of alcohol dependence and for the blockade of the effects of exogenously administered opioids.
REVIA has not been shown to provide any therapeutic benefit except as part of an appropriate plan of management for the addictions.

CONTRAINDICATIONS:

REVIA is contraindicated in:
1) Patients receiving opioid analgesics.
2) Patients currently dependent on opioids.
3) Patients in acute opioid withdrawal (see **WARNINGS**).
4) Any individual who has failed the naloxone challenge test or who has a positive urine screen for opioids.
5) Any individual with a history of sensitivity to REVIA or any other components of this product. It is not known if there is any cross-sensitivity with naloxone or the phenanthrene containing opioids.
6) Any individual with acute hepatitis or liver failure.

WARNINGS:

Hepatotoxicity:

REVIA has the capacity to cause hepatocellular injury when given in excessive doses.
REVIA is contraindicated in acute hepatitis or liver failure, and its use in patients with active liver disease must be carefully considered in light of its hepatotoxic effects.
The margin of separation between the apparently safe dose of REVIA and the dose causing hepatic injury appears to be only five-fold or less. REVIA does not appear to be a hepatotoxin at the recommended doses.
Patients should be warned of the risk of hepatic injury and advised to stop the use of REVIA and seek medical attention if they experience symptoms of acute hepatitis.

Evidence of the hepatotoxic potential of REVIA is derived primarily from a placebo controlled study in which REVIA was administered to obese subjects at a dose approximately five-fold that recommended for the blockade of opiate receptors (300 mg per day). In that study, 5 of 26 REVIA recipients developed elevations of serum transaminases (i.e., peak ALT values ranging from a low of 121 to a high of 532; or 3 to 19 times their baseline values) after three to eight weeks of treatment. Although the patients involved were generally clinically asymptomatic and the transaminase levels of all patients on whom follow-up was obtained returned to (or toward) baseline values in a matter of weeks, the lack of any transaminase elevations of similar magnitude in any of the 24 placebo patients in the same study is persuasive evidence that REVIA is a direct (i.e., not idiosyncratic) hepatotoxin.
This conclusion is also supported by evidence from other placebo controlled studies in which exposure to REVIA at doses above the amount recommended for the treatment of alcoholism or opiate blockade (50 mg/day) consistently produced more numerous and more significant elevations of serum transaminases than did placebo. Transaminase elevations in 3 of 9 patients with Alzheimer's Disease who received REVIA (at doses up to 300 mg/day) for 5 to 8 weeks in an open clinical trial have been reported.
Although no cases of hepatic failure due to REVIA administration have ever been reported, physicians are advised to consider this as a possible risk of treatment and to use the same care in prescribing REVIA as they would other drugs with the potential for causing hepatic injury.

Unintended Precipitation of Abstinence:
To prevent occurrence of an acute abstinence syndrome, or exacerbation of a pre-existing subclinical abstinence syndrome, patients must be opioid-free for a minimum of 7-10 days before starting REVIA. Since the absence of an opioid drug in the urine is often not sufficient proof that a patient is opioid-free, a naloxone challenge should be employed if the prescribing physician feels there is a risk of precipitating a withdrawal reaction following administration of REVIA. The naloxone challenge test is described in the DOSAGE AND ADMINISTRATION section.

Attempt to Overcome Blockade:
While REVIA is a potent antagonist with a prolonged pharmacologic effect (24 to 72 hours), the blockade produced by REVIA is surmountable. This is useful in patients who may

Continued on next page

ReVia—Cont.

require analgesia, but poses a potential risk to individuals who attempt, on their own, to overcome the blockade by administering large amounts of exogenous opioids. Indeed, any attempt by a patient to overcome the antagonism by taking opioids is very dangerous and may lead to a fatal overdose. Injury may arise because the plasma concentration of exogenous opioids attained immediately following their acute administration may be sufficient to overcome the competitive receptor blockade. As a consequence, the patient may be in immediate danger of suffering life endangering opioid intoxication (e.g., respiratory arrest, circulatory collapse). Patients should be told of the serious consequences of trying to overcome the opiate blockade (See **Information for Patients**).

There is also the possibility that a patient who had been treated with naltrexone will respond to lower doses of opioids than previously used, particularly if taken in such a manner that high plasma concentrations remain in the body beyond the time that naltrexone exerts its therapeutic effects. This could result in potentially life-threatening opioid intoxication (respiratory compromise or arrest, circulatory collapse, etc.). Patients should be aware that they may be more sensitive to lower doses of opioids after naltrexone treatment is discontinued.

Ultra Rapid Opioid Withdrawal:
Safe use of ReVia in ultra rapid opiate detoxification programs has not been established (see **ADVERSE REACTIONS**).

PRECAUTIONS:

General:

When Reversal of ReVia Blockade is Required: In an emergency situation in patients receiving fully blocking doses of ReVia, a suggested plan of management is regional analgesia, conscious sedation with a benzodiazepine, use of non-opioid analgesics or general anesthesia.

In a situation requiring opioid analgesia, the amount of opioid required may be greater than usual, and the resulting respiratory depression may be deeper and more prolonged.

A rapidly acting opioid analgesic which minimizes the duration of respiratory depression is preferred. The amount of analgesic administered should be titrated to the needs of the patient. Non-receptor mediated actions may occur and should be expected (e.g., facial swelling, itching, generalized erythema, or bronchoconstriction) presumably due to histamine release.

Irrespective of the drug chosen to reverse ReVia blockade, the patient should be monitored closely by appropriately trained personnel in a setting equipped and staffed for cardiopulmonary resuscitation.

Accidentally Precipitated Withdrawal: Severe opioid withdrawal syndromes precipitated by the accidental ingestion of ReVia have been reported in opioid-dependent individuals. Symptoms of withdrawal have usually appeared within five minutes of ingestion of ReVia and have lasted for up to 48 hours. Mental status changes including confusion, somnolence and visual hallucinations have occurred. Significant fluid losses from vomiting and diarrhea have required intravenous fluid administration. In all cases patients were closely monitored and therapy with non-opioid medications was tailored to meet individual requirements.

Use of ReVia does not eliminate or diminish withdrawal symptoms. If ReVia is initiated early in the abstinence process, it will not preclude the patient's experience of the full range of signs and symptoms that would be experienced if ReVia had not been started. Numerous adverse events are known to be associated with withdrawal.

Special Risk Patients:

Renal Impairment: ReVia and its primary metabolite are excreted primarily in the urine, and caution is recommended in administering the drug to patients with renal impairment.

Hepatic Impairment: Caution should be exercised when naltrexone hydrochloride is administered to patients with liver disease. An increase in naltrexone AUC of approximately 5- and 10-fold in patients with compensated and decompensated liver cirrhosis, respectively, compared with subjects with normal liver function has been reported. These data also suggest that alterations in naltrexone bioavailability are related to liver disease severity.

Suicide: The risk of suicide is known to be increased in patients with substance abuse with or without concomitant depression. This risk is not abated by treatment with ReVia (see **ADVERSE REACTIONS**).

Information for Patients: It is recommended that the prescribing physician relate the following information to patients being treated with ReVia:

You have been prescribed ReVia as part of the comprehensive treatment for your alcoholism or drug dependence. You should carry identification to alert medical personnel to the fact that you are taking ReVia. A ReVia medication card may be obtained from your physician and can be used for this purpose. Carrying the identification card should help to ensure that you can obtain adequate treatment in an emergency. If you require medical treatment, be sure to tell the treating physician that you are receiving ReVia therapy.

You should take ReVia as directed by your physician. If you attempt to self-administer heroin or any other opiate drug, in small doses while on ReVia, you will not perceive any effect. Most important, however, if you attempt to self-administer large doses of heroin or any other opioid while on ReVia, you may die or sustain serious injury, including coma. ReVia is well-tolerated in the recommended doses, but may cause liver injury when taken in excess or in people who develop liver disease from other causes. If you develop abdominal pain lasting more than a few days, white bowel movements, dark urine, or yellowing of your eyes, you should stop taking ReVia immediately and see your doctor as soon as possible.

Laboratory Tests: A high index of suspicion for drug-related hepatic injury is critical if the occurrence of liver damage induced by ReVia is to be detected at the earliest possible time. Evaluations, using appropriate batteries of tests to detect liver injury are recommended at a frequency appropriate to the clinical situation and the dose of ReVia.

ReVia (naltrexone hydrochloride) does not interfere with thin-layer, gas-liquid, and high pressure liquid chromatographic methods which may be used for the separation and detection of morphine, methadone or quinine in the urine. ReVia may or may not interfere with enzymatic methods for the detection of opioids depending on the specificity of the test. Please consult the test manufacturer for specific details.

Drug Interactions: Studies to evaluate possible interactions between ReVia and drugs other than opiates have not been performed. Consequently, caution is advised if the concomitant administration of ReVia and other drugs is required.

The safety and efficacy of concomitant use of ReVia and disulfiram is unknown, and the concomitant use of two potentially hepatotoxic medications is not ordinarily recommended unless the probable benefits outweigh the known risks.

Lethargy and somnolence have been reported following doses of ReVia and thioridazine.

Patients taking ReVia may not benefit from opioid containing medicines, such as cough and cold preparations, antidiarrheal preparations, and opioid analgesics. In an emergency situation when opioid analgesia must be administered to a patient receiving ReVia, the amount of opioid required may be greater than usual, and the resulting respiratory depression may be deeper and more prolonged (see **PRECAUTIONS**).

Carcinogenesis, Mutagenesis and Impairment of Fertility:
The following statements are based on the results of experiments in mice and rats. The potential carcinogenic, mutagenic and fertility effects of the metabolite 6-β-naltrexol are unknown.

In a two-year carcinogenicity study in rats, there were small increases in the numbers of testicular mesotheliomas in males and tumors of vascular origin in males and females. The incidence of mesothelioma in males given naltrexone at a dietary dose of 100 mg/kg/day (600 mg/m^2/day; 16 times the recommended therapeutic dose, based on body surface area) was 6%, compared with a maximum historical incidence of 4%. The incidence of vascular tumors in males and females given dietary doses of 100 mg/kg/day (600 mg/m^2/day) was 4%, but only the incidence in females was increased compared with a maximum historical control incidence of 2%. There was no evidence of carcinogenicity in a two-year dietary study with naltrexone in male and female mice.

There was limited evidence of a weak genotoxic effect of naltrexone in one gene mutation assay in a mammalian cell line, in the *Drosophila* recessive lethal assay, and in non-specific DNA repair tests with *E. coli*. However, no evidence of genotoxic potential was observed in a range of other *in vitro* tests, including assays for gene mutation in bacteria, yeast, or in a second mammalian cell line, a chromosomal aberration assay, and an assay for DNA damage in human cells. Naltrexone did not exhibit clastogenicity in an *in vivo* mouse micronucleus assay. Naltrexone (100 mg/kg/day [600 mg/m^2/day] PO; 16 times the recommended therapeutic dose, based on body surface area) caused a significant increase in pseudopregnancy in the rat. A decrease in the pregnancy rate of mated female rats also occurred. There was no effect on male fertility at this dose level. The relevance of these observations to human fertility is not known.

Pregnancy: Category C. Naltrexone has been shown to increase the incidence of early fetal loss when given to rats at doses ≥30 mg/kg/day (180 mg/m^2/day; 5 times the recommended therapeutic dose, based on body surface area) and to rabbits at oral doses ≥60 mg/kg/day (720 mg/m^2/day; 18 times the recommended therapeutic dose, based on body surface area). There was no evidence of teratogenicity when naltrexone was administered orally to rats and rabbits during the period of major organogenesis at doses up to 200 mg/kg/day (32 and 65 times the recommended therapeutic dose, respectively, based on body surface area).

Rats do not form appreciable quantities of the major human metabolite, 6-β-naltrexol; therefore, the potential reproductive toxicity of the metabolite in rats is not known.

There are no adequate and well-controlled studies in pregnant women. ReVia should be used during pregnancy only if the potential benefit justifies the potential risk to the fetus.

Labor and Delivery: Whether or not ReVia affects the duration of labor and delivery is unknown.

Nursing Mothers: In animal studies, naltrexone and 6-β-naltrexol were excreted in the milk of lactating rats dosed orally with naltrexone. Whether or not ReVia is excreted in human milk is unknown. Because many drugs are excreted in human milk, caution should be exercised when ReVia is administered to a nursing woman.

Pediatric Use: The safe use of ReVia in pediatric patients younger than 18 years old has not been established.

ADVERSE REACTIONS:

During two randomized, double-blind placebo-controlled 12 week trials to evaluate the efficacy of ReVia as an adjunctive treatment of alcohol dependence, most patients tolerated ReVia well. In these studies, a total of 93 patients received ReVia at a dose of 50 mg once daily. Five of these patients discontinued ReVia because of nausea. No serious adverse events were reported during these two trials.

While extensive clinical studies evaluating the use of ReVia in detoxified, formerly opioid-dependent individuals failed to identify any single, serious untoward risk of ReVia use, placebo-controlled studies employing up to five-fold higher doses of ReVia (up to 300 mg per day) than that recommended for use in opiate receptor blockade have shown that ReVia causes hepatocellular injury in a substantial proportion of patients exposed at higher doses (see **WARNINGS** and **PRECAUTIONS: Laboratory Tests**).

Aside from this finding, and the risk of precipitated opioid withdrawal, available evidence does not incriminate ReVia, used at any dose, as a cause of any other serious adverse reaction for the patient who is "opioid free." It is critical to recognize that ReVia can precipitate or exacerbate abstinence signs and symptoms in any individual who is not completely free of exogenous opioids.

Patients with addictive disorders, especially opioid addiction, are at risk for multiple numerous adverse events and abnormal laboratory findings, including liver function abnormalities. Data from both controlled and observational studies suggest that these abnormalities, other than the dose-related hepatotoxicity described above, are not related to the use of ReVia.

Among opioid free individuals, ReVia administration at the recommended dose has not been associated with a predictable profile of serious adverse or untoward events. However, as mentioned above, among individuals using opioids, ReVia may cause serious withdrawal reactions (see **CONTRAINDICATIONS, WARNINGS, DOSAGE AND ADMINISTRATION**).

Reported Adverse Events
ReVia has not been shown to cause significant increases in complaints in placebo-controlled trials in patients known to be free of opioids for more than 7–10 days. Studies in alcoholic populations and in volunteers in clinical pharmacology studies have suggested that a small fraction of patients may experience an opioid withdrawal-like symptom complex consisting of tearfulness, mild nausea, abdominal cramps, restlessness, bone or joint pain, myalgia, and nasal symptoms. This may represent the unmasking of occult opioid use, or it may represent symptoms attributable to naltrexone. A number of alternative dosing patterns have been recommended to try to reduce the frequency of these complaints (see **Individualization of Dosage**).

Alcoholism:
In an open label safety study with approximately 570 individuals with alcoholism receiving ReVia, the following new-onset adverse reactions occurred in 2% or more of the patients: nausea (10%), headache (7%), dizziness (4%), nervousness (4%), fatigue (4%), insomnia (3%), vomiting (3%), anxiety (2%) and somnolence (2%).

Depression, suicidal ideation, and suicidal attempts have been reported in all groups when comparing naltrexone, placebo, or controls undergoing treatment for alcoholism.

RATE RANGES OF NEW ONSET EVENTS

	Naltrexone	Placebo
Depression	0–15%	0–17%
Suicide Attempt/ Ideation	0–1%	0–3%

Although no causal relationship with ReVia is suspected, physicians should be aware that treatment with ReVia does not reduce the risk of suicide in these patients (see **PRECAUTIONS**).

Opioid Addiction:
The following adverse reactions have been reported both at baseline and during the ReVia clinical trials in opioid addiction at an incidence rate of more than 10%:

Difficulty sleeping, anxiety, nervousness, abdominal pain/cramps, nausea and/or vomiting, low energy, joint and muscle pain, and headache.

The incidence was less than 10% for:

Loss of appetite, diarrhea, constipation, increased thirst, increased energy, feeling down, irritability, dizziness, skin rash, delayed ejaculation, decreased potency, and chills.

The following events occurred in less than 1% of subjects:

Respiratory: nasal congestion, itching, rhinorrhea, sneezing, sore throat, excess mucus or phlegm, sinus trouble, heavy breathing, hoarseness, cough, shortness of breath.

Cardiovascular: nose bleeds, phlebitis, edema, increased blood pressure, non-specific ECG changes, palpitations, tachycardia.

Gastrointestinal: excessive gas, hemorrhoids, diarrhea, ulcer.

Musculoskeletal: painful shoulders, legs or knees; tremors, twitching.

Genitourinary: increased frequency of, or discomfort during, urination; increased or decreased sexual interest.

Dermatologic: oily skin, pruritus, acne, athlete's foot, cold sores, alopecia.

Psychiatric: depression, paranoia, fatigue, restlessness, confusion, disorientation, hallucinations, nightmares, bad dreams.

Special senses: eyes—blurred, burning, light sensitive, swollen, aching, strained; ears—"clogged", aching, tinnitus.
General: increased appetite, weight loss, weight gain, yawning, somnolence, fever, dry mouth, head "pounding", inguinal pain, swollen glands, "side" pains, cold feet, "hot spells."
Post-Marketing Experience: Data collected from post-marketing use of REVIA show that most events usually occur early in the course of drug therapy and are transient. It is not always possible to distinguish these occurences from those signs and symptoms that may result from a withdrawal syndrome. Events that have been reported include anorexia, asthenia, chest pain, fatigue, headache, hot flushes, malaise, changes in blood pressure, agitation, dizziness, hyperkinesia, nausea, vomiting, tremor, abdominal pain, diarrhea, elevations in liver enzymes or bilirubin, hepatic function abnormalities or hepatitis, palpitations, myalgia, anxiety, confusion, emphoria, hallucinations, insomnia, nervousness, somnolence, abnormal thinking, dyspnea, rash, increased sweating, and vision abnormalities.
Depression, suicide, attempted suicide and suicidal ideation have been reported in the post-marketing experience with REVIA used in the treatment of opioid dependence. No causal relationship has been demonstrated. In the literature, endogenous opioids have been theorized to contribute to a variety of conditions. In some individuals the use of opioid antagonists has been associated with a change in baseline levels of some hypothalamic, pituitary, adrenal, or gonadal hormones. The clinical significance of such changes is not fully understood.
Adverse events, including withdrawal symptoms and death, have been reported with the use of REVIA (naltrexone hydrochloride) in ultra rapid opiate detoxification programs. The cause of death in these cases is not known (see **WARNINGS**).
Laboratory Tests: With the exception of liver test abnormalities (see **WARNINGS** and **PRECAUTIONS**), results of laboratory tests, like adverse reaction reports, have not shown consistent patterns of abnormalities that can be attributed to treatment with REVIA.
Idiopathic thrombocytopenic purpura was reported in one patient who may have been sensitized to REVIA in a previous course of treatment with REVIA. The condition cleared without sequelae after discontinuation of REVIA and corticosteroid treatment.

DRUG ABUSE AND DEPENDENCE:

REVIA is a pure opioid antagonist. It does not lead to physical or psychological dependence. Tolerance to the opioid antagonist effect is not known to occur.

OVERDOSAGE:

There is limited clinical experience with REVIA overdosage in humans. In one study, subjects who received 800 mg daily REVIA for up to one week showed no evidence of toxicity.
In the mouse, rat and guinea pig, the oral LD50s were 1,100–1,550 mg/kg; 1,450 mg/kg; and 1,490 mg/kg; respectively. High doses of REVIA (generally ≥1,000 mg/kg) produced salivation, depression/reduced activity, tremors, and convulsions. Mortalities in animals due to high-dose REVIA administration usually were due to clonic-tonic convulsions and/or respiratory failure.
Treatment Of Overdosage: In view of the lack of actual experience in the treatment of REVIA overdose, patients should be treated symptomatically in a closely supervised environment. Physicians should contact a poison control center for the most up-to-date information.

DOSAGE AND ADMINISTRATION:

IF THERE IS ANY QUESTION OF OCCULT OPIOID DEPENDENCE, PERFORM A NALOXONE CHALLENGE TEST AND DO NOT INITIATE REVIA THERAPY UNTIL THE NALOXONE CHALLENGE IS NEGATIVE.
Treatment of Alcoholism:
A dose of 50 mg once daily is recommended for most patients (see **Individualization of Dosage**). The placebo-controlled studies that demonstrated the efficacy of REVIA as an adjunctive treatment of alcoholism used a dose regimen of REVIA 50 mg once daily for up to 12 weeks. Other dose regimens or durations of therapy were not evaluated in these trials.
A patient is a candidate for treatment with REVIA if:

- The patient is willing to take a medicine to help with alcohol dependence
- The patient is opioid free for 7–10 days
- The patient does not have severe or active liver or kidney problems (Typical guidelines suggest liver function tests no greater than 3 times the upper limits of normal, and bilirubin normal.)
- The patient is not allergic to REVIA, and no other contraindications are present

Refer to **CONTRAINDICATIONS**, **WARNINGS**, and **PRECAUTIONS** Sections for additional information.
REVIA should be considered as only one of many factors determining the success of treatment of alcoholism. Factors associated with a good outcome in the clinical trials with REVIA were the type, intensity, and duration of treatment; appropriate management of comorbid conditions; use of community-based support groups; and good medication compliance. To achieve the best possible treatment outcome, appropriate compliance-enhancing techniques should be implemented for all components of the treatment program, especially medication compliance.
Treatment of Opioid Dependence:
Initiate treatment with REVIA using the following guidelines:

1. Treatment should not be attempted unless the patient has remained opioid-free for at least 7–10 days. Self-reporting of abstinence from opioids in opioid addicts should be verified by analysis of the patient's urine for absence of opioids. The patient should not be manifesting withdrawal signs or reporting withdrawal symptoms.
2. If there is any question of occult opioid dependence, perform a naloxone challenge test. If signs of opioid withdrawal are still observed following naloxone challenge, treatment with REVIA should not be attempted. The naloxone challenge can be repeated in 24 hours.
3. Treatment should be initiated carefully, with an initial dose of 25 mg of REVIA. If no withdrawal signs occur, the patient may be started on 50 mg a day thereafter.

Naloxone Challenge Test: The naloxone challenge test should not be performed in a patient showing clinical signs or symptoms of opioid withdrawal, or in a patient whose urine contains opioids. The naloxone challenge test may be administered by either the intravenous or subcutaneous routes.
Intravenous:
Inject 0.2 mg naloxone.
Observe for 30 seconds for signs or symptoms of withdrawal.
If no evidence of withdrawal, inject 0.6 mg of naloxone.
Observe for an additional 20 minutes.
Subcutaneous:
Administer 0.8 mg naloxone.
Observe for 20 minutes for signs or symptoms of withdrawal.
Note: Individual patients, especially those with opioid dependence, may respond to lower doses of naloxone. In some cases, 0.1 mg IV naloxone has produced a diagnostic response.
Interpretation of the Challenge: Monitor vital signs and observe the patient for signs and symptoms of opioid withdrawal. These may include, but are not limited to: nausea, vomiting, dysphoria, yawning, sweating, tearing, rhinorrhea, stuffy nose, craving for opioids, poor appetite, abdominal cramps, sense of fear, skin erythema, disrupted sleep patterns, fidgeting, uneasiness, poor ability to focus, mental lapses, muscle aches or cramps, pupillary dilation, piloerection, fever, changes in blood pressure, pulse or temperature, anxiety, depression, irritability, back ache, bone or joint pains, tremors, sensations of skin crawling or fasciculations. If signs or symptoms of withdrawal appear, the test is positive and no additional naloxone should be administered.
Warning: If the test is positive, do NOT initiate REVIA therapy. Repeat the challenge in 24 hours. If the test is negative, REVIA therapy may be started if no other contraindictions are present. If there is any doubt about the result of the test, hold REVIA and repeat the challenge in 24 hours.
Alternative Dosing Schedules:
Once the patient has been started on REVIA, 50 mg every 24 hours will produce adequate clinical blockade of the actions of parenterally administered opioids (i.e., this dose will block the effects of a 25 mg intravenous heroin challenge). A flexible approach to a dosing regimen may need to be employed in cases of supervised administration. Thus, patients may receive 50 mg of REVIA every weekday with a 100 mg dose on Saturday, 100 mg every other day, or 150 mg every third day. The degree of blockade produced by REVIA may be reduced by these extended dosing intervals.
There may be a higher risk of hepatocellular injury with single doses above 50 mg, and use of higher doses and extended dosing intervals should balance the possible risks against the probable benefits (see **WARNINGS** and **Individualization of Dosage**).
Patient Compliance: REVIA should be considered as only one of many factors determining the success of treatment. To achieve the best possible treatment outcome, appropriate compliance-enhancing techniques should be implemented for all components of the treatment program, including medication compliance.

HOW SUPPLIED

REVIA (naltrexone hydrochloride) tablets are available in pale yellow 50 mg capsule-shaped film-coated tablets, scored and imprinted with "DuPont" on one side and "11" on the other, as follows:

Bottles of 30 Tablets	NDC 0056-0011-30
Bottles of 100 Tablets	NDC 0056-0011-70

Store at 25°C (77°F); excursions permitted to 15°–30°C (59°–86°F) [see USP Controlled Room Temperature].
DuPont Pharma
Wilmington, Delaware 19880
REVIA® is a Registered U.S. Trademark of DuPont Pharmaceuticals Co.

Made and Printed in U.S.A.
6430-03/Rev. May, 1999.
Shown in Product Identification Guide, page 311

SINEMET® (CARBIDOPA-LEVODOPA) TABLETS ℞

DESCRIPTION

SINEMET* (Carbidopa-Levodopa) is a combination of carbidopa and levodopa for the treatment of Parkinson's disease and syndrome.
Carbidopa, an inhibitor of aromatic amino acid decarboxylation, is a white, crystalline compound, slightly soluble in water, with a molecular weight of 244.3. It is designated chemically as (—)-L-α-hydrazino-α-methyl-β-(3,4-dihydroxybenzene) propanoic acid monohydrate. Its empirical formula is $C_{10}H_{14}N_2O_4 \cdot H_2O$, and its structural formula is:

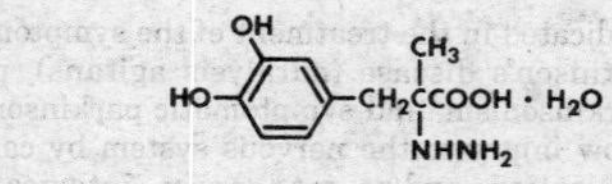

Tablet content is expressed in terms of anhydrous carbidopa which has a molecular weight of 226.3.
Levodopa, an aromatic amino acid, is a white, crystalline compound, slightly soluble in water, with a molecular weight of 197.2. It is designated chemically as (—)-L-α-amino-β-(3,4-dihydroxybenzene) propanoic acid. Its empirical formula is $C_9H_{11}NO_4$, and its structural formula is:

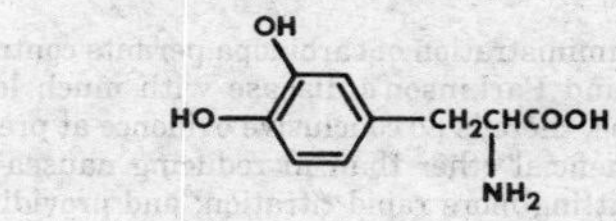

SINEMET is supplied as tablets in three strengths:
SINEMET 25-100, containing 25 mg of carbidopa and 100 mg of levodopa.
SINEMET 10-100, containing 10 mg of carbidopa and 100 mg of levodopa.
SINEMET 25-250, containing 25 mg of carbidopa and 250 mg of levodopa.
Inactive ingredients are cellulose, magnesium stearate, and starch. Tablets SINEMET 10-100 and 25-250 also contain FD&C Blue 2. Tablets SINEMET 25-100 also contain D&C Yellow 10 and FD&C Yellow 6.

CLINICAL PHARMACOLOGY

Parkinson's disease is a progressive, neurodegenerative disorder of the extrapyramidal nervous system affecting the mobility and control of the skeletal muscular system. Its characteristic features include resting tremor, rigidity, and bradykinetic moments. Symptomatic treatments, such as levodopa therapies, may permit the patient better mobility.
Mechanism of Action
Current evidence indicates that symptoms of Parkinson's disease are related to depletion of dopamine in the corpus striatum. Administration of dopamine is ineffective in the treatment of Parkinson's disease apparently because it does not cross the blood-brain barrier. However, levodopa, the metabolic precursor of dopamine, does cross the blood-brain barrier, and presumably is converted to dopamine in the brain. This is thought to be the mechanism whereby levodopa relieves symptoms of Parkinson's disease.
Pharmacodynamics
When levodopa is administered orally it is rapidly decarboxylated to dopamine in extracerebral tissues so that only a small portion of a given dose is transported unchanged to the central nervous system. For this reason, large doses of levodopa are required for adequate therapeutic effect and these may often be accompanied by nausea and other adverse reactions, some of which are attributable to dopamine formed in extracerebral tissues.
Since levodopa competes with certain amino acids for transport across the gut wall, the absorption of levodopa may be impaired in some patients on a high protein diet.
Carbidopa inhibits decarboxylation of peripheral levodopa. It does not cross the blood-brain barrier and does not affect the metabolism of levodopa within the central nervous system.
The incidence of levodopa-induced nausea and vomiting is less with SINEMET than with levodopa. In many patients, this reduction in nausea and vomiting will permit more rapid dosage titration.
Since its decarboxylase inhibiting activity is limited to extracerebral tissues, administration of carbidopa with levodopa makes more levodopa available for transport to the brain.
Pharmacokinetics
Carbidopa reduces the amount of levodopa required to produce a given response by about 75 percent and, when administered with levodopa, increases both plasma levels and the plasma half-life of levodopa, and decreases plasma and urinary dopamine and homovanillic acid.
The plasma half-life of levodopa is about 50 minutes, without carbidopa. When carbidopa and levodopa are administered together, the half-life of levodopa is increased to about 1.5 hours. At steady state, the bioavailability of carbidopa from SINEMET tablets is approximately 99% relative to the concomitant administration of carbidopa and levodopa.
In clinical pharmacologic studies, simultaneous administration of carbidopa and levodopa produced greater urinary excretion of levodopa in proportion to the excretion of dopamine than administration of the two drugs at separate times.
Pyridoxine hydrochloride (vitamin B_6), in oral doses of 10 mg to 25 mg, may reverse the effects of levodopa by increasing the rate of aromatic amino acid decarboxylation.
Continued on next page

Sinemet—Cont.

Carbidopa inhibits this action of pyridoxine; therefore, SINEMET can be given to patients receiving supplemental pyridoxine (vitamin B_6).

INDICATIONS AND USAGE

SINEMET is indicated in the treatment of the symptoms of idiopathic Parkinson's disease (paralysis agitans), postencephalitic parkinsonism, and symptomatic parkinsonism which may follow injury to the nervous system by carbon monoxide intoxication and/or manganese intoxication. SINEMET is indicated in these conditions to permit the administration of lower doses of levodopa with reduced nausea and vomiting, with more rapid dosage titration, with a somewhat smoother response, and with supplemental pyridoxine (vitamin B_6).

In some patients a somewhat smoother antiparkinsonian effect results from therapy with SINEMET than with levodopa. However, patients with markedly irregular ("on-off") responses to levodopa have not been shown to benefit from SINEMET.

Although the administration of carbidopa permits control of parkinsonism and Parkinson's disease with much lower doses of levodopa, there is no conclusive evidence at present that this is beneficial other than in reducing nausea and vomiting, permitting more rapid titration, and providing a somewhat smoother response to levodopa.

Certain patients who responded poorly to levodopa have improved when SINEMET was substituted. This is most likely due to decreased peripheral decarboxylation of levodopa which results from administration of carbidopa rather than to a primary effect of carbidopa on the nervous system. Carbidopa has not been shown to enhance the intrinsic efficacy of levodopa in parkinsonian syndromes.

In considering whether to give SINEMET to patients already on levodopa who have nausea and/or vomiting, the practitioner should be aware that, while many patients may be expected to improve, some do not. Since one cannot predict which patients are likely to improve, this can only be determined by a trial of therapy. It should be further noted that in controlled trials comparing SINEMET with levodopa, about half of the patients with nausea and/or vomiting on levodopa improved spontaneously despite being retained on the same dose of levodopa during the controlled portion of the trial.

CONTRAINDICATIONS

Nonselective monoamine oxidase (MAO) inhibitors are contraindicated for use with SINEMET. These inhibitors must be discontinued at least two weeks prior to initiating therapy with SINEMET. SINEMET may be administered concomitantly with the manufacturer's recommended dose of an MAO inhibitor with selectivity for MAO type B (e.g., selegiline HCl) (See PRECAUTIONS, *Drug Interactions*).

SINEMET is contraindicated in patients with known hypersensitivity to any component of this drug, and in narrow-angle glaucoma.

Because levodopa may activate a malignant melanoma, SINEMET should not be used in patients with suspicious, undiagnosed skin lesions or a history of melanoma.

WARNINGS

When SINEMET (Carbidopa-Levodopa) is to be given to patients who are being treated with levodopa, levodopa must be discontinued at least twelve hours before therapy with SINEMET (Carbidopa-Levodopa) is started. In order to reduce adverse reactions, it is necessary to individualize therapy. See DOSAGE AND ADMINISTRATION section before initiating therapy.

The addition of carbidopa with levodopa in the form of SINEMET reduces the peripheral effects (nausea, vomiting) due to decarboxylation of levodopa; however, carbidopa does not decrease the adverse reactions due to the central effects of levodopa. Because carbidopa permits more levodopa to reach the brain and more dopamine to be formed, certain adverse CNS effects, e.g., dyskinesias (involuntary movements), may occur at lower dosages and sooner with SINEMET than with levodopa alone.

Levodopa alone, as well as SINEMET, is associated with dyskinesias. The occurrence of dyskinesias may require dosage reduction.

As with levodopa, SINEMET may cause mental disturbances. These reactions are thought to be due to increased brain dopamine following administration of levodopa. All patients should be observed carefully for the development of depression with concomitant suicidal tendencies. Patients with past or current psychoses should be treated with caution.

SINEMET should be administered cautiously to patients with severe cardiovascular or pulmonary disease, bronchial asthma, renal, hepatic or endocrine disease.

As with levodopa, care should be exercised in administering SINEMET to patients with a history of myocardial infarction who have residual atrial, nodal, or ventricular arrhythmias. In such patients, cardiac function should be monitored with particular care during the period of initial dosage adjustment, in a facility with provisions for intensive cardiac care.

As with levodopa, treatment with SINEMET may increase the possibility of upper gastrointestinal hemorrhage in patients with a history of peptic ulcer.

Neuroleptic Malignant Syndrome (NMS): Sporadic cases of a symptom complex resembling NMS have been reported in association with dose reduction or withdrawal of therapy with SINEMET. Therefore, patients should be observed carefully when the dosage of SINEMET is reduced abruptly or discontinued, especially if the patient is receiving neuroleptics.

NMS is an uncommon but life-threatening syndrome characterized by fever or hyperthermia. Neurological findings, including muscle rigidity, involuntary movements, altered consciousness, mental status changes; other disturbances, such as autonomic dysfunction, tachycardia, tachypnea, sweating, hyper- or hypotension; laboratory findings, such as creatine phosphokinase elevation, leukocytosis, myoglobinuria, and increased serum myoglobin, have been reported.

The early diagnosis of this condition is important for the appropriate management of these patients. Considering NMS as a possible diagnosis and ruling out other acute illnesses (e.g., pneumonia, systemic infection, etc.) is essential. This may be especially complex if the clinical presentation includes both serious medical illness and untreated or inadequately treated extrapyramidal signs and symptoms (EPS). Other important considerations in the differential diagnosis include central anticholinergic toxicity, heat stroke, drug fever, and primary central nervous system (CNS) pathology.

The management of NMS should include: 1) intensive symptomatic treatment and medical monitoring and 2) treatment of any concomitant serious medical problems for which specific treatments are available. Dopamine agonists, such as bromocriptine, and muscle relaxants, such as dantrolene, are often used in the treatment of NMS, however, their effectiveness has not been demonstrated in controlled studies.

PRECAUTIONS

General

As with levodopa, periodic evaluations of hepatic, hematopoietic, cardiovascular, and renal function are recommended during extended therapy.

Patients with chronic wide-angle glaucoma may be treated cautiously with SINEMET provided the intraocular pressure is well controlled and the patient is monitored carefully for changes in intraocular pressure during therapy.

Information for Patients

The patient should be informed that SINEMET is an immediate-release formulation of carbidopa-levodopa that is designed to begin release of ingredients within 30 minutes. It is important that SINEMET be taken at regular intervals according to the schedule outlined by the physician. The patient should be cautioned not to change the prescribed dosage regimen and not to add any additional antiparkinson medications, including other carbidopa-levodopa preparations, without first consulting the physician.

Patients should be advised that sometimes a 'wearing-off' effect may occur at the end of the dosing interval. The physician should be notified if such response poses a problem to life-style.

Patients should be advised that occasionally, dark color (red, brown, or black) may appear in saliva, urine, or sweat after ingestion of SINEMET. Although the color appears to be clinically insignificant, garments may become discolored.

The patients should be advised that a change in diet to foods that are high in protein may delay the absorption of levodopa and may reduce the amount taken up in the circulation. Excessive acidity also delays stomach emptying, thus delaying the absorption of levodopa. Iron salts (such as in multi-vitamin tablets) may also reduce the amount of levodopa available to the body. The above factors may reduce the clinical effectiveness of the levodopa or carbidopa-levodopa therapy.

NOTE: The suggested advice to patients being treated with SINEMET is intended to aid in the safe and effective use of this medication. It is not a disclosure of all possible adverse or intended effects.

Laboratory Tests

Abnormalities in laboratory tests may include elevations of liver function tests such as alkaline phosphatase, SGOT (AST), SGPT (ALT), lactic dehydrogenase, and bilirubin. Abnormalities in blood urea nitrogen and positive Coombs test have also been reported. Commonly, levels of blood urea nitrogen, creatinine, and uric acid are lower during administration of SINEMET than with levodopa.

SINEMET may cause a false-positive reaction for urinary ketone bodies when a test tape is used for determination of ketonuria. This reaction will not be altered by boiling the urine specimen. False-negative tests may result with the use of glucose-oxidase methods of testing for glucosuria.

Cases of falsely diagnosed pheochromocytoma in patients on carbidopa-levodopa therapy have been reported very rarely. Caution should be exercised when interpreting the plasma and urine levels of catecholamines and their metabolites in patients on levodopa or carbidopa-levodopa therapy.

Drug Interactions

Caution should be exercised when the following drugs are administered concomitantly with SINEMET (Carbidopa-Levodopa).

Symptomatic postural hypotension has occurred when SINEMET is added to the treatment of a patient receiving antihypertensive drugs. Therefore, when therapy with SINEMET is started, dosage adjustment of the antihypertensive drug may be required.

For patients receiving MAO inhibitors (Type A or B), see CONTRAINDICATIONS. Concomitant therapy with selegiline and carbidopa-levodopa may be associated with severe orthostatic hypotension not attributable to carbidopa-levodopa alone (see CONTRAINDICATIONS).

There have been rare reports of adverse reactions, including hypertension and dyskinesia, resulting from the concomitant use of tricyclic antidepressants and SINEMET.

Dopamine D_2 receptor antagonists (e.g., phenothiazines, butyrophenones, risperidone) and isoniazid may reduce the therapeutic effects of levodopa. In addition, the beneficial effects of levodopa in Parkinson's disease have been reported to be reversed by phenytoin and papaverine. Patients taking these drugs with SINEMET should be carefully observed for loss of therapeutic response.

Iron salts may reduce the bioavailability of levodopa and carbidopa. The clinical relevance is unclear.

Although metoclopramide may increase the bioavailability of levodopa by increasing gastric emptying, metoclopramide may also adversely affect disease control by its dopamine receptor antagonistic properties.

Carcinogenesis, Mutagenesis, Impairment of Fertility

In a two-year bioassay of SINEMET, no evidence of carcinogenicity was found in rats receiving doses of approximately two times the maximum daily human dose of carbidopa and four times the maximum daily human dose of levodopa.

In reproduction studies with SINEMET, no effects on fertility were found in rats receiving doses of approximately two times the maximum daily human dose of carbidopa and four times the maximum daily human dose of levodopa.

Pregnancy

Pregnancy Category C. No teratogenic effects were observed in a study in mice receiving up to 20 times the maximum recommended human dose of SINEMET. There was a decrease in the number of live pups delivered by rats receiving approximately two times the maximum recommended human dose of carbidopa and approximately five times the maximum recommended human dose of levodopa during organogenesis. SINEMET caused both visceral and skeletal malformations in rabbits at all doses and ratios of carbidopa/levodopa tested, which ranged from 10 times/5 times the maximum recommended human dose of carbidopa/levodopa to 20 times/10 times the maximum recommended human dose of carbidopa/levodopa.

There are no adequate or well-controlled studies in pregnant women. It has been reported from individual cases that levodopa crosses the human placental barrier, enters the fetus, and is metabolized. Carbidopa concentrations in fetal tissue appeared to be minimal. Use of SINEMET in women of child-bearing potential requires that the anticipated benefits of the drug be weighed against possible hazards to mother and child.

Nursing Mothers

It is not known whether this drug is excreted in human milk. Because many drugs are excreted in human milk, caution should be exercised when SINEMET is administered to a nursing woman.

Pediatric Use

Safety and effectiveness in pediatric patients have not been established. Use of the drug in patients below the age of 18 is not recommended.

ADVERSE REACTIONS

The most common adverse reactions reported with SINEMET have included dyskinesias, such as choreiform, dystonic, and other involuntary movements and nausea.

The following other adverse reactions have been reported with SINEMET:

Body as a Whole: chest pain, asthenia.

Cardiovascular: cardiac irregularities, hypotension, orthostatic effects including orthostatic hypotension, hypertension, syncope, phlebitis, palpitation.

Gastrointestinal: dark saliva, gastrointestinal bleeding, development of duodenal ulcer, anorexia, vomiting, diarrhea, constipation, dyspepsia, dry mouth, taste alterations.

Hematologic: agranulocytosis, hemolytic and non-hemolytic anemia, thrombocytopenia, leukopenia.

Hypersensitivity: angioedema, urticaria, pruritus, Henoch-Schonlein purpura, bullous lesions (including pemphigus-like reactions).

Musculoskeletal: back pain, shoulder pain, muscle cramps.

Nervous System/Psychiatric: psychotic episodes including delusions, hallucinations, and paranoid ideation, neuroleptic malignant syndrome (see WARNINGS), bradykinetic episodes ("on-off" phenomenon), confusion, agitation, dizziness, somnolence, dream abnormalities including nightmares, insomnia, paresthesia, headache, depression with or without development of suicidal tendencies, dementia, increased libido. Convulsions also have occurred; however, a casual relationship with SINEMET has not been established.

Respiratory: dyspnea, upper respiratory infection.

Skin: rash, increased sweating, alopecia, dark sweat.

Urogenital: urinary tract infection, urinary frequency, dark urine.

Laboratory Tests: decreased hemoglobin and hematocrit; abnormalities in alkaline phosphatase, SGOT (AST), SGPT (ALT), lactic dehydrogenase, bilirubin, blood urea nitrogen (BUN), Coombs test; elevated serum glucose; white blood cells, bacteria, and blood in the urine.

Other adverse reactions that have been reported with levodopa alone and with various carbidopa-levodopa formulations, and may occur with SINEMET are:

Body as a Whole: abdominal pain and distress, fatigue.

Cardiovascular: myocardial infarction.

Gastrointestinal: gastrointestinal pain, dysphagia, sialorrhea, flatulence, bruxism, burning sensation of the tongue, heartburn, hiccups.
Metabolic: edema, weight gain, weight loss.
Musculoskeletal: leg pain.
Nervous System/Psychiatric: ataxia, extrapyramidal disorder, falling, anxiety, gait abnormalities, nervousness, decreased mental acuity, memory impairment, disorientation, euphoria, blepharospasm (which may be taken as an early sign of excess dosage; consideration of dosage reduction may be made at this time), trismus, increased tremor, numbness, muscle twitching, activation of latent Horner's syndrome, peripheral neuropathy.
Respiratory: pharyngeal pain, cough.
Skin: malignant melanoma (see also CONTRAINDICATIONS), flushing.
Special Senses: oculogyric crises, diplopia, blurred vision, dilated pupils.
Urogenital: urinary retention, urinary incontinence, priapism.
Miscellaneous: bizarre breathing patterns, faintness, hoarseness, malaise, hot flashes, sense of stimulation.
Laboratory Tests: decreased white blood cell count and serum potassium; increased serum creatinine and uric acid; protein and glucose in urine.

OVERDOSAGE

Management of acute overdosage with SINEMET is the same as management of acute overdosage with levodopa. Pyridoxine is not effective in reversing the actions of SINEMET.
General supportive measures should be employed, along with immediate gastric lavage. Intravenous fluids should be administered judiciously and an adequate airway maintained. Electrocardiographic monitoring should be instituted and the patient carefully observed for the development of arrhythmias; if required, appropriate anti-arrhythmic therapy should be given. The possibility that the patient may have taken other drugs as well as SINEMET should be taken into consideration. To date, no experience has been reported with dialysis; hence, its value in overdosage is not known.
Based on studies in which high doses of levodopa and/or carbidopa were administered, a significant proportion of rats and mice given single oral doses of levodopa of approximately 1500–2000 mg/kg are expected to die. A significant proportion of infant rats of both sexes are expected to die at a dose of 800 mg/kg. A significant proportion of rats are expected to die after treatment with similar doses of carbidopa. The addition of carbidopa in a 1:10 ratio with levodopa increases the dose at which a significant proportion of mice are expected to die to 3360 mg/kg.

DOSAGE AND ADMINISTRATION

The optimum daily dosage of SINEMET must be determined by careful titration in each patient. SINEMET tablets are available in a 1:4 ratio of carbidopa to levodopa (SINEMET 25-100) as well as 1:10 ratio (SINEMET 25-250 and SINEMET 10-100). Tablets of the two ratios may be given separately or combined as needed to provide the optimum dosage.
Studies show that peripheral dopa decarboxylase is saturated by carbidopa at approximately 70 to 100 mg a day. Patients receiving less than this amount of carbidopa are more likely to experience nausea and vomiting.
Usual Initial Dosage
Dosage is best initiated with one tablet of SINEMET 25-100 three times a day. This dosage schedule provides 75 mg of carbidopa per day. Dosage may be increased by one tablet every day or every other day, as necessary, until a dosage of eight tablets of SINEMET 25-100 a day is reached.
If SINEMET 10-100 is used, dosage may be initiated with one tablet three or four times a day. However, this will not provide an adequate amount of carbidopa for many patients. Dosage may be increased by one tablet every day or every other day until a total of eight tablets (2 tablets q.i.d.) is reached.
How to Transfer Patients from Levodopa
Levodopa must be discontinued at least twelve hours before starting SINEMET (Carbidopa-Levodopa). A daily dosage of SINEMET should be chosen that will provide approximately 25 percent of the previous levodopa dosage. Patients who are taking less than 1500 mg of levodopa a day should be started on one tablet of SINEMET 25-100 three or four times a day. The suggested starting dosage for most patients taking more than 1500 mg of levodopa is one tablet of SINEMET 25-250 three or four times a day.
Maintenance
Therapy should be individualized and adjusted according to the desired therapeutic response. At least 70 to 100 mg of carbidopa per day should be provided. When a greater proportion of carbidopa is required, one tablet of SINEMET 25-100 may be substituted for each tablet of SINEMET 10-100. When more levodopa is required, SINEMET 25-250 should be substituted for SINEMET 25-100 or SINEMET 10-100. If necessary, the dosage of SINEMET 25-250 may be increased by one-half or one tablet every day or every other day to a maximum of eight tablets a day. Experience with total daily dosages of carbidopa greater than 200 mg is limited.
Because both therapeutic and adverse responses occur more rapidly with SINEMET than with levodopa alone, patients should be monitored closely during the dose adjustment period. Specifically, involuntary movements will occur more rapidly with SINEMET than with levodopa. The occurrence of involuntary movements may require dosage reduction. Blepharospasm may be a useful early sign of excess dosage in some patients.
Addition of Other Antiparkinsonian Medications
Standard drugs for Parkinson's disease, other than levodopa without a decarboxylase inhibitor, may be used concomitantly while SINEMET is being administered, although dosage adjustments may be required.
Interruption of Therapy
Sporadic cases of a symptom complex resembling Neuroleptic Malignant Syndrome (NMS) have been associated with dose reductions and withdrawal of SINEMET. Patients should be observed carefully if abrupt reduction or discontinuation of SINEMET is required, especially if the patient is receiving neuroleptics. (See WARNINGS.)
If general anesthesia is required, SINEMET may be continued as long as the patient is permitted to take fluids and medication by mouth. If therapy is interrupted temporarily, the patient should be observed for symptoms resembling NMS, and the usual daily dosage may be administered as soon as the patient is able to take oral medication.

HOW SUPPLIED

Tablets SINEMET 25-100 are yellow, oval, uncoated tablets, that are scored and coded 650 on one side and SINEMET on the other side. They are supplied as follows:
NDC 0056-0650-68 bottles of 100
NDC 0056-0650-28 unit dose packages of 100.
Tablets SINEMET 10-100 are dark dapple-blue, oval, uncoated tablets, that are scored and coded 647 on one side and SINEMET on the other side. They are supplied as follows:
NDC 0056-0647-68 bottles of 100
NDC 0056-0647-28 unit dose packages of 100.
Tablets SINEMET 25-250 are light dapple-blue, oval, uncoated tablets, that are scored and coded 654 on one side and SINEMET on the other side. They are supplied as follows:
NDC 0056-0654-68 bottles of 100
NDC 0056-0654-28 unit dose packages of 100.
Storage
Tablets SINEMET 10-100 and Tablets SINEMET 25-250 must be protected from light.

Manufactured by:
MERCK & CO., INC.
WEST POINT, PA 19486, USA
For:
DuPont Pharma
Wilmington, Delaware 19880
6350-05/June, 1999

Shown in Product Identification Guide, page 311

*Registered trademark of MERCK & CO., INC.

SINEMET® CR ℞
(CARBIDOPA-LEVODOPA)
SUSTAINED-RELEASE TABLETS

DESCRIPTION

SINEMET* CR (Carbidopa-Levodopa) is a sustained-release combination of carbidopa and levodopa for the treatment of Parkinson's disease and syndrome.
Carbidopa, an inhibitor of aromatic amino acid decarboxylation, is a white, crystalline compound, slightly soluble in water, with a molecular weight of 244.3. It is designated chemically as (—)-L-α-hydrazino-α-methyl-β-(3,4-dihydroxybenzene) propanoic acid monohydrate. Its empirical formula is $C_{10}H_{14}N_2O_4 \cdot H_2O$ and its structural formula is:

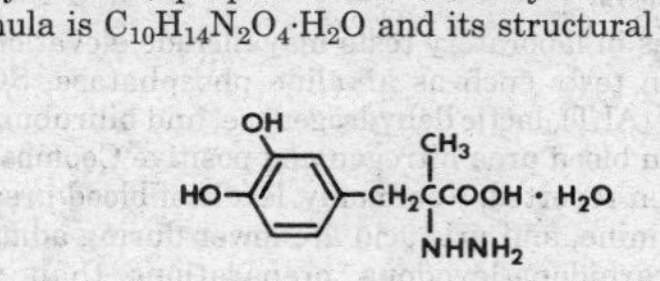

Tablet content is expressed in terms of anhydrous carbidopa, which has a molecular weight of 226.3.
Levodopa, an aromatic amino acid, is a white, crystalline compound, slightly soluble in water, with a molecular weight of 197.2. It is designated chemically as (—)-L-α-amino-β-(3,4-dihydroxybenzene) propanoic acid. Its empirical formula is $C_9H_{11}NO_4$ and its structural formula is:

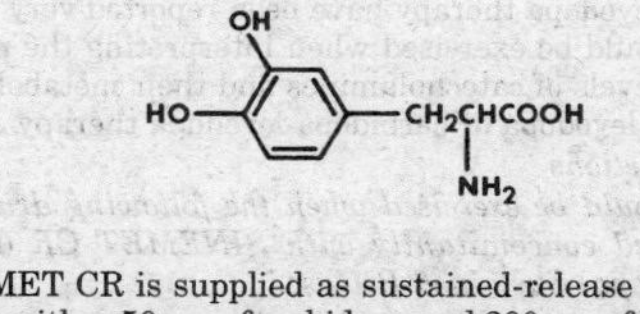

SINEMET CR is supplied as sustained-release tablets containing either 50 mg of carbidopa and 200 mg of levodopa, or 25 mg of carbidopa and 100 mg of levodopa. Inactive ingredients: hydroxypropyl cellulose, polyvinylacetate-crotonic acid copolymer, magnesium stearate and red ferric oxide. SINEMET CR 50–200 also contains D&C Yellow 10.
The 50–200 tablet is supplied as an oval, scored, biconvex, compressed tablet that is peach colored. The 25–100 tablet is supplied as an oval, biconvex, compressed tablet that is pink colored. The SINEMET CR tablet is a polymeric-based drug delivery system that controls the release of carbidopa and levodopa as it slowly erodes. SINEMET CR 25–100 is available to facilitate titration and as an alternative to the half-tablet of SINEMET CR 50–200.

CLINICAL PHARMACOLOGY

Mechanism of Action
Parkinson's disease is a progressive, neurodegenerative disorder of the extrapyramidal nervous system affecting the mobility and control of the skeletal muscular system. Its characteristic features include resting tremor, rigidity, and bradykinetic movements. Symptomatic treatments, such as levodopa therapies, may permit the patient better mobility.
Current evidence indicates that symptoms of Parkinson's disease are related to depletion of dopamine in the corpus striatum. Administration of dopamine is ineffective in the treatment of Parkinson's disease apparently because it does not cross the blood-brain barrier. However, levodopa, the metabolic precursor of dopamine, does cross the blood-brain barrier, and presumably is converted to dopamine in the brain. This is thought to be the mechanism whereby levodopa relieves symptoms of Parkinson's disease.
Pharmacodynamics
When levodopa is administered orally it is rapidly decarboxylated to dopamine in extracerebral tissues so that only a small portion of a given dose is transported unchanged to the central nervous system. For this reason, large doses of levodopa are required for adequate therapeutic effect and these may often be accompanied by nausea and other adverse reactions, some of which are attributable to dopamine formed in extracerebral tissues.
Since levodopa competes with certain amino acids for transport across the gut wall, the absorption of levodopa may be impaired in some patients on a high protein diet.
Carbidopa inhibits decarboxylation of peripheral levodopa. It does not cross the blood-brain barrier and does not affect the metabolism of levodopa within the central nervous system.
Since its decarboxylase inhibiting activity is limited to extracerebral tissues, administration of carbidopa with levodopa makes more levodopa available for transport to the brain.
Patients treated with levodopa therapy for Parkinson's disease may develop motor fluctuations characterized by end-of-dose failure, peak dose dyskinesia, and akinesia. The advanced form of motor fluctuations ('on-off' phenomenon) is characterized by unpredictable swings from mobility to immobility. Although the causes of the motor fluctuations are not completely understood, in some patients they may be attenuated by treatment regimens that produce steady plasma levels of levodopa.
SINEMET CR contains either 50 mg of carbidopa and 200 mg of levodopa, or 25 mg of carbidopa and 100 mg of levodopa in a sustained-release dosage form designed to release these ingredients over a 4- to 6-hour period. With SINEMET CR there is less variation in plasma levodopa levels than with SINEMET* (Carbidopa-Levodopa), the conventional formulation. *However, SINEMET CR (Carbidopa-Levodopa) Sustained-Release is less systemically bioavailable than SINEMET (Carbidopa-Levodopa) and may require increased daily doses to achieve the same level of symptomatic relief as provided by SINEMET (Carbidopa-Levodopa).*
In clinical trials, patients with moderate to severe motor fluctuations who received SINEMET CR *did not experience quantitatively significant reductions* in 'off' time when compared to SINEMET (Carbidopa-Levodopa). However, global ratings of improvement as assessed by both patient and physician were better during therapy with SINEMET CR than with SINEMET (Carbidopa-Levodopa). In patients without motor fluctuations, SINEMET CR, under controlled conditions, provided the same therapeutic benefit with less frequent dosing when compared to SINEMET (Carbidopa-Levodopa).
Pharmacokinetics
Carbidopa reduces the amount of levodopa required to produce a given response by about 75 percent and, when administered with levodopa, increases both plasma levels and the plasma half-life of levodopa, and decreases plasma and urinary dopamine and homovanillic acid.
Elimination half-life of levodopa in the presence of carbidopa is about 1.5 hours. Following SINEMET CR, the apparent half-life of levodopa may be prolonged because of continuous absorption.
In healthy elderly subjects (56–67 years old) the mean time-to-peak concentration of levodopa after a single dose of SINEMET CR 50–200 was about 2 hours as compared to 0.5 hours after standard SINEMET (Carbidopa-Levodopa). The maximum concentration of levodopa after a single dose of SINEMET CR was about 35% of the standard SINEMET (Carbidopa-Levodopa) (1151 vs 3256 ng/mL). The extent of availability of levodopa from SINEMET CR was about 70–75% relative to intravenous levodopa or standard SINEMET (Carbidopa-Levodopa) in the elderly. The absolute bioavailability of levodopa from SINEMET CR (relative to I.V.) in young subjects was shown to be only about 44%. The extent of availability and the peak concentrations of levodopa were comparable in the elderly after a single dose and at steady state after t.i.d. administration of SINEMET CR 50–200. In elderly subjects, the average

Continued on next page

Sinemet CR—Cont.

trough levels of levodopa at steady state after the CR tablet were about 2 fold higher than after the standard SINEMET (Carbidopa-Levodopa) (163 vs 74 ng/mL).
In these studies, using similar total daily doses of levodopa, plasma levodopa concentrations with SINEMET CR fluctuated in a narrower range than with SINEMET (Carbidopa-Levodopa). Because the bioavailability of levodopa from SINEMET CR relative to SINEMET (Carbidopa-Levodopa) is approximately 70–75%, the daily dosage of levodopa necessary to produce a given clinical response with the sustained-release formulation will usually be higher.
The extent of availability and peak concentrations of levodopa after a single dose of SINEMET CR 50–200 increased by about 50% and 25%, respectively, when administered with food.
At steady state, the bioavailability of carbidopa from SINEMET Tablets is approximately 99% relative to the concomitant administration of carbidopa and levodopa. At steady state, carbidopa bioavailability from SINEMET CR 50–200 is approximately 58% relative to that from SINEMET.
Pyridoxine hydrochloride (vitamin B_6), in oral doses of 10 mg to 25 mg, may reverse the effects of levodopa by increasing the rate of aromatic amino acid decarboxylation. Carbidopa inhibits this action of pyridoxine.

INDICATIONS AND USAGE

SINEMET CR is indicated in the treatment of the symptoms of idiopathic Parkinson's disease (paralysis agitans), postencephalitic parkinsonism, and symptomatic parkinsonism which may follow injury to the nervous system by carbon monoxide intoxication and/or manganese intoxication.

CONTRAINDICATIONS

Nonselective MAO inhibitors are contraindicated for use with SINEMET CR. These inhibitors must be discontinued at least two weeks prior to initiating therapy with SINEMET CR. SINEMET CR may be administered concomitantly with the manufacturer's recommended dose of an MAO inhibitor with selectivity for MAO type B (e.g., selegiline HCl) (See PRECAUTIONS, *Drug Interactions*).
SINEMET CR is contraindicated in patients with known hypersensitivity to any component of this drug and in patients with narrow-angle glaucoma.
Because levodopa may activate a malignant melanoma, SINEMET CR should not be used in patients with suspicious, undiagnosed skin lesions or a history of melanoma.

WARNINGS

When patients are receiving levodopa without a decarboxylase inhibitor, levodopa must be discontinued at least twelve hours before SINEMET CR is started. In order to reduce adverse reactions, it is necessary to individualize therapy. SINEMET CR should be substituted at a dosage that will provide approximately 25 percent of the previous levodopa dosage (see DOSAGE AND ADMINISTRATION).
Carbidopa does not decrease adverse reactions due to central effects of levodopa. By permitting more levodopa to reach the brain, particularly when nausea and vomiting is not a dose-limiting factor, certain adverse CNS effects, e.g., dyskinesias, will occur at lower dosages and sooner during therapy with SINEMET CR (Carbidopa-Levodopa) Sustained-Release than with levodopa alone.
Patients receiving SINEMET CR may develop increased dyskinesias compared to SINEMET (Carbidopa-Levodopa). Dyskinesias are a common side effect of carbidopa-levodopa treatment. The occurrence of dyskinesias may require dosage reduction.
As with levodopa, SINEMET CR may cause mental disturbances. These reactions are thought to be due to increased brain dopamine following administration of levodopa. All patients should be observed carefully for the development of depression with concomitant suicidal tendencies. Patients with past or current psychoses should be treated with caution.
SINEMET CR should be administered cautiously to patients with severe cardiovascular or pulmonary disease, bronchial asthma, renal, hepatic or endocrine disease.
As with levodopa, care should be exercised in administering SINEMET CR to patients with a history of myocardial infarction who have residual atrial, nodal, or ventricular arrhythmias. In such patients, cardiac function should be monitored with particular care during the period of initial dosage adjustment, in a facility with provisions for intensive cardiac care.
As with levodopa, treatment with SINEMET CR may increase the possibility of upper gastrointestinal hemorrhage in patients with a history of peptic ulcer.
Neuroleptic Malignant Syndrome (NMS): Sporadic cases of a symptom complex resembling NMS have been reported in association with dose reductions or withdrawal of SINEMET and SINEMET CR.
Therefore, patients should be observed carefully when the dosage of SINEMET CR is reduced abruptly or discontinued, especially if the patient is receiving neuroleptics.
NMS is an uncommon but life-threatening syndrome characterized by fever or hyperthermia. Neurological findings, including muscle rigidity, involuntary movements, altered consciousness, mental status changes; other disturbances, such as autonomic dysfunction, tachycardia, tachypnea, sweating, hyper- or hypotension; laboratory findings, such as creatine phosphokinase elevation, leukocytosis, myoglobinuria, and increased serum myoglobin have been reported.
The early diagnosis of this condition is important for the appropriate management of these patients. Considering NMS as a possible diagnosis and ruling out other acute illnesses (e.g., pneumonia, systemic infection, etc.) is essential. This may be especially complex if the clinical presentation includes both serious medical illness and untreated or inadequately treated extrapyramidal signs and symptoms (EPS). Other important considerations in the differential diagnosis include central anticholinergic toxicity, heat stroke, drug fever, and primary central nervous system (CNS) pathology.
The management of NMS should include: 1) intensive symptomatic treatment and medical monitoring and 2) treatment of any concomitant serious medical problems for which specific treatments are available. Dopamine agonists, such as bromocriptine, and muscle relaxants, such as dantrolene, are often used in the treatment of NMS; however, their effectiveness has not been demonstrated in controlled studies.

PRECAUTIONS

General
As with levodopa, periodic evaluations of hepatic, hematopoietic, cardiovascular, and renal function are recommended during extended therapy.
Patients with chronic wide-angle glaucoma may be treated cautiously with SINEMET CR provided the intraocular pressure is well controlled and the patient is monitored carefully for changes in intraocular pressure during therapy.
Information for Patients
The patient should be informed that SINEMET CR is a sustained-release formulation of carbidopa-levodopa which releases these ingredients over a 4- to 6-hour period. It is important that SINEMET CR be taken at regular intervals according to the schedule outlined by the physician. The patient should be cautioned not to change the prescribed dosage regimen and not to add any additional antiparkinson medications, including other carbidopa-levodopa preparations, without first consulting the physician.
If abnormal involuntary movements appear or get worse during treatment with SINEMET CR, the physician should be notified, as dosage adjustment may be necessary.
Patients should be advised that sometimes the onset of effect of the first morning dose of SINEMET CR may be delayed for up to 1 hour compared with the response usually obtained from the first morning dose of SINEMET (Carbidopa-Levodopa). The physician should be notified if such delayed responses pose a problem in treatment.
Patients should be advised that, occasionally, dark color (red, brown, or black) may appear in saliva, urine, or sweat after ingestion of SINEMET CR. Although the color appears to be clinically insignificant, garments may become discolored.
The patient should be informed that a change in diet to foods that are high in protein may delay the absorption of levodopa and may reduce the amount taken up in the circulation. Excessive acidity also delays stomach emptying, thus delaying the absorption of levodopa. Iron salts (such as in multi-vitamin tablets) may also reduce the amount of levodopa available to the body. The above factors may reduce the clinical effectiveness of the levodopa or carbidopa-levodopa therapy.
Patients must be advised that the whole or half tablet should be swallowed without chewing or crushing.
NOTE: The suggested advice to patients being treated with SINEMET CR is intended to aid in the safe and effective use of this medication. It is not a disclosure of all possible adverse or intended effects.
Laboratory Tests
Abnormalities in laboratory tests may include elevations of liver function tests such as alkaline phosphatase, SGOT (AST), SGPT (ALT), lactic dehydrogenase, and bilirubin. Abnormalities in blood urea nitrogen and positive Coombs test have also been reported. Commonly, levels of blood urea nitrogen, creatinine, and uric acid are lower during administration of carbidopa-levodopa preparations than with levodopa.
Carbidopa-levodopa preparations, such as SINEMET (Carbidopa-Levodopa) and SINEMET CR, may cause a false-positive reaction for urinary ketone bodies when a test tape is used for determination of ketonuria. This reaction will not be altered by boiling the urine specimen. False-negative tests may result with the use of glucose-oxidase methods of testing for glucosuria.
Cases of falsely diagnosed pheochromocytoma in patients on carbidopa-levodopa therapy have been reported very rarely. Caution should be exercised when interpreting the plasma and urine levels of catecholamines and their metabolites in patients on levodopa or carbidopa-levodopa therapy.
Drug Interactions
Caution should be exercised when the following drugs are administered concomitantly with SINEMET CR (Carbidopa-Levodopa) Sustained-Release.
Symptomatic postural hypotension has occurred when carbidopa-levodopa preparations were added to the treatment of patients receiving some antihypertensive drugs. Therefore, when therapy with SINEMET CR is started, dosage adjustment of the antihypertensive drug may be required.
For patients receiving monoamine oxidase (MAO) inhibitors (Type A or B), see CONTRAINDICATIONS. Concomitant therapy with selegiline and carbidopa-levodopa may be associated with severe orthostatic hypotension not attributable to carbidopa-levodopa alone (see CONTRAINDICATIONS).
There have been rare reports of adverse reactions, including hypertension and dyskinesia, resulting from the concomitant use of tricyclic antidepressants and carbidopa-levodopa preparations.
Dopamine D_2 receptor antagonists (e.g., phenothiazines, butyrophenones, risperidone) and isoniazid may reduce the therapeutic effects of levodopa. In addition, the beneficial effects of levodopa in Parkinson's disease have been reported to be reversed by phenytoin and papaverine. Patients taking these drugs with SINEMET CR should be carefully observed for loss of therapeutic response.
Iron salts may reduce the bioavailability of levodopa and carbidopa. The clinical relevance is unclear.
Although metoclopramide may increase the bioavailability of levodopa by increasing gastric emptying, metoclopramide may also adversely affect disease control by its dopamine receptor antagonsitic properties.
Carcinogenesis, Mutagenesis, Impairment of Fertility
In a two-year bioassay of SINEMET (Carbidopa-Levodopa), no evidence of carcinogenicity was found in rats receiving doses of approximately two times the maximum daily human dose of carbidopa and four times the maximum daily human dose of levodopa (equivalent to 8 SINEMET CR tablets).
In reproduction studies with SINEMET (Carbidopa-Levodopa), no effects on fertility were found in rats receiving doses of approximately two times the maximum daily human dose of carbidopa and four times the maximum daily human dose of levodopa (equivalent to 8 SINEMET CR tablets).
Pregnancy
Pregnancy Category C. No teratogenic effects were observed in a study in mice receiving up to 20 times the maximum recommended human dose of SINEMET (Carbidopa-Levodopa). There was a decrease in the number of live pups delivered by rats receiving approximately two times the maximum recommended human dose of carbidopa and approximately five times the maximum recommended human dose of levodopa during organogenesis. SINEMET (Carbidopa-Levodopa) caused both visceral and skeletal malformations in rabbits at all doses and ratios of carbidopa/levodopa tested, which ranged from 10 times/5 times the maximum recommended human dose of carbidopa/levodopa to 20 times/10 times the maximum recommended human dose of carbidopa/levodopa.
There are no adequate or well-controlled studies in pregnant women. It has been reported from individual cases that levodopa crosses the human placental barrier, enters the fetus, and is metabolized. Carbidopa concentrations in fetal tissue appeared to be minimal. Use of SINEMET CR in women of childbearing potential requires that the anticipated benefits of the drug be weighed against possible hazards to mother and child.
Nursing Mothers
It is not known whether this drug is excreted in human milk. Because many drugs are excreted in human milk, caution should be exercised when SINEMET CR is administered to a nursing woman.
Pediatric Use
Safety and effectiveness in pediatric patients have not been established. Use of the drug in patients below the age of 18 is not recommended.

ADVERSE REACTIONS

In controlled clinical trials, patients predominantly with moderate to severe motor fluctuations while on SINEMET (Carbidopa-Levodopa) were randomized to therapy with either SINEMET (Carbidopa-Levodopa) or SINEMET CR. The adverse experience frequency profile of SINEMET CR did not differ substantially from that of SINEMET (Carbidopa-Levodopa), as shown in Table I.

Table I.
Clinical Adverse Experiences Occurring in 1% or Greater of Patients

Adverse Experience	SINEMET CR n=491 %	SINEMET (Carbidopa-Levodopa) n=524 %
Dyskinesia	16.5	12.2
Nausea	5.5	5.7
Hallucinations	3.9	3.2
Confusion	3.7	2.3
Dizziness	2.9	2.3
Depression	2.2	1.3
Urinary tract infection	2.2	2.3
Headache	2.0	1.9
Dream abnormalities	1.8	0.8
Dystonia	1.8	0.8
Vomiting	1.8	1.9
Upper respiratory infection	1.8	1.0
Dyspnea	1.6	0.4
'On-Off' phenomena	1.6	1.1
Back pain	1.6	0.6
Dry mouth	1.4	1.1
Anorexia	1.2	1.1

Diarrhea	1.2	0.6
Insomnia	1.2	1.0
Orthostatic hypotension	1.0	1.1
Shoulder pain	1.0	0.6
Chest pain	1.0	0.8
Muscle cramps	0.8	1.0
Paresthesia	0.8	1.1
Urinary frequency	0.8	1.1
Dyspepsia	0.6	1.1
Constipation	0.2	1.5

Abnormal laboratory findings occurring at a frequency of 1% or greater in approximately 443 patients who received SINEMET CR and 475 who received SINEMET (Carbidopa-Levodopa) during controlled clinical trials included: decreased hemoglobin and hematocrit; elevated serum glucose; white blood cells, bacteria and blood in the urine.

The adverse experiences observed in patients in uncontrolled studies were similar to those seen in controlled clinical studies.

Other adverse experiences reported overall in clinical trials in 748 patients treated with SINEMET CR, listed by body system in order of decreasing frequency, include:

Body as a Whole: Asthenia, fatigue, abdominal pain, orthostatic effects.

Cardiovascular: Palpitation, hypertension, hypotension, myocardial infarction.

Gastrointestinal: Gastrointestinal pain, dysphagia, heartburn.

Metabolic: Weight loss.

Musculoskeletal: Leg pain.

Nervous System/Psychiatric: Chorea, somnolence, falling, anxiety, disorientation, decreased mental acuity, gait abnormalities, extrapyramidal disorder, agitation, nervousness, sleep disorders, memory impairment.

Respiratory: Cough, pharyngeal pain, common cold.

Skin: Rash.

Special Senses: Blurred vision.

Urogenital: Urinary incontinence.

Laboratory Tests: Decreased white blood cell count and serum potassium; increased BUN, serum creatinine and serum LDH; protein and glucose in the urine.

The following adverse experiences have been reported in post-marketing experience with SINEMET CR:

Cardiovascular: Cardiac irregularities, syncope.

Gasstrointestinal: Taste alterations, dark saliva.

Hypersensitivity: Angioedema, urticaria, pruritus, bullous lesions (including pemphigus-like reactions).

Nervous System/Psychiatric: Neuroleptic malignant syndrome (see WARNINGS), increased tremor, peripheral neuropathy, psychotic episodes including delusions and paranoid ideation, increased libido.

Skin: Alopecia, flushing, dark sweat.

Urogenital: Dark urine.

Other adverse reactions that have been reported with levodopa alone and with various carbidopa-levodopa formulations and may occur with SINEMET CR are:

Cardiovascular: Phlebitis.

Gastrointestinal: Gastrointestinal bleeding, development of duodenal ulcer, sialorrhea, bruxism, hiccups, flatulence, burning sensation of tongue.

Hematologic: Hemolytic and nonhemolytic anemia, thrombocytopenia, leukopenia, agranulocytosis.

Hypersensitivity: Henoch-Schonlein purpura.

Metabolic: Weight gain, edema.

Nervous System/Psychiatric: Ataxia, depression with suicidal tendencies, dementia, euphoria, convulsions (however, a causal relationship has not been established); bradykinetic episodes, numbness, muscle twitching, blepharospasm (which may be taken as an early sign of excess dosage; consideration of dosage reduction may be made at this time), trismus, activation of latent Horner's syndrome, nightmares.

Skin: Malignant melanoma (see also CONTRAINDICATIONS), increased sweating.

Special Senses: Oculogyric crises, mydriasis, diplopia.

Urogenital: Urinary retention, priapism.

Miscellaneous: Faintness, hoarseness, malaise, hot flashes, sense of stimulation bizare breathing patterns.

Laboratory Tests: Abnormalities in alkaline phosphatase, SGOT (AST), SGPT (ALT), bilirubin, Coombs test, uric acid.

OVERDOSAGE

Management of acute overdosage with SINEMET CR is the same as with levodopa. Pyridoxine is not effective in reversing the actions of SINEMET CR.

General supportive measures should be employed, along with immediate gastric lavage. Intravenous fluids should be administered judiciously and an adequate airway maintained. Electrocardiographic monitoring should be instituted and the patient carefully observed for the development of arrhythmias; if required, appropriate antiarrhythmic therapy should be given. The possibility that the patient may have taken other drugs as well as SINEMET CR should be taken into consideration. To date, no experience has been reported with dialysis; hence, its value in overdosage is not known.

Based on studies in which high doses of levodopa and/or carbidopa were administered, a significant proportion of rats and mice given single oral doses of levodopa of approximately 1500–2000 mg/kg are expected to die. A significant proportion of infant rats of both sexes are expected to die at a dose of 800 mg/kg. A significant proportion of rats are expected to die after treatment with similar doses of carbidopa. The addition of carbidopa in a 1:10 ratio with levodopa increases the dose at which a significant proportion of mice are expected to die to 3360 mg/kg.

TABLE II
Approximate Bioavailabilities at Steady State†

Tablet	Amount of Levodopa (mg) In Each Tablet	Approximate Bioavailability	Approximate Amount of Bioavailable Levodopa (mg) in Each Tablet
SINEMET CR 50–200	200	0.70–0.75‡	140–150
SINEMET 25–100	100	0.99†††	99

† This table is only a guide to bioavailabilities since other factors such as food, drugs, and inter-patient variabilities may affect the bioavailability of carbidopa and levodopa.

‡ The extent of availability of levodopa from SINEMET CR was about 70–75% relative to intravenous levodopa or standard SINEMET (Carbidopa-Levodopa) in the elderly.

††† The extent of availability of levodopa from SINEMET was 99% relative to intravenous levodopa in the healthy elderly.

Table III
Guidelines for Initial Conversion
from SINEMET (Carbidopa-Levodopa) to SINEMET CR

SINEMET (Carbidopa-Levodopa) Total Daily Dose* Levodopa (mg)	SINEMET CR Suggested Dosage Regimen
300–400	200 mg b.i.d.
500–600	300 mg b.i.d. or 200 mg t.i.d.
700–800	A total of 800 mg in 3 or more divided doses (e.g., 300 mg a.m., 300 mg early p.m., and 200 mg later p.m.)
900–1000	A total of 1000 mg in 3 or more divided doses (e.g., 400 mg a.m., 400 mg early p.m., and 200 mg later p.m.)

*For dosing ranges not shown in the table see DOSAGE AND ADMINISTRATION, *Initial Dosage—Patients currently treated with conventional carbidopa-levodopa preparations.*

DOSAGE AND ADMINISTRATION

SINEMET CR contains carbidopa and levodopa in a 1:4 ratio as either the 50–200 tablet or the 25–100 tablet. The daily dosage of SINEMET CR must be determined by careful titration. Patients should be monitored closely during the dose adjustment period, particularly with regard to appearance or worsening of involuntary movements, dyskinesias or nausea. SINEMET CR 50–200 may be administered as whole or as half-tablets which should not be chewed or crushed. SINEMET CR 25–100 may be used in combination with SINEMET CR 50–200 to titrate to the optimum dosage, or as an alternative to the 50–200 half tablet.

Standard drugs for Parkinson's disease, other than levodopa without a decarboxylase inhibitor, may be used concomitantly while SINEMET CR is being administered, although their dosage may have to be adjusted.

Since carbidopa prevents the reversal of levodopa effects caused by pyridoxine, SINEMET CR can be given to patients receiving supplemental pyridoxine (vitamin B_6).

Initial Dosage

Patients currently treated with conventional carbidopa-levodopa preparations: Studies show that peripheral dopa-decarboxylase is saturated by the bioavailable carbidopa at doses of 70 mg a day and greater. Because the bioavailabilities of carbidopa and levodopa in SINEMET and SINEMET CR are different, appropriate adjustments should be made, as shown in Table II.

[See table II above]

Dosage with SINEMET CR should be substituted at an amount that provides approximately 10% more levodopa per day, although this may need to be increased to a dosage that provides up to 30% more levodopa per day depending on clinical response (see DOSAGE AND ADMINISTRATION, *Titration*). The interval between doses of SINEMET CR should be 4–8 hours during the waking day. (See CLINICAL PHARMACOLOGY, *Pharmacodynamics*.)

A guideline for initiation of SINEMET CR is shown in Table III.

[See table III above]

Patients currently treated with levodopa without a decarboxylase inhibitor: Levodopa must be discontinued at least twelve hours before therapy with SINEMET CR is started. SINEMET CR should be substituted at a dosage that will provide approximately 25% of the previous levodopa dosage. In patients with mild to moderate disease, the initial dose is usually 1 tablet of SINEMET CR 50–200 b.i.d.

Patients not receiving levodopa: In patients with mild to moderate disease, the initial recommended dose is 1 tablet of SINEMET CR 50–200 b.i.d. Initial dosage should not be given at intervals of less than 6 hours.

Titration with SINEMET CR

Following initiation of therapy, doses and dosing intervals may be increased or decreased depending upon therapeutic response. Most patients have been adequately treated with doses of SINEMET CR that provide 400 to 1600 mg of levodopa per day, administered as divided doses at intervals ranging from 4 to 8 hours during the waking day. Higher doses of SINEMET CR (2400 mg or more of levodopa per day) and shorter intervals (less than 4 hours) have been used, but are not usually recommended.

When doses of SINEMET CR are given at intervals of less than 4 hours, and/or if the divided doses are not equal, it is recommended that the smaller doses be given at the end of the day.

An interval of at least 3 days between dosage adjustments is recommended.

Maintenance

Because Parkinson's disease is progressive, periodic clinical evaluations are recommended; adjustment of the dosage regimen of SINEMET CR may be required.

Addition of Other Antiparkinson Medications

Anticholinergic agents, dopamine agonists, and amantadine can be given with SINEMET CR. Dosage adjustment of SINEMET CR may be necessary when these agents are added.

A dose of SINEMET (Carbidopa-Levodopa) 25–100 or 10–100 (one half or a whole tablet) can be added to the dosage regimen of SINEMET CR in selected patients with advanced disease who need additional immediate-release levodopa for a brief time during daytime hours.

Interruption of Therapy

Sporadic cases of a symptom complex resembling Neuroleptic Malignant Syndrome (NMS) have been associated with dose reductions and withdrawal of SINEMET (Carbidopa-Levodopa) or SINEMET CR.

Patients should be observed carefully if abrupt reduction or discontinuation of SINEMET CR is required, especially if the patient is receiving neuroleptics. (See WARNINGS.)

If general anesthesia is required, SINEMET CR may be continued as long as the patient is permitted to take oral medication. If therapy is interrupted temporarily, the patient should be observed for symptoms resembling NMS, and the usual dosage should be administered as soon as the patient is able to take oral medication.

HOW SUPPLIED

SINEMET CR 50–200 (Carbidopa-Levodopa) Sustained-Release Tablets containing 50 mg of carbidopa and 200 mg of levodopa, are peach colored, oval, biconvex, compressed tablets, that are scored and coded 521 on one side and SINEMET CR on the other side. They are supplied as follows:

NDC 0056-0521-68 bottles of 100
NDC 0056-0521-28 unit dose package of 100
NDC 0056-0521-85 bottles of 500.

SINEMET CR 25–100 (Carbidopa-Levodopa) Sustained-Release Tablets containing 25 mg carbidopa and 100 mg of levodopa, are pink colored, oval, biconvex, compressed tablets, that are coded 601 (with bar) on one side and SINEMET CR on the other side. They are supplied as follows:

NDC 0056-0601-68 bottles of 100
NDC 0056-0601-28 unit dose packages of 100
NDC 0056-0601-85 bottles of 500.

Storage

Avoid temperatures above 30°C (86°F). Store in a tightly closed container.

Continued on next page

Sinemet CR—Cont.

Manufactured by:
MERCK & CO., INC.
West Point, PA 19486, USA
For:
DuPont Pharma
Wilmington, Delaware 19880
6351-06 Issued June 1999
Shown in Product Identification Guide, page 311

SUSTIVA™ ℞
(efavirenz) capsules
℞ only

DESCRIPTION

SUSTIVA (efavirenz) is an HIV-1 specific, non-nucleoside, reverse transcriptase inhibitor (NNRTI).

SUSTIVA is available as capsules for oral administration containing either 50 mg, 100 mg, or 200 mg of efavirenz and the following inactive ingredients: lactose monohydrate, magnesium stearate, sodium lauryl sulfate, and sodium starch glycolate. The capsule shell contains the following inactive ingredients and dyes: gelatin, sodium lauryl sulfate, titanium dioxide and/or yellow iron oxide. The capsule shells may also contain silicon dioxide. The capsules are printed with ink containing carmine 40 blue, FD&C Blue No. 2 and titanium dioxide.

Efavirenz is chemically described as (S) -6- chloro-4-(cyclopropylethynyl)-1,4-dihydro-4-(trifluoromethyl)-2H-3,1-benzoxazin-2-one.

Its empirical formula is $C_{14}H_9ClF_3NO_2$ and its structural formula is:

Efavirenz is a white to slightly pink crystalline powder with a molecular mass of 315.68. It is practically insoluble in water (<10 µg/mL).

MICROBIOLOGY

Mechanism of Action: Efavirenz is a non-nucleoside reverse transcriptase (RT) inhibitor of human immunodeficiency virus type 1 (HIV-1). Efavirenz activity is mediated predominantly by non-competitive inhibition of HIV-1 RT. HIV-2 RT and human cellular DNA polymerases alpha, beta, gamma, and delta are not inhibited by efavirenz.

***In vitro* HIV Susceptibility:** The clinical significance of *in vitro* susceptibility of HIV-1 to efavirenz has not been established. The *in vitro* antiviral activity of efavirenz was assessed in lymphoblastoid cell lines, peripheral blood mononuclear cells (PBMCs) and macrophage/monocyte cultures. The 90–95% inhibitory concentration (IC_{90-95}) of efavirenz for wild type laboratory adapted strains and clinical isolates ranged from 1.7 to 25 nM. Efavirenz demonstrated synergistic activity against HIV-1 in cell culture when combined with zidovudine (ZDV), didanosine, or indinavir (IDV).

Resistance: HIV-1 isolates with reduced susceptibility to efavirenz (>380-fold increase in IC_{90}) compared to baseline can emerge *in vitro*. Phenotypic (N=26) changes in evaluable HIV-1 isolates and genotypic (N=104) changes in plasma virus from selected patients treated with efavirenz in combination with IDV, or with ZDV plus lamivudine were monitored. One or more RT mutations at amino acid positions 98, 100, 101, 103, 106, 108, 188, 190 and 225, were observed in 102 of 104 patients with a frequency of at least 9% compared to baseline. The mutation at RT amino acid position 103 (lysine to asparagine) was the most frequently observed (≥90%). A mean loss in susceptibility (IC_{90}) to efavirenz of 47-fold was observed in 26 clinical isolates. Five clinical isolates were evaluated for both genotypic and phenotypic changes from baseline. Decreases in efavirenz susceptibility (range from 9 to >312-fold increase in IC_{90}) were observed for these isolates *in vitro* compared to baseline. All 5 isolates possessed at least one of the efavirenz-associated RT mutations. The clinical relevance of phenotypic and genotypic changes associated with efavirenz therapy is under evaluation.

Cross-Resistance: Rapid emergence of HIV-1 strains that are cross-resistant to non-nucleoside RT inhibitors has been observed *in vitro*. Thirteen clinical isolates previously characterized as efavirenz-resistant were also phenotypically resistant to nevirapine and delavirdine *in vitro* compared to baseline. Clinically derived ZDV-resistant HIV-1 isolates tested *in vitro* retained susceptibility to efavirenz. Cross-resistance between efavirenz and HIV protease inhibitors is unlikely because of the different enzyme targets involved.

CLINICAL PHARMACOLOGY

Pharmacokinetics

Absorption: Peak efavirenz plasma concentrations of 1.6–9.1 µM were attained by 5 hours following single oral doses of 100 mg to 1600 mg administered to uninfected volunteers. Dose-related increases in C_{max} and AUC were seen for doses up to 1600 mg; the increases were less than proportional suggesting diminished absorption at higher doses.

In HIV-infected patients at steady-state, mean C_{max}, mean C_{min}, and mean AUC were dose proportional following 200 mg, 400 mg, and 600 mg daily doses. Time-to-peak plasma concentrations were approximately 3–5 hours and steady-state plasma concentrations were reached in 6–10 days. In 35 patients receiving SUSTIVA 600 mg once daily, steady-state C_{max} was 12.9 ± 3.7 µM (mean ± S.D.), steady-state C_{min} was 5.6 ± 3.2 µM, and AUC was 184 ± 73 µM•h.

Effect of Food on Oral Absorption: In uninfected volunteers, meals of normal composition had no appreciable effect on the bioavailability of 100 mg of an investigational efavirenz formulation administered twice a day for 10 days with meals (Breakfast: 662 kcal, 13.8 g protein, 27.9 g fat, 94.6 g carbohydrate; Dinner: 567 kcal, 44.5 g protein, 12.5 g fat, 73.8 g carbohydrate). The relative bioavailability of a single 1200 mg dose of an investigational efavirenz formulation in uninfected volunteers (N=5) was increased 50% (range 11%–126%) following a high fat meal (1070 kcal, 82 g fat, 69% of calories from fat) (see **DOSAGE AND ADMINISTRATION**).

Distribution: Efavirenz is highly bound (approximately 99.5–99.75%) to human plasma proteins, predominantly albumin. In HIV-1 infected patients (N=9) who received SUSTIVA 200 to 600 mg once daily for at least one month, cerebrospinal fluid concentrations ranged from 0.26 to 1.19% (mean 0.69%) of the corresponding plasma concentration. This proportion is approximately 3-fold higher than the non-protein-bound (free) fraction of efavirenz in plasma.

Metabolism: Studies in humans and *in vitro* studies using human liver microsomes have demonstrated that efavirenz is principally metabolized by the cytochrome P450 system to hydroxylated metabolites with subsequent glucuronidation of these hydroxylated metabolites. These metabolites are essentially inactive against HIV-1. The *in vitro* studies suggest that CYP3A4 and CYP2B6 are the major isozymes responsible for efavirenz metabolism.

Efavirenz has been shown to induce P450 enzymes, resulting in the induction of its own metabolism. Multiple doses of 200–400 mg per day for 10 days resulted in a lower than predicted extent of accumulation (22–42% lower) and a shorter terminal half-life of 40–55 hours (single dose half-life 52–76 hours).

Elimination: Efavirenz has a terminal half-life of 52–76 hours after single doses and 40–55 hours after multiple doses. A one-month mass balance/excretion study was conducted using 400 mg per day with a ^{14}C-labeled dose administered on Day 8. Approximately 14–34% of the radiolabel was recovered in the urine and 16–61% was recovered in the feces. Nearly all of the urinary excretion of the radiolabeled drug was in the form of metabolites. Efavirenz accounted for the majority of the total radioactivity measured in feces.

Special Populations

Hepatic Impairment: The pharmacokinetics of efavirenz have not been adequately studied in patients with hepatic impairment (see **PRECAUTIONS; General**).

Renal Impairment: The pharmacokinetics of efavirenz have not been studied in patients with renal insufficiency; however, less than 1% of efavirenz is excreted unchanged in the urine, so the impact of renal impairment on efavirenz elimination should be minimal.

Gender and Race: The pharmacokinetics of efavirenz in patients appear to be similar between men and women and among the racial groups studied.

Geriatric: see **PRECAUTIONS; *Geriatric Use***

Pediatrics: see **PRECAUTIONS; *Pediatric Use***

Drug Interactions (see also CONTRAINDIATIONS and PRECAUTIONS; Drug Interactions)

Efavirenz has been shown *in vivo* to cause hepatic enzyme induction, thus increasing the biotransformation of some drugs metabolized by CYP3A4. *In vitro* studies have shown that efavirenz inhibited P450 isozymes 2C9, 2C19, and 3A4 with Ki values (8.5–17µM) in the range of observed efavirenz plasma concentrations. In *in vitro* studies, efavirenz did not inhibit CYP2E1 and inhibited CYP2D6 and CYP1A2 (Ki values 82–160 µM) only at concentrations well above those achieved clinically. The effects on CYP3A4 activity are expected to be similar between 200 mg, 400 mg and 600 mg doses of efavirenz. Coadministration of efavirenz with drugs primarily metabolized by 2C9, 2C19 and 3A4 isozymes may result in altered plasma concentrations of the coadministered drug. Drugs which induce CYP3A4 activity would be expected to increase the clearance of efavirenz resulting in lowered plasma concentrations.

Drug interaction studies were performed with efavirenz and other drugs likely to be coadministered or drugs commonly used as probes for pharmacokinetic interaction. The effects of coadministration of efavirenz on the AUC and C_{max} are summarized in Table 1 (effect of efavirenz on other drugs) and Table 2 (effect of other drugs on efavirenz). For information regarding clinical recommendations see **PRECAUTIONS; Drug Interactions.**

[See table 1 at left]
[See table 2 at top of next page]

INDICATIONS AND USAGE

SUSTIVA (efavirenz) in combination with other antiretroviral agents is indicated for the treatment of HIV-1 infection. This indication is based on two clinical trials of at least one year duration that demonstrated prolonged suppression of HIV-RNA.

Table 1
Effect of Efavirenz on Coadministered Drug Plasma C_{max} and AUC

Coadministered Drug:	Dose	Efavirenz Dose	Number of Subjects	Coadministered Drug (% change) C_{max} (mean [90% CI])	AUC (mean [90% CI])
Indinavir	800 mg q8h × 14 days× 14 days	200 mg × 14 days	17	↓ (16%) [–10–35%]	↓ (31%) [13–45%]
Nelfinavir	750 mg q8h × 7 days	600 mg × 7 days	10	↑ (21%) [10–33%]	↑ (20%) [8–34%]
Metabolite AG-1402				↓ (40%) [30–48%]	↓ (37%) [25–48%]
Ritonavir	500 mg q12h × 8 days After AM dose	600 mg × 10 days	11	↑ (24%) [12–38%]	↑ (18%) [6–33%]
	After PM dose			↔	↔
Saquinavir SGC*	1200 mg q8h × 10 days	600 mg × 10 days	12	↓ (50%) [28–66%]	↓ (62%) [45–74%]
Lamivudine	150 mg q12h × 14 days	600 mg × 14 days	9	↔	↔
Zidovudine	300 mg q12h × 14 days	600 mg × 14 days	9	↔	↔
Azithromycin	600 mg single dose	400 mg × 7 days	14	↑ (22%) [4–42%]	↔
Clarithromycin	500 mg q12h × 7 days	400 mg × 7 days	11	↓ (26%) [15–35%]	↓ (39%) [30–46%]
14-OH metabolite				↑ (49%) [32–69%]	↑ (34%) [18–53%]
Fluconazole	200 mg × 7 days	400 mg × 7 days	10	↔	↔
Ethinyl Estradiol	50 µg single dose	400 mg × 10 days	13	↔	↑ (37%) [25–51%]

↑ Indicates increase ↓ Indicates decrease ↔ Indicates no change
* Soft Gelatin Capsule

Continued on next page

Description of Studies

In the two principle studies described below (Study 006 and ACTG 364), the response was measured as the time to treatment failure (TTF). Plasma HIV-RNA levels were quantified using the AMPLICOR HIV-1 RNA MONITOR™ (assay limit 400 copies/mL in Study 006 and 500 copies/mL in ACTG 364).

Study 006, an ongoing, randomized, open-label trial, compares SUSTIVA (600 mg once daily) + indinavir (IDV, 1000 mg q8h) or SUSTIVA (600 mg once daily) + zidovudine (ZDV, 300 mg q12h) + lamivudine (LAM, 150 mg q12h) with indinavir (800 mg q8h) + zidovudine (300 mg q12h) + lamivudine (150 mg q12h). Twelve-hundred sixty-six patients (mean age 36.5 years [range 18–81], 60% Caucasian, 83% male) were enrolled. All patients were efavirenz, lamivudine, NNRTI-, and PI-naive at study entry. The mean baseline CD4 cell count was 341 cells/mm^3 and the mean baseline HIV-RNA level was 60,250 copies/mL. There was no significant difference in mean CD4 cell count among the treatment groups; the overall mean increase was approximately 200 cells at 48 weeks among patients who continued on study regimens. Treatment response and outcomes through 48 weeks are shown in Figure 1 and Table 3, respectively.

[See figure 1 at right]

[See table 3 at top of next page]

In addition to the complete 48-week follow-up data reported above, longer-term data are shown in Figure 2. This analysis allows for the inclusion of data beyond 48 weeks as Kaplan-Meier estimates by accounting for patients who have not reached 112 weeks of follow-up.

[See figure 2 on next page]

ACTG 364 is a randomized, double-blind, placebo-controlled 48-week study in NRTI-experienced patients who had completed two prior ACTG studies. One-hundred and ninety-six patients (mean age 41 years [range 18–76], 74% Caucasian, 88% male) received NRTIs in combination with SUSTIVA (efavirenz) (600 mg once daily), or nelfinavir (NFV, 750 mg TID), or SUSTIVA (600 mg once daily) + nelfinavir in a randomized double-blinded manner. The mean baseline CD4 cell count was 389 cells/mm^3 and mean baseline HIV-RNA level was 8,130 copies/mL. Upon entry into the study, all patients were assigned a new open label NRTI regimen, which was dependent on their previous NRTI treatment experience. There was no significant difference in the mean CD4 cell count among treatment groups; the overall mean increase was approximately 100 cells at 48 weeks among patients who continued on study regimens. Treatment response and outcomes are shown in Figure 3 and Table 4, respectively.

[See figure 3 on next page]

[See table 4 on next page]

In addition to the complete 48-week data reported above, longer-term data are shown in Figure 4. This analysis allows for the inclusion of data beyond 48 weeks as Kaplan-Meier estimates by accounting for patients who have not reached 72 weeks of follow-up.

[See figure 4 at top of page 1157]

CONTRAINDICATIONS

SUSTIVA (efavirenz) is contraindicated in patients with clinically significant hypersensitivity to any of its components.

SUSTIVA should not be administered concurrently with astemizole, cisapride, midazolam, triazolam, or ergot derivatives because competition for CYP3A4 by efavirenz could result in inhibition of metabolism of these drugs and create the potential for serious and/or life-threatening adverse events (e.g., cardiac arrhythmias, prolonged sedation or respiratory depression).

WARNINGS

SUSTIVA must not be used as a single agent to treat HIV or added on as a sole agent to a failing regimen. As with all other non-nucleoside reverse transcriptase inhibitors, resistant virus emerges rapidly when efavirenz is administered as monotherapy. The choice of new antiretroviral agents to be used in combination with efavirenz should take into consideration the potential for viral cross-resistance.

Psychiatric Symptoms: Serious psychiatric adverse experiences have been reported in patients treated with SUSTIVA. In controlled trials of 1,008 patients treated with regimens containing SUSTIVA and 635 patients treated with control regimens, the frequency of specific serious psychiatric events among patients who received SUSTIVA or control regimens, respectively, were: severe depression (0.9%, 0.5%), suicidal ideation/attempts (0.5%, 0.3%), aggressive behavior (0.3%, 0.3%), paranoid reactions (0.2%, 0.2%) and manic reactions (0.1%, 0%). Patients with a prior history of psychiatric disorders appear to be at greater risk for these serious psychiatric adverse experiences, with the frequency of each of the above events approximating 1%. There have also been occasional post-marketing reports of death by suicide, delusions and psychosis-like behavior, although a causal relationship to the use of SUSTIVA cannot be determined from these reports. Patients with serious psychiatric adverse experiences should seek immediate medical evaluation to assess the possibility that the symptoms may be related to the use of SUSTIVA, and if so, to determine whether the risks of continued therapy outweigh the benefits (see **ADVERSE REACTIONS**).

Nervous System Symptoms: Fifty-three percent of patients receiving SUSTIVA in controlled trials reported central nervous system symptoms compared to 25% of patients receiving control regimens. These symptoms included, but were not limited to, dizziness (28.1%), insomnia (16.3%), impaired concentration (8.3%), somnolence (7.0%), abnormal dreams (6.2%) and hallucinations (1.2%). These symptoms were severe in 2.0% of patients and 2.1% of patients discontinued therapy as a result. These symptoms usually begin during the first or second day of therapy and generally resolve after the first 2–4 weeks of therapy. After 4 weeks of therapy, the prevalence of nervous system symptoms of at least moderate severity ranged from 5–9% in patients treated with regimens containing SUSTIVA and from 3–5% in patients treated with a control regimen. Patients should be informed that these common symptoms were likely to improve with continued therapy and were not predictive of subsequent onset of the less frequent psychiatric symptoms (see **WARNINGS**; **Psychiatric Symptoms**). Dosing at bedtime improves the tolerability of these nervous system symptoms and is recommended during the first weeks of therapy and for patients who continue to experience these symptoms (see **ADVERSE REACTIONS**).

Patients receiving SUSTIVA should be alerted to the potential for additive central nervous system effects when SUSTIVA is used concomitantly with alcohol or psychoactive drugs.

Patients who experience central nervous system symptoms such as dizziness, impaired concentration and/or drowsiness should avoid potentially hazardous tasks such as driving or operating machinery.

Reproductive Risk Potential: Malformations have been observed in fetuses from efavirenz-treated monkeys that received doses which resulted in plasma drug concentrations similar to those in humans given 600 mg/day (see **PRECAUTIONS**; ***Pregnancy***); therefore, pregnancy should be avoided in women receiving SUSTIVA. Barrier contraception should always be used in combination with other methods of contraception (e.g., oral and or other hormonal contraceptives). Women of childbearing potential should undergo pregnancy testing prior to initiation of SUSTIVA.

Table 2
Effect of Coadministered Drug on Efavirenz Plasma C_{max} and AUC

Coadministered Drug:	Dose	Efavirenz Dose	Number of Subjects	Efavirenz (% change) C_{max} (mean [90% CI])	AUC (mean [90% CI])
Indinavir	800 mg q8h × 14 days	200 mg × 14 days	11	↔	↔
Nelfinavir	750 mg q8h × 7 days	600 mg × 7 days	10	↔	↔
Ritonavir	500 mg q12h × 8 days	600 mg × 10 days	9	↑ (14%) [4–26%]	↑ (21%) [10–34%]
Saquinavir SGC*	1200 mg q8h × 10 days	600 mg × 10 days	13	↓ (13%) [5–20%]	↓ (12%) [4–19%]
Rifampin	600 mg ×7 days	600 mg × 7 days	12	↓ (20%) [11–28%]	↓ (26%) [15–36%]
Azithromycin	600 mg single dose	400 mg × 7 days	14	↔	↔
Clarithromycin	500 mg q12h × 7 days	400 mg × 7 days	12	↑ (11%) [3–19%]	↔
Fluconazole	200 mg × 7 days	400 mg × 7 days	10	↔	↑ (16%) [6–26%]
Famotidine	40 mg single dose	400 mg single dose	17	↔	↔
Mylanta DS**	30 mL single dose	400 mg single dose	17	↔	↔
Ethinyl Estradiol	50 μg single dose	400 mg × 10 days	13	↔	↔

↑ Indicates increase ↓ Indicates decrease ↔ Indicates no change
* Soft Gelatin Capsule
** Contains aluminum hydroxide 400 mg, magnesium hydroxide 400 mg, plus simethicone 40 mg

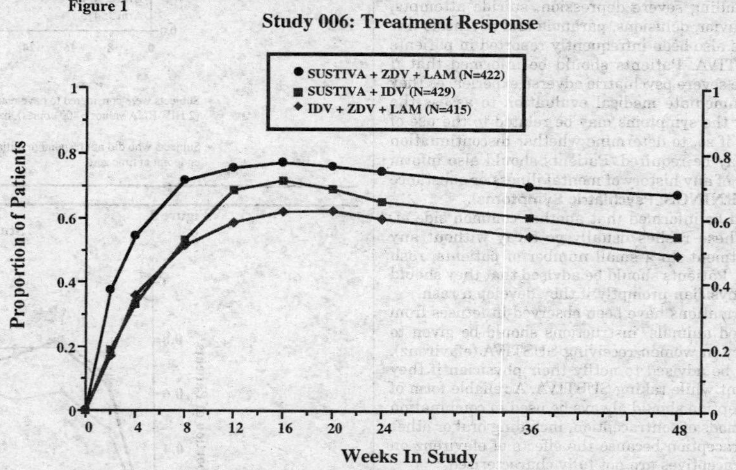

• Proportion of patients at each time point who have HIV-RNA <400 copies, are on their original study medication, and who have not experienced an AIDS-defining event.

PRECAUTIONS

General

Skin Rash: In controlled clinical trials, 26% (266/1008) of patients treated with 600 mg SUSTIVA experienced new onset skin rash compared with 17% (111/635) of patients treated in control groups. Rash associated with blistering, moist desquamation, or ulceration occurred in 0.9% (9/1008) of patients treated with SUSTIVA. The incidence of Grade 4 rash (e.g., erythema multiforme, Stevens-Johnson Syndrome) in patients treated with SUSTIVA in all studies and expanded access was 0.1%. The median time to onset of rash in adults was 11 days and the median duration, 16 days. The discontinuation rate for rash in clinical trials was 1.7% (17/1008). SUSTIVA should be discontinued in patients developing severe rash associated with blistering, desquamation, mucosal involvement or fever. Appropriate antihistamines and/or corticosteroids may improve the tolerability and hasten the resolution of rash.

Rash was reported in 23 of 57 pediatric patients (40%) treated with SUSTIVA. Two pediatric patients experienced Grade 3 rash (one confluent rash with fever; one urticaria), and two patients had Grade 4 rash (erythema multiforme). The median time to onset of rash in pediatric patients was eight days. Prophylaxis with appropriate antihistamines prior to initiating therapy with SUSTIVA in pediatric patients should be considered (see **ADVERSE REACTIONS**).

Liver Enzymes: In patients with known or suspected history of Hepatitis B or C infection and in patients treated with other medications associated with liver toxicity, monitoring of liver enzymes is recommended. In patients with persistent elevations of serum transaminases to greater than 5 times the upper limit of the normal range, the benefit of continued therapy with SUSTIVA needs to be weighed

Continued on next page

Sustiva—Cont.

against the unknown risks of significant liver toxicity (see **ADVERSE REACTIONS; Laboratory Abnormalities**).

Because of the extensive cytochrome P450-mediated metabolism of efavirenz and limited clinical experience in patients with hepatic impairment, caution should be exercised in administering SUSTIVA to these patients.

Cholesterol: Monitoring of cholesterol and triglycerides should be considered in patients treated with SUSTIVA (see **ADVERSE REACTIONS**).

Information for Patients

Patients should be informed that SUSTIVA is not a cure for HIV infection and that they may continue to develop opportunistic infections and other complications associated with HIV disease. Patients should be told that there are currently no data demonstrating that SUSTIVA therapy can reduce the risk of transmitting HIV to others through sexual contact or blood contamination.

Patients should be advised to take SUSTIVA every day as prescribed. SUSTIVA must always be used in combination with other antiretroviral drugs. Patients should remain under the care of a physician while taking SUSTIVA.

Patients should be informed that central nervous system symptoms including dizziness, insomnia, impaired concentration, drowsiness and abnormal dreams are commonly reported during the first weeks of therapy with SUSTIVA. Dosing at bedtime improves the tolerability of these symptoms, and these symptoms are likely to improve with continued therapy. Patients should be alerted to the potential for additive central nervous system effects when SUSTIVA is used concomitantly with alcohol or psychoactive drugs. Patients should be instructed that if they experience these symptoms they should avoid potentially hazardous tasks such as driving or operating machinery (see **WARNINGS; Nervous System Symptoms**). In clinical trials, patients who develop central nervous system symptoms were not more likely to subsequently develop psychiatric symptoms (see **WARNINGS; Psychiatric Symptoms**).

Patients should also be informed that serious psychiatric symptoms including severe depression, suicide attempts, aggressive behavior, delusions, paranoia and psychosis-like symptoms have also been infrequently reported in patients receiving SUSTIVA. Patients should be informed that if they experience severe psychiatric adverse experiences they should seek immediate medical evaluation to assess the possibility that the symptoms may be related to the use of SUSTIVA, and if so, to determine whether discontinuation of SUSTIVA may be required. Patients should also inform their physician of any history of mental illness or substance abuse (see **WARNINGS; Psychiatric Symptoms**).

Patients should be informed that another common side effect is rash. These rashes usually go away without any change in treatment. In a small number of patients, rash may be serious. Patients should be advised that they should contact their physician promptly if they develop a rash.

Because malformations have been observed in fetuses from efavirenz-treated animals, instructions should be given to avoid pregnancy in women receiving SUSTIVA (efavirenz). Women should be advised to notify their physician if they become pregnant while taking SUSTIVA. A reliable form of barrier contraception should always be used in combination with other methods of contraception, including oral or other hormonal contraception because the effects of efavirenz on hormonal contraceptives are not fully characterized.

SUSTIVA may interact with some drugs; therefore, patients should be advised to report the use of any prescription or non-prescription medication to their physician.

High fat meals may increase the absorption of SUSTIVA and should be avoided. SUSTIVA may be taken with meals of normal fat content (see **CLINICAL PHARMACOLOGY; *Effect of Food on Oral Absorption***).

Drug Interactions (see also CONTRAINDICATIONS and CLINICAL PHARMACOLOGY; Drug Interactions)

Efavirenz has been shown *in vivo* to induce CYP3A4. Other compounds that are substrates of CYP3A4 may have decreased plasma concentrations when coadministered with SUSTIVA. *In vitro* studies have demonstrated that efavirenz inhibits 2C9, 2C19 and 3A4 isozymes in the range of observed efavirenz plasma concentrations. Coadministration of efavirenz with drugs primarily metabolized by these isozymes may result in altered plasma concentrations of the coadministered drug. Therefore, appropriate dose adjustments may be necessary for these drugs.

Drugs which induce CYP3A4 activity (e.g., phenobarbital, rifampin, rifabutin) would be expected to increase the clearance of efavirenz resulting in lowered plasma concentrations. Drug interactions with SUSTIVA are summarized in Table 5.

[See table 5 on next page]

Concomitant Antiretroviral Agents:

Nelfinavir: The AUC and C_{max} of nelfinavir (750 mg q8h) are increased by 20% and 21%, respectively when given with SUSTIVA in uninfected volunteers. No dose adjustment is necessary when nelfinavir is administered in combination with SUSTIVA.

Indinavir: When indinavir (800 mg every 8 hours) was given with SUSTIVA (200 mg), the indinavir AUC and C_{max} were decreased by approximately 31% and 16%, respectively as a result of enzyme induction. Therefore, the dose of indinavir should be increased from 800 mg to 1000 mg every 8 hours when SUSTIVA and indinavir are coadministered. No adjustment of the dose of SUSTIVA is necessary when given with indinavir.

Table 3 Study 006 - Outcomes of Randomized Treatment Through 48 Weeks

Outcome	SUSTIVA +ZDV+LAM N=422	SUSTIVA +IDV N=429	IDV +ZDV+LAM N=415
HIV-RNA <400 copies/mL (<50† copies/mL)	68% (62%)	55% (49%)	49% (43%)
HIV-RNA ≥400 copies/mL ††	6%	14%	11%
CDC Category C Event ††	3%	2%	2%
Discontinuations for Adverse Events ††*	8%	8%	17%
Discontinuations for Other Reasons ††**	15%	22%	21%

† Ultrasensitive HIV-1 MONITOR™ assay
†† These rates reflect events that were counted as the initial reason for treatment failure in the analysis.
* See **ADVERSE RECTIONS** for a description of the safety profile of these regimens.
**Consent withdrawn, lost to follow-up, missing data or protocol violation

Figure 2

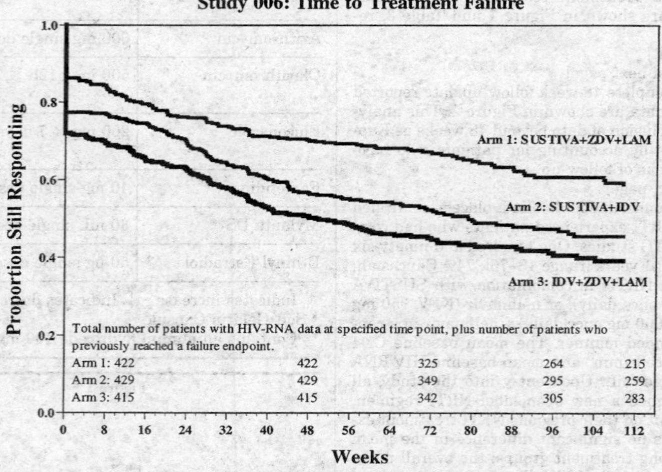

- Subjects were considered to have reached the study endpoint at the first time they either experienced virologic rebound (2 HIV-RNA values ≥400 copies), had an AIDS-defining clinical event, or discontinued study medication.
- Subjects who did not respond to initial treatment (no HIV-RNA values <400 copies) were considered to have reached this endpoint at time zero.

Figure 3

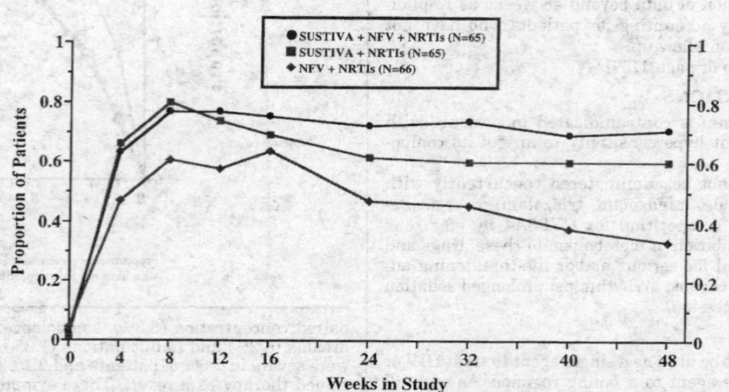

- Proportion of patients at each time point who have HIV-RNA <500 copies, are on their original study medication, and who have not experienced an AIDS-defining event.

Table 4 Study ACTG 364 - Outcomes of Randomized Treatment Through 48 Weeks

Outcome	SUSTIVA+NFV +NRTIs N=65	SUSTIVA +NRTIs N=65	NFV +NRTIs N=66
HIV-RNA <500 copies/mL	71%	60%	33%
HIV-RNA ≥500 copies/mL ††	17%	37%	62%
CDC Category C event ††	2%	0%	0%
Discontinuations for Adverse Events ††*	3%	3%	5%
Discontinuations for Other Reasons ††**	8%	0%	0%

†† These rates reflect events that were counted as the initial reason for treatment failure in the analysis.
* See **ADVERSE RECTIONS** for a description of the safety profile of these regimens.
**Consent withdrawn, lost to follow-up, missing data or protocol violation

Ritonavir: When SUSTIVA and ritonavir 500 mg (given every 12 hours) were studied in uninfected volunteers, the AUC for each drug was increased by approximately 20%. The combination was associated with a higher frequency of adverse clinical experiences (e.g., dizziness, nausea, paresthesia) and laboratory abnormalities (elevated liver enzymes). Monitoring of liver enzymes is recommended when SUSTIVA is used in combination with ritonavir.

Saquinavir: When saquinavir soft gelatin capsules (1200 mg q8h) were given with SUSTIVA to uninfected volunteers, saquinavir AUC and C_{max} were decreased by 62% and 50%, respectively. Use of SUSTIVA in combination with saquinavir as the sole protease inhibitor is not recommended.

Saquinavir/Ritonavir: No pharmacokinetic data are available on the potential interactions of SUSTIVA with the combination of saquinavir and ritonavir.

Amprenavir: SUSTIVA has the potential to decrease serum concentrations of amprenavir.

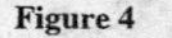

Figure 4

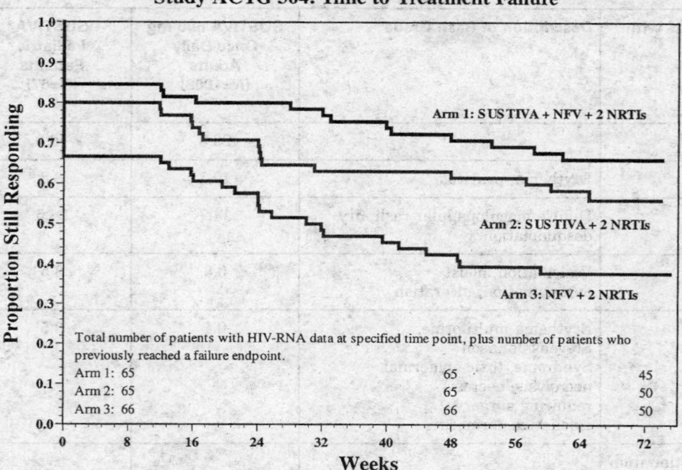

- Subjects were considered to have reached the study endpoint at the first time they either experienced virologic rebound (2 HIV-RNA values ≥500 copies), had an AIDS-defining clinical event, or discontinued study medication.
- Subjects who did not respond to initial treatment (no HIV-RNA values ≤500 copies) were considered to have reached this endpoint at time zero.
- The initial plateaus through Week 12 are due to the virologic testing schedule and the lack of dropouts during this interval.

Table 5*
Drugs That Should Not Be Coadministered With SUSTIVA

Drug Class	Drugs Within Class Not To Be Coadministered with SUSTIVA
Antihistamines	Astemizole
Benzodiazepines	midazolam, triazolam
GI Motility Agents	Cisapride
Anti-Migraine	ergot derivatives
Drugs That Require A Dose Adjustment When Coadministered With SUSTIVA	
Drug Class	**Drug Within Class Requiring Dose Increase**
Anti-HIV Protease Inhibitor	indinavir (increase dose from 800 mg to 1000 mg every 8 hours)
Other Potentially Clinically Significant Drug Interactions With SUSTIVA	
Anticoagulants: Warfarin	Plasma concentrations and effects potentially increased or decreased by SUSTIVA
Anti-HIV Protease Inhibitor: Saquinavir	Plasma concentrations decreased by SUSTIVA; should not be used as sole protease inhibitor in combination with SUSTIVA
Antimycobacterial Agents	
Clarithromycin	Plasma concentrations decreased by SUSTIVA; clinical significance unknown
Rifabutin	Effects unknown
Rifampin	Decreases efavirenz plasma concentrations; clinical significance unknown
Estrogens: Ethinyl Estradiol	Plasma concentrations increased by SUSTIVA; clinical significance unknown

* See Tables 1 and 2.

Table 6
Percent of Patients with One or More Selected Nervous System Symptoms[1,2]

Percent of Patients with:	SUSTIVA 600 mg Once Daily (N=1008)	Control Groups (N=635)
	%	%
Symptoms of Any Severity	52.7	24.6
Mild Symptoms[3]	33.3	15.6
Moderate Symptoms[4]	17.4	7.7
Severe Symptoms[5]	2.0	1.3
Treatment discontinuation as a result of symptoms	2.1	1.1

[1] Includes events reported regardless of causality.
[2] Data from Study 006 and three Phase 2/3 studies.
[3] "Mild" = Symptoms which do not interfere with patient's daily activities.
[4] "Moderate" = Symptoms which may interfere with daily activities.
[5] "Severe" = Events which interrupt patient's usual daily activities.

Nucleoside Analogue Reverse Transcriptase Inhibitors: Studies of the interaction between SUSTIVA and the combination of zidovudine (300 mg q12h) and lamivudine (150 mg q12h) were performed in HIV-infected patients. No clinically significant pharmacokinetic interactions were observed. Specific drug interaction studies have not been performed with SUSTIVA and other NRTIs. Clinically significant interactions would not be expected since the NRTIs are metabolized via a different route than efavirenz and would be unlikely to compete for the same metabolic enzymes and elimination pathways.

Non-Nucleoside Reverse Transcriptase Inhibitors: No studies have been performed with SUSTIVA in combination with other NNRTIs.

Antimicrobial Agents:

Rifamycins: Rifampin (600 mg daily) reduced efavirenz AUC by 26% and C_{max} by 20% in 12 uninfected volunteers. The clinical significance of the reduced efavirenz levels is not known. No dose adjustment of rifampin is recommended when given with SUSTIVA. Rifabutin has not been studied in combination with SUSTIVA; however, there is a potential for an interaction.

Macrolide Antibiotics:

Azithromycin: Coadministration of single 600 mg doses of azithromycin and multiple doses of SUSTIVA in uninfected volunteers did not result in any clinically significant pharmacokinetic interaction. No dosage adjustment is necessary when azithromycin is given in combination with SUSTIVA.

Clarithromycin: Coadministration of SUSTIVA with clarithromycin given as 500 mg every 12 hours for seven days resulted in a significant effect of efavirenz on the pharmacokinetics of clarithromycin. The AUC and C_{max} of clarithromycin decreased 39% and 26%, respectively, while the AUC and C_{max} of the clarithromycin hydroxymetabolite were increased 34% and 49%, respectively, when used in combination with SUSTIVA. The clinical significance of these changes in clarithromycin plasma levels is not known. In uninfected volunteers, 46% developed rash while receiving SUSTIVA and clarithromycin. No dose adjustment of SUSTIVA is recommended when given with clarithromycin. Alternatives to clarithromycin, such as azithromycin, should be considered.

Other macrolide antibiotics, such as erythromycin, have not been studied in combination with SUSTIVA.

Antifungal Agents:

No clinically significant pharmacokinetic interactions were seen when fluconazole (200 mg daily) and SUSTIVA were coadministered to uninfected volunteers. No dosage adjustment is necessary when the two drugs are used in combination. The potential for drug interactions with SUSTIVA and other imidazole and triazole antifungals, such as itraconazole and ketoconazole, has not been studied.

Other Drug Interactions:

Antacids/famotidine: Neither aluminum/magnesium hydroxide antacids (30 mL single dose) nor famotidine (40 mg single dose) altered the absorption of efavirenz in uninfected volunteers. These data suggest that alteration of gastric pH by other drugs would not be expected to affect efavirenz absorption.

Oral Contraceptives (ethinyl estradiol): Only the ethinyl estradiol component of oral contraceptives has been studied in combination with SUSTIVA. The AUC following a single dose of 50 µg ethinyl estradiol was increased (37%) by efavirenz. No significant changes were observed in C_{max} of ethinyl estradiol. The clinical significance of these effects is not known. No effect of a single dose of ethinyl estradiol on efavirenz C_{max} or AUC was observed. Because the potential interaction of efavirenz with oral contraceptives has not been fully characterized, a reliable method of barrier contraception should be used in addition to oral contraceptives.

Carcinogenesis, Mutagenesis and Impairment of Fertility:

Long-term carcinogenicity studies of efavirenz in rats and mice are in progress.

Efavirenz was not mutagenic or genotoxic in *in vitro* and *in vivo* genotoxicity assays which included bacterial mutation assays in *S. typhimurium* and *E. coli*, mammalian mutation assays in Chinese Hamster Ovary cells, chromosomal aberration assays in human peripheral blood lymphocytes or Chinese Hamster Ovary cells, and an *in vivo* mouse bone marrow micronucleus assay.

Efavirenz did not impair mating or fertility of male or female rats, and did not affect sperm of treated male rats. The reproductive performance of offspring born to female rats given efavirenz was not affected. As a result of the rapid clearance of efavirenz in rats, systemic drug exposures achieved in these studies were equivalent to or below those achieved in humans given therapeutic doses of efavirenz.

Pregnancy:

Pregnancy Category C: Malformations have been observed in 3 of 20 fetuses/infants from efavirenz-treated cynomolgus monkeys (versus 0 of 20 concomitant controls) in a developmental toxicity study. The pregnant monkeys were dosed throughout pregnancy (post coital days 20–150) with efavirenz 60 mg/kg daily, a dose which resulted in plasma drug concentrations similar to those in humans given 600 mg/day of SUSTIVA (efavirenz). Anencephaly and unilateral anophthalmia were observed in one fetus, microphthalmia was observed in another fetus, and cleft palate was observed in a third fetus. Efavirenz crosses the placenta in cynomolgus monkeys and produces fetal blood concentrations similar to maternal blood concentrations. Because teratogenic effects have been seen in primates at efavirenz exposures similar to those seen in the clinic at the recommended dose, pregnancy should be avoided in women receiving SUSTIVA. Barrier contraception should always be used in combination with other methods of contraception (e.g., oral or other hormonal contraceptives). Women of childbearing potential should undergo pregnancy testing prior to initiation of SUSTIVA (see **WARNINGS; Reproductive Risk Potential**).

Efavirenz has been shown to cross the placenta in rats and rabbits and produces fetal blood concentrations of efavirenz similar to maternal concentrations. An increase in fetal resorptions was observed in rats at efavirenz doses that produced peak plasma concentrations and AUC values in female rats equivalent to, or lower than those achieved in humans given 600 mg once daily of SUSTIVA. Efavirenz produced no reproductive toxicities when given to pregnant rabbits at doses that produced peak plasma concentrations similar to, and AUC values approximately half of those achieved in humans given 600 mg once daily of SUSTIVA. There are no adequate and well-controlled studies in pregnant women. SUSTIVA should be used during pregnancy

Continued on next page

Sustiva—Cont.

only if the potential benefit justifies the potential risk to the fetus, such as in pregnant women without other therapeutic options.

Antiretroviral Pregnancy Registry: To monitor fetal outcomes of pregnant women exposed to SUSTIVA, an Antiretroviral Pregnancy Registry has been established. Physicians are encouraged to register patients by calling (800) 258-4263.

Nursing Mothers:
The Centers for Disease Control and Prevention recommend that HIV-infected mothers not breast-feed their infants to avoid risking postnatal transmission of HIV infection. Studies in rats have demonstrated that efavirenz is excreted in milk. Mothers should be instructed not to breast-feed if they are receiving SUSTIVA.

Pediatric Use:
ACTG 382 is an ongoing open-label 48-week study in 57 NRTI-experienced pediatric patients to characterize the safety, pharmacokinetics, and antiviral activity of SUSTIVA in combination with nelfinavir (20–30 mg/kg TID) and NRTIs. Mean age was 8 years (range 3–16). SUSTIVA has not been studied in pediatric patients below 3 years of age or who weigh less than 13 Kg. The type and frequency of adverse experiences was generally similar to that of adult patients with the exception of a higher incidence of rash which was reported in 40% (23/57) of pediatric patients compared to 26% of adults, and a higher frequency of Grade 3 or 4 rash reported in 7% (4/57) of pediatric patients compared to 0.9% of adults (see **ADVERSE REACTIONS; Table 7**).
The starting dose of SUSTIVA was 600 mg once daily adjusted to body size, based on weight, targeting AUC levels in the range of 190–380 μM•h. The pharmacokinetics of efavirenz in pediatric patients were similar to the pharmacokinetics in adults who received 600 mg daily doses of SUSTIVA. In 48 pediatric patients receiving the equivalent of a 600 mg dose of SUSTIVA, steady-state C_{max} was 14.2±5.8 μM (mean ± S.D.), steady-state C_{min} was 5.6 ± 4.1 μM, and AUC was 218 ± 104 μM•h.

Geriatric Use:
Clinical studies of SUSTIVA did not include sufficient numbers of subjects aged 65 and over to determine whether they respond differently from younger subjects. In general, dose selection for an elderly patient should be cautious, reflecting the greater frequency of decreased hepatic, renal, or cardiac function and of concomitant disease or other therapy.

ADVERSE REACTIONS

The most significant adverse events observed in patients treated with SUSTIVA are nervous system symptoms, psychiatric symptoms, and rash.

Nervous System Symptoms: Fifty-three percent of patients receiving SUSTIVA reported central nervous system symptoms (see **WARNINGS; Nervous System Symptoms**). Table 6 lists the frequency of the symptoms of different degrees of severity, and gives the discontinuation rates, in clinical trials for one or more of the following nervous system symptoms: dizziness, insomnia, impaired concentration, somnolence, abnormal dreaming, euphoria, confusion, agitation, amnesia, hallucinations, stupor, abnormal thinking, and depersonalization. The frequencies of specific central and peripheral nervous system symptoms are provided in Table 8.
[See table 6 on previous page]

Psychiatric Symptoms: Serious psychiatric adverse experiences have been reported in patients treated with SUSTIVA. In controlled trials the frequency of specific serious psychiatric symptoms among patients who received SUSTIVA or control regimens, respectively, were: severe depression (0.9%, 0.5%), suicidal ideation or attempts (0.5%, 0.3%), aggressive behavior (0.3%, 0.3%), paranoid reactions (0.2%, 0.2%) and manic reactions (0.1%, 0%) (see **WARNINGS; Psychiatric Symptoms**). Additional psychiatric symptoms observed at a frequency of >2% among patients treated with SUSTIVA or control regimens, respectively, in controlled clinical trials were depression (10.0%, 8.2%), anxiety (8.2%, 5.5%), and nervousness (5.9%, 1.9%).

Skin Rash: Rashes are usually mild-to-moderate maculopapular skin eruptions that occur within the first two weeks of initiating therapy with SUSTIVA. In most patients, rash resolves with continuing SUSTIVA therapy within one month. SUSTIVA can be reinitiated in patients interrupting therapy because of rash. Use of appropriate antihistamines and/or corticosteroids may be considered when SUSTIVA is restarted. SUSTIVA should be discontinued in patients developing severe rash associated with blistering, desquamation, mucosal involvement or fever. The frequency of rash by NCI grade and the discontinuation rates as a result of rash are provided in Table 7.
[See table 7 above]

Table 7
Percent of Patients with Treatment-Emergent Rash[1,2]

Percent of Patients with:	Description of Rash Grade[3]	SUSTIVA 600 mg Once Daily Adults (N=1008) %	SUSTIVA Pediatric Patients (N=57) %	Control Groups Adults (N=635) %
Rash of Any Grade		26.3	40.3	17.5
Grade 1 Rash	Erythema, pruritus	10.7	8.8	9.8
Grade 2 Rash	Diffuse maculopapular rash, dry desquamation	14.7	24.5	7.4
Grade 3 Rash	Vesiculation, moist desquamation, ulceration	0.8	3.5	0.3
Grade 4 Rash	Erythema multiforme, Stevens-Johnson Syndrome, toxic epidermal necrolysis, necrosis requiring surgery, exfoliative dermatitis	0.1	3.5	0.0
Treatment discontinuation as a result of rash	—	1.7	8.8	0.3

[1] Includes events reported regardless of causality.
[2] Data from Study 006 and three Phase 2/3 studies.
[3] NCI Grading System.

As seen in Table 7, rash is more common in pediatric patients and more often of higher grade (i.e., more severe) (see **PRECAUTIONS; General**).
Experience with SUSTIVA in patients who discontinued other antiretroviral agents of the NNRTI class is limited. Nineteen patients who discontinued nevirapine because of rash have been treated with SUSTIVA. Nine of these patients developed mild-to-moderate rash while receiving therapy with SUSTIVA, and two of these patients discontinued because of rash.
A few cases of pancreatitis have been described, although a causal relationship with efavirenz has not been established. Asymptomatic increases in serum amylase levels were observed in a significantly higher number of patients treated with efavirenz 600 mg than in control patients (see **ADVERSE REACTIONS; Laboratory Abnormalities**).

Drug-related clinical adverse experiences of moderate or severe intensity observed in ≥2% of patients in two controlled clinical trials are presented in Table 8.
[See table 8 at top of next page]
In Study 006, lipodystrophy was reported in 2.3% of patients treated with SUSTIVA (efavirenz) + IDV, 0.7% of patients treated with SUSTIVA+ZDV+LAM and 1.0% of patients treated with IDV+ZDV+LAM.
Clinical adverse experiences of moderate to severe intensity observed in ≥10% of 57 pediatric patients aged 3 to 16 years who received SUSTIVA, nelfinavir, and one or more NRTIs were: rash (40%), diarrhea/loose stools (39%), fever (26%), cough (25%), and nausea/vomiting (16%). The incidence of nervous system symptoms was 9% (5/57). Two patients experienced Grade 3 rash, two patients had Grade 4 rash, and five patients (9%) discontinued because of rash (see also **PRECAUTIONS; *Pediatric Use***).

Post-Marketing Experience:
Body as a Whole: allergic reactions, asthenia
Central and Peripheral Nervous System: abnormal coordination, ataxia, convulsions, hypoesthesia, paresthesia, neuropathy, tremor
Endocrine: gynecomastia
Gastrointestinal: constipation, malabsorption
Cardiovascular: flushing, palpitations
Liver and Biliary System: hepatic enzyme increase, hepatic failure
Metabolic and Nutritional: hypercholesterolemia, hypertriglyceridemia
Musculoskeletal: arthralgia, myalgia, myopathy
Psychiatric: aggressive reactions, agitation, delusions, emotional lability, mania, neurosis, paranoia, psychosis, suicide
Respiratory: dyspnea
Skin and Appendages: erythema multiforme, nail disorders, skin discoloration, Stevens-Johnson Syndrome
Special Senses: abnormal vision, tinnitus

Laboratory Abnormalities:
Liver Enzymes: Among 1,008 patients treated with 600 mg efavirenz in controlled clinical trials, 3% developed AST levels and 3% developed ALT levels greater than five times the upper limit of normal. Similar elevations of AST and ALT were seen in patients treated with control regimens.
Liver function tests should be monitored in patients with a prior history of Hepatitis B and/or C. In 156 patients treated with 600 mg of SUSTIVA who were seropositive for Hepatitis B and/or C, 7% developed AST levels and 8% developed ALT levels greater than five times the upper limit of normal. In 91 patients seropositive for Hepatitis B and/or C treated with control regimens, 5% developed AST elevations and 4% developed ALT elevations to these levels. Elevations of GGT to greater than five times the upper limit of the normal range were observed in 4% of all patients treated with 600 mg of SUSTIVA and in 10% of patients seropositive for Hepatitis B or C. In patients treated with control regimens, the incidence of GGT elevations to this level was 1.5–2%, irrespective of Hepatitis B or C serology. Isolated elevations of GGT in patients receiving SUSTIVA may reflect enzyme induction not associated with liver toxicity (see **PRECAUTIONS; General**).
Lipids: Increases in total cholesterol of 10–20% have been observed in some uninfected volunteers receiving SUSTIVA. In patients treated with SUSTIVA+ZDV+LAM, increases in non-fasting total cholesterol and HDL of approximately 20% and 25%, respectively, were observed. In patients treated with SUSTIVA+IDV, increases in non-fasting cholesterol and HDL of approximately 40% and 35%, respectively, were observed. The effects of SUSTIVA on triglycerides and LDL were not well-characterized since samples were taken from non-fasting patients. The clinical significance of these findings is unknown (see **PRECAUTIONS; General**).
Serum Amylase: Asymptomatic elevations in serum amylase greater than 1.5 times the upper limit of normal were seen in 10% of patients treated with SUSTIVA and in 6% of patients treated with control regimens. The clinical significance of asymptomatic increases in serum amylase is unknown (see **ADVERSE REACTIONS**).
Cannabinoid Test Interaction: Efavirenz does not bind to cannabinoid receptors. False positive urine cannabinoid test results have been reported in uninfected volunteers who received SUSTIVA. False positive test results have only been observed with the CEDIA DAU Multi-Level THC assay, which is used for screening, and have not been observed with other cannabinoid assays tested including tests used for confirmation of positive results.

OVERDOSAGE

Some patients accidentally taking 600 mg twice daily have reported increased nervous system symptoms. One patient experienced involuntary muscle contractions.
Treatment of overdose with SUSTIVA should consist of general supportive measures, including monitoring of vital signs and observation of the patient's clinical status. Administration of activated charcoal may be used to aid removal of unabsorbed drug. There is no specific antidote for overdose with SUSTIVA. Since efavirenz is highly protein bound, dialysis is unlikely to significantly remove the drug from blood.

DOSAGE AND ADMINISTRATION

Adults: The recommended dosage of SUSTIVA is 600 mg orally, once daily, in combination with a protease inhibitor and/or nucleoside analogue reverse transcriptase inhibitors (NRTIs). SUSTIVA may be taken with or without food; however, a high fat meal may increase the absorption of SUSTIVA and should be avoided (see **CLINICAL PHARMACOLOGY; *Effect of Food on Oral Absorption***).
In order to improve the tolerability of nervous system side effects, bedtime dosing is recommended during the first two to four weeks of therapy and in patients who continue to experience these symptoms (see **PRECAUTIONS; General** and **ADVERSE REACTIONS**).

Concomitant Antiretrovial Therapy: SUSTIVA (efavirenz) must be given in combination with other antiretroviral medications (see **CLINICAL PHARMACOLOGY; Drug Interactions** and **PRECAUTIONS; Drug Interactions** and **INDICATIONS AND USAGE**).

Pediatric Patients: Table 9 describes the recommended dose of SUSTIVA for pediatric patients 3 years of age or older and weighing between 10 and 40 Kg. The recommended dosage of SUSTIVA for pediatric patients weighing greater than 40 Kg is 600 mg, once daily.

Table 9
Pediatric Dose to be Administered Once Daily

Body Weight		SUSTIVA
Kg	Lbs	Dose (mg)
10 to < 15	22 to < 33	200
15 to < 20	33 to < 44	250
20 to < 25	44 to < 55	300
25 to < 32.5	55 to < 71.5	350
32.5 to < 40	71.5 to < 88	400
≥ 40	≥ 88	600

HOW SUPPLIED

SUSTIVA capsules are available as follows:

Table 8
Percent of Patients with Treatment-Emergent[1] Adverse Events of Moderate or Severe Intensity Reported in ≥2% of Patients in Studies 006 and ACTG 364

Adverse Events	Study 006 LAN, NNRTI and Protease Inhibitor Naive Patients			Study ACTG 364 NRTI-experienced NNRTI and Protease Inhibitor Naive Patients		
	SUSTIVA[2] + ZDV/LAM (N=412)	SUSTIVA[2] + Indinavir (N=415)	Indinavir + ZDV/LAM (N=401)	SUSTIVA[2] + Nelfinavir + NRTIs (N=64)	SUSTIVA[2] + NRTIs (N=65)	Nelfinavir + NRTIs (N=66)
	%	%	%	%	%	%
Body as a Whole						
Fatigue	7	5	8	0	2	3
Pain	1	1	5	13	6	17
Central and Peripheral Nervous System						
Dizziness	8	8	3	2	6	6
Headache	7	4	4	5	2	3
Concentration Impaired	5	2	0	0	0	0
Insomnia	6	7	3	0	0	2
Abnormal Dreams	3	1	0	—	—	—
Somnolence	3	2	2	0	0	0
Anorexia	1	0	1	0	2	2
Gastrointestinal						
Nausea	12	7	25	3	2	2
Vomiting	7	6	14	—	—	—
Diarrhea	6	8	6	14	3	9
Dyspepsia	3	3	5	0	0	2
Abdominal Pain	1	2	4	3	3	3
Psychiatric						
Anxiety	1	3	0	—	—	—
Depression	2	1	0	3	0	5
Nervousness	2	2	0	2	0	2
Skin & Appendages						
Rash	13	20	7	9	5	9
Pruritus	0	1	1	9	5	9
Increased Sweating	2	1	0	0	0	0

[1] Includes adverse events at least possibly related to study drug or of unknown relationship for Study 006. Includes all adverse events regardless of relationship to study drug for Study ACTG 364.
[2] SUSTIVA provided as 600 mg Once Daily.
—= Not Specified.

Capsules 200 mg are gold color, reverse printed with "SUSTIVA" on the body and imprinted "200 mg" on the cap.
Bottles of 90 NDC 0056-0474-92
Capsules 100 mg are white, reverse printed with "SUSTIVA" on the body and imprinted "100 mg" on the cap.
Bottles of 30 NDC 0056-0473-30
Capsules 50 mg are gold color and white, printed with "SUSTIVA" on the gold color cap and reverse printed "50 mg" on the white body.
Bottles of 30 NDC 0056-0470-30
SUSTIVA capsules should be stored at 25°C (77°F); excursions permitted to 15°–30°C (59°–86°F) [see USP Controlled Room Temperature].
Distributed by:
DuPont Pharma
Wilmington, DE 19880
SUSTIVA™ is a trademark of DuPont Pharmaceuticals Company.

6495–03/Rev. February, 2000
Shown in Product Identification Guide, page 311

The following material is provided as an educational service to all healthcare professionals:

EDUCATIONAL MATERIAL

COUMADIN® (Warfarin Sodium Tablets, USP) Crystalline

Books/Booklets/Brochures
"COUMADIN ® Patient Aid". This booklet explains key points of anticoagulation therapy, how it affects the patient's lifestyle, warning signs, and Vitamin K information. It also includes a COUMADIN® ID card and a dosage calendar. Available in English and Spanish.
"Multilingual Patient Support". Important facts about COUMADIN® therapy are translated into 50 languages in this booklet. Key points include: reporting problems, having blood tested and following the prescribed weekly schedule.
"Atrial Fibriwhat ? Brochure". This easy-to-read patient brochure outlines what atrial fibrillation is, the risks associated with the disorder, and treatment plans available in English and Spanish.
Video/Audio
"COUMADIN ® Therapy and You". This 11 minute, ½-inch VHS video is designed to be shown by the physician to his/her patients on COUMADIN® in order to increase patient commitment and understanding of COUMADIN® therapy. An audiocassette of the same program, "COUMADIN® Therapy and You," is available for patients to take home.

Both items are available in English and Spanish.
Charts
"COUMADIN ® Patient Anticoagulation Flow Sheet". This laminated 8-½″ × 11″ chart provides a convenient way to record patient prothrombin times and COUMADIN® doses.
"COUMADIN ® Patient Education Easel Flip Chart". An easel that allows the physician or nurse to educate the patient about COUMADIN® therapy in a practical question-and-answer format. Available in English and Spanish.

All of the above material is available at no charge to physicians, pharmacists, and other healthcare professionals involved with the management of patients on COUMADIN® therapy by calling 1-800-COUMADIN or by visiting www.coumadin.com.

SINEMET®
(Carbidopa-Levodopa)
SINEMET® CR
(Carbidopa-Levodopa)
Sustained-Release Tablets
Booklets
"A Patient's Guide to Parkinson's Disease and Sinemet ® CR (Carbidopa-Levopoda) Sustained Release" (CR-31412-2)
"Tips on taking Sinemet ® CR" (CR-31414-02)
Available at no charge. Write DuPont Pharma and ask for materials by CR #, (302) 992-4240 or visit www.sinemetcr-.com.

REVIA® (naltrexone HCl tablets)
Booklets/Brochures
"REVIA® Patient Q & A". This booklet answers the most commonly asked questions about REVIA®.
"REVIA® Counselor Q & A". Answers most commonly asked question in a more detailed level for counselors. Provides information needed on how to use REVIA®.
"REVIA® Counselor Brochure". A practical implementation piece on what a counselor should see when using REVIA®. Effectively and completely communicates the features and benefits of REVIA®.
SUSTIVA™ (efavirenz). Please visit our website www.sustiva.com, or call 1-800-4-PHARMA to receive educational material in the management of HIV/AIDS for healthcare professionals.

Dura Pharmaceuticals, Inc.
7475 LUSK BOULEVARD
SAN DIEGO, CA 92121

For Medical Information and Adverse Drug Experiences Contact:
Medical Affairs Department
(888) 859-8583
FAX: 858-657-0977

For Sales Representatives requests Contact:
800-859-8586

AZACTAM® ℞
[a-zak 'tam]
(aztreonam for injection, USP)

Rx only

DESCRIPTION
AZACTAM (aztreonam for injection, USP) contains the active ingredient, aztreonam, a monobactam. It was originally isolated from *Chromobacterium violaceum*. It is a synthetic bactericidal antibiotic.
The monobactams, having a unique monocyclic beta-lactam nucleus, are structurally different from other beta-lactam antibiotics (e.g., penicillins, cephalosporins, cephamycins). The sulfonic acid substituent in the 1-position of the ring activates the beta-lactam moiety; an aminothiazolyl oxime side chain in the 3-position and a methyl group in the 4-position confer the specific antibacterial spectrum and beta-lactamase stability.
Aztreonam is designated chemically as (Z)-2-[[[(2-amino-4-thiazolyl)[[(2S,-3S)-2-methyl-4-oxo-1-sulfo-3-azetidinyl]carbamoyl]methylene]amino]oxy]-2-methylpropionic acid.
AZACTAM is a sterile, nonpyrogenic, sodium-free, white to yellowish-white lyophilized cake containing approximately 780 mg arginine per gram of aztreonam. Following constitution, the product is for intramuscular or intravenous use. Aqueous solutions of the product have a pH in the range of 4.5 to 7.5.

CLINICAL PHARMACOLOGY
Single 30-minute intravenous infusions of 500 mg, 1 g and 2 g doses of AZACTAM (aztreonam for injection, USP) in healthy subjects produced aztreonam peak serum levels of 54, 90 and 204 μg/mL, respectively, immediately after administration; at eight hours, serum levels were 1, 3 and 6 μg/mL, respectively (Figure 1). Single 3-minute intravenous injections of the same doses resulted in serum levels of 58, 125 and 242 μg/mL at five minutes following completion of injection.
Serum concentrations of aztreonam in healthy subjects following completion of single intramuscular injections of 500 mg and 1 g doses are depicted in Figure 1; maximum serum concentrations occur at about one hour. After identical single intravenous or intramuscular doses of AZACTAM, the serum concentrations of aztreonam are comparable at one hour (1.5 hours from start of intravenous infusion) with similar slopes of serum concentrations thereafter.
[See figure at top of next column]
The serum levels of aztreonam following single 500 mg or 1 g (intramuscular or intravenous) or 2 g (intravenous) doses

Continued on next page

Azactam—Cont.

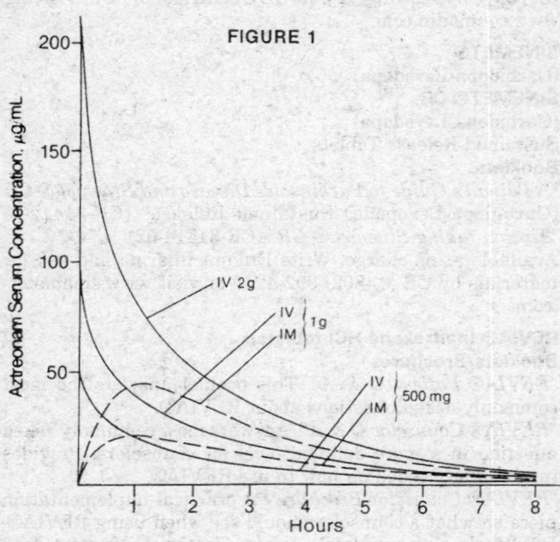

of AZACTAM exceed the MIC_{90} for *Neisseria* sp., *H. influenzae* and most genera of the *Enterobacteriaceae* for eight hours (for *Enterobacter* sp., the eight-hour serum levels exceed the MIC for 80 percent of strains). For *Ps. aeruginosa*, a single 2-g intravenous dose produces serum levels that exceed the MIC_{90} for approximately four to six hours. All of the above doses of AZACTAM result in average urine levels of aztreonam that exceed the MIC_{90} for the same pathogens for up to 12 hours.

When aztreonam pharmacokinetics were assessed for adult and pediatric patients, they were found to be comparable (down to 9 months old). The serum half-life of aztreonam averaged 1.7 hours (1.5 to 2.0) in subjects with normal renal function, independent of the dose and route of administration. In healthy subjects, based on a 70 kg person, the serum clearance was 91 mL/min and renal clearance was 56 mL/min; the apparent mean volume of distribution at steady-state averaged 12.6 liters, approximately equivalent to extracellular fluid volume.

In a study of healthy elderly male subjects (65 to 75 years of age), the average elimination half-life of aztreonam was slightly longer than in young healthy males.

In patients with impaired renal function, the serum half-life of aztreonam is prolonged (see **DOSAGE AND ADMINISTRATION, Renal Impairment in Adult Patients**). The serum half-life of aztreonam is only slightly prolonged in patients with hepatic impairment since the liver is a minor pathway of excretion.

Average urine concentrations of aztreonam were approximately 1100, 3500 and 6600 µg/mL within the first two hours following single 500 mg, 1-g and 2-g intravenous doses of AZACTAM (30-minute infusions), respectively. The range of average concentrations for aztreonam in the 8- to 12-hour urine specimens in these studies was 25 to 120 µg/mL. After intramuscular injection of single 500 mg and 1 g doses of AZACTAM (aztreonam for injection, USP), urinary levels were approximately 500 and 1200 µg/mL, respectively, within the first two hours, declining to 180 and 470 µg/mL in the six to eight hour specimens. In healthy subjects, aztreonam is excreted in the urine about equally by active tubular secretion and glomerular filtration. Approximately 60 to 70 percent of an intravenous or intramuscular dose was recovered in the urine by eight hours. Urinary excretion of a single parenteral dose was essentially complete by 12 hours after injection. About 12 percent of a single intravenous radiolabeled dose was recovered in the feces. Unchanged aztreonam and the inactive beta-lactam ring hydrolysis product of aztreonam were present in feces and urine.

Intravenous or intramuscular administration of a single 500 mg or 1 g dose of AZACTAM every eight hours for seven days to healthy subjects produced no apparent accumulation of aztreonam or modification of its disposition characteristics; serum protein binding averaged 56 percent and was independent of dose. An average of about 6 percent of a 1 g intramuscular dose was excreted as a microbiologically inactive open beta-lactam ring hydrolysis product (serum half-life approximately 26 hours) of aztreonam in the zero to eight hour urine collection on the last day of multiple dosing.

Renal function was monitored in healthy subjects given aztreonam; standard tests (serum creatinine, creatinine clearance, BUN, urinalysis and total urinary protein excretion) as well as special tests (excretion of N-acetyl-β-glucosaminidase, alanine aminopeptidase and β_2-microglobulin) were used. No abnormal results were obtained.

Aztreonam achieves measurable concentrations in the following body fluids and tissues:

[See table below]

The concentration of aztreonam in saliva at 30 minutes after a single 1 g intravenous dose (9 patients) was 0.2 µg/mL; in human milk at two hours after a single 1 g intravenous dose (6 patients), 0.2 µg/mL, and at six hours after a single 1 g intramuscular dose (6 patients), 0.3 µg/mL; in amniotic fluid at six to eight hours after a single 1 g intravenous dose (5 patients), 2 µg/mL. The concentration of aztreonam in peritoneal fluid obtained one to six hours after multiple 2 g intravenous doses ranged between 12 and 90 µg/mL in 7 of 8 patients studied.

Aztreonam given intravenously rapidly reaches therapeutic concentrations in peritoneal dialysis fluid; conversely, aztreonam given intraperitoneally in dialysis fluid rapidly produces therapeutic serum levels.

Concomitant administration of probenecid or furosemide and AZACTAM (aztreonam for injection, USP) causes clinically insignificant increases in the serum levels of aztreonam. Single-dose intravenous pharmacokinetic studies have not shown any significant interaction between aztreonam and concomitantly administered gentamicin, nafcillin sodium, cephradine, clindamycin or metronidazole. No reports of disulfiram-like reactions with alcohol ingestion have been noted; this is not unexpected since aztreonam does not contain a methyl-tetrazole side chain.

Microbiology

Aztreonam exhibits potent and specific activity *in vitro* against a wide spectrum of gram-negative aerobic pathogens including *Pseudomonas aeruginosa*. The bactericidal action of aztreonam results from the inhibition of bacterial cell wall synthesis due to a high affinity of aztreonam for penicillin binding protein 3 (PBP3). Aztreonam, unlike the majority of beta-lactam antibiotics, does not induce beta-lactamase activity and its molecular structure confers a high degree of resistance to hydrolysis by beta-lactamases (i.e., penicillinases and cephalosporinases) produced by most gram-negative and gram-positive pathogens; it is, therefore, usually active against gram-negative aerobic microorganisms that are resistant to antibiotics hydrolyzed by beta-lactamases. It is active against many strains that are multiply-resistant to other antibiotics, such as certain cephalosporins, penicillin, and aminoglycosides. Aztreonam maintains its antimicrobial activity over a pH range of 6 to 8 *in vitro*, as well as in the presence of human serum and under anaerobic conditions.

Aztreonam has been shown to be active against most strains of the following microorganisms, both *in vitro* and in clinical infections as described in the **INDICATIONS AND USAGE** section.

Aerobic gram-negative microorganisms:

Citrobacter species, including *C. freundii*
Enterobacter species, including *E. cloacae*
Escherichia coli
Haemophilus influenzae (including ampicillin-resistant and other penicillinase-producing strains)
Klebsiella oxytoca
Klebsiella pneumoniae
Proteus mirabilis
Pseudomonas aeruginosa
Serratia species, including *S. marcescens*

The following *in vitro* data are available, **but their clinical significance is unknown.**

Aztreonam exhibits *in vitro* minimal inhibitory concentrations (MIC's) of 8 µg/mL or less against most (≥90%) strains of the following microorganisms; however, the safety and effectiveness of aztreonam in treating clinical infections due to these microorganisms have not been established in adequate and well-controlled clinical trials.

Aerobic gram-negative microorganisms:

Aeromonas hydrophila
Morganella morganii
Neisseria gonorrhoeae (including penicillinase-producing strains)
Pasteurella multocida
Proteus vulgaris
Providencia stuartii
Providencia rettgeri
Yersinia enterocolitica

Aztreonam and aminoglycosides have been shown to be synergistic *in vitro* against most strains of *P. aeruginosa*, many strains of *Enterobacteriaceae*, and other gram-negative aerobic bacilli.

Alterations of the anaerobic intestinal flora by broad spectrum antibiotics may decrease colonization resistance, thus permitting overgrowth of potential pathogens, e.g., *Candida* and *clostridium* species. Aztreonam has little effect on the anaerobic intestinal microflora in *in vitro* studies. *Clostridium difficile* and its cytotoxin were not found in animal models following administration of aztreonam. (See **ADVERSE REACTIONS**, Gastrointestinal.)

Susceptibility Tests

Dilution Techniques: Quantitative methods are used to determine antimicrobial minimal inhibitory concentrations (MIC's). These MIC's provide estimates of the susceptibility of bacteria to antimicrobial compounds. The MIC's should be determined using a standardized procedure. Standardized procedures are based on a dilution method[1] (broth or agar) or equivalent with standardized inoculum concentrations and standardized concentrations of aztreonam powder. The MIC values should be interpreted according to the following criteria:

For testing aerobic microorganisms other than *Haemophilus influenzae:*

MIC (µg/mL)	Interpretation
≤8	Susceptible (S)
16	Intermediate (I)
≥32	Resistant (R)

When testing *Haemophilus influenzae*[a]:

MIC (µg/mL)	Interpretation[b]
≤2	Susceptible (S)

a. Interpretative criteria applicable only to tests performed by broth microdilution method using *Haemophilus* Test Medium (HTM)[1].

b. The current absence of data on resistant strains precludes defining any categories other than "Susceptible". Strains yielding MIC results suggestive of a "nonsusceptible" category should be submitted to a reference laboratory for further testing.

A report of "Susceptible" indicates that the pathogen is likely to be inhibited if the antimicrobial compound in the blood reaches the concentrations usually achievable. A report of "Intermediate" indicates that the result should be considered equivocal, and, if the microorganism is not fully susceptible to alternative, clinically feasible drugs, the test should be repeated. This category implies possible clinical applicability in body sites where the drug is physiologically concentrated or in situations where high dosage of drug can be used. This category also provides a buffer zone which prevents small uncontrolled technical factors from causing major discrepancies in interpretation. A report of "Resistant" indicates that the pathogen is not likely to be inhibited if the antimicrobial compound in the blood reaches the concentrations usually achievable; other therapy should be selected.

EXTRAVASCULAR CONCENTRATIONS OF AZTREONAM AFTER A SINGLE PARENTERAL DOSE[1]

Fluid or Tissue	Dose (g)	Route	Hours Postinjection	Number of Patients	Mean Concentration (µg/mL or µg/g)
Fluids					
bile	1	IV	2	10	39
blister fluid	1	IV	1	6	20
bronchial secretion	2	IV	4	7	5
cerebrospinal fluid (inflamed meninges)	2	IV	0.9–4.3	16	3
pericardial fluid	2	IV	1	6	33
pleural fluid	2	IV	1.1–3.0	3	51
synovial fluid	2	IV	0.8–1.9	11	83
Tissues					
atrial appendage	2	IV	0.9–1.6	12	22
endometrium	2	IV	0.7–1.9	4	9
fallopian tube	2	IV	0.7–1.9	8	12
fat	2	IV	1.3–2.0	10	5
femur	2	IV	1.0–2.1	15	16
gallbladder	2	IV	0.8–1.3	4	23
kidney	2	IV	2.4–5.6	5	67
large intestine	2	IV	0.8–1.9	9	12
liver	2	IV	0.9–2.0	6	47
lung	2	IV	1.2–2.1	6	22
myometrium	2	IV	0.7–1.9	9	11
ovary	2	IV	0.7–1.9	7	13
prostate	1	IM	0.8–3.0	8	8
skeletal muscle	2	IV	0.3–0.7	6	16
skin	2	IV	0.0–1.0	8	25
sternum	2	IV	1	6	6

[1]Tissue penetration is regarded as essential to therapeutic efficacy, but specific tissue levels have not been correlated with specific therapeutic effects.

Standardized susceptibility test procedures require the use of laboratory control microorganisms to control the technical aspects of the laboratory procedures. Standard aztreonam powder should provide the following MIC values:

Microorganism	MIC (µg/mL)
Escherichia coli ATCC 25922	0.06–0.25
Haemophilus influenzae[a] ATCC 49247	0.12–0.5
Pseudomonas aeruginosa ATCC 27853	2.0–8.0

a. Range applicable only to tests performed by broth microdilution method using *Haemophilus* Test Medium (HTM)[1].

Diffusion Techniques: Quantitative methods that require measurement of zone diameters also provide reproducible estimates of the susceptibility of bacteria to antimicrobial compounds. One such standardized procedure[2] requires the use of standardized inoculum concentrations. This procedure uses paper disks impregnated with 30-µg aztreonam to test the susceptibility of microorganisms to aztreonam.

Reports from the laboratory providing results of the standard single-disk susceptibility test with a 30-µg aztreonam disk should be interpreted according to the following criteria:

For testing aerobic microorganisms other than *Haemophilus influenzae:*

Zone diameter (mm)	Interpretation
≥22	Susceptible (S)
16–21	Intermediate (I)
≤15	Resistant (R)

When testing *Haemophilus influenzae*[a]:

Zone diameter (mm)	Interpretation[b]
≥26	Susceptible (S)

a. Interpretative criteria applicable only to tests performed by disk diffusion method using *Haemophilus* Test Medium (HTM)[2].

b. The current absence of data on resistant strains precludes defining any categories other than "Susceptible". Strains yielding zone diameter results suggestive of a "nonsusceptible" category should be submitted to a reference laboratory for further testing.

Interpretation should be as stated above for results using dilution techniques. Interpretation involves correlation of the diameter obtained in the disk test with the MIC for aztreonam.

As with standardized dilution techniques, diffusion methods require the use of laboratory control microorganisms that are used to control the technical aspects of the laboratory procedures. For the diffusion technique, the 30-µg aztreonam disk should provide the following zone diameters in these laboratory test quality control strains.

Microorganism	Zone diameter (mm)
Escherichia coli ATCC 25922	28–36 mm
Haemophilus influenzae[a] ATCC 49247	30–38 mm
Pseudomonas aeruginosa ATCC 27853	23–29 mm

a. Range applicable only to tests performed by disk diffusion method using *Haemophilus* Test Medium (HTM)[2].

INDICATIONS AND USAGE

Before initiating treatment with AZACTAM, appropriate specimens should be obtained for isolation of the causative organism(s) and for determination of susceptibility to aztreonam. Treatment with AZACTAM may be started empirically before results of the susceptibility testing are available; subsequently, appropriate antibiotic therapy should be continued.

AZACTAM (aztreonam for injection, USP) is indicated for the treatment of the following infections caused by susceptible gram-negative microorganisms:

Urinary Tract Infections (complicated and uncomplicated), including pyelonephritis and cystitis (initial and recurrent) caused by *Escherichia coli, Klebsiella pneumoniae, Proteus mirabilis, Pseudomonas aeruginosa, Enterobacter cloacae, Klebsiella oxytoca*, Citrobacter* species*and *Serratia marcescens**.

Lower Respiratory Tract Infections, including pneumonia and bronchitis caused by *Escherichia coli, Klebsiella pneumoniae, Pseudomonas aeruginosa, Haemophilus influenzae, Proteus mirabilis, Enterobacter* species and *Serratia marcescens**.

Septicemia caused by *Escherichia coli, Klebsiella pneumoniae, Pseudomonas aeruginosa, Proteus mirabilis*, Serratia marcescens** and *Enterobacter* species.

Skin and Skin-Structure Infections, including those associated with postoperative wounds, ulcers and burns caused by *Escherichia coli, Proteus mirabilis, Serratia marcescens, Enterobacter* species, *Pseudomonas aeruginosa, Klebsiella pneumoniae* and *Citrobacter* species*.

Intra-abdominal Infections, including peritonitis caused by *Escherichia coli, Klebsiella* species including *K. pneumoniae, Enterobacter* species including *E. cloacae*, Pseudomonas aeruginosa, Citrobacter* species* including *C. freundii** and *Serratia* species* including *S. marcescens**.

Gynecologic Infections, including endometritis and pelvic cellulitis caused by *Escherichia coli, Klebsiella pneumoniae*, Enterobacter* species* including *E. cloacae** and *Proteus mirabilis**.

*Efficacy for this organism in this organ system was studied in fewer than ten infections.

AZACTAM is indicated for adjunctive therapy to surgery in the management of infections caused by susceptible organisms, including abscesses, infections complicating hollow viscus perforations, cutaneous infections and infections of serous surfaces. AZACTAM is effective against most of the commonly encountered gram-negative aerobic pathogens seen in general surgery.

Concurrent Therapy

Concurrent initial therapy with other antimicrobial agents and AZACTAM (aztreonam for injection, USP) is recommended before the causative organism(s) is known in seriously ill patients who are also at risk of having an infection due to gram-positive aerobic pathogens. If anaerobic organisms are also suspected as etiologic agents, therapy should be initiated using an anti-anaerobic agent concurrently with AZACTAM (see **DOSAGE AND ADMINISTRATION**). Certain antibiotics (e.g., cefoxitin, imipenem) may induce high levels of beta-lactamase *in vitro* in some gram-negative aerobes such as *Enterobacter* and *Pseudomonas* species, resulting in antagonism to many beta-lactam antibiotics including aztreonam. These *in vitro* findings suggest that such beta-lactamase inducing antibiotics not be used concurrently with aztreonam. Following identification and susceptibility testing of the causative organism(s), appropriate antibiotic therapy should be continued.

CONTRAINDICATIONS

This preparation is contraindicated in patients with known hypersensitivity to aztreonam or any other component in the formulation.

WARNINGS

Both animal and human data suggest that AZACTAM is rarely cross-reactive with other beta-lactam antibiotics and weakly immunogenic. Treatment with aztreonam can result in hypersensitivity reactions in patients with or without prior exposure. (See **CONTRAINDICATIONS.**)

Careful inquiry should be made to determine whether the patient has any history of hypersensitivity reactions to any allergens.

While cross-reactivity of aztreonam with other beta-lactam antibiotics is rare, this drug should be administered with caution to any patient with a history of hypersensitivity to beta-lactams (e.g., penicillins, cephalosporins, and/or carbapenems). Treatment with aztreonam can result in hypersensitivity reactions in patients with or without prior exposure to aztreonam. If an allergic reaction to aztreonam occurs, discontinue the drug and institute supportive treatment as appropriate (e.g., maintenance of ventilation, pressor amines, antihistamines, corticosteroids). Serious hypersensitivity reactions may require epinephrine and other emergency measures. (See **ADVERSE REACTIONS.**)

Pseudomembranous colitis has been reported with nearly all antibacterial agents, including aztreonam, and may range in severity from mild to life-threatening. Therefore, it is important to consider this diagnosis in patients who present with diarrhea subsequent to the administration of antibacterial agents.

Treatment with antibacterial agents alters the normal flora of the colon and may permit overgrowth of Clostridia. Studies indicate that a toxin produced by *Clostridium difficile* is one primary cause of "antibiotic-associated colitis."

After the diagnosis of pseudomembranous colitis has been established, therapeutic measures should be initiated. Mild cases of pseudomembranous colitis usually respond to drug discontinuation alone. In moderate to severe cases, consideration should be given to management with fluids and electrolytes, protein supplementation, and treatment with an antibacterial drug clinically effective against *C. difficile* colitis.

Rare cases of toxic epidermal necrolysis have been reported in association with aztreonam in patients undergoing bone marrow transplant with multiple risk factors including sepsis, radiation therapy and other concomitantly administered drugs associated with toxic epidermal necrolysis.

PRECAUTIONS

General

In patients with impaired hepatic or renal function, appropriate monitoring is recommended during therapy.

If an aminoglycoside is used concurrently with aztreonam, especially if high dosages of the former are used or if therapy is prolonged, renal function should be monitored because of the potential nephrotoxicity and ototoxicity of aminoglycoside antibiotics.

The use of antibiotics may promote the overgrowth of nonsusceptible organisms, including gram-positive organisms (*Staphylococcus aureus* and *Streptococcus faecalis*) and fungi. Should superinfection occur during therapy, appropriate measures should be taken.

Carcinogenesis, Mutagenesis, Impairment of Fertility

Carcinogenicity studies in animals have not been performed.

Genetic toxicology studies performed *in vivo* and *in vitro* with aztreonam in several standard laboratory models revealed no evidence of mutagenic potential at the chromosomal or gene level.

Two-generation reproduction studies in rats at daily doses up to 20 times the maximum recommended human dose, prior to and during gestation and lactation, revealed no evidence of impaired fertility. There was a slightly reduced survival rate during the lactation period in the offspring of rats that received the highest dosage, but not in offspring of rats that received five times the maximum recommended human dose.

Pregnancy

Pregnancy Category B

Aztreonam crosses the placenta and enters the fetal circulation.

Studies in pregnant rats and rabbits, with daily doses up to 15 and 5 times, respectively, the maximum recommended human dose, revealed no evidence of embryo- or fetotoxicity or teratogenicity. No drug induced changes were seen in any of the maternal, fetal, or neonatal parameters that were monitored in rats receiving 15 times the maximum recommended human dose of aztreonam during late gestation and lactation.

There are no adequate and well-controlled studies in pregnant women. Because animal reproduction studies are not always predictive of human response, aztreonam should be used during pregnancy only if clearly needed.

Nursing Mothers

Aztreonam is excreted in breast milk in concentrations that are less than 1 percent of concentrations determined in simultaneously obtained maternal serum; consideration should be given to temporary discontinuation of nursing and use of formula feedings.

Pediatric Use

The safety and effectiveness of intravenous AZACTAM (aztreonam for injection, USP) have been established in the age groups 9 months to 16 years. Use of AZACTAM in these age groups is supported by evidence from adequate and well-controlled studies of AZACTAM in adults with additional efficacy, safety, and pharmacokinetic data from noncomparative clinical studies in pediatric patients. Sufficient data are not available for pediatric patients under 9 months of age or for the following treatment indications/pathogens: septicemia and skin and skin-structure infections (where the skin infection is believed or known to be due to *H. influenzae* type b). In pediatric patients with cystic fibrosis, higher doses of AZACTAM may be warranted. (See **CLINICAL PHARMACOLOGY, DOSAGE AND ADMINISTRATION,** and **CLINICAL STUDIES.**)

ADVERSE REACTIONS

Local reactions such as phlebitis/thrombophlebitis following IV administration, and discomfort/swelling at the injection site following IM administration occurred at rates of approximately 1.9 percent and 2.4 percent, respectively.

Systemic reactions (considered to be related to therapy or of uncertain etiology) occurring at an incidence of 1 to 1.3 percent include diarrhea, nausea and/or vomiting, and rash. Reactions occurring at an incidence of less than 1 percent are listed within each body system in order of decreasing severity:

Hypersensitivity—anaphylaxis, angioedema, bronchospasm.

Hematologic—pancytopenia, neutropenia, thrombocytopenia, anemia, eosinophilia, leukocytosis, thrombocytosis.

Gastrointestinal—abdominal cramps; rare cases of *C. difficile*-associated diarrhea, including pseudomembraneous colitis, or gastrointestinal bleeding have been reported. Onset of pseudomembranous colitis symptoms may occur during or after antibiotic treatment. (See **WARNINGS.**)

Dermatologic—toxic epidermal necrolysis (see **WARNINGS**), purpura, erythema multiforme, exfoliative dermatitis, urticaria, petechiae, pruritus, diaphoresis.

Cardiovascular—hypotension, transient ECG changes (ventricular bigeminy and PVC), flushing.

Respiratory—wheezing, dyspnea, chest pain.

Hepatobiliary—hepatitis, jaundice.

Nervous System—seizure, confusion, vertigo, paresthesia, insomnia, dizziness.

Musculoskeletal—muscular aches.

Special Senses—tinnitus, diplopia, mouth ulcer, altered taste, numb tongue, sneezing, nasal congestion, halitosis.

Other—vaginal candidiasis, vaginitis, breast tenderness.

Body as a Whole—weakness, headache, fever, malaise.

Pediatric Adverse Reactions

Of the 612 pediatric patients who were treated with AZACTAM in clinical trials, less than 1% required discontinuation of therapy due to adverse events. The following systemic adverse events, regardless of drug relationship, occurred in at least 1% of treated patients in domestic clinical trials: rash (4.3%), diarrhea (1.4%), and fever (1.0%). These adverse events were comparable to those observed in adult clinical trials.

In 343 pediatric patients receiving intravenous therapy, the following local reactions were noted: pain (12%), erythema (2.9%), induration (0.9%), and phlebitis (2.1%). In the US patient population, pain occurred in 1.5% of patients, while each of the remaining three local reactions had an incidence of 0.5%.

The following laboratory adverse events, regardless of drug relationship, occurred in at least 1% of treated patients: in-

Continued on next page

Azactam—Cont.

creased eosinophils (6.3%), increased platelets (3.6%), neutropenia (3.2%), increased AST (3.8%), increased ALT (6.5%), and increased serum creatinine (5.8%).

In US pediatric clinical trials, neutropenia (absolute neutrophil count less than 1000/mm^3) occurred in 11.3% of patients (8/71) younger than 2 years receiving 30 mg/kg q6h. AST and ALT elevations to greater than 3 times the upper limit of normal were noted in 15–20% of patients aged 2 years or above receiving 50 mg/kg q6h. The increased frequency of these reported laboratory adverse events may be due to either increased severity of illness treated or higher doses of AZACTAM (aztreonam for injection, USP) administered.

Adverse Laboratory Changes

Adverse laboratory changes without regard to drug relationship that were reported during clinical trials were:

Hepatic—elevations of AST (SGOT), ALT (SGPT), and alkaline phosphatase; signs or symptoms of hepatobiliary dysfunction occurred in less than 1 percent of recipients (see above).

Hematologic—increases in prothrombin and partial thromboplastin times, positive Coombs test.

Renal—increases in serum creatinine.

OVERDOSAGE

If necessary, aztreonam may be cleared from the serum by hemodialysis and/or peritoneal dialysis.

DOSAGE AND ADMINISTRATION

Dosage in Adult Patients

AZACTAM may be administered intravenously or by intramuscular injection. Dosage and route of administration should be determined by susceptibility of the causative organisms, severity and site of infection, and the condition of the patient.

The intravenous route is recommended for patients requiring single doses greater than 1 g or those with bacterial septicemia, localized parenchymal abscess (e.g., intra-abdominal abscess), peritonitis or other severe systemic or life-threatening infections.

The duration of therapy depends on the severity of infection. Generally, AZACTAM should be continued for at least 48 hours after the patient becomes asymptomatic or evidence of bacterial eradication has been obtained. Persistent infections may require treatment for several weeks. Doses smaller than those indicated should not be used.

Renal Impairment in Adult Patients

Prolonged serum levels of aztreonam may occur in patients with transient or persistent renal insufficiency. Therefore, the dosage of AZACTAM should be halved in patients with estimated creatinine clearances between 10 and 30 mL/min/1.73 m^2 after an initial loading dose of 1 g or 2 g.

When only the serum creatinine concentration is available, the following formula (based on sex, weight, and age of the patient) may be used to approximate the creatinine clearance (Clcr). The serum creatinine should represent a steady state of renal function.

$$\text{Males: Clcr} = \frac{\text{weight (kg)} \times \text{(140-age)}}{72 \times \text{serum creatinine (mg/dL)}}$$

Females: 0.85 × above value

In patients with severe renal failure (creatinine clearance less than 10 mL/min/1.73 m^2), such as those supported by hemodialysis, the usual dose of 500 mg, 1 g or 2 g should be given initially. The maintenance dose should be one-fourth of the usual initial dose given at the usual fixed interval of 6, 8 or 12 hours. For serious or life-threatening infections, in addition to the maintenance doses, one-eighth of the initial dose should be given after each hemodialysis session.

Dosage in The Elderly

Renal status is a major determinant of dosage in the elderly; these patients in particular may have diminished renal function. Serum creatinine may not be an accurate determinant of renal status. Therefore, as with all antibiotics eliminated by the kidneys, estimates of creatinine clearance should be obtained, and appropriate dosage modifications made if necessary.

Dosage in Pediatric Patients

AZACTAM (aztreonam for injection, USP) should be administered intravenously to pediatric patients with normal renal function. There are insufficient data regarding intramuscular administration to pediatric patients or dosing in pediatric patients with renal impairment. (See **PRECAUTIONS: Pediatric Use.**)

[See table below]

Because of the serious nature of infections due to *Pseudomonas aeruginosa*, dosage of 2 g every six or eight hours is recommended, at least upon initiation of therapy, in systemic infections caused by this organism in adults.

CLINICAL STUDIES

A total of 612 pediatric patients aged 1 month to 12 years were enrolled in uncontrolled clinical trials of aztreonam in the treatment of serious gram-negative infections, including urinary tract, lower respiratory tract, skin and skin-structure, and intra-abdominal infections.

Preparation Of Parenteral Solutions

General

Upon the addition of the diluent to the container, contents should be shaken **immediately** and **vigorously**. Constituted solutions are not for multiple-dose use; should the entire volume in the container not be used for a single-dose, the unused solution must be discarded.

Depending upon the concentration of aztreonam and diluent used, constituted AZACTAM yields a colorless to light straw yellow solution which may develop a slight pink tint on standing (potency is not affected). Parenteral drug products should be inspected visually for particulate matter and discoloration whenever solution and container permit.

Admixtures With Other Antibiotics

Intravenous infusion solutions of AZACTAM not exceeding 2% w/v prepared with Sodium Chloride Injection USP 0.9% or Dextrose Injection USP 5%, to which clindamycin phosphate, gentamicin sulfate, tobramycin sulfate, or cefazolin sodium have been added at concentrations usually used clinically, are stable for up to 48 hours at room temperature or seven days under refrigeration. Ampicillin sodium admixtures with aztreonam in Sodium Chloride Injection USP 0.9% are stable for 24 hours at room temperature and 48 hours under refrigeration; stability in Dextrose Injection USP 5% is two hours at room temperature and eight hours under refrigeration.

Aztreonam-cloxacillin sodium and aztreonam-vancomycin hydrochloride admixtures are stable in Dianeal® 137 (Peritoneal Dialysis Solution) with 4.25% Dextrose for up to 24 hours at room temperature.

Aztreonam is incompatible with nafcillin sodium, cephradine, and metronidazole.

Other admixtures are not recommended since compatibility data are not available.

Intravenous (IV) Solutions

For Bolus Injection: The contents of an AZACTAM (aztreonam for injection, USP) 15 mL or 30 mL capacity vial should be constituted with 6 to 10 mL Sterile Water for Injection USP. *For Infusion:* Contents of the 100 mL capacity bottle should be constituted to a final concentration not exceeding 2% w/v (at least 50 mL of any appropriate infusion solution listed below per gram aztreonam). These solutions may be frozen immediately after constitution in the original container. (See **Stability** below.)

If the contents of a 15 mL or 30 mL capacity vial are to be transferred to an appropriate infusion solution, each gram of aztreonam should be initially constituted with at least 3 mL Sterile Water for Injection USP. Further dilution may be obtained with one of the following intravenous infusion solutions:

Sodium Chloride Injection USP, 0.9%
Ringer's Injection USP
Lactated Ringer's Injection USP
Dextrose Injection USP, 5% or 10%
Dextrose and Sodium Chloride Injection USP, 5%:0.9%, 5%:0.45% or 5%:0.2%
Sodium Lactate Injection USP (M/6 Sodium Lactate)
Ionosol® B and 5% Dextrose
Isolyte® E
Isolyte® E with 5% Dextrose
Isolyte® M with 5% Dextrose
Normosol®-R
Normosol®-R and 5% Dextrose
Normosol®-M and 5% Dextrose
Mannitol Injection USP, 5% or 10%
Lactated Ringer's and 5% Dextrose Injection
Plasma-Lyte® M and 5% Dextrose
10% Travert® Injection
10% Travert® and Electrolyte No. 1 Injection
10% Travert® and Electrolyte No. 2 Injection
10% Travert® and Electrolyte No. 3 Injection

Intramuscular (IM) Solutions

The contents of an AZACTAM 15 mL or 30 mL capacity vial should be constituted with at least 3 mL of an appropriate diluent per gram aztreonam. The following diluents may be used:

Sterile Water for Injection USP
Sterile Bacteriostatic Water for Injection, USP (with benzyl alcohol or with methyl- and propylparabens)
Sodium Chloride Injection USP, 0.9%
Bacteriostatic Sodium Chloride Injection USP (with benzyl alcohol)

Stability Of IV And IM Solutions

AZACTAM solutions for IV infusion at concentrations not exceeding 2% w/v must be used within 48 hours following constitution if kept at controlled room temperature (59°–86° F/15°–30° C) or within seven days if refrigerated (36°–46° F/ 2°– 8° C).

Frozen aztreonam infusion solutions may be stored for up to three months at −4° F/−20° C; frozen solutions may be thawed at controlled room temperature or by overnight refrigeration. Solutions that have been thawed and maintained at controlled room temperature or under refrigeration should be used within 24 or 72 hours after removal from the freezer, respectively. Solutions should not be refrozen.

AZACTAM solutions at concentrations exceeding 2% w/v, except those prepared with Sterile Water for Injection USP or Sodium Chloride Injection USP, should be used promptly after preparation; the two excepted solutions must be used within 48 hours if stored at controlled room temperature or within seven days if refrigerated.

Intravenous Administration

Bolus Injection: A bolus injection may be used to initiate therapy. The dose should be **slowly** injected directly into a vein, or the tubing of a suitable administration set, over a period of three to five minutes (see next paragraph regarding flushing of tubing).

Infusion: With any intermittent infusion of aztreonam and another drug with which it is not pharmaceutically compatible, the common delivery tube should be flushed before and after delivery of aztreonam with any appropriate infusion solution compatible with both drug solutions; the drugs should not be delivered simultaneously. Any AZACTAM (aztreonam for injection, USP) infusion should be completed within a 20 to 60 minute period. With use of a *Y-type administration set*, careful attention should be given to the calculated volume of aztreonam solution required so that the entire dose will be infused. A volume control administration set may be used to deliver an initial dilution of AZACTAM (see **Preparation Of Parenteral Solutions, For Infusion**) into a compatible infusion solution during administration; in this case, the final dilution of aztreonam should provide a concentration not exceeding 2% w/v.

Intramuscular Administration

The dose should be given by deep injection into a large muscle mass (such as the upper outer quadrant of the gluteus maximus or lateral part of the thigh). Aztreonam is well tolerated and should not be admixed with any local anesthetic agent.

HOW SUPPLIED

AZACTAM® (aztreonam for injection, USP)-Lyophilized

Single-dose 15 mL capacity vials:
500 mg/vial: Packages of 10 (NDC 51479-050-05)
1 g/vial: Packages of 10 (NDC 51479-051-15)

Single-dose 30 mL capacity vial:
2 g/vial: Packages of 10 (NDC 51479-052-30)

Single-dose 100 mL capacity intravenous infusion bottles with bail bands:
1 g/bottle: Packages of 10 (NDC 51479-051-10)
2 g/bottle: Packages of 10 (NDC 51479-052-10)

Storage

Store original packages at room temperature; avoid excessive heat.

ALSO SUPPLIED AS:

AZACTAM® (aztreonam injection) in Galaxy® plastic container (PL 2040) as a frozen, 50 mL single-dose intravenous solution as follows:

1 g aztreonam/50 mL container: Packages of 24 (NDC 51479-048-01)
2 g aztreonam/50 mL container: Packages of 24 (NDC 51479-049-01)

REFERENCES:

1. National Committee for Clinical Laboratory Standards. *Methods for Dilution Antimicrobial Susceptibility Tests for Bacteria that Grow Aerobically*—Fourth Edition. Approved Standard NCCLS Document M7-A4, Vol. 17, No. 2, NCCLS, Villanova, PA, January 1997.
2. National Committee for Clinical Laboratory Standards. *Performance Standards for Antimicrobial disk susceptibility Tests*—Sixth Edition. Approved Standard NCCLS Document M2-A6, Vol. 17, No. 1, NCCLS, Villanova, PA, January 1997.

AZACTAM® is a registered trademark of Bristol-Myers Squibb Company

Manufactured by
Bristol-Myers Squibb Company
Princeton, NJ 08543 U.S.A.

AZACTAM DOSAGE GUIDELINES

Type of Infection	Dose	Frequency (hours)
ADULTS*		
Urinary tract infections	500 mg or 1 g	8 or 12
Moderately severe systemic infections	1 g or 2 g	8 or 12
Severe systemic or life-threatening infections	2 g	6 or 8
*Maximum recommended dose is 8 g per day		
PEDIATRIC PATIENTS**		
Mild to moderate infections	30 mg/kg	8
Moderate to severe infections	30 mg/kg	6 or 8
**Maximum recommended dose is 120 mg/kg/day.		

Distributed by
DURA Pharmaceuticals, Inc.
San Diego, CA 92121 U.S.A.

Revised March 1999
J4-671
AZL001A99

Shown in Product Identification Guide, page 311

CECLOR® CD ℞
(cefaclor extended release tablets)

DESCRIPTION

Cefaclor, USP, the active ingredient in Ceclor® CD (cefaclor extended release tablets), is a semisynthetic cephalosporin antibiotic for oral administration. Cefaclor, USP, is chemically designated as 3-chloro-7-D-(2-phenylglycinamido)-3-cephem-4-carboxylic acid monohydrate. The Ceclor CD formulation of cefaclor differs pharmacokinetically from the Ceclor® formulation of cefaclor. (*See* **CLINICAL PHARMACOLOGY**.) Cefaclor monohydrate has a molecular formula of $C_{15}H_{14}ClN_3O_4S \cdot H_2O$ and a molecular weight of 385.82.

[structural formula: COOH, Cl, H, O, C---CONH, NH₂, H, H, S, •H₂O]

Each Ceclor CD tablet contains cefaclor monohydrate equivalent to 375 mg (1.02 mmol) or 500 mg (1.36 mmol) anhydrous cefaclor. In addition, each extended release tablet contains the following inactive ingredients: celluloses; FD&C Blue No. 2; magnesium stearate; mannitol; methacrylic acid copolymer type C; propylene glycol; stearic acid; titanium dioxide; polyethylene glycol; talc; and edible black ink.

CLINICAL PHARMACOLOGY

Pharmacokinetics: The Ceclor CD formulation of cefaclor is pharmacokinetically different from the Ceclor® Pulvules® formulation. (*See* Table 1.) No direct comparisons with the suspension formulation of cefaclor have been conducted; therefore, there are no data with which to compare the pharmacokinetic properties of the CD formulation and the suspension formulation. Until further data are available, the pharmacokinetic equivalence of the CD and the suspension formulations should NOT be assumed.

Absorption and Metabolism: The extent of absorption (AUC) and the maximum plasma concentration (C_{max}) of cefaclor from Ceclor CD are greater when the extended release tablet is taken with food.

[NOTE: The extent of absorption (AUC) of cefaclor from Ceclor Pulvules is unaffected by food intake; however, when Ceclor Pulvules are taken with food, the C_{max} is decreased.]

There is no evidence of metabolism of cefaclor in humans.

Comparative Serum Pharmacokinetics—Serum pharmacokinetic parameters for Ceclor CD and Ceclor Pulvules are shown in the following table.

[See table 1 above]

Table 1
COMPARATIVE PHARMACOKINETICS OF CECLOR PULVULES VS CECLOR CD IN FASTING AND FED STATES

Parameter	Ceclor CD		Ceclor CD		Ceclor Pulvules	
	375 mg		500 mg		2 × 250 mg	
	fed	fast	fed	fast	fed	fast
	n = 10		n = 16	n = 16	n = 15	n = 16
C_{max}	3.7 (1.1)	NA	8.2 (4.2)	5.4 (1.6)	9.3 (2.7)	16.8 (4.7)
T_{max}	2.7 (1.0)	NA	2.5 (0.8)	1.5 (0.7)	1.5 (0.6)	0.9 (0.4)
AUC	9.9 (2.2)	NA	18.1 (4.2)	14.8 (4.0)	20.5 (2.8)	19.2 (5.0)

(± 1 standard deviation)
NA = data not available

No drug accumulation was noted when Ceclor CD was given twice daily.

The plasma half-life in healthy subjects is independent of dosage form and averages approximately 1 hour.

Food Effect on Pharmacokinetics: When Ceclor CD is taken with food, the AUC is 10% lower while the C_{max} is 12% lower and occurs 1 hour later compared to Ceclor Pulvules. In contrast, when Ceclor CD is taken without food, the AUC is 23% lower while the C_{max} is 67% lower and occurs 0.6 hours later, using an equivalent milligram dose of Ceclor Pulvules as a reference. **Therefore, Ceclor CD should be taken with food.**

Special Populations:

Renal Insufficiency—In patients with reduced renal function, the serum half-life of cefaclor is slightly prolonged. In those with complete absence of renal function, the plasma half-life of the intact molecule is 2.3 to 2.8 hours. Excretion pathways in patients with markedly impaired renal function have not been determined. Hemodialysis shortens the half-life by 25% to 30%.

Geriatric Patients—In elderly subjects (over age 65) with normal serum creatinine values, higher peak plasma concentrations and AUCs have been observed. This is considered to be primarily a result of an age-related decrement in renal function, and has no apparent clinical significance. Therefore, dosage adjustment is not necessary in elderly subjects with normal serum creatinine values.

Microbiology:

Cefaclor has *in vitro* activity against a broad range of gram-positive and gram-negative bacteria. The bactericidal action of cefaclor results from inhibition of cell-wall synthesis. Cefaclor is stable in the presence of some bacterial β-lactamases; consequently, some β-lactamase-producing organisms may be susceptible to cefaclor.

Ceclor CD has been shown to be active against most strains of the following microorganisms both *in vitro* and in clinical infections as described in the **INDICATIONS AND USAGE** section:

Gram-positive aerobes:
Staphylococcus aureus
Streptococcus pneumoniae
Streptococcus pyogenes

NOTE: Cefaclor is inactive against methicillin-resistant staphylococci.

Gram-negative aerobes:
Haemophilus influenzae (non-β-lactamase-producing strains only)
Moraxella catarrhalis (including β-lactamase-producing strains)

The following *in vitro* data are available, **but their clinical significance is unknown.** Cefaclor exhibits *in vitro* minimum inhibitory concentrations (MICs) of 8 μg/mL or less (systemic susceptibility breakpoint) against most (≥90%) strains of the following microorganisms; however, the safety and effectiveness of Ceclor CD in treating clinical infections due to these microorganisms have not been established in adequate and well-controlled trials.

Gram-positive aerobes:
Staphylococcus epidermidis

Gram-negative aerobes:
Haemophilus parainfluenzae
Klebsiella pneumoniae

Anaerobic bacteria:
Peptococcus niger
Peptostreptococci
Propionibacterium acnes

NOTE: *Acinetobacter calcoaceticus, Enterobacter* spp., *Enterococcus* spp., *Morganella morganii, Proteus vulgaris, Providencia* spp., *Pseudomonas* spp., and *Serratia* spp. are resistant to cefaclor.

Susceptibility Testing:Dilution Techniques—Quantitative methods are used to determine antimicrobial minimum inhibitory concentrations (MICs). These MICs provide estimates of the susceptibility of bacteria to antimicrobial compounds. The MICs should be determined using a standardized procedure. Standardized procedures are based on a dilution method[1] (broth, agar, or microdilution) or equivalent with standardized inoculum concentrations and standardized amounts of cefaclor powder. The MIC values should be interpreted according to the following criteria:

MIC (μg/mL)	Interpretation
≤8	Susceptible (S)
16	Intermediate (I)
≥32	Resistant (R)

A report of "Susceptible" indicates that the pathogen is likely to be inhibited if the antimicrobial compound in blood reaches the concentrations usually achievable. A report of "Intermediate" indicates that the result should be considered equivocal, and, if the microorganism is not fully susceptible to alternative, clinically feasible drugs, the test should be repeated. This category implies possible clinical applicability in body sites where the drug is physiologically concentrated or in situations where high dosage of drug can be used. This category also provides a buffer zone which prevents small uncontrolled technical factors from causing major discrepancies in interpretation. A report of "Resistant" indicates that the pathogen is not likely to be inhibited if the antimicrobial compound in the blood reaches the concentrations usually achievable; other therapy should be selected.

Standardized susceptibility test procedures require the use of laboratory control microorganisms to control the technical aspects of the laboratory procedures. Standard cefaclor powder should provide the following MIC values:

Microorganism		MIC range (μg/mL)
E. coli	ATCC 25922	1–4
E. faecalis	ATCC 29212	>32
S. aureus	ATCC 29213	1–4
H. influenzae	ATCC 49766*	1–4

*Broth microdilution tests performed using Haemophilus Test Medium (HTM)[1]

Diffusion Techniques: Quantitative methods that require measurement of zone diameters also provide reproducible estimates of the susceptibility of bacteria to antimicrobial compounds. One such standardized procedure[2] requires the use of standarized inoculum concentrations. This procedure uses paper disks impregnated with 30-μg cefaclor to test the susceptibility of microorganisms to cefaclor.

Reports from the laboratory providing results of the standard single-disk susceptibility test with a 30-μg cefaclor disk should be interpreted according to the following criteria:

Zone diameter (mm)	Interpretation
≥18	Susceptible (S)
15–17	Intermediate (I)
≤14	Resistant (R)

When testing* *H. Influenzae*, the following interpretive criteria should be used:

Zone diameter (mm)	Interpretation
≥20	Susceptible (S)
17–19	Intermediate (I)
≤16	Resistant (R)

*Disk susceptibility tests performed using Haemophilus Test Medium (HTM)[2]

Interpretation should be as stated above for results using dilution techniques. Interpretation involves correlation of the diameter obtained in the disk test with the MIC for cefaclor.

As with standardized dilution techniques, diffusion methods require the use of laboratory control microorganisms that are used to control the technical aspects of the laboratory procedures. For the diffusion technique, the 30-μg cefaclor disk should provide the following zone diameters in these laboratory test quality control strains:

Microorganisms		Zone Diameter (mm)
E. coli	ATCC 25922	23–27
S. aureus	ATCC 25923	27–31
*H. influenzae**	ATCC 49766	25–31

*Disk susceptibility tests performed using Haemophilus Test Medium (HTM)[2]

INDICATIONS AND USAGE

The safety and effectiveness of Ceclor CD in treating some of the indications and pathogens for which other formulations of cefaclor are approved have NOT been established. When administered at the recommended dosages and durations of therapy, Ceclor CD is indicated for the treatment of patients with the following mild to moderate infections when caused by susceptible strains of the designated organisms. (*See* **DOSAGE AND ADMINISTRATION** and **CLINICAL STUDIES** sections.)

Acute bacterial exacerbations of chronic bronchitis due to *Haemophilus influenzae* (non-β-lactamase-producing strains only), *Moraxella catarrhalis* (including β-lactamase-producing strains) or *Streptococcus pneumoniae.*

NOTE: In view of the insufficient numbers of isolates of β-lactamase-producing strains of *Haemophilus influenzae* that were obtained from clinical trials with Ceclor CD for patients with acute bacterial exacerbations of chronic bronchitis or secondary bacterial infections of acute bronchitis, it was not possible to adequately evaluate the effectiveness of Ceclor CD for bronchitis known, suspected, or considered potentially to be caused by β-lactamase-producing *H. influenzae.*

Secondary bacterial infections of acute bronchitis due to *Haemophilus influenzae* (non-β-lactamase-producing strains only), *Moraxella catarrhalis* (including β-lactamase-producing strains), or *Streptococcus pneumoniae*. (See above **NOTE.**)

Pharyngitis and tonsillitis due to *Streptococcus pyogenes.*

NOTE: Only penicillin by the intramuscular route of administration has been shown to be effective in the prophylaxis of rheumatic fever. Ceclor CD is generally effective in the eradication of *S. pyogenes* from the oropharynx; however, data establishing the efficacy of Ceclor CD for the prophylaxis of subsequent rheumatic fever are not available.

Uncomplicated skin and skin structure infections due to *Staphylococcus aureus* (methicillin-susceptible).

NOTE: In view of the insufficient numbers of isolates of *Streptococcus pyogenes* that were obtained from clinical trials with Ceclor CD for patients with uncomplicated skin and skin structure infections, it was not possible to ade-

Continued on next page

Ceclor CD—Cont.

quately evaluate the effectiveness of Ceclor CD for skin infections known, suspected, or considered potentially to be caused by *S. pyogenes*.

CONTRAINDICATIONS

Ceclor CD is contraindicated in patients with known hypersensitivity to cefaclor and other cephalosporins.

WARNINGS

BEFORE THERAPY WITH CECLOR CD IS INSTITUTED, CAREFUL INQUIRY SHOULD BE MADE TO DETERMINE WHETHER THE PATIENT HAS HAD PREVIOUS HYPERSENSITIVITY REACTIONS TO CEFACLOR, CEPHALOSPORINS, PENICILLINS, OR OTHER DRUGS. IF THIS PRODUCT IS TO BE GIVEN TO PENICILLIN-SENSITIVE PATIENTS, CAUTION SHOULD BE EXERCISED BECAUSE CROSS-SENSITIVITY AMONG BETA-LACTAM ANTIBIOTICS HAS BEEN CLEARLY DOCUMENTED AND MAY OCCUR IN UP TO 10% OF PATIENTS WITH A HISTORY OF PENICILLIN ALLERGY. IF AN ALLERGIC REACTION TO CECLOR CD OCCURS, DISCONTINUE THE DRUG. SERIOUS ACUTE HYPERSENSITIVITY REACTIONS MAY REQUIRE TREATMENT WITH EPINEPHRINE AND OTHER EMERGENCY MEASURES, INCLUDING OXYGEN, INTRAVENOUS FLUIDS, INTRAVENOUS ANTIHISTAMINES, CORTICOSTEROIDS, PRESSOR AMINES, AND AIRWAY MANAGEMENT, AS CLINICALLY INDICATED.

Pseudomembranous colitis has been reported with nearly all antibacterial agents, including cefaclor, and may range from mild to life-threatening. Therefore, it is important to consider this diagnosis in patients who present with diarrhea subsequent to the administration of antibacterial agents.

Treatment with antibacterial agents alters the normal flora of the colon and may permit overgrowth by clostridia. Studies indicate that a toxin produced by *Clostridium difficile* is a primary cause of "antibiotic-associated colitis."

After the diagnosis of pseudomembranous colitis has been established, therapeutic measures should be initiated. Mild cases of pseudomembranous colitis usually respond to discontinuation of the drug alone. In moderate to severe cases, consideration should be given to management with fluids and electrolytes, protein supplementation and treatment with an antibacterial drug clinically effective against *Clostridium difficile*.

PRECAUTIONS

General: Superinfection (overgrowth by non-susceptible organisms) should always be considered a possibility in a patient being treated with a broad-spectrum antimicrobial. Careful observation of the patient is essential. If superinfection occurs during therapy, appropriate measures should be taken.

Drug Interactions:

Antacids—The extent of absorption of Ceclor CD is diminished if magnesium or aluminum hydroxide-containing antacids are taken within 1 hour of administration; H_2 blockers do not alter either the rate or the extent of absorption of Ceclor CD.

Probenecid—The renal excretion of cefaclor is inhibited by probenecid.

Warfarin—There have been rare reports of increased prothrombin time with or without clinical bleeding in patients receiving cefaclor and warfarin concomitantly. No specific studies have been performed to rule in or rule out this potential drug/drug interaction.

Laboratory Test Interactions: Administration of Ceclor CD may result in a false-positive reaction for glucose in the urine. This phenomenon has been seen in patients taking cephalosporin antibiotics when the test is performed using Benedict's and Fehling's solutions and also with Clinitest®tablets.

Carcinogenesis, Mutagenesis, Impairment of Fertility: Studies in animals have not been performed to evaluate the carinogenic or mutagenic potential for cefaclor. Reproduction studies have revealed no evidence of impaired fertility.

Usage in Pregnancy—Teratogenic Effect: Pregnancy Category B: Reproduction studies using cefaclor have been performed in mice, rats, and ferrets at doses up to 3–5 times the maximum human dose (1500 mg/day) based on mg/m^2. These studies have revealed no harm to the fetus due to cefaclor. There are, however, no adequate and well-controlled studies in pregnant women. Because animal reproduction studies are not always predictive of human response. Ceclor CD should be used during pregnancy only if clearly needed.

Labor and Delivery: Ceclor CD has not been studied for use during labor and delivery. Treatment should be given only if clearly needed.

Nursing Mothers: No studies in lactating women have been performed with Ceclor CD. Small amounts of cefaclor (≤0.21 μg/mL) have been detected in human milk following administration of single 500-mg doses of Ceclor. The effect on nursing infants is not known. Caution should be exercised when Ceclor CD is administered to a nursing woman.

Pediatric Use: Safety and effectiveness of Ceclor CD in pediatric patients less than 16 years of age have not been established.

Geriatric Use: Healthy geriatric volunteers (≥65 years old) who received a single 750-mg dose of Ceclor CD had 40%–50% higher AUC and 20% lower renal clearance values when compared to healthy adult volunteers less than 45 years of age. These differences are considered to be primarily a result of age-related decreases in renal function. In clinical studies when geriatric patients received the usual recommended adult doses, clinical efficacy and safety were comparable to results in non-geriatric adult patients. No dosage changes are recommended for healthy geriatric patients.

Table 2
ADVERSE CLINICAL EVENTS
CECLOR CD MULTIPLE DOSE DOSING REGIMENS
CLINICAL TRIALS—NORTH AMERICA
(n = 1400)

	EVENT	INCIDENCE
Incidence Equal to or Greater Than 1%	Headache	4.9%
	Rhinitis	3.9%
	Diarrhea	3.8%
	Nausea	3.4%
	Vaginitis*	2.4%
	Vaginal Moniliasis*	2.2%
	Abdominal Pain	1.6%
	Cough Increased	1.5%
	Pharyngitis	1.4%
	Pruritus	1.4%
	Back Pain	1.0%

*n=934 for these events (subset of female participants).

Table 3
ADVERSE CLINICAL LABORATORY EVENTS
CECLOR CD MULTIPLE DOSE DOSING REGIMENS
CLINICAL TRIALS—NORTH AMERICA

	EVENT	INCIDENCE
Incidence Less Than 1%, But Greater Than 0.1%	Albumin decreased	0.3%
	Alkaline phosphatase increased	0.3%
	ALT/SGPT increased	0.3%
	Bilirubin total increased	0.3%
	Blood urea nitrogen (BUN) increased	0.2%
	Calcium decreased	0.7%
	Creatine phosphokinase increased	0.7%
	Creatinine increased	0.5%
	Eosinophils increased	0.3%
	Erythrocyte count decreased	0.3%
	GGT increased	0.2%
	Hemoglobin decreased	0.2%
	Lymphocytes decreased	0.3%
	Mean Cell Volume (MCV) increased	0.7%
	Neutrophils segmented decreased	0.3%
	Phosphorus increased	0.7%
	Platelet count decreased	0.3%
	Potassium increased	0.4%
	Sodium decreased	0.3%
	Sodium increased	0.4%

ADVERSE REACTIONS

Clinical Trials: There were 3272 patients treated with multiple doses of Ceclor CD in controlled clinical trials and an additional 211 subjects in pharmacology studies. There were no deaths in these trials thought to be related to toxicity from Ceclor CD. Treatment was discontinued in 1.7% of patients due to adverse events thought to be possibly or probably drug-related.

The following adverse clinical and laboratory events were reported during the Ceclor CD clinical trials conducted in North America at doses of 375 mg or 500 mg BID; however, relatedness of the adverse events to the drug was not assigned by clinical investigations during the trials (See Tables 2 and 3).

[See table 2 above]

Adverse reactions occurring during the clinical trials with cefaclor extended release tablets with an incidence of less than 1% but greater than 0.1% included the following (listed alphabetically):

Accidental injury, anorexia, anxiety, arthralgia, asthma, bronchitis, chest pain, chills, congestive heart failure, conjunctivitis, constipation, dizziness, dysmenorrhea, dyspepsia, dysuria, ear pain, edema, fever, flatulence, flu syndrome, gastritis, infection, insomnia, leukorrhea, lung disorder, maculopapular rash, malaise, menstrual disorder, myalgia, nausea and vomiting, neck pain, nervousness, nocturia, otitis media, pain, palpitation, peripheral edema, rash, respiratory disorder, sinusitis, somnolence, surgical procedure, sweating, tremor, urticaria, vomiting.

NOTE: One case of **serum-sickness-like** reaction was reported among the 3272 adult patients treated with Ceclor CD during the controlled clinical trials. These reactions have also been reported with the use of cefaclor in other oral formulations and are seen more frequently in pediatric patients than in adults. These reactions are characterized by findings of erythema multiforme, rash, and other skin manifestations accompanied by arthritis/arthralgia, with or without fever, and differ from classic serum sickness in that there is infrequently associated lymphadenopathy and proteinuria, no circulating immune complexes and no evidence to date of sequelae of the reaction. While further investigation is ongoing, **serum-sickness-like** reactions appear to be due to hypersensitivity and more often occur during or following a second (or subsequent) course of therapy with cefaclor. Such reactions have been reported with overall occurrence ranging from 1 in 200 (0.5%) in one focused trial; to 2 in 8346 (0.024%) in overall clinical trials (with an incidence in pediatric patients in clinical trials of 0.055%); to 1 in 38,000 (0.003%) in spontaneous event reports. Signs and symptoms usually occur a few days after initiation of therapy and subside within a few days after cessation of therapy. Occasionally these reactions have resulted in hospitalization, usually of short duration (median hospitalization = 2 to 3 days, based on postmarketing surveillance studies). In those patients requiring hospitalization, the symptoms have ranged from mild to severe at the time of admission with more of the severe reactions occurring in pediatric patients.

[See table 3 above]

In Postmarketing Experience: In addition to the events reported during clinical trials with Ceclor CD, the following adverse experiences are among those that have been reported during worldwide postmarketing surveillance: allergic reaction, anaphylactoid reaction, angioedema, face edema, hypotension, Stevens-Johnson syndrome, syncope, paresthesia, vasodilatation, and vertigo.

Other Adverse Reactions Associated With Other Formulations of Cefaclor: In addition to the above, the following other adverse reactions and altered laboratory tests have been associated with cefaclor in other oral formulations:

Clinical: Severe hypersensitivity reactions, including Stevens-Johnson syndrome, toxic epidermal necrolysis, and anaphylaxis, have been reported rarely. Anaphylactoid events may be manifested by solitary symptoms, including angioedema, edema (including face and limbs), parasthesias, syncope, or vasodilatation. Anaphylaxis may be more common in patients with a history of penicillin allergy. Rarely, hypersensitivity symptoms may persist for several months.

Symptoms of pseudomembranous colitis may appear either during or after antibiotic treatment. (*See* **WARNINGS**.)

Laboratory: Abnormal urinalysis, eosinophilia, leukopenia, neutropenia, transient elevations in AST, and transient thrombocytopenia have been reported.

Cephalosporin-Class Reactions: In addition to the adverse reactions listed above, the following adverse reactions and altered laboratory tests have been reported for cephalosporin-class antibiotics:

Clinical: Confusion, erythema multiforme, genital pruritus, hepatic dysfunction including cholestasis, hemolytic anemia, reversible hyperactivity, hypertonia, and reversible interstitial nephritis.

Laboratory—Positive direct Coombs' test.

OVERDOSAGE

The toxic symptoms following an overdose of cefaclor may include nausea, vomiting, epigastric distress, and diarrhea. The severity of the epigastric distress and the diarrhea are dose-related.

Absorption of drugs from the gastrointestinal tract may be decreased by giving activated charcoal, which, in many cases, is more effective than emesis or lavage. Consider charcoal instead of or in addition to gastric emptying. Repeated doses of charcoal over time may hasten elimination of some drugs that have been absorbed.

Adults (age 16 years and older): Type of Infection (as qualified in the **INDICATIONS AND USAGE** section of this labeling)	**Total Daily Dose**	**Dose and Frequency**	**Duration**
Acute Bacterial Exacerbations of Chronic Bronchitis due to *H. influenzae* (non-β-lactamase-producing strains only), *Moraxella catarrhalis* (including β-lactamase-producing strains), or *Streptococcus pneumoniae* (See **INDICATIONS and USAGE.**)	1000 mg	500 mg q12 hours	7 days
Secondary Bacterial Infections of Acute Bronchitis due to *H. influenzae* (non-β-lactamase-producing strains only), *M. catarrhalis* (including β-lactamase-producing strains), or *S. pneumoniae* (See **INDICATIONS and USAGE.**)	1000 mg	500 mg q12 hours	7 days
Pharyngitis and/or tonsillitis *due to S. pyogenes*	750 mg	375 mg q12 hours	10 days
Uncomplicated Skin and Skin Structure infections due to *S. aureus* (methicillin-susceptible strains) (See **INDICATIONS and USAGE.**)	750 mg	375 mg q12 hours	7–10 days

Although cefaclor is considered dialyzable, neither forced diuresis, peritoneal dialysis, hemodialysis, nor charcoal hemoperfusion have been demonstrated to be beneficial in an overdose of cefaclor.

DOSAGE AND ADMINISTRATION

The absorption of Ceclor CD is enhanced when it is administered with food. (*See* **CLINICAL PHARMACOLOGY.**) Therefore, **Ceclor CD should be administered with meals (i.e., at least within one hour of eating)**. The extended release tablets should not be cut, crushed, or chewed.

See INDICATIONS AND USAGE for information about patients for whom Ceclor CD is indicated.

NOTE: 500 mg BID of Ceclor CD is clinically equivalent to 250 mg TID of cefaclor as a pulvule in those indications listed in the **INDICATIONS AND USAGE** section of this label. **500 mg BID of Ceclor CD is NOT equivalent to 500 mg TID of other cefaclor formulations.**

[See table above]

Elderly patients with normal renal function do not require dosage adjustments.

HOW SUPPLIED

Tablets (extended release):
375 mg, blue (UC 5391)—(60s) NDC 51479-036-60
500 mg, blue (UC 5392)—(60s) NDC 51479-035-60
500 mg, blue (UC5392)—(14s) NDC 51479-035-03
(CDpak™, Tray of 3)

Store at controlled room temperature, 15° to 30°C (59° to 86°F).

CLINICAL STUDIES:

ACUTE BACTERIAL EXACERBATIONS OF CHRONIC BRONCHITIS AND SECONDARY BACTERIAL INFECTIONS OF ACUTE BRONCHITIS: In adequate and well-controlled clinical trials of Ceclor CD in the treatment of acute bacterial exacerbations of chronic bronchitis (ABECB) and secondary bacterial infections of acute bronchitis (SBIAB), only 4 evaluable patients with ABECB and no evaluable patients with SBIAB had infections caused by β-lactamase-producing *H. influenzae*. Four patients do not provide adequate data upon which to judge clinical efficacy of Ceclor CD against β-lactamase-producing *H. influenzae*.

UNCOMPLICATED SKIN AND SKIN STRUCTURE INFECTIONS: Ceclor CD (375 mg Q12H) (n=115) was compared to Ceclor Pulvules (250 mg TID) (n=106) for the treatment of patients with uncomplicated skin and skin structure infections, including cellulitis, pyoderma, abscess, and impetigo. Patients were treated for 7 to 10 days and were evaluated for clinical resolution and bacterial eradication approximately one week after completing therapy. To be evaluable, all patients had to have a recognized pathogen isolated from the skin infection just prior to the initiation of therapy. The results of this randomized, double-blinded, U.S. trial demonstrated:

(1) overall clinical cure rates were 72% (83 of 115 patients) and 75% (80 of 106 patients), respectively, for Ceclor CD and Ceclor Pulvules [95% CI around 3% difference = −16% to +9%],
(2) overall bacteriologic eradication rates against *Staphylococcus aureus* were comparable (*see* Table 4).

Table 4
CLINICAL RESPONSE* IN PATIENTS WITH SKIN AND SKIN STRUCTURE INFECTIONS

Outcome by Pathogen	CECLOR CD		CECLOR Pulvules	
Staphylococcus aureus	67/95	(71%)	58/81	(71%)
Streptococcus pyogenes	10/16	(63%)	8/9	(89%)
Other streptococci	7/11	(64%)	5/6	(83%)
Total	84/122	(69%)	71/96	(74%)

* Cure plus improvement

REFERENCES

1. National Committee for Clinical Laboratory Standards. Methods for Dilution Antimicrobial Susceptibility Tests for Bacteria that Grow Aerobically—Third edition; Approved Standard NCCLS Document M7-A3, Vol 13, No 25, NCCLS, Villanova, PA, December 1993
2. National Committee for Clinical Laboratory Standards. Performance Standards for Antimicrobial Disk Susceptibility Tests—Fifth edition; Approved Standard NCCLS Document M2-A5, Vol 13, No 24, NCCLS, Villanova, PA, December 1993

DURA PHARMACEUTICALS
Literature revised September 20, 1999

Manufactured by
Eli Lilly and Company
Indianapolis, IN 46285, USA
Distributed by DURA Pharmaceuticals, Inc.
San Diego, CA 92121
PV 2741 UCP CCD001B99

Shown in Product Identification Guide, page 311

ENTEX® capsules ℞
[n 'tex]
(phenylephrine hydrochloride/ phenylpropanolamine hydrochloride/guaifenesin)

DESCRIPTION

Each orange and white Entex capsule for oral administration contains
phenylephrine hydrochloride .... 5 mg
phenylpropanolamine hydrochloride .... 45 mg
guaifenesin .... 200 mg
This product contains ingredients of the following therapeutic classes: decongestant and expectorant.

HOW SUPPLIED

Orange and White Entex Capsules are imprinted "ENTEX" and "5147 9030".
NDC 51479-030-01 Bottles of 100
NDC 51479-030-05 Bottles of 500
Store below 77°F (25°C).
Rx only.

Manufactured by
WelPharm, Inc., Irvine, CA 92614
Manufactured for
DURA Pharmaceuticals, Inc.
San Diego, CA 92121
REVISED June, 1998 EC003C98

ENTEX® LIQUID ℞
[n 'tex]
(phenylephrine hydrochloride/ phenylpropanolamine hydrochloride/guaifenesin)

DESCRIPTION

Each 5 mL (one teaspoonful) for oral administration contains
phenylephrine hydrochloride .... 5 mg
phenylpropanolamine hydrochloride .... 20 mg
guaifenesin .... 100 mg
alcohol 5%

HOW SUPPLIED

Entex Liquid is available as an orange-colored, pleasant-tasting liquid.
NDC 51479-031-48 1 Pint (470 mL) bottle.
Store below 77°F (25°C). DO NOT REFRIGERATE.
Dispense in tight, light-resistant container as defined in USP.
Rx only.
Manufactured by
Schwarz Pharma Mfg., Inc.
Seymour, In 47274
Manufactured for
DURA Pharmaceuticals, Inc.
San Diego, CA 92121
Revised June, 1998 EL002C98

ENTEX® LA ℞
[n 'tex]
(phenylpropanolamine hydrochloride/guaifenesin)

DESCRIPTION

Each Entex LA orange, scored, long-acting tablet for oral administration contains
phenylpropanolamine hydrochloride .... 75 mg
guaifenesin .... 400 mg
in a special base to provide a prolonged therapeutic effect. This product contains ingredients of the following therapeutic classes: decongestant and expectorant.

Phenylpropanolamine hydrochloride is a decongestant having the chemical name, benzenemethanol, α-(1-aminoethyl)-, hydrochloride (R*, S*), (±), with the following structure:

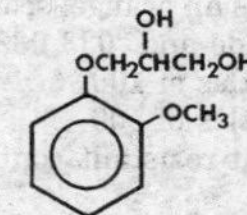

Guaifenesin is an expectorant having the chemical name, 1,2-propanediol, 3-(2-methoxyphenoxy)-, with the following structure:

Inactive Ingredients: Each tablet contains carbomer 934 P, compressible sugar, docusate sodium, FD&C Yellow No. 6 Aluminum Lake, hydroxypropyl cellulose, hydroxypropyl methylcellulose, polyethylene glycol, silicon dioxide, stearic acid, titanium dioxide, and zinc stearate.

CLINICAL PHARMACOLOGY

Phenylpropanolamine hydrochloride is an α-adrenergic receptor agonist (sympathomimetic) which produces vasoconstriction by stimulating α-receptors within the mucosa of the respiratory tract. Clinically, phenylpropanolamine shrinks swollen mucous membranes, reduces tissue hyperemia, edema, and nasal congestion, and increases nasal airway patency. Guaifenesin promotes lower respiratory tract drainage by thinning bronchial secretions, lubricates irritated respiratory tract membranes through increased mucous flow, and facilitates removal of viscous, inspissated mucus. As a result of these drugs, sinus and bronchial drainage is improved, and dry, nonproductive coughs become more productive and less frequent.

INDICATIONS AND USAGE

Entex LA is indicated for the symptomatic relief of sinusitis, bronchitis, pharyngitis, and coryza when these conditions are associated with nasal congestion and viscous mucus in the lower respiratory tract.

CONTRAINDICATIONS

Entex LA is contraindicated in individuals with known hypersensitivity to sympathomimetics, severe hypertension, or in patients receiving monoamine oxidase inhibitors.

WARNINGS

Sympathomimetic amines should be used with caution in patients with hypertension, diabetes mellitus, heart disease, peripheral vascular disease, increased intraocular pressure, hyperthyroidism, or prostatic hypertrophy.

PRECAUTIONS

Information for Patients: Do not crush or chew **Entex LA** tablets prior to swallowing.

Drug Interactions: **Entex LA** should not be used in patients taking monoamine oxidase inhibitors or other sympathomimetics.

Drug/Laboratory Test Interactions: Guaifenesin has been reported to interfere with clinical laboratory determinations of urinary 5-hydroxyindoleacetic acid (5-HIAA) and urinary vanillylmandelic acid (VMA).

Pregnancy: **Pregnancy Category C.** Animal reproduction studies have not been conducted with **Entex LA**. It is also

Continued on next page

Entex LA—Cont.

not known whether **Entex LA** can cause fetal harm when administered to a pregnant woman or can affect reproduction capacity. **Entex LA** should be given to a pregnant woman only if clearly needed.

Nursing Mothers: It is not known whether the drugs in **Entex LA** are excreted in human milk. Because many drugs are excreted in human milk and because of the potential for serious adverse reactions in nursing infants, a decision should be made whether to discontinue nursing or to discontinue the product, taking into account the importance of the drug to the mother.

Pediatric Use: Safety and effectiveness of **Entex LA** tablets in pediatric patients below the age of 6 have not been established.

ADVERSE REACTIONS

Possible adverse reactions include nervousness, insomnia, restlessness, headache, nausea, or gastric irritation. These reactions seldom, if ever, require discontinuation of therapy. Urinary retention may occur in patients with prostatic hypertrophy.

OVERDOSAGE

The treatment of overdosage should provide symptomatic and supportive care. If the amount ingested is considered dangerous or excessive, induce vomiting with ipecac syrup unless the patient is convulsing, comatose, or has lost the gag reflex, in which case perform gastric lavage using a large-bore tube. If indicated, follow with activated charcoal and a saline cathartic. Since the effects of **Entex LA** may last up to 12 hours, treatment should be continued for at least that length of time.

DOSAGE AND ADMINISTRATION

Adults and adolescents 12 years of age and older: one tablet twice daily (every 12 hours).

Children 6 to under 12 years: one-half (1/2) tablet twice daily (every 12 hours). **Entex LA** is not recommended for pediatric patients under 6 years of age.

Tablets may be broken in half for ease of administration without affecting release of medication but should not be crushed or chewed prior to swallowing.

HOW SUPPLIED

Entex LA is available as an orange, scored tablet coded with "ENTEX LA" on one side and "033 033" on the scored side.

NDC 51479-033-01 bottles of 100

NDC 51479-033-05 bottles of 500

Dispense in tight, light-resistant containers as defined in USP.

Store below 77°F (25°C).

Rx only.

Manufactured by
WelPharm, Inc.
Irvine, CA 92614
Manufactured for
DURA Pharmaceuticals, Inc.
San Diego, CA 92121
REVISED June, 1998 ELA 004C98

ENTEX® PSE ℞

[n 'tex P-S-E]
(pseudoephedrine hydrochloride/guaifenesin)

DESCRIPTION

Each **Entex PSE** yellow coated, scored, long-acting tablet for oral administration contains

pseudoephedrine hydrochloride .... 120 mg
guaifenesin .... 600 mg

in a special base to provide a prolonged therapeutic effect. This product contains ingredients of the following therapeutic classes: decongestant and expectorant.

Pseudoephedrine hydrochloride is a decongestant having the chemical name, benzenemethanol,α-[1-(methylamino-)ethyl]-[*S*-(*R**, *R**)]-, hydrochloride, with the following structure:

[Structure: C₆H₅–CH(OH)–CH(NHCH₃)–CH₃ · HCl]

Guaifenesin is an expectorant having the chemical name, 1,2-propanediol, 3-(2-methoxyphenoxy)-, with the following structure:

[Structure: 2-methoxyphenyl–OCH₂CH(OH)CH₂OH]

Inactive Ingredients: Each tablet contains compressible sugar, D&C Yellow No. 10 Aluminum Lake, dioctyl sodium sulfosuccinate, FD&C Yellow No. 6 Aluminum Lake, hydroxypropyl cellulose, hydroxypropyl methylcellulose, magnesium stearate, polyethylene glycol, purified water, silicon dioxide, sodium citrate, stearic acid, and titanium dioxide.

CLINICAL PHARMACOLOGY

Pseudoephedrine hydrochloride is an α-adrenergic receptor agonist (sympathomimetic) which produces vasoconstriction by stimulating α-receptors within the mucosa of the respiratory tract. Clinically, pseudoephedrine shrinks swollen mucous membranes, reduces tissue hyperemia, edema, and nasal congestion, and increases nasal airway patency. Guaifenesin promotes lower respiratory tract drainage by thinning bronchial secretions, lubricates irritated respiratory tract membranes through increased mucous flow, and facilitates removal of viscous, inspissated mucus. As a result of these drugs, sinus and bronchial drainage is improved, and dry, nonproductive coughs become more productive and less frequent.

INDICATIONS AND USAGE

Entex PSE tablets are indicated for the relief of nasal congestion due to the common cold, hay fever or other upper respiratory allergies, and nasal congestion associated with sinusitis. To promote nasal or sinus drainage; for the symptomatic relief of respiratory conditions characterized by dry nonproductive cough and in the presence of tenacious mucus and/or mucous plugs in the respiratory tract.

CONTRAINDICATIONS

Entex PSE tablets are contraindicated in patients with a known hypersensitivity to any of its ingredients, in nursing mothers, or in patients with severe hypertension, severe coronary artery disease, prostatic hypertrophy, or in patients on MAO inhibitor therapy.

WARNINGS

Sympathomimetic amines should be used with caution in patients with hypertension, diabetes mellitus, heart disease, peripheral vascular disease, increased intraocular pressure, hyperthyroidism, or prostatic hypertrophy.

PRECAUTIONS

General: Hypertensive patients should use **Entex PSE** tablets only with medical advice, as they may experience a change in blood pressure due to added vasoconstriction.

Information for Patients: Persistent cough may indicate a serious condition. If cough persists for more than one week, tends to recur, or is accompanied by a high fever, rash, or persistent headache, consult a physician.

Drug Interactions: MAO inhibitors and beta adrenergic blockers increase effects of sympathomimetics. Sympathomimetics may reduce the antihypertensive effects if methyldopa, guanethidine, mecamylamine, reserpine and veratrum alkaloids.

Drug/Laboratory Test Interactions: Guaifenesin has been reported to interfere with clinical laboratory determinations of urinary 5-hydroxyindoleacetic acid (5-HIAA) and urinary vanillylmandelic acid (VMA).

Pregnancy: Pregnancy Category C. Animal reproduction studies have not been conducted with **Entex PSE** tablets. It is also not known whether **Entex PSE** tablets can cause fetal harm when administered to a pregnant woman or can affect reproduction capacity. **Entex PSE** tablets should be given to a pregnant woman only if clearly needed.

Nursing Mothers: **Entex PSE** tablets are contraindicated in the nursing mother because of the higher than usual risks to infants from sympathomimetic agents.

Usage in Elderly: Patients 60 years and older are more likely to experience adverse reactions to sympathomimetics. Overdose may cause hallucinations, convulsions, CNS depression and death. Demonstrate safe use of a short-acting sympathomimetic before use of a sustained action formulation in elderly patients.

Pediatric Use: Safety and effectiveness of **Entex PSE** tablets in pediatric patients below the age of 6 have not been established.

ADVERSE REACTIONS

Gastrointestinal: nausea and vomiting.

Central Nervous System: nervousness, dizziness, sleeplessness, lightheadedness, tremor, hallucinations, convulsions, CNS depression, fear, anxiety, headache, increased irritability or excitement.

Cardiovascular: palpitations, tachycardia, cardiovascular collapse and death.

General: weakness.

Respiratory: respiratory difficulties.

OVERDOSAGE

Symptoms: Overdose may cause hallucinations, convulsions, CNS depression, cardiovascular collapse and death.

Treatment: Treatment of overdosage should provide symptomatic care. If the amount ingested is considered dangerous or excessive, induce vomiting with ipecac syrup unless the patient is convulsing, comatose, or has lost the gag reflex, in which case, perform gastric lavage using a large-bore tube. If indicated, follow with activated charcoal and a saline cathartic. Since the effects of **Entex PSE** tablets may last up to 12 hours, treatment should be continued for at least that length of time.

DOSAGE AND ADMINISTRATION

Adults and adolescents 12 years of age and older: one tablet twice daily (every 12 hours).

Children 6 to under 12 years: one-half (1/2) tablet twice daily (every 12 hours). **Entex PSE** tablets are not recommended for pediatric patients under 6 years of age.

Tablets may be broken in half for ease of administration without affecting release of medication but should not be crushed or chewed prior to swallowing.

HOW SUPPLIED

Entex PSE tablets are coated yellow, scored and coded with "Entex PSE" on one side and "032 032" on the scored side.

NDC 51479-032-01 bottles of 100

Store at controlled room temperature (59°–77°F or 15°–25°C).

Dispense in tight, light-resistant containers as defined in USP.

Rx only.

Manufactured by
WelPharm, Inc.
Irvine, CA 92614
Manufactured for
DURA Pharmaceuticals, Inc.
San Diego, CA 92121
REVISED June, 1998
EPSE003C98

MYAMBUTOL® ℞

[mī-ăm' būtol]
Ethambutol Hydrochloride
TABLETS
100 mg and 400 mg

DESCRIPTION

MYAMBUTOL ethambutol hydrochloride is an oral chemotherapeutic agent which is specifically effective against actively growing microorganisms of the genus *Mycobacterium*, including *M. tuberculosis*. The structural formula is:

[Structure: CH₃CH₂–CH(CH₂OH)–NHCH₂CH₂NH–CH(CH₂OH)–CH₂CH₃ · 2HCl]

(+)-2,2'(Ethylenediimino)-di-1-butanol dihydrochloride

MYAMBUTOL 100 and 400 mg tablets contain the following inactive ingredients: Gelatin, Hydroxypropyl Methylcellulose, Magnesium Stearate, Sodium Lauryl Sulfate, Sorbitol, Stearic Acid, Sucrose, Titanium Dioxide and other ingredients.

CLINICAL PHARMACOLOGY

MYAMBUTOL following a single oral dose of 25 mg/kg of body weight, attains a peak of 2 to 5 micrograms/mL in serum 2 to 4 hours after administration. When the drug is administered daily for longer periods of time at this dose, serum levels are similar. The serum level of MYAMBUTOL falls to undetectable levels by 24 hours after the last dose except in some patients with abnormal renal function. The intracellular concentrations of erythrocytes reach peak values approximately twice those of plasma and maintain this ratio throughout the 24 hours.

During the 24-hour period following oral administration of MYAMBUTOL approximately 50 percent of the initial dose is excreted unchanged in the urine, while an additional 8 to 15 percent appears in the form of metabolites. The main path of metabolism appears to be an initial oxidation of the alcohol to an aldehydic intermediate, followed by conversion to a dicarboxylic acid. From 20 to 22 percent of the initial dose is excreted in the feces as unchanged drug. No drug accumulation has been observed with consecutive single daily doses of 25 mg/kg in patients with normal kidney function, although marked accumulation has been demonstrated in patients with renal insufficiency.

MYAMBUTOL diffuses into actively growing *mycobacterium* cells such as tubercle bacilli. MYAMBUTOL appears to inhibit the synthesis of one or more metabolites, thus causing impairment of cell metabolism, arrest of multiplication, and cell death. No cross resistance with other available antimycobacterial agents has been demonstrated.

MYAMBUTOL has been shown to be effective against strains of *Mycobacterium tuberculosis* but does not seem to be active against fungi, viruses, or other bacteria. *Mycobacterium tuberculosis* strains previously unexposed to MYAMBUTOL have been uniformly sensitive to concentrations of 8 or less micrograms/mL, depending on the nature of the culture media. When MYAMBUTOL has been used alone for treatment of tuberculosis, tubercle bacilli from these patients have developed resistance to MYAMBUTOL ethambutol hydrochloride by *in vitro* susceptibility tests; the development of resistance has been unpredictable and appears to occur in a step-like manner. No cross resistance between MYAMBUTOL and other antituberculous drugs has been reported. MYAMBUTOL has reduced the incidence of the emergence of mycobacterial resistance to isoniazid when both drugs have been used concurrently.

An agar diffusion microbiologic assay, based upon inhibition of *Mycobacterium smegmatis* (ATCC 607) may be used to determine concentrations of MYAMBUTOL in serum and urine. This technique has not been published, but further information can be obtained upon inquiry to Lederle Laboratories.

ANIMAL PHARMACOLOGY

Toxicological studies in dogs on high prolonged doses produced evidence of myocardial damage and failure, and depigmentation of the tapetum lucidum of the eyes, the significance of which is not known. Degenerative changes in the central nervous system, apparently not dose-related, have also been noted in dogs receiving ethambutol hydrochloride over a prolonged period.

In the rhesus monkey, neurological signs appeared after treatment with high doses given daily over a period of several months. These were correlated with specific serum levels of ethambutol hydrochloride and with definite neuroanatomical changes in the central nervous system. Focal interstitial carditis was also noted in monkeys which received ethambutol hydrochloride in high doses for a prolonged period.

When pregnant mice or rabbits were treated with high doses of ethambutol hydrochloride, fetal mortality was slightly but not significantly (P>0.05) increased. Female rats treated with ethambutol hydrochloride displayed slight but insignificant (P>0.05) decreases in fertility and litter size.

In the fetuses born of mice treated with high doses of MYAMBUTOL during pregnancy, a low incidence of cleft palate, exencephaly and abnormality of the vertebral column were observed. More abnormalities of the cervical vertebra were seen in the newborn of rats treated with high doses of ethambutol hydrochloride during pregnancy. Rabbits receiving high doses of MYAMBUTOL during pregnancy gave birth to two fetuses with monophthalmia, one with a shortened right forearm accompanied by bilateral wrist-joint contracture and one with hare lip and cleft palate.

INDICATIONS

MYAMBUTOL is indicated for the treatment of pulmonary tuberculosis. It should not be used as the side antituberculous drug, but should be used in conjunction with at least one other antituberculous drug. Selection of the companion drug should be based on clinical experience, considerations of comparative safety and appropriate *in vitro* susceptibility studies. In patients who have not received previous antituberculous therapy, ie, initial treatment, the most frequently used regimens have been the following:

MYAMBUTOL plus isoniazid

MYAMBUTOL plus isoniazid plus streptomycin.

In patients who have received previous antituberculous therapy, mycobacterial resistance to other drugs used in initial therapy is frequent. Consequently, in such retreatment patients, MYAMBUTOL should be continued with at least one of the second line drugs not previously administered to the patient and to which bacterial susceptibility has been indicated by appropriate *in vitro* studies. Antituberculous drugs used with MYAMBUTOL have included cycloserine, ethionamide, pyrazinamide, viomycin and other drugs. Isoniazid, aminosalicylic acid, and streptomycin have also been used in multiple drug regimens. Alternating drug regimens have also been utilized.

CONTRAINDICATIONS

MYAMBUTOL is contraindicated in patients who are known to be hypersensitive to this drug. It is also contraindicated in patients with known optic neuritis unless clinical judgement determines that it may be used.

PRECAUTIONS

The effects of combinations of MYAMBUTOL ethambutol hydrochloride with other antituberculous drugs on the fetus is not known. While administration of this drug to pregnant human patients has produced no detectable effect upon the fetus, the possible teratogenic potential in women capable of bearing children should be weighed carefully against the benefits of therapy. There are published reports of five women who received the drug during pregnancy without apparent adverse effect upon the fetus.

MYAMBUTOL is not recommended for use in pediatric patients under thirteen years of age since safe conditions for use have not been established.

Patients with decreased renal function need the dosage reduced as determined by serum levels of MYAMBUTOL, since the main path of excretion of this drug is by the kidneys.

Because this drug may have adverse effects on vision, physical examination should include ophthalmoscopy, finger perimetry and testing of color discrimination. In patients with visual defects such as cataracts, recurrent inflammatory conditions of the eye, optic neuritis, and diabetic retinopathy, the evaluation of changes in visual acuity is more difficult, and care should be taken to be sure the variations in vision are not due to the underlying disease conditions. In such patients, consideration should be given to relationship between benefits expected and possible visual deterioration since evaluation of visual changes is difficult. (For recommended procedures, see next paragraphs under **ADVERSE REACTIONS**.)

As with any potent drug, periodic assessment of organ system functions, including renal, hepatic, and hematopoietic, should be made during long-term therapy.

ADVERSE REACTIONS

MYAMBUTOL may produce decreases in visual acuity which appear to be due to optic neuritis. This effect may be related to dose and duration of treatment. This effect is generally reversible when administration of the drug is discontinued promptly. In rare cases recovery may be delayed for up to one year or more. Irreversible blindness has been reported.

Optic neuropathy including optic neuritis or retrobulbar neuritis occurring in association with ethambutol therapy may be characterized by one or more of the following events: decreased visual acuity, scotoma, color blindness, and/or visual defect. These events have also been reported in the absence of a diagnosis of optic or retrobulbar neuritis.

Patients should be advised to report promptly to their physician any change of visual acuity.

The change in visual acuity may be unilateral or bilateral ahd hence *each eye must be tested separately and both eyes tested together.* Testing of visual acuity should be performed before beginning MYAMBUTOL therapy and periodically during drug administration, except that it should be done monthly when a patient is on a dosage of more than 15 mg per kilogram per day. Snellen eye charts are recommended for testing of visual acuity. Studies have shown that there are definite fluctuations of one or two lines of the Snellen chart in the visual acuity of many tuberculous patients *not* receiving MYAMBUTOL.

The following table may be useful in interpreting possible changes in visual acuity attributable to MYAMBUTOL.

[See table above]

Initial Snellen Reading	Reading Indicating Significant Decrease	Significant Number of Lines	Decrease Number of Points
20/13	20/25	3	12
20/15	20/25	2	10
20/20	20/30	2	10
20/25	20/40	2	15
20/30	20/50	2	20
20/40	20/70	2	30
20/50	20/70	1	20

In general, changes in visual acuity less than those indicated under "Significant Number of Lines" and "Decrease-Number of Points", may be due to chance variation, limitations of the testing method or physiologic variability. Conversely, changes in visual acuity equaling or exceeding those under "Significant Number of Lines" and "Decrease-Number of Points" indicate need for retesting and careful evaluation of the patient's visual status. If careful evaluation confirms the magnitude of visual change and fails to reveal another cause, MYAMBUTOL should be discontinued and the patient reevaluated at frequent intervals. Progressive decreases in visual acuity during therapy must be considered to be due to MYAMBUTOL.

If corrective glasses are used prior to treatment, these must be worn during visual acuity testing. During 1 to 2 years of therapy, a refractive error may develop which must be corrected in order to obtain accurate test results. Testing the visual acuity through a pinhole eliminates refractive errors.

Patients developing visual abnormality during MYAMBUTOL treatment may show subjective visual symptoms before or simultaneously with, the demonstration of decreases in visual acuity, and all patients receiving MYAMBUTOL should be questioned periodically about blurred vision and other subjective eye symptoms.

Recovery of visual acuity generally occurs over a period of weeks to months after the drug has been discontinued. Some patients have received MYAMBUTOL ethambutol hydrochloride again after such recovery without recurrence of loss of visual acuity.

Other adverse reactions reported include: anaphylactoid reactions, dermatitis, pruritus and joint pain; anorexia, nausea, vomiting, gastrointestinal upset, abdominal pain; fever, malaise, headache, and dizziness; mental confusion, disorientation and possible hallucinations. Numbness and tingling of the extremities due to peripheral neuritis have been reported infrequently.

Elevated serum uric acid levels occur and precipitation of acute gout has been reported. Pulmonary infiltrates and eosinophilia also have been reported during MYAMBUTOL therapy. Transient impairment of liver function as indicated by abnormal liver function tests is not an unusual finding. Since MYAMBUTOL is recommended for therapy in conjunction with one or more other antituberculous drugs, these changes may be related to the concurrent therapy.

DOSAGE AND ADMINISTRATION

MYAMBUTOL should not be used alone, in initial treatment or in retreatment. MYAMBUTOL should be administered on a once every 24-hour basis only. Absorption is not significantly altered by administration with food. Therapy, in general, should be continued until bacteriological conversion has become permanent and maximal clinical improvement has occurred.

MYAMBUTOL is not recommended for use in pediatric patients under thirteen years of age since safe conditions for use have not been established.

Initial Treatment: In patients who have not received previous antituberculous therapy, administer MYAMBUTOL 15 mg per kilogram (7 mg per pound) of body weight, as a single oral dose once every 24 hours. In the more recent studies, isoniazid has been administered concurrently in a single, daily, oral dose.

Retreatment: In patients who have received previous antituberculous therapy, administer MYAMBUTOL 25 mg per kilogram (11 mg per pound) of body weight, as a single oral dose once every 24 hours. Concurrently administer at least one other antituberculous drug to which the organisms have been demonstrated to be susceptible by appropriate *in vitro* tests. Suitable drugs usually consist of those not previously used in the treatment of the patient. After 60 days of MYAMBUTOL administration, decrease the dose to 15 mg per kilogram (7 mg per pound) of body weight, and administer as a single oral dose once every 24 hours.

During the period when a patient is on a daily dose of 25 mg/kg, monthly eye examinations are advised.

See Table for easy selection of proper weight-dose tablet(s).

Weight-Dose Table

15 mg/kg (7 mg/lb) Schedule

Weight Range Pounds	Kilograms	Daily Dose In mg
Under 85 lbs.	Under 37 Kg	500
85 – 94.5	37 – 43	600
95 – 109.5	43 – 50	700
110 – 124.5	50 – 57	800
125 – 139.5	57 – 64	900
140 – 154.5	64 – 71	1000
155 – 169.5	71 – 79	1100
170 – 184.5	79 – 84	1200
185 – 199.5	84 – 90	1200
200 – 214.5	90 – 97	1400
215 and Over	Over 97	1500

25 mg/kg (11 mg/lb) Schedule

Pounds	Kilograms	Daily Dose In mg
Under 85 lbs.	Under 38 kg	900
85 – 92.5	38 – 42	1000
93 – 101.5	42 – 45.5	1100
102 – 109.5	45.5 – 50	1200
110 – 118.5	50 – 54	1300
119 – 128.5	54 – 58	1400
129 – 136.5	58 – 62	1500
137 – 146.5	62 – 67	1600
147 – 155.5	67 – 71	1700
156 – 164.5	71 – 75	1800
165 – 173.5	75 – 79	1900
174 – 182.5	79 – 83	2000
183 – 191.5	83 – 87	2100
192 – 199.5	87 – 91	2200
200 – 209.5	91 – 95	2300
210 – 218.5	95 – 99	2400
219 and Over	Over 99	2500

HOW SUPPLIED

MYAMBUTOL® ethambutol hydrochloride Tablets

100 mg—round, convex, white, film coated tablets engraved M6 on one side and LL on the other, are supplied as follows:

NDC 51479-046-01—Bottle of 100

400 mg—round, convex, white, scored, film coated tablets engraved with LL on one side and M to the left and 7 to the right of the score on the other side, are supplied as follows:

NDC 51479-047-01—Bottle of 100

NDC 51479-047-10 —Bottle of 1000

NDC 51479-047-04 Unit dose 10 (2 × 5) Strips

Store at controlled room temperature 15°–30° C (59°–86° F).

Rx only

Manufactured by LEDERLE PHARMACEUTICAL DIVISION of

American Cyanamid Company, Pearl River, NY 10965

For DURA PHARMACEUTICALS, INC.

San Diego, CA 92121

CI 4544-4

Revised April 17, 2000

MY001B00

MAXIPIME® ℞

[*max-ə-pĭme*]

(Cefepime Hydrochloride) for Injection

For Intravenous or Intramuscular Use

Rx only

DESCRIPTION

Cefepime hydrochloride is a semi-synthetic, broad spectrum, cephalosporin antibiotic for parenteral administration. The chemical name is 1-[[(6R,7R)-7-[2-(2-amino-4-thiazolyl)-glyoxylamido]-2-carboxy-8-oxo-5-thia-1-azabicyclo-[4.2.0]oct-2-en-3-yl]methyl]-1-methylpyrrolidinium chloride, 7^2-(Z)- (O-methyloxime), monohydrochloride, monohydrate.

Cefepime hydrochloride is a white to pale yellow powder with a molecular formula of $C_{19}H_{25}ClN_6O_5S_2 \bullet HCl \bullet H_20$ and a molecular weight of 571.5. It is highly soluble in water.

MAXIPIME® (cefepime hydrochloride) for Injection, is supplied for intramuscular or intravenous administration in strengths equivalent to 500 mg, 1 g and 2 g of cefepime. (See **DOSAGE AND ADMINISTRATION**.) MAXIPIME is a sterile, dry mixture of cefepime hydrochloride and L-arginine. The L-arginine, at an approximate concentration of 725 mg/g of cefepime, is added to control the pH of the constituted solution at 4.0–6.0. Freshly constituted solutions of MAXIPIME will range in color from colorless to amber.

Continued on next page

Maxipime—Cont.

CLINICAL PHARMACOLOGY

Pharmacokinetics: The average plasma concentrations of cefepime observed in healthy adult male volunteers (n=9) at various times following single 30-minute infusions (IV) of cefepime 500 mg, 1 g, and 2 g are summarized in Table 1. Elimination of cefepime is principally via renal excretion with an average (± SD) half-life of 2.0 (±0.3) hours and total body clearance of 120.0 (± 8.0) mL/min in healthy volunteers. Cefepime pharmacokinetics are linear over the range 250 mg to 2 g. There is no evidence of accumulation in healthy adult male volunteers (n=7) receiving clinically relevant doses for a period of 9 days.

Absorption: The average plasma concentrations of cefepime and its derived pharmacokinetic parameters after intravenous administration are portrayed in Table 1.

TABLE 1
Average Plasma Concentrations in µg/mL of Cefepime and Derived Pharmacokinetic Parameters (±SD), Intravenous Administration

	MAXIPIME		
Parameter	500 mg IV	1 g IV	2 g IV
0.5 hr	38.2	78.7	163.1
1.0 hr	21.6	44.5	85.8
2.0 hr	11.6	24.3	44.8
4.0 hr	5.0	10.5	19.2
8.0 hr	1.4	2.4	3.9
12.0 hr	0.2	0.6	1.1
C_{max}, µg/mL	39.1 (3.5)	81.7 (5.1)	163.9 (25.3)
AUC, hr•µg/mL	70.8 (6.7)	148.5 (15.1)	284.8 (30.6)
Number of subjects (male)	9	9	9

Following intramuscular (IM) administration, cefepime is completely absorbed. The average plasma concentrations of cefepime at various times following a single IM injection are summarized in Table 2. The pharmacokinetics of cefepime are linear over the range of 500 mg to 2 g IM and do not vary with respect to treatment duration.

Table 2
Average Plasma Concentrations in µg/mL of Cefepime and Derived Pharmacokinetic Parameters (±SD), Intramuscular Administration

	MAXIPIME (cefepime hydrochloride)		
Parameter	500 mg IM	1 g IM	2 g IM
0.5 hr	8.2	14.8	36.1
1.0 hr	12.5	25.9	49.9
2.0 hr	12.0	26.3	51.3
4.0 hr	6.9	16.0	31.5
8.0 hr	1.9	4.5	8.7
12.0 hr	0.7	1.4	2.3
C_{max}, µg/mL	13.9 (3.4)	29.6 (4.4)	57.5 (9.5)
T_{max}, hr	1.4 (0.9)	1.6 (0.4)	1.5 (0.4)
AUC, hr•µg/mL	60.0 (8.0)	137.0 (11.0)	262.0 (23.0)
Number of subjects (male)	6	6	12

Distribution: The average steady state volume of distribution of cefepime is 18.0 (± 2.0)L. The serum protein binding of cefepime is approximately 20% and is independent of its concentration in serum.

Cefepime is excreted in human milk. A nursing infant consuming approximately 1000 mL of human milk per day would receive approximately 0.5 mg of cefepime per day. (See **PRECAUTIONS, Nursing Mothers.**)

Concentrations of cefepime achieved in specific tissues and body fluids are listed in Table 3.

[See table 3 above]

Table 3
Average Concentrations of Cefepime in Specific Body Fluids (µg/mL) or Tissues (µg/g)

Tissue or Fluid	Dose/Route	# of Patients	Average Time of Sample Post-Dose (hr)	Average Concentration
Blister Fluid	2 g IV	6	1.5	81.4 µg/mL
Bronchial Mucosa	2 g IV	20	4.8	24.1 µg/g
Sputum	2 g IV	5	4.0	7.4 µg/mL
Urine	500 mg IV	8	0-4	292 µg/mL
	1 g IV	12	0-4	926 µg/mL
	2 g IV	12	0-4	3120 µg/mL
Bile	2 g IV	26	9.4	17.8 µg/mL
Peritoneal Fluid	2 g IV	19	4.4	18.3 µg/mL
Appendix	2 g IV	31	5.7	5.2 µg/g
Gallbladder	2 g IV	38	8.9	11.9 µg/g
Prostate	2 g IV	5	1.0	31.5 µg/g

Data suggest that cefepime does cross the inflamed blood-brain barrier. **The clinical relevance of these data are uncertain at this time.**

Metabolism and Excretion: Cefepime is metabolized to N-methylpyrrolidine (NMP) which is rapidly converted to the N-oxide (NMP-N-oxide). Urinary recovery of unchanged cefepime accounts for approximately 85% of the administered dose. Less than 1% of the administered dose is recovered from urine as NMP, 6.8% as NMP-N-oxide, and 2.5% as an epimer of cefepime. Because renal excretion is a significant pathway of elimination, patients with renal dysfunction and patients undergoing hemodialysis require dosage adjustment. (See **DOSAGE AND ADMINISTRATION.**)

Special Populations: *Pediatric patients:* Cefepime pharmacokinetics have been evaluated in pediatric patients from 2 months to 11 years of age following single and multiple doses on q8h (n=29) and q12h (n=13) schedules. Following a single IV dose, total body clearance and the steady state volume of distribution averaged 3.3 (±1.0) mL/min/kg and 0.3 (±0.1) L/kg, respectively. The urinary recovery of unchanged cefepime was 60.4 (±30.4)% of the administered dose, and the average renal clearance was 2.0 (±1.1) mL/min/kg. There were no significant effects of age or gender (25 male vs. 17 female) on total body clearance or volume of distribution, corrected for body weight. No accumulation was seen when cefepime was given at 50 mg/kg q 12h (n=13), while C_{max}, AUC, and $t_{1/2}$ were increased about 15% at steady state after 50 mg/kg q8h. The exposure to cefepime following a 50 mg/kg IV dose in a pediatric patient is comparable to that in an adult treated with a 2 g IV dose. The absolute bioavailability of cefepime after an IM dose of 50 mg/kg was 82.3 (±15)% in eight patients.

Geriatric patients: Cefepime pharmacokinetics have been investigated in elderly (65 years of age and older) men (n=12) and women (n=12) whose creatinine clearance was 74.0 (± 15.0) mL/min. There appeared to be a decrease in cefepime total body clearance as a function of creatinine clearance. Therefore, dosage administration of cefepime in the elderly should be adjusted as appropriate if the patient's creatinine clearance is 60 mL/min or less. (See **DOSAGE AND ADMINISTRATION.**)

Renal Insufficiency: Cefepime pharmacokinetics have been investigated in patients with various degrees of renal insufficiency (n=30). The average half-life in patients requiring hemodialysis was 13.5 (± 2.7) hours and in patients requiring continuous peritoneal dialysis was 19.0 (± 2.0) hours. Cefepime total body clearance decreased proportionally with creatinine clearance in patients with abnormal renal function, which serves as the basis for dosage adjustment recommendations in this group of patients. (See **DOSAGE AND ADMINISTRATION.**)

Hepatic Insufficiency: The pharmacokinetics of cefepime were unaltered in patients with impaired hepatic function who received a single 1 g dose (n=11).

Microbiology: Cefepime is a bactericidal agent that acts by inhibition of bacterial cell wall synthesis. Cefepime has a broad spectrum of *in vitro* activity that encompasses a wide range of gram-positive and gram-negative bacteria. Cefepime has a low affinity for chromosomally-encoded beta-lactamases. Cefepime is highly resistant to hydrolysis by most beta-lactamases and exhibits rapid penetration into gram-negative bacterial cells. Within bacterial cells, the molecular targets of cefepime are the penicillin binding proteins (PBP).

Cefepime has been shown to be active against most strains of the following micro organisms, both *in vitro* and in clinical infections as described in the **INDICATIONS AND USAGE** section.

Aerobic Gram-Negative Microorganisms:
Enterobacter
Escherichia coli
Klebsiella pneumoniae
Proteus mirabilis
Pseudomonas aeruginosa

Aerobic Gram-Positive Microorganisms:
Staphylococcus aureus (methicillin-susceptible strains only)
Streptococcus pneumoniae
Streptococcus pyogenes (Lancefield's Group A streptococci)

The following *in vitro* data are available, **but their clinical significance is unknown**. Cefepime has been shown to have *in vitro* activity against most strains of the following microorganisms; however, the safety and effectiveness of cefepime in treating clinical infections due to these microorganisms have not been established in adequate and well-controlled trials.

Aerobic Gram-Positive Microorganisms:
Staphylococcus epidermidis (methicillin-susceptible strains only)
Staphylococcus saprophyticus
Streptococcus agalactiae (Lancefield's Group B streptococci)
Viridans group streptococci

NOTE: Most strains of enterococci, e.g. *Enterococcus faecalis*, and methicillin-resistant staphylococci are resistant to cefepime.

Aerobic Gram-Negative Microorganisms:
Acinetobacter calcoaceticus subsp. *lwoffi*
Citrobacter diversus
Citrobacter freundii
Enterobacter agglomerans
Haemophilus influenzae (including beta-lactamase producing strains)
Hafnia alvei
Klebsiella oxytoca
Moraxella catarrhalis (including beta-lactamase producing strains)
Morganella morganii
Proteus vulgaris
Providencia rettgeri
Providencia stuartii
Serratia marcescens

NOTE: Cefepime is inactive against many strains of *Stenotrophomonas* (formerly *Xanthomonas maltophilia* and *Pseudomonas maltophilia*).

Anaerobic Microorganisms:
NOTE: Cefepime is inactive against most strains of *Clostridium difficile*.

TABLE 4

Microorganism	MIC (µg/mL)		
	Susceptible (S)	Intermediate (I)	Resistant (R)
Microorganisms other than *Haemophilus* spp.* and *S. pneumoniae**	≤8	16	≥32
Haemophilus spp.*	≤2	—*	—*
*Streptococcus pneumoniae**	≤0.5	1	≥2

* NOTE: Isolates from these species should be tested for susceptibility using specialized dilution testing methods.[1] Also, strains of *Haemophilus* spp. with MIC's greater than 2 µg/mL should be considered equivocal and should be further evaluated.

Susceptibility Tests

Dilution Techniques: Quantitative methods are used to determine antimicrobial minimum inhibitory concentrations (MIC's). These MIC's provide estimates of the susceptibility of bacteria to antimicrobial compounds. The MIC's should be determined using a standardized procedure. Standardized procedures are based on a dilution method[1] (broth or agar) or equivalent with standardized inoculum concentrations and standardized concentrations of cefepime powder. The MIC values should be interpreted according to the following criteria:

[See table 4 on previous page]

A report of "Susceptible" indicates that the pathogen is likely to be inhibited if the antimicrobial compound in the blood reaches the concentrations usually achievable. A report of "Intermediate" indicates that the result should be considered equivocal, and, if the microorganism is not fully susceptible to alternative, clinically feasible drugs, the test should be repeated. This category implies possible clinical applicability in body sites where the drug is physiologically concentrated or in situations where high dosage of drug can be used. This category also provides a buffer zone which prevents small uncontrolled technical factors from causing major discrepancies in interpretation. A report of "Resistant" indicates that the pathogen is not likely to be inhibited if the antimicrobial compound in the blood reaches the concentrations usually achievable; other therapy should be selected.

Standardized susceptibility test procedures require the use of laboratory control microorganisms to control the technical aspects of the laboratory procedures. Laboratory control microorganisms are specific strains of microbiological assay organisms with intrinsic biological properties relating to resistance mechanisms and their genetic expression within bacteria; the specific strains are not clinically significant in their current microbiological status. Standard cefepime powder should provide the following MIC values (Table 5) when tested against the designated quality control strains:

TABLE 5

Microorganism	ATCC	MIC (μg/mL)
Escherichia coli	25922	0.015-0.06
Staphylococcus aureus	29213	1-4
Pseudomonas aeruginosa	27853	1-4
Haemophilus influenzae	49247	0.5-2
Streptococcus pneumoniae	49619	0.06-0.25

Diffusion Techniques: Quantitative methods that require measurement of zone diameters also provide reproducible estimates of the susceptibility of bacteria to antimicrobial compounds. One such standardized procedure[2] requires the use of standardized inoculum concentrations. This procedure uses paper disks impregnated with 30 μg of cefepime to test the susceptibility of microorganisms to cefepime. Interpretation is identical to that stated above for results using dilution techniques.

Reports from the laboratory providing results of the standard single-disk susceptibility test with a 30-μg cefepime disk should be interpreted according to the following criteria:

[See table 6 above]

As with standardized dilution techniques, diffusion methods require the use of laboratory control microorganisms to control the technical aspects of the laboratory procedures. Laboratory control microorganisms are specific strains of microbiological assay organisms with intrinsic biological properties relating to resistance mechanisms and their genetic expression within bacteria; the specific strains are not clinically significant in their current microbiological status. For the diffusion technique, the 30-μg cefepime disk should provide the following zone diameters in these laboratory test quality control strains (Table 7):

TABLE 7

Microorganism	ATCC	Zone Size Range (mm)
Escherichia coli	25922	29 - 35
Staphylococcus aureus	25923	23 - 29
Pseudomonas aeruginosa	27853	24 - 30
Haemophilus influenza	49247	25 - 31

TABLE 6

Microorganism	Zone Diameter (mm) Susceptible (S)	Intermediate (I)	Resistant (R)
Microorganisms other than *Haemophilus* spp.* and *S. pneumoniae**	≥ 18	15-17	≤ 14
Haemophilus spp.*	≥ 26	—*	—*

* NOTE: Isolates from these species should be tested for susceptibility using specialized diffusion testing methods[2]. Isolates of *Haemophilus* spp. with zones smaller than 26 mm should be considered equivocal and should be further evaluated. Isolates of *S. pneumoniae* should be tested against a 1 μg oxacillin disk; isolates with oxacillin zone sizes larger than or equal to 20 mm may be considered susceptible to cefepime.

TABLE 8
Demographics of Evaluable Patients (First Episodes Only)

	Cefepime	Ceftazidime
Total	**164**	**153**
Median age (yr)	56.0 (range, 18-82)	55.0 (range, 16-84)
Male	86 (52%)	85 (56%)
Female	78 (48%)	68 (44%)
Leukemia	65 (40%)	52 (34%)
Other hematologic malignancies	43 (26%)	36 (24%)
Solid tumor	54 (33%)	56 (37%)
Median ANC nadir (cells/μL)	20.0 (range, 0-500)	20.0 (range, 0-500)
Median duration of neutropenia (days)	6.0 (range, 0–39)	6.0 (range, 0-32)
Indwelling venous catheter	97 (59%)	86 (56%)
Prophylactic antibiotics	62 (38%)	64 (42%)
Bone marrow graft	9 (5%)	7 (5%)
SBP < 90 mm Hg at entry	7 (4%)	2 (1%)

ANC = absolute neutropil count; SBP = systolic blood pressure.

TABLE 9
Pooled Response Rates For Empiric Therapy of Febrile Neutropenic Patients

Outcome Measures	% Response Cefepime (N=164)	Ceftazidime (N=153)
Primary episode resolved with no treatment modification, no new febrile episodes or infection, and oral antibiotics allowed for completion of treatment	**51**	**55**
Primary episode resolved with no treatment modification, no new febrile episodes or infection, and no post-treatment oral antibiotics	**34**	**39**
Survival, any treatment modification allowed	93	97
Primary episode resolved with no treatment modification and oral antibiotics allowed for completion of treatment	62	67
Primary episode resoled with no treatment modification and no post-treatment oral antibiotics	46	51

TABLE 10
Adverse Clinical Reactions
Cefepime Multiple-Dose
Dosing Regimens Clinical Trials—North America

INCIDENCE EQUAL TO OR GREATER THAN 1%	Local reactions (3.0%), including phlebitis (1.3%), pain and/or inflammation (0.6%)*; rash (1.1%)
INCIDENCE LESS THAN 1% BUT GREATER THAN 0.1%	Colitis (including pseudomembranous colitis), diarrhea, fever, headache, nausea, oral moniliasis, pruritus, urticarial, vaginitis, vomiting

* local reactions, irrespective of relationship to cefepime in those patients who received intravenous infusion (n = 3048).

INDICATIONS AND USAGE

MAXIPIME (cefepime hydrochloride) is indicated in the treatment of the following infections caused by susceptible strains of the designated microorganisms (see also **PRECAUTIONS: Pediatric Use** and **DOSAGE AND ADMINISTRATION**):

Pneumonia (moderate to severe) caused by *Streptococcus pneumoniae*, including cases associated with concurrent bacteremia, *Pseudomonas aeruginosa*, *Klebsiella pneumoniae*, or *Enterobacter* species.

Empiric Therapy for Febrile Neutropenic Patients. Cefepime as monotherapy is indicated for empiric treatment of febrile neutropenic patients. In patients at high risk for severe infection (including patients with a history of recent bone marrow transplantation, with hypotension at presentation, with an underlying hematologic malignancy, or with severe or prolonged neutropenia), antimicrobial monotherapy may not be appropriate. Insufficient data exist to support the efficacy of cefepime monotherapy in such patients. (See **CLINICAL STUDIES**.)

Uncomplicated and Complicated Urinary Tract Infections (including pyelonephritis) caused by *Escherichia coli* or *Klebsiella pneumoniae*, when the infection is severe, or caused by *Escherichia coli*, *Klebsiella pneumoniae*, or *Proteus mirabilis*, when the infection is mild to moderate, including cases associated with concurrent bacteremia with these microorganisms.

Uncomplicated Skin and Skin Structure Infections caused by *Staphylococcus aureus* (methicillin-susceptible strains only) or *Streptococcus pyogenes*.

Complicated Intra-abdominal Infections (used in combination with metronidazole) caused by *Escherichia coli*, viridans group streptococci, *Pseudomonas aeruginosa*, *Klebsiella pneumoniae*, *Enterobacter* species, or *Bacteroides fragilis*. (See **CLINICAL STUDIES**.)

Culture and susceptibility testing should be performed where appropriate to determine the susceptibility of the causative microorganism(s) to cefepime.

Therapy with MAXIPIME may be instituted before results of susceptibility studies are known; however, once these results become available, the antibiotic treatment should be adjusted accordingly.

CLINICAL STUDIES

Febrile Neutropenic Patients

The safety and efficacy of empiric cefepime monotherapy of febrile neutropenic patients have been assessed in two multicenter, randomized trials, comparing cefepime monotherapy (at a dose of 2 g IV q8h) to ceftazidime monotherapy (at a dose of 2 g IV q8h). These studies comprised 317 evaluable patients. Table 8 describes the characteristics of the evaluable patient population.

[See table 8 above]

Table 9 describes the clinical response rates observed. For all outcome measures, cefepime was therapeutically equivalent to ceftazidime.

[See table 9 above]

Insufficient data exist to support the efficacy of cefepime monotherapy in patients at high risk for severe infection

Continued on next page

Maxipime—Cont.

(including patients with a history of recent bone marrow transplantation, with hypotension at presentation, with an underlying hematologic malignancy, or with severe or prolonged neutropenia). No data are available in patients with septic shock.

Complicated Intra-abdominal Infections

Patients hospitalized with complicated intra-abdominal infections participated in a randomized, double-blind, multicenter trial comparing the combination of cefepime (2 g q12h) plus intravenous metronidazole (500 mg q6h) versus imipenem/cilastatin (500 mg q6h) for a maximum duration of 14 days of therapy. The study was designed to demonstrate equivalence of the two therapies. The primary analyses were conducted on the protocol-valid population, which consisted of those with a surgically confirmed complicated infection, at least one pathogen isolated pretreatment, at least 5 days of treatment, and a 4–6 week follow-up assessment for cured patients. Subjects in the imipenem/cilastatin arm had higher APACHE II scores at baseline. The treatment groups were otherwise generally comparable with regard to their pretreatment characteristics. The overall clinical cure rate among the protocol-valid patients was 81% (51 cured/63 evaluable patients) in the cefepime plus metronidazole group and 66% (62/94) in the imipenem/cilastatin group. The observed differences in efficacy may have been due to a greater proportion of patients with high APACHE II scores in the imipenem/cilastatin group.

CONTRAINDICATIONS

MAXIPIME (cefepime hydrochloride) is contraindicated in patients who have shown immediate hypersensitivity reactions to cefepime or the cephalosporin class of antibiotics, penicillins or other beta-lactam antibiotics.

WARNINGS

BEFORE THERAPY WITH MAXIPIME (CEFEPIME HYDROCHLORIDE) FOR INJECTION IS INSTITUTED, CAREFUL INQUIRY SHOULD BE MADE TO DETERMINE WHETHER THE PATIENT HAS HAD PREVIOUS IMMEDIATE HYPERSENSITIVITY REACTIONS TO CEFEPIME, CEPHALOSPORINS, PENICILLINS, OR OTHER DRUGS. IF THIS PRODUCT IS TO BE GIVEN TO PENICILLIN-SENSITIVE PATIENTS, CAUTION SHOULD BE EXERCISED BECAUSE CROSS-HYPERSENSITIVITY AMONG BETA-LACTAM ANTIBIOTICS HAS BEEN CLEARLY DOCUMENTED AND MAY OCCUR IN UP TO 10% OF PATIENTS WITH A HISTORY OF PENICILLIN ALLERGY. IF AN ALLERGIC REACTION TO MAXIPIME OCCURS, DISCONTINUE THE DRUG. SERIOUS ACUTE HYPERSENSITIVITY REACTIONS MAY REQUIRE TREATMENT WITH EPINEPHRINE AND OTHER EMERGENCY MEASURES INCLUDING OXYGEN, CORTICOSTEROIDS, INTRAVENOUS FLUIDS, INTRAVENOUS ANTIHISTAMINES, PRESSOR AMINES, AND AIRWAY MANAGEMENT, AS CLINICALLY INDICATED.

Pseudomembranous colitis has been reported with nearly all antibacterial agents, including MAXIPIME, and may range in severity from mild to life-threatening. Therefore, it is important to consider this diagnosis in patients who present with diarrhea subsequent to the administration of antibacterial agents.

Treatment with antibacterial agents alters the normal flora of the colon and may permit overgrowth of clostridia. Studies indicate that a toxin produced by *Clostridium difficile* is a primary cause of "antibiotic-associated colitis".

After the diagnosis of pseudomembranous colitis has been established, therapeutic measures should be initiated. Mild cases of pseudomembranous colitis usually respond to drug discontinuation alone. In moderate-to-severe cases, consideration should be given to management with fluids and electrolytes, protein supplementation, and treatment with an antibacterial drug clinically effective against *Clostridium difficile* colitis.

PRECAUTIONS

General: As with other antimicrobials, prolonged use of MAXIPIME may result in overgrowth of nonsusceptible microorganisms. Repeated evaluation of the patient's condition is essential. Should superinfection occur during therapy, appropriate measures should be taken.

Many cephalosporins, including cefepime, have been associated with a fall in prothrombin activity. Those at risk include patients with renal or hepatic impairment, or poor nutritional state, as well as patients receiving a protracted course of antimicrobial therapy. Prothrombin time should be monitored in patients at risk, and exogenous vitamin K administered as indicated.

Positive direct Coombs' tests have been reported during treatment with MAXIPIME. In hematologic studies or in transfusion cross-matching procedures when antiglobulin tests are performed on the minor side or in Coombs' testing of newborns whose mothers have received cephalosporin antibiotics before parturition, it should be recognized that a positive Coombs' test may be due to the drug.

MAXIPIME (cefepime hydrochloride) should be prescribed with caution in individuals with a history of gastrointestinal disease, particularly colitis.

Arginine has been shown to alter glucose metabolism and elevate serum potassium transiently when administered at 33 times the amount provided by the maximum recommended human dose of MAXIPIME. The effect of lower doses is not presently known.

TABLE 11
Adverse Laboratory Changes
Cefepime Multiple-Dose Dosing Regimens
Clinical Trials—North America

INCIDENCE EQUAL TO OR GREATER THAN 1%	Positive Coombs' test (without hemolysis) (16.2%); decreased phosphorous (2.8%); increased ALT/SGPT (2.8%), AST/SGOT (2.4%), eosinophils (1.7%); abnormal PTT (1.6%), PT (1.4%)
INCIDENCE LESS THAN 1% BUT GREATER THAN 0.1%	Increased alkaline phosphatase, BUN, calcium, creatinine, phosphorous, potassium, total bilirubin; decreased calcium*, hematocrit, neutrophils, platelets, WBC

* Hypocalcemia was more common among elderly patients. Clinical consequences from changes in either calcium or phosphorus were not reported. A similar safety profile was seen in clinical trials of pediatric patients (see **PRECAUTIONS: Pediatric Use**).

Table 12
Recommended Dosage Schedule for MAXIPIME

Site and Type of Infection	Dose	Frequency	Duration (days)
Adults			
Moderate to Severe Pneumonia due to *S. pneumoniae**, *P. aeruginosa, K. pneumoniae*, or *Enterobacter* species	1–2 g IV	q12h	10
Empiric therapy for febrile neutropenic patients (See **INDICATIONS AND USAGE** and **CLINICAL STUDIES**.)	2 g IV	q8h	7**
Mild to Moderate Uncomplicated or Complicated Urinary Tract Infections, including pyelonephritis, due to *E. coli, K. pneumoniae*, or *P. mirabilis**	0.5–1 g IV/IM***	q12h	7–10
Severe Uncomplicated or Complicated Urinary Tract Infections, including pyelonephritis, due to *E. coli* or *K. pneumoniae**	2 g IV	q12h	10
Moderate to Severe Uncomplicated Skin and Skin Structure Infections due to *S. aureus* or *S. pyogenes*	2 g IV	q12h	10
Complicated Intra-abdominal Infections (used in combination with metronidazole) caused by *E. coli*, viridans group streptococci, *P. aeruginosa, K. pneumoniae, Enterobacter* species, or *B. fragilis*. (See **CLINICAL STUDIES**.)	2 g IV	q12h	7–10

Pediatric Patients (2 months up to 16 years)

The maximum dose for pediatric patients should not exceed the recommended adult dose. The usual recommended dosage in pediatric patients up to 40 kg in weight for uncomplicated and complicated urinary tract infections (including pyelonephritis), uncomplicated skin and skin structure infections, pneumonia, and as empiric therapy for febrile neutropenic patients is 50 mg/kg/dose, administered q12h (q8h for febrile neutropenic patients), for durations as given above.

* including cases associated with concurrent bacteremia

** or until resolution of neutropenia. In patients whose fever resolves but who remain neutropenic for more than 7 days, the need for continued antimicrobial therapy should be re-evaluated frequently.

***IM route of administration is indicated only for mild to moderate, uncomplicated or complicated UTI's due to *E. coli* when the IM route is considered to be a more appropriate route of drug administration.

TABLE 13
Recommended Maintenance Schedule in Adult Patients with Renal Impairment Relative to Normal Recommended Dosing Schedule

Creatinine Clearance (mL/min)	Recommended Maintenance Schedule			
> 60 Normal recommended dosing schedule	500 mg q12h	1 g q12h	2 g q12h	2 g q8h
30 – 60	500 mg q24h	1 g q24h	2 g q24h	2 g q12h
11 – 29	500 mg q24h	500 mg q24h	1 g q24h	2 g q24h
< 11	250 mg q24h	250 mg q24h	500 mg q24h	1 g q24h

When only serum creatinine is available, the following formula (Cockcroft and Gault equation)[3] may be used to estimate creatinine clearance. The serum creatinine should represent a steady state of renal function:

Males: Creatinine Clearance (mL/min) $= \dfrac{\text{Weight (kg)} \times (140 - \text{age})}{72 \times \text{serum creatinine (mg/dL)}}$

Females: $0.85 \times$ above value

In patients with impaired renal function (creatinine clearance ≤60 mL/min), the dose of MAXIPIME (cefepime hydrochloride) should be adjusted to compensate for the slower rate of renal elimination. Because high and prolonged serum antibiotic concentrations can occur from usual dosages in patients with renal insufficiency or other conditions that may compromise renal function, the maintenance dosage should be reduced when cefepime is administered to such patients. Serious adverse events including encephalopathy, myoclonus, seizures, and/or renal failure have been reported postmarketing in patients with renal impairment treated with unadjusted doses of cefepime (see **ADVERSE REACTIONS: In Postmarketing Experience and OVERDOSAGE**). Continued dosage should be determined by degree of renal impairment, severity of infection, and susceptibility of the causative organisms. (See specific recommendations for dosing adjustment in **DOSAGE AND ADMINISTRATION.**)

Drug Interactions

Renal function should be monitored carefully if high doses of aminoglycosides are to be administered with MAXIPIME because of the increased potential of nephrotoxicity and ototoxicity of aminoglycoside antibiotics. Nephrotoxicity has been reported following concomitant administration of other cephalosporins with potent diuretics such as furosemide.

Drug/Laboratory Test Interactions

The administration of cefepime may result in a false-positive reaction for glucose in the urine when using Clinitest® tablets. It is recommended that glucose tests based on enzymatic glucose oxidase reactions (such as Clinistix® or Tes-Tape®) be used.

Carcinogenesis, Mutagenesis, and Impairment of Fertility

No long-term animal carcinogenicity studies have been conducted with cefepime. A battery of *in vivo* and *in vitro* genetic toxicity tests, including the Ames Salmonella reverse mutation assay, CHO/HGPRT mammalian cell forward gene mutation assay, chromosomal aberration and sister chromatid exchange assays in human lymphocytes, CHO fibroblast clastogenesis assay, and cytogenetic and micronucleus assays in mice were conducted. The overall conclusion of these tests indicated no definitive evidence of genotoxic potential. No untoward effects on fertility or reproduction have been observed in rats, mice, and rabbits when cefepime is administered subcutaneously at 1 to 4 times the recommended maximum human dose calculated on a mg/m^2 basis.

Usage in Pregnancy—Teratogenic effects—Pregnancy Category B

Cefepime was not teratogenic or embryocidal when administered during the period of organogenesis to rats at doses up to 1000 mg/kg/day (4 times the recommended maximum human dose calculated on a mg/m^2 basis) or to mice at doses up to 1200 mg/kg (2 times the recommended maximum human dose calculated on a mg/m^2 basis) or to rabbits at a dose level of 100 mg/kg (approximately equal to the recommended maximum human dose calculated on a mg/m^2 basis).

There are, however, no adequate and well-controlled studies of cefepime use in pregnant women. Because animal reproduction studies are not always predictive of human response, this drug should be used during pregnancy only if clearly needed.

Nursing Mothers

Cefepime is excreted in human breast milk in very low concentrations [0.5 μg/mL]. Caution should be exercised when cefepime is administered to a nursing woman.

Labor and Delivery

Cefepime has not been studied for use during labor and delivery. Treatment should only be given if clearly indicated.

Pediatric Use

The safety and effectiveness of cefepime in the treatment of uncomplicated and complicated urinary tract infections (including pyelonephritis), uncomplicated skin and skin structure infections, pneumonia, and as empiric therapy for febrile neutropenic patients have been established in the age groups 2 months up to 16 years. Use of MAXIPIME in these age groups is supported by evidence from adequate and well-controlled studies of cefepime in adults with additional pharmacokinetic and safety data from pediatric trials (see **CLINICAL PHARMACOOGY**).

Safety and effectiveness in pediatric patients below the age of 2 months have not been established. There are insufficient clinical data to support the use of MAXIPIME in pediatric patients under 2 months of age or for the treatment of serious infections in the pediatric population where the suspected or proven pathogen is *Haemophilus influenzae* type b.

IN THOSE PATIENTS IN WHOM MENINGEAL SEEDING FROM A DISTANT INFECTION SITE OR IN WHOM MENINGITIS IS SUSPECTED OR DOCUMENTED, AN ALTERNATE AGENT WITH DEMONSTRATED CLINICAL EFFICACY IN THIS SETTING SHOULD BE USED.

Geriatric Use

In clinical studies, when geriatric patients received the usual recommended adult dose, clinical efficacy and safety were comparable to clinical efficacy and safety in non-geriatric adult patients.

In elderly patients, dosage and administration of cefepime should be adjusted in the presence of renal insufficiency. (See **DOSAGE and ADMINISTRATION**.)

ADVERSE REACTIONS

Clinical Trials: In clinical trials using multiple doses of cefepime, 4137 patients were treated with the recommended dosages of cefepime (500 mg to 2 g IV q12h). There were no deaths or permanent disabilities thought related to drug toxicity. Sixty-four (1.5%) patients discontinued medication due to adverse events thought by the investigators to be possibly, probably, or almost certainly related to drug toxicity. Thirty-three (51%) of these 64 patients who discontinued therapy did so because of rash. The percentage of cefepime-treated patients who discontinued study drug because of drug-related adverse events was very similar at daily doses of 500 mg, 1 g and 2 g q12h (0.8%, 1.1%, and 2.0%, respectively). However, the incidence of discontinuation due to rash increased with the higher recommended doses.

The following adverse events were thought to be probably related to cefepime during evaluation of the drug in clinical trials conducted in North America (n=3125 cefepime-treated patients).

[See table 10 on page 1169]

At the higher dose of 2 g q8h, the incidence of probably-related adverse events was higher among the 795 patients who received this dose of cefepime. They consisted of rash (4%), diarrhea (3%), nausea (2%), vomiting (1%), pruritus (1%), fever (1%), and headache (1%).

The following adverse laboratory changes, irrespective of relationship to therapy with cefepime, were seen during clinical trials conducted in North America.

[See table 11 at top of previous page]

In Postmarketing Experience: In addition to the events reported during North American clinical trials with cefepime, the following adverse experiences have been reported during worldwide postmarketing experience. Because of the uncontrolled nature of spontaneous reports, a causal relationship to MAXIPIME (cefepime hydrochloride) treatment has not been determined.

Encephalopathy, myoclonus, and seizures have been reported in renally impaired patients treated with unadjusted dosing regimens of cefepime. Several cephalosporins have been implicated in triggering seizures, particularly in patients with renal impairment when the dosage was not reduced. (See **DOSAGE AND ADMINISTRATION** and **OVERDOSAGE**.) If seizures associated with drug therapy occur, the drug should be discontinued. Anticonvulsant therapy can be given if clinically indicated. Precautions should be taken to adjust daily dosage in patients with renal insufficiency or other conditions that may compromise renal function to reduce antibiotic concentrations that can lead or contribute to these and other serious adverse events, including renal failure.

As with other cephalosporins, anaphylaxis including anaphylactic shock, transient leukopenia, neutropenia, agranulocytosis and thrombocytopenia have been reported.

Cephalosporin-class adverse reactions: In addition to the adverse reactions listed above that have been observed in patients treated with cefepime, the following adverse reactions and altered laboratory tests have been reported for cephalosporin-class antibiotics:

Stevens-Johnson syndrome, erythema multiforme, toxic epidermal necrolysis, renal dysfunction, toxic nephropathy, aplastic anemia, hemolytic anemia, hemorrhage, hepatic dysfunction including cholestasis, and pancytopenia.

TABLE 14
Preparation of Solutions of Maxipime

Single Dose Vials for Intravenous/Intramuscular Administration	Amount of Diluent to be added (mL)	Approximate Available Volume (mL)	Approximate Cefepime Concentration (mg/mL)
cefepime vial content			
500 mg (IV)	5.0	5.6	100
500 mg (IM)	1.3	1.8	280
1 g (IV)	10.0	11.3	100
1 g (IM)	2.4	3.6	280
2 g (IV)	10.0	12.5	160
Piggyback (100 mL)			
1 g bottle	50	50	20
1 g bottle	100	100	10
2 g bottle	50	50	40
2 g bottle	100	100	20
ADD-Vantage®			
1 g vial	50	50	20
1 g vial	100	100	10
2 g vial	50	50	40
2 g vial	100	100	20

Table 15
Cefepime Admixture Stability

Maxipime Concentration	Admixture and Concentration	IV Infusion Solutions	Stability Time for RT/L (20°–25° C)	Stability Time for Refrigeration (2°–8° C)
40 mg/mL	Amikacin 6 mg/mL	NS or D5W	24 hours	7 days
40 mg/mL	Ampicillin 1 mg/mL	D5W	8 hours	8 hours
40 mg/mL	Ampicillin 10 mg/mL	D5W	2 hours	8 hours
40 mg/mL	Ampicillin 1 mg/mL	NS	24 hours	48 hours
40 mg/mL	Ampicillin 10 mg/mL	NS	8 hours	48 hours
4 mg/mL	Ampicillin 40 mg/mL	NS	8 hours	8 hours
4–40 mg/mL	Clindamycin Phosphate 0.25–6 mg/mL	NS or D5W	24 hours	7 days
4 mg/mL	Heparin 10–50 units/mL	NS or D5W	24 hours	7 days
4 mg/mL	Potassium Chloride 10–40 mEq/L	NS or D5W	24 hours	7 days
4 mg/mL	Theophylline 0.8 mg/mL	D5W	24 hours	7 days
1–4 mg/mL	na	Aminosyn® II 4.25% with electrolytes and calcium	8 hours	3 days
0.125–0.25 mg/mL	na	Inpersol® with 4.25% dextrose	24 hours	7 days

NS = 0.9% Sodium Chloride Injection
D5W = 5% Dextrose Injection
na = not applicable
RT/L = Ambient room temperature and light

OVERDOSAGE

Patients who receive an overdose should be carefully observed and given supportive treatment. In the presence of renal insufficiency, hemodialysis, not peritoneal dialysis, is recommended to aid in the removal of cefepime from the body.

Accidental overdosing might occur if large doses are given to patients with reduced renal function. In clinical trials, MAXIPIME overdosage occurred in a patient with renal failure (creatinine clearance <11 mL/min) who received 2 g q24h for 7 days. The patient exhibited seizures, encephalopathy, and neuromuscular excitability. (See **PRECAUTIONS**, **ADVERSE REACTIONS**, and **DOSAGE AND ADMINISTRATION**.)

DOSAGE AND ADMINISTRATION

The recommended adult dosages and routes of administration are outlined in the following table. MAXIPIME (cefepime hydrochloride) should be administered intravenously over approximately 30 minutes.

[See table 12 on previous page]

Impaired Hepatic Function—No adjustment is necessary for patients with impaired hepatic function.

Continued on next page

Maxipime—Cont.

Impaired Renal Function—In patients with impaired renal function (creatinine clearance ≤60 mL/min), the dose of MAXIPIME (cefepime hydrochloride) should be adjusted to compensate for the slower rate of renal elimination. The recommended initial dose of MAXIPIME should be the same as in patients with normal renal function. The recommended maintenance doses of MAXIPIME in patients with renal insufficiency are presented in Table 13.

[See table 13 on page 1170]

In patients undergoing hemodialysis, approximately 68% of the total amount of cefepime present in the body at the start of dialysis will be removed during a 3-hour dialysis period. A repeat dose, equivalent to the initial dose, should be given at the completion of each dialysis session.

In patients undergoing continuous ambulatory peritoneal dialysis, MAXIPIME may be administered at normally recommended doses at a dosage interval of every 48 hours.

Data in pediatric patients with impaired renal function are not available; however, since cefepime pharmacokinetics are similar in adults and pediatric patients (see **CLINICAL PHARMACOLOGY**), changes in dosing regimen similar to those in adults (see Table 13) are recommended for pediatric patients.

Administration:

For Intravenous Infusion, constitute the 1 g or 2 g piggyback (100 mL) bottle with 50 or 100 mL of a compatible IV fluid listed in the **Compatibility and Stability** subsection. Alternatively, constitute the 500 mg, 1 g, or 2 g vial, and add an appropriate quantity of the resulting solution to an IV container with one of the compatible IV fluids. **THE RESULTING SOLUTION SHOULD BE ADMINISTERED OVER APPROXIMATELY 30 MINUTES.**

Intermittent IV infusion with a Y-type administration set can be accomplished with compatible solutions. However, during infusion of a solution containing cefepime, it is desirable to discontinue the other solution.

ADD-Vantage® vials are to be constituted only with 50 or 100 mL of 5% Dextrose Injection or 0.9% Sodium Chloride Injection in Abbott ADD-Vantage® flexible diluent containers. (See ADD-Vantage® Vial Instructions for Use.)

Intramuscular Administration: For IM administration, MAXIPIME (cefepime hydrochloride) should be constituted with one of the following diluents: Sterile Water for Injection, 0.9% Sodium Chloride, 5% Dextrose Injection, 0.5% or 1.0% Lidocaine Hydrochloride, or Sterile Bacteriostatic Water for Injection with Parabens or Benzyl Alcohol (refer to Table 14). Preparation of MAXIPIME solutions is summarized in Table 14.

[See table 14 at top of previous page]

Compatibility and Stability:

Intravenous: MAXIPIME is compatible at concentrations between 1 and 40 mg/mL with the following IV infusion fluids: 0.9% Sodium Chloride Injection, 5% and 10% Dextrose Injection, M/6 Sodium Lactate Injection, 5% Dextrose and 0.9% Sodium Chloride Injection, Lactated Ringers and 5% Dextrose Injection, Normosol-R®, and Normosol-M® in 5% Dextrose Injection. These solutions may be stored up to 24 hours at controlled room temperature 20°–25° C (68°–77° F) or 7 days in a refrigerator 2°–8° C (36°–46° F). MAXIPIME in ADD-Vantage® vials is stable at concentrations of 10–40 mg/mL in 5% Dextrose Injection or 0.9% Sodium Chloride Injection for 24 hours at controlled room temperature 20°–25° C or 7 days in a refrigerator 2°–8° C.

MAXIPIME admixture compatibility information is summarized in Table 15.

[See table 15 on previous page]

Solutions of MAXIPIME, like those of most beta-lactam antibiotics, should not be added to solutions of ampicillin at a concentration greater than 40 mg/mL, and should not be added to metronidazole, vancomycin, gentamicin, tobramycin, netilmicin sulfate or aminophylline because of potential interaction. However, if concurrent therapy with MAXIPIME is indicated, each of these antibiotics can be administered separately.

Intramuscular: MAXIPIME (cefepime hydrochloride) constituted as directed is stable for 24 hours at controlled room temperature 20°–25° C (68°–77° F) or for 7 days in a refrigerator 2°–8° C (36°–46° F) with the following diluents: Sterile Water for Injection, 0.9% Sodium Chloride Injection, 5% Dextrose Injection, Sterile Bacteriostatic Water for Injection with Parabens or Benzyl Alcohol, or 0.5% or 1% Lidocaine Hydrochloride.

NOTE: PARENTERAL DRUGS SHOULD BE INSPECTED VISUALLY FOR PARTICULATE MATTER BEFORE ADMINISTRATION.

As with other cephalosporins, the color of MAXIPIME powder, as well as its solutions, tend to darken depending on storage conditions; however, when stored as recommended, the product potency is not adversely affected.

HOW SUPPLIED

MAXIPIME® (cefepime hydrochloride) for Injection is supplied as follows:

[See table below]

NDC 51479-053-10	500 mg*	15 mL vial (tray of 10)
NDC 51479-054-10	1 g*	Piggyback bottle 100 mL (tray of 10)
NDC 51479-054-20	1 g*	ADD-Vantage® vial (tray of 10)
NDC 51479-054-30	1 g*	15 mL vial (tray of 10)
NDC 51479-055-20	2 g*	Piggyback bottle 100 mL (tray of 10)
NDC 51479-055-10	2 g*	ADD-Vantage® vial (tray of 10)
NDC 51479-055-30	2 g*	20 mL vial (tray of 10)

*Based on cefepime activity

Storage

MAXIPIME IN THE DRY STATE SHOULD BE STORED BETWEEN 2°–25° C (36°–77° F) AND PROTECTED FROM LIGHT.

U.S. Patent No. 4,406,899; 4,910,301; 4,994,451 and 5,244,891

REFERENCES

(1) National Committee for Clinical Laboratory *Standards. Methods for Dilution Antimicrobial Susceptibility Tests for Bacteria that Grow Aerobically*—Third Edition. Approved Standard NCCLS Document M7-A3, Vol. 13, No. 25, NCCLS, Villanova, PA, December, 1993.

(2) National Committee for Clinical Laboratory Standards. *Performance Standards for Antimicrobial Disk Susceptibility Tests*—Fifth Edition. Approved Standard NCCLS Document M2-A5, Vol. 13, No. 24, NCCLS, Villanova, PA, December, 1993.

(3) Cockcroft DW, Gault MH. Prediction of creatinine clearance from serum creatinine. *Nephron*. 1976; 16:31–41.

ADD-Vantage® is a registered trademark of Abbott Laboratories.
Normosol-R® is a registered trademark of Abbott Laboratories.
Normosol-M® is a registered trademark of Abbott Laboratories.
Aminosyn® is a registered trademark of Abbott Laboratories.
Inpersol® is a registered trademark of Abbott Laboratories.
Clinitest® and Clinistix® are registered trademarks of the Bayer Corporation.
Tes-Tape® is a registered trademark of Eli Lilly and Company.
MAXIPIME® is a registered trademark of Bristol-Myers Squibb Company

Manufactured by
Bristol-Myers Squibb Company
Princeton, NJ 08543 U.S.A.
Distributed by
DURA Pharmaceuticals, Inc.
San Diego, CA 92121 U.S.A.
0055DIM-02
Revised: April, 1999
E4-B001A-05-99
MAX001B99

Shown in Product Identification Guide, page 311

NASALIDE® ℞

[na 'ză-lide]
(flunisolide)
Nasal Spray, 25 mcg
For Nasal Use Only

DESCRIPTION

NASALIDE® (flunisolide) nasal spray is intended for administration as a spray to the nasal mucosa. Flunisolide, the active component of NASALIDE nasal spray, is an anti-inflammatory steroid with the chemical name: 6α-fluoro-11β,16α,17,21-tetrahydroxypregna-1,4-diene-3,20-dione cyclic 16,17-acetal with acetone (USAN).

It has the following chemical structure:

[Chemical structure: CH2OH, C=O, O, CH3, CH3, H, HO, CH3, H, CH3, H, H, H, O, F, H]

Flunisolide is a white to creamy white crystalline powder with a molecular weight of 434.49 and molecular formula of $C_{24}H_{31}FO_6$. It is soluble in acetone, sparingly soluble in chloroform, slightly soluble in methanol, and practically insoluble in water. It has a melting point of about 245°C.

Each 25 mL spray bottle contains flunisolide 6.25 mg (0.25 mg/mL) in a solution of propylene glycol, polyethylene glycol 3350, citric acid, sodium citrate, butylated hydroxyanisole, edetate disodium, benzalkonium chloride and purified water, with NaOH and/or HCl added to adjust the pH to a target of 5.3.

After initial priming (5 to 6 sprays), each spray of the unit delivers a metered droplet of 100 mg formulation spray containing 25 mcg of flunisolide. The size of the droplets produced by the unit is in excess of 8 microns to facilitate deposition on the nasal mucosa. The contents of one nasal spray bottle deliver 200 sprays.

CLINICAL PHARMACOLOGY

Flunisolide has demonstrated potent glucocorticoid and weak mineralocorticoid activity in classical animal test systems. As a glucocorticoid it is several hundred times more potent than the cortisol standard. Clinical studies with flunisolide have shown therapeutic activity on nasal mucous membranes with minimal evidence of systemic activity at the recommended doses.

A study in approximately 100 patients that compared the recommended dose of flunisolide nasal solution with an oral dose providing equivalent systemic amounts of flunisolide has shown that the clinical effectiveness of NASALIDE, when used topically as recommended, is due to its direct local effect and not to an indirect effect through systemic absorption.

Following administration of flunisolide to man, approximately half of the administered dose is recovered in the urine and half in the stool; 65% to 70% of the dose recovered in urine is the primary metabolite, which has undergone loss of the 6α fluorine and addition of a 6β hydroxy group. Flunisolide is well absorbed but is rapidly converted by the liver to the much less active primary metabolite and to glucuronate and/or sulfate conjugates. Because of first-pass liver metabolism, only 20% of the flunisolide reaches the systemic circulation when it is given orally whereas 50% of the flunisolide administered intranasally reaches the systemic circulation unmetabolized. The plasma half-life of flunisolide is 1 to 2 hours.

The effects of flunisolide on hypothalamic-pituitary-adrenal (HPA) axis function have been studied in adult volunteers. NASALIDE was administered intranasally as a spray in total doses over 7 times the recommended dose (2200 mcg, equivalent to 88 sprays/day) in 2 subjects for 4 days, about 3 times the recommended dose (800 mcg, equivalent to 32 sprays/day) in 4 subjects for 4 days, and over twice the recommended dose (700 mcg, equivalent to 28 sprays/day) in 6 subjects for 10 days. Early morning plasma cortisol concentrations and 24-hour urinary 17-ketogenic steroids were measured daily. There was evidence of decreased endogenous cortisol production at all three doses.

In controlled studies, NASALIDE was found to be effective in reducing symptoms of stuffy nose, runny nose and sneezing in most patients. These controlled clinical studies have been conducted in 488 adult patients at doses ranging from 8 to 16 sprays (200–400 mcg) per day and 127 pediatric patients at doses ranging from 6 to 8 sprays (150 to 200 mcg) per day for periods as long as 3 months. In 170 patients who had cortisol levels evaluated at baseline and after 3 months or more of flunisolide treatment, there was no unequivocal flunisolide-related depression of plasma cortisol levels.

Clinical studies have shown that improvement is usually apparent within a few days after starting NASALIDE.

The mechanisms responsible for the anti-inflammatory action of corticosteroids and for the activity of the aerosolized drug on the nasal mucosa are unknown.

INDICATIONS

NASALIDE is indicated for the nasal treatment of the symptoms of seasonal or perennial rhinitis.

NASALIDE should not be used in the presence of untreated localized infection involving nasal mucosa.

CONTRAINDICATIONS

Hypersensitivity to any of the ingredients.

WARNINGS

The replacement of a systemic corticosteroid with a topical corticoid can be accompanied by signs of adrenal insufficiency, and in addition some patients may experience symptoms of withdrawal, eg, joint and/or muscular pain, lassitude and depression. Patients previously treated for prolonged periods with systemic corticosteroids and transferred to NASALIDE should be carefully monitored to avoid acute adrenal insufficiency in response to stress.

When transferred to NASALIDE, careful attention must be given to patients previously treated for prolonged periods with systemic corticosteroids. This is particularly important in those patients who have associated asthma or other clinical conditions, where too rapid a decrease in systemic corticosteroids may cause a severe exacerbation of their symptoms.

The use of NASALIDE with alternate-day prednisone systemic treatment could increase the likelihood of HPA axis suppression compared to a therapeutic dose of either one alone. Therefore, NASALIDE treatment should be used with caution in patients already on alternate-day prednisone regimens for any disease.

Persons who are on drugs that suppress the immune system are more susceptible to infections than healthy individuals. Chicken pox and measles, for example, can have a more serious or even fatal course in nonimmune pediatric patients or adults on corticosteroids. In such pediatric patients or adults who have not had these diseases, particular care should be taken to avoid exposure. How the dose, route and duration of corticosteroid administration affects the risk of developing a disseminated infection is not known. The contribution of the underlying disease and/or prior corticosteroid treatment to the risk is also not known. If a nonimmune patient is exposed to chicken pox, prophylaxis with varicella zoster immune globulin (VZIG) may be indicated. If exposed to measles, prophylaxis with pooled intramuscular immunoglobulin (IG) may be indicated. (See the respective package insert for complete VZIG and IG prescribing information.) If chicken pox develops, treatment with antiviral agents may be considered.

PRECAUTIONS

General: Symptomatic relief may not occur in some patients for as long as 2 weeks. Although systemic effects are minimal at recommended doses, NASALIDE should not be continued beyond 3 weeks in the absence of significant symptomatic improvement. In clinical studies with flunisolide administered intranasally, the development of localized infections of the nose and pharynx with *Candida albicans* have occurred only rarely. When such an infection develops it may require treatment with appropriate local therapy or discontinuance of treatment with NASALIDE.

Flunisolide is absorbed into the circulation. Use of excessive doses of NASALIDE may suppress HPA axis function.

Flunisolide should be used with caution, if at all, in patients with active or quiescent tuberculosis infection of the respiratory tract or in untreated fungal, bacterial or systemic viral infections or ocular herpes simplex.

Because of the inhibitory effect of corticosteroids on wound healing, in patients who have experienced recent nasal septal ulcers, recurrent epistaxis, nasal surgery or trauma, a nasal corticosteroids should be used with caution until healing has occurred.

Although systemic effects have been minimal with recommended doses, this potential increases with excessive dosages. Therefore, larger than recommended doses should be avoided.

Information for Patients: Patients should use NASALIDE at regular intervals since its effectiveness depends on its regular use. The patient should take the medication as directed. It is not acutely effective and the prescribed dosage should not be increased. Instead, nasal vasoconstrictors or oral antihistamines may be needed until the effects of NASALIDE are fully manifested. One to 2 weeks may pass before full relief is obtained. The patient should contact the physician if symptoms do not improve, or if the condition worsens, or if sneezing or nasal irritation occurs.

Person who are on immunosuppressant doses of corticosteroids should be warned to avoid exposure to chicken pox or measles. Patients should also be advised that if they are exposed, medical advice should be sought without delay.

For the proper use of this unit and to attain maximum improvement, the patient should read and follow the accompanying patient leaflet of instructions carefully.

Patients should be advised to clear their nasal passages of secretions prior to use.

Carcinogenesis, Mutagenesis, Impairment of Fertility: In mice, flunisolide at an oral dose of 500 mcg/kg/day (approximately 6 times the maximum recommended daily intranasal dose in adults and children on a mg/m^2 basis) for 21 months was negative for carcinogenic effects. In rats, administration of flunisolide at an oral dose of 2.5 mcg/kg/day (less than the maximum recommended daily intranasal dose in adults and children on a mg/m^2 basis) for 24 months resulted in an increased incidence of mammary gland adenoma and islet cell adenoma of the pancreas in females. There were no significant increases in the incidence of any tumor type in rats at an oral dose of 1.0 mcg/kg (less than the maximum recommended daily intranasal dose in adults and children on a mg/m^2 basis).

Flunisolide showed no mutagenic activity in *in vitro* test systems including the Ames Assay and the Rec-Assay, and no clastogenic activity in either the *in vitro* chromosomal aberration assay in Chinese hamster lung fibroblast cells or the *in vivo* mouse bone marrow chromosomal aberration assay.

Flunisolide, at an oral dose of 200 mcg/kg/day (approximately 4 times the maximum recommended daily intranasal dose in adults on a mg/m^2 basis) produced impaired fertility in female rats, but was devoid of such effects at oral doses less than or equal to 40 mcg/kg/day (approximately equal to the maximum recommended daily intranasal dose in adults on a mg/m^2 basis).

Pregnancy: Pregnancy Category C. As with other corticosteroids, flunisolide has been shown to be teratogenic and fetotoxic in rabbits and rats at oral doses of 40 and 200 mcg/kg/day respectively. (approximately 2 and 4 times, respectively, the maximum recommended daily intranasal dose in adults on a mg/m^2 basis). There are no adequate and well-controlled studies in pregnant women. Flunisolide should be used during pregnancy only if the potential benefit justifies the potential risk to the fetus.

Nursing Mothers: It is not known whether this drug is excreted in human milk. Because other corticosteroids are excreted in human milk, caution should be exercised when flunisolide is administered to nursing women.

Pediatric Use: NASALIDE is not recommended for use in pediatric patients less than 6 years of age as safety and efficacy, including possible adverse effects on growth, have not been assessed in this age group.

ADVERSE REACTIONS

Adverse reactions reported in controlled clinical trials and long-term open studies in 595 patients treated with NASALIDE are described below. Of these patients, 409 were treated for 3 months or longer, 323 for 6 months or longer, 259 for 1 year or longer and 91 for 2 years or longer. In general, side effects elicited in the clinical studies have been primarily associated with the nasal mucous membranes. The most frequent complaints were those of mild transient nasal burning and stinging, which were reported in approximately 45% of the patients treated with NASALIDE in placebo-controlled and long-term studies. These complaints do not usually interfere with treatment; in only 3% of patients was it necessary to decrease dosage or stop treatment because of these symptoms. Approximately the same incidence of mild transient nasal burning and stinging was reported in patients on placebo as was reported in patients treated with NASALIDE in controlled studies, implying that these complaints may be related to the vehicle or the delivery system. The incidence of complaints of nasal burning and stinging decreased with increasing duration of treatment.

Other side effects reported at a frequency of 5% or less were: nasal congestion, sneezing, epistaxis and/or bloody mucus, nasal irritation, watery eyes, sore throat, nausea and/or vomiting and headaches. As with other nasally inhaled corticosteroids, nasal septal perforations have been reported in rare instances with the use of flunisolide nasal solutions. Temporary or permanent loss of the sense of smell and taste have also been reported with the use of flunisolide nasal solutions.

Systemic corticosteroid side effects were not reported during the controlled clinical trials. If recommended doses are exceeded, or if individuals are particularly sensitive, symptoms of hypercorticism, ie, Cushing's syndrome, could occur.

OVERDOSAGE

Flunisolide, infused intravenously, at doses up to 4 mg/kg in mice, rats and dogs (approximately 45, 300 and 90 times, respectively, the maximum recommended daily intranasal dose in adults and children on a mg/m^2 basis) was without lethality.

DOSAGE AND ADMINISTRATION

Adults: The recommended starting dose of NASALIDE is 2 sprays (50 mcg) in each nostril 2 times a day (total dose 200 mcg/day). If needed, this dose may be increased to 2 sprays in each nostril times a day (total dose 300 mcg/day).

Pediatric Patients 6 to 14 years: The recommended starting dose of NASALIDE is 1 spray (25 mcg) in each nostril 3 times a day or 2 sprays (50 mcg) in each nostril 2 times a day (total dose 150 to 200 mcg/day). NASALIDE is not recommended for use in pediatric patients less than 6 years of age as safety and efficacy studies, including possible adverse effects on growth, have not been conducted.

Maximum total daily doses should not exceed 8 sprays in each nostril for adults (total dose 400 mcg/day) and 4 sprays in each nostril for pediatric patients under 14 years of age (total dose 200 mcg/day). Since there is no evidence that exceeding the maximum recommended dosage is more effective and increased systemic absorption would occur, higher doses should be avoided.

After the desired clinical effect is obtained, the maintenance dose should be reduced to the smallest amount necessary to control the symptoms. Approximately 15% of patients with perennial rhinitis may be maintained on as little as 1 spray in each nostril per day.

For priming and repriming the nasal spray unit after storage: The patient should remove the green dust cover. Put two fingers on "shoulders" of preset pump unit, and place thumb on bottom of bottle. Push bottle with thumb FIRMLY and QUICKLY 5–6 times or until a fine spray appears. Now your preset pump is primed. The patient must prime the preset pump unit again if it has not been used for 5 days or more, or if it has been disassembled for cleaning.

DIRECTIONS FOR USE

A patient leaflet of instructions accompanies each package of NASALIDE Nasal Spray.

WARNING

Do not spray in eyes.

HOW SUPPLIED

NASALIDE is contained in a metered-dose, manual pump spray unit. Each 25 mL NASALIDE nasal spray white, HDPE bottle (NDC 51479-038-25) contains 6.25 mg (0.25 mg/mL), 200 sprays of flunisolide and is supplied in a nasal pump dispenser with green dust cover cap and with a patient leaflet of instructions.

Store at 15°–30°C (59°–86°F).

CONTENTS MADE IN CANADA

Rx only.

Revised: May, 2000

Manufactured for:
Dura Pharmaceuticals, Inc.
San Diego, CA 92121
Manufactured by:
PATHEON INC.
Mississauga, Ontario,
CANADA L5N 7K9

NIDE001C00
IN-5048/S

Shown in Product Identification Guide, page 311

NASAREL® ℞
[*Nā 'ză ril*]
(flunisolide)
Nasal Solution 0.025%
For Intranasal Use Only

DESCRIPTION

Flunisolide, the active component of NASAREL nasal solution, is an anti-inflammatory glucocorticosteroid with the chemical name: 6α-fluoro-11β,16α,17,21 tetrahydroxypregna-1,4-diene-3,20-dione cyclic 16, 17-acetal with acetone, hemihydrate.

It has the following chemical structure:

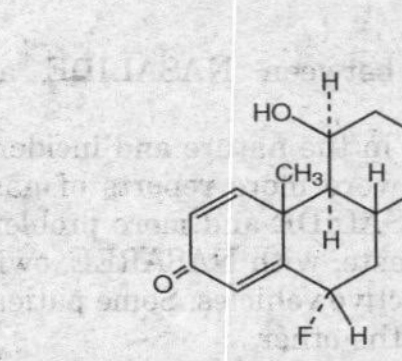

Flunisolide is a white to creamy white crystalline powder with a molecular weight of 443.51. It is soluble in acetone, sparingly soluble in chloroform, slightly soluble in methanol, and practically insoluble in water. It has a melting point of about 245°C. The octanol:water partition coefficient is 2.17 at neutral pH.

NASAREL is a metered dose manual pump spray unit containing 0.025% w/w flunisolide in an aqueous medium containing benzalkonium chloride, butylated hydroxytoluene, citric acid, edetate disodium, polyethylene glycol 400, polysorbate 20, propylene glycol, sodium citrate dihydrate, sorbitol, and purified water. Sodium hydroxide and/or hydrochloric acid may be added to adjust the pH to approximately 5.2. It contains no fluorocarbons. Each 25 mL spray bottle contains 6.25 mg of flunisolide.

After initial priming (5 to 6 actuations), each actuation of the pump spray unit delivers a metered spray containing approximately 25 mcg of flunisolide. The size of 99.5% of the droplets produced by the unit is greater than 8 microns. The contents of one nasal spray bottle deliver 200 sprays in addition to the priming sprays.

CLINICAL PHARMACOLOGY

General Pharmacology: Flunisolide nasal solution has demonstrated potent glucocorticoid and weak mineralocorticoid activity in classical animal test systems. As a glucocorticoid it was 180 times more potent than the cortisol standard in a rat anti-granuloma assay.

Pharmacokinetics: Flunisolide is well absorbed and is rapidly converted by the liver to the much less active primary metabolite and to glucuronide and sulfate conjugates. The primary metabolite results from the loss of the 6-alpha fluorine and addition of a 6-beta hydroxy group. Following administration of radiolabeled flunisolide to man, approximately half of the label is recovered in the urine and half in the stool. The primary metabolite accounts for 65% to 70% of the amount recovered in the urine. Due to first-pass liver metabolism, only 20% of an oral flunisolide dose reaches the systemic circulation unmetabolized as compared to 50% of an intranasal dose. The plasma half-life of flunisolide is 1 to 2 hours.

In a pharmacokinetic study comparing NASAREL with NASALIDE®, the original formulation, the two formulations were not bioequivalent. The total absorption of NASAREL was 25% less than that of NASALIDE, and the peak plasma concentration was 30% lower. The clinical significance of these differences is likely to be small, particularly since clinical efficacy is attributable to a local effect on the nasal mucosa. (see *Pharmacodynamics.*)

Pharmacodynamics: A study in approximately 100 patients compared control of hay fever symptoms by the recommended dose of flunisolide as NASALIDE (200 mcg/day) with control by an oral dose of flunisolide providing equivalent plasma levels. The results demonstrated that the clinical effectiveness was due to the direct topical effect of flunisolide and not to an indirect effect through systemic absorption.

The effects of flunisolide on hypothalamic-pituitary-adrenal (HPA) axis function have been studied in adult volunteers. Flunisolide as NASALIDE, the original nasal formulation, was administered to 20 subjects intranasally in average total daily doses ranging from approximately 350 mcg to 2200 mcg (equivalent to about 14 to 88 sprays per day) for 4 to 10 days. Early morning plasma cortisol concentrations and 24-hour urinary 17-ketogenic steroids were measured daily. There was no consistent effect on endogenous cortisol production, although evidence of mild adrenal suppression was seen in some subjects.

Controlled studies evaluated adult patients receiving average total daily doses ranging from approximately 50 to 400 mcg (equivalent to about 2 to 16 sprays per day) of NASALIDE, the original flunisolide nasal solution, for periods as long as 3 months. Three hundred and thirty-nine patients from these studies were entered into a long-term open label study. Morning plasma cortisol levels were available for 182 patients at baseline, 129 after 6 months, and 36 after 12 months of continuous treatment with flunisolide. No effect of flunisolide on cortisol production was detected.

The mechanisms responsible for the anti-inflammatory action of corticosteroids and for their effect on the nasal mucosa are not completely understood.

CLINICAL TRIALS

The effectiveness of NASAREL was tested in 289 patients for up to 6 weeks at doses up to 300 mcg per day. NASAREL was shown to be effective in treating the symptoms of allergic rhinitis, including rhinorrhea, nasal congestion and sneezing.

A pivotal, 3-center trial involved 196 patients with seasonal allergic rhinitis randomized to NASALIDE, the vehicle of NASALIDE, NASAREL and the vehicle of NASAREL. Both active treatments were statistically significantly more effective than the vehicles. There was not statistically signifi-

Continued on next page

Nasarel—Cont.

cant difference in efficacy between NASALIDE and NASAREL.

The two formulations do differ in the nature and incidence of adverse complaints. There were more reports of nasal burning and stinging with NASALIDE and more problems related to taste, such as aftertaste, with NASAREL, owing to the differences in their respective vehicles. Some patients may prefer one formulation to the other.

INDIVIDUALIZATION OF DOSAGE

The therapeutic effects of corticosteroid nasal sprays, unlike those of decongestants, are not immediate. This should be explained to the patient in advance in order to ensure cooperation and continuation of treatment with the prescribed dosage regimen. Full therapeutic benefit requires regular use and is usually evident within a few days. A longer period of therapy may be required for some patients. However, NASAREL should not be continued beyond 3 weeks in the absence of significant symptomatic improvement (see PRECAUTIONS, WARNINGS, *Information For Patients* and ADVERSE REACTIONS sections).

A starting dose of 2 sprays in each nostril twice daily is recommended. If greater control of symptoms is needed, the dose may be increased to 2 sprays in each nostril 3 times a day. For adults, maximum total daily doses should not exceed 8 sprays in each nostril per day (400 mcg/day).

After the desired clinical effect is obtained, the maintenance dose should be reduced to the smallest amount necessary to control the symptoms. Some patients with perennial rhinitis may be maintained on as little as 1 spray in each nostril per day. It is always desirable to titrate an individual patient to the minimum effective dose to reduce the possibility of side effects.

NASAREL and NASALIDE should not be considered to be identical. Physicians should consider the observed differences in the mean responses in terms of side effects (see ADVERSE REACTIONS) and flunisolide absorption (see *Pharmacokinetics*) in treating individual patients.

For pediatric patients 6 to 14 years of age, the recommended starting dose of NASAREL is one spray (25 mcg) in each nostril 3 times a day (total dose 150 mcg/day) or 2 sprays (50 mcg) in each nostril 2 times a day (total dose 200 mcg/day). Maximum daily doses should not exceed 4 sprays in each nostril per day (total dose 200 mcg/day) as the safety and efficacy of higher doses have not been established.

NASAREL is not recommended for use in pediatric patients less than 6 years of age as the safety and efficacy have not been assessed in this age-group.

INDICATIONS AND USAGE

NASAREL is indicated for the management of the symptoms of seasonal or perennial rhinitis.

CONTRAINDICATIONS

Hypersensitivity to any of the ingredients.

NASAREL should not be used in the presence of untreated localized infection involving the nasal mucosa.

WARNINGS

The replacement of a systemic corticosteroid with a topical corticoid can be accompanied by signs of adrenal insufficiency, and in addition some patients may experience symptoms of withdrawal, e.g., joint and/or muscular pain, lassitude and depression. Patients previously treated for prolonged periods with systemic corticosteroids and transferred to NASAREL should be carefully monitored to avoid acute adrenal insufficiency in response to stress.

Careful attention must also be given to patients who have associated asthma or other clinical conditions where too rapid a decrease in systemic corticosteroids may exacerbate their symptoms.

The use of NASAREL with systemic prednisone as alternate day therapy or with daily doses of less than 7.5 mg could increase the likelihood of hypothalamic-pituitary-adrenal axis suppression compared to a therapeutic dose of either one alone. Therefore, NASAREL treatment should be used with caution in patients already on prednisone regimens for any disease.

Persons who are on drugs which suppress the immune system are more susceptible to infections than healthy individuals. Chicken pox and measles, for example, can have a more serious or even fatal course in non-immune children or adults on corticosteroids. In such children or adults who have not had these diseases, particular care should be taken to avoid exposure. How the dose, route and duration of corticosteroid administration affects the risk of developing a disseminated infection is not known. The contribution of the underlying disease and/or prior corticosteroid treatment to the risk is also not known. If exposed to chicken pox, prophylaxis with varicella zoster immune globulin (VZIG) may be indicated. If exposed to measles, prophylaxis with pooled intramuscular immunoglobulin (IG) may be indicated. (See the respective package insert for complete VZIG and IG prescribing information). If chicken pox develops, treatment with antiviral agents may be considered.

PRECAUTIONS

General: In clinical studies with flunisolide administered intranasally, the development of localized infections of the nose and pharynx with *Candida albicans* has occurred only rarely. When such an infection develops it may require treatment with appropriate local therapy or discontinuance of treatment with NASAREL.

Since there is no evidence that exceeding the maximum recommended dose of NASAREL is more effective, higher doses should be avoided.

Patients should be advised to clear their nasal passages of secretions prior to use. NASAREL should not be used in the presence of untreated local infection involving the nasal mucosa.

Flunisolide should be used with caution, if at all, in patients with active or quiescent tuberculosis infections, fungal, bacterial or systemic viral infections or ocular herpes simplex.

As with other nasally inhaled corticosteroids, nasal septal perforations have been reported in rare instances with the use of flunisolide nasal solutions. Temporary or permanent loss of the sense of smell and taste have also been reported with the use of flunisolide nasal solutions.

Because of the inhibitory effect of corticosteroids on wound healing, a nasal corticosteroid should be used with caution in patients who have experienced recent nasal septal ulcers, recurrent epistaxis, nasal surgery or trauma, until healing has occurred.

Although systemic corticoid effects typical of Cushing's syndrome are minimal with recommended doses of topical steroids, this potential increases with excessive doses. If recommended doses are exceeded with long-term use, or if individuals are particularly sensitive, symptoms of hypercorticism could occur including suppression of hypothalamic-pituitary-adrenal function and/or retardation of growth in children or teenagers. Therefore, larger than recommended doses of NASAREL should be avoided.

Information for Patients: Patients should use NASAREL at regular intervals since its effectiveness depends on its regular use. Patients should take the medication as directed and should not exceed the prescribed dose. A decrease in symptoms can be expected to occur within a few days of initiating therapy in allergic rhinitis patients. Patients should contact their physician if the condition worsens, if sneezing or nasal irritation occurs, or if symptoms do not improve by three weeks.

Persons taking immunosuppressant doses of corticosteroids should be warned to avoid exposure to chicken pox or measles. Patients should also be advised that if they are exposed, medical advice should be sought without delay.

For the proper use of this unit and to attain maximum improvement, the patient should read and follow the accompanying Patient Instructions carefully.

Carcinogenesis: Long-term studies were conducted in mice and rats using oral administration to evaluate the carcinogenic potential of the drug. Flunisolide was administered to mice at doses of 5, 50 and 500 µg/kg/day (15, 150, and 1500 µg/m^2 respectively) and to rats at doses of 0.5, 1 and 2.5 µg/kg/day (3.0, 5.9 and 14.8 µg/m^2 respectively). There was an increase in the incidence of benign pulmonary adenomas in mice, but not in rats.

Female rats receiving the highest oral dose had an increased incidence of mammary adenocarcinoma compared to control rats. An increased incidence of this tumor type has been reported for other corticosteroids.

Impairment of Fertility: Female rats receiving high doses of flunisolide (200 µg/kg/day or 1180 µg/m^2 body surface area) showed some evidence of impaired fertility. Reproductive performance in the low (8 µg/kg/day or 47.2 µg/m^2) and mid-dose (40 µg/kg/day or 236 µg/m^2) groups was comparable to controls.

Pregnancy: Teratogenic effects: Pregnancy Category C. As with other corticosteroids, flunisolide has been shown to be teratogenic in rabbits and rats at doses of 40 and 200 mcg/kg/day (480 µg/m^2 and 1180 µg/m^2) respectively. It was also fetotoxic in these animals reproductive studies. There are no adequate and well-controlled studies in pregnant women. Flunisolide should be used during pregnancy only if the potential benefit justifies the potential risk to the fetus.

Nursing Mothers: It is not known whether this drug is excreted in human milk. Because other corticosteroids are excreted in human milk, caution should be exercised when flunisolide is administered to nursing women.

Pediatric Use: **NASAREL** is not recommended for use in pediatric patients less than 6 years of age as safety and efficacy, including possible adverse effects on growth, have not been assessed in this age group. For pediatric patients 6 years of age and over, recommended maximum daily doses should not be exceeded in order to minimize the risk of systemic corticoid effects, including potential growth retardation. (See INDIVIDUALIZATION OF DOSAGE and DOSAGE AND ADMINISTRATION.)

ADVERSE REACTIONS

The adverse event rates listed below are based on symptoms spontaneously reported in multidose controlled clinical trials in comparing NASAREL and NASALIDE for treatment of allergic rhinitis. In patients receiving NASAREL the most common adverse events were transient aftertaste (17%) and transient nasal burning and stinging (13%). These symptoms did not usually interfere with treatment.

Adverse Event Rates for NASAREL:

Incidence Greater than 1% (probably causally related)

Respiratory: Nasal burning/stinging (13%), epistaxis*, nasal dryness, pharyngitis, cough increased

Gastrointestinal: Nausea

Special Senses: Aftertaste (17%)

Incidence 1% or Less (probably causally related)

Respiratory: Hoarseness

Special Senses: Abnormal sense of smell

Incidence 1% or less (causal relationship unknown)†

Respiratory: Sinusitis

Adverse Event Rates for NASALIDE:

Incidence Greater than 1% (probably causally related)

Respiratory: Nasal burning/stinging (44%), epistaxis*, nasal dryness*, pharyngitis*, cough increased

Gastrointestinal: Nausea

Special Senses: Aftertaste (8%)

Incidence 1% or Less (probably causally related)

Respiratory: Hoarseness, nasal ulcer

Incidence 1% or Less (causal relationship unknown)†

Respiratory: Sinusitis

*Incidence of reported reaction between 3% and 9%. Those reactions occurring in less than 3% of the patients are unmarked.

†Reactions occurred under circumstances where the causal relationship has not been clearly established; they are presented as alerting information for physicians.

OVERDOSAGE

In mice, rats and dogs, intravenous flunisolide at doses up to 4 mg/kg showed no effect. One spray bottle contains 6.25 mg of flunisolide; therefore acute overdosage is unlikely.

DOSAGE AND ADMINISTRATION

For adults, the recommended starting dose of NASAREL is 2 sprays (50 mcg) in each nostril 2 times a day (total dose 200 mcg/day): the effect should be assessed in 4 to 7 days (See INDIVIDUALIZATION OF DOSAGE section). Some relief can be expected in approximately two-thirds of patients within that time. This dose may be increased to 2 sprays in each nostril 3 times a day (total dose 300 mcg/day) if greater effect is needed. For adults, maximum total daily doses should not exceed 8 sprays in each nostril per day (400 mcg/day). After the desired clinical effect is obtained, the maintenance dose should be reduced to the smallest amount necessary to control the symptoms (See INDIVIDUALIZATION OF DOSAGE section).

For pediatric patients 6 to 14 years of age, the recommended starting dose of NASAREL is 1 spray (25 mcg) in each nostril 3 times a day (total dose 150 mcg/day) or 2 sprays (50 mcg) in each nostril 2 times a day (total dose 200 mcg/day). For pediatric patients 6 to 14 years of age, maximum daily doses should not exceed 4 sprays in each nostril per day (total dose 200 mcg/day) as the safety and efficacy of higher doses have not been established.

NASAREL is not recommended for use in pediatric patients less than 6 years of age as safety and efficacy, including possible adverse effects on growth, have not been assessed in this age group.

NASAREL and NASALIDE should not be considered to be identical products. Physicians should consider the observed differences in the mean responses in terms of side effects (see ADVERSE REACTIONS) and flunisolide absorption (see *Pharmacokinetics*) in treating individual patients.

HOW SUPPLIED

Each 25 mL of NASAREL 0.025% nasal solution (6.25 mg flunisolide) is supplied in a spray bottle fitted with a meter pump, nasal adapter and a white protective cap (NDC 51479-037-25). The unit contains 200 metered sprays and comes with a patient instruction leaflet.

Store at 15°–30°C (59°–86°F).

CONTENTS MADE IN CANADA

Revised: August, 1997

Rx only.

Manufactured for:
Dura Pharmaceuticals, Inc.
San Diego, CA 92121

Manufactured by:
Patheon, Inc.
Mississauga, Ontatio CANADA L5N 7K9

NREL001B0897
IN-5011/S

Shown in Product Identification Guide, page 311

Duramed Pharmaceuticals, Inc.

5040 LESTER ROAD
CINCINNATI, OHIO 45213

Direct Inquiries to:
(513)-731-9900
(800)-543-8338

CENESTIN® ℞
(synthetic conjugated estrogens, A)
Tablets
Rx only

PRESCRIBING INFORMATION

ESTROGENS INCREASE THE RISK OF ENDOMETRIAL CARCINOMA.

Close clinical surveillance of all women taking estrogens is important. Adequate diagnostic measures, including endometrial sampling when indicated, should be undertaken to rule out malignancy in all cases of undiagnosed persistent or recurring abnormal vaginal bleeding. There is no evidence that natural estrogens are more or less hazardous than synthetic estrogens of equivalent estrogen doses.

DESCRIPTION

Synthetic conjugated estrogens, A tablets contain a blend of nine (9) synthetic estrogenic substances. The estrogenic substances are sodium estrone sulfate, sodium equilin sulfate, sodium 17α-dihydroequilin sulfate, sodium 17α-estradiol sulfate, sodium 17β-dihydroequilin sulfate, sodium 17α-dihydroequilenin sulfate, sodium 17β-dihydroequilenin sulfate, sodium equilenin sulfate and sodium 17β-estradiol sulfate.

The structural formulae for these estrogens are:

$C_{18}H_{21}NaO_5S$
372.42
Sodium Estrone Sulfate

$C_{18}H_{21}NaO_5S$
372.42
Sodium 17α-Dihydroequilin Sulfate

$C_{18}H_{23}NaO_5S$
374.44
Sodium 17α-Estradiol Sulfate

$C_{18}H_{17}NaO_5S$
368.39
Sodium Equilenin Sulfate

$C_{18}H_{19}NaO_5S$
370.41
Sodium 17β-Dihydroequilenin Sulfate

$C_{18}H_{19}NaO_5S$
370.41
Sodium Equilin Sulfate

$C_{18}H_{21}NaO_5S$
372.42
Sodium 17β-Dihydroequilin Sulfate

[See chemical structures in next column]

Tablets for oral administration, are available in 0.625 mg, 0.9 mg and 1.25 mg strengths of synthetic conjugated estrogens. Tablets also contain the following inactive ingredients: ethylcellulose, hydroxypropyl methylcellulose, lactose monohydrate, magnesium stearate, polyethylene glycol, polysorbate 80, pregelatinized starch, titanium dioxide, and triethyl citrate.

-0.625 mg tablets also contain: FD&C Red No. 40 aluminum lake.
-0.9 mg tablets do not contain any color additives.
-1.25 mg tablets also contain: FD&C Blue No. 2 aluminum lake.

Table 1
PHARMACOKINETIC PARAMETERS FOR UNCONJUGATED AND CONJUGATED ESTROGENS IN HEALTHY POSTMENOPAUSAL WOMEN UNDER FASTING CONDITIONS

Pharmacokinetic Parameters of Unconjugated Estrogens Following a Dose of 2 × 0.625 mg Cenestin

Drug	C_{max} (pg/mL) CV%	t_{max} (h) CV%	AUC_{0-72h} (pg•hr/mL) CV%
Baseline-corrected estrone	84.5 (41.7)	8.25 (35.6)	1749 (43.8)
Equilin	45.6 (47.3)	7.78 (28.8)	723 (67.9)

Pharmacokinetic Parameters of Conjugated Estrogens Following a Dose of 2 × 0.625 mg Cenestin

Drug	C_{max} (ng/mL) CV%	t_{max} (h) CV%	$t_{½}$ (h) CV%	AUC_{0-72h} (ng•hr/mL) CV%
Baseline-corrected estrone	4.43 (40.4)	7.7 (30.3)	10.6 (25.4)	69.89 (39.2)
Equilin	3.27 (43.5)	5.8 (31.1)	9.7 (23.0)	46.46 (47.5)

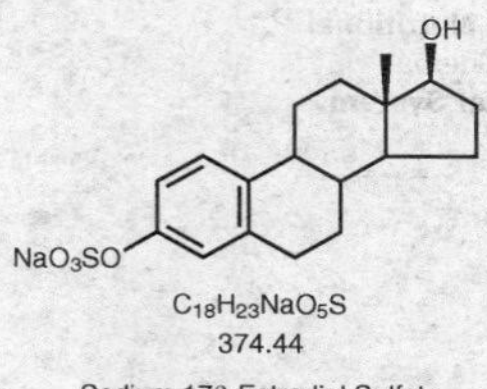

$C_{18}H_{23}NaO_5S$
374.44
Sodium 17β-Estradiol Sulfate

$C_{18}H_{19}NaO_5S$
370.41
Sodium 17α-Dihydroequilenin Sulfate

CLINICAL PHARMACOLOGY

Estrogens are largely responsible for the development and maintenance of the female reproductive system and secondary sexual characteristics. Although circulating estrogens exist in a dynamic equilibrium of metabolic interconversions, estradiol is the principal intracellular human estrogen and is substantially more potent than its metabolites, estrone and estriol at the receptor level. The primary source of estrogen in normally cycling adult women is the ovarian follicle, which secretes 70 to 500 µg of estradiol daily, depending on the phase of the menstrual cycle. After menopause, most endogenous estrogen is produced by conversion of androstenedione, secreted by the adrenal cortex, to estrone by peripheral tissues. Thus, estrone and the sulfate conjugated form, estrone sulfate, are the most abundant circulating estrogens in postmenopausal women.

Circulating estrogens modulate the pituitary secretion of the gonadotropins, leutinizing hormone (LH) and follicle stimulating hormone (FSH) through a negative feedback mechanism and estrogen replacement therapy acts to reduce the elevated levels of these hormones seen in postmenopausal women.

Pharmacokinetics

Absorption

Synthetic conjugated estrogens are soluble in water and are well absorbed from the gastrointestinal tract after release from the drug formulation. The Cenestin tablet releases the synthetic conjugated estrogens, A slowly over a period of several hours. Maximum plasma concentrations of conjugated estrogens are attained at about 8 hours and unconjugated estrogens are attained at about 9 hours after oral administration.

[See table 1 above]

[See figure in next column]

Food-Drug Interactions

The effect of food on the 0.625, 0.9 and 1.25 mg tablets has not been studied.

Distribution

The distribution of exogenous estrogens is similar to that of endogenous estrogens. Estrogens are widely distributed in the body and are generally found in higher concentrations in the sex hormone target organs. Estradiol and other naturally occurring estrogens are bound mainly to sex hormone binding globulin (SHBG), and to a lesser degree to albumin. Conjugated estrogens bind mainly to albumin while the unconjugated estrogens bind to both albumin and sex-hormone binding globulin (SHBG).

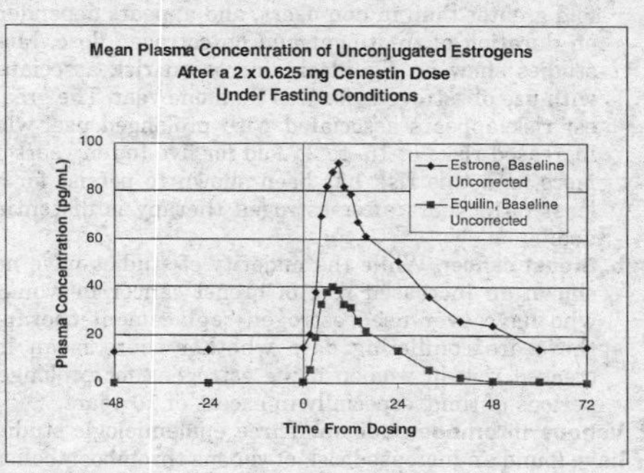

Metabolism

Exogenous estrogens are metabolized in the same manner as endogenous estrogens. Circulating estrogens exist in a dynamic equilibrium of metabolic interconversions. These transformations take place mainly in the liver. Estradiol is converted reversibly to estrone, and both can be converted to estriol, which is the major urinary metabolite. Estrogens also undergo enterohepatic recirculation via sulfate and glucuronide conjugation in the liver, biliary secretion of conjugates into the intestine, and hydrolysis in the gut followed by reabsorption. In postmenopausal women a significant portion of the circulating estrogens exist as sulfate conjugates, especially estrone sulfate, which serves as a circulating reservoir for the formation of more active estrogens.

Excretion

Estradiol, estrone, and estriol are excreted in the urine along with glucuronide and sulfate conjugates. The mean (SD) apparent terminal elimination half-life ($t_{½}$) of conjugated estrone is 15 (± 9) hours and conjugated equilin is 10 (± 3) hours.

Drug-Drug Interactions

There are no known drug interactions with estrogens.

Clinical Studies

A randomized, placebo-controlled multicenter clinical study was conducted evaluating the effectiveness of Cenestin for the treatment of vasomotor symptoms in 120 menopausal women. Patients were randomized to receive either placebo or 0.625 mg Cenestin daily for 12 weeks. Dose titration was allowed after one week of treatment. The starting dose was either doubled (2 × 0.625 mg Cenestin or placebo taken daily) or reduced (0.3 mg Cenestin or placebo taken daily), if necessary. Efficacy was assessed at 4, 8 and 12 weeks of treatment. By Week 12, 10% of the study participants remained on a single 0.625 mg Cenestin tablet daily while 77% required two (0.625 mg) tablets daily. The results in Table 2 indicate that compared to placebo, Cenestin produced a reduction in moderate-to-severe vasomotor symptoms at all time points (4, 8, and 12 weeks).

Table 2
Clinical Response*
Mean Change in Reduction of Vasomotor Symptoms

	Cenestin (n=70)	Placebo (n=47)	Difference
Baseline			
Mean # (SD)	96.8 (42.6)	94.1 (33.9)	-
Week 4			
Mean # (SD)	28.7 (28.8)	45.7 (36.8)	-
Mean Change	−68.1 (43.9)	−48.4 (46.2)	−19.9
Week 8			
Mean # (SD)	18.6 (25.0)	39.8 (39.1)	-
Mean Change	−78.3 (49.0)	−54.3 (49.2)	−24.6
Week 12			
Mean # (SD)	16.5 (25.7)	37.8 (38.7)	-
Mean Change	−80.3 (50.3)	−56.3 (48.0)	−24.7

Mean = Arithmetic Mean, SD = Standard Deviation
Difference = Difference between treatment LSMeans (Cenestin − Placebo).
*Intent-to-treat population = 117

Continued on next page

Cenestin—Cont.

INDICATIONS AND USAGE

Cenestin (synthetic conjugated estrogens, A) Tablets are indicated in the treatment of moderate to severe vasomotor symptoms associated with the menopause.

CONTRAINDICATIONS

Estrogens should not be used in individuals with any of the following conditions:

1. Known or suspected pregnancy (see PRECAUTIONS).
2. Undiagnosed abnormal genital bleeding.
3. Known or suspected cancer of the breast (except in appropriately selected patients being treated for metastatic disease).
4. Known or suspected estrogen-dependent neoplasia.
5. Active thrombophlebitis or thromboembolic disorders.

WARNINGS

1. Induction of malignant neoplasms.

a. Endometrial cancer. The reported endometrial cancer risk among unopposed estrogen users is about 2- to 12-fold greater than in non-users, and appears dependent on duration of treatment and on estrogen dose. Most studies show no significant increased risk associated with use of estrogens for less than one year. The greatest risk appears associated with prolonged use, with increased risks of 15- to 24-fold for five to ten years or more, and this risk has been shown to persist for at least 8–15 years after estrogen therapy is discontinued.

b. Breast cancer. While the majority of studies have not shown an increased risk of breast cancer in women who have ever used estrogen replacement therapy, there are conflicting data whether there is an increased risk in women using estrogens for prolonged periods of time, especially in excess of 10 years.

2. Venous thromboembolism. Three epidemiologic studies have found an increased risk of venous thromboembolism (VTE) in users of estrogen replacement therapy (ERT) who did not have predisposing conditions for VTE, such as past history of cardiovascular disease or a recent history of pregnancy, surgery, trauma, or serious illness. The increased risk was found only in current ERT users; it did not persist in former users. The findings were similar for ERT alone or with added progestin and pertain to commonly used ERT types and doses, including 0.625 mg or more per day orally of conjugated estrogens, 1 mg or more per day orally of estradiol, and 50 µg or more per day of transdermal estradiol. The studies found the VTE risk to be about one case per 10,000 women per year among women not using ERT and without predisposing conditions. The risk in current ERT users was increased to 2–3 cases per 10,000 women per year.

3. Cardiovascular disease. Large doses of estrogen (5 mg conjugated estrogens per day), comparable to those used to treat cancer of the prostate and breast, have been shown in large prospective clinical trial in men to increase the risks of nonfatal myocardial infarction, pulmonary embolism, and thrombophlebitis.

4. Hypercalcemia. Administration of estrogens may lead to severe hypercalcemia in patients with breast cancer and bone metastases. If this occurs, the drug should be stopped and appropriate measures taken to reduce the serum calcium level.

5. Gallbladder disease. A 2- to 4-fold increase in the risk of gallbladder disease requiring surgery in women receiving postmenopausal estrogens has been reported.

PRECAUTIONS

A. GENERAL

1. Addition of a progestin when a woman has not had a hysterectomy

Studies of the addition of a progestin for 10 or more days of a cycle of estrogen administration, or daily with estrogen in a continuous regimen, have reported a lowered incidence of endometrial hyperplasia than would be induced by estrogen treatment alone.

There are, however, possible risks which may be associated with the use of progestins in estrogen replacement regimens. These include:

(a) adverse effects on lipoprotein metabolism (lowering HDL and raising LDL)
(b) impairment of glucose tolerance; and
(c) possible enhancement of mitotic activity in breast epithelial tissue, although few epidemiological data are available to address this point.

The choice of progestin, its dose, and its regimen may be important in minimizing these adverse effects.

2. Elevated blood pressure

Substantial increases in blood pressure during estrogen replacement therapy have been attributed to idiosyncratic reactions to estrogens in a small number of case reports. A generalized effect of estrogen therapy on blood pressure was not found in the one randomized, placebo-controlled study that has been reported.

3. Familial hyperlipoproteinemia

Estrogen therapy may be associated with elevations of plasma triglycerides leading to pancreatitis and other complications in patients with familial defects of lipoprotein metabolism.

4. Impaired liver function

Estrogens may be poorly metabolized in patients with impaired liver function.

Table 3
Number (%) of Patients with Adverse Events With a Greater than 5% Occurrence Rate By Body System and Treatment Group

Body System / Adverse Event	Cenestin n (%)	Placebo n (%)	Total n (%)
Number of Patients Who Received Medication	72 (100)	48 (100)	120 (100)
Number of Patients With Adverse Events	68 (94)	43 (90)	111 (93)
Number of Patients Without Any Adverse Events	4 (6)	5 (10)	9 (8)
Body As A Whole			
Abdominal Pain	20 (28)	11 (23)	31 (26)
Asthenia	24 (33)	20 (42)	44 (37)
Back Pain	10 (14)	6 (13)	16 (13)
Fever	1 (1)	3 (6)	4 (3)
Headache	49 (68)	32 (67)	81 (68)
Infection	10 (14)	5 (10)	15 (13)
Pain	8 (11)	9 (19)	17 (14)
Cardiovascular System			
Palpitation	15 (21)	13 (27)	28 (23)
Digestive System			
Constipation	4 (6)	2 (4)	6 (5)
Diarrhea	4 (6)	0 (0)	4 (3)
Dyspepsia	7 (10)	3 (6)	10 (8)
Flatulence	21 (29)	14 (29)	35 (29)
Nausea	13 (18)	9 (19)	22 (18)
Vomiting	5 (7)	1 (2)	6 (5)
Metabolic and Nutritional			
Peripheral Edema	7 (10)	6 (13)	13 (11)
Musculoskeletal System			
Arthralgia	18 (25)	13 (27)	31 (26)
Myalgia	20 (28)	15 (31)	35 (29)
Nervous System			
Depression	20 (28)	18 (38)	38 (32)
Dizziness	8 (11)	5 (10)	13 (11)
Hypertonia	4 (6)	0 (0)	4 (3)
Insomnia	30 (42)	23 (48)	53 (44)
Leg Cramps	7 (10)	3 (6)	10 (8)
Nervousness	20 (28)	20 (42)	40 (33)
Paresthesia	24 (33)	15 (31)	39 (33)
Vertigo	12 (17)	12 (25)	24 (20)
Respiratory System			
Cough Increased	4 (6)	1 (2)	5 (4)
Pharyngitis	6 (8)	4 (8)	10 (8)
Rhinitis	6 (8)	7 (15)	13 (11)
Urogenital System			
Breast Pain	21 (29)	7 (15)	28 (23)
Dysmenorrhea	4 (6)	3 (6)	7 (6)
Metrorrhagia	10 (14)	3 (6)	13 (11)

B. INFORMATION FOR THE PATIENT

See text of PATIENT LABELING, below.

C. LABORATORY TESTS

Estrogen administration should generally be guided by clinical response at the smallest dose, rather than laboratory monitoring, for relief of symptoms for those indications in which symptoms are observable.

D. DRUG/LABORATORY TEST INTERACTIONS

1. Accelerated prothrombin time, partial thromboplastin time, and platelet aggregation time; increased platelet count; increased factors II, VII antigen, VIII antigen, VIII coagulant activity, IX, X, XII, VII-X complex, II-VII-X complex, and beta-thromboglobulin; decreased levels of anti-factor Xa and antithrombin III, decreased antithrombin III activity; increased levels of fibrinogen and fibrinogen activity; increased plasminogen antigen and activity.
2. Increased thyroid-binding globulin (TBG) leading to increased circulating total thyroid hormone, as measured by protein-bound iodine (PBI), T4 levels (by column or by radioimmunoassay) or T3 levels by radioimmunoassay. T3 resin uptake is decreased, reflecting the elevated TBG. Free T4 and free T3 concentrations are unaltered.
3. Other binding proteins may be elevated in serum, i.e., corticosteroid binding globulin (CGB), sex hormone-binding globulin (SHBG), leading to increased circulating corticosteroids and sex steroids respectively. Free or biologically active hormone concentrations are unchanged. Other plasma proteins may be increased (angiotensinogen/renin substrate, alpha-1-antitrypsin, ceruloplasmin).
4. Increased plasma HDL and HDL-2 subfraction concentrations, reduced LDL cholesterol concentration, increased triglycerides levels.
5. Impaired glucose tolerance.
6. Reduced response to metyrapone test.
7. Reduced serum folate concentration.

E. CARCINOGENESES, MUTAGENESIS, AND IMPAIRMENT OF FERTILITY

Long-term continuous administration of natural and synthetic estrogens in certain animal species increases the frequency of carcinomas of the breast, uterus, cervix, vagina, testis, and liver. See CONTRAINDICATIONS and WARNINGS.

F. PREGNANCY

Estrogens are not indicated for use during pregnancy or the immediate postpartum period. Estrogens are ineffective for the prevention or treatment of threatened or habitual abortion. Treatment with diethylstilbestrol (DES) during pregnancy has been associated with an increased risk of congenital defects and cancer in the reproductive organs of the fetus, and possibly other birth defects. The use of DES during pregnancy has also been associated with a subsequent increased risk of breast cancer in the mothers.

G. NURSING MOTHERS

As a general principle, the administration of any drug to nursing mothers should be done only when clearly necessary since many drugs are excreted in human milk. In addition, estrogen administration to nursing mothers has been shown to decrease the quantity and quality of the milk. Estrogens are not indicated for the prevention of postpartum breast engorgement.

H. PEDIATRIC USE

Safety and efficacy of Cenestin for the treatment of vasomotor symptoms due to hypoestrogenism in pediatric patients have not been established.

ADVERSE REACTIONS

See WARNINGS and PRECAUTIONS regarding the potential adverse effects on the fetus, the induction of malignant neoplasms, gallbladder disease, cardiovascular disease, elevated blood pressure and hypercalcemia. In a 12-week clinical trial that included 72 women treated with Cenestin and 48 women treated with placebo, the following adverse events occurred at a rate ≥ 5% (see Table 3).

[See table 3 above]

The following additional adverse reactions have been reported with estrogen therapy:

1. *Genitourinary system.* Changes in vaginal bleeding pattern and abnormal withdrawal bleeding or flow; breakthrough bleeding, spotting; increase in size of uterine leiomyomata; vaginal candidasis; change in amount of cervical secretion.
2. *Breasts.* Tenderness, enlargement.
3. *Gastrointestinal.* Nausea, vomiting; abdominal cramps, bloating; cholestatic jaundice; gallbladder disease.
4. *Skin.* Chloasma or melasma that may persist when drug is discontinued; erythema multiforme; erythema nodosum; hemorrhagic eruption; loss of scalp hair; hirsutism.
5. *Eyes.* Steepening of corneal curvature: intolerance to contact lenses.
6. *Central Nervous System.* Headache, migraine, dizziness; mental depression; chorea.
7. *Miscellaneous.* Increase or decrease in weight; reduced carbohydrate tolerance; aggravation or porphyria; edema; changes in libido.

OVERDOSAGE

Serious ill effects have not been reported following acute ingestion of large doses of estrogen-containing products by young children. Overdosage of estrogen may cause nausea and vomiting, and withdrawal bleeding may occur in females.

DOSAGE AND ADMINISTRATION

For treatment of moderate to severe vasomotor symptoms associated with the menopause, the lowest dose and regimen that will control symptoms should be chosen. Initial doses of 0.625 mg are recommended with titration up to 1.25 mg. Medication should be discontinued as promptly as possible. Attempts to discontinue or taper medication should be made at 3-month to 6-month intervals.

HOW SUPPLIED

Cenestin (synthetic conjugated estrogens, A) Tablets,
-0.625 mg tablets are available in containers of 30 (NDC 51285-442-30), 100 (NDC 51285-442-02), and 1000 (NDC 51285-442-05).
Tablets are round, red colored, film-coated, and are debossed with letters, **dp**, and number, 42.
-0.9 mg tablets are available in containers of 30 (NDC 51285-443-30), 100 (NDC 51285-443-02), and 1000 (NDC 51285-443-05).
Tablets are round, white, film-coated, and are debossed with letters, **dp**, and number, 43.
-1.25 mg tablets are available in containers of 30 (NDC 51285-444-30), 100 (NDC 51285-444-02), and 1000 (NDC 51285-444-05).
Tablets are round, blue colored, film-coated, and are debossed with letters, **dp**, and number, 44.
Store at 25°C (77°F); excursions are permitted to 15°–30°C (59°–86°F) [See USP Controlled Room Temperature]
Dispense in tight container as defined in USP.
Dispense in child-resistant packaging.
Dispenser: Include one "Information for the patient" leaflet with each package dispensed.

INFORMATION FOR THE PATIENT

Cenestin®
(synthetic conjugated estrogens, A) Tablets
PATIENT PACKAGE INSERT

INTRODUCTION

This leaflet describes when and how to use estrogens, and the risks and benefits of estrogen treatment.

Estrogens have important benefits but also some risks. You must decide, with your doctor, whether the risks are acceptable in comparison to the benefits. If you use estrogens, check with your doctor to be sure you are using the lowest possible dose that works, and that you don't use them longer than necessary. How long you need to use estrogens will depend on the reasons for use.

ESTROGENS INCREASE THE RISK OF CANCER OF THE UTERUS

If you use any drug that contains estrogen, it is important to visit your doctor regularly and report any unusual vaginal bleeding right away. Vaginal bleeding after menopause may be a warning sign of uterine cancer. Your doctor should evaluate any unusual vaginal bleeding to find out the cause.

USES OF CENESTIN

To reduce moderate or severe menopausal symptoms.

Estrogens are hormones made by the ovaries of normal women. Between ages 45 and 55, the ovaries normally stop making estrogens. This leads to a drop in body estrogen levels which causes the "change of life" or menopause (the end of monthly menstrual periods). If both ovaries are removed during an operation before natural menopause takes place, the sudden drop in estrogen levels causes "surgical menopause".

When estrogen levels begin dropping, some women develop very uncomfortable symptoms, such as feelings of warmth in the face, neck and chest or sudden intense episodes of heat and sweating ("hot flashes" or "hot flushes"). Using estrogen drugs can help the body adjust to lower estrogen levels and reduce these symptoms. Most women have only mild menopausal symptoms or none at all and do not need to use estrogen drugs for these symptoms. Others may need to take estrogens for a few months while their bodies adjust to lower estrogen levels. The majority of women do not need estrogen replacement for longer than six months for these symptoms.

WHO SHOULD NOT USE CENESTIN

Cenestin should not be used:

- **During pregnancy.**
  If you think you may be pregnant, do not use any form of estrogen-containing drug. Using some types of estrogens while you are pregnant may cause your unborn child to have birth defects. Estrogens do not prevent miscarriage.
- **If you have unusual vaginal bleeding which has not been evaluated by your doctor (see Boxed Warning).**
  Unusual vaginal bleeding can be a warning sign of cancer of the uterus, especially if it happens after menopause. Your doctor must find out the cause of the bleeding so that he or she can recommend the proper treatment.
- **If you have had cancer.**
  Since estrogens may increase the risk of certain types of breast and uterine cancer you should not use estrogens unless your doctor recommends that you take it. (For certain patients with breast or prostate cancer, estrogens may help.)
- **If you have circulation problems.**
  Men and women with abnormal blood clotting conditions should avoid estrogen use (see DANGERS OF ESTROGENS, below).
- **After childbirth or when breastfeeding a baby.**
  Estrogens should not be used to try to stop the breasts from filling with milk after a baby is born. Such treatment may increase the risk of developing blood clots (see DANGERS OF ESTROGENS, below).

DANGERS OF ESTROGENS

- **Cancer of the uterus.**
  Your risk of developing cancer of the uterus gets higher the longer you use estrogens and the larger doses you use. Because of this risk, it is important to take the lowest dose that works and to take it only as long as you need it.
  Using progestin therapy together with estrogen therapy may reduce the higher risk of uterine cancer related to estrogen use (see also OTHER INFORMATION, below).
  If you have had your uterus removed (total hysterectomy), there is no danger of developing cancer of the uterus.
- **Cancer of the breast.**
  Most studies have not shown a higher risk of breast cancer in women who have ever used estrogens. However, some studies have reported that breast cancer developed more often (up to twice the usual rate) in women who used estrogens for long periods of time (especially more than 10 years), or who used higher doses for shorter time periods.
  Regular breast examinations by a health professional and monthly self-examination are recommended for all women. Yearly mammography is recommended for women beginning at age 50.
- **Abnormal blood clotting.**
  Taking estrogens may cause changes in your blood clotting system. These changes allow the blood to clot more easily, possibly allowing clots to form in your bloodstream. If blood clots do form in your bloodstream, they can cut off the blood supply to vital organs, causing serious problems. These problems may include stroke (by cutting off blood to the brain), heart attack (by cutting off blood to the heart), a pulmonary clot (by cutting off blood to the lungs), or other problems. Any of these conditions may cause death or serious long term disability.
- **Gallbladder disease.**
  Women who use estrogens after menopause are more likely to develop gallbladder disease needing surgery than women who do not use estrogens.

SIDE EFFECTS

In addition to the risks listed above, the following side effects have been reported with estrogen use:
Nausea and vomiting.
Breast tenderness or enlargement.
Enlargement of benign tumors of the uterus (fibroids).
Retention of excess fluid.
Spotty darkening of the skin, particularly on the face.

USE IN CHILDREN

Cenestin has not been shown either effective or safe for use by infants, children, or adolescent boys or girls.

REDUCING THE RISKS OF ESTROGEN USE

If you use estrogens, you can reduce your risks by doing these things:

- **See your doctor regularly.**
  While you are using estrogens, it is important to visit your doctor at least once a year for a check-up. If you develop vaginal bleeding while taking estrogens, you may need further evaluation.
- **Reassess your need for estrogens.**
  You and your doctor should reevaluate whether or not you still need estrogens every three to six months.
- **Be alert for signs of trouble.**
  If any of these warning signals (or any other unusual symptoms) happen while you are using estrogens, call your doctor immediately.
  Abnormal bleeding from the vagina (possible uterine cancer)
  Pains in the calves or chest, sudden shortness of breath, or coughing blood (possible clot in the legs, heart, or lungs)
  Severe headache or vomiting, dizziness, faintness, changes in vision or speech, weakness or numbness of an arm or leg (possible clot in the brain or eye)
  Breast lumps (possible breast cancer; ask your doctor or health professional to show you how to examine your breasts monthly)
  Yellowing of the skin or eyes (possible liver problems)
  Pain, swelling, or tenderness in the abdomen (possible gallbladder problem)

OTHER INFORMATION

Estrogens increase the risk of developing a condition (endometrial hyperplasia) that may lead to cancer of the lining of the uterus. Taking progestins, another hormone drug, with estrogens lowers the risk of developing this condition. Therefore, if your uterus has not been removed, your doctor may prescribe a progestin for you to take together with the estrogen.

Your doctor has prescribed this drug for you and you alone. Do not give the drug to anyone else.

Keep this and all drugs out of the reach of children. In case of overdose, call your doctor, hospital or poison control center immediately.

HOW SUPPLIED

Cenestin (synthetic conjugated estrogens, A) Tablets,
-0.625 mg tablets are available in containers of 30 (NDC 51285-442-30), 100 (NDC 51285-442-02), and 1000 (NDC 51285-442-05).
Tablets are round, red colored, film-coated, and are debossed with letters, **dp**, and number, 42.
-0.9 mg tablets are available in containers of 30 (NDC 51285-443-30), 100 (NDC 51285-443-02), and 1000 (NDC 51285-443-05).
Tablets are round, white, film-coated, and are debossed with letters, **dp**, and number, 43.
-1.25 mg tablets are available in containers of 30 (NDC 51285-444-30), 100 (NDC 51285-444-02), and 1000 (NDC 51285-444-05).
Tablets are round, blue colored, film-coated, and are debossed with letters, **dp**, and number, 44.
Store at 25°C (77°F); excursions are permitted to 15°–30°C (59°–86°F). [See USP Controlled Room Temperature]

Manufactured by: Duramed Pharmaceuticals, Inc.
Cincinnati, OH 45213 USA

I00379B **REV. 01/00**

ECR Pharmaceuticals

Distributor of ECR &
Wm. P. Poythress Products
3969 DEEP ROCK ROAD
P. O. BOX 71600
RICHMOND, VA 23255

Direct Inquiries to:
Professional Services Department
(804) 527-1950
FAX: (804) 527-1959

For Medical Information Contact:
In Emergencies:
Professional Services Department
(804) 527-1950
FAX: (804) 527-1959

NDC 00095	Product	
—0131	**Anaplex DM Cough Syrup** Each teaspoon (5 ml) contains: Dextromethrophan Hydrobromide, 30 mg. Brompheniramine Maleate, 4 mg. Pseudoephedrine HCl, 60 mg. Sugar Free, Alcohol Free, Dye Free	℞
—0130	**Anaplex HD Cough Syrup** Each teaspoon (5 ml) contains: Hydrocodone Bitartrate, 1.7 mg; Pseudoephedrine HCl, 30 mg. Brompheniramine Maleate, 2 mg. Sugar Free. Alcohol Free, Dye Free.	℞ CIII
—0240	**Bupap Tablets** (Butalbital, 50 mg; Acetaminophen, 650 mg)	℞
—0016	**Bensulfoid Cream** (Sulfur, 8%; Resorcinol 2%; Alcohol, 10%)	OTC
—0086	**DEXPAK Taperpak** Weighted, tapered oral Corticosteroid Therapy. Each package contains 51 tablets, dexamethasone, USP 1.5 mg	℞
—6004	**Lodrane Liquid** Each teaspoon (5 ml) contains: Brompheniramine Maleate, 4 mg; Pseudoephedrine HCl, 60 mg. Sugar Free. Alcohol Free. Dye Free.	℞
—0006	**Lodrane Allergy Capsules** (Brompheniramine Maleate, 6 mg.) Sustained Release, Dye Free	℞
—6006	**Lodrane LD Capsules** (Brompheniramine Maleate, 6 mg; Pseudoephedrine HCl, 60 mg) Sustained Release, Dye Free	℞
—0225	**Nasatab LA Tablets** (Guaifenesin, 500 mg; Pseudoephedrine HCl, 120 mg) Sustained Release, Dye Free	℞
—0021	**Panalgesic Gold Cream** (Methyl Salicylate, 35%; Menthol, 4%)	OTC
—0120	**Panalgesic Gold Liniment** (Methyl Salicylate, 55%; Camphor, 3%; Menthol, 1%)	OTC
—0066	**Pneumotussin Tablets** (Guaifenesin, 300 mg; Hydrocodone Bitartrate, 2.5 mg)	℞ CIII
—0067	**Pneumotussin 2.5 Cough Syrup** Each teaspoon (5 ml) contains: (Guaifenesin, 200 mg; Hydrocodone Bitartrate, 2.5 mg)	℞ CIII

Eisai Inc.

500 FRANK W. BURR BOULEVARD
TEANECK, NJ 07666

Direct Inquiries to:
Eisai Medical Services
1 (888) 274-2378 (888-Aricept)
FAX: (201) 287-9744
Medical Emergency Contact:
Medical Emergencies:
24 hours/day, 7 days/week
1 (888) 274-2378 (888-Aricept)

ACIPHEX™ ℞

[*'ā-se-feks*]
(rabeprazole sodium)
Delayed-Release Tablets

DESCRIPTION

The active ingredient in ACIPHEX™ Delayed-Release Tablets is rabeprazole sodium, a substituted benzimidazole that inhibits gastric acid secretion. Rabeprazole sodium is known chemically as 2-[[[4-(3-methoxypropoxy)-3-methyl-2-pyridinyl]-methyl]sulfinyl]-1*H*–benzimidazole sodium salt. It has an empirical formula of $C_{18}H_{20}N_3NaO_3S$ and a molecular weight of 381.43. Rabeprazole sodium is a white to slightly yellowish-white solid. It is very soluble in water and methanol, freely soluble in ethanol, chloroform, and ethyl acetate and insoluble in ether and n-hexane. The stability of rabeprazole sodium is a function of pH; it is rapidly degraded in acid media, and is more stable under alkaline conditions. The structural formula is:

RABEPRAZOLE SODIUM

ACIPHEX™ is available for oral administration as delayed-release, enteric-coated tablets containing 20 mg of rabeprazole sodium. Inactive ingredients are mannitol, hydroxypropyl cellulose, magnesium oxide, low-substituted hydroxypropyl cellulose, magnesium stearate, ethylcellulose, hydroxypropyl methylcellulose phthalate, diacetylated monoglycerides, talc, titanium dioxide, carnauba wax, and ferric oxide (yellow) as a coloring agent.

CLINICAL PHARMACOLOGY

Pharmacokinetics and Metabolism
ACIPHEX™ delayed-release tablets are enteric-coated to allow rabeprazole sodium, which is acid labile, to pass through the stomach relatively intact. After oral administration of 20 mg ACIPHEX™, peak plasma concentrations (C_{max} of rabeprazole occur over a range of 2.0 to 5.0 hours (T_{max}). The rabeprazole C_{max} and AUC are linear over an oral dose range of 10 mg to 40 mg. There is no appreciable accumulation when doses of 10 mg to 40 mg are administered every 24 hours; the pharmacokinetics of rabeprazole are not altered by multiple dosing. The plasma half-life ranges from 1 to 2 hours.

Absorption: Following oral administration of 20 mg, rabeprazole is absorbed and can be detected in plasma by 1 hour. Absolute bioavailability for a 20 mg oral tablet of rabeprazole (compared to intravenous administration) is approximately 52%.

The effects of food on the absorption of rabeprazole have not been evaluated.

Distribution: Rabeprazole is 96.3% bound to human plasma proteins.

Metabolism: Rabeprazole is extensively metabolized. The thioether and sulphone are the primary metabolites measured in human plasma. These metabolites were not observed to have significant antisecretory activity. *In vitro* studies have demonstrated that rabeprazole is primarily metabolized in the liver by cytochromes P450 3A (sulphone metabolite) and 2C19 (desmethyl rabeprazole). The thioether metabolite is formed by reduction of rabeprazole.

Elimination: Following a single 20 mg oral dose of ^{14}C-labeled rabeprazole, approximately 90% of the drug was eliminated in the urine, primarily as thioether carboxylic acid; its glucuronide, and mercapturic acid metabolites. The remainder of the dose was recovered in the feces. Total recovery of radioactivity was 99.8%. No unchanged rabeprazole was recovered in the urine or feces.

Special Populations

Geriatric: In 20 healthy elderly subjects administered 20 mg rabeprazole once daily for seven days, AUC values approximately doubled and the C_{max} increased by 60% compared to values in a parallel younger control group. There was no evidence of drug accumulation after once daily administration. (see PRECAUTIONS).

Pediatric: The pharmacokinetics of rabeprazole in pediatric patients under the age of 18 years have not been studied.

Gender and Race: In analyses adjusted for body mass and height, rabeprazole pharmacokinetics showed no clinically significant differences between male and female subjects. In studies that used different formulations of rabeprazole, $AUC_{0-\infty}$ values for healthy Japanese men were approximately 50–60% greater than values derived from pooled data from healthy men in the United States.

Renal Disease: In 10 patients with stable end-stage renal disease requiring maintenance hemodialysis (creatinine clearance ≤5 mL/min/1.73 m^2), no clinically significant differences were observed in the pharmacokinetics of rabeprazole after a single 20 mg oral dose when compared to 10 healthy volunteers.

Hepatic Disease: In a single dose study of 10 patients with chronic mild to moderate compensated cirrhosis of the liver who were administered a 20 mg dose of rabeprazole, AUC_{0-24} was approximately doubled, the elimination half-life was 2- to 3-fold higher, and total body clearance was decreased to less than half compared to values in healthy men.

In a multiple dose study of 12 patients with mild to moderate hepatic impairment administered 20 mg rabeprazole once daily for eight days, $AUC_{0-\infty}$ and C_{max} values increased approximately 20% compared to values in healthy age- and gender-matched subjects. These increases were not statistically significant.

No information exists on rabeprazole disposition in patients with severe hepatic impairment. Please refer to the DOSAGE AND ADMINISTRATION section for information on dosage adjustment in patients with hepatic impairment.

PHARMACODYNAMICS

Mechanism of Action
Rabeprazole belongs to a class of antisecretory compounds (substituted benzimidazole proton-pump inhibitors) that do not exhibit anticholinergic or histamine H_2-receptor antagonist properties, but suppress gastric acid secretion by inhibiting the gastric H+, K+ATPase at the secretory surface of the gastric parietal cell. Because this enzyme is regarded as the acid (proton) pump within the parietal cell, rabeprazole has been characterized as a gastric proton-pump inhibitor. Rabeprazole blocks the final step of gastric acid secretion.

In gastric parietal cells, rabeprazole is protonated, accumulates, and is transformed to an active sulfenamide. When studied *in vitro*, rabeprazole is chemically activated at pH 1.2 with a half-life of 78 seconds. It inhibits acid transport in porcine gastric vesicles with a half-life of 90 seconds.

Antisecretory Activity
The anti-secretory effect begins within one hour after oral administration of 20 mg ACIPHEX™. The median inhibitory effect of ACIPHEX™ on 24 hour gastric acidity is 88% of maximal after the first dose. ACIPHEX™ 20 mg inhibits basal and peptone meal-stimulated acid secretion versus placebo by 86% and 95%, respectively, and increases the — percent of a 24-hour period that the gastric pH>3 from 10% to 65% (see table below). This relatively prolonged pharmacodynamic action compared to the short pharmacokinetic half-life (1–2 hours) reflects the sustained inactivation of the H+, K+ATPase.

Gastric Acid Parameters
ACIPHEX™ Versus Placebo After 7 Days of Once Daily Dosing

Parameter	ACIPHEX™ (20 mg QD)	Placebo
Basal Acid Output (mmol/hr)	0.4*	2.8
Stimulated Acid Output (mmol/hr)	0.6*	13.3
% Time Gastric pH>3	65*	10

*(p<0.01 versus placebo)

AUC Acidity (mmol•hr/L)
ACIPHEX™ Versus Placebo on Day 7 of Once Daily Dosing (mean±SD)

AUC interval (hrs)	Treatment: 10 mg RBP (N=24)	20 mg RBP (N=24)	40 mg RBP (N=24)	Placebo (N=24)
08:00 – 13:00	19.6±21.5*	12.9±23*	7.6±14.7*	91.1±39.7
13:00 – 19:00	5.6±9.7*	8.3±29.8*	1.3±5.2*	95.5±48.7
19:00 – 22:00	0.1±0.1*	0.1±0.06*	0.0±0.02*	11.9±12.5
22:00 – 08:00	129.2±84*	109.6±67.2*	76.9±58.4*	479.9±165
AUC 0-24 hours	155.5±90.6*	130.9±81*	85.8±64.3*	678.5±216

*(p<0.001 versus placebo)

Gastric Acid Parameters
ACIPHEX™ Once Daily Dosing Versus Placebo on Day 1 and Day 8

Parameter	ACIPHEX™ 20 mg QD Day 1	ACIPHEX™ 20 mg QD Day 8	Placebo Day 1	Placebo Day 8
Mean AUC_{0-24} Acidity	340.8*	176.9*	925.5	862.4
Median trough pH (23-hr)[a]	3.77	3.51	1.27	1.38
% Time Gastric pH>3[b]	54.6*	68.7*	19.1	21.7
% Time Gastric pH>4[b]	44.1*	60.3*	7.6	11.0

[a]No inferential statistics conducted for this parameter.
*(p<0.001 versus placebo)
[b]Gastric pH was measured every hour over a 24-hour period.

Compared to placebo, ACIPHEX™, 10 mg, 20 mg, and 40 mg, administered once daily for 7 days significantly decreased intragastric acidity with all doses for each of four meal-related intervals and the 24-hour time period overall. In this study, there were no statistically significant differences between doses; however, there was a significant dose-related decrease in intragastric acidity. The ability of rabeprazole to cause a dose-related decrease in mean intragastric acidity is illustrated below.

[See first table above]

After administration of 20 mg ACIPHEX™ once daily for eight days, the mean percent of time that gastric pH>3 or gastric pH>4 after a single dose (Day 1) and multiple doses (Day 8) was significantly greater than placebo (see table below). The decrease in gastric acidity and the increase in gastric pH observed with 20 mg ACIPHEX™ administered once daily for eight days were compared to the same parameters for placebo, as illustrated below:

[See second table above]

Effects on Esophageal Acid Exposure
In patients with gastroesophageal reflux disease (GERD) and moderate to severe esophageal acid exposure, ACIPHEX™ 20 mg and 40 mg per day decreased 24-hour esophageal acid exposure. After seven days of treatment, the percentage of time that esophageal pH<4 decreased from baselines of 24.7% for 20 mg and 23.7% for 40 mg, to 5.1% and 2.0%, respectively. Normalization of 24-hour intraesophageal acid exposure was correlated to gastric pH>4 for at least 35% of the 24-hour period; this level was achieved in 90% of subjects receiving ACIPHEX™ 20 mg and in 100% of subjects receiving ACIPHEX™ 40 mg. With ACIPHEX™ 20 mg and 40 mg per day, effects on gastric and esophageal pH were significant and substantial after one day of treatment, and more pronounced after seven days of treatment.

Effects on Serum Gastrin
In patients given daily doses of ACIPHEX™ for up to eight weeks to treat ulcerative or erosive esophagitis and in patients treated for up to 52 weeks to prevent recurrence of disease the median fasting gastrin level increased in a dose-related manner. The group median values stayed within the normal range.

Effects on Enterochromaffin-like (ECL) Cells
Increased serum gastrin secondary to antisecretory agents stimulates proliferation of gastric ECL cells which, over time, may result in ECL cell hyperplasia in rats and mice and gastric carcinoids in rats, especially in females (see Carcinogenesis, Mutagenesis, Impairment of Fertility).

In over 400 patients treated with ACIPHEX™ (10 or 20 mg/day) for up to one year, the incidence of ECL cell hyperplasia increased with time and dose, which is consistent with the pharmacological action of the proton-pump inhibitor. No patient developed the adenomatoid, dysplastic or neoplastic changes of ECL cells in the gastric mucosa. No patient developed the carcinoid tumors observed in rats.

Endocrine Effects
Studies in humans for up to one year have not revealed clinically significant effects on the endocrine system. In healthy male volunteers treated with ACIPHEX™ for 13 days, no clinically relevant changes have been detected in the following endocrine parameters examined: 17 β-estradiol, thyroid stimulating hormone, tri-iodothyronine, thyroxine, thyroxine-binding protein, parathyroid hormone, insulin, glucagon, renin, aldosterone, follicle-stimulating hormone, luteotrophic hormone, prolactin, somatotrophic hormone, dehy-

droepiandrosterone, cortisol-binding globulin, and urinary 6β-hydroxycortisol, serum testosterone and circadian cortisol profile.

Other Effects

In humans treated with ACIPHEX™ for up to one year, no systemic effects have been observed on the central nervous, lymphoid, hematopoietic, renal, hepatic, cardiovascular, or respiratory systems. No data are available on long-term treatment with ACIPHEX™ and ocular effects.

CLINICAL STUDIES

Healing of Erosive or Ulcerative Gastroesophageal Reflux Disease (GERD)

In a U.S., multicenter, randomized, double-blind, placebo-controlled study, 103 patients were treated for up to eight weeks with placebo, 10 mg, 20 mg or 40 mg ACIPHEX™ QD. For this and all studies of GERD healing, only patients with GERD symptoms and at least grade 2 esophagitis (modified Hetzel-Dent grading scale) were eligible for entry. Endoscopic healing was defined as grade 0 or 1. Each rabeprazole dose was significantly superior to placebo in producing endoscopic healing after four and eight weeks of treatment. The percentage of patients demonstrating endoscopic healing was as follows:

[See table above]

Healing of Erosive or Ulcerative Gastroesophageal Reflux Disease (GERD) Percentage of Patients Healed

Week	10 mg ACIPHEX™ QD N=27	20 mg ACIPHEX™ QD N=25	40 mg ACIPHEX™ QD N=26	Placebo N=25
4	63%*	56%*	54%*	0%
8	93%*	84%*	85%*	12%

*($p<0.001$ versus placebo)

In addition, there was a statistically significant difference in favor of the ACIPHEX™ 10 mg, 20 mg, and 40 mg doses compared to placebo at Weeks 4 and 8 regarding complete resolution of GERD heartburn frequency ($p\leq0.026$). All ACIPHEX™ groups reported significantly greater rates of complete resolution of GERD daytime heartburn severity compared to placebo at Weeks 4 and 8 ($p\leq0.036$). Mean reductions from baseline in daily antacid dose were statistically significant for all ACIPHEX™ groups when compared to placebo at both Weeks 4 and 8 ($p\leq0.007$).

In a North American multicenter, randomized, double-blind, active-controlled study of 336 patients, ACIPHEX™ was statistically superior to ranitidine with respect to the percentage of patients healed at endoscopy after four and eight weeks of treatment (see table below):

Healing of Erosive or Ulcerative Gastroesophageal Reflux Disease (GERD) Percentage of Patients Healed

Week	ACIPHEX™ 20 mg QD N=167	Ranitidine 150 mg QID N=169
4	59%*	36%
8	87%*	66%

*($p<0.001$ versus ranitidine)

ACIPHEX™ 20 mg once daily was significantly more effective than ranitidine 150 mg QID in the percentage of patients with complete resolution of heartburn at Weeks 4 and 8 ($p<0.001$). ACIPHEX™ 20 mg once daily was also more effective in complete resolution of daytime heartburn ($p<0.025$), and night time heartburn ($p\leq0.012$) at both Weeks 4 and 8, with significant differences by the end of the first week of the study.

Long-term Maintenance of Healing of Erosive or Ulcerative Gastroesophageal Reflux Disease (GERD Maintenance)

The long-term maintenance of healing in patients with erosive or ulcerative GERD previously healed with gastric antisecretory therapy was assessed in two U.S., multicenter, randomized, double-blind, placebo-controlled studies of identical design of 52 weeks duration. The two studies randomized 209 and 285 patients, respectively, to receive either 10 mg or 20 mg of ACIPHEX™ QD or placebo. As demonstrated in the tables below, ACIPHEX™ was significantly superior to placebo in both studies with respect to the maintenance of healing of GERD and the proportions of patients remaining free of heartburn symptoms at 52 weeks:

[See first table at top of next page]

[See second table on next page]

Healing of Duodenal Ulcers

In a U.S., randomized, double-blind, multi-center study assessing the effectiveness of 20 mg and 40 mg of ACIPHEX™ QD versus placebo for healing endoscopically defined duodenal ulcers, 100 patients were treated for up to four weeks. ACIPHEX™ was significantly superior to placebo in producing healing of duodenal ulcers. The percentages of patients with endoscopic healing are presented below:

Healing of Duodenal Ulcers Percentage of Patients Healed

Week	ACIPHEX™ 20 mg QD N=34	ACIPHEX™ 40 mg QD N=33	Placebo N=33
2	44%	42%	21%
4	79%*	91%*	39%

*$p\leq0.001$ versus placebo

At Weeks 2 and 4, significantly more patients in the ACIPHEX™ 20 and 40 mg groups reported complete resolution of ulcer pain frequency ($p\leq0.018$), daytime pain severity ($p\leq0.023$), and nighttime pain severity ($p\leq0.035$) compared with placebo patients. The only exception was the ACIPHEX™ 40 mg group versus placebo at Week 2 for duodenal ulcer pain frequency ($p=0.094$). Significant differences in resolution of daytime and nighttime pain were noted in both ACIPHEX™ groups relative to placebo by the end of the first week of the study. Significant reductions in daily antacid use were also noted in both ACIPHEX™ groups compared to placebo at Weeks 2 and 4 ($p<0.001$).

An international randomized, double-blind, active-controlled trial was conducted in 205 patients comparing 20 mg ACIPHEX™ QD with 20 mg omeprazole QD. The study was designed to provide at least 80% power to exclude a difference of at least 10% between ACIPHEX™ and omeprazole, assuming four-week healing response rates of 93% for both groups. In patients with endoscopically defined duodenal ulcers treated for up to four weeks, ACIPHEX™ was comparable to omeprazole in producing healing of duodenal ulcers. The percentages of patients with endoscopic healing at two and four weeks are presented below:

[See third table on next page]

ACIPHEX™ and omeprazole were comparable in providing complete resolution of symptoms.

Pathological Hypersecretory Conditions Including Zollinger-Ellison Syndrome

Twelve patients with idiopathic gastric hypersecretion or Zollinger-Ellison syndrome have been treated successfully with ACIPHEX™ at doses from 20 to 120 mg for up to 12 months. ACIPHEX™ produced satisfactory inhibition of gastric acid secretion in all patients and complete resolution of signs and symptoms of acid-peptic disease where present. ACIPHEX™ also prevented recurrence of gastric hypersecretion and manifestations of acid-peptic disease in all patients. The high doses of ACIPHEX™ used to treat this small cohort of patients with gastric hypersecretion were not associated with drug-related adverse effects.

INDICATIONS AND USAGE

Healing of Erosive or Ulcerative Gastroesophageal Reflux Disease (GERD)

ACIPHEX™ is indicated for short-term (4 to 8 weeks) treatment in the healing and symptomatic relief of erosive or ulcerative gastroesophageal reflux disease (GERD). For those patients who have not healed after 8 weeks of treatment, an additional 8-week course of ACIPHEX™ may be considered.

Maintenance of Healing of Erosive or Ulcerative Gastroesophageal Reflux Disease (GERD)

ACIPHEX™ is indicated for maintaining healing and reduction in relapse rates of heartburn symptoms in patients with erosive or ulcerative gastroesophageal reflux disease (GERD Maintenance).

Healing of Duodenal Ulcers

ACIPHEX™ is indicated for short-term (up to four weeks) treatment in the healing and symptomatic relief of duodenal ulcers. Most patients heal within four weeks.

Treatment of Pathological Hypersecretory Conditions, Including Zollinger-Ellison Syndrome

ACIPHEX™ is indicated for the long-term treatment of pathological hypersecretory conditions, including Zollinger-Ellison syndrome.

CONTRAINDICATIONS

Rabeprazole is contraindicated in patients with known hypersensitivity to rabeprazole, substituted benzimidazoles or to any component of the formulation.

PRECAUTIONS

General

Symptomatic response to therapy with rabeprazole does not preclude the presence of gastric malignancy.

Patients with healed GERD were treated for up to 40 months with rabeprazole and monitored with serial gastric biopsies. Patients without *H. pylori* infection (221 of 326 patients) had no clinically important pathologic changes in the gastric mucosa. Patients with *H. pylori* infection at baseline (105 of 326 patients) had mild or moderate inflammation in the gastric body or mild inflammation in the gastric antrum. Patients with mild grades of infection or inflammation in the gastric body tended to change to moderate, whereas those graded moderate at baseline tended to remain stable. Patients with mild grades of infection or inflammation in the gastric antrum tended to remain stable. At baseline 8% of patients had atrophy of glands in the gastric body and 15% had atrophy in the gastric antrum. At endpoint, 15% of patients had atrophy of glands in the gastric body and 11% had atrophy in the gastric antrum. Approximately 4% of patients had intestinal metaplasia at some point during follow-up, but no consistent changes were seen.

Information for Patients

Patients should be cautioned that ACIPHEX™ delayed-release tablets should be swallowed whole. The tablets should not be chewed, crushed, or split.

Drug Interactions

Rabeprazole is metabolized by the cytochrome P450 (CYP450) drug metabolizing enzyme system. Studies in healthy subjects have shown that rabeprazole does not have clinically significant interactions with other drugs metabolized by the CYP450 system, such as warfarin and theophylline given as single oral doses, diazepam as a single intravenous dose, and phenytoin given as a single intravenous dose (with supplemental oral dosing). *In vitro* incubations employing human liver microsomes indicated that rabeprazole inhibited cyclosporine metabolism with an IC_{50} of 62 micromolar, a concentration that is over 50 times higher than the C_{max} in healthy volunteers following 14 days of dosing with 20 mg of rabeprazole. This degree of inhibition is similar to that by omeprazole at equivalent concentrations.

Rabeprazole produces sustained inhibition of gastric acid secretion. An interaction with compounds which are dependent on gastric pH for absorption may occur due to the magnitude of acid suppression observed with rabeprazole. For example, in normal subjects, co-administration of rabeprazole 20 mg QD resulted in an approximately 30% decrease in the bioavailability of ketoconazole and increases in the AUC and C_{max} for digoxin of 19% and 29%, respectively. Therefore, patients may need to be monitored when such drugs are taken concomitantly with rabeprazole. Co-administration of rabeprazole and antacids produced no clinically relevant changes in plasma rabeprazole concentrations.

Carcinogenesis, Mutagenesis, Impairment of Fertility

In a 88/104-week carcinogenicity study in CD-1 mice, rabeprazole at oral doses up to 100 mg/kg/day did not produce any increased tumor occurrence. The highest tested dose produced a systemic exposure to rabeprazole (AUC) of 1.40 μg•hr/mL which is 1.6 times the human exposure (plasma $AUC_{0-\infty}$ = 0.88 μg•hr/mL) at the recommended dose for GERD (20 mg/day). In a 104-week carcinogenicity study in Sprague-Dawley rats, males were treated with oral doses of 5, 15, 30 and 60 mg/kg/day and females with 5, 15, 30, 60 and 120 mg/kg/day. Rabeprazole produced gastric enterochromaffin-like (ECL) cell hyperplasia in male and female rats and ECL cell carcinoid tumors in female rats at all doses including the lowest tested dose. The lowest dose (5 mg/kg/day) produced a systemic exposure to rabeprazole (AUC) of about 0.1 μg•hr/mL which is about 0.1 times the human exposure at the recommended dose for GERD. In male rats, no treatment related tumors were observed at doses up to 60 mg/kg/day producing a rabeprazole plasma exposure (AUC) of about 0.2 μg•hr/mL (0.2 times the human exposure at the recommended dose for GERD).

Rabeprazole was positive in the Ames test, the Chinese hamster ovary cell (CHO/HGPRT) forward gene mutation test and the mouse lymphoma cell (L5178Y/TK±) forward gene mutation test. Its demethylated-metabolite was also positive in the Ames test. Rabeprazole was negative in the *in vitro* Chinese hamster lung cell chromosome aberration test, the *in vitro* mouse micronucleus test, and the *in vivo* and *ex vivo* rat hepatocyte unscheduled DNA synthesis (UDS) tests.

Rabeprazole at intravenous doses up to 30 mg/kg/day (plasma AUC of 8.8 μg•hr/mL, about 10 times the human exposure at the recommended dose for GERD) was found to have no effect on fertility and reproductive performance of male and female rats.

Pregnancy

Teratogenic Effects. Pregnancy Category B: Teratology studies have been performed in rats at intravenous doses up to 50 mg/kg/day (plasma AUC of 11.8 μg•hr/mL, about 13 times the human exposure at the recommended dose for GERD) and rabbits at intravenous doses up to 30 mg/kg/day (plasma AUC of 7.3 μg•hr/mL, about 8 times the human exposure at the recommended dose for GERD) and have revealed no evidence of impaired fertility or harm to the fetus due to rabeprazole. There are, however, no adequate and well-controlled studies in pregnant women. Because animal reproduction studies are not always predictive of human response, this drug should be used during pregnancy only if clearly needed.

Nursing Mothers

Following intravenous administration of ^{14}C-labeled rabeprazole to lactating rats, radioactivity in milk reached levels that were 2- to 7-fold higher than levels in the blood. It is not known if unmetabolized rabeprazole is excreted in human breast milk. Administration of rabeprazole to rats in late gestation and during lactation at doses of 400 mg/kg/day (about 195-times the human dose based on mg/m^2) resulted in decreases in body weight gain of the pups.

Since many drugs are excreted in milk, and because of the potential for adverse reactions to nursing infants from rabeprazole, a decision should be made to discontinue nursing or discontinue the drug, taking into account the importance of the drug to the mother.

Pediatric Use

The safety and effectiveness of rabeprazole in pediatric patients have not been established.

Use in Women

Duodenal ulcer and erosive esophagitis healing rates in women are similar to those in men. Adverse events and laboratory test abnormalities in women occurred at rates similar to those in men.

Continued on next page

Aciphex—Cont.

Geriatric Use
Of the total number of subjects in clinical studies of ACIPHEX™, 19% were 65 years and over, while 4% were 75 years and over. No overall differences in safety or effectiveness were observed between these subjects and younger subjects, and other reported clinical experience has not identified differences in responses between the elderly and younger patients, but greater sensitivity of some older individuals cannot be ruled out.

ADVERSE REACTIONS
Worldwide, over 2900 patients have been treated with rabeprazole in Phase II-III clinical trials involving various dosages and durations of treatment. In general, rabeprazole treatment has been well-tolerated in both short-term and ling-term trials. The adverse events rates were generally similar between the 10 and 20 mg doses.

Incidence in Controlled North American and European Clinical Trials
In an analysis of adverse events assessed as possibly or probably related to treatment appearing in greater than 1% of ACIPHEX™ patients and appearing with greater frequency than placebo in controlled North American and European trials, the incidence of headache was 2.4% (n=1552) for ACIPHEX™ versus 1.6% (n=258) for placebo.
In short and long-term studies, the following adverse events, regardless of causality, were reported in ACIPHEX™-treated patients. Rare events are those reported in ≤1/1000 patients.
Body as a Whole: asthenia, fever, allergic reaction, chills, malaise, chest pain substernal, neck rigidity, photosensitivity reaction. Rare: abdomen enlarged, face edema, hangover effect. *Cardiovascular System:* hypertension, myocardial infarct, electrocardiogram abnormal, migraine, syncope, angina pectoris, bundle branch block, palpitation, sinus bradycardia, tachycardia. Rare: bradycardia, pulmonary embolus, supraventricular tachycardia, thrombophlebitis, vasodilation, QTC prolongation and ventricular tachycardia. *Digestive System:* diarrhea, nausea, abdominal pain, vomiting, dyspepsia, flatulence, constipation, dry mouth, eructation, gastroenteritis, rectal hemorrhage, melena, anorexia, cholelithiasis, mouth ulceration, stomatitis, dysphagia, gingivitis, cholecystitis, increased appetite, abnormal stools, colitis, esophagitis, glossitis, pancreatitis, proctitis. Rare: bloody diarrhea, cholangitis, duodenitis, gastrointestinal hemorrhage, hepatic encephalopathy, hepatitis, hepatoma, liver fatty deposit, salivary gland enlargement, thirst. *Endocrine System:* hyperthyroidism. *Hemic & Lymphatic System:* anemia, ecchymosis, lymphadenopathy, hypochromic anemia. *Metabolic & Nutritional Disorders:* peripheral edema, edema, weight gain, gout, dehydration, weight loss. *Musculo-Skeletal System:* myalgia, arthritis, leg cramps, bone pain, arthrosis, bursitis. Rare: twitching. *Nervous System:* insomnia, anxiety, dizziness, depression, nervousness, somnolence, hypertonia, neuralgia, vertigo, convulsion, abnormal dreams, libido decreased, neuropathy, paresthesia, tremor. Rare: agitation, amnesia, confusion, extrapyramidal syndrome, hyperkinesia. *Respiratory System:* dyspnea, asthma, epistaxis, laryngitis, hiccup, hyperventilation. Rare: apnea, hypoventilation. *Skin and Appendages:* rash, pruritus, sweating, urticaria, alopecia. Rare: dry skin, herpes zoster, psoriasis, skin discoloration. *Special Senses:* cataract, amblyopia, glaucoma, dry eyes, abnormal vision, tinnitus, otitis media. Rare: corneal opacity, blurry vision, diplopia, deafness, eye pain, retinal degeneration, strabismus. *Urogenital System:* cystitis, urinary frequency, dysmenorrhea, dysuria, kidney calculus, metrorrhagia, polyuria. Rare: breast enlargement, hematuria, impotence, leukorrhea, menorrhagia, orchitis, urinary incontinence.
Laboratory Values: The following changes in laboratory parameters were reported as adverse events: abnormal platelets, albuminuria, creatine phosphokinase increased, erythrocytes abnormal, hypercholesteremia, hyperglycemia, hyperlipemia, hypokalemia, hyponatremia, leukocytosis, leukorrhea, liver function tests abnormal, prostatic specific antigen increase, SGPT increased, urine abnormality, WBC abnormal.
In controlled clinical studies, 3/1456 (0.2%) patients treated with rabeprazole and 2/237 (0.8%) patients treated with placebo developed treatment-emergent abnormalities (which were either new on study or present at study entry with an increase of 1.25 × baseline value) in SGOT (AST), SGPT (ALT), or both. None of the three rabeprazole patients experienced chills, fever, right upper quadrant pain, nausea or jaundice.
Post-Marketing Adverse Events: Additional adverse events reported from worldwide marketing experience with rabeprazole sodium are: sudden death, coma and hyperammonemia, jaundice, rhabdomyolysis, disorientation and delirium, bullous and other drug eruptions of the skin, interstitial pneumonia, and TSH elevations. In most instances, the relationship to rabeprazole sodium was unclear. In addition, agranulocytosis, hemolytic anemia, leukopenia, pancytopenia, and thrombocytopenia have been reported.

OVERDOSAGE
Because strategies for the management of overdose are continually evolving, it is advisable to contact a Poison Control Center to determine the latest recommendations for the management of an overdose of any drug. There has been no experience with large overdoses with rabeprazole.

Long-term Maintenance of Healing of Erosive or Ulcerative Gastroesophageal Reflux Disease (GERD Maintenance) Percent of Patients in Endoscopic Remission

	ACIPHEX™ 10 mg	ACIPHEX™ 20 mg	Placebo
Study 1	N=66	N=67	N=70
Week 4	83%*	96%*	44%
Week 13	79%*	93%*	39%
Week 26	77%*	93%*	31%
Week 39	76%*	91%*	30%
Week 52	73%*	90%*	29%
Study 2	N=93	N=93	N=99
Week 4	89%*	94%*	40%
Week 13	86%*	91%*	33%
Week 26	85%*	89%*	30%
Week 39	84%*	88%*	29%
Week 52	77%*	86%*	29%
COMBINED STUDIES	N=159	N=160	N=169
Week 4	87%*	94%*	42%
Week 13	83%*	92%*	36%
Week 26	82%*	91%*	31%
Week 39	81%*	89%*	30%
Week 52	75%*	87%*	29%

*($p<0.001$ versus placebo)

Long-term Maintenance of Healing of Erosive or Ulcerative Gastroesophageal Reflux Disease (GERD Maintenance): Percent of Patients Without Relapse in Heartburn Frequency and Daytime and Nighttime Heartburn Severity at Week 52

	ACIPHEX™ 10 mg	ACIPHEX™ 20 mg	Placebo
Heartburn Frequency			
Study 1	46/55 (84%)*	48/52 (92%)*	17/45 (38%)
Study 2	50/72 (69%)*	57/72 (79%)*	22/79 (28%)
Daytime Heartburn Severity			
Study 1	61/64 (95%)*	60/62 (97%)*	42/61 (69%)
Study 2	73/84 (87%)†	82/87 (94%)*	67/90 (74%)
Nighttime Heartburn Severity			
Study 1	57/61 (93%)*	60/61 (98%)*	37/56 (66%)
Study 2	67/80 (84%)	79/87 (91%)†	64/87 (74%)

* $p\leq0.001$ versus placebo
† $0.001<p<0.05$ versus placebo

Healing of Duodenal Ulcers Percentage of Patients Healed

Week	ACIPHEX™ 20 mg QD N=102	Omeprazole 20 mg QD N=103	95% Confidence Interval for the Treatment Difference (ACIPHEX™ - Omeprazole)
2	69%	61%	(−6%, 22%)
4	98%	93%	(−3%, 15%)

Seven reports of accidental overdosage with rabeprazole have been received. The maximum reported overdose was 80 mg. There were no clinical signs or symptoms associated with any reported overdose. Patients with Zollinger-Ellison syndrome have been treated with up to 120 mg rabeprazole QD. No specific antidote for rabeprazole is known. Rabeprazole is extensively protein bound and is not readily dialyzable. In the event of overdosage, treatment should be symptomatic and supportive.
Single oral doses of rabeprazole at 786 mg/kg and 1024 mg/kg were lethal to mice and rats, respectively. The single oral dose of 2000 mg/kg was not lethal to dogs. The major symptoms of acute toxicity were hypoactivity, labored respiration, lateral or prone position and convulsion in mice and rats and watery diarrhea, tremor, convulsion and coma in dogs.

DOSAGE AND ADMINISTRATION
Healing of Erosive or Ulcerative Gastroesophageal Reflux Disease (GERD)
The recommended adult oral dose is one ACIPHEX™ 20 mg delayed-release tablet to be taken once daily for four to eight weeks. (See INDICATIONS AND USAGE). For those patients who have not healed after 8 weeks of treatment, an additional 8-week course of ACIPHEX™ may be considered.

Maintenance of Healing of Erosive or Ulcerative Gastroesophageal Reflux Disease (GERD Maintenance)
The recommended adult oral dose is one ACIPHEX™ 20 mg delayed-release tablet to be taken once daily. (See INDICATIONS AND USAGE).

Healing of Duodenal Ulcers
The recommended adult oral dose is one ACIPHEX™ 20 mg delayed-release tablet to be taken once daily after the morning meal for a period up to four weeks. (See INDICATIONS AND USAGE). Most patients with duodenal ulcer heal within four weeks. A few patients may require additional therapy to achieve healing.

Treatment of Pathological Hypersecretory Conditions Including Zollinger-Ellison Syndrome
The dosage of ACIPHEX™ in patients with pathologic hypersecretory conditions varies with the individual patient. The recommended adult oral starting dose is 60 mg once a day. Doses should be adjusted to individual patient needs and should continue for as long as clinically indicated. Some patients may require divided doses. Doses up to 100 mg QD

and 60 mg BID have been administered. Some patients with Zollinger-Ellison syndrome have been treated continuously with ACIPHEX™ for up to one year.

No dosage adjustment is necessary in elderly patients, in patients with renal disease or in patients with mild to moderate hepatic impairment. Administration of rabeprazole to patients with mild to moderate liver impairment resulted in increased exposure and decreased elimination. Due to the lack of clinical data on rabeprazole in patients with severe hepatic impairment, caution should be exercised in those patients.

ACIPHEX™ tablets should be swallowed whole. The tablets should not be chewed, crushed, or split.

HOW SUPPLIED

ACIPHEX™ 20 mg is supplied as delayed-release light yellow enteric-coated tablets. The medication code number (E243) is imprinted on one side.

Bottles of 30 (NDC#62856-243-30)

Unit Dose Blisters Package of 100 (10 × 10) (NDC#62856-243-41)

Store at 25°C (77°F); excursions permitted to 15–30°C (59–86°F). Protect from moisture.

Rx only.

ACIPHEX™ is a trademark of Eisai Co., Ltd., Tokyo, Japan.

Manufactured by Eisai Co., Ltd.
Misato, Japan
Made in Japan
Marketed by Eisai Inc., Teaneck, NJ 07666
and
Janssen Pharmaceutica Inc., Titusville, NJ 08560-0200

Revised October 1999

Shown in Product Identification Guide, page 311

ARICEPT® ℞
(Donepezil Hydrochloride Tablets)

DESCRIPTION

ARICEPT® (donepezil hydrochloride) is a reversible inhibitor of the enzyme acetylcholinesterase, known chemically as (±)-2,3-dihydro-5,6-dimethoxy-2-[[1-(phenylmethyl)-4-piperidinyl]methyl]-1*H*-inden-1-one hydrochloride. Donepezil hydrochloride is commonly referred to in the pharmacological literature as E2020. It has an empirical formula of $C_{24}H_{29}NO_3HCl$ and a molecular weight of 415.96. Donepezil hydrochloride is a white crystalline powder and is freely soluble in chloroform, soluble in water and in glacial acetic acid, slightly soluble in ethanol and in acetonitrile and practically insoluble in ethyl acetate and in n-hexane.

ARICEPT® is available for oral administration in film-coated tablets containing 5 or 10 mg of donepezil hydrochloride. Inactive ingredients are lactose monohydrate, corn starch, microcrystalline cellulose, hydroxypropyl cellulose, and magnesium stearate. The film coating contains talc, polyethylene glycol, hydroxypropyl methylcellulose and titanium dioxide. Additionally, the 10 mg tablet contains yellow iron oxide (synthetic) as a coloring agent.

CLINICAL PHARMACOLOGY

Current theories on the pathogenesis of the cognitive signs and symptoms of Alzheimer's Disease attribute some of them to a deficiency of cholinergic neurotransmission.

Donepezil hydrochloride is postulated to exert its therapeutic effect by enhancing cholinergic function. This is accomplished by increasing the concentration of acetylcholine through reversible inhibition of its hydrolysis by acetylcholinesterase. If this proposed mechanism of action is correct, donepezil's effect may lessen as the disease process advances and fewer cholinergic neurons remain functionally intact. There is no evidence that donepezil alters the course of the underlying dementing process.

Clinical Trial Data

The effectiveness of ARICEPT® as a treatment for Alzheimer's Disease is demonstrated by the results of two randomized, double-blind, placebo-controlled clinical investigations in patients with Alzheimer's disease (diagnosed by NINCDS and DSM III-R criteria, Mini-Mental State Examination ≥ 10 and ≤ 26 and Clinical Dementia Rating of 1 or 2). The mean age of patients participating in ARICEPT® trials was 73 years with a range of 50 to 94. Approximately 62% of patients were women and 38% were men. The racial distribution was white 95%, black 3% and other races 2%.

Study Outcome Measures: In each study, the effectiveness of treatment with ARICEPT® was evaluated using a dual outcome assessment strategy.

The ability of ARICEPT® to improve cognitive performance was assessed with the cognitive subscale of the Alzheimer's Disease Assessment Scale (ADAS-cog), a multi-item instrument that has been extensively validated in longitudinal cohorts of Alzheimer's Disease patients. The ADAS-cog examines selected aspects of cognitive performance including elements of memory, orientation, attention, reasoning, language and praxis. The ADAS-cog scoring range is from 0 to 70, with higher scores indicating greater cognitive impairment. Elderly normal adults may score as low as 0 or 1, but it is not unusual for non-demented adults to score slightly higher.

The patients recruited as participants in each study had mean scores on the Alzheimer's Disease Assessment Scale (ADAS-cog) of approximately 26 units, with a range from 4 to 61. Experience gained in longitudinal studies of ambulatory patients with mild to moderate Alzheimer's Disease suggest that they gain 6 to 12 units a year on the ADAS-cog. However, lesser degrees of change are seen in patients with very mild or very advanced disease because the ADAS-cog is not uniformly sensitive to change over the course of the disease. The annualized rate of decline in the placebo patients participating in ARICEPT® trials was approximately 2 to 4 units per year.

The ability of ARICEPT® to produce an overall clinical effect was assessed using a Clinician's Interview Based Impression of Change that required the use of caregiver information, the CIBIC plus. The CIBIC plus is not a single instrument and is not a standardized instrument like the ADAS-cog. Clinical trials for investigational drugs have used a variety of CIBIC formats, each different in terms of depth and structure.

As such, results from a CIBIC plus reflect clinical experience from the trial or trials in which it was used and cannot be compared directly with the results of CIBIC plus evaluations from other clinical trials. The CIBIC plus used in ARICEPT® trials was a semi-structured instrument that was intended to examine four major areas of patient function: General, Cognitive, Behavioral and Activities of Daily Living. It represents the assessment of a skilled clinician based upon his/her observations at an interview with the patient, in combination with information supplied by a caregiver familiar with the behavior of the patient over the interval rated. The CIBIC plus is scored as a seven point categorical rating, ranging from a score of 1, indicating "markedly improved," to a score of 4, indicating "no change" to a score of 7, indicating "markedly worse." The CIBIC plus has not been systematically compared directly to assessments not using information from caregivers (CIBIC) or other global methods.

Thirty-Week Study

In a study of 30 weeks duration, 473 patients were randomized to receive single daily doses of placebo, 5 mg/day or 10 mg/day of ARICEPT®. The 30-week study was divided into a 24-week double-blind active treatment phase followed by a 6-week single-blind placebo washout period. The study was designed to compare 5 mg/day or 10 mg/day fixed doses of ARICEPT® to placebo. However, to reduce the likelihood of cholinergic effects, the 10 mg/day treatment was started following an initial 7-day treatment with 5 mg/day doses.

Effects on the ADAS-cog: Figure 1 illustrates the time course for the change from baseline in ADAS-cog scores for all three dose groups over the 30 weeks of the study. After 24 weeks of treatment, the mean differences in the ADAS-cog change scores for ARICEPT® treated patients compared to the patients on placebo were 2.8 and 3.1 units for the 5 mg/day and 10 mg/day treatments, respectively. These differences were statistically significant. While the treatment effect size may appear to be slightly greater for the 10 mg/day treatment, there was no statistically significant difference between the two active treatments.

Following 6 weeks of placebo washout, scores on the ADAS-cog for both the ARICEPT® treatment groups were indistinguishable from those patients who had received only placebo for 30 weeks. This suggests that the beneficial effects of ARICEPT® abate over 6 weeks following discontinuation of treatment and do not represent a change in the underlying disease. There was no evidence of a rebound effect 6 weeks after abrupt discontinuation of therapy.

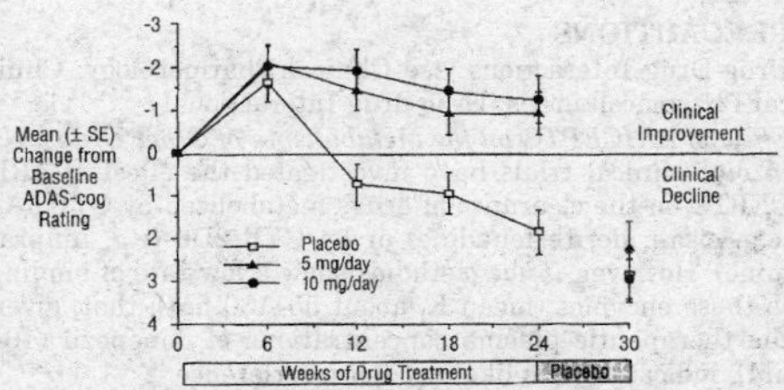

Figure 1. Time-course of the Change from Baseline in ADAS-cog Score for Patients Completing 24 Weeks of Treatment.

Figure 2 illustrates the cumulative percentages of patients from each of the three treatment groups who had attained the measure of improvement in ADAS-cog score shown on the X axis. Three change scores, (7-point and 4-point reductions from baseline or no change in score) have been identified for illustrative purposes and the percent of patients in each group achieving that result is shown in the inset table. The curves demonstrate that both patients assigned to placebo and ARICEP® have a wide range of responses, but that the active treatment groups are more likely to show the greater improvements. A curve for an effective treatment would be shifted to the left of the curve for placebo, while an ineffective or deleterious treatment would be superimposed upon or shifted to the right of the curve for placebo, respectively.

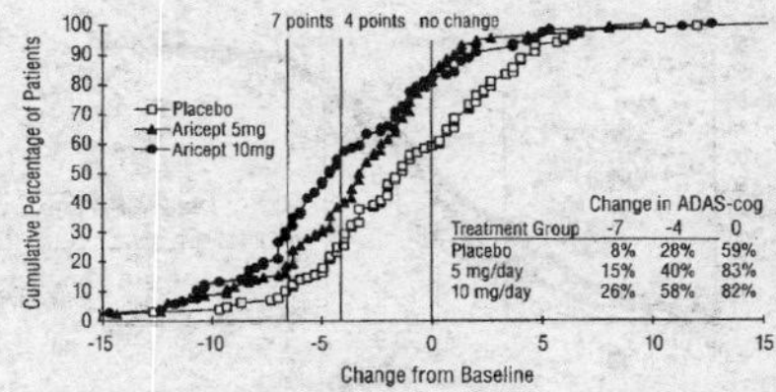

Figure 2. Cumulative Percentage of Patients Completing 24 Weeks of Double-blind Treatment with Specified Changes from Baseline ADAS-cog Scores. The Percentages of Randomized Patients who Completed the Study were: Placebo 80%, 5 mg/day 85% and 10 mg/day 68%.

Effects on the CIBIC plus: Figure 3 is a histogram of the frequency distribution of CIBIC plus scores attained by patients assigned to each of the three treatment groups who completed 24 weeks of treatment. The mean drug-placebo differences for these groups of patients were 0.35 units and 0.39 units for 5 mg/day and 10 mg/day of ARICEPT®, respectively. These differences were statistically significant. There was no statistically significant difference between the two active treatments.

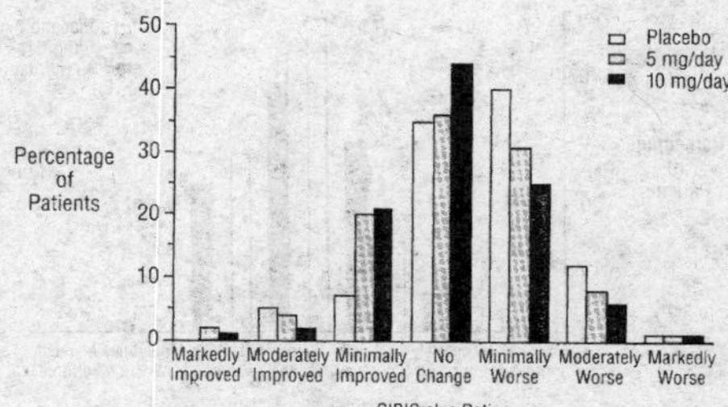

Figure 3. Frequency Distribution of CIBIC plus Scores at Week 24

Fifteen-Week Study

In a study of 15 weeks duration, patients were randomized to receive single daily doses of placebo or either 5 mg/day or 10 mg/day of ARICEPT® for 12 weeks, followed by a 3-week placebo washout period. As in the 30-week study, to avoid acute cholinergic effects, the 10 mg/day treatment followed an initial 7-day treatment with 5 mg/day doses.

Effects on the ADAS-Cog: Figure 4 illustrates the time course of the change from baseline in ADAS-cog scores for all three dose groups over the 15 weeks of the study. After 12 weeks of treatment, the differences in the mean ADAS-cog change scores for the ARICEPT® treated patients compared to the patients on placebo were 2.7 and 3.0 units each, for the 5 and 10 mg/day ARICEPT® treatment groups respectively. These differences were statistically significant. The effect size for the 10 mg/day group may appear to be slightly larger than that for 5 mg/day. However, the differences between active treatments were not statistically significant.

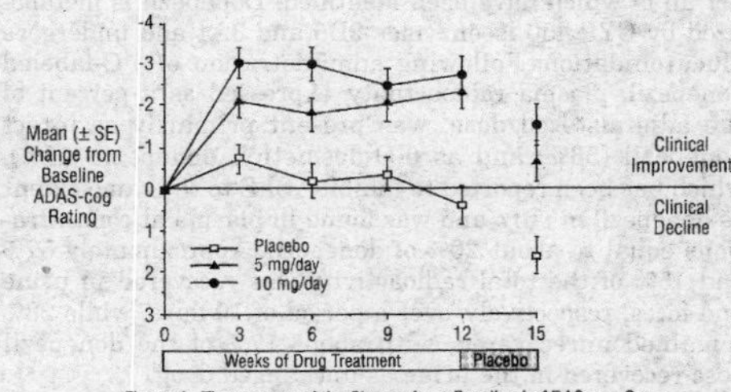

Figure 4. Time-course of the Change from Baseline in ADAS-cog Score for Patients Completing the 15-week Study.

Following 3 weeks of placebo washout, scores on the ADAS-cog for both the ARICEPT® treatment groups increased, indicating that discontinuation of ARICEPT® resulted in a loss of its treatment effect. The duration of this placebo washout period was not sufficient to characterize the rate of loss of the treatment effect, but, the 30-week study (see above) demonstrated that treatment effects associated with the use of ARICEPT® abate within 6 weeks of treatment discontinuation.

Figure 5 illustrates the cumulative percentages of patients from each of the three treatment groups who attained the measure of improvement in ADAS-cog score shown on the X axis. The same three change scores, (7-point and 4-point reductions from baseline or no change in score) as selected for the 30-week study have been used for this illustration. The percentages of patients achieving those results are shown in the inset table.

As observed in the 30-week study, the curves demonstrate that patients assigned to either placebo or to ARICEPT® have a wide range of responses, but that the ARICEPT® treated patients are more likely to show the greater improvements in cognitive performance.

[See figure 5 at top of next column]

Continued on next page

Aricept—Cont.

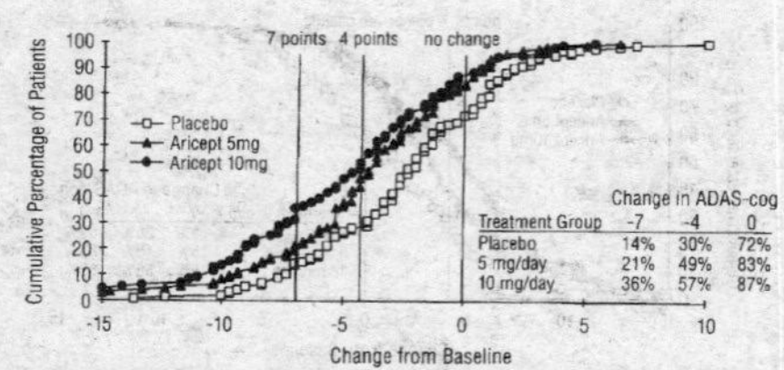

Figure 5. Cumulative Percentage of Patients with Specified Changes from Baseline ADAS-cog Scores. The Percentages of Randomized Patients Within Each Treatment Group Who Completed the Study Were: Placebo 93%, 5 mg/day 90% and 10 mg/day 82%.

Effects on the CIBIC plus: Figure 6 is a histogram of the frequency distribution of CIBIC plus scores attained by patients assigned to each of the three treatment groups who completed 12 weeks of treatment. The differences in mean scores for ARICEPT® treated patients compared to the patients on placebo at Week 12 were 0.36 and 0.38 units for the 5 mg/day and 10 mg/day treatment groups, respectively. These differences were statistically significant.

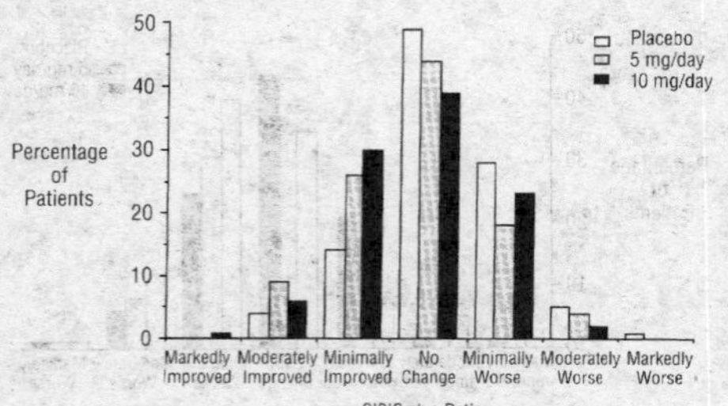

Figure 6. Frequency Distribution of CIBIC plus Scores at Week 12

In both studies, patient age, sex and race were not found to predict the clinical outcome of ARICEPT® treatment.

Clinical Pharmacokinetics

Donepezil is well absorbed with a relative oral bioavailability of 100% and reaches peak plasma concentrations in 3 to 4 hours. Pharmacokinetics are linear over a dose range of 1–10 mg given once daily. Neither food nor time of administration (morning vs. evening dose) influences the rate or extent of absorption. The elimination half life of donepezil is about 70 hours and the mean apparent plasma clearance (Cl/F) is 0.13 L/hr/kg. Following multiple dose administration, donepezil accumulates in plasma by 4–7 fold and steady state is reached within 15 days. The steady state volume of distribution is 12 L/kg. Donepezil is approximately 96% bound to human plasma proteins, mainly to albumins (about 75%) and alpha$_1$ - acid glycoprotein (about 21%) over the concentration range of 2–1000 ng/mL.

Donepezil is both excreted in the urine intact and extensively metabolized to four major metabolites, two of which are known to be active, and a number of minor metabolites, not all of which have been identified. Donepezil is metabolized by CYP 450 isoenzymes 2D6 and 3A4 and undergoes glucuronidation. Following administration of ^{14}C-labeled donepezil, plasma radioactivity, expressed as a percent of the administered dose, was present primarily as intact donepezil (53%) and as 6-O-desmethyl donepezil (11%), which has been reported to inhibit AChE to the same extent as donepezil *in vitro* and was found in plasma at concentrations equal to about 20% of donepezil. Approximately 57% and 15% of the total radioactivity was recovered in urine and feces, respectively, over a period of 10 days, while 28% remained unrecovered, with about 17% of the donepezil dose recovered in the urine as unchanged drug.

Special Populations:

Hepatic Disease: In a study of 10 patients with stable alcoholic cirrhosis, the clearance of ARICEPT® was decreased by 20% relative to 10 healthy age and sex matched subjects.

Renal Disease: In a study of 4 patients with moderate to severe renal impairment (Cl_{Cr} < 22 mL/min/1.73 m^2) the clearance of ARICEPT® did not differ from 4 age and sex matched healthy subjects.

Age: No formal pharmacokinetic study was conducted to examine age related differences in the pharmacokinetics of ARICEPT®. However, mean plasma ARICEPT® concentrations measured during therapeutic drug monitoring of elderly patients with Alzheimer's Disease are comparable to those observed in young healthy volunteers.

Gender and Race: No specific pharmacokinetic study was conducted to investigate the effects of gender and race on the disposition of ARICEPT®. However, retrospective pharmacokinetic analysis indicates that gender and race (Japanese and Caucasians) did not affect the clearance of ARICEPT®.

Drug-Drug Interactions

Drugs Highly Bound to Plasma Proteins: Drug displacement studies have been performed *in vitro* between this highly bound drug (96%) and other drugs such as furosemide, digoxin, and warfarin. ARICEPT® at concentrations of 0.3–10 µg/mL did not affect the binding of furosemide (5 µg/mL), digoxin (2 ng/mL), and warfarin (3 µg/mL) to human albumin. Similarly, the binding of ARICEPT® to human albumin was not affected by furosemide, digoxin and warfarin.

Effect of ARICEPT® on the Metabolism of Other Drugs: No *in vivo* clinical trials have investigated the effect of ARICEPT® on the clearance of drugs metabolized by CYP 3A4 (e.g. cisapride, terfenadine) or by CYP 2D6 (e.g. imipramine). However, *in vitro* studies show a low rate of binding to these enzymes (mean K_i about 50–130 µM), that, given the therapeutic plasma concentrations of donepezil (164 nM), indicates little likelihood of interference.

Whether ARICEPT® has any potential for enzyme induction is not known.

Formal pharmacokinetic studies evaluated the potential of ARICEPT® for interaction with theophylline, cimetidine, warfarin and digoxin. No significant effects on the pharmacokinetics of these drugs were observed.

Effect of Other Drugs on the Metabolism of ARICEPT®: Ketoconazole and quinidine, inhibitors of CYP450, 3A4 and 2D6, respectively, inhibit donepezil metabolism *in vitro.* Whether there is a clinical effect of these inhibitors is not known. Inducers of CYP 2D6 and CYP 3A4 (e.g., phenytoin, carbamazepine, dexamethasone, rifampin, and phenobarbital) could increase the rate of elimination of ARICEPT®. Formal pharmacokinetic studies demonstrated that the metabolism of ARICEPT® is not significantly affected by concurrent administration of digoxin or cimetidine.

INDICATIONS AND USAGE

ARICEPT® is indicated for the treatment of mild to moderate dementia of the Alzheimer's type.

CONTRAINDICATIONS

ARICEPT® is contraindicated in patients with known hypersensitivity to donepezil hydrochloride or to piperidine derivatives.

WARNINGS

Anesthesia: ARICEPT®, as a cholinesterase inhibitor, is likely to exaggerate succinylcholine-type muscle relaxation during anesthesia.

Cardiovascular Conditions: Because of their pharmacological action, cholinesterase inhibitors may have vagotonic effects on heart rate (e.g., bradycardia). The potential for this action may be particularly important to patients with "sick sinus syndrome" or other supraventricular cardiac conduction conditions. Syncopal episodes have been reported in association with the use of ARICEPT®.

Gastrointestinal Conditions: Through their primary action, cholinesterase inhibitors may be expected to increase gastric acid secretion due to increased cholinergic activity. Therefore, patients should be monitored closely for symptoms of active or occult gastrointestinal bleeding, especially those at increased risk for developing ulcers, e.g., those with a history of ulcer disease or those receiving concurrent nonsteroidal anti-inflammatory drugs (NSAIDS). Clinical studies of ARICEPT® have shown no increase, relative to placebo, in the incidence of either peptic ulcer disease or gastrointestinal bleeding.

ARICEPT®, as a predictable consequence of its pharmacological properties, has been shown to produce diarrhea, nausea and vomiting. These effects, when they occur, appear more frequently with the 10 mg/day dose than with the 5 mg/day dose. In most cases, these effects have been mild and transient, sometimes lasting one to three weeks, and have resolved during continued use of ARICEPT®.

Genitourinary: Although not observed in clinical trials of ARICEPT®, cholinomimetics may cause bladder outflow obstruction.

Neurological Conditions: Seizures: Cholinomimetics are believed to have some potential to cause generalized convulsions. However, seizure activity also may be a manifestation of Alzheimer's Disease.

Pulmonary Conditions: Because of their cholinomimetic actions, cholinesterase inhibitors should be prescribed with care to patients with a history of asthma or obstructive pulmonary disease.

PRECAUTIONS

Drug-Drug Interactions (see Clinical Pharmacology: Clinical Pharmacolkinetis: Drug-drug Interactions)

Effect of ARICEPT® on the Metabolismn of Other Drugs: No *in vivo* clinical trials have investigated the effect of ARICEPT® on the clearance of drugs metabolized by CYP 3A4 (e.g. cisapride, terfenadine) or by CYP 2D6 (e.g. imipramine). However, *in vitro* studies show a low rate of binding to these enzymes (mean K_i about 50–130 µM), that, given the therapeutic plasma concentrations of donepezil (164 nM), indicates little likelihood of interference.

Whether ARICEPT® has any potential for enzyme induction is not known.

Effect of Other Drugs on the Metabolism of ARICEPT®: Ketoconazole and quinidine, inhibitors of CYP450, 3A4 and 2D6, respectively, inhibit donepezil metabolism *in vitro.* Whether there is a clinical effect of these inhibitors is not known. Inducers of CYP 2D6 and CYP 3A4 (e.g., phenytoin, carbamazepine, dexamethasone, rifampin, and phenobarbital) could increase the rate of elimination of ARICEPT®.

Use with Anticholinergics: Because of their mechanism of action, cholinesterase inhibitors have the potential to interfere with the activity of anticholinergic medications.

Use with Cholinomimetics and Other Cholinesterase Inhibitors: A synergistic effect may be expected when cholinesterase inhibitors are given concurrently with succinylcholine, similar neuromuscular blocking agents or cholinergic agonists such as bethanechol.

Carcinogenesis, Mutagenesis, Impairment of Fertility

Carcinogenicity studies of donepezil have not been completed.

Donepezil was not mutagenic in the Ames reverse mutation assay in bacteria. In the chromosome aberration test in cultures of Chinese hamster lung (CHL) cells, some clastogenic effects were observed. Donepezil was not clastogenic in the *in vivo* mouse micronucleus test.

Donepezil had no effect on fertility in rats at doses up to 10 mg/kg/day (approximately 8 times the maximum recommended human dose on a mg/m^2 basis).

Pregnancy

Pregnancy Category C: Teratology studies conducted in pregnant rats at doses up to 16 mg/kg/day (approximately 13 times the maximum recommended human dose on a mg/m^2 basis) and in pregnant rabbits at doses up to 10 mg/kg/day (approximately 16 times the maximum recommended human dose on a mg/m^2 basis) did not disclose any evidence for a teratogenic potential of donepezil. However, in a study in which pregnant rats were given up to 10 mg/kg/day (approximately 8 times the maximum recommended human dose on a ng/m^2 basis) from day 17 of gestation through day 20 postpartum, there was a slight increase in still births and a slight decrease in pup survival through day 4 postpartum at this dose; the next lower dose tested was 3 mg/kg/day. There are no adequate or well-controlled studies in pregnant women. ARICEPT® should be used during pregnancy only if the potential benefit justifies the potential risk to the fetus.

Nursing Mothers

It is not known whether donepezil is excreted in human breast milk. ARICEPT® has no indication for use in nursing mothers.

Pediatric Use

There are no adequate and well-controlled trials to document the safety and efficacy of ARICEPT® in any illness occurring in children.

ADVERSE REACTIONS

Adverse Events Leading to Discontinuation

The rates of discontinuation from controlled clinical trials of ARICEPT® due to adverse events for the ARICEPT® 5 mg/day treatment groups were comparable to those of placebo-treatment groups at approximately 5%. The rate of discontinuation of patients who received 7-day escalations from 5 mg/day to 10 mg/day, was higher at 13%.

The most common adverse events leading to discontinuation, defined as those occurring in at least 2% of patients and at twice the incidence seen in placebo patients, are shown in Table 1.

Table 1. Most Frequent Adverse Events Leading to Withdrawal from Controlled Clinical Trials by Dose Group

Dose Group	Placebo	5 mg/day ARICEPT®	10 mg/day ARICEPT®
Patients Randomized	355	350	315
Event/% Discontinuing			
Nausea	1%	1%	3%
Diarrhea	0%	<1%	3%
Vomiting	<1%	<1%	2%

Most Frequent Adverse Clinical Events Seen in Association with the Use of ARICEPT®

The most common adverse events, defined as those occurring at a frequency of at least 5% in patients receiving 10 mg/day and twice the placebo rate, are largely predicted by ARICEPT®'s cholinomimetic effects. These include nausea, diarrhea, insomnia, vomiting, muscle cramp, fatigue and anorexia. These adverse events were often of mild intensity and transient, resolving during continued ARICEPT® treatment without the need for dose modification.

There is evidence to suggest that the frequency of these common adverse events may be affected by the rate of titration. An open-label study was conducted with 269 patients who received placebo in the 15 and 30–week studies. These patients were titrated to a dose of 10 mg/day over a 6-week period. The rates of common adverse events were lower than those seen in patients titrated to 10 mg/day over one week in the controlled clinical trials and were comparable to those seen in patients on 5 mg/day.

See Table 2 for a comparison of the most common adverse events following one and six week titration regimens.

Table 2. Comparison of rates of adverse events in patients titrated to 10 mg/day over 1 and 6 weeks

	No titration		One week titration	Six week titration
Adverse Event	Placebo (n=315)	5 mg/day (n=311)	10 mg/day (n=315)	5 mg/day (n=269)
Nausea	6%	5%	19%	6%
Diarrhea	5%	8%	15%	9%

Insomnia	6%	6%	14%	6%
Fatigue	3%	4%	8%	3%
Vomiting	3%	3%	8%	5%
Muscle cramps	2%	6%	8%	3%
Anorexia	2%	3%	7%	3%

Adverse Events Reported in Controlled Trials
The events cited reflect experience gained under closely monitored conditions of clinical trials in a highly selected patient population. In actual clinical practice or in other clinical trials, these frequency estimates may not apply, as the conditions of use, reporting behavior, and the kinds of patients treated may differ. Table 3 lists treatment emergent signs and symptoms that were reported in at least 2% of patients in placebo-controlled trials who received ARICEPT® and for which the rate of occurrence was greater for ARICEPT® assigned than placebo assigned patients. In general, adverse events occurred more frequently in female patients and with advancing age.

Table 3. Adverse Events Reported in Controlled Clinical Trials in at Least 2% of Patients Receiving ARICEPT® and at a Higher Frequency than Placebo-treated Patients

Body System/Adverse Event	Placebo (n=355)	ARICEPT® (n=747)
Percent of Patients with any Adverse Event	72	74
Body as a Whole		
Headache	9	10
Pain, various locations	8	9
Accident	6	7
Fatigue	3	5
Cardiovascular System		
Syncope	1	2
Digestive System		
Nausea	6	11
Diarrhea	5	10
Vomiting	3	5
Anorexia	2	4
Hemic and Lymphatic System		
Ecchymosis	3	4
Metabolic and Nutritional Systems		
Weight Decrease	1	3
Musculoskeletal System		
Muscle Cramps	2	6
Arthritis	1	2
Nervous System		
Insomnia	6	9
Dizziness	6	8
Depression	<1	3
Abnormal Dreams	0	3
Somnolence	<1	2
Urogenital System		
Frequent Urination	1	2

Other Adverse Events Observed During Clinical Trials
ARICEPT® has been administered to over 1700 individuals during clinical trials worldwide. Approximately 1200 of these patients have been treated for at least 3 months and more than 100 patients have been treated for at least 6 months. Controlled and uncontrolled trials in the United States included approximately 900 patients. In regards to the highest dose of 10 mg/day, this population includes 650 patients treated for 3 months, 475 patients treated for 6 months and 116 patients treated for over 1 year. The range of patient exposure is from 1 to 1214 days.
Treatment emergent signs and symptoms that occurred during 3 controlled clinical trials and two open-label trials in the United States were recorded as adverse events by the clinical investigators using terminology of their own choosing. To provide an overall estimate of the proportion of individuals having similar types of events, the events were grouped into a smaller nuber of standardized categories using a modified COSTART dictionary and event frequencies were calculated across all studies. These categories are used in the listing below. The frequencies represent the proportion of 900 patients from these trials who experienced that event while receiving ARICEPT®. All adverse events occurring at least twice are included, except for those already listed in Tables 2 or 3, COSTART terms too general to be informative, or events less likely to be drug caused. Events are classified by body system and listed using the following definitions: *frequent adverse events*—those occurring in at least 1/100 patients; *infrequent adverse events*—those occurring in 1/100 to 1/1000 patients. These adverse events are not necessarily related to ARICEPT® treatment and in most cases were observed at a similar frequency in placebo-treated patients in the controlled studies. No important additional adverse events were seen in studies conducted outside the United States.
Body as a Whole: *Frequent:* influenza, chest pain, toothache; *Infrequent:* fever, edema face, periorbital edema, hernia hiatal, abscess, cellulitis, chills, generalized coldness, head fullness, listlessness.
Cardiovascular System: *Frequent:* hypertension, vasodilation, atrial fibrillation, hot flashes, hypotension; *Infrequent:* angina pectoris, postural hypotension, myocardial infarction, AV block (first degree), congestive heart failure, arteritis, bradycardia, peripheral vascular disease, supraventricular tachycardia, deep vein thrombosis.
Digestive System: *Frequent:* fecal incontinence, gastrointestinal bleeding, bloating, epigastric pain; *Infrequent:* eructation, gingivitis, increased appetite, flatulence, periodontal abscess, cholelithiasis, diverticulitis, drooling, dry mouth, fever sore, gastritis, irritable colon, tongue edema, epigastric distress, gastroenteritis, increased transaminases, hemorrhoids, ileus, increased thirst, jaundice, melena, polydipsia, duodenal ulcer, stomach ulcer.
Endocrine System: *Infrequent:* diabetes mellitus, goiter.
Hemic and Lymphatic System: *Infrequent:* anemia, thrombocythemia, thrombocytopenia, eosinophilia, erythrocytopenia.
Metabolic and Nutritional Disorders: *Frequent:* dehydration; *Infrequent:* gout, hypokalemia, increased creatine kinase, hyperglycemia, weight increase, increased lactate dehydrogenase.
Musculoskeletal System: *Frequent:* bone fracture; *Infrequent:* muscle weakness, muscle fasciculation.
Nervous System: *Frequent:* delusions, tremor, irritability, paresthesia, aggression, vertigo, ataxia, increased libido, restlessness, abnormal crying, nervousness, aphasia; *Infrequent:* cerebrovascular accident, intracranial hemorrhage, transient ischemic attack, emotional lability, neuralgia, coldness (localized), muscle spasm, dysphoria, gait abnormality, hypertonia, hypokinesia, neurodermatitis, numbness (localized), paranoia, dysarthria, dysphasia, hostility, decreased libido, melancholia, emotional withdrawal, nystagmus, pacing.
Respiratory System: *Frequent:* dyspnea, sore throat, bronchitis; *Infrequent:* epistaxis, post nasal drip, pneumonia, hyperventilation, pulmonary congestion, wheezing hypoxia, pharyngitis, pleurisy, pulmonary collapse, sleep apnea, snoring.
Skin and Appendages: *Frequent:* pruritus, diaphoresis, urticaria; *Infrequent:* dermatitis, erythema, skin discoloration, hyperkeratosis, alopecia, fungal dermatitis, herpes zoster, hirsutism, skin striae, night sweats, skin ulcer.
Special Senses: *Frequent:* cataract, eye irritation, vision blurred; *Infrequent:* dry eyes, glaucoma, earache, tinnitus, blepharitis, decreased hearing, retinal hemorrhage, otitis externa, otitis media, bad taste, conjunctival hemorrhage, ear buzzing, motion sickness, spots before eyes.
Urogenital System: *Frequent:* urinary incontinence, nocturia; *Infrequent:* dysuria, hematuria, urinary urgency, metrorrhagia, cystitis, enuresis, prostate hypertrophy, pyelonephritis, inability to empty bladder, breast fibroadenosis, fibrocystic breast, mastitis, pyuria, renal failure, vaginitis.
Postintroduction Reports
Voluntary reports of adverse events temporally associated with ARICEPT® that have been received since market introduction that are not listed above, and that there is inadequate data to determine the causal relationship with the drug include the following: abdominal pain, agitation, cholecystitis, confusion, convulsions, hallucinations, heart block (all types), hemolytic anemia, hepatitis, hyponatremia, pancreatitis, and rash.

OVERDOSAGE

Because strategies for the management of overdose are continually evolving, it is advisable to contact a Poison Control Center to determine the latest recommendations for the management of an overdose of any drug.
As in any case of overdose, general supportive measures should be utilized. Overdosage with cholinesterase inhibitors can result in cholinergic crisis characterized by severe nausea, vomiting, salivation, sweating, bradycardia, hypotension, respiratory depression, collapse and convulsions. Increasing muscle weakness is a possibility and may result in death if respiratory muscles are involved. Tertiary anticholinergics such as atropine may be used as an antidote for ARICEPT® overdosage. Intravenous atropine sulfate titrated to effect is recommended: an initial dose of 1.0 to 2.0 mg IV with subsequent doses based upon clinical response. Atypical responses in blood pressure and heart rate have been reported with other cholinomimetics when co-administered with quaternary anticholinergics such as glycopyrrolate. It is not known whether ARICEPT® and/or its metabolites can be removed by dialysis (hemodialysis, peritoneal dialysis, or hemofiltration).
Dose-related signs of toxicity in animals included reduced spontaneous movement, prone position, staggering gait, lacrimation, clonic convulsions, depressed respiration, salivation, miosis, tremors, fasciculation and lower body surface temperature.

DOSAGE AND ADMINISTRATION

The dosages of ARICEPT® shown to be effective in controlled clinical trials are 5 mg and 10 mg administered once per day.
The higher dose of 10 mg did not provide a statistically significantly greater clinical benefit than 5 mg. There is a suggestion, however, based upon order of group mean scores and dose trend analyses of data from these clinical trials, that a daily dose of 10 mg of ARICEPT® might provide additional benefit for some patients. Accordingly, whether or not to employ a dose of 10 mg is a matter of prescriber and patient preference.
Evidence from the controlled trials indicates that the 10 mg dose, with a one week titration, is likely to be associated with a higher incidence of cholinergic adverse events than the 5 mg dose. In open label trials using a 6 week titration, the frequency of these same adverse events was similar between the 5 mg and 10 mg dose groups. Therefore, because steady state is not achieved for 15 days and because the incidence of untoward effects may be influenced by the rate of dose escalation, treatment with a dose of 10 mg should not be contemplated until patients have been on a daily dose of 5 mg for 4 to 6 weeks.
ARICEPT® should be taken in the evening, just prior to retiring. ARICEPT® can be taken with or without food.

HOW SUPPLIED

ARICEPT® is supplied as film-coated, round tablets containing either 5 mg or 10 mg of donepezil hydrochloride.
The 5 mg tablets are white. The strength, in mg (5), is debossed on one side and ARICEPT is debossed on the other side.
The 10 mg tablets are yellow. The strength, in mg (10), is debossed on one side and ARICEPT is debossed on the other side.

5 mg (White)	Bottles of 30 (NDC# 62856-245-30)
	Bottles of 90 (NDC# 62856-245-90)
	Unit Dose Blister Package 100 (10x10) (NDC# 62856-245-41)
10 mg (Yellow)	Bottles of 30 (NDC# 62856-246-30)
	Bottles of 90 (NDC# 62856-246-90)
	Unit Dose Blister Package 100 (10x10) (NDC# 62856-246-41)

Storage: Store at controlled room temperature, 15°C to 30°C (59°F to 86°F).

Rx only

ARICEPT® is a registered trademark of Eisai Co., Ltd, Tokyo, Japan
Manufactured and Marketed by
Eisai Inc., Teaneck, NJ 07666
Distributed/Marketed by
Roerig Division of Pfizer Inc., New York, NY 10017

Printed in U.S.A.
200142 Revised February 2000

Shown in Product Identification Guide, page 312

Available to physicians through Eisai Medical Sales Specialists and Representatives, free of charge.

Learning About Alzheimer's Disease Brochure
Managing Alzheimers Disease Brochure
(both are disease specific brochures)
Know your Medicine Brochure
(for patients on Aricept)
26 week patient diary
(also for patients on Aricept)

Elan Pharma

800 GATEWAY BOULEVARD
SOUTH SAN FRANCISCO, CA 94080

For Medical Information Contact:
(888) NEURO-05
(888) 638-7605
To Report Adverse Events Contact:
(877) ELAN GSS
(877) 352–6477

The products below are distributed by Elan Pharma, a business unit of Elan Pharmaceuticals, Inc.

DIASTAT® Rectal Delivery System ℂⅣ ℞

[*dī 'ă-stat*]
(diazepam rectal gel)
Rx only

DESCRIPTION

Diastat* rectal delivery system is a non-sterile diazepam gel provided in a prefilled, unit-dose, rectal delivery system. Diastat contains 5 mg/mL diazepam, propylene glycol, ethyl alcohol (10%), hydroxypropyl methylcellulose, sodium benzoate, benzyl alcohol (1.5%), benzoic acid and water. Diastat is clear to slightly yellow and has a pH between 6.5–7.2.

Diazepam, the active ingredient of Diastat, is a benzodiazepine anticonvulsant with the chemical name 7-chloro-1,3-dihydro-1-methyl-5-phenyl-2H-1,4-benzodiazepin-2-one. The structural formula is as follows:

* Registered trademark of Elan Pharmaceuticals, Inc.

CLINICAL PHARMACOLOGY

Mechanism of Action

Although the precise mechanism by which diazepam exerts its antiseizure effects is unknown, animal and *in vitro* studies suggest that diazepam acts to suppress seizures through an interaction with γ-aminobutyric acid (GABA) receptors of the A-type ($GABA_A$). GABA, the major inhibitory neurotransmitter in the central nervous system, acts at this receptor to open the membrane channel allowing chloride ions to flow into neurons. Entry of chloride ions causes an inhibitory potential that reduces the ability of neurons to depolarize to the threshold potential necessary to produce action potentials. Excessive depolarization of neurons is implicated in the generation and spread of seizures. It is believed that diazepam enhances the actions of GABA by causing GABA to bind more tightly to the $GABA_A$ receptor.

Pharmacokinetics

Pharmacokinetic information of diazepam following rectal administration was obtained from studies conducted in healthy adult subjects. No pharmacokinetic studies were conducted in pediatric patients. Therefore, information from the literature is used to define pharmacokinetic labeling in the pediatric population.

Diastat is well absorbed following rectal administration, reaching peak plasma concentrations in 1.5 hours. The absolute bioavailability of Diastat relative to Valium® injectable is 90%. The volume of distribution of Diastat is calculated to be approximately 1 L/kg. The mean elimination half-life of diazepam and desmethyldiazepam following administration of a 15 mg dose of Diastat was found to be about 46 hours (CV=43%) and 71 hours (CV=37%), respectively. Both diazepam and its major active metabolite desmethyldiazepam bind extensively to plasma proteins (95–98%).

[See figure 1 above]

Metabolism and Elimination: It has been reported in the literature that diazepam is extensively metabolized to one major active metabolite (desmethyldiazepam) and two minor active metabolites, 3-hydroxydiazepam (temazepam) and 3-hydroxy-N-diazepam (oxazepam) in plasma. At therapeutic doses, desmethyldiazepam is found in plasma at concentrations equivalent to those of diazepam while oxazepam and temazepam are not usually detectable. The metabolism of diazepam is primarily hepatic and involves demethylation (involving primarily CYP2C19 and CYP3A4) and 3-hydroxylation (involving primarily CYP3A4), followed by glucuronidation. The marked inter-individual variability in the clearance of diazepam reported in the literature is probably attributable to variability of CYP2C19 (which is known to exhibit genetic polymorphism; about 3–5% of Caucasians have little or no activity and are "poor metabolizers") and CYP3A4. No inhibition was demonstrated in the presence of inhibitors selective for CYP2A6, CYP2C9, CYP2D6, CYP2E1, or CYP1A2, indicating that these enzymes are not significantly involved in metabolism of diazepam.

Special Populations

Hepatic Impairment: No pharmacokinetic studies were conducted with Diastat in hepatically impaired subjects. Literature review indicates that following administration of 0.1 to 0.15 mg/kg of diazepam intravenously, the half-life of diazepam was prolonged by two to five-fold in subjects with alcoholic cirrhosis (n=24) compared to age-matched control subjects (n=37) with a corresponding decrease in clearance by half: however, the exact degree of hepatic impairment in these subjects was not characterized in this literature (see PRECAUTIONS section).

Renal Impairment: The pharmacokinetics of diazepam have not been studied in renally impaired subjects (see PRECAUTIONS section).

Pediatrics: No pharmacokinetic studies were conducted with Diastat in the pediatric population. However, literature review indicates that following IV administration (0.33 mg/kg), diazepam has a longer half-life in neonates (birth up to one month; approximately 50–95 hours) and infants (one month up to two years; about 40–50 hours), whereas it has a shorter half-life in children (two to 12 years; approximately 15–21 hours) and adolescents (12 to 16 years; about 18–20 years) (see PRECAUTIONS section).

Elderly: A study of single dose IV administration of diazepam (0.1 mg/kg) indicates that the elimination half-life of diazepam increases linearly with age, ranging from about 15 hours at 18 years (healthy young adults) to about 100 hours at 95 years (healthy elderly) with a corresponding decrease in clearance of free diazepam (see PRECAUTIONS and DOSAGE AND ADMINISTRATION sections).

Effect of Gender, Race, and Cigarette Smoking: No targeted pharmacokinetic studies have been conducted to evaluate the effect of gender, race, and cigarette smoking on the pharmacokinetics of diazepam. However, covariate analysis of a population of treated patients following administration of Diastat indicated that neither gender nor cigarette smoking had any effect on the pharmacokinetics of diazepam.

Clinical Studies

The effectiveness of Diastat has been established in two adequate and well-controlled clinical studies in children and adults exhibiting the seizure pattern described below under INDICATIONS.

A randomized, double-blind study compared sequential doses of Diastat and placebo in 91 patients (47 children, 44 adults) exhibiting the appropriate seizure profile. The first dose was given at the onset of an identified episode. Children were dosed again four hours after the first dose and were observed for a total of 12 hours. Adults were dosed at four and 12 hours after the first dose and were observed for a total of 24 hours. Primary outcomes for this study were seizure frequency during the period of observation and a global assessment that took into account the severity and nature of the seizures as well as their frequency.

The median seizure frequency for the Diastat treated group was zero seizures per hour, compared to a median seizure frequency of 0.3 seizures per hour for the placebo group, a difference that was statistically significant ($p < 0.0001$). All three categories of the global assessment (seizure frequency, seizure severity, and "overall") were also found to be statistically significant in favor of Diastat ($p < 0.0001$). The following histogram displays the results for the "overall" category of the global assessment.

[See figure 2 above]

Patients treated with Diastat experienced prolonged time-to-next-seizure compared to placebo (p = 0.0002) as shown in the following graph.

[See figure 3 above]

FIGURE 1: Plasma Concentrations of Diazepam and Dimethyldiazepam Following Diastat or IV Diazepam

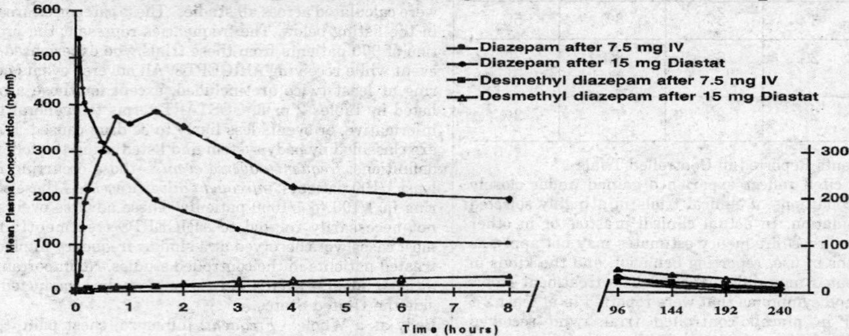

FIGURE 2: Caregiver Overall Global Assessment of the Efficacy of Diastat

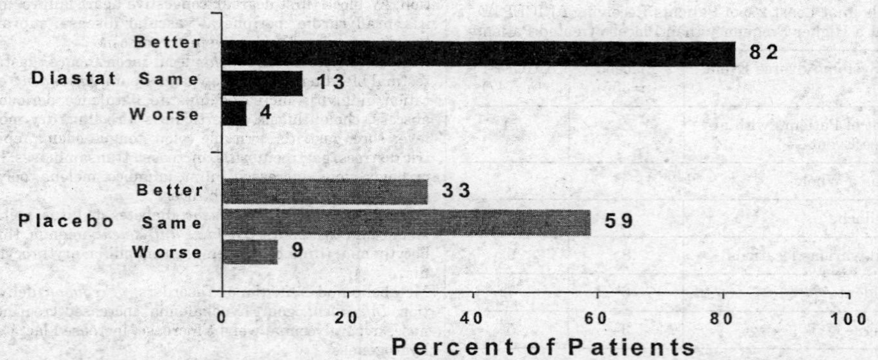

FIGURE 3: Kaplan-Meier Survival Analysis of Time-to-Next-Seizure - First Study

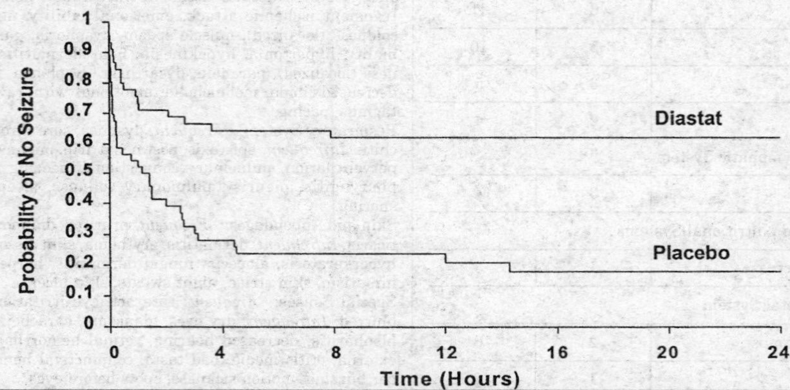

In addition, 62% of patients treated with Diastat were seizure-free during the observation period compared to 20% of placebo patients.
Analysis of response by gender and age revealed no substantial differences between treatment in either of these subgroups. Analysis of response by race was considered unreliable, due to the small percentage of non-Caucasions.
A second double-blind study compared single doses of Diastat and placebo in 114 patients (53 children, 61 adults). The dose was given at the onset of the identified episode and patients were observed for a total of 12 hours. The primary outcome in this study was seizure frequency. The median seizure frequency for the Diastat-treated group was zero seizures per 12 hours, compared to a median seizure frequency of 2.0 seizures per 12 hours for the placebo group, a difference that was statistically significant ($p < 0.03$). Patients treated with Diastat experienced prolonged time-to-next-seizure compared to placebo ($p = 0.0072$) as shown in the following graph.
[See figure 4 above]
In addition, 55% of patients treated with Diastat were seizure-free during the observation period compared to 34% of patients receiving placebo. Overall, caregivers judged Diastat to be more effective than placebo (p=0.018), based on a 10 centimeter visual analog scale. In addition, investigators also evaluated the effectiveness of Diastat and judged Diastat to be more effective than placebo ($p < 0.001$).
An analysis of response by gender revealed a statistically significant difference between treatments in females but not in males in this study, and the difference between the 2 genders in response to the treatments reached borderline statistical significance. Analysis of response by race was considered unreliable, due to the small percentage of non-Caucasions.

FIGURE 4: Kaplan-Meier Survival Analysis of Time-to-Next-Seizure - Second Study

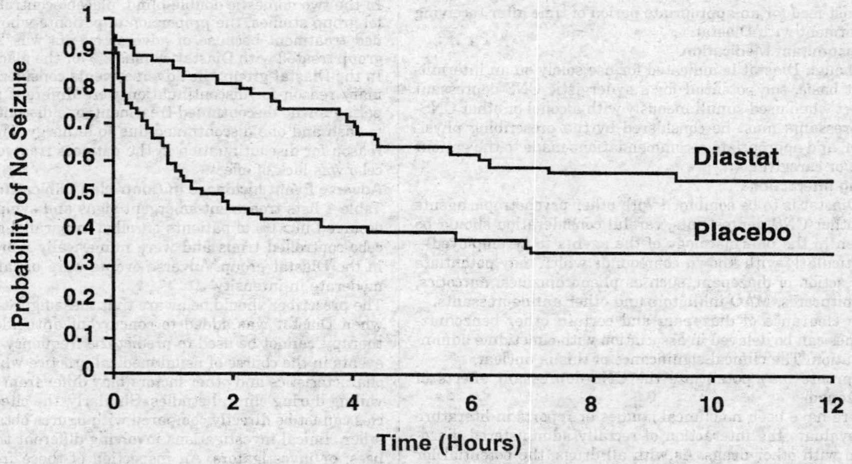

INDICATIONS AND USAGE
Diastat is a gel formulation of diazepam intended for rectal administration in the management of selected, refractory, patients with epilepsy, on stable regimens of AEDs, who require intermittent use of diazepam to control bouts of increased seizure activity.
Evidence to support the use of Diastat was adduced in two controlled trials (see CLINICAL PHARMACOLOGY, CLINICAL STUDIES subsection) that enrolled patients with partial onset or generalized convulsive seizures who were identified jointly by their caregivers and physicians as suffering intermittent and periodic episodes of markedly increased seizure activity, sometimes heralded by non-convulsive symptoms, that for the individual patient were characteristic and were deemed by the prescriber to be of a kind for which a benzodiazepine would ordinarily be administered acutely. Although these clusters or bouts of seizures differed among patients, for any individual patient the clusters of seizure activity were not only stereotypic but were judged by those conducting and participating in these studies to be distinguishable from other seizures suffered by that patient. The conclusion that a patient experienced such unique episodes of seizure activity was based on historical information.

CONTRAINDICATIONS
Diastat is contraindicated in patients with a known hypersensitivity to diazepam. Diastat may be used in patients with open angle glaucoma who are receiving appropriate therapy but is contraindicated in acute narrow angle glaucoma.

WARNINGS
General
Diastat should only be administered by caregivers who in the opinion of the prescribing physician 1) are able to distinguish the distinct cluster of seizures (and/or the events presumed to herald their onset) from the patient's ordinary seizure activity, 2) have been instructed and judged to be competent to administer the treatment rectally, 3) understand explicitly which seizure manifestations may or may not be treated with Diastat, and 4) are able to monitor the clinical response and recognize when that response is such that immediate professional medical evaluation is required.
CNS Depression
Because Diastat produces CNS depression, patients receiving this drug who are otherwise capable and qualified to do so should be cautioned against engaging in hazardous occupations requiring mental alertness, such as operating machinery, driving a motor vehicle, or riding a bicycle until they have completely returned to their level of baseline functioning.
Although Diastat is indicated for use solely on an intermittent basis, the potential for a synergistic CNS-depressant effect when used simultaneously with alcohol or other CNS depressants must be considered by the prescribing physician, and appropriate recommendations made to the patient and/or caregiver.
Prolonged CNS depression has been observed in neonates treated with diazepam. Therefore, Diastat is not recommended for use in children under six months of age.
Pregnancy Risks
No clinical studies have been conducted with Diastat in pregnant women. Data from several sources raise concerns about the use of diazepam during pregnancy.
Animal Findings: Diazepam has been shown to be teratogenic in mice and hamsters when given orally at single doses of 100 mg/kg or greater (approximately eight times the maximum recommended human dose [MRHD=1 mg/kg/day] or greater on a mg/m^2 basis). Cleft palate and exencephaly are the most common and consistently reported malformations produced in these species by administration of high, maternally-toxic doses of diazepam during organogenesis. Rodent studies have indicated that prenatal exposure to diazepam doses similar to those used clinically can produce long-term changes in cellular immune responses, brain neurochemistry, and behavior.
General Concerns and Considerations About Anticonvulsants: Reports suggest an association between the use of anticonvulsant drugs by women with epilepsy and an elevated incidence of birth defects in children born to these women. Data are more extensive with respect to phenytoin and phenobarbital, but a smaller number of systematic or anecdotal reports suggest a possible similar association with the use of all known anticonvulsant drugs.
The reports suggesting an elevated incidence of birth defects in children of drug-treated epileptic women cannot be regarded as adequate to prove a definite cause and effect relationship. There are intrinsic methodologic problems in obtaining adequate data on drug teratogenicity in humans; the possibility also exists that other factors, e.g., genetic factors or the epileptic condition itself, may be more important than drug therapy in leading to birth defects. The great majority of mothers on anticonvulsant medication deliver normal infants. It is important to note that anticonvulsant drugs should not be discontinued in patients in whom the drug is administered to prevent seizures because of the strong possibility of precipitating *status epilepticus* with attendant hypoxia and threat to life. In individual cases where the severity and frequency of the seizure disorder are such that the removal of medication does not pose a serious threat to the patient, discontinuation of the drug may be considered prior to and during pregnancy, although it cannot be said with any confidence that even mild seizures do not pose some hazards to the developing embryo or fetus.
General Concerns About Benzodiazepines: An increased risk of congenital malformations associated with the use of benzodiazepine drugs has been suggested in several studies.
There may also be non-teratogenic risks associated with the use of benzodiazepines during pregnancy. There have been reports of neonatal flaccidity, respiratory and feeding difficulties, and hypothermia in children born to mothers who have been receiving benzodiazepines late in pregnancy. In addition, children born to mothers receiving benzodiazepines on a regular basis late in pregnancy may be at some risk of experiencing withdrawal symptoms during the postnatal period.
Advice Regarding the Use of Diastat in Women of Childbearing Potential: In general, the use of Diastat in women of childbearing potential, and more specifically during known pregnancy, should be considered only when the clinical situation warrants the risk to the fetus.
The specific considerations addressed above regarding the use of anticonvulsants in epileptic women of childbearing potential should be weighed in treating or counseling these women.
Because of experience with other members of the benzodiazepine class, Diastat is assumed to be capable of causing an increased risk of congenital abnormalities when administered to a pregnant woman during the first trimester. The possibility that a woman of childbearing potential may be pregnant at the time of institution of therapy should be considered. If this drug is used during pregnancy, or if the patient becomes pregnant while taking this drug, the patient should be apprised of the potential hazard to the fetus. Patients should also be advised that if they become pregnant during therapy or intend to become pregnant they should communicate with their physician about the desirability of discontinuing the drug.
Withdrawal Symptoms
Withdrawal symptoms of the barbiturate type have occurred after the discontinuation regular use of benzodiazepines (see DRUG ABUSE AND DEPENDENCE section).
Chronic Use
Diastat is not recommended for chronic, daily use as an anticonvulsant because of the potential for development of tolerance to diazepam. Chronic daily use of diazepam may increase the frequency and/or severity of tonic clonic seizures, requiring an increase in the dosage of standard anticonvulsant medication. In such cases, abrupt withdrawal of chronic diazepam may also be associated with a temporary increase in the frequency and/or severity of seizures.
Use in Patients with Petit Mal Status
Tonic *status epilepticus* has been precipitated in patients treated with IV diazepam for petit mal status or petit mal variant status.

PRECAUTIONS
Caution in Renally Impaired Patients
Metabolites of Diastat are excreted by the kidneys; to avoid their excess accumulation, caution should be exercised in the administration of the drug to patients with impaired renal function.
Caution in Hepatically Impaired Patients
Concomitant liver disease is known to decrease the clearance of diazepam (see CLINICAL PHARMACOLOGY, Special Populations, Hepatic Impairment). Therefore, Diastat should be used with caution in patients with liver disease.
Use in Pediatrics
The controlled trials demonstrating the effectiveness of Diastat included children two years of age and older. Clinical studies have not been conducted to establish the efficacy and safety of Diastat in children under two years of age.
Use in Patients with Compromised Respiratory Function
Diastat should be used with caution in patients with compromised respiratory function related to a concurrent disease process (e.g., asthma, pneumonia) or neurologic damage.
Use in Elderly
In elderly patients Diastat should be used with caution due to an increase in half-life with a corresponding decrease in the clearance of free diazepam. It is also recommended that the dosage be decreased to reduce the likelihood of ataxia or oversedation.
Information to be Communicated by the Prescriber to the Caregiver
Prescribers are strongly advised to take all reasonable steps to ensure that caregivers fully understand their role and obligations vis a vis the administration of Diastat to individuals in their care. Prescribers should routinely discuss the steps in the Patient/Caregiver Package Insert (see Patient/Caregiver Insert printed at the end of the product labeling and also included in the product carton). The successful and safe use of Diastat depends in large measure on the competence and performance of the caregiver.
Prescribers should advise caregivers that they expect to be informed immediately if a patient develops any new findings which are not typical of the patient's characteristic seizure episode.
Interference With Cognitive and Motor Performance: Because benzodiazepines have the potential to impair judgment, thinking, or motor skills, patients should be cautioned about operating hazardous machinery, including automobiles, until they are reasonably certain that Diastat therapy does not affect them adversely.
Pregnancy: Patients should be advised to notify their physician if they become pregnant or intend to become pregnant during therapy with Diastat (see WARNINGS section).

Continued on next page

Diastat—Cont.

Nursing: Because diazepam and its metabolites may be present in human breast milk for prolonged periods of time after acute use of Diastat, patients should be advised not to breast-feed for an appropriate period of time after receiving treatment with Diastat.

Concomitant Medication

Although Diastat is indicated for use solely on an intermittent basis, the potential for a synergistic CNS-depressant effect when used simultaneously with alcohol or other CNS-depressants must be considered by the prescribing physician, and appropriate recommendations made to the patient and/or caregiver.

Drug Interactions

If Diastat is to be combined with other psychotropic agents or other CNS depressants, careful consideration should be given to the pharmacology of the agents to be employed—particularly with known compounds which may potentiate the action of diazepam, such as phenothiazines, narcotics, barbiturates, MAO inhibitors and other antidepressants.

The clearance of diazepam and certain other benzodiazepines can be delayed in association with cimetidine administration. The clinical significance of this is unclear.

Valproate may potentiate the CNS-depressant effects of diazepam.

There have been no clinical studies or reports in literature to evaluate the interaction of rectally administered diazepam with other drugs. As with all drugs, the potential for interaction by a variety of mechanisms is a possibility.

Effect of Other Drugs On Diazepam Metabolism: *In vitro* studies using human liver preparations suggest that CYP2C19 and CYP3A4 are the principal isozymes involved in the initial oxidative metabolism of diazepam. Therefore, potential interactions may occur when diazepam is given concurrently with agents that affect CYP2C19 and CYP3A4 activity. Potential inhibitors of CYP2C19 (e.g., cimetidine, quinidine, and tranylcypromine) and CYP3A4 (e.g., ketoconazole, troleandomycin, and clotrimazole) could decrease the rate of diazepam elimination, while inducers of CYP2C19 (e.g., rifampin) and CYP3A4 (e.g., carbamazepine, phenytoin, dexamethasone and phenobarbital) could increase the rate of elimination of diazepam.

Effect of Diazepam On the Metabolism of Other Drugs: There are no reports as to which isozymes could be inhibited or induced by diazepam. But, based on the fact that diazepam is a substrate for CYP2C19 and CYP3A4, it is possible that diazepam may interfere with the metabolism of drugs which are substrates for CYP2C19, (e.g. omeprazole, propranolol, and imipramine) and CYP3A4 (e.g. cyclosporine, paclitaxel, terfenadine, theophylline, and warfarin) leading to a potential drug-drug interaction.

Carcinogenesis, Mutagenesis, Impairment of Fertility

The carcinogenic potential of rectal diazepam has not been evaluated. In studies in which mice and rats were administered diazepam in the diet at a dose of 75 mg/kg/day (approximately six and 12 times, respectively, the maximum recommended human dose [MRHD=1 mg/kg/day] on a mg/m^2 basis) for 80 and 104 weeks, respectively, an increased incidence of liver tumors was observed in males of both species.

The data currently available are inadequate to determine the mutagenic potential of diazepam.

Reproduction studies in rats showed decreases in the number of pregnancies and in the number of surviving offspring following administration of an oral dose of 100 mg/kg/day (approximately 16 times the MRHD on a mg/m^2 basis) prior to and during mating and throughout gestation and lactation. No adverse effects on fertility or offspring viability were noted at a dose of 80 mg/kg/day (approximately 13 times the MRHD on a mg/m^2 basis).

Pregnancy—Category D (see WARNINGS section.)

Labor and Delivery

In humans, measurable amounts of diazepam have been found in maternal and cord blood, indicating placental transfer of the drug. Until additional information is available, Diastat is not recommended for obstetrical use.

Nursing Mothers

Because diazepam and its metabolites may be present in human breast milk for prolonged periods of time after acute use of Diastat, patients should be advised not to breast-feed for an appropriate period of time after receiving treatment with Diastat.

ADVERSE REACTIONS

Diastat adverse event data were collected from double-blind, placebo-controlled studies and open-label studies. The majority of adverse events were mild to moderate in severity and transient in nature.

Two patients who received Diastat died seven to 15 weeks following treatment; neither of these deaths was deemed related to Diastat.

The most frequent adverse event reported to be related to Diastat in the two double-blind, placebo-controlled studies was somnolence (23%). Less frequent adverse events were dizziness, headache, pain, abdominal pain, nervousness, vasodilatation, diarrhea, ataxia, euphoria, incoordination, asthma, rhinitis, and rash, which occurred in approximately 2–5% of patients.

Approximately 1.4% of the 573 patients who received Diastat in clinical trials of epilepsy discontinued treatment because of an adverse event. The adverse event most frequently associated with discontinuation (occurring in three patients) was somnolence. Other adverse events most commonly associated with discontinuation and occurring in two patients were hypoventilation and rash. Adverse events occurring in one patient were asthenia, hyperkinesia, incoordination, vasodilatation and urticaria. These events were judged to be related to Diastat.

In the two domestic double-blind, placebo-controlled, parallel-group studies, the proportion of patients who discontinued treatment because of adverse events was 2% for the group treated with Diastat, versus 2% for the placebo group. In the Diastat group, the adverse events considered the primary reason for discontinuation were different in the two patients who discontinued treatment; one discontinued due to rash and one discontinued due to lethargy. The primary reason for discontinuation in the patients treated with placebo was lack of effect.

Adverse Event Incidence in Controlled Clinical Trials

Table 1 lists treatment-emergent signs and symptoms that occurred in >1% of patients enrolled in parallel-group, placebo-controlled trials and were numerically more common in the Diastat group. Adverse events were usually mild or moderate in intensity.

The prescriber should be aware that these figures, obtained when Diastat was added to concurrent antiepileptic drug therapy, cannot be used to predict the frequency of adverse events in the course of usual medical practice when patient characteristics and other factors may differ from those prevailing during clinical studies. Similarly, the cited frequencies cannot be directly compared with figures obtained from other clinical investigations involving different treatments, uses, or investigators. An inspection of these frequencies, however, does provide the prescribing physician with one basis to estimate the relative contribution of drug and non-drug factors to the adverse event incidences in the population studied.

TABLE 1: Treatment-Emergent Signs And Symptoms That Occurred In >1% Of Patients Enrolled In Parallel-Group, Placebo-Controlled Trials And Were Numerically More Common In The Diastat Group

Body System	COSTART Term	Diastat N = 101 %	Placebo N = 104 %
Body As A Whole	Headache	5%	4%
Cardiovascular	Vasodilatation	2%	0%
Digestive	Diarrhea	4%	<1%
Nervous	Ataxia	3%	<1%
	Dizziness	3%	2%
	Euphoria	3%	0%
	Incoordination	3%	0%
	Somnolence	23%	8%
Respiratory	Asthma	2%	0%
Skin and Appendages	Rash	3%	0%

Other events reported by 1% or more of patients treated in controlled trials but equally or more frequent in the placebo group than in the Diastat group were abdominal pain, pain, nervousness, and rhinitis. Other events reported by fewer than 1% of patients were infection, anorexia, vomiting, anemia, lymphadenopathy, grand mal convulsion, hyperkinesia, cough increased, pruritis, sweating, mydriasis, and urinary tract infection.

The pattern of adverse events was similar for different age, race and gender groups.

Other Adverse Events Observed During All Clinical Trials: Diastat has been administered to 573 patients with epilepsy during all clinical trials, only some of which were placebo-controlled. During these trials, all adverse events were recorded by the clinical investigators using terminology of their own choosing. To provide a meaningful estimate of the proportion of individuals having adverse events, similar types of events were grouped into a smaller number of standardized categories using modified COSTART dictionary terminology. These categories are used in the listing below. All of the events listed below occurred in at least 1% of the 573 individuals exposed to Diastat. All reported events are included except those already listed above, events unlikely to be drug-related, and those too general to be informative. Events are included without regard to determination of a causal relationship to diazepam.

BODY AS A WHOLE: Asthenia

CARDIOVASCULAR: Hypotension, vasodilatation

NERVOUS: Agitation, Confusion convulsion, dysarthria, emotional lability, speech disorder, thinking abnormal, vertigo

RESPIRATORY: Hiccup

The following infrequent adverse events were not seen with Diastat but have been reported previously with diazepam use: depression, slurred speech, syncope, constipation, changes in libido, urinary retention, bradycardia, cardiovascular collapse, nystagmus, urticaria, neutropenia and jaundice.

Paradoxical reactions such as acute hyperexcited states, anxiety, hallucinations, increased muscle spasticity, insomnia, rage, sleep disturbances and stimulation have been reported with diazepam; should these occur, use of Diastat should be discontinued.

DRUG ABUSE AND DEPENDENCE

Diazepam is a Schedule IV controlled substance and can produce drug dependence. It is recommended that patients be treated with Diastat no more frequently than every five days and no more than five times per month.

Addiction-prone individuals (such as drug addicts or alcoholics) should be under careful surveillance when receiving diazepam or other psychotropic agents because of the predisposition of such patients to habituation and dependence.

Abrupt discontinuation of diazepam following chronic regular use has resulted in withdrawal symptoms, similar in character to those noted with barbiturates and alcohol (convulsions, tremor, abdominal and muscle cramps, vomiting and sweating). The more severe withdrawal symptoms have usually been limited to those patients who had received excessive doses over an extended period of time. Generally milder withdrawal symptoms (e.g., dysphoria and insomnia) have been reported following abrupt discontinuation of benzodiazepines taken continuously at therapeutic levels for several months.

OVERDOSAGE

Two patients in the clinical studies received more than twice the target dose; no adverse events were reported.

Previous reports of diazepam overdosage have shown that manifestations of diazepam overdosage include somnolence, confusion, coma, and diminished reflexes. Respiration, pulse and blood pressure should be monitored, as in all cases of drug overdosage, although, in general, these effects have been minimal. General supportive measures should be employed, along with intravenous fluids, and an adequate airway maintained. Hypotension may be combated by the use of levarterenol or metaraminol. Dialysis is of limited value.

Flumazenil, a specific benzodiazepine-receptor antagonist, is indicated for the complete or partial reversal of the sedative effects of benzodiazepines and may be used in situations when an overdose with a benzodiazepine is known or suspected. Prior to the administration of flumazenil, necessary measures should be instituted to secure airway, ventilation and intravenous access. Flumazenil is intended as an adjunct to, not as a substitute for, proper management of benzodiazepine overdose. Patients treated with flumazenil should be monitored for resedation, respiratory depression and other residual benzodiazepine effects for an appropriate period after treatment. **The prescriber should be aware of a risk of seizure in association with flumazenil treatment, particularly in long-term benzodiazepine users and in cyclic antidepressant overdose.** The complete flumazenil package insert, including CONTRAINDICATIONS, WARNINGS and PRECAUTIONS, should be consulted prior to use.

DOSAGE AND ADMINISTRATION (see Also Patient/Caregiver Package Insert)

This section is intended primarily for the prescriber; however, the prescriber should also be aware of the dosing information and directions for use provided in the patient package insert.

A decision to prescribe Diastat involves more than the diagnosis and the selection of the correct dose for the patient.

First, the prescriber must be convinced from historical reports and/or personal observations that the patient exhibits the characteristic identifiable seizure cluster that can be distinguished from the patient's usual seizure activity by the caregiver who will be responsible for administering Diastat.

Second, because Diastat is only intended for adjunctive use, the prescriber must ensure that the patient is receiving an optimal regimen of standard anti-epileptic drug treatment and is, nevertheless, continuing to experience these characteristic episodes.

Third, because a non-health professional will be obliged to identify episodes suitable for treatment, make the decision to administer treatment upon that identification, administer the drug, monitor the patient, and assess the adequacy of the response to treatment, a major component of the prescribing process involves the necessary instruction of this individual.

Fourth, the prescriber and caregiver must have a common understanding of what is and is not an episode of seizures that is appropriate for treatment, the timing of administration in relation to the onset of the episode, the mechanics of administering the drug, how and what to observe following administration, and what would constitute an outcome requiring immediate and direct medical attention.

Calculating Prescribed Dose

The Diastat dose should be individualized for maximum beneficial effect. The recommended dose of Diastat is 0.2–0.5 mg/kg depending on age. See the dosing table for specific recommendations.

Age (years)	Recommended Dose
2 through 5	0.5 mg/kg
6 through 11	0.3 mg/kg
12 and older	0.2 mg/kg

Because Diastat is provided in fixed, unit-doses of 5, 10, 15 and 20 mg, the prescribed dose is obtained by rounding upward to the next available dose. The following table provides acceptable weight ranges for each dose and age category, such that patients will receive between 90% and 180% of the calculated recommended dose. The safety of this strategy has been established in clinical trials.

2-5 Years 0.5 mg/kg		6-11 Years 0.3 mg/kg		12+ Years 0.2 mg/kg	
Weight (kg)	Dose (mg)	Weight (kg)	Dose (mg)	Weight (kg)	Dose (mg)

6 to 11	5	10 to 18	5	14 to 27	5
12 to 22	10	19 to 37	10	28 to 50	10
23 to 33	15	38 to 55	15	51 to 75	15
34 to 44	20	56 to 74	20	76 to 111	20

The rectal delivery system includes a plastic applicator with a flexible, molded tip available in two lengths, designated for convenience as "Pediatric", "Universal" and "Adult". The 2.5 and 5 mg dosages are available with a 4.4 cm Pediatric tip, the 10 mg dosage is available with a 4.4 cm Universal tip and the 15 and 20 mg dosages are available with a 6.0 cm Adult tip.

It is important to note that if a 15 mg dose is to be administered to a pediatric patient utilizing the plastic applicator with a pediatric tip, prescriptions must be written for 2 different twin packs, one for the 5 mg dosage and one for the 10 mg dosage (see HOW SUPPLIED section).

In elderly and debilitated patients, it is recommended that the dosage be adjusted downward to reduce the likelihood of ataxia or oversedation.

The prescribed dose of Diastat should be adjusted by the physician periodically to reflect changes in the patient's age or weight. It is recommended that dosage be reviewed at six month intervals.

A 2.5 mg dose is available for use as a supplemental dose. This dose may be prescribed at the discretion of the physician for patients who require more precise dose titration than is achieved using one of the four standard doses provided. The 2.5 mg dose may also be used as a partial replacement dose for patients who may expel a portion of the first dose.

Additional Dose

The prescriber may wish to prescribe a second dose of Diastat. A second dose, when required, may be given 4–12 hours after the first dose.

Treatment Frequency

It is recommended that Diastat be used to treat no more than five episodes per month and no more than one episode every five days.

HOW SUPPLIED

Diastat (diazepam rectal gel) rectal delivery system is a non-sterile diazepam gel provided in a prefilled, unit-dose, rectal delivery system. The rectal delivery system includes a plastic applicator with a flexible, molded tip available in two lengths, designated for convenience as "Pediatric", "Universal" or "Adult". Diastat is available in the following five presentations:

Dosage Strength	Rectal Tip Size	NDC Number
2.5 mg Twin Pack	Pediatric (4.4 cm)	NDC 59075-650-20
5 mg Twin Pack	Pediatric	NDC 59075-651-20
10 mg Twin Pack	Universal (4.4 cm)	NDC 59075-652-20
15 mg Twin Pack	Adult (6.0 cm)	NDC 59075-654-20
20 mg Twin Pack	Adult	NDC 59075-655-20

Each Twin Pack contains two Diastat rectal delivery systems, two packets of lubricating jelly, and Patient/Caregiver Package Insert.

Store at controlled room temperature 15–30°C (59–86°F).

CAUTION: Federal law prohibits dispensing without prescription.

CAUTION: Federal law prohibits the transfer of this drug to any person other than the patient for whom it was prescribed.

Distributed by:
Elan Pharma, a business unit of Elan Pharmaceuticals, Inc.
South San Francisco, California 94080
Manufactured by:
DPT Laboratories, Inc.
San Antonio, Texas 78215

Dia*stat*™ ADMINISTRATION INSTRUCTIONS

(diazepam rectal gel)

IMPORTANT

Read first before using

To the caregiver:

Please do not give DIASTAT® until:

1. you have thoroughly read these instructions,
2. reviewed administration steps with the doctor,
3. understand the directions.

Please do not administer DIASTAT until you feel comfortable with how to use DIASTAT. The doctor will tell you exactly when to use DIASTAT. When you use DIASTAT correctly and safely you will help bring seizures under control. Be sure to discuss every aspect of your role with the doctor. If you are not comfortable, then discuss your role with the doctor again.

To help the person with seizures:

- ✓You must be able to tell the difference between a cluster and ordinary seizures.
- ✓You must be comfortable and satisfied that you are able to give DIASTAT.
- ✓You need to agree with the doctor on the exact conditions when to treat with DIASTAT.
- ✓You must know how and for how long you should check the person after giving DIASTAT.

To know what responses to expect:

- ✓You need to know how soon seizures should stop or decrease in frequency after giving DIASTAT.
- ✓You need to know what you should do if the seizures do not stop or there is a change in the person's breathing, behavior or condition that alarms you.

If you have any questions or feel unsure about using the treatment, CALL THE DOCTOR before using DIASTAT.

Where can I find more information and support?

The two best places to go for information and support are:

ASAP™ (Appropriate Seizure Action Program) sponsored by Elan Pharmaceuticals, Inc. You can reach ASAP by calling 1-888-801-ASAP (2727).

EF (Epilepsy Foundation). You can reach EF by calling 800-EFA-1000 or www.efa.org.

When to treat. *Based on the doctor's directions or prescription.*

______

Special considerations.

DIASTAT should be used with caution:

- In people with respiratory (breathing) difficulties (e.g., asthma or pneumonia)
- In the elderly
- In women of child bearing potential, pregnancy or nursing mothers

Discuss beforehand with the doctor any additional steps you may need to take if there is leakage of DIASTAT or a bowel movement.

Patient's DIASTAT dosage is: ______ **mg**

Patient's resting breathing rate ______ Patient's current weight ______

Check expiration date and always remove cap and seal pin before using.

TREATMENT 1

Important things to tell the doctor.

Seizures Before DIASTAT			
Date	Time	Seizure Type	No. of Seizures
______	______	______	______

Seizures After DIASTAT		
Time	Seizure Type	No. of Seizures
______	______	______

Things to do after treatment with DIASTAT.

Stay with the person for 4 hours and make notes of the following:

- Changes in breathing rate ______
- Changes in color ______
- Confirm current weight is still the same as when DIASTAT was prescribed ______
- Possible side effects from treatment ______

TREATMENT 2

Important things to tell the doctor.

Seizures Before DIASTAT			
Date	Time	Seizure Type	No. of Seizures
______	______	______	______

Seizures After DIASTAT		
Time	Seizure Type	No. of Seizures

Things to do after treatment with DIASTAT.

- Changes in resting breathing rate ______
- Changes in color ______
- Confirm current weight is still the same as when DIASTAT was prescribed ______
- Possible side effects from treatment ______

Disposal

- Discard all used material in the garbage can.
- Do not reuse.
- Discard in a safe place away from children.

DIASTAT is a registered trademark of Elan Pharmaceuticals, Inc.

HOW TO ADMINISTER Dia*stat*™

(diazepam rectal gel)

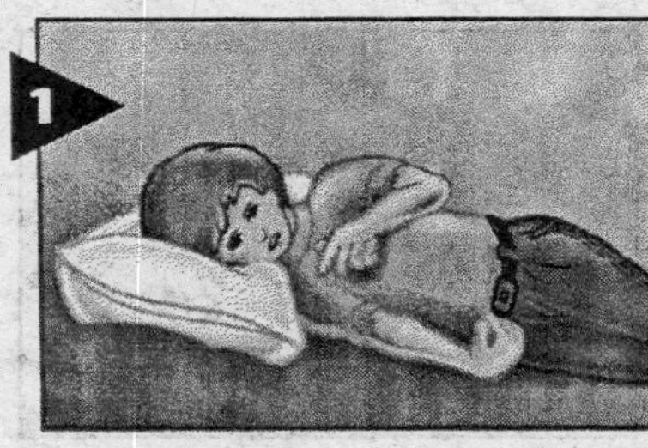

Put person on their side where they can't fall

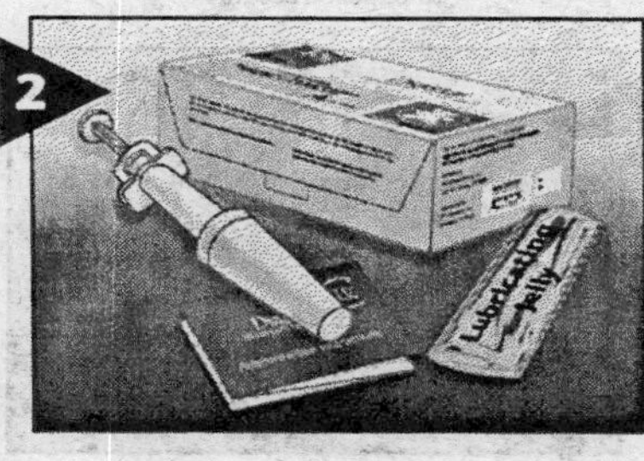

Get medicine

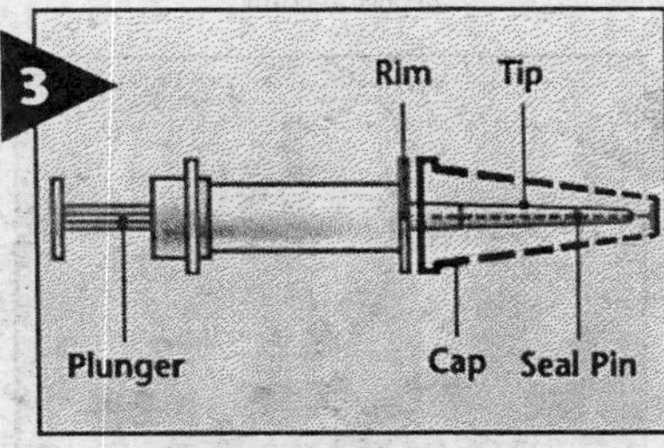

Get syringe

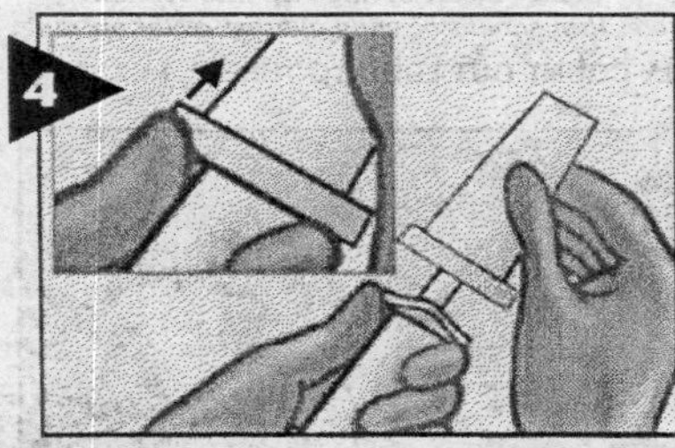

Push up with thumb and pull to remove protective cover from syringe

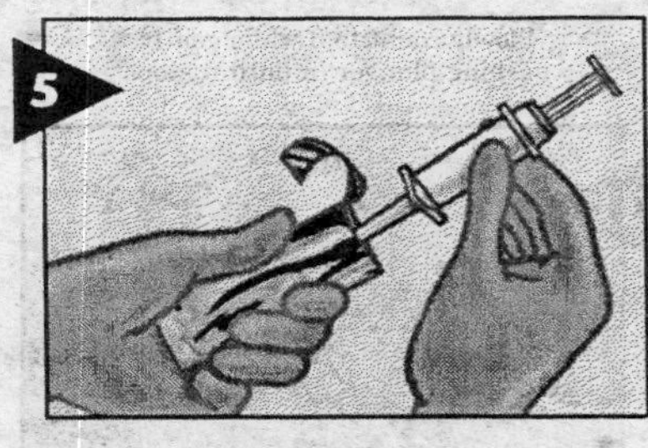

Lubricate rectal tip with lubricating jelly

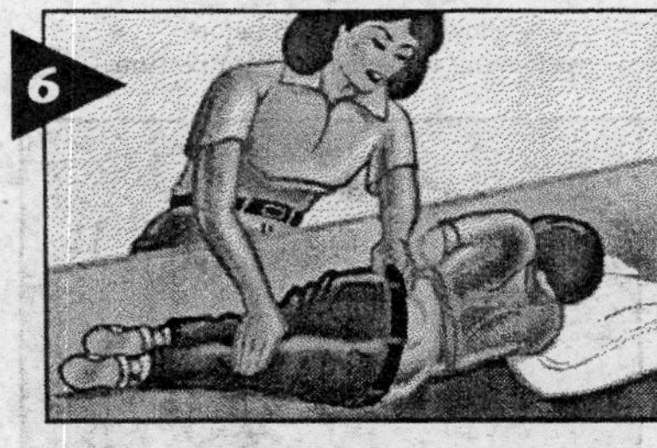

Turn person on side facing you

Continued on next page

Diastat—Cont.

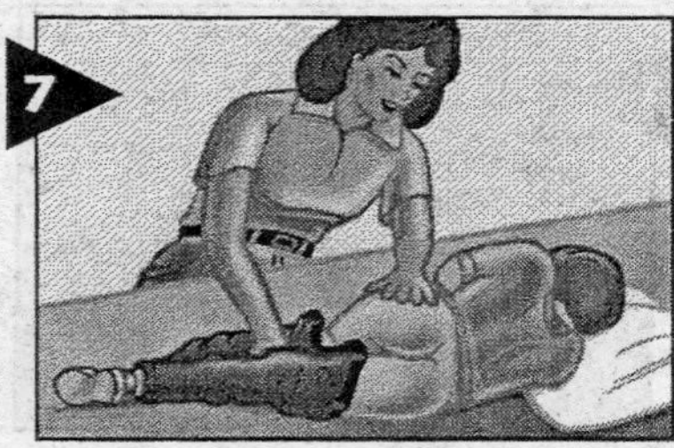

Bend upper leg forward
to expose rectum

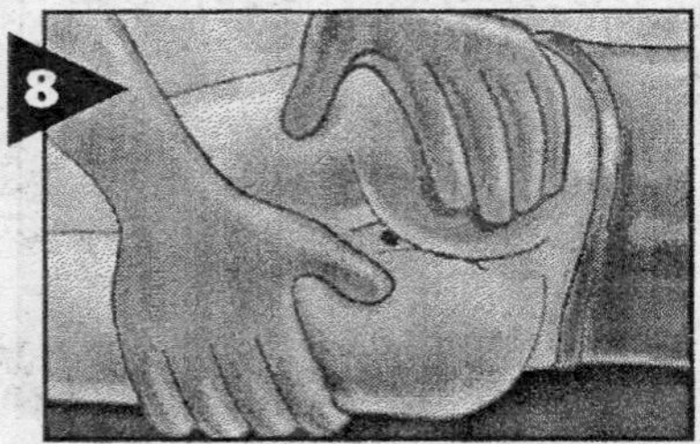

Separate buttocks to
expose rectum

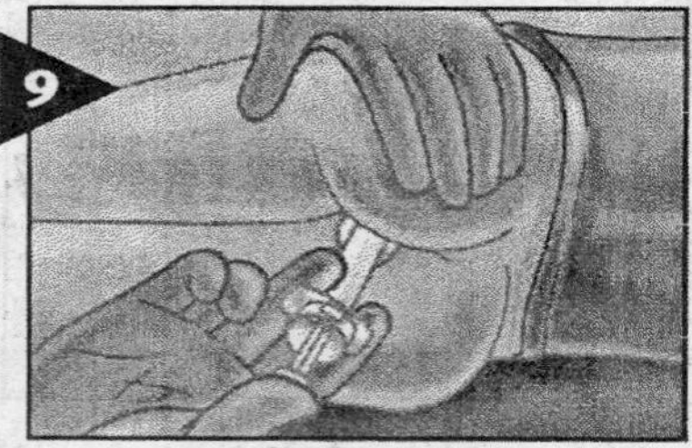

Gently insert syringe tip into rectum
Note: Rim should be snug against rectal opening.

SLOWLY COUNT OUT LOUD TO THREE...1...2...3

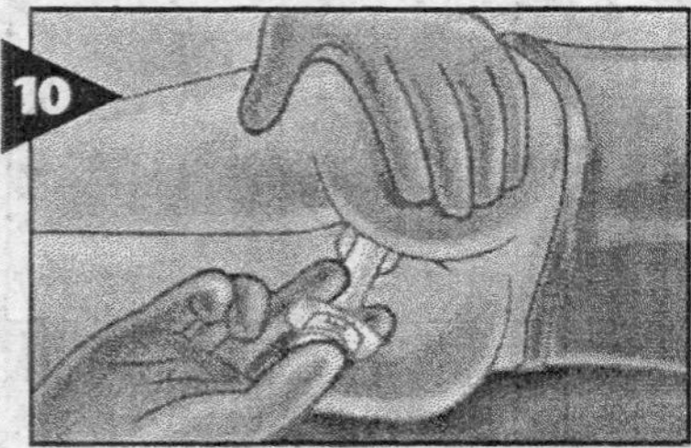

Slowly count to 3 while gently
pushing plunger in until it stops

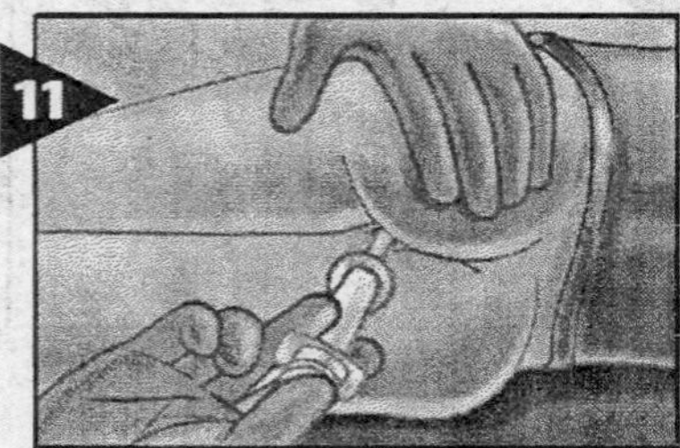

Slowly count to 3 before
removing the syringe from rectum

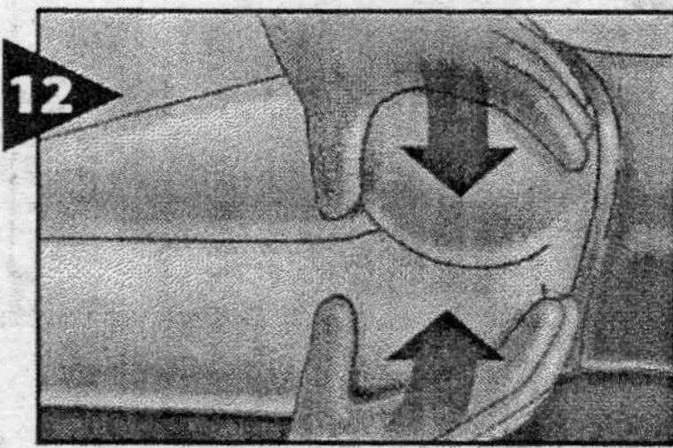

Slowly count to 3 while holding
buttocks together to prevent leakage

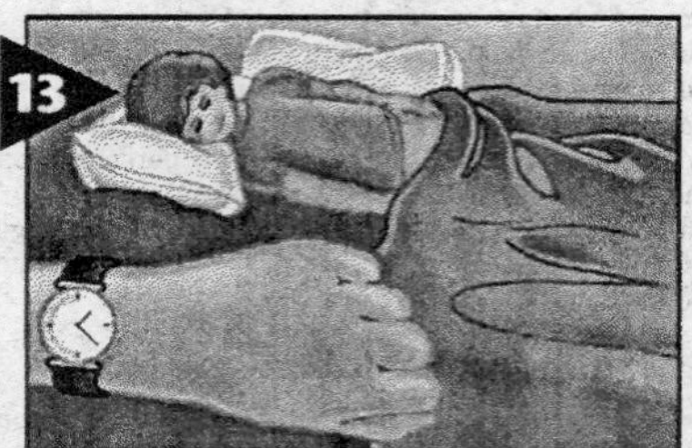

Keep person on side facing you, note
time given and continue to observe

CALL FOR HELP IF ANY OF THE FOLLOWING OCCUR

- Seizure(s) continues 15 minutes after giving DIASTAT or per the doctor's instructions.
- Seizure behavior is different from other episodes.
- You are alarmed by the frequency or severity of the seizure(s).
- You are alarmed by the color or breathing of the person.
- The person is having unusual or serious problems.

Local Emergency Number: **Doctor's Number:**

(please be sure to note if your area has 911)

Information for Emergency Squad: *Time DIASTAT given:* ________ *Dose:*________

DIASTAT is a registered trademark of Elan Pharmaceuticals, Inc.
ASAP is a trademark of Elan Pharmaceuticals, Inc.
 Rev 7/99
Shown in Product Identification Guide, page 312

MYSOLINE® ℞

[mī 'sō-lēn]
(primidone)
Anticonvulsant

Rx Only

DESCRIPTION

Chemical name: 5-ethyldihydro-5-phenyl-4,6 (1H, 5H) pyrimidinedione.
Structural formula:

H
O N
C_2H_5 NH
O

Mysoline* (primidone) is a white, crystalline, highly stable substance, M.P. 279–284°C. It is poorly soluble in water (60 mg per 100 mL at 37°C) and in most organic solvents. It possesses no acidic properties, in contrast to its barbiturate analog.
Mysoline 50 mg and 250 mg tablets contain the following inactive ingredients: Microcrystalline Cellulose, NF; Lactose, USP; Methylcellulose, USP; Sodium Starch Glycolate, NF; Talc, USP; Sodium Lauryl Sulfate, NF; Magnesium Stearate, NF; Water, USP, Purified.
Mysoline 250 mg tablets also contain Yellow Iron Oxide, NF.
Mysoline suspension contains these inactive ingredients: Ammonia Solution, Diluted; Citric Acid, USP; D&C Yellow No. 10; FD&C Yellow No. 6; Magnesium Aluminum Silicate; Methylparaben, NF; Propylparaben, NF; Saccharin Sodium, NF; Sodium Alginate; Sodium Citrate; Sodium Hypochlorite Solution, USP; Sorbic Acid, NF; Sorbitan Monolaurate; Water, USP, Purified; Flavors.

* Registered trademark of Elan Pharmaceuticals, Inc.

ACTIONS

Mysoline raises electro- or chemoshock seizure thresholds or alters seizure patterns in experimental animals. The mechanism(s) of primidone's antiepileptic action is not known.
Primidone *per se* has anticonvulsant activity as do its two metabolites, phenobarbital and phenylethylmalonamide (PEMA). In addition to its anticonvulsant activity, PEMA potentiates the anticonvulsant activity of phenobarbital in experimental animals.

INDICATIONS

Mysoline, used alone or concomitantly with other anticonvulsants, is indicated in the control of grand mal, psychomotor, and focal epileptic seizures. It may control grand mal seizures refractory to other anticonvulsant therapy.

CONTRAINDICATIONS

Primidone is contraindicated in: 1) patients with porphyria and 2) patients who are hypersensitive to phenobarbital (see ACTIONS).

WARNINGS

The abrupt withdrawal of antiepileptic medication may precipitate status epilepticus.
The therapeutic efficacy of a dosage regimen takes several weeks before it can be assessed.

Usage In Pregnancy
The effects of Mysoline in human pregnancy and nursing infants are unknown.
Recent reports suggest an association between the use of anticonvulsant drugs by women with epilepsy and an elevated incidence of birth defects in children born to these women. Data are more extensive with respect to diphenylhydantoin and phenobarbital, but these are also the most commonly prescribed anticonvulsants; less systematic or anecdotal reports suggest a possible similar association with the use of all known anticonvulsant drugs.
The reports suggesting an elevated incidence of birth defects in children of drug-treated epileptic women cannot be regarded as adequate to prove a definite cause-and-effect relationship. There are intrinsic methodologic problems in obtaining adequate data on drug teratogenicity in humans: the possibility also exists that other factors leading to birth defects, e.g., genetic factors or the epileptic condition itself, may be more important than drug therapy. The majority of mothers on anticonvulsant medication deliver normal infants. It is important to note that anticonvulsant drugs should not be discontinued in patients in whom the drug is administered to prevent major seizures because of the strong possibility of precipitating status epilepticus with attendant hypoxia and threat to life. In individual cases where the severity and frequency of the seizure disorders are such that the removal of medication does not pose a serious threat to the patient, discontinuation of the drug may be considered prior to and during pregnancy, although it cannot be said with any confidence that even minor seizures do not pose some hazard to the developing embryo or fetus. The prescribing physician will wish to weigh these considerations in treating or counseling epileptic women of childbearing potential.
Neonatal hemorrhage, with a coagulation defect resembling vitamin K deficiency, has been described in newborns whose mothers were taking primidone and other anticonvulsants. Pregnant women under anticonvulsant therapy should receive prophylactic vitamin K_1 therapy for one month prior to, and during, delivery.

PRECAUTIONS

The total daily dosage should not exceed 2 g. Since Mysoline therapy generally extends over prolonged periods, a complete blood count and a sequential multiple analysis-12 (SMA-12) test should be made every six months.

In Nursing Mothers
There is evidence that in mothers treated with primidone, the drug appears in the milk in substantial quantities. Since tests for the presence of primidone in biological fluids are too complex to be carried out in the average clinical laboratory, it is suggested that the presence of undue somnolence and drowsiness in nursing newborns of Mysoline-treated mothers be taken as an indication that nursing should be discontinued.

ADVERSE REACTIONS

The most frequently occurring early side effects are ataxia and vertigo. These tend to disappear with continued therapy, or with reduction of initial dosage. Occasionally, the following have been reported: nausea, anorexia, vomiting, fatigue, hyperirritability, emotional disturbances, sexual impotency, diplopia, nystagmus, drowsiness, and morbilliform skin eruptions. Granulocytopenia, agranulocytosis, and red-cell hypoplasia and aplasia, have been reported rarely. These and, occasionally, other persistent or severe side effects may necessitate withdrawal of the drug. Megaloblastic anemia may occur as a rare idiosyncrasy to Mysoline and to other anticonvulsants. The anemia responds to folic acid without necessity of discontinuing medication.

DOSAGE AND ADMINISTRATION

Adult Dosage
Patients 8 years of age and older who have received no previous treatment may be started on Mysoline according to the following regimen using either 50 mg or scored 250 mg Mysoline tablets.

Days 1 to 3: 100 to 125 mg at bedtime
Days 4 to 6: 100 to 125 mg b.i.d.
Days 7 to 9: 100 to 125 mg t.i.d.
Day 10 to maintenance: 250 mg t.i.d.

For most adults and children 8 years of age and over, the usual maintenance dosage is three to four 250 mg Mysoline tablets daily in divided doses (250 mg t.i.d. or q.i.d.). If required, an increase to five or six 250 mg tablets daily may be made but daily doses should not exceed 500 mg q.i.d.

INITIAL: ADULTS AND CHILDREN OVER 8

KEY: ·=50 mg tablet •=250 mg tablet

DAY	1	2	3	4	5	6
AM				··	··	··
NOON						
PM	··	··	··	··	··	··

DAY	7	8	9	10	11	12
AM	··	··	··	•		
NOON	··	··	··	•	Adjust to	
PM	··	··	··	•	Maintenance	

Dosage should be individualized to provide maximum benefit. In some cases, serum blood level determinations of primidone may be necessary for optimal dosage adjustment. The clinically effective serum level for primidone is between 5 to 12 μg/mL.

In Patients Already Receiving Other Anticonvulsants

Mysoline should be started at 100 to 125 mg at bedtime and gradually increased to maintenance level as the other drug is gradually decreased. This regimen should be continued until satisfactory dosage level is achieved for the combination, or the other medication is completely withdrawn. When therapy with Mysoline alone is the objective, the transition from concomitant therapy should not be completed in less than two weeks.

Pediatric Dosage

For children under 8 years of age, the following regimen may be used:

Days 1 to 3: 50 mg at bedtime
Days 4 to 6: 50 mg b.i.d.
Days 7 to 9: 100 mg b.i.d.
Day 10 to maintenance: 125 mg t.i.d. to 250 mg t.i.d.

For children under 8 years of age, the usual maintenance dosage is 125 to 250 mg three times daily or, 10 to 25 mg/kg/day in divided doses.

HOW SUPPLIED

Mysoline Tablets

Each square-shaped, scored, yellow tablet, identified by "MYSOLINE 250" and an embossed M, contains 250 mg of primidone, in bottles of 100 (NDC 59075-691-10) and 1,000 (NDC 59075-691-11).

Also available in a unit-dose package of 100 (NDC 59075-691-81).

Each square-shaped, scored, white tablet, identified by "MYSOLINE 50" and an embossed M, contains 50 mg of primidone, in bottles of 100 (NDC 59075-690-10) and 500 (NDC 59075-690-50).

The appearance of these tablets is a trademark of Elan Pharmaceuticals, Inc.

Mysoline Suspension

Each 5 mL (teaspoonful) contains 250 mg of primidone, in bottles of 8 fluid ounces (NDC 59075-692-50).

Store at room temperature, approximately 25° C (77° F).

Dispense in a tight, light-resistant container as defined in the U.S.P.

Distributed by:
Elan Pharmaceuticals
South San Francisco, CA 94080

Issued 4/21/99

Shown in Product Identification Guide, page 312

ZONEGRAN™ ℞

[*zän' ə-grăn*]
(zonisamide)
Capsules
Rx only

DESCRIPTION

ZONEGRAN™ (zonisamide) is an antiseizure drug chemically classified as a sulfonamide and unrelated to other antiseizure agents. The active ingredient is zonisamide, 1,2-benzisoxazole-3-methanesulfonamide. The empirical formula is $C_8H_8N_2O_3S$ with a molecular weight of 212.23. Zonisamide is a white powder, pKa = 10.2, and is moderately soluble in water (0.80 mg/mL) and 0.1 N HCl (0.50 mg/mL). The chemical structure is:

$CH_2SO_2NH_2$

ZONEGRAN is supplied for oral administration as capsules containing 100 mg zonisamide. Each capsule contains the labeled amount of zonisamide plus the following inactive ingredients: microcrystalline cellulose, hydrogenated vegetable oil, sodium laurel sulfate, gelatin, and colorants.

CLINICAL PHARMACOLOGY

Mechanism of Action: The precise mechanism(s) by which zonisamide exerts its antiseizure effect is unknown. Zonisamide demonstrated anticonvulsant activity in several experimental models. In animals, zonisamide was effective against tonic extension seizures induced by maximal electroshock but ineffective against clonic seizures induced by subcutaneous pentylenetetrazol. Zonisamide raised the threshold for generalized seizures in the kindled rat model and reduced the duration of cortical focal seizures induced by electrical stimulation of the visual cortex in cats. Furthermore, zonisamide suppressed both interictal spikes and the secondarily generalized seizures produced by cortical application of tungstic acid gel in rats or by cortical freezing in cats. The relevance of these models to human epilepsy is unknown.

Zonisamide may produce these effects through action at sodium and calcium channels. *In vitro* pharmacological studies suggest that zonisamide blocks sodium channels and reduces voltage-dependent, transient inward currents (T-type Ca^{2+} currents), consequently stabilizing neuronal membranes and suppressing neuronal hypersynchronization. *In vitro* binding studies have demonstrated that zonisamide binds to the GABA/benzodiazepine receptor ionophore complex in an allosteric fashion which does not produce changes in chloride flux. Other *in vitro* studies have demonstrated that zonisamide (10–30 μg/mL) suppresses synaptically-driven electrical activity without affecting postsynaptic GABA or glutamate responses (cultured mouse spinal cord neurons) or neuronal or glial uptake of [^{3}H]-GABA (rat hippocampal slices). Thus, zonisamide does not appear to potentiate the synaptic activity of GABA. *In vivo* microdialysis studies demonstrated that zonisamide facilitates both dopaminergic and serotonergic neurotransmission. Zonisamide also has weak carbonic anhydrase inhibiting activity, but this pharmacologic effect is not thought to be a major contributing factor in the antiseizure activity of zonisamide.

Pharmacokinetics: Following a 200–400 mg oral zonisamide dose, peak plasma concentrations (range: 2–5 μg/mL) in normal volunteers occur within 2–6 hours. In the presence of food, the time to maximum concentration is delayed, occurring at 4–6 hours, but food has no effect on the bioavailability of zonisamide. Zonisamide extensively binds to erythrocytes, resulting in an eight-fold higher concentration of zonisamide in red blood cells (RBC) than in plasma. The pharmacokinetics of zonisamide are dose proportional in the range of 200–400 mg, but the C_{max} and AUC increase disproportionately at 800 mg, perhaps due to saturable binding of zonisamide to RBC. Once a stable dose is reached, steady state is achieved within 14 days. The elimination half-life of zonisamide in plasma is about 63 hours. The elimination half-life of zonisamide in RBC is approximately 105 hours. The apparent volume of distribution (V/F) of zonisamide is about 1.45 L/kg following a 400 mg oral dose. Zonisamide, at concentrations of 1.0–7.0 μg/mL, is approximately 40% bound to human plasma proteins. Protein binding of zonisamide is unaffected in the presence of therapeutic concentrations of phenytoin, phenobarbital or carbamazepine.

Metabolism and Excretion: Following oral administration of ^{14}C-zonisamide to healthy volunteers, only zonisamide was detected in plasma. Zonisamide is excreted primarily in urine as parent drug and as the glucuronide of a metabolite. Following multiple dosing, 62% of the ^{14}C dose was recovered in the urine, with 3% in the feces by day 10. Zonisamide undergoes acetylation to form N-acetyl zonisamide and reduction to form the open ring metabolite, 2-sulfamoylacetyl phenol (SMAP). Of the excreted dose, 35% was recovered as zonisamide, 15% as N-acetyl zonisamide, and 50% as the glucuronide of SMAP. Reduction of zonisamide to SMAP is mediated by cytochrome P450 isozyme 3A4 (CYP3A4). Zonisamide does not induce its own metabolism. Plasma clearance of zonisamide is approximately 0.30–0.35 mL/min/kg in patients not receiving enzyme-inducing antiepilepsy drugs (AEDs). The clearance of zonisamide is increased to 0.5 mL/min/kg in patients concurrently on enzyme-inducing AEDs.

Renal clearance is about 3.5 mL/min. The clearance of an oral dose of zonisamide from RBC is 2 mL/min.

Special Populations:

Renal Insufficiency: Single 300 mg zonisamide doses were administered to three groups of volunteers. Group 1 was a healthy group with a creatinine clearance ranging from 70–152 mL/min. Group 2 and Group 3 had creatinine clearances ranging from 14.5–59 mL/min and 10–20 mL/min, respectively. Zonisamide renal clearance decreased with decreasing renal function (3.42, 2.50, 2.23 mL/min, respectively). Marked renal impairment (creatinine clearance < 20 mL/min) was associated with an increase in zonisamide AUC of 35% (see **DOSAGE AND ADMINISTRATION** section).

Hepatic Disease: The pharmacokinetics of zonisamide in patients with impaired liver function have not been studied (see **DOSAGE AND ADMINISTRATION** section).

Age: The pharmacokinetics of a 300 mg single dose of zonisamide was similar in young (mean age 28 years) and elderly subjects (mean age 69 years).

Gender and Race: Information on the effect of gender and race on the pharmacokinetics of zonisamide is not available.

Interactions of Zonisamide with Other Antiepilepsy Drugs (AEDs): Concurrent medication with drugs that either induce or inhibit CYP3A4 may alter serum concentrations of zonisamide. Concomitant administration of phenytoin and carbamazepine increases zonisamide plasma clearance from 0.30–0.35 mL/min/kg to 0.35–0.5 mL/min/kg. The half-life of zonisamide is decreased to 27 hours by phenytoin, to 38 hours by phenobarbital and carbamazepine, and to 46 hours by valproate. Plasma protein binding of phenytoin and carbamazepine was not affected by zonisamide administration (see **PRECAUTIONS, Drug Interactions** subsection).

Clinical Studies: The effectiveness of ZONEGRAN as adjunctive therapy (added to other antiepilepsy drugs) has been established in three multicenter, placebo-controlled, double blind, 3-month clinical trials (two domestic, one European) in 499 patients with refractory partial onset seizures with or without secondary generalization. Each patient had a history of at least four partial onset seizures per month in spite of receiving one or two antiepilepsy drugs at therapeutic concentrations. The 499 patients (209 women, 290 men) ranged in age from 13–68 years with a mean age of about 35 years. In the two US studies, over 80% of the patients were Caucasian; 100% of patients in the European study were Caucasian. ZONEGRAN or placebo was added to the existing therapy. The primary measure of effectiveness was median percent reduction from baseline in partial seizure frequency. The secondary measure was proportion of patients achieving a 50% or greater seizure reduction from baseline (responders). The results described below are for all partial seizures in the intent-to-treat populations.

In the first study (n = 203), all patients had a 1-month baseline observation period, then received placebo or ZONEGRAN in one of two dose escalation regimens; either 1) 100 mg/day for five weeks, 200 mg/day for one week, 300 mg/day for one week, and then 400 mg/day for five weeks; or 2) 100 mg/day for one week, followed by 200 mg/day for five weeks, then 300 mg/day for one week, then 400 mg/day for five weeks. This design allowed a 100 mg vs. placebo comparison over weeks 1–5, and a 200 mg vs. placebo comparison over weeks 2–6; the primary comparison was 400 mg (both escalation groups combined) vs. placebo over weeks 8–12. The total daily dose was given as twice a day dosing. Statistically significant treatment differences favoring ZONEGRAN were seen for doses of 100, 200, and 400 mg/day.

In the second (n=152) and third (n=138) studies, patients had a 2–3 month baseline, then were randomly assigned to placebo or ZONEGRAN for three months. ZONEGRAN was introduced by administering 100 mg/day for the first week, 200 mg/day the second week, then 400 mg/day for two weeks, after which the dose (ZONEGRAN or placebo) could be adjusted as necessary to a maximum dose of 20 mg/kg/day or a maximum plasma level of 40 μg/mL. In the second study, the total daily dose was given as twice a day dosing; in the third study, it was given as a single daily dose. The average final maintenance doses received in the studies were 530 and 430 mg/day in the second and third studies, respectively. Both studies demonstrated statistically significant differences favoring ZONEGRAN for doses of 400–600 mg/day, and there was no apparent difference between once daily and twice daily dosing (in different studies). Analysis of the data (first 4 weeks) during titration demonstrated statistically significant differences favoring ZONEGRAN at doses between 100 and 400 mg/day. The primary comparison in both trials was for any dose over Weeks 5–12.

[See table 1 above]

[See table 2 above]

Table 1. Median % Reduction in All Partial Seizures and % Responders in Primary Efficacy Analyses: Intent-To-Treat Analysis

Study	Median % reduction in partial seizures ZONEGRAN	Placebo	%Responders ZONEGRAN	Placebo
Study 1:	n=98	n=72	n=98	n=72
Weeks 8–12:	40.5%*	9.0%	41.8%*	22.2%
Study 2:	n=69	n=72	n=69	n=72
Weeks 5–12:	29.6%*	-3.2%	29.0%	15.0%
Study 3:	n=67	n=66	n=67	n=66
Weeks 5–12:	27.2%*	-1.1%	28.0%*	12.0%

*p<0.05 compared to placebo

Table 2. Median % Reduction in All Partial Seizures and % Responders for Dose Analyses in Study 1: Intent-To-Treat Analysis

Dose Group	Median % reduction in partial seizures ZONEGRAN	Placebo	%Responders ZONEGRAN	Placebo
100–400 mg/day:	n=112	n=83	n=112	n=83
Weeks 1–12:	32.3%*	5.6%	32.1%*	9.6%
100 mg/day:	n=56	n=80	n=56	n=80
Weeks 1–5:	24.7%*	8.3%	25.0%*	11.3%
200 mg/day:	n=55	n=82	n=55	n=82
Weeks 2–6:	20.4%*	4.0%	25.5%*	9.8%

*p<0.05 compared to placebo

Figure 1 presents the proportion of patients (X-axis) whose percentage reduction from baseline in the all partial seizure rate was at least as great as that indicated on the Y-axis in the second and third placebo-controlled trials. A positive

Continued on next page

Zonegran—Cont.

value on the Y-axis indicates an improvement from baseline (i.e., a decrease in seizure rate), while a negative value indicates a worsening from baseline (i.e., an increase in seizure rate). Thus, in a display of this type, the curve for an effective treatment is shifted to the left of the curve for placebo. The proportion of patients achieving any particular level of reduction in seizure rate was consistenly higher for the ZONEGRAN groups compared to the placebo groups. For example, Figure 1 indicates that approximately 27% of patients treated with ZONEGRAN experienced a 75% or greater reduction, compared to approximately 12% in the placebo groups.

Figure 1 Proportion of Patients Achieving Differing Levels of Seizure Reduction in ZONEGRAN and Placebo Groups in Studies 2 and 3

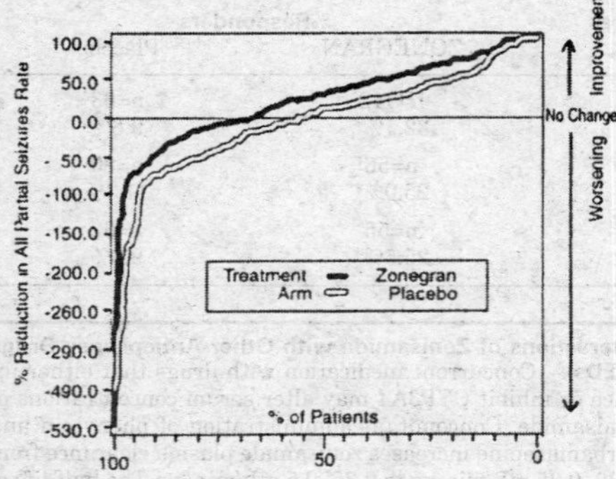

No differences in efficacy based on age, sex or race, as measured by a change in seizure frequency from baseline, were detected.

INDICATIONS AND USAGE

ZONEGRAN is indicated as adjunctive therapy in the treatment of partial seizures in adults with epilepsy.

CONTRAINDICATIONS

ZONEGRAN is contraindicated in patients who have demonstrated hypersensitivity to sulfonamides or zonisamide.

WARNINGS

Potentially Fatal Reactions to Sulfonamides: Fatalities have occurred, although rarely, as a result of severe reactions to sulfonamides (zonisamide is a sulfonamide) including Stevens-Johnson syndrome, toxic epidermal necrolysis, fulminant hepatic necrosis, agranulocytosis, aplastic anemia, and other blood dyscrasias. Such reactions may occur when a sulfonamide is readministered irrespective of the route of administration. If signs of hypersensitivity or other serious reactions occur, discontinue zonisamide immediately. Specific experience with sulfonamide-type adverse reaction to zonisamide is described below.

Serious Skin Reactions: Consideration should be given to discontinuing ZONEGRAN in patients who develop an otherwise unexplained rash. If the drug is not discontinued, patients should be observed frequently. Seven deaths from severe rash [i.e. Stevens-Johnson syndrome (SJS) and toxic epidermal necrolysis (TEN)] were reported in the first 11 years of marketing in Japan. All of the patients were receiving other drugs in addition to zonisamide. In post-marketing experience from Japan, a total of 49 cases of SJS or TEN have been reported, a reporting rate of 46 per million patient-years of exposure. Although this rate is greater than background, it is probably an underestimate of the true incidence because of under-reporting. There were no confirmed cases of SJS or TEN in the US, European, or Japanese development programs.

In the US and European randomized controlled trials, 6 of 269 (2.2%) zonisamide patients discontinued treatment because of rash compared to none on placebo. Across all trials during the US and European development, rash that led to discontinuation of zonisamide was reported in 1.4% of patients (12.0 events per 1000 patient-years of exposure). During Japanese development, serious rash or rash that led to study drug discontinuation was reported in 2.0% of patients (27.8 events per 1000 patient-years). Rash usually occurred early in treatment, with 85% reported within 16 weeks in the US and European studies and 90% reported within two weeks in the Japanese studies. There was no apparent relationship of dose to the occurrence of rash.

Serious Hematologic Events: Two confirmed cases of aplastic anemia and one confirmed case of agranulocytosis were reported in the first 11 years of marketing in Japan, rates greater than generally accepted background rates. There were no cases of aplastic anemia and two confirmed cases of agranulocytosis in the US, European, or Japanese development programs. There is inadequate information to assess the relationship, if any, between dose and duration of treatment and these events.

Oligohydrosis and Hyperthermia in Pediatric Patients: Thirteen cases of oligohydrosis among patients 1.6–17 years of age were reported in the first 11 years of marketing in Japan, a reported rate of 12 per million patient-years of exposure. Temperatures in these patients ranged from 37–42°C. Two of these cases were diagnosed as heatstroke requiring hospitalization. There were no reported cases of oligohydrosis in the US and European development program. During Japanese development, one case (0.1%) was reported among 1008 patients. Doses ranged from 5.0–15.0 mg/kg/day in these patients. Because decreased sweating may be accompanied by elevated body temperature, especially in the summer, body temperature should be carefully monitored. Safety and effectiveness of ZONEGRAN in pediatric patients have not been established. ZONEGRAN is not approved for pediatric use.

Seizures on Withdrawal: As with other AEDs, abrupt withdrawal of ZONEGRAN in patients with epilepsy may precipitate increased seizure frequency or status epilepticus. Dose reduction or discontinuation of zonisamide should be done gradually.

Teratogenicity: Women of child bearing potential who are given zonisamide should be advised to use effective contraception. Zonisamide was teratogenic in mice, rats, and dogs and embryolethal in monkeys when administered during the period of organogenesis. A variety of fetal abnormalities, including cardiovascular defects, and embryo-fetal deaths, occurred at maternal plasma levels similar to or lower than therapeutic levels in humans. These findings suggest that the use of ZONEGRAN during pregnancy in humans may present a significant risk to the fetus (see **PRECAUTIONS, Pregnancy** subsection). It cannot be said with any confidence, however, that even mild seizures do not pose some hazards to the developing fetus. Zonisamide should be used during pregnancy only if the potential benefit justifies the potential risk to the fetus.

Cognitive/Neuropsychiatric Adverse Events: Use of ZONEGRAN was frequently associated with central nervous system-related adverse events. The most significant of these can be classified into three general categories: 1) psychiatric symptoms, including depression and psychosis, 2) psychomotor slowing, difficulty with concentration, and speech or language problems, in particular, word-finding difficulties, and 3) somnolence or fatigue.

In placebo-controlled trials, 2.2% of patients discontinued ZONEGRAN or were hospitalized for depression compared to 0.4% of placebo patients, while 1.1% of ZONEGRAN and 0.4% of placebo patients attempted suicide. Among all epilepsy patients treated with ZONEGRAN, 1.4% were discontinued and 1.0% were hospitalized because of reported depression or suicide attempts. In placebo-controlled trials, 2.2% of patients discontinued ZONEGRAN or were hospitalized due to psychosis or psychosis-related symptoms compared to none of the placebo patients. Among all epilepsy patients treated with ZONEGRAN, 0.9% were discontinued and 1.4% were hospitalized because of reported psychosis or related symptoms.

Psychomotor slowing and difficulty with concentration occurred in the first month of treatment and were associated with doses above 300 mg/day. Speech and language problems tended to occur after 6–10 weeks of treatment and at doses above 300 mg/day. Although in most cases these events were of mild to moderate severity, they at times led to withdrawal from treatment.

Somnolence and fatigue were frequently reported CNS adverse events during clinical trials with ZONEGRAN. Although in most cases these events were of mild to moderate severity, they led to withdrawal from treatment in 0.2% of the patients enrolled in controlled trials. Somnolence and fatigue tended to occur within the first month of treatment. Somnolence and fatigue occurred most frequently at doses of 300–500 mg/day. **Patients should be cautioned about this possibility and special care should be taken by patients if they drive, operate machinery, or perform any hazardous task.**

PRECAUTIONS

General: Somnolence is commonly reported, especially at higher doses of ZONEGRAN (see **WARNINGS: Cognitive/Neuropsychiatric Adverse Events** subsection). Zonisamide is metabolized by the liver and eliminated by the kidneys; caution should therefore be exercised when administering ZONEGRAN to patients with hepatic and renal dysfunction (see **CLINICAL PHARMACOLOGY, Special Populations** subsection).

Kidney Stones: Among 991 patients treated during the development of ZONEGRAN, 40 patients (4.0%) with epilepsy receiving ZONEGRAN developed clinically possible or confirmed kidney stones (e.g. clinical symptomatology, sonography, etc.), a rate of 34 per 1000 patients-years of exposure (40 patients with 1168 years of exposure). Of these, 12 were symptomatic, and 28 were described as possible kidney stones based on sonographic detection. In nine patients, the diagnosis was confirmed by a passage of a stone or by a definitive sonographic finding. The rate of occurrence of kidney stones was 28.7 per 1000 patient-years of exposure in the first six months, 62.6 per 1000 patient-years of exposure between 6 and 12 months, and 24.3 per 1000 patient-years of exposure after 12 months of use. There are no normative sonographic data available for either the general population or patients with epilepsy. The clinical significance of the sonographic finding is unknown. The analyzed stones were composed of calcium or urate salts. In general, increasing fluid intake and urine output can help reduce the risk of stone formation, particularly in those with predisposing risk factors. It is unknown, however, whether these measures will reduce the risk of stone formation in patients treated with ZONEGRAN.

Effect on Renal Function: In several clinical studies, zonisamide was associated with a statistically significant 8% mean increase from baseline of serum creatinine and blood urea nitrogen (BUN) compared to essentially no change in the placebo patients. The increase appeared to persist over time but was not progressive; this has been interpreted as an effect on glomerular filtration rate (GFR). There were no episodes of unexplained acute renal failure in clinical development in the US, Europe, or Japan. The decrease in GFR appeared within the first 4 weeks of treatment. In a 30-day study, the GFR returned to baseline within 2–3 weeks of drug discontinuation. There is no information about reversibility, after drug discontinuation of the effects on GFR after long-term use. ZONEGRAN should be discontinued in patients who develop acute renal failure or a clinically significant sustained increase in the creatinine/BUN concentration. ZONEGRAN should not be used in patients with renal failure (estimated GFR <50 mL/min) as there has been insufficient experience concerning drug dosing and toxicity.

Sudden Unexplained Death in Epilepsy: During the development of ZONEGRAN, nine sudden unexplained deaths occurred among 991 patients with epilepsy receiving ZONEGRAN for whom accurate exposure data are available. This represents an incidence of 7.7 deaths per 1000 patient years. Although this rate exceeds that expected in a healthy population, it is within the range of estimates for the incidence of sudden unexplained deaths in patients with refractory epilepsy not receiving ZONEGRAN (ranging from 0.5 per 1000 patient years for the general population of patients with epilepsy, to 2–5 per 1000 patient years for patients with refractory epilepsy; higher incidences range from 9–15 per 1000 patient years among surgical candidates and surgical failures). Some of the deaths could represent seizure-related deaths in which the seizure was not observed.

Status Epilepticus: Estimates of the incidence of treatment-emergent status epilepticus in ZONEGRAN-treated patients are difficult because a standard definition was not employed. Nonetheless, in controlled trials, 1.1% of patients treated with ZONEGRAN had an event labeled as status epilepticus compared to none of the patients treated with placebo. Among patients treated with ZONEGRAN across all epilepsy studies (controlled and uncontrolled), 1.0% of patients had an event reported as status epilepticus.

Information for Patients: Patients should be advised as follows:

1. **ZONEGRAN may produce drowsiness, especially at higher doses. Patients should be advised not to drive a car or operate other complex machinery until they have gained experience on ZONEGRAN sufficient to determine whether it affects their performance.**
2. Patients should contact their physician immediately if a skin rash develops or seizures worsen.
3. Patients should contact their physician immediately if they develop signs or symptoms, such as sudden back pain, abdominal pain, and/or blood in the urine, that could indicate a kidney stone. Increasing fluid intake and urine output may reduce the risk of stone formation, particularly in those with predisposing risk factors for stones.
4. Patients should contact their physician immediately if a child has been taking ZONEGRAN and is not sweating as usual with or without a fever.
5. Because zonisamide can cause hematological complications, patients should contact their physician immediately if they develop a fever, sore throat, oral ulcers, or easy bruising.
6. As with other AEDs, patients should contact their physician if they intend to become pregnant or are pregnant during ZONEGRAN therapy. Patients should notify their physician if they intend to breast-feed or are breast-feeding an infant.

Laboratory Tests: In several clinical studies, zonisamide was associated with a mean increase in the concentration of serum creatinine and blood urea nitrogen (BUN) of approximately 8% over the baseline measurement. Consideration should be given to monitoring renal function periodically (see **PRECAUTIONS, Effect on Renal Function** subsection).

Zonisamide was associated with an increase in serum alkaline phosphatase. In the randomized, controlled trials, a mean increase of approximately 7% over baseline was associated with zonisamide compared to a 3% mean increase in placebo-treated patients. These changes were not statistically significant. The clinical relevance of these changes is unknown.

Drug Interactions: *Effects of ZONEGRAN on the pharmacokinetics of other antiepilepsy drugs (AEDs):* Zonisamide had no appreciable effect on the steady state plasma concentrations of phenytoin, carbamazepine, or valproate during clinical trials. Zonisamide did not inhibit mixed-function liver oxidase enzymes (cytochrome P450), as measured in human liver microsomal preparations, *in vitro*. Zonisamide is not expected to interfere with the metabolism of other drugs that are metabolized by cytochrome P450 isozymes.

Effects of other drugs on ZONEGRAN pharmacokinetics: Drugs that induce liver enzymes increase the metabolism and clearance of zonisamide and decrease its half-life. The half-life of zonisamide following a 400 mg dose in patients concurrently on enzyme-inducing AEDs such as phenytoin, carbamazepine, or phenobarbital was between 27–38 hours; the half-life of zonisamide in patients concurrently on the non-enzyme inducing AED, valproate, was 46 hours. Concurrent medication with drugs that either induce or inhibit CYP3A4 would be expected to alter serum concentrations of zonisamide.

Interaction with cimetidine: Zonisamide single dose pharmacokinetic parameters were not affected by cimetidine (300 mg four times a day for 12 days).

Carcinogenicity, Mutagenesis, Impairment of Fertility: No evidence of cacinogenicity was found in mice or rats following dietary administration of zonisamide for two years at doses of up to 80 mg/kg/day. In mice, this dose is approximately equivalent to the maximum recommended human dose (MRHD) of 400 mg/day on a mg/m^2 basis. In rats, this dose is 1–2 times the MRHD on a mg/m^2 basis.

Zonisamide increased mutation frequency in Chinese hamster lung cells in the absence of metabolic activation. Zonisamide was not mutagenic or clastogenic in the Ames test, mouse lymphoma assay, sister chromatid exchange test, and human lymphocyte cytogenetics assay *in vitro*, and the rat bone marrow cytogenetics assay *in vivo*.

Rats treated with zonisamide (20, 60, or 200 mg/kg) before mating and during the initial gestation phase showed signs of reproductive toxicity (decreased corpora lutea, implantations, and live fetuses) at all doses. The low dose in this study is approximately 0.5 times the maximum recommended human dose (MRHD) on a mg/m^2 basis. The effect of zonisamide on human fertility is unknown.

Pregnancy: Pregnancy Category C (see **WARNINGS, Teratogenicity** subsection):

Zonisamide was teratogenic in mice, rats, and dogs and embryolethal in monkeys when administered during the period of organogenesis. Fetal abnormalities or embryo-fetal deaths occurred in these species at zonisamide dosage and maternal plasma levels similar to or lower than therapeutic levels in humans, indicating that use of this drug in pregnancy entails a significant risk to the fetus. A variety of external, visceral, and skeletal malformations was produced in animals by prenatal exposure to zonisamide. Cardiovascular defects were prominent in both rats and dogs.

Following administration of zonisamide (10, 30, or 60 mg/kg/day) to pregnant dogs during organogenesis, increased incidences of fetal cardiovascular malformations (ventricular septal defects, cardiomegaly, various valvular and arterial anomalies) were found at doses of 30 mg/kg/day or greater. The low effect dose for malformations produced peak maternal plasma zonisamide levels (25 µg/mL) about 0.5 times the highest plasma levels measured in patients receiving the maximum recommended human dose (MRHD) of 400 mg/day. In dogs, cardiovascular malformations were found in approximately 50% of all fetuses exposed to the high dose, which was associated with maternal plasma levels (44 µg/mL) approximately equal to the highest levels measured in humans receiving the MRHD. Incidences of skeletal malformations were also increased at the high dose, and fetal growth retardation and increased frequencies of skeletal variations were seen at all doses in this study. The low dose produced maternal plasma levels (12 µg/mL) about 0.25 times the highest human levels.

In cynomolgus monkeys, administration of zonisamide (10 or 20 mg/kg/day) to pregnant animals during organogenesis resulted in embryo-fetal deaths at both doses. The possibility that these deaths were due to malformations cannot be ruled out. The lowest embryolethal dose in monkeys was associated with peak maternal plasma zonisamide levels (5 µg/mL) approximately 0.1 times the highest levels measured in patients at the MRHD.

In a mouse embryo-fetal development study, treatment of pregnant animals with zonisamide (125, 250, or 500 mg/kg/day) during the period of organogenesis resulted in increased incidences of fetal malformations (skeletal and/or craniofacial defects) at all doses tested. The low dose in this study is approximately 1.5 times the MRHD on a mg/m^2 basis. In rats, increased frequencies of malformations (cardiovascular defects) and variations (persistence cords of thymic tissue, decreased skeletal ossification) were observed among the offspring of dams treated with zonisamide (20, 60, or 200 mg/kg/day) throughout organogenesis at all doses. The low effect dose is approximately 0.5 times the MRHD on a mg/m^2 basis.

Perinatal death was increased among the offspring of rats treated with zonisamide (10, 30, or 60 mg/kg/day) from the latter part of gestation up to weaning at the high dose, or approximately 1.4 times the MRHD on a mg/m^2 basis. The no effect level of 30 mg/kg/day is approximately 0.7 times the MRHD on a mg/m^2 basis.

There are no adequate and well-controlled studies in pregnant women. ZONEGRAN should be used during pregnancy only if the potential benefit justifies the potential risk to the fetus.

Labor and Delivery: The effect of ZONEGRAN on labor and delivery in humans is not known.

Use in Nursing Mothers: It is not known whether zonisamide is excreted in human milk. Because many drugs are excreted in human milk and because of the potential for serious adverse reactions in nursing infants from zonisamide, a decision should be made whether to discontinue nursing or to discontinue drug, taking into account the importance of the drug to the mother. ZONEGRAN should be used in nursing mothers only if the benefits outweigh the risks.

Pediatric Use: The safety and effectiveness of ZONEGRAN in children under age 16 have not been established. Cases of oligohydrosis and hyperpyrexia have been reported (see **WARNINGS, Oligohydrosis and Hyperthermia in Pediatric Patients** subsection).

Geriatric Use: Single dose pharmacokinetic parameters are similar in elderly and young healthy volunteers (see **CLINICAL PHARMACOLOGY, Special Populations** subsection). Clinical studies of zonisamide did not include sufficient numbers of subjects aged 65 and over to determine whether they respond differently from younger subjects. Other reported clinical experience has not identified differences in responses between the elderly and younger patients. In general, dose selection for an elderly patient should be cautious, usually starting at the low end of the dosing range, reflecting the greater frequency of decreased hepatic, renal, or cardiac function, and of concomitant disease or other drug therapy.

TABLE 3: Incidence (%) of Treatment-Emergent Adverse Events in Placebo-Controlled, Add-On Trials (Events that occurred in at least 2% of ZONEGRAN-treated patients and occurred more frequently in ZONEGRAN-treated than placebo-treated patients)

BODY SYSTEM/ PREFERRED TERM	ZONEGRAN (n=269) %	Placebo (n=230) %
BODY AS A WHOLE		
Headache	10	8
Abdominal Pain	6	3
Flu Syndrome	4	3
DIGESTIVE		
Anorexia	13	6
Nausea	9	6
Diarrhea	5	2
Dyspepsia	3	1
Constipation	2	1
Dry Mouth	2	1
HEMATOLOGIC AND LYMPHATIC		
Ecchymosis	2	1
METABOLIC AND NUTRITIONAL		
Weight Loss	3	2
NERVOUS SYSTEM		
Dizziness	13	7
Ataxia	6	1
Nystagmus	4	2
Paresthesia	4	1
NEUROPSYCHIATRIC AND COGNITIVE DYSFUNCTION-ALTERED COGNITIVE FUNCTION		
Confusion	6	3
Difficulty Concentrating	6	2
Difficulty with Memory	6	2
Mental Slowing	4	2
NEUROPSYCHIATRIC AND COGNITIVE DYSFUNCTION-ALTERED BEHAVIORAL ABNORMALITIES (NON-PSYCHOSIS-RELATED)		
Agitation/Irritability	9	4
Depression	6	3
Insomnia	6	3
Anxiety	3	2
Nervousness	2	1
NEUROPSYCHIATRIC AND COGNITIVE DYSFUNCTION-BEHAVIORAL ABNORMALITIES (PSYCHOSIS-RELATED)		
Schizophrenic/Schizophreniform Behavior	2	0
NEUROPSYCHIATRIC AND COGNITIVE DYSFUNCTION-CNS DEPRESSION		
Somnolence	17	7
Fatigue	8	6
Tiredness	7	5
NEUROPSYCHIATRIC AND COGNITIVE DYSFUNCTION-SPEECH AND LANGUAGE ABNORMALITIES		
Speech Abnormalities	5	2
Difficulties in Verbal Expression	2	<1
RESPIRATORY		
Rhinitis	2	1
SKIN AND APPENDAGES		
Rash	3	2
SPECIAL SENSES		
Diplopia	6	3
Taste Perversion	2	0

ADVERSE REACTIONS

The most commonly observed adverse events associated with the use of ZONEGRAN in controlled clinical trials that were not seen at an equivalent frequency among placebo-treated patients were somnolence, anorexia, dizziness, headache, nausea, and agitation/irritability.

In controlled clinical trials, 12% of patients receiving ZONEGRAN as adjunctive therapy discontinued due to an adverse event compared to 6% receiving placebo. Approximately 21% of the 1,336 patients with epilepsy who received ZONEGRAN in clinical studies discontinued treatment because of an adverse event. The adverse events most commonly associated with discontinuation were somnolence, fatigue and/or ataxia (6%), anorexia (3%), difficulty concentrating (2%), difficulty with memory, mental slowing, nausea/vomiting (2%), and weight loss (1%). Many of these adverse events were dose-related (see **WARNINGS** and **PRECAUTIONS**).

Adverse Event Incidence in Controlled Clinical Trials: Table 3 lists treatment-emergent adverse events that occurred in

Continued on next page

Zonegran—Cont.

at least 2% of patients treated with ZONEGRAN in controlled clinical trials that were numerically more common in the ZONEGRAN group. In these studies, either ZONEGRAN or placebo was added to the patient's current AED therapy. Adverse events were usually mild or moderate in intensity.

The prescriber should be aware that these figures, obtained when ZONEGRAN was added to concurrent AED therapy, cannot be used to predict the frequency of adverse events in the course of usual medical practice when patient characteristics and other factors may differ from those prevailing during clinical studies. Similarly, the cited frequencies cannot be directly compared with figures obtained from other clinical investigations involving different treatments, uses, or investigators. An inspection of these frequencies, however, does provide the prescriber with one basis by which to estimate the relative contribution of drug and non-drug factors to the adverse event incidences in the population studied.

[See table 3 on previous page]

Other Adverse Events Observed During Clinical Trials: ZONEGRAN has been administered to 1,598 individuals during all clinical trials, only some of which were placebo-controlled. During these trials, all events were recorded by the investigators using their own terms. To provide a useful estimate of the proportion of individuals having adverse events, similar events have been grouped into a smaller number of standardized categories using a modified COSTART dictionary. The frequencies represent the proportion of the 1,598 individuals exposed to ZONEGRAN who experienced an event on at least one occasion. All events are included except those already listed in the previous table or discussed in **WARNINGS** or **PRECAUTIONS**, trivial events, those too general to be informative, and those not reasonably associated with ZONEGRAN.

Events further classified within each category and listed in order of decreasing frequency as follows: frequent occurring in at least 1:100 patients; infrequent occurring in 1:100 to 1:1000 patients; rare occurring in fewer than 1:1000 patients.

Body as a Whole: *Frequent:* Accidental injury, asthenia. *Infrequent:* Chest pain, flank pain, malaise, allergic reaction, face edema, neck rigidity. *Rare:* Lupus erythematosus.

Cardiovascular: *Infrequent:* Palpitation, tachycardia, vascular insufficiency, hypotension, hypertension, thrombophlebitis, syncope, bradycardia. *Rare:* Atrial fibrillation, heart failure, pulmonary embolus, ventricular extrasystoles.

Digestive: *Frequent:* Vomiting. *Infrequent:* Flatulence, gingivitis, gum hyperplasia, gastritis, gastroenteritis, stomatitis, cholelithiasis, glossitis, melena, rectal hemorrhage, ulcerative stomatitis, gastro-duodenal ulcer, dysphagia, gum hemorrhage. *Rare:* Cholangitis, hematemesis, cholecystitis, cholestatic jaundice, colitis, duodenitis, esophagitis, fecal incontinence, mouth ulceration.

Hematologic and Lymphatic: *Infrequent:* Leukopenia, anemia, immunodeficiency, lymphadenopathy. *Rare:* Thrombocytopenia, microcytic anemia, petechia.

Metabolic and Nutritional: *Infrequent:* Peripheral edema, weight gain, edema, thirst, dehydration. *Rare:* Hypoglycemia, hyponatremia, lactic dehydrogenase increased, SGOT increased, SGPT increased.

Musculoskeletal: *Infrequent:* Leg cramps, myalgia, myasthenia, arthralgia, arthritis.

Nervous System: *Frequent:* Tremor, convulsion, abnormal gait, hyperesthesia, incoordination. *Infrequent:* Hypertonia, twitching, abnormal dreams, vertigo, libido decreased, neuropathy, hyperkinesia, movement disorder, dysarthria, cerebrovascular accident, hypotonia, peripheral neuritis, paresthesia, reflexes increased. *Rare:* Circumoral paresthesia, dyskinesia, dystonia, encephalopathy, facial paralysis, hypokinesia, hyperesthesia, myoclonus, oculogyric crisis.

Behavioral Abnormalities—Non-Psychosis-Related: *Infrequent:* Euphoria.

Respiratory: *Frequent:* Pharyngitis, cough increased. *Infrequent:* Dyspnea. *Rare:* Apnea, hemoptysis.

Skin and Appendages: *Frequent:* Pruritus. *Infrequent:* Maculopapular rash, acne, alopecia, dry skin, sweating, eczema, urticaria, hirsutism, pustular rash, vesiculobullous rash.

Special Senses: *Frequent:* Ambylopia, tinnitus. *Infrequent:* Conjuctivitis, parosmia, deafness, visual field defect, glaucoma. *Rare:* Photophobia, iritis.

Urogenital: *Infrequent:* Urinary frequency, dysuria, urinary incontinence, hematura, impotence, urinary retention, urinary urgency, amenorrhea, polyuria, nocturia. *Rare:* Albuninuria, enuresis, bladder pain, bladder calculus, gynocomastia, mastitis, menorrhagia.

DRUG ABUSE AND DEPENDENCE

The abuse and dependence potential of ZONEGRAN has not been evaluated in human studies (see **WARNINGS, Cognitive/Neuropsychiatric Adverse Events** subsection). In a series of animal studies, zonisamide did not demonstrate abuse liability and dependence potential. Monkeys did not self-administer zonisamide in a standard reinforcing paradigm. Rats exposed to zonisamide did not exhibit signs of physical dependence of the CNS-depressant type. Rats did not generalize the effects of diazepam to zonisamide in a standard discrimination paradigm after training, suggesting that zonisamide does not have abuse potential of the benzodiazepine-CNS depressant type.

OVERDOSAGE

Human Experience: Experience with ZONEGRAN daily doses over 800 mg/day is limited. During ZONEGRAN clinical development, three patients ingested unknown amounts of ZONEGRAN as suicide attempts, and all three were hospitalized with CNS symptoms. One patient became comatose and developed bradycardia, hypotension, and respiratory depression; the zonisamide plasma level was 100.1 μg/mL measured 31 hours post-ingestion. Zonisamide plasma levels fell with a half-life of 57 hours, and the patient became alert five days later.

Management: No specific antidotes for ZONEGRAN overdosage are available. Following a suspected recent overdosage, emesis should be induced or gastric lavage performed with the usual precautions to protect the airway. General supportive care is indicated, including frequent monitoring of vital signs and close observation.

Zonisamide has a long half-life (see **CLINICAL PHARMACOLOGY** section). Due to the low protein binding of zonisamide (40%), renal dialysis may not be effective. A poison control center should be contacted for information on the management of ZONEGRAN overdosage.

DOSAGE AND ADMINISTRATION

ZONEGRAN (zonisamide) is recommended as adjunctive therapy for the treatment of partial seizures in adults. Safety and efficacy in pediatric patients below the age of 16 have not been established. ZONEGRAN should be administered once or twice daily, except for the daily dose of 100 mg at the initiation of therapy. ZONEGRAN is given orally and can be taken with or without food. Capsules should be swallowed whole.

Adults over Age 16: The prescriber should be aware that, because of the long half-life of zonisamide, up to two weeks may be required to achieve steady state levels upon reaching a stable dose or following dosage adjustment. Although the regimen described below is one that has been shown to be tolerated, the prescriber may wish to prolong the duration of treatment at the lower doses in order to fully assess the effects of zonisamide at steady state, noting that many of the side effects of zonisamide are more frequent at doses of 300 mg per day and above. Although there is some evidence of greater response at doses above 100–200 mg/day, the increase appears small and formal dose-response studies have not been conducted.

The initial dose should be 100 mg daily. After two weeks, the dose may be increased to 200 mg/day for at least two weeks. It can be increased to 300 mg/day and 400 mg/day, with the dose stable for at least two weeks to achieve steady state at each level. Evidence from controlled trials suggests that ZONEGRAN doses of 100–600 mg/day are effective, but there is no suggestion of increasing response above 400 mg/day (see **CLINICAL PHARMACOLOGY, Clinical Studies** subsection). There is little experience with doses greater than 600 mg/day.

Patients with Renal or Hepatic Disease: Because zonisamide is metabolized in the liver and excreted by the kidneys, patients with renal or hepatic disease should be treated with caution, and might require slower titration and more frequent monitoring (see **CLINICAL PHARMACOLOGY** and **PRECAUTIONS**).

HOW SUPPLIED

ZONEGRAN is available as a 100 mg two-piece hard gelatin capsule consisting of a white opaque body with a red opaque cap. The capsules are printed with a company logo and "ZONEGRAN 100" in black. They are supplied in:

Bottles of 100 NDC #59075-680-10

Store at 25°C (77°F), excursions permitted to 15–30° C (59–86°F) [see USP Controlled Room Temperature], in a dry place and protected from light.

US Patent #4,172,896.

ANIMAL TOXICOLOGY

In dogs treated with zonisamide (10, 30, or 75 mg/kg/day) for 1 year, dark brown discoloration of the liver and concentric lamellar bodies in the cytoplasm of hepatocytes were observed in association with clinical chemistry changes indicative of liver damage (elevated alkaline phosphatase, gamma glutamyl transferase, and alanine amino transferase; decreased albumin) and altered drug metabolism at the highest dose, which is approximately 6 times the maximum recommended human dose (MRHD) of 400 mg/day on a mg/m^2 basis. Gross liver changes not clearly accompanied by biochemical evidence of hepatotoxicity were noted at 30 mg/kg/day, or approximately 2.4 times the MRHD on mg/m^2 basis. The no effect dose of 10 mg/kg/day is slightly less than the MRHD on mg/m^2 basis. The significance of these findings for humans is not known.

Distributed by:
Elan Pharma,
a business unit of Elan Pharmaceuticals.
South San Francisco, CA 94080
ZONEGRAN is a trademark licensed exclusively to Elan Pharmaceuticals, Inc.

March 30, 2000

PATIENT INFORMATION LEAFLET
Questions and Answers about ZONEGRAN™ (zonisamide) capsules

What is the most important information I should know about ZONEGRAN?

Some people taking ZONEGRAN (ZON-uh-gran) can get serious reactions. **If you get any of the following symptoms, call your doctor right away:**

- Rash (may be a sign of a dangerous condition)
- Fever, sore throat, sores in your mouth, or bruising easily (may be signs of a blood problem)
- Sudden back pain, abdominal (stomach area) pain, pain when urinating, bloody or dark urine (may be signs of a kidney stone)
- Decreased sweating or a rise in body temperature (especially in patients under 17 years old)
- Depression
- Thoughts that are unusual for you
- Speech or language problems

ZONEGRAN can cause drowsiness and coordination problems. **Do not drive or operate dangerous machinery until you know how ZONEGRAN affects you.**

What is ZONEGRAN?

ZONEGRAN is a medicine to treat partial seizures in adults. It is taken with other seizure medicines to help control your seizures.

Who should not take ZONEGRAN?

Talk to your doctor first before stopping ZONEGRAN.

Tell your doctor if you are allergic to sulfa drugs. Do not take ZONEGRAN if you are allergic to any sulfa drugs (for example, Bactrim™ or Septra®) or ZONEGRAN.

How should I take ZONEGRAN?

Be sure to follow your doctor's directions. Starting a new medicine can be confusing. If you have any questions, call your doctor.

Start with one ZONEGRAN capsule each day (100 mg). Swallow the capsule whole. Do not bite into or break the capsule. You may take this medicine with or without food. After a week or so, your doctor may increase your dose of ZONEGRAN. This may occur more than once. It is done to get the best control for your seizures. Take only the number of ZONEGRAN capsules you were told to take.

Talk to your doctor about what to do if you miss a dose.

If you think you have overdosed on your medicine, call your local poison control center or emergency room right away.

Drink 6–8 glasses of water a day. This may help prevent kidney stones.

Talk to your doctor before stopping ZONEGRAN or any other seizure medicine. Stopping a seizure medicine all at once can cause status epilepticus, a serious problem.

What should I avoid while taking ZONEGRAN?

ZONEGRAN may make you drowsy. Do not drive a car or operate complex machinery until you know how ZONEGRAN may affect you.

Tell your doctor about any other medicines you may be taking, including non-prescription medicines.

Tell your doctor right away if you are pregnant or plan to become pregnant. You and your doctor can decide if the benefits of taking ZONEGRAN outweigh the risks. ZONEGRAN may cause birth defects.

It is not known whether ZONEGRAN is passed through breast milk to the baby. Before taking ZONEGRAN, tell your doctor if you are nursing or planning to nurse your baby.

What are the possible or reasonably likely side effects of ZONEGRAN?

The most common side effects are drowsiness, loss of appetite, dizziness, headache, nausea, agitation, and irritability. These side effects could occur at any time, but most often occur in the first 4 weeks.

Contact your doctor right away if:

- you develop skin rash
- your seizures worsen
- you develop signs of kidney stones (sudden back pain, abdominal pain, blood in your urine)
- you develop signs of a blood problem (fever, sore throat, sores in your mouth, or bruising easily)
- you get depressed
- you start having thoughts that are unusual for you
- you are very drowsy, have difficulty concentrating, or have coordination problems
- you develop speech or language problems

Other information about ZONEGRAN:

Medicines are sometimes prescribed for purposes other than those listed in a patient leaflet. Use ZONEGRAN only for the reason your doctor told you. Do not use it for another reason. Do not share your ZONEGRAN with others.

This is a summary of information about ZONEGRAN. Call your healthcare professional with any questions. Your doctor or pharmacist can give you the complete information about ZONEGRAN that is written for health professionals. You can also get information about ZONEGRAN at www.elanpharma.com. You can get information and help from the Epilepsy Foundation at 800-EFA-1000 or www.efa.org.

Distributed by:
Elan Pharma,
a business unit of Elan Pharmaceuticals.
South San Francisco, CA 94080
ZONEGRAN is a trademark licensed exclusively to Elan Pharmaceuticals, Inc.
All other product names may be trademarks of the respective companies with which they are associated.

Shown in Product Identification Guide, page 312

Elkins-Sinn, Inc.

2 ESTERBROOK LANE
CHERRY HILL, NJ 08003-4099

Direct Inquiries to:
Professional Service
(610) 688-4400

For Emergency Medical Information Contact:
Day: (800) 934–5556 8:30 AM to 4:30 PM (Eastern Standard Time), Weekdays only
Night: (610) 688-4400 (Emergencies only; non-emergencies should wait until the next day)

For Medical/Pharmacy Inquiries on Marketed Products Call:
(800) 934-5556 8:30 AM to 4:30 PM
(Eastern Standard Time), Weekdays only

Elkins-Sinn's DOSETTE® line offers a broad spectrum of injectable products in a variety of unit-of-use containers—DOSETTE® vials, DOSETTE® ampuls, DOSETTE® syringes, and DOSETTE® cartridge-needle units. Easily adaptable to any hospital pharmacy set-up, the DOSETTE® system combines easily identifiable, clearly printed product labeling with space-conserving packaging. Each DOSETTE® container is characterized by product name and strength in large, bold-faced type, important usage and storage data, lot identification number, and expiration date.
Elkins-Sinn also produces a vast number of multiple dose vials. Listed below are the major ESI products. For prescribing information on products listed, write to Professional Service, Wyeth-Ayerst Laboratories, P.O. Box 8299, Philadelphia, PA 19101, or contact your local Wyeth-Ayerst representative.

AMIKACIN SULFATE INJECTION, USP
250 mg/mL 2 mL Dosette Vial
250 mg/mL 4 mL Vial

ATROPINE SULFATE INJECTION, USP
400 mcg/mL (0.4 mg, 1/150 gr) 1 mL Dosette Ampul
400 mcg/mL (0.4 mg, 1/150 gr) 20 mL Multiple Dose Vial

CHLORPROMAZINE HYDROCHLORIDE INJECTION, USP
25 mg/mL 1 mL Dosette Ampul
50 mg/2 mL 2 mL Dosette Ampul

CYANOCOBALAMIN INJECTION, USP
1 mg/mL (1000 mcg) 1 mL Dosette Vial
1 mg/mL (1000 mcg) 30 mL Multiple Dose Vial

DEXAMETHASONE SODIUM PHOSPHATE INJECTION, USP
4 mg/mL 5 mL Multiple Dose Vial
10 mg/mL 1 mL Dosette Vial
10 mg/mL 10 mL Multiple Dose Vial

DIAZEPAM INJECTION, USP (CIV)
5 mg/mL 1 mL Dosette Vial
5 mg/mL 10 mL Multiple Dose Vial
5 mg/mL 1 mL Dosette Syringe
10 mg/2 mL 2 mL Dosette Vial
10 mg/2 mL 2 mL Dosette Ampul
10 mg/2 mL 2 mL Dosette Syringe

DIGOXIN INJECTION, USP
500 mcg/2 mL (0.5 mg) 2 mL Dosette Ampul

DIPHENHYDRAMINE HYDROCHLORIDE INJECTION, USP
50 mg/mL 1 mL Dosette Vial

DIPYRIDAMOLE INJECTION, USP
5 mg/mL 2 mL Syringe
5 mg/mL 10 mL Multiple Dose Vial

DURAMORPH® (Morphine Sulfate Injection, USP) (CII) (Preservative-Free for Epidural & Intrathecal Administration)
5 mg/10 mL (0.5 mg/mL) 10 mL Dosette Ampul
10 mg/10 mL (1 mg/mL) 10 mL Dosette Ampul

EPINEPHRINE INJECTION, USP
1 mg/mL (1:1000) 1 mL Dosette Ampul

FENTANYL CITRATE INJECTION, USP (Preservative-Free) (CII)
100 mcg/2 mL (0.05 mg/mL) 2 mL Dosette Ampul
250 mcg/5 mL (0.05 mg/mL) 5 mL Dosette Ampul
500 mcg/10 mL (0.05 mg/mL) 10 mL Dosette Ampul
1000 mcg/20 mL (0.05 mg/mL) 20 mL Dosette Ampul
1500 mcg/30 mL Single Dose Vial
2500 mcg/50 mL Single Dose Vial

GENTAMICIN SULFATE INJECTION, USP
20 mg/2 mL (10 mg/mL—Pediatric) 2 mL Dosette Vial
80 mg/2 mL (40 mg/mL) 2 mL Dosette Vial
800 mg/20 mL (40 mg/mL) 20 mL Multiple Dose Vial

GENTAMICIN SULFATE INJECTION, USP DOSETTE CARTRIDGE NEEDLE UNITS
60 mg/1.5 mL 1.5 mL Dosette Cartridge
80 mg/2 mL 2 mL Dosette Cartridge

HEPARIN SODIUM INJECTION, USP (Porcine Derived)
1,000 Units/mL 1 mL Dosette Vial
5,000 Units/mL 1 mL Dosette Vial
5,000 Units/mL 10 mL Multiple Dose Vial
10,000 Units/mL 1 mL Dosette Vial

HEP-LOCK® (Heparin Lock Flush Solution, USP)
10 Units/mL 1 mL Dosette Vial
10 Units/mL 2 mL Dosette Vial
10 Units/mL 10 mL Multiple Dose Vial
10 Units/mL 30 mL Multiple Dose Vial
100 Units/mL 1 mL Dosette Vial
100 Units/mL 2 mL Dosette Vial
100 Units/mL 10 mL Multiple Dose Vial
100 Units/mL 30 mL Multiple Dose Vial

HEP-LOCK® (Preservative-Free Heparin Lock Flush Solution, USP)
10 Units/mL 1 mL Dosette Vial
100 Units/mL 1 mL Dosette Vial

HYDROMORPHONE HYDROCHLORIDE INJECTION, USP (CII)
2 mg/mL 1 mL Dosette Vial
2 mg/mL 20 mL Multiple Dose Vial

HYDROXYZINE HYDROCHLORIDE I.M. INJECTION, USP
50 mg/mL 1 mL Dosette Vial
100 mg/2 mL 2 mL Dosette Vial
50 mg/mL 10 mL Multiple Dose Vial

INFUMORPH® 200 (Preservative-free Morphine Sulfate Sterile Solution) (CII) For Use in Continuous Microinfusion Devices
200 mg/20 mL (10 mg/mL) 20 mL Dosette Ampul

INFUMORPH® 500 (Preservative-free Morphine Sulfate Sterile Solution) (CII) For Use in Continuous Microinfusion Devices
500 mg/20 mL (25 mg/mL) 20 mL Dosette Ampul

ISOPROTERENOL HYDROCHLORIDE INJECTION, USP (Refrigeration not required)
0.2 mg/mL (1:5000) 5 mL Dosette Ampul

LEUCOVORIN CALCIUM FOR INJECTION (Lyophilized)
50 mg Single Use Vial
100 mg Single Use Vial

LIDOCAINE HYDROCHLORIDE INJECTION, USP (Preserved)
1% (10 mg/mL) 30 mL Multiple Dose Vial
1% (10 mg/mL) 50 mL Multiple Dose Vial
2% (20 mg/mL) 30 mL Multiple Dose Vial
2% (20 mg/mL) 50 mL Multiple Dose Vial

LIDOCAINE HYDROCHLORIDE INJECTION, USP (Preservative-Free, Single Use)
1% (10 mg/mL) 5 mL Single Use Vial

LIDOCAINE HYDROCHLORIDE AND EPINEPHRINE INJECTION, USP (1:100,000) (Refrigeration not required)
1% (10 mg/mL) 30 mL Multiple Dose Vial
2% (20 mg/mL) 30 mL Multiple Dose Vial

LORAZEPAM INJECTION, USP (CIV)
2 mg/mL 1 mL Dosette Cartridge
4 mg/mL 1 mL Dosette Cartridge

MEPERIDINE HYDROCHLORIDE INJECTION, USP (CII)
25 mg/mL 1 mL Dosette Vial
50 mg/mL 1 mL Dosette Vial
75 mg/mL 1 mL Dosette Vial
75 mg/mL 1 mL Dosette Ampul
100 mg/mL 1 mL Dosette Vial

MORPHINE SULFATE INJECTION, USP (CII)
1 mg/mL 60 mL Single Use Vial
5 mg/mL ($^1/_{12}$ gr) 1 mL Dosette Vial
8 mg/mL ($^1/_8$ gr) 1 mL Dosette Vial
8 mg/mL ($^1/_8$ gr) 1 mL Dosette Ampul
10 mg/mL ($^1/_6$ gr) 1 mL Dosette Vial
10 mg/mL ($^1/_6$ gr) 1 mL Dosette Ampul
10 mg/mL ($^1/_6$ gr) 10 mL Multiple Dose Vial
15 mg/mL ($^1/_4$ gr) 1 mL Dosette Vial
15 mg/mL ($^1/_4$ gr) 1 mL Dosette Ampul
15 mg/mL ($^1/_4$ gr) 20 mL Multiple Dose Vial

NALOXONE HYDROCHLORIDE INJECTION, USP
400 mcg/mL (0.4 mg/mL) 1 mL Dosette Ampul
400 mcg/mL (0.4 mg/mL) 10 mL Multiple Dose Vial

NEOSTIGMINE METHYLSULFATE INJECTION, USP
1:1000 (1 mg/mL) 10 mL Multiple Dose Vial
1:2000 (0.5 mg/mL) 10 mL Multiple Dose Vial

PANCURONIUM BROMIDE INJECTION
1 mg/mL 10 mL Multiple Dose Vial
2 mg/mL 2 mL Dosette Vial
2 mg/mL 2 mL Dosette Ampul
2 mg/mL 5 mL Dosette Ampul
2 mg/mL 5 mL Single Use Vial

PHENOBARBITAL SODIUM INJECTION, USP (CIV)
65 mg/mL (1 gr) 1 mL Dosette Vial
130 mg/mL (2 gr) 1 mL Dosette Vial

PHENYLEPHRINE HYDROCHLORIDE INJECTION, USP
10 mg/mL 1 mL Dosette Vial

PHENYTOIN SODIUM INJECTION, USP
100 mg/2 mL (50 mg/mL) 2 mL Dosette Vial
250 mg/5 mL (50 mg/mL) 5 mL Single Use Vial

PROCAINAMIDE HYDROCHLORIDE INJECTION, USP
100 mg/mL (1 gram/10 mL) 10 mL Multiple Dose Vial
500 mg/mL (1 gram/2 mL) 2 mL Multiple Dose Vial

PROCHLORPERAZINE EDISYLATE INJECTION, USP
10 mg/2 mL 2 mL Dosette Vial

PROMETHAZINE HYDROCHLORIDE INJECTION, USP
25 mg/mL 1 mL Dosette Ampul
50 mg/mL 1 mL Dosette Ampul

PROTAMINE SULFATE INJECTION, USP (Preservative-Free) (Refrigeration not required)
50 mg/5 mL 5 mL Dosette Ampul
250 mg/25 mL 25 mL Single Use Vial

SODIUM CHLORIDE INJECTION, USP (Preservative-Free, Single Use)
0.9% 2 mL Dosette Vial
0.9% 5 mL Dosette Ampul
0.9% 10 mL Dosette Ampul

SODIUM CHLORIDE INJECTION, BACTERIOSTATIC, USP (Preserved with 0.9% Benzyl Alcohol)
0.9% 30 mL Multiple Dose Vial
0.9% 2 mL Dosette Cartridge

SOTRADECOL® (Sodium Tetradecyl Sulfate Injection)
1% 2 mL Dosette Ampul
3% 2 mL Dosette Ampul

SUFENTANIL CITRATE INJECTION, USP
500 mcg/mL 1 mL Dosette Ampul
100 mcg/2 mL 2 mL Dosette Ampul
250 mcg/5 mL 5 mL Dosette Ampul

SULFAMETHOXAZOLE & TRIMETHOPRIM CONCENTRATE FOR INJECTION, USP
80 mg/mL Sulfamethoxazole with 16 mg/mL Trimethoprim 5 mL Single Use Vial
80 mg/mL Sulfamethoxazole with 16 mg/mL Trimethoprim 10 mL Single Use Vial
80 mg/mL Sulfamethoxazole with 16 mg/mL Trimethoprim 30 mL Multiple Dose Vial

THIAMINE HYDROCHLORIDE INJECTION, USP
100 mg/mL 1 mL Dosette Vial

AMIKACIN ℞
[*ă 'mĭ-că-sĭn*]
SULFATE INJECTION, USP

WARNINGS

Patients treated with parenteral aminoglycosides should be under close clinical observation because of the potential ototoxicity and nephrotoxicity associated with their use. Safety for treatment periods which are longer than 14 days has not been established.
Neurotoxicity, manifested as vestibular and permanent bilateral auditory ototoxicity, can occur in patients with preexisting renal damage and in patients with normal renal function treated at higher doses and/or for periods longer than those recommended. The risk of aminoglycoside-induced ototoxicity is greater in patients with renal damage. High frequency deafness usually occurs first and can be detected only by audiometric testing. Vertigo may occur and may be evidence of vestibular injury. Other manifestations of neurotoxicity may include numbness, skin tingling, muscle twitching and convulsions. The risk of hearing loss due to aminoglycosides increases with the degree of exposure to either high peak or high trough serum concentrations. Patients developing cochlear damage may not have symptoms during therapy to warn them of developing eighth-nerve toxicity, and total or partial irreversible bilateral deafness may occur after the drug has been discontinued. Aminoglycoside-induced ototoxicity is usually irreversible.
Aminoglycosides are potentially nephrotoxic. The risk of nephrotoxicity is greater in patients with impaired renal function and in those who receive high doses or prolonged therapy.
Neuromuscular blockade and respiratory paralysis have been reported following parenteral injection, topical instillation (as in orthopedic and abdominal irrigation or in local treatment of empyema) and following oral use of aminoglycosides. The possibility of these phenomena should be considered if aminoglycosides are administered by any route, especially in patients receiving anesthetics; neuromuscular blocking agents such as tubocurarine, succinylcholine, decamethonium; or in patients receiving massive transfusions of citrate-anticoagulated blood. If blockage occurs, calcium salts may reverse these phenomena, but mechanical respiratory assistance may be necessary.
Renal and eighth-nerve function should be closely monitored especially in patients with known or suspected renal impairment at the onset of therapy and also in those whose renal function is initially normal but who develop signs of renal dysfunction during therapy. Serum concentrations of amikacin should be monitored when feasible to assure adequate levels and to avoid potentially toxic levels and prolonged peak concentrations above 35 micrograms per mL. Urine should be examined for decreased specific gravity, increased excretion of proteins and the presence of cells or casts. Blood urea nitrogen, serum creatinine or creatinine clearance should be measured periodically. Serial audiograms should be obtained where feasible in patients old enough to be tested, particularly high risk patients. Evidence of ototoxicity (dizziness, vertigo, tinnitus, roaring in the ears and hearing loss) or nephrotoxicity requires discontinuation of the drug or dosage adjustment.
Concurrent and/or sequential systemic, oral or topical use of other neurotoxic or nephrotoxic products, particularly bacitracin, cisplatin, amphotericin B, cephaloridine, paromomycin, viomycin, polymyxin B, colistin, vancomycin or other aminoglycosides should be avoided. Other factors that may increase risk of toxicity are advanced age and dehydration.
The concurrent use of amikacin with potent diuretics (ethacrynic acid or furosemide) should be avoided since diuretics by themselves may cause ototoxicity. In addi-

Continued on next page

Amikacin—Cont.

tion, when administered intravenously, diuretics may enhance aminoglycoside toxicity by altering antibiotic concentrations in serum and tissue.

DESCRIPTION

Amikacin sulfate, a semi-synthetic aminoglycoside antibiotic derived from kanamycin, has the following structural formula:

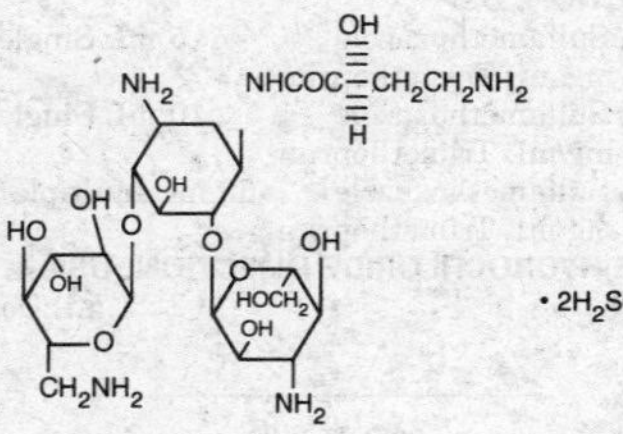

D-Streptamine, *O*-3-amino-3-deoxy-α-D-glucopyranosyl-(1→6)-*O* - [6-amino-6-deoxy-α-D-glucopyranosyl-(1→4)] - *N* [1]-(4-amino-2-hydroxy-1-oxobutyl)-2-deoxy-, (*S*)-, sulfate (1:2) (salt)

$C_{22}H_{43}N_5O_{13} \cdot 2H_2SO_4$ **Molecular weight 781.75**

The dosage form is supplied as a sterile, colorless to light straw-colored solution for IM or IV use.

Each mL contains 250 mg amikacin as the sulfate, sodium citrate (dihydrate) 28.5 mg and sodium metabisulfite 6.6 mg in Water for Injection. pH 3.5–5.5; sodium hydroxide and/or sulfuric acid added, if needed, for pH adjustment. Sealed under nitrogen.

CLINICAL PHARMACOLOGY

INTRAMUSCULAR ADMINISTRATION

Amikacin is rapidly absorbed after intramuscular administration. In normal adult volunteers, average peak serum concentrations of about 12, 16 and 21 mcg/mL are obtained 1 hour after intramuscular administration of 250 mg (3.7 mg/kg), 375 mg (5 mg/kg), 500 mg (7.5 mg/kg), single doses, respectively. At 10 hours, serum levels are about 0.3 mcg/mL, 1.2 mcg/mL and 2.1 mcg/mL, respectively.

Tolerance studies in normal volunteers reveal that amikacin is well tolerated locally following repeated intramuscular dosing, and when given at maximally recommended doses, no ototoxicity or nephrotoxicity has been reported. There is no evidence of drug accumulation with repeated dosing for 10 days when administered according to recommended doses.

With normal renal function, about 91.9% of an intramuscular dose is excreted unchanged in the urine in the first 8 hours and 98.2% within 24 hours. Mean urine concentrations for 6 hours are 563 mcg/mL following a 250 mg dose, 697 mcg/mL following a 375 mg dose and 832 mcg/mL following a 500 mg dose.

Preliminary intramuscular studies in newborns of different weights (less than 1.5 kg, 1.5 to 2 kg, over 2 kg) at a dose of 7.5 mg/kg revealed that, like other aminoglycosides, serum half-life values were correlated inversely with post-natal age and renal clearances of amikacin. The volume of distribution indicates that amikacin, like other aminoglycosides, remains primarily in the extracellular fluid space of neonates. Repeated dosing every 12 hours in all the above groups did not demonstrate accumulation after 5 days.

INTRAVENOUS ADMINISTRATION

Single doses of 500 mg (7.5 mg/kg) administered to normal adults as an infusion over a period of 30 minutes produced a mean peak serum concentration of 38 mcg/mL at the end of the infusion and levels of 24 mcg/mL, 18 mcg/mL and 0.75 mcg/mL at 30 minutes, 1 hour and 10 hours post-infusion, respectively. Eighty-four percent of the administered dose was excreted in the urine in 9 hours and about 94% within 24 hours.

Repeat infusions of 7.5 mg/kg every 12 hours in normal adults were well tolerated and caused no drug accumulation.

GENERAL

Pharmacokinetic studies in normal adult subjects reveal the mean serum half-life to be slightly over 2 hours with a mean total apparent volume of distribution of 24 liters (28% of the body weight). By the ultrafiltration technique, reports of serum protein binding range from 0 to 11%. The mean serum clearance rate is about 100 mL/min and the renal clearance rate is 94 mL/min in subjects with normal renal function.

Amikacin is excreted primarily by glomerular filtration. Patients with impaired renal function or diminished glomerular filtration pressure excrete the drug much more slowly (effectively prolonging the serum half-life). Therefore, renal function should be monitored carefully and dosage adjusted accordingly (see suggested dosage schedule under **DOSAGE AND ADMINISTRATION).**

Following administration at the recommended dose, therapeutic levels are found in bone, heart, gallbladder and lung tissue in addition to significant concentrations in urine; bile; sputum; bronchial secretions; interstitial, pleural and synovial fluids.

Spinal fluid levels in normal infants are approximately 10 to 20% of the serum concentrations and may reach 50% when the meninges are inflamed. Amikacin has been demonstrated to cross the placental barrier and yield significant concentrations in amniotic fluid. The peak fetal serum concentration is about 16% of the peak maternal serum concentration and maternal and fetal serum half-life values are about 2 and 3.7 hours, respectively.

MICROBIOLOGY

Gram-negative—Amikacin is active *in vitro* against *Pseudomonas* species, *Escherichia coli, Proteus* species (indole-positive and indole-negative), *Providencia* species, *Klebsiella-Enterobacter-Serratia* species, *Acinetobacter* (formerly *Mima-Herellea*) species and *Citrobacter freundii.*

When strains of the above organisms are found to be resistant to other aminoglycosides, including gentamicin, tobramycin and kanamycin, many are susceptible to amikacin *in vitro.*

Gram-positive—Amikacin is active *in vitro* against penicillinase and non-penicillinase-producing *Staphylococcus* species, including methicillin-resistant strains. However, aminoglycosides in general have a low order of activity against other gram-positive organisms, viz., *Streptococcus pyogenes*, enterococci and *Streptococcus pneumoniae* (formerly *Diplococcus pneumoniae).*

Amikacin resists degradation by most aminoglycoside inactivating enzymes known to affect gentamicin, tobramycin and kanamycin.

In vitro studies have shown that amikacin sulfate combined with a beta-lactam antibiotic acts synergistically against many clinically significant gram-negative organisms.

Disc Susceptibility Tests—Quantitative methods that require measurement of zone diameters give the most precise estimates of antibiotic susceptibility. One such procedure* has been recommended for use with discs to test susceptibility to amikacin. Interpretation involves correlation of the diameters obtained in the disc test with MIC values for amikacin. When the causative organism is tested by the Kirby-Bauer method of disc susceptibility, a 30 mcg amikacin disc should give a zone of 17 mm or greater to indicate susceptibility. Zone sizes of 14 mm or less indicate resistance. Zone sizes of 15 to 16 mm indicate intermediate susceptibility. With this procedure, a report from the laboratory of "susceptible" indicates that the infecting organism is likely to respond to therapy. A report of "resistant" indicates that the infecting organism is not likely to respond to therapy. A report of "intermediate susceptibility" suggests that the organism would be susceptible if the infection is confined to tissues and fluids (e.g., urine) in which high antibiotic levels are attained.

INDICATIONS AND USAGE

Amikacin Sulfate Injection is indicated in the short-term treatment of serious infections due to susceptible strains of gram-negative bacteria, including *Pseudomonas* species, *Escherichia coli,* species of indole-positive and indole-negative *Proteus, Providencia* species, *Klebsiella-Enterobacter-Serratia* species and *Acinetobacter (Mima-Herellea)* species.

Clinical studies have shown Amikacin Sulfate Injection to be effective in bacterial septicemia (including neonatal sepsis); in serious infections of the respiratory tract, bones and joints, central nervous system (including meningitis) and skin and soft tissue; intra-abdominal infections (including peritonitis); and in burns and post-operative infections (including post-vascular surgery). Clinical studies have shown amikacin also to be effective in serious complicated and recurrent urinary tract infections due to these organisms. Aminoglycosides, including amikacin, are not indicated in uncomplicated initial episodes of urinary tract infections unless the causative organisms are not susceptible to antibiotics having less potential toxicity.

Bacteriologic studies should be performed to identify causative organisms and their susceptibilities to amikacin. Amikacin may be considered as initial therapy in suspected gram-negative infections, and therapy may be instituted before obtaining the results of susceptibility testing. Clinical trials demonstrated that amikacin was effective in infections caused by gentamicin- and/or tobramycin-resistant strains of gram-negative organisms, particularly *Proteus rettgeri, Providencia stuartii, Serratia marcescens* and *Pseudomonas aeruginosa.* The decision to continue therapy with the drug should be based on results of the susceptibility tests, the severity of the infection and the response of the patient, as well as important additional considerations (see **WARNINGS** box).

Amikacin has also been shown to be effective in staphylococcal infections and may be considered as initial therapy under certain conditions in the treatment of known or suspected staphylococcal disease such as severe infections where the causative organism may be either a gram-negative bacterium or a staphylococcus, infections due to susceptible strains of staphylococci in patients allergic to other antibiotics and in mixed staphylococcal/gram-negative infections.

In certain severe infections such as neonatal sepsis, concomitant therapy with a penicillin-type drug may be indicated because of the possibility of infections due to gram-positive organisms such as streptococci or pneumococci.

CONTRAINDICATIONS

A history of hypersensitivity to amikacin is a contraindication for its use. A history of hypersensitivity or serious toxic reactions to aminoglycosides may contraindicate the use of any other aminoglycoside because of the known cross-sensitivities of patients to drugs in this class.

WARNINGS

See **WARNINGS** box above.

Aminoglycosides can cause fetal harm when administered to a pregnant woman. Aminoglycosides cross the placenta and there have been several reports of total irreversible, bilateral congenital deafness in children whose mothers received streptomycin during pregnancy. Although serious side effects to the fetus or newborns have not been reported in the treatment of pregnant women with other aminoglycosides, the potential for harm exists. Reproduction studies of amikacin have been performed in rats and mice and revealed no evidence of impaired fertility or harm to the fetus due to amikacin. There are no well-controlled studies in pregnant women, but investigational experience does not include any positive evidence of adverse effects to the fetus. If this drug is used during pregnancy, or if the patient becomes pregnant while taking this drug, the patient should be apprised of the potential hazard to the fetus.

Contains sodium metabisulfite, a sulfite that may cause allergic-type reactions including anaphylactic symptoms and life-threatening or less severe asthmatic episodes in certain susceptible people. The overall prevalence of sulfite sensitivity in the general population is unknown and probably low. Sulfite sensitivity is seen more frequently in asthmatic than nonasthmatic people.

PRECAUTIONS

Aminoglycosides are quickly and almost totally absorbed when they are applied topically, except to the urinary bladder, in association with surgical procedures. Irreversible deafness, renal failure and death due to neuromuscular blockade have been reported following irrigation of both small and large surgical fields with an aminoglycoside preparation.

Amikacin Sulfate Injection is potentially nephrotoxic, ototoxic and neurotoxic. The concurrent or serial use of other ototoxic or nephrotoxic agents should be avoided either systemically or topically because of the potential for additive effects. Increased nephrotoxicity has been reported following concomitant parenteral administration of aminoglycoside antibiotics and cephalosporins. Concomitant cephalosporins may spuriously elevate creatinine determinations.

Since amikacin is present in high concentrations in the renal excretory system, patients should be well-hydrated to minimize chemical irritation of the renal tubules. Kidney function should be assessed by the usual methods prior to starting therapy and daily during the course of treatment.

If signs of renal irritation appear (casts, white or red cells or albumin), hydration should be increased. A reduction in dosage (see **DOSAGE AND ADMINISTRATION**) may be desirable if other evidence of renal dysfunction occurs such as decreased creatinine clearance; decreased urine specific gravity; increased BUN, creatinine or oliguria. If azotemia increases or if a progressive decrease in urinary output occurs, treatment should be stopped.

Note: When patients are well hydrated and kidney function is normal, the risk of nephrotoxic reactions with amikacin is low if the dosage recommendations (see **DOSAGE AND ADMINISTRATION**) are not exceeded.

Elderly patients may have reduced renal function which may not be evident in routine screening tests such as BUN or serum creatinine. A creatinine clearance determination may be more useful. Monitoring of renal function during treatment with aminoglycosides is particularly important.

Aminoglycosides should be used with caution in patients with muscular disorders such as myasthenia gravis or parkinsonism since these drugs may aggravate muscle weakness because of their potential curare-like effect on the neuromuscular junction.

In vitro mixing of aminoglycosides with beta-lactam antibiotics (penicillin or cephalosporins) may result in a significant mutual inactivation. A reduction in serum half-life or serum level may occur when an aminoglycoside or penicillin-type drug is administered by separate routes. Inactivation of the aminoglycoside is clinically significant only in patients with severely impaired renal function. Inactivation may continue in specimens of body fluids collected for assay, resulting in inaccurate aminoglycoside readings. Such specimens should be properly handled (assayed promptly, frozen or treated with beta-lactamase).

Cross-allergenicity among aminoglycosides has been demonstrated.

As with other antibiotics, the use of amikacin may result in overgrowth of non-susceptible organisms. If this occurs, appropriate therapy should be instituted.

Aminoglycosides should not be given concurrently with potent diuretics (see **WARNINGS** box).

CARCINOGENESIS, MUTAGENESIS, IMPAIRMENT OF FERTILITY

Studies in humans have not been performed with the aminoglycosides to determine their effect on carcinogenesis, mutagenesis or impairment of fertility.

PREGNANCY

Pregnancy Category D (see **WARNINGS** section).

NURSING MOTHERS

It is not known whether this drug is excreted in human milk. As a general rule, nursing should not be undertaken while a patient is on a drug since many drugs are excreted in human milk.

PEDIATRIC USE

Aminoglycosides should be used with caution in premature and neonatal infants because of the renal immaturity of these patients and the resulting prolongation of serum half-life of these drugs.

ADVERSE REACTIONS

All aminoglycosides have the potential to induce auditory, vestibular and renal toxicity and neuromuscular blockade (see **WARNINGS** box). They occur more frequently in patients with present or past history of renal impairment, of treatment with other ototoxic or nephrotoxic drugs and in patients treated for longer periods and/or with higher doses than recommended.

Neurotoxicity-Ototoxicity—Toxic effects on the eighth cranial nerve can result in hearing loss, loss of balance or both. Amikacin primarily affects auditory function. Cochlear damage includes high frequency deafness and usually occurs before clinical hearing loss can be detected.

Neurotoxicity-Neuromuscular Blockage—Acute muscular paralysis and apnea can occur following treatment with aminoglycoside drugs.

Nephrotoxicity—Elevation of serum creatinine, albuminuria, presence of red and white cells, casts, azotemia and oliguria have been reported. Renal function changes are usually reversible when the drug is discontinued.

Other—In addition to those described above, other adverse reactions which have been reported on rare occasions are skin rash, drug fever, headache, paresthesia, tremor, nausea and vomiting, eosinophilia, arthralgia, anemia and hypotension.

OVERDOSAGE

In the event of overdosage or toxic reaction, peritoneal dialysis or hemodialysis will aid in the removal of amikacin from the blood. In the newborn infant, exchange transfusion may also be considered.

DOSAGE AND ADMINISTRATION

The patient's pretreatment body weight should be obtained for calculation of correct dosage. Amikacin Sulfate Injection may be given intramuscularly or intravenously.

The status of renal function should be estimated by measurement of the serum creatinine concentration or calculation of the endogenous creatinine clearance rate. The blood urea nitrogen (BUN) is much less reliable for this purpose. Reassessment of renal function should be made periodically during therapy.

Whenever possible, amikacin concentrations in serum should be measured to assure adequate but not excessive levels. It is desirable to measure both peak and trough serum concentrations intermittently during therapy. Peak concentrations (30–90 minutes after injection) above 35 micrograms per mL and trough concentrations (just prior to the next dose) above 10 micrograms per mL should be avoided. Dosage should be adjusted as indicated.

INTRAMUSCULAR ADMINISTRATION FOR PATIENTS WITH NORMAL RENAL FUNCTION

The recommended dosage for adults, children and older infants (see **WARNINGS** box) with normal renal function is 15 mg/kg/day divided into 2 or 3 equal doses administered at equally divided intervals, i.e., 7.5 mg/kg q12h or 5 mg/kg q8h. Treatment of patients in the heavier weight classes should not exceed 1.5 gram/day.

When amikacin is indicated in newborns (see **WARNINGS** box), it is recommended that a loading dose of 10 mg/kg be administered initially to be followed with 7.5 mg/kg every 12 hours.

The usual duration of treatment is 7 to 10 days. It is desirable to limit the duration of treatment to short-term whenever feasible. The total daily dose by all routes of administration should not exceed 15 mg/kg/day. In difficult and complicated infections where treatment beyond 10 days is considered, the use of amikacin should be reevaluated. If continued, amikacin serum levels and renal, auditory and vestibular functions should be monitored. At the recommended dosage level, uncomplicated infections due to amikacin-sensitive organisms should respond in 24 to 48 hours. If definite clinical response does not occur within 3 to 5 days, therapy should be stopped and the antibiotic susceptibility pattern of the invading organism should be rechecked. Failure of the infection to respond may be due to resistance of the organism or to the presence of septic foci requiring surgical drainage.

When amikacin is indicated in uncomplicated urinary tract infections, a dose of 250 mg twice daily may be used.

DOSAGE GUIDELINES
ADULTS AND CHILDREN WITH NORMAL RENAL FUNCTION

Patient Weight		Dosage		
lbs	kg	7.5 mg/kg q12h	OR	5 mg/kg q8h
99	45	337.5 mg		225 mg
110	50	375 mg		250 mg
121	55	412.5 mg		275 mg
132	60	450 mg		300 mg
143	65	487.5 mg		325 mg
154	70	525 mg		350 mg
165	75	562.5 mg		375 mg
176	80	600 mg		400 mg
187	85	637.5 mg		425 mg
198	90	675 mg		450 mg
209	95	712.5 mg		475 mg
220	100	750 mg		500 mg

INTRAMUSCULAR ADMINISTRATION FOR PATIENTS WITH IMPAIRED RENAL FUNCTION

Whenever possible, serum amikacin concentrations should be monitored by appropriate assay procedures. Doses may be adjusted in patients with impaired renal function either by administering normal doses at prolonged intervals or by administering reduced doses at a fixed interval.

Both methods are based on the patient's creatinine clearance or serum creatinine values since these have been found to correlate with aminoglycoside half-lives in patients with diminished renal function. These dosage schedules must be used in conjunction with careful clinical and laboratory observations of the patient and should be modified as necessary. Neither method should be used when dialysis is being performed.

Normal Dosage at Prolonged Intervals—If the creatinine clearance rate is not available and the patient's condition is stable, a dosage interval in hours for the normal dose can be calculated by multiplying the patient's serum creatinine by 9, e.g., if the serum creatinine concentration is 2 mg/100 mL, the recommended single dose (7.5 mg/kg) should be administered every 18 hours.

Reduced Dosage at Fixed Time Intervals—When renal function is impaired and it is desirable to administer amikacin at a fixed time interval, dosage must be reduced. In these patients, serum amikacin concentrations should be measured to assure accurate administration of amikacin and to avoid concentrations above 35 mcg/mL. If serum assay determinations are not available and the patient's condition is stable, serum creatinine and creatinine clearance values are the most readily available indicators of the degree of renal impairment to use as a guide for dosage.

First, initiate therapy by administering a normal dose, 7.5 mg/kg, as a loading dose. This loading dose is the same as the normally recommended dose which would be calculated for a patient with a normal renal function as described above.

To determine the size of maintenance doses administered every 12 hours, the loading dose should be reduced in proportion to the reduction in the patient's creatinine clearance rate:

$$\text{Maintenance Dose Every 12 hours} = \frac{\text{observed CC in mL/min}}{\text{normal CC in mL/min}} \times \text{calculated loading dose in mg}$$

(CC—creatinine clearance rate)

An alternate rough guide for determining reduced dosage at 12-hour intervals (for patients whose steady state serum creatinine values are known) is to divide the normally recommended dose by the patient's serum creatinine.

The above dosage schedules are not intended to be rigid recommendations but are provided as guides to dosage when the measurement of amikacin serum levels is not feasible.

INTRAVENOUS ADMINISTRATION

The individual dose, the total daily dose and the total cumulative dose of amikacin sulfate are identical to the dose recommended for intramuscular administration. The solution for intravenouis use is prepared by adding the contents of a 500 mg vial to 100–200 mL of sterile diluent such as Normal Saline or 5% Dextrose in Water or any other compatible solution.

The solution is administered to adults over a 30 to 60 minute period. The total daily dose should not exceed 15 mg/kg/day and may be divided into either 2 or 3 equally divided doses at equally divided intervals.

In pediatric patients, the amount of fluid used will depend on the amount ordered for the patient. It should be a sufficient amount to infuse the amikacin over a 30 to 60 minute period. Infants should receive a 1 to 2 hour infusion.

Amikacin should not be physically premixed with other drugs but should be administered separately according to the recommended dose and route.

Stability in IV Fluids—Amikacin sulfate is stable for 24 hours at room temperature at concentrations of 0.25 and 5 mg/mL in the following solutions:

5% Dextrose Injection, USP
5% Dextrose and 0.2% Sodium Chloride Injection, USP
5% Dextrose and 0.45% Sodium Chloride Injection, USP
0.9% Sodium Chloride Injection, USP
Lactated Ringer's Injection, USP
Normosol® M in 5% Dextrose Injection (or Plasma-Lyte 56 Injection in 5% Dextrose in Water)
Normosol® R in 5% Dextrose Injection (or Plasma-Lyte 148 Injection in 5% Dextrose in Water)

Aminoglycosides administered by any of the above routes should not be physically premixed with other drugs but should be administered separately.

Because of the potential toxicity of aminoglycosides, "fixed dosage" recommendations which are not based upon body weight are not advised. Rather, it is essential to calculate the dosage to fit the needs of each patient.

Parenteral drug products should be inspected visually for particulate matter and discoloration prior to administration whenever the solution and container permit.

HOW SUPPLIED

Amikacin Sulfate Injection, USP is available in the following packages:

250 mg/mL
2 mL (500 mg) DOSETTE® vials packaged in 10s (*NDC* 0641-0123-23)
4 mL (1 gram) vials packaged in 10s (*NDC* 0641-2357-43)

STORAGE

Amikacin Sulfate Injection, USP is supplied as a colorless solution which requires no refrigeration. Store at controlled room temperature 15°–30°C (59°–86°F).

Store solutions for intravenous use as directed in **DOSAGE AND ADMINISTRATION.**

At times, the solution may become a very pale yellow; this does not indicate a decrease in potency.

*Bauer, AW; Kirby, WMM; Sherris, JC and Turck, M: Antibiotic Testing by a Standardized Single Disc Method, AM J CLIN PATHOL, 45:493, 1966; Standardized Disc Susceptibility Test, *FEDERAL REGISTER*, 37:20527-29, 1972.

Manufactured by
ELKINS-SINN, INC.
Cherry Hill, NJ 08003-4099
A subsidiary of A.H. Robins Company
J-0122C Revised January 1993

DURAMORPH® Ⓒ

[*dūr "a 'mŏrf*]
(morphine sulfate injection, USP)
Preservative-Free

Warning: May be habit forming.

DESCRIPTION

Morphine is the most important alkaloid of opium and is a phenanthrene derivative. It is available as the sulfate salt, having the following structural formula:

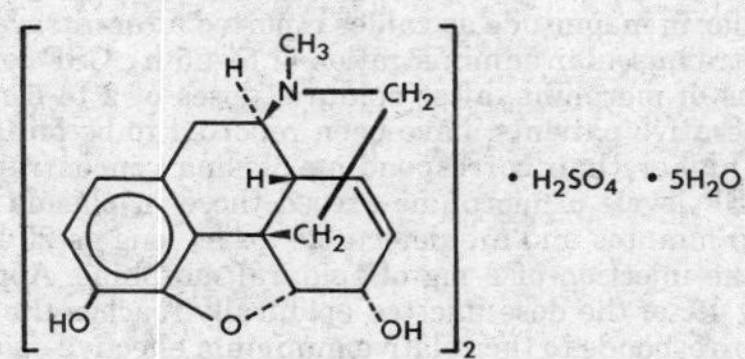

7,8 Didehydro-4,5-epoxy-17-methyl-(5α,6α)-morphinan-3,6-diol sulfate (2:1) (salt), pentahydrate

$(C_{17}H_{19}NO_3)_2 \cdot H_2SO_4 \cdot 5H_2O$ Molecular weight is 758.83

Preservative-free DURAMORPH® (Morphine Sulfate Injection, USP) is a sterile, nonpyrogenic, isobaric solution of morphine sulfate, free of antioxidants, preservatives or other potentially neurotoxic additives and is intended for intravenous, epidural or intrathecal administration as a narcotic analgesic. Each milliliter contains morphine sulfate 0.5 mg or 1 mg and sodium chloride 9 mg in Water for Injection. pH range is 2.5–6.5. Ampuls are sealed under nitrogen. Each Dosette® ampul of DURAMORPH® is intended for **SINGLE USE ONLY.** *Discard any unused portion.* DO NOT HEAT-STERILIZE.

CLINICAL PHARMACOLOGY

Morphine produces a wide spectrum of pharmacologic effects including analgesia, dysphoria, euphoria, somnolence, respiratory depression, diminished gastrointestinal motility and physical dependence. Opiate analgesia involves at least three anatomical areas of the central nervous system: the periaqueductal-periventricular gray matter, the ventromedial medulla and the spinal cord. A systemically administered opiate may produce analgesia by acting at any, all or some combination of these distinct regions. Morphine interacts predominantly with the μ-receptor. The μ-binding sites of opioids are very discretely distributed in the human brain, with high densities of sites found in the posterior amygdala, hypothalamus, thalamus, nucleus caudatus, putamen and certain cortical areas. They are also found on the terminal axons of primary afferents within laminae I and II (substantia gelatinosa) of the spinal cord and in the spinal nucleus of the trigeminal nerve.

Morphine has an apparent volume of distribution ranging from 1.0 to 4.7 L/kg after *intravenous* dosage. Protein binding is low, about 36%, and muscle tissue binding is reported as 54%. A blood-brain barrier exists, and when morphine is introduced outside of the CNS (e.g. *intravenously*), plasma concentrations of morphine remain higher than the corresponding CSF morphine levels. Conversely, when morphine is injected into the *intrathecal space*, it diffuses out into the systemic circulation slowly, accounting for the long duration of action of morphine administered by this route. Morphine has a total plasma clearance which ranges from 0.9 to 1.2 L/kg/h (liters/kilogram/hour) in postoperative patients, but shows considerable interindividual variation. The major pathway of clearance is hepatic glucuronidation to morphine-3-glucuronide, which is pharmacologically inactive. The major excretion path of the conjugate is through the kidneys, with about 10% in the feces. Morphine is also eliminated by the kidneys, 2 to 12% being excreted unchanged in the urine. Terminal half-life is commonly reported to vary from 1.5 to 4.5 hours, although the longer half-lives were obtained when morphine levels were monitored over protracted periods with very sensitive radioimmunoassay methods. The accepted elimination half-life in normal subject is 1.5 to 2 hours.

"Selective" blockade of pain sensation is possible by neuraxial application of morphine. In addition, duration of analge-

Continued on next page

Duramorph—Cont.

sia may be much longer by this route compared to systemic administration. However, CNS effects, associated with systemic administration, are still seen. These include respiratory depression, sedation, nausea and vomiting, pruritus and urinary retention. In particular, both early and late respiratory depression (up to 24 hours post dosing) have been reported following neuraxial administration. Circulation of the spinal fluid may also result in high concentrations of morphine reaching the brain stem directly.

The incidence of unwanted CNS effects, including delayed respiratory depression, associated with neuraxial application of morphine, is related to the circulatory dynamics of the epidural venous plexus and the spinal fluid. The lipid solubility and degree of ionization of morphine plays an important part in both the onset and duration of analgesia and the CNS effects. Morphine has a pK_a 7.9, with an octanol/water partition coefficient of 1.42 at pH 7.4. At this pH, the tertiary amino group in each of the opioids is mostly ionized, making the molecule water soluble. Morphine, with additional hydroxyl groups on the molecule, is significantly more water soluble than any other opioid in clinical use.

Morphine, injected into the *epidural space*, is rapidly absorbed into the general circulation. Absorption is so rapid that the plasma concentration-time profiles closely resemble those obtained after intravenous or intramuscular administration. Peak plasma concentrations averaging 33–40 ng/mL (range 5–62 ng/mL) are achieved within 10 to 15 minutes after administration of 3 mg of morphine. Plasma concentrations decline in a multiexponential fashion. The terminal half-life is reported to range from 39 to 249 minutes (mean of 90±34.3 min) and, though somewhat shorter, is similar in magnitude as values reported after intravenous and intramuscular administration (1.5–4.5 h). CSF concentrations of morphine, after epidural doses of 2 to 6 mg in postoperative patients, have been reported to be 50 to 250 times higher than corresponding plasma concentrations. The CSF levels of morphine exceed those in plasma after only 15 minutes and are detectable for as long as 20 hours after the injection of 2 mg of epidural morphine. Approximately 4% of the dose injected epidurally reaches the CSF. This corresponds to the relative minimum effective epidural and intrathecal doses of 5 mg and 0.25 mg, respectively. The disposition of morphine in the CSF follows a biphasic pattern, with an early half-life of 1.5 h and a late phase half-life of about 6 h. Morphine crosses the dura slowly, with an absorption half-life across the dura averaging 22 minutes. Maximum CSF concentrations are seen 60–90 minutes after injection. Minimum effective CSF concentrations for postoperative analgesia average 150 ng/mL (range <1–380 ng/mL).

The *intrathecal route* of administration circumvents meningeal diffusion barriers and, therefore, lower doses of morphine produce comparable analgesia to that induced by the epidural route. After intrathecal bolus injection of morphine, there is a rapid initial distribution phase lasting 15–30 minutes and a half-life in the CSF of 42–136 min (mean 90±16 min). Derived from limited data, it appears that the disposition of morphine in the CSF, from 15 minutes postintrathecal administration to the end of a six-hour observation period, represents a combination of the distribution and elimination phases. Morphine concentrations in the CSF averaged 332±137 ng/mL at 6 hours, following a bolus dose of 0.3 mg of morphine. The apparent volume of distribution of morphine in the intrathecal space is about 22±8 mL.

Time-to-peak plasma concentrations, however, are similar (5–10 min) after either epidural or intrathecal bolus administration of morphine. Maximum plasma morphine concentrations after 0.3 mg intrathecal morphine have been reported from <1 to 7.8 ng/mL. The minimum analgesic morphine plasma concentration during Patient-Controlled Analgesia (PCA) has been reported as 20–40 ng/mL, suggesting that any analgesic contribution from systemic redistribution would be minimal after the first 30–60 minutes with epidural administration and virtually absent with intrathecal administration of morphine.

INDICATIONS AND USAGE

DURAMORPH® is a systemic narcotic analgesic for administration by the intravenous, epidural or intrathecal routes. It is used for the management of pain not responsive to non-narcotic analgesics. DURAMORPH®, administered epidurally or intrathecally, provides pain relief for extended periods without attendant loss of motor, sensory or sympathetic function.

CONTRAINDICATIONS

DURAMORPH® is contraindicated in those medical conditions which would preclude the administration of opioids by the intravenous route—allergy to morphine or other opiates, acute bronchial asthma, upper airway obstruction.

WARNINGS

Morphine sulfate may be habit forming. (See DRUG ABUSE AND DEPENDENCE.)

DURAMORPH® administration should be limited to use by those familiar with the management of respiratory depression. Rapid intravenous administration may result in chest wall rigidity.

Prior to any epidural or intrathecal drug administration, the physician should be familiar with patient conditions (such as infection at the injection site, bleeding diathesis, anticoagulant therapy, etc.) which call for special evaluation of the benefit versus risk potential.

In the case of epidural or intrathecal administration, DURAMORPH® should be administered by or under the direction of a physician experienced in the techniques and familiar with the patient management problems associated with epidural or intrathecal drug administration. Because epidural administration has been associated with less potential for immediate or late adverse effects than intrathecal administration, the epidural route should be used whenever possible.

SEVERE RESPIRATORY DEPRESSION UP TO 24 HOURS FOLLOWING EPIDURAL OR INTRATHECAL ADMINISTRATION HAS BEEN REPORTED.

BECAUSE OF THE RISK OF SEVERE ADVERSE EFFECTS WHEN THE EPIDURAL OR INTRATHECAL ROUTE OF ADMINISTRATION IS EMPLOYED, PATIENTS MUST BE OBSERVED IN A FULLY EQUIPPED AND STAFFED ENVIRONMENT FOR AT LEAST 24 HOURS AFTER THE INITIAL DOSE.

THE FACILITY MUST BE EQUIPPED TO RESUSCITATE PATIENTS WITH SEVERE OPIATE OVERDOSAGE, AND THE PERSONNEL MUST BE FAMILIAR WITH THE USE AND LIMITATIONS OF SPECIFIC NARCOTIC ANTAGONISTS (NALOXONE, NALTREXONE) IN SUCH CASES.

TOLERANCE AND MYOCLONIC ACTIVITY

PATIENTS SOMETIMES MANIFEST UNUSUAL ACCELERATION OF NEURAXIAL MORPHINE REQUIREMENTS, WHICH MAY CAUSE CONCERN REGARDING SYSTEMIC ABSORPTION AND THE HAZARDS OF LARGE DOSES; THESE PATIENTS MAY BENEFIT FROM HOSPITALIZATION AND DETOXIFICATION. TWO CASES OF MYOCLONIC-LIKE SPASM OF THE LOWER EXTREMITIES HAVE BEEN REPORTED IN PATIENTS RECEIVING MORE THAN 20 MG/DAY OF INTRATHECAL MORPHINE. AFTER DETOXIFICATION, IT MIGHT BE POSSIBLE TO RESUME TREATMENT AT LOWER DOSES, AND SOME PATIENTS HAVE BEEN SUCCESSFULLY CHANGED FROM CONTINUOUS EPIDURAL MORPHINE TO CONTINUOUS INTRATHECAL MORPHINE. REPEAT DETOXIFICATION MAY BE INDICATED AT A LATER DATE. THE UPPER DAILY DOSAGE LIMIT FOR EACH PATIENT DURING CONTINUING TREATMENT MUST BE INDIVIDUALIZED.

PRECAUTIONS

GENERAL

Control of pain by neuraxial opiate delivery is always accompanied by considerable risk to the patients and requires a high level of skill to be successfully accomplished. The task of treating these patients must be undertaken by experienced clinical teams, well-versed in patient selection, evolving technology and emerging standards of care. For safety reasons, it is recommended that administration of DURAMORPH® by the epidural or intrathecal routes be limited to the lumbar area. Intrathecal use has been associated with a higher incidence of respiratory depression than epidural use.

Seizures may result from high doses. Patients with known seizure disorders should be carefully observed for evidence of morphine-induced seizure activity.

USE IN PATIENTS WITH INCREASED INTRACRANIAL PRESSURE OR HEAD INJURY

DURAMORPH® should be used with extreme caution in patients with head injury or increased intracranial pressure. Pupillary changes (miosis) from morphine may obscure the existence, extent and course of intracranial pathology. High doses of neuraxial morphine may produce myoclonic events (see WARNINGS and ADVERSE REACTIONS). Clinicians should maintain a high index of suspicion for adverse drug reactions when evaluating altered mental status or movement abnormalities in patients receiving this modality of treatment.

USE IN CHRONIC PULMONARY DISEASE

Care is urged in using this drug in patients who have a decreased respiratory reserve (e.g., emphysema, severe obesity, kyphoscoliosis or paralysis of the phrenic nerve). DURAMORPH® should not be given in cases of chronic asthma, upper airway obstruction or in any other chronic pulmonary disorder without due consideration of the known risk of acute respiratory failure following morphine administration in such patients.

USE IN HEPATIC OR RENAL DISEASE

The elimination half-life of morphine may be prolonged in patients with reduced metabolic rates and with hepatic and/or renal dysfunction. Hence, care should be exercised in administering DURAMORPH® epidurally to patients with these conditions, since high blood morphine levels, due to reduced clearance, may take several days to develop.

USE IN BILIARY SURGERY OR DISORDERS OF THE BILIARY TRACT

As significant morphine is released into the systemic circulation from neuraxial administration, the ensuring smooth muscle hypertonicity may result in biliary colic.

USE WITH DISORDERS OF THE URINARY SYSTEM

Initiation of neuraxial opiate analgesia is frequently associated with disturbances of micturition, especially in males with prostatic enlargement. Early recognition of difficulty in urination and prompt intervention in cases of urinary retention is indicated.

USE IN AMBULATORY PATIENTS

Patients with reduced circulating blood volume, impaired myocardial function or on sympatholytic drugs should be monitored for the possible occurrence of orthostatic hypotension, a frequent complication in single-dose neuraxial morphine analgesia.

USE WITH OTHER CENTRAL NERVOUS SYSTEM DEPRESSANTS

The depressant effects of morphine are potentiated by the presence of other CNS depressants such as alcohol, sedatives, antihistaminics or psychotropic drugs. Use of neuroleptics in conjunction with neuraxial morphine may increase the risk of respiratory depression.

CARCINOGENESIS, MUTAGENESIS, IMPAIRMENT OF FERTILITY

Morphine is without known carcinogenic or mutagenic effects and is not known to impair fertility at non-narcotic doses in animals, but studies of the carcinogenic and mutagenic potential or the effect on fertility of DURAMORPH® have not been conducted.

PREGNANCY

Teratogenic Effects—Pregnancy Category C. Morphine sulfate is not teratogenic in rats at 35 mg/kg/day (thirty-five times the usual human dose) but does result in increased pup mortality and growth retardation at doses that narcotize the animal (>10 mg/kg/day, ten times the usual human dose). DURAMORPH® should only be given to pregnant women when no other method of controlling pain is available and means are at hand to manage the delivery and perinatal care of the opiate-dependent infant.

Nonteratogenic Effects. Infants born to mothers who have been taking morphine chronically may exhibit withdrawal symptoms.

LABOR AND DELIVERY

Intravenous morphine readily passes into the fetal circulation and may result in respiratory depression in the neonate. Naloxone and resuscitative equipment should be available for reversal of narcotic-induced respiratory depression in the neonate. In addition, intravenous morphine may reduce the strength, duration and frequency of uterine contraction resulting in prolonged labor.

Epidurally and intrathecally administered morphine readily passes into the fetal circulation and may result in respiratory depression of the neonate. Controlled clinical studies have shown that *epidural* administration has little or no effect on the relief of labor pain.

NURSING MOTHERS

Morphine is excreted in maternal milk. Effects on the nursing infant are not known.

PEDIATRIC USE

Adequate studies, to establish the safty and effectiveness of spinal morphine in children, have not been performed, and usage in this population is not recommended.

USE IN THE AGED

The pharmacodynamic effects of neuraxial morphine in the aged are more variable than in the younger population. Patients will vary widely in the effective initial dose, rate of development of tolerance and the frequency and magnitude of associated adverse effects as the dose is increased. Initial doses should be based on careful clinical obsrvation following "test doses", after making due allowances for the effects of the patient's age and infirmity on his/her ability to clear the drug, particularly in patients receiving epidural morphine.

ADVERSE REACTIONS

The most serious adverse experience encountered during administration of DURAMORPH® is respiratory depression. This depression may be severe and could require intervention. (See WARNINGS AND OVERDOSAGE.) Because of delay in maximum CNS effect with intravenously administered drug (30 min), rapid administration may result in overdosing. Single-dose neuraxial administration may result in acute or delayed respiratory depression for periods at least as long as 24 hours.

Tolerance and myoclonus: See **WARNINGS** for discussion of these and related hazards.

While low doses of intravenously administered morphine have little effect on cardiovascular stability, high doses are excitatory, resulting from **sympathetic hyperactivity** and increase in circulating catecholamines. Excitation of the central nervous system, resulting in **convulsions**, may accompany high doses of morphine given intravenously. **Dysphoric reactions** may occur after any size dose and **toxic psychoses** have been reported.

Pruritus: Single-dose epidural or intrathecal administration is accompanied by a high incidence of *pruritus* that is dose-related but not confined to the site of administration. Pruritus, following continuous infusion of epidural or intrathecal morphine, is occasionally reported in the literature; these reactions are poorly understood as to their cause.

Urinary retention: Urinary retention, which may persist 10 to 20 hours following single epidural or intrathecal administration, is a frequent side effect and must be anticipated primarily in male patients, with a somewhat lower incidence in females. Also frequently reported in the literature is the occurrence of urinary retention during the first several days of hospitalization for the initiation of continuous intrathecal or epidural morphine therapy. Patients who develop urinary retention have responded to cholinomimetic treatment and/or judicious use of catheters (see PRECAUTIONS).

Constipation: Constipation is frequently encountered during continuous infusion of morphine; this can usually be managed by conventional therapy.

Headache: Lumbar puncture-type headache is encountered in a significant minority of cases for several days following intrathecal catheter implantation; this, generally, responds to bed rest and/or other conventional therapy.

Other: Other adverse experiences reported following morphine therapy include—**Dizziness, euphoria, anxiety, depression of cough reflex, interference with thermal regulation and oliguria.** Evidence of histamine release such as **urticaria, wheals** and/or **local tissue irritation** may occur. **Nausea** and **vomiting** are frequently seen in patients following morphine administration.

Pruritus, nausea/vomiting and urinary retention, if associated with continuous infusion therapy, may respond to intravenous administration of a low dose of naloxone (0.2 mg). The risks of using narcotic antagonists in patients chronicially receiving narcotic therapy should be considered.

In general, side effects are amenable to reversal by narcotic antagonists.

NALOXONE INJECTION AND RESUSCITATIVE EQUIPMENT SHOULD BE IMMEDIATELY AVAILABLE FOR ADMINISTRATION IN CASE OF LIFE-THREATENING OR INTOLERABLE SIDE EFFECTS AND WHENEVER DURAMORPH® THERAPY IS BEING INITIATED.

DRUG ABUSE AND DEPENDENCE

CONTROLLED SUBSTANCE

Morphine sulfate is a Schedule II narcotic under the United States Controlled Substance Act (21 U.S.C. 801–886).

Morphine is the most commonly cited prototype for narcotic substances that possess an addiction-forming or addiction-sustaining liability. A patient may be at risk for developing a dependence to morphine if used improperly or for overly long periods of time. As with all potent opioids which are μ-agonists, tolerance as well as psychological and physicial dependence to morphine may develop irrespective of the route of administration (intravenous, intramuscular, intrathecal, epidural or oral). Individuals with a prior history of opioid or other substance abuse or dependence, being more apt to respond to the euphorogenic and reinforcing properties of morphine, would be considered to be at greater risk. Care must be taken to avert withdrawal in those patients who have been maintained on parenteral/oral narcotics when epidural or intrathecal administration is considered. Withdrawal symptoms may occur when morphine is discontinued abruptly or upon administration of a narcotic antagonist.

OVERDOSAGE

PARENTERAL ADMINISTRATION OF NARCOTICS IN PATIENTS RECEIVING EPIDURAL OR INTRATHECAL MORPHINE MAY RESULT IN OVERDOSAGE.

Overdosage of morphine is characterized by respiratory depression, with or without concomitant CNS depression. Since respiratory arrest may result either through direct depression of the respiratory center or as the result of hypoxia, primary attention should be given to the establishment of adequate respiratory exchange through provision of a patent airway and institution of assisted, or controlled, ventilation. The narcotic antagonist, naloxone, is a specific antidote. An initial dose of 0.4 to 2 mg of naloxone should be administered intravenously, simultaneously with respiratory resuscitation. If the desired degree of counteraction and improvement in respiratory function is not obtained, naloxone may be repeated at 2- to 3-minute intervals. If no response is observed after 10 mg of naloxone has been administered, the diagnosis of narcotic-induced, or partial narcotic-induced, toxicity should be questioned. Intramuscular or subcutaneous administration may be used if the intravenous route is not available.

As the duration of effect of naloxone is considerably shorter than that of epidural or intrathecal morphine, repeated administration may be necessary. Patients should be closely observed for evidence of renarcotization.

DOSAGE AND ADMINISTRATION

DURAMORPH® is intended for intravenous, epidural or intrathecal administration.

INTRAVENOUS ADMINISTRATION

Dosage: The initial dose of morphine should be 2 mg to 10 mg/70 kg of body weight. No information is available regarding the use of DURAMORPH® in patients under the age of 18.

EPIDURAL ADMINISTRATION

DURAMORPH® SHOULD BE ADMINISTERED EPIDURALLY BY OR UNDER THE DIRECTION OF A PHYSICIAN EXPERIENCED IN THE TECHNIQUE OF EPIDURAL ADMINISTRATION AND WHO IS THOROUGHLY FAMILIAR WITH THE LABELING. IT SHOULD BE ADMINISTERED ONLY IN SETTINGS WHERE ADEQUATE PATIENT MONITORING IS POSSIBLE. RESUSCITATIVE EQUIPMENT AND A SPECIFIC ANTAGONIST (NALOXONE INJECTION) SHOULD BE IMMEDIATELY AVAILABLE FOR THE MANAGEMENT OF RESPIRATORY DEPRESSION AS WELL AS COMPLICATIONS WHICH MIGHT RESULT FROM INADVERTENT INTRATHECAL OR INTRAVASCULAR INJECTION. (NOTE: INTRATHECAL DOSAGE IS USUALLY 1/10 THAT OF EPIDURAL DOSAGE.) **PATIENT MONITORING SHOULD BE CONTINUED FOR AT LEAST 24 HOURS AFTER EACH DOSE, SINCE DELAYED RESPIRATORY DEPRESSION MAY OCCUR.**

Proper placement of a needle or catheter in the epidural space should be verified before DURAMORPH® is injected. Acceptable techniques for verifying proper placement include: a) aspiration to check for absence of blood or cerebrospinal fluid, or b) administration of 5 mL (3 mL in obstetric patients) of 1.5% PRESERVATIVE-FREE Lidocaine and Epinephrine (1:200,000) Injection and then observe the patient for lack of tachycardia (this indicates that vascular injection has *not* been made) and lack of sudden onset of segmental anesthesia (this indicates that intrathecal injection has *not* been made).

Epidural Adult Dosage: Initial injection of 5 mg in the lumbar region may provide satisfactory pain relief for up to 24 hours. If adequate pain relief is not achieved within one hour, careful administration of incremental doses of 1 to 2 mg at intervals sufficient to assess effectiveness may be given. No more than 10 mg/24 hr should be administered.

Thoracic administration has been shown to dramatically increase the incidence of early and late respiratory depression even at doses of 1 to 2 mg.

For continuous infusion, an initial dose of 2 to 4 mg/24 hours is recommended. Further doses of 1 to 2 mg may be given if pain relief is not achieved initially.

Aged patients—Administer with extreme caution. (See PRECAUTIONS.)

Epidural Pediatric Use: No information on use in pediatric patients is available. (See PRECAUTIONS.)

INTRATHECAL ADMINISTRATION

NOTE: INTRATHECAL DOSAGE IS USUALLY 1/10 THAT OF EPIDURAL DOSAGE.

DURAMORPH® SHOULD BE ADMINISTERED INTRATHECALLY BY OR UNDER THE DIRECTION OF A PHYSICIAN EXPERIENCED IN THE TECHNIQUE OF INTRATHECAL ADMINISTRATION AND WHO IS THOROUGHLY FAMILIAR WITH THE LABELING. IT SHOULD BE ADMINISTERED ONLY IN SETTINGS WHERE ADEQUATE PATIENT MONITORING IS POSSIBLE. RESUSCITATIVE EQUIPMENT AND A SPECIFIC ANTAGONIST (NALOXONE INJECTION) SHOULD BE IMMEDIATELY AVAILABLE FOR THE MANAGEMENT OF RESPIRATORY DEPRESSION AS WELL AS COMPLICATIONS WHICH MIGHT RESULT FROM INADVERTENT INTRAVASCULAR INJECTION. **PATIENT MONITORING SHOULD BE CONTINUED FOR AT LEAST 24 HOURS AFTER EACH DOSE, SINCE DELAYED RESPIRATORY DEPRESSION MAY OCCUR.** RESPIRATORY DEPRESSION (BOTH EARLY AND LATE ONSET) HAS OCCURRED MORE FREQUENTLY FOLLOWING INTRATHECAL ADMINISTRATION THAN EPIDURAL ADMINISTRATION.

Intrathecal Adult Dosage: A single injection of 0.2 to 1 mg may provide satisfactory pain relief for up to 24 hours. (CAUTION: THIS IS ONLY 0.4 TO 2 ML OF THE 5 MG/10 ML AMPUL OR 0.2 TO 1 ML OF THE 10 MG/10 ML AMPUL OF DURAMORPH®). DO NOT INJECT INTRATHECALLY MORE THAN 2 ML OF THE 5 MG/10 ML AMPUL OR 1 ML OF THE 10 MG/10 ML AMPUL. USE IN THE LUMBAR AREA ONLY IS RECOMMENDED. Repeated intrathecal injections of DURAMORPH® are not recommended. A constant intravenous infusion of naloxone, 0.6 mg/hr, for 24 hours after intrathecal injection may be used to reduce the incidence of potential side effects.

Aged patients—Administer with extreme caution. (See PRECAUTIONS.)

Repeat Dosage: If pain recurs, alternative routes of administration should be considered, since experience with repeated doses of morphine by the intrathecal route is limited.

Intrathecal Pediatric Use: No information on use in pediatric patients is available. (See PRECAUTIONS.)

SAFETY AND HANDLING INSTRUCTIONS

DURAMORPH® is supplied in sealed ampuls. Accidental dermal exposure should be treated by the removal of any contaminated clothing and rinsing the affected area with water.

Each ampul of DURAMORPH® contains a potent narcotic which has been associated with abuse and dependence among health care providers. **Due to the limited indications for this product, the risk of overdosage and the risk of its diversion and abuse, it is recommended that special measures be taken to control this product within the hospital or clinic. DURAMORPH® should be subject to rigid accounting, rigorous control of wastage and restricted access.**

Parenteral drug products should be inspected for particulate matter and discoloration prior to administration, whenever solution and container permit. DO NOT USE IF COLOR IS DARKER THAN PALE YELLOW, IF IT IS DISCOLORED IN ANY OTHER WAY OR IF IT CONTAINS A PRECIPITATE.

HOW SUPPLIED

Preservative-free DURAMORPH® (Morphine Sulfate Injection, USP) is available in amber DOSETTE® ampuls for intravenous, epidural or intrathecal administration:

5 mg/10 mL (0.5 mg/mL) packaged in 10s (NDC 0641-1112-33)

10 mg/10 mL (1 mg/1 mL) packaged in 10s (NDC 0641-1114-33)

Also available from Elkins-Sinn: INFUMORPH® (Preservative-free Morphine Sulfate Sterile Solution) 200 mg/20 mL (10 mg/mL) and 500 mg/20 mL (25 mg/mL) for epidural and intrathecal administration via a continuous microinfusion device. See insert J-1131.

STORAGE

Protect from light. Store in carton at controlled room temperature, 15° to 30°C (59° to 86°F) until ready to use. DO NOT FREEZE.

DURAMORPH® contains no preservative or antioxidant. DISCARD ANY UNUSED PORTION. DO NOT HEAT-STERILIZE.

* * * *

Manufactured by
ELKINS-SINN, INC., Cherry Hill, NJ 08003-4099
A division of A.H. Robins Company

J-1113J Revised June 1994

INFUMORPH® 200 Ⓒ
INFUMORPH® 500 Ⓒ

(Preservative-free Morphine Sulfate Sterile Solution)
WARNING: May be habit forming.
For Use in Continuous Microinfusion Devices

DESCRIPTION

Morphine is the most important alkaloid of opium and is a phenanthrene derivative. It is available as the sulfate salt, having the following structural formula:

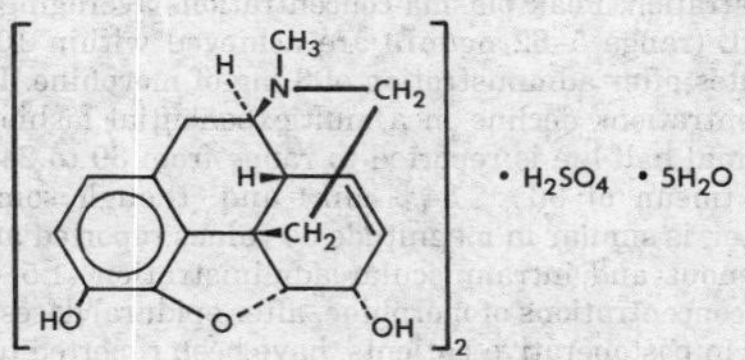

7,8-Didehydro-4,5-epoxy-17-methyl-(5α,6α)-morphinan-3,6-diol sulfate (2:1) (salt), pentahydrate
$(C_{17}H_{19}NO_3)_2 \cdot H_2SO_4 \cdot 5H_2O$) MW 758.83.

INFUMORPH® is a sterile, nonpyrogenic, isobaric, **high potency solution of morphine sulfate,** free of antioxidants, preservatives or other potentially neurotoxic additives. **INFUMORPH® is intended for use in continuous microinfusion devices for intraspinal administration in the management of pain.**

Each 20 mL ampul of **INFUMORPH® 200** contains morphine sulfate, USP 200 mg or 10 mg/mL and sodium chloride 8 mg/mL in Water for Injection, USP. Each 20 mL ampul of **INFUMORPH® 500** contains morphine sulfate, USP 500 mg or 25 mg/mL and sodium chloride 6.25 mg/mL in Water for Injection, USP. If needed, sodium hydroxide and/or sulfuric acid are added for pH adjustment to 4.5. Ampuls are sealed under nitrogen. Each 20 mL DOSETTE® ampul of **INFUMORPH®** is intended for **single use only.** *Discard any unused portion.* DO NO HEAT-STERILIZE.

CLINICAL PHARMACOLOGY

Morphine produces a wide spectrum of pharmacologic effects including analgesia, dysphoria, euphoria, somnolence, respiratory depression, diminished gastrointestinal motility and physical dependence. Opiate analgesia involves at least three anatomical areas of the central nervous system: the periaqueductal-periventricular gray matter, the ventromedial medulla and the spinal cord. A systemically administered opiate may produce analgesia by acting at any, all or some combination of these distinct regions. Morphine interacts predominantly with the μ-receptor. The μ-binding sites of opioids are very discretely distributed in the human brain, with high densities of sites found in the posterior amygdala, hypothalamus, thalamus, nucleus caudatus, putamen and certain cortical areas. They are also found on the terminal axons of primary afferents within laminae I and II (substantia gelatinosa) of the spinal cord and in the spinal nucleus of the trigeminal nerve.

Morphine has an apparent volume of distribution ranging from 1.0 to 4.7 L/kg after *intravenous* dosage. Protein binding is low, about 36%, and muscle tissue binding is reported as 54%. A blood-brain barrier exists, and when morphine is introduced outside of the CNS (e.g., *intravenously*), plasma concentrations of morphine remain higher than the corresponding CSF morphine levels. Conversely, when morphine is injected into the *intrathecal space,* it diffuses out into the systemic circulation slowly, accounting for the long duration of action of morphine administered by this route.

Morphine has a total plasma clearance which ranges from 0.9 to 1.2 L/kg/h (liters/kilogram/hour) in postoperative patients, but shows considerable interindividual variation. The major pathway of clearance is hepatic glucuronidation to morphine-3-glucuronide, which is pharmacologically inactive. The major excretion path of the conjugate is through the kidneys, with about 10% in the feces. Morphine is also eliminated by the kidneys, 2 to 12% being excreted unchanged in the urine. Terminal half-life is commonly reported to vary from 1.5 to 4.5 hours, although the longer half-lives were obtained when morphine levels were monitored over protracted periods with very sensitive radioimmunoassay methods. The accepted elimination half-life in normal subjects is 1.5 to 2 hours.

"Selective" blockade of pain sensation is possible by neuraxial application of morphine. In addition, duration of analge-

Continued on next page

Infumorph 200/500—Cont.

sia may be much longer by this route compared to systemic administration. However, CNS effects, associated with systemic administration, are still seen. These include respiratory depression, sedation, nausea and vomiting, pruritis and urinary retention. In particular, both early and late respiratory depression (up to 24 hours post dosing) have been reported following neuraxial administration. Circulation of the spinal fluid may also result in high concentrations of morphine reaching the brain stem directly.

The incidence of unwanted CNS effects, including delayed respiratory depression, associated with neuraxial application of morphine, is related to the circulatory dynamics of the epidural venous plexus and the spinal fluid. The lipid solubility and degree of ionization of morphine plays an important part in both the onset and duration of analgesia and the CNS effects. Morphine has a pK_a 7.9, with an octanol/water partition coefficient of 1.42 at pH 7.4. At this pH, the tertiary amino group in each of the opioids is mostly ionized, making the molecule water soluble. Morphine, with additional hydroxyl groups on the molecule, is significantly more water soluble than any other opioid in clinical use.

Morphine, injected into the *epidural space,* is rapidly absorbed into the general circulation. Absorption is so rapid that the plasma concentration-time profiles closely resembled those obtained after intravenous or intramuscular administration. Peak plasma concentrations averaging 33–40 ng/mL (range 5–62 ng/mL) are achieved within 10 to 15 minutes after administration of 3 mg of morphine. Plasma concentrations decline in a multiexponential fashion. The terminal half-life is reported to range from 39 to 249 minutes (mean of 90 ± 34.3 min) and, though somewhat shorter, is similar in magnitude as values reported after intravenous and intramuscular administration (1.5–4.5 h). CSF concentrations of morphine, after epidural doses of 2 to 6 mg in postoperative patients, have been reported to be 50 to 250 times higher than corresponding plasma concentrations. The CSF levels of morphine exceed those in plasma after only 15 minutes and are detectable for as long as 20 hours after the injection of 2 mg of epidural morphine. Approximately 4% of the dose injected epidurally reaches the CSF. This corresponds to the relative minimum effective epidural and intrathecal doses of 5 mg and 0.25 mg, respectively. The disposition of morphine in the CSF follows a biphasic pattern, with an early half-life of 1.5 h and a late phase half-life of about 6 h. Morphine crosses the dura slowly, with an absorption half-life across the dura averaging 22 minutes. Maximum CSF concentrations are seen 60–90 minutes after injection. Minimum effective CSF concentrations for postoperative analgesia average 150 ng/mL (range <1–380 ng/mL).

The *intrathecal route* of administration circumvents meningeal diffusion barriers and, therefore, lower doses of morphine produce comparable analgesia to that induced by the epidural route. After intrathecal bolus injection of morphine, there is a rapid initial distribution phase lasting 15–30 minutes and a half-life in the CSF of 42–136 min (mean 90 ± 16 min). Derived from limited data, it appears that the disposition of morphine in the CSF, from 15 minutes postintrathecal administration to the end of a six-hour observation period, represents a combination of the distribution and elimination phases. Morphine concentrations in the CSF averaged 332 ± 137 ng/mL at 6 hours, following a bolus dose of 0.3 mg of morphine. The apparent volume of distribution of morphine in the intrathecal space is about 22 ± 8 mL.

Time-to-peak plasma concentrations, however, is similar (5–10 min) after either epidural or intrathecal bolus administration of morphine. Maximum plasma morphine concentrations after 0.3 mg intrathecal morphine have been reported from <1 to 7.8 ng/mL. The minimum analgesic morphine plasma concentration during Patient-Controlled Analgesia (PCA) has been reported as 20–40 ng/mL, suggesting that any analgesic contribution from systemic redistribution would be minimal after the first 30–60 minutes with epidural administration and virtually absent with intrathecal administration of morphine.

INDICATION AND USAGE

INFUMORPH® (Preservative-free Morphine Sulfate Sterile Solution) is indicated only for intrathecal or epidural infusion in the treatment of intractable chronic pain. It was developed for use in continuous microinfusion devices and may require dilution before use as dictated by the characteristics of the device and the dosage requirements of the individual patient.

INFUMORPH® IS NOT RECOMMENDED FOR SINGLE-DOSE INTRAVENOUS, INTRAMUSCULAR OR SUBCUTANEOUS ADMINISTRATION DUE TO THE VERY LARGE AMOUNT OF MORPHINE IN THE AMPUL AND THE ASSOCIATED RISK OF OVERDOSAGE.

CONTRAINDICATIONS

The only absolute contraindication to the use of INFUMORPH® is known allergy to morphine. Contraindications to the use of neuraxial analgesia include: the presence of infection at the injection microinfusion site, concomitant anticoagulant therapy, uncontrolled bleeding diathesis and the presence of any other concomitant therapy or medical condition which would render epidural or intrathecal administration of medication especially hazardous.

WARNINGS

THIS PRODUCT WAS DEVELOPED FOR USE (AFTER APPROPRIATE DILUTION, IF NECESSARY) IN CONTINUOUS MICROINFUSION DEVICES FOR INTRATHECAL OR EPIDURAL INFUSION OF NARCOTICS TO CONTROL SEVERE CANCER PAIN. CHRONIC NEURAXIAL OPIOID ANALGESIA IS APPROPRIATE ONLY WHEN LESS INVASIVE MEANS OF CONTROLLING PAIN HAVE FAILED AND SHOULD ONLY BE UNDERTAKEN BY THOSE WHO ARE EXPERIENCED IN APPLYING THE TREATMENT IN A SETTING WHERE ITS COMPLICATIONS CAN BE ADEQUATELY MANAGED.

BECAUSE OF THE RISK OF SEVERE ADVERSE EFFECTS, PATIENTS MUST BE OBSERVED IN A FULLY EQUIPPED AND STAFFED ENVIRONMENT FOR AT LEAST 24 HOURS AFTER THE INITIAL (SINGLE) TEST DOSE AND, AS APPROPRIATE, FOR THE FIRST SEVERAL DAYS AFTER CATHETER IMPLANTATION.

THE FACILITY MUST BE EQUIPPED TO RESUSCITATE PATIENTS WITH SEVERE OPIATE OVERDOSAGE, AND THE PERSONNEL MUST BE FAMILIAR WITH THE USE AND LIMITATIONS OF SPECIFIC NARCOTIC ANTAGONISTS (NALOXONE, NALTREXONE) IN SUCH CASES.

RESERVOIR FILLING MUST BE PERFORMED BY FULLY TRAINED AND QUALIFIED PERSONNEL, FOLLOWING THE DIRECTIONS PROVIDED BY THE DEVICE MANUFACTURER. CARE SHOULD BE TAKEN IN SELECTING THE PROPER REFILL FREQUENCY TO PREVENT DEPLETION OF THE RESERVOIR, WHICH WOULD RESULT IN EXACERBATION OF SEVERE PAIN AND/OR REFLUX OF CSF INTO SOME DEVICES. STRICT ASEPTIC TECHNIQUE IN FILLING IS REQUIRED TO AVOID BACTERIAL CONTAMINATION AND SERIOUS INFECTION. **EXTREME CARE MUST BE TAKEN TO ENSURE THAT THE NEEDLE IS PROPERLY IN THE FILLING PORT OF THE DEVICE BEFORE ATTEMPTING TO REFILL THE RESERVOIR. INJECTING THE SOLUTION INTO THE TISSUE AROUND THE DEVICE OR (IN THE CASE OF DEVICES THAT HAVE MORE THAN ONE PORT) ATTEMPTING TO INJECT THE REFILL DOSE INTO THE DIRECT INJECTION PORT WILL RESULT IN A LARGE, CLINICALLY SIGNIFICANT, OVERDOSAGE TO THE PATIENT.**

A PERIOD OF OBSERVATION APPROPRIATE TO THE CLINICAL SITUATION SHOULD FOLLOW EACH REFILL OR MANIPULATION OF THE DRUG RESERVOIR. BEFORE DISCHARGE, THE PATIENT AND ATTENDANT(S) SHOULD RECEIVE INSTRUCTION IN THE PROPER HOME CARE OF THE DEVICE AND INSERTION SITE AND IN THE RECOGNITION AND PRACTICAL TREATMENT OF AN OVERDOSE OF NEURAXIAL MORPHINE.

TOLERANCE AND MYOCLONIC ACTIVITY

PATIENTS SOMETIMES MANIFEST UNUSUAL ACCELERATION OF NEURAXIAL MORPHINE REQUIREMENTS, WHICH MAY CAUSE CONCERN REGARDING SYSTEMIC ABSORPTION AND THE HAZARDS OF LARGE DOSES; THESE PATIENTS MAY BENEFIT FROM HOSPITALIZATION AND DETOXIFICATION. TWO CASES OF MYOCLONIC-LIKE SPASM OF THE LOWER EXTREMITIES HAVE BEEN REPORTED IN PATIENTS RECEIVING MORE THAN 20 MG/DAY OF INTRATHECAL MORPHINE. AFTER DETOXIFICATION, IT MIGHT BE POSSIBLE TO RESUME TREATMENT AT LOWER DOSES, AND SOME PATIENTS HAVE BEEN SUCCESSFULLY CHANGED FROM CONTINUOUS EPIDURAL MORPHINE TO CONTINUOUS INTRATHECAL MORPHINE. REPEAT DETOXIFICATION MAY BE INDICATED AT A LATER DATE. THE UPPER DAILY DOSAGE LIMIT FOR EACH PATIENT DURING CONTINUING TREATMENT MUST BE INDIVIDUALIZED.

PRECAUTIONS

Control of pain by neuraxial opiate delivery, using a continuous microinfusion device, is always accompanied by considerable risk to the patients and requires a high level of skill to be successfully accomplished. The task of treating these patients must be undertaken by experienced clinical teams, well-versed in patient selection, evolving technology and emerging standards of care. For reasons of safety, it is recommended that administration of INFUMORPH® 200 and 500 (10 and 25 mg/mL, respectively) by the intrathecal route be limited to the lumber area.

USE IN PATIENTS WITH INCREASED INTRACRANIAL PRESSURE OR HEAD INJURY

INFUMORPH® (Preservative-free Morphine Sulfate Sterile Solution) should be used with extreme caution in patients with head injury or increased intracranial pressure. Pupillary changes (miosis) from morphine may obscure the existence, extent and course of intracranial pathology. High doses of neuraxial morphine may produce myoclonic events (see WARNINGS and ADVERSE REACTIONS). Clinicians should maintain a high index of suspicion for adverse drug reactions when evaluating altered mental status or movement abnormalities in patients receiving this modality of treatment.

USE IN CHRONIC PULMONARY DISEASE

Care is urged in using this drug in patients who have a decreased respiratory reserve (e.g., emphysema, severe obesity, kyphoscoliosis or paralysis of the phrenic nerve). INFUMORPH® should not be given in cases of chronic asthma, upper airway obstruction or in any other chronic pulmonary disorder without due consideration of the known risk of acute respiratory failure following morphine administration in such patients.

USE IN HEPATIC OR RENAL DISEASE

The elimination half-life of morphine may be prolonged in patients with reduced metabolic rate and with hepatic and/or renal dysfunction. Hence, care should be exercised in administering INFUMORPH® epidurally to patients with these conditions, since high-blood morphine levels, due to reduced clearance, may take several days to develop.

USE IN BILIARY SURGERY OR DISORDERS OF THE BILIARY TRACT

As significant morphine is released into the systemic circulation from neuraxial administration, the ensuing smooth muscle hypertonicity may result in biliary colic.

USE WITH DISORDERS OF THE URINARY SYSTEM

Initiation of neuraxial opiate analgesia is frequently associated with disturbances of micturition, especially in males with prostatic enlargement. Early recognition of difficulty in urination and prompt intervention in cases of urinary retention is indicated.

USE IN AMBULATORY PATIENTS

Patients with reduced circulating blood volume, impaired myocardial function or on sympatholytic drugs should be monitored for the possible occurrence of orthostatic hypotension, a frequent complication in single-dose neuraxial morphine analgesia.

USE WITH OTHER CENTRAL NERVOUS SYSTEM DEPRESSANTS

The depressant effects of morphine are potentiated by the presence of other CNS depressants such as alcohol, sedatives, antihistaminics or psychotropic drugs. Use of neuroleptics in conjunction with neuraxial morphine may increase the risk of respiratory depression.

CARCINOGENESIS, MUTAGENESIS, IMPAIRMENT OF FERTILITY

Morphine is without known carcinogenic or mutagenic effects and is not known to impair fertility at non-narcotic doses in animals, but studies of the carcinogenic and mutagenic potential or the effect on fertility of INFUMORPH® have not been conducted.

PREGNANCY CATEGORY C

Morphine sulfate is not teratogenic in rats at 35 mg/kg/day (thirty-five times the usual human dose) but does result in increased pup mortality and growth retardation at doses that narcotize the animal (>10 mg/kg/day, ten times the usual human dose). INFUMORPH® should only be given to pregnant women when no other method of controlling pain is available and means are at hand to manage the delivery and perinatal care of the opiate-dependent infant.

LABOR AND DELIVERY

INFUMORPH® 200 and 500 (10 and 25 mg/mL, respectively) are too highly concentrated for routine use in obstetric neuraxial analgesia.

NURSING MOTHERS

Morphine is excreted in maternal milk. Effects on the nursing infant are not known.

PEDIATRIC USE

Adequate studies, to establish the safety and effectiveness of spinal morphine in children, have not been performed, and usage in this population is not recommended.

USE IN THE AGED

The pharmacodynamic effects of neuraxial morphine in the aged are more variable than in the younger population. Patients will vary widely in the effective initial dose, rate of development of tolerance and the frequency and magnitude of associated adverse effects as the dose is increased. Initial doses should be based on careful clinical observation following "test doses", after making due allowances for the effects of the patient's age and infirmity on their ability to clear the drug, particularly in patients receiving epidural morphine.

ADVERSE REACTIONS

IMPROPER OR ERRONEOUS SUBSTITUTION OF INFUMORPH® 200 or 500 (10 or 25 mg/mL, respectively) FOR REGULAR DURAMORPH® (0.5 or 1 mg/mL) IS LIKELY TO RESULT IN SERIOUS OVERDOSAGE, LEADING TO SEIZURES, RESPIRATORY DEPRESSION AND, POSSIBLY, FATAL OUTCOME.

The most serious adverse experiences encountered during continuous intrathecal or epidural infusion of INFUMORPH® are respiratory depression and myoclonus.

1. Single-dose neuraxial administration may result in acute or delayed respiratory depression for periods at least as long as 24 hours. **Severe respiratory depression, potentially life-threatening, can result from technical errors during refill, e.g., injection of INFUMORPH® outside the filling port, unintentional injection into the direct bypass-dosing port featured on some devices or local infiltration.**
2. **Tolerance and myoclonus:** See **WARNINGS** for discussion of these and related hazards.

While low doses of intravenously administered morphine have little effect on cardiovascular stability, high doses are excitatory, resulting from **sympathetic hyperactivity** and increase in circulatory catecholamines. Excitation of the central nervous system, resulting in **convulsions**, may accompany high doses of morphine given intravenously.

Dysphoric reactions may occur after any size dose and **toxic psychoses** have been reported.

Pruritus: Single-dose epidural or intrathecal administration is accompanied by a high incidence of **pruritus** that is dose-related but not confined to the site of administration. Pruritus, following continuous infusion of epidural or intrathecal morphine, is occasionally reported in the literature; these reactions are poorly understood as to their cause.

Urinary retention: Urinary retention, which may persist 10 to 20 hours following single epidural or intrathecal administration, is a frequent side effect and must be anticipated primarily in male patients, with a somewhat lower incidence in females. Also frequently reported in the literature is the occurrence of urinary retention during the first several days of hospitalization for the initiation of continuous intrathecal or epidural morphine therapy. Patients who develop urinary retention have responded to cholinomimetic treatment and/or judicious use of catheters (see PRECAUTIONS).

Constipation: Constipation is frequently encountered during continuous infusion of morphine; this can usually be managed by conventional therapy.

Headache: Lumbar puncture-type headache is encountered in a significant minority of cases for several days following intrathecal catheter implantation; this, generally, responds to bed rest and/or other conventional therapy.

Peripheral edema: There are several reports of peripheral edema, including unexplained genital swelling in male patients, following infusion-device implant surgery.

Other: Other adverse experiences reported following morphine therapy include—**Dizziness, euphoria, anxiety, depression of cough reflex, interference with thermal regulation** and **oliguria**. Evidence of histamine release such as **urticaria, wheals** and/or **local tissue irritation** may occur.

Pruritus, nausea/vomiting and urinary retention, if associated with continuous infusion therapy, may respond to intravenous administration of a low dose of naloxone (0.2 mg). The risks of using narcotic antagonists in patients chronically receiving narcotic therapy should be considered.

NALOXONE INJECTION AND RESUSCITATIVE EQUIPMENT SHOULD BE IMMEDIATELY AVAILABLE FOR USE IN CASE OF LIFE-THREATENING OR INTOLERABLE SIDE EFFECTS AND WHENEVER INFUMORPH® THERAPY IS BEING INITIATED, THE RESERVOIR IS BEING REFILLED OR ANY MANIPULATION OF THE RESERVOIR SYSTEM IS TAKING PLACE.

DRUG ABUSE AND DEPENDENCE

CONTROLLED SUBSTANCE

Morphine sulfate is a Schedule II narcotic under the United States Controlled Substance Act (21 U.S.C. 801–886).

Morphine is the most commonly cited prototype for narcotic substances that possess an addiction-forming or addiction-sustaining liability. A patient may be at risk for developing a dependence to morphine if used improperly or for overly long periods of time. As with all potent opioids which are μ-agonists, tolerance as well as psychological and physical dependence to morphine may develop irrespective of the route of administration (intravenous, intramuscular, intrathecal, epidural or oral). Individuals with a prior history of opioid or other substance abuse or dependence, being more apt to respond to the euphorogenic and reinforcing properties of morphine, would be considered to be a greater risk. Care must be taken to avert withdrawal in patients who have been maintained on parenteral/oral narcotics when epidural or intrathecal administration is considered. Withdrawal symptoms may occur when morphine is discontinued abruptly or upon administration of a narcotic antagonist.

OVERDOSAGE

PARENTERAL ADMINISTRATION OF NARCOTICS IN PATIENTS RECEIVING EPIDURAL OR INTRATHECAL MORPHINE MAY RESULT IN OVERDOSAGE.

Overdosage of morphine is characterized by respiratory depression, with or without concomitant CNS depression. Since respiratory arrest may result either through direct depression of the respiratory center, or as the result of hypoxia, primary attention should be given to the establishment of adequate respiratory exchange through provision of a patent airway and institution of assisted, or controlled, ventilation. The narcotic antagonist, naloxone, is a specific antidote. An initial dose of 0.4 to 2 mg of naloxone should be administered intravenously, simultaneously with respiratory resuscitation. If the desired degree of counteraction and improvement in respiratory function is not obtained, naloxone may be repeated at 2- to 3-minute intervals. If no response is observed after 10 mg of naloxone has been administered, the diagnosis of narcotic-induced, or partial narcotic-induced, toxicity should be questioned. Intramuscular or subcutaneous administration may be used if the intravenous route is not available.

As the duration of effect of naloxone is considerably shorter than that of epidural or intrathecal morphine, repeated administration may be necessary. Patients should be closely observed for evidence of renarcotization.

DOSAGE AND ADMINISTRATION

INFUMORPH® 200 AND 500 (10 AND 25 MG/ML, RESPECTIVELY) SHOULD NOT BE USED FOR SINGLE-DOSE NEURAXIAL INJECTION BECAUSE LOWER DOSES CAN BE MORE RELIABLY ADMINISTERED WITH THE STANDARD PREPARATION OF DURAMORPH® (0.5 AND 1 MG/ML).

CANDIDATES FOR NEURAXIAL ADMINISTRATION OF INFUMORPH® IN A CONTINUOUS MICROINFUSION DEVICE SHOULD BE HOSPITALIZED TO PROVIDE FOR ADEQUATE PATIENT MONITORING DURING ASSESSMENT OF RESPONSE TO SINGLE DOSES OF INTRATHECAL OR EPIDURAL MORPHINE. HOSPITALIZATION SHOULD BE MAINTAINED FOR SEVERAL DAYS AFTER SURGERY INVOLVING THE INFUSION DEVICE FOR ADDITIONAL MONITORING AND ADJUSTMENT OF DAILY DOSAGE. THE FACILITY MUST BE EQUIPPED WITH RESUSCITATIVE EQUIPMENT, OXYGEN, NALOXONE INJECTION AND OTHER RESUSCITATIVE DRUGS. BECAUSE OF THE RISK OF DELAYED RESPIRATORY DEPRESSION, PATIENTS SHOULD BE OBSERVED IN A FULLY EQUIPPED AND STAFFED ENVIRONMENT FOR AT LEAST 24 HOURS AFTER EACH TEST DOSE AND, AS INDICATED, FOR THE FIRST SEVERAL DAYS AFTER SURGERY.

Familiarization with the continuous microinfusion device is essential. The desired amount of morphine should be withdrawn from the ampul through a microfilter. **To minimize risk from glass or other particles, the product must be filtered through a 5 μ (or smaller) microfilter before injecting into the microinfusion device.** If dilution is required, 0.9% Sodium Chloride Injection is recommended.

Intrathecal Dosage: The starting dose must be individualized, based upon in-hospital evaluation of the response to serial single-dose intrathecal bolus injections of regular DURAMORPH® (Morphine Sulfate Injection, USP) 0.5 mg/mL or 1 mg/mL, with close observation of the analgesic efficacy and adverse effects *prior* to surgery involving the continuous microinfusion device.

The recommended initial lumbar intrathecal dose range in patients with no tolerance to opioids is 0.2 to 1 mg/day. The published range of doses for individuals who have some degree of opioid tolerance varies from 1 to 10 mg/day. The upper daily dosage limit for each patient must be individualized.

Limited experience with continuous intrathecal infusion of morphine has shown that the daily doses have to be increased over time. Although the rate of increase, over time, in the dose required to sustain analgesia is highly variable, an estimate of the expected rate of increase is shown in the following Figure.

Figure: Dose Trend in Continuous Infusions of Intrathecal Morphine
(Mean and 95% Confidence Intervals)

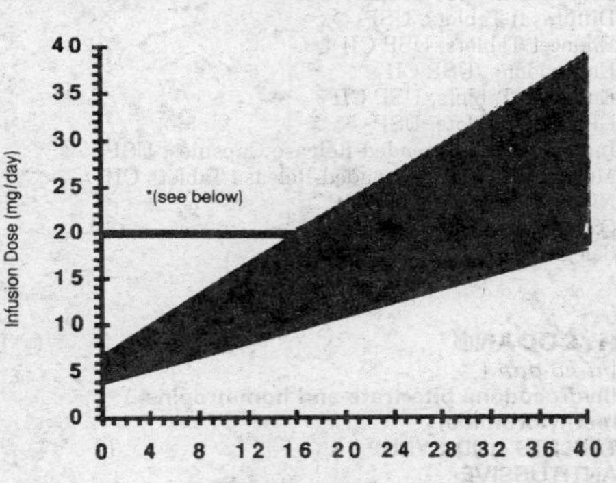

*20 mg/day is the lowest dose for which regional myoclonus has been reported.
The rate of occurrence cannot be estimated.

Doses above 20 mg/day should be employed with caution since they may be associated with a higher likelihood of serious side effects (see WARNINGS concerning potential neurological hazards and ADVERSE REACTIONS).

Epidural Dosage: The starting dose must be individualized, based upon in-hospital evaluation of the response to serial single-dose epidural bolus injections of regular DURAMORPH® (Morphine Sulfate Injection, USP) 0.5 mg/mL or 1 mg/mL, with dose observation for analgesic efficacy and adverse effects *prior* to surgery involving the continuous microinfusion device.

The recommended initial epidural dose in patients who are not tolerant to opioids ranges from 3.5 to 7.5 mg/day. The usual starting dose for continuous epidural infusion, based upon limited data in patients who have some degree of opioid tolerance, is 4.5 to 10 mg/day. The dose requirements may increase significantly during treatment, frequently to 20–30 mg/day. The upper daily limit for each patient must be individualized.

SAFETY AND HANDLING INFORMATION

INFUMORPH® is supplied in sealed ampuls. Accidental dermal exposure should be treated by the removal of any contaminated clothing and rinsing the affected area with water.

Each ampul of INFUMORPH® contains a large amount of potent narcotic which has been associated with abuse and dependence among health care providers. **Due to the limited indications for this product, the risk of overdosage and the risk of its diversion and abuse, it is recommended that special measures be taken to control this product within the hospital or clinic. *INFUMORPH® should be subject to rigid accounting, rigorous control of wastage and restricted access.***

This parenteral drug product must be inspected for particulate matter before opening the amber ampul and again for color after removing contents from the ampul. Do not use if the solution in the unopened ampul contains a precipitate which does not disappear upon shaking. After removal, do not use unless the solution is colorless or pale yellow.

HOW SUPPLIED

Amber DOSETTE® ampuls for epidural or intrathecal administration via a continuous microinfusion device.

INFUMORPH® 200 (Preservative-free Morphine Sulfate Sterile Solution) 200 mg/20 mL (10 mg/mL) packaged individually (*NDC* 0641-1131-31)

INFUMORPH® 500 (Preservative-free Morphine Sulfate Sterile Solution) 500 mg/20 mL (25 mg/mL) packaged individually (*NDC* 0641-1132-31)

Also available from Elkins-Sinn, Inc. DURAMORPH® (Morphine Sulfate Injection, USP) 5 mg/10 mL (0.5 mg/mL) and 10 mg/10 mL (1 mg/mL). See insert J-1113.

STORAGE

Protect from light. Store in carton at controlled room temperature 15°–30°C (59°–86°F) until ready to use. DO NOT FREEZE. INFUMORPH® contains no preservative or antioxidant. DISCARD ANY UNUSED PORTION. DO NOT HEAT-STERILIZE.

Manufactured by
ELKINS-SINN, INC. Cherry Hill, NJ 08003-4099
A subsidiary of A.H. Robins Company

J-1131B Revised June 1993

SOTRADECOL® ℞

[*sō 'trah "de 'kol "*]
(Sodium Tetradecyl Sulfate Injection)
For Intravenous Use Only

DESCRIPTION

Sodium tetradecyl sulfate is an anionic surfactant which occurs as a white, waxy solid. The structural formula is as follows:

$$CH_3(CH_2)_3CH(C_2H_5)(CH_2)_2CH(CH_2CH(CH_3)_2)OSO_2ONa$$

$C_{14}H_{29}NaSO_4$
7-Ethyl-2-methyl-4-hendecanol sulfate sodium salt
M.W. 316.44

Sotradecol® (Sodium Tetradecyl Sulfate Injection) is a sterile nonpyrogenic solution for intravenous use as a sclerosing agent. Each mL contains sodium tetradecyl sulfate 10 mg or 30 mg, benzyl alcohol 0.02 mL and dibasic sodium phosphate, anhydrous 0.72 mg in Water for Injection. pH 7.9; monobasic sodium phosphate and/or sodium hydroxide added, if needed, for pH adjustment.

CLINICAL PHARMACOLOGY

Sotradecol® (Sodium Tetradecyl Sulfate Injection) is a mild sclerosing agent. Intravenous injection causes intima inflammation and thrombus formation. This usually occludes the injected vein. Subsequent formation of fibrous tissue results in partial or complete vein obliteration.

INDICATIONS AND USAGE

Indicated in the treatment of small uncomplicated varicose veins of the lower extremities that show simple dilation with competent valves. The benefit-to-risk ratio should be considered in selected patients who are great surgical risks.

CONTRAINDICATIONS

Contraindicated in previous hypersensitivity reactions to the drug; in acute superficial thrombophlebitis; significant valvular or deep vein incompetence; huge superficial veins with wide open communications to deeper veins; phlebitis migrans; acute cellulitis; allergic conditions; acute infections; varicosities caused by abdominal and pelvic tumors unless the tumor has been removed; bedridden patients; such uncontrolled systemic diseases as diabetes, toxic hyperthyroidism, tuberculosis, asthma, neoplasm, sepsis, blood dyscrasias and acute respiratory or skin diseases.

WARNINGS

Since severe adverse local effects, including tissue necrosis, may occur following extravasation, Sotradecol® (Sodium Tetradecyl Sulfate Injection), should be administered only by a physician familiar with proper injection technique. Extreme care in needle placement and using the minimal effective volume at each injection site are, therefore, important.

Allergic reactions, including anaphylaxis, have been reported that led to death. Therefore, as a precaution against anaphylactic shock, it is recommended that 0.5 mL of Sotradecol® be injected into a varicosity, followed by observation of the patient for several hours before administration of a second or larger dose. The possibility of an anaphylactic reaction should be kept in mind, and the physician should be prepared to treat it appropriately. In extreme emergencies, 0.25 mL of 1:1000 Epinephrine Injection (0.25 mg) intravenously should be used and side reactions controlled with antihistamines.

Continued on next page

Sotradecol—Cont.

PRECAUTIONS

GENERAL

The drug should only be administered by physicians who are familiar with an acceptable injection technique. Because of the danger of thrombosis extension into the deep venous system, thorough preinjection evaluation for valvular competency should be carried out and slow injections with a small amount (not over 2 mL) of the preparation should be injected into the varicosity. In particular, deep venous patency must be determined by angiography and/or the Perthes test before sclerotherapy is undertaken. Venous sclerotherapy should not be undertaken if tests, such as the Trendelenberg and Perthes, and angiography show significant valvular or deep venous incompetence. The physician should bear in mind that injection necrosis is likely to result from extravascular injection of sclerosing agents.

Extreme caution must be exercised in the presence of underlying arterial disease such as marked peripheral arteriosclerosis or thromboangiitis obliterans (Buerger's Disease). Embolism may occur as long as four weeks after injection of sodium tetradecyl sulfate. The incidence of recurrence is low if the patient wears elastic stockings.

DRUG INTERACTIONS

No well-controlled studies have been performed on patients taking antiovulatory agents. The physician must use judgment and evaluate any patient taking antiovulatory drugs prior to initiating treatment with Sotradecol®. (See ADVERSE REACTIONS.)

Heparin should not be included in the same syringe as Sotradecol®, since the two are incompatible.

CARCINOGENESIS, MUTAGENESIS, IMPAIRMENT OF FERTILITY

When tested in the L5178YTK$^{+/-}$ mouse lymphoma assay, sodium tetradecyl sulfate did not induce a dose-related increase in the frequency of thymidine kinase-deficient mutants and, therefore, was judged to be nonmutagenic in this system. However, no long-term animal carcinogenicity studies with sodium tetradecyl sulfate have been performed.

PREGNANCY

Teratogenic Effects—Pregnancy Category C. Animal reproduction studies have not been conducted with Sotradecol®. It is also not known whether Sotradecol® can cause fetal harm when administered to a pregnant woman or can affect reproduction capacity. Sotradecol® should be given to a pregnant woman only if clearly needed.

NURSING MOTHERS

It is not known whether this drug is excreted in human milk. Because many drugs are excreted in human milk, caution should be exercised when Sotradecol® is administered to a nursing woman.

PEDIATRIC USE

Safety and effectiveness in pediatric patients have not been established.

ADVERSE REACTIONS

Local reactions consisting of pain, urticaria or ulceration may occur at the site of injection. A permanent discoloration, usually small and hardly noticeable but which may be objectionable from a cosmetic viewpoint, may remain along the path of the sclerosed vein segment. Sloughing and necrosis of tissue may occur following extravasation of the drug.

Allergic reactions such as hives, asthma, hayfever and anaphylactic shock have been reported. Mild systemic reactions that have been reported include headache, nausea and vomiting. (See WARNINGS.)

Four deaths have been reported with the use of Sotradecol®. One death has been reported in a patient who received Sotradecol® and who had been receiving an antiovulatory agent. Another death (fatal pulmonary embolism) has been reported in a 36-year-old female treated with sodium tetradecyl *acetate* and who was **not** taking oral contraceptives. Two cases of anaphylactic shock leading to death have been reported in patients who received Sotradecol®. One of the patients reported a medical history of asthma, a contraindication to the administration of Sotradecol®.

DOSAGE AND ADMINISTRATION

For intravenous use only. Do not use if precipitated or discolored. The strength of solution required depends on the size and degree of varicosity. In general, the 1% solution will be found most useful with the 3% solution preferred for larger varicosities. The dosage should be kept small, using 0.5 to 2 mL (preferably 1 mL maximum) for each injection, and the maximum single treatment should not exceed 10 mL.

Parenteral drug products should be inspected visually for particulate matter and discoloration prior to administration, whenever solution and container permit.

HOW SUPPLIED

Sotradecol® (Sodium Tetradecyl Sulfate Injection)

1%—2 mL DOSETTE® ampuls packaged in 5s (NDC 0641-1514-34)

3%—2 mL DOSETTE® ampuls packaged in 5s (NDC 0641-1516-34)

STORAGE

Store at controlled room temperature 15°–30°C (59°–86°F).

ANIMAL TOXICOLOGY

The intravenous LD_{50} of sodium tetradecyl sulfate in mice was reported to be 90 ± 5 mg/kg.

In the rat, the acute intravenous LD_{50} of sodium tetradecyl sulfate was estimated to be between 72 mg/kg and 108 mg/kg.

Purified sodium tetradecyl sulfate was found to have an LD_{50} of 2 g/kg when administered orally by stomach tube as a 25% aqueous solution to rats. In rats given 0.15 g/kg in drinking water for 30 days, no appreciable toxicity was seen, although some growth inhibition was discernible.

* * * *

Manufactured by
ELKINS-SINN, INC., Cherry Hill, NJ 08003-4099
A division of A.H. Robins Company
J-1514H Revised November 1996

ENDO PHARMACEUTICALS INC.

223 Wilmington West Chester Pike
Chadds Ford, PA 19317
Endo Laboratories
Endo Generic Products

Direct Inquiries to:
Customer Service:
(800) 462-3636
Fax: 877-329-3636

For Medical Information/Adverse Drug Experience Reporting Contact:
(800) 462-3636

Other Products Available:

Amantadine HCl Syrup, USP
Amiloride HCl and HCTZ Tablets, USP
Butalbital, Aspirin, Caffeine, and Codeine Phosphate Capsules, USP
Captopril/HCTZ Tablets, USP
Carbidopa and Levodopa Tablets, USP
Cimetidine HCl Injection
Cimetidine HCl Oral Solution
Cimetidine Tablets, USP
Dicyclomine HCl Capsules, USP
Dicyclomine HCl Tablets, USP
Diflunisal Tablets, USP
Endocet Tablets, USP CII
Endocodone, USP CII
Endodan Tablets, USP CII
Glipizide Tablets, USP
Indomethacin Extended-Release Capsules, USP
Morphine Sulfate Extended-Release Tablets CII
Nitroglycerin Tablets, USP
Oxycodone/APAP Capsules
Selegiline HCl Tablets, USP

HYCODAN® Ⓒ℞

[*hī-kō-dan*]
(hydrocodone bitartrate and homatropine methylbromide)
TABLETS AND SYRUP
ANTITUSSIVE
Rx only

DESCRIPTION

HYCODAN contains hydrocodone (dihydrocodeinone) bitartrate, a semisynthetic centrally-acting narcotic antitussive. Homatropine methylbromide is included in a subtherapeutic amount to discourage deliberate overdosage.

Each HYCODAN tablet or teaspoonful (5 mL) contains:

Hydrocodone bitartrate, USP	5 mg
Homatropine methylbromide, USP	1.5 mg

HYCODAN tablets also contain: calcium phosphate dibasic, colloidal silicon dioxide, lactose, magnesium stearate, starch and stearic acid.

HYCODAN syrup also contains: caramel coloring, FD&C Red 40, liquid sugar, methylparaben, propylparaben, sorbitol solution and wild cherry imitation flavor.

The hydrocodone component is 4,5α-epoxy-3-methoxy-17-methylmorphinan-6-one tartrate (1:1) hydrate (2:5), a fine white crystal or crystalline powder, which is derived from the opium alkaloid, thebaine, has a molecular weight of (494.50), and may be represented by the following structural formula:

$C_{18}H_{21}NO_3 \cdot C_4H_6O_6 \cdot 2\ ^1/_2H_2O$
HYDROCODONE BITARTRATE

[See chemical structure at top of next column]

Homatropine methylbromide is 8-Azoniabicyclo [3.2.1] octane,3-[(hydroxyphenylacetyl)oxy]-8,8-dimethyl-,bromide, endo-; a white crystal or fine white crystalline powder, with a molecular weight of (370.29).

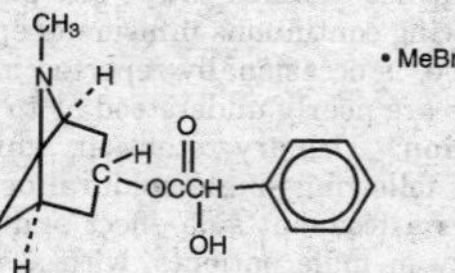

$C_{17}H_{24}BrNO_3$
HOMATROPINE METHYLBROMIDE

CLINICAL PHARMACOLOGY

Hydrocodone is a semisynthetic narcotic antitussive and analgesic with multiple actions qualitatively similar to those of codeine. The precise mechanism of action of hydrocodone and other opiates is not known; however, hydrocodone is believed to act directly on the cough center. In excessive doses, hydrocodone, like other opium derivatives, will depress respiration. The effects of hydrocodone in therapeutic doses on the cardiovascular system are insignificant. Hydrocodone can produce miosis, euphoria, physical and physiological dependence.

Following a 10 mg oral dose of hydrocodone administered to five adult male subjects, the mean peak concentration was 23.6 ± 5.2 ng/mL. Maximum serum levels were achieved at 1.3 ± 0.3 hours and the half-life was determined to be 3.8 ± 0.3 hours. Hydrocodone exhibits a complex pattern of metabolism including O-demethylation, N-demethylation and 6-keto reduction to the corresponding 6-α- and 6-β-hydroxymetabolites.

INDICATIONS AND USAGE

HYCODAN (hydrocodone bitartrate and homatropine methylbromide) is indicated for the symptomatic relief of cough.

CONTRAINDICATIONS

HYCODAN should not be administered to patients who are hypersensitive to hydrocodone or homatropine methylbromide.

WARNINGS

Hydrocodone can produce drug dependence of the morphine type and, therefore, has the potential for being abused. Psychic dependence, physical dependence and tolerance may develop upon repeated administration of HYCODAN and it should be prescribed and administered with the same degree of caution appropriate to the use of other narcotic drugs (see DRUG ABUSE AND DEPENDENCE).

Respiratory Depression: HYCODAN produces dose-related respiratory depression by directly acting on brain stem respiratory centers. If respiratory depression occurs, it may be antagonized by the use of naloxone hydrochloride and other supportive measures when indicated.

Head Injury And Increased Intracranial Pressure: The respiratory depression properties of narcotics and their capacity to elevate cerebrospinal fluid pressure may be markedly exaggerated in the presence of head injury, other intracranial lesions or a pre-existing increase in intracranial pressure. Furthermore, narcotics produce adverse reactions which may obscure the clinical course of patients with head injuries.

Acute Abdominal Conditions: The administration of HYCODAN or other narcotics may obscure the diagnosis or clinical course of patients with acute abdominal conditions.

Pediatric Use: In young pediatric patients, as well as adults, the respiratory center is sensitive to the depressant action of narcotic cough suppressants in a dose-dependent manner. Benefit to risk ratio should be carefully considered especially in the pediatric population with respiratory embarrassment (e.g., croup).

PRECAUTIONS

General: Before prescribing medication to suppress or modify cough, it is important to ascertain that the underlying cause of cough is identified, that modification of cough does not increase the risk of clinical or physiological complications, and that appropriate therapy for the primary disease is provided.

Special Risk Patients: HYCODAN should be given with caution to certain patients such as the elderly or debilitated, and those with severe impairment of hepatic or renal functions, hypothyroidism, Addison's disease, prostatic hypertrophy or urethral stricture, asthma, and narrow-angle glaucoma.

Information for Patients: Hydrocodone may impair the mental and/or physical abilities required for the performance of potentially hazardous tasks such as driving a car or operating machinery. The patient using HYCODAN (hydrocodone bitartrate and homatropine methylbromide) should be cautioned accordingly.

Drug Interactions: Patients receiving narcotics, antihistamines, antipsychotics, antianxiety agents or other CNS depressants (including alcohol) concomitantly with HYCODAN may exhibit an additive CNS depression. When combined therapy is contemplated, the dose of one or both agents should be reduced. The use of MAO inhibitors or tricyclic antidepressants with hydrocodone preparations may increase the effect of either the antidepressant or hydrocodone.

Carcinogenesis, Mutagenesis, Impairment of Fertility: Studies of HYCODAN in animals to evaluate the carcinogenic and mutagenic potential and the effect on fertility have not been conducted.

Pregnancy

Teratogenic Effects: Pregnancy Category C; Animal reproduction studies have not been conducted with HYCODAN.

It is also not known whether HYCODAN can cause fetal harm when administered to a pregnant woman or can affect reproduction capacity. HYCODAN should be given to a pregnant woman only if clearly needed.

Nonteratogenic Effects: Babies born to mothers who have been taking opioids regularly prior to delivery will be physically dependent. The withdrawal signs include irritability and excessive crying, tremors, hyperactive reflexes, increased respiratory rate, increased stools, sneezing, yawning, vomiting and fever. The intensity of the syndrome does not always correlate with the duration of maternal opioid use or dose.

Labor and Delivery: As with all narcotics, administration of HYCODAN to the mother shortly before delivery may result in some degree of respiratory depression in the newborn, especially if higher doses are used.

Nursing Mothers: It is not known whether this drug is excreted in human milk. Because many drugs are excreted in human milk and because of the potential for serious adverse reactions in nursing infants from HYCODAN, a decision should be made whether to discontinue nursing or to discontinue the drug, taking into account the importance of the drug to the mother.

Pediatric Use: Safety and effectiveness of HYCODAN in pediatric patients under six have not been established.

ADVERSE REACTIONS

Central Nervous System: Sedation, drowsiness, mental clouding, lethargy, impairment of mental and physical performance, anxiety, fear, dysphoria, dizziness, psychic dependence, mood changes.

Gastrointestinal System: Nausea and vomiting may occur; they are more frequent in ambulatory than in recumbent patients. Prolonged administration of HYCODAN may produce constipation.

Genitourinary System: Ureteral spasm, spasm of vesicle sphincters and urinary retention have been reported with opiates.

Respiratory Depression: HYCODAN may produce dose-related respiratory depression by acting directly on brain stem respiratory centers (see OVERDOSAGE).

Dermatological: Skin rash, pruritus.

DRUG ABUSE AND DEPENDENCE

HYCODAN is a Schedule III narcotic. Psychic dependence, physical dependence and tolerance may develop upon repeated administration of narcotics; therefore, HYCODAN (hydrocodone bitartrate and homatropine methylbromide) should be prescribed and administered with caution. However, psychic dependence is unlikely to develop when HYCODAN is used for a short time for the treatment of cough. Physical dependence, the condition in which continued administration of the drug is required to prevent the appearance of a withdrawal syndrome, assumes clinically significant proportions only after several weeks of continued oral narcotic use, although some mild degree of physical dependence may develop after a few days of narcotic therapy.

OVERDOSAGE

Signs and Symptoms: Serious overdosage with hydrocodone is characterized by respiratory depression (a decrease in respiratory rate and/or tidal volume, Cheyne-Stokes respiration, cyanosis), extreme somnolence progressing to stupor or coma, skeletal muscle flaccidity, cold and clammy skin, and sometimes bradycardia and hypotension. In severe overdosage, apnea, circulatory collapse, cardiac arrest and death may occur. The ingestion of very large amounts of HYCODAN may, in addition, result in acute homatropine intoxication.

Treatment: Primary attention should be given to the reestablishment of adequate respiratory exchange through provision of a patent airway and the institution of assisted or controlled ventilation. The narcotic antagonist naloxone hydrochloride is a specific antidote for respiratory depression which may result from overdosage or unusual sensitivity to narcotics including hydrocodone. Therefore, an appropriate dose of naloxone hydrochloride should be administered, preferably by the intravenous route, simultaneously with efforts at respiratory resuscitation. For further information, see full prescribing information for naloxone hydrochloride. An antagonist should not be administered in the absence of clinically significant respiratory depression. Oxygen, intravenous fluids, vasopressors and other supportive measures should be employed as indicated. Gastric emptying may be useful in removing unabsorbed drug.

DOSAGE AND ADMINISTRATION

Adults: One (1) tablet or one (1) teaspoonful (5 mL) of the syrup every 4 to 6 hours as needed; do not exceed six (6) tablets or six (6) teaspoonfuls in 24 hours.

Children 6 to 12 years of age: One-half ($^1/_2$) tablet or one-half ($^1/_2$) teaspoonful (2.5 mL) of the syrup every 4 to 6 hours as needed; do not exceed three (3) tablets or three (3) teaspoonfuls in 24 hours.

HOW SUPPLIED

HYCODAN is supplied as a white, biconvex tablet, one face bisected and debossed with "HYCODAN," and the other face plain, available in:

Bottles of 100	NDC 63481-042-70
Bottles of 500	NDC 63481-042-85

Store tablets at controlled room temperature 15°–30°C (59°–86°F).

HYCODAN is also available as a clear red colored, wild cherry flavored syrup in:

Bottles of one pint	NDC 63481-234-16

Store syrup at 25°C (77°F); excursions permitted to 15°–30°C (59°–86°F). (See USP Controlled Room Temperature).

Oral prescription where permitted by State law.

HYCODAN® is a Registered Trademark of Endo Pharmaceuticals Inc.

6479-02/Rev. Sept., 1998

Shown in Product Identification Guide, page 312

HYCOMINE® COMPOUND Ⓒ℞

[*hī-ko-mēn kom 'pound*]

DESCRIPTION

HYCOMINE Compound tablets contain hydrocodone (dihydrocodeinone) bitartrate, a semi-synthetic centrally-acting narcotic antitussive; chlorpheniramine maleate, an antihistamine; phenylephrine hydrochloride, a sympathomimetic amine decongestant; acetaminophen, an analgesic/antipyretic; and caffeine, a centrally-acting stimulant, for oral administration.

HYDROCODONE BITARTRATE

HYDROCODONE BITARTRATE

CHLORPHENIRAMINE MALEATE

PHENYLEPHRINE HYDROCHLORIDE

ACETAMINOPHEN

CAFFEINE

Each HYCOMINE Compound tablet contains:

Hydrocodone bitartrate, USP	5 mg
WARNING: May be habit forming	
Chlorpheniramine maleate, USP	2 mg
Phenylephrine hydrochloride, USP	10 mg
Acetaminophen, USP	250 mg
Caffeine, anhydrous, USP	30 mg

HYCOMINE Compound tablets also contain: cherry flavor, colloidal silicon dioxide, FD&C Red 40, magnesium stearate, microcrystalline cellulose, povidone and starch.

CLINICAL PHARMACOLOGY

Clinical trials have proven hydrocodone bitartrate to be an effective antitussive agent which is pharmacologically 2 to 8 times as potent as codeine. At equi-effective doses, its sedative action is greater than codeine. The precise mechanism of action of hydrocodone and other opiates is not known, however, hydrocodone is believed to act by directly depressing the cough center. In excessive doses hydrocodone, like other opium derivatives, will depress respiration. The effects of hydrocodone in therapeutic doses on the cardiovascular system is insignificant. The constipation effects of hydrocodone are much weaker than that of morphine and no stronger than that of codeine. Hydrocodone can produce miosis, euphoria, physical and psychological dependence. At therapeutic antitussive doses, it does exert analgesic effects. Following a 10 mg oral dose of hydrocodone administered to five adult male human subjects, the mean peak concentration was 23.6 ± 5.2 ng/mL. Maximum serum levels were achieved at 1.3 ± 0.3 hours and the half-life was determined to be 3.8 ± 0.3 hours. Hydrocodone exhibits a complex pattern of metabolism including O-demethylation, N-demethylation and 6-keto reduction to the corresponding 6-α- and 6-β-hydroxymetabolites.

Chlorpheniramine maleate is a competitive H_1-receptor histamine blocking drug, thereby counteracting the effects of histamine release associated with allergic manifestations of upper respiratory tract inflammatory disorders. H_1-blocking drugs inhibit the actions of histamine on smooth muscle, capillary permeability, and can both stimulate and depress the central nervous system. Phenylephrine hydrochloride effects its vasoconstrictor activity by releasing noradrenaline from sympathetic nerve endings, and from direct stimulation of α-adrenoreceptors in blood vessels. Acetaminophen is an antipyretic and peripherally acting analgesic. Caffeine is a central nervous system stimulant.

INDICATIONS AND USAGE

HYCOMINE Compound is indicated for the symptomatic relief of cough, nasal congestion, and discomfort associated with upper respiratory tract infections.

CONTRAINDICATIONS

HYCOMINE Compound is contraindicated in patients hypersensitive to any component of the drug, and concurrent MAO inhibitor therapy. Patients known to be hypersensitive to other opioids, antihistamines, or sympathomimetic amines may exhibit cross sensitivity with HYCOMINE Compound. Phenylephrine is contraindicated in patients with heart disease, hypertension, diabetes or hyperthyroidism. Hydrocodone is contraindicated in the presence of an intracranial lesion associated with increased intracranial pressure, and whenever ventilatory function is depressed.

WARNINGS

May be habit forming. Hydrocodone can produce drug dependence of the morphine type and therefore has the potential for being abused. Psychic dependence, physical dependence and tolerance may develop upon repeated administration of HYCOMINE Compound and it should be prescribed and administered with the same degree of caution appropriate to the use of other narcotic drugs. (See DRUG ABUSE AND DEPENDENCE.)

Respiratory Depression: HYCOMINE Compound produces dose-related respiratory depression by directly acting on brain stem respiratory centers. If respiratory depression occurs, it may be antagonized by the use of NARCAN® (naloxone hydrochloride) and other supportive measures when indicated.

Head Injury and Increased Intracranial Pressure: The respiratory depressant properties of narcotics and their capacity to elevate cerebrospinal fluid pressure may be markedly exaggerated in the presence of head injury, other intracranial lesions or a pre-existing increase in intracranial pressure. Furthermore, narcotics produce adverse reactions which may obscure the clinical course of patients with head injuries.

Acute Abdominal Conditions: The administration of HYCOMINE Compound or other narcotics may obscure the diagnosis or clinical course of patients with acute abdominal conditions.

Phenylephrine: Hypertensive crises can occur with concurrent use of phenylephrine and monoamine oxidase (MAO) inhibitors, indomethacin or with beta-blockers and methyldopa.

If a hypertensive crisis occurs these drugs should be discontinued immediately and therapy to lower blood pressure should be instituted immediately. Fever should be managed by means of external cooling.

Chlorpheniramine: Antihistamines may produce drowsiness or excitation, particularly in children and elderly patients.

PRECAUTIONS

Before prescribing medication to suppress or modify cough, it is important to ascertain that the underlying cause of cough is identified, that modification of cough does not increase the risk of clinical or physiologic complications, and that appropriate therapy for the primary disease is provided.

Usage in Ambulatory Patients: Hydrocodone, like all narcotics, and antihistamines such as chlorpheniramine maleate, may impair the mental and/or physical abilities required for the performance of potentially hazardous tasks such as driving a car or operating machinery; phenylephrine may produce a rapid pulse, dizziness or palpitations; patients should be cautioned accordingly.

Drug Interactions: Patients receiving other narcotic analgesics, general anesthetics, phenothiazines, other tranquilizers, sedative-hypnotics or other CNS depressants (including alcohol) concomitantly with hydrocodone may exhibit an additive CNS depression. When such combined therapy is contemplated, the dose of one or both agents should be reduced. The use of phenylephrine with other sympathomimetic amines and MAO inhibitors may produce an additive elevation of blood pressure. MAO inhibitors may prolong the anticholinergic effects of antihistamines. (See WARNINGS.)

Carcinogenesis, Mutagenesis, Impairment of Fertility: Carcinogenicity, mutagenicity, and reproduction studies have not been conducted with HYCOMINE Compound.

Usage in Pregnancy: Pregnancy Category C. Animal reproduction studies have not been conducted with HYCOMINE Compound. It is also not known whether HYCOMINE

Continued on next page

Hycomine Compound—Cont.

Compound can cause fetal harm when administered to a pregnant woman or can affect reproductive capacity. HYCOMINE Compound should be given to a pregnant woman only if clearly needed.

Nonteratogenic Effects: Babies born to mothers who have been taking opioids regularly prior to delivery will be physically dependent. The withdrawal signs include irritability and excessive crying, tremors, hyperactive reflexes, increased respiratory rate, increased stools, sneezing, yawning, vomiting and fever. The intensity of the syndrome does not always correlate with the duration of maternal opioid use or dose. Chlorpromazine 0.7–1.0 mg/kg q 6 h, phenobarbital 2 mg/kg q 6 h, and paregoric 2–4 drops/kg q 4 h, have been used to treat withdrawal symptoms in infants. The duration of therapy is 4 to 28 days, with the dosages decreased as tolerated.

Nursing Mothers: It is not known whether this drug is excreted in human milk. Because many drugs are excreted in human milk and because of the potential for serious adverse reactions in nursing infants from HYCOMINE Compound, a decision should be made whether to discontinue nursing or discontinue the drug, taking into account the importance of the drug to the mother.

Pediatric Use: Safety and effectiveness in pediatric patients below the age of 2 years have not been established.

ADVERSE REACTIONS

Respiratory System: Hydrocodone produces dose-related respiratory depression by acting directly on brain stem respiratory centers.

Cardiovascular System: Hypertension, postural hypotension, tachycardia and palpitations.

Genitourinary System: Ureteral spasm, spasm of vesical sphincters and urinary retention have been reported with opiates.

Central Nervous System: Sedation, drowsiness, mental clouding, lethargy, impairment of mental and physical performance, anxiety, fear, dysphoria, dizziness, psychic dependence, mood changes, and blurred vision.

Gastrointestinal System: Nausea and vomiting occur more frequently in ambulatory than in recumbent patients.

DRUG ABUSE AND DEPENDENCE

Special care should be exercised in prescribing hydrocodone for emotionally unstable patients and for those with a history of drug misuse. Such patients should be closely supervised when long-term therapy is contemplated.

HYCOMINE Compound is a Schedule III narcotic. Psychic dependence, physical dependence, and tolerance may develop upon repeated administration of narcotics; therefore, HYCOMINE Compound should always be prescribed and administered with caution. Physical dependence is the condition in which continued administration of the drug is required to prevent the appearance of a withdrawal syndrome.

Patients physically dependent on opioids will develop an abstinence syndrome upon abrupt discontinuation of the opioid or following the administration of a narcotic antagonist. The character and severity of the withdrawal symptoms are related to the degree of physical dependence. Manifestations of opioid withdrawal are similar to but milder than that of morphine and include lacrimation, rhinorrhea, yawning, sweating, restlessness, dilated pupils, anorexia, gooseflesh, irritability and tremor. In more severe forms, nausea, vomiting, intestinal spasm and diarrhea, increased heart rate and blood pressure, chills, and pains in bones and muscles of the back and extremities may occur. Peak effects will usually be apparent at 48 to 72 hours.

Treatment of withdrawal is usually managed by providing sufficient quantities of an opioid to suppress **severe** withdrawal symptoms and then gradually reducing the dose of opioid over a period of several days.

OVERDOSAGE

The signs and symptoms of overdosage of the individual components of HYCOMINE Compound may be modified in varying degrees by the presence of other active ingredients. Overdosage with phenylephrine alone may result in tremor, restlessness, increased motor activity, agitation and hallucinations.

Acetaminophen

Signs and Symptoms: In acute acetaminophen overdosage, dose-dependent, potentially fatal hepatic necrosis is the most serious adverse effect. Renal tubular necrosis, hypoglycemic coma and thrombocytopenia may also occur.

Acetaminophen in massive overdosage may cause hepatic toxicity in some patients. In cases of suspected overdose, you may wish to call your regional poison center for assistance in diagnosis and for directions in the use of N-acetylcysteine as an antidote.

In adults, hepatic toxicity has rarely been reported with acute overdoses of less than 10 grams and fatalities with less than 15 grams. Importantly, young children seem to be more resistant than adults to the hepatotoxic effect of an acetaminophen overdose. Despite this, the measures outlined below should be initiated in any adult or child suspected of having ingested an acetaminophen overdose.

Early symptoms following a potentially hepatotoxic overdose may include nausea, vomiting, diaphoresis and general malaise. Clinical and laboratory evidence of hepatic toxicity may not be apparent until 48 to 72 hours post-ingestion.

Treatment: The stomach should be emptied promptly by lavage or by induction of emesis with syrup of ipecac. Patient's estimates of the quantity of a drug ingested are notoriously unreliable. Therefore, if an acetaminophen overdose is suspected, a serum acetaminophen assay should be obtained as early as possible, but no sooner than four hours following ingestion. Liver function studies should be obtained initially and repeated at 24-hour intervals.

The antidote, N-acetylcysteine should be administered as early as possible, preferably within 16 hours of the overdose ingestions for optimal results, but in any case, within 24 hours. Following recovery, there are no residual structural or functional hepatic abnormalities.

Hydrocodone

Signs and Symptoms: Serious overdosage with hydrocodone is characterized by respiratory depression (a decrease in respiratory rate and/or tidal volume, Cheyne-Stokes respiration, cyanosis), extreme somnolence progressing to stupor or coma, skeletal muscle flaccidity, cold and clammy skin, and sometimes bradycardia and hypotension. In severe overdosage, apnea, circulatory collapse, cardiac arrest and death may occur.

Treatment: Primary attention should be given to the reestablishment of adequate respiratory exchange through provision of a patent airway and the institution of assisted or controlled ventilation. The narcotic antagonist naloxone hydrochloride is a specific antidote for respiratory depression which may result from overdosage or unusual sensitivity to narcotics including hydrocodone. Therefore, an appropriate dose of naloxone hydrochloride should be administered, preferably by the intravenous route, simultaneously with efforts at respiratory resuscitation. For further information, see full prescribing information for naloxone hydrochloride. An antagonist should not be administered in the absence of clinically significant respiratory depression. Oxygen, intravenous fluids, vasopressors and other supportive measures should be employed as indicated. Gastric emptying may be useful in removing unabsorbed drug. Activated charcoal may be of benefit.

DOSAGE AND ADMINISTRATION

Usual dosage, not less than 4 hours apart:
Adults: 1 tablet 4 times a day
Children: 6 to 12 years: 1/2 tablet 4 times a day

HOW SUPPLIED

HYCOMINE® Compound is available as a coral pink, scored tablet in bottles as follows:

Bottles of 100	NDC 63481-048-70
Bottles of 500	NDC 63481-048-85

CAUTION: Federal (USA) law prohibits dispensing without prescription.

Oral prescription where permitted by State Law.

Store at controlled room temperature 15°–30°C (59°–86°F).

Dispense in a tight, light-resistant container as defined in the USP.

HYCOMINE® is a Registered Trademark of Endo Pharmaceuticals Inc.

NARCAN® is a Registered Trademark of Endo Pharmaceuticals Inc.

6491-00/November, 1997

Shown in Product Identification Guide, page 312

HYCOMINE® Ⓒ℞
[hī-co-mēn]
(hydrocodone bitartrate and phenylpropanolamine hydrochloride)
Pediatric Syrup

HYCOMINE® Ⓒ℞
[hī-co-mēn]
(hydrocodone bitartrate and phenylpropanolamine hydrochloride)
Syrup

DESCRIPTION

HYCOMINE contains hydrocodone (dihydrocodeinone) bitartrate, a semisynthetic centrally-acting narcotic antitussive and phenylpropanolamine hydrochloride, a sympathomimetic amine decongestant for oral administration.

The pH of HYCOMINE and HYCOMINE Pediatric Syrup is 3.2–4.2. The hydrocodone component is (5α)-4,5-epoxy-3-methoxy-17-methylmorphinan-6-one [R-(R*,R*)]-2,3-dihydroxybutanedioate (1:1) hydrate (2:5), a fine white crystal or crystalline powder, which is derived from the opium alkaloid, thebaine, and has a molecular weight of 494.50. The phenylpropanolamine component is (±)-(R*,S*)-α-(1-aminoethyl) benzenemethanol hydrochloride and has a molecular weight of 187.67. These may be represented by the following structural formulas:

HYDROCODONE BITARTRATE

[See chemical structure at top of next column]

PHENYLPROPANOLAMINE HYDROCHLORIDE

HYCOMINE
<u>Pediatric Syrup</u>
Each teaspoonful (5 mL) contains:

Hydrocodone bitartrate, USP	2.5 mg
WARNING: May be habit forming	
Phenylpropanolamine hydrochloride, USP	12.5 mg

<u>HYCOMINE Syrup</u>
Each teaspoonful (5 mL) contains:

Hydrocodone bitartrate, USP	5 mg
WARNING: May be habit forming	
Phenylpropanolamine hydrochloride, USP	25 mg

Also, HYCOMINE, both strengths, contain: artificial cherry flavor, glycerin, methylparaben, propylparaben, saccharin sodium, and sorbitol solution. HYCOMINE Pediatric Syrup contains: D&C Yellow 10 and FD&C Green 3. HYCOMINE Syrup: FD&C Red 40 and FD&C Yellow 6.

CLINICAL PHARMACOLOGY

Hydrocodone is a semisynthetic narcotic antitussive and analgesic with multiple actions qualitatively similar to those of codeine. The precise mechanism of action of hydrocodone and other opiates is not known; however, hydrocodone is believed to act directly on the cough center. In excessive doses, hydrocodone, like other opium derivatives, will depress respiration. The effects of hydrocodone in therapeutic doses on the cardiovascular system are insignificant. Hydrocodone can produce miosis, euphoria, physical and physiological dependence.

Following a 10 mg oral dose of hydrocodone administered to five adult male subjects, the mean peak concentration was 23.6 ± 5.2 ng/mL. Maximum serum levels were achieved at 1.3 ± 0.3 hours and the half-life was determined to be 3.8 ± 0.3 hours. Hydrocodone exhibits a complex pattern of metabolism including O-demethylation, N-demethylation and 6-keto reduction to the corresponding 6-α- and 6-β-hydroxymetabolites.

Phenylpropanolamine effects its vasoconstrictor activity by releasing noradrenaline from sympathetic nerve endings, and from direct stimulation of α-adrenoreceptors of blood vessels.

INDICATIONS AND USAGE

HYCOMINE (hydrocodone bitartrate and phenylpropanolamine hydrochloride) is indicated for the symptomatic relief of cough and nasal congestion.

CONTRAINDICATIONS

HYCOMINE is contraindicated in patients hypersensitive to hydrocodone or phenylpropanolamine, and in patients on concurrent MAO inhibitor therapy. Patients known to be hypersensitive to other opioids or sympathomimetic amines may exhibit cross sensitivity to HYCOMINE. Phenylpropanolamine is contraindicated in patients with heart disease, hypertension, diabetes or hyperthyroidism. Hydrocodone is contraindicated in the presence of an intracranial lesion associated with increased intracranial pressure; and whenever ventilatory function is depressed.

WARNINGS

May be habit forming. Hydrocodone can produce drug dependence of the morphine type and, therefore, has the potential for being abused. Psychic dependence, physical dependence and tolerance may develop upon repeated administration of HYCOMINE and it should be prescribed and administered with the same degree of caution appropriate to the use of other narcotic drugs (see DRUG ABUSE AND DEPENDENCE).

Respiratory Depression: HYCOMINE produces dose-related respiratory depression by directly acting on brain stem respiratory centers. If respiratory depression occurs, it may be antagonized by the use of naloxone hydrochloride and other supportive measures when indicated.

Head Injury and Increased Intracranial Pressure: The respiratory depression properties of narcotics and their capacity to elevate cerebrospinal fluid pressure may be markedly exaggerated in the presence of head injury, other intracranial lesions or a preexisting increase in intracranial pressure. Furthermore, narcotics produce adverse reactions which may obscure the clinical course of patients with head injuries.

Acute Abdominal Conditions: The administration of HYCOMINE or other narcotics may obscure the diagnosis or clinical course of patients with acute abdominal conditions.

Pediatric Use: In young children, as well as adults, the respiratory center is sensitive to the depressant action of narcotic cough suppressants in a dose-dependent manner. Benefit to risk ratio should be carefully considered especially in children with respiratory embarrassment (e.g., croup).

Phenylpropanolamine: Hypertensive crises can occur with concurrent use of phenylpropanolamine and monoamine oxidase (MAO) inhibitors, indomethacin or with beta-blockers and methyldopa.

If a hypertensive crisis occurs, these drugs should be discontinued immediately and therapy to lower blood pressure should be instituted immediately. Fever should be managed by means of external cooling.

PRECAUTIONS

General: Before prescribing medication to suppress or modify cough, it is important to ascertain that the underlying cause of cough is identified, that modification of cough does not increase the risk of clinical or physiologic complications, and that appropriate therapy for the primary disease is provided.

Special Risk Patients: HYCOMINE should be given with caution to certain patients such as the elderly or debilitated, and those with severe impairment of hepatic or renal functions, hypothyroidism, Addison's disease, prostatic hypertrophy or urethral stricture, asthma, narrow-angle glaucoma, and uncontrolled hypertension.

Information for Patients: Hydrocodone may impair the mental and/or physical abilities required for the performance of potentially hazardous tasks such as driving a car or operating machinery; phenylpropanolamine may produce a rapid pulse, dizziness or palpitations. The patient using HYCOMINE (hydrocodone bitartrate and phenylpropanolamine hydrochloride) should be cautioned accordingly.

Drug Interactions: Patients receiving other narcotic analgesics, general anesthetics, phenothiazines, other tranquilizers, sedative-hypnotics or other CNS depressants (including alcohol) concomitantly with hydrocodone may exhibit an additive CNS depression. When such combined therapy is contemplated, the dose of one or both agents should be reduced. The use of phenylpropanolamine with other sympathomimetic amines and MAO inhibitors may produce an additive elevation of blood pressure (see WARNINGS).

Carcinogenesis, Mutagenesis, Impairment of Fertility: Carcinogenicity, mutagenicity and reproduction studies have not been conducted with HYCOMINE.

Pregnancy:

Teratogenic Effects: Pregnancy Category C: Animal reproduction studies have not been conducted with HYCOMINE. It is also not known whether HYCOMINE can cause fetal harm when administered to a pregnant woman or can affect reproductive capacity. HYCOMINE should be given to a pregnant woman only if clearly needed.

Nonteratogenic Effects: Babies born to mothers who have been taking opioids regularly prior to delivery will be physically dependent. The withdrawal signs include irritability and excessive crying, tremors, hyperactive reflexes, increased respiratory rate, increased stools, sneezing, yawning, vomiting and fever. The intensity of the syndrome does not always correlate with the duration of maternal opioid use or dose.

Labor and Delivery: As with all narcotics, administration of HYCOMINE to the mother shortly before delivery may result in some degree of respiratory depression in the newborn, especially if higher doses are used.

Nursing Mothers: It is not known whether this drug is excreted in human milk. Because many drugs are excreted in human milk and because of the potential for serious adverse reactions in nursing infants from HYCOMINE, a decision should be made whether to discontinue nursing or discontinue the drug, taking into account the importance of the drug to the mother.

Pediatric Use: Safety and effectiveness of HYCOMINE in pediatric patients under six have not been established.

ADVERSE REACTIONS

Respiratory System: Hydrocodone produces dose-related respiratory depression by acting directly on brain stem respiratory centers (see OVERDOSAGE).

Cardiovascular System: Hypertension, postural hypotension, tachycardia and palpitations.

Genitourinary System: Ureteral spasm, spasm of vesical sphincters and urinary retention have been reported with opiates.

Central Nervous System: Sedation, drowsiness, mental clouding, lethargy, impairment of mental and physical performance, anxiety, fear, dysphoria, dizziness, psychic dependence, mood changes and blurred vision.

Gastrointestinal System: Nausea and vomiting occur more frequently in ambulatory than in recumbent patients. Prolonged administration of HYCOMINE may produce constipation.

Dermatological: Skin rash, pruritus.

DRUG ABUSE AND DEPENDENCE

HYCOMINE is a Schedule III narcotic. Psychic dependence, physical dependence, and tolerance may develop upon repeated administration of narcotics; therefore, HYCOMINE should be prescribed and administered with caution. However, psychic dependence is unlikely to develop when HYCOMINE is used for a short time for the treatment of cough. Physical dependence, the condition in which continued administration of the drug is required to prevent the appearance of a withdrawal syndrome, assumes clinically significant proportions only after several weeks of continued oral narcotic use, although some mild degree of physical dependence may develop after a few days of narcotic therapy.

OVERDOSAGE

Signs and Symptoms: Serious overdosage with HYCOMINE is characterized by respiratory depression (a decrease in respiratory rate and/or tidal volume, Cheyne-Stokes respiration, cyanosis), extreme somnolence progressing to stupor or coma, skeletal muscle flaccidity, cold and clammy skin, and sometimes bradycardia and hypotension. In severe overdosage, apnea, circulatory collapse, cardiac arrest, and death may occur.

The signs and symptoms of overdosage of the individual components of HYCOMINE (hydrocodone bitartrate and phenylpropanolamine hydrochloride) may be modified in varying degrees by the presence of other active ingredients. Overdosage with phenylpropanolamine alone may result in tremor, restlessness, increased motor activity, agitation and hallucinations.

Treatment: Primary attention should be given to the reestablishment of adequate respiratory exchange through provision of a patent airway and the institution of assisted or controlled ventilation. The narcotic antagonist naloxone hydrochloride is a specific antidote for respiratory depression which may result from overdosage or unusual sensitivity to narcotics including hydrocodone. Therefore, an appropriate dose of naloxone hydrochloride should be administered, preferably by the intravenous route, simultaneously with efforts at respiratory resuscitation. For further information, see full prescribing information for naloxone hydrochloride. An antagonist should not be administered in the absence of clinically significant respiratory depression. Oxygen, intravenous fluids, vasopressors and other supportive measures should be employed as indicated. Gastric emptying may be useful in removing unabsorbed drug.

DOSAGE AND ADMINISTRATION

Adults: The usual dose for adults is one teaspoonful HYCOMINE Syrup (hydrocodone bitartrate 5 mg and phenylpropanolamine hydrochloride 25 mg/5 cc) every four hours as needed, not to exceed six teaspoonfuls in a 24 hour period.

Children 6 to 12 years of age: The usual dose for children 6 to 12 years of age is one teaspoonful HYCOMINE Pediatric Syrup (hydrocodone bitartrate 2.5 mg and phenylpropanolamine hydrochloride 12.5 mg/5 cc) every four hours as needed, not to exceed six teaspoonfuls in a 24 hour period.

HOW SUPPLIED

HYCOMINE Syrup (5 mg hydrocodone bitartrate, USP and 25 mg phenylpropanolamine hydrochloride, USP—per 5 mL teaspoonful) is available as an orange-colored, cherry-flavored syrup in bottles as follows:

One Pint (473.2 mL): NDC 63481-246-16

HYCOMINE Pediatric Syrup (2.5 mg hydrocodone bitartrate, USP and 12.5 mg phenylpropanolamine hydrochloride, USP—per 5 mL teaspoonful) is available as a green-colored, cherry-flavored syrup in bottles as follows:

One Pint (473.2 mL): NDC 63481-247-16

Store at controlled room temperature 15°–30°C (59°–86°F).

Oral prescription where permitted by State law.

CAUTION: Federal (USA) law prohibits dispensing without a prescription.

HYCOMINE® is a Registered Trademark of Endo Pharmaceuticals Inc.

6480/August, 1997

HYCOTUSS® CIII ℞

[hī-kō-tus]

(hydrocodone bitartrate and guaifenesin)
Expectorant

DESCRIPTION

HYCOTUSS Expectorant Syrup contains hydrocodone (dihydrocodeinone) bitartrate, a semi-synthetic centrally-acting narcotic antitussive and guaifenesin, an expectorant for oral administration.

HYDROCODONE BITARTRATE

GUAIFENESIN

Each teaspoonful (5 mL) contains:

Hydrocodone bitartrate, USP .... 5 mg
WARNING: May be habit forming
Guaifenesin, USP .... 100 mg
Alcohol, USP .... 10% v/v

HYCOTUSS Expectorant Syrup also contains: artificial butterscotch flavor, FD&C Red 40, FD&C Yellow 6, glycerin, liquid sugar, methylparaben, propylparaben, saccharin sodium, and sorbitol solution.

CLINICAL PHARMACOLOGY

Clinical trials have proven hydrocodone bitartrate to be an effective antitussive agent which is pharmacologically 2 to 8 times as potent as codeine. At equi-effective doses, its sedative action is greater than codeine. The precise mechanism of action of hydrocodone and other opiates is not known, however, hydrocodone is believed to act by directly depressing the cough center. In excessive doses hydrocodone, like other opium derivatives, can depress respiration. The effects of hydrocodone in therapeutic doses on the cardiovascular system is insignificant. The constipation effects of hydrocodone are much weaker than that of morphine and no stronger than that of codeine. Hydrocodone can produce miosis, euphoria, physical and psychological dependence. At therapeutic antitussive doses, it does exert analgesic effects. Following a 10 mg oral dose of hydrocodone administered to five male human subjects, the mean peak concentration was 23.6 ± 5.2 ng/mL. Maximum serum levels were achieved at 1.3 ± 0.3 hours and half-life was determined to be 3.8 ± 0.3 hours. Hydrocodone exhibits a complex pattern of metabolism including O-demethylation, N-demethylation and 6-keto reduction to the corresponding 6-α- and 6-β-hydroxymetabolites.

The exact mechanism of action is not established but guaifenesin is believed to act by stimulating receptors in the gastric mucosa that initiates a reflex secretion of respiratory tract fluid, thereby increasing the volume and decreasing the viscosity of bronchial secretions. Studies with guaifenesin indicate that it is rapidly absorbed from the gastrointestinal tract and has a half-life of one hour.

INDICATIONS AND USAGE

HYCOTUSS (hydrocodone bitartrate and guaifenesin) Expectorant is indicated for the symptomatic relief of irritating non-productive cough associated with upper and lower respiratory tract congestion.

CONTRAINDICATIONS

HYCOTUSS Expectorant is contraindicated in patients hypersensitive to hydrocodone or guaifenesin. Patients known to be hypersensitive to other opioids may exhibit cross sensitivity to HYCOTUSS Expectorant. Hydrocodone is contraindicated in the presence of an intracranial lesion associated with increased intracranial pressure; and whenever ventilatory function is depressed.

WARNINGS

May be habit forming. Hydrocodone can produce drug dependence of the morphine type and therefore has the potential for being abused. Psychic dependence, physical dependence and tolerance may develop upon repeated administration of HYCOTUSS Expectorant and it should be prescribed and administered with the same degree of caution appropriate to the use of other narcotic drugs (See DRUG ABUSE AND DEPENDENCE).

Respiratory Depression: HYCOTUSS Expectorant produces dose-related respiratory depression by directly acting on the brain stem respiratory centers. If respiratory depression occurs, it may be antagonized by the use of NARCAN® (naloxone hydrochloride) and other supportive measures when indicated.

Head Injury and Increased Intracranial Pressure: The respiratory depressant properties of narcotics and their capacity to elevate cerebrospinal fluid pressure may be markedly exaggerated in the presence of head injury, other intracranial lesions or a pre-existing increase in intracranial pressure. Furthermore, narcotics produce adverse reactions which may obscure the clinical course of patients with head injuries.

Acute Abdominal Conditions: The administration of HYCOTUSS Expectorant or other opioids may obscure the diagnosis or clinical course of patients with acute abdominal conditions.

PRECAUTIONS

Before prescribing medication to suppress or modify cough, it is important to ascertain that the underlying cause of cough is identified, that modification of cough does not increase the risk of clinical or physiologic complications, and that appropriate therapy for the primary disease is provided.

Usage in Ambulatory Patients: Hydrocodone, like all narcotics, may impair the mental and/or physical abilities required for the performance of potentially hazardous tasks such as driving a car or operating machinery, and patients should be warned accordingly.

Drug Interactions: Patients receiving other narcotics, analgesics, general anesthetics, phenothiazines, other tranquilizers, sedative hypnotics or other CNS depressants (including alcohol) concomitantly with hydrocodone may exhibit an additive CNS depression. When such combined therapy is contemplated, the dose of one or both agents should be reduced (see WARNINGS).

Laboratory Interactions: The metabolite of guaifenesin has been found to produce an apparent increase in urinary 5-hydroxyindoleacetic acid, and guaifenesin therefore may interfere with the interpretation of this test for the diagnosis of carcinoid syndrome. Guaifenesin administration should be discontinued 24 hours prior to the collection of urine specimens for the determination of 5-hydroxyindoleacetic acid.

Carcinogenesis, Mutagenesis, Impairment of Fertility: Carcinogenicity, mutagenicity and reproduction studies have not been conducted with HYCOTUSS (hydrocodone bitartrate and guaifenesin) Expectorant.

Usage in Pregnancy: Pregnancy Category C. Animal reproduction studies have not been conducted with HYCOTUSS Expectorant. It is also not known whether HYCOTUSS Expectorant can cause fetal harm when administered to a pregnant woman or can affect reproductive capacity. HYCOTUSS Expectorant should be given to a pregnant woman only if clearly needed.

Continued on next page

Hycotuss—Cont.

Nonteratogenic Effects: Babies born to mothers who have been taking opioids regularly prior to delivery will be physically dependent. The withdrawal signs include irritability and excessive crying, tremors, hyperactive reflexes, increased respiratory rate, increased stools, sneezing, yawning, vomiting and fever. The intensity of the syndrome does not always correlate with the duration of maternal opioid use or dose. There is no consensus on the best method of managing withdrawal. Chlorpromazine 0.7–1.0 mg/kg q 6 h, phenobarbital 2 mg/kg q 6 h, and paregoric 2–4 drops/kg q 4 h, have been used to treat withdrawal symptoms in infants. The duration of therapy is 4 to 28 days, with the dosages decreased as tolerated.

Nursing Mothers: It is not known whether this drug is excreted in human milk. Because many drugs are excreted in human milk and because of the potential for serious adverse reactions in nursing infants from HYCOTUSS Expectorant, a decision should be made whether to discontinue nursing or discontinue the drug, taking into account the importance of the drug to the mother.

ADVERSE REACTIONS

Respiratory System: Hydrocodone produces dose-related respiratory depression by acting directly on brain stem respiratory centers.

Cardiovascular System: Hypertension, postural hypotension and palpitations.

Genitourinary System: Ureteral spasm, spasm of vesical sphincters and urinary retention have been reported with opiates.

Central Nervous System: Sedation, drowsiness, mental clouding, lethargy, impairment of mental and physical performance, anxiety, fear, dysphoria, dizziness, psychic dependence, mood changes and blurred vision.

Gastrointestinal System: Nausea and vomiting occur more frequently in ambulatory than in recumbent patients.

DRUG ABUSE AND DEPENDENCE

Special care should be exercised in prescribing hydrocodone for emotionally unstable patients and for those with a history of drug misuse. Such patients should be closely supervised when long-term therapy is contemplated.

HYCOTUSS Expectorant is a Schedule III narcotic. Psychic dependence, physical dependence and tolerance may develop upon repeated administration of narcotics; therefore, HYCOTUSS Expectorant should always be prescribed and administered with caution. Physical dependence is the condition in which continued administration of the drug is required to prevent the appearance of a withdrawal syndrome.

Patients physically dependent on opioids will develop an abstinence syndrome upon abrupt discontinuation of the opioid or following the administration of a narcotic antagonist. The character and severity of the withdrawal symptoms are related to the degree of physical dependence. Manifestations of opioid withdrawal are similar to but milder than that of morphine and include lacrimation, rhinorrhea, yawning, sweating, restlessness, dilated pupils, anorexia, gooseflesh, irritability and tremor. In more severe forms, nausea, vomiting, intestinal spasm and diarrhea, increased heart rate and blood pressure, chills, and pains in bones and muscles of the back and extremities may occur. Peak effects will usually be apparent at 48 to 72 hours.

Treatment of withdrawal is usually managed by providing sufficient quantities of an opioid to suppress **severe** withdrawal symptoms and then gradually reducing the dose of opioid over a period of several days.

OVERDOSAGE

Signs and Symptoms: Serious overdosage with HYCOTUSS (hydrocodone bitartrate and guaifenesin) Expectorant is characterized by respiratory depression (a decrease in respiratory rate and/or tidal volume, Cheyne-Stokes respiration, cyanosis), extreme somnolence progressing to stupor or coma, skeletal muscle flaccidity, cold and clammy skin, and sometimes bradycardia and hypotension. In severe overdosage, apnea, circulatory collapse, cardiac arrest, and death may occur.

Treatment: Primary attention should be given to the reestablishment of adequate respiratory exchange through provision of a patent airway and the institution of assisted or controlled ventilation. The narcotic antagonist naloxone hydrochloride is a specific antidote for respiratory depression which may result from overdosage or unusual sensitivity to narcotics including hydrocodone. Therefore, an appropriate dose of naloxone hydrochloride should be administered, preferably by the intravenous route, simultaneously with efforts at respiratory resuscitation. For further information, see full prescribing information for naloxone hydrochloride. An antagonist should not be administered in the absence of clinically significant respiratory depression. Oxygen, intravenous fluids, vasopressors, and other supportive measures should be employed as indicated. Gastric emptying may be useful in removing unabsorbed drug. Activated charcoal may be of benefit.

DOSAGE AND ADMINISTRATION

Usual Adult Dose: One teaspoonful (5 mL) after meals and at bedtime, not less than 4 hours apart (not to exceed 6 teaspoonsful in a 24 hour period). Treatment should be initiated with one teaspoonful and subsequent doses, up to a maximum single dose of 3 teaspoonsful, adjusted if required.

Usual Children's Dose:
Over 12 years: Initial dose 1 teaspoonful; maximum single dose, 2 teaspoonsful.
6 to 12 years: Initial dose $^1/_2$ teaspoonful; maximum single dose, 1 teaspoonful.

HOW SUPPLIED

HYCOTUSS Expectorant is available as an orange-colored, butterscotch flavored syrup in bottles as follows:
One pint: NDC 63481-235-16
Store at controlled room temperature 15°–30°C (59°–86°F).
Oral prescription where permitted by State Law.
CAUTION: Federal (USA) law prohibits dispensing without prescription.
HYCOTUSS® is a Registered Trademark of Endo Pharmaceuticals Inc.
NARCAN® is a Registered Trademark of Endo Pharmaceuticals Inc.

6481-00/November, 1997

LIDODERM® ℞

[lī-dō-dĕrm]
(lidocaine patch 5%)
Rx only

DESCRIPTION

LIDODERM (lidocaine patch 5%) is comprised of an adhesive material containing 5% lidocaine, which is applied to a non-woven polyester felt backing and covered with a polyethylene terephthalate (PET) film release liner. The release liner is removed prior to application to the skin. The size of the patch is 10 cm × 14 cm.

Lidocaine is chemically designated as acetamide, 2-(diethylamino)-N-(2,6-dimethylphenyl), has an octanol:water partition ratio of 43 at pH 7.4, and has the following structure:

[Structure: 2,6-dimethylphenyl ring (two CH_3) –NH–CO–CH_2–N(C_2H_5)(C_2H_5)]

Each adhesive patch contains 700 mg of lidocaine (50 mg per gram adhesive) in an aqueous base. It also contains the following inactive ingredients: dihydroxyaluminum aminoacetate, disodium edetate, gelatin, glycerin, kaolin, methylparaben, polyacrylic acid, polyvinyl alcohol, propylene glycol, propylparaben, sodium carboxymethylcellulose, sodium polyacrylate, D-sorbitol, tartaric acid, and urea.

CLINICAL PHARMACOLOGY

Pharmacodynamics:
Lidocaine is an amide-type local anesthetic agent and is suggested to stabilize neuronal membranes by inhibiting the ionic fluxes required for the initiation and conduction of impulses.

The penetration of lidocaine into intact skin after application of LIDODERM is sufficient to produce an analgesic effect, but less than the amount necessary to produce a complete sensory block.

Pharmacokinetics:
Absorption:
The amount of lidocaine systemically absorbed from LIDODERM is directly related to both the duration of application and the surface area over which it is applied. In a pharmacokinetic study, three LIDODERM patches were applied over an area of 420 cm^2 of intact skin on the back of normal volunteers for 12 hours. Blood samples were withdrawn for determination of lidocaine concentration during the application and for 12 hours after removal of patches. The results are summarized in Table 1.
[See table 1 below]

When LIDODERM is used according to the recommended dosing instructions, only 3 ± 2% of the dose applied is expected to be absorbed. At least 95% (665 mg) of lidocaine will remain in a used patch. Mean peak blood concentration of lidocaine is about 0.13 µg/mL (about 1/10 of the therapeutic concentration required to treat cardiac arrhythmias). Repeated application of three patches simultaneously for 12 hours (recommended maximum daily dose), once per day for three days, indicated that the lidocaine concentration does not increase with daily use. The mean plasma pharmacokinetic profile for the 15 healthy volunteers is shown in Figure 1.
[See figure 1 at top of next column]

Distribution:
When lidocaine is administered intravenously to healthy volunteers, the volume of distribution is 0.7 to 2.7 L/kg

Figure 1
Mean lidocaine blood concentrations after three consecutive daily applications of three LIDODERM patches simultaneously for 12 hours per day in healthy volunteers (n = 15).

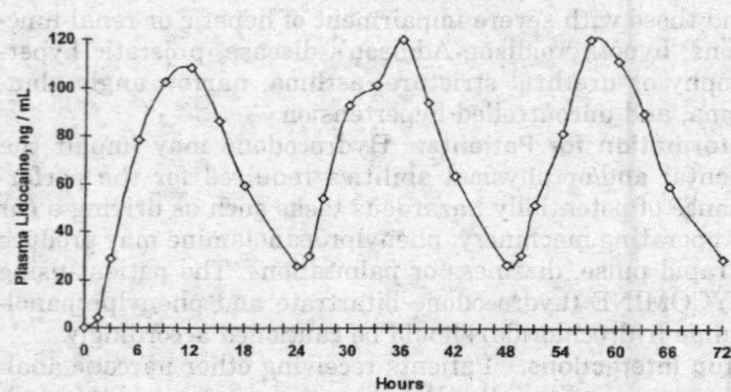

(mean 1.5 ± 0.6 SD, n = 15). At concentrations produced by application of LIDODERM, lidocaine is approximately 70% bound to plasma proteins, primarily alpha-1-acid glycoprotein. At much higher plasma concentrations (1 to 4 µg/mL of free base), the plasma protein binding of lidocaine is concentration dependent. Lidocaine crosses the placental and blood brain barriers, presumably by passive diffusion.

Metabolism:
It is not known if lidocaine is metabolized in the skin. Lidocaine is metabolized rapidly by the liver to a number of metabolites, including monoethylglycinexylidide (MEGX) and glycinexylidide (GX), both of which have pharmacologic activity similar to, but less potent than that of lidocaine. A minor metabolite, 2,6-xylidine, has unknown pharmacologic activity but is carcinogenic in rats. The blood concentration of this metabolite is negligible following application of LIDODERM (lidocaine patch 5%). Following intravenous administration, MEGX and GX concentrations in serum range from 11 to 36% and from 5 to 11% of lidocaine concentrations, respectively.

Excretion:
Lidocaine and its metabolites are excreted by the kidneys. Less than 10% of lidocaine is excreted unchanged. The half-life of lidocaine elimination from the plasma following IV administration is 81 to 149 minutes (mean 107 ± 22 SD, n = 15). The systemic clearance is 0.33 to 0.90 L/min (mean 0.64 ± 0.18 SD, n = 15).

CLINICAL STUDIES

Single-dose treatment with LIDODERM was compared to treatment with vehicle patch (without lidocaine), and to no treatment (observation only) in a double-blind, crossover clinical trial with 35 post-herpetic neuralgia patients. Pain intensity and pain relief scores were evaluated periodically for 12 hours. LIDODERM performed statistically better than vehicle patch in terms of pain intensity from 4 to 12 hours.

Multiple-dose, two-week treatment with LIDODERM was compared to vehicle patch (without lidocaine) in a double-blind, crossover clinical trial of withdrawal-type design conducted in 32 patients, who were considered as responders to the open-label use of LIDODERM prior to the study. The constant type of pain was evaluated but not the pain induced by sensory stimuli (dysesthesia). Statistically significant differences favoring LIDODERM were observed in terms of time to exit from the trial (14 versus 3.8 days at p-value <0.001), daily average pain relief, and patient's preference of treatment. About half of the patients also took oral medication commonly used in the treatment of post-herpetic neuralgia. The extent of use of concomitant medication was similar in the two treatment groups.

INDICATION AND USAGE

LIDODERM is indicated for relief of pain associated with post-herpetic neuralgia. It should be applied only to **intact skin.**

CONTRAINDICATIONS

LIDODERM is contraindicated in patients with a known history of sensitivity to local anesthetics of the amide type, or to any other component of the product.

WARNINGS

Accidental Exposure in Children:
Even a *used* LIDODERM patch contains a large amount of lidocaine (at least 665 mg). The potential exists for a small child or a pet to suffer serious adverse effects from chewing or ingesting a new or used LIDODERM patch, although the risk with this formulation has not been evaluated. It is important for patients to **store and dispose of LIDODERM out of the reach of children and pets.**

Excessive Dosing:
Excessive dosing by applying LIDODERM to larger areas or for longer than the recommended wearing time could result in increased absorption of lidocaine and high blood concen-

Table 1
Absorption of lidocaine from LIDODERM
Normal volunteers (n = 15, 12-hour wearing time)

LIDODERM Patch	Application Site	Area (cm^2)	Dose Absorbed (mg)	C_{max} (µg/mL)	T_{max} (hr)
3 patches (2100 mg)	Back	420	64 ± 32	0.13 ± 0.06	11 hr

trations, leading to serious adverse effects (see ADVERSE REACTIONS, Systemic Reactions). Lidocaine toxicity could be expected at lidocaine blood concentrations above 5 µg/mL. The blood concentration of lidocaine is determined by the rate of systemic absorption and elimination. Longer duration of application, application of more than the recommended number of patches, smaller patients, or impaired elimination may all contribute to increasing the blood concentration of lidocaine. With recommended dosing of LIDODERM, the average peak blood concentration is about 0.13 µg/mL, but concentrations higher than 0.25 µg/mL have been observed in some individuals.

PRECAUTIONS

General:

Hepatic Disease:

Patients with severe hepatic disease are at greater risk of developing toxic blood concentrations of lidocaine, because of their inability to metabolize lidocaine normally.

Allergic Reactions:

Patients allergic to para-aminobenzoic acid derivatives (procaine, tetracaine, benzocaine, etc.) have not shown cross sensitivity to lidocaine. However, LIDODERM should be used with caution in patients with a history of drug sensitivities, especially if the etiologic agent is uncertain.

Non-intact Skin:

Application to broken or inflamed skin, although not tested, may result in higher blood concentrations of lidocaine from increased absorption. LIDODERM is only recommended for use on intact skin.

Eye Exposure:

The contact of LIDODERM with eyes, although not studied, should be avoided based on the findings of severe eye irritation with the use of similar products in animals. If eye contact occurs, immediately wash out the eye with water or saline and protect the eye until sensation returns.

Drug Interactions:

Antiarrhythmic Drugs:

LIDODERM should be used with caution in patients receiving Class I antiarrhythmic drugs (such as tocainide and mexiletine) since the toxic effects are additive and potentially synergistic.

Local Anesthetics:

When LIDODERM is used concomitantly with other products containing local anesthetic agents, the amount absorbed from all formulations must be considered.

Carcinogenesis, Mutagenesis, Impairment of Fertility:

Carcinogenesis:

A minor metabolite, 2,6-xylidine, has been found to be carcinogenic in rats. The blood concentration of this metabolite is negligible following application of LIDODERM.

Mutagenesis:

Lidocaine HCl is not mutagenic in Salmonella/mammalian microsome test nor clastogenic in chromosome aberration assay with human lymphocytes and mouse micronucleus test.

Impairment of Fertility:

The effect of LIDODERM on fertility has not been studied.

Pregnancy:

Teratogenic Effects: Pregnancy Category B.

LIDODERM (lidocaine patch 5%) has not been studied in pregnancy. Reproduction studies with lidocaine have been performed in rats at doses up to 30 mg/kg subcutaneously and have revealed no evidence of harm to the fetus due to lidocaine. There are, however, no adequate and well-controlled studies in pregnant women. Because animal reproduction studies are not always predictive of human response, LIDODERM should be used during pregnancy only if clearly needed.

Labor and Delivery:

LIDODERM has not been studied in labor and delivery. Lidocaine is not contraindicated in labor and delivery. Should LIDODERM be used concomitantly with other products containing lidocaine, total doses contributed by all formulations must be considered.

Nursing Mothers:

LIDODERM has not been studied in nursing mothers. Lidocaine is excreted in human milk, and the milk:plasma ratio of lidocaine is 0.4. Caution should be exercised when LIDODERM is administered to a nursing woman.

Pediatric Use:

Safety and effectiveness in pediatric patients have not been established.

ADVERSE REACTIONS

Localized Reactions:

During or immediately after treatment with LIDODERM (lidocaine patch 5%), the skin at the site of treatment may develop erythema or edema or may be the locus of abnormal sensation. These reactions are generally mild and transient, resolving spontaneously within a few minutes to hours. In clinical studies with LIDODERM, there were no serious reactions reported. One out of 150 subjects in a three-week study was discontinued from treatment because of a skin reaction (erythema and hives).

Allergic Reactions:

Allergic and anaphylactoid reactions associated with lidocaine, although rare, can occur. They are characterized by urticaria, angioedema, bronchospasm, and shock. If they occur, they should be managed by conventional means. The detection of sensitivity by skin testing is of doubtful value.

Systemic (Dose-Related) Reactions:

Systemic adverse reactions following appropriate use of LIDODERM are unlikely, due to the small dose absorbed (see CLINICAL PHARMACOLOGY, Pharmacokinetics). Systemic adverse effects of lidocaine are similar in nature to those observed with other amide local anesthetic agents, including CNS excitation and/or depression (light-headedness, nervousness, apprehension, euphoria, confusion, dizziness, drowsiness, tinnitus, blurred or double vision, vomiting, sensations of heat, cold or numbness, twitching, tremors, convulsions, unconsciousness, respiratory depression and arrest). Excitatory CNS reactions may be brief or not occur at all, in which case the first manifestation may be drowsiness merging into unconsciousness. Cardiovascular manifestations may include bradycardia, hypotension and cardiovascular collapse leading to arrest.

OVERDOSAGE

Lidocaine overdose from cutaneous absorption is rare, but could occur. If there is any suspicion of lidocaine overdose (see ADVERSE REACTIONS, Systemic Reactions), drug blood concentration should be checked. The management of overdose includes close monitoring, supportive care, and symptomatic treatment. Dialysis is of negligible value in the treatment of acute overdose with lidocaine.

In the absence of massive topical overdose or oral ingestion, evaluation of symptoms of toxicity should include consideration of other etiologies for the clinical effects, or overdosage from other sources of lidocaine or other local anesthetics.

The oral LD_{50} of lidocaine HCl is 459 (346–773) mg/kg (as the salt) in non-fasted female rats and 214 (159–324) mg/kg (as the salt) in fasted female rats, which are equivalent to roughly 4000 mg and 2000 mg, respectively, in a 60 to 70 kg man based on the equivalent surface area dosage conversion factors between species.

DOSAGE AND ADMINISTRATION

Apply LIDODERM to intact skin to cover the most painful area. Apply up to three patches, only once for up to 12 hours within a 24-hour period. Patches may be cut into smaller sizes with scissors prior to removal of the release liner. Clothing may be worn over the area of application. Smaller areas of treatment are recommended in a debilitated patient, or a patient with impaired elimination.

If irritation or a burning sensation occurs during application, remove the patch(es) and do not reapply until the irritation subsides.

When LIDODERM is used concomitantly with other products containing local anesthetic agents, the amount absorbed from all formulations must be considered.

HANDLING AND DISPOSAL

Hands should be washed after the handling of LIDODERM, and eye contact with LIDODERM should be avoided. The used patch should be immediately disposed of in such a way as to prevent its access by children or pets.

HOW SUPPLIED

LIDODERM (lidocaine patch 5%) is available as the following:

NDC 63481-687-06 resealable envelope, containing 5 patches (10 cm × 14 cm), box of 6 envelopes

KEEP ENVELOPE SEALED AT ALL TIMES WHEN NOT IN USE.

Store at 25°C (77°F); excursions permitted to 15°–30°C (59°–86°F). [See USP Controlled Room Temperature].

LIDODERM® is a Registered Trademark of Hind Health Care, Inc.

6524-02/July, 1999

MOBAN® ℞

[mō 'ban]

(molindone hydrochloride)

DESCRIPTION

MOBAN (molindone hydrochloride) is a dihydroindolone compound which is not structurally related to the phenothiazines, the butyrophenones or the thioxanthenes.

MOBAN is 3-ethyl-6, 7-dihydro-2-methyl-5-(morpholinomethyl) indol-4 (5H)-one hydrochloride. It is a white to off-white crystalline powder, freely soluble in water and alcohol and has a molecular weight of 312.67.

MOBAN Tablets also contain:

All strengths:	calcium sulfate, lactose, magnesium stearate, microcrystalline cellulose and povidone.
5 mg:	alginic acid, colloidal silicon dioxide and FD&C Yellow 6.
10 mg:	alginic acid, colloidal silicon dioxide, FD&C Blue 2 and FD&C Red 40.
25 mg:	alginic acid, colloidal silicon dioxide, D&C Yellow 10, FD&C Blue 2, and FD&C Yellow 6.
50 mg:	FD&C Blue 2 and sodium starch glycolate.
100 mg:	FD&C Blue 2, FD&C Yellow 6 and sodium starch glycolate.

MOBAN Concentrate contains: alcohol, artificial cherry flavor, artificial cover flavor, edetate disodium, glycerin, liquid sugar, methylparaben, propylparaben, sodium metabisulfite, sorbitol solution, and hydrochloric acid reagent grade for pH adjustment.

N-CH2 O CH2-CH3 •HCl CH3 N H

MOLINDONE HYDROCHLORIDE

ACTIONS

MOBAN has a pharmacological profile in laboratory animals which predominantly resembles that of major tranquilizers causing reduction of spontaneous locomotion and aggressiveness, suppression of a conditioned response and antagonism of the bizarre stereotyped behavior and hyperactivity induced by amphetamines. In addition, MOBAN antagonizes the depression caused by the tranquilizing agent tetrabenazine.

In human clinical studies tranquilization is achieved in the absence of muscle relaxing or incoordinating effects. Based on EEG studies, MOBAN exerts its effect on the ascending reticular activating system.

Human metabolic studies show MOBAN to be rapidly absorbed and metabolized when given orally. Unmetabolized drug reached a peak blood level at 1.5 hours. Pharmacological effect from a single oral dose persists for 24–36 hours. There are 36 recognized metabolites with less than 2–3% unmetabolized MOBAN being excreted in urine and feces.

INDICATIONS

MOBAN is indicated for the management of the manifestations of psychotic disorders. The antipsychotic efficacy of MOBAN was established in clinical studies which enrolled newly hospitalized and chronically hospitalized, acutely ill, schizophrenic patients as subjects.

CONTRAINDICATIONS

MOBAN is contraindicated in severe central nervous system depression (alcohol, barbiturates, narcotics, etc.) or comatose states, and in patients with known hypersensitivity to the drug.

WARNINGS

Tardive Dyskinesia

Tardive dyskinesia, a syndrome consisting of potentially irreversible, involuntary, dyskinetic movements may develop in patients treated with neuroleptic (antipsychotic) drugs. Although the prevalence of the syndrome appears to be highest among the elderly, especially elderly women, it is impossible to rely upon prevalence estimates to predict, at the inception of neuroleptic treatment, which patients are likely to develop the syndrome. Whether neuroleptic drug products differ in their potential to cause tardive dyskinesia is unknown.

Both the risk of developing the syndrome and the likelihood that it will become irreversible are believed to increase as the duration of treatment and the total cumulative dose of neuroleptic drugs administered to the patient increase. However, the syndrome can develop, although much less commonly, after relatively brief treatment periods at low doses.

There is no known treatment for established cases of tardive dyskinesia, although the syndrome may remit, partially or completely, if neuroleptic treatment is withdrawn. Neuroleptic treatment, itself, however, may suppress (or partially suppress) the signs and symptoms of the syndrome and thereby may possibly mask the underlying disease process. The effect that symptomatic suppression has upon the long-term course of the syndrome is unknown.

Given these considerations, neuroleptics should be prescribed in a manner that is most likely to minimize the occurrence of tardive dyskinesia. Chronic neuroleptic treatment should generally be reserved for patients who suffer from a chronic illness that, 1) is known to respond to neuroleptic drugs, and 2) for whom alternative, equally effective, but potentially less harmful treatments are not available or appropriate. In patients who do require chronic treatment, the smallest dose and the shortest duration of treatment producing a satisfactory clinical response should be sought. The need for continued treatment should be reassessed periodically.

If signs and symptoms of tardive dyskinesia appear in a patient on neuroleptics, drug discontinuation should be considered. However, some patients may require treatment despite the presence of the syndrome.

(For further information about the description of tardive dyskinesia and its clinical detection, please refer to the section on Adverse Reactions.)

Neuroleptic Malignant Syndrome (NMS)

A potentially fatal symptom complex sometimes referred to as Neuroleptic Malignant Syndrome (NMS) has been reported in association with antipsychotic drugs. Clinical manifestations of NMS are hyperpyrexia, muscle rigidity, altered mental status and evidence of autonomic instability (irregular pulse or blood pressure, tachycardia, diaphoresis, and cardiac dysrhythmias).

The diagnostic evaluation of patients with this syndrome is complicated. In arriving at a diagnosis, it is important to identify cases where the clinical presentation includes both serious medical illness (e.g., pneumonia, systemic infection,

Continued on next page

Moban—Cont.

etc.) and untreated or inadequately treated extrapyramidal signs and symptoms (EPS). Other important considerations in the differential diagnosis include central anticholinergic toxicity, heat stroke, drug fever and primary central nervous system (CNS) pathology.

The management of NMS should include, 1) immediate discontinuation of antipsychotic drugs and other drugs not essential to concurrent therapy, 2) intensive symptomatic treatment and medical monitoring, and 3) treatment of any concomitant serious medical problems for which specific treatments are available. There is no general agreement about specific pharmacological treatment regimens for uncomplicated NMS.

If a patient requires antipsychotic drug treatment after recovery from NMS, the potential reintroduction of drug therapy should be carefully considered. The patient should be carefully monitored, since recurrences of NMS have been reported.

Usage in Pregnancy: Studies in pregnant patients have not been carried out. Reproduction studies have been performed in the following animals:

Pregnant Rats oral dose—	
no adverse effect	20 mg/kg/day—10 days
no adverse effect	40 mg/kg/day—10 days
Pregnant Mice oral dose—	
slight increase resorptions	20 mg/kg/day—10 days
slight increase resorptions	40 mg/kg/day—10 days
Pregnant Rabbits oral dose—	
no adverse effect	5 mg/kg/day—12 days
no adverse effect	10 mg/kg/day—12 days
no adverse effect	20 mg/kg/day—12 days

Animal reproductive studies have not demonstrated a teratogenic potential. The anticipated benefits must be weighed against the unknown risks to the fetus if used in pregnant patients.

Nursing Mothers: Data are not available on the content of MOBAN (molindone hydrochloride) in the milk of nursing mothers.

Pediatric Use: Use of MOBAN in pediatric patients below the age of twelve years is not recommended because safe and effective conditions for its usage have not been established.

MOBAN has not been shown effective in the management of behavioral complications in patients with mental retardation.

Sulfites Sensitivity: MOBAN Concentrate contains sodium metabisulfite, a sulfite that may cause allergic-type reactions including anaphylactic symptoms and life-threatening or less severe asthmatic episodes in certain susceptible people. The overall prevalence of sulfite sensitivity in the general population is unknown and probably low. Sulfite sensitivity is seen more frequently in asthmatic than in nonasthmatic people.

PRECAUTIONS

Some patients receiving MOBAN may note drowsiness initially and they should be advised against activities requiring mental alertness until their response to the drug has been established.

Increased activity has been noted in patients receiving MOBAN. Caution should be exercised where increased activity may be harmful.

MOBAN does not lower the seizure threshold in experimental animals to the degree noted with more sedating antipsychotic drugs. However, in humans convulsive seizures have been reported in a few instances.

The physician should be aware that this tablet preparation contains calcium sulfate as an excipient and that calcium ions may interfere with the absorption of preparations containing phenytoin sodium and tetracyclines.

MOBAN has an antiemetic effect in animals. A similar effect may occur in humans and may obscure signs of intestinal obstruction or brain tumor.

Neuroleptic drugs elevate prolactin levels; the elevation persists during chronic administration. Tissue culture experiments indicate that approximately one-third of human breast cancers are prolactin dependent *in vitro*, a factor of potential importance if the prescription of these drugs is contemplated in a patient with a previously detected breast cancer. Although disturbances such as galactorrhea, amenorrhea, gynecomastia, and impotence have been reported, the clinical significance of elevated serum prolactin levels is unknown for most patients. An increase in mammary neoplasms has been found in rodents after chronic administration of neuroleptic drugs. Neither clinical studies nor epidemiologic studies conducted to date, however, have shown an association between chronic administration of these drugs and mammary tumorigenesis; the available evidence is considered too limited to be conclusive at this time.

ADVERSE REACTIONS

CNS EFFECTS

The most frequently occurring effect is initial drowsiness that generally subsides with continued usage of the drug or lowering of the dose.

Noted less frequently were depression, hyperactivity and euphoria.

Neurological

Extrapyramidal Reactions

Extrapyramidal reactions noted below may occur in susceptible individuals and are usually reversible with appropriate management.

Akathisia

Motor restlessness may occur early.

Parkinson Syndrome

Akinesia, characterized by rigidity, immobility and reduction of voluntary movements and tremor, have been observed. Occurrence is less frequent than akathisia.

Dystonic Syndrome

Prolonged abnormal contractions of muscle groups occur infrequently. These symptoms may be managed by the addition of a synthetic antiparkinson agent (other than L-dopa), small doses of sedative drugs, and/or reduction in dosage.

Tardive Dyskinesia

Neuroleptic drugs are known to cause a syndrome of dyskinetic movements commonly referred to as tardive dyskinesia. The movements may appear during treatment or upon withdrawal of treatment and may be either reversible or irreversible (i.e., persistent) upon cessation of further neuroleptic administration.

The syndrome is known to have a variable latency for development and the duration of the latency cannot be determined reliably. It is thus wise to assume that any neuroleptic agent has the capacity to induce the syndrome and act accordingly until sufficient data has been collected to settle the issue definitively for a specific drug product. In the case of neuroleptics known to produce the irreversible syndrome, the following has been observed.

Tardive dyskinesia has appeared in some patients on long-term therapy and has also appeared after drug therapy has been discontinued. The risk appears to be greater in elderly patients on high-dose therapy, especially females. The symptoms are persistent and in some patients appear to be irreversible. The syndrome is characterized by rhythmical involuntary movements of the tongue, face, mouth or jaw (e.g., protrusion of tongue, puffing of cheeks, puckering of mouth, chewing movements). There may be involuntary movements of extremities.

There is no known effective treatment of tardive dyskinesia; antiparkinsonism agents usually do not alleviate the symptoms of this syndrome. It is suggested that all antipsychotic agents be discontinued if these symptoms appear. Should it be necessary to reinstitute treatment, or increase the dosage of the agent, or switch to a different antipsychotic agent, the syndrome may be masked. It has been reported that fine vermicular movements of the tongue may be an early sign of the syndrome and if the medication is stopped at that time the syndrome may not develop (See WARNINGS).

Autonomic Nervous System

Occasionally blurring of vision, tachycardia, nausea, dry mouth and salivation have been reported. Urinary retention and constipation may occur particularly if anticholinergic drugs are used to treat extrapyramidal symptoms. One patient being treated with MOBAN (molindone hydrochloride) experienced priapism which required surgical intervention, apparently resulting in residual impairment of erectile function.

Laboratory Tests

There have been rare reports of leucopenia and leucocytosis. If such reactions occur, treatment with MOBAN may continue if clinical symptoms are absent. Alterations of blood glucose, B.U.N., and red blood cells have not been considered clinically significant.

Metabolic and Endocrine Effects

Alteration of thyroid function has not been significant. Amenorrhea has been reported infrequently. Resumption of menses in previously amenorrheic women has been reported. Initially heavy menses may occur. Galactorrhea and gynecomastia have been reported infrequently. Increase in libido has been noted in some patients. Impotence has not been reported. Although both weight gain and weight loss have been in the direction of normal or ideal weight, excessive weight gain has not occurred with MOBAN.

Hepatic Effects

There have been rare reports of clinically significant alterations in liver function in association with MOBAN use.

Cardiovascular

Rare, transient, non-specific T wave changes have been reported on E.K.G. Association with a clinical syndrome has not been established. Rarely has significant hypotension been reported.

Ophthalmological

Lens opacities and pigmentary retinopathy have not been reported where patients have received MOBAN. In some patients, phenothiazine induced lenticular opacities have resolved following discontinuation of the phenothiazine while continuing therapy with MOBAN.

Skin

Early, non-specific skin rash, probably of allergic origin, has occasionally been reported. Skin pigmentation has not been seen with MOBAN usage alone.

MOBAN has certain pharmacological similarities to other antipsychotic agents. Because adverse reactions are often extensions of the pharmacological activity of a drug, all of the known pharmacological effects associated with other antipsychotic drugs should be kept in mind when MOBAN is used. Upon abrupt withdrawal after prolonged high dosage an abstinence syndrome has not been noted.

DOSAGE AND ADMINISTRATION

Initial and maintenance doses of MOBAN (molindone hydrochloride) should be individualized.

Initial Dosage Schedule

The usual starting dosage is 50–75 mg/day.

— Increase to 100 mg/day in 3 or 4 days.

— Based on severity of symptomatology, dosage may be titrated up or down depending on individual patient response.

— An increase to 225 mg/day may be required in patients with severe symptomatology.

Elderly and debilitated patients should be started on lower dosage.

Maintenance Dosage Schedule

1. Mild-5 mg-15 mg three or four times a day.
2. Moderate-10 mg-25 mg three or four times a day.
3. Severe-225 mg/day may be required.

DRUG INTERACTIONS

Potentiation of drugs administered concurrently with MOBAN has not been reported. Additionally, animal studies have not shown increased toxicity when MOBAN is given concurrently with representative members of three classes of drugs (i.e., barbiturates, chloral hydrate and antiparkinson drugs).

MANAGEMENT OF OVERDOSAGE

Symptomatic, supportive therapy should be the rule.

Gastric lavage is indicated for the reduction of absorption of MOBAN which is freely soluble in water.

Since the adsorption of MOBAN by activated charcoal has not been determined, the use of this antidote must be considered of theoretical value.

Emesis in a comatose patient is contraindicated. Additionally, while the emetic effect of apomorphine is blocked by MOBAN in animals, this blocking effect has not been determined in humans.

A significant increase in the rate of removal of unmetabolized MOBAN from the body by forced diuresis, peritoneal or renal dialysis would not be expected. (Only 2% of a single ingested dose of MOBAN is excreted unmetabolized in the urine). However, poor response of the patient may justify use of these procedures.

While the use of laxatives or enemas might be based on general principles, the amount of unmetabolized MOBAN in feces is less than 1%. Extrapyramidal symptoms have responded to the use of diphenhydramine (Benadryl*), Amantadine HCl (Symmetrel®*) and the synthetic anticholinergic antiparkinson agents, (i.e., Artane*, Cogentin*, Akineton*).

HOW SUPPLIED

As tablets in bottles of 100 with potencies and colors as follows:

[See table below]

As a concentrate (clear, colorless to straw-yellow syrup) containing 20 mg molindone hydrochloride per mL in 4 oz. (120 mL) bottles, NDC 63481-460-04.

Store at controlled room temperature 15°–30°C (59°–86°F). Protect from light.

*Benadryl-Trademark, Parke Davis and Co.
*Artane-Trademark, Lederle Laboratories
*Cogentin-Trademark, Merck Sharp & Dohme
*Akineton-Trademark, Knoll Pharmaceutical Co.
*Symmetrel-Trademark, Endo Pharmaceuticals Inc.

MOBAN® is a Registered trademark of Endo Pharmaceuticals Inc.

6500-00/January, 1998

Shown in Product Identification Guide, page 312

5 mg	Orange, round, biconvex tablet, one face inscribed with "Moban 5", and the other face plain.	NDC 63481-072-70
10 mg	Lavender, round, biconvex tablet, one face inscribed with "Moban 10", and the other face plain.	NDC 63481-073-70
25 mg	Green, round, biconvex tablet, one face scored and inscribed with "Moban 25", and the other face plain with partial bisect.	NDC 63481-074-70
50 mg	Blue, round, biconvex tablet, one face scored and inscribed with "Moban 50", and the other face plain.	NDC 63481-076-70
100 mg	Tan, round, biconvex tablet, one face scored and inscribed with "Moban 100", and the other face plain.	NDC 63481-077-70

NARCAN® ℞

[*nar'kan*]

(naloxone hydrochloride injection, USP)

Opioid Antagonist

DESCRIPTION

NARCAN (naloxone hydrochloride injection, USP), an opioid antagonist, is a synthetic congener of oxymorphone.

In structure it differs from oxymorphone in that the methyl group on the nitrogen atom is replaced by an allyl group.

NALOXONE HYDROCHLORIDE
(-)-17-Allyl-4, 5α-epoxy-3, 14 - dihydroxy morphinan-6-one hydrochloride

Naloxone hydrochloride occurs as a white to slightly off-white powder, and is soluble in water, in dilute acids, and in strong alkali; slightly soluble in alcohol; practically insoluble in ether and in chloroform.

NARCAN injection is available as a sterile solution for intravenous, intramuscular and subcutaneous administration in three concentrations: 0.02 mg, 0.4 mg and 1.0 mg of naloxone hydrochloride per mL. One mL of the 0.02 mg and 0.4 mg strengths contains 8.6 mg of sodium chloride. One mL of the 1.0 mg strength contains 8.35 mg of sodium chloride. In the 10 mL multiple dose vial, one mL of the 0.4 mg and 1.0 mg strengths also contains 2.0 mg of methylparaben and propylparaben as preservatives in a ratio of 9 to 1. pH is adjusted to 3.5 ± 0.5 with hydrochloric acid.

NARCAN injection is also available in a paraben-free formulation in three concentrations: 0.02 mg. 0.4 mg and 1.0 mg of naloxone hydrochloride per mL. One mL of each strength contains 9.0 mg of sodium chloride. pH is adjusted to 3.5 ± 0.5 with hydrochloric acid.

CLINICAL PHARMACOLOGY

Complete or Partial Reversal of Opioid Depression NARCAN prevents or reverses the effects of opioids including respiratory depression, sedation and hypotension. Also, it can reverse the psychotomimetic and dysphoric effects of agonist-antagonists such as pentazocine.

NARCAN is an essentially pure opioid antagonist, i.e., it does not possess the "agonistic" or morphine-like properties characteristic of other opioid antagonists; NARCAN does not produce respiratory depression, psychotomimetic effects or pupillary constriction. In the absence of opioids or agonistic effects of other opioid antagonists, it exhibits essentially no pharmacologic activity.

NARCAN has not been shown to produce tolerance or cause physical or psychological dependence.

In the presence of physical dependence on opioids NARCAN will produce withdrawal symptoms.

While the mechanism of action of NARCAN is not fully understood, the preponderance of evidence suggests that NARCAN antagonizes opioid effects by competing for the same receptor sites.

When NARCAN is administered intravenously, the onset of action is generally apparent within two minutes; the onset of action is only slightly less rapid when it is administered subcutaneously or intramuscularly. The duration of action is dependent upon the dose and route of administration of NARCAN. Intramuscular administration produces a more prolonged effect than intravenous administration. The requirement for repeat doses of NARCAN, however, will also be dependent upon the amount, type and route of administration of the opioid being antagonized.

Following parenteral administration, NARCAN is rapidly distributed in the body. It is metabolized in the liver, primarily by glucuronide conjugation and excreted in urine. In one study the serum half-life in adults ranged from 30 to 81 minutes (mean 64 ± 12 minutes). In a neonatal study the mean plasma half-life was observed to be 3.1 ± 0.5 hours.

Adjunctive Use in Septic Shock Although the mechanism of action is not completely understood, NARCAN appears to block endorphin-mediated hypotension in septic shock patients.

NARCAN has been shown in some cases of septic shock to produce a rise in blood pressure that may last up to several hours; however, this pressor response has not been demonstrated to improve patient survival.

Patients who have responded to NARCAN received the drug early in the course of treatment of septic shock. Because of the limited number of patients who have been treated, optimal dosage and treatment regimens have not been established. Published reports demonstrating a pressor effect have evaluated single bolus injections of 0.4 mg over three (3) to five (5) minutes, which have been repeated for 3–5 doses depending on the response. Bolus infusion doses ranging from 0.03 mg/kg to 0.2 mg/kg over five (5) minutes have also been reported. If a response was elicited, treatment was continued by intravenous infusion of concentrations of 0.03 mg/kg/hour to 0.3 mg/kg/hour for 1–24 hours or more depending upon the clinical response.

INDICATIONS AND USAGE

NARCAN is indicated for the complete or partial reversal of opioid depression, including respiratory depression, induced by natural and synthetic opioids, including propoxyphene, methadone and certain mixed agonist-antagonist analgesics: nalbuphine, pentazocine and butorphanol. NARCAN is also indicated for the diagnosis of suspected opioid tolerance or acute opioid overdosage.

NARCAN may be useful as an adjunctive agent to increase blood pressure in the management of septic shock (see **CLINICAL PHARMACOLOGY; Adjunctive Use in Septic Shock**).

CONTRAINDICATIONS

NARCAN is contraindicated in patients known to be hypersensitive to naloxone hydrochloride or to any of the other ingredients in NARCAN.

WARNINGS

NARCAN should be administered cautiously to persons including newborns of mothers who are known or suspected to be physically dependent on opioids. In such cases an abrupt and complete reversal of opioid effects may precipitate an acute withdrawal syndrome.

The signs and symptoms of opioid withdrawal in a patient physically dependent on opioids may include, but are not limited to, the following: body aches, diarrhea, tachycardia, fever, runny nose, sneezing, piloerection, sweating, yawning, nausea or vomiting, nervousness, restlessness or irritability, shivering or trembling, abdominal cramps, weakness, and increased blood pressure. In the neonate, opioid withdrawal may also include: convulsions, excessive crying, and hyperactive reflexes.

The patient who has satisfactorily responded to NARCAN should be kept under continued surveillance and repeated doses of NARCAN should be administered, as necessary, since the duration of action of some opioids may exceed that of NARCAN.

NARCAN is not effective against respiratory depression due to non-opioid drugs. Reversal of buprenorphine-induced respiratory depression may be incomplete. If an incomplete response occurs, respirations should be mechanically assisted.

PRECAUTIONS

General In addition to NARCAN, other resuscitative measures such as maintenance of a free airway, artificial ventilation, cardiac massage, and vasopressor agents should be available and employed when necessary to counteract acute opioid poisoning.

Abrupt postoperative reversal of opioid depression may result in nausea, vomiting, sweating, tremulousness, tachycardia, increased blood pressure, seizures, ventricular tachycardia and fibrillation, pulmonary edema, and cardiac arrest which may result in death.

Several instances of hypotension, hypertension, ventricular tachycardia and fibrillation, pulmonary edema, and cardiac arrest have been reported in postoperative patients. Death, coma, and encephalopathy have been reported as sequelae of these events. These have occurred in patients most of whom had pre-existing cardiovascular disorders or received other drugs which may have similar adverse cardiovascular effects. Although a direct cause and effect relationship has not been established, NARCAN should be used with caution in patients with pre-existing cardiac disease or patients who have received medications with potential adverse cardiovascular effects, such as hypotension, ventricular tachycardia or fibrillation, and pulmonary edema. It has been suggested that the pathogenesis of pulmonary edema associated with the use of NARCAN is similar to neurogenic pulmonary edema, i.e., a centrally mediated massive catecholamine response leading to a dramatic shift of blood volume into the pulmonary vascular bed resulting in increased hydrostatic pressures.

Carcinogenesis, Mutagenesis, Impairment of Fertility Studies in animals to assess the carcinogenic potential of NARCAN have not been conducted. NARCAN was weakly positive in the Ames mutagenicity and *in vitro* human lymphocyte chromosome aberration tests and was negative in the *in vitro* Chinese hamster V79 cell HGPRT mutagenicity assay and in an *in vivo* rat bone marrow chromosome aberration study. Reproduction studies conducted in mice and rats at doses as high as 50 times the usual human dose (10 mg/day) demonstrated no impairment of fertility.

Use in Pregnancy

Teratogenic Effects Pregnancy Category B: Reproduction studies performed in mice and rats at doses as high as 50 times the usual human dose (10 mg/day), revealed no evidence of impaired fertility or harm to the fetus due to NARCAN. There are, however, no adequate and well controlled studies in pregnant women. Because animal reproduction studies are not always predictive of human response, NARCAN should be used during pregnancy only if clearly needed.

Non-teratogenic Effects Risk-benefit must be considered before NARCAN is administered to a pregnant woman who is known or suspected to be opioid-dependent since maternal dependence may often be accompanied by fetal dependence. Naloxone crosses the placenta and may precipitate withdrawal in the fetus as well as in the mother.

Use in Labor and Delivery It is not known if NARCAN affects the duration of labor and/or delivery.

Nursing Mothers It is not known whether NARCAN is excreted in human milk. Because many drugs are excreted in human milk, caution should be exercised when NARCAN is administered to a nursing woman.

Usage in Pediatric Patients and Neonates for Septic Shock The safety and effectiveness of NARCAN in the treatment of hypotension in pediatric patients and neonates with septic shock have not been established.

Renal Insufficiency/Failure The safety and effectiveness of NARCAN in patients with renal insufficiency/failure have not been established in well-controlled clinical trials. Caution should be exercised when NARCAN is administered to this patient population.

Liver Disease The safety and effectiveness of NARCAN in patients with liver disease have not been established in well-controlled clinical trials. In one small study in patients with liver cirrhosis, plasma naloxone concentrations were approximately six times higher than in patients without liver disease. NARCAN was well tolerated and no adverse events were reported. Caution should be exercised when NARCAN is administered to patients with liver disease.

ADVERSE REACTIONS

Postoperative The following adverse events have been associated with the use of NARCAN in postoperative patients: hypotension, hypertension, ventricular tachycardia and fibrillation, dyspnea, pulmonary edema, and cardiac arrest. Death, coma, and encephalopathy have been reported as sequelae of these events. Excessive doses of NARCAN in postoperative patients may result in significant reversal of analgesia and may cause agitation (see **PRECAUTIONS** and **DOSAGE AND ADMINISTRATION; Usage in Adults; Postoperative Opioid Depression**).

Opioid Depression Abrupt reversal of opioid depression may result in nausea, vomiting, sweating, tachycardia, increased blood pressure, tremulousness, seizures, ventricular tachycardia and fibrillation, pulmonary edema, and cardiac arrest which may result in death (see **PRECAUTIONS**).

Opioid Dependence Abrupt reversal of opioid effects in persons who are physically dependent on opioids may precipitate an acute withdrawal syndrome which may include, but is not limited to, the following signs and symptoms: body aches, fever, sweating, runny nose, sneezing, piloerection, yawning, weakness, shivering or trembling, nervousness, restlessness or irritability, diarrhea, nausea or vomiting, abdominal cramps, increased blood pressure, tachycardia. In the neonate, opioid withdrawal may also include: convulsions; excessive crying; hyperactive reflexes (see **WARNINGS**).

Agitation and paresthesias have been infrequently reported with the use of NARCAN (naloxone hydrochloride injection, USP).

DRUG ABUSE AND DEPENDENCE

NARCAN is an opioid antagonist. Physical dependence associated with the use of NARCAN has not been reported. Tolerance to the opioid antagonist effect of NARCAN is not known to occur.

OVERDOSAGE

There is limited clinical experience with NARCAN overdosage in humans.

Adult Patients In one study, volunteers and morphine-dependent subjects who received 24 mg/70 kg did not demonstrate toxicity.

In another study, 36 patients with acute stroke received a loading dose of 4 mg/kg (10 mg/m^2/min) of NARCAN followed immediately by 2 mg/kg/hr for 24 hours. There were a few reports of serious adverse events: seizures (2 patients), severe hypertension (1), and hypotension and/or bradycardia(3).

At doses of 2 mg/kg in normal subjects, memory impairment has been reported.

Pediatric Patients Up to 11 doses of 0.2 mg of naloxone (2.2 mg) have been administered to children following overdose of diphenoxylate hydrochloride with atropine sulfate. Pediatric reports include a 2-1/2 year old child who inadvertently received a dose of 20 mg of naloxone and a 4-1/2 year-old who received 11 doses during a 12-hour period, both of whom had no adverse sequelae.

Patient Management Patients who experience a NARCAN overdose should be treated symptomatically in a closely-supervised environment. Physicians should contact a poison control center for the most up-to-date patient management information.

Animal Data The intravenous single-dose LD_{50} (95% confidence limits) in rats and mice is 150 (135–165) mg/kg and 109 (97–121) mg/kg, respectively. In newborn rats, the subcutaneous single-dose LD_{50} (95% confidence limits) is 260 (228–296) mg/kg. Subcutaneous injection in rats at 100 mg/kg/day for three weeks produced only transiently increased salivation and partial ptosis; no drug-related effects were seen at 10 mg/kg/day for three weeks.

Some chemical impurities in naloxone, i.e., noroxymorphone and bisnaloxone, have been shown to produce emesis in dogs when administered alone at i.v. doses equivalent to impurity levels present in naloxone at 60 times the usual human dose (10 mg/day).

DOSAGE AND ADMINISTRATION

NARCAN may be administered intravenously, intramuscularly, or subcutaneously. The most rapid onset of action is achieved by intravenous administration, which is recommended in emergency situations.

Since the duration of action of some opioids may exceed that of NARCAN, the patient should be kept under continued surveillance. Repeated doses of NARCAN should be administered, as necessary.

Intravenous Infusion NARCAN may be diluted for intravenous infusion in normal saline or 5% dextrose solutions. The addition of 2 mg of NARCAN in 500 mL of either solution provides a concentration of 0.004 mg/mL. Mixtures should be used within 24 hours. After 24 hours, the remaining unused mixture must be discarded. The rate of administration should be titrated in accordance with the patient's response.

NARCAN should not be mixed with preparations containing bisulfite, metabisulfite, long-chain or high molecular weight anions, or any solution having an alkaline pH. No drug or

Continued on next page

Narcan—Cont.

chemical agent should be added to NARCAN unless its effect on the chemical and physical stability of the solution has first been established.

General Parenteral drug products should be inspected visually for particulate matter and discoloration prior to administration whenever solution and container permit.

Usage in Adults

Opioid Overdose - Known or Suspected An initial dose of 0.4 mg to 2 mg of NARCAN may be administered intravenously. If the desired degree of counteraction and improvement in respiratory functions are not obtained, it may be repeated at two- to three-minute intervals. If no response is observed after 10 mg of NARCAN have been administered, the diagnosis of opioid-induced or partial opioid-induced toxicity should be questioned. Intramuscular or subcutaneous administration may be necessary if the intravenous route is not available.

Postoperative Opioid Depression For the partial reversal of opioid depression following the use of opioids during surgery, smaller doses of NARCAN are usually sufficient. The dose of NARCAN should be titrated according to the patient's response. For the initial reversal of respiratory depression, NARCAN should be injected in increments of 0.1 to 0.2 mg intravenously at two- to three-minute intervals to the desired degree of reversal i.e., adequate ventilation and alertness without significant pain or discomfort. Larger than necessary dosage of NARCAN may result in significant reversal of analgesia and increase in blood pressure. Similarly, too rapid reversal may induce nausea, vomiting, sweating or circulatory stress.

Repeat doses of NARCAN may be required within one- to two-hour intervals depending upon the amount, type (i.e., short or long acting) and time interval since last administration of an opioid. Supplemental intramuscular doses have been shown to produce a longer lasting effect.

NARCAN Challenge Test Used for the diagnosis of suspected opioid tolerance or acute opioid overdosage. The NARCAN challenge test should not be performed in a patient showing clinical signs or symptoms of opioid withdrawal, or in a patient whose urine contains opioids. The NARCAN challenge test may be administered by either the intravenous or subcutaneous routes.

Intravenous:

Inject 0.2 mg NARCAN.

Observe for 30 seconds for signs or symptoms of withdrawal.

If no evidence of withdrawal, inject 0.6 mg NARCAN.

Observe for an additional 20 minutes.

Subcutaneous:

Administer 0.8 mg NARCAN.

Observe for 20 minutes for signs or symptoms of withdrawal.

Note: Individual patients, especially those with opioid dependence, may respond to lower doses of NARCAN. In some cases, 0.1 mg I.V. NARCAN has produced a diagnostic response.

Interpretation of the Challenge Monitor vital signs and observe the patient for signs and symptoms of opioid withdrawal. These may include, but are not limited to: nausea, vomiting, dysphoria, yawning, sweating, tearing, rhinorrhea, stuffy nose, craving for opioid, poor appetite, abdominal cramps, sense of fear, skin erythema, disrupted sleep patterns, fidgeting, uneasiness, poor ability to focus, mental lapses, muscle aches or cramps, pupillary dilation, piloerection, fever, changes in blood pressure, pulse or temperature, anxiety, depression, irritability, back ache, bone or joint pains, tremors, sensations of skin crawling or fasciculations. If signs or symptoms of withdrawal appear, the test is positive and no additional NARCAN should be administered.

Septic Shock The optimal dosage of NARCAN or duration of therapy for the treatment of hypotension in septic shock patients has not been established (see **CLINICAL PHARMACOLOGY**).

Usage in Children

Opioid Overdose - Known or Suspected The usual initial dose in children is 0.01 mg/kg body weight given I.V. If this dose does not result in the desired degree of clinical improvement, a subsequent dose of 0.1 mg/kg body weight may be administered. If an I.V. route of administration is not available, NARCAN may be administered I.M. or S.C. in divided doses. If necessary, NARCAN can be diluted with sterile water for injection.

Postoperative Opioid Depression Follow the recommendations and cautions under **Adult Postoperative Depression**. For the initial reversal of respiratory depression, NARCAN should be injected in increments of 0.005 mg to 0.01 mg intravenously at two- to three-minute intervals to the desired degree of reversal.

Usage in Neonates

Opioid-induced Depression The usual initial dose is 0.01 mg/kg body weight administered I.V., I.M., or S.C. This dose may be repeated in accordance with adult administration guidelines for postoperative opioid depression.

HOW SUPPLIED

NARCAN (naloxone hydrochloride injection, USP) for intravenous, intramuscular and subcutaneous administration is available as:

[See table below]

Store at controlled room temperature 15°–30°C (59°–86°F). Protect from excessive light.

Store in carton until contents have been used.

CAUTION: Federal (USA) law prohibits dispensing without prescription.

NARCAN® is a Registered Trademark of Endo Pharmaceuticals Inc.

6487-00/January, 1998

0.4 mg/mL	10 mL multiple dose vial-box of 1	NDC 63481-365-05
0.4 mg/mL (paraben-free)	1 mL ampul-box of 10	NDC 63481-358-10
1.0 mg/mL	10 mL multiple dose vial-box of 1	NDC 63481-368-05
1.0 mg/mL (paraben-free)	2 mL ampul-box of 10	NDC 63481-377-10
0.02 mg/mL (paraben-free)	2 mL ampul-box of 10	NDC 63481-359-10

NUBAIN® ℞

[*nū 'bān*]

(nalbuphine hydrochloride)

Rx only

DESCRIPTION

NUBAIN (nalbuphine hydrochloride) is a synthetic narcotic agonist-antagonist analgesic of the phenanthrene series. It is chemically related to both the widely used narcotic antagonist, naloxone, and the potent narcotic analgesic, oxymorphone.

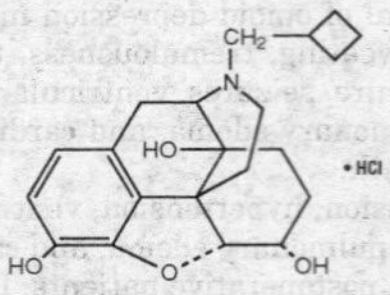

• HCl **NALBUPHINE HYDROCHLORIDE** (-)-17-(cyclobutylmethyl)-4, 5α-epoxymorphinan-3, 6α,14-triol, hydrochloride

NUBAIN is a sterile solution suitable for subcutaneous, intramuscular, or intravenous injection. NUBAIN is available in two concentrations, 10 mg and 20 mg of nalbuphine hydrochloride per mL. Both strengths in 10 mL vials contain 0.94% sodium citrate hydrous, 1.26% citric acid anhydrous, and 0.2% of a 9:1 mixture of methylparaben and propylparaben as preservatives; pH is adjusted, if necessary, to 3.5 to 3.7 with hydrochloric acid. The 10 mg/mL strength contains 0.2% sodium chloride.

NUBAIN is also available in ampuls in a sterile, paraben-free formulation in two concentrations, 10 mg and 20 mg of nalbuphine hydrochloride per mL. One mL of each strength contains 0.94% sodium citrate hydrous, and 1.26% citric acid anhydrous; pH is adjusted, if necessary, to 3.5 to 3.7 with hydrochloric acid. The 10 mg/mL strength contains 0.2% sodium chloride.

CLINICAL PHARMACOLOGY

NUBAIN is a potent analgesic. Its analgesic potency is essentially equivalent to that of morphine on a milligram basis. Receptor studies show that NUBAIN binds to mu, kappa, and delta receptors, but not to sigma receptors. NUBAIN is primarily a kappa agonist/partial mu antagonist analgesic.

The onset of action of NUBAIN occurs within 2 to 3 minutes after intravenous administration, and in less than 15 minutes following subcutaneous or intramuscular injection. The plasma half-life of nalbuphine is 5 hours, and in clinical studies the duration of analgesic activity has been reported to range from 3 to 6 hours.

The narcotic antagonist activity of NUBAIN is one-fourth as potent as nalorphine and 10 times that of pentazocine.

NUBAIN may produce the same degree of respiratory depression as equianalgesic doses of morphine. However, NUBAIN exhibits a ceiling effect such that increases in dose greater than 30 mg do not produce further respiratory depression.

NUBAIN by itself has potent narcotic antagonist activity at doses equal to or lower than its analgesic dose. When administered following or concurrent with mu agonist opioid analgesics (e.g., morphine, oxymorphone, fentanyl), NUBAIN may partially reverse or block narcotic-induced respiratory depression from the mu agonist analgesic. NUBAIN may precipitate withdrawal in patients dependent on opioid narcotic drugs. NUBAIN should be used with caution in patients who have been receiving mu opioid analgesics on a regular basis.

INDICATIONS AND USAGE

NUBAIN is indicated for the relief of moderate to severe pain. NUBAIN can also be used as a supplement to balanced anesthesia, for preoperative and postoperative analgesia, and for obstetrical analgesia during labor and delivery.

CONTRAINDICATIONS

NUBAIN should not be administered to patients who are hypersensitive to nalbuphine hydrochloride, or to any of the other ingredients in NUBAIN.

WARNINGS

NUBAIN should be administered as a supplement to general anesthesia only by persons specifically trained in the use of intravenous anesthetics and management of the respiratory effects of potent opioids.

Naloxone, resuscitative and intubation equipment and oxygen should be readily available.

Drug Abuse Caution should be observed in prescribing NUBAIN for emotionally unstable patients, or for individuals with a history of narcotic abuse. Such patients should be closely supervised when long-term therapy is contemplated (see **DRUG ABUSE AND DEPENDENCE**).

Use in Ambulatory Patients NUBAIN may impair the mental or physical abilities required for the performance of potentially dangerous tasks such as driving a car or operating machinery. Therefore, NUBAIN should be administered with caution to ambulatory patients who should be warned to avoid such hazards.

Use in Emergency Procedures Maintain patient under observation until recovered from NUBAIN effects that would affect driving or other potentially dangerous tasks.

Use in Pregnancy (other than labor) Safe use of NUBAIN in pregnancy has not been established. Although animal reproductive studies have not revealed teratogenic or embryotoxic effects, nalbuphine should be administered to pregnant women only if clearly needed.

Use During Labor and Delivery The placental transfer of nalbuphine is high, rapid, and variable with a maternal to fetal ratio ranging from 1:0.37 to 1:1.6. Fetal and neonatal adverse effects that have been reported following the administration of nalbuphine to the mother during labor include fetal bradycardia, respiratory depression at birth, apnea, cyanosis and hypotonia. Maternal administration of naloxone during labor has normalized these effects in some cases. Severe and prolonged fetal bradycardia has been reported. Permanent neurological damage attributed to fetal bradycardia has occurred. A sinusoidal fetal heart rate pattern associated with the use of nalbuphine has also been reported. NUBAIN should be used with caution in women during labor and delivery, and newborns should be monitored for respiratory depression, apnea, bradycardia, and arrhythmias if NUBAIN has been used.

Head Injury and Increased Intracranial Pressure The possible respiratory depressant effects and the potential of potent analgesics to elevate cerebrospinal fluid pressure (resulting from vasodilation following CO_2 retention) may be markedly exaggerated in the presence of head injury, intracranial lesions or a pre-existing increase in intracranial pressure. Furthermore, potent analgesics can produce effects which may obscure the clinical course of patients with head injuries. Therefore, NUBAIN should be used in these circumstances only when essential, and then should be administered with extreme caution.

Interaction With Other Central Nervous System Depressants Although NUBAIN possesses narcotic antagonist activity, there is evidence that in nondependent patients it will not antagonize a narcotic analgesic administered just before, concurrently, or just after an injection of NUBAIN. Therefore, patients receiving a narcotic analgesic, general anesthetics, phenothiazines, or other tranquilizers, sedatives, hypnotics, or other CNS depressants (including alcohol) concomitantly with NUBAIN may exhibit an additive effect. When such combined therapy is contemplated, the dose of one or both agents should be reduced.

PRECAUTIONS

General

Impaired Respiration At the usual adult dose of 10 mg/70 kg, NUBAIN causes some respiratory depression approximately equal to that produced by equal doses of morphine. However, in contrast to morphine, respiratory depression is not appreciably increased with higher doses of NUBAIN. Respiratory depression induced by NUBAIN can be reversed by NARCAN® (naloxone hydrochloride) when indicated. NUBAIN should be administered with caution at low doses to patients with impaired respiration (e.g., from other medication, uremia, bronchial asthma, severe infection, cyanosis, or respiratory obstructions).

Impaired Renal or Hepatic Function Because NUBAIN is metabolized in the liver and excreted by the kidneys, NUBAIN should be used with caution in patients with renal or liver dysfunction and administered in reduced amounts.

Myocardial Infarction As with all potent analgesics, NUBAIN should be used with caution in patients with myocardial infarction who have nausea or vomiting.

Biliary Tract Surgery As with all narcotic analgesics, NUBAIN should be used with caution in patients about to undergo surgery of the biliary tract since it may cause spasm of the sphincter of Oddi.

Cardiovascular System During evaluation of NUBAIN in anesthesia, a higher incidence of bradycardia has been reported in patients who did not receive atropine pre-operatively.

Information for Patients

Patients should be advised of the following information:

— NUBAIN is associated with sedation and may impair mental and physical abilities required for the perfor-

mance of potentially dangerous tasks such as driving a car or operating machinery.
— NUBAIN is to be used as prescribed by a physician. Dose or frequency should not be increased without first consulting with a physician since NUBAIN may cause psychological or physical dependence.
— The use of NUBAIN with other narcotics can cause signs and symptoms of withdrawal.
— Abrupt discontinuation of NUBAIN after prolonged usage may cause signs and symptoms of withdrawal.

Laboratory Tests
NUBAIN may interfere with enzymatic methods for the detection of opioids depending on the specificity/sensitivity of the test. Please consult the test manufacturer for specific details.

Carcinogenesis, Mutagenesis, Impairment of Fertility
No evidence of carcinogenicity was found in a 24-month carcinogenicity study in rats and an 18-month carcinogenicity study in mice at oral doses as high as the equivalent of approximately three times the maximum recommended therapeutic dose.
No evidence of a mutagenic/genotoxic potential to NUBAIN was found in the Ames, Chinese Hamster Ovary HGPRT, and Sister Chromatid Exchange, mouse micronucleus, and rat bone marrow cytogenicity assays. Nalbuphine induced an increased frequency of mutation in mouse lymphoma cells.

Usage in Pregnancy
Teratogenic Effects
Pregnancy Category B—Reproduction studies have been performed in rabbits and in rats at dosages as high as approximately 14 and 31 times respectively the maximum recommended daily dose and revealed no evidence of impaired fertility or harm to the fetus due to NUBAIN. There are, however, no adequate and well-controlled studies in pregnant women. Because animal reproduction studies are not always predictive of human response, this drug should be used during pregnancy only if clearly needed (see **WARNINGS**).

Non-teratogenic Effects
Neonatal body weight and survival was reduced when NUBAIN was subcutaneously administered to female rats prior to mating and throughout gestation and lactation or to pregnant rats during the last third of gestation and throughout lactation at doses approximately 8 to 17 times the maximum recommended therapeutic dose. The clinical significance of this effect is unknown.

Use During Labor and Delivery
See **WARNINGS**.

Nursing Mothers
Limited data suggest that NUBAIN (nalbuphine hydrochloride) is excreted in maternal milk but only in a small amount (less than 1% of the administered dose) and with a clinically insignificant effect. Caution should be exercised when NUBAIN is administered to a nursing woman.

Pediatric Use
Safety and effectiveness in pediatric patients below the age of 18 years have not been established.

ADVERSE REACTIONS

The most frequent adverse reaction in 1066 patients treated in clinical studies with NUBAIN was sedation 381 (36%).
Less frequent reactions were: sweaty/clammy 99 (9%), nausea/vomiting 68 (6%), dizziness/vertigo 58 (5%), dry mouth 44 (4%), and headache 27 (3%).
Other adverse reactions which occurred (reported incidence of 1% or less) were:
CNS Effects Nervousness, depression, restlessness, crying, euphoria, floating, hostility, unusual dreams, confusion, faintness, hallucinations, dysphoria, feeling of heaviness, numbness, tingling, unreality. The incidence of psychotomimetic effects, such as unreality, depersonalization, delusions, dysphoria and hallucinations has been shown to be less than that which occurs with pentazocine.
Cardiovascular Hypertension, hypotension, bradycardia, tachycardia.
Gastrointestinal Cramps, dyspepsia, bitter taste.
Respiratory Depression, dyspnea, asthma.
Dermatologic Itching, burning, urticaria.
Miscellaneous Speech difficulty, urinary urgency, blurred vision, flushing and warmth.
Allergic Reactions Anaphylactic/anaphylactoid and other serious hypersensitivity reactions have been reported following the use of nalbuphine and may require immediate, supportive medical treatment. These reactions may include shock, respiratory distress, respiratory arrest, bradycardia, cardiac arrest, hypotension, or laryngeal edema. Other allergic-type reactions reported include stridor, bronchospasm, wheezing, edema, rash, pruritus, nausea, vomiting, diaphoresis, weakness, and shakiness.
Post-marketing Other reports include pulmonary edema, agitation and injection site reactions such as pain, swelling, redness, burning, and hot sensations.

DRUG ABUSE AND DEPENDENCE

NUBAIN has been shown to have a low abuse potential. When compared with drugs which are not mixed agonist-antagonists, it has been reported that nalbuphine's potential for abuse would be less than that of codeine and propoxyphene. Drug abuse has been reported infrequently. Psychological and physical dependence and tolerance may follow the abuse or misuse of nalbuphine (see **WARNINGS**).
Care should be taken to avoid increases in dosage or frequency of administration which in susceptible individuals might result in physical dependence.
Abrupt discontinuation of NUBAIN following prolonged use has been followed by symptoms of narcotic withdrawal, i.e., abdominal cramps, nausea and vomiting, rhinorrhea, lacrimation, restlessness, anxiety, elevated temperature and piloerection.

OVERDOSAGE

The immediate intravenous administration of NARCAN® (naloxone hydrochloride) is a specific antidote. Oxygen, intravenous fluids, vasopressors and other supportive measures should be used as indicated.
The administration of single doses of 72 mg of NUBAIN subcutaneously to eight normal subjects has been reported to have resulted primarily in symptoms of sleepiness and mild dysphoria.

DOSAGE AND ADMINISTRATION

The usual recommended adult dose is 10 mg for a 70 kg individual, administered subcutaneously, intramuscularly or intravenously; this dose may be repeated every 3 to 6 hours as necessary. Dosage should be adjusted according to the severity of the pain, physical status of the patient, and other medications which the patient may be receiving. (See **Interaction with Other Central Nervous System Depressants** under **WARNINGS**). In non-tolerant individuals, the recommended single maximum dose is 20 mg, with a maximum total daily dose of 160 mg.
The use of NUBAIN as a supplement to balanced anesthesia requires larger doses than those recommended for analgesia. Induction doses of NUBAIN range from 0.3 mg/kg to 3 mg/kg intravenously to be administered over a 10 to 15 minute period with maintenance doses of 0.25 to 0.5 mg/kg in single intravenous administrations as required. The use of NUBAIN may be followed by respiratory depression which can be reversed with the narcotic antagonist NARCAN® (naloxone hydrochloride).
NUBAIN is physically incompatible with nafcillin and ketorolac.
Patients Dependent on Narcotics Patients who have been taking narcotics chronically may experience withdrawal symptoms upon the administration of NUBAIN. If unduly troublesome, narcotic withdrawal symptoms can be controlled by the slow intravenous administration of small increments of morphine, until relief occurs. If the previous analgesic was morphine, meperidine, codeine, or other narcotic with similar duration of activity, one-fourth of the anticipated dose of NUBAIN can be administered initially and the patient observed for signs of withdrawal, i.e., abdominal cramps, nausea and vomiting, lacrimation, rhinorrhea, anxiety, restlessness, elevation of temperature or piloerection. If untoward symptoms do not occur, progressively larger doses may be tried at appropriate intervals until the desired level of analgesia is obtained with NUBAIN.

HOW SUPPLIED

NUBAIN® (nalbuphine hydrochloride) injection for intramuscular, subcutaneous, or intravenous use is a sterile solution available in:
NDC 63481-508-05 (sulfite-free) 10 mg/mL, 10 mL multiple dose vials (box of 1)
NDC 63481-432-10 (sulfite/paraben-free) 10 mg/mL, 1 mL ampuls (box of 10)
NDC 63481-509-05 (sulfite-free) 20 mg/mL, 10 mL multiple dose vials (box of 1)
NDC 63481-433-10 (sulfite/paraben-free) 20 mg/mL, 1 mL ampuls (box of 10)
Store at controlled room temperature 15°–30°C (59°–86°F). Protect from excessive light. Store in carton until contents have been used.
Parenteral drug products should be inspected visually for particulate matter and discoloration prior to administration whenever solution and container permit.
NUBAIN® is a Registered Trademark of Endo Pharmaceuticals Inc.
NARCAN® is a Registered Trademark of Endo Pharmaceuticals Inc.

6494-01/Rev. April, 1999

NUMORPHAN® Ⓒ ℞

[nū-mor 'fan]
(Oxymorphone Hydrochloride Injection, USP)
(Oxymorphone Hydrochloride Suppositories, USP)
Opioid Analgesic
℞ only

DESCRIPTION

NUMORPHAN (oxymorphone hydrochloride, USP), a semi-synthetic opioid substitute for morphine, is a potent analgesic.
[See chemical structure at top of next column]
Oxymorphone hydrochloride is a white or slightly off-white, odorless powder, which is sparingly soluble in alcohol and ether, but freely soluble in water. The molecular weight of oxymorphone hydrochloride is 337.80. The pK_{a1} and pK_{a2} of oxymorphone at 37°C are 8.17 and 9.54, respectively. The octanol/aqueous partition coefficient at 37°C and pH 7.4 is 0.98.
NUMORPHAN Injection is available in two concentrations, 1 mg/mL, 1 mL ampul and 1.5 mg/mL, 10 mL vial of oxy-

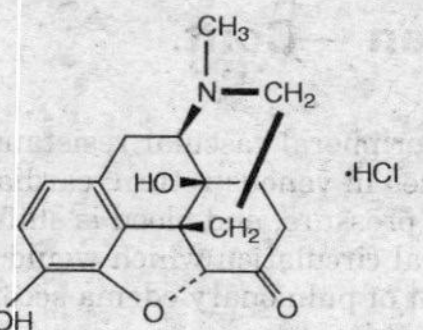

4,5α -Epoxy-3, 14-dihydroxy-17-methylmorphinan-6-one hydrochloride

morphone hydrochloride. In addition, each 1 mg/mL ampul contains 8.0 mg/mL sodium chloride. Each 1.5 mg/mL vial contains 8.0 mg/mL sodium chloride, 1.8 mg/mL methylparaben and 0.2 mg/mL propylparaben. pH for both the ampul and vial is adjusted with hydrochloric acid.
The NUMORPHAN Rectal Suppository is available in a concentration of 5 mg of oxymorphone hydrochloride in a base consisting of polyethylene glycol 1000 and polyethylene glycol 3350.

CLINICAL PHARMACOLOGY

NUMORPHAN is a potent opioid analgesic. Administered parenterally, 1 mg of NUMORPHAN is approximately equivalent in analgesic activity to 10 mg of morphine sulfate.
Many of the effects described below are common to the class of opioid analgesics, including NUMORPHAN.
Central Nervous System (CNS): Opioid analgesics exert their principal pharmacologic effects on the CNS and the gastrointestinal tract. The principal actions of therapeutic value are analgesia and sedation. The precise mechanism of the analgesic action is unknown. However, specific CNS opiate receptors have been identified and likely play a role in the expression of analgesic effects.
Opioids produce respiratory depression by direct action on brain stem respiratory centers. The mechanism of respiratory depression involves a reduction in the responsiveness of the brain stem respiratory centers to increases in carbon dioxide tension and to electrical stimulation. Opioids depress the cough reflex by direct action on the cough center in the medulla. Opioids cause miosis. Pinpoint pupils are a common sign of opioid overdose but are not pathognomonic. Marked mydriasis may be seen with worsening hypoxia.
Gastrointestinal Tract and Other Smooth Muscle: Opioids decrease gastric, biliary, and pancreatic secretions. These drugs cause a reduction in motility associated with an increase in tone in the antrum of the stomach and duodenum. Digestion of food in the small intestine is delayed and propulsive contractions are decreased. Propulsive peristaltic waves in the colon are decreased while tone is increased to the point of spasm. The end result is constipation. Opioids can cause a marked increase in biliary tract pressure as a result of spasm of the sphincter of Oddi.
Opioids increase smooth muscle tone in the urinary tract and can induce spasms. Urinary urgency and difficulty with urination may result. These effects, in conjunction with the central effect of these drugs on release of vasopressin, may produce oliguria.

Pharmacokinetics
The onset of action of parenterally administered NUMORPHAN is rapid; initial effects are usually perceived within 5 to 10 minutes. Its duration of action is approximately 3 to 6 hours.
Distribution: After an IV dose, the steady state volume of distribution was 3.08 ± 1.14 L/kg in healthy male and female subjects.
Metabolism: Oxymorphone undergoes extensive hepatic metabolism in humans. After a 10 mg oral dose, 49% was excreted over a five-day period in the urine. Of this, 82% was excreted in the first 24 hours after administration. The recovered drug-related products contained the oxymorphone (1.9%), the conjugate of oxymorphone (44.1%), the 6β-carbinol produced by 6-keto reduction of oxymorphone (0.3%), and the conjugates of 6β-carbinol (2.6%) and 6α-carbinol (0.1%).
Elimination: In healthy subjects, the mean terminal half-life of oxymorphone was 1.3 ± 0.7 hours. The mean systemic clearance was 2.0 ± 0.5 L/min.

INDICATIONS AND USAGE

NUMORPHAN Suppository is indicated for the relief of moderate to severe pain.
NUMORPHAN Injection is indicated for the relief of moderate to severe pain. It is also indicated for preoperative medication, for support of anesthesia, for obstetrical analgesia, and for relief of anxiety in patients with dyspnea associated with pulmonary edema secondary to acute left ventricular dysfunction.

CONTRAINDICATIONS

NUMORPHAN should not be administered to patients who are hypersensitive to oxymorphone hydrochloride or to any of the other ingredients in NUMORPHAN, or hypersensitive to morphine analogs.
NUMORPHAN should not be administered to individuals during an acute asthmatic attack or to patients with severe respiratory depression, upper airway obstruction, or any patient who has or is suspected of having a paralytic ileus.
NUMORPHAN should not be used in the treatment of pulmonary edema secondary to a chemical respiratory irritant.
Opioid analgesics cause pooling of blood in the extremities

Continued on next page

Numorphan —Cont.

by decreasing peripheral vascular resistance. This effect results in decreases in venous return, cardiac work, and pulmonary venous pressure, and blood is shifted from the central to peripheral circulation which would not be beneficial in the treatment of pulmonary edema secondary to a chemical respiratory irritant.

WARNINGS

Interactions with Other Central Nervous System Depressants: Patients receiving other opioid analgesics, general anesthetics, phenothiazines, other tranquilizers, sedatives, hypnotics or other CNS depressants (including alcohol) concomitantly with NUMORPHAN may exhibit an additive CNS depression (See PRECAUTIONS; Drug Interactions).

Respiratory Depression: NUMORPHAN should be administered with extreme caution to patients with conditions accompanied by hypoxia, hypercapnia or decreased respiratory reserve such as: asthma, chronic obstructive pulmonary disease or cor pulmonale, severe obesity, sleep apnea syndrome, myxedema, kyphoscoliosis, CNS depression or coma.

Head Injury and Increased Intracranial Pressure: The possible respiratory depressant effects of potent analgesics and their potential to elevate cerebrospinal fluid pressure (resulting from vasodilation following CO_2 retention) may be markedly exaggerated in the presence of head injury, intracranial lesions or a preexisting increase in intracranial pressure. Furthermore, potent analgesics can produce effects which may obscure the clinical course of patients with head injuries. Therefore, NUMORPHAN should be used in these circumstances only when essential, and then should be administered with extreme caution.

Acute Abdominal Conditions: The administration of opioids may obscure the diagnosis or clinical course of patients with acute abdominal conditions.

Drug Dependence: NUMORPHAN, as with other opioid drugs, can produce tolerance, psychological dependence, and physical dependence and has the potential for being abused (See DRUG ABUSE AND DEPENDENCE).

Pregnancy: Safe use in pregnancy has not been established (relative to possible adverse effects on fetal development). As with other analgesics, the use of NUMORPHAN in pregnancy, in nursing mothers, or in women of child-bearing potential requires that the possible benefits of the drug be weighed against the possible hazards to the mother and the child (See PRECAUTIONS).

PRECAUTIONS

General

Special Risk Patients: NUMORPHAN should be used with caution in elderly and debilitated patients and in patients who are known to be sensitive to central nervous system depressants, such as those with cardiovascular, pulmonary, renal or hepatic disease. Caution should also be exercised in patients with hypothyroidism, acute alcoholism, delirium tremens, convulsive disorders, Addison's disease, gallbladder disease or gallstones, prostatic hypertrophy or urethral stricture, recent gastrointestinal or genitourinary tract surgery, inflammatory bowel disease, diarrhea secondary to poisoning until the toxin is eliminated, diarrhea secondary to pseudomembranous colitis, cardiac arrhythmias, increased ocular pressure, and toxic psychosis. Debilitated and elderly patients and those with severe liver disease should receive smaller doses of NUMORPHAN.

Hypotensive Effect: Opioid analgesics may cause severe hypotension in patients whose ability to maintain blood pressure has been compromised by a depleted blood volume or coadministration of drugs such as phenothiazines or general anesthetics. Administer with caution to patients in circulatory shock, since vasodilatation produced by the drug may further reduce cardiac output and blood pressure. Orthostatic hypotension may occur in ambulatory patients.

Information for Patients

Patients should be cautioned regarding the following:

Drowsiness, dizziness, or lightheadedness related to the use of this medication may impair mental and/or physical abilities required for the performance of potentially hazardous tasks, such as driving a car, operating machinery, etc.

This medication, like other opioid analgesics, will add to the effect of alcohol and other CNS depressants [such as antihistamines, sedatives, hypnotics, tranquilizers, general anesthetics, phenothiazines, other opioids, tricyclic antidepressants, and monoamine oxidase (MAO) inhibitors]. Alcohol should not be consumed while taking NUMORPHAN.

Withdrawal side effects may be precipitated by suddenly stopping this drug after prolonged use (regular use for several weeks or more). The medication should be gradually reduced before completely discontinuing use.

Elderly patients are more sensitive to opioid analgesics, especially the respiratory depressant effects and opioid induced urinary retention. Lower doses or longer dosing intervals may be required.

Orthostatic hypotension may occur with the use of this medication, especially in ambulatory patients. Patients should get up slowly from a lying or sitting position.

NUMORPHAN may be habit forming and has the potential for being abused. Tolerance, psychological and physical dependence can occur.

Safe use in pregnancy has not been established. Prolonged use of opioid analgesics during pregnancy may cause fetal-neonatal physical dependence, and neonatal withdrawal may occur.

Laboratory Tests

Opioids may increase biliary tract pressure with resultant increases in plasma amylase or lipase.

Drug Interactions

The concomitant use of other CNS depressants including sedatives, hypnotics, tranquilizers, general anesthetics, phenothiazines, other opioids, tricyclic antidepressants, monoamine oxidase (MAO) inhibitors, and alcohol may produce additive CNS depressant effects. When such combined therapy is contemplated, the dose of one or both agents should be reduced (See WARNINGS).

Anticholinergics or other medications with anticholinergic activity when used concurrently with opioid analgesics may result in increased risk of urinary retention and/or severe constipation, which may lead to paralytic ileus.

It has been reported that the incidence of bradycardia was increased when oxymorphone was combined with propofol for induction of anesthesia.

In addition, CNS toxicity has been reported (confusion, disorientation, respiratory depression, apnea, seizures) following coadministration of cimetidine with opioid analgesics; no clear-cut cause and effect relationship was established.

Carcinogenesis, Mutagenesis, Impairment of Fertility

Long-term studies have not been performed in animals to evaluate the carcinogenic potential of NUMORPHAN (oxymorphone hydrochloride, USP). Studies to evaluate the mutagenic potential of NUMORPHAN have not been conducted. There have been no studies to evaluate the effect of NUMORPHAN on fertility.

Usage in Pregnancy

Teratogenic Effects

Pregnancy Category C—NUMORPHAN was reported to produce malformations in offspring of hamsters that received 1,500 times the recommended dose on Day 8 of gestation. There have been no adequate and well-controlled studies of reproductive toxicity in other laboratory animals or in pregnant women. It is not known whether NUMORPHAN can cause fetal harm when administered to a pregnant woman or can affect reproductive capacity. As with other opioid analgesics, the use of NUMORPHAN in pregnancy or in women of child-bearing potential requires that the possible benefits of the drug be weighed against the possible hazards to the mother and the child.

Non-teratogenic Effects—Prolonged use of opioid analgesics during pregnancy may cause fetal-neonatal physical dependence. Neonatal withdrawal may occur. Symptoms usually appear during the first days of life and may include convulsions, irritability, excessive crying, tremors, hyperactive reflexes, fever, vomiting, diarrhea, sneezing, yawning, and increased respiratory rate.

Labor and Delivery

NUMORPHAN should be used with caution during labor. Sinusoidal fetal heart rate patterns may occur with the use of opioid analgesics.

Opioid analgesics in therapeutic doses may prolong labor. Generally, the effect of opioids on the pregnant uterus appears to depend on the time of administration; administration of the drugs during the latent phase of the first stage of labor, or before cervical dilation of 4–5 cm has occurred, may hamper the progress of labor.

Opioid analgesics, including NUMORPHAN, may cause respiratory depression in the newborn. The effect of NUMORPHAN, if any, on the later growth, development, and functional maturation of the child is unknown.

Nursing Mothers

It is not known whether NUMORPHAN is excreted in human milk. Because many drugs, including some opioids, are excreted in human milk, caution should be exercised when NUMORPHAN is administered to a nursing woman.

Pediatric Use

Safety and effectiveness of NUMORPHAN in pediatric patients below the age of 18 years have not been established.

ADVERSE REACTIONS

As with all potent opioid analgesics, possible side effects when using NUMORPHAN include:

Central Nervous System: Drowsiness, sedation, lightheadedness, unusual tiredness or weakness, headache, dysphoria, euphoria, miosis, diplopia, blurred vision, nervousness, restlessness, confusion, mental clouding, trouble sleeping, paradoxical CNS stimulation, hallucinations, mental depression.

Gastrointestinal System: Nausea, vomiting, dry mouth, constipation, biliary tract spasm, cramps or pain, loss of appetite, paralytic ileus or toxic megacolon in patients with inflammatory bowel disease.

Cardiovascular System: Hypotension, orthostatic hypotension particularly in ambulatory patients, tachycardia, bradycardia, palpitations, flushing.

Respiratory System: Respiratory depression, atelectasis, allergic bronchospastic reaction, allergic laryngeal edema, allergic laryngospasm.

Genitourinary System: Ureteral spasm, urinary hesitancy or retention, antidiuretic effect.

Dermatologic: Itching, sweating, injection site reaction, allergic reaction (such as skin rash, hives, and/or itching, swelling of the face).

DRUG ABUSE AND DEPENDENCE

NUMORPHAN is a Schedule II opioid and is subject to the Federal Controlled Substances Act.

NUMORPHAN, as with other opioid drugs, can produce tolerance, psychological dependence, and physical dependence and has the potential for being abused. The addiction potential of the drug appears to be about the same as for morphine.

Withdrawal symptoms may occur when opioids are abruptly discontinued after prolonged use. Withdrawal symptoms may be characterized by some or all of the following: restlessness, lacrimation, rhinorrhea, yawning, perspiration, gooseflesh, restless sleep, and mydriasis during the first 24 hours. These symptoms often increase in severity and over the next 72 hours may be accompanied by increasing irritability, anxiety, weakness, twitching, and spasms of muscles; kicking movements; severe backaches; abdominal and leg pains; abdominal and muscle cramps; hot and cold flashes; insomnia; nausea, anorexia, vomiting, intestinal spasm, diarrhea, coryza, and repetitive sneezing; increase in body temperature, blood pressure, respiratory rate and heart rate. Because of excessive loss of fluids through sweating, vomiting and diarrhea, there is usually marked weight loss, dehydration, ketosis, and disturbances in acid-base balance. Cardiovascular collapse can occur. Without treatment most observable symptoms disappear in 5–14 days; however, there appears to be a phase of secondary or chronic abstinence which may last for 2–6 months characterized by decreasing insomnia, irritability, and muscular aches. In addition, the patient may have miosis and a slight lowering of blood pressure, pulse rate, and body temperature; respiratory centers exhibit a decreased response to the stimulatory effects of carbon dioxide.

The dose of NUMORPHAN should be gradually reduced before discontinuation in those patients who require treatment for physical dependence.

Infants born to mothers physically dependent on opioids will also be physically dependent and may exhibit respiratory difficulties and withdrawal symptoms (See PRECAUTIONS; Usage in Pregnancy).

OVERDOSAGE

Signs and Symptons: Serious overdosage with NUMORPHAN is characterized by respiratory depression, (a decrease in respiratory rate and/or tidal volume, Cheyne-Stokes respiration, cyanosis), extreme somnolence progressing to stupor or coma, skeletal muscle flaccidity, cold and clammy skin, and sometimes bradycardia and hypotension. In severe overdosage, apnea, circulatory collapse, cardiac arrest and death may occur.

Treatment: Primary attention should be given to the reestablishment of adequate respiratory exchange through provision of a patent airway and the institution of assisted or controlled ventilation. The opioid antagonist naloxone hydrochloride (NARCAN®) is a specific antidote against respiratory depression which may result from overdosage or unusual sensitivity to opioids including oxymorphone. Therefore, an appropriate dose of naloxone hydrochloride should be administered (usual initial adult dose 0.4 mg–2 mg) preferably by the intravenous route and simultaneously with efforts at respiratory resuscitation. Since the duration of action of oxymorphone may exceed that of the antagonist, the patient should be kept under continued surveillance and repeated doses of the antagonist should be administered as needed to maintain adequate respiration.

Naloxone hydrochloride should not be administered in the absence of clinically significant respiratory or cardiovascular depression. In addition, it should be considered that the use of an opioid antagonist in patients physically dependent on opioids may precipitate an acute withdrawal syndrome that cannot be readily suppressed while the action of the antagonist persists. If respiratory depression is associated with muscular rigidity, administration of a neuromuscular blocking agent may be necessary to facilitate assisted or controlled ventilation. Muscular rigidity may also respond to opioid antagonist therapy.

Oxygen, intravenous fluids, vasopressors and other supportive measures should be employed as indicated.

DOSAGE AND ADMINISTRATION

Smaller doses of NUMORPHAN than those recommended below should be used for debilitated and elderly patients and those with severe liver disease.

Usual Adult Dosage of NUMORPHAN Injection: Subcutaneous or intramuscular administration: initially 1 mg to 1.5 mg, repeated every 4 to 6 hours as needed. Intravenous: 0.5 mg initially. In nondebilitated patients the dose can be cautiously increased until satisfactory pain relief is obtained. For analgesia during labor 0.5 mg to 1 mg intramuscularly is recommended.

Parenteral drug products should be inspected visually for particulate matter and discoloration prior to administration whenever solution and container permit.

Usual Adult Dosage of NUMORPHAN Rectal Suppositories: One suppository, 5 mg, every 4 to 6 hours. In nondebilitated patients the dose can be cautiously increased until satisfactory pain relief is obtained.

HOW SUPPLIED

For Injection: DEA Order Form Required

1 mg/mL 1 mL ampuls (paraben/sodium dithionite-free) (box of 10) NDC 63481-444-10

1.5 mg/mL 10 mL multiple dose vials (sodium dithionite-free) (box of 1) NDC 63481-445-01

Store at 25°C (77°F); excursions permitted to 15°–30°C (59°–86°F). [See USP Controlled Room Temperature].

Protect from light.

For Rectal Suppositories: DEA Order Form Required

5 mg Wrapped in gold foil (box of 6) NDC 63481-761-06

Store under refrigeration 2°–8°C (36°–46°F).

NUMORPHAN® is a Registered Trademark of Endo Pharmaceuticals Inc.

NARCAN® is a Registered Trademark of Endo Pharmaceuticals Inc.

6477-01/Rev. September, 1999

PERCOCET® Ⓒ℞
(Oxycodone HCl and Acetaminophen Tablets, USP)
2.5/325mg • 5/325mg • 7.5/500mg • 10/650mg
Rx only

DESCRIPTION

Each tablet, for oral administration, contains oxycodone hydrochloride and acetaminophen in the following strengths:

Oxycodone Hydrochloride	2.5 mg*
Acetaminophen, USP	325 mg
Oxycodone Hydrochloride	5 mg*
Acetaminophen, USP	325 mg
Oxycodone Hydrochloride	7.5 mg*
Acetaminophen, USP	500 mg
Oxycodone Hydrochloride	10 mg*
Acetaminophen, USP	650 mg

*2.5 mg oxycodone HCl is equivalent to 2.2409 mg of oxycodone.
5 mg oxycodone HCl is equivalent to 4.4815 mg of oxycodone.
7.5 mg oxycodone HCl is equivalent to 6.7228 mg of oxycodone.
10 mg oxycodone HCl is equivalent to 8.9637 mg of oxycodone.

All strengths of PERCOCET also contain the following inactive ingredients: Colloidal silicon dioxide, croscarmellose sodium, crospovidone, microcrystalline cellulose, povidone, pregelatinized starch, and stearic acid. In addition, the 2.5 mg/325 mg strength contains FD&C Red No. 40 Aluminum Lake, the 5 mg/325 mg strength contains FD&C Blue No. 1 Aluminum Lake, the 7.5 mg/500 mg strength contains FD&C Yellow No. 6 Aluminum Lake and the 10 mg/650 mg strength contains D&C Yellow No. 10 Aluminum Lake.
Acetaminophen, 4′-hydroxyacetanilide, is a non-opiate, non-salicylate analgesic and antipyretic which occurs as a white, odorless, crystalline powder, possessing a slightly bitter taste. The molecular formula for acetaminophen is $C_8H_9NO_2$ and the molecular weight is 151.17. It may be represented by the following structural formula:

CH_3CONH — OH

Oxycodone, 14-hydroxydihydrocodeinone, is a semisynthetic pure opioid agonist which occurs as a white, odorless, crystalline powder having a saline, bitter taste. The molecular formula for oxycodone hydrochloride is $C_{18}H_{21}NO_4$•HCl and the molecular weight 351.83. It is derived from the opium alkaloid thebaine, and may be represented by the following structural formula:

CH_3 N HO CH_3O O O

CLINICAL PHARMACOLOGY

The principal ingredient, oxycodone, is a semisynthetic opioid analgesic with multiple actions qualitatively similar to those of morphine; the most prominent involves the central nervous system and organs composed of smooth muscle. The principal actions of therapeutic value of the oxycodone in PERCOCET are analgesia and sedation.
Oxycodone is similar to codeine and methadone in that it retains at least one-half of its analgesic activity when administered orally.
Acetaminophen is a non-opiate, non-salicylate analgesic and antipyretic.

INDICATIONS AND USAGE

PERCOCET (Oxycodone HCl and Acetaminophen Tablets, USP) is indicated for the relief of moderate to moderately severe pain.

CONTRAINDICATIONS

PERCOCET should not be administered to patients who are hypersensitive to oxycodone, acetaminophen, or any other components of this product.

WARNINGS

Drug Dependence: Oxycodone can produce drug dependence of the morphine type and, therefore, has the potential for being abused. Psychic dependence, physical dependence and tolerance may develop upon repeated administration of PERCOCET, and it should be prescribed and administered with the same degree of caution appropriate to the use of other oral opioid-containing medications. Like other opioid-containing medications, PERCOCET is subject to the Federal Controlled Substances Act (Schedule II).

PRECAUTIONS

General
Head Injury and Increased Intracranial Pressure: The respiratory depressant effects of opioids and their capacity to elevate cerebrospinal fluid pressure may be markedly exaggerated in the presence of head injury, other intracranial lesions or a pre-existing increase in intracranial pressure. Furthermore, opioids produce adverse reactions which may obscure the clinical course of patients with head injuries.
Acute Abdominal Conditions: The administration of PERCOCET or other opioids may obscure the diagnosis or clinical course in patients with acute abdominal conditions.
Special Risk Patients: PERCOCET should be given with caution to certain patients such as the elderly or debilitated, and those with severe impairment of hepatic or renal function, hypothyroidism, Addison's disease, and prostatic hypertrophy or urethral stricture.
Information for Patients
Oxycodone may impair the mental and/or physical abilities required for the performance of potentially hazardous tasks such as driving a car or operating machinery. The patient using PERCOCET should be cautioned accordingly.
Drug Interactions
Patients receiving other opioid analgesics, general anesthetics, phenothiazines, other tranquilizers, sedative-hypnotics or other CNS depressants (including alcohol) concomitantly with PERCOCET may exhibit an additive CNS depression. When such combined therapy is contemplated, the dose of one or both agents should be reduced.
The use of MAO inhibitors or tricyclic antidepressants with oxycodone preparations may increase the effect of either the antidepressant or oxycodone.
The concurrent use of anticholinergics with opioids may produce paralytic ileus.
Usage in Pregnancy
Teratogenic Effects; Pregnancy Category C: Animal reproductive studies have not been conducted with PERCOCET. It is also not known whether PERCOCET can cause fetal harm when administered to a pregnant woman or can affect reproductive capacity. PERCOCET should not be given to a pregnant woman unless in the judgment of the physician, the potential benefits outweigh the possible hazards.
Nonteratogenic Effects: Use of opioids during pregnancy may produce physical dependence in the neonate.
Labor and Delivery: As with all opioids, administration of PERCOCET to the mother shortly before delivery may result in some degree of respiratory depression in the newborn and the mother, especially if higher doses are used.
Nursing Mothers
It is not known whether PERCOCET is excreted in human milk. Because many drugs are excreted in human milk, caution should be exercised when PERCOCET is administered to a nursing woman.
Pediatric Use
Safety and effectiveness in pediatric patients have not been established.

ADVERSE REACTIONS

The most frequently observed adverse reactions include lightheadedness, dizziness, sedation, nausea and vomiting. These effects seem to be more prominent in ambulatory than in nonambulatory patients, and some of these adverse reactions may be alleviated if the patient lies down.
Other adverse reactions include euphoria, dysphoria, constipation, skin rash and pruritus. At higher doses, oxycodone has most of the disadvantages of morphine including respiratory depression.

DRUG ABUSE AND DEPENDENCE

PERCOCET (Oxycodone HCl and Acetaminophen Tablets, USP) is a Schedule II controlled substance.
Oxycodone can produce drug dependence and has the potential for being abused (See WARNINGS).

OVERDOSAGE

Acetaminophen
Signs and Symptoms: In acute acetaminophen overdosage, dose-dependent, potentially fatal hepatic necrosis is the most serious adverse effect. Renal tubular necrosis, hypoglycemic coma and thrombocytopenia may also occur.
In adults, hepatic toxicity has rarely been reported with acute overdoses of less than 10 grams and fatalities with less than 15 grams. Importantly, young children seem to be more resistant than adults to the hepatotoxic effect of an acetaminophen overdose. Despite this, the measures outlined below should be initiated in any adult or child suspected of having ingested an acetaminophen overdose.
Early symptoms following a potentially hepatotoxic overdose may include: nausea, vomiting, diaphoresis and general malaise. Clinical and laboratory evidence of hepatic toxicity may not be apparent until 48 to 72 hours post-ingestion.
Treatment: The stomach should be emptied promptly by lavage or by induction of emesis with syrup of ipecac. Patient's estimates of the quantity of a drug ingested are notoriously unreliable. Therefore, if an acetaminophen overdose is suspected, a serum acetaminophen assay should be obtained as early as possible, but no sooner than four hours following ingestion. Liver function studies should be obtained initially and repeated at 24-hour intervals.
The antidote, N-acetylcysteine, should be administered as early as possible, preferably within 16 hours of the overdose ingestion for optimal results, but in any case, within 24 hours. Following recovery, there are no residual, structural, or functional hepatic abnormalities.
Oxycodone
Signs and Symptoms: Serious overdosage with oxycodone is characterized by respiratory depression (a decrease in respiratory rate and/or tidal volume, Cheyne-Stokes respiration, cyanosis), extreme somnolence progressing to stupor or coma, skeletal muscle flaccidity, cold and clammy skin, and sometimes bradycardia and hypotension. In severe overdosage, apnea, circulatory collapse, cardiac arrest and death may occur.
Treatment: Primary attention should be given to the reestablishment of adequate respiratory exchange through provision of a patent airway and the institution of assisted or controlled ventilation. The opioid antagonist naloxone hydrochloride is a specific antidote against respiratory depression which may result from overdosage or unusual sensitivity to opioids, including oxycodone. Therefore, an appropriate dose of naloxone hydrochloride (usual initial adult dose 0.4 mg to 2 mg) should be administered preferably by the intravenous route, and simultaneously with efforts at respiratory resuscitation (see package insert). Since the duration of action of oxycodone may exceed that of the antagonist, the patient should be kept under continued surveillance and repeated doses of the antagonist should be administered as needed to maintain adequate respiration.
An antagonist should not be administered in the absence of clinically significant respiratory or cardiovascular depression. Oxygen, intravenous fluids, vasopressors and other supportive measures should be employed as indicated.
Gastric emptying may be useful in removing unabsorbed drug.

DOSAGE AND ADMINISTRATION

Dosage should be adjusted according to the severity of the pain and the response of the patient. It may occasionally be necessary to exceed the usual dosage recommended below in cases of more severe pain or in those patients who have become tolerant to the analgesic effect of opioids. PERCOCET is given orally.
Percocet 2.5 mg/325 mg
The usual adult dosage is one or two tablets every six hours. The total daily dose of acetaminophen should not exceed 4 grams.
Percocet 5 mg/325 mg; Percocet 7.5 mg/500 mg; Percocet 10 mg/650 mg
The usual adult dosage is one tablet every 6 hours as needed for pain. The total daily dose of acetaminophen should not exceed 4 grams.

Strength	Maximal Daily Dose
2.5 mg/325 mg	12 Tablets
5 mg/325 mg	12 Tablets
7.5 mg/500 mg	8 Tablets
10 mg/650 mg	6 Tablets

HOW SUPPLIED

PERCOCET (Oxycodone HCl and Acetaminophen Tablets, USP) is supplied as follows:
2.5 mg/325 mg
Pink oval tablet embossed with "PERCOCET" on one side and "2.5" on the other.

Bottles of 100	NDC 63481-627-70
Bottles of 500	NDC 63481-627-85
Unit dose package of 100 tablets	NDC 63481-627-75

5 mg/325 mg
Blue round tablet embossed with "PERCOCET" and "5" on one side and bisect on the other.

Bottles of 100	NDC 63481-623-70
Bottles of 500	NDC 63481-623-85
Unit dose package of 100 tablets	NDC 63481-623-75

7.5 mg/500 mg
Peach capsule-shaped tablet embossed with "PERCOCET" on one side and "7.5" on the other.

Bottles of 100	NDC 63481-621-70
Bottles of 500	NDC 63481-621-85
Unit dose package of 100 tablets	NDC 63481-621-75

10 mg/650 mg
Yellow oval tablet embossed with "PERCOCET" on one side and "10" on other.

Bottles of 100	NDC 63481-622-70
Bottles of 500	NDC 63481-622-85
Unit dose package of 100 tablets	NDC 63481-622-75

Store at controlled room temperature 15°–30°C (59°–86°F).
Dispense in a tight, light-resistant container as defined in the USP, with a child-resistant closure (as required).
DEA Order Form Required.

Manufactured for:
Endo Pharmaceuticals Inc.
Chadds Ford, Pennsylvania 19317

Manufactured by:
DuPont Pharma
Wilmington, Delaware 19880
PERCOCET® is a Registered Trademark of Endo Pharmaceuticals Inc.

PM-0062R/Rev. Jan., 2000

PERCODAN® Ⓒ℞
[*perk 'o-dan*]
(Oxycodone and Aspirin Tablets, USP)
Rx only

DESCRIPTION

Each tablet of PERCODAN contains:

Oxycodone Hydrochloride	4.50 mg*
Oxycodone Terephthalate	0.38 mg**
Aspirin, USP	325 mg

*4.50 mg oxycodone HCl is equivalent to 4.0338 mg of oxycodone.
**0.38 mg oxycodone terephthalate is equivalent to 0.3008 mg of oxycodone.

Continued on next page

Percodan—Cont.

PERCODAN Tablets also contain: D&C Yellow 10, FD&C Yellow 6, microcrystalline cellulose and starch.
The oxycodone component is 14-hydroxydihydrocodeinone, a white odorless crystalline powder which is derived from the opium alkaloid, thebaine, and may be represented by the following structural formula:

CH_3 N, HO, CH_3O, O, O

CLINICAL PHARMACOLOGY

The principal ingredient, oxycodone, is a semisynthetic opioid analgesic with multiple actions qualitatively similar to those of morphine; the most prominent of these involve the central nervous system and organs composed of smooth muscle. The principal actions of therapeutic value of the oxycodone in PERCODAN are analgesia and sedation.
Oxycodone is similar to codeine and methadone in that it retains at least one-half of its analgesic activity when administered orally.
PERCODAN also contains the non-opioid antipyretic-analgesic, aspirin.

INDICATIONS

For the relief of moderate to moderately severe pain.

CONTRAINDICATIONS

Hypersensitivity to oxycodone or aspirin.

WARNINGS

Drug Dependence: Oxycodone can produce drug dependence of the morphine type and, therefore, has the potential for being abused. Psychic dependence, physical dependence and tolerance may develop upon repeated administration of PERCODAN, and it should be prescribed and administered with the same degree of caution appropriate to the use of other oral opioid-containing medications. Like other opioid-containing medications, PERCODAN is subject to the Federal Controlled Substances Act.
Usage in Ambulatory Patients: Oxycodone may impair the mental and/or physical abilities required for the performance of potentially hazardous tasks such as driving a car or operating machinery. The patient using PERCODAN should be cautioned accordingly.
Interaction with Other Central Nervous System Depressants: Patients receiving other opioid analgesics, general anesthetics, phenothiazines, other tranquilizers, sedative-hypnotics or other CNS depressants (including alcohol) concomitantly with PERCODAN may exhibit an additive CNS depression. When such combined therapy is contemplated, the dose of one or both agents should be reduced.
Usage in Pregnancy: Safe use in pregnancy has not been established relative to possible adverse effects on fetal development. Therefore, PERCODAN should not be used in pregnant women unless, in the judgment of the physician, the potential benefits outweigh the possible hazards.
Pediatric Use: PERCODAN should not be administered to pediatric patients. PERCODAN®-Demi, containing half the amount of oxycodone, can be considered. (See product prescribing information for PERCODAN-Demi.)
Reye Syndrome is a rare but serious disease which can follow flu or chicken pox in children and teenagers. While the cause of Reye Syndrome is unknown, some reports claim aspirin (or salicylates) may increase the risk of developing this disease.
Salicylates should be used with caution in the presence of peptic ulcer or coagulation abnormalities.

PRECAUTIONS

Head Injury and Increased Intracranial Pressure: The respiratory depressant effects of opioids and their capacity to elevate cerebrospinal fluid pressure may be markedly exaggerated in the presence of head injury, other intracranial lesions or a pre-existing increase in intracranial pressure. Furthermore, opioids produce adverse reactions which may obscure the clinical course of patients with head injuries.
Acute Abdominal Conditions: The administration of PERCODAN or other opioids may obscure the diagnosis or clinical course in patients with acute abdominal conditions.
Special Risk Patients: PERCODAN should be given with caution to certain patients such as the elderly or debilitated, and those with severe impairment of hepatic or renal function, hypothyroidism, Addison's disease, and prostatic hypertrophy or urethral stricture.

ADVERSE REACTIONS

The most frequently observed adverse reactions include lightheadedness, dizziness, sedation, nausea and vomiting. These effects seem to be more prominent in ambulatory than in nonambulatory patients, and some of these adverse reactions may be alleviated if the patient lies down.
Other adverse reactions include euphoria, dysphoria, constipation and pruritus.

DRUG ABUSE AND DEPENDENCE

PERCODAN (oxycodone and aspirin) tablets are a Schedule II controlled substance. Oxycodone can produce drug dependence and has the potential for being abused (See WARNINGS).

DOSAGE AND ADMINISTRATION

Dosage should be adjusted according to the severity of the pain and the response of the patient. It may occasionally be necessary to exceed the usual dosage recommended below in cases of more severe pain or in those patients who have become tolerant to the analgesic effect of opioids. PERCODAN is given orally. The usual adult dosage is one tablet every 6 hours as needed for pain. The total daily dose of aspirin should not exceed 4 grams or 12 tablets.

DRUG INTERACTIONS

The CNS depressant effects of PERCODAN may be additive with that of other CNS depressants (See WARNINGS).
Aspirin may enhance the effect of anticoagulants and inhibit the uricosuric effects of uricosuric agents.

MANAGEMENT OF OVERDOSAGE

Signs and Symptoms: Serious overdose with PERCODAN is characterized by respiratory depression (a decrease in respiratory rate and/or tidal volume, Cheyne-Stokes respiration, cyanosis), extreme somnolence progressing to stupor or coma, skeletal muscle flaccidity, cold and clammy skin, and sometimes bradycardia and hypotension. In severe overdosage, apnea, circulatory collapse, cardiac arrest and death may occur. The ingestion of very large amounts of PERCODAN may, in addition, result in acute salicylate intoxication.
Treatment: Primary attention should be given to the reestablishment of adequate respiratory exchange through provision of a patent airway and the institution of assisted or controlled ventilation. The opioid antagonist naloxone hydrochloride (NARCAN®) is a specific antidote against respiratory depression which may result from overdosage or unusual sensitivity to opioids including oxycodone. Therefore, an appropriate dose of naloxone hydrochloride should be administered (usual initial adult dose 0.4 mg–2 mg) preferably by the intravenous route, simultaneously with efforts at respiratory resuscitation. Since the duration of action of oxycodone may exceed that of the antagonist, the patient should be kept under continued surveillance and repeated doses of the antagonist should be administered as needed to maintain adequate respiration.
Oxygen, intravenous fluids, vasopressors and other supportive measures should be employed as indicated.
Gastric emptying may be useful in removing unabsorbed drug.

HOW SUPPLIED

PERCODAN (4.50 mg oxycodone hydrochloride, 0.38 mg oxycodone terephthalate, 325 mg Aspirin, USP), supplied as a yellow tablet, with one face scored and inscribed "PERCODAN" and plain on the other side is available in:

Bottles of 100	NDC 63481-135-70
Bottles of 500	NDC 63481-135-85
Hospital blister pack of 25 (in units of 100 tablets)	NDC 63481-135-75

Store at 25°C (77°F); excursions permitted to 15°–30°C (59°–86°F). [See USP Controlled Room Temperature].
Dispense in a tight, light-resistant container as defined in the USP, with a child-resistant closure (as required).
DEA Order Form Required.
PERCODAN® is a Registered Trademark of Endo Pharmaceuticals Inc.
NARCAN® is a Registered Trademark of Endo Pharmaceuticals Inc.

6483-01/Rev. November, 1999
Shown in Product Identification Guide, page 312

PERCODAN®-DEMI Ⓒ℞
[*perk 'o-dan*]
(oxycodone and aspirin)

DESCRIPTION

Each tablet of PERCODAN-Demi contains:

Oxycodone hydrochloride	2.25 mg*
Oxycodone terephthalate	0.19 mg**
Aspirin, USP	325 mg

*2.25 mg oxycodone HCl is equivalent to 2.0169 mg of oxycodone.
**0.19 mg oxycodone terephthalate is equivalent to 0.1504 mg of oxycodone.

PERCODAN-Demi Tablets also contain: microcrystalline cellulose and starch.
The oxycodone component is 14-hydroxydihydrocodeinone, a white odorless crystalline powder which is derived from the opium alkaloid, thebaine, and may be represented by the following structural formula:

CH_3 N, HO, CH_3O, O, O

ACTIONS

The principal ingredient, oxycodone, is a semisynthetic narcotic analgesic with multiple actions qualitatively similar to those of morphine; the most prominent of these involve the central nervous system and organs composed of smooth muscle. The principal actions of therapeutic value of the oxycodone in PERCODAN-Demi are analgesia and sedation.
Oxycodone is similar to codeine and methadone in that it retains at least one half of its analgesic activity when administered orally.
PERCODAN-Demi also contains the non-narcotic antipyretic-analgesic, aspirin.

INDICATIONS

For the relief of moderate to moderately severe pain.

CONTRAINDICATIONS

Hypersensitivity to oxycodone or aspirin.

WARNINGS

Drug Dependence: Oxycodone can produce drug dependence of the morphine type and, therefore, has the potential for being abused. Psychic dependence, physical dependence and tolerance may develop upon repeated administration of PERCODAN-Demi, and it should be prescribed and administered with the same degree of caution appropriate to the use of other oral narcotic-containing medications. Like other narcotic-containing medications, PERCODAN-Demi is subject to the Federal Controlled Substances Act.
Usage in ambulatory patients: Oxycodone may impair the mental and/or physical abilities required for the performance of potentially hazardous tasks such as driving a car or operating machinery. The patient using PERCODAN-Demi should be cautioned accordingly.
Interaction with other central nervous system depressants: Patients receiving other narcotic analgesics, general anesthetics, phenothiazines, other tranquilizers, sedative-hypnotics or other CNS depressants (including alcohol) concomitantly with PERCODAN-Demi may exhibit an additive CNS depression. When such combined therapy is contemplated, the dose of one or both agents should be reduced.
Usage in pregnancy: Safe use in pregnancy has not been established relative to possible adverse effects on fetal development. Therefore, PERCODAN-Demi should not be used in pregnant women unless, in the judgment of the physician, the potential benefits outweigh the possible hazards.
Reye Syndrome is a rare but serious disease which can follow flu or chicken pox in children and teenagers. While the cause of Reye Syndrome is unknown, some reports claim aspirin (or salicylates) may increase the risk of developing this disease.
Salicylates should be used with caution in the presence of peptic ulcer or coagulation abnormalities.

PRECAUTIONS

Head injury and increased intracranial pressure: The respiratory depressant effects of narcotics and their capacity to elevate cerebrospinal fluid pressure may be markedly exaggerated in the presence of head injury, other intracranial lesions or a pre-existing increase in intracranial pressure. Furthermore, narcotics produce adverse reactions which may obscure the clinical course of patients with head injuries.
Acute abdominal conditions: The administration of PERCODAN-Demi (oxycodone and aspirin) or other narcotics may obscure the diagnosis or clinical course in patients with acute abdominal conditions.
Special risk patients: PERCODAN-Demi should be given with caution to certain patients such as the elderly or debilitated, and those with severe impairment of hepatic or renal function, hypothyroidism, Addison's disease, and prostatic hypertrophy or urethral stricture.

ADVERSE REACTIONS

The most frequently observed adverse reactions include lightheadedness, dizziness, sedation, nausea and vomiting. These effects seem to be more prominent in ambulatory than in non-ambulatory patients, and some of these adverse reactions may be alleviated if the patient lies down.
Other adverse reactions include euphoria, dysphoria, constipation and pruritus.

DRUG ABUSE AND DEPENDENCE

PERCODAN-Demi tablets are a Schedule II controlled substance. Oxycodone can produce drug dependence and has the potential for being abused (See WARNINGS).

DOSAGE AND ADMINISTRATION

Dosage should be adjusted according to the severity of the pain and the response of the patient. It may occasionally be necessary to exceed the usual dosage recommended below in cases of more severe pain or in those patients who have become tolerant to the analgesic effect of narcotics. PERCODAN-Demi is given orally.
Dosage: Adults—One or two tablets every six hours.
Children 12 years and older—One-half tablet every six hours.
Children 6 to 12 years—One-quarter tablet every six hours.
PERCODAN-Demi is not indicated for children under 6 years of age.

DRUG INTERACTIONS

The CNS depressant effects of PERCODAN-Demi may be additive with that of other CNS depressants (See WARNINGS).
Aspirin may enhance the effect of anticoagulants and inhibit the uricosuric effect of uricosuric agents.

MANAGEMENT OF OVERDOSAGE

Signs and Symptoms: Serious overdose with PERCODAN-Demi is characterized by respiratory depression (a decrease in respiratory rate and/or tidal volume, Cheyne-Stokes respiration, cyanosis), extreme somnolence progressing to stupor or coma, skeletal muscle flaccidity, cold and clammy skin, and sometimes bradycardia and hypotension. In severe overdosage, apnea, circulatory collapse, cardiac arrest and death may occur. The ingestion of very large amounts of PERCODAN-Demi may, in addition, result in acute salicylate intoxication.

Treatment: Primary attention should be given to the reestablishment of adequate respiratory exchange through provision of a patent airway and the institution of assisted or controlled ventilation. The narcotic antagonist naloxone hydrochloride (NARCAN®) is a specific antidote against respiratory depression which may result from overdosage or unusual sensitivity to narcotics including oxycodone. Therefore, an appropriate dose of naloxone hydrochloride should be administered (usual initial adult dose 0.4 mg–2 mg) preferably by the intravenous route, simultaneously with efforts at respiratory resuscitation. Since the duration of action of oxycodone may exceed that of the antagonist, the patient should be kept under continued surveillance and repeated doses of the antagonist should be administered as needed to maintain adequate respiration.

Oxygen, intravenous fluids, vasopressors and other supportive measures should be employed as indicated.

Gastric emptying may be useful in removing unabsorbed drug.

HOW SUPPLIED

As white, scored tablets available in:

Bottles of 100 NDC 63481-166-70

Store at controlled room temperature 15°–30°C (59°–86°F).

DEA Order Form Required.

Rx only

PERCODAN® is a Registered Trademark of Endo Pharmaceuticals Inc.

NARCAN® is a Registered Trademark of Endo Pharmaceuticals Inc.

6484-00/April, 1998

Shown in Product Identification Guide, page 312

PERCOLONE® Ⓒ℞

[*perk 'ō-lōne*]

(Oxycodone Hydrochloride Tablets, USP)

Rx only

DESCRIPTION

Each PERCOLONE tablet contains:

Oxycodone Hydrochloride, USP .... 5 mg*

*5 mg oxycodone HCl is equivalent to 4.4815 mg of oxycodone.

Inactive ingredients: Microcrystalline cellulose and stearic acid.

Oxycodone is 14-hydroxydihydrocodeinone, a white odorless crystalline powder which is derived from the opium alkaloid, thebaine, and may be represented by the following structural formula:

CLINICAL PHARMACOLOGY

The analgesic ingredient, oxycodone, is a semisynthetic opioid with multiple actions qualitatively similar to those of morphine; the most prominent of these involve the central nervous system and organs composed of smooth muscle. The principal actions of therapeutic value of PERCOLONE are analgesia and sedation.

PERCOLONE is similar to codeine and methadone in that it retains at least one half of its analgesic activity when administered orally.

INDICATIONS

For the relief of moderate to moderately severe pain.

CONTRAINDICATIONS

Hypersensitivity to PERCOLONE.

WARNINGS

Drug Dependence: PERCOLONE can produce drug dependence of the morphine type, and therefore, has the potential for being abused. Psychic dependence, physical dependence and tolerance may develop upon repeated administration of this drug, and it should be prescribed and administered with the same degree of caution appropriate to the use of other oral opioid-containing medications. Like other opioid-containing medications, this drug is subject to the Federal Controlled Substances Act.

Usage in Ambulatory Patients: PERCOLONE may impair the mental and/or physical abilities required for the performance of potentially hazardous tasks such as driving a car or operating machinery. The patient using this drug should be cautioned accordingly.

Interaction with Other Central Nervous System Depressants: Patients receiving other opioid analgesics, general anesthetics, phenothiazines, other tranquilizers, sedative-hypnotics or other CNS depressants (including alcohol) concomitantly with PERCOLONE may exhibit an additive CNS depression. When such combined therapy is contemplated, the dose of one or both agents should be reduced.

Usage in Pregnancy: Safe use in pregnancy has not been established relative to possible adverse effects on fetal development. Therefore, this drug should not be used in pregnant women unless, in the judgment of the physician, the potential benefits outweigh the possible hazards.

Pediatric Use: This drug should not be administered to pediatric patients.

PRECAUTIONS

Head Injury and Increased Intracranial Pressure: The respiratory depressant effects of opioids and their capacity to elevate cerebrospinal fluid pressure may be markedly exaggerated in the presence of head injury, other intracranial lesions or a pre-existing increase in intracranial pressure. Furthermore, opioids produce adverse reactions which may obscure the clinical course of patients with head injuries.

Acute Abdominal Conditions: The administration of this drug or other opioids may obscure the diagnosis or clinical course in patients with acute abdominal conditions.

Special Risk Patients: This drug should be given with caution to certain patients such as the elderly, or debilitated, and those with severe impairment of hepatic or renal function, hypothyroidism, Addison's disease and prostatic hypertrophy or urethral stricture.

ADVERSE REACTIONS

The most frequently observed adverse reactions include lightheadedness, dizziness, sedation, nausea and vomiting. These effects seem to be more prominent in ambulatory than in nonambulatory patients, and some of these adverse reactions may be alleviated if the patient lies down.

Other adverse reactions include euphoria, dysphoria, constipation, skin rash and pruritus.

DOSAGE AND ADMINISTRATION

The usual adult oral dose is 10 to 30 mg every 4 hours as needed for pain or as directed by physician. The dose must be individually adjusted according to severity of pain, patient response and patient size. More severe pain may require 30 mg or more every 4 hours. If the pain increases in severity, analgesia is not adequate or tolerance occurs, a gradual increase in dosage may be required.

For control of severe, chronic pain in patients with certain terminal diseases, this drug should be administered on a regularly scheduled basis, every 4 hours, at the lowest dosage level that will achieve adequate analgesia.

DRUG INTERACTIONS

The CNS depressant effects of PERCOLONE (oxycodone hydrochloride) may be additive with that of other CNS depressants. See WARNINGS.

MANAGEMENT OF OVERDOSAGE

Signs and Symptoms: Serious overdose of PERCOLONE is characterized by respiratory depression (a decrease in respiratory rate and/or tidal volume, Cheyne-Stokes respiration, cyanosis), extreme somnolence progressing to stupor or coma, skeletal muscle flaccidity, cold and clammy skin, and sometimes bradycardia and hypotension. In severe overdosage, apnea, circulatory collapse, cardiac arrest and death may occur.

Treatment: Primary attention should be given to the reestablishment of adequate respiratory exchange through provision of a patent airway and the institution of assisted or controlled ventilation. The opioid antagonist naloxone is a specific antidote against respiratory depression which may result from overdosage or unusual sensitivity to opioids, including PERCOLONE. Therefore, an appropriate dose of naloxone (usual initial adult dose: 0.4 mg) should be administered, preferably by the intravenous route, simultaneously with efforts at respiratory resuscitation. Since the duration of action of PERCOLONE may exceed that of the antagonist, the patient should be kept under continued surveillance and repeated doses of the antagonist should be administered as needed to maintain adequate respiration.

An antagonist should not be administered in the absence of clinically significant respiratory or cardiovascular depression.

Oxygen, intravenous fluids, vasopressors and other supportive measures should be employed as indicated.

Gastric emptying may be useful in removing unabsorbed drug.

HOW SUPPLIED

PERCOLONE is supplied as 5 mg white, round, biconvex tablets, bisected and debossed with "EPI" over "132" on one side and debossed with "5" on the other side as follows:

Bottles of 100 NDC 63481-132-70

Blister Packs of 25 NDC 63481-132-75

(in units of 100 Tablets)

DEA Order Form Required.

Dispense in a well-closed container as defined in the USP/NF. Protect from moisture. Store at 25°C (77°F); excursions permitted to 15°–30°C (59°–86°F). [See USP Controlled Room Temperature].

PERCOLONE® is a Registered Trademark of Endo Pharmaceuticals Inc.

6450-02/Rev. September, 1999

Shown in Product Identification Guide, page 312

SYMMETREL® ℞

[*sim 'e-trel*]

(amantadine hydrochloride)

Tablets and Syrup, USP

DESCRIPTION

SYMMETREL is designated generically as amantadine hydrochloride and chemically as 1-adamantanamine hydrochloride.

Amantadine hydrochloride is a stable white or nearly white crystalline powder, freely soluble in water and soluble in alcohol and in chloroform.

Amantadine hydrochloride has pharmacological actions as both an anti-Parkinson and an antiviral drug.

SYMMETREL is available in tablets and syrup.

Each tablet intended for oral administration contains 100 mg amantadine hydrochloride and has the following inactive ingredients: hydroxypropyl methylcellulose, magnesium stearate, microcrystalline cellulose, sodium starch glycolate, FD&C Yellow No. 6.

SYMMETREL syrup contains 50 mg of amantadine hydrochloride per 5 mL and has the following inactive ingredients: artificial raspberry flavor, citric acid, methylparaben, propylparaben, and sorbitol solution.

CLINICAL PHARMACOLOGY

Pharmacodynamics

Mechanism of Action: Antiviral The mechanism by which amantadine exerts its antiviral activity is not clearly understood. It appears to mainly prevent the release of infectious viral nucleic acid into the host cell by interfering with the function of the transmembrane domain of the viral M2 protein. In certain cases, amantadine is also known to prevent virus assembly during virus replication. It does not appear to interfere with the immunogenicity of inactivated influenza A virus vaccine.

Antiviral Activity: Amantadine inhibits the replication of influenza A virus isolates from each of the subtypes, i.e., H1N1, H2N2 and H3N2. It has very little or no activity against influenza B virus isolates. A quantitative relationship between the *in vitro* susceptibility of influenza A virus to amantadine and the clinical response to therapy has not been established in man. Sensitivity test results, expressed as the concentration of amantadine required to inhibit by 50% the growth of virus (ED_{50}) in tissue culture vary greatly (from 0.1 μg/mL to 25.0 μg/mL) depending upon the assay protocol used, size of virus inoculum, isolates of influenza A virus strains tested, and the cell type used. Host cells in tissue culture readily tolerated amantadine up to a concentration of 100 μg/mL.

Drug Resistance: Influenza A variants with reduced *in vitro* sensitivity to amantadine have been isolated from epidemic strains in areas where adamantane derivatives are being used. Influenza viruses with reduced *in vitro* sensitivity have been shown to be transmissible and to cause typical influenza illness. The quantitative relationship between the *in vitro* sensitivity of influenza A variants to amantadine and the clinical response to therapy has not been established.

Mechanism of Action: Parkinson's Disease The mechanism of action of amantadine in the treatment of Parkinson's disease and drug-induced extrapyramidal reactions is not known. Data from animal studies have either shown or suggested SYMMETREL:

(a) To enhance extracellular concentrations of dopamine by increasing dopamine release or decreasing reuptake of dopamine into presynaptic neurons;

(b) To stimulate the dopamine receptor itself or drive the post synaptic dopaminergic system to a more dopamine sensitive status.

However, doses employed in the animal studies were often of a magnitude greater than the clinically therapeutic doses. More recent work using doses in the low clinically therapeutic range (low μM) showed amantadine to inhibit the N-methyl-D-aspartic acid (NMDA) receptor-mediated stimulation of acetylcholine release from rat striatum, most likely at the MK-801 site. Although amantadine does not possess anticholinergic activity in dogs at doses of 31.5 mg/kg, equivalent to an approximate human dose of 15.8 mg/kg (based on body surface area conversions), clinically, it exhibits its anticholinergic-like side effects such as dry mouth, urinary retention, and constipation.

Pharmacokinetics: SYMMETREL is well absorbed orally. Maximum plasma concentrations are directly related to dose for doses up to 200 mg/day. Doses above 200 mg/day may result in a greater than proportional increase in maximum plasma concentrations. It is primarily excreted unchanged in the urine by glomerular filtration and tubular secretion. Eight metabolites of amantadine have been identified in human urine. One metabolite, an N-acetylated compound, was quantified in human urine and accounted for 5–15% of the administered dose. Plasma acetylamantadine

Continued on next page

Symmetrel —Cont.

accounted for up to 80% of the concurrent amantadine plasma concentration in 5 of 12 healthy volunteers following the ingestion of a 200 mg dose of amantadine. Acetylamantadine was not detected in the plasma of the remaining seven volunteers. The contribution of this metabolite to efficacy or toxicity is not known.

There appears to be a relationship between plasma amantadine concentrations and toxicity. As concentration increases, toxicity seems to be more prevalent, however, absolute values of amantadine concentrations associated with adverse effects have not been fully defined.

Amantadine pharmacokinetics were determined in 24 normal adult male volunteers after the oral administration of a single amantadine hydrochloride 100 mg soft gel capsule. The mean ± SD maximum plasma concentration was 0.22 ± 0.03 μg/mL (range: 0.18 to 0.32 μg/mL). The time to peak concentration was 3.3 ± 1.5 hours (range: 1.5 to 8.0 hours). The apparent oral clearance was 0.28 ± 0.11 L/hr/kg (range: 0.14 to 0.62 L/hr/kg). The half-life was 17 ± 4 hours (range: 10 to 25 hours). Across other studies, amantadine plasma half-life has averaged 16 ± 6 hours (range: 9 to 31 hours) in 19 healthy volunteers.

After oral administration of a single dose of 100 mg amantadine syrup to five healthy volunteers, the mean ± SD maximum plasma concentration C_{max} was 0.24 ± 0.04 μg/mL and ranged from 0.18 to 0.28 μg/mL. After 15 days of amantadine 100 mg b.i.d., the C_{max} was 0.47 ± 0.11 μg/mL in four of the five volunteers. The administration of amantadine tablets as a 200 mg single dose to 6 healthy subjects resulted in a C_{max} of 0.51 ± 0.14 μg/mL. Across studies, the time to C_{max} (T_{max}) averaged about 2 to 4 hours.

Plasma amantadine clearance ranged from 0.2 to 0.3 L/hr/kg after the administration of 5 mg to 25 mg intravenous doses of amantadine to 15 healthy volunteers.

In six healthy volunteers, the ratio of amantadine renal clearance to apparent oral plasma clearance was 0.79 ± 0.17 (mean ± SD).

The volume of distribution determined after the intravenous administration of amantadine to 15 healthy subjects was 3 to 8 L/kg, suggesting tissue binding. Amantadine, after single oral 200 mg doses to 6 healthy young subjects and to 6 healthy elderly subjects has been found in nasal mucus at mean ± SD concentrations of 0.15 ± 0.16, 0.28 ± 0.26, and 0.39 ± 0.34 μg/g at 1, 4, and 8 hours after dosing, respectively. These concentrations represented 31 ± 33%, 59 ± 61%, and 95 ± 86% of the corresponding plasma amantadine concentrations. Amantadine is approximately 67% bound to plasma proteins over a concentration range of 0.1 to 2.0 μg/mL. Following the administration of amantadine 100 mg as a single dose, the mean ± SD red blood cell to plasma ratio ranged from 2.7 ± 0.5 in 6 healthy subjects to 1.4 ± 0.2 in 8 patients with renal insufficiency.

The apparent oral plasma clearance of amantadine is reduced and the plasma half-life and plasma concentrations are increased in healthy elderly individuals age 60 and older. After single dose administration of 25 to 75 mg to 7 healthy, elderly male volunteers, the apparent plasma clearance of amantadine was 0.10 ± 0.04 L/hr/kg (range 0.06 to 0.17 L/hr/kg) and the half-life was 29 ± 7 hours (range 20 to 41 hours). Whether these changes are due to decline in renal function or other age related factors is not known.

In a study of young healthy subjects (n=20), mean renal clearance of amantadine, normalized for body mass index, was significantly higher in males compared to females ($p<0.032$).

Compared with otherwise healthy adult individuals, the clearance of amantadine is significantly reduced in adult patients with renal insufficiency. The elimination half-life increases two to three fold or greater when creatinine clearance is less than 40 mL/min/1.73 m^2 and averages eight days in patients on chronic maintenance hemodialysis. Amantadine is removed in negligible amounts by hemodialysis.

The pH of the urine has been reported to influence the excretion rate of SYMMETREL. Since the excretion rate of SYMMETREL increases rapidly when the urine is acidic, the administration of urine acidifying drugs may increase the elimination of the drug from the body.

INDICATIONS AND USAGE

SYMMETREL is indicated for the prophylaxis and treatment of signs and symptoms of infection caused by various strains of influenza A virus. SYMMETREL (amantadine hydrochloride) is also indicated in the treatment of parkinsonism and drug-induced extrapyramidal reactions.

Influenza A Prophylaxis: SYMMETREL is indicated for chemoprophylaxis against signs and symptoms of influenza A virus infection when early vaccination is not feasible or when the vaccine is contraindicated or not available. In the prophylaxis of influenza, early vaccination on an annual basis as recommended by the Centers for Disease Control's Immunization Practices Advisory Committee is the method of choice. Because SYMMETREL does not completely prevent the host immune response to influenza A infection, individuals who take this drug may still develop immune responses to natural disease or vaccination and may be protected when later exposed to antigenically related viruses. Following vaccination during an influenza A outbreak, SYMMETREL prophylaxis should be considered for the 2- to 4-week time period required to develop an antibody response.

Influenza A Treatment: SYMMETREL is also indicated in the treatment of uncomplicated respiratory tract illness caused by influenza A virus strains especially when administered early in the course of illness. There are no well-controlled clinical studies demonstrating that treatment with SYMMETREL will avoid the development of influenza A virus pneumonitis or other complications in high risk patients.

There is no clinical evidence indicating that SYMMETREL is effective in the prophylaxis or treatment of viral respiratory tract illnesses other than those caused by influenza A virus strains.

Parkinson's Disease/Syndrome: SYMMETREL is indicated in the treatment of idiopathic Parkinson's disease (Paralysis Agitans), postencephalitic parkinsonism, and symptomatic parkinsonism which may follow injury to the nervous system by carbon monoxide intoxication. It is indicated in those elderly patients believed to develop parkinsonism in association with cerebral arteriosclerosis. In the treatment of Parkinson's disease, SYMMETREL is less effective than levodopa, (-)-3-(3,4-dihydroxyphenyl)-L-alanine, and its efficacy in comparison with the anticholinergic antiparkinson drugs has not yet been established.

Drug-Induced Extrapyramidal Reactions: SYMMETREL is indicated in the treatment of drug-induced extrapyramidal reactions. Although anticholinergic-type side effects have been noted with SYMMETREL when used in patients with drug-induced extrapyramidal reactions, there is a lower incidence of these side effects than that observed with the anticholinergic antiparkinson drugs.

CONTRAINDICATIONS

SYMMETREL is contraindicated in patients with known hypersensitivity to amantadine hydrochloride or to any of the other ingredients in SYMMETREL.

WARNINGS

Deaths: Deaths have been reported from overdose with SYMMETREL. The lowest reported acute lethal dose was 2 grams. Acute toxicity may be attributable to the anticholinergic effects of amantadine. Drug overdose has resulted in cardiac, respiratory, renal or central nervous system toxicity. Cardiac dysfunction includes arrhythmia, tachycardia and hypertension (see OVERDOSAGE).

Suicide Attempts: Suicide attempts, some of which have been fatal, have been reported in patients treated with SYMMETREL, many of whom received short courses for influenza treatment or prophylaxis. The incidence of suicide attempts is not known and the pathophysiologic mechanism is not understood. Suicide attempts and suicidal ideation have been reported in patients with and without prior history of psychiatric illness. SYMMETREL can exacerbate mental problems in patients with a history of psychiatric disorders or substance abuse. Patients who attempt suicide may exhibit abnormal mental states which include disorientation, confusion, depression, personality changes, agitation, aggressive behavior, hallucinations, paranoia, other psychotic reactions, and somnolence or insomnia. Because of the possibility of serious adverse effects, caution should be observed when prescribing SYMMETREL to patients being treated with drugs having CNS effects, or for whom the potential risks outweigh the benefit of treatment.

CNS Effects: Patients with a history of epilepsy or other "seizures" should be observed closely for possible increased seizure activity.

Patients receiving SYMMETREL who note central nervous system effects or blurring of vision should be cautioned against driving or working in situations where alertness and adequate motor coordination are important.

Other: Patients with a history of congestive heart failure or peripheral edema should be followed closely as there are patients who developed congestive heart failure while receiving SYMMETREL.

Patients with Parkinson's disease improving on SYMMETREL should resume normal activities gradually and cautiously, consistent with other medical considerations, such as the presence of osteoporosis or phlebothrombosis.

Because SYMMETREL has anticholinergic effects and may cause mydriasis, it should not be given to patients with untreated angle closure glaucoma.

PRECAUTIONS

SYMMETREL should not be discontinued abruptly in patients with Parkinson's disease since a few patients have experienced a parkinsonian crisis, i.e., a sudden marked clinical deterioration, when this medication was suddenly stopped. The dose of anticholinergic drugs or of SYMMETREL should be reduced if atropine-like effects appear when these drugs are used concurrently.

Neuroleptic Malignant Syndrome (NMS): Sporadic cases of possible Neuroleptic Malignant Syndrome (NMS) have been reported in association with dose reduction or withdrawal of SYMMETREL therapy. Therefore, patients should be observed carefully when the dosage of SYMMETREL is reduced abruptly or discontinued, especially if the patient is receiving neuroleptics.

NMS is an uncommon but life-threatening syndrome characterized by fever or hyperthermia; neurologic findings including muscle rigidity, involuntary movements, altered consciousness; mental status changes; other disturbances such as autonomic dysfunction, tachycardia, tachypnea, hyper- or hypotension; laboratory findings such as creatine phosphokinase elevation, leukocytosis, myoglobinuria, and increased serum myoglobin.

The early diagnosis of this condition is important for the appropriate management of these patients. Considering NMS as a possible diagnosis and ruling out other acute illnesses (e.g., pneumonia, systemic infection, etc.) is essential. This may be especially complex if the clinical presentation includes both serious medical illness and untreated or inadequately treated extrapyramidal signs and symptoms (EPS). Other important considerations in the differential diagnosis include central anticholinergic toxicity, heat stroke, drug fever and primary central nervous system (CNS) pathology.

The management of NMS should include: 1) intensive symptomatic treatment and medical monitoring, and 2) treatment of any concomitant serious medical problems for which specific treatments are available. Dopamine agonists, such as bromocriptine, and muscle relaxants, such as dantrolene are often used in the treatment of NMS, however, their effectiveness has not been demonstrated in controlled studies.

Renal disease: Because SYMMETREL is mainly excreted in the urine, it accumulates in the plasma and in the body when renal function declines. Thus, the dose of SYMMETREL should be reduced in patients with renal impairment and in individuals who are 65 years of age or older. Hemodialysis does not remove significant amounts of SYMMETREL; in patients with renal failure, a 4-hour hemodialysis removed 7 to 15 mg after a single 300 mg oral dose[1] (see DOSAGE AND ADMINISTRATION; Dosage for Impaired Renal Function).

Liver disease: Care should be exercised when administering SYMMETREL to patients with liver disease. Rare instances of reversible elevation of liver enzymes have been reported in patients receiving SYMMETREL, though a specific relationship between the drug and such changes has not been established.

Other: The dose of SYMMETREL may need careful adjustment in patients with congestive heart failure, peripheral edema, or orthostatic hypotension. Care should be exercised when administering SYMMETREL to patients with a history of recurrent eczematoid rash, or to patients with psychosis or severe psychoneurosis not controlled by chemotherapeutic agents.

Information for Patients:

Patients should be advised of the following information:

Blurry vision and/or impaired mental acuity may occur.

Gradually increase physicial activity as the symptoms of Parksinson's disease improve.

Avoid excessive alcohol usage, since it may increase the potential for CNS effects such as dizziness, confusion, lightheadedness and orthostatic hypotension.

Avoid getting up suddenly from a sitting or lying position. If dizziness or lightheadedness occurs, notify physician.

Notify physician if mood/mental changes, swelling of extremities, difficulty urinating and/or shortness of breath occur.

Do not take more medication than prescribed because of the risk of overdose. If there is no improvement in a few days, or if medication appears less effective after a few weeks, discuss with a physician.

Consult physician before discontinuing medication.

Seek medical attention immediately if it is suspected that an overdose of medication has been taken.

Drug Interactions: Careful observation is required when SYMMETREL is administered concurrently with central nervous system stimulants.

Agents with anticholinergic properties may potentiate the anticholinergic-like side effects of amantadine.

Coadministration of thioridazine has been reported to worsen the tremor in elderly patients with Parkinson's disease, however, it is not known if other phenothiazines produce a similar response.

Coadministration of Dyazide (triamterene/hydrochlorothiazide) resulted in a higher plasma amantadine concentration in a 61-year-old man receiving SYMMETREL (amantadine hydrochloride) 100 mg TID for Parkinson's disease.[2] It is not known which of the components of Dyazide contributed to the observation or if related drugs produce a similar response.

Coadministration of trimethoprim-sulfamethoxazole may impair renal clearance of amantadine resulting in higher plasma concentrations.

Coadministration of quinine or quinidine with amantadine was shown to reduce the renal clearance of amantadine.

Carcinogenesis and Mutagenesis: Long-term *in vivo* animal studies designed to evaluate the carcinogenic potential of SYMMETREL have not been performed. In several *in vitro* assays for gene mutation, SYMMETREL did not increase the number of spontaneously observed mutations in four strains of *Salmonella typhimurium* (Ames Test) or in a mammalian cell line (Chinese Hamster Ovary cells) when incubations were performed either with or without a liver metabolic activation extract. Further, there was no evidence of chromosome damage observed in an *in vitro* test using freshly derived and stimulated human peripheral blood lymphocytes (with and without metabolic activation) or in an *in vivo* mouse bone marrow micronucleus test (140–550 mg/kg; estimated human equivalent doses of 11.7–45.8 mg/kg based on body surface area conversion).

Impairment of Fertility: In a three litter reproduction study in rats, SYMMETREL at a dose of 32 mg/kg/day (estimated human equivalent dose of 4.5 mg/kg/day, based on body surface area conversions) administered to both males and females slightly impaired fertility. There were no effects on fertility at a dose level of 10 mg/kg/day (estimated human equivalent dose of 1.4 mg/kg/day); intermediate doses were not tested.

Failed fertility has been reported during human *in vitro* fertilization (IVF) when the sperm donor ingested amantadine 2 weeks prior to, and during the IVF cycle.

Pregnancy Category C: SYMMETREL has been reported to be teratogenic in rats at 50 mg/kg/day and embryotoxic at 100 mg/kg/day (estimated human equivalent dose of 7.1 mg/kg/day and 14.2 mg/kg/day, respectively, based on body surface area conversion). A dose of 37 mg/kg/day (estimated human equivalent dose of 5.3 mg/kg/day) did not produce a teratogenic or embryotoxic effect in the rat. Embryotoxic and teratogenic effects were not seen in rabbits that received 32 mg/kg/day (estimated human equivalent dose of 9.6 mg/kg/day, based on body surface area conversion). There are no adequate and well-controlled studies in pregnant women. Human data regarding teratogenicity after maternal use of amantadine is scarce. Tetralogy of Fallot and tibial hemimelia (normal karyotype) occurred in an infant exposed to amantadine during the first trimester of pregnancy (100 mg P.O. for 7 days during the 6th and 7th week of gestation). Cardiovascular maldevelopment (single ventricle with pulmonary atresia) was associated with maternal exposure to amantadine (100 mg/d) administered during the first 2 weeks of pregnancy. SYMMETREL should be used during pregnancy only if the potential benefit justifies the potential risk to the embryo or fetus.

Nursing Mothers: SYMMETREL is excreted in human milk. Use is not recommended in nursing mothers.

Pediatric Use: The safety and efficacy of SYMMETREL in newborn infants and infants below the age of 1 year have not been established.

Usage in the Elderly: Because SYMMETREL is primarily excreted in the urine, it accumulates in the plasma and in the body when renal function declines. Thus, the dose of SYMMETREL should be reduced in patients with renal impairment and in individuals who are 65 years of age or older. The dose of SYMMETREL may need reduction in patients with congestive heart failure, peripheral edema, or orthostatic hypotension (see DOSAGE AND ADMINISTRATION).

ADVERSE REACTIONS

The adverse reactions reported most frequently at the recommended dose of SYMMETREL (5–10%) are: nausea, dizziness (lightheadedness), and insomnia.

Less frequently (1–5%) reported adverse reactions are: depression, anxiety and irritability, hallucinations, confusion, anorexia, dry mouth, constipation, ataxia, livedo reticularis, peripheral edema, orthostatic hypotension, headache, somnolence, nervousness, dream abnormality, agitation, dry nose, diarrhea and fatigue.

Infrequently (0.1–1%) occurring adverse reactions are: congestive heart failure, psychosis, urinary retention, dyspnea, skin rash, vomiting, weakness, slurred speech, euphoria, thinking abnormality, amnesia, hyperkinesia, hypertension, decreased libido, and visual disturbance, including punctate subepithelial or other corneal opacity, corneal edema, decreased visual acuity, sensitivity to light, and optic nerve palsy.

Rare (less than 0.1%) occurring adverse reactions are: instances of convulsion, leukopenia, neutropenia, eczematoid dermatitis, oculogyric episodes, suicidal attempt, suicide, and suicidal ideation (see WARNINGS).

Other adverse reactions reported during postmarketing experience with SYMMETREL usage include:

Nervous System/Psychiatric—coma, stupor, delirium, hypokinesia, hypertonia, delusions, aggressive behavior, paranoid reaction, manic reaction, involuntary muscle contractions, gait abnormalities, paresthesia, EEG changes, and tremor;

Cardiovascular—cardiac arrest, arrhythmias including malignant arrhythmias, hypotension, and tachycardia;

Respiratory—acute respiratory failure, pulmonary edema, and tachypnea;

Gastrointestinal—dysphagia;

Hematologic—leukocytosis;

Special Senses—keratitis and mydriasis;

Skin and Appendages—pruritus and diaphoresis;

Miscellaneous—neuroleptic malignant syndrome (see WARNINGS), allergic reactions including anaphylactic reactions, edema, and fever;

Laboratory Test—elevated: CPK, BUN, serum creatinine, alkaline phosphatase, LDH, bilirubin, GGT, SGOT, and SGPT.

OVERDOSAGE

Deaths have been reported from overdose with SYMMETREL. The lowest reported acute lethal dose was 2 grams. Because some patients have attempted suicide by overdosing with amantadine, prescriptions should be written for the smallest quantity consistent with good patient management.

Acute toxicity may be attributable to the anticholinergic effects of amantadine. Drug overdose has resulted in cardiac, respiratory, renal or central nervous system toxicity. Cardiac dysfunction includes arrhythmia, tachycardia and hypertension. Pulmonary edema and respiratory distress (including adult respiratory distress syndrome—ARDS) have been reported; renal dysfunction including increased BUN, decreased creatinine clearance and renal insufficiency can occur. Central nervous system effects that have been reported include insomnia, anxiety, agitation, aggressive behavior, hypertonia, hyperkinesia, ataxia, gait abnormality, tremor, confusion, disorientation, depersonalization, fear, delirium, hallucinations, psychotic reactions, lethargy, somnolence and coma. Seizures may be exacerbated in patients with prior history of seizure disorders. Hyperthermia has also been observed in cases where a drug overdose has occurred.

There is no specific antidote for an overdose of SYMMETREL. However, slowly administered intravenous physostigmine in 1 and 2 mg doses in an adult[3] at 1- to 2-hour intervals and 0.5 mg doses in a child[4] at 5- to 10-minute intervals up to a maximum of 2 mg/hour have been reported to be effective in the control of central nervous system toxicity caused by amantadine hydrochloride. For acute overdosing, general supportive measures should be employed along with immediate gastric lavage or induction of emesis. Fluids should be forced, and if necessary, given intravenously. Hemodialysis does not remove significant amounts of SYMMETREL; in patients with renal failure, a 4-hour hemodialysis removed 7 to 15 mg after a single 300 mg oral dose.[1] The pH of the urine has been reported to influence the excretion rate of SYMMETREL. Since the excretion rate of SYMMETREL increases rapidly when the urine is acidic, the administration of urine acidifying drugs may increase the elimination of the drug from the body. The blood pressure, pulse, respiration and temperature should be monitored. The patient should be observed for hyperactivity and convulsions; if required, sedation, and anticonvulsant therapy should be administered. The patient should be observed for the possible development of arrhythmias and hypotension; if required, appropriate antiarrhythmic and antihypotensive therapy should be given. Electrocardiographic monitoring may be required after ingestion, since malignant tachyarrhythmias can appear after overdose.

Care should be exercised when administering adrenergic agents, such as isoproterenol, to patients with a SYMMETREL overdose, since the dopaminergic activity of SYMMETREL has been reported to induce malignant arrhythmias. The blood electrolytes, urine pH and urinary output should be monitored. If there is no record of recent voiding, catheterization should be done.

DOSAGE AND ADMINISTRATION

The dose of SYMMETREL may need reduction in patients with congestive heart failure, peripheral edema, orthostatic hypotension, or impaired renal function (see Dosage for Impaired Renal Function).

Dosage for Prophylaxis and Treatment of Uncomplicated Influenza A Virus Illness:

Adult: The adult daily dosage of SYMMETREL (amantadine hydrochloride) is 200 mg; two 100 mg tablets (or four teaspoonfuls of syrup) as a single daily dose. The daily dosage may be split into one tablet of 100 mg (or two teaspoonfuls of syrup) twice a day. If central nervous system effects develop in once-a-day dosage, a split dosage schedule may reduce such complaints. In persons 65 years of age or older, the daily dosage of SYMMETREL is 100 mg.

A 100 mg daily dose has also been shown in experimental challenge studies to be effective as prophylaxis in healthy adults who are not at high risk for influenza-related complications. However, it has not been demonstrated that a 100 mg daily dose is as effective as a 200 mg daily dose for prophylaxis, nor has the 100 mg daily dose been studied in the treatment of acute influenza illness. In recent clinical trials, the incidence of central nervous system (CNS) side effects associated with the 100 mg daily dose was at or near the level of placebo. The 100 mg dose is recommended for persons who have demonstrated intolerance to 200 mg of SYMMETREL daily because of CNS or other toxicities.

Pediatric Patients: 1 yr.–9 yrs. of age: The total daily dose should be calculated on the basis of 2 to 4 mg/lb/day (4.4 to 8.8 mg/kg/day), but not to exceed 150 mg per day.

9 yrs.–12 yrs. of age: The total daily dose is 200 mg given as one tablet of 100 mg (or two teaspoonfuls of syrup) twice a day. The 100 mg daily dose has not been studied in this pediatric population. Therefore, there are no data which demonstrate that this dose is as effective as or is safer than the 200 mg daily dose in this patient population.

Prophylactic dosing should be started in anticipation of an influenza A outbreak and before or after contact with individuals with influenza A virus respiratory tract illness.

SYMMETREL should be continued daily for at least 10 days following a known exposure. If SYMMETREL is used chemoprophylactically in conjunction with inactivated influenza A virus vaccine until protective antibody responses develop, then it should be administered for 2 to 4 weeks after the vaccine has been given. When inactivated influenza A virus vaccine is unavailable or contraindicated, SYMMETREL should be administered for the duration of known influenza A in the community because of repeated and unknown exposure.

Treatment of influenza A virus illness should be started as soon as possible, preferably within 24 to 48 hours after onset of signs and symptoms, and should be continued for 24 to 48 hours after the disappearance of signs and symptoms.

Dosage for Parkinsonism:

Adult: The usual dose of SYMMETREL is 100 mg twice a day when used alone. SYMMETREL has an onset of action usually within 48 hours.

The initial dose of SYMMETREL is 100 mg daily for patients with serious associated medical illnesses or who are receiving high doses of other antiparkinson drugs. After one to several weeks at 100 mg once daily, the dose may be increased to 100 mg twice daily, if necessary.

Occasionally, patients whose responses are not optimal with SYMMETREL at 200 mg daily may benefit from an increase up to 400 mg daily in divided doses. However, such patients should be supervised closely by their physicians.

Patients initially deriving benefit from SYMMETREL not uncommonly experience a fall-off of effectiveness after a few months. Benefit may be regained by increasing the dose to 300 mg daily. Alternatively, temporary discontinuation of SYMMETREL for several weeks, followed by reinitiation of the drug, may result in regaining benefit in some patients. A decision to use other antiparkinson drugs may be necessary.

Dosage for Concomitant Therapy: Some patients who do not respond to anticholinergic antiparkinson drugs may respond to SYMMETREL. When SYMMETREL or anticholinergic antiparkinson drugs are each used with marginal benefit, concomitant use may produce additional benefit.

When SYMMETREL and levodopa are initiated concurrently, the patient can exhibit rapid therapeutic benefits. SYMMETREL should be held constant at 100 mg daily or twice daily while the daily dose of levodopa is gradually increased to optimal benefit.

When SYMMETREL is added to optimal well-tolerated doses of levodopa, additional benefit may result, including smoothing out the fluctuations in improvement which sometimes occur in patients on levodopa alone. Patients who require a reduction in their usual dose of levodopa because of development of side effects may possibly regain lost benefit with the addition of SYMMETREL.

Dosage for Drug-Induced Extrapyramidal Reactions:

Adult: The usual dose of SYMMETREL is 100 mg twice a day. Occasionally, patients whose responses are not optimal with SYMMETREL at 200 mg daily may benefit from an increase up to 300 mg daily in divided doses.

Dosage for Impaired Renal Function:

Depending upon creatinine clearance, the following dosage adjustments are recommended:

CREATININE CLEARANCE (mL/min/1.73m^2)	SYMMETREL DOSAGE
30–50	200 mg 1st day and 100 mg each day thereafter
15–29	200 mg 1st day followed by 100 mg on alternate days
<15	200 mg every 7 days

The recommended dosage for patients on hemodialysis is 200 mg every 7 days.

HOW SUPPLIED

SYMMETREL is available in light orange, convex curved, triangular shaped 100 mg tablets with "SYMMETREL" debossed on one side and plain on the other side as follows:

Bottles of 100	NDC 63481-108-70
Bottles of 500	NDC 63481-108-85

As a clear, colorless syrup [each 5 mL (1 teaspoonful) contains 50 mg amantadine hydrochloride] in:

16 oz. (480 mL) bottles	NDC 63481-205-16

Store at controlled room temperature 15°–30°C (59°–86°F).

Dispense in a tight container as defined in the USP.

REFERENCES

1. V.W. Horadam, et al., *Ann. Intern. Med.* 94:454, 1981.
2. W.W. Wilson and A.H. Rajput, Amantadine-Dyazide Interaction, *Can. Med. Assoc. J.* 129:974–975, 1983.
3. D.F. Casey, *N. Engl. J. Med.* 298:516, 1978.
4. C.D. Berkowitz, *J. Pediatr.* 95:144, 1979.

Caution: Federal (USA) law prohibits dispensing without prescription.

6486-01/Rev. February, 1998

Shown in Product Identification Guide, page 312

ZYDONE® Ⓒ℞

[zī ʺdōn]

(Hydrocodone Bitartrate and Acetaminophen Tablets, USP)

Rx only

DESCRIPTION

ZYDONE Tablets, for oral administration, contain hydrocodone bitartrate and acetaminophen in the following strengths:

Hydrocodone Bitartrate, USP	5 mg
Acetaminophen, USP	400 mg
Hydrocodone Bitartrate, USP	7.5 mg
Acetaminophen, USP	400 mg
Hydrocodone Bitartrate, USP	10 mg
Acetaminophen, USP	400 mg

In addition, each tablet contains the following inactive ingredients: colloidal silicon dioxide, croscarmellose sodium, crospovidone, microcrystalline cellulose, povidone, pregelatinized starch, and stearic acid. The 5 mg/400 mg strength contains FD&C Yellow No. 10; 7.5 mg/400 mg contains FD&C Blue No. 2; and 10 mg/400 mg contains FD&C Red No. 40.

Hydrocodone bitartrate is an opioid analgesic and antitussive and occurs as fine, white crystals or as a crystalline

Continued on next page

Zydone—Cont.

powder. It is affected by light. The chemical name is 4,5α-Epoxy-3-methoxy-17-methylmorphinan-6-one tartrate (1:1) hydrate (2:5). It has the following structural formula:

$C_{18}H_{21}NO_3 \cdot C_4H_6O_6 \cdot 2\frac{1}{2} H_2O$ MW = 494.50

Acetaminophen, 4'-Hydroxyacetanilide, a slightly bitter, white, odorless, crystalline powder, is a non-opiate, non-salicylate analgesic and antipyretic. It has the following structural formula:

$C_8H_9NO_2$ MW = 151.17

CLINICAL PHARMACOLOGY

Hydrocodone is a semisynthetic opioid analgesic and antitussive with multiple actions qualitatively similar to those of codeine. Most of these involve the central nervous system and smooth muscle. The precise mechanism of action of hydrocodone and other opiates is not known, although it is believed to relate to the existence of opiate receptors in the central nervous system. In addition to analgesia, opioids may produce drowsiness, changes in mood and mental clouding.

The analgesic action of acetaminophen involves peripheral influences, but the specific mechanism is as yet undetermined. Antipyretic activity is mediated through hypothalamic heat-regulating centers. Acetaminophen inhibits prostaglandin synthetase. Therapeutic doses of acetaminophen have negligible effects on the cardiovascular or respiratory systems; however, toxic doses may cause circulatory failure and rapid, shallow breathing.

Pharmacokinetics: The behavior of the individual components is described below.

Hydrocodone: Following a 10 mg oral dose of hydrocodone administered to five adult male subjects, the mean peak concentration was 23.6 ± 5.2 ng/mL. Maximum serum levels were achieved at 1.3 ± 0.3 hours and the half-life was determined to be 3.8 ± 0.3 hours. Hydrocodone exhibits a complex pattern of metabolism including O-demethylation, N-demethylation and 6-keto reduction to the corresponding 6-α- and 6-β-hydroxymetabolites.

See OVERDOSAGE for toxicity information.

Acetaminophen: Acetaminophen is rapidly absorbed from the gastrointestinal tract and is distributed throughout most body tissues. The plasma half-life is 1.25 to 3 hours, but may be increased by liver damage and following overdosage. Elimination of acetaminophen is principally by liver metabolism (conjugation) and subsequent renal excretion of metabolites. Approximately 85% of an oral dose appears in the urine within 24 hours of administration, most as the glucuronide conjugate, with small amounts of other conjugates and unchanged drug.

See OVERDOSAGE for toxicity information.

INDICATIONS AND USAGE

ZYDONE (hydrocodone bitartrate and acetaminophen tablets) is indicated for the relief of moderate to moderately severe pain.

CONTRAINDICATIONS

ZYDONE tablets should not be administered to patients who have previously exhibited hypersensitivity to hydrocodone, acetaminophen, or any other component of this product.

WARNINGS

Respiratory Depression: At high doses or in sensitive patients, hydrocodone may produce dose-related respiratory depression by acting directly on the brain stem respiratory center. Hydrocodone also affects the center that controls respiratory rhythm, and may produce irregular and periodic breathing.

Head Injury and Increased Intracranial Pressure: The respiratory depressant effects of opioids and their capacity to elevate cerebrospinal fluid pressure may be markedly exaggerated in the presence of head injury, other intracranial lesions or a preexisting increase in intracranial pressure. Furthermore, opioids produce adverse reactions which may obscure the clinical course of patients with head injuries.

Acute Abdominal Conditions: The administration of opioids may obscure the diagnosis or clinical course of patients with acute abdominal conditions.

PRECAUTIONS

General:

Special Risk Patients: As with any opioid analgesic agent, ZYDONE tablets should be used with caution in elderly or

5 mg/400 mg Yellow, elongated octagonal, convex tablets debossed with "E" on one side and "5" on the other.	Bottles of 100 Bottles of 500 Unit dose package of 100 tablets	NDC 63481-668-70 NDC 63481-668-85 NDC 63481-668-75
7.5 mg/400 mg Blue, elongated octagonal, convex tablets debossed with "E" on one side and "7.5" on the other.	Bottles of 100 Bottles of 500 Unit dose package of 100 tablets	NDC 63481-669-70 NDC 63481-669-85 NDC 63481-669-75
10 mg/400 mg Red, elongated octagonal, convex tablets debossed with "E" on one side and "10" on the other.	Bottles of 100 Bottles of 500 Unit dose package of 100 tablets	NDC 63481-698-70 NDC 63481-698-85 NDC 63481-698-75

debilitated patients, and those with severe impairment of hepatic or renal function, hypothyroidism, Addison's disease, prostatic hypertrophy or urethral stricture. The usual precautions should be observed and the possibility of respiratory depression should be kept in mind.

Cough Reflex: Hydrocodone suppresses the cough reflex; as with all opioids, caution should be exercised when ZYDONE tablets are used postoperatively and in patients with pulmonary disease.

Information for Patients: Hydrocodone, like all opioids, may impair mental and/or physical abilities required for the performance of potentially hazardous tasks such as driving a car or operating machinery; patients should be cautioned accordingly.

Alcohol and other CNS depressants may produce an additive CNS depression, when taken with this combination product, and should be avoided.

Hydrocodone may be habit-forming. Patients should take the drug only for as long as it is prescribed, in the amounts prescribed, and no more frequently than prescribed.

Laboratory Tests: In patients with severe hepatic or renal disease, effects of therapy should be monitored with serial liver and/or renal function tests.

Drug Interactions: Patients receiving opioids, antihistamines, antipsychotics, antianxiety agents, or other CNS depressants (including alcohol) concomitantly with hydrocodone bitartrate and acetaminophen tablets may exhibit an additive CNS depression. When combined therapy is contemplated, the dose of one or both agents should be reduced. The use of MAO inhibitors or tricyclic antidepressants with hydrocodone preparations may increase the effect of either the antidepressant or hydrocodone.

Drug/Laboratory Test Interactions: Acetaminophen may produce false-positive test results for urinary 5-hydroxyindoleacetic acid.

Carcinogenesis, Mutagenesis, Impairment of Fertility: No adequate studies have been conducted in animals to determine whether hydrocodone or acetaminophen have a potential for carcinogenesis, mutagenesis, or impairment of fertility.

Pregnancy:

Teratogenic Effects: Pregnancy Category C: There are no adequate and well-controlled studies in pregnant women. ZYDONE tablets should be used during pregnancy only if the potential benefit justifies the potential risk to the fetus.

Nonteratogenic Effects: Babies born to mothers who have been taking opioids regularly prior to delivery will be physically dependent. The withdrawal signs include irritability and excessive crying, tremors, hyperactive reflexes, increased respiratory rate, increased stools, sneezing, yawning, vomiting, and fever. The intensity of the syndrome does not always correlate with the duration of maternal opioid use or dose. There is no consensus on the best method of managing withdrawal.

Labor and Delivery: As with all opioids, administration of this product to the mother shortly before delivery may result in some degree of respiratory depression in the newborn, especially if higher doses are used.

Nursing Mothers: Acetaminophen is excreted in breast milk in small amounts, but the significance of its effects on nursing infants is not known. It is not known whether hydrocodone is excreted in human milk. Because many drugs are excreted in human milk and because of the potential for serious adverse reactions in nursing infants from hydrocodone and acetaminophen, a decision should be made whether to discontinue nursing or to discontinue the drug, taking into account the importance of the drug to the mother.

Pediatric Use: Safety and effectiveness in the pediatric patients have not been established.

ADVERSE REACTIONS

The most frequently reported adverse reactions are lightheadedness, dizziness, sedation, nausea and vomiting. These effects seem to be more prominent in ambulatory than in non-ambulatory patients, and some of these adverse reactions may be alleviated if the patient lies down.

Other adverse reactions include:

Central Nervous System: Drowsiness, mental clouding, lethargy, impairment of mental and physical performance, anxiety, fear, dysphoria, psychic dependence, mood changes.

Gastrointestinal System: Prolonged administration of ZYDONE (hydrocodone bitartrate and acetaminophen tablets) may produce constipation.

Genitourinary System: Ureteral spasm, spasm of vesical sphincters and urinary retention have been reported with opiates.

Respiratory Depression: Hydrocodone bitartrate may produce dose-related respiratory depression by acting directly on brain stem respiratory centers (see OVERDOSAGE).

Dermatological: Skin rash, pruritus.

The following adverse drug events may be borne in mind as potential effects of acetaminophen: allergic reactions, rash, thrombocytopenia, agranulocytosis.

Potential effects of high dosage are listed in the OVERDOSAGE section.

DRUG ABUSE AND DEPENDENCE

Controlled Substance: ZYDONE Tablets are classified as a Schedule III controlled substance.

Abuse and Dependence: Psychic dependence, physical dependence, and tolerance may develop upon repeated administration of opioids; therefore, this product should be prescribed and administered with caution. However, psychic dependence is unlikely to develop when hydrocodone bitartrate and acetaminophen tablets are used for a short time for the treatment of pain.

Physical dependence, the condition in which continued administration of the drug is required to prevent the appearance of a withdrawal syndrome, assumes clinically significant proportions only after several weeks of continued opioid use, although some mild degree of physical dependence may develop after a few days of opioid therapy. Tolerance, in which increasingly large doses are required in order to produce the same degree of analgesia, is manifested initially by a shortened duration of analgesic effect, and subsequently by decreases in the intensity of analgesia. The rate of development of tolerance varies among patients.

OVERDOSAGE

Following an acute overdosage, toxicity may result from hydrocodone or acetaminophen.

Signs and Symptoms:

Hydrocodone: Serious overdose with hydrocodone is characterized by respiratory depression (a decrease in respiratory rate and/or tidal volume, Cheyne-Stokes respiration, cyanosis) extreme somnolence progressing to stupor or coma, sketetal muscle flaccidity, cold and clammy skin, and sometimes bradycardia and hypotension. In severe overdosage, apnea, circulatory collapse, cardiac arrest and death may occur.

Acetaminophen: In acetaminophen overdosage: dose-dependent, potentially fatal hepatic necrosis is the most serious adverse effect. Renal tubular necrosis, hypoglycemic coma and thrombocytopenia may also occur.

Early symptoms following a potentially hepatotoxic overdose may include: nausea, vomiting, diaphoresis and general malaise. Clinical and laboratory evidence of hepatic toxicity may not be apparent until 48 to 72 hours post-ingestion.

In adults, hepatic toxicity has rarely been reported with acute overdoses of less than 10 grams or fatalities with less than 15 grams.

Treatment: A single or multiple overdose with hydrocodone and acetaminophen is a potentially lethal polydrug overdose, and consultation with a regional poison control center is recommended.

Immediate treatment includes support of cardiorespiratory function and measures to reduce drug absorption. Vomiting should be induced mechanically, or with syrup of ipecac, if the patient is alert (adequate pharyngeal and laryngeal reflexes). Oral activated charcoal (1 g/kg) should follow gastric emptying. The first dose should be accompanied by an appropriate cathartic. If repeated doses are used, the cathartic might be included with alternate doses as required. Hypotension is usually hypovolemic and should respond to fluids. Vasopressors and other supportive measures should be employed as indicated. A cuffed endotracheal tube should be inserted before gastric lavage of the unconscious patient and, when necessary, to provide assisted respiration.

Meticulous attention should be given to maintaining adequate pulmonary ventilation. In severe cases of intoxication, pertitoneal dialysis, or preferably hemodialysis may be considered. If hypoprothrombinemia occurs due to acetaminophen overdose, vitamin K should be administered intravenously.

Naloxone, an opioid antagonist, can reverse respiratory depression and coma associated with opioid overdose. NARCAN® (naloxone hydrochloride) 0.4 mg to 2 mg is given parenterally. Since the duration of action of hydrocodone may

exceed that of naloxone, the patient should be kept under continuous surveillance and repeated doses of the antagonist should be administered as needed to maintain adequate respiration. An opioid antagonist should not be administered in the absence of clinically significant respiratory or cardiovascular depression.
If the dose of acetaminophen may have exceeded 140 mg/kg, acetylcysteine should be administered as early as possible. Serum acetaminophen levels should be obtained, since levels four or more hours following ingestion help predict acetaminophen toxicity. Do not await acetaminophen assay results before initiating treatment. Hepatic enzymes should be obtained initially, and repeated at 24-hour intervals.
Methemoglobinemia over 30% should be treated with methylene blue by slow intravenous administration.
The toxic dose for adults for acetaminophen is 10 grams.

DOSAGE AND ADMINISTRATION

Dosage should be adjusted according to the severity of pain and response of the patient. However, it should be kept in mind that tolerance to hydrocodone can develop with continued use and that the incidence of untoward effects is dose related.

5 mg/400 mg: The usual adult dose is one or two tablets every four to six hours as needed for pain. The total daily dosage should not exceed eight tablets.

7.5 mg/400 mg: The usual adult dosage is one tablet every four to six hours as needed for pain. The total daily dosage should not exceed six tablets.

10 mg/400 mg: The usual adult dosage is one tablet every four to six hours as needed for pain. The total daily dosage should not exceed six tablets.

HOW SUPPLIED

ZYDONE (Hydrocodone Bitartrate and Acetaminophen Tablets, USP) is supplied as follows:
[See table at top of previous page]
Store at controlled room temperature 15°–30°C (59°–86°F).
Dispense in a tight, light-resistant container as defined in the USP, with a child-resistant closure (as required).
A Schedule III Opioid. Oral prescription where permitted by State law.
ZYDONE® is a Registered Trademark of Endo Pharmaceuticals Inc.
NARCAN® is Registered Trademark of Endo Pharmaceuticals Inc.

6476-00/December, 1998
Shown in Product Identification Guide, page 312

Enzon, Inc.

20 KINGSBRIDGE RD.
PISCATAWAY, NJ 08854

Direct Inquiries to:
Toni L. Klich
(732) 980-4619
FAX: (732) 980-5911

For Medical Information Contact:
In Emergencies:
(732) 980-4560
FAX: (732) 980-4566

ADAGEN® ℞
[*ad-a-jen*]
(pegademase bovine)
Injection

PRODUCT OVERVIEW

KEY FACTS

ADAGEN® (pegademase bovine) Injection is a modified enzyme used to provide direct and specific replacement of adenosine deaminase (ADA), an enzyme that is deficient in some patients with severe combined immunodeficiency disease (SCID). While regular administration of the compound can improve immune function and reduce the incidence of opportunistic infections in patients with ADA-deficient SCID, it is of no value in patients with immunodeficiency due to other causes. Further, it is not intended as a replacement for HLA-identical bone marrow transplant therapy.

MAJOR USES

ADAGEN® is to be used as enzyme replacement therapy in patients who have SCID associated with a deficiency of ADA, and who are not suitable candidates for-or who have failed-bone marrow transplantation. ADAGEN® should be used in infants from birth or in children of any age at the time of diagnosis.

SAFETY INFORMATION

ADAGEN® should be administered with caution to patients with thrombocytopenia and should not be given if thrombocytopenia is severe.

PRESCRIBING INFORMATION

ADAGEN® ℞
[*ad-a-jen*]
(pegademase bovine) Injection

DESCRIPTION

ADAGEN® (pegademase bovine) Injection is a modified enzyme used for enzyme replacement therapy for the treatment of severe combined immunodeficiency disease (SCID) associated with a deficiency of adenosine deaminase.
ADAGEN® (pegademase bovine) Injection is supplied in an isotonic, pyrogen free, sterile solution, pH 7.2–7.4, for intramuscular injection only. The solution is clear and colorless. It is supplied in 1.5 mL single-dose vials.
The chemical name for **ADAGEN®** (pegademase bovine) Injection is (monomethoxypolyethylene glycol succinimidyl)$_{11-17}$-adenosine deaminase. It is a conjugate of numerous strands of monomethoxypolyethylene glycol (PEG), molecular weight 5,000, covalently attached to the enzyme adenosine deaminase (ADA). ADA (adenosine deaminase EC 3.5.4.4) used in the manufacture of **ADAGEN®** (pegademase bovine) Injection is derived from bovine intestine.
The structural formula of **ADAGEN®** (pegademase bovine) Injection is:

$$[CH_3-(OCH_2CH_2)_x-O-\underset{\underset{O}{\|}}{C}-CH_2CH_2-\underset{\underset{O}{\|}}{C}-NH]_y-\text{adenosine deaminase}$$

x = 114 oxyethylene groups per PEG strand.
y = 11–17 primary amino groups of lysine onto which succinyl PEG is attached.

Each milliliter of **ADAGEN®** (pegademase bovine) Injection contains:

Pegademase bovine	250 units*
Monobasic sodium phosphate, USP	1.20 mg
Dibasic sodium phosphate, USP	5.58 mg
Sodium Chloride, USP	8.50 mg
Water for Injection, USP	q.s. to 1.0 mL

*One unit of activity is defined as the amount of ADA that converts 1 µM of adenosine to inosine per minute at 25°C and pH 7.3.

CLINICAL PHARMACOLOGY

Severe Combined Immunodeficiency Disease Associated with ADA Deficiency

Severe combined immunodeficiency disease (SCID) associated with a deficiency of ADA is a rare, inherited, and often fatal disease. In the absence of the ADA enzyme, the purine substrates adenosine and 2′-deoxyadenosine accumulate, causing metabolic abnormalities that are directly toxic to lymphocytes.
The immune deficiency can be cured by bone marrow transplantation. When a suitable bone marrow donor is unavailable or when bone marrow transplantation fails, non-selective replacement of the ADA enzyme has been provided by periodic irradiated red blood cell transfusions. However, transmission of viral infections and iron overload are serious risks associated with irradiated red blood cell transfusions, and relatively few ADA deficient patients have benefitted from chronic transfusion therapy.
ADAGEN® (pegademase bovine) Injection provides specific and direct replacement of the deficient enzyme, but will not benefit patients with immunodeficiency due to other causes.
In patients with ADA deficiency, rigorous adherence to a schedule of **ADAGEN®** (pegademase bovine) Injection administration can eliminate the toxic metabolites of ADA deficiency and result in improved immune function. It is imperative that treatment with **ADAGEN®** (pegademase bovine) Injection be carefully monitored by measurement of the level of ADA activity in plasma. Monitoring of the level of deoxyadenosine triphosphate (dATP) in erythrocytes is also helpful in determining that the dose of **ADAGEN®** (pegademase bovine) Injection is adequate.

Actions

ADAGEN® (pegademase bovine) Injection provides specific replacement of the deficient enzyme.
In the absence of the enzyme ADA, the purine substrates adenosine, 2′-deoxyadenosine and their metabolites are toxic to lymphocytes. The direct action of **ADAGEN®** (pegademase bovine) Injection is the correction of these metabolic abnormalities. Improvement in immune function and diminished frequency of opportunistic infections compared with the natural history of combined immunodeficiency due to ADA deficiency only occurs after metabolic abnormalities are corrected. There is a lag between the correction of the metabolic abnormalities and improved immune function. This period of time is variable, and has been reported to be from a few weeks to as long as 6 months. In contrast to the natural history of combined immunodeficiency disease due to ADA deficiency, a trend toward diminished frequency of opportunistic infections and fewer complications of infections has occurred in patients receiving **ADAGEN®** (pegademase bovine) Injection.

Pharmacokinetics

The pharmacokinetics and biochemical effects of **ADAGEN®** (pegademase bovine) Injection have been studied in six children ranging in age from 6 weeks to 12 years with SCID associated with ADA deficiency.
After the intramuscular injection of **ADAGEN®** (pegademase bovine) Injection, peak plasma levels of ADA activity were reached 2 to 3 days following administration. The plasma elimination half-life of ADA following the administration of **ADAGEN®** (pegademase bovine) Injection was variable, even for the same child. The range was 3 to >6 days. Following weekly injections of **ADAGEN®** (pegademase bovine) Injection at 15 U/kg, the average trough level of ADA activity in plasma was between 20 and 25 µmol/hr/mL.

Biochemical Effects

The changes in red blood cell deoxyadenosine nucleotide (dATP) and S-adenosylhomocysteine hydrolase (SAHase) have been evaluated. In patients with ADA deficiency, inadequate elimination of 2′-deoxyadenosine caused a marked elevation in dATP and a decrease in SAHase level in red blood cells. Prior to treatment with **ADAGEN®** (pegademase bovine) Injection, the levels of dATP in the red blood cells ranged from 0.056 to 0.899 µmol/mL of erythrocytes. After 2 months of maintenance treatment with **ADAGEN®** (pegademase bovine) Injection, the levels decreased to a range of 0.007 to 0.015 µmol/mL. The normal value of dATP is below 0.001 µmol/mL. In the same period of time, the levels of SAHase increased from the pretreatment range of 0.09 to 0.22 nmol/hr/mg protein to a range of 2.37 to 5.16 nmol/hr/mg protein. The normal value for SAHase is 4.18± 1.9 nmol/hr/mg protein.
The optimal dosage and schedule of administration of **ADAGEN®** (pegademase bovine) Injection should be established for each patient, based on monitoring of plasma ADA activity levels (trough levels before maintenance injection), biochemical markers of ADA deficiency (primarily red cell dATP content), and parameters of immune function. Since improvement in immune function follows correction of metabolic abnormalities, maintenance dosage in individual patients should be aimed at achieving the following biochemical goals: 1) maintain plasma ADA activity (trough levels) in the range of 15–35 µmol/hr/mL (assayed at 37°C); and 2) decline in erythrocyte dATP to ≤ 0.005–0.015 µmol/mL packed erythrocytes, or ≤ 1% of the total erythrocyte adenine nucleotide (ATP + dATP) content, with a normal ATP level, as measured in a pre-injection sample.
In vitro immunologic data (lymphocyte response to mitogens and lymphocyte surface antigens) were obtained, but their clinical significance is unknown. Prior to treatment with **ADAGEN®** (pegademase bovine) Injection, immune status was significantly below normal, as indicated by <10% of normal mitogen responses and circulating mononuclear cells bearing T-cell surface antigens. These parameters improved, though not always to normal, within 2 to 6 months of therapy.

INDICATIONS AND USAGE

ADAGEN® (pegademase bovine) Injection is indicated for enzyme replacement therapy for adenosine deaminase (ADA) deficiency in patients with severe combined immunodeficiency disease (SCID) who are not suitable candidates for—or who have failed—bone marrow transplantation. **ADAGEN®** (pegademase bovine) Injection is recommended for use in infants from birth or in children of any age at the time of diagnosis. **ADAGEN®** (pegademase bovine) Injection is not intended as a replacement for HLA indentical bone marrow transplant therapy. **ADAGEN®** (pegademase bovine) Injection is also not intended to replace continued close medical supervision and the initiation of appropriate diagnostic tests and therapy (e.g., antibiotics, nutrition, oxygen, gammaglobulin) as indicated for intercurrent illnesses.

CONTRAINDICATIONS

There is no evidence to support the safety and efficacy of **ADAGEN®** (pegademase bovine) Injection as preparatory or support therapy for bone marrow transplantation. Since **ADAGEN®** (pegademase bovine) Injection is administered by intramuscular injection, it should be used with caution in patients with thrombocytopenia and should not be used if thrombocytopenia is severe.

PRECAUTIONS

Warnings

At present, testing prior to distribution may not assure the initial and continuing potency of each new lot of **ADAGEN®** (pegademase bovine) Injection. Any laboratory or clinical indication of a decrease in potency of **ADAGEN®** (pegademase bovine) Injection should be reported immediately by telephone to ENZON, Inc. Telephone 732 980-4560. Fax 732 980-4566.

General

There have been no reports of hypersensitivity reactions in patients who have been treated with **ADAGEN®** (pegademase bovine) Injection.
One of 12 patients showed an enhanced rate of clearance of plasma ADA activity after 5 months of therapy at 15 U/kg/week. Enhanced clearance was correlated with the appearance of an antibody that directly inhibited both unmodified ADA and **ADAGEN®** (pegademase bovine) Injection. Subsequently, the patient was treated with twice weekly intramuscular injections at an increased dose of 20 U/kg, or a total weekly dose of 40 U/kg. No adverse effects were observed at the higher dose and effective levels of plasma ADA were restored. After 4 months, the patient returned to a weekly dosage schedule of 20 U/kg and effective plasma levels have been maintained.
Appropriate care to protect immune deficient patients should be maintained until improvement in immune function has been documented. The degree of immune function improvement may vary from patient to patient and, therefore, each patient will require appropriate care consistent with immunologic status.

Laboratory Tests

The treatment of SCID associated with ADA deficiency with **ADAGEN®]** (pegademase bovine) Injection should be monitored by measuring plasma ADA activity and red blood cell dATP levels.

Continued on next page

Adagen—Cont.

Plasma ADA activity and red cell dATP should be determined prior to treatment. Once treatment with **ADAGEN®** (pegademase bovine) Injection has been initiated, a desirable range of plasma ADA activity (trough level before maintenance injection) should be 15–35 µmol/hr/mL. This minimum trough level will ensure that plasma ADA activity from injection to injection is maintained above the level of total erythrocyte ADA activity in the blood of normal individuals.
Plasma ADA activity (pre-injection) should be determined every 1–2 weeks during the first 8–12 weeks of treatment in order to establish an effective dose of **ADAGEN®** (pegademase bovine) Injection. After two months of maintenance treatment with **ADAGEN®** (pegademase bovine) Injection, red cell dATP levels should decrease to a range of ≤0.005 to 0.015 µmol/mL. The normal value of dATP is below 0.001 µmol/mL. Once the level of dATP has fallen adequately, it should be measured 2–4 times a year during the remainder of the first year and 2–3 times a year thereafter, assuming no interruption in therapy.
Between 3 and 9 months, plasma ADA should be determined twice a month, then monthly until after 18–24 months of treatment with **ADAGEN®** (pegademase bovine) Injection.
Patients who have successfully been maintained on therapy for two years should continue to have plasma ADA measured every 2–4 months and red cell dATP measured twice yearly. More frequent monitoring would be necessary if therapy were interrupted or if an enhanced rate of clearance of plasma ADA activity develops.
Once effective ADA plasma levels have been established, should a patient's plasma ADA activity level fall below 10 µmol/hr/mL (which cannot be attributed to improper dosing, sample handling or antibody development) then all patients receiving this lot of **ADAGEN®** (pegademase bovine) Injection will be required to have a blood sample for plasma ADA determination taken prior to their next injection of **ADAGEN®** (pegademase bovine) Injection. The index patient will require re-testing for determination of plasma ADA activity prior to his/her next injection of **ADAGEN®** (pegademase bovine) Injection. If this value, as well as the value from one of the other patients from a different site, is less than 10 µmol/hr/mL then the lot in use will be recalled and replaced with a new clinical lot by ENZON, Inc.
Immune function, including the ability to produce antibodies, generally improves after 2–6 months of therapy, and matures over a longer period. Compared with the natural history of combined immunodeficiency disease due to ADA deficiency, a trend toward diminished frequency of opportunistic infections and fewer complications of infections has occurred in patients receiving **ADAGEN®** (pegademase bovine) Injection. However, the lag between the correction of the metabolic abnormalities and improved immune function with a trend toward diminished frequency of infections and complications of infection is variable, and has ranged from a few weeks to approximately 6 months. Improvement in the general clinical status of the patient may be gradual (as evidenced by improvement in various clinical parameters) but should be apparent by the end of the first year of therapy.
Antibody to **ADAGEN®** (pegademase bovine) Injection may develop in patients and may result in more rapid clearance of **ADAGEN®** (pegademase bovine) Injection. Antibody to **ADAGEN®** (pegademase bovine) Injection should be suspected if a persistent fall in pre-injection levels of plasma ADA to ≤10 µmol/hr/mL occurs. If other causes for a decline in plasma ADA levels can be ruled out [such as improper storage of **ADAGEN®** (pegademase bovine) Injection vials (freezing or prolonged storage at temperatures above 8°C), or improper handling of plasma samples (e.g., repeated freezing and thawing during transport to laboratory)], then a specific assay for antibody to ADA and **ADAGEN®** (pegademase bovine) Injection (ELISA, enzyme inhibition) should be performed.
In patients undergoing treatment with **ADAGEN®** (pegademase bovine) Injection, a decline in immune function, with increased risk of opportunistic infections and complications of infection, will result from failure to maintain adequate levels of plasma ADA activity [whether due to the development of antibody to **ADAGEN®** (pegademase bovine) Injection, to improper calculation of **ADAGEN®** (pegademase bovine) Injection dosage, to interruption of treatment or to improper storage of **ADAGEN®** (pegademase bovine) Injection with subsequent loss of activity]. If a persistent decline in plasma ADA activity occurs, immune function and clinical status should be monitored closely and precautions should be taken to minimize the risk of infection. If antibody to ADA or **ADAGEN®** (pegademase bovine) Injection is found to be the cause of a persistent fall in plasma ADA activity, then adjustment in the dosage of **ADAGEN®** (pegademase bovine) Injection and other measures may be taken to induce tolerance and restore adequate ADA activity.

Drug Interactions
There are no known drug interactions with **ADAGEN®** (pegademase bovine) Injection. However, Vidarabine is a substrate for ADA and 2′-deoxycoformycin is a potent inhibitor of ADA. Thus, the activities of these drugs and **ADAGEN®** (pegademase bovine) Injection could be substantially altered if they are used in combination with one another.

Carcinogenesis, Mutagenesis, Impairment of Fertility
Long-term carcinogenic studies in animals have not been performed with **ADAGEN®** (pegademase bovine) Injection nor have studies been performed on impairment of fertility. **ADAGEN®** (pegademase bovine) Injection did not exhibit a mutagenic effect when tested against Salmonella typhimurium strains in the Ames assay.

Pregnancy
Pregnancy Category C. Animal reproduction studies have not been conducted with **ADAGEN®** (pegademase bovine) Injection. It is also not known whether **ADAGEN®** (pegademase bovine) Injection can cause fetal harm when administered to a pregnant woman or can affect reproduction capacity. **ADAGEN®** (pegademase bovine) Injection should be given to a pregnant woman only if clearly needed.

Nursing Mothers
It is not known whether **ADAGEN®** (pegademase bovine) Injection is excreted in human milk. Because many drugs are excreted in human milk, caution should be exercised when **ADAGEN®** (pegademase bovine) Injection is administered to a nursing woman.

ADVERSE REACTIONS

Clinical experience with **ADAGEN®** (pegademase bovine) Injection has been limited. The following adverse reactions have been reported: headache in one patient and pain at the injection site in two patients.

OVERDOSAGE

There is no documented experience with **ADAGEN®** (pegademase bovine) Injection overdosage. An intraperitoneal dose of 50,000 U/kg of **ADAGEN®** (pegademase bovine) Injection in mice resulted in weight loss up to 9%.

DOSAGE AND ADMINISTRATION

Before prescribing **ADAGEN®** (pegademase bovine) Injection the physician should be thoroughly familiar with the details of this prescribing information. For further information concerning the essential monitoring of **ADAGEN®** (pegademase bovine) Injection therapy, the prescribing physician should contact ENZON, Inc., 20 Kingsbridge Road, Piscataway, NJ 08854. Telephone 732 980-4560. Fax 732 980-4566.
ADAGEN® (pegademase bovine) Injection is recommended for use in infants from birth or in children of any age at the time of diagnosis.
Parenteral drug products should be inspected visually for particulate matter and discoloration prior to administration, whenever solution and container permits.
ADAGEN® (pegademase bovine) Injection should not be diluted nor mixed with any other drug prior to administration.
ADAGEN® (pegademase bovine) Injection should be administered every 7 days as an intramuscular injection. The dosage of **ADAGEN®** (pegademase bovine) Injection should be individualized. The recommended dosing schedule is 10 U/kg for the first dose, 15 U/kg for the second dose, and 20 U/kg for the third dose. The usual maintenance dose is 20 U/kg per week. Further increases of 5 U/kg/week may be necessary, but a maximum single dose of 30 U/kg should not be exceeded. Plasma levels of ADA more than twice the upper limit of 35 µmol/hr/mL have occurred on occasion in several patients, and have been maintained for several weeks in one patient who received twice weekly injections (20 U/kg per dose) of **ADAGEN®** (pegademase bovine) Injection. No adverse effects have been observed at these higher levels; there is no evidence that maintaining pre-injection plasma ADA above 35 µmol/hr/mL produces any additional clinical benefits.
Dose proportionality has not been established and patients should be closely monitored when the dosage is increased.
ADAGEN® (pegademase bovine) Injection is not recommended for intravenous administration. The optimal dosage and schedule of administration should be established for each patient based on monitoring of plasma ADA activity levels (trough levels before maintenance injection) and biochemical markers of ADA deficiency (primarily red cell dATP content). Since improvement in immune function follows correction of metabolic abnormalities, maintenance dosage in individual patients should be aimed at achieving the following biochemical goals: 1) maintain plasma ADA activity (trough levels before maintenance injection) in the range of 15–35 µmol/hr/mL (assayed at 37°C); and 2) decline in erythrocyte dATP to ≤0.005–0.015 µmol/mL packed erythrocytes, or ≤1% of the total erythrocyte adenine nucleotide (ATP + dATP) content, with a normal ATP level, as measured in a pre-injection sample. In addition, continued monitoring of immune function and clinical status is essential in any patient with a primary immunodeficiency disease and should be continued in patients undergoing treatment with **ADAGEN®** (pegademase bovine) Injection.

HOW SUPPLIED

ADAGEN® (pegademase bovine) Injection is a clear, colorless solution for intramuscular injection. Each vial contains 250 units/mL and is supplied as a 1.5 mL single-use vial, in boxes of 4 vials (NDC-57665-001-01).
Refrigerate. Store between +2°C and +8°C (36°F and 46°F). DO NOT FREEZE. **ADAGEN®** (pegademase bovine) Injection should not be stored at room temperature. This product should not be used if there are any indications that it may have been frozen.

REFERENCES

1. Hershfield MS, Buckley RH, Greenberg ML, et al. Treatment of adenosine deaminase deficiency with polyethylene glycol-modified adenosine deaminase. N Engl J Med 1987; 316:589–96.
2. Levy Y, Hershfield MS, Fernandez-Mejia C, Polmar ST, Scudiery D, Berger M, Sorensen RU. Adenosine deaminase deficiency with late onset of recurrent infections: response to treatment with polyethylene glycol-modified adenosine deaminase. J. Pediatr 1988; 113:312–17.
3. Kredich NM, Hershfield MS. Immunodeficiency diseases caused by adenosine deaminase deficiency and purine nucleoside phosphorylase deficiency. 6th ed. In: Scriver CR, Beaudet AL, Sly WS, Valle D, eds. The metabolic basis of inherited disease. New York: McGraw Hill, 1989; 1045–75.
4. Hirschhorn R. Inherited enzyme deficiencies and immunodeficiency: adenosine deaminase (ADA) and purine nucleoside phosphorylase (PNP) deficiencies. Clin Immunol Immunopathol 1986; 40:157–65.
5. Hirschhorn R, Roegner-Maniscalco V, Kuritsky L, Rosen FS. Bone marrow transplantation only partially restores purine metabolites to normal adenosine deaminase-deficient patients. J Clin Invest 1981; 68:1387–93.
6. Polmar AH, Stern RC, Schwartz AL, Wetzler EM, Chase PA, Hirschhorn R. Enzyme replacement therapy for adenosine deaminase deficiency and severe combined immunodeficiency. N Engl J Med 1976; 295:1337–43.
7. Rubinstein A, Hirschhorn R, Sicklick M, Murphy RA. In vivo and in vitro effects of thymosin and adenosine deaminase on adenosine-deaminase-deficient lymphocytes. N Engl J Med 1979; 300:387–92.
8. Hirschhorn R, Papageorgiou PS, Kesarwala HH, Taft LT. Amelioration of neurologic abnormalities after "enzyme replacement" in adenosine deaminase deficiency. N Engl J Med 1980; 303:377–80.
9. Hirshhorn R, Ratech H, Rubinstein A, et al. Increased excretion of modified adenine nucleosides by children with adenosine deaminase deficiency. Pediatr Res 1982; 16:362–9.
10. Polmar SH. Enzyme replacement and other biochemical approaches to the therapy of adenosine deaminase deficiency. In: Elliott K, Whelan J, eds. Enzyme defects and immune dysfunction. Amsterdam: Excerpta Medica, 1979; 213–30.

ESI Lederle Inc.

P.O. BOX 41502
PHILADELPHIA, PA 19101

Direct Inquiries to:
Professional Service
(610) 688-4400

For Emergency Medical Information Contact:
Day: (800) 934–5556 8:30 AM to 4:30 PM (Eastern Standard Time), Weekdays only
Night: (610) 688-4400 (Emergencies only; non-emergencies should wait until the next day)

For Medical/Pharmacy Inquiries on Marketed Products Call:
(800) 934–5556 8:30 AM to 4:30 PM
(Eastern Standard Time), Weekdays only

ESI Lederle Inc. was formerly known as ESI Pharma, Inc. Products previously listed under the ESI Pharma, Inc. heading are now products of ESI Lederle Inc. and are described below.

AYGESTIN® ℞

[ā-jĕs 'tĭn]
(norethindrone acetate tablets, USP)

Caution: Federal law prohibits dispensing without prescription.

WARNING:
THE USE OF Aygestin DURING THE FIRST FOUR MONTHS OF PREGNANCY IS NOT RECOMMENDED.
Progestational agents have been used beginning with the first trimester of pregnancy in an attempt to prevent habitual abortion. There is no adequate evidence that such use is effective when such drugs are given during the first four months of pregnancy. Furthermore, in the vast majority of women, the cause of abortion is a defective ovum which progestational agents could not be expected to influence. In addition, the use of progestational agents, with their uterine-relaxant properties, in patients with fertilized defective ova may cause a delay in spontaneous abortion. Therefore, the use of such drugs during the first four months of pregnancy is not recommended.
Several reports suggest an association between intrauterine exposure to progestational drugs in the first trimester of pregnancy and genital abnormalities in male and female fetuses. The risk of hypospadias, 5 to 8 per 1,000 male births in the general population, may be approximately doubled with exposure to these drugs. There are insufficient data to quantify the risk to exposed female fetuses, but insofar as some of these drugs induce mild virilization of the external genitalia of the female fetus, and because of the increased association of hypospadias in the male fetus, it is prudent to avoid the use of these drugs during the first trimester of pregnancy.

If the patient is exposed to Aygestin (norethindrone acetate tablets, USP) during the first four months of pregnancy or if she becomes pregnant while taking this drug, she should be apprised of the potential risks to the fetus.

DESCRIPTION

Aygestin (norethindrone acetate tablets, USP)—5 mg oral tablets.

Aygestin, (17-hydroxy-19-nor-17α-pregn-4-en-20-yn-3-one acetate), a synthetic, orally active progestin, is the acetic acid ester of norethindrone. It is a white, or creamy white, crystalline powder.

Aygestin Tablets contain the following inactive ingredients: lactose, magnesium stearate, and microcrystalline cellulose.

CLINICAL PHARMACOLOGY

Norethindrone acetate induces secretory changes in an estrogen-primed endometrium. It acts to inhibit the secretion of pituitary gonadotropins which, in turn, prevent follicular maturation and ovulation. On a weight basis, it is twice as potent as norethindrone.

INDICATIONS AND USAGE

Aygestin is indicated for the treatment of secondary amenorrhea, endometriosis, and abnormal uterine bleeding due to hormonal imbalance in the absence of organic pathology, such as submucous fibroids or uterine cancer.

CONTRAINDICATIONS

Thrombophlebitis, thromboembolic disorders, cerebral apoplexy, or a past history of these conditions.
Markedly impaired liver function or liver disease.
Known or suspected carcinoma of the breast.
Undiagnosed vaginal bleeding.
Missed abortion.
As a diagnostic test for pregnancy.

WARNINGS

1. Discontinue medication pending examination if there is a sudden partial or complete loss of vision or if there is sudden onset of proptosis, diplopia, or migraine. If examination reveals papilledema or retinal vascular lesions, medication should be withdrawn.
2. Because of the occasional occurrence of thrombophlebitis and pulmonary embolism in patients taking progestogens, the physician should be alert to the earliest manifestations of the disease.
3. Masculinization of the female fetus has occurred when progestogens have been used in pregnant women.

PRECAUTIONS

GENERAL PRECAUTIONS.

1. The pretreatment physical examination should include special reference to breasts and pelvic organs, as well as a Papanicolaou smear.
2. Because this drug may cause some degree of fluid retention, conditions which might be influenced by this factor, such as epilepsy, migraine, asthma, cardiac or renal dysfunctions, require careful observation.
3. In cases of breakthrough bleeding, as in all cases of irregular bleeding per vaginam, nonfunctional causes should be borne in mind. In cases of undiagnosed vaginal bleeding, adequate diagnostic measures are indicated.
4. Patients who have a history of psychic depression should be carefully observed and the drug discontinued if the depression recurs to a serious degree.
5. Any possible influence of prolonged progestogen therapy on pituitary, ovarian, adrenal, hepatic, or uterine functions awaits further study.
6. Concomitant Use in Estrogen Replacement Therapy: In postmenopausal estrogen replacement therapy, studies of the addition of a progestin for 7 or more days of a cycle of estrogen administration have reported a lowered incidence of endometrial hyperplasia. Morphological and biochemical studies of the endometrium suggest that 10 to 13 days of progestin are needed to provide maximal maturation of the endometrium and to eliminate any hyperplastic changes. Whether this will provide protection from endometrial carcinoma has not been clearly established. There are possible additional risks which may be associated with the inclusion of progestin in estrogen replacement regimens. Progestin therapy may have an adverse effect on lipid metabolism.
7. A decrease in glucose tolerance has been observed in a small percentage of patients on estrogen-progestogen combination drugs. The mechanism of this decrease is obscure. For this reason, diabetic patients should be carefully observed while receiving progestogen therapy.
8. The age of the patient constitutes no absolute limiting factor, although treatment with progestogens may mask the onset of the climacteric.
9. The pathologist should be advised of progestogen therapy when relevant specimens are submitted.

INFORMATION FOR THE PATIENT.

See text which appears at the end of this insert.

CARCINOGENESIS, MUTAGENESIS, AND IMPAIRMENT OF FERTILITY.

Some beagle dogs treated with medroxyprogesterone acetate developed mammary nodules. Although nodules occasionally appeared in control animals, they were intermittent in nature, whereas nodules in treated animals were larger and more numerous, and persisted. There is no general agreement as to whether the nodules are benign or malignant. Their significance with respect to humans has not been established.

PREGNANCY CATEGORY X.

See Boxed Warning.

NURSING MOTHERS.

Detectable amounts of progestogens have been identified in the milk of mothers receiving them. The effect of this on the nursing infant has not been determined.

PEDIATRIC USE.

Safety and effectiveness in pediatric patients have not been established.

ADVERSE REACTIONS

The following adverse reactions have been observed in women taking progestins:
Breakthrough bleeding.
Spotting.
Change in menstrual flow.
Amenorrhea.
Edema.
Changes in weight (decreases, increases).
Changes in cervical erosion and cervical secretions.
Cholestatic jaundice.
Rash (allergic) with and without pruritus.
Melasma or chloasma.
Mental depression.

Progestins may alter the result of pregnanediol determinations. The following laboratory results may be altered by the concomitant use of estrogens with progestins:
Hepatic function.
Coagulation tests—increase in prothrombin, factors VII, VIII, IX, and X.
Increase in PBI, BEI, and a decrease in T^3 uptake.
Reduced response to metyrapone test.

A statistically significant association has been demonstrated between use of estrogen-progestogen combination drugs and the following serious adverse reactions: thrombophlebitis, pulmonary embolism, and cerebral thrombosis and embolism. For this reason, patients on progestogen therapy should be carefully observed. Although available evidence is suggestive of an association, such a relationship has been neither confirmed nor refuted for the following serious adverse reactions:
Neuro-ocular lesions, *e.g.*, retinal thrombosis and optic neuritis.

The following adverse reactions have been observed in patients receiving estrogen-progestogen combination drugs:

1. Rise in blood pressure in susceptible individuals.
2. Premenstrual-like syndrome.
3. Changes in libido.
4. Changes in appetite.
5. Cystitis-like syndrome.
6. Headache.
7. Nervousness.
8. Dizziness.
9. Fatigue.
10. Backache.
11. Hirsutism.
12. Loss of scalp hair.
13. Erythema multiforme.
14. Erythema nodosum.
15. Hemorrhagic eruption.
16. Itching.

In view of these observations, patients on progestogen therapy should be carefully observed.

DOSAGE AND ADMINISTRATION

Therapy with Aygestin must be adapted to the specific indications and therapeutic response of the individual patient. This dosage schedule assumes the interval between menses to be 28 days.

Secondary amenorrhea, abnormal uterine bleeding due to hormonal imbalance in the absence of organic pathology: 2.5 to 10 mg Aygestin may be given daily for 5 to 10 days during the second half of the theoretical menstrual cycle to produce an optimum secretory transformation of an endometrium that has been adequately primed with either endogenous or exogenous estrogen.

Progestin withdrawal bleeding usually occurs within three to seven days after discontinuing Aygestin therapy. Patients with a past history of recurrent episodes of abnormal uterine bleeding may benefit from planned menstrual cycling with Aygestin.

Endometriosis: Initial daily dosage of 5 mg Aygestin for two weeks. Dosage should be increased by 2.5 mg per day every two weeks until 15 mg per day of Aygestin is reached. Therapy may be held at this level for six to nine months or until annoying breakthrough bleeding demands temporary termination.

HOW SUPPLIED

Each white, scored Aygestin® Tablet contains 5 mg norethindrone acetate, USP, in bottles of 50 (NDC 59911-5894-1).
Store at room temperature (approximately 25° C)
Dispense in a well-closed container as defined in the USP

INFORMATION FOR THE PATIENT

Your doctor has prescribed Aygestin (norethindrone acetate tablets, USP), a progestin, for you. Aygestin is similar to the progesterone hormones naturally produced by the body. Progestins are used to treat menstrual disorders and to test if the body is producing certain hormones.

Warning

Progesterone or progesterone-like drugs have been used to prevent miscarriage in the first few months of pregnancy. No adequate evidence is available to show that they are effective for this purpose. Furthermore, most cases of early miscarriage are due to causes which could not be helped by these drugs.

There is an increased risk of minor birth defects in children whose mothers take this drug during the first four months of pregnancy. Several reports suggest an association between mothers who take these drugs in the first trimester of pregnancy and genital abnormalities in male and female babies. The risk to the male baby is the possibility of being born with a condition in which the opening of the penis is on the underside rather than the tip of the penis (hypospadias). Hypospadias occurs in about 5 to 8 per 1,000 male births and is about doubled with exposure to these drugs. There is not enough information to quantify the risk to exposed female fetuses, but enlargement of the clitoris and fusion of the labia may occur, although rarely.

Therefore, since drugs of this type may induce mild masculinization of the external genitalia of the female fetus, as well as hypospadias in the male fetus, it is wise to avoid using the drug during the first trimester of pregnancy.

These drugs have been used as a test for pregnancy but such use is no longer considered safe because of possible damage to a developing baby. Also, more rapid methods for testing for pregnancy are now available.

If you take Aygestin (norethindrone acetate tablets, USP) and later find you were pregnant when you took it, be sure to discuss this with your doctor as soon as possible.

HOW SUPPLIED

Aygestin® (norethindrone acetate tablets, USP)—white, scored 5 mg tablets, in bottles of 50, for oral administration.
ESI Lederle Inc.
Philadelphia, PA 19101
CI 4835-1 Revised March 6, 1996

Shown in Product Identification Guide, page 312

ESI Pharma, Inc.

P.O. BOX 41502
PHILADELPHIA, PA 19101

The name ESI Pharma, Inc. has been changed to ESI Lederle Inc. All products listed under the ESI Pharma company heading can now be found under ESI Lederle Inc. Please turn to page 1218 of this 2001 PDR.

Everett Laboratories, Inc.

29 SPRING STREET
WEST ORANGE, NEW JERSEY 07052

Direct Inquiries to:
Professional Service Department
Phone: (973) 324-0200
Fax: (973) 324-0795

CORTIC ear drops ℞

Each 1 ml contains:

Chloroxylenol	1 mg
Pramoxine HCl	10 mg
Hydrocortisone	10 mg

SUPPLIED

Plastic dropper vials of 10 ml.

RENAX® CAPLET ℞

Vitamin-Mineral formulation to meet the Nutritional Needs of the Renal Patient.

Each caplet contains:

Vitamin E	35 IU
Vitamin C	50 mg
Vitamin B_1 (Thiamine)	3 mg
Vitamin B_2 (Riboflavin)	2 mg
Niacin (as Niacinamide)	20 mg
Folic Acid	2.5 mg
Vitamin B_6	15 mg
Vitamin B_{12}	12 mcg
Biotin	300 mcg
Pantothenic Acid	10 mg
Zinc	20 mg

Continued on next page

Renax—Cont.

Selenium	70 mcg
Chromium (as Chromium Chloride)	200 mcg

SUPPLIED

Bottles of 90 imprinted EV0300

STROVITE® FORTE CAPLETS ℞

Therapeutic Multi-vitamin/Mineral Supplement
Sugar Free and Sodium Free

SUPPLIED

Bottles of 100 imprinted EV0204

STROVITE FORTE SYRUP ℞

Vitamin Mineral Supplement
Sugar, Sodium, and Yeast Free

SUPPLIED

Bottle 16 Oz.—Unit Dose 15 ml

TUSSAFED®-EX DROPS ℞

Sugar Free—Alcohol Free

Each dropperful (1 ml) contains:

Guaifenesin	50 mg
Dextromethorphan HBR	5 mg
Phenylephrine HCL	2.5 mg

SUPPLIED

Bottles of 1 fl. oz. (30 ml)

TUSSAFED®-EX SYRUP ℞

SUGAR Free – ALCOHOL Free

Each 5 mL contains:

Dextromethorphan HBR	10 MG
Guaifenesin	200 MG
Phenylephrine HCL	30 MG

SUPPLIED

16 oz

TUSSAFED-HC SYRUP ℂⅢ

Each 5 ml Contains:

Hydrocodone Bitarate	2.5 mg
(WARNING: MAY BE HABIT FORMING)	
Phenylephrine HCL	7.5 mg
Guaifenesin	50 mg

SUPPLIED

Bottle 16 Oz.

TUSSAFED®-LA CAPLETS ℞

Dye Free—Sugar Free
Lactose Free—Sodium Free

Each LA Caplet contains:

Guaifenesin	600 mg
Dextromethorphan HBR	30 mg
Pseudoephedrine HCL	60 mg

DOSAGE

6–12 yrs 1 Caplet every 12 hrs
12 yrs & older 1–2 Caplets every 12 hrs.

SUPPLIED

Bottle of 100 caplets—Imprinted EV 0650

VITAFOL Caplets ℞

Vitamins, Minerals, Iron, Folic Acid Supplement
Sugar Free

SUPPLIED

Boxes of 100 (10×10) Unit Dose Pack
Imprinted EV-0072

VITAFOL® — PN CAPLETS ℞

(PRENATAL)
Sugar, Sodium, Yeast Free

Vitamins, Minerals, Iron 65 MG
Folic Acid 1 MG,

SUPPLIED

Boxes of 100 (10×10) Unit Dose Pack
Imprinted EV0078

VITAFOL Syrup ℞

Vitamins, Minerals, Iron, Folic Acid Supplement
Sodium, Alcohol, and Yeast Free

SUPPLIED

Bottles of 16 oz.

FARO Pharmaceuticals, Inc.

135 ROUTE 202/206
BEDMINSTER, NJ 07921

Direct Inquiries to:
Customer Service
877-994-3276
Fax:
877-280-6677

IMURAN® ℞

[ĭm′ū-ran″]
(azathioprine)
50-mg Scored Tablets
100 mg (as the sodium salt) for I.V. injection, equivalent to 100 mg azathioprine sterile lyophilized material.

> **WARNING:** Chronic immunosuppression with this purine antimetabolite increases *risk of neoplasia* in humans. Physicians using this drug should be very familiar with this risk as well as with the mutagenic potential to both men and women and with possible hematologic toxicities. See WARNINGS.

DESCRIPTION

IMURAN (azathioprine), an immunosuppressive antimetabolite, is available in tablet form for oral administration and 100-mg vials for intravenous injection. Each scored tablet contains 50 mg azathioprine and the inactive ingredients lactose, magnesium stearate, potato starch, povidone, and stearic acid. Each 100-mg vial contains azathioprine, as the sodium salt, equivalent to 100 mg azathioprine sterile lyophilized material and sodium hydroxide to adjust pH.
Azathioprine is chemically 6-[(1-methyl-4-nitro-1*H*-imidazol-5-yl)thio]-1*H*-purine. The structural formula of azathioprine is:

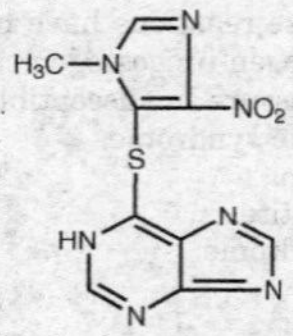

It is an imidazolyl derivative of 6-mercaptopurine and many of its biological effects are similar to those of the parent compound.
Azathioprine is insoluble in water, but may be dissolved with addition of one molar equivalent of alkali. The sodium salt of azathioprine is sufficiently soluble to make a 10 mg/mL water solution which is stable for 24 hours at 59° to 77°F (15° to 25°C). Azathioprine is stable in solution at neutral or acid pH but hydrolysis to mercaptopurine occurs in excess sodium hydroxide (0.1N), especially on warming. Conversion to mercaptopurine also occurs in the presence of sulfhydryl compounds such as cysteine, glutathione, and hydrogen sulfide.

CLINICAL PHARMACOLOGY

Metabolism:[1] Azathioprine is well absorbed following oral administration. Maximum serum radioactivity occurs at 1 to 2 hours after oral ^{35}S-azathioprine and decays with a half-life of 5 hours. This is not an estimate of the half-life of azathioprine itself, but is the decay rate for all ^{35}S-containing metabolites of the drug. Because of extensive metabolism, only a fraction of the radioactivity is present as azathioprine. Usual doses produce blood levels of azathioprine, and of mercaptopurine derived from it, which are low ($<$1 mcg/mL). Blood levels are of little predictive value for therapy since the magnitude and duration of clinical effects correlate with thiopurine nucleotide levels in tissues rather than with plasma drug levels. Azathioprine and mercaptopurine are moderately bound to serum proteins (30%) and are partially dialyzable.
Azathioprine is cleaved in vivo to mercaptopurine. Both compounds are rapidly eliminated from blood and are oxidized or methylated in erythrocytes and liver; no azathioprine or mercaptopurine is detectable in urine after 8 hours. Conversion to inactive 6-thiouric acid by xanthine oxidase is an important degradative pathway, and the inhibition of this pathway in patients receiving allopurinol (ZYLOPRIM®) is the basis for the azathioprine dosage reduction required in these patients (see PRECAUTIONS: Drug Interactions). Proportions of metabolites are different in individual patients, and this presumably accounts for variable magnitude and duration of drug effects. Renal clearance is probably not important in predicting biological effectiveness or toxicities, although dose reduction is practiced in patients with poor renal function.
Homograft Survival:[1,2] Summary information from transplant centers and registries indicates relatively universal use of IMURAN with or without other immunosuppressive agents.[3,4,5] Although the use of azathioprine for inhibition of renal homograft rejection is well established, the mechanism(s) for this action are somewhat obscure. The drug suppresses hypersensitivities of the cell-mediated type and causes variable alterations in antibody production. Suppression of T-cell effects, including ablation of T-cell suppression, is dependent on the temporal relationship to antigenic stimulus or engraftment. This agent has little effect on established graft rejections or secondary responses.
Alterations in specific immuno responses or immunologic functions in transplant recipients are difficult to relate specifically to immunosuppression by azathioprine. These patients have subnormal responses to vaccines, low numbers of T-cells, and abnormal phagocytosis by peripheral blood cells, but their mutogenic responses, serum immunoglobulins, and secondary antibody responses are usually normal.
Immunoinflammatory Response: Azathioprine suppresses disease manifestations as well as underlying pathology in animal models of autoimmune disease. For example, the severity of adjuvant arthritis is reduced by azathioprine.
The mechanisms whereby azathioprine affects autoimmune diseases are not known. Azathioprine is immunosuppressive, delayed hypersensitivity and cellular cytotoxicity tests being suppressed to a greater degree than are antibody responses. In the rat model of adjuvant arthritis, azathioprine has been shown to inhibit the lymph node hyperplasia which precedes the onset of the signs of the disease. Both the immunosuppressive and therapeutic effects in animal models are dose-related. Azathioprine is considered a slow-acting drug and effects may persist after the drug has been discontinued.

INDICATIONS AND USAGE

IMURAN is indicated as an adjunct for the prevention of rejection in renal homotransplantation. It is also indicated for the management of severe, active rheumatoid arthritis unresponsive to rest, aspirin, or other nonsteroidal anti-inflammatory drugs, or to agents in the class of which gold is an example.
Renal Homotransplantation: IMURAN is indicated as an adjunct for the prevention of rejection in renal homotransplantation. Experience with over 16,000 transplants shows a 5-year patient survival of 35% to 55%, but this is dependent on donor, match for HLA antigens, anti-donor or anti-B-cell alloantigen antibody, and other variables. The effect of IMURAN on these variables has not been tested in controlled trials.
Rheumatoid Arthritis:[8,7] IMURAN is indicated only in adult patients meeting criteria for classic or definite rheumatoid arthritis as specified by the American Rheumatism Association.[8] IMURAN should be restricted to patients with severe, active and erosive disease not responsive to conventional management including rest, aspirin, or other nonsteroidal drugs, or to agents in the class of which gold is an example. Rest, physiotherapy, and salicylates should be continued while IMURAN is given, but it may be possible to reduce the dose of corticosteroids in patients on IMURAN. The combined use of IMURAN with gold, antimalarials, or penicillamine has not been studied for either added benefit or unexpected adverse effects. The use of IMURAN with these agents cannot be recommended.

CONTRAINDICATIONS

IMURAN should not be given to patients who have shown hypersensitivity to the drug.
IMURAN should not be used for treating rheumatoid arthritis in pregnant women.
Patients with rheumatoid arthritis previously treated with alkylating agents (cyclophosphamide, chlorambucil, melphalan, or others) may have a prohibitive risk of neoplasia if treated with IMURAN.[9]

WARNINGS

Severe *leukopenia and/or thrombocytopenia* may occur in patients on IMURAN. Macrocytic anemia and severe bone marrow depression may also occur. Hematologic toxicities are dose-related and may be more severe in renal transplant patients whose homograft is undergoing rejection. It is suggested that patients on IMURAN have complete blood counts, including platelet counts, weekly during the first month, twice monthly for the second and third months of treatment, then monthly or more frequently if dosage alterations or other therapy changes are necessary. Delayed hematologic suppression may occur. Prompt reduction in dosage or temporary withdrawal of the drug may be necessary if there is a rapid fall in or persistently low leukocyte count, or other evidence of bone marrow depression. Leukopenia does not correlate with therapeutic effect; therefore the dose should not be increased intentionally to lower the white blood cell count.
Serious infections are a constant hazard for patients receiving chronic immunosuppression, especially for homograft recipients. Fungal, viral, bacterial, and protozoal infections may be fatal and should be treated vigorously. Reduction of azathioprine dosage and/or use of other drugs should be considered.

IMURAN is mutagenic in animals and humans, carcinogenic in animals, and may increase the patient's *risk of neoplasia*. Renal transplant patients are known to have an increased risk of malignancy, predominantly skin cancer and reticulum cell or lymphomatous tumors.[10] The risk of post-transplant lymphomas may be increased in patients who receive aggressive treatment with immunosuppressive drugs.[11] The degree of immunosuppression is determined, not only by the immunosuppressive regimen, but also by a number of other patient factors. The number of immunosuppressive agents may not necessarily increase the risk of post-transplant lymphomas. However, transplant patients who receive multiple immunosuppressive agents may be at risk for over-immunosuppression; therefore, immunosuppressive drug therapy should be maintained at the lowest effective levels. Information is available on the spontaneous neoplasia risk in rheumatoid arthritis,[12,13] and on neoplasia following immunosuppressive therapy of other autoimmune diseases.[14,15] It has not been possible to define the precise risk of neoplasia due to IMURAN.[16] The data suggest the risk may be elevated in patients with rheumatoid arthritis, though lower than for renal transplant patients.[11,13] However, acute myelogenous leukemia as well as solid tumors have been reported in patients with rheumatoid arthritis who have received azathioprine. Data on neoplasia in patients receiving IMURAN can be found under ADVERSE REACTIONS.

IMURAN has been reported to cause temporary depression in spermatogenesis and reduction in sperm viability and sperm count in mice at doses 10 times the human therapeutic dose;[17] a reduced percentage of fertile matings occurred when animals received 5 mg/kg.[18]

Pregnancy: Pregnancy Category D. IMURAN can cause fetal harm when administered to a pregnant woman. IMURAN should not be given during pregnancy without careful weighing of risk versus benefit. Whenever possible, use of IMURAN in pregnant patients should be avoided. This drug should not be used for treating rheumatoid arthritis in pregnant women.[19]

IMURAN is teratogenic in rabbits and mice when given in doses equivalent to the human dose (5 mg/kg daily). Abnormalities included skeletal malformations and visceral anomalies.[18]

Limited immunologic and other abnormalities have occurred in a few infants born of renal allograft recipients on IMURAN. In a detailed case report,[20] documented lymphopenia, diminished IgG and IgM levels, CMV infection, and a decreased thymic shadow were noted in an infant born to a mother receiving 150 mg azathioprine and 30 mg prednisone daily throughout pregnancy. At 10 weeks most features were normalized. DeWitte et al[21] reported pancytopenia and severe immune deficiency in a preterm infant whose mother received 125 mg azathioprine and 12.5 mg prednisone daily. There have been two published reports of abnormal physical findings. Williamson and Karp[22] described an infant born with preaxial polydactyly whose mother received azathioprine 200 mg daily and prednisone 20 mg every other day during pregnancy. Tallent et al[23] described an infant with a large myelomeningocele in the upper lumbar region, bilateral dislocated hips, and bilateral tallpes equinovarus. The father was on long-term azathioprine therapy.

Benefit versus risk must be weighed carefully before use of IMURAN in patients of reproductive potential. There are no adequate and well-controlled studies in pregnant women. If this drug is used during pregnancy or if the patient becomes pregnant while taking this drug, the patient should be apprised of the potential hazard to the fetus. Women of childbearing age should be advised to avoid becoming pregnant.

PRECAUTIONS

General: A gastrointestinal hypersensitivity reaction characterized by severe nausea and vomiting has been reported.[24,25,26] These symptoms may also be accompanied by diarrhea, rash, fever, malaise, myalgias, elevations in liver enzymes, and occasionally, hypotension. Symptoms of gastrointestinal toxicity most often develop within the first several weeks of therapy with IMURAN and are reversible upon discontinuation of the drug. The reaction can recur within hours after rechallenge with a single dose of IMURAN.

Information for Patients: Patients being started on IMURAN should be informed of the necessity of periodic blood counts while they are receiving the drug and should be encouraged to report any unusual bleeding or bruising to their physician. They should be informed of the danger of infection while receiving IMURAN and asked to report signs and symptoms of infection to their physician. Careful dosage instructions should be given to the patient, especially when IMURAN is being administered in the presence of impaired renal function or concomitantly with allopurinol (see Drug Interactions subsection and DOSAGE AND ADMINISTRATION). Patients should be advised of the potential risks of the use of IMURAN during pregnancy and during the nursing period. The increased risk of neoplasia following therapy with IMURAN should be explained to the patient.

Laboratory Tests: See WARNINGS and ADVERSE REACTIONS sections.

Drug Interactions: ***Use with Allopurinol:*** The principal pathway for detoxification of IMURAN is inhibited by allopurinol. Patients receiving IMURAN and allopurinol concomitantly should have a dose reduction of IMURAN, to approximately $^1/_2$ to $^1/_4$ the usual dose.

Use with Other Agents Affecting Myelopoesis: Drugs which may affect leukocyte production, including cotrimoxazole, may lead to exaggerated leukopenia, especially in renal transplant recipients.[27]

Use with Angiotensin-Converting Enzyme Inhibitors: The use of angiotensin-converting enzyme inhibitors to control hypertension in patients on azathioprine has been reported to induce anemia and severe leukopenia.[28]

Use with Warfarin: IMURAN may inhibit the anticoagulant effect of warfarin.

Carcinogenesis, Mutagenesis, Impairment of Fertility: See WARNINGS section.

Pregnancy: ***Teratogenic Effects:*** Pregnancy Category D. See WARNINGS section.

Nursing Mothers: The use of IMURAN in nursing mothers is not recommended. Azathioprine or its metabolites are transferred at low levels, both transplacentally and in breast milk.[29,30,31] Because of the potential for tumorigenicity shown for azathioprine, a decision should be made whether to discontinue nursing or discontinue the drug, taking into account the importance of the drug to the mother.

Pediatric Use: Safety and efficacy of azathioprine in pediatric patients have not been established.

ADVERSE REACTIONS

The principal and potentially serious toxic effects of IMURAN are hematologic and gastrointestinal. The risks of secondary infection and neoplasia are also significant (see WARNINGS). The frequency and severity of adverse reactions depend on the dose and duration of IMURAN as well as on the patient's underlying disease or concomitant therapies. The incidence of hematologic toxicities and neoplasia encountered in groups of renal homograft recipients is significantly higher than that in studies employing IMURAN for rheumatoid arthritis. The relative incidences in clinical studies are summarized below:

Toxicity	Renal Homograft	Rheumatoid Arthritis
Leukopenia (any degree)	>50%	28%
<2500 cells/mm^3	16%	5.3%
Infections	20%	<1%
Neoplasia		*
Lymphoma	0.5%	
Others	2.8%	

*Data on the rate and risk of neoplasia among persons with rheumatoid arthritis treated with azathioprine are limited. The incidence of lymphoproliferative disease in patients with RA appears to be significantly higher than that in the general population.[12] In one completed study, the rate of lymphoproliferative disease in RA patients receiving higher than recommended doses of azathioprine (5 mg/kg per day) was 1.8 cases per 1000 patient-years of follow-up, compared with 0.8 cases per 1000 patient-years of follow-up in those not receiving azathioprine.[13] However, the proportion of the increased risk attributable to the azathioprine dosage or to other therapies (i.e., alkylating agents) received by patients treated with azathioprine cannot be determined.

Hematologic: Leukopenia and/or thrombocytopenia are dose-dependent and may occur late in the course of therapy with IMURAN. Dose reduction or temporary withdrawal allows reversal of these toxicities. Infection may occur as a secondary manifestation of bone marrow suppression or leukopenia, but the incidence of infection in renal homotransplantation is 30 to 60 times that in rheumatoid arthritis. Macrocytic anemia and/or bleeding have been reported.

There are rare individuals with an inherited deficiency of the enzyme thiopurine methyltransferase (TPMT) who may be unusually sensitive to the myelosuppressive effect of azathioprine and prone to developing rapid bone marrow suppression following the initiation of treatment with IMURAN.

Gastrointestinal: Nausea and vomiting may occur within the first few months of therapy with IMURAN, and occurred in approximately 12% of 676 rheumatoid arthritis patients. The frequency of gastric disturbance often can be reduced by administration of the drug in divided doses and/or after meals. However, in some patients, nausea and vomiting may be severe and may be accompanied by symptoms such as diarrhea, fever, malaise, and myalgias (see PRECAUTIONS). Vomiting with abdominal pain may occur rarely with a hypersensitivity pancreatitis. Hepatotoxicity manifest by elevation of serum alkaline phosphatase, bilirubin, and/or serum transaminases is known to occur following azathioprine use, primarily in allograft recipients. Hepatotoxicity has been uncommon (less than 1%) in rheumatoid arthritis patients. Hepatotoxicity following transplantation most often occurs within 6 months of transplantation and is generally reversible after interruption of IMURAN. A rare, but life-threatening hepatic veno-occlusive disease associated with chronic administration of azathioprine has been described in transplant patients and in one patient receiving IMURAN for panuveitis.[32,33,34] Periodic measurement of serum transaminases, alkaline phosphatase, and bilirubin is indicated for early detection of hepatotoxicity. If hepatic veno-occlusive disease is clinically suspected, IMURAN should be permanently withdrawn.

Others: Additional side effects of low frequency have been reported. These include skin rashes, alopecia, fever, arthralgias, diarrhea, steatorrhea, negative nitrogen balance, and reversible interstitial pneumonitis.

OVERDOSAGE

The oral LD_{50}s for single doses of IMURAN in mice and rats are 2500 mg/kg and 400 mg/kg, respectively. Very large doses of this antimetabolite may lead to marrow hypoplasia, bleeding, infection, and death. About 30% of IMURAN is bound to serum proteins, but approximately 45% is removed during an 8-hour hemodialysis.[35] A single case has been reported of a renal transplant patient who ingested a single dose of 7500 mg IMURAN. The immediate toxic reactions were nausea, vomiting, and diarrhea, followed by mild leukopenia and mild abnormalities in liver function. The white blood cell count, SGOT, and bilirubin returned to normal 6 days after the overdose.

DOSAGE AND ADMINISTRATION

Renal Homotransplantation: The dose of IMURAN required to prevent rejection and minimize toxicity will vary with individual patients; this necessitates careful management. The initial dose is usually 3 to 5 mg/kg daily, beginning at the time of transplant. IMURAN is usually given as a single daily dose on the day of, and in a minority of cases 1 to 3 days before, transplantation. IMURAN is often initiated with the intravenous administration of the sodium salt, with subsequent use of labels (at the same dose level) after the postoperative period. Intravenous administration of the sodium salt is indicated only in patients unable to tolerate oral medications. Dose reduction to maintenance levels of 1 to 3 mg/kg daily is usually possible. The dose of IMURAN should not be increased to toxic levels because of threatened rejection. Discontinuation may be necessary for severe hematologic or other toxicity, even if rejection of the homograft may be a consequence of drug withdrawal.

Rheumatoid Arthritis: IMURAN is usually given on a daily basis. The initial dose should be approximately 1.0 mg/kg (50 to 100 mg) given as a single dose or on a twice-daily schedule. The dose may be increased, beginning at 6 to 8 weeks and thereafter by steps at 4-week intervals, if there are no serious toxicities and if initial response is unsatisfactory. Dose increments should be 0.5 mg/kg daily, up to a maximum dose of 2.5 mg/kg per day. Therapeutic response occurs after several weeks of treatment, usually 6 to 8; an adequate trial should be a minimum of 12 weeks. Patients not improved after 12 weeks can be considered refractory. IMURAN may be continued long-term in patients with clinical response, but patients should be monitored carefully, and gradual dosage reduction should be attempted to reduce risk of toxicities.

Maintenance therapy should be at the lowest effective dose, and the dose given can be lowered decrementally with changes of 0.5 mg/kg or approximately 25 mg daily every 4 weeks while other therapy is kept constant. The optimum duration of maintenance IMURAN has not been determined. IMURAN can be discontinued abruptly, but delayed effects are possible.

Use in Renal Dysfunction: Relatively oliguric patients, especially those with tubular necrosis in the immediate postcadaveric transplant period, may have delayed clearance of IMURAN or its metabolites, may be particularly sensitive to this drug, and are usually given lower doses.

Parenteral Administration: Add 10 mL of Sterile Water for Injection, and swirl until a clear solution results. This solution, equivalent to 100 mg azathioprine, is for intravenous use only; it has a pH of approximately 9.6, and it should be used within 24 hours. Further dilution into sterile saline or dextrose is usually made for infusion; the final volume depends on time for the infusion, usually 30 to 60 minutes, but as short as 5 minutes and as long as 8 hours for the daily dose.

Parenteral drug products should be inspected visually for particulate matter and discoloration prior to administration, whenever solution and container permit.

Procedures for proper handling and disposal of this immunosuppressive antimetabolite drug should be considered. Several guidelines on this subject have been published.[36–42] There is no general agreement that all of the procedures recommended in the guidelines are necessary or appropriate.

HOW SUPPLIED

50 mg overlapping circle-shaped, yellow to off-white, scored tablets imprinted with "IMURAN" and "50" on each tablet; bottle of 100 (NDC 60976-597-55).

Store at 15° to 25°C (59° to 77°F) in a dry place and protect from light.

20-mL vial, each containing the equivalent of 100 mg azathioprine (as the sodium salt) (NDC 60976-598-71).

Store at 15° to 25°C (59° to 77°F) and protect from light.

The sterile, lyophilized sodium salt is yellow, and should be dissolved in Sterile Water for Injection (see DOSAGE AND ADMINISTRATION: Parenteral Administration).

REFERENCES

1. Elion GB, Hitchings GH. Azathioprine. In: Sartonelli AC, Johns DG, eds. *Antineoplastic and Immunosuppressive Agents Pt II*. New York, NY: Springer Verlag; 1975: chap 48.
2. McIntosh J, Hansen P, Ziegler J, et al. Defective immune and phagocytic functions in uraemia and renal

Continued on next page

Imuran—Cont.

transplantation. *Int Arch Allergy Appl Immunol.* 1976;15:544–549.
3. Renal Transplant Registry Advisory Committee. The 12th report of the Human Renal Transplant Registry, *JAMA*. 1975;233:787–796.
4. McGeown M. Immunosuppression for kidney transplantation. *Lancet.* 1973;2:310–312.
5. Simmons RL, Thompson EJ, Yunis EJ, et al. 115 patients with first cadaver kidney transplants followed two to seven and a half years: a multifactorial analysis. *Am J Med.* 1977;62:234–242.
6. Fye K, Talal N. Cytotoxic drugs in the treatment of rheumatoid arthritis. *Ration Drug Ther.* 1975;9:1–5.
7. Davis JD, Muss HB, Turner RA. Cytotoxic agents in the treatment of rheumatoid arthritis. *South Med J.* 1978;71:58–64.
8. McEwen C. The diagnosis and differential diagnosis of rheumatoid arthritis. In: Hollander JL, ed. *Arthritis and Allied Conditions: A Textbook of Rheumatology*. 8th ed. Philadelphia, PA: Lea and Feblger; 1972;403–418.
9. Hoover R, Fraumenl JF, Drug-induced cancer. *Cancer.* 1981;47:1071–1080.
10. Hoover R, Fraumenl JF Jr. Risk of cancer in renal transplant recipients. *Lancet.* 1973;2:55–57.
11. Wilkinson AH, Smith JL, Hunsiker LG, et al. Increased frequency of post-transplant lymphomas in patients treated with cyclosporine, azathioprine, and prednisone. *Transplantation.* 1989;47:293–296.
12. Prior P, Symmons DPM, Hawkins CF, et al. Cancer morbidity in rheumatoid arthritis. *Ann Rheum Dis.* 1984;43: 128–131.
13. Silman AJ, Petrie J, Hazelman B, et al. Lymphoproliferative cancer and other malignancy in patients with rheumatoid arthritis treated with azathioprine: a 20 year follow up study. *Ann Rheum Dis.* 1988;47:988–992.
14. Louie S, Schwartz RS. Immunodeficiency and pathogenesis of lymphoma and leukemia. *Semin Hematol.* 1978;15:117–138.
15. Wang KK, Czaja AJ, Beaver SJ, et al. Extra hepatic malignancy following long-term immunosuppressive therapy of severe hepatitis B surface antigen-negative chronic active hepatitis. *Hepatology.* 1989;10:39–43.
16. Sieber SM, Adamson RH. Toxicity of antineoplastic agents in man: chromosomal aberrations, antifertility effects, congenital malformations, and carcinogenic potential. In: Klein G, Weinhouse S, eds. *Advances In Cancer Research*, New York, NY: Academic Press; 1975;22: 57–155.
17. Clark JM. The mutagenicity of azathioprine in mice. *Drosophila Melanogaster and Neurospora Crassa. Mut Res.* 1975;28:87–99.
18. Data on file, Glaxo Wellcome Inc.
19. Tagatz GE, Simmons RL. Pregnancy after renal transplantation. *Ann Intern Med.* 1975;82:113–114. Editorial Notes.
20. Coté CJ, Meuwissen HJ, Pickering RJ. Effects on the neonate of prednisone and azathioprine administered to the mother during pregnancy. *J. Pediatr.* 1974;85:324–328.
21. DeWitte DB, Buick MK, Stephen EC, et al. Neonatal pancytopenia and severe combined immunodeficiency associated with antenatal administration of azathioprine and prednisone. *J Pediatr.* 1984;105:625–628.
22. Williamson RA, Karp LE. Azathioprine teratogenicity; review of the literature and case report. *Obstet Gynecol.* 1981;58:247–250.
23. Tallent MB, Simmons RL, Najarian JS. Birth defects in child of male recipient of kidney transplant. *JAMA.* 1970;211:1854–1855.
24. Assini JF, Hamilton R, Strosberg JM. Adverse reactions to azathioprine mimicking gastroenteritis. *J. Rheumatol.* 1986;13:1117–1118.
25. Cochran D, Adamson AR, Halsey JP. Adverse reactions to azathioprine mimicking gastroenteritis. *J. Rheumatol.* 1987;14:1075.
26. Cox J, Daneshmend JK, Hawkey CJ, et al. Devastating diarrhoea caused by azathioprine: management difficulty in inflammatory bowel disease. *Gut.* 1988;29:686–688.
27. Bradley PP, Warden GD, Maxwell JG, et al. Neutropenia and thrombocytopenia in renal allograft recipients treated with trimethoprim-sulfamethoxazole. *Ann Int Med.* 1980;93:560–562.
28. Kirchertz EJ, Grone HJ, Rieger J, et al. Successful low dose captopril rechallenge following drug-induced leucopenia. *Lancet.* 1981;1:1362–1363.
29. Nelson D, Bugge C. Data on file, Glaxo Wellcome Inc.
30. Saarikowski S, Seppälä M. Immunosuppression during pregnancy: transmission of azathioprine and its metabolites from the mother to the fetus. *Am J Obstet Gynecol.* 1973;115:1100–1106.
31. Coulam CB, Moyer TP, Jiang NS, et al. Breast-feeding after renal transplantation. *Transplant Proc.* 1982;14: 605–609.
32. Read AE, Wiesner RH, LaBrecque DR, et al. Hepatic veno-occlusive disease associated with renal transplantation and azathioprine therapy. *Ann Intern Med.* 1986;104:651–655.
33. Katzka DA, Saul SH, Jorkasky D, et al. Azathioprine and hepatic venocclusive disease in renal transplant patients. *Gastroenterology.* 1986;90:446–454.
34. Weitz H, Gokel JM, Loeschke K, et al. Veno-occlusive disease of the liver in patients receiving immunosuppressive therapy. *Virchows Arch A.* 1982;395:245–255.
35. Schusziarra V, Zlekursch V, Schlamp R, et al. Pharmacokinetics of azathioprine under haemodialysis. *Int J Clin Pharmacol Biopharm.* 1976;14:298–302.
36. Recommendations for the safe handling of parenteral antineoplastic drugs. Washington, DC: Division of Safety. National Institutes of Health; 1983. US Dept of Health and Human Services, Public Health Service publication NIH 83-2621.
37. AMA Council on Scientific Affairs. Guidelines for handling parenteral antineoplastics. *JAMA.* 1985;253:1590–1591.
38. National Study Commission on Cytotoxic Exposure. Recommendation for handling cytotoxic agents. 1987. Available from Louis P. Jeffrey, Chairman, National Study Commission on Cytotoxic Exposure. Massachusetts College of Pharmacy and Allied Health Sciences, 179 Longwood Avenue, Boston, MA 02115.
39. Clinical Oncological Society of Australia. Guidelines and recommendations for safe handling of antineoplastic agents. *Med J Australia.* 1983;1:426–428.
40. Jones RB, Frank R, Mass T. Safe handling of chemotherapeutic agents: a report from the Mount Sinai Medical Center. *CA-A Cancer J for Clin.* 1983;33:258–263.
41. American Society of Hospital Pharmacists. ASHP technical assistance bulletin on handling cytotoxic and hazardous drugs. *Am J Hosp Pharm.* 1990;47:1033–1049.
42. Yodalken RE, Bennett D. OSHA work-practice guidelines for personnel dealing with cytotoxic (antineoplastic) drugs. *Am J Hosp Pharm.* 1986;43:1193–1204.

Manufactured by
Catalyticá Pharmaceuticals, Inc.
Greenville, NC 27834
For FARO Pharmaceuticals, Inc.
Bedminster, NJ 07921

Feb. 1999

Shown in Product Identification Guide, page 312

TRANDATE® ℞
(labetalol hydrochloride) Tablets

DESCRIPTION

TRANDATE Tablets are adrenergic receptor blocking agents that have both selective alpha$_1$-adrenergic and nonselective beta-adrenergic receptor blocking actions in a single substance.

Labetalol hydrochloride (HCl) is a racemate chemically designated as 2-hydroxy-5-[1-hydroxy-2-[(1-methyl-3-phenylpropyl)amino]ethyl]benzamide monohydrochloride, and it has the following structure:

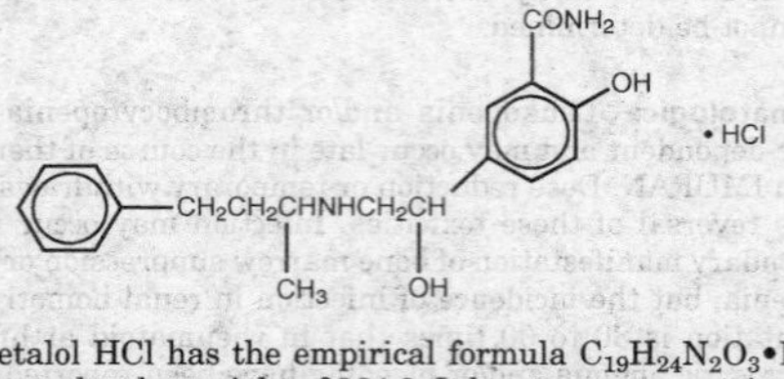

CONH$_2$
OH
• HCl
CH$_2$CH$_2$CHNHCH$_2$CH
CH$_3$ OH

Labetalol HCl has the empirical formula $C_{19}H_{24}N_2O_3$•HCl and a molecular weight of 364.9. It has two asymmetric centers and therefore exists as a molecular complex of two diastereoisomeric pairs. Dilevalol, the R,R′ stereoisomer, makes up 25% of racemic labetalol.

Labetalol HCl is a white or off-white crystalline powder, soluble in water.

TRANDATE Tablets contain 100, 200, or 300 mg of labetalol HCl and are taken orally. The tablets also contain the inactive ingredients corn starch, FD&C Yellow No. 6 (100- and 300-mg tablets only), hydroxypropyl methylcellulose, lactose, magnesium stearate, methylparaben, pregelatinized corn starch, propylparaben, sodium benzoate (200-mg tablet only), talc (100-mg tablet only), and titanium dioxide.

CLINICAL PHARMACOLOGY

Labetalol HCl combines both selective, competitive, alpha$_1$-adrenergic blocking and nonselective, competitive, beta-adrenergic blocking activity in a single substance. In man, the ratios of alpha- to beta-blockade have been estimated to be approximately 1:3 and 1:7 following oral and intravenous (IV) administration, respectively. Beta$_2$-agonist activity has been demonstrated in animals with minimal beta$_1$-agonist (ISA) activity detected. In animals, at doses greater than those required for alpha- or beta-adrenergic blockade, a membrane stabilizing effect has been demonstrated.

Pharmacodynamics: The capacity of labetalol HCl to block alpha receptors in man has been demonstrated by attenuation of the pressor effect of phenylephrine and by a significant reduction of the pressor response caused by immersing the hand in ice-cold water ("cold-pressor test"). Labetalol HCl's beta$_1$-receptor blockade in man was demonstrated by a small decrease in the resting heart rate, attenuation of tachycardia produced by isoproterenol or exercise, and by attenuation of the reflex tachycardia to the hypotension produced by amyl nitrite. Beta$_2$-receptor blockade was demonstrated by inhibition of the isoproterenol-induced fall in diastolic blood pressure. Both the alpha- and beta-blocking actions of orally administered labetalol HCl contribute to a decrease in blood pressure in hypertensive patients. Labetalol HCl consistently, in dose-related fashion, blunted increases in exercise-induced blood pressure and heart rate, and in their double product. The pulmonary circulation during exercise was not affected by labetalol HCl dosing.

Single oral doses of labetalol HCl administered to patients with coronary artery disease had no significant effect on sinus rate, intraventricular conduction, or QRS duration. The atrioventricular (A-V) conduction time was modestly prolonged in two of seven patients. In another study, IV labetalol HCl slightly prolonged A-V nodal conduction time and atrial effective refractory period with only small changes in heart rate. The effects on A-V nodal refractoriness were inconsistent.

Labetalol HCl produces dose-related falls in blood pressure without reflex tachycardia and without significant reduction in heart rate, presumably through a mixture of its alpha- and beta-blocking effects. Hemodynamic effects are variable, with small, nonsignificant changes in cardiac output seen in some studies but not others, and small decreases in total peripheral resistance. Elevated plasma renins are reduced.

Doses of labetalol HCl that controlled hypertension did not affect renal function in mildly to severely hypertensive patients with normal renal function.

Due to the alpha$_1$-receptor blocking activity of labetalol HCl, blood pressure is lowered more in the standing than in the supine position, and symptoms of postural hypotension (2%), including rare instances of syncope, can occur. Following oral administration, when postural hypotension has occurred, it has been transient and is uncommon when the recommended starting dose and titration increments are closely followed (see DOSAGE AND ADMINISTRATION). Symptomatic postural hypotension is most likely to occur 2 to 4 hours after a dose, especially following the use of large initial doses or upon large changes in dose.

The peak effects of single oral doses of labetalol HCl occur within 2 to 4 hours. The duration of effect depends upon dose, lasting at least 8 hours following single oral doses of 100 mg and more than 12 hours following single oral doses of 300 mg. The maximum, steady-state blood pressure response upon oral, twice-a-day dosing occurs within 24 to 72 hours.

The antihypertensive effect of labetalol has a linear correlation with the logarithm of labetalol plasma concentration, and there is also a linear correlation between the reduction in exercise-induced tachycardia occurring at 2 hours after oral administration of labetalol HCl and the logarithm of the plasma concentration.

About 70% of the maximum beta-blocking effect is present for 5 hours after the administration of a single oral dose of 400 mg with suggestion that about 40% remains at 8 hours.

The antianginal efficacy of labetalol HCl has not been studied. In 37 patients with hypertension and coronary artery disease, labetalol HCl did not increase the incidence or severity of angina attacks.

Exacerbation of angina and, in some cases, myocardial infarction and ventricular dysrhythmias have been reported after abrupt discontinuation of therapy with beta-adrenergic blocking agents in patients with coronary artery disease. Abrupt withdrawal of these agents in patients without coronary artery disease has resulted in transient symptoms, including tremulousness, sweating, palpitation, headache, and malaise. Several mechanisms have been proposed to explain these phenomena, among them increased sensitivity to catecholamines because of increased number of beta receptors.

Although beta-adrenergic receptor blockade is useful in the treatment of angina and hypertension, there are also situations in which sympathetic stimulation is vital. For example, in patients with severely damaged hearts, adequate ventricular function may depend on sympathetic drive. Beta-adrenergic blockade may worsen A-V block by preventing the necessary facilitating effects of sympathetic activity on conduction. Beta$_2$-adrenergic blockade results in passive bronchial constriction by interfering with endogenous adrenergic bronchodilator activity in patients subject to bronchospasm, and it may also interfere with exogenous bronchodilators in such patients.

Pharmacokinetics and Metabolism: Labetalol HCl is completely absorbed from the gastrointestinal tract with peak plasma levels occurring 1 to 2 hours after oral administration. The relative bioavailability of labetalol HCl tablets compared to an oral solution is 100%. The absolute bioavailability (fraction of drug reaching systemic circulation) of labetalol when compared to an IV infusion is 25%; this is due to extensive "first pass" metabolism. Despite "first-pass" metabolism, there is a linear relationship between oral doses of 100 to 3000 mg and peak plasma levels. The absolute bioavailability of labetalol is increased when administered with food.

The plasma half-life of labetalol following oral administration is about 6 to 8 hours. Steady-state plasma levels of labetalol during repetitive dosing are reached by about the third day of dosing. In patients with decreased hepatic or renal function, the elimination half-life of labetalol is not altered; however, the relative bioavailability in hepatically impaired patients is increased due to decreased "first-pass" metabolism.

The metabolism of labetalol is mainly through conjugation to glucuronide metabolites. These metabolites are present in plasma and are excreted in the urine and, via the bile, into the feces. Approximately 55% to 60% of a dose appears in the urine as conjugates or unchanged labetalol within the first 24 hours of dosing.

Labetalol has been shown to cross the placental barrier in humans. Only negligible amounts of the drug crossed the blood-brain barrier in animal studies. Labetalol is approximately 50% protein bound. Neither hemodialysis nor peritoneal dialysis removes a significant amount of labetalol HCl from the general circulation (<1%).

Elderly Patients: Some pharmacokinetic studies indicate that the elimination of labetalol is reduced in elderly patients. Therefore, although elderly patients may initiate therapy at the currently recommended dosage of 100 mg b.i.d., elderly patients will generally require lower maintenance dosages than nonelderly patients.

INDICATIONS AND USAGE

TRANDATE Tablets are indicated in the management of hypertension. TRANDATE Tablets may be used alone or in combination with other antihypertensive agents, especially thiazide and loop diuretics.

CONTRAINDICATIONS

TRANDATE Tablets are contraindicated in bronchial asthma, overt cardiac failure, greater-than-first-degree heart block, cardiogenic shock, severe bradycardia, other conditions associated with severe and prolonged hypotension, and in patients with a history of hypersensitivity to any component of the product (see WARNINGS).

Beta-blockers, even those with apparent cardioselectivity, should not be used in patients with a history of obstructive airway disease, including asthma.

WARNINGS

Hepatic Injury: Severe hepatocellular injury, confirmed by rechallenge in at least one case, occurs rarely with labetalol therapy. The hepatic injury is usually reversible, but hepatic necrosis and death have been reported. Injury has occurred after both short- and long-term treatment and may be slowly progressive despite minimal symptomatology. Similar hepatic events have been reported with a related research compound, dilevalol HCl, including two deaths. Dilevalol HCl is one of the four isomers of labetalol HCl. Thus, for patients taking labetalol, periodic determination of suitable hepatic laboratory tests would be appropriate. Appropriate laboratory testing should be done at the first symptom/sign of liver dysfunction (e.g., pruritus, dark urine, persistent anorexia, jaundice, right upper quadrant tenderness, or unexplained "flu-like" symptoms). If the patient has laboratory evidence of liver injury or jaundice, labetalol should be stopped and not restarted.

Cardiac Failure: Sympathetic stimulation is a vital component supporting circulatory function in congestive heart failure. Beta-blockade carries a potential hazard of further depressing myocardial contractility and precipitating more severe failure. Although beta-blockers should be avoided in overt congestive heart failure, if necessary, labetalol HCl can be used with caution in patients with a history of heart failure who are well compensated. Congestive heart failure has been observed in patients receiving labetalol HCl. Labetalol HCl does not abolish the inotropic action of digitalis on heart muscle.

In Patients Without a History of Cardiac Failure: In patients with latent cardiac insufficiency, continued depression of the myocardium with beta-blocking agents over a period of time can, in some cases, lead to cardiac failure. At the first sign or symptom of impending cardiac failure, patients should be fully digitalized and/or be given a diuretic, and the response should be observed closely. If cardiac failure continues despite adequate digitalization and diuretic, therapy with TRANDATE Tablets should be withdrawn (gradually, if possible).

Exacerbation of Ischemic Heart Disease Following Abrupt Withdrawal: Angina pectoris has not been reported upon labetalol HCl discontinuation. However, hypersensitivity to catecholamines has been observed in patients withdrawn from beta-blocker therapy; exacerbation of angina and, in some cases, myocardial infarction have occurred after *abrupt* discontinuation of such therapy. When discontinuing chronically administered TRANDATE Tablets, particularly in patients with ischemic heart disease, the dosage should be gradually reduced over a period of 1 to 2 weeks and the patient should be carefully monitored. If angina markedly worsens or acute coronary insufficiency develops, therapy with TRANDATE Tablets should be reinstituted promptly, at least temporarily, and other measures appropriate for the management of unstable angina should be taken. Patients should be warned against interruption or discontinuation of therapy without the physician's advice. Because coronary artery disease is common and may be unrecognized, it may be prudent not to discontinue therapy with TRANDATE Tablets abruptly in patients being treated for hypertension.

Nonallergic Bronchospasm (e.g., Chronic Bronchitis and Emphysema): Patients with bronchospastic disease should, in general, not receive beta-blockers. TRANDATE Tablets may be used with caution, however, in patients who do not respond to, or cannot tolerate, other antihypertensive agents. It is prudent, if TRANDATE Tablets are used, to use the smallest effective dose, so that inhibition of endogenous or exogenous beta-agonists is minimized.

Pheochromocytoma: Labetalol HCl has been shown to be effective in lowering blood pressure and relieving symptoms

	Labetalol HCl (n = 227) %	Placebo (n = 98) %	Propranolol (n = 84) %	Metoprolol (n = 49) %
Body as a whole				
Fatigue	5	0	12	12
Asthenia	1	1	1	0
Headache	2	1	1	2
Gastrointestinal				
Nausea	6	1	1	2
Vomiting	<1	0	0	0
Dyspepsia	3	1	1	0
Abdominal pain	0	0	1	2
Diarrhea	<1	0	2	0
Taste distortion	1	0	0	0
Central and peripheral nervous systems				
Dizziness	11	3	4	4
Paresthesia	<1	0	0	0
Drowsiness	<1	2	2	2
Autonomic nervous system				
Nasal stuffiness	3	0	0	0
Ejaculation failure	2	0	0	0
Impotence	1	0	1	3
Increased sweating	<1	0	0	0
Cardiovascular				
Edema	1	0	0	0
Postural hypotension	1	0	0	0
Bradycardia	0	0	5	12
Respiratory				
Dyspnea	2	0	1	2
Skin				
Rash	1	0	0	0
Special senses				
Vision abnormality	1	0	0	0
Vertigo	2	1	0	0

in patients with pheochromocytoma. However, paradoxical hypertensive responses have been reported in a few patients with this tumor; therefore, use caution when administering labetalol HCl to patients with pheochromocytoma.

Diabetes Mellitus and Hypoglycemia: Beta-adrenergic blockade may prevent the appearance of premonitory signs and symptoms (e.g., tachycardia) of acute hypoglycemia. This is especially important with labile diabetics. Beta-blockade also reduces the release of insulin in response to hyperglycemia; it may therefore be necessary to adjust the dose of antidiabetic drugs.

Major Surgery: The necessity or desirability of withdrawing beta-blocking therapy before major surgery is controversial. Protracted severe hypotension and difficulty in restarting or maintaining a heartbeat have been reported with beta-blockers. The effect of labetalol HCl's alpha-adrenergic activity has not been evaluated in this setting.

A synergism between labetalol HCl and halothane anesthesia has been shown (see PRECAUTIONS: Drug Interactions).

PRECAUTIONS

General: ***Impaired Hepatic Function***: TRANDATE Tablets should be used with caution in patients with impaired hepatic function since metabolism of the drug may be diminished.

Jaundice or Hepatic Dysfunction: (see WARNINGS).

Information for Patients: As with all drugs with beta-blocking activity, certain advice to patients being treated with labetalol HCl is warranted. This information is intended to aid in the safe and effective use of this medication. It is not a disclosure of all possible adverse or intended effects. While no incident of the abrupt withdrawal phenomenon (exacerbation of angina pectoris) has been reported with labetalol HCl, dosing with TRANDATE Tablets should not be interrupted or discontinued without a physician's advice. Patients being treated with TRANDATE Tablets should consult a physician at any signs or symptoms of impending cardiac failure or hepatic dysfunction (see WARNINGS). Also, transient scalp tingling may occur, usually when treatment with TRANDATE Tablets is initiated (see ADVERSE REACTIONS).

Laboratory Tests: As with any new drug given over prolonged periods, laboratory parameters should be observed over regular intervals. In patients with concomitant illnesses, such as impaired renal function, appropriate tests should be done to monitor these conditions.

Drug Interactions: In one survey, 2.3% of patients taking labetalol HCl in combination with tricyclic antidepressants experienced tremor, as compared to 0.7% reported to occur with labetalol HCl alone. The contribution of each of the treatments to this adverse reaction is unknown, but the possibility of a drug interaction cannot be excluded.

Drugs possessing beta-blocking properties can blunt the bronchodilator effect of beta-receptor agonist drugs in patients with bronchospasm; therefore, doses greater than the normal antiasthmatic dose of beta-agonist bronchodilator drugs may be required.

Cimetidine has been shown to increase the bioavailability of labetalol HCl. Since this could be explained either by enhanced absorption or by an alteration of hepatic metabolism of labetalol HCl, special care should be used in establishing the dose required for blood pressure control in such patients.

Synergism has been shown between halothane anesthesia and intravenously administered labetalol HCl. During controlled hypotensive anesthesia using labetalol HCl in association with halothane, high concentrations (3% or above) of halothane should not be used because the degree of hypotension will be increased and because of the possibility of a large reduction in cardiac output and an increase in central venous pressure. The anesthesiologist should be informed when a patient is receiving labetalol HCl.

Labetalol HCl blunts the reflex tachycardia produced by nitroglycerin without preventing its hypotensive effect. If labetalol HCl is used with nitroglycerin in patients with angina pectoris, additional antihypertensive effects may occur. Care should be taken if labetalol is used concomitantly with calcium antagonists of the verapamil type.

Risk of Anaphylactic Reaction: While taking beta-blockers, patients with a history of severe anaphylactic reaction to a variety of allergens may be more reactive to repeated challenge, either accidental, diagnostic, or therapeutic. Such patients may be unresponsive to the usual doses of epinephrine used to treat allergic reaction.

Drug/Laboratory Test Interactions: The presence of labetalol metabolites in the urine may result in falsely elevated levels of urinary catecholamines, metanephrine, normetanephrine, and vanillylmandelic acid when measured by fluorimetric or photometric methods. In screening patients suspected of having a pheochromocytoma and being treated with labetalol HCl, a specific method, such as a high performance liquid chromatographic assay with solid phase extraction (e.g., *J Chromatogr* 385:241, 1987) should be employed in determining levels of catecholamines.

Labetalol HCl has also been reported to produce a false-positive test for amphetamine when screening urine for the presence of drugs using the commercially available assay methods Toxi-Lab A® (thin-layer chromatographic assay) and Emit-d.a.u.® (radioenzymatic assay). When patients being treated with labetalol have a positive urine test for amphetamine using these techniques, confirmation should be made by using more specific methods, such as a gas chromatographic-mass spectrometer technique.

Carcinogenesis, Mutagenesis, Impairment of Fertility: Long-term oral dosing studies with labetalol HCl for 18 months in mice and for 2 years in rats showed no evidence of carcinogenesis. Studies with labetalol HCl using dominant lethal assays in rats and mice and exposing microorganisms according to modified Ames tests showed no evidence of mutagenesis.

Pregnancy: ***Teratogenic Effects***: ***Pregnancy Category C***: Teratogenic studies were performed with labetalol in rats and rabbits at oral doses up to approximately six and four times the maximum recommended human dose (MRHD), respectively. No reproducible evidence of fetal malformations was observed. Increased fetal resorptions were seen in both species at doses approximating the MRHD. A teratology study performed with labetalol in rabbits at IV doses up to 1.7 times the MRHD revealed no evidence of drug-related harm to the fetus. There are no adequate and well-controlled studies in pregnant women. Labetalol should be used during pregnancy only if the potential benefit justifies the potential risk to the fetus.

Nonteratogenic Effects: Hypotension, bradycardia, hypoglycemia, and respiratory depression have been reported in infants of mothers who were treated with labetalol HCl for hypertension during pregnancy. Oral administration of labetalol to rats during late gestation through weaning at

Continued on next page

Trandate—Cont.

doses of two to four times the MRHD caused a decrease in neonatal survival.

Labor and Delivery: Labetalol HCl given to pregnant women with hypertension did not appear to affect the usual course of labor and delivery.

Nursing Mothers: Small amounts of labetalol (approximately 0.004% of the maternal dose) are excreted in human milk. Caution should be exercised when TRANDATE Tablets are administered to a nursing woman.

Pediatric Use: Safety and effectiveness in pediatric patients have not been established.

Elderly Patients: As in the general population, some elderly patients (60 years of age and older) have experienced orthostatic hypotension, dizziness, or lightheadedness during treatment with labetalol. Because elderly patients are generally more likely than younger patients to experience orthostatic symptoms, they should be cautioned about the possibility of such side effects during treatment with labetalol.

ADVERSE REACTIONS

Most adverse effects are mild and transient and occur early in the course of treatment. In controlled clinical trials of 3 to 4 months' duration, discontinuation of TRANDATE Tablets due to one or more adverse effects was required in 7% of all patients. In these same trials, other agents with solely beta-blocking activity used in the control groups led to discontinuation in 8% to 10% of patients, and a centrally acting alpha-agonist led to discontinuation in 30% of patients.

The incidence rates of adverse reactions listed in the following table were derived from multicenter, controlled clinical trials comparing labetalol HCl, placebo, metoprolol, and propranolol over treatment periods of 3 and 4 months. Where the frequency of adverse effects for labetalol HCl and placebo is similar, causal relationship is uncertain. The rates are based on adverse reactions considered probably drug related by the investigator. If all reports are considered, the rates are somewhat higher (e.g., dizziness, 20%; nausea, 14%; fatigue, 11%), but the overall conclusions are unchanged.

[See table at top of previous page]

The adverse effects were reported spontaneously and are representative of the incidence of adverse effects that may be observed in a properly selected patient population, i.e., a group excluding patients with bronchospastic disease, overt congestive heart failure, or other contraindications to beta-blocker therapy.

Clinical trials also included studies utilizing daily doses up to 2400 mg in more severely hypertensive patients. Certain of the side effects increased with increasing dose, as shown in the following table that depicts the entire US therapeutic trials data base for adverse reactions that are clearly or possibly dose related.

[See table below]

In addition, a number of other less common adverse events have been reported:

Body as a Whole: Fever.

Cardiovascular: Hypotension, and rarely, syncope, bradycardia, heart block.

Central and Peripheral Nervous System: Paresthesia, most frequently described as scalp tingling. In most cases, it was mild and transient and usually occurred at the beginning of treatment.

Collagen Disorders: Systemic lupus erythematosus, positive antinuclear factor.

Eyes: Dry eyes.

Immunological System: Antimitochondrial antibodies.

Liver and Biliary System: Hepatic necrosis, hepatitis, cholestatic jaundice, elevated liver function tests.

Musculoskeletal System: Muscle cramps, toxic myopathy.

Respiratory System: Bronchospasm.

Skin and Appendages: Rashes of various types, such as generalized maculopapular, lichenoid, urticarial, bullous lichen planus, psoriaform, and facial erythema; Peyronie's disease; reversible alopecia.

Urinary System: Difficulty in micturition, including acute urinary bladder retention.

Hypersensitivity: Rare reports of hypersensitivity (e.g., rash, urticaria, pruritus, angioedema, dyspnea) and anaphylactoid reactions.

Following approval for marketing in the United Kingdom, a monitored release survey involving approximately 6800 patients was conducted for further safety and efficacy evaluation of this product. Results of this survey indicate that the type, severity, and incidence of adverse effects were comparable to those cited above.

Potential Adverse Effects: In addition, other adverse effects not listed above have been reported with other beta-adrenergic blocking agents.

Central Nervous System: Reversible mental depression progressing to catatonia, an acute reversible syndrome characterized by disorientation for time and place, short-term memory loss, emotional lability, slightly clouded sensorium, and decreased performance on psychometrics.

Cardiovascular: Intensification of A-V block (see CONTRAINDICATIONS).

Allergic: Fever combined with aching and sore throat, laryngospasm, respiratory distress.

Hematologic: Agranulocytosis, thrombocytopenic or nonthrombocytopenic purpura.

Gastrointestinal: Mesenteric artery thrombosis, ischemic colitis.

The oculomucocutaneous syndrome associated with the beta-blocker practolol has not been reported with labetalol HCl.

Clinical Laboratory Tests: There have been reversible increases of serum transaminases in 4% of patients treated with labetalol HCl and tested and, more rarely, reversible increases in blood urea.

OVERDOSAGE

Overdosage with labetalol HCl causes excessive hypotension that is posture sensitive and, sometimes, excessive bradycardia. Patients should be placed supine and their legs raised if necessary to improve the blood supply to the brain. If overdosage with labetalol HCl follows oral ingestion, gastric lavage or pharmacologically induced emesis (using syrup of ipecac) may be useful for removal of the drug shortly after ingestion. The following additional measures should be employed if necessary: **Excessive bradycardia**—administer atropine or epinephrine. **Cardiac failure**—administer a digitalis glycoside and a diuretic. Dopamine or dobutamine may also be useful. **Hypotension**—administer vasopressors, e.g., norepinephrine. There is pharmacologic evidence that norepinephrine may be the drug of choice. **Bronchospasm**—administer epinephrine and/or an aerosolized beta$_2$-agonist. **Seizures**—administer diazepam.

In severe beta-blocker overdose resulting in hypotension and/or bradycardia, glucagon has been shown to be effective when administered in large doses (5 to 10 mg rapidly over 30 seconds, followed by continuous infusion of 5 mg per hour that can be reduced as the patient improves).

Neither hemodialysis nor peritoneal dialysis removes a significant amount of labetalol HCl from the general circulation (<1%).

The oral LD_{50} value of labetalol HCl in the mouse is approximately 600 mg/kg and in the rat is >2 g/kg. The IV LD_{50} in these species is 50 to 60 mg/kg.

DOSAGE AND ADMINISTRATION

DOSAGE MUST BE INDIVIDUALIZED.

The recommended *initial* dosage is 100 mg *twice* daily whether used alone or added to a diuretic regimen. After 2 or 3 days, using standing blood pressure as an indicator, dosage may be titrated in increments of 100 mg b.i.d. every 2 or 3 days. The usual *maintenance* dosage of labetalol HCl is between 200 and 400 mg *twice* daily.

Since the full antihypertensive effect of labetalol HCl is usually seen within the first 1 to 3 hours of the initial dose or dose increment, the assurance of a lack of an exaggerated hypotensive response can be clinically established in the office setting. The antihypertensive effects of continued dosing can be measured at subsequent visits, approximately 12 hours after a dose, to determine whether further titration is necessary.

Patients with severe hypertension may require from 1200 to 2400 mg per day, with or without thiazide diuretics. Should side effects (principally nausea or dizziness) occur with these doses administered twice daily, the same total daily dose administered three times daily may improve tolerability and facilitate further titration. Titration increments should not exceed 200 mg twice daily.

When a diuretic is added, an additive antihypertensive effect can be expected. In some cases this may necessitate a labetalol HCl dosage adjustment. As with most antihypertensive drugs, optimal dosages of TRANDATE Tablets are usually lower in patients also receiving a diuretic.

When transferring patients from other antihypertensive drugs, TRANDATE Tablets should be introduced as recommended and the dosage of the existing therapy progressively decreased.

Elderly Patients: As in the general population, labetalol therapy may be initiated at 100 mg twice daily and titrated upwards in increments of 100 mg b.i.d. as required for control of blood pressure. Since some elderly patients eliminate labetalol more slowly, however, adequate control of blood pressure may be achieved at a lower maintenance dosage compared to the general population. The majority of elderly patients will require between 100 and 200 mg b.i.d.

Labetalol HCl Daily Dose (mg)	200	300	400	600	800	900	1200	1600	2400
Number of patients	522	181	606	608	503	117	411	242	175
Dizziness (%)	2	3	3	3	5	1	9	13	16
Fatigue	2	1	4	4	5	3	7	6	10
Nausea	<1	0	1	2	4	0	7	11	19
Vomiting	0	0	<1	<1	<1	0	1	2	3
Dyspepsia	1	0	2	1	1	0	2	2	4
Paresthesia	2	0	2	2	1	1	2	5	5
Nasal stuffiness	1	1	2	2	2	2	4	5	6
Ejaculation failure	0	2	1	2	3	0	4	3	5
Impotence	1	1	1	1	2	4	3	4	3
Edema	1	0	1	1	1	0	1	2	2

HOW SUPPLIED

TRANDATE Tablets, 100 mg, light orange, round, scored, film-coated tablets engraved on one side with "TRANDATE 100," bottles of 100 (NDC 60976-346-43) and 500 (NDC 60976-346-44) and unit dose packs of 100 tablets (NDC 60976-346-47).

TRANDATE Tablets, 200 mg, white, round, scored, film-coated tablets engraved on one side with "TRANDATE 200," bottles of 100 (NDC 60976-347-43) and 500 (NDC 60976-347-44) and unit dose packs of 100 tablets (NDC 60976-347-47).

TRANDATE Tablets, 300 mg, peach, round, scored, film-coated tablets engraved on one side with "TRANDATE 300," bottles of 100 (NDC 60976-348-43) and 500 (NDC 60976-348-44) and unit dose packs of 100 tablets (NDC 60976-348-47).

TRANDATE Tablets should be stored between 2° and 30°C (36° and 86°F). TRANDATE Tablets in the unit dose boxes should be protected from excessive moisture.

FARO™ Pharmaceuticals, Inc.

Manufactured by
Glaxo Wellcome Inc.
Research Triangle Park, NC 27709
For FARO Pharmaceuticals, Inc.
Bedminster, NJ 07921

Feb. 1999

Shown in Product Identification Guide, page 312

ZYLOPRIM® ℞

(allopurinol)
100-mg Scored Tablets and
300-mg Scored Tablets

DESCRIPTION

ZYLOPRIM (allopurinol) has the following structural formula:

ZYLOPRIM is known chemically as 1,5-dihydro-4*H*-pyrazolo [3,4-*d*]pyrimidin-4-one. It is a xanthine oxidase inhibitor which is administered orally. Each scored white tablet contains 100 mg allopurinol and the inactive ingredients lactose, magnesium stearate, potato starch, and povidone. Each scored peach tablet contains 300 mg allopurinol and the inactive ingredients corn starch, FD&C Yellow No. 6 Lake, lactose, magnesium stearate, and povidone. Its solubility in water at 37°C is 80.0 mg/dL and is greater in an alkaline solution.

CLINICAL PHARMACOLOGY

ZYLOPRIM acts on purine catabolism, without disrupting the biosynthesis of purines. It reduces the production of uric acid by inhibiting the biochemical reactions immediately preceding its formation.

ZYLOPRIM is a structural analogue of the natural purine base, hypoxanthine. It is an inhibitor of xanthine oxidase, the enzyme responsible for the conversion of hypoxanthine to xanthine and of xanthine to uric acid, the end product of purine metabolism in man. ZYLOPRIM is metabolized to the corresponding xanthine analogue, oxipurinol (alloxanthine), which also is an inhibitor of xanthine oxidase.

Zyloprim (allopurinol) 1,5-dihydro-4*H*-pyrazolo-[3,4-*d*]pyrimidin-4-one — Oxipurinol 1*H*-pyrazolo [3,4-d] pyrimidine 4,6 (5*H*,7*H*)-dione

Hypoxanthine purin-6(1*H*)-one — Xanthine 3,7-dihydro-1*H*-purine-2,6-dione — Uric Acid 7,9-dihydro-1*H*-purine-2,6,8(3*H*)-trione

It has been shown that reutilization of both hypoxanthine and xanthine for nucleotide and nucleic acid synthesis is markedly enhanced when their oxidations are inhibited by

ZYLOPRIM and oxipurinol. This reutilization does not disrupt normal nucleic acid anabolism, however, because feedback inhibition is an integral part of purine biosynthesis. As a result of xanthine oxidase inhibition, the serum concentration of hypoxanthine plus xanthine in patients receiving ZYLOPRIM for treatment of hyperuricemia is usually in the range of 0.3 to 0.4 mg/dL compared to a normal level of approximately 0.15 mg/dL. A maximum of 0.9 mg/dL of these oxypurines has been reported when the serum urate was lowered to less than 2 mg/dL by high doses of ZYLOPRIM. These values are far below the saturation levels at which point their precipitation would be expected to occur (above 7 mg/dL).

The renal clearance of hypoxanthine and xanthine is at least 10 times greater than that of uric acid. The increased xanthine and hypoxanthine in the urine have not been accompanied by problems of nephrolithiasis. Xanthine crystalluria has been reported in only three patients. Two of the patients had Lesch-Nyhan syndrome, which is characterized by excessive uric acid production combined with a deficiency of the enzyme, hypoxanthineguanine phosphoribosyltransferase (HGPRTase). This enzyme is required for the conversion of hypoxanthine, xanthine, and guanine to their respective nucleotides. The third patient had lymphosarcoma and produced an extremely large amount of uric acid because of rapid cell lysis during chemotherapy.

ZYLOPRIM is approximately 90% absorbed from the gastrointestinal tract. Peak plasma levels generally occur at 1.5 hours and 4.5 hours for ZYLOPRIM and oxipurinol respectively, and after a single oral dose of 300 mg ZYLOPRIM, maximum plasma levels of about 3 mcg/mL of ZYLOPRIM and 6.5 mcg/mL of oxipurinol are produced.

Approximately 20% of the ingested ZYLOPRIM is excreted in the feces. Because of its rapid oxidation to oxipurinol and a renal clearance rate approximately that of glomerular filtration rate, ZYLOPRIM has a plasma half-life of about 1 to 2 hours. Oxipurinol, however, has a longer plasma half-life (approximately 15 hours) and therefore effective xanthine oxidase inhibition is maintained over a 24-hour period with single daily doses of ZYLOPRIM. Whereas ZYLOPRIM is cleared essentially by glomerular filtration, oxipurinol is reabsorbed in the kidney tubules in a manner similar to the reabsorption of uric acid.

The clearance of oxipurinol is increased by uricosuric drugs, and as a consequence, the addition of a uricosuric agent reduces to some degree the inhibition of xanthine oxidase by oxipurinol and increases to some degree the urinary excretion of uric acid. In practice, the net effect of such combined therapy may be useful in some patients in achieving minimum serum uric acid levels provided the total urinary uric acid load does not exceed the competence of the patient's renal function.

Hyperuricemis may be primary, as in gout, or secondary to diseases such as acute and chronic leukemia, polycythemia vera, multiple myeloma, and psoriasis. It may occur with the use of diuretic agents, during renal dialysis, in the presence of renal damage, during starvation or reducing diets, and in the treatment of neoplastic disease where rapid resolution of tissue masses may occur. Asymptomatic hyperuricemia is not an indication for treatment with ZYLOPRIM (see INDICATIONS AND USAGE).

Gout is a metabolic disorder which is characterized by hyperuricemia and resultant deposition of monosodium urate in the tissues, particularly the joints and kidneys. The etiology of this hyperuricemia is the overproduction of uric acid in relation to the patient's ability to excrete it. If progressive deposition of urates is to be arrested or reversed, it is necessary to reduce the serum uric acid level below the saturation point to suppress urate precipitation.

Administration of ZYLOPRIM generally results in a fall in both serum and urinary uric acid within 2 to 3 days. The degree of this decrease can be manipulated almost at will since it is dose-dependent. A week or more of treatment with ZYLOPRIM may be required before its full effects are manifested; likewise, uric acid may return to pretreatment levels slowly (usually after a period of 7 to 10 days following cessation of therapy). This reflects primarily the accumulation and slow clearance of oxipurinol. In some patients a dramatic fall in urinary uric acid excretion may not occur, particularly in those with severe tophaceous gout. It has been postulated that this may be due to the mobilization of urate from tissue deposits as the serum uric acid level begins to fall.

The action of ZYLOPRIM differs from that of uricosuric agents, which lower the serum uric acid level by increasing urinary excretion of uric acid. ZYLOPRIM reduces both the serum and urinary uric acid levels by inhibiting the formation of uric acid. The use of ZYLOPRIM to block the formation of urates avoids the hazard of increased renal excretion of uric acid posed by uricosuric drugs.

ZYLOPRIM can substantially reduce serum and urinary uric acid levels in previously refractory patients even in the presence of renal damage serious enough to render uricosuric drugs virtually ineffective. Salicylates may be given conjointly for their antirheumatic effect without compromising the action of ZYLOPRIM. This is in contrast to the nullifying effect of salicylates on uricosuric drugs.

ZYLOPRIM also inhibits the enzymatic oxidation of mercaptopurine, the sulfur-containing analogue of hypoxanthine, to 6-thiouric acid. This oxidation, which is catalyzed by xanthine oxidase, inactivates mercaptopurine. Hence, the inhibition of such oxidation by ZYLOPRIM may result in as much as a 75% reduction in the therapeutic dose requirement of mercaptopurine when the two compounds are given together.

INDICATIONS AND USAGE

THIS IS NOT AN INNOCUOUS DRUG. IT IS NOT RECOMMENDED FOR THE TREATMENT OF ASYMPTOMATIC HYPERURICEMIA.

ZYLOPRIM reduces serum and urinary uric acid concentrations. Its use should be individualized for each patient and requires an understanding of its mode of action and pharmacokinetics (see CLINICAL PHARMACOLOGY, CONTRAINDICATIONS, WARNINGS, and PRECAUTIONS).

ZYLOPRIM is indicated in:

1) the management of patients with signs and symptoms of primary or secondary gout (acute attacks, tophi, joint destruction, uric acid lithiasis, and/or nephropathy).
2) the management of patients with leukemia, lymphoma and malignancies who are receiving cancer therapy which causes elevations of serum and urinary uric acid levels. Treatment with ZYLOPRIM should be discontinued when the potential for overproduction of uric acid is no longer present.
3) the management of patients with recurrent calcium oxalate calculi whose daily uric acid excretion exceeds 800 mg/day in male patients and 750 mg/day in female patients. Therapy in such patients should be carefully assessed initially and reassessed periodically to determine in each case that treatment is beneficial and that the benefits outweigh the risks.

CONTRAINDICATIONS

Patients who have developed a severe reaction to ZYLOPRIM should not be restarted on the drug.

WARNINGS

ZYLOPRIM SHOULD BE DISCONTINUED AT THE FIRST APPEARANCE OF SKIN RASH OR OTHER SIGNS WHICH MAY INDICATE AN ALLERGIC REACTION. In some instances a skin rash may be followed by more severe hypersensitivity reactions such as exfoliative, urticarial, and purpuric lesions, as well as Stevens-Johnson syndrome (erythema multiforme exudativum), and/or generalized vasculitis, irreversible hepatotoxicity, and, on rare occasions, death.

In patients receiving mercaptopurine or IMURAN® (azathioprine), the concomitant administration of 300 to 600 mg of ZYLOPRIM per day will require a reduction in dose to approximately one-third to one-fourth of the usual dose of mercaptopurine or azathioprine. Subsequent adjustment of doses of mercaptopurine or azathioprine should be made on the basis of therapeutic response and the appearance of toxic effects (see CLINICAL PHARMACOLOGY).

A few cases of reversible clinical hepatotoxicity have been noted in patients taking ZYLOPRIM, and in some patients, asymptomatic rises in serum alkaline phosphatase or serum transaminase have been observed. If anorexia, weight loss, or pruritus develop in patients on ZYLOPRIM, evaluation of liver function should be part of their diagnostic workup. In patients with pre-existing liver disease, periodic liver function tests are recommended during the early stages of therapy.

Due to the occasional occurrence of drowsiness, patients should be alerted to the need for due precaution when engaging in activities where alertness is mandatory.

The occurrence of hypersensitivity reactions to ZYLOPRIM may be increased in patients with decreased renal function receiving thiazides and ZYLOPRIM concurrently. For this reason, in this clinical setting, such combinations should be administered with caution and patients should be observed closely.

PRECAUTIONS

General: An increase in acute attacks of gout has been reported during the early stages of administration of ZYLOPRIM, even when normal or subnormal serum uric acid levels have been attained. Accordingly, maintenance doses of colchicine generally should be given prophylactically when ZYLOPRIM is begun. In addition, it is recommended that the patient start with a low dose of ZYLOPRIM (100 mg daily) and increase at weekly intervals by 100 mg until a serum uric acid level of 6 mg/dL or less is attained but without exceeding the maximum recommended dose (800 mg per day). The use of colchicine or anti-inflammatory agents may be required to suppress gouty attacks in some cases. The attacks usually become shorter and less severe after several months of therapy. The mobilization of urates from tissue deposits which cause fluctuations in the serum uric acid levels may be a possible explanation for these episodes. Even with adequate therapy with ZYLOPRIM, it may require several months to deplete the uric acid pool sufficiently to achieve control of the acute attacks.

A fluid intake sufficient to yield a daily urinary output of at least 2 liters and the maintenance of a neutral or, preferably, slightly alkaline urine are desirable to (1) avoid the theoretical possibility of formation of xanthine calculi under the influence of therapy with ZYLOPRIM and (2) help prevent renal precipitation of urates in patients receiving concomitant uricosuric agents.

Some patients with pre-existing renal disease or poor urate clearance have shown a rise in BUN during administration of ZYLOPRIM. Although the mechanism responsible for this has not been established, patients with impaired renal function should be carefully observed during the early stages of administration of ZYLOPRIM and the dosage decreased or the drug withdrawn if increased abnormalities in renal function appear and persist.

Renal failure in association with administration of ZYLOPRIM has been observed among patients with hyperuricemia secondary to neoplastic diseases. Concurrent conditions such as multiple myeloma and congestive myocardial disease were present among those patients whose renal dysfunction increased after ZYLOPRIM was begun. Renal failure is also frequently associated with gouty nephropathy and rarely with hypersensitivity reactions associated with ZYLOPRIM. Albuminuria has been observed among patients who developed clinical gout following chronic glomerulonephritis and chronic pyelonephritis.

Patients with decreased renal function require lower doses of ZYLOPRIM than those with normal renal function. Lower than recommended doses should be used to initiate therapy in any patients with decreased renal function and they should be observed closely during the early stages of administration of ZYLOPRIM. In patients with severely impaired renal function or decreased urate clearance, the half-life of oxipurinol in the plasma is greatly prolonged. Therefore, a dose of 100 mg per day or 300 mg twice a week, or perhaps less, may be sufficient to maintain adequate xanthine oxidase inhibition to reduce serum urate levels.

Bone marrow depression has been reported in patients receiving ZYLOPRIM, most of whom received concomitant drugs with the potential for causing this reaction. This has occurred as early as 6 weeks to as long as 6 years after the initiation of therapy of ZYLOPRIM. Rarely, a patient may develop varying degrees of bone marrow depression, affecting one or more cell lines, while receiving ZYLOPRIM alone.

Information for Patients: Patients should be informed of the following:

(1) They should be cautioned to discontinue ZYLOPRIM and to consult their physician immediately at the first sign of a skin rash, painful urination, blood in the urine, irritation of the eyes, or swelling of the lips or mouth. (2) They should be reminded to continue drug therapy prescribed for gouty attacks since optimal benefit of ZYLOPRIM may be delayed for 2 to 6 weeks. (3) They should be encouraged to increase fluid intake during therapy to prevent renal stones. (4) If a single dose of ZYLOPRIM is occasionally forgotten, there is no need to double the dose at the next scheduled time. (5) There may be certain risks associated with the concomitant use of ZYLOPRIM and dicumarol, sulfinpyrazone, mercaptopurine, azathioprine, ampicillin, amoxicillin, and thiazide diuretics, and they should follow the instructions of their physician. (6) Due to the occasional occurrence of drowsiness, patients should take precautions when engaging in activities where alertness is mandatory. (7) Patients may wish to take ZYLOPRIM after meals to minimize gastric irritation.

Laboratory Tests: The correct dosage and schedule for maintaining the serum uric acid within the normal range is best determined by using the serum uric acid as an index. In patients with pre-existing liver disease, periodic liver tests are recommended during the early stages of therapy (see WARNINGS).

ZYLOPRIM and its primary active metabolite, oxipurinol, are eliminated by the kidneys; therefore, changes in renal function have a profound effect on dosage. In patients with deceased renal function or who have concurrent illnesses which can affect renal function such as hypertension and diabetes mellitus, periodic laboratory parameters of renal function, particularly BUN and serum creatinine or creatinine clearance, should be performed and the patient's dosage of ZYLOPRIM reassessed.

The prothrombin time should be reassessed periodically in the patients receiving dicumarol who are given ZYLOPRIM.

Drug Interactions: In patients receiving mercaptopurine or IMURAN (azathioprine), the concomitant administration of 300 to 600 mg of ZYLOPRIM per day will require a reduction in dose to approximately one third to one fourth of the usual dose of mercaptopurine or azathioprine. Subsequent adjustment of doses of mercaptopurine or azathioprine should be made on the basis of therapeutic response and the appearance of toxic effects (see CLINICAL PHARMACOLOGY).

It has been reported that ZYLOPRIM prolongs the half-life of the anticoagulant, dicumarol. The clinical basis of this drug interaction has not been established but should be noted when ZYLOPRIM is given to patients already on dicumarol therapy.

Since the excretion of oxipurinol is similar to that of urate, uricosuric agents, which increase the excretion of urate, are also likely to increase the excretion of oxipurinol and thus lower the degree of inhibition of xanthine oxidase. The concomitant administration of uricosuric agents and ZYLOPRIM has been associated with a decrease in the excretion of oxypurines (hypoxanthine and xanthine) and an increase in urinary uric acid excretion compared with that observed with ZYLOPRIM alone. Although clinical evidence to date has not demonstrated renal precipitation of oxypurines in patients either on ZYLOPRIM alone or in combination with uricosuric agents, the possibility should be kept in mind.

The reports that the concomitant use of ZYLOPRIM and thiazide diuretics may contribute to the enhancement of allopurinol toxicity in some patients have been reviewed in an attempt to establish a cause-and-effect relationship and a

Continued on next page

Zyloprim—Cont.

mechanism of causation. Review of these case reports indicates that the patients were mainly receiving thiazide diuretics for hypertension and that tests to rule out decreased renal function secondary to hypertensive nephropathy were not often performed. In those patients in whom renal insufficiency was documented, however, the recommendation to lower the dose of ZYLOPRIM was not followed. Although a causal mechanism and a cause-and-effect relationship have not been established, current evidence suggests that renal function should be monitored in patients on thiazide diuretics and ZYLOPRIM even in the absence of renal failure, and dosage levels should be even more conservatively adjusted in those patients on such combined therapy if diminished renal function is detected.

An increase in the frequency of skin rash has been reported among patients receiving ampicillin or amoxicillin concurrently with ZYLOPRIM compared to patients who are not receiving both drugs. The cause of the reported association has not been established.

Enhanced bone marrow suppression by cyclophosphamide and other cytotoxic agents has been reported among patients with neoplastic disease, except leukemia, in the presence of ZYLOPRIM. However, in a well-controlled study of patients with lymphoma on combination therapy, ZYLOPRIM did not increase the marrow toxicity of patients treated with cyclophosphamide, doxorubicin, bleomycin, procarbazine, and/or mechlorethamine.

Tolbutamide's conversion to inactive metabolites has been shown to be catalyzed by xanthine oxidase from rat liver. The clinical significance, if any, of these observations is unknown.

Chlorpropamide's plasma half-life may be prolonged by ZYLOPRIM, since ZYLOPRIM and chlorpropamide may compete for excretion in the renal tubule. The risk of hypoglycemia secondary to this mechanism may be increased if ZYLOPRIM and chlorpropamide are given concomitantly in the presence of renal insufficiency.

Rare reports indicate that cyclosporine levels may be increased during concomitant treatment with ZYLOPRIM. Monitoring of cyclosporine levels and possible adjustment of cyclosporine dosage should be considered when these drugs are co-administered.

Drug/Laboratory Tests Interactions: ZYLOPRIM is not known to alter the accuracy of laboratory tests.

Pregnancy: ***Teratogenic Effects:*** Pregnancy Category C. Reproductive studies have been performed in rats and rabbits at doses up to twenty times the usual human dose (5 mg/kg per day), and it was concluded that there was no impaired fertility or harm to the fetus due to allopurinol. There is a published report of a study in pregnant mice given 50 or 100 mg/kg allopurinol intraperitoneally on gestation days 10 or 13. There were increased numbers of dead fetuses in dams given 100 mg/kg allopurinol but not in those given 50 mg/kg. There were increased numbers of external malformations in fetuses at both doses of allopurinol on gestation day 10 and increased numbers of skeletal malformations in fetuses at both doses on gestation day 13. It cannot be determined whether this represented a fetal effect or an effect secondary to maternal toxicity. There are, however, no adequate or well-controlled studies in pregnant women. Because animal reproduction studies are not always predictive of human response, this drug should be used during pregnancy only if clearly needed.

Experience with ZYLOPRIM during human pregnancy has been limited partly because women of reproductive age rarely require treatment with ZYLOPRIM. There are two unpublished reports and one published paper of women giving birth to normal offspring after receiving ZYLOPRIM during pregnancy.

Nursing Mothers: Allopurinol and oxipurinol have been found in the milk of a mother who was receiving ZYLOPRIM. Since the effect of allopurinol on the nursing infant is unknown, caution should be exercised when ZYLOPRIM is administered to a nursing woman.

Pediatric Use: ZYLOPRIM is rarely indicated for use in children with the exception of those with hyperuricemia secondary to malignancy or to certain rare inborn errors of purine metabolism (see INDICATIONS AND USAGE and DOSAGE AND ADMINISTRATION).

ADVERSE REACTIONS

Data upon which the following estimates of incidence of adverse reactions are made are derived from experiences reported in the literature, unpublished clinical trials and voluntary reports since marketing of ZYLOPRIM (allopurinol) began. Past experience suggested that the most frequent event following the initiation of allopurinol treatment was an increase in acute attacks of gout (average 6% in early studies). An analysis of current usage suggests that the incidence of acute gouty attacks has diminished to less than 1%. The explanation for this decrease has not been determined but may be due in part to initiating therapy more gradually (see PRECAUTIONS and DOSAGE AND ADMINISTRATION).

The most frequent adverse reaction to ZYLOPRIM is skin rash. Skin reactions can be severe and sometimes fatal. Therefore, treatment with ZYLOPRIM should be discontinued immediately if a rash develops (see WARNINGS). Some patients with the most severe reaction also had fever, chills, arthralgias, cholestatic jaundice, eosinophilia and mild leukocytosis or leukopenia. Among 55 patients with gout treated with ZYLOPRIM for 3 to 34 months (average greater than 1 year) and followed prospectively, Rundles observed that 3% of patients developed a type of drug reaction which was predominantly a pruritic maculopapular skin eruption, sometimes scaly or exfoliative. However, with current usage, skin reactions have been observed less frequently than 1%. The explanation for this decrease is not obvious. The incidence of skin rash may be increased in the presence of renal insufficiency. The frequency of skin rash among patients receiving ampicillin or amoxicillin concurrently with ZYLOPRIM has been reported to be increased (see PRECAUTIONS).

Most Common Reactions* Probably Causally Related:

Gastrointestinal: Diarrhea, nausea, alkaline phosphatase increase, SGOT/SGPT increase.

Metabolic and Nutritional: Acute attacks of gout.

Skin and Appendages: Rash, maculopapular rash.

* Early clinical studies and incidence rates from early clinical experience with ZYLOPRIM suggested that these adverse reactions were found to occur at a rate of greater than 1%. The most frequent event observed was acute attacks of gout following the initiation of therapy. Analyses of current usage suggest that the incidence of these adverse reactions is now less than 1%. The explanation for this decrease has not been determined, but it may be due to following recommended usage (see ADVERSE REACTIONS introduction, INDICATIONS AND USAGE, PRECAUTIONS, and DOSAGE AND ADMINISTRATION).

Incidence Less Than 1% Probably Causally Related:

Body As a Whole: Ecchymosis, fever, headache.

Cardiovascular: Necrotizing angiitis, vasculitis.

Gastrointestinal: Hepatic necrosis, granulomatous hepatitis, hepatomegaly, hyperbilirubinemia, cholestatic jaundice, vomiting, intermittent abdominal pain, gastritis, dyspepsia.

Hemic and Lymphatic: Thrombocytopenia, eosinophilia, leukocytosis, leukopenia.

Musculoskeletal: Myopathy, arthralgias.

Nervous: Peripheral neuropathy, neuritis, paresthesia, somnolence.

Respiratory: Epistaxis.

Skin and Appendages: Erythema multiforme exudativum (Stevens-Johnson syndrome), toxic epidermal necrolysis (Lyell's syndrome), hypersensitivity vasculitis, purpura, vesicular bullous dermatitis, exfoliative dermatitis, eczematoid dermatitis, pruritus, urticaria, alopecia, onycholysis, lichen planus.

Special Senses: Taste loss/perversion.

Urogenital: Renal failure, uremia (see PRECAUTIONS).

Incidence Less Than 1% Causal Relationship Unknown:

Body As a Whole: Malaise.

Cardiovascular: Pericarditis, peripheral vascular disease, thrombophlebitis, bradycardia, vasodilation.

Endocrine: Infertility (male), hypercalcemia, gynecomastia (male).

Gastrointestinal: Hemorrhagic pancreatitis, gastrointestinal bleeding, stomatitis, salivary gland swelling, hyperlipidemia, tongue edema, anorexia.

Hemic and Lymphatic: Aplastic anemia, agranulocytosis, eosinophilic fibrohistiocytic lesion of bone marrow, pancytopenia, prothrombin decrease, anemia, hemolytic anemia, reticulocytosis, lymphadenopathy, lymphocytosis.

Musculoskeletal: Myalgia.

Nervous: Optic neuritis, confusion, dizziness, vertigo, foot drop, decrease in libido, depression, amnesia, tinnitus, asthenia, insomnia.

Respiratory: Bronchospasm, asthma, pharyngitis, rhinitis.

Skin and Appendages: Furunculosis, facial edema, sweating, skin edema.

Special Senses: Cataracts, macular retinitis, iritis, conjunctivitis, amblyopia.

Urogenital: Nephritis, impotence, primary hematuria, albuminuria.

OVERDOSAGE

Massive overdosing or acute poisoning by ZYLOPRIM has not been reported.

In mice, the 50% lethal dose (LD_{50}) is 160 mg/kg given intraperitoneally (IP) with deaths delayed up to 5 days and 700 mg/kg orally (PO) (approximately 140 times the usual human dose) with deaths delayed up to 3 days. In rats, the acute LD_{50} is 750 mg/kg IP and 6000 mg/kg PO (approximately 1200 times the human dose).

In the management of overdosage there is no specific antidote for ZYLOPRIM. There has been no clinical experience in the management of a patient who has taken massive amounts of ZYLOPRIM.

Both ZYLOPRIM and oxipurinol are dialyzable; however, the usefulness of hemodialysis or peritoneal dialysis in the management of an overdose of ZYLOPRIM is unknown.

DOSAGE AND ADMINISTRATION

The dosage of ZYLOPRIM to accomplish full control of gout and to lower serum uric acid to normal or near-normal levels varies with the severity of the disease. The average is 200 to 300 mg/day for patients with mild gout and 400 to 600 mg/day for those with moderately severe tophaceous gout. The appropriate dosage may be administered in divided doses or as a single equivalent dose with the 300 mg-tablet. Dosage requirements in excess of 300 mg should be administered in divided doses. The minimal effective dosage is 100 to 200 mg daily and the maximal recommended dosage is 800 mg daily. To reduce the possibility of flare-up of acute gouty attacks, it is recommended that the patient start with a low dose of ZYLOPRIM (100 mg daily) and increase at weekly intervals by 100 mg until a serum uric acid level of 6 mg/dL or less is attained but without exceeding the maximal recommended dosage.

Normal serum urate levels are usually achieved in 1 to 3 weeks. The upper limit of normal is about 7 mg/dL for men and postmenopausal women and 6 mg/dL for premenopausal women. Too much reliance should not be placed on a single serum uric acid determination since, for technical reasons, estimation of uric acid may be difficult. By selecting the appropriate dosage and, in certain patients, using uricosuric agents concurrently, it is possible to reduce serum uric acid to normal or, if desired, to as low as 2 to 3 mg/dL and keep it there indefinitely.

While adjusting the dosage of ZYLOPRIM in patients who are being treated with colchicine and/or anti-inflammatory agents, it is wise to continue the latter therapy until serum uric acid has been normalized and there has been freedom from acute gouty attacks for several months.

In transferring a patient from a uricosuric agent to ZYLOPRIM, the dose of the uricosuric agent should be gradually reduced over a period of several weeks and the dose of ZYLOPRIM gradually increased to the required dose needed to maintain a normal serum uric acid level.

It should also be noted that ZYLOPRIM is generally better tolerated if taken following meals. A fluid intake sufficient to yield a daily urinary output of at least 2 liters and the maintenance of a neutral or, preferably, slightly alkaline urine are desirable.

Since ZYLOPRIM and its metabolites are primarily eliminated only by the kidney, accumulation of the drug can occur in renal failure, and the dose of ZYLOPRIM should consequently be reduced. With a creatinine clearance of 10 to 20 mL/min, a daily dosage of 200 mg of ZYLOPRIM is suitable. When the creatinine clearance is less than 10 mL/min, the daily dosage should not exceed 100 mg. With extreme renal impairment (creatinine clearance less than 3 mL/min) the interval between doses may also need to be lengthened.

The correct size and frequency of dosage for maintaining the serum uric acid just within the normal range is best determined by using the serum uric acid level as an index.

For the prevention of uric acid nephropathy during the vigorous therapy of neoplastic disease, treatment with 600 to 800 mg daily for 2 or 3 days is advisable together with a high fluid intake. Otherwise similar considerations to the above recommendations for treating patients with gout govern the regulation of dosage for maintenance purposes in secondary hyperuricemia.

The dose of ZYLOPRIM recommended for management of recurrent calcium oxalate stones in hyperuricosuric patients is 200 to 300 mg/day in divided doses or as the single equivalent. This dose may be adjusted up or down depending upon the resultant control of the hyperuricosuria based upon subsequent 24 hour urinary urate determinations. Clinical experience suggests that patients with recurrent calcium oxalate stones may also benefit from dietary changes such as the reduction of animal protein, sodium, refined sugars, oxalate-rich foods, and excessive calcium intake, as well as an increase in oral fluids and dietary fiber.

Children, 6 to 10 years of age, with secondary hyperuricemia associated with malignancies may be given 300 mg ZYLOPRIM daily while those under 6 years are generally given 150 mg daily. The response is evaluated after approximately 48 hours of therapy and a dosage adjustment is made if necessary.

HOW SUPPLIED

100-mg (white) scored, flat cylindrical tablets imprinted with "ZYLOPRIM 100" on a raised hexagon, bottles of 100 (NDC 60976-996-55).

Store at 15° to 25°C (59° to 77°F) in a dry place.

300-mg (peach) scored, flat, cylindrical tablets imprinted with "ZYLOPRIM 300" on a raised hexagon, bottles of 100 (NDC 60976-998-55) and 500 (NDC 60976-998-70).

Store at 15° to 25°C (59° to 77°F) in a dry place and protect from light.

FARO™ Pharmaceuticals, Inc.
Manufactured by
Catalytica Pharmaceuticals, Inc.
Greenville, NC 27834
For FARO Pharmaceuticals, Inc.
Bedminster, NJ 07921

Feb. 1999

IDENTIFICATION PROBLEM?
Turn to the **Product Identification Guide,**
where you'll find more than
1600 products pictured in actual
size and full color.

Faulding Laboratories Inc.
5511 CAPITAL CENTER DRIVE
SUITE 550
RALEIGH, NC 27606

(919) 233-5788
Direct Inquiries to:
Customer Service
(800) 432-8534

KADIAN® Ⓒ℞
Morphine Sulfate Sustained Release
KADIAN® 20 mg Capsules
KADIAN® 50 mg Capsules
KADIAN® 100 mg Capsules

DESCRIPTION
KADIAN® capsules 20, 50 and 100 mg contain identical polymer coated sustained release pellets of morphine sulfate for oral administration.
Chemically, morphine sulfate is 7,8-didehydro-4,5 α- epoxy-17-methyl-morphinan-3,6 α- diol sulfate (2:1) (salt) pentahydrate and has the following structural formula:

$\cdot H_2SO_4 \cdot 5H_2O$

Morphine sulfate is an odorless, white, crystalline powder with a bitter taste and a molecular weight of 758 (as the sulfate). It has a solubility of 1 in 21 parts of water and 1 in 1000 parts of alcohol, but is practically insoluble in chloroform or ether. The octanol: water partition coefficient of morphine is 1.42 at physiologic pH and the pK_b is 7.9 for the tertiary nitrogen (mostly ionized at pH 7.4).
Each KADIAN® sustained release capsule contains either 20, 50, or 100 mg of Morphine Sulfate USP and the following inactive ingredients common to all strengths: hydroxypropyl methylcellulose, ethylcellulose, methacrylic acid copolymer, polyethylene glycol, diethyl phthalate, talc, corn starch, and sucrose. The 20 mg capsule shell contains gelatin, silicon dioxide, sodium lauryl sulfate, D&C yellow #10, titanium dioxide, and black ink SW-9009. The 50 mg capsule shell contains gelatin, silicon dioxide, sodium lauryl sulfate, D&C red #28, FD&C red #40, FD&C blue #1, titanium dioxide, and black ink SW-9009. The 100 mg capsule shell contains gelatin, silicon dioxide, sodium lauryl sulfate, D&C yellow #10, FD&C blue #1, titanium dioxide, and black ink SW-9009.

CLINICAL PHARMACOLOGY
Morphine is a natural product that is the prototype for the class of natural and synthetic opioid analgesics. Opioids produce a wide spectrum of pharmacologic effects including analgesia, dysphoria, euphoria, somnolence, respiratory depression, diminished gastrointestinal motility, altered circulatory dynamics, histamine release and physical dependence.
Morphine produces both its therapeutic and its adverse effects by interaction with one or more classes of specific opioid receptors located throughout the body. Morphine acts as a pure agonist, binding with and activating opioid receptors at sites in the peri-aqueductal and peri-ventricular grey matter, the ventro-medial medulla and the spinal cord to produce analgesia.
Effects on the Central Nervous System
The principal therapeutic actions of morphine are analgesia, sedation and alterations of mood. Opioids of this class do not usually eliminate pain, but they do reduce the perception of pain by the central nervous system.
Morphine produces respiratory depression by reducing the responsiveness of the brain stem respiratory centers to increases in carbon dioxide tension (or to direct electrical stimulation).
Morphine depresses the cough reflex by direct effect on the cough center in the medulla. Antitussive effects may occur with doses lower than those usually required for analgesia. Morphine causes miosis, even in total darkness, and little tolerance develops to this effect. Pinpoint pupils are a sign of opioid overdose but are not pathognomonic (e.g. pontine lesions of hemorrhagic or ischemic origins may produce similar findings). Marked mydriasis rather than miosis may be seen due to severe hypoxia in overdose situations.
Effects on the Gastrointestinal Tract
Gastric, biliary and pancreatic secretions are decreased by morphine. Morphine causes a reduction in motility associated with an increase in tone in the antrum of the stomach and duodenum. Digestion of food in the small intestine is delayed and propulsive contractions are decreased. Propulsive peristaltic waves in the colon are decreased, while tone is increased to the point of spasm. The end result is constipation. Morphine can cause a marked increase in biliary tract pressure as a result of spasm of the sphincter of Oddi.
Effects on the Cardiovascular System
Morphine produces peripheral vasodilation which may result in orthostatic hypotension or syncope. Release of histamine may be induced by morphine and can contribute to opioid-induced hypotension. Manifestations of histamine release and/or peripheral vasodilation may include pruritus, flushing, red eyes and sweating.

Table 1: Mean pharmacokinetic parameters (% coefficient variation) resulting from a fasting single dose study in normal volunteers and a multiple dose study in patients with cancer pain.

Regimen/ Dosage Form	AUC#,+ (ng.h/mL)	C_{max}+ (ng/mL)	T_{max} (h)	C_{min}+ (ng/mL)	Fluctuation*
Single Dose (n=24)					
KADIAN® Capsule	271.0 (19.4)	15.6 (24.4)	8.6 (41.1)	na^	na
Controlled-Release Tablet	304.3 (19.1)	30.5 (32.1)	2.5 (52.6)	na	na
Morphine Solution	362.4 (42.6)	64.4 (38.2)	0.9 (55.8)	na	na
Multiple Dose (n=24)					
KADIAN® Capsule q24h	500.9 (38.6)	37.3 (37.7)	10.3 (32.2)	9.9 (52.3)	3.0 (45.5)
Controlled-Release Tablet q12h	457.3 (40.2)	36.9 (42.0)	4.4 (53.0)	7.6 (60.3)	4.1 (51.5)

For single dose AUC = $AUC_{0\text{-}48h}$, for multiple dose AUC = $AUC_{0\text{-}24h}$ at steady state
\+ For single dose parameter normalized to 100 mg, for multiple dose parameter normalized to 100 mg per 24 hours
* Steady-state fluctuation in plasma concentrations = C_{max}–C_{min}/C_{min}
^ Not applicable

Pharmacodynamics
The relationship between the blood level of morphine and the analgesic response will depend on the patient's age, state of health, medical condition, and the extent of previous opioid treatment.
A minimum effective concentration (MEC) of morphine for pain relief has been reported as 27.2 ± 14.5 ng/mL (mean ± SD) in cancer patients treated with morphine solution. These results compare with the MEC for plasma morphine reported as 14.7 ± 4.8 ng/mL (mean ± SD) in patients with postoperative pain. The high degree of variation is of clinical significance as it may result in either under-dosing or over-dosing if the dosage is not adjusted to the patient's clinical status and analgesic response (see **PRECAUTIONS** and **DOSAGE AND ADMINISTRATION**).
For opioid-tolerant patients the situation is much more complex. Some patients will become rapidly tolerant to the analgesic effects of morphine, and will require high daily oral morphine doses for adequate pain control. Since the development of tolerance to both the therapeutic and adverse effects of opioids is highly individualized, the dose of morphine should be individualized to the patient's condition and should not be based on an arbitrary choice of a dose or blood level to be achieved.
Pharmacokinetics
KADIAN® capsules contain polymer coated sustained release pellets of morphine sulfate that release morphine significantly more slowly than from morphine sulfate tablets and shorter-acting controlled-release oral morphine sulfate preparations. KADIAN® activity is primarily due to morphine. One metabolite, morphine-6-glucuronide, has been shown to have analgesic activity, but poorly crosses the blood-brain barrier.
Following oral administration, the extent of absorption is essentially the same for immediate or sustained release formulations, although the time to peak blood level (T_{max}) will be longer and the C_{max} will be lower for formulations that delay the release of morphine in the gastrointestinal tract. Elimination of morphine is primarily via hepatic metabolism to glucuronide metabolites (55 to 65%) which are then renally excreted. The terminal half-life of morphine is 2 to 4 hours, however, a longer term half-life of about 15 hours has been reported in studies where blood has been sampled up to 48 hours.
The single-dose pharmacokinetics of KADIAN® are linear over the dosage range of 30 to 100 mg. The single dose and multiple dose pharmacokinetic parameters of KADIAN® in normal volunteers are summarized in Table 1.
[See table 1 above]
Absorption
Following the administration of oral morphine solution, approximately 50% of the morphine absorbed reaches the systemic circulation within 30 minutes. However, following the administration of an equal amount of KADIAN® to healthy volunteers, this occurs, on average, after 8 hours. As with most forms of oral morphine, because of pre-systemic elimination, only about 20 to 40% of the administered dose reaches the systemic circulation.
Food Effects: While concurrent administration of food slows the rate of absorption of KADIAN®, the extent of absorption is not affected and KADIAN® can be administered without regard to meals.
Steady State: When KADIAN® is given on a fixed dosing regimen to patients with chronic pain due to malignancy, steady state is achieved in about two days. At steady state, KADIAN® will have a significantly lower C_{max} and a higher C_{min} than equivalent doses of oral morphine solution and some other controlled-release preparations (see Graph 1).
[See graph 1 in next column]
When given once-daily (every 24 hours) to 24 patients with malignancy, KADIAN® had a similar C_{max} and higher C_{min} at steady state in clinical usage, when compared to twice-daily (every 12 hours) controlled-release morphine tablets (MS Contin®), given at an equivalent total daily dosage (see Graph 2 and Table 1). Drug-disease interactions are frequently seen in the older and more gravely ill patients, and may result in both altered absorption and reduced clearance as compared to normal volunteers (see **Geriatric, Hepatic Failure,** and **Renal Insufficiency** sections).
[See graph 2 in next column]

Graph 1 (Study # MOB-1/90):
Mean steady state plasma morphine concentrations for KADIAN® (twice a day), controlled-release morphine tablet (twice a day) and oral morphine solution (every 4 hours); plasma concentrations are normalized to 100 mg every 24 hours, (n=24).

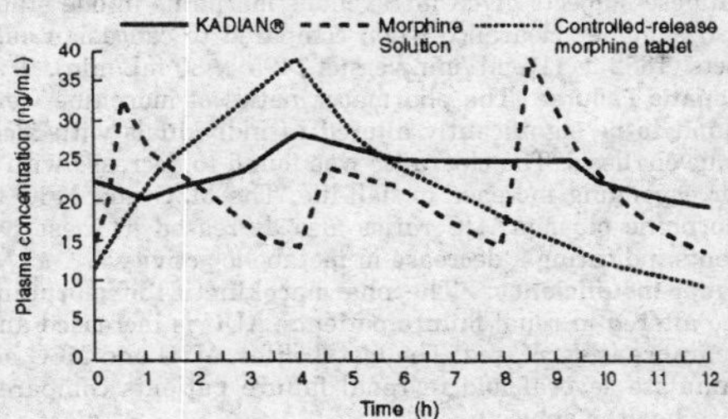

Graph 2 (Study # MOR-9/92):
Dose normalized mean steady state plasma morphine concentrations for KADIAN® (once a day), and an equivalent dose of a 12-hour, controlled-release morphine tablet given twice a day. Plasma concentrations are normalized to 100 mg every 24 hours, (n=24).

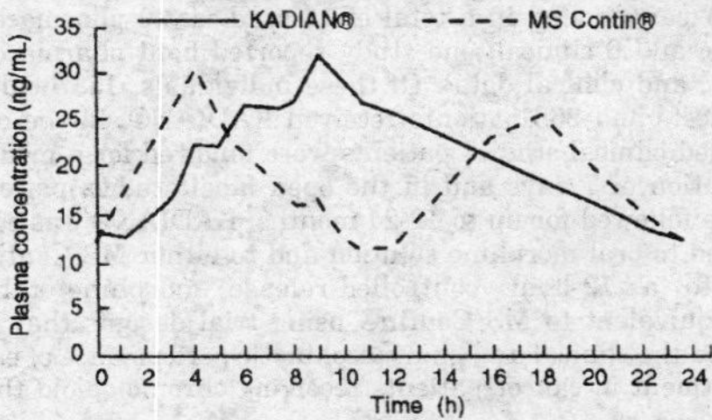

Distribution
Once absorbed, morphine is distributed to skeletal muscle, kidneys, liver, intestinal tract, lungs, spleen and brain.
The volume of distribution of morphine is approximately 3 to 4 L/kg. Morphine is 30 to 35% reversibly bound to plasma proteins.
Although the primary site of action of morphine is in the CNS, only small quantities pass the blood-brain barrier. Morphine also crosses the placental membranes (see **PRECAUTIONS - Pregnancy**) and has been found in breast milk (see **PRECAUTIONS - Nursing Mothers**).
Metabolism
The major pathway of the detoxification of morphine is conjugation, either with D-glucuronic acid in the liver to produce glucuronides or with sulfuric acid to give morphine-3-etheral sulfate. Although a small fraction (less than 5%) of morphine is demethylated, for all practical purposes, virtually all morphine is converted to glucuronide metabolites including morphine-3-glucuronide, M3G (about 50%) and morphine-6-glucuronide, M6G (about 5 to 15%). Studies in healthy subjects and cancer patients have shown that the glucuronide metabolite to morphine mean molar ratios (based on AUC) are similar after both single doses and at steady state for KADIAN®, 12-hour controlled-release morphine sulfate tablets and morphine sulfate solution.
M3G has no significant analgesic activity. M6G has been shown to have opioid agonist and analgesic activity in humans.
Excretion
Approximately 10% of morphine dose is excreted unchanged in the urine. Most of the dose is excreted in the urine as M3G and M6G. A small amount of the glucuronide metabolites is excreted in the bile and there is some minor enterohepatic cycling. Seven to 10% of administered morphine is excreted in the feces.
The mean adult plasma clearance is about 20-30 mL/minute/kg. The effective terminal half-life of morphine after IV administration is reported to be approximately 2.0 hours. Longer plasma sampling in some studies suggests a longer terminal half-life of morphine of about 15 hours.
Special Populations
Geriatric: The elderly may have increased sensitivity to morphine and may achieve higher and more variable serum levels than younger patients. In adults, the duration of analgesia increases progressively with age, though the degree of analgesia remains unchanged. KADIAN® pharmacokinetics have not been investigated in elderly patients (>65

Continued on next page

Kadian—Cont.

years) although such patients were included in the clinical studies.

Nursing Mothers: Morphine is excreted in the maternal milk, and the milk to plasma morphine AUC ratio is about 2.5:1. The amount of morphine received by the infant depends on the maternal plasma concentration, amount of milk ingested by the infant, and the extent of first pass metabolism.

Pediatric: Infants under 1 month of age have a prolonged elimination half-life and decreased clearance relative to older infants and pediatric patients. The clearance of morphine and its elimination half-life begin to approach adult values by the second month of life. Pediatric patients old enough to take capsules should have pharmacokinetic parameters similar to adults, dosed on a per kilogram basis (see **PRECAUTIONS - Pediatric Use**).

Gender: No meaningful differences between male and female patients were demonstrated in the analysis of the pharmacokinetic data from clinical studies.

Race: Pharmacokinetic differences due to race may exist. Chinese subjects given intravenous morphine in one study had a higher clearance when compared to caucasian subjects (1852 ± 116 mL/min versus 1495 ± 80 mL/min).

Hepatic Failure: The pharmacokinetics of morphine were found to be significantly altered in individuals with alcoholic cirrhosis. The clearance was found to decrease with a corresponding increase in half-life. The M3G and M6G to morphine plasma AUC ratios also decreased in these patients indicating a decrease in metabolic activity.

Renal Insufficiency: The pharmacokinetics of morphine are altered in renal failure patients. AUC is increased and clearance is decreased. The metabolites, M3G and M6G accumulate several fold in renal failure patients compared with healthy subjects.

Drug-Drug Interactions: The known drug interactions involving morphine are pharmacodynamic, not pharmacokinetic (see **PRECAUTIONS - Drug Interactions**).

Clinical Studies

A total of 177 healthy subjects and 337 patients with cancer pain participated in a total of 15 studies (10 pharmacokinetic and 6 clinical; one study reported both pharmacokinetic and clinical data). Of these individuals, 158 healthy subjects and 268 patients received KADIAN®. In the controlled clinical studies patients were followed for a median duration of 7 days and in the open label studies patients were followed for up to 12-24 months. KADIAN® was compared to oral morphine solution and to either MS Contin® or to a 12-hour controlled-release morphine tablet bioequivalent to MS Contin® using trial designs that followed the clinical and pharmacokinetic performance of each treatment in cancer patients receiving chronic opioid therapy.

In two controlled studies, patients with moderate to severe cancer pain were titrated with immediate-release morphine (IRM) solution or tablets to a stable total daily dose of morphine for at least three consecutive days, then randomized to KADIAN® or 12-hour controlled-release morphine for seven days of observation. KADIAN® given once a day proved similar to the same total dose of morphine given in divided doses in a 12-hour dosage form, with respect to pain relief, use of rescue medication, patient and investigator global assessment, and quality of sleep. Individual patient differences in the pattern of pain control emphasize the need to individualize both dose and dosing interval (see **DOSAGE AND ADMINISTRATION**).

INDICATIONS AND USAGE

KADIAN® is indicated for the management of moderate to severe pain where treatment with an opioid analgesic is indicated for more than a few days (see **CLINICAL PHARMACOLOGY; Clinical Studies**).

KADIAN® was developed for use in patients with chronic pain who require repeated dosing with a potent opioid analgesic, and has been tested in patients with pain due to malignant conditions. KADIAN® has not been tested as an analgesic for the treatment of acute pain or in the postoperative setting and is not recommended for such use.

CONTRAINDICATIONS

KADIAN® is contraindicated in patients with a known hypersensitivity to morphine, morphine salts or any of the capsule components.

KADIAN® is contraindicated in patients with respiratory depression in the absence of resuscitative equipment, and in patients with acute or severe bronchial asthma.

KADIAN® is contraindicated in any patient who has or is suspected of having paralytic ileus.

WARNINGS (See also CLINICAL PHARMACOLOGY)

Impaired Respiration

Respiratory depression is the chief hazard of all morphine preparations. Respiratory depression occurs more frequently in elderly and debilitated patients, and those suffering from conditions accompanied by hypoxia, hypercapnia, or upper airway obstruction (when even moderate therapeutic doses may significantly decrease pulmonary ventilation).

Morphine should be used with extreme caution in patients with chronic obstructive pulmonary disease or cor pulmonale, and in patients having a substantially decreased respiratory reserve (e.g. severe kyphoscoliosis), hypoxia, hypercapnia, or pre-existing respiratory depression. In such patients, even usual therapeutic doses of morphine may increase airway resistance and decrease respiratory drive to the point of apnea.

Head Injury and Increased Intracranial Pressure

The respiratory depressant effects of morphine with carbon dioxide retention and secondary elevation of cerebrospinal fluid pressure may be markedly exaggerated in the presence of head injury, other intracranial lesions, or a pre-existing increase in intracranial pressure. Morphine produces effects which may obscure neurologic signs of further increases in pressure in patients with head injuries. Morphine should only be administered under such circumstances when considered essential and then with extreme care.

Hypotensive Effect

KADIAN®, like all opioid analgesics, may cause severe hypotension in an individual whose ability to maintain blood pressure has already been compromised by a reduced blood volume, or a concurrent administration of drugs such as phenothiazines or general anesthetics. (see also **PRECAUTIONS - Drug Interactions**). KADIAN® may produce orthostatic hypotension and syncope in ambulatory patients.

KADIAN®, like all opioid analgesics, should be administered with caution to patients in circulatory shock, as vasodilation produced by the drug may further reduce cardiac output and blood pressure.

Gastrointestinal Obstruction

KADIAN® should not be given to patients with gastrointestinal obstruction, particularly paralytic ileus, as there is a risk of the product remaining in the stomach for an extended period and the subsequent release of a bolus of morphine when normal gut motility is restored. As with other solid morphine formulations diarrhea may reduce morphine absorption.

PRECAUTIONS (See also CLINICAL PHARMACOLOGY)

General

KADIAN® is intended for use in patients who require continuous treatment with a potent opioid analgesic. As with any potent opioid, it is critical to adjust the dosing regimen for KADIAN® for each patient, taking into account the patient's prior analgesic treatment experience. Although it is clearly impossible to enumerate every consideration that is important to the selection of the initial dose of KADIAN®, attention should be given to the points under **DOSAGE AND ADMINISTRATION.**

Cordotomy

Patients taking KADIAN® who are scheduled for cordotomy or other interruption of pain transmission pathways should have KADIAN® ceased 24 hours prior to the procedure and the pain controlled by parenteral short-acting opioids. In addition, the post-procedure titration of analgesics for such patients should be individualized to avoid either oversedation or withdrawal syndromes.

Use in Pancreatic/Biliary Tract Disease

KADIAN® may cause spasm of the sphincter of Oddi and should be used with caution in patients with biliary tract disease, including acute pancreatitis. Opioids may cause increases in the serum amylase level.

Special risk groups

KADIAN® should be administered with caution, and in reduced dosages in elderly or debilitated patients; patients with severe renal or hepatic insufficiency; patients with Addison's disease; myxedema; hypothyroidism; prostatic hypertrophy or urethral stricture.

Caution should also be exercised in the administration of KADIAN® to patients with CNS depression, toxic psychosis, acute alcoholism and delirium tremens, and convulsive disorders.

Driving and operating machinery

Morphine may impair the mental and/or physical abilities needed to perform potentially hazardous activities such as driving a car or operating machinery. Patients must be cautioned accordingly. Patients should also be warned about the potential combined effects of morphine with other CNS depressants, including other opioids, phenothiazines, sedative/hypnotics and alcohol (see **Drug Interactions**).

Information for Patients

If clinically advisable, patients receiving KADIAN® should be given the following instructions by the physician:

1. KADIAN® capsules should be swallowed whole (not chewed, crushed, or dissolved). Alternatively, KADIAN® capsules may be opened and the entire contents sprinkled on a small amount of applesauce immediately prior to ingestion. The pellets should NOT be chewed, crushed, or dissolved due to risk of overdose. When prescribing KADIAN® by the sprinkle method, details of proper technique should be explained to the patient. KADIAN® capsules may also be opened and the entire contents sprinkled over about 10 mL of water in a beaker then flushed with swirling through a pre-wetted 16-French gastrostomy tube fitted with a plastic funnel at the port end. The beaker is rinsed with additional aliquots of water as necessary to transfer all of the pellets to flush the tube. **NASOGASTRIC TUBES SHOULD NOT BE USED.** (also see **DOSAGE AND ADMINISTRATION**)
2. The dose of KADIAN® should not be adjusted without consulting the physician.
3. Morphine may impair mental and/or physical ability required for the performance of potentially hazardous tasks (e.g. driving, operating machinery). Patients started on KADIAN® or whose dose has been changed should refrain from dangerous activity until it is established that they are not adversely affected.
4. Morphine should not be taken with alcohol or other CNS depressants (sleeping medication, tranquilizers) because additive effects including CNS depression may occur. A physician should be consulted if other medications are currently being used or are prescribed for future use.
5. Women of childbearing potential who become or are planning to become pregnant, should consult a physician.
6. Upon completion of therapy, it may be appropriate to taper the morphine dose, rather than abruptly discontinuing it.
7. While psychological dependence ("addiction") to morphine used in the treatment of pain is very rare, morphine is one of a class of drugs known to be abused and should be handled accordingly.
8. As with other opioids, patients taking KADIAN® should be advised that severe constipation could occur and appropriate laxatives, stool softeners and other appropriate treatments should be initiated from the beginning of opioid therapy.

Drug Interactions

<u>CNS Depressants:</u> Morphine should be used with great caution and in reduced dosage in patients who are concurrently receiving other central nervous system (CNS) depressants including sedatives, hypnotics, general anesthetics, antiemetics, phenothiazines, other tranquilizers and alcohol because of the risk of respiratory depression, hypotension and profound sedation or coma. When such combined therapy is contemplated, the initial dose of one or both agents should be reduced by at least 50%.

<u>Muscle Relaxants:</u> Morphine may enhance the neuromuscular blocking action of skeletal relaxants and produce an increased degree of respiratory depression.

<u>Mixed Agonist/Antagonist Opioid Analgesics:</u> From a theoretical perspective, mixed agonist/antagonist analgesics (i.e. pentazocine, nalbuphine and butorphanol) should NOT be administered to patients who have received or are receiving a course of therapy with a pure opioid agonist analgesic. In these patients, mixed agonist/antagonist analgesics may reduce the analgesic effect and/or may precipitate withdrawal symptoms.

<u>Monoamine Oxidase Inhibitors (MAOIs):</u> MAOIs have been reported to intensify the effects of at least one opioid drug causing anxiety, confusion and significant depression of respiration or coma. We do not recommend the use of KADIAN® in patients taking MAOIs or within 14 days of stopping such treatment.

<u>Cimetidine:</u> There is an isolated report of confusion and severe respiratory depression when a hemodialysis patient was concurrently administered morphine and cimetidine.

<u>Diuretics:</u> Morphine can reduce the efficacy of diuretics by inducing the release of antidiuretic hormone. Morphine may also lead to acute retention of urine by causing spasm of the sphincter of the bladder, particularly in men with prostatism.

<u>Food:</u> KADIAN® capsules should be swallowed whole (not chewed, crushed, or dissolved). Alternatively, KADIAN® capsules may be opened and the entire contents sprinkled on a small amount of applesauce immediately prior to ingestion. The pellets in KADIAN® should NOT be chewed, crushed, or dissolved due to risk of overdose. (see **DOSAGE AND ADMINISTRATION,** and **INFORMATION FOR PATIENTS**)

Carcinogenicity/Mutagenicity/Impairment of Fertility

Long-term studies in animals to evaluate the carcinogenic potential of morphine have not been conducted. There are no reports of carcinogenic effects in humans.

In vitro studies have reported that morphine is non-mutagenic in the Ames test with *Salmonella*, and induces chromosomal aberrations in human leukocytes and lethal mutation induction in *Drosophila*. Morphine was found to be mutagenic *in vitro* in human T-cells, increasing the DNA fragmentation. *In vivo*, morphine was mutagenic in the mouse micronucleus test and induced chromosomal aberrations in spermatids and murine lymphocytes.

Chronic opioid abusers (e.g., heroin abusers) and their offspring display higher rates of chromosomal damage. However, the rates of chromosomal abnormalities were similar in nonexposed individuals and in heroin users enrolled in long term opioid maintenance programs.

Pregnancy

Teratogenic effects (Pregnancy Category C)

Teratogenic effects of morphine have been reported in the animal literature. High parental doses during the second trimester were teratogenic in neurological, soft and skeletal tissue. The abnormalities included encephalopathy and axial skeletal fusions. These doses were often maternally toxic and were 0.3 to 3-fold the maximum recommended human dose (MRHD) on a mg/m^2 basis. The relative contribution of morphine-induced maternal hypoxia and malnutrition, each of which can be teratogenic, has not been clearly defined. Treatment of male rats with approximately 3-fold the MRHD for 10 days prior to mating decreased litter size and viability.

Nonteratogenic effects

Morphine given subcutaneously, at non-maternally toxic doses, to rats during the third trimester with approximately 0.15-fold the MRHD caused reversible reductions in brain and spinal cord volume, and testes size and body weight in the offspring, and decreased fertility in female offspring. The offspring of rats and hamsters treated orally or intraperitoneally throughout pregnancy with 0.04- to 0.3-fold the MRHD of morphine have demonstrated delayed growth, motor and sexual maturation and decreased male fertility. Chronic morphine exposure of fetal animals resulted in mild

withdrawal, altered reflex and motor skill development, and altered responsiveness to morphine that persisted into adulthood.
There are no well-controlled studies of chronic *in utero* exposure to morphine sulfate in human subjects. However, uncontrolled retrospective studies of human neonates chronically exposed to other opioids *in utero*, demonstrated reduced brain volume which normalized over the first month of life. Infants born to opioid-abusing mothers are more often small for gestational age, have a decreased ventilatory response to CO_2 and increased risk of sudden infant death syndrome.
Morphine should only be used during pregnancy if the need for strong opioid analgesia justifies the potential risk to the fetus.

Labor and Delivery
KADIAN® is not recommended for use in women during and immediately prior to labor, where shorter acting analgesics or other analgesic techniques are more appropriate. Occasionally, opioid analgesics may prolong labor through actions which temporarily reduce the strength, duration and frequency of uterine contractions. However, this effect is not consistent and may be offset by an increased rate of cervical dilatation which tends to shorten labor.
Neonates whose mothers received opioid analgesics during labor should be observed closely for signs of respiratory depression. A specific opioid antagonist, such as naloxone or nalmefene, should be available for reversal of opioid-induced respiratory depression in the neonate.

Neonatal Withdrawal Syndrome
Chronic maternal use of opiates or opioids during pregnancy coexposes the fetus. The newborn may experience subsequent neonatal withdrawal syndrome (NWS). Manifestations of NWS include irritability, hyperactivity, abnormal sleep pattern, high-pitched cry, tremor, vomiting, diarrhea, weight loss, and failure to gain weight. The onset, duration, and severity of the disorder differ based on such factors as the addictive drug used, time and amount of mother's last dose, and rate of elimination of the drug from the newborn. Approaches to the treatment of this syndrome have included supportive care and, when indicated, drugs such as paragoric or phenobarbital.

Nursing Mothers
Low levels of morphine sulfate have been detected in human milk. Withdrawal symptoms can occur in breast-feeding infants when maternal administration of morphine sulfate is stopped. Because of the potential for adverse reactions in nursing infants from KADIAN®, a decision should be made whether to discontinue nursing or discontinue the drug, taking into account the importance of the drug to the mother.

Pediatric Use
There are studies from the literature reporting the safe and effective use of both immediate and sustained release oral morphine preparations for analgesia in pediatric patients who were dosed on a per kilogram basis. However, the safety of KADIAN®, both the entire capsule and the pellets sprinkled on applesauce, have not been directly investigated in pediatric patients below the age of 18 years. The range of doses available is not suitable for the treatment of very young pediatric patients or those who are not old enough to take capsules safely. The applesauce sprinkling method is not an appropriate alternative for these patients.

ADVERSE REACTIONS

Serious adverse reactions that may be associated with KADIAN® therapy in clinical use are those observed with other opioid analgesics and include: respiratory depression, respiratory arrest, circulatory depression, cardiac arrest, hypotension, and/or shock (see **OVERDOSAGE, WARNINGS**).
The less severe adverse events seen on initiation of therapy with KADIAN® are also typical opioid side effects. These events are dose dependent, and their frequency depends on the clinical setting, the patient's level of opioid tolerance, and host factors specific to the individual. They should be expected and managed as a part of opioid analgesia. The most frequent of these include drowsiness, dizziness, constipation and nausea. In many cases, the frequency of these events during initiation of therapy may be minimized by careful individualization of starting dosage, slow titration, and the avoidance of large rapid swings in plasma concentrations of the opioid. Many of these adverse events, will cease or decrease as KADIAN® therapy is continued and some degree of tolerance is developed, but others may be expected to remain troublesome throughout therapy.

Management of Excessive Drowsiness
Most patients receiving morphine will experience initial drowsiness. This usually disappears within 3–5 days and is not a cause of concern unless it is excessive, or accompanied by unsteadiness or confusion. Dizziness and unsteadiness may be associated with postural hypotension, particularly in elderly or debilitated patients, and has been associated with syncope and falls in non-tolerant patients started on opioids.
Excessive or persistent sedation should be investigated. Factors to be considered should include: concurrent sedative medications, the presence of hepatic or renal insufficiency, hypoxia or hypercapnia due to exacerbated respiratory failure, intolerance to the dose used (especially in older patients), disease severity and the patient's general condition.
The dosage should be adjusted according to individual needs, but additional care should be used in the selection of initial doses for the elderly patient, the cachectic or gravely ill patient, or in patients not already familiar with opioid analgesic medications to prevent excessive sedation at the onset of treatment.

Management of Nausea and Vomiting
Nausea and vomiting are common after single doses of morphine or as an early undesirable effect of chronic opioid therapy. The prescription of a suitable antiemetic should be considered, with the awareness that sedation may result (see **Drug Interactions**). The frequency of nausea and vomiting usually decreases within a week or so but may persist due to opioid-induced gastric stasis. Metoclopramide is often useful in such patients.

Management of Constipation
Virtually all patients suffer from constipation while taking opioids on a chronic basis. Some patients, particularly elderly, debilitated or bedridden patients may become impacted. Tolerance does not usually develop for the constipating effects of opioids. Patients must be cautioned accordingly and laxatives, softeners and other appropriate treatments should be used prophylactically from the beginning of opioid therapy.

Adverse Events Probably Related to KADIAN® Administration
In controlled clinical trials in patients with chronic cancer pain the most common adverse events reported by patients at least once during therapy were drowsiness (9%), constipation (9%), nausea (7%), dizziness (6%), and anxiety (6%). Other less common side effects expected from morphine or seen in less than 3% of patients in the clinical trials were:
Body as a Whole: Asthenia, accidental injury, fever, pain, chest pain, headache, diaphoresis, chills, flu syndrome, back pain, malaise, withdrawal syndrome
Cardiovascular: Tachycardia, atrial fibrillation, hypotension, hypertension, pallor, facial flushing, palpitations, bradycardia, syncope
Central Nervous System: Confusion, dry mouth, anxiety, abnormal thinking, abnormal dreams, lethargy, depression, tremor, loss of concentration, insomnia, amnesia, paresthesia, agitation, vertigo, foot drop, ataxia, hypesthesia, slurred speech, hallucinations, vasodilation, euphoria, apathy, seizures, myoclonus
Endocrine: Hyponatremia due to inappropriate ADH secretion, gynecomastia
Gastrointestinal: Vomiting, anorexia, dysphagia, dyspepsia, diarrhea, abdominal pain, stomach atony disorder, gastro-esophageal reflux, delayed gastric emptying, biliary colic
Hemic & Lymphatic: Anemia, leukopenia, thrombocytopenia
Metabolic & Nutritional: Peripheral edema, hyponatremia, edema
Musculoskeletal: Back pain, bone pain, arthralgia
Respiratory: Hiccup, rhinitis, atelectasis, asthma, hypoxia, dyspnea, respiratory insufficiency, voice alteration, depressed cough reflex, non-cardiogenic pulmonary edema
Skin and Appendages: Rash, decubitus ulcer, pruritus, skin flush
Special Senses: Amblyopia, conjunctivitis, miosis, blurred vision, nystagmus, diplopia
Urogenital: Urinary abnormality, amenorrhea, urinary retention, urinary hesitancy, reduced libido, reduced potency, prolonged labor

DRUG ABUSE AND DEPENDENCE

Morphine is the prototype of opioid agonist drugs, and may be subject to misuse, abuse and addiction. Addiction to opioids prescribed for pain management is rare, but requests for opioids from patients addicted to opioids are common and physicians should take appropriate care in prescribing this controlled substance.
Opioid analgesics may cause physical dependence. Physical dependence results in withdrawal symptoms in patients who abruptly discontinue the drug. Withdrawal also may be precipitated through the administration of drugs with opioid antagonist activity, e.g. naloxone, nalmefene, or mixed agonist/antagonist analgesics (pentazocine, butorphanol, nalbuphine), (see also **OVERDOSAGE**).
Physical dependence usually does not occur to a clinically significant degree until after several weeks of continued opioid usage. Tolerance, in which increasingly large doses are required in order to produce the same degree of analgesia, is initially manifested by a shortened duration of analgesic effect, and subsequently, by decreases in the intensity of analgesia.
In chronic pain patients, and in opioid-tolerant cancer patients, the administration of KADIAN® should be guided by the degree of tolerance manifested. Physical dependence, per se, is not ordinarily a concern when one is dealing with a patient in pain, and fear of tolerance should not deter using adequate doses to adequately relieve pain.
If morphine is abruptly discontinued an abstinence syndrome may occur. This is usually mild and is characterized by rhinitis, myalgia, abdominal cramping and occasional diarrhea. Most observable symptoms disappear in 5–14 days without treatment; however, there may be a phase of secondary or chronic abstinence which may last for 2–6 months characterized by insomnia, irritability and muscular aches.
If treatment of physical dependence of patients taking morphine is necessary, the patient may be detoxified by gradual reduction of the dose. Gastrointestinal disturbances or dehydration should be treated with supportive care.
KADIAN® has no role in the management of opioid addiction.

OVERDOSAGE

Symptoms
Acute overdosage with morphine is manifested by respiratory depression, somnolence progressing to stupor or coma, skeletal muscle flaccidity, cold and clammy skin, constricted pupils, and, sometimes, pulmonary edema, bradycardia, hypotension and death. Marked mydriasis rather than miosis may be seen due to severe hypoxia in overdose situations.

Treatment
Primary attention should be given to the re-establishment of a patent airway and institution of assisted or controlled ventilation. Gastric contents may need to be emptied to remove unabsorbed drug when a sustained release formulation such as KADIAN® has been taken. Care should be taken to secure the airway before attempting treatment by gastric emptying or activated charcoal.
The pure opioid antagonists, naloxone or nalmefene, are specific antidotes to respiratory depression which results from opioid overdose. Since the duration of reversal would be expected to be less than the duration of action of KADIAN®, the patient must be carefully monitored until spontaneous respiration is reliably re-established. KADIAN® will continue to release and add to the morphine load for up to 24 hours after administration and the management of an overdose should be monitored accordingly. If the response to opioid antagonists is suboptimal or not sustained, additional antagonist should be given as directed by the manufacturer of the product.
Opioid antagonists should not be administered in the absence of clinically significant respiratory or circulatory depression secondary to morphine overdose. Such agents should be administered cautiously to persons who are known, or suspected to be physically dependent on KADIAN®. In such cases, an abrupt or complete reversal of opioid effects may precipitate an acute abstinence syndrome.
Opioid Tolerant Individuals: In an individual physically dependent on opioids, administration of the usual dose of the antagonist will precipitate an acute withdrawal. The severity of the withdrawal produced will depend on the degree of physical dependence and the dose of the antagonist administered. Use of an opioid antagonist should be reserved for cases where such treatment is clearly needed. If it is necessary to treat serious respiratory depression in the physically dependent patient, administration of the antagonist should be begun with care and by titration with smaller than usual doses.
Supportive measures (including oxygen, vasopressors) should be employed in the management of circulatory shock and pulmonary edema as indicated. Cardiac arrest or arrhythmias may require cardiac massage or defibrillation.

DOSAGE AND ADMINISTRATION

KADIAN® CAPSULES SHOULD BE SWALLOWED WHOLE (NOT CHEWED, CRUSHED, OR DISSOLVED).
ALTERNATIVELY, KADIAN® CAPSULES MAY BE OPENED AND THE ENTIRE CONTENTS SPRINKLED ON A SMALL AMOUNT OF APPLESAUCE IMMEDIATELY PRIOR TO INGESTION. THE PELLETS IN KADIAN® CAPSULES SHOULD NOT BE CHEWED, CRUSHED, OR DISSOLVED DUE TO RISK OF OVERDOSE.
TAKING CHEWED OR CRUSHED KADIAN® CAPSULES OR PELLETS WILL LEAD TO THE RAPID RELEASE AND ABSORPTION OF A POTENTIALLY TOXIC DOSE OF MORPHINE.
KADIAN® CAPSULES MAY BE OPENED AND THE ENTIRE CONTENTS SPRINKLED OVER ABOUT 10 ML OF WATER AND FLUSHED WITH SWIRLING THROUGH A PRE-WETTED 16 FRENCH GASTROSTOMY TUBE FITTED WITH FUNNEL AT THE PORT END. ADDITIONAL ALIQUOTS OF WATER ARE USED TO TRANSFER ALL PELLETS AND TO FLUSH THE TUBE. THE ADMINISTRATION OF KADIAN® PELLETS THROUGH A NASOGASTRIC TUBE SHOULD NOT BE ATTEMPTED.
The sustained release nature of KADIAN® allows it to be administered on **either** a once-a-day or twice-a-day schedule. KADIAN® produces analgesia similar to that produced by conventional immediate-release and controlled-release formulations for the same total daily dose of morphine. However, peak and trough blood levels depend on the release characteristics of each specific formulation, and other oral morphines may not be therapeutically equivalent to KADIAN® for an individual patient.
KADIAN® capsules have the same extent of absorption (AUC) as immediate-release oral formulations and controlled-release oral formulations of morphine sulfate. However, key pharmacokinetic parameters (e.g. C_{max}, T_{max}) for KADIAN® are significantly different from other controlled-release oral formulations.
As with any potent opioid drug product, it is critical to adjust the dosing regimen for each patient individually, taking into account the patient's prior analgesic treatment experience. In the selection of the initial dose of KADIAN®, attention should be given to:

1) the total daily dose, potency and kind of opioid the patient has been taking previously;
2) the reliability of the relative potency estimate used to calculate the equivalent dose of morphine needed;
3) the patient's degree of opioid tolerance;
4) the general condition and medical status of the patient;
5) concurrent medication;
6) the type and severity of the patient's pain.

Continued on next page

Kadian—Cont.

The following dosing recommendations, therefore, can only be considered suggested approaches to what is actually a series of clinical decisions over time in the management of the pain of an individual patient.

Conversion from Other Oral Morphine Formulations to KADIAN®

Patients on other oral morphine formulations may be converted to KADIAN® by administering one-half of the patient's total daily oral morphine dose as KADIAN® capsules every 12 hours (twice-a-day) or by administering the total daily oral morphine dose as KADIAN® capsules every 24 hours (once-a-day). KADIAN® should not be given more frequently than every 12 hours.

Conversion from Parenteral Morphine or Other Parenteral or Oral Opioids to KADIAN®

KADIAN® can be administered to patients previously receiving treatment with parenteral morphine or other opioids. While there are useful tables of oral and parenteral equivalents in cancer analgesia, there is substantial interpatient variation in the relative potency of different opioid drugs and formulations. For these reasons, it is better to underestimate the patient's 24 hour oral morphine requirement and provide rescue medication, than to overestimate and manage an adverse event. The following general points should be considered:

Parenteral to oral morphine ratio: It may take anywhere from 2–6 mg of oral morphine to provide analgesia equivalent to 1 mg of parenteral morphine. A dose of oral morphine three times the daily parenteral morphine requirement may be sufficient in chronic use settings.

Other parenteral or oral opioids to oral morphine sulfate: Physicians are advised to refer to published relative potency data, keeping in mind that such ratios are only approximate. In general, it is safest to give half of the estimated daily morphine demand as the initial dose, and to manage inadequate analgesia by supplementation with immediate-release morphine. (See discussion which follows.)

The first dose of KADIAN® may be taken with the last dose of any immediate-release (short-acting) opioid medication due to the long delay until the peak effect after administration of KADIAN®.

Use of KADIAN® as the First Opioid Analgesic

There has been no evaluation of KADIAN® as an initial opioid analgesic in the management of pain. Because it may be more difficult to titrate a patient to adequate analgesia using a sustained release morphine, it is ordinarily advisable to begin treatment using an immediate-release morphine formulation.

Individualization of Dosage

The best use of opioid analgesics in the management of chronic malignant and non-malignant pain is challenging, and is well described in materials published by the World Health Organization and the Agency for Health Care Policy and Research which are available from Faulding Laboratories upon request. KADIAN® is a third step drug which is most useful when the patient requires a constant level of opioid analgesia as a "floor" or "platform" from which to manage breakthrough pain. When a patient has reached the point where comfort cannot be provided with a combination of non-opioid medications (NSAIDs and acetaminophen) and intermittent use of moderate or strong opioids, the patient's total opioid therapy should be converted into a 24 hour oral morphine equivalent.

KADIAN® should be started by administering one-half of the estimated total daily oral morphine dose every 12 hours (twice-a-day) or by administering the total daily oral morphine dose every 24 hours (once-a-day). The dose should be titrated no more frequently than every-other-day to allow the patients to stabilize before escalating the dose. If breakthrough pain occurs, the dose may be supplemented with a small dose (less than 20% of the total daily dose) of a short-acting analgesic. Patients who are excessively sedated after a once-a-day dose or who regularly experience inadequate analgesia before the next dose should be switched to twice-a-day dosing.

Patients who do not have a proven tolerance to opioids should be started only on the 20 mg strength, and usually should be increased at a rate not greater than 20 mg every-other-day. Most patients will rapidly develop some degree of tolerance, requiring dosage adjustment until they have achieved their individual best balance between baseline analgesia and opioid side effects such as confusion, sedation and constipation. No guidance can be given as to the recommended maximal dose, especially in patients with chronic pain of malignancy. In such cases the total dose of KADIAN® should be advanced until the desired therapeutic endpoint is reached or clinically significant opioid-related adverse reactions intervene.

Alternative Methods of Administration

In a study of healthy volunteers, KADIAN® pellets sprinkled over applesauce were found to be bioequivalent to KADIAN® capsules swallowed whole with applesauce under fasting conditions. Other foods have not been tested. Patients who have difficulty swallowing whole capsules or tablets may benefit from this alternative method of administration.

1) Sprinkle the pellets onto a small amount of applesauce. Applesauce should be room temperature or cooler.
2) Use immediately.
3) Rinse mouth to ensure all pellets have been swallowed.
4) Patients should consume entire portion and should not divide applesauce into separate doses.

The entire capsule contents may be administered through a 16 French gastrostomy tube.

1) Flush the gastrostomy tube with water to ensure that it is wet.
2) Sprinkle the KADIAN® Pellets into 10 mL of water.
3) Use a swirling motion to pour the pellets and water into the gastrostomy tube through a funnel.
4) Rinse the beaker with a further 10 mL of water and pour this into the funnel.
5) Repeat rinsing until no pellets remain in the beaker.

THE ADMINISTRATION OF KADIAN® PELLETS THROUGH A NASOGASTRIC TUBE SHOULD NOT BE ATTEMPTED.

Considerations in the Adjustment of Dosing Regimens

If signs of excessive opioid effects are observed early in the dosing interval, the next dose should be reduced. If this adjustment leads to inadequate analgesia, that is, if breakthrough pain occurs when KADIAN® is administered on an every 24 hours dosing regimen, consideration should be given to dosing every 12 hours. If breakthough pain occurs on a 12 hour dosing regimen a supplemental dose of short-acting analgesic may be given. As experience is gained, adjustments in both dose and dosing interval can be made to obtain an appropriate balance between pain relief and opioid side effects. To avoid accumulation the dosing interval of KADIAN® should not be reduced below 12 hours.

Conversion from KADIAN® to Other Controlled-Release Oral Morphine Formulations

KADIAN® is not bioequivalent to other controlled-release morphine preparations. Although for a given dose the same total amount of morphine is available from KADIAN® as from morphine solution or controlled-release morphine tablets, the slower release of morphine from KADIAN® results in reduced maximum and increased minimum plasma morphine concentrations than with shorter acting morphine products. Conversion from KADIAN® to the same total daily dose of controlled-release morphine preparations may lead to either excessive sedation at peak or inadequate analgesia at trough and close observation and appropriate dosage adjustments are recommended.

Conversion from KADIAN® to Parenteral Opioids

When converting a patient from KADIAN® to parenteral opioids, it is best to calculate an equivalent parenteral dose, and then initiate treatment at half of this calculated value. For example, to estimate the required 24 hour dose of parenteral morphine for a patient taking KADIAN®, one would take the 24 hour KADIAN® dose, divide by an oral to parenteral conversion ratio of 3, divide the estimated 24 hour parenteral dose into six divided doses (for a four hour dosing interval), then halve this dose as an initial trial.

For example, to estimate the required parenteral morphine dose for a patient taking 360 mg of KADIAN® a day, divide the 360 mg daily oral morphine dose by a conversion ratio of 1 mg of parenteral morphine for every 3 mg of oral morphine. The estimated 120 mg daily parenteral requirement is then divided into six 20 mg doses, and half of this, or 10 mg, is then given every 4 hours as an initial trial dose.

This approach is likely to require a dosage increase in the first 24 hours for many patients, but is recommended because it is less likely to cause overdose than trying to establish an equivalent dose without titration.

Opioid analgesic agents may not effectively relieve dysesthetic pain, post-herpetic neuralgia, stabbing pains, activity-related pain, and some forms of headache. This does not mean that patients suffering from these types of pain should not be given an adequate trial of opioid analgesics. However, such patients may need to be promptly evaluated for other types of pain therapy.

Safety and Handling

KADIAN® consists of closed hard gelatin capsules containing polymer coated morphine sulfate pellets that pose no known handling risk to health care workers. Oral morphine products are not known to be associated with a high risk of diversion, but all strong opioids are liable to diversion and misuse both by the general public and health care workers, and should be handled accordingly.

HOW SUPPLIED

KADIAN® capsules contain white to off-white or tan colored polymer coated sustained release pellets of morphine sulfate and are available in three dose strengths:

20 mg size 4 capsule, yellow opaque cap imprinted KADIAN and yellow opaque body imprinted 20 mg. Capsules are supplied in bottles of 30 (NDC 63857-322-03), 60 (NDC 63857-322-06) and 100 (NDC 63857-322-11).

50 mg size 2 capsule, blue opaque cap imprinted KADIAN and blue opaque body imprinted with 50 mg. Capsules are supplied in bottles of 30 (NDC 63857-323-03), 60 (NDC 63857-323-06) and 100 (NDC 63857-323-11).

100 mg size 0 capsule, green opaque cap imprinted KADIAN and green opaque body imprinted with 100 mg. Capsules are supplied in bottles of 30 (NDC 63857-324-03), 60 (NDC 63857-324-06) and 100 (NDC 63857-324-11).

Store at 25°C (77°F); excursions permitted to 15°–30°C (59°–86°F). Protect from light and moisture.

Dispense in a sealed, tamper-evident, childproof, light-resistant container.

CAUTION

DEA Order Form Required.

Rx only

KADIAN® is a registered trademark of F H Faulding & Co Limited

MS Contin® is a registered trademark of The Purdue Frederick Company

Manufactured for: **FAULDING LABORATORIES INC.**
Raleigh, NC 27606
by: Purepac Pharmaceutical Co.
Elizabeth, NJ 07207 USA
40-8838 Revised—March 2000

Shown in Product Identification Guide, page 312

Ferndale Laboratories, Inc.

780 W. EIGHT MILE ROAD
FERNDALE, MI 48220

Direct Inquiries to:
Mr. Thayer McMillan
(248) 548-0900
FAX: (248) 548-8427

For Medical Information Contact:
In Emergencies:
Mr. Pravin M. Patel
(248) 548-0900
FAX: (248) 548-0708

ANALPRAM–HC® CREAM 1% or 2.5% ℞
Rectal Cream
ANALPRAM–HC® LOTION 2.5% ℞

DESCRIPTION

ANALPRAM-HC® CREAM: Contains Hydrocortisone Acetate 1% or 2.5% and Pramoxine HCl 1% in a hydrophilic cream base containing stearic acid, cetyl alcohol, aquaphor, isopropylpalmitate, polyoxyl-40 stearate, propylene glycol, potassium sorbate, sorbic acid, triethanolamine lauryl sulfate and water.

ANALPRAM–HC® LOTION 2.5%: Contains Hydrocortisone Acetate 2.5% and Pramoxine Hydrochloride 1% in a hydrophilic lotion base containing stearic acid, cetyl alcohol, forlan-L, glycerin, triethanolamine, polyoxyl 40 stearate, diisopropyl adipate, povidone, silicone, potassium sorbate, sorbic acid, and purified water.

Topical corticosteroids are anti-inflammatory and antipruritic agents. The structural formula, the chemical name, molecular formula and molecular weight for active ingredients are presented below.

Hydrocortisone acetate
(Pregn-4-ene-3,20-dione,21 - (acetyloxy)-11, 17-dihydroxy-,(11 β)-.)
$C_{23}H_{32}O_6$; mol wt: 404.50

Pramoxine hydrochloride
(4-(3-(p-butoxyphenoxy)propyl)morpholine hydrochloride)
$C_{17}H_{27}NO_3.HCl$; mol wt: 329.87

CLINICAL PHARMACOLOGY

Topical corticosteroids share anti-inflammatory, anti-pruritic and vasoconstrictive actions.

The mechanism of anti-inflammatory activity of the topical corticosteroids is unclear. Various laboratory methods, including vasoconstrictor assays, are used to compare and predict potencies and/or clinical efficacies of the topical corticosteroids. There is some evidence to suggest that a recognizable correlation exists between vasoconstrictor potency and therapeutic efficacy in man.

Pramoxine hydrochloride is a topical anesthetic agent which provides temporary relief from itching and pain. It acts by stabilizing the neuronal membrane of nerve endings with which it comes into contact.

Pharmacokinetics: The extent of percutaneous absorption of topical corticosteroids is determined by many factors including the vehicle, the integrity of the epidermal barrier, and the use of occlusive dressings.

Topical corticosteroids can be absorbed from normal intact skin. Inflammation and/or other disease processes in the skin increase percutaneous absorption. Occlusive dressings substantially increase the percutaneous absorption of topical corticosteroids. Thus, occlusive dressings may be a valuable therapeutic adjunct for treatment of resistant dermatoses (See DOSAGE AND ADMINISTRATION).

Once absorbed through the skin, topical corticosteroids are handled through pharmacokinetic pathways similar to systemically administered corticosteroids. Corticosteroids are bound to plasma proteins in varying degrees. Corticosteroids are metabolized primarily in the liver and are then excreted by the kidneys. Some of the topical corticosteroids and their metabolites are also excreted into the bile.

INDICATIONS AND USAGE

Topical corticosteroids are indicated for the relief of the inflammatory and pruritic manifestations of corticosteroid-responsive dermatoses of the anal region.

CONTRAINDICATIONS

Topical corticosteroids are contraindicated in those patients with a history of hypersensitivity to any of the components of the preparation.

PRECAUTIONS

General: Systemic absorption of topical corticosteroids has produced reversible hypothalamic-pituitary-adrenal (HPA) axis suppression, manifestations of Cushing's syndrome, hyperglycemia, and glucosuria in some patients.

Conditions which augment systemic absorption include the application of the more potent steroids, use over large surface areas, prolonged use, and the addition of occlusive dressings.

Therefore, patients receiving a large dose of a potent topical steroid applied to a large surface area and under an occlusive dressing should be evaluated periodically for evidence of HPA axis suppression by using the urinary free cortisol and ACTH stimulation tests. If HPA axis suppression is noted, an attempt should be made to withdraw the drug, to reduce the frequency of application, or to substitute a less potent steroid.

Recovery of HPA axis function is generally prompt and complete upon discontinuation of the drug. Infrequently, signs and symptoms of steroid withdrawal may occur, requiring supplemental systemic corticosteroids.

Children may absorb proportionally larger amounts of topical corticosteroids and thus be more susceptible to systemic toxicity. (See PRECAUTIONS—Pediatric Use).

If irritation develops, topical corticosteroids should be discontinued and appropriate therapy instituted.

In the presence of dermatological infections, the use of an appropriate antifungal or antibacterial agent should be instituted. If a favorable response does not occur promptly, the corticosteroid should be discontinued until the infection has been adequately controlled.

Information for the Patient: Patients using topical corticosteroids should receive the following information and instructions:

1. This medication is to be used as directed by the physician. It is for external use only. Avoid contact with the eyes.
2. Patients should be advised not to use this medication for any disorder other than for which it was prescribed.
3. The treated skin area should not be bandaged or otherwise covered or wrapped as to be occlusive unless directed by the physician.
4. Patients should report any signs of local adverse reactions especially under occlusive dressing.
5. Parents of pediatric patients should be advised not to use tightfitting diapers or plastic pants on a child being treated in the diaper area, as these garments may constitute occlusive dressings.

Laboratory Tests: The following tests may be helpful in evaluating the HPA axis suppression:

Urinary free cortisol test
ACTH stimulation test

Carcinogenesis, Mutagenesis, and Impairment of Fertility: Long-term animal studies have not been performed to evaluate the carcinogenic potential or the effect on fertility of topical corticosteroids.

Studies to determine mutagenicity with prednisolone and hydrocortisone have revealed negative results.

Pregnancy Category C: Corticosteroids are generally teratogenic in laboratory animals when administered systemically at relatively low dosage levels. The more potent corticosteroids have been shown to be teratogenic after dermal application in laboratory animals. There are no adequate and well-controlled studies in pregnant women on teratogenic effects from topically applied corticosteroids. Therefore, topical corticosteroids should be used during pregnancy only if the potential benefit justifies the potential risk to the fetus. Drugs of this class should not be used extensively on pregnant patients, in large amounts, or for prolonged periods of time.

Nursing Mothers: It is not known whether topical administration of corticosteroids could result in sufficient systemic absorption to produce detectable amounts in breast milk. Systemically administered corticosteroids are secreted into breast milk in quantities NOT likely to have a deleterious effect on the infant. Nevertheless, caution should be exercised when topical corticosteroids are administered to a nursing woman.

Pediatric Use: PEDIATRIC PATIENTS MAY DEMONSTRATE GREATER SUSCEPTIBILITY TO TOPICAL CORTICOSTEROID-INDUCED HPA AXIS SUPPRESSION AND CUSHING'S SYNDROME THAN MATURE PATIENTS BECAUSE OF A LARGER SKIN SURFACE AREA TO BODY WEIGHT RATIO.

Hypothalamic-pituitary-adrenal (HPA) axis suppression, Cushing's syndrome, and intracranial hypertension have been reported in children receiving topical corticosteroids. Manifestations of adrenal suppression in children include linear growth retardation, delayed weight gain, low plasma cortisol levels, and absence of response to ACTH stimulation. Manifestations of intracranial hypertension include bulging fontanelles, headaches, and bilateral papilledema.

Administration of topical corticosteroids to children should be limited to the least amount compatible with an effective therapeutic regimen. Chronic corticosteroid therapy may interfere with the growth and development of children.

ADVERSE REACTIONS

The following local adverse reactions are reported infrequently with topical corticosteroids, but may occur more frequently with the use of occlusive dressings. These reactions are listed in an approximate decreasing order of occurrence:

Burning	Hypopigmentation
Itching	Perioral dermatitis
Irritation	Allergic contact dermatitis
Dryness	Maceration of the skin
Folliculitis	Secondary infection
Hypertrichosis	Skin Atrophy
Acneiform eruptions	Striae
	Miliaria

OVERDOSAGE

Topically applied corticosteroids can be absorbed in sufficient amounts to produce systemic effects (See PRECAUTIONS).

DOSAGE AND ADMINISTRATION

Topical corticosteroids are generally applied to the affected area as a thin film three or four times daily depending on the severity of the condition.

Occlusive dressings may be used for the management of psoriasis or recalcitrant conditions. If an infection develops, the use of occlusive dressings should be discontinued and appropriate antimicrobial therapy instituted.

For cleansing of anogenital area, spread Analpram HC® Lotion 2.5% on cotton or tissue and wipe affected area.

HOW SUPPLIED

ANALPRAM-HC® CREAM 1% is supplied in 1 oz tube with rectal applicator. NDC 0496–0778–04

ANALPRAM-HC® CREAM 2.5% is supplied in 1 oz tube with rectal applicator. NDC 0496-0800-04

ANALPRAM-HC® LOTION 2.5% is supplied in 2 fl oz bottle. NDC 0496–0829–04

Dispense in a tight container as defined in the official compendium.

Store at controlled room temperature 15°– 30°C (59°– 86°F).

DECUBITENE™ Oxygenated Oil — OTC

[*dĕ-cū-bĭ-tēne*]

Decubitene is a specially formulated preparation consisting of 99% oxygenated triglycerides of corn oil origin designed specifically as a first response to dermal warning lesions (Stage I pressure ulcers) on mobility restricted patients.

HOW SUPPLIED

Decubitene™ is supplied in spray bottles containing 20 ml UPC 7-34118-0845-2-1

DERMAMIST™ — OTC

[*dĕrm-a-mīst*]

Dermamist™ is a skin protectant spray designed to prevent the loss of vital moisture after showering.

HOW SUPPLIED

Dermamist™ is supplied in aerosol cans containing 125 ml NDC 0496-0847-04

ELA-*Max*® Topical Anesthetic Cream — OTC

[*elă-măx*]

(lidocaine 4%)

DESCRIPTION

ELA-Max® Cream (lidocaine 4%) is a topical anesthetic cream. Lidocaine is chemically designated as acetamide, 2-(diethylamino)-N-(2,6–dimethylphenyl), has an octanol: water partition ratio of 43 at pH 7.4, and has the following structure:

CH_3 — $NHCOCH_2N(C_2H_5)_2$ — CH_3

$C_{14}H_{22}N_2O$ Mol. wt. 234.33

Each gram of ELA-Max Cream contains lidocaine 40 mg, lecithin, propylene glycol, benzyl alcohol, vitamin E acetate, cholesterol, carbomer 940, triethanolamine, polysorbate 80, purified water.

CLINICAL PHARMACOLOGY

Mechanism of Action: ELA-Max Cream (lidocaine 4%) applied to intact skin provides dermal analgesia by a release of lidocaine from the cream into the epidermal and dermal layers of the skin, and by the accumulation of lidocaine in the vicinity of pain receptors and nerve endings. Lidocaine is an amide-type local anesthetic agent which stabilizes neuronal membranes by inhibiting the ionic fluxes required for the initiation and conduction of impulses, thereby effecting local anesthetic action. The onset, depth and duration of dermal analgesia provided by ELA-Max Cream depends primarily on the duration of application.

Dermal application of ELA-Max Cream may cause a transient, local blanching followed by a transient, local redness or erythemia.

Pharmacokinetics: The amount of lidocaine systemically absorbed from ELA-Max Cream is directly related to both the duration of application and to the area over which it is applied.

It is not known if lidocaine is metabolized in the skin. Lidocaine is metabolized rapidly by the liver to a number of metabolites including monoethylglycinexylidide (MEGX) and glycinexylidide (GX), both of which have pharmacologic activity similar to, but less potent than that of lidocaine. The metabolite, 2,6–xylidine, has unknown pharmacologic activity but is carcinogenic in rats (see Carcinogenesis subsection of PRECAUTIONS).

Following intravenous administration, MEGX and GX concentrations in serum range from 11 to 36% and from 5 to 11% of lidocaine concentrations, respectively.

The half-life of lidocaine elimination from the plasma following IV administration is approximately 65 to 150 minutes (mean 110,±24 SD, n = 13). This half-life may be increased in cardiac or hepatic dysfunction. More than 98% of an absorbed dose of lidocaine can be recovered in the urine as metabolites or parent drug. The systemic clearance is 10 to 20 mL/min/kg (mean 13,±3 SD, n = 13).

INDICATION AND USAGE

ELA-Max Cream (lidocaine 4%) is indicated for the temporary relief of pain associated with minor cuts and abrasions of the skin, minor burns, including sunburn, minor skin irritation and insect bites.

ELA-Max Cream is not recommended on mucous membranes because limited studies show greater absorption of lidocaine than through intact skin. Safe dosing recommendations for use on mucous membranes cannot be made because it has not been studied adequately. ELA-Max Cream is not recommended in any clinical situation in which penetration or migration beyond the tympanic membrane into the middle ear is possible because of ototoxic effects observed in animal studies (see WARNINGS).

CONTRAINDICATIONS

ELA-Max Cream (lidocaine 4%) is contraindicated in patients with a known history of sensitivity to local anesthetics of the amide type or to any other component of the product.

WARNINGS

For external use only. Avoid contact with eyes. Do not apply to irritated skin or if excessive irritation develops. If condition worsens, or if symptoms persist unaltered for more than seven days or clear up and occur again within only a few days, discontinue use of this product and consult a doctor. Do not use in large quantities, particularly over raw or blistered areas. As with any drug, if you are pregnant or nursing a baby, seek the advice of a health professional before using this product. In case of accidental ingestion, seek professional help or contact a poison control center immediately. Keep this and all medicines out of the reach of children.

Application of ELA-Max Cream to larger areas or for longer times than those recommended could result in sufficient absorption of lidocaine resulting in serious adverse effects (see DOSAGE AND ADMINISTRATION).

Studies in laboratory animals (guinea pigs) have shown that lidocaine cream has an ototoxic effect when instilled into the middle ear. In these same studies, animals exposed to lidocaine cream in the external auditory canal only, showed no abnormality. ELA-Max Cream should not be used in any clinical situation in which its penetration or migration beyond the tympanic membrane into the middle ear is possible.

PRECAUTIONS

General: Repeated doses of ELA-Max Cream may increase blood levels of lidocaine. ELA-Max Cream should be used with caution in patients who may be more sensitive to the systemic effects of lidocaine including acutely ill, debilitated, or elderly patients.

ELA-Max Cream coming in contact with the eye should be avoided because animal studies have demonstrated severe eye irritation. Also the loss of protective reflexes can permit corneal irritation and potential abrasion. Absorption of lidocaine cream in conjunctival tissues has not been determined. If eye contact occurs, immediately wash out the eye with water or saline and protect the eye until sensation returns.

Patients allergic to para-aminobenzoic acid derivatives (procaine, tetracaine, benzocaine, etc.) have not shown cross sensitivity to lidocaine; however, ELA-Max Cream should be used with caution in patients with a history of drug sensitivities, especially if the etiologic agent is uncertain. Patients with severe hepatic disease, because of their inability to metabolize local anesthetics normally, are at greater risk of developing toxic plasma concentrations of lidocaine.

Information for Patients: When ELA-Max Cream is used, the patient should be aware that the production of dermal analgesia may be accompanied by the block of all sensations in the treated skin. For this reason, the patient should avoid inadvertant trauma to the treated area by scratching, rub-

Continued on next page

ELA-Max—Cont.

bing, or exposure to extreme hot or cold temperatures until complete sensation has returned.

Drug Interactions: ELA-Max® Cream should be used with caution in patients receiving Class 1 antiarrhythmic drugs (such as tocainide and mexiletine) since the toxic effects are additive and generally synergistic.

Carcinogenesis, Mutagenesis, Impairment of Fertility:

Carcinogenesis: Metabolites of lidocaine have been shown to be carcinogenic in laboratory animals.

Mutagenesis: The mutagenic potential of lidocaine HCl has been tested in the Ames Salmonella/mammalian microsome test and by analysis of structural chromosome aberrations in human lymphocytes *in vitro*, and by mouse micronucleus test *in vivo*. There was no indication in these tests of any mutagenic effects.

The mutagenicity of 2,6-xylidine, a metabolite of lidocaine, has been studied in different tests with mixed results. The compound was found to be weakly mutagenic in the Ames test only under metabolic activation conditions. In addition, 2,6-xylidine was observed to be mutagenic at the thymidine kinase locus, with or without activation, and induced chromosome aberrations and sister chromatid exchanges at concentrations at which the drug precipitated out of the solution (1.2 mg/mL). No evidence of genotoxicity was found in the *in vivo* assays measuring unscheduled DNA synthesis in rat hepatocytes, chromosome damage in polychromatic erythrocytes or preferential killing of DNA repair-deficient bacteria in liver, lung, kidney, testes and blood extracts from mice. However, covalent binding studies of DNA from liver and ethmoid turbinates in rats indicate that 2,6-xylidine may be genotoxic under certain conditions *in vivo*.

Impairment of Fertility: See Use in Pregnancy

Use in Pregnancy:

Teratogenic Effects: Pregnancy Category B: There are no adequate and well-controlled studies in pregnant women. Because animal reproduction studies are not always predictive of human response, ELA-Max Cream should be used during pregnancy only if clearly needed.

Labor and Delivery: Lidocaine is not contraindicated in labor and delivery. Should ELA-Max Cream be used concomitantly with other products containing lidocaine, total doses contributed by all formulations must be considered.

Nursing Mothers: Lidocaine is excreted in human milk. Therefore, caution should be exercised when ELA-Max Cream is administered to a nursing mother since the milk: plasma ration of lidocaine is 0.4.

Pediatric Use: Consult a doctor prior to use on children under 2 years of age. When using ELA-Max Cream in young children, care must be taken to insure that application of the cream is limited to the intended site (See DOSAGE AND ADMINISTRATION). Accidental ingestion may lead to dose related toxicity.

ADVERSE REACTIONS

Localized reactions: During or immediately after treatment with ELA-Max Cream, the skin at the site of treatment may develop erythema or edema or may be the locus of abnormal sensation.

Allergic Reactions: Allergic and anaphylactoid reactions associated with lidocaine can occur. They are characterized by urticaria, angioedema, bronchospasm, and shock. If they occur they should be managed by conventional means. The detection of sensitivity by skin testing is of doubtful value.

System (Dose Related) Reactions: Systemic adverse reactions following appropriate use of ELA-Max Cream are unlikely due to the small dose absorbed. Systemic adverse reactions of lidocaine are similar in nature to those observed with other amide local anesthetic agents including CNS excitation and/or depression (light-headedness, nervousness, apprehension, euphoria, confusion, dizziness, drowsiness, tinnitus, blurred or double vision, vomiting, sensations of heat, cold or numbness, twitching, tremors, convulsions, unconsciousness, respiratory depression and arrest). Excitatory CNS reactions may be brief or not occur at all, in which case the first manifestation may be drowsiness merging into unconsciousness. Cardiovascular manifestations may include bradycardia, hypotension, and cardiovascular collapse leading to arrest.

OVERDOSAGE

Peak blood levels following a 60g application to 400 cm^2 for 3 hours are 0.05 to 0.16 µg/mL for lidocaine. Toxic levels of lidocaine (>5 µg/mL) cause decreases in cardiac output, total peripheral resistance and mean arterial pressure. These changes may be attributable to direct depressant effects of these local anesthetic agents on the cardiovascular system. In the absence of massive topical overdose or oral ingestion, evaluation should include other etiologies for the clinical effects of overdosage from other sources of lidocaine or other local anesthetics.

DOSAGE AND ADMINISTRATION

A thick layer of ELA-Max Cream is applied to intact skin. A single application of ELA-Max Cream in a child weighing less than 10 kg should not be applied over an area larger than 100 cm^2. A single application of ELA-Max Cream in children weighing between 10 kg and 20 kg should not be applied over an area larger than 200 cm^2.

When applying ELA-Max Cream to young children, care must be taken to maintain careful observation of the child to prevent accidental ingestion of ELA-Max Cream.

When ELA-Max Cream (lidocaine 4%) is used concomitantly with other products containing local anesthetic agents, the amount absorbed from all formulations must be considered. The amount absorbed in the case of ELA-Max Cream is determined by the area over which it is applied and the duration of application. Although the incidence of systemic adverse reactions with ELA-Max Cream is very low, caution should be exercised, particularly when applying it over large areas and leaving it on for longer than 2 hours. The incidence of systemic adverse reactions can be expected to be directly proportional to the area and time of exposure.

HOW SUPPLIED

ELA-Max Cream is available as the following:
NDC 0496-0823-06 5 gram tube, box of 5
NDC 0496-0823-30 30 gram tube
Store between 15° and 30°C (59° – 86°F).
NOT FOR OPHTHALMIC USE.
KEEP CONTAINER TIGHTLY CLOSED AT ALL TIMES WHEN NOT IS USE.
Manufactured Jointly by:
Ferndale Laboratories, Inc.
Ferndale, MI 48220 and
BioZone Laboratories, Inc.
Pittsburg, CA 94565
ELA-MAX is a Registered trademark of Ferndale Laboratories, Inc.
©Ferndale Laboratories, Inc.
MG #13350 Iss: 10/98

ELA-Max®5 Anorectal Cream OTC

[*elă 'măx-five*]
(lidocaine 5%)

DESCRIPTION

ELA-Max®5 Anorectal Cream (lidocaine 5%) is a topical anesthetic cream. Lidocaine is chemically designated as acetamide, 2-(diethylamino)-N-(2,6-dimethylphenyl), has an octanol:water partition ratio of 43 at pH 7.4, and has the following structure:

CH_3
$NHCOCH_2N(C_2H_5)_2$
CH_3
$C_{14}H_{22}N_2O$ Mol. wt. 234.33

Each gram of ELA-Max 5 Anorectal Cream contains lidocaine 50 mg, lecithin, propylene glycol, benzyl alcohol, vitamin E acetate, cholesterol, isopropyl myristate, carbomer 940, triethanolamine, polysorbate 80, purified water.

CLINICAL PHARMACOLOGY

Mechanism of Action: ELA-Max 5 Anorectal Cream (lidocaine 5%) applied to intact skin provides dermal analgesia by a release of lidocaine from the cream into the epidermal and dermal layers of the skin, and by the accumulation of lidocaine in the vicinity of pain receptors and nerve endings. Lidocaine is an amide-type local anesthetic agent which stabilizes neuronal membranes by inhibiting the ionic fluxes required for the initiation and conduction of impulses, thereby effecting local anesthetic action. The onset, depth and duration of dermal analgesia provided by ELA-Max 5 Anorectal Cream depends primarily on the duration of application.

Dermal application of ELA-Max 5 Anorectal Cream may cause a transient, local blanching followed by a transient, local redness or erythemia.

Pharmacokinetics: The amount of lidocaine systemically absorbed from ELA-Max 5 Anorectal Cream is directly related to both the duration of application and to the area over which it is applied.

It is not known if lidocaine is metabolized in the skin. Lidocaine is metabolized rapidly by the liver to a number of metabolites including monoethylglycinexylidide (MEGX) and glycinexylidide (GX), both of which have pharmacologic activity similar to, but less potent than that of lidocaine. The metabolite, 2,6-xylidine, has unknown pharmacologic activity but is carcinogenic in rats (see Carcinogenesis subsection of PRECAUTIONS). Following intravenous administration, MEGX and GX concentrations in serum range from 11 to 36% and from 5 to 11% of lidocaine concentrations, respectively.

The half-life of lidocaine elimination from the plasma following IV administration is approximately 65 to 150 minutes (mean 110, ±24 SD, n=13). This half-life may be increased in cardiac or hepatic dysfunction. More than 98% of an absorbed dose of lidocaine can be recovered in the urine as metabolites or parent drug. The systemic clearance is 10 to 20 mL/min/kg (mean 13, ±3 SD, n=13).

INDICATION AND USAGE

ELA-Max 5 Anorectal Cream (lidocaine 5%) is indicated for the temporary relief of local discomfort, including pain and itching, soreness or burning associated with anorectal disorders. ELA-Max 5 Anorectal Cream is not recommended on mucous membranes because limited studies show greater absorption of lidocaine than through intact skin. Safe dosing recommendations for use on mucous membranes cannot be made because it has not been studied adequately.

ELA-Max 5 Anorectal Cream is not recommended in any clinical situation in which penetration or migration beyond the tympanic membrane into the middle ear is possible because of ototoxic effects observed in animal studies (see WARNINGS).

CONTRAINDICATIONS

ELA-Max 5 Anorectal Cream (lidocaine 5%) is contraindicated in patients with a known history of sensitivity to local anesthetics of the amide type or to any other component of the product.

WARNINGS

For external use only. Avoid contact with eyes. Do not apply to irritated skin or if excessive irritation develops. If condition worsens, or if symptoms persist unaltered for seven days, or clear up and occur again within only a few days, discontinue use of this product and consult a doctor. Do not exceed the recommended daily dosage unless directed by a doctor. Do not apply to raw or blistered areas. In case of bleeding, consult a doctor promptly. Do not put this product into the rectum using fingers or any mechanical device or applicator. Certain persons can develop allergic reactions to ingredients in this product. If redness, irritation, swelling, pain or other symptoms develop or increase, discontinue use and consult a doctor. As with any drug, if you are pregnant or nursing a baby, seek the advice of a health professional before using this product. In case of accidental ingestion, seek professional help or contact a poison control center immediately. Keep this and all medicines out of the reach of children.

Application of ELA-Max 5 Anorectal Cream to larger areas or for longer times than those recommended could result in sufficient absorption of lidocaine resulting in serious adverse effects (see DOSAGE AND ADMINISTRATION). Studies in laboratory animals (guinea pigs) have shown that lidocaine cream has an ototoxic effect when instilled into the middle ear. In these same studies, animals exposed to lidocaine cream in the external auditory canal only, showed no abnormality.

ELA-Max 5 Anorectal Cream should not be used in any clinical situation in which its penetration or migration beyond the tympanic membrane into the middle ear is possible.

PRECAUTIONS

General: Repeated doses of ELA-Max 5 Anorectal Cream may increase blood levels of lidocaine.

ELA-Max 5 Anorectal Cream should be used with caution in patients who may be more sensitive to the systemic effects of lidocaine including acutely ill, debilitated, or elderly patients.

ELA-Max 5 Anorectal Cream coming in contact with the eye should be avoided because animal studies have demonstrated severe eye irritation. Also the loss of protective reflexes can permit corneal irritation and potential abrasion. Absorption of lidocaine cream in conjunctival tissues has not been determined. If eye contact occurs, immediately wash out the eye with water or saline and protect the eye until sensation returns. Patients allergic to para-aminobenzoic acid derivatives (procaine, tetracaine, benzocaine, etc.) have not shown cross-sensitivity to lidocaine; however, ELA-Max 5 Anorectal Cream should be used with caution in patients with a history of drug sensitivities, especially if the etiologic agent is uncertain. Patients with severe hepatic disease, because of their inability to metabolize local anesthetics normally, are at greater risk of developing toxic plasma concentrations of lidocaine.

Information for Patients: When ELA-Max®5 Anorectal Cream is used, the patient should be aware that the production of dermal analgesia may be accompanied by the block of all sensations in the treated skin. For this reason, the patient should avoid inadvertant trauma to the treated area by scratching, rubbing, or exposure to extreme hot or cold temperatures until complete sensation has returned.

Drug Interactions: ELA-Max 5 Anorectal Cream should be used with caution in patients receiving Class I antiarrhythmic drugs (such as tocainide and mexiletine) since the toxic effects are additive and generally synergistic.

Carcinogenesis, Mutagenesis, Impairment of Fertility:

Carcinogenesis: Metabolites of lidocaine have been shown to be carcinogenic in laboratory animals.

Mutagenesis: The mutagenic potential of lidocaine HCl has been tested in the Ames Salmonella/mammalian microsome test and by analysis of structural chromosome aberrations in human lymphocytes *in vitro*, and by mouse micronucleus test *in vivo*. There was no indication in these tests of any mutagenic effects. The mutagenicity of 2,6-xylidine, a metabolite of lidocaine, has been studied in different tests with mixed results. The compound was found to be weakly mutagenic in the Ames test only under metabolic activation conditions. In addition, 2,6-xylidine was observed to be mutagenic at the thymidine kinase locus, with or without activation, and induced chromosome aberrations and sister chromatid exchanges at concentrations at which the drug precipitated out of the solution (1.2 mg/mL). No evidence of genotoxicity was found in the *in vivo* assays measuring unscheduled DNA synthesis in rat hepatocytes, chromosome damage in polychromatic erythrocytes or preferential killing of DNA repair-deficient bacteria in liver, lung, kidney, testes and blood extracts from mice. However, covalent binding studies of DNA from liver and ethmoid turbinates in rats indicate that 2,6-xylidine may be genotoxic under certain conditions *in vivo*.

Impairment of Fertility: See Use in Pregnancy

Use in Pregnancy:

Teratogenic Effects: Pregnancy Category B. There are no adequate and well-controlled studies in pregnant women.

Because animal reproduction studies are not always predictive of human response, ELA-Max 5 Anorectal Cream should be used during pregnancy only if clearly needed.

Labor and Delivery: Lidocaine is not contraindicated in labor and delivery. Should ELA-Max 5 Anorectal Cream be used concomitantly with other products containing lidocaine, total doses contributed by all formulations must be considered.

Nursing Mothers: Lidocaine is excreted in human milk. Therefore, caution should be exercised when ELA-Max 5 Anorectal Cream is administered to a nursing mother since the milk:plasma ratio of lidocaine is 0.4.

Pediatric Use: Consult a doctor prior to use on children under 12 years of age. When using ELA-Max 5 Anorectal Cream in young children, care must be taken to insure that application of the cream is limited to the intended site (see DOSAGE AND ADMINISTRATION). Accidental ingestion may lead to dose related toxicity.

ADVERSE REACTIONS

Localized reactions: During or immediately after treatment with ELA-Max 5 Anorectal Cream, the skin at the site of treatment may develop erythema or edema or may be the locus of abnormal sensation.

Allergic Reactions: Allergic and anaphylactoid reactions associated with lidocaine can occur. They are characterized by urticaria, angioedema, bronchospasm, and shock. If they occur they should be managed by conventional means. The detection of sensitivity by skin testing is of doubtful value.

System (Dose Related) Reactions: Systemic adverse reactions following appropriate use of ELA-Max 5 Anorectal Cream are unlikely due to the small dose absorbed. Systemic adverse reactions of lidocaine are similar in nature to those observed with other amide local anesthetic agents including CNS excitation and/or depression (light-headedness, nervousness, apprehension, euphoria, confusion, dizziness, drowsiness, tinnitus, blurred or double vision, vomiting, sensations of heat, cold or numbness, twitching, tremors, convulsions, unconsciousness, respiratory depression and arrest). Excitatory CNS reactions may be brief or not occur at all, in which case the first manifestation may be drowsiness merging into unconsciousness. Cardiovascular manifestations may include bradycardia, hypotension, and cardiovascular collapse leading to arrest.

OVERDOSAGE

Peak blood levels following a 60g application to 400 cm^2 for 3 hours are 0.05 to 0.16 µg/mL for lidocaine. Toxic levels of lidocaine (>5 µg/mL) cause decreases in cardiac output, total peripheral resistance and mean arterial pressure. These changes may be attributable to direct depressant effects of these local anesthetic agents on the cardiovascular system. In the absence of massive topical overdose or oral ingestion, evaluation should include other etiologies for the clinical effects of overdosage from other sources of lidocaine or other local anesthetics.

DOSAGE AND ADMINISTRATION

A thick layer of ELA-Max 5 Anorectal Cream is applied to intact skin. A single application of ELA-Max 5 Anorectal Cream in a child weighing less than 10 kg should not be applied over an area larger than 100 cm^2 A single application of ELA-Max 5 Anorectal Cream in children weighing between 10 kg and 20 kg should not be applied over an area larger than 200 cm^2.

When applying ELA-Max 5 Anorectal Cream to young children, care must be taken to maintain careful observation of the child to prevent accidental ingestion of ELA-Max 5 Anorectal Cream.

When ELA-Max 5 Anorectal Cream (lidocaine 5%) is used concomitantly with other products containing local anesthetic agents, the amount absorbed from all formulations must be considered. The amount absorbed in the case of ELA-Max 5 Anorectal Cream is determined by the area over which it is applied and the duration of application. Although the incidence of systemic adverse reactions with ELA-Max 5 Anorectal Cream is very low, caution should be exercised, particularly when applying it over large areas and leaving it on for longer than 2 hours. The incidence of systemic adverse reactions can be expected to be directly proportional to the area and time of exposure.

HOW SUPPLIED

ELA-Max 5 Anorectal Cream is available as the following:
NDC 0496-0824-15 15 gram tube
NDC 0496-0824-30 30 gram tube
Store between 15° and 30°C (59°–86°F).
NOT FOR OPHTHALMIC USE.
KEEP CONTAINER TIGHTLY CLOSED AT ALL TIMES WHEN NOT IN USE.
Manufactured Jointly by:
Ferndale Laboratories, Inc.
Ferndale, MI 48220 and
BioZone Laboratories, Inc.
Pittsburg, CA 94565
ELA-MAX is a R]egistered trademark of
Ferndale Laboratories, Inc.
©Ferndale Laboratories, Inc.
MG #13351 Iss: 10/98

KRONOFED–A® Kronocaps ℞
KRONOFED–A–JR® Kronocaps ℞

Each sustained release Kronofed A®, white and clear capsule contains:

Pseudoephedrine HCl .... 120 mg
Chlorpheniramine Maleate .... 8 mg

Each sustained release Kronofed-A-Jr®, white and clear capsule contains:

Pseudoephedrine HCl .... 60 mg
Chlorpheniramine Maleate .... 4 mg

INDICATIONS

For temporary relief of upper respiratory and nasal congestion associated with the common cold, hay fever and allergies, sinusitis and vasomotor and allergic rhinitis.

CONTRAINDICATIONS

Severe hypertension or severe cardiac disease. Sensitivity to antihistamines or sympathomimetic agents.

PRECAUTIONS

Use with caution in patients with hyperthyroidism. Patients susceptible to the soporific effects of chlorpheniramine should be warned against driving or operating of machinery which requires complete mental alertness.

PREGNANCY

Pregnancy Category C: Animal reproduction studies have not been conducted with **KRONOFED-A®** medications. It is also not known whether **KRONOFED-A®** medications can cause fetal harm when administered to a pregnant woman or can affect reproduction capacity. **KRONOFED-A®** medications should be given to a pregnant woman only if clearly needed.

Nursing Mothers: Due to the possible passage of pseudoephedrine and chlorpheniramine into breast milk, and, because of the higher than usual risk for infants from sympathomimetic amines and antihistamines, the benefit to the mother vs. the potential risk should be considered and a decision should be made whether to discontinue nursing or to discontinue the drug.

CAUTION

Federal law prohibits dispensing without prescription.

DOSAGE

Kronofed-A® Capsules: Adults and children over 12 years of age—1 capsule every 12 hours. **Kronofed-A-JR®** Capsules: Children 6–12 years of age—1 capsule every 12 hours. Adults 1 or 2 capsules every 12 hours.

HOW SUPPLIED

Kronofed-A® Kronocaps
Bottles of 100 NDC 0496–0382–02
Bottles of 500 NDC 0496–0382–10

Kronofed-A-Jr® Kronocaps
Bottles of 100 NDC 0496–0434–02
Bottles of 500 NDC 0496–0434–10

LOCOID® ℞
(hydrocortisone butyrate)
Cream 0.1%
Ointment 0.1%
Topical Solution 0.1%

CAUTION: Federal law prohibits dispensing without prescription.

DESCRIPTION

LOCOID® cream, ointment and topical solution contain the topical corticosteroid, hydrocortisone butyrate, a non-fluorinated hydrocortisone ester. It has the chemical name: pregn-4-ene-3, 20-dione, 11, 21-dihydroxy-17-[(1-oxobutyl)oxy-,(11β)-; the molecular formula: $C_{25}H_{36}O_6$; the molecular weight: 432.54; and the CAS registry number: 13609-67-1. Its structural formula is:

LOCOID® Cream 0.1%
Each gram of LOCOID® cream contains 1 mg of hydrocortisone butyrate in a hydrophilic base consisting of cetostearyl alcohol, ceteth-20, mineral oil, white petrolatum, citric acid, sodium citrate, propylparaben and butylparaben (preservatives) and purified water.

LOCOID® Ointment 0.1%
Each gram of LOCOID® ointment contains 1 mg of hydrocortisone butyrate in a base consisting of mineral oil and polyethylene.

LOCOID® Solution 0.1%
Each mL of LOCOID® solution contains 1 mg of hydrocortisone butyrate in a vehicle consisting of isopropyl alcohol (50%), glycerin, povidone, citric acid, sodium citrate and purified water.

CLINICAL PHARMACOLOGY

Topical corticosteroids share anti-inflammatory, anti-pruritic and vasoconstrictive actions.

The mechanism of anti-inflammatory activity of the topical corticosteroids is unclear. Various laboratory methods, including vasoconstrictor assays, are used to compare and predict potencies and/or clinical efficacies of the topical corticosteroids. There is some evidence to suggest that a recognizable correlation exists between vasoconstrictor potency and therapeutic efficacy in man.

Pharmacokinetics
The extent of percutaneous absorption of topical corticosteroids is determined by many factors including the vehicle, the integrity of the epidermal barrier, and the use of occlusive dressings.

Topical corticosteroids can be absorbed from normal intact skin. Inflammation and/or other disease processes in the skin increase percutaneous absorption. Occlusive dressings substantially increase the percutaneous absorption of topical corticosteroids. Thus, occlusive dressings may be a valuable therapeutic adjunct for treatment of resistant dermatoses. (See DOSAGE AND ADMINISTRATION.)

Once absorbed through the skin, topical corticosteroids are handled through pharmacokinetic pathways similar to systemically administered corticosteroids. Corticosteroids are bound to plasma proteins in varying degrees. Corticosteroids are metabolized primarily in the liver and are then excreted by the kidneys. Some of the topical corticosteroids and their metabolites are also excreted into the bile.

INDICATIONS AND USAGE

LOCOID® cream 0.1% and ointment 0.1% (hydrocortisone butyrate) are indicated for the relief of the inflammatory and pruritic manifestations of corticosteroid-responsive dermatoses.

LOCOID® solution 0.1% (hydrocortisone butyrate) is indicated for the relief of the inflammatory and pruritic manifestations of seborrheic dermatitis.

CONTRAINDICATIONS

Topical corticosteroids are contraindicated in those patients with a history of hypersensitivity to any of the components of the preparation.

PRECAUTIONS

General: Systemic absorption of topical corticosteroids has produced reversible hypothalamic-pituitary-adrenal (HPA) axis suppression, manifestations of Cushing's syndrome, hyperglycemia, and glucosuria in some patients. Conditions which augment systemic absorption include the application of the more potent steroids, use over large surface areas, prolonged use, and the addition of occlusive dressings.

Therefore, patients receiving a large dose of a potent topical steroid applied to a large surface area or under an occlusive dressing should be evaluated periodically for evidence of HPA axis suppression by using the urinary free cortisol and ACTH stimulation tests. If HPA axis suppression is noted, an attempt should be made to withdraw the drug, to reduce the frequency of application, or to substitute a less potent steroid.

Recovery of HPA axis function is generally prompt and complete upon discontinuation of the drug. Infrequently, signs and symptoms of steroid withdrawal may occur, requiring supplemental systemic corticosteroids.

Children may absorb proportionally larger amounts of topical corticosteroids and thus be more susceptible to systemic toxicity (See PRECAUTIONS—PEDIATRIC USE.)

If irritation develops, topical corticosteroids should be discontinued and appropriate therapy instituted. In the presence of dermatological infections, the use of an appropriate antifungal or antibacterial agent should be instituted. If a favorable response does not occur promptly, the corticosteroid should be discontinued until the infection has been adequately controlled.

Information for the patient
Patients using topical corticosteroids should receive the following information and instructions:

1. This medication is to be used as directed by the physician. It is for external use only. Avoid contact with the eyes.
2. Patients should be advised not to use this medication for any disorder other than for which it was prescribed.
3. The treated skin area should not be bandaged or otherwise covered or wrapped as to be occlusive unless directed by the physician.
4. Patients should report any signs of local adverse reactions especially under occlusive dressing.
5. Parents of pediatric patients should be advised not to use tight-fitting diapers or plastic pants on a child being treated in the diaper area, as these garments may constitute occlusive dressings.

Laboratory tests
The following tests may be helpful in evaluating the HPA axis suppression:
Urinary free cortisol test
ACTH stimulation test

Carcinogenesis, Mutagenesis, and Impairment of Fertility
Long-term animal studies have not been performed to evaluate the carcinogenic potential or the effect on fertility of topical corticosteroids.

Studies to determine mutagenicity with prednisolone and hydrocortisone have revealed negative results.

Pregnancy Category C
Corticosteroids are generally teratogenic in laboratory animals when administered systemically at relatively low dosage levels. The more potent corticosteroids have been shown to be teratogenic after dermal application in laboratory animals. There are no adequate and well-controlled studies in

Continued on next page

Locoid—Cont.

pregnant women on teratogenic effects from topically applied corticosteroids. Therefore, topical corticosteroids should be used during pregnancy only if the potential benefit justifies the potential risk to the fetus. Drugs of this class should not be used extensively on pregnant patients, in large amounts, or for prolonged periods of time.

Nursing Mothers

It is not known whether topical administration of corticosteroids could result in sufficient systemic absorption to produce detectable quantities in breast milk. Systemically administered corticosteroids are secreted into breast milk, in quantities not likely to have a deleterious effect on the infant. Nevertheless, caution should be exercised when topical corticosteroids are administered to a nursing woman.

Pediatric Use

Pediatric patients may demonstrate greater susceptibility to topical corticosteroid-induced HPA axis suppression and Cushing's syndrome than mature patients because of a larger skin surface area to body weight ratio.
Hypothalamic-pituitary-adrenal (HPA) axis suppression, Cushing's syndrome, and intracranial hypertension have been reported in children receiving topical corticosteroids. Manifestations of adrenal suppression in children include linear growth retardation, delayed weight gain, low plasma cortisol levels, and absence of response to ACTH stimulation. Manifestations of intracranial hypertension include bulging fontanelles, headaches, and bilateral papilledema. Administration of topical corticosteroids to children should be limited to the least amount compatible with an effective therapeutic regimen. Chronic corticosteroid therapy may interfere with the growth and development of children.

ADVERSE REACTIONS

The following local adverse reactions are reported infrequently with topical corticosteroids, but may occur more frequently with the use of occlusive dressings. These reactions are listed in an approximate decreasing order of occurrence: burning, itching, irritation, dryness, folliculitis, hypertrichosis, acneiform eruptions, hypopigmentation, perioral dermatitis, allergic contact dermatitis, maceration of the skin, secondary infection, skin atrophy, striae, miliaria.

OVERDOSAGE

Topically applied corticosteroids can be absorbed in sufficient amounts to produce systemic effects. (See PRECAUTIONS.)

DOSAGE AND ADMINISTRATION

LOCOID® cream 0.1% or LOCOID® ointment 0.1% (hydrocortisone butyrate) should be applied to the affected area as a thin film two to three times daily depending on the severity of the condition.
Occlusive dressings may be used for the management of psoriasis or recalcitrant conditions.
If an infection develops, the use of occlusive dressings should be discontinued and appropriate antimicrobial therapy instituted.
LOCOID® solution 0.1% (hydrocortisone butyrate) should be applied to the affected area as a thin film from two to three times daily depending on the severity of the condition.

HOW SUPPLIED

LOCOID® cream 0.1% (hydrocortisone butyrate) is supplied in tubes containing:
15 g NDC 0496-0802-15
45 g NDC 0496-0802-45
LOCOID® ointment 0.1% (hydrocortisone butyrate) is supplied in tubes containing:
15 g NDC 0496-0803-15
45 g NDC 0496-0803-45
LOCOID® solution 0.1% (hydrocortisone butyrate) is supplied in polyethylene bottles:
30 mL NDC 0496-0804-30
60 mL NDC 0496-0804-60

STORAGE

LOCOID® cream 0.1%: Store between 59° and 77°F (15° and 25°C).
LOCOID® ointment 0.1%: Store between 36°and 86°F (2°and 30°C).
LOCOID® solution 0.1%: Store between 41°and 77°F (5°and 25°C).

MARKETED BY:
FERNDALE LABORATORIES, INC.
FERNDALE, MICHIGAN 48220
MANUFACTURED BY:
Yamanouchi Europe bv
Leiderdorp/Netherlands
Revised: October 1996

LOCOID LIPOCREAM® CREAM, 0.1% ℞

[lō'coĭd lĭpō '-cream]
(hydrocortisone butyrate cream)

For Dermatological Use Only

DESCRIPTION

LOCOID Lipocream® Cream contains the topical corticosteroid hydrocortisone butyrate, a hydrocortisone ester. It has the chemical name: (11β)-11,21-dihydroxy-17-[(1-oxobutyl)oxy]-pregn-4-ene-3,20-dione; the molecular formula: $C_{25}H_{36}O_6$; the molecular weight: 432.54; and the CAS registry number: 13609-67-1. The structural formula is:

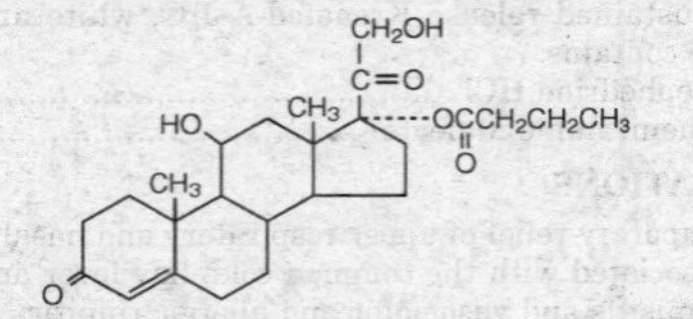

LOCOID Lipocream® Cream, 0.1%

Each gram of LOCOID Lipocream® Cream contains 1 mg of hydrocortisone butyrate in a hydrophilic base consisting of cetostearyl alcohol, ceteth-20, mineral oil, white petrolatum, citric acid, sodium citrate, propylparaben and butylparaben (preservatives) and purified water.

CLINICAL PHARMACOLOGY

Topical corticosteroids share anti-inflammatory, anti-pruritic and vasoconstrictive actions. The mechanism of anti-inflammatory activity of the topical corticosteroids is unclear. Various laboratory methods, including vasoconstrictor assays, are used to compare and predict potencies and/or clinical efficacies of the topical corticosteroids. There is some evidence to suggest that a recognizable correlation exists between vasoconstrictor potency and therapeutic efficacy in man.

PHARMACOKINETICS

The extent of percutaneous absorption of topical corticosteroids is determined by many factors including the vehicle, the integrity of the epidermal barrier, and the use of occlusive dressings.
Topical corticosteroids can be absorbed from normal intact skin. Inflammation and/or other disease processes in the skin increase percutaneous absorption. Occlusive dressings or widespread application may increase the possibility of hypothalamic-pituitary-adrenal (HPA) axis suppression.
The vasoconstrictor assay showed that LOCOID Lipocream® Cream has a more pronounced skin blanching effect than LOCOID® Cream, suggesting greater percutaneous absorption from the former. At the present time, no adequate HPA axis suppression studies have been conducted for LOCOID Lipocream® Cream. Once absorbed through the skin, topical corticosteroids are handled through pharmacokinetic pathways similar to systemically administered corticosteroids. Corticosteroids are bound to plasma proteins in varying degrees.
Corticosteroids are metabolized primarily in the liver and are then excreted by the kidneys. Some of the topical corticosteroids and their metabolites are also excreted in the bile.

INDICATIONS AND USAGE

LOCOID Lipocream® Cream 0.1% (hydrocortisone butyrate cream) is indicated for the relief of the inflammatory and pruritic manifestations of corticosteroid-responsive dermatoses.

CONTRAINDICATIONS

Topical corticosteroids are contraindicated in those patients with a history of hypersensitivity to any of the components of the preparation.

PRECAUTIONS

General

Systemic absorption of topical corticosteroids has produced reversible HPA axis suppression, manifestations of Cushing's syndrome, hyperglycemia, and glucosuria in some patients.
Conditions which increase the risk of systemic toxicity include the application of the more potent steroids, use over large surface areas, prolonged use, and the addition of occlusive dressings.
Children may absorb proportionally larger amounts of topical corticosteroids and thus be more susceptible to systemic toxicity. (See PRECAUTIONS — PEDIATRIC USE).
If irritation develops, topical corticosteroids should be discontinued and appropriate therapy instituted. In the presence of dermatological infections, the use of an appropriate antifungal or antibacterial agent should be instituted. If a favorable response does not occur promptly, the corticosteroid should be discontinued until the infection has been adequately controlled.

Information for the Patient

Patients using topical corticosteroids should receive the following information and instructions:

1. This medication is to be used as directed by the physician. It is for external use only. Avoid contact with the eyes.
2. Patients should be advised not to use this medication for any disorder other than for which it was prescribed.
3. The treated skin area should not be bandaged or otherwise covered or wrapped as to be occlusive.
4. Patients should report any signs of local adverse reactions.
5. Parents of pediatric patients should be advised not to use tight-fitting diapers or plastic pants on a child being treated in the diaper area, as these garments may constitute occlusive dressings.

Laboratory Tests

The following tests may be helpful in evaluating the HPA axis suppression:
Urinary free cortisol test
ACTH stimulation test

Carcinogenesis, Mutagenesis, and Impairment of Fertility

Long-term animal studies have not been performed to evaluate the carcinogenic potential or the effect on fertility of topical corticosteroids.
Studies to determine mutagenicity in *Salmonella ryphimurium* strains TA98, TA100, and TA92 with prednisolone and hydrocortisone have revealed negative results.

Pregnancy: Teratogenic Effects:

Pregnancy Category C:

Corticosteroids are generally teratogenic in laboratory animals when administered systemically at relatively low dosage levels. Some corticosteroids have been shown to be teratogenic after dermal application in laboratory animals. In teratogenicity studies, topical administration of 1% or 10% hydrocortisone butyrate in a ointment to pregnant Wistar rats (gestational days 6–15) or New Zealand white rabbits (gestational days 6–18) resulted in no teratogenic findings. However, a dose-dependent increase in fetal resorptions was reported in rabbits, and fetal resorptions were observed in rats treated with 10% hydrocortisone butyrate.
The doses given to rats are approximately 8 to 80 times the human topical dose based on a body surface area comparison (assuming 100% absorption). For rabbits, the doses given were approximately 0.2 and 2 times the human topical dose. Increased resorptions were also noted in Wistar rats given subcutaneous administrations of hydrocortisone butyrate (9mg/kg/day; 3 times the human topical dose) on gestational days 9 through 15. In CS mice given subcutaneously administrations of 1mg/kg/day (0.2 times the human topical dose), an increased number of cervical ribs and one fetus with clubbed legs was reported. There are no adequate and well-controlled studies in pregnant women on teratogenic effects from topically applied corticosteroids. Therefore, topical corticosteroids should be used during pregnancy only if the potential benefit justifies the potential risk to the fetus. LOCOID Lipocream® Cream 0.1% (hydrocortisone butyrate cream) should not be used extensively on pregnant patients, in large amounts, or for longer than two weeks.

Nursing Mothers

It is not known whether topical administration of corticosteroids could result in sufficient systemic absorption to produce detectable quantities in breast milk.
Systemically administered corticosteroids are secreted into breast milk in quantities *not* likely to have a deleterious effect on the infant. Nevertheless, caution should be exercised when topical corticosteroids are administered to a nursing woman.

Pediatric Use

Safety and effectiveness in pediatric patients have not been established.
Pediatric patients may demonstrate greater susceptibility to topical corticosteroid-induced HPA axis suppression and Cushing's syndrome than mature patients because of a larger skin surface area to body weight ratio.
HPA axis suppression, Cushing's syndrome, and intracranial hypertension have been reported in children receiving topical corticosteroids.
Manifestations of adrenal suppression in children include linear growth retardation, delayed weight gain, low plasma cortisol levels, and absence of response to ACTH stimulation. Manifestations of intracranial hypertension include bulging fontanelles, headaches, and bilateral papilledema. Chronic corticosteroid therapy may interfere with the growth and development of children.

ADVERSE REACTIONS

The following local adverse reactions are reported infrequently with topical corticosteroids but may occur more frequently with the use of occlusive dressings. These reactions are listed in an approximate decreasing order of occurrence: burning, itching, irritation, dryness, folliculitis, hypertrichosis, acneiform eruptions, hypopigmentation, perioral dermatitis, allergic contact dermatitis, maceration of the skin, secondary infection, skin atrophy, striae and miliaria.

OVERDOSAGE

Topically applied corticosteroids can be absorbed in sufficient amounts to produce systemic effects. (See PRECAUTIONS).

DOSAGE AND ADMINISTRATION

LOCOID Lipocream® Cream 0.1% (hydrocortisone butyrate cream) should be applied to the affected area as a thin film two or three times daily (depending on the severity of the condition) and for no longer than two weeks.
If an infection develops, appropriate antimicrobial therapy should be instituted.

HOW SUPPLIED

LOCOID Lipocream® Cream 0.1% (hydrocortisone butyrate cream) is supplied in tubes containing:
15 g NDC 0496-0821-15
45 g NDC 0496-0821-45

STORAGE

Store at controlled room temperature between 59° and 77°F (15° and 25°C).

CAUTION

Federal law prohibits dispensing without prescription.

Marketed by:
FERNDALE LABORATORIES, INC.
Ferndale, Michigan 48220 USA
U.S. Patent No. 5,635,497

Manufactured by:
Yamanouchi Europe B.V.
Leiderdorp/The Netherlands
12143004/1
(010997)

PRAMOSONE® CREAM, LOTION AND OINTMENT ℞

DESCRIPTION

Pramosone® Cream: Contains Hydrocortisone acetate 1% or 2.5% and Pramoxine HCl 1% in a hydrophilic base containing stearic acid, cetyl alcohol, aquaphor, isopropyl palmitate, polyoxyl 40 stearate, propylene glycol, potassium sorbate, sorbic acid, triethanolamine lauryl sulfate and water.
Pramosone® Lotion: Contains Hydrocortisone acetate 1% or 2.5% and Pramoxine HCl 1% in a base containing forlan-L, cetyl alcohol, stearic acid, di-isopropyl adipate, polyoxyl 40 stearate, silicone, triethanolamine, glycerine, polyvinylpyrolidone, potassium sorbate, sorbic acid and water.
Pramosone® Ointment: Contains Hydrocortisone acetate 1% or 2.5% and Pramoxine HCl 1% in an emollient ointment base containing sorbitan sesquioleate, water, aquaphor and white petrolatum.
Topical corticosteroids are anti-inflammatory and antipruritic agents. The structural formula, the chemical name, molecular formula and molecular weight for active ingredients are presented below.

Hydrocortisone acetate
(Pregn-4-ene-3,20-dione,21 - (acetyloxy)-11, 17-dihydroxy-,(11 β)-.)
$C_{23}H_{32}O_6$; mol wt: 404.50

Pramoxine hydrochloride
(4-(3-(p-butoxyphenoxy)propyl)morpholine hydrochloride)
$C_{17}H_{27}NO_3$.HCl; mol wt: 329.87

CLINICAL PHARMACOLOGY

Topical corticosteroids share anti-inflammatory, anti-pruritic and vasoconstrictive actions.
The mechanism of anti-inflammatory activity of the topical corticosteroids is unclear. Various laboratory methods, including vasoconstrictor assays, are used to compare and predict potencies and/or clinical efficacies of the topical corticosteroids. There is some evidence to suggest that a recognizable correlation exists between vasoconstrictor potency and therapeutic efficacy in man.
Pramoxine hydrochloride is a topical anesthetic agent which provides temporary relief from itching and pain. It acts by stabilizing the neuronal membrane of nerve endings with which it comes into contact.
Pharmacokinetics: The extent of percutaneous absorption of topical corticosteroids is determined by many factors including the vehicle, the integrity of the epidermal barrier, and the use of occlusive dressings.
Topical corticosteroids can be absorbed from normal intact skin. Inflammation and/or other disease processes in the skin increase percutaneous absorption. Occlusive dressings substantially increase the percutaneous absorption of topical corticosteroids. Thus, occlusive dressings may be a valuable therapeutic adjunct for treatment of resistant dermatoses (See DOSAGE AND ADMINISTRATION).
Once absorbed through the skin, topical corticosteroids are handled through pharmacokinetic pathways similar to systemically administered corticosteroids. Corticosteroids are bound to plasma proteins in varying degrees. Corticosteroids are metabolized primarily in the liver and are then excreted by the kidneys. Some of the topical corticosteroids and their metabolites are also excreted into the bile.

INDICATIONS AND USAGE

Topical corticosteroids are indicated for the relief of the inflammatory and pruritic manifestations of corticosteroid-responsive dermatoses.

CONTRAINDICATIONS

Topical corticosteroids are contraindicated in those patients with a history of hypersensitivity to any of the components of the preparation.

PRECAUTIONS

General: Systemic absorption of topical corticosteroids has produced reversible hypothalamic-pituitary-adrenal (HPA) axis suppression, manifestations of Cushing's syndrome, hyperglycemia, and glucosuria in some patients.
Conditions which augment systemic absorption include the application of the more potent steroids, use over large surface areas, prolonged use, and the addition of occlusive dressings.
Therefore, patients receiving a large dose of a potent topical steroid applied to a large surface area and under an occlusive dressing should be evaluated periodically for evidence of HPA axis suppression by using the urinary free cortisol and ACTH stimulation tests. If HPA axis suppression is noted, an attempt should be made to withdraw the drug, to reduce the frequency of application, or to substitute a less potent steroid.
Recovery of HPA axis function is generally prompt and complete upon discontinuation of the drug. Infrequently, signs and symptoms of steroid withdrawal may occur, requiring supplemental systemic corticosteroids.
Children may absorb proportionally larger amounts of topical corticosteroids and thus be more susceptible to systemic toxicity. (See PRECAUTIONS—Pediatric Use).
If irritation develops, topical corticosteroids should be discontinued and appropriate therapy instituted.
In the presence of dermatological infections, the use of an appropriate antifungal or antibacterial agent should be instituted. If a favorable response does not occur promptly, the corticosteroid should be discontinued until the infection has been adequately controlled.
Information for the Patient: Patients using topical corticosteroids should receive the following information and instructions:
1. This medication is to be used as directed by the physician. It is for external use only. Avoid contact with the eyes.
2. Patients should be advised not to use this medication for any disorder other than for which it was prescribed.
3. The treated skin area should not be bandaged or otherwise covered or wrapped as to be occlusive unless directed by the physician.
4. Patients should report any signs of local adverse reactions especially under occlusive dressing.
5. Parents of pediatric patients should be advised not to use tightfitting diapers or plastic pants on a child being treated in the diaper area, as these garments may constitute occlusive dressings.
Laboratory Tests: The following tests may be helpful in evaluating the HPA axis suppression:
Urinary free cortisol test
ACTH stimulation test
Carcinogenesis, Mutagenesis, and Impairment of Fertility: Long-term animal studies have not been performed to evaluate the carcinogenic potential or the effect on fertility of topical corticosteroids.
Studies to determine mutagenicity with prednisolone and hydrocortisone have revealed negative results.
Pregnancy Category C: Corticosteroids are generally teratogenic in laboratory animals when administered systemically at relatively low dosage levels. The more potent corticosteroids have been shown to be teratogenic after dermal application in laboratory animals. There are no adequate and well-controlled studies in pregnant women on teratogenic effects from topically applied corticosteroids. Therefore, topical corticosteroids should be used during pregnancy only if the potential benefit justifies the potential risk to the fetus. Drugs of this class should not be used extensively on pregnant patients, in large amounts, or for prolonged periods of time.
Nursing Mothers: It is not known whether topical administration of corticosteroids could result in sufficient systemic absorption to produce detectable amounts in breast milk. Systemically administered corticosteroids are secreted into breast milk in quantities NOT likely to have a deleterious effect on the infant. Nevertheless, caution should be exercised when topical corticosteroids are administered to a nursing woman.
Pediatric Use: PEDIATRIC PATIENTS MAY DEMONSTRATE GREATER SUSCEPTIBILITY TO TOPICAL CORTICOSTEROID-INDUCED HPA AXIS SUPPRESSION AND CUSHING'S SYNDROME THAN MATURE PATIENTS BECAUSE OF A LARGER SKIN SURFACE AREA TO BODY WEIGHT RATIO.
Hypothalamic-pituitary-adrenal (HPA) axis suppression, Cushing's syndrome, and intracranial hypertension have been reported in children receiving topical corticosteroids. Manifestations of adrenal suppression in children include linear growth retardation, delayed weight gain, low plasma cortisol levels, and absence of response to ACTH stimulation. Manifestations of intracranial hypertension include bulging fontanelles, headaches, and bilateral papilledema. Administration of topical corticosteroids to children should be limited to the least amount compatible with an effective therapeutic regimen. Chronic corticosteroid therapy may interfere with the growth and development of children.

ADVERSE REACTIONS

The following local adverse reactions are reported infrequently with topical corticosteroids, but may occur more frequently with the use of occlusive dressings. These reactions are listed in an approximate decreasing order of occurrence:

Burning	Hypopigmentation
Itching	Perioral dermatitis
Irritation	Allergic contact dermatitis
Dryness	Maceration of the skin
Folliculitis	Secondary infection
Hypertrichosis	Skin Atrophy
Acneiform eruptions	Striae
	Miliaria

OVERDOSAGE

Topically applied corticosteroids can be absorbed in sufficient amounts to produce systemic effects (See PRECAUTIONS).

DOSAGE AND ADMINISTRATION

Topical corticosteroids are generally applied to the affected area as a thin film three or four times daily depending on the severity of the condition.
Occlusive dressings may be used for the management of psoriasis or recalcitrant conditions. If an infection develops, the use of occlusive dressings should be discontinued and appropriate antimicrobial therapy instituted.

HOW SUPPLIED

CREAM:	1%	1 oz Tube	NDC 0496-0716-04
		2 oz Tube	NDC 0496-0716-03
	2.5%	1 oz Tube	NDC 0496-0717-04
		2 oz Tube	NDC 0496-0717-03
LOTION:	1%	2 fl oz	NDC 0496-0729-06
		4 fl oz	NDC 0496-0729-04
		8 fl oz	NDC 0496-0729-03
	2.5%	2 fl oz	NDC 0496-0726-06
		4 fl oz	NDC 0496-0726-04
OINTMENT:	1%	1 oz Tube	NDC 0496-0763-04
	2.5%	1 oz Tube	NDC 0496-0777-04

Dispense in a tight container as defined in the official compendium.
Store at controlled room temperature 15°–30°C (59°–86°F).

PRAX® LOTION* OTC

(Pramoxine HCl 1% in an emollient hydrophilic base)

HOW SUPPLIED

Prax® Lotion is supplied in dispenser bottles containing
4 fl oz NDC 0496-0748-04
8 fl oz NDC 0496-0748-03

*Additional information available upon request.

PRO-Q™ Skin Protectant OTC

Pro-Q™ is a revolutionary topical preparation designed to fortify the skin's natural capacity to protect the body from the destructive effects of external irritants and sensitizers.

HOW SUPPLIED

Pro-Q™ is supplied in canisters containing
35 ml NDC 0496-0842-01
75 ml NDC 0496-0842-02
161 ml NDC 0496-0842-05

SBR-LIPOCREAM™ OTC

SBR-Lipocream™ is specially designed to help repair and maintain the body's natural skin barrier function. SBR-Lipocream™ is for patients with sensitive skin or skin that is predisposed to chronic skin disease and irritation.

HOW SUPPLIED

SBR-Lipocream™ is supplied in tubes containing
100 g NDC 0496-0819-01

Ferring Pharmaceuticals Inc.

120 WHITE PLAINS ROAD, SUITE #400
TARRYTOWN, NY 10591

Direct Inquiries to:
Ferring Pharmaceuticals Inc.
Customer Service Department
120 White Plains Road, Suite #400
Tarrytown, NY 10591
1-(888)-FERRING (337-7464)

For Medical Information Contact:
In Emergencies:
Ferring Pharmaceuticals Inc.
Professional Services Department
120 White Plains Road, Suite #400
Tarrytown, NY 10591
(800) 822-8214

ACTHREL® ℞

(corticorelin ovine triflutate for injection)
For intravenous injection only
DIAGNOSTIC USE ONLY

HOW SUPPLIED

As a 5 mL, amber, single-dose vial (NDC 55566-0302-1). Each vial contains a sterile, nonpyrogenic, lyophilized white cake containing 100 mcg corticorelin ovine (as the trifluroacetate), 0.88 mg ascorbic acid, 10 mg lactose, and 26 mg cysteine hydrochloride monohydrate.
Store refrigerated at 2°C to 8°C (36°F to 45°F) and protect from light.
Please see full prescribing information in the Diagnostic Product Information section.

Continued on next page

DESMOPRESSIN ACETATE ℞

Injection 4 µg/mL

DESCRIPTION

DESMOPRESSIN ACETATE Injection 4 µg/mL is a synthetic analogue of the natural pituitary hormone 8-arginine vasopressin (ADH), an antidiuretic hormone affecting renal water conservation. It is chemically defined as follows:

Mol.Wt. 1183.3

Empirical Formula: $C_{46}H_{64}N_{14}O_{12}S_2 \cdot C_2H_4O_2 \cdot 3H_2O$

$SCH_2CH_2C(=O)$-Tyr-Phe-Gln-Asn-Cys-Pro-D-Arg-Gly-$NH_2 \cdot CH_3COOH \cdot 3H_2O$ (S of residue 1 linked to Cys 6)

1 2 3 4 5 6 7 8 9

1-(3-mercaptopropionic acid)-8-D-arginine vasopressin monoacetate (salt) trihydrate.

DESMOPRESSIN ACETATE Injection 4 µg/mL is provided as a sterile, aqueous solution for injection.

Each mL provides:	Desmopressin acetate	4.0 µg
	Sodium chloride	9.0 mg
	Hydrochloric acid to adjust pH to 4	

The 10 mL vial contains chlorobutanol as a preservative (5.0 mg/mL).

CLINICAL PHARMACOLOGY

DESMOPRESSIN ACETATE Injection 4 µg/mL contains as active substance, desmopressin acetate, a synthetic analogue of the natural hormone arginine vasopressin. One mL (4 µg) of DESMOPRESSIN ACETATE solution has an antidiuretic activity of about 16 IU; 1 µg of DESMOPRESSIN ACETATE is equivalent to 4 IU.

DESMOPRESSIN ACETATE has been shown to be more potent than arginine vasopressin in increasing plasma levels of factor VIII activity in patients with hemophilia and von Willebrand's disease Type I.

Dose-response studies were performed in healthy persons, using doses of 0.1 to 0.4 µg/kg body weight, infused over a 10-minute period. Maximal dose response occurred at 0.3 to 0.4 µg/kg. The response to DESMOPRESSIN ACETATE of factor VIII activity and plasminogen activator is dose-related, with maximal plasma levels of 300 to 400 percent of initial concentrations obtained after infusion of 0.4 µg/kg body weight. The increase is rapid and evident within 30 minutes, reaching a maximum at a point ranging from 90 minutes to two hours. The factor VIII related antigen and ristocetin cofactor activity were also increased to a smaller degree, but still are dose-dependent.

1. The biphasic half-lives of DESMOPRESSIN ACETATE were 7.8 and 75.5 minutes for the fast and slow phases, respectively, compared with 2.5 and 14.5 minutes for lysine vasopressin, another form of the hormone. As a result, DESMOPRESSIN ACETATE provides a prompt onset of antidiuretic action with a long duration after each administration.
2. The change in structure of arginine vasopressin to DESMOPRESSIN ACETATE has resulted in a decreased vasopressor action and decreased actions on visceral smooth muscle relative to the enhanced antidiuretic activity, so that clinically effective antidiuretic doses are usually below threshold levels for effects on vascular or visceral smooth muscle.
3. When administered by injection, DESMOPRESSIN ACETATE has an antidiuretic effect about ten times that of an equivalent dose administered intranasally.
4. The bioavailability of the subcutaneous route of administration was determined qualitatively using urine output data. The exact fraction of drug absorbed by that route of administration has not been quantitatively determined.
5. The percentage increase of factor VIII levels in patients with mild hemophilia A and von Willebrand's disease was not significantly different from that observed in normal healthy individuals when treated with 0.3 µg/kg of DESMOPRESSIN ACETATE infused over 10 minutes.
6. Plasminogen activator activity increases rapidly after DESMOPRESSIN ACETATE infusion, but there has been no clinically significant fibrinolysis in patients treated with DESMOPRESSIN ACETATE.
7. The effect of repeated DESMOPRESSIN ACETATE administration when doses were given every 12 to 24 hours has generally shown a gradual diminution of the factor VIII activity increase noted with a single dose. The initial response is reproducible in any particular patient if there are 2 or 3 days between administrations.

INDICATIONS AND USAGE

Hemophilia A: DESMOPRESSIN ACETATE Injection 4 µg/mL is indicated for patients with hemophilia A with factor VIII coagulant activity levels greater than 5%.

DESMOPRESSIN ACETATE will often maintain hemostasis in patients with hemophilia A during surgical procedures and postoperatively when administered 30 minutes prior to scheduled procedure.

DESMOPRESSIN ACETATE will also stop bleeding in hemophilia A patients with episodes of spontaneous or trauma-induced injuries such as hemarthroses, intramuscular hematomas or mucosal bleeding.

DESMOPRESSIN ACETATE is not indicated for the treatment of hemophilia A with factor VIII coagulant activity levels equal to or less than 5%, or for the treatment of hemophilia B, or in patients who have factor VIII antibodies.

In certain clinical situations, it may be justified to try DESMOPRESSIN ACETATE in patients with factor VIII levels between 2% to 5%; however, these patients should be carefully monitored.

von Willebrand's Disease (Type I): DESMOPRESSIN ACETATE Injection 4 µg/mL is indicated for patients with mild to moderate classic von Willebrand's disease (Type I) with factor VIII levels greater than 5%. DESMOPRESSIN ACETATE will often maintain hemostasis in patients with mild to moderate von Willebrand's disease during surgical procedures and postoperatively when administered 30 minutes prior to the scheduled procedure.

DESMOPRESSIN ACETATE will usually stop bleeding in mild to moderate von Willebrand's patients with episodes of spontaneous or trauma-induced injuries such as hemarthroses, intramuscular hematomas or mucosal bleeding.

Those von Willebrand's disease patients who are least likely to respond are those with severe homozygous von Willebrand's disease with factor VIII coagulant activity and factor VIII von Willebrand factor antigen levels less than 1%. Other patients may respond in a variable fashion depending on the type of molecular defect they have. Bleeding time and factor VIII coagulant activity, ristocetin cofactor activity, and von Willebrand factor antigen should be checked during administration of DESMOPRESSIN ACETATE to ensure that adequate levels are being achieved.

DESMOPRESSIN ACETATE is not indicated for the treatment of severe classic von Willebrand's disease (Type I) and when there is evidence of an abnormal molecular form of factor VIII antigen. (See **WARNINGS**.)

Diabetes Insipidus: DESMOPRESSIN ACETATE Injection 4 µg/mL is indicated as antidiuretic replacement therapy in the management of central (cranial) diabetes insipidus and for the management of the temporary polyuria and polydipsia following head trauma or surgery in the pituitary region. DESMOPRESSIN ACETATE is ineffective for the treatment of nephrogenic diabetes insipidus.

DESMOPRESSIN ACETATE is also available as an intranasal preparation. However, this means of delivery can be compromised by a variety of factors that can make nasal insufflation ineffective or inappropriate. These include poor intranasal absorption, nasal congestion and blockage, nasal discharge, atrophy of nasal mucosa, and severe atrophic rhinitis. Intranasal delivery may be inappropriate where there is an impaired level of consciousness. In addition, cranial surgical procedures, such as transsphenoidal hypophysectomy, create situations where an alternative route of administration is needed as in cases of nasal packing or recovery from surgery.

CONTRAINDICATIONS

DESMOPRESSIN ACETATE Injection 4 µg/mL is contraindicated in individuals with known hypersensitivity to desmopressin acetate or to any of the components of **DESMOPRESSIN ACETATE Injection 4 µg/mL.**

WARNINGS

Patients who do not have need of antidiuretic hormone for its antidiuretic effect, in particular those who are young or elderly, should be cautioned to ingest only enough fluid to satisfy thirst, in order to decrease the potential occurrence of water intoxication and hyponatremia.

Fluid intake should be adjusted downward, particularly in very young and elderly patients, in order to decrease the potential occurrence of water intoxication and hyponatremia. Particular attention should be paid to the possibility of the rare occurrence of an extreme decrease in plasma osmolality that may result in seizures which could lead to coma.

DESMOPRESSIN ACETATE should not be used to treat patients with Type IIB von Willebrand's disease since platelet aggregation may be induced.

PRECAUTIONS

General: For injection use only.

DESMOPRESSIN ACETATE Injection 4 µg/mL has infrequently produced changes in blood pressure causing either a slight elevation in blood pressure or a transient fall in blood pressure and a compensatory increase in heart rate. The drug should be used with caution in patients with coronary artery insufficiency and/or hypertensive cardiovascular disease.

DESMOPRESSIN ACETATE should be used with caution in patients with conditions associated with fluid and electrolyte imbalance, such as cystic fibrosis, because these patients are prone to hyponatremia.

There have been rare reports of thrombotic events following **DESMOPRESSIN ACETATE Injection 4 µg/mL** in patients predisposed to thrombus formation. No causality has been determined, however, the drug should be used with caution in these patients.

Severe allergic reactions have been reported rarely. Fatal anaphylaxis has been reported in one patient who received intravenous DESMOPRESSIN ACETATE. It is not known whether antibodies to **DESMOPRESSIN ACETATE Injection 4 µg/mL** are produced after repeated injections.

Hemophilia A: Laboratory tests for assessing patient status include levels of factor VIII coagulant, factor VIII antigen and factor VIII ristocetin cofactor (von Willebrand factor) as well as activated partial thromboplastin time. Factor VIII coagulant activity should be determined before giving DESMOPRESSIN ACETATE for hemostasis. If factor VIII coagulant activity is present at less than 5% of normal, DESMOPRESSIN ACETATE should not be relied on.

von Willebrand's Disease: Laboratory tests for assessing patient status include levels of factor VIII coagulant activity, factor VIII ristocetin cofactor activity, and factor VIII von Willebrand factor antigen. The skin bleeding time may be helpful in following these patients.

Diabetes Insipidus: Laboratory tests for monitoring the patient include urine volume and osmolality. In some cases, plasma osmolality may be required.

Drug Interactions: Although the pressor activity of DESMOPRESSIN ACETATE is very low compared with the antidiuretic activity, use of doses as large as 0.3 µg/kg of DESMOPRESSIN ACETATE with other pressor agents should be done only with careful patient monitoring.

DESMOPRESSIN ACETATE has been used with epsilon aminocaproic acid without adverse effects.

Carcinogenicity, Mutagenicity, Impairment of Fertility: Studies with DESMOPRESSIN ACETATE have not been performed to evaluate carcinogenic potential, mutagenic potential or effects on fertility.

Pregnancy Category B: Fertility studies have not been done. Teratology studies in rats and rabbits at doses from 0.05 to 10 µg/kg/day (approximately 0.1 times the maximum systemic human exposure in rats and up to 38 times the maximum systemic human exposure in rabbits based on surface area, mg/m^2) revealed no harm to the fetus due to DESMOPRESSIN ACETATE. There are, however, no adequate and well controlled studies in pregnant women. Because animal reproduction studies are not always predictive of human response, this drug should be used during pregnancy only if clearly needed.

Several publications of desmopressin acetate's use in the management of diabetes insipidus during pregnancy are available; these include a few anecdotal reports of congenital anomalies and low birth weight babies. However, no causal connection between these events and desmopressin acetate has been established. A fifteen year, Swedish epidemiologic study of the use of desmopressin acetate in pregnant women with diabetes insipidus found the rate of birth defects to be no greater than that in the general population; however the statistical power of this study is low. As opposed to preparations containing natural hormones, desmopressin acetate in antidiuretic doses has no uterotonic action and the physician will have to weigh the therapeutic advantages against the possible risks in each case.

Nursing Mothers: There have been no controlled studies in nursing mothers. A single study in postpartum women demonstrated a marked change in plasma, but little if any change in assayable DESMOPRESSIN ACETATE in breast milk following an intranasal dose of 10 µg. It is not known whether this drug is excreted in human milk. Because many drugs are excreted in human milk, caution should be exercised when DESMOPRESSIN ACETATE is administered to a nursing woman.

Pediatric Use: Use in infants and pediatric patients will require careful fluid intake restriction to prevent possible hyponatremia and water intoxication. **DESMOPRESSIN ACETATE Injection 4 µg/mL** *should not be used in infants less than three months of age* in the treatment of hemophilia A or von Willebrand's disease; safety and effectiveness in pediatric patients under 12 years of age with diabetes insipidus have not been established.

ADVERSE REACTIONS

Infrequently, DESMOPRESSIN ACETATE has produced transient headache, nausea, mild abdominal cramps and vulval pain. These symptoms disappeared with reduction in dosage. Occasionally, injection of DESMOPRESSIN ACETATE has produced local erythema, swelling or burning pain. Occasional facial flushing has been reported with the administration of DESMOPRESSIN ACETATE. **DESMOPRESSIN ACETATE Injection** has infrequently produced changes in blood pressure causing either a slight elevation or a transient fall and a compensatory increase in heart rate. Severe allergic reactions including anaphylaxis have been reported rarely with **DESMOPRESSIN ACETATE Injection.**

See **WARNINGS** for the possibility of water intoxication and hyponatremia.

There have been rare reports of thrombotic events (acute cerebrovascular thrombosis, acute myocardial infarction) following **DESMOPRESSIN ACETATE Injection** in patients predisposed to thrombus formation.

OVERDOSAGE

(See **ADVERSE REACTIONS.**) In case of overdosage, the dosage should be reduced, frequency of administration decreased, or the drug withdrawn according to the severity of the condition.

There is no known specific antidote for desmopressin acetate or **DESMOPRESSIN ACETATE Injection 4 µg/mL.**

An oral LD_{50} has not been established. An intravenous dose of 2 mg/kg in mice demonstrated no effect.

DOSAGE AND ADMINISTRATION

Hemophilia A and von Willebrand's Disease (Type I): DESMOPRESSIN ACETATE Injection 4 µg/mL is administered as an intravenous infusion at a dose of 0.3 µg DESMOPRESSIN ACETATE/kg body weight diluted in sterile physiological saline and infused slowly over 15 to 30 minutes. In adults and children weighing more than 10 kg, 50 mL of diluent is recommended; in children weighing 10 kg or less, 10 mL of diluent is recommended. Blood pressure and pulse should be monitored during infusion. If **DESMOPRESSIN ACETATE Injection 4 µg/mL** is used preoperatively, it should be administered 30 minutes prior to the scheduled procedure.

The necessity for repeat administration of DESMOPRESSIN ACETATE or use of any blood products for hemostasis should be determined by laboratory response as well as the clinical condition of the patient. The tendency toward

tachyphylaxis (lessening of response) with repeated administration given more frequently than every 48 hours should be considered in treating each patient.
Diabetes Insipidus: This formulation is administered subcutaneously or by direct intravenous injection. **DESMOPRESSIN ACETATE Injection 4 μg/mL** dosage must be determined for each patient and adjusted according to the pattern of response. Response should be estimated by two parameters: adequate duration of sleep and adequate, not excessive, water turnover.
The usual dosage range in adults is 0.5 mL (2.0 μg) to 1 mL (4.0 μg) daily, administered intravenously or subcutaneously, usually in two divided doses. The morning and evening doses should be separately adjusted for an adequate diurnal rhythm of water turnover. For patients who have been controlled on intranasal DESMOPRESSIN ACETATE and who must be switched to the injection form, either because of poor intranasal absorption or because of the need for surgery, the comparable antidiuretic dose of the injection is about one-tenth the intranasal dose.
Parenteral drug products should be inspected visually for particulate matter and discoloration prior to administration whenever solution and container permit.

HOW SUPPLIED

DESMOPRESSIN ACETATE Injection 4 μg/mL is available as a sterile solution in cartons of ten 1 mL single-dose ampules (NDC 55566-5030-1) and in 10 mL multiple-dose vials (NDC 55566-5040-1), each containing 4.0 μg DESMOPRESSIN ACETATE per mL.
Store refrigerated 2 to 8°C (36 to 46°F).
Rx only
Keep out of the reach of children.
Manufactured for
FERRING PHARMACEUTICALS INC.
TARRYTOWN, NY 10591
By Ferring Pharmaceuticals, Malmö, Sweden
Rev. 8/98 6018-01

ADVERSE REACTION	PLACEBO (N=59) %	DESMOPRESSIN ACETATE 20 μg (N=60) %	DESMOPRESSIN ACETATE 40 μg (N=61) %
BODY AS A WHOLE			
Abdominal Pain	0	2	2
Asthenia	0	0	2
Chills	0	0	2
Headache	0	2	5
Throat Pain	2	0	0
NERVOUS SYSTEM			
Depression	2	0	0
Dizziness	0	0	3
RESPIRATORY SYSTEM			
Epistaxis	2	3	0
Nostril Pain	0	2	0
Respiratory Infection	2	0	0
Rhinitis	2	8	3
CARDIOVASCULAR SYSTEM			
Vasodilation	2	0	0
DIGESTIVE SYSTEM			
Gastrointestinal Disorder	0	2	0
Nausea	0	0	2
SKIN & APPENDAGES			
Leg Rash	2	0	0
Rash	2	0	0
SPECIAL SENSES			
Conjunctivitis	0	2	0
Edema Eyes	0	2	0
Lachrymation Disorder	0	0	2

DESMOPRESSIN ACETATE Rhinal Tube

℞

DESCRIPTION

Desmopressin Acetate Rhinal Tube is a synthetic analogue of the natural pituitary hormone 8-arginine vasopressin (ADH), an antidiuretic hormone affecting renal water conservation. It is chemically defined as follows:

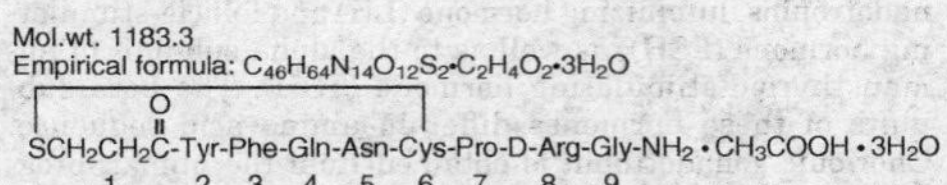

1-(3-mercaptopropionic acid)-8-D-arginine vasopressin monoacetate (salt) trihydrate.
Desmopressin Acetate Rhinal Tube is provided as an aqueous solution for intranasal use.
Each mL contains:

Desmopressin acetate	0.1 mg
Chlorobutanol	5.0 mg
Sodium Chloride	9.0 mg
Hydrochloric acid to adjust pH to approximately 4	

CLINICAL PHARMACOLOGY

Desmopressin Acetate Rhinal Tube contains as active substance desmopressin acetate, a synthetic analogue of the natural hormone arginine vasopressin. One mL (0.1 mg) of intranasal Desmopressin acetate has an antidiuretic activity of about 400 IU; 10 μg of desmopressin acetate is equivalent to 40 IU.

1. The biphasic half-lives for intranasal Desmopressin acetate were 7.8 and 75.5 minutes for the fast and slow phases, compared with 2.5 and 14.5 minutes for lysine vasopressin, another form of the hormone used in this condition. As a result, intranasal Desmopressin acetate provides a prompt onset of antidiuretic action with a long duration after each administration.
2. The change in structure of arginine vasopressin to Desmopressin acetate has resulted in a decreased vasopressor action and decreased actions on visceral smooth muscle relative to the enhanced antidiuretic activity, so that clinically effective antidiuretic doses are usually below threshold levels for effects on vascular or visceral smooth muscle.
3. Desmopressin acetate administered intranasally has an antidiuretic effect about one-tenth that of an equivalent dose administered by injection.

INDICATIONS AND USAGE

Primary Nocturnal Enuresis: Desmopressin Acetate Rhinal Tube is indicated for the management of primary nocturnal enuresis. It may be used alone or adjunctive to behavioral conditioning or other non-pharmacological intervention. It has been shown to be effective in some cases that are refractory to conventional therapies.
Central Cranial Diabetes Insipidus: Desmopressin Acetate Rhinal Tube is indicated as antidiuretic replacement therapy in the management of central cranial diabetes insipidus and for management of the temporary polyuria and polydipsia following head trauma or surgery in the pituitary region. It is ineffective for the treatment of nephrogenic diabetes insipidus.
The use of **Desmopressin Acetate Rhinal Tube** in patients with an established diagnosis will result in a reduction in urinary output with increase in urine osmolality and a decrease in plasma osmolality. This will allow the resumption of a more normal life-style with a decrease in urinary frequency and nocturia.
There are reports of an occasional change in response with time, usually greater than 6 months. Some patients may show a decreased responsiveness, others a shortened duration of effect. There is no evidence this effect is due to the development of binding antibodies but may be due to a local inactivation of the peptide.
Patients are selected for therapy by establishing the diagnosis by means of the water deprivation test, the hypertonic saline infusion test, and/or the response to antidiuretic hormone. Continued response to intranasal Desmopressin acetate can be monitored by urine volume and osmolality.
Desmopressin acetate is also available as a solution for injection when the intranasal route may be compromised. These situations include nasal congestion and blockage, nasal discharge, atrophy of nasal mucosa, and severe atrophic rhinitis. Intranasal delivery may also be inappropriate where there is an impaired level of consciousness. In addition, cranial surgical procedures, such as transsphenoidal hypophysectomy create situations where an alternative route of administration is needed as in cases of nasal packing or recovery from surgery.

CONTRAINDICATIONS

Desmopressin Acetate Rhinal Tube is contraindicated in individuals with known hypersensitivity to desmopressin acetate or to any of the components of **Desmopressin Acetate Rhinal Tube.**

WARNINGS

1. For intranasal use only.
2. In very young and elderly patients in particular, fluid intake should be adjusted downward in order to decrease the potential occurrence of water intoxication and hyponatremia. Particular attention should be paid to the possibility of the rare occurrence of an extreme decrease in plasma osmolality that may result in seizures which could lead to coma.

PRECAUTIONS

General: Intranasal Desmopressin acetate at high dosage has infrequently produced a slight elevation of blood pressure, which disappeared with a reduction in dosage. The drug should be used with caution in patients with coronary artery insufficiency and/or hypertensive cardiovascular disease because of possible rise in blood pressure.
Desmopressin acetate should be used with caution in patients with conditions associated with fluid and electrolyte imbalance, such as cystic fibrosis, because these patients are prone to hyponatremia.
Rare severe allergic reactions have been reported with Desmopressin acetate. Anaphylaxis has been reported with intravenous administration of Desmopressin acetate Injection, but not with Desmopressin Acetate Intranasal.
Central Cranial Diabetes Insipidus: Since **Desmopressin Acetate Rhinal Tube** is used intranasally, changes in the nasal mucosa such as scarring, edema, or other disease may cause erratic, unreliable absorption in which case intranasal Desmopressin acetateshould not be used. For such situations, Desmopressin Acetate Injection should be considered.
Primary Nocturnal Enuresis: If changes in the nasal mucosa have occurred, unreliable absorption may result. **Desmopressin Acetate Rhinal Tube** should be discontinued until the nasal problems resolve.
Laboratory Tests: Laboratory tests for following the patient with central cranial diabetes insipidus or post-surgical or head trauma-related polyuria and polydipsia include urine volume and osmolality. In some cases plasma osmolality measurements may be required. For the healthy patient with primary nocturnal enuresis, serum electrolytes should be checked at least once if therapy is continued beyond 7 days.
Drug Interactions: Although the pressor activity of Desmopressin acetate is very low compared to the antidiuretic activity, use of large doses of intranasal Desmopressin acetate with other pressor agents should only be done with careful patient monitoring.
Carcinogenesis, Mutagenesis, Impairment of Fertility: Studies with Desmopressin acetate have not been performed to evaluate carcinogenic potential, mutagenic potential or effects on fertility.
Pregnancy Category B: Fertility studies have not been done. Teratology studies in rats and rabbits at doses from 0.05 to 10 μg/kg/day (approximately 0.1 times the maximum systemic human exposure in rats and up to 38 times the maximum systemic human exposure in rabbits based on surface area, mg/m^2) revealed no harm to the fetus due to Desmopressin acetate. There are, however, no adequate and well controlled studies in pregnant women. Because animal reproduction studies are not always predictive of human response, this drug should be used during pregnancy only if clearly needed.
Several publications of desmopressin acetate's use in the management of diabetes insipidus during pregnancy are available; these include a few anecdotal reports of congenital anomalies and low birth weight babies. However, no causal connection between these events and desmopressin acetate has been established. A fifteen year, Swedish epidemiologic study of the use of desmopressin acetate in pregnant women with diabetes insipidus found the rate of birth defects to be no greater than that in the general population; however the statistical power of this study is low. As opposed to preparations containing natural hormones, desmopressin acetate in antidiuretic doses has no uterotonic action and the physician will have to weigh the therapeutic advantages against the possible risks in each case.
Nursing Mothers: There have been no controlled studies in nursing mothers. A single study in postpartum women demonstrated a marked change in plasma, but little if any change in assayable Desmopressin acetate in breast milk following an intranasal dose of 10 μg. It is not known whether this drug is excreted in human milk. Because many drugs are excreted in human milk, caution should be exercised when Desmopressin acetate is administered to a nursing woman.
Pediatric Use: *Primary Nocturnal Enuresis:* **Desmopressin Acetate Rhinal Tube** has been used in childhood nocturnal enuresis. Short-term (4-8 weeks) **Desmopressin Acetate Rhinal Tube** administration has been shown to be safe and modestly effective in pediatric patients aged 6 years or older with severe childhood nocturnal enuresis. Adequately controlled studies with intranasal Desmopressin acetatein primary nocturnal enuresis have not been conducted beyond 4-8 weeks. The dose should be individually adjusted to achieve the best results.
Central Cranial Diabetes Insipidus: **Desmopressin Acetate Rhinal Tube** has been used in pediatric patients with diabetes insipidus. Use in infants and pediatric patients will require careful fluid intake restriction to prevent possible hyponatremia and water intoxication. The dose must be individually adjusted to the patient with attention in the very young to the danger of an extreme decrease in plasma osmolality with resulting convulsions. Dose should start at 0.05 mL or less.

Continued on next page

Desmopressin Acetate—Cont.

There are reports of an occasional change in response with time, usually greater than 6 months. Some patients may show a decreased responsiveness, others a shortened duration of effect. There is no evidence this effect is due to the development of binding antibodies but may be due to a local inactivation of the peptide.

ADVERSE REACTIONS

Infrequently, high dosages of intranasal Desmopressin acetate have produced transient headache and nausea. Nasal congestion, rhinitis and flushing have also been reported occasionally along with mild abdominal cramps. These symptoms disappeared with reduction in dosage. Nosebleed, sore throat, cough and upper respiratory infections have also been reported.
The following table lists the percent of patients having adverse experiences without regard to relationship to study drug from the pooled pivotal study data for nocturnal enuresis.
[See table at top of previous page]
See **WARNINGS** for the possibility of water intoxication and hyponatremia.

OVERDOSAGE

(See **ADVERSE REACTIONS**.) In case of overdosage, the dose should be reduced, frequency of administration decreased, or the drug withdrawn according to the severity of the condition. There is no known specific antidote for desmopressin acetate or **Desmopressin Acetate Rhinal Tube**.
An oral LD_{50} has not been established. An intravenous dose of 2 mg/kg in mice demonstrated no effect.

DOSAGE AND ADMINISTRATION

Primary Nocturnal Enuresis: Dosage should be adjusted according to the individual. The recommended initial dose for those 6 years of age and older is 20 µg or 0.2 mL solution intranasally at bedtime. Adjustment up to 40 µg is suggested if the patient does not respond. Some patients may respond to 10 µg and adjustment to that lower dose may be done if the patient has shown a response to 20 µg. It is recommended that one-half of the dose be administered per nostril. Adequately controlled studies with intranasal Desmopressin acetate in primary nocturnal enuresis have not been conducted beyond 4–8 weeks.
Central Cranial Diabetes Insipidus: This drug is administered into the nose through a soft, flexible plastic rhinal tube which has four graduation marks on it that measure 0.2, 0.15, 0.1 and 0.05 mL. **Desmopressin Acetate Rhinal Tube** dosage must be determined for each individual patient and adjusted according to the diurnal pattern of response. Response should be estimated by two parameters: adequate duration of sleep and adequate, not excessive, water turnover. Patients with nasal congestion and blockage have often responded well to intranasal Desmopressin acetate. The usual dosage range in adults is 0.1 to 0.4 mL daily, either as a single dose or divided into two or three doses. Most adults require 0.2 mL daily in two divided doses. The morning and evening doses should be separately adjusted for an adequate diurnal rhythm of water turnover. For children aged 3 months to 12 years, the usual dosage range is 0.05 to 0.3 mL daily, either as a single dose or divided into two doses. About 1/4 to 1/3 of patients can be controlled by a single daily dose of Desmopressin acetate administered intranasally.

HOW SUPPLIED

Desmopressin Acetate Rhinal Tube is available in a 2.5 mL vial, packaged with two rhinal tube applicators per carton (NDC 55566-5020-1). Also available in a shelf packs of 10 × 2.5 mL vials (NDC 55566-5020-2).
Store refrigerated 2 to 8°C (36 to 46°F). When traveling, closed bottles will maintain stability for 3 weeks when stored at controlled room temperature, 20 to 25°C (68 to 77°F).
Rx only
Keep out of the reach of children.
Manufactured for
FERRING PHARMACEUTICALS INC.
TARRYTOWN, NY 10591
By Ferring Pharmaceuticals, Malmö, Sweden
Rev. 8/98 6026-01

PATIENT INSTRUCTION GUIDE

DESMOPRESSIN
acetate
RHINAL TUBE

1. Pull plastic tag on neck of bottle.

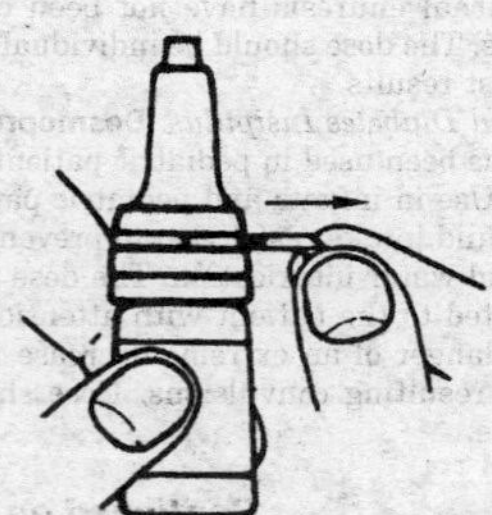

2. Break security seal and remove plastic cap.

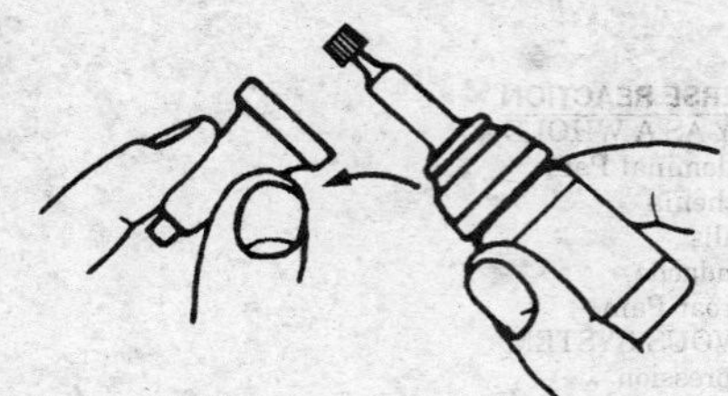

3. Twist off the small knurled seal from the dropper. **Use the same seal reversed to prevent subsequent leakage,** especially if the bottle is not stored upright.

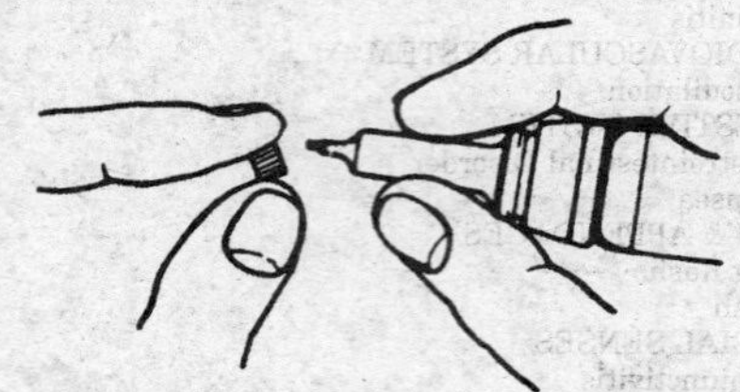

4. The drug is administered by a soft, flexible, plastic rhinal tube which has dose marks at 0.2, 0.15, 0.1 and 0.05 mL. Take the arrow-marked part of the tube in one hand and place the fingers of the other hand around the cylindrical part of the closure. Insert the top of the dropper in a downward position into the arrow-marked end of the tube and squeeze the dropper until the solution has reached the desired calibration mark. The dose is measured from the arrow-marked end of the tube to the appropriate calibration. Disconnect the tube from the bottle by withdrawing the bottle quickly downwards. In order to prevent air bubbles from forming in the tube, maintain constant pressure on the dropper. If difficulty is experienced in filling the tube, a diabetic or tuberculin syringe may be used to draw up the dose and load the tube.

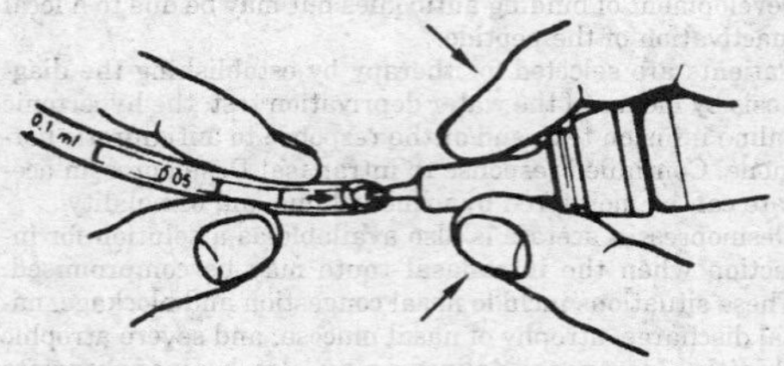

5. Hold the tube with the fingers approximately 3/4 inch from the end and insert into a nostril until the tips of the fingers reach the nostril.

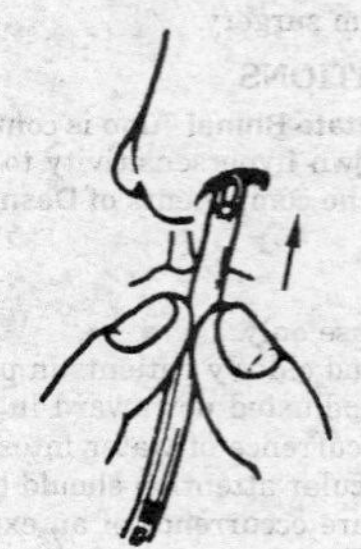

6. Put the other end of the tube into the mouth. Hold the breath, tilt the head back and then blow with a short, strong puff through the tube so that the solution reaches the right place in the nasal cavity. Through this procedure, medication is limited to the nasal cavity and the preparation does not pass down into the throat.
In very young patients, it may be necessary for an adult to blow the solution into the child's nose. In such cases, the tube will not need to be put into the nose as far as in the older child or adult. The tube should be placed in the nose gently just far enough so that the solution does not run out. A baby must be held firmly and securely.

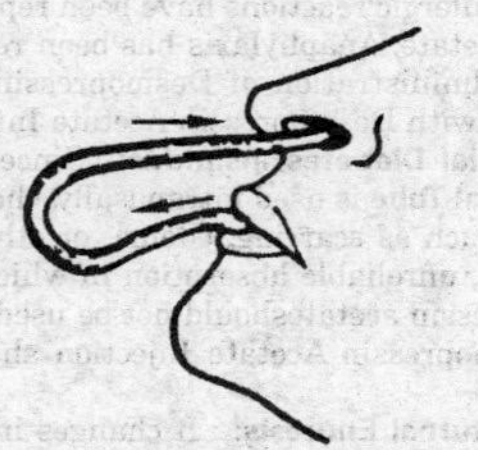

7. **After use, reseal dropper tip and close the bottle with the plastic cap.** Wash the tube in water and shake thoroughly, until no more water is left. The tube can then be used for the next application.

IMPORTANT:
Replace Knurled Seal

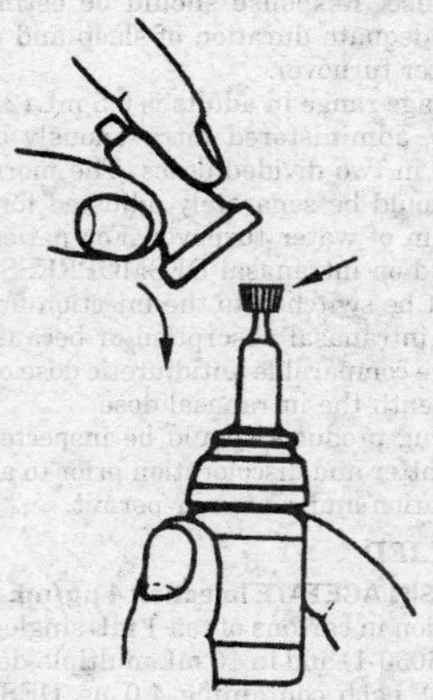

Store refrigerated 2 to 8°C (36 to 46°F). When traveling, closed bottles will maintain stability for 3 weeks when stored at controlled room temperature, 20 to 25°C (68 to 77°F).
Manufactured for
FERRING PHARMACEUTICALS INC.
TARRYTOWN, NY 10591
By Ferring Pharmaceuticals, Malmö, Sweden 6026-01

NOVAREL™ ℞
(Chorionic Gonadotropin for Injection, USP)

DESCRIPTION

Human chorionic gonadotropin (HCG), a polypeptide hormone produced by the human placenta, is composed of an alpha and a beta sub-unit. The alpha sub-unit is essentially identical to the alpha sub-units of the human pituitary gonadotropins, luteinizing hormone (LH) and follicle-stimulating hormone (FSH), as well as to the alpha sub-unit of human thyroid-stimulating hormone (TSH). The beta subunits of these hormones differ in amino acid sequence.
Chorionic gonadotropin is obtained from the human pregnancy urine. It is standardized by a biological assay procedure.
Chorionic Gonadotropin for Injection, USP is available in multiple dose vials containing 10,000 USP Units with accompanying Bacteriostatic Water for Injection for reconstitution. When reconstituted with 10 mL of the accompanying diluent each vial contains:

Chorionic gonadotropin	10,000 Units
Mannitol	100 mg
Benzyl alcohol	0.9%
Water for Injection	q.s.

Buffered with dibasic sodium phosphate and monobasic sodium phosphate. Hydrochloric acid and/or sodium hydroxide may have been used for pH adjustment (6.0-8.0). Nitrogen gas is used in the freeze drying process.

CLINICAL PHARMACOLOGY

The action of HCG is virtually identical to that of pituitary LH, although HCG appears to have a small degree of FSH activity as well. It stimulates production of gonadal steroid hormones by stimulating the interstitial cells (Leydig cells) of the testis to produce androgens and the corpus luteum of the ovary to produce progesterone. Androgen stimulation in the male leads to the development of secondary sex characteristics and may stimulate testicular descent when no anatomical impediment to descent is present. This descent is usually reversible when HCG is discontinued. During the normal menstrual cycle, LH participates with FSH in the development and maturation of the normal ovarian follicle, and the mid-cycle LH surge triggers ovulation. HCG can substitute for LH in this function. During a normal pregnancy, HCG secreted by the placenta maintains the corpus luteum after LH secretion decreases, supporting continued secretion of estrogen and progesterone and preventing menstruation. HCG HAS NO KNOWN EFFECT ON FAT MOBILIZATION, APPETITE OR SENSE OF HUNGER, OR BODY FAT DISTRIBUTION.

INDICATIONS AND USAGE

HCG HAS NOT BEEN DEMONSTRATED TO BE EFFECTIVE ADJUNCTIVE THERAPY IN THE TREATMENT OF OBESITY. THERE IS NO SUBSTANTIAL EVIDENCE THAT IT INCREASES WEIGHT LOSS BEYOND THAT RESULTING FROM CALORIC RESTRICTION, THAT IT CAUSES A MORE ATTRACTIVE OR "NORMAL" DISTRIBUTION OF FAT, OR THAT IT DECREASES THE HUNGER AND DISCOMFORT ASSOCIATED WITH CALORIE-RESTRICTED DIETS.

1. Prepubertal cryptorchidism not due to anatomical obstruction. In general, HCG is thought to induce testicular descent in situations when descent would have occurred at puberty. HCG thus may help predict whether or not orchiopexy will be needed in the future. Although, in some cases, descent following HCG administration is permanent, in most cases, the response is temporary. Therapy is usually instituted between the ages four and nine.
2. Selected cases of hypogonadotropic hypogonadism (hypogonadism secondary to a pituitary deficiency) in males.
3. Induction of ovulation and pregnancy in the anovulatory, infertile woman in whom the cause of anovulation is secondary and not due to primary ovarian failure, and who has been appropriately pretreated with human menotropins.

CONTRAINDICATIONS

Precocious puberty, prostatic carcinoma or other androgen-dependent neoplasm, prior allergic reaction to HCG.

WARNINGS

HCG should be used in conjunction with human menopausal gonadotropins only by physicians experienced with infertility problems who are familiar with the criteria for patient selection, contraindications, warnings, precautions and adverse reactions described in the package insert for menotropins. The principal serious adverse reactions are: (1) Ovarian hyperstimulation, a syndrome of sudden ovarian enlargement, ascites with or without pain and/or pleural effusion, (2) Rupture of ovarian cysts with resultant hemoperitoneum, (3) Multiple births and (4) Arterial thromboembolism.

PRECAUTIONS

General

Induction of androgen secretion by HCG may induce precocious puberty in patients treated for cryptorchidism. Therapy should be discontinued if signs of precocious puberty occur.

Since androgens may cause fluid retention, HCG should be used with caution in patients with cardiac or renal disease, epilepsy, migraine or asthma.

Drug/Laboratory Test Interactions

Chorionic gonadotropin may interfere with radioimmunoassay for gonadotropins, particularly luteinizing hormone.

Carcinogenesis, Mutagenesis, Impairment of Fertility

Long-term studies in animals have not been performed to evaluate the carcinogenic or mutagenic potential of chorionic gonadotropin.

Pediatric Use

Safety and effectiveness of chorionic gonadotropin in children below the age of four have not been established.

Pregnancy

Teratogenic Effects: Pregnancy Category C—Chorionic gonadotropin may cause fetal harm when administered to a pregnant woman. Defects of forelimbs and central nervous system and alterations in sex ratio have been reported in mice receiving combined gonadotropin and chorionic gonadotropin therapy in dosages to induce superovulation. Multiple ovulations with resulting plural gestations (mostly twins) have been reported to occur in approximately 20% of pregnancies when conception has followed chorionic gonadotropin therapy.

Nursing Mothers

It is not known whether chorionic gonadotropin is excreted in human milk. Because many drugs are excreted in human milk, caution should be exercised when chorionic gonadotropin is administered to a nursing woman.

ADVERSE REACTIONS

Headache, irritability, restlessness, depression, fatigue, edema, precocious puberty, gynecomastia and pain at the site of injection.

DOSAGE AND ADMINISTRATION

Intramuscular Use Only

The dosage regimen employed in any particular case will depend upon the indication for use, the age and weight of the patient and the physician's preference. The following regimens have been advocated by various authorities.

Prepubertal Cryptorchidism Not Due To Anatomical Obstruction

1. 4,000 USP Units three times weekly for three weeks.
2. 5,000 USP Units every second day for four injections.
3. 15 injections of 500 to 1,000 USP Units over a period of six weeks.
4. 500 USP Units three times weekly for four to six weeks. If this course of treatment is not successful, another is begun one month later giving 1,000 USP Units per injection.

Selected Cases Of Hypogonadotropic Hypogonadism In Males

1. 500 to 1,000 USP Units three times a week for three weeks, followed by the same dose twice a week for three weeks.
2. 4,000 USP Units three times weekly for six to nine months, following which the dosage may be reduced to 2,000 USP Units three times weekly for an additional three months.

Induction of ovulation and pregnancy in the anovulatory, infertile woman in whom the cause of anovulation is secondary and not due to primary ovarian failure and who has been appropriately pretreated with human menotropins (see prescribing information for menotropins for dosage and administration for that drug product). 5,000 to 10,000 USP Units one day following the last dose of menotropins. (A dosage of 10,000 Units is recommended in the labeling for menotropins.)

IMPORTANT: USE COMPLETELY WITHIN 60 DAYS AFTER RECONSTITUTION. REFRIGERATE AFTER RECONSTITUTION.

DIRECTIONS FOR RECONSTITUTION:

Two-Vial Package

Withdraw sterile air from lyophilized vial and inject into diluent vial. Remove 10 mL from diluent vial and add to lyophilized vial; agitate gently until solution is complete.

HOW SUPPLIED

Chorionic Gonadotropin for Injection, USP, lyophilized, is supplied in two-vial packages including Bacteriostatic Water for Injection as diluent as follows:

Product	NDC No.	
No. F25021	55566-1501-1	Chorionic Gonadotropin for Injection, USP, 10,000 USP Units in a 10 mL multiple dose vial with accompanying diluent in packages of 10.

The product is assayed in accord with the USP method and potencies refer to USP Units (International Units) defined in terms of the USP Chorionic Gonadotropin Reference Standard.

Store at controlled room temperature 15°–30°C (59°–86°F).

Rx only

6007-02

NSN 6505-01-145-6377

Manufactured for:
Ferring Pharmaceuticals Inc.
Tarrytown, NY 10591
By: American Pharmaceutical Partners, Inc.
Los Angeles, CA 90024
45761A
Revised: September 1999

REPRONEX® ℞

(MENOTROPINS FOR INJECTION, USP) FOR SUBCUTANEOUS INECTION AND INTRAMUSCULAR INJECTION

DESCRIPTION

Repronex® (menotropins for injection, USP) is a purified preparation of gonadotropins extracted from the urine of postmenopausal women. Each vial of Repronex® contains 75 International Units (IU) or 150 IU of follicle-stimulating hormone (FSH) activity and 75 IU or 150 IU of luteinizing hormone (LH) activity, respectively, plus 20 mg lactose monohydrate in a sterile, lyophilized form. The final product may contain sodium phosphate buffer (sodium phosphate tribasic and phosphoric acid). Repronex® is administered by subcutaneous or intramuscular injection. Human Chorionic Gonadotropin (hCG), a naturally occurring hormone in post-menopausal urine, is detected in Repronex®.

Repronex® is biologically standardized for FSH and LH (ICSH) gonadotropin activities in terms of the Second International Reference Preparation for Human Menopausal Gonadotropins established in September, 1964 by the Expert Committee on Biological Standards of the World Health Organization.

Both FSH and LH are glycoproteins that are acidic and water soluble. Therapeutic class: Infertility.

CLINICAL PHARMACOLOGY

Menotropins administered for 7 to 12 days produces ovarian follicular growth in women who do not have primary ovarian failure. Treatment with menotropins in most instances results only in follicular growth and maturation. When sufficient follicular maturation has occurred, hCG must be given to induce ovulation.

PHARMACOKINETICS

Single doses of 300 IU menotropins (Menogon®, Ferring's European formulation) were administered subcutaneously (SC) and intramuscularly (IM) in a 2-period crossover study to 16 healthy female subjects while their endogenous FSH and LH were being suppressed. Serum FSH concentrations were determined. Based on the ratio of FSH C_{max} and $AUC_{0-\infty}$, SC and IM administration of menotropins are not bioequivalent. Compared to IM administration, the SC administration of menotropins results in an increase of FSH C_{max} and $AUC_{0-\infty}$ by 35 and 20%, respectively.

Based on two subjects who received either the highest SC or IM Repronex® dose, FSH pharmacokinetics (PK) appears to be linear up to 450 IU menotropins. The mean accumulation factors for FSH upon six doses of SC or IM 150 to 450 IU/day Repronex® are 1.6 and 1.4, respectively. Upon six doses of SC or IM 150 IU/day Repronex®, the observed serum FSH concentrations range from 1.7 to 15.9 mIU/mL and 0.5 to 10.1 mIU/mL, respectively. The FSH pharmacokinetic parameters from population modeling for these two studies are in Table 1.

[See table 1 at top of next page]

Serum LH concentrations upon multiple dose SC or IM Repronex® are low and variable. No recognizable trend in the increase in serum LH concentrations from SC or IM 150 to 450 IU/day Repronex® doses was observed. After the 6th dose of SC or IM 150 IU/day Repronex®, the range of baseline-corrected serum LH concentrations is 0 to 3.2 mIU/mL for both routes of administration.

Absorption

The geometric mean of FSH C_{max} and $AUC_{0-\infty}$ upon single dose SC administration of menotropins is 5.62 mIU/mL and 385.2 mIU·h/mL, respectively; the corresponding geometric median of FSH t_{max} is 12 hours. The geometric mean of FSH C_{max} and $AUC_{0-\infty}$ upon single dose IM administration of menotropins is 4.15 mIU/mL and 320.1 mIU·h/mL, respectively; the corresponding geometric median of FSH t_{max} is 18 hours.

Distribution

Human tissue or organ distribution of FSH and LH have not been studied for Repronex®.

Metabolism

Metabolism of FSH and LH have not been studied for Repronex® in humans.

Excretion

The mean elimination half-lives of FSH upon single dose SC and IM administration of menotropins are 53.7 and 59.2 hours, respectively.

Pediatric Populations

Repronex® is not used in pediatric populations.

Geriatric Populations

Repronex® is not used in geriatric populations.

Special Populations

The safety and efficacy of Repronex® in renal and hepatic insufficiency have not been studied.

Drug Interactions

No drug/drug interaction studies have been conducted for Repronex® in humans.

CLINICAL STUDIES

Efficacy results for two randomized, active controlled, multicenter studies in *in vitro* fertilization (IVF) and ovulation induction (OI) are summarized in tables 2 and 3. The patients underwent pituitary suppression with a GnRH agonist before starting Repronex® administration. The first study evaluated 186 patients undergoing IVF who received 225 IU Repronex® daily for 5 days. This was followed by individual titration of the dose from 75 to 450 IU daily based on ultrasound and estradiol (E_2) levels. The total duration of dosing did not exceed 12 days. The second study evaluated 108 patients who received 150 IU Repronex® daily for 5 days. This was followed by individual titration of the dose from 75 to 450 IU daily based on ultrasound and estradiol (E_2) levels. The total duration of dosing did not exceed 12 days.

[See table 2 on next page]
[See table 3 on next page]

INDICATIONS AND USAGE

Repronex®, in conjunction with hCG, is indicated for multiple follicular development (controlled ovarian stimulation) and ovulation induction in patients who have previously received pituitary suppression.

Selection of Patients

1. Before treatment with Repronex® is instituted, a thorough gynecologic and endocrinologic evaluation must be performed. Except for those patients enrolled in an *in vitro* fertilization program, this should include a hysterosalpingogram (to rule out uterine and tubal pathology) and documentation of anovulation by means of basal body temperature, serial vaginal smears, examination of cervical mucus, determination of serum (or urine) progesterone, urinary pregnanediol and endometrial biopsy. Patients with tubal pathology should receive menotropins only if enrolled in an *in vitro* fertilization program.
2. Primary ovarian failure should be excluded by the determination of gonadotropin levels.
3. Careful examination should be made to rule out the presence of an early pregnancy.
4. Patients in late reproductive life have a greater predilection to endometrial carcinoma as well as a higher incidence of anovulatory disorders. Cervical dilation and curettage should always be done for diagnosis before starting Repronex® therapy in such patients who demonstrate abnormal uterine bleeding or other signs of endometrial abnormalities.
5. Evaluation of the husband's fertility potential should be included in the workup.

CONTRAINDICATIONS

Repronex® is contraindicated in women who have:

1. A high FSH level indicating primary ovarian failure.
2. Uncontrolled thyroid and adrenal dysfunction.
3. An organic intracranial lesion such as a pituitary tumor.
4. The presence of any cause of infertility other than anovulation unless they are candidates for *in vitro*-fertilization.
5. Abnormal bleeding of undetermined origin.
6. Ovarian cysts or enlargement not due to polycystic ovary syndrome.
7. Prior hypersensitivity to menotropins.
8. Repronex® is not indicated in women who are pregnant. There are limited human data on the effects of menotropins when administered during pregnancy.

WARNINGS

Repronex® is a drug that should only be used by physicians who are thoroughly familiar with infertility problems. It is a potent gonadotropic substance capable of causing mild to severe adverse reactions in women. Gonadotropin therapy requires a certain time commitment by physicians and supportive health professionals, and its use requires the avail-

Continued on next page

Repronex—Cont.

ability of appropriate monitoring facilities (see **PRECAUTIONS—Laboratory Tests**). In female patients it must be used with a great deal of care.

Overstimulation of the Ovary During Repronex® Therapy

Ovarian Enlargement: Mild to moderate uncomplicated ovarian enlargement which may be accompanied by abdominal distension and/or abdominal pain occurs in approximately 5 to 10% of those treated with Repronex® menotropins and hCG, and generally regresses without treatment within two or three weeks.

In order to minimize the hazard associated with the occasional abnormal ovarian enlargement which may occur with Repronex® hCG therapy, the lowest dose consistent with expectation of good results, should be used. Careful monitoring of ovarian response can further minimize the risk of overstimulation.

If the ovaries are abnormally enlarged on the last day of Repronex® therapy, hCG should not be administered in this course of therapy; this will reduce the chances of development of the Ovarian Hyperstimulation Syndrome.

The Ovarian Hyperstimulation Syndrome (OHSS): OHSS is a medical event distinct from uncomplicated ovarian enlargement. OHSS may progress rapidly to become a serious medical event. It is characterized by an apparent dramatic increase in vascular permeability which can result in a rapid accumulation of fluid in the peritoneal cavity, thorax, and potentially, the pericardium. The early warning signs of development of OHSS are severe pelvic pain, nausea, vomiting, and weight gain. The following symptomatology has been seen with cases of OHSS: abdominal pain, abdominal distension, gastrointestinal symptoms including nausea, vomiting and diarrhea, severe ovarian enlargement, weight gain, dyspnea, and oliguria. Clinical evaluation may reveal hypovolemia, hemoconcentration, electrolyte imbalances, ascites, hemoperitoneum, pleural effusions, hydrothorax, acute pulmonary distress, and thromboembolic events (see "Pulmonary and Vascular Complications" below). Transient liver function test abnormalities suggestive of hepatic dysfunction, which may be accompanied by morphologic changes on liver biopsy, have been reported in association with the Ovarian Hyperstimulation Syndrome (OHSS).

OHSS occured in 3 of 125 (2.4%) Repronex® treated women during ART clinical studies. None of these cases was classified as severe. In Ovulation Induction clinical studies, 4 of 72 (5.5%) Repronex® treated women developed OHSS and of this number one case was classified as severe (1.4%). Cases of OHSS are more common, more severe and more protracted if pregnancy occurs. OHSS develops rapidly; therefore patients should be followed for at least two weeks after hCG administration. Most often, OHSS occurs after treatment has been discontinued and reaches its maximum at about seven to ten days following treatment. Usually, OHSS resolves spontaneously with the onset of menses. If there is evidence that OHSS may be developing prior to hCG administration (see **PRECAUTIONS—Laboratory Tests**), the hCG should be withheld.

If OHSS occurs, treatment should be stopped and the patient hospitalized. Treatment is primarily symptomatic, consisting of bed rest, fluid and electrolyte management, and analgesics if needed. The phenomenon of hemoconcentration associated with fluid loss into the peritoneal cavity, pleural cavity, and the pericardial cavity has been seen to occur and should be thoroughly assessed in the following manner: 1) fluid intake and output, 2) weight, 3) hematocrit, 4) serum and urinary electrolytes, 5) urine specific gravity, 6) BUN and creatinine, and 7) abdominal girth. These determinations are to be performed daily or more often if the need arises.

With OHSS there is an increased risk of injury to the ovary. The ascitic, pleural, and pericardial fluid should not be removed unless absolutely necessary to relieve symptoms such as pulmonary distress or cardiac tamponade. Pelvic examination may cause rupture of an ovarian cyst, which may result in hemoperitoneum, and should therefore be avoided. If this does occur, and if bleeding becomes such that surgery is required, the surgical treatment should be designed to control bleeding and to retain as much ovarian tissue as possible. Intercourse should be prohibited in those patients in whom significant ovarian enlargement occurs after ovulation because of the danger of hemoperitoneum resulting from ruptured ovarian cysts.

The management of OHSS may be divided into three phases: the acute, the chronic, and the resolution phases. Because the use of diuretics can accentuate the diminished intravascular volume, diuretics should be avoided except in the late phase of resolution as described below.

Acute Phase: Management during the acute phase should be designed to prevent hemoconcentration due to loss of intravascular volume to the third space and to minimize the risk of thromboembolic phenomena and kidney damage. Treatment is designed to normalize electrolytes while maintaining an acceptable but somewhat reduced intravascular volume. Full correction of the intravascular volume deficit may lead to an unacceptable increase in the amount of third space fluid accumulation. Management includes administration of limited intravenous fluids, electrolytes, and human serum albumin. Monitoring for the development of hyperkalemia is recommended.

Chronic Phase: After stabilizing the patient during the acute phase, excessive fluid accumulation in the third space should be limited by instituting severe potassium, sodium, and fluid restriction.

Table 1. FSH Pharmacokinetic Parameters† Upon Menotropins Administration

	Single Dose‡		Multiple Dose¶	
FSH Parameter	SC	IM	SC	IM
$K_a(h^{-1})$	0.128 (42.1)	0.117 (21.3)	0.076 (46.3)	0.064 (63.2)
Cl/F (L/h)	0.770 (17.1)	0.94 (6.9)	1.11 (39.5)	1.44 (43.5)
V/F (L)	39.37 (14.1)	57.68 (11.4)	23.09 (8.3)	23.5 (2.5)

† mean (CV%)
‡ Menogon® (Ferring's European formulation of menotropins)
¶ Repronex

Table 2. Efficacy Outcomes by Treatment Group for IVF (one cycle of treatment)

Parameter	Repronex® IM	Repronex® SC
	N=65	N=60
Total oocytes Retrieved	13.6	12.7
Mature oocytes Retrieved	9.4	8.6
Pts w/oocyte Retrieval (%)	61(93.8)	55(91.7)
Pts w/Embryo Transfer (%)	58(89.2)	51(85.0)
Pts w/Chemical Pregnancy (%)	31(47.7)	35(58.3)
Pts w/Clinical Pregnancy (%)	25(38.5)	30(50.0)
Pts w/Continuing Pregnancy (%)	24(36.9) [1]	29(48.3) [2]
Pts. w/Live Births (%)	22(33.8) [3]	25(41.7) [4]

1. Continuing pregnancies included 14 single, 7 twins, and 3 triplet pregnancies.
2. Continuing pregnancies included 14 single, 9 twins, 3 triplets, and 3 quadruplet pregnancies.
3. Total of 34 live births. One spontaneous abortion. The follow-up data is not available for one patient.
4. Total of 39 live births. Two spontaneous abortions. The follow-up data is not available for two patients.

Table 3. Efficacy Outcomes by Treatment Groups in Ovulation Induction (one cycle of treatment)

Parameter	Repronex® IM	Repronex® SC
	N=36	N=36
Ovulation (%)	23 (63.9)	25 (69.4)
Received (hCG) %	25 (69.4)	27 (75.0)
Mean Peak Serum E2 (SD)	1158.5 (742.3)	1452.6* (1270.6)
Chemical Pregnancy (%)	4 (11.1)	11 (30.6)
Clinical Pregnancy (%)	4 (11.1)	6 (16.7)
Continuing Pregnancy (%)	4 (11.1) [1]	6 (16.7) [2]
Pts. w/Live Births (%)	4(11.1) [3]	4(11.1) [4]

* Fisher's Exact/Chi-Squared Tests—significant for Repronex® SC vs. Repronex® IM
1. Continuing pregnancies included 2 single and 2 triplet pregnancies.
2. Continuing pregnancies included 3 single, 1 twin and 2 quadruplet pregnancies.
3. Total of 6 live births.
4. Total of 6 live births. One spontaneous abortion. The follow-up data is not available for one patient.

Resolution Phase: A fall in hematocrit and an increasing urinary output without an increased intake are observed due to the return of third space fluid to the intravascular compartment. Peripheral and/or pulmonary edema may result if the kidneys are unable to excrete third space fluid as rapidly as it is mobilized. Diuretics may be indicated during the resolution phase if necessary to combat pulmonary edema.

Pulmonary and Vascular Complications

Serious pulmonary conditions (e.g., atelectasis, acute respiratory distress syndrome) have been reported. In addition, thromboembolic events both in association with, and separate from, the Ovarian Hyperstimulation Syndrome have been reported following menotropins therapy. Intravascular thrombosis and embolism, which may originate in venous or arterial vessels, can result in reduced blood flow to critical organs or the extremities. Sequelae of such events have included venous thrombophlebitis, pulmonary embolism, pulmonary infarction, cerebral vascular occlusion (stroke), and arterial occlusion resulting in loss of limb. In rare cases, pulmonary complications and/or thromboembolic events have resulted in death.

Multiple Pregnancies

Multiple pregnancies have occurred following treatment with Repronex® IM and SC. In a clinical trial for ovulation induction in which Repronex® IM and Repronex® SC were directly compared, the rates of multiple pregnancies were as follows. Of the four clinical pregnancies with Repronex® IM, two were single and two were multiple pregnancies. Both multiple pregnancies were triplet pregnancies. Of the six clinical pregnancies with Repronex® SC, three were single and three were multiple pregnancies. The three multiple pregnancies included one twin pregnancy and two quadruplet pregnancies.

In a clinical trial of IVF patients in which Repronex® IM and Repronex® SC were directly compared, the rates of multiple pregnancies were as follows. Of the 24 continuing pregnancies on Repronex® IM, 14 were single and 10 were multiple pregnancies. The ten multiple pregnancies included three triplet and seven twin pregnancies. Of the 29 continuing pregnancies on Repronex® SC, 14 were single and 15 were multiple pregnancies. The 15 multiple pregnancies included three quadruplet, three triplet and nine twin pregnancies. The patient and her partner should be advised of the potential risk of multiple births before starting treatment.

Hypersensitivity/Anaphylactic Reactions

Hypersensitivity/anaphylactic reactions associated with menotropins administration have been reported in some patients. These reactions presented as generalized urticaria, facial edema, angioneurotic edema, and/or dyspnea suggestive of laryngeal edema. The relationship of these symptoms to uncharacterized urinary proteins is uncertain.

PRECAUTIONS

General

Careful attention should be given to diagnosis in the selection of candidates for menotropins therapy (see "**INDICATIONS AND USAGE —Selection of Patients**").

Information for Patients

Prior to therapy with Repronex®, patients should be informed of the duration of treatment and the monitoring of their condition that will be required. Possible adverse reactions (see **ADVERSE REACTIONS** section) and the risk of multiple births should also be discussed.

Laboratory Tests

Treatment for Induction of ovulation

The combination of both estradiol levels and ultrasonography are useful for monitoring the growth and development of follicles, timing hCG administration, as well as minimizing the risk of the Ovarian Hyperstimulation Syndrome and multiple gestation.

The clinical confirmation of ovulation, is determined by:

a) A rise in basal body temperature;

b) Increase in serum progesterone; and

Table 4. Patients with Adverse Events ≥ 1%

	Repronex® IM (N=101)	Repronex® SC (N=96)
Adverse Events	n (%)	n (%)
INJECTION SITE AEs		
Injection Site Edema	1 (1.0)	8 (8.3)*
Injection Site Reaction	2 (2.0)	8 (8.3)*
GENITOURINARY/REPRODUCTIVE AEs		
OHSS	2 (2.0)	5 (5.2)
Vaginal Hemorrhage	8 (7.9)	3 (3.1)
Ovarian Disease	3 (3.0)	8 (8.3)
Ectopic Pregnancy	1 (1.0)	1 (1.0)
Pelvic Pain	3 (3.0)	1 (1.0)
Breast Tenderness	2 (2.0)	2 (2.1)
GASTROINTESTINAL AEs		
Nausea	4 (4.0)	7(7.3)
Vomiting	0 (0)	3 (3.1)
Diarrhea	0 (0)	2(2.1)
Abdominal Cramping	7(6.9)	5(5.2)
Abdominal Pain	5(5.0)	7(7.3)
Enlarged Abdomen	6(6.0)	2 (2.1)
OTHER BODY SYSTEM AEs		
Headache	6 (6.0)	5 (5.2)
Infection	1(1.0)	0 (0)
Dyspnea	1(1.0)	2(2.1)

* Fisher's Exact/Chi-Squared Tests—significant for Repronex® SC vs. Repronex® IM.

c) Menstruation following the shift in basal body temperature.

When used in conjunction with indices of progesterone production, sonographic visualization of the ovaries will assist in determining if ovulation has occurred. Sonographic evidence of ovulation may include the following:

a) Fluid in the cul-de-sac;
b) Ovarian stigmata; and
c) Collapsed follicle.

Because of the subjectivity of the various tests for the determination of follicular maturation and ovulation, it cannot be overemphasized that the physician should choose tests with which he/she is thoroughly familiar.

Carcinogenesis and Mutagenesis

Long-term toxicity studies in animals have not been performed to evaluate the carcinogenic potential of menotropins.

Pregnancy

Pregnancy Category X: See **CONTRAINDICATIONS** section.

Nursing Mothers

It is not known whether this drug is excreted in human milk. Because many drugs are excreted in human milk, caution should be exercised if menotropins are administered to a nursing woman.

Pediatric Patients

Safety and effectiveness in pediatric patients have not been established.

Geriatric Patients

Safety and effectiveness in geriatric patients have not been established.

ADVERSE REACTIONS

The following adverse reactions, reported during menotropins therapy, are listed in decreasing order of potential severity:

1. Pulmonary and vascular complications (see **WARNINGS**)
2. Ovarian Hyperstimulation Syndrome (see **WARNINGS**)
3. Hemoperitoneum
4. Adnexal torsion (as a complication of ovarian enlargement)
5. Mild to moderate ovarian enlargement
6. Ovarian cysts
7. Abdominal pain
8. Sensitivity to menotropins (Febrile reactions suggestive of allergic response have been reported following the administration of menotropins. Reports of flu-like symptoms including fever, chills, musculoskeletal aches, joint pains, nausea, headaches, and malaise have also been reported).
9. Gastrointestinal symptoms (nausea, vomiting, diarrhea, abdominal cramps, bloating)
10. Pain, rash, swelling and/or irritation at the site of injection
11. Body rashes
12. Dizziness, tachycardia, dyspnea, tachypnea

The following medical events have been reported subsequent to pregnancies resulting from menotropins therapy:

1. Ectopic pregnancy
2. Congenital abnormalities

With menotropin therapy congenital abnormalities have been reported. One infant was shown to have multiple congenital anomalies consisting of aplasia of the sigmoid colon, cecovesicle fistula, bifid scrotum, meningocele, bilateral internal tibial torsion, and right metatarsus adductus. Other reported anomalies include imperforate anus, congenital heart lesions, supernumerary digits, hypospadias, extrophy of the bladder, Down's syndrome and hydrocephalus. The incidence of congenital abnormalities does not exceed that found in the general population.

There have been infrequent reports of ovarian neoplasms, both benign and malignant, in women who have undergone multiple drug regimens for ovulation induction; however, a causal relationship has not been established.

Adverse events occurring in ≥1% of patients exposed to Repronex® IM or Repronex® SC are described in Table 4. [See table 4 above]

DRUG ABUSE AND DEPENDENCE

There have been no reports of abuse or dependence with menotropins.

OVERDOSAGE

Aside from possible ovarian hyperstimulation (see **WARNINGS**), little is known concerning the consequences of acute overdosage with menotropins.

DOSAGE AND ADMINISTRATION

1. Dosage:

Infertile patients with oligo-anovulation:

The dose of Repronex® to stimulate development of ovarian follicles must be individualized for each patient. The lowest dose consistent with achieving good results based on clinical experience and reported clinical data should be used.

The recommended initial dose of Repronex® for patients who have received GnRH agonist or antagonist pituitary suppression is 150 IU daily for the first 5 days of treatment. Based on clinical monitoring (including serum estradiol levels and vaginal ultrasound results) subsequent dosing should be adjusted according to individual patient response. Adjustments in dose should not be made more frequently than once every 2 days and should not exceed more than 75 to 150 IU per adjustment. The maximum daily dose of Repronex® should not exceed 450 IU and dosing beyond 12 days is not recommended.

If patient response to Repronex® is appropriate, hCG (5000 to 10,000 USP units) should be given 1 day following the last dose of Repronex®. The hCG should be withheld if the serum estradiol is greater than 2000 pg/mL, if the ovaries are abnormally enlarged or if abdominal pain occurs, and the patient should be advised to refrain from intercourse. These precautions may reduce the risk of Ovarian Hyperstimulation Syndrome and multiple gestation. Patients should be followed closely for at least 2 weeks after hCG administration. If there is inadequate follicle development or ovulation without subsequent pregnancy, the course of treatment with Repronex® may be repeated. The couple should be encouraged to have intercourse daily, beginning on the day prior to the administration of hCG until ovulation becomes apparent from the indices employed for the determination of progestational activity. In the light of the foregoing indices and parameters mentioned, it should become obvious that, unless a physician is willing to devote considerable time to these patients and be familiar with and conduct the necessary laboratory studies, he/she should not use Repronex®.

Assisted Reproductive Technologies:

The recommended initial dose of Repronex® for patients who have received GnRH agonist or antagonist pituitary suppression is 225 IU. Based on clinical monitoring (including serum estradiol levels and vaginal ultrasound results) subsequent dosing should be adjusted according to individual patient response. Adjustments in dose should not be made more frequently than once every 2 days and should not exceed more than 75 to 150 IU per adjustment. The maximum daily dose of Repronex® given should not exceed 450 IU and dosing beyond 12 days is not recommended.

Once adequate follicular development is evident, hCG (5000 – 10,000 USP units) should be administered to induce final follicular maturation in preparation for oocyte retrieval. The administration of hCG must be withheld in cases where the ovaries are abnormally enlarged on the last day of therapy. This should reduce the chance of developing OHSS.

2. Administration:

Dissolve the contents of one to 6 vials of Repronex® in one to two mL of sterile saline and **ADMINISTER SUBCUTANEOUSLY OR INTRAMUSCULARLY** immediately. Any unused reconstituted material should be discarded.

Parenteral drug products should be inspected visually for particulate matter and discoloration prior to administration, whenever solution and container permit.

The lower abdomen (alternating sides) should be used for subcutaneous administration.

HOW SUPPLIED

Repronex® (menotropins for injection, USP) is available in vials as a sterile, lyophilized, white to off-white powder or pellet.

Each vial is available with an accompanying vial of sterile diluent containing 2 mL of 0.9% Sodium Chloride Injection, USP:

75 IU FSH and 75 IU of LH activity, supplied as:
NDC 55566-7185-1—Box of 1 vial + 1 vial diluent.
NDC 55566-7185-2—Box of 5 vials + 5 vials diluent.
150 IU FSH and 150 IU of LH activity, supplied as:
NDC 55566-7125-1—Box of 1 vial + 1 vial diluent.

By biological assay, one IU of LH for the Second International Reference Preparation (2nd-IRP) for hMG is biologically equivalent to approximately 0.5 U of hCG.

Lyophilized powder may be stored refrigerated or at room temperature (3° to 25°C/37° to 77°F). Protect from light. Use immediately after reconstitution. Discard unused material.

℞ only

Vials of sterile diluent of 0.9% Sodium Chloride Injection, USP manufactured for Ferring Pharmaceuticals Inc.

Manufactured for:
FERRING PHARMACEUTICALS INC.
TARRYTOWN, NY 10591
By: LEDERLE PARENTERALS, INC.
Carolina, Puerto Rico 00987
CI 6098-1
6039-01
8/99

THYREL® TRH ℞
(protirelin)
Injection
FOR INTRAVENOUS ADMINISTRATION

HOW SUPPLIED

As 1 mL ampuls—boxes of 5 (NDC 55566-0081-5). Each mL contains Thyrel TRH 0.50 mg (500 µg), sodium chloride 9.0 mg for isotonicity, hydrochloric acid and sodium hydroxide as needed to adjust pH.

Store at controlled room temperature 15° to 30°C (59° to 86°F).

Please see full prescribing information in the Diagnostic Product Information section.

For EMERGENCY telephone numbers, consult the **Manufacturers' Index**.

Fielding Pharmaceutical Company

11551 ADIE ROAD
MARYLAND HEIGHTS, MO 63043

Direct Inquires to:
Professional Services Department
(314) 567-5462
For Medical Information Contact:
In Emergencies:
(314) 567-5462

GYNODIOL™ ℞
(estradiol tablets, USP)
Rx only

DESCRIPTION

Gynodiol™ (estradiol tablets, USP) is a white, crystalline solid, chemically described as estra-1,3,5(10)-triene-3,17β-diol. It has a molecular formula of $C_{18}H_{24}O_2$ and molecular weight of 272.39. The structural formula is:

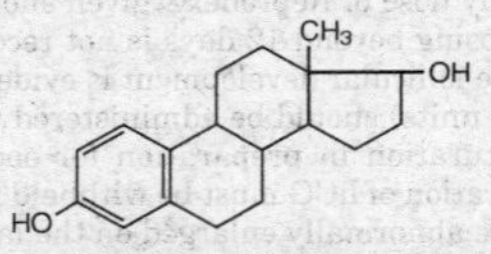

Gynodiol™ (estradiol tablets, USP) for oral administration, contain: 0.5 mg, 1 mg, 1.5 mg, or 2 mg of micronized estradiol per tablet.

Gynodiol™ (estradiol tablets, USP) 0.5 mg contain the following inactive ingredients: lactose monohydrate, croscarmellose sodium, carboxymethylcellulose sodium, pregelatinized starch, magnesium stearate, polysorbate 80, FD&C Blue No. 1 Aluminum Lake, D&C Red No. 27 Aluminum Lake.

Gynodiol™ (estradiol tablets, USP) 1 mg contain the following inactive ingredients: lactose monohydrate, croscarmellose sodium, carboxymethylcellulose sodium, pregelatinized starch, magnesium stearate, polysorbate 80, D&C Red No. 27 Aluminum Lake.

Gynodiol™ (estradiol tablets, USP) 1.5 mg contain the following inactive ingredients: lactose monohydrate, croscarmellose sodium, carboxymethylcellulose sodium, pregelatinized starch, magnesium stearate, polysorbate 80, FD&C Blue No. 1 Aluminum Lake, D&C Yellow No. 10 Aluminum Lake.

Gynodiol™ (estradiol tablets, USP) 2 mg contain the following inactive ingredients: lactose monohydrate, croscarmellose sodium, carboxymethylcellulose sodium, pregelatinized starch, magnesium stearate, FD&C Blue No. 2 Aluminum Lake, polysorbate 80.

HOW SUPPLIED

Gynodiol™ (estradiol tablets, USP) 0.5 mg; round, lavender colored tablet with bisect, debossed with ◇ and 0768. Available in containers of 30 (NDC 0421-0768-00), and 100 (NDC 0421-0768-01).

Gynodiol™ (estradiol tablets, USP) 1 mg; round, rose colored tablet with bisect, debossed with ◇ and 1259: Available in containers of 30 (NDC 0421-1259-00), and 100 (NDC 0421-1259-01).

Gynodiol™ (estradiol tablets, USP) 1.5 mg; round, aqua colored tablet with bisect, debossed with ◇ and 0158: Available in containers of 30 (NDC 0421-0158-00), and 100 (NDC 0421-0158-01).

Gynodiol™ (estradiol tablets, USP) 2 mg; round, blue colored tablet with bisect, debossed with ◇ and 0748: Available in containers of 30 (NDC 0421-0748-00), and 100 (NDC 0421-0748-01).

Store at controlled room temperature 15°–30°C (59°–86°F).

NESTABS® CBF ℞
Prenatal Multi-vitamin/Mineral Tablets

DESCRIPTION

Nestabs® CBF is a white film-coated tablet with "CBF" debossed on one side and scored on the opposite side.
Each tablet contains:

Vitamin A (beta carotene)	4,000 IU
Vitamin D (D_3)	400 IU
Vitamin E (dl-alpha-tocopheryl acetate)	30 IU
Vitamin C (ascorbic acid)	120 mg
Folic Acid	1 mg
Vitamin B_1 (thiamine mononitrate)	3 mg
Vitamin B_2 (riboflavin)	3 mg
Niacin (niacinamide)	20 mg
Vitamin B_6 (pyridoxine hcl)	3 mg
Vitamin B_{12} (cyanocobalamin)	8 mcg
Calcium (calcium carbonate)	200 mg
Iodine (potassium iodide)	150 mcg
Zinc (zinc oxide)	15 mg
Iron (carbonyl iron)	50 mg

INDICATIONS AND USAGE

Nestabs® CBF is indicated for use in improving the nutritional status of women throughout pregnancy and in the postnatal period for both lactating and nonlactating mothers. Nestabs® CBF is also beneficial in improving the nutritional status of women prior to conception.

CONTRAINDICATIONS

This product is contraindicated in patients with a known hypersensitivity to any of the ingredients.

WARNINGS

Folic acid alone is improper therapy in the treatment of pernicious anemia and other megaloblasitc anemias where vitamin B_{12} is deficient.

> WARNING: Accidental overdose of iron-containing products is a leading cause of fatal poisoning in children under 6. Keep this product out of reach of children. In case of accidental overdose, call a doctor or poison control center immediately.

PRECAUTIONS

Folic acid in doses above 0.1 mg daily may obscure pernicious anemia in that hematologic remission can occur while neurological manifestations remain progressive.

ADVERSE REACTIONS

Allergic sensitization has been reported following both oral and parenteral administration of folic acid.

DOSAGE AND ADMINISTRATION

One tablet daily or as directed by a physician.

HOW SUPPLIED

Nestabs® CBF tablets for oral administration are supplied as white elliptical film-coated tablets with "CBF" debossed on one side and scored on the opposite side in child-resistant packages of 90 tablets (9 cards of 2 × 5 blisters). NDC 0421-2001-01.

Store at controlled room temperature 15°–30° (59°–86°F)
RX only

NESTABS® RX ℞
Prenatal Multi-vitamin/Mineral Tablets

DESCRIPTION

Nestabs® RX is a light blue film-coated tablet with "NRX" debossed on one side and score on the opposite side.
Each tablet contains:

Vitamin A (beta carotene)	4,000 IU
Vitamin D (D_3)	400 IU
Vitamin E (dl-alpha tocopheryl acetate)	30 IU
Vitamin C (ascorbic acid)	120 mg
Folic Acid	1 mg
Vitamin B_1 (thiamine mononitrate)	3 mg
Vitamin B_2 (riboflavin)	3 mg
Niacin (niacinamide)	20 mg
Vitamin B_6 (pyridoxine hcl)	3 mg
Vitamin B_{12} (cyanocobalamin)	8 mcg
Biotin	30 mcg
Pantothenic Acid	7 mg
Calcium (calcium carbonate)	200 mg
Iodine (potassium iodide)	150 mcg
Zinc (zinc oxide)	15 mg
Magnesium	100 mg
Iron (carbonyl iron)	29 mg
Copper	3 mg

INDICATIONS AND USAGE

Nestabs® RX is indicated for use in improving the nutritional status of women throughout pregnancy and in the postnatal period for both lactating and nonlactating mothers. Nestabs® RX is also beneficial in improving the nutritional status of women prior to conception.

CONTRAINDICATIONS

This product is contraindicated in patients with a known hypersensitivity to any of the ingredients.

WARNINGS

Folic acid alone is improper therapy in the treatment of pernicious anemia and other megaloblastic anemias where vitamin B_{12} is deficient.

> WARNING: Accidental overdose of iron-containing products is a leading cause of fatal poisoning in children under 6. Keep this product out of reach of children. In case of accidental overdose, call a doctor or poison control center immediately.

PRECAUTIONS

Folic acid in doses above 0.1mg daily may obscure pernicious anemia in that hematologic remission can occur while neurological manifestations remain progressive.

ADVERSE REACTIONS

Allergic sensitization has been reported following both oral and parenteral administration of folic acid.

DOSAGE AND ADMINISTRATION

One tablet daily or as directed by a physician.

HOW SUPPLIED

Nestabs® RX tablets for oral administration are supplied as light blue elliptical film-coated tablets with "NRX" debossed on one side and scored on the opposite side in bottles of 90's (NDC 0421-1317-01).

Store at controlled room temperature 15°–30°C (59°–86°F)
RX only

First Horizon Pharmaceutical Corporation

660 HEMBREE PARKWAY
SUITE 106
ROSWELL, GA 30076

Direct Inquiries to:
Alan Roberts
(770) 442-9707
FAX: (770) 442-9594
Medical Emergency Contact:
800-849-9707
FAX: (770) 442-9594

COGNEX® ℞
(Tacrine Hydrochloride Capsules)

DESCRIPTION

Cognex® (tacrine hydrochloride) is a reversible cholinesterase inhibitor, known chemically as 1,2,3,4-tetrahydro-9-acridinamine monohydrochloride monohydrate. Tacrine hydrochloride is commonly referred to in the clinical and pharmacological literature as THA. It has an empirical formula of $C_{13}H_{14}N_2 \cdot HCl \cdot H_2O$ and a molecular weight of 252.74.

Tacrine hydrochloride is a white solid and is freely soluble in distilled water, 0.1N hydrochloric acid, acetate buffer (pH 4.0), phosphate buffer (pH 7.0 to 7.4), methanol, dimethylsulfoxide (DMSO), ethanol, and propylene glycol. The compound is sparingly soluble in linoleic acid and PEG 400.

Each capsule of Cognex® contains tacrine as the hydrochloride. Inactive ingredients are hydrous lactose, magnesium stearate, and microcrystalline cellulose. The hard gelatin capsules contain gelatin, NF; silicon dioxide, NF; sodium lauryl sulfate, NF; and the following dyes: 10 mg: D&C Yellow #10, FD&C Green #3, titanium dioxide; 20 mg: D&C Yellow #10, FD&C Blue #1, titanium dioxide; 30 mg: D&C Yellow #10, FD&C Blue #1, FD&C Red #40, titanium dioxide; 40 mg: D&C Yellow #10, FD&C Blue #1, FD&C Red #40, D&C Red #28, titanium dioxide.

Each 10-, 20-, 30-, and 40-mg Cognex® capsule for oral administration contains 12.75, 25.50, 38.25, and 51.00 mg of tacrine HCl, respectively.

CLINICAL PHARMACOLOGY

Although widespread degeneration of multiple CNS neuronal systems eventually occurs, early pathological changes in Alzheimer's Disease involve, in a relatively selective manner, cholinergic neuronal pathways that project from the basal forebrain to the cerebral cortex and hippocampus. The resulting deficiency of cortical acetylcholine is believed to account for some of the clinical manifestations of mild to moderate dementia. Tacrine, an orally bioavailable, centrally active, reversible cholinesterase inhibitor, presumably acts by elevating acetylcholine concentrations in the cerebral cortex by slowing the degradation of acetylcholine released by still intact cholinergic neurons. If this theoretical mechanism of action is correct, tacrine's effects may lessen as the disease process advances and fewer cholinergic neurons remain functionally intact. There is no evidence that tacrine alters the course of the underlying dementing process.

Clinical Trial Data

The conclusion that Cognex® is an effective treatment for Alzheimer's Disease derives from two adequate and well controlled clinical investigations that evaluated tacrine's effects in patients with probable Alzheimer's disease of mild to moderate severity (NINCDS criteria, Mini-Mental State Examination (MMSE) of Folstein, Folstein and McHugh scores of 10 to 26).

In each study, outcomes during treatment with tacrine and placebo were assessed on two primary measures: (1) the cognitive subscale of the Alzheimer's Disease Assessment Scale (ADAS cog) of Rosen, Mohs, and Davis and (2) a clinician's rated clinical global impression of change.

Study Endpoints

The ADAS cog is a multi-item test battery administered by a psychometrician that examines aspects of memory, attention, praxis, reason, and language. The worst possible score is 70. Elderly, normal adults may score as low as 0 or 1 unit, but individuals judged not to be demented can score higher. The mean score of patients entering each study was approximately 28 units (range 7 to 62). The ADAS cog score is reported to deteriorate at a rate of about 6 to 10 units per year for untreated patients at this stage of dementia.

The clinician's global assessments used in the two studies relied on a clinician's judgment about the overall clinical change observed in patients over the course of the study. Although the conditions for obtaining the clinical assessment differed in each study, the global assessment was rated on a

7-point scale in both studies. A rating of four (4) represents no change; lower ratings indicate improvement from baseline and higher ratings deterioration.

Twelve-Week Study

In one study of 12 weeks duration, patients were randomized to sequences that provided a comparison between placebo, 20, 40, and 80 mg/day by study's end. Statistically significant drug-placebo differences were detected on both primary outcome measures for the group titrated to 80 mg/day. Estimates of the size of the treatment effect varied between 2 and 4 ADAS cog units. The imprecision in these estimates reflects the fact that different analyses, conducted in attempts to account for the effects of the failure of a substantial fraction of the patients randomized to complete the full 12 weeks of the study, yielded different results.

The placebo-80 mg/day comparison also achieved statistical significance on the clinician's global impression of change (CGIC) with a 0.3 to 0.4 unit mean difference. The following diagram illustrates the percentages of patients falling into each global category at trial's end for the patients given placebo or 80 mg/day.

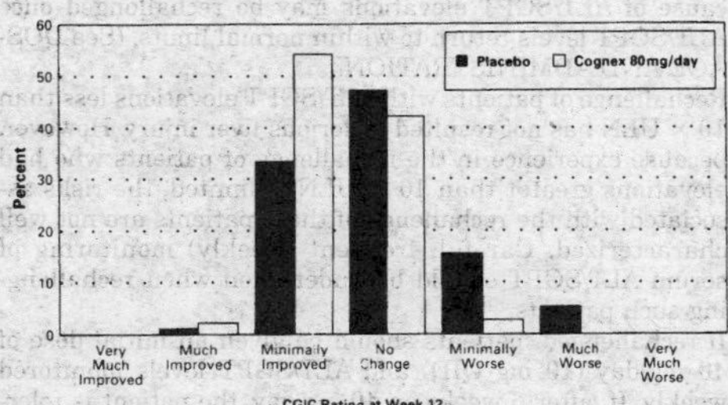

FIGURE 1 Percent of Patients in Each of the Seven Outcome Categories on the Clinician-Rated CGIC for Patients Completing 12 Weeks of Treatment (83% of patients randomized to placebo completed 12 weeks of treatment and are represented above; 56% of those randomized to the 80 mg/day Cognex® sequence completed 12 weeks).

Thirty-Week Study

The second study was 30 weeks long. Six hundred sixty-three patients were randomized to 4 treatment sequences (placebo and 3 drug groups) that called for the daily dose of tacrine to be increased at 6-week intervals, starting with a 40-mg/day dose. By study's end, a comparison between placebo, 80, 120, and 160 mg/day was possible. Patients in the 160 mg group received this dose for the final 12 weeks; the 120 mg group received that dose for 18 weeks.

The study showed statistically significant drug-placebo differences for the 80 and 120 mg/day groups at 18 weeks and for the 120 and 160 mg/day groups at 30 weeks on both a performance-based test of cognitive function (the ADAS cog) and a clinician's assessment of global change (Clinician Interview Based Impression: CIBI). Because many patients failed to complete 30 weeks on treatment, analyses that used each patient's last on-study value or retrieved patients' (see below) 30-week value, even if they were no longer in the study ("intent-to-treat" analysis) were also carried out. All analyses confirmed the effectiveness of tacrine, although the estimated mean treatment effect was different in each analysis.

Effects on ADAS Cog: The results for the ADAS cog are shown in Figure 2 for the subset of patients actually completing the full 30 weeks of the study. They show that individual patients, whether assigned to tacrine or to placebo, had a wide range of responses. This variability in response is illustrated in the display that follows (Figure 2).

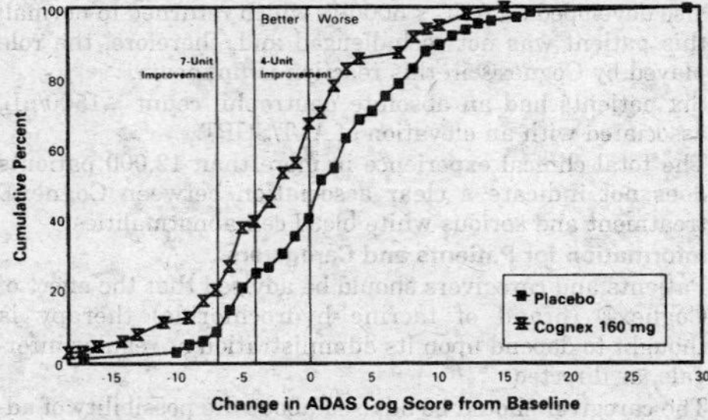

FIGURE 2 Cumulative Percent of Patients Completing 30 Weeks of Treatment Who Attained a Change in ADAS Cog Score From Baseline at Least as Large as the Value on the X Axis. The display is based on scores obtained from a subset of patients (ie, 64% of the 184 randomized to placebo and 27% of the 239 randomized to the 160 mg/day treament group).

Figure 2 presents the cumulative percentage (Y axis) of patients assigned to placebo or 160 mg/day who actually completed 30 weeks on treatment and who attained a change in ADAS cog score from baseline at least as large as the ADAS cog change score value given on the X axis. A negative change from baseline represents improvement; a positive change deterioration. Thus, in a display of this type, the curve for an effective treatment is shifted to the left of the curve for placebo. The frequency in each group of any response, e.g., an improvement of 7 ADAS cog units, can be found by plotting the change on the X axis, then reading upward along the Y axis. The variability of response is apparent from the fact that the distribution of responses under both treatment conditions range from large negative to large positive values. Nonetheless, the mean drug-placebo ADAS cog difference for the 30-week 160 mg/day completer patients is 4.8 units, a statistically significant difference.

Table 1. Proportion of Patients Attaining ≥7 Unit Improvement on the ADAS Cog at the Week 30 Assessment

Treatment Group N Randomized	I N (%) of Those Randomized	II N (%) of Those Completing Week 30	III N (%) of Those With Week 30 Assessments
Placebo (N = 184)	10/184(5.4)	10/117(8.5)	11/143[1](7.7)
160 mg/day (N = 239)	13/239(5.4)	13/64 (20.3)	25/172[2](14.5)

[1]: 13 of the 143 were receiving tacrine when evaluated.
[2]: 41 of the 172 were not receiving tacrine when evaluated.

Effects on CIBI: The results on the CIBI are shown in Figure 3.

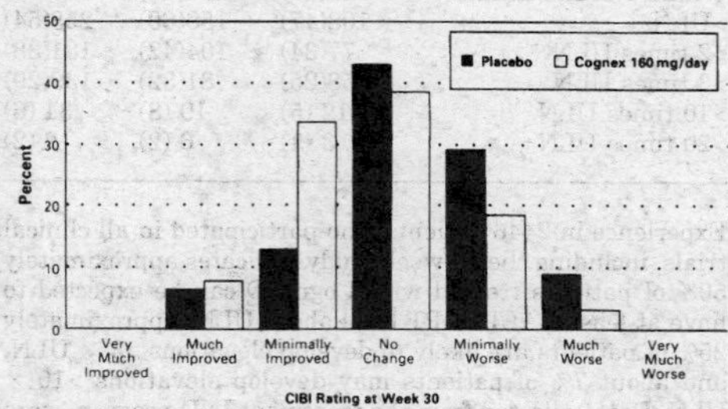

FIGURE 3 Percent of Patients in Each of the Seven Outcome Categories of the CIBI Among Those Completing 30 Weeks. The display is based on scores obtained from the same subset of patients as Figure 2.

Figure 3 is a histogram of the frequency distribution of CIBI scores attained by patients assigned to placebo or to the 160 mg/day tacrine dose group who actually completed the full 30 weeks of the study. The mean tacrine-placebo difference for this group of patients on the CIBI was 0.5 units and was statistically significant.

Expected Responses in Newly Treated Patients: Although the results described clearly document tacrine's effectiveness, they are based on only a fraction of the patients initially randomized to tacrine, those who could tolerate tacrine and remain on treatment uninterrupted for the full 30 weeks. In considering the expected outcome in a group of patients newly started on tacrine, account must be taken both of the likelihood of staying on therapy and the responses in patients who do so.

Table 1 provides 3 different estimates of the proportion of patients assigned to treatment with tacrine at 160 mg a day or with placebo who attained a particular measure of improvement (i.e., a 7 point improvement from baseline in ADAS cog score). The criterion has been chosen entirely for illustrative purposes.

[See table 1 above]

The first column of the table is based on all patients participating in the study. The proportion provides an estimate of the likelihood that a patient entering the study will (1) still be on his or her assigned treatment at week 30 **and** (2) will improve 7 or more ADAS cognitive points over his or her baseline score. The estimate of response derived in this manner is conservative because the rules under which the 30-week study was conducted required the withdrawal of patients with relatively low (>3 × ULN), asymptomatic, transaminase elevations. In actual clinical practice under the conditions of treatment recommended in the Dosage and Administration Section, a larger fraction of these patients would be able to remain on tacrine and the proportion of those improving 7 or more points on tacrine would be expected, therefore, to be increased (the third column illustrates this).

The second column of the table presents the proportion of 7 unit responders based on the number of patients who (1) were able to complete the full 30 weeks of the study and (2) attained an ADAS cognitive score at week 30 that was 7 or more points better than their baseline score. This analysis provides an optimistic estimate of tacrine's effects because it reflects experience gained only with the minority of patients who were able to remain on treatment to the study's end. The comparison between the proportions of placebo and 160 mg patients attaining a 7 or more point improvement is complicated further by the fact that a larger proportion of tacrine assigned patients withdrew prematurely.

The third column of the table presents the proportion of patients who had evaluations made at 30 weeks and had a 7-point or greater response. The analysis includes data from patients still on their assigned treatment at week 30 as well as patients who withdrew from the study prior to that time, but were retrieved for a week 30 evaluation. Because patients who withdrew prior to week 30 were permitted to receive tacrine under "open label" conditions, retrieved patients included in this analysis could be receiving either no treatment or treatment with tacrine. In this analysis, patients are considered under the treatment to which they were randomized, regardless of the treatment they were actually receiving at week 30. Thus, some placebo patients could have received tacrine and some tacrine patients could have been receiving no tacrine. Like the analysis based on percent randomized (column I), this analysis, therefore, tends to provide a conservative view of the expected effects of tacrine treatment.

Effects of Cognex® Over Time: Figure 4 shows for each dose group the time course of change from baseline in ADAS cog scores for patients completing 30 weeks of treatment. There appears to be a persistent difference between groups, but all groups, after initial improvement, deteriorate with time.

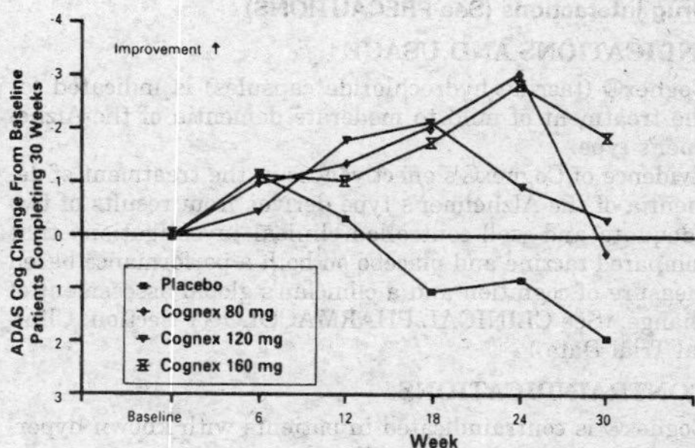

FIGURE 4 ADAS Cog Change From Baseline Over Time for the Subset of Patients Completing 30 Weeks of Treatment. In all tacrine treatment groups dosing was initiated at 40 mg/day and increased in increments of 40 mg every 6 weeks until the target dose was achieved.

Patient age, gender, and other baseline patient characteristics were not found to predict clinical outcome.

Clinical Pharmacokinetics (Absorption, Distribution, Metabolism, and Elimination)

Absorption: Cognex® is rapidly absorbed after oral administration; maximal plasma concentrations occur within 1 to 2 hours. The rate and extent of tacrine absorption following administration of tacrine capsules and solution are virtually indistinguishable. Absolute bioavailability of tacrine is approximately 17 (SD ± 13) %. Food reduces tacrine bioavailability by approximately 30–40%; however, there is no food effect if tacrine is administered at least an hour before meals. The effect of achlorhydria on the absorption of tacrine is unknown.

Distribution: Mean volume of distribution of tacrine is approximately 349 (SD ± 193) L. Tacrine is about 55% bound to plasma proteins. The extent and degree of tacrine's distribution within various body compartments has not been systematically studied. However, 336 hours after the administration of a single radiolabeled dose, approximately 25% of the radiolabel was not recovered in a mass balance study, suggesting the possibility that tacrine and/or one or more of its metabolites may be retained.

Metabolism: Tacrine is extensively metabolized by the cytochrome P450 system to multiple metabolites, not all of which have been identified. The vast majority of radiolabeled species present in the plasma following a single dose of ^{14}C radiolabeled tacrine are unidentified (ie, only 5% of radioactivity in plasma has been identified [tacrine and 3-hydroxylated metabolites; 1-, 2-, and 4-hydroxytacrine]). Studies utilizing human liver preparations demonstrated that cytochrome P450 IA2 is the principal isozyme involved in tacrine metabolism. These findings are consistent with the observation that tacrine and/or one of its metabolites inhibits the metabolism of theophylline in humans (see PRECAUTIONS: Drug-Drug Interactions: theophylline). Results from a study utilizing quinidine to inhibit cytochrome P450 IID6 indicate that tacrine is not metabolized extensively by this enzyme system.

Following aromatic ring hydroxylation, tacrine's metabolites undergo glucuronidation. Whether tacrine and/or its metabolites undergo biliary excretion or entero-hepatic circulation is unknown.

Special Populations: *Age:* Based on pooled pharmacokinetic studies (n = 192), there is no clinically relevant influence of age (50 to 84 years) on tacrine clearance. *Gender:* Average tacrine plasma concentrations are approximately 50% higher in females than in males. This is not explained by differences in body surface area or elimination half-life. The difference is probably due to higher systemic availability after oral dosing and may reflect the known lower activity of cytochrome P450 IA2 in women. *Race:* The effect of race on tacrine clearance has not been studied. *Smoking:* Mean plasma tacrine concentrations in current smokers are approximately one third the concentrations in nonsmokers. Cigarette smoking is known to induce cytochrome P450 IA2. *Renal disease:* Renal disease does not appear to affect the clearance of tacrine. *Liver disease:* Although studies in patients with liver disease have not been done, it is likely that functional hepatic impairment will reduce the clearance of tacrine and its metabolites.

Presystemic Clearance/Elimination/Excretion: Tacrine undergoes presystemic clearance (ie, first pass metabolism). The extent of this first pass metabolism depends upon the dose of tacrine administered. Because the enzyme system

Continued on next page

Cognex—Cont.

involved can be saturated at relatively low doses, a larger fraction of a high dose of tacrine will escape first pass elimination than of a smaller dose. Thus, when a 40 mg daily dose is increased by 40 mg, the average plasma concentration will be increased by approximately 6 ng/mL. However, when a daily dose of 80 or 120 mg is increased by 40 mg, the increment in average plasma concentration is approximately 10 ng/mL.
Elimination of tacrine from the plasma, however, is not dose dependent (ie, the half-life is independent of dose or plasma concentration). The elimination half-life is approximately 2 to 4 hours. Following initiation of therapy or a change in daily dose, steady state tacrine plasma concentration should be attained within 24 to 36 hours.

Drug Interactions (See PRECAUTIONS)

INDICATIONS AND USAGE

Cognex® (tacrine hydrochloride capsules) is indicated for the treatment of mild to moderate dementia of the Alzheimer's type.
Evidence of Cognex®'s effectiveness in the treatment of dementia of the Alzheimer's type derives from results of two adequate and well-controlled clinical investigations that compared tacrine and placebo on both a performance based measure of cognition and a clinician's global assessment of change. (See CLINICAL PHARMACOLOGY Section: Clinical Trial Data.)

CONTRAINDICATIONS

Cognex® is contraindicated in patients with known hypersensitivity to tacrine or acridine derivatives.
Cognex® is contraindicated in patients previously treated with Cognex® who developed treatment-associated jaundice: a serum bilirubin >3 mg/dL; and/or those exhibiting clinical signs or symptoms of hypersensitivity (eg, rash or fever) in association with ALT/SGPT elevations.

WARNINGS

Anesthesia

Cognex®, as a cholinesterase inhibitor, is likely to exaggerate succinylcholine-type muscle relaxation during anesthesia.

Cardiovascular Conditions

Because of its cholinomimetic action, Cognex® may have vagotonic effects on the heart rate (eg, bradycardia). This action may be particularly important to patients with conduction abnormalities, bradyarrhythmia, or a sick sinus syndrome.

Gastrointestinal Disease and Dysfunction

Cognex® is an inhibitor of cholinesterase and may be expected to increase gastric acid secretion due to increased cholinergic activity. Therefore, patients are at increased risk for developing ulcers. Those with a history of ulcer disease or those receiving concurrent nonsteroidal antiinflammatory drugs (NSAIDS) should be monitored closely for symptoms of active or occult gastrointestinal disease.
Cognex®, also as a predictable consequence of its pharmacological properties, can cause nausea, vomiting, and loose stools at recommended doses.

Liver Injury

Cognex® should be prescribed with care in patients with current evidence or history of abnormal liver function indicated by significant abnormalities in serum transaminase (ALT/SGPT; AST/SGOT), bilirubin, and gamma-glutamyl transpeptidase (GGT) levels (see PRECAUTIONS and DOSAGE AND ADMINISTRATION sections).
The use of tacrine in patients without a prior history of liver disease is commonly associated with serum aminotransferase elevations, some to levels ordinarily considered to indicate clinically important hepatic injury (see Table 2).
Experience gained in more than 12,000 patients who received tacrine in clinical studies and the treatment IND program indicates that if tacrine is promptly withdrawn following detection of these elevations, clinically evident signs and symptoms of liver injury are rare.
Long-term follow up of patients who experience transaminase elevations, however, is limited and it is impossible, therefore, to exclude, with certainty, the possibility of chronic sequelae.

Controlled Clinical Trials, Treatment IND and Post Marketing Experience:

Experience with tacrine in controlled trials and in a large, less closely monitored experience (a treatment IND) is summarized below:
Clinically evident liver toxicity: One of more than 12,000 patients exposed to tacrine in clinical studies and the treatment IND program had documented elevated bilirubin (5.3 × Upper Limit of Normal, ULN) and jaundice with transaminase levels (AST/SGOT) nearly 20 × ULN.
Rare cases of liver toxicity associated with jaundice, raised serum bilirubin, pyrexia, hepatitis and liver failure have been reported in post-marketing experience. Most of these cases have been reversible but some deaths have occurred. Since there was multiple pathology including infection, gallstones and carcinoma it was not possible to clearly establish the relationship to Cognex® treatment.
Blood chemistry signs of liver injury: Experience from the 30-week clinical study (described earlier) provides a representative estimate of the frequency of ALT/SGPT elevations expected for patients whose transaminase levels are monitored weekly and who receive Cognex® according to the recommended regimen for dose introduction and titration (Table 2). A dosing regimen employing a more rapid escalation of the daily dose of tacrine may be associated with more serious clinical events (see *Monitoring of Liver function and the Management of the patient who develops transaminase elevations*).

Table 2. Cumulative Incidence of ALT/SGPT Elevations Based on Maximum Values with Weekly Monitoring During the 30-Week Study
[Number and (%) of Patients]

Maximum ALT	Males N=229	Females N=250	Total N=479
Within Normal Limits	121(53)	100(40)	221(46)
>ULN	108(47)	150(60)	258(54)
>2 times ULN	77(34)	104(42)	181(38)
>3 times ULN	58(25)	81(32)	139(29)
>10 times ULN	12 (5)	19 (8)	31 (6)
>20 times ULN	3 (1)	6 (2)	9 (2)

Experience in 2446 patients who participated in all clinical trials, including the 30-week study, indicates approximately 50% of patients treated with Cognex® can be expected to have at least 1 ALT/SGPT level above ULN; approximately 25% of patients are likely to develop elevations >3 × ULN, and about 7% of patients may develop elevations >10 × ULN. Data collected from the treatment IND program were consistent with those obtained during clinical studies, and showed 3% of 5665 patients experiencing an ALT/SGPT elevation >10 × ULN.
In clinical trials where transaminases were monitored weekly, the median time to onset of the first ALT/SGPT elevation above ULN was approximately 6 weeks, with maximum ALT/SGPT occurring 1 week later, even in instances when Cognex® treatment was stopped. Under the conditions of forced slow upwards dose titration (increases of 40 mg a day every 6 weeks) employed in clinical studies, 95% of transaminase elevations >3 × ULN occurred within the first 18 weeks of Cognex® therapy, and 99% of the 10-fold elevations occurred by the 12th week and on not more than 80 mg; note, however, that for most patients ALT was monitored weekly and Cognex® was stopped when liver enzymes exceeded 3 × ULN. A total of 276 patients were monitored for ALT/SGPT levels every other week in two double-blind clinical studies, an open-label study, and amended treatment IND. The incidence, severity, time to onset, peak and recovery of ALT/SGPT levels were similar to weekly monitoring. With less frequent monitoring than every other week or the less stringent discontinuation criteria recommended below (see DOSAGE AND ADMINISTRATION), it is possible that marked elevations might be more common. It must also be appreciated that experience with prolonged exposure to the high dose (160 mg/day) is limited. In all cases, transaminase levels returned to within normal limits upon discontinuation of Cognex® treatment or following dosage reduction, usually within 4 to 6 weeks.
This relatively benign experience may be the consequence of careful laboratory monitoring that facilitated the discontinuation of patients early on after the onset of their transaminase elevations. Consequently, frequent monitoring of serum transaminase levels is recommended (see DOSAGE AND ADMINISTRATION, WARNINGS: Liver Injury: Monitoring of Liver Function and the Management of the Patient Who Develops Transaminase Elevations, and PRECAUTIONS: Laboratory Tests).
Liver biopsy experience: Liver biopsy results in 7 patients who received tacrine (1 in a Parke-Davis sponsored study and 6 in studies reported in the literature) revealed hepatocellular necrosis in 6 patients, and granulomatous changes in the seventh. In all cases, liver function tests returned to normal with no evidence of persisting hepatic dysfunction.
Experience with the Rechallenge of Patients with Transaminase Elevations following recovery: Two hundred and twelve patients among the 866 patients assigned to tacrine in the 12 and 30 week studies were withdrawn because they developed transaminase elevations >3 × ULN. One hundred and forty-five of these patients were subsequently rechallenged with weekly monitoring of ALT/SGPT. During their initial exposure to tacrine, 20 of these 145 had experienced initial elevations >10 times ULN, while the remainder had experienced elevations between 3 and 10 × ULN.
Upon rechallenge with an initial dose of 40 mg/day, only 48 (33%) of the 145 patients developed transaminase elevations greater than 3 × ULN. Of these patients, 44 had elevations that were between 3 and 10 × ULN and 4 had elevations that were >10 × ULN.
The mean time to onset of elevations occurred earlier on rechallenge than on initial exposure (22 versus 48 days). Of the 145 patients rechallenged, 127 (88%) were able to continue Cognex® treatment, and 91 of these 127 patients titrated to doses higher than those associated with the initial transaminase elevation.
Predictors of the risk of transaminase elevations: The incidence of transaminase elevations is higher among females. There are no other known predictors of the risk of hepatocellular injury.
***Monitoring of Liver function and the Management of the patient who develops transaminase elevations.* (See also DOSAGE AND ADMINISTRATION and PRECAUTIONS: Laboratory Tests.)**
Blood chemistries: Serum transaminase levels (specifically ALT/SGPT) should be monitored every other week from at least week 4 to week 16 following initiation of treatment, after which monitoring may be decreased to every 3 months. For patients who develop ALT/SGPT elevations greater than two times the upper limit of normal, the dose and monitoring regimen should be modified as described in Table 4 (see DOSAGE AND ADMINISTRATION).
A full monitoring sequence should be repeated in the event that a patient suspends treatment with tacrine for more than 4 weeks.
If ALT/SGPT elevations occur, the frequency of monitoring and the dose of Cognex® should be modified according to the table shown below in DOSAGE AND ADMINISTRATION.
Rechallenge: **Patients with clinical jaundice confirmed by a significant elevation in total bilirubin (>3 mg/dL) and/or those exhibiting clinical signs and/or symptoms of hypersensitivity (e.g. rash or fever) in association with ALT/SGPT elevations should immediately and permanently discontinue Cognex® and not be rechallenged.** Other patients who are required to discontinue Cognex® treatment because of ALT/SGPT elevations may be rechallenged once ALT/SGPT levels return to within normal limits. (See DOSAGE AND ADMINISTRATION.)
Rechallenge of patients with ALT/SGPT elevations less than 10 × ULN has not resulted in serious liver injury. However, because experience in the rechallenge of patients who had elevations greater than 10 × ULN is limited, the risks associated with the rechallenge of these patients are not well characterized. Careful, frequent (weekly) monitoring of serum ALT/SGPT should be undertaken when rechallenging such patients.
If rechallenged, patients should be given an initial dose of 40 mg/day (10 mg QID) and ALT/SGPT levels monitored weekly. If, after 6 weeks on 40 mg/day, the patient is tolerating the dosage with no unacceptable elevations in ALT/SGPT, recommended dose-titration may be resumed. Weekly monitoring of the ALT/SGPT levels should continue for a total of 16 weeks after which monitoring may be decreased to monthly for 2 months and every 3 months thereafter.
Liver biopsy: Liver biopsy is not indicated in cases of uncomplicated transaminase elevation.

Genitourinary

Cholinomimetics may cause bladder outflow obstruction.

Neurological Conditions

Seizures: Cholinomimetics are believed to have some potential to cause generalized convulsions; seizure activity may, however, also be a manifestation of Alzheimer's disease.
Sudden worsening of the degree of cognitive impairment: Worsening of cognitive function has been reported following abrupt discontinuation of Cognex® or after a large reduction in total daily dose (80 mg/day or more).

Pulmonary Conditions

Because of its cholinomimetic action, Cognex® should be prescribed with care to patients with a history of asthma.

PRECAUTIONS

General

Liver Injury: see WARNINGS

Hematology

An absolute neutrophil count (ANC) less than 500/µL occurred in 4 patients who received Cognex® during the course of clinical trials. Three of the 4 patients had concurrent medical conditions commonly associated with a low ANC; 2 of these patients remained on Cognex®. The fourth patient, who had a history of hypersensitivity (penicillin allergy), withdrew from the study as a result of a rash and also developed an ANC <500/µL, which returned to normal; this patient was not rechallenged and, therefore, the role played by Cognex® in this reaction is unknown.
Six patients had an absolute neutrophil count ≤1500/µL, associated with an elevation of ALT/SGPT.
The total clinical experience in more than 12,000 patients does not indicate a clear association between Cognex® treatment and serious white blood cell abnormalities.

Information for Patients and Caregivers

Patients and caregivers should be advised that the effect of Cognex® (brand of tacrine hydrochloride) therapy is thought to depend upon its administration at regular intervals, as directed.
The caregiver should be advised about the possibility of adverse effects. Two types should be distinguished: (1) those occurring in close temporal association with the initiation of treatment or an increase in dose (eg, nausea, vomiting, loose stools, diarrhea, etc) and (2) those with a delayed onset (eg, rash, jaundice, changes in the color of stool—black, very dark or light [ie, acholic]).
Patients and caregivers should be encouraged to inform the physician about the emergence of new events or any increase in the severity of existing adverse clinical events.
Caregivers should be advised that abrupt discontinuation of Cognex® or a large reduction in total daily dose (80 mg/day or more) may cause a decline in cognitive function and behavioral disturbances. Unsupervised increases in the dose of tacrine may also have serious consequences. Consequently, changes in dose should not be undertaken in the absence of direct instruction of a physician.

Laboratory Tests (see WARNINGS: Liver Injury and DOSAGE AND ADMINISTRATION)

Serum transaminase levels (specifically ALT/SGPT) should be monitored in patients given Cognex® (see WARNINGS: Liver Injury).

Drug-Drug Interactions

Possible metabolic basis for interactions: Tacrine is primarily eliminated by hepatic metabolism via cytochrome P450 drug metabolizing enzymes. Drug-drug interactions may occur when Cognex® is given concurrently with agents such as theophylline that undergo extensive metabolism via cytochrome P450 IA2.

Theophylline. **Coadministration of tacrine with theophylline increased theophylline elimination half-life and average plasma theophylline concentrations by approximately 2-fold. Therefore, monitoring of plasma theophylline concentrations and appropriate reduction of theophylline dose are recommended in patients receiving tacrine and theophylline concurrently. The effect of theophylline on tacrine pharmacokinetics has not been assessed.**

Cimetidine. Cimetidine increased the Cmax and AUC of tacrine by approximately 54% and 64%, respectively.

Anticholinergics. Because of its mechanism of action, Cognex® has the potential to interfere with the activity of anticholinergic medications.

Cholinomimetics and Cholinesterase Inhibitors. A synergistic effect is expected when Cognex® is given concurrently with succinylcholine (see WARNINGS), cholinesterase inhibitors, or cholinergic agonists such as bethanechol.

Fluvoxamine. In a study of 13 healthy, male volunteers, a single 40 mg dose of tacrine added to fluvoxamine 100 mg/day administered at steady-state was associated with five- and eight-fold increases in tacrine Cmax and AUC, respectively, compared to the administration of tacrine alone. Five subjects experienced nausea, vomiting, sweating, and diarrhea following coadministration, consistent with the cholinergic effects of tacrine.

Other Interactions. Rate and extent of tacrine absorption were not influenced by the coadministration of an antacid containing magnesium and aluminum. Tacrine had no major effect on digoxin or diazepam pharmacokinetics or the anticoagulant activity of warfarin.

Carcinogenesis, Mutagenesis, Impairment of Fertility

Tacrine was mutagenic to bacteria in the Ames test. Unscheduled DNA synthesis was induced in rat and mouse hepatocytes *in vitro*. Results of cytogenetic (chromosomal aberration) studies were equivocal. Tacrine was not mutagenic in an *in vitro* mammalian mutation test. Overall, the results of these tests, along with the fact that tacrine belongs to a chemical class (acridines) containing some members which are animal carcinogens, suggest that tacrine may be carcinogenic.

Studies of the effects of tacrine on fertility have not been performed.

Pregnancy

Category C: Animal reproduction studies have not been conducted with tacrine. It is also not known whether Cognex® can cause fetal harm when administered to a pregnant woman or can affect reproductive capacity.

Nursing Mothers

It is not known whether this drug is excreted in human milk.

Pediatric Use

There are no adequate and well-controlled trials to document the safety and efficacy of tacrine in any dementing illness occurring in pediatric patients.

ADVERSE REACTIONS

Common Adverse Events Leading to Discontinuation

In clinical trials, approximately 17% of the 2706 patients who received Cognex® and 5% of the 1886 patients who received placebo withdrew permanently because of adverse events. It should be noted that some of the placebo-treated patients were exposed to Cognex® prior to receiving placebo due to the variety of study designs used, including crossover studies. Transaminase elevations were the most common reason for withdrawals during Cognex® treatment (8% of all Cognex®-treated patients, or 212 of 456 patients withdrawn). The controlled clinical trial protocols required that any patient with an ALT/SGPT elevation >3 × ULN be withdrawn, because of concern about potential hepatotoxicity. Apart from withdrawals due to transaminase elevations, 244 patients (9%) withdrew for adverse events while receiving Cognex®.

Other adverse events that most frequently led to the withdrawal of tacrine-treated patients in clinical trials were nausea and/or vomiting (1.5%), agitation (0.9%), rash (0.7%), anorexia (0.7%), and confusion (0.5%). These adverse events also most frequently led to the withdrawal of placebo-treated patients, although at lower frequencies (0.1% to 0.2%).

Most Frequent Adverse Clinical Events Seen in Association With the Use of Tacrine

The events identified here are those that occurred at an absolute incidence of at least 5% of patients treated with Cognex®, and at a rate at least 2-fold higher in patients treated with Cognex® than placebo.

The most common adverse events associated with the use of Cognex® were elevated transaminases, nausea and/or vomiting, diarrhea, dyspepsia, myalgia, anorexia, and ataxia. Of these events, nausea and/or vomiting, diarrhea, dyspepsia, and anorexia appeared to be dose-dependent.

Adverse Events Reported in Controlled Trials

The events cited in the tables below reflect experience gained under closely monitored conditions of clinical trials with a highly selective patient population. In actual clinical practice or in other clinical trials, these frequency estimates may not apply, as the conditions of use, reporting behavior, and the kinds of patients treated may differ.

Table 3 lists treatment-emergent signs and symptoms that occurred in at least 2% of patients with Alzheimer's disease in placebo-controlled trials and who received the recommended regimen for dose introduction and titration of Cognex® (see DOSAGE AND ADMINISTRATION).

Table 3. Adverse Events Occurring in at Least 2% of Patients Receiving Cognex® at a Starting Dose of 40 mg/day with Titration in 40 mg/day Increments Every 6 Weeks

BODY SYSTEM/ Adverse Events	Cognex® N = 634		Placebo N = 342	
LABORATORY DEVIATIONS				
Elevated Transaminase[a]	184	(29)	5	(2)
BODY AS A WHOLE				
Headache	67	(11)	52	(15)
Fatigue	26	(4)	9	(3)
Chest Pain	24	(4)	18	(5)
Weight Decrease	21	(3)	4	(1)
Back Pain	15	(2)	14	(4)
Asthenia	15	(2)	7	(2)
DIGESTIVE SYSTEM				
Nausea and/or Vomiting	178	(28)	29	(9)
Diarrhea	99	(16)	18	(5)
Dyspepsia	57	(9)	22	(6)
Anorexia	54	(9)	11	(3)
Abdominal Pain	48	(8)	24	(7)
Flatulence	22	(4)	5	(2)
Constipation	24	(4)	8	(2)
HEMIC AND LYMPHATIC SYSTEM				
Purpura	15	(2)	8	(2)
MUSCULOSKELETAL SYSTEM				
Myalgia	54	(9)	18	(5)
NERVOUS SYSTEM				
Dizziness	73	(12)	39	(11)
Confusion	42	(7)	24	(7)
Ataxia	36	(6)	12	(4)
Insomnia	37	(6)	18	(5)
Somnolence	22	(4)	11	(3)
Tremor	14	(2)	2	(<1)
PSYCHOBIOLOGIC FUNCTION				
Agitation	43	(7)	30	(9)
Depression	22	(4)	14	(4)
Thinking Abnormal	17	(3)	14	(4)
Anxiety	16	(3)	7	(2)
Hallucination	15	(2)	12	(4)
Hostility	15	(2)	5	(2)
RESPIRATORY SYSTEM				
Rhinitis	51	(8)	22	(6)
Upper Respiratory Infection	18	(3)	11	(3)
Coughing	17	(3)	18	(5)
SKIN AND APPENDAGES				
Rash[b]	46	(7)	18	(5)
Facial Flushing, Skin Flushing	16	(3)	3	(<1)
UROGENITAL SYSTEM				
Urination Frequency	21	(3)	12	(4)
Urinary Tract Infection	21	(3)	20	(6)
Urinary Incontinence	16	(3)	9	(3)

[a] ALT or AST value of approximately 3 × ULN or greater or that resulted in a change in patient management. Patients were monitored weekly.

[b] Includes COSTART terms: rash, rash-erythematous, rash-maculopapular, urticaria, petechial rash, rash-vesiculobullous, and pruritus.

Other Adverse Events Observed During All Clinical Trials

Cognex® has been administered to 2706 individuals during clinical trials. A total of 1471 patients were treated for at least 3 months, 1137 for at least 6 months, and 773 for at least 1 year. Any untoward reactions that occurred during these trials were recorded as adverse events by the clinical investigators using terminology of their own choosing. To provide a meaningful estimate of the proportion of individuals having similar types of events, the events were grouped into a smaller number of standardized categories using a modified COSTART dictionary. These categories are used in the listing below. The frequencies represent the proportion of the 2706 individuals exposed to Cognex® who experienced that event while receiving Cognex®. All adverse events are included except those already listed on the previous table and those COSTART terms too general to be informative. Events are further classified by body system categories and listed using the following definitions: frequent adverse events are defined as those occurring in at least 1/100 patients; infrequent adverse events are those occurring in 1/100 to 1/1000 patients; and rare adverse events are those occurring in less than 1/1000 patients. These adverse events are not necessarily related to Cognex® treatment. Only rare adverse events deemed to be potentially important are included.

Body As a Whole: *Frequent:* Chill, fever, malaise, peripheral edema. *Infrequent:* Face edema, dehydration, weight increase, cachexia, edema (generalized), lipoma. *Rare:* Heat exhaustion, sepsis, cholingeric crisis, death.

Cardiovascular System: *Frequent:* Hypotension, hypertension. *Infrequent:* Heart failure, myocardial infarction, angina pectoris, cerebrovascular accident, transient ischemic attack, phlebitis, venous insufficiency, abdominal aortic aneurysm, atrial fibrillation or flutter, palpitation, tachycardia, bradycardia, pulmonary embolus, migraine, hypercholesterolemia. *Rare:* Heart arrest, premature atrial contractions, A-V block, bundle branch block.

Digestive System: *Infrequent:* Glossitis, gingivitis, mouth or throat dry, stomatitis, increased salivation, dysphagia, esophagitis, gastritis, gastroenteritis, GI hemorrhage, stomach ulcer, hiatal hernia, hemorrhoids, stools bloody, diverticulitis, fecal impaction, fecal incontinence, hemorrhage (rectum), cholelithiasis, cholecystitis, increased appetite. *Rare:* Duodenal ulcer, bowel obstruction.

Endocrine System: *Infrequent:* Diabetes. *Rare:* Hyperthyroid, hypothyroid.

Hemic and Lymphatic: *Infrequent:* Anemia, lymphadenopathy. *Rare:* Leukopenia, thrombocytopenia, hemolysis, pancytopenia.

Musculoskeletal: *Frequent:* Fracture, arthralgia, arthritis, hypertonia. *Infrequent:* Osteoporosis, tendinitis, bursitis, gout. *Rare:* Myopathy.

Nervous System: *Frequent:* Convulsions, vertigo, syncope, hyperkinesia, paresthesia. *Infrequent:* Dreaming abnormal, dysarthria, aphasia, amnesia, wandering, twitching, hypesthesia, delirium, paralysis, bradykinesia, movement disorder, cogwheel rigidity, paresis, neuritis, hemiplegia, Parkinson's disease, neuropathy, extrapyramidal syndrome, reflexes decreased/absent. *Rare:* Tardive dyskinesia, dysesthesia, dystonia, encephalitis, coma, apraxia, oculogyric crisis, akathisia, oral facial dyskinesia, Bell's palsy, exacerbation of Parkinson's disease.

Psychobiologic Function: *Frequent:* Nervousness. *Infrequent:* Apathy, increased libido, paranoia, neurosis. *Rare:* Suicidal, psychosis, hysteria.

Respiratory System: *Frequent:* Pharyngitis, sinusitis, bronchitis, pneumonia, dyspnea. *Infrequent:* Epistaxis, chest congestion, asthma, hyperventilation, lower respiratory infection. *Rare:* Hemoptysis, lung edema, lung cancer, acute epiglottitis.

Skin and Appendages: *Frequent:* Sweating increased. *Infrequent:* Acne, alopecia, dermatitis, eczema, skin dry, herpes zoster, psoriasis, cellulitis, cyst, furunculosis, herplex simplex, hyperkeratosis, basal cell carcinoma, skin cancer. *Rare:* Desquamation, seborrhea, squamous cell carcinoma, ulcer (skin), skin necrosis, melanoma.

Urogenital System: *Infrequent:* Hematuria, renal stone, kidney infection, glycosuria, dysuria, polyuria, nocturia, pyuria, cystitis, urinary retention, urination urgency, vaginal hemorrhage, pruritus (genital), breast pain, impotence, prostate cancer. *Rare:* Bladder tumor, renal tumor, renal failure, urinary obstruction, breast cancer, epididymitis, carcinoma (ovary).

Special Senses: *Frequent:* Conjunctivitis. *Infrequent:* Cataract, eyes dry, eye pain, visual field defect, diplopia, amblyopia, glaucoma, hordeolum, deafness, earache, tinnitus, inner ear infection, otitis media, unusual taste. *Rare:* Vision loss, ptosis, blepharitis, labyrinthitis, inner ear disturbance.

Postintroduction Reports

Voluntary reports of adverse events temporarily associated with Cognex® that have been received since market introduction, that are not listed above, and that may have no causal relationship with the drug include the following: pancreatitis, perforated peptic ulcer, and falling.

OVERDOSAGE

As in any case of overdose, general supportive measures should be utilized. Overdosage with cholinesterase inhibitors can cause a cholinergic crisis characterized by severe nausea/vomiting, salivation, sweating, bradycardia, hypotension, collapse, and convulsions. Increasing muscle weakness is a possibility and may result in death if respiratory muscles are involved.

Tertiary anticholinergics such as atropine may be used as an antidote for Cognex® overdosage. Intravenous atropine sulfate titrated to effect is recommended: in adults, initial dose of 1.0 to 2.0 mg IV with subsequent doses based on clinical response. In children, the usual IM or IV dose is 0.05 mg/kg, repeated every 10–30 minutes until muscarinic signs and symptoms subside and repeated if they reappear. Atypical increases in blood pressure and heart rate have been reported with other cholinomimetics when coadministered with quaternary anticholinergics such as glycopyrrolate.

It is not known whether Cognex® or its metabolites can be eliminated by dialysis (hemodialysis, peritoneal dialysis, or hemofiltration).

The estimated median lethal dose of tacrine following a single oral dose in rats is 40 mg/kg, or approximately 12 times the maximum recommended human dose of 160 mg/day. Dose-related signs of cholinergic stimulation were observed in animals and included vomiting, diarrhea, salivation, lacrimation, ataxia, convulsions, tremor, and stereotypic head and body movements.

DOSAGE AND ADMINISTRATION

The recommendations for dose titration are based on experience from clinical trials. The rate of dose escalation may be slowed if a patient is intolerant to the titration schedule recommended below. It is not advisable, however, to accelerate the dose incrementation plan.

Following initiation of therapy, or any dosage increase, patients should be observed carefully for adverse effects. Cognex® should be taken between meals whenever possible; however, if minor GI upset occurs, Cognex® may be taken with meals to improve tolerability. Taking Cognex® with meals can be expected to reduce plasma levels approximately 30% to 40%.

Continued on next page

Cognex—Cont.

The initial dose of Cognex® brand of tacrine hydrochloride is 40 mg/day (10 mg Q.I.D.). This dose should be maintained for a minimum of 4 weeks with every other week monitoring of transaminase levels beginning 4 weeks after initiation of treatment. It is important that the dose not be increased during this period because of the potential for delayed onset of transaminase elevations.

Dose Titration

Following 4 weeks of treatment at 40 mg/day (10 mg Q.I.D.), the dose of Cognex® should then be increased to 80 mg/day (20 mg Q.I.D.), providing there are no significant transaminase elevations and the patient is tolerating treatment. Patients should be titrated to higher doses (120 and 160 mg/day, in divided doses on a Q.I.D. schedule) at 4-week intervals on the basis of tolerance.

Dose Adjustment

Serum ALT/SGPT should be monitored every other week from at least week 4 to week 16 following initiation of treatment, after which monitoring may be decreased to every 3 months. For patients who develop ALT/SGPT elevations greater than two times the upper limit of normal, the dose and monitoring regimen should be modified as described in Table 4.

A full monitoring and dose titration sequence must be repeated in the event that a patient suspends treatment with tacrine for more than 4 weeks.

Table 4. Recommended Dose amd Monitoring Regimen Modification in Response to ALT/SGPT Elevations

ALT/SGPT Level	Treatment and Monitoring Regimen
≤2 × ULN	Continue treatment according to recommended titration and monitoring schedule.
>2 to ≤3 × ULN	Continue treatment according to recommended titration. Monitor ALT/SGPT levels weekly until levels return to normal limits.
>3 to ≤5 × ULN	Reduce the daily dose of Cognex® by 40 mg/day. Monitor ALT/SGPT levels weekly. Resume dose titration and every other week monitoring when the levels of the ALT/SGPT return to normal limits.
>5 × ULN	Stop Cognex® treatment. Monitor the patient closely for signs and symptoms associated with hepatitis and follow ALT/SGPT levels until within normal limits. See Rechallenge section below. Experience is limited in patients with ALT/SGPT >10 × ULN. The risk of rechallenge must be considered against demonstrated clinical benefit. **Patients with clinical jaundice confirmed by a significant elevation in total bilirubin (>3 mg/dL) and/or those exhibiting clinical signs and/or symptoms of hypersensitivity (e.g. rash or fever) in association with ALT/SGPT elevations should immediately and permanently discontinue Cognex® and not be rechallenged.**

Rechallenge

Patients who are required to discontinue Cognex® treatment because of ALT/SGPT elevations may be rechallenged once ALT/SGPT levels return to normal limits.

Rechallenge of patients exposed to ALT/SGPT elevations less than 10 × ULN has not resulted in serious liver injury. However, because experience in the rechallenge of patients who had elevations greater than 10 × ULN is limited, the risks associated with the rechallenge of these patients are not well characterized. Careful, frequent (weekly) monitoring of serum ALT/SGPT should be undertaken when rechallenging such patients.

If rechallenged, patients should be given an initial dose of 40 mg/day (10 mg QID) and ALT/SGPT levels monitored weekly. If, after 6 weeks on 40 mg/day, the patient is tolerating the dosage with no unacceptable elevations in ALT/SGPT, the recommended dose-titration may be resumed. Weekly monitoring of the ALT/SGPT levels should continue for a total of 16 weeks after which monitoring may be decreased to monthly for 2 months and every 3 months thereafter.

HOW SUPPLIED

Cognex® is supplied as capsules of tacrine hydrochloride containing 10, 20, 30, and 40 mg of tacrine. The capsule logo is Cognex®, with the strength (eg, 10, 20, 30, or 40) printed underneath.

10 mg (yellow/dark green)	Bottles of 120 (N 0071-0096-25) Unit-dose package of 100 (10 × 10) (N 0071-0096-40)
20 mg (yellow/light blue)	Bottles of 120 (N 0071-0097-25) Unit-dose package of 100 (10 × 10) (N 0071-0097-40)
30 mg (yellow/swedish orange)	Bottles of 120 (N 0071-0095-25) Unit-dose package of 100 (10 × 10) (N 0071-0095-40)
40 mg (yellow/lavender)	Bottles of 120 (N 0071-0098-25) Unit-dose package of 100 (10 × 10) (N 0071-0098-40)

Storage

Store at controlled room temperature 15°C to 30°C (59°F to 86°F) away from moisture.

Rx only

Manufactured by:
Parke Davis Pharmaceuticals, Ltd.
Vega Baja, PR 00694
Distributed by:
First Horizon Pharmaceutical™ Corporation
Roswell, GA 30076
©1997-2000 FHPC
Revised April 2000 0096G025

DEFEN—L.A. Tablets ℞
[*dē-fĕn*]

DESCRIPTION

Each dye-free, film-coated tablet imprinted DEFEN and scored contains:

Pseudoephedrine HCl	60 mg
Guaifenesin	600 mg

HOW SUPPLIED

Bottles of 100

MESCOLOR® TABLETS ℞
[*mĕs-cō-lŏr*]

DESCRIPTION

Each dye-free, film-coated, tablet imprinted HP 15 and scored contains:

Chlorpheniramine Maleate	8.0 mg
Pseudoephedrine HCl	120.0 mg
Methscopolamine Nitrate	2.5 mg

HOW SUPPLIED

Bottles of 100

NITROLINGUAL® PUMPSPRAY ℞
[*nī-trō lĭng uəl*]
(nitroglycerin lingual spray)
400 mcg per spray, 75 or 200 Metered Sprays

DESCRIPTION

Nitroglycerin, an organic nitrate, is a vasodilator which has effects on both arteries and veins. The chemical name for nitroglycerin is 1,2,3-propanetriol trinitrate ($C_3H_5N_3O_9$). The compound has a molecular weight of 227.09. The chemical structure is:

$$\begin{array}{l} CH_2{-}ONO_2 \\ | \\ CH{-}ONO_2 \\ | \\ CH_2{-}ONO_2 \end{array}$$

Nitrolingual® Pumpspray (nitroglycerin lingual spray 400 mcg) is a metered dose spray containing nitroglycerin. This product delivers nitroglycerin (400 mcg per spray, 75 or 200 metered sprays) in the form of spray droplets onto or under the tongue. Inactive ingredients: medium-chain triglycerides, dehydrated alcohol, medium-chain partial glycerides, peppermint oil.

CLINICAL PHARMACOLOGY

The principal pharmacological action of nitroglycerin is relaxation of vascular smooth muscle, producing a vasodilator effect on both peripheral arteries and veins with more prominent effects on the latter. Dilation of the post-capillary vessels, including large veins, promotes peripheral pooling of blood and decreases venous return to the heart, thereby reducing left ventricular end-diastolic pressure (pre-load). Arteriolar relaxation reduces systemic vascular resistance and arterial pressure (after-load).

The mechanism by which nitroglycerin relieves angina pectoris is not fully understood. Myocardial oxygen consumption or demand (as measured by the pressure-rate product, tension-time index, and stroke-work index) is decreased by both the arterial and venous effects of nitroglycerin and presumably, a more favorable supply-demand ratio is achieved. While the large epicardial coronary arteries are also dilated by nitroglycerin, the extent to which this action contributes to relief of exertional angina is unclear.

Nitroglycerin is rapidly metabolized *in vivo*, with a liver reductase enzyme having primary importance in the formation of glycerol nitrate metabolites and inorganic nitrate. Two active major metabolites, 1,2- and 1,3-dinitroglycerols, the products of hydrolysis, although less potent as vasodilators, have longer plasma half-lives than the parent compound. The dinitrates are further metabolized to mononitrates (considered biologically inactive with respect to cardiovascular effects) and ultimately glycerol and carbon dioxide.

Therapeutic doses of nitroglycerin may reduce systolic, diastolic and mean arterial blood pressure. Effective coronary perfusion pressure is usually maintained, but can be compromised if blood pressure falls excessively or increased heart rate decreases diastolic filling time.

Elevated central venous and pulmonary capillary wedge pressures, pulmonary vascular resistance and systemic vascular resistance are also reduced by nitroglycerin therapy. Heart rate is usually slightly increased, presumably a reflex response to the fall in blood pressure. Cardiac index may be increased, decreased, or unchanged. Patients with elevated left ventricular filling pressure and systemic vascular resistance values in conjunction with a depressed cardiac index are likely to experience an improvement in cardiac index. On the other hand, when filling pressures and cardiac index are normal, cardiac index may be slightly reduced.

In a pharmacokinetic study when a single 0.8 mg dose of Nitrolingual® Pumpspray was administered to healthy volunteers (n = 24), the mean C_{max} and t_{max}, were 1,041pg/mL · min and 7.5 minutes, respectively. Additionally, in these subjects the mean area-under-the-curve (AUC) was 12,769 pg/mL · min.

In a randomized, double-blind single-dose, 5-period crossover study in 51 patients with exertional angina pectoris significant dose-related increases in exercise tolerance, time to onset of angina and ST-segment depression were seen following doses of 0.2, 0.4, 0.8 and 1.6 mg of nitroglycerin delivered by metered pumpspray as compared to placebo. Additionally the drug was well tolerated as evidenced by a profile of generally mild to moderate adverse events.

INDICATIONS AND USAGE

Nitrolingual® Pumpspray is indicated for acute relief of an attack or prophylaxis of angina pectoris due to coronary artery disease.

CONTRAINDICATIONS

Nitrolingual® Pumpspray is contraindicated in patients who have shown purported hypersensitivity or idiosyncrasy to it or other nitrates or nitrites.

WARNINGS

Amplification of the vasodilatory effects of Nitrolingual® Pumpspray by sildenafil can result in severe hypotension. The time course and dose dependence of this interaction have not been studied. Appropriate supportive care has not been studied, but it seems reasonable to treat this as a nitrate overdose, with elevation of the extremities and with central volume expansion. The use of any form of nitroglycerin during the early days of acute myocardial infarction requires particular attention to hemodynamic monitoring and clinical status.

PRECAUTIONS

(General)

Severe hypotension, particularly with upright posture, may occur even with small doses of nitroglycerin. The drug, therefore, should be used with caution in subjects who may have volume depletion from diuretic therapy or in patients who have low systolic blood pressure (*e.g.*, below 90 mm Hg). Paradoxical bradycardia and increased angina pectoris may accompany nitroglycerin-induced hypotension.

Nitrate therapy may aggravate the angina caused by hypertrophic cardiomyopathy.

Tolerance to this drug and cross-tolerance to other nitrates, and nitrites may occur. Tolerance to the vascular and antianginal effects of nitrates has been demonstrated in clinical trials, experience through occupational exposure, and in isolated tissue experiments in the laboratory.

In industrial workers continuously exposed to nitroglycerin, tolerance clearly occurs. Moreover, physical dependence also occurs since chest pain, acute myocardial infarction, and even sudden death have occurred during temporary withdrawal of nitroglycerin from the workers. In various clinical trials in angina patients, there are reports of anginal attacks being more easily provoked and of rebound in the hemodynamic effects soon after nitrate withdrawal. The relative importance of these observations to the routine, clinical use of nitroglycerin is not known.

PRECAUTIONS

(INFORMATION FOR PATIENTS)

Physicians should discuss with patients the contraindication of Nitrolingual® Pumpspray with concurrent sildenafil (Viagra®).

DRUG INTERACTIONS: Alcohol may enhance sensitivity to the hypotensive effects of nitrates. Nitroglycerin acts directly on vascular muscle. Therefore, any other agents that depend on vascular smooth muscle as the final common path can be expected to have decreased or increased effect depending upon the agent.

Marked symptomatic orthostatic hypotension has been reported when calcium channel blockers and oral controlled-release nitroglycerin were used in combination. Dose adjustments of either class of agents may be necessary.

CARCINOGENESIS, MUTAGENESIS, IMPAIRMENT OF FERTILITY: Animal carcinogenicity studies with sublingual nitroglycerin have not been performed.

Rats receiving up to 434 mg/kg/day of dietary nitroglycerin for 2 years developed dose-related fibrotic and neoplastic changes in liver, including carcinomas, and interstitial cell tumors in testes. At high dose, the incidences of hepatocellular carcinomas in both sexes were 52% *vs.* 0% in controls, and incidences of testicular tumors were 52% *vs.* 8% in controls. Lifetime dietary administration of up to 1058 mg/kg/day of nitroglycerin was not tumorigenic in mice.

Nitroglycerin was weakly mutagenic in Ames tests performed in two different laboratories. Nevertheless, there was no evidence of mutagenicity in an *in vivo* dominant lethal assay with male rats treated with doses up to about 363 mg/kg/day, p.o., or in *in vitro* cytogenic tests in rat and dog tissues.

In a three-generation reproduction study, rats received dietary nitroglycerin at doses up to about 434 mg/kg/day for six months prior to mating of the F_0 generation with treatment continuing through successive F_1 and F_2 generations. The high dose was associated with decreased feed intake and body weight gain in both sexes at all matings. No specific effect on the fertility of the F_0 generation was seen. Infertility noted in subsequent generations, however, was attributed to increased interstitial cell tissue and aspermatogenesis in the high-dose males. In this three-generation study there was no clear evidence of teratogenicity.

PREGNANCY: Pregnancy Category C—Animal teratology studies have not been conducted with nitroglycerin-pumpspray. Teratology studies in rats and rabbits, however, were conducted with topically applied nitroglycerin ointment at doses up to 80 mg/kg/day and 240 mg/kg/day, respectively. No toxic effects on dams or fetuses were seen at any dose tested. There are no adequate and well-controlled studies in pregnant women.. Nitroglycerin should be given to pregnant women only if clearly needed.

NURSING MOTHERS: It is not known whether nitroglycerin is excreted in human milk. Because many drugs are excreted in human milk, caution should be exercised when Nitrolingual® Pumpspray is administered to a nursing woman.

PEDIATRIC USE: Safety and effectiveness of nitroglycerin in pediatric patients have not been established.

ADVERSE REACTIONS

Adverse reactions to oral nitroglycerin dosage forms, particularly headache and hypotension, are generally dose-related. In clinical trials at various doses of nitroglycerin, the following adverse effects have been observed:

Headache, which may be severe and persistent, is the most commonly reported side effect of nitroglycerin with an incidence on the order of about 50% in some studies. Cutaneous vasodilation with flushing may occur. Transient episodes of dizziness and weakness, as well as other signs of cerebral ischemia associated with postural hypotension, may occasionally develop. Occasionally, an individual may exhibit marked sensitivity to the hypotensive effects of nitrates and severe responses (nausea, vomiting, weakness, restlessness, pallor, perspiration and collapse) may occur even with therapeutic doses. Drug rash and/or exfoliative dermatitis have been reported in patients receiving nitrate therapy. Nausea and vomiting appear to be uncommon.

Nitrolingual® Pumpspray given to 51 chronic stable angina patients in single doses of 0.4, 0.8 and 1.6 mg as part of a double-blind, 5-period single-dose cross-over study exhibited an adverse event profile that was generally mild to moderate. Adverse events occurring at a frequency greater than 2% included: headache, dizziness, and paresthesia. Less frequently reported events in this trial included (≤2%): dyspnea, pharyngitis, rhinitis, vasodilation, peripheral edema, asthenia, and abdominal pain.

OVERDOSAGE

Signs and Symptoms:

Nitrate overdosage may result in: severe hypotension, persistent throbbing headache, vertigo, palpitation, visual disturbance, flushing and perspiring skin (later becoming cold and cyanotic), nausea and vomiting (possibly with colic and even bloody diarrhea), syncope (especially in the upright posture), methemoglobinemia with cyanosis and anorexia, initial hyperpnea, dyspnea and slow breathing, slow pulse (dicrotic and intermittent), heart block, increased intracranial pressure with cerebral symptoms of confusion and moderate fever, paralysis and coma followed by clonic convulsions, and possibly death due to circulatory collapse.

Methemoglobinemia:

Case reports of clinically significant methemoglobinemia are rare at conventional doses of organic nitrates. The formation of methemoglobin in dose-related and in the case of genetic abnormalities of hemoglobin that favor methemoglobin formation, even conventional doses of organic nitrates could produce harmful concentrations of methemoglobin.

Treatment of Overdosage:

Keep the patient recumbent in a shock position and comfortably warm. Passive movement of the extremities may aid venous return. Administer oxygen and artificial ventilation, if necessary. If methemoglobinemia is present, administration of methylene blue (1% solution), 1–2 mg per kilogram of body weight intravenously, may be required. If an excessive of Nitrolingual® Pumpspray has been recently swallowed gastric lavage may be of use.

WARNING

Epinephrine is ineffective in reversing the severe hypotensive events associated with overdosage. It and related compounds are contraindicated in this situation.

DOSAGE AND ADMINISTRATION

At the onset of an attack, one or two metered sprays should be administered onto or under the tongue. No more than three metered sprays are recommended within a 15-minute period. If the chest pain persists, prompt medical attention is recommended. Nitrolingual® Pumpspray may be used prophylactically five to ten minutes prior to engaging in activities which might precipitate an acute attack.

Each metered spray of Nitrolingual® Pumpspray delivers 48 mg of solution containing 400 mcg of nitroglycerin after an initial priming of 1 spray. It will remain adequately primed for 6 weeks. If the product is not used within 6 weeks it can be adequately reprimed with 1 spray. There are 75 or 200 metered sprays per bottle. The total number of available doses is dependent, however, on the number of sprays per use (1 or 2 sprays), and the frequency of repriming.

During application the patient should rest, ideally in the sitting position. The container should be held vertically with the valve head uppermost and the spray orifice as close to the mouth as possible. The dose should preferably be sprayed onto the tongue by pressing the button firmly and the mouth should be closed immediately after each dose. THE SPRAY SHOULD NOT BE INHALED. The medication should not be expectorated or the mouth rinsed for 5 to 10 minutes following administration. Patients should be instructed to familiarize themselves with the position of the spray orifice, which can be identified by the finger rest on top of the valve, or order to facilitate orientation for administration at night.

HOW SUPPLIED

Each box of Nitrolingual® Pumpspray, contains one clear glass bottle coated with red transparent plastic which assists in containing the glass and medication should the bottle be shattered. Each unit contains 5.7 g (NDC 59630-300-75) or 12 g (NDC 59630-300-20) (Net Content) of nitroglycerin lingual spray which will deliver 75 or 200 metered sprays containing 400 mcgs of nitroglycerin per spray.

Store at 25 °C (77 °F); excursions permitted to 15–30 °C (59–86 °F) [see USP Controlled Room Temperature].

Note: Nitrolingual® Pumpspray contains 20% alcohol. Do not forcefully open or burn container after use. Do not spray toward flames.

Rx Only.

Manufactured for FIRST HORIZON PHARMACEUTICAL CORPORATION, ROSWELL, GA 30076 by G. Pohl-Boskamp GmbH & Co., D-25551 Hohenlockstedt, Germany.

220420026/2 Rev. 6/00

Shown in Product Identification Guide, page 312

PONSTEL® ℞

[*pŏn 'stĕl"*]
(mefenamic acid)

DESCRIPTION

Ponstel® (mefenamic acid) is a member of the fenamate group of nonsteroidal anti-inflammatory drugs (NSAIDs). Each blue-banded, ivory capsule contains 250 mg of mefenamic acid for oral administration. Mefenamic acid is a white to greyish-white, odorless, microcrystalline powder with a melting point of 230°–231°C and water solubility of 0.004% at pH 7.1. The chemical name is 2-[(2,3-dimethylphenyl) amino-N-2,3-xylylanthranilic acid. The molecular weight is 241.29. Its molecular formula is $C_{15}H_{15}NO_2$ and the structural formula of mefenamic acid is:

COOH
NH
CH_3 CH_3

Each capsule also contains lactose, NF. The capsule shell and/or band contains citric acid, USP; D&C yellow No. 10; FD&C blue No. 1; FD&C red No. 3; FD&C yellow No. 6; gelatin, NF; glycerol monooleate; silicon dioxide, NF; sodium benzoate, NF; sodium lauryl sulfate, NF; titanium dioxide, USP.

CLINICAL PHARMACOLOGY

Pharmacodynamics

Ponstel is a nonsteroidal anti-inflammatory drug (NSAID) that exhibits anti-inflammatory, analgesic, and antipyretic activities in animal models. The mechanism of action of Ponstel, like that of other NSAIDs, is not completely understood but may be related to prostaglandin synthetase inhibition.

Pharmacokinetics

Absorption: Mefenamic acid is rapidly absorbed after oral administration. In two 500-mg single oral dose studies, the mean extent of absorption was 30.5 mcg/hr/mL (17%CV).[1,2] The bioavailability of the capsule relative to an IV dose or an oral solution has not been studied.

Following a single 1-gram oral dose, mean peak plasma levels ranging from 10–20 mcg/mL[3] have been reported. Peak plasma levels are attained in 2 to 4 hours and the elimination half-life approximates 2 hours. Following multiple doses, plasma levels are proportional to dose with no evidence of drug accumulation. In a multiple dose trial of normal adult subjects (n=6) receiving 1-gram doses of mefenamic acid four times daily, steady-state concentrations of 20 mcg/mL were reached on the second day of administration, consistent with the short half-life.

The effect of food on the rate and extent of absorption of mefenamic acid has not been studied. Concomitant ingestion of antacids containing magnesium hydroxide has been shown to significantly increase the rate and extent of mefenamic acid absorption (see PRECAUTIONS, Drug Interactions).[1]

Distribution: Mefenamic acid has been reported as being greater than 90% bound to albumin.[9] The relationship of unbound fraction to drug concentration has not been studied. The apparent volume of distribution (Vz_{ss}/F) estimated following a 500-mg oral dose of mefenamic acid was 1.06 L/kg.[2]

Based on its physical and chemical properties, Ponstel is expected to be excreted in human breast milk.

Metabolism: Mefenamic acid is metabolized by cytochrome P450 enzyme CYP2C9 to 3-hydroxymethyl mefenamic acid (Metabolite I). Further oxidation to a 3-carboxymefenamic acid (Metabolite II) may occur.[10] The activity of these metabolites has not been studied. The metabolites may undergo glucuronidation and mefenamic acid is also glucuronidated directly. A peak plasma level approximating 20 mcg/mL was observed at 3 hours for the hydroxy metabolite and its glucuronide (n=6) after a single 1-gram dose. Similarly, a peak plasma level of 8 mcg/mL was observed at 6–8 hours for the carboxy metabolite and its glucuronide.[3]

Excretion: Approximately fifty-two percent of a mefenamic acid dose is excreted into the urine primarily as glucuronides of mefenamic acid (6%), 3-hydroxymefenamic acid (25%) and 3-carboxymefenamic acid (21%). The fecal route of elimination accounts for up to 20% of the dose, mainly in the form of unconjugated 3-carboxymefenamic acid.[3]

The elimination half-life of mefenamic acid is approximately two hours. Half-lives of metabolites I and II have not been precisely reported, but appear to be longer than the parent compound.[3] The metabolites may accumulate in patients with renal or hepatic failure. The mefenamic acid glucuronide may bind irreversibly to plasma proteins. Because both renal and hepatic excretion are significant pathways of elimination, dosage adjustments in patients with renal or hepatic dysfunction may be necessary. Ponstel should not be administered to patients with preexisting renal disease or in patients with significantly impaired renal function.

TABLE 1. Pharmacokinetic Parameter Estimates for Mefenamic Acid

PK Parameters	Normal Healthy Adults (18–45 yr)	
	Value	CV
Tmax(hr)	2	66
Oral clearance (L/hr)	21.23	38
Apparent volume of distribution; Vz/F (L/kg)	1.06	60
Half-life; $t^1/_2$ (hrs)	2 to 4	NA

Special Populations

Pediatric: Ponstel has not been adequately investigated in pediatric patients less than 14 years of age. A study in 17 preterm infants administered 2 mg/kg indicated that the half-life was about five times as long as adults, consistent with the low activity of metabolic enzymes in newborn infants. The mean Cmax in this study was 4 mcg/mL (range 2.9–6.1). The mean time to maximum concentration (Tmax) was 8 hours (range 2–18 hrs).[11]

Race: Pharmacokinetic differences due to race have not been identified.

Hepatic Insufficiency: Mefenamic acid pharmacokinetics have not been studied in patients with hepatic dysfunction. As hepatic metabolism is a significant pathway of mefenamic acid elimination, patients with acute and chronic hepatic disease may require reduced doses of Ponstel compared to patients with normal hepatic function.

Renal Insufficiency: Mefenamic acid pharmacokinetics have not been investigated in subjects with renal insufficiency. Given that mefenamic acid, its metabolites and conjugates are primarily excreted by the kidneys, the potential exists for mefenamic acid metabolites to accumulate. Ponstel should not be administered to patients with preexisting renal disease or in patients with significantly impaired renal function.

Clinical Studies

In controlled, double-blind, clinical trials, Ponstel was evaluated for the treatment of primary spasmodic dysmenorrhea. The parameters used in determining efficacy included pain assessment by both patient and investigator; the need for concurrent analgesic medication; and evaluation of change in frequency and severity of symptoms characteristic of spasmodic dysmenorrhea. Patients received either Ponstel, 500 mg (2 capsules) as an initial dose of 250 mg every 6 hours, or placebo at onset of bleeding or of pain, whichever began first. After three menstrual cycles, patients were crossed over to the alternate treatment for an additional three cycles. Ponstel was significantly superior to placebo in all parameters, and both treatments (drug and placebo) were equally tolerated.

INDICATIONS AND USAGE

Ponstel is indicated:

- For relief of mild to moderate pain in patients ≥14 years of age, when therapy will not exceed one week (7 days).

Continued on next page

Ponstel—Cont.

• For treatment of primary dysmenorrhea.

CONTRAINDICATIONS

Ponstel is contraindicated in patients with known hypersensitivity to mefenamic acid. Ponstel should not be given to patients who have experienced asthma, urticaria, or allergic-type reactions after taking aspirin or other NSAIDs. Severe, rarely fatal, anaphylactic-like reactions to NSAIDs have been reported in such patients (see WARNINGS—Anaphylactoid Reactions, and PRECAUTIONS—Preexisting Asthma).

Ponstel is contraindicated in patients with active ulceration or chronic inflammation of either the upper or lower gastrointestinal tract.

Ponstel should not be used in patients with preexisting renal disease.

WARNINGS

Gastrointestinal (GI) Effects—Risk of GI Ulceration, Bleeding, and Perforation

Serious gastrointestinal toxicity, such as inflammation, bleeding, ulceration, and perforation of the stomach, small intestine or large intestine, can occur at any time, with or without warning symptoms, in patients treated with nonsteroidal anti-inflammatory drugs (NSAIDs). Minor upper gastrointestinal problems, such as dyspepsia, are common and may also occur at any time during NSAID therapy. Therefore, physicians and patients should remain alert for ulceration and bleeding, even in the absence of previous GI tract symptoms. Patients should be informed about the signs and/or symptoms of serious GI toxicity and the steps to take if they occur. The utility of periodic laboratory monitoring has not been demonstrated, nor has it been adequately assessed. Only one in five patients, who develop a serious upper GI adverse event on NSAID therapy, is symptomatic. It has been demonstrated that upper GI ulcers, gross bleeding or perforation, caused by NSAIDs, appear to occur in approximately 1% of patients treated for 3–6 months, and in about 2–4% of patients treated for one year. These trends continue, thus increasing the likelihood of developing a serious GI event at some time during the course of therapy. However, even short-term therapy is not without risk.

NSAIDs should be prescribed with extreme caution in those with a prior history of ulcer disease or gastrointestinal bleeding. Most spontaneous reports of fatal GI events are in elderly or debilitated patients and therefore special care should be taken in treating this population. To minimize the potential risk for an adverse GI event, the lowest effective dose should be used for the shortest possible duration. For high risk patients, alternate therapies that do not involve NSAIDs should be considered.

Studies have shown that patients with a *prior history of peptic ulcer disease and/or gastrointestinal bleeding* and who use NSAIDs, have a greater than 10-fold risk for developing a GI bleed than patients with neither of these risk factors. In addition to a past history of ulcer disease, pharmacoepidemiological studies have identified several other cotherapies or comorbid conditions that may increase the risk for GI bleeding such as: treatment with oral corticosteroids, treatment with anticoagulants, longer duration of NSAID therapy, smoking, alcoholism, older age, and poor general health status.

Anaphylactoid Reactions

As with other NSAIDs, anaphylactoid reactions may occur in patients without known prior exposure to Ponstel. Ponstel should not be given to patients with the aspirin triad. This symptom complex typically occurs in asthmatic patients who experience rhinitis with or without nasal polyps, or who exhibit severe, potentially fatal bronchospasm after taking aspirin or other NSAIDs (see CONTRAINDICATIONS and PRECAUTIONS—Preexisting Asthma). Emergency help should be sought in cases where an anaphylactoid reaction occurs.

Advanced Renal Disease

In cases with preexisting advanced kidney disease, treatment with Ponstel is not recommended (see CONTRAINDICATIONS).

Pregnancy

In late pregnancy, as with other NSAIDs, Ponstel should be avoided because it may cause premature closure of the ductus arteriosus.

PRECAUTIONS

General

Ponstel cannot be expected to substitute for corticosteroids or to treat corticosteroid insufficiency. Abrupt discontinuation of corticosteroids may lead to disease exacerbation. Patients on prolonged corticosteroid therapy should have their therapy tapered slowly if a decision is made to discontinue corticosteroids.

Because Ponstel reduces inflammation, it may diminish the diagnostic signs for detecting complications of presumed noninfectious, painful conditions.

Hepatic Effects

Borderline elevations of one or more liver function tests may occur in up to 15% of patients taking NSAIDs, including Ponstel. These laboratory abnormalities may progress, may remain unchanged, or may be transient with continuing therapy. Notable elevations of ALT or AST (approximately three or more times the upper limit of normal) have been reported in approximately 1% of patients in clinical trials with NSAIDs. In addition, rare cases of severe hepatic reactions, including jaundice and fatal fulminant hepatitis, liver necrosis and hepatic failure, some of them with fatal outcomes have been reported.

A patient with symptoms and/or signs suggesting liver dysfunction, or in whom an abnormal liver test has occurred, should be evaluated for evidence of the development of a more severe hepatic reaction while on therapy with Ponstel. If clinical signs and symptoms consistent with liver disease develop, or if systemic manifestations occur (eg, eosinophilia, rash, etc.), Ponstel should be discontinued.

Renal Effects

Caution should be used when initiating treatment with Ponstel in patients with considerable dehydration. It is advisable to rehydrate patients first and then start therapy with Ponstel. Ponstel is not recommended in patients with pre-existing kidney disease (see CONTRAINDICATIONS). Long-term administration of Ponstel has resulted in renal papillary necrosis and other renal medullary changes. Renal toxicity has also been seen in patients in which renal prostaglandins have a compensatory role in the maintenance of renal perfusion. In these patients, administration of a nonsteroidal anti-inflammatory drug may cause a dose-dependant reduction in prostaglandin formation and, secondarily, in renal blood flow, which may precipitate overt renal decompensation. Patients at greatest risk of this reaction are those with impaired renal function, heart failure, liver dysfunction, those taking diuretics and ACE inhibitors, and the elderly. Discontinuation of nonsteroidal anti-inflammatory drug therapy is usually followed by recovery to the pretreatment state.

Ponstel metabolites are eliminated primarily by the kidneys. The extent to which the metabolites may accumulate in patients with renal failure has not been studied.

Hematological Effects

Anemia is sometimes seen in patients receiving NSAIDs, including Ponstel. This may be due to fluid retention, GI loss, or an effect upon erythropoiesis. Patients on long-term treatment with NSAIDs, including Ponstel, should have their hemoglobin or hematocrit checked if they exhibit any signs or symptoms of anemia.

All drugs which inhibit the biosynthesis of prostaglandins may interfere to some extent with platelet function and vascular responses to bleeding.

NSAIDs inhibit platelet aggregation and have been shown to prolong bleeding time in some patients. Unlike aspirin, their effect on platelet function is quantitatively less, or shorter duration, and reversible. Ponstel does not generally affect platelet counts, or partial thromboplastin time (PTT), but may prolong prothrombin time (PT). Patients receiving Ponstel who may be adversely affected by alterations in platelet function, such as those with coagulation disorders or patients receiving anticoagulants, should be carefully monitored.

Fluid Retention and Edema

Fluid retention and edema have been observed in some patients taking NSAIDs. Therefore, as with other NSAIDs, Ponstel should be used with caution in patients with fluid retention, hypertension, or heart failure.

Preexisting Asthma

Patients with asthma may have aspirin-sensitive asthma. The use of aspirin in patients with aspirin-sensitive asthma has been associated with severe bronchospasm which can be fatal. Since cross reactivity, including bronchospasm, between aspirin and other nonsteroidal anti-inflammatory drugs has been reported in such aspirin-sensitive patients, Ponstel should not be administered to patients with this form of aspirin sensitivity and should be used with caution in patients with preexisting asthma.

Information for Patients

Ponstel, like other drugs of its class, can cause discomfort and, rarely, more serious side effects, such as gastrointestinal bleeding, which may result in hospitalization and even fatal outcomes. Although serious GI tract ulcerations and bleeding can occur without warning symptoms, patients should be alert for the signs and symptoms of ulcerations and bleeding, and should ask for medical advice when observing any indicative sign or symptoms. Patients should be apprised of the importance of this follow-up (see WARNING, Risk of Gastrointestinal Ulceration, Bleeding and Perforation).

Patients should report to their physicians signs or symptoms of gastrointestinal ulceration or bleeding, skin rash, weight gain, or edema.

Patients should be informed of the warning signs and symptoms of hepatotoxicity (eg, nausea, fatigue, lethargy, pruritus, jaundice, right upper quadrant tenderness, and "flu-like" symptoms). If these occur, patients should be instructed to stop therapy and seek immediate medical therapy.

Patients should also be instructed to seek immediate emergency help in the case of an anaphylactoid reaction (see WARNINGS).

In late pregnancy, as with other NSAIDs, Ponstel should be avoided because it may cause premature closure of the ductus arteriosus.

NSAIDs are often essential agents in the management of arthritis and have a major role in the treatment of pain, but they also may be commonly employed for conditions which are less serious.

Physicians may wish to discuss with their patients the potential risks (see WARNINGS, PRECAUTIONS, and ADVERSE REACTIONS sections) and likely benefits of NSAID treatment, particularly when the drugs are used for less serious conditions where treatment without NSAIDs may represent an acceptable alternative to both the patient and physician.

Laboratory Tests

Patients on long-term treatment with NSAIDs should have their CBC and a chemistry profile checked periodically. If clinical signs and symptoms consistent with liver or renal disease develop, systemic manifestations occur (eg, eosinophilia, rash, etc.) or if abnormal liver tests persist or worsen, Ponstel should be discontinued.

Drug Interactions

Aspirin: As with other NSAIDs, concomitant administration of Ponstel and aspirin is not generally recommended because of the potential of increased adverse effects.

Methotrexate: NSAIDs have been reported to competitively inhibit methotrexate accumulation in rabbit kidney slices. This may indicate that they could enhance the toxicity of methotrexate. Caution should be used when NSAIDs are administered concomitantly with methotrexate.

ACE inhibitors: Reports suggest that NSAIDs may diminish the antihypertensive effect of ACE inhibitors. This interaction should be given consideration in patients taking NSAIDs concomitantly with ACE inhibitors.

Furosemide: Clinical studies, as well as post-marketing observations, have shown that NSAIDs can reduce the natriuretic effect of furosemide and thiazides in some patients. This response has been attributed to inhibition of renal prostaglandin synthesis. During concomitant therapy of Ponstel with furosemide, the patient should be observed closely for signs of renal failure (see PRECAUTIONS, Renal Effects), as well as to assure diuretic efficacy.

Lithium: NSAIDs have produced an elevation of plasma lithium levels and a reduction in renal lithium clearance. The mean minimum lithium concentration increased 15% and the renal clearance was decreased by approximately 20%. These effects have been attributed to inhibition of renal prostaglandin synthesis by the NSAID. Thus, when NSAIDs and lithium are administered concurrently, subjects should be observed carefully for signs of lithium toxicity.

Warfarin: The effects of warfarin and NSAIDs on GI bleeding are synergistic, such that users of both drugs together have a risk of serious GI bleeding higher than users of either drug alone.

Antacids: In a single dose study (n=6), ingestion of an antacid containing 1.7-gram of magnesium hydroxide with 500-mg of mefenamic acid increased the Cmax and AUC of mefenamic acid by 125% and 36%, respectively.[1]

A number of compounds are inhibitors of CYP2C9 including fluconazole, lovastatin and trimethoprim. Drug interaction studies of mefenamic acid of these compounds have not been conducted. The possibility of altered safety and efficacy should be considered when Ponstel is used concomitantly with these drugs.

Drug/Laboratory Test Interactions

Ponstel may prolong prothrombin time.[4] Therefore, when the drug is administered to patients receiving oral anticoagulant drugs, frequent monitoring of prothrombin time is necessary.

A false-positive reaction for urinary bile, using the diazo tablet test, may result after mefenamic acid administration. If biliuria is suspected, other diagnostic procedures, such as the Harrison spot test, should be performed.

Pregnancy

Teratogenic Effects: *Pregnancy Category C.* Reproduction studies have been performed in rats, rabbits, and dogs. Rats given up to 10 times the human dose showed decreased fertility, delay in parturition, and a decreased rate of survival to weaning. Rabbits at 2.5 times the human dose showed an increase in the number of resorptions. There were no fetal anomalies observed in these studies nor in dogs at up to 10 times the human dose.[4]

However, animal reproduction studies are not always predictive of human response. There are no adequate and well-controlled studies in pregnant women. Ponstel should be used during pregnancy only if the potential benefit justifies the potential risk to the fetus.

Nonteratogenic Effects: Because of the known effects of nonsteroidal anti-inflammatory drugs on the fetal cardiovascular system (closure of ductus arteriosus), use during pregnancy (particularly late pregnancy) should be avoided.

Labor and Delivery

In rat studies with NSAIDs, as with other drugs known to inhibit prostaglandin synthesis, an increased incidence of dystocia, delayed parturition, and decreased pup survival occurred. The effects of Ponstel on labor and delivery in pregnant women are unknown.

Nursing Mothers

Trace amounts of Ponstel may be present in breast milk and transmitted to the nursing infant.[7] Because of the potential for serious adverse reactions in nursing infants from Ponstel, a decision should be made whether to discontinue nursing or to discontinue the drug, taking into account the importance of the drug to the mother.

Pediatric Use

Safety and effectiveness in pediatric patients below the age of 14 have not been established.

Geriatric Use

As with any NSAID, caution should be exercised in treating the elderly (65 years and older).

ADVERSE REACTIONS

In patients taking Ponstel or other NSAIDs, the most frequently reported adverse experiences occurring in approximately 1–10% of patients are:

Gastrointestinal experiences including—abdominal pain, constipation, diarrhea, dyspepsia, flatulence, gross bleeding/perforation, heartburn, nausea, GI ulcers (gastric/duodenal), vomiting, abnormal renal function, anemia, dizziness, edema, elevated liver enzymes, headaches, increased bleeding time, pruritus, rashes, tinnitus

Additional adverse experiences reported occasionally and listed here by body system include:

Body as a whole—fever, infection, sepsis

Cardiovascular system—congestive heart failure, hypertension, tachycardia, syncope

Digestive system—dry mouth, esophagitis, gastric/peptic ulcers, gastritis, gastrointestinal bleeding, glossitis, hematemesis, hepatitis, jaundice

Hemic and lymphatic system—ecchymosis, eosinophilia, leukopenia, melena, purpura, rectal bleeding, stomatitis, thrombocytopenia

Metabolic and nutritional—weight changes

Nervous system—anxiety, asthenia, confusion, depression, dream abnormalities, drowsiness, insomnia, malaise, nervousness, paresthesia, somnolence, tremors, vertigo

Respiratory system—asthma, dyspnea

Skin and appendages—alopecia, photosensitivity, pruritus, sweat

Special senses—blurred vision

Urogenital system—cystitis, dysuria, hematuria, interstitial nephritis, oliguria/polyuria, proteinuria, renal failure

Other adverse reactions, which occur rarely are:

Body as a whole—anaphylactoid reactions, appetite changes, death

Cardiovascular system—arrhythmia, hypotension, myocardial infarction, palpitations, vasculitis

Digestive system—eructation, liver failure, pancreatitis

Hemic and lymphatic system—agranulocytosis, hemolytic anemia, aplastic anemia, lymphadenopathy, pancytopenia

Metabolic and nutritional—hyperglycemia

Nervous system—convulsions, coma, hallucinations, meningitis

Respiratory—respiratory depression, pneumonia

Skin and appendages—angioedema, toxic epidermal necrosis, erythema multiforme, exfoliative dermatitis, Stevens-Johnson syndrome, urticaria

Special senses—conjunctivitis, hearing impairment

OVERDOSAGE

Symptoms following acute NSAIDs overdoses are usually limited to lethargy, drowsiness, nausea, vomiting, and epigastric pain, which are generally reversible with supportive care. Gastrointestinal bleeding can occur. Hypertension, acute renal failure, respiratory depression and coma may occur, but are rare. Anaphylactoid reactions have been reported with therapeutic ingestion of NSAIDs, and may occur following an overdose.

Patients should be managed by symptomatic and supportive care following a NSAID overdose. There are no specific antidotes. Emesis and/or activated charcoal (60 to 100 g in adults, 1 to 2 g/kg in children) and/or osmotic cathartic may be indicated in patients seen within 4 hours of ingestion with symptoms or following a large overdose (5 to 10 times the usual dose). Forced diuresis, alkalinization of urine, hemodialysis, or hemoperfusion may not be useful due to high protein binding.

DOSAGE AND ADMINISTRATION

As with other NSAIDs, the lowest dose should be sought for each patient. Therefore, after observing the response to initial therapy with Ponstel, the dose and frequency should be adjusted to suit an individual patient's needs.

Administration is by the oral route, preferably with food.

For relief of acute pain in adults and adolescents ≥14 years of age, the recommended dose is 500 mg as an initial dose followed by 250 mg every 6 hours as needed, usually not to exceed one week.[4]

For the treatment of primary dysmenorrhea, the recommended dose is 500 mg as an initial dose followed by 250 mg every 6 hours, starting with the onset of bleeding and associated symptoms. Clinical studies indicate that effective treatment can be initiated with the start of menses and should not be necessary for more than 2 to 3 days.[5]

HOW SUPPLIED

Ponstel (mefenamic acid) is available as 250 mg blue-banded, ivory capsules, imprinted with "FHPC 400."

Bottles of 100 N 59630-0400-10

Storage

Store at controlled room temperature 15°–30°C (59°–86°F). Protect from moisture.

REFERENCES

1. Neuvonen PJ, Kivisto KT: Enhancement of drug absorption by antacids. An unrecognized drug interation. *Clin Pharmacokinet.* 27: 120–8, Aug 1994.
2. Tall AR, Mistilits SP: Studies on Ponstan (mefenamic acid): I. Gastro-intestinal blood loss; II. Absorption and excretion of a new formulation. *J Int Med Res* (UK). 1975, 3 (3) p176-82.
3. Winder CV, Kaump DH, Glazko et al: Experimental observations of flufenamic, mefenamic, and meclofenamic acids. *AnnPhys Med* (Eng), Suppl p7–49. 1967.
4. Glazko AJ: Experimental observations of flufenamic, mefenamic, and meclofenamic acids. Part III. Metabolic disposition, in *Fenamates in Medicine.* A Symposium, London, 1966. *Annals of Physical Medicine,* Supplement, pp 23–36, 1967.
5. Data on file, Medical Affairs Dept, Parke-Davis.
6. Budoff PW: Use of mefenamic acid in the treatment of primary dysmenorrhea. *JAMA.* 241:2713–2716, 1979.
7. Buchanan RA, et al. The breast milk excretion of mefenamic acid. *Curr Ther Res.* 10:592, 1968.
8. Corby DG, Decker WJ: Management of acute poisioning with activated charcoal. *Pediatrics.* 54:324, 1974.
9. Champion GD, Graham GG: Pharmacokinetics of non-steroidal anti-inflammatory agents. *Aust NZ J Med.* 8 (Supp 1): 94–100, Jun 1978.
10. McGurk KA, Remmel RP, Hosagrahara VP, Tosh D, Burchell B: Reactivity of mefenamic acid 1-o- acyl glucuronide with proteins in vitro and ex vivo. *Drug Metab Dispos.* Aug 1996, 24 (8) p842–9.
11. Ito K, Niida Y, Sato J et al: Pharmacokinetics of mefenamic acid in preterm infants with patent ductus arteriosus. *Acta Paediatr JPN.* 36 (4): 387-91, 1994.

Rx only

Revised May 2000

Manufactured by

PARKE-DAVIS

Div or Warner-Lambert Co

Morris Plains, NJ 07950 USA

Distributed by

First Horizon Pharmaceutical Corporation

Roswell, GA 30076

PROTUSS® LIQUID Ⓒ℞

[prō-təs]

DESCRIPTION

Each teaspoonful (5 mL) grape flavored liquid contains:

Hydrocodone Bitartrate	5 mg
(Warning: May be habit forming)	
Potassium Guaiacolsulfonate	300 mg

HOW SUPPLIED

Bottles of 4 oz and 16 oz.

PROTUSS®-D LIQUID Ⓒ℞

[prō-təs-D]

DESCRIPTION

Each teaspoonful (5 mL) contains:

Hydrocodone Bitartrate	5 mg
(Warning: May be habit forming)	
Potassium Guaiacolsulfonate	300 mg
Pseudoephedrine HCl	30 mg

HOW SUPPLIED

Bottles of 4 oz and 16 oz

PROTUSS®-DM TABLETS ℞

[prō-təs-DM]

DESCRIPTION

Each dye-free, film-coated tablet imprinted PRO DM and scored contains:

Dextromethorphan HBr	30 mg
Pseudoephedrine HCl	60 mg
Guaifenesin	600 mg

HOW SUPPLIED

Bottles of 100

ROBINUL® and ROBINUL® FORTE ℞

(glycopyrrolate tablets, USP)

CI 4859-2

DESCRIPTION

Robinul® and Robinul® Forte tablets contain the synthetic anticholinergic, glycopyrrolate. Glycopyrrolate is a quaternary ammonium compound with the following chemical name: 3-[(cyclopentylhydroxyphenylacetyl)oxy]-1,1-dimethylpyrrolidinium bromide.

Robinul® tablets are scored, compressed white tablets engraved HPC 200. Each tablet contains:

Glycopyrrolate, USP .... 1 mg

Robinul® Forte tablets are scored, compressed white tablets engraved HORIZON 205. Each tablet contains:

Glycopyrrolate, USP .... 2 mg

Inactive Ingredients: Dibasic Calcium Phosphate, Lactose, Magnesium Stearate, Povidone, Sodium Starch Glycolate.

ACTIONS

Glycopyrrolate, like other anticholinergic (antimuscarinic) agents, inhibits the action of acetylcholine on structures innervated by postganglionic cholinergic nerves and on smooth muscles that respond to acetylcholine but lack cholinergic innervation. These peripheral cholinergic receptors are present in the autonomic effector cells of smooth muscle, cardiac muscle, the sino-atrial node, the atrioventricular node, exocrine glands, and, to a limited degree, in the autonomic ganglia. Thus, it diminishes the volume and free acidity of gastric secretions and controls excessive pharyngeal, tracheal, and bronchial secretions.

Glycopyrrolate antagonizes muscarinic symptoms (e.g., bronchorrhea, bronchospasm, bradycardia, and intestinal hypermotility) induced by cholinergic drugs such as the anticholinesterases.

The highly polar quaternary ammonium group of glycopyrrolate limits its passage across lipid membranes, such as the blood-brain barrier, in contrast to atropine sulfate and scopolamine hydrobromide, which are non-polar tertiary amines which penetrate lipid barriers easily.

INDICATIONS

For use as adjunctive therapy in the treatment of peptic ulcer.

CONTRAINDICATIONS

Glaucoma; obstructive uropathy (for example, bladder neck obstruction due to prostatic hypertrophy); obstructive disease of the gastrointestinal tract (as in achalasia, pyloroduodenal stenosis, etc.); paralytic ileus; intestinal atony of the elderly or debilitated patient; unstable cardiovascular status in acute hemorrhage; severe ulcerative colitis; toxic megacolon complicating ulcerative colitis; myasthenia gravis. Robinul® (glycopyrrolate) tablets are contraindicated in those patients with a hypersensitivity to glycopyrrolate.

WARNINGS

In the presence of a high environmental temperature, heat prostration (fever and heat stroke due to decreased sweating) can occur with use of Robinul®.

Diarrhea may be an early symptom of incomplete intestinal obstruction, especially in patients with ileostomy or colostomy. In this instance treatment with this drug would be inappropriate and possibly harmful.

Robinul® (glycopyrrolate) may produce drowsiness or blurred vision. In this event, the patient should be warned not to engage in activities requiring mental alertness such as operating a motor vehicle or other machinery, or performing hazardous work while taking this drug.

Theoretically, with overdosage, a curare-like action may occur, i.e., neuromuscular blockade leading to muscular weakness and possible paralysis.

Pregnancy

The safety of this drug during pregnancy has not been established. The use of any drug during pregnancy requires that the potential benefits of the drug be weighed against possible hazards to mother and child. Reproduction studies in rats revealed no teratogenic effects from glycopyrrolate; however, the potent anti-cholinergic action of this agent resulted in diminished rates of conception and of survival at weaning, in a dose-related manner. Other studies in dogs suggest that this may be due to diminished seminal secretion which is evident at high doses of glycopyrrolate. Information on possible adverse effects in the pregnant female is limited to uncontrolled data derived from marketing experience. Such experience has revealed no reports of teratogenic or other fetus-damaging potential. No controlled studies to establish the safety of the drug in pregnancy have been performed.

Nursing Mothers

It is not known whether this drug is excreted in human milk. As a general rule, nursing should not be undertaken while a patient is on a drug since many drugs are excreted in human milk.

Pediatric Use

Since there is no adequate experience in pediatric patients who have received this drug, safety and efficacy in pediatric patients have not been established.

PRECAUTIONS

Use Robinul® with caution in the elderly and in all patients with:

- Autonomic neuropathy.
- Hepatic or renal disease.
- Ulcerative colitis—large doses may suppress intestinal motility to the point of producing a paralytic ileus and for this reason may precipitate or aggravate "toxic megacolon," a serious complication of the disease.
- Hyperthyroidism, coronary heart disease, congestive heart failure, cardiac tachyarrhythmias, tachycardia, hypertension and prostatic hypertrophy.
- Hiatal hernia associated with reflux esophagitis, since anticholinergic drugs may aggravate this condition.

ADVERSE REACTIONS

Anticholinergics produce certain effects, most of which are extensions of their fundamental pharmacological actions. Adverse reactions to anticholinergics in general may include xerostomia; decreased sweating; urinary hesitancy and retention; blurred vision; tachycardia; palpitations; dilatation of the pupil; cycloplegia; increased ocular tension; loss of taste; headaches; nervousness; mental confusion; drowsiness; weakness; dizziness; insomnia; nausea; vomiting; constipation; bloated feeling; impotence; suppression of lactation; severe allergic reaction or drug idiosyncrasies including anaphylaxis, urticaria and other dermal manifestations.

Robinul® (glycopyrrolate) is chemically a quaternary ammonium compound; hence, its passage across lipid membranes, such as the blood-brain barrier, is limited in contrast to atropine sulfate and scopolamine hydrobromide. For this reason the occurrence of CNS related side effects is

Continued on next page

Robinul—Cont.

lower, in comparison to their incidence following administration of anticholinergics which are chemically tertiary amines that can cross this barrier readily.

OVERDOSAGE

The symptoms of overdosage of glycopyrrolate are peripheral in nature rather than central.

1. To guard against further absorption of the drug—use gastric lavage, cathartics and/or enemas.
2. To combat peripheral anticholinergic effects (residual mydriasis, dry mouth, etc.)—utilize a quaternary ammonium anticholinesterase, such as neostigmine methylsulfate.
3. To combat hypotension—use pressor amines (norepinephrine, metaraminol) i.v.; and supportive care.
4. To combat respiratory depression—administer oxygen; utilize a respiratory stimulant such as Dopram® i.v.; artificial respiration.

DOSAGE AND ADMINISTRATION

The dosage of Robinul® or Robinul® Forte should be adjusted to the needs of the individual patient to assure symptomatic control with a minimum of adverse reactions. The presently recommended maximum daily dosage of glycopyrrolate is 8 mg.

Robinul® (glycopyrrolate, 1 mg) tablets. The recommended initial dosage of Robinul® for adults is one tablet three times daily (in the morning, early afternoon, and at bedtime). Some patients may require two tablets at bedtime to assure overnight control of symptoms. For maintenance, a dosage of one tablet twice a day is frequently adequate.

Robinul® Forte (glycopyrrolate, 2 mg) tablets. The recommended dosage of Robinul® Forte for adults is one tablet two or three times daily at equally spaced intervals.

Robinul® tablets are not recommended for use in pediatric patients under the age of 12 years.

Drug Interactions

There are no known drug interactions.

HOW SUPPLIED

Robinul® (glycopyrrolate, 1 mg) tablets in bottles of 100 (NDC 59630-200-10).

Robinul® Forte (glycopyrrolate, 2 mg) tablets in bottles of 100 (NDC 59630-205-10).

Store at controlled room temperature, 20°–25° C (68°–77° F).

Dispense in tight container.

Rx only

Manufactured By Pharmaceutical Division
A.H. Robins Company
Richmond, VA 23220
Manufactured for:
First Horizon Pharmaceutical™ Corporation
CI 4859-2 Revised May 2, 2000

TANAFED® SUSPENSION ℞
[tan-ă-fed]

DESCRIPTION

Each teaspoonful (5 mL) strawberry/banana flavored suspension contains:

Chlorpheniramine Tannate	4.5 mg
Pseudoephedrine Tannate	75.0 mg

HOW SUPPLIED

Bottles of 4 oz and 16 oz

ZEBUTAL™ CAPSULES ℞
[zĕb "ūt 'al]

DESCRIPTION:

Each Salmon/red capsule imprinted "◆ HPC" and "170" white ink contains:

Butalbital, USP 50 mg
Acetaminophen, USP 500 mg
Caffeine, USP 40 mg

HOW SUPPLIED

Bottles of 100 capsules
Bottles of 500 capsules

ZOTO®-HC EAR DROPS ℞
[zō-tō]

DESCRIPTION

Each 1 mL contains:

Chloroxylenol	1 mg
Pramoxine HCl	10 mg
Hydrocortisone	10 mg

HOW SUPPLIED

Plastic dropper vials of 10 mL.

C. B. Fleet Co., Inc.
4615 MURRAY PL.
LYNCHBURG, VA 24506-1349

Direct Inquiries to:
David Vaughan
Director of Quality Assurance:
(804) 528-4000

FLEET® GLYCERIN LAXATIVES: SUPPOSITORIES AND LIQUID GLYCERIN SUPPOSITORIES OTC
(glycerin USP)

COMPOSITION

FLEET® Babylax®—Each rectal applicator delivers 2.3g of glycerin USP

FLEET® Liquid Glycerin Suppositories for Adults and Children 6 years of age and over—Each rectal applicator delivers 5.6g of glycerin USP

FLEET® Maximum-Strength Glycerin Suppositories for Adults—Each suppository contains 3g of glycerin USP

FLEET® Glycerin Suppositories for Adults—Each suppository contains 2g of glycerin USP

FLEET® Glycerin Suppositories for Children 2 years to under 6—Each suppository contains 1g of glycerin USP

ACTIONS AND USES

Glycerin is a hyperosmotic laxative, which is given rectally, and usually produces a bowel movement within 15 minutes to 1 hour. The laxative effect of glycerin is due to the local irritant effect of sodium stearate and glycerin's osmotic effect. However, rectal irritation may occur with its use. The hyperosmotic laxative effect of glycerin attracts water into the stool. These products are used for fast, predictable relief of occasional constipation.

GENERAL LAXATIVE WARNINGS

Do not use a laxative product when nausea, vomiting, or abdominal pain is present unless directed by a physician. If you notice a sudden change in bowel habits that persists over a period of 2 weeks, consult a physician before using a laxative. Rectal bleeding or failure to have a bowel movement after use of a laxative may indicate a serious condition. Discontinue use and consult a physician. Laxative products should not be used longer than 1 week unless directed by a physician. This product may cause rectal discomfort or a burning sensation. Keep this and all drugs out of the reach of children. In case of accidental overdose or ingestion, seek professional assistance or contact a Poison Control Center immediately.

DOSAGE AND ADMINISTRATION

FLEET® Babylax®—Children 2 to under 6 years: 1 unit or as directed by a physician. Children under 2 years: Consult a physician.

Preferred position: Place child on left side with knees bent and arms resting comfortably, or have child kneel, then lower head and chest forward until left side of face is resting on surface with left arm folded comfortably.

CAUTION: REMOVE ORANGE PROTECTIVE SHIELD FROM TIP BEFORE INSERTING. Hold unit upright, grasping bulb of unit with fingers. Grasp orange protective shield with other hand, pull gently to remove. With steady pressure, gently insert tip into rectum with a slight side-to-side movement, with tip pointing towards navel. **DISCONTINUE USE IF RESISTANCE IS ENCOUNTERED. FORCING THE TIP CAN RESULT IN INJURY.** Insertion may be easier if child receiving suppository bears down as if having a bowel movement. This helps relax the muscles around the anus. Squeeze the bulb until nearly all liquid has been expelled. While continuing to squeeze the bulb, remove tip from rectum and discard unit. It is not necessary to empty unit completely. The unit contains more than the amount of liquid needed for effective use. A small amount of liquid will remain in the unit after squeezing.

FLEET® Liquid Glycerin Suppositories for Adults and Children 6 years of age and older: One unit or as directed by a physician.

Preferred position: Lie on left side with right knee bent and arms resting comfortably, or kneel, then lower head and chest forward until left side of face is resting on surface with left arm folded comfortably.

CAUTION: REMOVE ORANGE PROTECTIVE SHIELD BEFORE INSERTING. Hold unit upright, grasping bulb of unit with fingers. Grasp orange protective shield with other hand, pull gently to remove. With steady pressure, insert tip into rectum with a slight side-to-side movement, with tip pointing toward navel. **DISCONTINUE USE IF RESISTANCE IS ENCOUNTERED. FORCING THE TIP CAN RESULT IN INJURY.** Insertion may be easier if person receiving suppository bears down as if having a bowel movement. This helps relax the muscles around the anus. Squeeze the bulb until nearly all liquid has been expelled. While continuing to squeeze the bulb, remove tip from rectum and discard unit. It is not necessary to empty unit completely. The unit contains more than the amount of liquid needed for use. A small amount of liquid will remain in the unit after squeezing.

FLEET® Maximum-Strength Glycerin Suppositories—Adults and Children 6 years of age and older: One suppository.

Remove foil wrapper and insert one suppository well up into rectum. Suppository need not melt completely to produce laxative action. Keep away from excessive heat.

FLEET® Glycerin Suppositories—Adults and Children 6 years of age and older: One suppository.

If foil-wrapped, remove foil wrapper. Insert one suppository well up into rectum. Suppository need not melt to produce laxative action. Store container tightly closed and keep away from excessive heat.

FLEET® Glycerin Suppositories Child Size—Children 2 to under 6 years: One suppository.

Children under 2 years: Consult a physician.

Insert suppository well up into rectum. Suppository need not melt completely to produce laxative action. Store container tightly closed and keep away from excessive heat.

HOW SUPPLIED

FLEET® Babylax®—Each box contains 6 child rectal applicators (4 mL each).

FLEET® Liquid Glycerin Suppositories for Adults and Children 6 years of age and over—Each box contains 4 adult rectal applicators (7.5 mL each).

FLEET® Maximum-Strength Glycerin Suppositories—Each box contains 18 individually foil-wrapped adult suppositories.

FLEET® Glycerin Suppositories—Available in jars of 12, 24, and 50 adult suppositories as well as a box containing 12 individually foil-wrapped adult suppositories.

FLEET® Glycerin Suppositories Child Size—Available in jars of 12

IS THIS PRODUCT OTC?

Yes.

FLEET® BISACODYL LAXATIVES: ENEMA, SUPPOSITORIES, AND TABLETS OTC
(bisacodyl USP)

COMPOSITION

Latex free FLEET® Bisacodyl Enema - 10 mg bisacodyl USP enema solution in a 37 mL ready-to-use squeeze bottle with a 2-inch, pre-lubricated Comfortip®. Disposable after single use.

FLEET® Stimulant Laxative Tablets - Enteric coated 5 mg bisacodyl USP tablets.

FLEET® Laxative Suppositories - 10 mg bisacodyl USP suppositories.

ACTION AND USES

Bisacodyl is a stimulant laxative, given either orally or rectally, acting directly on the colonic mucosa where it stimulates sensory nerve endings to produce parasympathetic reflexes resulting in increased peristaltic contractions of the colon. The contact action of the drug is restricted to the colon and motility in the small intestine is not appreciably influenced. FLEET® Stimulant Laxative Tablets usually work within 6–12 hours. FLEET® Laxative Suppositories produce a bowel movement within 15 minutes to 1 hour and the **latex free** FLEET® Bisacodyl Enema produces a bowel movement within 15–20 minutes. Bisacodyl is useful as a laxative for occasional relief of constipation, in bowel cleansing in preparation for X-ray and endoscopic examination. May be used as a laxative in postoperative, antepartum, or postpartum care or in preparation for delivery.

GENERAL LAXATIVE WARNINGS

Do not use a laxative product when nausea, vomiting, or abdominal pain is present unless directed by a physician. If you notice a sudden change in bowel habits that persists over a period of 2 weeks, consult a physician before using a laxative. Rectal bleeding or failure to have a bowel movement after use of a laxative may indicate a serious condition. Discontinue use and consult a physician. Laxative products should not be used longer than 1 week unless directed by a physician. As with any drug, if you are pregnant or nursing a baby, seek the advice of a health professional before using this product. This product may cause abdominal discomfort, faintness, and cramps. Keep this and all drugs out of the reach of children. In case of accidental overdose or ingestion, seek professional assistance or contact a Poison Control Center immediately.

DOSAGE AND ADMINISTRATION

Enema

SHAKE BEFORE USING.

REMOVE ORANGE PROTECTIVE SHIELD FROM TIP BEFORE ADMINISTERING.

Dosage:

Adults and children 12 years of age and over: Use one 1.25 fl. oz. bottle (30 mL delivered dose) in a single daily dose.

Children under 12 years of age: DO NOT USE.

Preferred position: Lie on left side with left knee slightly bent and the right leg drawn up, or knee-chest position. Diaphragm at base of tube prevents accidental leakage and assures controlled flow of the enema solution. May be used at room temperature.

Tablets

Adults and children 12 years of age and over: Take 2 to 3 tablets (usually 2) in a single dose once daily.

Children 6 to under 12 years of age: Take 1 tablet once daily.

Expect results in 6–12 hours if taken at bedtime or within 6 hours if taken before breakfast. Swallow tablets whole. Do not chew or crush tablets. Do not administer tablets within 1 hour after taking an antacid, milk, or milk products.

Children under 6 years of age: Consult your physician.
Suppositories
Adults and children 12 years of age and over: Use 1 suppository once daily. Remove foil wrapper. Lie on your side and, with pointed end first, push suppository high into the rectum so it will not slip out. Retain it for 15 to 20 minutes. If you feel the suppository must come out immediately, it was not inserted high enough and should be pushed higher.
Children 6 to under 12 years of age: One half of one 10 mg suppository once daily.
Children under 6 years of age: Consult your physician.

PROFESSIONAL ADMINISTRATION

See FLEET® Ready-to-Use Enema and FLEET® Prep Kits.

HOW SUPPLIED
Enema
FLEET® Bisacodyl Enema is supplied in a 1.25 fl. oz. (37 mL) ready-to-use squeeze bottle.
IMPORTANT: FLEET® Bisacodyl Enema IS NOT INTENDED FOR ORAL CONSUMPTION, in any dosage size.
Tablets
FLEET® Stimulant Laxative Tablets are supplied in cartons of 25 tablets (5 mg each tablet) wrapped in a foil seal.
Suppositories
FLEET® Bisacodyl Suppositories are supplied in cartons of 4 individually foil-wrapped suppositories (10 mg each).
IS THIS PRODUCT OTC?
Yes.

FLEET® ENEMA, A SALINE LAXATIVE — OTC
FLEET® ENEMA FOR CHILDREN, A SALINE LAXATIVE

COMPOSITION

FLEET® ENEMA: Each 118 mL (delivered dose) contains 19 g monobasic sodium phosphate monohydrate and 7 g dibasic sodium phosphate heptahydrate. The **latex free** FLEET® Enema unit, with a 2-inch, pre-lubricated Comfortip®, contains 4.5 fl. oz. (133 mL) of enema solution in a ready-to-use squeeze bottle. FLEET® ENEMA FOR CHILDREN: Each 59 mL (delivered dose) contains 9.5 g monobasic sodium phosphate monohydrate and 3.5 g dibasic sodium phosphate heptahydrate. The **latex free** FLEET® Enema for Children unit, with a 2-inch, pre-lubricated Comfortip® contains 2.25 fl. oz. (66 mL) of enema solution in a ready-to-use squeeze bottle. Designed for quick, convenient administration by nurse or patient according to instructions. Disposable after single use.

ELEMENTAL & ELECTROLYTIC CONTENT

mEq Phosphate (PO_4) per mL	4.15
mEq Sodium (Na) per mL	1.61
mmole Phosphorus (P) per mL	1.38

ACTION AND USES

FLEET® Enema is useful as a laxative in the relief of occasional constipation, and as part of a bowel cleansing regimen in preparing the patient for surgery or for preparing the colon for x-ray and endoscopic examination. Used as directed, FLEET® Enema provides thorough yet safe cleansing action and induces complete emptying of the left colon usually within 2 to 5 minutes without pain or spasm. Also used for general postoperative care and to help relieve fecal or barium impaction.

GENERAL LAXATIVE WARNINGS

Using more than one enema in 24 hours can be harmful.
Do not use laxative products when nausea, vomiting, or abdominal pain is present unless directed by a physician. If you notice a sudden change in bowel habits that persists over a period of 2 weeks, consult a physician. Rectal bleeding or failure to have a bowel movement after use of a laxative may indicate a serious condition. Discontinue use and consult a physician. Laxative products should not be used longer than 1 week unless directed by a physician. As with any drug, if you are pregnant or nursing a baby, seek the advice of a health professional before using this product. Keep this and all drugs out of the reach of children. In case of accidental overdose or ingestion, seek professional assistance or contact a Poison Control Center immediately.

PROFESSIONAL USE WARNINGS

Do not use in patients with congenital megacolon, bowel obstruction, imperforate anus or congestive heart failure. Use with caution in patients with impaired renal function, pre-existing electrolyte disturbances or in patients on diuretics or other medications which may affect electrolyte levels—or where colostomy exists.
Since FLEET® Enema contains sodium phosphates, there is a risk of elevated serum levels of sodium and phosphate and decreased levels of calcium and potassium and consequently hypocalcemia, hyperphosphatemia, hypernatremia, and acidosis may occur. This is of particular concern in children with megacolon or any other condition where there is retention of enema solution.
Additional fluids by mouth are recommended with all bowel cleansing dosages.
SINCE FLEET® BRAND ENEMAS ARE AVAILABLE IN ADULT AND CHILDREN'S SIZES, PRESCRIBE CAREFULLY.

PRECAUTIONS

DO NOT ADMINISTER 4.5 OZ. ADULT SIZE TO CHILDREN UNDER 12 YEARS OF AGE. DO NOT ADMINISTER A FULL 2.25 OZ. CHILDREN'S SIZE TO CHILDREN UNDER 5 YEARS OF AGE. FOR CHILDREN 2 TO UNDER 5 YEARS, USE ONE-HALF BOTTLE (SEE **DOSAGE AND ADMINISTRATION**). DO NOT USE WITH CHILDREN UNDER 2 YEARS OF AGE. IF AFTER THE ENEMA SOLUTION IS ADMINISTERED THERE IS NO RETURN OF LIQUID, CONTACT A PHYSICIAN IMMEDIATELY AS DEHYDRATION COULD OCCUR.

OVERDOSAGE

Overdosage or retention of FLEET® Enema may cause hypocalcemia, hyperphosphatemia, hypernatremia, hypernatremic dehydration and acidosis.
Calcium, phosphate, potassium and sodium levels should be carefully monitored. Immediate corrective action should be taken to restore electrolyte balance with appropriate fluid replacements. Prompt parenteral administration of fluids with lower concentrations of sodium and chloride than extracellular fluid (40–50 mEq/liter) and moderate concentration of potassium (20–30 mEq/liter) administered at a rate of 3,000 to 4,000 cc/sq. m of body surface during the first 12 to 24 hours is dependent on the severity of dehydration and the clinical response.

DOSAGE AND ADMINISTRATION
Dosage: FLEET® Enema for Adults:
Do not use more unless directed by a doctor. See Warnings.

Adults and Children 12 years and over	One Bottle
Children 2 to 11 years	Use Fleet® Enema for Children
Children under 2 years	DO NOT USE

Sodium Content—4.4 g (191 mEq) in each 118 mL.
REMOVE ORANGE PROTECTIVE SHIELD FROM TIP BEFORE INSERTING.
Preferred position: Lie on left side with knee slightly bent and the right leg drawn up, or knee-chest position.
Diaphragm at base of tube prevents accidental leakage and assures controlled flow of the enema solution. May be used at room temperature.
Dosage: FLEET® Enema for Children:
Do not use more unless directed by a doctor. See Warnings.

Children 5 to 11 years	One Bottle or as directed by a doctor
Children 2 to under 5 years	One-Half Bottle (See Below)
Children under 2 years	DO NOT USE

One-half bottle preparation: Unscrew cap and remove 2 tablespoons of liquid with a measuring spoon. Replace cap and follow DIRECTIONS on back of carton.
Sodium Content—2.2 g (95.5 mEq) in each 59 mL.
REMOVE ORANGE PROTECTIVE SHIELD FROM TIP BEFORE INSERTING.
Preferred position: Lie on left side with knee slightly bent and the right leg drawn up, or knee-chest position.
Diaphragm at base of tube prevents accidental leakage and assures controlled flow of the enema solution. May be used at room temperature.

PROFESSIONAL DOSAGE AND ADMINISTRATION

FLEET® Enema for Adults should not be used in children under 12 years of age. In those cases where complications are reported, infants and young children are often involved. FLEET® Enema for Children should be used with caution in children of any age. Careful consideration of the use of enemas in general in children is recommended. See DOSAGE AND ADMINISTRATION for dosing detail.
Proper and safe use of FLEET® Enema also requires that the product be administered according to the Directions. Health care professionals should remember, when administering the product, to gently insert the enema into the rectum with the tip pointing toward the navel. Insertion may be made easier by having the patient bear down as they would in having a bowel movement. Care during insertion is necessary due to lack of sensory innervation of the rectum and due to possibility of bowel perforation. Once inserted, squeeze the bottle until nearly all the liquid is expelled. If resistance is encountered on insertion of the nozzle or in administering the solution, the procedure should be discontinued. Forcing the enema can result in perforation and/or abrasion of the rectum.
If an enema containing phosphate or sodium is not advised, use FLEET® Bisacodyl Enema.

HOW SUPPLIED

FLEET® Enema is supplied in a 4.5 fl. oz. (133 mL) ready-to-use squeeze bottle. Children's size, 2.25 fl. oz. (66 mL).
IMPORTANT: FLEET® Enema, Adult and children size, ARE NOT INTENDED FOR ORAL CONSUMPTION in any dosage size.

IS THIS PRODUCT OTC?

Yes.

FLEET® MINERAL OIL ENEMA — OTC
A LUBRICANT LAXATIVE

COMPOSITION

The **latex free** FLEET® Mineral Oil Enema unit, with a 2-inch, pre-lubricated Comfortip®, delivers 118 mL of mineral oil USP in a ready-to-use squeeze bottle. FLEET® Mineral Oil Enema is sodium free. Disposable after single use.

ACTION AND USES

FLEET® Mineral Oil Enema serves to soften and lubricate hard stools, easing their passage without irritating the mucosa. Results approximate a normal bowel movement in that only the rectum, sigmoid, and part or all of the descending colon are evacuated. Indicated for relief of fecal impaction; valuable in relief of occasional constipation when straining must be avoided (in hypertension, coronary occlusion, proctologic procedures, postoperative care); for removal of barium sulfate residues from the colon after barium administration for GI series or outlining the left atrium; to obtain the laxative benefits of mineral oil while avoiding possible untoward effects of oral administration such as (1) interference with intestinal absorption of fat-soluble vitamins A, D, E and K and other nutrients (2) danger of systemic absorption (3) possible risk of lipid pneumonia due to aspiration. Generally effective in 2 to 15 minutes.

GENERAL LAXATIVE WARNINGS

Do not use laxative products when nausea, vomiting, or abdominal pain is present unless directed by a physician. If you notice a sudden change in bowel habits that persists over a period of 2 weeks, consult a physician before using a laxative. Rectal bleeding or failure to have a bowel movement after use of a laxative may indicate a serious condition. Discontinue use and consult a physician. Laxative products should not be used longer than 1 week unless directed by a physician. As with any drug, if you are pregnant or nursing a baby, seek the advice of a health professional before using this product. Keep this and all drugs out of the reach of children. In case of accidental overdose or ingestion, seek professional assistance or contact a Poison Control Center immediately.

PRECAUTIONS

DO NOT ADMINISTER TO CHILDREN UNDER 2 YEARS OF AGE.

DOSAGE AND ADMINISTRATION

Dosage: Adults and Children 12 years of age and over—one 4.5 fl. oz. bottle (118 mL delivered dose) in a single daily dose. Children 2 to under 12 years of age—½ bottle (59 mL delivered dose) in a single daily dose.
REMOVE ORANGE PROTECTIVE SHIELD FROM TIP BEFORE INSERTING.
Preferred position: Lie on left side with knee slightly bent and the right leg drawn up, or knee-chest position.
Diaphragm at base of tube prevents accidental leakage and assures controlled flow of the enema solution. May be used at room temperature. For more thorough cleansing, follow with regular FLEET® Enema—**according to dosage instructions contained in PDR.**

PROFESSIONAL DOSAGE AND ADMINISTRATION

FLEET® Mineral Oil Enema should not be used in children under 2 years of age and should be used with caution in children of any age. Careful consideration of the use of enemas in general in children is recommended.
Proper and safe use of FLEET® Mineral Oil Enema also requires that the product be administered according to the Directions. Health care professionals should remember, when administering the product, to gently insert the enema into the rectum with the tip pointing toward the naval. Insertion may be made easier by having the patient bear down as they would in having a bowel movement. Care during insertion is necessary due to lack of sensory innervation of the rectum and due to possibility of bowel perforation. Once inserted, squeeze the bottle until nearly all the liquid is expelled. If resistance is encountered on insertion of the nozzle or in administering the solution, the procedure should be discontinued. Forcing the enema can result in perforation and/or abrasion of the rectum.

HOW SUPPLIED

FLEET® Mineral Oil Enema is supplied in 4.5 fl.oz. (133 mL) ready-to-use squeeze bottle.

IS THIS PRODUCT OTC?

Yes.

FLEET® PHOSPHO-SODA® — OTC
AN ORAL SALINE LAXATIVE

COMPOSITION

Each 5 mL of Unflavored or Ginger-lemon flavor FLEET® Phospho-soda® contains 2.4 g monobasic sodium phosphate monohydrate and 0.9 g dibasic sodium phosphate heptahydrate in a stable, buffered aqueous solution.

Elemental and Electrolytic Content

mEq Phosphate (PO_4) per mL	12.45
mEq Sodium (Na) per mL	4.82
mmole Phosphorus (P) per mL	4.15

INDICATIONS

As a laxative, for the relief of occasional constipation. As a purgative, for use as part of a bowel cleansing regimen in preparing the patient for surgery or for preparing the colon for x-ray or endoscopic examination. See PROFESSIONAL DOSAGE AND ADMINISTRATION.

Continued on next page

Fleet Phospho-Soda—Cont.

ACTION AND USES

Versatile in action as a gentle laxative or purgative, according to dosage. This product produces a bowel movement in $^{1}/_{2}$ to 6 hours, depending on dosage. Especially useful as a bowel prep for colonoscopy, surgery, and radiology procedures.

CONTRAINDICATIONS

DO NOT USE THIS PRODUCT IF YOU HAVE KIDNEY DISEASE OR ARE ON A SODIUM RESTRICTED DIET UNLESS DIRECTED BY A PHYSICIAN. EACH TEASPOONFUL (5 ML) CONTAINS 556 MG (24.17 MILLIEQUIVALENTS) SODIUM.

PROFESSIONAL USE WARNINGS

Do not use in patients with congenital megacolon, bowel obstruction, ascites or congestive heart failure.
Use with caution in patients with impaired renal function, pre-existing electrolyte imbalances or with debilitated patients.
Since FLEET® Phospho-soda® contains sodium phosphates, there is a risk of elevated serum levels of sodium and phosphate and decreased levels of calcium and potassium and consequent hypocalcemia, hypokalemia, hyperphosphatemia, hypernatremia, and acidosis may occur.
Additional fluids by mouth are recommended with all bowel cleansing dosages.

WARNINGS

TAKING MORE THAN THE RECOMMENDED DOSE IN 24 HOURS CAN BE HARMFUL. IF THERE IS NO BOWEL MOVEMENT AFTER MAXIMUM DOSAGE, CONTACT A PHYSICIAN AS DEHYDRATION COULD OCCUR.
SINCE FLEET® PHOSPHO-SODA® IS AVAILABLE IN TWO SIZES, PRESCRIBE BY VOLUMES. DO NOT PRESCRIBE "BY THE BOTTLE" AS SERIOUS SIDE EFFECTS FROM OVERDOSAGE MAY OCCUR.
Ask a doctor before using this product if you are on a sodium restricted diet, have a kidney disease or are pregnant or nursing a baby. Ask a doctor before using any laxative if you have nausea, vomiting, abdominal pain, have a sudden change in bowel habits lasting more than 2 weeks or have already used a laxative for more than 1 week. Stop using this product and consult a doctor if you have rectal bleeding or have no bowel movement after use as dehydration may occur. These symptoms may indicate a serious condition.
Keep this and all drugs out of the reach of children. In case of overdose or accidental ingestion, seek professional assistance or contact a Poison Control Center immediately.

OVERDOSAGE

Overdosage or retention of FLEET® Phospho-soda® may cause hypocalcemia, hyperphosphatemia, hypernatremia, hypernatremic dehydration and acidosis.
Calcium, phosphate, potassium and sodium levels should be carefully monitored. Immediate corrective action should be taken to restore electrolyte balance with appropriate fluid replacements. Prompt parenteral administration of fluids with lower concentrations of sodium and chloride than extracellular fluid (40–50 mEq/liter) and moderate concentration of potassium (20–30 mEq/liter) administered at a rate of 3,000 to 4,000 cc/sq. m of body surface during the first 12 to 24 hours is dependent on the severity of dehydration and the clinical response.

DOSAGE AND ADMINISTRATION

For best results, take on an empty stomach. Most effective when taken upon rising, at least 30 minutes before a meal, or at bedtime for overnight action. **Dilute recommended dosage with one-half glass (4 fl. oz.) clear Liquid. Drink, then follow with one glass (8 fl. oz.) clear liquid.**
DOSAGE: SINCE FLEET® PHOSPHO-SODA® IS AVAILABLE IN TWO SIZES, PRESCRIBE BY VOLUMES; DO NOT PRESCRIBE "BY THE BOTTLE". DO NOT EXCEED RECOMMENDED DOSAGE AS SERIOUS SIDE EFFECTS MAY OCCUR.
SINGLE DAILY DOSAGE: DO NOT TAKE MORE UNLESS DIRECTED BY A DOCTOR. SEE WARNINGS.

Adults and children 12 years and older	20 to 45 mL* (4 to 9 teaspoons*)
Children 10 and 11 years	10 to 20 mL* (2 to 4 teaspoons*)
Children 5 to 9 years	5 to 10 mL* (1 to 2 teaspoons*)
Children under 5 years	Ask a doctor

* DO NOT TAKE MORE THAN THIS AMOUNT IN A 24-HOUR PERIOD.

PROFESSIONAL DOSAGE AND ADMINISTRATION

For use as a bowel cleansing regimen prior to surgery or x-ray and endoscopic examinations:
Hydration and Diet:
On the day before the procedure, drink only clear liquids [e.g., soft drinks, strained fruit juices, tea, coffee, bouillon/broths, Jell-O®, Popsicles®—nothing colored red or purple] for breakfast, lunch and dinner. Drink as much clear liquid as possible throughout the day. Drink 3 additional glasses of clear liquids after the first dose of Fleet Phospho-soda.
Dosing:
Two—1.5 oz. doses of **diluted** Fleet Phospho-soda (see below). See References. Dosage timing as directed by the physician.
Dilution Alternatives:
1) Mix 1.5 oz. (3 tablespoons) Fleet Phospho-soda with 4 oz. of cold clear liquid. Then follow with at least 8 oz. of clear liquid.

OR

2) Mix 1.5 oz. (3 tablespoons) Fleet Phospho-Soda with three 8 oz. glasses cold clear liquid (One tablespoon of Fleet Phospho-soda per glass). Drink all three glasses within 30 minutes.

The taste of Fleet Phospho-soda is improved by mixing it with ginger ale, apple juice or lemon-lime type drinks.

HOW SUPPLIED

Unflavored or Ginger-lemon flavor, in bottles of 1.5 fl. oz. and 3 fl. oz. FLEET® Phospho-soda® should not be confused with FLEET® Enema, a sodium phosphates disposable ready-to-use enema. FLEET® Enema, Adult and Children size, ARE NOT INTENDED FOR ORAL CONSUMPTION in any dosage size.

IS THIS PRODUCT OTC?

Yes.

REFERENCES

1. Cohen, Stephen M. et al. Prospective, Randomized, Endoscopic-Blinded Trial Comparing Precolonoscopy Bowel Cleansing Methods. Diseases of the Colon & Rectum. 1994; 37(7):689.
2. Frommer, D. Cleansing Ability and Tolerance of Three Bowel Preparations for Colonoscopy. Diseases of the Colon & Rectum. 1997; 40(1):100.
3. Golub, R. W. et al. Colonoscopic Bowel Preparations—Which One? Diseases of the Colon & Rectum. 1995; 38(6): 594.
4. Kolts, B. E. et al. A Comparison of the Effectiveness and Patient Tolerance of Oral Sodium Phosphate, Castor Oil, and Standard Electrolyte Lavage for Colonoscopy or Sigmoidoscopy Preparation. The American Journal of Gastroenterology. 1993; 88(8):1218.
5. Oliveira, Lucia et al. Mechanical Bowel Preparation for Elective Colorectal Surgery. Diseases of the Colon & Rectum. 1997; 40(5):585.
6. Vanner, S. J. et al. A Randomized Prospective Trial Comparing Oral Sodium Phosphate with Standard Polyethylene Glycol-Based Lavage Solution (Golytely) in the Preparation of Patients for Colonoscopy. The American Journal of Gastroenterology. 1990; 85(4):422.

FLEET® PREP KITS OTC
Bowel Evacuant

COMPOSITION

FLEET® Prep Kit 1 contains:
1. FLEET® Phospho-soda®—1.5 fl. oz. (45 mL) Active Ingredients: Each teaspoon (5 mL) contains monobasic sodium phosphate monohydrate 2.4g and dibasic sodium phosphate heptahydrate 0.9g.
2. FLEET® Bisacodyl Tablets—4 laxative tablets. Active Ingredient: Each enteric-coated tablet contains bisacodyl, USP, 5 mg.
3. FLEET® Bisacodyl Suppository—1 laxative suppository. Active Ingredient: Each suppository contains bisacodyl, USP, 10 mg.
4. 1 Patient Instruction Sheet.

FLEET® Prep Kit 2 contains:
1. FLEET® Phospho-soda®—1.5 fl. oz. (45 mL).
2. FLEET® Bisacodyl Tablets—4 tablets.
3. FLEET® Bagenema—1.
4. 1 Patient Instruction Sheet.

FLEET® Prep Kit 3 contains:
1. FLEET® Phospho-soda® —1.5 fl. oz. (45 mL)
2. FLEET® Bisacodyl Tablets—4 tablets.
3. FLEET® Bisacodyl Enema 1.25 fl. oz. (37 mL)—1 laxative enema. Active Ingredient: Each 30 mL delivered dose contains bisacodyl, USP 10 mg.
4. 1 Patient Instruction Sheet.

ACTIONS AND USES

Bowel Cleansing System

INDICATIONS

For use as part of a bowel cleansing regimen in preparation of the colon for radiology (prior to barium enemas or I.V.P.'s), surgery, and many endoscopic and colonoscopic procedures.

WARNINGS

DO NOT EXCEED RECOMMENDED DOSE UNLESS DIRECTED BY A PHYSICIAN. SERIOUS SIDE EFFECTS MAY OCCUR FROM EXCESS DOSAGE.
Each recommended dose (1.5 fl. oz.) (45 mL) of FLEET® Phospho-soda® contains 5004 mg sodium. **Persons on a sodium restricted diet or with kidney disease should consult a health professional before use.**
Bisacodyl products may cause abdominal discomfort, faintness, and cramps.
Swallow tablets whole. Do not chew tablets or give to persons who cannot swallow without chewing unless directed by a physician. Do not take tablets within 1 hour after taking antacids, milk, or milk products.
Keep this and all drugs out of the reach of children. In case of accidental overdose or ingestion, seek professional assistance or contact a Poison Control Center immediately.

PROFESSIONAL USE WARNINGS

Do not use in patients with congenital megacolon, bowel obstruction, ascites or congestive heart failure.
Use with caution in patients with impaired renal function, pre-existing electrolyte imbalances or with debilitated patients.
Since FLEET® Phospho-soda® contains sodium phosphates, there is a risk of elevated serum levels of sodium and phosphate and decreased levels of calcium and potassium and consequent hypocalcemia, hyperphosphatemia, hypernatremia, and acidosis may occur.
Additional fluids by mouth are recommended with all bowel cleansing dosages.
If any of these complications occur following administration of FLEET® Phospho-soda®, immediate corrective action should be taken to restore electrolyte balance with appropriate fluid replacements. Calcium, magnesium, and phosphorus levels should be carefully monitored. **See individual listings FLEET® Phospho-soda®, and FLEET® Bisacodyl Laxatives for additional warnings.**
THESE KITS SHOULD NOT BE USED BY PATIENTS UNDER 12 YEARS OF AGE.

PRECAUTIONS

DO NOT EXCEED RECOMMENDED DOSE UNLESS DIRECTED BY A PHYSICIAN, AS SERIOUS SIDE EFFECTS MAY OCCUR. IF THERE IS NO BOWEL MOVEMENT AFTER MAXIMUM DOSAGE, CONTACT A PHYSICIAN AS DEHYDRATION COULD OCCUR.

DOSAGE AND ADMINISTRATION

SEE PATIENT INSTRUCTION SHEET FOR 18, 24, AND 48 HOUR PREPARATION SCHEDULE IN EACH KIT. The patient should open and read the enclosed directions and labels at least 48 hours in advance of examination.

HOW SUPPLIED

See "Description" for contents of each kit.
Shipping Unit: 48 FLEET® Prep Kits per carton.
For full prescribing information on specific products, see individual listings (FLEET® Phospho-soda®, FLEET® Bisacodyl Laxatives).

IS THIS PRODUCT OTC?

Yes.

Fleming & Company
1600 FENPARK DR.
FENTON, MO 63026

Direct Inquiries to:
H.C. Mansmann, Jr. MD
PH: 636-343-8200
FAX: 636-343-5322
email: info@flemingcompany.com

AEROLATE SR & JR Capsules ℞
(theophylline, anhydrous T.D.)

AEROLATE LIQUID
(theophylline, anhydrous)

COMPOSITION

Contains theophylline 4 grs. (260 mg) as SR, 2 grs (130 mg) as JR, in red/clear capsules. Liquid has 150 mg theophylline/15cc in a non-sugar, non-alcoholic, non-saccharin tangerine flavored base.

ACTION AND USES

Timed action pellets by-pass stomach to prevent gastric upset. Bronchodilation is achieved through bowel absorption only. Liquid is for the acute attack primarily.

ADMINISTRATION AND DOSAGE

One capsule every 12 hours. Every 8 hours in severe attacks. Liquid—adults—40 ml (2.5 tablespoonfuls) for acute attack. Children—0.25 ml/lb. Maintainance therapy—adults—for the first 6 doses, 25 ml (1.5 tablespoonfuls) before breakfast, at 3 p.m., at bedtime. Then 15 ml doses at above times. Children—0.15 ml/lb at these times, then 0.1 ml/lb per dose.

SIDE EFFECTS

Nausea, vomiting, epigastric or substernal pain, palpitation, headache, dizziness may occur.

HOW SUPPLIED

Capsules in bottles of 100.
Liquid in pints.

ALUMADRINE Tablets ℞

DESCRIPTION
Each flat, quadri-scored, embossed "107", purple tablet, 6mm thick and 10mm in diameter contains:

Acetaminophen	**500 mg**
Phenylpropanolamine HCl	**25 mg**
Chlorpheniramine maleate	**4 mg**

OTHER INGREDIENTS
Pregelatinized Starch, crospovidone, povidone, stearic acid, magnesium stearate, FD&C blue #1, aluminum lake and D&C red #27 aluminum lake.

CLINICAL PHARMACOLOGY
Acetaminophen produces analgesia by elevation of the pain threshold and antipyresis through action on the hypothalamic heat-regulating center. Phenylpropanolamine HCl is a sympathomimetic and is a vasoconstrictor with decongestive action on nasal and upper respiratory tract mucous membranes. Chlorpheniramine maleate is an alkylamine antihistamine which possesses anticholinergic and sedative effects.

INDICATIONS AND USAGE
Symptomatic relief and reduction of fever or relief of pain in common upper respiratory infections; allergic rhinitis; vasomotor rhinitis. *Pediatric use:* Safety and effectiveness in pediatric patients have not been established.

CONTRAINDICATIONS
Hypersensitivity to any of the ingredients; cardiac disease; hypertension; patients receiving MAO inhibitors; hyperthyroidism.

WARNINGS
Alumadrine tablets may increase the effects of alcohol and other CNS depressants. Do not take simultaneously with other products containing Phenylpropanolamine HCl.

PRECAUTIONS
General: Use cautiously in patients with glaucoma, stenosing peptic ulcer, pyloroduodenal obstruction, prostatic hypertrophy, bladder neck obstruction, diabetes. Withdraw medication if restlessness or nervousness occurs or if high fever persists. *Information for patients:* Because this product may cause drowsiness or blurring of vision, patients should be cautioned against driving or operating machinery. Also caution patients of the added effects of alcohol and other CNS depressants. *Pregnancy: Pregnancy Category C.* It is not known whether this product can cause fetal harm when administered to a pregnant woman or can affect reproduction capacity. This product should be given to a pregnant woman only if clearly needed. *Nursing Mothers:* It is not known whether these drugs are excreted in human milk. Because many drugs are excreted in human milk, caution should be exercised when this product is administered to a nursing woman.

ADVERSE REACTIONS
General: Urticaria, drug rash, anaphylactic shock, photosensitivity, excessive perspiration, chills, dryness of mouth, nose and throat. *Cardiovascular:* Hypotension, hypertension, headache, palpitations, tachycardia, extrasystoles and angina pain. *Hematologic:* Hemolytic anemia, thrombocytopenia, agranulocytosis, leukopenia. *CNS:* Sedation, dizziness, disturbed coordination, fatigue, confusion, restlessness, excitation, nervousness, tremor, irritability, insomnia, euphoria, paresthesias, blurred vision, diplopia, vertigo, tinnitus, acute labyrinthitis, hysteria neuritis and convulsions. *GI:* Epigastric distress, anorexia, nausea, vomiting, diarrhea, constipation. *GU:* Urinary frequency, urinary difficulty or retention, early menses. *Respiratory:* Thickening of bronchial secretions, tightness of chest and wheezing, nasal stuffiness.

OVERDOSAGE
The stomach should be emptied promptly by lavage or by induction of emesis.

DOSAGE AND ADMINISTRATION
Adults—Two tablets initially, then one tablet every four hours. Do not exceed 6 tablets in 24 hours.

HOW SUPPLIED
Supplied as quadri-scored, embossed "107", purple tablets, in bottles of 100, NDC 0256-0107-01.

Rev. 8/99

CHLOR-3 OTC

DESCRIPTION
Medical condiment containing sodium chloride 50%; potassium chloride 30%; magnesium chloride 20%.

INDICATIONS AND USAGE
To reduce sodium intake for patients on diuretics; for potential hypertensives and cardiacs.
To encourage physicians to recommend a condiment to replace "table salt" for family use and gourmet cooking.

HOW SUPPLIED
Shaker 8 oz. plastic bottles.

Each dose contains:

	Phenylephrine HCl	Chlorpheniramine Maleate	Methscopolamine Nitrate
Extendryl SR Capsule	20 mg	8 mg	2.50 mg
Extendryl JR Capsule	10 mg	4 mg	1.25 mg
Extendryl Chewable Tablet (Root beer flavored)	10 mg	2 mg	1.25 mg
Extendryl Syrup (5 mL) (Root beer flavored)	10 mg	2 mg	1.25 mg

EXTENDRYL SR/JR EXTENDED-RELEASE CAPSULES, SYRUP, CHEWABLE TABLETS ℞
Decongestant, antihistamine, anticholinergic

DESCRIPTION
[See table above]

CLINICAL PHARMACOLOGY
Chlorpheniramine maleate is an alkylamine antihistamine which possesses anticholinergic and sedative effects. Phenylephrine HCl is a sympathomimetic which acts predominantly on alpha receptors and has little action on beta receptors, with a mild central stimulant effect. Methscopolamine nitrate is a derivative of scopolamine, which possesses the peripheral actions of the belladonna alkaloids, but does not exhibit the central actions because of its inability to cross the blood-brain barrier.

INDICATIONS AND USAGE
Relief of respiratory congestion, allergic rhinitis, vasomotor rhinitis, and allergic skin reactions of urticaria and angioedema.

CONTRAINDICATIONS
Contraindicated in patients receiving MAO inhibitors, in patients with a known hypersensitivity to any of the ingredients, and in patients with glaucoma, hypertension, cardiac disease, or hyperthyroidism.

PRECAUTIONS
General: Use cautiously, if at all, in the presence of pyloric obstruction. Use with caution in those over 40 years of age, in the presence of diabetes mellitus or urinary retention, and in men with prostatic hypertrophy or a history of bladder difficulty. If disturbances in urination occur, medication should be discontinued for 1 or 2 days and then resumed at a lower dosage. Antihistamines may cause excitability, especially in children. *Information for patients:* Because this product may cause blurring of vision or drowsiness, patients should be cautioned against driving or operating machinery. *Drug interactions:* MAO inhibitors and beta adrenergic blockers increase the effects of sympathomimetics. Sympathomimetics may reduce the antihypertensive effects of methyldopa, guanethidine, mecamylamine, reserpine and veratrum alkaloids. Concomitant use of antihistamines with alcohol or other CNS depressants may have an additive effect. *Pregnancy:* Pregnancy Category C. It is also not known whether the product can cause fetal harm when administered to a pregnant woman or can affect reproduction capacity. The product should be given to a pregnant woman only if clearly needed. *Nursing mothers:* It is not known whether these drugs are excreted in human milk. Because many drugs are excreted in human milk, caution should be exercised when this product is administered to a nursing woman. *Pediatric use:* Safety and effectiveness in children below the age of 6 have not been established.
Geriatric use: Anticholinergic and CNS stimulant effects more likely to occur in older patients; danger of precipitating undiagnosed glaucoma; possible impairment of memory.

ADVERSE REACTIONS
Side effects include xerostomia, blurred vision, bradycardia, mydriasis, flushing, palpitation, dizziness, constipation, urinary retention, drowsiness, increased irritability or excitability, nausea or dysphagia.

OVERDOSAGE
The stomach should be emptied promptly by lavage or by induction of emesis (syrup of ipecac recommended). The installation of activated charcoal into the stomach also should be considered. If respiratory depression is present, treat promptly with oxygen and/or mechanical support of ventilation. If convulsions or marked CNS excitement occurs, only short-acting benzodiazepine-type drugs should be used.

DOSAGE AND ADMINISTRATION
Extended-Release Capsules: Adults and children 12 years of age and older: One SR. capsule every 12 hours. Children 6 to under 12 years of age: One JR. capsule every 12 hours. *Syrup:* Adults and children 12 years of age and older: 1 or 2 teaspoonfuls every 3 or 4 hours. Children 6 to under 12 years of age: $^1/_2$ to 1 teaspoonful depending on age and body weight, may be repeated every 4 hours. *Tablets:* Adults and children 12 years of age and older: 1 or 2 tablets every 4 hours. Children 6 to under 12 years of age: 1 tablet every 4 hours. Do not exceed 4 doses in 24 hours.

HOW SUPPLIED
Capsules and tablets in bottles of 100, syrup in pints.
Supplied as green/red Extendryl Extended-Release Sr/Jr capsules in bottles of 100: "Sr," NDC 0256-0111-01; "Jr," NDC 0256-0177-01.
Extendryl Syrup as root beer flavored syrup in pints, NDC 0256-0127-01.
Extendryl Chewable Tablets: convex, tan colored, scored on one side in bottles of 100, NDC 0256-0133-01.

Rev. 8/99

MAGONATE® Tablets
MAGONATE® Liquid
MAGONATE NATAL Liquid
Magnesium Gluconate (Dihydrate), USP (Dietary Supplement)

DESCRIPTION
Each 2 tablets contain magnesium 54 mgs (from 1000 mg magnesium gluconate dihydrate) calcium 175 mg and phosphorous 182 mg (from 752 mg dibasic calcium phosphate dihydrate). Each 5 mL of MAGONATE® liquid contains magnesium (elemental) 54 mgs. (Each 5 ml contains the same amount of magnesium as contained in 1000 mgs of magnesium gluconate dihydrate). Each ml of MAGONATE NATAL Liquid (magnesium gluconate) contains 3.52 mg (0.29 mEq) of magnesium as the gluconate in a sugarless and flavor free isotonic base.

SUGGESTED USES
Magonate® Tablets and Liquid are indicated to maintain magnesium levels when the dietary intake of magnesium is inadequate or when excretion and loss are excessive.
Magonate® is recommended during and for three weeks after a course in chemotherapy, then monitored regularly. MAGONATE NATAL Liquid is indicated for newborns with magnesium deficiency and for the restoration of magnesium in infants.

PRECAUTIONS
Excessive dosage may cause loose stools.

CONTRAINDICATIONS
Patients with kidney disease should not take magnesium supplements without the supervision of a physician.

DOSAGES AND ADMINISTRATION
Two Magonate® tablets or 1 teaspoon Magonate® Liquid three times a day (mid-morning, mid-afternoon and bedtime) on an empty stomach with a glass of water. MAGONATE Natal Liquid usual dose is 1 ml per kg of body weight daily, divided into two doses or 10 drops per kg twice a day.

HOW SUPPLIED
Magonate® Tablets are orange scored, and supplied in bottles of 100 (NDC 256-0172-01), and 1000 (NDC 256-0172-02) tablets. Magonate® Liquid is supplied in pints, (NDC 256-0184-01). MAGONATE NATAL Liquid is supplied in pints.

Rev. 7/00

MARBLEN Antacid OTC
(calcium and magnesium carbonates)
ANTACID SUSPENSION

(See PDR For Nonprescription Drugs.)

NEPHROCAPS® ℞
Dialysis/Stress Vitamin Supplement

DESCRIPTION
Each black softgel contains:
Vitamin C 100 mg (ascorbic acid); folate 1 mg; niacin 20 mg (niacinamide) thiamin 1.5 mg (thiamine mononitrate); riboflavin 1.7 mg; Vitamin B-6 10 mg (pyridoxine HCl); Vitamin B-12 6 mcg (cyanocobalamin); pantothenic acid 5 mg (calcium pantothenate); and biotin 150 mcg.

INDICATIONS AND USAGE
In the wasting syndrome in chronic renal failure; uremia; impaired metabolic functions of the kidney and to maintain levels when the dietary intake of vitamins is inadequate or excretion and loss are excessive. **Also, highly effective as a stress vitamin.**

PRECAUTIONS
Folic acid may mask the symptoms of pernicious anemia in that hematologic remission may occur while neurologic manifestations remain progressive.

DOSAGE AND ADMINISTRATION
One softgel daily or as directed by a physician. If on dialysis, take after treatment.

HOW SUPPLIED
Plastic bottles of 100 black, oval softgels, NDC 0256-0185-01.
Contains FD&C yellow # 6.

Rev. 8/99

NICOTINEX Elixir OTC
Niacin Dietary Supplement

(See PDR For Nonprescription Drugs.)

Continued on next page

OBEGYN® Prenatal Supplement ℞
Multivitamin/multimineral powder for reconstitution

DESCRIPTION
OBEGYN® Prenatal Supplement is a daily multivitamin & multimineral supplement in powder form to be reconstituted with water, producing a good tasting orange flavored drink.
Each dose (4 level teaspoonsful of powder, [8.25g]) contains:

Vitamin A (as palmitate)	2,500 IU
Vitamin A (from beta carotene)	2,500 IU
Vitamin C (as ascorbic acid)	120 mg
Vitamin D (as cholecalciferol)	400 IU
Vitamin E (as dl-alpha tocopheryl acetate)	60 IU
Vitamin B1 (as thiamine mononitrate)	1.7 mg
Vitamin B2 (riboflavin)	2 mg
Niacin (as niacinamide)	20 mg
Vitamin B6 (as pyridoxine hydrochloride)	10 mg
FOLIC ACID	1 mg
Vitamin B12 (as cyanocobalamin)	12 mcg
BIOTIN	300 mcg
Pantothenic acid (as calcium pantothenate)	10 mg
CALCIUM (from calcium lactate)	455 mg
IRON (from ferrous gluconate)	18 mg
Iodine (from potassium iodide)	150 mcg
MAGNESIUM (from magnesium gluconate)	150 mg
Zinc (from zinc oxide)	25 mg
Copper (from cupric sulfate)	2 mg
ORANGE FLAVORED	
DYE FREE	

INDICATIONS AND USAGE
OBEGYN™ Prenatal Supplement is a multi-vitamin & mineral supplement for use before, during and/or after pregnancy for the lactating or non-lactating mother.

WARNING
Accidental overdoses of iron-containing products is a leading cause of fatal poisoning in children under 6. Keep this product out of reach of children. In case of accidental overdose call a doctor or poison control center immediately.

PRECAUTIONS
Folic acid may mask the symptoms of pernicious anemia in that hematologic remission may occur while neurologic manifestations remain progressive. The calcium content should be considered before prescribing for patients with kidney stones. Phenylketonurics: contains phenylalanine 84 mg per 8.25 g.

ADVERSE REACTIONS
Allergic sensitization has been reported following oral administration of folic acid.

DOSAGE AND ADMINISTRATION
Reconstitute in 4–5 oz. tap water, one level scoop (8.25 g) daily (preferably at bedtime) or in divided doses for ages four through adult. Use two level tsps (4.125g) for ages two and three. Can be chilled with ice to enhance taste. Drink entire mixture immediately after preparation. Use only as directed.

HOW SUPPLIED
OBEGYN™ is available as a slightly orange-colored powder in bottles containing 495 g (60 doses). NDC 256-0200-01.
Store at room temperature. Keep container tightly closed and protected from heat and moisture at all times. Do not shake this container.

CAUTION
Federal law prohibits dispensing without prescription.

Rev. 7/97

OCEAN® Nasal Mist OTC
(buffered isotonic saline)

USE
Upright delivers a spray; horizontally a stream; upside down a drop.
(See PDR For Nonprescription Drugs.)

5/99

PIMA Syrup ℞
potassium iodide, not USP
(expectorant, radiation protection)

DESCRIPTION
Each teaspoonful (5ml) contains iodide 249 mg (1.95 mEq) as the potassium salt in a black raspberry flavored syrup.

ACTION
Potassium iodide expectorant to liquefy mucus. When administered prior to and following administration of radioactive isotopes and in radiation emergencies involving the release of radioactive iodine, potassium iodide protects the thyroid gland by blocking the thyroidal uptake of radioactive isotopes of iodine.

INDICATIONS AND USAGE
As an expectorant in the symptomatic treatment of chronic pulmonary diseases where tenacious mucus complicates the problem, including bronchial asthma, bronchitis and pulmonary emphysema.
Potassium iodide is indicated as a radiation protectant (thyroid gland) prior to and following oral administration or inhalation of radioactive isotopes of iodine or in radiation emergencies.

ADMINISTRATION AND DOSAGE
Children—one half to one tsps. and adults one or two tsps. every 4–6 hours.

CONTRAINDICATIONS
In patients sensitive to iodides, hyperthyroidism, rare cases of iodine-induced goiter and patients with renal disorders.

SIDE EFFECTS
Allergic reactions, specifically angioedema, arthralgia, eosinophilia, swelling of lymph nodes and urticaria may require medical attention. Nausea, vomiting, minor skin eruptions, gastrointestinal upset, epigastric pain. Iodism and potassium toxicity may occur with prolonged use. Metallic after-taste has been reported.

WARNING
Discontinue use if skin rash or other evidence of hypersensitivity appears.

DOSAGE AND ADMINISTRATION
As an expectorant, children under three—1/2 tsp. three times daily. Children over three—one tsp. three times daily. Adults—one or two tsps. three times daily. Take at least 4–6 oz. of water with each dose.
As a Radiation Protectant, infants up to 1 year of age: 1 ml once a day 24 hours prior to and for ten days following administration of, or exposure to, radioactive isotopes of iodine. Children over 1 year of age: 2 ml once a day 24 hours prior to and for ten days following administration of, or exposure to, radioactive isotopes of iodine. Adults: 3 ml once a day 24 hours prior to and for ten days following administration of, or exposure to, radioactive isotopes of iodine.

HOW SUPPLIED
Plastic pint bottles, NDC 0256-0139-01

Rev. 12/99

PURGE OTC
(flavored castor oil)
STIMULANT LAXATIVE

(See PDR For Nonprescription Drugs.)

RUM–K ℞
(potassium chloride 15% conc, not USP)

DESCRIPTION
Each two teaspoonfuls supply 20 mEq. of potassium and chloride in a butter/rum flavored base that is alcohol and sugar free.

OTHER INGREDIENTS
Filtered water, glycerin, sorbitol, sodium saccharin and artificial flavor.

ACTION
Electrolyte replenisher

INDICATIONS AND USAGE
For the treatment of hypokalemia, with or without metabolic alkalosis and for the prophylaxis of hypokalemia in patients who would be at particular risk if hypokalemia were to develop. It may be used in the treatment of cardiac arrhythmias due to digitalis intoxication.

CONTRAINDICATIONS
Severe renal impairment with oliguria or azotemia, diarrhea resulting in severe dehydration, untreated Addison's disease, heat cramps and hyperkalemia from any cause.

WARNINGS:
Do not administer full strength. Potassium chloride 15% conc. can cause gastrointestinal irritation. See Dosage and Administration.

PRECAUTIONS
In response to a rise in the concentration of body potassium, renal excretion of the ion is increased. With normal kidney function, it is difficult, therefore, to produce potassium intoxication by oral administration. However, potassium supplements must be administered with caution, since the amount of the deficiency or daily dosage is not accurately known. Frequent checks of the clinical status of the patient, and periodic ECG and/or serum potassium levels should be made. High serum concentrations of potassium ion may cause death through cardiac depression, arrhythmias or arrest. This drug should be used with caution in the presence of cardiac disease. If the basic disturbance produces metabolic acidosis, as in some renal tubular disorders, an organic salt such as potassium gluconate may be more advantageous.

ADVERSE REACTIONS
Vomiting, nausea, abdominal discomfort, diarrhea may occur. Symptoms and signs of potassium overdose include paresthesias of extremities, flaccid paralysis, listlessness, fall in blood pressure, weakness and heaviness of the legs, cardiac arrhythmias and heart block. Hyperkalemia may cause ECG changes as disappearance of the P wave, widening and slurring of QRS complex, changes of the S-T segment, tall peaked T waves.

DOSAGE AND ADMINISTRATION
Adults—two teaspoonsful (10ml) in 6 or more oz water 2 to 4 times daily after meals to supply 40–80 mEq of elemental potassium and chloride. Larger doses may be required and administered under close supervision.

OVERDOSE
Potassium intoxication may result from overdosage of potassium or from therapeutic dosage in conditions stated under "Contraindications". Hyperkalemia, when detected, must be treated immediately because lethal levels can be reached in a few hours.

HOW SUPPLIED
Pint bottles NDC 0256-0160-01

Rev. 12/99

Forest Pharmaceuticals, Inc.
(Subsidiary of Forest Laboratories, Inc.)
13600 SHORELINE DRIVE
ST. LOUIS, MO 63045

Direct Inquiries to:
Professional Affairs Department
13600 Shoreline Drive
St. Louis, MO 63045
(800) 678-1605

AEROBID® ℞
AEROBID®-M
(flunisolide)
Inhaler System
For oral inhalation only

DESCRIPTION
Flunisolide, the active component of **AEROBID** Inhaler System, is an anti-inflammatory steroid having the chemical name 6α-fluoro-11β, 16α, 17, 21-tetrahydroxypregna-1, 4-diene-3, 20-dione cyclic-16, 17-acetal with acetone.
It has the following structure:

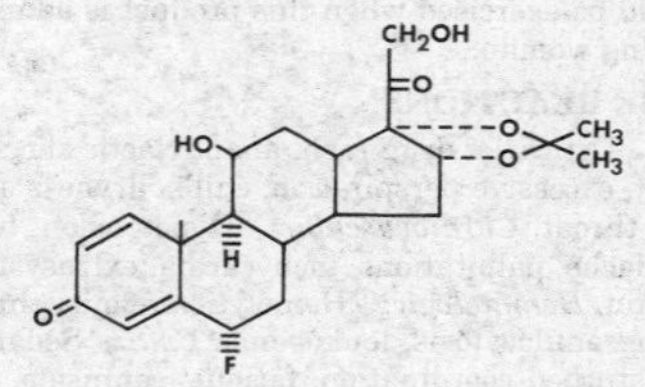

Flunisolide is a white to creamy white crystalline powder with a molecular weight of 434.49. It is soluble in acetone, sparingly soluble in chloroform, slightly soluble in methanol, and practically insoluble in water. It has a melting point of about 245°C.
AEROBID Inhaler is delivered in a metered-dose aerosol system containing a microcrystalline suspension of flunisolide as the hemihydrate in propellants (trichloromonofluoromethane, dichlorodifluoromethane and dichlorotetrafluoroethane) with sorbitan trioleate as a dispersing agent. **AEROBID-M** also contains menthol as a flavoring agent. Each activation delivers approximately 250 mcg of flunisolide to the patient. One **AEROBID** Inhaler System is designed to deliver at least 100 metered inhalations.

CLINICAL PHARMACOLOGY
Flunisolide has demonstrated marked anti-inflammatory and anti-allergic activity in classical test systems. It is a corticosteroid that is several hundred times more potent in animal anti-inflammatory assays than the cortisol standard. The molar dose of each activation of flunisolide in this preparation is approximately 2.5 to 7 times that of comparable inhaled corticosteroid products marketed for the same indication. The dose of flunisolide delivered per activation in this preparation is 10 times that per activation of Nasalide® (flunisolide) nasal solution. Clinical studies have shown therapeutic activity on bronchial mucosa with minimal evidence of systemic activity at recommended doses.
After oral inhalation of 1 mg flunisolide, total systemic availability was 40%. The flunisolide that is swallowed is rapidly and extensively converted to the 6β-OH metabolite and to water-soluble conjugates during the first pass through the liver. This offers a metabolic explanation for the low systemic activity of oral flunisolide itself since the metabolite has the low corticosteroid potency (on the order of the cortisol standard). The inhaled flunisolide absorbed through the bronchial tree is converted to the same metab-

olites. Repeated inhalation of 2.0 mg of flunisolide per day (the maximum recommended dose) for 14 days did not show accumulation of the drug in plasma. The plasma half-life of flunisolide is approximately 1.8 hours.

The following observations relevant to systemic absorption were made in clinical studies. In one uncontrolled study a statistically significant decrease in responsiveness to metyrapone was noted in 15 adult steroid-independent patients treated with 2.0 mg of flunisolide per day (the maximum recommended dose) for 3 months. A small but statistically significant drop in eosinophils from 11.5% to 7.4% of total circulating leucocytes was noted in another study in children who were not taking oral corticosteroids simultaneously. A 5% incidence of menstrual disturbances was reported during open studies, in which there were no control groups for comparison.

Aerosol administration of flunisolide 2.0 mg twice daily for one week to 6 healthy male subjects revealed neither suppression of adrenal function as measured by early morning cortisol levels nor impairment of HPA axis function as determined by insulin hypoglycemia tests.

Controlled clinical studies have included over 500 patients with asthma, among them 150 children age 6 and over. More than 120 patients have been treated in open trials for two years or more. No significant adrenal suppression attributed to flunisolide was seen in these studies.

Significant decreases of systemic steroid dosages have been possible in flunisolide-treated patients. Recommended doses of flunisolide appear to be the therapeutic equivalent of an average of 10 mg/day of oral prednisone. Asthma patients have had further symptomatic improvement with flunisolide treatment even while reducing concomitant medication.

INDICATIONS AND USAGE

AEROBID (flunisolide) Inhaler is indicated in the maintenance treatment of asthma as prophylactic therapy. **AEROBID** is also indicated for asthma patients who require systemic corticosteroid administration, where adding **AEROBID** may reduce or eliminate the need for the systemic corticosteroids.

AEROBID Inhaler is NOT indicated for the relief of acute bronchospasm.

CONTRAINDICATIONS

AEROBID (flunisolide) Inhaler is contraindicated in the primary treatment of status asthmaticus or other acute episodes of asthma where intensive measures are required.

Hypersensitivity to any of the ingredients of this preparation contraindicates its use.

WARNINGS

Particular care is needed in patients who are transferred from systemically active corticosteroids to **AEROBID** Inhaler because deaths due to adrenal insufficiency have occurred in asthmatic patients during and after transfer from systemic corticosteroids to aerosol corticosteroids. After withdrawal from systemic corticosteroids, a number of months are required for recovery of hypothalamic-pituitary-adrenal (HPA) function. During this period of HPA suppression, patients may exhibit signs and symptoms of adrenal insufficiency when exposed to trauma, surgery or infections, particularly gastroenteritis. Although **AEROBID** Inhaler may provide control of asthmatic symptoms during these episodes, it does NOT provide the systemic steroid that is necessary for coping with these emergencies. During periods of stress or a severe asthmatic attack, patients who have been withdrawn from systemic corticosteroids should be instructed to resume systemic steroids (in large doses) immediately and to contact their physician for further instruction. These patients should also be instructed to carry a warning card indicating that they may need supplementary systemic steroids during periods of stress or a severe asthma attack. To assess the risk of adrenal insufficiency in emergency situations, routine tests of adrenal cortical function, including measurement of early morning resting cortisol levels, should be performed periodically in all patients. An early morning resting cortisol level may be accepted as normal if it falls at or near the normal mean level.

Localized infections with *Candida albicans* or *Aspergillus niger* have occurred in the mouth and pharynx and occasionally in the larynx. Positive cultures for oral *Candida* may be present in up to 34% of patients. Although the frequency of clinically apparent infection is considerably lower, these infections may require treatment with appropriate antifungal therapy or discontinuance of treatment with **AEROBID** Inhaler.

AEROBID Inhaler is not to be regarded as a bronchodilator and is not indicated for rapid relief of bronchospasm.

Patients should be instructed to contact their physician immediately when episodes of asthma that are not responsive to bronchodilators occur during the course of treatment. During such episodes, patients may require therapy with systemic corticosteroids. Theoretically, the use of inhaled corticosteroids with alternate day prednisone systemic treatment should be accompanied by more HPA suppression than a therapeutically equivalent regimen of either alone.

Transfer of patients from systemic steroid therapy to **AEROBID** Inhaler may unmask allergic conditions previously suppressed by the systemic steroid therapy, e.g. rhinitis, conjunctivitis, and eczema.

Persons who are on drugs which suppress the immune system are more susceptible to infections than healthy individuals. Chicken pox and measles, for example, can have a more serious or even fatal course in non-immune children or adults on corticosteroids. In such children or adults who have not had these diseases, particular care should be taken to avoid exposure. How the dose, route and duration of corticosteriod administration affects the risk of developing a disseminated infection is not known. The contribution of the underlying disease and/or prior corticosteroid treatment to the risk is also not known. If exposed to chicken pox, prophylaxis with varicella zoster immune globulin (VZIG) may be indicated. If exposed to measles, prophylaxis with pooled intramuscular immunoglobulin (IG) may be indicated. (See the respective package inserts for complete VZIG and IG prescribing information). If chicken pox develops, treatment with antiviral agents may be considered.

PRECAUTIONS

General: Because of the relatively high molar dose of flunisolide per activation in this preparation, and because of the evidence suggesting higher levels of systemic absorption with flunisolide than with other comparable inhaled corticosteroids (see CLINICAL PHARMACOLOGY section), patients treated with **AEROBID** (flunisolide) should be observed carefully for any evidence of systemic corticosteroid effect, including suppression of bone growth in children. Particular care should be taken in observing patients postoperatively or during periods of stress for evidence of a decrease in adrenal function. During withdrawal from oral steroids, some patients may experience symptoms of systemically active steroid withdrawal, e.g., joint and/or muscular pain, lassitude and depression, despite maintenance or even improvement of respiratory function. (See DOSAGE AND ADMINISTRATION for details.)

In responsive patients, flunisolide may permit control of asthmatic symptoms without suppression of HPA function. Since flunisolide is absorbed into the circulation and can be systemically active, the beneficial effects of **AEROBID** Inhaler in minimizing or preventing HPA dysfunction may be expected only when recommended dosages are not exceeded. The long-term local and systemic effects of **AEROBID** (flunisolide) in human subjects are still not fully known. In particular, the effects resulting from chronic use of **AEROBID** on developmental or immunologic processes in the mouth, pharynx, trachea, and lung are unknown.

Inhaled corticosteroids should be used with caution, if at all, in patients with active or quiescent tuberculosis infection of the respiratory tract; untreated systemic fungal, bacterial, parasitic or viral infections; or ocular herpes simplex.

Pulmonary infiltrates with eosinophilia may occur in patients on **AEROBID** Inhaler therapy. Although it is possible that in some patients this state may become manifest because of systemic steroid withdrawal when inhalational steroids are administered, a causative role for the drug and/or its vehicle cannot be ruled out.

Information for Patients:

Since the relief from **AEROBID** Inhaler depends on its regular use and on proper inhalation technique, patients must be instructed to take inhalations at regular intervals. They should also be instructed in the correct method of use (See Patient Instruction Leaflet).

Patients whose systemic corticosteroids have been reduced or withdrawn should be instructed to carry a warning card indicating that they may need supplemental systemic steroids during periods of stress or a severe asthmatic attack that is not responsive to bronchodilators.

Persons who are on immunosuppressant doses of corticosteroids should be warned to avoid exposure to chicken pox or measles. Patients should also be advised that if they are exposed, medical advice should be sought without delay.

An illustrated leaflet of patient instructions for proper use accompanies each **AEROBID** Inhaler System.

CONTENTS UNDER PRESSURE

Do not puncture. Do not use or store near heat or open flame. Exposure to temperatures above 120°F (49°C) may cause container to explode. Never throw container into fire or incinerator. Keep out of reach of children.

Carcinogenesis: Long-term studies were conducted in mice and rats using oral administration to evaluate the carcinogenic potential of the drug. There was an increase in the incidence of pulmonary adenomas in mice, but not in rats. Female rats receiving the highest oral dose had an increased incidence of mammary adenocarcinoma compared to control rats. An increased incidence of this tumor type has been reported for other corticosteroids.

Impairment of Fertility: Female rats receiving high doses of flunisolide (200 mcg/kg/day) showed some evidence of impaired fertility. Reproductive performance in the low-(8 mcg/kg/day) and mid-dose (40 mcg/kg/day) groups was comparable to controls.

Pregnancy: Pregnancy Category C. As with other corticosteroids, flunisolide has been shown to be teratogenic in rabbits and rats at doses of 40 and 200 mcg/kg/day respectively. It was also fetotoxic in these animal reproductive studies. There are no adequate and well-controlled studies in pregnant women. Flunisolide should be used during pregnancy only if the potential benefit justifies the potential risk to the fetus.

Nursing Mothers: It is not known whether this drug is excreted in human milk. Because other corticosteroids are excreted in human milk, caution should be exercised when flunisolide is administered to nursing women.

Pediatric Use: Safety and effectiveness have not been established in children below the age of 6. Oral corticoids have been shown to cause growth suppression in children and adolescents, particularly with higher doses over extended periods. If a child or adolescent on any corticoid appears to have growth suppression, the possibility that they are particularly sensitive to this effect of steroids should be considered.

ADVERSE REACTIONS

Adverse events reported in controlled clinical trials and long-term open studies in 514 patients treated with **AEROBID** (flunisolide) are described below. Of those patients, 463 were treated for 3 months or longer, 407 for 6 months or longer, 287 for 1 year or longer, and 122 for 2 years or longer.

Musculoskeletal reactions were reported in 35% of steroid-dependent patients in whom the dose of oral steroid was being tapered. This is a well-known effect of steroid withdrawal.

Incidence 10% or greater:

Gastrointestinal: diarrhea (10%), nausea and/or vomiting (25%), upset stomach (10%)

General: flu (10%)

Mouth and Throat: sore throat (20%)

Nervous System: headache (25%)

Respiratory: cold symptoms (15%), nasal congestion (15%), upper respiratory infection (25%)

Special Senses: unpleasant taste (10%)

Incidence 3–9%

Cardiovascular: palpitations

Gastrointestinal: abdominal pain, heartburn

General: chest pain, decreased appetite, edema, fever

Mouth and Throat: *Candida* infection

Nervous System: dizziness, irritability, nervousness, shakiness

Reproductive: menstrual disturbances

Respiratory: chest congestion, cough*, hoarseness, rhinitis, runny nose, sinus congestion, sinus drainage, sinus infection, sinusitis, sneezing, sputum, wheezing*

Skin: eczema, itching (pruritus), rash

Special Senses: ear infection, loss of smell or taste

Incidence 1–3%

General: chills, increased appetite and weight gain, malaise, peripheral edema, sweating, weakness

Cardiovascular: hypertension, tachycardia

Gastrointestinal: constipation, dyspepsia, gas

Hemic/Lymph: capillary fragility, enlarged lymph nodes

Mouth and Throat: dry throat, glossitis, mouth irritation, pharyngitis, phlegm, throat irritation

Nervous System: anxiety, depression, faintness, fatigue, hyperactivity, hypoactivity, insomnia, moodiness, numbness, vertigo

Respiratory: bronchitis, chest tightness*, dyspnea, epistaxis, head stuffiness, laryngitis, nasal irritation, pleurisy, pneumonia, sinus discomfort

Skin: acne, hives or urticaria

Special Senses: blurred vision, earache, eye discomfort, eye infection

Incidence less than 1%, judged by investigators as possibly or probably drug related: abdominal fullness, shortness of breath.

*The incidences as shown of cough, wheezing, and chest tightness were judged by investigators to be possibly or probably drug-related. In placebo-controlled trials, the *overall* incidences of these adverse events (regardless of investigators' judgment of drug relationship) were similar for drug and placebo-treated groups. They may be related to the vehicle or delivery system.

DOSAGE AND ADMINISTRATION

The **AEROBID** (flunisolide) Inhaler System is for oral inhalation only.

Adults: The recommended starting dose is 2 inhalations twice daily, morning and evening, for a total daily dose of 1 mg. The maximum daily dose should not exceed 4 inhalations twice a day for a total daily dose of 2 mg. When the drug is used chronically at 2 mg/day, patients should be monitored periodically for effects on the hypothalamic-pituitary-adrenal (HPA) axis.

Pediatric Patients: For children and adolescents 6–15 years of age, two inhalations may be administered twice daily for a total daily dose of 1 mg. Higher doses have not been studied. Insufficient information is available to warrant use in children under age 6. With chronic use, pediatric patients should be monitored for growth as well as for effects on the HPA axis.

Rinsing the mouth after inhalation is advised.

Different considerations must be given to the following groups of patients in order to obtain the full therapeutic benefit of **AEROBID** *(flunisolide) Inhaler.*

Patients Not Receiving Systemic Corticosteroids:

Patients who require maintenance therapy of their asthma may benefit from treatment with **AEROBID** at the doses recommended above. In patients who respond to **AEROBID**, improvement in pulmonary function is usually apparent within one to four weeks after the start of therapy. Once the desired effect is achieved, consideration should be given to tapering to the lowest effective dose.

Patients Maintained on Systemic Corticosteroids:

Clinical studies have shown that **AEROBID** may be effective in the management of asthmatics dependent or maintained on systemic corticosteroids and may permit replacement or significant reduction in the dosage of systemic corticosteroids.

Continued on next page

Aerobid—Cont.

The patient's asthma should be reasonably stable before treatment with **AEROBID** is started. Initially, **AEROBID** should be used concurrently with the patient's usual maintenance dose of systemic corticosteroid. After approximately one week, gradual withdrawal of the systemic corticosteroid is started by reducing the daily or alternate daily dose. Reductions may be made after an interval of one or two weeks, depending on the response of the patient. A slow rate of withdrawal is strongly recommended. Generally, these decrements should not exceed 2.5 mg of prednisone or its equivalent. During withdrawal, some patients may experience symptoms of systemic corticosteroid withdrawal; e.g., joint and/or muscular pain, lassitude and depression, despite maintenance or even improvement of pulmonary function. Such patients should be encouraged to continue with the inhaler but should be monitored for objective signs of adrenal insufficiency. If evidence of adrenal insufficiency occurs, the systemic corticosteroid doses should be increased temporarily and thereafter withdrawal should continue more slowly. During periods of stress or a severe asthma attack, transfer patients may require supplementary treatment with systemic corticosteroids.

HOW SUPPLIED

AEROBID (flunisolide) Inhaler Systems are available in canisters of 100 metered inhalations.
NDC 0456-0672-99 **AEROBID**
NDC 0456-0670-99 **AEROBID-M**
"Note: The indented statement below is required by the Federal government's Clean Air Act for all products containing or manufactured with chlorofluorocarbons (CFC's)."

WARNING: Contains trichloromonofluoromethane, dichlorodifluoromethane and dichlorotetrafluoroethane, substances which harm public health and environment by destroying ozone in the upper atmosphere.

"A notice similar to the above WARNING has been placed in the information for the patient of this product pursuant to EPA regulations."

Caution: Federal Law prohibits dispensing without prescription.

Revised 4/96

mfd for
FOREST PHARMACEUTICALS, INC.
St. Louis, MO 63045
mfd by
3M Pharmaceuticals
St. Paul, MN

605301

Shown in Product Identification Guide, page 312

AeroChamber® ℞
AeroChamber® with *Mask—Small*
AeroChamber® with *Mask*
AeroChamber® with *Mask—Large*
Valved Aerosol Holding Chamber/Aerosol Holding Chamber with *Mask* for Use With Metered Dose Inhalers.

Before using AeroChamber/AeroChamber with *Mask*, it is important to read these instructions very carefully, including the CAUTION sections that follow:

CAUTION

1. When cleaning, the only part of the AeroChamber/AeroChamber with Mask to be removed is the rubber-like ring that holds the Metered Dose Inhaler and the protective mouthpiece cap from the AeroChamber. Do not remove the mouthpiece/face mask from the AeroChamber body.
2. Except as stated in 1 above, do not disassemble the AeroChamber/AeroChamber with Mask, as the overall reliability and safety of the product may be affected.
3. Replace AeroChamber/AeroChamber with Mask at once and do not use if the one-way valve becomes dislodged (partially or fully) or begins to harden or curl.
4. Running water through the AeroChamber/AeroChamber with Mask at high pressure may harm the valve. Examine AeroChamber/AeroChamber with Mask visually before and after cleaning to make sure the one-way valve and other parts are properly secured.
5. Disassembly may loosen or dislodge the one-way valve. Examine the AeroChamber/AeroChamber with Mask visually before and after use to make sure the one-way valve and other parts are properly secured.
6. Do not allow children to play with the AeroChamber/AeroChamber with Mask—allowing them to do so may alter its function and/or overall reliability. The mask membrane, the one-way valve, and the exhalation valve (Mask-Small) can be damaged as a result of pulling or poking.
7. As indicated, your AeroChamber/AeroChamber with Mask should be inspected visually before and after daily use and may need to be replaced after 6 to 12 months of use.

INTRODUCTION

The AeroChamber/AeroChamber with Mask line is a family of valved aerosol holding chambers available from Forest Pharmaceuticals, Inc., designed to be used with virtually all Metered Dose Inhalers [MDI's]. When you release a puff of aerosol into the AeroChamber/AeroChamber with Mask, the puff will be held there for a few seconds. The valved holding chamber selectively removes most large aerosol-drug particles that normally deposit in the mouth and throat, while allowing the smaller, therapeutic particles to pass through the patented one-way valve into the lungs. This provides effective treatment and helps to reduce unwanted side effects. In addition, the AeroChamber/AeroChamber with Mask is designed to make Metered Dose Inhalers easier to use.

CLEANING INSTRUCTIONS

The AeroChamber/AeroChamber with Mask is made of durable plastic materials and has one or two moving parts; the one-way valve and, in the AeroChamber with Mask-Small, an exhalation valve. With repeated use, residue may accumulate inside the AeroChamber/AeroChamber with Mask and around the one-way valve. This may eventually interfere with effective use. We suggest cleaning the Metered Dose Inhaler as instructed by the manufacturer and AeroChamber/AeroChamber with Mask about once a week or more often depending on your usage of the product.

To clean the AeroChamber/AeroChamber with Mask:

1. Remove the rubber-like ring from the end that holds the Metered Dose Inhaler and the protective mouthpiece cap from the AeroChamber. Do not remove the mouthpiece/face mask from the AeroChamber body.
2. Soak AeroChamber/AeroChamber with Mask, rubber-like ring, and the protective mouthpiece cap from the AeroChamber in basin filled with warm water, using mild detergent to dislodge or loosen any residue.
3. Rinse AeroChamber/AeroChamber with Mask, rubber-like ring, and the protective mouthpiece cap from the AeroChamber in basin filled with clean warm water, using a gentle motion.
4. Lightly shake away excess water droplets and leave on clean surface to air-dry.
5. Be sure the AeroChamber/AeroChamber with Mask is completely dry before use.
6. Replace the rubber-like ring on the AeroChamber/AeroChamber with Mask.

TECHNICAL INFORMATION

This apparently simple device is a product of considerable medical research and engineering. It was developed in a leading medical center.

The valved holding chamber selectively removes large aerosol particles that normally deposit in the mouth and throat, while allowing the smaller treatment particles to pass into the lungs. This provides effective treatment and helps reduce unwanted side effects.

AeroChamber

INSTRUCTIONS FOR USE

Please discuss the use of the AeroChamber with your physician, pharmacist, or other healthcare professional.

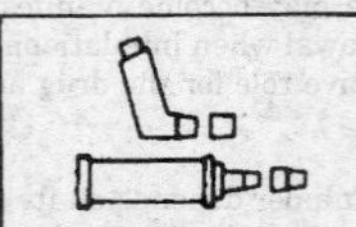

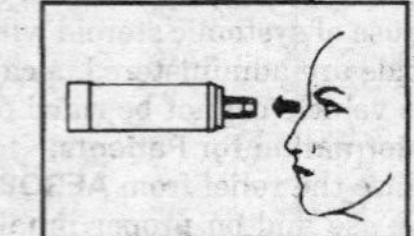

1. Remove the protective cap from Metered-Dose Inhaler [MDI]. Remove the protective cap from the mouthpiece of AeroChamber.
2. Visually check the AeroChamber for foreign objects. Ensure that all parts are secure, including the one-way valve.

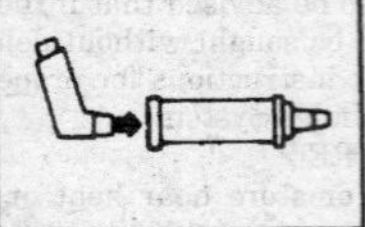

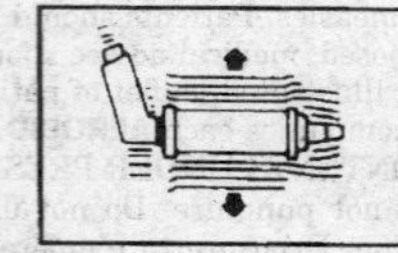

3. Insert inhaler mouth-piece into the round opening in the rubber-like ring at the end of the AeroChamber.
4. Holding the AeroChamber and Inhaler [MDI] firmly, shake vigorously 3 or 4 times.

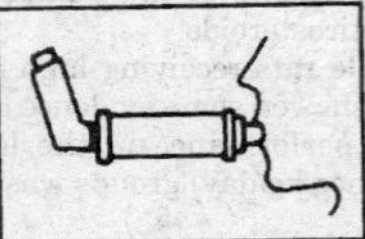

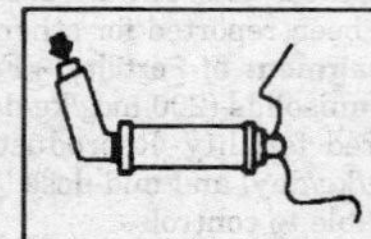

5. Exhale normally. Place the AeroChamber mouthpiece in mouth and close lips.
6. Spray only one puff from the inhaler [MDI] into the AeroChamber per inhalation maneuver. Spraying more than one puff into the AeroChamber before or during an inhalation maneuver will result in delivery of improper dose of medication.

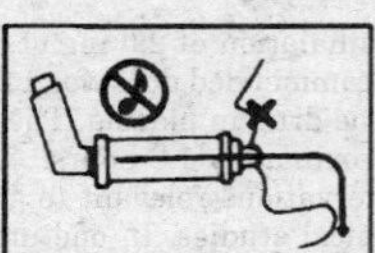

7. Breathe in slowly and deeply through mouth until you have taken a full breath. Do not breathe in so fast as to activate the flow signal whistle. A whistling sound from the flow signal indicates that you are breathing in too quickly.
8. Hold breath for 5 to 10 seconds.
9. Repeat steps 4 to 8 as prescribed by your physician.
10. Remove inhaler and examine the AeroChamber to make certain that the one-way valve is properly secured.
11. Replace protective cap on AeroChamber and MDI.

HELPFUL HINTS:

1. In order to obtain the maximum benefit from your Metered Dose Inhaler, it is extremely important to fill your lungs during inhalation by taking a *slow*, deep breath. If the flow signal makes a whistling sound, it is an indication that you are breathing in too quickly.
2. The one-way valve allows you to inhale at your own rate so that coordination of inhalation with the actuation of the inhaler is not a problem.
3. If you have trouble inhaling through your mouth, with the AeroChamber mouthpiece between your lips, it may be necessary to gently pinch your nose while inhaling the medication.
4. For the elderly and small children who may have difficulty using the AeroChamber, there is also an AeroChamber available with Mask which allows another person to assist with coordination.
5. When using the AeroChamber with a corticosteroid Metered Dose Inhaler, it is recommended by the manufacturer of these drugs to rinse your mouth with water to remove any medication residue.

> **IMPORTANT INFORMATION**
> Package insert dosing instructions should be consulted for all Metered Dose Inhalers [MDIs] when used with AeroChamber. Dosage and administration recommendations vary for different MDIs, and the limitations and conditions of use for each product should be considered before utilizing this device, particularly for younger and older patients.

This device helps deliver aerosol medication to the lungs more reliably. Should you have any problem using the AeroChamber please contact your doctor.

CAUTION: Federal law restricts this device to sale by, or on the order of, a physician.

Manufactured by Monaghan Medical Corporation, Plattsburgh, NY 12901

Assembled in USA of Canadian Components covered by one or more of the following patent numbers: 4,470,412; 5,042,467; 5,012,803; 4,809,692; 4,832,015; 5,012,804

AeroChamber with *Mask—Small*

INSTRUCTIONS FOR USE

Please discuss the use of the AeroChamber with Mask-Small with your physician, pharmacist, or other healthcare professional.

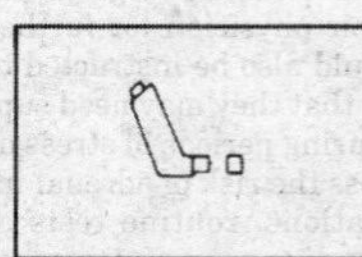

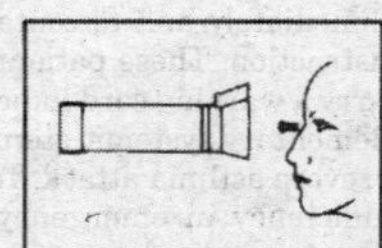

1. Remove the protective cap from Metered Dose Inhaler [MDI].
2. Visually check the AeroChamber with Mask-Small for foreign objects. Ensure that all parts are secure.

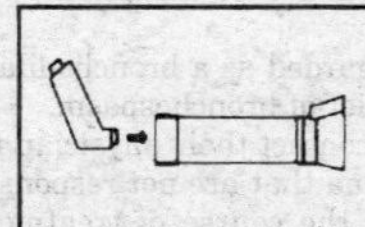

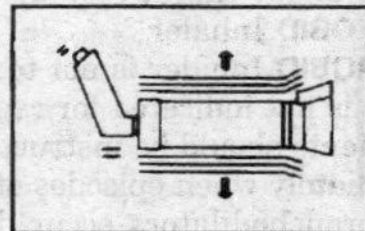

3. Insert inhaler mouthpiece into the round opening in the rubber-like end of the AeroChamber with Mask-Small.
4. Holding the AeroChamber with Mask-Small and inhaler firmly, shake vigorously 3 or 4 times.

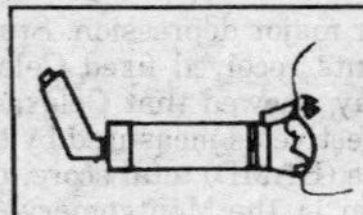

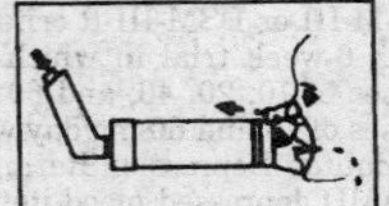

5. Place the soft mask gently to the face so that the mouth and nose are covered. Be certain to create a good seal; leaks will inhibit the delivery of the medication. The exhalation valve allows the patient to exhale comfortably while the mask is held firmly around their mouth and nose.

6. While the patient is exhaling, spray only one puff from the inhaler into the AeroChamber with Mask-Small. Spraying more than one puff into the AeroChamber with Mask-Small before or during an inhalation maneuver will result in delivery of improper dose of medication.

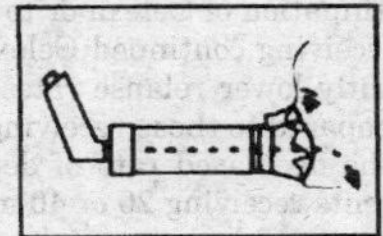

7. Hold the mask firmly to the patient's face for at least six (6) breaths.
8. Repeat steps 4 to 7 as prescribed by your physician, waiting at least 30 seconds between puffs.
9. Remove inhaler and replace its protective cap.

AeroChamber with *Mask*

INSTRUCTIONS FOR USE

Please discuss the use of the AeroChamber with Mask with your physician, pharmacist, or other healthcare professional.

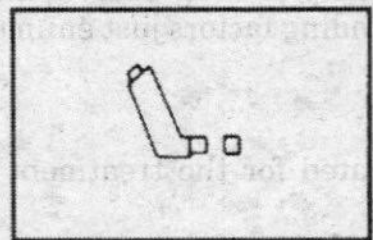

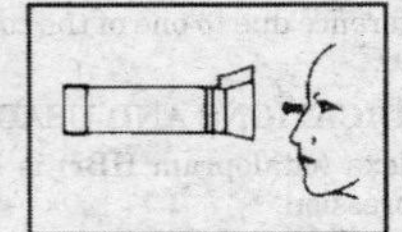

1. Remove the protective cap from Metered Dose Inhaler (MDI).

2. Visually check the AeroChamber with Mask for foreign objects. Ensure that all parts are secure.

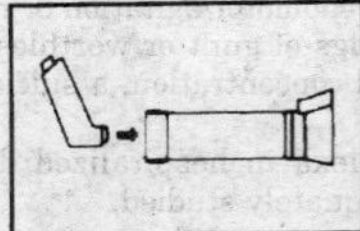

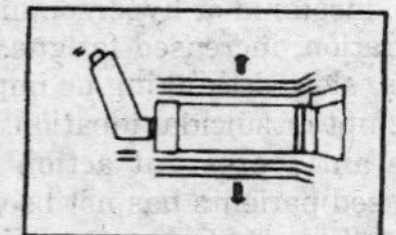

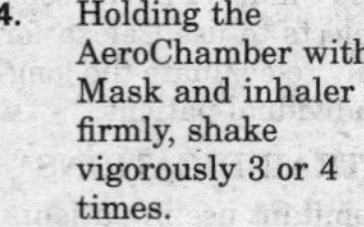

3. Insert inhaler mouthpiece into the opening in the soft rubber-like end of the AeroChamber with Mask.

4. Holding the AeroChamber with Mask and inhaler firmly, shake vigorously 3 or 4 times.

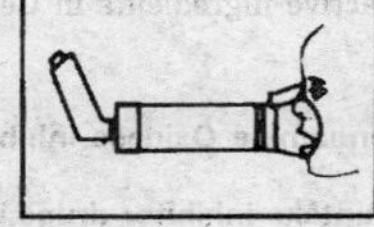

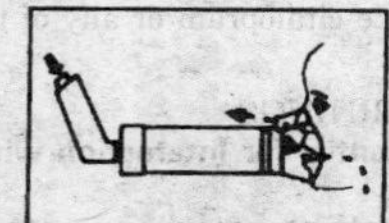

5. Place the soft mask gently to the face so that the mouth and nose are covered. Be certain to create a good seal: leaks will inhibit the delivery of the medication. The exhalation valve allows the patient to exhale comfortably while the mask is held firmly around their mouth and nose.

6. While the patient is exhaling, spray only one puff from the inhaler into the AeroChamber with Mask. Spraying more than one puff into the AeroChamber with Mask before or during an inhalation maneuver will result in delivery of improper dose of medication.

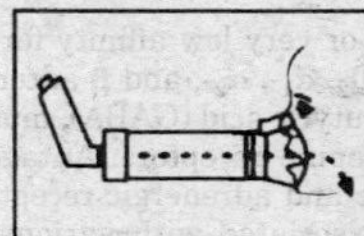

7. Hold the mask firmly to the patient's face for at least six (6) breaths.
8. Repeat steps 4 to 7 as prescribed by your physician, waiting at least 30 seconds between puffs.
9. Remove inhaler and replace its protective cap.

HELPFUL HINTS

1. Some children may resist their treatment by grabbing at the mask. Place the child on your lap and wrap one arm around the child to simplify placing the mask on the child's face.
2. In the case of a smaller child it may be more comfortable to lay the child on a bed while administering the medication.
3. If the child seems frightened by the AeroChamber with Mask-Small or AeroChamber with Mask, familiarize the child with the device by stroking his or her cheek with the soft mask. If the child cries during treatment with the AeroChamber with Mask-Small or AeroChamber with Mask, the medication will still be delivered as long as there is a good seal between the mask and the child's face. Remember, the child will inhale after crying or screaming.
4. When using the AeroChamber with Mask-Small or AeroChamber with Mask with a corticosteroid Metered Dose Inhaler, it is recommended that the patient's face be cleaned with soap and water to remove any medication residue.

IMPORTANT INFORMATION:
Package insert dosing instructions should be consulted for all Metered Dose Inhalers [MDIs] when used with AeroChamber with Mask-Small or AeroChamber with Mask. Dosage and administration recommendations vary for different MDIs, and the limitations and conditions of use for each product should be considered before utilizing this device, particularly for younger and older patients.

This device helps deliver aerosol medication to the lungs more reliably. Should you have any problem using the AeroChamber with Mask-Small or AeroChamber with Mask, please contact your doctor.

CAUTION: Federal law restricts this device to sale by, or on the order of, a physician.
Manufactured by Monaghan Medical corporation, Plattsburgh, NY 12901
Assembled in USA of Canadian components covered by one or more of the following patent numbers: 4,470,412; 5,042,467; 5,012,803; 4,809,692; 4,832,015; 5,012,804

AeroChamber with *Mask—Large*

INSTRUCTIONS FOR USE:

Please discuss the use of the AeroChamber with Mask-Large with your physician, pharmacist, or other healthcare professional.

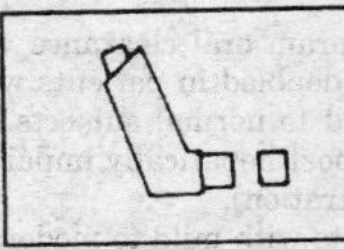

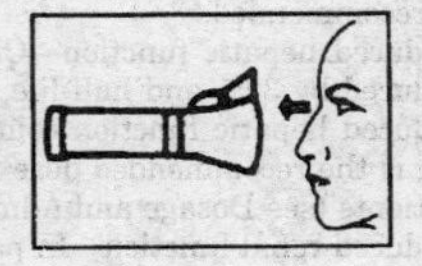

1. Remove the protective cap from Metered Dose Inhaler [MDI].

2. Visually check the AeroChamber with Mask-Large for foreign objects. Ensure that all parts are secure, including the one-way valve.

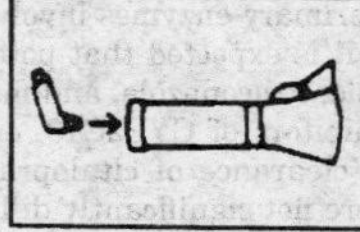

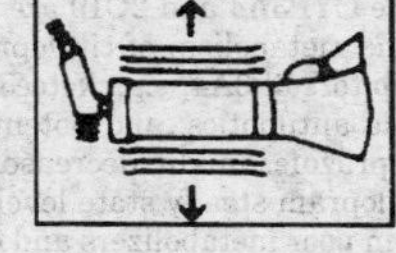

3. Insert inhaler mouthpiece into the round opening in the rubber-like ring at the end of the AeroChamber with Mask-Large.

4. Holding the AeroChamber with Mask-Large and inhaler [MDI] firmly, shake vigorously 3 or 4 times.

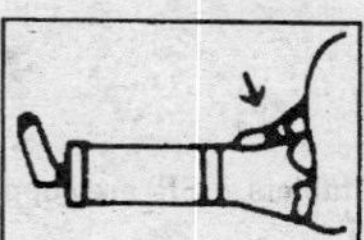

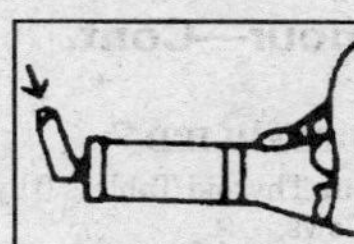

5. Place the soft mask gently to the face so that the mouth and nose are covered. Be certain to create a good seal. Leaks will inhibit the delivery of the medication. Seeing the diaphragm move is a helpful indication of a good seal.

6. Spray only one puff from the inhaler [MDI] into the AeroChamber with Mask-Large per inhalation maneuver. Spraying more than one puff into the AeroChamber with Mask-Large before or during an inhalation maneuver will result in delivery of improper dose of medication.

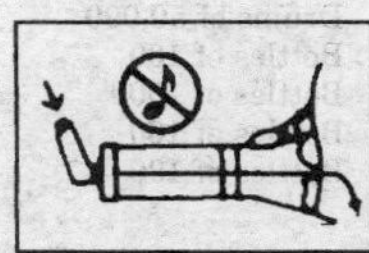

7. Breathe in slowly and deeply until you have taken a full breath. Do not breathe in so fast as to activate the flow signal whistle. A whistle sound from the flow signal indicates that you are breathing in too quickly.
8. Repeat steps 4 to 7 as prescribed by your physician.
9. Remove inhaler and examine the AeroChamber with Mask-Large to make certain that the one-way valve is properly secured.

HELPFUL HINTS

1. In order to obtain the maximum benefit from your Metered Dose Inhaler, it is extremely important to fill your lungs during inhalation by taking a *slow*, deep breath. If the flow signal makes a whistling sound, it is an indication that you are breathing in too quickly.
2. The one-way valve allows you to inhale at your own rate so that coordination of inhalation with the actuation of the inhaler is not a problem.
3. When using the AeroChamber with Mask-Large with a corticosteroid Metered Dose Inhaler, it is recommended that the patient's face be cleaned with soap and water to remove any medication residue.

IMPORTANT INFORMATION
Package insert dosing instructions should be consulted for all Metered Dose Inhalers [MDIs] when used with AeroChamber with Mask-Large. Dosage and administration recommendations vary for different MDIs and the limitations and conditions of use for each product should be considered before utilizing this device, particularly for younger and older patients.

This device helps deliver aerosol medication to the lungs more reliably. Should you have any problem using the AeroChamber with Mask-Large, please contact your doctor.

CAUTION: Federal law restricts this device to sale by, or on the order of, a physician.
Manufactured by Monaghan Medical Corporation, Plattsburgh, NY 12901
Assembled in USA of Canadian components covered by one or more of the following patent numbers: 4,470,412; 5,042,467; 5,012,803; 4,809,692; 4,832,015; 5,012,804
Distributed by:
FOREST PHARMACEUTICALS, INC.
UAD LABORATORIES
St. Louis, Missouri 63045
REV 7/96 ACL
Shown in Product Identification Guide, page 312

ARMOUR® THYROID Tablets ℞
[thī 'roid]
(THYROID TABLETS, U.S.P.)

DESCRIPTION

Armour® Thyroid (thyroid tablets, USP) for oral use is a natural preparation derived from porcine thyroid glands and has a strong, characteristic odor. (T_3 liothyronine is approximately four times as potent as T_4 levothyroxine on a microgram for microgram basis.) They provide 38 mcg levothyroxine (T_4) and 9 mcg liothyronine (T_3) per grain of thyroid. The inactive ingredients are calcium stearate, dextrose microcrystalline cellulose, sodium starch glycolate and opadry white.

Continued on next page

Armour—Cont.

HOW SUPPLIED

Armour Thyroid Tablets (thyroid tablets, USP) are supplied as follows:

Size	Available in	NDC No.
15 mg (1/4 gr)	Bottles of 100	0456-0457-01
30 mg (1/2 gr)	Bottles of 100	0456-0458-01
	Bottles of 1000	0456-0458-00
	Drums of 50,000	0456-0458-69
	Unit dose cartons of 100	0456-0458-63
60 mg (1 gr)	Bottles of 100	0456-0459-01
	Bottles of 1000	0456-0459-00
	Bottles of 5000	0456-0459-51
	Drums of 50,000	0456-0459-69
	Unit dose cartons of 100	0456-0459-63
90 mg (1 1/2 gr)	Bottles of 100	0456-0460-01
120 mg (2 gr)	Bottles of 100	0456-0461-01
	Bottles of 1000	0456-0461-00
	Drums of 50,000	0456-0461-69
180 mg (3 gr)	Bottles of 100	0456-0462-01
	Bottles of 1000	0456-0462-00
240 mg (4 gr)	Bottles of 100	0456-0463-01
300 mg (5 gr)	Bottles of 100	0456-0464-01

The bottles of 100 are special dispensing bottles with child-resistant closures.

Note: (T_3 liothyronine is approximately four times as potent as T_4 levothyroxine on a microgram-for-microgram basis.)

Tablets should be stored at controlled room temperature, 59°–86°F (15°–30°C), in capped bottles or unbroken plastic strip packing.

Forest Pharmaceuticals, Inc.
A Subsidiary of Forest Laboratories, Inc.
St. Louis, MO 63045
REV 4/00 11840400

Shown in Product Identification Guide, page 312

CELEXA™ ℞
(citalopram hydrobromide)

DESCRIPTION

Celexa™ (citalopram HBr) is an orally administered selective serotonin reuptake inhibitor (SSRI) with a chemical structure unrelated to that of other SSRI's or of tricyclic, tetracyclic, or other available antidepressant agents. Citalopram HBr is a racemic bicyclic phthalane derivative designated (±)-1-(3-dimethylaminopropyl)-1-(4-fluorophenyl)-1,3-dihydroisobenzofuran-5-carbonitrile, HBr with the following structural formula:

The molecular formula is $C_{20}H_{22}BrFN_2O$ and its molecular weight is 405.35.

Citalopram HBr occurs as a fine white to off-white powder. Citalopram HBr is sparingly soluble in water and soluble in ethanol.

Celexa (citalopram hydrobromide) is available as tablets or as an oral solution.

Celexa tablets are film coated, oval, scored tablets containing citalopram HBr in strengths equivalent to 20 mg or 40 mg citalopram base. The tablets also contain the following inactive ingredients: Copolyvidone, Corn Starch, Crosscarmellose Sodium, Glycerin, Lactose Monohydrate, Magnesium Stearate, Hydroxypropyl Methyl Cellulose, Microcrystalline Cellulose, Polyethylene Glycol, and Titanium Dioxide. Iron Oxides are used as coloring agents in the pink (20 mg) tablets.

Celexa oral solution contains citalopram HBr equivalent to 2 mg/mL citalopram base. It also contains the following inactive ingredients: Sorbitol, Purified Water, Propylene Glycol, Methylparaben, Natural Peppermint Flavor, and Propylparaben.

CLINICAL PHARMACOLOGY

Pharmacodynamics

The mechanism of action of citalopram HBr as an antidepressant is presumed to be linked to potentiation of serotonergic activity in the central nervous system resulting from its inhibition of CNS neuronal reuptake of serotonin (5-HT). *In vitro* and *in vivo* studies in animals suggest that citalopram is a highly selective serotonin reuptake inhibitor (SSRI) with minimal effects on norepinephrine (NE) and dopamine (DA) neuronal reuptake. Tolerance to the inhibition of 5-HT uptake is not induced by long term (14 day) treatment of rats with citalopram. Citalopram is a racemic mixture (50/50), and the inhibition of 5-HT reuptake by citalopram is primarily due to the (S)-enantiomer.

Citalopram has no or very low affinity for $5\text{-}HT_{1A}$, $5\text{-}HT_{2A}$, dopamine D_1 and D_2, α_1-, α_2-, and β-adrenergic, histamine H_1, gamma aminobutyric acid (GABA), muscarinic cholinergic, and benzodiazepine receptors. Antagonism of muscarinic, histaminergic and adrenergic receptors has been hypothesized to be associated with various anticholinergic, sedative and cardiovascular effects of other psychotropic drugs.

Pharmacokinetics

The single- and multiple-dose pharmacokinetics of citalopram are linear and dose-proportional in a dose range of 10–60 mg/day. Biotransformation of citalopram is mainly hepatic, with a mean terminal half-life of about 35 hours. With once daily dosing, steady state plasma concentrations are achieved within approximately one week. At steady state, the extent of accumulation of citalopram in plasma, based on the half-life, is expected to be 2.5 times the plasma concentrations observed after a single dose. The tablet and oral solution dosage forms of citalopram HBr are bioequivalent.

Absorption and Distribution

Following a single oral dose (40 mg tablet) of citalopram, peak blood levels occur at about 4 hours. The absolute bioavailability of citalopram was about 80% relative to an intravenous dose and absorption is not affected by food. The volume of distribution of citalopram is about 12 L/kg and the binding of citalopram (CT), demethylcitalopram (DCT) and didemethylcitalopram (DDCT) to human plasma proteins is about 80%.

Metabolism and Elimination

Following intravenous administrations of citalopram, the fraction of drug recovered in the urine as citalopram and DCT was about 10% and 5%, respectively. The systemic clearance of citalopram was 330 mL/min, with approximately 20% of that due to renal clearance.

Citalopram is metabolized to demethylcitalopram (DCT), didemethylcitalopram (DDCT), citalopram-N-oxide and a deaminated propionic acid derivative. In humans, unchanged citalopram is the predominant compound in plasma. At steady state, the concentrations of citalopram's metabolites, DCT and DDCT, in plasma are approximately one-half and one-tenth, respectively, that of the parent drug. *In vitro* studies show that citalopram is at least 8 times more potent than its metabolites in the inhibition of serotonin reuptake, suggesting that the metabolites evaluated do not likely contribute significantly to the antidepressant actions of citalopram.

In vitro studies using human liver microsomes indicated that CYP3A4 and CYP2C19 are the primary isozymes involved in the N-demethylation of citalopram.

Population Subgroups

Age—Citalopram pharmacokinetics in subjects ≥ 60 years of age were compared to younger subjects in two normal volunteer studies. In a single dose study, citalopram AUC and half-life were increased in the elderly subjects by 30% and 50%, respectively, whereas in a multiple dose study they were increased by 23% and 30% respectively. 20 mg is the recommended dose for most elderly patients (See Dosage and Administration).

Gender—In three pharmacokinetic studies (total N=32), citalopram AUC in women was one and a half to two times that in men. This difference was not observed in five other pharmacokinetic studies (total N=114). In clinical studies, no differences in steady state serum citalopram levels were seen between men (N=237) and women (N=388). There were no gender differences in the pharmacokinetics of DCT and DDCT. No adjustment of dosage on the basis of gender is recommended.

Reduced hepatic function—Citalopram oral clearance was reduced by 37% and half-life was doubled in patients with reduced hepatic function compared to normal subjects. 20 mg is the recommended dose for most hepatically impaired patients (see Dosage and Administration).

Reduced renal function—In patients with mild to moderate renal function impairment, oral clearance of citalopram was reduced by 17% compared to normal subjects. No adjustment of dosage for such patients is recommended. No information is available about the pharmacokinetics of citalopram in patients with severely reduced renal function (creatinine clearance < 20 mL/min).

Drug-Drug Interactions

In vitro enzyme inhibition data did not reveal an inhibitory effect of citalopram on CYP3A4, but did suggest that it is a weak inhibitor of CYP-1A2, -2D6, and -2C19. Citalopram would be expected to have little inhibitory effect on *in vivo* metabolism mediated by these cytochromes. However, *in vivo* data to address this question are very limited.

Since CYP3A4 and 2C19 are the primary enzymes involved in the metabolism of citalopram, it is expected that potent inhibitors of 3A4, e.g., ketoconazole, itraconazole, and macrolide antibiotics, and potent inhibitors of CYP2C19, e.g., omeprazole, might decrease the clearance of citalopram. Citalopram steady state levels were not significantly different in poor metabolizers and extensive 2D6 metabolizers after multiple dose administration of Celexa, suggesting that coadministration, with Celexa, of a drug that inhibits CYP2D6, is unlikely to have clinically significant effects on citalopram metabolism. See Drug Interactions under Precautions for more detailed information on available drug interaction data.

Clinical Efficacy Trials

The efficacy of Celexa as a treatment for depression was established in two placebo-controlled studies (of 4 to 6 weeks in duration) in adult outpatients (ages 18–66) meeting DSM-III or DSM-III-R criteria for major depression. Study 1, a 6-week trial in which patients received fixed Celexa doses of 10, 20, 40, and 60 mg/day, showed that Celexa at doses of 40 and 60 mg/day was effective as measured by the Hamilton Depression Rating Scale (HAMD) total score, the HAMD depressed mood item (Item 1), the Montgomery Asberg Depression Rating Scale, and the Clinical Global Impression (CGI) Severity scale. This study showed no clear effect of the 10 and 20 mg/day doses, and the 60 mg/day dose was not more effective than the 40 mg/day dose. In study 2, a 4-week, placebo-controlled trial in depressed patients, of whom 85% met criteria for melancholia, the initial dose was 20 mg/day, followed by titration to the maximum tolerated dose or a maximum dose of 80 mg/day. Patients treated with Celexa showed significantly greater improvement than placebo patients on the HAMD total score, HAMD item 1, and the CGI Severity score. In three additional placebo-controlled depression trials, the difference in response to treatment between patients receiving Celexa and patients receiving placebo was not statistically significant, possibly due to high spontaneous response rate, smaller sample size, or, in the case of one study, too low a dose.

In two long-term studies, depressed patients who had responded to Celexa during an initial 6 or 8 weeks of acute treatment (fixed doses of 20 or 40 mg/day in one study and flexible doses of 20–60 mg/day in the second study) were randomized to continuation of Celexa or to placebo. In both studies, patients receiving continued Celexa treatment experienced significantly lower relapse rates over the subsequent 6 months compared to those receiving placebo. In the fixed dose study, the decreased rate of depression relapse was similar in patients receiving 20 or 40 mg/day of Celexa.

Analyses of the relationship between treatment outcome and age, gender, and race did not suggest any differential responsiveness on the basis of these patient characteristics.

Comparison of Clinical Trial Results

Highly variable results have been seen in the clinical development of all antidepressant drugs. Furthermore, in those circumstances when the drugs have not been studied in the same controlled clinical trial(s), comparisons among the results of studies evaluating the effectiveness of different antidepressant drug products are inherently unreliable. Because conditions of testing (e.g., patient samples, investigators, doses of the treatments administered and compared, outcome measures, etc.) vary among trials, it is virtually impossible to distinguish a difference in drug effect from a difference due to one of the confounding factors just enumerated.

INDICATIONS AND USAGE

Celexa (citalopram HBr) is indicated for the treatment of depression.

The efficacy of Celexa in the treatment of depression was established in 4–6 week controlled trials of outpatients whose diagnosis corresponded most closely to the DSM-III and DSM-III-R category of major depressive disorder (see Clinical Pharmacology).

A major depressive episode (DSM-IV) implies a prominent and relatively persistent (nearly every day for at least 2 weeks) depressed or dysphoric mood that usually interferes with daily functioning, and includes at least five of the following nine symptoms: depressed mood, loss of interest in usual activities, significant change in weight and/or appetite, insomnia or hypersomnia, psychomotor agitation or retardation, increased fatigue, feelings of guilt or worthlessness, slowed thinking or impaired concentration, a suicide attempt or suicidal ideation.

The antidepressant action of Celexa in hospitalized depressed patients has not been adequately studied.

The efficacy of Celexa in maintaining an antidepressant response for up to 24 weeks following 6 to 8 weeks of acute treatment was demonstrated in two placebo-controlled trials (see Clinical Pharmacology). Nevertheless, the physician who elects to use Celexa for extended periods should periodically re-evaluate the long-term usefulness of the drug for the individual patient.

CONTRAINDICATIONS

Concomitant use in patients taking monoamine oxidase inhibitors (MAOI's) is contraindicated (see Warnings).

Celexa is contraindicated in patients with a hypersensitivity to citalopram or any of the inactive ingredients in Celexa.

WARNINGS

Potential for Interaction with Monoamine Oxidase Inhibitors

In patients receiving serotonin reuptake inhibitor drugs in combination with a monoamine oxidase inhibitor (MAOI), there have been reports of serious, sometimes fatal, reactions including hyperthermia, rigidity, myoclonus, autonomic instability with possible rapid fluctuations of vital signs, and mental status changes that include extreme agitation progressing to delirium and coma. These reactions have also been reported in patients who have recently discontinued SSRI treatment and have been started on a MAOI. Some cases presented with features resembling neuroleptic malignant syndrome. Furthermore, limited animal data on the effects of combined use of SSRI's and MAOI's suggest that these drugs may act synergistically to elevate blood pressure and evoke behavioral excitation. Therefore, it is recommended that Celexa should not be used in combination with a MAOI, or within 14 days of discontinuing treatment with a MAOI. Similarly, at least 14 days should be allowed after stopping Celexa before starting a MAOI.

PRECAUTIONS

General

Hyponatremia

Several cases of hyponatremia and SIADH (syndrome of inappropriate antidiuretic hormone secretion) have been reported in association with Celexa treatment. All patients with these events have recovered with discontinuation of Celexa and/or medical intervention.

Activation of Mania/Hypomania

In placebo-controlled trials of Celexa, some of which included patients with bipolar disorder, activation of mania/hypomania was reported in 0.2% of 1063 patients treated with Celexa and in none of the 446 patients treated with placebo. Activation of mania/hypomania has also been reported in a small proportion of patients with major affective disorders treated with other marketed antidepressants. As with all antidepressants, Celexa should be used cautiously in patients with a history of mania.

Seizures

Although anticonvulsant effects of citalopram have been observed in animal studies, Celexa has not been systematically evaluated in patients with a seizure disorder. These patients were excluded from clinical studies during the product's premarketing testing. In clinical trials of Celexa, seizures occurred in 0.3% of patients treated with Celexa (a rate of one patient per 98 years of exposure) and 0.5% of patients treated with placebo (a rate of one patient per 50 years of exposure). Like other antidepressants, Celexa should be introduced with care in patients with a history of seizure disorder.

Suicide

The possibility of a suicide attempt is inherent in depression and may persist until significant remission occurs. Close supervision of high risk patients should accompany initial drug therapy. Prescriptions for Celexa should be written for the smallest quantity of tablets consistent with good patient management, in order to reduce the risk of overdose.

Interference with Cognitive and Motor Performance

In studies in normal volunteers, Celexa in doses of 40 mg/day did not produce impairment of intellectual function or psychomotor performance. Because any psychoactive drug may impair judgment, thinking, or motor skills, however, patients should be cautioned about operating hazardous machinery, including automobiles, until they are reasonably certain that Celexa therapy does not affect their ability to engage in such activities.

Use in Patients with Concomitant Illness

Clinical experience with Celexa in patients with certain concomitant systemic illnesses is limited. Caution is advisable in using Celexa in patients with diseases or conditions that produce altered metabolism or hemodynamic responses.

Celexa has not been systematically evaluated in patients with a recent history of myocardial infarction or unstable heart disease. Patients with these diagnoses were generally excluded from clinical studies during the product's premarketing testing. However, the electrocardiograms of 1116 patients who received Celexa in clinical trials were evaluated and the data indicate that Celexa is not associated with the development of clinically significant ECG abnormalities.

In subjects with hepatic impairment, citalopram clearance was decreased and plasma concentrations were increased. The use of Celexa in hepatically impaired patients should be approached with caution and a lower maximum dosage is recommended (see Dosage and Administration).

Because citalopram is extensively metabolized, excretion of unchanged drug in urine is a minor route of elimination. Until adequate numbers of patients with severe renal impairment have been evaluated during chronic treatment with Celexa, however, it should be used with caution in such patients (see Dosage and Administration).

Information for Patients

Physicians are advised to discuss the following issues with patients for whom they prescribe Celexa.

Although in controlled studies Celexa has not been shown to impair psychomotor performance, any psychoactive drug may impair judgment, thinking or motor skills, and so patients should be cautioned about operating hazardous machinery, including automobiles, until they are reasonably certain that Celexa therapy does not affect their ability to engage in such activities.

Patients should be told that, although Celexa has not been shown in experiments with normal subjects to increase the mental and motor skill impairments caused by alcohol, the concomitant use of Celexa and alcohol in depressed patients is not advised.

Patients should be advised to inform their physician if they are taking, or plan to take, any prescription or over-the-counter drugs, as there is a potential for interactions.

Patients should be advised to notify their physician if they become pregnant or intend to become pregnant during therapy.

Patients should be advised to notify their physician if they are breast feeding an infant.

While patients may notice improvement with Celexa therapy in 1 to 4 weeks, they should be advised to continue therapy as directed.

Laboratory Tests

There are no specific laboratory tests recommended.

Drug Interactions

CNS Drugs—Given the primary CNS effects of citalopram, caution should be used when it is taken in combination with other centrally acting drugs.

Alcohol—Although citalopram did not potentiate the cognitive and motor effects of alcohol in a clinical trial, as with other psychotropic medications, the use of alcohol by depressed patients taking Celexa is not recommended.

Monoamine Oxidase Inhibitors (MAOI's)—See Contraindications and Warnings.

Cimetidine—In subjects who had received 21 days of 40 mg/day Celexa, combined administration of 400 mg/day cimetidine for 8 days resulted in an increase in citalopram AUC and C_{max} of 43% and 39%, respectively. The clinical significance of these findings is unknown.

Digoxin—In subjects who had received 21 days of 40 mg/day Celexa, combined administration of Celexa and digoxin (single dose of 1 mg) did not significantly affect the pharmacokinetics of either citalopram or digoxin.

Lithium—Coadministration of Celexa (40 mg/day for 10 days) and lithium (30 mmol/day for 5 days) had no significant effect on the pharmacokinetics of citalopram or lithium. Nevertheless, plasma lithium levels should be monitored with appropriate adjustment to the lithium dose in accordance with standard clinical practice. Because lithium may enhance the serotonergic effects of citalopram, caution should be exercised when Celexa and lithium are coadministered.

Sumatriptan—There have been rare postmarketing reports describing patients with weakness, hyperreflexia, and incoordination following the use of a selective serotonin reuptake inhibitor (SSRI) and sumatriptan. If concomitant treatment with sumatriptan and an SSRI (e.g., fluoxetine, fluvoxamine, paroxetine, sertraline, citalopram) is clinically warranted, appropriate observation of the patient is advised.

Warfarin—Administration of 40 mg/day Celexa for 21 days did not affect the pharmacokinetics of warfarin, a CYP3A4 substrate. Prothrombin time was increased by 5%, the clinical significance of which is unknown.

Carbamazepine—Combined administration of Celexa (40 mg/day for 14 days) and carbamazepine (titrated to 400 mg/day for 35 days) did not significantly affect the pharmacokinetics of carbamazepine, a CYP3A4 substrate. Although trough citalopram plasma levels were unaffected, given the enzyme inducing properties of carbamazepine, the possibility that carbamazepine might increase the clearance of citalopram should be considered if the two drugs are coadministered.

CYP3A4 and 2C19 Inhibitors—*In vitro* studies indicated that CYP3A4 and 2C19 are the primary enzymes involved in the metabolism of citalopram. As data are not available from clinical pharmacokinetic studies, the possibility that the clearance of citalopram will be decreased when citalopram is administered with a potent inhibitor of CYP3A4 (e.g., ketoconazole, intraconazole, fluconazole, or erythromycin), or a potent inhibitor of CYP2C19 (e.g., omeprazole), should be considered.

Metoprolol—Administration of 40 mg/day Celexa for 22 days resulted in a two-fold increase in the plasma levels of the beta-adrenergic blocker metoprolol. Increased metoprolol plasma levels have been associated with decreased cardioselectivity. Coadministration of Celexa and metoprolol had no clinically significant effects on blood pressure or heart rate.

Imipramine and Other Tricyclic Antidepressants (TCAs)—*In vitro* studies suggest that citalopram is a relatively weak inhibitor of CYP2D6. Coadministration of Celexa (40 mg/day for 10 days) with the tricyclic antidepressant imipramine (single dose of 100 mg), a substrate for CYP2D6, did not significantly affect the plasma concentrations of imipramine or citalopram. However, the concentration of the imipramine metabolite desipramine was increased by approximately 50%. The clinical significance of the desipramine change is unknown. Nevertheless, caution is indicated in the coadministration of TCA's with Celexa.

Electroconvulsive Therapy (ECT)—There are no clinical studies of the combined use of electroconvulsive therapy (ECT) and Celexa.

Carcinogenesis, Mutagenesis, Impairment of Fertility

Carcinogenesis

Citalopram was administered in the diet to NMRI/BOM strain mice and COBS WI strain rats for 18 and 24 months, respectively. There was no evidence for carcinogenicity of citalopram in mice receiving up to 240 mg/kg/day, which is equivalent to 20 times the maximum recommended human daily dose (MRHD) of 60 mg on a surface area (mg/m^2) basis. There was an increased incidence of small intestine carcinoma in rats receiving 8 or 24 mg/kg/day, doses which are approximately 1.3 and 4 times the MRHD, respectively, on a mg/m^2 basis. A no-effect dose of this finding was not established. The relevance of these findings to humans is unknown.

Mutagenesis

Citalopram was mutagenic in the *in vitro* bacterial reverse mutation assay (Ames test) in 2 of 5 bacterial strains (Salmonella TA98 and TA1537) in the absence of metabolic activation. It was clastogenic in the *in vitro* Chinese hamster lung cell assay for chromosomal aberrations in the presence and absence of metabolic activation. Citalopram was not mutagenic in the *in vitro* mammalian forward gene mutation assay (HPRT) in mouse lymphoma cells or in a coupled *in vitro*/*in vivo* unscheduled DNA synthesis (UDS) assay in rat liver. It was not clastogenic in the *in vitro* chromosomal aberration assay in human lymphocytes or in two *in vivo* mouse micronucleus assays.

Impairment of Fertility

When citalopram was administered orally to male and female rats prior to and throughout mating and gestation at doses of 16/24 (males/females), 32, 48, and 72 mg/kg/day, mating was decreased at all doses, and fertility was decreased at doses ≥32 mg/kg/day, approximately 5 times the maximum recommended human dose (MRHD) of 60 mg/day on a body surface area (mg/m^2) basis. Gestation duration was increased at 48 mg/kg/day, approximately 8 times the MRHD.

Pregnancy

Pregnancy Category C

In animal reproduction studies, citalopram has been shown to have adverse effects on embryo/fetal and postnatal development, including teratogenic effects, when administered at doses greater than human therapeutic doses.

In two rat embryo/fetal development studies, oral administration of citalopram (32, 56, or 112 mg/kg/day) to pregnant animals during the period of organogenesis resulted in decreased embryo/fetal growth and survival and an increased incidence of fetal abnormalities (including cardiovascular and skeletal defects) at the high dose, which is approximately 18 times the maximum recommended human dose (MRHD) of 60 mg/day on a body surface area (mg/m^2) basis. This dose was also associated with maternal toxicity (clinical signs, decreased BW gain). The developmental no effect dose of 56 mg/kg/day is approximately 9 times the MRHD on a mg/m^2 basis. In a rabbit study, no adverse effects on embryo/fetal development were observed at doses of up to 16 mg/kg/day, or approximately 5 times the MRHD on a mg/m^2 basis. Thus, teratogenic effects were observed at a maternally toxic dose in the rat and were not observed in the rabbit.

When female rats were treated with citalopram (4.8, 12.8, or 32 mg/kg/day) from late gestation through weaning, increased offspring mortality during the first 4 days after birth and persistent offspring growth retardation were observed at the highest dose, which is approximately 5 times the MRHD on a mg/m^2 basis. The no effect dose of 12.8 mg/kg/day is approximately 2 times the MRHD on a mg/m^2 basis. Similar effects on offspring mortality and growth were seen when dams were treated throughout gestation and early lactation at doses ≥24 mg/kg/day, approximately 4 times the MRHD on a mg/m^2 basis. A no effect dose was not determined in that study.

There are no adequate and well-controlled studies in pregnant women; therefore, citalopram should be used during pregnancy only if the potential benefit justifies the potential risk to the fetus.

Labor and Delivery

The effect of Celexa on labor and delivery in humans is unknown.

Nursing Mothers

As has been found to occur with many other drugs, citalopram is excreted in human breast milk. There have been two reports of infants experiencing excessive somnolence, decreased feeding, and weight loss in association with breast feeding from a citalopram-treated mother; in one case, the infant was reported to recover completely upon discontinuation of citalopram by its mother, and in the second case, no follow up information was available. The decision whether to continue or discontinue either nursing or Celexa therapy should take into account the risks of citalopram exposure for the infant and the benefits of Celexa treatment for the mother.

Pediatric Use

Safety and effectiveness in pediatric patients have not been established.

Geriatric Use

Of 4422 patients in clinical studies of Celexa, 1357 were 60 and over, 1034 were 65 and over, and 457 were 75 and over. No overall differences in safety or effectiveness were observed between these subjects and younger subjects, and other reported clinical experience has not identified differences in responses between the elderly and younger patients, but greater sensitivity of some older individuals cannot be ruled out. Most elderly patients treated with Celexa in clinical trials received daily doses between 20 and 40 mg (see Dosage and Administration).

In two pharmacokinetic studies, citalopram AUC was increased by 23% and 30%, respectively, in elderly subjects as compared to younger subjects, and its half-life was increased by 30% and 50%, respectively (see Clinical Pharmacology).

20 mg/day is the recommended dose for most elderly patients (see Dosage and Administration).

ADVERSE REACTIONS

The premarketing development program for Celexa included citalopram exposures in patients and/or normal subjects from 3 different groups of studies: 429 normal subjects in clinical pharmacology/pharmacokinetic studies; 4422 exposures from patients in controlled and uncontrolled clinical trials, corresponding to approximately 1370 patient exposure years. There were, in addition, over 19,000 exposures from mostly open-label, European postmarketing studies. The conditions and duration of treatment with Celexa varied greatly and included (in overlapping categories) open-label and double-blind studies, inpatient and outpatient studies, fixed-dose and dose-titration studies, and short-term and long-term exposure. Adverse reactions were as-

Continued on next page

Celexa—Cont.

sessed by collecting adverse events, results of physical examinations, vital signs, weights, laboratory analyses, ECGs, and results of ophthalmologic examinations.

Adverse events during exposure were obtained primarily by general inquiry and recorded by clinical investigators using terminology of their own choosing. Consequently, it is not possible to provide a meaningful estimate of the proportion of individuals experiencing adverse events without first grouping similar types of events into a smaller number of standardized event categories. In the tables and tabulations that follow, standard World Health Organization (WHO) terminology has been used to classify reported adverse events.

The stated frequencies of adverse events represent the proportion of individuals who experienced, at least once, a treatment-emergent adverse event of the type listed. An event was considered treatment-emergent if it occurred for the first time or worsened while receiving therapy following baseline evaluation.

Adverse Findings Observed in Short-Term, Placebo-Controlled Trials

Adverse Events Associated with Discontinuation of Treatment

Among 1063 depressed patients who received Celexa at doses ranging from 10 to 80 mg/day in placebo-controlled trials of up to 6 weeks in duration, 16% discontinued treatment due to an adverse event, as compared to 8% of 446 patients receiving placebo. The adverse events associated with discontinuation and considered drug-related (i.e., associated with discontinuation in at least 1% of Celexa-treated patients at a rate at least twice that of placebo) are shown in TABLE 1. It should be noted that one patient can report more than one reason for discontinuation and be counted more than once in this table.

[See table 1 at right]

TABLE 1
Adverse Events Associated with Discontinuation of Treatment in Short-Term, Placebo-Controlled, Depression Trials

Body System/Adverse Event	Percentage of Patients Discontinuing Due to Adverse Event: Citalopram (N=1063)	Placebo (N=446)
General		
Asthenia	1%	<1%
Gastrointestinal Disorders		
Nausea	4%	0%
Dry Mouth	1%	<1%
Vomiting	1%	0%
Central and Peripheral Nervous System Disorders		
Dizziness	2%	<1%
Psychiatric Disorders		
Insomnia	3%	1%
Somnolence	2%	1%
Agitation	1%	<1%

Adverse Events Occurring at an Incidence of 2% or More Among Celexa-Treated Patients

Table 2 enumerates the incidence, rounded to the nearest percent, of treatment emergent adverse events that occurred among 1063 depressed patients who received Celexa at doses ranging from 10 to 80 mg/day in placebo-controlled trials of up to 6 weeks in duration. Events included are those occurring in 2% or more of patients treated with Celexa and for which the incidence in patients treated with Celexa was greater than the incidence in placebo-treated patients.

The prescriber should be aware that these figures cannot be used to predict the incidence of adverse events in the course of usual medical practice where patient characteristics and other factors differ from those which prevailed in the clinical trials. Similarly, the cited frequencies cannot be compared with figures obtained from other clinical investigations involving different treatments, uses, and investigators. The cited figures, however, do provide the prescribing physician with some basis for estimating the relative contribution of drug and non-drug factors to the adverse event incidence rate in the population studied.

The only commonly observed adverse event that occurred in Celexa patients with an incidence of 5% or greater and at least twice the incidence in placebo patients was ejaculation disorder (primarily ejaculatory delay) in male patients (see TABLE 2)

[See table 2 at right]

TABLE 2
Treatment-Emergent Adverse Events: Incidence in Placebo-Controlled Clinical Trials*

Body System/Adverse Event	(Percentage of Patients Reporting Event) Celexa (N=1063)	Placebo (N=446)
Autonomic Nervous System Disorders		
Dry Mouth	20%	14%
Sweating Increased	11%	9%
Central & Peripheral Nervous System Disorders		
Tremor	8%	6%
Gastrointestinal Disorders		
Nausea	21%	14%
Diarrhea	8%	5%
Dyspepsia	5%	4%
Vomiting	4%	3%
Abdominal Pain	3%	2%
General		
Fatigue	5%	3%
Fever	2%	<1%
Musculoskeletal System Disorders		
Arthralgia	2%	1%
Myalgia	2%	1%
Psychiatric Disorders		
Somnolence	18%	10%
Insomnia	15%	14%
Anxiety	4%	3%
Anorexia	4%	2%
Agitation	3%	1%
Dysmenorrhea[1]	3%	2%
Libido Decreased	2%	<1%
Yawning	2%	<1%
Respiratory System Disorders		
Upper Respiratory Tract Infection	5%	4%
Rhinitis	5%	3%
Sinusitis	3%	<1%
Urogenital		
Ejaculation Disorder[2,3]	6%	1%
Impotence[3]	3%	<1%

*Events reported by at least 2% of patients treated with Celexa are reported, except for the following events which had an incidence on placebo ≥ Celexa: headache, asthenia, dizziness, constipation, palpitation, vision abnormal, sleep disorder, nervousness, pharyngitis, micturition disorder, back pain.

[1]Denominator used was for females only (N=638 Celexa; N=252 placebo).

[2]Primarily ejaculatory delay.

[3]Denominator used was for males only (N=425 Celexa; N=194 placebo).

Dose Dependency of Adverse Events

The potential relationship between the dose of Celexa administered and the incidence of adverse events was examined in a fixed dose study in depressed patients receiving placebo or Celexa 10, 20, 40, and 60 mg. Jonckheere's trend test revealed a positive dose response ($p<0.05$) for the following adverse events: fatigue, impotence, insomnia, sweating increased, somnolence, and yawning.

Male and Female Sexual Dysfunction with SSRIs

Although changes in sexual desire, sexual performance and sexual satisfaction often occur as manifestations of a psychiatric disorder, they may also be a consequence of pharmacologic treatment. In particular, some evidence suggests that selective serotonin reuptake inhibitors (SSRIs) can cause such untoward sexual experiences.

Reliable estimates of the incidence and severity of untoward experiences involving sexual desire, performance and satisfaction are difficult to obtain, however, in part because patients and physicians may be reluctant to discuss them. Accordingly, estimates of the incidence of untoward sexual experience and performance cited in product labeling, are likely to underestimate their actual incidence.

The table below displays the incidence of sexual side effects reported by a least 2% of patients taking Celexa in a pool of placebo-controlled clinical trials in patients with depression.

[See third table above]

Treatment	Celexa (425 males)	Placebo (194 males)
Abnormal Ejaculation (mostly ejaculatory delay)	6.1% (males only)	1% (males only)
Decreased Libido	3.8% (males only)	<1% (males only)
Impotence	2.8% (males only)	<1% (males only)

In female depressed patients receiving Celexa, the reported incidence of decreased libido and anorgasmia was 1.3% (n=638 females) and 1.1% (n=252 females), respectively.

There are no adequately designed studies examining sexual dysfunction with citalopram treatment.

Priapism has been reported with all SSRIs.

While it is difficult to know the precise risk of sexual dysfunction associated with the use of SSRIs, physicians should routinely inquire about such possible side effects.

Vital Sign Changes

Celexa and placebo groups were compared with respect to (1) mean change from baseline in vital signs (pulse, systolic blood pressure, and diastolic blood pressure) and (2) the incidence of patients meeting criteria for potentially clinically significant changes from baseline in these variables. These analyses did not reveal any clinically important changes in vital signs associated with Celexa treatment. In addition, a comparison of supine and standing vital sign measures for Celexa and placebo treatments indicated that Celexa treatment is not associated with orthostatic changes.

Weight Changes

Patients treated with Celexa in controlled trials experienced a weight loss of about 0.5 kg compared to no change for placebo patients.

Laboratory Changes

Celexa and placebo groups were compared with respect to (1) mean change from baseline in various serum chemistry, hematology, and urinalysis variables and (2) the incidence of patients meeting criteria for potentially clinically significant changes from baseline in these variables. These analyses revealed no clinically important changes in laboratory test parameters associated with Celexa treatment.

ECG Changes

Electrocardiograms from Celexa (N=802) and placebo (N=241) groups were compared with respect to (1) mean change from baseline in various ECG parameters and (2) the incidence of patients meeting criteria for potentially clinically significant changes from baseline in these variables. The only statistically significant drug-placebo difference observed was a decrease in heart rate for Celexa of 1.7 bpm compared to no change in heart rate for placebo. There were no observed differences in QT or other ECG intervals.

Other Events Observed During the Premarketing Evaluation of Celexa (citalopram HBr)

Following is a list of WHO terms that reflect treatment-emergent adverse events, as defined in the introduction to the ADVERSE REACTIONS section, reported by patients treated with Celexa at multiple doses in a range of 10 to 80 mg/day during any phase of a trial within the premarketing database of 4422 patients. All reported events are included except those already listed in Table 2 or elsewhere in labeling, those events for which a drug cause was remote, those event terms which were so general as to be uninformative, and those occurring in only one patient. It is important to emphasize that, although the events reported occurred during treatment with Celexa, they were not necessarily caused by it.

Events are further categorized by body system and listed in order of decreasing frequency according to the following definitions: frequent adverse events are those occurring on one or more occasions in at least 1/100 patients; infrequent adverse events are those occurring in less than 1/100 patients but at least 1/1000 patients; rare events are those occurring in fewer than 1/1000 patients.

Cardiovascular—*Frequent:* tachycardia, postural hypotension, hypotension. *Infrequent:* hypertension, bradycardia, edema (extremities), angina pectoris, extrasystoles, cardiac failure, flushing, myocardial infarction, cerebrovascular accident, myocardial ischemia. *Rare:* transient ischemic attack, phlebitis, atrial fibrillation, cardiac arrest, bundle branch block.

Central and Peripheral Nervous System Disorders—*Frequent:* paresthesia, migraine. *Infrequent:* hyperkinesia, vertigo, hypertonia, extrapyramidal disorder, leg cramps, involuntary muscle contractions, hypokinesia, neuralgia, dystonia, abnormal gait, hypesthesia, ataxia. *Rare:* abnormal coordination, hyperesthesia, ptosis, stupor.

Endocrine Disorders—*Rare:* hypothyroidism, goiter, gynecomastia.

Gastrointestinal Disorders—*Frequent:* saliva increased, flatulence. *Infrequent:* gastritis, gastroenteritis, stomatitis, eructation, hemorrhoids, dysphagia, teeth grinding, gingivitis, esophagitis. *Rare:* colitis, gastric ulcer, cholecystitis, cholelithiasis, duodenal ulcer, gastroesophageal reflux, glossitis, jaundice, diverticulitis, rectal hemorrhage, hiccups.

General—*Infrequent:* hot flushes, rigors, alcohol intolerance, syncope, influenza-like symptoms. *Rare:* hayfever.

Hemic and Lymphatic Disorders—*Infrequent:* purpura, anemia, epistaxis, leukocytosis, leucopenia, lymphadenopathy. *Rare:* pulmonary embolism, granulocytopenia, lymphocytosis, lymphopenia, hypochromic anemia, coagulation disorder, gingival bleeding.

Metabolic and Nutritional Disorders—*Frequent:* decreased weight, increased weight. *Infrequent:* increased hepatic enzymes, thirst, dry eyes, increased alkaline phosphatase, abnormal glucose tolerance. *Rare:* bilirubinemia, hypokalemia, obesity, hypoglycemia, hepatitis, dehydration.

Musculoskeletal System Disorders—*Infrequent:* arthritis, muscle weakness, skeletal pain. *Rare:* bursitis, osteoporosis.

Psychiatric Disorders—*Frequent:* impaired concentration, amnesia, apathy, depression, increased appetite, aggravated depression, suicide attempt, confusion. *Infrequent:* increased libido, aggressive reaction, paroniria, drug dependence, depersonalization, hallucination, euphoria, psychotic depression, delusion, paranoid reaction, emotional lability, panic reaction, psychosis. *Rare:* catatonic reaction, melancholia.

Reproductive Disorders/Female*—*Frequent:* amenorrhea. *Infrequent:* galactorrhea, breast pain, breast enlargement, vaginal hemorrhage.

---

*% based on female subjects only: 2955

Respiratory System Disorders—*Frequent:* coughing. *Infrequent:* bronchitis, dyspnea, pneumonia. *Rare:* asthma, laryngitis, bronchospasm, pneumonitis, sputum increased.

Skin and Appendages Disorders—*Frequent:* rash, pruritus. *Infrequent:* photosensitivity reaction, urticaria, acne, skin discoloration, eczema, alopecia, dermatitis, skin dry, psoriasis. *Rare:* hypertrichosis, decreased sweating, melanosis, keratitis, cellulitis, pruritus ani.

Special Senses—*Frequent:* accommodation abnormal, taste perversion. *Infrequent:* tinnitus, conjunctivitis, eye pain. *Rare:* mydriasis, photophobia, diplopia, abnormal lacrimation, cataract, taste loss.

Urinary System Disorders—*Frequent:* polyuria. *Infrequent:* micturition frequency, urinary incontinence, urinary retention, dysuria. *Rare:* facial edema, hematuria, oliguria, pyelonephritis, renal calculus, renal pain.

Other Events Observed During the Non-US Postmarketing Evaluation of Celexa (citalopram HBr)

It is estimated that approximately 8 million patients have been treated with Celexa since market introduction. Although no causal relationship to Celexa treatment has been found, the following adverse events have been reported to be temporally associated with Celexa treatment in at least 3 patients (unless otherwise noted) and are not described elsewhere in labeling: angioedema, choreoathetosis, epidermal necrolysis (3 cases), erythema multiforme, hepatic necrosis (2 cases), neuroleptic malignant syndrome, pancreatitis, serotonin syndrome, spontaneous abortion, thrombocytopenia, ventricular arrhythmia, Torsades de pointes, priapism, and withdrawal syndrome.

DRUG ABUSE AND DEPENDENCE

Controlled Substance Class

Celexa (citalopram HBr) is not a controlled substance.

Physical and Psychological Dependence

Animal studies suggest that the abuse liability of Celexa is low. Celexa has not been systematically studied in humans for its potential for abuse, tolerance, or physical dependence. The premarketing clinical experience with Celexa did not reveal any drug seeking behavior. However, these observations were not systematic and it is not possible to predict on the basis of this limited experience the extent to which a CNS-active drug will be misused, diverted, and/or abused once marketed. Consequently, physicians should carefully evaluate Celexa patients for history of drug abuse and follow such patients closely, observing them for signs of misuse or abuse (e.g., development of tolerance, incrementations of dose, drug seeking behavior).

OVERDOSAGE

Human Experience

Although there were no reports of fatal citalopram overdose in clinical trials involving overdoses of up to 2000 mg, postmarketing reports of drug overdoses involving citalopram have included 12 fatalities, 10 in combination with other drugs and/or alcohol and 2 with citalopram alone (3920 mg and 2800 mg), as well as non-fatal overdoses of up to 6000 mg. Symptoms most often accompanying citalopram overdose, alone or in combination with other drugs and/or alcohol, included dizziness, sweating, nausea, vomiting, tremor, somnolence, and sinus tachycardia. In more rare cases, observed symptoms included amnesia, confusion, coma, convulsions, hyperventilation, cyanosis, rhabdomyolysis, and ECG changes (including QTc prolongation, nodal rhythm, ventricular arrhythmia, and one possible case of Torsades de pointes).

Management of Overdose

Establish and maintain an airway to ensure adequate ventilation and oxygenation. Gastric evacuation by lavage and use of activated charcoal should be considered. Careful observation and cardiac and vital sign monitoring are recommended, along with general symptomatic and supportive care. Due to the large volume of distribution of citalopram, forced diuresis, dialysis, hemoperfusion, and exchange transfusion are unlikely to be of benefit. There are no specific antidotes for Celexa.

In managing overdose, consider the possibility of multiple drug involvement. The physician should consider contacting a poison control center for additional information on the treatment of any overdose.

DOSAGE AND ADMINISTRATION

Initial Treatment

Celexa (citalopram HBr) should be administered at an initial dose of 20 mg once daily, generally with an increase to a dose of 40 mg/day. Dose increases should usually occur in increments of 20 mg at intervals of no less than one week. Although certain patients may require a dose of 60 mg/day, the only study pertinent to dose response for effectiveness did not demonstrate an advantage for the 60 mg/day dose over the 40 mg/day dose; doses above 40 mg are therefore not ordinarily recommended.

Celexa should be administered once daily, in the morning or evening, with or without food.

Special Populations

20 mg/day is the recommended dose for most elderly patients and patients with hepatic impairment, with titration to 40 mg/day only for nonresponding patients.

No dosage adjustment is necessary for patients with mild or moderate renal impairment. Celexa should be used with caution in patients with severe renal impairment.

Maintenance Treatment

It is generally agreed that acute episodes of depression require several months or longer of sustained pharmacologic therapy. Systematic evaluation of Celexa in two studies has shown that its antidepressant efficacy is maintained for periods of up to 24 weeks following 6 or 8 weeks of initial treatment (32 weeks total). In one study, patients were assigned randomly to placebo or to the same dose of Celexa (20–60 mg/day) during maintenance treatment as they had received during the acute stabilization phase, while in the other study, patients were assigned randomly to continuation of Celexa 20 or 40 mg/day, or placebo, for maintenance treatment. In the latter study, the rates of relapse to depression were similar for the two dose groups (see Clinical Trials under Clinical Pharmacology). Based on these limited data, it is not known whether the dose of citalopram needed to maintain euthymia is identical to the dose needed to induce remission. If adverse reactions are bothersome, a decrease in dose to 20 mg/day can be considered.

Switching Patients To or From a Monoamine Oxidase Inhibitor

At least 14 days should elapse between discontinuation of an MAOI and initiation of Celexa therapy. Similarly, at least 14 days should be allowed after stopping Celexa before starting a MAOI (see Contraindications and Warnings).

HOW SUPPLIED

Tablets:

20 mg	Bottle of 100	NDC # 0456-4020-01
	10 × 10 Unit Dose	NDC # 0456-4020-63

Pink, oval, scored film coated.

Imprint on scored side with "F" on the left side and "P" on the right side.

Imprint on the non-scored side with "20 mg".

40 mg	Bottle of 100	NDC # 0456-4040-01
	10 × 10 Unit Dose	NDC # 0456-4040-63

White, oval, scored film coated.

Imprint on scored side with "F" on the left side and "P" on the right side.

Imprint on the non-scored side with "40 mg".

Oral Solution:

10 mg/5 mL, peppermint flavor – (120 mL) NDC 0456-4130-04

Store at 25°C (77°F); excursions permitted to 15–30°C (59–86°F).

ANIMAL TOXICOLOGY

Retinal Changes in Rats

Pathologic changes (degeneration/atrophy) were observed in the retinas of albino rats in the 2-year carcinogenicity study with citalopram. There was an increase in both incidence and severity of retinal pathology in both male and female rats receiving 80 mg/kg/day (13 times the maximum recommended daily human dose of 60 mg on a mg/m^2 basis). Similar findings were not present in rats receiving 24 mg/kg/day for two years, in mice treated for 18 months at doses up to 240 mg/kg/day or in dogs treated for one year at doses up to 20 mg/kg/day (4, 20 and 10 times, respectively, the maximum recommended daily human dose on a mg/m^2 basis). Additional studies to investigate the mechanism for this pathology have not been performed, and the potential significance of this effect in humans has not been established.

Cardiovascular Changes in Dogs

In a one-year toxicology study, 5 of 10 beagle dogs receiving oral doses of 8 mg/kg/day (4 times the maximum recommended daily human dose of 60 mg on a mg/m^2 basis) died suddenly between weeks 17 and 31 following initiation of treatment. Although appropriate data from that study are not available to directly compare plasma levels of citalopram (CT) and its metabolites, demethylcitalopram (DCT) and didemethylcitalopram (DDCT), to levels that have been achieved in humans, pharmacokinetic data indicate that the relative dog to human exposure was greater for the metabolites than for citalopram. Sudden deaths were not observed in rats at doses up to 120 mg/kg/day, which produced plasma levels of CT, DCT and DDCT similar to those observed in dogs at doses of 8 mg/kg/day. A subsequent intravenous dosing study demonstrated that in beagle dogs, DDCT caused QT prolongation, a known risk factor for the observed outcome in dogs. This effect occurred in dogs at doses producing peak DDCT plasma levels of 810 to 3250 nM (39–155 times the mean steady state DDCT plasma level measured at the maximum recommended human daily dose of 60 mg). In dogs, peak DDCT plasma concentrations are approximately equal to peak CT plasma concentrations, whereas in humans, steady state DDCT plasma concentrations are less than 10% of steady state CT plasma concentrations. Assays of DDCT plasma concentrations in 2,020 citalopram treated individuals demonstrated that DDCT levels rarely exceeded 70 nM; the highest measured level of DDCT in human overdose was 138 nM. While DDCT is ordinarily present in humans at lower levels than in dogs, it is unknown whether there are individuals who may achieve higher DDCT levels. The possibility that DCT, a principal metabolite in humans, may prolong the QT interval in the dog has not been directly examined because DCT is rapidly converted to DDCT in that species.

Rx only

Tablets Mfg. by:
Forest Laboratories Ireland Ltd.
Clonshaugh Industrial Estate
Dublin 17 Ireland

Made in Ireland

Oral Solution Mfg. By:
Forest Pharmaceuticals, Inc.
Subsidiary of Forest Laboratories, Inc.
St. Louis, MO 63045 USA

Tablets and Oral Solution Distributed and Marketed by:
Forest Pharmaceuticals, Inc.
Subsidiary of Forest Laboratories, Inc.
St. Louis, MO 63045 USA

Licensed from H. Lundbeck A/S

Rev. 5/00

Shown in Product Identification Guide, page 312

CERVIDIL® ℞

Brand of dinoprostone vaginal insert

Rx only

DESCRIPTION

Dinoprostone vaginal insert is a thin, flat, polymeric slab which is rectangular in shape with rounded corners contained within the pouch of a knitted polyester retrieval system, an integral part of which is a long tape. Each slab is buff colored, semitransparent and contains 10 mg of dinoprostone. The hydrogel insert is contained within the pouch of an off-white knitted polyester retrieval system designed to aid retrieval at the end of the dosing interval. The finished product is a controlled release formulation which has been found to release dinoprostone *in vivo* at a rate of approximately 0.3 mg/hr.

The chemical name for dinoprostone (commonly known as prostaglandin E_2 or PGE_2) is 11α, 15S-dihydroxy-9-oxo-prosta-5Z, 13E-dien-1-oic acid and the structural formula is represented below:

The molecular formula is $C_{20}H_{32}O_5$ and its molecular weight is 352.5. Dinoprostone occurs as a white to off-white crystalline powder. It has a melting point within the range of 65° to 69°C. Dinoprostone is soluble in ethanol and in 25% ethanol in water. Each insert contains 10 mg of dinoprostone in 241 mg of a cross-linked polyethylene oxide/urethane polymer which is a semi-opaque, beige colored, flat rectangular slab measuring 29 mm by 9.5 mm and 0.8 mm in thickness. The insert and its retrieval system, made of

Continued on next page

Cervidil—Cont.

polyester yarn, are non-toxic and when placed in a moist environment, absorb water, swell, and release dinoprostone.

CLINICAL PHARMACOLOGY

Dinoprostone (PGE_2) is a naturally-occurring biomolecule. It is found in low concentrations in most tissues of the body and functions as a local hormone (1–3). As with any local hormone, it is very rapidly metabolized in the tissues of synthesis (the half-life estimated to be 2.5–5 minutes). The rate limiting step for inactivation is regulated by the enzyme 15-hydroxyprostaglandin dehydrogenase (PGDH) (1,4). Any PGE_2 that escapes local inactivation is rapidly cleared to the extent of 95% on the first pass through the pulmonary circulation (1,2).

In pregnancy, PGE_2 is secreted continuously by the fetal membranes and placenta and plays an important role in the final events leading to the initiation of labor (1,2). It is known that PGE_2 stimulates the production of $PGF_2\alpha$ which in turn sensitizes the myometrium to endogenous or exogenously administrated oxytocin. Although PGE_2 is capable of initiating uterine contractions and may interact with oxytocin to increase uterine contractility, the available evidence indicates that, in the concentrations found during the early part of labor, PGE_2 plays an important role in cervical ripening without affecting uterine contractions (5–7). This distinction serves as the basis for considering cervical ripening and induction of labor, usually by the use of oxytocin (8–10), as two separate processes.

PGE_2 plays an important role in the complex set of biochemical and structural alterations involved in cervical ripening. Cervical ripening involves a marked relaxation of the cervical smooth muscle fibers of the uterine cervix which must be transformed from a rigid structure to a softened, yielding and dilated configuration to allow passage of the fetus through the birth canal (11–13). This process involves activation of the enzyme collagenase, which is responsible for digestion of some of the structural collagen network of the cervix (1,14). This is associated with a concomitant increase in the amount of hydrophilic glycosaminoglycan, hyaluronic acid, and a decrease in dermatan sulfate (1). Failure of the cervix to undergo these natural physiologic changes, usually assessed by the method described by Bishop (15,16), prior to the onset of effective uterine contractions, results in an unfavorable outcome for successful vaginal delivery and may result in fetal compromise. It is estimated that in approximately 5% of pregnancies the cervix does not ripen normally (17). In an additional 10–11% of pregnancies, labor must be induced for medical or obstetric reasons prior to the time of cervical ripening (17).

The delivery rate of PGE_2 *in vivo* is about 0.3 mg/hour over a period of 12 hours. The controlled release of PGE_2 from the hydrogel insert is an attempt to provide sufficient quantities of PGE_2 to the local receptors to satisfy hormonal requirements. In the majority of patients, these local effects are manifested by changes in the consistency, dilatation and effacement of the cervix as measured by the Bishop score. Although some patients experience uterine hyperstimulation as a result of direct PGE_2- or $PGF_2\alpha$-mediated sensitization of the myometrium to oxytocin, systemic effects of PGE_2 are rarely encountered. The insert is fitted with a biocompatible retrieval system which facilitates removal at the conclusion of therapy or in the event of an adverse reaction.

No correlation could be established between PGE_2 release and plasma concentrations of PGE_m. The relative contributions of endogenously and exogenously released PGE_2 to the plasma levels of the metabolite PGE_m could not be determined. Moreover, it is uncertain as to whether the measured concentrations of PGE_m reflect the natural progression of PGE_m concentrations in blood as birth approaches or to what extent the measured concentrations following PGE_2 administration represent an increase over basal levels that might be measured in control patients.

INDICATIONS AND USAGE

Cervidil Vaginal Insert (dinoprostone, 10 mg) is indicated for the initiation and/or continuation of cervical ripening in patients at or near term in whom there is a medical or obstetrical indication for the induction of labor.

CONTRAINDICATIONS

Cervidil is contraindicated in:

- Patients with known hypersensitivity to prostaglandins.
- Patients in whom there is clinical suspicion or definite evidence of fetal distress where delivery is not imminent.
- Patients with unexplained vaginal bleeding during this pregnancy.
- Patients in whom there is evidence or strong suspicion of marked cephalopelvic disproportion.
- Patients in whom oxytocic drugs are contraindicated or when prolonged contraction of the uterus may be detrimental to fetal safety or uterine integrity, such as previous cesarean section or major uterine surgery (see **PRECAUTIONS** and **ADVERSE REACTIONS**).
- Patients already receiving intravenous oxytocic drugs.
- Multipara with 6 or more previous term pregnancies.

WARNINGS

For hospital use only

Cervidil should be administered only by trained obstetrical personnel in a hospital setting with appropriate obstetrical care facilities.

Table 1

Total Cervidil-Treated Drug Related Adverse Events

	Controlled Studies[1]		STUDY 101–801[2]	
	Active	Placebo	Active	Placebo
Uterine hyperstimulation with fetal distress	2.8%	0.3%	2.9%	0%
Uterine hyperstimulation without fetal distress	4.7%	0%	2.0%	0%
Fetal Distress without uterine hyperstimulation	3.8%	1.2%	2.9%	1.0%
N	320	338	102	104

[1] Controlled Studies (with and without retrieval system)
[2] Controlled Study (with retrieval system)

Table 2

Efficacy of Cervidil in Double Blind Studies

		Primip/Nullip		Multip		
Parameter	**Study #**	**Cervidil**	**Placebo**	**Cervidil**	**Placebo**	**P-Value**
Treatment	101–103 (N=81)	65%	28%	87%	29%	<0.001
Success*	101–003 (N=371)	68%	24%	77%	24%	<0.001
	101–801 (N=206)	72%	48%	55%	41%	0.003
Time to Delivery (hours)						
Average	101–103 (N=81)	33.7	48.6	14.0	28.6	
Median		25.7	34.5	12.3	24.6	0.001
Average	101–801 (N=206)	31.1	51.8	52.3	45.9	
Median		25.5	37.2	20.8	27.4	<0.001
Time to Onset of Labor (hours)						
Average	101–103 (N=81)	19.9	39.4	6.8	22.4	
Median		12.0	19.2	6.9	18.3	<0.001

* Treatment success was defined as Bishop score increase at 12 hours of ≥3, vaginal delivery within 12 hours or Bishop score at 12 hours ≥6. These studies were not designed with the power to show differences in cesarean section rates between Cervidil and placebo groups and none were noted.

PRECAUTIONS

1. General Precautions: Since prostaglandins potentiate the effect of oxytocin, Cervidil must be removed before oxytocin administration is initiated and the patient's uterine activity carefully monitored for uterine hyperstimulation. If uterine hyperstimulation is encountered or if labor commences, the vaginal insert should be removed. Cervidil should also be removed prior to amniotomy.

Cervidil is contraindicated when prolonged contraction of the uterus may be detrimental to fetal safety and uterine integrity. Therefore, Cervidil should not be administered to patients with a history of previous cesarean section or uterine surgery given the potential risk for uterine rupture and associated obstetrical complications.

Caution should be exercised in the administration of Cervidil for cervical ripening in patients with ruptured membranes, in cases of non-vertex, or non-singleton presentation, and in patients with a history of previous uterine hypertony, glaucoma, or a history of childhood asthma, even though there have been no asthma attacks in adulthood.

Uterine activity, fetal status and the progression of cervical dilatation and effacement should be carefully monitored whenever the dinoprostone vaginal insert is in place. Any evidence of uterine hyperstimulation, sustained uterine contractions, fetal distress, or other fetal or maternal adverse reactions, should be a cause for consideration of removal of the insert.

2. Drug Interactions: Cervidil may augment the activity of oxytocic agents and their concomitant use is not recommended. A dosing interval of at least 30 minutes is recommended for the sequential use of oxytocin following the removal of the dinoprostone vaginal insert. No other drug interactions have been identified.

3. Carcinogenesis, Mutagenesis, Impairment of Fertility: Long-term carcinogenicity and fertility studies have not been conducted with Cervidil (dinoprostone) Vaginal Insert. No evidence of mutagenicity has been observed with prostaglandin E_2 in the Unscheduled DNA Synthesis Assay, the Micronucleus Test, or Ames Assay.

4. Pregnancy, Teratogenic Effects:
Pregnancy Category C:
Prostaglandin E_2 has produced an increase in skeletal anomalies in rats and rabbits. No effect would be expected clinically, when used as indicated, since Cervidil (dinoprostone) Vaginal Insert is administered after the period of organogenesis. Prostaglandin E_2 has been shown to be embryotoxic in rats and rabbits, and any dose that produces sustained increased uterine tone could put the embryo or fetus at risk.

5. Pediatric Use: The safety and efficacy of Cervidil has been established in women of a reproductive age and women who are pregnant. Although safety and efficacy has not been established in pediatric patients, safety and efficacy are expected to be the same for adolescents.

ADVERSE REACTIONS

Cervidil is well tolerated. In placebo-controlled trials in which 658 women were entered and 320 received active therapy (218 without retrieval system, 102 with retrieval system), the following events were reported.
[See table 1 above]
In Postmarketing Experience Reports, uterine rupture has been reported in association with the use of Cervidil.

Drug related fever, nausea, vomiting, diarrhea, and abdominal pain were noted in less than 1% of patients who received Cervidil.

In study 101–801 (with the retrieval system) cases of hyperstimulation reversed within 2 to 13 minutes of removal of the product. Tocolytics were required in one of the five cases.

In cases of fetal distress, when product removal was thought advisable there was a return to normal rhythm and no neonatal sequelae.

Five minute Apgar scores were 7 or above in 98.2% (646/658) of studied neonates whose mothers received Cervidil. In a report of a 3 year pediatric follow-up study in 121 infants, 51 of whose mothers received Cervidil, there were no deleterious effects on physical examination or psychomotor evaluation (18).

DRUG ABUSE AND DEPENDENCE

No drug abuse or dependence has been seen with the use of Cervidil.

OVERDOSAGE

Cervidil is used as a single dosage in a single application. Overdosage is usually manifested by uterine hyperstimulation which may be accompanied by fetal distress and is responsive to removal of the insert. Other treatment must be symptomatic since, to date, clinical experience with prostaglandin antagonists is insufficient.

The use of beta-adrenergic agents should be considered in the event of undesirable increased uterine activity.

DOSAGE AND ADMINISTRATION

The dosage of dinoprostone in the vaginal insert is 10 mg designed to be released at approximately 0.3 mg/hour over a 12 hour period. Cervidil should be removed upon onset of active labor or 12 hours after insertion.

One Cervidil is placed transversely in the posterior fornix of the vagina immediately after removal from its foil package. The insertion of the vaginal insert does not require sterile conditions. The vaginal insert must not be used without its retrieval system. There is no need for previous warming of the product. A minimal amount of K-Y® jelly (or other water-miscible lubricant) may be used to assist in insertion of Cervidil. Care should be taken not to permit excess contact or coating with the lubricant and thus prevent optimal swelling and release of dinoprostone from the vaginal insert. Patients should remain in the supine position for 2 hours following insertion, but thereafter may be ambulatory.

HOW SUPPLIED

Cervidil (NDC 0456-4123-63) contains 10 mg dinoprostone. The product is wound and enclosed in an aluminum sleeve which is contained in an aluminum/polyethylene pack.

Store in a freezer: between −20°C and −10°C (−4°F and 14°F). Cervidil is packed in foil and is stable when stored in a freezer for a period of three years. Vaginal inserts exposed to high humidity will absorb moisture from the air and thereby alter the release characteristics of dinoprostone. Once used, the vaginal insert should be discarded.

Rx only

CLINICAL STUDIES

[See table 2 above]

REFERENCES

1. Physiology of Labor. In: Williams Obstetrics. Eds. Pritchard, J.A., MacDonald, P.C., and Gant, N.F. Appleton-Century-Crofts, Conn, Pp 295-321, (1985).

2. Rall, T.W. and Schliefer, L.S. Oxytocin, prostaglandin, ergot alkaloids, and other drugs; tocolytics agents, In: The Pharmacological Basis of Therapeutics. Eds. Gilman, A.G., Goodman, L.S., Rall, T.W., and Murad, F. MacMillan Publ. Co., New York, Pp 926-945, (1985).
3. Casey, M.L. and MacDonald, P.C. The initiation of labor in women: Regulation of phospholipid and arachidonic acid metabolism and of prostaglandin production. Semin. Perinat. 10: 270-275, (1986).
4. Casey, M.L., MacDonald, P.C. and Mitchell, M.D. Stimulation of prostaglandin E_2 production in amnion cells in culture by a substance(s) in human fetal urine. Biochem. Biophys. Res. Comm. 114:1056, (1983).
5. Olson, C.M., Lye, S.J., Skinner, K., and Challis, J.R.G. Prostanoid concentrations in maternal/fetal plasma and amniotic fluid and intrauterine tissue prostanoid output in relation to myometrial contractility during the onset of Endocrinology. 116: 389-397, (1985).
6. Ledger, W.L., Ellwood, D.A., and Taylor, M.J. Cervical softening in late pregnant sheep by infusion of prostaglandin E-2 into cervical artery. J. Reprod. Fert. 69, 511-515, (1983).
7. Olson, D.M., Lye, S.J., Skinner, K., and Challis, J.R.G. Early changes in prostaglandin concentrations in ovine maternal and fetal plasma, amniotic fluid and from dispersed cells of intrauterine tissues before the onset of ACTH-induced pre-term labor. J. Reprod. Fert. 71: 45-55, (1984).
8. Caldero-Garcia, R. and Posiero, J. Oxytocin and the contractility of the human uterus, Ann, N.Y. Acad. Sci. 75: 813, (1959).
9. Posiero, J. and Noriega-Guerra, L. Dose-response relationships in uterine effects of oxytocin infusion. Oxytocin. Eds., Caldero-Garcia, R. and Heller, J. Pergamon Press, New York, (1961).
10. Cibils, L. Enhancement of induction of labor. In: Risks in the Practice of Modern Obstetrics. Aldjem, S. Ed. Mosby Publishing, St. Louis, (1972).
11. Bryman, I., Lindblom, B., and Norstrom, A. Extreme sensitivity of cervical musculature to prostaglandin E_2 in early pregnancy. Lancet, 2:1471, (1982).
12. Thiery, M. Induction of labor with prostaglandins. In: Human Parturition. Eds. Keirse, M.J.N.C., Anderson, A.B.M.; and Gravenhorst, J.B. Martinus Nijhoff Publ., Boston, 155-164, (1979).
13. Thiery, M. and Amy, J.J. Induction of labor with prostaglandins. In: Advances in Prostaglandin Research. Prostaglandin and Reproduction. Karim, S.M.M., Ed., MTP, Lancaster, Pp. 149-228, (1975).
14. MacLennan, A.H., Katz, M., and Creasey, R. The morphologic characteristics of cervical ripening induced by the hormones relaxin and prostaglandin F_2 in a rabbit model. Am. J. Obstet. Gynecol, 152: 910696, (1985).
15. Bishop, E. Elective induction of labor. Obstet. & Gynecol. 5: 519-527, (1955).
16. Bishop, E. Pelvic scoring for elective induction. Obstet. & Gynecol. 24: 266-268. (1969).
17. Thiery, M. Preinduction cervical ripening. In: Obstetrics and Gynecology Annual, Vol. 12 Ed. Wynn, R.M. Appleton-Century-Crofts, New York, Pp. 103-146, (1983).
18. MacKenzie, I.; Information on File: Controlled Therapeutics (Scotland).

Mfg by:
Controlled Therapeutics
East Kilbride, Scotland G74 5PB

Made in the U.K.

Distributed by:
FOREST PHARMACEUTICALS, INC.
Subsidiary of Forest Laboratories, Inc.
St. Louis, MO 63045 USA
Rev. 2/00 RMC226

Shown in Product Identification Guide, page 312

ENDAL™-HD ℂ℞
[*ĕn dăl-HD*]

DESCRIPTION

Each 5mL contains:

Hydrocodone Bitartrate	1.67 mg
(WARNING: May Be Habit Forming)	
Phenylephrine Hydrochloride	5 mg
Chlorpheniramine Maleate	2 mg

HOW SUPPLIED

Endal-HD is supplied in bottles of one pint (473 mL) NDC# 0785-6200-16.

ESGIC® Capsules ℞
[*es 'jik*]
(Butalbital, Acetaminophen and Caffeine Capsules, USP)
50 mg/325 mg/40 mg

ESGIC® Tablets ℞
(Butalbital, Acetaminophen and Caffeine Tablets, USP)
50 mg/325 mg/40 mg

ESGIC-PLUS™ Tablets ℞
(Butalbital, Acetaminophen and Caffeine Tablets, USP)
50 mg/500 mg/40 mg

DESCRIPTION

Each Esgic-Plus Tablet contains:

Butalbital*	50 mg
(*Warning: May be habit forming)	
Acetaminophen	500 mg
Caffeine	40 mg

In addition, each tablet contains the following inactive ingredients: colloidal silicon dioxide, croscarmellose sodium, crospovidone, microcrystalline cellulose, povidone, pregelatinized cornstarch, and stearic acid.

HOW SUPPLIED

Esgic-Plus Tablets, containing butalbital* 50 mg (*Warning: May be habit forming), acetaminophen 500 mg and caffeine 40 mg, are white, capsule-shaped, single-scored, and are debossed "FOREST" on the upper side and "678" on one side of the score on the lower side. They are supplied in bottles of 100, NDC 0456-0678-01, and in bottles of 500, NDC 0456-0678-02.

Storage: Store at controlled room temperature 15°–30°C (59°–86°F).

Dispense in a tight, light-resistant container with a child-resistant closure.

CAUTION: Federal law prohibits dispensing without prescription.

Manufactured by:
MIKART, INC.
Atlanta, GA 30318
Distributed by:
FOREST PHARMACEUTICALS, INC.
Subsidiary of
Forest Laboratories, Inc.
St. Louis, Missouri 63045
Rev. 7/97 Code 719A00

Shown in Product Identification Guide, page 312

FLUMADINE® TABLETS ℞
[*flu 'mă-dīne*]
(rimantadine hydrochloride tablets)

FLUMADINE® SYRUP ℞
(rimantadine hydrochloride syrup)

DESCRIPTION

Flumadine® (rimantadine hydrochloride) is a synthetic antiviral drug available as a 100 mg film-coated tablet and as a syrup for oral administration. Each film-coated tablet contains 100 mg of rimantadine hydrochloride plus hydroxypropyl methylcellulose, magnesium stearate, microcrystalline cellulose, sodium starch glycolate, FD&C Yellow No. 6 Lake and FD&C Yellow No. 6. The film coat contains hydroxypropyl methylcellulose and polyethylene glycol. Each teaspoonful (5 mL) of the syrup contains 50 mg of rimantadine hydrochloride in an aqueous solution containing citric acid, parabens (methyl and propyl), saccharin sodium, sorbitol, D&C Red No. 33 and flavors.

Rimantadine hydrochloride is a white to off-white crystalline powder which is freely soluble in water (50 mg/mL at 20°C). Chemically, rimantadine hydrochloride is alpha-methyltricyclo-[3.3.1.1/3.7]decane-1-methanamine hydrochloride, with an empirical formula of $C_{12}H_{21}N \cdot HCl$, a molecular weight of 215.77 and the following structural formula:

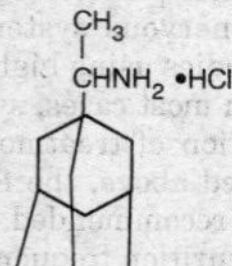

CLINICAL PHARMACOLOGY

MECHANISM OF ACTION: The mechanism of action of rimantadine is not fully understood. Rimantadine appears to exert its inhibitory effect early in the viral replicative cycle, possibly inhibiting the uncoating of the virus. Genetic studies suggest that a virus protein specified by the virion M_2 gene plays an important role in the susceptibility of influenza A virus to inhibition by rimantadine.

MICROBIOLOGY: Rimantadine is inhibitory to the *in vitro* replication of influenza A virus isolates from each of the three antigenic subtypes, *i.e.*, H1N1, H2N2 and H3N2, that have been isolated from man. Rimantadine has little or no activity against influenza B virus (Ref. 1,2). Rimantadine does not appear to interfere with the immunogenicity of inactivated influenza A vaccine.

A quantitative relationship between the *in vitro* susceptibility of influenza A virus to rimantadine and clinical response to therapy has not been established.

Susceptibility test results, expressed as the concentration of the drug required to inhibit virus replication by 50% or more in a cell culture system, vary greatly (from 4 ng/mL to 20 μg/mL) depending upon the assay protocol used, size of the virus inoculum, isolates of the influenza A virus strains tested, and the cell types used (Ref. 2).

Rimantadine-resistant strains of influenza A virus have emerged among freshly isolated epidemic strains in closed settings where rimantadine has been used. Resistant viruses have been shown to be transmissible and to cause typical influenza illness. (Ref. 3).

PHARMACOKINETICS: Although the pharmacokinetic profile of Flumadine has been described, no pharmacodynamic data establishing a correlation between plasma concentration and its antiviral effect are available.

The tablet and syrup formulations of Flumadine are equally absorbed after oral administration. The mean ± SD peak plasma concentration after a single 100 mg dose of Flumadine was 74 ± 22 ng/mL (range: 45 to 138 ng/mL). The time to peak concentration was 6 ± 1 hours in healthy adults (age 20 to 44 years). The single dose elimination half-life in this population was 25.4 ± 6.3 hours (range: 13 to 65 hours). The single dose elimination half-life in a group of healthy 71 to 79 year-old subjects was 32 ± 16 hours (range: 20 to 65 hours).

After the administration of rimantadine 100 mg twice daily to healthy volunteers (age 18 to 70 years) for 10 days, area under the curve (AUC) values were approximately 30% greater than predicted from a single dose. Plasma trough levels at steady state ranged between 118 and 468 ng/mL. In these patients no age-related differences in pharmacokinetics were detected. However, in a comparison of three groups of healthy older subjects (age 50–60, 61–70 and 71–79 years), the 71 to 79 year-old group had average AUC values, peak concentrations and elimination half-life values at steady state that were 20 to 30% higher than the other two groups. Steady-state concentrations in elderly nursing home patients (age 68 to 102 years) were 2- to 4-fold higher than those seen in healthy young and elderly adults.

The pharmacokinetic profile of rimantadine in children has not been established. In a group (n=10) of children 4 to 8 years old who were given a single dose (6.6 mg/kg) of Flumadine syrup, plasma concentrations of rimantadine ranged from 446 to 988 ng/mL at 5 to 6 hours and from 170 to 424 ng/mL at 24 hours. In some children drug was detected in plasma 72 hours after the last dose.

Following oral administration, rimantadine is extensively metabolized in the liver with less than 25% of the dose excreted in the urine as unchanged drug. Three hydroxylated metabolites have been found in plasma. These metabolites, an additional conjugated metabolite and parent drug account for 74 ± 10% (n=4) of a single 200 mg dose of rimantadine excreted in urine over 72 hours.

In a group (n=14) of patients with chronic liver disease, the majority of whom were stabilized cirrhotics, the pharmacokinetics of rimantadine were not appreciably altered following a single 200 mg oral dose compared to 6 healthy subjects who were sex, age and weight matched to 6 of the patients with liver disease. After administration of a single 200 mg dose to patients (n=10) with severe hepatic dysfunction, AUC was approximately 3-fold larger, elimination half-life was approximately 2-fold longer and apparent clearance was about 50% lower when compared to historic data from healthy subjects.

Studies of the effects of renal insufficiency on the pharmacokinetics of rimantadine have given inconsistent results. Following administration of a single 200 mg oral dose of rimantadine to 8 patients with a creatinine clearance (CLcr) of 31–50 mL/min and 6 patients with a CLcr of 11–30 mL/min, the apparent clearance was 37% and 16% lower, respectively, and plasma metabolite concentrations were higher when compared to weight-, age-, and sex-matched healthy subjects (n=9, CLcr > 50 mL/min). After a single 200 mg oral dose of rimantadine was given to 8 hemodialysis patients (CLcr 0–10 mL/min), there was a 1.6-fold increase in the elimination half-life and a 40% decrease in apparent clearance compared to age-matched healthy subjects. Hemodialysis did not contribute to the clearance of rimantadine.

The in vitro human plasma protein binding of rimantadine is about 40% over typical plasma concentrations. Albumin is the major binding protein.

INDICATIONS AND USAGE

Flumadine is indicated for the prophylaxis and treatment of illness caused by various strains of influenza A virus in adults.

Flumadine is indicated for prophylaxis against influenza A virus in children.

PROPHYLAXIS: In controlled studies of children over the age of 1 year, healthy adults and elderly patients, Flumadine has been shown to be safe and effective in preventing signs and symptoms of infection caused by various strains of influenza A virus. Early vaccination on an annual basis as recommended by the Centers of Disease Control's Immunization Practices Advisory Committee is the method of choice in the prophylaxis of influenza unless vaccination is contraindicated, not available or not feasible. Since Flumadine does not completely prevent the host immune response to influenza A infection, individuals who take this drug may still develop immune responses to natural disease or vaccination and may be protected when later exposed to antigenically-related viruses. Following vaccination during an influenza outbreak, Flumadine prophylaxis should be considered for the 2 to 4 week time period required to develop an antibody response. However, the safety and effectiveness of Flumadine prophylaxis have not been demonstrated for longer than 6 weeks.

TREATMENT: Flumadine therapy should be considered for adults who develop an influenza-like illness during

Continued on next page

Flumadine—Cont.

known or suspected influenza A infection in the community. When administered within 48 hours after onset of signs and symptoms of infection caused by influenza A virus strains, Flumadine has been shown to reduce the duration of fever and systemic symptoms.

CONTRAINDICATIONS

Flumadine is contraindicated in patients with known hypersensitivity to drugs of the adamantane class, including rimantadine and amantadine.

PRECAUTIONS

GENERAL: An increased incidence of seizures has been reported in patients with a history of epilepsy who received the related drug amantadine. In clinical trials of Flumadine, the occurrence of seizure-like activity was observed in a small number of patients with a history of seizures who were not receiving anticonvulsant medication while taking Flumadine. If seizures develop, Flumadine should be discontinued.

The safety and pharmacokinetics of rimantadine in renal and hepatic insufficiency have only been evaluated after single-dose administration. In a single dose study of patients with anuric renal failure, the apparent clearance of rimantadine was approximately 40% lower and the elimination half-life was 1.6-fold greater than that in healthy age-matched controls. In a study of 14 persons with chronic liver disease (mostly stabilized cirrhotics), no alterations in the pharmacokinetics were observed after the administration of a single dose of rimantadine. However, the apparent clearance of rimantadine following a single dose to 10 patients with severe liver dysfunction was 50% lower than reported for healthy subjects. Because of the potential for accumulation of rimantadine and its metabolites in plasma, caution should be exercised when patients with renal or hepatic insufficiency are treated with rimantadine.

Transmission of rimantadine resistant virus should be considered when treating patients whose contacts are at high risk for influenza A illness. Influenza A virus strains resistant to rimantadine can emerge during treatment and such resistant strains have been shown to be transmissible and to cause typical influenza illness (Ref. 3). Although the frequency, rapidity, and clinical significance of the emergence of drug-resistant virus are not yet established, several small studies have demonstrated that 10% to 30% of patients with initially sensitive-virus, upon treatment with rimantadine, shed rimantadine resistant virus. (Ref. 3, 4, 5, 6)

Clinical response to rimantadine, although slower in those patients who subsequently shed resistant virus, was not significantly different from those who did not shed resistant virus. (Ref. 3) No data are available in humans that address the activity or effectiveness of rimantadine therapy in subjects infected with resistant virus.

DRUG INTERACTIONS: Cimetidine: The effects of chronic cimetidine use on the metabolism of rimantadine are not known. When a single 100 mg dose of Flumadine was administered one hour after the initiation of cimetidine (300 mg four times a day), the apparent total rimantadine clearance of this single dose in mormal healthy adults was reduced by 18% (compared to the apparent total rimantadine clearance in the same subjects in the absence of cimetidine).

Acetaminophen: Flumadine, 100 mg, was given twice daily for 13 days to 12 healthy volunteers. On day 11, acetaminophen (650 mg four times daily) was started and continued for 8 days. The pharmacokinetics of rimantadine were assessed on days 11 and 13. Coadministration with acetaminophen reduced the peak concentration and AUC values for rimantadine by approximately 11%.

Aspirin: Flumadine, 100 mg, was given twice daily for 13 days to 12 healthy volunteers. On day 11, aspirin (650 mg, four times daily) was started and continued for 8 days. The pharmacokinetics of rimantadine were assessed on days 11 and 13. Peak plasma concentrations and AUC of rimantadine were reduced approximately 10% in the presence of aspirin.

CARCINOGENESIS, MUTAGENESIS, AND IMPAIRMENT OF FERTILITY: Carcinogenesis: Carcinogenicity studies in animals have not been performed.

Mutagenesis: No mutagenic effects were seen when rimantadine was evaluated in several standard assays for mutagenicity.

Impairment of Fertility: A reproduction study in male and female rats did not show detectable impairment of fertility at dosages up to 60 mg/kg/day (3 times the maximum human dose based on body surface area comparisons).

PREGNANCY: Teratogenic Effects: Pregnancy Category C. There are no adequate and well-controlled studies in pregnant women. Rimantadine is reported to cross the placenta in mice. Rimantadine has been shown to be embryotoxic in rats when given at a dose of 200 mg/kg/day (11 times the recommended human dose based on body surface area comparisons). At this dose the embryotoxic effect consisted of increased fetal resorption in rats; this dose also produced a variety of maternal effects including ataxia, tremors, convulsions and significantly reduced weight gain. No embryotoxicity was observed when rabbits were given doses up to 50 mg/kg/day (5 times the recommended human dose based on body surface area comparisons). However, there was evidence of a developmental abnormality in the form of a change in the ratio of fetuses with 12 or 13 ribs. This ratio is normally about 50:50 in a litter but was 80:20 after rimantadine treatment.

Nonteratogenic Effects: Rimantadine was administered to pregnant rats in a peri- and postnatal reproduction toxicity study at doses of 30, 60 and 120 mg/kg/day (1.7, 3.4 and 6.8 times the recommended human dose based on body surface area comparisons). Maternal toxicity during gestation was noted at the two higher doses of rimantadine, and at the highest dose, 120 mg/kg/day, there was an increase in pup mortality during the first 2 to 4 days postpartum. Decreased fertility of the F1 generation was also noted for the two higher doses.

For these reasons, Flumadine should be used during pregnancy only if the potential benefit justifies the risk to the fetus.

NURSING MOTHERS: Flumadine should not be administered to nursing mothers because of the adverse effects noted in offspring of rats treated with rimantadine during the nursing period. Rimantadine is concentrated in rat milk in a dose-related manner: 2 to 3 hours following administration of rimantadine, rat breast milk levels were approximately twice those observed in the serum.

PEDIATRIC USE: In children, Flumadine is recommended for the prophylaxis of influenza A. The safety and effectiveness of Flumadine in the treatment of symptomatic influenza infection in children have not been established. Prophylaxis studies with Flumadine have not been performed in children below the age of 1 year.

ADVERSE REACTIONS

In 1,027 patients treated with Flumadine in controlled clinical trials at the recommended dose of 200 mg daily, the most frequently reported adverse events involved the gastrointestinal and nervous systems.

Incidence >1%: Adverse events reported most frequently (1–3%) at the recommended dose in controlled clinical trials are shown in the table below.

	Rimantadine (n=1027)	Control (n=986)
Nervous System		
Insomnia	2.1%	0.9%
Dizziness	1.9%	1.1%
Headache	1.4%	1.3%
Nervousness	1.3%	0.6%
Fatigue	1.0%	0.9%
Gastrointestinal System		
Nausea	2.8%	1.6%
Vomiting	1.7%	0.6%
Anorexia	1.6%	0.8%
Dry mouth	1.5%	0.6%
Abdominal Pain	1.4%	0.8%
Body as a Whole		
Asthenia	1.4%	0.5%

Less frequent adverse events (0.3 to 1%) at the recommended dose in controlled clinical trials were: *Gastrointestinal System:* diarrhea, dyspepsia; *Nervous System:* impairment of concentration, ataxia, somnolence, agitation, depression; *Skin and Appendages:* rash; *Hearing and Vestibular:* tinnitus; *Respiratory:* dyspena.

Additional adverse events (less than 0.3%) reported at recommended doses in controlled clinical trials were: Nervous System: gait abnormality, euphoria, hyperkinesia, tremor, hallucination, confusion, convulsions; *Respiratory:* bronchospasm, cough; *Cardiovascular:* pallor, palpitation, hypertension, cerebrovascular disorder, cardiac failure, pedal edema, heart block, tachycardia, syncope; *Reproduction:* non-puerperal lactation; *Special Senses:* taste loss/change, parosmia.

Rates of adverse events, particularly those involving the gastrointestinal and nervous systems, increased significantly in controlled studies using higher than recommended doses of Flumadine. In most cases, symptoms resolved rapidly with discontinuation of treatment. In addition to the adverse events reported above, the following were also reported at higher than recommended doses: increased lacrimation, increased micturition frequency, fever, rigors, agitation, constipation, diaphoresis, dysphagia, stomatitis, hypesthesia and eye pain.

Adverse Reactions in Trials of Rimantadine and Amantadine: In a six-week prophylaxis study of 436 healthy adults comparing rimantadine with amantadine and placebo, the following adverse reactions were reported with an incidence >1%.

	Rimantadine 200 mg/day (n=145)	Placebo (n=143)	Amantadine 200 mg/day (n=148)
Nervous System			
Insomnia	3.4%	0.7%	7.0%
Nervousness	2.1%	0.7%	2.8%
Impaired Concentration	2.1%	1.4%	2.1%
Dizziness	0.7%	0.0%	2.1%
Depression	0.7%	0.7%	3.5%
Total % of subjects with adverse reactions	6.9%	4.1%	14.7%
Total % of subjects withdrawn due to adverse reactions	6.9%	3.4%	14.0%

USAGE IN THE ELDERLY: In general, the incidence of adverse events in controlled clinical trials in the elderly was higher in both the Flumadine and placebo-treated groups compared to younger adults and children. In a placebo-controlled study of 83 nursing home patients with influenza, 10.6% of those treated with Flumadine compared with 8.3% in the placebo group experienced events related to the central nervous system. The profile of these events was similar to that for the most frequent adverse events reported in other controlled trials (see list above).

Pooled data from controlled studies of prophylaxis and treatment of influenza with Flumadine in persons over 65 years of age showed an increase in adverse clinical events associated with the recommended dose of Flumadine (100 mg twice a day) compared to controls as follows: central and peripheral nervous systems, 12.5% for Flumadine versus 8.7% for control patients; gastrointestinal system, 17.0% for Flumadine versus 11.3% for controls.

OVERDOSAGE

As with any overdose, supportive therapy should be administered as indicated. Overdoses of a related drug, amantadine, have been reported with adverse reactions consisting of agitation, hallucinations, cardiac arrhythmia and death. The administration of intravenous physostigmine (a cholinergic agent) at doses of 1 to 2 mg in adults (Ref. 7) and 0.5 mg in children (Ref. 8) repeated as needed as long as the dose did not exceed 2 mg/hour has been reported anecdotally to be beneficial in patients with central nervous system effects from overdoses of amantadine.

DOSAGE AND ADMINISTRATION

FOR PROPHYLAXIS IN ADULTS AND CHILDREN:

Adults: The recommended adult dose of Flumadine is 100 mg twice a day. In patients with severe hepatic dysfunction, renal failure (CrCl ≤ 10 mL/min.) and elderly nursing home patients, a dose reduction to 100 mg daily is recommended. There are currently no data available regarding the safety of rimantadine during multiple dosing in subjects with renal or hepatic impairment. Because of the potential for accumulation of rimantadine metabolites during multiple dosing, patients with any degree of renal insufficiency should be monitored for adverse effects, with dosage adjustments being made as necessary.

Children: In children less than 10 years of age, Flumadine should be administered once a day, at a dose of 5 mg/kg but not exceeding 150 mg. For children 10 years of age or older, use the adult dose.

FOR TREATMENT IN ADULTS: The recommended adult dose of Flumadine is 100 mg twice a day. In patients with severe hepatic dysfunction, renal failure (CrCl ≤ 10 mL/min) and elderly nursing home patients, a dose reduction to 100 mg daily is recommended. There are currently no data available regarding the safety of rimantadine during multiple dosing in subjects with renal or hepatic impairment. Because of the potential for accumulation of rimantadine metabolites during multiple dosing, patients with any degree of renal insufficiency should be monitored for adverse effects, with dosage adjustments being made as necessary. Flumadine therapy should be initiated as soon as possible, preferably within 48 hours after onset of signs and symptoms of influenza A infection. Therapy should be continued for approximately seven days from the initial onset of symptoms.

HOW SUPPLIED

Flumadine® tablets (rimantadine hydrochloride tablets) are supplied as 100 mg tablets (orange, oval-shaped, film-coated) in bottles of 100 (NDC 0456-0521-01). Imprint on tablets: (Front) FLUMADINE 100; (Back) FOREST.

Flumadine® syrup (rimantadine hydrochloride syrup) containing 50 mg of rimantadine hydrochloride per teaspoonful (5 mL) (purplish-red, raspberry-flavored) is supplied in bottles of 8 oz (NDC 0456-0527-08).

Tablets and syrup should be stored at 15°–30°C (59°–86°F).

Rx only

REFERENCES

1. Belshe, R.B., Burk, B., Newman, F., Cerruti, R.L. and Sim, I.S. (1989) J. Infect. Dis. 159, 430–435.
2. Sim, I.S., Cerruti, R.L. and Connell, E.V., (1989) J. Resp. Dis. (Suppl.), S46–S51.
3. Hayden, F.G., Belshe, R.B., Clover, R.D. et al (1989) N.Engl. J. Med. 321 (25), 1696–1702.
4. Hall, C.B., Dolin, R., Gala, C.L., et al (1987) Pediatrics 80, 275–282.
5. Thompson, J., Fleet, W., Lawrence, E. et al (1987) J.Med. Vir. 21, 249–255.
6. Belshe, R.B., Smith, M.H., Hall, C.B., et al (1988) J. Virol. 62, 1508–1512.
7. Casey, D.F. N. Engl. J. Med. 1978:298:516.
8. Berkowitz, C.D. J. Pediatrics. 1979:95:144.

Rev. 3/99
MG #9040 (07)

FOREST PHARMACEUTICALS, INC.
Subsidiary of Forest Laboratories, Inc.
St Louis, MO 63045

Shown in Product Identification Guide, page 312

INFASURF® for Neonatal RDS

℞

[in 'fă-surf]
(calfactant)
Intratracheal Suspension
Sterile Suspension for Intratracheal Use Only

Rx only

DESCRIPTION

Infasurf® (calfactant) Intratracheal Suspension is a sterile, non-pyrogenic lung surfactant intended for intratracheal instillation only. It is an extract of natural surfactant from calf lungs which includes phospholipids, neutral lipids, and hydrophobic surfactant-associated proteins B and C (SP-B and SP-C). It contains no preservatives.

Infasurf is an off-white suspension of calfactant in 0.9% aqueous sodium chloride solution. It has a pH of 5.0 – 6.0. Each milliliter of Infasurf contains 35 mg total phospholipids (including 26 mg phosphatidylcholine of which 16 mg is disaturated phosphatidylcholine) and 0.65 mg proteins including 0.26 mg of SP-B.

CLINICAL PHARMACOLOGY

Endogenous lung surfactant is essential for effective ventilation because it modifies alveolar surface tension thereby stabilizing the alveoli. Lung surfactant deficiency is the cause of Respiratory Distress Syndrome (RDS) in premature infants. Infasurf restores surface activity to the lungs of these infants.

Activity: Infasurf adsorbs rapidly to the surface of the air-liquid interface and modifies surface tension similarly to natural lung surfactant. A minimum surface tension of ≤ 3 mN/m is produced *in vitro* by Infasurf as measured on a pulsating bubble surfactometer. *Ex vivo*, Infasurf restores the pressure volume mechanics and compliance of surfactant-deficient rat lungs. *In vivo*, Infasurf improves lung compliance, respiratory gas exchange, and survival in preterm lambs with profound surfactant deficiency.

Animal Metabolism: Infasurf is administered directly to the lung lumen surface, its site of action. No human studies of absorption, biotransformation or excretion of Infasurf have been performed. The administration of Infasurf with radiolabeled phospholipids into the lungs of adult rabbits results in the persistence of 50% of radioactivity in the lung alveolar lining and 25% of radioactivity in the lung tissue 24 hours later. Less than 5% of the radioactivity is found in other organs. In premature lambs with lethal surfactant deficiency, less than 30% of instilled Infasurf is present in the lung lining after 24 hours.

Clinical Studies: The efficacy of infasurf was demonstrated in two multiple-dose controlled clinical trials involving approximately 2,000 infants treated with Infasurf (approximately 100 mg phospholipid/kg) or Exosurf Neonatal®. In addition, two controlled trials on Infasurf versus Survanta®, and four uncontrolled trials were conducted that involved approximately 15,500 patients treated with Infasurf.

Infasurf versus Exosurf Neonatal®

Treatment Trial

A total of 1,126 infants ≤ 72 hours of age with RDS who required endotracheal intubation and had an a/A PO_2 < 0.22 were enrolled into a multiple-dose, randomized, double-blind treatment trial comparing Infasurf (3 mL/kg) and Exosurf Neonatal® (5 mL/kg). Patients were given an initial dose and one repeat dose 12 hours later if intubation was still required. The dose was instilled in two aliquots through a side-port adapter into the proximal end of the endotracheal tube. Each aliquot was given in small bursts over 20–30 inspiratory cycles. After each aliquot was instilled, the infant was positioned with either the right or the left side dependent. Results for efficacy parameters evaluated at 28 days or to discharge for all treated patients from this treatment trial are shown in Table 1.

Table 1 — Infasurf vs Exosurf Neonatal® Treatment Trial:

Efficacy	Infasurf (N=570)	Exosurf Neonatal® (N=556)	
Parameter	%	%	p-value
Incidence of air leaks[a]	11	22	≥0.001
Death due to RDS	4	4	0.95
Any death to 28 day	8	10	0.21
Any death before discharge	9	12	0.07
BPD[b]	5	6	0.41
Crossover to other surfactant[c]	4	4	1

[a] Pneumothorax and/or pulmonary interstitial emphysema.
[b] BPD is bronchopulmonary dysplasia, diagnosed by positive X-ray and oxygen dependence at 28 days.
[c] Protocol permitted use of comparator surfactant in patients who failed to respond to therapy with the initial randomized surfactant if the infant was < 96 hours of age, had received a full course of the randomized surfactant, and had an a/A PO_2 ratio < 0.10

Prophylaxis Trial

A total of 853 infants < 29 weeks gestation were enrolled into a multiple-dose, randomized, double-blind prophylaxis trial comparing Infasurf (3 mL/kg) and Exosurf Neonatal® (5 mL/kg). The initial dose was administered within 30 minutes of birth. Repeat doses were administered at 12 and 24 hours if the patient remained intubated. Each dose was administered divided in 2 equal aliquots, and given through a side port adapter into the proximal end of the endotracheal tube. Each aliquot was given in small bursts over 20–30 inspiratory cycles. After each aliquot was instilled, the infant was positioned with either the right or the left side dependent. Results for efficacy parameters evaluated to day 28 or to discharge for all treated patients from this prophylaxis trial are shown in Table 2.

Table 3 — Common Complications of Prematurity and RDS in Controlled Trials:

Complication	Infasurf (N=1001) %	Exosurf Neonatal® (N=978) %	Infasurf (N=553) %	Survanta® (N=566) %
Apnea	61	61	76	76
Patient ductus arteriosus	47	48	45	48
Intracranial hemorrhage	29	31	36	36
Severe intracranial hemorrhage[a]	12	10	9	7
IVH and PVL[b]	7	3	5	5
Sepsis	20	22	28	27
Pulmonary air leaks	12	22	15	15
Pulmonary interstitial emphysema	7	17	10	10
Pulmonary hemorrhage	7	7	7	6
Necrotizing enterocolitis	5	5	17	18

[a] Grade III and IV by the method of Papile.
[b] Patients with both intraventricular hemorrhage and periventricular leukomalacia.

Table 2 — Infasurf vs Exosurf Neonatal® Prophylaxis Trial:

Efficacy	Infasurf (N=431)	Exosurf Neonatal® (N=422)	
Parameter	%	%	p-value
Incidence of RDS	15	47	≤0.001
Incidence of air leaks[a]	10	15	0.01
Death due to RDS	2	5	≤0.01
Any death to 28 days	12	16	0.10
Any death before discharge	18	19	0.56
BPD[b]	16	17	0.60
Crossover to other surfactant[c]	0.2	3	≤0.001

[a] Pneumothorax and/or pulmonary interstitial emphysema.
[b] BPD is bronchopulmonary dysplasia, diagnosed by positive X-ray and oxygen dependence at 28 days.
[c] Protocol permitted use of comparator surfactant in patients who failed to respond to therapy with the initial randomized surfactant if the infant was < 72 hours of age, had received a full course of the randomized surfactant, and had an a/A PO_2 ratio was < 0.10

Infasurf versus Survanta®

Treatment Trial

A total of 662 infants with RDS who required endotracheal intubation and had an a/A PO_2 < 0.22 were enrolled into a multiple-dose, randomized, double-blind treatment trial comparing Infasurf (4 mL/kg of a formulation that contained 25 mg of phospholipids/mL rather than the 35 mg/mL in the marketed formulation) and Survanta® (4 mL/kg). Repeat doses were allowed ≥ 6 hours following the previous treatment (for up to three doses before 96 hours of age) if the patient required ≥ 30% oxygen. The surfactant was given through a 5 French feeding catheter inserted into the endotracheal tube. The total dose was instilled in four equal aliquots with the catheter removed between each of the instillations and mechanical ventilation resumed for 0.5 to 2 minutes. Each of the aliquots was administered with the patient in one of four different positions (prone, supine, right, and left lateral) to facilitate even distribution of the surfactant. Results for the major efficacy parameters evaluated at 28 days or to discharge (incidence of air leaks, death due to respiratory causes or to any cause, BPD, or treatment failure) for all treated patients from this treatment trial were not significantly different between Infasurf and Survanta®.

Prophylaxis Trial

A total of 457 infants ≤ 30 weeks gestation and < 1251 grams birth weight were enrolled into a multiple-dose, randomized, double-blind trial comparing Infasurf (4 mL/kg of a formulation that contained 25 mg of phospholipids/mL rather than the 35 mg/mL in the marketed formulation) and Survanta® (4 mL/kg). The initial dose was administered within 15 minutes of birth and repeat doses were allowed ≥ 6 hours following the previous treatment (for up to three doses before 96 hours of age) if the patient required ≥ 30% oxygen. The surfactant was given through a 5 French feeding catheter inserted into the endotracheal tube. The total dose was instilled in four equal aliquots with the catheter removed between each of the instillations and mechanical ventilation resumed for 0.5 to 2 minutes. Each of the aliquots was administered with the patient in one of four different positions: prone, supine, right, and left lateral.

Results for efficacy endpoints evaluated at 28 days or to discharge for all treated patients from this prophylaxis trial showed an increase in mortality from any cause at 28 days (p=0.03) and in death due to respiratory causes (p=0.005) in Infasurf-treated infants. For evaluable patients (patients who met the protocol-defined entry criteria), mortality from any cause and mortality due to respiratory causes were also higher in the Infasurf group (p=0.07 and 0.03, respectively). However, these observations have not been replicated in other adequate and well-controlled trials and their relevance to the intended population is unknown. All other efficacy outcomes (incidence of RDS, air leaks, BPD, and treatment failure) were not significantly different between Infasurf and Survanta® when analyzed for all treated patients and for evaluable patients.

Acute Clinical Effects: As with other surfactants, marked improvements in oxygenation and lung compliance may occur shortly after the administration of Infasurf. All controlled clinical trials with Infasurf demonstrated significant improvements in fraction of inspired oxygen (F_IO_2) and mean airway pressure (MAP) during the first 24 to 48 hours following initiation of Infasurf therapy.

INDICATIONS AND USAGE

Infasurf is indicated for the prevention of Respiratory Distress Syndrome (RDS) in premature infants at high risk for RDS and for the treatment ("rescue") of premature infants who develop RDS. Infasurf decreases the incidence of RDS, mortality due to RDS, and air leaks associated with RDS.

Prophylaxis

Prophylaxis therapy at birth with Infasurf is indicated for premature infants < 29 weeks of gestational age at significant risk for RDS. Infasurf prophylaxis should be administered as soon as possible, preferably within 30 minutes after birth.

Treatment

Infasurf therapy is indicated for infants ≤ 72 hours of age with RDS (confirmed by clinical and radiologic findings) and requiring endotracheal intubation.

WARNINGS

Infasurf is intended for intratracheal use only.

THE ADMINISTRATION OF EXOGENOUS SURFACTANTS, INCLUDING INFASURF, OFTEN RAPIDLY IMPROVES OXYGENATION AND LUNG COMPLIANCE. Following administration of Infasurf, patients should be carefully monitored so that oxygen therapy and ventilatory support can be modified in response to changes in respiratory status.

Infasurf therapy is not a substitute for neonatal intensive care. Optimal care of premature infants at risk for RDS and newborn infants with RDS who need endotracheal intubation requires an acute care unit organized, staffed, equipped, and experienced with intubation, ventilator management, and general care of these patients.

TRANSIENT EPISODES OF REFLUX OF INFASURF INTO THE ENDOTRACHEAL TUBE, CYANOSIS, BRADYCARDIA, OR AIRWAY OBSTRUCTION HAVE OCCURRED DURING THE DOSING PROCEDURES. These events require stopping Infasurf administration and taking appropriate measures to alleviate the condition. After the patient is stable, dosing can proceed with appropriate monitoring.

PRECAUTIONS

When repeat dosing was given at fixed 12-hour intervals in the Infasurf vs. Exosurf Neonatal® trials, transient episodes of cyanosis, bradycardia, reflux of surfactant into the endotracheal tube, and airway obstruction were observed more frequently among infants in the Infasurf-treated group.

An increased proportion of patients with both intraventricular hemorrhage (IVH) and periventricular leukomalacia (PVL) was observed in Infasurf-treated infants in the Infasurf-Exosurf Neonatal® controlled trials. These observations were not associated with increased mortality.

No data are available on the use of Infasurf in conjunction with experimental therapies of RDS, e.g., high-frequency ventilation.

Data from controlled trials on the efficacy of Infasurf are limited to doses of approximately 100 mg phospholipid/kg body weight and up to a total of 4 doses.

Carcinogenesis, Mutagenesis, Impairment of Fertility

Carcinogenesis studies and animal reproduction studies have not been performed with Infasurf. A single mutagenicity study (Ames assay) was negative.

ADVERSE REACTIONS

The most common adverse reactions associated with Infasurf dosing procedures in the controlled trials were: cyanosis (65%), airway obstruction (39%), bradycardia (34%), reflux of surfactant into the endotracheal tube (21%), require-

Continued on next page

Infasurf—Cont.

ment for manual ventilation (16%), and reintubation (3%). These events were generally transient and not associated with serious complications or death.
The incidence of common complications of prematurity and RDS in the four controlled Infasurf trials are presented in Table 3. Prophylaxis and treatment study results for each surfactant are combined.
[See table 3 at top of previous page]

Follow-up Evaluations
Two year follow-up data of neurodevelopmental outcomes in 415 infants enrolled in 5 centers that participated in the Infasurf vs. Exosurf Neonatal® controlled trials demonstrated significant developmental delays in equal percentages of Infasurf and Exosurf Neonatal® patients.

OVERDOSAGE

There have been no reports of overdosage with Infasurf. While there are no known adverse effects of excess lung surfactant, overdosage would result in overloading the lungs with an isotonic solution. Ventilation should be supported until clearance of the liquid is accomplished.

DOSAGE AND ADMINISTRATION

FOR INTRATRACHEAL ADMINISTRATION ONLY
Infasurf should be administered under the supervision of clinicians experienced in the acute care of newborn infants with respiratory failure who require intubation.
Rapid and substantial increases in blood oxygenation and improved lung compliance often follow Infasurf instillation. Close clinical monitoring and surveillance following administration may be needed to adjust oxygen therapy and ventilator pressures appropriately.

Dosage
Each dose of Infasurf is 3 mL/kg body weight at birth. Infasurf has been administered every 12 hours for a total of up to 3 doses.

Directions for Use
Infasurf is a suspension which settles during storage. Gentle swirling or agitation of the vial is often necessary for redispersion. DO NOT SHAKE. Visible flecks in the suspension and foaming at the surface are normal for Infasurf.
Infasurf should be stored at refrigerated temperature 2°–8°C (36° to 46°F). Warning of Infasurf before administration is not necessary.
Unopened, unused vials of Infasurf that have warmed to room temperature can be returned to refrigerated storage within 24 hours for future use. Repeated warming to room temperature should be avoided. Each single-use vial should be entered only once and the vial with any unused material should be discarded after the initial entry.

INFASURF DOES NOT REQUIRE RECONSTITUTION. DO NOT DILUTE OR SONICATE.

Dosing Procedures

General
Infasurf should only be administered intratracheally through an endotracheal tube. The dose of Infasurf is 3 mL/kg birth weight. The dose is drawn into a syringe from the single-use vial using a 20-gauge or larger needle with care taken to avoid excessive foaming. Administration is made by instillation of the Infasurf suspension into the endotracheal tube.

Administration for Treatment of RDS

Initial Dose
Infasurf should be administered intratracheally through a side-port adapter into the endotracheal tube. Two attendants, one to instill the Infasurf, the other to monitor the patient and assist in positioning, facilitate the dosing. The dose (3 mL/kg) sould be administered in two aliquots of 1.5 mL/kg each. After each aliquot is instilled, the infant should be positioned with either the right or the left side dependent. Administration is made while ventilation is continued over 20–30 breaths for each aliquot, with small bursts timed only during the inspiratory cycles. A pause followed by evaluation of the respiratory status and repositioning should separate the two aliquots.

Repeat Doses
Repeat doses of 3 mL/kg of birth weight, up to a total of 3 doses 12 hours apart, have been given in the Infasurf controlled clinical trials if the patient was still intubated.
In the Infasurf versus Survanta® trials, Infasurf was administered through a 5 French feeding catheter inserted into the endotracheal tube. The total dose was instilled in four equal aliquots with the catheter removed between each of the installations and mechanical ventilation resumed for 0.5 to 2 minutes. Each of the aliquots was administered with the patient in one of four different positions (prone, supine, right, and left lateral) to facilitate even distribution of the surfactant. Repeat doses were administered as early as 6 hours after the previous dose for a total of up to 4 doses if the infant was still intubated and required at least 30% inspired oxygen to maintain a $P_aO_2 \leq 80$ torr.

Administration for Prophylaxis of RDS at Birth
The amount of a prophylaxis dose of Infasurf should be based on the infant's birth weight. Administration of Infasurf should be given as soon as possible after birth. Usually the immediate care and stabilization of the premature infant born with hypoxemia and/or bradycardia should precede Infasurf prophylaxis.
The dosing procedures are described under Administration for Treatment of RDS.

Dosing Precautions
During administration of Infasurf liquid suspension into the airway, infants often experience bradycardia, reflux of Infasurf into the endotracheal tube, airway obstruction, cyanosis, dislodgement of the endotracheal tube, or hypoventilation. If any of these events occur, the administration should be interrupted and the infant's condition should be stabilized using appropriate interventions before the administration of Infasurf is resumed. Endotracheal suctioning or reintubation is sometimes needed when there are signs of airway obstruction during the administration of the surfactant.

HOW SUPPLIED

Infasurf (calfactant) Intratracheal Suspension is supplied sterile in single-use, rubber-stoppered glass vials containing 6 mL off-white suspension (NDC 0456-4600-06).
Store Infasurf (calfactant) Intratracheal Suspension at refrigerated temperature 2° to 8°C (36° to 46°F) and protect from light. Vials are for single use only. After opening, discard unused drug.
Manufactured for:
FOREST PHARMACEUTICALS, INC.
Subsidiary of Forest Laboratories, Inc.
St. Louis, MO 63045
Manufactured by:
ONY, Inc.
Amherst, NY 14228
RMC 235 Rev. 07/98
Shown in Product Identification Guide, page 312

LEVOTHROID® Tablets ℞

[lēv 'o-throid"]
(levothyroxine sodium tablets, USP)

Dist. by
FOREST PHARMACEUTICALS, INC.
A Subsidiary of Forest Laboratories, Inc.
St. Louis, MO 63045

DESCRIPTION

LEVOTHROID TABLETS (levothyroxine sodium tablets, USP) provide crystalline sodium levothyroxine (T_4), a potent thyroid hormone, in twelve different strengths to permit easy, convenient dosage adjustment.
The structural formula for sodium levothyroxine as contained in Levothroid Tablets is:

Sodium L-3, 3′, 5, 5′-tetraiodothyronine

Inactive Ingredients (Levothroid Tablets): Lactose Monohydrate, NF; Magnesium Stearate, NF; Colloidal Silicon Dioxide, NF; Microcrystalline Cellulose, NF.
The following are the color additives listed by strength:

Strength	Color Additive
25 mcg	FD&C Red # 40, D&C Yellow #10
50 mcg	None
75 mcg	FD&C Red # 40, D&C Yellow #10 FD&C Blue #1
88 mcg	FD&C Red # 40, D&C Yellow #10 FD&C Blue #1
100 mcg	FD&C Red # 40, D&C Yellow #10
112 mcg	FD&C Red # 40
125 mcg	FD&C Red #40, FD&C Blue #1
137 mcg	FD&C Blue #1
150 mcg	FD&C Blue #1
175 mcg	FD&C Red #40, D&C Yellow #10 FD&C Blue #1
200 mcg	FD&C Red #40
300 mcg	FD&C Red # 40, D&C Yellow #10 FD&C Blue #1

CLINICAL PHARMACOLOGY

The major thyroid hormones are L-thyroxine (T_4) and L-triiodothyronine (T_3). The amounts of T_4 and T_3 released into the circulation from the normally functioning thyroid gland are regulated by the amount of thyrotropin (TSH) secreted from the anterior pituitary gland. TSH secretion is in turn regulated by the levels of circulating T_4 and T_3 and by secretion of thyrotropin releasing factor (TRH) from the hypothalamus. Recognition of this complex feedback system is important in the diagnosis and treatment of thyroid dysfunction.
The principal effect of exogenous thyroid hormone is to increase the metabolic rate of body tissues.
The thyroid hormones are also concerned with growth and differentiation of tissues. In deficiency states in the young there is retardation of growth and failure of maturation of the skeletal and other body systems, especially in failure of ossification in the epiphyses and in the growth and development of the brain.
The precise mechanism of action by which thyroid hormones affect thermogenesis and cellular growth and differentiation is not known. It is recognized that these physiologic effects are mediated at the cellular level primarily by T_3, a large part of which is derived from T_4 by deiodination in the peripheral tissues. Thyroxine (T_4) is the major component of normal secretions of the thyroid gland and is thus the primary determinant of normal thyroid function.
Levothroid tablets are rapidly absorbed after oral administration. Maximum observed plasma concentrations are reached within 1.5 to 3 hours of oral dosing. Following a single dose of 600 mcg or Levothroid to healthy volunteers, peak plasma concentrations of T_4 averaged 12.2 mcg/dL, where as T_3 plasma levels were indistinguishable from the baseline values. Peak plasma concentration of T_4 increased proportionally with increases in dose from 50 to 300 mcg.
Depending on other factors, absorption has varied from 48 to 79 percent of the administered dose. Fasting increases absorption. Malabsorption syndromes, as well as dietary factors, (children's soybean formula, concomitant use of anionic exchange resins such as cholestyramine) cause excessive fecal loss.
More than 99 percent of circulating hormones are bound to serum proteins, including thyroid-binding globulin (TBg), thyroid-binding prealbumin (TBPA), and albumin (TBa), whose capacities and affinities vary for the hormones. L-thyroxine displays greater binding affinity than L-triiodothyronine, both in the circulation and at the cellular level, which explains its longer duration of action. The half-life of T_4 in normal plasma is 6–7 days while that of T_3 is about 1 day. The plasma half-lives of T_4 and T_3 are decreased in hyperthyroidism and increased in hypothyroidism.

INDICATIONS AND USAGE

Levothroid Tablets (levothyroxine sodium tablets, USP) are indicated as replacement or substitution therapy for diminished or absent thyroid function (e.g., cretinism, myxedema, non-toxic goiter or hypothyroidism generally, including the hypothyroid state in children, in pregnancy and in the elderly) resulting from functional deficiency, primary atrophy, from partial or complete absence of the gland or from the effects of surgery, radiation or antithyroid agents. Therapy must be maintained continuously to control the symptoms of hypothyroidism.
It may also be used to suppress the secretion of thyrotropin (TSH), action which may be beneficial in simple nonendemic goiter and in chronic lymphocytic thyroiditis. This may cause a reduction in the goiter size. In addition, Levothroid, in conjunction with surgery and radioactive iodine therapy, is indicated as a pituitary TSH suppressant in the management of TSH-dependent well-differentiated papillary or follicular carcinoma of the thyroid.
Thyroid hormone drugs are indicated as a diagnostic agent in suppression tests to differentiate suspected mild hyperthyroidism or thyroid gland autonomy.
Thyroid hormones may also be used with antithyroid drugs to treat thyrotoxicosis. This combination has been used to prevent goitrogenesis and hypothyroidism.

CONTRAINDICATIONS

Levothroid Tablets administration is contraindicated in untreated thyrotoxicosis, in acute myocardial infarction, and apparent hypersensitivity to thyroid hormones. There is no well-documented evidence of allergic reactions to thyroid hormones. Levothroid Tablets are contraindicated in the presence of uncorrected adrenal insufficiency because it increases the tissue demands for adrenocortical hormones and may cause an acute adrenal crisis in such patients. (See PRECAUTIONS).

WARNINGS

> Drugs with thyroid hormone activity, alone or together with other therapeutic agents, have been used for the treatment of obesity. In euthyroid patients, doses within the range of daily hormonal requirements are ineffective for weight reduction. Larger doses may produce serious or even life-threatening manifestations of toxicity, particularly when given in association with sympathomimetic amines such as those used for their anorectic effects.

The use of thyroid hormones in the therapy of obesity, alone or combined with other drugs, is unjustified and has been shown to be ineffective. Neither is their use justified for the treatment of male or female infertility unless this condition is accompanied by hypothyroidism.

PRECAUTIONS

GENERAL—Levothroid Tablets should be used with caution in patients with cardiovascular disease, including hypertension. The development of chest pain or other aggravation of cardiovascular disease will require a decrease in dosage.
Thyroid hormone therapy in patients with concomitant diabetes mellitus or diabetes insipidus or adrenal cortical insufficiency aggravates the intensity of their symptoms. Ap-

propriate adjustments of the various therapeutic measures directed at these concomitant endocrine diseases are required. The therapy of myxedema coma requires simultaneous administration of glucocorticoids. (See DOSAGE AND ADMINISTRATION).

In infants, excessive doses of thyroid hormone preparations may produce craniosynostosis.

INFORMATION FOR THE PATIENT—Patients on thyroid preparations and parents of children on thyroid therapy should be informed that:

1. Replacement therapy is to be taken essentially for life, with the exception of cases of transient hypothyroidism, usually associated with thyroiditis, and in those patients receiving a therapeutic trial of the drug.

2. They should immediately report during the course of therapy any signs or symptoms of thyroid hormone toxicity, e.g., chest pain, increased pulse rate, palpitations, excessive sweating, heat intolerance, nervousness, or any other unusual event.

3. In case of concomitant diabetes mellitus, the daily dosage of antidiabetic medication may need readjustment as thyroid hormone replacement is achieved. If thyroid medication is stopped, a downward readjustment of the dosage of insulin or oral hypoglycemic agent may be necessary to avoid hypoglycemia. At all times, close monitoring of urinary glucose levels is mandatory in such patients.

4. In case of concomitant oral anticoagulant therapy, the prothrombin time should be measured frequently to determine if the dosage of oral anticoagulants is to be readjusted.

5. Partial loss of hair may be experienced by children in the first few months of thyroid therapy, but this is usually a transient phenomenon and later recovery is usually the rule.

LABORATORY TESTS—The patient's response to thyroid replacement may be followed by laboratory tests such as serum thyroxine (T_4), serum triiodothyronine (T_3), free thyroxine index and thyroid stimulating hormone (TSH) blood levels. In hypopituitarism, the serum TSH level is not usually useful and monitoring should be done with measurement of serum total or free T_4. In euthyroid goiter patients or those with thyroid cancer the serum TSH should be suppressed below the reference range.

DRUG INTERACTIONS—Antidiabetic Agents—In patients with diabetes mellitus, addition of thyroid hormone therapy may cause an increase in the required dosage of insulin or oral hypoglycemic agents. Conversely, decreasing the dose of thyroid hormone may possibly cause hypoglycemic reactions if the dosage of insulin or oral hypoglycemic agents is not adjusted.

Anticoagulants—Thyroid replacement may potentiate anticoagulant effects with agents such as warfarin or bishydroxycoumarin and reduction of one-third in anticoagulant dosage should be undertaken upon initiation of Levothroid Tablets therapy. Subsequent anticoagulant dosage adjustment should be made on the basis of frequent prothrombin determinations.

Sympathetic interactions—Injection of epinephrine in patients with coronary artery disease may precipitate an episode of coronary insufficiency. This may be enhanced in patients receiving thyroid preparations. Careful observation is required if catecholamines are administered to patients in this category.

Cholestyramine or colestipol binds both T_4 and T_3 in the intestine, thus impairing absorption of these thyroid hormones. *In vitro* studies indicate that the binding is not easily removed. Therefore, four to five hours should elapse between administration of cholestyramine or colestipol and thyroid hormones.

Estrogens tend to increase serum thyroxine-binding globulin (TBg). In a patient with a non-functioning thyroid gland who is receiving thyroid replacement therapy, free levothyroxine may be decreased when estrogens are started thus increasing thyroid requirements. However, if the patient's thyroid gland has sufficient function the decreased free thyroxine will result in a compensatory increase in thyroxine output by the thyroid. Therefore, patients without a functioning thyroid gland who are on thyroid replacement therapy may need to increase their thyroxine dose if estrogens or estrogen-containing oral contraceptives are given.

DRUG/LABORATORY TEST INTERACTIONS—The following drugs or moieties are known to interfere with laboratory tests performed in patients on thyroid hormone therapy: androgens, corticosteroids, estrogens, oral contraceptives containing estrogens, iodine-containing preparations, and the numerous preparations containing salicylates. In some instances, for example, the use of androgens, estrogens, or oral contraceptives, a patient's thyroid status may be affected and monitoring with serum TSH measurements may be suggested.

1. Changes in TBg concentration should be taken into consideration in the interpretation of T_4 and T_3 values. In such cases, the unbound (free) hormone should be measured. Pregnancy, estrogens, and estrogen-containing oral contraceptives increase TBg concentrations. TBg may also be increased during infectious hepatitis. Decreases in TBg concentrations are observed in nephrosis, acromegaly, and after androgen or corticosteroid therapy. Familial hyper- or hypothyroxine-binding-globulinemias have been described. The incidence of TBg deficiency approximates 1 in 9000. The binding of thyroxine by thyroid-binding prealbumin (TBPA) is inhibited by salicylates.

2. Medical or dietary iodine interferes with all *in vivo* tests of radioiodine uptake, producing low uptakes which may not be reflective of a true decrease in hormone synthesis.

3. The persistence of clinical and laboratory evidence of hypothyroidism in spite of adequate dosage replacement indicates either poor patient compliance, poor absorption, excessive fecal loss, or inactivity of the preparation. Intracellular resistance to thyroid hormone is quite rare.

CARCINOGENESIS, MUTAGENESIS, AND IMPAIRMENT OF FERTILITY—A reportedly apparent association between prolonged thyroid therapy and breast cancer has not been confirmed and patients on thyroxine for established indications should not discontinue therapy. No confirmatory long-term studies in animals have been performed to evaluate carcinogenic potential, mutagenicity, or impairment of fertility in either males or females.

PREGNANCY-CATEGORY A—Thyroid hormones do not readily cross the placental barrier. The clinical experience to date does not indicate any adverse effect on fetuses when thyroid hormones are administered to pregnant women. On the basis of current knowledge, thyroid replacement therapy to hypothyroid women should not be discontinued during pregnancy, but the requirements for dosage may increase and should not be measured periodically with measurements of serum TSH concentration.

NURSING MOTHERS—Minimal amounts of thyroid hormones are excreted in human milk. Thyroid hormone is not associated with serious adverse reactions and does not have a known tumorigenic potential. However, caution should be exercised when thyroid is administered to a nursing woman.

GERIATRIC USE—Sufficient numbers of subjects have been studied to indicate that the administration of levothyroxine to the elderly may require adjustment of dosing or monitoring.

In one study, the average full replacement dose of levothyroxine of 23 elderly (average age 75.5 years) ambulatory patients with primary hypothyroidism was 75% of the mean full replacement dose of 44 younger (average age 48.1 years) patients. In another study, levothyroxine replacement dose in elderly patients (mean age, 66.1 years) was found to be 33% less than that formerly recommended.

The decrease in replacement dose in the elderly may be due to the reduction in the fractional thyroxine degradation rate. The reduction in thyroxine turnover in the elderly may be a function of age-related decline in lean body mass.

Optimal daily levothyroxine dosage may not decline universally in all elderly patients, but be dependent on the etiology of the disorder causing the hypothyroidism. Therefore, it should not be assumed that all elderly patients require smaller maintenance doses of Levothroid than younger patients. At any age, titration of dose to restoration of euthyroidism should be based on the clinical response of the patient and normalization of serum TSH concentration.

PEDIATRIC USE—The diagnosis and institution of therapy for cretinism should be done as soon after birth as feasible to prevent developmental deficiency. Screening tests for serum T_4 and TSH will identify this group of newborn patients.

ADVERSE REACTIONS

Patients who are sensitive to lactose may show intolerance to Levothroid Tablets since this substance is used in the manufacture of the product.

Adverse reactions other than those indicative of hyperthyroidism because of therapeutic overdosage, either initially or during the maintenance period, are rare. (See OVERDOSAGE).

OVERDOSAGE

Excessive dosage of thyroid medication may result in symptoms of hyperthyroidism. Since, however, the effects do not appear at once, the symptoms may not appear for one to three weeks after the dosage regimen is begun. The most common signs and symptoms of overdosage are menstrual changes, increase in blood pressure, increase in appetite, weight loss, palpitation, nervousness, diarrhea or abdominal cramps, sweating, tachycardia, cardiac arrhythmias, angina pectoris, tremors, headache, insomnia, intolerance to heat and fever. If symptoms of overdosage appear, discontinue medication for several days and reinstitute treatment at a lower dosage level.

Laboratory tests such as serum T_4, and serum T_3 and the free thyroxine index will be elevated during the period of overdosage.

Complications as a result of the induced hypermetabolic state may include cardiac failure and death due to arrhythmia or failure.

TREATMENT OF OVERDOSAGE—Dosage should be reduced or therapy temporarily discontinued if signs and symptoms of overdosage appear. Treatment may be reinstituted at a lower dosage. In normal individuals, normal hypothalamic-pituitary-thyroid axis function is restored in 6 to 8 weeks after thyroid suppression.

Treatment of acute massive thyroid hormone overdosage is aimed at reducing gastrointestinal absorption of the drugs and counteracting central and peripheral effects, mainly those of increased sympathetic activity. Vomiting may be induced initially if further gastrointestinal absorption can reasonably be prevented and barring contraindications such as coma, convulsions, or loss of the gagging reflex. Treatment is symptomatic and supportive. Oxygen may be administered and ventilation maintained. Cardiac glycosides may be indicated if congestive heart failure develops. Measures to control fever, hypoglycemia, or fluid loss should be instituted if needed. Antiadrenergic agents, particularly propranolol, have been used advantageously in the treatment of increased sympathetic activity. Propranolol may be administered intravenously at a dosage of 1 to 3 mg over a 10-minute period or orally, 80 to 160 mg/day, initially, especially when no contraindications exist for its use. Other adjunctive measures may include administration of cholestyramine to interfere with thyroxine absorption, and glucocorticoids to inhibit conversion of T_4 to T_3.

DOSAGE AND ADMINISTRATION

The goal of therapy should be the restoration of euthyroidism as judged by clinical response and confirmed by appropriate laboratory values. In adults with no complicating endocrine or cardiovascular disease, the predicted full maintenance dose may be achieved immediately with adjustments made as indicated by clinical evaluation. The usual maintenance dose of Levothroid Tablets is 100 to 200 mcg.

In patients with known complications or in case of doubt, individual dose titration at 2- to 4-week intervals is recommended. The usual starting dose is 50 mcg with increases of 50 mcg at 2- to 4-week intervals until the patient is euthyroid or symptoms ensue which preclude further dose increase.

In adult myxedema or hypothyroid patients with angina, the starting dose should be 25 mcg with increases at 2- to 4-week intervals of 25 to 50 mcg as determined by clinical response.

Myxedema coma is usually precipitated in the hypothyroid patient of long-standing by intercurrent illness or drugs such as sedatives and anesthetics and should be considered a medical emergency. Therapy should be directed at the correction of electrolyte disturbances and possible infection besides the administration of thyroid hormones. Corticosteroids should be administered routinely. T_4 and T_3 may be administered via a nasogastric tube, but the preferred route of administration of both hormones is intravenous. Sodium levothyroxine (T_4) is given at a starting dose of 200–500 mcg (100 mcg/mL given rapidly), and is usually well tolerated, even in the elderly. This initial dose is followed by daily supplements of 100 to 200 mcg given IV. Normal T_4 levels are achieved in 24 hours followed in 3 days by threefold increase of T_3. Oral therapy with Levothroid Tablets should be resumed as soon as the clinical situation has been stabilized and the patient is able to take oral medication.

Pediatric dosage should follow the recommendations summarized in Table I. In infants with congenital hypothyroidism, therapy with full doses should be instituted as soon as the diagnosis has been made. Levothroid Tablets may be given to infants and children who cannot swallow intact tablets by crushing the tablet and suspending the freshly crushed tablet in a small amount of water (5 to 10 ml), breast milk or formula (non-soybean). The suspension can be given by spoon or dropper. DO NOT STORE THE SUSPENSION FOR ANY PERIOD OF TIME. The crushed tablet may also be sprinkled over a small amount of food, such as cooked cereal or apple sauce. Foods or formulas containing large amounts of iron, soybean, or fiber should not be used to administer Levothroid.

TABLE I
Recommended Pediatric Dosage For Congenital Hypothyroidism*

LEVOTHROID TABLETS
(levothyroxine sodium tablets, USP)

Age	Dose per day	Daily dose per kg of body weight
0–6 mos	25–50 mcg	10–15 mcg
6–12 mos	50–75 mcg	6–8 mcg
1–5 yrs	75–100 mcg	5–6 mcg
6–12 yrs	100–150 mcg	4–5 mcg

* To be adjusted on the basis of clinical response and laboratory tests (See **Laboratory Tests**).

HOW SUPPLIED

Strength	Package Size	NDC Number
25 mcg	bottle of 100	0456-0320-01
25 mcg	bottle of 1000	0456-0320-00
25 mcg	bottle of 5000	0456-0320-51
25 mcg	unit dose carton of 100	0456-0320-63
50 mcg	bottle of 100	0456-0321-01
50 mcg	bottle of 1000	0456-0321-00
50 mcg	bottle of 5000	0456-0321-51
50 mcg	unit dose carton of 100	0456-0321-63
75 mcg	bottle of 100	0456-0322-01
75 mcg	bottle of 1000	0456-0322-00
75 mcg	bottle of 5000	0456-0322-51
75 mcg	unit dose carton of 100	0456-0322-63

Continued on next page

Levothroid—Cont.

88 mcg	bottle of 100	0456-0329-01
88 mcg	bottle of 1000	0456-0329-00
88 mcg	bottle of 5000	0456-0329-51
88 mcg	unit dose carton of 100	0456-0329-63
100 mcg	bottle of 100	0456-0323-01
100 mcg	bottle of 1000	0456-0323-00
100 mcg	bottle of 5000	0456-0323-51
100 mcg	unit dose carton of 100	0456-0323-63
112 mcg	bottle of 100	0456-0330-01
112 mcg	bottle of 1000	0456-0330-00
112 mcg	bottle of 5000	0456-0330-51
112 mcg	unit dose carton of 100	0456-0330-63
125 mcg	bottle of 100	0456-0324-01
125 mcg	bottle of 1000	0456-0324-00
125 mcg	bottle of 5000	0456-0324-51
125 mcg	unit dose carton of 100	0456-0324-63
137 mcg	bottle of 100	0456-0331-01
137 mcg	bottle of 1000	0456-0331-00
137 mcg	bottle of 5000	0456-0331-51
137 mcg	unit dose carton of 100	0456-0331-63
150 mcg	bottle of 100	0456-0325-01
150 mcg	bottle of 1000	0456-0325-00
150 mcg	bottle of 5000	0456-0325-51
150 mcg	unit dose carton of 100	0456-0325-63
175 mcg	bottle of 100	0456-0326-01
175 mcg	bottle of 1000	0456-0326-00
175 mcg	bottle of 5000	0456-0326-51
175 mcg	unit dose carton of 100	0456-0326-63
200 mcg	bottle of 100	0456-0327-01
200 mcg	bottle of 1000	0456-0327-00
200 mcg	bottle of 5000	0456-0327-51
200 mcg	unit dose carton of 100	0456-0327-63
300 mcg	bottle of 100	0456-0328-01
300 mcg	bottle of 1000	0456-0328-00
300 mcg	bottle of 5000	0456-0328-51
300 mcg	unit dose carton of 100	0456-0328-63

Strength	Tablet Color	Markings
25 mcg	Orange	25
50 mcg	White	50
75 mcg	Grey	75
88 mcg	Mint Green	88
100 mcg	Yellow	100
112 mcg	Rose	112
125 mcg	Purple	125
137 mcg	Blue	137
150 mcg	Light Blue	150
175 mcg	Turquoise	175
200 mcg	Pink	200
300 mcg	Lime Green	300

Tablets should be stored at controlled room temperature, 59°–86°F (15°–30°C) in capped bottles or unbroken plastic strip packing. Levothroid Tablets should be protected from light and moisture.

Rev. 7/99 03690799

Shown in Product Identification Guide, page 312

LORCET®-HD Ⓒ℞

[*lōr-sét h d*]

DESCRIPTION

Each Lorcet-HD capsule contains 5 mg Hydrocodone* Bitartrate *(WARNING: May be habit forming) and 500 mg Acetaminophen.

HOW SUPPLIED

Lorcet-HD capsules are opaque maroon capsules imprinted with the UAD logo; 1120 and are supplied in bottles of 100 capsules. Each capsule contains Hydrocodone* Bitartrate, 5mg *(WARNING: May Be Habit Forming) and Acetaminophen (APAP), 500 mg. NDC# 0785-1120-01.

Mfd. by:
Mallinckrodt
Hobart, NY 13788

Mfd. for:
Forest Pharmaceuticals, Inc.
St. Louis, MO 63045

LORCET® PLUS Ⓒ℞

[*lōr-sét plus*]

Hydrocodone Bitartrate and Acetaminophen Tablets USP 7.5 mg/650 mg

DESCRIPTION

Each Lorcet Plus tablet contains:
Hydrocodone* Bitartrate .... 7.5 mg
*(**WARNING**: May be habit forming)
Acetaminophen .... 650 mg

HOW SUPPLIED

Lorcet Plus, Hydrocodone Bitartrate and Acetaminophen Tablets USP, each tablet of which contains hydrocodone* bitartrate 7.5 mg *(WARNING: May be habit forming) and acetaminophen 650 mg, are white, capsule-shaped, scored tablets, debossed "U" on one side and "201" on the other side, and are supplied in containers of 100 tablets, NDC #0785-1122-01, containers of 500 tablets, NDC #0785-1122-50, and in unit-dose cartons of 100 tablets (4 cards of 25 tablets per card), NDC #0785-1122-63.

Shown in Product Identification Guide, page 312

LORCET® 10/650 Ⓒ℞

[*lōr sēt*]

HYDROCODONE* BITARTRATE AND ACETAMINOPHEN TABLETS USP 10 mg/650 mg

DESCRIPTION

Each Lorcet 10/650 tablet contains:
Hydrocodone*
Bitartrate .... 10 mg
*(**WARNING**: May be habit forming)
Acetaminophen .... 650 mg

In addition, each tablet contains the following inactive ingredients: colloidal silicon dioxide, croscarmellose sodium, crospovidone, microcrystalline cellulose, povidone, pregelatinized starch, stearic acid and FD&C Blue #1 Lake.

HOW SUPPLIED

Lorcet 10/650, Hydrocodone* Bitartrate and Acetaminophen Tablets, each tablet of which contains hydrocodone* bitartrate 10 mg *(**WARNING**: May be habit forming) and acetaminophen 650 mg, are light-blue, capsule-shaped, scored tablets, debossed "UAD" on one side and "63 50" on the other side, and are supplied in containers of 100 tablets, NDC 0785-6350-01 and in containers of 500 tablets, NDC 0785-6350-50, and in containers of unit dose (4 × 25's), NDC 0785-6350-63.

Shown in Product Identification Guide, page 313

MONUROL® ℞

[*mon' ur ol*]

(fosfomycin tromethamine)
SACHET
Rx only

DESCRIPTION

MONUROL (fosfomycin tromethamine) sachet contains fosfomycin tromethamine, a synthetic, broad-spectrum, bactericidal antibiotic for oral administration. It is available as a single-dose sachet which contains white granules consisting of 5.631 grams of fosfomycin tromethamine (equivalent to 3 grams of fosfomycin), and the following inactive ingredients: mandarin flavor, orange flavor, saccharin, and sucrose. The contents of the sachet must be dissolved in water. Fosfomycin tromethamine, a phosphonic acid derivative, is available as (1*R*,2*S*)-(1,2-epoxypropyl)phosphonic acid, compound with 2-amino-2-(hydroxymethyl)-1,3-propanediol (1:1). It is a white granular compound with a molecular weight of 259.2. Its empirical formula is $C_3H_7O_4P \cdot C_4H_{11}NO_3$, and its chemical structure is as follows:

H_3C–(epoxide, H, H)–P(=O)(OH)–$OH \cdot H_2N$–C(CH_2OH)(CH_2OH)–CH_2OH

CLINICAL PHARMACOLOGY

Absorption: Fosfomycin tromethamine is rapidly absorbed following oral administration and converted to the free acid, fosfomycin. Absolute oral bioavailability under fasting conditions is 37%. After a single 3-gm dose of MONUROL, the mean (± 1 SD) maximum serum concentration (C_{max}) achieved was 26.1 (± 9.1) μg/mL within 2 hours. The oral bioavailability of fosfomycin is reduced to 30% under fed conditions. Following a single 3-gm oral dose of MONUROL with a high-fat meal, the mean C_{max} achieved was 17.6 (± 4.4) μg/mL within 4 hours.

Cimetidine does not affect the pharmacokinetics of fosfomycin when coadministered with MONUROL. Metoclopramide lowers the serum concentrations and urinary excretion of fosfomycin when coadministered with MONUROL. (See **PRECAUTIONS, Drug Interactions.**)

Distribution: The mean apparent steady-state volume of distribution (V_{SS}) is 136.1 (±44.1) L following oral administration of MONUROL. Fosfomycin is not bound to plasma proteins.

Fosfomycin is distributed to the kidneys, bladder wall, prostate, and seminal vesicles. Following a 50 mg/Kg dose of fosfomycin to patients undergoing urological surgery for bladder carcinoma, the mean concentration of fosfomycin in the bladder, taken at a distance from the neoplastic site, was 18.0 μg per gram of tissue at 3 hours after dosing. Fosfomycin has been shown to cross the placental barrier in animals and man.

Excretion: Fosfomycin is excreted unchanged in both urine and feces. Following oral administration of MONUROL, the mean total body clearance (CL_{TB}) and mean renal clearance (CL_R) of fosfomycin were 16.9 (± 3.5) L/hr and 6.3 (± 1.7) L/hr, respectively. Approximately 38% of a 3-gm dose of MONUROL is recovered from urine, and 18% is recovered from feces. Following intravenous administration, the mean CL_{TB} and mean CL_R of fosfomycin were 6.1 (± 1.0) L/hr and 5.5 (± 1.2) L/hr, respectively.

A mean urine fosfomycin concentration of 706 (± 466) μg/mL was attained within 2–4 hours after a single oral 3-gm dose of MONUROL under fasting conditions. The mean urinary concentration of fosfomycin was 10 μg/mL in samples collected 72–84 hours following a single oral dose of MONUROL.

Following a 3-gm dose of MONUROL administered with a high fat meal, a mean urine fosfomycin concentration of 537 (± 252) μg/mL was attained within 6–8 hours. Although the rate of urinary excretion of fosfomycin was reduced under fed conditions, the cumulative amount of fosfomycin excreted in the urine was the same, 1118 (± 201) mg (fed) vs. 1140 mg (±238) (fasting). Further, urinary concentrations equal to or greater than 100 μg/mL were maintained for the same duration, 26 hours, indicated that MONUROL can be taken without regard to food.

Following oral administration of MONUROL, the mean half-life for elimination ($t_{1/2}$) is 5.7 (± 2.8) hours.

Special Populations:

Geriatric: Based on limited data regarding 24-hour urinary drug concentrations, no differences in urinary excretion of fosfomycin have been observed in elderly subjects. No dosage adjustment is necessary in the elderly.

Gender: There are no gender differences in the pharmacokinetics of fosfomycin.

Renal Insufficiency: In 5 anuric patients undergoing hemodialysis, the $t_{1/2}$ of fosfomycin during hemodialysis was 40 hours. In patients with varying degrees of renal impairment (creatinine clearances varying from 54 mL/min to 7 mL/min), the $t_{1/2}$ of fosfomycin increased from 11 hours to 50 hours. The percent of fosfomycin recovered in urine decreased from 32% to 11% indicating that renal impairment significantly decreases the excretion of fosfomycin.

Microbiology

Fosfomycin (the active component of fosfomycin tromethamine) has *in vitro* activity against a broad range of gram-positive and gram-negative aerobic microorganisms which are associated with uncomplicated urinary tract infections. Fosfomycin is bactericidal in urine at therapeutic doses. The bactericidal action of fosfomycin is due to its inactivation of the enzyme enolpyruvyl transferase, thereby irreversibly blocking the condensation of uridine diphosphate-N-acetylglucosamine with p-enolpyruvate, one of the first steps in bacterial cell wall synthesis. It also reduces adherence of bacteria to uroepithelial cells.

There is generally no cross-resistance between fosfomycin and other classes of antibacterial agents such as beta-lactams and aminoglycosides.

Fosfomycin has been shown to be active against most strains of the following microorganisms, both *in vitro* and in clinical infections as described in the **INDICATIONS AND USAGE** section:

Aerobic gram-positive microorganisms
Enterococcus faecalis

Aerobic gram-negative microorganisms
Escherichia coli

The following *in vitro* data are available, **but their clinical significance is unknown.**

Fosfomycin exhibits *in vitro* minimum inhibitory concentrations (MIC's) of 64 μg/mL or less against most (≥ 90%) strains of the following microorganisms; however, the safety and effectiveness of fosfomycin in treating clinical infections due to these microorganisms has not been established in adequate and well-controlled clinical trials:

Aerobic gram-positive microorganisms
Enterococcus faecium

Aerobic gram-negative microorganisms
Citrobacter diversus
Citrobacter freundii
Enterobacter aerogenes

Treatment Arm	Treatment Duration (days)	Microbiologic Eradication Rate		Clinical Success Rate	Outcome (based on difference in microbiologic eradication rates at 5–11 days post therapy)
		5–11 days post therapy	Study day 12–21		
Fosfomycin	1	630/771 (82%)	591/771 (77%)	542/771 (70%)	
Ciprofloxacin	7	219/222 (98%)	219/222 (98%)	213/222 (96%)	Fosfomycin inferior to ciprofloxacin
Trimethoprim/ sulfamethoxazole	10	194/197 (98%)	194/197 (98%)	186/197 (94%)	Fosfomycin inferior to trimethoprim/ sulfamethoxazole
Nitrofurantoin	7	180/238 (76%)	180/238 (76%)	183/238 (77%)	Fosfomycin equivalent to nitrofurantoin

Klebsiella oxytoca
Klebsiella pneumoniae
Proteus mirabilis
Proteus vulgaris
Serratia marcescens

SUSCEPTIBILITY TESTING

Dilution Techniques:

Quantitative methods are used to determine minimum inhibitory concentrations (MIC's). These MIC's provide estimates of the susceptibility of bacteria to antimicrobial compounds. One such standardized procedure uses a standardized agar dilution method[1] or equivalent with standardized inoculum concentrations and standardized concentrations of fosfomycin tromethamine (in terms of fosfomycin base content) powder supplemented with 25 µg/mL of glucose-6-phosphate. **BROTH DILUTION METHODS SHOULD NOT BE USED TO TEST SUSCEPTIBILITY TO FOSFOMYCIN.** The MIC values obtained should be interpreted according to the following criteria:

MIC (µg/mL)	Interpretation
≤ 64	Susceptible (S)
128	Intermediate (I)
≥ 256	Resistant (R)

A report of "susceptible" indicates that the pathogen is likely to be inhibited by usually achievable concentrations of the antimicrobial compound in the urine. A report of "intermediate" indicates that the result should be considered equivocal, and, if the microorganism is not fully susceptible to alternative, clinically feasible drugs, the test should be repeated. This category provides a buffer zone that prevents small uncontrolled technical factors from causing major discrepancies in interpretation. A report of "resistant" indicates that usually achievable concentrations of the antimicrobial compound in the urine are unlikely to be inhibitory and that other therapy should be selected.
Standardized susceptibility test procedures require the use of laboratory control microorganisms. Standard fosfomycin tromethamine powder should provide the following MIC values for agar dilution testing in media containing 25 µg/mL of glucose-6-phosphate. **[Broth dilution testing should not be performed].**

Microorganism	MIC (µg/mL)
Enterococcus faecalis ATCC 29212	32–128
Escherichia coli ATCC 25922	0.5–2
Pseudomonas aeruginosa ATCC 27853	2–8
Staphylcoccus aureus ATCC 29213	0.5–4

Diffusion Techniques:

Quantitative methods that require measurement of zone diameters also provide reproducible estimates of the susceptibility of bacteria to antimicrobial agents. One such standardized procedure[2] requires the use of standardized inoculum concentrations. This procedure uses paper disks impregnated with 200-µg fosfomycin and 50-µg of glucose-6-phosphate to test the susceptibility of microorganisms to fosfomycin.
Reports from the laboratory providing results of the standard single-disk susceptibility test with disks containing 200 µg of fosfomycin and 50 µg of glucose-6-phosphate should be interpreted according to the following criteria:

Zone Diameter (mm)	Interpretation
≥16	Susceptible (S)
13–15	Intermediate (I)
≤12	Resistant (R)

Interpretation should be stated as above for results using dilution techniques. Interpretation involves correlation of the diameter obtained in the disk test with the MIC for fosfomycin.
As with standardized dilution techniques, diffusion methods require use of laboratory control microorganisms that are used to control the technical aspects of the laboratory procedures. For the diffusion technique, the 200-µg fosfomycin disk with the 50-µg of glucose-6-phosphate should provide the following zone diameters in these laboratory quality control strains:

Microorganism	Zone Diameter (mm)
Escherichia coli ATCC 25922	22–30
Staphylococcus aureus ATCC 25923	25–33

INDICATIONS AND USAGE

MONUROL is indicated only for the treatment of uncomplicated urinary tract infections (acute cystitis) in women due to susceptible strains of *Escherichia coli* and *Enterococcus faecalis.* MONUROL is not indicated for the treatment of pyelonephritis or perinephric abscess.
If persistence or reappearance of bacteriuria occurs after treatment with MONUROL, other therapeutic agents should be selected. (See **PRECAUTIONS** and **CLINICAL STUDIES** section.)

CONTRAINDICATIONS

MONUROL is contraindicated in patients with known hypersensitivity to the drug.

PRECAUTIONS

General

Do not use more than one single dose of MONUROL to treat a single episode of acute cystitis. Repeated daily doses of MONUROL did not improve the clinical success or microbiological eradication rates compared to single dose therapy, but did increase the incidence of adverse events.
Urine specimens for culture and susceptibility testing should be obtained before and after completion of therapy.

Information for Patients

Patients should be informed:

- That MONUROL (fosfomycin tromethamine) can be taken with or without food.
- That their symptoms should improve in two to three days after taking MONUROL; if not improved, the patient should contact her health care provider.

Drug Interactions

Metoclopramide: When coadministered with MONUROL, metoclopramide, a drug which increases gastrointestinal motility, lowers the serum concentration and urinary excretion of fosfomycin. Other drugs that increase gastrointestinal motility may produce similar effects.
Cimetidine: Cimetidine does not affect the pharmacokinetics of fosfomycin when coadministered with MONUROL.

Carcinogenesis, Mutagenesis, Impairment of Fertility

Long term carcinogenicity studies in rodents have not been conducted because MONUROL is intended for single dose treatment in humans. MONUROL was not mutagenic or genotoxic in the *in vitro* Ames' bacterial reversion test, in cultured human lymphocytes, in Chinese hamster V79 cells, and the *in vivo* mouse micronucleus assay. MONUROL did not affect fertility or reproductive performance in male and female rats.

Pregnancy: Teratogenic Effects
Pregnancy Category B
When administered intramuscularly as the sodium salt at a dose of 1 gm to pregnant women, fosfomycin crosses the placental barrier. MONUROL crosses the placental barrier of rats; it does not produce teratogenic effects in pregnant rats at dosages as high as 1000 mg/kg/day (approximately 9 and 1.4 times the human dose based on body weight and mg/m^2, respectively). When administered to pregnant female rabbits at dosages as high as 1000 mg/kg/day (approximately 9 and 2.7 times the human dose based on body weight and mg/m^2, respectively), fetotoxicities were observed. However, these toxicities were seen at maternally toxic doses and were considered to be due to the sensitivity of the rabbit to changes in the intestinal microflora resulting from the antibiotic administration. There are, however, no adequate and well-controlled studies in pregnant women. Because animal reproduction studies are not always predictive of human response, this drug should be used during pregnancy only if clearly needed.

Nursing Mothers

It is not known whether fosfomycin tromethamine is excreted in human milk. Because many drugs are excreted in human milk and because of the potential for serious adverse reactions in nursing infants from MONUROL, a decision should be made whether to discontinue nursing or to not administer the drug, taking into account the importance of the drug to the mother.

Pediatric Use

Safety and effectiveness in children age 12 years and under have not been established in adequate and well-controlled studies.

Use in the Elderly

There were no clinically significant differences in the bacteriological effectiveness or safety profiles of MONUROL for women 65 years of age or younger compared to women over 65 years of age.

ADVERSE REACTIONS

Clinical Trials:

In clinical studies, drug related adverse events which were reported in greater than 1% of the fosfomycin-treated study population are listed below:

Drug-Related Adverse Events (%) in Fosfomycin and Comparator Populations

Adverse Events	Fosfomycin N=1233	Nitrofurantoin N=374	Trimethoprim / sulfamethoxazole N=428	Ciprofloxacin N=445
Diarrhea	9.0	6.4	2.3	3.1
Vaginitis	5.5	5.3	4.7	6.3
Nausea	4.1	7.2	8.6	3.4
Headache	3.9	5.9	5.4	3.4
Dizziness	1.3	1.9	2.3	2.2
Asthenia	1.1	0.3	0.5	0.0
Dyspepsia	1.1	2.1	0.7	1.1

In clinical trials, the most frequently reported adverse events occurring in >1% of the study population regardless of drug relationship, were:
diarrhea 10.4%, headache 10.3%, vaginitis 7.6%, nausea 5.2%, rhinitis 4.5%, back pain 3.0%, dysmenorrhea 2.6%, pharyngitis 2.5%, dizziness 2.3%, abdominal pain 2.2%, pain 2.2%, dyspepsia 1.8%, asthenia 1.7%, and rash 1.4%.
The following adverse events occurred in clinical trials at a rate of less than 1%, regardless of drug relationship:
abnormal stools, anorexia, constipation, dry mouth, dysuria, ear disorder, fever, flatulence, flu syndrome, hematuria, infection, insomnia, lymphadenopathy, menstrual disorder, migraine, myalgia, nervousness, paresthesia, pruritus, SGPT increased, skin disorder, somnolence, and vomiting.
One patient developed unilateral optic neuritis, an event considered possibly related to MONUROL therapy.

Post-marketing Experience:

Serious adverse events from the marketing experience with MONUROL outside of the United States have been rarely reported and include:
angioedema, aplastic anemia, asthma (exacerbation), cholestatic jaundice, hepatic necrosis, and toxic megacolon.

Laboratory Changes:

Significant laboratory changes reported in U.S. clinical trials of MONUROL without regard to drug relationship include: increased eosinophil count, increased or decreased WBC count, increased bilirubin, increased SGPT, increased SGOT, increased alkaline phosphatase, decreased hematocrit, decreased hemoglobin, increased and decreased platelet count. The changes were generally transient and were not clinically significant.

OVERDOSAGE

In acute toxicology studies, oral administration of high doses of MONUROL up to 5 gm/kg were well-tolerated in mice and rats, produced transient and minor incidences of watery stool in rabbits, and produced diarrhea with anorexia in dogs occurring in 2–3 days after single dose administration. These doses represent 50–125 times the human therapeutic dose.
There have been no reported cases of overdosage. In the event of overdosage, treatment should be symptomatic and supportive.

DOSAGE AND ADMINISTRATION

The recommended dosage for women 18 years of age and older for uncomplicated urinary tract infection (acute cystitis) is one sachet of MONUROL. MONUROL may be taken with or without food.
MONUROL should not be taken in its dry form. Always mix MONUROL with water before ingesting. (See PREPARATION section.)

PREPARATION

MONUROL should be taken orally. Pour the entire contents of a single-dose sachet of MONUROL into 3 to 4 ounces of water (1/2 cup) and stir to dissolve. Do not use hot water. MONUROL should be taken immediately after dissolving in water.

HOW SUPPLIED

MONUROL is available as a single-dose sachet containing the equivalent of 3 grams of fosfomycin.
NDC # 0456-4300-08

Store at controlled room temperature 15° to 30° C (59° to 86°F).

Rx only

Keep this and all drugs out of the reach of children.
Manufactured by:
Inpharzam S.A.
Division of Zambon Group, SpA
Via Industria
6814 Cadempino, Switzerland
Made in Switzerland
Distributed by:
Forest Pharmaceuticals, Inc.
Subsidiary of Forest Laboratories, Inc.
St. Louis, MO 63045

Continued on next page

Monurol—Cont.

REFERENCES

1. National Committee for Clinical Laboratory Standards, Methods for Dilution. Antimicrobial Susceptibility Tests for Bacteria that Grow Aerobically — Third Edition; Approved Standard NCCLS Document M7-A3, Vol. 13, No. 25 NCCLS, Villanova, PA, December, 1993.
2. National Committee for Clinical Laboratory Standards, Performance Standard for Antimicrobial Disk Susceptibility Tests — Fifth Edition; Approved Standard NCCLS Document M2-A5, Vol. 13, No. 24 NCCLS, Villanova, PA, December, 1993.

CLINICAL STUDIES

In controlled, double-blind studies of acute cystitis performed in the United States, a single-dose of MONUROL was compared to three other oral antibiotics (See table below). The study population consisted of patients with symptoms and signs of acute cystitis of less than 4 days duration, no manifestations of upper tract infection (e.g., flank pain, chills, fever), no history of recurrent urinary tract infections (20% of patients in the clinical studies had a prior episode of acute cystitis within the preceding year), no known structural abnormalities, and no clinical or laboratory evidence of hepatic dysfunction, and no known or suspected CNS disorders, such as epilepsy, or other factors which would predispose to seizures. In these studies, the following clinical success (resolution of symptoms) and microbiologic eradication rates were obtained:

[See table at top left of previous page]

Pathogen	Fosfomycin 3 gm single dose	Ciprofloxacin 250 mg bid × 7d	Trimethoprim/sulfamethoxazole 160 mg/800 mg bid × 10d	Nitrofurantoin 100mg bid × 7d
E. coli	509/644 (79%)	184/187 (98%)	171/174 (98%)	146/187 (78%)
E. faecalis	10/10 (100%)	0/0	4/4 (100%)	1/2 (50%)

Rev. 4/99 RMC 237

Shown in Product Identification Guide, page 313

TESSALON® ℞

100 mg/200 mg
(benzonatate, USP)

DESCRIPTION

TESSALON, a non-narcotic oral antitussive agent, is 2, 5, 8, 11, 14, 17, 20, 23, 26-nonaoxaoctacosan-28-yl p-(butylamino) benzoate; with a molecular weight of 603.7.

$CH_3(CH_2)_2CH_2NH$—[benzene ring]—$COOCH_2CH_2(OCH_2CH_2)_nOCH_3$

$C_{30}H_{53}NO_{11}$

Each TESSALON Perle contains:
Benzonatate, USP 100 mg
Each TESSALON Capsule contains:
Benzonatate, USP 200 mg
TESSALON Capsules also contain: D&C Yellow 10, gelatin, glycerin, methylparaben and propylparaben.

CLINICAL PHARMACOLOGY

TESSALON acts peripherally by anesthetizing the stretch receptors located in the respiratory passages, lungs, and pleura by dampening their activity and thereby reducing the cough reflex at its source. It begins to act within 15 to 20 minutes and its effect lasts for 3 to 8 hours. TESSALON has no inhibitory effect on the respiratory center in recommended dosage.

INDICATIONS AND USAGE

TESSALON is indicated for the symptomatic relief of cough.

CONTRAINDICATIONS

Hypersensitivity to benzonatate or related compounds.

WARNINGS

Severe hypersensitivity reactions (including bronchospasm, laryngospasm and cardiovascular collapse) have been reported which are possibly related to local anesthesia from sucking or chewing the perle instead of swallowing it. Severe reactions have required intervention with vasopressor agents and supportive measures.
Isolated instances of bizarre behavior, including mental confusion and visual hallucinations, have also been reported in patients taking TESSALON in combination with other prescribed drugs.

PRECAUTIONS

Benzonatate is chemically related to anesthetic agents of the para-amino-benzoic acid class (e.g., procaine; tetracaine) and has been associated with adverse CNS effects possibly related to a prior sensitivity to related agents or interaction with concomitant medication.

Information for Patients: Release of TESSALON from the capsule in the mouth can produce a temporary local anesthesia of the oral mucosa and choking could occur. Therefore, the capsules should be swallowed without chewing.

Usage in Pregnancy: Pregnancy Category C. Animal reproduction studies have not been conducted with TESSALON. It is also not known whether TESSALON can cause fetal harm when administered to a pregnant woman or can affect reproduction capacity. TESSALON should be given to a pregnant woman only if clearly needed.

Nursing Mothers: It is not known whether this drug is excreted in human milk. Because many drugs are excreted in human milk caution should be exercised when TESSALON is administered to a nursing woman.

Carcinogenesis, Mutagenesis, Impairment of Fertility: Carcinogenicity, mutagenicity, and reproduction studies have not been conducted with TESSALON.

Pediatric Use: Safety and effectiveness in children below the age of 10 has not been established.

ADVERSE REACTIONS

Potential Adverse Reactions to TESSALON may include:
Hypersensitivity reactions including bronchospasm, laryngospasm, cardiovascular collapse possibly related to local anesthesia from chewing or sucking the capsule.

CNS: sedation; headache; dizziness; mental confusion; visual hallucinations.

GI: constipation, nausea, GI upset.

Dermatologic: pruritus; skin eruptions.

Other: nasal congestion; sensation of burning in the eyes; vague "chilly" sensation; numbness of the chest; hypersensitivity.

Rare instances of deliberate or accidental overdose have resulted in death.

OVERDOSAGE

Overdose may result in death.
The drug is chemically related to tetracaine and other topical anesthetics and shares various aspects of their pharmacology and toxicology. Drugs of this type are generally well absorbed after ingestion.

Signs and Symptoms:
If capsules are chewed or dissolved in the mouth, oropharyngeal anesthesia will develop rapidly. CNS stimulation may cause restlessness and tremors which may proceed to clonic convulsions followed by profound CNS depression.

Treatment:
Evacuate gastric contents and administer copious amounts of activated charcoal slurry. Even in the conscious patient, cough and gag reflexes may be so depressed as to necessitate special attention to protection against aspiration of gastric contents and orally administered materials. Convulsions should be treated with a short-acting barbiturate given intravenously and carefully titrated for the smallest effective dosage. Intensive support of respiration and cardiovascular-renal function is an essential feature of the treatment of severe intoxication from overdosage.
Do not use CNS stimulants.

DOSAGE AND ADMINISTRATION

Adults and Children over 10: Usual dose is one 100 mg or 200 mg capsule t.i.d. as required. If necessary, up to 600 mg daily may be given.

HOW SUPPLIED

Perles, 100 mg (yellow); bottles of 100
NDC 0456-0688-01 Imprint: T.
Perles, 100 mg (yellow); bottles of 500
NDC 0456-0688-02 Imprint: T.
Capsules, 200 mg (yellow); bottles of 100
NDC 0456-0698-01 Imprint: 0698.
Capsules, 200 mg (yellow); bottles of 500
NDC 0456-0698-02 Imprint: 0698.
Store at controlled room temperature 15°–30°C (59°–86°F).

Rev. 8/99(02)
MG #11385

Mfd by
R.P. Scherer-North America
St. Petersburg, Florida 33716

for
FOREST PHARMACEUTICALS, INC.
SUBSIDIARY OF FOREST LABORATORIES, INC.
ST. LOUIS, MISSOURI 63045

Shown in Product Identification Guide, page 313

THYROLAR® Tablets

Name	Composition (T_3/T_4 per tablet)	Color	Armacode®
Thyrolar—1/4(0456–0040–01)	3.1 mcg/12.5 mcg	Violet/White	YC
Thyrolar—1/2(0456–0045–01)	6.25 mcg/25 mcg	Peach/White	YD
Thyrolar—1 (0456–0050–01)	12.5 mcg/50 mcg	Pink/White	YE
Thyrolar—2 (0456–0055–01)	25 mcg/100 mcg	Green/White	YF
Thyrolar—3 (0456–0060–01)	37.5 mcg/150 mcg	Yellow/White	YH

THYROLAR® Tablets ℞

[thī-rō-lär]
(Liotrix Tablets, USP)

DESCRIPTION

Thyrolar Tablets (Liotrix Tablets, USP) contain triiodothyronine (T_3 liothyronine) sodium and tetraiodothyronine (T_4 levothyroxine) sodium in the amounts listed in the "How Supplied" section. (T_3 liothyronine sodium is approximately four times as potent as T_4 thyroxine on a microgram for microgram basis.)
The inactive ingredients are calcium phosphate, colloidal silicon dioxide, corn starch, lactose, and magnesium stearate. The tablets also contain the following dyes: Thyrolar 1/4-FD&C Blue #1 and FD&C Red #40; Thyrolar 1/2-FD&C Red #40 and D&C Yellow #10; Thyrolar 1-FD&C Red #40; Thyrolar 2-FD&C Blue #1, FD&C Red #40, and D&C Yellow #10; Thyrolar 3-FD&C Red #40 and D&C Yellow #10.

STRUCTURAL FORMULAS

Liothyronine (T_3) Sodium

HO—[ring]—O—[ring]—CH_2—C(NH_2)(H)—COONa

Levothyroxine (T_4) Sodium

HO—[ring]—O—[ring]—CH_2—C(NH_2)(H)—COONa · xH_2O

HOW SUPPLIED

Thyrolar Tablets (Liotrix Tablets, USP) are available in five potencies, coded as follows:
[See table above]
Supplied in bottles of 100, two-layered compressed tablets.
Tablets should be stored at cold temperature, between 36° and 46°F (2° and 8°C) in a tight, light-resistant container.
Note: (T_3 liothyronine sodium is approximately four times as potent as T_4 thyroxine on a microgram for microgram basis.)
Rev. 07/96 14360796
FOREST PHARMACEUTICALS, INC.
A Subsidiary of Forest Laboratories, Inc.
St. Louis, MO 63045

Shown in Product Identification Guide, page 313

TIAZAC® ℞

(diltiazem hydrochloride)
Extended Release Capsules

DESCRIPTION

Tiazac (diltiazem hydrochloride) is a calcium ion cellular influx inhibitor (slow channel blocker). Chemically, diltiazem hydrochloride is 1,5-Benzothiazepin-4(5H)-one,3-(acetyloxy)-5[2-(dimethylamino)ethyl]-2,-3-dihydro-2(4-methoxyphenyl)-, monohydrochloride, (+)-cis. The chemical structure is:

[Structure: benzothiazepinone ring with OCH_3-phenyl, $OOCCH_3$, $CH_2CH_2N(CH_3)_2$ · HCl]

Diltiazem hydrochloride is a white to off-white crystalline powder with a bitter taste. It is soluble in water, methanol and chloroform and has a molecular weight of 450.98.
Tiazac capsules contain diltiazem hydrochloride in extended release beads at doses of 120, 180, 240, 300, 360 and 420 mg.
Tiazac also contains: Microcrystalline Cellulose NF, Sucrose Stearate, Eudragit, Povidone USP, Talc USP, Magnesium Stearate NF, Hydroxypropylmethylcellulose USP, Titanium Dioxide USP, Polysorbate NF, Simethicone USP, Gelatin NF, FD&C Blue #1, FD&C Red #40, D&C Red #28, FD&C Green #3, Black Iron Oxide USP, and other solids.

For oral administration.

CLINICAL PHARMACOLOGY

The therapeutic effects of diltiazem hydrochloride are believed to be related to its ability to inhibit the cellular influx of calcium ions during membrane depolarization of cardiac and vascular smooth muscle.

Mechanisms of Action.

Hypertension: Diltiazem produces its antihypertensive effect primarily by relaxation of vascular smooth muscle and the resultant decrease in peripheral vascular resistance. The magnitude of blood pressure reduction is related to the degree of hypertension: thus hypertensive individuals experience an antihypertensive effect, whereas there is only a modest fall in blood pressure in normotensives.

Angina: Diltiazem HCl has been shown to produce increases in exercise tolerance, probably due to its ability to reduce myocardial oxygen demand. This is accomplished via reductions in heart rate and systemic blood pressure at submaximal and maximal work loads.

Diltiazem has been shown to be a potent dilator of coronary arteries, both epicardial and subendocardial. Spontaneous and ergonovine-induced coronary artery spasm are inhibited by diltiazem.

In animal models, diltiazem interferes with the slow inward (depolarizing) current in excitable tissue. It causes excitation-contraction uncoupling in various myocardial tissues without changes in the configuration of the action potential. Diltiazem produces relaxation of the coronary vascular smooth muscle and dilation of both large and small coronary vascular smooth muscle and dilation of both large and small coronary arteries at drug levels which cause little or no negative inotropic effect. The resultant increases in coronary blood flow (epicardial and subendocardial) occur in ischemic and nonischemic models and are accompanied by dose-dependent decreases in systemic blood pressure and decreases in peripheral resistance.

Hemodynamic and Electrophysiologic Effects. Like other calcium channel antagonists, diltiazem decreases sinoatrial and atrioventricular conduction in isolated tissues and has a negative inotropic effect in isolated preparations. In the intact animal, prolongation of the AH interval can be seen at higher doses.

In man, diltiazem prevents spontaneous and ergonovine-provoked coronary artery spasm. It causes a decrease in peripheral vascular resistance and a modest fall in blood pressure in normotensive individuals and, in exercise tolerance studies in patients with ischemic heart disease, reduces the heart rate-blood pressure product for any given work load. Studies to date, primarily in patients with good ventricular function, have not revealed evidence of a negative inotropic effect; cardiac output, ejection fraction, and left ventricular end diastolic pressure have not been affected. Such data have no predictive value with respect to effects in patients with poor ventricular function, and increased heart failure has been reported in patients with preexisting impairment of ventricular function. There are as yet few data on the interaction of diltiazem and beta-blockers in patients with poor ventricular function. Resting heart rate is usually slightly reduced by diltiazem.

Tiazac produces antihypertensive effects both in the supine and standing positions. Postural hypotension is infrequently noted upon suddenly assuming an upright position. No reflex tachycardia is associated with the chronic antihypertensive effects.

Diltiazem hydrochloride decreases vascular resistance, increases cardiac output (by increasing stroke volume), and produces a slight decrease or no change in heart rate. During dynamic exercise, increases in diastolic pressure are inhibited while maximum achievable systolic pressure is usually reduced. Chronic therapy with diltiazem hydrochloride produces no change or an increase in plasma catecholamines. No increased activity of the renin-angiotensin-aldosterone axis has been observed. Diltiazem hydrochloride reduces the renal and peripheral effects of angiotensin II. Hypertensive animal models respond to diltiazem with reductions in blood pressure and increased urinary output and natriuresis without a change in urinary sodium/potassium ratio. In man, transient natriuresis and kaliuresis have been reported, but only in high intravenous doses of 0.5 mg/kg of body weight.

Diltiazem-associated prolongation of the AH interval is not more pronounced in patients with first degree heart block. In patients with sick sinus syndrome, diltiazem significantly prolongs sinus cycle length (up to 50% in some cases). Intravenous diltiazem in doses of 20 mg prolongs AH conduction time and AV node functional and effective refractory periods by approximately 20%.

In two short-term, double-blind, placebo-controlled studies in 256 hypertensive patients with doses up to 540 mg/day, Tiazac showed a clinically unimportant but statistically significant, dose-related increase in PR interval (0.008 seconds). There were no instances of greater than first-degree AV block in any of the clinical trials (see WARNINGS).

Pharmacodynamics.

Hypertension: In short-term, double-blind, placebo-controlled clinical trials Tiazac demonstrated a dose-related antihypertensive response among patients with mild to moderate hypertension. In one parallel-group study of 198 patients Tiazac was given for four weeks. The changes in diastolic blood pressure measured at trough (24 hours after the dose) for placebo, 90mg, 180mg, 360mg and 540mg were -5.4, -6.3, -6.2, -8.2, and -11.8mm Hg, respectively. Supine diastolic blood pressure as well as standing diastolic and systolic blood pressures also showed statistically significant linear dose response effects.

In another clinical trial that followed a dose-escalation design, Tiazac also reduced blood pressure in a linear dose-related manner. Supine diastolic blood pressure measured following two week intervals of treatment was reduced by -3.7mm Hg with 120 mg/day versus -2.0mm Hg with placebo, by -7.6mm Hg after escalation to 240 mg/day versus -2.3mm Hg with placebo, by -8.1mm Hg after escalation to 360 mg/day versus -0.9mm Hg with placebo, and by -10.8mm Hg after escalation to 480/540 mg/day versus -2.2mm Hg with placebo.

Angina: In a double-blind, parallel-group, placebo-controlled trial (approximately 50 patients/group, in patients with chronic stable angina), Tiazac at doses of 120–540/day increased exercise tolerance time. At trough, 24 hours after dosing, exercise tolerance times using a Bruce exercise protocol, increased by 14, 26, 41, 33 and 32 seconds over baseline for placebo and the 120 mg, 240 mg, 360 mg, and 540 mg/day treated patient groups, respectively. At peak, 8 hours after dosing, exercise tolerance times relative to baseline were statistically significantly increased by 13, 38, 64, 55 and 42 seconds for placebo and 120 mg, 240 mg, 360 mg, and 540 mg/day Tiazac treated patients, respectively. Compared to baseline, Tiazac treated patients experienced statistically significant reductions in anginal attacks and decreased nitroglycerin requirements when compared to placebo treated patients.

Pharmacokinetics and Metabolism. Diltiazem is well absorbed from the gastrointestinal tract but undergoes substantial hepatic first-pass effect. The absolute bioavailability of an oral dose of an immediate release formulation (compared to intravenous administration) is approximately 40%. Only 2% to 4% of unchanged diltiazem appears in the urine. The plasma elimination half-life of diltiazem is approximately 3.0–4.5 h. Drugs which induce or inhibit hepatic microsomal enzymes may alter diltiazem disposition. Therapeutic blood levels of diltiazem appear to be in the range of 40–200 ng/mL. There is a departure from linearity when dose strengths are increased; the half-life is slightly increased with dose.

The two primary metabolites of diltiazem are desacetyldiltiazem and desmethyldiltiazem. The desacetyl metabolite is approximately 25% to 50% as potent a coronary vasodilator as diltiazem and is present in plasma at concentrations of 10% to 20% of parent diltiazem. However, recent studies employing sensitive and specific analytical methods have confirmed the existence of several sequential metabolic pathways of diltiazem. As many as nine diltiazem metabolites have been identified in the urine of humans. Total radioactivity measurements following single intravenous dose administration in healthy volunteers suggest the presence of other unidentified metabolites. These metabolites are more slowly excreted, (with a half-life of total radioactivity of approximately 20 hours) and attain concentrations in excess of diltiazem.

In vitro binding studies show diltiazem HCl is 70% to 80% bound to plasma proteins. Competitive *in vitro* ligand binding studies have also shown diltiazem HCl binding is not altered by therapeutic concentrations of digoxin, hydrochlorothiazide, phenylbutazone, propranolol, salicylic acid, or warfarin. A study that compared patients with normal hepatic function to patients with cirrhosis who received immediate release diltiazem found an increase in diltiazem elimination half-life and a 69% increase in bioavailability in the hepatically impaired patients. Patients with severely impaired renal function (creatinine clearance <50 mL/min) who received immediate release diltiazem had modestly increased diltiazem concentrations compared to patients with normal renal function.

Tiazac® Capsules. When compared to a regimen of immediate-release tablets at steady-state, approximately 93% of drug is absorbed from the Tiazac formulation. When Tiazac was coadministered with a high fat content breakfast, the extent of diltiazem absorption was not affected; T_{max}, however, occurred slightly earlier. The apparent elimination half-life after single or multiple dosing is 4 to 9.5 hours (mean 6.5 hours).

Tiazac demonstrates non-linear pharmacokinetics. As the daily dose of Tiazac capsules is increased from 120 to 540 mg, there was a more than proportional increase in diltiazem plasma concentrations as evidenced by an increase of AUC, C_{max} and C_{min} of 6.8, 6 and 8.6 times, respectively, for a 4.5 times increase in dose.

INDICATIONS AND USAGE

Hypertension:

Tiazac is indicated for the treatment of hypertension. It may be used alone or in combination with other antihypertensive medications.

Chronic Stable Angina:

Tiazac is indicated for the treatment of chronic stable angina.

CONTRAINDICATIONS

Diltiazem is contraindicated in (1) patients with sick sinus syndrome except in the presence of a functioning ventricular pacemaker, (2) patients with second- or third-degree AV block except in the presence of a functioning ventricular pacemaker, (3) patients with severe hypotension (less than 90 mm Hg systolic), (4) patients who have demonstrated hypersensitivity to the drug, and (5) patients with acute myocardial infarction and pulmonary congestion documented by x-ray on admission.

WARNINGS

1. Cardiac Conduction. Diltiazem hydrochloride prolongs AV node refractory periods without significantly prolonging sinus node recovery time, except in patients with sick sinus syndrome. This effect may rarely result in abnormally slow heart rates (particularly in patients with sick sinus syndrome) or second- or third-degree AV block (13 of 3007 patients or 0.43%). Concomitant use of diltiazem with beta-blockers or digitalis may result in additive effects on cardiac conduction. A patient with Prinzmetal's angina developed periods of asystole (2 to 5 seconds) after a single dose of 60 mg of diltiazem.

2. Congestive Heart Failure. Although diltiazem has a negative inotropic effect in isolated animal tissue preparations, hemodynamic studies in humans with normal ventricular function have not shown a reduction in cardiac index nor consistent negative effects on contractility (dp/dt). An acute study of oral diltiazem in patients with impaired ventricular function (ejection fraction 24% ± 6%) showed improvement in indices of ventricular function without significant decrease in contractile function (dp/dt). Worsening of congestive heart failure has been reported in patients with preexisting impairment of ventricular function. Experience with the use of diltiazem hydrochloride in combination with beta-blockers in patients with impaired ventricular function is limited. Caution should be exercised when using this combination.

3. Hypotension. Decreases in blood pressure associated with diltiazem hydrochloride therapy may occasionally result in symptomatic hypotension.

4. Acute Hepatic Injury. Mild elevations of transaminases with and without concomitant elevation in alkaline phosphatase and bilirubin have been observed in clinical studies. Such elevations were usually transient and frequently resolved even with continued diltiazem treatment. In rare instances, significant elevations in enzymes such as alkaline phosphatase, LDH, SGOT, and SGPT, and other phenomena consistent with acute hepatic injury have been noted. These reactions tended to occur early after therapy initiation (1 to 8 weeks) and have been reversible upon discontinuation of drug therapy. The relationship to diltiazem hydrochloride is uncertain in some cases, but probable in some (see PRECAUTIONS).

PRECAUTIONS

General. Diltiazem hydrochloride is extensively metabolized by the liver and excreted by the kidneys and in bile. As with any drug given over prolonged periods, laboratory parameters of renal and hepatic function should be monitored at regular intervals. The drug should be used with caution in patients with impaired renal or hepatic function. In subacute and chronic dog and rat studies designed to produce toxicity, high doses of diltiazem were associated with hepatic damage. In special subacute hepatic studies, oral doses of 125 mg/kg and higher in rats were associated with histological changes in the liver which were reversible when the drug was discontinued. In dogs, doses of 20 mg/kg were also associated with hepatic changes; however, these changes were reversible with continued dosing.

Dermatological events (see ADVERSE REACTIONS section) may be transient and may disappear despite continued use of diltiazem hydrochloride. However, skin eruptions progressing to erythema multiforme and/or exfoliative dermatitis have also been infrequently reported. Should a dermatologic reaction persist, the drug should be discontinued.

Drug Interactions. Due to the potential for additive effects, caution and careful titration are warranted in patients receiving diltiazem hydrochloride concomitantly with other agents known to affect cardiac contractility and/or conduction (see WARNINGS). Pharmacologic studies indicate that there may be additive effects in prolonging AV conduction when using beta-blockers or digitalis concomitantly with Tiazac (see WARNINGS). As with all drugs, care should be exercised when treating patients with multiple medications. Diltiazem is both a substrate and an inhibitor of the cytochrome P-450 3A4 enzyme system. Other drugs that are specific substrates, inhibitors, or inducers of the enzyme system may have a significant impact on the efficacy and side effect profile of diltiazem. Patients taking other drugs that are substrates of CYP450 3A4 , especially patients with renal and/or hepatic impairment, may require dosage adjustment when starting or stopping concomitantly administered diltiazem in order to maintain optimum therapeutic blood levels.

Beta Blockers. Controlled and uncontrolled domestic studies suggest that concomitant use of diltiazem hydrochloride and beta-blockers is usually well tolerated, but available data are not sufficient to predict the effects of concomitant treatment in patients with left ventricular dysfunction or cardiac conduction abnormalities. Administration of diltiazem hydrochloride concomitantly with propranolol in five normal volunteers resulted in increased propranolol levels in all subjects and bioavailability of propranolol was increased approximately 50%. *In vitro*, propranolol appears to be displaced from its binding sites by diltiazem. If combination therapy is initiated or withdrawn in conjunction with propranolol, an adjustment in the propranolol dose may be warranted (see WARNINGS).

Cimetidine. A study in six healthy volunteers has shown a significant increase in peak diltiazem plasma levels (58%) and area-under-the-curve (53%) after a 1-week course of cimetidine 1200 mg per day and a single dose of diltiazem 60

Continued on next page

Tiazac—Cont.

mg. Ranitidine produced smaller, nonsignificant increases. The effect may be mediated by cimetidine's known inhibition of hepatic cytochrome P-450, the enzyme system responsible for the first-pass metabolism of diltiazem. Patients currently receiving diltiazem therapy should be carefully monitored for a change in pharmacological effect when initiating and discontinuing therapy with cimetidine. An adjustment in the diltiazem dose may be warranted.

Digitalis. Administration of diltiazem hydrochloride with digoxin in 24 healthy male subjects increased plasma digoxin concentrations approximately 20%. Another investigator found no increase in digoxin levels in 12 patients with coronary artery disease. Since there have been conflicting results regarding the effect of digoxin levels, it is recommended that digoxin levels be monitored when initiating, adjusting, and discontinuing diltiazem hydrochloride therapy to avoid possible over- or under-digitalization (see WARNINGS).

Anesthetics. The depression of cardiac contractility, conductivity, and automaticity as well as the vascular dilation associated with anesthetics may be potentiated by calcium channel blockers. When used concomitantly, anesthetics and calcium blockers should be titrated carefully.

Cyclosporine. A pharmacokinetic interaction between diltiazem and cyclosporine has been observed during studies involving renal and cardiac transplant patients. In renal and cardiac transplant recipients, a reduction of cyclosporine dose ranging from 15% to 48% was necessary to maintain cyclosporine trough concentrations similar to those seen prior to the addition of diltiazem. If these agents are to be administered concurrently, cyclosporine concentrations should be monitored, especially when diltiazem therapy is initiated, adjusted, or discontinued.

The effect of cyclosporine on diltiazem plasma concentrations has not been evaluated.

Carbamazepine. Concomitant administration of diltiazem with carbamazepine has been reported to result in elevated serum levels of carbamazepine (40% to 72% increase), resulting in toxicity in some cases. Patients receiving these drugs concurrently should be monitored for a potential drug interaction.

Benzodiazepines. Studies showed that diltiazem increased the AUC of midazolam and triazolam by 3–4 fold and the C_{max} by 2–fold, compared to placebo. The elimination half life of midazolam and triazolam also increased (1.5–2.5 fold) during coadministration with diltiazem. These pharmacokinetic effects seen during diltiazem coadministration can result in increased clinical effects (e.g., prolonged sodation) of both midazolam and triazolam.

Lovastatin. In a ten-subject study, coadministration of diltiazem (120 mg bid) with lovastatin resulted in a 3–4 times increase in mean lovastatin AUC and C_{max} vs. lovastatin alone; no change in pravastatin AUC and C_{max} was observed during diltiazem coadministration. Diltiazem plasma levels were not significantly affected by lovastatin or pravastatin.

Rifampin. Coadministration of rifampin with diltiazem lowered the diltiazem plasma concentrations to undetectable levels. Coadministration of diltiazem with rifampin or any known CYP3A4 inducer should be avoided when possible, and alternative therapy considered.

Carcinogenesis, Mutagenesis, Impairment of Fertility. A 24-month study in rats at oral dosage levels of up to 100 mg/kg/day and a 21-month study in mice at oral dosage levels of up to 30 mg/kg/day showed no evidence of carcinogenicity. There was also no mutagenic response *in vitro* or *in vivo* in mammalian cell assays or *in vitro* in bacteria. No evidence of impaired fertility was observed in a study performed in male and female rats at oral dosages of up to 100 mg/kg/day.

Pregnancy. Category C. Reproduction studies have been conducted in mice, rats, and rabbits. Administration of doses ranging from 4 to 6 times (depending on species) the upper limit of the optimum dosage range in clinical trials (480 mg q.d. or 8 mg/kg q.d. for a 60 kg patient) resulted in embryo and fetal lethality. These studies revealed, in one species or another, a propensity to cause abnormalities of the skeleton, heart, retina, and tongue. Also observed were reductions in early individual pup weights and pup survival, prolonged delivery and increased incidence of stillbirths. There are no well-controlled studies in pregnant women; therefore, use diltiazem hydrochloride in pregnant women only if the potential benefit justifies the potential risk to the fetus.

Nursing Mothers. Diltiazem is excreted in human milk. One report suggests that concentrations in breast milk may approximate serum levels. If use of Tiazac is deemed essential, an alternative method of infant feeding should be instituted.

Pediatric Use. Safety and effectiveness in children have not been established.

Geriatric Use. Clinical studies of diltiazem did not include sufficient numbers of subjects aged 65 and over to determine whether they respond differently from younger subjects. Other reported clinical experience has not identified differences in responses between the elderly and younger patients. In general, dose selection for an elderly patient should be cautious, usually starting at the low end of the dosing range, reflecting the greater frequency of decreased hepatic, renal, or cardiac function, and of concomitant disease or other drug therapy.

MOST COMMON ADVERSE EVENTS IN DOUBLE-BLIND PLACEBO-CONTROLLED HYPERTENSION TRIALS*

	Placebo	Tiazac®			Placebo	Tiazac®	
		Up to 360 mg	480–540 mg			Up to 360 mg	480–540 mg
Adverse Events (COSTART Term)	n = 57 # pts(%)	n = 149 # pts(%)	n = 48 # pts(%)	Adverse Events (COSTART Term)	n = 57 # pts(%)	n = 149 # pts(%)	n = 48 # pts(%)
edema, peripheral	1 (2)	8 (5)	7 (15)	rash	0 (0)	3 (2)	0 (0)
dizziness	4 (7)	6 (4)	2 (4)	infection	2 (4)	2 (1)	3 (6)
vasodilation	1 (2)	5 (3)	1 (2)	diarrhea	0 (0)	2 (1)	1 (2)
dyspepsia	0 (0)	7 (5)	0 (0)	palpitations	0 (0)	2 (1)	1 (2)
pharyngitis	2 (4)	3 (2)	3 (6)	nervousness	0 (0)	3 (2)	0 (0)

MOST COMMON ADVERSE EVENTS IN DOUBLE-BLIND PLACEBO-CONTROLLED ANGINA TRIALS*

	Placebo	Tiazac®			Placebo	Tiazac®	
		Up to 360 mg	540 mg			Up to 360 mg	540 mg
Adverse Events (COSTART Term)	n = 50 # pts(%)	n = 158 # pts(%)	n = 49 # pts(%)	Adverse Events (COSTART Term)	n = 50 # pts(%)	n = 158 # pts(%)	n = 49 # pts(%)
headache	1 (2)	13 (8)	4 (8)	flu syndrome	0 (0)	0 (0)	1 (2)
edema, peripheral	1 (2)	3 (2)	5 (10)	cough increase	0 (0)	2 (1)	1 (2)
pain	1 (2)	10 (6)	3 (6)	extrasystoles	0 (0)	0 (0)	1 (2)
dizziness	0 (0)	5 (3)	5 (10)	gout	0 (0)	2 (1)	1 (2)
asthenia	0 (0)	1 (1)	2 (4)	myalgia	0 (0)	0 (0)	1 (2)
dyspepsia	0 (0)	2 (1)	3 (6)	impotence	0 (0)	0 (0)	1 (2)
dyspnea	0 (0)	1 (1)	3 (6)	conjunctivitis	0 (0)	0 (0)	1 (2)
bronchitis	0 (0)	1 (1)	2 (4)	rash	0 (0)	2 (1)	1 (2)
AV block	0 (0)	0 (0)	2 (4)	abdominal enlargement	0 (0)	0 (0)	1 (2)
infection	0 (0)	2 (1)	1 (2)				

* Adverse events occurring in treated patients at 2% or more than placebo-treated patients.

Strength	Description	Quantity	NDC#
120 mg	#3 lavender/lavender capsule imprinted: Tiazac 120	7's	0456-2612-07
		30's	0456-2612-30
		90's	0456-2612-90
		1000's	0456-2612-00
		HUD's	0456-2612-63
180 mg	#2 white/blue-green capsule imprinted: Tiazac 180	7's	0456-2613-07
		30's	0456-2613-30
		90's	0456-2613-90
		1000's	0456-2613-00
		HUD's	0456-2613-63
240 mg	#1 blue-green/lavender capsule imprinted: Tiazac 240	7's	0456-2614-07
		30's	0456-2614-30
		90's	0456-2614-90
		1000's	0456-2614-00
		HUD's	0456-2614-63
300 mg	#0 white/lavender capsule imprinted: Tiazac 300	7's	0456-2615-07
		30's	0456-2615-30
		90's	0456-2615-90
		1000's	0456-2615-00
		HUD's	0456-2615-63
360 mg	#0 blue-green/blue-green capsule imprinted: Tiazac 360	7's	0456-2616-07
		30's	0456-2616-30
		90's	0456-2616-90
		1000's	0456-2616-00
		HUD's	0456-2616-63
420 mg	#00 white/white capsule imprinted: Tiazac 420	7's	0456-2617-07
		30's	0456-2617-30
		90's	0456-2617-90
		1000's	0456-2617-00

ADVERSE REACTIONS

Serious adverse reactions have been rare in studies with Tiazac, as well as with other diltiazem formulations. It should be recognized that patients with impaired ventricular function and cardiac conduction abnormalities have usually been excluded from these studies. A total of 256 hypertensives were treated for between 4 and 8 weeks; a total of 207 patients with chronic stable angina were treated for 3 weeks with doses of Tiazac ranging from 120–540 mg once daily. Two patients experienced first-degree AV block at 540 mg dose. The following table presents the most common adverse reactions, whether or not drug-related, reported in placebo-controlled trials in patients receiving Tiazac up to 360 mg and up to 540 mg with rates in placebo patients shown for comparison.

[See first table above]

[See second table above]

In addition, the following events have been reported infrequently (less than 2%) in clinical trials with other diltiazem products:

Cardiovascular. Angina, arrhythmia, AV block (second- or third-degree), bundle branch block, congestive heart failure, ECG abnormalities, hypotension, palpitations, syncope, tachycardia, ventricular extrasystoles.

Nervous System. Abnormal dreams, amnesia, depression, gait abnormality, hallucinations, insomnia, nervousness, paresthesia, personality change, somnolence, tinnitus, tremor.

Gastrointestinal. Anorexia, constipation, diarrhea, dry mouth, dysgeusia, mild elevations of SGOT, SGPT, LDH, and alkaline phosphatase (see hepatic warnings), nausea, thirst, vomiting, weight increase.

Dermatological. Petechiae, photosensitivity, pruritus.

Other. Albuminuria, allergic reaction, amblyopia, asthenia, CPK increase, crystalluria, dyspnea, edema, epistaxis, eye irritation, headache, hyperglycemia, hyperuricemia, impotence, muscle cramps, nasal congestion, neck rigidity, nocturia, osteoarticular pain, pain, polyuria, rhinitis, sexual difficulties, gynecomastia.

In addition, the following postmarketing events have been reported infrequently in patients receiving diltiazem hydrochloride: alopecia, erythema multiforme, exfoliative dermatitis, Stevens-Johnson syndrome, toxic epidermal necrolysis, extrapyramidal symptoms, gingival hyperplasia, hemolytic anemia, increased bleeding time, leukopenia, purpura, retinopathy, and thrombocytopenia. In addition, events such as myocardial infarction have been observed which are not readily distinguishable from the natural history of the disease in these patients. A number of well-documented cases of generalized rash, characterized as leukocytoclastic vasculitis, have been reported. However, a definitive cause and effect relationship between these events and diltiazem hydrochloride therapy is yet to be established.

OVERDOSAGE

The oral LD50's in mice and rats range from 415 to 740 mg/kg and from 560 to 810 mg/kg, respectively. The intravenous LD50's in these species were 60 and 38 mg/kg, respectively. The oral LD50 in dogs is considered to be in excess of 50 mg/kg, while lethality was seen in monkeys at 360 mg/kg.

The toxic dose in man is not known. Due to extensive metabolism, blood levels after a standard dose of diltiazem can vary over tenfold, limiting the usefulness of blood levels in overdose cases. There have been 29 reports of diltiazem overdose in doses ranging from less than 1 gm to 10.8 gm. Sixteen of these reports involved multiple drug ingestions. Twenty-two reports indicated patients had recovered from diltiazem overdose ranging from less than 1 gm to 10.8 gm. There were seven reports with a fatal outcome; although the amount of diltiazem ingested was unknown, multiple drug ingestions were confirmed in six of the seven reports.
Events observed following diltiazem overdose included bradycardia, hypotension, heart block, and cardiac failure. Most reports of overdose described some supportive medical measure and/or drug treatment. Bradycardia frequently responded favorably to atropine as did heart block, although cardiac pacing was also frequently utilized to treat heart block. Fluids and vasopressors were used to maintain blood pressure, and in cases of cardiac failure, inotropic agents were administered. In addition, some patients received treatment with ventilatory support, activated charcoal, and/or intravenous calcium. Evidence of the effectiveness of intravenous calcium administration to reverse the pharmacological effects of diltiazem overdose was conflicting.
In the event of overdose or exaggerated response, appropriate supportive measures should be employed in addition to gastrointestinal decontamination. Diltiazem does not appear to be removed by peritoneal or hemodialysis. Based on the known pharmacological effects of diltiazem and/or reported clinical experiences, the following measures may be considered:
Bradycardia: Administer atropine (0.60 to 1.0 mg). If there is no response to vagal blockage, administer isoproterenol cautiously.
High-Degree AV Block: Treat as for bradycardia above. Fixed high-degree AV block should be treated with cardiac pacing.
Cardiac Failure: Administer inotropic agents (isoproterenol, dopamine, or dobutamine) and diuretics.
Hypotension: Vasopressors (e.g., dopamine or levarterenol bitartrate). Actual treatment and dosage should depend on the severity of the clinical situation and the judgment and experience of the treating physician.
In a few reported cases, overdose with calcium channel blockers has been associated with hypotension and bradycardia, initially refractory to atropine but becoming more responsive to this treatment when the patients received large doses (close to 1 gram/hour for more than 24 hours) of calcium chloride.
Due to extensive metabolism, plasma concentrations after a standard dose of diltiazem can vary over tenfold, which significantly limits their value in evaluation cases of overdosage.
Charcoal hemoperfusion has been used successfully as an adjunct therapy to hasten drug elimination. Overdoses with as much as 10.8 gm of oral diltiazem have been successfully treated using appropriate supportive care.

DOSAGE AND ADMINISTRATION
Hypertension: Dosage needs to be adjusted by titration to individual patient needs. When used as monotherapy, usual starting doses are 120 to 240 mg once daily. Maximum antihypertensive effect is usually observed by 14 days of chronic therapy; therefore, dosage adjustments should be scheduled accordingly. The usual dosage range studied in clinical trials was 120 to 540 mg once daily. Current clinical experience with 540 mg dose is limited; however, the dose may be increased to 540 mg once daily.
Angina: Dosages for the treatment of angina should be adjusted to each patient's needs, starting with a dose of 120 mg to 180 mg once daily. Individual patients may respond to higher doses of up to 540 mg once daily. When necessary, titration should be carried out over 7 to 14 days.
Concomitant use with Other Cardiovascular Agents.
1. Sublingual Nitroglycerin may be taken as required to abort acute anginal attacks during diltiazem hydrochloride therapy.
2. Prophylactic Nitrate Therapy — Diltiazem hydrochloride may be safely co-administered with short- and long-acting nitrates.
3. Beta-blockers. (See WARNINGS and PRECAUTIONS.)
4. Antihypertensives — Diltiazem hydrochloride has an additive antihypertensive effect when used with other antihypertensive agents. Therefore, the dosage of diltiazem hydrochloride or the concomitant antihypertensives may need to be adjusted when adding one to the other.
Hypertensive or anginal patients who are treated with other formulations of diltiazem can safely be switched to Tiazac capsules at the nearest equivalent total daily dose. Subsequent titration to higher or lower doses may, however, be necessary and should be initiated as clinically indicated.

HOW SUPPLIED
Tiazac (diltiazem hydrochloride) Extended-Release Capsules
[See third table on previous page]
Storage conditions: Store at controlled room temperature 20°–25°C (68°–77°F). Avoid excessive humidity.
℞ Only.
Manufactured by:
Biovail Corporation International
Mississauga, Ontario CANADA L5L 1J9
Manufactured for:
Forest Pharmaceuticals, Inc.
Subsidiary of Forest Laboratories, Inc.
St. Louis, Missouri 63045
Rev: 10/99 LB-0001-06
Shown in Product Identification Guide, page 313

Fujisawa Healthcare, Inc.
PARKWAY NORTH CENTER
THREE PARKWAY NORTH
DEERFIELD, IL 60015-2548

For Medical Information Contact:
Generally:
Medical and Scientific Information
(800) 727-7003
In Emergencies:
Medical and Scientific Information
(800) 727-7003

ADENOCARD® IV ℞
(adenosine)
FOR RAPID BOLUS INTRAVENOUS USE

DESCRIPTION
Adenosine is an endogenous nucleoside occurring in all cells of the body. It is chemically 6-amino-9-β-D-ribofuranosyl-9-H-purine and has the following structural formula:

$C_{10}H_{13}N_5O_4$ **267.24**

Adenosine is a white crystalline powder. It is soluble in water and practically insoluble in alcohol. Solubility increases by warming and lowering the pH. Adenosine is not chemically related to other antiarrhythmic drugs. Adenocard® (adenosine) is a sterile solution for rapid bolus intravenous injection. Each mL contains 3 mg adenosine and 9 mg sodium chloride in Water for Injection. The pH of the solution is between 4.5 and 7.5.

CLINICAL PHARMACOLOGY
Mechanism of Action
Adenocard (adenosine) slows conduction time through the A-V node, can interrupt the reentry pathways through the A-V node, and can restore normal sinus rhythm in patients with paroxysmal supraventricular tachycardia (PSVT), including PSVT associated with Wolff-Parkinson-White Syndrome.
Adenocard is antagonized competitively by methylxanthines such as caffeine and theophylline, and potentiated by blockers of nucleoside transport such as dipyridamole. Adenocard is not blocked by atropine.
Hemodynamics
The intravenous bolus dose of 6 or 12 mg Adenocard (adenosine) usually has no systemic hemodynamic effects. When larger doses are given by infusion, adenosine decreases blood pressure by decreasing peripheral resistance.
Pharmacokinetics
Intravenously administered adenosine is rapidly cleared from the circulation via cellular uptake, primarily by erythrocytes and vascular endothelial cells. This process involves a specific transmembrane nucleoside carrier system that is reversible, nonconcentrative, and bidirectionally symmetrical. Intracellular adenosine is rapidly metabolized either via phosphorylation to adenosine monophosphate by adenosine kinase, or via deamination to inosine by adenosine deaminase in the cytosol. Since adenosine kinase has a lower K_m and V_{max} than adenosine deaminase, deamination plays a significant role only when cytosolic adenosine saturates the phosphorylation pathway. Inosine formed by deamination of adenosine can leave the cell intact or can be degraded to hypoxanthine, xanthine, and ultimately uric acid. Adenosine monophosphate formed by phosphorylation of adenosine is incorporated into the high-energy phosphate pool. While extracellular adenosine is primarily cleared by cellular uptake with a half-life of less than 10 seconds in whole blood, excessive amounts may be deaminated by an ecto-form of adenosine deaminase. As Adenocard requires no hepatic or renal function for its activation or inactivation, hepatic and renal failure would not be expected to alter its effectiveness or tolerability.
Clinical Trial Results
In controlled studies in the United States, bolus doses of 3, 6, 9, and 12 mg were studied. A cumulative 60% of patients with paroxysmal supraventricular tachycardia had converted to normal sinus rhythm within one minute after an intravenous bolus dose of 6 mg Adenocard (some converted on 3 mg and failures were given 6 mg), and a cumulative 92% converted after a bolus dose of 12 mg. Seven to sixteen percent of patients converted after 1–4 placebo bolus injections. Similar responses were seen in a variety of patient subsets, including those using or not using digoxin, those with Wolff-Parkinson-White Syndrome, males, females, blacks, Caucasians, and Hispanics.
Adenosine is not effective in converting rhythms other than PSVT, such as atrial flutter, atrial fibrillation, or ventricular tachycardia, to normal sinus rhythm. To date, such patients have not had adverse consequences following administration of adenosine.

INDICATIONS AND USAGE
Intravenous Adenocard (adenosine) is indicated for the following.
Conversion to sinus rhythm of paroxysmal supraventricular tachycardia (PSVT), including that associated with accessory bypass tracts (Wolff-Parkinson-White Syndrome). When clinically advisable, appropriate vagal maneuvers (e.g., Valsalva maneuver), should be attempted prior to Adenocard administration.
It is important to be sure the Adenocard solution actually reaches the systemic circulation (see **DOSAGE AND ADMINISTRATION**).
Adenocard does not convert atrial flutter, atrial fibrillation, or ventricular tachycardia to normal sinus rhythm. In the presence of atrial flutter or atrial fibrillation, a transient modest slowing of ventricular response may occur immediately following Adenocard administration.

CONTRAINDICATIONS
Intravenous Adenocard (adenosine) is contraindicated in:
1. Second- or third-degree A-V block (except in patients with a functioning artificial pacemaker).
2. Sinus node disease, such as sick sinus syndrome or symptomatic bradycardia (except in patients with a functioning artificial pacemaker).
3. Known hypersensitivity to adenosine.

WARNINGS
Heart Block
Adenocard (adenosine) exerts its effect by decreasing conduction through the A-V node and may produce a short lasting first-, second- or third-degree heart block. Appropriate therapy should be instituted as needed. Patients who develop high-level block on one dose of Adenocard should not be given additional doses. Because of the very short half-life of adenosine, these effects are generally self-limiting.
Transient or prolonged episodes of asystole have been reported with fatal outcomes in some cases.
Rarely, ventricular fibrillation has been reported following Adenocard administration, including both resuscitated and fatal events. In most instances, these cases were associated with the concomitant use of digoxin and, less frequently with digoxin and verapamil. Although no causal relationship or drug-drug interaction has been established, Adenocard should be used with caution in patients receiving digoxin or digoxin and verapamil in combination. Appropriate resuscitative measures should be available.
Arrhythmias at Time of Conversion
At the time of conversion to normal sinus rhythm, a variety of new rhythms may appear on the electrocardiogram. They generally last only a few seconds without intervention, and may take the form of premature ventricular contractions, atrial premature contractions, sinus bradycardia, sinus tachycardia, skipped beats, and varying degrees of A-V nodal block. Such findings were seen in 55% of patients.
Bronchoconstriction
Adenocard (adenosine) is a respiratory stimulant (probably through activation of carotid body chemoreceptors) and intravenous administration in man has been shown to increase minute ventilation (Ve) and reduce arterial PCO_2 causing respiratory alkalosis.
Adenosine administered by inhalation has been reported to cause bronchoconstriction in asthmatic patients, presumably due to mast cell degranulation and histamine release. These effects have not been observed in normal subjects. Adenocard has been administered to a limited number of patients with asthma and mild to moderate exacerbation of their symptoms has been reported. Respiratory compromise has occurred during adenosine infusion in patients with obstructive pulmonary disease. Adenocard should be used with caution in patients with obstructive lung disease not associated with bronchoconstriction (e.g., emphysema, bronchitis, etc.) and should be avoided in patients with bronchoconstriction or bronchospasm (e.g., asthma). Adenocard should be discontinued in any patient who develops severe respiratory difficulties.

PRECAUTIONS
Drug Interactions
Intravenous Adenocard (adenosine) has been effectively administered in the presence of other cardioactive drugs, such as quinidine, beta-adrenergic blocking agents, calcium channel blocking agents, and angiotensin converting enzyme inhibitors, without any change in the adverse reaction profile. Digoxin and verapamil use may be rarely associated with ventricular fibrillation when combined with Adenocard (see **WARNINGS**). Because of the potential for additive or synergistic depressant effects on the SA and AV nodes, however, Adenocard should be used with caution in the presence of these agents. The use of Adenocard in patients receiving digitalis may be rarely associated with ventricular fibrillation (see **WARNINGS**).

Continued on next page

Adenocard—Cont.

The effects of adenosine are antagonized by methylxanthines such as caffeine and theophylline. In the presence of these methylxanthines, larger doses of adenosine may be required or adenosine may not be effective. Adenosine effects are potentiated by dipyridamole. Thus, smaller doses of adenosine may be effective in the presence of dipyridamole. Carbamazepine has been reported to increase the degree of heart block produced by other agents. As the primary effect of adenosine is to decrease conduction through the A-V node, higher degrees of heart block may be produced in the presence of carbamazepine.

Carcinogenesis, Mutagenesis, Impairment of Fertility

Studies in animals have not been performed to evaluate the carcinogenic potential of Adenocard (adenosine). Adenosine was negative for genotoxic potential in the Salmonella (Ames Test) and Mammalian Microsome Assay.

Adenosine, however, like other nucleosides at millimolar concentrations present for several doubling times of cells in culture, is known to produce a variety of chromosomal alterations. Fertility studies in animals have not been conducted with adenosine.

Pregnancy Category C

Animal reproduction studies have not been conducted with adenosine; nor have studies been performed in pregnant women. As adenosine is a naturally occurring material, widely dispersed throughout the body, no fetal effects would be anticipated. However, since it is not known whether Adenocard can cause fetal harm when administered to pregnant women, Adenocard should be used during pregnancy only if clearly needed.

Pediatric Use

No controlled studies have been conducted in pediatric patients to establish the safety and efficacy of Adenocard for the conversion of paroxysmal supraventricular tachycardia (PSVT). However, intravenous adenosine has been used for the treatment of PSVT in neonates, infants, children and adolescents (see **DOSAGE AND ADMINISTRATION**).[1]

Geriatric Use

Clinical studies of Adenocard did not include sufficient numbers of subjects aged 65 and over to determine whether they respond differently from younger subjects. Other reported clinical experience has not identified differences in responses between elderly and younger patients. In general, Adenocard in geriatric patients should be used with caution since this population may have a diminished cardiac function, nodal dysfunction, concomitant diseases or drug therapy that may alter hemodynamic function and produce severe bradycardia or AV block.

ADVERSE REACTIONS

The following reactions were reported with intravenous Adenocard (adenosine) used in controlled U.S. clinical trials. The placebo group had a less than 1% rate of all of these reactions.

Cardiovascular	Facial flushing (18%), headache (2%), sweating, palpitations, chest pain, hypotension (less than 1%).
Respiratory	Shortness of breath/ dyspnea (12%), chest pressure (7%), hyperventilation, head pressure (less than 1%).
Central Nervous System	Lightheadedness (2%), dizziness, tingling in arms, numbness (1%), apprehension, blurred vision, burning sensation, heaviness in arms, neck and back pain (less than 1%).
Gastrointestinal	Nausea (3%), metallic taste, tightness in throat, pressure in groin (less than 1%).

Also, in post-market clinical experience with Adenocard, cases of prolonged asystole, ventricular tachycardia, ventricular fibrillation, transient increase in blood pressure, bradycardia, atrial fibrillation, and bronchospasm, in association with Adenocard use, have been reported (see **WARNINGS**).

OVERDOSAGE

The half-life of Adenocard (adenosine) is less than 10 seconds. Thus, adverse effects are generally rapidly self-limiting. Treatment of any prolonged adverse effects should be individualized and be directed toward the specific effect. Methylxanthines, such as caffeine and theophylline, are competitive antagonists of adenosine.

DOSAGE AND ADMINISTRATION

For rapid bolus intravenous use only.

Adenocard (adenosine) Injection should be given as a rapid bolus by the peripheral intravenous route. To be certain the solution reaches the systemic circulation, it should be administered either directly into a vein or, if given into an IV line, it should be given as close to the patient as possible and followed by a rapid saline flush.

Adult Patients

The dose recommendation is based on clinical studies with peripheral venous bolus dosing. Central venous (CVP or other) administration of Adenocard has not been systematically studied.

The recommended intravenous doses for adults are as follows:

Initial dose: 6 mg given as a rapid intravenous bolus (administered over a 1–2 second period).

Repeat administration: If the first dose does not result in elimination of the supraventricular tachycardia within 1–2 minutes, 12 mg should be given as a rapid intravenous bolus. This 12 mg dose may be repeated a second time if required.

Pediatric Patients

The dosages used in neonates, infants, children and adolescents were equivalent to those administered to adults on a weight basis.

Pediatric Patients with a Body Weight <50 kg:

Initial dose: Give 0.05 to 0.1 mg/kg as a rapid IV bolus given either centrally or peripherally. A saline flush should follow.

Repeat administration: If conversion of PSVT does not occur within 1–2 minutes, additional bolus injections of adenosine can be administered at incrementally higher doses, increasing the amount given by 0.05 to 0.1 mg/kg. Follow each bolus with a saline flush. This process should continue until sinus rhythm is established or a maximum single dose of 0.3 mg/kg is used.

Pediatric Patients with a Body Weight ≥50 kg:

Administer the adult dose.

Doses greater than 12 mg are not recommended for adult and pediatric patients.

NOTE: Parenteral drug products should be inspected visually for particulate matter and discoloration prior to administration.

HOW SUPPLIED

Adenocard® (adenosine) Injection is supplied as a sterile solution in normal saline.

NDC 0469-0872-02 Product Code 87102 6 mg/2 mL (3mg/mL) in 2 mL flip-top vials, packaged in 10's.

NDC 0469-7234-12 Product Code 723412 6 mg/2 mL (3mg/mL) in a 2 mL disposable syringe, in a package of five.

NDC 0469-7234-14 Product Code 723414 12 mg/4 mL (3mg/mL) in a 5 mL disposable syringe, in a package of five.

Store at controlled room temperature 15°–30°C (59°–86°F).

DO NOT REFRIGERATE as crystallization may occur. If crystallization has occurred, dissolve crystals by warming to room temperature. The solution must be clear at the time of use.

Contains no preservatives. Discard unused portion.

Rx only

REFERENCE

1. Paul T., Pfammatter. J-P. Adenosine: an effective and safe antiarrhythmic drug in pediatrics. Pediatric Cardiology 1997; 18:118–126.

Manufactured for:
Fujisawa Healthcare, Inc., Deerfield IL 60015
45514L
Revised: May 1999

Shown in Product Identification Guide, page 313

ADENOSCAN® ℞

adenosine
For Intravenous Infusion Only

DESCRIPTION

Adenosine is an endogenous nucleoside occurring in all cells of the body. It is chemically 6-amino-9-beta-D-ribofuranosyl-9-H-purine and has the following structural formula:

$C_{10}H_{13}N_5O_4$ **267.24**

Adenosine is a white crystalline powder. It is soluble in water and practically insoluble in alcohol. Solubility increases by warming and lowering the pH of the solution.

Each Adenoscan vial contains a sterile, nonpyrogenic solution of adenosine 3 mg/mL and sodium chloride 9 mg/mL in Water for Injection, q.s. The pH of the solution is between 4.5 and 7.5.

CLINICAL PHARMACOLOGY

Mechanism of Action

Adenosine is a potent vasodilator in most vascular beds, except in renal afferent arterioles and hepatic veins where it produces vasoconstriction. Adenosine is thought to exert its pharmacological effects through activation of purine receptors (cell-surface A_1 and A_2 adenosine receptors). Although the exact mechanism by which adenosine receptor activation relaxes vascular smooth muscle is not known, there is evidence to support both inhibition of the slow inward calcium current reducing calcium uptake, and activation of adenylate cyclase through A_2 receptors in smooth muscle cells. Adenosine may also lessen vascular tone by modulating sympathetic neurotransmission. The intracellular uptake of adenosine is mediated by a specific transmembrane nucleoside transport system. Once inside the cell, adenosine is rapidly phosphorylated by adenosine kinase to adenosine monophosphate, or deaminated by adenosine deaminase to inosine. These intracellular metabolites of adenosine are not vasoactive.

Myocardial uptake of thallium-201 is directly proportional to coronary blood flow. Since Adenoscan significantly increases blood flow in normal coronary arteries with little or no increase in stenotic arteries, Adenoscan causes relatively less thallium-201 uptake in vascular territories supplied by stenotic coronary arteries i.e., a greater difference is seen after Adenoscan between areas served by normal and areas served by stenotic vessels than is seen prior to Adenoscan.

Hemodynamics

Adenosine produces a direct negative chronotropic, dromotropic and inotropic effect on the heart, presumably due to A_1-receptor agonism, and produces peripheral vasodilation, presumably due to A_2-receptor agonism. The net effect of Adenoscan in humans is typically a mild to moderate reduction in systolic, diastolic and mean arterial blood pressure associated with a reflex increase in heart rate. Rarely, significant hypotension and tachycardia have been observed.

Pharmacokinetics

Intravenously administered adenosine is rapidly cleared from the circulation via cellular uptake, primarily by erythrocytes and vascular endothelial cells. This process involves a specific transmembrane nucleoside carrier system that is reversible, nonconcentrative, and bidirectionally symmetrical. Intracellular adenosine is rapidly metabolized either via phosphorylation to adenosine monophosphate by adenosine kinase, or via deamination to inosine by adenosine deaminase in the cytosol. Since adenosine kinase has a lower K_m and V_{max} than adenosine deaminase, deamination plays a significant role only when cytosolic adenosine saturates the phosphorylation pathway. Inosine formed by deamination of adenosine can leave the cell intact or can be degraded to hypoxanthine, xanthine, and ultimately uric acid. Adenosine monophosphate formed by phosphorylation of adenosine is incorporated into the high-energy phosphate pool. While extracellular adenosine is primarily cleared by cellular uptake with a half-life of less than 10 seconds in whole blood, excessive amounts may be deaminated by an ectoform of adenosine deaminase. As Adenoscan requires no hepatic or renal function for its activation or inactivation, hepatic and renal failure would not be expected to alter its effectiveness or tolerability.

Clinical Trials

In two crossover comparative studies involving 319 subjects who could exercise (including 106 healthy volunteers and 213 patients with known or suspected coronary disease), Adenoscan and exercise thallium images were compared by blinded observers. The images were concordant for the presence of perfusion defects in 85.5% of cases by global analysis (patient by patient) and up to 93% of cases based on vascular territories. In these two studies, 193 patients also had recent coronary arteriography for comparison (healthy volunteers were not catheterized). The sensitivity (true positive Adenoscan divided by the number of patients with positive (abnormal) angiography) for detecting angiographically significant disease (≥50% reduction in the luminal diameter of at least one major vessel) was 64% for Adenoscan and 64% for exercise testing, while the specificity (true negative divided by the number of patients with negative angiograms) was 54% for Adenoscan and 65% for exercise testing. The 95% confidence limits for Adenoscan sensitivity were 56% to 78% and for specificity were 37% to 71%.

Intracoronary Doppler flow catheter studies have demonstrated that a dose of intravenous Adenoscan of 140 mcg/kg/min produces maximum coronary hyperemia (relative to intracoronary papaverine) in approximately 95% of cases within two to three minutes of the onset of the infusion. Coronary blood flow velocity returns to basal levels within one to two minutes of discontinuing the Adenoscan infusion.

INDICATIONS AND USAGE

Intravenous Adenoscan is indicated as an adjunct to thallium-201 myocardial perfusion scintigraphy in patients unable to exercise adequately (See **WARNINGS**).

CONTRAINDICATIONS

Intravenous Adenoscan (adenosine) should not be administered to individuals with:

1. Second- or third-degree AV block (except in patients with a functioning artificial pacemaker).
2. Sinus node disease, such as sick sinus syndrome or symptomatic bradycardia (except in patients with a functioning artificial pacemaker).
3. Known or suspected bronchoconstrictive or bronchospastic lung disease (e.g., asthma).
4. Known hypersensitivity to adenosine.

WARNINGS

Fatal Cardiac Arrest, Life Threatening Ventricular Arrhythmias, and Myocardial Infarction.

Fatal cardiac arrest, sustained ventricular tachycardia (requiring resuscitation), and nonfatal myocardial infarction have been reported coincident with Adenoscan infusion. Patients with unstable angina may be at greater risk. Appropriate resuscitative measures should be available.

Sinoatrial and Atrioventricular Nodal Block

Adenoscan (adenosine) exerts a direct depressant effect on the SA and AV nodes and has the potential to cause first-, second- or third-degree AV block, or sinus bradycardia. Approximately 6.3% of patients develop AV block with Adenoscan, including first-degree (2.9%), second-degree (2.6%) and third-degree (0.8%) heart block. All episodes of AV block have been asymptomatic, transient, and did not require intervention. Adenoscan can cause sinus bradycardia. Adenoscan should be used with caution in patients with pre-existing first-degree AV block or bundle branch block and should be avoided in patients with high-grade AV block or sinus node dysfunction (except in patients with a functioning artificial pacemaker). Adenoscan should be discontinued in any patient who develops persistent or symptomatic high-grade AV block. Sinus pause has been rarely observed with adenosine infusions.

Hypotension

Adenoscan (adenosine) is a potent peripheral vasodilator and can cause significant hypotension. Patients with an intact baroreceptor reflex mechanism are able to maintain blood pressure and tissue perfusion in response to Adenoscan by increasing heart rate and cardiac output. However, Adenoscan should be used with caution in patients with autonomic dysfunction, stenotic valvular heart disease, pericarditis or pericardial effusions, stenotic carotid artery disease with cerebrovascular insufficiency, or uncorrected hypovolemia, due to the risk of hypotensive complications in these patients. Adenoscan should be discontinued in any patient who develops persistent or symptomatic hypotension.

Hypertension

Increases in systolic and diastolic pressure have been observed (as great as 140 mm Hg systolic in one case) concomitant with Adenoscan infusion; most increases resolved spontaneously within several minutes, but in some cases, hypertension lasted for several hours.

Bronchoconstriction

Adenoscan (adenosine) is a respiratory stimulant (probably through activation of carotid body chemoreceptors) and intravenous administration in man has been shown to increase minute ventilation (Ve) and reduce arterial PCO_2 causing respiratory alkalosis. Approximately 28% of patients experience breathlessness (dyspnea) or an urge to breathe deeply with Adenoscan. These respiratory complaints are transient and only rarely require intervention. Adenosine administered by inhalation has been reported to cause bronchoconstriction in asthmatic patients, presumably due to mast cell degranulation and histamine release. These effects have not been observed in normal subjects. Adenoscan has been administered to a limited number of patients with asthma and mild to moderate exacerbation of their symptoms has been reported. Respiratory compromise has occurred during adenosine infusion in patients with obstructive pulmonary disease. Adenoscan should be used with caution in patients with obstructive lung disease not associated with bronchoconstriction (e.g., emphysema, bronchitis, etc.) and should be avoided in patients with bronchoconstriction or bronchospasm (e.g., asthma). Adenoscan should be discontinued in any patient who develops severe respiratory difficulties.

PRECAUTIONS

Drug Interactions

Intravenous Adenoscan (adenosine) has been given with other cardioactive drugs (such as beta adrenergic blocking agents, cardiac glycosides, and calcium channel blockers) without apparent adverse interactions, but its effectiveness with these agents has not been systematically evaluated. Because of the potential for additive or synergistic depressant effects on the SA and AV nodes, however, Adenoscan should be used with caution in the presence of these agents. The vasoactive effects of the Adenoscan are inhibited by adenosine receptor antagonists, such as alkylxanthines (e.g., caffeine and theophylline). The safety and efficacy of Adenoscan in the presence of these agents has not been systematically evaluated.

The vasoactive effects of Adenoscan are potentiated by nucleoside transport inhibitors, such as dipyridamole. The safety and efficacy of Adenoscan in the presence of dipyridamole has not been systematically evaluated.

Whenever possible, drugs that might inhibit or augment the effects of adenosine should be withheld for at least five half-lives prior to the use of Adenoscan.

Carcinogenesis, Mutagenesis, Impairment of Fertility

Studies in animals have not been performed to evaluate the carcinogenic potential of Adenoscan (adenosine). Adenosine was negative for genotoxic potential in the Salmonella (Ames Test) and Mammalian Microsome Assay.

Adenosine, however, like other nucleosides at millimolar concentrations present for several doubling times of cells in culture, is known to produce a variety of chromosomal alterations. In rats and mice, adenosine administered intraperitoneally once a day for five days at 50, 100, and 150 mg/kg [10-30 (rats) and 5-15 (mice) times human dosage on a mg/M^2 basis] caused decreased spermatogenesis and increased numbers of abnormal sperm, a reflection of the ability of adenosine to produce chromosomal damage.

Pregnancy Category C

Animal reproduction studies have not been conducted with adenosine; nor have studies been performed in pregnant women. Because it is not known whether Adenoscan can cause fetal harm when administered to pregnant women, Adenoscan should be used during pregnancy only if clearly needed.

Pediatric Use

The safety and effectiveness of Adenoscan in patients less than 18 years of age have not been established.

ADVERSE REACTIONS

The following reactions with an incidence of at least 1% were reported with intravenous Adenoscan among 1421 patients enrolled in controlled and uncontrolled U.S. clinical trials. Despite the short half-life of adenosine, 10.6% of the side effects occurred not with the infusion of Adenoscan but several hours after the infusion terminated. Also, 8.4% of the side effects that began coincident with the infusion persisted for up to 24 hours after the infusion was complete. In many cases, it is not possible to know whether these late adverse events are the result of Adenoscan infusion.

Flushing	44%
Chest discomfort	40%
Dyspnea or urge to breathe deeply	28%
Headache	18%
Throat, neck or jaw discomfort	15%
Gastrointestinal discomfort	13%
Lightheadedness/dizziness	12%
Upper extremity discomfort	4%
ST segment depression	3%
First-degree AV block	3%
Second-degree AV block	3%
Paresthesia	2%
Hypotension	2%
Nervousness	2%
Arrhythmias	1%

Adverse experiences of any severity reported in less than 1% of patients include:

Body as a Whole: back discomfort; lower extremity discomfort; weakness.

Cardiovascular System: nonfatal myocardial infarction; life-threatening ventricular arrhythmia; third-degree AV block; bradycardia; palpitation; sinus exit block; sinus pause; sweating; T-wave changes, hypertension (systolic blood pressure >200 mm Hg).

Central Nervous System: drowsiness; emotional instability; tremors.

Genital/Urinary System: vaginal pressure; urgency.

Respiratory System: cough.

Special Senses: blurred vision; dry mouth; ear discomfort; metallic taste; nasal congestion; scotomas; tongue discomfort.

OVERDOSAGE

The half-life of adenosine is less than 10 seconds and side effects of Adenoscan (when they occur) usually resolve quickly when the infusion is discontinued, although delayed or persistent effects have been observed. Methylxanthines, such as caffeine and theophylline, are competitive adenosine receptor antagonists and theophylline has been used to effectively terminate persistent side effects. In controlled U.S. clinical trials, theophylline (50-125 mg slow intravenous injection) was needed to abort Adenoscan side effects in less than 2% of patients.

DOSAGE AND ADMINISTRATION

For intravenous infusion only.

Adenoscan should be given as a continuous peripheral intravenous infusion.

The recommended intravenous dose for adults is 140 mcg/kg/min infused for six minutes (total dose of 0.84 mg/kg).

The required dose of thallium-201 should be injected at the midpoint of the Adenoscan infusion (i.e., after the first three minutes of Adenoscan). Thallium-201 is physically compatible with Adenoscan and may be injected directly into the Adenoscan infusion set.

The injection should be as close to the venous access as possible to prevent an inadvertent increase in the dose of Adenoscan (the contents of the IV tubing) being administered.

There are no data on the safety or efficacy of alternative Adenoscan infusion protocols.

The safety and efficacy of Adenoscan administered by the intracoronary route have not been established.

The following Adenoscan infusion nomogram may be used to determine the appropriate infusion rate corrected for total body weight:

Patient Weight		*Infusion Rate*
kg	*lbs*	*mL/min*
45	99	2.1
50	110	2.3
55	121	2.6
60	132	2.8
65	143	3.0
70	154	3.3
75	165	3.5
80	176	3.8
85	187	4.0
90	198	4.2

This nomogram was derived from the following general formula:

$$\frac{0.140\ (\text{mg/kg/min}) \times \text{total body weight (kg)}}{\text{Adenoscan concentration (3 mg/mL)}} = \text{infusion rate (mL/min)}$$

Note: Parenteral drug products should be inspected visually for particulate matter and discoloration prior to administration.

HOW SUPPLIED

Adenoscan (adenosine) is supplied as 20 mL and 30 mL vials of sterile nonpyrogenic solution in normal saline.

Product Code	NDC No.	
87120	0469-0871-20	60 mg/20 mL (3 mg/mL) in a 20 mL single-dose, flip-top glass vial, packaged individually and in packages of ten.
87130	0469-0871-30	90 mg/30 mL (3mg/mL) in a 30 mL single-dose, flip-top glass vial, packaged individually and in packages of ten.

Store at controlled room temperature 15°-30°C (59°-86°F). Do not refrigerate as crystallization may occur. If crystallization has occurred, dissolve crystals by warming to room temperature. The solution must be clear at the time of use. Contains no preservative. Discard unused portion.

Rx only

Manufactured for:
Fujisawa Healthcare, Inc.
Deerfield, IL 60015
45558F/Revised: January 1999

Shown in Product Identification Guide, page 313

AMBISOME® ℞

[*ăm-bĭ-sōme*]

(amphotericin B) liposome for injection

DESCRIPTION

AmBisome for Injection is a sterile, non-pyrogenic lyophilized product for intravenous infusion. Each vial contains 50 mg of amphotericin B, USP, intercalated into a liposomal membrane consisting of approximately 213 mg hydrogenated soy phosphatidylcholine; 52 mg cholesterol, NF; 84 mg distearoylphosphatidylglycerol; 0.64 mg alpha tocopherol, USP; together with 900 mg sucrose, NF; and 27 mg disodium succinate hexahydrate as buffer. Following reconstitution with Sterile Water for Injection, USP, the resulting pH of the suspension is between 5.0–6.0.

AmBisome is a true single bilayer liposomal drug delivery system. Liposomes are closed, spherical vesicles created by mixing specific proportions of amphophilic substances such as phospholipids and cholesterol so that they arrange themselves into multiple concentric bilayer membranes when hydrated in aqueous solutions. Single bilayer liposomes are then formed by microemulsification of multilamellar vesicles using a homogenizer. AmBisome consists of these unilamellar bilayer liposomes with amphotericin B intercalated within the membrane. Due to the nature and quantity of amphophilic substances used, and the lipophilic moiety in the amphotericin B molecule, the drug is an integral part of the overall structure of the AmBisome liposomes. AmBisome contains true liposomes that are less than 100 nm in diameter. A schematic depiction of the liposome is presented below.

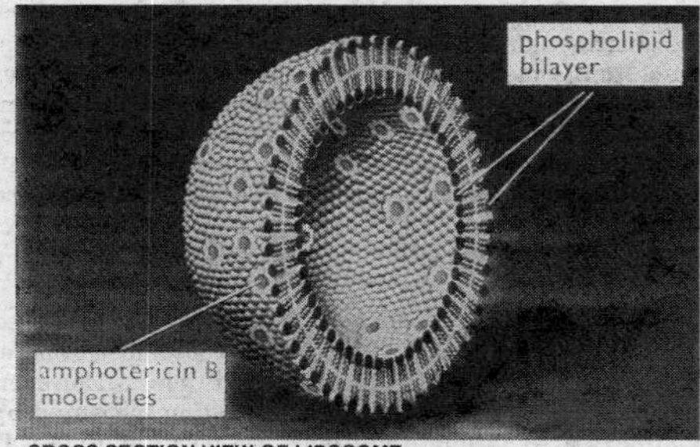

CROSS SECTION VIEW OF LIPOSOME

Note: Liposomal encapsulation or incorporation into a lipid complex can substantially affect a drug's functional properties relative to those of the unencapsulated drug or non-lipid associated drug. In addition, different liposomal or lipid-complex products with a common active ingredient may vary from one another in the chemical composition and physical form of the lipid component. Such differences may affect the functional properties of these drug products.

Amphotericin B is a macrocyclic, polyene, antifungal antibiotic produced from a strain of *Streptomyces nodosus.*

Amphotericin B is designated chemically as:
[1R-(1R*,3S*,5R*,6R*,9R*,11R*,15S*,16R*,17R*,18S*,19E,21E,23E,25E,27E,29E,31E,33R*,35S*,36R*,37S*)]-33-[(3-Amino-3,6-dideoxy-β-D-mannopyranosyl)oxy]-1,3,5,6,9,11,17,37-octahydroxy-15,16,18-trimethyl-13-oxo-14,39-dioxabicyclo[33.3.1]nonatriaconta-19,21,23,25,27,29,31-heptaene-36-carboxylic acid (CAS No. 1397-89-3).

Amphotericin B has a molecular formula of $C_{47}H_{73}NO_{17}$ and a molecular weight of 924.09.

The structure of amphotericin B is shown below:

[See chemical structure at top of next column]

MICROBIOLOGY

Mechanism of Action

Amphotericin B, the active ingredient of AmBisome, acts by binding to the sterol component of a cell membrane leading

Continued on next page

Ambisome—Cont.

Pharmacokinetic Parameters of AmBisome

Dose (mg/kg/day):	1.0		2.5		5.0	
Day	1 n = 8	Last n = 7	1 n = 7	Last n = 7	1 n = 12	Last n = 9
Parameters						
C_{max} (mcg/mL)	7.3 ± 3.8	12.2 ± 4.9	17.2 ± 7.1	31.4 ± 17.8	57.6 ± 21.0	83.0 ± 35.2
AUC_{0-24} (mcg•hr/mL)	27 ± 14	60 ± 20	65 ± 33	197 ± 183	269 ± 96	555 ± 311
$t_{½}$(hr)	10.7 ± 6.4	7.0 ± 2.1	8.1 ± 2.3	6.3 ± 2.0	6.4 ± 2.1	6.8 ± 2.1
V_{ss}(L/kg)	0.44 ± 0.27	0.14 ± 0.05	0.40 ± 0.37	0.16 ± 0.09	0.16 ± 0.10	0.10 ± 0.07
Cl (mL/hr/kg)	39 ± 22	17 ± 6	51 ± 44	22 ± 15	21 ± 14	11 ± 6

Empirical Therapy in Febrile Neutropenic Patients: Randomized, Double-Blind Study in 687 Patients

	AmBisome	Amphotericin B
Number of patients receiving at least one dose of study drug	343	344
Overall Success	171 (49.9%)	169 (49.1%)
Fever resolution during neutropenic period	199 (58.0%)	200 (58.1%)
No treatment emergent fungal infection	300 (87.5%)	301 (87.7%)
Survival through 7 days post study drug	318 (92.7%)	308 (89.5%)
Study drug not prematurely discontinued due to toxicity or lack of efficacy*	294 (85.7%)	280 (81.4%)

* 8 and 10 patients, respectively, were treated as failures due to premature discontinuation alone.

Empirical Therapy in Febrile Neutropenic Patients: Emergent Fungal Infections

	AmBisome	Amphotericin B
Number of patients receiving at least one dose of study drug	343	344
Mycologically confirmed fungal infection	11 (3.2%)	27 (7.8%)
Clinically diagnosed fungal infection	32 (9.3%)	16 (4.7%)
Total emergent fungal infections	43 (12.5%)	43 (12.5%)

AmBisome Efficacy in Visceral Leishmaniasis

Immunocompetent Patients

No. of Patients	Parasite (%) Clearance at EOT	Overall Success (%) at F/U
87	86/87 (98.9)	83/86 (96.5)

Immunocompromised Patients

Regimen	Total Dose	Parasite (%) Clearance at EOT	Overall Success (%) at FU
100 mg/day X 21 days	29.0-38.9 mg/kg	10/10 (100)	2/10 (20.0)
4 mg/kg/day, days 1-5, and 10, 17, 24, 31, 38	40 mg/kg	8/9 (88.9)	0/7 (0.0)
TOTAL		18/19 (94.7)	2/17 (11.8)

to alterations in cell permeability and cell death. While amphotericin B has a higher affinity for the ergosterol component of the fungal cell membrane, it can also bind to the cholesterol component of the mammalian cell leading to cytotoxicity. AmBisome, the liposomal preparation of amphotericin B, has been shown to penetrate the cell wall of both extracellular and intracellular forms of susceptible fungi.

Activity *In Vitro* and *In Vivo*

AmBisome has shown *in vitro* activity comparable to amphotericin B against the following organisms: *Aspergillus* species (*A. fumigatus, A. flavus*), *Candida* species (*C. albicans, C. krusei, C. lusitaniae, C. parapsilosis, C. tropicalis*), *Cryptococcus neoformans*, and *Blastomyces dermatitidis*. However, standardized techniques for susceptibility testing of antifungal agents have not been established and results of such studies do not necessarily correlate with clinical outcome.

AmBisome is active in animal models against *Aspergillus fumigatus, Candida albicans, Candida krusei, Candida lusitaniae, Cryptococcus neoformans, Blastomyces dermatitidis, Coccidioides immitis, Histoplasma capsulatum, Paracoccidioides brasiliensis, Leishmania donovani* and *Leishmania infatum*. The administration of AmBisome in these animal models demonstrated prolonged survival of infected animals, reduction of microorganisms from target organs, or a decrease in lung weight.

Drug Resistance

Mutants with decreased susceptibility to amphotericin B have been isolated from several fungal species after serial passage in culture media containing the drug, and from some patients receiving prolonged therapy. Drug combination studies *in vitro* and *in vivo* suggest that imidazoles may induce resistance to amphotericin B. However, the clinical relevance to drug resistance has not been established.

CLINICAL PHARMACOLOGY

Pharmacokinetics

The assay used to measure amphotericin B in the serum after administration of AmBisome does not distinguish amphotericin B that is complexed with the phospholipids of AmBisome from amphotericin B that is uncomplexed. The pharmacokinetic profile of amphotericin B after administration of AmBisome is based upon total serum concentrations of amphotericin B. The pharmacokinetic profile of amphotericin B was determined in febrile neutropenic cancer and bone marrow transplant patients who received 1–2 hour infusions of 1.0 to 5.0 mg/kg/day AmBisome for 3 to 20 days. The pharmacokinetics of amphotericin B after administration of AmBisome are nonlinear such that there is a greater than proportional increase in serum concentrations with an increase in dose from 1.0 to 5.0 mg/kg/day. The pharmacokinetic parameters of total amphotericin B (mean ± SD) after the first dose and at steady state are shown in the table below.

[See first table above]

Distribution

Based on total amphotericin B concentrations measured within a dosing interval (24 hours) after administration of AmBisome, the mean half-life was 7–10 hours. However, based on total amphotericin B concentration measured up to 49 days after dosing AmBisome, the mean half-life was 100–153 hours. The long terminal elimination half-life is probably a slow redistribution from tissues. Steady state concentrations were generally achieved within 4 days of dosing.

Although variable, mean trough concentrations of amphotericin B remained relatively constant with repeated administration of the same dose over the range of 1.0 to 5.0 mg/kg/day, indicating no significant drug accumulation in the serum.

Metabolism

The metabolic pathways of AmBisome are not known.

Excretion

The mean clearance at steady state was independent of dose. The excretion of amphotericin B after administration of AmBisome has not been studied.

Pharmacokinetics in Special Populations

Renal Impairment

The effect of renal impairment on the disposition of AmBisome has not been studied. However, AmBisome has been successfully administered to patients with pre-existing renal impairment (see **DESCRIPTION OF CLINICAL STUDIES**).

Hepatic Impairment

The effect of hepatic impairment on the disposition of AmBisome is not known.

Pediatric and Elderly Patients

The pharmacokinetics of amphotericin B after administration of AmBisome in pediatric and elderly patients have not been studied; however, AmBisome has been used in pediatric and elderly patients (see **DESCRIPTION OF CLINICAL STUDIES**).

Gender and Ethnicity

The effect of gender or ethnicity on the pharmacokinetics of amphotericin B after administration of AmBisome is not known.

INDICATIONS AND USAGE

AmBisome is indicated for the following:

- Empirical therapy for presumed fungal infection in febrile, neutropenic patients.
- Treatment of patients with *Aspergillus* species, *Candida* species and/or *Cryptococcus* species infections refractory to amphotericin B deoxycholate, or in patients where renal impairment or unacceptable toxicity precludes the use of amphotericin B deoxycholate.
- Treatment of visceral leishmaniasis. In immunocompromised patients with visceral leishmaniasis treated with AmBisome, relapse rates were high following initial clearance of parasites (see **DESCRIPTION OF CLINICAL STUDIES**).

See **DOSAGE AND ADMINISTRATION** for recommended doses by indication.

DESCRIPTION OF CLINICAL STUDIES

Ten clinical studies supporting the efficacy and safety of AmBisome were conducted. This clinical program included both controlled and uncontrolled clinical studies. These studies, which involved 1904 patients, included patients with confirmed systemic mycoses, empirical therapy, and visceral leishmaniasis.

Seventeen hundred and fifty episodes were evaluable for efficacy, of which 1145 (302 pediatric and 843 adults) were treated with AmBisome.

Three controlled empirical therapy trials compared the efficacy and safety of AmBisome to amphotericin B. One of these studies was conducted in a pediatric population, one in adults, and a third in patients aged 2 years or more. In addition, a controlled empirical therapy trial comparing the safety of AmBisome to Abelcet® (amphotericin B lipid complex) was conducted in patients aged 2 years or more.

One compassionate use study enrolled patients who had failed amphotericin B deoxycholate therapy or who were unable to receive amphotericin B deoxycholate because of renal insufficiency.

Empirical Therapy in Febrile Neutropenic Patients

Study 94-0-002, a randomized, double-blind, comparative multi-center trial, evaluated the efficacy of AmBisome (1.5–6.0 mg/kg/day) compared with amphotericin B deoxycholate (0.3–1.2 mg/kg/day) in the empirical treatment of 687 adult and pediatric neutropenic patients who were febrile despite having received at least 96 hours of broad spectrum antibacterial therapy. Therapeutic success required (a) resolution of fever during the neutropenic period, (b) absence of an

emergent fungal infection, (c) patient survival for at least 7 days post therapy, (d) no discontinuation of therapy due to toxicity or lack of efficacy, and (e) resolution of any study-entry fungal infection.
The overall therapeutic success rates for AmBisome and amphotericin B deoxycholate were equivalent. Results are summarized in the following table. Note: The categories presented below are not mutually exclusive.
[See second table on previous page]
This therapeutic equivalence had no apparent relationship to the use of prestudy antifungal prophylaxis or concomitant granulocytic colony stimulating factors.
The incidence of mycologically confirmed and clinically diagnosed, emergent fungal infections are presented in the following table. AmBisome and amphotericin B were found to be equivalent with respect to the total number of emergent fungal infections.
[See third table on previous page]
Mycologically confirmed fungal infections at study-entry were cured in 8 of 11 patients in the AmBisome group and 7 of 10 in the amphotericin B group.
Study 97-0-034, a randomized, double-blind, comparative multi-center trial, evaluated the safety of AmBisome (3.0 and 5.0 mg/kg/day) compared with amphotericin B lipid complex (5 mg/kg/day) in the empirical treatment of 202 adult and 42 pediatric neutropenic patients. One hundred and sixty-six patients received AmBisome (85 patients received 3 mg/kg/day and 81 received 5 mg/kg/day) and 78 patients received amphotericin B lipid complex. The study patients were febrile despite having received at least 72 hours of broad spectrum antibacterial therapy. The primary endpoint of this study was safety. The study was not designed to draw statistically meaningful conclusions related to comparative efficacy, and in fact, Abelcet is not labeled for this indication.
Two supportive prospective randomized, open label, comparative multi-center studies examined the efficacy of two dosages of AmBisome (1 and 3 mg/kg/day) compared to amphotericin B deoxycholate (1 mg/kg/day) in the treatment of neutropenic patients with presumed fungal infections. These patients were undergoing chemotherapy as part of a bone marrow transplant or had hematological disease. Study 104–10 enrolled adult patients (n=134). Study 104–14 enrolled pediatric patients (n=214). Both studies support the efficacy equivalence of AmBisome and amphotericin B as empirical therapy in febrile neutropenic patients.

Treatment of Patients with *Aspergillus* Species, *Candida* Species and/or *Cryptococcus* Species Infections Refractory to Amphotericin B Deoxycholate, or in Patients Where Renal Impairment or Unacceptable Toxicity Precludes the Use of Amphotericin B Deoxycholate

AmBisome was evaluated in a compassionate use study in hospitalized patients with systemic fungal infections. These patients either had fungal infections refractory to amphotericin B deoxycholate, were intolerant to the use of amphotericin B deoxycholate, or had pre-existing renal insufficiency. Patient recruitment involved 140 infectious episodes in 133 patients, with 53 episodes evaluable for mycological response and 91 episodes evaluable for clinical outcome. Clinical success and mycological eradication occurred in some patients with documented aspergillosis, candidiasis, and cryptococcus.

Treatment of Visceral Leishmaniasis

AmBisome was studied in patients with visceral leishmaniasis who were infected in the Mediterranean basin with documented or presumed *Leishmaniasis infantum*. Clinical studies have not provided conclusive data regarding efficacy against *L. donovani* and *L. chagasi*.
AmBisome achieved high rates of acute parasite clearance in immunocompetent patients when total doses of 12–30 mg/kg were administered. Most of these immunocompetent patients remained relapse-free during follow-up periods of 6 months or longer. While acute parasite clearance was achieved in most of the immunocompromised patients who received total doses of 30–40 mg/kg, the majority of these patients were observed to relapse in the 6 months following the completion of therapy. Of the 21 immunocompromised patients studied, 17 were coinfected with HIV; approximately half of the HIV infected patients had AIDS. The following table presents a comparison of efficacy rates among immunocompetent and immunocompromised patients infected in the Mediterranean basin who had no prior treatment or remote prior treatment for visceral leishmaniasis. Efficacy is expressed as both acute parasite clearance at the end of therapy (EOT) and as overall success (clearance with no relapse) during the follow-up period (F/U) of greater than 6 months for immunocompetent and immunocompromised patients:
[See fourth table on previous page]
When followed for 6 months or more after treatment, the overall success rate among immunocompetent patients was 96.5% and the overall success rate among immunocompromised patients was 11.8% due to relapse in the majority of patients. While case reports have suggested there may be a role for long-term therapy to prevent relapses in HIV coinfected patients (Lopez-Dupla, et al. *J. Antimicrob Chemother* 1993;32:657-659), there are no data to date documenting the efficacy or safety of repeat courses of AmBisome or of maintenance therapy with this drug among immunocompromised patients.

CONTRAINDICATIONS

AmBisome is contraindicated in those patients who have demonstrated or have known hypersensitivity to amphotericin B deoxycholate or any other constituents of the product unless, in the opinion of the treating physician, the benefit of therapy outweighs the risk.

WARNINGS

Anaphylaxis has been reported with amphotericin B deoxycholate and other amphotericin B-containing drugs, including AmBisome. If a severe anaphylactic reaction occurs, the infusion should be immediately discontinued and the patient should not receive further infusions of AmBisome.

PRECAUTIONS

General

As with any amphotericin B-containing product the drug should be administered by medically trained personnel. During the initial dosing period, patients should be under close clinical observation. AmBisome has been shown to be significantly less toxic than amphotericin B deoxycholate; however, adverse events may still occur.

Laboratory Tests

Patient management should include laboratory evaluation of renal, hepatic and hematopoietic function, and serum electrolytes (particularly magnesium and potassium).

Drug Interactions

No formal clinical studies of drug interactions have been conducted with AmBisome. However, the following drugs are known to interact with amphotericin B and may interact with AmBisome.

Antineoplastic agents: Concurrent use of antineoplastic agents may enhance the potential for renal toxicity, bronchospasm, and hypotension. Antineoplastic agents should be given concomitantly with caution.
Corticosteroids and corticotropin (ACTH): Concurrent use of corticosteroids and ACTH may potentiate hypokalemia which could predispose the patient to cardiac dysfunction. If used concomitantly, serum electrolytes and cardiac function should be closely monitored.
Digitalis glycosides: Concurrent use may induce hypokalemia and may potentiate digitalis toxicity. When administered concomitantly, serum potassium levels should be closely monitored.
Flucytosine: Concurrent use of flucytosine may increase the toxicity of flucytosine by possibly increasing its cellular uptake and/or impairing its renal excretion.
Azoles (e.g. ketoconazole, miconazole, clotrimazole, fluconazole, etc.): *In vitro* and *in vivo* animal studies of the combination of amphotericin B and imidazoles suggest that imidazoles may induce fungal resistance to amphotericin B. Combination therapy should be administered with caution, especially in immunocompromised patients.
Leukocyte transfusions: Acute pulmonary toxicity has been reported in patients simultaneously receiving intravenous amphotericin B and leukocyte transfusions.
Other nephrotoxic medications: Concurrent use of amphotericin B and other nephrotoxic medications may enhance

Continued on next page

Empirical Therapy Study 94-0-002 Common Adverse Events

Adverse Event by Body System	AmBisome n=343 %	Amphotericin B n=344 %
Body as a Whole		
Abdominal pain	19.8	21.8
Asthenia	13.1	10.8
Back pain	12.0	7.3
Blood product transfusion react.	18.4	18.6
Chills	47.5	75.9
Infection	11.1	9.3
Pain	14.0	12.8
Sepsis	14.0	11.3
Cardiovascular System		
Chest pain	12.0	11.6
Hypertension	7.9	16.3
Hypotension	14.3	21.5
Tachycardia	13.4	20.9
Digestive System		
Diarrhea	30.3	27.3
Gastrointestinal hemorrhage	9.9	11.3
Nausea	39.7	38.7
Vomiting	31.8	43.9
Metabolic and Nutritional Disorders		
Alkaline phosphatase increased	22.2	19.2
ALT (SGPT) increased	14.6	14.0
AST (SGOT) increased	12.8	12.8
Bilirubinemia	18.1	19.2
BUN increased	21.0	31.1
Creatinine increased	22.4	42.2
Edema	14.3	14.8
Hyperglycemia	23.0	27.9
Hypernatremia	4.1	11.0
Hypervolemia	12.2	15.4
Hypocalcemia	18.4	20.9
Hypokalemia	42.9	50.6
Hypomagnesemia	20.4	25.6
Peripheral edema	14.6	17.2
Nervous System		
Anxiety	13.7	11.0
Confusion	11.4	13.4
Headache	19.8	20.9
Insomnia	17.2	14.2
Respiratory System		
Cough increased	17.8	21.8
Dyspnea	23.0	29.1
Epistaxis	14.9	20.1
Hypoxia	7.6	14.8
Lung disorder	17.8	17.4
Pleural effusion	12.5	9.6
Rhinitis	11.1	11.0
Skin and Appendages		
Pruritus	10.8	10.2
Rash	24.8	24.4
Sweating	7.0	10.8
Urogenital System		
Hematuria	14.0	14.0

Ambisome—Cont.

the potential for drug-induced renal toxicity. Intensive monitoring of renal function is recommended in patients requiring any combination of nephrotoxic medications.

Skeletal muscle relaxants: Amphotericin B-induced hypokalemia may enhance the curariform effect of skeletal muscle relaxants (e.g. tubocurarine) due to hypokalemia. When administered concomitantly, serum potassium levels should be closely monitored.

Carcinogenesis, Mutagenesis, Impairment of Fertility

No long term studies in animals have been performed to evaluate carcinogenic potential of AmBisome. AmBisome has not been tested to determine its mutagenic potential. A Segment I Reproductive Study in rats found an abnormal estrous cycle (prolonged diestrus) and decreased number of corpora lutea in the high dose groups (10 and 15 mg/kg, doses equivalent to human doses of 1.6 and 2.4 mg/kg based on body surface area considerations). AmBisome did not affect fertility or days to copulation. There were no effects on male reproductive function.

Pregnancy Category B

There have been no adequate and well-controlled studies of AmBisome in pregnant women. Systemic fungal infections have been successfully treated in pregnant women with amphotericin B deoxycholate, but the number of cases reported has been small.

Segment II studies in both rats and rabbits have concluded that AmBisome had no teratogenic potential in these species. In rats, the maternal non-toxic dose of AmBisome was estimated to be 5 mg/kg (equivalent to 0.16 to 0.8 times the recommended human clinical dose range of 1 to 5 mg/kg) and in rabbits, 3 mg/kg (equivalent to 0.2 to 1 times the recommended human clinical dose range), based on body surface area correction. Rabbits receiving the higher doses, (equivalent to 0.5 to 2 times the recommended human dose) of AmBisome experienced a higher rate of spontaneous abortions than did the control groups. AmBisome should only be used during pregnancy if the possible benefits to be derived outweigh the potential risks involved.

Nursing Mothers

Many drugs are excreted in human milk. However, it is not known whether AmBisome is excreted in human milk. Due to the potential for serious adverse reactions in breast-fed infants, a decision should be made whether to discontinue nursing or whether to discontinue the drug, taking into account the importance of the drug to the mother.

Pediatric Use

Pediatric patients, age 1 month to 16 years, with presumed fungal infection (empirical therapy), confirmed systemic fungal infections or with visceral leishmaniasis have been successfully treated with AmBisome. In studies which included 302 pediatric patients administered AmBisome, there was no evidence of any differences in efficacy or safety of AmBisome compared to adults. Since pediatric patients have received AmBisome at doses comparable to those used in adults on a per kilogram body weight basis, no dosage adjustment is required in this population. Safety and effectiveness in pediatric patients below the age of one month has not been established.

(See **DESCRIPTION OF CLINICAL STUDIES—Empirical Therapy in Febrile Neutropenic Patients** and **DOSAGE AND ADMINISTRATION**.)

Elderly Patients

Experience with AmBisome in the elderly (65 years or older) comprised 71 patients. It has not been necessary to alter the dose of AmBisome for this population. As with most other drugs, elderly patients receiving AmBisome should be carefully monitored.

ADVERSE REACTIONS

The following adverse events are based on the experience of 592 adult patients (295 treated with AmBisome and 297 treated with amphotericin B deoxycholate) and 95 pediatric patients (48 treated with AmBisome and 47 treated with amphotericin B deoxycholate) in Study 94-0-002, a randomized, double-blind, multi-center study in febrile, neutropenic patients. AmBisome and amphotericin B were infused over two hours.

The incidence of common adverse events (incidence of 10% or greater) occurring with AmBisome compared to amphotericin B deoxycholate, regardless of relationship to study drug, is shown in the following table:

[See table at top of previous page]

AmBisome was well tolerated. AmBisome had a lower incidence of chills, hypertension, hypotension, tachycardia, hypoxia, hypokalemia, and various events related to decreased kidney function as compared to amphotericin B deoxycholate.

In pediatric patients (16 years of age or less) in this double-blind study, AmBisome compared to amphotericin B deoxycholate had a lower incidence of hypokalemia (37% versus 55%), chills (29% versus 68%), vomiting (27% versus 55%), and hypertension (10% versus 21%). Similar trends, although with a somewhat lower incidence, were observed in open-label, randomized Study 104-14 involving 205 febrile neutropenic pediatric patients (141 treated with AmBisome and 64 treated with amphotericin B deoxycholate). Pediatric patients appear to have more tolerance than older individuals for the nephrotoxic effects of amphotericin B deoxycholate.

Empirical Therapy Study 97-0-034
Common Adverse Events

Adverse Event by Body System	AmBisome 3 mg/kg/day n=85 %	AmBisome 5 mg/kg/day n=81 %	Amphotericin B Lipid Complex 5 mg/kg/day n=78 %
Body as a Whole			
Abdominal pain	12.9	9.9	11.5
Asthenia	8.2	6.2	11.5
Chills/rigors	40.0	48.1	89.7
Sepsis	12.9	7.4	11.5
Transfusion reaction	10.6	8.6	5.1
Cardiovascular System			
Chest pain	8.2	11.1	6.4
Hypertension	10.6	19.8	23.1
Hypotension	10.6	7.4	19.2
Tachycardia	9.4	18.5	23.1
Digestive System			
Diarrhea	15.3	17.3	14.1
Nausea	25.9	29.6	37.2
Vomiting	22.4	25.9	30.8
Metabolic and Nutritional Disorders			
Alkaline phosphatase increased	7.1	8.6	12.8
Bilirubinemia	16.5	11.1	11.5
BUN increased	20.0	18.5	28.2
Creatinine increased	20.0	18.5	48.7
Edema	12.9	12.3	12.8
Hyperglycemia	8.2	8.6	14.1
Hypervolemia	8.2	11.1	14.1
Hypocalcemia	10.6	4.9	5.1
Hypokalemia	37.6	43.2	39.7
Hypomagnesemia	15.3	25.9	15.4
Liver function tests abnormal	10.6	7.4	11.5
Nervous System			
Anxiety	10.6	7.4	9.0
Confusion	12.9	8.6	3.8
Headache	9.4	17.3	10.3
Respiratory System			
Dyspnea	17.6	22.2	23.1
Epistaxis	10.6	8.6	14.1
Hypoxia	7.1	6.2	20.5
Lung disorder	14.1	13.6	15.4
Skin and Appendages			
Rash	23.5	22.2	14.1

Incidence of Day 1 Infusion Related Reactions (IRR) By Patient Age

	Pediatric Patients (≤ 16 years of age)		Adult Patients (> 16 years of age)	
	AmBisome	Amphotericin B	AmBisome	Amphotericin B
Total number of patients receiving at least one dose of study drug	48	47	295	297
Patients with fever† Increase ≥ 1.0°C	6 (13%)	22 (47%)	52 (18%)	128 (43%)
Patients with chills/rigors	4 (8%)	22 (47%)	59 (20%)	165 (56%)
Patients with nausea	4 (8%)	4 (9%)	38 (13%)	31 (10%)
Patients with vomiting	2 (4%)	7 (15%)	19 (6%)	21 (7%)
Patients with other reactions	10 (21%)	13 (28%)	47 (16%)	69 (23%)

†Day 1 body temperature increased above the temperature taken within 1 hour prior to infusion (preinfusion temperature) or above the lowest infusion value (no preinfusion temperature recorded).

The incidence of adverse events occurring in more than 10% of subjects in one or more arms regardless of relationship to study drug are summarized in the following table:

[See first table above]

Infusion Related Reactions

In Study 94-0-002, the large, double-blind study of pediatric and adult febrile neutropenic patients, no premedication to prevent infusion related reaction was administered prior to the first dose of study drug (Day 1). AmBisome-treated patients had a lower incidence of infusion related fever (17% versus 44%), chills/rigors (18% versus 54%), and vomiting (6% versus 8%) on Day 1 as compared to amphotericin B deoxycholate-treated patients.

The incidence of infusion related reactions on Day 1 in pediatric and adult patients is summarized in the following table:

[See second table above]

Cardiorespiratory events, except for vasodilatation (flushing), during all study drug infusions were more frequent in amphotericin B-treated patients as summarized in the following table:

Incidence of Infusion Related Cardiorespiratory Events

Event	AmBisome n=343	Amphotericin B n=344
Hypotension	12 (3.5%)	28 (8.1%)
Tachycardia	8 (2.3%)	43 (12.5%)
Hypertension	8 (2.3%)	39 (11.3%)
Vasodilatation	18 (5.2%)	2 (0.6%)

Dyspnea	16 (4.7%)	25 (7.3%)
Hyperventilation	4 (1.2%)	17 (4.9%)
Hypoxia	1 (0.3%)	22 (6.4%)

The percentage of patients who received drugs either for the treatment or prevention of infusion related reactions (e.g., acetaminophen, diphenhydramine, meperidine and hydrocortisone) was lower in AmBisome-treated patients compared with amphotericin B deoxycholate-treated patients.

In the empirical therapy study 97-0-034, on Day 1, where no premedication was administered, the overall incidence of infusion related events of chills/rigors was signifcantly lower for patients administered AmBisome compared with amphotericin B lipid complex. Fever, chills/rigors and hypoxia were significantly lower for each AmBisome group compared with the amphotericin B lipid complex group. The infusion related event hypoxia was reported for 11.5% of amphotericin B lipid complex-treated patients compared with 0% of patients administered 3 mg/kg per day AmBisome and 1.2% of patients treated with 5 mg/kg per day AmBisome.

[See first table at right]

Day 1 body temperature increased above the temperature taken within 1 hour prior to infusion (preinfusion temperature) or above the lowest infusion value (no preinfusion temperature recorded).

Patients were not administered premedications to prevent infusion related reactions prior to the Day 1 study drug infusion.

There have been a few reports of flushing, back pain with or without chest tightness, and chest pain associated with AmBisome administration; on occasion this has been severe. Where these symptoms were noted, the reaction developed within a few minutes after the start of infusion and disappeared rapidly when the infusion was stopped. The symptoms do not occur with every dose and usually do not recur on subsequent administrations when the infusion rate is slowed.

Toxicity and Discontinuation of Dosing

In Study 94-0-002, a significantly lower incidence of grade 3 or 4 toxicity was observed in the AmBisome group compared with the amphotericin B group. In addition, nearly three times as many patients administered amphotericin B required a reduction in dose due to toxicity or discontinuation of study drug due to an infusion related reaction compared with those administered AmBisome.

In empirical therapy study 97-0-034, a greater proportion of patients in the amphotericin B lipid complex group discontinued the study drug due to an adverse event than in the AmBisome groups.

Less Common Adverse Events

The following adverse events also have been reported in 2% to 10% of AmBisome-treated patients receiving chemotherapy or bone marrow transplantation in five comparative, clinical trials:

Body as a Whole—abdomen enlarged, allergic reaction, cellulitis, cell mediated immunological reaction, face edema, graft versus host disease, malaise, neck pain, and procedural complication.

Cardiovascular System—arrhythmia, atrial fibrillation, bradycardia, cardiac arrest, cardiomegaly, hemorrhage, postural hypotension, valvular heart disease, vascular disorder, and vasodilatation (flushing).

Digestive System—anorexia, constipation, dry mouth/nose, dyspepsia, dysphagia, eructation, fecal incontinence, flatulence, hemorrhoids, gum/oral hemorrhage, hematemesis, hepatocellular damage, hepatomegaly, liver function test abnormal, ileus, mucositis, rectal disorder, stomatitis, ulcerative stomatitis, and veno-occlusive liver disease.

Hemic & Lymphatic System—anemia, coagulation disorder, ecchymosis, fluid overload, petechia, prothrombin decreased, prothrombin increased, and thrombocytopenia.

Metabolic & Nutritional Disorders—acidosis, amylase increased, hyperchloremia, hyperkalemia, hypermagnesemia, hyperphosphatemia, hyponatremia, hypophosphatemia, hypoproteinemia, lactate dehydrogenase increased, nonprotein nitrogen (NPN) increased, and respiratory alkalosis.

Musculoskeletal System—arthralgia, bone pain, dystonia, myalgia, and rigors.

Nervous System—agitation, coma, convulsion, cough, depression, dysesthesia, dizziness, hallucinations, nervousness, paresthesia, somnolence, thinking abnormality, and tremor.

Respiratory System—asthma, atelectasis, hemoptysis, hiccup, hyperventilation, influenza-like symptoms, lung edema, pharyngitis, pneumonia, respiratory insufficiency, respiratory failure, and sinusitis.

Skin & Appendages—alopecia, dry skin, herpes simplex, injection site inflammation, maculopapular rash, purpura, skin discoloration, skin disorder, skin ulcer, urticaria, and vesiculobullous rash.

Special Senses—conjunctivitis, dry eyes, and eye hemorrhage.

Urogenital System—abnormal renal function, acute kidney failure, acute renal failure, dysuria, kidney failure, toxic nephropathy, urinary incontinence, and vaginal hemorrhage.

The following infrequent adverse experience have been reported in post-marketing surveillance, in addition to those mentioned above: angioedema, erythema, urticaria, cyanosis/hypoventilation, pulmonary edema, agranulocytosis, hemorrhagic cystitis.

Incidence of Day 1 Infusion Related Reactions (IRR) Chills/Rigors Empirical Therapy Study 97-0-034

	AmBisome			Amphotericin B lipid complex 5 mg/kg/day
	3 mg/kg/day	5 mg/kg/day	BOTH	
Total number of patients	85	81	166	78
Patients with Chills/Rigors (Day 1)	16 (18.8%)	19 (23.5%)	35 (21.1%)	62 (79.5%)
Patients with other notable reactions:				
Fever (≥ 1.0°C increase in temperature)	20 (23.5%)	16 (19.8%)	36 (21.7%)	45 (57.7%)
Nausea	9 (10.6%)	7 (8.6%)	16 (9.6%)	9 (11.5%)
Vomiting	5 (5.9%)	5 (6.2%)	10 (6.0%)	11 (14.1%)
Hypertension	4 (4.7%)	7 (8.6%)	11 (6.6%)	12 (15.4%)
Tachycardia	2 (2.4%)	8 (9.9%)	10 (6.0%)	14 (17.9%)
Dyspnea	4 (4.7%)	8 (9.9%)	12 (7.2%)	8 (10.3%)
Hypoxia	0	1 (1.2%)	1 (<1%)	9 (11.5%)

Incidence of Nephrotoxicity Empirical Therapy Study 97-0-034

	AmBisome			Amphotericin B lipid complex 5 mg/kg/day
	3 mg/kg/day	5 mg/kg/day	BOTH	
Total number of patients	85	81	166	78
Number with nephrotoxicity				
1.5× baseline serum creatinine value	25 (29.4%)	21 (25.9%)	46 (27.7%)	49 (62.8%)
2× baseline serum creatinine value	12 (14.1%)	12 (14.8%)	24 (14.5%)	33 (42.3%)

Clinical Laboratory Values

The effect of AmBisome on renal and hepatic function and on serum electrolytes was assessed from laboratory values measured repeatedly in Study 94-0-002. The frequency and magnitude of hepatic test abnormalities were similar in the AmBisome and amphotericin B groups. Nephrotoxicity was defined as creatinine values increasing 100% or more over pretreatment levels in pediatric patients, and creatinine values increasing 100% or more over pretreatment levels in adult patients provided the peak creatinine concentration was >1.2 mg/dL. Hypokalemia was defined as potassium levels ≤2.5 mmol/L any time during treatment.

Incidence of nephrotoxicity, mean peak serum creatinine concentration, mean change from baseline in serum creatinine, and, incidence of hypokalemia in the double-blind randomized study were lower in the AmBisome group as summarized in the following table:

Study 94-0-002 Laboratory Evidence of Nephrotoxicity

	AmBisome	Amphotericin B
Total number of patients receiving at least one dose of study drug	343	344
Nephrotoxicity	64 (18.7%)	116 (33.7%)
Mean peak creatinine	1.24 mg/dL	1.52 mg/dL
Mean change from baseline in creatinine	0.48 mg/dL	0.77 mg/dL
Hypokalemia	23 (6.7%)	40 (11.6%)

The effect of AmBisome (3 mg/kg/day) vs. amphotericin B (0.6 mg/kg/day) on renal function in adult patients enrolled in this study is illustrated in the following figure:

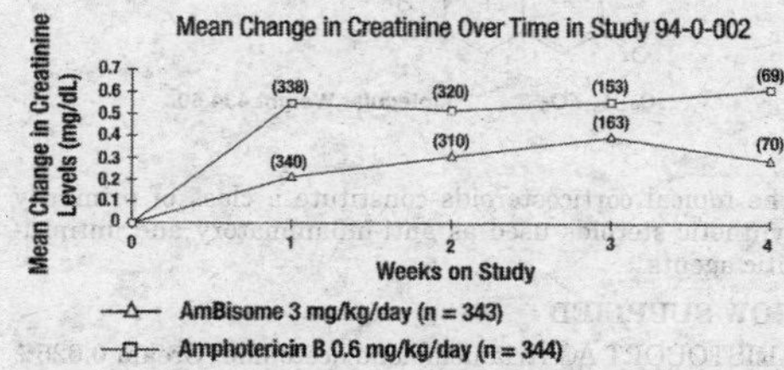

In empirical therapy study 97-0-034, the incidence of nephrotoxicity as measured by increases of serum creatinine from baseline was significantly lower for patients administered AmBisome (individual dose groups and combined) compared with amphotericin B lipid complex.

[See second table above right]

The following graph shows the average serum creatinine concentrations in the compassionate use study and shows that there is a drop from pretreatment concentrations for all patients, especially those with elevated (greater than 1.7 mg/dL) pretreatment creatinine concentrations.

[See figure at top of next column]

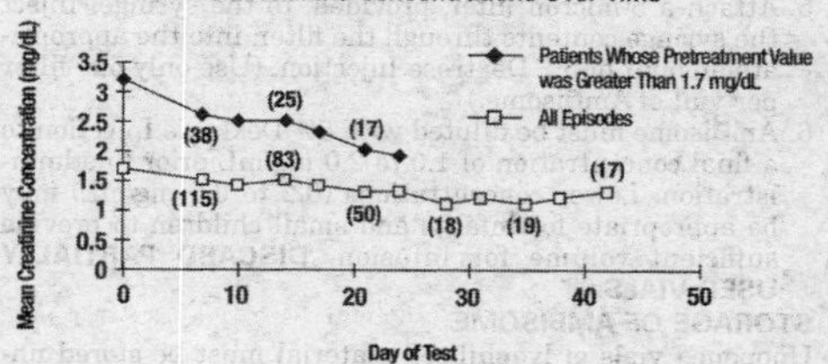

OVERDOSAGE

The toxicity of AmBisome due to overdose has not been defined. Repeated daily doses up to 7.5 mg/kg have been administered in clinical trials with no reported dose-related toxicity.

Management—If overdosage should occur, cease administration immediately. Symptomatic supportive measures should be instituted. Particular attention should be given to monitoring renal function.

DOSAGE AND ADMINISTRATION

AmBisome should be administered by intravenous infusion, using a controlled infusion device, over a period of approximately 120 minutes.

An in-line membrane filter may be used for the intravenous infusion of AmBisome; provided **THE MEAN PORE DIAMETER OF THE FILTER IS NOT LESS THAN 1.0 MICRON.**

NOTE: An existing intravenous line must be flushed with 5% Dextrose Injection prior to infusion of AmBisome. If this is not feasible, AmBisome must be administered through a separate line.

Infusion time may be reduced to approximately 60 minutes in patients in whom the treatment is well-tolerated. If the patient experiences discomfort during infusion, the duration of infusion may be increased.

The recommended initial dose of AmBisome for each indication for adult and pediatric patients is as follows:

Indication	Dose (mg/kg/day)
Empirical therapy	3.0
Systemic fungal infections: *Aspergillus* *Candida* *Cryptococcus*	3.0-5.0

Dosing and rate of infusion should be individualized to the needs of the specific patient to ensure maximum efficacy while minimizing systemic toxicities or adverse events.

Doses recommended for visceral leishmaniasis are presented below:

Continued on next page

Ambisome—Cont.

Visceral Leishmaniasis	Dose (mg/kg/day)
Immunocompetent patients	3.0 (days 1-5) and 3.0 on days 14, 21
Immunocompromised patients	4.0 (days 1-5) and 4.0 on days 10, 17, 24, 31, 38

For immunocompetent patients who do not achieve parasitic clearance with the recommended dose, a repeat course of therapy may be useful.
For immunocompromised patients who do not clear parasites or who experience relapses, expert advice regarding further treatment is recommended. For additional information see **DESCRIPTION OF CLINICAL STUDIES.**

Directions for Reconstitution, Filtration and Dilution

Read This Entire Section Carefully Before Beginning Reconstitution

AmBisome **must** be reconstituted using Sterile Water for Injection, USP (without a bacteriostatic agent). Vials of AmBisome containing 50 mg of amphotericin B are prepared as follows:

Reconstitution

1. Aseptically add 12 mL of Sterile Water for Injection, USP to each AmBisome vial to yield a preparation containing 4 mg amphotericin B/mL.

CAUTION: DO NOT RECONSTITUTE WITH SALINE OR ADD SALINE TO THE RECONSTITUTED CONCENTRATION, OR MIX WITH OTHER DRUGS. The use of any solution other than those recommended, or the presence of a bacteriostatic agent in the solution, may cause precipitation of AmBisome.

2. **Immediately after the addition of water, SHAKE THE VIAL VIGOROUSLY** for 30 seconds to completely disperse the AmBisome. AmBisome forms a yellow, translucent suspension. Visually inspect the vial for particulate matter and continue shaking until completely dispersed.

Filtration and Dilution

3. Calculate the amount of reconstituted (4 mg/mL) AmBisome to be further diluted.
4. Withdraw this amount of reconstituted AmBisome into a sterile syringe.
5. Attach a 5-micron filter, provided, to the syringe. Inject the syringe contents through the filter, into the appropriate amount of 5% Dextrose Injection. (Use only one filter per vial of AmBisome.)
6. AmBisome must be diluted with 5% Dextrose Injection to a final concentration of 1.0 to 2.0 mg/mL prior to administration. Lower concentrations (0.2 to 0.5 mg/mL) may be appropriate for infants and small children to provide sufficient volume for infusion. **DISCARD PARTIALLY USED VIALS.**

STORAGE OF AMBISOME

Unopened vials of lyophilized material must be stored under refrigeration at 2°–8° C (36°–46° F).

Storage of Reconstituted Product Concentrate

The reconstituted product concentrate may be stored for up to 24 hours at 2°–8° C (36°–46° F) following reconstitution with Sterile Water for Injection, USP. Do not freeze.

Storage of Diluted Product

Injection of AmBisome should commence within 6 hours of dilution with 5% Dextrose Injection.
As with all parenteral drug products, the reconstituted AmBisome should be inspected visually for particulate matter and discoloration prior to administration, whenever solution and container permit. Do not use material if there is any evidence of precipitation or foreign matter. Aseptic technique must be strictly observed in all handling since no preservative or bacteriostatic agent is present in AmBisome or in the materials specified for reconstitution and dilution.

HOW SUPPLIED

AmBisome for Injection is available as single 50 mg vial cartons and in packs of ten individual vial cartons (NDC 0469-3051-30).
Each carton contains one pre-packaged, disposable sterile 5 micron filter.
Rx only
Manufactured for:
Fujisawa Healthcare, Inc.
Deerfield, IL 60015-2548
http://www.AmBisome.com
by:
Gilead Sciences, Inc.
San Dimas, CA 91773
AmBisome® is a registered trademark of Gilead Sciences, Inc.
003 Revised February 2000
Abelcet® is a registered trademark of the Liposome Company, Inc.

Shown in Product Identification Guide, page 313

ARISTOCORT® ℞

[*a-ris-tō-cort*]
sterile triamcinolone diacetate
Suspension 25 mg/mL
Intralesional
NOT FOR INTRAVENOUS USE

DESCRIPTION

ARISTOCORT triamcinolone diacetate possesses glucocorticoid properties while being essentially devoid of mineralocorticoid activity thus causing little or no sodium retention. Supplied as a sterile suspension of 25 mg/mL micronized triamcinolone diacetate in the following vehicle:

Polysorbate 80	0.20%
Polyethylene Glycol 3350	3%
Sodium Chloride	0.85%
Benzyl Alcohol (preservative)	0.90%
Water for Injection q.s.	100%

Hydrochloric acid and/or sodium hydroxide may be used during manufacture to adjust pH of suspension to approximately 6.
Chemically triamcinolone diacetate is 9-Fluoro-11β,16α, 17,21-tetrahydroxypregna-1,4-diene-3,20-dione 16,21-diacetate.
Molecular weight is 478.51. Its structural formula is:

HOW SUPPLIED

ARISTOCORT® (sterile triamcinolone diacetate) suspension, 25 mg/mL, Intralesional, NOT FOR INTRAVENOUS USE.
NDC 0469-5117-05 Product Code 511705
5 mL Vial
Store at Controlled Room Temperature 15°–30°C (59°–86°F).
DO NOT FREEZE.
Rx only
Manufactured for Fujisawa Healthcare, Inc., Deerfield, IL 60015,
by
Lederle Parenterals, Inc.,
Carolina, Puerto Rico 00987
CI 6023-1 Issued April 2, 1999

ARISTOCORT A® ℞

[*a-ris-tō-cort*]
(triamcinolone acetonide)
0.025% CREAM
with AQUATAIN™ hydrophilic base

DESCRIPTION

0.025% TOPICAL CREAM
Each gram of ARISTOCORT A Topical Cream contains 0.25 mg of the highly active steroid Triamcinolone Acetonide (a derivative of triamcinolone) in AQUATAIN, a specially formulated cream base composed of Emulsifying Wax, Isopropyl Palmitate, Glycerin, Sorbitol Solution, Lactic Acid, 2% Benzyl Alcohol and Purified Water. AQUATAIN is non-staining, water-washable, paraben-free, spermaceti-free and has a light texture and consistency.
Triamcinolone acetonide is (11β, 16α)-9-fluoro-11, 21-dihydroxy-16,17-[(1-methylethylidene)bis(oxy)]pregna-1, 4-diene-3,20-dione. Its structural formula is:

$C_{24}H_{31}FO_6$ Molecular Weight 434.50

The topical corticosteroids constitute a class of primarily synthetic steroids used as anti-inflammatory and antipruritic agents.

HOW SUPPLIED

ARISTOCORT A® (triamcinolone acetonide) Cream 0.025% (0.25 mg/g) with AQUATAIN™ hydrophilic base.
NDC 0469-5101-15 Product Code 510115
15 g tube
NDC 0469-5101-60 Product Code 510160
60 g tube
Store at Controlled Room Temperature 15°–30°C (59°–86°F).
Rx only
DO NOT FREEZE.
Manufactured for Fujisawa Healthcare, Inc., Deerfield, IL 60015,
Revised: July 1998/127458

ARISTOCORT® Forte ℞

[*a-ris-tō-cort*]
(sterile triamcinolone diacetate)
Suspension 40 mg/mL
Parenteral
NOT FOR INTRAVENOUS USE

DESCRIPTION

A sterile suspension of 40 mg/mL of triamcinolone diacetate (micronized) suspended in a vehicle consisting of:

Polysorbate 80	0.20%
Polyethylene Glycol 3350	3%
Sodium Chloride	0.85%
Benzyl Alcohol (preservative)	0.90%
Water for Injection q.s.	100%

Hydrochloric acid and/or sodium hydroxide may be used during manufacture to adjust pH of suspension to approximately 6.
This preparation is a slightly soluble suspension suitable for parenteral administration through a 24-gauge needle (or larger), but NOT suitable for intravenous use. It may be administered by the intramuscular, intra-articular, or intrasynovial routes, depending upon the situation. The response to each glucocorticoid varies considerably with each type of disease indication and each corticosteroid prescribed.
Irreversible clumping occurs when product is frozen.
Chemically triamcinolone diacetate is 9-Fluoro-11β, 16α, 17,21-tetrahydroxypregna-1,4-diene-3,20-dione 16,21-diacetate.
Molecular weight is 478.51. Its structural formula is:

HOW SUPPLIED

ARISTOCORT® FORTE (sterile triamcinolone diacetate) suspension, 40 mg/mL, Parenteral, NOT FOR INTRAVENOUS USE.
NDC 0469-5116-01 Product Code 511601
1 mL Vial
NDC 0469-5116-05 Product Code 511605
5 mL Vial
Store at Controlled Room Temperature 15°–30°C (59°–86°F).
DO NOT FREEZE.
Irreversible clumping occurs when product is frozen.
Rx only
Manufactured for Fujisawa Healthcare, Inc.,
Deerfield, IL 60015,
by
Lederle Parenterals, Inc.,
Carolina, Puerto Rico 00987
CI 6022-1 Issued April 2, 1999

ARISTOCORT A® ℞

[*a-ris-tō-cort*]
(triamcinolone acetonide)
0.1% OINTMENT
with PROPYLENE GLYCOL

DESCRIPTION

0.1% TOPICAL OINTMENT
Each gram of ARISTOCORT A Topical Ointment contains 1 mg of the highly active steroid Triamcinolone Acetonide (a derivative of triamcinolone) in a specially formulated ointment base composed of White Petrolatum, USP, Propylene Glycol, Emulsifying Wax, Tenox II (butylated hydroxyanisole, propyl gallate, citric acid, propylene glycol) and Lactic Acid.
Triamcinolone acetonide is (11β,16α)-9-fluoro-11,21-dihydroxy -16,17-[(1-methylethylidene)bis (oxy)] pregna-1,4 - diene-3,20-dione.
Its structural formula is:

$C_{24}H_{31}FO_6$ Molecular Weight 434.50

The topical corticosteroids constitute a class of primarily synthetic steroids used as anti-inflammatory and antipruritic agents.

HOW SUPPLIED

ARISTOCORT A® (triamcinolone acetonide) Ointment 0.1% (1 mg/g) with Propylene Glycol
NDC 0469-5105-15 Product Code 510515
15 g tube

NDC 0469-5105-60 Product Code 510560
60 g tube
Store at Controlled Room Temperature 15°–30°C (59–86°F).
Rx only
Manufactured for Fujisawa Healthcare, Inc., Deerfield, IL 60015,
Revised: December 1998/127453

ARISTOCORT A® ℞

[*a-ris-tō-cort*]
(triamcinolone acetonide)
0.1% CREAM
with AQUATAIN™ hydrophilic base

DESCRIPTION

0.1% TOPICAL CREAM
Each gram of ARISTOCORT A Topical Cream contains 1 mg of the highly active steroid Triamcinolone Acetonide (a derivative of triamcinolone) in AQUATAIN, a specially formulated cream base composed of Emulsifying Wax, Isopropyl Palmitate, Glycerin, Sorbitol Solution, Lactic Acid, 2% Benzyl Alcohol and Purified Water. AQUATAIN is non-staining, water-washable, paraben-free, spermaceti-free and has a light texture and consistency.
Triamcinolone acetonide is (11β,16α)-9-fluoro-11,21-dihydroxy-16,17- [(1-methylethylidene)bis(oxy)]pregna-1,4-diene-3,20-dione. Its structural formula is:

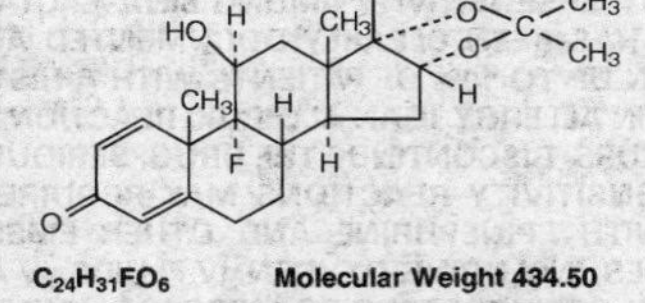

$C_{24}H_{31}FO_6$ Molecular Weight 434.50

The topical corticosteroids constitute a class of primarily synthetic steroids used as anti-inflammatory and antipruritic agents.

HOW SUPPLIED

ARISTOCORT A® (triamcinolone acetonide) Cream 0.1% (1 mg/g) with AQUATAIN™ hydrophilic base
NDC 0469-5102-15 Product Code 510215
15 g tube
NDC 0469-5102-60 Product Code 510260
60 g tube
NDC 0469-5102-24 Product Code 510324
240 g jar
Store at Controlled Room Temperature 15°–30°C (59°–86°F).
Rx only
DO NOT FREEZE.
Manufactured for Fujisawa Healthcare, Inc., Deerfield, IL 60015,
Revised: July 1998/127451

ARISTOCORT A® ℞

[*a-ris-tō-cort*]
(triamcinolone acetonide)
0.5% CREAM with AQUATAIN™ hydrophilic base

DESCRIPTION

0.5% TOPICAL CREAM
Each gram of ARISTOCORT A Topical Cream contains 5 mg of the highly active steroid Triamcinolone Acetonide (a derivative of triamcinolone) in AQUATAIN, a specially formulated cream base composed of Emulsifying Wax, Isopropyl Palmitate, Glycerin, Sorbitol Solution, Lactic Acid, 2% Benzyl Alcohol and Purified Water. AQUATAIN is non-staining, water-washable, paraben-free, spermaceti-free and has a light texture and consistency.
Triamcinolone acetonide is (11β, 16α)-9-fluoro-11,21-dihydroxy-16, 17-[(1-methylethylidene)bis(oxy)]pregna-1,4-diene-3,20-dione. Its structural formula is:

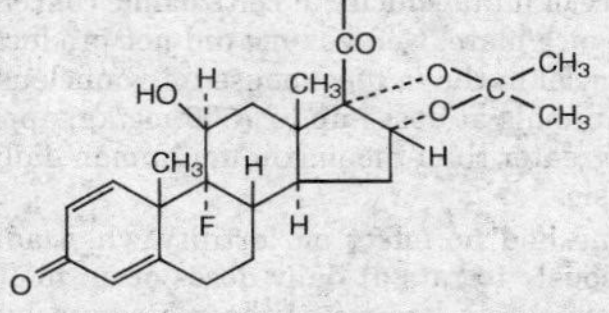

$C_{24}H_{31}FO_6$ Molecular Weight 434.50

The topical corticosteroids constitute a class of primarily synthetic steroids used as anti-inflammatory and antipruritic agents.

HOW SUPPLIED

ARISTOCORT A® (triamcinolone acetonide) Cream 0.5% (5 mg/g) with AQUATAIN™ hydrophilic base
NDC 0469-5104-15 Product Code 510415
15 g tube
Store at Controlled Room Temperature 15°–30°C (59°–86°F).
Rx only
DO NOT FREEZE.
Manufactured for Fujisawa Healthcare, Inc., Deerfield, IL 60015,
Revised: July 1998/127452

ARISTOSPAN® ℞

[*a-ris-tō-span*]
(sterile triamcinolone hexacetonide)
Suspension 5 mg/mL
Parenteral For Intralesional Use
NOT FOR INTRAVENOUS USE

DESCRIPTION

A sterile suspension containing 5 mg/mL of micronized triamcinolone hexacetonide in the following inactive ingredients:

Polysorbate 80	0.20%
Sorbitol Solution	50%
Benzyl Alcohol (preservative)	0.90%
Water for Injection q.s.	100%

Hydrochloric Acid and Sodium Hydroxide, if required, to adjust pH to 4.5–6.5.
The hexacetonide ester of the potent glucocorticoid triamcinolone is relatively insoluble (0.0002% at 25°C in water). When injected intralesionally or sublesionally, it can be expected to be absorbed slowly from the injection site.
Chemically triamcinolone hexacetonide is 9-Fluoro-11β, 16α, 17,21- tetrahydroxypregna-1,4-diene-3,20-dione cyclic 16,17-acetal with acetone 21-(3,3-dimethylbutyrate). Molecular weight is 532.65. The structural formula is:

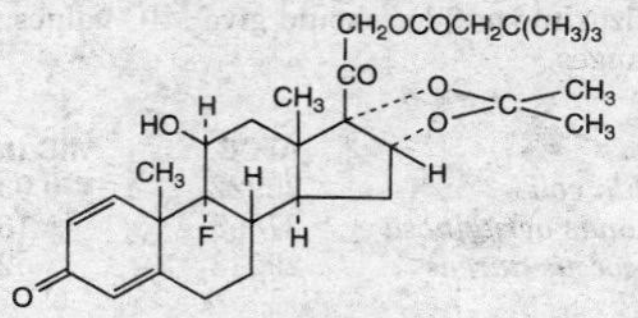

HOW SUPPLIED

ARISTOSPAN® (sterile triamcinolone hexacetonide) suspension, 5 mg/mL, for Intralesional Use. NOT FOR INTRAVENOUS USE.
NDC 0469-5118-05 Product Code 511805
5 mL Vial
Store at Controlled Room Temperature 15–30°C (59–86°F).
DO NOT FREEZE.
Rx only
Manufactured for Fujisawa Healthcare, Inc., Deerfield, IL 60015,
by
Lederle Parenterals, Inc.,
Carolina, Puerto Rico 00987
CI 6024-1 Issued April 2, 1999

ARISTOSPAN® ℞

[*a-ris-tō-span*]
(sterile triamcinolone hexacetonide)
Suspension 20 mg/mL
Parenteral For Intra-articular Use
NOT FOR INTRAVENOUS USE

DESCRIPTION

A sterile suspension containing 20 mg/mL of micronized triamcinolone hexacetonide in the following inactive ingredients:

Polysorbate 80	0.40%
Sorbitol Solution	50%
Benzyl Alcohol (preservative)	0.90%
Water for Injection q.s.	100%

Hydrochloric Acid and Sodium Hydroxide, if required, to adjust pH to 4.5–6.5.
The hexacetonide ester of the potent glucocorticoid triamcinolone is relatively insoluble (0.0002% at 25°C in water). When injected intra-articularly, it can be expected to be absorbed slowly from the injection site.
Chemically triamcinolone hexacetonide is 9-Fluoro-11β, 16α, 17,21-tetrahydroxypregna-1,4-diene-3,20-dione cyclic 16,17-acetal with acetone 21-(3,3-dimethylbutyrate). Molecular weight is 532.65. The structural formula is:

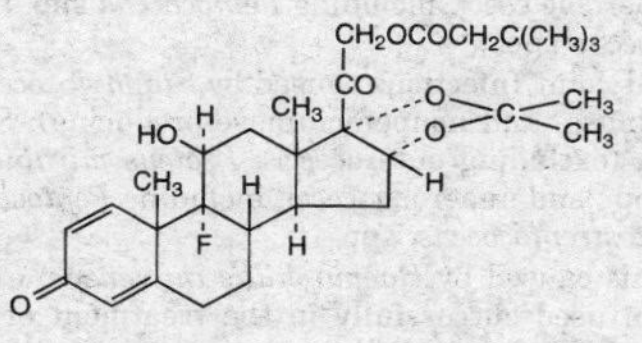

HOW SUPPLIED

ARISTOSPAN® (sterile triamcinolone hexacetonide) suspension 20 mg/mL, for Intra-articular Use. NOT FOR INTRAVENOUS USE.
NDC 0469-5119-01 Product Code 511901
1 mL Vial
NDC 0469-5119-05 Product Code 511905
5 mL vial
Store at Controlled Room Temperature 15–30°C (59–86°F).
DO NOT FREEZE.
Rx only
Manufactured for Fujisawa Healthcare, Inc.,
Deerfield, IL 60015,
by
Lederle Parenterals, Inc.,
Carolina, Puerto Rico 00987
CI 6025-1 Issued April 2, 1999

CEFIZOX® ℞

(CEFTIZOXIME FOR INJECTION, USP)
FOR INTRAMUSCULAR OR INTRAVENOUS USE

DESCRIPTION

Cefizox® (ceftizoxime for injection, USP) is a sterile, semisynthetic, broad-spectrum, beta-lactamase resistant cephalosporin antibiotic for parenteral (IV, IM) administration. It is the sodium salt of [6R-[6a, 7β(Z)]]-7-[[(2,3-dihydro-2-imino-4-thiazolyl) (methoxyimino) acetyl] amino]-8-oxo-5-thia-1-azabicyclo [4.2.0] oct-2-ene-2-carboxylic acid. Its sodium content is approximately 60 mg (2.6 mEq) per gram of ceftizoxime activity.
It has the following structural formula:

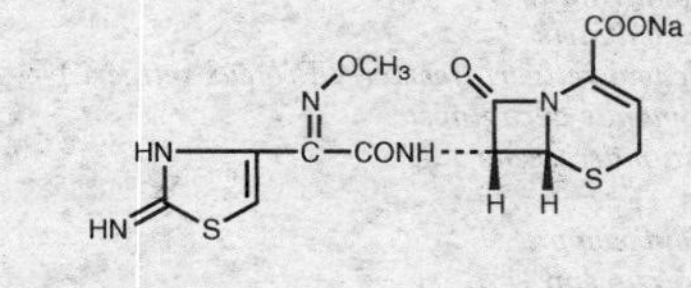

$C_{13}H_{12}N_5NaO_5S_2$ 405.38

Ceftizoxime for injection, USP is a white to pale yellow crystalline powder.
Cefizox is supplied in vials equivalent to 500 mg, 1 gram or 2 grams of ceftizoxime, and in Piggyback Vials for IV admixture equivalent to 1 gram or 2 grams of ceftizoxime.

CLINICAL PHARMACOLOGY

The table below demonstrates the serum levels and duration of Cefizox (ceftizoxime for injection, USP) following IM administration of 500 mg and 1 gram doses, respectively, to normal volunteers.

Serum Concentrations After Intramuscular Administration
Serum Concentration (mcg/mL)

Dose	½ hr	1 hr	2 hr	4 hr	6 hr	8 hr
500 mg	13.3	13.7	9.2	4.8	1.9	0.7
1 gm	36.0	39.0	31.0	15.0	6.0	3.0

Following intravenous administration of 1, 2, and 3 gram doses of Cefizox to normal volunteers, the following serum levels were obtained.

Serum Concentrations After Intravenous Administration
Serum Concentration (mcg/mL)

Dose	5 min	10 min	30 min	1 hr	2 hr	4 hr	8 hr
1 gram	ND	ND	60.5	38.9	21.5	8.4	1.4
2 grams	131.8	110.9	77.5	53.6	33.1	12.1	2.0
3 grams	221.1	174.0	112.7	83.9	47.4	26.2	4.8

ND=Not Done

A serum half-life of approximately 1.7 hours was observed after IV or IM administration.
Cefizox is 30% protein bound.
Cefizox is not metabolized, and is excreted virtually unchanged by the kidneys in 24 hours. This provides a high urinary concentration. Concentrations greater than 6000 mcg/mL have been achieved in the urine by 2 hours after a 1 gram dose of Cefizox intravenously. Probenecid slows tubular secretion and produces even higher serum levels, increasing the duration of measurable serum concentrations.
Cefizox achieves therapeutic levels in various body fluids, e.g., cerebrospinal fluid (in patients with inflamed meninges), bile, surgical wound fluid, pleural fluid, aqueous humor, ascitic fluid, peritoneal fluid, prostatic fluid and saliva, and in the following body tissues: heart, gallbladder, bone, biliary, peritoneal, prostatic, and uterine.
In clinical experience to date, no disulfiram-like reactions have been reported with Cefizox.

Microbiology

The bactericidal action of Cefizox (ceftizoxime for injection, USP) results from inhibition of cell-wall synthesis. Cefizox is highly resistant to a broad spectrum of beta-lactamases

Continued on next page

Cefizox for IM/IV Use—Cont.

(penicillinase and cephalosporinase), including Richmond types I, II, III, TEM, and IV, produced by both aerobic and anaerobic gram-positive and gram-negative organisms. Cefizox is active against a wide range of gram-positive and gram-negative organisms, and is usually active against the following organisms *in vitro* and in clinical situations (see **INDICATIONS AND USAGE**).

Gram-Positive Aerobes
- *Staphylococcus aureus* (including penicillinase- and nonpenicillinase-producing strains)
- NOTE: Methicillin-resistant staphylococci are resistant to cephalosporins, including ceftizoxime.
- *Staphylococcus epidermidis* (including penicillinase- and nonpenicillinase-producing strains)
- *Streptococcus agalactiae*
- *Streptococcus pneumoniae*
- *Streptococcus pyogenes*
- NOTE: Ceftizoxime is usually inactive against most strains of *Enterococcus faecalis* (formerly *S. faecalis*).

Gram-Negative Aerobes
- *Acinetobacter spp.*
- *Enterobacter spp.*
- *Escherichia coli*
- *Haemophilus influenzae* (including ampicillin-resistant strains)
- *Klebsiella pneumoniae*
- *Morganella morganii (formerly Proteus morganii*)
- *Neisseria gonorrhoeae*
- *Proteus mirabilis*
- *Proteus vulgaris*
- *Providencia rettgeri (formerly Proteus rettgeri*)
- *Pseudomonas aeruginosa*
- *Serratia marcescens*

Anaerobes
- *Bacteroides spp.*
- *Peptococcus spp.*
- *Peptostreptococcus spp.*

Ceftizoxime is usually active against the following organisms *in vitro*, but the clinical significance of these data is unknown.

Gram-Positive Aerobes
- *Corynebacterium diphtheriae*

Gram-Negative Aerobes
- *Aeromonas hydrophila*
- *Citrobacter spp.*
- *Moraxella spp.*
- *Neisseria meningitidis*
- *Pasteurella multocida*
- *Providencia stuartii*
- *Salmonella spp.*
- *Shigella spp.*
- *Yersinia enterocolitica*

Anaerobes
- *Actinomyces spp.*
- *Bifidobacterium spp.*
- *Clostridium spp.*
- NOTE: Most strains of *Clostridium difficile* are resistant.
- *Eubacterium spp.*
- *Fusobacterium spp.*
- *Propionibacterium spp.*
- *Veillonella spp.*

Susceptibility Testing: Diffusion Techniques

Quantitative methods that require measurement of zone diameters give the most precise estimate of the susceptibility of bacteria to antimicrobial agents. One such standard procedure[1] has been recommended for use with disks to test susceptibility of organisms to ceftizoxime. Interpretation involves the correlation of the diameters obtained in the disk test with the minimum inhibitory concentration (MIC) for ceftizoxime.

Organisms should be tested with the ceftizoxime disk, since ceftizoxime has been shown by *in vitro* tests to be active against certain strains found resistant when other beta-lactam disks are used.

Reports from the laboratory giving results of the standard single-disk susceptibility test with a 30 mcg ceftizoxime disk should be interpreted according to the following criteria (with the exception of *Pseudomonas aeruginosa*).

Zone Diameter (mm)	Interpretation
≥20	(S) Susceptible
15–19	(MS) Moderately Susceptible
≤14	(R) Resistant

A report of "Susceptible" indicates that the pathogen is likely to be inhibited by generally achievable blood levels. A report of "Moderately Susceptible" suggests that the organism would be susceptible if high dosage is used or if the infection is confined to tissue and fluids (e.g., urine) in which high antibiotic levels are attained. A report of "Resistant" indicates that achievable concentrations of the antibiotic are unlikely to be inhibitory and other therapy should be selected.

Standardized procedures require the use of laboratory control organisms. The 30 mcg ceftizoxime disk should give the following zone diameters.

Organism	ATCC	Zone Diameter (mm)
Escherichia coli	25922	30–36
Pseudomonas aeruginosa	27853	12–17
Staphylococcus aureus	25923	27–35

Susceptibility Testing for Pseudomonas in Urinary Tract Infections

Most strains of *Pseudomonas aeruginosa* are moderately susceptible to ceftizoxime. Ceftizoxime achieves high levels in the urine (greater than 6000 mcg/mL at 2 hours with 1 gram IV) and, therefore, the following zone sizes should be used when testing ceftizoxime for treatment of urinary tract infections caused by *Pseudomonas aeruginosa.*

Susceptible organisms produce zones of 20 mm or greater, indicating that the test organism is likely to respond to therapy.

Organisms that produce zones of 11 to 19 mm are expected to be susceptible when the infection is confined to the urinary tract (in which high antibiotic levels are attained).

Resistant organisms produce zones of 10 mm or less, indicating that other therapy should be selected.

Susceptibility Testing: Dilution Techniques

When using the NCCLS agar dilution or broth dilution (including microdilution) method[2] or equivalent, the following MIC data should be used for interpretation.

MIC (mcg/mL)	Interpretation
≤8	(S) Susceptible
16–32	(MS) Moderately Susceptible
≥64	(R) Resistant

As with standard disk diffusion methods, dilution procedures require the use of laboratory control organisms. Standard ceftizoxime powder should give MIC values in the following ranges.

Organism	ATCC	MIC (mcg/mL)
Escherichia coli	25922	0.03–0.12
Pseudomonas aeruginosa	27853	16–64
Staphylococcus aureus	29213	2–8

INDICATIONS AND USAGE

Cefizox (ceftizoxime for injection, USP) is indicated in the treatment of infections due to susceptible strains of the microorganisms listed below.

Lower Respiratory Tract Infections caused by *Klebsiella* spp.; *Proteus mirabilis; Escherichia coli; Haemophilus influenzae* including ampicillin-resistant strains; *Staphylococcus aureus* (penicillinase- and nonpenicillinase-producing); *Serratia* spp.; *Enterobacter* spp.; *Bacteroides* spp.; and *Streptococcus* spp. including *S. pneumoniae,* but excluding enterococci.

Urinary Tract Infections caused by *Staphylococcus aureus* (penicillinase- and nonpenicillinase-producing); *Escherichia coli; Pseudomonas* spp. including *P. aeruginosa; Proteus mirabilis; P. vulgaris; Providencia rettgeri* (formerly *Proteus rettgeri*) and *Morganella morganii* (formerly *Proteus morganii*); *Klebsiella* spp.; *Serratia* spp. including *S. marcescens;* and *Enterobacter* spp.

Gonorrhea including uncomplicated cervical and urethral gonorrhea caused by *Neisseria gonorrhoeae.*

Pelvic Inflammatory Disease caused by *Neisseria gonorrhoeae, Escherichia coli* or *Streptococcus agalactiae.*

NOTE: Ceftizoxime, like other cephalosporins, has no activity against *Chlamydia trachomatis.* Therefore, when cephalosporins are used in the treatment of patients with pelvic inflammatory disease and *C. trachomatis* is one of the suspected pathogens, appropriate anti-chlamydial coverage should be added.

Intra-Abdominal Infections caused by *Escherichia coli; Staphylococcus epidermidis; Streptococcus* spp. (excluding enterococci); *Enterobacter* spp.; *Klebsiella* spp.; *Bacteroides* spp. including *B. fragilis;* and anaerobic cocci, including *Peptococcus* spp. and *Peptostreptococcus* spp.

Septicemia caused by *Streptococcus* spp. including *S. pneumoniae* (but excluding enterococci); *Staphylococcus aureus* (penicillinase- and nonpenicillinase-producing); *Escherichia coli; Bacteroides* spp. including *B. fragilis; Klebsiella* spp.; and *Serratia* spp.

Skin and Skin Structure Infections caused by *Staphylococcus aureus* (penicillinase- and nonpenicillinase-producing); *Staphylococcus epidermidis; Escherichia coli; Klebsiella* spp.; *Streptococcus* spp. including *Streptococcus pyogenes* (but excluding enterococci); *Proteus mirabilis; Serratia* spp.; *Enterobacter* spp.; *Bacteroides* spp. including *B. fragilis;* and anaerobic cocci, including *Peptococcus* spp. and *Peptostreptococcus* spp.

Bone and Joint Infections caused by *Staphylococcus aureus* (penicillinase- and nonpenicillinase-producing); *Streptococcus* spp. (excluding enterococci); *Proteus mirabilis; Bacteroides* spp.; and anaerobic cocci, including *Peptococcus* spp. and *Peptostreptococcus* spp.

Meningitis caused by *Haemophilus influenzae.* Cefizox has also been used successfully in the treatment of a limited number of pediatric and adult cases of meningitis caused by *Streptococcus pneumoniae.*

Cefizox has been effective in the treatment of seriously ill, compromised patients, including those who were debilitated, immunosuppressed, or neutropenic.

Infections caused by aerobic gram-negative and by mixtures of organisms resistant to other cephalosporins, aminoglycosides, or penicillins have responded to treatment with Cefizox.

Because of the serious nature of some urinary tract infections due to *P. aeruginosa* and because many strains of *Pseudomonas* species are only moderately susceptible to Cefizox, higher dosage is recommended. Other therapy should be instituted if the response is not prompt.

Susceptibility studies on specimens obtained prior to therapy should be used to determine the response of causative organisms to Cefizox. Therapy with Cefizox may be initiated pending results of the studies; however, treatment should be adjusted according to study findings. In serious infections, Cefizox has been used concomitantly with aminoglycosides (see **PRECAUTIONS**). Before using Cefizox concomitantly with other antibiotics, the prescribing information for those agents should be reviewed for contraindications, warnings, precautions, and adverse reactions. Renal function should be carefully monitored.

CONTRAINDICATIONS

Cefizox (ceftizoxime for injection, USP) is contraindicated in patients who have known allergy to the drug.

WARNINGS

BEFORE THERAPY WITH CEFIZOX IS INSTITUTED, CAREFUL INQUIRY SHOULD BE MADE TO DETERMINE WHETHER THE PATIENT HAS HAD PREVIOUS HYPERSENSITIVITY REACTIONS TO CEFIZOX, OTHER CEPHALOSPORINS, PENICILLINS, OR OTHER DRUGS. IF THIS PRODUCT IS TO BE GIVEN TO PENICILLIN–SENSITIVE PATIENTS, CAUTION SHOULD BE EXERCISED BECAUSE CROSS HYPERSENSITIVITY AMONG BETA–LACTAM ANTIBIOTICS HAS BEEN CLEARLY DOCUMENTED AND MAY OCCUR IN UP TO 10% OF PATIENTS WITH A HISTORY OF PENICILLIN ALLERGY. IF AN ALLERGIC REACTION TO CEFIZOX OCCURS, DISCONTINUE THE DRUG. SERIOUS ACUTE HYPERSENSITIVITY REACTIONS MAY REQUIRE TREATMENT WITH EPINEPHRINE AND OTHER EMERGENCY MEASURES, INCLUDING OXYGEN, IV FLUIDS, IV ANTIHISTAMINES, CORTICOSTEROIDS, PRESSOR AMINES, AND AIRWAY MANAGEMENT, AS CLINICALLY INDICATED.

Pseudomembranous colitis has been reported with nearly all antibacterial agents, including ceftizoxime, and may range in severity from mild to life threatening. Therefore, it is important to consider this diagnosis in patients who present with diarrhea subsequent to the administration of antibacterial agents.

Treatment with antibacterial agents alters the normal flora of the colon and may permit overgrowth of clostridia. Studies indicate that a toxin produced by *Clostridium difficile* is a primary cause of "antibiotic-associated" colitis.

After the diagnosis of pseudomembranous colitis has been established, appropriate therapeutic measures should be initiated. Mild cases of pseudomembranous colitis usually respond to drug discontinuation alone. In moderate to severe cases, consideration should be given to management with fluids and electrolytes, protein supplementation, and treatment with an antibacterial drug clinically effective against *Clostridium difficile* colitis.

PRECAUTIONS

General

As with all broad-spectrum antibiotics, Cefizox (ceftizoxime for injection, USP) should be prescribed with caution in individuals with a history of gastrointestinal disease, particularly colitis.

Although Cefizox has not been shown to produce an alteration in renal function, renal status should be evaluated, especially in seriously ill patients receiving maximum dose therapy. As with any antibiotic, prolonged use may result in overgrowth of nonsusceptible organisms. Careful observation is essential; appropriate measures should be taken if superinfection occurs.

Drug Interactions

Although the occurrence has not been reported with Cefizox, nephrotoxicity has been reported following concomitant administration of other cephalosporins and aminoglycosides.

Carcinogenesis, Mutagenesis, Impairment of Fertility

Long-term studies in animals to evaluate the carcinogenic potential of ceftizoxime have not been conducted.

In an *in vitro* bacterial cell assay (i.e., Ames test), there was no evidence of mutagenicity at ceftizoxime concentrations of 0.001–0.5 mcg/plate. Ceftizoxime did not produce increases in micronuclei in the *in vivo* mouse micronucleus test when given to animals at doses up to 7500 mg/kg, approximately six times greater than the maximum human daily dose on a mg/M^2 basis.

Ceftizoxime had no effect on fertility when administered subcutaneously to rats at daily doses of up to 1000 mg/kg/day, approximately two times the maximum human daily dose on a mg/M^2 basis. Ceftizoxime produced no histological changes in the sexual organs of male and female dogs when given intravenously for thirteen weeks at a dose of 1000 mg/kg/day, approximately five times greater than the maximum human daily dose on a mg/M^2 basis.

Pregnancy: Teratogenic Effects: Pregnancy Category B.

Reproduction studies performed in rats and rabbits have revealed no evidence of impaired fertility or harm to the fetus due to Cefizox. There are, however, no adequate and well-controlled studies in pregnant women. Because animal reproduction studies are not always predictive of human effects, this drug should be used during pregnancy only if clearly needed.

Labor and Delivery

Safety of Cefizox use during labor and delivery has not been established.

Nursing Mothers

Cefizox is excreted in human milk in low concentrations. Caution should be exercised when Cefizox is administered to a nursing woman.

Pediatric Use

Safety and efficacy in pediatric patients from birth to six months of age have not been established. In pediatric patients six months of age and older, treatment with Cefizox has been associated with transient elevated levels of eosinophils, AST (SGOT), ALT (SGPT), and CPK (creatine phosphokinase). The CPK elevation may be related to IM administration.

The potential for the toxic effect in pediatric patients from chemicals that may leach from the single-dose IV preparation in plastic has not been determined.

ADVERSE REACTIONS

Cefizox® (ceftizoxime for injection, USP) is generally well tolerated. The *most* frequent adverse reactions (*greater* than 1% but *less* than 5%) are:

Hypersensitivity—Rash, pruritus, fever.

Hepatic—Transient elevation in AST (SGOT), ALT (SGPT), and alkaline phosphatase.

Hematologic—Transient eosinophilia, thrombocytosis. Some individuals have developed a positive Coombs test.

Local—Injection site—Burning, cellulitis, phlebitis with IV administration, pain, induration, tenderness, paresthesia.

The *less* frequent adverse reactions (*less* than 1%) are:

Hypersensitivity—Numbness and anaphylaxis have been reported rarely.

Hepatic—Elevation of bilirubin has been reported rarely.

Renal—Transient elevations of BUN and creatinine have been occasionally observed with Cefizox.

Hematologic—Anemia, including hemolytic anemia with occasional fatal outcome, leukopenia, neutropenia, and thrombocytopenia have been reported rarely.

Urogenital—Vaginitis has occurred rarely.

Gastrointestinal—Diarrhea; nausea and vomiting have been reported occasionally.

Symptoms of pseudomembranous colitis can appear during or after antibiotic treatment (see **WARNINGS**).

In addition to the adverse reactions listed above which have been observed in patients treated with ceftizoxime, the following adverse reactions and altered laboratory tests have been reported for cephalosporin-class antibiotics:

Stevens-Johnson syndrome, erythema multiforme, toxic epidermal necrolysis, serum-sickness like reaction, toxic nephropathy, aplastic anemia, hemorrhage, prolonged prothrombin time, elevated LDH, pancytopenia, and agranulocytosis.

Several cephalosporins have been implicated in triggering seizures, particularly in patients with renal impairment, when the dosage was not reduced. (See **DOSAGE AND ADMINISTRATION**.) If seizures associated with drug therapy occur, the drug should be discontinued. Anticonvulsant therapy can be given if clinically indicated.

DOSAGE AND ADMINISTRATION

The usual adult dosage is 1 or 2 grams of Cefizox (ceftizoxime for injection, USP) every 8 to 12 hours. Proper dosage and route of administration should be determined by the condition of the patient, severity of the infection, and susceptibility of the causative organisms.

General Guidelines for Dosage of Cefizox

Type of Infection	Daily Dose (Grams)	Frequency and Route
Uncomplicated Urinary Tract	1	500 mg q12h IM or IV
Other Sites	2–3	1 gram q8–12h IM or IV
Severe or Refractory	3–6	1 gram q8h IM or IV 2 grams q8–12h IM[a] or IV
PID[b]	6	2 grams q8h IV
Life-Threatening[c]	9–12	3–4 grams q8h IV

a) When administering 2 gram IM doses, the dose should be divided and given in different large muscle masses.

b) If *C. trachomatis* is a suspected pathogen, appropriate anti-chlamydial coverage should be added, because ceftizoxime has no activity against this organism.

c) In life-threatening infections, dosages up to 2 grams every 4 hours have been given.

Because of the serious nature of urinary tract infections due to *P. aeruginosa* and because many strains of *Pseudomonas* species are only moderately susceptible to Cefizox, higher dosage is recommended. Other therapy should be instituted if the response is not prompt.

A single, 1 gram IM dose is the usual dose for treatment of uncomplicated gonorrhea.

The IV route may be preferable for patients with bacterial septicemia, localized parenchymal abscesses (such as intra-abdominal abscess), peritonitis, or other severe or life-threatening infections.

In those with normal renal function, the IV dosage for such infections is 2 to 12 grams of Cefizox (ceftizoxime for injection, USP) daily. In conditions such as bacterial septicemia, 6 to 12 grams/day may be given initially by the IV route for several days, and the dosage may then be gradually reduced according to clinical response and laboratory findings.

Pediatric Dosage Schedule

	Unit Dose	Frequency
Pediatric patients 6 months or older	50 mg/kg	q6-8h

Dosage may be increased to a total daily dose of 200 mg/kg (not to exceed the maximum adult dose for serious infection).

Impaired Renal Function

Modification of Cefizox dosage is necessary in patients with impaired renal function. Following an initial loading dose of 500 mg–1 gram IM or IV, the maintenance dosing schedule shown below should be followed. Further dosing should be determined by therapeutic monitoring, severity of the infection, and susceptibility of the causative organisms.

When only the serum creatinine level is available, creatinine clearance may be calculated from the following formula. The serum creatinine level should represent current renal function at the steady state.

Males

$$\text{Clcr} = \frac{\text{Weight (kg)} \times (140 - \text{age})}{72 \times \text{serum creatinine (mg/100 mL)}}$$

Females are 0.85 of the calculated clearance values for males.

In patients undergoing hemodialysis, no additional supplemental dosing is required following hemodialysis; however, dosing should be timed so that the patient receives the dose (according to the table below) at the end of the dialysis.

Dosage in Adults with Reduced Renal Function

Creatinine Clearance mL/min	Renal Function	Less Severe Infections	Life-Threatening Infections
79–50	Mild impairment	500 mg q8h	0.75–1.5 grams q8h
49–5	Moderate to severe impairment	250–500 mg q12h	0.5–1 gram q12h
4–0	Dialysis patients	500 mg q48h or 250 mg q24h	0.5–1 gram q48h or 0.5 gram q24h

Preparation of Parenteral Solution

RECONSTITUTION

IM Administration: Reconstitute with Sterile Water for Injection. SHAKE WELL.

Vial Size	Diluent to Be Added	Approx. Avail. Vol.	Approx. Avg. Concentration	Room Temp. Stability
500 mg	1.5 mL	1.8 mL	280 mg/mL	16 hours
1 gram	3.0 mL	3.7 mL	270 mg/mL	16 hours
2 grams*	6.0 mL	7.4 mL	270 mg/mL	16 hours

*When administering 2 gram IM doses, the dose should be divided and given in different large muscle masses.

IV Administration: Reconstitute with Sterile Water for Injection. SHAKE WELL.

Vial Size	Diluent to Be Added	Approx. Avail. Vol.	Approx. Avg. Concentration	Room Temp. Stability
500 mg	5 mL	5.3 mL	95 mg/mL	24 hours
1 gram	10 mL	10.7 mL	95 mg/mL	24 hours
2 grams	20 mL	21.4 mL	95 mg/mL	24 hours

These solutions of Cefizox are stable 24 hours at room temperature or 96 hours if refrigerated (5°C).

Parenteral drug products should be inspected visually for particulate matter prior to administration. If particulate matter is evident in reconstituted fluids, then the drug solution should be discarded. Reconstituted solutions may range from yellow to amber without changes in potency.

Piggyback Vials: Reconstitute with 50 to 100 mL of Sodium Chloride Injection or any other IV solution listed below. SHAKE WELL

Administer with primary IV fluids, as a single dose. These Piggyback vial solutions of Cefizox are stable 24 hours at room temperature or 96 hours if refrigerated (5°C).

A solution of 1 gram Cefizox in 13 mL Sterile Water for Injection is isotonic.

IM Injection

Inject well within the body of a relatively large muscle. Aspiration is necessary to avoid inadvertent injection into a blood vessel. When administering 2 gram IM doses, the dose should be divided and given in different large muscle masses.

IV Administration

Direct (bolus) injection, slowly over 3 to 5 minutes, directly or through tubing for patients receiving parenteral fluids (see list below). Intermittent or continuous infusion, dilute reconstituted Cefizox in 50 to 100 mL of one of the following solutions:

- Sodium Chloride Injection
- 5% or 10% Dextrose Injection
- 5% Dextrose and 0.9%, 0.45%, or 0.2% Sodium Chloride Injection
- Ringer's Injection
- Lactated Ringer's Injection
- Invert Sugar 10% in Sterile Water for Injection
- 5% Sodium Bicarbonate in Sterile Water for Injection
- 5% Dextrose in Lactated Ringer's Injection (only when reconstituted with 4% Sodium Bicarbonate Injection)

In these fluids, Cefizox is stable 24 hours at room temperature or 96 hours if refrigerated (5°C).

HOW SUPPLIED

Cefizox® (ceftizoxime for injection, USP)

NDC 0469-7250-01 Product No. 725001
Equivalent to 500 mg ceftizoxime in 10 mL, single-dose, flip-top vials, individually packaged

NDC 0469-7251-01 Product No. 725101
Equivalent to 1 gram ceftizoxime in 20 mL, single-dose, flip-top vials, individually packaged

NDC 0469-7252-01 Product No. 725201
Equivalent to 1 gram ceftizoxime in 100 mL, single-dose, Piggyback, flip-top vials, packaged in tens

NDC 0469-7253-02 Product No. 725302
Equivalent to 2 grams ceftizoxime in 20 mL, single-dose, flip-top vials, individually packaged

NDC 0469-7254-02 Product No. 725402
Equivalent to 2 grams ceftizoxime in 100 mL, single-dose, Piggyback, flip-top vials, packaged in tens

Unreconstituted Cefizox should be protected from excessive light, and stored at controlled room temperature (59°– 86°F) in the original package until used.

Rx only

REFERENCES

1. National Committee for Clinical Laboratory Standards, Approved Standard. *Performance Standards for Antimicrobial Disk Susceptibility Test,* 4th Edition, Vol 10 (7): M2-A4. Villanova, PA, April 1990.
2. National Committee for Clinical Laboratory Standards, Approved Standard. *Methods for Dilution Antimicrobial Susceptibility Tests for Bacteria that Grow Aerobically,* 2nd Edition, Vol 10 (8):M7-A2. Villanova, PA, April 1990.

Product of Japan

Manufactured for: Fujisawa Healthcare, Inc.

Deerfield, IL 60015

Revised July 1998

CEFIZOX® ℞

(CEFTIZOXIME FOR INJECTION, USP)

PHARMACY BULK PACKAGE—Not For Direct Infusion

DESCRIPTION

Cefizox® (ceftizoxime for injection, USP) pharmacy bulk vial is a sterile dosage form which contains many single doses for use in a pharmacy admixture program in the preparation of parenteral fluids. Cefizox is a sterile, semi-synthetic, broad-spectrum, beta-lactamase resistant cephalosporin antibiotic for parenteral (I.V., I.M.) administration. It is the sodium salt of [6R-[6a, 7β(Z)]]-7-[[(2,3-dihydro-2-imino-4-thiazolyl) (methoxyimino) acetyl] amino]-8-oxo-5-thia-1-azabicyclo [4.2.0] oct-2-ene-2-carboxylic acid. Its sodium content is approximately 60 mg (2.6 mEq) per gram of ceftizoxime activity.

It has the following structural formula:

$C_{13}H_{12}N_5NaO_5S_2$ 405.38

$C_{13}H_{12}N_5NaO_5S_2$ 405.38

Ceftizoxime for injection, USP is a white to pale yellow crystalline powder. Cefizox is supplied in vials equivalent to 10 grams of ceftizoxime in pharmacy bulk packaging.

HOW SUPPLIED

Cefizox® (ceftizoxime for injection, USP)

NDC 0469-7255-10 Product No. 725510
Equivalent to 10 grams ceftizoxime in 100 mL, Pharmacy Bulk Package, packaged in tens

Unreconstituted Cefizox should be protected from excessive light, and stored at controlled room temperature (59°–86°F) in the original package until used.

Rx only

Product of Japan

Manufactured for: Fujisawa Healthcare, Inc.

Deerfield, IL 60015

Revised July 1998

Continued on next page

CEFIZOX® ℞

(ceftizoxime for injection, USP)
For Intravenous Infusion

DESCRIPTION

Cefizox® (ceftizoxime for injection, USP) is a sterile, semisynthetic, broad-spectrum, beta-lactamase resistant cephalosporin antibiotic for parenteral (I.V., I.M.) administration. It is the sodium salt of [6R-[6a, 7β(Z)]]-7-[[(2,3-dihydro-2-imino-4-thiazolyl) (methoxyimino) acetyl] amino]-8-oxo-5-thia-1-azabicyclo [4.2.0] oct-2-ene-2-carboxylic acid. Its sodium content is approximately 60 mg (2.6 mEq) per gram of ceftizoxime activity.

It has the following structural formula:

$C_{13}H_{12}N_5NaO_5S_2$ 405.38

$C_{13}H_{12}N_5NaO_5S_2$ 405.38

Ceftizoxime for injection is a white to pale yellow crystalline powder.

Cefizox is supplied in ADD-Vantage® vials as ceftizoxime sodium equivalent to 1 gram or 2 grams ceftizoxime.

HOW SUPPLIED

Cefizox® (ceftizoxime for injection, USP) in ADD-Vantage® Vials

NDC 0469-7271-01 Product No. 727101
equivalent to 1 gram ceftizoxime, packaged in tens

NDC 0469-7272-02 Product No. 727202
equivalent to 2 grams ceftizoxime, packaged in tens

Unreconstituted Cefizox should be protected from excessive light, and stored at controlled room temperature 15°–30°C (59°–86°F) in the original package until used.

ADD-Vantage® is a registered trademark of Abbott Laboratories.

U.S. Patent 4,427,674

Product of Japan Printed in USA

Manufactured for Fujisawa Healthcare, Inc., Deerfield, IL 60015, by SmithKline Beecham, Philadelphia, PA 19101.

685560-A Revised December 1998

Rx Only

CEFIZOX® ℞

(ceftizoxime injection)
in Galaxy® Plastic Container (PL 2040)
For Intravenous Use

DESCRIPTION

Cefizox® (ceftizoxime injection) in the Galaxy® plastic container (PL 2040) contains ceftizoxime as ceftizoxime sodium. It is a sterile, semisynthetic, broad spectrum, cephalosporin antibiotic for intravenous administration. Chemically, it is sodium (*6R,7R*) - 7 - [2- (2 - imino - 4 - thiazolin-4-yl) glyoxylamido]-8-oxo-5-thia-1-azabicyclo [4.2.0.]oct-2-ene-2-carboxylate 7^2-(*Z*)-(*O*–methyloxime). The molecular formula is $C_{13}H_{12}N_5NaO_5S_2$ and the molecular weight is 405.38. The structural formula of ceftizoxime sodium is as follows:

Cefizox (ceftizoxime injection) in the Galaxy® plastic container is a frozen iso-osmotic, sterile, nonpyrogenic premixed 50 mL solution containing 1 g or 2 g of ceftizoxime as ceftizoxime sodium. Dextrose, USP has been added to these dosages to adjust osmolality (approximately 1.9 g and 950 mg to the 1 g and 2 g dosages as dextrose hydrous, respectively). Thawed solutions range from very pale yellow to yellow. The pH of thawed solutions range from 5.5 to 8.0. After thawing to room temperature, the solution is intended for intravenous use only.

The Galaxy® container is fabricated from a specially designed multilayer plastic (PL 2040). Solutions are in contact with the polyethylene layer of this container and can leach out certain chemical components of the plastic in very small amounts within the expiration dating period. The suitability of the plastic has been confirmed in tests in animals according to the USP biological tests for plastic containers, as well as by tissue culture toxicity studies.

HOW SUPPLIED

Cefizox® (ceftizoxime injection) is supplied as a frozen, iso-osmotic, sterile, nonpyrogenic solution in 50 mL single dose Galaxy® plastic containers (PL 2040) as follows:

NDC 0469-7220-01 Product No. 722001
1 g ceftizoxime/50 mL container

NDC 0469-7221-02 Product No. 722102
2 g ceftizoxime/50 mL container

Store at or below –20°C/–4°F.

Rx only

See DIRECTIONS FOR USE OF CEFIZOX® (ceftizoxime injection) IN GALAXY® PLASTIC CONTAINER (PL 2040).

Galaxy® is a registered trademark of Baxter International Inc.

Ceftizoxime sodium is a product of Japan.

Manufactured for Fujisawa Healthcare, Inc.
Deerfield, IL 60015 by
Baxter Healthcare Corporation, Deerfield, IL 60015,
45621F/Revised June 1998

CYCLOCORT® ℞

[amcinonide]

DESCRIPTION

The topical corticosteroids constitute a class of primarily synthetic steroids used as anti-inflammatory and antipruritic agents.

TOPICAL LOTION 0.1%

Each gram of CYCLOCORT (amcinonide) Topical Lotion contains 1 mg of the active steroid amcinonide in AQUATAIN,* a white, smooth, homogeneous, opaque emulsion composed of Benzyl Alcohol 1% (wt/wt) as preservative, Emulsifying Wax, Glycerin, Isopropyl Palmitate, Lactic Acid, Purified Water, and Sorbitol Solution. In addition, contains Polyethylene Glycol 400.

Sodium hydroxide may be used to adjust pH to approximately 4.4 during manufacture.

TOPICAL CREAM 0.1%

Each gram of CYCLOCORT (amcinonide) Topical Cream contains 1 mg of the active steroid amcinonide in AQUATAIN,* a white, smooth, homogeneous, opaque emulsion composed of Benzyl Alcohol 2% (wt/wt) as preservative, Emulsifying Wax, Glycerin, Isopropyl Palmitate, Lactic Acid, Purified Water, and Sorbitol Solution.

*AQUATAIN™ is non-staining, water-washable, paraben-free, spermaceti-free, and has a light texture and consistency.

TOPICAL OINTMENT 0.1%

Each gram of CYCLOCORT (amcinonide) Topical Ointment contains 1 mg of the active steroid amcinonide in a specially formulated base composed of Benzyl Alcohol 2% (wt/wt) as preservative, White Petrolatum, USP, Emulsifying Wax, and Tenox II (Butylated Hydroxyanisole, Propyl Gallate, Citric Acid, Propylene Glycol).

Chemically, amcinonide is:

$C_{28}H_{35}FO_7$ Molecular Weight 502.58

Pregna-1,4-diene-3,20-dione, 21-(acetyloxy)-16,17-[cyclopentylidenebis (oxy)]-9-fluoro-11-hydroxy-, (11β, 16α).

HOW SUPPLIED

CYCLOCORT® (amcinonide) Topical Lotion 0.1% (1 mg/g) with AQUATAIN™ hydrophilic base

NDC 0469-7404-20 Product Code 740420
20 mL (19.6 g) Bottle

NDC 0469-7404-60 Product Code 740460
60 mL (58.8 g) Bottle

CYCLOCORT® (amcinonide) Topical Cream 0.1% (1 mg/g) with AQUATAIN™ hydrophilic base

NDC 0469-7054-15 Product Code 705415
15 gram Tube

NDC 0469-7054-30 Product Code 705430
30 gram Tube

NDC 0469-7054-60 Product Code 705460
60 gram Tube

CYCLOCORT® (amcinonide) Topical Ointment 0.1% (1 mg/g)

NDC 0469-7115-15 Product Code 711515
15 gram Tube

NDC 0469-7115-30 Product Code 711530
30 gram Tube

NDC 0469-7115-60 Product Code 711560
60 gram Tube

Store at controlled room temperature 15°–30°C (59°–86°F). DO NOT FREEZE.

Rx only

Manufactured for Fujisawa Healthcare, Inc., Deerfield, IL 60015

Revised: September 1998/127457

PROGRAF® ℞

tacrolimus capsules
tacrolimus injection (for intravenous infusion only)

WARNING

Increased susceptibility to infection and the possible development of lymphoma may result from immunosuppression. Only physicians experienced in immunosuppressive therapy and management of organ transplant patients should prescribe Prograf. Patients receiving the drug should be managed in facilities equipped and staffed with adequate laboratory and supportive medical resources. The physician responsible for maintenance therapy should have complete information requisite for the follow-up of the patient.

DESCRIPTION

Prograf is available for oral administration as capsules (tacrolimus capsules) containing the equivalent of 0.5 mg, 1 mg, or 5 mg of anhydrous tacrolimus. Inactive ingredients include lactose, hydroxypropyl methylcellulose, croscarmellose sodium, and magnesium stearate. The 0.5 mg capsule shell contains gelatin, titanium dioxide and ferric oxide, the 1 mg capsule shell contains gelatin and titanium dioxide, and the 5 mg capsule shell contains gelatin, titanium dioxide and ferric oxide.

Prograf is also available as a sterile solution (tacrolimus injection) containing the equivalent of 5 mg anhydrous tacrolimus in 1 mL for administration by intravenous infusion only. Each mL contains polyoxyl 60 hydrogenated castor oil (HCO-60), 200 mg, and dehydrated alcohol, USP, 80.0% v/v. Prograf injection must be diluted with 0.9% Sodium Chloride Injection or 5% Dextrose Injection before use.

Tacrolimus, previously known as FK506, is the active ingredient in Prograf. Tacrolimus is a macrolide immunosuppressant produced by *Streptomyces tsukubaensis*. Chemically, tacrolimus is designated as [3*S*–[3*R**[*E*(1*S**,3*S**,4*S**)], 4*S**,5*R**,8*S**,9*E*,12*R**,14*R**,15*S**,16*R**,18*S**,19*S**,26a*R**]]-5,6,8,11,12,13,14,15,16,17,18,19,24,25,26,26a-hexadecahydro-5,19-dihydroxy-3-[2-(4-hydroxy-3-methoxycyclohexyl)-1-methylethenyl]-14,16-dimethoxy-4,10,12,18-tetramethyl-8-(2-propenyl)-15,19-epoxy-3H-pyrido[2,1-c][1,4] oxaazacyclotricosine-1,7,20,21(4H,23H)-tetrone, monohydrate.

The chemical structure of tacrolimus is:

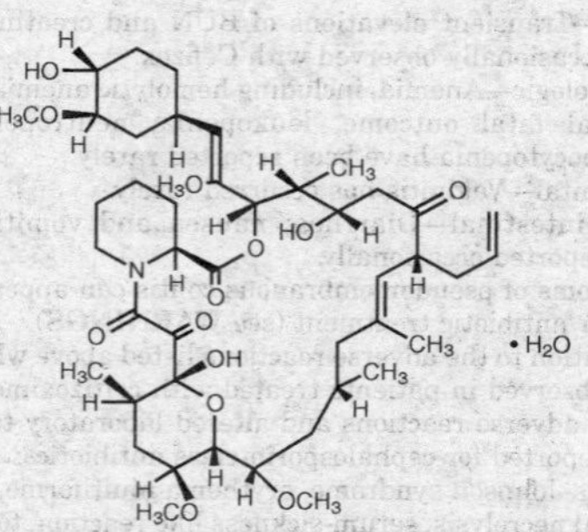

Tacrolimus has an empirical formula of $C_{44}H_{69}NO_{12} \cdot H_2O$ and a formula weight of 822.05. Tacrolimus appears as white crystals or crystalline powder. It is practically insoluble in water, freely soluble in ethanol, and very soluble in methanol and chloroform.

CLINICAL PHARMACOLOGY

Mechanism of Action

Tacrolimus prolongs the survival of the host and transplanted graft in animal transplant models of liver, kidney, heart, bone marrow, small bowel and pancreas, lung and trachea, skin, cornea, and limb.

In animals, tacrolimus has been demonstrated to suppress some humoral immunity and, to a greater extent, cell-mediated reactions such as allograft rejection, delayed type hypersensitivity, collagen-induced arthritis, experimental allergic encephalomyelitis, and graft versus host disease.

Tacrolimus inhibits T-lymphocyte activation, although the exact mechanism of action is not known. Experimental evidence suggests that tacrolimus binds to an intracellular protein, FKBP-12. A complex of tacrolimus-FKBP-12, calcium, calmodulin, and calcineurin is then formed and the phosphatase activity of calcineurin inhibited. This effect may prevent the dephosphorylation and translocation of nuclear factor of activated T-cells (NF-AT), a nuclear component thought to initiate gene transcription for the formation of lymphokines (such as interleukin-2, gamma interferon). The net result is the inhibition of T-lymphocyte activation (i.e., immunosuppression).

Pharmacokinetics

Tacrolimus activity is primarily due to the parent drug. The pharmacokinetic parameters (means ± S.D.) of tacrolimus have been determined following intravenous (IV) and oral (PO) administration in healthy volunteers, liver transplant and kidney transplant patients. (See table below.)

[See table at top of next page]

Due to intersubject variability in tacrolimus pharmacokinetics, individualization of dosing regimen is necessary for optimal therapy. (See **DOSAGE AND ADMINISTRATION**). Pharmacokinetic data indicate that whole blood concentrations rather than plasma concentrations serve as the more appropriate sampling compartment to describe tacrolimus pharmacokinetics.

Absorption

Absorption of tacrolimus from the gastrointestinal tract after oral administration is incomplete and variable. The absolute bioavailability of tacrolimus was 17 ± 10% in adult kidney transplant patients (N = 26), 22 ± 6% in adult liver transplant patients (N = 17), and 18 ± 5% in healthy volunteers (N = 16).

A single dose study conducted in 32 healthy volunteers established the bioequivalence of the 1 mg and 5 mg capsules. Another single dose study in 32 healthy volunteers established the bioequivalence of the 0.5 mg and 1 mg capsules. Tacrolimus maximum blood concentration (C_{max}) and area under the curve (AUC) appeared to increase in a dose-proportional fashion in 18 fasted healthy volunteers receiving a single oral dose of 3, 7 and 10 mg.

In 18 kidney transplant patients, tacrolimus trough concentrations from 3 to 30 ng/mL measured at 10–12 hours post-dose (C_{min}) correlated well with the AUC (correlation coefficient 0.93). In 24 liver transplant patients over a concentration range of 10 to 60 ng/mL, the correlation coefficient was 0.94.

Food Effects: The rate and extent of tacrolimus absorption were greatest under fasted conditions. The presence and composition of food decreased both the rate and extent of tacrolimus absorption when administered to 15 healthy volunteers.

The effect was most pronounced with a high-fat meal (848 kcal, 46% fat): mean AUC and C_{max} were decreased 37% and 77%, respectively; T_{max} was lengthened 5-fold. A high-carbohydrate meal (668 kcal, 85% carbohydrate) decreased mean AUC and mean C_{max} by 28% and 65%, respectively.

In healthy volunteers (N = 16), the time of the meal also affected tacrolimus bioavailability. When given immediately following the meal, mean C_{max} was reduced 71%, and mean AUC was reduced 39%, relative to the fasted condition. When administered 1.5 hours following the meal, mean C_{max} was reduced 63%, and mean AUC was reduced 39%, relative to the fasted condition.

In 11 liver transplant patients, Prograf administered 15 minutes after a high fat (400 kcal, 34% fat) breakfast, resulted in decreased AUC (27 ± 18%) and C_{max} (50 ± 19%), as compared to a fasted state.

Distribution

The plasma protein binding of tacrolimus is approximately 99% and is independent of concentration over a range of 5–50 ng/mL. Tacrolimus is bound mainly to albumin and alpha-1-acid glycoprotein, and has a high level of association with erythrocytes. The distribution of tacrolimus between whole blood and plasma depends on several factors, such as hematocrit, temperature at the time of plasma separation, drug concentration, and plasma protein concentration. In a U.S. study, the ratio of whole blood concentration to plasma concentration averaged 35 (range 12 to 67).

Metabolism

Tacrolimus is extensively metabolized by the mixed-function oxidase system, primarily the cytochrome P-450 system (CYP3A). A metabolic pathway leading to the formation of 8 possible metabolites has been proposed. Demethylation and hydroxylation were identified as the primary mechanisms of biotransformation *in vitro*. The major metabolite identified in incubations with human liver microsomes is 13-demethyl tacrolimus. In *in vitro* studies, a 31-demethyl metabolite has been reported to have the same activity as tacrolimus.

Excretion

The mean clearance following IV administration of tacrolimus is 0.040, 0.083 and 0.053 L/hr/kg in healthy volunteers, adult kidney transplant patients and adult liver transplant patients, respectively. In man, less than 1% of the dose administered is excreted unchanged in urine.

In a mass balance study of IV administered radiolabeled tacrolimus to 6 healthy volunteers, the mean recovery of radiolabel was 77.8 ± 12.7%. Fecal elimination accounted for 92.4 ± 1.0% and the elimination half-life based on radioactivity was 48.1 ± 15.9 hours whereas it was 43.5 ± 11.6 hours based on tacrolimus concentrations. The mean clearance of radiolabel was 0.029 ± 0.015 L/hr/kg and clearance of tacrolimus was 0.029 ± 0.009 L/hr/kg.

When administered PO, the mean recovery of the radiolabel was 94.9 ± 30.7%. Fecal elimination accounted for 92.6 ± 30.7%, urinary elimination accounted for 2.3 ± 1.1% and the elimination half-life based on radioactivity was 31.9 ± 10.5 hours whereas it was 48.4 ± 12.3 hours based on tacrolimus concentrations. The mean clearance of radiolabel was 0.226 ± 0.116 L/hr/kg and clearance of tacrolimus 0.172 ± 0.088 L/hr/kg.

Special Populations

Pediatric

Pharmacokinetics of tacrolimus have been studied in liver transplantation patients, 0.7 to 13.2 years of age. Following IV administration of a 0.037 mg/kg/day dose to 12 pediatric patients, mean terminal half-life, volume of distribution and clearance were 11.5 ± 3.8 hours, 2.6 ± 2.1 L/kg and 0.138 ± 0.071 L/hr/kg, respectively. Following oral administration to 9 patients, mean AUC and C_{max} were 337 ± 167 ng·hr/mL and 43.4 ± 27.9 ng/mL, respectively. The absolute bioavailability was 31 ± 21%.

Whole blood trough concentrations from 31 patients less than 12 years old showed that pediatric patients needed higher doses than adults to achieve similar tacrolimus trough concentrations. (See **DOSAGE AND ADMINISTRATION**).

Renal and Hepatic Insufficiency

The mean pharmacokinetic parameters for tacrolimus following single administrations to patients with renal and hepatic impairment are given in the following table.

[See second table above]

Renal Insufficiency:

Tacrolimus pharmacokinetics following a single IV administration were determined in 12 patients (7 not on dialysis and 5 on dialysis, serum creatinine of 3.9 ± 1.6 and 12.0 ± 2.4 mg/dL, respectively) prior to their kidney transplant. The pharmacokinetic parameters obtained were similar for both groups.

Population	N	Route (Dose)	Parameters: C_{max} (ng/mL)	T_{max} (hr)	AUC (ng·hr/mL)	$t_{1/2}$ (hr)	Cl (L/hr/kg)	V (L/kg)
Healthy Volunteers	8	IV (0.025 mg/kg/4hr)	—	—	598* ± 125	34.2 ± 7.7	0.040 ± 0.009	1.91 ± 0.31
	16	PO (5 mg)	29.7 ± 7.2	1.6 ± 0.7	243** ± 73	34.8 ± 11.4	0.041† ± 0.008	1.94† ± 0.53
Kidney Transplant Pts	26	IV (0.02 mg/kg/12hr)	—	—	294*** ± 262	18.8 ± 16.7	0.083 ± 0.050	1.41 ± 0.66
		PO (0.2 mg/kg/day)	19.2 ± 10.3	3.0	203*** ± 42	#	#	#
		PO (0.3 mg/kg/day)	24.2 ± 15.8	1.5	288*** ± 93	#	#	#
Liver Transplant Pts	17	IV (0.05 mg/kg/12 hr)	—	—	3300*** ± 2130	11.7 ± 3.9	0.053 ± 0.017	0.85 ± 0.30
		PO (0.3 mg/kg/day)	68.5 ± 30.0	2.3 ± 1.5	519*** ± 179	#	#	#

† Corrected for individual bioavailability
* AUC_{0-120}
** AUC_{0-72}
*** AUC_{0-inf}
— not applicable
\# not available

Population (No. of Patients)	Dose	AUC_{0-t} (ng·hr/mL)	$t_{1/2}$ (hr)	V (L/kg)	Cl (L/hr/kg)
Renal Impairment (n=12)	0.02 mg/kg/4hr IV	393±123*	26.3±9.2	1.07 ±0.20	0.038 ±0.014
Mild Hepatic Impairment (n=6)	0.02 mg/kg/4hr IV	367±107**	60.6±43.8 Range: 27.8–141	3.1 ±1.6	0.042 ±0.02
	7.7 mg PO	488±320**	66.1±44.8 Range: 29.5–138	3.7 ±4.7***	0.034 ±0.019***

* 0–60 hr.
** 0–72 hr.
*** corrected for bioavailability

The mean clearance of tacrolimus in patients with renal dysfunction was similar to that in normal volunteers (see previous table).

Hepatic Insufficiency:

Tacrolimus pharmacokinetics have been determined in six patients with mild hepatic dysfunction (mean Pugh score: 6.2) following single IV and oral administrations. The mean clearance of tacrolimus in patients with mild hepatic dysfunction was not substantially different from that in normal volunteers (see previous table).

Race

A formal study to evaluate the pharmacokinetic disposition of tacrolimus in Black transplant patients has not been conducted. However, a retrospective comparison of Black and Caucasian kidney transplant patients indicated that Black patients required higher tacrolimus doses to attain similar trough concentrations. (See **DOSAGE AND ADMINISTRATION**).

Gender

The effect of gender on tacrolimus pharmacokinetics has not been evaluated, however, there was no difference in dosing by gender in the kidney transplant trial.

Clinical Studies

Liver Transplantation

The safety and efficacy of Prograf-based immunosuppression following orthotopic liver transplantation were assessed in two prospective, randomized, non-blinded multicenter studies. The active control groups were treated with a cyclosporine-based immunosuppressive regimen. Both studies used concomitant adrenal corticosteroids as part of the immunosuppressive regimens. These studies were designed to evaluate whether the two regimens were therapeutically equivalent, with patient and graft survival at 12 months following transplantation as the primary endpoints. The Prograf-based immunosuppressive regimen was found to be equivalent to the cyclosporine-based immunosuppressive regimens.

In one trial, 529 patients were enrolled at 12 clinical sites in the United States; prior to surgery, 263 were randomized to the Prograf-based immunosuppressive regimen and 266 to a cyclosporine-based immunosuppressive regimen (CBIR). In 10 of the 12 sites, the same CBIR protocol was used, while 2 sites used different control protocols. This trial excluded patients with renal dysfunction, fulminant hepatic failure with Stage IV encephalopathy, and cancers; pediatric patients (≤ 12 years old) were allowed.

In the second trial, 545 patients were enrolled at 8 clinical sites in Europe; prior to surgery, 270 were randomized to the Prograf-based immunosuppressive regimen and 275 to CBIR. In this study, each center used its local standard CBIR protocol in the active-control arm. This trial excluded pediatric patients, but did allow enrollment of subjects with renal dysfunction, fulminant hepatic failure in Stage IV encephalopathy, and cancers other than primary hepatic with metastases.

One-year patient survival and graft survival in the Prograf-based treatment groups were equivalent to those in the CBIR treatment groups in both studies. The overall one-year patient survival (CBIR and Prograf-based treatment groups combined) was 88% in the U.S. study and 78% in the European study. The overall one-year graft survival (CBIR and Prograf-based treatment groups combined) was 81% in the U.S. study and 73% in the European study. In both studies, the median time to convert from IV to oral Prograf dosing was 2 days.

Because of the nature of the study design, comparisons of differences in secondary endpoints, such as incidence of acute rejection, refractory rejection or use of OKT3 for steroid-resistant rejection, could not be reliably made.

Kidney Transplantation

Prograf-based immunosuppression following kidney transplantation was assessed in a randomized, multicenter, non-blinded, prospective study. There were 412 kidney transplant patients enrolled at 19 clinical sites in the United States. Study therapy was initiated when renal function was stable as indicated by a serum creatinine ≤ 4 mg/dL (median of 4 days after transplantation, range 1 to 14 days). Patients less than 6 years of age were excluded.

There were 205 patients randomized to Prograf-based immunosuppression and 207 patients were randomized to cyclosporine-based immunosuppression. All patients received prophylactic induction therapy consisting of an antilymphocyte antibody preparation, corticosteroids and azathioprine. Overall one year patient and graft survival was 96.1% and 89.6%, respectively and was equivalent between treatment arms.

Because of the nature of the study design, comparisons of differences in secondary endpoints, such as incidence of acute rejection, refractory rejection or use of OKT3 for steroid-resistant rejection, could not be reliably made.

INDICATIONS AND USAGE

Prograf is indicated for the prophylaxis of organ rejection in patients receiving allogeneic liver or kidney transplants. It is recommended that Prograf be used concomitantly with adrenal corticosteroids. Because of the risk of anaphylaxis, Prograf injection should be reserved for patients unable to take Prograf capsules orally.

CONTRAINDICATIONS

Prograf is contraindicated in patients with a hypersensitivity to tacrolimus. Prograf injection is contraindicated in patients with a hypersensitivity to HCO-60 (polyoxyl 60 hydrogenated castor oil).

WARNINGS

(See boxed **WARNING.**)

Continued on next page

Prograf—Cont.

Insulin-dependent post-transplant diabetes mellitus (PTDM) was reported in 20% of Prograf-treated kidney transplant patients (See Table). The median time to onset of PTDM was 68 days. Insulin dependence was reversible in 15% of these patients at one year and in 50% at two years post transplant. Black and Hispanic kidney transplant patients were at an increased risk of development of PTDM.

Incidence of Post Transplant Diabetes Mellitus (PTDM)* and Insulin Use at 24 Months in Kidney Transplant Recipients

	Prograf	CBIR
Patients without pretransplant history of diabetes mellitus	151	151
New onset PTDM*, 1st Year	30/151 (20%)	6/151 (4%)
Still insulin dependent at one year in those without prior history of diabetes	25/151 (17%)	5/151 (3%)
New onset PTDM* post 1 year	1	0
Patients with PTDM* at 24 months	16/151 (11%)	5/151 (3%)

* use of insulin for 30 or more consecutive days, with < 5 day gap, without a prior history of insulin dependent diabetes mellitus or non insulin dependent diabetes mellitus.

Development of Post Transplant Diabetes Mellitus (PTDM) by Race and by Treatment Group during First Year Post Kidney Transplantation

	Prograf		CBIR	
Patient Race	No. of Patients at Risk	Patients Who Developed PTDM*	No. of Patients at Risk	Patients Who Developed PTDM*
Black	41	15 (37%)	36	3 (8%)
Hispanic	17	5 (29%)	18	1 (6%)
Caucasian	82	10 (12%)	87	1 (1%)
Other	11	0 (0%)	10	1 (10%)
Total	151	30 (20%)	151	6 (4%)

* use of insulin for 30 or more consecutive days, with < 5 day gap, without a prior history of insulin dependent diabetes mellitus or non insulin dependent diabetes mellitus.

Incidence of Post Transplant Diabetes Mellitus (PTDM)* and Insulin Use at One Year in Liver Transplant Recipients

	US Study		European Study	
Status of PTDM*	**Prograf**	**CBIR**	**Prograf**	**CBIR**
Patients at risk**	239	236	239	249
New Onset PTDM*	42 (18%)	30 (13%)	26 (11%)	12 (5%)
Patients still on insulin at 1 year	23 (10%)	19 (8%)	18 (8%)	6 (2%)

*use of insulin for 30 or more consecutive days, with < 5 day gap, without a prior history of insulin dependent diabetes mellitus or non insulin dependent diabetes mellitus.
**Patients without pretransplant history of diabetes mellitus.

Drugs That May Increase Tacrolimus Blood Concentrations:

Calcium Channel Blockers	Antifungal Agents	Macrolide Antibiotics	Gastrointestinal Prokinetic Agents	Other Drugs
diltiazem	clotrimazole	clarithromycin	cisapride	bromocriptine
nicardipine	fluconazole	erythromycin	metoclopramide	cimetidine
nifedipine	itraconazole	troleandomycin		cyclosporine
verapamil	ketoconazole			danazol
				methylprednisolone
				protease inhibitors

Drugs That May Decrease Tacrolimus Blood Concentrations:

Anticonvulsants	Antibiotics
carbamazepine	rifabutin
phenobarbital	rifampin
phenytoin	

*This table is not all inclusive

[See first table above]

Insulin-dependent post-transplant diabetes mellitus was reported in 18% and 11% of Prograf-treated liver transplant patients and was reversible in 45% and 31% of these patients at one year post transplant, in the U.S. and European randomized studies, respectively (See Table below). Hyperglycemia was associated with the use of Prograf in 47% and 33% of liver transplant recipients in the U.S. and European randomized studies, respectively, and may require treatment (see **ADVERSE REACTIONS**).

[See second table above]

Prograf can cause neurotoxicity and nephrotoxicity, particularly when used in high doses. Nephrotoxicity was reported in approximately 52% of kidney transplantation patients and in 40% and 36% of liver transplantation patients receiving Prograf in the U.S. and European randomized trials, respectively (see **ADVERSE REACTIONS**). More overt nephrotoxicity is seen early after transplantation, characterized by increasing serum creatinine and a decrease in urine output. Patients with impaired renal function should be monitored closely as the dosage of Prograf may need to be reduced. In patients with persistent elevations of serum creatinine who are unresponsive to dosage adjustments, consideration should be given to changing to another immunosuppressive therapy. Care should be taken in using tacrolimus with other nephrotoxic drugs. **In particular, to avoid excess nephrotoxicity, Prograf should not be used simultaneously with cyclosporine. Prograf or cyclosporine should be discontinued at least 24 hours prior to initiating the other. In the presence of elevated Prograf or cyclosporine concentrations, dosing with the other drug usually should be further delayed.**

Mild to severe hyperkalemia was reported in 31% of kidney transplant receipients and in 45% and 13% of liver transplant recipients treated with Prograf in the U.S. and European randomized trials, respectively, and may require treatment (see **ADVERSE REACTIONS**). **Serum potassium levels should be monitored and potassium-sparing diuretics should not be used during Prograf therapy (see PRECAUTIONS).**

Neurotoxicity, including tremor, headache, and other changes in motor function, mental status, and sensory function were reported in approximately 55% of liver transplant recipients in the two randomized studies. Tremor occurred more often in Prograf-treated kidney transplant patients (54%) compared to cyclosporine-treated patients. The incidence of other neurological events in kidney transplant patients was similar in the two treatment groups (see **ADVERSE REACTIONS**). Tremor and headache have been associated with high whole-blood concentrations of tacrolimus and may respond to dosage adjustment. Seizures have occurred in adult and pediatric patients receiving Prograf (see **ADVERSE REACTIONS**). Coma and delirium also have been associated with high plasma concentrations of tacrolimus.

As in patients receiving other immunosuppressants, patients receiving Prograf are at increased risk of developing lymphomas and other malignancies, particularly of the skin. The risk appears to be related to the intensity and duration of immunosuppression rather than to the use of any specific agent. A lymphoproliferative disorder (LPD) related to Epstein-Barr Virus (EBV) infection has been reported in immunosuppressed organ transplant recipients. The risk of LPD appears greatest in young children who are at risk for primary EBV infection while immunosuppressed or who are switched to Prograf following long-term immunosuppression therapy. Because of the danger of oversuppression of the immune system which can increase susceptibility to infection, combination immunosuppressant therapy should be used with caution.

A few patients receiving Prograf injection have experienced anaphylactic reactions. Although the exact cause of these reactions is not known, other drugs with castor oil derivatives in the formulation have been associated with anaphylaxis in a small percentage of patients. Because of this potential risk of anaphylaxis, Prograf injection should be reserved for patients who are unable to take Prograf capsules. **Patients receiving Prograf injection should be under continuous observation for at least the first 30 minutes following the start of the infusion and at frequent intervals thereafter. If signs or symptoms of anaphylaxis occur, the infusion should be stopped. An aqueous solution of epinephrine should be available at the bedside as well as a source of oxygen.**

PRECAUTIONS

General

Hypertension is a common adverse effect of Prograf therapy (see **ADVERSE REACTIONS**). Mild or moderate hypertension is more frequently reported than severe hypertension. Antihypertensive therapy may be required; the control of blood pressure can be accomplished with any of the common antihypertensive agents. Since tacrolimus may cause hyperkalemia, potassium-sparing diuretics should be avoided. While calcium-channel blocking agents can be effective in treating Prograf-associated hypertension, care should be taken since interference with tacrolimus metabolism may require a dosage reduction (see ***Drug Interactions***).

Renally and Hepatically Impaired Patients

For patients with renal insufficiency some evidence suggests that lower doses should be used (see **DOSAGE AND ADMINISTRATION**).

The use of Prograf in liver transplant recipients experiencing post-transplant hepatic impairment may be associated with increased risk of developing renal insufficiency related to high whole-blood levels of tacrolimus. These patients should be monitored closely and dosage adjustments should be considered. Some evidence suggests that lower doses should be used in these patients (see **DOSAGE AND ADMINISTRATION**).

Myocardial Hypertrophy

Myocardial hypertrophy has been reported in association with the administration of Prograf, and is generally manifested by echocardiographically demonstrated concentric increases in left ventricular posterior wall and interventricular septum thickness. Hypertrophy has been observed in infants, children and adults. This condition appears reversible in most cases following dose reduction or discontinuance of therapy. In a group of 20 patients with pre- and post-treatment echocardiograms who showed evidence of myocardial hypertrophy, mean tacrolimus whole blood concentrations during the period prior to diagnosis of myocardial hypertrophy ranged from 11 to 53 ng/mL in infants (N = 10, age 0.4 to 2 years), 4 to 46 ng/mL in children (N = 7, age 2 to 15 years) and 11 to 24 ng/mL in adults (N = 3, age 37 to 53 years).

In patients who develop renal failure or clinical manifestations of ventricular dysfunction while receiving Prograf therapy, echocardiographic evaluation should be considered. If myocardial hypertrophy is diagnosed, dosage reduction or discontinuation of Prograf should be considered.

Information for Patients

Patients should be informed of the need for repeated appropriate laboratory tests while they are receiving Prograf. They should be given complete dosage instructions, advised of the potential risks during pregnancy, and informed of the increased risk of neoplasia. Patients should be informed that changes in dosage should not be undertaken without first consulting their physician.

Patients should be informed that Prograf can cause diabetes mellitus and should be advised of the need to see their physician if they develop frequent urination, increased thirst or hunger.

Laboratory Tests

Serum creatinine, potassium, and fasting glucose should be assessed regularly. Routine monitoring of metabolic and hematologic systems should be performed as clinically warranted.

Drug Interactions

Drug interaction studies with tacrolimus have not been conducted. Due to the potential for additive or synergistic impairment of renal function, care should be taken when administering Prograf with drugs that may be associated with renal dysfunction. These include, but are not limited to, aminoglycosides, amphotericin B, and cisplatin. Initial clinical experience with the co-administration of Prograf and cyclosporine resulted in additive/synergistic nephrotoxicity. Patients switched from cyclosporine to Prograf should receive the first Prograf dose no sooner than 24 hours after the last cyclosporine dose. Dosing may be further delayed in the presence of elevated cyclosporine levels.

Drugs that May Alter Tacrolimus Concentrations

Since tacrolimus is metabolized mainly by the CYP3A enzyme systems, substances known to inhibit these enzymes may decrease the metabolism of tacrolimus with resultant increases in whole blood or plasma concentrations. Drugs known to induce these enzyme systems may result in an increased metabolism of tacrolimus and decreased whole blood or plasma concentrations. Monitoring of blood concentrations and appropriate dosage adjustments are essential when such drugs are used concomitantly.

[See third table above]

Interaction studies with drugs used in HIV therapy have not been conducted. However, care should be exercised when drugs that are nephrotoxic (e.g., ganciclovir) or that are metabolized by CYP3A (e.g., ritonavir) are administered concomitantly with tacrolimus. Grapefruit juice affects CYP3A-mediated metabolism and should be avoided **(See DOSAGE AND ADMINISTRATION)**.

Other Drug Interactions

Immunosuppressants may affect vaccination. Therefore, during treatment with Prograf, vaccination may be less effective. The use of live vaccines should be avoided; live vaccines may include, but are not limited to measles, mumps, rubella, oral polio, BCG, yellow fever, and TY21a typhoid.[1]

Carcinogenesis, Mutagenesis and Impairment of Fertility

An increased incidence of malignancy is a recognized complication of immunosuppression in recipients of organ transplants. The most common forms of neoplasms are non-Hodgkin's lymphomas and carcinomas of the skin. As with other immunosuppressive therapies, the risk of malignancies in Prograf recipients may be higher than in the normal, healthy population. Lymphoproliferative disorders associated with Epstein-Barr Virus infection have been seen. It has been reported that reduction or discontinuation of immunosuppression may cause the lesions to regress.

No evidence of genotoxicity was seen in bacterial (Salmonella and E. coli) or mammalian (Chinese hamster lung-derived cells) *in vitro* assays of mutagenicity, the *in vitro* CHO/HGPRT assay of mutagenicity, or *in vivo,* clastogenicity assays performed in mice; tacrolimus did not cause unscheduled DNA synthesis in rodent hepatocytes.

Carcinogenicity studies were carried out in male and female rats and mice. In the 80-week mouse study and in the 104-week rat study no relationship of tumor incidence to tacrolimus dosage was found. The highest doses used in the mouse and rat studies were 0.8–2.5 times (mice) and 3.5–7.1 times (rats) the recommended clinical dose range of 0.1–0.2 mg/kg/day when corrected for body surface area.

No impairment of fertility was demonstrated in studies of male and female rats. Tacrolimus, given orally at 1.0 mg/kg (0.7–1.4× the recommended clinical dose range of 0.1–0.2 mg/kg/day based on body surface area corrections) to male and female rats, prior to and during mating, as well as to dams during gestation and lactation, was associated with embryolethality and with adverse effects on female reproduction. Effects on female reproductive function (parturition) and embryolethal effects were indicated by a higher rate of pre-implantation loss and increased numbers of undelivered and nonviable pups. When given at 3.2 mg/kg (2.3–4.6× the recommended clinical dose range based on body surface area correction), tacrolimus was associated with maternal and paternal toxicity as well as reproductive toxicity including marked adverse effects on estrus cycles, parturition, pup viability, and pup malformations.

Pregnancy: Category C

In reproduction studies in rats and rabbits, adverse effects on the fetus were observed mainly at dose levels that were toxic to dams. Tacrolimus at oral doses of 0.32 and 1.0 mg/kg during organogenesis in rabbits was associated with maternal toxicity as well as an increase in incidence of abortions; these doses are equivalent to 0.5–1× and 1.6–3.3× the recommended clinical dose range (0.1–0.2 mg/kg) based on body surface area corrections. At the higher dose only, an increased incidence of malformations and developmental variations was also seen. Tacrolimus, at oral doses of 3.2 mg/kg during organogenesis in rats, was associated with maternal toxicity and caused an increase in late resorptions, decreased numbers of live births, and decreased pup weight and viability. Tacrolimus, given orally at 1.0 and 3.2 mg/kg (equivalent to 0.7–1.4× and 2.3–4.6× the recommended clinical dose range based on body surface area corrections) to pregnant rats after organogenesis and during lactation, was associated with reduced pup weights.

No reduction in male or female fertility was evident.

There are no adequate and well-controlled studies in pregnant women. Tacrolimus is transferred across the placenta. The use of tacrolimus during pregnancy has been associated with neonatal hyperkalemia and renal dysfunction. Prograf should be used during pregnancy only if the potential benefit to the mother justifies potential risk to the fetus.

Nursing Mothers

Since tacrolimus is excreted in human milk, nursing should be avoided.

Pediatric Patients

Experience with Prograf in pediatric kidney transplant patients is limited. Successful liver transplants have been performed in pediatric patients (ages up to 16 years) using Prograf. The two randomized active-controlled trials of Prograf in primary liver transplantation included 56 pediatric patients. Thirty-one patients were randomized to Prograf-based and 25 to cyclosporine-based therapies. Additionally, a minimum of 122 pediatric patients were studied in an uncontrolled trial of tacrolimus in living related donor liver transplantation. Pediatric patients generally required higher doses of Prograf to maintain blood trough concentrations of tacrolimus similar to adult patients (see **DOSAGE AND ADMINISTRATION**).

ADVERSE REACTIONS

Liver Transplantation

The principal adverse reactions of Prograf are tremor, headache, diarrhea, hypertension, nausea, and renal dysfunction. These occur with oral and IV administration of Prograf and may respond to a reduction in dosing. Diarrhea was sometimes associated with other gastrointestinal complaints such as nausea and vomiting.

LIVER TRANSPLANTATION: ADVERSE EVENTS OCCURRING IN ≥ 15% OF PROGRAF-TREATED PATIENTS

	U.S. STUDY (%)		EUROPEAN STUDY (%)	
	Prograf (N=250)	CBIR (N=250)	Prograf (N=264)	CBIR (N=265)
Nervous System				
Headache (see **WARNINGS**)	64	60	37	26
Tremor (see **WARNINGS**)	56	46	48	32
Insomnia	64	68	32	23
Paresthesia	40	30	17	17
Gastrointestinal				
Diarrhea	72	47	37	27
Nausea	46	37	32	27
Constipation	24	27	23	21
LFT Abnormal	36	30	6	5
Anorexia	34	24	7	5
Vomiting	27	15	14	11
Cardiovascular				
Hypertension (see **PRECAUTIONS**)	47	56	38	43
Urogenital				
Kidney Function Abnormal (see **WARNINGS**)	40	27	36	23
Creatinine Increased (see **WARNINGS**)	39	25	24	19
BUN Increased (see **WARNINGS**)	30	22	12	9
Urinary Tract Infection	16	18	21	19
Oliguria	18	15	19	12

	U.S. STUDY (%)		EUROPEAN STUDY (%)	
	Prograf (N=250)	CBIR (N=250)	Prograf (N=264)	CBIR (N=265)
Metabolic and Nutritional				
Hyperkalemia (see **WARNINGS**)	45	26	13	9
Hypokalemia	29	34	13	16
Hyperglycemia (see **WARNINGS**)	47	38	33	22
Hypomagnesemia	48	45	16	9
Hemic and Lymphatic				
Anemia	47	38	5	1
Leukocytosis	32	26	8	8
Thrombocytopenia	24	20	14	19
Miscellaneous				
Abdominal Pain	59	54	29	22
Pain	63	57	24	22
Fever	48	56	19	22
Asthenia	52	48	11	7
Back Pain	30	29	17	17
Ascites	27	22	7	8
Peripheral Edema	26	26	12	14
Respiratory System				
Pleural Effusion	30	32	36	35
Atelectasis	28	30	5	4
Dyspnea	29	23	5	4
Skin and Appendages				
Pruritus	36	20	15	7
Rash	24	19	10	4

KIDNEY TRANSPLANTATION: ADVERSE EVENTS OCCURRING IN ≥ 15% OF PROGRAF-TREATED PATIENTS

	Prograf (N=205)	CBIR (N=207)
Nervous System		
Tremor (See WARNINGS)	54	34
Headache (See WARNINGS)	44	38
Insomnia	32	30
Paresthesia	23	16
Dizziness	19	16
Gastrointestinal		
Diarrhea	44	41
Nausea	38	36
Constipation	35	43
Vomiting	29	23
Dyspepsia	28	20
Cardiovascular		
Hypertension (See PRECAUTIONS)	50	52
Chest pain	19	13

	Prograf (N=205)	CBIR (N=207)
Urogenital		
Creatinine increased (See WARNINGS)	45	42
Urinary tract infection	34	35
Metabolic and Nutritional		
Hypophosphatemia	49	53
Hypomagnesemia	34	17
Hyperlipemia	31	38
Hyperkalemia (See WARNINGS)	31	32
Diabetes mellitus (See WARNINGS)	24	9
Hypokalemia	22	25
Hyperglycemia (See WARNINGS)	22	16
Edema	18	19

	Prograf (N=205)	CBIR (N=207)
Hemic and Lymphatic		
Anemia	30	24
Leukopenia	15	17
Miscellaneous		
Infection	45	49
Peripheral edema	36	48
Asthenia	34	30
Abdominal pain	33	31
Pain	32	30
Fever	29	29
Back pain	24	20
Respiratory System		
Dyspnea	22	18
Cough increased	18	15
Musculoskeletal		
Arthralgia	25	24
Skin		
Rash	17	12
Pruritus	15	7

Hyperkalemia and hypomagnesemia have occurred in patients receiving Prograf therapy. Hyperglycemia has been noted in many patients; some may require insulin therapy (see **WARNINGS**).

The incidence of adverse events was determined in two randomized comparative liver transplant trials among 514 patients receiving tacrolimus and steroids and 515 patients receiving a cyclosporine-based regimen (CBIR). The proportion of patients reporting more than one adverse event was 99.8% in the tacrolimus group and 99.6% in the CBIR group. Precautions must be taken when comparing the incidence of adverse events in the U.S. study to that in the European study. The 12–month posttransplant information from the U.S. study and from the European study is presented below. The two studies also included different patient populations and patients were treated with immunosuppressive regimens of differing intensities. Adverse events reported in ≥ 15% in tacrolimus patients (combined study results) are presented below for the two controlled trials in liver transplantation:

[See first table above]

Less frequently observed adverse reactions in both liver transplantation and kidney transplantation patients are described under the subsection **Less Frequently Reported Adverse Reactions** below.

Kidney Transplantation

The most common adverse reactions reported were infection, tremor, hypertension, decreased renal function, constipation, diarrhea, headache, abdominal pain and insomnia. Adverse events that occurred in ≥ 15% of Prograf-treated kidney transplant patients are presented below:

[See second table above]

Less frequently observed adverse reactions in both liver transplantation and kidney transplantation patients are described under the subsection **Less Frequently Reported Adverse Reactions** below.

Less Frequently Reported Adverse Reactions

The following adverse events were reported in the range of 3% to less than 15% incidence in either liver or kidney transplant recipients who were treated with tacrolimus in the Phase 3 comparative trials.

NERVOUS SYSTEM: (see **WARNINGS**) abnormal dreams, agitation, amnesia, anxiety, confusion, convulsion, depression, dizziness, emotional lability, encephalopathy, hallucinations, hypertonia, incoordination, myoclonus, nervousness, neuropathy, psychosis, somnolence, thinking abnormal; SPECIAL SENSES: abnormal vision, amblyopia, ear pain, otitis media, tinnitus; GASTROINTESTINAL: anorexia, cholangitis, cholestatic jaundice, dyspepsia, dysphagia, esophagitis, flatulence, gastritis, gastrointestinal hemorrhage, GGT increase, GI perforation, hepatitis, ileus, increased appetite, jaundice, liver damage, liver function test abnormal, oral moniliasis, rectal disorder, stomatitis; CARDIOVASCULAR: angina pectoris, chest pain, deep thrombophlebitis, abnormal ECG, hemorrhage, hypotension, postural hypotension, peripheral vascular disorder, phlebitis, tachycardia, thrombosis, vasodilatation; UROGENITAL: (see **WARNINGS**) albuminuria, cystitis, dysuria, hematuria, hydronephrosis, kidney failure, kidney tubular necrosis, nocturia, pyuria, toxic nephropathy, oliguria, urinary frequency, urinary incontinence, vaginitis; METABOLIC/NUTRITIONAL: acidosis, alkaline phosphatase increased, alkalosis, ALT (SGPT) increased, AST (SGOT) increased, bicarbonate decreased, bilirubinemia, BUN increased, dehydration, GGT increased, healing abnormal, hypercalcemia, hypercholesterolemia, hyperlipemia, hyperphosphatemia, hyperuricemia, hypervolemia, hypocalcemia, hypoglycemia, hyponatremia, hypophophatemia, hypoproteinemia, lactic dehydrogenase increase, weight gain; ENDOCRINE: (see **PRECAUTIONS**) Cushing's syndrome, diabetes mellitus; HEMIC/LYMPHATIC: coagulation disorder, ecchymosis, hypochromic anemia, leukocytosis, leukopenia, polycythemia, prothrombin decreased, serum iron decreased, thrombocytopenia; MISCELLANEOUS: abdomen enlarged, abscess, accidental injury, allergic reaction, cellulitis, chills, flu syndrome, generalized edema, hernia, peritonitis, photosensitivity reaction, sepsis; MUSCULOSKELETAL: arthralgia, cramps, generalized spasm, joint disorder, leg cramps, myalgia, myasthenia, osteoporosis; RESPIRATORY: asthma, bronchitis, cough increased, lung

Continued on next page

Prograf—Cont.

disorder, pneumothorax, pulmonary edema, pharyngitis, pneumonia, respiratory disorder, rhinitis, sinusitis, voice alteration; SKIN: acne, alopecia, exfoliative dermatitis, fungal dermatitis, herpes simplex, hirsutism, skin discoloration, skin disorder, skin ulcer, sweating.

There have been rare spontaneous reports of myocardial hypertrophy associated with clinically manifested ventricular dysfunction in patients receiving Prograf therapy (see **PRECAUTIONS**-*Myocardial Hypertrophy*).

OVERDOSAGE

Limited overdosage experience is available. Acute overdosages of up to 30 times the intended dose have been reported. Almost all cases have been asymptomatic and all patients recovered with no sequelae. Occasionally, acute overdosage has been followed by adverse reactions consistent with those listed in the **ADVERSE REACTIONS** section except in one case where transient urticaria and lethargy were observed. Based on the poor aqueous solubility and extensive erythrocyte and plasma protein binding, it is anticipated that tacrolimus is not dialyzable to any significant extent; there is no experience with charcoal hemoperfusion. The oral use of activated charcoal has been reported in treating acute overdoses, but experience has not been sufficient to warrant recommending its use. General supportive measures and treatment of specific symptoms should be followed in all cases of overdosage.

In acute oral and IV toxicity studies, mortalities were seen at or above the following doses: in adult rats, 52X the recommended human oral dose; in immature rats, 16X the recommended oral dose; and in adult rats, 16X the recommended human IV dose (all based on body surface area corrections).

DOSAGE AND ADMINISTRATION

Prograf Injection (tacrolimus injection)

For IV Infusion Only

NOTE: Anaphylactic reactions have occurred with injectables containing castor oil derivatives. See WARNINGS.

In patients unable to take oral Prograf capsules, therapy may be initiated with Prograf injection. The initial dose of Prograf should be administered no sooner than 6 hours after transplantation. The recommended starting dose of Prograf injection is 0.03–0.05 mg/kg/day as a continuous IV infusion. Adult patients should receive doses at the lower end of the dosing range. Concomitant adrenal corticosteroid therapy is recommended early post-transplantation. Continuous IV infusion of Prograf injection should be continued only until the patient can tolerate oral administration of Prograf capsules.

Preparation for Administration/Stability

Prograf injection must be diluted with 0.9% Sodium Chloride Injection or 5% Dextrose Injection to a concentration between 0.004 mg/mL and 0.02 mg/mL prior to use. Diluted infusion solution should be stored in glass or polyethylene containers and should be discarded after 24 hours. The diluted infusion solution should not be stored in a PVC container due to decreased stability and the potential for extraction of phthalates. In situations where more dilute solutions are utilized (e.g., pediatric dosing, etc.), PVC-free tubing should likewise be used to minimize the potential for significant drug adsorption onto the tubing. Parenteral drug products should be inspected visually for particulate matter and discoloration prior to administration, whenever solution and container permit. Due to the chemical instability of tacrolimus in alkaline media, Prograf injection should not be mixed or co-infused with solutions of pH 9 or greater (e.g., ganciclovir or acyclovir).

Prograf capsules (tacrolimus capsules)

[See first table above]

Liver Transplantation

It is recommended that patients initiate oral therapy with Prograf capsules if possible. If IV therapy is necessary, conversion from IV to oral Prograf is recommended as soon as oral therapy can be tolerated. This usually occurs within 2–3 days. The initial dose of Prograf should be administered no sooner than 6 hours after transplantation. In a patient receiving an IV infusion, the first dose of oral therapy should be given 8–12 hours after discontinuing the IV infusion. The recommended starting oral dose of Prograf capsules is 0.10–0.15 mg/kg/day administered in two divided daily doses every 12 hours. Co-administered grapefruit juice has been reported to increase tacrolimus blood trough concentrations in liver transplant patients. (See ***Drugs that May Alter Tacrolimus Concentrations***).

Dosing should be titrated based on clinical assessments of rejection and tolerability. Lower Prograf dosages may be sufficient as maintenance therapy. Adjunct therapy with adrenal corticosteroids is recommended early post transplant.

Dosage and typical tacrolimus whole blood trough concentrations are shown in the table above; blood concentration details are described in **Blood Concentration Monitoring: *Liver Transplantation*** below.

Kidney Transplantation

The recommended starting oral dose of Prograf is 0.2 mg/kg/day administered every 12 hours in two divided doses. The initial dose of Prograf may be administered within 24 hours of transplantation, but should be delayed until renal function has recovered (as indicated for example by a serum creatinine ≤ 4 mg/dL). Black patients may require higher doses to achieve comparable blood concentrations. Dosage

Summary of Initial Oral Dosage Recommendations and Typical Whole Blood Trough Concentrations

Patient Population	Recommended Initial Oral Dose*	Typical Whole Blood Trough Concentrations
Adult kidney transplant patients	0.2 mg/kg/day	month 1–3 : 7–20 ng/mL month 4–12 : 5–15 ng/mL
Adult liver transplant patients	0.10–0.15 mg/kg/day	month 1–12 : 5–20 ng/mL
Pediatric liver transplant patients	0.15–0.20 mg/kg/day	month 1–12 : 5–20 ng/mL

*Note: two divided doses, q12h

	Caucasian n = 114		Black n = 56	
Time After Transplant	**Dose (mg/kg)**	**Trough Concentrations (ng/mL)**	**Dose (mg/kg)**	**Trough Concentrations (ng/mL)**
Day 7	0.18	12.0	0.23	10.9
Month 1	0.17	12.8	0.26	12.9
Month 6	0.14	11.8	0.24	11.5
Month 12	0.13	10.1	0.19	11.0

and typical tacrolimus whole blood trough concentrations are shown in the table above; blood concentration details are described in **Blood Concentration Monitoring: *Kidney Transplantation*** below.

The data in kidney transplant patients indicate that the Black patients required a higher dose to attain comparable trough concentrations compared to Caucasian patients.

[See second table above]

Pediatric Patients

Pediatric liver transplantation patients without pre-existing renal or hepatic dysfunction have required and tolerated higher doses than adults to achieve similar blood concentrations. Therefore, it is recommended that therapy be initiated in pediatric patients at a starting IV dose of 0.03–0.05 mg/kg/day and a starting oral dose of 0.15–0.20 mg/kg/day. Dose adjustments may be required. Experience in pediatric kidney transplantation patients is limited.

Patients with Hepatic or Renal Dysfunction

Due to the potential for nephrotoxicity, patients with renal or hepatic impairment should receive doses at the lowest value of the recommended IV and oral dosing ranges. Further reductions in dose below these ranges may be required. Prograf therapy usually should be delayed up to 48 hours or longer in patients with post-operative oliguria.

Conversion from One Immunosuppressive Regimen to Another

Prograf should not be used simultaneously with cyclosporine. Prograf or cyclosporine should be discontinued at least 24 hours before initiating the other. In the presence of elevated Prograf or cyclosporine concentrations, dosing with the other drug usually should be further delayed.

Blood Concentration Monitoring

Monitoring of tacrolimus blood concentrations in conjunction with other laboratory and clinical parameters is considered an essential aid to patient management for the evaluation of rejection, toxicity, dose adjustments and compliance. Factors influencing frequency of monitoring include but are not limited to hepatic or renal dysfunction, the addition or discontinuation of potentially interacting drugs and the posttransplant time. Blood concentration monitoring is not a replacement for renal and liver function monitoring and tissue biopsies.

Two methods have been used for the assay of tacrolimus, a microparticle enzyme immunoassay (MEIA) and an ELISA. Both methods have the same monoclonal antibody for tacrolimus. Comparison of the concentrations in published literature to patient concentrations using the current assays must be made with detailed knowledge of the assay methods and biological matrices employed. Whole blood is the matrix of choice and specimens should be collected into tubes containing ethylene diamine tetraacetic acid (EDTA) anti-coagulant. Heparin anti-coagulation is not recommended because of the tendency to form clots on storage. Samples which are not analyzed immediately should be stored at room temperature or in a refrigerator and assayed within 7 days; if samples are to be kept longer they should be deep frozen at −20°C for up to 12 months.

Liver Transplantation

Although there is a lack of direct correlation between tacrolimus concentrations and drug efficacy, data from Phase II and III studies of liver transplant patients have shown an increasing incidence of adverse events with increasing trough blood concentrations. Most patients are stable when trough whole blood concentrations are maintained between 5 to 20 ng/mL. Long term posttransplant patients often are maintained at the low end of this target range.

Data from the U.S. clinical trial show that tacrolimus whole blood concentrations, as measured by ELISA, were most variable during the first week post-transplantation. After this early period, the median trough blood concentrations, measured at intervals from the second week to one year post-transplantation, ranged from 9.8 ng/mL to 19.4 ng/mL.

Therapeutic Drug Monitoring, 1995, Volume 17, Number 6 contains a consensus document and several position papers regarding the therapeutic monitoring of tacrolimus from the 1995 International Consensus Conference on Immunosuppressive Drugs. Refer to these manuscripts for further discussions of tacrolimus monitoring.

Kidney Transplantation

Data from the U.S. study indicates that trough concentrations of tacrolimus in whole blood, as measured by IMx®, were most variable during the first week of dosing. During the first three months, 80% of the patients maintained trough concentrations between 7–20 ng/mL, and then between 5–15 ng/mL, through one-year.

The relative risk of toxicity is increased with higher trough concentrations. Therefore, monitoring of whole blood trough concentrations is recommended to assist in the clinical evaluation of toxicity.

HOW SUPPLIED

Prograf capsules (tacrolimus capsules) 0.5 mg

Oblong, light yellow, branded with red "0.5 mg" on the capsule cap and "607" on the capsule body, supplied in 60-count bottles (NDC 0469-0607-67) and 10 blister cards of 10 capsules (NDC 0469-0607-10), containing the equivalent of 0.5 mg anhydrous tacrolimus.

Prograf capsules (tacrolimus capsules) 1 mg

Oblong, white, branded with red "1 mg" on the capsule cap and "617" on the capsule body, supplied in 100–count bottles (NDC 0469-0617-71) and 10 blister cards of 10 capsules (NDC 0469-0617-10), containing the equivalent of 1 mg anhydrous tacrolimus.

Prograf capsules (tacrolimus capsules) 5 mg

Oblong, grayish/red, branded with white "5 mg" on the capsule cap and "657" on the capsule body, supplied in 100–count bottles (NDC 0469-0657-71) and 10 blister cards of 10 capsules (NDC 0469-0657-10), containing the equivalent of 5 mg anhydrous tacrolimus.

Store and Dispense

Store at 25°C (77°F); excursion permitted to 15°C–30°C (59°F–86°F).

Prograf injection (tacrolimus injection) 5 mg (for IV infusion only)

Supplied as a sterile solution in 1 mL ampules containing the equivalent of 5 mg of anhydrous tacrolimus per mL, in boxes of 10 ampules (NDC 0469-3016-01).

Store and Dispense

Store between 5°C and 25°C (41°F and 77°F).

Rx only

Made in Ireland
for Fujisawa Healthcare, Inc.
Deerfield, IL 60015–2548
by Fujisawa Ireland, Ltd.
Killorglin, Co. Kerry, Ireland

REFERENCE

1. CDC: Recommendations of the Advisory Committee on Immunization Practices: Use of vaccines and immune globulins in persons with altered immunocompetence. MMWR 1993;42(RR-4):1–18.

Shown in Product Identification Guide, page 313

For information on over-the-counter drugs, consult **PDR For Nonprescription Drugs**.

Galderma Laboratories, L. P.
P.O. BOX 331329
FT. WORTH, TX 76163

Direct Inquiries to:
(800) 582-8225
8:00 am—5:00 pm Central
Monday through Friday
or www.galderma.com

BENZAC AC® $2^1/_2$, 5 & 10 ℞
(benzoyl peroxide gel)
BENZAC AC® Wash $2^1/_2$, 5 & 10 ℞
(benzoyl peroxide)

DESCRIPTION

Benzac AC® $2^1/_2$, **5** and **10** (benzoyl peroxide gel), **Benzac AC® Wash** $2^1/_2$, **5** and **10** (benzoyl peroxide), are topical, water-base, benzoyl peroxide containing preparations for use in the treatment of acne vulgaris. Benzoyl peroxide is an oxidizing agent which possesses antibacterial properties and is classified as a keratolytic. Benzoyl peroxide ($C_{14}H_{10}O_4$) is represented by the following chemical structure:

O = C – O – O – C = O

Benzac AC® $2^1/_2$, **Benzac AC® 5**, and **Benzac AC® 10** contain, respectively, benzoyl peroxide $2^1/_2$%, 5% and 10% as the active ingredient in a gel base containing docusate sodium, edetate disodium, poloxamer 182, carbomer 940, propylene glycol, acrylates copolymer, glycerin, silicon dioxide, sodium hydroxide and purified water. May contain citric acid to adjust pH.

Benzac AC® Wash $2^1/_2$, **Benzac AC® Wash 5** and **Benzac AC® Wash 10** contain, respectively, benzoyl peroxide $2^1/_2$%, 5% and 10% as the active ingredient in a vehicle consisting of purified water, sodium C14–16 olefin sulfonate, acrylates copolymer, glycerin, sodium hydroxide, and carbomer 940. May contain citric acid to adjust pH.

CLINICAL PHARMACOLOGY

The mechanism of action of benzoyl peroxide is not totally understood but its antibacterial activity against *Propionibacterium acnes* is thought to be a major mode of action. In addition, patients treated with benzoyl peroxide show a reduction in lipids and free fatty acids and mild desquamation (drying and peeling activity) with a simultaneous reduction in comedones and acne lesions.

Little is known about the percutaneous penetration, metabolism, and excretion of benzoyl peroxide, although it has been shown that benzoyl peroxide absorbed by the skin is metabolized to benzoic acid and then excreted as benzoate in the urine. There is no evidence of systemic toxicity caused by benzoyl peroxide in humans.

INDICATIONS AND USAGE

Benzac AC® $2^1/_2$, **5** and **10** and **Benzac AC® Wash** $2^1/_2$, **5** and **10** are indicated for the topical treatment of acne vulgaris.

CONTRAINDICATIONS

These preparations are contraindicated in patients with a history of hypersensitivity to any of their components.

PRECAUTIONS

General: For external use only. If severe irritation develops, discontinue use and institute appropriate therapy. After the reaction clears, treatment may often be resumed with less frequent application. These preparations should not be used in or near the eyes or on mucous membranes.

Information for patients: Avoid contact with eyes, eyelids, lips and mucous membranes. If accidental contact occurs, rinse with water. Contact with any colored material (including hair and fabric) may result in bleaching or discoloration. If excessive irritation develops, discontinue use and consult your physician.

Carcinogenesis, Mutagenesis, Impairment of Fertility: Data from several studies employing a strain of mice that are highly susceptible to developing cancer suggest that benzoyl peroxide acts as a tumor promotor. The clinical significance of these findings to humans is unknown. Benzoyl peroxide has not been found to be mutagenic (Ames Test) and there are no published data indicating it impairs fertility.

Pregnancy: Teratogenic Effects: *Pregnancy Category C:* Animal reproduction studies have not been conducted with benzoyl peroxide. It is not known whether benzoyl peroxide can cause fetal harm when administered to a pregnant woman or can affect reproduction capacity. Benzoyl peroxide should be used by a pregnant woman only if clearly needed. There are no available data on the effect of benzoyl peroxide on the later growth, development and functional maturation of the unborn child.

Nursing Mothers: It is not known whether this drug is excreted in human milk. Because many drugs are excreted in human milk, caution should be exercised when benzoyl peroxide is administered to a nursing woman.

Pediatric Use: Safety and effectiveness in children have not been established.

ADVERSE REACTIONS

Allergic contact dermatitis and dryness have been reported with topical benzoyl peroxide therapy.

OVERDOSAGE

If excessive scaling, erythema or edema occur, the use of this preparation should be discontinued. To hasten resolution of the adverse effects, cool compresses may be used. After symptoms and signs subside, a reduced dosage schedule may be cautiously tried if the reaction is judged to be due to excessive use and not allergenicity.

DOSAGE AND ADMINISTRATION

Benzac AC® $2^1/_2$, **5** or **10** should be applied once or twice daily to cover affected areas after washing with a mild cleanser and water.

Benzac AC® Wash $2^1/_2$, **5** or **10**. Wash once or twice daily avoiding contact with the eyes and mucous membranes. Wet the area of application. Apply **Benzac AC® Wash** $2^1/_2$, **5** or **10** to the hands and wash the affected areas. Rinse with water and pat dry.

HOW SUPPLIED

Benzac AC® $2^1/_2$ Water Base Gel
60 g tubes—**NDC** 0299-3620-60
90 g tubes—**NDC** 0299-3620-90
Benzac AC® 5 Water Base Gel
60 g tubes—**NDC** 0299-3625-60
90 g tubes—**NDC** 0299-3625-90
Benzac AC® 10 Water Base Gel
60 g tubes—**NDC** 0299-3630-60
90 g tubes—**NDC** 0299-3630-90
Benzac AC® Wash $2^1/_2$
8 oz plastic bottles—**NDC** 0299-3635-08
Benzac AC® Wash 5
8 oz plastic bottles—**NDC** 0299-3640-08
Benzac AC® Wash 10
8 oz plastic bottles—**NDC** 0299-3645-08

STORAGE

Store Benzac AC® and **Benzac AC® Wash** at controlled room temperature (59°–86°F).

CAUTION

Federal law prohibits dispensing without prescription.
Revised: March 1994

DESOWEN® ℞
(desonide cream, ointment and lotion)
Cream 0.05%
Ointment 0.05%
and Lotion 0.05%

For Dermatologic Use Only–
Not for Ophthalmic Use–

DESCRIPTION

DesOwen® Cream 0.05%, Ointment 0.05%, and Lotion 0.05% contain desonide (Pregna-1,4-diene-3,20-dione,11, 21-dihydroxy-16,17-[(1-methylethylidene)bis(oxy)]-,(11β, 16α-) a synthetic nonfluorinated corticosteroid for topical dermatologic use. The corticosteroids constitute a class of primarily synthetic steroids used topically as anti-inflammatory and anti-pruritic agents.

Chemically, desonide is $C_{24}H_{32}O_6$. It has the following structural formula:

Desonide has the molecular weight of 416.51. It is a white to off white odorless powder which is soluble in methanol and practically insoluble in water.

Each gram of **DesOwen®** Cream contains 0.5 mg of desonide in a base of purified water, emulsifying wax, propylene glycol, stearic acid, isopropyl palmitate, synthetic beeswax, polysorbate 60, potassium sorbate, sorbic acid, propyl gallate, citric acid, and sodium hydroxide.

Each gram of **DesOwen®** Ointment contains 0.5 mg of desonide in a base of mineral oil and polyethylene.

Each gram of **DesOwen®** Lotion contains 0.5 mg of desonide in a base of sodium lauryl sulfate, light mineral oil, cetyl alcohol, stearyl alcohol, propylene glycol, methylparaben, propylparaben, sorbitan monostearate, glyceryl stearate SE, edetate sodium and purified water. May contain citric acid and/or sodium hydroxide for pH adjustment.

CLINICAL PHARMACOLOGY

Like other topical corticosteroids, desonide has anti-inflammatory, antipruritic and vasoconstrictive properties. The mechanism of the anti-inflammatory activity of the topical steroids, in general, is unclear. However corticosteroids are thought to act by the induction of phospholipase A_2 inhibitory proteins, collectively called lipocortins. It is postulated that these proteins control the biosynthesis of potent mediators of inflammation such as prostaglandins and leukotrienes by inhibiting the release of their common precursor arachidonic acid. Arachidonic acid is released from membrane phospholipids by phospholipase A_2.

Pharmacokinetics: The extent of percutaneous absorption of topical corticosteroids is determined by many factors including the vehicle and the integrity of the epidermal barrier. Occlusive dressings with hydrocortisone for up to 24 hours have not been demonstrated to increase penetration; however, occlusion of hydrocortisone for 96 hours markedly enhances penetration. Topical corticosteroids can be absorbed from normal intact skin. Inflammation and/or other disease processes in the skin may increase percutaneous absorption.

Studies performed with **DesOwen®** (desonide cream, ointment and lotion) Cream, Ointment, and Lotion indicate that they are in the low to medium range of potency as compared with other topical corticosteroids.

INDICATION AND USAGE

DesOwen® Cream, Ointment and Lotion are low to medium potency corticosteroids indicated for the relief of the inflammatory and pruritic manifestations of corticosteroid responsive dermatoses.

CONTRAINDICATIONS

DesOwen® Cream, Ointment and Lotion are contraindicated in those patients with a history of hypersensitivity to any of the components of the preparations.

PRECAUTIONS

General: Systemic absorption of topical corticosteroids can produce reversible hypothalamic-pituitary-adrenal (HPA) axis suppression with the potential for glucocorticosteroid insufficiency after withdrawal of treatment. Manifestations of Cushing's syndrome, hyperglycemia, and glucosuria can also be produced in some patients by systemic absorption of topical corticosteroids while on treatment.

Patients applying a topical steroid to a large surface area or to areas under occlusion should be evaluated periodically for evidence of HPA axis suppression. This may be done by using the ACTH stimulation, A.M. plasma cortisol, and urinary free cortisol tests. Patients receiving superpotent corticosteroids should not be treated for more than 2 weeks at a time and only small areas should be treated at any one time due to the increased risk of HPA axis suppression.

If HPA axis suppression is noted, an attempt should be made to withdraw the drug, to reduce the frequency of application, or to substitute a less potent corticosteroid. Recovery of HPA axis function is generally prompt and complete upon discontinuation of topical corticosteroids. Infrequently, signs and symptoms of glucocorticosteroid insufficiency may occur requiring supplemental systemic corticosteroids. For information on systemic supplementation, see prescribing information for those products.

Pediatric patients may be more susceptible to systemic toxicity from equivalent doses due to their larger skin surface to body mass ratios. (See PRECAUTIONS—Pediatric use).

If irritation develops, **DesOwen®** Cream, Ointment or Lotion should be discontinued and appropriate therapy instituted. Allergic contact dermatitis with corticosteroids is usually diagnosed by observing *failure to heal* rather than noting a clinical exacerbation as with most topical products not containing corticosteroids. Such an observation should be corroborated with appropriate diagnostic patch testing.

If concomitant skin infections are present or develop, an appropriate antifungal or antibacterial agent should be used. If a favorable response does not occur promptly, use of **DesOwen®** (desonide cream, ointment and lotion) Cream, Ointment or Lotion should be discontinued until the infection has been adequately controlled.

Information for patients: Patients using topical corticosteroids should receive the following information and instructions:

1. This medication is to be used as directed by the physician. It is for external use only. Avoid contact with the eyes.
2. This medication should not be used for any disorder other than that for which it was prescribed.
3. The treated skin area should not be bandaged or otherwise covered or wrapped so as to be occlusive unless directed by the physician.
4. Patients should report to their physician any signs of local adverse reactions.

Laboratory tests: The following tests may be helpful in evaluating patients for HPA axis suppression:
ACTH stimulation test
A.M. plasma cortisol test
Urinary free cortisol test

Carcinogenesis, mutagenesis, and impairment of fertility: Long-term animal studies have not been performed to evaluate the carcinogenic potential or the effect on reproduction with the use of **DesOwen®** Cream, Ointment, and Lotion.

Pregnancy: *Teratogenic effects: Pregnancy category C:* Corticosteroids have been shown to be teratogenic in laboratory animals when administered systemically at relatively low dosage levels. Some corticosteroids have been shown to be teratogenic after dermal application in laboratory animals. Animal reproduction studies have not been conducted with **DesOwen®** Cream, Ointment or Lotion. It is also not known whether **DesOwen®** Cream, Ointment or Lotion can cause fetal harm when administered to a preg-

Continued on next page

Desowen—Cont.

nant woman or can affect reproduction capacity. **DesOwen®** Cream, Ointment and Lotion should be given to a pregnant woman only if clearly needed.

Nursing mothers: Systemically administered corticosteroids appear in human milk and could suppress growth, interfere with endogenous corticosteroid production, or cause other untoward effects. It is not known whether topical administration of corticosteroids could result in sufficient systemic absorption to produce detectable quantities in human milk. Because many drugs are excreted in human milk, caution should be exercised when **DesOwen®** Cream, Ointment or Lotion is administered to a nursing woman.

Pediatric use: Safety and effectiveness in pediatric patients have not been established. Because of a higher ratio of skin surface area to body mass, pediatric patients are at a greater risk than adults of HPA axis suppression when they are treated with topical corticosteroids. They are therefore also at greater risk of glucocorticosteroid insufficiency after withdrawal of treatment and of Cushing's syndrome while on treatment. Adverse effects including striae have been reported with inappropriate use of topical corticosteroids in infants and children.

HPA axis suppression, Cushing's syndrome, linear growth retardation, delayed weight gain and intracranial hypertension have been reported in children receiving topical corticosteroids. Manifestations of adrenal suppression in children include low plasma cortisol levels, and absence of response to ACTH stimulation. Manifestations of intracranial hypertension include bulging fontanelles, headaches, and bilateral papilledema.

ADVERSE REACTIONS

In controlled clinical trials, the total incidence of adverse reactions associated with the use of desonide was approximately 8%. These were: stinging and burning approximately 3%, irritation, contact dermatitis, condition worsened, peeling of skin, itching, intense transient erythema, and dryness/scaliness, each less than 2%.

The following additional local adverse reactions have been reported infrequently with other topical corticosteroids, and they may occur more frequently with the use of occlusive dressings, especially with higher potency corticosteroids. These reactions are listed in an approximate decreasing order of occurrence: folliculitis, acneiform eruptions, hypopigmentation, perioral dermatitis, secondary infection, skin atrophy, striae, and miliaria.

OVERDOSAGE

Topically applied **DesOwen®** (desonide cream, ointment, and lotion) Cream, Ointment and Lotion can be absorbed in sufficient amounts to produce systemic effects (See PRECAUTIONS).

DOSAGE AND ADMINISTRATION

DesOwen® Cream, Ointment or Lotion should be applied to the affected areas as a thin film two or three times daily depending on the severity of the condition. SHAKE LOTION WELL BEFORE USING.

As with other corticosteroids, therapy should be discontinued when control is achieved. If no improvement is seen within 2 weeks, reassessment of diagnosis may be necessary.

DesOwen® Cream, Ointment and Lotion should not be used with occlusive dressings.

HOW SUPPLIED

DesOwen® (desonide cream) Cream 0.05% is supplied in tubes containing:

15 g **NDC** 0299-5770-15
60 g **NDC** 0299-5770-60

DesOwen® (desonide ointment) Ointment 0.05% is supplied in tubes containing:

15 g **NDC** 0299-5775-15
60 g **NDC** 0299-5775-60

DesOwen® (desonide lotion) Lotion 0.05% is supplied in bottles containing:

2 fl oz **NDC** 0299-5765-02
4 fl oz **NDC** 0299-5765-04

Storage Conditions: Store between 2° and 30°C (36° and 86°F).

CAUTION: Federal law prohibits dispensing without prescription.

225025-0395 Revised: March 1995

DIFFERIN® ℞
(adapalene gel)
Gel, 0.1%

DESCRIPTION

Differin® Gel, containing adapalene, is used for the topical treatment of acne vulgaris. Each gram of **Differin®** Gel contains adapalene 0.1% (1mg) in a vehicle consisting of propylene glycol, carbomer 940, poloxamer 182, edetate disodium, methylparaben, sodium hydroxide, and purified water. May contain hydrochloric acid to adjust pH.

The chemical name of adapalene is 6-[3-(1-adamantyl)-4-methoxyphenyl]-2-naphthoic acid. Adapalene is a white to off-white powder which is soluble in tetrahydrofuran, sparingly soluble in ethanol, and practically insoluble in water. The molecular formula is $C_{28}H_{28}O_3$ and molecular weight is 412.52. Adapalene is represented by the following structural formula:

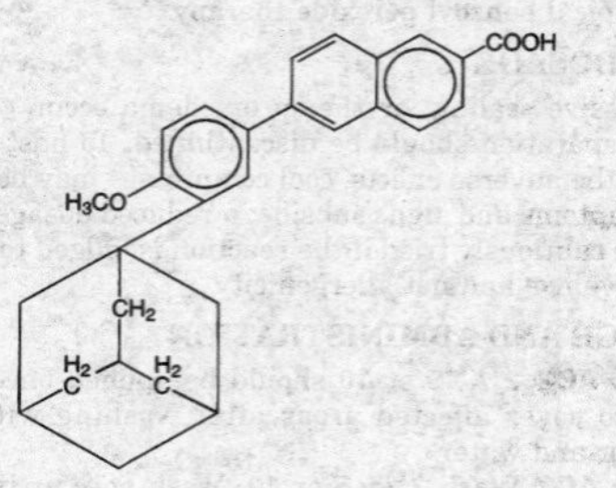

CLINICAL PHARMACOLOGY

Adapalene is a chemically stable, retinoid-like compound. Biochemical and pharmacological profile studies have demonstrated that adapalene is a modulator of cellular differentiation, keratinization, and inflammatory processes all of which represent important features in the pathology of acne vulgaris.

Mechanistically, adapalene binds to specific retinoic acid nuclear receptors but does not bind to the cytosolic receptor protein. Although the exact mode of action of adapalene is unknown, it is suggested that topical adapalene may normalize the differentiation of follicular epithelial cells resulting in decreased microcomedone formation.

Pharmacokinetics: Absorption of adapalene through human skin is low. Only trace amounts (<0.25 ng/mL) of parent substance have been found in the plasma of acne patients following chronic topical application of adapalene in controlled clinical trials. Excretion appears to be primarily by the biliary route.

INDICATIONS AND USAGE

Differin® Gel is indicated for the topical treatment of acne vulgaris.

CONTRAINDICATIONS

Differin® Gel should not be administered to individuals who are hypersensitive to adapalene or any of the components in the vehicle gel.

WARNINGS

Use of **Differin®** Gel should be discontinued if hypersensitivity to any of the ingredients is noted. Patients with sunburn should be advised not to use the product until fully recovered.

PRECAUTIONS

General: If a reaction suggesting sensitivity or chemical irritation occurs, use of the medication should be discontinued. Exposure to sunlight, including sunlamps, should be minimized during the use of adapalene. Patients who normally experience high levels of sun exposure, and those with inherent sensitivity to sun, should be warned to exercise caution. Use of sunscreen products and protective clothing over treated areas is recommended when exposure cannot be avoided. Weather extremes, such as wind or cold, also may be irritating to patients under treatment with adapalene.

Avoid contact with the eyes, lips, angles of the nose, and mucous membranes. The product should not be applied to cuts, abrasions, eczematous skin, or sunburned skin.

Certain cutaneous signs and symptoms such as erythema, dryness, scaling, burning, or pruritus may be experienced during treatment. These are most likely to occur during the first two to four weeks and will usually lessen with continued use of the medication. Depending upon the severity of adverse events, patients should be instructed to reduce the frequency of application or discontinue use.

Drug Interactions: As **Differin®** Gel has the potential to produce local irritation in some patients, concomitant use of other potentially irritating topical products (medicated or abrasive soaps and cleansers, soaps and cosmetics that have a strong drying effect, and products with high concentrations of alcohol, astringents, spices, or lime) should be approached with caution. Particular caution should be exercised in using preparations containing sulfur, resorcinol, or salicylic acid in combination with **Differin®** Gel. If these preparations have been used, it is advisable not to start therapy with **Differin®** Gel until the effects of such preparations in the skin have subsided.

Carcinogenesis, Mutagenesis, Impairment of Fertility: Carcinogenicity studies with adapalene have been conducted in mice at topical doses of 0.3, 0.9, and 2.6 mg/kg/day and in rats at oral doses of 0.15, 0.5, and 1.5 mg/kg/day, approximately 4–75 times the maximal daily human topical dose. In the oral study, positive linear trends were observed in the incidence of follicular cell adenomas and carcinomas in the thyroid glands of female rats, and in the incidence of benign and malignant pheochromocytomas in the adrenal medullas of male rats.

No photocarcinogenicity studies were conducted. Animal studies have shown an increased tumorigenic risk with the use of pharmacologically similar drugs (e.g., retinoids) when exposed to UV irradiation in the laboratory or to sunlight. Although the significance of these studies to human use is not clear, patients should be advised to avoid or minimize exposure to either sunlight or artificial UV irradiation sources.

In a series of *in vivo* and *in vitro* studies, adapalene did not exhibit mutagenic or genotoxic activities.

Pregnancy: Teratogenic effects. Pregnancy Category C. No teratogenic effects were seen in rats at oral doses of adapalene 0.15 to 5.0 mg/kg/day, up to 120 times the maximal daily human topical dose. Cutaneous route teratology studies conducted in rats and rabbits at doses of 0.6, 2.0, and 6.0 mg/kg/day, up to 150 times the maximal daily human topical dose exhibited no fetotoxicity and only minimal increases in supernumerary ribs in rats. There are no adequate and well-controlled studies in pregnant women. Adapalene should be used during pregnancy only if the potential benefit justifies the potential risk to the fetus.

Nursing Mothers: It is not known whether this drug is excreted in human milk. Because many drugs are excreted in human milk, caution should be exercised when **Differin®** Gel is administered to a nursing woman.

Pediatric Use: Safety and effectiveness in pediatric patients below the age of 12 have not been established.

ADVERSE REACTIONS

Some adverse effects such as erythema, scaling, dryness, pruritus, and burning will occur in 10–40% of patients. Pruritus or burning immediately after application also occurs in approximately 20% of patients. The following additional adverse experiences were reported in approximately 1% or less of patients: skin irritation, burning/stinging, erythema, sunburn, and acne flares. These are most commonly seen during the first month of therapy and decrease in frequency and severity thereafter. All adverse effects with use of **Differin®** Gel during clinical trials were reversible upon discontinuation of therapy.

OVERDOSAGE

Differin® Gel is intended for cutaneous use only. If the medication is applied excessively, no more rapid or better results will be obtained and marked redness, peeling, or discomfort may occur. The acute oral toxicity of **Differin®** Gel in mice and rats is greater than 10 mL/kg. Chronic ingestion of the drug may lead to the same side effects as those associated with excessive oral intake of Vitamin A.

DOSAGE AND ADMINISTRATION

Differin® Gel should be applied once a day to affected areas after washing in the evening before retiring. A thin film of the gel should be applied, avoiding eyes, lips, and mucous membranes.

During the early weeks of therapy, an apparent exacerbation of acne may occur. This is due to the action of the medication on previously unseen lesions and should not be considered a reason to discontinue therapy. Therapeutic results should be noticed after eight to twelve weeks of treatment.

HOW SUPPLIED

Differin® (adapalene gel) Gel, 0.1% is supplied in the following sizes:

15 g laminate tube-**NDC** 0299-5910-15
45 g laminate tube-**NDC** 0299-5910-45

Storage: Store at controlled room temperature 20°–25°C (68°–77°F).

CAUTION: Federal law prohibits dispensing without prescription.

225022-0596
Revised: May 1996

DIFFERIN® ℞
(adapalene solution)
Solution, 0.1%

DESCRIPTION

DIFFERIN® Solution, containing adapalene, is used for the topical treatment of acne vulgaris. Each mL of DIFFERIN® Solution contains adapalene 0.1% (1 mg) in a vehicle consisting of polyethylene glycol 400 and SD alcohol 40-B, 30% (w/v).

The chemical name of adapalene is 6-[3-(1-adamantyl)-4-methoxyphenyl]-2-naphthoic acid. Adapalene is a white to off-white powder which is soluble in tetrahydrofuran, sparingly soluble in ethanol, and practically insoluble in water. The molecular formula is $C_{28}H_{28}O_3$ and molecular weight is 412.52. Adapalene is represented by the following structural formula:

COOH
H₃CO
CH₂
H₂C H₂C

CLINICAL PHARMACOLOGY

Adapalene is a chemically stable, retinoid-like compound. Biochemical and pharmacological profile studies have demonstrated that adapalene is a modulator of cellular differentiation, keratinization, and inflammatory processes all of which represent important features in the pathology of acne vulgaris. Mechanistically, adapalene binds to specific retinoic acid nuclear receptors but does not bind to the cytosolic receptor protein. Although the exact mode of action of adapalene is unknown, it is suggested that topical adapalene may normalize the differentiation of follicular epithelial cells resulting in decreased microcomedone formation.

Pharmacokinetics: Absorption of adapalene through human skin is low. Only trace amounts (< 0.25 ng/mL) of parent substance have been found in the plasma of acne patients following chronic topical application of adapalene in controlled clinical trials. Excretion appears to be primarily by the biliary route.

INDICATIONS AND USAGE

DIFFERIN® Solution is indicated for the topical treatment of acne vulgaris.

CONTRAINDICATIONS

DIFFERIN® Solution should not be administered to individuals who are hypersensitive to adapalene or any of the components in the vehicle solution.

WARNINGS

Use of DIFFERIN® Solution should be discontinued if hypersensitivity to any of the ingredients is noted. Patients with sunburn should be advised not to use the product until fully recovered.

PRECAUTIONS

General: If a reaction suggesting sensitivity or chemical irritation occurs, use of the medication should be discontinued. Exposure to sunlight, including sunlamps, should be minimized during the use of adapalene. Patients who normally experience high levels of sun exposure, and those with inherent sensitivity to sun, should be warned to exercise caution. Use of sunscreen products and protective clothing over treated areas is recommended when exposure cannot be avoided. Weather extremes, such as wind or cold, also may be irritating to patients under treatment with adapalene.

Avoid contact with the eyes, lips, angles of the nose, and mucous membranes. The product should not be applied to cuts, abrasions, eczematous skin, or sunburned skin.

Certain cutaneous signs and symptoms such as erythema, dryness, scaling, burning, or pruritus may be experienced during treatment. These are most likely to occur during the first two to four weeks and will usually lessen with continued use of the medication. Depending upon the severity of adverse events, patients should be instructed to reduce the frequency of application or discontinue use.

Drug Interactions: As DIFFERIN® Solution has the potential to produce local irritation in some patients, concomitant use of other potentially irritating topical products (medicated or abrasive soaps and cleansers, soaps and cosmetics that have a strong drying effect, and products with high concentrations of alcohol, astringents, spices, or lime) should be approached with caution. Particular caution should be exercised in using preparations containing sulfur, resorcinol, or salicylic acid in combination with DIFFERIN® Solution. If these preparations have been used, it is advisable not to start therapy with DIFFERIN® Solution until the effects of such preparations in the skin have subsided.

Carcinogenesis, Mutagenesis, Impairment of Fertility: Carcinogenicity studies with adapalene have been conducted in mice at topical doses of 0.3, 0.9, and 2.6 mg/kg/day and in rats at oral doses of 0.15, 0.5, and 1.5 mg/kg/day, approximately 4–75 times the maximal daily human topical dose. In the oral study, positive linear trends were observed in the incidence of follicular cell adenomas and carcinomas in the thyroid glands of female rats, and in the incidence of benign and malignant pheochromocytomas in the adrenal medullas of male rats.

No photocarcinogenicity studies were conducted. Animal studies have shown an increased tumorigenic risk with the use of pharmacologically similar drugs (e.g., retinoids) when exposed to UV irradiation in the laboratory or to sunlight. Although the significance of these studies to human use is not clear, patients should be advised to avoid or minimize exposure to either sunlight or artificial UV irradiation sources.

In a series of *in vivo* and *in vitro* studies, adapalene did not exhibit mutagenic or genotoxic activities.

Pregnancy: Teratogenic effects. Pregnancy Category C. No teratogenic effects were seen in rats at oral doses of adapalene 0.15 to 5.0 mg/kg/day, up to 120 times the maximal daily human topical dose. Cutaneous route teratology studies conducted in rats and rabbits at doses of 0.6, 2.0, and 6.0 mg/kg/day, up to 150 times the maximal daily human topical dose exhibited no fetotoxicity and only minimal increases in supernumerary ribs in rats. There are no adequate and well-controlled studies in pregnant women. Adapalene should be used during pregnancy only if the potential benefit justifies the potential risk to the fetus.

Nursing Mothers: It is not known whether this drug is excreted in human milk. Because many drugs are excreted in human milk, caution should be exercised when DIFFERIN® Solution is administered to a nursing woman.

Pediatric Use: Safety and effectiveness in pediatric patients below the age of 12 have not been established.

ADVERSE REACTIONS

Some adverse effects such as erythema, scaling, dryness, pruritus, and burning will occur in 30–60% of patients. Pruritus or burning immediately after application also occurs in approximately 30% of patients. The following additional adverse experiences were reported in approximately 1% or less of patients: skin irritation, burning/stinging, erythema, sunburn, and acne flares. These are most commonly seen during the first month of therapy and decrease in frequency and severity thereafter. All adverse effects with use of DIFFERIN® Solution during clinical trials were reversible upon discontinuation of therapy.

OVERDOSAGE

DIFFERIN® Solution is intended for cutaneous use only. If the medication is applied excessively, no more rapid or better results will be obtained and marked redness, peeling, or discomfort may occur. The acute oral toxicity of DIFFERIN® Solution in mice and rats is greater than 10 mL/kg. Chronic ingestion of the drug may lead to the same side effects as those associated with excessive oral intake of Vitamin A.

DOSAGE AND ADMINISTRATION

1. DIFFERIN® Solution should be applied once a day to affected areas.
2. Before retiring in the evening, wash and dry areas to be treated.
3. Apply a thin film of medication to the affected areas. Avoid the eyes, lips, and mucous membranes.

Pledget: Remove pledget from foil just before using. Discard pledget after single use. Do not use if seal is broken.

Glass bottle: Replace cap after each use.

During the early weeks of therapy, an apparent exacerbation of acne may occur. This is due to the action of the medication on previously unseen lesions and should not be considered a reason to discontinue therapy. Therapeutic results should be noticed after eight to twelve weeks of treatment.

HOW SUPPLIED

DIFFERIN® (adapalene solution) Solution, 0.1% is supplied in the following sizes:

30 mL glass bottle with applicator – **NDC** 0299-5905-30
60-count unit-of-use pledget – **NDC** 0299-5905-16

The applicator is designed so that the solution may be applied directly to the involved skin.

Storage: Store at controlled room temperature 20° – 25°C (68° – 77°F). Keep container tightly closed and store upright.

CAUTION: Federal law prohibits dispensing without prescription.

225050-0100
Revised: January 2000

METROCREAM® ℞

(metronidazole topical cream)
Topical Cream, 0.75%

FOR TOPICAL USE ONLY
(NOT FOR OPHTHALMIC USE)

DESCRIPTION

MetroCream® Topical Cream contains metronidazole, USP, at a concentration of 7.5 mg per gram (0.75%) in an emollient cream consisting of emulsifying wax, sorbitol solution, glycerin, isopropyl palmitate, benzyl alcohol, lactic acid and/or sodium hydroxide to adjust pH, and purified water. Metronidazole is a member of the imidazole class of antibacterial agents and is classified therapeutically as an antiprotozoal and antibacterial agent. Chemically, metronidazole is 2-methyl-5-nitro-1*H*-imidazole-1-ethanol. The molecular formula is $C_6H_9N_3O_3$ and molecular weight is 171.16. Metronidazole is represented by the following structural formula:

CH_2CH_2OH / O_2N / N / CH_3 / N

CLINICAL PHARMACOLOGY

The mechanisms by which metronidazole acts in the treatment of rosacea are unknown, but appear to include an anti-inflammatory effect.

INDICATIONS AND USAGE

MetroCream® (metronidazole topical cream) Topical Cream is indicated for topical application in the treatment of inflammatory papules and pustules of rosacea.

CONTRAINDICATIONS

MetroCream® (metronidazole topical cream) Topical Cream is contraindicated in individuals with a history of hypersensitivity to metronidazole, or other ingredients of the formulation.

PRECAUTIONS

General: Topical metronidazole has been reported to cause tearing of the eyes. Therefore, contact with the eyes should be avoided. If a reaction suggesting local irritation occurs, patients should be directed to use the medication less frequently or discontinue use. Metronidazole is a nitroimidazole and should be used with care in patients with evidence of, or history of blood dyscrasia.

Information for patients: This medication is to be used as directed by the physician. It is for external use only. Avoid contact with the eyes.

Drug Interactions: Oral metronidazole has been reported to potentiate the anticoagulant effect of warfarin and coumarin anticoagulants, resulting in a prolongation of prothrombin time. The effect of topical metronidazole on prothrombin time is not known.

Carcinogenesis, mutagenesis, impairment of fertility: Metronidazole has shown evidence of carcinogenic activity in a number of studies involving chronic, oral administration in mice and rats but not in studies involving hamsters. Metronidazole has shown evidence of mutagenic activity in several *in vitro* bacterial assay systems. In addition, a dose-response increase in the frequency of micronuclei was observed in mice after intraperitoneal injections and an increase in chromosome aberrations have been reported in patients with Crohn's disease who were treated with 200-1200 mg/day of metronidazole for 1 to 24 months. However, no excess chromosomal aberrations in circulating human lymphocytes have been observed in patients treated for 8 months.

Pregnancy: *Teratogenic effects: Pregnancy category B*

There are no adequate and well-controlled studies with the use of **MetroCream®** (metronidazole topical cream) Topical Cream in pregnant women. Metronidazole crosses the placental barrier and enters the fetal circulation rapidly. No fetotoxicity was observed after oral metronidazole in rats or mice. However, because animal reproduction studies are not always predictive of human response and since oral metronidazole has been shown to be a carcinogen in some rodents, this drug should be used during pregnancy only if clearly needed.

Nursing Mothers: After oral administration, metronidazole is secreted in breast milk in concentrations similar to those found in the plasma. Even though blood levels are significantly lower with topically applied metronidazole than those achieved after oral administration of metronidazole, a decision should be made whether to discontinue nursing or to discontinue the drug, taking into account the importance of the drug to the mother.

Pediatric Use: Safety and effectiveness in pediatric patients have not been established.

ADVERSE REACTIONS

In controlled clinical trials, the total incidence of adverse reactions associated with the use of **MetroCream®** Topical Cream was approximately 10%. Skin discomfort (burning and stinging) was the most frequently reported event followed by erythema, skin irritation, pruritus and worsening of rosacea. All individual events occurred in less than 3% of patients.

The following additional adverse experiences have been reported with the topical use of metronidazole: dryness, transient redness, metallic taste, tingling or numbness of extremities and nausea.

DOSAGE AND ADMINISTRATION

Apply and rub in a thin layer of **MetroCream®** (metronidazole topical cream) Topical Cream twice daily, morning and evening, to entire affected areas after washing.

Areas to be treated should be washed with a mild cleanser before application. Patients may use cosmetics after application of **MetroCream®** Topical Cream.

HOW SUPPLIED

MetroCream® (metronidazole topical cream) Topical Cream, 0.75% is supplied in a 45 g aluminum tube–**NDC** 0299-3836-45.

Storage conditions: STORE AT CONTROLLED ROOM TEMPERATURE: 59° to 86°F (15° to 30°C).

Caution: Federal law prohibits dispensing without prescription.

225029-0695
Revised: June 1995

METROGEL® ℞

(metronidazole topical gel)
Topical Gel, 0.75%
FOR TOPICAL USE ONLY
(NOT FOR OPHTHALMIC USE)

DESCRIPTION

MetroGel® Topical Gel contains metronidazole, USP, at a concentration of 7.5 mg per gram (0.75%) in a gel consisting of purified water, methylparaben, propylparaben, propylene glycol, carbomer 940, sodium hydroxide, and edetate disodium. Metronidazole is classified therapeutically as an antiprotozoal and antibacterial agent. Chemically, metronidazole is named 2-methyl-5-nitro-1*H* -imidazole-1-ethanol and has the following structure:

CH_2CH_2OH / O_2N / N / CH_3 / N

CLINICAL PHARMACOLOGY

Bioavailability studies on the topical administration of 1 gram of **MetroGel®** Topical Gel (7.5 mg of metronidazole) to

Continued on next page

Metrogel—Cont.

the face of 10 rosacea patients showed a maximum serum concentration of 66 nanograms per milliliter in one patient. This concentration is approximately 100 times less than concentrations afforded by a single 250 mg oral tablet. The serum metronidazole concentrations were below the detectable limits of the assay at the majority of time points in all patients. Three of the patients had no detectable serum concentrations of metronidazole at any time point. The mean dose of gel applied during clinical studies was 600 mg which represents 4.5 mg of metronidazole per application. Therefore, under normal usage levels, the formulation affords minimal serum concentrations of metronidazole. The mechanisms by which **MetroGel®** (metronidazole topical gel) Topical Gel acts in the treatment of rosacea are unknown, but appear to include an anti-inflammatory effect.

INDICATIONS AND USAGE

MetroGel® Topical Gel is indicated for topical application in the treatment of inflammatory papules and pustules of rosacea.

CONTRAINDICATIONS

MetroGel® Topical Gel is contraindicated in individuals with a history of hypersensitivity to metronidazole, parabens, or other ingredients of the formulation.

PRECAUTIONS

General: **MetroGel®** Topical Gel has been reported to cause tearing of the eyes. Therefore, contact with the eyes should be avoided. If a reaction suggesting local irritation occurs, patients should be directed to use the medication less frequently or discontinue use. Metronidazole is a nitroimidazole and should be used with care in patients with evidence of, or history of blood dyscrasia.

Information for patients: This medication is to be used as directed by the physician. It is for external use only. Avoid contact with the eyes.

Drug Interactions: Oral metronidazole has been reported to potentiate the anticoagulant effect of coumarin and warfarin resulting in a prolongation of prothrombin time. The effect of topical metronidazole on prothrombin time is not known.

Carcinogenesis, mutagenesis, impairment of fertility: Metronidazole has shown evidence of carcinogenic activity in a number of studies involving chronic, oral administration in mice and rats but not in studies involving hamsters. Metronidazole has shown evidence of mutagenic activity in several *in vitro* bacterial assay systems. In addition, a dose-response increase in the frequency of micronuclei was observed in mice after intraperitoneal injections and an increase in chromosome aberrations have been reported in patients with Crohn's disease who were treated with 200–1200 mg/day of metronidazole for 1 to 24 months. However, no excess chromosomal aberrations in circulating human lymphocytes have been observed in patients treated for 8 months.

Pregnancy: ***Teratogenic effects: Pregnancy category B:*** There has been no experience to date with the use of **MetroGel®** (metronidazole topical gel) Topical Gel in pregnant patients. Metronidazole crosses the placental barrier and enters the fetal circulation rapidly. No fetotoxicity was observed after oral metronidazole in rats or mice. However, because animal reproduction studies are not always predictive of human response and since oral metronidazole has been shown to be a carcinogen in some rodents, this drug should be used during pregnancy only if clearly needed.

Nursing mothers: After oral administration, metronidazole is secreted in breast milk in concentrations similar to those found in the plasma. Even though **MetroGel®** Topical Gel blood levels are significantly lower than those achieved after oral metronidazole, a decision should be made whether to discontinue nursing or to discontinue the drug, taking into account the importance of the drug to the mother.

Pediatric use: Safety and effectiveness in pediatric patients have not been established.

ADVERSE REACTIONS

The following adverse experiences have been reported with the topical use of metronidazole: burning, skin irritation, dryness, transient redness, metallic taste, tingling or numbness of extremities and nausea.

DOSAGE AND ADMINISTRATION

Apply and rub in a thin film of **MetroGel®** Topical Gel twice daily, morning and evening, to entire affected areas after washing.

Areas to be treated should be cleansed before application of **MetroGel®** (metronidazole topical gel) Topical Gel. Patients may use cosmetics after application of **MetroGel®** Topical Gel.

HOW SUPPLIED

MetroGel® (metronidazole topical gel) Topical Gel is supplied in a 1 oz (28.4 g) aluminum tube—**NDC** 0299-3835-28 and a 45 g aluminum tube—**NDC** 0299-3835-45.

Storage conditions: STORE AT CONTROLLED ROOM TEMPERATURE: 59° to 86°F (15° to 30°C).

Caution: Federal law prohibits dispensing without prescription.

225032-0895

Revised: August 1995

METROLOTION® ℞

(metronidazole lotion)
Topical Lotion, 0.75%
Rx only

FOR TOPICAL USE ONLY
(NOT FOR OPHTHALMIC USE)

DESCRIPTION

MetroLotion® (metronidazole lotion) Topical Lotion contains metronidazole, USP, at a concentration of 7.5 mg per gram (0.75% w/w) in a lotion consisting of benzyl alcohol, carbomer 941, cyclomethicone, glycerin, glyceryl stearate, light mineral oil, PEG-100 stearate, polyethylene glycol 400, potassium sorbate, purified water, steareth-21, stearyl alcohol, and sodium hydroxide and/or lactic acid to adjust pH.

Metronidazole is an imidazole and is classified therapeutically as an antiprotozoal and antibacterial agent. Chemically, metronidazole is 2-methyl-5-nitro-1*H*-imidazole-1-ethanol. The molecular formula is $C_6H_9N_3O_3$ and molecular weight is 171.16. Metronidazole is represented by the following structural formula:

CH_2CH_2OH; O_2N; N; CH_3; N

CLINICAL PHARMACOLOGY

The mechanisms by which metronidazole acts in the treatment of rosacea are unknown, but appear to include an anti-inflammatory effect.

Pharmacokinetics: Absorption of metronidazole after topical application of MetroLotion® Topical Lotion is less complete and more prolonged than after oral administration. Detectable plasma levels were found in all subjects following the administration of a single 1 gram dose of MetroLotion® Topical Lotion (containing 7.5 mg of metronidazole) to the faces of 12 healthy volunteers. The highest concentration (64 ng/mL) seen was approximately 100 times lower than the peak concentrations produced by a single 250 mg tablet of metronidazole. The mean relative bioavailability of metronidazole from MetroLotion® Topical Lotion was 47.4%.

INDICATIONS AND USAGE

MetroLotion® Topical Lotion is indicated for topical application in the treatment of inflammatory papules and pustules of rosacea.

CLINICAL STUDIES

A controlled clinical study was conducted in 144 patients with moderate to severe rosacea, in which MetroLotion® Topical Lotion was compared with its vehicle. Applications were made twice daily for 12 weeks during which patients were instructed to avoid spicy foods, thermally hot foods and drinks, alcoholic beverages, and caffeine. Patients were also provided samples of a soapless cleansing lotion and, if requested, a moisturizer. MetroLotion® Topical Lotion was significantly more effective than its vehicle in mean percent reduction of inflammatory lesions associated with rosacea and in the investigators' global assessment of improvement. The results of the mean percent reduction in inflammatory lesion counts from baseline after 12 weeks of treatment and the investigators' global assessment of improvement at week 12 are presented in the following table:

[See table below]

The scale is based on the following definitions:

Worse:
: Exacerbation of either erythema or quantitative assessment of papules and/or pustules.

No Change:
: Condition remains the same.

Minimal Improvement:
: Slight improvement in the quantitative assessment of papules and/or pustules, and/or slight improvement in erythema.

Definite Improvement:
: More pronounced improvement in the quantitative assessment of papules and/or pustules, and/or more pronounced improvement in erythema.

Marked Improvement:
: Obvious improvement in the quantitative assessment of papules and/or pustules, and/or obvious improvement in erythema.

Clear:
: No papules or pustules and minimal residual or no erythema.

CONTRAINDICATIONS

MetroLotion® Topical Lotion is contraindicated in individuals with a history of hypersensitivity to metronidazole or to other ingredients of the formulation.

PRECAUTIONS

General: Topical metronidazole formulations have been reported to cause tearing of the eyes. Therefore, contact with the eyes should be avoided. If a reaction suggesting local irritation occurs, patients should be directed to use the medication less frequently or discontinue use. Metronidazole is a nitroimidazole and should be used with care in patients with evidence or history of blood dyscrasia.

Information for Patients: Patients using MetroLotion® Topical Lotion should receive the following information and instructions:

1. This medication is to be used only as directed by the physician.
2. It is for external use only.
3. Avoid contact with the eyes.
4. Cleanse affected area(s) before applying this medication.
5. Patients should report any adverse reaction to their physician.

Drug Interactions: Oral metronidazole has been reported to potentiate the anticoagulant effect of warfarin and coumarin anticoagulants, resulting in a prolongation of prothrombin time. The effect of topical metronidazole on prothrombin time is not known.

Carcinogenesis, Mutagenesis, Impairment of Fertility: Metronidazole has shown evidence of carcinogenic activity in a number of studies involving chronic, oral administration in mice and rats but not in studies involving hamsters. Neither carcinogenicity nor photocarcinogenicity studies have been performed by the topical route with MetroLotion® Topical Lotion or any marketed metronidazole formulations.

In several long-term studies in mice, oral doses of approximately 198 mg/m²/day or greater (approximately 29 to 71 times the human topical dose on a mg/m² basis) were associated with an increase in lung tumors in male mice and lymphomas in female mice.

Several long-term studies by the oral route in rats have shown statistically significant increases in mammary and hepatic tumors in female rats and testicular tumors and pituitary adenomas in male rats at doses (in feed) of 1593 mg/m²/day or greater (approximately 230 to 573 times the human topical dose on a mg/m² basis). In another oral study (by gavage), mammary tumors in female rats were observed with a dose of 177 mg/m²/day (approximately 26 to 64 times the human topical dose on a mg/m² basis).

In a published study, the ultraviolet radiation-induced carcinogenesis was enhanced in albino hairless mice by intraperitoneal administration of 45 mg/m² metronidazole, as shown by a decreased latency period to the development of skin neoplasms. The concentration of metronidazole in the skin following the intraperitoneal administration was not determined. This study did not distinguish whether metronidazole must be present during the exposure to ultraviolet radiation in order to enhance tumor formation or whether metronidazole could promote tumor formation from preexisting ultraviolet radiation-initiated cells. The significance of these results in the topical use of metronidazole for the treatment of rosacea is unclear.

Metronidazole has shown evidence of mutagenic activity in several *in vitro* bacterial assay systems. In addition, a dose-response increase in the frequency of micronuclei was observed in mice after intraperitoneal injections. An increase in chromosome aberrations in peripheral blood lymphocytes was reported in patients with Crohn's disease who were treated with 200–1200 mg/day of metronidazole for 1 to 24

Efficacy Outcomes at Week 12

Mean Percent Reduction in Inflammatory Lesion Counts from Baseline

MetroLotion® Topical Lotion N=65	Vehicle Lotion N=60
55%	20%

Investigators' Global Assessment of Improvement (percent change from baseline)

	Worse	No Change	Minimal Improvement	Definite Improvement	Marked Improvement	Clear
MetroLotion® Topical Lotion N=65	5%	12%	11%	32%	32%	8%
Vehicle Lotion N=60	15%	27%	23%	15%	20%	0%

months. However, in another study, no excess chromosomal aberrations in circulating human lymphocytes were observed in patients treated for 8 months.
In rats, oral metronidazole at doses of 1770 mg/m^2/day (approximately 255 to 637 times the human topical dose on a mg/m^2 basis) induced inhibition of spermatogenesis and severe testicular degeneration. In two strains of mice (ICR and CF1), conflicting results have been reported indicating either no effect or a similar effect to that reported in rats.
Pregnancy: *Teratogenic Effects: Pregnancy Category B:* There are no adequate and well-controlled studies with the use of MetroLotion® Topical Lotion in pregnant women. Metronidazole crosses the placental barrier and enters the fetal circulation rapidly. No fetotoxicity was observed after oral administration of metronidazole in rats or mice. However, because animal reproduction studies are not always predictive of human response and since oral metronidazole has been shown to be a carcinogen in some rodents, this drug should be used during pregnancy only if clearly needed.
Nursing Mothers: After oral administration, metronidazole is secreted in breast milk in concentrations similar to those found in the plasma. Even though blood levels are significantly lower with topically applied metronidazole than those achieved after oral administration of metronidazole, a decision should be made whether to discontinue nursing or to discontinue the drug, taking into account the importance of the drug to the mother.
Pediatric Use: Safety and effectiveness in pediatric patients have not been established.

ADVERSE REACTIONS

In a controlled clinical trial, safety data from 141 patients who used MetroLotion® Topical Lotion (n=71), or the lotion vehicle (n=70), twice daily and experienced a local cutaneous adverse event which may or may not have been related to the treatments include: local allergic reaction, MetroLotion® Topical Lotion 2 (3%), lotion vehicle 0; contact dermatitis, MetroLotion® Topical Lotion 2 (3%), lotion vehicle 1 (1%); pruritus, MetroLotion® Topical Lotion 1 (1%), lotion vehicle 0; skin discomfort (burning and stinging), MetroLotion® Topical Lotion 1 (1%), lotion vehicle 2 (3%); erythema, MetroLotion® Topical Lotion 4 (6%), lotion vehicle 0; dry skin, MetroLotion® Topical Lotion 0, lotion vehicle 1 (1%); and worsening of rosacea, MetroLotion® Topical Lotion 1 (1%), lotion vehicle 7 (10%).
The following additional adverse experiences have been reported with the topical use of metronidazole: skin irritation, transient redness, metallic taste, tingling or numbness of extremities, and nausea.

DOSAGE AND ADMINISTRATION

Apply a thin layer to entire affected areas after washing. Use morning and evening or as directed by physician. Avoid application close to the eyes.
Patients may use cosmetics after waiting for the MetroLotion® Topical Lotion to dry (not less than 5 minutes).

HOW SUPPLIED

MetroLotion® (metronidazole lotion) Topical Lotion, 0.75% is supplied in the following size:
2 fl. oz. (59 mL) plastic bottle—**NDC** 0299-3838-02
Storage: Store at controlled room temperature 68° to 77°F (20°–25°C). Protect from freezing.
225044-1198
Revised: November 1998

GATE Pharmaceuticals
Div. of TEVA Pharmaceuticals USA
650 CATHILL ROAD
SELLERSVILLE, PA 18960

Direct Inquiries to:
1090 Horsham Road
P. O. Box 1090
North Wales, PA 19454
(800) 292-4283

ADIPEX-P® Ⓒ ℞
(phentermine HCl 37.5 mg)

DESCRIPTION

Phentermine hydrochloride USP has the chemical name of α,α-Dimethylphenethylamine hydrochloride. The structural formula is as follows:

$C_6H_5-CH_2-C(CH_3)_2-NH_2 \cdot HCl$

$C_{10}H_{15}N \cdot HCl$ M.W. 185.7

Phentermine hydrochloride is a white, odorless, hygroscopic, crystalline powder which is soluble in water and lower alcohols, slightly soluble in chloroform and insoluble in ether.
ADIPEX-P®, an anorectic agent for oral administration, is available as a capsule or tablet containing 37.5 mg of phentermine hydrochloride (equivalent to 30 mg of phentermine base).
ADIPEX-P® Capsules contain the inactive ingredients Corn Starch, Gelatin, Lactose Monohydrate, Magnesium Stearate, Titanium Dioxide, Black Iron Oxide, FD&C Blue #1, FD&C Red #40 and D&C Red #33.
ADIPEX-P® Tablets contain the inactive ingredients Corn Starch, Lactose (Anhydrous), Magnesium Stearate, Microcrystalline Cellulose, Pregelatinized Starch, Sucrose, and FD&C Blue #1.

CLINICAL PHARMACOLOGY

ADIPEX-P® is a sympathomimetic amine with pharmacologic activity similar to the prototype drugs of this class used in obesity, the amphetamines. Actions include central nervous system stimulation and elevation of blood pressure. Tachyphylaxis and tolerance have been demonstrated with all drugs of this class in which these phenomena have been looked for.
Drugs of this class used in obesity are commonly known as "anorectics" or "anorexigenics." It has not been established that the action of such drugs in treating obesity is primarily one of appetite suppression. Other central nervous system actions, or metabolic effects, may be involved, for example. Adult obese subjects instructed in dietary management and treated with "anorectic" drugs lose more weight on the average than those treated with placebo and diet, as determined in relatively short-term clinical trials.
The magnitude of increased weight loss of drug-treated patients over placebo-treated patients is only a fraction of a pound a week. The rate of weight loss is greatest in the first week of therapy for both drug and placebo subjects and tends to decrease in succeeding weeks. The possible origins of the increased weight loss due to the various drug effects are not established. The amount of weight loss associated with the use of an "anorectic" drug varies from trial to trial, and the increased weight loss appears to be related in part to variables other than the drugs prescribed, such as the physician-investigator, the population treated and the diet prescribed. Studies do not permit conclusions as to the relative importance of the drug and non-drug factors on weight loss.
The natural history of obesity is measured in years, whereas the studies cited are restricted to a few weeks' duration; thus, the total impact of drug-induced weight loss over that of diet alone must be considered clinically limited.

INDICATIONS AND USAGE

ADIPEX-P® (phentermine hydrochloride) is indicated as a short-term (a few weeks) adjunct in a regimen of weight reduction based on exercise, behavioral modification and caloric restriction in the management of exogenous obesity for patients with an initial body mass index ≥30 kg/m^2, or ≥27 kg/m^2 in the presence of other risk factors (e.g., hypertension, diabetes, hyperlipidemia).
Below is a chart of Body Mass Index (BMI) based on various heights and weights.
BMI is calculated by taking the patient's weight, in kilograms (kg), divided by the patient's height, in meters (m), squared. Metric conversions are as follows: pounds ÷ 2.2 = kg; inches × 0.0254 = meters.

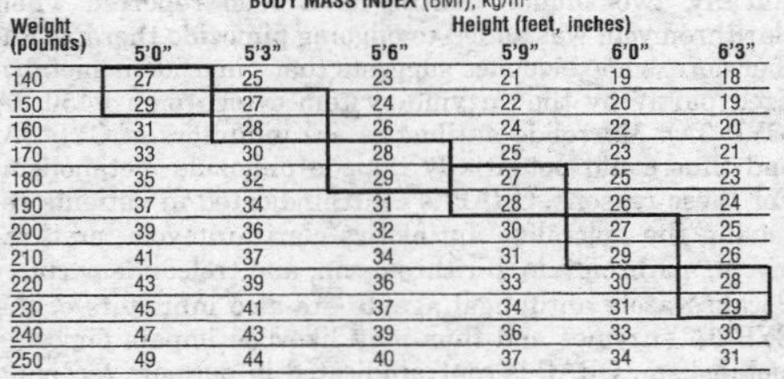

BODY MASS INDEX (BMI), kg/m^2

Weight (pounds)	Height (feet, inches) 5'0"	5'3"	5'6"	5'9"	6'0"	6'3"
140	27	25	23	21	19	18
150	29	27	24	22	20	19
160	31	28	26	24	22	20
170	33	30	28	25	23	21
180	35	32	29	27	25	23
190	37	34	31	28	26	24
200	39	36	32	30	27	25
210	41	37	34	31	29	26
220	43	39	36	33	30	28
230	45	41	37	34	31	29
240	47	43	39	36	33	30
250	49	44	40	37	34	31

The limited usefulness of agents of this class (see **CLINICAL PHARMACOLOGY**) should be measured against possible risk factors inherent in their use such as those described below.

CONTRAINDICATIONS

Advanced arteriosclerosis, cardiovascular disease, moderate to severe hypertension, hyperthyroidism, known hypersensitivity or idiosyncrasy to the sympathomimetic amines, glaucoma.
Agitated states.
Patients with a history of drug abuse.
During or within 14 days following the administration of monoamine oxidase inhibitors (hypertensive crises may result).

WARNINGS

ADIPEX-P® is indicated only as short-term monotherapy for the management of exogenous obesity. The safety and efficacy of combination therapy with phentermine and any other drug products for weight loss, including selective serotonin reuptake inhibitors (e.g., fluoxetine, sertraline, fluvoxamine, paroxetine), have not been established. Therefore, coadministration of these drug products for weight loss is not recommended.
Primary Pulmonary Hypertension (PPH)—a rare, frequently fatal disease of the lungs—has been reported to occur in patients receiving a combination of phentermine with fenfluramine or dexfenfluramine. The possibility of an association between PPH and the use of phentermine alone cannot be ruled out; there have been rare cases of PPH in patients who reportedly have taken phentermine alone. The initial symptom of PPH is usually dyspnea. Other initial symptoms include: angina pectoris, syncope or lower extremity edema. Patients should be advised to report immediately any deterioration in exercise tolerance. Treatment should be discontinued in patients who develop new, unexplained symptoms of dyspnea, angina pectoris, syncope or lower extremity edema.
Valvular Heart Disease: Serious regurgitant cardiac valvular disease, primarily affecting the mitral, aortic and/or tricuspid valves, has been reported in otherwise health persons who had taken a combination of phentermine with fenfluramine or dexfenfluramine for weight loss. The etiology of these valvulopathies has not been established and their course in individuals after the drugs are stopped is not known. The possibility of an association between valvular heart disease and the use of phentermine alone cannot be ruled out; there have been rare cases of valvular heart disease in patients who reportedly have taken phentermine alone.
Tolerance to the anorectic effect usually develops within a few weeks. When this occurs, the recommended dose should not be exceeded in an attempt to increase the effect; rather, the drug should be discontinued.
ADIPEX-P® may impair the ability of the patient to engage in potentially hazardous activities such as operating machinery or driving a motor vehicle; the patient should therefore be cautioned accordingly.

DRUG ABUSE AND DEPENDENCE

ADIPEX-P® is related chemically and pharmacologically to the amphetamines. Amphetamines and related stimulant drugs have been extensively abused, and the possibility of abuse of ADIPEX-P® should be kept in mind when evaluating the desirability of including a drug as part of a weight reduction program. Abuse of amphetamines and related drugs may be associated with intense psychological dependence and severe social dysfunction. There are reports of patients who have increased the dosage to many times that recommended. Abrupt cessation following prolonged high dosage administration results in extreme fatigue and mental depression; changes are also noted on the sleep EEG. Manifestations of chronic intoxication with anorectic drugs include severe dermatoses, marked insomnia, irritability, hyperactivity and personality changes. The most severe manifestation of chronic intoxications is psychosis, often clinically indistinguishable from schizophrenia.
Usage with Alcohol: Concomitant use of alcohol with ADIPEX-P® may result in an adverse drug interaction.

PRECAUTIONS

General
Caution is to be exercised in prescribing ADIPEX-P® (phentermine hydrochloride) for patients with even mild hypertension.
Insulin requirements in diabetes mellitus may be altered in association with the use of ADIPEX-P® and the concomitant dietary regimen.
ADIPEX-P® may decrease the hypotensive effect of guanethidine.
The least amount feasible should be prescribed or dispensed at one time in order to minimize the possibility of overdosage.
Carcinogenesis, Mutagenesis, Impairment of Fertility: Studies have not been performed with ADIPEX-P® (phentermine hydrochloride) to determine the potential for carcinogenesis, mutagenesis or impairment of fertility.
Pregnancy—Teratogenic Effects: Pregnancy Category C. Animal reproduction studies have not been conducted with ADIPEX-P®. It is also not known whether ADIPEX-P® can cause fetal harm when administered to a pregnant woman or can affect reproductive capacity. ADIPEX-P® should be given to pregnant woman only if clearly needed.
Nursing Mothers
Because of the potential for serious adverse reactions in nursing infants, a decision should be made whether to discontinue nursing or to discontinue the drug, taking into account the importance of the drug to the mother.
Pediatric Use
Safety and effectiveness in pediatric patients have not been established.

ADVERSE REACTIONS

Cardiovascular: Primary pulmonary hypertension and/or regurgitant cardiac valvular disease (see **WARNINGS**), palpitation, tachycardia, elevation of blood pressure.
Central Nervous System:
Overstimulation, restlessness, dizziness, insomnia, euphoria, dysphoria, tremor, headache; rarely psychotic episodes at recommended doses.
Gastrointestinal: Dryness of the mouth, unpleasant taste, diarrhea, constipation, other gastrointestinal disturbances.
Allergic: Urticaria.
Endocrine: Impotence, changes in libido.

OVERDOSAGE

Manifestations of actue overdosage with phentermine include restlessness, tremor, hyperreflexia, rapid respiration, confusion, assaultiveness, hallucinations, panic states. Fatigue and depression usually follow the central stimulation. Cardiovascular effects include arrhythmia, hypertension or hypotension, and circulatory collapse. Gastrointestinal symptoms include nausea, vomiting, diarrhea and abdominal cramps. Fatal poisoning usually terminates in convulsions and coma.

Continued on next page

Adipex-P—Cont.

Management of acute phentermine intoxication is largely symptomatic and includes lavage and sedation with a barbiturate. Experience with hemodialysis or peritoneal dialysis is inadequate to permit recommendations in this regard. Acidification of the urine increases phentermine excretion. Intravenous phentolamine (Regitine®, CIBA) has been suggested for possble acute, severe hypertension, if this complicates phentermine overdosage.

DOSAGE AND ADMINISTRATION

Exogenous Obesity: Dosage should be individualized to obtain an adequate response with the lowest effective dose. The usual adult dose is one capsule or tablet (37.5 mg) daily, administered before breakfast or 1–2 hours after breakfast. For tablets, the dosage may be adjusted to the patient's need. For some patients $^1/_2$ tablet (18.75 mg) daily may be adequate, while in some cases it may be desirable to give $^1/_2$ tablet (18.75 mg) two times a day.
Late evening medication should be avoided because of the possibility of resulting insomnia.
Phentermine is not recommended for use in patients sixteen (16) years of age and under.

HOW SUPPLIED

Available in tablets and capsules containing 37.5 mg phentermine hydrochloride (equivalent to 30 mg phentermine base). Each blue and white, oblong, scored tablet is debossed with "ADIPEX-P" and "9"- "9". The #3 capsule has an opaque white body and an opaque bright blue cap. Each capsule is imprinted with "ADIPEX-P" - "37.5" on the cap and two stripes on the body using dark blue ink.
Tablets are packaged in bottles of 100 (NDC 57844-009-01); 400 (NDC 57844-009-26); and 1000 (NDC 57844-009-10).
Capsules are packaged in bottles of 100 (NDC 57844-019-01).
Store at controlled room temperature 15°–30°C (59°–86°F).
Dispense in a tight container as defined in the USP, with a child-resistant closure (as required).
Manufactured for:
GATE PHARMACEUTICALS
Div. of Teva Pharmaceuticals USA
Sellersville, PA 18960
Manufactured by:
TEVA PHARMACEUTICALS USA
Sellersville, PA 18960

Rev. O 10/98

Shown in Product Identification Guide, page 313

ORAP® ℞
(pimozide)
Tablets

DESCRIPTION

ORAP® (pimozide) is an orally active antipsychotic agent of the diphenylbutylpiperidine series. The structural formula of pimozide, 1-[1-[4,4-bis(4-fluorophenyl)butyl]-4-piperidinyl]-1, 3-dihydro-2H-benzimidazole-2-one is:

The solubility of pimozide in water is less than 0.01 mg/mL; it is slightly soluble in most organic solvents.
Each white ORAP tablet contains either 1 mg or 2 mg of pimozide and the following inactive ingredients: calcium stearate, microcrystalline cellulose, lactose anhydrous and corn starch.

CLINICAL PHARMACOLOGY

Pharmacodynamic Actions
ORAP (pimozide) is an orally active antipsychotic drug product which shares with other antipsychotics the ability to blockade dopaminergic receptors on neurons in the central nervous system. Although its exact mode of action has not been established, the ability of pimozide to suppress motor and phonic tics in Tourette's Disorder is thought to be a function of its dopaminergic blocking activity. However, receptor blockade is often accompanied by a series of secondary alterations in central dopamine metabolism and function which may contribute to both pimozide's therapeutic and untoward effects. In addition, pimozide, in common with other antipsychotic drugs, has various effects on other central nervous system receptor systems which are not fully characterized.
Metabolism and Pharmacokinetics
More than 50% of a dose of pimozide is absorbed after oral administration. Based on the pharmacokinetic and metabolic profile, pimozide appears to undergo significant first pass metabolism. Peak serum levels occur generally six to eight hours (range 4–12 hours) after dosing.
Pimozide is extensively metabolized, primarily by N-dealkylation in the liver. This metabolism is catalyzed mainly by the cytochrome P450 3A (CYP 3A) enzymatic system and to a lesser extent, by cytochrome P450 1A2 (CYP 1A2). Two major metabolites have been identified, 1-(4-piperidyl)-2-benzimidazolinone and 4,4-bis(4-florophenyl) butyric acid. The antipsychotic activity of these metabolites is undermined. The major route of elimination of pimozide and its metabolites is through the kidney.
The mean serum elimination half-life of pimozide in schizophrenic patients was approximately 55 hours. There was a 13-fold interindividual difference in the area under the serum pimozide level-time curve and an equivalent degree of variation in peak serum levels among patients studied. The significance of this is unclear since there are few correlations between plasma levels and clinical findings.
Effects of food and disease upon the absorption, distribution, metabolism and elimination of pimozide are not known. Effects of concomitant medication on pimozide metabolism are described in the **CONTRAINDICATIONS** section.

INDICATIONS AND USAGE

ORAP (pimozide) is indicated for the suppression of motor and phonic tics in patients with Tourette's Disorder who have failed to respond satisfactorily to standard treatment. ORAP is not intended as a treatment of first choice nor is it intended for the treatment of tics that are merely annoying or cosmetically troublesome. ORAP should be reserved for use in Tourette's Disorder patients whose development and/or daily life function is severely compromised by the presence of motor and phonic tics.
Evidence supporting approval of pimozide for use in Tourette's Disorder was obtained in two controlled clinical investigations which enrolled patients between the ages of 8 and 53 years. Most subjects in the two trials were 12 or older.

CONTAINDICATIONS

1. ORAP (pimozide) is contraindicated in the treatment of simple tics or tics other than those associated with Tourette's Disorder.
2. ORAP should not be used in patients taking drugs that may, themselves, cause motor and phonic tics (e.g., pemoline, methylphenidate and amphetamines) until such patients have been withdrawn from these drugs to determine whether or not the drugs, rather than Tourette's Disorder, are responsible for the tics.
3. Because ORAP prolongs the QT interval of the electrocardiogram it is contraindicated in patients with congenital long QT syndrome, patients with a history of cardiac arrhythmias, or patients taking other drugs which prolong the QT interval of the electrocardiogram (see **PRECAUTIONS—Drug Interactions**).
4. ORAP is contraindicated in patients with severe toxic central nervous system depression or comatose states from any cause.
5. ORAP is contraindicated in patients with hyper-sensitivity to it. As it is not known whether cross-sensitivity exists among the antipsychotics, pimozide should be used with appropriate caution in patients who have demonstrated hypersensitivity to other antipsychotic drugs.
6. Ventricular arrhythmias have been rarely associated with the use of macrolide antibiotics in patients with prolonged QT intervals, as might be produced by ORAP. Specifically, two sudden deaths have been reported when clarithromycin was added to ongoing pimozide therapy. Futhermore, some evidence suggests that pimozide is metabolized partly by the enzyme system cytochrome P450 3A (CYP 3A). Macrolide antibiotics are inhibitors of CYP 3A, and thus could potentially impede pimozide metabolism. For these reasons, ORAP is contraindicated in patients receiving the macrolide antibiotics clarithromycin, erythromycin, azithromycin, dirithromycin, and troleandomycin.
Because azole antifungal agents are also inhibitors of the CYP 3A enzymes and thus may likewise impair pimozide metabolism, ORAP is contraindicated in patients receiving the azole antifungal agents itraconazole and ketoconazole.
Similarly, protease inhibitor drugs are also inhibitors of CYP 3A, and thus ORAP is contraindicated in patients receiving protease inhibitors such as ritonavir, saquinovir, indinavir, and nelfinavir. (See **PRECAUTIONS—Drug Interactions**.)
Nefazodone is a potent inhibitor of CYP 3A, and its concomitant use with ORAP is also contraindicated.
Other drugs that are relatively less potent inhibitors of CYP 3A should also be avoided, in view of the risks e.g. zileuton

WARNINGS

The use of ORAP (pimozide) in the treatment of Tourette's Disorder involves different risk/benefit considerations than when antipsychotic drugs are used to treat other conditions. Consequently, a decision to use ORAP should take into consideration the following (see also **PRECAUTIONS—Information for Patients**).
Tardive Dyskinesia
A syndrome consisting of potentially irreversible, involuntary, dyskinetic movements may develop in patients treated with antipsychotic drugs. Although the prevalence of the syndrome appears to be highest among the elderly, especially elderly women, it is impossible to rely upon prevalence estimates to predict, at the inception of antipsychotic treatment, which patients are likely to develop the syndrome. Whether antipsychotic drug products differ in their potential to cause tardive dyskinesia in unknown.
Both the risk of developing tardive dyskinesia and the likelihood that it will become irreversible are believed to increase as the duration of treatment and the total cumulative dose of antipsychotic drugs administered to the patient increase. However, the syndrome can develop, although much less commonly, after relatively brief treatment periods at low doses.
There is no known treatment for established cases of tardive dyskinesia, although the syndrome may remit, partially or completely, if antipsychotic treatment is withdrawn. Antipsychotic treatment itself, however, may suppress (or partially suppress) the signs and symptoms of the syndrome and thereby may possibly mask the underlying process. The effect that symptomatic suppression has upon the long-term course of the syndrome is unknown.
Given these considerations, antipsychotic drugs should be prescribed in a manner that is most likely to minimize the occurrence of tardive dyskinesia. Chronic antipsychotic treatment should generally be reserved for patients who suffer from a chronic illness that, 1) is known to respond to antipsychotic drugs, and 2) for whom alternative, equally effective, but potentially less harmful treatments are not available or appropriate. In patients who do require chronic treatment, the smallest dose and the shortest duration of treatment producing a satisfactory clinical response should be sought. The need for continued treatment should be reassessed periodically.
If signs and symptoms of tardive dyskinesia appear in a patient on antipsychotics, drug discontinuation should be considered. However, some patients may require treatment despite the presence of the syndrome.
(For further information about the description of tardive dyskinesia and its clinical detection, please refer to **ADVERSE REACTIONS** and **PRECAUTIONS—Information for Patients**.)
Neuroleptic Malignant Syndrome (NMS)
A potentially fatal symptom complex sometimes referred to as Neuroleptic Malignant Syndrome (NMS) has been reported in association with antipsychotic drugs. Clinical manifestations of NMS are hyperpyrexia, muscle rigidity, altered mental status (including catatonic signs) and evidence of autonomic instability (irregular pulse or blood pressure, tachycardia, diaphoresis, and cardiac dysrhythmias). Additional signs may include elevated creatine phosphokinase, myoglobinuria (rhabdomyolysis) and acute renal failure.
The diagnostic evaluation of patients with this syndrome is complicated. In arriving at a diagnosis, it is important to identify cases where the clinical presentation includes both serious medical illness (e.g., pneumonia, systemic infection, etc.) and untreated or inadequately treated extrapyramidal signs and symptoms (EPS). Other important considerations in the differential diagnosis include central anticholinergic toxicity, heat stroke, drug fever and primary central nervous system (CNS) pathology.
The management of NMS should include 1) immediate discontinuation of antipsychotic drugs and other drugs not essential to concurrent therapy, 2) intensive symptomatic treatment and medical monitoring, and 3) treatment of any concomitant serious medical problems for which specific treatments are available. There is no general agreement about specific pharmacological treatment regimens for uncomplicated NMS.
If a patient requires antipsychotic drug treatment after recovery from NMS, the potential reintroduction of drug therapy should be carefully considered. The patient should be carefully monitored, since recurrences of NMS have been reported.
Hyperpyrexia, not associated with the above symptom complex, has been reported with other antipsychotic drugs.
Other
Sudden, unexpected deaths have occurred in experimental studies of conditions other than Tourette's Disorder. These deaths occurred while patients were receiving dosages in the range of 1 mg per kg. One possible mechanism for such deaths is prolongation of the QT interval predisposing patients to ventricular arrhythmia. An electrocardiogram should be performed before ORAP treatment is initiated and periodically thereafter, especially during the period of dose adjustment.
ORAP may have a tumorigenic potential. Based on studies conducted in mice, it is known that pimozide can produce a dose-related increase in pituitary tumors. The full significance of this finding is not known, but should be taken into consideration in the physician's and patient's decisions to use this drug product. This finding should be given special consideration when the patient is young and chronic use of pimozide is anticipated (see **PRECAUTIONS—Carcinogenesis, Mutagenesis, Impairment of Fertility**).

PRECAUTIONS

General
ORAP (pimozide) may impair the mental and/or physical abilities required for the performance of potentially hazardous tasks, such as driving a car or operating machinery, especially during the first few days of therapy.
ORAP produces anticholinergic side effects and should be used with caution in individuals whose conditions may be aggravated by anticholinergic activity.
ORAP should be administered cautiously to patients with impairment of liver or kidney function, because it is metabolized by the liver and excreted by the kidneys.
Antipsychotics should be administered with caution to patients receiving anticonvulsant medication, with a history of seizures, or with EEG abnormalities, because they may lower the convulsive threshold. If indicated, adequate anticonvulsant therapy should be maintained concomitantly.

Information for Patients

Treatment with ORAP exposes the patients to serious risks. A decision to use ORAP chronically in Tourette's Disorder is one that deserves full consideration by the patient (or patient's family) as well as by the treating physician. Because the goal of treatment is symptomatic improvement, the patient's view of the need for treatment and assessment of response are critical in evaluating the impact of therapy and weighing its benefits against the risks. Since the physician is the primary source of information about the use of a drug in any disease, it is recommended that the following information be discussed with patients and/or their families.

ORAP is intended only for use in patients with Tourette's Disorder whose symptoms are severe and who cannot tolerate, or who do not respond to HALDOL* (haloperidol).

Given the likelihood that a proportion of patients exposed chronically to antipsychotics will develop tardive dyskinesia, it is advised that all patients in whom chronic use is contemplated be given, if possible, full information about this risk. The decision to inform patients and/or their guardians must obviously take into account the clinical circumstances and the competency of the patient to understand the information provided.

There is limited information available on the use of ORAP in children under 12 years of age.

The information available on ORAP from foreign marketing experience and from U.S. clinical trials indicates that ORAP has a side effect profile similar to that of other antipsychotic drugs. Patients should be informed that all types of side effects associated with the use of antipsychotics may be associated with the use of ORAP.

In addition, sudden, unexpected deaths have occurred in patients taking high doses of ORAP for conditions other than Tourette's Disorder. These deaths may have been the result of an effect of ORAP upon the heart. Therefore, patients should be instructed not to exceed the prescribed dose of ORAP and they should realize the need for the initial ECG and for follow-up ECGs during treatment.

Also, pimozide, at a dose about 15 times that given humans, caused an increase in the number of benign tumors of the pituitary gland in female mice, it is not possible to say how important this is. Similar tumors were not seen in rats given pimozide, nor at lower doses in mice, which is reassuring. However, any such finding must be considered to suggest a possible risk of long term use of the drug.

Because substances in grapefruit juice may inhibit the metabolism of pimozide by CYP 3A, patients should be advised to avoid grapefruit juice.

Laboratory Tests

An ECG should be done at baseline and periodically thereafter throughout the period of dose adjustment. Any indication of prolongation of QTc interval beyond an absolute limit of 0.47 seconds (children) or 0.52 seconds (adults), or more than 25% above the patient's original baseline should be considered a basis for stopping further dose increase (see **CONTRAINDICATIONS**) and considering a lower dose.

Since hypokalemia has been associated with ventricular arrhythmias, potassium insufficiency, secondary to diuretics, diarrhea, or other cause, should be corrected before ORAP therapy is initiated and normal potassium maintained during therapy.

Drug Interactions

Because ORAP prolongs the QT interval of the electrocardiogram, an additive effect on QT interval would be anticipated if administered with other drugs, such as phenothiazines, tricyclic antidepressants or antiarrhythmic agents, which prolong the QT interval. Also, the use of macrolide antibiotics in patients with prolonged QT intervals has been rarely associated with ventricular arrhythmias. Such concomitant administration should not be undertaken (see **CONTRAINDICATIONS**).

Since ORAP is partly metabolized via CYP 3A, it should not be administered concomitantly with inhibitors of this metabolic system, such as azole antifungal agents and protease inhibitor drugs (see CONTRAINDICATIONS).

As CYP 1A2 may also contribute to the metabolism of ORAP, prescribers should be aware of the theoretical potential of drug interactions with inhibitors of this enzymatic system.

ORAP may be capable of potentiating CNS depressants, including analgesics, sedatives, anxiolytics, and alcohol.

A single case report has suggested possible additive effects of pimozide and fluoxetine leading to bradycardia.

Interaction with Food

Patients should avoid grapefruit juice because it may inhibit the metabolism of pimozide by CYP 3A.

Carcinogenesis, Mutagenesis, Impairment of Fertility

Carcinogenicity studies were conducted in mice and rats. In mice, pimozide causes a dose-related increase in pituitary and mammary tumors.

When mice were treated for up to 18 months with pimozide, pituitary gland changes developed in females only. These changes were characterized as hyperplasia at doses approximating the human dose and adenoma at doses about fifteen times the maximum recommended human dose on a mg per kg basis. The mechanism for the induction of pituitary tumors in mice is not known.

Mammary gland tumors in female mice were also increased, but these tumors are expected in rodents treated with antipsychotic drugs which elevate prolactin levels. Chronic administration of an antipsychotic also causes elevated prolactin levels in humans. Tissue culture experiments indicate that approximately one-third of human breast cancers are prolactin-dependent in *vitro*, a factor of potential importance if the prescription of these drugs is contemplated in a patient with a previously detected breast cancer. Although disturbances such as galactorrhea, amenorrhea, gynecomastia, and impotence have been reported with antipsychotic drugs, the clinical significance of elevated serum prolactin levels is unknown for most patients. Neither clinical studies nor epidemiologic studies conducted to date have shown an association between chronic administration of these drugs and mammary tumorigenesis. The available evidence, however, is considered too limited to be conclusive at this time.

In a 24-month carcinogenicity study in rats, animals received up to 50 times the maximum recommended human dose. No increased incidence of overall tumors or tumors at any site was observed in either sex. Because of the limited number of animals surviving this study, the meaning of these results is unclear.

Pimozide did not have mutagenic activity in the Ames test with four bacterial test strains, in the mouse dominant lethal test or in the micronucleus test is rats.

Reproduction studies in animals were not adequate to assess all aspects of fertility. Nevertheless, female rats administered pimozide had prolonged estrus cycles, an effect also produced by other antipsychotic drugs.

Pregnancy

Category C. Reproduction studies performed in rats and rabbits at oral doses up to 8 times the maximum human dose did not reveal evidence of teratogenicity. In the rat, however, this multiple of the human dose resulted in decreased pregnancies and in the retarded development of fetuses. These effects are thought to be due to an inhibition or delay in implantation which is also observed in rodents administered other antipsychotic drugs. In the rabbit, maternal toxicity, mortality, decreased weight gain, and embryotoxicity including increased resorptions were dose-related. Because animal reproduction studies are not always predictive of human response, pimozide should be given to a pregnant women only if the potential benefits of treatment clearly outweigh the potential risks.

Labor and Delivery

This drug has no recognized use in labor or delivery.

Nursing Mothers

It is not known whether pimozide is excreted in human milk. Because many drugs are excreted in human milk and because of the potential for tumorigenicity and unknown cardiovascular effects in the infant, a decision should be made whether to discontinue nursing or to discontinue the drug, taking into account the importance of the drug to the mother.

Pediatric Use

Although Tourette's Disorder most often has its onset between the ages of 2 and 15 years, information on the use and efficacy of ORAP in patients less than 12 years of age is limited. A 24-week open label study in 36 children between the ages of 2 and 12 demonstrated that pimozide has a similar safety profile in this age group as in older patients and there were no safety findings that would preclude its use in this age group.

Because its use and safety have not been evaluated in other childhood disorders, ORAP is not recommended for use in any condition other than Tourette's Disorder.

ADVERSE REACTIONS

General

Extrapyramidal Reactions: Neuromuscular (extrapyramidal) reactions during the administration of ORAP (pimozide) have been reported frequently, often during the first few days of treatment. In most patients, these reactions involved Parkinson-like symptoms which, then first observed, were usually mild to moderately severe and usually reversible.

Other types of neuromuscular reactions (motor restlessness, dystonia, akathisia, hyperreflexia, opisthotonos, oculgyric crises) have been reported far less frequently. Severe extrapyramidal reactions have been reported to occur at relatively low doses. Generally the occurrence and severity of most extrapyramidal symptoms are dose-related since they occur at relatively high doses and have been shown to disappear or become less severe when the dose is reduced. Administration of antiparkinson drugs such as benztropine mesylate or trihexphenidyl hydrochloride may be required for control of such reactions. It should be noted that persistent extrapyramidal reactions have been reported and that the drug may have to be discontinued in such cases.

Withdrawal Emergent Neurological Signs: Generally, patients receiving short term therapy experience no problems with abrupt discontinuation of antipsychotic drugs. However, some patients on maintenance treatment experience transient dyskinetic signs after abrupt withdrawal. In certain of these cases the dyskinetic movements are indistinguishable from the syndrome described below under "Tardive Dyskinesia" except for duration. It is not known whether gradual withdrawal of antipsychotic drugs with reduce the rate of occurrence of withdrawal emergent neurological signs, but until further evidence becomes available, it seems reasonable to gradually withdraw use of ORAP.

Tardive Dyskinesia: ORAP may be associated with persistent dyskinesias. Tardive dyskinesia, a syndrome consisting of potentially irreversible, involuntary, dyskinetic movements, may appear in some patients on long-term therapy or may occur after drug therapy has been discontinued. The risk appears to be greater in elderly patients on high-dose therapy, especially females. The symptoms are persistent and in some patients appear irreversible. The syndrome is characterized by rhythmical unvoluntary movements of tongue, face, mouth or jaw (e.g., protrusions of tongue, puffing of cheeks, puckering of mouth, chewing movements). Sometimes these may be accompanied by involuntary movements of extremities and the trunk.

There is no known effective treatment for tardive dyskinesia; antiparkinson agents usually do not alleviate the symptoms of this syndrome. It is suggested that all antipsychotic agents be discontinued if these symptoms appear. Should it be necessary to reinstitute treatment, or increase the dosage of the agent, or switch to a different antipsychotic agent, this syndrome may be masked.

It has been reported that fine vermicular movement of the tongue may be an early sign of tardive dyskinesia and if the medication is stopped at that time the syndrome may not develop.

Electrocardiographic Changes: Electrocardiographic changes have been observed in clinical trials of ORAP in Tourette's Disorder and schizophrenia. These have included prolongation of the QT interval, flattening, notching and inversion of the T wave and the appearance of U waves. Sudden, unexpected deaths and grand mal seizure have occurred at doses above 20 mg/day.

Neuroleptic Malignant Syndrome: Neuroleptic malignant syndrome (NMS) has been reported with ORAP. (See **WARNINGS** for further information concerning NMS.)

Hyperpyrexia: Hyperpyrexia has been reported with other antipsychotic drugs.

Clinical Trials

The following adverse reaction tabulation was derived from 20 patients in a 6-week long placebo-controlled clinical trial of ORAP in Tourette's Disorder.

Body System/ Adverse Reaction	Pimozide (N = 20)	Placebo (N = 20)
Body as a Whole		
Headache	1	2
Gastrointestinal		
Dry Mouth	5	1
Diarrhea	1	0
Nausea	0	2
Vomiting	0	1
Constipation	4	2
Eructations	0	1
Thirsty	1	0
Appetite increase	1	0
Endocrine		
Menstrual disorder	0	1
Breast secretions	0	1
Musculoskeletal		
Muscle cramps	0	1
Muscle tightness	3	0
Stooped posture	2	0
CNS		
Drowsiness	7	3
Sedation	14	5
Insomnia	2	2
Dizziness	0	1
Akathisia	8	0
Rigidity	2	0
Speech disorder	2	0
Handwriting change	1	0
Akinesia	8	0
Psychiatric		
Depression	2	3
Excitement	0	1
Nervous	1	0
Adverse behavior effect	5	0
Special Senses		
Visual disturbance	4	0
Taste change	1	0
Sensitivity of eyes to light	1	0
Decrease accommodation	4	1
Spots before eyes	0	1
Urogenital		
Impotence	3	0

The following adverse event tabulation was derived from 36 children (age 2 to 12) in a 24-week open trial of ORAP in Tourette's Disorder.

Body System/ Adverse Reaction	Number of Patients Experiencing Each Event (%) All Events (N=36)	Drug-Related Events (N=36)
Body as a Whole		
Asthenia	9 (25.0)	5 (13.8)
Headache	8 (22.2)	1 (2.7)
Gastrointestinal		
Dysphagia	1 (2.7)	1 (2.7)
Increased Salivation	5 (13.8)	2 (5.5)
Musculoskeletal		
Myalgia	1 (2.7)	1 (2.7)

Continued on next page

Orap—Cont.

Central Nervous System		
Dreaming Abnormal	1 (2.7)	1 (2.7)
Hyperkinesia	2 (5.5)	1 (2.7)
Somnolence	10 (27.7)	9 (25.0)
Torticollis	1 (2.7)	1 (2.7)
Tremor, Limbs	1 (2.7)	1 (2.7)
Psychiatric		
Adverse Behavior Effect	10 (27.7)	8 (22.2)
Nervous	3 (8.3)	2 (5.5)
Skin		
Rash	3 (8.3)	1 (2.7)
Special Senses		
Visual disturbance	2 (5.5)	1 (2.7)
Cardiovascular		
ECG Abnormal	1 (2.7)*	1 (2.7)

Because clinical investigational experience with ORAP in Tourette's Disorder is limited, uncommon adverse reactions may not have been detected. The physician should consider that other adverse reactions associated with antipsychotics may occur.

Other Adverse Reactions

In addition to the adverse reactions listed above, those listed below have been reported in U.S. clinical trails of ORAP in conditions other than Tourette's Disorder.

Body as a Whole: Asthenia, chest pain, periorbital edema
Cardiovascular/Respiratory: Postural hypotension, hypotension, hypertension, tachycardia, palpitations
Gastrointestinal: Increased salivation, nausea, vomiting, anorexia, GI distress
Endocrine: Loss of libido
Metabolic/Nutritional: Weight gain, weight loss
Central Nervous System: Dizziness, tremor, parkinsonism, fainting, dyskinesia
Psychiatric: Excitement
Skin: Rash, sweating, skin irritation
Special Senses: Blurred vision, cataracts
Urogenital: Nocturia, urinary frequency

Postmarketing Reports

The following experiences were described in spontaneous postmarketing reports. These reports do not provide sufficient information to establish a clear causal relationship will the use of ORAP.

Gastrointestinal: Gingival hyperplasia in one patient
Hematologic: Hemolytic anemia
Metabolic/Nutritional: Hyponatremia
Other: Seizure

OVERDOSAGE

In general, the signs and symptoms of overdosage with ORAP (pimozide) would be an exaggeration of known pharmacologic effects and adverse reactions, the most prominent of which would be: 1) electrocardiographic abnormalities, 2) severe extrapyramidal reactions, 3) hypotension, 4) a comatose state with respiratory depression.

In the event of overdosage, gastric lavage, establishment of a patent airway and, if necessary, mechanically-assisted respiration are advised. Electrocardiographic monitoring should commence immediately and continue until the ECG parameters are within the normal range. Hypotension and circulatory collapse may be counteracted by use of intravenous fluids, plasma, or concentrated albumin, and vasopressor agents such as metaraminol, phenylephrine and norepinephrine. Epinephrine should not be used. In case of severe extrapyramidal reactions, antiparkinson medication should be administered. Because of the long half-life of pimozide, patients who take an overdose should be observed for at least 4 days. As with all drugs, the physician should consider contacting a poison control center for additional information on the treatment of overdose.

DOSAGE AND ADMINISTRATION

General

The suppression of tics by ORAP requires a slow and gradual introduction of the drug. The patient's dose should be carefully adjusted to a point where the suppression of tics and the relief afforded is balanced against the untoward side effects of the drug.

An ECG should be done at baseline and periodically thereafter especially during the period of dose adjustment (see **WARNINGS** and **PRECAUTIONS—Laboratory Tests**).

Periodic attempts should be made to reduce the dosage of ORAP to see whether or not tics persist at the level and extent first identified. In attempts to reduce the dosage of ORAP, consideration should be given to the possibility that increases of tic intensity and frequency may represent a transient, withdrawal-related phenomenon rather than a return of disease symptoms. Specifically, one to two weeks should be allowed to elapse before one concludes that an increase in tic manifestations is a function of the underlying disease syndrome rather than a response to drug withdrawal. A gradual withdrawal is recommended in any case.

Children

Reliable dose response data for the effects of ORAP (pimozide) on tic manifestation in Tourette's Disorder patients below the age of twelve are not available.

Treatment should be initiated at a dose of 0.05 mg/kg preferably taken once at bedtime. The dose may be increased every third day to a maximum of 0.2 mg/kg not to exceed 10 mg/kg.

Adults

In general, treatment with ORAP should be initiated with a dose of 1 to 2 mg a day in divided doses. The dose may be increased thereafter every other day. Most patients are maintained at less than 0.2 mg/kg per day, or 10 mg/day, whichever is less. Doses greater than 0.2 mg/kg/day or 10 mg/day are not recommended.

ANIMAL PHARMACOLOGY

A chronic study in dogs indicated that pimozide caused gingival hyperplasia when administered for several months at about 5 times the maximum recommended human dose. This condition was reversible after withdrawal.

HOW SUPPLIED

ORAP® (pimozide) 1 mg tablets are white, oval, scored tablets, debossed "ORAP 1". They are available in bottles of 100 (NDC 57844-151-01).

ORAP® (pimozide) 2 mg tablets are white, oval, scored tablets, debbosed "LEMMON" on one side and "ORAP 2" on the other. They are available in bottles of 100 (NDC 57844-187-01).

Store at controlled room temperature 15°–30°C (59°–86°F).

Dispense in a tight, light-resistant container as defined in the official compendum.

Pharmacist: Dispense in child-resistant container.

Manufactured for:
GATE PHARMACEUTICALS
Div. of TEVA Pharmaceuticals USA
Sellersville, PA 18960

Manufactured by:
TEVA PHARMACEUTICALS USA
Sellersville, PA 18960
Rev. J 8/99

Shown in Product Identification Guide, page 313

Gebauer Company

9410 ST. CATHERINE AVE.
CLEVELAND, OH 44104

Direct Inquiries to:
(800) 321-9348
(216) 271-5252
www.gebauerco.com

For Medical Information Contact:
In Emergencies:
(800) 321-9348
(216) 271-5252
www.gebauerco.com

After Hours and Weekend Emergencies:
Chemtrac:
(800) 424-9300

Gebauer's ETHYL CHLORIDE* ℞

(Chloroethane)

***As packaged, may not meet USP specifications for nonvolatile residue.**

INDICATIONS FOR USE

Gebauer's Ethyl Chloride is a vapocoolant (skin refrigerant) intended for topical application to control pain associated with injections, minor surgical procedures (such as lancing boils or incision and drainage of small abscesses) and the temporary relief of minor sports injuries.

It is also intended for the treatment of restricted motion associated with myofascial pain caused by trigger points.

PRECAUTIONS

Inhalation of Ethyl Chloride should be avoided as it may produce narcotic and general anesthetic effects, deep anesthesia or fatal coma with respiratory or cardiac arrest.

Ethyl Chloride is FLAMMABLE and should never be used in the presence of an open flame, or electrical cautery equipment.

When used to produce local freezing of tissues, adjacent skin areas should be protected by an application of petrolatum. The thawing process may be painful, and freezing may lower local resistance to infections and delay healing.

CONTRAINDICATIONS

Ethyl Chloride is contraindicated in individuals with a history of hypersensitivity to it.

WARNINGS

For external use only. Do not spray in eyes.

Skin Absorption of Ethyl Chloride can occur; no cases of chronic poisoning have been reported. Ethyl Chloride is known as a liver and kidney toxin; long term exposure may cause liver or kidney damage.

Contents under pressure. Do not store above 120°F. Best stored at room temperature.

WARNING: This product contains a chemical known to the State of California to cause cancer.

ADVERSE REACTIONS

Cutaneous sensitization may occur, but appears to be extremely rare. Freezing can occasionally alter pigmentation.

CAUTION

Federal law restricts this device to sale by or on the order of a physician or other practitioner licensed by state law to use or order the use of the device.

PRESCRIBING INFORMATION

DIRECTIONS FOR USE

Hold the bottle inverted while spraying. Open the dispenseal spring valve completely allowing the Gebauer's Ethyl Chloride to flow from the amber bottle. To apply Gebauer's Ethyl Chloride from mist spray aerosol can, hold can upright. Depress valve completely.

1. TOPICAL ANESTHESIA IN MINOR SURGERY
   Clean the operative site with a suitable antiseptic. Apply petrolatum to protect the adjacent areas. Spray Gebauer's Ethyl Chloride on the target area continuously for 3 to 7 seconds from a distance of 3 to 9 inches (8 – 23 cm.). Spray until the skin just begins to turn white; do not frost the skin. Swab the target area with antiseptic and promptly make the incision.
2. MINOR SPORTS INJURIES
   The pain of bruises, contusions, abrasions, swelling and minor sprains may be controlled with Gebauer's Ethyl Chloride.
   The amount of cooling depends on the dosage. Dosage varies with duration of application. The anesthetic effect of Gebauer's Ethyl Chloride rarely lasts more than a few seconds to a minute. Avoid spraying the skin beyond this point.
3. PRE-INJECTION ANESTHESIA
   Prepare the syringe. Spray the target area with Gebauer's Ethyl Chloride continuously for 3 to 7 seconds from a distance of 3 to 9 inches (8 – 23 cm.). Spray the area until the skin just turns white; do not frost the skin. Swab the target area with antiseptic and quickly introduce the needle with the skin taut.
4. SPRAY AND STRETCH TECHNIQUE FOR MYOFASCIAL PAIN
   Gebauer's Ethyl Chloride may be used as a counterirritant in the management of myofascial pain, restricted motion and muscle tension. Clinical conditions that may respond to Gebauer's Ethyl Chloride include low back pain (due to tight muscles), acute stiff neck, torticollis, acute bursitis of the shoulder, tight muscles associated with osteoarthritis, tight hamstrings, sprained ankle, tight masseter muscles, certain types of headaches, and referred pain due to irritated trigger points. Relief of pain facilitates early mobilization and the restoration of muscle function.
   The Spray and Stretch technique is a therapeutic system which involves three stages: EVALUATION, SPRAYING AND STRETCHING. The therapeutic value of Spray and Stretch becomes most effective when the practitioner has mastered all stages and applies them in the proper sequence.

a. Evaluation
The evaluation phase determines if the cause of pain is an active irritated trigger point. A trigger point is a deep hypersensitive localized spot in a muscle. An active trigger point, not the muscle causes a referred pain pattern. With trigger points, the source of pain is seldom the site of pain. A trigger point may be detected by a snapping palpation over the muscle causing the muscle in which the irritated trigger point is situated to twitch.

b. Spraying
1) Have the patient assume a comfortable position.
2) Take precautions to cover the patient's eyes, nose and mouth if spraying near the face.
3) Hold the bottle inverted. From a distance of approximately 12 to 18 inches (30 - 46 cm.), aim the pinpoint stream so that it meets the skin at an acute angle to lessen the shock of impact.
4) Direct the spray in parallel sweeps 1.5 to 2 cm. apart at the rate of approximately 4 in./sec. (10 cm./sec.). Continue until the entire muscle has been covered. The number of sweeps is determined by the size of the muscle. The spray should be applied from the muscle attachment over the trigger point, through and over the reference zone.

c. Stretching
Passively stretch the muscle during spray applications. Gradually increase the force with successive sweeps. As the muscle relaxes, smoothly take up the slack by establishing a new stretch length. It is necessary to reach the full normal length of the muscle to completely inactivate the trigger point and relieve the pain. Rewarm the muscle. If necessary, repeat the procedure. Apply moist heat for 10 to 15 minutes following treatment. For lasting benefit, eliminate any factors that perpetuate the trigger mechanism.

HOW SUPPLIED

3.5 fl. oz.

Fine Nozzle glass bottle	P/N 0386-0001-04
Medium Nozzle glass bottle	P/N 0386-0001-03
Mist Nozzle can	P/N 0386-0001-02

GEBAUER'S FLUORI-METHANE® ℞

Vapocoolant (Skin Refrigerant)
Dichlorodifluoromethane, N.F., 15%
Trichloromonofluoromethane, N.F., 85%

INDICATIONS FOR USE

Gebauer's Fluori-Methane is a topical anesthetic intended to treat restricted motion associated with myofascial pain caused by trigger points. It will also control pain associated with injections and provide temporary relief of minor sports injuries.

ADVERSE REACTIONS

Cutaneous sensitization may occur but appears to be extremely rare. Freezing can occasionally alter pigmentation.

CONTRAINDICATIONS

Fluori-Methane is contraindicated in individuals with a history of hypersensitivity to dichlorodifluoromethane and/or trichloromonofluoromethane. This product should not be used on patients having vascular impairment of the extremities.

WARNINGS

For external use only. Contents under pressure. Store at controlled room temperature. Do not store above 120°F. Do not store on or near high frequency ultrasound equipment.

PRECAUTIONS

Avoid contact with eyes. Do not apply to the point of frost formation.

CAUTION:

Federal law restricts this device to sale by or on the order of a physician or other practitioner licensed by state law to use or order use of the device.

HOW SUPPLIED

3.5 fl. oz. (103 ml)

DIRECTIONS FOR USE

To apply Gebauer's Fluori-Methane, invert the bottle over the treatment area. Open the dispenseal valve completely, allowing the liquid to flow in a stream from the bottle.

1. TEMPORARY RELIEF OF MINOR SPORTS INJURIES:

The pain of bruises, contusions, swelling and minor sprains may be controlled with Fluori-Methane.

The amount of cooling depends on the dosage. Dosage varies with duration of application. The anesthetic effect of Gebauer's Fluori-Methane rarely lasts more than a few seconds to a minute. This time interval is usually sufficient to help reduce or relieve the initial trauma of the injury.

Spray the affected area from a distance of 3" to 9" (8–23 cm) for 3 to 7 seconds until the skin just turns white. Avoid spraying the skin beyond this point.

2. PRE-INJECTION ANESTHESIA:

Prepare the syringe. Spray the target area with Gebauer's Fluori-Methane continuously for 3 to 7 seconds from a distance of 3" to 9" (8–23 cm). Spray the area until the skin just turns white; do not frost the skin. Swab the target area with antiseptic and quickly introduce the needle with the skin taut.

3. SPRAY AND STRETCH TECHNIQUE FOR MYOFASCIAL PAIN:

Gebauer's Fluori-Methane may be used as a counterirritant in the management of myofascial pain, restricted motion and muscle tension. Clinical conditions that may respond to Gebauer's Fluori-Methane include low back pain (due to tight muscles), acute stiff neck, torticollis, acute bursitis of the shoulder, tight hamstrings, sprained ankle, tight masseter muscles, certain types of headache and referred pain due to irritated trigger joints. Relief of pain facilitates early mobilization and the restoration of muscle function.

The Spray and Stretch technique is a therapeutic system involving three stages:

EVALUATION, SPRAYING AND STRETCHING:

The therapeutic value of Spray and Stretch becomes most effective when the practitioner has mastered all stages and applies them in the proper sequence.

a. Evaluation

If the patient has been evaluated to have pain caused by an active, irritated trigger point, then proceed as follows:

b. Spraying

1) Have the patient assume a comfortable position.
2) Take precautions to cover the patient's eyes, nose and mouth if spraying near the face.
3) Invert the bottle and open the dispenseal valve. From a distance of approximately 12" to 18" (30–46 cm), aim the jet stream so that it meets the skin at an acute angle to lessen the shock of impact.
4) Direct the spray in parallel sweeps 1.5 to 2 cm apart at the rate of approximately 4 in/sec (10cm/sec). Continue until the entire muscle has been covered. The number of sweeps is determined by the size of the muscle. The spray should be applied from the muscle attachment over the trigger point through and over the reference zone.

c. Stretching

Passively stretch the muscle during the spray application. Gradually increase the force with successive sweeps. As the muscle relaxes, smoothly take up the slack by establishing a new stretch length. It is necessary to reach the full normal length of the muscle to completely inactivate the trigger point and relieve the pain.

Rewarm the muscle. If necessary, repeat the procedure. Apply moist heat for 10 to 15 minutes following the treatment. For lasting benefit, eliminate any factors that perpetuate the trigger mechanism.

NOTE: The indented statement below is required by the Federal Government's Clean Air Act for all products containing or manufactured with chlorofluorocarbons (CFCs):

> Warning: Contains Dichlorodifluoromethane and Trichloromonofluoromethane, substances which harm public health and environment by destroying ozone in the upper atmosphere.

Your physician has determined that this product is likely to help your personal health. USE THIS PRODUCT AS DIRECTED UNLESS INSTRUCTED TO DO OTHERWISE BY YOUR PHYSICIAN. If you have any questions about alternatives, consult with your physician.

Manufactured by:
Gebauer Company
Cleveland, OH 44104
800-321-9348
www.gebauerco.com

Rev. 8/00

Genentech, Inc.

1 DNA Way
SOUTH SAN FRANCISCO, CA 94080-4990

For Medical Information Contact:

Medical Information or Drug Safety Departments (24 hours):
(800) 821-8590
(650) 225-1000
E-mail: medinfo@gene.com

Or write:
Medical Information or Drug Safety Departments
Genentech, Inc.
1 DNA Way
South San Francisco, CA 94080-4990

ACTIVASE®

℞

Alteplase
recombinant

DESCRIPTION

Activase, Alteplase, is a tissue plasminogen activator produced by recombinant DNA technology. It is a sterile, purified glycoprotein of 527 amino acids. It is synthesized using the complementary DNA (cDNA) for natural human tissue-type plasminogen activator obtained from a human melanoma cell line. The manufacturing process involves the secretion of the enzyme alteplase into the culture medium by an established mammalian cell line (Chinese Hamster Ovary cells) into which the cDNA for alteplase has been genetically inserted. Fermentation is carried out in a nutrient medium containing the antibiotic gentamycin, 100 mg/L. However, the presence of the antibiotic is not detectable in the final product.

Phosphoric acid and/or sodium hydroxide may be used prior to lyophilization for pH adjustment.

Activase is a sterile, white to off-white, lyophilized powder for intravenous administration after reconstitution with Sterile Water for Injection, USP.

Quantitative Composition of the Lyophilized Product

	100 mg Vial	50 mg Vial
Alteplase	100 mg (58 million IU)	50 mg (29 million IU)
L-Arginine	3.5 g	1.7 g
Phosphoric Acid	1 g	0.5 g
Polysorbate 80	≤ 11 mg	≤ 4 mg
Vacuum	No	Yes

Biological potency is determined by an in vitro clot lysis assay and is expressed in International Units as tested against the WHO standard. The specific activity of Activase is 580,000 IU/mg.

CLINICAL PHARMACOLOGY

Activase is an enzyme (serine protease) which has the property of fibrin-enhanced conversion of plasminogen to plasmin. It produces limited conversion of plasminogen in the absence of fibrin. When introduced into the systemic circulation at pharmacologic concentration, Activase binds to fibrin in a thrombus and converts the entrapped plasminogen to plasmin. This initiates local fibrinolysis with limited systemic proteolysis. Following administration of 100 mg Activase, there is a decrease (16%–36%) in circulating fibrinogen.[1,2] In a controlled trial, 8 of 73 patients (11%) receiving Activase (1.25 mg/kg body weight over 3 hours) experienced a decrease in fibrinogen to below 100 mg/dL.[2]

The clearance of Alteplase in AMI patients has shown that it is rapidly cleared from the plasma with an initial half-life of less than 5 minutes. There is no difference in the dominant initial plasma half-life between the 3-Hour and accelerated regimens for AMI. The plasma clearance of Alteplase is 380–570 mL/min.[3,4] The clearance is mediated primarily by the liver. The initial volume of distribution approximates plasma volume.

Acute Myocardial Infarction (AMI) Patients

Coronary occlusion due to a thrombus is present in the infarct-related coronary artery in approximately 80% of patients experiencing a transmural myocardial infarction evaluated within 4 hours of onset of symptoms.[5,6]

Two Activase dose regimens have been studied in patients experiencing acute myocardial infarction. (Please see DOSAGE AND ADMINISTRATION.) The comparative efficacy of these two regimens has not been evaluated.

Accelerated Infusion in AMI Patients

Accelerated infusion of Activase was studied in an international, multi-center trial (GUSTO) that randomized 41,021 patients with acute myocardial infarction to four thrombolytic regimens. Entry criteria included onset of chest pain within 6 hours of treatment and ST-segment elevation of ECG. The regimens included accelerated infusion of Activase (≤ 100 mg over 90 minutes, see DOSAGE AND ADMINISTRATION) plus intravenous (IV) heparin (accelerated infusion of Alteplase, n=10,396), or the Kabikinase brand of Streptokinase (1.5 million units over 60 minutes) plus IV heparin (SK [IV], n=10,410), or Streptokinase (as above) plus subcutaneous (SQ) heparin (SK [SQ], n=9841). A fourth regimen combined Alteplase and Streptokinase. Aspirin and heparin use was directed by the GUSTO study protocol as follows: All patients were to receive 160 mg chewable aspirin administered as soon as possible, followed by 160–325 mg daily. IV heparin was directed to be a 5000 U IV bolus initiated as soon as possible, followed by a 1000 U/hour continuous IV infusion for at least 48 hours; subsequent heparin therapy was at the discretion of the attending physician. SQ heparin was directed to be 12,500 U administered 4 hours after initiation of SK therapy, followed by 12,500 U twice daily for 7 days or until discharge, whichever came first. Many of the patients randomized to receive SQ heparin received some IV heparin, usually in response to recurrent chest pain and/or the need for a medical procedure. Some received IV heparin on arrival to the emergency room prior to enrollment and randomization.

Results for the primary endpoint of the study, 30-day mortality, are shown in Table 1. The incidence of 30-day mortality for accelerated infusion of Alteplase was 1.0% lower than for SK (IV) and 1.0% lower than for SK (SQ). The secondary endpoints of combined 30-day mortality or nonfatal stroke, and 24-hour mortality, as well as the safety endpoints of total stroke and intracerebral hemorrhage are also shown in Table 1. The incidence of combined 30-day mortality or nonfatal stroke for the Alteplase accelerated infusion was 1.0% lower than for SK (IV) and 0.8% lower than for SK (SQ).

[See table 1 at top of next page]

Subgroup analysis of patients by age, infarct location, time from symptom onset to thrombolytic treatment, and treatment in the U.S. or elsewhere showed consistently lower 30-day mortality for the Alteplase accelerated infusion group. For patients who were over 75 years of age, a predefined subgroup consisting of 12% of patients enrolled, the incidence of stroke was 4.0% for the Alteplase accelerated infusion group, 2.8% for SK (IV), and 3.2% for SK (SQ); the incidence of combined 30-day mortality or nonfatal stroke was 20.6% for accelerated infusion of Alteplase, 21.5% for SK (IV), and 22.0% for SK (SQ).

An angiographic substudy of the GUSTO trial provided data on infarct-related artery patency. Table 2 presents 90-minute, 180-minute, 24-hour, and 5–7 day patency values by TIMI flow grade for the three treatment regimens. Reocclusion rates were similar for all three treatment regimens.

[See table 2 on next page]

The exact relationship between coronary artery patency and clinical activity has not been established.

The safety and efficacy of the accelerated infusion of Alteplase have not been evaluated using antithrombotic or antiplatelet regimens other than those used in the GUSTO trial.

3-Hour Infusion in AMI Patients

In patients studied in a controlled trial with coronary angiography at 90 and 120 minutes following infusion of Activase, infarct artery patency was observed in 71% and 85% of patients (n=85), respectively.[2] In a second study, where patients received coronary angiography prior to and following infusion of Activase within 6 hours of the onset of symptoms, reperfusion of the obstructed vessel occurred within 90 minutes after the commencement of therapy in 71% of 83 patients.[1]

The exact relationship between coronary artery patency and clinical activity has not been established.

In a double-blind, randomized trial (138 patients) comparing Activase to placebo, patients infused with Activase within 4 hours of onset of symptoms experienced improved left ventricular function at Day 10 compared to the placebo group, when ejection fraction was measured by gated blood pool scan (53.2% vs 46.4%, p=0.018). Relative to baseline (Day 1) values, the net changes in ejection fraction were +3.6% and −4.7% for the treated and placebo groups, respectively (p=0.0001). Also documented was a reduced incidence of clinical congestive heart failure in the treated group (14%) compared to the placebo group (33%) (p=0.009).[7]

In a double-blind, randomized trial (145 patients) comparing Activase to placebo, patients infused with Activase within 2.5 hours of onset of symptoms experienced improved left ventricular function at a mean of 21 days compared to the placebo group, when ejection fraction was measured by gated blood pool scan (52% vs 48%, p=0.08) and by contrast ventriculogram (61% vs 54%, p=0.006). Although the contribution of Activase alone is unclear, the incidence of nonischemic cardiac complications when taken as a group (i.e., congestive heart failure, pericarditis, atrial fibrillation, and conduction disturbance) was reduced when compared to those patients treated with placebo ($p < 0.01$).[8]

In a double-blind, randomized trial (5013 patients) comparing Activase to placebo (ASSET study), patients infused

Continued on next page

Activase—Cont.

with Activase within 5 hours of the onset of symptoms of acute myocardial infarction experienced improved 30-day survival compared to those treated with placebo. At 1 month, the overall mortality rates were 7.2% for the Activase-treated group and 9.8% for the placebo-treated group (p=0.001).[9,10] This benefit was maintained at 6 months for Activase-treated patients (10.4%) compared to those treated with placebo (13.1%, p=0.008).[10]

In a double-blind, randomized trial (721 patients) comparing Activase to placebo, patients infused with Activase within 5 hours of the onset of symptoms experienced improved ventricular function 10–22 days after treatment compared to the placebo group, when global ejection fraction was measured by contrast ventriculography (50.7% vs 48.5%, p=0.01). Patients treated with Activase had a 19% reduction in infarct size, as measured by cumulative release of HBD (α-hydroxybutyrate dehydrogenase) activity compared to placebo-treated patients (p=0.001). Patients treated with Activase had significantly fewer episodes of cardiogenic shock (p=0.02), ventricular fibrillation ($p < 0.04$) and pericarditis (p=0.01) compared to patients treated with placebo. Mortality at 21 days in Activase-treated patients was reduced to 3.7% compared to 6.3% in placebo-treated patients (1-sided p=0.05).[11] Although these data do not demonstrate unequivocally a significant reduction in mortality for this study, they do indicate a trend that is supported by the results of the ASSET study.

Acute Ischemic Stroke Patients

Two placebo-controlled, double-blind trials (The NINDS t-PA Stroke Trial, Part 1 and Part 2) have been conducted in patients with acute ischemic stroke.[12] Both studies enrolled patients with measurable neurological deficit who could complete screening and begin study treatment within 3 hours from symptom onset. A cranial computerized tomography (CT) scan was performed prior to treatment to rule out the presence of intracranial hemorrhage (ICH). Patients were also excluded for the presence of conditions related to risks of bleeding (see CONTRAINDICATIONS), for minor neurological deficit, for rapidly improving symptoms prior to initiating study treatment, or for blood glucose of < 50 mg/dL or > 400 mg/dL.

Patients were randomized to receive either 0.9 mg/kg Activase (maximum of 90 mg), or placebo. Activase was administered as a 10% initial bolus over 1 minute followed by continuous intravenous infusion of the remainder over 60 minutes (see DOSAGE AND ADMINISTRATION). In patients without recent use of oral anticoagulants or heparin, study treatment was initiated prior to the availability of coagulation study results. However, the infusion was discontinued if either a pretreatment prothrombin time (PT) > 15 seconds or an elevated activated partial thromboplastin time (aPTT) was identified. Although patients with or without prior aspirin use were enrolled, administration of anticoagulants and antiplatelet agents was prohibited for the first 24 hours following symptom onset.

The initial study (NINDS-Part 1, n=291) evaluated neurological improvement at 24 hours after stroke onset. The primary endpoint, the proportion of patients with a 4 or more point improvement in the National Institutes of Health Stroke Scale (NIHSS) score or complete recovery (NIHSS score = 0), was not significantly different between treatment groups. A secondary analysis suggested improved 3-month outcome associated with Activase treatment using the following stroke assessment scales: Barthel Index, Modified Rankin Scale, Glasgow Outcome Scale, and the NIHSS.

A second study (NINDS-Part 2, n=333) assessed clinical outcome at 3 months as the primary outcome. A favorable outcome was defined as minimal or no disability using the four stroke assessment scales: Barthel Index (score ≥ 95), Modified Rankin Scale (score ≤ 1), Glasgow Outcome Scale (score = 1), and NIHSS (score ≤ 1). The results comparing Activase- and placebo-treated patients for the four outcome scales together (Generalized Estimating Equations) and individually are presented in Table 3. In this study, depending upon the scale, the favorable outcome of minimal or no disability occurred in at least 11 per 100 more patients treated with Activase than those receiving placebo. Secondary analyses demonstrated consistent functional and neurological improvement within all four stroke scales as indicated by median scores. These results were highly consistent with the 3-month outcome treatment effects observed in the Part 1 study.

[See table 3 above]

The incidences of all-cause 90-day mortality, ICH, and new ischemic stroke following Activase treatment compared to placebo are presented in Table 4 as a combined safety analysis (n=624) for Parts 1 and 2. These data indicated a significant increase in ICH following Activase treatment, particularly symptomatic ICH within 36 hours. In Activase-treated patients, there were no increases compared to placebo in the incidences of 90-day mortality or severe disability.

[See table 4 above]

In a prespecified subgroup analysis in patients receiving aspirin prior to onset of stroke symptoms, there was preserved favorable outcome for Activase-treated patients.

Exploratory, multivariate analyses of both studies combined (n=624) to investigate potential predictors of ICH and treatment effect modifiers were performed. In Activase-treated patients presenting with severe neurological deficit (e.g., NIHSS > 22) or of advanced age (e.g., > 77 years of age), the

Table 1

Event	Accelerated Activase	SK (IV)	p-Value[1]	SK (SQ)	p-Value[1]
30-Day Mortality	6.3%	7.3%	0.003	7.3%	0.007
30-Day Mortality or Nonfatal Stroke	7.2%	8.2%	0.006	8.0%	0.036
24-Hour Mortality	2.4%	2.9%	0.009	2.8%	0.029
Any Stroke	1.6%	1.4%	0.32	1.2%	0.03
Intracerebral Hemorrhage	0.7%	0.6%	0.22	0.5%	0.02

[1] *Two-tailed p-value is for comparison of Accelerated Activase to the respective SK control arm.*

Table 2

Patency (TIMI 2 or 3)	Accelerated Activase	SK (IV)	p-Value	SK (SQ)	p-Value
90-Minute	n=272 81.3%	n=261 59.0%	< 0.0001	n=260 53.5%	< 0.0001
180-Minute	n=80 76.3%	n=76 72.4%	0.58	n=95 71.6%	0.48
24-Hour	n=81 88.9%	n=72 87.5%	0.24	n=67 82.1%	0.79
5–7 Day	n=72 83.3%	n=77 90.9%	0.47	n=75 78.7%	0.17

Table 3
The NINDS t-PA Stroke Trial, Part 2
3-Month Efficacy Outcomes

	Frequency of Favorable Outcome[1]				
Analysis	Placebo (n=165)	Activase (n=168)	Absolute Difference (95% CI)	Relative Frequency[2] (95% CI)	p-Value[3]
Generalized Estimating Equations (Multivariate)	—	—	—	1.34 (1.05, 1.72)	0.02
Barthel Index	37.6%	50.0%	12.4% (3.0, 21.9)	1.33 (1.04, 1.71)	0.02
Modified Rankin Scale	26.1%	38.7%	12.6% (3.7, 21.6)	1.48 (1.08, 2.04)	0.02
Glasgow Outcome Scale	31.5%	44.0%	12.5% (3.3, 21.8)	1.40 (1.05, 1.85)	0.02
NIHSS	20.0%	31.0%	11.0% (2.6, 19.3)	1.55 (1.06, 2.26)	0.02

[1]*Favorable Outcome is defined as recovery with minimal or no disability.*
[2]*Value > 1 indicates frequency of recovery in favor of Activase treatment.*
[3]*p-Value for Relative Frequency is from Generalized Estimating Equations with log link.*

Table 4
The NINDS t-PA Stroke Trial
Safety Outcome

	Part 1 and Part 2 Combined		
	Placebo (n=312)	Activase (n=312)	p-Value[2]
All-Cause 90-day Mortality	64 (20.5%)	54 (17.3%)	0.36
Total ICH[1]	20 (6.4%)	48 (15.4%)	< 0.01
Symptomatic	4 (1.3%)	25 (8.0%)	< 0.01
Asymptomatic	16 (5.1%)	23 (7.4%)	0.32
Symptomatic ICH within 36 hours	2 (0.6%)	20 (6.4%)	< 0.01
New Ischemic Stroke (3-months)	17 (5.4%)	18 (5.8%)	1.00

[1] *Within trial follow-up period. Symptomatic ICH was defined as the occurrence of sudden clinical worsening followed by subsequent verification of ICH on CT scan. Asymptomatic ICH was defined as ICH detected on a routine repeat CT scan without preceding clinical worsening.*
[2]*Fisher's Exact Test*

trends toward increased risk for symptomatic ICH within the first 36 hours were more prominent. Similar trends were also seen for total ICH and for all-cause 90-day mortality in these patients. When risk was assessed by the combination of death and severe disability in these patients, there was no difference between placebo and Activase groups. Analyses for efficacy suggested a reduced but still favorable clinical outcome for Activase-treated patients with severe neurological deficit or advanced age at presentation.

Pulmonary Embolism Patients

In a comparative randomized trial (n=45),[13] 59% of patients (n=22) treated with Activase (100 mg over 2 hours) experienced moderate or marked lysis of pulmonary emboli when assessed by pulmonary angiography 2 hours after treatment initiation. Activase-treated patients also experienced a significant reduction in pulmonary embolism-induced pulmonary hypertension within 2 hours of treatment (p=0.003). Pulmonary perfusion at 24 hours, as assessed by radionuclide scan, was significantly improved (p=0.002).

INDICATIONS AND USAGE

Acute Myocardial Infarction

Activase is indicated for use in the management of acute myocardial infarction in adults for the improvement of ventricular function following AMI, the reduction of the incidence of congestive heart failure, and the reduction of mortality associated with AMI. Treatment should be initiated as soon as possible after the onset of AMI symptoms (see CLINICAL PHARMACOLOGY).

Acute Ischemic Stroke

Activase is indicated for the management of acute ischemic stroke in adults for improving neurological recovery and reducing the incidence of disability. **Treatment should only be initiated within 3 hours after the onset of stroke symptoms, and after exclusion of intracranial hemorrhage by a cranial computerized tomography (CT) scan or other diagnostic imaging method sensitive for the presence of hemorrhage (see CONTRAINDICATIONS).**

Pulmonary Embolism

Activase is indicated in the management of acute massive pulmonary embolism (PE) in adults:

— For the lysis of acute pulmonary emboli, defined as obstruction of blood flow to a lobe or multiple segments of the lungs.

— For the lysis of pulmonary emboli accompanied by unstable hemodynamics, e.g., failure to maintain blood pressure without supportive measures.

The diagnosis should be confirmed by objective means, such as pulmonary angiography or noninvasive procedures such as lung scanning.

CONTRAINDICATIONS

Acute Myocardial Infarction or Pulmonary Embolism

Activase therapy in patients with acute myocardial infarction or pulmonary embolism is contraindicated in the following situations because of an increased risk of bleeding:

- **Active internal bleeding**
- **History of cerebrovascular accident**

- **Recent intracranial or intraspinal surgery or trauma (see WARNINGS)**
- **Intracranial neoplasm, arteriovenous malformation, or aneurysm**
- **Known bleeding diathesis**
- **Severe uncontrolled hypertension**

Acute Ischemic Stroke

Activase therapy in patients with acute ischemic stroke is contraindicated in the following situations because of an increased risk of bleeding, which could result in significant disability or death:

- **Evidence of intracranial hemorrhage on pretreatment evaluation**
- **Suspicion of subarachnoid hemorrhage on pretreatment evaluation**
- **Recent (within 3 months) intracranial or intraspinal surgery, serious head trauma, or previous stroke**
- **History of intracranial hemorrhage**
- **Uncontrolled hypertension at time of treatment (e.g., > 185 mm Hg systolic or > 110 mm Hg diastolic)**
- **Seizure at the onset of stroke**
- **Active internal bleeding**
- **Intracranial neoplasm, arteriovenous malformation, or aneurysm**
- **Known bleeding diathesis including but not limited to:**
  - **— Current use of oral anticoagulants (e.g., warfarin sodium) or an International Normalized Ratio (INR) >1.7 or a prothrombin time (PT) > 15 seconds**
  - **— Administration of heparin within 48 hours preceding the onset of stroke and have an elevated activated partial thromboplastin time (aPTT) at presentation**
  - **— Platelet count < 100,000/mm^3**

WARNINGS

Bleeding

The most common complication encountered during Activase therapy is bleeding. The type of bleeding associated with thrombolytic therapy can be divided into two broad categories:

- Internal bleeding, involving intracranial and retroperitoneal sites, or the gastrointestinal, genitourinary, or respiratory tracts.
- Superficial or surface bleeding, observed mainly at invaded or disturbed sites (e.g., venous cutdowns, arterial punctures, sites of recent surgical intervention).

The concomitant use of heparin anticoagulation may contribute to bleeding. Some of the hemorrhage episodes occurred 1 or more days after the effects of Activase had dissipated, but while heparin therapy was continuing.

As fibrin is lysed during Activase therapy, bleeding from recent puncture sites may occur. Therefore, thrombolytic therapy requires careful attention to all potential bleeding sites (including catheter insertion sites, arterial and venous puncture sites, cutdown sites, and needle puncture sites).

Intramuscular injections and nonessential handling of the patient should be avoided during treatment with Activase. Venipunctures should be performed carefully and only as required.

Should an arterial puncture be necessary during an infusion of Activase, it is preferable to use an upper extremity vessel that is accessible to manual compression. Pressure should be applied for at least 30 minutes, a pressure dressing applied, and the puncture site checked frequently for evidence of bleeding.

Should serious bleeding (not controllable by local pressure) occur, the infusion of Activase and any concomitant heparin should be terminated immediately.

Each patient being considered for therapy with Activase should be carefully evaluated and anticipated benefits weighed against potential risks associated with therapy.

In the following conditions, the risks of Activase therapy for all approved indications may be increased and should be weighed against the anticipated benefits:

- Recent major surgery, e.g., coronary artery bypass graft, obstetrical delivery, organ biopsy, previous puncture of noncompressible vessels
- Cerebrovascular disease
- Recent gastrointestinal or genitourinary bleeding
- Recent trauma
- Hypertension: systolic BP ≥175 mm Hg and/or diastolic BP ≥110 mm Hg
- High likelihood of left heart thrombus, e.g., mitral stenosis with atrial fibrillation
- Acute pericarditis
- Subacute bacterial endocarditis
- Hemostatic defects including those secondary to severe hepatic or renal disease
- Significant hepatic dysfunction
- Pregnancy
- Diabetic hemorrhagic retinopathy, or other hemorrhagic ophthalmic conditions
- Septic thrombophlebitis or occluded AV cannula at seriously infected site
- Advanced age (e.g., over 75 years old)
- Patients currently receiving oral anticoagulants, e.g., warfarin sodium
- Any other condition in which bleeding constitutes a significant hazard or would be particularly difficult to manage because of its location

Cholesterol Embolization

Cholesterol embolism has been reported rarely in patients treated with all types of thrombolytic agents; the true incidence is unknown. This serious condition, which can be lethal, is also associated with invasive vascular procedures (e.g., cardiac catheterization, angiography, vascular surgery) and/or anticoagulant therapy. Clinical features of cholesterol embolism may include livedo reticularis, "purple toe" syndrome, acute renal failure, gangrenous digits, hypertension, pancreatitis, myocardial infarction, cerebral infarction, spinal cord infarction, retinal artery occlusion, bowel infarction, and rhabdomyolysis.

Use in Acute Myocardial Infarction

In a small subgroup of AMI patients who are at low risk for death from cardiac causes (i.e., no previous myocardial infarction, Killip class I) and who have high blood pressure at the time of presentation, the risk for stroke may offset the survival benefit produced by thrombolytic therapy.[14]

Arrhythmias

Coronary thrombolysis may result in arrhythmias associated with reperfusion. These arrhythmias (such as sinus bradycardia, accelerated idioventricular rhythm, ventricular premature depolarizations, ventricular tachycardia) are not different from those often seen in the ordinary course of acute myocardial infarction and may be managed with standard antiarrhythmic measures. It is recommended that antiarrhythmic therapy for bradycardia and/or ventricular irritability be available when infusions of Activase are administered.

Use in Acute Ischemic Stroke

In addition to the previously listed conditions, the risks of Activase therapy to treat acute ischemic stroke may be increased in the following conditions and should be weighed against the anticipated benefits:

- Patients with severe neurological deficit (e.g., NIHSS > 22) at presentation. There is an increased risk of intracranial hemorrhage in these patients.
- Patients with major early infarct signs on a computerized cranial tomography (CT) scan (e.g., substantial edema, mass effect, or midline shift).

In patients without recent use of oral anticoagulants or heparin, Activase treatment can be initiated prior to the availability of coagulation study results. However, infusion should be discontinued if either a pretreatment International Normalized Ratio (INR) > 1.7 or a prothrombin time (PT) > 15 seconds or an elevated activated partial thromboplastin time (aPTT) is identified.

Treatment should be limited to facilities that can provide appropriate evaluation and management of ICH.

In acute ischemic stroke, neither the incidence of intracranial hemorrhage nor the benefits of therapy are known in patients treated with Activase more than 3 hours after the onset of symptoms. **Therefore, treatment of patients with acute ischemic stroke more than 3 hours after symptom onset is not recommended.**

Due to the increased risk for misdiagnosis of acute ischemic stroke, special diligence is required in making this diagnosis in patients whose blood glucose values are < 50 mg/dL or > 400 mg/dL. The safety and efficacy of treatment with Activase in patients with minor neurological deficit or with rapidly improving symptoms prior to the start of Activase administration has not been evaluated. **Therefore, treatment of patients with minor neurological deficit or with rapidly improving symptoms is not recommended.**

Use in Pulmonary Embolism

It should be recognized that the treatment of pulmonary embolism with Activase has not been shown to constitute adequate clinical treatment of underlying deep vein thrombosis. Furthermore, the possible risk of reembolization due to the lysis of underlying deep venous thrombi should be considered.

PRECAUTIONS

General

Standard management of myocardial infarction or pulmonary embolism should be implemented concomitantly with Activase treatment. Noncompressible arterial puncture must be avoided and internal jugular and subclavian venous punctures should be avoided to minimize bleeding from noncompressible sites. Arterial and venous punctures should be minimized. In the event of serious bleeding, Activase and heparin should be discontinued immediately. Heparin effects can be reversed by protamine.

Readministration

There is no experience with readministration of Activase. If an anaphylactoid reaction occurs, the infusion should be discontinued immediately and appropriate therapy initiated.

Although sustained antibody formation in patients receiving one dose of Activase has not been documented, readministration should be undertaken with caution. Detectable levels of antibody (a single point measurement) were reported in one patient, but subsequent antibody test results were negative.

Drug/Laboratory Test Interactions

During Activase therapy, if coagulation tests and/or measures of fibrinolytic activity are performed, the results may be unreliable unless specific precautions are taken to prevent in vitro artifacts. Activase is an enzyme that when present in blood in pharmacologic concentrations remains active under in vitro conditions. This can lead to degradation of fibrinogen in blood samples removed for analysis. Collection of blood samples in the presence of aprotinin (150–200 units/mL) can to some extent mitigate this phenomenon.

Drug Interactions

The interaction of Activase with other cardioactive or cerebroactive drugs has not been studied. In addition to bleeding associated with heparin and vitamin K antagonists, drugs that alter platelet function (such as acetylsalicylic acid, dipyridamole and Abciximab) may increase the risk of bleeding if administered prior to, during, or after Activase therapy.

Use of Antithrombotics

Aspirin and heparin have been administered concomitantly with and following infusions of Activase in the management of acute myocardial infarction or pulmonary embolism. Because heparin, aspirin, or Activase may cause bleeding complications, careful monitoring for bleeding is advised, especially at arterial puncture sites.

The concomitant use of heparin or aspirin during the first 24 hours following symptom onset were prohibited in The NINDS t-PA Stroke Trial. The safety of such concomitant use with Activase for the management of acute ischemic stroke is unknown.

Blood Pressure Control

Blood pressure should be monitored frequently and controlled during and following Activase administration in the management of acute ischemic stroke. In The NINDS t-PA Stroke Trial, blood pressure was actively controlled (≤ 185/110 mm Hg) for 24 hours. Blood pressure was monitored during the hospital stay.

Carcinogenesis, Mutagenesis, Impairment of Fertility

Long-term studies in animals have not been performed to evaluate the carcinogenic potential or the effect on fertility. Short-term studies, which evaluated tumorigenicity of Activase and effect on tumor metastases in rodents, were negative.

Studies to determine mutagenicity (Ames test) and chromosomal aberration assays in human lymphocytes were negative at all concentrations tested. Cytotoxicity, as reflected by a decrease in mitotic index, was evidenced only after prolonged exposure and only at the highest concentrations tested.

Pregnancy (Category C)

Activase has been shown to have an embryocidal effect in rabbits when intravenously administered in doses of approximately two times (3 mg/kg) the human dose for AMI. No maternal or fetal toxicity was evident at 0.65 times (1 mg/kg) the human dose in pregnant rats and rabbits dosed during the period of organogenesis. There are no adequate and well-controlled studies in pregnant women. Activase should be used during pregnancy only if the potential benefit justifies the potential risk to the fetus.

Nursing Mothers

It is not known whether Activase is excreted in human milk. Because many drugs are excreted in human milk, caution should be exercised when Activase is administered to a nursing woman.

Pediatric Use

Safety and effectiveness of Activase in pediatric patients have not been established.

ADVERSE REACTIONS

Bleeding

The most frequent adverse reaction associated with Activase in all approved indications is bleeding (see WARNINGS).[15,16]

Should serious bleeding in a critical location (intracranial, gastrointestinal, retroperitoneal, pericardial) occur, Activase therapy should be discontinued immediately, along with any concomitant therapy with heparin. Death and permanent disability are not uncommonly reported in patients that have experienced stroke (including intracranial bleeding) and other serious bleeding episodes.

In the GUSTO trial for the treatment of acute myocardial infarction, using the accelerated infusion regimen the incidence of all strokes for the Activase-treated patients was 1.6%, while the incidence of nonfatal stroke was 0.9%. The incidence of hemorrhagic stroke was 0.7%, not all of which were fatal. The incidence of all strokes, as well as that for hemorrhagic stroke, increased with increasing age (see CLINICAL PHARMACOLOGY: Accelerated Infusion in AMI Patients). Data from previous trials utilizing a 3-hour infusion of ≤ 100 mg indicated that the incidence of total stroke in six randomized, double-blind, placebo-controlled trials[2,7–11,17] was 1.2% (37/3161) in Alteplase-treated patients compared with 0.9% (27/3092) in placebo-treated patients.

For the 3-hour infusion regimen, the incidence of significant internal bleeding (estimated as > 250 cc blood loss) has been reported in studies in over 800 patients. These data do not include patients treated with the Alteplase accelerated infusion.

	Total Dose ≤ 100 mg
gastrointestinal	5%
genitourinary	4%
ecchymosis	1%
retroperitoneal	< 1%
epistaxis	< 1%
gingival	< 1%

The incidence of intracranial hemorrhage (ICH) in acute myocardial infarction patients treated with Activase is as follows:

Dose	Number of Patients	ICH (%)
100 mg, 3-hour	3272	0.4
≤ 100 mg, accelerated	10,396	0.7

Continued on next page

Activase—Cont.

150 mg	1779	1.3
1–1.4 mg/kg	237	0.4

These data indicate that a dose of 150 mg of Activase should not be used in the treatment of AMI because it has been associated with an increase in intracranial bleeding.[18]

For acute massive pulmonary embolism, bleeding events were consistent with the general safety profile observed with Activase in acute myocardial infarction patients receiving the 3-hour infusion regimen.

The incidence of ICH, especially symptomatic ICH, in patients with acute ischemic stroke was higher in Activase-treated patients than placebo patients (see CLINICAL PHARMACOLOGY).

A study of another alteplase product, Actilyse, in acute ischemic stroke, suggested that doses greater than 0.9 mg/kg may be associated with an increased incidence of ICH.[19]

Doses greater than 0.9 mg/kg (maximum 90 mg) should not be used in the management of acute ischemic stroke.

Bleeding events other than ICH were noted in the studies of acute ischemic stroke and were consistent with the general safety profile of Activase. In The NINDS t-PA Stroke Trial (Parts 1 and 2), the frequency of bleeding requiring red blood cell transfusions was 6.4% for Activase-treated patients compared to 3.8% for placebo (p=0.19, using Mantel-Haenszel Chi-Square).

Fibrin which is part of the hemostatic plug formed at needle puncture sites will be lysed during Activase therapy. Therefore, Activase therapy requires careful attention to potential bleeding sites, e.g., catheter insertion sites, and arterial puncture sites.

Allergic Reactions

Allergic-type reactions, e.g., anaphylactoid reaction, laryngeal edema, rash, and urticaria have been reported very rarely (< 0.02%). A cause and effect relationship to Activase therapy has not been established. When such reactions occur, they usually respond to conventional therapy.

Other Adverse Reactions

The following adverse reactions have been reported among patients receiving Activase in clinical trials and in postmarketing experience. These reactions are frequent sequelae of the underlying disease and the effect of Activase on the incidence of these events is unknown.

Use in Acute Myocardial Infarction: Arrhythmias, AV block, cardiogenic shock, heart failure, cardiac arrest, recurrent ischemia, myocardial reinfarction, myocardial rupture, electromechanical dissociation, pericardial effusion, pericarditis, mitral regurgitation, cardiac tamponade, thromboembolism, pulmonary edema. These events may be life threatening and may lead to death. Nausea and/or vomiting, hypotension and fever have also been reported.

Use in Pulmonary Embolism: Pulmonary reembolization, pulmonary edema, pleural effusion, thromboembolism, hypotension. These events may be life threatening and may lead to death. Fever has also been reported.

Use in Acute Ischemic Stroke: Cerebral edema, cerebral herniation, seizure, new ischemic stroke. These events may be life threatening and may lead to death.

DOSAGE AND ADMINISTRATION

Activase is for intravenous administration only. Extravasation of Activase infusion can cause ecchymosis and/or inflammation. Management consists of terminating the infusion at that IV site and application of local therapy.

Acute Myocardial Infarction

Administer Activase as soon as possible after the onset of symptoms. There are two Activase dose regimens for use in the management of acute myocardial infarction; controlled studies to compare clinical outcomes with these regimens have not been conducted.

A DOSE OF 150 mg OF ACTIVASE SHOULD NOT BE USED FOR THE TREATMENT OF ACUTE MYOCARDIAL INFARCTION BECAUSE IT HAS BEEN ASSOCIATED WITH AN INCREASE IN INTRACRANIAL BLEEDING.

Accelerated Infusion

The recommended total dose is based upon patient weight, not to exceed 100 mg. For patients weighing > 67 kg, the recommended dose administered is 100 mg as a 15 mg intravenous bolus, followed by 50 mg infused over the next 30 minutes, and then 35 mg infused over the next 60 minutes. For patients weighing ≤ 67 kg, the recommended dose is administered as a 15 mg intravenous bolus, followed by 0.75 mg/kg infused over the next 30 minutes not to exceed 50 mg, and then 0.50 mg/kg over the next 60 minutes not to exceed 35 mg.

The safety and efficacy of this accelerated infusion of Alteplase regimen has only been investigated with concomitant administration of heparin and aspirin as described in CLINICAL PHARMACOLOGY.

a. The bolus dose may be prepared in one of the following ways:
   1. By removing 15 mL from the vial of reconstituted (1 mg/mL) Activase using a syringe and needle. If this method is used with the 50 mg vials, the syringe should not be primed with air and the needle should be inserted into the Activase vial stopper. If the 100 mg vial is used, the needle should be inserted away from the puncture mark made by the transfer device.
   2. By removing 15 mL from a port (second injection site) on the infusion line after the infusion set is primed.
   3. By programming an infusion pump to deliver a 15 mL (1 mg/mL) bolus at the initiation of the infusion.

b. The remainder of the Activase dose may be administered as follows:

   50 mg vials—administer using either a polyvinyl chloride bag or glass vial and infusion set.

   100 mg vial—insert the spike end of an infusion set through the same puncture site created by the transfer device in the stopper of the vial of reconstituted Activase. Hang the Activase vial from the plastic molded capping attached to the bottom of the vial.

3-Hour Infusion

The recommended dose is 100 mg administered as 60 mg in the first hour (of which 6 to 10 mg is administered as a bolus), 20 mg over the second hour, and 20 mg over the third hour. For smaller patients (< 65 kg), a dose of 1.25 mg/kg administered over 3 hours, as described above, may be used.[15]

Although the value of the use of anticoagulants during and following administration of Activase has not been fully studied, heparin has been administered concomitantly for 24 hours or longer in more than 90% of patients.

Aspirin and/or dipyridamole have been given to patients receiving Alteplase during and/or following heparin treatment.

a. The bolus dose may be prepared in one of the following ways:
   1. By removing 6 to 10 mL from the vial of reconstituted (1 mg/mL) Activase using a syringe and needle. If this method is used with the 50 mg vials, the syringe should not be primed with air and the needle should be inserted into the Activase vial stopper. If the 100 mg vial is used, the needle should be inserted away from the puncture mark made by the transfer device.
   2. By removing 6 to 10 mL from a port (second injection site) on the infusion line after the infusion set is primed.
   3. By programming an infusion pump to deliver a 6 to 10 mL (1 mg/mL) bolus at the initiation of the infusion.

b. The remainder of the Activase dose may be administered as follows:

   50 mg vials—administer using either a polyvinyl chloride bag or glass vial and infusion set.

   100 mg vial—insert the spike end of an infusion set through the same puncture site created by the transfer device in the stopper of the vial of reconstituted Activase. Hang the Activase vial from the plastic molded capping attached to the bottom of the vial.

Acute Ischemic Stroke

THE TOTAL DOSE FOR TREATMENT OF ACUTE ISCHEMIC STROKE SHOULD NOT EXCEED 90 mg.

The recommended dose is 0.9 mg/kg (not to exceed 90 mg total dose) infused over 60 minutes with 10% of the total dose administered as an initial intravenous bolus over 1 minute.

The safety and efficacy of this regimen with concomitant administration of heparin and aspirin during the first 24 hours after symptom onset has not been investigated.

a. The bolus dose may be prepared in one of the following ways:
   1. By removing the appropriate volume from the vial of reconstituted (1 mg/mL) Activase using a syringe and needle. If this method is used with the 50 mg vials, the syringe should not be primed with air and the needle should be inserted into the Activase vial stopper. If the 100 mg vial is used, the needle should be inserted away from the puncture mark made by the transfer device.
   2. By removing the appropriate volume from a port (second injection site) on the infusion line after the infusion set is primed.
   3. By programming an infusion pump to deliver the appropriate volume as a bolus at the initiation of the infusion.

b. The remainder of the Activase dose may be administered as follows:

   50 mg vials—administer using either a polyvinyl chloride bag or glass vial and infusion set.

   100 mg vial—remove from the vial any quantity of drug in excess of that specified for patient treatment. Insert the spike end of an infusion set through the same puncture site created by the transfer device in the stopper of the vial of reconstituted Activase. Hang the Activase vial from the plastic molded capping attached to the bottom of the vial.

Pulmonary Embolism

The recommended dose is 100 mg administered by intravenous infusion over 2 hours. Heparin therapy should be instituted or reinstituted near the end of or immediately following the Activase infusion when the partial thromboplastin time or thrombin time returns to twice normal or less.

The Activase dose may be administered as follows:

50 mg vials—administer using either a polyvinyl chloride bag or glass vial and infusion set.

100 mg vial—insert the spike end of an infusion set through the same puncture site created by the transfer device in the stopper of the vial of reconstituted Activase. Hang the Activase vial from the plastic molded capping attached to the bottom of the vial.

Reconstitution and Dilution

Activase should be reconstituted by aseptically adding the appropriate volume of the accompanying Sterile Water for Injection, USP, to the vial. It is important that Activase be reconstituted only with Sterile Water for Injection, USP, without preservatives. Do not use Bacteriostatic Water for Injection, USP. The reconstituted preparation results in a colorless to pale yellow transparent solution containing Activase 1mg/mL at approximately pH 7.3. The osmolality of this solution is approximately 215 mOsm/kg.

Because Activase contains no antibacterial preservatives, it should be reconstituted immediately before use. The solution may be used for intravenous administration within 8 hours following reconstitution when stored between 2–30°C (36–86°F). Before further dilution or administration, the product should be visually inspected for particulate matter and discoloration prior to administration whenever solution and container permit.

Activase may be administered as reconstituted at 1 mg/mL. As an alternative, the reconstituted solution may be diluted further immediately before administration in an equal volume of 0.9% Sodium Chloride Injection, USP, or 5% Dextrose Injection, USP, to yield a concentration of 0.5 mg/mL. Either polyvinyl chloride bags or glass vials are acceptable. Activase is stable for up to 8 hours in these solutions at room temperature. Exposure to light has no effect on the stability of these solutions. Excessive agitation during dilution should be avoided; mixing should be accomplished with gentle swirling and/or slow inversion. Do not use other infusion solutions, e.g., Sterile Water for Injection, USP, or preservative-containing solutions for further dilution.

50 mg Vials

Reconstitution should be carried out using a large bore needle (e.g., 18 gauge) and a syringe, directing the stream of Sterile Water for Injection, USP, into the lyophilized cake. **DO NOT USE IF VACUUM IS NOT PRESENT.** Slight foaming upon reconstitution is not unusual; standing undisturbed for several minutes is usually sufficient to allow dissipation of any large bubbles.

No other medication should be added to infusion solutions containing Activase. Any unused infusion solution should be discarded.

100 mg Vial

Reconstitution should be carried out using the transfer device provided, adding the contents of the accompanying 100 mL vial of Sterile Water for Injection, USP, to the contents of the 100 mg vial of Activase powder. Slight foaming upon reconstitution is not unusual; standing undisturbed for several minutes is usually sufficient to allow dissipation of any large bubbles. Please refer to the accompanying Instructions for Reconstitution and Administration. **100 mg VIALS DO NOT CONTAIN VACUUM.**

100 mg VIAL RECONSTITUTION

1. Use aseptic technique throughout.
2. Remove the protective flip-caps from one vial of Activase and one vial of Sterile Water for Injection, USP (SWFI).
3. Open the package containing the transfer device by peeling the paper label off the package.
4. Remove the protective cap from one end of the transfer device and keeping the vial of SWFI upright, insert the piercing pin vertically into the center of the stopper of the vial of SWFI.
5. Remove the protective cap from the other end of the transfer device. **DO NOT INVERT THE VIAL OF SWFI.**
6. Holding the vial of Activase upside-down, position it so that the center of the stopper is directly over the exposed piercing pin of the transfer device.
7. Push the vial of Activase down so that the piercing pin is inserted through the center of the Activase vial stopper.
8. Invert the two vials so that the vial of Activase is on the bottom (upright) and the vial of SWFI is upside-down, allowing the SWFI to flow down through the transfer device. Allow the entire contents of the vial of SWFI to flow into the Activase vial (approximately 0.5 cc of SWFI will remain in the diluent vial). Approximately 2 minutes are required for this procedure.
9. Remove the transfer device and the empty SWFI vial from the Activase vial. Safely discard both the transfer device and the empty diluent vial according to institutional procedures.
10. Swirl gently to dissolve the Activase powder. **DO NOT SHAKE.**

No other medication should be added to infusion solutions containing Activase.

Any unused infusion solution should be discarded.

HOW SUPPLIED

Activase is supplied as a sterile, lyophilized powder in 50 mg vials containing vacuum and in 100 mg vials without vacuum.

Each 50 mg Activase vial (29 million IU) is packaged with diluent for reconstitution (50 mL Sterile Water for Injection, USP): NDC 50242-044-13.

Each 100 mg Activase vial (58 million IU) is packaged with diluent for reconstitution (100 mL Sterile Water for Injection, USP), and one transfer device: NDC 50242-085-27.

Storage

Store lyophilized Activase at controlled room temperature not to exceed 30°C (86°F), or under refrigeration (2–8°C/36–46°F). Protect the lyophilized material during extended storage from excessive exposure to light.

Do not use beyond the expiration date stamped on the vial.

REFERENCES

1. Mueller H, Rao AK, Forman SA, et al. Thrombolysis in myocardial infarction (TIMI): comparative studies of coronary reperfusion and systemic fibrinogenolysis with two forms of recombinant tissue-type plasminogen activator. *J Am Coll Cardiol.* 1987;10:479–90.
2. Topol EJ, Morriss DC, Smalling RW, et al. A multicenter, randomized, placebo-controlled trial of a new form of in-

travenous recombinant tissue-type plasminogen activator (Activase®) in acute myocardial infarction. *J Am Coll Cardiol.* 1987;9:1205–13.
3. Seifried E, Tanswell P, Ellbrück D, et al. Pharmacokinetics and haemostatic status during consecutive infusions of recombinant tissue-type plasminogen activator in patients with acute myocardial infarction. *Thromb Haemostas.* 1989;61:497–501.
4. Tanswell P, Tebbe U, Neuhaus K-L, et al. Pharmacokinetics and fibrin specificity of Alteplase during accelerated infusions in acute myocardial infarction. *J Am Coll Cardiol.* 1992;19:1071–5.
5. De Wood MA, Spores J, Notske R, et al. Prevalence of total coronary occlusion during the early hours of transmural myocardial infarction. *New Engl J Med.* 1980;303:897–902.
6. Chesebro JH, Knatterud G, Roberts R, et al. Thrombolysis in myocardial infarction (TIMI) trial, Phase I: a comparison between intravenous tissue plasminogen activator and intravenous streptokinase. *Circulation.* 1987;76(1):142–54.
7. Guerci AD, Gerstenblith G, Brinker JA, et al. A randomized trial of intravenous tissue plasminogen activator for acute myocardial infarction with subsequent randomization to elective coronary angioplasty. *New Engl J Med.* 1987;317:1613-18.
8. O'Rourke M, Baron D, Keogh A, et al. Limitation of myocardial infarction by early infusion of recombinant tissue-plasminogen activator. *Circulation.* 1988;77:1311–15.
9. Wilcox RG, von der Lippe G, Olsson CG, et al. Trial of tissue plasminogen activator for mortality reduction in acute myocardial infarction: ASSET. *Lancet.* 1988;2:525–30.
10. Hampton JR, The University of Nottingham. Personal communication.
11. Van de Werf F, Arnold AER, et al. Effect of intravenous tissue-plasminogen activator on infarct size, left ventricular function and survival in patients with acute myocardial infarction. *Br Med J.* 1988;297:1374–9.
12. The National Institute of Neurological Disorders and Stroke t-PA Stroke Study Group. Tissue plasminogen activator for acute ischemic stroke. *New Engl J Med.* 1995;333:1581–7.
13. Goldhaber SZ, Kessler CM, Heit J, et al. A randomized controlled trial of recombinant tissue plasminogen activator versus urokinase in the treatment of acute pulmonary embolism. *Lancet.* 1988;2:293–8.
14. Aylward P, Wilcox R, Horgan J, White H, Granger C, Califf R, et al. for the GUSTO-I Investigators. Relation of increased arterial blood pressure to mortality and stroke in the context of contemporary thrombolytic therapy for acute myocardial infarction: a randomized trial. *Ann Int Med.* 1996;125:891–900.
15. Califf RM, Topol EJ, George BS, et al. Hemorrhagic complications associated with the use of intravenous tissue plasminogen activator in treatment of acute myocardial infarction. *Am J Med.* 1988;85:353–9.
16. Bovill EG, Terrin ML, Stump DC, et al. Hemorrhagic events during therapy with recombinant tissue-type plasminogen activator, heparin, and aspirin for acute myocardial infarction: results from the thrombolysis in myocardial infarction (TIMI), Phase II trial. *Ann Int Med.* 1991;115(4):256–65.
17. National Heart Foundation of Australia Coronary Thrombolysis Group. Coronary thrombolysis and myocardial infarction salvage by tissue plasminogen activator given up to 4 hours after onset of myocardial infarction. *Lancet.* 1988;1:203–7.
18. Gore JM, Sloan M, Price TR, et al. and the TIMI Investigators. Intracerebral hemorrhage, cerebral infarction, and subdural hematoma after acute myocardial infarction and thrombolytic therapy in the thrombolysis in myocardial infarction study. *Circulation.* 1991;83:448–59.
19. Hacke W, Kaste M, Fieschi C, Toni D, Lesaffre E, von Kummer R, et al. for the ECASS Study Group. Intravenous thrombolysis with recombinant tissue plasminogen activator for acute hemispheric stroke. The European Cooperative Acute Stroke Study (ECASS). *JAMA.* 1995;274:1017–25.

Activase®, Alteplase, recombinant 4800510

Manufactured by
GENENTECH, INC. Revised April 1999
1 DNA Way

South San Francisco, CA 94080-4990

Shown in Product Identification Guide, page 313

HERCEPTIN® ℞
Trastuzumab

WARNING

CARDIOMYOPATHY:

HERCEPTIN administration can result in the development of ventricular dysfunction and congestive heart failure. Left ventricular function should be evaluated in all patients prior to and during treatment with HERCEPTIN. Discontinuation of HERCEPTIN treatment should be strongly considered in patients who develop a clinically significant decrease in left ventricular function. The incidence and severity of cardiac dysfunction was particularly high in patients who received HERCEPTIN in combination with anthracyclines and cyclophosphamide. (See WARNINGS.)

Table 1
Phase III Clinical Efficacy in First-Line Treatment

	Combined Results		Paclitaxel subgroup		AC subgroup	
	HERCEPTIN + All Chemotherapy (n = 235)	All Chemotherapy (n = 234)	HERCEPTIN + Paclitaxel (n = 92)	Paclitaxel (n = 96)	HERCEPTIN + AC[a] (n = 143)	AC (n = 138)
Primary Endpoint						
Time to Progression[b,c]						
Median (months)	7.2	4.5	6.7	2.5	7.6	5.7
95% confidence interval	6.9, 8.2	4.3, 4.9	5.2, 9.9	2.0, 4.3	7.2, 9.1	4.6, 7.1
p-value (log rank)	<0.0001		<0.0001		0.002	
Secondary Endpoints						
Overall Response Rate[b]						
Rate (percent)	45	29	38	15	50	38
95% confidence interval	39, 51	23, 35	28, 48	8, 22	42, 58	30, 46
p-value ($_x$2-test)	<0.001		<0.001		0.10	
Duration of Response[b,c]						
Median (months)	8.3	5.8	8.3	4.3	8.4	6.4
25%, 75% quantile	5.5, 14.8	3.9, 8.5	5.1, 11.0	3.7, 7.4	5.8, 14.8	4.5, 8.5
1-Year Survival[c]						
Percent alive	79	68	73	61	83	73
95% confidence interval	74, 84	62, 74	66, 80	51, 71	77, 89	66, 82
p-value (Z-test)	<0.01		0.08		0.04	

[a]AC = anthracycline (doxorubicn or epirubicin) and cyclophosphamide.
[b]Assessed by an independent Response Evaluation Committee
[c]Kaplan-Meier Estimate

DESCRIPTION

HERCEPTIN (Trastuzumab) is a recombinant DNA-derived humanized monoclonal antibody that selectively binds with high affinity in a cell-based assay (Kd = 5 nM) to the extracellular domain of the human epidermal growth factor receptor 2 protein, HER2.[1,2] The antibody is an IgG_1 kappa that contains human framework regions with the complementarity-determining regions of a murine antibody (4D5) that binds to HER2.

The humanized antibody against HER2 is produced by a mammalian cell (Chinese Hamster Ovary) [CHO] suspension culture in a nutrient medium containing the antibiotic gentamicin. Gentamicin is not detectable in the final product.

HERCEPTIN is a sterile, white to pale yellow, preservative-free lyophilized powder for intravenous (IV) administration. The nominal content of each HERCEPTIN vial is 440 mg Trastuzumab, 9.9 mg L-histidine HCl, 6.4 mg L-histidine, 400 mg α,α-trehalose dihydrate, and 1.8 mg polysorbate 20, USP. Reconstitution with **only 20 mL of the supplied Bacteriostatic Water for Injection (BWFI)**, USP, containing 1.1% benzyl alcohol as a preservative, yields a multi-dose solution containing 21 mg/mL Trastuzumab, at a pH of approximately 6.

CLINICAL PHARMACOLOGY

General

The HER2 (or c-erbB2) proto-oncogene encodes a transmembrane receptor protein of 185 kDa, which is structurally related to the epidermal growth factor receptor.[1] HER2 protein overexpression is observed in 25%–30% of primary breast cancers. HER2 protein overexpression can be determined using an immunohistochemistry-based assessment of fixed tumor blocks.[3]

Trastuzumab has been shown, in both *in vitro* assays and in animals, to inhibit the proliferation of human tumor cells that overexpress HER2.[4–6]

Trastuzumab is a mediator of antibody-dependent cellular cytotoxicity (ADCC).[7,8] *In vitro*, HERCEPTIN-mediated ADCC has been shown to be preferentially exerted on HER2 overexpressing cancer cells compared with cancer cells that do not overexpress HER2.

Pharmacokinetics

The pharmacokinetics of Trastuzumab were studied in breast cancer patients with metastatic disease. Short duration intravenous infusions of 10 to 500 mg once weekly demonstrated dose-dependent pharmacokinetics. Mean half-life increased and clearance decreased with increasing dose level. The half-life averaged 1.7 and 12 days at the 10 and 500 mg dose levels, respectively. Trastuzumab's volume of distribution was approximately that of serum volume (44 mL/kg). At the highest weekly dose studied (500 mg), mean peak serum concentrations were 377 microgram/mL.

In studies using a loading dose of 4 mg/kg followed by a weekly maintenance dose of 2 mg/kg, a mean half-life of 5.8 days (range = 1 to 32 days) was observed. Between weeks 16 and 32, Trastuzumab serum concentrations reached a steady-state with a mean trough and peak concentrations of approximately 79 microgram/mL and 123 microgram/mL, respectively.

Detectable concentrations of the circulating extracellular domain of the HER2 receptor (shed antigen) are found in the serum of some patients with HER2 overexpressing tumors. Determination of shed antigen in baseline serum samples revealed that 64% (286/447) of patients had detectable shed antigen, which ranged as high as 1880 ng/mL (median = 11 ng/mL). Patients with higher baseline shed antigen levels were more likely to have lower serum trough concentrations. However, with weekly dosing, most patients with elevated shed antigen levels achieved target serum concentrations of Trastuzumab by week 6.

Data suggest that the disposition of Trastuzumab is not altered based on age or serum creatinine (up to 2.0 mg/dL). No formal interaction studies have been performed.

Mean serum trough concentrations of Trastuzumab, when administered in combination with paclitaxel, were consistently elevated approximately 1.5-fold as compared with serum concentrations of Trastuzumab used in combination with anthracycline plus cyclophosphamide. In primate studies, administration of Trastuzumab with paclitaxel resulted in a reduction in Trastuzumab clearance. Serum levels of Trastuzumab in combination with cisplatin, doxorubicin or epirubicin plus cyclophosphamide did not suggest any interactions; no formal drug interaction studies were performed.

CLINICAL STUDIES

The safety and efficacy of HERCEPTIN were studied in a randomized, controlled clinical trial in combination with chemotherapy (469 patients) and an open-label single agent clinical trial (222 patients). Both trials studied patients with metastatic breast cancer whose tumors overexpress the HER2 protein. Patients were eligible if they had 2+ or 3+ levels of overexpression (based on a 0–3+ scale) by immunohistochemical assessment of tumor tissue performed by a central testing lab.

A multicenter, randomized, controlled clinical trial was conducted in 469 patients with metastatic breast cancer who had not been previously treated with chemotherapy for metastatic disease. Patients were randomized to receive chemotherapy alone or in combination with HERCEPTIN given intravenously as a 4 mg/kg loading dose followed by weekly doses of HERCEPTIN at 2 mg/kg. For those who had received prior anthracycline therapy in the adjuvant setting, chemotherapy consisted of paclitaxel (175 mg/m^2 over 3 hours every 21 days for at least six cycles); for all other patients, chemotherapy consisted of anthracycline plus cyclophosphamide (AC: doxorubicin 60 mg/m^2 or epirubicin 75 mg/m^2 plus 600 mg/m^2 cyclophosphamide every 21 days for six cycles). Compared with patients in the AC subgroups (n = 281), patients in the paclitaxel subgroups (n = 188) were more likely to have had the following: poor prognostic factors (premenopausal status, estrogen or progesterone receptor negative tumors, positive lymph nodes), prior therapy (adjuvant chemotherapy, myeloablative chemotherapy, radiotherapy), and a shorter disease-free interval.

Compared with patients randomized to chemotherapy alone, the patients randomized to HERCEPTIN and chemotherapy experienced a significantly longer time to disease progression, a higher overall response rate (ORR), a longer median duration of response, and a higher one-year survival rate. (See Table 1.) These treatment effects were observed both in patients who received HERCEPTIN plus paclitaxel and in those who received HERCEPTIN plus AC, however the magnitude of the effects was greater in the paclitaxel subgroup. The degree of HER2 overexpression was a predictor of treatment effect. (See CLINICAL STUDIES: *HER2 protein overexpression.*)

[See table 1 above]

HERCEPTIN was studied as a single agent in a multicenter, open-label, single-arm clinical trial in patients with HER2 overexpressing metastatic breast cancer who had relapsed following one or two prior chemotherapy regimens for metastatic disease. Of 222 patients enrolled, 66% had received prior adjuvant chemotherapy, 68% had received two prior chemotherapy regimens for metastatic disease, and 25% had received prior myeloablative treatment with

Continued on next page

Herceptin—Cont.

hematopoietic rescue. Patients were treated with a loading dose of 4 mg/kg IV followed by weekly doses of HERCEPTIN at 2 mg/kg IV. The ORR (complete response + partial response), as determined by an independent Response Evaluation Committee, was 14%, with a 2% complete response rate and a 12% partial response rate. Complete responses were observed only in patients with disease limited to skin and lymph nodes. The degree of HER2 overexpression was a predictor of treatment effect. (See CLINICAL STUDIES: *HER2 protein overexpression.*)

HER2 protein overexpression

Relationship to Response: In the clinical studies described, patient eligibility was determined by testing tumor specimens for overexpression of HER2 protein. Specimens were tested with a research-use-only immunohistochemical assay (referred to as the Clinical Trial Assay, CTA) and scored as 0, 1+, 2+, or 3+ with 3+ indicating the strongest positivity. Only patients with 2+ or 3+ positive tumors were eligible (about 33% of those screened).

Data from both efficacy trials suggest that the beneficial treatment effects were largely limited to patients with the highest level of HER2 protein overexpression (3+). (See Table 2.)

[See table 2 at right]

Immunohistochemical Detection: In clinical trials, the Clinical Trial Assay (CTA) was used for immunohistochemical detection of HER2 protein overexpression. The DAKO HercepTest™, another immunohistochemical test for HER2 protein overexpression, has not been directly studied for its ability to predict HERCEPTIN treatment effect, but has been compared to the CTA on over 500 breast cancer histology specimens obtained from the National Cancer Institute Cooperative Breast Cancer Tissue Resource. Based upon these results and an expected incidence of 33% of 2+ or 3+ HER2 overexpression in tumors from women with metastatic breast cancer, one can estimate the correlation of the HercepTest™ results with CTA results. Of specimens testing 3+ (strongly positive) on the HercepTest™, 94% would be expected to test at least 2+ on the CTA (i.e., meeting the study entry criterion) including 82% which would be expected to test 3+ on the CTA (i.e., the reading most associated with clinical benefit). Of specimens testing 2+ (weakly positive) on the HercepTest™, only 34% would be expected to test at least 2+ on the CTA, including 14% which would be expected to test 3+ on the CTA.

INDICATIONS AND USAGE

HERCEPTIN as a single agent is indicated for the treatment of patients with metastatic breast cancer whose tumors overexpress the HER2 protein and who have received one or more chemotherapy regimens for their metastatic disease. HERCEPTIN in combination with paclitaxel is indicated for treatment of patients with metastatic breast cancer whose tumors overexpress the HER2 protein and who have not received chemotherapy for their metastatic disease. HERCEPTIN should only be used in patients whose tumors have HER2 protein overexpression. (See CLINICAL STUDIES: *HER2 protein overexpression* for information regarding HER2 protein testing and the relationship between the degree of overexpression and the treatment effect.)

CONTRAINDICATIONS

None known.

WARNINGS

Cardiotoxicity:

Signs and symptoms of cardiac dysfunction, such as dyspnea, increased cough, paroxysmal nocturnal dyspnea, peripheral edema, S_3 gallop, or reduced ejection fraction, have been observed in patients treated with HERCEPTIN. Congestive heart failure associated with HERCEPTIN therapy may be severe and has been associated with disabling cardiac failure, death, and mural thrombosis leading to stroke. The clinical status of patients in the trials who developed congestive heart failure were classified for severity using the New York Heart Association classification system (I–IV, where IV is the most severe level of cardiac failure). (See Table 3.)

[See table 3 above]

Candidates for treatment with HERCEPTIN should undergo thorough baseline cardiac assessment including history and physical exam and one or more of the following: EKG, echocardiogram, and MUGA scan. There are no data regarding the most appropriate method of evaluation for the identification of patients at risk for developing cardiotoxicity. Monitoring may not identify all patients who will develop cardiac dysfunction.

Extreme caution should be exercised in treating patients with pre-existing cardiac dysfunction.

Patients receiving HERCEPTIN should undergo frequent monitoring for deteriorating cardiac function.

The probability of cardiac dysfunction was highest in patients who received HERCEPTIN concurrently with anthracyclines. The data suggest that advanced age may increase the probability of cardiac dysfunction.

Pre-existing cardiac disease or prior cardiotoxic therapy (e.g., anthracycline or radiation therapy to the chest) may decrease the ability to tolerate HERCEPTIN therapy; however, the data are not adequate to evaluate the correlation between HERCEPTIN-induced cardiotoxicity and these factors.

Table 2
Treatment Effect versus Level of HER2 Expression

	Single-Arm Trial	Treatment Subgroups in Randomized Trial			
	HERCEPTIN	HERCEPTIN + Paclitaxel	Paclitaxel	HERCEPTIN + AC	AC
Overall Response Rate					
2+ overexpression	4% (2/50)	21% (5/24)	16% (3/19)	40% (14/35)	43% (18/42)
3+ overexpression	17% (29/172)	44% (30/68)	14% (11/77)	53% (57/108)	36% (35/96)
Median time to progression (months) (95% CI)					
2+ overexpression	N/A[a]	4.4 (2.2, 6.6)	3.2 (2.0, 5.6)	7.8 (6.4, 10.1)	7.1 (4.8, 9.8)
3+ overexpression	N/A[a]	7.1 (6.2, 12.0)	2.2 (1.8, 4.3)	7.3 (7.1, 9.2)	4.9 (4.5, 6.9)

[a]N/A = Not Assessed

Table 3
Incidence and Severity of Cardiac Dysfunction

	HERCEPTIN[a] alone n = 213	HERCEPTIN+ Paclitaxel[b] n = 91	Paclitaxel[b] n = 95	HERCEPTIN+ Anthracycline+ cyclophosphamide[b] n = 143	Anthracycline+ cyclophosphamide[b] n = 135
Any Cardiac Dysfunction	7%	11%	1%	28%	7%
Class III-IV	5%	4%	1%	19%	3%

[a] Open-label, single-agent Phase 2 study (94% received prior anthracyclines).
[b] Randomized Phase III study comparing chemotherapy plus HERCEPTIN to chemotherapy alone, where chemotherapy is either anthracycline/cyclophosphamide or paclitaxel

Discontinuation of HERCEPTIN therapy should be strongly considered in patients who develop clinically significant congestive heart failure. In the clinical trials, most patients with cardiac dysfunction responded to appropriate medical therapy often including discontinuation of HERCEPTIN. The safety of continuation or resumption of HERCEPTIN in patients who have previously experienced cardiac toxicity has not been studied. There are insufficient data regarding discontinuation of HERCEPTIN therapy in patients with asymptomatic decreases in ejection fraction; such patients should be closely monitored for evidence of clinical deterioration.

PRECAUTIONS

General: HERCEPTIN therapy should be used with caution in patients with known hypersensitivity to Trastuzumab, Chinese Hamster Ovary cell proteins, or any component of this product.

Drug Interactions: There have been no formal drug interaction studies performed with HERCEPTIN in humans. Administration of paclitaxel in combination with HERCEPTIN resulted in a two-fold decrease in HERCEPTIN clearance in a non-human primate study and in a 1.5-fold increase in HERCEPTIN serum levels in clinical studies (see Pharmacokinetics).

Benzyl Alcohol: For patients with a known hypersensitivity to benzyl alcohol (the preservative in Bacteriostatic Water for Injection) reconstitute HERCEPTIN with Sterile Water for Injection (SWFI), USP. DISCARD THE SWFI-RECONSTITUTED HERCEPTIN VIAL FOLLOWING A SINGLE USE.

Immunogenicity: Of 903 patients who have been evaluated, human anti-human antibody (HAHA) to Trastuzumab was detected in one patient, who had no allergic manifestations.

Carcinogenesis, Mutagenesis, Impairment of Fertility:

Carcinogenesis: HERCEPTIN has not been tested for its carcinogenic potential.

Mutagenesis: No evidence of mutagenic activity was observed in Ames tests using six different test strains of bacteria, with and without metabolic activation, at concentrations of up to 5000 μg/mL Trastuzumab. Human peripheral blood lymphocytes treated *in vitro* at concentrations of up to 5000 μg/plate Trastuzumab, with and without metabolic activation, revealed no evidence of mutagenic potential. In an *in vivo* mutagenic assay (the micronucleus assay), no evidence of chromosomal damage to mouse bone marrow cells was observed following bolus intravenous doses of up to 118 mg/kg Trastuzumab.

Impairment of Fertility: A fertility study has been conducted in female cynomolgus monkeys at doses up to 25 times the weekly human maintenance dose of 2 mg/kg HERCEPTIN and has revealed no evidence of impaired fertility.

Pregnancy Category B: Reproduction studies have been conducted in cynomolgus monkeys at doses up to 25 times the weekly human maintenance dose of 2 mg/kg HERCEPTIN and have revealed no evidence of impaired fertility or harm to the fetus. However, HER2 protein expression is high in many embryonic tissues including cardiac and neural tissues; in mutant mice lacking HER2, embryos died in early gestation.[9] Placental transfer of HERCEPTIN during the early (Days 20–50 of gestation) and late (Days 120–150 of gestation) fetal development period was observed in monkeys. There are, however, no adequate and well-controlled studies in pregnant women. Because animal reproduction studies are not always predictive of human response, this drug should be used during pregnancy only if clearly needed.

Nursing Mothers: A study conducted in lactating cynomolgus monkeys at doses 25 times the weekly human maintenance dose of 2 mg/kg HERCEPTIN demonstrated that Trastuzumab is secreted in the milk. The presence of Trastuzumab in the serum of infant monkeys was not associated with any adverse effects on their growth or development from birth to 3 months of age. It is not known whether HERCEPTIN is excreted in human milk. Because human IgG is excreted in human milk, and the potential for absorption and harm to the infant is unknown, women should be advised to discontinue nursing during HERCEPTIN therapy and for 6 months after the last dose of HERCEPTIN.

Pediatric Use: The safety and effectiveness of HERCEPTIN in pediatric patients have not been established.

Geriatric Use: HERCEPTIN has been administered to 133 patients who were 65 years of age or over. The risk of cardiac dysfunction may be increased in geriatric patients. The reported clinical experience is not adequate to determine whether older patients respond differently from younger patients.

ADVERSE REACTIONS

A total of 958 patients have received HERCEPTIN alone or in combination with chemotherapy. Data in Table 4 are based on the experience with the recommended dosing regimen for HERCEPTIN in the randomized controlled clinical trial in 234 patients who received HERCEPTIN in combination with chemotherapy and four open-label studies of HERCEPTIN as a single agent in 352 patients at doses of 10–500 mg administered weekly.

Cardiac Failure/Dysfunction: For a description of cardiac toxicities, see WARNINGS.

Anemia and Leukopenia: An increased incidence of anemia and leukopenia was observed in the treatment group receiving HERCEPTIN and chemotherapy, especially in the HERCEPTIN and AC subgroup, compared with the treatment group receiving chemotherapy alone. The majority of these cytopenic events were mild or moderate in intensity, reversible, and none resulted in discontinuation of therapy with HERCEPTIN.

Hematologic toxicity is infrequent following the administration of HERCEPTIN as a single agent, with an incidence of Grade III toxicities for WBC, platelets, hemoglobin all <1%. No grade IV toxicities were observed.

Diarrhea: Of patients treated with HERCEPTIN as a single agent, 25% experienced diarrhea. An increased incidence of diarrhea, primarily mild to moderate in severity, was observed in patients receiving HERCEPTIN in combination with chemotherapy.

Infection: An increased incidence of infections, primarily mild upper respiratory infections of minor clinical significance or catheter infections, was observed in patients receiving HERCEPTIN in combination with chemotherapy.

Infusion-Associated Symptoms: During the first infusion with HERCEPTIN, a symptom complex most commonly consisting of chills and/or fever was observed in about 40% of patients. The symptoms were usually mild to moderate in severity and were treated with acetaminophen, diphenhydramine, and meperidine (with or without reduction in the rate of HERCEPTIN infusion). HERCEPTIN discontinuation was infrequent. Other signs and/or symptoms may include nausea, vomiting, pain (in some cases at tumor sites), rigors, headache, dizziness, dyspnea, hypotension, rash, and asthenia. The symptoms occurred infrequently with subsequent HERCEPTIN infusions.

[See table 4 at right]

Other serious adverse events

The following other serious adverse events occurred in at least one of the 958 patients treated with HERCEPTIN:

Body as a Whole: cellulitis, anaphylactoid reaction, ascites, hydrocephalus, radiation injury, deafness, amblyopia

Cardiovascular: vascular thrombosis, pericardial effusion, heart arrest, hypotension, syncope, hemorrhage, shock arrhythmia

Digestive: hepatic failure, gastroenteritis, hematemesis, ileus, intestinal obstruction, colitis, esophageal ulcer, stomatitis, pancreatitis, hepatitis

Endocrine: hypothyroidism

Hematological: pancytopenia, acute leukemia, coagulation disorder, lymphangitis

Metabolic: hypercalcemia, hypomagnesemia, hyponatremia, hypoglycemia, growth retardation, weight loss

Musculoskeletal: pathological fractures, bone necrosis, myopathy

Nervous: convulsion, ataxia, confusion, manic reaction

Respiratory: apnea, pneumothorax, asthma, hypoxia, laryngitis

Skin: herpes zoster, skin ulceration

Urogenital: hydronephrosis, kidney failure, cervical cancer, hematuria, hemorrhagic cystitis, pyelonephritis

OVERDOSAGE

There is no experience with overdosage in human clinical trials. Single doses higher than 500 mg have not been tested.

DOSAGE AND ADMINISTRATION

Usual Dose

The recommended initial loading dose is 4 mg/kg Trastuzumab administered as a 90-minute infusion. The recommended weekly maintenance dose is 2 mg/kg Trastuzumab and can be administered as a 30-minute infusion if the initial loading dose was well tolerated. HERCEPTIN may be administered in an outpatient setting. HERCEPTIN is to be diluted in saline for IV infusion. **DO NOT ADMINISTER AS AN IV PUSH OR BOLUS** (see ADMINISTRATION).

Preparation for Administration

The diluent provided has been formulated to maintain the stability and sterility of HERCEPTIN for up to 28 days. Other diluents have not been shown to contain effective preservatives for HERCEPTIN. Each vial of HERCEPTIN should be reconstituted with **ONLY 20 mL of BWFI, USP, 1.1% benzyl alcohol preserved, as supplied,** to yield a multi-dose solution containing 21 mg/mL Trastuzumab. Use of all 30 mL of diluent results in a lower-than-intended dose of HERCEPTIN. THE REMAINDER (approximately 10 mL) OF THE DILUENT SHOULD BE DISCARDED. Immediately upon reconstitution with BWFI, the vial of HERCEPTIN must be labeled in the area marked "Do not use after:" with the future date that is 28 days from the date of reconstitution.

If the patient has known hypersensitivity to benzyl alcohol, HERCEPTIN must be reconstituted with Sterile Water for Injection (see PRECAUTIONS). HERCEPTIN WHICH HAS BEEN RECONSTITUTED WITH SWFI MUST BE USED IMMEDIATELY AND ANY UNUSED PORTION DISCARDED. USE OF OTHER RECONSTITUTION DILUENTS SHOULD BE AVOIDED.

Shaking the reconstituted HERCEPTIN or causing excessive foaming during the addition of diluent may result in problems with dissolution and the amount of HERCEPTIN that can be withdrawn from the vial.

Use appropriate aseptic technique when performing the following reconstitution steps:

a. Using a sterile syringe, slowly inject **20 mL** of the diluent into the vial containing the lyophilized cake of Trastuzumaub. The stream of diluent should be directed into the lyophilized cake.
b. Swirl the vial gently to aid reconstitution. Trastuzumaub may be sensitive to shear-induced stress, e.g., agitation or rapid expulsion from a syringe. **DO NOT SHAKE.**
c. Slight foaming of the product upon reconstitution is not unusual. Allow the vial to stand undisturbed for approximately 5 minutes. The solution should be essentially free of visible particulates, clear to slightly opalescent, and colorless to pale yellow.

Determine the number of mg of Trastuzumab needed, based on a loading dose of 4 mg Trastuzumab/kg body weight or a maintenance dose of 2 mg Trastuzumab/kg body weight. Calculate the volume of 21 mg/mL Trastuzumab solution and withdraw this amount from the vial and add it to an infusion bag containing 250 mL of 0.9% Sodium Chloride Injection, USP. **DEXTROSE (5%) SOLUTION SHOULD NOT BE USED.** Gently invert the bag to mix the solution. The reconstituted preparation results in a colorless to pale yellow transparent solution. Parenteral drug products should be inspected visually for particulates and discoloration prior to administration.

No incompatibilities between HERCEPTIN and polyvinylchloride or polyethylene bags have been observed.

Administration

Treatment may be administered in an outpatient setting by administration of a 4 mg/kg Trastuzumab loading dose by

Table 4

Adverse Events Occurring in ≥ 5% of Patients or at Increased Incidence in the HERCEPTIN Arm of the Randomized Study (Percent of Patients)

	Single Agent n = 352	HERCEPTIN + Paclitaxel n = 91	Paclitaxel Alone n = 95	HERCEPTIN + AC n = 143	AC Alone n = 135
Body as a Whole					
Pain	47	61	62	57	42
Asthenia	42	62	57	54	55
Fever	36	49	23	56	34
Chills	32	41	4	35	11
Headache	26	36	28	44	31
Abdominal pain	22	34	22	23	18
Back pain	22	34	30	27	15
Infection	20	47	27	47	31
Flu syndrome	10	12	5	12	6
Accidental injury	6	13	3	9	4
Allergic reaction	3	8	2	4	2
Cardiovascular					
Tachycardia	5	12	4	10	5
Congestive heart failure	7	11	1	28	7
Digestive					
Nausea	33	51	9	76	77
Diarrhea	25	45	29	45	26
Vomiting	23	37	28	53	49
Nausea and vomiting	8	14	11	18	9
Anorexia	14	24	16	31	26
Heme & Lymphatic					
Anemia	4	14	9	36	26
Leukopenia	3	24	17	52	34
Metabolic					
Peripheral edema	10	22	20	20	17
Edema	8	10	8	11	5
Musculoskeletal					
Bone pain	7	24	18	7	7
Arthralgia	6	37	21	8	9
Nervous					
Insomnia	14	25	13	29	15
Dizziness	13	22	24	24	18
Paresthesia	9	48	39	17	11
Depression	6	12	13	20	12
Peripheral neuritis	2	23	16	2	2
Neuropathy	1	13	5	4	4
Respiratory					
Cough increased	26	41	22	43	29
Dyspnea	22	27	26	42	25
Rhinitis	14	22	5	22	16
Pharyngitis	12	22	14	30	18
Sinusitis	9	21	7	13	6
Skin					
Rash	18	38	18	27	17
Herpes simplex	2	12	3	7	9
Acne	2	11	3	3	<1
Urogenital					
Urinary tract infection	5	18	14	13	7

intravenous (IV) infusion over 90 minutes. **DO NOT ADMINISTER AS AN IV PUSH OR BOLUS.** Patients should be observed for fever and chills or other infusion-associated symptoms (see ADVERSE REACTIONS). If prior infusions are well tolerated, subsequent weekly doses of 2 mg/kg Trastuzumab may be administered over 30 minutes.

HERCEPTIN should not be mixed or diluted with other drugs. HERCEPTIN infusions should not be administered or mixed with Dextrose solutions.

Stability and Storage

Vials of HERCEPTIN are stable at 2–8°C (36–46°F) prior to reconstitution. Do not use beyond the expiration date stamped on the vial. A vial of HERCEPTIN reconstituted with BWFI, as supplied, is stable for 28 days after reconstitution when stored refrigerated at 2–8°C (36–46°F), and the solution is preserved for multiple use. Discard any remaining multi-dose reconstituted solution after 28 days. If unpreserved SWFI (not supplied) is used, the reconstituted HERCEPTIN solution should be used immediately and any unused portion must be discarded. DO NOT FREEZE HERCEPTIN THAT HAS BEEN RECONSTITUTED.

The solution of HERCEPTIN for infusion diluted in polyvinylchloride or polyethylene bags containing 0.9% Sodium Chloride for Injection, USP, may be stored at 2–8°C (36–46°F) for up to 24 hours prior to use. Diluted HERCEPTIN has been shown to be stable for up to 24 hours at room temperature (2–25°C). However, since diluted HERCEPTIN contains no effective preservative, the reconstituted and diluted solution should be stored refrigerated (2–8°C).

HOW SUPPLIED

HERCEPTIN is supplied as a lyophilized, sterile powder nominally containing 440 mg Trastuzumab per vial under vacuum.

Each carton contains one vial of 440 mg HERCEPTIN (Trastuzumab) and one 30 mL vial of Bacteriostatic Water for Injection, USP, 1.1% benzyl alcohol. NDC 50242-134-60.

REFERENCES

1. Coussens L, Yang-Feng TL, Liao Y-C, Chen E, Gray A, McGrath J, et al. Tyrosine kinase receptor with extensive homology to EGF receptor shares chromosomal location with *neu* oncogene. Science 1985; 230:1132–9
2. Slamon DJ, Godolphin W, Jones LA, Holt JA, Wong SG, Keith DE, et al. Studies of the HER2/*neu* proto-oncogene in human breast and ovarian cancer. Science 1989; 244: 707–12.
3. Press MF, Pike MC, Chazin VR, Hung G, Udove JA, Markowicz M, et al. Her2/*neu* expression in node-negative breast cancer: direct tissue quantitation by computerized image analysis and association of overexpression with increased risk of recurrent disease. Cancer Res 1993; 53:4960–70.
4. Hudziak RM, Lewis GD, Winget M, Fendly BM, Shepard HM, Ullrich A. p185^{HER2} monoclonal antibody has antiproliferative effects *in vitro* and sensitizes human breast tumor cells to tumor necrosis factor. Mol Cell Biol 1989; 9:1165–72.
5. Lewis GD, Figari I, Fendly B, Wong WL, Carter P, Gorman C, et al. Differential responses of human tumor cell lines to anti-p185HER2 monoclonal antibodies. Cancer Immunol Immunother 1993; 37:255–63.
6. Baselga J, Norton L, Albanell J, Kim Y-M, Mendelsohn J. Recombinant humanized anti-HER2 antibody (Herceptin™) enhances the antitumor activity of paclitaxel and doxorubicin against HER2/*neu* overexpressing human breast cancer xenografts. Cancer Res. 1998; 58: 2825–2831.
7. Hotaling TE, Reitz B, Wolfgang-Kimball D, Bauer K, Fox JA. The humanized anti-HER2 antibody rhuMAb HER2 mediates antibody dependent cell-mediated cytotoxicity via fcγR III [abstract]. Proc Annu Meet Am Assoc Cancer Res 1996; 37:471.
8. Pegram MD, Baly D, Wirth C, Gilkerson E, Slamon DJ, Sliwkowski MX, et al. Antibody dependent cell-mediated cytotoxicity in breast cancer patients in Phase III clinical trials of a humanized anti-HER2 antibody [abstract]. Proc Am Assoc Cancer Res 1997; 38:602.
9. Lee, KS. Requirement for neuregulin receptor, erbB2, in neural and cardiac development. Nature 1995; 379: 394–96.

HERCEPTIN® (Trastuzumab)

Manufactured by: 4817401
Genentech, Inc. Revised January 2000

Continued on next page

Herceptin—Cont.

1 DNA Way
South San Francisco, CA 94080-4990

Shown in Product Identification Guide, page 313

NUTROPIN® ℞
[somatropin (rDNA origin) for injection]

DESCRIPTION

Nutropin® [somatropin (rDNA origin) for injection] is a human growth hormone (hGH) produced by recombinant DNA technology. Nutropin has 191 amino acid residues and a molecular weight of 22,125 daltons. The amino acid sequence of the product is identical to that of pituitary-derived human growth hormone. The protein is synthesized by a specific laboratory strain of *E. coli* as a precursor consisting of the rhGH molecule preceded by the secretion signal from an *E. coli* protein. This precursor is directed to the plasma membrane of the cell. The signal sequence is removed and the native protein is secreted into the periplasm so that the protein is folded appropriately as it is synthesized.

Nutropin is a highly purified preparation. Biological potency is determined using a cell proliferation bioassay.

Nutropin is a sterile, white, lyophilized powder intended for subcutaneous administration after reconstitution with Bacteriostatic Water for Injection, USP (benzyl alcohol preserved). The reconstituted product is nearly isotonic at a concentration of 5 mg/mL growth hormone (GH) and has a pH of approximately 7.4.

Each 5 mg Nutropin vial contains 5 mg (approximately 15 IU) somatropin, lyophilized with 45 mg mannitol, 1.7 mg sodium phosphates (0.4 mg sodium phosphate monobasic and 1.3 mg sodium phosphate dibasic), and 1.7 mg glycine.

Each 10 mg Nutropin vial contains 10 mg (approximately 30 IU) somatropin, lyophilized with 90 mg mannitol, 3.4 mg sodium phosphates (0.8 mg sodium phosphate monobasic and 2.6 mg sodium phosphate dibasic), and 3.4 mg glycine.

Bacteriostatic Water for Injection, USP, is sterile water containing 0.9 percent benzyl alcohol per mL as an antimicrobial preservative packaged in a multidose vial. The diluent pH is 4.5–7.0.

CLINICAL PHARMACOLOGY

General

In vitro and in vivo preclinical and clinical testing have demonstrated that Nutropin is therapeutically equivalent to pituitary-derived human GH (hGH). Pediatric patients who lack adequate endogenous GH secretion, patients with chronic renal insufficiency, and patients with Turner syndrome that were treated with Nutropin resulted in an increase in growth rate and an increase in insulin-like growth factor-I (IGF-I) levels similar to that seen with pituitary-derived hGH.

Actions that have been demonstrated for Nutropin, somatrem, and/or pituitary-derived hGH include:

A. Tissue Growth—1) Skeletal Growth: GH stimulates skeletal growth in pediatric patients with growth failure due to a lack of adequate secretion of endogenous GH or secondary to chronic renal insufficiency and in patients with Turner syndrome. Skeletal growth is accomplished at the epiphyseal plates at the ends of a growing bone. Growth and metabolism of epiphyseal plate cells are directly stimulated by GH and one of its mediators, IGF-I. Serum levels of IGF-I are low in children and adolescents who are GH deficient, but increase during treatment with GH. In pediatric patients, new bone is formed at the epiphyses in response to GH and IGF-I. This results in linear growth until these growth plates fuse at the end of puberty. 2) Cell Growth: Treatment with hGH results in an increase in both the number and the size of skeletal muscle cells. 3) Organ Growth: GH influences the size of internal organs, including kidneys, and increases red cell mass. Treatment of hypophysectomized or genetic dwarf rats with GH results in organ growth that is proportional to the overall body growth. In normal rats subjected to nephrectomy-induced uremia, GH promoted skeletal and body growth.

B. Protein Metabolism—Linear growth is facilitated in part by GH-stimulated protein synthesis. This is reflected by nitrogen retention as demonstrated by a decline in urinary nitrogen excretion and blood urea nitrogen during GH therapy.

C. Carbohydrate Metabolism—GH is a modulator of carbohydrate metabolism. For example, patients with inadequate secretion of GH sometimes experience fasting hypoglycemia that is improved by treatment with GH. GH therapy may decrease insulin sensitivity. Untreated patients with chronic renal insufficiency and Turner syndrome have an increased incidence of glucose intolerance. Administration of hGH to adults or children resulted in increases in serum fasting and postprandial insulin levels, more commonly in overweight or obese individuals. In addition, mean fasting and postprandial glucose and hemoglobin A_{Ic} levels remained in the normal range.

D. Lipid Metabolism—In GH-deficient patients, administration of GH resulted in lipid mobilization, reduction in body fat stores, increased plasma fatty acids, and decreased plasma cholesterol levels.

Last Measured Height* by Sex and Nutropin Dose

	Age (yr) Mean±SD (range)	Last Measured Height* (cm) 0.3 mg/kg/wk Mean±SD	0.7 mg/kg/wk Mean±SD	Height Difference Between Groups (cm) Mean±SE
Male	17.2±1.3 (13.6 to 19.4)	170.9±7.9 (n=42)	174.5±7.9 (n=41)	3.6±1.7
Female	15.8±1.8 (11.9 to 19.3)	154.7±6.3 (n=7)	157.6±6.3 (n=7)	2.9±3.4

*Adjusted for baseline height

E. Mineral Metabolism—The retention of total body potassium in response to GH administration apparently results from cellular growth. Serum levels of inorganic phosphorus may increase slightly in patients with inadequate secretion of endogenous GH, chronic renal insufficiency, or patients with Turner syndrome during GH therapy due to metabolic activity associated with bone growth as well as increased tubular reabsorption of phosphate by the kidney. Serum calcium is not significantly altered in these patients. Sodium retention also occurs. Adults with childhood-onset GH deficiency show low bone mineral density (BMD). GH therapy results in increases in serum alkaline phosphatase. (See PRECAUTIONS: Laboratory Tests.)

F. Connective Tissue Metabolism—GH stimulates the synthesis of chondroitin sulfate and collagen as well as the urinary excretion of hydroxyproline.

Pharmacokinetics

Subcutaneous Absorption—The absolute bioavailability of recombinant human growth hormone (rhGH) after subcutaneous administration in healthy adult males has been determined to be 81±20%. The mean terminal $t_{1/2}$ after subcutaneous administration is significantly longer than that seen after intravenous administration (2.1±0.43 hr vs. 19.5±3.1 min) indicating that the subcutaneous absorption of the compound is slow and rate-limiting.

Distribution—Animal studies with rhGH showed that GH localizes to highly perfused organs, particularly the liver and kidney. The volume of distribution at steady state for rhGH in healthy adult males is about 50 mL/kg body weight, approximating the serum volume.

Metabolism—Both the liver and kidney have been shown to be important metabolizing organs for GH. Animal studies suggest that the kidney is the dominant organ of clearance. GH is filtered at the glomerulus and reabsorbed in the proximal tubules. It is then cleaved within renal cells into its constituent amino acids, which return to the systemic circulation.

Elimination—The mean terminal $t_{1/2}$ after intravenous administration of rhGH in healthy adult males is estimated to be 19.5±3.1 minutes. Clearance of rhGH after intravenous administration in healthy adults and children is reported to be in the range of 116–174 mL/hr/kg.

Bioequivalence of Formulations—Nutropin has been determined to be bioequivalent to Nutropin AQ® [somatropin (rDNA origin) injection] based on the statistical evaluation of AUC and C_{max}.

Special Populations

Pediatric—Available literature data suggest that rhGH clearances are similar in adults and children.

Gender—No data are available for exogenously administered rhGH. Available data for methionyl recombinant GH, pituitary-derived GH, and endogenous GH suggest no consistent gender-based differences in GH clearance.

Geriatrics—Limited published data suggest that the plasma clearance and average steady-state plasma concentration of rhGH may not be different between young and elderly patients.

Race—Reported values for half-lives for endogenous GH in normal adult black males are not different from observed values for normal adult white males. No data for other races are available.

Growth Hormone Deficiency (GHD)—Reported values for clearance of rhGH in adults and children with GHD range 138–245 mL/hr/kg and are similar to those observed in healthy adults and children. Mean terminal $t_{1/2}$ values following intravenous and subcutaneous administration in adult and pediatric GHD patients are also similar to those observed in healthy adult males.

Renal Insufficiency—Children and adults with chronic renal failure (CRF) and end-stage renal disease (ESRD) tend to have decreased clearance compared to normals. Endogenous GH production may also increase in some individuals with ESRD. However, no rhGH accumulation has been reported in children with CRF or ESRD dosed with current regimens.

Turner Syndrome—No pharmacokinetic data are available for exogenously administered rhGH. However, reported half-lives, absorption, and elimination rates for endogenous GH in this population are similar to the ranges observed for normal subjects and GHD populations.

Hepatic Insufficiency—A reduction in rhGH clearance has been noted in patients with severe liver dysfunction. The clinical significance of this decrease is unknown.

Summary of Nutropin Pharmacokinetic Parameters in Healthy Adult Males
0.1 mg (approximately 0.3 IU[a])/kg SC

	C_{max} (μg/L)	T_{max} (hr)	$t_{1/2}$ (hr)	$AUC_{0-\infty}$ (μg•hr/L)	CL/F_{SC} (mL/[hr•kg])
MEAN[b]	67.2	6.2	2.1	643	158
CV%	29	37	20	12	12

Abbreviations: C_{max}=maximum concentration; $t_{1/2}$ =half life; $AUC_{0-\infty}$=area under the curve; CL/F_{SC}=systemic clearance; F_{SC}=subcutaneous bioavailability (not determined); CV%=coefficient of variation in %; SC=subcutaneous

[a]Based on current International Standard of 3 IU=1 mg
[b]n=36

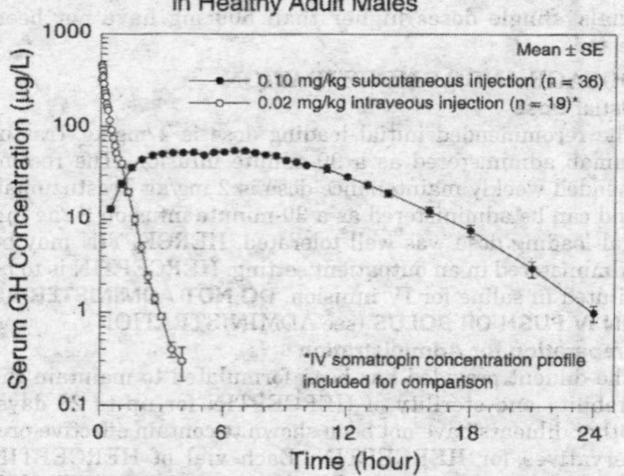

Efficacy Studies

Growth Hormone Deficiency (GHD) in Pubertal Patients

One open-label, multicenter, randomized clinical trial of two dosages of Nutropin was performed in pubertal patients with GHD. Ninety-seven patients (mean age 13.9 years, 83 male, 14 female) currently being treated with approximately 0.3 mg/kg/wk of GH were randomized to 0.3 mg/kg/wk or 0.7 mg/kg/wk Nutropin doses. All patients were already in puberty (Tanner stage ≥2) and had bone ages ≤14 yr in males or ≤12 yr in females. Mean baseline height standard deviation (SD) score was −1.3.

The mean last measured height in all 97 patients after a mean duration of 2.7±1.2 years, by analysis of covariance (ANCOVA) adjusting for baseline height, is shown below.

[See table at top of page]

The mean height SD score at last measured height (n=97) was −0.7±1.0 in the 0.3 mg/kg/wk group and −0.1±1.2 in the 0.7 mg/kg/wk group. For patients completing 3.5 or more years (mean 4.1 years) of Nutropin treatment (15/49 patients in the 0.3 mg/kg/wk group and 16/48 patients in the 0.7 mg/kg/wk group), the mean last measured height was 166.1±8.0 cm in the 0.3 mg/kg/wk group and 171.8±7.1 cm in the 0.7 mg/kg/wk group, adjusting for baseline height and sex.

The mean change in bone age was approximately one year for each year in the study in both dose groups. Patients with baseline height SD scores above −1.0 were able to attain normal adult heights with the 0.3 mg/kg/wk dose of Nutropin (mean height SD score at near-adult height = −0.1, n=15).

Thirty-one patients had bone mineral density (BMD) determined by dual energy x-ray absorptiometry (DEXA) scans at study conclusion. The two dose groups did not differ significantly in mean SD score for total body BMD (−0.9±1.9 in the 0.3 mg/kg/wk group vs. −0.8±1.2 in the 0.7 mg/kg/wk group, n=20) or lumbar spine BMD (−1.0±1.0 in the 0.3 mg/kg/wk group vs. −0.2±1.7 in the 0.7 mg/kg/wk group, n=21).

Over a mean duration of 2.7 years, patients in the 0.7 mg/kg/wk group were more likely to have IGF-I values above the normal range than patients in the 0.3 mg/kg/wk group (27.7% vs. 9.0% of IGF-I measurements for individual patients). The clinical significance of elevated IGF-I values is unknown.

Effects of Nutropin on Growth Failure Due to Chronic Renal Insufficiency (CRI)

Two multicenter, randomized, controlled clinical trials were conducted to determine whether treatment with Nutropin prior to renal transplantation in patients with chronic renal insufficiency could improve their growth rates and height deficits. One study was a double-blind, placebo-controlled trial and the other was an open-label, randomized trial. The dose of Nutropin in both controlled studies was 0.05 mg/kg/day (0.35 mg/kg/wk) administered daily by subcutaneous injection. Combining the data from those patients completing two years in the two controlled studies results in 62 patients treated with Nutropin and 28 patients in the control groups (either placebo-treated or untreated). The mean first year growth rate was 10.8 cm/yr for Nutropin-treated patients, compared with a mean growth rate of 6.5 cm/yr for placebo/untreated controls ($p<0.00005$). The mean second year growth rate was 7.8 cm/yr for the Nutropin-treated group, compared with 5.5 cm/yr for controls ($p<0.00005$). There was a significant increase in mean height standard deviation (SD) score in the Nutropin group (–2.9 at baseline to –1.5 at Month 24, n=62) but no significant change in the controls (–2.8 at baseline to –2.9 at Month 24, n=28). The mean third year growth rate of 7.6 cm/yr in the Nutropin-treated patients (n=27) suggests that Nutropin stimulates growth beyond two years. However, there are no control data for the third year because control patients crossed over to Nutropin treatment after two years of participation. The gains in height were accompanied by appropriate advancement of skeletal age. These data demonstrate that Nutropin therapy improves growth rate and corrects the acquired height deficit associated with chronic renal insufficiency. Currently there are insufficient data regarding the benefit of treatment beyond three years. Although predicted final height was improved during Nutropin therapy, the effect of Nutropin on final adult height remains to be determined.

Post-Transplant Growth

The North American Pediatric Renal Transplant Cooperative Study (NAPRTCS) has reported data for growth post-transplant in children who did not receive GH. The average change in height SD score during the initial two years post-transplant was 0.18 (n=300, J Pediatr. 1993;122:397–402). Controlled studies of GH treatment for the short stature associated with CRI were not designed to compare the growth of treated or untreated patients after they received renal transplants. However, growth data are available from a small number of patients who have been followed for at least 11 months. Of the 7 control patients, 4 increased their height SD score and 3 had either no significant change or a decrease in height SD score. The 13 patients treated with Nutropin prior to transplant had either no significant change or an increase in height SD score after transplantation, indicating that the individual gains achieved with GH therapy prior to transplant were maintained after transplantation. The differences in the height deficit narrowed between the treated and untreated groups in the post-transplant period.

Turner Syndrome

One long-term, randomized, open-label, multicenter, concurrently controlled study, two long-term, open-label, multicenter, historically controlled studies and one long-term, randomized, dose-response study were conducted to evaluate the efficacy of GH for the treatment of girls with short stature due to Turner syndrome.

In the randomized study GDCT, comparing GH-treated patients to a concurrent control group who received no GH, the GH-treated patients who received a dose of 0.3 mg/kg/week given 6 times per week from a mean age of 11.7 years for a mean duration of 4.7 years attained a mean near final height of 146.0 cm (n=27) as compared to the control group who attained a near final height of 142.1 cm (n=19). By analysis of covariance, the effect of GH therapy was a mean height increase of 5.4 cm (p=0.001).

In two of the studies (85-023 and 85-044), the effect of long-term GH treatment (0.375 mg/kg/week given either 3 times per week or daily) on adult height was determined by comparing adult heights in the treated patients with those of age-matched historical controls with Turner syndrome who never received any growth-promoting therapy. In Study 85-023, estrogen treatment was delayed until patients were at least age 14. GH therapy resulted in a mean adult height gain of 7.4 cm (mean duration of GH therapy of 7.6 years) vs. matched historical controls by analysis of covariance.

In Study 85-044, patients treated with early GH therapy were randomized to receive estrogen-replacement therapy (conjugated estrogens, 0.3 mg escalating to 0.625 mg daily) at either age 12 or 15 years. Compared with matched historical controls, early GH therapy (mean duration of GH therapy 5.6 years) combined with estrogen replacement at age 12 years resulted in an adult height gain of 5.9 cm (n=26), whereas girls who initiated estrogen at age 15 years (mean duration of GH therapy 6.1 years) had a mean adult height gain of 8.3 cm (n=29). Patients who initiated GH therapy after age 11 (mean age 12.7 years; mean duration of GH therapy 3.8 years) had a mean adult height gain of 5.0 cm (n=51).

Thus, in both studies, 85-023 and 85-044, the greatest improvement in adult height was observed in patients who received early GH treatment and estrogen after age 14 years.

In a randomized, blinded, dose-response study, GDCI, patients were treated from a mean age of 11.1 years for a mean duration of 5.3 years with a weekly dose of either 0.27 mg/kg or 0.36 mg/kg administered 3 or 6 times weekly. The mean near final height of patients receiving growth hormone was 148.7 cm (n=31). This represents a mean gain in adult height of approximately 5 cm compared with previous observations of untreated Turner syndrome girls.

In these studies, Turner syndrome patients (n=181) treated to final adult height achieved statistically significant average estimated adult height gains ranging 5.0–8.3 cm.

[See table above]

Study/Group	Study Design[a]	N at Adult Height	GH Age (yr)	Estrogen Age (yr)	GH Duration (yr)	Adult Height Gain (cm)[b]
GDCT	RCT	27	11.7	13	4.7	5.4
85-023	MHT	17	9.1	15.2	7.6	7.4
85-044: A*	MHT	29	9.4	15.0	6.1	8.3
B*		26	9.6	12.3	5.6	5.9
C*		51	12.7	13.7	3.8	5.0
GDCI	RDT	31	11.1	8–13.5	5.3	~5[c]

[a] RCT: randomized controlled trial; MHT: matched historical controlled trial; RDT: randomized dose-response trial.
[b] Analysis of covariance vs. controls
[c] Compared with historical data
*A: GH age <11 yr, estrogen age 15 yr
B: GH age <11 yr, estrogen age 12 yr
C: GH age >11 yr, estrogen at Month 12

Adult Growth Hormone Deficiency (GHD)

Two multicenter, double-blind, placebo-controlled clinical trials were conducted using Nutropin in GH-deficient adults. One study was conducted in subjects with adult-onset GHD, mean age 48.3 years, n=166, at doses of 0.0125 or 0.00625 mg/kg/day; doses of 0.025 mg/kg/day were not tolerated in these subjects. A second study was conducted in previously treated subjects with childhood-onset GHD, mean age 23.8 years, n=64, at randomly assigned doses of 0.025 or 0.0125 mg/kg/day. The studies were designed to assess the effects of replacement therapy with GH on body composition.

Significant changes from baseline to Month 12 of treatment in body composition (i.e., total body % fat mass, trunk % fat mass, and total body % lean mass by DEXA scan) were seen in all Nutropin groups in both studies ($p<0.0001$ for change from baseline and vs. placebo), whereas no statistically significant changes were seen in either of the placebo groups. In the adult-onset study, the Nutropin group improved mean total body fat from 35.0% to 31.5%, mean trunk fat from 33.9% to 29.5%, and mean lean body mass from 62.2% to 65.7%, whereas the placebo group had mean changes of 0.2% or less (p=not significant). Due to the possible effect of GH-induced fluid retention on DEXA measurements of lean body mass, DEXA scans were repeated approximately 3 weeks after completion of therapy; mean % lean body mass in the Nutropin group was 65.0%, a change of 2.8% from baseline, compared with a change of 0.4% in the placebo group ($p<0.0001$ between groups).

In the childhood-onset study, the high-dose Nutropin group improved mean total body fat from 38.4% to 32.1%, mean trunk fat from 36.7% to 29.0%, and mean lean body mass from 59.1% to 65.5%; the low-dose Nutropin group improved mean total body fat from 37.1% to 31.3%, mean trunk fat from 37.9% to 30.6%, and mean lean body mass from 60.0% to 66.0%; the placebo group had mean changes of 0.6% or less (p=not significant).

[See table at bottom of next page]

In the adult-onset study, significant decreases from baseline to Month 12 in LDL cholesterol and LDL:HDL ratio were seen in the Nutropin group compared to the placebo group, $p<0.02$; there were no statistically significant between-group differences in change from baseline to Month 12 in total cholesterol, HDL cholesterol, or triglycerides. In the childhood-onset study, significant decreases from baseline to Month 12 in total cholesterol, LDL cholesterol, and LDL:HDL ratio were seen in the high-dose Nutropin group only, compared to the placebo group, $p<0.05$. There were no statistically significant between-group differences in HDL cholesterol or triglycerides from baseline to Month 12.

In the childhood-onset study, 55% of the patients had decreased spine bone mineral density (BMD) (z-score <-1) at baseline. The administration of Nutropin (n=16) (0.025 mg/kg/day) for two years resulted in increased spine BMD from baseline when compared to placebo (n=13) (4.6% vs. 1.0%, respectively, $p<0.03$); a transient decrease in spine BMD was seen at six months in the Nutropin-treated patients. Thirty-five percent of subjects treated with this dose had supraphysiological levels of IGF-I at some point during the study, which may carry unknown risks. No significant improvement in total body BMD was found when compared to placebo. A lower GH dose (0.0125 mg/kg/day) did not show significant increments in either of these bone parameters when compared to placebo. No statistically significant effects on BMD were seen in the adult-onset study where patients received GH (0.0125 mg/kg/day) for one year.

Muscle strength, physical endurance, and quality of life measurements were not markedly abnormal at baseline, and no statistically significant effects of Nutropin therapy were observed in the two studies.

INDICATIONS AND USAGE

Pediatric Patients

Nutropin® [somatropin (rDNA origin) for injection] is indicated for the long-term treatment of growth failure due to a lack of adequate endogenous GH secretion.

Nutropin® [somatropin (rDNA origin) for injection] is also indicated for the treatment of growth failure associated with chronic renal insufficiency up to the time of renal transplantation. Nutropin therapy should be used in conjunction with optimal management of chronic renal insufficiency.

Nutropin® [somatropin (rDNA origin) for injection] is also indicated for the long-term treatment of short stature associated with Turner syndrome.

Adult Patients

Nutropin® [somatropin (rDNA origin) for injection] is indicated for the replacement of endogenous GH in patients with adult GH deficiency who meet both of the following two criteria:

1. Biochemical diagnosis of adult GH deficiency by means of a subnormal response to a standard growth hormone stimulation test (peak GH≤5 μg/L), and
2. Adult-onset: Patients who have adult GH deficiency either alone or with multiple hormone deficiencies (hypopituitarism) as a result of pituitary disease, hypothalamic disease, surgery, radiation therapy, or trauma; or

Childhood-onset: Patients who were GH deficient during childhood, confirmed as an adult before replacement therapy with Nutropin is started.

CONTRAINDICATIONS

Growth hormone should not be initiated to treat patients with acute critical illness due to complications following open heart or abdominal surgery, multiple accidental trauma or to patients having acute respiratory failure. Two placebo-controlled clinical trials in non-growth hormone–deficient adult patients (n=522) with these conditions revealed a significant increase in mortality (41.9% vs. 19.3%) among somatropin-treated patients (doses 5.3–8 mg/day) compared to those receiving placebo (see WARNINGS).

Nutropin should not be used for growth promotion in pediatric patients with closed epiphyses.

Nutropin should not be used in patients with active neoplasia. GH therapy should be discontinued if evidence of neoplasia develops.

Nutropin, when reconstituted with Bacteriostatic Water for Injection, USP (benzyl alcohol preserved), should not be used in patients with a known sensitivity to benzyl alcohol.

WARNINGS

See CONTRAINDICATIONS for information on increased mortality in patients with acute critical illnesses in intensive care units due to complications following open heart or abdominal surgery, multiple accidental trauma or with acute respiratory failure. The safety of continuing growth hormone treatment in patients receiving replacement doses for approved indications who concurrently develop these illnesses has not been established. Therefore, the potential benefit of treatment continuation with growth hormone in patients having acute critical illnesses should be weighed against the potential risk.

Benzyl alcohol as a preservative in Bacteriostatic Water for Injection, USP, has been associated with toxicity in newborns. When administering Nutropin to newborns, reconstitute with Sterile Water for Injection, USP. USE ONLY ONE DOSE PER NUTROPIN VIAL AND DISCARD THE UNUSED PORTION.

PRECAUTIONS

General: Nutropin should be prescribed by physicians experienced in the diagnosis and management of patients with GH deficiency, Turner syndrome, or chronic renal insufficiency. No studies have been completed of Nutropin therapy in patients who have received renal transplants. Currently, treatment of patients with functioning renal allografts is not indicated.

Experience with prolonged rhGH treatment in adults is limited.

Geriatric Usage: Clinical studies of Nutropin did not include sufficient numbers of subjects aged 65 and over to determine whether they respond differently from younger subjects. Other reported clinical experience has not identified differences in responses between the elderly and younger patients. In general, dose selection for an elderly patient should be cautious, usually starting at the low end of the dosing range, reflecting the greater frequency of decreased hepatic, renal, or cardiac function, and of concomitant disease or other drug therapy.

Patients with epiphyseal closure who were treated with GH-replacement therapy in childhood should be re-evaluated according to the criteria in the INDICATIONS AND USAGE SECTION before continuation of GH therapy at the reduced dose level recommended for GH-deficient adults.

Because Nutropin may reduce insulin sensitivity, patients should be monitored for evidence of glucose intolerance.

For patients with diabetes mellitus, the insulin dose may require adjustment when GH therapy is instituted. Because GH may reduce insulin sensitivity, particularly in obese individuals, patients should be observed for evidence of glucose intolerance. Patients with diabetes or glucose intolerance should be monitored closely during GH therapy.

Continued on next page

Nutropin—Cont.

Nutropin therapy in adults with GHD of adult onset was associated with an increase of median fasting insulin in the Nutropin 0.0125 mg/kg/day group from 9.0 µU/mL at baseline to 13.0 µU/mL at Month 12 with a return to the baseline median after a 3-week post-washout period off GH therapy. In the placebo group there was no change from 8.0 µU/mL at baseline to Month 12, and after the post-washout the median was 9.0 µU/mL. The between-treatment-groups difference in change from baseline to Month 12 was significant, $p<0.0001$. In childhood-onset subjects, there was a change of median fasting insulin in the Nutropin 0.025 mg/kg/day group from 11.0 µU/mL at baseline to 20.0 µU/mL at Month 12, in the Nutropin 0.0125 mg/kg/day group from 8.5 µU/mL to 11.0 µU/mL, and in the placebo group from 7.0 µU/mL to 8.0 µU/mL. The between-treatment-groups difference for these changes was significant, p=0.0007.

In subjects with adult-onset GHD, there was no between-treatment-group difference in changes from baseline to Month 12 in mean HbA_{1c}, p=0.08. In childhood-onset, mean HbA_{1c} increased in the Nutropin 0.025 mg/kg/day group from 5.2% at baseline to 5.5% at Month 12, and did not change in the Nutropin 0.0125 mg/kg/day group from 5.1% at baseline or in the placebo group from 5.3% at baseline. The between-treatment-groups difference was significant, p=0.009.

Patients with a history of an intracranial lesion should be examined frequently for progression or recurrence of the lesion. In pediatric patients, clinical literature has demonstrated no relationship between GH-replacement therapy and CNS tumor recurrence or new extracranial tumors. In adults, it is unknown whether there is any relationship between GH-replacement therapy and CNS tumor recurrence.

Patients with growth failure secondary to chronic renal insufficiency should be examined periodically for evidence of progression of renal osteodystrophy. Slipped capital femoral epiphysis or avascular necrosis of the femoral head may be seen in children with advanced renal osteodystrophy, and it is uncertain whether these problems are affected by GH therapy. X-rays of the hip should be obtained prior to initiating GH therapy for CRI patients. Physicians and parents should be alert to the development of a limp or complaints of hip or knee pain in patients treated with Nutropin.

Slipped capital femoral epiphysis may occur more frequently in patients with endocrine disorders or in patients undergoing rapid growth.

Progression of scoliosis can occur in patients who experience rapid growth. Because GH increases growth rate, patients with a history of scoliosis who are treated with GH should be monitored for progression of scoliosis. GH has not been shown to increase the incidence of scoliosis. Skeletal abnormalities including scoliosis are commonly seen in untreated Turner syndrome patients. Physicians should be alert to these abnormalities, which may manifest during GH therapy.

Patients with Turner syndrome should be evaluated carefully for otitis media and other ear disorders since these patients have an increased risk of ear or hearing disorders. In a randomized, controlled trial, there was a statistically significant increase, as compared to untreated controls, in otitis media (43% vs. 26%) and ear disorders (18% vs. 5%) in patients receiving GH. In addition, patients with Turner syndrome should be monitored closely for cardiovascular disorders (e.g., stroke, aortic aneurysm, hypertension) as these patients are also at risk for these conditions.

Intracranial hypertension (IH) with papilledema, visual changes, headache, nausea, and/or vomiting has been reported in a small number of patients treated with GH products. Symptoms usually occurred within the first eight (8) weeks of the initiation of GH therapy. In all reported cases, IH-associated signs and symptoms resolved after termination of therapy or a reduction of the GH dose. Funduscopic examination of patients is recommended at the initiation and periodically during the course of GH therapy. Patients with CRI and Turner syndrome may be at increased risk for development of IH.

See WARNINGS for use of Bacteriostatic Water for Injection, USP (benzyl alcohol preserved), in newborns.

As with any protein, local or systemic allergic reactions may occur. Parents/Patient should be informed that such reactions are possible and that prompt medical attention should be sought if allergic reactions occur.

Laboratory Tests: Serum levels of inorganic phosphorus, alkaline phosphatase, and parathyroid hormone (PTH) may increase with Nutropin therapy.

Untreated hypothyroidism prevents optimal response to Nutropin. Patients with Turner syndrome have an inherently increased risk of developing autoimmune thyroid disease. Changes in thyroid hormone laboratory measurements may develop during Nutropin treatment. Therefore, patients should have periodic thyroid function tests and should be treated with thyroid hormone when indicated.

Drug Interactions: Excessive glucocorticoid therapy will inhibit the growth-promoting effect of human GH. Patients with ACTH deficiency should have their glucocorticoid-replacement dose carefully adjusted to avoid an inhibitory effect on growth.

The use of Nutropin in patients with chronic renal insufficiency receiving glucocorticoid therapy has not been evaluated. Concomitant glucocorticoid therapy may inhibit the growth-promoting effect of Nutropin. If glucocorticoid-replacement is required, the glucocorticoid dose should be carefully adjusted.

There was no evidence in the controlled studies of Nutropin's interaction with drugs commonly used in chronic renal insufficiency patients. Limited published data indicate that GH treatment increases cytochrome P450 (CP450) mediated antipyrine clearance in man. These data suggest that GH administration may alter the clearance of compounds known to be metabolized by CP450 liver enzymes (e.g., corticosteroids, sex steroids, anticonvulsants, cyclosporin). Careful monitoring is advisable when GH is administered in combination with other drugs known to be metabolized by CP450 liver enzymes.

Carcinogenesis, Mutagenesis, Impairment of Fertility: Carcinogenicity, mutagenicity, and reproduction studies have not been conducted with Nutropin.

Pregnancy: Pregnancy (Category C). Animal reproduction studies have not been conducted with Nutropin. It is also not known whether Nutropin can cause fetal harm when administered to a pregnant woman or can affect reproduction capacity. Nutropin should be given to a pregnant woman only if clearly needed.

Nursing Mothers: It is not known whether Nutropin is excreted in human milk. Because many drugs are excreted in human milk, caution should be exercised when Nutropin is administered to a nursing mother.

Information for Patients: Patients being treated with GH and/or their parents should be informed of the potential benefits and risks associated with treatment. If home use is determined to be desirable by the physician, instructions on appropriate use should be given, including a review of the contents of the Patient Information Insert. This information is intended to aid in the safe and effective administration of the medication. It is not a disclosure of all possible adverse or intended effects.

If home use is prescribed, a puncture-resistant container for the disposal of used syringes and needles should be recommended to the patient. Patients and/or parents should be thoroughly instructed in the importance of proper disposal and cautioned against any reuse of needles and syringes (see Patient Information Insert).

ADVERSE REACTIONS

As with all protein pharmaceuticals, a small percentage of patients may develop antibodies to the protein. GH antibody binding capacities below 2 mg/L have not been associated with growth attenuation. In some cases when binding capacity exceeds 2 mg/L, growth attenuation has been observed. In clinical studies of pediatric patients that were treated with Nutropin for the first time, 0/107 growth hormone–deficient (GHD) patients, 0/125 CRI patients, and 0/112 Turner syndrome patients screened for antibody production developed antibodies with binding capacities ≥2 mg/L at six months.

Additional short-term immunologic and renal function studies were carried out in a group of patients with chronic renal insufficiency after approximately one year of treatment to detect other potential adverse effects of antibodies to GH. Testing included measurements of C1q, C3, C4, rheumatoid factor, creatinine, creatinine clearance, and BUN. No adverse effects of GH antibodies were noted.

In addition to an evaluation of compliance with the prescribed treatment program and thyroid status, testing for antibodies to GH should be carried out in any patient who fails to respond to therapy.

In studies in patients treated with Nutropin, injection site pain was reported infrequently.

Leukemia has been reported in a small number of GHD patients treated with GH. It is uncertain whether this increased risk is related to the pathology of GH deficiency itself, GH therapy, or other associated treatments such as radiation therapy for intracranial tumors. On the basis of current evidence, experts cannot conclude that GH therapy is responsible for these occurrences. The risk to GHD, CRI, or Turner syndrome patients, if any, remains to be established.

Other adverse drug reactions that have been reported in GH-treated patients include the following: 1) Metabolic: mild, transient peripheral edema. In GHD adults, edema or peripheral edema was reported in 41% of GH-treated patients and 25% of placebo-treated patients. 2) Musculoskeletal: arthralgias; carpal tunnel syndrome. In GHD adults, arthralgias and other joint disorders were reported in 27% of GH-treated patients and 15% of placebo-treated patients. 3) Skin: rare increased growth of pre-existing nevi; patients should be monitored for malignant transformation. 4) Endocrine: gynecomastia. Rare pancreatitis.

OVERDOSAGE

Acute overdosage could lead to hyperglycemia. Long-term overdosage could result in signs and symptoms of gigantism and/or acromegaly consistent with the known effects of excess GH. (See recommended and maximal dosage instructions given below.)

DOSAGE AND ADMINISTRATION

The Nutropin dosage and administration schedule should be individualized for each patient. Response to growth hormone therapy in pediatric patients tends to decrease with time. However, in pediatric patients failure to increase growth rate, particularly during the first year of therapy, suggests the need for close assessment of compliance and evaluation of other causes of growth failure, such as hypothyroidism, under-nutrition, and advanced bone age.

Dosage

Pediatric Growth Hormone Deficiency (GHD)

A weekly dosage of up to 0.30 mg/kg of body weight divided into daily subcutaneous injection is recommended. In pubertal patients, a weekly dosage of up to 0.7 mg/kg divided daily may be used.

Adult Growth Hormone Deficiency (GHD)

The recommended dosage at the start of therapy is not more than 0.006 mg/kg given as a daily subcutaneous injection. The dose may be increased according to individual patient requirements to a maximum of 0.025 mg/kg daily in patients under 35 years and to a maximum of 0.0125 mg/kg daily in patients over 35 years.

To minimize the occurrence of adverse events in older or overweight patients, lower doses may be necessary. During therapy, dosage should be decreased if required by the occurrence of side effects or excessive IGF-I levels.

Mean Changes from Baseline to Month 12 in Proportion of Fat and Lean by DEXA for Studies M0431g and M0381g (Adult-onset and Childhood-onset GHD, respectively)

	M0431g			M0381g			
Proportion	Placebo (n=62)	Nutropin (n=63)	Between-groups t-test p-value	Placebo (n=13)	Nutropin 0.0125 mg/kg/day (n=15)	Nutropin 0.025 mg/kg/day (n=15)	Placebo vs. pooled Nutropin t-test p-value
Total body percent fat							
Baseline	36.8	35.0	0.38	35.0	37.1	38.4	0.45
Month 12	36.8	31.5		35.2	31.3	32.1	
Baseline to Month 12 change	**−0.1**	**−3.6**	<0.0001	**+0.2**	**−5.8**	**−6.3**	<0.0001
Post-washout	36.4	32.2		N/A	N/A	N/A	
Baseline to post-washout change	**−0.4**	**−2.8**	<0.0001	N/A	N/A	N/A	
Trunk percent fat							
Baseline	35.3	33.9	0.50	32.5	37.9	36.7	0.23
Month 12	35.4	29.5		33.1	30.6	29.0	
Baseline to Month 12 change	**0.0**	**−4.3**	<0.0001	**+0.6**	**−7.3**	**−7.6**	<0.0001
Post-washout	34.9	30.5		N/A	N/A	N/A	
Baseline to post-washout change	**−0.3**	**−3.4**		N/A	N/A	N/A	
Total body percent lean							
Baseline	60.4	62.2	0.37	62.0	60.0	59.1	0.48
Month 12	60.5	65.7		61.8	66.0	65.5	
Baseline to Month 12 change	**+0.2**	**+3.6**	<0.0001	**−0.2**	**+6.0**	**+6.4**	<0.0001
Post-washout	60.9	65.0		N/A	N/A	N/A	
Baseline to post-washout change	**+0.4**	**+2.8**	<0.0001	N/A	N/A	N/A	

Chronic Renal Insufficiency (CRI)
A weekly dosage of up to 0.35 mg/kg of body weight divided into daily subcutaneous injection is recommended.
Nutropin therapy may be continued up to the time of renal transplantation.
In order to optimize therapy for patients who require dialysis, the following guidelines for injection schedule are recommended:

1. Hemodialysis patients should receive their injection at night just prior to going to sleep or at least 3–4 hours after their hemodialysis to prevent hematoma formation due to the heparin.
2. Chronic Cycling Peritoneal Dialysis (CCPD) patients should receive their injection in the morning after they have completed dialysis.
3. Chronic Ambulatory Peritoneal Dialysis (CAPD) patients should receive their injection in the evening at the time of the overnight exchange.

Turner Syndrome
A weekly dosage of up to 0.375 mg/kg of body weight divided into equal doses 3 to 7 times per week by subcutaneous injection is recommended.

Administration
After the dose has been determined, reconstitute as follows: each 5 mg vial should be reconstituted with 1–5 mL of Bacteriostatic Water for Injection, USP (benzyl alcohol preserved); or each 10 mg vial should be reconstituted with 1–10 mL of Bacteriostatic Water for Injection, USP (benzyl alcohol preserved), only. For use in newborns see WARNINGS. The pH of Nutropin after reconstitution with Bacteriostatic Water for Injection, USP (benzyl alcohol preserved), is approximately 7.4.
To prepare the Nutropin solution, inject the Bacteriostatic Water for Injection, USP (benzyl alcohol preserved), into the Nutropin vial, aiming the stream of liquid against the glass wall. Then swirl the product vial with a **GENTLE** rotary motion until the contents are completely dissolved. **DO NOT SHAKE**. Because Nutropin is a protein, shaking can result in a cloudy solution. The Nutropin solution should be clear immediately after reconstitution. Occasionally, after refrigeration, you may notice that small colorless particles of protein are present in the Nutropin solution. This is not unusual for solutions containing proteins. If the solution is cloudy immediately after reconstitution or refrigeration, the contents **MUST NOT** be injected.
Before needle insertion, wipe the septum of both the Nutropin and diluent vials with rubbing alcohol or an antiseptic solution to prevent contamination of the contents by microorganisms that may be introduced by repeated needle insertions. It is recommended that Nutropin be administered using sterile, disposable syringes and needles. The syringes should be of small enough volume that the prescribed dose can be drawn from the vial with reasonable accuracy.

STABILITY AND STORAGE
Before Reconstitution—Nutropin® [somatropin (rDNA origin) for injection] and Bacteriostatic Water for Injection, USP (benzyl alcohol preserved), must be stored at 2–8°C/36–46°F (under refrigeration). **Avoid freezing the vials of Nutropin and Bacteriostatic Water for Injection, USP (benzyl alcohol preserved).** Expiration dates are stated on the labels.
After Reconstitution—Vial contents are stable for 14 days when reconstituted with Bacteriostatic Water for Injection, USP (benzyl alcohol preserved), and stored at 2–8°C/36–46°F (under refrigeration). Store the unused portion of Bacteriostatic Water for Injection, USP (benzyl alcohol preserved), at 2–8°C/36–46°F (under refrigeration). **Avoid freezing the reconstituted vial of Nutropin and the Bacteriostatic Water for Injection, USP (benzyl alcohol preserved).**

HOW SUPPLIED

Nutropin is supplied as 5 mg (approximately 15 IU) or 10 mg (approximately 30 IU) of lyophilized, sterile somatropin per vial.
Each 5 mg carton contains two vials of Nutropin® [somatropin (rDNA origin) for injection] (5 mg per vial) and one 10 mL multiple dose vial of Bacteriostatic Water for Injection, USP (benzyl alcohol preserved). NDC 50242-072-02
Each 10 mg carton contains two vials of Nutropin® [somatropin (rDNA origin) for injection] (10 mg per vial) and two 10 mL multiple dose vials of Bacteriostatic Water for Injection, USP (benzyl alcohol preserved).
NDC 50242-018-20
Nutropin® [somatropin (rDNA origin) for injection] manufactured by:
Genentech, Inc.
1 DNA Way
South San Francisco, CA 94080-4990
Bacteriostatic Water for Injection, USP (benzyl alcohol preserved), manufactured for:
Genentech, Inc.

4808607

 Revised April 2000

Shown in Product Identification Guide, page 313

NUTROPIN AQ® ℞
[somatropin (rDNA origin) injection]

DESCRIPTION

Nutropin AQ® [somatropin (rDNA origin) injection] is a human growth hormone (hGH) produced by recombinant DNA technology. Nutropin AQ has 191 amino acid residues and a molecular weight of 22,125 daltons. The amino acid sequence of the product is identical to that of pituitary-derived human growth hormone. The protein is synthesized by a specific laboratory strain of *E. coli* as a precursor consisting of the rhGH molecule preceded by the secretion signal from an *E. coli* protein. This precursor is directed to the plasma membrane of the cell. The signal sequence is removed and the native protein is secreted into the periplasm so that the protein is folded appropriately as it is synthesized.
Nutropin AQ is a highly purified preparation. Biological potency is determined using a cell proliferation bioassay. Nutropin AQ may contain not more than fifteen percent deamidated growth hormone (GH) at expiration. The deamidated form of GH has been extensively characterized and has been shown to be safe and fully active.
Nutropin AQ is a sterile liquid intended for subcutaneous administration. The product is nearly isotonic at a concentration of 5 mg of GH per mL and has a pH of approximately 6.0.
Each 2 mL vial contains 10 mg (approximately 30 IU) somatropin, formulated in 17.4 mg sodium chloride, 5 mg phenol, 4 mg polysorbate 20, and 10 mM sodium citrate.

Summary of Nutropin AQ Pharmacokinetic Parameters
in Healthy Adult Males
0.1 mg (approximately 0.3 IU[a])/kg SC

	C_{max} (μg/L)	T_{max} (hr)	$t_{½}$ (hr)	$AUC_{0-\infty}$ (μg•hr/L)	CL/F_{sc} (mL/[hr•kg])
MEAN[b]	71.1	3.9	2.3	677	150
CV%	17	56	18	13	13

Abbreviations: C_{max}=maximum concentration; $t_{1/2}$ =half-life; $AUC_{0-\infty}$=area under the curve; CL/F_{sc}=systemic clearance; F_{sc}=subcutaneous bioavailability (not determined); CV%=coefficient of variation in %; SC=subcutaneous

[a] Based on current International Standard of 3 IU=1 mg
[b] n=36

CLINICAL PHARMACOLOGY

General
In vitro and in vivo preclinical and clinical testing have demonstrated that Nutropin AQ is therapeutically equivalent to pituitary-derived human GH (hGH). Pediatric patients who lack adequate endogenous GH secretion, patients with chronic renal insufficiency, and patients with Turner syndrome that were treated with Nutropin AQ or Nutropin® [somatropin (rDNA origin) for injection] resulted in an increase in growth rate and an increase in insulin-like growth factor-I (IGF-I) levels similar to that seen with pituitary-derived hGH.
Actions that have been demonstrated for Nutropin AQ, somatropin, somatrem, and/or pituitary-derived hGH include:

A. **Tissue Growth**—1) Skeletal Growth: GH stimulates skeletal growth in pediatric patients with growth failure due to a lack of adequate secretion of endogenous GH or secondary to chronic renal insufficiency and in patients with Turner syndrome. Skeletal growth is accomplished at the epiphyseal plates at the ends of a growing bone. Growth and metabolism of epiphyseal plate cells are directly stimulated by GH and one of its mediators, IGF-I. Serum levels of IGF-I are low in children and adolescents who are GH deficient, but increase during treatment with GH. In pediatric patients, new bone is formed at the epiphyses in response to GH and IGF-I. This results in linear growth until these growth plates fuse at the end of puberty. 2) Cell Growth: Treatment with hGH results in an increase in both the number and the size of skeletal muscle cells. 3) Organ Growth: GH influences the size of internal organs, including kidneys, and increases red cell mass. Treatment of hypophysectomized or genetic dwarf rats with GH results in organ growth that is proportional to the overall body growth. In normal rats subjected to nephrectomy-induced uremia, GH promoted skeletal and body growth.
B. **Protein Metabolism**—Linear growth is facilitated in part by GH-stimulated protein synthesis. This is reflected by nitrogen retention as demonstrated by a decline in urinary nitrogen excretion and blood urea nitrogen during GH therapy.
C. **Carbohydrate Metabolism**—GH is a modulator of carbohydrate metabolism. For example, patients with inadequate secretion of GH sometimes experience fasting hypoglycemia that is improved by treatment with GH. GH therapy may decrease insulin sensitivity. Untreated patients with chronic renal insufficiency and Turner syndrome have an increased incidence of glucose intolerance. Administration of hGH to adults or children resulted in increases in serum fasting and postprandial insulin levels, more commonly in overweight or obese individuals. In addition, mean fasting and postprandial glucose and hemoglobin A_{Ic} levels remained in the normal range.
D. **Lipid Metabolism**—In GH-deficient patients, administration of GH resulted in lipid mobilization, reduction in body fat stores, increased plasma fatty acids, and decreased plasma cholesterol levels.
E. **Mineral Metabolism**—The retention of total body potassium in response to GH administration apparently results from cellular growth. Serum levels of inorganic phosphorus may increase slightly in patients with inadequate secretion of endogenous GH, chronic renal insufficiency, or patients with Turner syndrome during GH therapy due to metabolic activity associated with bone growth as well as increased tubular reabsorption of phosphate by the kidney. Serum calcium is not significantly altered in these patients. Sodium retention also occurs. Adults with childhood-onset GH deficiency show low bone mineral density (BMD). GH therapy results in increases in serum alkaline phosphatase. (See PRECAUTIONS: Laboratory Tests.)
F. **Connective Tissue Metabolism**—GH stimulates the synthesis of chondroitin sulfate and collagen as well as the urinary excretion of hydroxyproline.

Pharmacokinetics
Subcutaneous Absorption—The absolute bioavailability of recombinant human growth hormone (rhGH) after subcutaneous administration in healthy adult males has been determined to be 81±20%. The mean terminal $t_{1/2}$ after subcutaneous administration is significantly longer than that seen after intravenous administration (2.1±0.43 hr vs. 19.5±3.1 min) indicating that the subcutaneous absorption of the compound is slow and rate-limiting.
Distribution—Animal studies with rhGH showed that GH localizes to highly perfused organs, particularly the liver and kidney. The volume of distribution at steady state for rhGH in healthy adult males is about 50 mL/kg body weight, approximating the serum volume.
Metabolism—Both the liver and kidney have been shown to be important metabolizing organs for GH. Animal studies suggest that the kidney is the dominant organ of clearance. GH is filtered at the glomerulus and reabsorbed in the proximal tubules. It is then cleaved within renal cells into its constituent amino acids, which return to the systemic circulation.
Elimination—The mean terminal $t_{1/2}$ after intravenous administration of rhGH in healthy adult males is estimated to be 19.5±3.1 minutes. Clearance of rhGH after intravenous administration in healthy adults and children is reported to be in the range of 116–174 mL/hr/kg.
Bioequivalence of Formulations—Nutropin AQ® [somatropin (rDNA origin) injection] has been determined to be bioequivalent to Nutropin® [somatropin (rDNA origin) for injection] based on the statistical evaluation of AUC and C_{max}.

Special Populations
Pediatric—Available literature data suggest that rhGH clearances are similar in adults and children.
Gender—No data are available for exogenously administered rhGH. Available data for methionyl recombinant GH, pituitary-derived GH, and endogenous GH suggest no consistent gender-based differences in GH clearance.
Geriatrics—Limited published data suggest that the plasma clearance and average steady-state plasma concentration of rhGH may not be different between young and elderly patients.
Race—Reported values for half-lives for endogenous GH in normal adult black males are not different from observed values for normal adult white males. No data for other races are available.
Growth Hormone Deficiency (GHD)—Reported values for clearance of rhGH in adults and children with GHD range 138–245 mL/hr/kg and are similar to those observed in healthy adults and children. Mean terminal $t_{1/2}$ values following intravenous and subcutaneous administration in adult and pediatric GHD patients are also similar to those observed in healthy adult males.
Renal Insufficiency—Children and adults with chronic renal failure (CRF) and end-stage renal disease (ESRD) tend to have decreased clearance compared to normals. Endogenous GH production may also increase in some individuals with ESRD. However, no rhGH accumulation has been reported in children with CRF or ESRD dosed with current regimens.
Turner Syndrome—No pharmacokinetic data are available for exogenously administered rhGH. However, reported half-lives, absorption, and elimination rates for endogenous GH in this population are similar to the ranges observed for normal subjects and GHD populations.
Hepatic Insufficiency—A reduction in rhGH clearance has been noted in patients with severe liver dysfunction. The clinical significance of this decrease is unknown.
[See table above]
[See figure at top of next column]

Efficacy Studies
Growth Hormone Deficiency (GHD) in Pubertal Patients
One open-label, multicenter, randomized clinical trial of two dosages of Nutropin® [somatropin (rDNA origin) for injection] was performed in pubertal patients with GHD. Ninety-seven patients (mean age 13.9 years, 83 male, 14 female)

Continued on next page

Nutropin AQ—Cont.

Single Dose Mean Growth Hormone Concentrations in Healthy Adult Males

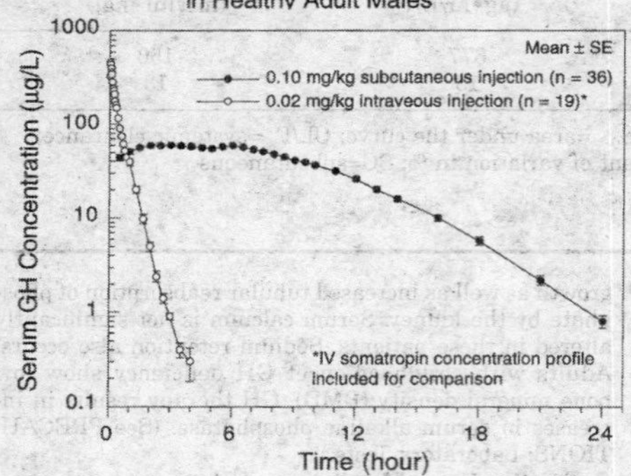

currently being treated with approximately 0.3 mg/kg/wk of GH were randomized to 0.3 mg/kg/wk or 0.7 mg/kg/wk Nutropin doses. All patients were already in puberty (Tanner stage ≥2) and had bone ages ≤14 yr in males or ≤12 yr in females. Mean baseline height standard deviation (SD) score was −1.3.

The mean last measured height in all 97 patients after a mean duration of 2.7±1.2 years, by analysis of covariance (ANCOVA) adjusting for baseline height, is shown below.

[See table above]

Last Measured Height* by Sex and Nutropin Dose

	Age (yr) Mean±SD (range)	Last Measured Height* (cm) 0.3 mg/kg/wk Mean±SD	0.7 mg/kg/wk Mean±SD	Between Groups (cm) Mean±SE
Male	17.2±1.3 (13.6 to 19.4)	170.9±7.9 (n=42)	174.5±7.9 (n=41)	3.6±1.7
Female	15.8±1.8 (11.9 to 19.3)	154.7±6.3 (n=7)	157.6±6.3 (n=7)	2.9±3.4

*Adjusted for baseline height

The mean height SD score at last measured height (n=97) was −0.7±1.0 in the 0.3 mg/kg/wk group and −0.1±1.2 in the 0.7 mg/kg/wk group. For patients completing 3.5 or more years (mean 4.1 years) of Nutropin treatment (15/49 patients in the 0.3 mg/kg/wk group and 16/48 patients in the 0.7 mg/kg/wk group), the mean last measured height was 166.1±8.0 cm in the 0.3 mg/kg/wk group and 171.8±7.1 cm in the 0.7 mg/kg/wk group, adjusting for baseline height and sex.

The mean change in bone age was approximately one year for each year in the study in both dose groups. Patients with baseline height SD scores above −1.0 were able to attain normal adult heights with the 0.3 mg/kg/wk dose of Nutropin (mean height SD score at near-adult height = −0.1, n=15).

Thirty-one patients had bone mineral density (BMD) determined by dual energy x-ray absorptiometry (DEXA) scans at study conclusion. The two dose groups did not differ significantly in mean SD score for total body BMD (−0.9±1.9 in the 0.3 mg/kg/wk group vs. −0.8±1.2 in the 0.7 mg/kg/wk group, n=20) or lumbar spine BMD (−1.0±1.0 in the 0.3 mg/kg/wk group vs. −0.2±1.7 in the 0.7 mg/kg/wk group, n=21). Over a mean duration of 2.7 years, patients in the 0.7 mg/kg/wk group were more likely to have IGF-I values above the normal range than patients in the 0.3 mg/kg/wk group (27.2% vs. 9.0% of IGF-I measurements for individual patients). The clinical significance of elevated IGF-I values is unknown.

Effects of Nutropin® [somatropin (rDNA origin) for injection] on Growth Failure Due to Chronic Renal Insufficiency (CRI)

Two multicenter, randomized, controlled clinical trials were conducted to determine whether treatment with Nutropin prior to renal transplantation in patients with chronic renal insufficiency could improve their growth rates and height deficits. One study was a double-blind, placebo-controlled trial and the other was an open-label, randomized trial. The dose of Nutropin in both controlled studies was 0.05 mg/kg/day (0.35 mg/kg/wk) administered daily by subcutaneous injection. Combining the data from those patients completing two years in the two controlled studies results in 62 patients treated with Nutropin and 28 patients in the control groups (either placebo-treated or untreated). The mean first year growth rate was 10.8 cm/yr for Nutropin-treated patients, compared with a mean growth rate of 6.5 cm/yr for placebo/untreated controls (p<0.00005). The mean second year growth rate was 7.8 cm/yr for the Nutropin-treated group, compared with 5.5 cm/yr for controls (p<0.00005). There was a significant increase in mean height standard deviation (SD) score in the Nutropin group (−2.9 at baseline to −1.5 at Month 24, n=62) but no significant change in the controls (−2.8 at baseline to −2.9 at Month 24, n=28). The mean third year growth rate of 7.6 cm/yr in the Nutropin-treated patients (n=27) suggests that Nutropin stimulates growth beyond two years. However, there are no control data for the third year because control patients crossed over to Nutropin treatment after two years of participation. The gains in height were accompanied by appropriate advancement of skeletal age. These data demonstrate that Nutropin therapy improves growth rate and corrects the acquired height deficit associated with chronic renal insufficiency. Currently there are insufficient data regarding the benefit of treatment beyond three years. Although predicted final height was improved during Nutropin therapy, the effect of Nutropin on final adult height remains to be determined.

Post-Transplant Growth

The North American Pediatric Renal Transplant Cooperative Study (NAPRTCS) has reported data for growth post-transplant in children who did not receive GH. The average change in height SD score during the initial two years post-transplant was 0.18 (n=300, J Pediatr. 1993;122:397–402). Controlled studies of GH treatment for the short stature associated with CRI were not designed to compare the growth of treated or untreated patients after they received renal transplants. However, growth data are available from a small number of patients who have been followed for at least 11 months. Of the 7 control patients, 4 increased their height SD score and 3 had either no significant change or a decrease in height SD score. The 13 patients treated with Nutropin® [somatropin (rDNA origin) for injection] prior to transplant had either no significant change or an increase in height SD score after transplantation, indicating that the individual gains achieved with GH therapy prior to transplant were maintained after transplantation. The differences in the height deficit narrowed between the treated and untreated groups in the post-transplant period.

Turner Syndrome

One long-term, randomized, open-label, multicenter, concurrently controlled study, two long-term, open-label, multicenter, historically controlled studies and one long-term, randomized, dose-response study were conducted to evaluate the efficacy of GH for the treatment of girls with short stature due to Turner syndrome.

In the randomized study GDCT, comparing GH-treated patients to a concurrent control group who received no GH, the GH-treated patients who received a dose of 0.3 mg/kg/week given 6 times per week from a mean age of 11.7 years for a mean duration of 4.7 years attained a mean near final height of 146.0 cm (n=27) as compared to the control group who attained a near final height of 142.1 cm (n=19). By analysis of covariance, the effect of GH therapy was a mean height increase of 5.4 cm (p=0.001).

In two of the studies (85-023 and 85-044), the effect of long-term GH treatment (0.375 mg/kg/week given either 3 times per week or daily) on adult height was determined by comparing adult heights in the treated patients with those of age-matched historical controls with Turner syndrome who never received any growth-promoting therapy. In Study 85-023, estrogen treatment was delayed until patients were at least age 14. GH therapy resulted in a mean adult height gain of 7.4 cm (mean duration of GH therapy of 7.6 years) vs. matched historical controls by analysis of covariance.

In Study 85-044, patients treated with early GH therapy were randomized to receive estrogen-replacement therapy (conjugated estrogens, 0.3 mg escalating to 0.625 mg daily) at either age 12 or 15 years. Compared with matched historical controls, early GH therapy (mean duration of GH therapy 5.6 years) combined with estrogen replacement at age 12 years resulted in an adult height gain of 5.9 cm (n=26), whereas girls who initiated estrogen at age 15 years (mean duration of GH therapy 6.1 years) had a mean adult height gain of 8.3 cm (n=29). Patients who initiated GH therapy after age 11 (mean age 12.7 years; mean duration of GH therapy 3.8 years) had a mean adult height gain of 5.0 cm (n=51).

Thus, in both studies, 85-023 and 85-044, the greatest improvement in adult height was observed in patients who received early GH treatment and estrogen after age 14 years.

In a randomized, blinded, dose-response study, GDCI, patients were treated from a mean age of 11.1 years for a mean duration of 5.3 years with a weekly dose of either 0.27 mg/kg or 0.36 mg/kg administered 3 or 6 times weekly. The mean near final height of patients receiving growth hormone was 148.7 cm (n=31). This represents a mean gain in adult height of approximately 5 cm compared with previous observations of untreated Turner syndrome girls.

In these studies, Turner syndrome patients (n=181) treated to final adult height achieved statistically significant average estimated adult height gains ranging 5.0–8.3 cm.

[See table above]

Study/ Group	Study Design[a]	N at Adult Height	GH Age (yr)	Estrogen Age (yr)	GH Duration (yr)	Adult Height Gain (cm)[b]
GDCT	RCT	27	11.7	13	4.7	5.4
85-023	MHT	17	9.1	15.2	7.6	7.4
85-044: A*	MHT	29	9.4	15.0	6.1	8.3
B*		26	9.6	12.3	5.6	5.9
C*		51	12.7	13.7	3.8	5.0
GDCI	RDT	31	11.1	8–13.5	5.3	~5[c]

[a]RCT: randomized controlled trial; MHT: matched historical controlled trial; RDT: randomized dose-response trial.
[b] Analysis of convariance vs. controls
[c] Compared with historical data
* A: GH age <11 yr, estrogen age 15 yr
B: GH age <11 yr, estrogen age 12 yr
C: GH age >11 yr, estrogen at Month 12

Adult Growth Hormone Deficiency (GHD)

Two multicenter, double-blind, placebo-controlled clinical trials were conducted using Nutropin® [somatropin (rDNA origin) for injection] in GH-deficient adults. One study was conducted in subjects with adult-onset GHD, mean age 48.3 years, n=166, at doses of 0.0125 or 0.00625 mg/kg/day; doses of 0.025 mg/kg/day were not tolerated in these subjects. A second study was conducted in previously treated subjects with childhood-onset GHD, mean age 23.8 years, n=64, at randomly assigned doses of 0.025 or 0.0125 mg/kg/day. The studies were designed to assess the effects of replacement therapy with GH on body composition.

Significant changes from baseline to Month 12 of treatment in body composition (i.e., total body % fat mass, trunk % fat mass, and total body % lean mass by DEXA scan) were seen in all Nutropin groups in both studies (p<0.0001 for change from baseline and vs. placebo), whereas no statistically significant changes were seen in either of the placebo groups. In the adult-onset study, the Nutropin group improved mean total body fat from 35.0% to 31.5%, mean trunk fat from 33.9% to 29.5%, and mean lean body mass from 62.2% to 65.7%, whereas the placebo group had mean changes of 0.2% or less (p=not significant). Due to the possible effect of GH-induced fluid retention on DEXA measurements of lean body mass, DEXA scans were repeated approximately 3 weeks after completion of therapy; mean % lean body mass in the Nutropin group was 65.0%, a change of 2.8% from baseline, compared with a change of 0.4% in the placebo group (p<0.0001 between groups).

In the childhood-onset study, the high-dose Nutropin group improved mean total body fat from 38.4% to 32.1%, mean trunk fat from 36.7% to 29.0%, and mean lean body mass from 59.1% to 65.5%; the low-dose Nutropin group improved mean total body fat from 37.1% to 31.3%, mean trunk fat from 37.9% to 30.6%, and mean lean body mass from 60.0% to 66.0%; the placebo group had mean changes of 0.6% or less (p=not significant).

[See table at top of next page]

In the adult-onset study, significant decreases from baseline to Month 12 in LDL cholesterol and LDL:HDL ratio were seen in the Nutropin group compared to the placebo group, p<0.02; there were no statistically significant between-group differences in change from baseline to Month 12 in total cholesterol, HDL cholesterol, or triglycerides. In the childhood-onset study, significant decreases from baseline to Month 12 in total cholesterol, LDL cholesterol, and LDL:HDL ratio were seen in the high-dose Nutropin group only, compared to the placebo group, p<0.05. There were no statistically significant between-group differences in HDL cholesterol or triglycerides from baseline to Month 12.

In the childhood-onset study, 55% of the patients had decreased spine bone mineral density (BMD) (z-score <−1) at baseline. The administration of Nutropin (n=16) (0.025 mg/kg/day) for two years resulted in increased spine BMD from baseline when compared to placebo (n=13) (4.6% vs. 1.0%, respectively, p<0.03); a transient decrease in spine BMD was seen at six months in the Nutropin-treated patients. Thirty-five percent of subjected treated with this dose had supraphysiological levels of IGF-I at some point during the study, which may carry unknown risks. No significant improvement in total body BMD was found when compared to placebo. A lower GH dose (0.0125 mg/kg/day) did not show significant increments in either of these bone parameters when compared to placebo. No statistically signifiant effects on BMD were seen in the adult-onset study where patients received GH (0.0125 mg/kg/day) for one year.

Muscle strength, physical endurance, and quality of life measurements were not markedly abnormal at baseline, and no statistically significant effects of Nutropin therapy were observed in the two studies.

INDICATIONS AND USAGE

Pediatric Patients

Nutropin AQ® [somatropin (rDNA origin) injection] is indicated for the long-term treatment of growth failure due to a lack of adequate endogenous GH secretion.

Nutropin AQ® [somatropin (rDNA origin) injection] is also indicated for the treatment of growth failure associated

Mean Changes from Baseline to Month 12 in Proportion of Fat and Lean by DEXA for Studies M0431g and M0381g (Adult-onset and Childhood-onset GHD, Respectively)

	M0431g			M0381g			
Proportion	Placebo (n=62)	Nutropin (n=63)	Between-groups t-test p-value	Placebo (n=13)	Nutropin 0.0125 mg/kg/day (n=15)	Nutropin 0.025 mg/kg/day (n=15)	Placebo vs. pooled Nutropin t-test p-value
Total body percent fat							
Baseline	36.8	35.0	0.38	35.0	37.1	38.4	0.45
Month 12	36.8	31.5		35.2	31.3	32.1	
Baseline to Month 12 change	**−0.1**	**−3.6**	<0.0001	**+0.2**	**−5.8**	**−6.3**	<0.0001
Post-washout	36.4	32.2		N/A	N/A	N/A	
Baseline to post-washout change	**−0.4**	**−2.8**	<0.0001	N/A	N/A	N/A	
Trunk percent fat							
Baseline	35.3	33.9	0.50	32.5	37.9	36.7	0.23
Month 12	35.4	29.5		33.1	30.6	29.0	
Baseline to Month 12 change	**0.0**	**−4.3**	<0.0001	**+0.6**	**−7.3**	**−7.6**	<0.0001
Post-washout	34.9	30.5		N/A	N/A	N/A	
Baseline to post-washout change	**−0.3**	**−3.4**		N/A	N/A	N/A	
Total body percent lean							
Baseline	60.4	62.2	0.37	62.0	60.0	59.1	0.48
Month 12	60.5	65.7		61.8	66.0	65.5	
Baseline to Month 12 change	**+0.2**	**+3.6**	<0.0001	**−0.2**	**+6.0**	**+6.4**	<0.0001
Post-washout	60.9	65.0		N/A	N/A	N/A	
Baseline to post-washout change	**+0.4**	**+2.8**	<0.0001	N/A	N/A	N/A	

with chronic renal insufficiency up to the time of renal transplantation. Nutropin AQ therapy should be used in conjunction with optimal management of chronic renal insufficiency.

Nutropin AQ® [somatropin (rDNA origin) injection] is also indicated for the long-term treatment of short stature associated with Turner syndrome.

Adult Patients

Nutropin AQ® [somatropin (rDNA origin) injection] is indicated for the replacement of endogenous GH in patients with adult GH deficiency who meet both of the following two criteria:

1. Biochemical diagnosis of adult GH deficiency by means of a subnormal response to a standard growth hormone stimulation test (peak GH≤5 µg/L), and
2. Adult-onset: Patients who have adult GH deficiency either alone or with multiple hormone deficiencies (hypopituitarism) as a result of pituitary disease, hypothalamic disease, surgery, radiation therapy, or trauma; or

Childhood-onset: Patients who were GH deficient during childhood, confirmed as an adult before replacement therapy with Nutropin AQ is started.

CONTRAINDICATIONS

Growth hormone should not be initiated to treat patients with acute critical illness due to complications following open heart or abdominal surgery, multiple accidental trauma or to patients having acute respiratory failure. Two placebo-controlled clinical trials in non-growth hormone–deficient adult patients (n=522) with these conditions revealed a significant increase in mortality (41.9% vs. 19.3%) among somatropin-treated patients (doses 5.3–8 mg/day) compared to those receiving placebo (see WARNINGS).

Nutropin AQ should not be used for growth promotion in pediatric patients with closed epiphyses.

Nutropin AQ should not be used in patients with active neoplasia. GH therapy should be discontinued if evidence of neoplasia develops.

WARNINGS

See CONTRAINDICATIONS for information on increased mortality in patients with acute critical illnesses in intensive care units due to complications following open heart or abdominal surgery, multiple accidental trauma or with acute respiratory failure. The safety of continuing growth hormone treatment in patients receiving replacement doses for approved indications who concurrently develop these illnesses has not been established. Therefore, the potential benefit of treatment continuation with growth hormone in patients having acute critical illnesses should be weighed against the potential risk.

PRECAUTIONS

General: Nutropin AQ should be prescribed by physicians experienced in the diagnosis and management of patients with GH deficiency, Turner syndrome, or chronic renal insufficiency. No studies have been completed of Nutropin AQ therapy in patients who have received renal transplants. Currently, treatment of patients with functioning renal allografts is not indicated.

Experience with prolonged rhGH treatment in adults is limited.

Geriatric Usage: Clinical studies of Nutropin AQ did not include sufficient numbers of subjects aged 65 and over to determine whether they respond differently from younger subjects. Other reported clinical experience has not identified differences in responses between the elderly and younger patients. In general, dose selection for an elderly patient should be cautious, usually starting at the low end of the dosing range, reflecting the greater frequency of decreased hepatic, renal, or cardiac function, and of concomitant disease or other drug therapy.

Patients with epiphyseal closure who were treated with GH-replacement therapy in childhood should be re-evaluated according to the criteria in the INDICATIONS AND USAGE SECTION before continuation of GH therapy at the reduced dose level recommended for GH-deficient adults.

Because Nutropin AQ may reduce insulin sensitivity, patients should be monitored for evidence of glucose intolerance.

For patients with diabetes mellitus, the insulin dose may require adjustment when GH therapy is instituted. Because GH may reduce insulin sensitivity, particularly in obese individuals, patients should be observed for evidence of glucose intolerance. Patients with diabetes or glucose intolerance should be monitored closely during GH therapy.

Nutropin therapy in adults with GH deficiency of adult onset was associated with an increase of median fasting insulin in the Nutropin 0.0125 mg/kg/day group from 9.0 µU/mL at baseline to 13.0 µU/mL at Month 12 with a return to the baseline median after a 3-week post-washout period off GH therapy. In the placebo group there was no change from 8.0 µU/mL at baseline to Month 12, and after the post-washout the median was 9.0 µU/mL. The between-treatment-groups difference in change from baseline to Month 12 was significant, p<0.0001. In childhood-onset subjects there was a change of median fasting insulin in the Nutropin 0.025 mg/kg/day group from 11.0 µU/mL at baseline to 20.0 µU/mL at Month 12, in the Nutropin 0.0125 mg/kg/day group from 8.5 µU/mL to 11.0 µU/mL, and in the placebo group from 7.0 µU/mL to 8.0 µU/mL. The between-treatment-groups difference for these changes was significant, p=0.0007.

In subjects with adult-onset GH deficiency, there was no between-treatment-group difference in changes from baseline to Month 12 in mean HbA_{1c}, p=0.08. In childhood-onset mean HbA_{1c} increased in the Nutropin 0.025 mg/kg/day group from 5.2% at baseline to 5.5% at Month 12, and did not change in the Nutropin 0.0125 mg/kg/day group from 5.1% at baseline or in the placebo group from 5.3% at baseline. The between-treatment-groups difference was significant, p=0.009.

Patients with a history of an intracranial lesion should be examined frequently for progression or recurrence of the lesion. In pediatric patients, clinical literature has demonstrated no relationship between GH-replacement therapy and CNS tumor recurrence or new extracranial tumors. In adults, it is unknown whether there is any relationship between GH-replacement therapy and CNS tumor recurrence.

Patients with growth failure secondary to chronic renal insufficiency should be examined periodically for evidence of progression of renal osteodystrophy. Slipped capital femoral epiphysis or avascular necrosis of the femoral head may be seen in children with advanced renal osteodystrophy, and it is uncertain whether these problems are affected by GH therapy. X-rays of the hip should be obtained prior to initiating GH therapy for CRI patients. Physicians and parents should be alert to the development of a limp or complaints of hip or knee pain in patients treated with Nutropin AQ.

Slipped capital femoral epiphysis may occur more frequently in patients with endocrine disorders or in patients undergoing rapid growth.

Progression of scoliosis can occur in patients who experience rapid growth. Because GH increases growth rate, patients with a history of scoliosis who are treated with GH should be monitored for progression of scoliosis. GH has not been shown to increase the incidence of scoliosis. Skeletal abnormalities including scoliosis are commonly seen in untreated Turner syndrome patients. Physicians should be alert to these abnormalities, which may manifest during GH therapy.

Patients with Turner syndrome should be evaluated carefully for otitis media and other ear disorders since these patients have an increased risk of ear or hearing disorders. In a randomized, controlled trial, there was a statistically significant increase, as compared to untreated controls, in otitis media (43% vs. 26%) and ear disorders (18% vs. 5%) in patients receiving GH. In addition, patients with Turner syndrome should be monitored closely for cardiovascular disorders (e.g., stroke, aortic aneurysm, hypertension) as these patients are also at risk for these conditions.

Intracranial hypertension (IH) with papilledema, visual changes, headache, nausea, and/or vomiting has been reported in a small number of patients treated with GH products. Symptoms usually occurred within the first eight (8) weeks of the initiation of GH therapy. In all reported cases, IH-associated signs and symptoms resolved after termination of therapy or a reduction of the GH dose. Funduscopic examination of patients is recommended at the initiation and periodically during the course of GH therapy. Patients with CRI and Turner syndrome may be at increased risk for development of IH.

As with any protein, local or systemic allergic reactions may occur. Parents/Patient should be informed that such reactions are possible and that prompt medical attention should be sought if allergic reactions occur.

Laboratory Tests: Serum levels of inorganic phosphorus, alkaline phosphatase, and parathyroid hormone (PTH) may increase with Nutropin AQ therapy.

Untreated hypothyroidism prevents optimal response to Nutropin AQ. Patients with Turner syndrome have an inherently increased risk of developing autoimmune thyroid disease. Changes in thyroid hormone laboratory measurements may develop during Nutropin AQ treatment. Therefore, patients should have periodic thyroid function tests and should be treated with thyroid hormone when indicated.

Drug Interactions: Excessive glucocorticoid therapy will inhibit the growth-promoting effect of human GH. Patients with ACTH deficiency should have their glucocorticoid-replacement dose carefully adjusted to avoid an inhibitory effect on growth.

The use of Nutropin AQ in patients with chronic renal insufficiency receiving glucocorticoid therapy has not been evaluated. Concomitant glucocorticoid therapy may inhibit the growth-promoting effect of Nutropin AQ. If glucocorticoid replacement is required, the glucocorticoid dose should be carefully adjusted.

There was no evidence in the controlled studies of GH's interaction with drugs commonly used in chronic renal insufficiency patients. Limited published data indicate that GH treatment increases cytochrome P450 (CP450) mediated antipyrine clearance in man. These data suggest that GH administration may alter the clearance of compounds known to be metabolized by CP450 liver enzymes (e.g., corticosteroids, sex steroids, anticonvulsants, cyclosporin). Careful monitoring is advisable when GH is administered in combination with other drugs known to be metabolized by CP450 liver enzymes.

Carcinogenesis, Mutagenesis, Impairment of Fertility: Carcinogenicity, mutagenicity, and reproduction studies have not been conducted with Nutropin AQ.

Pregnancy: Pregnancy (Category C). Animal reproduction studies have not been conducted with Nutropin AQ. It is also not known whether Nutropin AQ can cause fetal harm when administered to a pregnant woman or can affect reproduction capacity. Nutropin AQ should be given to a pregnant woman only if clearly needed.

Nursing Mothers: It is not known whether Nutropin AQ is excreted in human milk. Because many drugs are excreted in human milk, caution should be exercised when Nutropin AQ is administered to a nursing mother.

Information for Patients: Patients being treated with GH and/or their parents should be informed of the potential benefits and risks associated with treatment. If home use is determined to be desirable by the physician, instructions on

Continued on next page

Nutropin AQ—Cont.

appropriate use should be given, including a review of the contents of the Patient Information Insert. This information is intended to aid in the safe and effective administration of the medication. It is not a disclosure of all possible adverse or intended effects.

If home use is prescribed, a puncture-resistant container for the disposal of used syringes and needles should be recommended to the patient. Patients and/or parents should be thoroughly instructed in the importance of proper disposal and cautioned against any reuse of needles and syringes (see Patient Information Insert).

ADVERSE REACTIONS

As with all protein pharmaceuticals, a small percentage of patients may develop antibodies to the protein. GH antibody binding capacities below 2 mg/L have not been associated with growth attenuation. In some cases when binding capacity exceeds 2 mg/L, growth attenuation has been observed. In clinical studies of pediatric patients that were treated with Nutropin® [somatropin (rDNA origin) for injection] for the first time, 0/107 growth hormone—deficient (GHD) patients, 0/125 CRI patients, and 0/112 Turner syndrome patients screened for antibody production developed antibodies with binding capacities ≥2 mg/L at six months. In a clinical study of patients that were treated with Nutropin AQ® [somatropin (rDNA origin) injection] for the first time, 0/38 GHD patients screened for antibody production for up to 15 months developed antibodies with binding capacities ≥2 mg/L.

Additional short-term immunologic and renal function studies were carried out in a group of patients with chronic renal insufficiency after approximately one year of treatment to detect other potential adverse effects of antibodies to GH. Testing included measurements of C1q, C3, C4, rheumatoid factor, creatinine, creatinine clearance, and BUN. No adverse effects of GH antibodies were noted.

In addition to an evaluation of compliance with the prescribed treatment program and thyroid status, testing for antibodies to GH should be carried out in any patient who fails to respond to therapy.

Injection site discomfort has been reported. This is more commonly observed in children switched from another GH product to Nutropin AQ. Experience with Nutropin AQ in adults is limited.

Leukemia has been reported in a small number of GHD patients treated with GH. It is uncertain whether this increased risk is related to the pathology of GH deficiency itself, GH therapy, or other associated treatments such as radiation therapy for intracranial tumors. On the basis of current evidence, experts cannot conclude that GH therapy is responsible for these occurrences. The risk to GHD, CRI, or Turner syndrome patients, if any, remains to be established.

Other adverse drug reactions that have been reported in GH-treated patients include the following: 1) Metabolic: mild, transient peripheral edema. In GHD adults, edema or peripheral edema was reported in 41% of GH-treated patients and 25% of placebo-treated patients. 2) Musculoskeletal: arthralgias; carpal tunnel syndrome. In GHD adults, arthralgias and other joint disorders were reported in 27% of GH-treated patients and 15% of placebo-treated patients. 3) Skin: rare increased growth of pre-existing nevi; patients should be monitored for malignant transformation. 4) Endocrine: gynecomastia. Rare pancreatitis.

OVERDOSAGE

Acute overdosage could lead to hyperglycemia. Long-term overdosage could result in signs and symptoms of gigantism and/or acromegaly consistent with the known effects of excess GH. (See recommended and maximal dosage instructions given below.)

DOSAGE AND ADMINISTRATION

The Nutropin AQ dosage and administration schedule should be individualized for each patient. Response to GH therapy in pediatric patients tends to decrease with time. However, in pediatric patients failure to increase growth rate, particularly during the first year of therapy, suggests the need for close assessment of compliance and evaluation of other causes of growth failure, such as hypothyroidism, under-nutrition, and advanced bone age.

Dosage

Pediatric Growth Hormone Deficiency (GHD)

A weekly dosage of up to 0.30 mg/kg of body weight divided into daily subcutaneous injection is recommended. In pubertal patients, a weekly dosage of up to 0.7 mg/kg divided daily may be used.

Adult Growth Hormone Deficiency (GHD)

The recommended dosage at the start of therapy is not more than 0.006 mg/kg given as a daily subcutaneous injection. The dose may be increased according to individual patient requirements to a maximum of 0.025 mg/kg daily in patients under 35 years and to a maximum of 0.0125 mg/kg daily in patients over 35 years.

To minimize the occurrence of adverse events in older or overweight patients, lower doses may be necessary. During therapy, dosage should be decreased if required by the occurrence of side effects or excessive IGF-I levels.

Chronic Renal Insufficiency (CRI)

A weekly dosage of up to 0.35 mg/kg of body weight divided into daily subcutaneous injection is recommended.

Nutropin AQ therapy may be continued up to the time of renal transplantation.

In order to optimize therapy for patients who require dialysis, the following guidelines for injection schedule are recommended:

1. Hemodialysis patients should receive their injection at night just prior to going to sleep or at least 3–4 hours after their hemodialysis to prevent hematoma formation due to the heparin.
2. Chronic Cycling Peritoneal Dialysis (CCPD) patients should receive their injection in the morning after they have completed dialysis.
3. Chronic Ambulatory Peritoneal Dialysis (CAPD) patients should receive their injection in the evening at the time of the overnight exchange.

Turner Syndrome

A weekly dosage of up to 0.375 mg/kg of body weight divided into equal doses 3 to 7 times per week by subcutaneous injection is recommended.

Administration

The solution should be clear immediately after removal from the refrigerator. Occasionally, after refrigeration, you may notice that small colorless particles of protein are present in the solution. This is not unusual for solutions containing proteins. Allow the vial to come to room temperature and gently swirl. If the solution is cloudy, the contents **MUST NOT** be injected.

Before needle insertion, wipe the septum of the Nutropin AQ vial with rubbing alcohol or an antiseptic solution to prevent contamination of the contents by microorganisms that may be introduced by repeated needle insertions. It is recommended that Nutropin AQ be administered using sterile, disposable syringes and needles. The syringes should be of small enough volume that the prescribed dose can be drawn from the vial with reasonable accuracy.

STABILITY AND STORAGE

Vial contents are stable for 28 days after initial use when stored at 2–8°C/36–46°F (under refrigeration). **Avoid freezing the vial of Nutropin AQ.**

HOW SUPPLIED

Nutropin AQ is supplied as 10 mg (approximately 30 IU) of sterile liquid somatropin per vial.

Each carton contains six single vial cartons containing one 2 mL vial of Nutropin AQ® [somatropin (rDNA origin) injection] (5 mg/mL). NDC 50242-114-11.

Nutropin AQ® [somatropin (rDNA origin) injection] manufactured by:

Genentech, Inc.
1 DNA Way
South San Francisco, CA 94080-4990

4810905

 Revised April 2000

Shown in Product Identification Guide, page 313

NUTROPIN DEPOT™ ℞

[somatropin (rDNA origin) for injectable suspension]

DESCRIPTION

Nutropin Depot™ [somatropin (rDNA origin) for injectable suspension] is a long-acting dosage form of recombinant human growth hormone (rhGH). Somatropin has 191 amino acid residues and a molecular weight of 22,125 daltons. The amino acid sequence of the product is identical to that of pituitary-derived human growth hormone. The protein is synthesized by a specific laboratory strain of *E. coli* as a precursor consisting of the rhGH molecule preceded by the secretion signal from an *E. coli* protein. This precursor is directed to the plasma membrane of the cell. The signal sequence is removed and the native protein is secreted into the periplasm so that the protein is folded appropriately as it is synthesized.

Somatropin is a highly purified preparation. Biological potency is determined using a cell proliferation bioassay.

The Nutropin Depot formulation consists of micronized particles of rhGH embedded in biocompatible, biodegradable polylactide-coglycolide (PLG) microspheres. Nutropin Depot is packaged in vials as a sterile, white to off-white, preservative-free, free-flowing powder. Before administration, the powder is suspended in Diluent for Nutropin Depot (a sterile aqueous solution).

Each 13.5 mg 3 cc single-use vial of Nutropin Depot contains 13.5 mg somatropin, 1.2 mg zinc acetate, 0.8 mg zinc carbonate, and 68.9 mg PLG.

Each 18 mg 3 cc single-use vial of Nutropin Depot contains 18 mg somatropin, 1.6 mg zinc acetate, 1.1 mg zinc carbonate, and 91.8 mg PLG.

Each 22.5 mg 3 cc single-use vial of Nutropin Depot contains 22.5 mg somatropin, 2.0 mg zinc acetate, 1.4 mg zinc carbonate, and 114.8 mg PLG.

Each dosage size contains an overage of rhGH microspheres to ensure delivery of labeled contents.

Each 1.5 mL single-use vial of Diluent for Nutropin Depot contains 30 mg/mL carboxymethylcellulose sodium salt, 1 mg/mL polysorbate 20, 9 mg/mL sodium chloride, and sterile water for injection; pH 5.8–7.2.

CLINICAL PHARMACOLOGY

General

In vivo preclinical and clinical testing has demonstrated that growth hormone (GH) stimulates longitudinal bone growth and elevates insulin-like growth factor-I (IGF-I) levels.

Actions that have been demonstrated for hGH include:

A. Tissue Growth—1) Skeletal Growth: GH stimulates skeletal growth in pediatric patients with growth failure due to a lack of adequate secretion of endogenous GH. Skeletal growth is accomplished at the epiphyseal plates at the ends of a growing bone. Growth and metabolism of epiphyseal plate cells are directly stimulated by GH and one of its mediators, IGF-I. Serum levels of IGF-I are low in children and adolescents who are growth hormone deficient (GHD), but increase during treatment with GH. In pediatric patients, new bone is formed at the epiphyses in response to GH and IGF-I. This results in linear growth until these growth plates fuse at the end of puberty. 2) Cell Growth: Treatment with hGH results in an increase in both the number and the size of skeletal muscle cells. 3) Organ Growth: GH increases the size of internal organs, including kidneys, and increases red cell mass. Treatment of hypophysectomized or genetic dwarf rats with GH results in increases in organ and overall body growth. In normal rats subjected to nephrectomy-induced uremia, GH promoted skeletal and body growth.

B. Protein Metabolism—Linear growth is facilitated in part by GH-stimulated protein synthesis. This is reflected by nitrogen retention as demonstrated by a decline in urinary nitrogen excretion and blood urea during GH therapy.

C. Carbohydrate Metabolism—GH is a modulator of carbohydrate metabolism. Patients with inadequate endogenous secretion of GH sometimes experience fasting hypoglycemia that is improved by treatment with GH. GH therapy may decrease insulin sensitivity. Administration of hGH formulated for daily dosing resulted in increased mean fasting and postprandial insulin levels, more commonly in overweight or obese individuals. Mean trough levels for fasting and postprandial insulin were unchanged after 3 or 6 months of Nutropin Depot therapy in GHD children. As with daily GH, mean trough levels for fasting glucose, postprandial glucose, and hemoglobin A_{1c} remained unchanged after 3 or 6 months of Nutropin Depot therapy.

D. Lipid Metabolism—In GHD patients, administration of GH formulated for daily dosing resulted in lipid mobilization, reduction in body fat stores, increased plasma fatty acids, and decreased plasma cholesterol levels.

E. Mineral Metabolism—The retention of total body potassium in response to GH administration apparently results from cellular growth. Serum levels of inorganic phosphorus may increase slightly in patients with inadequate secretion of endogenous GH due to metabolic activity associated with bone growth as well as increased tubular reabsorption of phosphate by the kidney. Serum calcium is not significantly altered in these patients. Sodium retention also occurs. (See PRECAUTIONS: Laboratory Tests.) GH therapy results in increases in serum alkaline phosphatase.

F. Connective Tissue Metabolism—GH stimulates the synthesis of chondroitin sulfate and collagen as well as the urinary excretion of hydroxyproline.

Pharmacokinetics

Nutropin Depot is a long-acting dosage form of somatropin designed to be administered by subcutaneous (SC) injection once or twice monthly. Following the injection, bioactive rhGH is released from the microspheres into the SC environment initially by diffusion, followed by both polymer degradation and diffusion. Although no studies have been performed that address the distribution, elimination, or metabolism of Nutropin Depot, once released and absorbed the rhGH is believed to be distributed and eliminated in a manner similar to somatropin formulated for daily administration.

The serum hGH concentration-time profiles of single doses of 0.75 mg/kg and 1.5 mg/kg of Nutropin Depot have been characterized in pediatric GHD patients (refer to Figure 1). The in vivo profiles are characterized by an initial rapid release followed by a slow decline in GH concentration. Both the maximum concentrations achieved (C_{max}) and total exposure ($AUC_{0-28\ days}$) appear to be proportional to dose. Serum hGH levels greater than 1 μg/L persist for approximately 11–14 days postdose for the two doses. Repeated dosing of Nutropin Depot over 6 months showed no progressive accumulation of GH.

Absorption—In a study of Nutropin Depot in pediatric patients with GHD, an SC dose of 0.75 mg/kg (n=12) or 1.5 mg/kg (n=8) was administered. The mean ±SD hGH C_{max} values were 48±26 μg/L and 90±23 μg/L, respectively, at 12–13 hours postdose. The corresponding $AUC_{0-28\ days}$ values were 83±49 μg • day/L and 140±34 μg • day/L, respectively, for the two doses. For the 0.75 mg/kg and 1.5 mg/kg doses, the $AUC_{0-2\ days}$ accounted for approximately 52±16 percent and 61±10 percent of the total $AUC_{0-28\ days}$, respectively. Estimates of relative bioavailability in GHD children for a single dose of Nutropin Depot ranged from 33% to 38% when compared to a single dose of Nutropin AQ® [somatropin (rDNA origin) injection] in healthy adults, and from 48% to 55% when compared to chronically dosed Protropin® (somatrem for injection) in GHD children.

Distribution—Animal studies with rhGH formulated for daily administration showed that GH localizes to highly perfused organs, particularly the liver and kidney. The volume of distribution at steady state for rhGH formulated for

daily administration in healthy adult males is about 50 mL/kg body weight, approximating the serum volume.
Metabolism—Both the liver and kidney have been shown to be important metabolizing organs for GH. Animal studies using rhGH formulated for daily administration suggest that the kidney is the dominant organ of clearance. GH is filtered at the glomerulus and reabsorbed in the proximal tubules. It is then cleaved within renal cells into its constituent amino acids, which return to the systemic circulation.
Elimination—The mean terminal $t_{1/2}$ after intravenous (IV) administration of rhGH formulated for daily administration in healthy adult males is estimated to be 19.5±3.1 minutes. Clearance of rhGH after IV administration in healthy adults and children is reported to be in the range of 116–174 mL/hr/kg.

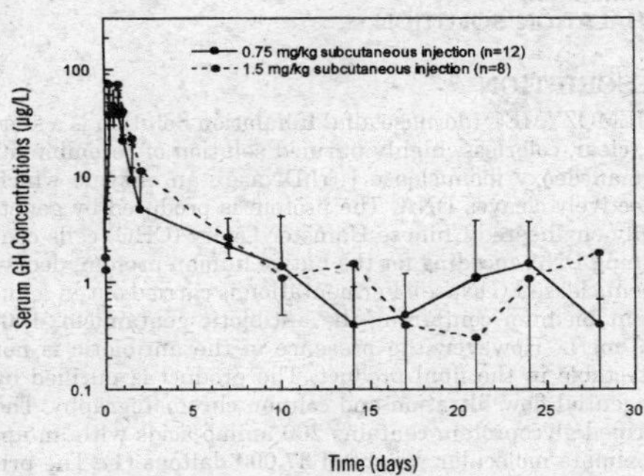

Figure 1
Single-Dose Mean (SD) GH Concentrations in Pediatric GHD Patients

Special Populations
Pediatric—Available literature data suggest that rhGH clearances are similar in adults and children.
Gender—Following administration of either 0.75 mg/kg or 1.5 mg/kg Nutropin Depot, Day 1 GH levels were higher in females compared to males. No relationship was observed between gender and pharmacodynamic marker (IGF-I and IGFBP-3) levels.
Race—The effect of race on Nutropin Depot disposition is unknown due to the limited number of non-Caucasian patients in the Nutropin Depot studies.
Growth Hormone Deficiency—Nutropin Depot has not been studied in healthy adults or children. However, reported values for clearance of rhGH formulated for daily administration in adults and children were GHD range 138–245 mL/hr/kg and are similar to those observed in healthy adults and children. Mean terminal $t_{1/2}$ values following IV and SC administration in adult and pediatric patients with GHD are also similar to those observed in healthy adult males.
Renal Insufficiency—Nutropin Depot has not been studied in patients with renal insufficiency. Children and adults with chronic renal failure (CRF) and end-stage renal disease (ESRD) tend to have decreased clearance of rhGH formulated for daily administration compared with normals. Endogenous GH production may also increase in some individuals with ESRD. However, no GH accumulation has been reported in children with CRF or ESRD dosed with daily regimens.
Hepatic Insufficiency—Nutropin Depot has not been studied in patients with hepatic insufficiency. A reduction in clearance of rhGH formulated for daily administration has been noted in patients with severe liver dysfunction. The clinical significance of this decrease is unknown.

Pharmacodynamics
IGF-I levels peaked between 1.5 and 3.5 days postdose and remained above baseline for approximately 16 to 20 days, confirming GH activity for an extended period. Repeated dosing of Nutropin Depot over 6 months showed no progressive accumulation of IGF-I (as shown in Figure 2) or IGF-binding protein 3 (IGFBP-3).

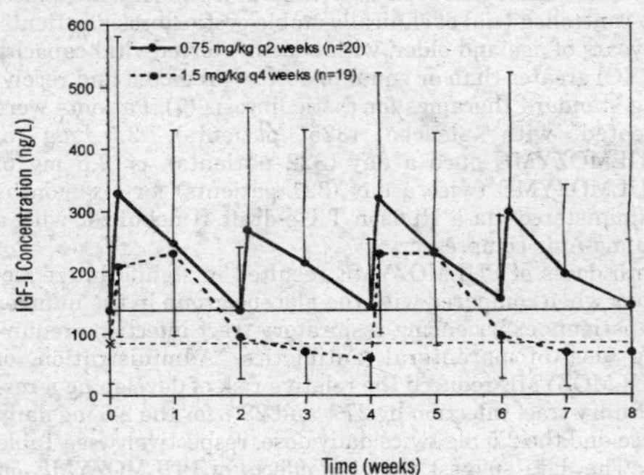

Figure 2
Repeated-Dose Mean (SD) IGF-I Concentrations in Pediatric GHD Patients

EFFICACY STUDIES

Pediatric Growth Hormone Deficiency (GHD)
In two multicenter, open-label clinical studies in prepubertal children (mean age (±SD) 7.4±2.8) with idiopathic or organic GHD previously untreated with rhGH, 91 patients were treated with Nutropin Depot at 1.5 mg/kg once monthly or 0.75 mg/kg twice monthly by subcutaneous injection for up to six months. (See DOSAGE AND ADMINISTRATION for the number of injections required per dose.) The mean prestudy growth rate was 4.8±2.4 cm/yr (n=89). The dose-pooled, mean 6-month annualized growth rate on Nutropin Depot therapy was 8.4±2.2 cm/yr (n=89).
Seventy-six patients continued treatment in an extension study. For patients who completed 12 months the mean growth rate was 7.8±1.9 cm/yr for the two dose groups combined (n=69). Mean height SD score changed from –3.0±1.0 prestudy to –2.5±0.9 at Month 12 (n=69). The mean 0 to 12 month change in bone age was 1.0±0.4 years (n=63). During the long-term extension study, fourteen of seventy-five (19%) patients discontinued due to dissatisfaction with growth response. Historical studies of GHD children treated with daily Protropin® (somatrem for injection) or Nutropin® [somatropin (rDNA origin) for injection] injections for 12 months at 0.3 mg/kg weekly had the following mean values: baseline growth rate 3.6 to 4.8 cm/yr; first year growth rate 10.1 to 11.3 cm/yr; first year change in bone age 1.1 to 1.5 years.
In a dose-ranging study, 24 patients previously treated with daily GH (mean age 9.6±2.2 years; mean duration of prior GH therapy 2.8±1.6 yr, range 0.9 to 6.1 yr) were switched to Nutropin Depot therapy at the above doses. The mean growth rate on previous treatment was 8.2±3.0 cm/yr (range 3.2 to 13.1 cm/yr) and on Nutropin Depot was 5.1±2.0 cm/yr (range 2.4 to 9.6 cm/yr). During a long-term extension study, four of ten previously treated patients discontinued due to dissatisfaction with growth response. Historical studies of GHD children (n=181) treated with daily Protropin® (somatrem for injection) or Nutropin® [somatropin (rDNA origin) for injection] at a dose of 0.3 mg/kg weekly had the following mean growth rates: first year growth rate 9.7 to 11.4 cm/yr; second year growth rate 8.1 to 8.9 cm/yr; third year growth rate 7.5 to 7.8 cm/yr; fourth year growth rate 6.6 to 7.1 cm/yr.

INDICATIONS AND USAGE

Nutropin Depot™ [somatropin (rDNA origin) for injectable suspension] is indicated for the long-term treatment of growth failure due to a lack of adequate endogenous GH secretion.
Considerations for use:—As with any GH treatment, patients should be monitored closely throughout therapy for growth response to Nutropin Depot. Failure to respond adequately requires careful assessment, as described under DOSAGE AND ADMINISTRATION. Patients for whom no discernible cause is found should be considered for a course of treatment with a daily form of rhGH. Experience in patients who were treated with daily GH and switched to Nutropin Depot is limited.

CONTRAINDICATIONS

Growth hormone should not be initiated to treat patients with acute critical illness due to complications following open heart or abdominal surgery, multiple accidental trauma, or to patients having acute respiratory failure. Two placebo-controlled clinical trials in non-growth hormone-deficient adult patients (n=522) with these conditions revealed a significant increase in mortality (41.9% vs. 19.3%) among somatropin-treated patients (doses 5.3–8 mg/day) compared to those receiving placebo (see WARNINGS).
Nutropin Depot should not be used for growth promotion in pediatric patients with closed epiphyses.
Nutropin Depot should not be used in patients with active neoplasia. GH therapy should be discontinued if evidence of neoplasia develops.

WARNINGS

See CONTRAINDICATIONS for information on increased mortality in patients with acute critical illnesses in intensive care units due to complications following open heart or abdominal surgery, multiple accidental trauma, or with acute respiratory failure. The safety of continuing growth hormone treatment in patients receiving replacement doses for approved indications who concurrently develop these illnesses has not been established. Therefore, the potential benefit of treatment continuation with growth hormone in patients having acute critical illnesses should be weighed against the potential risk.

PRECAUTIONS

General: Nutropin Depot should be prescribed by physicians experienced in the diagnosis and management of patients with GHD.
Because GH may reduce insulin sensitivity, patients should be monitored for evidence of glucose intolerance.
For patients with diabetes mellitus, the insulin dose may require adjustment when GH therapy is instituted. Because GH may reduce insulin sensitivity, particularly in obese individuals, patients should be observed for evidence of glucose intolerance. Patients with diabetes or glucose intolerance should be monitored closely during GH therapy.
Patients with symptomatic hypoglycemia associated with GHD should be closely monitored.
Patients with a history of an intracranial lesion should be examined frequently for progression or recurrence of the lesion. In pediatric patients, clinical literature has demonstrated no relationship between GH replacement therapy and CNS tumor recurrence or new extracranial tumors.
Slipped capital femoral epiphysis may occur more frequently in patients with endocrine disorders or in patients undergoing rapid growth.
Progression of scoliosis can occur in patients who experience rapid growth. Because GH increases growth rate, patients with a history of scoliosis who are treated with GH should be monitored for progression of scoliosis. GH has not been shown to increase the incidence of scoliosis.
Intracranial hypertension (IH) with papilledema, visual changes, headache, nausea, and/or vomiting has been reported in a small number of patients treated with GH products. Symptoms usually occurred within the first 8 weeks of the initiation of GH therapy. In all reported cases, IH-associated signs and symptoms resolved after termination of therapy or a reduction of the GH dose. Funduscopic examination of patients is recommended at the initiation and periodically during the course of GH therapy.
As with any protein, local or systemic allergic reactions may occur. Parents/Patients should be informed that such reactions are possible and that prompt medical attention should be sought if allergic reactions occur (see ADVERSE REACTIONS).
Laboratory Tests: Serum levels of inorganic phosphorus, alkaline phosphatase, and parathyroid hormone (PTH) may increase with GH therapy.
Untreated hypothyroidism prevents optimal response to GH. Changes in thyroid hormone laboratory measurements may develop during GH treatment. Therefore, patients should have periodic thyroid function tests and should be treated with thyroid hormone when indicated.
Drug Interactions: Excessive glucocorticoid therapy will inhibit the growth-promoting effect of human GH. Patients with ACTH deficiency should have their glucocorticoid-replacement dose carefully adjusted to avoid an inhibitory effect on growth.
Limited published data indicate that GH treatment increases cytochrome P450 (CP450) mediated antipyrine clearance in humans. These data suggest that GH administration may alter the clearance of compounds known to be metabolized by CP450 liver enzymes (e.g., corticosteroids, sex steroids, anticonvulsants, cyclosporin). Careful monitoring is advisable when GH is administered in combination with other drugs known to be metabolized by CP450 liver enzymes.
Carcinogenesis, Mutagenesis, Impairment of Fertility: Carcinogenicity, mutagenicity, and fertility studies have not been conducted with Nutropin Depot.
Pregnancy Category C: Animal reproduction studies have not been conducted with Nutropin Depot. It is also not known whether Nutropin Depot can cause fetal harm when administered to a pregnant woman or can affect reproduction capacity. Nutropin Depot should be given to a pregnant woman only if clearly needed.
Nursing Mothers: It is not known whether GH is excreted in human milk. Because many drugs are excreted in human milk, caution should be exercised when Nutropin Depot is administered to a nursing mother.
Information for Patients: Patients being treated with Nutropin Depot and/or their parents should be informed of the potential benefits and risks associated with treatment. If home use is determined to be desirable by the physician, instructions on appropriate use should be given, including a review of the contents of the Patient Information Insert. This information is intended to aid in the safe and effective administration of the medication. It is not a disclosure of all possible adverse or intended effects.
If home use is prescribed, a puncture-resistant container for the disposal of used syringes and needles should be recommended to the patient. Patients and/or parents should be thoroughly instructed in the importance of proper disposal and cautioned against any reuse of needles and syringes (see Patient Information Insert).

ADVERSE REACTIONS

As with all protein pharmaceuticals, patients may develop antibodies to the protein. GH antibody-binding capacities below 2 mg/L have not been associated with growth attenuation. In some cases when binding capacity exceeds 2

Continued on next page

Patient Weight (kg)	Number of Injections Per Dose	
	0.75 mg/kg twice monthly	1.5 mg/kg once monthly
≤15	1	1
>15–30	1	2
>30–45	2	3
>45–60	2	*
>60	3	*

*Twice-monthly dosing recommended

Nutropin Depot—Cont.

mg/L, growth attenuation has been observed. In clinical studies of pediatric patients who were treated with Nutropin Depot, 0/138 patients with GHD screened for antibody production developed antibodies with binding capacities ≥2 mg/L at any time during a treatment period of up to 17.4 months.
In addition to an evaluation of compliance with the prescribed treatment program and thyroid status, testing for antibodies to GH should be carried out in any patient who fails to respond to therapy.
In studies involving 138 pediatric patients treated with Nutropin Depot, the most frequent adverse reactions were injection-site reactions, which occurred in nearly all patients. On average, 2 to 3 injection-site adverse reactions were reported per injection. These reactions included nodules (61% of injections), erythema (53%), pain post-injection (47%), pain during injection (43%), bruising (20%), itching (13%), lipoatrophy (13%), and swelling or puffiness (8%). The intensity of these reactions was generally rated mild to moderate, with pain during injection occasionally rated as severe (7%).
Adverse reactions observed less frequently in the Nutropin Depot studies which were considered possibly, probably, or definitely related to the drug by the treating physician (usually occurring 1–3 days postdose) included: headache (13% of subjects), nausea (8%), lower extremity pain (7%), fever (7%), and vomiting (5%). These symptoms were generally self-limited and well-tolerated. One patient experienced a generalized body rash that was most likely an allergic reaction to Nutropin Depot.
Leukemia has been reported in a small number of GHD patients treated with GH. It is uncertain whether this increased risk is related to the pathology of GH deficiency itself, GH therapy, or other associated treatments such as radiation therapy for intracranial tumors. On the basis of current evidence, experts cannot conclude that GH therapy is responsible for these occurrences.
Other adverse drug reactions that have been reported in GH-treated patients include the following: 1) Metabolic: mild, transient peripheral edema; 2) Musculoskeletal: arthralgia, carpal tunnel syndrome; 3) Skin: rare increased growth of pre-existing nevi; patients should be monitored for malignant transformation; 4) Endocrine: gynecomastia; and 5) Rare pancreatitis. Of these reactions, only edema (<1% of patients) and arthralgia (4%) were reported as related to drug in the Nutropin Depot studies.

OVERDOSAGE

The recommended dosage of Nutropin Depot should not be exceeded. Acute overdosage could lead to fluid retention, headache, nausea, vomiting, and/or hyperglycemia. Long-term overdosage could result in signs and symptoms of gigantism and/or acromegaly, consistent with the known effects of excess GH. (See recommended dosage instructions given below.)

DOSAGE AND ADMINISTRATION

The Nutropin Depot dosage and administration schedule should be individualized for each patient. Reponse to GH therapy in pediatric patients tends to decrease over time. However in pediatric patients, failure to increase growth rate, particularly during the first year of therapy, suggests the need for close assessment of compliance and evaluation of other causes of growth failure, such as hypothyroidism, undernutrition, and advanced bone age.
Once-Monthly Injection—It is recommended that an SC injection at a dosage of 1.5 mg/kg body weight be administered on the same day of each month. Dosages above the recommended once-monthly regimen have not been studied in clinical trials. Note: subjects over 15 kg will require more than one injection per dose.
Twice-Monthly Injections—It is recommended that an SC injection at a dosage of 0.75 mg/kg body weight be administered twice each month on the same days of each month (e.g., Days 1 and 15 of each month). Dosages above the recommended twice-monthly regimen have not been studied in clinical trials. Note: subjects over 30 kg will require more than one injection per dose.
The table below indicates the required number of injections per dose.
[See table at top of previous page]

Preparation of Dose

Nutropin Depot powder may **only** be suspended in Diluent for Nutropin Depot supplied in the kit and administered with the supplied needles.

1. Using the chart below, determine the volume of diluent needed to suspend Nutropin Depot. Withdraw the diluent into a 3 cc syringe using the needle supplied in the kit. Only the diluent supplied in the kit should be used for reconstitution, and any remaining diluent should be discarded.

Vial Size (mg somatropin)	Volume of Diluent to Be Added (mL)
13.5	0.8
18	1.0
22.5	1.2

Note: Since the suspension is viscous and prevents complete withdrawal of the entire vial contents, the vials are overfilled to ensure delivery of the labeled amount of somatropin. Using these diluent volumes for final suspension results in a final concentration of 19 mg/mL somatropin in each vial size.

2. Inject the diluent into the vial against the vial wall. Swirl the vial vigorously for up to 2 minutes to disperse the powder in the diluent. Mixing is complete when the suspension appears uniform, thick, and milky, and all the powder is fully dispersed. Do not store the vial after reconstitution or the suspension may settle.
3. Withdraw the required dose. Only one vial should be used for each injection. Replace the needle with a new needle from the kit and administer the dose immediately to avoid settling of the suspension in the syringe. Deliver the dose from the syringe at a continuous rate over not more than 5 seconds. Discard unused vial contents as the product contains no preservative. An extra needle has been provided in the kit.

Stability and Storage

Before Suspension—Nutropin Depot and diluent vials must be stored at 2–8°C/36–46°F (under refrigeration). **Avoid freezing the vials of Nutropin Depot and Diluent for Nutropin Depot.** Do not expose the Nutropin Depot vial to temperatures above 25°C (77°F). Expiration dates are stated on the labels.
After Suspension—Because Nutropin Depot contains no preservatives, all injections must be given immediately. Do not allow the suspension to settle prior to withdrawal of the dose. Suspended solution cannot be stored or used to suspend another vial of Nutropin Depot.

HOW SUPPLIED

Nutropin Depot is supplied as single-use vials with 13.5 mg, 18 mg, or 22.5 mg sterile, preservative-free somatropin powder per vial.
Each 13.5 mg kit contains one single-use 13.5 mg vial of Nutropin Depot™ [somatropin (rDNA origin) for injectable suspension], one 1.5 mL single-use vial of Diluent for Nutropin Depot, and three 21-gauge, 1/2" needles: NDC 50242-032-35.
Each 18 mg kit contains one single-use 18 mg vial of Nutropin Depot™ [somatropin (rDNA origin) for injectable suspension], one 1.5 mL single-use vial of Diluent for Nutropin Depot, and three 21-gauge, 1/2" needles: NDC 50242-034-41.
Each 22.5 mg kit contains one single-use 22.5 mg vial of Nutropin Depot™ [somatropin (rDNA origin) for injectable suspension], one 1.5 mL single-use vial of Diluent for Nutropin Depot, and three 21-gauge, 1/2" needles: NDC 50242-036-54.
Nutropin Depot™ [somatropin (rDNA origin) for injectable suspension] and **Diluent for Nutropin Depot** are manufactured for:
Genentech, Inc.
1 DNA Way
South San Francisco, CA 94080-4990 4819500
 December 1999
Shown in Product Identification Guide, page 313

PROTROPIN® ℞
(somatrem for injection)

DESCRIPTION

Protropin® (somatrem for injection), is a polypeptide hormone produced by recombinant DNA technology. Protropin has 192 amino acid residues and a molecular weight of about 22,000 daltons. The product contains the identical sequence of 191 amino acids constituting pituitary-derived human growth hormone plus an additional amino acid, methionine, on the N-terminus of the molecule. Protropin is synthesized in a special laboratory strain of *E. coli* bacteria which has been modified by the addition of the gene for human growth hormone production.
Protropin is a highly purified preparation. Biological potency is determined using a cell proliferation bioassay.
Protropin is a sterile, white, lyophilized powder intended for intramuscular or subcutaneous administration after reconstitution with Bacteriostatic Water for Injection, USP (benzyl alcohol preserved).
Each 5 mg Protropin vial contains 5 mg (approximately 15 IU) somatrem, lyophilized with 40 mg mannitol, and 1.7 mg sodium phosphates (0.1 mg sodium phosphate monobasic and 1.6 mg sodium phosphate dibasic).
Each 10 mg Protropin vial contains 10 mg (approximately 30 IU) somatrem, lyophilized with 80 mg mannitol, and 3.4 mg sodium phosphates (0.2 mg sodium phosphate monobasic and 3.2 mg sodium phosphate dibasic).
Phosphoric acid may be used for pH adjustment.
Bacteriostatic Water for Injection, USP, is a sterile water containing 0.9 percent benzyl alcohol per mL as an antimicrobial preservative packaged in a multi-dose vial. The diluent pH is 4.5–7.0.

HOW SUPPLIED

Protropin® (somatrem for injection) is supplied as 5 mg (approximately 15 IU) or 10 mg (approximately 30 IU) of lyophilized, sterile, somatrem per vial.
Each 5 mg carton contains two vials of Protropin® (somatrem for injection) (5 mg per vial) and one 10 mL multiple dose vial of Bacteriostatic Water for Injection, USP (benzyl alcohol preserved). NDC 50242-015-02
Each 10 mg carton contains two vials of Protropin® (somatrem for injection) (10 mg per vial) and two 10 mL multiple dose vials of Bacteriostatic Water for Injection, USP (benzyl alcohol preserved). NDC 50242-016-20
Protropin® (somatrem for injection) manufactured by:
Genentech, Inc.
1 DNA Way
South Francisco, CA 94080-4990
Bacteriostatic Water for Injection, USP (benzyl alcohol preserved), manufactured for: **Genentech, Inc.**
4005310
 Revised January 1999
Shown in Product Identification Guide, page 313

PULMOZYME® ℞
(dornase alfa)
recombinant
INHALATION SOLUTION

DESCRIPTION

PULMOZYME® (dornase alfa) Inhalation Solution is a sterile, clear, colorless, highly purified solution of recombinant human deoxyribonuclease I (rhDNase), an enzyme which selectively cleaves DNA. The protein is produced by genetically engineered Chinese Hamster Ovary (CHO) cells containing DNA encoding for the native human protein, deoxyribonuclease I (DNase). Fermentation is carried out in a nutrient medium containing the antibiotic gentamicin, 100-200 mg/L. However, the presence of the antibiotic is not detectable in the final product. The product is purified by tangential flow filtration and column chromatography. The purified glycoprotein contains 260 amino acids with an approximate molecular weight of 37,000 daltons (1). The primary amino acid sequence is identical to that of the native human enzyme.
PULMOZYME is administered by inhalation of an aerosol mist produced by a compressed air driven nebulizer system (see Clinical Experience; DOSAGE AND ADMINISTRATION). Each PULMOZYME single-use ampule will deliver 2.5 mL of the solution to the nebulizer bowl. The aqueous solution contains 1.0 mg/mL dornase alfa, 0.15 mg/mL calcium chloride dihydrate and 8.77 mg/mL sodium chloride. The solution contains no preservative. The nominal pH of the solution is 6.3.

CLINICAL PHARMACOLOGY

General

In cystic fibrosis (CF) patients, retention of viscous purulent secretions in the airways contributes both to reduced pulmonary function and to exacerbations of infection (2,3).
Purulent pulmonary secretions contain very high concentrations of extracellular DNA released by degenerating leukocytes that accumulate in response to infection (4). In vitro, PULMOZYME hydrolyzes the DNA in sputum of CF patients and reduces sputum viscoelasticity (1).

Pharmacokinetics

When 2.5 mg PULMOZYME was administered by inhalation to eighteen CF patients, mean sputum concentrations of 3 µg/mL DNase were measurable within 15 minutes. Mean sputum concentrations declined to an average of 0.6 µg/mL two hours following inhalation. Inhalation of up to 10 mg TID of PULMOZYME by 4 CF patients for six consecutive days, did not result in a significant elevation of serum concentrations of DNase above normal endogenous levels (5,6). After administration of up to 2.5 mg of PULMOZYME twice daily for six months to 321 CF patients, no accumulation of serum DNase was noted.
PULMOZYME, 2.5 mg by inhalation, was administered daily to 98 patients aged 3 months to ≤10 years, and bronchoalveolar lavage (BAL) fluid was obtained within 90 minutes of the first dose. BAL DNase concentrations were detectable in all patients but showed a broad range, from 0.007 to 1.8 mcg/mL. Over an average of 14 days of exposure, serum DNase concentrations (mean ± s.d.) increased by 1.3 ± 1.3 ng/mL for the 3 months to <5 year age group and by 0.8 ± 1.2 ng/mL for the 5 to ≤10 year age group. The relationship between BAL or serum DNase concentration and adverse experiences and clinical outcomes is unknown.

Clinical Experience

PULMOZYME has been evaluated in a randomized, placebo-controlled trial of clinically stable cystic fibrosis patients, 5 years of age and older, with baseline forced vital capacity (FVC) greater than or equal to 40% of predicted and receiving standard therapies for cystic fibrosis (7). Patients were treated with placebo (325 patients), 2.5 mg of PULMOZYME once a day (322 patients), or 2.5 mg of PULMOZYME twice a day (321 patients) for six months administered via a Hudson T Up-draft II nebulizer with a Pulmo-Aide compressor.
Both doses of PULMOZYME resulted in significant reductions when compared with the placebo group in the number of patients experiencing respiratory tract infections requiring use of parenteral antibiotics. Administration of PULMOZYME reduced the relative risk of developing a respiratory tract infection by 27% and 29% for the 2.5 mg daily dose and the 2.5 mg twice daily dose, respectively (see Table 1). The data suggest that the effects of PULMOZYME on respiratory tract infections in older patients (>21 years) may be smaller than in younger patients, and that twice daily dosing may be required in the older patients. Patients with baseline FVC>85% may also benefit from twice a day dosing (see Table 1). The reduced risk of respiratory infec-

tion observed in PULMOZYME treated patients did not directly correlate with improvement in FEV_1 during the initial two weeks of therapy.

Within 8 days of the start of treatment with PULMOZYME, mean FEV_1 increased 7.9% in those treated once a day and 9.0% in those treated twice a day compared to the baseline values. The overall mean FEV_1 during long-term therapy increased 5.8% from baseline at the 2.5 mg daily dose level and 5.6% from baseline at the 2.5 mg twice daily dose level. Placebo recipients did not show significant mean changes in pulmonary function testing (see Figure 1).

For patients 5 years of age or older, with baseline FVC greater than or equal to 40%, administration of PULMOZYME decreased the incidence of occurrence of first respiratory tract infection requiring parenteral antibiotics, and improved mean FEV_1, regardless of age or baseline FVC.

[See table 1 at right]

Figure 1: Mean Percent Change from Baseline FEV_1 in Patients with FVC≥ 40% of Predicted

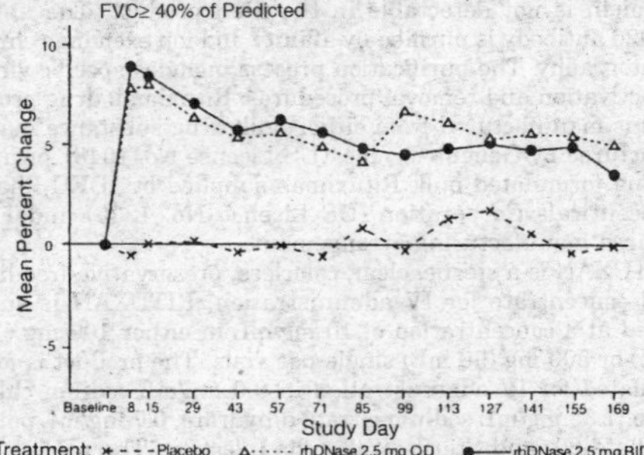

PULMOZYME has also been evaluated in a second randomized, placebo-controlled study in clinically stable patients with baseline FVC <40% of predicted (8). Patients were enrolled and treated with placebo (162 patients) or PULMOZYME 2.5 mg QD (158 patients) for twelve weeks. In patients who received PULMOZYME, there was an increase in mean change (as percent of baseline) compared to placebo in FEV_1 (9.4% vs. 2.1%, p< 0.001) and in FVC (12.4% vs. 7.3% p<0.01). PULMOZYME did not significantly reduce the risk of developing a respiratory tract infection requiring parenteral antibiotics (54% of PULMOZYME patients vs 55% of placebo patients had experienced a respiratory tract infection by 12 weeks, relative risk = .93, p=0.62).

Other Studies

Clinical trials have indicated that PULMOZYME therapy can be continued or initiated during an acute respiratory exacerbation.

Short-term dose ranging studies demonstrated that doses in excess of 2.5 mg BID did not provide further improvement in FEV_1. Patients who have received drug on a cyclical regimen (ie, administration of PULMOZYME 10 mg BID for 14 days, followed by a 14 day wash out period) showed rapid improvement in FEV_1 with the initiation of each cycle and a return to baseline with each PULMOZYME withdrawal.

INDICATIONS AND USAGE

Daily administration of PULMOZYME in conjunction with standard therapies is indicated in the management of cystic fibrosis patients to improve pulmonary function. In patients with an FVC ≥40% of predicted, daily administration of PULMOZYME has also been shown to reduce the risk of respiratory tract infections requiring parenteral antibiotics. Safety and efficacy of daily administration have not been demonstrated in patients for longer than twelve months.

CONTRAINDICATIONS

PULMOZYME is contraindicated in patients with known hypersensitivity to dornase alfa, Chinese Hamster Ovary cell products, or any component of the product.

WARNINGS

None.

PRECAUTIONS

General

PULMOZYME should be used in conjunction with standard therapies for CF.

Information for Patients

PULMOZYME must be stored in the refrigerator at 2–8°C (36–46°F) and protected from strong light. It should be kept refrigerated during transport and should not be exposed to room temperatures for a total time of 24 hours. The solution should be discarded if it is cloudy or discolored. PULMOZYME contains no preservative and, once opened, the entire contents of the ampule must be used or discarded. Patients should be instructed in the proper use and maintenance of the nebulizer and compressor system used in its delivery.

PULMOZYME should not be diluted or mixed with other drugs in the nebulizer. Mixing of PULMOZYME with other drugs could lead to adverse physicochemical and/or functional changes in PULMOZYME or the admixed compound.

Drug Interactions

Clinical trials have indicated that PULMOZYME can be effectively and safely used in conjunction with standard cystic fibrosis therapies including oral, inhaled and/or parenteral antibiotics, bronchodilators, enzyme supplements, vitamins, oral or inhaled corticosteroids, and analgesics. No formal drug interaction studies have been performed.

Table 1
Incidence of First Respiratory Tract Infection
Requiring Parenteral Antibiotics in Patients with FVC ≥40% of Predicted

	Placebo N=325	2.5 mg QD N=322	2.5 mg BID N=321
Percent of Patients Infected	43%	34%	33%
Relative Risk (vs placebo)		0.73	0.71
p-value (vs placebo)		0.015	0.007
Subgroup by Age and Baseline FVC	**Placebo (N)**	**2.5 mg QD (N)**	**2.5 mg BID (N)**
Age			
5–20 years	42% (201)	25% (199)	28% (184)
21 years and older	44% (124)	48% (123)	39% (137)
Baseline FVC			
40–85% Predicted	54% (194)	41% (201)	44% (203)
>85% Predicted	27% (131)	21% (121)	14% (118)

Table 2
Adverse Events Increased 3% or More in PULMOZYME Treated Patients Over Placebo in CF Clinical Trials

	Trial in Mild to Moderate CF Patients (FVC ≥40% of predicted) treated for 24 weeks			Trial in Advanced CF Patients (FVC <40% of predicted) treated for 12 weeks	
Adverse Event (of any severity or seriousness)	Placebo n=325	PULMOZYME QD n=322	PULMOZYME BID n=321	Placebo n=159	PULMOZYME QD n=161
Voice alteration	7%	12%	16%	6%	18%
Pharyngitis	33%	36%	40%	28%	32%
Rash	7%	10%	12%	1%	3%
Laryngitis	1%	3%	4%	1%	3%
Chest Pain	16%	18%	21%	23%	25%
Conjunctivitis	2%	4%	5%	0%	1%
Rhinitis	Differences were less than 3% for these adverse events in the Trial in mild to moderate CF patients			24%	30%
FVC decrease of ≥10% of predicted°				17%	22%
Fever				28%	32%
Dyspepsia				0%	3%
Dyspnea (when reported as serious)	Difference was less than 3% for this adverse event in the Trial in mild to moderate CF patients			12%†	17%†

°Single measurement only, does not reflect overall FVC changes
†Total reports of dyspnea (regardless of severity or seriousness) had a difference of less than 3% for the Trial in advanced CF patients

Carcinogenesis, Mutagenesis, Impairment of Fertility

Carcinogenesis: Lifetime studies in Sprague Dawley rats showed no carcinogenic effect when PULMOZYME was administered at doses up to 246 µg/kg body weight per day. PULMOZYME was administered to rats as an aerosol for up to 30 minutes per day, daily for two years, with resulting lower respiratory tract doses of up to 246 µg/kg per day, which represents up to a 28.8-fold multiple of the clinical dose. There was no increase in the development of benign or malignant neoplasms and no occurrence of unusual tumor types in rats after lifetime exposure.

Mutagenesis: Ames tests using six different tester strains of bacteria (4 of S. typhimurium and 2 of E. coli) at concentrations up to 5000 µg/plate, a cytogenetic assay using human peripheral blood lymphocytes at concentrations up to 2000 µg/plate, and a mouse lymphoma assay at concentrations up to 1000 µg/plate, with and without metabolic activation, revealed no evidence of mutagenesis potential. PULMOZYME was tested in a micronucleus (in vivo) assay for its potential to produce chromosome damage in bone marrow cells of mice following a bolus intravenous dose of 10 mg/kg on two consecutive days. No evidence of chromosomal damage was noted.

Impairment of Fertility: In studies with rats receiving up to 10 mg/kg/day, a dose representing systemic exposures greater than 600 times that expected following the recommended human dose, fertility and reproductive performance of both males and females was not affected.

Pregnancy (Category B)

Reproduction studies have been performed in rats and rabbits with intravenous doses up to 10 mg/kg/day, representing systemic exposures greater than 600 times that expected following the recommended human dose. These studies have revealed no evidence of impaired fertility, harm to the fetus, or effects on development due to PULMOZYME. There are, however, no adequate and well-controlled studies in pregnant women. Because animal reproductive studies are not always predictive of the human response, this drug should be used during pregnancy only if clearly needed.

Nursing Mothers

It is not known whether PULMOZYME is excreted in human milk. Small amounts of dornase alfa were detected in maternal milk of cynomolgus monkeys when administered a bolus dose (100 µg/kg) of dornase alfa followed by a six hour intravenous infusion (80 µg/kg/hr). Little or no measurable dornase alfa would be expected in human milk after chronic aerosol administration of recommended doses. Because many drugs are excreted in human milk, caution should still be exercised when PULMOZYME is administered to a nursing woman.

Pediatric Use

Because of the limited experience with the administration of Pulmozyme to patients younger than 5 years of age, its use should be considered only for those patients in whom there is a potential for benefit in pulmonary function or in risk of respiratory tract infection.

ADVERSE REACTIONS

Patients have been exposed to PULMOZYME for up to 12 months in clinical trials.

In a randomized, placebo-controlled clinical trial in patients with FVC ≥40% of predicted, over 600 patients received PULMOZYME once or twice daily for six months; most adverse events were not more common on PULMOZYME than on placebo and probably reflected the sequelae of the underlying lung disease. In most cases events that were increased were mild, transient in nature, and did not require alterations in dosing. Few patients experienced adverse events resulting in permanent discontinuation from PULMOZYME, and the discontinuation rate was similar for

Continued on next page

Pulmozyme—Cont.

placebo (2%) and PULMOZYME (3%). Events that were more frequent (greater than 3%) in PULMOZYME treated patients than in placebo-treated patients are listed in Table 2.

In a randomized, placebo-controlled trial of patients with advanced disease (FVC <40% of predicted) the safety profile for most adverse events was similar to that reported for the trial in patients with mild to moderate disease. For this study, adverse events that were reported with a higher frequency (greater than 3%) in the PULMOZYME treated patients, are also listed in Table 2.

[See table 2 on previous page]

Events Observed at Similar Rates in PULMOZYME® (dornase alfa) Inhalation Solution and Placebo Treated Patients with FVC ≥40% of Predicted

Body as a Whole	Abdominal pain, Asthenia, Fever, Flu syndrome, Malaise, Sepsis
Digestive System	Intestinal Obstruction, Gall Bladder disease, Liver disease, Pancreatic disease
Metabolic Nutritional System	Diabetes Mellitus, Hypoxia, Weight Loss
Respiratory System	Apnea, Bronchiectasis, Bronchitis, Change in Sputum, Cough Increase, Dyspnea, Hemoptysis, Lung Function Decrease, Nasal Polyps, Pneumonia, Pneumothorax, Rhinitis, Sinusitis, Sputum Increase, Wheeze

Mortality rates observed in controlled trials were similar for the placebo and PULMOZYME treated patients. Causes of death were consistent with progression of cystic fibrosis and included apnea, cardiac arrest, cardiopulmonary arrest, cor pulmonale, heart failure, massive hemoptysis, pneumonia, pneumothorax, and respiratory failure.

The safety of Pulmozyme, 2.5 mg by inhalation, was studied with 2 weeks of daily administration in 98 patients with cystic fibrosis (65 aged 3 months to <5 years, 33 aged 5 to ≤10 years). The PARI BABY™ reusable nebulizer (which uses a facemask instead of a mouthpiece) was utilized in patients unable to demonstrate the ability to inhale or exhale orally throughout the entire treatment period (54/65, 83% of the younger and 2/33, 6% of the older patients). The number of patients reporting cough was higher in the younger age group as compared to the older age group (29/65, 45% compared to 10/33, 30%) as was the number reporting moderate to severe cough (24/65, 37% as compared to 6/33, 18%). Other events tended to be of mild to moderate severity. The number of patients reporting rhinitis was higher in the younger age group as compared to the older age group (23/65, 35% compared to 9/33, 27%) as was the number reporting rash (4/65, 6% as compared to 0/33). The nature of adverse events was similar to that seen in the larger trials of Pulmozyme.

Allergic Reactions

There have been no reports of anaphylaxis attributed to the administration of PULMOZYME to date. Skin rash and urticaria have been observed, and were mild and transient in nature. Within all of the studies, a small percentage (average of 2-4%) of patients treated with PULMOZYME developed serum antibodies to PULMOZYME. None of these patients developed anaphylaxis, and the clinical significance of serum antibodies to PULMOZYME is unknown.

OVERDOSAGE

Single-dose inhalation studies in rats and monkeys at doses up to 180-times higher than doses routinely used in clinical studies are well tolerated. Single dose oral administration of PULMOZYME in doses up to 200 mg/kg are also well tolerated by rats.

Cystic fibrosis patients have received up to 20 mg BID for up to 6 days and 10 mg BID intermittently (2 weeks on/2 weeks off drug) for 168 days. These doses were well tolerated.

DOSAGE AND ADMINISTRATION

The recommended dose for use in most cystic fibrosis patients is one 2.5 mg single-use ampule inhaled once daily using a recommended nebulizer. Some patients may benefit from twice daily administration (see Clinical Experience, Table 1). Clinical trials have been performed with the following nebulizers and compressors: the disposable jet nebulizer Hudson T Up-draft II and disposable jet nebulizer Marquest Acorn II in conjunction with a Pulmo-Aide compressor, and the reusable PARI LC Jet+ nebulizer, in conjunction with the PARI PRONEB compressor. Safety and efficacy have been demonstrated only with these recommended nebulizer systems.

In the two-week trial of deposition and safety in patients 3 months to ≤10 years of age, those patients who were unable to demonstrate the ability to inhale or exhale orally throughout the entire treatment period used the PARI BABY™ reusable nebulizer. The PARI BABY™ nebulizer is identical to the PARI LC Jet+ system except that the mouthpiece is replaced by a tight fitting facemask connected to an elbow piece.

No clinical data are currently available that support the safety and efficacy of administration of PULMOZYME with other nebulizer systems. The patient should follow the manufacturer's instructions on the use and maintenance of the equipment.

PULMOZYME should not be diluted or mixed with other drugs in the nebulizer. Mixing of PULMOZYME with other drugs could lead to adverse physicochemical and/or functional changes in PULMOZYME or the admixed compound.

HOW SUPPLIED

PULMOZYME® (dornase alfa) Inhalation Solution is supplied in single-use ampules. Each ampule delivers 2.5 mL of a sterile, clear, colorless, aqueous solution containing 1.0 mg/mL dornase alfa, 0.15 mg/mL calcium chloride dihydrate and 8.77 mg/mL sodium chloride with no preservative. The nominal pH of the solution is 6.3.

PULMOZYME is supplied in:

- 14 unit cartons, containing 14 single-use ampules in single-unit foil pouches: NDC 50242-100-38
- 30 unit cartons containing 5 foil pouches of 6 single-use ampules: NDC 50242-100-40.

Storage

PULMOZYME® (dornase alfa) Inhalation Solution should be stored under refrigeration (2–8°C/36–46°F). Ampules should be protected from strong light. Do not use beyond the expiration date stamped on the ampule. Unused ampules should be stored in their protective foil pouch under refrigeration.

REFERENCES

1. Shak S, Capon DJ, Hellmiss R, Marsters SA, Baker CL. Recombinant human DNase I reduces the viscosity of cystic fibrosis sputum. Proc Natl Acad Sci USA 1990;87: 9188–92.
2. Boat TF. Cystic Fibrosis. In: Murray JF, Nadel JA, editors. Textbook of respiratory medicine. Philadelphia: Saunders WB, 1988;1:1126-52.
3. Collins FS. Cystic Fibrosis: molecular biology and therapeutic implications. Science 1992;256:774–9.
4. Potter JL, Spector S, Matthews LW, Lemm J. Studies of pulmonary secretions. Am Rev of Respir Dis 1969;99: 909–15.
5. Hubbard RC, McElvaney NG, Birrer P, Shak S, Robinson WW, Jolley C, et al. A preliminary study of aerosolized recombinant human deoxyribonuclease I in the treatment of cystic fibrosis. N Eng J Med 1992;326: 812–5.
6. Aitken ML, Burke W, McDonald G, Shak S, Montgomery AB, Smith A. Recombinant human DNase inhalation in normal subjects and patients with cystic fibrosis. JAMA 1992;267(14):1947–51.
7. Fuchs HJ, Borowitz DS, Christiansen DH, Morris EM, Nash ML, Ramsey BW, et al. Effect of aerosolized recombinant human DNase on exacerbations of respiratory symptoms and on pulmonary function in patients with cystic fibrosis. N Engl J Med 1994;331:637-42.
8. McCoy K, Hamilton S, Johnson C. Effects of 12-week administration of dornase alfa in patients with advanced cystic fibrosis lung disease. Chest 1996;110:889-95.

PULMOZYME® 4812403
(dornase alfa) Revised February 1998
recombinant
INHALATION SOLUTION
Manufactured by
GENENTECH, Inc.
1 DNA Way
South San Francisco, CA 94080-4990

Shown in Product Identification Guide, page 313

RITUXAN® ℞
Rituximab

WARNINGS

Infusion-related reactions: Infusion-related deaths (death within 24 hours of infusion) have been reported at a rate of approximately 0.04–0.07% (4–7 per 10,000 patients treated). These events appear as manifestations of an infusion-related complex and include hypoxia, pulmonary infiltrates, adult respiratory distress syndrome, myocardial infarction, ventricular fibrillation or cardiogenic shock. Nearly all fatal infusion-related events occurred in association with the first infusion. In the reported cases, the following factors were more frequently associated with fatal outcomes: women, patients with pulmonary infiltrates, and patients with CLL or mantle cell lymphoma (see WARNINGS).

Regarding the management of infusion-related reactions:

- Patients who develop clinically significant cardiopulmonary events should have RITUXAN infusion discontinued and receive medical treatment.
- Patients with pre-existing cardiac and pulmonary conditions or those with prior clinically significant cardiopulmonary adverse events should be monitored during and after subsequent infusions of RITUXAN.
- Patients with high numbers of circulating malignant cells (≥25,000/mm^3) with or without other evidence of high tumor burden should be more closely monitored for infusion reactions and tumor lysis syndrome.

Tumor Lysis Syndrome (TLS): Acute renal failure requiring dialysis with instances of fatal outcome has been reported in the setting of TLS. Assessment of serum electrolytes and renal function is indicated in patients with rapid decreases in tumor volume (see WARNINGS).

DESCRIPTION

The RITUXAN (Rituximab) antibody is a genetically engineered chimeric murine/human monoclonal antibody directed against the CD20 antigen found on the surface of normal and malignant B lymphocytes. The antibody is an IgG_1 kappa immunoglobulin containing murine light- and heavy-chain variable region sequences and human constant region sequences. Rituximab is composed of two heavy chains of 451 amino acids and two light chains of 213 amino acids (based on cDNA analysis) and has an approximate molecular weight of 145 kD. Rituximab has a binding affinity for the CD20 antigen of approximately 8.0 nM.

The chimeric anti-CD20 antibody is produced by mammalian cell (Chinese Hamster Ovary) suspension culture in a nutrient medium containing the antibiotic gentamicin. Gentamicin is not detectable in the final product. The anti-CD20 antibody is purified by affinity and ion exchange chromatography. The purification process includes specific viral inactivation and removal procedures. Rituximab drug product is manufactured from either bulk drug substance manufactured by Genentech, Inc. (US License No. 1048), or utilizing formulated bulk Rituximab supplied by IDEC Pharmaceuticals Corporation (US License No. 1235) under a shared manufacturing arrangement.

RITUXAN is a sterile, clear, colorless, preservative-free liquid concentrate for IV administration. RITUXAN is supplied at a concentration of 10 mg/mL in either 100 mg (10 mL) or 500 mg (50 mL) single-use vials. The product is formulated for IV administration in 9.0 mg/mL sodium chloride, 7.35 mg/mL sodium citrate dihydrate, 0.7 mg/mL polysorbate 80, and Sterile Water for Injection. The pH is adjusted to 6.5.

CLINICAL PHARMACOLOGY

General

Rituximab binds specifically to the antigen CD20 (human B-lymphocyte-restricted differentiation antigen, Bp35), a hydrophobic transmembrane protein with a molecular weight of approximately 35 kD located on pre-B and mature B lymphocytes.[1,2] The antigen is also expressed on >90% of B-cell non-Hodgkin's lymphomas (NHL)[3] but is not found on hematopoietic stem cells, pro-B cells, normal plasma cells or other normal tissues.[4] CD20 regulates an early step(s) in the activation process for cell cycle initiation and differentiation,[4] and possibly functions as a calcium ion channel.[5] CD20 is not shed from the cell surface and does not internalize upon antibody binding.[6] Free CD20 antigen is not found in the circulation.[2]

Preclinical Pharmacology and Toxicology

Mechanism of Action: The Fab domain of Rituximab binds to the CD20 antigen on B lymphocytes, and the Fc domain recruits immune effector functions to mediate B-cell lysis in vitro. Possible mechanisms of cell lysis include complement-dependent cytotoxicity (CDC)[7] and antibody-dependent cell mediated cytotoxicity (ADCC). The antibody has been shown to induce apoptosis in the DHL-4 human B-cell lymphoma line.[8]

Normal Tissue Cross-reactivity: Rituximab binding was observed on lymphoid cells in the thymus, the white pulp of the spleen, and a majority of B lymphocytes in peripheral blood and lymph nodes. Little or no binding was observed in the non-lymphoid tissues examined.

Human Pharmacokinetics/Pharmacodynamics

In patients given single doses at 10, 50, 100, 250 or 500 mg/m^2 as an IV infusion, serum levels and the half-life of Rituximab were proportional to dose. In nine patients given 375 mg/m^2 as an IV infusion for four doses, the mean serum half-life was 59.8 hours (range 11.1 to 104.6 hours) after the first infusion and 174 hours (range 26 to 442 hours) after the fourth infusion. The wide range of half-lives may reflect the variable tumor burden among patients and the changes in CD20 positive (normal and malignant) B-cell populations upon repeated administrations.

Rituximab at a dose of 375 mg/m^2 was administered as an IV infusion at weekly intervals for four doses to 166 patients. The peak and trough serum levels of Rituximab were inversely correlated with baseline values for the number of circulating CD20 positive B cells and measures of disease burden. Median steady-state serum levels were higher for responders compared to nonresponders; however, no difference was found in the rate of elimination as measured by serum half-life. Serum levels were higher in patients with International Working Formulation (IWF) subtypes B, C, and D as compared to those with subtype A. Rituximab was detectable in the serum of patients three to six months after completion of treatment.

The pharmacokinetic profile of Rituximab when administered as six infusions of 375 mg/m^2 in combination with six cycles of CHOP chemotherapy was similar to that seen with Rituximab alone.

Administration of RITUXAN resulted in a rapid and sustained depletion of circulating and tissue-based B cells. Lymph node biopsies performed 14 days after therapy showed a decrease in the percentage of B cells in seven of eight patients who had received single doses of Rituximab ≥100 mg/m^2.[9] Among the 166 patients in the pivotal study, circulating B cells (measured as CD19 positive cells) were depleted within the first three doses with sustained depletion for up to 6 to 9 months posttreatment in 83% of patients. One of the responding patients (1%), failed to show significant depletion of CD19 positive cells after the third infusion of Rituximab as compared to 19% of the nonresponding patients. B-cell recovery began at approximately six months following completion of treatment. Median B-cell levels returned to normal by twelve months following completion of treatment.

There were sustained and statistically significant reductions in both IgM and IgG serum levels observed from 5 through 11 months following Rituximab administration. However, only 14% of patients had reductions in IgM and/or IgG serum levels, resulting in values below the normal range.

CLINICAL STUDIES

A multicenter, open-label, single-arm study was conducted in 166 patients with relapsed or refractory low-grade or follicular B-cell NHL who received 375 mg/m^2 of RITUXAN given as an IV infusion weekly for four doses. Patients with tumor masses >10 cm or with >5,000 lymphocytes/µL in the peripheral blood were excluded from the study. The overall response rate (ORR) was 48% (80/166) with a 6% (10/166) complete response (CR) and a 42% (70/166) partial response (PR) rate. Disease-related signs and symptoms (including B-symptoms) were present in 23% (39/166) of patients at study entry and resolved in 64% (25/39) of those patients. The median time to onset of response was 50 days and the median duration of response is projected to be 10 to 12 months.

In a multivariate analysis, the ORR was higher in patients with IWF B, C, and D histologic subtypes as compared to IWF subtype A (58% vs. 12%), higher in patients whose largest lesion was <5 cm vs. >7 cm in greatest diameter (53% vs. 38%), and higher in patients with chemosensitive relapse as compared to chemoresistant (defined as duration of response <3 months) relapse (53% vs. 36%). ORR in patients previously treated with autologous bone marrow transplant was 78% (18/23). The following factors were not associated with a lower response rate: age ≥60 years, extranodal disease, prior anthracycline therapy, and bone marrow involvement.

In a second multicenter, multiple-dose study, 37 patients with relapsed or refractory B-cell NHL received 375 mg/m^2 of RITUXAN as an IV infusion once weekly for four doses.[10,11] The ORR was 46% with a median duration of response of 8.6 months (range 2.6 to 26.2+). Single doses of up to 500 mg/m^2 were well tolerated.[9]

Twenty patients have received two courses and one patient has received three courses of RITUXAN as four weekly infusions of 375 mg/m^2 per infusion. The percentage of patients reporting adverse events upon retreatment was similar to that reported following the first course, although the incidence of specific adverse events differed (see ADVERSE REACTIONS). All patients had obtained an objective clinical response (CR or PR) to the first course of RITUXAN; upon retreatment, 6 of 12 patients evaluable for response obtained a complete or partial remission.

Twenty-nine patients with relapsed or refractory, bulky (single lesion of >10 cm in diameter), low-grade NHL received 375 mg/m^2 of RITUXAN as four weekly infusions. The overall incidence of adverse events and the incidence of Grade 3 and 4 adverse events was higher in patients with bulky disease than in patients with non-bulky disease (see ADVERSE REACTIONS). Ten of 21 patients evaluable for response have obtained a complete or partial remission.

INDICATIONS AND USAGE

RITUXAN is indicated for the treatment of patients with relapsed or refractory low-grade or follicular, CD20 positive, B-cell non-Hodgkin's lymphoma.

CONTRAINDICATIONS

RITUXAN is contraindicated in patients with known Type I hypersensitivity or anaphylactic reactions to murine proteins or to any component of this product. (See WARNINGS.)

WARNINGS (see BOXED WARNINGS)

Infusion-Related Events (see BOXED WARNING): An infusion-related symptom complex consisting of fever and chills/rigors occurred in the majority of patients during the first RITUXAN infusion. Other frequent infusion-related symptoms included nausea, urticaria, fatigue, headache, pruritus, bronchospasm, dyspnea, sensation of tongue or throat swelling (angioedema), rhinitis, vomiting, hypotension, flushing, and pain at disease sites. These reactions generally occurred within 30 minutes to 2 hours of beginning the first infusion, and resolved with slowing or interruption of the RITUXAN infusion and with supportive care (diphenhydramine, acetaminophen, IV saline, and vasopressors). RITUXAN infusion should be interrupted for severe reactions. In most cases, the infusion can be resumed at a 50% reduction in rate (e.g., from 100 mg/hr to 50 mg/hr) when symptoms have completely resolved. In clinical studies, the incidence of infusion-related events decreased from 80% (7% Grade 3/4) during the first infusion to approximately 40% (5% to 10% Grade 3/4) with subsequent infusions. Mild to moderate hypotension requiring interruption of RITUXAN infusion with or without the administration of IV saline occurred in 32 (10%) patients. Angioedema was reported in 41 (13%) patients and was serious in one patient. Bronchospasm occurred in 24 (8%) patients; one-quarter of these patients were treated with bronchodilators.

Tumor Lysis Syndrome (see BOXED WARNING): TLS, characterized by rapid reduction in tumor volume, renal insufficiency, hyperkalemia, hypocalcemia, hyperuricemia, or hyperphosphatasemia, has been reported within 12 to 24 hours after the first RITUXAN infusion at a reported rate of 0.04%–0.05%. The risks of TLS appear to be higher in patients with high numbers of circulating malignant cells. Correction of electrolytes abnormalities, monitoring of renal function and fluid balance, and supportive care, including dialysis, should be initiated as indicated. Following complete resolution of the complications of TLS, RITUXAN has been tolerated when re-administered in conjunction with prophylactic therapy for TLS in a limited number of cases.

General

RITUXAN is associated with hypersensitivity reactions which may respond to adjustments in the infusion rate. Hypotension, bronchospasm, and angioedema have occurred in association with RITUXAN infusion as part of an infusion-related symptom complex. RITUXAN infusion should be interrupted for severe reactions and can be resumed at a 50% reduction in rate (e.g., from 100 mg/hr to 50 mg/hr) when symptoms have completely resolved. Treatment of these symptoms with diphenhydramine and acetaminophen is recommended; additional treatment with bronchodilators or IV saline may be indicated. In most cases, patients who have experienced non-life-threatening reactions have been able to complete the full course of therapy. (See DOSAGE and ADMINISTRATION.) Medications for the treatment of hypersensitivity reactions, e.g., epinephrine, antihistamines and corticosteroids, should be available for immediate use in the event of a reaction during administration.

Cardiovascular

Infusions should be discontinued in the event of serious or life-threatening cardiac arrhythmias. Patients who develop clinically significant arrhythmias should undergo cardiac monitoring during and after subsequent infusions of RITUXAN. Patients with preexisting cardiac conditions including arrhythmias and angina have had recurrences of these events during RITUXAN therapy and should be monitored throughout the infusion and immediate post-infusion period.

PRECAUTIONS

Laboratory Monitoring: Complete blood counts (CBC) and platelet counts should be obtained at regular intervals during RITUXAN therapy and more frequently in patients who develop cytopenias (see ADVERSE REACTIONS).

Drug/Laboratory Interactions: There have been no formal drug interaction studies performed with RITUXAN.

HAMA/HACA Formation: Human anti-murine antibody (HAMA) was not detected in 67 patients evaluated. Less than 1.0% (3/355) of patients evaluated for human antichimeric antibody (HACA) were positive. Patients who develop HAMA/HACA titers may have allergic or hypersensitivity reactions when treated with this or other murine or chimeric monoclonal antibodies.

Immunization: The safety of immunization with any vaccine, particularly live viral vaccines, following RITUXAN therapy has not been studied. The ability to generate a primary or anamnestic humoral response to any vaccine has also not been studied.

Carcinogenesis, Mutagenesis, Impairment of Fertility: No long-term animal studies have been performed to establish the carcinogenic or mutagenic potential of RITUXAN, or to determine its effects on fertility in males or females. Individuals of childbearing potential should use effective contraceptive methods during treatment and for up to 12 months following RITUXAN therapy.

Pregnancy Category C: Animal reproduction studies have not been conducted with RITUXAN. It is not known whether RITUXAN can cause fetal harm when administered to a pregnant woman or whether it can affect reproductive capacity. Human IgG is known to pass the placental barrier, and thus may potentially cause fetal B-cell depletion; therefore, RITUXAN should be given to a pregnant woman only if clearly needed.

Nursing Mothers: It is not known whether RITUXAN is excreted in human milk. Because human IgG is excreted in human milk and the potential for absorption and immunosuppression in the infant is unknown, women should be advised to discontinue nursing until circulating drug levels are no longer detectable. (See CLINICAL PHARMACOLOGY.)

Pediatric Use: The safety and effectiveness of RITUXAN in pediatric patients have not been established.

ADVERSE REACTIONS

Safety data, except where indicated, are based on 315 patients treated in five single-agent studies of RITUXAN. These include patients with bulky disease (lesions >10 cm), those who have received more than one course of RITUXAN, and patients receiving 375 mg/m^2 for eight doses.

Infusion-Related Events: (See BOXED WARNING and WARNINGS.)

Immunologic Events: RITUXAN induced B-cell depletion in 70 to 80% of patients and was associated with decreased serum immunoglobulins in a minority of patients. The incidence of infection did not appear to be increased. During the treatment period, 50 out of 166 patients (30%) in the pivotal trial developed 68 infectious events; six (9%) were Grade 3 in severity and none were Grade 4 events. Of the six serious infectious events, none were associated with neutropenia. The serious bacterial events included sepsis due to *Listeria* (n=1), *Staphylococcal* bacteremia (n=1), and polymicrobial sepsis (n=1). In the posttreatment period (30 days to 11 months following the last dose), bacterial infections included sepsis (n=1); significant viral infections included *Herpes simplex* infections (n=2) and *Herpes zoster* (n=3). Additional reports of focal bacterial infections, sepsis, and viral infections have been received in the postmarketing setting. Serious infections, including sepsis, have been reported in patients with and without neutropenia.

Retreatment Events: Twenty-one patients have received more than one course of RITUXAN. The percentage of patients reporting any adverse event upon retreatment was similar to the percentage of patients reporting adverse events upon initial exposure. The following adverse events were reported more frequently in retreated subjects: asthenia, throat irritation, flushing, tachycardia, anorexia, leukopenia, thrombocytopenia, anemia, peripheral edema, dizziness, depression, respiratory symptoms, night sweats, and pruritus.

Hematologic Events: Severe cytopenias were reported including thrombocytopenia (1.3%), neutropenia (1.9%), and anemia (1.0%). A single occurrence of transient aplastic anemia (pure red cell aplasia) and two occurrences of hemolytic anemia following RITUXAN therapy were reported. In addition, there have been rare postmarketing reports of prolonged pancytopenia and marrow hypoplasia.

Cardiac Events (see BOXED WARNING): Four patients developed ventricular or supraventricular arrhythmias and one patient developed angina in association with the RITUXAN infusion. Rare, fatal cardiac failure with symptomatic onset weeks after RITUXAN has also been reported. Patients who develop clinically significant cardiopulmonary events should have RITUXAN infusion discontinued.

Pulmonary Events (see BOXED WARNING): Three pulmonary events have been reported in temporal association with RITUXAN infusion as a single agent: acute, infusion-related bronchospasm, an acute pneumonitis presenting 1–4 weeks post-RITUXAN infusion, and bronchiolitis obliterans. The bronchiolitis obliterans was associated with progressive pulmonary symptoms and culminated in death several months following the last RITUXAN infusion. The safety of resumption or continued administration of RITUXAN in patients with pneumonitis or bronchiolitis obliterans is unknown.

Table 1
Adverse Events ≥5% of Patients (N=315)

	Incidence All Grades N	%
Any Adverse Event	**275**	**87**
Body As A Whole		
Fever	154	49
Chills	102	32
Asthenia	49	16
Headache	43	14
Throat Irritation	19	6
Abdominal Pain	18	6
Cardiovascular System		
Hypotension	32	10
Digestive System		
Nausea	55	18
Vomiting	23	7
Hemic and Lymphatic System		
Leukopenia	33	11
Thrombocytopenia	25	8
Neutropenia	21	7
Metabolic and Nutritional System		
Angioedema	41	13
Musculo-Skeletal System		
Myalgia	21	7
Nervous System		
Dizziness	23	7
Respiratory System		
Rhinitis	25	8
Bronchospasm	24	8
Skin and Appendages		
Pruritus	32	10
Rash	31	10
Urticaria	24	8

Severe and life-threatening (Grade 3 and 4) events were reported in 10% (32/315) of patients. The following Grade 3 and 4 adverse events were reported: neutropenia (1.9%), chills (1.6%), leukopenia and thrombocytopenia (1.3% for each), hypotension, anemia, bronchospasm, and urticaria (1.0% for each), headache, abdominal pain, and arrhythmia (0.6% for each), asthenia, hypertension, nausea, vomiting, coagulation disorder, angioedema, arthralgia, pain, rhinitis, increased cough, dyspnea, bronchiolitis obliterans, hypoxia, asthma, pruritus, and rash (one patient each, 0.3%).

The following adverse events occurred in ≥1.0% but <5.0% of patients, in order of decreasing incidence: flushing, arthralgia, diarrhea, anemia, cough increase, hypertension, lacrimation disorder, pain, hyperglycemia, back pain, peripheral edema, paresthesia, dyspepsia, chest pain, anorexia, anxiety, malaise, tachycardia, agitation, insomnia, sinusitis, conjunctivitis, abdominal enlargement, postural hypotension, LDH increase, hypocalcemia, hypesthesia, respiratory disorder, tumor pain, pain at injection site, bradycardia, hypertonia, nervousness, bronchitis, and taste perversion.

Multisystem adverse events—The following serious adverse reactions have been reported at a frequency of less than 0.1% in the postmarketing setting:

Body as a Whole: Lupus-like syndrome and serum sickness
Cardiovascular System: Systemic vasculitis

Continued on next page

Rituxan—Cont.

Musculoskeletal System: Polyarticular arthritis
Respiratory System: Pleuritis
Skin and Appendages: Severe bullous skin reactions (including toxic epidermal necrolysis) and pemphigus; some with fatal outcome
Special Senses: Optic neuritis and uveitis
Several of these events were reported as individual components of multisystem processes (e.g., optic neuritis in a patient with systemic vasculitis, pleuritis in association with lupus-like syndrome, etc.) and often in conjunction with rash and polyarthritis.
The proportion of patients reporting any adverse event was similar in patients with bulky disease and those with lesions <10 cm in diameter. However, the incidence of dizziness, neutropenia, thrombocytopenia, myalgia, anemia, and chest pain was higher in patients with lesions >10 cm. The incidence of any Grade 3 and 4 event was higher (31% vs. 13%) and the incidence of Grade 3 or 4 neutropenia, anemia, hypotension, and dyspnea was also higher in patients with bulky disease compared with patients with lesions <10 cm.

OVERDOSAGE

There has been no experience with overdosage in human clinical trials. Single doses higher than 500 mg/m^2 have not been tested.

DOSAGE AND ADMINISTRATION

Usual Dose:
The recommended dosage of RITUXAN is 375 mg/m^2 given as an IV infusion once weekly for four doses (Days 1, 8, 15, and 22). RITUXAN may be administered in an outpatient setting. **DO NOT ADMINISTER AS AN INTRAVENOUS PUSH OR BOLUS. (See Administration.)**
Instructions for Administration
Preparation for Administration: Use appropriate aseptic technique. Withdraw the necessary amount of RITUXAN and dilute to a final concentration of 1 to 4 mg/mL into an infusion bag containing either 0.9% Sodium Chloride, USP, or 5% Dextrose in Water, USP. Gently invert the bag to mix the solution. Discard any unused portion left in the vial. Parenteral drug products should be inspected visually for particulate matter and discoloration prior to administration.
RITUXAN solutions for infusion are stable at 2–8°C (36–46°F) for 24 hours and at room temperature for an additional 12 hours. No incompatibilities between RITUXAN and polyvinylchloride or polyethylene bags have been observed.
Administration: DO NOT ADMINISTER AS AN INTRAVENOUS PUSH OR BOLUS. Hypersensitivity reactions may occur (see WARNINGS). Premedication consisting of acetaminophen and diphenhydramine should be considered before each infusion of RITUXAN. Premedication may attenuate infusion-related events. Since transient hypotension may occur during RITUXAN infusion, consideration should be given to withholding anti-hypertensive medications 12 hours prior to RITUXAN infusion.
First Infusion: The RITUXAN solution for infusion should be administered intravenously at an initial rate of 50 mg/hr. RITUXAN should not be mixed or diluted with other drugs. If hypersensitivity or infusion-related events do not occur, escalate the infusion rate in 50 mg/hr increments every 30 minutes, to a maximum of 400 mg/hr. If hypersensitivity or an infusion-related event develops, the infusion should be temporarily slowed or interrupted (see WARNINGS). The infusion can continue at one-half the previous rate upon improvement of patient symptoms.
Subsequent Infusions: Subsequent RITUXAN infusions can be administered at an initial rate of 100 mg/hr, and increased by 100 mg/hr increments at 30-minute intervals, to a maximum of 400 mg/hr as tolerated.
Stability and Storage: RITUXAN vials are stable at 2–8°C (36–46°F). Do not use beyond expiration date stamped on carton. RITUXAN vials should be protected from direct sunlight.

HOW SUPPLIED

RITUXAN is supplied as 100 mg and 500 mg of sterile, preservative-free, single-use vials.
Single unit 100 mg carton: Contains one 10 mL vial of RITUXAN (10 mg/mL).
NDC 50242-051-21
Single unit 500 mg carton: Contains one 50 mL vial of RITUXAN (10 mg/mL).
NDC 50242-053-06

REFERENCES

1. Valentine MA, Meier KE, Rossie S, et al. Phosphorylation of the CD20 phosphoprotein in resting B lymphocytes. *J Biol Chem* 1989 264(19): 11282–11287.
2. Einfeld DA, Brown JP, Valentine MA, et al. Molecular cloning of the human B cell CD20 receptor predicts a hydrophobic protein with multiple transmembrane domains. *EMBO J* 1988 7(3):711–717.
3. Anderson KC, Bates MP, Slaughenhoupt BL, et al. Expression of human B cell-associated antigens on leukemias and lymphomas: A model of human B cell differentiation. *Blood* 1984 63(6):1424–1433.
4. Tedder TF, Boyd AW, Freedman AS, et al. The B cell surface molecule B1 is functionally linked with B cell activation and differentiation. *J Immunol* 1985 135(2):973–979.
5. Tedder TF, Zhou LJ, Bell PD, et al. The CD20 surface molecule of B lymphocytes functions as a calcium channel. *J Cell Biochem* 1990 14D:195.
6. Press OW, Applebaum F, Ledbetter JA, Martin PJ, Zarling J, Kidd P, et al. Monoclonal antibody 1F5 (anti-CD20) serotherapy of human B-cell lymphomas. *Blood* 1987 69(2):584–591.
7. Reff ME, Carner C, Chambers KS, Chinn PC, Leonard JE, Raab R, et al. Depletion of B cells in vivo by a chimeric mouse human monoclonal antibody to CD20. *Blood* 1994 83(2):435–445.
8. Demidem A, Lam T, Alas S, Hariharan K, Hanna N, and Bonavida B. Chimeric anti-CD20 (IDEC-C2B8) monoclonal antibody sensitizes a B cell lymphoma cell line to cell killing by cytotoxic drugs. *Cancer Biotherapy & Radiopharmaceuticals* 1997 12(3):177–186.
9. Maloney DG, Liles TM, Czerwinski C, Waldichuk J, Rosenberg J, Grillo-López A, et al. Phase I clinical trial using escalating single-dose infusion of chimeric anti-CD20 monoclonal antibody (IDEC-C2B8) in patients with recurrent B-cell lymphoma. *Blood* 1994 84(8):2457–2466.
10. Maloney DG, Grillo-López AJ, Bodkin D, White CA, Liles T-M, Royston I, et al. IDEC-C2B8: Results of a phase I multiple-dose trial in patients with relapsed non-Hodgkin's lymphoma. *J Clin Oncol* 1997 15(10): 3266–3274.
11. Maloney DG, Grillo-López AJ, White CA, Bodkin D, Schilder RJ, Neidhart JA, et al. IDEC-C2B8 (Rituximab) anti-CD20 monoclonal antibody therapy in patients with relapsed low-grade non-Hodgkin's lymphoma. *Blood* 1997 90(6):2188–2195.

Jointly Marketed by:
IDEC Pharmaceuticals Corporation
11011 Torreyana Road
San Diego, CA 92121
7141404 LJ0069
Genentech, Inc.
1 DNA Way
South San Francisco, CA 94080-4990
(4809703 Revised July 1999)

Shown in Product Identification Guide, page 313

TNKase™ ℞
(Tenecteplase)
Full Prescribing Information

DESCRIPTION

Tenecteplase is a tissue plasminogen activator (tPA) produced by recombinant DNA technology using an established mammalian cell line (Chinese Hamster Ovary cells). Tenecteplase is a 527 amino acid glycoprotein developed by introducing the following modifications to the complementary DNA (cDNA) for natural human tPA: a substitution of threonine 103 with asparagine, and a substitution of asparagine 117 with glutamine, both within the kringle 1 domain, and a tetra-alanine substitution at amino acids 296–299 in the protease domain. Cell culture is carried out in nutrient medium containing the antibiotic gentamicin (65 mg/L). However, the presence of the antibiotic is not detectable in the final product (limit of detection is 0.67 µg/vial). TNKase is a sterile, white to off-white, lyophilized powder for single intravenous (IV) bolus administration after reconstitution with Sterile Water for Injection (SWFI), USP. Each vial of TNKase nominally contains 52.5 mg Tenecteplase, 0.55 g L-arginine, 0.17 g phosphoric acid, and 4.3 mg polysorbate 20, which includes a 5% overfill. Each vial will deliver 50 mg of Tenecteplase.

CLINICAL PHARMACOLOGY

General
Tenecteplase is a modified form of human tissue plasminogen activator (tPA) that binds to fibrin and converts plasminogen to plasmin. In the presence of fibrin, *in vitro* studies demonstrate that Tenecteplase conversion of plasminogen to plasmin is increased relative to its conversion in the absence of fibrin. This fibrin specificity decreases systemic activation of plasminogen and the resulting degradation of circulating fibrinogen as compared to a molecule lacking this property. Following administration of 30, 40, or 50 mg of TNKase, there are decreases in circulating fibrinogen (4%–15%) and plasminogen (11%–24%). The clinical significance of fibrin-specificity on safety (e.g., bleeding) or efficacy has not been established. Biological potency is determined by an *in vitro* clot lysis assay and is expressed in Tenecteplase-specific units. The specific activity of Tenecteplase has been defined as 200 units/mg.
Pharmacokinetics
In patients with acute myocardial infarction (AMI), TNKase administered as a single bolus exhibits a biphasic disposition from the plasma. Tenecteplase was cleared from the plasma with an initial half-life of 20 to 24 minutes. The terminal phase half-life of Tenecteplase was 90 to 130 minutes. In 99 of 104 patients treated with Tenecteplase, mean plasma clearance ranged from 99 to 119 mL/min.
The initial volume of distribution is weight related and approximates plasma volume. Liver metabolism is the major clearance mechanism for Tenecteplase.

CLINICAL STUDIES

ASSENT-2 was an international, randomized, double-blind trial that compared 30-day mortality rates in 16,949 patients assigned to receive an IV bolus dose of TNKase or an accelerated infusion of Activase® (Alteplase, recombinant).[1] Eligibility criteria included onset of chest pain within 6 hours of randomization and ST-segment elevation or left bundle branch block on electrocardiogram (ECG). Patients were to be excluded from the trial if they received GP IIb/IIIa inhibitors within the previous 12 hours. TNKase was dosed using actual or estimated weight in a weight-tiered fashion as described in DOSAGE AND ADMINISTRATION. All patients were to receive 150–325 mg of aspirin administered as soon as possible, followed by 150–325 mg daily. Intravenous heparin was to be administered as soon as possible: for patients weighing ≤ 67 kg, heparin was administered as a 4000 unit IV bolus followed by infusion at 800 U/hr; for patients weighing > 67 kg, heparin was administered as a 5000 unit IV bolus followed by infusion at 1000 U/hr. Heparin was continued for 48 to 72 hours with infusion adjusted to maintain aPTT at 50–75 seconds. The use of GP IIb/IIIa inhibitors was discouraged for the first 24 hours following randomization. The results of the primary endpoint (30-day mortality rates with non-parametric adjustment for the covariates of age, Killip class, heart rate, systolic blood pressure and infarct location) along with selected other 30-day endpoints are shown in Table 1.
[See table 1 below]
Rates of mortality and the combined endpoint of death or stroke among pre-specified subgroups, including age, gender, time to treatment, infarct location, and history of previous myocardial infarction, demonstrate consistent relative risks across these subgroups. There was insufficient enrollment of non-Caucasian patients to draw any conclusions regarding relative efficacy in racial subsets.
Rates of in-hospital procedures, including percutaneous transluminal coronary angioplasty (PTCA), stent placement, intra-aortic balloon pump (IABP) use, and coronary artery bypass graft (CABG) surgery, were similar between the TNKase and Activase groups.
TIMI 10B was an open-label, controlled, randomized, dose-ranging, angiography study which utilized a blinded core laboratory for review of coronary arteriograms.[2] Patients (n = 837) presenting within 12 hours of symptom onset were treated with fixed doses of 30, 40, or 50 mg of TNKase or the accelerated infusion of Activase and underwent coronary arteriography at 90 minutes. The results showed that the 40 mg and 50 mg doses were similar to accelerated infusion of Activase in restoring patency. TIMI grade 3 flow and TIMI grade 2/3 flow at 90 minutes are shown in Table 2. The exact relationship between coronary artery patency and clinical activity has not been established.
[See table 2 at top of next page]
The angiographic results from TIMI 10B and the safety data from ASSENT-1, an additional uncontrolled safety study of 3,235 TNKase-treated patients, provided the framework to develop a weight-tiered TNKase dose regimen.[3] Exploratory analyses suggested that a weight-adjusted dose of 0.5 mg/kg to 0.6 mg/kg of TNKase resulted in a better patency to bleeding relationship than fixed doses of TNKase across a broad range of patient weights.

INDICATIONS AND USAGE

TNKase is indicated for use in the reduction of mortality associated with acute myocardial infarction (AMI). Treatment should be initiated as soon as possible after the onset of AMI symptoms (see CLINICAL STUDIES).

Table 1
ASSENT-2
Mortality, Stroke, and Combined Outcome of Death or Stroke Measured at Thirty Days

30-day Events	TNKase (N=8461)	Accelerated Activase (N=8488)	Relative Risk TNKase/Activase (95% CI)
Mortality	6.2%	6.2%	1.00 (0.89, 1.12)
Intracranial Hemorrhage (ICH)	0.9%	0.9%	0.99 (0.73, 1.35)
Any Stroke	1.8%	1.7%	1.07 (0.86, 1.35)
Death or Nonfatal Stroke	7.1%	7.0%	1.01 (0.91, 1.13)

CONTRAINDICATIONS

TNKase therapy in patients with acute myocardial infarction is contraindicated in the following situations because of an increased risk of bleeding (see WARNINGS):

- **Active internal bleeding**
- **History of cerebrovascular accident**
- **Intracranial or intraspinal surgery or trauma within 2 months**
- **Intracranial neoplasm, arteriovenous malformation, or aneurysm**
- **Known bleeding diathesis**
- **Severe uncontrolled hypertension**

WARNINGS

Bleeding

The most common complication encountered during TNKase therapy is bleeding. The type of bleeding associated with thrombolytic therapy can be divided into two broad categories:

- Internal bleeding, involving intracranial and retroperitoneal sites, or the gastrointestinal, genitourinary, or respiratory tracts.
- Superficial or surface bleeding, observed mainly at vascular puncture and access sites (e.g., venous cutdowns, arterial punctures) or sites of recent surgical intervention.

Should serious bleeding (not controlled by local pressure) occur, any concomitant heparin or antiplatelet agents should be discontinued immediately.

In clinical studies of TNKase, patients were treated with both aspirin and heparin. Heparin may contribute to the bleeding risks associated with TNKase. The safety of the use of TNKase with other antiplatelet agents has not been adequately studied (see PRECAUTIONS: Drug Interactions). Intramuscular injections and nonessential handling of the patient should be avoided for the first few hours following treatment with TNKase. Venipunctures should be performed and monitored carefully.

Should an arterial puncture be necessary during the first few hours following TNKase therapy, it is preferable to use an upper extremity vessel that is accessible to manual compression. Pressure should be applied for at least 30 minutes, a pressure dressing applied, and the puncture site checked frequently for evidence of bleeding.

Each patient being considered for therapy with TNKase should be carefully evaluated and anticipated benefits weighed against potential risks associated with therapy. In the following conditions, the risk of TNKase therapy may be increased and should be weighed against the anticipated benefits:

- Recent major surgery, e.g., coronary artery bypass graft, obstetrical delivery, organ biopsy, previous puncture of noncompressible vessels
- Cerebrovascular disease
- Recent gastrointestinal or genitourinary bleeding
- Recent trauma
- Hypertension: systolic BP ≥ 180 mm Hg and/or diastolic BP ≥ 110 mm Hg
- High likelihood of left heart thrombus, e.g., mitral stenosis with atrial fibrillation
- Acute pericarditis
- Subacute bacterial endocarditis
- Hemostatic defects, including those secondary to severe hepatic or renal disease
- Severe hepatic dysfunction
- Pregnancy
- Diabetic hemorrhagic retinopathy or other hemorrhagic ophthalmic conditions
- Septic thrombophlebitis or occluded AV cannula at seriously infected site
- Advanced age (see PRECAUTIONS: Geriatric Use)
- Patients currently receiving oral anticoagulants, e.g., warfarin sodium
- Recent administration of GP IIb/IIIa inhibitors
- Any other condition in which bleeding constitutes a significant hazard or would be particularly difficult to manage because of its location

Cholesterol Embolization

Cholesterol embolism has been reported rarely in patients treated with all types of thrombolytic agents; the true incidence is unknown. This serious condition, which can be lethal, is also associated with invasive vascular procedures (e.g., cardiac catheterization, angiography, vascular surgery) and/or anticoagulant therapy. Clinical features of cholesterol embolism may include livedo reticularis, "purple toe" syndrome, acute renal failure, gangrenous digits, hypertension, pancreatitis, myocardial infarction, cerebral infarction, spinal cord infarction, retinal artery occlusion, bowel infarction, and rhabdomyolysis.

Arrhythmias

Coronary thrombolysis may result in arrhythmias associated with reperfusion. These arrhythmias (such as sinus bradycardia, accelerated idioventricular rhythm, ventricular premature depolarizations, ventricular tachycardia) are not different from those often seen in the ordinary course of acute myocardial infarction and may be managed with standard anti-arrhythmic measures. It is recommended that anti-arrhythmic therapy for bradycardia and/or ventricular irritability be available when TNKase is administered.

PRECAUTIONS

General

Standard management of myocardial infarction should be implemented concomitantly with TNKase treatment. Arterial and venous punctures should be minimized. Noncompressible arterial puncture must be avoided and internal jugular and subclavian venous punctures should be avoided to minimize bleeding from the noncompressible sites. In the event of serious bleeding, heparin and antiplatelet agents should be discontinued immediately. Heparin effects can be reversed by protamine.

Table 2
TIMI 10B Patency Rates
TIMI Grade Flow at 90 Minutes

	Activase ≤ 100 mg (n=311)	TNKase 30 mg (n=302)	TNKase 40 mg (n=148)	TNKase 50 mg (n=76)
TIMI Grade 3 Flow	63%	54%	63%	66%
TIMI Grade 2/3 Flow	82%	77%	79%	88%
95% CI (TIMI 2/3 Flow)	(77%, 86%)	(72%, 81%)	(72%, 85%)	(79%, 94%)

Table 3
ASSENT-2
Non-ICH Bleeding Events

	TNKase (N=8461)	Accelerated Activase (N=8488)	Relative Risk TNKase/Activase (95% CI)
Major bleeding[a]	4.7%	5.9%	0.78 (0.69, 0.89)
Minor bleeding	21.8%	23.0%	0.94 (0.89, 1.00)
Units of transfused blood			
Any	4.3%	5.5%	0.77 (0.67, 0.89)
1–2	2.6%	3.2%	
> 2	1.7%	2.2%	

[a]Major bleeding is defined as bleeding requiring blood transfusion or leading to hemodynamic compromise.

The B-D® 10 cc Syringe with TwinPak™ Dual Cannula Device

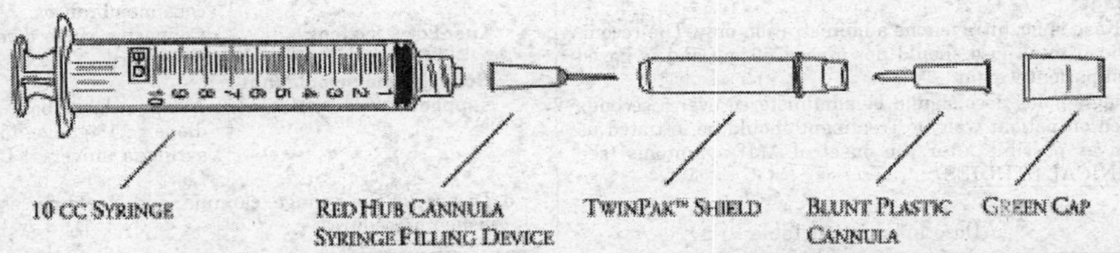

Readministration

Readministration of plasminogen activators, including TNKase, to patients who have received prior plasminogen activator therapy has not been systematically studied. Three of 487 patients tested for antibody formation to TNKase had a positive antibody titer at 30 days. The data reflect the percentage of patients whose test results were considered positive for antibodies to TNKase in a radioimmunoprecipitation assay, and are highly dependent on the sensitivity and specificity of the assay. Additionally, the observed incidence of antibody positivity in an assay may be influenced by several factors including sample handling, concomitant medications, and underlying disease. For these reasons, comparison of the incidence of antibodies to TNKase with the incidence of antibodies to other products may be misleading. Although sustained antibody formation in patients receiving one dose of TNKase has not been documented, readministration should be undertaken with caution. If an anaphylactic reaction occurs, appropriate therapy should be administered.

Drug Interactions

Formal interaction studies of TNKase with other drugs have not been performed. Patients studied in clinical trials of TNKase were routinely treated with heparin and aspirin. Anticoagulants (such as heparin and vitamin K antagonists) and drugs that alter platelet function (such as acetylsalicylic acid, dipyridamole, and GP IIb/IIIa inhibitors) may increase the risk of bleeding if administered prior to, during, or after TNKase therapy.

Drug/Laboratory Test Interactions

During TNKase therapy, results of coagulation tests and/or measures of fibrinolytic activity may be unreliable unless specific precautions are taken to prevent *in vitro* artifacts. Tenecteplase is an enzyme that, when present in blood in pharmacologic concentrations, remains active under *in vitro* conditions. This can lead to degradation of fibrinogen in blood samples removed for analysis.

Carcinogenesis, Mutagenesis, Impairment of Fertility

Studies in animals have not been performed to evaluate the carcinogenic potential, mutagenicity, or the effect on fertility.

Pregnancy (Category C)

TNKase has been shown to elicit maternal and embryo toxicity in rabbits given multiple IV administrations. In rabbits administered 0.5, 1.5 and 5.0 mg/kg/day, vaginal hemorrhage resulted in maternal deaths. Subsequent embryonic deaths were secondary to maternal hemorrhage and no fetal anomalies were observed. TNKase does not elicit maternal and embryo toxicity in rabbits following a single IV administration. Thus, in developmental toxicity studies conducted in rabbits, the no observable effect level (NOEL) of a single IV administration of TNKase on maternal or developmental toxicity was 5 mg/kg (approximately 8–10 times the human dose). There are no adequate and well-controlled studies in pregnant women. TNKase should be given to pregnant women only if the potential benefits justify the potential risk to the fetus.

Nursing Mothers

It is not known if TNKase is excreted in human milk. Because many drugs are excreted in human milk, caution should be exercised when TNKase is administered to a nursing woman.

Pediatric Use

The safety and effectiveness of TNKase in pediatric patients have not been established.

Geriatric Use

Of the patients in ASSENT-2 who received TNKase, 4,958 (59%) were under the age of 65; 2,256 (27%) were between the ages of 65 and 74; and 1,244 (15%) were 75 and over. The 30-day mortality rates by age were 2.5% in patients under the age of 65, 8.5% in patients between the ages of 65 and 74, and 16.2% in patients age 75 and over. The ICH rates were 0.4% in patients under the age of 65, 1.6% in patients between the ages of 65 and 74, and 1.7% in patients age 75 and over. The rates of any stroke were 1.0% in patients under the age of 65, 2.9% in patients between the ages of 65 and 74, and 3.0% in patients age 75 and over. Major bleeding rates, defined as bleeding requiring blood transfusion or leading to hemodynamic compromise, were 3.1% in patients under the age of 65, 6.4% in patients between the ages of 65 and 74, and 7.7% in patients age 75 and over. In elderly patients, the benefits of TNKase on mortality should be carefully weighed against the risk of increased adverse events, including bleeding.

ADVERSE REACTIONS

Bleeding

The most frequent adverse reaction associated with TNKase is bleeding (see WARNINGS).

Should serious bleeding occur, concomitant heparin and antiplatelet therapy should be discontinued. Death or permanent disability can occur in patients who experience stroke or serious bleeding episodes.

For TNKase-treated patients in ASSENT-2, the incidence of intracranial hemorrhage was 0.9% and any stroke was 1.8%. The incidence of all strokes, including intracranial bleeding, increases with increasing age (see PRECAUTIONS: Geriatric Use).

In the ASSENT-2 study, the following bleeding events were reported (see Table 3).

[See table 3 above]

Non-intracranial major bleeding and the need for blood transfusions were lower in patients treated with TNKase.

Continued on next page

TNKase—Cont.

Types of major bleeding reported in 1% or more of the patients were hematoma (1.7%) and gastrointestinal tract (1%). Types of major bleeding reported in less than 1% of the patients were urinary tract, puncture site (including cardiac catheterization site), retroperitoneal, respiratory tract, and unspecified. Types of minor bleeding reported in 1% or more of the patients were hematoma (12.3%), urinary tract (3.7%), puncture site (including cardiac catheterization site) (3.6%), pharyngeal (3.1%), gastrointestinal tract (1.9%), epistaxis (1.5%), and unspecified (1.3%).

Allergic Reactions

Allergic-type reactions (e.g., anaphylaxis, angioedema, laryngeal edema, rash, and urticaria) have rarely (< 1%) been reported in patients treated with TNKase. Anaphylaxis was reported in < 0.1% of patients treated with TNKase; however, causality was not established. When such reactions occur, they usually respond to conventional therapy.

Other Adverse Reactions

The following adverse reactions have been reported among patients receiving TNKase in clinical trials. These reactions are frequent sequelae of the underlying disease, and the effect of TNKase on the incidence of these events is unknown. These events include cardiogenic shock, arrhythmias, atrioventricular block, pulmonary edema, heart failure, cardiac arrest, recurrent myocardial ischemia, myocardial reinfarction, myocardial rupture, cardiac tamponade, pericarditis, pericardial effusion, mitral regurgitation, thrombosis, embolism, and electromechanical dissociation. These events can be life-threatening and may lead to death. Nausea and/or vomiting, hypotension, and fever have also been reported.

DOSAGE AND ADMINISTRATION

Dosage

TNKase is for intravenous administration only. The recommended total dose should not exceed 50 mg and is based upon patient weight.

A single bolus dose should be administered over 5 seconds based on patient weight. Treatment should be initiated as soon as possible after the onset of AMI symptoms (see CLINICAL STUDIES).

Dose Information Table

Patient Weight (kg)	TNKase (mg)	Volume TNKase* to be administered (mL)
< 60	30	6
≥ 60 to < 70	35	7
≥ 70 to < 80	40	8
≥ 80 to < 90	45	9
≥ 90	50	10

*From one vial of TNKase reconstituted with 10 mL SWFI.

The safety and efficacy of TNKase has only been investigated with concomitant administration of heparin and aspirin as described in CLINICAL STUDIES.

[See graphic third from top on previous page]

Reconstitution

NOTE: Read all instructions completely before beginning reconstitution and administration.

1. Remove the shield assembly from the supplied B-D® 10 cc syringe with TwinPak™ Dual Cannula Device (see figure) and aseptically withdraw 10 mL of Sterile Water for Injection (SWFI), USP, from the supplied diluent vial using the red hub cannula syringe filling device. Do not use Bacteriostatic Water for Injection, USP.
   Note: Do not discard the shield assembly.
2. Inject the entire contents of the syringe (10 mL) into the TNKase vial directing the diluent stream into the powder. Slight foaming upon reconstitution is not unusual; any large bubbles will dissipate if the product is allowed to stand undisturbed for several minutes.
3. Gently swirl until contents are completely dissolved. DO NOT SHAKE. The reconstituted preparation results in a colorless to pale yellow transparent solution containing TNKase at 5 mg/mL at a pH of approximately 7.3. The osmolality of this solution is approximately 290 mOsm/kg.
4. Determine the appropriate dose of TNKase (see Dose Information Table) and withdraw this volume (in milliliters) from the reconstituted vial with the syringe. **Any unused solution should be discarded.**
5. Once the appropriate dose of TNKase is drawn into the syringe, stand the shield vertically on a flat surface (with green side down) and passively recap the red hub cannula.
6. Remove the entire shield assembly, including the red hub cannula, by twisting counterclockwise. Note: The shield assembly also contains the clear-ended blunt plastic cannula; retain for split septum IV access.

Administration

1. The product should be visually inspected prior to administration for particulate matter and discoloration. TNKase may be administered as reconstituted at 5 mg/mL.
2. Precipitation may occur when TNKase is administered in an IV line containing dextrose. Dextrose-containing lines should be flushed with a saline-containing solution prior to and following single bolus administration of TNKase.
3. Reconstituted TNKase should be administered as a single IV bolus over 5 seconds.
4. Because TNKase contains no antibacterial preservatives, it should be reconstituted immediately before use. If the reconstituted TNKase is not used immediately, refrigerate the TNKase vial at 2–8°C (36–46°F) and use within 8 hours.
5. Although the supplied syringe is compatible with a conventional needle, this syringe is designed to be used with needleless IV systems. From the information below, follow the instructions applicable to the IV system in use.

Split septum IV system:
- Remove the green cap.
- Attach the clear-ended blunt plastic cannula to the syringe.
- Remove the shield and use the blunt plastic cannula to access the split septum injection port.
- Because the blunt plastic cannula has two side ports, air or fluid expelled through the cannula will exit in two sideways directions; direct away from face or mucous membranes.

Luer-Lok® system: Connect syringe directly to IV port.

Conventional needle (not supplied in this kit): Attach a large bore needle, e.g., 18 gauge, to the syringe's universal Luer-Lok®.

6. Dispose of the syringe, cannula, and shield per established procedures.

HOW SUPPLIED

TNKase is supplied as a sterile, lyophilized powder in a 50 mg vial under partial vacuum. Each 50 mg vial of TNKase is packaged with one 10 mL vial of Sterile Water for Injection, USP, for reconstitution, The B-D® 10 cc Syringe with TwinPak™ Dual Cannula Device, and three alcohol prep pads. NDC 50242-038-61.

Stability and Storage

Store lyophilized TNKase at controlled room temperature not to exceed 30°C (86°F) or under refrigeration 2–8°C (36–46°F). Do not use beyond the expiration date stamped on the vial.

REFERENCES

1. ASSENT-2 Investigators. Single-bolus tenecteplase compared with front-loaded alteplase in acute myocardial infarction: the ASSENT-2 double-blind randomised trial. Lancet 1999;354:716-22.
2. Cannon CP, Gibson CM, McCabe CH, Adgey AAJ, Schweiger MJ, Sequeira RF, et al. TNK-tissue plasminogen activator compared with front-loaded alteplase in acute myocardial infarction. Results of the TIMI 10B trial. Circulation 1998;98:2805-14.
3. Van de Werf F, Cannon CP, Luyten A, Houbracken K, McCabe CH, Berioli S, et al. Safety assessment of a single bolus administration of TNK-tissue plasminogen activator in acute myocardial infarction: the ASSENT-1 trial. Am Heart J 1999;137:786-91.

TNKase™
Tenecteplase

Manufactured by:
Genentech, Inc. 4819900
1 DNA Way June 2000
South San Francisco, CA 94080-4990

Shown in Product Identification Guide, page 313

IDENTIFICATION PROBLEM?
Turn to the **Product Identification Guide,**
where you'll find more than
1600 products pictured in actual
size and full color.

Genetics Institute

87 CAMBRIDGE PARK DRIVE
CAMBRIDGE, MA 02140

A Subsidiary of American Home Products
Direct Inquiries to:
1-888-638-6342

BENEFIX™ ℞
COAGULATION FACTOR IX (RECOMBINANT)

DESCRIPTION

BeneFɪx,™ Coagulation Factor IX (Recombinant), is a purified protein produced by recombinant DNA technology for use in therapy of factor IX deficiency, known as hemophilia B or Christmas disease. Coagulation Factor IX (Recombinant) is a glycoprotein with an approximate molecular mass of 55,000 Da consisting of 415 amino acids in a single chain. It has a primary amino acid sequence that is identical to the Ala^{148} allelic form of plasma-derived factor IX, and has structural and functional characteristics similar to those of endogenous factor IX.

BeneFɪx™ is produced by a genetically engineered Chinese hamster ovary (CHO) cell line that is extensively characterized and shown to be free of infectious agents. The stored cell banks are free of blood or plasma products. The CHO cell line secretes recombinant factor IX into a defined cell culture medium that does not contain any proteins derived from animal or human sources, and the recombinant factor IX is purified by a chromatography purification process that does not require a monoclonal antibody step and yields a high-purity, active product. A membrane filtration step that has the ability to retain molecules with apparent molecular weights >70,000 (such as large proteins and viral particles) is included for additional viral safety. BeneFɪx™ is predominantly a single component by SDS-polyacrylamide gel electrophoresis evaluation. The potency (in international units, I.U.) is determined using an in vitro one-stage clotting assay against the World Health Organization (WHO) International Standard for Factor IX concentrate. One international unit is the amount of factor IX activity present in 1 mL of pooled, normal human plasma. The specific activity of BeneFɪx™ is greater than or equal to 200 I.U. per milligram of protein. BeneFɪx™ is not derived from human blood and contains no preservatives or added animal or human components.

BeneFɪx™ is inherently free from the risk of transmission of human blood-borne pathogens such as HIV, hepatitis viruses, and parvovirus.

BeneFɪx™ is formulated as a sterile, nonpyrogenic, lyophilized powder preparation. BeneFɪx™ is intended for intravenous (IV) injection. It is available in single use vials containing the labeled amount of factor IX activity, expressed in international units (I.U.). Each vial contains nominally 250, 500, or 1000 I.U. of Coagulation Factor IX (Recombinant). After reconstitution of the lyophilized drug product, the concentrations of excipients in the 500 and 1000 I.U. dosage strengths are 10 mM L-histidine, 1% sucrose, 260 mM glycine, 0.005% polysorbate 80. The concentrations after reconstitution in the 250 I.U. dosage strength are half those of the other two dosage strengths. The 500 and 1000 I.U. dosage strengths are isotonic after reconstitution, and the 250 I.U. dosage strength has half the tonicity of the other two dosage strengths after reconstitution. All dosage strengths yield a clear, colorless solution upon reconstitution.

CLINICAL PHARMACOLOGY

Factor IX is activated by factor VII/tissue factor complex in the extrinsic coagulation pathway as well as by factor XIa in the intrinsic coagulation pathway. Activated factor IX, in combination with activated factor VIII, activates factor X. This results ultimately in the conversion of prothrombin to thrombin. Thrombin then converts fibrinogen to fibrin, and a clot can be formed.

Factor IX is the specific clotting factor deficient in patients with hemophilia B and in patients with acquired factor IX deficiencies. The administration of BeneFɪx,™ Coagulation Factor IX (Recombinant), increases plasma levels of factor IX and can temporarily correct the coagulation defect in these patients.

After single intravenous (IV) doses of 50 I.U./kg of BeneFɪx™ in 36 patients, each given as a 10-minute infusion, the mean increase in circulating factor IX activity was 0.8 ± 0.2 I.U./dL per I.U./kg infused (ranged from 0.4 to 1.4) and the mean biologic half-life was 19.4 ± 5.4 hours (ranged from 11 to 36). The in vivo recovery using BeneFɪx™ was statistically significantly less (28% lower) than the recovery using a highly purified plasma-derived factor IX product. There was no significant difference in biological half-life. In subsequent evaluations at 6 and 12 months, the pharmacokinetic parameters were similar to the initial results.

In clinical studies of BeneFɪx™ involving a total of 64 patients (44 previously treated patients [PTPs], 11 previously untreated patients [PUPs], and the 9 patients participating only in the surgical study), more than 7 million I.U. were administered over a period of up to 18 months. This includes 57 HIV-negative and 7 HIV-positive patients. Forty-five patients were evaluated for efficacy, all of whom were treated successfully for bleeding episodes on an on-demand basis or for the prevention of bleeds. Bleeding episodes that were managed successfully include hemarthroses and bleeding in soft tissue and muscle.

Management of hemostasis was evaluated in the surgical setting. Thirteen surgical procedures have been performed in 12 patients, with a cumulative dose ranging from 10,000 to 348,000 I.U. The 10 major procedures were performed using a pulse replacement regimen (N=7) or a continuous infusion regimen (N=3), and included a liver transplantation, a hernia repair, six orthopedic surgeries, and two dental extractions. Circulatory factor IX levels targeted to restore and maintain hemostasis were achieved with both pulse replacement and continuous infusion regimens. Hemostasis was maintained throughout the surgical period, and there was no clinical evidence of thrombotic complications in any of these patients. In four patients for whom fibrinopeptide A and prothrombin fragment 1 + 2 were measured preinfusion, at 4 to 8 hours, and then daily up to 96 hours, there was no evidence of significant increase in coagulation activation. Data from two additional patients were judged to be not evaluable.

A study of BeneFIX™ has been initiated in patients who had not been treated previously with plasma-derived factor IX concentrate (PUPs). In preliminary data, 11 of the 20 patients enrolled in the study received at least one infusion of BeneFIX.™ These 11 patients received a total of 27,208 I.U. in 42 infusions. Thirty to 50 patients will be enrolled and followed for up to 5 years to complete evaluation of BeneFIX™ in this patient population for safety, efficacy, and immunogenicity.

A low-level inhibitor developed in 1 of 44 BeneFIX™ patients who had previously received plasma-derived products. This patient had an extensive previous history of exposure to plasma-derived factor IX products, including a single subcutaneous exposure, without history of inhibitor development. Antibodies were detected in this patient after 9 months of treatment (39 exposure days) with BeneFIX.™ This patient was able to continue treatment with BeneFIX™ with no anamnestic rise in inhibitor or anaphylaxis.

Twelve days after a dose of BeneFIX™ for a bleeding episode, one hepatitis C antibody positive patient developed a renal infarct. The relationship of the infarct to prior administration of BeneFIX™ is uncertain but was judged to be unlikely by the investigator. The patient continued to be treated with BeneFIX.™

INDICATIONS AND USAGE

BeneFIX,™ Coagulation Factor IX (Recombinant), is indicated for the control and prevention of hemorrhagic episodes in patients with hemophilia B (congenital factor IX deficiency or Christmas disease), including control and prevention of bleeding in surgical settings.

BeneFIX™ is not indicated for the treatment of other factor deficiencies (e.g., factors II, VII, and X), nor for the treatment of hemophilia A patients with inhibitors to factor VIII, nor for the reversal of coumarin-induced anticoagulation, nor for the treatment of bleeding due to low levels of liver-dependent coagulation factors.

CONTRAINDICATIONS

Because BeneFIX,™ Coagulation Factor IX (Recombinant), is produced in a Chinese hamster ovary cell line, it may be contraindicated in patients with a known history of hypersensitivity to hamster protein.

WARNINGS

As with any intravenous protein product, allergic type hypersensitivity reactions are possible. Patients should be informed of the early signs of hypersensitivity reactions including hives, generalized urticaria, tightness of the chest, wheezing, hypotension, and anaphylaxis. Patients should be advised to discontinue use of the product and contact their physician if these symptoms occur.

Since the use of factor IX complex concentrates has historically been associated with the development of thromboembolic complications, the use of factor IX-containing products may be potentially hazardous in patients with signs of fibrinolysis and in patients with disseminated intravascular coagulation (DIC).

PRECAUTIONS

General

Historically, the administration of factor IX complex concentrates derived from human plasma, containing factors II, VII, IX and X, has been associated with the development of thromboembolic complications.[1] Although BeneFIX™ contains no coagulation factor other than factor IX, the potential risk of thrombosis and DIC observed with other products containing factor IX should be recognized. Because of the potential risk of thromboembolic complications, caution should be exercised when administering this product to patients with liver disease, to patients postoperatively, to neonates, or to patients at risk of thromboembolic phenomena or DIC. In each of these situations, the benefit of treatment with BeneFIX™ should be weighed against the risk of these complications.

Activity-neutralizing antibodies (inhibitors) have been detected in patients receiving factor IX– containing products. As with all factor IX products, patients using BeneFIX™ should be monitored for the development of factor IX inhibitors (see **Clinical Pharmacology**). It has been reported[2] that patients dosed with high-purity plasma-derived factor IX products who develop inhibitors to factor IX are at increased risk of anaphylaxis upon subsequent challenge with factor IX.

Type of Hemorrhage	Circulating Factor IX Activity Required (%)	Frequency of Doses (h)	Duration of Therapy (d)
Minor			
Uncomplicated hemarthroses, superficial muscle, or soft tissue	20–30	12–24	1–2
Moderate			
Intramuscle or soft tissue with dissection, mucous membranes, dental extractions, or hematuria	25–50	12–24	Treat until bleeding stops and healing begins; about 2 to 7 days
Major			
Pharynx, retropharynx, retroperitoneum, CNS, surgery	50–100	12–24	7–10

Source: Roberts and Eberst[3]

Dosing of BeneFIX™ may differ from that of plasma-derived factor IX products (see **Clinical Pharmacology** and **Dosage and Administration**).

Carcinogenesis, Mutagenesis, Impairment of Fertility

BeneFIX,™ Coagulation Factor IX (Recombinant), has been shown to be nonmutagenic in the Ames assay and nonclastogenic in a chromosomal aberrations assay. No investigations on carcinogenesis or impairment of fertility have been conducted.

Pregnancy Category C

Animal reproduction and lactation studies have not been conducted with BeneFIX,™ Coagulation Factor IX (Recombinant). It is not known whether BeneFIX™ can affect reproductive capacity or cause fetal harm when given to pregnant women. BeneFIX™ should be administered to pregnant and lactating women only if clearly indicated.

Pediatric Use

Safety and efficacy studies are ongoing in previously treated children and adolescents and in previously untreated children (see **Clinical Pharmacology**, **Warnings**, and **Precautions**). During clinical studies conducted in PUPs, no adverse reactions related to therapy were reported in 42 infusions.

ADVERSE REACTIONS

As with the intravenous administration of any product, the following reactions may be observed after administration: headache, fever, chills, flushing, nausea, vomiting, lethargy, or other manifestations of allergic reactions. During clinical studies with BeneFIX,™ Coagulation Factor IX (Recombinant), conducted in previously treated patients (PTPs), 60 mild adverse reactions definitely, probably, or possibly related to therapy were reported for 2548 infusions. These were nausea (16), discomfort at the IV site (13), altered taste (10), burning sensation in jaw and skull (6), allergic rhinitis (3), lightheadedness (2), headache (2), dizziness (1), chest tightness (1), fever (1), phlebitis/cellulitis at IV site (1), drowsiness (1), dry cough/sneeze (1), rash (1), and a single hive (1). Twelve days after a dose of BeneFIX™ for a bleeding episode, one hepatitis C antibody positive patient developed a renal infarct. The relationship of the infarct to prior administration of BeneFIX™ is uncertain but was judged to be unlikely by the investigator. The patient continued to be treated with BeneFIX.™

If any adverse reaction takes place that is thought to be related to the administration of BeneFIX,™ the rate of infusion should be decreased or the infusion stopped.

DOSAGE AND ADMINISTRATION

Treatment with BeneFIX,™ Coagulation Factor IX (Recombinant), should be initiated under the supervision of a physician experienced in the treatment of hemophilia B.

Dosage and duration of treatment for all factor IX products depend on the severity of the factor IX deficiency, the location and extent of bleeding, and the patient's clinical condition, age and recovery of factor IX. For all these reasons, doses administered should be titrated to the patient's clinical response and, when clinically indicated, factor IX activity recovery levels.

In an eleven patient crossover, randomized PK evaluation of BeneFIX™ and a single lot of high-purity plasma-derived factor IX, the recovery was lower for BeneFIX™ (see **Clinical Pharmacology**). On average, on international unit of BeneFIX™ per kilogram of body weight increased the circulating activity of factor IX by 0.8 ± 0.2 (ranged from 0.4 to 1.4) I.U./dL.

Dosing should be based on the reported clinical trial pharmacokinetic results for BeneFIX.™ The following formula provides a guide to empirical dosage calculations:

$$\text{number of factor IX IU required} = \text{body weight (in kg)} \times \text{desired factor IX increase (\%)} \times 1.2\ \text{IU/kg}$$

In the presence of an inhibitor, higher doses may be required.

The following chart[3] may be used to guide dosing in bleeding episodes and surgery:

[See table above]

In the clinical efficacy studies, patients were initially administered the same dose previously used for plasma-derived Factor IX. Even in the absence of Factor IX inhibitor, several patients required increased doses in these studies. To ensure that the desired Factor IX activity level has been achieved, precise monitoring using the Factor IX activity assay is advised, in particular, for surgical interventions.

BeneFIX™ is administered by IV infusion over several minutes after reconstitution of the lyophilized powder with Sterile Water for Injection (USP).

INSTRUCTIONS FOR USE

Reconstitution

Always wash your hands before performing the following procedures. Aseptic technique should be used during the reconstitution procedure.

BeneFIX,™ Coagulation Factor IX (Recombinant), will be administered by intravenous (IV) infusion after reconstitution with Sterile Water for Injection (diluent).

1. Allow the vials of lyophilized BeneFIX™ and diluent to reach room temperature.
2. Remove the plastic flip-top caps from the BeneFIX™ vial and the diluent vial to expose the central portions of the rubber stoppers.
3. Wipe the tops of both vials with the alcohol swab provided, or use another antiseptic solution, and allow to dry.
4. Remove the protective cover from the short end of the sterile double-ended needle and insert the short end into the diluent vial at the center of the stopper.
5. Remove the protective cover from the long end of the needle and insert the long end into the BeneFIX™ vial at the center of the stopper.
   Note: Point the double-ended needle toward the wall of the BeneFIX™ vial to prevent excessive foaming.
6. Fully invert the diluent vial to the vertical position and allow the diluent to run completely into the BeneFIX™ vial.
7. Once the transfer is complete, remove the long end of the needle from the BeneFIX™ vial, recap, and properly discard the needle with the diluent vial.
   Note: If the diluent does not transfer completely into the BeneFIX™ vial, DO NOT USE the contents of the vial. Note that it is acceptable for a small amount of fluid to remain in the diluent vial after transfer.
8. Gently rotate the vial to dissolve the powder.
9. Parenteral drug products should be inspected visually for particulate matter and discoloration prior to administration, whenever solution and container permit. Reconstituted BeneFIX™ should appear clear and colorless.

BeneFIX™ should be administered within 3 hours after reconstitution. The reconstituted solution may be stored at room temperature prior to administration.

Administration (Intravenous Injection)

BeneFIX,™ Coagulation Factor IX (Recombinant), should be administered using a single sterile disposable plastic syringe. In addition, the solution should be withdrawn from the vial using the sterile filter spike.

1. Using aseptic technique, attach the sterile filter spike to the sterile disposable syringe.
   Note: Do NOT inject air into the BeneFIX™ vial. This may cause partial loss of product.
2. Insert the filter spike end into the stopper of the BeneFIX™ vial.
3. Invert the vial and withdraw the reconstituted solution into the syringe.
4. Remove and discard the filter spike.
   Note: If you use more than one vial of BeneFIX,™ the contents of multiple vials may be drawn into the same syringe through a separate, unused filter spike.
5. Attach the syringe to the Luer end of the infusion set tubing and perform venipuncture as instructed by your physician.

After reconstitution, BeneFIX™ should be injected intravenously over several minutes. The rate of administration should be determined by the patient's comfort level (see **Adverse Reactions**).

Dispose of all unused solution, empty vials, and used needles and syringes in an appropriate container for throwing away waste that might hurt others if not handled properly.

Storage

Product as packaged for sale: BeneFIX™ Coagulation Factor IX (Recombinant), should be stored under refrigeration at a temperature of 2 to 8°C (36 to 46°F). Prior to the expiration date, BeneFIX™ may also be stored at room temperature not to exceed 25°C (77°F) for up to 6 months. The patient should make note of the date the product was placed at room temperature in the space provided on the outer carton. Freezing should be avoided to prevent damage to the diluent vial. Do not use BeneFIX™ after the expiry date on the label.

Continued on next page

Benefix—Cont.

Product after reconstitution: The product does not contain a preservative and should be used within 3 hours.

HOW SUPPLIED

BeneFix,™ Coagulation Factor IX (Recombinant), is supplied in single use vials which contain nominally 250, 500, or 1000 I.U. per vial (NDC # 58394-003-01, 58394-002-01, and 58394-001-01, respectively) with sterile diluent, sterile double-ended needle for reconstitution, sterile filter spike for withdrawal, sterile infusion set, and two (2) alcohol swabs. Actual factor IX activity in I.U. is stated on the label of each vial.

REFERENCES

1. Lusher JM. Thrombogenicity associated with factor IX complex concentrates. *Semin Hematol.* 1991;28 (3 Suppl. 6):3–5.
2. Shapiro AD, Ragni MV, Lusher JM, et al. Safety and efficacy of monoclonal antibody purified factor IX concentrate in previously untreated patients with hemophilia B. *Thromb Haemost.* 1996;75(1):30–35.
3. Roberts HR, Eberst ME. Current management of hemophilia B. *Hematol Oncol Clin North Am.* 1993;7(6):1269–1280.

GENETICS INSTITUTE®
87 Cambridge Park Drive
Cambridge, MA 02140-2387
1-888-237-3200
FIX00003.04
6/97
Shown in Product Identification Guide, page 313

NEUMEGA® ℞
[nĕu-mĕga]
(Oprelvekin)

DESCRIPTION

Interleukin eleven (IL-11) is a thrombopoietic growth factor that directly stimulates the proliferation of hematopoietic stem cells and megakaryocyte progenitor cells and induces megakaryocyte maturation resulting in increased platelet production. IL-11 is a member of a family of human growth factors which includes human growth hormone, granulocyte colony-stimulating factor (G-CSF), and other growth factors.

Oprelvekin, the active ingredient in Neumega, is produced in *Escherichia coli (E. coli)* by recombinant DNA methods. The protein has a molecular mass of approximately 19,000 daltons, and is non-glycosylated. The polypeptide is 177 amino acids in length and differs from the 178 amino acid length of native IL-11 only in lacking the amino-terminal proline residue. This alteration has not resulted in measurable differences in bioactivity either *in vitro* or *in vivo*.

Neumega is available for subcutaneous administration in single-use vials containing 5 mg of Oprelvekin (specific activity approximately 8×10^6 Units/mg) as a sterile, lyophilized powder with 23 mg Glycine, USP, 1.6 mg Dibasic Sodium Phosphate Heptahydrate, USP, and 0.55 mg Monobasic Sodium Phosphate Monohydrate, USP. When reconstituted with 1 mL of Sterile Water for Injection, USP, the resulting solution has a pH of 7.0 and a concentration of 5 mg/mL.

CLINICAL PHARMACOLOGY

The primary hematopoietic activity of Neumega is stimulation of megakaryocytopoiesis and thrombopoiesis. Neumega has shown potent thrombopoietic activity in animal models of compromised hematopoiesis, including moderately to severely myelosuppressed mice and nonhuman primates. In these models, Neumega improved platelet nadirs and accelerated platelet recoveries compared to controls.

Preclinical studies have shown that mature megakaryocytes which develop during *in vivo* treatment with Neumega are ultrastructurally normal. Platelets produced in response to Neumega were morphologically and functionally normal and possessed a normal life-span.

IL-11 has also been shown to have non-hematopoietic activities in animals including: the regulation of intestinal epithelium growth (enhanced healing of gastrointestinal lesions), the inhibition of adipogenesis, the induction of acute phase protein synthesis, inhibition of pro-inflammatory cytokine production by macrophages, and the stimulation of osteoclastogenesis and neurogenesis.

IL-11 is produced by bone marrow stromal cells and is part of the cytokine family that shares the gp130 signal transducer. Primary osteoblasts and mature osteoclasts express mRNAs for both IL-11 receptor (IL-11R alpha) and gp130. Both bone-forming and bone-resorbing cells are potential targets of IL-11. (1)

Pharmacokinetics

The pharmacokinetics of Neumega have been evaluated in studies in healthy, adult subjects and oncology patients receiving chemotherapy. In a study in which a single 50 μg/kg subcutaneous dose was administered to eighteen men, the peak serum concentration (Cmax) of 17.4±5.4 ng/mL (mean ± S.D.) was reached at 3.2±2.4 hrs (Tmax) following dosing. The terminal half life was 6.9±1.7 hrs. In a second study in which single 75 μg/kg subcutaneous and intravenous doses were administered to twenty-four healthy subjects, the pharmacokinetic profiles were similar between men and women. The absolute bioavailability of Neumega was >80%. In a study in which multiple, subcutaneous doses of both 25 and 50 μg/kg were administered to cancer patients receiving chemotherapy, Neumega did not accumulate and clearance of Neumega was not impaired following multiple doses.

Neumega was also administered to twenty-eight infants, children, and adolescents receiving ICE (ifosfamide, carboplatin, etoposide) chemotherapy. Analysis of data from twenty-three pediatric patients showed that Cmax and Tmax were comparable to the adult population. The mean ± S.D. area under the concentration-time curve (AUC) for pediatric patients (8 months to 17 years), receiving 50 μg/kg or 100 μg/kg was 137±56 ng*hr/mL or 237±20 ng*hr/mL, respectively, compared with 189±41 ng*hr/mL in adults receiving 50 μg/kg. Available data suggest that clearance of IL-11 decreases with patient age, and that clearance in infants and children (8 months to 11 years) is approximately 1.2 to 1.6 fold higher than adults and adolescents (ages 12 and over).

In preclinical studies in rats, radiolabeled Neumega was rapidly cleared from the serum and distributed to highly perfused organs. The kidney was the primary route of elimination. The amount of intact Neumega in urine was low, indicating that the molecule was metabolized before excretion. In a clinical study, a single dose of Neumega was administered to subjects with severely impaired renal function (creatinine clearance < 15 mL/min). The mean ± S.D. values for Cmax and AUC were 30.8 ± 8.6 ng/mL and 373 ± 106 ng*hr/mL, respectively. When compared with control subjects in this study with normal renal function, the mean Cmax was 2.2 fold higher and the mean AUC was 2.6 fold (95% confidence interval 1.7–3.8) higher in the subjects with severe renal impairment. In the subjects with severe renal impairment, clearance was approximately 40% of the value seen in subjects with normal renal function. The average terminal half-life was similar in subjects with severe renal impairment and those with normal renal function.

Pharmacodynamics

In a study in which Neumega was administered to non-myelosuppressed cancer patients, daily subcutaneous dosing for 14 days with Neumega increased the platelet count in a dose-dependent manner. Platelet counts began to increase relative to baseline between 5 and 9 days after the start of dosing with Neumega. After cessation of treatment, platelet counts continued to increase for up to 7 days then returned toward baseline within 14 days. No change in platelet reactivity as measured by platelet activation in response to ADP, and platelet aggregation in response to ADP, epinephrine, collagen, ristocetin and arachidonic acid has been observed in association with Neumega treatment.

In a randomized, double-blind, placebo-controlled study in normal volunteers, subjects receiving Neumega had a mean increase in plasma volume of >20%, and all subjects receiving Neumega had at least a 10% increase in plasma volume. Red blood cell volume decreased similarly (due to repeated phlebotomy) in the Neumega and placebo groups. As a result, whole blood volume increased approximately 10% and hemoglobin concentration decreased approximately 10% in subjects receiving Neumega compared with subjects receiving placebo. Mean 24 hour sodium excretion decreased, and potassium excretion did not increase, in subjects receiving Neumega compared with subjects receiving placebo.

CLINICAL STUDIES

Two randomized, double-blind, placebo-controlled trials studied Neumega for the prevention of severe thrombocytopenia following single or repeated sequential cycles of various myelosuppressive chemotherapy regimens.

One study evaluated the effectiveness of Neumega in eliminating the need for platelet transfusions in patients who had recovered from an episode of severe chemotherapy-induced thrombocytopenia (defined as a platelet count ≤20,000/μL), and were to receive one additional cycle of the same chemotherapy without dose reduction. Patients had various underlying non-myeloid malignancies, and were undergoing dose-intensive chemotherapy with a variety of regimens. Patients were randomized to receive Neumega at a dose of 25 μg/kg or 50 μg/kg, or placebo. The primary endpoint was whether the patient required one or more platelet transfusions in the subsequent chemotherapy cycle. Ninety-three patients were randomized. Five patients withdrew from the study prior to receiving study drug. As a result, eighty-eight patients were included in a modified intent-to-treat analysis. The results for the Neumega 50 μg/kg and placebo groups are summarized in Table 1. The placebo group includes one patient who underwent chemotherapy dose reduction and who avoided platelet transfusions.

[See table 1 below]

In the primary efficacy analysis, more patients avoided platelet transfusion in the Neumega 50 μg/kg arm than in the placebo arm (p=0.04, Fisher's Exact test, 2-tailed). The difference in the proportion of patients avoiding platelet transfusions in the Neumega 50 μg/kg and placebo groups was 21% (95% confidence interval 2 to 40%). The results observed in patients receiving 25 μg/kg of Neumega were intermediate between those of the placebo and the 50 μg/kg groups.

A second study evaluated the effectiveness of Neumega in eliminating platelet transfusions over two dose-intensive chemotherapy cycles in breast cancer patients who had not previously experienced severe chemotherapy-induced thrombocytopenia. All patients received the same chemotherapy regimen (cyclophosphamide 3,200 mg/m^2 and doxorubicin 75 mg/m^2). All patients received concomitant Filgrastim (G-CSF) in all cycles. The patients were stratified by whether or not they had received prior chemotherapy, and randomized to receive Neumega 50 μg/kg or placebo. The primary endpoint was whether or not a patient required one or more platelet transfusions in the two study cycles. Seventy-seven patients were randomized. Thirteen patients failed to complete both study cycles—eight of these had insufficient data to be evaluated for the primary endpoint. The results of this trial are summarized in Table 2.

[See table 2 at top of next page]

This study showed a trend in favor of Neumega, particularly in the subgroup of patients with prior chemotherapy. Open-label treatment with Neumega has been continued for up to four consecutive chemotherapy cycles without evidence of any adverse effect on the rate of neutrophil recovery or red blood cell transfusion requirements. Some patients continued to maintain platelet nadirs >20,000 cells/μL for at least four sequential cycles of chemotherapy without the need for transfusions, chemotherapy dose reduction, or changes in treatment schedules.

Platelet activation studies done on a limited number of patients showed no evidence of abnormal spontaneous platelet activation, or an abnormal response to ADP. In an unblinded, retrospective analysis of the two placebo-controlled studies, 19 of 69 patients (28%) receiving Neumega 50 μg/kg and 34 of 67 patients (51%) receiving placebo reported at least one hemorrhagic adverse event which involved bleeding.

In a randomized, double-blind, placebo-controlled, phase 2 study conducted in patients who received autologous bone marrow transplantation following myeloablative chemotherapy, the incidence of platelet transfusions and time to neutrophil and platelet engraftment were similar in the Neumega and placebo-treated arms.

In long term follow-up of patients, the distribution of survival and progression-free survival times was similar between patients randomized to Neumega therapy and those randomized to receive placebo.

INDICATIONS AND USAGE

Neumega is indicated for the prevention of severe thrombocytopenia and the reduction of the need for platelet transfusions following myelosuppressive chemotherapy in patients with nonmyeloid malignancies who are at high risk of severe thrombocytopenia. Efficacy was demonstrated in patients who had experienced severe thrombocytopenia following the previous chemotherapy cycle. Neumega is not indicated following myeloablative chemotherapy.

CONTRAINDICATIONS

Neumega is contraindicated in patients with a history of hypersensitivity to Neumega or any component of the product.

WARNINGS

Neumega is known to cause fluid retention (see CLINICAL PHARMACOLOGY: Pharmacodynamics), and it should be used with caution in patients with clinically evident congestive heart failure, patients who may be susceptible to developing congestive heart failure, and patients with a history of heart failure who are well-compensated and receiving appropriate medical therapy (see PRECAUTIONS: Fluid Retention).

Close monitoring of fluid and electrolyte status should be performed in patients receiving chronic diuretic therapy. Sudden deaths have occurred in Oprelvekin-treated patients receiving chronic diuretic therapy and ifosfamide who developed severe hypokalemia (see ADVERSE REACTIONS).

PRECAUTIONS

General

Dosing with Neumega should begin 6 to 24 hours following the completion of chemotherapy dosing. The safety and efficacy of Neumega given immediately prior to or concurrently with cytotoxic chemotherapy have not been established (see DOSAGE AND ADMINISTRATION).

TABLE 1
STUDY RESULTS

	Placebo n=30	Neumega 50 μg/kg n=29
Number (%) of patients avoiding platelet transfusion	2 (7%)	8 (28%)
Number (%) of patients requiring platelet transfusion	28 (93%)	21 (72%)
Median (mean) number of platelet transfusion events	2.5 (3.3)	1 (2.2)

Neumega has not been evaluated in patients receiving chemotherapy regimens of greater than 5 days duration or regimens associated with delayed myelosuppression (e.g., nitrosoureas, mitomycin-C).
The parenteral administration of Neumega should be attended by appropriate precautions in case allergic reactions occur (see CONTRAINDICATIONS).

Fluid Retention

Patients receiving Neumega have commonly experienced mild to moderate fluid retention as indicated by peripheral edema or dyspnea on exertion. Weight gain has been uncommon. The fluid retention is reversible within several days following discontinuation of Neumega. In some patients, preexisting pleural effusions have increased during administration of Neumega. Preexisting fluid collections, including pericardial effusions or ascites, should be monitored. Drainage should be considered if medically indicated. Capillary leak syndrome has not been observed following treatment with Neumega.
Moderate decreases in hemoglobin concentration, hematocrit, and red blood cell count (~10–15%) without a decrease in red blood cell mass have been observed. These changes are predominantly due to an increase in plasma volume (dilutional anemia) that is primarily related to renal sodium and water retention. The decrease in hemoglobin concentration typically begins within 3–5 days of the initiation of Neumega, and is reversible over approximately a week following discontinuation of Neumega.
During dosing with Neumega, fluid balance should be monitored and appropriate medical management is advised. If a diuretic is used, fluid and electrolyte balance should be carefully monitored. Neumega should be used with caution in patients who may develop fluid retention as a result of associated medical conditions or whose medical condition may be exacerbated by fluid retention.

Cardiovascular Events

Neumega should be used with caution in patients with a history of atrial arrhythmia, and only after consideration of the potential risks in relation to anticipated benefit. Transient atrial arrhythmias (atrial fibrillation or atrial flutter) have occurred in approximately 10% of patients following treatment with Neumega. In some patients this may be due to increased plasma volume associated with fluid retention (See PRECAUTIONS: Fluid Retention); Neumega has been shown not to be directly arrhythmogenic. Arrhythmias have usually been brief in duration and usually without clinical sequelae; however sequelae including stroke have been observed in patients receiving Neumega who experienced atrial arrhythmias. Conversion to sinus rhythm typically occurred spontaneously or after rate-control drug therapy. Most patients have continued to receive Neumega without recurrence of atrial arrhythmia. A retrospective analysis of data from clinical studies of Neumega suggests that advancing age and other conditions associated with an increased risk of atrial arrhythmias such as use of cardiac medications and a history of doxorubicin exposure are risk factors for the development of atrial fibrillation or atrial flutter in patients receiving Neumega. Ventricular arrhythmias have not been attributed to the use of Neumega.

Ophthalmologic Events

Transient, mild visual blurring has occasionally been reported by patients treated with Neumega. Papilledema has been reported in approximately 1.5% of patients treated with Neumega following repeated cycles of exposure. Nonhuman primates treated with Neumega at a dose of 1,000 µg/kg SC once daily for 4 to 13 weeks developed papilledema which was not associated with inflammation or any other histologic abnormality and was reversible after dosing was discontinued. Neumega should be used with caution in patients with preexisting papilledema, or with tumors involving the central nervous system since it is possible that papilledema could worsen or develop during treatment.

Antibody Formation/Allergic Reactions

A small proportion (1%) of patients receiving Neumega in clinical studies developed antibodies to Oprelvekin and transient rashes were occasionally observed at the injection site following Neumega administration. The presence of these antibodies or injection site reactions have not been correlated with clinical symptoms such as anaphylactoid reactions or a loss of clinical response to Neumega. No anaphylactoid or other severe adverse allergic reactions were reported in clinical studies following single or repeated doses of Neumega.

Chronic Administration

Neumega has been administered safely using the recommended dosing schedule (see DOSAGE AND ADMINISTRATION) for up to 6 cycles following chemotherapy. The safety and efficacy of chronic administration of Neumega have not been established. Continuous dosing (2–13 weeks) in nonhuman primates produced joint capsule and tendon fibrosis and periosteal hyperostosis (see PRECAUTIONS: Pediatric Use). The relevance of these findings to humans is unclear.

Information for Patients

In situations when the physician determines that Neumega may be used outside of the hospital or office setting, persons who will be administering Neumega should be instructed as to the proper dose, and the method for reconstituting and administering Neumega (See DOSAGE AND ADMINISTRATION and Patient Information at the end of this insert). If home use is prescribed, patients should be instructed in the importance of proper disposal and cautioned against the reuse of needles, syringes, drug product, and diluent. A puncture resistant container should be used by the patient for the disposal of used needles.
Patients should be informed of the most common adverse reactions associated with Neumega administration, including those symptoms related to fluid retention (see ADVERSE REACTIONS and PRECAUTIONS). Mild to moderate peripheral edema and shortness of breath on exertion can occur within the first week of treatment and may continue for the duration of administration of Neumega. Patients who have preexisting pleural or other effusions or a history of congestive heart failure should be advised to contact their physician for worsening of dyspnea. Most patients who receive Neumega develop some anemia. Patients who are older or who have other risk factors for the development of atrial arrhythmias should be cautioned to contact their physician if symptoms attributable to atrial arrhythmia develop and are not transient. Female patients of childbearing potential should be advised of the possible risks to the fetus of Neumega (see PRECAUTIONS: Pregnancy).

TABLE 2
STUDY RESULTS

	Overall n=77		No Prior Chemotherapy n=54		Prior Chemotherapy n=23	
	Placebo n=37	Neumega n=40	Placebo n=27	Neumega n=27	Placebo n=10	Neumega n=13
Number (%) of patients avoiding platelet transfusion	15 (41%)	26 (65%)	14 (52%)	19 (70%)	1 (10%)	7 (54%)
Number (%) of patients requiring platelet transfusion	16 (43%)	12 (30%)	9 (33%)	7 (26%)	7 (70%)	5 (38%)
Number (%) of patients not evaluable	6 (16%)	2 (5%)	4 (15%)	1 (4%)	2 (20%)	1 (8%)

Laboratory Monitoring

A complete blood count should be obtained prior to chemotherapy and at regular intervals during Neumega therapy (see DOSAGE AND ADMINISTRATION). Platelet counts should be monitored during the time of the expected nadir and until adequate recovery has occurred (post-nadir counts ≥50,000).

Drug Interactions

Most patients in trials evaluating Neumega were treated concomitantly with Filgrastim (granulocyte colony-stimulating factor[G-CSF]) with no adverse effect of Neumega on the activity of G-CSF. No information is available on the clinical use of Sargramostim (granulocyte-macrophage colony-stimulating factor [GM-CSF]) with Neumega. However, in a study in nonhuman primates in which Neumega and GM-CSF were coadministered, there were no adverse interactions between Neumega and GM-CSF and no apparent difference in the pharmacokinetic profile of Neumega.
Drug interactions between Neumega and other drugs have not been fully evaluated. Based on *in vitro* and nonclinical *in vivo* evaluations of Neumega, drug-drug interactions with known substrates of P450 enzymes would not be predicted.

Carcinogenesis, Mutagenesis, Impairment of Fertility

No studies have been performed to assess the carcinogenic potential of Neumega. *In vitro*, Neumega did not stimulate the growth of tumor colony-forming cells harvested from patients with a variety of human malignancies. Neumega has been shown to be non-genotoxic in *in vitro* studies. These data suggest that Neumega is not mutagenic. Although prolonged estrus cycles have been noted at 2 to 20 times the human dose, no effects on fertility have been observed in rats treated with Neumega at doses up to 1000 µg/kg/day.

Pregnancy Category C

Neumega has been shown to have embryocidal effects in pregnant rats and rabbits when given in doses of 0.2 to 20 times the human dose. There are no adequate and well-controlled studies of Neumega in pregnant women. Neumega should be used during pregnancy only if the potential benefit justifies the potential risk to the fetus.
Neumega has been tested in studies of fertility and early embryonic development in rats and in studies of organogenesis (teratogenicity) in rats and rabbits. Parental toxicity has been observed when Neumega is given at doses of 2 to 20 times the human dose (≥100 µg/kg/day) in the rat and when given in doses of 0.02 to 2.0 times the human dose (≥1 µg/kg/day) in the rabbit. Findings in the rat consisted of transient hypoactivity and dyspnea after administration, as well as prolonged estrus cycle, increased early embryonic deaths and decreased numbers of live fetuses. In addition, low fetal body weights and a reduced number of ossified sacral and caudal vertebrae (i.e., retarded fetal development) occurred in rats at 20 times the human dose, but no long-term behavioral or developmental abnormalities were evident. Findings in the rabbits consisted of decreased (fecal/urine) eliminations (the only toxicity noted at 1 µg/kg/day) as well as decreased food consumption, body weight loss, abortion, increased embryonic and fetal deaths, and decreased numbers of live fetuses. There have been no teratogenic effects of Neumega observed in rabbits.

Nursing Mothers

It is not known if Neumega is excreted in human milk. Because many drugs are excreted in human milk and because of the potential for serious adverse reactions in nursing infants from Neumega, a decision should be made whether to discontinue nursing or to discontinue the drug, taking into account the importance of the drug to the mother.

Pediatric Use

Efficacy trials have not been conducted in a pediatric population. Preliminary data are available from an ongoing pharmacokinetic study in twenty-eight patients ages 8 months to 17 years who have been treated with Neumega at doses of 25 to 100 µg/kg following ICE (ifosfamide, etoposide, carboplatin) chemotherapy. Neumega treatment was given once daily for a maximum of 28 days in up to eight cycles. Based upon this study, a dose of 75 to 100 µg/kg in the pediatric population will produce plasma levels consistent with those obtained in adults given 50 µg/kg (see CLINICAL PHARMACOLOGY: Pharmacokinetics).
Adverse events in this pediatric open-label, non-comparative study were generally similar to those observed using Neumega at a dose of 50 µg/kg in the randomized chemotherapy studies in adults. Most adverse events that were associated with Neumega in adults occurred either with similar or lower frequency in the pediatric study compared with adults. The incidences of tachycardia (46% [13/28]) and conjunctival injection (50% [14/28]) in the pediatric study were higher than in adults (see ADVERSE REACTIONS). There was no evidence of a dose-response relationship for any of the Neumega-associated adverse events among the pediatric patients.
No studies have been performed to assess the long-term effects of Neumega on growth and development. In growing rodents treated with 100, 300, or 1000 µg/kg/day for a minimum of 28 days, thickening of femoral and tibial growth plates was noted, which did not completely resolve after a 28-day non-treatment period. In a nonhuman primate toxicology study of Neumega, animals treated for 2 to 13 weeks at doses of 10 to 1000 µg/kg showed partially reversible joint capsule and tendon fibrosis and periosteal hyperostosis. The clinical significance of these findings is not known. An asymptomatic, laminated periosteal reaction in the diaphyses of the femur, tibia and fibula has been observed in one patient during pediatric trials involving multiple courses of Neumega treatment. The relationship of these findings to treatment with Neumega is unclear.

Use in Patients with Renal Impairment

Neumega is eliminated primarily by the kidneys. The pharmacokinetics of Neumega have not been studied in patients with mild or moderate renal impairment (creatinine clearance ≥ 15 mL/min). Fluid retention associated with Neumega treatment has not been studied in patients with renal impairment, but fluid balance should be carefully monitored in these patients (See PRECAUTIONS: Fluid Retention).

ADVERSE REACTIONS

Three hundred eight subjects, with ages ranging from 8 months to 75 years, have been exposed to Neumega treatment. Subjects have received up to six (eight in pediatric patients) sequential courses of Neumega treatment, with each course lasting from 1 to 28 days. Apart from the sequelae of the underlying malignancy or cytotoxic chemotherapy, most adverse events were mild or moderate in severity and reversible after discontinuation of Neumega dosing.
In general, the incidence and type of adverse events were similar between Neumega 50 µg/kg and placebo groups. The following adverse events, occurring in ≥10% of patients, were observed at equal or greater frequency in placebo-treated patients: asthenia, pain, chills, abdominal pain, infection, anorexia, constipation, dyspepsia, ecchymosis, myalgia, bone pain, nervousness, and alopecia. Selected adverse events that occurred in Neumega-treated patients are listed in Table 3.
[See table 3 at bottom of next page]
The following adverse events also occurred more frequently in cancer patients receiving Neumega than in those receiving placebo: amblyopia, paresthesia, dehydration, skin discoloration, exfoliative dermatitis, and eye hemorrhage; a statistically significant association of Neumega to these events has not been established. Other than a higher incidence of severe asthenia in Neumega treated patients (10 [14%] in Neumega patients versus 2 [3%] in placebo patients), the incidence of severe or life-threatening adverse events was comparable in the Neumega and placebo treatment groups.
The incidence of fever, neutropenic fever, flu-like symptoms, thrombocytosis, thrombotic events, the average number of units of red blood cells transfused per patient, and the duration of neutropenia <500 cells/µL were similar in the Neumega 50 µg/kg and placebo groups.
Two patients with cancer treated with Neumega experienced sudden death which the investigator considered possibly or probably related to Neumega. Both deaths occurred in patients with severe hypokalemia (<3.0 mEq/L) who had received high doses of ifosfamide and were receiving daily doses of a diuretic. The relationship of these deaths to Neumega remains unclear.

Abnormal Laboratory Values

The most common laboratory abnormality reported in patients in clinical trials was a decrease in hemoglobin con-

Continued on next page

Neumega—Cont.

centration predominantly as a result of expansion of the plasma volume (see PRECAUTIONS: Fluid Retention). The increase in plasma volume is also associated with a decrease in the serum concentration of albumin and several other proteins (e.g., transferrin and gamma globulins). A parallel decrease in calcium without clinical effects has been documented.
After daily SC injections, treatment with Neumega resulted in a two-fold increase in plasma fibrinogen. Other acute-phase proteins also increased. These protein levels returned to normal after dosing with Neumega was discontinued. Von Willebrand factor (vWF) concentrations increased with a normal multimer pattern in healthy subjects receiving Neumega.

OVERDOSAGE

Doses of Neumega above 100 µg/kg have not been administered to humans. While clinical experience is limited, doses of Neumega greater than 50 µg/kg may be associated with an increased incidence of cardiovascular events in adult patients (see PRECAUTIONS: Fluid Retention/Cardiovascular). If an overdose of Neumega is administered, Neumega should be discontinued, and the patient should be closely observed for signs of toxicity (see PRECAUTIONS and ADVERSE REACTIONS). Reinstitution of Neumega therapy should be based upon individual patient factors (e.g., evidence of toxicity, continued need for therapy).

DOSAGE AND ADMINISTRATION

The recommended dose of Neumega in adults is 50 µg/kg given once daily. Neumega should be administered subcutaneously as a single injection in either the abdomen, thigh, or hip (or upper arm if not self-injecting). Based upon a pharmacokinetic study, a dose of 75 to 100 µg/kg in the pediatric population will produce plasma levels consistent with those obtained in adults given 50 µg/kg (see CLINICAL PHARMACOLOGY: Pharmacokinetics).
Dosing should be initiated 6 to 24 hours after the completion of chemotherapy. Platelet counts should be monitored periodically to assess the optimal duration of therapy. Dosing should be continued until the post-nadir platelet count is ≥50,000 cells/µL. In controlled clinical studies, doses were administered in courses of 10 to 21 days. Dosing beyond 21 days per treatment course is not recommended.
Treatment with Neumega should be discontinued at least 2 days before starting the next planned cycle of chemotherapy.

Preparation of Neumega

1. Neumega is a sterile, white, preservative-free, lyophilized powder for subcutaneous injection upon reconstitution. Neumega (5 mg vials) should be reconstituted aseptically with 1.0 mL of Sterile Water for Injection, USP (without preservative). The reconstituted Neumega solution is clear, colorless, isotonic, with a pH of 7.0, and contains 5 mg/mL of Neumega. The single-use vial should not be re-entered or reused. Any unused portion of either reconstituted Neumega solution or Sterile Water for Injection, USP should be discarded.
2. During reconstitution, the Sterile Water for Injection, USP should be directed at the side of the vial and the contents gently swirled. EXCESSIVE OR VIGOROUS AGITATION SHOULD BE AVOIDED.
3. Parenteral drug products should be inspected visually for particulate matter and discoloration prior to administration, whenever solution and container permit. If particulate matter is present or the solution is discolored, the vial should not be used.
4. Because neither Neumega powder for injection nor its accompanying diluent, Sterile Water for Injection, USP contains a preservative, Neumega should be used as soon as possible following reconstitution. Neumega may be used within 3 hours of reconstitution when stored either at 2 to 8°C (36 to 46°F) or at room temperature up to 25°C (77°F). DO NOT FREEZE OR SHAKE THE RECONSTITUTED SOLUTION.

HOW SUPPLIED

Neumega is supplied as a sterile, white, preservative-free, lyophilize powder in vials containing 5 mg Oprelvekin. Neumega is available in boxes containing one single-dose Neumega vial and one 5-mL vial of diluent for Neumega (Sterile Water for Injection, USP) – NDC 58394-004-01; and boxes containing seven single-dose Neumega vials and seven 5-mL vials of diluent for Neumega (Sterile Water for Injection, USP) – NDC 58394-004-02.

Storage

Lyophilized Neumega and diluent should be stored in a refrigerator at 2 to 8°C (36 to 46°F). DO NOT FREEZE. Reconstituted Neumega must be used within 3 hours of reconstitution and can be stored in the vial either at 2 to 8°C (36 to 46°F) or at room temperature up to 25°C (77°F).

REFERENCES

(1) Du, X, and Williams, D., Interleukin 11: Review of Molecular, Cell Biology and Clinical Use. Blood. 89(11): 3897-3908, 1997.

GENETICS INSTITUTE

Genetics Institute, Inc.
Cambridge, MA 02140-2387, USA
US License Number 1163
Telephone: 1-888-446-3344
IL1131.00 Rev. 12/97

NEUMEGA®

(Oprelvekin)

PATIENT INFORMATION

General Information

Neumega is intended for use under the guidance and supervision of a health care professional. If, however, your physician recommends self-injection, you should be instructed in the preparation of Neumega, the proper method for self-injection, and the correct dose to use. You should not try self-administration until you are certain that you understand your health care professional's instructions. Each dose should be given at about the same time each day. If you miss a dose, continue with the next scheduled dose.

Possible Side Effects

As with any medication, use of Neumega may be associated with side effects. In clinical studies, these effects were generally mild or moderate and stopped after treatment. The most common side effects seen in studies of Neumega were edema (swelling) of the arms and/or legs, shortness of breath when moving about, and anemia. These side effects are probably related to water retention. Edema and shortness of breath on exertion can occur within the first week of treatment and may continue for the duration of administration of Neumega. It is also possible that you may experience irregular heartbeats. If you experience chest pain, shortness of breath, fatigue, blurred vision, or an irregular pulse that persists, contact your physician. If you have any other problems, whether or not you think they are related to Neumega, you should tell your doctor.
If you are a woman of child-bearing potential, you should be aware that use of Neumega poses possible risks of the fetus. If you become pregnant or wish to become pregnant during treatment with Neumega, consult your physician about continuing to use Neumega.

Dosage and Administration

The Neumega vial contains a powder which must be reconstituted prior to injection in 1 mL of Sterile Water for Injection, USP provided with Neumega. Powdered Neumega and Sterile Water for Injection, USP should be stored in a refrigerator at 2 to 8°C (36 to 46°F). DO NOT FREEZE.
A new vial of Neumega and Sterile Water for Injection, USP should be used to prepare each dose. Do not use Neumega or Sterile Water for Injection, USP beyond the expiration date printed on the vial. Any unused portion of reconstituted Neumega medication or Sterile Water for Injection, USP remaining in the vial should be discarded. Because neither Neumega powder for injection nor its accompanying Sterile Water for Injection, USP contain a preservative, the single-use vials should not be reentered or reused.
Neumega should be used as soon as possible following reconstitution and must be used within 3 hours of reconstitution. The reconstituted Neumega solution can be stored in the vial for up to 3 hours either at room temperature up to 25°C (77°F), or in the refrigerator at 2 to 8°C (36 to 46°F) THE RECONSTITUTED SOLUTION SHOULD NOT BE STORED IN A SYRINGE.

NOTE: Follow aseptic technique in reconstitution and administration as demonstrated by the health care professional.

Reconstituting Neumega

1. Have all supplies (four sterile alcohol swabs, syringe, needle, Neumega vial, and "Sterile Water for Injection, USP") available before starting procedure. Wash hands thoroughly with soap and water before preparing the medication.
2. Flip off the protective cap from the vial labeled "Sterile Water for Injection, USP" and the vial labeled "Neumega." Wipe the top of each vial with a sterile alcohol swab, using a different swab for each vial. Leave the swabs on top of the vials.
3. Remove syringe and needle from sterile packaging. Attach needle to syringe (if needle is not already attached). Remove protective cover from the tip of the syringe. Do not touch the needle with your hand or allow it to come in contact with other surfaces.
4. Pull the plunger of the syringe back to the 1.2 mL mark.
5. Remove the alcohol swab from the top of vial labeled "Sterile Water for Injection, USP." Keep the vial upright and push the needle through the center of the rubber stopper. Inject the air from the syringe into the vial.
6. Keep the needle in the vial and gently turn the vial with the needle in it upside down. Withdraw 1.0 mL of Sterile Water for Injection, USP by slowly pulling back on the plunger. Make sure that the tip of the needle remains in the fluid at all times.
7. Remove syringe from the vial of Sterile Water for Injection, USP. Discard used vial. Remove the alcohol swab from the Neumega vial. Keep the vial of Neumega upright and push the needle of the syringe containing Sterile Water for Injection, USP through the center of the rubber stopper. Press the plunger of the syringe SLOWLY. Direct the stream of Sterile Water down the inside wall of the vial.

Without removing the syringe, **GENTLY** swirl the vial until the powder is dissolved.

DO NOT SHAKE THE VIAL. (Shaking will cause foaming.) Once mixed, the solution should be colorless and clear of any particles. **DO NOT** inject if any cloudiness or particles are seen.

8. Turn the vial and syringe upside down. Keep needle tip in the solution and slowly pull back on the plunger to fill the syringe to the mark specified for the dosage being administered. If bubbles appear in the syringe, push bubbles back into the vial. Withdraw additional medication to specified mark.

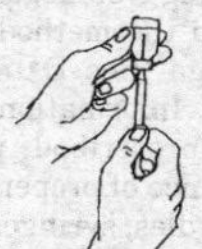

9. Withdraw needle from vial. Hold syringe and needle straight up and lightly tap the side of the syringe to bring any air bubbles to the top.

TABLE 3
SELECTED ADVERSE EVENTS

Body System / Adverse Event	Placebo n=67	(%)	50 µg/kg n=69	(%)
Body as a Whole				
Edema*	10	(15)	41	(59)
Neutropenic fever	28	(42)	33	(48)
Headache	24	(36)	28	(41)
Fever	19	(28)	25	(36)
Cardiovascular System				
Tachycardia*	2	(3)	14	(20)
Vasodilatation	6	(9)	13	(19)
Palpitations*	2	(3)	10	(14)
Syncope	4	(6)	9	(13)
Atrial fibrillation/flutter*	1	(1)	8	(12)
Digestive System				
Nausea/vomiting	47	(70)	53	(77)
Mucositis	25	(37)	30	(43)
Diarrhea	22	(33)	30	(43)
Oral moniliasis*	1	(1)	10	(14)
Nervous System				
Dizziness	19	(28)	26	(38)
Insomnia	18	(27)	23	(33)
Respiratory System				
Dyspnea*	15	(22)	33	(48)
Rhinitis	21	(31)	29	(42)
Cough increased	15	(22)	20	(29)
Pharyngitis	11	(16)	17	(25)
Pleural effusions*	0	(0)	7	(10)
Skin and Appendages				
Rash	11	(16)	17	(25)
Special Senses				
Conjunctival injection*	2	(3)	13	(19)

*Occurred in significantly more Neumega-treated patients than in placebo-treated patients.

10. Hold syringe upright and press plunger slightly to push air out through the needle. A small amount of solution may exit the syringe. This will ensure that all air is removed from the syringe.

Injecting Neumega

1. Identify the area on the abdomen, thigh, or hip (or upper arm if not self-injecting). Select a different site each time Neumega is injected. This will help avoid soreness in one area.

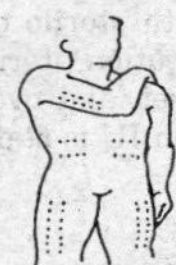

2. Cleanse the skin where the injection is to be made with an alcohol swab. Hold the syringe "like a dart" between the thumb and first finger close to the syringe/needle connection.
3. With the other hand, pinch about an inch of skin between thumb and forefinger, forming a bulge in the skin at the injection site.
4. Insert the needle quickly into the skin at a 45 degree angle. Release pinched skin.

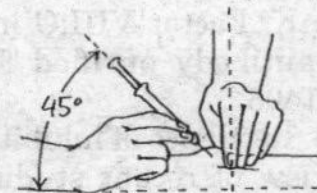

5. GENTLY pull back on the syringe plunger. If blood comes into the syringe, do not inject. Withdraw the needle from skin and inject at a different cleaned site.
6. Inject Neumega by slowly pushing the plunger all the way down in one continuous motion.
7. Hold a new alcohol swab near the needle and pull the needle straight out of the skin. Press the alcohol swab over the injection site for several seconds. DO NOT RUB SITE.
8. DO NOT RECAP NEEDLE. Immediately after use discard used syringe and needle into "Sharps Container."

Genetics Institute, Inc.
Rev. 12/97 Cambridge, MA 02140-2387, USA

Shown in Product Identification Guide, page 313

REFACTO® ℞
[*rē-făk 'tō*]
Antihemophilic Factor, Recombinant

DESCRIPTION

ReFacto® Antihemophilic Factor (Recombinant) is a purified protein produced by recombinant DNA technology for use in therapy of factor VIII deficiency. ReFacto is a glycoprotein with an approximate molecular mass of 170 kDa consisting of 1438 amino acids. It has an amino acid sequence that is comparable to the 90 + 80 kDa form of factor VIII, and post-translational modifications that are similar to those of the plasma-derived molecule. ReFacto has *in vitro* functional characteristics comparable to those of endogenous factor VIII.

ReFacto is produced by a genetically engineered Chinese hamster ovary (CHO) cell line. The CHO cell line secretes B-domain deleted recombinant factor VIII into a defined cell culture medium that contains human serum albumin and recombinant insulin, but does not contain any proteins derived from animal sources. The protein is purified by a chromatography purification process that yields a high-purity, active product. The potency expressed in international units (IU) is determined using the European Pharmacopoeial chromogenic assay against the WHO standard. The specific activity of ReFacto is 11,200–15,500 IU per milligram of protein. ReFacto is not purified from human blood and contains no preservatives or added human components in the final formulation.

ReFacto is formulated as a sterile, nonpyrogenic, lyophilized powder preparation for intravenous (IV) injection. It is available in single-use vials containing the labeled amount of factor VIII activity (IU). Each vial contains nominally 250, 500, or 1000 IU of ReFacto per vial. The formulated product is a clear colorless solution upon reconstitution and contains sodium chloride, sucrose, L-histidine, calcium chloride, and polysorbate 80.

CLINICAL PHARMACOLOGY

Factor VIII is the specific clotting factor deficient in patients with hemophilia A (classical hemophilia). The administration of ReFacto® Antihemophilic Factor (Recombinant) increases plasma levels of factor VIII activity and can temporarily correct the *in vitro* coagulation defect in these patients.

Activated factor VIII acts as a cofactor for activated factor IX accelerating the conversion of factor X to activated factor X. Activated factor X converts prothrombin into thrombin. Thrombin then converts fibrinogen into fibrin and a clot is formed. Factor VIII activity is greatly reduced in patients with hemophilia A and therefore replacement therapy is necessary.

In a crossover pharmacokinetic study of eighteen (18) previously treated patients **using the chromogenic assay,** the circulating mean half-life for Re-Facto was 14.5 ± 5.3 hours (ranged from 7.6–27.7 hours), which was not statistically significantly different from plasma-derived Antihemophilic Factor (Human) (pdAHF), which had a mean half-life of 13.7 ± 3.4 hours (ranged from 8.8–23.7 hours). Mean incremental recovery (K-value) of ReFacto in plasma was 2.4 ± 0.4 IU/dL per IU/kg (ranged from 1.9–3.3 IU/dL per IU/kg). This was comparable to the mean incremental recovery observed in plasma for pdAHF which was 2.3 ± 0.3 IU/dL per IU/kg (ranged from 1.7–2.9 IU/dL per IU/kg). **Results obtained from this controlled pharmacokinetic study, which used a central laboratory for the analysis of all plasma samples, showed that the one-stage factor VII clotting assay gave results which were approximately 50% of the values obtained with the chromogenic assay.**

In two additional clinical studies, pharmacokinetic parameters were evaluated for previously treated patients [PTPs] and previously untreated patients [PUPs]. In PTPs (n=87) ReFacto had a mean incremental recovery of 2.4 ± 0.4 IU/dL per IU/kg (ranged from 1.1–3.8 IU/dL per IU/kg) and an elimination half-life (n=67) of 10.7 ± 2.8 hours. In PUPs (n=45) ReFacto had a lower mean incremental recovery of 1.7 ± 0.4 IU/dL per IU/kg (ranged from 0.2–2.8 IU/dL per IU/kg) as compared to PTPs. Population pharmacokinetic modeling using data from 44 PUPs led to a mean estimated half-life of ReFacto in PUPs of 8.0 ± 2.2 hours. These parameters did not change over time (12 months) for PTPs or PUPs.

In clinical studies of ReFacto involving a total of 218 patients (117 PTPs including 4 who participated in the surgery study only, and 101 PUPs), more than 84 million IU were administered over a period of up to 54 months. The 117 PTPs were given a median of 230 injections (range of 4–1530 injections) over a median of 1200 days (range of 31–1640 days). The 101 PUPs were given a median of 26 injections (range of 1–490 injections) over a median of 830 days (range of 1–1298 days). One hundred thirteen PTPs and 99 PUPs were evaluated for efficacy in bleeding episodes. The 113 PTPs experienced a median of 54 bleeding episodes and the 99 PUPs experienced a median of 12 bleeding episodes. All were treated successfully on an on-demand basis or for the reduction of bleeding episodes except for one PTP and two PUPs who discontinued ReFacto treatment and switched to another product after the development of inhibitors. Bleeding episodes included hemarthroses, and bleeding in soft tissue, muscle, and other anatomical sites.

ReFacto has been studied in short-term routine prophylaxis. In uncontrolled clinical trials, an average dose of 27 ± 10 IU/kg in PTPs (n=77) and an average dose of 57 ± 20 IU/kg in PUPs (n=17) was given repeatedly at variable intervals longer than 2 weeks. In 64 patients who had both on-demand and prophylactic periods during their time on study, the mean rate of spontaneous musculoskeletal bleeding episodes was less during periods of routine prophylaxis. There were an average of 10 bleeding episodes per year during the prophylactic periods compared to an average of 37 bleeding episodes per year during the on-demand periods. The clinical trial experience with routine prophylaxis in PUPs is limited (n=17). These non-randomized trial results should be interpreted with caution, as the investigators exercised their own discretion in deciding when and in whom prophylaxis was to be initiated and terminated.

Management of hemostasis was evaluated in the surgical setting where 28 surgical procedures have been performed in 25 patients. The average preoperative dose in PTPs was 59 IU/kg. Procedures included orthopedic procedures, inguinal hernia repair, epidural hematoma evacuation, transposition ulnar nerve, and other minor procedures (e.g., venous access catheter placement and explantation, toenail removal). Circulatory factor VIII levels targeted to restore and maintain hemostasis were achieved. While the one-stage clotting assay was used most frequently in the surgical setting (24 versus 4 surgeries), hemostasis was maintained throughout the surgical period regardless of which assay was used. Hemostasis efficacy was rated as excellent or good in all procedures.

The occurrence of neutralizing antibody (inhibitors) is well known in the treatment of patients with hemophilia A[1,2,3] Thirty out of 101 PUPs (30%) developed an inhibitor: 16 out of 101 (16%) with a high titer (≥ 5 BU) (11 of the 16 patients had peak values ≥10 BU/mL) and 14 out of 101 (14%) with a low titer (<5 BU). In this study the incidence of inhibitor development to factor VIII using ReFacto is similar to that reported for other factor VIII products.[1,2,3,5]

One of 113 PTPs (0.9%) developed a low titer inhibitor after 107 exposure days with ReFacto. In this study the incidence of inhibitor development to factor VIII using ReFacto is similar to that reported for other factor VIII products[4].

INDICATIONS AND USAGE

ReFacto® Antihemophilic Factor (Recombinant) is indicated for the control and prevention of hemorrhagic episodes and for surgical prophylaxis in patients with hemophilia A (congenital factor VIII deficiency or classic hemophilia).

ReFacto is indicated for short-term routine prophylaxis to reduce the frequency of spontaneous bleeding episodes. The effect of regular routine prophylaxis on long-term morbidity and mortality is unknown.

ReFacto can be of a signficiant therapeutic value for treatment of hemophilia A in certain patients with inhibitors to factor VIII[6]. In clinical studies of ReFacto, patients who develop inhibitors on study continued to manifest a clinical response when inhibitor titers were < 10 BU/mL. When an inhibitor is present, the dosage requirement of factor VIII is variable. The dosage can be determined only by a clinical response and by monitoring of circulating factor VIII levels after treatment (see **DOSAGE AND ADMINISTRATION**).

ReFacto does not contain von Willebrand factor and therefore is not indicated in von Willebrand's disease.

CONTRAINDICATIONS

Known hypersensitivity to mouse, hamster, or bovine proteins may be a contraindication to the use of ReFacto® Antihemophilic Factor (Recombinant).

WARNINGS

As with any intravenous protein product, allergic type hypersensitivity reactions are possible. Patients should be informed of the early signs of hypersensitivity reactions including hives, generalized urticaria, tightness of the chest, wheezing, hypotension, and anaphylaxis. Patients should be advised to discontinue use of the product and contact their physicians if these symptoms occur.

PRECAUTIONS

General

Activity-neutralizing antibodies (inhibitors) have been detected in patients receiving factor VIII-containing products. There is no evidence that ReFacto® Antihemophilic Factor (Recombinant) is associated with a higher-than-historical incidence of inhibitors. As with all coagulation factor VIII products, patients should be monitored for the development of inhibitors that should be titrated in Bethesda Units using appropriate biological testing.

Formation of Antibodies to Mouse and Hamster Protein

As Antihemophilic Factor (Recombinant), ReFacto contains trace amounts of mouse protein (maximum of 5 ng/1000 IU) and hamster protein (maximum of 30 ng/1000 IU), the remote possibility exists that patients treated with this product may develop hypersensitivity to these non-human mammalian proteins.

Carcinogenicity, Mutagenicity, Impairment of Fertility

ReFacto® Antihemophilic Factor (Recombinant) has been shown to be nonmutagenic in the mouse micronucleus assay. No other mutagenicity studies and no investigations on carcinogenesis or impairment of fertility have been conducted.

Pregnancy Category C

Animal reproduction and lactation studies have not been conducted with ReFacto® Antihemophilic Factor (Recombinant). It is not known whether ReFacto can affect reproductive capacity or cause fetal harm when given to pregnant women. ReFacto should be administered to pregnant and lactating women only if clearly indicated.

Pediatric Use

ReFacto® Antihemophilic Factor (Recombinant) is appropriate for use in children of all ages, including newborns. Safety and efficacy studies have been performed both in previously treated children and adolescents (N=22, ages 8–15 years) and in previously untreated neonates, infants, and children (N=101, ages 0–52 months) (see **CLINICAL PHARMACOLOGY** and **PRECAUTIONS**).

Geriatric Use

Clinical studies of ReFacto did not include sufficient numbers of subjects aged 65 and over to determine whether they respond differently from younger subjects. Other reported clinical experience has not identified differences in responses between the elderly and younger patients. As with any patient receiving ReFacto, dose selection for an elderly patient should be individualized.

ADVERSE REACTIONS

As with the intravenous administration of any protein product, the following reactions may be observed after administration: headache, fever, chills, flushing, nausea, vomiting, lethargy, or manifestations of allergic reactions. During clinical studies with ReFacto® Antihemophilic Factor (Recombinant), 77 adverse reactions in 43 or 218 patients (20%) probably or possibly-related to therapy were reported for 64,363 infusions (0.12%). These were anaphylaxis (1), dyspnea (6), urticaria (1), nausea (11), headache (4), vasodilation (5), dizziness (4), permanent venous access catheter complications (3), asthenia (3), fever (3), taste perversion [altered taste] (3), bleeding/hematoma (3), infected hematoma (1), anorexia (2), diarrhea (2), injection site reaction (2), somnolence (2), rash (2), pruritus (2), angina pectoris (1), tachycardia (1), perspiration increased (1), chills (1), increased amino transferase (1), increased bilirubin (1), pain in finger (1), muscle weakness (1), CPK increase (1), cold sensation (1), eye disorder-vision abnormal (1), coughing (1), myalgia (1), gastroenteritis (1), abdominal pain (1), acne (1), and forehead bruises (1). If any adverse reaction takes place that is thought to be related to administration of ReFacto, the rate of infusion should be decreased or stopped.

In addition, inhibitor development is a known adverse event associated with the treatment of patients with hemophilia A (see **CLINIAL PHARMACOLOGY**).

A total of 182 adverse reactions in 54 of 218 patients (25%) who received 32,013 infusions (0.6%) were reported by the investigator to have an "unlikely" or "not assessable" relationship to ReFacto administration. The study sponsor con-

Continued on next page

Refacto—Cont.

sidered that the events may be of possible or of unknown relationship to therapy because of the temporal relationship to the infusion and/or the frequency of the event for a given patient and/or because insufficient information was available to assign another causality. In this category, 25 patients experienced the following 38 events which are different from the events described above: pain (10), rhinitis (10), vomiting (4), insomnia (3), constipation (2), pharyngitis (2), flushing (1), palpitation (1), sinusitis (1), gastritis (1), dyspepsia (1), hypotension (1), and URI (1).

Other adverse experiences that were reported during the clinical trials, but which were assessed by both the investigator and the sponsor as "unlikely" to be related to ReFacto administration included: dyspnea (3), rash (2), pruritus (1), neuropathy (1), arm weakness (1), and thrombophlebitis of upper arm (1).

DOSAGE AND ADMINISTRATION

Treatment with ReFacto® Antihemophilic Factor (Recombinant) should be initiated under the supervision of a physician experienced in the treatment of hemophilia A.

Dosage and duration of treatment depend on the severity of the factor VIII deficiency, the location and extent of bleeding, and the patient's clinical condition. Doses administered should be titrated to the patient's clinical response. In the presence of an inhibitor, higher doses may be required.

One international unit (IU) of factor VIII activity corresponds approximately to the quantity of factor VIII in one mL of normal human plasma. The calculation of the required dosage of factor VIII is based upon the empirical finding that, on average, 1 IU of factor VIII per kg body weight raises the plasm factor VIII activity by approximately 2 IU/dL per IU/kg administered. The required dosage is determined using the following formula:

Required units = body weight (kg)
× desired factor VIII rise (IU/dL or % of normal)
× 0.5 (IU/kg per IU/dL)

The following chart can be used to guide dosing in bleeding episodes and surgery:

[See table at bottom of page 1252]

Precise monitoring of the replacement therapy by means of coagulation analysis (plasma factor VIII activity) is recommended, particularly for surgical intervention.

Product is labeled on the basis of the chromogenic assay. The available clinical trial data suggest either the one-stage clotting assay or the chromogenic assay may be used to help follow patients clinically. Most clinical trial subjects were monitored with the one-stage clotting assay. It must be noted that the one-stage clotting assay yields results which are lower than the values obtained with the chromogenic assay (see **CLINICAL PHARMACOLOGY**).

For short-term routine prophylaxis to prevent or reduce the frequency of spontaneous musculoskeletal hemorrhage in patients with hemophilia A, ReFacto should be given at least twice a week. In some cases, especially pediatric patients, shorter dosage intervals or higher doses may be necessary. Pharmacokinetic/pharmacodynamic modeling, based on pharmacokinetic data from 185 infusions in 102 PTPs, predicts that routine prophylactic dosing 3 times per week may be associated with a lower bleeding risk than with dosing twice weekly. No randomized comparison of different doses or frequency regimens of ReFacto for routine prophylaxis has been performed. In clinical studies in PTPs (ages 8–73 years) and PUPs (ages 9–52 months), the mean dose used for routine prophylaxis was 27 ± 10 IU/kg and 57 ± 20 IU/kg, respectively.

Patients using ReFacto should be monitored for the development of factor VIII inhibitors. If expected factor VIII activity plasma levels are not attained, or if bleeding is not controlled with an appropriate dose, an assay should be performed to determine if a factor VIII inhibitor is present. If the inhibitor is present at levels less than 10 Bethesda Units per mL, administration of additional antihemophilic factor may neutralize the inhibitor.

ReFacto is administered by IV infusion after reconstitution of the lyophilized powder with Sodium Chloride Diluent (provided).

INSTRUCTIONS FOR USE

Patients should follow the specific reconstitution and administration procedures provided by their physicians. The procedures below are provided as general guidelines for the reconstitution and administration of ReFacto.

Reconstitution

Always wash your hands before performing the following procedures. Aseptic technique should be used during the reconstitution procedure.

ReFacto® Antihemophilic Factor (Recombinant) is administered by intravenous (IV) infusion after reconstitution with the supplied Sodium Chloride Diluent.

1. Allow the vials of lyophilized ReFacto and diluent to reach room temperature.
2. Remove the plastic flip-top caps from the ReFacto vial and the diluent vial to expose the central portions of the rubber stoppers.
3. Wipe the tops of both vials with the alcohol swab provided, or use another antiseptic solution, and allow to dry.
4. Remove the transparent protective cover from the short end of the sterile double-ended needle and insert that end into the diluent vial at the center of the stopper.
5. Remove the colored protective cover from the long end of the sterile double-ended needle. Invert the diluent vial and, to minimize leakage, quickly insert the long end of the needle through the center of the stopper of the upright ReFacto vial.

Note: Point the double-ended needle toward the wall of the ReFacto vial to prevent excessive foaming.

6. The vacuum will draw the diluent into the ReFacto vial.
7. Once the transfer is complete, remove the double-ended needle from the ReFacto vial, and properly discard the needle with the diluent vial.

Note: If the diluent does not transfer completely into the ReFacto vial, DO NOT USE the contents of the vial. Note that it is acceptable for a small amount of fluid to remain in the solvent vial after transfer.

8. Gently rotate the vial to dissolve the powder.
9. The final solution should be inspected visually for particulate matter before administration. The solution should appear clear and colorless.

ReFacto should be administered with 3 hours after reconstitution. The reconstituted solution may be stored at room temperature prior to administration.

Administration (Intravenous Infection)

ReFacto® Antihemophilic Factor (Recombinant) should be administered using a single sterile disposable plastic syringe. In addition, the solution should be withdrawn from the vial using the sterile filter needle.

1. Using aseptic technique, attach the sterile filter needle to the sterile disposable syringe. Pull back the syringe plunger to the 5 mL mark.
2. Insert the filter needle into the stopper of the ReFacto vial. Push plunger forward to inject air into the vial.
3. Invert the vial and withdraw the reconstituted solution into the syringe.
4. Remove and discard the filter needle.

Note: If you use more than one vial of ReFacto, the contents of multiple vials may be drawn into the same syringe through a separate, unused filter needle.

5. Attach the syringe to the luer end of the infusion set tubing and perform venipuncture as instructed by your physician.

After reconstitution, ReFacto should be injected intravenously over several minutes. The rate of administration should be determined by the patient's comfort level.

Dispose of all unused solution, empty vials, and used needles and syringes in an appropriate container for throwing away waste that might hurt others if not handled properly.

Storage

Product as packaged for sale: ReFacto® Antihemophilic Factor (Recombinant) should be stored under refrigeration at a temperature of 2 to 8 °C (36 to 46 °F). ReFacto may also be stored at room temperature not to exceed 25 °C (77 °F) for up to 3 months. Freezing should be avoided to prevent damage to the diluent vial. During storage, avoid prolonged exposure of ReFacto® vial to light. Do not use ReFacto after the expiry date on the label.

Product after reconstitution: The product does not contain a preservative and should be used within 3 hours.

HOW SUPPLIED

ReFacto® Antihemophilic Factor (Recombinant) is supplied in single-use vials which contain nominally 250, 500, or 1000 IU per vial (NDC 58394-007-01, 58394-006-01, 58394-005-01, respectively) with sterile diluent, sterile double-ended needle for reconstitution, sterile filter needle for withdrawal, sterile infusion set, and two (2) alcohol swabs. Actual factor VIII activity in IU is stated on the label of each vial.

REFERENCES

1. Ehrenforth S, Kreuz W, Scharrer I, et al. Incidence of development of factor VIII and factor IX inhibitors in hemophiliacs. Lancet. 1992;339:594–598.
2. Bray GL, Gomperts ED, Courter S, et al. A multicenter study of recombinant factor VIII (Recombinate): safety, efficacy, and inhibitor risk in previously untreated patients with hemophilia A. Blood. 1994;83(9):2428–2435.
3. Lusher J, Arkin S, Abildgaard CF, Schwartz RS, Group TKPUPS. Recombinant factor VIII for the treatment of previously untreated patients with hemophilia A. N Engl J Med. 1993;328:453–459.
4. Kessler C, Sachse K. Factor VIII:C inhibitor associated with monoclonal-antibody purified FVIII concentrate. Lancet 1990; 335:1403.
5. Scharrer I, Bray G. Incidence of inhibitors in haemophilia A patients—a review of recent studies of recombinant and plasma-derived factor VIII concentrates. Hemophilia 1999; 5:145.
6. Kessler CM. An Introduction to Factor VIII Inhibitors: The Detection and Quantitation. American Journal of Medicine 91 1991, (Supplement 5A): 1S–5S.

Manufactured by:
Pharmacia & Upjohn AB
Stockholm, Sweden
Manufactored for:
KEY CODE 3704 Genetics Institute, Inc.
Cambridge MA 02140-2387, USA
Rev. 3/00 US License Number 1163
Telephone: 1-800-934-5556

Type of Hemorrhage	Factor VIII Level Required (IU/dL or % of normal)	Frequency of Doses (h)/ Duration of Therapy (d)
Minor		
Early hemarthrosis, minor muscle or oral bleeds.	20–40	Repeat every 12 to 24 hours as necessary until resolved. At least 1 day, depending upon the severity of the hemorrhage.
Moderate		
Hemorrhages into muscle. Mild trauma capitis. Minor operations including tooth extraction. Hemorrhages into the oral cavity.	30–60	Repeat infusion every 12–24 hours for 3–4 or until adequate local hemostatis is achieved. For tooth extraction a single infusion plus oral antifibrinolytic therapy within 1 hour may be sufficient.
Major		
Gastrointestinal bleeding. intracranial, intra-abdominal or intrathoracic hemorrhages. Fractures. Major operations.	60–100	Repeat infusion every 8–24 hours until threat is resolved or in the case of surgery, until adequate local hemostatis is acheived.

Geneva Pharmaceuticals, Inc.

2655 WEST MIDWAY BLVD.
P.O. BOX 446
BROOMFIELD, CO 80038–0446

Direct Inquiries to:
Customer Support Department
(800) 525–8747
(303) 466–2400
FAX: (303) 727–4656

GENEVA PHARMACEUTICALS

NDC # 00781-	Product/Strength	℞ OTC
1671	Albuterol Tablets USP 2mg	℞
1672	Albuterol Tablets USP 4mg	℞
1061	Alprazolam Tablets USP .25mg	℞ C-IV
1077	Alprazolam Tablets USP .50mg	℞ C-IV
1079	Alprazolam Tablets USP 1.0mg	℞ C-IV
1089	Alprazolam Tablets USP 2.0 mg	℞ C-IV
1486	Amitriptyline HCl Tablets USP 10mg	℞
1487	Amitriptyline HCl Tablets USP 25mg	℞
1488	Amitriptyline HCl Tablets USP 50mg	℞
1489	Amitriptyline HCl Tablets USP 75mg	℞
1490	Amitriptyline HCl Tablets USP 100mg	℞
1491	Amitriptyline HCl Tablets USP 150mg	℞
1844	Amoxapine Tablets USP 25mg	℞
1845	Amoxapine Tablets USP 50mg	℞
1846	Amoxapine Tablets USP 100mg	℞
1847	Amoxapine Tablets USP 150mg	℞
1078	Atenolol Tablets USP 25mg	℞
1506	Atenolol Tablets USP 50mg	℞
1507	Atenolol Tablets USP 100mg	℞
2819	Bromocriptine Mesylate Capsules USP 5mg	℞
1817	Bromocriptine Mesylate Tablets USP 2.5mg	℞
1053	Bupropion HCl Tablets 75mg	℞
1064	Bupropion HCl Tablets 100mg	℞
1050	Carisoprodol Tablets USP 350mg	℞
1715	Chlorpromazine HCl Tablets USP 10mg	℞
1716	Chlorpromazine HCl Tablets USP 25mg	℞
1717	Chlorpromazine HCl Tablets USP 50mg	℞
1718	Chlorpromazine HCl Tablets USP 100mg	℞
1719	Chlorpromazine HCl Tablets USP 200mg	℞
1447	Cimetidine Tablets USP 200mg	℞
1448	Cimetidine Tablets USP 300mg	℞
1449	Cimetidine Tablets USP 400mg	℞
1444	Cimetidine Tablets USP 800mg	℞
1358	Clemastine Fumarate Tablets USP 1.34mg	OTC
1359	Clemastine Fumarate Tablets USP 2.68mg	℞
6131	Clemastine Fumarate Syrup .5mg/5ml	℞

2027 Clomipramine HCl Capsules 25mg ℞
2037 Clomipramine HCl Capsules 50mg ℞
2047 Clomipramine HCl Capsules 75mg ℞
1324 Cyclobenzaprine HCl Tablets USP 10mg ℞
1971 Desipramine HCl Tablets USP 10mg ℞
1972 Desipramine HCl Tablets USP 25mg ℞
1973 Desipramine HCl Tablets USP 50mg ℞
1974 Desipramine HCl Tablets USP 75mg ℞
1975 Desipramine HCl Tablets USP 100mg ℞
1976 Desipramine HCl Tablets USP 150mg ℞
1297 Diclofenac Potassium Immediate Release Tablets USP 50mg ℞
1785 Diclofenac Sodium Delayed-Release Tablets 25mg ℞
1787 Diclofenac Sodium Delayed-Release Tablets 50mg ℞
1789 Diclofenac Sodium Delayed-Release Tablets 75mg ℞
1381 Diclofenoc Sodium Extended Release Tablets 100mg
2120 Fiortal (Butalbital/Aspirin/Caffeine Capsules USP 50/325/40mg) ℞ CIII
2221 Fiortal with Codeine (Butalbital/Aspirin/Caffeine/Codeine) Capsules USP 50/325/40/30mg ℞ CIII
1129 Flurbiprofen Tablets 100mg ℞
1436 Fluphenazine HCl Tablets USP 1mg ℞
1437 Fluphenazine HCl Tablets USP 2.5mg ℞
1438 Fluphenazine HCl Tablets USP 5mg ℞
1439 Fluphenazine HCl Tablets USP 10mg ℞
1818 Furosemide Tablets USP 20mg ℞
1966 Furosemide Tablets USP 40mg ℞
1446 Furosemide Tablets USP 80mg ℞
1452 Glipizide Tablets USP 5mg ℞
1453 Glipizide Tablets USP 10mg ℞
1391 Haloperidol Tablets USP 0.5mg ℞
1392 Haloperidol Tablets USP 1mg ℞
1393 Haloperidol Tablets USP 2mg ℞
1396 Haloperidol Tablets USP 5mg ℞
1397 Haloperidol Tablets USP 10mg ℞
1398 Haloperidol Tablets USP 20mg ℞
1407 Hydroxychloroquine Sulfate Tablets USP 200mg ℞
1762 Imipramine HCl Tablets USP 10mg ℞
1764 Imipramine HCl Tablets USP 25mg ℞
1766 Imipramine HCl Tablets USP 50mg ℞
1635 Isosorbide Dinitrate Tablets USP 5mg ℞
1556 Isosorbide Dinitrate Tablets USP 10mg ℞
1695 Isosorbide Dinitrate Tablets USP 20mg ℞
1840 Isoxsuprine HCl Tablets USP 10mg ℞
1842 Isoxsuprine HCl Tablets USP 20mg ℞
1262 Lonox Tablets 2.5mg/0.025mg (Diphenoxylate HCl and Atropine Sulfate Tablets USP) ℞ CV
2761 Loperamide HCl Capsules USP 2mg ℞
1403 Lorazepam Tablets USP 0.5mg ℞ CIV
1404 Lorazepam Tablets USP 1.0mg ℞ CIV
1405 Lorazepam Tablets USP 2.0mg ℞ CIV
1345 Meclizine HCl Tablets USP 12.5mg OTC
1375 Meclizine HCl Tablets USP 25mg OTC
1542 Meclizine HCl Tablets USP 12.5mg ℞
1544 Meclizine HCl Tablets USP 25mg ℞
1072 Methazolamide Tablets USP 25mg ℞
1071 Methazolamide Tablets USP 50mg ℞
1760 Methocarbamol Tablets USP 500mg ℞
1750 Methocarbamol Tablets USP 750mg ℞
1748 Methylphenidate HCl Tablets USP 5mg ℞ CII
1749 Methylphenidate HCl Tablets USP 10mg ℞ CII
1753 Methylphenidate HCl Tablets USP 20mg ℞ CII
1754 Methylphenidate Sustained Release Tablets USP 20mg ℞ CII
3070 Metoprolol Injectable USP 5mg/mL ℞
1223 Metoprolol Tartrate Tablets USP 50mg ℞
1228 Metoprolol Tartrate Tablets USP 100mg ℞
2130 Mexiletine HCl Capsules USP 150mg ℞
2131 Mexiletine HCl Capsules USP 200mg ℞
2132 Mexiletine HCl Capsules USP 250mg ℞
1163 Naproxen Tablets USP 250mg ℞
1164 Naproxen Tablets USP 375mg ℞
1165 Naproxen Tablets USP 500mg ℞
1187 Naproxen Sodium Tablets USP 275mg ℞
1188 Naproxen Sodium Tablets USP 550mg ℞
2630 Nortriptyline HCl Capsules USP 10mg ℞
2631 Nortriptyline HCl Capsules USP 25mg ℞
2632 Nortriptyline HCl Capsules USP 50mg ℞
2633 Nortriptyline HCl Capsules USP 75mg ℞
1649 Orphenadrine Citrate Extended Release Tablets 100mg
2809 Oxazepam Capsules USP 10mg ℞ CIV
2810 Oxazepam Capsules USP 15mg ℞ CIV
2811 Oxazepam Capsules USP 30mg ℞ CIV
1731 Pemoline Tablets 18.75mg
1741 Pemoline Tablets 37.5mg
1751 Pemoline Tablets 75mg
1265 Perphenazine and Amitriptyline HCl Tablets USP 2mg/10mg ℞
1266 Perphenazine and Amitriptyline HCl Tablets USP 4mg/10mg ℞
1267 Perphenazine and Amitriptyline HCl Tablets USP 4mg/25mg ℞
1268 Perphenazine and Amitriptyline HCl Tablets USP 4mg/50mg ℞
1273 Perphenazine and Amitriptyline HCl Tablets USP 2mg/25mg ℞
1046 Perphenazine Tablets USP 2mg ℞
1047 Perphenazine Tablets USP 4mg ℞
1048 Perphenazine Tablets USP 8mg ℞
1049 Perphenazine Tablets USP 16mg ℞
1168 Pindolol Tablets 5mg USP ℞
1169 Pindolol Tablets 10mg USP ℞
1830 Promethazine HCl Tablets USP 25mg ℞
1832 Promethazine HCl Tablets USP 50mg ℞
1533 Pseudoephedrine HCl Tablets USP 30mg OTC
1535 Pseudoephedrine HCl Tablets USP 60mg OTC
1883 Ranitidine HCl Tablets USP 150mg ℞
1884 Ranitidine HCl Tablets USP 300mg ℞
2855 Ranitidine HCl Capsules USP 150mg ℞
2865 Ranitidine HCl Capsules USP 300mg ℞
2018 Rimactane® Capsules 300mg ℞
1599 Spironolactone Tablets USP 25mg ℞
1811 Sulindac Tablets USP 150mg ℞
1812 Sulindac Tablets USP 200mg ℞
2209 Temazepam Capsules USP 7.5mg ℞ CIV
2201 Temazepam Capsules USP 15mg ℞ CIV
2202 Temazepam Capsules USP 30mg ℞ CIV
2051 Terazosin Capsules 1mg
2052 Terazosin Capsules 2mg
2053 Terazosin Capsules 5mg
2054 Terazosin Capsules 10mg
1551 Terazosin Tablets 1mg
1561 Terazosin Tablets 2mg
1571 Terazosin Tablets 5mg
1541 Terazosin Tablets 10mg
1604 Thioridazine HCl Tablets USP 10mg ℞
1614 Thioridazine HCl Tablets USP 15mg ℞
1624 Thioridazine HCl Tablets USP 25mg ℞
1634 Thioridazine HCl Tablets USP 50mg ℞
1644 Thioridazine HCl Tablets USP 100mg ℞
1664 Thioridazine HCl Tablets USP 150mg ℞
1674 Thioridazine HCl Tablets USP 200mg ℞
2226 Thiothixene Capsules USP 1mg ℞
2227 Thiothixene Capsules USP 2mg ℞
2228 Thiothixene Capsules USP 5mg ℞
2229 Thiothixene Capsules USP 10mg ℞
1807 Trazodone HCl Tablets USP 50mg ℞
1808 Trazodone HCl Tablets USP 100mg ℞
7045 Tretinoin Cream USP 0.025% ℞
7047 Tretinoin Cream USP 0.05% ℞
7049 Tretinoin Cream USP 0.1% ℞
7061 Tretinoin Gel USP 0.025%
1123 Triamterene and Hydrochlorothiazide Tablets USP 37.5mg/25mg ℞
2074 Triamterene and Hydrochlorothiazide Capsules USP 37.5mg/25mg ℞
2715 Triamterene and Hydrochlorothiazide Red Capsules USP 50mg/25mg ℞
2540 Triamterene and Hydrochlorothiazide White Capsules USP 50mg/25mg ℞
1008 Triamterene and Hydrochlorothiazide Tablets USP 75mg/50mg ℞
1030 Trifluoperazine HCl Tablets USP 1mg ℞
1032 Trifluoperazine HCl Tablets USP 2mg ℞
1034 Trifluoperazine HCl Tablets USP 5mg ℞
1036 Trifluoperazine HCl Tablets USP 10mg ℞
1014 Verapamil HCl Tablets USP 40mg ℞
1016 Verapamil HCl Tablets USP 80mg ℞
1017 Verapamil HCl Tablets USP 120mg ℞

Genzyme Corporation

ONE KENDALL SQUARE
CAMBRIDGE, MA 02139

Direct Inquiries to:
Clinical Services
(800) 745-4447
FAX: (617) 252-7700

For Medical Information Contact:
In Emergencies:
(800) 745-4447

CEREZYME® ℞

[*sĕr 'ĕ-zīm*]
imiglucerase for injection
200 UNITS
400 UNITS

DESCRIPTION

Cerezyme® (imiglucerase for injection) is an analogue of the human enzyme, β-glucocerebrosidase produced by recombinant DNA technology. β-Glucocerebrosidase (β-D-glucosyl-N-acylsphingosine glucohydrolase, E.C. 3.2.1.45) is a lysosomal glycoprotein enzyme which catalyzes the hydrolysis of the glycolipid glucocerebroside to glucose and ceramide. **Cerezyme®** is produced by recombinant DNA technology using mammalian cell culture (Chinese hamster ovary). Purified imiglucerase is a monomeric glycoprotein of 497 amino acids, containing 4 N-linked glycosylation sites (Mr = 60,430). Imiglucerase differs from placental glucocerebrosidase by one amino acid at position 495 where histidine is substituted for arginine. The oligosaccharide chains at the glycosylation sites have been modified to terminate in mannose sugars. The modified carbohydrate structures on imiglucerase are somewhat different from those on placental glucocerebrosidase. These mannose-terminated oligosaccharide chains of imiglucerase are specifically recognized by endocytic carbohydrate receptors on macrophages, the cells that accumulate lipid in Gaucher disease.

Cerezyme® is supplied as a sterile, non-pyrogenic, white to off-white lyophilized product. The quantitative composition of the lyophilized drug is provided in the following table:

[See first table at bottom of next page]

An enzyme unit (U) is defined as the amount of enzyme that catalyzes the hydrolysis of one micromole of the synthetic substrate para-nitrophenyl-β-D-glucopyranoside (pNP-Glc) per minute at 37°C. The product is stored at 2–8°C (36–46°F). After reconstitution with Sterile Water for Injection, USP, the imiglucerase concentration is 40 U/mL (see **DOSAGE AND ADMINISTRATION** for final concentrations and volumes). Reconstituted solutions have a pH of approximately 6.1.

In addition, Haemaccel® (cross-linked gelatin polypeptides), which is used as a stabilizing agent during the manufacturing process, may also be present in very small amounts in the final product.

CLINICAL PHARMACOLOGY

Mechanism of Action/Pharmacodynamics

Gaucher disease is characterized by a deficiency of β-glucocerebrosidase activity, resulting in accumulation of glucocerebroside in tissue macrophages which become engorged and are typically found in the liver, spleen, and bone marrow and occasionally in lung, kidney, and intestine. Secondary hematologic sequelae include severe anemia and thrombocytopenia in addition to the characteristic progressive hepatosplenomegaly, skeletal complications, including osteonecrosis and osteopenia with secondary pathological fractures. **Cerezyme®** (imiglucerase for injection) catalyzes the hydrolysis of glucocerebroside to glucose and ceramide. In clinical trials, **Cerezyme®** improved anemia and thrombocytopenia, reduced spleen and liver size, and decreased cachexia to a degree similar to that observed with Ceredase®.

Pharmacokinetics

During one hour intravenous infusions of four doses (7.5, 15, 30, 60 U/kg) of **Cerezyme®** (imiglucerase for injection) steady-state enzymatic activity was achieved by 30 minutes. Following infusion, plasma enzymatic activity declined rapidly with a half-life ranging from 3.6 to 10.4 minutes. Plasma clearance ranged from 9.8 to 20.3 mL/min/kg, (mean ± S.D., 14.5 ± 4.0 mL/min/kg). The volume of distribution corrected for weight ranged from 0.09 to 0.15 L/kg (0.12 ± 0.02 L/kg). These variables do not appear to be influenced by dose or duration of infusion. However, only one or two patients were studied at each dose level and infusion rate. The pharmacokinetics of **Cerezyme®** do not appear to be different from placental-derived alglucerase (Ceredase®). In patients who developed IgG antibody to **Cerezyme®**, an apparent effect on serum enzyme levels resulted in diminished volume of distribution and clearance and increased elimination half-life compared to patients without antibody (see **WARNINGS**).

INDICATIONS AND USAGE

Cerezyme® (imiglucerase for injection) is indicated for long-term enzyme replacement therapy for patients with a confirmed diagnosis of Type 1 Gaucher disease that results in one or more of the following conditions:

a. anemia
b. thrombocytopenia
c. bone disease
d. hepatomegaly or splenomegaly

CONTRAINDICATIONS

There are no known contraindications to the use of **Cerezyme®** (imiglucerase for injection). Treatment with **Cerezyme®** should be carefully re-evaluated if there is significant clinical evidence of hypersensitivity to the product.

WARNINGS

Approximately 15% of patients treated and tested to date have developed IgG antibody to **Cerezyme®** (imiglucerase for injection) during the first year of therapy. Patients who developed IgG antibody largely did so within 6 months of treatment and rarely developed antibodies to **Cerezyme®** after 12 months of therapy. Approximately 46% of patients with detectable IgG antibodies experienced symptoms of hypersensitivity.

Patients with antibody to **Cerezyme®** have a higher risk of hypersentivity reaction. Conversely, not all patients with symptoms of hypersensitivity have detectable IgG antibody. It is suggested that patients be monitored periodically for IgG antibody formation during the first year of treatment. Treatment with **Cerezyme®** should be approached with caution in patients who have exhibited symptoms of hypersensitivity to the product.

Anaphylactoid reaction has been reported in less than 1% of the patient population. Further treatment with imiglucerase should be conducted with caution. Most patients have successfully continued therapy after a reduction in rate of infusion and pretreatment with antihistamines and/or corticosteroids.

Continued on next page

Cerezyme—Cont.

PRECAUTIONS

General

In less than 1% of the patient population, pulmonary hypertension has also been observed during treatment with **Cerezyme®**. Pulmonary hypertension is a known complication of Gaucher disease, and has been observed both in patients receiving and not receiving **Cerezyme®**. No causal relationship with **Cerezyme®** has been established. Patients with respiratory symptoms should be evaluated for the presence of pulmonary hypertension.

Therapy with **Cerezyme®** (imiglucerase for injection) should be directed by physicians knowledgeable in the management of patients with Gaucher disease.

Caution may be advisable in administration of **Cerezyme®** to patients previously treated with Ceredase® and who have developed antibody to Ceredase® or who have exhibited symptoms of hypersensitivity to Ceredase®.

Carcinogenesis, Mutagenesis, Impairment of Fertility

Studies have not been conducted in either animals or humans to assess the potential effects of **Cerezyme®** (imiglucerase for injection) on carcinogenesis, mutagenesis, or impairment of fertility.

Teratogenic Effects: Pregnancy Category C

Animal reproduction studies have not been conducted with **Cerezyme®** (imiglucerase for injection). It is also not known whether **Cerezyme®** can cause fetal harm when administered to a pregnant woman, or can affect reproductive capacity. **Cerezyme®** should not be administered during pregnancy except when the indication and need are clear and the potential benefit is judged by the physician to substantially justify the risk.

Nursing Mothers

It is not known whether this drug is excreted in human milk. Because many drugs are excreted in human milk, caution should be exercised when **Cerezyme®** (imiglucerase for injection) is administered to a nursing woman.

ADVERSE REACTIONS

Experience in patients treated with **Cerezyme®** (imiglucerase for injection) has revealed that approximately 9.8% of patients experienced adverse events which were judged to be related to **Cerezyme®** administration and which occurred with an increase in frequency. Some of the adverse events were related to the route of administration. These include discomfort, pruritus, burning, swelling or sterile abscess at the site of venipuncture. Each of these events were found to occur in < 1% of the total patient population.

Symptoms suggestive of hypersensitivity have been noted in approximately 4.4% of patients. Onset of such symptoms has occurred during or shortly after infusions; these symptoms include pruritus, flushing, urticaria/angioedema, chest discomfort, respiratory symptoms, cyanosis and hypotension. Anaphylactoid reaction has also been reported. (see **WARNINGS**). Each of these events were found to occur in < 1% of the total patient population. Pre-treatment with antihistamines and/or corticosteroids and reduced rate of infusion have allowed continued use of **Cerezyme®** in most patients.

Additional adverse reactions that have been reported in approximately 5.4% of patients treated with **Cerezyme®** include: nausea, abdominal pain, diarrhea, rash, fatigue, headache, fever, dizziness, chills, backache, and tachycardia. Each of these events were found to occur in < 1% of the total patient population.

In addition to the adverse reactions that have been observed in patients treated with **Cerezyme®**, the following adverse reactions have been reported for this therapeutic class of drug: transient peripheral edema and vomiting.

OVERDOSE

Experience with doses up to 240 U/kg every two weeks have been reported. At that dose there have been no reports of obvious toxicity.

DOSAGE AND ADMINISTRATION

Cerezyme® (imiglucerase for injection) is administered by intravenous infusion over 1–2 hours. Dosage should be individualized to each patient. Initial dosages range from 2.5 U/kg of body weight 3 times a week to 60 U/kg once every 2 weeks. 60 units/kg every 2 weeks is the dosage for which the most data are available. Disease severity may dictate that treatment be initiated at a relatively high dose or relatively frequent administration. Dosage adjustments should be made on an individual basis, and may increase or decrease, based on achievement of therapeutic goals as assessed by routine comprehensive evaluations of the patients's clinical manifestations.

Cerezyme® should be stored at 2–8°C (36–46°F). Each vial, after reconstitution with Sterile Water for Injection, USP, should be inspected visually for particulate matter and discoloration before use. Any vials exhibiting particulate matter or discoloration should not be used. DO NOT USE **Cerezyme®** after the expiration date on the vial.

On the day of use, after the correct amount of **Cerezyme®** to be administered to the patient has been determined, the appropriate number of vials are each reconstituted with Sterile Water for Injection, USP. The final concentrations and administration volumes are provided in the following table:

[See second table below]

A nominal 5.0 mL for the 200 unit vial (10.0 mL for the 400 unit vial) is withdrawn from each vial. The appropriate amount of **Cerezyme®** for each patient is diluted with 0.9% Sodium Chloride Injection, USP, to a final volume of 100 to 200 mL. **Cerezyme®** is administered by intravenous infusion over 1 to 2 hours—or at a rate between 0.5–1.0 unit per kg body weight per minute. Aseptic techniques should be used when diluting the dose. Since **Cerezyme®** does not contain any preservative, after reconstitution, vials should be promptly diluted and not stored for subsequent use. **Cerezyme®**, after reconstitution, has been shown to be stable for up to 12 hours when stored at room temperature (25°C) and at 2–8°C. **Cerezyme®**, when diluted, has been shown to be stable for up to 24 hours when stored at 2–8°C. Relatively low toxicity, combined with the extended time course of response, allows small dosage adjustments to be made occasionally to avoid discarding partially used bottles. Thus, the dosage administered in individual infusions may be slightly increased or decreased to utilize fully each vial as long as the monthly administered dosage remains substantially unaltered.

HOW SUPPLIED

Cerezyme® (imiglucerase for injection) is supplied as a sterile, non-pyrogenic, lyophilized product. It is available as follows:

200 Units per Vial NDC 58468-1983-1
400 Units per Vial NDC 58468-4663-1
Store at 2–8°C (36–46°F).

Rx only

U.S. Patent Numbers: 5,236,838
5,549,892

Cerezyme® (imiglucerase for injection) is manufactured by:
Genzyme Corporation
One Kendall Square
Cambridge, MA 02139 USA

Certain manufacturing operations may have been performed by other firms.

4668 (9/99)

Ingredient	200 Unit Vial	400 Unit Vial
Imiglucerase (total amount)*	212 units	424 units
Mannitol	170 mg	340 mg
Sodium Citrates (Trisodium Citrate) (Disodium Hydrogen Citrate)	70 mg (52 mg) (18 mg)	140 mg (104 mg) (36 mg)
Polysorbate 80, NF	0.53 mg	1.06 mg
Citric Acid and/or Sodium Hydroxide may have been added at the time of manufacture to adjust pH.		

*This provides a respective withdrawal dose of 200 and 400 units of imigulcerase.

	200 Unit Vial	400 Unit Vial
Sterile water for reconstitution	5.1 mL	10.2 mL
Final volume of reconstituted product	5.3 mL	10.6 mL
Concentration after reconstitution	40 U/mL	40 U/mL
Withdrawal volume	5.0 mL	10.0 mL
Units of enzyme within final volume	200 Units	400 units

RENAGEL® TABLETS ℞

[rĕn ə gĕl]

(sevelamer hydrochloride)

400 and 800 mg

RENAGEL® CAPSULES ℞

[se vel' a mer]

(sevelamer hydrochloride)

403 mg

DESCRIPTION

The active ingredient in Renagel* Tablets and Capsules is sevelamer hydrochloride, a polymeric phosphate binder intended for oral administration. Sevelamer hydrochloride is poly(allylamine hydrochloride) crosslinked with epichlorohydrin in which forty percent of the amines are protonated. It is known chemically as poly(allylamine-co-N,N'-diallyl-1,3-diamino-2-hydroxypropane) hydrochloride. Sevelamer hydrochloride is hydrophilic, but insoluble in water. The structure is represented below:

Chemical Structure of Sevelamer Hydrochloride

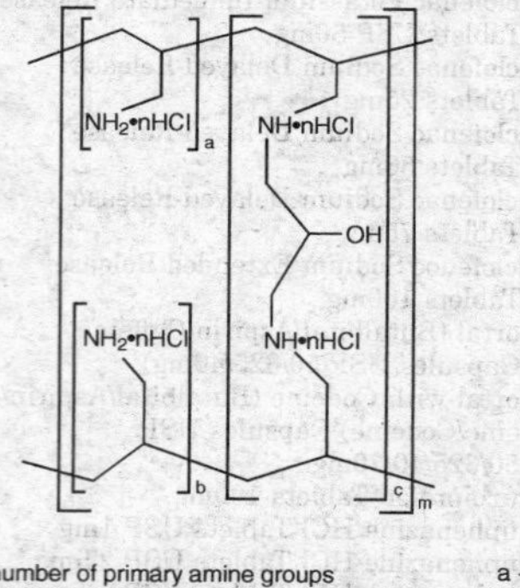

a, b = number of primary amine groups a + b = 9
c = number of crosslinking groups c = 1
n = fraction of protonated amines n = 0.4
m = large number to indicate extended polymer network

The primary amine groups shown in the structure are derived directly from poly(allylamine hydrochloride). The crosslinking groups consist of two secondary amine groups derived from poly(allylamine hydrochloride) and one molecule of epichlorohydrin.

Renagel® Tablets: Each film-coated tablet of Renagel contains either 800 mg or 400 mg of sevelamer hydrochloride on an anhydrous basis. The inactive ingredients are hydroxypropyl methylcellulose, diacetylated monoglyceride, colloidal silicon dioxide, and stearic acid. The tablet imprint contains iron oxide black ink.

Renagel® Capsules: Each hard-gelatin capsule of Renagel contains 403 mg of sevelamer hydrochloride on an anhydrous basis. The inactive ingredients are colloidal silicon dioxide and stearic acid. The capsule and imprint contain titanium dioxide and indigo carmine ink.

* Registered trademark of GelTex Pharmaceuticals, Inc.

CLINICAL PHARMACOLOGY

Patients with end-stage renal disease (ESRD) retain phosphorus and can develop hyperphosphatemia. High serum phosphorus can precipitate serum calcium resulting in ectopic calcification. When the product of serum calcium and phosphorus concentrations (Ca × P) exceeds 66, there is an increased risk that ectopic calcification will occur. Hyperphosphatemia plays a role in the development of secondary hyperparathyroidism in renal insufficiency. An increase in parathyroid hormone (PTH) levels is characteristic of patients with chronic renal failure. Increased levels of PTH can lead to osteitis fibrosa, a bone disease. A decrease in serum phosphorus may decrease serum PTH levels.

Treatment of hyperphosphatemia includes reduction in dietary intake of phosphate, inhibition of intestinal phosphate absorption with phosphate binders, and removal of phosphate with dialysis. Renagel taken with meals has been shown to decrease serum phosphorus concentrations in patients with ESRD who are on hemodialysis. All clinical studies were conducted with Renagel Capsules. *In vitro* studies have shown that the capsule and tablet formulations bind phosphate to a similar extent. Since Renagel does not contain aluminum, it does not cause aluminum intoxication. Renagel treatment also results in a lowering of low-density lipoprotein (LDL) and total serum cholesterol levels.

Pharmacokinetics: A mass balance study using ^{14}C-sevelamer hydrochloride in 16 healthy male and female volunteers showed that sevelamer hydrochloride is not systemically absorbed. No absorption studies have been performed in patients with renal disease.

Clinical trials: The ability of Renagel Capsules to lower serum phosphorus in ESRD patients on hemodialysis was demonstrated in three Phase 2 studies with treatment duration ranging from 2 to 12 weeks and two Phase 3 studies with treatment duration of 8 weeks. Four of the 5 studies were open-label dose-titration studies. One of the Phase 2 studies was a placebo-controlled study. The Phase 3 crossover study, described below, had a control arm. About half the patients from these studies (N=192) were treated with Renagel Capsules in a long-term open-label extension study of 44 weeks.

Cross-over study of Renagel Capsules and calcium acetate: Eighty-four ESRD patients on hemodialysis who were hyperphosphatemic (serum phosphorus >6.0 mg/dL) following a two-week phosphate binder washout period were randomized to receive either Renagel Capsules for eight weeks followed by calcium acetate for eight weeks or calcium acetate for eight weeks followed by Renagel Capsules for eight weeks. Treatment periods were separated by a two-week phosphate binder washout period. Patients started on Renagel Capsules or calcium acetate tablets three times per day

Table 3. Starting Dose for Patients Not Taking a Phosphate Binder

SERUM PHOSPHORUS	RENAGEL® 800 MG	RENAGEL® 400 MG OR RENAGEL® CAPSULES
≥ 6.0 and < 7.5 mg/dL	1 tablet three times daily with meals	2 tablets or capsules three times daily with meals
≥ 7.5 and < 9.0 mg/dL	2 tablets three times daily with meals	3 tablets or capsules three times daily with meals
≥ 9.0 mg/dL	2 tablets three times daily with meals	4 tablets or capsules three times daily with meals

Table 4. Starting Dose for Patients Switching From Calcium Acetate to Renagel

CALCIUM ACETATE 667 MG (TABLETS PER MEAL)	RENAGEL® 800 MG (TABLETS PER MEAL)	RENAGEL® 400 MG OR RENAGEL® CAPSULES (TABLETS OR CAPSULES PER MEAL)
1 tablet	1 tablet	2 tablets or capsules
2 tablets	2 tablets	3 tablets or capsules
3 tablets	3 tablets	5 tablets or capsules

with meals. Over each eight-week treatment period, at three separate time points the dose of either agent could be titrated up 1 capsule or tablet per meal (3 per day) to control serum phosphorus. Renagel Capsules and calcium acetate both significantly decreased mean serum phosphorus by about 2 mg/dL (Table 1).

Table 1. Mean Serum Phosphorus (mg/dL) at Baseline and Endpoint

	Renagel (N=81)	Ca Acetate (N=83)
Baseline at End of Washout	8.4	8.0
Change from Baseline at Endpoint (95% Confidence Interval)	-2.0* (-2.5, -1.5)	-2.1* (-2.6, -1.7)

*$p<0.0001$, within treatment group comparison

Figure 1 illustrates that the proportion of patients achieving a given level of serum phosphorus lowering is comparable between the two treatment groups. For example, about half the patients in each group had a decrease of at least 2 mg/dL at endpoint.

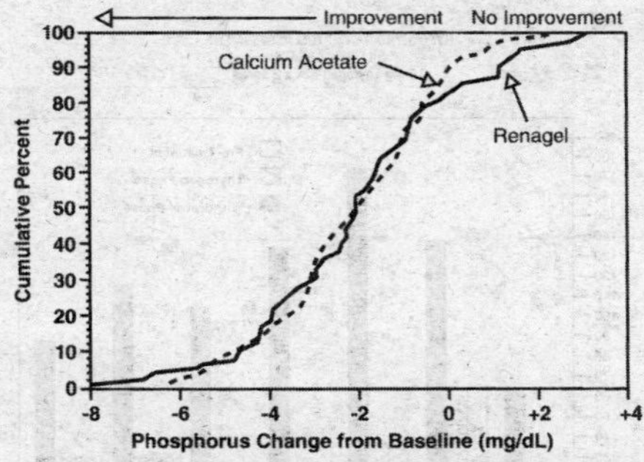

Figure 1. Cumulative percent of patients (Y-axis) attaining a phosphorus change from baseline at least as great as the value on the X-axis. A shift to the left of a curve indicates a better response.

Average daily consumption at the end of treatment was 4.9 g sevelamer hydrochloride (range of 0.0 to 12.6 g) and 5.0 g of calcium acetate (range of 0.0 to 17.8 g). During calcium acetate treatment, 22% of patients developed serum calcium ≥ 11.0 mg/dL on at least one occasion versus 5% for Renagel ($p < 0.05$). Thus the risk of developing hypercalcemia is less with Renagel Capsules compared to calcium acetate.

Mean LDL cholesterol and mean total cholesterol declined significantly on Renagel Capsules treatment (-24% and -15%, respectively). Neither LDL nor total cholesterol changed on calcium acetate treatment. Triglycerides, high-density lipoprotein (HDL) cholesterol, and albumin did not change on either treatment.

Similar reductions in serum phosphorus and LDL cholesterol were observed in an eight-week open-label, uncontrolled study of 172 end stage renal disease patients on hemodialysis.

INDICATIONS AND USAGE

Renagel is indicated for the reduction of serum phosphorus in patients with end-stage renal disease (ESRD). The safety and efficacy of Renagel in ESRD patients who are not on hemodialysis have not been studied. In hemodialysis patients, Renagel decreases the incidence of hypercalcemic episodes relative to patients on calcium acetate treatment.

CONTRAINDICATIONS

Renagel is contraindicated in patients with hypophosphatemia or bowel obstruction. Renagel is contraindicated in patients known to be hypersensitive to sevelamer hydrochloride or any of its constituents.

PRECAUTIONS

General: The safety and efficacy of Renagel in patients with dysphagia, swallowing disorders, severe gastrointestinal (GI) motility disorders, or major GI tract surgery have not been established. Consequently, caution should be exercised when Renagel is used in patients with these GI disorders.

Renagel does not contain calcium or alkali supplementation; serum calcium, bicarbonate, and chloride levels should be monitored.

In preclinical studies in rats and dogs, sevelamer hydrochloride reduced vitamin D, E, K, and folic acid levels at doses of 6–100 times the recommended human dose. In clinical trials, there was no evidence of reduction in serum levels of vitamins. Most (approximately 75%) patients in Renagel clinical trials received vitamin supplements, which is typical of patients on hemodialysis.

Information for the patient: The prescriber should inform patients to take Renagel with meals and adhere to their prescribed diets. Instructions should be given on concomitant medications that should be dosed apart from Renagel. Because the contents of Renagel expand in water, tablets and capsules should be swallowed intact and should not be crushed, chewed, broken into pieces, or taken apart prior to administration.

Drug interactions: Renagel Capsules were studied in human drug-drug interaction studies with digoxin, warfarin, enalapril and metoprolol.

Digoxin: In 19 healthy subjects receiving 6 Renagel capsules three times a day with meals for 2 days, Renagel did not alter the pharmacokinetics of a single dose of digoxin.

Warfarin: In 14 healthy subjects receiving 6 Renagel capsules three times a day with meals for 2 days, Renagel did not alter the pharmacokinetics of a single dose of warfarin.

Enalapril: In 28 healthy subjects a single dose of 6 Renagel capsules did not alter the pharmacokinetics of a single dose of enalapril.

Metoprolol: In 31 healthy subjects a single dose of 6 Renagel capsules did not alter the pharmacokinetics of a single dose of metoprolol.

However, when administering any other oral medication where a reduction in the bioavailability of that medication would have a clinically significant effect on safety or efficacy, the drug should be administered at least one hour before or three hours after Renagel, or the physician should consider monitoring blood levels of the drug. Patients taking anti-arrhythmic and anti-seizure medications were excluded from the clinical trials. Special precautions should be taken when prescribing Renagel to patients also taking these medications.

Carcinogenesis, mutagenesis, and impairment of fertility: Long-term studies in animals to evaluate carcinogenic potential have not been completed. In an in vitro mammalian cytogenetics test with metabolic activation, sevelamer hydrochloride caused a statistically significant increase in the number of structural chromosome aberrations. Sevelamer hydrochloride was not mutagenic in the Ames bacterial mutation assay. Sevelamer hydrochloride did not impair fertility in male or female rats.

Pregnancy:

Pregnancy Category C

In rats, at doses of 1.5 and 4.5 g/kg/day (approximately 15 and 45 times the recommended human dose based on mg/kg), sevelamer hydrochloride caused reduced or irregular ossification of fetal bones, probably due to a reduced absorption of fat-soluble vitamin D. In rabbits, sevelamer hydrochloride slightly increased prenatal mortality due to an increased incidence of early resorptions at a dose of 1 g/kg/day (approximately 10 times the recommended human dose based on mg/kg). Requirements for vitamins and other nutrients are increased in pregnancy. The effect of Renagel on the absorption of vitamins and other nutrients has not been studied in pregnant women. There are no adequate and well-controlled studies in pregnant women or nursing mothers.

Geriatric use: There is no evidence for special considerations when Renagel is administered to elderly patients.

Pediatric use: The safety and efficacy of Renagel has not been established in pediatric patients.

ADVERSE REACTIONS

In a placebo-controlled study with a treatment duration of two weeks, the adverse events reported for Renagel Capsules (N=24) were similar to those reported for placebo (N=12). In a cross-over study with treatment durations of eight weeks each, the adverse events reported for Renagel Capsules (N=82) were similar to those reported for calcium acetate (N=82) (Table 2).

Table 2. Treatment-Emergent Adverse Events ≥10% from a Cross-Over Trial of Renagel Capsules versus Calcium Acetate for Eight Weeks of Treatment (N=82)

	Renagel	Ca Acetate
Adverse Event	N (%)	N (%)
Any	64 (78)	65 (79)
Body As A Whole	36 (44)	38 (46)
Headache	8 (10)	9 (11)
Infection	12 (15)	9 (11)
Pain	11 (13)	13 (16)
Cardiovascular	24 (29)	29 (35)
Hypertension	7 (9)	8 (10)
Hypotension	9 (11)	10 (12)
Thrombosis	8 (10)	5 (6)
Digestive	28 (34)	23 (28)
Diarrhea	13 (16)	8 (10)
Dyspepsia	9 (11)	3 (4)
Vomiting	10 (12)	4 (5)
Respiratory	8 (10)	18 (22)
Cough Increased	3 (4)	9 (11)

In a long-term, open-label extension trial, adverse events possibly related to Renagel Capsules and which were not dose-related, included nausea (7%), constipation (2%), diarrhea (4%), flatulence (4%), and dyspepsia (5%).

OVERDOSAGE

Renagel Capsules have been given to normal healthy volunteers in doses of up to 14 grams per day for eight days with no adverse effects. There are no reported overdosages of Renagel in patients. Since Renagel is not absorbed, the risk of systemic toxicity is low.

DOSAGE AND ADMINISTRATION

Patients Not Taking a Phosphate Binder. The recommended starting dose of Renagel is 800 to 1600 mg, which can be administered as one to two Renagel® 800 mg Tablets, two to four Renagel® 400 mg Tablets, or two to four Renagel® Capsules with each meal based on serum phosphorus level. Table 3 provides recommended starting doses of Renagel for patients not taking a phosphate binder.

[See table 3 above]

Patients Switching From Calcium Acetate. In a study in 84 ESRD patients on hemodialysis, a similar reduction in serum phosphorus was seen with equivalent doses (mg for mg) of Renagel Capsules and calcium acetate. Table 4 gives recommended starting doses of Renagel based on a patient's current calcium acetate dose.

[See table 4 above]

Dose Titration for All Patients Taking Renagel. Dosage should be adjusted based on the serum phosphorus concentration with a goal of lowering serum phosphorus to 6.0 mg/dL or less. The dose may be increased or decreased by one tablet or capsule per meal at two week intervals as necessary. Table 5 gives a dose titration guideline. The average dose in Phase 3 clinical trials was four 403 mg capsules per meal. The maximum dose studied was 10 Renagel capsules per meal (the equivalent of 5 Renagel® 800 mg Tablets per meal or 10 Renagel® 400 mg Tablets per meal).

Table 5. Dose Titration Guideline

Serum Phosphorus	Renagel Dose
>6.0 mg/dL	Increase 1 tablet/capsule per meal at 2 week intervals
3.5–6.0 mg/dL	Maintain current dose
<3.5 mg/dL	Decrease 1 tablet/capsule per meal

Continued on next page

Renagel—Cont.

Drug interaction studies have demonstrated that Renagel Capsules have no effect on the bioavailability of digoxin, warfarin, enalapril, or metoprolol. When administering any other oral drug for which alteration in blood levels could have a clinically significant effect on safety or efficacy, the drug should be administered at least one hour before or three hours after Renagel, or the physician should consider monitoring blood levels of the drug. (See PRECAUTIONS: Drug interactions.)
Do not use Renagel after the expiration date on the bottle.

HOW SUPPLIED

Renagel® 800 mg Tablets are supplied as oval, film-coated, compressed tablets, imprinted with "RENAGEL 800," containing 800 mg of sevelamer hydrochloride on an anhydrous basis, hydroxypropyl methylcellulose, diacetylated monoglyceride, colloidal silicon dioxide, and stearic acid. Renagel® 800 mg Tablets are packaged in bottles of 180 tablets.
NDC 58468-0021-1 Bottle of 180 Tablets
Renagel® 400 mg Tablets are supplied as oval, film-coated, compressed tablets, imprinted with "RENAGEL 400," containing 400 mg of sevelamer hydrochloride on an anhydrous basis, hydroxypropyl methylcellulose, diacetylated monoglyceride, colloidal silicon dioxide, and stearic acid. Renagel® 400 mg Tablets are packaged in bottles of 360 tablets.
NDC 58468-0020-1 Bottle of 360 Tablets
Renagel® Capsules are supplied as hard-gelatin capsules, axially imprinted with "G403," containing 403 mg of sevelamer hydrochloride on an anhydrous basis, colloidal silicon dioxide, and stearic acid. Renagel® Capsules are packaged in bottles of 200 capsules.
NDC 58468-4709-1 Bottle of 200 Capsules

Storage

Store at 25°C (77°F): excursions permitted to 15–30°C (59–86°F).
[See USP controlled room temperature]
Protect from moisture.
Rx Only
Manufactured for GelTex Pharmaceuticals, Inc., Waltham, MA
Distributed by:
Genzyme Corporation
One Kendall Square
Cambridge, MA 02139
USA
Tel. (800) 847-0069
4712 (7/00)
Issued 7/00
Shown in Product Identification Guide, page 314

THYROGEN® ℞

[thī'rō-gen]
(thyrotropin alfa for injection)

DESCRIPTION

Thyrogen® (thyrotropin alfa for injection) contains a highly purified recombinant form of human thyroid stimulating hormone (TSH), a glycoprotein which is produced by recombinant DNA technology. Thyrotropin alfa is synthesized in a genetically modified Chinese hamster ovary cell line.
Thyrotropin alfa is a heterodimeric glycoprotein comprised of two non-covalently linked subunits, an alpha subunit of 92 amino acid residues containing two N-linked glycosylation sites and a beta subunit of 118 residues containing one N-linked glycosylation site. The amino acid sequence of thyrotropin alfa is identical to that of human pituitary thyroid stimulating hormone.
Both thyrotropin alfa and naturally occurring human pituitary thyroid stimulating hormone are synthesized as a mixture of glycosylation variants. Unlike pituitary TSH, which is secreted as a mixture of sialylated and sulfated forms, thyrotropin alfa is sialylated but not sulfated. The biological activity of thyrotropin alfa is determined using both an *in vivo* bioassay and an *in vitro* bioassay. The *in vivo* bioassay measures an increase in thyroxine (T_4) level in response to the intraperitoneal injection of thyrotropin alfa after suppression of endogenous TSH levels in mice. The *in vitro* assay measures the amount of cAMP produced by a bovine thyroid-derived microsome preparation in response to thyrotropin alfa. The specific activity of thyrotropin alfa is calibrated against the World Health Organization (WHO) human pituitary derived TSH reference standard, NIBSC 84/703. The biological activity of thyrotropin alfa has been determined to be no less than 4 IU/mg by the *in vitro* bioassay.

Thyrogen is supplied as a sterile, non-pyrogenic, white to off-white lyophilized product, intended for intramuscular (IM) administration after reconstitution with Sterile Water for Injection, USP. Each vial of Thyrogen contains 1.1 mg thyrotropin alfa (≥ 4 IU), 36 mg Mannitol, 5.1 mg Sodium Phosphate, and 2.4 mg Sodium Chloride.
After reconstitution with 1.2 mL of Sterile Water for Injection, USP, the thyrotropin alfa concentration is 0.9 mg/mL. The pH of the reconstituted solution is approximately 7.0.

CLINICAL PHARMACOLOGY

Pharmacodynamics

Thyrotropin alfa (recombinant human thyroid stimulating hormone) is a heterodimeric glycoprotein produced by recombinant DNA technology. It has comparable biochemical properties to the human pituitary TSH. Binding of thyrotropin alfa to TSH receptors on normal thyroid epithelial cells or on well-differentiated thyroid cancer tissue stimulates iodine uptake and organification, and synthesis and secretion of thyroglobulin (Tg), triiodothyronine (T_3) and thyroxine (T_4).
In patients with thyroid cancer, a near total or total thyroidectomy is performed and patients are placed on synthetic thyroid hormone supplements to replace endogenous hormone and to suppress serum levels of TSH in order to avoid TSH-stimulated tumor growth. Thereafter, patients are followed up for the presence of remnants or of residual or recurred cancer by thyroglobulin (Tg) testing while they remain on thyroid hormone suppressive therapy and are euthyroid, or by Tg testing and radioiodine imaging after thyroid hormone withdrawal. Thyrogen is an exogenous source of human TSH that offers an additional diagnostic tool in the follow-up of patients with a history of well-differentiated thyroid cancer.

Pharmacokinetics

The pharmacokinetics of Thyrogen were studied in 16 patients with well-differentiated thyroid cancer given a single 0.9 mg IM dose. Mean peak concentrations of 116 ± 38 mU/L were reached between 3 and 24 hours after injection (median of 10 hours). The mean apparent elimination half-life was 25 ± 10 hours. The organ(s) of TSH clearance in man have not been identified, but studies of pituitary-derived TSH suggest the involvement of the liver and kidneys.

Clinical Trials

Two phase 3 clinical trials were conducted in 358 evaluable patients with well-differentiated thyroid cancer to compare 48-hour radioiodine (^{131}I) whole body scans obtained after Thyrogen to whole body scans after thyroid hormone withdrawal. One of these trials also compared Tg levels obtained after Thyrogen to those on thyroid hormone suppressive therapy, and to those after thyroid hormone withdrawal. All Tg testing was performed in a central laboratory using a radioimmunoassay (RIA) with a functional sensitivity of 2.5 ng/mL. Only successfully ablated patients (defined as patients who have undergone total or near total thyroidectomy with or without radioiodine ablation, and with < 1% uptake in the thyroid bed on a scan after thyroid hormone withdrawal) without detectable anti-thyroglobulin antibodies were included in the Tg data analysis. The maximum Thyrogen Tg value was obtained 72 hours after the final Thyrogen injection, and this value was used in the analysis (see DOSAGE AND ADMINISTRATION).

Radioiodine Whole Body Scan Results

The following table summarizes the scan data in patients with positive scans after withdrawal of thyroid hormone from the phase 3 studies:
[See table below]
Across the two clinical studies, the Thyrogen scan failed to detect remnant and/or cancer localized to the thyroid bed in 16% (20/124) of patients in whom it was detected by a scan after thyroid hormone withdrawal. In addition, the Thyrogen scan failed to detect metastatic disease in 24% (9/38) of patients in whom it was detected by a scan after thyroid hormone withdrawal.

Thyroglobulin (Tg) Results:

Thyrogen Tg Testing Alone and in Combination with Radioiodine Imaging: Comparison with Results after Thyroid Hormone Withdrawal:

In Tg antibody negative patients with a thyroid remnant or cancer as defined by a withdrawal Tg ≥2.5 ng/mL or a positive scan (after thyroid hormone withdrawal or after radioiodine therapy), the Thyrogen Tg was ≥ 2.5 ng/mL in 69% (40/58) of patients after 2 doses of Thyrogen, and in 80% (53/66) of patients after 3 doses of Thyrogen. Across both dosage groups, 45% had a Tg ≥ 2.5 ng/mL on thyroid hormone suppressive therapy.
In these same patients, adding the whole body scan increased the detection rate of thyroid remnant or cancer to 84% (49/58) of patients after 2 doses of Thyrogen and 94% (62/66) of patients after 3 doses of Thyrogen.

Thyrogen Tg Testing Alone and in Combination with Radioiodine Imaging in Patients with Confirmed Metastatic Disease:

Metastatic disease was confirmed by a post-treatment scan or by lymph node biopsy in 35 patients. Thyrogen Tg was ≥ 2.5 ng/mL in all 35 patients while Tg on thyroid hormone suppressive therapy was ≥ 2.5 ng/mL in 79% of these patients.
In this same cohort of 35 patients with confirmed metastatic disease, the Thyrogen Tg levels were below 10 ng/mL in 27% (3/11) of patients after 2 doses of Thyrogen and in 13% (3/24) of patients after 3 doses of Thyrogen. The corresponding thyroid hormone withdrawal Tg levels in these 6 patients were 15.6–137 ng/mL. The Thyrogen scan detected metastatic disease in 1 of these 6 patients (see INDICATIONS AND USAGE, Considerations in the Use of Thyrogen).
As with thyroid hormone withdrawal, the intra-patient reproducibility of Thyrogen testing with regard to both Tg stimulation and radioiodine imaging has not been studied.

Quality of Life:

Following Thyrogen, no change was observed in any of the 8 domains of the SF-36 Health Survey, a patient-administered quality-of-life measurement instrument. Following thyroid hormone withdrawal, statistically significant negative changes in quality of life parameters were observed in 4 of the 8 SF-36 domains. These 4 domains were: physical functioning, physical role, bodily pain and emotional role. No change was observed in the following scales: general health, vitality, social functioning and mental health.

Hypothyroid Signs and Symptoms:

Thyrogen administration was not associated with the signs and symptoms of hypothyroidism that accompanied thyroid hormone withdrawal as measured by the Billewicz scale. Statistically significant worsening in all signs and symptoms were observed during the hypothyroid phase (p<0.01).

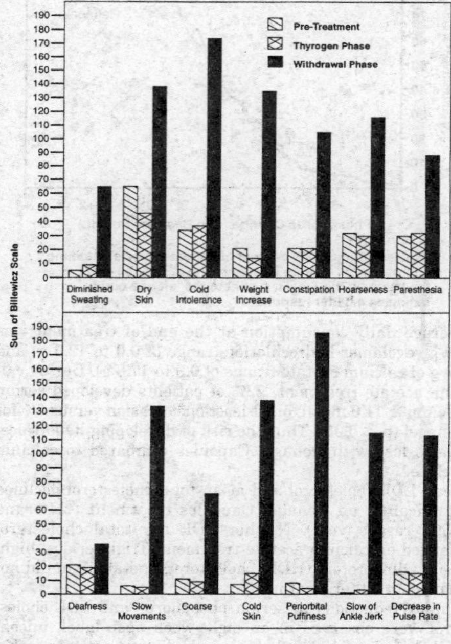

	# scan pairs by disease category	#(%) scan pairs in which Thyrogen scan detected disease seen on withdrawal scan	#(%) scan pairs in which Thyrogen scan did not detect disease seen on withdrawal scan
First Phase 3 Study (0.9 mg IM qd x 2)			
positive for remnant or cancer in thyroid bed	48	39(81)	9(19)
metastatic disease	15	11(73)	4(27)
total positive withdrawal scans*	63	50(79)	13(21)
Second Phase 3 Study (0.9 mg IM qd x 2)			
positive for remnant or cancer in thyroid bed	35	30(86)	5(14)
metastatic disease	9	6(67)	3(33)
total positive withdrawal scans*	44	36(82)	8(18)
Second Phase 3 Study (0.9 mg IM q 72 hrs x 3)			
positive for remnant or cancer in thyroid bed	41	35(85)	6(15)
metastatic disease	14	12(86)	2(14)
total positive withdrawal scans*	55	47(85)	8(15)

* Across all studies, uptake was detected on the Thyrogen scan but not observed on the scan after thyroid hormone withdrawal in 5 patients with remnant or cancer in the thyroid bed.

INDICATIONS AND USAGE

Thyrogen (thyrotropin alfa for injection) is indicated for use as an adjunctive diagnostic tool for serum thyroglobulin (Tg) testing with or without radioiodine imaging in the follow-up of patients with well-differentiated thyroid cancer.

Potential Clinical Uses:

1) Thyrogen Tg testing may be used in patients with an undetectable Tg on thyroid hormone suppressive therapy to

exclude the diagnosis of residual or recurrent thyroid cancer (see CLINICAL PHARMACOLOGY, Clinical Trials, Thyroglobulin (Tg) Results).

2) Thyrogen testing may be used in patients requiring serum Tg testing and radioiodine imaging who are unwilling to undergo thyroid hormone withdrawal testing and whose treating physician believes that use of a less sensitive test is justified.
3) Thyrogen testing may be used in patients who are either unable to mount an adequate endogenous TSH response to thyroid hormone withdrawal or in whom withdrawal is medically contraindicated.

Considerations in the Use of Thyrogen:

1) **Even when Thyrogen-stimulated Tg testing is performed in combination with radioiodine imaging, there remains a meaningful risk of missing a diagnosis of thyroid cancer or of underestimating the extent of disease. Therefore, thyroid hormone withdrawal Tg testing with radioiodine imaging remains the standard diagnostic modality to assess the presence, location and extent of thyroid cancer.**
2) Thyrogen Tg levels are generally lower than, and do not correlate with Tg levels after thyroid hormone withdrawal (see CLINICAL PHARMACOLOGY, Thyroglobulin (Tg) Results).
3) A newly detectable Tg level or a Tg level rising over time after Thyrogen, or a high index of suspicion of metastatic disease, even in the setting of a negative or low-stage Thyrogen radioiodine scan, should prompt further evaluation such as thyroid hormone withdrawal to definitively establish the location and extent of thyroid cancer. On the other hand, none of the 31 patients studied with undetectable Thyrogen Tg levels (< 2.5 ng/mL) had metastatic disease. Therefore, an undetectable Thyrogen Tg level suggests the absence of clinically significant disease (see CLINICAL PHARMACOLOGY, Clinical Trials).
4) The decisions whether to perform a Thyrogen radioiodine scan in conjunction with a Thyrogen serum Tg test and whether and when to withdraw a patient from thyroid hormone are complex. Pertinent factors in these decisions include the sensitivity of the Tg assay used, the Thyrogen Tg level obtained, and the index of suspicion of recurrent or persistent local or metastatic disease. In the clinical trials, combination Tg and scan testing did enhance the diagnostic accuracy of Thyrogen in some cases (see CLINICAL PHARMACOLOGY Clinical Trials).
5) Thyrogen is not recommended to stimulate radioiodine uptake for the purposes of ablative radiotherapy of thyroid cancer.
6) The signs and symptoms of hypothyroidism which accompany thyroid hormone withdrawal are avoided with Thyrogen (see CLINICAL PHARMACOLOGY, Clinical Trials, Quality of Life, Hypothyroid Signs and Symptoms).

PRECAUTIONS

(see INDICATIONS AND USAGE, Considerations in the Use of Thyrogen)

General

The use of Thyrogen (thyrotropin alfa for injection) should be directed by physicians knowledgeable in the management of patients with thyroid cancer.

Thyroglobulin (Tg) antibodies may confound the Tg assay and render Tg levels uninterpretable. Therefore, in such cases, even with a negative or low-stage Thyrogen radioiodine scan, consideration should be given to evaluating patients further with, for example, a confirmatory thyroid hormone withdrawal scan to determine the location and extent of thyroid cancer.

Thyrogen should be administered intramuscularly only. It should not be administered intravenously.

TSH antibodies have not been reported in patients treated with Thyrogen in the clinical trials, although only 27 patients received Thyrogen on more than one occasion.

Caution should be exercised when Thyrogen is administered to patients who have been previously treated with bovine TSH and, in particular, to those patients who have experienced hypersensitivity reactions to bovine TSH.

Thyrogen is known to cause a transient but significant rise in serum thyroid hormone concentration. Therefore, caution should be exercised in patients with a known history of heart disease and with significant residual thyroid tissue (see ADVERSE REACTIONS).

Drug-Drug Interactions

Formal interaction studies between Thyrogen and other medicinal products have not been performed. In clinical trials, no interactions were observed between Thyrogen and the thyroid hormones triiodothyronine (T_3) and thyroxine (T_4) when administered concurrently.

The use of Thyrogen allows for radioiodine imaging while patients are euthyroid on triiodothyronine (T_3) and/or thyroxine (T_4). Data on radioiodine ^{131}I kinetics indicate that the clearance of radioiodine is approximately 50% greater in euthyroid patients than in hypothyroid patients, who have decreased renal function. Thus radioiodine retention is less in euthyroid patients at the time of imaging and this factor should be considered when selecting the activity of radioiodine for use in radioiodine imaging.

Carcinogenesis, Mutagenesis, Impairment of Fertility

Long-term toxicity studies in animals have not been performed with Thyrogen to evaluate the carcinogenic potential of the drug. Thyrogen was not mutagenic in the bacterial reverse mutation assay. Studies have not been performed with Thyrogen to evaluate the effects on fertility.

Pregnancy Category C

Animal reproduction studies have not been conducted with Thyrogen.

It is also not known whether Thyrogen can cause fetal harm when administered to a pregnant woman or can affect reproductive capacity. Thyrogen should be given to a pregnant woman only if clearly needed.

Nursing Mothers

It is not known whether the drug is excreted in human milk. Because many drugs are excreted in human milk, caution should be exercised when Thyrogen is administered to a nursing woman.

Pediatric Use

Safety and effectiveness in pediatric patients below the age of 16 years have not been established.

Geriatric Use

Results from controlled trials indicate no difference in the safety and efficacy of Thyrogen between adult patients less than 65 years and those greater than 65 years of age.

ADVERSE REACTIONS

Adverse reaction data are derived from the two clinical trials in which 381 patients were treated with Thyrogen (thyrotropin alfa for injection) and from post-marketing surveillance.

The most common adverse events (> 5%) reported in clinical trials were: nausea (10.5%) and headache (7.3%). Events reported in ≥ 1% of patients in the trials are summarized in the following table:

Summary of Adverse Events During Clinical Studies (≥ 1%)

	% of Patients with Adverse Events (n) (n = 381)
Body as a Whole	
Headache	7.3%(28)
Asthenia	3.4%(13)
Chills	1.0%(4)
Fever	1.0%(4)
Flu Syndrome	1.0%(4)
Digestive System	
Nausea	10.5%(40)
Vomiting	2.1%(8)
Nausea and Vomiting	1.3%(5)
Nervous System	
Dizziness	1.6%(6)
Paresthesia	1.6%(6)

There have been several reports of hypersensitivity reactions including urticaria, rash, pruritus and flushing. However, in clinical trials no patients have developed antibodies to thyrotropin alfa, either after single or repeated (27 patients) use of the product.

Four patients out of 55 (7.3%) with CNS metastases who were followed in a special treatment protocol experienced acute hemiplegia, hemiparesis or pain one to three days after Thyrogen administration. The symptoms were attributed to local edema and/or focal hemorrhage at the site of the cerebral or spinal cord metastases. In addition, one case each of acute visual loss and of dysphagia secondary to laryngeal edema, requiring tracheotomy, have been reported 24 hours after Thyrogen administration in patients with metastases to the optic nerve and paratracheal areas, respectively. Pre-treatment with corticosteroids may be considered under such circumstances.

A 77 year-old non-thyroidectomized patient with a history of heart disease and spinal metastases who received 4 Thyrogen injections over 6 days in a special treatment protocol experienced a fatal MI 24 hours after he received the last Thyrogen injection. The event was likely related to Thyrogen-induced hyperthyroidism.

OVERDOSAGE

There has been no reported experience of overdose in humans. However, in clinical trials, three patients experienced symptoms after receiving Thyrogen doses higher than those recommended. Two patients had nausea after a 2.7 mg IM dose, and in one of these patients, the event was accompanied by weakness, dizziness and headache. Another patient experienced nausea, vomiting and hot flashes after a 3.6 mg IM dose.

In addition, one patient experienced symptoms after receiving Thyrogen intravenously. This patient received 0.3 mg Thyrogen as a single intravenous bolus and, 15 minutes later experienced severe nausea, vomiting, diaphoresis, hypotension (BP decreased from 115/66 mm Hg to 81/44 mm Hg) and tachycardia (pulse increased from 75 to 117 bpm).

DOSAGE AND ADMINISTRATION

Thyrogen 0.9 mg intramuscularly may be administered every 24 hours for two doses or every 72 hours for three doses.

After reconstitution with 1.2 mL Sterile Water for Injection, a 1.0 mL solution (0.9 mg thyrotropin alfa) is administered by intramuscular injection to the buttock.

For radioiodine imaging, radioiodine administration should be given 24 hours following the final Thyrogen injection. Scanning should be performed 48 hours after radioiodine administration (72 hours after the final injection of Thyrogen).

The following parameters utilized in the second Phase 3 study are recommended for radioiodine scanning with Thyrogen:

- A diagnostic activity of 4 mCi (148 MBq) ^{131}I should be used.
- Whole body images should be acquired for a minimum of 30 minutes and/or should contain a minimum of 140,000 counts.
- Scanning times for single (spot) images of body regions should be 10–15 minutes or less if the minimum number of counts is reached sooner (i.e., 60,000 for a large field of view camera, 35,000 counts for a small field of view).

For serum Tg testing, the serum sample should be obtained 72 hours after the final injection of Thyrogen.

INSTRUCTIONS FOR USE

Thyrogen (thyrotropin alfa for injection) is for intramuscular injection to the buttock. The powder should be reconstituted immediately prior to use with 1.2 mL of the diluent provided. Each vial of Thyrogen and each vial of diluent is intended for single use. Discard unused portion of the diluent.

Thyrogen should be stored at 2–8°C (36–46°F). Each vial, after reconstitution with 1.2 mL of the accompanying Sterile Water for Injection, USP, should be inspected visually for particulate matter or discoloration before use. Any vials exhibiting particulate matter or discoloration should not be used.

If necessary, the reconstituted solution can be stored for up to 24 hours at a temperature between 2°C and 8°C, while avoiding microbial contamination.

DO NOT USE Thyrogen after the expiration date on the vial. Protect from light.

HOW SUPPLIED

Thyrogen (thyrotropin alfa for injection) is supplied as a sterile, non-pyrogenic, lyophilized product. It is available as a kit containing two 1.1 mg vials (≥ 4 IU) of Thyrogen® (thyrotropin alfa for injection) and two 10 mL vials of Sterile Water for Injection, USP.

NDC 58468-1849-4

Store at 2–8°C.

Rx ONLY

Thyrogen® (thyrotropin alfa for injection)

Manufactured and Distributed by:

Genzyme Corporation
One Kendall Square
Cambridge, MA 02139
(800) 745-4447

Marketed by:

Knoll Pharmaceutical Company

Genzyme Corporation

Issued August 1999 4728 (8/99)

Gilead Sciences, Inc.

333 LAKESIDE DRIVE
FOSTER CITY, CA 94404

Direct Inquiries To:
Customer Service
(800) GILEAD5

Medical Emergency Contact:
Director, Medical Information
(800) GILEAD5
FAX: (650) 522-5477

DAUNOXOME® ℞

(daunorubicin citrate liposome injection)

WARNINGS

1. Cardiac function should be monitored regularly in patients receiving DaunoXome because of the potential risk for cardiac toxicity and congestive heart failure. Cardiac monitoring is advised especially in those patients who have received prior anthracyclines or who have pre-existing cardiac disease or who have had prior radiotherapy encompassing the heart.
2. Severe myelosuppression may occur.
3. DaunoXome should be administered only under the supervision of a physician who is experienced in the use of cancer chemotherapeutic agents.
4. Dosage should be reduced in patients with impaired hepatic function. **(See DOSAGE AND ADMINISTRATION)**
5. A triad of back pain, flushing, and chest tightness has been reported in 13.8% of the patients (16/116) treated with DaunoXome in the Phase III clinical trial, and in 2.7% of treatment cycles (27/994). This triad generally occurs during the first five minutes of the infusion, subsides with interruption of the infusion, and generally does not recur if the infusion is then resumed at a slower rate.

DESCRIPTION

DaunoXome is a sterile, pyrogen-free, preservative-free product in a single use vial for intravenous infusion.

DaunoXome contains an aqueous solution of the citrate salt of daunorubicin encapsulated within lipid vesicles (liposomes) composed of a lipid bilayer of distearoylphosphati-

Continued on next page

DaunoXome—Cont.

dylcholine and cholesterol (2:1 molar ratio), with a mean diameter of about 45 nm. The lipid to drug weight ratio is 18.7:1 (total lipid:daunorubicin base), equivalent to a 10:5:1 molar ratio of distearoylphosphatidylcholine: cholesterol: daunorubicin. Daunorubicin is an anthracycline antibiotic with antineoplastic activity, originally obtained from *Streptomyces peucetius*. Daunorubicin has a 4-ring anthracycline moiety linked by a glycosidic bond to daunosamine, an amino sugar. Daunorubicin may also be isolated from *Streptomyces coeruleorubidus* and has the following chemical name: (8S-*cis*)-8-acetyl-10-[(3-amino-2,3,6-trideoxy-α-L-*lyxo*-hexopyranosyl)oxy]-7,8,9,10-tetrahydro-6,8,11-trihydroxy-1-methoxy-5,12-naphthacenedione hydrochloride.

Daunorubicin citrate has the following chemical structure:

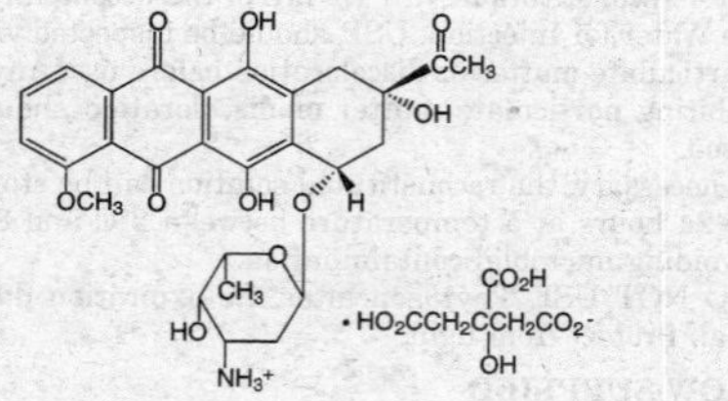

DSPC (distearoylphosphatidylcholine) has the following chemical structure:

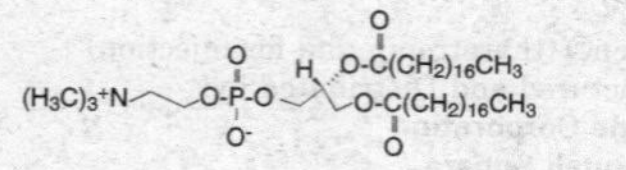

The following represents the idealized, spherical morphology of a liposome:

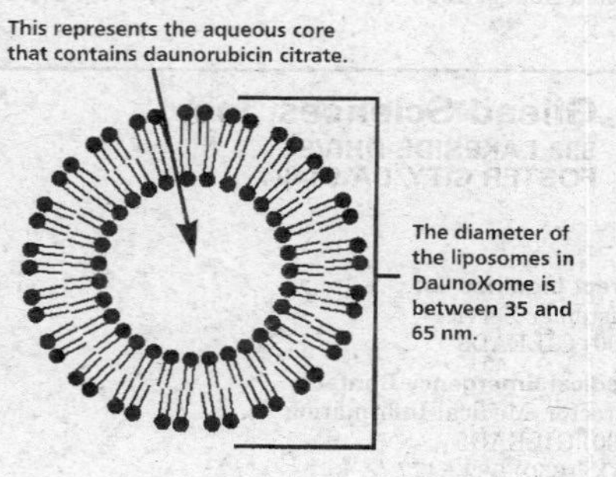
This represents the aqueous core that contains daunorubicin citrate.
The diameter of the liposomes in DaunoXome is between 35 and 65 nm.
represents a molecule of DSPC.

Note: Liposomal encapsulation can substantially affect a drug's functional properties relative to those of the unencapsulated drug.

In addition, different liposomal drug products may vary from one another in the chemical composition and physical form of the liposomes. Such differences can substantially affect the functional properties of liposomal drug products.

Each vial contains daunorubicin citrate equivalent to 50 mg of daunorubicin base, encapsulated in liposomes consisting of 704 mg distearoylphosphatidylcholine and 168 mg cholesterol. The liposomes encapsulating daunorubicin are dispersed in an aqueous medium containing 2,125 mg sucrose, 94 mg glycine, and 7 mg calcium chloride dihydrate in a total volume of 25 mL/vial. The pH of the dispersion is between 4.9 and 6.0. The liposome dispersion should appear red and translucent.

CLINICAL PHARMACOLOGY

Mechanism of Action

DaunoXome is a liposomal preparation of daunorubicin formulated to maximize the selectivity of daunorubicin for solid tumors *in situ*. While in the circulation, the DaunoXome formulation helps to protect the entrapped daunorubicin from chemical and enzymatic degradation, minimizes protein binding, and generally decreases uptake by normal (non-reticuloendothelial system) tissues. The specific mechanism by which DaunoXome is able to deliver daunorubicin to solid tumors *in situ* is not known. However, it is believed to be a function of increased permeability of the tumor neovasculature to some particles in the size range of DaunoXome. In animal studies, daunorubicin has been shown to accumulate in tumors to a greater extent when administered as DaunoXome than when administered as daunorubicin. Once within the tumor environment, daunorubicin is released over time enabling it to exert its antineoplastic activity.

Pharmacokinetics

Following intravenous injection of DaunoXome, plasma clearance of daunorubicin shows monoexponential decline. The pharmacokinetic parameter values for total daunorubicin following a single 40 mg/m^2 dose of DaunoXome administered over a 30–60 minute period to patients with AIDS-related Kaposi's sarcoma and following a single rapid intravenous, 80 mg/m^2 dose of conventional daunorubicin to patients with disseminated solid malignancies are shown in Table I.

TABLE 1
PHARMACOKINETIC PARAMETERS OF DaunoXome IN AIDS PATIENTS WITH KAPOSI'S SARCOMA AND REPORTED PARAMETERS FOR CONVENTIONAL DAUNORUBICIN

Parameter (units)	[a]DaunoXome	[b]Conventional Daunorubicin
Plasma Clearance (mL/min)	17.3 ± 6.1	[c]236 ± 181
Volume of Distribution (L)	6.4 ± 1.5	1006 ± 622
Distribution Half-Life (h)	4.41 ± 2.33	0.77 ± 0.3
Elimination Half-Life (h)	—	55.4 ± 13.7

[a]N=30; [b]N=4; [c]Calculated

The plasma pharmacokinetics of DaunoXome differ significantly from the results reported for conventional daunorubicin hydrochloride. DaunoXome has a small steady-state volume of distribution 6.4 L, (probably because it is confined to vascular fluid volume), and clearance of 17 mL/min. These differences in the volume of distribution and clearance result in a higher daunorubicin exposure (in terms of plasma AUC) from DaunoXome than with conventional daunorubicin hydrochloride. The apparent elimination half-life of DaunoXome is 4.4 hours, far shorter than that of daunorubicin, and probably represents a distribution half-life. Although preclinical biodistribution data in animals suggest that DaunoXome crosses the normal blood-brain barrier, it is unknown whether DaunoXome crosses the blood-brain barrier in humans.

Metabolism: Daunorubicinol, the major active metabolite of daunorubicin, was detected at low levels in the plasma following intravenous administration of DaunoXome.

No formal assessments of pharmacokinetic drug—drug interactions between DaunoXome and other agents have been conducted.

Special Populations: The pharmacokinetics of DaunoXome have not been evaluated in women, in different ethnic groups, or in subjects with renal and hepatic insufficiency.

Clinical Study

In an open-label, randomized, controlled clinical study conducted at 13 centers in the U.S.A. and Canada in advanced (25 or more mucocutaneous lesions; the development of 10 or more lesions in a one month period of time; symptomatic visceral involvement; or tumor-associated edema) HIV-related Kaposi's sarcoma, two treatment regimens were compared as first line cytotoxic therapy: DaunoXome 40 mg/m^2 and ABV (doxorubicin (Adriamycin®*) 10 mg/m^2, bleomycin 15 U, and vincristine 1.0 mg). All drugs were administered intravenously every 2 weeks. Responses were assessed using the AIDS Clinical Trials Group Oncology Committee of the National Institute of Allergy and Infectious Diseases (ACTG) criteria (a response required at least one of any of the following for at least 28 days: a. ≥ 50% reduction in the number; b. ≥ 50% reduction in the sums of the products of the largest perpendicular diameters of bidimensionally measurable marker lesions; or c. complete flattening of ≥ 50% of all previously raised lesions). Table II summarizes the efficacy results.

*Adriamycin is a registered trademark of Pharmacia Upjohn, Kalamazoo, MI.

TABLE II
EFFICACY DATA
FIRST LINE CYTOTOXIC THERAPY FOR ADVANCED KAPOSI'S SARCOMA

	DaunoXome n=116	ABV n=111
Response Rate	23%*	30%
Duration of Response, Median	110 days**	113 days
Time to Progression, Median	92 days***	105 days
Survival	342 days****	291 days

* The 95% confidence interval for difference in the response rates (ABV - DaunoXome) was (−5%, 18%)

** The hazard ratio (ABV/DaunoXome) for duration of response was 0.80, and the 95% confidence intervals were (0.44, 1.46).

*** The hazard ratio (ABV/DaunoXome) for time to progression was 0.78, and the 95% confidence intervals were (0.57, 1.07).

**** The hazard ratio for mortality (ABV/DaunoXome) was 1.29, and 95% confidence intervals were (0.92, 1.79).

Twenty of the 33 ABV responders responded to therapy by criteria more stringent than flattening of lesions (i.e., shrinkage of lesions and/or reduction in the number of lesions). Eleven of the 27 DaunoXome responders responded to therapy by criteria other than flattening of lesions. Photographic evidence of tumor response to DaunoXome and ABV was comparable across all anatomic sites (e.g., face, oral cavity, trunk, legs, and feet).

INDICATIONS AND USAGE

DaunoXome is indicated as a first line cytotoxic therapy for advanced HIV-associated Kaposi's sarcoma. DaunoXome is not recommended in patients with less than advanced HIV-related Kaposi's sarcoma.

CONTRAINDICATIONS

Therapy with DaunoXome is contraindicated in patients who have experienced a serious hypersensitivity reaction to previous doses of DaunoXome or to any of its constituents.

WARNINGS

DaunoXome is intended for administration under the supervision of a physician who is experienced in the use of cancer chemotherapeutic agents.

The primary toxicity of DaunoXome is myelosuppression, especially of the granulocytic series, which may be severe, and associated with fever and may result in infection. Effects on the platelets and erythroid series are much less marked. Careful hematologic monitoring is required and since patients with HIV infection are immunocompromised, patients must be observed carefully for evidence of intercurrent or opportunistic infections.

Special attention must be given to the potential cardiac toxicity of DaunoXome. Although there is no reliable means of predicting congestive heart failure, cardiomyopathy induced by anthracyclines is usually associated with a decrease of the left ventricular ejection fraction (LVEF). Cardiac function should be evaluated in each patient by means of a history and physical examination before each course of DaunoXome and determination of LVEF should be performed at total cumulative doses of DaunoXome of 320 mg/m^2, and every 160 mg/m^2 thereafter.

Patients who have received prior therapy with anthracyclines (doxorubicin >300 mg/m^2 or equivalent), have pre-existing cardiac disease, or have received previous radiotherapy encompassing the heart may be less "cardiac" tolerant to treatment with DaunoXome. Therefore, monitoring of LVEF at cumulative DaunoXome doses should occur prior to therapy and every 160 mg/m^2 of DaunoXome.

In patients with Kaposi's sarcoma, congestive heart failure has been reported in one patient at a cumulative dose of 340 mg/m^2 of DaunoXome. In eight Kaposi's sarcoma patients, LVEF decreases were reported at cumulative doses ranging from 200 mg/m^2 to 2100 mg/m^2 (median dose 320 mg/m^2) of DaunoXome. In clinical studies in malignancies other than Kaposi's sarcoma and treated with doses of DaunoXome greater than the recommended dose of 40 mg/m^2, congestive heart failure has been reported at a cumulative dose as low as 200 mg/m^2 of DaunoXome; seven patients have been reported with LVEF decreases. The proportion of patients at risk for cardiotoxicity is unknown because the denominator is uncertain since there were several instances of missing repeat cardiac evaluations.

A triad of back pain, flushing, and chest tightness has been reported in 13.8% of the patients (16/116) treated with DaunoXome in the randomized clinical trial and in 2.7% of treatment cycles (27/994). This triad generally occurs during the first five minutes of the infusion, subsides with interruption of the infusion, and generally does not recur if the infusion is then resumed at a slower rate. This combination of symptoms appears to be related to the lipid component of DaunoXome, as a similar set of signs and symptoms has been observed with other liposomal products not containing daunorubicin.

Daunorubicin has been associated with local tissue necrosis at the site of drug extravasation. Although no such local tissue necrosis has been observed with DaunoXome, care should be taken to ensure that there is no extravasation of drug when DaunoXome is administered.

Dosage should be reduced in patients with impaired hepatic function. **(See DOSAGE AND ADMINISTRATION)**

Pregnancy Category D

DaunoXome can cause fetal harm when administered to a pregnant woman. DaunoXome was administered to rats on gestation days 6 through 15 at 0.3, 1.0 or 2.0 mg/kg/day, (about 1/20th, 1/6th, or 1/3rd the recommended human dose on a mg/m2 basis). DaunoXome produced severe maternal toxicity and embryolethality at 2.0 mg/kg/day and was embryotoxic and caused fetal malformations (anophthalmia, microphthalmia, incomplete ossification) at 0.3 mg/kg/day. Embryotoxicity was characterized by increased embryo-fetal deaths, reduced number of litters, and reduced litter sizes.

There are no studies of DaunoXome in pregnant women. If DaunoXome is used during pregnancy, or if the patient becomes pregnant while taking DaunoXome, the patient must be warned of the potential hazard to the fetus. Patients should be advised to avoid becoming pregnant while taking DaunoXome.

PRECAUTIONS

Drug Interactions

In the patient population studied, DaunoXome has been administered to patients receiving a variety of concomitant medications (e.g., antiretroviral agents, antiviral agents, antiinfective agents). Although interactions of DaunoXome with other drugs have not been observed, no systematic studies of interactions have been conducted.

Carcinogenesis, Mutagenesis, and Impairment of Fertility

No carcinogenesis, mutagenesis, or impairment of fertility studies were conducted with DaunoXome.

Carcinogenesis: Carcinogenicity and mutagenicity studies have been conducted with daunorubicin, the active component of DaunoXome. A high incidence of mammary tumors was observed about 120 days after a single intravenous dose of 12.5 mg/kg daunorubicin in rats (about 2 times the human dose on a mg/m^2 basis). Mutagenesis: Daunorubicin was mutagenic in *in vitro* tests (Amest assay, V79 hamster cell assay), and clastogenic in *in vitro* (CCRF-CEM human lymphoblasts) and in *in vivo* (SCE assay in mouse bone marrow) tests. Impairment of Fertility: Daunorubicin intravenous doses of 0.25 mg/kg/day (about 8 times the human dose on a mg/m^2 basis) in male dogs caused testicular atrophy and total aplasia of spermatocytes in the seminiferous tubules.

Pregnancy

Pregnancy "Category D". See Warnings Section.

Pediatric Use

Safety and effectiveness in pediatric patients have not been established.

Use in the Elderly

Safety and effectiveness in the elderly have not been established.

Special Populations

Safety has not been established in patients with pre-existing hepatic or renal dysfunction.

ADVERSE REACTIONS

DaunoXome contains daunorubicin, encapsulated within a liposome. Conventional daunorubicin has acute myelosuppression as its dose limiting side effect, with the greatest effect on the granulocytic series. In addition, daunorubicin causes alopecia, and nausea and vomiting in a significant number of patients treated. Extravasation of conventional daunorubicin can cause severe local tissue necrosis. Chronic therapy at total doses above 300 mg/m^2 causes a cumulative-dose-related cardiomyopathy with congestive heart failure.

Administered as DaunoXome, daunorubicin has substantially altered pharmacokinetics and some differences in toxicity. The most important acute toxicity of DaunoXome remains myelosuppression, principally of the granulocytic series, with much less marked effects on the platelets and erythroid series.

In an open-label, randomized, controlled clinical trial conducted in 13 centers in the U.S.A. and Canada in advanced HIV-related Kaposi's sarcoma, two treatment regimens were compared as first line cytotoxic therapy: DaunoXome and ABV (doxorubicin (Adriamycin®), bleomycin, and vincristine). All drugs were administered intravenously every 2 weeks. The safety data presented below include all reported or observed adverse experiences, including those not considered to be drug related. Patients with advanced HIV-associated Kaposi's sarcoma are seriously ill due to their underlying infection and are receiving several concomitant medications including potentially toxic antiviral and antiretroviral agents. The contribution of the study drugs to the adverse experience profile is therefore difficult to establish.

Table III summarizes the important safety data.

TABLE III
SUMMARY OF IMPORTANT SAFETY DATA

	DaunoXome (N=116) % of patients	ABV (N=111) % of patients
Neutropenia (<1000 cells/mm^3)	36%	35%
Neutropenia (<500 cells/mm^3)	15%	5%
Opportunistic Infections/ Illnesses, % of patients	40%	27%
Median time to first Opportunistic Infections/ Illnesses	214 days	412 days**
Number of cases with absolute reduction in ejection fraction of 20–25%*	3	1
Number of cases removed from therapy due to cardiac causes*	2	0
Alopecia All grades % of patients	8%	36%***
Neuropathy All grades % of patients	13%	41%***

* The denominator is uncertain since there were several instances of missing repeat cardiac evaluations.
** p=0.21
*** p<0.001

A triad of back pain, flushing and chest tightness was reported in 13.8% of the patients (16/116) treated with DaunoXome in the Phase III clinical trial and in 2.7% of treatment cycles (27/994). Most of the episodes were mild to moderate in severity (12% of patients and 2.5% of treatment cycles).

Mild alopecia was reported in 6% of patients treated with DaunoXome and moderate alopecia in 2% of patients. Mild nausea was reported in 35% of DaunoXome patients, moderate nausea in 16% of patients and severe nausea in 3% of patients. For patients treated with DaunoXome, mild vomiting was reported in 10%, moderate in 10%, and severe in 3% of patients. Although grade 3–4 injection site inflammation was reported in 2 patients treated with DaunoXome, no intances of local tissue necrosis were observed with extravasation.

Table IV is a listing of all the mild-moderate and severe adverse events reported on both treatment arms in Protocol 103-09 in ≥ 5% of DaunoXome patients.

TABLE IV
ADVERSE EXPERIENCES: PROTOCOL 103–09

	DaunoXome (N=116)		ABV (N=111)	
	Mild Moderate	Severe	Mild Moderate	Severe
Nausea	51%	3%	45%	5%
Fatigue	43%	6%	44%	7%
Fever	42%	5%	49%	5%
Diarrhea	34%	4%	29%	6%
Cough	26%	2%	19%	0%
Dyspnea	23%	3%	17%	3%
Headache	22%	3%	23%	2%
Allergic Reactions	21%	3%	19%	2%
Abdominal Pain	20%	3%	23%	4%
Anorexia	21%	2%	26%	2%
Vomiting	20%	3%	26%	2%
Rigors	19%	0%	23%	0%
Back Pain	16%	0%	8%	0%
Increased Sweating	12%	2%	12%	0%
Neuropathy	12%	1%	38%	3%
Rhinitis	12%	0%	6%	0%
Edema	9%	2%	8%	1%
Chest Pain	9%	1%	7%	0%
Depression	7%	3%	6%	0%
Malaise	9%	1%	11%	1%
Stomatitis	9%	1%	8%	0%
Alopecia	8%	0%	36%	0%
Dizziness	8%	0%	9%	0%
Sinusitis	8%	0%	5%	1%
Arthralgia	7%	0%	6%	0%
Constipation	7%	0%	18%	0%
Myalgia	7%	0%	12%	0%
Pruritus	7%	0%	14%	0%
Insomnia	6%	0%	14%	0%
Influenza-like symptoms	5%	0%	5%	0%
Tenesmus	4%	1%	1%	0%
Abnormal vision	3%	2%	3%	0%

The following adverse events were reported in ≤ 5% of patients treated with DaunoXome, tabulated by body system.

Body As A Whole: Injection site inflammation

Cardiovascular: Hot flushes, hypertension, palpitation, syncope, tachycardia. In other follow-up clinical trials of DaunoXome used in treatment of Kaposi's sarcoma or other malignancies, the following serious cardiac events were reported: Pericardial effusion, pericardial tamponade, ventricular extrasystoles, cardiac arrest, sinus tachycardia, atrial fibrillation, pulmonary hypertension, myocardial infarction, supraventricular tachycardia, angina pectoris (see **WARNINGS** section)

Digestive: Increased appetite, dysphagia, GI hemorrhage, gastritis, gingival bleeding, hemorrhoids, hepatomegaly, melena, dry mouth, tooth caries

Hemic and Lymphatic: Lymphadenopathy, splenomegaly

Metabolic and Nutritional: Dehydration, thirst

Nervous: Amnesia, anxiety, ataxia, confusion, convulsions, emotional lability, abnormal gait, hallucination, hyperkinesia, hypertonia, meningitis, somnolence, abnormal thinking, tremor

Respiratory: Hemoptysis, hiccups, pulmonary infiltration, increased sputum

Skin: Folliculitis, seborrhea, dry skin

Special Senses: Conjunctivitis, deafness, earache, eye pain, taste perversion, tinnitus

Urogenital: Dysuria, nocturia, polyuria

OVERDOSAGE

The symptoms of acute overdosage are increased severities of the observed dose-limiting toxicities of therapeutic doses of DaunoXome, myelosuppression (especially granulocytopenia), fatigue, and nausea and vomiting.

DOSAGE AND ADMINISTRATION

DaunoXome should be administered intravenously over a 60 minute period at a dose of 40 mg/m^2, with doses repeated every two weeks. Blood counts should be repeated prior to each dose, and therapy withheld if the absolute granulocyte count is less than 750 cells/mm^3. Treatment should be continued until there is evidence of progressive disease (e.g., based on best response achieved: new visceral sites of involvement, or progression of visceral disease; development of 10 or more new, cutaneous lesions or a 25% increase in the number of lesions compared to baseline; a change in the character of 25% or more of all previously counted flat lesions to raised; increase in surface area of the indicator lesions), or until other intercurrent complications of HIV disease preclude continuation of therapy.

Patients with Impaired Hepatic and Renal Function

Limited clinical experience exists in treating hepatically and renally impaired patients with DaunoXome.

Therefore, based on experience with daunorubicin HCl, it is recommended that the dosage of DaunoXome be reduced if the bilirubin or creatinine is elevated as follows: Serum bilirubin 1.2 to 3 mg/dL, give 3/4 the normal dose; serum bilirubin or creatinine > 3 mg/dL, give 1/2 the normal dose.

Do not mix DaunoXome with other drugs.

Preparation Of Solution

DaunoXome should be diluted 1:1 with 5% Dextrose Injection (D5W) before administration. Each vial of DaunoXome contains daunorubicin citrate equivalent to 50 mg daunorubicin base, at a concentration of 2 mg/mL. The recommended concentration after dilution is 1 mg daunorubicin/mL of solution.

Use aseptic technique.

Aseptic technique must be strictly observed in all handling, since no preservative or bacteriostatic agent is present in DaunoXome or in the materials recommended for dilution. Withdraw the calculated volume of DaunoXome from the vial into a sterile syringe, and transfer it into a sterile infusion bag containing an equivalent amount of D5W. Administer diluted DaunoXome immediately. If not used immediately, diluted DaunoXome should be refrigerated at 2°–8°C (36°–46°F). for a maximum of 6 hours.

Caution: The only fluid which may be mixed with DaunoXome is D5W; DaunoXome must not be mixed with saline, bacteriostatic agents such as benzyl alcohol, or any other solution.

Do not use an in-line filter for the intravenous infusion of DaunoXome.

All parenteral drug products should be inspected visually for particulate matter and discoloration prior to administration, whenever solution and container permit. DaunoXome is a translucent dispersion of liposomes that scatters light to some degree. Do not use DaunoXome if it appears opaque, or has precipitate or foreign matter present.

Procedures for proper handling and disposal of anticancer drugs should be followed.[1–7]

HOW SUPPLIED

DaunoXome is a translucent, red, liposomal dispersion supplied in single use vials, each sealed with a synthetic rubber stopper and aluminum sealing ring with a plastic cap. DaunoXome provides daunorubicin citrate equivalent to 50 mg of daunorubicin base, at a concentration of 2 mg/mL. DaunoXome is supplied under NDC 56146-0301-1 for a single unit pack, NDC 56146-0301-4 for a 4-unit pack, and NDC 56146-0301-0 for a 10-unit pack.

Rx only

Storage

Store DaunoXome in a refrigerator, 2°–8°C (36°–46°F).
Do not freeze. Protect from light.

U.S. PATENT NUMBERS

The United States Patent Numbers applicable to DaunoXome are: 5,441,745; 5,435,989; 5,019,369; 4,946,683; 4,753,788; and additional patents pending.

REFERENCES

1. Recommendations for the Safe Handling of Parenteral Antineoplastic Drugs. NIH Publication No. 83-2621. For sale by the Superintendent of Documents, US Government Printing Office, Washington, DC 20402.

Continued on next page

DaunoXome—Cont.

2. AMA Council Report, Guidelines for Handling Parenteral Antineoplastics. JAMA 1985; 253 (11): 1590–1592.
3. National Study Commission on Cytotoxic Exposure—Recommendations for Handling Cytotoxic Agents. Available from Louis P. Jeffrey, Sc.D., Chairman, National Study Commission on Cytotoxic Exposure. Massachusetts College of Pharmacy and Allied Health Sciences, 179 Longwood Avenue, Boston, Massachusetts 02115.
4. Clinical Oncological Society of Australia. Guidelines and Recommendations for Safe Handling of Antineoplastic Agents. Med. J. Australia 1983; 1: 426–428.
5. Jones RB, et al.; Safe Handling of Chemotherapeutic Agents: A report from the Mount Sinai Medical Center. CA-A Cancer Journal for Clinicians 1983; (Sept/Oct) 258–263.
6. American Society of Hospital Pharmacists Technical Assistance Bulletin on Handling Cytotoxic and Hazardous Drugs. Am. J. Hosp. Pharm. 1990; 47: 1033–1049.
7. OSHA Work-Practice Guidelines for Personnel Dealing with Cytotoxic (Antineoplastic) Drugs. Am. J. Hosp. Pharm. 1986; 43: 1193–1204.

Gilead Sciences, Inc.
650 Cliffside Drive • San Dimas, CA 91773 USA

For medical information about DaunoXome (daw-nuh-zome), call 800-403-3945.

Rev. 4/99

VISTIDE® ℞
(cidofovir injection)
FOR INTRAVENOUS INFUSION ONLY.
NOT FOR INTRAOCULAR INJECTION.

WARNING:
RENAL IMPAIRMENT IS THE MAJOR TOXICITY OF VISTIDE. CASES OF ACUTE RENAL FAILURE RESULTING IN DIALYSIS AND/OR CONTRIBUTING TO DEATH HAVE OCCURRED WITH AS FEW AS ONE OR TWO DOSES OF VISTIDE. TO REDUCE POSSIBLE NEPHROTOXICITY, INTRAVENOUS PREHYDRATION WITH NORMAL SALINE AND ADMINISTRATION OF PROBENECID MUST BE USED WITH EACH VISTIDE INFUSION. RENAL FUNCTION (SERUM CREATININE AND URINE PROTEIN) MUST BE MONITORED WITHIN 48 HOURS PRIOR TO EACH DOSE OF VISTIDE AND THE DOSE OF VISTIDE MODIFIED FOR CHANGES IN RENAL FUNCTION AS APPROPRIATE (SEE DOSAGE AND ADMINISTRATION). VISTIDE IS CONTRAINDICATED IN PATIENTS WHO ARE RECEIVING OTHER NEPHROTOXIC AGENTS. NEUTROPENIA HAS BEEN OBSERVED IN ASSOCIATION WITH VISTIDE TREATMENT. THEREFORE, NEUTROPHIL COUNTS SHOULD BE MONITORED DURING VISTIDE THERAPY.
VISTIDE IS INDICATED ONLY FOR THE TREATMENT OF CMV RETINITIS IN PATIENTS WITH ACQUIRED IMMUNODEFICIENCY SYNDROME.
IN ANIMAL STUDIES CIDOFOVIR WAS CARCINOGENIC, TERATOGENIC AND CAUSED HYPOSPERMIA (SEE CARCINOGENESIS, MUTAGENESIS, & IMPAIRMENT OF FERTILITY).

DESCRIPTION
VISTIDE® is the brand name for cidofovir injection. The chemical name of cidofovir is 1-[(*S*)-3-hydroxy-2-(phosphonomethoxy)propyl]cytosine dihydrate (HPMPC), with the molecular formula of $C_8H_{14}N_3O_6P \bullet 2H_2O$ and a molecular weight of 315.22 (279.19 for anhydrous). The chemical structure is:

Cidofovir is a white crystalline powder with an aqueous solubility of ≥170 mg/mL at pH 6-8 and a log P (octanol/aqueous buffer, pH 7.1) value of -3.3.
VISTIDE is a sterile, hypertonic aqueous solution for intravenous infusion only. The solution is clear and colorless. It is supplied in clear glass vials, each containing 375 mg of anhydrous cidofovir in 5 mL aqueous solution at a concentration of 75 mg/mL. The formulation is pH-adjusted to 7.4 with sodium hydroxide and/or hydrochloric acid and contains no preservatives. The appropriate volume of VISTIDE must be removed from the single-use vial and diluted prior to administration (see DOSAGE AND ADMINISTRATION).

Table 2. Cidofovir Pharmacokinetic Parameters Following 3.0 and 5.0 mg/kg Infusions, Without and With Probenecid*

PARAMETERS	VISTIDE ADMINISTERED WITHOUT PROBENECID		VISTIDE ADMINISTERED WITH PROBENECID	
	3 mg/kg (n = 10)	5 mg/kg (n = 2)	3 mg/kg (n = 12)	5 mg/kg (n = 6)
AUC (μg·hr/mL)	20.0 ± 2.3	28.3	25.7 ± 8.5	40.8 ± 9.0
Cmax (end of infusion) (μg/mL)	7.3 ± 1.4	11.5	9.8 ± 3.7	19.6 ± 7.2
Vdss (mL/kg)	537 ± 126 (n = 12)		410 ± 102 (n = 18)	
Clearance (mL/min/1.73 m²)	179 ± 23.1 (n = 12)		148 ± 38.8 (n = 18)	
Renal Clearance (mL/min/1.73 m²)	150 ± 26.9 (n = 12)		98.6 ± 27.9 (n = 11)	

* See DOSAGE AND ADMINISTRATION

MICROBIOLOGY
Mechanism of Action: Cidofovir suppresses cytomegalovirus (CMV) replication by selective inhibition of viral DNA synthesis. Biochemical data support selective inhibition of CMV DNA polymerase by cidofovir diphosphate, the active intracellular metabolite of cidofovir. Cidofovir diphosphate inhibits herpesvirus polymerases at concentrations that are 8- to 600-fold lower than those needed to inhibit human cellular DNA polymerase alpha, beta, and gamma[1,2,3]. Incorporation of cidofovir into the growing viral DNA chain results in reductions in the rate of viral DNA synthesis.
In Vitro Susceptibility: Cidofovir is active *in vitro* against a variety of laboratory and clinical isolates of CMV and other herpesviruses (Table 1). Controlled clinical studies of efficacy have been limited to patients with AIDS and CMV retinitis.

Table 1. Cidofovir Inhibition of Virus Multiplication in Cell Culture

Virus	IC_{50} (μM)
Wild-type CMV Isolates	0.5–2.8
HSV-1, HSV-2	12.7–31.7

Resistance: CMV isolates with reduced susceptibility to cidofovir have been selected *in vitro* in the presence of high concentrations of cidofovir[4]. IC_{50} values for selected resistant isolates ranged from 7–15 μM.
There are insufficient data at this time to assess the frequency or the clinical significance of the development of resistant isolates following VISTIDE administration to patients.
The possibility of viral resistance should be considered for patients who show a poor clinical response or experience recurrent retinitis progression during therapy.
Cross Resistance: Cidofovir-resistant isolates selected *in vitro* following exposure to increasing concentrations of cidofovir were assessed for susceptibility to ganciclovir and foscarnet[4]. All were cross resistant to ganciclovir, but remained susceptible to foscarnet. Ganciclovir- or ganciclovir/foscarnet-resistant isolates that are cross resistant to cidofovir have been obtained from drug naive patients and from patients following ganciclovir or ganciclovir/foscarnet therapy. To date, the majority of ganciclovir-resistant isolates are UL97 gene product (phosphokinase) mutants and remain susceptible to cidofovir[5]. Reduced susceptibility to cidofovir, however, has been reported for DNA polymerase mutants of CMV which are resistant to ganciclovir[6–9]. To date, all clinical isolates which exhibit high level resistance to ganciclovir, due to mutations in both the DNA polymerase and UL97 genes, have been shown to be cross resistant to cidofovir. Cidofovir is active against some, but not all, CMV isolates which are resistant to foscarnet[10–12]. The incidence of foscarnet-resistant isolates that are resistant to cidofovir is not known.
A few triple-drug resistant isolates have been described. Genotypic analysis of two of these triple-resistant isolates revealed several point mutations in the CMV DNA polymerase gene. The clinical significance of the development of these cross-resistant isolates is not known.

CLINICAL PHARMACOLOGY
PHARMACOKINETICS
VISTIDE must be administered with probenecid. The pharmacokinetics of cidofovir, administered both without and with probenecid, are described below.
The pharmacokinetics of cidofovir without probenecid were evaluated in 27 HIV-infected patients with or without asymptomatic CMV infection. Dose-independent pharmacokinetics were demonstrated after one hr infusions of 1.0 (n = 5), 3.0 (n = 10), 5.0 (n = 2) and 10.0 (n = 8) mg/kg (See Table 2 for pharmacokinetic parameters). There was no evidence of cidofovir accumulation after 4 weeks of repeated administration of 3 mg/kg/week (n = 5) without probenecid. In patients with normal renal function, approximately 80 to 100% of the VISTIDE dose was recovered unchanged in urine within 24 hr (n = 27). The renal clearance of cidofovir was greater than creatinine clearance, indicating renal tubular secretion contributes to the elimination of cidofovir.
The pharmacokinetics of cidofovir administered with probenecid were evaluated in 12 HIV-infected patients with or without asymptomatic CMV infection and 10 patients with relapsing CMV retinitis. Dose-independent pharmacokinetics were observed for cidofovir, administered with probenecid, after one hr infusions of 3.0 (n = 12), 5.0 (n = 6), and 7.5 (n = 4) mg/kg (See Table 2). Approximately 70 to 85% of the VISTIDE dose administered with concomitant probenecid was excreted as unchanged drug within 24 hr. When VISTIDE was administered with probenecid, the renal clearance of cidofovir was reduced to a level consistent with creatinine clearance, suggesting that probenecid blocks active renal tubular secretion of cidofovir.
[See table 2 above]
In vitro, cidofovir was less than 6% bound to plasma or serum proteins over the cidofovir concentration range 0.25 to 25 μg/mL. CSF concentrations of cidofovir following intravenous infusion of VISTIDE 5 mg/kg with concomitant probenecid and intravenous hydration were undetectable (< 0.1 μg/mL, assay detection threshold) at 15 minutes after the end of a 1 hr infusion in one patient whose corresponding serum concentration was 8.7 μg/mL.

DRUG-DRUG INTERACTIONS
Zidovudine
The pharmacokinetics of zidovudine were evlaluated in 10 patients receiving zidovudine alone or with intravenous cidofovir (without probenecid). There was no evidence of an effect of cidofovir on the pharmacokinetics of zidovudine.

SPECIAL POPULATIONS
Renal Insufficiency
Pharmacokinetic data collected from subjects with creatinine clearance values as low as 11 mL/min indicate that cidofovir clearance decreases proportionally with creatinine clearance.
High-flux hemodialysis has been shown to reduce the serum levels of cidofovir by approximately 75%.
Initiation of therapy with VISTIDE is contraindicated in patients with serum creatinine > 1.5 mg/dL, a calculated creatinine clearance ≤ 55 mL/min, or a urine protein ≥ 100 mg/dL (equivalent to ≥ 2+ proteinuria) (See CONTRAINDICATIONS).
Geriatric/Gender/Race
The effects of age, gender, and race on cidofovir pharmacokinetics have not been investigated.

INDICATION AND USAGE
VISTIDE is indicated for the treatment of CMV retinitis in patients with acquired immunodeficiency syndrome (AIDS). THE SAFETY AND EFFICACY OF VISTIDE HAVE NOT BEEN ESTABLISHED FOR TREATMENT OF OTHER CMV INFECTIONS (SUCH AS PNEUMONITIS OR GASTROENTERITIS), CONGENITAL OR NEONATAL CMV DISEASE, OR CMV DISEASE IN NON-HIV-INFECTED INDIVIDUALS.

DESCRIPTION OF CLINICAL TRIALS
Three phase II/III controlled trials of VISTIDE have been conducted in HIV-infected patients with CMV retinitis.
Delayed Versus Immediate Therapy (Study 105): In stage 1 of this open-label trial, conducted by the Studies of the Ocular Complications of AIDS (SOCA) Clinical Research Group, 29 previous untreated patients with peripheral CMV retinitis were randomized to either immediate treatment with VISTIDE (5 mg/kg once a week for 2 weeks, then 3 mg/kg every other week) or to have VISTIDE delayed until progression of CMV retinitis[13]. In stage 2 of this trial, an additional 35 previously untreated patients with peripheral CMV retinitis were randomized to either immediate treatment with VISTIDE (5 mg/kg once a week for 2 weeks, then 5 mg/kg every other week), immediate treatment with VISTIDE (5 mg/kg once a week for 2 weeks, then 3 mg/kg every other week), or to have VISTIDE delayed until progression of CMV retinitis. Of the 64 patients in this study, 12 were randomized to 5 mg/kg maintenance therapy, 26 to 3 mg/kg maintenance therapy, and 26 to delayed therapy. Of the 12 patients enrolled in the 5 mg/kg maintenance group, 5 patients progressed, 5 patients discontinued therapy and 2 patients had no progression at study completion. Based on masked readings of retinal photographs, the median [95% confidence interval (CI)] time to retinitis progression was not reached (25, not reached) for the 5 mg/kg maintenance

group. Median (95% CI) time to the alternative endpoint of retinitis progression or study drug discontinuation was 44 days (24, 207) for the 5 mg/kg maintenance group. Patients receiving 5 mg/kg maintenance had delayed time to retinitis progression compared to patients receiving 3 mg/kg maintenance or deferred therapy.

Delayed Versus Immediate Therapy (Study 106): In an open-label trial, 48 previously untreated patients with peripheral CMV retinitis were randomized to either immediate treatment with VISTIDE (5 mg/kg once a week for 2 weeks, then 5 mg/kg every other week), or to have VISTIDE delayed until progression of CMV retinitis[14]. Patient baseline characteristics and disposition are shown in Table 3. Of 25 and 23 patients in the immediate and delayed groups respectively, 23 and 21 were evaluated for retinitis progression as determined by retinal photography. Based on masked readings of retinal photographs, the median [95% confidence interval (CI)] times to retinitis progression were 120 days (40, 134) and 22 days (10, 27) for the immediate and delayed therapy groups, respectively. This difference was statistically significant. However, because of the limited number of patients remaining on treatment over time (3 of 25 patients received VISTIDE for 120 days or longer), the median time to progression for the immediate therapy group was difficult to precisely estimate. Median (95% CI) times to the alternative endpoint of retinitis progression or study discontinuation (including adverse events, withdrawn consent, and systemic CMV disease) were 52 days (37, 85) and 22 days (13, 27) for the immediate and delayed therapy groups, respectively. This difference was statistically significant. Time to progression estimates from this study may not be directly comparable to estimates reported for other therapies.

Table 3. Patient Characteristics and Disposition (Study 106)

	Immediate Therapy (n = 25)	Delayed Therapy (n = 23)
Baseline Characteristics		
Age (years)	38	38
Sex (M/F)	24/1	22/1
Median CD4 Cell Count	6	9
Endpoints		
CMV Retinitis Progression	10	18
Discontinued Due to Adverse Event	6	0
Withdrew Consent	3[a]	1
Discontinued Due to Intercurrent Illness	2[b]	1[b]
Discontinued Based on Ophthalmological Examination	1[c]	1[c]
No Progression at Study Completion	1	0
Not Evaluable at Baseline	2	2

[a] One patient died 2 weeks after withdrawing consent.
[b] Two patients on immediate therapy were diagnosed with CMV disease and discontinued from study. One patient on delayed therapy was diagnosed with CMV gastrointestinal disease.
[c] CMV retinitis progression not confirmed by retinal photography.

Dose-response study of VISTIDE (Study 107): In an open-label trial, 100 patients with relapsing CMV retinitis were randomized to receive 5 mg/kg once a week for 2 weeks and then either 5 mg/kg (n = 49) or 3 mg/kg (n = 51) every other week. Enrolled patients had been diagnosed with CMV retinitis an average of 390 days prior to randomization and had received a median of 3.8 prior courses of systemic CMV therapy. Eighty-four of the 100 patients were considered evaluable for progression by serial retinal photographs (43 randomized to 5 mg/kg and 41 randomized to 3 mg/kg). Twenty-six and 21 patients discontinued therapy due to either an adverse event, intercurrent illness, excluded medication, or withdrawn consent in the 5 mg/kg and 3 mg/kg groups, respectively. Thirty-eight of the 100 randomized patients had progressed according to masked assessment of serial retinal photographs (13 randomized to 5 mg/kg and 25 randomized to 3 mg/kg). Using retinal photographs, the median (95% CI) times to retinitis progression for the 5 mg/kg and 3 mg/kg groups were 115 days (70, not reached) and 49 days (35, 52), respectively. This difference was statistically significant. Similar to Study 106, the median time to retinitis progression for the 5 mg/kg group was difficult to precisely estimate due to the limited number of patients remaining on treatment over time (4 of the 49 patients in the 5 mg/kg group were treated for 115 days or longer). Median 95% CI) times to the alternative endpoint of retinitis progression or study drug discontinuation were 49 days (38, 63) and 35 days (27, 39) for the 5 mg/kg and 3 mg/kg groups, respectively. This difference was statistically significant.

CONTRAINDICATIONS

Initiation of therapy with VISTIDE is contraindicated in patients with a serum creatinine > 1.5 mg/dL, a calculated creatinine clearance ≤ 55 mL/min, or a urine protein ≥ 100 mg/dL (equivalent to ≥ 2+ proteinuria).

VISTIDE is contraindicated in patients receiving agents with nephrotoxic potential. Such agents must be discontinued at least seven days prior to starting therapy with VISTIDE.

VISTIDE is contraindicated in patients with hypersensitivity to cidofovir.

VISTIDE is contraindicated in patients with a history of clinically severe hypersensitivity to probenecid or other sulfa-containing medications.

Direct intraocular injection of VISTIDE is contraindicated; direct injection of cidofovir has been associated with iritis, ocular hypotony, and permanent impairment of vision.

WARNINGS

Nephrotoxicity: Dose-dependent nephrotoxicity is the major dose-limiting toxicity related to VISTIDE administration. Cases of acute renal failure resulting in dialysis and/or contributing to death have occurred with as few as one or two doses of VISTIDE. Renal function (serum creatinine and urine protein) must be monitored within 48 hours prior to each dose of VISTIDE. Dose adjustment or discontinuation is required for changes in renal function (serum creatinine and/or urine protein) while on therapy. Proteinuria, as measured by urinalysis in a clinical laboratory, may be an early indicator of VISTIDE-related nephrotoxicity. Continued administration of VISTIDE may lead to additional proximal tubular cell injury, which may result in glycosuria, decreases in serum phosphate, uric acid, and bicarbonate, elevations in serum creatinine, and/or acute renal failure, in some cases, resulting in the need for dialysis. Patients with these adverse events occurring concurrently and meeting a criteria of Fanconi's syndrome have been reported. Renal function that did not return to baseline after drug discontinuation has been observed in clinical studies of VISTIDE. Intravenous normal saline hydration and oral probenecid must accompany each VISTIDE infusion. Probenecid is known to interact with the metabolism or renal tubular excretion of many drugs (see PRECAUTIONS). The safety of VISTIDE has not been evaluated in patients receiving other known potentially nephrotoxic agents, such as intravenous aminoglycosides (e.g., tobramycin, gentamicin, and amikacin), amphotericin B, foscarnet, intravenous pentamidine, vancomycin, and non-steroidal anti-inflammatory agents (see DOSAGE AND ADMINISTRATION).

Preexisting Renal Impairment: Initiation of therapy with VISTIDE is contraindicated in patients with a baseline serum creatinine > 1.5 mg/dL, a creatinine clearance ≤ 55 mL/min, or a urine protein ≥ 100 mg/dL (equivalent to ≥ 2+ proteinuria).

Hematological Toxicity: Neutropenia may occur during VISTIDE therapy. Neutrophil count should be monitored while receiving VISTIDE therapy.

Decreased Intraocular Pressure/Ocular Hypotony: Decreased intraocular pressure may occur during VISTIDE therapy, and in some instances has been associated with decreased visual acuity. Intraocular pressure should be monitored during VISTIDE therapy.

Metabolic Acidosis: Decreased serum bicarbonate associated with proximal tubule injury and renal wasting syndrome (including Fanconi's syndrome) have been reported in patients receiving VISTIDE (see ADVERSE REACTIONS). Cases of metabolic acidosis in association with liver dysfunction and pancreatitis resulting in death have been reported in patients receiving VISTIDE.

PRECAUTIONS

General

Due to the potential for increased nephrotoxicity, doses greater than the recommended dose must not be administered and the frequency or rate of administration must not be exceeded (see DOSAGE AND ADMINISTRATION).

VISTIDE is formulated for intravenous infusion only and must not be administered by intraocular injection. Administration of VISTIDE by infusion must be accompanied by oral probenecid and intravenous saline prehydration (see DOSAGE AND ADMINISTRATION).

Uveitis/Iritis

Uveitis or iritis was reported in clinical trials and during postmarketing in patients receiving VISTIDE therapy. Treatment with topical corticosteroids with or without topical cycloplegic agents should be considered. Patients should be monitored for signs and symptoms of uveitis/iritis during VISTIDE therapy.

Information for Patients

Patients should be advised that VISTIDE is not a cure for CMV retinitis, and that they may continue to experience progression of retinitis during and following treatment. Patients receiving VISTIDE should be advised to have regular follow-up ophthalmologic examinations. Patients may also experience other manifestations of CMV disease despite VISTIDE therapy.

HIV-infected patients may continue taking antiretroviral therapy, but those taking zidovudine should be advised to temporarily discontinue zidovudine administration or decrease their zidovudine dose by 50%, on days of VISTIDE administration only, because probenecid reduces metabolic clearance of zidovudine.

Patients should be informed on the major toxicity of VISTIDE, namely renal impairment, and that dose modification, including reduction, interruption, and possibly discontinuation, may be required. Close monitoring of renal function (routine urinalysis and serum creatinine) while on therapy should be emphasized.

The importance of completing a full course of probenecid with each VISTIDE dose should be emphasized. Patients should be warned of potential adverse events caused by probenecid (e.g., headache, nausea, vomiting, and hypersensitivity reactions). Hypersensitivity/allergic reactions may include rash, fever, chills and anaphylaxis. Administration of probenecid after a meal or use of antiemetics may decrease the nausea. Prophylatic or therapeutic antihistamines and/or acetaminophen can be used to ameliorate hypersensitivity reactions.

Patients should be advised that cidofovir causes tumors, primarily mammary adenocarcinomas, in rats. VISTIDE should be considered a potential carcinogen in humans (See Carcinogenesis, Mutagenesis, & Impairment of Fertility). Women should be advised of the limited enrollment of women in clinical trials of VISTIDE.

Patients should be advised that VISTIDE caused reduced testes weight and hypospermia in animals. Such changes may occur in humans and cause infertility. Women of childbearing potential should be advised that cidofovir is embryotoxic in animals and should not be used during pregnancy. Women of childbearing potential should be advised to use effective contraception during and for 1 month following treatment with VISTIDE. Men should be advised to practice barrier contraceptive methods during and for 3 months after treatment with VISTIDE.

Drug Interactions

Probenecid: Probenecid is known to interact with the metabolism or renal tubular excretion of many drugs (e.g., acetaminophen, acyclovir, angiotensin-converting enzyme inhibitors, aminosalicylic acid, barbiturates, benzodiazepines, bumetanide, clofibrate, methotrexate, famotidine, furosemide, nonsteroidal anti-inflammatory agents, theophylline, and zidovudine). Concomitant medications should be carefully assessed. Zidovudine should either be temporarily discontinued or decreased by 50% when coadministered with probenecid on the day of VISTIDE infusion.

Nephrotoxic agents: Concomitant administration of VISTIDE and agents with nephrotoxic potential [e.g., intravenous aminoglycosides (e.g., tobramycin, gentamicin, and amikacin), amphotericin B, foscarnet, intravenous pentamidine, vancomycin, and non-steroidal anti-inflammatory agents] is contraindicated. Such agents must be discontinued at least seven days prior to starting therapy with VISTIDE.

Carcinogenesis, Mutagenesis, & Impairment of Fertility

Chronic, two-year carcinogenicity studies in rats and mice have not been carried out to evaluate the carcinogenic potential of cidofovir. However, a 26-week toxicology study evaluating once weekly subscapular subcutaneous injections of cidofovir in rats was terminated at 19 weeks because of the induction, in females, of palpable masses, the first of which was detected after six doses. The masses were diagnosed as mammary adenocarcinomas which developed at doses as low as 0.6 mg/kg/week, equivalent to 0.04 times the human systemic exposure at the recommended intravenous VISTIDE dose based on AUC comparisons.

In a 26-week intravenous toxicology study in which rats received 0.6, 3, or 15 mg/kg cidofovir once weekly, a significant increase in mammary adenocarcinomas in female rats as well as a significant incidence of Zymbal's gland carcinomas in male and female rats were seen at the high dose but not at the lower two doses. The high dose was equivalent to 1.1 times the human systemic exposure at the recommended dose of VISTIDE, based on comparisons of AUC measurements. In light of the results of these studies, cidofovir should be considered to be a carcinogen in rats as well as a potential carcinogen in humans.

Cynomolgus monkeys received intravenous cidofovir, alone and in conjunction with concomitant oral probenecid, intravenously once weekly for 52 weeks at doses resulting in exposures of approximately 0.7 times the human systemic exposure at the recommended dose of VISTIDE. No tumors were detected. However, the study was not designed as a carcinogenicity study due to the small number of animals at each dose and the short duration of treatment.

No mutagenic response was observed in microbial mutagenicity assays involving *Salmonella typhimurium* (Ames) and *Escherichia coli* in the presence and absence of metabolic activation. An increase in micronucleated polychromatic erythrocytes *in vivo* was seen in mice receiving ≥ 2000 mg/kg, a dosage approximately 65-fold higher than the maximum recommended clinical intravenous VISTIDE dose based on body surface area estimations. Cidofovir induced chromosomal aberrations in human peripheral blood lymphocytes *in vitro* without metabolic activation. At the 4 cidofovir levels tested, the percentage of damaged metaphases and number of aberrations per cell increased in a concentration-dependent manner.

Studies showed that cidofovir caused inhibition of spermatogenesis in rats and monkeys. However, no adverse effects on fertility or reproduction were seen following once weekly intravenous injections of cidofovir in male rats for 13 consecutive weeks at doses up to 15 mg/kg/week (equivalent to 1.1 times the recommended human dose based on AUC comparisons). Female rats dosed intravenously once weekly at 1.2 mg/kg/week (equivalent to 0.09 times the recommended human dose based on AUC) or higher, for up to 6 weeks prior to mating and for 2 weeks post mating had decreased litter sizes and live births per litter and increased early resorptions per litter. Peri- and post-natal development studies in which female rats received subcutaneous injections of cidofovir once daily at doses up to 1.0 mg/kg/day from day 7 of gestation through day 21 postpartum (approximately 5 weeks) resulted in no adverse effects on viability, growth, behavior, sexual maturation or reproductive capacity in the offspring.

Continued on next page

Vistide—Cont.

Pregnancy: Category C
Cidofovir was embryotoxic (reduced fetal body weights) in rats at 1.5 mg/kg/day and in rabbits at 1.0 mg/kg/day, doses which were also maternally toxic, following daily intravenous dosing during the period of organogenesis. The no-observable-effect levels for embryotoxicity in rats (0.5 mg/kg/day) and in rabbits (0.25 mg/kg/day) were approximately 0.04 and 0.05 times the clinical dose (5 mg/kg every other week) based on AUC, respectively. An increased incidence of fetal external, soft tissue and skeletal anomalies (meningocele, short snout, and short maxillary bones) occurred in rabbits at the high dose (1.0 mg/kg/day) which was also maternally toxic. There are no adequate and well-controlled studies in pregnant women. VISTIDE should be used during pregnancy only if the potential benefit justifies the potential risk to the fetus.

Nursing Mothers
It is not known whether cidofovir is excreted in human milk. Since many drugs are excreted in human milk and because of the potential for adverse reactions as well as the potential for tumorigenicity shown for cidofovir in animal studies, VISTIDE should not be administered to nursing mothers. The U.S. Public Health Service Centers for Disease Control and Prevention advises HIV-infected women not to breastfeed to avoid postnatal transmission of HIV to a child who may not yet be infected.

Pediatric Use
Safety and effectiveness in children have not been studied. The use of VISTIDE in children with AIDS warrants extreme caution due to the risk of long-term carcinogenicity and reproductive toxicity. Administration of VISTIDE to children should be undertaken only after careful evaluation and only if the potential benefits of treatment outweigh the risks.

Geriatric Use
No studies of the safety or efficacy of VISTIDE in patients over the age of 60 have been conducted. Since elderly individuals frequently have reduced glomerular filtration, particular attention should be paid to assessing renal function before and during VISTIDE administration (see DOSAGE AND ADMINISTRATION).

ADVERSE REACTIONS

1. ***Nephrotoxicity***: Renal toxicity, as manifested by ≥ 2+ proteinuria, serum creatinine elevations of ≥ 0.4 mg/dL, or decreased creatinine clearance ≤ 55 mL/min, occurred in 79 of 135 (59%) patients receiving VISTIDE at a maintenance dose of 5 mg/kg every other week. Maintenance dose reductions from 5 mg/kg to 3 mg/kg due to proteinuria or serum creatinine elevations were made in 12 to 41 (29%) patients who had not received prior therapy for CMV retinitis (Study 106) and in 19 of 74 (26%) patients who had received prior therapy for CMV retinitis (Study 107). Prior foscarnet use has been associated with an increased risk of nephrotoxicity; therefore, such patients must be monitored closely (see CONTRAINDICATIONS, WARNINGS, DOSAGE AND ADMINISTRATION).
2. ***Neutropenia***: In clinical trials, at the 5 mg/kg maintenance dose, a decrease in absolute neutrophil count to ≤ 500 cells/mm^3 occurred in 24% of patients. Granulocyte colony stimulating factor (GCSF) was used in 39% of patients.
3. ***Decreased Intraocular Pressure/Ocular Hypotony***: Among the subset of patients monitored for intraocular pressure changes, a ≥ 50% decrease from baseline intraocular pressure was reported in 17 of 70 (24%) patients at the 5 mg/kg maintenance dose. Severe hypotony (intraocular pressure of 0–1 mm Hg) has been reported in 3 patients. Risk of ocular hypotony may be increased in patients with preexisting diabetes mellitus.
4. ***Anterior Uveitis/Iritis***: Uveitis or iritis has been reported in clinical trials and during postmarketing in patients receiving VISTIDE therapy. Uveitis or iritis was reported in 15 of 135 (11%) patients receiving 5 mg/kg maintenance dosing. Treatment with topical corticosteroids with or without topical cycloplegic agents may be considered. Patients should be monitored for signs and symptoms of uveitis/iritis during VISTIDE therapy.
5. ***Metabolic Acidosis***: A diagnosis of Fanconi's syndrome, as manifested by multiple abnormalities of proximal renal tubular function, was reported in 1% of patients. Decreases in serum bicarbonate to ≤ 16 mEq/L occurred in 16% of cidofovir-treated patients. Cases of metabolic acidosis in association with liver dysfunction and pancreatitis resulting in death have been reported in patients receiving VISTIDE.

In clinical trials, VISTIDE was withdrawn due to adverse events in approximately 39% of patients treated with 5 mg/kg every other week as maintenance therapy.
The incidence of adverse reactions reported as serious in three controlled clinical studies in patients with CMV retinitis, regardless of presumed relationship to drug, is listed in Table 4.

Table 4. Serious Clinical Adverse Events or Laboratory Abnormalities Occurring in >5% of Patients

	N = 135[a] # patients	(%)
Proteinuria (≥100 mg/dL)	68	(50)
Neutropenia (≤500 cells/mm^3)	33	(24)
Decreased Intraocular Pressure[b]	17	(24)
Decreased Serum Bicarbonate (≤16 mEq/L)	21	(16)
Fever	19	(14)
Infection	16	(12)
Creatinine Elevation (≥2.0 mg/dL)	16	(12)
Pneumonia	12	(9)
Dyspnea	11	(8)
Nausea with Vomiting	10	(7)

[a] Patients receiving 5 mg/kg maintenance regimen in Studies 105, 106 and 107.
[b] Defined as decreased intraocular pressure (IOP) to ≤ 50% that at baseline. Based on 70 patients receiving 5 mg/kg maintenance dosing (Studies 105, 106 and 107), for whom baseline and follow-up IOP determinations were recorded.

The most frequently reported adverse events regardless of relationship to study drugs (cidofovir or probenecid) or severity are shown in Table 5.
The following additional list of adverse events/intercurrent illnesses have been observed in clinical studies of VISTIDE and are listed below regardless of causal relationship to VISTIDE. Evaluation of these reports was difficult because of the diverse manifestations of the underlying disease and because most patients received numerous concomitant medicines.
Body as a Whole: abdominal pain, accidental injury, AIDS, allergic reaction, back pain, catheter blocked, cellulitis, chest pain, chills and fever, cryptococcosis, cyst, death, face edema, flu-like syndrome, hypothermia, injection site reaction, malaise, mucous membrane disorder, neck pain, overdose, photosensitivity reaction, sarcoma, sepsis
Cardiovascular System: cardiomyopathy, cardiovascular disorder, congestive heart failure, hypertension, hypotension, migraine, pallor, peripheral vascular disorder, phlebitis, postural hypotension, shock, syncope, tachycardia, vascular disorder, edema
Digestive System: cholangitis, colitis, constipation, esophagitis, dyspepsia, dysphagia, fecal incontinence, flatulence, gastritis, gastrointestinal hemorrhage, gingivitis, hepatitis, hepatomegaly, hepatosplenomegaly, jaundice, abnormal liver function, liver damage, liver necrosis, melena, pancreatitis, proctitis, rectal disorder, stomatitis, aphthous stomatitis, tongue discoloration, mouth ulceration, tooth caries
Endocrine System: adrenal cortex insufficiency
Hemic & Lymphatic System: hypochromic anemia, leukocytosis, leukopenia, lymphadenopathy, lymphoma like reaction, pancytopenia, splenic disorder, splenomegaly, thrombocytopenia, thrombocytopenic purpura
Metabolic & Nutritional System: cachexia, dehydration, edema, hypercalcemia, hyperglycemia, hyperkalemia, hyperlipemia, hypocalcemia, hypoglycemia, hypoglycemic reaction, hypokalemia, hypomagnesemia, hyponatremia, hypophosphatemia, hypoproteinemia, increased alkaline phosphatase, increased BUN, increased lactic dehydrogenase, increased SGOT, increased SGPT, peripheral edema, respiratory alkalosis, thirst, weight loss, weight gain
Musculoskeletal System: arthralgia, arthrosis, bone necrosis, bone pain, joint disorder, leg cramps, myalgia, myasthenia, pathological fracture
Nervous System: abnorml dreams, abnormal gait, acute brain syndrome, agitation, amnesia, anxiety, ataxia, cerebrovascular disorder, confusion, convulsion, delirium, dementia, depression, dizziness, drug dependence, dry mouth, encephalopathy, facial paralysis, hallucinations, hemiplegia, hyperesthesia, hypertonia, hypotony, incoordination, increased libido, insomnia, myoclonus, nervousness, neuropathy, paresthesia, personality disorder, somnolence, speech disorder, tremor, twitching, vasodilation, vertigo
Respiratory System: asthma, bronchitis, epistaxis, hemoptysis, hiccup, hyperventilation, hypoxia, increased sputum, larynx edema, lung disorder, pharyngitis, pneumothorax, rhinitis, sinusitis
Skin & Appendages: acne, angioedema, dry skin, eczema, exfoliative dermatitis, furunculosis, herpes simplex, nail disorder, pruritus, rash, seborrhea, skin discoloration, skin disorder, skin hypertorphy, skin ulcer, sweating, urticaria
Special Senses: abnormal vision, amblyopia, blindness, cataract, conjunctivitis, corneal lesion, corneal opacity, diplopia, dry eyes, ear disorder, ear pain, eye disorder, eye pain, hyperacusis, iritis, keratitis, miosis, otitis externa, otitis media, refraction disorder, retinal detachment, retinal disorder, taste perversion, tinnitus, uveitis, visual field defect, hearing loss
Urogenital System: decreased creatinine clearance, dysuria, glycosuria, hematuria, kidney stone, mastitis, metorrhagia, nocturia, polyuria, prostatic disorder, toxic nephropathy, urethritis, urinary casts, urinary incontinence, urinary retention, urinary tract infection

Table 5. All Clinical Adverse Events, Laboratory Abnormalities or Intercurrent Illnesses Regardless of Severity Occurring in >15% of Patients

	N = 115[a] # patients	(%)
Any Adverse Event	115	(100)
Proteinuria (≥ 30 mg/dL)	101	(88)
Nausea +/− Vomiting	79	(69)
Fever	67	(58)
Neutropenia (<750 cells/mm^3)	50	(43)
Asthenia	50	(43)
Headache	34	(30)
Rash	34	(30)
Infection	32	(28)
Alopecia	31	(27)
Diarrhea	30	(26)
Pain	29	(25)
Creatinine Elevation (>1.5 mg/dL)	28	(24)
Anemia	28	(24)
Anorexia	26	(23)
Dyspnea	26	(23)
Chills	25	(22)
Increased Cough	22	(19)
Oral Moniliasis	21	(18)

[a] Patients receiving 5 mg/kg maintenance regimen in Studies 106 and 107.

Reporting of Adverse Reactions
Malignancies or serious adverse reactions that occur in patients who have received VISTIDE should be reported to Gilead in writing to the Director of Clinical Research, Gilead Sciences, Inc., 333 Lakeside Drive, Foster City, CA 94404 or by calling 1-800-GILEAD-5 (445-3235), or to FDA MedWatch 1-800-FDA-1088/fax 1-800-FDA-0178.

OVERDOSAGE

Two cases of cidofovir overdose have been reported. These patients received single doses of VISTIDE at 16.3 mg/kg and 17.4 mg/kg, respectively, with concomitant oral probenecid and intravenous hydration. In both cases, the patients were hospitalized and received oral probenecid (one gram three times daily) and vigorous intravenous hydration with normal saline for 3 to 5 days. Significant changes in renal function were not observed in either patient.

DOSAGE AND ADMINISTRATION

VISTIDE MUST NOT BE ADMINISTERED BY INTRAOCULAR INJECTION.

Dosage
THE RECOMMENDED DOSAGE, FREQUENCY, OR INFUSION RATE MUST NOT BE EXCEEDED. VISTIDE MUST BE DILUTED IN 100 MILLILITERS 0.9% (NORMAL) SALINE PRIOR TO ADMINISTRATION. TO MINIMIZE POTENTIAL NEPHROTOXICITY, PROBENECID AND INTRAVENOUS SALINE PREHYDRATION MUST BE ADMINISTERED WITH EACH VISTIDE INFUSION.

Induction Treatment The recommended induction dose of VISTIDE for patients with a serum creatinine of ≤ 1.5 mg/dL, a calculated creatinine clearance > 55 mL/min, and a urine protein < 100 mg/dL (equivalent to < 2+ proteinuria) is 5 mg/kg body weight (given as an intravenous infusion at a constant rate over 1 hr) administered once weekly for two consecutive weeks. Because serum creatinine in patients with advanced AIDS and CMV retinitis may not provide a complete picture of the patient's underlying renal status, it is important to utilize the Cockcroft-Gault formula to more precisely estimate creatinine clearance (CrCl). As creatinine clearance is dependent on serum creatinine and patient weight, it is necessary to calculate clearance prior to initiation of VISTIDE CrCl (mL/min) should be calculated according to the following formula:
[See formula at left]

$$\text{Creatinine clearance for males} = \frac{[140\text{-age (years)}] \times [\text{body wt (kg)}]}{72 \times [\text{serum creatinine (mg/dL)}]}$$

$$\text{Creatinine clearance for females} = \frac{[140\text{-age (years)}] \times [\text{body wt (kg)}] \times 0.85}{72 \times [\text{serum creatinine (mg/dL)}]}$$

Maintenance Treatment The recommended maintenance dose of VISTIDE is 5 mg/kg body weight (given as an intravenous infusion at a constant rate over 1 hr), administered once every 2 weeks.

Dose Adjustment

Changes in Renal Function during VISTIDE Therapy: The maintenance dose of VISTIDE must be reduced from 5 mg/kg to 3 mg/kg for an increase in serum creatinine of 0.3–0.4 mg/dL above baseline. VISTIDE therapy must be discontinued for an increase in serum creatinine of ≥ 0.5 mg/dL above baseline or development of ≥ 3+ proteinuria.

Preexisting Renal Impairment: VISTIDE is contraindicated in patients with a serum creatinine concentration > 1.5 mg/dL, a calculated creatinine clearance ≤ 55 mL/min, or a urine protein ≥ 100 mg/dL (equivalent to ≥ 2+ proteinuria).

Probenecid Probenecid must be administered orally with each VISTIDE dose. Two grams must be administered 3 hr prior to the VISTIDE dose and one gram administered at 2 and again at 8 hr after completion of the 1 hr VISTIDE infusion (for a total of 4 grams).

Ingestion of food prior to each dose of probenecid may reduce drug-related nausea and vomiting. Administration of an antiemetic may reduce the potential for nausea associated with probenecid ingestion. In patients who develop allergic or hypersensitivity symptoms to probenecid, the use of an appropriate prophylactic or therapeutic antihistamine and/or acetaminophen should be considered (see CONTRAINDICATIONS).

Hydration Patients must receive at least one liter of 0.9% (normal) saline solution intravenously with each infusion of VISTIDE. The saline solution should be infused over a 1–2 hr period immediately before the VISTIDE infusion. Patients who can tolerate the additional fluid load should receive a second liter. If administered, the second liter of saline should be initiated either at the start of the VISTIDE infusion or immediately afterwards, and infused over a 1 to 3 hr period.

Method of Preparation and Administration

Inspect vial visually for particulate matter and discoloration prior to administration. If particulate matter or discoloration is observed, the vial should not be used. With a syringe, extract the appropriate volume of VISTIDE from the vial and transfer the dose to an infusion bag containing 100 mL 0.9% (normal) saline solution. Infuse the entire volume intravenously into the patient at a constant rate over a 1 hr period. Use of a standard infusion pump for administration is recommended.

It is recommended that VISTIDE infusion admixtures be administered within 24 hr of preparation and that refrigerator or freezer storage not be used to extend this 24 hr limit. If admixtures are not intended for immediate use, they may be stored under refrigeration (2–8°C) for no more than 24 hr. Refrigerate admixtures should be allowed to equilibrate to room temperature prior to use.

The chemical stability of VISTIDE admixtures was demonstrated in polyvinyl chloride composition and ethylene/propylene copolymer composition commercial infusion bags, and in glass bottles. **No data are available to support the addition of other drugs or supplements to the cidofovir admixture for concurrent administration.**

VISTIDE is supplied in single-use vials. Partially used vials should be discarded (see Handling and Disposal).

Compatibility with Ringer's solution, Lactated Ringer's solution or bacteriostatic infusion fluids has not been evaluated.

Handling and Disposal

Due to mutagenic properties of cidofovir, adequate precautions including the use of appropriate safety equipment are recommended for the preparation, administration, and disposal of VISTIDE. The National Institutes of Health presently recommends that such agents be prepared in a Class II laminar flow biological safety cabinet and that personnel preparing drugs of this class wear surgical gloves and a closed front surgical-type gown with knit cuffs. If VISTIDE contacts the skin, wash membranes and flush thoroughly with water. Excess VISTIDE and all other materials used in the admixture preparation and administration should be placed in a leak-proof, puncture-proof container. The recommended method of disposal is high temperature incineration.

Patient Monitoring

Serum creatinine and urine protein must be monitored within 48 hours prior to each dose. White blood cell counts with differential should be monitored prior to each dose. In patients with proteinuria, intravenous hydration should be administered and the test repeated. Intraocular pressure, visual acuity and ocular symptoms should be monitored periodically.

HOW SUPPLIED

VISTIDE (cidofovir injection) 75 mg/mL for intravenous infusion, is supplied as a non-preserved solution in single-use clear glass vials as follows:

NDC 61958-0101-1 375 mg in a 5 mL vial in a single-unit carton

VISTIDE should be stored at controlled room temperature 20°–25°C (68°–77°F).

CAUTION: Federal law prohibits dispensing without prescription.

Manufactured by:
Ben Venue Laboratories, Inc.
Bedford, OH 44146-0568

Manufactured for and distributed by:
Gilead Sciences, Inc.
333 Lakeside Drive
Foster City, CA 94404

VISTIDE® (cidofovir injection) is covered by U.S. Patent No. 5,142,051 and its foreign counterparts. Other patents pending.

REFERENCES

1. Ho HT, Woods KL, Bronson JJ, De Boeck H, Martin JC and Hitchcock MJM. Intracellular Metabolism of the Antiherpervirus Agent (S)-1-[3-hydroxy-2-(phosphonylmethoxy)propyl]cytosine. *Mol Pharmacol*, **41**:197-202, 1992.
2. Cherrington JM, Allen SJW, McKee BH, and Chen MS. Kinetic Analysis of the Interaction Between the Diphosphate of (S)-1-(3-hydroxy-2-phosphonylmethoxypropyl) cystosine, zalcibatine TP, zidovudineTP, and FIAUTP with Human DNA Polymerases b and g. *Biochem Pharmacol*, **48**:1986-1988, 1994.
3. Xiong X, Smith JL, Kim C, Huang E, and Chen MS. Kinetic Analysis of the Interaction of Cidofovir Diphosphate with Human Cytomegalovirus DNA Polymerase. *Biochem Pharmacol*, **51**:1563-1567, 1996.
4. Cherrington JM, Mulato AS, Fuller MD, Chen MS. *In Vitro* Selection of a Human Cytomegalovirus (HCMV) that is Resistant to Cidofovir. 35th International Conference on Antimicrobial Agents and Chemotherapy (ICAAC), San Francisco, CA. Abstract H117, 1995.
5. Stanat SC, Reardon JE, Erice A, Jordan MC, Drew WL, and Biron KK. Ganciclovir-Resistant Cytomegalovirus Clinical Isolates: Mode of Resistance to Ganciclovir. *Antimicrob Agents Chemother*, **35**:2191-2197, 1991.
6. Sullivan V, Biron KK, Talarico C, Stanat SC, Davis M, Pozzi M, and Coen DM. A Point Mutation in the Human Cytomegalovirus DNA Polymerase Gene Confers Resistance to Ganciclovir and phosphonylmethoxyalkyl Derivatives. *Antimicrob Agents Chemother*, **37**:19-25, 1993.
7. Tatarowicz WA, Lurain NS, and Thompson KD. A Ganciclovir-Resistant Clinical Isolate of Human Cytomegalovirus Exhibiting Cross-Resistance to other DNA Polymerase Inhibitors. *J Infect Dis*, **166**:904-907, 1992.
8. Lurain NS, Thompson KD, Holmes EW, and Read GS. Point Mutations in the DNA Polymerase Gene of Human Cytomegalovirus that Result in Resistance to Antiviral Agents. *J Virol*, **66**:7146-7152, 1992.
9. Smith IL, Cherrington JM, Jiles RE, Fuller MD, Freeman WR, Spector SA. High-level Resistance of Cytomegalovirus to Ganciclovir is Associated with Alterations in both the UL97 and DNA Polymerase Genes. *J Infect Dis* **176**:69-77, 1997.
10. Sullivan V and Coen DM. Isolation of Foscarnet-Resistant Human Cytomegalovirus Patterns of Resistance and Sensitivity to Other Antiviral Drugs. *J Infect Dis*, **164**:781-784, 1991.
11. Snoeck R, Andrei G, and De Clercq E. Patterns of Resistance and Sensitivity to Antiviral Compounds of Drug-Resistant Strains of Human Cytomegalovirus Selected *in Vitro*. *Eur J Clin Microbiol Infect Dis* **15**:574-579, 1996.
12. Baldanti F, Underwood MR, Stanat SC, Biron KK, Chou S, Sarasini A, Silini E, and Gerna G. Single Amino Acid Changes in the DNA Polymerase Confer Foscarnet Resistance and Slow-Growth Phenotype, White Mutations in the UL-97-Encoded Phosphotransferase Confer Ganciclovir Resistance in Three Double-Resistant Human Cytomegalovirus Strains Recovered from Patients with AIDS. *J Virol*, **70**:1390-1395, 1996.
13. The Studies of Ocular Complications of AIDS Research Group in Collaboration with the AIDS Clinical Trials Group. Cidofovir (HPMPC) for the Treatment of Cytomegalovirus Retinitis in Patients with AIDS: the HPMPC Peripheral Cytomegalovirus Retinitis Trial. *Ann Intern Med* **126**:264-274, 1997.
14. Lalezari JP, Stagg RJ, Kupperman BD, et al. Intravenous Cidofovir for Peripheral Cytomegalovirus Retinitis in Patients with AIDS. A Randomized, Controlled Trial. *Ann Intern Med* **126**:257-263, 1997.

Part Number: RM-1176 March 1999

Glaxo Wellcome Inc.

FIVE MOORE DRIVE
RESEARCH TRIANGLE PARK, NC 27709

For Medical Information for Healthcare Professionals Contact:
1-888-825-5249

In Emergencies:
Medical Information: 1-800-334-0089

For Consumer inquiries Contact:
1-888-825-5249

ACLOVATE® ℞

[*a'klō-vāt''*]

(alclometasone dipropionate cream)
Cream, 0.05%

ACLOVATE® ℞

(alclometasone dipropionate ointment)
Ointment, 0.05%

For Dermatologic Use Only—
Not for Ophthalmic Use.

DESCRIPTION

ACLOVATE Cream and Ointment contain alclometasone dipropionate (7α-chloro- 11β,17,21-trihydroxy -16α- methylpregna-1,4-diene-3,20-dione 17,21-dipropionate), a synthetic corticosteroid for topical dermatologic use. The corticosteroids constitute a class of primarily synthetic steroids used topically as anti-inflammatory and antipruritic agents. Chemically, alclometasone dipropionate is $C_{28}H_{37}ClO_7$.

Alclometasone dipropionate has the molecular weight of 521. It is a white powder, insoluble in water, slightly soluble in propylene glycol, and moderately soluble in hexylene glycol.

Each gram of ACLOVATE Cream contains 0.5 mg of alclometasone dipropionate in a hydrophilic, emollient cream base of propylene glycol, white petrolatum, cetearyl alcohol, glyceryl stearate, PEG 100 stearate, Ceteth-20, monobasic sodium phosphate, chlorocresol, phosphoric acid, and purified water.

Each gram of ACLOVATE Ointment contains 0.5 mg of alclometasone dipropionate in an ointment base of hexylene glycol, white wax, propylene glycol stearate, and white petrolatum.

CLINICAL PHARMACOLOGY

Like other topical corticosteroids, alclometasone dipropionate has anti-inflammatory, antipruritic, and vasoconstrictive properties. The mechanism of the anti-inflammatory activity of the topical steroids, in general, is unclear. However, corticosteroids are thought to act by the induction of phospholipase A_2 inhibitory proteins, collectively called lipocortins. It is postulated that these proteins control the biosynthesis of potent mediators of inflammation such as prostaglandins and leukotrienes by inhibiting the release of their common precursor, arachidonic acid. Arachidonic acid is released from membrane phospholipids by phospholipase A_2.

Pharmacokinetics: The extent of percutaneous absorption of topical corticosteroids is determined by many factors, including the vehicle and the integrity of the epidermal barrier. Occlusive dressings with hydrocortisone for up to 24 hours have not been demonstrated to increase penetration; however, occlusion of hydrocortisone for 96 hours markedly enhances penetration. Topical corticosteroids can be absorbed from normal intact skin. Inflammation and/or other disease processes in the skin may increase percutaneous absorption. A study utilizing a radiolabeled alclometasone dipropionate ointment formulation was performed to measure systemic absorption and excretion. Results indicated that approximately 3% of the steroid was absorbed during 8 hours of contact with intact skin of normal volunteers.

Studies performed with ACLOVATE Cream and Ointment indicate that these products are in the low to medium range of potency as compared with other topical corticosteroids.

INDICATIONS AND USAGE

ACLOVATE Cream and Ointment are low to medium potency corticosteroids indicated for the relief of the inflammatory and pruritic manifestations of corticosteroid-responsive dermatoses. ACLOVATE Cream and Ointment may be used in pediatric patients 1 year of age or older, although the safety and efficacy of drug use for longer than 3 weeks have not been established (see PRECAUTIONS: Pediatric Use). Since the safety and efficacy of ACLOVATE Cream and Ointment have not been established in pediatric patients below 1 year of age, their use in this age-group is not recommended.

CONTRAINDICATIONS

ACLOVATE Cream and Ointment are contraindicated in those patients with a history of hypersensitivity to any of the components in these preparations.

PRECAUTIONS

General: Systemic absorption of topical corticosteroids can produce reversible hypothalamic-pituitary-adrenal (HPA) axis suppression with the potential for glucocorticosteroid insufficiency after withdrawal of treatment. Manifestations of Cushing's syndrome, hyperglycemia, and glucosuria can also be produced in some patients by systemic absorption of topical corticosteroids while on treatment.

Patients applying a topical steroid to a large surface area or to areas under occlusion should be evaluated periodically for evidence of HPA axis suppression. This may be done by using the ACTH stimulation, A.M. plasma cortisol, and urinary free cortisol tests.

The effects of ACLOVATE Cream and Ointment on the HPA axis have been evaluated. In one study, ACLOVATE Cream and Ointment were applied to 30% of the body twice daily for 7 days, and occlusive dressings were used in selected patients either 12 hours or 24 hours daily. In another study, ACLOVATE Cream was applied to 80% of the body surface of normal subjects twice daily for 21 days with daily 12-hour periods of whole body occlusion. Average plasma and urinary free cortisol levels and urinary levels of 17-hydroxysteroids were decreased (about 10%), suggesting suppression of the HPA axis under these conditions. Plasma cortisol

Continued on next page

This product information is based on labeling in effect on June 23, 2000. For further information, contact via direct mail, phone, or web site. Medical Information, Glaxo Wellcome Inc., PO Box 13398, Research Triangle Park, NC 27709. Healthcare Professionals (Medical Information): 800-334-0089. Patients (Customer Response Center): 1-888-825-5249. Glaxo Wellcome Corporate Web Site: www.glaxowellcome.com

Aclovate—Cont.

levels have also been demonstrated to decrease in pediatric patients treated twice daily for 3 weeks without occlusion. If HPA axis suppression is noted, an attempt should be made to withdraw the drug, to reduce the frequency of application, or to substitute a less potent corticosteroid. Recovery of HPA axis function is generally prompt upon discontinuation of topical corticosteroids. Infrequently, signs and symptoms of glucocorticosteroid insufficiency may occur, requiring supplemental systemic corticosteroids. For information on systemic supplementation, see prescribing information for those products.

Pediatric patients may be more susceptible to systemic toxicity from equivalent doses due to their larger skin surface area to body mass ratios (see PRECAUTIONS: Pediatric Use).

If irritation develops, ACLOVATE Cream or Ointment should be discontinued and appropriate therapy instituted. Allergic contact dermatitis with corticosteroids is usually diagnosed by observing *a failure to heal* rather than noting a clinical exacerbation, as with most topical products not containing corticosteroids. Such an observation should be corroborated with appropriate diagnostic patch testing.

If concomitant skin infections are present or develop, an appropriate antifungal or antibacterial agent should be used. If a favorable response does not occur promptly, use of ACLOVATE Cream or Ointment should be discontinued until the infection has been adequately controlled.

Information for Patients: Patients using topical corticosteroids should receive the following information and instructions:

1. This medication is to be used as directed by the physician. It is for external use only. Avoid contact with the eyes.
2. This medication should not be used for any disorder other than that for which it was prescribed.
3. The treated skin area should not be bandaged, otherwise covered or wrapped so as to be occlusive, unless directed by the physician.
4. Patients should report to their physician any signs of local adverse reactions.
5. Parents of pediatric patients should be advised not to use ACLOVATE Cream or Ointment in the treatment of diaper dermatitis. ACLOVATE Cream or Ointment should not be applied in the diaper area as diapers or plastic pants may constitute occlusive dressing (see DOSAGE AND ADMINISTRATION).
6. This medication should not be used on the face, underarms, or groin areas unless directed by the physician.
7. As with other corticosteroids, therapy should be discontinued when control is achieved. If no improvement is seen within 2 weeks, contact the physician.

Laboratory Tests: The following tests may be helpful in evaluating patients for HPA axis suppression:

ACTH stimulation test
A.M. plasma cortisol test
Urinary free cortisol test

Carcinogenesis, Mutagenesis, Impairment of Fertility: Long-term animal studies have not been performed to evaluate the carcinogenic potential or the effect on fertility of topical corticosteroids.

Pregnancy: *Teratogenic Effects: Pregnancy Category C*: Corticosteroids have been shown to be teratogenic in laboratory animals when administered systemically at relatively low dosage levels. Some corticosteroids have been shown to be teratogenic after dermal application in laboratory animals. There are no adequate and well-controlled studies in pregnant women. ACLOVATE Cream or Ointment should be used during pregnancy only if the potential benefit justifies the potential risk to the fetus.

Nursing Mothers: Systemically administered corticosteroids appear in human milk and could suppress growth, interfere with endogenous corticosteroid production, or cause other untoward effects. It is not known whether topical administration of topical corticosteroids could result in sufficient systemic absorption to produce detectable quantities in human milk. Because many drugs are excreted in human milk, caution should be exercised when ACLOVATE Cream or Ointment is administered to a nursing woman.

Pediatric Use: ACLOVATE Cream and Ointment may be used with caution in pediatric patients 1 year of age or older, although the safety and efficacy of drug use for longer than 3 weeks have not been established. Use of ACLOVATE Cream and Ointment is supported by results from adequate and well-controlled studies in pediatric patients with corticosteroid-responsive dermatoses. Since the safety and efficacy of ACLOVATE Cream and Ointment have not been established in pediatric patients below 1 year of age, its use in this age-group is not recommended. Because of a higher ratio of skin surface area to body mass, pediatric patients are at a greater risk than adults of HPA axis suppression and Cushing's syndrome when they are treated with topical corticosteroids. They are therefore also at greater risk of adrenal insufficiency during and/or after withdrawal of treatment. Adverse effects, including striae, have been reported with inappropriate use of topical corticosteroids in infants and children. Pediatric patients applying ACLOVATE Cream or Ointment to >20% of the body surface area are at higher risk for HPA axis suppression.

HPA axis suppression, Cushing's syndrome, linear growth retardation, delayed weight gain, and intracranial hypertension have been reported in pediatric patients receiving topical corticosteroids. Manifestations of adrenal suppression in pediatric patients include low plasma cortisol levels and absence of response to ACTH stimulation. Manifestations of intracranial hypertension include bulging fontanelles, headaches, and bilateral papilledema.

ACLOVATE Cream or Ointment should not be used in the treatment of diaper dermatitis.

ADVERSE REACTIONS

The following local adverse reactions have been reported with ACLOVATE Cream in approximately 2% of patients: itching and burning, erythema, dryness, irritation, and papular rashes.

The following local adverse reactions have been reported with ACLOVATE Ointment in approximately 1% of patients: itching, burning, and erythema.

The following additional local adverse reactions have been reported infrequently with topical corticosteroids, but may occur more frequently with the use of occlusive dressings. These reactions are listed in approximate decreasing order of occurrence: folliculitis, acneiform eruptions, hypopigmentation, perioral dermatitis, allergic contact dermatitis, secondary infection, skin atrophy, striae, and miliaria.

OVERDOSAGE

Topically applied ACLOVATE Cream and Ointment can be absorbed in sufficient amounts to produce systemic effects (see PRECAUTIONS).

DOSAGE AND ADMINISTRATION

Apply a thin film of ACLOVATE Cream or Ointment to the affected skin areas two or three times daily; massage gently until the medication disappears.

ACLOVATE Cream and Ointment may be used in pediatric patients 1 year of age or older. Safety and effectiveness of ACLOVATE Cream or Ointment in pediatric patients for more than 3 weeks of use have not been established. Use in pediatric patients under 1 year of age is not recommended.

As with other corticosteroids, therapy should be discontinued when control is achieved. If no improvement is seen within 2 weeks, reassessment of diagnosis may be necessary.

ACLOVATE Cream or Ointment should not be used with occlusive dressings unless directed by a physician.

ACLOVATE Cream or Ointment should not be applied in the diaper area if the child still requires diapers or plastic pants as these garments may constitute occlusive dressing.

HOW SUPPLIED

ACLOVATE Cream, 0.05% is supplied in 15-g (NDC 0173-0401-00), 45-g (NDC 0173-0401-01), and 60-g (NDC 0173-0401-06) tubes.

ACLOVATE Ointment, 0.05% is supplied in 15-g (NDC 0173-0402-00), 45-g (NDC 0173-0402-01), and 60-g (NDC 0173-0402-06) tubes.

Store between 2° and 30°C (36° and 86°F).

Manufactured for Glaxo Wellcome Inc.
Research Triangle Park, NC 27709
by Schering Corporation, Kenilworth, NJ 07033
August 1997/RL-452

Shown in Product Identification Guide, page 314

AGENERASE® ℞
[*ă-jin 'ə-rās*]
(amprenavir)
Capsules

> AGENERASE (amprenavir) in combination with other antiretroviral agents is indicated for the treatment of HIV-1 infection. This indication is based on analyses of plasma HIV RNA levels and CD4 cell counts in controlled studies of up to 24 weeks in duration. At present, there are no results from controlled trials evaluating long-term suppression of HIV RNA or disease progression with AGENERASE.
>
> Because of the potential risk of toxicity from the large amount of the excipient propylene glycol contained in **AGENERASE Oral Solution**, that formulation is contraindicated in certain patient populations and should be used with caution in others. Consult the complete prescribing information for **AGENERASE Oral Solution** for full information.

DESCRIPTION

AGENERASE (amprenavir) is an inhibitor of the human immunodeficiency virus (HIV) protease. The chemical name of amprenavir is (3*S*)-tetrahydro-3-furyl *N*-[(1*S*,2*R*)-3-(4-amino-*N*-isobutylbenzenesulfonamido)-1-benzyl-2-hydroxypropyl]carbamate. Amprenavir is a single stereoisomer with the (3*S*)(1*S*,2*R*) configuration. It has a molecular formula of $C_{25}H_{35}N_3O_6S$.

Amprenavir is a white to cream-colored solid with a solubility of approximately 0.04 mg/mL in water at 25°C.

AGENERASE Capsules are available for oral administration in strengths of 50 and 150 mg. Each 50-mg capsule contains the inactive ingredients d-alpha tocopheryl polyethylene glycol 1000 succinate (TPGS), polyethylene glycol 400 (PEG 400) 246.7 mg, and propylene glycol 19 mg. Each 150-mg capsule contains the inactive ingredients TPGS, polyethylene glycol (PEG 400) 740 mg, and propylene glycol 57 mg. The capsule shell contains the inactive ingredients d-sorbitol and sorbitans solution, gelatin, glycerin, and titanium dioxide. The soft gelatin capsules are printed with edible red ink. Each 150-mg AGENERASE Capsule contains 109 IU vitamin E in the form of d-alpha tocopheryl polyethylene glycol 1000 succinate (TPGS). The total amount of vitamin E in the recommended daily adult dose of AGENERASE is 1744 IU.

MICROBIOLOGY

Mechanism of Action: Amprenavir is an inhibitor of HIV-1 protease. Amprenavir binds to the active site of HIV-1 protease and thereby prevents the processing of viral gag and gag-pol polyprotein precursors, resulting in the formation of immature non-infectious viral particles.

Antiviral Activity *in Vitro*: The *in vitro* antiviral activity of amprenavir was evaluated against HIV-1 IIIB in both acutely and chronically infected lymphoblastic cell lines (MT-4, CEM-CCRF, H9) and in peripheral blood lymphocytes. The 50% inhibitory concentration (IC_{50}) of amprenavir ranged from 0.012 to 0.08 µM in acutely infected cells and was 0.41 µM in chronically infected cells (1 µM = 0.50 mcg/mL). Amprenavir exhibited synergistic anti-HIV-1 activity in combination with abacavir, zidovudine, didanosine, or saquinavir, and additive anti-HIV-1 activity in combination with indinavir, nelfinavir, and ritonavir *in vitro*. These drug combinations have not been adequately studied in humans. The relationship between *in vitro* anti-HIV-1 activity of amprenavir and the inhibition of HIV-1 replication in humans has not been defined.

Resistance: HIV-1 isolates with a decreased susceptibility to amprenavir have been selected *in vitro* and were also obtained from patients treated with amprenavir. Genotypic analysis of isolates from amprenavir-treated patients showed mutations in the HIV-1 protease gene resulting in amino acid substitutions primarily at positions M46I/L, I47V, I50V, I54L/V, and I84V as well as mutations in the viral protease p1/p6 cleavage site. Phenotypic analysis of HIV-1 isolates from some patients on amprenavir monotherapy for 8 to 12 weeks showed a 5- to 10-fold decrease in susceptibility to amprenavir *in vitro* compared to baseline. Phenotypic analysis of HIV-1 isolates from 28 patients treated with amprenavir in combination with zidovudine and lamivudine for 16 to 36 weeks identified isolates from 6 patients that exhibited a 5- to 11-fold decrease in susceptibility to amprenavir *in vitro* compared to wild-type virus. Clinical isolates that exhibited a decrease in amprenavir susceptibility harbored amprenavir-associated mutations. The clinical relevance of the genotypic and phenotypic changes associated with amprenavir therapy has not been established.

Cross-Resistance: Varying degrees of HIV-1 cross resistance among protease inhibitors have been observed. The potential for protease inhibitor cross-resistance in HIV-1 isolates from amprenavir-treated patients has not been fully evaluated.

CLINICAL PHARMACOLOGY

Pharmacokinetics in Adults: The pharmacokinetic properties of amprenavir have been studied in asymptomatic, HIV-infected adult patients after administration of single oral doses of 150 to 1200 mg and multiple oral doses of 300 to 1200 mg twice daily.

Absorption and Bioavailability: Amprenavir was rapidly absorbed after oral administration in HIV-1-infected patients with a time to peak concentration (t_{max}) typically between 1 and 2 hours after a single oral dose. The absolute oral bioavailability of amprenavir in humans has not been established.

Increases in the area under the plasma concentration versus time curve (AUC) after single oral doses between 150 and 1200 mg were slightly greater than dose-proportional. Increases in AUC were dose-proportional after 3 weeks of dosing with doses from 300 to 1200 mg twice daily. The pharmacokinetic parameters after administration of amprenavir 1200 mg b.i.d. for 3 weeks to HIV-infected subjects are shown in Table 1.

[See table 1 below]

The relative bioavailability of AGENERASE Capsules and Oral Solution was assessed in healthy adults. AGENERASE Oral Solution was 14% less bioavailable compared to the capsules.

Effects of Food on Oral Absorption: The relative bioavailability of AGENERASE Capsules was assessed in the fasting and fed states in healthy volunteers (standardized high-fat meal: 967 kcal, 67 grams fat, 33 grams protein, 58 grams carbohydrate). Administration of a single 1200-mg dose of amprenavir in the fed state compared to the fasted state was associated with changes in C_{max} (fed: 6.18 ± 2.92 mcg/

Table 1: Average (%CV) Pharmacokinetic Parameters After 1200 mg b.i.d. of Amprenavir Capsules (n = 5)

C_{max} (mcg/mL)	t_{max} (hours)	AUC_{0-12} (mcg•h/mL)	C_{avg} (mcg/mL)	C_{min} (mcg/mL)	CL/F (mL/min/kg)
5.36 (62%)	1.9 (51%)	18.5 (63%)	1.54 (63%)	0.28 (52%)	31 (132%)

mL, fasted: 9.72 ± 2.75 mcg/mL), t_{max} (fed: 1.51 ± 0.68, fasted: 1.05 ± 0.63), and $AUC_{0-\infty}$ (fed: 22.06 ± 11.6 mcg•h/mL, fasted: 28.05 ± 10.1 mcg•h/mL). AGENERASE may be taken with or without food, but should not be taken with a high-fat meal (see DOSAGE AND ADMINISTRATION).

Distribution: The apparent volume of distribution (V_z/F) is approximately 430 L in healthy adult subjects. *In vitro* binding is approximately 90% to plasma proteins. The high affinity binding protein for amprenavir is alpha$_1$-acid glycoprotein (AAG). The partitioning of amprenavir into erythrocytes is low, but increases as amprenavir concentrations increase, reflecting the higher amount of unbound drug at higher concentrations.

Metabolism: Amprenavir is metabolized in the liver by the cytochrome P450 CYP3A4 enzyme system. The 2 major metabolites result from oxidation of the tetrahydrofuran and aniline moieties. Glucuronide conjugates of oxidized metabolites have been identified as minor metabolites in urine and feces.

Elimination: Excretion of unchanged amprenavir in urine and feces is minimal. Approximately 14% and 75% of an administered single dose of ^{14}C-amprenavir can be accounted for as radiocarbon in urine and feces, respectively. Two metabolites accounted for >90% of the radiocarbon in fecal samples. The plasma elimination half-life of amprenavir ranged from 7.1 to 10.6 hours.

Special Populations: ***Hepatic Insufficiency:*** AGENERASE has been studied in adult patients with impaired hepatic function using a single 600-mg oral dose. The $AUC_{0-\infty}$ was significantly greater in patients with moderate cirrhosis (25.76 ± 14.68 mcg•h/mL) compared with healthy volunteers (12.00 ± 4.38 mcg•h/mL). The $AUC_{0-\infty}$ and C_{max} were significantly greater in patients with severe cirrhosis ($AUC_{0-\infty}$: 38.66 ± 16.08 mcg•h/mL; C_{max}: 9.43 ± 2.61 mcg/mL) compared with healthy volunteers ($AUC_{0-\infty}$: 12.00 ± 4.38 mcg•h/mL; C_{max}: 4.90 ± 1.39 mcg/mL). Patients with impaired hepatic function require dosage adjustment (see DOSAGE AND ADMINISTRATION).

Renal Insufficiency: The impact of renal impairment on amprenavir elimination in adult patients has not been studied. The renal elimination of unchanged amprenavir represents <3% of the administered dose.

Pediatric Patients: The pharmacokinetics of amprenavir have been studied after either single or repeat doses of AGENERASE Capsules or Oral Solution in 84 pediatric patients. Twenty HIV-1-infected children ranging in age from 4 to 12 years received single doses from 5 mg/kg to 20 mg/kg using 25-mg or 150-mg capsules. The C_{max} of amprenavir increased less than proportionally with dose. The $AUC_{0-\infty}$ increased proportionally at doses between 5 and 20 mg/kg. Amprenavir is 14% less bioavailable from the liquid formulation than from the capsules; therefore **AGENERASE Capsules and AGENERASE Oral Solution are not interchangeable on a milligram per milligram basis.**

AGENERASE Oral Solution is contraindicated in infants and children below the age of 4 years due to the potential risk of toxicity from the large amount of the excipient propylene glycol. Please see the complete prescribing information for **AGENERASE Oral Solution** for full information.

[See table 2 above]

Geriatric Patients: The pharmacokinetics of amprenavir have not been studied in patients over 65 years of age.

Gender: The pharmacokinetics of amprenavir do not differ between males and females.

Race: The pharmacokinetics of amprenavir do not differ between Blacks and non-Blacks.

Drug Interactions: See also CONTRAINDICATIONS, WARNINGS, and PRECAUTIONS: Drug Interactions.

Amprenavir is metabolized in the liver by the cytochrome P450 enzyme system. Amprenavir inhibits CYP3A4. Caution should be used when coadministering medications that are substrates, inhibitors, or inducers of CYP3A4, or potentially toxic medications that are metabolized by CYP3A4. Amprenavir does not inhibit CYP2D6, CYP1A2, CYP2C9, CYP2C19, CYP2E1, or uridine glucuronosyltransferase (UDPGT).

Drug interaction studies were performed with amprenavir capsules and other drugs likely to be coadministered or drugs commonly used as probes for pharmacokinetic interactions. The effects of coadministration of amprenavir on the AUC, C_{max}, and C_{min} are summarized in Table 3 (effect of other drugs on amprenavir) and Table 4 (effect of amprenavir on other drugs). For information regarding clinical recommendations, see PRECAUTIONS.

[See table 3 above]

[See table 4 at top of next page]

Nucleoside Reverse Transcriptase Inhibitors (NRTIs): There was no effect of amprenavir on abacavir in subjects receiving both agents based on historical data.

HIV Protease Inhibitors: The effect of amprenavir on total drug concentrations of other HIV protease inhibitors in subjects receiving both agents was evaluated using comparisons to historical data. Indinavir steady-state C_{max}, AUC, and C_{min} were decreased by 22%, 38%, and 27%, respectively, by concomitant amprenavir. Similar decreases in C_{max} and AUC were seen after the first dose. Saquinavir steady-state C_{max}, AUC, and C_{min} were increased 21%, decreased 19%, and decreased 48%, respectively, by concomitant amprenavir. Nelfinavir steady-state C_{max}, AUC, and C_{min} were increased by 12%, 15%, and 14%, respectively, by concomitant amprenavir.

For information regarding clinical recommendations, see PRECAUTIONS: Drug Interactions.

Table 2: Average (%CV) Pharmacokinetic Parameters in Children Ages 4 to 12 Years Receiving 20 mg/kg b.i.d. or 15 mg/kg t.i.d. of AGENERASE Oral Solution

Dose	n	C_{max} (mcg/mL)	t_{max} (hours)	AUC_{ss}* (mcg•h/mL)	C_{avg} (mcg/mL)	C_{min} (mcg/mL)	CL/F (mL/min/kg)
20 mg/kg b.i.d.	20	6.77 (51%)	1.1 (21%)	15.46 (59%)	1.29 (59%)	0.24 (98%)	29 (58%)
15 mg/kg t.i.d.	17	3.99 (37%)	1.4 (90%)	8.73 (36%)	1.09 (36%)	0.27 (95%)	32 (34%)

*AUC is 0 to 12 hours for b.i.d. and 0 to 8 hours for t.i.d., therefore the C_{avg} is a better comparison of the exposures.

Table 3: Drug Interactions: Pharmacokinetic Parameters for Amprenavir in the Presence of the Coadministered Drug

Co-administered Drug	Dose of Coadministered Drug	Dose of AGENERASE	n	% Change in **Amprenavir** Pharmacokinetic Parameters* (90% CI)		
				C_{max}	AUC	C_{min}
Abacavir	300 mg b.i.d. for 3 weeks	900 mg b.i.d. for 3 weeks	4	↑47 (↓15 to ↑154)	↑29 (↓18 to ↑103)	↑27 (↓46 to ↑197)
Clarithromycin	500 mg b.i.d. for 4 days	1200 mg b.i.d. for 4 days	12	↑15 (↑1 to ↑31)	↑18 (↑8 to ↑29)	↑39 (↑31 to ↑47)
Indinavir	800 mg t.i.d. for 2 weeks (fasted)	750 or 800 mg t.i.d. for 2 weeks (fasted)	9	↑18 (↓13 to ↑58)	↑33 (↑2 to ↑73)	↑25 (↓27 to ↑116)
Ketoconazole	400 mg single dose	1200 mg single dose	12	↓16 (↓25 to ↓6)	↑31 (↑20 to ↑42)	NA
Lamivudine	150 mg single dose	600 mg single dose	11	⇔ (↓17 to ↑9)	⇔ (↓15 to ↑14)	NA
Nelfinavir	750 mg t.i.d. for 2 weeks (fed)	750 or 800 mg t.i.d. for 2 weeks (fed)	6	↓14 (↓38 to ↑20)	⇔ (↓19 to ↑47)	↑189 (↑52 to ↑448)
Rifabutin	300 mg q.d. for 10 days	1200 mg b.i.d. for 10 days	5	⇔ (↓21 to ↑10)	↓15 (↓28 to 0)	↓15 (↓38 to ↑17)
Rifampin	300 mg q.d. for 4 days	1200 mg b.i.d. for 4 days	11	↓70 (↓76 to ↓62)	↓82 (↓84 to ↓78)	↓92 (↓95 to ↓89)
Saquinavir	800 mg t.i.d. for 2 weeks (fed)	750 or 800 mg t.i.d. for 2 weeks (fed)	7	↓37 (↓54 to ↓14)	↓32 (↓49 to ↓9)	↓14 (↓52 to ↑54)
Zidovudine	300 mg single dose	600 mg single dose	12	⇔ (↓5 to ↑24)	↑13 (↓2 to ↑31)	NA

*Based on total-drug concentrations.
↑ = Increase; ↓ = Decrease; ⇔ = No change (↑ or ↓ <10%); NA = C_{min} not calculated for single-dose study.

INDICATIONS AND USAGE

AGENERASE (amprenavir) in combination with other antiretroviral agents is indicated for the treatment of HIV-1 infection. This indication is based on analyses of plasma HIV RNA levels and CD4 cell counts in controlled studies of up to 24 weeks in duration. At present, there are no results from controlled trials evaluating long-term suppression of HIV RNA or disease progression with AGENERASE (see Description of Clinical Studies).

Description of Clinical Studies: ***Therapy-Naive Adults:*** PROAB3001, an ongoing, randomized, double-blind, placebo-controlled, multicenter study, compared treatment with AGENERASE Capsules (1200 mg twice daily) plus lamivudine (150 mg twice daily) plus zidovudine (300 mg twice daily) versus lamivudine (150 mg twice daily) plus zidovudine (300 mg twice daily) in 232 patients, median age 37 years (range 18 to 63 years), 75% Caucasian, 89% male, with a median CD4 cell count of 416 cells/mm^3 (range 139 to 1800 cells/mm^3) and a median plasma HIV-1 RNA of 4.67 log_{10} copies/mL) (range 3.06 to 6.31 log_{10} copies/mL) at baseline. Through 24 weeks of therapy, there was no significant difference in the median CD4 cell count between the treatment arms. Figure 1 shows the proportions of patients with plasma HIV-1 RNA levels <400 copies/mL through 24 weeks.

[See figure 1 in next column]

HIV-1 RNA status and reasons for discontinuation of randomized treatment at 24 weeks are summarized (Table 5).

[See table 5 on next page]

Therapy-Experienced Adults: PROAB3006, an ongoing, randomized, open-label multicenter study, compared treatment with AGENERASE Capsules (1200 mg twice daily) plus NRTIs versus indinavir (800 mg every 8 hours) plus NRTIs in 504 NRTI- and non-nucleoside reverse transcriptase inhibitor- (NNRTI) experienced, protease inhibitor-naive patients, median age 37 years (range 20 to 71 years), 72% Caucasian, 80% male, with a median CD4 cell count of 399 cells/mm^3 (range 9 to 1706 cells/mm^3) and a median plasma HIV-1 RNA level of 3.93 log_{10} copies/mL (range 2.60 to 7.01 log_{10} copies/mL) at baseline. Through 24 weeks of therapy, there was a smaller increase in median CD4 cell count from baseline for the amprenavir group than for the indinavir group. Figure 2 shows the proportions of patients with plasma HIV-1 RNA levels <400 copies/mL through 24 weeks.

[See figure 2 at top of next page]

Figure 1: Virologic Response Through Week 24, PROAB3001[1,2]

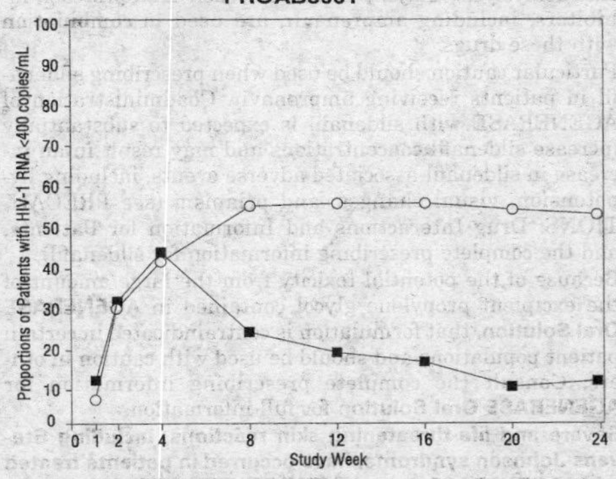

○ AGENERASE/Lamivudine/Zidovudine (n = 116)
■ Lamivudine/Zidovudine (n = 116)
[1]Roche AMPLICOR HIV-1 MONITOR assay.
[2]Discontinuations and missing data were considered as HIV-1 RNA ≥400 copies/mL.

HIV-1 RNA status and reasons for discontinuation of randomized treatment at 24 weeks are summarized (Table 6).

[See table 6 on next page]

CONTRAINDICATIONS

AGENERASE should not be administered concurrently with astemizole, bepridil, cisapride, dihydroergotamine, ergotamine, midazolam, and triazolam. Although these drugs have not been specifically studied, coadministration may result in competitive inhibition of metabolism of these

Continued on next page

This product information is based on labeling in effect on June 23, 2000. For further information, contact via direct mail, phone, or web site. Medical Information, Glaxo Wellcome Inc., PO Box 13398, Research Triangle Park, NC 27709. Healthcare Professionals (Medical Information): 800-334-0089. Patients (Customer Response Center): 1-888-825-5249. Glaxo Wellcome Corporate Web Site: www.glaxowellcome.com

Agenerase Capsules—Cont.

Figure 2: Virologic Response Through Week 24, PROAB3006[3,4]

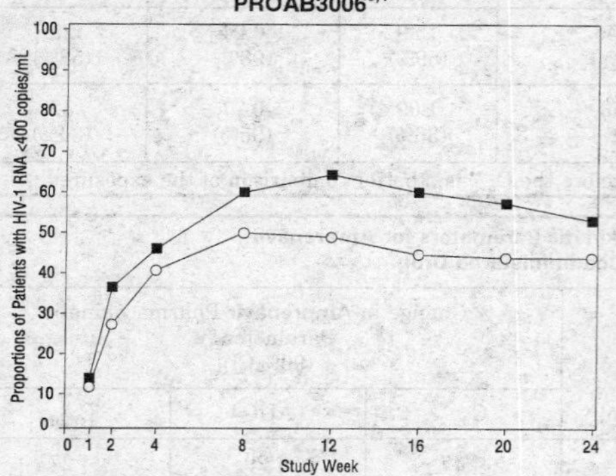

○ AGENERASE plus NRTIs (n = 254)
■ Indinavir plus NRTIs (n = 250)
[3]Roche AMPLICOR HIV-1 MONITOR assay.
[4]Discontinuations and missing data were considered as HIV-1 RNA ≥400 copies/mL.

products and may cause serious or life-threatening adverse events. (See WARNINGS for agents whose coadministration may result in competitive inhibition of metabolism but for which concentration monitoring is recommended.)
Because of the potential toxicity from the large amount of the excipient propylene glycol contained in **AGENERASE Oral Solution,** that formulation is contraindicated in certain patient populations and should be used with caution in others. Consult the complete prescribing information for **AGENERASE Oral Solution** for full information.
AGENERASE is contraindicated in patients with previously demonstrated clinically significant hypersensitivity to any of the components of this product.

WARNINGS

Serious and/or life-threatening drug interactions could occur between amprenavir and amiodarone, lidocaine (systemic), tricyclic antidepressants, and quinidine. Concentration monitoring of these agents is recommended if these agents are used concomitantly with AGENERASE (see CONTRAINDICATIONS).
Rifampin should not be used in combination with amprenavir because it reduces plasma concentrations and AUC of amprenavir by about 90%.
Concomitant use of AGENERASE with lovastatin or simvastatin is not recommended. Caution should be exercised if HIV protease inhibitors, including AGENERASE, are used concurrently with other HMG-CoA reductase inhibitors that are also metabolized by the CYP3A4 pathway (e.g., atorvastatin or cerivastatin). The risk of myopathy, including rhabdomyolysis, may be increased when HIV protease inhibitors, including amprenavir, are used in combination with these drugs.
Particular caution should be used when prescribing sildenafil in patients receiving amprenavir. Coadministration of AGENERASE with sildenafil is expected to substantially increase sildenafil concentrations and may result in an increase in sildenafil-associated adverse events, including hypotension, visual changes, and priapism (see PRECAUTIONS: Drug Interactions and Information for Patients, and the complete prescribing information for sildenafil).
Because of the potential toxicity from the large amount of the excipient propylene glycol contained in **AGENERASE Oral Solution,** that formulation is contraindicated in certain patient populations and should be used with caution in others. Consult the complete prescribing information for **AGENERASE Oral Solution** for full information.
Severe and life-threatening skin reactions, including Stevens-Johnson syndrome, have occurred in patients treated with AGENERASE (see ADVERSE REACTIONS). Acute hemolytic anemia has been reported in a patient treated with AGENERASE.
New onset diabetes mellitus, exacerbation of pre-existing diabetes mellitus, and hyperglycemia have been reported during post-marketing surveillance in HIV-infected patients receiving protease inhibitor therapy. Some patients required either initiation or dose adjustments of insulin or oral hypoglycemic agents for treatment of these events. In some cases, diabetic ketoacidosis has occurred. In those patients who discontinued protease inhibitor therapy, hyperglycemia persisted in some cases. Because these events have been reported voluntarily during clinical practice, estimates of frequency cannot be made and causal relationships between protease inhibitor therapy and these events have not been established.

PRECAUTIONS

General: AGENERASE Capsules and AGENERASE Oral Solution are not interchangeable on a milligram per milligram basis (see CLINICAL PHARMACOLOGY: Pediatric Patients).
Amprenavir is a sulfonamide. The potential for cross-sensitivity between drugs in the sulfonamide class and amprenavir is unknown. Patients with a known sulfonamide allergy should be treated with caution.

Table 4: Drug Interactions: Pharmacokinetic Parameters for Coadministered Drug in the Presence of Amprenavir

Co-administered Drug	Dose of Coadministered Drug	Dose of AGENERASE	n	% Change in Pharmacokinetic Parameters of **Coadministered Drug** (90% CI)		
				C_{max}	AUC	C_{min}
Clarithromycin	500 mg b.i.d. for 4 days	1200 mg b.i.d. for 4 days	12	↓10 (↓24 to ↑7)	⇔ (↓17 to ↑11)	⇔ (↓13 to ↑20)
Ketoconazole	400 mg single dose	1200 mg single dose	12	↑19 (↑8 to ↑33)	↑44 (↑31 to ↑59)	NA
Lamivudine	150 mg single dose	600 mg single dose	11	⇔ (↓17 to ↑3)	⇔ (↓11 to 0)	NA
Rifabutin	300 mg q.d. for 10 days	1200 mg b.i.d. for 10 days	5	↑119 (↑82 to ↑164)	↑193 (↑156 to ↑235)	↑271 (↑171 to ↑409)
Rifampin	300 mg q.d. for 4 days	1200 mg b.i.d. for 4 days	11	⇔ (↓13 to ↑12)	⇔ (↓10 to ↑13)	ND
Zidovudine	300 mg single dose	600 mg single dose	12	↑40 (↑14 to ↑71)	↑31 (↑19 to ↑45)	NA

↑ = Increase; ↓ = Decrease; ⇔ = No change (↑ or ↓<10%); NA = C_{min} not calculated for single-dose study; ND = Interaction cannot be determined as C_{min} was below the lower limit of quantitation.

Table 5: Outcomes of Randomized Treatment Through Week 24 (PROAB3001)

Outcome	AGENERASE (n = 116)	Placebo (n = 116)
HIV RNA <400 copies/mL*	53%	11%
HIV RNA ≥400 copies/mL[†,‡]	13%	62%
CDC Class C event[‡]	0%	0%
Discontinued due to adverse events[‡]	15%	3%
Discontinued due to other reasons[‡,§]	19%	22%
On treatment with missing HIV RNA value[‡]	0%	1%
TOTAL	100%	100%

*Corresponds to rates at Week 24 in Figure 1.
[†]Includes discontinuations due to virological failure at or before Week 24.
[‡]Treatment failure in the analysis.
[§]Consent withdrawn, lost to follow-up, and protocol violation.

Table 6: Outcomes of Randomized Treatment Through Week 24 (PROAB3006)

Outcome	AGENERASE (n = 254)	Indinavir (n = 250)
HIV RNA <400 copies/mL*	43%	53%
HIV RNA ≥400 copies/mL[†,‡]	22%	18%
CDC Class C event[‡]	<1%	2%
Discontinued due to adverse events[‡]	16%	8%
Discontinued due to other reasons[‡,§]	14%	12%
On treatment with missing HIV RNA value[‡]	4%	7%
TOTAL	100%	100%

*Corresponds to rates at Week 24 in Figure 2.
[†]Includes discontinuations due to virological failure at or before Week 24.
[‡]Treatment failure in the analysis.
[§]Consent withdrawn, lost to follow-up, and protocol violation.

AGENERASE is principally metabolized by the liver; therefore caution should be exercised when administering this drug to patients with hepatic impairment (see DOSAGE AND ADMINISTRATION).
Formulations of AGENERASE provide high daily doses of vitamin E (see Information for Patients, DESCRIPTION, and DOSAGE AND ADMINISTRATION). The effects of long-term, high-dose vitamin E administration is humans is not well characterized and has not been specifically studied in HIV-infected individuals. High vitamin E doses may exacerbate the blood coagulation defect of vitamin K deficiency caused by anticoagulant therapy or malabsorption.
Patients with Hemophilia: There have been reports of spontaneous bleeding in patients with hemophilia A and B treated with protease inhibitors. In some patients, additional factor VIII was required. In many of the reported cases, treatment with protease inhibitors was continued or restarted. A causal relationship between protease inhibitor therapy and these episodes has not been established.
Fat Redistribution: Redistribution/accumulation of body fat including central obesity, dorsocervical fat enlargement (buffalo hump), peripheral wasting, breast enlargement, and "cushingoid appearance" have been observed in patients receiving protease inhibitors. The mechanism and long-term consequences of these events are currently unknown. A causal relationship has not been established.
Resistance/Cross-Resistance: Because the potential for HIV cross-resistance among protease inhibitors has not been fully explored, it is unknown what effect amprenavir therapy will have on the activity of subsequently administered protease inhibitors (see MICROBIOLOGY).

Information for Patients: A Patient Package Insert (PPI) for AGENERASE Capsules is available for patient information.
Patients treated with AGENERASE Capsules should be cautioned against switching to **AGENERASE Oral Solution** because of the increased risk of adverse events from the large amount of propylene glycol in **AGENERASE Oral Solution.** Please see the complete prescribing information for **AGENERASE Oral Solution** for full information.
Patients should be informed that AGENERASE is not a cure for HIV infection and that they may continue to develop opportunistic infections and other complications associated with HIV disease. The long-term effects of AGENERASE (amprenavir) are unknown at this time. Patients should be told that there are currently no data demonstrating that therapy with AGENERASE can reduce the risk of transmitting HIV to others through sexual contact.
Patients should remain under the care of a physician while using AGENERASE. Patients should be advised to take AGENERASE every day as prescribed. AGENERASE must always be used in combination with other antiretroviral drugs. Patients should not alter the dose or discontinue therapy without consulting their physician. If a dose is missed, patients should take the dose as soon as possible and then return to their normal schedule. However, if a dose is skipped, the patient should not double the next dose.
Patients should inform their doctor if they have a sulfa allergy. The potential for cross-sensitivity between drugs in the sulfonamide class and amprenavir is unknown.
Some drugs should not be used with AGENERASE. Therefore, patients should be advised that they must report to their doctor the use of any other prescription or nonprescription medication.

Patients taking antacids (or didanosine) should take AGENERASE at least 1 hour before or after antacid (or didanosine) use.
Patients receiving sildenafil should be advised that they may be at an increased risk of sildenafil-associated adverse events including hypotension, visual changes, and priapism, and should promptly report any symptoms to their doctor.
Patients receiving hormonal contraceptives should be instructed that alternate contraceptive measures should be used during therapy with AGENERASE.
High-fat meals may decrease the absorption of AGENERASE and should be avoided. AGENERASE may be taken with meals of normal fat content.
Patients should be informed that redistribution or accumulation of body fat may occur in patients receiving protease inhibitors and that the cause and long-term health effects of these conditions are not known at this time.
Adult and pediatric patients should be advised not to take supplemental vitamin E since the vitamin E content of AGENERASE Capsules and Oral Solution exceeds the Reference Daily Intake (adults 30 IU, pediatrics approximately 10 IU).

Drug Interactions: See also CONTRAINDICATIONS, WARNINGS, and CLINICAL PHARMACOLOGY: Drug Interactions.
AGENERASE is an inhibitor of cytochrome P450 CYP3A4 metabolism and therefore should not be administered concurrently with medications with narrow therapeutic windows that are substrates of CYP3A4. There are other agents that may result in serious and/or life-threatening drug interactions (see CONTRAINDICATIONS and WARNINGS). [See table 7 at right]

Antimycobacterials: Rifampin: Rifampin should not be used in combination with amprenavir since it reduces plasma concentrations and AUC of amprenavir by about 90%.

Rifabutin: Coadministration of amprenavir with rifabutin results in a 15% decrease in amprenavir plasma AUC and a 193% increase in rifabutin plasma AUC. A dosage reduction of rifabutin to at least half the recommended dose is required when AGENERASE and rifabutin are coadministered (see CLINICAL PHARMACOLOGY: Drug Interactions). A complete blood count should be performed weekly and as clinically indicated in order to monitor for neutropenia in patients receiving amprenavir and rifabutin.

Other Potentially Significant Drug Interactions: Other medications that interact at CYP3A4, either as substrates, inhibitors, or inducers of the enzyme, could have potential interactions when used concomitantly. The clinical significance of these potential interactions is unknown and has not been studied.

Antibiotics: Dapsone and erythromycin may have their plasma concentrations increased by AGENERASE. Erythromycin may also increase amprenavir serum concentrations.

Antifungals: Itraconazole may have its plasma concentrations increased by AGENERASE. Itraconazole may increase serum concentrations of amprenavir.

Benzodiazepines: Alprazolam, clorazepate, diazepam, and flurazepam may have their serum concentrations increased by AGENERASE, which could increase their activity.

Calcium Channel Blockers: Diltiazem, nicardipine, nifedipine, and nimodipine may have their serum concentrations increased by AGENERASE, which could increase their activity.

Cholesterol-Lowering Agents: Atorvastatin, cerivastatin, lovastatin, pravastatin, and simvastatin may have their serum concentration increased by AGENERASE, which could increase their activity or toxicity. Concomitant use of AGENERASE with lovastatin or simvastatin is not recommended. Caution should be exercised if HIV protease inhibitors, including AGENERASE, are used concurrently with other HMG-CoA reductase inhibitors that are also metabolized by the CYP3A4 pathway (e.g., atorvastatin or cerivastatin). The risk of myopathy, including rhabdomyolysis, may be increased when HIV protease inhibitors, including amprenavir, are used in combination with these drugs.

Erectile Dysfunction Agents: Particular caution should be used when prescribing sildenafil in patients receiving amprenavir. Because amprenavir is a cytochrome P4503A4 inhibitor, coadministration of AGENERASE with sildenafil is likely to result in an increase of sildenafil concentrations by competitive inhibition of metabolism. The magnitude of this interaction has not been determined. Results from drug interaction studies in healthy volunteers indicate that coadministration of saquinavir soft gelatin capsules (1200 mg t.i.d.) increases sildenafil (100 mg single dose) AUC by 210% (3.1-fold) and coadministration of ritonavir (500 mg b.i.d.) increases sildenafil (100 mg single dose) AUC by 1000% (11-fold). Providers should consult the sildenafil prescribing information for dose reductions of sildenafil in patients receiving ritonavir. Patients receiving amprenavir and sildenafil should be advised that they may be at an increased risk for sildenafil-associated adverse events, including hypotension, visual changes, and priapism, and should report these symptoms promptly to their doctor.

NNRTIs: NNRTIs have the potential to increase (delavirdine) or decrease (efavirenz, nevirapine) serum concentrations of amprenavir.

Steroids: Estrogens, progestogens, and some glucocorticoids may have an interaction with AGENERASE, but there is insufficient information to predict the nature of the interaction. Because of this potential for metabolic interactions with amprenavir, the efficacy of hormonal contraceptives may be reduced. Alternate or additional reliable barrier methods of contraception are recommended for women of childbearing potential.

Table 7: Drug Interactions with AGENERASE

Should Not Be Coadministered

Drug Class	Drug Within Class Not To Be Coadministered
Antihistamines	Astemizole
Antimycobacterials	Rifampin*
Benzodiazepines	Midazolam, triazolam
Cardiovascular	Bepridil
Ergot derivatives	Dihydroergotamine, ergotamine
GI motility agents	Cisapride

*Decreases plasma concentrations of amprenavir and should not be coadministered as it is likely to reduce antiviral activity.

Coadministration Requires Concentration Monitoring

Drug Class	Drug Within Class to Monitor
Antiarrhythmics	Amiodarone, lidocaine (systemic), quinidine
Anticoagulants	Warfarin*
Antidepressants	Tricyclic antidepressants

*Monitor INR (International Normalized Ratio).

Dosage Adjustment Required

Drug Class	Drug Within Class Requiring a Dosage Adjustment
Antimycobacterials	Rifabutin (reduce dose to at least half that recommended)*

*A complete blood count should be performed weekly and as clinically indicated in order to monitor for neutropenia in patients receiving amprenavir and rifabutin.

Other Potentially Significant Drug Interactions

Anticonvulsants: phenobarbital, phenytoin, carbamazepine	Induce CYP3A4 and may decrease amprenavir concentrations.
Cholesterol-lowering agents: atorvastatin, cerivastatin, lovastatin, pravastatin, and simvastatin	May have their serum concentrations increased by AGENERASE, which could increase their activity or toxicity (see WARNINGS).
Erectile dysfunction agents: sildenafil	Expected to substantially increase sildenafil concentrations (consult sildenafil prescribing information for dose reduction of sildenafil in patients receiving ritonavir).

Other Agents: There are other agents that may have their plasma concentrations increased by AGENERASE, and include, but are not limited to: clozapine, carbamazepine, loratadine, pimozide, and warfarin.
Cimetidine and ritonavir may increase amprenavir plasma concentrations.
Antacids (and didanosine secondary to the antacid content) have not been specifically studied. Based upon data with other protease inhibitors, it is advisable that antacids not be taken at the same time as AGENERASE because of potential interference with absorption. It is recommended that their administration be separated by at least an hour.

Carcinogenesis and Mutagenesis: Long-term carcinogenicity studies of amprenavir in rodents are in progress. Amprenavir was not mutagenic or genotoxic in a battery of *in vitro* and *in vivo* assays including bacterial reverse mutation (Ames), mouse lymphoma, rat micronucleus, and chromosome aberrations in human lymphocytes.

Fertility: The effects of amprenavir on fertility and general reproductive performance were investigated in male rats (treated for 28 days before mating, at doses producing up to twice the expected clinical exposure based on AUC comparisons) and female rats (treated for 15 days before mating through day 17 of gestation at doses producing up to 2 times the expected clinical exposure). Amprenavir did not impair mating or fertility of male or female rats and did not affect the development and maturation of sperm from treated rats. The reproductive performance of the F1 generation born to female rats given amprenavir was not different from control animals.

Pregnancy and Reproduction: Pregnancy Category C. Embryo/fetal development studies were conducted in rats (dosed from 15 days before pairing to day 17 of gestation) and rabbits (dosed from day 8 to day 20 of gestation). In pregnant rabbits, amprenavir administration was associated with abortions and an increased incidence of 3 minor skeletal variations resulting from deficient ossification of the femur, humerus trochlea, and humerus. Systemic exposure at the highest tested dose was approximately one-twentieth of the exposure seen at the recommended human dose. In rat fetuses, thymic elongation and incomplete ossification of bones were attributed to amprenavir. Both findings were seen at systemic exposures that were one half of that associated with the recommended human dose.
Pre- and post-natal developmental studies were performed in rats dosed from day 7 of gestation to day 22 of lactation. Reduced body weights (10% to 20%) were observed in the offspring. The systemic exposure associated with this finding was approximately twice the exposure in humans following administration of the recommended human dose. The subsequent development of these offspring, including fertility and reproductive performance, was not affected by the maternal administration of amprenavir.
There are no adequate and well-controlled studies in pregnant women. AGENERASE should be used during pregnancy only if the potential benefit justifies the potential risk to the fetus.
AGENERASE Oral Solution is contraindicated during pregnancy due to the potential risk of toxicity to the fetus from the high propylene glycol content.

Antiretroviral Pregnancy Registry: To monitor maternal-fetal outcomes of pregnant women exposed to AGENERASE, an Antiretroviral Pregnancy Registry has been established. Physicians are encouraged to register patients by calling 1-800-258-4263.

Nursing Mothers: The Centers for Disease Control and Prevention recommend that HIV-infected mothers not breastfeed their infants to avoid risking postnatal transmission of HIV. Although it is not known if amprenavir is excreted in human milk, amprenavir is secreted into the milk of lactating rats. Because of both the potential for HIV transmission and any possible adverse effects of amprenavir, **mothers should be instructed not to breastfeed if they are receiving AGENERASE.**

Pediatric Use: One hundred eighteen patients 4 to 17 years of age have received amprenavir as single or multiple doses in studies. An adverse event profile similar to that seen in adults was seen in pediatric patients.
AGENERASE Oral Solution is contraindicated in infants and children below the age of 4 years due to the potential risk of toxicity from the large amount of the excipient propylene glycol. Please see the complete prescribing information for **AGENERASE Oral Solution** for full information.
The safety, effectiveness, and pharmacokinetics of amprenavir have not been evaluated in pediatric patients below the age of 4 years (see CLINICAL PHARMACOLOGY and DOSAGE AND ADMINISTRATION).

Continued on next page

This product information is based on labeling in effect on June 23, 2000. For further information, contact via direct mail, phone, or web site. Medical Information, Glaxo Wellcome Inc., PO Box 13398, Research Triangle Park, NC 27709. Healthcare Professionals (Medical Information): 800-334-0089. Patients (Customer Response Center): 1-888-825-5249. Glaxo Wellcome Corporate Web Site: www.glaxowellcome.com

Agenerase Capsules—Cont.

Geriatric Use: Clinical studies of AGENERASE did not include sufficient numbers of patients aged 65 and over to determine whether they respond differently from younger adults. In general, dose selection for an elderly patient should be cautious, reflecting the greater frequency of decreased hepatic, renal, or cardiac function, and of concomitant disease or other drug therapy.

ADVERSE REACTIONS

Rates of discontinuation of randomized therapy due to adverse events were 15% in amprenavir vs 3% in placebo recipients from Study 3001, and 16% in amprenavir vs 8% in indinavir recipients from Study 3006. In these studies, adverse events leading to amprenavir discontinuation included gastrointestinal events (11%), rash (3%), and paresthesias (<1%).

Most gastrointestinal events (nausea, vomiting, diarrhea, and abdominal pain) that led to amprenavir discontinuation were graded as mild or moderate in severity.

In all multidose studies in HIV-infected patients, skin rash occurred in 28% of patients treated with amprenavir. Rashes were usually maculopapular and of mild or moderate intensity, some with pruritus. Rashes had onsets ranging from 7 to 73 days (median: 10 days) after amprenavir initiation. With mild or moderate rash, amprenavir dosing was often continued without interruption; if interrupted, reintroduction of amprenavir generally did not result in rash recurrence (Phase 3 studies).

Severe or life-threatening rash, including Stevens-Johnson syndrome, occurred in 1% of recipients of AGENERASE (4% of recipients who developed rash) (see WARNINGS). Amprenavir therapy should be discontinued for severe or life-threatening rashes and for moderate rashes accompanied by systemic symptoms.

[See table 8 above]

In Phase 3 studies, 1 patient experienced diabetes mellitus *de novo,* and another developed a dorsocervical fat enlargement (buffalo hump).

[See table 9 above]

In studies 3001 and 3006, no increased frequency of Grade 3 or 4 AST, ALT, amylase, or bilirubin elevations was seen compared to controls.

Pediatric Patients: An adverse event profile similar to that seen in adults was seen in pediatric patients.

Table 8: Selected Clinical Adverse Events Grades 1-4 (≥5% Frequency)

	PROAB3001 Therapy-Naive Patients		PROAB3006 NRTI-Experienced Patients	
Adverse Event	AGENERASE/ Lamivudine/ Zidovudine (n = 113)	Lamivudine/ Zidovudine (n = 109)	AGENERASE/ NRTI (n = 245)	Indinavir/NRTI (n = 241)
Digestive				
Nausea	73%	50%	38%	26%
Vomiting	29%	17%	20%	11%
Diarrhea or loose stools	33%	34%	56%	32%
Taste disorders	10%	5%	1%	7%
Skin				
Rash	25%	6%	18%	10%
Nervous				
Paresthesia, oral/perioral	26%	5%	30%	2%
Paresthesia (including peripheral)	8%	3%	12%	9%
Psychiatric				
Depressive or mood disorders	15%	4%	4%	6%

Table 9: Selected Laboratory Abnormalities Grades 1-4 Reported in ≥5% of Patients

	PROAB3001 Therapy-Naive Patients		PROAB3006 NRTI-Experienced Patients	
Laboratory Abnormality (non-fasting specimens)	AGENERASE/ Lamivudine/ Zidovudine (n = 113)	Lamivudine/ Zidovudine (n = 109)	AGENERASE/ NRTI (n = 245)	Indinavir/NRTI (n = 241)
Hyperglycemia (>116 mg/dL)	37%	29%	41%	44%
Hypertriglyceridemia (>213 mg/dL)	36%	22%	47%	40%
Hypercholesterolemia (>283 mg/dL)	4%	3%	9%	10%

OVERDOSAGE

There is no known antidote for AGENERASE. It is not known whether amprenavir can be removed by peritoneal dialysis or hemodialysis. If overdosage occurs, the patient should be monitored for evidence of toxicity and standard supportive treatment applied as necessary.

DOSAGE AND ADMINISTRATION

AGENERASE may be taken with or without food; however, a high-fat meal decreases the absorption of amprenavir and should be avoided (see CLINICAL PHARMACOLOGY: Effects of Food on Oral Absorption). **Adult and pediatric patients should be advised not to take supplemental vitamin E since the vitamin E content of AGENERASE Capsules exceeds the Reference Daily Intake (adults 30 IU, pediatrics approximately 10 IU) (see DESCRIPTION).**

Adults: The recommended oral dose of AGENERASE Capsules for adults is 1200 mg (8 150-mg capsules) twice daily in combination with other antiretroviral agents.

Pediatric Patients: For adolescents (13 to 16 years), the recommended oral dose of AGENERASE Capsules is 1200 mg (8 150-mg capsules) twice daily in combination with other antiretroviral agents. For patients between 4 and 12 years of age or for patients 13 to 16 years of age with weight of <50 kg, the recommended oral dose of AGENERASE Capsules is 20 mg/kg twice daily or 15 mg/kg 3 times daily (to a maximum daily dose of 2400 mg) in combination with other antiretroviral agents.

Before using **AGENERASE Oral Solution,** the complete prescribing information should be consulted.

AGENERASE Capsules and AGENERASE Oral Solution are not interchangeable on a milligram per milligram basis (see CLINICAL PHARMACOLOGY).

Patients with Hepatic Impairment: AGENERASE Capsules should be used with caution in patients with moderate or severe hepatic impairment. Patients with a Child-Pugh score ranging from 5 to 8 should receive a reduced dose of AGENERASE Capsules of 450 mg twice daily, and patients with a Child-Pugh score ranging from 9 to 12 should receive a reduced dose of AGENERASE Capsules of 300 mg twice daily (see CLINICAL PHARMACOLOGY: Hepatic Insufficiency).

HOW SUPPLIED

AGENERASE Capsules, 50 mg, are oblong, opaque, off-white to cream-colored soft gelatin capsules printed with "GX CC1" on the side.

Bottles of 480 with child-resistant closures (NDC 0173-0679-00).

AGENERASE Capsules, 150 mg, are oblong, opaque, off-white to cream-colored soft gelatin capsules printed with "GX CC2" on one side.

Bottles of 240 with child-resistant closures (NDC 0173-0672-00).

Store at controlled room temperature of 25°C (77°F) (see USP).

PATIENT INFORMATION

AGENERASE® (amprenavir) Capsules

Please read this information before you start taking AGENERASE (pronounced ah-GEN-er-ase) Capsules, and re-read it each time you receive your prescription, just in case something has changed. Remember that this information does not take the place of careful discussions with your doctor when you start this medication and at checkups. You should not change or stop your anti-HIV treatment without first talking with your doctor. **You should tell your doctor about any drug you are taking or planning to take because taking AGENERASE Capsules with some medications can result in serious or life-threatening problems.**

You should not switch from AGENERASE Capsules to **AGENERASE Oral Solution** without talking with your doctor.

What are AGENERASE Capsules?

AGENERASE Capsules are a medication used to treat HIV infection. HIV is the virus that causes AIDS (acquired immune deficiency syndrome). AGENERASE Capsules are taken by mouth as soft gel capsules. AGENERASE belongs to a class of anti-HIV medicines call protease inhibitors.

How do AGENERASE Capsules work?

AGENERASE Capsules are used only in combination with other anti-HIV medicines. When used in combination therapy, AGENERASE Capsules may help lower the amount of HIV found in your blood, raise CD4 (T) cell count, and keep your immune system as healthy as possible so that it can help fight infection. However, AGENERASE Capsules do not have these effects in all patients.

What are the side effects of AGENERASE Capsules?

Common side effects of AGENERASE Capsules are nausea, vomiting, diarrhea, rash, and a tingling sensation around the mouth. Severe or life-threatening rash has been reported.

Contact your doctor if you have nausea, vomiting, diarrhea, or rash. Your doctor may be able to help you manage these symptoms. Your doctor will advise you whether your symptoms can be managed on therapy or whether AGENERASE Capsules should be stopped.

This list of side effects is not complete. Your doctor or pharmacist can discuss with you a more complete list of possible side effects with AGENERASE Capsules. Talk to your doctor promptly about any side effects you have.

How should I take AGENERASE Capsules?

Take AGENERASE Capsules exactly as your doctor prescribes them. The usual dosage for adults and adolescents (at least 13 years of age) is 8 150-mg soft gel capsules twice a day (morning and night), in combination with other anti-HIV medicines.

AGENERASE Capsules can be taken with or without food. However, you should not take AGENERASE with a high-fat meal because this could reduce the effectiveness of AGENERASE Capsules.

What should I do if I miss a dose of AGENERASE Capsules?

To help make sure that your anti-HIV therapy is as effective as possible, be very careful to take all of your medication exactly as your doctor prescribed it and do not skip any doses.

If you miss a dose of AGENERASE Capsules by more than 4 hours, wait and take the next dose at the regularly scheduled time. However, if you miss a dose by fewer than 4 hours, take your missed dose immediately. Then take your next dose at the regularly scheduled time. Do not take more or less than your prescribed dose of AGENERASE Capsules at any one time.

When your supply of AGENERASE Capsules or other anti-HIV drugs starts to run low, arrange to get more from your doctor or pharmacy. It is very important that you take anti-HIV drugs as prescribed by your doctor because the amount of virus in your blood may increase if one or more of the drugs is stopped, even for a short time.

Can AGENERASE Capsules be taken with other medications?

Protease inhibitors, including AGENERASE, may interact with other drugs, including those you take without a prescription. Before you take AGENERASE, tell your doctor about any drugs that you are taking or planning to take, including non-prescription drugs.

- **You should not take any of the following medications with AGENERASE Capsules because serious or life-threatening problems could occur.***
  HALCION® (triazolam)
  HISMANAL® (astemizole)
  Ergot medications (CAFERGOT® and others)
  PROPULSID® (cisapride)
  VERSED® (midazolam)
  VASCOR® (bepridil)
- **You should also not take rifampin** with AGENERASE Capsules because this drug reduces the effectiveness of AGENERASE. Rifampin is also known as: RIFADIN®, RIFAMATE®, RIFATER®, and RIMACTANE®.
- **Serious and/or life-threatening drug interactions can also occur if you take AGENERASE Capsules with any of the following drugs.*** If you need to take any of these drugs, your doctor may closely monitor the amount of drug in your blood to minimize potential problems.
  CORDARONE® (amiodarone)
  Phenobarbital
  DILANTIN® (phenytoin)
  Lidocaine
  COUMADIN® (warfarin)
  (quinidine) QUINAGLUTE®, CARDIOQUIN®, QUINIDEX®
  Antidepressants such as ELAVIL® (amitriptyline), NORPRAMIN® (desipramine), PAMELOR® (nortriptyline), TOFRANIL® (imipramine)
- Tell your doctor about any drugs that you are taking or planning to take, including non-prescription drugs.
- Before you take VIAGRA® (sildenafil) with AGENERASE, talk to your doctor about possible drug interactions and side effects. If you take VIAGRA and AGENERASE together, you may be at increased risk of side effects of VIAGRA such as low blood pressure, visual changes, and penile erection lasting more than 4 hours. If an erection lasts longer than 4 hours, your should seek immediate medical assistance to avoid permanent damage to your penis. Your doctor can explain these symptoms to you.
- If you use birth control pills, talk to your doctor about choosing a different type of contraceptive, since AGENERASE may reduce the effectiveness of some birth control pills.
- Because AGENERASE Capsules and Oral Solution contain large amounts of vitamin E, you should not take additional vitamin E while take AGENERASE.

- It is not recommended that you take AGENERASE with the cholesterol-lowering drugs MEVACOR® (lovastatin) or ZOCOR® (simvastatin) because of the possible drug interactions. There is also an increased risk of drug interactions between AGENERASE and LIPITOR® (atorvastatin) and BAYCOL® (cerivastatin) Talk to your doctor if you are taking or are planning to take these or other drugs for lowering cholesterol.
- **Special considerations:***
  If you take AGENERASE Capsules with MYCOBUTIN® (rifabutin), your doctor will lower the dose of MYCOBUTIN.
  If you take AGENERASE Capsules with VIDEX® (didanosine, ddl), take them at least 1 hour apart.
  If you take AGENERASE Capsules with antacids, take them at least 1 hour apart.

Do AGENERASE Capsules cure HIV infection or AIDS?
AGENERASE Capsules do not cure HIV infection or AIDS. At this time we do not know if AGENERASE will help you live longer or have fewer of the medical problems (opportunistic infections) that are associated with HIV infection or AIDS. Because of this, you must be sure to be seen regularly by your healthcare professional.

Do AGENERASE Capsules reduce the risk of passing HIV to others?
No. AGENERASE Capsules, as well as other anti-HIV medications, have not been shown to reduce the risk of passing HIV to others through sexual contact or blood contamination. Continue to practice safe sex and do not use or share dirty needles.

Who should not take AGENERASE Capsules?
Do not take AGENERASE Capsules if you have had a serious allergic reaction to AGENERASE or any of its ingredients. If you have liver disease, your dosage of AGENERASE may have to be adjusted.
If you are allergic to sulfa drugs, you should inform your doctor.

Can children take AGENERASE Capsules?
Children from 4 to 12 years of age can take AGENERASE Capsules. Your doctor will tell you if the oral solution or capsule is best for your child. Your child's doctor will decide the right dose based on your child's weight and age. **AGENERASE Oral Solution** should not be used in infants and children below 4 years of age.

Can pregnant women and nursing mothers take AGENERASE?
AGENERASE Capsules have not been studied in pregnant women and the risk to the unborn child is not known. Talk to your doctor if you are pregnant or if you become pregnant while taking AGENERASE.
AGENERASE Oral Solution should not be used in pregnant women.
Mothers with HIV should not breastfeed their infants because HIV in the breast milk can infect the infant.

What other medical conditions should I discuss with my doctor?
Talk to your doctor if you are pregnant or if you become pregnant while you are taking AGENERASE. Also talk to your doctor if you have hemophilia or problems with your liver or kidneys.

How should I store AGENERASE Capsules?
AGENERASE Capsules should be stored at room temperature and should not be refrigerated.

Other information:
This medication is prescribed for a particular condition. Do not use it for any other condition or give it to anybody else. Keep AGENERASE Capsules and all medicines out of the reach of children.
Ask a healthcare professional any questions you may have about AGENERASE.
AGENERASE is a registered trademark of the Glaxo Wellcome group of companies.
*The brands listed are trademarks of their respective owners and are not trademarks of the Glaxo Wellcome group of companies. The markers of these brands are not affiliated with and do not endorse Glaxo Wellcome or its products.
AGENERASE Capsules are manufactured by
R.P. Scherer, Beinheim, France
for Glaxo Wellcome Inc., Research Triangle Park, NC 27709
Licensed from Vertex Pharmaceuticals Incorporated
Cambridge, MA 02139
US Patent Nos. 5,585,397; 5,723,490; and 5,646,180

May 2000/RL-824

Shown in Product Identification Guide, page 314

AGENERASE® ℞

[*ă-jin 'ə-rās*]
(amprenavir)
Oral Solution

AGENERASE (amprenavir) in combination with other antiretroviral agents is indicated for the treatment of HIV-1 infection. This indication is based on analyses of plasma HIV RNA levels and CD4 cell counts in controlled studies of up to 24 weeks in duration. At present, there are no results from controlled trials evaluating long-term suppression of HIV RNA or disease progression with AGENERASE.

Because of the potential risk of toxicity from the large amount of the excipient propylene glycol, AGENERASE Oral Solution is contraindicated in infants and children below the age of 4 years, pregnant women, patients with hepatic or renal failure, and patients treated with disulfiram or metronidazole (see CONTRAINDICATIONS AND WARNINGS).
AGENERASE Oral Solution should be used only when AGENERASE Capsules or other protease inhibitor formulations are not therapeutic options.

Table 1: Average (%CV) Pharmacokinetic Parameters After 1200 mg b.i.d. of Amprenavir Capsules (n = 5)

C_{max} (mcg/mL)	t_{max} (hours)	AUC_{0-12} (mcg•h/mL)	C_{avg} (mcg/mL)	C_{min} (mcg/mL)	CL/F (mL/min/kg)
5.36 (62%)	1.9 (51%)	18.5 (63%)	1.54 (63%)	0.28 (52%)	31 (132%)

DESCRIPTION

AGENERASE (amprenavir) is an inhibitor of the human immunodeficiency virus (HIV) protease. The chemical name of amprenavir is (3*S*)-tetrahydro-3-furyl *N*-[(1*S*,2*R*)-3-(4-amino-*N*-isobutylbenzenesulfonamido)-1-benzyl-2-hydroxypropyl]carbamate. Amprenavir is a single stereoisomer with the (3*S*)(1*S*,2*R*) configuration. It has a molecular formula of $C_{25}H_{35}N_3O_6S$ and a molecular weight of 505.64. Amprenavir is a white to cream-colored solid with a solubility of approximately 0.04 mg/mL in water at 25°C.
AGENERASE Oral Solution is for oral administration. One milliliter (1 mL) of AGENERASE Oral Solution contains 15 mg of amprenavir in solution and the inactive ingredients acesulfame potassium, artificial grape bubblegum flavor, citric acid (anhydrous), d-alpha tocopheryl polyethylene glycol 1000 succinate (TPGS), menthol, natural peppermint flavor, polyethylene glycol 400 (PEG 400) (170 mg), propylene glycol (550 mg), saccharin sodium, sodium chloride, and sodium citrate (dihydrate). Solutions of sodium hydroxide and/or diluted hydrochloric acid may have been added to adjust pH. Each mL of AGENERASE Oral Solution contains 46 IU vitamin E in the form of d-alpha tocopheryl polyethylene glycol 1000 succinate. Propylene glycol is in the formulation to achieve adequate solubility of amprenavir. The recommended daily dose of AGENERASE Oral Solution of 22.5 mg/kg twice daily corresponds to a propylene glycol intake of 1650 mg/kg per day. Acceptable intake of propylene glycol for pharmaceuticals has not been established.

MICROBIOLOGY

Mechanism of Action: Amprenavir is an inhibitor of HIV-1 protease. Amprenavir binds to the active site of HIV-1 protease and thereby prevents the processing of viral gag and gag-pol polyprotein precursors, resulting in the formation of immature non-infectious viral particles.
Antiviral Activity *in Vitro*: The *in vitro* antiviral activity of amprenavir was evaluated against HIV-1 IIIB in both acutely and chronically infected lymphoblastic cell lines (MT-4, CEM-CCRF, H9) and in peripheral blood lymphocytes. The 50% inhibitory concentration (IC_{50}) of amprenavir ranged from 0.012 to 0.08 µM in acutely infected cells and was 0.41 µM in chronically infected cells (1 µM = 0.50 mcg/mL). Amprenavir exhibited synergistic anti-HIV-1 activity in combination with abacavir, zidovudine, didanosine, or saquinavir, and additive anti-HIV-1 activity in combination with indinavir, nelfinavir, and ritonavir *in vitro*. These drug combinations have not been adequately studied in humans. The relationship between *in vitro* anti-HIV-1 activity of amprenavir and the inhibition of HIV-1 replication in humans has not been defined.
Resistance: HIV-1 isolates with a decreased susceptibility to amprenavir have been selected *in vitro* and were also obtained from patients treated with amprenavir. Genotypic analysis of isolates from amprenavir-treated patients showed mutations in the HIV-1 protease gene resulting in amino acid substitutions primarily at positions M46I/L, I47V, I50V, I54L/V, and I84V as well as mutations in the viral protease p1/p6 cleavage site. Phenotypic analysis of HIV-1 isolates from some patients on amprenavir monotherapy for 8 to 12 weeks showed a 5- to 10-fold decrease in susceptibility to amprenavir *in vitro* compared to baseline. Phenotypic analysis of HIV-1 isolate from 28 patients treated with amprenavir in combination with zidovudine and lamivudine for 16 to 36 weeks identified isolates from 6 patients that exhibited a 5- to 11-fold decrease in susceptibility to amprenavir *in vitro* compared to wild-type virus. Clinical isolates that exhibited a decrease in amprenavir susceptibility harbored amprenavir-associated mutations. The clinical relevance of the genotypic and phenotypic changes associated with amprenavir therapy has not been established.
Cross-Resistance: Varying degrees of HIV-1 cross-resistance among protease inhibitors have been observed. The potential for protease inhibitor cross-resistance in HIV-1 isolates from amprenavir-treated patients has not been fully evaluated.

CLINICAL PHARMACOLOGY

Pharmacokinetics in Adults: The pharmacokinetic properties of amprenavir have been studied in asymptomatic, HIV-infected adult patients after administration of single oral doses of 150 to 1200 mg and multiple oral doses of 300 to 1200 mg twice daily.
Absorption and Bioavailability: Amprenavir was rapidly absorbed after oral administration in HIV-1-infected patients with a time to peak concentration (t_{max}) typically between 1 and 2 hours after a single oral dose. The absolute oral bioavailability of amprenavir in humans has not been established.
Increases in the area under the plasma concentration versus time curve (AUC) after single oral doses between 150 and 1200 mg were slightly greater than dose-proportional. Increases in AUC were dose-proportional after 3 weeks of dosing with doses from 300 to 1200 mg twice daily. The pharmacokinetic parameters after administration of amprenavir 1200 mg b.i.d. for 3 weeks to HIV-infected subjects are shown in Table 1.
[See table 1 above]
The relative bioavailability of AGENERASE Capsules and Oral Solution was assessed in healthy adults. AGENERASE Oral Solution was 14% less bioavailable compared to the capsules.
Effects of Food on Oral Absorption: The relative bioavailability of AGENERASE Capsules was assessed in the fasting and fed states in healthy volunteers (standardized high-fat meal: 967 kcal, 6 grams fat, 33 grams protein, 58 grams carbohydrate). Administration of a single 1200-mg dose of amprenavir in the fed state compared to the fasted state was associated with changes in C_{max} (fed: 6.18 ± 2.92 mcg/mL, fasted: 9.72 ± 2.75 mcg/mL), t_{max} (fed: 1.51 ± 0.68, fasted: 1.05 ± 0.63), and $AUC_{0-\infty}$ (fed: 22.06 ± 11.6 mcg•h/mL, fasted: 28.05 ± 10.1 mcg•h/mL). AGENERASE may be taken with or without food, but should not be taken with a high-fat meal (see DOSAGE AND ADMINISTRATION).
Distribution: The apparent volume of distribution (V_z/F) is approximately 430 L in healthy adult subjects. *In vitro* binding is approximately 90% to plasma proteins. The high affinity binding protein for amprenavir is alpha$_1$-acid glycoprotein (AAG). The partitioning of amprenavir into erythrocytes is low, but increases as amprenavir concentrations increase, reflecting the higher amount of unbound drug at higher concentrations.
Metabolism: Amprenavir is metabolized in the liver by the cytochrome P450 CYP3A4 enzyme system. The two major metabolites result from oxidation of the tetrahydrofuran and aniline moieties. Glucuronide conjugates of oxidized metabolites have been identified as minor metabolites in urine and feces.
AGENERASE Oral Solution contains a large amount of propylene glycol, which is hepatically metabolized by the alcohol and aldehyde dehydrogenase enzyme pathway. Alcohol dehydrogenase (ADH) is present in the human fetal liver at 2 months of gestational age, but at only 3% of adult activity. Although the data are limited, it appears that by 12 to 30 months of postnatal age, ADH activity is equal to or greater than that observed in adults. Additionally, certain patient groups (females, Asians, Eskimos, Native Americans) may be at increased risk of propylene glycol-associated adverse events due to diminished ability to metabolize propylene glycol (see CLINICAL PHARMACOLOGY: Special Populations: Gender and Race).
Elimination: Excretion of unchanged amprenavir in urine and feces is minimal. Approximately 14% and 75% of an administered single dose of ^{14}C-amprenavir can be accounted for as radiocarbon in urine and feces, respectively. Two metabolites accounted for >90% of the radiocarbon in fecal samples. The plasma elimination half-life of amprenavir ranged from 7.1 to 10.6 hours.
Special Populations: *Hepatic Insufficiency:* AGENERASE Oral Solution is contraindicated in patients with hepatic failure.
Patients with hepatic impairment are at increased risk of propylene glycol-associated adverse events (see WARNINGS). AGENERASE Oral Solution should be used with caution in patients with hepatic impairment. AGENERASE Capsules have been studied in adult patients with impaired hepatic function using a single 600-mg oral dose. The $AUC_{0-\infty}$ was significantly greater in patients with moderate cirrhosis (25.76 ± 14.68 mcg•h/mL) compared with healthy volunteers (12.00 ± 4.38 mcg•h/mL). The $AUC_{0-\infty}$ and C_{max} were significantly greater in patients with severe cirrhosis ($AUC_{0-\infty}$: 38.66 ± 16.08 mcg•h/mL; C_{max}: 9.43 ± 2.61 mcg/mL) compared with healthy volunteers ($AUC_{0-\infty}$: 12.00 ± 4.38 mcg•h/mL; C_{max}: 4.90 ± 1.39 mcg/mL). Patients with impaired hepatic function require dosage adjustment (see DOSAGE AND ADMINISTRATION).
Renal Insufficiency: AGENERASE Oral Solution is contraindicated in patients with renal failure.
Patients with renal impairment are at increased risk of propylene glycol-associated adverse events. Additionally, be-

Continued on next page

This product information is based on labeling in effect on June 23, 2000. For further information, contact via direct mail, phone, or web site. Medical Information, Glaxo Wellcome Inc., PO Box 13398, Research Triangle Park, NC 27709. Healthcare Professionals (Medical Information): 800-334-0089. Patients (Customer Response Center): 1-888-825-5249. Glaxo Wellcome Corporate Web Site: www.glaxowellcome.com

Agenerase Oral Solution—Cont.

cause metabolites of the excipient propylene glycol in AGENERASE Oral Solution may alter acid-base balance, patients with renal impairment should be monitored for potential adverse events (see WARNINGS). AGENERASE Oral Solution should be used with caution in patients with renal impairment. The impact of renal impairment on amprenavir elimination has not been studied. The renal elimination of unchanged amprenavir represents <3% of the administered dose.

Pediatric Patients: AGENERASE Oral Solution is contraindicated in infants and children below 4 years of age (see CONTRAINDICATIONS and WARNINGS).

The pharmacokinetics of amprenavir have been studied after either single or repeat doses of AGENERASE Capsules or Oral Solution in 84 pediatric patients. Twenty HIV-1-infected children ranging in age from 4 to 12 years received single doses from 5 mg/kg to 20 mg/kg using 25-mg or 150-mg capsules. The C_{max} of amprenavir increased less than proportionally with dose. The $AUC_{0-\infty}$ increased proportionally at doses between 5 and 20 mg/kg. Amprenavir is 14% less bioavailable from the liquid formulation than from the capsules; therefore **AGENERASE Capsules and AGENERASE Oral Solution are not interchangeable on a milligram per milligram basis.**

[See table 2 at right]

Geriatric Patients: The pharmacokinetics of amprenavir have not been studied in patients over 65 years of age.

Gender: The pharmacokinetics of amprenavir do not differ between males and females. Females may have a lower amount of alcohol dehydrogenase compared with males and may be at increased risk of propylene glycol-associated adverse events; no data are available on propylene glycol metabolism in females.

Race: The pharmacokinetics of amprenavir do not differ between Blacks and non-Blacks. Certain ethnic populations (Asians, Eskimos, and Native Americans) may be at increased risk of propylene glycol-associated adverse events because of alcohol dehydrogenase polymorphisms; no data are available on propylene glycol metabolism in these groups.

Drug Interactions: See also CONTRAINDICATIONS, WARNINGS, and PRECAUTIONS: Drug Interactions.

Amprenavir is metabolized in the liver by the cytochrome P450 enzyme system. Amprenavir inhibits CYP3A4. Caution should be used when coadministering medications that are substrates, inhibitors, or inducers of CYP3A4, or potentially toxic medications that are metabolized by CYP3A4. Amprenavir does not inhibit CYP2D6, CYP1A2, CYP2C9, CYP2C19, CYP2E1, or uridine glucuronosyltransferase (UDPGT).

Drug interaction studies were performed with amprenavir capsules and other drugs likely to be coadministered or drugs commonly used as probes for pharmacokinetic interactions. The effects of coadministration of amprenavir on the AUC, C_{max}, and C_{min} are summarized in Table 3 (effect of other drugs on amprenavir) and Table 4 (effect of amprenavir on other drugs). For information regarding clinical recommendations, see PRECAUTIONS.

[See table 3 at right]

[See table 4 at right]

Nucleoside Reverse Transcriptase Inhibitors (NRTIs): There was no effect of amprenavir on abacavir in subjects receiving both agents based on historical data.

HIV Protease Inhibitors: The effect of amprenavir on total drug concentrations of other HIV protease inhibitors in subjects receiving both agents was evaluated using comparisons to historical data. Indinavir steady-state C_{max}, AUC, and C_{min} were decreased by 22%, 38%, and 27%, respectively, by concomitant amprenavir. Similar decreases in C_{max} and AUC were seen after the first dose. Saquinavir steady-state C_{max}, AUC, and C_{min} were increased 21%, decreased 19%, and decreased 48%, respectively, by concomitant amprenavir. Nelfinavir steady-state C_{max}, AUC, and C_{min} were increased by 12%, 15%, and 14%, respectively, by concomitant amprenavir.

For information regarding clinical recommendations, see PRECAUTIONS: Drug Interactions.

Table 2: Average (%CV) Pharmacokinetic Parameters in Children Ages 4 to 12 Years Receiving 20 mg/kg b.i.d. or 15 mg/kg t.i.d. of AGENERASE Oral Solution

Dose	n	C_{max} (mcg/mL)	t_{max} (hours)	AUC_{ss}* (mcg•h/mL)	C_{avg} (mcg/mL)	C_{min} (mcg/mL)	CL/F (mL/min/kg)
20 mg/kg b.i.d.	20	6.77 (51%)	1.1 (21%)	15.46 (59%)	1.29 (59%)	0.24 (98%)	29 (58%)
15 mg/kg t.i.d.	17	3.99 (37%)	1.4 (90%)	8.73 (36%)	1.09 (36%)	0.27 (95%)	32 (34%)

*AUC is 0 to 12 hours for b.i.d. and 0 to 8 hours for t.i.d., therefore the C_{avg} is a better comparison of the exposures.

Table 3: Drug Interactions: Pharmacokinetic Parameters for Amprenavir in the Presence of the Coadministered Drug

Co-administered Drug	Dose of Coadministered Drug	Dose of AGENERASE	n	% Change in **Amprenavir** Pharmacokinetic Parameters* (90% CI)		
				C_{max}	AUC	C_{min}
Abacavir	300 mg b.i.d. for 3 weeks	900 mg b.i.d. for 3 weeks	4	↑47 (↓15 to ↑154)	↑29 (↓18 to ↑103)	↑27 (↓46 to ↑197)
Clarithromycin	500 mg b.i.d. for 4 days	1200 mg b.i.d. for 4 days	12	↑15 (↑1 to ↑31)	↑18 (↑8 to ↑29)	↑39 (↑31 to ↑47)
Indinavir	800 mg t.i.d. for 2 weeks (fasted)	750 or 800 mg t.i.d. for 2 weeks (fasted)	9	↑18 (↓13 to ↑58)	↑33 (↑2 to ↑73)	↑25 (↓27 to ↑116)
Ketoconazole	400 mg single dose	1200 mg single dose	12	↓16 (↓25 to ↓6)	↑31 (↑20 to ↑42)	NA
Lamivudine	150 mg single dose	600 mg single dose	11	⇔ (↓17 to ↑9)	⇔ (↓15 to ↑14)	NA
Nelfinavir	750 mg t.i.d. for 2 weeks (fed)	750 or 800 mg t.i.d. for 2 weeks (fed)	6	↓14 (↓38 to ↑20)	⇔ (↓19 to ↑47)	↑189 (↑52 to ↑448)
Rifabutin	300 mg q.d. for 10 days	1200 mg b.i.d. for 10 days	5	⇔ (↓21 to ↑10)	↓15 (↓28 to 0)	↓15 (↓38 to ↑17)
Rifampin	300 mg q.d. for 4 days	1200 mg b.i.d. for 4 days	11	↓70 (↓76 to ↓62)	↓82 (↓84 to ↓78)	↓92 (↓95 to ↓89)
Saquinavir	800 mg t.i.d. for 2 weeks (fed)	750 or 800 mg t.i.d. for 2 weeks (fed)	7	↓37 (↓54 to ↓14)	↓32 (↓49 to ↓9)	↓14 (↓52 to ↑54)
Zidovudine	300 mg single dose	600 mg single dose	12	⇔ (↓5 to ↑24)	↑13 (↓2 to ↑31)	NA

*Based on total-drug concentrations.
↑ = Increase; ↓ = Decrease; ⇔ = No change (↑ or ↓<10%); NA = C_{min} not calculated for single-dose study.

Table 4: Drug Interactions: Pharmacokinetic Parameters for Coadministered Drug in the Presence of Amprenavir

Co-administered Drug	Dose of Co-administered Drug	Dose of AGENERASE	n	% Change in Pharmacokinetic Parameters of **Coadministered Drug** (90% CI)		
				C_{max}	AUC	C_{min}
Clarithromycin	500 mg b.i.d. for 4 days	1200 mg b.i.d. for 4 days	12	↑10 (↓24 to ↑7)	⇔ (↓17 to ↑11)	⇔ (↓13 to ↑20)
Ketoconazole	400 mg single dose	1200 mg single dose	12	↑19 (↑8 to ↑33)	↑44 (↑31 to ↑59)	NA
Lamivudine	150 mg single dose	600 mg single dose	11	⇔ (↓17 to ↑3)	⇔ (↓11 to 0)	NA
Rifabutin	300 mg q.d. for 10 days	1200 mg b.i.d. for 10 days	5	↑119 (↑82 to ↑164)	↑193 (↑156 to ↑235)	↑271 (↑171 to ↑409)
Rifampin	300 mg q.d. for 4 days	1200 mg b.i.d. for 4 days	11	⇔ (↓13 to ↑12)	⇔ (↓10 to ↑13)	ND
Zidovudine	300 mg single dose	600 mg single dose	12	↑40 (↑14 to ↑71)	↑31 (↑19 to ↑45)	NA

↑ = Increase; ↓ = Decrease; ⇔ = No change (↑ or ↓<10%); NA = C_{min} not calculated for single-dose study; ND = Interaction cannot be determined as C_{min} was below the lower limit of quantitation.

INDICATIONS AND USAGE

AGENERASE (amprenavir) in combination with other antiretroviral agents is indicated for the treatment of HIV-1 infection. This indication is based on analyses of plasma HIV RNA levels and CD4 cell counts in controlled studies of up to 24 weeks in duration. At present, there are no results from controlled trials evaluating long-term suppression of HIV RNA or disease progression with AGENERASE (see Description of Clinical Studies).

AGENERASE Oral Solution should be used only when AGENERASE Capsules or other protease inhibitor formulations are not therapeutic options.

Description of Clinical Studies: ***Therapy-Naive Adults:*** PROAB3001, an ongoing, randomized, double-blind, placebo-controlled, multicenter study, compared treatment with AGENERASE Capsules (1200 mg twice daily) plus lamivudine (150 mg twice daily) plus zidovudine (300 mg twice daily) versus lamivudine (150 mg twice daily) plus zidovudine (300 mg twice daily) in 232 patients, median age 37 years (range 18 to 63 years), 75% Caucasian, 89% male, with a median CD4 cell count of 416 cells/mm^3 (range 139 to 1800 cells/mm^3) and a median plasma HIV-1 RNA of 4.67 log_{10} copies/mL (range 3.06 to 6.31 log_{10} copies/mL) at baseline. Through 24 weeks of therapy, there was no significant difference in the median CD4 cell count between the treatment arms. Figure 1 shows the proportions of patients with plasma HIV-1 RNA levels <400 copies/mL through 24 weeks.

[See figure 1 at top of next page]

HIV-1 RNA status and reasons for discontinuation of randomized treatment at 24 weeks are summarized (Table 5).

[See table 5 at bottom of next page]

Therapy-Experienced Adults: PROAB3006, an ongoing, randomized, open-label multicenter study, compared treatment with AGENERASE Capsules (1200 mg twice daily) plus NRTIs versus indinavir (800 mg every 8 hours) plus NRTIs in 504 NRTI- and non-nucleoside reverse transcriptase inhibitor- (NNRTI) experienced, protease inhibitor-naive patients, median age 37 years (range 20 to 71 years), 72% Caucasian, 80% male, with a median CD4 cell count of 399 cells/mm^3 (range 9 to 1706 cells/mm^3) and a median plasma HIV-1 RNA level of 3.93 log_{10} copies/mL (range 2.60 to 7.01 log_{10} copies/mL) at baseline. Through 24 weeks of therapy, there was a smaller increase in median CD4 cell count from baseline for the amprenavir group than for the indinavir group. Figure 2 shows the proportions of patients with plasma HIV-1 RNA levels <400 copies/mL through 24 weeks.

[See figure 2 in next column]

HIV-1 RNA status and reasons for discontinuation of randomized treatment at 24 weeks are summarized (Table 6).

[See table 6 at bottom of next page]

CONTRAINDICATIONS

Because of the potential risk of toxicity from the large amount of the excipient propylene glycol, AGENERASE

Figure 1: Virologic Response Through Week 24, PROAB3001[1,2]

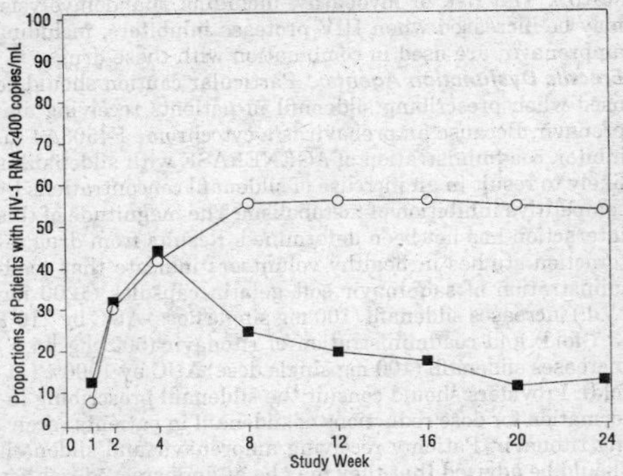

○ AGENERASE/Lamivudine/Zidovudine (n = 116)
■ Lamivudine/Zidovudine (n = 116)
[1]Roche AMPLICOR HIV-1 MONITOR assay.
[2]Discontinuations and missing data were considered as HIV-1 RNA ≥400 copies/mL.

Figure 2: Virologic Response Through Week 24, PROAB3006[3,4]

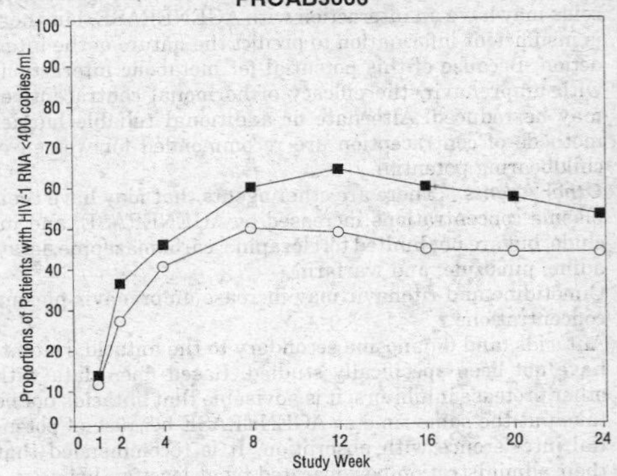

○ AGENERASE plus NRTIs (n = 254)
■ Indinavir plus NRTIs (n = 250)
[3]Roche AMPLICOR HIV-1 MONITOR assay.
[4]Discontinuations and missing data were considered as HIV-1 RNA ≥400 copies/mL.

Oral Solution is contraindicated in infants and children below the age of 4 years, pregnant women, patients with hepatic or renal failure, and patients treated with disulfiram or metronidazole (see WARNINGS and PRECAUTIONS). AGENERASE also should not be administered concurrently with astemizole, bepridil, cisapride, dihydroergotamine, ergotamine, midazolam, and triazolam. Although these drugs have not been specifically studied, coadministration may result in competitive inhibition of metabolism of these products and may cause serious or life-threatening adverse events. (See WARNINGS for agents whose coadministration may result in competitive inhibition of metabolism but for which concentration monitoring is recommended.)

AGENERASE is contraindicated in patients with previously demonstrated clinically significant hypersensitivity to any of the components of this product.

WARNINGS

Because of the potential risk of toxicity from the large amount of the excipient propylene glycol, AGENERASE Oral Solution is contraindicated in infants and children below the age of 4 years, pregnant women, patients with hepatic or renal failure, and patients treated with disulfiram or metronidazole (see CLINICAL PHARMACOLOGY, CONTRAINDICATIONS, and PRECAUTIONS).

Because of the possible toxicity associated with the large amount of propylene glycol and the lack of information on chronic exposure to large amounts of propylene glycol, AGENERASE Oral Solution should be used only when AGENERASE Capsules or other protease inhibitor formulations are not therapeutic options. Certain ethnic populations (Asians, Eskimos, Native Americans) and women may be at increased risk of propylene glycol-associated adverse events due to diminished ability to metabolize propylene glycol; no data are available on propylene glycol metabolism in these groups (see CLINICAL PHARMACOLOGY: Special Populations: Gender and Race).

If patients require treatment with AGENERASE Oral Solution, they should be monitored closely for propylene glycol-associated adverse events, including seizures, stupor, tachycardia, hyperosmolality, lactic acidosis, renal toxicity, and hemolysis. Patients should be switched from AGENERASE Oral Solution to AGENERASE Capsules as soon as they are able to take the capsule formulation.

Use of alcoholic beverages is not recommended in patients treated with AGENERASE Oral Solution.

Serious and/or life-threatening drug interactions could occur between amprenavir and amiodarone, lidocaine (systemic), tricyclic antidepressants, and quinidine. Concentration monitoring of these agents is recommended if these agents are used concomitantly with AGENERASE (see CONTRAINDICATIONS).

Rifampin should not be used in combination with amprenavir because it reduces plasma concentrations and AUC of amprenavir by about 90%.

Concomitant use of AGENERASE with lovastatin or simvastatin is not recommended. Caution should be exercised if HIV protease inhibitors, including AGENERASE, are used concurrently with other HMG-CoA reductase inhibitors that are also metabolized by the CYP3A4 pathway (e.g., atorvastatin or cerivastatin). The risk of myopathy, including rhabdomyolysis, may be increased when HIV protease inhibitors, including amprenavir, are used in combination with these drugs.

Particular caution should be used when prescribing sildenafil in patients receiving amprenavir. Coadministration of AGENERASE with sildenafil is expected to substantially increase sildenafil concentrations and may result in an increase in sildenafil-associated adverse events, including hypotension, visual changes, and priapism (see PRECAUTIONS: Drug Interactions and Information for Patients, and the complete prescribing information for sildenafil).

Severe and life-threatening skin reactions, including Stevens-Johnson syndrome, have occurred in patients treated with AGENERASE (see ADVERSE REACTIONS).

Acute hemolytic anemia has been reported in a patient treated with AGENERASE.

New onset diabetes mellitus, exacerbation of pre-existing diabetes mellitus, and hyperglycemia have been reported during post-marketing surveillance in HIV-infected patients receiving protease inhibitor therapy. Some patients required either initiation or dose adjustments of insulin or oral hypoglycemic agents for treatment of these events. In some cases, diabetic ketoacidosis has occurred. In those patients who discontinued protease inhibitor therapy, hyperglycemia persisted in some cases. Because these events have been reported voluntarily during clinical practice, estimates of frequency cannot be made and causal relationships between protease inhibitor therapy and these events have not been established.

PRECAUTIONS

General: AGENERASE Capsules and AGENERASE Oral Solution are not interchangeable on a milligram per milligram basis (see CLINICAL PHARMACOLOGY: Pediatric Patients and CONTRAINDICATIONS).

Amprenavir is a sulfonamide. The potential for cross-sensitivity between drugs in the sulfonamide class and amprenavir is unknown. Patients with a known sulfonamide allergy should be treated with caution.

AGENERASE is principally metabolized by the liver; therefore caution should be exercised when administering this drug to patients with hepatic impairment (see DOSAGE AND ADMINISTRATION).

Formulations of AGENERASE provide high daily doses of vitamin E (see Information for Patients, DESCRIPTION, and DOSAGE AND ADMINISTRATION). The effects of long-term, high-dose vitamin E administration in humans is not well characterized and has not been specifically studied in HIV-infected individuals. High vitamin E doses may exacerbate the blood coagulation defect of vitamin K deficiency caused by anticoagulant therapy or malabsorption.

Patients with Hemophilia: There have been reports of spontaneous bleeding in patients with hemophilia A and B treated with protease inhibitors. In some patients, additional factor VIII was required. In many of the reported cases, treatment with protease inhibitors was continued or restarted. A causal relationship between protease inhibitor therapy and these episodes has not been established.

Fat Redistribution: Redistribution/accumulation of body fat including central obesity, dorsocervical fat enlargement (buffalo hump), peripheral wasting, breast enlargement, and "cushingoid appearance" have been observed in patients receiving protease inhibitors. The mechanism and long-term consequences of these events are currently unknown. A causal relationship has not been established.

Resistance/Cross-Resistance: Because of the potential for HIV cross-resistance among protease inhibitors has not been fully explored, it is unknown what effect amprenavir therapy will have on the activity of subsequently administered protease inhibitors (see MICROBIOLOGY).

Information for Patients: A Patient Package Insert (PPI) for AGENERASE Oral Solution is available for patient information.

AGENERASE Oral Solution is contraindicated in infants and children below the age of 4 years, pregnant women, patients with hepatic or renal failure, and patients treated with disulfiram or metronidazole. AGENERASE Oral Solution should be used only when AGENERASE Capsules or other protease inhibitor formulations are not therapeutic options.

Patients treated with AGENERASE Capsules should be cautioned against switching to AGENERASE Oral Solution because of the increased risk of adverse events from the large amount of propylene glycol in AGENERASE Oral Solution.

Women, Asians, Eskimos, or Native Americans, as well as patients who have hepatic or renal insufficiency, should be informed that they may be at increased risk of adverse events from the large amount of propylene glycol in AGENERASE Oral Solution.

Patients should be informed that AGENERASE is not a cure for HIV infection and that they may continue to develop opportunistic infections and other complications associated with HIV disease. The long-term effects of AGENERASE (amprenavir) are unknown at this time. Patients should be told that there are currently no data demonstrating that therapy with AGENERASE can reduce the risk of transmitting HIV to others through sexual contact. Patients should remain under the care of a physician while using AGENERASE. Patients should be advised to take AGENERASE every day as prescribed. AGENERASE must always be used in combination with other antiretroviral drugs. Patients should not alter the dose or discontinue therapy without consulting their physician. If a dose is

Continued on next page

Table 5: Outcomes of Randomized Treatment Through Week 24 (PROAB3001)

Outcome	AGENERASE (n = 116)	Placebo (n = 116)
HIV RNA <400 copies/mL*	53%	11%
HIV RNA ≥400 copies/mL†,‡	13%	62%
CDC Class C event‡	0%	0%
Discontinued due to adverse events‡	15%	3%
Discontinued due to other reasons‡,§	19%	22%
On treatment with missing HIV RNA value‡	0%	1%
TOTAL	100%	100%

*Corresponds to rates at Week 24 in Figure 1.
†Includes discontinuations due to virological failure at or before Week 24.
‡Treatment failure in the analysis.
§Consent withdrawn, lost to follow-up, and protocol violation.

Table 6: Outcomes of Randomized Treatment Through Week 24 (PROAB3006)

Outcome	AGENERASE (n = 254)	Indinavir (n = 250)
HIV RNA <400 copies/mL*	43%	53%
HIV RNA ≥400 copies/mL†,‡	22%	18%
CDC Class C event‡	<1%	2%
Discontinued due to adverse events‡	16%	8%
Discontinued due to other reasons‡,§	14%	12%
On treatment with missing HIV RNA value‡	4%	7%
TOTAL	100%	100%

*Corresponds to rates at Week 24 in Figure 2.
†Includes discontinuations due to virological failure at or before Week 24.
‡Treatment failure in the analysis.
§Consent withdrawn, lost to follow-up, and protocol violation.

This product information is based on labeling in effect on June 23, 2000. For further information, contact via direct mail, phone, or web site. Medical Information, Glaxo Wellcome Inc., PO Box 13398, Research Triangle Park, NC 27709. Healthcare Professionals (Medical Information): 800-334-0089. Patients (Customer Response Center): 1-888-825-5249. Glaxo Wellcome Corporate Web Site: www.glaxowellcome.com

Agenerase Oral Solution—Cont.

missed, patients should take the dose as soon as possible and then return to their normal schedule. However, if a dose is skipped, the patient should not double the next dose.
Patients should inform their doctor if they have a sulfa allergy. The potential for cross-sensitivity between drugs in the sulfonamide class and amprenavir is unknown.
Some drugs should not be used with AGENERASE. Therefore, patients should be advised that they must report to their doctor the use of any other prescription or nonprescription medication.
Patients taking antacids (or didanosine) should take AGENERASE at least 1 hour before or after antacid (or didanosine) use.
Patients should be advised that drinking alcoholic beverages is not recommended while taking AGENERASE Oral Solution.
Patients receiving sildenafil should be advised that they may be at an increased risk of sildenafil-associated adverse events including hypotension, visual changes, and priapism, and should promptly report any symptoms to their doctor.
Patients receiving hormonal contraceptives should be instructed that alternate contraceptive measures should be used during therapy with AGENERASE.
High-fat meals may decrease the absorption of AGENERASE and should be avoided. AGENERASE may be taken with meals of normal fat content.
Patients should be informed that redistribution or accumulation of body fat may occur in patients receiving protease inhibitors and that the cause and long-term health effects of these conditions are not known at this time.
Adult and pediatric patients should be advised not to take supplemental vitamin E since the vitamin E content of AGENERASE exceeds the Reference Daily Intake (adults 30 IU, pediatrics approximately 10 IU).

Drug Interactions: See also CONTRAINDICATIONS, WARNINGS, and CLINICAL PHARMACOLOGY: Drug Interactions.
AGENERASE is an inhibitor of cytochrome P450 CYP3A4 metabolism and therefore should not be administered concurrently with medications with narrow therapeutic windows that are substrates of CYP3A4. There are other agents that may result in serious and/or life-threatening drug interactions (see CONTRAINDICATIONS and WARNINGS). [See table 7 below]
Antimycobacterials: Rifampin: Rifampin should not be used in combination with amprenavir since it reduces plasma concentrations and AUC of amprenavir by about 90%.
Rifabutin: Coadministration of amprenavir with rifabutin results in a 15% decrease in amprenavir plasma AUC and a 193% increase in rifabutin plasma AUC. A dosage reduction of rifabutin to at least half the recommended dose is required when AGENERASE and rifabutin are coadministered (see CLINICAL PHARMACOLOGY: Drug Interactions). A complete blood count should be performed weekly and as clinically indicated in order to monitor for neutropenia in patients receiving amprenavir and rifabutin.
Other Potentially Significant Drug Interactions: Other medications that interact at CYP3A4, either as substrates, inhibitors, or inducers of the enzyme, could have potential interactions when used concomitantly. The clinical significance of these potential interactions is unknown and has not been studied.
Antibiotics: Dapsone and erythromycin may have their plasma concentrations increased by AGENERASE. Erythromycin may also increase amprenavir serum concentrations.
Antifungals: Itraconazole may have its plasma concentrations increased by AGENERASE. Itraconazole may increase serum concentrations of amprenavir.
Benzodiazepines: Alprazolam, clorazepate, diazepam, and flurazepam may have their serum concentrations increased by AGENERASE, which could increase their activity.
Calcium Channel Blockers: Diltiazem, nicardipine, nifedipine, and nimodipine may have their serum concentrations increased by AGENERASE, which could increase their activity.
Cholesterol-Lowering Agents: Atorvastatin, cerivastatin, lovastatin, pravastatin, and simvastatin may have their serum concentration increased by AGENERASE, which could increase their activity or toxicity. Concomitant use of AGENERASE with lovastatin or simvastatin is not recommended. Caution should be exercised if HIV protease inhibitors, including AGENERASE, are used concurrently with other HMG-CoA reductase inhibitors that are also metabolized by the CYP3A4 pathway (e.g., atorvastatin or cerivastatin). The risk of myopathy, including rhabdomyolysis, may be increased when HIV protease inhibitors, including amprenavir, are used in combination with these drugs.
Erectile Dysfunction Agents: Particular caution should be used when prescribing sildenafil in patients receiving amprenavir. Because amprenavir is a cytochrome P4503A4 inhibitor, coadministration of AGENERASE with sildenafil is likely to result in an increase of sildenafil concentrations by competitive inhibition of metabolism. The magnitude of this interaction has not been determined. Results from drug interaction studies in healthy volunteers indicate that coadministration of saquinavir soft gelatin capsules (1200 mg t.i.d.) increases sildenafil (100 mg single dose) AUC by 210% (3.1-fold) and coadministration of ritonavir (500 mg b.i.d.) increases sildenafil (100 mg single dose) AUC by 1000% (11-fold). Providers should consult the sildenafil prescribing information for dose reductions of sildenafil in patients receiving ritonavir. Patients receiving amprenavir and sildenafil should be advised that they may be at an increased risk for sildenafil-associated adverse events, including hypotension, visual changes, and priapism, and should report these symptoms promptly to their doctor.
NNRTIs: NNRTIs have the potential to increase (delavirdine) or decrease (efavirenz, nevirapine) serum concentrations of amprenavir.
Steroids: Estrogens, progestogens, and some glucocorticoids may have an interaction with AGENERASE, but there is insufficient information to predict the nature of the interaction. Because of this potential for metabolic interactions with amprenavir, the efficacy of hormonal contraceptives may be reduced. Alternate or additional reliable barrier methods of contraception are recommended for women of childbearing potential.
Other Agents: There are other agents that may have their plasma concentrations increased by AGENERASE, and include, but are not limited to: clozapine, carbamazepine, loratadine, pimozide, and warfarin.
Cimetidine and ritonavir may increase amprenavir plasma concentrations.
Antacids (and didanosine secondary to the antacid content) have not been specifically studied. Based upon data with other protease inhibitors, it is advisable that antacids not be taken at the same time as AGENERASE because of potential interference with absorption. It is recommended that their administration be separated by at least an hour.
Use of alcoholic beverages is not recommended in patients treated with AGENERASE Oral Solution.

Table 7: Drug Interactions with AGENERASE

Should Not Be Coadministered

Drug Class	Drug Within Class Not To Be Coadministered
Alcohol dependence treatment	Disulfiram (do not administer with AGENERASE Oral Solution)
Antibiotics	Metronidazole (do not administer with AGENERASE Oral Solution)
Antihistamines	Astemizole
Antimycobacterials	Rifampin*
Benzodiazepines	Midazolam, triazolam
Cardiovascular	Bepridil
Ergot derivatives	Dihydroergotamine, ergotamine
GI motility agents	Cisapride

*Decreases plasma concentrations of amprenavir and should not be coadministered as it is likely to reduce antiviral activity.

Coadministration Requires Concentration Monitoring

Drug Class	Drug Within Class to Monitor
Antiarrhythmics	Amiodarone, lidocaine (systemic), quinidine
Anticoagulants	Warfarin*
Antidepressants	Tricyclic antidepressants

*Monitor INR (International Normalized Ratio).

Dosage Adjustment Required

Drug Class	Drug Within Class Requiring a Dosage Adjustment
Antimycobacterials	Rifabutin (reduce dose to at least half that recommended)*

*A complete blood count should be performed weekly and as clinically indicated in order to monitor for neutropenia in patients receiving amprenavir and rifabutin.

Other Potentially Significant Drug Interactions

Anticonvulsants: phenobarbital, phenytoin, carbamazepine	Induce CYP3A4 and may decrease amprenavir concentrations.
Cholesterol-lowering agents: atorvastatin, cerivastatin, lovastatin, pravastatin, and simvastatin	May have their serum concentrations increased by AGENERASE, which could increase their activity or toxicity (see WARNINGS).
Erectile dysfunction agents: sildenafil	Expected to substantially increase sildenafil concentrations (consult sildenafil prescribing information for dose reduction of sildenafil in patients receiving ritonavir).

Carcinogenesis and Mutagenesis: Long-term carcinogenicity studies of amprenavir in rodents are in progress. Amprenavir was not mutagenic or genotoxic in a battery of *in vitro* and *in vivo* assays including bacterial reverse mutation (Ames), mouse lymphoma, rat micronucleus, and chromosome aberrations in human lymphocytes.
Fertility: The effects of amprenavir on fertility and general reproductive performance were investigated in male rats (treated for 28 days before mating, at doses producing up to twice the expected clinical exposure based on AUC comparisons) and female rats (treated for 15 days before mating through day 17 of gestation at doses producing up to 2 times the expected clinical exposure). Amprenavir did not impair mating or fertility of male or female rats and did not affect the development and maturation of sperm from treated rats. The reproductive performance of the F1 generation born to female rats given amprenavir was not different from control animals.
Pregnancy and Reproduction: AGENERASE Oral Solution is contraindicated during pregnancy due to the potential risk of toxicity to the fetus from the high propylene glycol content. Therefore, if AGENERASE is used in pregnant women, the AGENERASE Capsules formulation should be used (see complete prescribing information for AGENERASE Capsules).
Antiretroviral Pregnancy Registry: To monitor maternal-fetal outcomes of pregnant women exposed to AGENERASE, an Antiretroviral Pregnancy Registry has been established. Physicians are encouraged to register patients by calling 1-800-258-4263.
Nursing Mothers: The Centers for Disease Control and Prevention recommend that HIV-infected mothers not breastfeed their infants to avoid risking postnatal transmission of HIV. Although it is not known if amprenavir is excreted in human milk, amprenavir is secreted into the milk of lactating rats. Because of both the potential for HIV transmission and any possible adverse effects of amprenavir, **mothers should be instructed not to breastfeed if they are receiving AGENERASE.**
Pediatric Use: AGENERASE Oral Solution is contraindicated in infants and children below the age of 4 years due to the potential risk of toxicity from the excipient propylene glycol (see CONTRAINDICATIONS and WARNINGS). Alcohol dehydrogenase (ADH), which metabolizes propylene glycol, is present in the human fetal liver at 2 months of gestational age, but at only 3% of adult activity. Although the data are limited, it appears that by 12 to 30 months of postnatal age, ADH activity is equal to or greater than that observed in adults.
One hundred eighteen patients 4 to 17 years of age have received amprenavir as single or multiple doses in studies. An adverse event profile similar to that seen in adults was seen in pediatric patients.
Geriatric Use: Clinical studies of AGENERASE did not include sufficient numbers of patients aged 65 and over to de-

termine whether they respond differently from younger adults. In general, dose selection for an elderly patient should be cautious, reflecting the greater frequency of decreased hepatic, renal, or cardiac function, and of concomitant disease or other drug therapy.

ADVERSE REACTIONS

Rates of discontinuation of randomized therapy due to adverse events were 15% in amprenavir vs 3% in placebo recipients from Study 3001, and 16% in amprenavir vs 8% in indinavir recipients from Study 3006. In these studies, adverse events leading to amprenavir discontinuation included gastrointestinal events (11%), rash (3%), and paresthesias (<1%).

Most gastrointestinal events (nausea, vomiting, diarrhea, and abdominal pain) that led to amprenavir discontinuation were graded as mild or moderate in severity.

In all multidose studies in HIV-infected patients, skin rash occurred in 28% of patients treated with amprenavir. Rashes were usually maculopapular and of mild or moderate intensity, some with pruritus. Rashes had onsets ranging from 7 to 73 days (median: 10 days) after amprenavir initiation. With mild or moderate rash, amprenavir dose was often continued without interruption; if interrupted, reintroduction of amprenavir generally did not result in rash recurrence (Phase 3 studies).

Severe or life-threatening rash, including Stevens-Johnson syndrome, occurred in 1% of recipients of AGENERASE (4% of recipients who developed rash) (see WARNINGS). Amprenavir therapy should be discontinued for severe or life-threatening rashes and for moderate rashes accompanied by systemic symptoms.

[See table 8 at right]

In Phase 3 studies, 1 patient experienced diabetes mellitus *de novo*, and another developed a dorsocervical fat enlargement (buffalo hump).

[See table 9 at right]

In studies 3001 and 3006, no increased frequency of Grade 3 or 4 AST, ALT, amylase, or bilirubin elevations was seen compared to controls.

Pediatric Patients: An adverse event profile similar to that seen in adults was seen in pediatric patients.

OVERDOSAGE

There is no known antidote for AGENERASE. It is not known whether amprenavir can be removed by peritoneal dialysis or hemodialysis. If overdosage occurs, the patient should be monitored for evidence of toxicity and standard supportive treatment applied as necessary.

AGENERASE Oral Solution contains large amounts of propylene glycol. In the event of overdosage, monitoring and management of acid-base abnormalities is recommended. Propylene glycol can be removed by hemodialysis.

DOSAGE AND ADMINISTRATION

AGENERASE may be taken with or without food; however, a high-fat meal decreases the absorption of amprenavir and should be avoided (see CLINICAL PHARMACOLOGY: Effects of Food on Oral Absorption). **Adult and pediatric patients should be advised not to take supplemental vitamin E since the vitamin E content of AGENERASE Oral Solution exceeds the Reference Daily Intake (adults 30 IU, pediatrics approximately 10 IU) (see DESCRIPTION).**

The recommended dose of AGENERASE Oral Solution based on body weight and age is shown in Table 10. **Consideration should be given to switching patients from AGENERASE Oral Solution to AGENERASE Capsules as soon as they are able to take the capsule formulation (see WARNINGS).**

[See table 10 at right]

Patients with Hepatic Impairment: AGENERASE Oral Solution is contraindicated in patients with hepatic failure (see CONTRAINDICATIONS).

Patients with hepatic impairment are at increased risk of propylene glycol-associated adverse events (see WARNINGS). AGENERASE Oral Solution should be used with caution in patients with hepatic impairment. Based on a study with AGENERASE Capsules, adult patients with a Child-Pugh score ranging from 5 to 8 should receive a reduced dose of AGENERASE Oral Solution of 513 mg (34 mL) twice daily, and adult patients with a Child-Pugh score ranging from 9 to 12 should receive a reduced dose of AGENERASE Oral Solution of 342 mg (23 mL) twice daily (see CLINICAL PHARMACOLOGY: Hepatic Insufficiency). AGENERASE Oral Solution has not been studied in children with hepatic impairment.

Renal Insufficiency: AGENERASE Oral Solution is contraindicated in patients with renal failure (see CONTRAINDICATIONS).

Patients with renal impairment are at increased risk of propylene glycol-associated adverse events. AGENERASE Oral Solution should be used with caution in patients with renal impairment (see WARNINGS).

AGENERASE Capsules and AGENERASE Oral Solution are not interchangeable on a milligram per milligram basis (see CLINICAL PHARMACOLOGY).

HOW SUPPLIED

AGENERASE Oral Solution, a clear, pale yellow to yellow, grape bubblegum-peppermint-flavored liquid, contains 15 mg of amprenavir in each 1 mL.

Bottles of 240 mL with child-resistant closures (NDC 0173-0687-00). This product does not require reconstitution.

Store at controlled room temperature of 25°C (77°F) (see USP).

Table 8: Selected Clinical Adverse Events Grades 1-4 (≥5% Frequency)

Adverse Event	PROAB3001 Therapy-Naive Patients		PROAB3006 NRTI-Experienced Patients	
	AGENERASE*/ Lamivudine/ Zidovudine (n = 113)	Lamivudine/ Zidovudine (n = 109)	AGENERASE*/ NRTI (n = 245)	Indinavir/NRTI (n = 241)
Digestive				
Nausea	73%	50%	38%	26%
Vomiting	29%	17%	20%	11%
Diarrhea or loose stools	33%	34%	56%	32%
Taste disorders	10%	5%	1%	7%
Skin				
Rash	25%	6%	18%	10%
Nervous				
Paresthesia, oral/perioral	26%	5%	30%	2%
Paresthesia (including peripheral)	8%	3%	12%	9%
Psychiatric				
Depressive or mood disorders	15%	4%	4%	6%

*AGENERASE Capsules

Table 9: Selected Laboratory Abnormalities Grades 1-4 Reported in ≥5% of Patients

Laboratory Abnormality (non-fasting specimens)	PROAB3001 Therapy-Naive Patients		PROAB3006 NRTI-Experienced Patients	
	AGENERASE*/ Lamivudine/ Zidovudine (n = 113)	Lamivudine/ Zidovudine (n = 109)	AGENERASE*/ NRTI (n = 245)	Indinavir/NRTI (n = 241)
Hyperglycemia (>116 mg/dL)	37%	29%	41%	44%
Hypertriglyceridemia (>213 mg/dL)	36%	22%	47%	40%
Hypercholesterolemia (>283 mg/dL)	4%	3%	9%	10%

*AGENERASE Capsules

Table 10: Recommended Dosages of AGENERASE Oral Solution

Age/Weight Criteria	Dose	
	b.i.d.	t.i.d.
4 - 12 years or 13 - 16 years and <50 kg	22.5 mg/kg (1.5 mL/kg) (maximum dose 2800 mg per day)	17 mg/kg (1.1 mL/kg) (maximum dose 2800 mg per day)
13 - 16 years and ≥50 kg or >16 years	1400 mg	NA

PATIENT INFORMATION

AGENERASE® (amprenavir) Oral Solution

Please read this information before you start taking AGENERASE (pronounced ah-GEN-er-ase) Oral Solution, and re-read it each time you receive your prescription, just in case something has changed. Remember that this information does not take the place of careful discussions with your doctor when you start this medication and at checkups. You should not change or stop your anti-HIV treatment without first talking with your doctor. **You should tell your doctor about any drug you are taking or planning to take because taking AGENERASE Oral Solution with some medications can result in serious or life-threatening problems.**

What is AGENERASE Oral Solution?

AGENERASE Oral Solution is a medication used to treat HIV infection. HIV is the virus that causes AIDS (acquired immune deficiency syndrome). AGENERASE Oral Solution is taken by mouth as an oral solution. It belongs to a class of anti-HIV medicines called protease inhibitors.

What is the Important Safety Information on AGENERASE Oral Solution?

AGENERASE Oral Solution should not be used in infants and children below the age of 4 years, pregnant women, patients with liver or kidney failure, and patients receiving disulfiram (ANTABUSE®) or metronidazole (FLAGYL®).

AGENERASE Oral Solution contains a large amount of propylene glycol, a liquid needed to dissolve amprenavir. Because of the possible side effects of the large amount of propylene glycol, AGENERASE Oral Solution should be used only when AGENERASE Capsules or other protease inhibitor formulations are not options. You should not switch from AGENERASE Capsules to AGENERASE Oral Solution without talking to your doctor.

If you are a woman or an Asian, Eskimo, or Native American, or if you have liver or kidney disease, you may be at increased risk of side effects from the large amount of propylene glycol in AGENERASE Oral Solution.

How does AGENERASE Oral Solution work?

AGENERASE Oral Solution is used only in combination with other anti-HIV medicines. When used in combination therapy, AGENERASE Oral Solution may help lower the amount of HIV found in your blood, raise CD4 (T) cell count, and keep your immune system as healthy as possible so that it can help fight infection. However, AGENERASE Oral Solution does not have these effects in all patients.

What are the side effects of AGENERASE Oral Solution?

Common side effects of AGENERASE Oral Solution are nausea, vomiting, diarrhea, rash, and a tingling sensation around the mouth. Severe or life-threatening rash has been reported.

Possible side effects from the large amount of propylene glycol in AGENERASE Oral Solution include seizures, drowsiness, fast heart rate, and kidney and blood abnormalities. Contact your doctor if you have nausea, vomiting, diarrhea, or rash. Your doctor may be able to help you manage these symptoms. Your doctor will advise you whether your symptoms can be managed on therapy or whether AGENERASE Oral Solution should be stopped.

This list of side effects is not complete. Your doctor or pharmacist can discuss with you a more complete list of possible side effects with AGENERASE Oral Solution. Talk to your doctor promptly about any side effects you have.

How should I take AGENERASE Oral Solution?

Take AGENERASE Oral Solution exactly as your doctor prescribes it. AGENERASE Oral Solution can be taken with or without food. However, you should not take AGENERASE with a high-fat meal because this could reduce the effectiveness of AGENERASE Oral Solution.

What should I do if I miss a dose of AGENERASE Oral Solution?

To help make sure that your anti-HIV therapy is as effective as possible, be very careful to take all of your medication exactly as your doctor prescribed it and do not skip any doses.

If you miss a dose of AGENERASE Oral Solution by more than 4 hours, wait and take the next dose at the regularly scheduled time. However, if you miss a dose by fewer than 4 hours, take your missed dose immediately. Then take your next dose at the regularly scheduled time. Do not take more or less than your prescribed dose of AGENERASE Oral Solution at any one time.

Continued on next page

This product information is based on labeling in effect on June 23, 2000. For further information, contact via direct mail, phone, or web site. Medical Information, Glaxo Wellcome Inc., PO Box 13398, Research Triangle Park, NC 27709. Healthcare Professionals (Medical Information): 800-334-0089. Patients (Customer Response Center): 1-888-825-5249. Glaxo Wellcome Corporate Web Site: www.glaxowellcome.com

Agenerase Oral Solution—Cont.

When your supply of AGENERASE Oral Solution or other anti-HIV drugs starts to run low, arrange to get more from your doctor or pharmacy. It is very important that you take anti-HIV drugs as prescribed by your doctor because the amount of virus in your blood may increase if one or more of the drugs is stopped, even for a short time.

Can AGENERASE Oral Solution be taken with other medications?

Protease inhibitors, including AGENERASE, may interact with other drugs, including those you take without a prescription. Before you take AGENERASE, tell your doctor about any drugs that you are taking or planning to take, including non-prescription drugs.

- **AGENERASE Oral Solution should not be taken with ANTABUSE (disulfiram) or FLAGYL (metronidazole).**
- Drinking alcoholic beverages is not recommended while taking AGENERASE Oral Solution because it may increase side effects related to propylene glycol content.
- **You should not take any of the following medications with AGENERASE Oral Solution because serious or life-threatening problems could occur.***
  HALCION® (triazolam)
  HISMANAL® (astemizole)
  Ergot medications (CAFERGOT® and others)
  PROPULSID® (cisapride)
  VERSED® (midazolam)
  VASCOR® (bepridil)
- **You should also not take rifampin** with AGENERASE Oral Solution because this drug reduces the effectiveness of AGENERASE. Rifampin is also known as: RIFADIN®, RIFAMATE®, RIFATER®, and RIMACTANE®.
- **Serious and/or life-threatening drug interactions can also occur if you take AGENERASE Oral Solution with any of the following drugs.*** If you need to take any of these drugs, your doctor may closely monitor the amount of drug in your blood to minimize potential problems.
  CORDARONE® (amiodarone)
  Phenobarbital
  DILANTIN® (phenytoin)
  Lidocaine
  COUMADIN® (warfarin)
  (quinidine) QUINAGLUTE®, CARDIOQUIN®, QUINIDEX®
  Antidepressants such as ELAVIL® (amitriptyline), NORPRAMIN® (desipramine), PAMELOR® (nortriptyline), TOFRANIL® (imipramine)
- Tell your doctor about any drugs that you are taking or planning to take, including non-prescription drugs.
- Before you take VIAGRA® (sildenafil) with AGENERASE Oral Solution, talk to your doctor about possible drug interactions and side effects. If you take VIAGRA and AGENERASE Oral Solution together, you may be at increased risk of side effects of VIAGRA such as low blood pressure, visual changes, and penile erection lasting more than 4 hours. If an erection lasts longer than 4 hours, you should seek immediate medical assistance to avoid permanent damage to your penis. Your doctor can explain these symptoms to you.
- If you use birth control pills, talk to your doctor about choosing a different type of contraceptive, since AGENERASE Oral Solution may reduce the effectiveness of some birth control pills.
- Because AGENERASE Oral Solution contains large amounts of vitamin E, you should not take additional vitamin E while taking AGENERASE Oral Solution.
- It is not recommended that you take AGENERASE with the cholesterol-lowering drugs MEVACOR® (lovastatin) or ZOCOR® (simvastatin) because of the possible drug interactions. There is also an increased risk of drug interactions between AGENERASE and LIPITOR® (atorvastatin) and BAYCOL® (cerivastatin). Talk to your doctor if you are taking or are planning to take these or other drugs for lowering cholesterol.
- **Special considerations:***
  If you take AGENERASE Oral Solution with MYCOBUTIN® (rifabutin), your doctor will lower the dose of MYCOBUTIN.
  If you take AGENERASE Oral Solution with VIDEX® (didanosine, ddl), take them at least 1 hour apart.
  If you take AGENERASE Oral Solution with antacids, take them at least 1 hour apart.

Does AGENERASE Oral Solution cure HIV infection or AIDS?

AGENERASE Oral Solution does not cure HIV infection or AIDS. At this time we do not know if AGENERASE will help you live longer or have fewer of the medical problems (opportunistic infections) that are associated with HIV infection or AIDS. Because of this, you must be sure to be seen regularly by your healthcare professional.

Does AGENERASE Oral Solution reduce the risk of passing HIV to others?

No. AGENERASE Oral Solution, as well as other anti-HIV medications, has not been shown to reduce the risk of passing HIV to others through sexual contact or blood contamination. Continue to practice safe sex and do not use or share dirty needles.

Who should not take AGENERASE Oral Solution?

AGENERASE Oral Solution should not be used in infants and children below 4 years of age, pregnant women, patients with liver or kidney failure, or patients on disulfiram (ANTABUSE) or metronidazole (FLAGYL).

Do not take AGENERASE Oral Solution if you have had a serious allergic reaction to AGENERASE Oral Solution or any of its ingredients. If you have liver disease, your dosage of AGENERASE Oral Solution may have to be adjusted.
If you are allergic to sulfa drugs, you should inform your doctor.

Can children take AGENERASE Oral Solution?

AGENERASE Oral Solution should not be used in infants and children below 4 years of age.
Children from 4 to 12 years of age can take AGENERASE Oral Solution. Your doctor will tell you if the oral solution or capsule is best for your child. Your child's doctor will decide the right dose based on your child's weight and age.

Can pregnant women and nursing mothers take AGENERASE Oral Solution?

AGENERASE Oral Solution should not be used by pregnant women. Talk to your doctor if you are pregnant or if you become pregnant while taking AGENERASE Oral Solution. Mothers with HIV should not breastfeed their infants because HIV in the breast milk can infect the infant.

What other medical conditions should I discuss with my doctor?

Talk to your doctor if you are pregnant or if you become pregnant while you are taking AGENERASE Oral Solution. Also talk to your doctor if you have hemophilia or problems with your liver or kidneys.

How should I store AGENERASE Oral Solution?

AGENERASE Oral Solution should be stored at room temperature and should not be refrigerated.

Other information:

This medication is prescribed for a particular condition. Do not use it for any other condition or give it to anybody else. Keep AGENERASE Oral Solution and all medicines out of the reach of children.
Ask a healthcare professional any questions you may have about AGENERASE Oral Solution.
AGENERASE is a registered trademark of the Glaxo Wellcome group of companies.
*The brands listed are trademarks of their respective owners and are not trademarks of the Glaxo Wellcome group of companies. The makers of these brands are not affiliated with and do not endorse Glaxo Wellcome or its products.
Glaxo Wellcome Inc., Research Triangle Park, NC 27709
Licensed from Vertex Pharmaceuticals Incorporated
Cambridge, MA 02139
AGENERASE is a registered trademark of the Glaxo Wellcome group of companies.
US Patent Nos. 5,585,397; 5,723,490; and 5,646,180

May 2000/RL-825

Shown in Product Identification Guide, page 314

ALKERAN® ℞

[ăl 'kur-ăn]
(melphalan hydrochloride)
for Injection

> **WARNING:** Melphalan should be administered under the supervision of a qualified physician experienced in the use of cancer chemotherapeutic agents. Severe bone marrow suppression with resulting infection or bleeding may occur. Controlled trials comparing intravenous (IV) to oral melphalan have shown more myelosuppression with the IV formulation. Hypersensitivity reactions, including anaphylaxis, have occurred in approximately 2% of patients who received the IV formulation. Melphalan is leukemogenic in humans. Melphalan produces chromosomal aberrations in vitro and in vivo and, therefore, should be considered potentially mutagenic in humans.

DESCRIPTION

Melphalan, also known as L-phenylalanine mustard, phenylalanine mustard, L-PAM, or L-sarcolysin, is a phenylalanine derivative of nitrogen mustard. Melphalan is a bifunctional alkylating agent that is active against selected human neoplastic diseases. It is known chemically as 4-[bis(2-chloroethyl)amino]-*L*-phenylalanine. The molecular formula is $C_{13}H_{18}Cl_2N_2O_2$ and the molecular weight is 305.20.
Melphalan is the active L-isomer of the compound and was first synthesized in 1953 by Bergel and Stock; the D-isomer, known as medphalan, is less active against certain animal tumors, and the dose needed to produce effects on chromosomes is larger than that required with the L-isomer. The racemic (DL-) form is known as merphalan or sarcolysin.
Melphalan is practically insoluble in water and has a pKa_1 of ~2.5.
ALKERAN for Injection is supplied as a sterile, nonpyrogenic, freeze-dried powder. Each single-use vial contains melphalan hydrochloride equivalent to 50 mg melphalan and 20 mg povidone. ALKERAN for Injection is reconstituted using the sterile diluent provided. Each vial of sterile diluent contains sodium citrate 0.2 g, propylene glycol 6.0 mL, ethanol (96%) 0.52 mL, and Water for Injection to a total of 10 mL. ALKERAN for Injection is administered intravenously.

CLINICAL PHARMACOLOGY

Melphalan is an alkylating agent of the bischloroethylamine type. As a result, its cytotoxicity appears to be related to the extent of its interstrand cross-linking with DNA, probably by binding at the N^7 position of guanine. Like other bifunctional alkylating agents, it is active against both resting and rapidly dividing tumor cells.
Pharmacokinetics: The pharmacokinetics of melphalan after IV administration has been extensively studied in adult patients. Following injection, drug plasma concentrations declined rapidly in a biexponential manner with distribution phase and terminal elimination phase half-lives of approximately 10 and 75 minutes, respectively. Estimates of average total body clearance varied among studies, but typical values of approximately 7 to 9 mL/min per kg (250 to 325 mL/min per m^2) were observed. One study has reported that on repeat dosing of 0.5 mg/kg every 6 weeks, the clearance of melphalan decreased from 8.1 mL/min per kg after the first course, to 5.5 mL/min per kg after the third course, but did not decrease appreciably after the third course. Mean (±SD) peak melphalan plasma concentrations in myeloma patients given IV melphalan at doses of 10 or 20 mg/m^2 were 1.2±0.4 and 2.8±1.9 ng/mL, respectively.
The steady-state volume of distribution of melphalan is 0.5 L/kg. Penetration into cerebrospinal fluid (CSF) is low. The extent of melphalan binding to plasma proteins ranges from 60% to 90%. Serum albumin is the major binding protein, while α_1-acid glycoprotein appears to account for about 20% of the plasma protein binding. Approximately 30% of the drug is (covalently) irreversibly bound to plasma proteins. Interactions with immunoglobulins have been found to be negligible.
Melphalan is eliminated from plasma primarily by chemical hydrolysis to monohydroxymelphalan and dihydroxymelphalan. Aside from these hydrolysis products, no other melphalan metabolites have been observed in humans. Although the contribution of renal elimination to melphalan clearance appears to be low, one study noted an increase in the occurrence of severe leukopenia in patients with elevated BUN after 10 weeks of therapy.
Clinical Trial: A randomized trial compared prednisone plus IV melphalan to prednisone plus oral melphalan in the treatment of myeloma. As discussed below, overall response rates at week 22 were comparable; however, because of changes in trial design, conclusions as to the relative activity of the two formulations after week 22 are impossible to make.
Both arms received oral prednisone starting at 0.8 mg/kg per day with doses tapered over 6 weeks. Melphalan doses in each arm were:
Arm 1 Oral melphalan 0.15 mg/kg per day × 7 followed by 0.05 mg/kg per day when WBC began to rise.
Arm 2 IV melphalan 16 mg/m^2 q 2 weeks × 4 (over 6 weeks) followed by the same dose every 4 weeks.
Doses of melphalan were adjusted according to the following criteria:

Table 1: Criteria for Dosage Adjustment in a Randomized Clinical Trial

WBC/mm³	Platelets	Percent of Full Dose
≥4000	≥100,000	100
≥3000	≥75,000	75
≥2000	≥50,000	50
<2000	<50,000	0

One hundred seven patients were randomized to the oral melphalan arm and 203 patients to the IV melphalan arm. More patients had a poor-risk classification (58% versus 44%) and high tumor load (51% versus 34%) on the oral compared to the IV arm (P<0.04). Response rates at week 22 are shown in the following table:

Table 2: Response Rates at Week 22

Initial Arm	Evaluable Patients	Responders n (%)	P
Oral melphalan	100	44 (44%)	P>0.2
IV melphalan	195	74 (38%)	

Because of changes in protocol design after week 22, other efficacy parameters such as response duration and survival cannot be compared.
Severe myelotoxicity (WBC ≤1000 and/or platelets ≤25,000) was more common in the IV melphalan arm (28%) than in the oral melphalan arm (11%).
An association was noted between poor renal function and myelosuppression; consequently, an amendment to the protocol required a 50% reduction in IV melphalan dose if the BUN was ≥30 mg/dL. The rate of severe leukopenia in the IV arm in the patients with BUN over 30 mg/dL decreased from 50% (8/16) before protocol amendment to 11% (3/28) (P = .01) after the amendment.
Before the dosing amendment, there was a 10% (8/77) incidence of drug-related death in the IV arm. After the dosing amendment, this incidence was 3% (3/108). This compares to an overall 1% (1/100) incidence of drug-related death in the oral arm.

INDICATIONS AND USAGE

ALKERAN for Injection is indicated for the palliative treatment of patients with multiple myeloma for whom oral therapy is not appropriate.

CONTRAINDICATIONS

Melphalan should not be used in patients whose disease has demonstrated prior resistance to this agent. Patients who have demonstrated hypersensitivity to melphalan should not be given the drug.

WARNINGS

Melphalan should be administered in carefully adjusted dosage by or under the supervision of experienced physicians who are familiar with the drug's actions and the possible complications of its use.

As with other nitrogen mustard drugs, excessive dosage will produce marked bone marrow suppression. Bone marrow suppression is the most significant toxicity associated with ALKERAN for Injection in most patients. Therefore, the following tests should be performed at the start of therapy and prior to each subsequent dose of ALKERAN: platelet count, hemoglobin, white blood cell count, and differential. Thrombocytopenia and/or leukopenia are indications to withhold further therapy until the blood counts have sufficiently recovered. Frequent blood counts are essential to determine optimal dosage and to avoid toxicity. Dose adjustment on the basis of blood counts at the nadir and day of treatment should be considered.

Hypersensitivity reactions including anaphylaxis have occurred in approximately 2% of patients who received the IV formulation (see ADVERSE REACTIONS). These reactions usually occur after multiple courses of treatment. Treatment is symptomatic. The infusion should be terminated immediately, followed by the administration of volume expanders, pressor agents, corticosteroids, or antihistamines at the discretion of the physician. If a hypersensitivity reaction occurs, IV or oral melphalan should not be readministered since hypersensitivity reactions have also been reported with oral melphalan.

Carcinogenesis: Secondary malignancies, including acute nonlymphocytic leukemia, myeloproliferative syndrome, and carcinoma, have been reported in patients with cancer treated with alkylating agents (including melphalan). Some patients also received other chemotherapeutic agents or radiation therapy. Precise quantitation of the risk of acute leukemia, myeloproliferative syndrome, or carcinoma is not possible. Published reports of leukemia in patients who have received melphalan (and other alkylating agents) suggest that the risk of leukemogenesis increases with chronicity of treatment and with cumulative dose. In one study, the 10-year cumulative risk of developing acute leukemia or myeloproliferative syndrome after oral melphalan therapy was 19.5% for cumulative doses ranging from 730 to 9652 mg. In this same study, as well as in an additional study, the 10-year cumulative risk of developing acute leukemia or myeloproliferative syndrome after oral melphalan therapy was less than 2% for cumulative doses under 600 mg. This does not mean that there is a cumulative dose below which there is no risk of the induction of secondary malignancy. The potential benefits from melphalan therapy must be weighed on an individual basis against the possible risk of the induction of a second malignancy.

Adequate and well-controlled carcinogenicity studies have not been conducted in animals. However, intraperitoneal (IP) administration of melphalan in rats (5.4 to 10.8 mg/m^2) and in mice (2.25 to 4.5 mg/m^2) three times per week for 6 months followed by 12 months post-dose observation produced peritoneal sarcoma and lung tumors, respectively.

Mutagenesis: Melphalan has been shown to cause chromatid or chromosome damage in humans. Intramuscular administration of melphalan at 6 and 60 mg/m^2 produced structural aberrations of the chromatid and chromosomes in bone marrow cells of Wistar rats.

Impairment of Fertility: Melphalan causes suppression of ovarian function in premenopausal women, resulting in amenorrhea in a significant number of patients. Reversible and irreversible testicular suppression have also been reported.

Pregnancy: Pregnancy Category D. Melphalan may cause fetal harm when administered to a pregnant woman. While adequate animal studies have not been conducted with IV melphalan, oral (6 to 18 mg/m^2 per day for 10 days) and IP (18 mg/m^2) administration in rats was embryolethal and teratogenic. Malformations resulting from melphalan included alterations of the brain (underdevelopment, deformation, meningocele, and encephalocele) and eye (anophthalmia and microphthalmos), reduction of the mandible and tail, as well as hepatocele (exomphaly). There are no adequate and well-controlled studies in pregnant women. If this drug is used during pregnancy, or if the patient becomes pregnant while taking this drug, the patient should be apprised of the potential hazard to the fetus. Women of childbearing potential should be advised to avoid becoming pregnant.

PRECAUTIONS

General: In all instances where the use of ALKERAN for Injection is considered for chemotherapy, the physician must evaluate the need and usefulness of the drug against the risk of adverse events. Melphalan should be used with extreme caution in patients whose bone marrow reserve may have been compromised by prior irradiation or chemotherapy or whose marrow function is recovering from previous cytotoxic therapy.

Dose reduction should be considered in patients with renal insufficiency receiving IV melphalan. In one trial, increased bone marrow suppression was observed in patients with BUN levels ≥30 mg/dL. A 50% reduction in the IV melphalan dose decreased the incidence of severe bone marrow suppression in the latter portion of this study.

Information for Patients: Patients should be informed that the major acute toxicities of melphalan are related to bone marrow suppression, hypersensitivity reactions, gastrointestinal toxicity, and pulmonary toxicity. The major long-term toxicities are related to infertility and secondary malignancies. Patients should never be allowed to take the drug without close medical supervision and should be advised to consult their physicians if they experience skin rash, signs or symptoms of vasculitis, bleeding, fever, persistent cough, nausea, vomiting, amenorrhea, weight loss, or unusual lumps/masses. Women of childbearing potential should be advised to avoid becoming pregnant.

Laboratory Tests: Periodic complete blood counts with differentials should be performed during the course of treatment with melphalan. At least one determination should be obtained prior to each dose. Patients should be observed closely for consequences of bone marrow suppression, which include severe infections, bleeding, and symptomatic anemia (see WARNINGS).

Drug Interactions: The development of severe renal failure has been reported in patients treated with a single dose of IV melphalan followed by standard oral doses of cyclosporine. Cisplatin may affect melphalan kinetics by inducing renal dysfunction and subsequently altering melphalan clearance. IV melphalan may also reduce the threshold for BCNU lung toxicity. When nalidixic acid and IV melphalan are given simultaneously, the incidence of severe hemorrhagic necrotic enterocolitis has been reported to increase in pediatric patients.

Carcinogenesis, Mutagenesis, Impairment of Fertility: See WARNINGS section.

Pregnancy: ***Teratogenic Effects:*** Pregnancy Category D: See WARNINGS section.

Nursing Mothers: It is not known whether this drug is excreted in human milk. IV melphalan should not be given to nursing mothers.

Pediatric Use: The safety and effectiveness in pediatric patients have not been established.

Geriatric Use: Clinical experience with ALKERAN has not identified differences in responses between the elderly and younger patients. In general, dose selection for an elderly patient should be cautious, reflecting the greater frequency of decreased hepatic, renal, or cardiac function, and of concomitant disease or other drug therapy.

ADVERSE REACTIONS (see OVERDOSAGE)

The following information on adverse reactions is based on data from both oral and IV administration of melphalan as a single agent, using several different dose schedules for treatment of a wide variety of malignancies.

Hematologic: The most common side effect is bone marrow suppression. White blood cell count and platelet count nadirs usually occur 2 to 3 weeks after treatment, with recovery in 4 to 5 weeks after treatment. Irreversible bone marrow failure has been reported.

Gastrointestinal: Gastrointestinal disturbances such as nausea and vomiting, diarrhea, and oral ulceration occur infrequently. Hepatic toxicity, including veno-occlusive disease, has been reported.

Hypersensitivity: Acute hypersensitivity reactions including anaphylaxis were reported in 2.4% of 425 patients receiving ALKERAN for Injection for myeloma (see WARNINGS). These reactions were characterized by urticaria, pruritus, edema, and in some patients, tachycardia, bronchospasm, dyspnea, and hypotension. These patients appeared to respond to antihistamine and corticosteroid therapy. If a hypersensitivity reaction occurs, IV or oral melphalan should not be readministered since hypersensitivity reactions have also been reported with oral melphalan.

Miscellaneous: Other reported adverse reactions include skin hypersensitivity, skin ulceration at injection site, skin necrosis rarely requiring skin grafting, vasculitis, alopecia, hemolytic anemia, allergic reaction, pulmonary fibrosis, and interstitial pneumonitis.

OVERDOSAGE

Overdoses resulting in death have been reported. Overdoses, including doses up to 290 mg/m^2, have produced the following symptoms: severe nausea and vomiting, decreased consciousness, convulsions, muscular paralysis, and cholinomimetic effects. Severe mucositis, stomatitis, colitis, diarrhea, and hemorrhage of the gastrointestinal tract occur at high doses (>100 mg/m^2). Elevations in liver enzymes and veno-occlusive disease occur infrequently. Significant hyponatremia caused by an associated inappropriate secretion of ADH syndrome has been observed. Nephrotoxicity and adult respiratory distress syndrome have been reported rarely. The principal toxic effect is bone marrow suppression. Hematologic parameters should be closely followed for 3 to 6 weeks. An uncontrolled study suggests that administration of autologous bone marrow or hematopoietic growth factors (i.e., sargramostim, filgrastim) may shorten the period of pancytopenia. General supportive measures together with appropriate blood transfusions and antibiotics should be instituted as deemed necessary by the physician. This drug is not removed from plasma to any significant degree by hemodialysis or hemoperfusion. A pediatric patient survived a 254-mg/m^2 overdose treated with standard supportive care.

DOSAGE AND ADMINISTRATION

The usual IV dose is 16 mg/m^2. Dosage reduction of up to 50% should be considered in patients with renal insufficiency (BUN ≥30 mg/dL) (see PRECAUTIONS: General). The drug is administered as a single infusion over 15 to 20 minutes. Melphalan is administered at 2-week intervals for four doses, then, after adequate recovery from toxicity, at 4-week intervals. Available evidence suggests about one third to one half of the patients with multiple myeloma show a favorable response to the drug. Experience with oral melphalan suggests that repeated courses should be given since improvement may continue slowly over many months, and the maximum benefit may be missed if treatment is abandoned prematurely. Dose adjustment on the basis of blood cell counts at the nadir and day of treatment should be considered.

Administration Precautions: As with other toxic compounds, caution should be exercised in handling and preparing the solution of ALKERAN. Skin reactions associated with accidental exposure may occur. The use of gloves is recommended. If the solution of ALKERAN contacts the skin or mucosa, immediately wash the skin or mucosa thoroughly with soap and water.

Procedures for proper handling and disposal of anticancer drugs should be considered. Several guidelines on this subject have been published.[1–7] There is no general agreement that all of the procedures recommended in the guidelines are necessary or appropriate.

Parenteral drug products should be visually inspected for particulate matter and discoloration prior to administration whenever solution and container permit. If either occurs, do not use this product.

Preparation for Administration/Stability:

1. ALKERAN for Injection must be reconstituted by rapidly injecting 10 mL of the supplied diluent directly into the vial of lyophilized powder using a sterile needle (20-gauge or larger needle diameter) and syringe. Immediately shake vial vigorously until a clear solution is obtained. This provides a 5-mg/mL solution of melphalan. Rapid addition of the diluent followed by immediate vigorous shaking is important for proper dissolution.
2. **Immediately** dilute the dose to be administered in 0.9% Sodium Chloride Injection, USP, to a concentration not greater than 0.45 mg/mL.
3. Administer the diluted product over a minimum of 15 minutes.
4. Complete administration within 60 minutes of reconstitution.

The time between reconstitution/dilution and administration of ALKERAN should be kept to a minimum because reconstituted and diluted solutions of ALKERAN are unstable. Over as short a time as 30 minutes, a citrate derivative of melphalan has been detected in reconstituted material from the reaction of ALKERAN with Sterile Diluent for ALKERAN. Upon further dilution with saline, nearly 1% label strength of melphalan hydrolyzes every 10 minutes.

A precipitate forms if the reconstituted solution is stored at 5°C. DO NOT REFRIGERATE THE RECONSTITUTED PRODUCT.

HOW SUPPLIED

ALKERAN for Injection is supplied in a carton containing one single-use clear glass vial of freeze-dried melphalan hydrochloride equivalent to 50 mg melphalan and one 10-mL clear glass vial of sterile diluent (NDC 0173-0130-93).

Store at controlled room temperature 15° to 30°C (59° to 86°F) and protect from light.

REFERENCES

1. Recommendations for the safe handling of parenteral antineoplastic drugs. Washington, DC: Division of Safety, National Institutes of Health; 1983. US Dept of Health and Human Services, Public Health Service publication NIH 83-2621.
2. AMA Council on Scientific Affairs. Guidelines for handling parenteral antineoplastics. *JAMA.* 1985; 253:1590-1591.
3. National Study Commission on Cytotoxic Exposure. Recommendations for handling cytotoxic agents. 1987. Available from Louis P. Jeffrey, Chairman, National Study Commission on Cytotoxic Exposure. Massachusetts College of Pharmacy and Allied Health Sciences, 179 Longwood Avenue, Boston, MA 02115.
4. Clinical Oncological Society of Australia. Guidelines and recommendations for safe handling of antineoplastic agents. *Med J Australia.* 1983;1:426-428.
5. Jones RB, Frank R, Mass T. Safe handling of chemotherapeutic agents: a report from the Mount Sinai Medical Center. *CA-A Cancer J for Clin.* 1983;33:258-263.
6. American Society of Hospital Pharmacists. ASHP technical assistance bulletin on handling cytotoxic and hazardous drugs. *Am J Hosp Pharm.* 1990;47:1033-1049.

Continued on next page

This product information is based on labeling in effect on June 23, 2000. For further information, contact via direct mail, phone, or web site. Medical Information, Glaxo Wellcome Inc., PO Box 13398, Research Triangle Park, NC 27709. Healthcare Professionals (Medical Information): 800-334-0089. Patients (Customer Response Center): 1-888-825-5249. Glaxo Wellcome Corporate Web Site: www.glaxowellcome.com

Alkeran for Injection—Cont.

7. Yodaiken RE, Bennett D. OSHA work-practice guidelines for personnel dealing with cytotoxic (antineoplastic) drugs. *Am J Hosp Pharm.* 1986;43:1193-1204.

US Patent No. 4,997,651
Glaxo Wellcome Inc., Research Triangle Park, NC 27709

August 1998/RL-610
Shown in Product Identification Guide, page 314

ALKERAN® ℞

[*ăl-kur 'ăn*]
(melphalan)
2-mg Scored Tablets

WARNING: ALKERAN (melphalan) should be administered under the supervision of a qualified physician experienced in the use of cancer chemotherapeutic agents. Severe bone marrow suppression with resulting infection or bleeding may occur. Melphalan is leukemogenic in humans.
Melphalan produces chromosomal aberrations in vitro and in vivo and, therefore, should be considered potentially mutagenic in humans.

DESCRIPTION

ALKERAN (melphalan), also known as L-phenylalanine mustard, phenylalanine mustard, L-PAM, or L-sarcolysin, is a phenylalanine derivative of nitrogen mustard. Melphalan is a bifunctional alkylating agent which is active against selective human neoplastic diseases. It is known chemically as 4-[bis(2-chloroethyl)amino]-*L*-phenylalanine. The molecular formula is $C_{13}H_{18}Cl_2N_2O_2$ and the molecular weight is 305.20.

Melphalan is the active L-isomer of the compound and was first synthesized in 1953 by Bergel and Stock; the D-isomer, known as medphalan, is less active against certain animal tumors, and the dose needed to produce effects on chromosomes is larger than that required with the L-isomer. The racemic (DL–) form is known as merphalan or sarcolysin. Melphalan is practically insoluble in water and has a pKa_1 of ~2.5.

ALKERAN (melphalan) is available in tablet form for oral administration. Each scored tablet contains 2 mg melphalan and the inactive ingredients lactose, magnesium stearate, potato starch, povidone, and sucrose.

CLINICAL PHARMACOLOGY

Melphalan is an alkylating agent of the bischloroethylamine type. As a result, its cytotoxicity appears to be related to the extent of its interstrand cross-linking with DNA, probably by binding at the N^7 position of guanine. Like other bifunctional alkylating agents, it is active against both resting and rapidly dividing tumor cells.

Pharmacokinetics: The pharmacokinetics of ALKERAN after oral administration has been extensively studied in adult patients. Plasma melphalan levels are highly variable after oral dosing, both with respect to the time of the first appearance of melphalan in plasma (range 0 to 336 minutes) and to the peak plasma concentration (range 0.166 to 3.741 mcg/mL) achieved. These results may be due to incomplete intestinal absorption, a variable "first pass" hepatic metabolism, or to rapid hydrolysis. Five patients were studied after both oral and intravenous (IV) dosing with 0.6 mg/kg as a single bolus dose by each route. The areas under the plasma concentration-time curves after oral administration averaged 61% ± 26% (± standard deviation; range 25% to 89%) of those following IV administration. In 18 patients given a single oral dose of 0.6 mg/kg of ALKERAN, the terminal plasma half-disappearance time of parent drug was 89.5 ± 50 minutes. The 24-hour urinary excretion of parent drug in these patients was 10% ± 4.5%, suggesting that renal clearance is not a major route of elimination of parent drug.

One study using universally labeled ^{14}C-melphalan, found substantially less radioactivity in the urine of patients given the drug by mouth (30% of administered dose in 9 days) than in the urine of those given it intravenously (35% to 65% in 7 days). Following either oral or IV administration, the pattern of label recovery was similar, with the majority being recovered in the first 24 hours. Following oral administration, peak radioactivity occurred in plasma at 2 hours and then disappeared with a half-life of approximately 160 hours. In one patient where parent drug (rather than just radiolabel) was determined, the melphalan half-disappearance time was 67 minutes.

The steady-state volume of distribution of melphalan is 0.5 L/kg. Penetration into cerebrospinal fluid (CSF) is low. The extent of melphalan binding to plasma proteins ranges from 60% to 90%. Serum albumin is the major binding protein, while α_1-acid glycoprotein appears to account for about 20% of the plasma protein binding. Approximately 30% of melphalan is (covalently) irreversibly bound to plasma proteins. Interactions with immunoglobulins have been found to be negligible.

Melphalan is eliminated from plasma primarily by chemical hydrolysis to monohydroxymelphalan and dihydroxymelphalan. Aside from these hydrolysis products, no other melphalan metabolites have been observed in humans. Although the contribution of renal elimination to melphalan clearance appears to be low, one pharmacokinetic study showed a significant positive correlation between the elimination rate constant for melphalan and renal function and a significant negative correlation between renal function and the area under the plasma melphalan concentration/time curve.

INDICATIONS AND USAGE

ALKERAN Tablets are indicated for the palliative treatment of multiple myeloma and for the palliation of non-resectable epithelial carcinoma of the ovary.

CONTRAINDICATIONS

ALKERAN should not be used in patients whose disease has demonstrated a prior resistance to this agent. Patients who have demonstrated hypersensitivity to melphalan should not be given the drug.

WARNINGS

ALKERAN should be administered in carefully adjusted dosage by or under the supervision of experienced physicians who are familiar with the drug's actions and the possible complications of its use.

As with other nitrogen mustard drugs, excessive dosage will produce marked bone marrow suppression. Bone marrow suppression is the most significant toxicity associated with ALKERAN in most patients. Therefore, the following tests should be performed at the start of therapy and prior to each subsequent course of ALKERAN: platelet count, hemoglobin, white blood cell count, and differential. Thrombocytopenia and/or leukopenia are indications to withhold further therapy until the blood counts have sufficiently recovered. Frequent blood counts are essential to determine optimal dosage and to avoid toxicity (see PRECAUTIONS: Laboratory Tests). Dose adjustment on the basis of blood counts at the nadir and day of treatment should be considered.

Hypersensitivity reactions, including anaphylaxis, have occurred rarely (see ADVERSE REACTIONS). These reactions have occurred after multiple courses of treatment and have recurred in patients who experienced a hypersensitivity reaction to IV ALKERAN. If a hypersensitivity reaction occurs, oral or IV ALKERAN should not be readministered.

Carcinogenesis: Secondary malignancies, including acute nonlymphocytic leukemia, myeloproliferative syndrome, and carcinoma have been reported in patients with cancer treated with alkylating agents (including melphalan). Some patients also received other chemotherapeutic agents or radiation therapy. Precise quantitation of the risk of acute leukemia, myeloproliferative syndrome, or carcinoma is not possible. Published reports of leukemia in patients who have received melphalan (and other alkylating agents) suggest that the risk of leukemogenesis increases with chronicity of treatment and with cumulative dose. In one study, the 10-year cumulative risk of developing acute leukemia or myeloproliferative syndrome after melphalan therapy was 19.5% for cumulative doses ranging from 730 mg to 9652 mg. In this same study, as well as in an additional study, the 10-year cumulative risk of developing acute leukemia or myeloproliferative syndrome after melphalan therapy was less than 2% for cumulative doses under 600 mg. This does not mean that there is a cumulative dose below which there is no risk of the induction of secondary malignancy. The potential benefits from melphalan therapy must be weighed on an individual basis against the possible risk of the induction of a second malignancy.

Adequate and well-controlled carcinogenicity studies have not been conducted in animals. However, i.p. administration of melphalan in rats (5.4 to 10.8 mg/m^2) and in mice (2.25 to 4.5 mg/m^2) three times per week for 6 months followed by 12 months post-dose observation produced peritoneal sarcoma and lung tumors, respectively.

Mutagenesis: ALKERAN has been shown to cause chromatid or chromosome damage in humans. Intramuscular administration of ALKERAN at 6 and 60 mg/m^2 produced structural aberrations of the chromatid and chromosomes in bone marrow cells of Wistar rats.

Impairment of Fertility: ALKERAN causes suppression of ovarian function in premenopausal women, resulting in amenorrhea in a significant number of patients. Reversible and irreversible testicular suppression have also been reported.

Pregnancy: Pregnancy Category D. ALKERAN may cause fetal harm when administered to a pregnant woman. Melphalan was embryolethal and teratogenic in rats following oral (6 to 18 mg/m^2 per day for 10 days) and intraperitoneal (18 mg/m^2 per kg single dose) administration. Malformations resulting from melphalan included alterations of the brain (underdevelopment, deformation, meningocele, and encephalocele) and eye (anophthalmia and microphthalmos), reduction of the mandible and tail, as well as hepatocele (exomphaly).

There are no adequate and well-controlled studies in pregnant women. If this drug is used during pregnancy, or if the patient becomes pregnant while taking this drug, the patient should be apprised of the potential hazard to the fetus. Women of childbearing potential should be advised to avoid becoming pregnant.

PRECAUTIONS

General: In all instances where the use of ALKERAN is considered for chemotherapy, the physician must evaluate the need and usefulness of the drug against the risk of adverse events. ALKERAN should be used with extreme caution in patients whose bone marrow reserve may have been compromised by prior irradiation or chemotherapy, or whose marrow function is recovering from previous cytotoxic therapy. If the leukocyte count falls below 3,000 cells/mcL, or the platelet count below 100,000 cells/mcL, ALKERAN should be discontinued until the peripheral blood cell counts have recovered.

A recommendation as to whether or not dosage reduction should be made routinely in patients with renal insufficiency cannot be made because:

(a) There is considerable inherent patient-to-patient variability in the systemic availability of melphalan in patients with normal renal function.
(b) Only a small amount of the administered dose appears as parent drug in the urine of patients with normal renal function.

Patients with azotemia should be closely observed, however, in order to make dosage reductions, if required, at the earliest possible time.

Information for Patients: Patients should be informed that the major toxicities of ALKERAN are related to bone marrow suppression, hypersensitivity reactions, gastrointestinal toxicity, and pulmonary toxicity. The major long-term toxicities are related to infertility and secondary malignancies. Patients should never be allowed to take the drug without close medical supervision and should be advised to consult their physician if they experience skin rash, vasculitis, bleeding, fever, persistent cough, nausea, vomiting, amenorrhea, weight loss, or unusual lumps/masses. Women of childbearing potential should be advised to avoid becoming pregnant.

Laboratory Tests: Periodic complete blood counts with differentials should be performed during the course of treatment with ALKERAN. At least one determination should be obtained prior to each treatment course. Patients should be observed closely for consequences of bone marrow suppression, which include severe infections, bleeding, and symptomatic anemia (see WARNINGS).

Drug Interactions: There are no known drug/drug interactions with oral ALKERAN.

Carcinogenesis, Mutagenesis, Impairment of Fertility: See WARNINGS section.

Pregnancy: ***Teratogenic Effects:*** Pregnancy Category D: See WARNINGS section.

Nursing Mothers: It is not known whether this drug is excreted in human milk. ALKERAN should not be given to nursing mothers.

Pediatric Use: The safety and effectiveness of ALKERAN in pediatric patients have not been established.

Geriatric Use: Clinical experience with ALKERAN has not identified differences in responses between the elderly and younger patients. In general, dose selection for an elderly patient should be cautious, reflecting the greater frequency of decreased hepatic, renal, or cardiac function, and of concomitant disease or other drug therapy.

ADVERSE REACTIONS

Hematologic: The most common side effect is bone marrow suppression. Although bone marrow suppression frequently occurs, it is usually reversible if melphalan is withdrawn early enough. However, irreversible bone marrow failure has been reported.

Gastrointestinal: Gastrointestinal disturbances such as nausea and vomiting, diarrhea, and oral ulceration occur infrequently. Hepatic toxicity has been reported rarely.

Miscellaneous: Other reported adverse reactions include: pulmonary fibrosis and interstitial pneumonitis, skin hypersensitivity, vasculitis, alopecia, and hemolytic anemia. Allergic reactions, including rare anaphylaxis, have occurred after multiple courses of treatment.

OVERDOSAGE

Overdoses, including doses up to 50 mg/day for 16 days, have been reported. Immediate effects are likely to be vomiting, ulceration of the mouth, diarrhea, and hemorrhage of the gastrointestinal tract. The principal toxic effect is bone marrow suppression. Hematologic parameters should be closely followed for 3 to 6 weeks. An uncontrolled study suggests that administration of autologous bone marrow or hematopoietic growth factors (i.e., sargramostim, filgrastim) may shorten the period of pancytopenia. General supportive measures, together with appropriate blood transfusions and antibiotics, should be instituted as deemed necessary by the physician. This drug is not removed from plasma to any significant degree by hemodialysis.[1]

DOSAGE AND ADMINISTRATION

Multiple Myeloma: The usual oral dose is 6 mg (3 tablets) daily. The entire daily dose may be given at one time. The dose is adjusted, as required, on the basis of blood counts done at approximately weekly intervals. After 2 to 3 weeks of treatment, the drug should be discontinued for up to 4 weeks during which time the blood count should be followed carefully. When the white blood cell and platelet counts are rising, a maintenance dose of 2 mg daily may be instituted. Because of the patient-to-patient variation in melphalan plasma levels following oral administration of the drug, several investigators have recommended that the dosage of ALKERAN be cautiously escalated until some myelosuppression is observed in order to assure that potentially therapeutic levels of the drug have been reached.

Other dosage regimens have been used by various investigators. Osserman and Takatsuki have used an initial course of 10 mg/day for 7 to 10 days.[2,3] They report that maximal suppression of the leukocyte and platelet counts occurs within 3 to 5 weeks and recovery within 4 to 8 weeks. Continuous maintenance therapy with 2 mg/day is instituted when the white blood cell count is greater than 4,000 cells/mcL and the platelet count is greater than 100,000 cells/mcL. Dosage is adjusted to between 1 and 3 mg/day depending upon the hematological response. It is desirable to try to maintain a significant degree of bone marrow depression so as to keep the leukocyte count in the range of 3,000 to 3,500 cells/mcL.

Hoogstraten et al have started treatment with 0.15 mg/kg per day for 7 days.[4] This is followed by a rest period of at least 14 days, but it may be as long as 5 to 6 weeks. Maintenance therapy is started when the white blood cell and platelet counts are rising. The maintenance dose is 0.05 mg/kg per day or less and is adjusted according to the blood count.

Available evidence suggests that about one third to one half of the patients with multiple myeloma show a favorable response to oral administration of the drug.

One study by Alexanian et al has shown that the use of ALKERAN in combination with prednisone significantly improves the percentage of patients with multiple myeloma who achieve palliation.[5] One regimen has been to administer courses of ALKERAN at 0.25 mg/kg per day for 4 consecutive days (or, 0.20 mg/kg per day for 5 consecutive days) for a total dose of 1 mg/kg per course. These 4- to 5-day courses are then repeated every 4 to 6 weeks if the granulocyte count and the platelet count have returned to normal levels.

It is to be emphasized that response may be very gradual over many months; it is important that repeated courses or continuous therapy be given since improvement may continue slowly over many months, and the maximum benefit may be missed if treatment is abandoned too soon.

In patients with moderate to severe renal impairment, currently available pharmacokinetic data do not justify an absolute recommendation on dosage reduction to those patients, but it may be prudent to use a reduced dose initially.

Epithelial Ovarian Cancer: One commonly employed regimen for the treatment of ovarian carcinoma has been to administer ALKERAN at a dose of 0.2 mg/kg daily for 5 days as a single course. Courses are repeated every 4 to 5 weeks depending upon hematologic tolerance.[6,7]

Administration Precautions: Procedures for proper handling and disposal of anticancer drugs should be considered. Several guidelines on this subject have been published.[8-14] There is no general agreement that all of the procedures recommended in the guidelines are necessary or appropriate.

HOW SUPPLIED

ALKERAN is supplied as white, scored tablets containing 2 mg melphalan, imprinted with "ALKERAN" and "A2A"; in bottles of 50 (NDC 0173-0045-35).

Store at 15° to 25°C (59° to 77°F) in a dry place, protect from light, and dispense in glass.

REFERENCES

1. Pallante SL, Fenselau C, Mennel RG, et al. Quantitation by gas chromatography-chemical ionization-mass spectrometry of phenylalanine mustard in plasma of patients. *Cancer Res.* 1980;40:2268-2272.
2. Osserman EF. Therapy of plasma cell myeloma with melphalan (1-phenylalanine mustard). *Proc Am Assoc Cancer Res.* 1963;4:50. Abstract.
3. Osserman EF, Takatsuki K. Plasma cell myeloma: gamma globulin synthesis and structure. A review of biochemical and clinical data, with the description of a newly-recognized and related syndrome. "H-gamma-2-chain" (Franklin's) disease. *Medicine* (Balt). 1963;42:357-384.
4. Hoogstraten B, Sheehe PR, Cuttner J, et al. Melphalan in multiple myeloma. *Blood.* 1967;30:74-83.
5. Alexanian R, Haut A, Khan AU, et al. Treatment for multiple myeloma; combination chemotherapy with different melphalan dose regimens. *JAMA.* 1969;208:1680-1685.
6. Smith JP, Rutledge FN: Chemotherapy in advanced ovarian cancer. *Natl Cancer Inst Monogr.* 1975; 42:141-143.
7. Young RC, Chabner BA, Hubbard SP, et al. Advanced ovarian adenocarcinoma: a prospective clinical trial of melphalan (L-PAM) versus combination chemotherapy. *N Engl J Med.* 1978;299:1261-1266.
8. Recommendations for the safe handling of parenteral antineoplastic drugs. Washington, DC: Division of Safety, National Institutes of Health; 1983. US Dept of Health and Human Services, Public Health Service publication NIH 83-2621.
9. AMA Council on Scientific Affairs. Guidelines for handling parenteral antineoplastics. *JAMA.* 1985;253:1590-1591.
10. National Study Commission on Cytotoxic Exposure. Recommendations for handling cytotoxic agents. 1987. Available from Louis P. Jeffrey, Chairman, National Study Commission on Cytotoxic Exposure. Massachusetts College of Pharmacy and Allied Health Sciences, 179 Longwood Avenue, Boston, MA 02115.
11. Clinical Oncological Society of Australia. Guidelines and recommendations for safe handling of antineoplastic agents. *Med J Australia.* 1983;1:426-428.
12. Jones RB, Frank R, Mass T. Safe handling of chemotherapeutic agents: a report from the Mount Sinai Medical Center. *CA-A Cancer J for Clin.* 1983;33:258-263.
13. American Society of Hospital Pharmacists. ASHP technical assistance bulletin on handling cytotoxic and hazardous drugs. *Am J Hosp Pharm.* 1990;47:1033-1049.
14. Yodaiken RE, Bennett D. OSHA work-practice guidelines for personnel dealing with cytotoxic (antineoplastic) drugs. *Am J Hosp Pharm.* 1986;43:1193-1204.

Manufactured by Catalytica Pharmaceuticals, Inc.
Greenville, NC 27834
for Glaxo Wellcome Inc., Research Triangle Park, NC 27709

September 1997/RL-467

Shown in Product Identification Guide, page 314

AMERGE® ℞

[*ə-merge'*]
(naratriptan hydrochloride)
Tablets

DESCRIPTION

AMERGE Tablets contain naratriptan as the hydrochloride, which is a selective 5-hydroxytryptamine$_1$ receptor subtype agonist. Naratriptan hydrochloride is chemically designated as N-methyl-3-(1-methyl-4-piperidinyl)-1H-indole-5-ethanesulfonamide monohydrochloride.

The empirical formula is $C_{17}H_{25}N_3O_2S \bullet HCl$, representing a molecular weight of 371.93. Naratriptan hydrochloride is a white to pale yellow powder that is readily soluble in water. Each AMERGE Tablet for oral administration contains 1.11 or 2.78 mg of naratriptan hydrochloride equivalent to 1 or 2.5 mg of naratriptan, respectively. Each tablet also contains the inactive ingredients croscarmellose sodium; hydroxypropyl methylcellulose; lactose; magnesium stearate; microcrystalline cellulose; triacetin; and titanium dioxide, iron oxide yellow, and indigo carmine aluminum lake (FD&C Blue No. 2) for coloring.

CLINICAL PHARMACOLOGY

Mechanism of Action: Naratriptan binds with high affinity to 5-HT$_{1D}$ and 5-HT$_{1B}$ receptors and has no significant affinity or pharmacological activity at 5-HT$_{2-4}$ receptor subtypes or at adrenergic α_1, α_2, or β; dopaminergic D_1 or D_2; muscarinic; or benzodiazepine receptors.

The therapeutic activity of naratriptan in migraine is generally attributed to its agonist activity at 5-HT$_{1D/1B}$ receptors. Two current theories have been proposed to explain the efficacy of 5-HT$_{1D/1B}$ receptor agonists in migraine. One theory suggests that activation of 5-HT$_{1D/1B}$ receptors located on intracranial blood vessels, including those on the arteriovenous anastomoses, leads to vasoconstriction, which is correlated with the relief of migraine headache. The other hypothesis suggests that activation of 5-HT$_{1D/1B}$ receptors on sensory nerve endings in the trigeminal system results in the inhibition of pro-inflammatory neuropeptide release.

In the anesthetized dog, naratriptan has been shown to reduce the carotid arterial blood flow with little or no effect on arterial blood pressure or total peripheral resistance. While the effect on blood flow was selective for the carotid arterial bed, increases in vascular resistance of up to 30% were seen in the coronary arterial bed. Naratriptan has also been shown to inhibit trigeminal nerve activity in rat and cat. In 10 human subjects with suspected coronary artery disease (CAD) undergoing coronary artery catheterization, there was a 1% to 10% reduction in coronary artery diameter following subcutaneous injection of 1.5 mg of naratriptan.

Pharmacokinetics: Naratriptan tablets are well absorbed, with about 70% oral bioavailability. Following administration of a 2.5-mg tablet orally, the peak concentrations are obtained in 2 to 3 hours. After administration of 1- or 2.5-mg tablets, the C_{max} is somewhat (about 50%) higher in women (not corrected for milligram-per-kilogram dose) than in men. During a migraine attack, absorption was slower, with a t_{max} of 3 to 4 hours. Food does not affect the pharmacokinetics of naratriptan. Naratriptan displays linear kinetics over the therapeutic dose range.

The steady-state volume of distribution of naratriptan is 170 L. Plasma protein binding is 28% to 31% over the concentration range of 50 to 1000 ng/mL.

Naratriptan is predominantly eliminated in urine, with 50% of the dose recovered unchanged and 30% as metabolites in urine. In vitro, naratriptan is metabolized by a wide range of cytochrome P450 isoenzymes into a number of inactive metabolites.

The mean elimination half-life of naratriptan is 6 hours. The systemic clearance of naratriptan is 6.6 mL/min/kg. The renal clearance (220 mL/min) exceeds glomerular filtration rate, indicating active tubular secretion. Repeat administration of naratriptan tablets does not result in drug accumulation.

Special Populations: ***Age:*** A small decrease in clearance (approximately 26%) was observed in healthy elderly subjects (65 to 77 years) compared to younger patients, resulting in slightly higher exposure (see PRECAUTIONS).

Race: The effect of race on the pharmacokinetics of naratriptan has not been examined.

Renal Impairment: Clearance of naratriptan was reduced by 50% in patients with moderate renal impairment (creatinine clearance: 18 to 39 mL/min) compared to the normal group. Decrease in clearances resulted in an increase of mean half-life from 6 hours (healthy) to 11 hours (range: 7 to 20 hours). The mean C_{max} increased by approximately 40%. The effects of severe renal impairment (creatinine clearance $\leq$15 mL/min) on the pharmacokinetics of naratriptan has not been assessed. (See CONTRAINDICATIONS and DOSAGE AND ADMINISTRATION.)

Hepatic Impairment: Clearance of naratriptan was decreased by 30% in patients with moderate hepatic impairment (Child-Pugh grade A or B). This resulted in an approximately 40% increase in the half-life (range: 8 to 16 hours). The effects of severe hepatic impairment (Child-Pugh grade C) on the pharmacokinetics of naratriptan have not been assessed. (See CONTRAINDICATIONS and DOSAGE AND ADMINISTRATION.)

Drug Interactions: In normal volunteers, coadministration of single doses of naratriptan tablets and alcohol did not result in substantial modification of naratriptan pharmacokinetic parameters.

From population pharmacokinetic analyses, coadministration of naratriptan and fluoxetine, beta-blockers, or tricyclic antidepressants did not affect the clearance of naratriptan. Naratriptan does not inhibit monoamine oxidase (MAO) enzymes and is a poor inhibitor of P450; metabolic interactions between naratriptan and drugs metabolized by P450 or MAO are therefore unlikely.

Oral Contraceptives: Oral contraceptives reduced clearance by 32% and volume of distribution by 22%, resulting in slightly higher concentrations of naratriptan. Hormone replacement therapy had no effect on pharmacokinetics in older female patients.

Smoking increased the clearance of naratriptan by 30%.

CLINICAL TRIALS

The efficacy of AMERGE Tablets in the acute treatment of migraine headaches was evaluated in 6 randomized, double-blind, placebo-controlled studies of which 4 used the recommended dosing regimen and were conducted as outpatient trials. Three of these studies enrolled adult patients who were predominantly female (86%) and Caucasian (96%) with a mean age of 41 (range: 18 to 65). One study enrolled adolescents with a mean age of 14 (range: 12 to 17). In the adolescent study, 54% of the patients were female and 89% were Caucasian. In all studies, patients were instructed to treat at least 1 moderate to severe headache. Headache response, defined as a reduction in headache severity from moderate or severe pain to mild or no pain, was assessed up to 4 hours after dosing. Associated symptoms such as nausea, vomiting, photophobia, and phonophobia were also assessed. Maintenance of response was assessed for up to 24 hours postdose. A second dose of AMERGE Tablets or other medication was allowed 4 to 24 hours after the initial treatment for recurrent headache. The frequency and time to use of these additional treatments were also determined.

In all 3 trials in adults utilizing the recommended dosage regimen and outpatient use, the percentage of patients achieving headache response 4 hours after treatment, the primary outcome measure, was significantly greater among patients receiving AMERGE compared to those who received placebo. In all studies, response to 2.5 mg was numerically greater than response to 1 mg and in the largest of the 3 studies, there was a statistically significant greater percentage of patients with headache response at 4 hours in the 2.5-mg group compared to the 1-mg group. The results are summarized in Table 1.

[See table 1 above]

Table 1: Percentage of Adult Patients With Headache Response (Mild or No Headache) 4 Hours Following Treatment

	Placebo	AMERGE 1.0 mg	AMERGE 2.5 mg
Study 1	34% (n = 122)	50%* (n = 117)	60%* (n = 127)
Study 2	27% (n = 104)	52%* (n = 208)	66%*† (n = 199)
Study 3	32% (n = 169)	54%* (n = 166)	65%* (n = 167)

* P<0.05 in comparison with placebo.
† P<0.05 in comparison with 1 mg.

In the single study in adolescents, there were no statistically significant differences between any of the treatment groups. The headache response rates at 4 hours (n) were 65% (n = 74), 67% (n = 78), and 64% (n = 70) for placebo, 1-mg, and 2.5-mg groups, respectively.

Continued on next page

This product information is based on labeling in effect on June 23, 2000. For further information, contact via direct mail, phone, or web site. Medical Information, Glaxo Wellcome Inc., PO Box 13398, Research Triangle Park, NC 27709. Healthcare Professionals (Medical Information): 800-334-0089. Patients (Customer Response Center): 1-888-825-5249. Glaxo Wellcome Corporate Web Site: www.glaxowellcome.com

Amerge—Cont.

Comparisons of drug performance based upon results obtained in different clinical trials are never reliable. Because studies are conducted at different times, with different samples of patients, by different investigators, employing different criteria and/or different interpretations of the same criteria, under different conditions (dose, dosing regimen, etc.), quantitative estimates of treatment response and the timing of response may be expected to vary considerably from study to study.

The estimated probability of achieving an initial headache response in adults over the 4 hours following treatment is depicted in Figure 1.

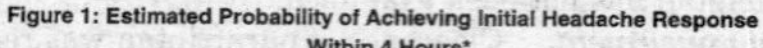

Figure 1: Estimated Probability of Achieving Initial Headache Response Within 4 Hours*

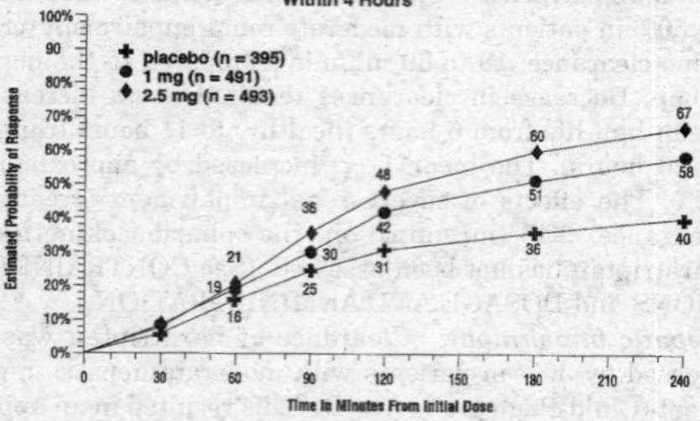

*The figure shows the probability over time of obtaining headache response (no or mild pain) following treatment with naratriptan tablets. The averages displayed are based on pooled data from the 3 controlled clinical trials providing evidence of efficacy (Studies 1, 2, and 3). In this Kaplan-Meier plot, patients not achieving response within 240 minutes were censored at 240 minutes.

For patients with migraine-associated nausea, photophobia, and phonophobia at baseline, there was a lower incidence of these symptoms 4 hours following administration of 1- and 2.5-mg AMERGE Tablets compared to placebo.

Four to 24 hours following the initial dose of study treatment, patients were allowed to use additional treatment for pain relief in the form of a second dose of study treatment or other medication. The estimated probability of patients taking a second dose or other medication for migraine over the 24 hours following the initial dose of study treatment is summarized in Figure 2.

Figure 2: Estimated Probability of Patients Taking a Second Dose of AMERGE Tablets or Other Medication for Migraine Over the 24 Hours Following the Initial Dose of Study Treatment*

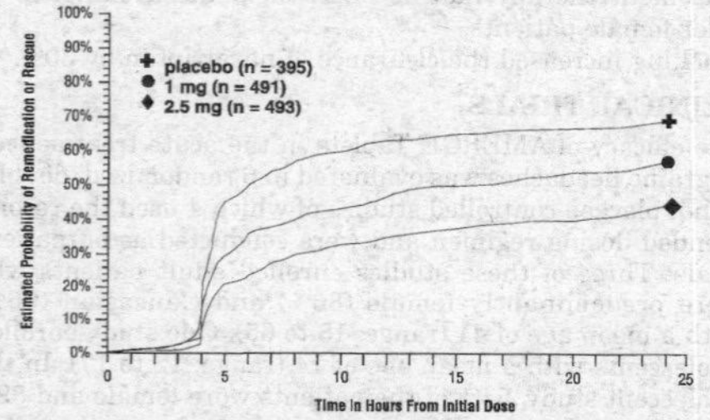

*Kaplan-Meier plot based on data obtained in the 3 controlled clinical trials (Studies 1, 2, and 3) providing evidence of efficacy with patients not using additional treatments censored at 24 hours. The plot also includes patients who had no response to the initial dose. Remedication was discouraged prior to 4 hours postdose.

There is no evidence that doses of 5 mg provide a greater effect than 2.5 mg. There was no evidence to suggest that treatment with AMERGE was associated with an increase in the severity or frequency of migraine attacks. The efficacy of AMERGE Tablets was unaffected by presence of aura; gender, age, or weight of the patient; oral contraceptive use; or concomitant use of common migraine prophylactic drugs (e.g., beta-blockers, calcium channel blockers, tricyclic antidepressants). There was insufficient data to assess the impact of race on efficacy.

INDICATIONS AND USAGE

AMERGE Tablets are indicated for the acute treatment of migraine attacks with or without aura in adults.

AMERGE Tablets are not intended for the prophylactic therapy of migraine or for use in the management of hemiplegic or basilar migraine (see CONTRAINDICATIONS). Safety and effectiveness of AMERGE Tablets have not been established for cluster headache, which is present in an older, predominantly male population.

CONTRAINDICATIONS

AMERGE Tablets should not be given to patients with history, symptoms, or signs of ischemic cardiac, cerebrovascular, or peripheral vascular syndromes. In addition, patients with other significant underlying cardiovascular diseases should not receive AMERGE Tablets. Ischemic cardiac syndromes include, but are not limited to, angina pectoris of any type (e.g., stable angina of effort and vasospastic forms of angina such as the Prinzmetal variant), all forms of myocardial infarction, and silent myocardial ischemia. Cerebrovascular sydromes include, but are not limited to, strokes of any type as well as transient ischemic attacks. Peripheral vascular disease includes, but is not limited to, ischemic bowel disease (see WARNINGS).

Because AMERGE Tablets may increase blood pressure, they should not be given to patients with uncontrolled hypertension (see WARNINGS).

AMERGE Tablets are contraindicated in patients with severe renal impairment (creatinine clearance: <15 mL/min) (see CLINICAL PHARMACOLOGY and DOSAGE AND ADMINISTRATION).

AMERGE Tablets are contraindicated in patients with severe hepatic impairment (Child-Pugh grade C) (see CLINICAL PHARMACOLOGY and DOSAGE AND ADMINISTRATION).

AMERGE Tablets should not be administered to patients with hemiplegic or basilar migraine.

AMERGE Tablets should not be used within 24 hours of treatment with another 5-HT$_1$ agonist, an ergotamine-containing or ergot-type medication like dihydroergotamine or methysergide.

AMERGE Tablets are contraindicated in patients with hypersensitivity to naratriptan or any of the components.

WARNINGS

AMERGE Tablets should only be used where a clear diagnosis of migraine has been established.

Risk of Myocardial Ischemia and/or Infarction and Other Adverse Cardiac Events: Because of the potential of this class of compounds (5-HT$_{1B/1D}$ agonists) to cause coronary vasospasm, naratriptan should not be given to patients with documented ischemic or vasospastic coronary artery disease (CAD) (see CONTRAINDICATIONS). It is strongly recommended that 5-HT$_1$ agonists (including naratriptan) not be given to patients in whom unrecognized CAD is predicted by the presence of risk factors (e.g., hypertension, hypercholesterolemia, smoker, obesity, diabetes, strong family history of CAD, female with surgical or physiological menopause, or male over 40 years of age) unless a cardiovascular evaluation provides satisfactory clinical evidence that the patient is reasonably free of coronary artery and ischemic myocardial disease or other significant underlying cardiovascular disease. The sensitivity of cardiac diagnostic procedures to detect cardiovascular disease or predisposition to coronary artery vasospasm is modest, at best. If, during the cardiovascular evaluation, the patient's medical history, electrocardiographic, or other investigations reveal findings indicative of, or consistent with, coronary artery vasospasm or myocardial ischemia, naratriptan should not be administered (see CONTRAINDICATIONS).

For patients with risk factors predictive of CAD, who are determined to have a satisfactory cardiovascular evaluation, it is strongly recommended that administration of the first dose of naratriptan take place in the setting of a physician's office or similar medically staffed and equipped facility. Because cardiac ischemia can occur in the absence of clinical symptoms, consideration should be given to obtaining on the first occasion of use an electrocardiogram (ECG) during the interval immediately following administration of AMERGE Tablets, in these patients with risk factors.

It is recommended that patients who are intermittent long-term users of 5-HT$_1$ agonists, including AMERGE Tablets, and who have or acquire risk factors predictive of CAD, as described above, undergo periodic cardiovascular evaluation as they continue to use AMERGE Tablets.

The systematic approach described above is intended to reduce the likelihood that patients with unrecognized cardiovascular disease will be inadvertently exposed to naratriptan.

Cardiac Events and Fatalities Associated With 5-HT$_1$ Agonists: Naratriptan can cause coronary artery vasospasm (see CLINICAL PHARMACOLOGY). Serious adverse cardiac events, including acute myocardial infarction, life-threatening disturbances of cardiac rhythm, and death have been reported within a few hours following the administration of 5-HT$_1$ agonists. Considering the extent of use of 5-HT$_1$ agonists in patients with migraine, the incidence of these events is extremely low.

Premarketing Experience With AMERGE Tablets: Among approximately 3500 patients with migraine who participated in premarketing clinical trials of naratriptan tablets, 4 patients treated with single oral doses of naratriptan ranging from 1 to 10 mg experienced asymptomatic ischemic ECG changes with at least 1, who took 7.5 mg, likely due to coronary vasospasm.

Cerebrovascular Events and Fatalities With 5-HT$_1$ Agonists: Cerebral hemorrhage, subarachnoid hemorrhage, stroke, and other cerebrovascular events have been reported in patients treated with 5-HT$_1$ agonists, and some have resulted in fatalities. In a number of cases, it appears possible that the cerebrovascular events were primary, the agonist having been administered in the incorrect belief that the symptoms experienced were a consequence of migraine, when they were not. It should be noted that patients with migraine may be at increased risk of certain cerebrovascular events (e.g., stroke, hemorrhage, transient ischemic attack).

Other Vasospasm-Related Events: 5-HT$_1$ agonists may cause vasospastic reactions other than coronary artery spasm. Both peripheral vascular ischemia and colonic ischemia with abdominal pain and bloody diarrhea have been reported with 5-HT$_1$ agonists.

Increase in Blood Pressure: In healthy volunteers, dose-related increases in systemic blood pressure have been observed after administration of up to 20 mg of oral naratriptan. At the recommended doses, the elevations are generally small, although an increase of systolic pressure of 32 mmHg was seen in 1 patient following a single 2.5-mg dose. The effect may be more pronounced in the elderly and hypertensive patients. A patient who was mildly hypertensive (the baseline blood pressure was 150/98) experienced a significant increase in blood pressure to 204/144 mmHg 225 minutes after administration of a 10-mg oral dose. Significant elevation in blood pressure, including hypertensive crisis, has been reported on rare occasions in patients receiving 5-HT$_1$ agonists with and without a history of hypertension. Naratriptan is contraindicated in patients with uncontrolled hypertension (see CONTRAINDICATIONS).

An 18% increase in mean pulmonary artery pressure and an 8% increase in mean aortic pressure was seen following dosing with 1.5 mg of subcutaneous naratriptan in a study evaluating 10 subjects with suspected CAD undergoing cardiac catheterization.

Hypersensitivity: Hypersensitivity (anaphylaxis/anaphylactoid) reactions may occur in patients receiving naratriptan. Such reactions can be life threatening or fatal. In general, hypersensitivity reactions to drugs are more likely to occur in individuals with a history of sensitivity to multiple allergens (see CONTRAINDICATIONS).

PRECAUTIONS

General: Chest discomfort (including pain, pressure, heaviness, tightness) has been reported after administration of 5-HT$_1$ agonists, including AMERGE Tablets. These events have not been associated with arrhythmias or ischemic ECG changes in clinical trials with AMERGE Tablets. Because naratriptan may cause coronary artery vasospasm, patients who experience signs or symptoms suggestive of angina following naratriptan should be evaluated for the presence of CAD or a predisposition to Prinzmetal variant angina before receiving additional doses of naratriptan, and should be monitored electrocardiographically if dosing is resumed and similar symptoms recur. Similarly, patients who experience other symptoms or signs suggestive of decreased arterial flow, such as ischemic bowel syndrome or Raynaud syndrome following naratriptan administration should be evaluated for atherosclerosis or predisposition to vasospasm (see CONTRAINDICATIONS and WARNINGS).

AMERGE Tablets should also be administered with caution to patients with diseases that may alter the absorption, metabolism, or excretion of drugs, such as impaired renal or hepatic function (see CLINICAL PHARMACOLOGY, CONTRAINDICATIONS, and DOSAGE AND ADMINISTRATION).

Care should be taken to exclude other potentially serious neurological conditions before treating headache in patients not previously diagnosed with migraine or who experience a headache that is atypical for them. There have been rare reports where patients received 5-HT$_1$ agonists for severe headaches that were subsequently shown to have been secondary to an evolving neurologic lesion (see WARNINGS).

For a given attack, if a patient has no response to the first dose of naratriptan, the diagnosis of migraine should be reconsidered before administration of a second dose.

Binding to Melanin-Containing Tissues: In rats treated with a single oral dose (10 mg/kg) of radiolabeled naratriptan, the elimination half-life of radioactivity from the eye was 90 days, suggesting that naratriptan and/or its metabolites may bind to the melanin of the eye. Because there could be accumulation in melanin-rich tissues over time, this raises the possibility that naratriptan could cause toxicity in these tissues after extended use. Although no systematic monitoring of ophthalmologic function was undertaken in clinical trials, and no specific recommendations for ophthalmologic monitoring are offered, prescribers should be aware of the possibility of long-term ophthalmologic effects.

Changes in the Precorneal Tear Film: Dogs receiving oral naratriptan showed transient changes in the precorneal tear film. Corneal stippling was seen at the lowest dose tested, 1 mg/kg per day, and occurred intermittently from day 1 throughout the first 2 to 3 weeks of treatment. Although a no-effect dose was not established, the exposure at the lowest dose tested was approximately 5 times the human exposure after a 5-mg oral dose.

Information for Patients: See PATIENT INFORMATION at the end of this labeling for the text of the separate leaflet provided for patients.

Laboratory Tests: No specific laboratory tests are recommended for monitoring patients prior to and/or after treatment with AMERGE Tablets.

Drug Interactions: Ergot-containing drugs have been reported to cause prolonged vasospastic reactions. Because there is a theoretical basis that these effects may be additive, use of ergotamine-containing or ergot-type medications (like dihydroergotamine or methysergide) and naratriptan within 24 hours is contraindicated (see CONTRAINDICATIONS).

The administration of naratriptan with other 5-HT$_1$ agonists has not been evaluated in migraine patients. Because their vasospastic effects may be additive, coadministration of naratriptan and other 5-HT$_1$ agonists within 24 hours of each other is not recommended (see CONTRAINDICATIONS).

Selective serotonin reuptake inhibitors (SSRIs) (e.g., fluoxetine, fluvoxamine, paroxetine, sertraline) have been reported, rarely, to cause weakness, hyperreflexia, and incoordination when coadministered with 5-HT$_1$ agonists. If concomitant treatment with naratriptan and an SSRI is clinically warranted, appropriate observation of the patient is advised.

Drug/Laboratory Test Interactions: AMERGE Tablets are not known to interfere with commonly employed clinical laboratory tests.

Carcinogenesis, Mutagenesis, Impairment of Fertility: ***Carcinogenesis:*** Lifetime carcinogenicity studies, 104 weeks in duration, were carried out in mice and rats by oral gavage. There was no evidence of an increase in tumors related to naratriptan administration in mice receiving up to 200 mg/kg/day. That dose was associated with a plasma AUC exposure that was 110 times the exposure in humans receiving the maximum recommended daily dose of 5 mg. Two rat studies were conducted, 1 using a standard diet and the other a nitrite-supplemented diet (naratriptan can be nitrosated in vitro to form a mutagenic product that has been detected in the stomachs of rats fed a high nitrite diet). Doses of 5, 20, and 90 mg/kg were associated with week 13 AUC exposures that in the standard diet study were 7, 40, and 236 times, and in the nitrite-supplemented diet study were 7, 29, and 180 times, the exposure attained in humans given the maximum recommended daily dose of 5 mg. In both studies, there was an increase in the incidence of thyroid follicular hyperplasia in high-dose males and females and in thyroid follicular adenomas in high-dose males. In the standard diet study only, there was also an increase in the incidence of benign c-cell adenomas in the thyroid of high-dose males and females. The exposures achieved at the no-effect dose for thyroid tumors were 40 (standard diet) and 29 (nitrite-supplemented diet) times the exposure achieved in humans receiving the maximum recommended daily dose of 5 mg. In the nitrite-supplemented diet study only, the incidence of benign lymphocytic thymoma was increased in all treated groups of females. It was not determined if the nitrosated product is systemically absorbed. However, no changes were seen in the stomachs of rats in that study.

Mutagenesis: Naratriptan was not mutagenic when tested in 2 gene mutation assays, the Ames test and the in vitro thymidine locus mouse lymphoma assay. It was not clastogenic in 2 cytogenetics assays, the in vitro human lymphocyte assay and the in vivo mouse micronucleus assay. Naratriptan can be nitrosated in vitro to form a mutagenic product (WHO nitrosation assay) that has been detected in the stomachs of rats fed a nitrite-supplemented diet.

Impairment of Fertility: In a reproductive toxicity study in which male and female rats were dosed prior to and throughout the mating period with 10, 60, 170, or 340 mg/kg/day (plasma exposures [AUC] approximately 11, 70, 230, and 470 times, respectively, the human exposure at the maximum recommended daily dose [MRDD] of 5 mg), there was a treatment-related decrease in the number of females exhibiting normal estrous cycles at doses of 170 mg/kg/day or greater and an increase in preimplantation loss at 60 mg/kg/day or greater. In high-dose group males, testicular/epididymal atrophy accompanied by spermatozoa depletion reduced mating success and may have contributed to the observed preimplantation loss. The exposures achieved at the no-effect doses for preimplantation loss, anestrus, and testicular effects were approximately 11, 70, and 230 times, respectively, the exposures in humans receiving the MRDD.

In a study in which rats were dosed orally with 10, 60, or 340 mg/kg/day for 6 months, changes in the female reproductive tract including atrophic or cystic ovaries and anestrus were seen at the high dose. The exposure at the no-effect dose of 60 mg/kg was approximately 85 times the exposure in humans receiving the MRDD.

Pregnancy: Pregnancy Category C. There are no adequate and well-controlled studies in pregnant women; therefore, naratriptan should be used during pregnancy only if the potential benefit justifies the potential risk to the fetus.

To monitor fetal outcomes of pregnant women exposed to AMERGE, Glaxo Wellcome Inc. maintains a Naratriptan Pregnancy Registry. Health care providers are encouraged to register patients by calling (800) 336-2176.

In reproductive toxicity studies in rats and rabbits, oral administration of naratriptan was associated with developmental toxicity (embryolethality, fetal abnormalities, pup mortality, offspring growth retardation) at doses producing maternal plasma drug exposures as low as 11 and 2.5 times, respectively, the exposure in humans receiving the maximum recommended daily dose (MRDD) of 5 mg.

When pregnant rats were administered naratriptan during the period of organogenesis at doses of 10, 60, or 340 mg/kg/day, there was a dose-related increase in embryonic death, with a statistically significant difference at the highest dose, and incidences of fetal structural variations (incomplete/irregular ossification of skull bones, sternebrae, ribs) were increased at all doses. The maternal plasma exposures (AUC) at these doses were approximately 11, 70, and 470 times the exposure in humans at the MRDD. The high dose was maternally toxic, as evidenced by decreased maternal body weight gain during gestation. A no-effect dose for developmental toxicity in rats exposed during organogenesis was not established.

When doses of 1, 5, or 30 mg/kg/day were given to pregnant Dutch rabbits throughout organogenesis, the incidence of a specific fetal skeletal malformation (fused sternebrae) was increased at the high dose, and increased incidences of embryonic death and fetal variations (major blood vessel variations, supernumerary ribs, incomplete skeletal ossification) were observed at all doses (4, 20, and 120 times, respectively, the MRDD on a body surface area basis). Maternal toxicity (decreased body weight gain) was evident at the high dose in this study. In a similar study in New Zealand White rabbits (1, 5, or 30 mg/kg/day throughout organogenesis), decreased fetal weights and increased incidences of fetal skeletal variations were observed at all doses (maternal exposures equivalent to 2.5, 19, and 140 times exposure in humans receiving the MRDD), while maternal body weight gain was reduced at 5 mg/kg or greater. A no-effect dose for developmental toxicity in rabbits exposed during organogenesis was not established.

When female rats were treated with 10, 60, or 340 mg/kg/day during late gestation and lactation, offspring behavioral impairment (tremors) and decreased offspring viability and growth were observed at doses of 60 mg/kg or greater, while maternal toxicity occurred only at the highest dose. Maternal exposures at the no-effect dose for developmental effects in this study were approximately 11 times the exposure in humans receiving the MRDD.

Nursing Mothers: Naratriptan-related material is excreted in the milk of rats. Therefore, caution should be exercised when considering the administration of AMERGE Tablets to a nursing woman.

Pediatric Use: Safety and effectiveness of AMERGE Tablets in pediatric patients (less than 18 years of age) have not been established.

One randomized, placebo-controlled clinical trial evaluating oral naratriptan (0.25 to 2.5 mg) in pediatric patients aged 12 to 17 years evaluated a total of 300 adolescent migraineurs. This study did not establish the efficacy of oral naratriptan compared to placebo in the treatment of migraine in adolescents (see CLINICAL TRIALS). Adverse events observed in this clinical trial were similar in nature to those reported in clinical trials in adults.

Geriatric Use: The use of naratriptan in elderly patients is not recommended.

AMERGE Tablets are known to be substantially excreted by the kidney, and the risk of adverse reactions to this drug may be greater in elderly patients who have reduced renal function. In addition, elderly patients are more likely to have decreased hepatic function; they are at higher risk for CAD; and blood pressure increases may be more pronounced in the elderly. Clinical studies of AMERGE Tablets did not include patients over 65 years of age.

ADVERSE REACTIONS

Serious cardiac events, including some that have been fatal, have occurred following the use of 5-HT$_1$ agonists. These events are extremely rare and most have been reported in patients with risk factors predictive of CAD. Events reported have included coronary artery vasospasm, transient myocardial ischemia, myocardial infarction, ventricular tachycardia, and ventricular fibrillation (see CONTRAINDICATIONS, WARNINGS, and PRECAUTIONS).

Incidence in Controlled Clinical Trials: The most common adverse events were paresthesias, dizziness, drowsiness, malaise/fatigue, and throat/neck symptoms, which occurred at a rate of 2% and at least 2 times placebo rate. Since patients treated only 1 to 3 headaches in the controlled clinical trials, the opportunity for discontinuation of therapy in response to an adverse event was limited. In a long-term, open label study where patients were allowed to treat multiple migraine attacks for up to 1 year, 15 patients (3.6%) discontinued treatment due to adverse events.

Table 2 lists adverse events that occurred in 5 placebo-controlled clinical trials of approximately 1752 exposures to placebo and AMERGE Tablets in adult migraine patients. The events cited reflect experience gained under closely monitored conditions of clinical trials in a highly selected patient population. In actual clinical practice or in other clinical trials, these frequency estimates may not apply, as the conditions of use, reporting behavior, and the kinds of patients treated may differ. Only events that occurred at a frequency of 2% or more in the AMERGE Tablets 2.5-mg treatment group and were more frequent in that group than in the placebo group are included in Table 2. From this table, it appears that many of these adverse events are dose related.

[See table 2 above]

Table 2: Treatment-Emergent Adverse Events Reported by at Least 2% of Patients in Placebo-Controlled Migraine Trials

Adverse Event Type	Placebo (n = 498)	AMERGE 1 mg (n = 627)	AMERGE 2.5 mg (n = 627)
Atypical sensation	1%	2%	4%
Paresthesias (all types)	<1%	1%	2%
Gastrointestinal	5%	6%	7%
Nausea	4%	4%	5%
Neurologial	3%	4%	7%
Dizziness	1%	1%	2%
Drowsiness	<1%	1%	2%
Malaise/fatigue	1%	2%	2%
Pain and pressure sensation	2%	2%	4%
Throat/neck symptoms	1%	1%	2%

One event present in more than 1% of patients receiving AMERGE Tablets (vomiting) occurred more frequently on placebo than on naratriptan 2.5 mg.

AMERGE Tablets are generally well tolerated. Most adverse reactions were mild and transient.

The incidence of adverse events in placebo-controlled clinical trials was not affected by age or weight of the patients, duration of headache prior to treatment, presence of aura, use of prophylactic medications, or tobacco use. There was insufficient data to assess the impact of race on the incidence of adverse events.

Other Events Observed in Association With the Administration of AMERGE Tablets: In the paragraphs that follow, the frequencies of less commonly reported adverse clinical events are presented. Because the reports include events observed in open and uncontrolled studies, the role of AMERGE Tablets in their causation cannot be reliably determined. Furthermore, variability associated with adverse event reporting, the terminology used to describe adverse events, etc. limit the value of the quantitative frequency estimates provided. Event frequencies are calculated as the number of patients reporting an event divided by the total number of patients (n = 3557) exposed to oral naratriptan doses up to 10 mg. All reported events are included except those already listed in the previous table, those too general to be informative, and those not reasonably associated with the use of the drug. Events are further classified within body system categories and enumerated in order of decreasing frequency using the following definitions: frequent adverse events are those occurring in at least 1/100 patients, infrequent adverse events are those occurring in 1/100 to 1/1000 patients, and rare adverse events are those occurring in fewer than 1/1000 patients.

Atypical Sensations: Frequent were warm/cold temperature sensations. Infrequent were feeling strange and burning/stinging sensation.

Cardiovascular: Infrequent were palpitations, increased blood pressure, tachyarrhythmias, and abnormal ECG (PR prolongation, QT$_c$ prolongation, ST/T wave abnormalities, premature ventricular contractions, atrial flutter, or atrial fibrillation), and syncope. Rare were bradycardia, varicosities, hypotension, and heart murmurs.

Ear, Nose, and Throat: Frequent were ear, nose, and throat infections. Infrequent were phonophobia, sinusitis, upper respiratory inflammation, and tinnitus. Rare were allergic rhinitis; labyrinthitis; ear, nose, and throat hemorrhage; and hearing difficulty.

Endocrine and Metabolic: Infrequent were thirst and polydipsia, dehydration, and fluid retention. Rare were hyperlipidemia, hypercholesterolemia, hypothyroidism, hyperglycemia, glycosuria and ketonuria, and parathyroid neoplasm.

Eye: Frequent was photophobia. Infrequent was blurred vision. Rare were eye pain and discomfort, sensation of eye pressure, eye hemorrhage, dry eyes, difficulty focusing, and scotoma.

Gastrointestinal: Frequent were hyposalivation and vomiting. Infrequent were dyspeptic symptoms, diarrhea, gastrointestinal discomfort and pain, gastroenteritis, and constipation. Rare were abnormal liver function tests, abnormal bilirubin levels, hemorrhoids, gastritis, esophagitis, salivary gland inflammation, oral itching and irritation, regurgitation and reflux, and gastric ulcers.

Hematological Disorders: Infrequent was increased white cells. Rare were thrombocytopenia, quantitative red cell or hemoglobin defects, anemia, and purpura.

Lower Respiratory Tract: Infrequent were bronchitis, cough, and pneumonia. Rare were tracheitis, asthma, pleuritis, and airway constriction and obstruction.

Musculoskeletal: Infrequent were muscle pain, arthralgia and articular rheumatism, muscle cramps and spasms, joint and muscle stiffness, tightness, and rigidity. Rare were bone and skeletal pain.

Neurological: Frequent was vertigo. Infrequent were tremors, cognitive function disorders, sleep disorders, and disorders of equilibrium. Rare were compressed nerve syndromes, confusion, sedation, hyperesthesia, coordination disorders, paralysis of cranial nerves, decreased consciousness, dreams, altered sense of taste, neuralgia, neuritis, aphasia, hypoesthesia, motor retardation, muscle twitching

Continued on next page

This product information is based on labeling in effect on June 23, 2000. For further information, contact via direct mail, phone, or web site. Medical Information, Glaxo Wellcome Inc., PO Box 13398, Research Triangle Park, NC 27709. Healthcare Professionals (Medical Information): 800-334-0089. Patients (Customer Response Center): 1-888-825-5249. Glaxo Wellcome Corporate Web Site: www.glaxowellcome.com

Amerge—Cont.

and fasciculation, psychomotor restlessness, and convulsions.

Non-Site Specific: Infrequent were chills and/or fever, descriptions of odor or taste, edema and swelling, allergies, and allergic reactions. Rare were spasms and mobility disorders.

Pain and Pressure Sensations: Frequent were pressure/tightness/heaviness sensations.

Psychiatry: Infrequent were anxiety, depressive disorders, and detachment. Rare were aggression and hostility, agitation, hallucinations, panic, and hyperactivity.

Reproduction: Rare were lumps of female reproductive tract, breast inflammation, inflammation of vagina, inflammation of fallopian tube, breast discharge, endometrium disorders, decreased libido, and lumps of breast.

Skin: Infrequent were sweating, skin rashes, pruritus, and urticaria. Rare were skin erythema, dermatitis and dermatosis, hair loss and alopecia, pruritic skin rashes, acne and folliculitis, allergic skin reactions, macular skin/rashes, skin photosensitivity, photodermatitis, skin flakiness, and dry skin.

Urology: Infrequent were bladder inflammation and polyuria and diuresis. Rare were urinary tract hemorrhage, urinary urgency, pyelitis, and urinary incontinence.

Observed During Clinical Practice: The following section enumerates potentially important adverse events that have occurred in clinical practice and that have been reported spontaneously to various surveillance systems. The events enumerated represent reports arising from both domestic and nondomestic use of naratriptan. These events do not include those already listed in the ADVERSE REACTIONS section above. Because the reports cite events reported spontaneously from worldwide postmarketing experience, frequency of events and the role of AMERGE in their causation cannot be reliably determined.

Cardiovascular: Angina, myocardial infarction (see WARNINGS).

Gastrointestinal: Colonic ischemia (see WARNINGS).

Lower Respiratory: Dyspnea.

Neurologic: Cerebral vascular accident, including transient ischemic attack, subarachnoid hemorrhage, and cerebral infarction (see WARNINGS).

General: Hypersensitivity, including anaphylaxis/anaphylactoid reactions, in come cases severe (e.g., circulatory collapse) (see WARNINGS).

DRUG ABUSE AND DEPENDENCE

In one clinical study enrolling 12 subjects, all of whom had experience using oral opiates and other psychoactive drugs, AMERGE Tablets produced less intense subjective responses ordinarily associated with many drugs of abuse than did codeine (30 to 90 mg).

OVERDOSAGE

A patient who was mildly hypertensive experienced a significant increase in blood pressure after administration of a 10-mg dose starting at 30 minutes (baseline value of 150/98 to 204/144 mmHg 225 minutes). This event resolved after treatment with antihypertensive therapy. Oral administration of 25 mg of naratriptan in 1 healthy young male subject increased blood pressure from 120/67 mmHg pretreatment up to 191/113 mmHg at approximately 6 hours postdose and resulted in adverse events including lightheadedness, tension in the neck, tiredness, and loss of coordination. Blood pressure returned to near baseline by 8 hours after dosing without any pharmacological intervention.

Another subject experienced asymptomatic ischemic ECG changes likely due to coronary artery vasospasm approximately 2 hours following a 7.5-mg oral dose.

The elimination half-life of naratriptan is about 6 hours (see CLINICAL PHARMACOLOGY), and therefore monitoring of patients after overdose with AMERGE Tablets should continue for at least 24 hours or while symptoms or signs persist. There is no specific antidote to naratriptan. Standard supportive treatment should be applied as required. If the patient presents with chest pain or other symptoms consistent with angina pectoris, ECG monitoring should be performed for evidence of ischemia. It is unknown what effect hemodialysis or peritoneal dialysis has on the serum concentrations of naratriptan.

DOSAGE AND ADMINISTRATION

In controlled clinical trials, single doses of 1 and 2.5 mg of AMERGE Tablets taken with fluid were effective for the acute treatment of migraines in adults. A greater proportion of patients had headache response following a 2.5-mg dose than following a 1-mg dose (see CLINICAL TRIALS). Individuals may vary in response to doses of AMERGE Tablets. The choice of dose should therefore be made on an individual basis, weighing the possible benefit of the 2.5-mg dose with the potential for a greater risk of adverse events. If the headache returns or if the patient has only partial response, the dose may be repeated once after 4 hours, for a maximum dose of 5 mg in a 24-hour period. There is evidence that doses of 5 mg do not provide a greater effect than 2.5 mg. The safety of treating, on average, more than 4 headaches in a 30-day period has not been established.

Renal Impairment: The use of AMERGE is contraindicated in patients with severe renal impairment (creatinine clearance <15 mL/min) because of decreased clearance of the drug. (See CONTRAINDICATIONS and CLINICAL PHARMACOLOGY.) In patients with mild to moderate renal impairment, the maximum daily dose should not exceed 2.5 mg over a 24-hour period and a lower starting dose should be considered.

Hepatic Impairment: The use of AMERGE is contraindicated in patients with severe hepatic impairment (Child-Pugh grade C) because of decreased clearance (see CONTRAINDICATIONS and CLINICAL PHARMACOLOGY). In patients with mild or moderate hepatic impairment, the maximum daily dose should not exceed 2.5 mg over a 24-hour period and a lower starting dose should be considered (see CLINICAL PHARMACOLOGY).

HOW SUPPLIED

AMERGE Tablets 1 and 2.5 mg of naratriptan (base) as the hydrochloride. AMERGE Tablets, 1 mg, are white, D-shaped, film-coated tablets embossed with "GX CE3" on one side in blister packs of 9 tablets (NDC 0173-0561-00). AMERGE Tablets, 2.5 mg, are green, D-shaped, film-coated tablets embossed with "GX CE5" on one side in blister packs of 9 tablets (NDC 0173-0562-00).

Store at controlled room temperature, 20° to 25°C (68° to 77°F) (see USP).

PATIENT INFORMATION

The following wording is contained in a separate leaflet provided for patients.

Information for the Patient
AMERGE® (naratriptan hydrochloride) Tablets

Please read this leaflet carefully before you take AMERGE Tablets. This leaflet provides a summary of the information available about your medicine. Please do not throw away this leaflet until you have finished your medicine. You may need to read this leaflet again. This leaflet does not contain all the information on AMERGE Tablets. For further information or advice, ask your doctor or pharmacist.

Information About Your Medicine:

The name of your medicine is AMERGE (naratriptan hydrochloride) Tablets. It can be obtained only by prescription from your doctor. The decision to use AMERGE Tablets is one that you and your doctor should make jointly, taking into account your individual preferences and medical circumstances. If you have risk factors for heart disease (such as high blood pressure, high cholesterol, obesity, diabetes, smoking, strong family history of heart disease, or you are postmenopausal or a male over 40), you should tell your doctor, who should evaluate you for heart disease in order to determine if AMERGE is appropriate for you. The majority of those who have taken AMERGE Tablets have not experienced any significant side effects. Rarely, deaths and/or serious heart problems have been reported with this class of medicines; in all but a few instances, however, these deaths and/or serious heart problems occurred in people with heart disease and it was not clear whether these medications were a contributing factor.

1. The Purpose of Your Medicine:

AMERGE Tablets are intended to relieve your migraine, but not to prevent or reduce the number of attacks you experience. Use AMERGE Tablets only to treat an actual migraine attack.

2. Important Questions to Consider Before Taking AMERGE Tablets:

If the answer to any of the following questions is **YES** or if you do not know the answer, then please discuss it with your doctor before you use AMERGE Tablets.

- Are you pregnant? Do you think you might be pregnant? Are you trying to become pregnant? Are you not using adequate contraception? Are you breastfeeding?
- Do you have any chest pain, heart disease, shortness of breath, or irregular heartbeats? Have you had a heart attack?
- Do you have risk factors for heart disease (such as high blood pressure, high cholesterol, obesity, diabetes, smoking, strong family history of heart disease, or you are postmenopausal or a male over 40)?
- Have you had a stroke, transient ischemic attacks or "TIAs", or Raynaud syndrome?
- Do you have high blood pressure?
- Have you ever had to stop taking this or any other medication because of an allergy or other problems?
- Are you taking any other migraine medications, including other 5-HT_1 agonists such as IMITREX® (sumatriptan), or medications containing ergotamine, dihydroergotamine, or methysergide?
- Are you taking any medication for depression such as selective serotonin reuptake inhibitors [SSRIs])?
- Have you had, or do you have, any disease of the kidney or liver?
- Is this headache different from your usual migraine attacks?

Remember, if you answered **YES** to any of the above questions, then discuss it with your doctor.

3. The Use of AMERGE Tablets During Pregnancy:

Do not use AMERGE Tablets if you are pregnant, think you might be pregnant, are trying to become pregnant, or are not using adequate contraception, unless you have discussed this with your doctor.

4. How to Use AMERGE Tablets:

For adults, the usual dose is a single tablet taken whole with fluids. It may be given at any time after the headache starts. For an individual attack, if you have no response to the first tablet, do not take a second tablet without first talking to your doctor. If you need more relief due to a partial response or return of your headache after the first tablet, a second tablet may be taken but not sooner than 4 hours following the first tablet. Do not take more than a total of 2 AMERGE Tablets in any 24-hour period. If you have kidney or liver disease, take as directed by your doctor.

5. Side Effects to Watch for:

- Some patients experience pain or tightness in the chest or throat when using AMERGE Tablets. If this happens to you, then discuss it with your doctor before using any more AMERGE Tablets. If the chest pain, tightness, or pressure is severe or does not go away, call your doctor immediately.
- If you have sudden and/or severe abdominal pain following AMERGE Tablets, call your doctor immediately.
- Shortness of breath; wheeziness; heart throbbing, swelling of eyelids, face, or lips; or a skin rash, skin lumps, or hives happens rarely. If it happens to you, then tell your doctor immediately. Do not take any more AMERGE Tablets unless your doctor tells you to do so.
- Some people may have feelings of tingling, heat, flushing (redness of face lasting a short time), heaviness or pressure after treatment with AMERGE Tablets. A few people may feel drowsy, dizzy, tired, or sick. Tell your doctor of these symptoms at your next visit.
- If you feel unwell in any other way or have any symptoms that you do not understand, you should contact your doctor immediately.

6. What to Do if an Overdose is Taken:

If you have taken more medication than you have been told, contact either your doctor, hospital emergency department, or nearest poison control center immediately.

7. Storing Your Medicine:

Keep your medicine in a safe place where children cannot reach it. It may be harmful to children. Store your medication away from heat and light. Do not store at temperatures above 77°F (25°C). If your medication has expired (the expiration date is printed on the treatment pack), throw it away as instructed. If your doctor decides to stop your treatment, do not keep any leftover medicine unless your doctor tells you to. Throw away your medicine as instructed.

Glaxo Wellcome Inc., Research Triangle Park, NC 27709
US Patent No. 4,997,841

September 1999/RL-747

Shown in Product Identification Guide, page 314

ANECTINE® ℞

[*ă-nĕk 'tēn*]
(succinylcholine chloride)
Injection, USP

WARNING

RISK OF CARDIAC ARREST FROM HYPERKALEMIC RHABDOMYOLYSIS

There have been rare reports of acute rhabdomyolysis with hyperkalemia followed by ventricular dysrhythmias, cardiac arrest, and death after the administration of succinylcholine to apparently healthy children who were subsequently found to have undiagnosed skeletal muscle myopathy, most frequently Duchenne's muscular dystrophy.

This syndrome often presents as peaked T-waves and sudden cardiac arrest within minutes after the administration of the drug in healthy appearing children (usually, but not exclusively, males, and most frequently 8 years of age or younger). There have also been reports in adolescents.

Therefore, when a healthy appearing infant or child develops cardiac arrest soon after administration of succinylcholine not felt to be due to inadequate ventilation, oxygenation, or anesthetic overdose, immediate treatment for hyperkalemia should be instituted. This should include administration of intravenous calcium, bicarbonate, and glucose with insulin, with hyperventilation. Due to the abrupt onset of this syndrome, routine resuscitative measures are likely to be unsuccessful. However, extraordinary and prolonged resuscitative efforts have resulted in successful resuscitation in some reported cases. In addition, in the presence of signs of malignant hyperthermia, appropriate treatment should be instituted concurrently.

Since there may be no signs or symptoms to alert the practitioner to which patients are at risk, it is recommended that the use of succinylcholine in children should be reserved for emergency intubation or instances where immediate securing of the airway is necessary, e.g., laryngospasm, difficult airway, full stomach, or for intramuscular use when a suitable vein is inaccessible (see PRECAUTIONS: Pediatric Use and DOSAGE AND ADMINISTRATION).

This drug should be used only by individuals familiar with its actions, characteristics, and hazards.

DESCRIPTION

ANECTINE (succinylcholine chloride) is an ultra short-acting depolarizing-type, skeletal muscle relaxant for intravenous (IV) administration.

Succinylcholine chloride is a white, odorless, slightly bitter powder and very soluble in water. The drug is unstable in alkaline solutions but relatively stable in acid solutions, depending upon the concentration of the solution and the stor-

age temperature. Solutions of succinylcholine chloride should be stored under refrigeration to preserve potency. ANECTINE Injection is a sterile nonpyrogenic solution for IV injection, containing 20 mg succinylcholine chloride in each mL and made isotonic with sodium chloride. The pH is adjusted to 3.5 with hydrochloric acid. Methylparaben (0.1%) is added as a preservative.
The chemical name for succinylcholine chloride is 2,2'-[(1,4-dioxo-1,4-butanediyl) bis(oxy)] bis [*N,N,N*-trimethylethanaminium] dichloride.

CLINICAL PHARMACOLOGY

Succinylcholine is a depolarizing skeletal muscle relaxant. As does acetylcholine, it combines with the cholinergic receptors of the motor end plate to produce depolarization. This depolarization may be observed as fasciculations. Subsequent neuromuscular transmission is inhibited so long as adequate concentration of succinylcholine remains at the receptor site. Onset of flaccid paralysis is rapid (less than 1 minute after IV administration), and with single administration lasts approximately 4 to 6 minutes.
Succinylcholine is rapidly hydrolyzed by plasma cholinesterase to succinylmonocholine (which possesses clinically insignificant depolarizing muscle relaxant properties) and then more slowly to succinic acid and choline (see PRECAUTIONS). About 10% of the drug is excreted unchanged in the urine. The paralysis following administration of succinylcholine is progressive, with differing sensitivities of different muscles. This initially involves consecutively the levator muscles of the face, muscles of the glottis, and finally, the intercostals and the diaphragm and all other skeletal muscles.
Succinylcholine has no direct action on the uterus or other smooth muscle structures. Because it is highly ionized and has low fat solubility, it does not readily cross the placenta.
Tachyphylaxis occurs with repeated administration (see PRECAUTIONS).
Depending on the dose and duration of succinylcholine administration, the characteristic depolarizing neuromuscular block (Phase I block) may change to a block with characteristics superficially resembling a nondepolarizing block (Phase II block). This may be associated with prolonged respiratory muscle paralysis or weakness in patients who manifest the transition to Phase II block. When this diagnosis is confirmed by peripheral nerve stimulation, it may sometimes be reversed with anticholinesterase drugs such as neostigmine (see PRECAUTIONS). Anticholinesterase drugs may not always be effective. If given before succinylcholine is metabolized by cholinesterase, anticholinesterase drugs may prolong rather than shorten paralysis.
Succinylcholine has no direct effect on the myocardium. Succinylcholine stimulates both autonomic ganglia and muscarinic receptors which may cause changes in cardiac rhythm, including cardiac arrest. Changes in rhythm, including cardiac arrest, may also result from vagal stimulation, which may occur during surgical procedures, or from hyperkalemia, particularly in children (see PRECAUTIONS: Pediatric Use). These effects are enhanced by halogenated anesthetics.
Succinylcholine causes an increase in intraocular pressure immediately after its injection and during the fasciculation phase, and slight increases which may persist after onset of complete paralysis (see WARNINGS).
Succinylcholine may cause slight increases in intracranial pressure immediately after its injection and during the fasciculation phase (see PRECAUTIONS).
As with other neuromuscular blocking agents, the potential for releasing histamine is present following succinylcholine administration. Signs and symptoms of histamine-mediated release such as flushing, hypotension, and bronchoconstriction are, however, uncommon in normal clinical usage.
Succinylcholine has no effect on consciousness, pain threshold, or cerebration. It should be used only with adequate anesthesia (see WARNINGS).

INDICATIONS AND USAGE

Succinylcholine chloride is indicated as an adjunct to general anesthesia, to facilitate tracheal intubation, and to provide skeletal muscle relaxation during surgery or mechanical ventilation.

CONTRAINDICATIONS

Succinylcholine is contraindicated in persons with personal or familial history of malignant hyperthermia, skeletal muscle myopathies, and known hypersensitivity to the drug. It is also contraindicated in patients after the acute phase of injury following major burns, multiple trauma, extensive denervation of skeletal muscle, or upper motor neuron injury, because succinylcholine administered to such individuals may result in severe hyperkalemia which may result in cardiac arrest (see WARNINGS). The risk of hyperkalemia in these patients increases over time and usually peaks at 7 to 10 days after the injury. The risk is dependent on the extent and location of the injury. The precise time of onset and the duration of the risk period are not known.

WARNINGS

SUCCINYLCHOLINE SHOULD BE USED ONLY BY THOSE SKILLED IN THE MANAGEMENT OF ARTIFICIAL RESPIRATION AND ONLY WHEN FACILITIES ARE INSTANTLY AVAILABLE FOR TRACHEAL INTUBATION AND FOR PROVIDING ADEQUATE VENTILATION OF THE PATIENT, INCLUDING THE ADMINISTRATION OF OXYGEN UNDER POSITIVE PRESSURE AND THE ELIMINATION OF CARBON DIOXIDE. THE CLINICIAN MUST BE PREPARED TO ASSIST OR CONTROL RESPIRATION.
TO AVOID DISTRESS TO THE PATIENT, SUCCINYLCHOLINE SHOULD NOT BE ADMINISTERED BEFORE UNCONSCIOUSNESS HAS BEEN INDUCED. IN EMERGENCY SITUATIONS, HOWEVER, IT MAY BE NECESSARY TO ADMINISTER SUCCINYLCHOLINE BEFORE UNCONSCIOUSNESS IS INDUCED.
SUCCINYLCHOLINE IS METABOLIZED BY PLASMA CHOLINESTERASE AND SHOULD BE USED WITH CAUTION, IF AT ALL, IN PATIENTS KNOWN TO BE OR SUSPECTED OF BEING HOMOZYGOUS FOR THE ATYPICAL PLASMA CHOLINESTERASE GENE.

Hyperkalemia: (SEE BOX WARNING.) Succinylcholine should be administered with **GREAT CAUTION** to patients suffering from electrolyte abnormalities and those who may have massive digitalis toxicity, because in these circumstances succinylcholine may induce serious cardiac arrhythmias or cardiac arrest due to hyperkalemia.
GREAT CAUTION should be observed if succinylcholine is administered to patients during the acute phase of injury following major burns, multiple trauma, extensive denervation of skeletal muscle, or upper motor neuron injury (see CONTRAINDICATIONS). The risk of hyperkalemia in these patients increases over time and usually peaks at 7 to 10 days after the injury. The risk is dependent on the extent and location of the injury. The precise time of onset and the duration of the risk period are undetermined. Patients with chronic abdominal infection, subarachnoid hemorrhage, or conditions causing degeneration of central and peripheral nervous systems should receive succinylcholine with **GREAT CAUTION** because of the potential for developing severe hyperkalemia.

Malignant Hyperthermia: Succinylcholine administration has been associated with acute onset of malignant hyperthermia, a potentially fatal hypermetabolic state of skeletal muscle. The risk of developing malignant hyperthermia following succinylcholine administration increases with the concomitant administration of volatile anesthetics. Malignant hyperthermia frequently presents as intractable spasm of the jaw muscles (masseter spasm) which may progress to generalized rigidity, increased oxygen demand, tachycardia, tachypnea, and profound hyperpyrexia. Successful outcome depends on recognition of early signs, such as jaw muscle spasm, acidosis, or generalized rigidity to initial administration of succinylcholine for tracheal intubation, or failure of tachycardia to respond to deepening anesthesia. Skin mottling, rising temperature, and coagulopathies may occur later in the course of the hypermetabolic process. Recognition of the syndrome is a signal for discontinuance of anesthesia, attention to increased oxygen consumption, correction of acidosis, support of circulation, assurance of adequate urinary output, and institution of measures to control rising temperature. Intravenous dantrolene sodium is recommended as an adjunct to supportive measures in the management of this problem. Consult literature references and the dantrolene prescribing information for additional information about the management of malignant hyperthermic crisis. Continuous monitoring of temperature and expired CO_2 is recommended as an aid to early recognition of malignant hyperthermia.

Other: In both adults and children, the incidence of bradycardia, which may progress to asystole, is higher following a second dose of succinylcholine. The incidence and severity of bradycardia is higher in children than in adults. Pretreatment with anticholinergic agents (e.g., atropine) may reduce the occurrence of bradyarrhythmias.
Succinylcholine causes an increase in intraocular pressure. It should not be used in instances in which an increase in intraocular pressure is undesirable (e.g., narrow angle glaucoma, penetrating eye injury) unless the potential benefit of its use outweighs the potential risk.
Succinylcholine is acidic (pH = 3.5) and should not be mixed with alkaline solutions having a pH greater than 8.5 (e.g., barbiturate solutions).

PRECAUTIONS: (SEE BOX WARNING.)

General: When succinylcholine is given over a prolonged period of time, the characteristic depolarization block of the myoneural junction (Phase I block) may change to a block with characteristics superficially resembling a nondepolarizing block (Phase II block). Prolonged respiratory muscle paralysis or weakness may be observed in patients manifesting this transition to Phase II block. The transition from Phase I to Phase II block has been reported in seven of seven patients studied under halothane anesthesia after an accumulated dose of 2 to 4 mg/kg succinylcholine (administered in repeated, divided doses). The onset of Phase II block coincided with the onset of tachyphylaxis and prolongation of spontaneous recovery. In another study, using balanced anesthesia (N_2O/O_2/narcotic-thiopental) and succinylcholine infusion, the transition was less abrupt, with great individual variability in the dose of succinylcholine required to produce Phase II block. Of 32 patients studied, 24 developed Phase II block. Tachyphylaxis was not associated with the transition to Phase II block, and 50% of the patients who developed Phase II block experienced prolonged recovery.
When Phase II block is suspected in cases of prolonged neuromuscular blockade, positive diagnosis should be made by peripheral nerve stimulation prior to administration of any anticholinesterase drug. Reversal of Phase II block is a medical decision which must be made upon the basis of the individual, clinical pharmacology, and the experience and judgment of the physician. The presence of Phase II block is indicated by fade of responses to successive stimuli (preferably "train-of-four"). The use of an anticholinesterase drug to reverse Phase II block should be accompanied by appropriate doses of an anticholinergic drug to prevent disturbances of cardiac rhythm. After adequate reversal of Phase II block with an anticholinesterase agent, the patient should be continually observed for at least 1 hour for signs of return of muscle relaxation. Reversal should not be attempted unless: (1) a peripheral nerve stimulator is used to determine the presence of Phase II block (since anticholinesterase agents will potentiate succinylcholine-induced Phase I block), and (2) spontaneous recovery of muscle twitch has been observed for at least 20 minutes and has reached a plateau with further recovery proceeding slowly; this delay is to ensure complete hydrolysis of succinylcholine by plasma cholinesterase prior to administration of the anticholinesterase agent. Should the type of block be misdiagnosed, depolarization of the type initially induced by succinylcholine (i.e., Phase I block) will be prolonged by an anticholinesterase agent.
Succinylcholine should be employed with caution in patients with fractures or muscle spasm because the initial muscle fasciculations may cause additional trauma.
Succinylcholine may cause a transient increase in intracranial pressure; however, adequate anesthetic induction prior to administration of succinylcholine will minimize this effect.
Succinylcholine may increase intragastric pressure, which could result in regurgitation and possible aspiration of stomach contents.
Neuromuscular blockade may be prolonged in patients with hypokalemia or hypocalcemia.

Reduced Plasma Cholinesterase Activity: Succinylcholine should be used carefully in patients with reduced plasma cholinesterase (pseudocholinesterase) activity. The likelihood of prolonged neuromuscular block following administration of succinylcholine must be considered in such patients (see DOSAGE AND ADMINISTRATION).
Plasma cholinesterase activity may be diminished in the presence of genetic abnormalities of plasma cholinesterase (e.g., patients heterozygous or homozygous for atypical plasma cholinesterase gene), pregnancy, severe liver or kidney disease, malignant tumors, infections, burns, anemia, decompensated heart disease, peptic ulcer, or myxedema. Plasma cholinesterase activity may also be diminished by chronic administration of oral contraceptives, glucocorticoids, or certain monoamine oxidase inhibitors, and by irreversible inhibitors of plasma cholinesterase (e.g., organophosphate insecticides, echothiophate, and certain antineoplastic drugs).
Patients homozygous for atypical plasma cholinesterase gene (1 in 2500 patients) are extremely sensitive to the neuromuscular blocking effect of succinylcholine. In these patients, a 5- to 10-mg test dose of succinylcholine may be administered to evaluate sensitivity to succinylcholine, or neuromuscular blockade may be produced by the cautious administration of a 1-mg/mL solution of succinylcholine by slow IV infusion. Apnea or prolonged muscle paralysis should be treated with controlled respiration.

Drug Interactions: Drugs which may enhance the neuromuscular blocking action of succinylcholine include: promazine, oxytocin, aprotinin, certain non-penicillin antibiotics, quinidine, β-adrenergic blockers, procainamide, lidocaine, trimethaphan, lithium carbonate, magnesium salts, quinine, chloroquine, diethylether, isoflurane, desflurane, metoclopramide, and terbutaline. The neuromuscular blocking effect of succinylcholine may be enhanced by drugs that reduce plasma cholinesterase activity (e.g., chronically administered oral contraceptives, glucocorticoids, or certain monoamine oxidase inhibitors) or by drugs that irreversibly inhibit plasma cholinesterase (see PRECAUTIONS).
If other neuromuscular blocking agents are to be used during the same procedure, the possibility of a synergistic or antagonistic effect should be considered.

Carcinogenesis, Mutagenesis, Impairment of Fertility: There have been no long-term studies performed in animals to evaluate carcinogenic potential.

Pregnancy: *Teratogenic Effects:* Pregnancy Category C. Animal reproduction studies have not been conducted with succinylcholine chloride. It is also not known whether succinylcholine can cause fetal harm when administered to a pregnant woman or can affect reproduction capacity. Succinylcholine should be given to a pregnant woman only if clearly needed.

Nonteratogenic Effects: Plasma cholinesterase levels are decreased by approximately 24% during pregnancy and for several days postpartum. Therefore, a higher proportion of patients may be expected to show increased sensitivity (prolonged apnea) to succinylcholine when pregnant than when nonpregnant.

Continued on next page

This product information is based on labeling in effect on June 23, 2000. For further information, contact via direct mail, phone, or web site. Medical Information, Glaxo Wellcome Inc., PO Box 13398, Research Triangle Park, NC 27709. Healthcare Professionals (Medical Information): 800-334-0089. Patients (Customer Response Center): 1-888-825-5249. Glaxo Wellcome Corporate Web Site: www.glaxowellcome.com

Anectine—Cont.

Labor and Delivery: Succinylcholine is commonly used to provide muscle relaxation during delivery by cesarean section. While small amounts of succinylcholine are known to cross the placental barrier, under normal conditions the quantity of drug that enters fetal circulation after a single dose of 1 mg/kg to the mother should not endanger the fetus. However, since the amount of drug that crosses the placental barrier is dependent on the concentration gradient between the maternal and fetal circulations, residual neuromuscular blockade (apnea and flaccidity) may occur in the neonate after repeated high doses to, or in the presence of atypical plasma cholinesterase in, the mother.

Nursing Mothers: It is not known whether succinylcholine is excreted in human milk. Because many drugs are excreted in human milk, caution should be exercised following succinylcholine administration to a nursing woman.

Pediatric Use: There are rare reports of ventricular dysrhythmias and cardiac arrest secondary to acute rhabdomyolysis with hyperkalemia in apparently healthy children who receive succinylcholine (see BOX WARNING). Many of these children were subsequently found to have a skeletal muscle myopathy such as Duchenne's muscular dystrophy whose clinical signs were not obvious. The syndrome often presents as sudden cardiac arrest within minutes after the administration of succinylcholine. These children are usually, but not exclusively, males, and most frequently 8 years of age or younger. There have also been reports in adolescents. There may be no signs or symptoms to alert the practitioner to which patients are at risk. A careful history and physical may identify developmental delays suggestive of a myopathy. A preoperative creatine kinase could identify some but not all patients at risk. Due to the abrupt onset of this syndrome, routine resuscitative measures are likely to be unsuccessful. Careful monitoring of the electrocardiogram may alert the practitioner to peaked T-waves (an early sign). Administration of IV calcium, bicarbonate, and glucose with insulin, with hyperventilation have resulted in successful resuscitation in some of the reported cases. Extraordinary and prolonged resuscitative efforts have been effective in some cases. In addition, in the presence of signs of malignant hyperthermia, appropriate treatment should be initiated concurrently (see WARNINGS). Since it is difficult to identify which patients are at risk, it is recommended that the use of succinylcholine in children should be reserved for emergency intubation or instances where immediate securing of the airway is necessary, e.g., laryngospasm, difficult airway, full stomach, or for intramuscular use when a suitable vein is inaccessible.

As in adults, the incidence of bradycardia in children is higher following the second dose of succinylcholine. The incidence and severity of bradycardia is higher in children than in adults. Pretreatment with anticholinergic agents, e.g., atropine, may reduce the occurrence of bradyarrhythmias.

ADVERSE REACTIONS

Adverse reactions to succinylcholine consist primarily of an extension of its pharmacological actions. Succinylcholine causes profound muscle relaxation resulting in respiratory depression to the point of apnea; this effect may be prolonged. Hypersensitivity reactions, including anaphylaxis, may occur in rare instances. The following additional adverse reactions have been reported: cardiac arrest, malignant hyperthermia, arrhythmias, bradycardia, tachycardia, hypertension, hypotension, hyperkalemia, prolonged respiratory depression or apnea, increased intraocular pressure, muscle fasciculation, jaw rigidity, postoperative muscle pain, rhabdomyolysis with possible myoglobinuric acute renal failure, excessive salivation, and rash.

OVERDOSAGE

Overdosage with succinylcholine may result in neuromuscular block beyond the time needed for surgery and anesthesia. This may be manifested by skeletal muscle weakness, decreased respiratory reserve, low tidal volume, or apnea. The primary treatment is maintenance of a patent airway and respiratory support until recovery of normal respiration is assured. Depending on the dose and duration of succinylcholine administration, the characteristic depolarizing neuromuscular block (Phase I) may change to a block with characteristics superficially resembling a nondepolarizing block (Phase II) (see PRECAUTIONS).

DOSAGE AND ADMINISTRATION

The dosage of succinylcholine should be individualized and should always be determined by the clinician after careful assessment of the patient (see WARNINGS).

Parenteral drug products should be inspected visually for particulate matter and discoloration prior to administration whenever solution and container permit. Solutions which are not clear and colorless should not be used.

Adults: ***For Short Surgical Procedures:*** The average dose required to produce neuromuscular blockade and to facilitate tracheal intubation is 0.6 mg/kg ANECTINE Injection given intravenously. The optimum dose will vary among individuals and may be from 0.3 to 1.1 mg/kg for adults. Following administration of doses in this range, neuromuscular blockade develops in about 1 minute; maximum blockade may persist for about 2 minutes, after which recovery takes place within 4 to 6 minutes. However, very large doses may result in more prolonged blockade. A 5- to 10-mg test dose may be used to determine the sensitivity of the patient and the individual recovery time (see PRECAUTIONS).

For Long Surgical Procedures: The dose of succinylcholine administered by infusion depends upon the duration of the surgical procedure and the need for muscle relaxation. The average rate for an adult ranges between 2.5 and 4.3 mg per minute.

Solutions containing from 1 to 2 mg per mL succinylcholine have commonly been used for continuous infusion. The more dilute solution (1 mg per mL) is probably preferable from the standpoint of ease of control of the rate of administration of the drug and, hence, of relaxation. This IV solution containing 1 mg per mL may be administered at a rate of 0.5 mg (0.5 mL) to 10 mg (10 mL) per minute to obtain the required amount of relaxation. The amount required per minute will depend upon the individual response as well as the degree of relaxation required. Avoid overburdening the circulation with a large volume of fluid. It is recommended that neuromuscular function be carefully monitored with a peripheral nerve stimulator when using succinylcholine by infusion in order to avoid overdose, detect development of Phase II block, follow its rate of recovery, and assess the effects of reversing agents (see PRECAUTIONS).

Intermittent IV injections of succinylcholine may also be used to provide muscle relaxation for long procedures. An IV injection of 0.3 to 1.1 mg/kg may be given initially, followed, at appropriate intervals, by further injections of 0.04 to 0.07 mg/kg to maintain the degree of relaxation required.

Pediatrics: For emergency tracheal intubation or in instances where immediate securing of the airway is necessary, the IV dose of succinylcholine is 2 mg/kg for infants and small children; for older children and adolescents the dose is 1 mg/kg (see BOX WARNING and PRECAUTIONS: Pediatric Use).

Rarely, IV bolus administration of succinylcholine in infants and children may result in malignant ventricular arrhythmias and cardiac arrest secondary to acute rhabdomyolysis with hyperkalemia. In such situations, an underlying myopathy should be suspected.

Intravenous bolus administration of succinylcholine in infants or children may result in profound bradycardia or, rarely, asystole. As in adults, the incidence of bradycardia in children is higher following a second dose of succinylcholine. The occurrence of bradyarrhythmias may be reduced by pretreatment with atropine (see PRECAUTIONS: Pediatric Use).

Intramuscular Use: If necessary, succinylcholine may be given intramuscularly to infants, older children, or adults when a suitable vein is inaccessible. A dose of up to 3 to 4 mg/kg may be given, but not more than 150 mg total dose should be administered by this route. The onset of effect of succinylcholine given intramuscularly is usually observed in about 2 to 3 minutes.

Compatibility and Admixtures: Succinylcholine is acidic (pH 3.5) and should not be mixed with alkaline solutions having a pH greater than 8.5 (e.g., barbiturate solutions). ANECTINE Injection is stable for 24 hours after dilution to a final concentration of 1 to 2 mg/mL in 5% Dextrose Injection, USP or 0.9% Sodium Chloride Injection, USP. Aseptic techniques should be used to prepare the diluted product. Admixtures of ANECTINE should be prepared for single patient use only. The unused portion of diluted ANECTINE should be discarded.

HOW SUPPLIED

For immediate injection of single doses for short procedures: ANECTINE (succinylcholine chloride) Injection, 20 mg in each mL.

Multiple-dose vials of 10 mL, box of 12 vials (NDC 0173-0071-95).

Store in refrigerator at 2° to 8°C (36° to 46°F). The multi-dose vials are stable for up to 14 days at room temperature without significant loss of potency.

Manufactured by Catalytica Pharmaceuticals, Inc.
Greenville, NC 27834
for Glaxo Wellcome Inc., Research Triangle Park, NC 27709

May 1999/RL-710

Shown in Product Identification Guide, page 314

BECLOVENT® ℞

[*be 'klō-vent"*]
(beclomethasone dipropionate, USP)
Inhalation Aerosol

For Oral Inhalation Only

DESCRIPTION

Beclomethasone dipropionate, USP, the active component of BECLOVENT Inhalation Aerosol, is an anti-inflammatory corticosteroid having the chemical name 9-chloro-11β,17,21-trihydroxy-16β-methylpregna-1,4-diene-3,20-dione 17,21-dipropionate.

Beclomethasone 17,21-dipropionate is a diester of beclomethasone, a synthetic halogenated corticosteroid. Beclomethasone dipropionate is a white to creamy-white, odorless powder with a molecular formula of $C_{28}H_{37}ClO_7$ and a molecular weight of 521.05. It is very slightly soluble in water, very soluble in chloroform, and freely soluble in acetone and in alcohol.

BECLOVENT Inhalation Aerosol is a pressurized metered-dose aerosol unit containing a microcrystalline suspension of beclomethasone dipropionate-trichloromonofluoromethane clathrate in a mixture of propellants (trichloromonofluoromethane and dichlorodifluoromethane) with oleic acid. Each canister contains beclomethasone dipropionate-trichloromonofluoromethane clathrate having a molecular proportion of beclomethasone dipropionate to trichloromonofluoromethane between 3:1 and 3:2. Each actuation delivers a quantity of clathrate equivalent to 42 mcg of beclomethasone dipropionate, USP from the mouthpiece and 50 mcg from the valve. The contents of one 6.7-g canister provide 80 oral inhalations, and the contents of one 16.8-g canister provide 200 oral inhalations.

CLINICAL PHARMACOLOGY

Animal studies show that beclomethasone dipropionate has potent anti-inflammatory activity. When beclomethasone dipropionate was administered systemically to mice, the anti-inflammatory activity was accompanied by other features typical of glucocorticoid action, including thymic involution, liver glycogen deposition, and pituitary-adrenal suppression. After systemic administration of beclomethasone dipropionate to rats, the anti-inflammatory action was associated with little or no effect on other tests of glucocorticoid activity.

Beclomethasone dipropionate is sparingly soluble and is poorly mobilized from subcutaneous or intramuscular injection sites. However, systemic absorption occurs after all routes of administration. When given to animals in the form of an aerosolized suspension of the trichloromonofluoromethane clathrate, the drug is deposited in the mouth and nasal passages, the trachea and principal bronchi, and the lung; a considerable portion of the drug is also swallowed. Absorption occurs rapidly from all respiratory and gastrointestinal tissues, as indicated by the rapid clearance of radioactively labeled drug from local tissues and appearance of tracer in the circulation. There is no evidence of tissue storage of beclomethasone dipropionate or its metabolites. Lung slices can metabolize beclomethasone dipropionate rapidly to beclomethasone 17-monopropionate and more slowly to free beclomethasone (which has very weak anti-inflammatory activity). However, irrespective of the route of administration (injection, oral, or aerosol), the principal route of excretion of the drug and its metabolites is the feces. Less than 10% of the drug and its metabolites is excreted in the urine. In humans, 12% to 15% of an orally administered dose of beclomethasone dipropionate was excreted in the urine as both conjugated and free metabolites of the drug.

The precise mechanisms of glucocorticoid action in asthma are unknown. Inflammation is recognized as an important component in the pathogenesis of asthma. Glucocorticoids have been shown to inhibit multiple cell types (e.g., mast cells, eosinophils, basophils, lymphocytes, macrophages, and neutrophils) and mediator production or secretion (e.g., histamine, eicosanoids, leukotrienes, and cytokines) involved in the asthmatic response. These anti-inflammatory actions of glucocorticoids may contribute to their efficacy in asthma.

Clinical Trials: The effects of beclomethasone dipropionate on HPA function have been evaluated in adult volunteers. There was no suppression of early morning plasma cortisol concentrations when beclomethasone dipropionate was administered in a dose of 840 mcg/day for 1 month as an aerosol or 1000 mcg/day for 3 days by intramuscular injection. However, partial suppression of plasma cortisol concentration was observed when beclomethasone dipropionate was administered in doses of 2000 mcg/day intramuscularly or 1680 mcg/day by aerosol. Immediate suppression of plasma cortisol concentrations was observed after single doses of 4000 mcg of beclomethasone dipropionate.

In one study the effects of beclomethasone dipropionate on HPA function were examined in patients with asthma. There was no change in basal early morning plasma cortisol concentrations or in the cortisol responses to tetracosactrin (ACTH 1:24) stimulation after daily aerosol administration of 336, 672, or 1008 mcg of beclomethasone dipropionate for 28 days. After daily aerosol administration of 1344 mcg for 28 days, there was slight reduction in basal cortisol concentrations and a statistically significant (P<.01) reduction in plasma cortisol responses to tetracosactrin stimulation. Following 52 weeks of aerosol treatment with 840 mcg of beclomethasone dipropionate daily, 7/115 (6%) of patients exhibited a plasma cortisol measurement below the lower limit of normal (150 $nmol^{-1}$).

Clinical experience has shown that some patients with asthma who require corticosteroid therapy for control of symptoms can be partially or completely withdrawn from systemic corticosteroids if therapy with beclomethasone dipropionate aerosol is substituted. Beclomethasone dipropionate aerosol is not effective for all patients with asthma or at all stages of the disease in a given patient.

INDICATIONS

BECLOVENT Inhalation Aerosol is indicated in the maintenance treatment of asthma as prophylactic therapy. BECLOVENT Inhalation Aerosol is also indicated for asthma patients who require systemic corticosteroid administration, where adding BECLOVENT Inhalation Aerosol may reduce or eliminate the need for the systemic corticosteroids.

BECLOVENT Inhalation Aerosol is NOT indicated for the relief of acute bronchospasm.

CONTRAINDICATIONS

BECLOVENT Inhalation Aerosol is contraindicated in the primary treatment of status asthmaticus or other acute episodes of asthma where intensive measures are required.

Hypersensitivity to any of the ingredients of this preparation contraindicates its use.

WARNINGS

Particular care is needed in patients who are transferred from systemically active corticosteroids to BECLOVENT Inhalation Aerosol because deaths due to adrenal insufficiency have occurred in asthmatic patients during and after transfer from systemic corticosteroids to aerosol beclomethasone dipropionate. After withdrawal from systemic corticosteroids, a number of months are required for recovery of hypothalamic-pituitary-adrenal (HPA) function. During this period of HPA suppression, patients may exhibit signs and symptoms of adrenal insufficiency when exposed to trauma, surgery, or infections, particularly gastroenteritis. Although BECLOVENT Inhalation Aerosol may provide control of asthmatic symptoms during these episodes, it does NOT provide the systemic steroid that is necessary for coping with these emergencies.

During periods of stress or a severe asthmatic attack, patients who have been withdrawn from systemic corticosteroids should be instructed to resume systemic steroids (in large doses) immediately and to contact their physician for further instruction. These patients should also be instructed to carry a warning card indicating that they may need supplementary systemic steroids during periods of stress or a severe asthma attack. To assess the risk of adrenal insufficiency in emergency situations, routine tests of adrenal cortical function, including measurement of early morning resting cortisol levels, should be performed periodically in all patients. An early morning resting cortisol level may be accepted as normal only if it falls at or near the normal mean level.

Localized infections with *Candida albicans* or *Aspergillus niger* have occurred in the mouth and pharynx and occasionally in the larynx. Positive cultures for oral *Candida* may be present in up to 75% of patients. Although the frequency of clinically apparent infection is considerably lower, these infections can develop with any inhaled corticosteroid and may require treatment with appropriate antifungal therapy or discontinuation of treatment with BECLOVENT Inhalation Aerosol.

BECLOVENT Inhalation Aerosol is not a bronchodilator and is not indicated for rapid relief of bronchospasm.

Patients should be instructed to contact their physicians immediately when episodes of asthma that are not responsive to bronchodilators occur during the course of treatment with BECLOVENT Inhalation Aerosol. During such episodes, patients may require therapy with systemic corticosteroids.

Transfer of patients from systemic corticosteroid therapy to BECLOVENT Inhalation Aerosol may unmask allergic conditions previously suppressed by the systemic corticosteroid therapy, e.g., rhinitis, conjunctivitis, and eczema.

Persons who are on drugs that suppress the immune system are more susceptible to infections than healthy individuals. Chickenpox and measles, for example, can have a more serious or even fatal course in nonimmune children or adults on corticosteroids. In such children or adults who have not had these diseases, particular care should be taken to avoid exposure. How the dose, route, and duration of corticosteroid administration affect the risk of developing a disseminated infection is not known. The contribution of the underlying disease and/or prior corticosteroid treatment to the risk is also not known. If exposed to chickenpox, prophylaxis with varicella zoster immune globulin (VZIG) may be indicated. If exposed to measles, prophylaxis with pooled intramuscular immunoglobulin (IG) may be indicated. (See the respective package inserts for complete VZIG and IG prescribing information.) If chickenpox develops, treatment with antiviral agents may be considered.

Avoid spraying in eyes.

PRECAUTIONS

During withdrawal from oral corticosteroids, some patients may experience symptoms of systemically active corticosteroid withdrawal, e.g., joint and/or muscular pain, lassitude, and depression, despite maintenance or even improvement of respiratory function (see DOSAGE AND ADMINISTRATION).

In responsive patients, beclomethasone dipropionate may permit control of asthmatic symptoms without suppression of HPA function, as discussed above (see CLINICAL PHARMACOLOGY). Since beclomethasone dipropionate is absorbed into the circulation and can be systemically active, the beneficial effects of BECLOVENT Inhalation Aerosol in minimizing or preventing HPA dysfunction may be expected only when recommended dosages are not exceeded.

Because of the possibility of systemic absorption of orally inhaled corticosteroids, including beclomethasone, patients should be monitored for symptoms of systemic effects such as mental disturbances, increased bruising, weight gain, cushingoid features, acneiform lesions, and cataracts. Therefore, if such changes occur, BECLOVENT Inhalation Aerosol should be discontinued slowly, consistent with accepted procedures for discontinuing oral steroids.

A reduction of growth velocity in children or teenagers may occur as a result of inadequate control of chronic diseases such as asthma or from use of corticosteroids for treatment. Physicians should closely follow the growth of adolescents taking corticosteroids by any route and weigh the benefits of corticosteroid therapy and asthma control against the possibility of growth suppression if an adolescent's growth appears slowed.

The long-term local and systemic effects of BECLOVENT Inhalation Aerosol in human subjects are still not fully known. In particular, the effects resulting from chronic use of BECLOVENT Inhalation Aerosol on developmental or immunologic processes in the mouth, pharynx, trachea, and lung are unknown.

Inhaled corticosteroids should be used with caution, if at all, in patients with active or quiescent tuberculosis infection of the respiratory tract; untreated systemic fungal, bacterial, parasitic, or viral infections; or ocular herpes simplex.

Pulmonary infiltrates with eosinophilia may occur in patients on BECLOVENT Inhalation Aerosol therapy. Although it is possible that in some patients this state may become manifest because of systemic corticosteroid withdrawal when inhalational corticosteroids are administered, a causative role for beclomethasone dipropionate and/or its vehicle cannot be ruled out.

Information for Patients: Patients being treated with BECLOVENT Inhalation Aerosol should receive the following information and instructions. This information is intended to aid in the safe and effective use of this medication. It is not a disclosure of all possible adverse or intended effects.

Patients should use BECLOVENT Inhalation Aerosol at regular intervals as directed. Results of clinical trials indicated significant improvement may occur within the first day or two of treatment; however, the full benefit may not be achieved until treatment has been administered 1 or 2 weeks or longer. The patient should not increase the prescribed dosage but should contact the physician if symptoms do not improve or if the condition worsens.

Patients should be advised that BECLOVENT Inhalation Aerosol is not intended for use in the treatment of acute asthma. Patients should be made aware of the prophylactic nature of therapy with inhaled beclomethasone dipropionate and that it should be taken regularly even when they are asymptomatic. Patients should be instructed to contact their physicians immediately if there is any deterioration of their asthma.

BECLOVENT Inhalation Aerosol should not be stopped abruptly. If discontinuing use of BECLOVENT Inhalation Aerosol is necessary, the patient's physician should be contacted immediately.

Each patient should be advised to rinse his/her mouth each time after using BECLOVENT Inhalation Aerosol.

Patients should be warned to avoid exposure to chickenpox or measles. Patients should also be advised that if they are exposed, medical advice should be sought without delay.

Carcinogenesis, Mutagenesis, Impairment of Fertility: The carcinogenicity of beclomethasone dipropionate was evaluated in rats that were exposed for a total of 95 weeks, 13 weeks at inhalation doses up to 0.4 mg/kg and the remaining 82 weeks at combined oral and inhalation doses up to 2.4 mg/kg. There was no evidence of carcinogenicity in this study at the highest dose, approximately 20 or 36 times the maximum recommended daily inhalation dose in adults and children, respectively, on a mg/m^2 basis.

Beclomethasone dipropionate did not induce gene mutation in bacterial cells or mammalian Chinese Hamster ovary (CHO) cells in vitro. No significant clastogenic effect was seen in cultured CHO cells in vitro or in the mouse micronucleus test in vivo.

In rats, beclomethasone dipropionate caused decreased conception rates at an oral dose of 16 mg/kg (approximately 130 times the maximum recommended daily inhalation dose in adults on a mg/m^2 basis). Inhibition of the estrous cycle in dogs was observed following oral dosing at 0.5 mg/kg (approximately 15 times the maximum recommended daily inhalation dose in adults on a mg/m^2 basis). No inhibition of the estrous cycle in dogs was seen following 12 months' exposure at an estimated daily inhalation dose of 0.33 mg/kg (approximately 9 times the maximum recommended daily inhalation dose in adults on a mg/m^2 basis).

Pregnancy: Teratogenic Effects: Pregnancy Category C. Like other corticosteroids, beclomethasone dipropionate was teratogenic and embryocidal in the mouse and rabbit at a subcutaneous dose of 0.1 mg/kg in mice or 0.025 mg/kg in rabbits (approximately 1/2 the maximum recommended daily inhalation dose in adults on a mg/m^2 basis). No teratogenicity or embryocidal effects were seen in rats when exposed to an inhalation dose of 0.1 mg/kg plus oral doses of up to 10 mg/kg per day for a combined dose of 10.1 mg/kg (approximately 80 times the maximum recommended daily inhalation dose in adults on a mg/m^2 basis). There are no adequate and well-controlled studies in pregnant women. BECLOVENT Inhalation Aerosol should be used during pregnancy only if the potential benefit justifies the potential risk to the fetus.

Nursing Mothers: Corticosteroids are secreted in human milk. Because of the potential for serious adverse reactions in nursing infants for BECLOVENT Inhalation Aerosol, a decision should be made whether to discontinue nursing or to discontinue the drug, taking into account the importance of the drug to the mother.

Pediatric Use: The safety and effectiveness of BECLOVENT Inhalation Aerosol have been established in children aged 6 years and above. The safety and effectiveness of BECLOVENT Inhalation Aerosol in children below 6 years of age have not been established. Corticosteroids have been shown to cause a reduction in growth velocity in children and teenagers with extended use. If a child or teenager on any corticosteroid appears to have growth suppression, the possibility that they are particularly sensitive to this effect of corticosteroids should be considered (see PRECAUTIONS).

ADVERSE REACTIONS

Deaths due to adrenal insufficiency have occurred in asthmatic patients during and after transfer from systemic corticosteroids to aerosol beclomethasone dipropionate (see WARNINGS).

Suppression of HPA function (reduction of early morning plasma cortisol levels) has been reported in adult patients who received 1344-mcg daily doses of BECLOVENT Inhalation Aerosol for 1 month. A few patients on BECLOVENT Inhalation Aerosol have complained of hoarseness or dry mouth.

In addition, the following adverse events have been reported spontaneously during worldwide postmarketing surveillance. Therefore, the frequency of events and causality cannot be reliably determined. The adverse events reported in association with BECLOVENT Inhalation Aerosol include:

General: Immediate and delayed hypersensitivity reactions including anaphylactic/anaphylactoid reactions, angioedema, bronchospasm, rash, urticaria.

Ear, Nose, and Throat: Dryness and irritation of the nose, throat, and mouth; hoarseness; localized infections with *Candida* or *Aspergillus*; unpleasant taste and smell; loss of taste and smell.

Endocrine and Metabolic: Cushingoid features, growth velocity reduction in children/adolescents, weight gain.

Eye: Cataracts, glaucoma, increased intraocular pressure.

Gastrointestinal: Nausea, vomiting.

Nervous: Dizziness, headache, lightheadedness.

Psychiatry: Agitation, depression, mental disturbances.

Respiratory: Paradoxical bronchospasm, wheezing.

Skin: Acneiform lesions, atrophy, bruising, pruritus, purpura, striae.

OVERDOSAGE

For maximum doses studied in humans, see the Clinical Trials subsection. Chronic overdosage may result in signs/symptoms of hypercorticism (see PRECAUTIONS). No deaths occurred when beclomethasone dipropionate was given as single oral doses of 3000 mg/kg to mice and 2000 mg/kg to rats (approximately 12 000 and 16 000 times, respectively, the maximum recommended human daily inhalation dose on a mg/m^2 basis).

DOSAGE AND ADMINISTRATION

BECLOVENT Inhalation Aerosol should be test sprayed into the air before using for the first time and in cases where the product has not been used for a prolonged period of time.

Adults and Children 12 Years of Age and Older: The usual recommended dosage is two inhalations (84 mcg) given three or four times a day. Alternatively, four inhalations (168 mcg) given twice daily have been shown to be effective in some patients. In patients with severe asthma, it is advisable to start with 12 to 16 inhalations a day (504 to 672 mcg) and adjust the dosage downward according to the response of the patient. The maximal daily intake should not exceed 20 inhalations, 840 mcg (0.84 mg), in adults.

Children 6 to 12 Years of Age: The usual recommended dosage is one or two inhalations (42 to 84 mcg) given three or four times a day according to the response of the patient. Alternatively, four inhalations (168 mcg) given twice daily have been shown to be effective in some patients. The maximal daily intake should not exceed 10 inhalations, 420 mcg (0.42 mg), in children 6 to 12 years of age. Insufficient clinical data exist with respect to the administration of BECLOVENT Inhalation Aerosol in children below the age of 6.

Rinsing the mouth after inhalation is advised.

Different considerations must be given to the following groups of patients in order to obtain the full therapeutic benefit of BECLOVENT Inhalation Aerosol.

Patients Not Receiving Systemic Corticosteroids: Patients who require maintenance therapy of their asthma may benefit from treatment with BECLOVENT Inhalation Aerosol at the doses recommended above. In patients who respond to BECLOVENT Inhalation Aerosol, improvement in pulmonary function is usually apparent within 1 to 4 weeks after the start of therapy. Once the desired effect is achieved, consideration should be given to tapering to the lowest effective dose.

Patients Maintained on Systemic Corticosteroids: Clinical studies have shown that BECLOVENT Inhalation Aerosol may be effective in the management of asthmatics dependent or maintained on systemic corticosteroids and may permit replacement or significant reduction in the dosage of systemic corticosteroids.

Continued on next page

This product information is based on labeling in effect on June 23, 2000. For further information, contact via direct mail, phone, or web site. Medical Information, Glaxo Wellcome Inc., PO Box 13398, Research Triangle Park, NC 27709. Healthcare Professionals (Medical Information): 800-334-0089. Patients (Customer Response Center): 1-888-825-5249. Glaxo Wellcome Corporate Web Site: www.glaxowellcome.com

Beclovent—Cont.

The patient's asthma should be reasonably stable before treatment with BECLOVENT Inhalation Aerosol is started. Initially, BECLOVENT Inhalation Aerosol should be used concurrently with the patient's usual maintenance dose of systemic corticosteroid. After approximately 1 week, gradual withdrawal of the systemic corticosteroid is started by reducing the daily or alternate-daily dose. Reductions may be made after an interval of 1 or 2 weeks, depending on the response of the patient. Generally, these decrements should not exceed 2.5 mg of prednisone or its equivalent. During withdrawal, some patients may experience symptoms of systemic corticosteroid withdrawal, e.g., joint and/or muscular pain, lassitude, and depression, despite maintenance or even improvement in pulmonary function. Such patients should be encouraged to continue with the inhaler but should be monitored for objective signs of adrenal insufficiency. If evidence of adrenal insufficiency occurs, the systemic corticosteroid doses should be increased temporarily and thereafter withdrawal should continue more slowly.

During periods of stress or a severe asthma attack, transfer patients may require supplementary treatment with systemic corticosteroids.

Directions for Use: Illustrated Patient's Instructions for Use accompany each package of BECLOVENT Inhalation Aerosol.

CONTENTS UNDER PRESSURE: Do not puncture. Do not use or store near heat or open flame. Exposure to temperatures above 120°F may cause bursting. Never throw container into fire or incinerator. Keep out of reach of children.

HOW SUPPLIED

BECLOVENT Inhalation Aerosol is supplied in a 6.7-g canister containing 80 metered inhalations with oral adapter and patient's instructions (NDC 0173-0469-00) and in a 16.8-g canister containing 200 metered inhalations with oral adapter and patient's instructions (NDC 0173-0312-88). Also available, BECLOVENT Inhalation Aerosol Refill 16.8-g canister only with patient's instructions (NDC 0173-0312-98). Each actuation delivers a quantity of clathrate equivalent to 42 mcg of beclomethasone dipropionate, USP from the mouthpiece and 50 mcg from the valve.

The BECLOVENT Inhalation Aerosol canister should only be used with the tan BECLOVENT Inhalation Aerosol mouthpiece, and this mouthpiece should not be used with any other inhalation product. A dark brown cap fits over the mouthpiece when not in use.

The correct amount of medication in each inhalation cannot be assured after 80 inhalations from the 6.7-g canister or 200 inhalations from the 16.8-g canister even though the canister is not completely empty. The canister should be discarded when the labeled number of actuations has been used.

Store between 2° and 30°C (36° and 86°F). As with most inhaled medications in aerosol canisters, the therapeutic effect of this medication may decrease when the canister is cold. For optimal results, the canister should be at room temperature before use. Shake well before using.

Glaxo Wellcome Inc., Research Triangle Park, NC 27709
December 1997/RL-536

Shown in Product Identification Guide, page 314

BECONASE® ℞

[be 'kō-nāz"]
(beclomethasone dipropionate, USP)
Inhalation Aerosol

For Nasal Inhalation Only

DESCRIPTION

Beclomethasone dipropionate, USP, the active component of BECONASE Inhalation Aerosol, is an anti-inflammatory steroid having the chemical name 9-chloro-11β,17,21-trihydroxy-16β-methylpregna-1,4-diene-3,20-dione 17,21-dipropionate.

Beclomethasone dipropionate is a white to creamy-white, odorless powder with a molecular weight of 521.25. It is very slightly soluble in water, very soluble in chloroform, and freely soluble in acetone and in alcohol.

BECONASE Inhalation Aerosol is a metered-dose aerosol unit containing a microcrystalline suspension of beclomethasone dipropionate-trichloromonofluoromethane clathrate in a mixture of propellants (trichloromonofluoromethane and dichlorodifluoromethane) with oleic acid. Each canister contains beclomethasone dipropionate-trichloromonofluoromethane clathrate having a molecular proportion of beclomethasone dipropionate to trichloromonofluoromethane between 3:1 and 3:2. Each actuation delivers from the compact actuator a quantity of clathrate equivalent to 42 mcg of beclomethasone dipropionate, USP. The contents of one 6.7-g canister provide at least 80 metered doses, and the contents of one 16.8-g canister provide at least 200 metered doses.

CLINICAL PHARMACOLOGY

Beclomethasone 17,21-dipropionate is a diester of beclomethasone, a synthetic halogenated corticosteroid. Animal studies show that beclomethasone dipropionate has potent glucocorticoid and weak mineralocorticoid activity.

The mechanisms responsible for the anti-inflammatory action of beclomethasone dipropionate are unknown. The precise mechanism of the aerosolized drug's action in the nose is also unknown. Biopsies of nasal mucosa obtained during clinical studies showed no histopathologic changes when beclomethasone dipropionate was administered intranasally.

The effects of beclomethasone dipropionate on hypothalamic-pituitary-adrenal (HPA) function have been evaluated in adult volunteers by other routes of administration. Studies with beclomethasone dipropionate by the intranasal route may demonstrate that there is more or that there is less absorption by this route of administration. There was no suppression of early morning plasma cortisol concentrations when beclomethasone dipropionate was administered in a dose of 1,000 mcg per day for 1 month as an oral aerosol or for 3 days by intramuscular injection. However, partial suppression of plasma cortisol concentrations was observed when beclomethasone dipropionate was administered in doses of 2,000 mcg per day either by oral aerosol or intramuscular injection. Immediate suppression of plasma cortisol concentrations was observed after single doses of 4,000 mcg of beclomethasone dipropionate. Suppression of HPA function (reduction of early morning plasma cortisol levels) has been reported in adult patients who received 1,600-mcg daily doses of oral beclomethasone dipropionate for 1 month. In clinical studies using beclomethasone dipropionate intranasally, there was no evidence of adrenal insufficiency.

Beclomethasone dipropionate is sparingly soluble. When given by nasal inhalation in the form of an aqueous or aerosolized suspension, the drug is deposited primarily in the nasal passages. A portion of the drug is swallowed. Absorption occurs rapidly from all respiratory and gastrointestinal tissues. There is no evidence of tissue storage of beclomethasone dipropionate or its metabolites. *In vitro* studies have shown that tissue other than the liver (lung slices) can rapidly metabolize beclomethasone dipropionate to beclomethasone 17-monopropionate and more slowly to free beclomethasone (which has very weak anti-inflammatory activity).

However, irrespective of the route of entry, the principal route of excretion of the drug and its metabolites is the feces. In humans, 12% to 15% of an orally administered dose of beclomethasone dipropionate is excreted in the urine as both conjugated and free metabolites of the drug.

Studies have shown that the degree of binding to plasma proteins is 87%.

INDICATIONS AND USAGE

BECONASE Inhalation Aerosol is indicated for the relief of the symptoms of seasonal or perennial rhinitis in those cases poorly responsive to conventional treatment.

BECONASE Inhalation Aerosol is also indicated for the prevention of recurrence of nasal polyps following surgical removal.

Clinical studies in patients with seasonal or perennial rhinitis have shown that improvement is usually apparent within a few days. However, symptomatic relief may not occur in some patients for as long as 2 weeks. Although systemic effects are minimal at recommended doses, BECONASE Inhalation Aerosol should not be continued beyond 3 weeks in the absence of significant symptomatic improvement. BECONASE Inhalation Aerosol should not be used in the presence of untreated localized infection involving the nasal mucosa.

Clinical studies have shown that treatment of the symptoms associated with nasal polyps may have to be continued for several weeks or more before a therapeutic result can be fully assessed. Recurrence of symptoms due to polyps can occur after stopping treatment, depending on the severity of the disease.

CONTRAINDICATIONS

Hypersensitivity to any of the ingredients of this preparation contraindicates its use.

WARNINGS

The replacement of a systemic corticosteroid with BECONASE Inhalation Aerosol can be accompanied by signs of adrenal insufficiency.

Careful attention must be given when patients previously treated for prolonged periods with systemic corticosteroids are transferred to BECONASE Inhalation Aerosol. This is particularly important in those patients who have associated asthma or other clinical conditions where too rapid a decrease in systemic corticosteroids may cause a severe exacerbation of their symptoms.

Studies have shown that the combined administration of alternate-day prednisone systemic treatment and orally inhaled beclomethasone increases the likelihood of HPA suppression compared to a therapeutic dose of either one alone. Therefore, BECONASE Inhalation Aerosol treatment should be used with caution in patients already on alternate-day prednisone regimens for any disease.

If recommended doses of intranasal beclomethasone are exceeded or if individuals are particularly sensitive or predisposed by virtue of recent systemic steroid therapy, symptoms of hypercorticism may occur, including very rare cases of menstrual irregularities, acneiform lesions, cataracts, and cushingoid features. If such changes occur, BECONASE Inhalation Aerosol should be discontinued slowly consistent with accepted procedures for discontinuing oral steroid therapy.

Persons who are on drugs that suppress the immune system are more susceptible to infections than healthy individuals. Chickenpox and measles, for example, can have a more serious or even fatal course in nonimmune children or adults on corticosteroids. In such children or adults who have not had these diseases, particular care should be taken to avoid exposure. How the dose, route, and duration of corticosteroid administration affects the risk of developing a disseminated infection is not known. The contribution of the underlying disease and/or prior corticosteroid treatment to the risk is also not known. If exposed to chickenpox, prophylaxis with varicella zoster immune globulin (VZIG) may be indicated. If exposed to measles, prophylaxis with pooled intramuscular immunoglobulin (IG) may be indicated. (See the respective package inserts for complete VZIG and IG prescribing information.) If chickenpox develops, treatment with antiviral agents may be considered.

PRECAUTIONS

General: During withdrawal from oral steroids, some patients may experience symptoms of withdrawal, e.g., joint and/or muscular pain, lassitude, and depression.

Rare instances of nasal septum perforation have been spontaneously reported.

Rare instances of wheezing, cataracts, glaucoma, and increased intraocular pressure have been reported following the intranasal use of beclomethasone dipropionate.

In clinical studies with beclomethasone dipropionate administered intranasally, the development of localized infections of the nose and pharynx with *Candida albicans* has occurred only rarely. When such an infection develops, it may require treatment with appropriate local therapy or discontinuation of treatment with BECONASE Inhalation Aerosol.

Beclomethasone dipropionate is absorbed into the circulation. Use of excessive doses of BECONASE Inhalation Aerosol may suppress HPA function.

BECONASE Inhalation Aerosol should be used with caution, if at all, in patients with active or quiescent tuberculous infections of the respiratory tract; untreated fungal, bacterial, or systemic viral infections; or ocular herpes simplex.

For BECONASE Inhalation Aerosol to be effective in the treatment of nasal polyps, the aerosol must be able to enter the nose. Therefore, treatment of nasal polyps with BECONASE Inhalation Aerosol should be considered adjunctive therapy to surgical removal and/or the use of other medications that will permit effective penetration of BECONASE Inhalation Aerosol into the nose. Nasal polyps may recur after any form of treatment.

As with any long-term treatment, patients using BECONASE Inhalation Aerosol over several months or longer should be examined periodically for possible changes in the nasal mucosa.

Because of the inhibitory effect of corticosteroids on wound healing, patients who have experienced recent nasal septum ulcers, nasal surgery, or trauma should not use a nasal corticosteroid until healing has occurred.

Although systemic effects have been minimal with recommended doses, this potential increases with excessive doses. Therefore, larger than recommended doses should be avoided.

Information for Patients: Patients should use BECONASE Inhalation Aerosol at regular intervals since its effectiveness depends on its regular use. The patient should take the medication as directed. It is not acutely effective, and the prescribed dosage should not be increased. Instead, nasal vasoconstrictors or oral antihistamines may be needed until the effects of BECONASE Inhalation Aerosol are fully manifested. One to 2 weeks may pass before full relief is obtained. The patient should contact the physician if symptoms do not improve, if the condition worsens, or if sneezing or nasal irritation occurs. For the proper use of this unit and to attain maximum improvement, the patient should read and follow carefully the patient's instructions section of the package insert.

Persons who are on immunosuppressant doses of corticosteroids should be warned to avoid exposure to chickenpox or measles. Patients should also be advised that if they are exposed, medical advice should be sought without delay.

Carcinogenesis, Mutagenesis, Impairment of Fertility: Treatment of rats for a total of 95 weeks, 13 weeks by inhalation and 82 weeks by the oral route, resulted in no evidence of carcinogenic activity. Mutagenic studies have not been performed.

Impairment of fertility, as evidenced by inhibition of the estrous cycle in dogs, was observed following treatment by the oral route. No inhibition of the estrous cycle in dogs was seen following treatment with beclomethasone dipropionate by the inhalation route.

Pregnancy: *Teratogenic Effects: Pregnancy Category C:* Like other corticoids, parenteral (subcutaneous) beclomethasone dipropionate has been shown to be teratogenic and embryocidal in the mouse and rabbit when given in doses approximately 10 times the human dose. In these studies, beclomethasone was found to produce fetal resorption, cleft palate, agnathia, microstomia, absence of tongue, delayed ossification, and agenesis of the thymus. No teratogenic or embryocidal effects have been seen in the rat when beclomethasone dipropionate was administered by inhalation at 10 times the human dose or orally at 1,000 times the human dose. There are no adequate and well-controlled studies in pregnant women. Beclomethasone dipropionate should be used during pregnancy only if the potential benefit justifies the potential risk to the fetus.

Nonteratogenic Effects: Hypoadrenalism may occur in infants born of mothers receiving corticosteroids during pregnancy. Such infants should be carefully observed.

Nursing Mothers: It is not known whether beclomethasone dipropionate is excreted in human milk. Because other corticosteroids are excreted in human milk, caution should be exercised when BECONASE Inhalation Aerosol is administered to a nursing woman.

Pediatric Use: Safety and effectiveness in children below 6 years of age have not been established.

ADVERSE REACTIONS

In general, side effects in clinical studies have been primarily associated with the nasal mucous membranes.

Adverse reactions reported in controlled clinical trials and long-term open studies in patients treated with BECONASE Inhalation Aerosol are described below.

Sensations of irritation and burning in the nose (11 per 100 patients) following the use of BECONASE Inhalation Aerosol have been reported. Also, occasional sneezing attacks (10 per 100 adult patients) have occurred immediately following the use of the intranasal inhaler. This symptom may be more common in children. Rhinorrhea may occur occasionally (1 per 100 patients).

Localized infections of the nose and pharynx with *Candida albicans* have occurred rarely (see PRECAUTIONS).

Transient episodes of epistaxis have been reported in 2 per 100 patients.

Rare cases of ulceration of the nasal mucosa and instances of nasal septum perforation have been spontaneously reported (see PRECAUTIONS).

Reports of headache, light-headedness, dryness and irritation of the nose and throat, and unpleasant taste and smell have been received. There are rare reports of loss of taste and smell.

Rare instances of wheezing, cataracts, glaucoma, and increased intraocular pressure have been reported following the use of intranasal beclomethasone dipropionate (see PRECAUTIONS).

Rare cases of immediate and delayed hypersensitivity reactions, including urticaria, angioedema, rash, and bronchospasm, have been reported following the oral and intranasal inhalation of beclomethasone.

Systemic corticosteroid side effects were not reported during the controlled clinical trials. If recommended doses are exceeded, however, or if individuals are particularly sensitive, symptoms of hypercorticism, i.e., Cushing's syndrome, could occur.

OVERDOSAGE

When used at excessive doses, systemic corticosteroid effects such as hypercorticism and adrenal suppression may appear. If such changes occur, BECONASE Inhalation Aerosol should be discontinued slowly consistent with accepted procedures for discontinuing oral steroid therapy. The oral LD_{50} of beclomethasone dipropionate is greater than 1 g/kg in rodents. One canister of BECONASE Inhalation Aerosol contains 8.4 mg of beclomethasone dipropionate; therefore, acute overdosage is unlikely.

DOSAGE AND ADMINISTRATION

Adults and Children 12 Years of Age and Older: The usual dosage is one inhalation (42 mcg) in each nostril two to four times a day (total dose, 168 to 336 mcg per day). Patients can often be maintained on a maximum dose of one inhalation in each nostril three times a day (252 mcg per day).

Children 6 to 12 Years of Age: The usual dosage is one inhalation in each nostril three times a day (252 mcg per day). BECONASE Inhalation Aerosol is *not* recommended for children below 6 years of age since safety and efficacy studies have not been conducted in this age-group.

In patients who respond to BECONASE Inhalation Aerosol, an improvement of the symptoms of seasonal or perennial rhinitis usually becomes apparent within a few days after the start of BECONASE Inhalation Aerosol therapy. However, symptomatic relief may not occur in some patients for as long as 2 weeks. BECONASE Inhalation Aerosol should not be continued beyond 3 weeks in the absence of significant symptomatic improvement.

The therapeutic effects of corticosteroids, unlike those of decongestants, are not immediate. This should be explained to the patient in advance in order to ensure cooperation and continuation of treatment with the prescribed dosage regimen.

In the presence of excessive nasal mucus secretion or edema of the nasal mucosa, the drug may fail to reach the site of intended action. In such cases it is advisable to use a nasal vasoconstrictor during the first 2 to 3 days of BECONASE Inhalation Aerosol therapy.

Directions for Use: Illustrated Patient's Instructions for Use accompany each package of BECONASE Inhalation Aerosol.

CONTENTS UNDER PRESSURE: Do not puncture. Do not use or store near heat or open flame. Exposure to temperatures above 120°F may cause bursting. Never throw container into fire or incinerator. Keep out of reach of children.

HOW SUPPLIED

BECONASE Inhalation Aerosol is supplied in a 6.7-g canister containing 80 metered doses (NDC 0173-0468-00) and in a 16.8-g canister containing 200 metered doses (NDC 0173-0336-02), each with beige compact actuator and patient's instructions.

Store between 2° and 30°C (36° and 86°F). As with most inhaled medications in aerosol canisters, the therapeutic effect of this medication may decrease when the canister is cold. Shake well before using.

Glaxo Wellcome Inc., Research Triangle Park, NC 27709
May 1997/RL-424
Shown in Product Identification Guide, page 314

BECONASE AQ® ℞
(beclomethasone dipropionate, monohydrate)
Nasal Spray, 0.042%*

***Calculated on the dried basis.** **SHAKE WELL**
For Intranasal Use Only **BEFORE USE.**

DESCRIPTION

Beclomethasone dipropionate, monohydrate, the active component of BECONASE AQ Nasal Spray, is an anti-inflammatory steroid having the chemical name 9-chloro-11β,17,21-trihydroxy-16β-methylpregna-1,4-diene-3,20-dione 17,21-dipropionate, monohydrate.

Beclomethasone dipropionate, monohydrate is a white to creamy-white, odorless powder with a molecular weight of 539.06. It is very slightly soluble in water, very soluble in chloroform, and freely soluble in acetone and in alcohol.

BECONASE AQ Nasal Spray is a metered-dose, manual pump spray unit containing a microcrystalline suspension of beclomethasone dipropionate, monohydrate equivalent to 0.042% w/w beclomethasone dipropionate, calculated on the dried basis, in an aqueous medium containing microcrystalline cellulose, carboxymethylcellulose sodium, dextrose, benzalkonium chloride, polysorbate 80, and 0.25% v/w phenylethyl alcohol. Hydrochloric acid may be added to adjust pH. The pH is between 4.5 and 7.0.

After initial priming (three to four actuations), each actuation of the pump delivers from the nasal adapter 100 mg of suspension containing beclomethasone dipropionate, monohydrate equivalent to 42 mcg of beclomethasone dipropionate. Each bottle of BECONASE AQ Nasal Spray will provide at least 200 metered doses.

CLINICAL PHARMACOLOGY

Beclomethasone 17,21-dipropionate is a diester of beclomethasone, a synthetic halogenated corticosteroid. Animal studies show that beclomethasone dipropionate has potent glucocorticoid and weak mineralocorticoid activity.

The mechanisms responsible for the anti-inflammatory action of beclomethasone dipropionate are unknown. The precise mechanism of the aerosolized drug's action in the nose is also unknown. Biopsies of nasal mucosa obtained during clinical studies showed no histopathologic changes when beclomethasone dipropionate was administered intranasally.

The effects of beclomethasone dipropionate on hypothalamic-pituitary-adrenal (HPA) function have been evaluated in adult volunteers by other routes of administration. Studies with beclomethasone dipropionate by the intranasal route may demonstrate that there is more or that there is less absorption by this route of administration. There was no suppression of early morning plasma cortisol concentrations when beclomethasone dipropionate was administered in a dose of 1000 mcg/day for 1 month as an oral aerosol or for 3 days by intramuscular injection. However, partial suppression of plasma cortisol concentrations was observed when beclomethasone dipropionate was administered in doses of 2000 mcg/day either by oral aerosol or intramuscular injection. Immediate suppression of plasma cortisol concentrations was observed after single doses of 4000 mcg of beclomethasone dipropionate. Suppression of HPA function (reduction of early morning plasma cortisol levels) has been reported in adult patients who received 1600-mcg daily doses of oral beclomethasone dipropionate for 1 month. In clinical studies using beclomethasone dipropionate aerosol intranasally, there was no evidence of adrenal insufficiency. The effect of BECONASE AQ Nasal Spray on HPA function was not evaluated but would not be expected to differ from intranasal beclomethasone dipropionate aerosol.

In one study in asthmatic children, the administration of inhaled beclomethasone at recommended daily doses for at least 1 year was associated with a reduction in nocturnal cortisol secretion. The clinical significance of this finding is not clear. It reinforces other evidence, however, that topical beclomethasone may be absorbed in amounts that can have systemic effects and that physicians should be alert for evidence of systemic effects, especially in chronically treated patients (see PRECAUTIONS).

Beclomethasone dipropionate is sparingly soluble. When given by nasal inhalation in the form of an aqueous or aerosolized suspension, the drug is deposited primarily in the nasal passages. A portion of the drug is swallowed. Absorption occurs rapidly from all respiratory and gastrointestinal tissues. There is no evidence of tissue storage of beclomethasone dipropionate or its metabolites. In vitro studies have shown that tissue other than the liver (lung slices) can rapidly metabolize beclomethasone dipropionate to beclomethasone 17-monopropionate and more slowly to free beclomethasone (which has very weak anti-inflammatory activity). However, irrespective of the route of entry, the principal route of excretion of the drug and its metabolites is the feces. In humans, 12% to 15% of an orally administered dose of beclomethasone dipropionate is excreted in the urine as both conjugated and free metabolites of the drug.

Studies have shown that the degree of binding to plasma proteins is 87%.

INDICATIONS AND USAGE

BECONASE AQ Nasal Spray is indicated for the relief of the symptoms of seasonal or perennial allergic and nonallergic (vasomotor) rhinitis.

Results from two clinical trials have shown that significant symptomatic relief was obtained within 3 days. However, symptomatic relief may not occur in some patients for as long as 2 weeks. BECONASE AQ Nasal Spray should not be continued beyond 3 weeks in the absence of significant symptomatic improvement. BECONASE AQ Nasal Spray should not be used in the presence of untreated localized infection involving the nasal mucosa.

BECONASE AQ Nasal Spray is also indicated for the prevention of recurrence of nasal polyps following surgical removal.

Clinical studies have shown that treatment of the symptoms associated with nasal polyps may have to be continued for several weeks or more before a therapeutic result can be fully assessed. Recurrence of symptoms due to polyps can occur after stopping treatment, depending on the severity of the disease.

CONTRAINDICATIONS

Hypersensitivity to any of the ingredients of this preparation contraindicates its use.

WARNINGS

The replacement of a systemic corticosteroid with BECONASE AQ Nasal Spray can be accompanied by signs of adrenal insufficiency.

Careful attention must be given when patients previously treated for prolonged periods with systemic corticosteroids are transferred to BECONASE AQ Nasal Spray. This is particularly important in those patients who have associated asthma or other clinical conditions where too rapid a decrease in systemic corticosteroids may cause a severe exacerbation of their symptoms.

Studies have shown that the combined administration of alternate-day prednisone systemic treatment and orally inhaled beclomethasone increases the likelihood of HPA suppression compared to a therapeutic dose of either one alone. Therefore, BECONASE AQ Nasal Spray treatment should be used with caution in patients already on alternate-day prednisone regimens for any disease.

If recommended doses of intranasal beclomethasone are exceeded or if individuals are particularly sensitive or predisposed by virtue of recent systemic steroid therapy, symptoms of hypercorticism may occur, including very rare cases of menstrual irregularities, acneiform lesions, cataracts, and cushingoid features. If such changes occur, BECONASE AQ Nasal Spray should be discontinued slowly consistent with accepted procedures for discontinuing oral steroid therapy.

Persons who are on drugs that suppress the immune system are more susceptible to infections than healthy individuals. Chickenpox and measles, for example, can have a more serious or even fatal course in nonimmune children or adults on corticosteroids. In such children or adults who have not had these diseases, particular care should be taken to avoid exposure. How the dose, route, and duration of corticosteroid administration affect the risk of developing a disseminated infection is not known. The contribution of the underlying disease and/or prior corticosteroid treatment to the risk is also not known. If exposed to chickenpox, prophylaxis with varicella zoster immune globulin (VZIG) may be indicated. If exposed to measles, prophylaxis with pooled intramuscular immunoglobulin (IG) may be indicated. (See the respective package inserts for complete VZIG and IG prescribing information.) If chickenpox develops, treatment with antiviral agents may be considered.

PRECAUTIONS

General: During withdrawal from oral steroids, some patients may experience symptoms of withdrawal, e.g., joint and/or muscular pain, lassitude, and depression.

Rarely, immediate hypersensitivity reactions may occur after the intranasal administration of beclomethasone (see ADVERSE REACTIONS).

Rare instances of nasal septum perforation have been spontaneously reported.

Rare instances of wheezing, cataracts, glaucoma, and increased intraocular pressure have been reported following the use of intranasal beclomethasone.

In clinical studies with beclomethasone dipropionate administered intranasally, the development of localized infections of the nose and pharynx with *Candida albicans* has occurred only rarely. When such an infection develops, it may require treatment with appropriate local therapy or discontinuation of treatment with BECONASE AQ Nasal Spray.

If persistent nasopharyngeal irritation occurs, it may be an indication for stopping BECONASE AQ Nasal Spray.

Beclomethasone dipropionate is absorbed into the circulation. Use of excessive doses of BECONASE AQ Nasal Spray may suppress HPA function.

BECONASE AQ Nasal Spray should be used with caution, if at all, in patients with active or quiescent tuberculous infections of the respiratory tract; untreated fungal, bacterial, or systemic viral infections; or ocular herpes simplex.

Continued on next page

This product information is based on labeling in effect on June 23, 2000. For further information, contact via direct mail, phone, or web site. Medical Information, Glaxo Wellcome Inc., PO Box 13398, Research Triangle Park, NC 27709. Healthcare Professionals (Medical Information): 800-334-0089. Patients (Customer Response Center): 1-888-825-5249. Glaxo Wellcome Corporate Web Site: www.glaxowellcome.com

Beconase AQ—Cont.

For BECONASE AQ Nasal Spray to be effective in the treatment of nasal polyps, the spray must be able to enter the nose. Therefore, treatment of nasal polyps with BECONASE AQ Nasal Spray should be considered adjunctive therapy to surgical removal and/or the use of other medications that will permit effective penetration of BECONASE AQ Nasal Spray into the nose. Nasal polyps may recur after any form of treatment.

As with any long-term treatment, patients using BECONASE AQ Nasal Spray over several months or longer should be examined periodically for possible changes in the nasal mucosa.

Because of the inhibitory effect of corticosteroids on wound healing, patients who have experienced recent nasal septum ulcers, nasal surgery, or trauma should not use a nasal corticosteroid until healing has occurred.

Although systemic effects have been minimal with recommended doses, this potential increases with excessive doses. Therefore, larger than recommended doses should be avoided.

Information for Patients: Patients being treated with BECONASE AQ Nasal Spray should receive the following information and instructions. This information is intended to aid in the safe and effective use of this medication. It is not a disclosure of all possible adverse or intended effects. Patients should use BECONASE AQ Nasal Spray at regular intervals since its effectiveness depends on its regular use. The patient should take the medication as directed. It is not acutely effective, and the prescribed dosage should not be increased. Instead, nasal vasoconstrictors or oral antihistamines may be needed until the effects of BECONASE AQ Nasal Spray are fully manifested. One to 2 weeks may pass before full relief is obtained. The patient should contact the physician if symptoms do not improve, if the condition worsens, or if sneezing or nasal irritation occurs. For the proper use of the unit and to attain maximum improvement, the patient should read and follow carefully the patient's instructions section of the full prescribing information.

Persons who are on immunosuppressant doses of corticosteroids should be warned to avoid exposure to chickenpox or measles. Patients should also be advised that if they are exposed, medical advice should be sought without delay.

Carcinogenesis, Mutagenesis, Impairment of Fertility: Treatment of rats for a total of 95 weeks, 13 weeks by inhalation and 82 weeks by the oral route, resulted in no evidence of carcinogenic activity. Mutagenic studies have not been performed.

Impairment of fertility, as evidenced by inhibition of the estrous cycle in dogs, was observed following treatment by the oral route. No inhibition of the estrous cycle in dogs was seen following treatment with beclomethasone dipropionate by the inhalation route.

Pregnancy: ***Teratogenic Effects:*** Pregnancy Category C. Like other corticoids, parenteral (subcutaneous) beclomethasone dipropionate has been shown to be teratogenic and embryocidal in the mouse and rabbit when given in doses approximately 10 times the human dose. In these studies, beclomethasone was found to produce fetal resorption, cleft palate, agnathia, microstomia, absence of tongue, delayed ossification, and agenesis of the thymus. No teratogenic or embryocidal effects have been seen in the rat when beclomethasone dipropionate was administered by inhalation at 10 times the human dose or orally at 1000 times the human dose. There are no adequate and well-controlled studies in pregnant women. Beclomethasone dipropionate should be used during pregnancy only if the potential benefit justifies the potential risk to the fetus.

Nonteratogenic Effects: Hypoadrenalism may occur in infants born of mothers receiving corticosteroids during pregnancy. Such infants should be carefully observed.

Nursing Mothers: It is not known whether beclomethasone dipropionate is excreted in human milk. Because other corticosteroids are excreted in human milk, caution should be exercised when BECONASE AQ Nasal Spray is administered to a nursing woman.

Pediatric Use: The safety and effectiveness of BECONASE AQ Nasal Spray have been established in children aged 6 years and above through evidence from extensive clinical use in adult and pediatric patients. The safety and effectiveness of BECONASE AQ Nasal Spray in children below 6 years of age have not been established.

Glucocorticoids have been shown to cause a reduction in growth velocity in children and teenagers with extended use. If a child or teenager on any glucocorticoid appears to have growth suppression, the possibility that they are particularly sensitive to this effect of glucocorticoids should be considered.

ADVERSE REACTIONS

In general, side effects in clinical studies have been primarily associated with irritation of the nasal mucous membranes. Rare cases of immediate and delayed hypersensitivity reactions, including urticaria, angioedema, rash, and bronchospasm, have been reported following the oral and intranasal inhalation of beclomethasone dipropionate.

Adverse reactions reported in controlled clinical trials and open studies in patients treated with BECONASE AQ Nasal Spray are described below.

Mild nasopharyngeal irritation following the use of beclomethasone aqueous nasal spray has been reported in up to 24% of patients treated, including occasional sneezing attacks (about 4%) occurring immediately following use of the spray. In patients experiencing these symptoms, none had to discontinue treatment. The incidence of transient irritation and sneezing was approximately the same in the group of patients who received placebo in these studies, implying that these complaints may be related to vehicle components of the formulation.

Fewer than 5 per 100 patients reported headache, nausea, or lightheadedness following the use of BECONASE AQ Nasal Spray. Fewer than 3 per 100 patients reported nasal stuffiness, nosebleeds, rhinorrhea, or tearing eyes.

Rare cases of ulceration of the nasal mucosa and instances of nasal septum perforation have been spontaneously reported (see PRECAUTIONS).

Reports of dryness and irritation of the nose and throat, and unpleasant taste and smell have been received. There are rare reports of loss of taste and smell.

Rare instances of wheezing, cataracts, glaucoma, and increased intraocular pressure have been reported following the use of intranasal beclomethasone dipropionate (see PRECAUTIONS).

OVERDOSAGE

When used at excessive doses, systemic corticosteroid effects such as hypercorticism and adrenal suppression may appear. If such changes occur, BECONASE AQ Nasal Spray should be discontinued slowly consistent with accepted procedures for discontinuing oral steroid therapy. The oral LD_{50} of beclomethasone dipropionate is greater than 1 g/kg in rodents. One bottle of BECONASE AQ Nasal Spray contains beclomethasone dipropionate, monohydrate equivalent to 10.5 mg of beclomethasone dipropionate; therefore, acute overdosage is unlikely.

DOSAGE AND ADMINISTRATION

Adults and Children 12 Years of Age and Older: The usual dosage is one or two inhalations (42 to 84 mcg) in each nostril twice a day (total dose, 168 to 336 mcg/day).

Children 6 to 12 Years of Age: Patients should be started with one inhalation in each nostril twice a day; patients not adequately responding to 168 mcg or those with more severe symptoms may use 336 mcg (two inhalations in each nostril). BECONASE AQ Nasal Spray is *not* recommended for children below 6 years of age.

In patients who respond to BECONASE AQ Nasal Spray, an improvement of the symptoms of seasonal or perennial rhinitis usually becomes apparent within a few days after the start of BECONASE AQ Nasal Spray therapy. However, symptomatic relief may not occur in some patients for as long as 2 weeks. BECONASE AQ Nasal Spray should not be continued beyond 3 weeks in the absence of significant symptomatic improvement.

The therapeutic effects of corticosteroids, unlike those of decongestants, are not immediate. This should be explained to the patient in advance in order to ensure cooperation and continuation of treatment with the prescribed dosage regimen.

In the presence of excessive nasal mucous secretion or edema of the nasal mucosa, the drug may fail to reach the site of intended action. In such cases it is advisable to use a nasal vasoconstrictor during the first 2 to 3 days of BECONASE AQ Nasal Spray therapy.

Directions for Use: Illustrated Patient's Instructions for Use accompany each package of BECONASE AQ Nasal Spray.

HOW SUPPLIED

BECONASE AQ Nasal Spray, 0.042%* is supplied in an amber glass bottle fitted with a metering atomizing pump and nasal adapter in a box of one (NDC 0173-0388-79) with patient's instructions for use. Each bottle contains 25 g of suspension.

Store between 15° and 30°C (59° and 86°F).

*Calculated on the dried basis.

Glaxo Wellcome Inc., Research Triangle Park, NC 27709

April 1998/RL-561

Shown in Product Identification Guide, page 314

CEFTIN® Tablets ℞

[sef 'tin]

(cefuroxime axetil tablets)

CEFTIN® for Oral Suspension

(cefuroxime axetil powder for oral suspension)

DESCRIPTION

CEFTIN Tablets and CEFTIN for Oral Suspension contain cefuroxime as cefuroxime axetil. CEFTIN is a semisynthetic, broad-spectrum cephalosporin antibiotic for oral administration.

Chemically, cefuroxime axetil, the 1-(acetyloxy) ethyl ester of cefuroxime, is (*RS*)-1-hydroxyethyl (6*R*,7*R*)-7-[2-(2-furyl) glyoxylamido] -3-(hydroxymethyl) -8-oxo-5-thia-1-azabicyclo[4.2.0]oct-2-ene-2-carboxylate,7^2-(*Z*)-(*O*-methyl-oxime), 1-acetate 3-carbamate. Its molecular formula is $C_{20}H_{22}N_4O_{10}S$, and it has a molecular weight of 510.48.

Cefuroxime axetil is in the amorphous form.

CEFTIN Tablets are film-coated and contain the equivalent of 125, 250, or 500 mg of cefuroxime as cefuroxime axetil. CEFTIN Tablets contain the inactive ingredients colloidal silicon dioxide, croscarmellose sodium, FD&C Blue No. 1 (250- and 500-mg tablets only), hydrogenated vegetable oil, hydroxypropyl methylcellulose, methylparaben, microcrystalline cellulose, propylene glycol, propylparaben, sodium benzoate (125-mg tablets only), sodium lauryl sulfate, and titanium dioxide.

CEFTIN for Oral Suspension, when reconstituted with water, provides the equivalent of 125 mg or 250 mg of cefuroxime (as cefuroxime axetil) per 5 mL of suspension. CEFTIN for Oral Suspension contains the inactive ingredients povidone K30, stearic acid, sucrose, and tutti-frutti flavoring.

CLINICAL PHARMACOLOGY

Absorption and Metabolism: After oral administration, cefuroxime axetil is absorbed from the gastrointestinal tract and rapidly hydrolyzed by nonspecific esterases in the intestinal mucosa and blood to cefuroxime. Cefuroxime is subsequently distributed throughout the extracellular fluids. The axetil moiety is metabolized to acetaldehyde and acetic acid.

Pharmacokinetics: Approximately 50% of serum cefuroxime is bound to protein. Serum pharmacokinetic parameters for CEFTIN Tablets and CEFTIN for Oral Suspension are shown in Tables 1 and 2.

[See table 1 at top of next page]

[See table 2 on next page]

Comparative Pharmacokinetic Properties: A 250 mg/5 mL-dose of CEFTIN Suspension is bioequivalent to two times 125 mg/5 mL-dose of CEFTIN Suspension when administered with food (see table below). **CEFTIN for Oral Suspension was not bioequivalent to CEFTIN Tablets when tested in healthy adults. The tablet and powder for oral suspension formulations are NOT substitutable on a mg/mg basis.** The area under the curve for the suspension averaged 91% of that for the tablet, and the peak plasma concentration for the suspension averaged 71% of the peak plasma concentration of the tablets. Therefore, the safety and effectiveness of both the tablet and oral suspension formulations had to be established in separate clinical trials.

[See table 3 on next page]

Food Effect on Pharmacokinetics: Absorption of the tablet is greater when taken after food (absolute bioavailability of CEFTIN Tablets increases from 37% to 52%). Despite this difference in absorption, the clinical and bacteriologic responses of patients were independent of food intake at the time of tablet administration in two studies where this was assessed.

All pharmacokinetic and clinical effectiveness and safety studies in pediatric patients using the suspension formulation were conducted in the fed state. No data are available on the absorption kinetics of the suspension formulation when administered to fasted pediatric patients.

Renal Excretion: Cefuroxime is excreted unchanged in the urine; in adults, approximately 50% of the administered dose is recovered in the urine within 12 hours. The pharmacokinetics of cefuroxime in the urine of pediatric patients have not been studied at this time. Until further data are available, the renal pharmacokinetic properties of cefuroxime axetil established in adults should not be extrapolated to pediatric patients.

Because cefuroxime is renally excreted, the serum half-life is prolonged in patients with reduced renal function. In a study of 20 elderly patients (mean age = 83.9 years) having a mean creatinine clearance of 34.9 mL/min, the mean serum elimination half-life was 3.5 hours. Despite the lower elimination of cefuroxime in geriatric patients, dosage adjustment based on age is not necessary (see PRECAUTIONS: Geriatric Use).

Microbiology: The *in vivo* bactericidal activity of cefuroxime axetil is due to cefuroxime's binding to essential target proteins and the resultant inhibition of cell-wall synthesis.

Cefuroxime has bactericidal activity against a wide range of common pathogens, including many beta-lactamase–producing strains. Cefuroxime is stable to many bacterial beta-lactamases, especially plasmid-mediated enzymes that are commonly found in enterobacteriaceae.

Cefuroxime has been demonstrated to be active against most strains of the following microorganisms both *in vitro* and in clinical infections as described in the INDICATIONS AND USAGE section (see INDICATIONS AND USAGE section).

Aerobic Gram-positive Microorganisms:

Staphylococcus aureus (including beta-lactamase–producing strains)
Streptococcus pneumoniae
Streptococcus pyogenes

Aerobic Gram-negative Microorganisms:

Escherichia coli
Haemophilus influenzae (including beta-lactamase–producing strains)
Haemophilus parainfluenzae
Klebsiella pneumoniae
Moraxella catarrhalis (including beta-lactamase–producing strains)
Neisseria gonorrhoeae (including beta-lactamase–producing strains)

Spirochetes:

Borrelia burgdorferi.

Cefuroxime has been shown to be active *in vitro* against most strains of the following microorganisms; however, the clinical significance of these findings is unknown.

Cefuroxime exhibits *in vitro* minimum inhibitory concentrations (MICs) of 4.0 mcg/mL or less (systemic susceptible breakpoint) against most (≥90%) strains of the following microorganisms; however, the safety and effectiveness of ce-

Table 1: Postprandial Pharmacokinetics of Cefuroxime Administered as CEFTIN Tablets to Adults*

Dose† (Cefuroxime Equivalent)	Peak Plasma Concentration (mcg/mL)	Time of Peak Plasma Concentration (h)	Mean Elimination Half-Life (h)	AUC (mcg-h mL)
125 mg	2.1	2.2	1.2	6.7
250 mg	4.1	2.5	1.2	12.9
500 mg	7.0	3.0	1.2	27.4
1000 mg	13.6	2.5	1.3	50.0

*Mean values of 12 healthy adult volunteers.
†Drug administered immediately after a meal.

Table 2: Postprandial Pharmacokinetics of Cefuroxime Administered as CEFTIN for Oral Suspension to Pediatric Patients*

Dose† (Cefuroxime Equivalent)	n	Peak Plasma Concentration (mcg/mL)	Time of Peak Plasma Concentration (h)	Mean Elimination Half-Life (h)	AUC (mcg-h mL)
10 mg/kg	8	3.3	3.6	1.4	12.4
15 mg/kg	12	5.1	2.7	1.9	22.5
20 mg/kg	8	7.0	3.1	1.9	32.8

*Mean age = 23 months.
†Drug administered with milk or milk products.

Table 3: Pharmacokinetics of Cefuroxime Administered as 250 mg/5 mL or 2 × 125 mg/5 mL CEFTIN for Oral Suspension to Adults* With Food

Dose (Cefuroxime Equivalent)	Peak Plasma Concentration (mcg/mL)	Time of Peak Plasma Concentration (h)	Mean Elimination Half-Life (h)	AUC (mcg-h mL)
250 mg/5 mL	2.23	3	1.40	8.92
2 × 125 mg/5 mL	2.37	3	1.44	9.75

*Mean values of 18 healthy adult volunteers.

furoxime in treating clinical infections due to these microorganisms have not been established in adequate and well-controlled trials.

Aerobic Gram-positive Microorganisms:
Staphylococcus epidermidis
Staphylococcus saprophyticus
Streptococcus agalactiae
NOTE: Certain strains of enterococci, e.g., *Enterococcus faecalis* (formerly *Streptococcus faecalis*), are resistant to cefuroxime. Methicillin-resistant staphylococci are resistant to cefuroxime.

Aerobic Gram-negative Microorganisms:
Morganella morganii
Proteus inconstans
Proteus mirabilis
Providencia rettgeri
NOTE: *Pseudomonas* spp., *Campylobacter* spp., *Acinetobacter calcoaceticus*, and most strains of *Serratia* spp. and *Proteus vulgaris* are resistant to most first- and second-generation cephalosporins. Some strains of *Morganella morganii, Enterobacter cloacae*, and *Citrobacter* spp. have been shown by *in vitro* tests to be resistant to cefuroxime and other cephalosporins.

Anaerobic Microorganisms:
Peptococcus niger
NOTE: Most strains of *Clostridium difficile* and *Bacteroides fragilis* are resistant to cefuroxime.

Susceptibility Tests: *Dilution Techniques:* Quantitative methods that are used to determine MICs provide reproducible estimates of the susceptibility of bacteria to antimicrobial compounds. One such standardized procedure uses a standardized dilution method[1] (broth, agar, or microdilution) or equivalent with cefuroxime powder. The MIC values obtained should be interpreted according to the following criteria:

MIC (mcg/mL)	Interpretation
≤4	(S) Susceptible
8–16	(I) Intermediate
≥32	(R) Resistant

A report of "Susceptible" indicates that the pathogen, if in the blood, is likely to be inhibited by usually achievable concentrations of the antimicrobial compound in blood. A report of "Intermediate" indicates that inhibitory concentrations of the antibiotic may be achieved if high dosage is used or if the infection is confined to tissues or fluids in which high antibiotic concentrations are attained. This category also provides a buffer zone that prevents small, uncontrolled technical factors from causing major discrepancies in interpretation. A report of "Resistant" indicates that usually achievable concentrations of the antimicrobial compound in the blood are unlikely to be inhibitory and that other therapy should be selected.
Standardized susceptibility test procedures require the use of laboratory control microorganisms. Standard cefuroxime powder should give the following MIC values:

Microorganism	MIC (mcg/mL)
Escherichia coli ATCC 25922	2–8
Staphylococcus aureus ATCC 29213	0.5–2

Diffusion Techniques: Quantitative methods that require measurement of zone diameters provide estimates of the susceptibility of bacteria to antimicrobial compounds. One such standardized procedure[2] that has been recommended (for use with disks) to test the susceptibility of microorganisms to cefuroxime uses the 30-mcg cefuroxime disk. Interpretation involves correlation of the diameter obtained in the disk test with the MIC for cefuroxime.
Reports from the laboratory providing results of the standard single-disk susceptibility test with a 30-mcg cefuroxime disk should be interpreted according to the following criteria:

Zone Diameter (mm)	Interpretation
≥23	(S) Susceptible
15–22	(I) Intermediate
≤14	(R) Resistant

Interpretation should be as stated above for results using dilution techniques.
As with standard dilution techniques, diffusion methods require the use of laboratory control microorganisms. The 30-mcg cefuroxime disk provides the following zone diameters in these laboratory test quality control strains:

Microorganism	Zone Diameter (mm)
Escherichia coli ATCC 25922	20–26
Staphylococcus aureus ATCC 25923	27–35

INDICATIONS AND USAGE

NOTE: CEFTIN TABLETS AND CEFTIN FOR ORAL SUSPENSION ARE NOT BIOEQUIVALENT AND ARE NOT SUBSTITUTABLE ON A MG/MG BASIS (SEE CLINICAL PHARMACOLOGY).
CEFTIN Tablets: CEFTIN Tablets are indicated for the treatment of patients with mild to moderate infections caused by susceptible strains of the designated microorganisms in the conditions listed below:

1. **Pharyngitis/Tonsillitis** caused by *Streptococcus pyogenes.* **NOTE:** The usual drug of choice in the treatment and prevention of streptococcal infections, including the prophylaxis of rheumatic fever, is penicillin given by the intramuscular route. CEFTIN Tablets are generally effective in the eradication of streptococci from the nasopharynx; however, substantial data establishing the efficacy of cefuroxime in the subsequent prevention of rheumatic fever are not available. Please also note that in all clinical trials, all isolates had to be sensitive to both penicillin and cefuroxime. There are no data from adequate and well-controlled trials to demonstrate the effectiveness of cefuroxime in the treatment of penicillin-resistant strains of *Streptococcus pyogenes.*
2. **Acute Bacterial Otitis Media** caused by *Streptococcus pneumoniae, Haemophilus influenzae* (including beta-lactamase–producing strains), *Moraxella catarrhalis* (including beta-lactamase–producing strains), or *Streptococcus pyogenes.*
3. **Acute Bacterial Maxillary Sinusitis** caused by *Streptococcus pneumoniae* or *Haemophilus influenzae* (non-beta-lactamase–producing strains only). (See CLINICAL STUDIES section.)
   NOTE: In view of the insufficient numbers of isolates of beta-lactamase–producing strains of *Haemophilus influenzae* and *Moraxella catarrhalis* that were obtained from clinical trials with CEFTIN Tablets for patients with acute bacterial maxillary sinusitis, it was not possible to adequately evaluate the effectiveness of CEFTIN Tablets for sinus infections known, suspected, or considered potentially to be caused by beta-lactamase–producing *Haemophilus influenzae* or *Moraxella catarrhalis.*
4. **Acute Bacterial Exacerbations of Chronic Bronchitis and Secondary Bacterial Infections of Acute Bronchitis** caused by *Streptococcus pneumoniae, Haemophilus influenzae* (beta-lactamase negative strains), or *Haemophilus parainfluenzae* (beta-lactamase negative strains). (See DOSAGE AND ADMINISTRATION section and CLINICAL STUDIES section).
5. **Uncomplicated Skin and Skin-Structure Infections** caused by *Staphylococcus aureus* (including beta-lactamase–producing strains) or *Streptococcus pyogenes.*
6. **Uncomplicated Urinary Tract Infections** caused by *Escherichia coli* or *Klebsiella pneumoniae.*
7. **Uncomplicated Gonorrhea,** urethral and endocervical, caused by penicillinase-producing and non-penicillinase–producing strains of *Neisseria gonorrhoeae* and uncomplicated gonorrhea, rectal, in females, caused by non-penicillinase–producing strains of *Neisseria gonorrhoeae.*
8. **Early Lyme Disease (erythema migrans)** caused by *Borrelia burgdorferi.*

CEFTIN for Oral Suspension: CEFTIN for Oral Suspension is indicated for the treatment of pediatric patients 3 months to 12 years of age with mild to moderate infections caused by susceptible strains of the designated microorganisms in the conditions listed below. The safety and effectiveness of CEFTIN for Oral Suspension in the treatment of infections other than those specifically listed below have not been established either by adequate and well-controlled trials or by pharmacokinetic data with which to determine an effective and safe dosing regimen.

1. **Pharyngitis/Tonsillitis** caused by *Streptococcus pyogenes.* **NOTE:** The usual drug of choice in the treatment and prevention of streptococcal infections, including the prophylaxis of rheumatic fever, is penicillin given by the intramuscular route. CEFTIN for Oral Suspension is generally effective in the eradication of streptococci from the nasopharynx; however, substantial data establishing the efficacy of cefuroxime in the subsequent prevention of rheumatic fever are not available. Please also note that in all clinical trials, all isolates had to be sensitive to both penicillin and cefuroxime. There are no data from adequate and well-controlled trials to demonstrate the effectiveness of cefuroxime in the treatment of penicillin-resistant strains of *Streptococcus pyogenes.*
2. **Acute Bacterial Otitis Media** caused by *Streptococcus pneumoniae, Haemophilus influenzae* (including beta-lactamase–producing strains), *Moraxella catarrhalis* (including beta-lactamase–producing strains), or *Streptococcus pyogenes.*
3. **Impetigo** caused by *Staphylococcus aureus* (including beta-lactamase–producing strains) or *Streptococcus pyogenes.*

Culture and susceptibility testing should be performed when appropriate to determine susceptibility of the causative microorganism(s) to cefuroxime. Therapy may be started while awaiting the results of this testing. Antimicrobial therapy should be appropriately adjusted according to the results of such testing.

CONTRAINDICATIONS

CEFTIN products are contraindicated in patients with known allergy to the cephalosporin group of antibiotics.

WARNINGS: CEFTIN TABLETS AND CEFTIN FOR ORAL SUSPENSION ARE NOT BIOEQUIVALENT AND ARE THEREFORE NOT SUBSTITUTABLE ON A MG/MG BASIS (SEE CLINICAL PHARMACOLOGY).

BEFORE THERAPY WITH CEFTIN PRODUCTS IS INSTITUTED, CAREFUL INQUIRY SHOULD BE MADE TO DETERMINE WHETHER THE PATIENT HAS HAD PREVIOUS HYPERSENSITIVITY REACTIONS TO CEFTIN PRODUCTS, OTHER CEPHALOSPORINS, PENICILLINS, OR OTHER DRUGS. IF THIS PRODUCT IS TO BE GIVEN TO PENICILLIN-SENSITIVE PATIENTS, CAUTION SHOULD BE EXERCISED BECAUSE CROSS-HYPERSENSITIVITY AMONG BETA-LACTAM ANTIBIOTICS HAS BEEN CLEARLY DOCUMENTED AND MAY OCCUR IN UP TO 10% OF PATIENTS WITH A HISTORY OF PENICILLIN ALLERGY. IF A CLINICALLY SIGNIFICANT ALLERGIC REACTION TO CEFTIN PRODUCTS OCCURS, DISCONTINUE THE DRUG AND INSTITUTE APPROPRIATE THERAPY. SERIOUS ACUTE HYPERSENSITIVITY REACTIONS MAY REQUIRE TREATMENT WITH EPINEPHRINE AND OTHER EMERGENCY MEASURES, INCLUDING OXYGEN, INTRAVENOUS FLUIDS, INTRAVENOUS ANTIHISTAMINES, CORTICOSTEROIDS, PRESSOR AMINES, AND AIRWAY MANAGEMENT, AS CLINICALLY INDICATED.
Pseudomembranous colitis has been reported with nearly all antibacterial agents, including cefuroxime, and may range from mild to life threatening. Therefore, it is important to consider this diagnosis in patients who present with diarrhea subsequent to the administration of antibacterial agents.

Continued on next page

This product information is based on labeling in effect on June 23, 2000. For further information, contact via direct mail, phone, or web site. Medical Information, Glaxo Wellcome Inc., PO Box 13398, Research Triangle Park, NC 27709. Healthcare Professionals (Medical Information): 800-334-0089. Patients (Customer Response Center): 1-888-825-5249. Glaxo Wellcome Corporate Web Site: www.glaxowellcome.com

Ceftin Tablets/O.S.—Cont.

Treatment with antibacterial agents alters normal flora of the colon and may permit overgrowth of clostridia. Studies indicate that a toxin produced by *Clostridium difficile* is one primary cause of antibiotic-associated colitis.
After the diagnosis of pseudomembranous colitis has been established, appropriate therapeutic measures should be initiated. Mild cases of pseudomembranous colitis usually respond to drug discontinuation alone. In moderate to severe cases, consideration should be given to management with fluids and electrolytes, protein supplementation, and treatment with an antibacterial drug effective against *Clostridium difficile*.

PRECAUTIONS

General: As with other broad-spectrum antibiotics, prolonged administration of cefuroxime axetil may result in overgrowth of nonsusceptible microorganisms. If superinfection occurs during therapy, appropriate measures should be taken.
Cephalosporins, including cefuroxime axetil, should be given with caution to patients receiving concurrent treatment with potent diuretics because these diuretics are suspected of adversely affecting renal function.
Cefuroxime axetil, as with other broad-spectrum antibiotics, should be prescribed with caution in individuals with a history of colitis. The safety and effectiveness of cefuroxime axetil have not been established in patients with gastrointestinal malabsorption. Patients with gastrointestinal malabsorption were excluded from participating in clinical trials of cefuroxime axetil.
Information for Patients/Caregivers (Pediatric): 1. During clinical trials, the tablet was tolerated by pediatric patients old enough to swallow the cefuroxime axetil tablet whole. The crushed tablet has a strong, persistent, bitter taste and should not be administered to pediatric patients in this manner. Pediatric patients who cannot swallow the tablet whole should receive the oral suspension.
2. Discontinuation of therapy due to taste and/or problems of administering this drug occurred in 1.4% of pediatric patients given the oral suspension. Complaints about taste (which may impair compliance) occurred in 5% of pediatric patients.
Drug/Laboratory Test Interactions: A false-positive reaction for glucose in the urine may occur with copper reduction tests (Benedict's or Fehling's solution or with CLINITEST® tablets), but not with enzyme-based tests for glycosuria (e.g., CLINISTIX®, TES-TAPE®). As a false-negative result may occur in the ferricyanide test, it is recommended that either the glucose oxidase or hexokinase method be used to determine blood/plasma glucose levels in patients receiving cefuroxime axetil. The presence of cefuroxime does not interfere with the assay of serum and urine creatinine by the alkaline picrate method.
Drug/Drug Interactions: Concomitant administration of probenecid with cefuroxime axetil tablets increases the area under the serum concentration versus time curve by 50%. The peak serum cefuroxime concentration after a 1.5-g single dose is greater when taken with 1 g of probenecid (mean = 14.8 mcg/mL) than without probenecid (mean = 12.2 mcg/mL).
Drugs that reduce gastric acidity may result in a lower bioavailability of CEFTIN compared with that of fasting state and tend to cancel the effect of postprandial absorption.
Carcinogenesis, Mutagenesis, Impairment of Fertility: Although lifetime studies in animals have not been performed to evaluate carcinogenic potential, no mutagenic potential was found for cefuroxime axetil in the micronucleus test and a battery of bacterial mutation tests. Reproduction studies in rats at doses up to 1000 mg/kg per day (nine times the recommended maximum human dose based on mg/m^2) have revealed no evidence of impaired fertility.
Pregnancy: ***Teratogenic Effects:*** Pregnancy Category B. Reproduction studies have been performed in rats and mice at doses up to 3200 mg/kg per day (23 times the recommended maximum human dose based on mg/m^2) and have revealed no evidence of harm to the fetus due to cefuroxime axetil. There are, however, no adequate and well-controlled studies in pregnant women. Because animal reproduction studies are not always predictive of human response, this drug should be used during pregnancy only if clearly needed.
Labor and Delivery: Cefuroxime axetil has not been studied for use during labor and delivery.
Nursing Mothers: Because cefuroxime is excreted in human milk, consideration should be given to discontinuing nursing temporarily during treatment with cefuroxime axetil.
Pediatric Use: The safety and effectiveness of CEFTIN have been established for pediatric patients aged 3 months to 12 years for acute bacterial maxillary sinusitis based upon its approval in adults. Use of CEFTIN in pediatric patients is supported by pharmacokinetic and safety data in adults and pediatric patients, and by clinical and microbiological data from adequate and well-controlled studies of the treatment of acute bacterial maxillary sinusitis in adults and of acute otitis media with effusion in pediatric patients. It is also supported by post-marketing adverse events surveillance (see CLINICAL PHARMACOLOGY, INDICATIONS AND USAGE, ADVERSE REACTIONS, DOSAGE AND ADMINISTRATION, and CLINICAL STUDIES).

Table 4: Adverse Reactions
CEFTIN Tablets
Multiple-Dose Dosing Regimens—Clinical Trials

Incidence ≥1%	Diarrhea/loose stools	3.7%
	Nausea/vomiting	3.0%
	Transient elevation in AST	2.0%
	Transient elevation in ALT	1.6%
	Eosinophilia	1.1%
	Transient elevation in LDH	1.0%
Incidence <1% but >0.1%	Abdominal pain	
	Abdominal cramps	
	Flatulence	
	Indigestion	
	Headache	
	Vaginitis	
	Vulvar itch	
	Rash	
	Hives	
	Itch	
	Dysuria	
	Chills	
	Chest pain	
	Shortness of breath	
	Mouth ulcers	
	Swollen tongue	
	Sleepiness	
	Thirst	
	Anorexia	
	Positive Coombs' test	

Table 5: Adverse Reactions
CEFTIN Tablets
1-g Single-Dose Regimen for Uncomplicated Gonorrhea—Clinical Trials

Incidence ≥1%	Nausea/vomiting	6.8%
	Diarrhea	4.2%
Incidence <1% but >0.1%	Abdominal pain	
	Dyspepsia	
	Erythema	
	Rash	
	Pruritus	
	Vaginal candidiasis	
	Vaginal itch	
	Vaginal discharge	
	Headache	
	Dizziness	
	Somnolence	
	Muscle cramps	
	Muscle stiffness	
	Muscle spasm of neck	
	Tightness/pain in chest	
	Bleeding/pain in urethra	
	Kidney pain	
	Tachycardia	
	Lockjaw-type reaction	

Geriatric Use: In clinical trials when 12- to 64-year-old patients and geriatric patients (65 years of age or older) were treated with usual recommended dosages (i.e., 125 to 500 mg b.i.d., depending on type of infections), no overall differences in effectiveness were observed between the two age-groups. The geriatric patients reported somewhat fewer gastrointestinal events and less frequent vaginal candidiasis compared with patients aged 12 to 64 years old; however, no clinically significant differences were reported between the two age-groups. Therefore, no adjustment of the usual adult dose is necessary based on age alone.

ADVERSE REACTIONS

CEFTIN TABLETS IN CLINICAL TRIALS: Multiple-Dose Dosing Regimens: ***7 to 10 Days Dosing:*** Using multiple doses of cefuroxime axetil tablets, 912 patients were treated with the recommended dosages of cefuroxime axetil (125 to 500 mg twice a day). There were no deaths or permanent disabilities thought related to drug toxicity. Twenty (2.2%) patients discontinued medication due to adverse events thought by the investigators to be possibly, probably, or almost certainly related to drug toxicity. Seventeen (85%) of the 20 patients who discontinued therapy did so because of gastrointestinal disturbances, including diarrhea, nausea, vomiting, and abdominal pain. The percentage of cefuroxime axetil tablet-treated patients who discontinued study drug because of adverse events was very similar at daily doses of 1000, 500, and 250 mg (2.3%, 2.1%, and 2.2%, respectively). However, the incidence of gastrointestinal adverse events increased with the higher recommended doses.
The following adverse events were thought by the investigators to be possibly, probably, or almost certainly related to cefuroxime axetil tablets in multiple-dose clinical trials (n = 912 cefuroxime axetil-treated patients).
[See table 4 above]
5-Day Experience (see CLINICAL STUDIES section): In clinical trials using CEFTIN in a dose of 250 mg b.i.d. in the treatment of secondary bacterial infections of acute bronchitis, 399 patients were treated for 5 days and 402 patients were treated for 10 days. No difference in the occurrence of adverse events was found between the two regimens.
In Clinical Trials for Early Lyme Disease With 20 Days Dosing: Two multicenter trials assessed cefuroxime axetil tablets 500 mg twice a day for 20 days. The most common drug-related adverse experiences were diarrhea (10.6% of patients), Jarisch-Herxheimer's reaction (5.6%), and vaginitis (5.4%). Other adverse experiences occurred with frequencies comparable to those reported with 7 to 10 days dosing.
Single-Dose Regimen for Uncomplicated Gonorrhea: In clinical trials using a single dose of cefuroxime axetil tablets, 1061 patients were treated with the recommended dosage of cefuroxime axetil (1000 mg) for the treatment of uncomplicated gonorrhea. There were no deaths or permanent disabilities thought related to drug toxicity in these studies.
The following adverse events were thought by the investigators to be possibly, probably, or almost certainly related to cefuroxime axetil in 1000-mg single-dose clinical trials of cefuroxime axetil tablets in the treatment of uncomplicated gonorrhea conducted in the US.
[See table 5 above]
CEFTIN FOR ORAL SUSPENSION IN CLINICAL TRIALS: In clinical trials using multiple doses of cefuroxime axetil powder for oral suspension, pediatric patients (96.7% of whom were younger than 12 years of age) were treated with the recommended dosages of cefuroxime axetil (20 to 30 mg/kg per day divided twice a day up to a maximum dose of 500 or 1000 mg/day, respectively). There were no deaths or permanent disabilities in any of the patients in these studies. Eleven US patients (1.2%) discontinued medication due to adverse events thought by the investigators to be possibly, probably, or almost certainly related to drug toxicity. The discontinuations were primarily for gastrointestinal disturbances, usually diarrhea or vomiting. During clinical trials, discontinuation of therapy due to the taste and/or problems with administering this drug occurred in 13 (1.4%) pediatric patients enrolled at centers in the US.
The following adverse events were thought by the investigators to be possibly, probably, or almost certainly related to cefuroxime axetil for oral suspension in multiple-dose clinical trials (n = 931 cefuroxime axetil-treated US patients).
[See table 6 at top of next page]
OBSERVED DURING CLINICAL PRACTICE: In addition to adverse events reported from clinical trials, the following events have been identified during post-approval use of CEFTIN. Because they are reported voluntarily from a population of unknown size, estimates of frequency cannot be made. These events have been chosen for inclusion due to combination of their seriousness, frequency of reporting, or potential causal connection of CEFTIN.

Blood and Lymphatic: Increased prothrombin time.
General: The following hypersensitivity reactions have been reported: anaphylaxis, angioedema, pruritus, rash, serum sickness-like reaction, and urticaria.
Gastrointestinal: Pseudomembranous colitis (see WARNINGS).
Hematologic: Hemolytic anemia, leukopenia, pancytopenia, and thrombocytopenia.
Hepatobiliary Tract and Pancreas: Hepatic impairment including hepatitis and cholestasis, jaundice.
Neurologic: Seizure.
Skin: Erythema multiforme, Stevens-Johnson syndrome, and toxic epidermal necrolysis.
Urologic: Renal dysfunction.

CEPHALOSPORIN-CLASS ADVERSE REACTIONS

In addition to the adverse reactions listed above that have been observed in patients treated with cefuroxime axetil, the following adverse reactions and altered laboratory tests have been reported for cephalosporin-class antibiotics: renal dysfunction, toxic nephropathy, hepatic cholestasis, aplastic anemia, hemolytic anemia, hemorrhage, increased prothrombin time, increased BUN, increased creatinine, false-positive test for urinary glucose, increased alkaline phosphatase, neutropenia, thrombocytopenia, leukopenia, elevated bilirubin, pancytopenia, and agranulocytosis.
Several cephalosporins have been implicated in triggering seizures, particularly in patients with renal impairment when the dosage was not reduced (see DOSAGE AND ADMINISTRATION and OVERDOSAGE). If seizures associated with drug therapy occur, the drug should be discontinued. Anticonvulsant therapy can be given if clinically indicated.

OVERDOSAGE

Overdosage of cephalosporins can cause cerebral irritation leading to convulsions. Serum levels of cefuroxime can be reduced by hemodialysis and peritoneal dialysis.

DOSAGE AND ADMINISTRATION

NOTE: CEFTIN TABLETS AND CEFTIN FOR ORAL SUSPENSION ARE NOT BIOEQUIVALENT AND ARE NOT SUBSTITUTABLE ON A MG/MG BASIS (SEE CLINICAL PHARMACOLOGY).
[See table 7 at right]
CEFTIN for Oral Suspension: CEFTIN for Oral Suspension may be administered to pediatric patients ranging in age from 3 months to 12 years, according to dosages in Table 8:
[See table 8 at right]
Patients With Renal Failure: The safety and efficacy of cefuroxime axetil in patients with renal failure have not been established. Since cefuroxime is renally eliminated, its half-life will be prolonged in patients with renal failure.
Directions for Mixing CEFTIN for Oral Suspension: Prepare a suspension at the time of dispensing as follows:

1. Shake the bottle to loosen the powder.
2. Remove the cap.
3. Add the total amount of water for reconstitution (see Table 9) and replace the cap.
4. Invert the bottle and vigorously rock the bottle from side to side so that water rises through the powder.
5. Once the sound of the powder against the bottle disappears, turn the bottle upright and vigorously shake it in a diagonal direction.

[See table 9 at right]
NOTE: SHAKE THE ORAL SUSPENSION WELL BEFORE EACH USE. Replace cap securely after each opening. The reconstituted suspension should be stored between 2° and 25°C (36° and 77°F) (either in the refrigerator or at room temperature). DISCARD AFTER 10 DAYS.

HOW SUPPLIED

CEFTIN Tablets: CEFTIN Tablets, 125 mg of cefuroxime (as cefuroxime axetil), are white, capsule-shaped, film-coated tablets engraved with "395" on one side and "Glaxo" on the other side as follows:

20 Tablets/Bottle	NDC 0173-0395-00
60 Tablets/Bottle	NDC 0173-0395-01
Unit Dose Packs of 100	NDC 0173-0395-02

CEFTIN Tablets, 250 mg of cefuroxime (as cefuroxime axetil), are light blue, capsule-shaped, film-coated tablets engraved with "387" on one side and "Glaxo" on the other side as follows:

20 Tablets/Bottle	NDC 0173-0387-00
60 Tablets/Bottle	NDC 0173-0387-42
Unit Dose Packs of 100	NDC 0173-0387-01

CEFTIN Tablets, 500 mg of cefuroxime (as cefuroxime axetil), are dark blue, capsule-shaped, film-coated tablets engraved with "394" on one side and "Glaxo" on the other side as follows:

20 Tablets/Bottle	NDC 0173-0394-00
60 Tablets/Bottle	NDC 0173-0394-42
Unit Dose Packs of 50	NDC 0173-0394-01

Store the tablets between 15° and 30°C (59° and 86°F). Replace cap securely after each opening. Protect unit dose packs from excessive moisture.
CEFTIN for Oral Suspension: CEFTIN for Oral Suspension is provided as dry, white to pale yellow, tutti-frutti–flavored powder. When reconstituted as directed, CEFTIN for Oral Suspension provides the equivalent of 125 mg or 250 mg of cefuroxime (as cefuroxime axetil) per 5 mL of suspension. It is supplied in amber glass bottles as follows:
125 mg/5 mL:

50-mL Suspension	NDC 0173-0406-01
100-mL Suspension	NDC 0173-0406-00

Table 6: Adverse Reactions CEFTIN for Oral Suspension Multiple-Dose Dosing Regimens— Clinical Trials

Incidence ≥1%	Diarrhea/loose stools	8.6%
	Dislike of taste	5.0%
	Diaper rash	3.4%
	Nausea/vomiting	2.6%
Incidence <1% but >0.1%	Abdominal pain	
	Flatulence	
	Gastrointestinal infection	
	Candidiasis	
	Vaginal irritation	
	Rash	
	Hyperactivity	
	Irritable behavior	
	Eosinophilia	
	Positive direct Coombs' test	
	Elevated liver enzymes	
	Viral illness	
	Upper respiratory infection	
	Sinusitis	
	Cough	
	Urinary tract infection	
	Joint swelling	
	Arthralgia	
	Fever	
	Ptyalism	

Table 7: CEFTIN Tablets (May be administered without regard to meals.)

Population/Infection	Dosage	Duration (days)
Adolescents and Adults (13 years and older)		
Pharyngitis/tonsillitis	250 mg b.i.d.	10
Acute bacterial maxillary sinusitis	250 mg b.i.d.	10
Acute bacterial exacerbations of chronic bronchitis	250 or 500 mg b.i.d.	10*
Secondary bacterial infections of acute bronchitis	250 or 500 mg b.i.d.	5–10
Uncomplicated skin and skin-structure infections	250 or 500 mg b.i.d.	10
Uncomplicated urinary tract infections	125 or 250 mg b.i.d.	7–10
Uncomplicated gonorrhea	1000 mg once	single dose
Early Lyme disease	500 mg b.i.d.	20
Pediatric Patients (who can swallow tablets whole)		
Pharyngitis/tonsillitis	125 mg b.i.d.	10
Acute otitis media	250 mg b.i.d.	10
Acute bacterial maxillary sinusitis	250 mg b.i.d.	10

*The safety and effectiveness of CEFTIN administered for less than 10 days in patients with acute exacerbations of chronic bronchitis have not been established.

Table 8: CEFTIN for Oral Suspension (Must be administered with food. Shake well each time before using.)

Population/Infection	Dosage	Daily Maximum Dose	Duration (days)
Pediatric Patients (3 months to 12 years)			
Pharyngitis/tonsillitis	20 mg/kg/day divided b.i.d.	500 mg	10
Acute otitis media	30 mg/kg/day divided b.i.d.	1000 mg	10
Acute bacterial maxillary sinusitis	30 mg/kg/day divided b.i.d.	1000 mg	10
Impetigo	30 mg/kg/day divided b.i.d.	1000 mg	10

Table 9: Amount of Water Required for Reconstitution of Labeled Volumes of CEFTIN for Oral Suspension

CEFTIN for Oral Suspension	Labeled Volume After Reconstitution	Amount of Water Required for Reconstitution
125 mg/5 mL	50 mL	20 mL
	100 mL	37 mL
250 mg/5 mL	50 mL	19 mL
	100 mL	35 mL

250 mg/5 mL:

50-mL Suspension	NDC 0173-0554-00
100-mL Suspension	NDC 0173-0555-00

Before reconstitution, store dry powder between 2° and 30°C (36° and 86°F).
After reconstitution, store suspension between 2° and 25°C (36° and 77°F), in a refrigerator or at room temperature. DISCARD AFTER 10 DAYS.

CLINICAL STUDIES

CEFTIN Tablets: ***Acute Bacterial Maxillary Sinusitis:*** One adequate and well-controlled study was performed in patients with acute bacterial maxillary sinusitis. In this study each patient had a maxillary sinus aspirate collected by sinus puncture before treatment was initiated for presumptive acute bacterial sinusitis. All patients had to have radiographic and clinical evidence of acute maxillary sinusitis. As shown in the following summary of the study, the general clinical effectiveness of CEFTIN Tablets was comparable to an oral antimicrobial agent that contained a specific beta-lactamase inhibitor in treating acute maxillary sinusitis. However, sufficient microbiology data were obtained to demonstrate the effectiveness of CEFTIN Tablets in treating acute bacterial maxillary sinusitis due only to *Streptococcus pneumoniae* or non-beta-lactamase–producing *Haemophilus influenzae.* An insufficient number of beta-lactamase–producing *Haemophilus influenzae* and *Moraxella catarrhalis* isolates were obtained in this trial to adequately evaluate the effectiveness of CEFTIN Tablets in the treatment of acute bacterial maxillary sinusitis due to these two organisms.
This study enrolled 317 adult patients, 132 patients in the United States and 185 patients in South America. Patients were randomized in a 1:1 ratio to cefuroxime axetil 250 mg b.i.d. or an oral antimicrobial agent that contained a specific beta-lactamase inhibitor. An intent-to-treat analysis of the submitted clinical data yielded the following results:

Continued on next page

This product information is based on labeling in effect on June 23, 2000. For further information, contact via direct mail, phone, or web site. Medical Information, Glaxo Wellcome Inc., PO Box 13398, Research Triangle Park, NC 27709. Healthcare Professionals (Medical Information): 800-334-0089. Patients (Customer Response Center): 1-888-825-5249. Glaxo Wellcome Corporate Web Site: www.glaxowellcome.com

Ceftin Tablets/O.S.—Cont.

[See table 10 at right]
In this trial and in a supporting maxillary puncture trial, 15 evaluable patients had non-beta-lactamase–producing *Haemophilus influenzae* as the identified pathogen. Ten (10) of these 15 patients (67%) had their pathogen (non-beta-lactamase–producing *Haemophilus influenzae*) eradicated. Eighteen (18) evaluable patients had *Streptococcus pneumoniae* as the identified pathogen. Fifteen (15) of these 18 patients (83%) had their pathogen (*Streptococcus pneumoniae*) eradicated.

Safety: The incidence of drug-related gastrointestinal adverse events was statistically significantly higher in the control arm (an oral antimicrobial agent that contained a specific beta-lactamase inhibitor) versus the cefuroxime axetil arm (12% versus 1%, respectively; $P<0.001$), particularly drug-related diarrhea (8% versus 1%, respectively; $P = 0.001$).

Early Lyme Disease: Two adequate and well-controlled studies were performed in patients with early Lyme disease. In these studies all patients had to present with physician-documented erythema migrans, with or without systemic manifestations of infection. Patients were randomized in a 1:1 ratio to a 20-day course of treatment with cefuroxime axetil 500 mg b.i.d. or doxycycline 100 mg t.i.d. Patients were assessed at 1 month posttreatment for success in treating early Lyme disease (Part I) and at 1 year posttreatment for success in preventing the progression to the sequelae of late Lyme disease (Part II).

A total of 355 adult patients (181 treated with cefuroxime axetil and 174 treated with doxycycline) were enrolled in the two studies. In order to objectively validate the clinical diagnosis of early Lyme disease in these patients, two approaches were used: 1) blinded expert reading of photographs, when available, of the pretreatment erythema migrans skin lesion; and 2) serologic confirmation (using enzyme-linked immunosorbent assay [ELISA] and immunoblot assay ["Western" blot]) of the presence of antibodies specific to *Borrelia burgdorferi*, the etiologic agent of Lyme disease. By these procedures, it was possible to confirm the physician diagnosis of early Lyme disease in 281 (79%) of the 355 study patients. The efficacy data summarized below are specific to this "validated" patient subset, while the safety data summarized below reflect the entire patient population for the two studies.

Analysis of the submitted clinical data for evaluable patients in the "validated" patient subset yielded the following results:

[See table 11 at right]
CEFTIN and doxycycline were effective in prevention of the development of sequelae of late Lyme disease.

Safety: Drug-related adverse events affecting the skin were reported significantly more frequently by patients treated with doxycycline than by patients treated with cefuroxime axetil (12% versus 3%, respectively; $P = 0.002$), primarily reflecting the statistically significantly higher incidence of drug-related photosensitivity reactions in the doxycycline arm versus the cefuroxime axetil arm (9% versus 0%, respectively; $P<0.001$). While the incidence of drug-related gastrointestinal adverse events was similar in the two treatment groups (cefuroxime axetil - 13%; doxycycline - 11%), the incidence of drug-related diarrhea was statistically significantly higher in the cefuroxime axetil arm versus the doxycycline arm (11% versus 3%, respectively; $P = 0.005$).

Secondary Bacterial Infections of Acute Bronchitis: Four randomized, controlled clinical studies were performed comparing 5 days versus 10 days of CEFTIN for the treatment of patients with secondary bacterial infections of acute bronchitis. These studies enrolled a total of 1253 patients (CAE-516 n = 360; CAE-517 n = 177; CAEA4001 n = 362; CAEA4002 n = 354). The protocols for CAE-516 and CAE-517 were identical and compared CEFTIN 250 mg b.i.d. for 5 days, CEFTIN 250 mg b.i.d. for 10 days, and AUGMENTIN® 500 mg t.i.d. for 10 days. These two studies were conducted simultaneously. CAEA4001 and CAEA4002 compared CEFTIN 250 mg b.i.d. for 5 days, CEFTIN 250 mg b.i.d. for 10 days, and CECLOR® 250 mg t.i.d. for 10 days. They were otherwise identical to CAE-516 and CAE-517 and were conducted over the following two years. Patients were required to have polymorphonuclear cells present on the Gram stain of their screening sputum specimen, but isolation of a bacterial pathogen from the sputum culture was not required for inclusion. The following table demonstrates the results of the clinical outcome analysis of the pooled studies CAE-516/CAE-517 and CAEA4001/CAEA4002, respectively:

[See table 12 above]
The response rates for patients who were both clinically and bacteriologically evaluable were consistent with those reported for the clinically evaluable patients.

Safety: In these clinical trials, 399 patients were treated with CEFTIN for 5 days and 402 patients with CEFTIN for 10 days. No difference in the occurrence of adverse events was observed between the two regimens.

REFERENCES:

1. National Committee for Clinical Laboratory Standards. *Methods for Dilution Antimicrobial Susceptibility Tests for Bacteria that Grow Aerobically.* 3rd ed. Approved Standard NCCLS Document M7-A3, Vol. 13, No. 25. Villanova, Pa: NCCLS; 1993.
2. National Committee for Clinical Laboratory Standards. *Performance Standards for Antimicrobial Disk Susceptibility Tests.* 4th ed. Approved Standard NCCLS Document M2-A4, Vol. 10, No. 7. Villanova, Pa: NCCLS; 1990.

Table 10: Clinical Effectiveness of CEFTIN Tablets Compared to Beta-Lactamase Inhibitor-Containing Control Drug in the Treatment of Acute Bacterial Maxillary Sinusitis

	US Patients*		South American Patients†	
	CEFTIN n = 49	Control n = 43	CEFTIN n = 87	Doxycycline n = 89
Clinical success (cure + improvement)	65%	53%	77%	74%
Clinical cure	53%	44%	72%	64%
Clinical improvement	12%	9%	5%	10%

*95% Confidence interval around the success difference [-0.08, +0.32].
†95% Confidence interval around the success difference [-0.10, +0.16].

Table 11: Clinical Effectiveness of CEFTIN Tablets Compared to Doxycycline in the Treatment of Early Lyme Disease

	Part I (1 Month Posttreatment)*		Part II (1 Year Posttreatment)†	
	CEFTIN n = 125	Doxycycline n = 108	CEFTIN n = 105‡	Doxycycline n = 83‡
Satisfactory clinical outcome§	91%	93%	84%	87%
Clinical cure/success	72%	73%	73%	73%
Clinical improvement	19%	19%	10%	13%

*95% confidence interval around the satisfactory difference for Part I (-0.08, +0.05).
†95% confidence interval around the satisfactory difference for Part II (-0.13, +0.07).
‡n's include patients assessed as unsatisfactory clinical outcomes (failure + recurrence) in Part I (CEFTIN - 11 [5 failure, 6 recurrence]; doxycycline - 8 [6 failure, 2 recurrence]).
§Satisfactory clinical outcome includes cure + improvement (Part I) and success + improvement (Part II).

Table 12: Clinical Effectiveness of CEFTIN Tablets 250 mg b.i.d. in Secondary Bacterial Infections of Acute Bronchitis: Comparison of 5 Versus 10 Days' Treatment Duration

	CAE-516 and CAE-517*		CAEA4001 and CAEA4002†	
	5 Day (n = 127)	10 Day (n = 139)	5 Day (n = 173)	10 Day (n = 192)
Clinical success (cure + improvement)	80%	87%	84%	82%
Clinical cure	61%	70%	73%	72%
Clinical improvement	19%	17%	11%	10%

*95% Confidence interval around the success difference [-0.164, +0.029].
†95% Confidence interval around the success difference [-0.061, +0.103].

Glaxo Wellcome Inc., Research Triangle Park, NC 27709
CEFTIN is a registered trademark of Glaxo Wellcome.
CLINITEST and CLINISTIX are registered trademarks of Ames Division, Miles Laboratories, Inc.
TES-TAPE is a registered trademark of Eli Lilly and Company.
US Patent Nos. 4,267,320; 4,562,181; 4,865,851; and 4,897,270

August 1999/RL-743
Shown in Product Identification Guide, page 314

CEPTAZ® ℞

[*sĕp ' tăz*]
(ceftazidime for injection)
L-arginine formulation

For Intravenous or Intramuscular Use

DESCRIPTION

Ceftazidime is a semisynthetic, broad-spectrum, beta-lactam antibiotic for parenteral administration. It is the pentahydrate of pyridinium, 1-[[7-[[(2-amino-4-thiazolyl)[(1-carboxy-1-methylethoxy) imino]acetyl] amino]-2-carboxy-8-oxo-5-thia -1- azabicyclo[4.2.0]oct-2-en-3-yl]methyl]-, hydroxide, inner salt, [6R-[6α,7β(Z)]].

The empirical formula is $C_{22}H_{32}N_6O_{12}S_2$, representing a molecular weight of 636.6.

CEPTAZ is a sterile, dry mixture of ceftazidime pentahydrate and L-arginine. The L-arginine is at a concentration of 349 mg/g of ceftazidime activity. CEPTAZ dissolves without the evolution of gas. The product contains no sodium ion. Solutions of CEPTAZ range in color from light yellow to amber, depending on the diluent and volume used. The pH of freshly constituted solutions usually ranges from 5 to 7.5.

CLINICAL PHARMACOLOGY

After intravenous (IV) administration of 500-mg and 1-g doses of ceftazidime over 5 minutes to normal adult male volunteers, mean peak serum concentrations of 45 and 90 mcg/mL, respectively, were achieved. After IV infusion of 500-mg, 1-g, and 2-g doses of ceftazidime over 20 to 30 minutes to normal adult male volunteers, mean peak serum concentrations of 42, 69, and 170 mcg/mL, respectively, were achieved. The average serum concentrations following IV infusion of 500-mg, 1-g, and 2-g doses to these volunteers over an 8-hour interval are given in Table 1.

Table 1

Ceftazidime IV Dose	Serum Concentrations (mcg/mL) 0.5 h	1 h	2 h	4 h	8 h
500 mg	42	25	12	6	2
1 g	60	39	23	11	3
2 g	129	75	42	13	5

The absorption and elimination of ceftazidime were directly proportional to the size of the dose. The half-life following IV administration was approximately 1.9 hours. Less than 10% of ceftazidime was protein bound. The degree of protein binding was independent of concentration. There was no evidence of accumulation of ceftazidime in the serum in individuals with normal renal function following multiple IV doses of 1 and 2 g every 8 hours for 10 days.

Following intramuscular (IM) administration of 500-mg and 1-g doses of ceftazidime to normal adult volunteers, the mean peak serum concentrations were 17 and 39 mcg/mL, respectively, at approximately 1 hour. Serum concentrations remained above 4 mcg/mL for 6 and 8 hours after the IM administration of 500-mg and 1-g doses, respectively. The half-life of ceftazidime in these volunteers was approximately 2 hours.

The presence of hepatic dysfunction had no effect on the pharmacokinetics of ceftazidime in individuals administered 2 g intravenously every 8 hours for 5 days. Therefore, a dosage adjustment from the normal recommended dosage is not required for patients with hepatic dysfunction, provided renal function is not impaired.

Approximately 80% to 90% of an IM or IV dose of ceftazidime is excreted unchanged by the kidneys over a 24-hour period. After the IV administration of single 500-mg or 1-g doses, approximately 50% of the dose appeared in the urine in the first 2 hours. An additional 20% was excreted between 2 and 4 hours after dosing, and approximately another 12% of the dose appeared in the urine between 4 and 8 hours later. The elimination of ceftazidime by the kidneys resulted in high therapeutic concentrations in the urine.

The mean renal clearance of ceftazidime was approximately 100 mL/min. The calculated plasma clearance of approximately 115 mL/min indicated nearly complete elimination of ceftazidime by the renal route. Administration of probenecid before dosing had no effect on the elimination kinetics of ceftazidime. This suggested that ceftazidime is eliminated by glomerular filtration and is not actively secreted by renal tubular mechanisms.

Since ceftazidime is eliminated almost solely by the kidneys, its serum half-life is significantly prolonged in pa-

tients with impaired renal function. Consequently, dosage adjustments in such patients as described in the DOSAGE AND ADMINISTRATION section are suggested.
Ceftazidime concentrations achieved in specific body tissues and fluids are depicted in Table 2.
[See table 2 at right]
Microbiology: Ceftazidime is bactericidal in action, exerting its effect by inhibition of enzymes responsible for cell-wall synthesis. A wide range of gram-negative organisms is susceptible to ceftazidime *in vitro*, including strains resistant to gentamicin and other aminoglycosides. In addition, ceftazidime has been shown to be active against gram-positive organisms. It is highly stable to most clinically important beta-lactamases, plasmid or chromosomal, which are produced by both gram-negative and gram-positive organisms and, consequently, is active against many strains resistant to ampicillin and other cephalosporins.
Ceftazidime has been shown to be active against the following organisms both *in vitro* and in clinical infections (see INDICATIONS AND USAGE).
Aerobes, Gram-negative: *Citrobacter* spp., including *Citrobacter freundii* and *Citrobacter diversus; Enterobacter* spp., including *Enterobacter cloacae* and *Enterobacter aerogenes; Escherichia coli; Haemophilus influenzae*, including ampicillin-resistant strains; *Klebsiella* spp. (including *Klebsiella pneumoniae); Neisseria meningitidis; Proteus mirabilis; Proteus vulgaris; Pseudomonas* spp. (including *Pseudomonas aeruginosa*); and *Serratia* spp.
Aerobes, Gram-positive: *Staphylococcus aureus*, including penicillinase- and non–penicillinase-producing strains; *Streptococcus agalactiae* (group B streptococci); *Streptococcus pneumoniae;* and *Streptococcus pyogenes* (group A beta-hemolytic streptococci).
Anaerobes: *Bacteroides* spp. (NOTE: many strains of *Bacteroides fragilis* are resistant).
Ceftazidime has been shown to be active *in vitro* against most strains of the following organisms; however, the clinical significance of this activity is unknown: *Acinetobacter* spp., *Clostridium* spp. (not including *Clostridium difficile), Haemophilus parainfluenzae, Morganella morganii* (formerly *Proteus morganii), Neisseria gonorrhoeae, Peptococcus* spp., *Peptostreptococcus* spp., *Providencia* spp. (including *Providencia rettgeri*, formerly *Proteus rettgeri*), *Salmonella* spp., *Shigella* spp., *Staphylococcus epidermidis*, and *Yersinia enterocolitica.*
Ceftazidime and the aminoglycosides have been shown to be synergistic *in vitro* against *Pseudomonas aeruginosa* and the enterobacteriaceae. Ceftazidime and carbenicillin have also been shown to be synergistic *in vitro* against *Pseudomonas aeruginosa.*
Ceftazidime is not active *in vitro* against methicillin-resistant staphylococci, *Streptococcus faecalis* and many other enterococci, *Listeria monocytogenes, Campylobacter* spp., or *Clostridium difficile.*
Susceptibility Tests: ***Diffusion Techniques:*** Quantitative methods that require measurement of zone diameters give an estimate of antibiotic susceptibility. One such procedure[1–3] has been recommended for use with disks to test susceptibility to ceftazidime.
Reports from the laboratory giving results of the standard single-disk susceptibility test with a 30-mcg ceftazidime disk should be interpreted according to the following criteria:
Susceptible organisms produce zones of 18 mm or greater, indicating that the test organism is likely to respond to therapy.
Organisms that produce zones of 15 to 17 mm are expected to be susceptible if high dosage is used or if the infection is confined to tissues and fluids (e.g., urine) in which high antibiotic levels are attained.
Resistant organisms produce zones of 14 mm or less, indicating that other therapy should be selected.
Organisms should be tested with the ceftazidime disk since ceftazidime has been shown by *in vitro* tests to be active against certain strains found resistant when other beta-lactam disks are used.
Standardized procedures require the use of laboratory control organisms. The 30-mcg ceftazidime disk should give zone diameters between 25 and 32 mm for *Escherichia coli* ATCC 25922. For *Pseudomonas aeruginosa* ATCC 27853, the zone diameters should be between 22 and 29 mm. For *Staphylococcus aureus* ATCC 25923, the zone diameters should be between 16 and 20 mm.
Dilution Techniques: In other susceptibility testing procedures, e.g., ICS agar dilution or the equivalent, a bacterial isolate may be considered susceptible if the minimum inhibitory concentration (MIC) value for ceftazidime is not more than 16 mcg/mL. Organisms are considered resistant to ceftazidime if the MIC is ≥64 mcg/mL. Organisms having an MIC value of <64 mcg/mL but >16 mcg/mL are expected to be susceptible if high dosage is used or if the infection is confined to tissues and fluids (e.g., urine) in which high antibiotic levels are attained.
As with standard diffusion methods, dilution procedures require the use of laboratory control organisms. Standard ceftazidime powder should give MIC values in the range of 4 to 16 mcg/mL for *Staphylococcus aureus* ATCC 25923. For *Escherichia coli* ATCC 25922, the MIC range should be between 0.125 and 0.5 mcg/mL. For *Pseudomonas aeruginosa* ATCC 27853, the MIC range should be between 0.5 and 2 mcg/mL.

INDICATIONS AND USAGE

CEPTAZ is indicated for the treatment of patients with infections caused by susceptible strains of the designated organisms in the following diseases:

Table 2: Ceftazidime Concentrations in Body Tissues and Fluids

Tissue or Fluid	Dose/Route	No. of Patients	Time of Sample Postdose	Average Tissue or Fluid Level (mcg/mL or mcg/g)
Urine	500 mg IM	6	0–2 h	2,100.0
	2 g IV	6	0–2 h	12,000.0
Bile	2 g IV	3	90 min	36.4
Synovial fluid	2 g IV	13	2 h	25.6
Peritoneal fluid	2 g IV	8	2 h	48.6
Sputum	1 g IV	8	1 h	9.0
Cerebrospinal fluid	2 g q8h IV	5	120 min	9.8
(inflamed meninges)	2 g q8h IV	6	180 min	9.4
Aqueous humor	2 g IV	13	1–3 h	11.0
Blister fluid	1 g IV	7	2–3 h	19.7
Lymphatic fluid	1 g IV	7	2–3 h	23.4
Bone	2 g IV	8	0.67 h	31.1
Heart muscle	2 g IV	35	30–280 min	12.7
Skin	2 g IV	22	30–180 min	6.6
Skeletal muscle	2 g IV	35	30–280 min	9.4
Myometrium	2 g IV	31	1–2 h	18.7

1. **Lower Respiratory Tract Infections,** including pneumonia, caused by *Pseudomonas aeruginosa* and other *Pseudomonas* spp.; *Haemophilus influenzae*, including ampicillin-resistant strains; *Klebsiella* spp.; *Enterobacter* spp.; *Proteus mirabilis; Escherichia coli; Serratia* spp.; *Citrobacter* spp.; *Streptococcus pneumoniae;* and *Staphylococcus aureus* (methicillin-susceptible strains).
2. **Skin and Skin-Structure Infections** caused by *Pseudomonas aeruginosa; Klebsiella* spp.; *Escherichia coli; Proteus* spp., including *Proteus mirabilis* and indole-positive *Proteus; Enterobacter* spp.; *Serratia* spp.; *Staphylococcus aureus* (methicillin-susceptible strains); and *Streptococcus pyogenes* (group A beta-hemolytic streptococci).
3. **Urinary Tract Infections,** both complicated and uncomplicated, caused by *Pseudomonas aeruginosa; Enterobacter* spp.; *Proteus* spp., including *Proteus mirabilis* and indole-positive *Proteus; Klebsiella* spp.; and *Escherichia coli.*
4. **Bacterial Septicemia** caused by *Pseudomonas aeruginosa, Klebsiella* spp., *Haemophilus influenzae, Escherichia coli, Serratia* spp., *Streptococcus pneumoniae*, and *Staphylococcus aureus* (methicillin-susceptible strains).
5. **Bone and Joint Infections** caused by *Pseudomonas aeruginosa, Klebsiella* spp., *Enterobacter* spp., and *Staphylococcus aureus* (methicillin-susceptible strains).
6. **Gynecologic Infections,** including endometritis, pelvic cellulitis, and other infections of the female genital tract caused by *Escherichia coli.*
7. **Intra-abdominal Infections,** including peritonitis caused by *Escherichia coli, Klebsiella* spp., and *Staphylococcus aureus* (methicillin-susceptible strains) and polymicrobial infections caused by aerobic and anaerobic organisms and *Bacteroides* spp. (many strains of *Bacteroides fragilis* are resistant).
8. **Central Nervous System Infections,** including meningitis, caused by *Haemophilus influenzae* and *Neisseria meningitidis.* Ceftazidime has also been used successfully in a limited number of cases of meningitis due to *Pseudomonas aeruginosa* and *Streptococcus pneumoniae.*

Specimens for bacterial cultures should be obtained before therapy in order to isolate and identify causative organisms and to determine their susceptibility to ceftazidime. Therapy may be instituted before results of susceptibility studies are known; however, once these results become available, the antibiotic treatment should be adjusted accordingly.
CEPTAZ may be used alone in cases of confirmed or suspected sepsis. Ceftazidime has been used successfully in clinical trials as empiric therapy in cases where various concomitant therapies with other antibiotics have been used.
CEPTAZ may also be used concomitantly with other antibiotics, such as aminoglycosides, vancomycin, and clindamycin; in severe and life-threatening infections; and in the immunocompromised patient (see COMPATIBILITY AND STABILITY). When such concomitant treatment is appropriate, prescribing information in the labeling for the other antibiotics should be followed. The dosage depends on the severity of the infection and the patient's condition.

CONTRAINDICATIONS

CEPTAZ is contraindicated in patients who have shown hypersensitivity to ceftazidime or the cephalosporin group of antibiotics.

WARNINGS

BEFORE THERAPY WITH CEPTAZ IS INSTITUTED, CAREFUL INQUIRY SHOULD BE MADE TO DETERMINE WHETHER THE PATIENT HAS HAD PREVIOUS HYPERSENSITIVITY REACTIONS TO CEFTAZIDIME, CEPHALOSPORINS, PENICILLINS, OR OTHER DRUGS. IF THIS PRODUCT IS GIVEN TO PENICILLIN-SENSITIVE PATIENTS, CAUTION SHOULD BE EXERCISED BECAUSE CROSS-HYPERSENSITIVITY AMONG BETA-LACTAM ANTIBIOTICS HAS BEEN CLEARLY DOCUMENTED AND MAY OCCUR IN UP TO 10% OF PATIENTS WITH A HISTORY OF PENICILLIN ALLERGY. IF AN ALLERGIC REACTION TO CEPTAZ OCCURS, DISCONTINUE THE DRUG. SERIOUS ACUTE HYPERSENSITIVITY REACTIONS MAY REQUIRE TREATMENT WITH EPINEPHRINE AND OTHER EMERGENCY MEASURES, INCLUDING OXYGEN, IV FLUIDS, IV ANTIHISTAMINES, CORTICOSTEROIDS, PRESSOR AMINES, AND AIRWAY MANAGEMENT, AS CLINICALLY INDICATED.
Pseudomembranous colitis has been reported with nearly all antibacterial agents, including ceftazidime, and may range from mild to life threatening. Therefore, it is important to consider this diagnosis in patients who present with diarrhea subsequent to the administration of antibacterial agents.
Treatment with antibacterial agents alters the normal flora of the colon and may permit overgrowth of clostridia. Studies indicate that a toxin produced by *Clostridium difficile* is one primary cause of "antibiotic-associated colitis."
After the diagnosis of pseudomembranous colitis has been established, appropriate therapeutic measures should be initiated. Mild cases of pseudomembranous colitis usually respond to drug discontinuation alone. In moderate to severe cases, consideration should be given to management with fluids and electrolytes, protein supplementation, and treatment with an antibacterial drug clinically effective against *Clostridium difficile* colitis.
Elevated levels of ceftazidime in patients with renal insufficiency can lead to seizures, encephalopathy, asterixis, neuromuscular excitability, and myoclonia (see PRECAUTIONS).

PRECAUTIONS

General: High and prolonged serum ceftazidime concentrations can occur from usual dosages in patients with transient or persistent reduction of urinary output because of renal insufficiency. The total daily dosage should be reduced when ceftazidime is administered to patients with renal insufficiency (see DOSAGE AND ADMINISTRATION). Elevated levels of ceftazidime in these patients can lead to seizures, encephalopathy, asterixis, neuromuscular excitability, and myoclonia. Continued dosage should be determined by degree of renal impairment, severity of infection, and susceptibility of the causative organisms.
As with other antibiotics, prolonged use of CEPTAZ may result in overgrowth of nonsusceptible organisms. Repeated evaluation of the patient's condition is essential. If superinfection occurs during therapy, appropriate measures should be taken.
Inducible type I beta-lactamase resistance has been noted with some organisms (e.g., *Enterobacter* spp., *Pseudomonas* spp., and *Serratia* spp.). As with other extended-spectrum beta-lactam antibiotics, resistance can develop during therapy, leading to clinical failure in some cases. When treating infections caused by these organisms, periodic susceptibility testing should be performed when clinically appropriate. If patients fail to respond to monotherapy, an aminoglycoside or similar agent should be considered.
Cephalosporins may be associated with a fall in prothrombin activity. Those at risk include patients with renal or hepatic impairment, or poor nutritional state, as well as patients receiving a protracted course of antimicrobial therapy. Prothrombin time should be monitored in patients at risk and exogenous vitamin K administered as indicated.
CEPTAZ should be prescribed with caution in individuals with a history of gastrointestinal disease, particularly colitis.
Arginine has been shown to alter glucose metabolism and elevate serum potassium transiently when administered at 50 times the recommended dose. The effect of lower dosing is not known.
Distal necrosis can occur after inadvertent intra-arterial administration of ceftazidime.

Continued on next page

This product information is based on labeling in effect on June 23, 2000. For further information, contact via direct mail, phone, or web site. Medical Information, Glaxo Wellcome Inc., PO Box 13398, Research Triangle Park, NC 27709. Healthcare Professionals (Medical Information): 800-334-0089. Patients (Customer Response Center): 1-888-825-5249. Glaxo Wellcome Corporate Web Site: www.glaxowellcome.com

Ceptaz—Cont.

Drug Interactions: Nephrotoxicity has been reported following concomitant administration of cephalosporins with aminoglycoside antibiotics or potent diuretics such as furosemide. Renal function should be carefully monitored, especially if higher dosages of the aminoglycosides are to be administered or if therapy is prolonged, because of the potential nephrotoxicity and ototoxicity of aminoglycosidic antibiotics. Nephrotoxicity and ototoxicity were not noted when ceftazidime was given alone in clinical trials.

Chloramphenicol has been shown to be antagonistic to beta-lactam antibiotics, including ceftazidime, based on *in vitro* studies and time kill curves with enteric gram-negative bacilli. Due to the possibility of antagonism *in vivo,* particularly when bactericidal activity is desired, this drug combination should be avoided.

Drug/Laboratory Test Interactions: The administration of ceftazidime may result in a false-positive reaction for glucose in the urine when using CLINITEST® tablets, Benedict's solution, or Fehling's solution. It is recommended that glucose tests based on enzymatic glucose oxidase reactions (such as CLINISTIX® or TES-TAPE®) be used.

Carcinogenesis, Mutagenesis, Impairment of Fertility: Long-term studies in animals have not been performed to evaluate carcinogenic potential. However, a mouse Micronucleus test and an Ames test were both negative for mutagenic effects.

Pregnancy: ***Teratogenic Effects:*** Pregnancy Category B. Reproduction studies have been performed in mice and rats at doses up to 40 times the human dose and have revealed no evidence of impaired fertility or harm to the fetus due to ceftazidime. CEPTAZ at 23 times the human dose was not teratogenic or embryotoxic in a rat reproduction study. There are, however, no adequate and well-controlled studies in pregnant women. Because animal reproduction studies are not always predictive of human response, this drug should be used during pregnancy only if clearly needed.

Nursing Mothers: Ceftazidime is excreted in human milk in low concentrations. It is not known whether the arginine component of this product is excreted in human milk. Because many drugs are excreted in human milk and because safety of the arginine component of CEPTAZ in nursing infants has not been established, a decision should be made whether to discontinue nursing or to discontinue the drug, taking into account the importance of the drug to the mother.

Pediatric Use: Safety of the arginine component of CEPTAZ in neonates, infants, and children has not been established. This product is for use in patients 12 years and older. If treatment with ceftazidime is indicated for neonates, infants, or children, a sodium carbonate formulation should be used.

ADVERSE REACTIONS

The following adverse effects from clinical trials were considered to be either related to ceftazidime therapy or were of uncertain etiology. The most common were local reactions following IV injection and allergic and gastrointestinal reactions. No disulfiramlike reactions were reported.

Local Effects, reported in fewer than 2% of patients, were phlebitis and inflammation at the site of injection (1 in 69 patients).

Hypersensitivity Reactions, reported in 2% of patients, were pruritus, rash, and fever. Immediate reactions, generally manifested by rash and/or pruritus, occurred in 1 in 285 patients. Toxic epidermal necrolysis, Stevens-Johnson syndrome, and erythema multiforme have also been reported with cephalosporin antibiotics, including ceftazidime. Angioedema and anaphylaxis (bronchospasm and/or hypotension) have been reported very rarely.

Gastrointestinal Symptoms, reported in fewer than 2% of patients, were diarrhea (1 in 78), nausea (1 in 156), vomiting (1 in 500), and abdominal pain (1 in 416). The onset of pseudomembranous colitis symptoms may occur during or after treatment (see WARNINGS).

Central Nervous System Reactions (fewer than 1%) included headache, dizziness, and paresthesia. Seizures have been reported with several cephalosporins, including ceftazidime. In addition, encephalopathy, asterixis, neuromuscular excitability, and myoclonia have been reported in renally impaired patients treated with unadjusted dosage regimens of ceftazidime (see PRECAUTIONS: General).

Less Frequent Adverse Events (fewer than 1%) were candidiasis (including oral thrush) and vaginitis.

Hematologic: Rare cases of hemolytic anemia have been reported.

Laboratory Test Changes noted during ceftazidime clinical trials were transient and included: eosinophilia (1 in 13), positive Coombs' test without hemolysis (1 in 23), thrombocytosis (1 in 45), and slight elevations in one or more of the hepatic enzymes, aspartate aminotransferase (AST, SGOT) (1 in 16), alanine aminotransferase (ALT, SGPT) (1 in 15), LDH (1 in 18), GGT (1 in 19), and alkaline phosphatase (1 in 23). As with some other cephalosporins, transient elevations of blood urea, blood urea nitrogen, and/or serum creatinine were observed occasionally. Transient leukopenia, neutropenia, agranulocytosis, thrombocytopenia, and lymphocytosis were seen very rarely.

Observed During Clinical Practice: In addition to the adverse events reported from clinical trials, the following events have been identified during post-approval use of CEPTAZ. Because they are reported voluntarily from a population of unknown size, estimates of frequency cannot be made. These events have been chosen for inclusion due to a combination of their seriousness, frequency of reporting, or potential causal connection to CEPTAZ.

General: Anaphylactic or anaphylactoid reactions, which, in rare instances, were severe (e.g., cardiopulmonary arrest), including laryngeal edema, stridor, and urticaria; pain at injection site.

Hepatobiliary Tract and Pancreas: Hyperbilirubinemia.

Renal and Genitourinary: Renal impairment.

Cephalosporin-Class Adverse Reactions: In addition to the adverse reactions listed above that have been observed in patients treated with ceftazidime, the following adverse reactions and altered laboratory tests have been reported for cephalosporin-class antibiotics:

Adverse Reactions: Colitis, toxic nephropathy, hepatic dysfunction including cholestasis, aplastic anemia, hemorrhage.

Altered Laboratory Tests: Prolonged prothrombin time, false-positive test for urinary glucose, pancytopenia.

OVERDOSAGE

Ceftazidime overdosage has occurred in patients with renal failure. Reactions have included seizure activity, encephalopathy, asterixis, neuromuscular excitability, and coma. Patients who receive an acute overdosage should be carefully observed and given supportive treatment. In the presence of renal insufficiency, hemodialysis or peritoneal dialysis may aid in the removal of ceftazidime from the body.

DOSAGE AND ADMINISTRATION

Dosage: The usual adult dosage is 1 gram administered intravenously or intramuscularly every 8 to 12 hours. The dosage and route should be determined by the susceptibility of the causative organisms, the severity of infection, and the condition and renal function of the patient.

The guidelines for dosage of CEPTAZ are listed in Table 3. The following dosage schedule is recommended.

[See table 3 below]

Table 3: Recommended Dosage Schedule

	Dose	Frequency
Patients 12 years and older*		
Usual recommended dosage	**1 gram IV or IM**	**q8–12h**
Uncomplicated urinary tract infections	250 mg IV or IM	q12h
Bone and joint infections	2 grams IV	q12h
Complicated urinary tract infections	500 mg IV or IM	q8–12h
Uncomplicated pneumonia; mild skin and skin-structure infections	500 mg–1 gram IV or IM	q8h
Serious gynecologic and intra-abdominal infections	2 grams IV	q8h
Meningitis	2 grams IV	q8h
Very severe life-threatening infections, especially in immunocompromised patients	2 grams IV	q8h
Lung infections caused by *Pseudomonas* spp. in patients with cystic fibrosis with normal renal function†	30–50 mg/kg IV to a maximum of 6 grams per day	q8h

* This product is for use in patients 12 years and older. If treatment with ceftazidime is indicated for patients less than 12 years old, a sodium carbonate formulation should be used.

† Although clinical improvement has been shown, bacteriologic cures cannot be expected in patients with chronic respiratory disease and cystic fibrosis.

Impaired Hepatic Function: No adjustment in dosage is required for patients with hepatic dysfunction.

Impaired Renal Function: Ceftazidime is excreted by the kidneys, almost exclusively by glomerular filtration. Therefore, in patients with impaired renal function (glomerular filtration rate [GFR] <50 mL/min), it is recommended that the dosage of ceftazidime be reduced to compensate for its slower excretion. In patients with suspected renal insufficiency, an initial loading dose of 1 gram of CEPTAZ may be given. An estimate of GFR should be made to determine the appropriate maintenance dosage. The recommended dosage is presented in Table 4.

Table 4: Recommended Maintenance Dosages of CEPTAZ in Renal Insufficiency

NOTE: IF THE DOSE RECOMMENDED IN TABLE 3 ABOVE IS LOWER THAN THAT RECOMMENDED FOR PATIENTS WITH RENAL INSUFFICIENCY AS OUTLINED IN TABLE 4, THE LOWER DOSE SHOULD BE USED.

Creatinine Clearance (mL/min)	Recommended Unit Dose of CEPTAZ	Frequency of Dosing
50–31	1 gram	q12h
30–16	1 gram	q24h
15–6	500 mg	q24h
<5	500 mg	q48h

When only serum creatinine is available, the following formula (Cockcroft's equation)[4] may be used to estimate creatinine clearance. The serum creatinine should represent a steady state of renal function:

Males:

$$\text{Creatinine clearance (mL/min)} = \frac{\text{Weight (kg)} \times (140-\text{age})}{72 \times \text{serum creatinine (mg/dL)}}$$

Females: 0.85 × male value

In patients with severe infections who would normally receive 6 grams of CEPTAZ daily were it not for renal insufficiency, the unit dose given in the table above may be increased by 50% or the dosing frequency may be increased appropriately. Further dosing should be determined by therapeutic monitoring, severity of the infection, and susceptibility of the causative organism.

In patients undergoing hemodialysis, a loading dose of 1 gram is recommended, followed by 1 gram after each hemodialysis period.

CEPTAZ can also be used in patients undergoing intraperitoneal dialysis and continuous ambulatory peritoneal dialysis. In such patients, a loading dose of 1 gram of CEPTAZ may be given, followed by 500 mg every 24 hours. It is not known whether or not CEPTAZ can be safely incorporated into dialysis fluid.

Note: Generally CEPTAZ should be continued for 2 days after the signs and symptoms of infection have disappeared, but in complicated infections longer therapy may be required.

Administration: CEPTAZ may be given intravenously or by deep IM injection into a large muscle mass such as the upper outer quadrant of the gluteus maximus or lateral part of the thigh. Intra-arterial administration should be avoided (see PRECAUTIONS).

Intramuscular Administration: For IM administration, CEPTAZ should be constituted with one of the following diluents: Sterile Water for Injection, Bacteriostatic Water for Injection, or 0.5% or 1% Lidocaine Hydrochloride Injection. Refer to Table 5.

Intravenous Administration: The IV route is preferable for patients with bacterial septicemia, bacterial meningitis, peritonitis, or other severe or life-threatening infections, or for patients who may be poor risks because of lowered resistance resulting from such debilitating conditions as malnutrition, trauma, surgery, diabetes, heart failure, or malignancy, particularly if shock is present or pending.

For direct intermittent IV administration, constitute CEPTAZ as directed in Table 5 with Sterile Water for Injection, 5% Dextrose Injection, or 0.9% Sodium Chloride Injection. Slowly inject directly into the vein over a period of 3 to 5 minutes or give through the tubing of an administration set while the patient is also receiving one of the compatible IV fluids (see COMPATIBILITY AND STABILITY).

For IV infusion, constitute the 1- or 2-gram infusion pack with 100 mL of Sterile Water for Injection or one of the compatible IV fluids listed under the COMPATIBILITY AND STABILITY section. Alternatively, constitute the 1- or 2-gram vial and add an appropriate quantity of the resulting solution to an IV container with one of the compatible IV fluids.

Intermittent IV infusion with a Y-type administration set can be accomplished with compatible solutions. However, during infusion of a solution containing ceftazidime, it is desirable to discontinue the other solution.

[See table 5 at bottom of next page]

Solutions of CEPTAZ, like those of most beta-lactam antibiotics, should not be added to solutions of aminoglycoside antibiotics because of potential interaction.

However, if concurrent therapy with CEPTAZ and an aminoglycoside is indicated, each of these antibiotics can be administered separately to the same patient.

Instructions for Constitution: Vials of CEPTAZ as supplied are under a slightly reduced pressure. This may assist entry of the diluent. No gas-relief needle is required when adding the diluent, except for the infusion pack where it is required during the latter stages of addition (in order to preserve product sterility, a gas-relief needle should not be inserted until an overpressure is produced in the vial). No evolution of gas occurs on constitution. When the vial contents are dissolved, vials other than infusion packs may still be under a reduced pressure. This reduced pressure is particularly noticeable for the 10-gram pharmacy bulk package.

COMPATIBILITY AND STABILITY

Intramuscular: CEPTAZ , when constituted as directed with Sterile Water for Injection, Bacteriostatic Water for Injection, or 0.5% or 1% Lidocaine Hydrochloride Injection, maintains satisfactory potency for 18 hours at room temperature or for 7 days under refrigeration. Solutions in Sterile Water for Injection that are frozen immediately after constitution in the original container are stable for 6 months when stored at −20°C. Components of the solution may precipitate in the frozen state and will dissolve on reaching room temperature with little or no agitation. Potency is not affected. Frozen solutions should only be thawed at room temperature. Do not force thaw by immersion in water baths or by microwave irradiation. Once thawed, solutions should not be refrozen. Thawed solutions may be stored for up to 12 hours at room temperature or for 7 days in a refrigerator.

Intravenous: ***Ceftazidime concentration greater than 100 mg/mL (2-g vial or 10-g pharmacy bulk package):*** CEPTAZ, when constituted as directed with Sterile Water for Injection, 0.9% Sodium Chloride Injection, or 5% Dextrose Injection, maintains satisfactory potency for 18 hours at room temperature or for 7 days under refrigeration. Solutions of a similar concentration in Sterile Water for Injection that are frozen immediately after constitution in the original container are stable for 6 months when stored at −20°C. Components of the solution may precipitate in the frozen state and will dissolve upon reaching room temperature with little or no agitation. Potency is not affected. Frozen solutions should only be thawed at room temperature. Do not force thaw by immersion in water baths or by microwave irradiation. Once thawed, solutions should not be refrozen. Thawed solutions may be stored for up to 12 hours at room temperature or for 7 days in a refrigerator.

Ceftazidime concentration of 100 mg/mL or less (1-g vial or infusion packs): CEPTAZ, when constituted as directed with Sterile Water for Injection, 0.9% Sodium Chloride Injection, or 5% Dextrose Injection, maintains satisfactory potency for 24 hours at room temperature or for 7 days under refrigeration. Solutions, prepared by a pharmacist, of the approved arginine formulation of ceftazidime of a similar concentration in Sterile Water for Injection, 0.9% Sodium Chloride Injection, or 5% Dextrose Injection in the original container or in 0.9% Sodium Chloride Injection in VIAFLEX® (PL 146® Plastic) small-volume containers that are frozen immediately after constitution by the pharmacist are stable for 6 months when stored at −20°C. Solutions in the PL 146 Plastic small-volume containers are in contact with the polyvinyl chloride layer of this container and can leach out certain chemical components of the plastic in very small amounts within the expiration period. The suitability of the plastic has been confirmed in tests in animals according to USP biological tests for plastic containers as well as by tissue culture toxicity studies. Stability of the frozen solution in other containers has not been confirmed. Frozen solutions should only be thawed at room temperature. Do not force thaw by immersion in water baths or by microwave irradiation. For the larger volumes of IV infusion solutions where it may be necessary to warm the frozen product, care should be taken to avoid heating after thawing is complete. Once thawed, solutions should not be refrozen. Thawed solutions may be stored for up to 18 hours at room temperature or for 7 days in a refrigerator.

Components of the solution may precipitate in the frozen state and will dissolve on reaching room temperature with little or no agitation. Potency is not affected. Check for minute leaks in plastic containers by squeezing bag firmly. Discard bag if leaks are found as sterility may be impaired. Do not add supplementary medication to bags. Do not use unless solution is clear and seal is intact.

Use sterile equipment.

Caution: Do not use plastic containers in series connections. Such use could result in air embolism due to residual air being drawn from the primary container before administration of the fluid from the secondary container is complete.

Preparation for Administration:

1. Suspend container from eyelet support.
2. Remove protector from outlet port at bottom of container.
3. Attach administration set. Refer to complete directions accompanying set.

CEPTAZ is compatible with the more commonly used IV infusion fluids. Solutions at concentrations between 1 and 40 mg/mL in 0.9% Sodium Chloride Injection; 1/6 M Sodium Lactate Injection; 5% Dextrose Injection; 5% Dextrose and 0.225% Sodium Chloride Injection; 5% Dextrose and 0.45% Sodium Chloride Injection; 5% Dextrose and 0.9% Sodium Chloride Injection; 10% Dextrose Injection; Ringer's Injection, USP; Lactated Ringer's Injection, USP; 10% Invert Sugar in Sterile Water for Injection; and Normosol®-M in 5% Dextrose Injection may be stored for up to 24 hours at room temperature or for 7 days if refrigerated.

CEPTAZ is less stable in Sodium Bicarbonate Injection than in other IV fluids. It is not recommended as a diluent. Solutions of CEPTAZ in 5% Dextrose Injection and 0.9% Sodium Chloride Injection are stable for at least 6 hours at room temperature in plastic tubing, drip chambers, and volume control devices of common IV infusion sets.

Ceftazidime at a concentration of 4 mg/mL has been found compatible for 24 hours at room temperature or for 7 days under refrigeration in 0.9% Sodium Chloride Injection or 5% Dextrose Injection when admixed with: cefuroxime sodium (ZINACEF®) 3 mg/mL; heparin sodium in concentrations up to 50 U/mL; or potassium chloride in concentrations up to 40 mEq/L. Ceftazidime may be constituted at a concentration of 20 mg/mL with metronidazole injection 5 mg/mL, and the resultant solution may be stored for 24 hours at room temperature or for 7 days under refrigeration. Ceftazidime at a concentration of 20 mg/mL has been found compatible for 24 hours at room temperature or for 7 days under refrigeration in 0.9% Sodium Chloride Injection or 5% Dextrose Injection when admixed with 6 mg/mL clindamycin (as clindamycin phosphate).

Vancomycin solution exhibits a physical incompatibility when mixed with a number of drugs, including ceftazidime. The likelihood of precipitation with ceftazidime is dependent on the concentrations of vancomycin and ceftazidime present. It is therefore recommended, when both drugs are to be administered by intermittent IV infusion, that they be given separately, flushing the IV lines (with one of the compatible IV fluids) between the administration of these two agents.

Note: Parenteral drug products should be inspected visually for particulate matter before administration whenever solution and container permit.

As with other cephalosporins, CEPTAZ powder as well as solutions tend to darken, depending on storage conditions; within the stated recommendations, however, product potency is not adversely affected.

Directions for Dispensing: ***Pharmacy Bulk Package—Not for Direct Infusion:*** The pharmacy bulk package is for use in a pharmacy admixture service only under a laminar flow hood. Entry into the vial must be made with a sterile transfer set or other sterile dispensing device, and the contents dispensed in aliquots using aseptic technique. The use of syringe and needle is not recommended as it may cause leakage (see DOSAGE AND ADMINISTRATION). GOOD PHARMACY PRACTICE DICTATES THAT THE CLOSURE BE PENETRATED ONLY ONE TIME AFTER CONSTITUTION. AFTER INITIAL PENETRATION OF THE CLOSURE, USE ENTIRE CONTENTS OF VIAL PROMPTLY. ANY UNUSED PORTION MUST BE DISCARDED WITHIN 18 HOURS OF CONSTITUTION.

HOW SUPPLIED

CEPTAZ in the dry state should be stored between 15° and 30°C (59° and 86°F) and protected from light. CEPTAZ is a dry, white to off-white powder supplied in vials and infusion packs as follows:

NDC 0173-0414-00 1-g* Vial (Tray of 25)
NDC 0173-0415-00 2-g* Vial (Tray of 25)
NDC 0173-0416-00 1-g* Infusion Pack (Tray of 10)
NDC 0173-0417-00 2-g* Infusion Pack (Tray of 10)
NDC 0173-0418-00 10-g* Pharmacy Bulk Package (Tray of 6)

*Equivalent to anhydrous ceftazidime.

REFERENCES

1. Bauer AW, Kirby WMM, Sherris JC, Turck M. Antibiotic susceptibility testing by a standardized single disk method. *Am J Clin Pathol.* 1966;45:493-496.
2. National Committee for Clinical Laboratory Standards. *Approved Standard: Performance Standards for Antimicrobial Disc Susceptibility Tests.* (M2-A3). December 1984.
3. Certification procedure for antibiotic sensitivity discs (21 CFR 460.1). *Federal Register.* May 30, 1974;39:19182-19184.
4. Cockcroft DW, Gault MH. Prediction of creatinine clearance from serum creatinine. *Nephron.* 1976;16:31-41.

Glaxo Wellcome Inc., Research Triangle Park, NC 27709

CEPTAZ and ZINACEF are registered trademarks of Glaxo Wellcome.

CLINITEST and CLINISTIX are registered trademarks of Ames Division, Miles Laboratories, Inc.

TES-TAPE is a registered trademark of Eli Lilly and Company.

VIAFLEX and PL 146 Plastic are registered trademarks of Baxter International Inc.

US Patent Nos. 4,258,041; 4,329,453; and 4,582,830

November 1998/RL-644

Shown in Product Identification Guide, page 314

Table 5: Preparation of Solutions of CEPTAZ

Size	Amount of Diluent to Be Added (mL)	Volume to Be Withdrawn (mL)	Approximate Ceftazidime Concentration (mg/mL)
Intramuscular			
1-gram vial	3.0	Total	250
Intravenous			
1-gram vial	10.0	Total	90
2-gram vial	10.0	Total	170
Infusion pack			
1-gram vial	100	—	10
2-gram vial	100	—	20
Pharmacy bulk package			
10-gram vial	40	Amount needed	200

COMBIVIR® Tablets ℞

[*kom 'bə-vir*]

(lamivudine/zidovudine tablets)

WARNING: ZIDOVUDINE, ONE OF THE TWO ACTIVE INGREDIENTS IN COMBIVIR, HAS BEEN ASSOCIATED WITH HEMATOLOGIC TOXICITY INCLUDING NEUTROPENIA AND SEVERE ANEMIA, PARTICULARLY IN PATIENTS WITH ADVANCED HIV DISEASE (SEE WARNINGS). PROLONGED USE OF ZIDOVUDINE HAS BEEN ASSOCIATED WITH SYMPTOMATIC MYOPATHY.
LACTIC ACIDOSIS AND SEVERE HEPATOMEGALY WITH STEATOSIS, INCLUDING FATAL CASES, HAVE BEEN REPORTED WITH THE USE OF NUCLEOSIDE ANALOGUES ALONE OR IN COMBINATION, INCLUDING LAMIVUDINE, ZIDOVUDINE, AND OTHER ANTIRETROVIRALS (SEE WARNINGS).

DESCRIPTION

COMBIVIR: COMBIVIR Tablets are combination tablets containing lamivudine and zidovudine. Lamivudine (EPIVIR®, 3TC®) and zidovudine (RETROVIR®, azidothymidine, AZT, or ZDV) are synthetic nucleoside analogues with activity against human immunodeficiency virus (HIV). COMBIVIR Tablets are for oral administration. Each film-coated tablet contains 150 mg of lamivudine, 300 mg of zidovudine, and the inactive ingredients colloidal silicon dioxide, magnesium stearate, microcrystalline cellulose, and sodium starch glycolate. The film-coating solution contains Opadry YS-1-7706-G White and purified water.

Lamivudine: The chemical name of lamivudine is (2R,cis)-4-amino-1-(2-hydroxymethyl-1,3-oxathiolan-5-yl)-(1H)-pyrimidin-2-one. Lamivudine is the (-)enantiomer of a dideoxy analogue of cytidine. Lamivudine has also been referred to as (-)2′,3′-dideoxy, 3′-thiacytidine. It has a molecular formula of $C_8H_{11}N_3O_3S$ and a molecular weight of 229.3.

Lamivudine is a white to off-white crystalline solid with a solubility of approximately 70 mg/mL in water at 20°C.

Zidovudine: The chemical name of zidovudine is 3′-azido-3′-deoxythymidine. It has a molecular formula of $C_{10}H_{13}N_5O_4$ and a molecular weight of 267.24.

Zidovudine is a white to beige, odorless, crystalline solid with a solubility of 20.1 mg/mL in water at 25°C.

MICROBIOLOGY

Mechanism of Action: ***Lamivudine:*** Lamivudine is a synthetic nucleoside analogue. Intracellularly, lamivudine is phosphorylated to its active 5′-triphosphate metabolite, lamivudine triphosphate (L-TP). The principal mode of action of L-TP is inhibition of reverse transcriptase (RT) via DNA chain termination after incorporation of the nucleoside analogue. L-TP is a weak inhibitor of mammalian DNA polymerases α and β, and mitochondrial DNA polymerase-γ.

Zidovudine: Zidovudine is a synthetic nucleoside analogue. Intracellularly, zidovudine is phosphorylated to its active 5′-triphosphate metabolite, zidovudine triphosphate (ZDV-TP). The principal mode of action of ZDV-TP is inhibition of RT via DNA chain termination after incorporation of the nucleoside analogue. ZDV-TP is a weak inhibitor of the mammalian DNA polymerase-α and mitochondrial DNA polymerase-γ and has been reported to be incorporated into the DNA of cells in culture.

Antiviral Activity In Vitro: The relationship between in vitro susceptibility of HIV to lamivudine or zidovudine and the inhibition of HIV replication in humans has not been established.

Lamivudine Plus Zidovudine: In HIV-1–infected MT-4 cells, lamivudine in combination with zidovudine had synergistic antiretroviral activity. Synergistic activity of lamivudine and zidovudine was also shown in a variable-ratio study.

Lamivudine: In vitro activity of lamivudine against HIV-1 was assessed in a number of cell lines (including monocytes and fresh human peripheral blood lymphocytes). IC_{50} and IC_{90} values (50% and 90% inhibitory concentrations) for lamivudine were 0.0006 mcg/mL to 0.034 mcg/mL and 0.015 to 0.321 mcg/mL, respectively. Lamivudine had anti–HIV-1 activity in all acute virus-cell infections tested.

Zidovudine: In vitro activity of zidovudine against HIV-1 was assessed in a number of cell lines (including monocytes

Continued on next page

This product information is based on labeling in effect on June 23, 2000. For further information, contact via direct mail, phone, or web site. Medical Information, Glaxo Wellcome Inc., PO Box 13398, Research Triangle Park, NC 27709. Healthcare Professionals (Medical Information): 800-334-0089. Patients (Customer Response Center): 1-888-825-5249. Glaxo Wellcome Corporate Web Site: www.glaxowellcome.com

Combivir—Cont.

and fresh human peripheral blood lymphocytes). The IC_{50} and IC_{90} values for zidovudine were 0.003 to 0.013 mcg/mL and 0.03 to 0.13 mcg/mL, respectively. Zidovudine had anti-HIV-1 activity in all acute virus-cell infections tested. However, zidovudine activity was substantially less in chronically infected cell lines. In cell culture drug combination studies with zidovudine, interferon-alpha demonstrated additive activity and zalcitabine, didanosine, saquinavir, indinavir, ritonavir, nelfinavir, nevirapine, and delavirdine demonstrated synergistic activity.

Drug Resistance: Lamivudine Plus Zidovudine Administered As Separate Formulations: In patients receiving lamivudine monotherapy or combination therapy with lamivudine plus zidovudine, HIV-1 isolates from most patients became phenotypically and genotypically resistant to lamivudine within 12 weeks. In some patients harboring zidovudine-resistant virus at baseline, phenotypic sensitivity to zidovudine was restored by 12 weeks of treatment with lamivudine and zidovudine. Combination therapy with lamivudine plus zidovudine delayed the emergence of mutations conferring resistance to zidovudine.

HIV-1 strains resistant to both lamivudine and zidovudine have been isolated from patients after prolonged lamivudine/zidovudine therapy. Dual resistance required the presence of multiple mutations, the most essential of which may be at codon 333 (Gly→Glu). The incidence of dual resistance and the duration of combination therapy required before dual resistance occurs are unknown.

Lamivudine: Lamivudine-resistant isolates of HIV-1 have been selected in vitro and have also been recovered from patients treated with lamivudine or lamivudine plus zidovudine. Genotypic analysis of the resistant isolates showed that the resistance was due to mutations in the HIV-1 reverse transcriptase gene at codon 184 from methionine to either isoleucine or valine.

Zidovudine: HIV isolates with reduced susceptibility to zidovudine have been selected in vitro and were also recovered from patients treated with zidovudine. Genotypic analyses of the isolates showed mutations which result in five amino acid substitutions (Met41→Leu, Asp67→Asn, Lys70→Arg, Thr215→Tyr or Phe, and Lys219→Gln) in the HIV-1 reverse transcriptase gene. In general, higher levels of resistance were associated with greater number of mutations.

Cross-Resistance: Cross-resistance among certain reverse transcriptase inhibitors has been recognized.

Lamivudine Plus Zidovudine: Cross-resistance between lamivudine and zidovudine has not been reported. In some patients treated with lamivudine alone or in combination with zidovudine, isolates have emerged with a mutation at codon 184 which confers resistance to lamivudine. In the presence of the 184 mutation, cross-resistance to didanosine and zalcitabine has been seen in some patients; the clinical significance is unknown. In some patients treated with zidovudine plus didanosine or zalcitabine, isolates resistant to multiple drugs, including lamivudine, have emerged (see under Zidovudine below).

Lamivudine: See Lamivudine Plus Zidovudine (above).

Zidovudine: HIV isolates with multidrug resistance to zidovudine, didanosine, zalcitabine, stavudine, and lamivudine were recovered from a small number of patients treated for ≥1 year with zidovudine plus didanosine or zidovudine plus zalcitabine. The pattern of genotypic resistant mutations with such combination therapies was different (Ala62→Val, Val75→Ile, Phe77→Leu, Phe116→Tyr, and Gln151→Met) from the pattern with zidovudine monotherapy, with the 151 mutation being most commonly associated with multidrug resistance. The mutation at codon 151 in combination with the mutations at 62, 75, 77, and 116 results in a virus with reduced susceptibility to zidovudine, didanosine, zalcitabine, stavudine, and lamivudine. Multiple drug resistance has been observed in two of 39 (5%) patients receiving zidovudine and didanosine combination therapy for 2 years.

CLINICAL PHARMACOLOGY

Pharmacokinetics in Adults: *COMBIVIR:* One COMBIVIR Tablet was bioequivalent to one EPIVIR Tablet (150 mg) plus one RETROVIR Tablet (300 mg) following single-dose administration to fasting healthy subjects (n = 24).

Lamivudine: The pharmacokinetic properties of lamivudine in fasting patients are summarized in Table 1. Following oral administration, lamivudine is rapidly absorbed and extensively distributed. Binding to plasma protein is low. Approximately 70% of an intravenous dose of lamivudine is recovered as unchanged drug in the urine. Metabolism of lamivudine is a minor route of elimination. In humans, the only known metabolite is the trans-sulfoxide metabolite (approximately 5% of an oral dose after 12 hours).

Zidovudine: The pharmacokinetic properties of zidovudine in fasting patients are summarized in Table 1. Following oral administration, zidovudine is rapidly absorbed and extensively distributed. Binding to plasma protein is low. Zidovudine is eliminated primarily by hepatic metabolism. The major metabolite of zidovudine is 3′-azido-3′-deoxy-5′-*O*-β-*D*-glucopyranuronosylthymidine (GZDV). GZDV area under the curve (AUC) is about three-fold greater than the zidovudine AUC. Urinary recovery of zidovudine and GZDV accounts for 14% and 74% of the dose following oral administration, respectively. A second metabolite, 3′-amino-3′-deoxythymidine (AMT), has been identified in plasma. The AMT AUC was one fifth of the zidovudine AUC.

Table 1: Pharmacokinetic Parameters* for Lamivudine and Zidovudine in Adults

Parameter	Lamivudine		Zidovudine	
Oral bioavailability (%)	86 ± 16	n = 12	64 ± 10	n = 5
Apparent volume of distribution (L/kg)	1.3 ± 0.4	n = 20	1.6 ± 0.6	n = 8
Plasma protein binding (%)	<36		<38	
CSF:plasma ratio**	0.12 [0.04 to 0.47]	n = 38†	0.60 [0.04 to 2.62]	n = 39‡
Systemic clearance (L/h/kg)	0.33 ± 0.06	n = 20	1.6 ± 0.6	n = 6
Renal clearance (L/h/kg)	0.22 ± 0.06	n = 20	0.34 ± 0.05	n = 9
Elimination half-life (h)§	5 to 7		0.5 to 3	

* Data presented as mean ± standard deviation except where noted.
** Median [range].
† Children.
‡ Adults.
§ Approximate range.

Table 2: Effect of Coadministered Drugs on Lamivudine and Zidovudine AUC*

Note: ROUTINE DOSE MODIFICATION OF LAMIVUDINE AND ZIDOVUDINE IS NOT WARRANTED WITH COADMINISTRATION OF THE FOLLOWING DRUGS.

Drugs That May Alter Lamivudine Blood Concentrations

Coadministered Drug and Dose	Lamivudine Dose	n	Lamivudine Concentrations: AUC	Lamivudine Concentrations: Variability	Concentration of Coadministered Drug
Nelfinavir 750 mg q 8 hr × 7 to 10 days	single 150 mg	11	↑ AUC 10%	95% CI: 1% to 20%	↔
Trimethoprim 160 mg/ Sulfamethoxazole 800 mg daily× 5 days	single 300 mg	14	↑ AUC 43%	90% CI: 32% to 55%	↔

Drugs That May Alter Zidovudine Blood Concentrations

Coadministered Drug and Dose	Zidovudine Dose	n	Zidovudine Concentrations: AUC	Zidovudine Concentrations: Variability	Concentration of Coadministered Drug
Atovaquone 750 mg q 12 h with food	200 mg q 8 h	14	↑ AUC 31%	Range 23% to 78%**	↔
Fluconazole 400 mg daily	200 mg q 8 h	12	↑AUC 74%	95% CI: 54% to 98%	Not Reported
Methadone 30 to 90 mg daily	200 mg q 4 h	9	↑AUC 43%	Range 16% to 64%**	↔
Nelfinavir 750 mg q 8 hr × 7 to 10 days	single 200 mg	11	↓AUC 35%	Range 28% to 41%	↔
Probenecid 500 mg q 6 h × 2 days	2 mg/kg q 8 h × 3 days	3	↑AUC 106%	Range 100% to 170%**	Not Assessed
Ritonavir 300 mg q 6 h × 4 days	200 mg q 8 h × 4 days	9	↓AUC 25%	95% CI: 15% to 34%	↔
Valproic acid 250 mg or 500 mg q 8 h × 4 days	100 mg q 8 h × 4 days	6	↑AUC 80%	Range 64% to 130%**	Not Assessed

↑ = Increase; ↓ = Decrease; ↔ = no significant change; AUC = area under the concentration versus time curve; CI =confidence interval.
* This table is not all inclusive.
** Estimated range of percent difference.

[See table 1 above]

Effect of Food on Absorption of COMBIVIR: COMBIVIR may be administered with or without food. The extent of lamivudine and zidovudine absorption (AUC) following administration of COMBIVIR with food was similar when compared to fasting healthy subjects (n = 24).

Special Populations: *Impaired Renal Function: COMBIVIR:* Because lamivudine and zidovudine require dose adjustment in the presence of renal insufficiency, COMBIVIR is not recommended for patients with impaired renal function (see PRECAUTIONS).

Pregnancy: See PRECAUTIONS: Pregnancy.

COMBIVIR: No data are available.

Zidovudine: Zidovudine pharmacokinetics has been studied in a Phase 1 study of eight women during the last trimester of pregnancy. As pregnancy progressed, there was no evidence of drug accumulation. The pharmacokinetics of zidovudine was similar to that of nonpregnant adults. Consistent with passive transmission of the drug across the placenta, zidovudine concentrations in neonatal plasma at birth were essentially equal to those in maternal plasma at delivery. Although data are limited, methadone maintenance therapy in five pregnant women did not appear to alter zidovudine pharmacokinetics. In a nonpregnant adult population, a potential for interaction has been identified (see CLINICAL PHARMACOLOGY: Drug Interactions).

Nursing Mothers: See PRECAUTIONS: Nursing Mothers.

COMBIVIR: No data are available.

Zidovudine: After administration of a single dose of 200 mg zidovudine to 13 HIV-infected women, the mean concentration of zidovudine was similar in human milk and serum.

Pediatric Patients: COMBIVIR: COMBIVIR should not be administered to pediatric patients less than 12 years of age because it is a fixed-dose combination that cannot be adjusted for this patient population.

Geriatric Patients: Lamivudine and zidovudine pharmacokinetics have not been studied in patients over 65 years of age.

Gender: COMBIVIR: A pharmacokinetic study in healthy male (n = 12) and female (n = 12) subjects showed no gender differences in zidovudine exposure (AUC∞) or lamivudine AUC∞ normalized for body weight.

Race: Lamivudine: There are no significant racial differences in lamivudine pharmacokinetics.

Drug Interactions: See PRECAUTIONS: Drug Interactions.

COMBIVIR: No drug interaction studies have been conducted using COMBIVIR Tablets.

Lamivudine Plus Zidovudine: No clinically significant alterations in lamivudine or zidovudine pharmacokinetics were observed in 12 asymptomatic HIV-infected adult patients given a single dose of zidovudine (200 mg) in combination with multiple doses of lamivudine (300 mg q 12 h).

[See table 2 above]

INDICATIONS AND USAGE

COMBIVIR in combination with other antiretroviral agents is indicated for the treatment of HIV infection.

Description of Clinical Studies: ***COMBIVIR:*** There have been no clinical trials conducted with COMBIVIR. See CLINICAL PHARMACOLOGY for information about bioequivalence. One COMBIVIR Tablet given twice a day is an alternative regimen to EPIVIR Tablets 150 mg twice a day plus RETROVIR 600 mg per day in divided doses.

Lamivudine Plus Zidovudine: The NUCB3007 (CAESAR) study was conducted using EPIVIR 150-mg Tablets (150 mg b.i.d.) and RETROVIR 100-mg Capsules (2 × 100 mg t.i.d.). CAESAR was a multicenter, double-blind, placebo-controlled study comparing continued current therapy [zidovudine alone (62% of patients) or zidovudine with didanosine or zalcitabine (38% of patients)] to the addition of EPIVIR or EPIVIR plus an investigational non-nucleoside reverse transcriptase inhibitor, randomized 1:2:1. A total of 1816 HIV-infected adults with 25 to 250 (median 122) CD4 cells/mm^3 at baseline were enrolled: median age was 36 years, 87% were male, 84% were nucleoside-experienced, and 16% were therapy-naive. The median duration on study was 12 months. Results are summarized in Table 3.

[See table 3 at right]

Table 3: Number of Patients (%) With At Least One HIV Disease-Progression Event or Death

Endpoint	Current Therapy (n = 460)	EPIVIR plus Current Therapy (n = 896)	EPIVIR plus a NNRTI* plus Current Therapy (n = 460)
HIV progression or death	90 (19.6%)	86 (9.6%)	41 (8.9%)
Death	27 (5.9%)	23 (2.6%)	14 (3.0%)

*An investigational non-nucleoside reverse transcriptase inhibitor not approved in the United States.

CONTRAINDICATIONS

COMBIVIR Tablets are contraindicated in patients with previously demonstrated clinically significant hypersensitivity to any of the components of the product.

WARNINGS

COMBIVIR is a fixed-dose combination of lamivudine and zidovudine. Ordinarily, COMBIVIR should not be administered concomitantly with either lamivudine or zidovudine. The complete prescribing information for all agents being considered for use with COMBIVIR should be consulted before combination therapy with COMBIVIR is initiated.

Bone Marrow Suppression: COMBIVIR should be used with caution in patients who have bone marrow compromise evidenced by granulocyte count <1000 cells/mm^3 or hemoglobin <9.5 g/dL (see ADVERSE REACTIONS).

Frequent blood counts are strongly recommended in patients with advanced HIV disease who are treated with COMBIVIR. For HIV-infected individuals and patients with asymptomatic or early HIV disease, periodic blood counts are recommended.

Lactic Acidosis/Severe Hepatomegaly with Steatosis: Lactic acidosis and severe hepatomegaly with steatosis, including fatal cases, have been reported with the use of nucleoside analogues alone or in combination, including lamivudine, zidovudine, and other antiretrovirals. A majority of these cases have been in women. Obesity and prolonged nucleoside exposure may be risk factors. Particular caution should be exercised when administering COMBIVIR to any patient with known risk factors for liver disease; however, cases have also been reported in patients with no known risk factors. Treatment with COMBIVIR should be suspended in any patient who develops clinical or laboratory findings suggestive of lactic acidosis or pronounced hepatotoxicity (which may include hepatomegaly and steatosis even in the absence of marked transaminase elevations).

Myopathy: Myopathy and myositis, with pathological changes similar to that produced by HIV disease, have been associated with prolonged use of zidovudine and therefore may occur with therapy with COMBIVIR.

PRECAUTIONS

Patients With HIV and Hepatitis B Virus Coinfection: In clinical trials and postmarketing experience, some patients with HIV infection who have chronic liver disease due to hepatitis B virus infection experienced clinical or laboratory evidence of recurrent hepatitis upon discontinuation of lamivudine. Consequences may be more severe in patients with decompensated liver disease.

Patients With Impaired Renal Function: Reduction of the dosages of lamivudine and zidovudine is recommended for patients with impaired renal function. Patients with creatinine clearance ≤50 mL/min should not receive COMBIVIR.

Information for Patients: COMBIVIR is not a cure for HIV infection and patients may continue to experience illnesses associated with HIV infection, including opportunistic infections. Patients should be advised that the use of COMBIVIR has not been shown to reduce the risk of transmission of HIV to others through sexual contact or blood contamination. Patients should be informed that the major toxicities of COMBIVIR are neutropenia and/or anemia. They should be told of the extreme importance of having their blood counts followed closely while on therapy, especially for patients with advanced HIV disease. Patients should be advised of the importance of taking COMBIVIR as it is prescribed.

Drug Interactions: Coadministration of ganciclovir, interferon-alpha, and other bone marrow suppressive or cytotoxic agents may increase the hematologic toxicity of zidovudine (see CLINICAL PHARMACOLOGY).

Carcinogenesis, Mutagenesis, and Impairment of Fertility:

Carcinogenicity:

Lamivudine: Lamivudine long-term carcinogenicity studies in mice and rats showed no evidence of carcinogenic potential at exposures up to 10 times (mice) and 58 times (rats) those observed in humans at the recommended therapeutic dose.

Zidovudine: Zidovudine was administered orally at three dosage levels to separate groups of mice and rats (60 females and 60 males in each group). Initial single daily doses were 30, 60, and 120 mg/kg per day in mice and 80, 220, and 600 mg/kg per day in rats. The doses in mice were reduced to 20, 30, and 40 mg/kg per day after day 90 because of treatment-related anemia, whereas in rats only the high dose was reduced to 450 mg/kg per day on day 91 and then to 300 mg/kg per day on day 279.

In mice, seven late-appearing (after 19 months) vaginal neoplasms (five nonmetastasizing squamous cell carcinomas, one squamous cell papilloma, and one squamous polyp) occurred in animals given the highest dose. One late-appearing squamous cell papilloma occurred in the vagina of a middle-dose animal. No vaginal tumors were found at the lowest dose.

In rats, two late-appearing (after 20 months), nonmetastasizing vaginal squamous cell carcinomas occurred in animals given the highest dose. No vaginal tumors occurred at the low or middle dose in rats. No other drug-related tumors were observed in either sex of either species.

At doses that produced tumors in mice and rats, the estimated drug exposure (as measured by AUC) was approximately three times (mouse) and 24 times (rat) the estimated human exposure at the recommended therapeutic dose of 100 mg every 4 hours.

Two transplacental carcinogenicity studies were conducted in mice. One study administered zidovudine at doses of 20 mg/kg per day or 40 mg/kg per day from gestation day 10 through parturition and lactation with dosing continuing in offspring for 24 months postnatally. The doses of zidovudine employed in this study produced zidovudine exposures approximately three times the estimated human exposure at recommended doses. After 24 months, at the highest dose, an increase in incidence of vaginal tumors was noted with no increase in tumors in the liver or lung or any other organ in either gender. These findings are consistent with results of the standard oral carcinogenicity study in mice, as described earlier. A second study administered zidovudine at maximum tolerated doses of 12.5 mg/day or 25 mg/day (~1000 mg/kg nonpregnant body weight or ~450 mg/kg of term body weight) to pregnant mice from days 12 through 18 of gestation. There was an increase in the number of tumors in the lung, liver, and female reproductive tracts in the offspring of mice receiving the higher dose level of zidovudine.

It is not known how predictive the results of rodent carcinogenicity studies may be for humans.

Mutagenicity: Lamivudine: Lamivudine was negative in a microbial mutagenicity screen, in an in vitro cell transformation assay, in a rat micronucleus test, in a rat bone marrow cytogenetic assay, and in an assay for unscheduled DNA synthesis in rat liver. It was mutagenic in a L5178Y/TK$^{+/-}$ mouse lymphoma assay and clastogenic in a cytogenetic assay using cultured human lymphocytes.

Continued on next page

Table 4: Selected Clinical Adverse Events (≥5% Frequency) in Four Controlled Clinical Trials With EPIVIR 300 mg/day and RETROVIR 600 mg/day

Adverse Event	EPIVIR plus RETROVIR (n = 251)
Body as a whole	
Headache	35%
Malaise & fatigue	27%
Fever or chills	10%
Digestive	
Nausea	33%
Diarrhea	18%
Nausea & vomiting	13%
Anorexia and/or decreased appetite	10%
Abdominal pain	9%
Abdominal cramps	6%
Dyspepsia	5%
Nervous system	
Neuropathy	12%
Insomnia & other sleep disorders	11%
Dizziness	10%
Depressive disorders	9%
Respiratory	
Nasal signs & symptoms	20%
Cough	18%
Skin	
Skin rashes	9%
Musculoskeletal	
Musculoskeletal pain	12%
Myalgia	8%
Arthralgia	5%

Table 5: Frequencies of Selected Laboratory Abnormalities Among Adults in Four Controlled Clinical Trials of EPIVIR 300 mg/day plus RETROVIR 600 mg/day*

Test (Abnormal Level)	EPIVIR plus RETROVIR % (n)
Neutropenia (ANC<750/mm^3)	7.2% (237)
Anemia (Hgb<8.0 g/dL)	2.9% (241)
Thrombocytopenia (platelets<50,000/mm^3)	0.4% (240)
ALT (>5.0 × ULN)	3.7% (241)
AST (>5.0 × ULN)	1.7% (241)
Bilirubin (>2.5 × ULN)	0.8% (241)
Amylase (>2.0 × ULN)	4.2% (72)

ULN = Upper limit of normal.
ANC = Absolute neutrophil count.
n = Number of patients assessed.
* Frequencies of these laboratory abnormalities were higher in patients with mild laboratory abnormalities at baseline.

This product information is based on labeling in effect on June 23, 2000. For further information, contact via direct mail, phone, or web site. Medical Information, Glaxo Wellcome Inc., PO Box 13398, Research Triangle Park, NC 27709. Healthcare Professionals (Medical Information): 800-334-0089. Patients (Customer Response Center): 1-888-825-5249. Glaxo Wellcome Corporate Web Site: www.glaxowellcome.com

Combivir—Cont.

Zidovudine: Zidovudine was mutagenic in a L5178Y/TK$^{+/-}$ mouse lymphoma assay, positive in an in vitro cell transformation assay, clastogenic in a cytogenetic assay using cultured human lymphocytes, and positive in mouse and rat micronucleus tests after repeated doses. It was negative in a cytogenetic study in rats given a single dose.
Impairment of Fertility: Lamivudine: In a study of reproductive performance, lamivudine, administered to male and female rats at doses up to 130 times the usual adult dose based on body surface area considerations, revealed no evidence of impaired fertility (judged by conception rates) and no effect on the survival, growth, and development to weaning of the offspring.
Zidovudine: Zidovudine, administered to male and female rats at doses up to 7 times the usual adult dose based on body surface area considerations, had no effect on fertility judged by conception rates.
Pregnancy: Pregnancy Category C.
COMBIVIR: There are no adequate and well-controlled studies of COMBIVIR in pregnant women. Reproduction studies with lamivudine and zidovudine have been performed in animals (see Lamivudine and Zidovudine sections below). COMBIVIR should be used during pregnancy only if the potential benefits outweigh the risks.
Lamivudine: Reproduction studies with orally administered lamivudine have been performed in rats and rabbits at 130 and 60 times, respectively, the usual adult dose (based on relative body surface area) and have revealed no evidence of teratogenicity. Some evidence of early embryolethality was seen in the rabbit at doses similar to those produced by the usual adult dose and higher, but there was no indication of this effect in the rat at orally administered doses up to 130 times the usual adult dose. Studies in pregnant rats and rabbits showed that lamivudine is transferred to the fetus through the placenta.
Zidovudine: Reproduction studies with orally administered zidovudine in the rat and in the rabbit at doses up to 500 mg/kg per day revealed no evidence of teratogenicity with zidovudine. Zidovudine treatment resulted in embryo/fetal toxicity as evidenced by an increase in the incidence of fetal resorptions in rats given 150 or 450 mg/kg per day and rabbits given 500 mg/kg per day. The doses used in the teratology studies resulted in peak zidovudine plasma concentrations (after one-half of the daily dose) in rats 66 to 226 times, and in rabbits 12 to 87 times, mean steady-state peak human plasma concentrations (after one-sixth of the daily dose) achieved with the recommended daily dose (100 mg every 4 hours). In an additional teratology study in rats, a dose of 3000 mg/kg per day (very near the oral median lethal dose in rats of 3683 mg/kg) caused marked maternal toxicity and an increase in the incidence of fetal malformations. This dose resulted in peak zidovudine plasma concentrations 350 times peak human plasma concentrations. No evidence of teratogenicity was seen in this experiment at doses of 600 mg/kg per day or less. Two rodent carcinogenicity studies were conducted (see Carcinogenesis, Mutagenesis, Impairment of Fertility).
Antiretroviral Pregnancy Registry: To monitor maternal-fetal outcomes of pregnant women exposed to COMBIVIR and other antiretroviral agents, an Antiretroviral Pregnancy Registry has been established. Physicians are encouraged to register patients by calling 1-800-258-4263.
Nursing Mothers: The Centers for Disease Control and Prevention recommend that HIV-infected mothers not breastfeed their infants to avoid risking postnatal transmission of HIV infection.
COMBIVIR: Zidovudine is excreted in breast milk (see CLINICAL PHARMACOLOGY: Pharmacokinetics: Nursing Mothers); however, no data are available on COMBIVIR or lamivudine. Therefore, there is a potential for adverse effects in nursing infants. **Mothers should be instructed not to breastfeed if they are receiving COMBIVIR.**
Pediatric Use: COMBIVIR should not be administered to pediatric patients less than 12 years of age because it is a fixed-dose combination that cannot be adjusted for this patient population.

ADVERSE REACTIONS

Lamivudine Plus Zidovudine Administered As Separate Formulations: In four randomized, controlled trials of EPIVIR 300 mg per day plus RETROVIR 600 mg per day, the following selected clinical and laboratory adverse events were observed (see Tables 4 and 5).
[See table 4 on previous page]
Pancreatitis was observed in three of the 656 adult patients (<0.5%) who received EPIVIR in controlled clinical trials. Selected laboratory abnormalities observed during therapy are listed in Table 5.
[See table 5 on previous page]
Observed During Clinical Practice: In addition to adverse events reported from clinical trials, the following events have been identified during post-approval use of EPIVIR and/or RETROVIR. Because they are reported voluntarily from a population of unknown size, estimates of frequency cannot be made. These events have been chosen for inclusion due to a combination of their seriousness, frequency of reporting, or potential causal connection to EPIVIR and/or RETROVIR.
Endocrine and Metabolic: Hyperglycemia.
General: Sensitization reactions (including anaphylaxis), vasculitis.
Hepatobiliary Tract and Pancreas: Lactic acidosis and hepatic steatosis (see WARNINGS), pancreatitis.
Musculoskeletal: Muscle weakness, CPK elevation, rhabdomyolysis.
Nervous: Seizures.
Skin: Alopecia, erythema multiforme, Stevens-Johnson syndrome, urticaria.

OVERDOSAGE

COMBIVIR: There is no known antidote for COMBIVIR.
Lamivudine: One case of an adult ingesting 6 grams of lamivudine was reported; there were no clinical signs or symptoms noted and hematologic tests remained normal. It is not known whether lamivudine can be removed by peritoneal dialysis or hemodialysis.
Zidovudine: Acute overdoses of zidovudine have been reported in pediatric patients and adults. These involved exposures up to 50 grams. The only consistent findings were nausea and vomiting. Other reported occurrences included headache, dizziness, drowsiness, lethargy, confusion, and one report of a grand mal seizure. Hematologic changes were transient. All patients recovered. Hemodialysis and peritoneal dialysis appear to have a negligible effect on the removal of zidovudine while elimination of its primary metabolite, GZDV, is enhanced.

DOSAGE AND ADMINISTRATION

The recommended oral dose of COMBIVIR for adults and adolescents (at least 12 years of age) is one tablet (containing 150 mg of lamivudine and 300 mg of zidovudine) twice daily.
Dose Adjustment: Because it is a fixed-dose combination, COMBIVIR should not be prescribed for patients requiring dosage adjustment such as those with reduced renal function (creatinine clearance ≤50 mL/min) or those experiencing dose-limiting adverse events.

HOW SUPPLIED

COMBIVIR Tablets, containing 150 mg lamivudine and 300 mg zidovudine, are white, film-coated, modified-capsule-shaped tablets engraved with "GXFC3" on one side. They are available as follows:
60 Tablets/Bottle (NDC 0173-0595-00)
Store between 2° and 30°C (36° and 86°F).
Unit Dose Pack of 120 (NDC 0173-0595-02)
Store between 2° and 30°C (36° and 86°F).
Glaxo Wellcome Inc., Research Triangle Park, NC 27709
Lamivudine is manufactured under agreement from BioChem Pharma Inc.
Laval, Quebec, Canada
U.S. Patent Nos. 5,047,407; 4,818,538; 4,828,838; 4,724,232; 4,833,130; 4,837,208; and 5,859,021
January 2000/RL-794
Shown in Product Identification Guide, page 314

CUTIVATE® ℞

[*kyoot' ə-vāt*]
(fluticasone propionate cream)
Cream, 0.05%

For Dermatologic Use Only—
Not for Ophthalmic Use.

DESCRIPTION

CUTIVATE (fluticasone propionate cream) Cream, 0.05% contains fluticasone propionate [(6α,11β,16α,17α)-6,9,-difluoro-11-hydroxy-16-methyl-3-oxo-17-(1-oxopropoxy) androsta-1,4-diene-17-carbothioic acid, S-fluoromethyl ester], a synthetic fluorinated corticosteroid, for topical dermatologic use. The topical corticosteroids constitute a class of primarily synthetic steroids used as anti-inflammatory and antipruritic agents.
Fluticasone propionate has a molecular weight of 500.6. It is a white to off-white powder and is insoluble in water.
Each gram of CUTIVATE Cream contains fluticasone propionate 0.5 mg in a base of propylene glycol, mineral oil, cetostearyl alcohol, Ceteth-20, isopropyl myristate, dibasic sodium phosphate, citric acid, purified water, and imidurea as preservative.

CLINICAL PHARMACOLOGY

Like other topical corticosteroids, fluticasone propionate has anti-inflammatory, antipruritic, and vasoconstrictive properties. The mechanism of the anti-inflammatory activity of the topical steroids, in general, is unclear. However, corticosteroids are thought to act by the induction of phospholipase A_2 inhibitory proteins, collectively called lipocortins. It is postulated that these proteins control the biosynthesis of potent mediators of inflammation such as prostaglandins and leukotrienes by inhibiting the release of their common precursor, arachidonic acid. Arachidonic acid is released from membrane phospholipids by phospholipase A_2.
Fluticasone propionate is lipophilic and has a strong affinity for the glucocorticoid receptor. It has weak affinity for the progesterone receptor, and virtually no affinity for the mineralocorticoid, estrogen, or androgen receptors. The therapeutic potency of glucocorticoids is related to the half-life of the glucocorticoid-receptor complex. The half-life of the fluticasone propionate-glucocorticoid receptor complex is approximately 10 hours.
Studies performed with CUTIVATE Cream indicate that it is in the medium range of potency as compared with other topical corticosteroids.
Pharmacokinetics: *Absorption:* The activity of CUTIVATE is due to the parent drug, fluticasone propionate. The extent of percutaneous absorption of topical corticosteroids is determined by many factors, including the vehicle and the integrity of the epidermal barrier. Occlusive dressing enhances penetration. Topical corticosteroids can be absorbed from normal intact skin. Inflammation and/or other disease processes in the skin increase percutaneous absorption.
In a human study of 12 healthy males receiving 12.5 g of 0.05% fluticasone propionate cream twice daily for 3 weeks, plasma levels were generally below the level of quantification (0.05 ng/mL). In another study of 6 healthy males administered 25 g of 0.05% fluticasone propionate cream under occlusion for 5 days, plasma levels of fluticasone ranged from 0.07 to 0.39 ng/mL.
In an animal study using radiolabeled 0.05% fluticasone propionate cream and ointment preparations, rats received a topical dose of 1 g/kg for a 24-hour period. Total recovery of radioactivity was approximately 80% at the end of 7 days. The majority of the dose (73%) was recovered from the surface of the application site. Less than 1% of the dose was recovered in the skin at the application site. Approximately 5% of the dose was absorbed systemically through the skin. Absorption from the skin continued for the duration of the study (7 days), indicating a long retention time at the application site.
Distribution: Following intravenous administration of 1 mg fluticasone propionate in healthy volunteers, the initial disposition phase for fluticasone propionate was rapid and consistent with its high lipid solubility and tissue binding. The apparent volume of distribution averaged 4.2 L/kg (range, 2.3 to 16.7 L/kg). The percentage of fluticasone propionate bound to human plasma proteins averaged 91%. Fluticasone propionate is weakly and reversibly bound to erythrocytes. Fluticasone propionate is not significantly bound to human transcortin.
Metabolism: No metabolites of fluticasone propionate were detected in an in vitro study of radiolabeled fluticasone propionate incubated in a human skin homogenate. The total blood clearance of systemically absorbed fluticasone propionate averages 1093 mL/min (range, 618 to 1702 mL/min) after a 1-mg intravenous dose, with renal clearance accounting for less than 0.02% of the total. Fluticasone propionate is metabolized in the liver by cytochrome P450 3A4-mediated hydrolysis of the 5-fluoromethyl carbothioate grouping. This transformation occurs in 1 metabolic step to produce the inactive 17-β-carboxylic acid metabolite, the only known metabolite detected in man. This metabolite has approximately 2000 times less affinity than the parent drug for the glucocorticoid receptor of human lung cytosol in vitro and negligible pharmacological activity in animal studies. Other metabolites detected in vitro using cultured human hepatoma cells have not been detected in man.
Excretion: Following intravenous dose of 1 mg in healthy volunteers, fluticasone propionate showed polyexponential kinetics and had an average terminal half-life of 7.2 hours (range, 3.2 to 11.2 hours).

INDICATIONS AND USAGE

CUTIVATE Cream is a medium potency corticosteroid indicated for the relief of the inflammatory and pruritic manifestations of corticosteroid-responsive dermatoses. CUTIVATE Cream may be used with caution in pediatric patients 3 months of age or older. The safety and efficacy of drug use for longer than 4 weeks in this population have not been established. The safety and efficacy of CUTIVATE Cream in pediatric patients below 3 months of age have not been established.

CONTRAINDICATIONS

CUTIVATE Cream is contraindicated in those patients with a history of hypersensitivity to any of the components in the preparation.

PRECAUTIONS

General: Systemic absorption of topical corticosteroids can produce reversible hypothalamic-pituitary-adrenal (HPA) axis suppression with the potential for glucocorticosteroid insufficiency after withdrawal from treatment. Manifestations of Cushing's syndrome, hyperglycemia, and glucosuria can also be produced in some patients by systemic absorption of topical corticosteroids while on treatment.
Patients applying a potent topical steroid to a large surface area or to areas under occlusion should be evaluated periodically for evidence of HPA axis suppression. This may be done by using the ACTH stimulation, A.M. plasma cortisol, and urinary free cortisol tests.
If HPA axis suppression is noted, an attempt should be made to withdraw the drug, to reduce the frequency of application, or to substitute a less potent steroid. Recovery of HPA axis function is generally prompt upon discontinuation of topical corticosteroids. Infrequently, signs and symptoms of glucocorticosteroid insufficiency may occur requiring supplemental systemic corticosteroids. For information on systemic supplementation, see prescribing information for those products.
Fluticasone propionate cream, 0.05% caused depression of A.M. plasma cortisol levels in 1 of 6 adult patients when used daily for 7 days in patients with psoriasis or eczema involving at least 30% of the body surface. After 2 days of treatment, this patient developed a 60% decrease from pretreatment values in the A.M. plasma cortisol level.
There was some evidence of corresponding decrease in the 24-hour urinary free cortisol levels. The A.M. plasma corti-

sol level remained slightly depressed for 48 hours but recovered by day 6 of treatment.

Fluticasone propionate cream, 0.05%, caused HPA axis suppression in 2 of 43 pediatric patients, ages 2 and 5 years old, who were treated for 4 weeks covering at least 35% of the body surface area. Follow-up testing 12 days after treatment discontinuation, available for 1 of the 2 subjects, demonstrated a normally responsive HPA axis (see PRECAUTIONS: Pediatric Use).

Pediatric patients may be more susceptible to systemic toxicity from equivalent doses due to their larger skin surface to body mass ratios (see PRECAUTIONS: Pediatric Use).

Fluticasone propionate cream, 0.05% may cause local cutaneous adverse reactions (see ADVERSE REACTIONS).

If irritation develops, CUTIVATE Cream should be discontinued and appropriate therapy instituted. Allergic contact dermatitis with corticosteroids is usually diagnosed by observing failure to heal rather than noting a clinical exacerbation as with most topical products not containing corticosteroids. Such an observation should be corroborated with appropriate diagnostic patch testing.

If concomitant skin infections are present or develop, an appropriate antifungal or antibacterial agent should be used. If a favorable response does not occur promptly, use of CUTIVATE Cream should be discontinued until the infection has been adequately controlled.

CUTIVATE Cream should not be used in the presence of preexisting skin atrophy and should not be used where infection is present at the treatment site. CUTIVATE Cream should not be used in the treatment of rosacea and perioral dermatitis.

Information for Patients: Patients using topical corticosteroids should receive the following information and instructions:

1. This medication is to be used as directed by the physician. It is for external use only. Avoid contact with the eyes.
2. This medication should not be used for any disorder other than that for which it was prescribed.
3. The treated skin area should not be bandaged or otherwise covered or wrapped so as to be occlusive unless directed by the physician.
4. Patients should report to their physician any signs of local adverse reactions.
5. Parents of pediatric patients should be advised not to use this medication in the treatment of diaper dermatitis. CUTIVATE Cream should not be applied in the diaper areas as diapers or plastic pants may constitute occlusive dressing (see DOSAGE AND ADMINISTRATION).
6. This medication should not be used on the face, underarms, or groin areas unless directed by a physician.
7. As with other corticosteroids, therapy should be discontinued when control is achieved. If no improvement is seen within 2 weeks, contact the physician.

Laboratory Tests: The following tests may be helpful in evaluating patients for HPA axis suppression:

ACTH stimulation test
A.M. plasma cortisol test
Urinary free cortisol test

Carcinogenesis, Mutagenesis, and Impairment of Fertility: Two 18-month studies were performed in mice to evaluate the carcinogenic potential of fluticasone propionate when given topically (as an 0.05% ointment) and orally. No evidence of carcinogenicity was found in either study.

Fluticasone propionate was not mutagenic in the standard Ames test, *E. coli* fluctuation test, *S. cerevisiae* gene conversion test, or Chinese Hamster ovarian cell assay. It was not clastogenic in mouse micronucleus or cultured human lymphocyte tests.

In a fertility and general reproductive performance study in rats, fluticasone propionate administered subcutaneously to females at up to 50 mcg/kg per day and to males at up to 100 mcg/kg per day (later reduced to 50 mcg/kg per day) had no effect upon mating performance or fertility. These doses are approximately 15 and 30 times, respectively, the human systemic exposure following use of the recommended human topical dose of fluticasone propionate cream, 0.05%, assuming human percutaneous absorption of approximately 3% and the use in a 70-kg person of 15 g/day.

Pregnancy: *Teratogenic Effects:* Pregnancy Category C. Corticosteroids have been shown to be teratogenic in laboratory animals when administered systemically at relatively low dosage levels. Some corticosteroids have been shown to be teratogenic after dermal application in laboratory animals. Teratology studies in the mouse demonstrated fluticasone propionate to be teratogenic (cleft palate) when administered subcutaneously in doses of 45 mcg/kg per day and 150 mcg/kg per day. This dose is approximately 14 and 45 times, respectively, the human topical dose of fluticasone propionate cream, 0.05%. There are no adequate and well-controlled studies in pregnant women. CUTIVATE Cream should be used during pregnancy only if the potential benefit justifies the potential risk to the fetus.

Nursing Mothers: Systemically administered corticosteroids appear in human milk and could suppress growth, interfere with endogenous corticosteroid production, or cause other untoward effects. It is not known whether topical administration of corticosteroids could result in sufficient systemic absorption to produce detectable quantities in human milk. Because many drugs are excreted in human milk, caution should be exercised when CUTIVATE Cream is administered to a nursing woman.

Pediatric Use: CUTIVATE Cream may be used with caution in pediatric patients as young as 3 months of age. The safety and efficacy of drug use for longer than 4 weeks in this population have not been established. The safety and efficacy of CUTIVATE Cream in pediatric patients below 3 months of age have not been established.

Fluticasone propionate cream, 0.05%, caused HPA axis suppression in 2 of 43 pediatric patients, ages 2 and 5 years old, who were treated for 4 weeks covering at least 35% of the body surface area. Follow-up testing 12 days after treatment discontinuation, available for 1 of the 2 subjects, demonstrated a normally responsive HPA axis (see ADVERSE REACTIONS). Adverse effects including striae have been reported with use of topical corticosteroids in pediatric patients.

HPA axis suppression, Cushing's syndrome, linear growth retardation, delayed weight gain, and intracranial hypertension have been reported in pediatric patients receiving topical corticosteroids. Manifestations of adrenal suppression in pediatric patients include low plasma cortisol levels to an absence of response to ACTH stimulation. Manifestations of intracranial hypertension include bulging fontanelles, headaches, and bilateral papilledema.

ADVERSE REACTIONS

In controlled clinical trials of twice-daily administration, the total incidence of adverse reactions associated with the use of CUTIVATE Cream was approximately 4%. These adverse reactions were usually mild; self-limiting; and consisted primarily of pruritus, dryness, numbness of fingers, and burning. These events occurred in 2.9%, 1.2%, 1.0%, and 0.6% of patients, respectively.

Two clinical studies compared once- to twice-daily administration of CUTIVATE Cream for the treatment of moderate to severe eczema. The local drug-related adverse events for the 491 patients enrolled in both studies are shown in Table 1. In the study enrolling both adult and pediatric patients, the incidence of local adverse events in the 119 pediatric patients ages 1 to 12 years was comparable to the 140 patients ages 13 to 62 years.

Fifty-one pediatric patients ages 3 months to 5 years, with moderate to severe eczema, were enrolled in an open-label HPA axis safety study. CUTIVATE Cream was applied twice daily for 3 to 4 weeks over an arithmetic mean body surface

Continued on next page

Table 1: Drug-Related Adverse Events—Skin

Adverse Events	Fluticasone Once Daily (n = 210)	Fluticasone Twice Daily (n = 203)	Vehicle Twice Daily (n = 78)
Skin infection	1 (0.5%)	0	0
Infected eczema	1 (0.5%)	2 (1.0%)	0
Viral warts	0	1 (0.5%)	0
Herpes simplex	0	1 (0.5%)	0
Impetigo	1 (0.5%)	0	0
Atopic dermatitis	1 (0.5%)	0	0
Eczema	1 (0.5%)	0	0
Exacerbation of eczema	4 (1.9%)	1 (0.5%)	1 (1.3%)
Erythema	0	2 (1.0%)	0
Burning	2 (1.0%)	2 (1.0%)	2 (2.6%)
Stinging	0	2 (1.0%)	1 (1.3%)
Skin irritation	6 (2.9%)	2 (1.0%)	0
Pruritus	2 (1.0%)	4 (1.9%)	4 (5.1%)
Exacerbation of pruritus	4 (1.9%)	1 (0.5%)	1 (1.3%)
Folliculitis	1 (0.5%)	1 (0.5%)	0
Blisters	0	1 (0.5%)	0
Dryness of skin	3 (1.4%)	1 (0.5%)	0

Table 2: Adverse Events* From Pediatric Open-Label Trial (n = 51)

Adverse Events	Fluticasone Twice Daily
Burning	1 (2.0%)
Dusky erythema	1 (2.0%)
Erythematous rash	1 (2.0%)
Facial telangiectasia†	2 (4.9%)
Non-facial telangiectasia	1 (2.0%)
Urticaria	1 (2.0%)

*See text for additional detail.
†n = 41.

Table 3: Physician's Assessment of Clinical Response

	CUTIVATE Cream		Vehicle	
	Study 1 (n = 59)	Study 2 (n = 74)	Study 1 (n = 66)	Study 2 (n = 75)
Cleared	8%	1%	3%	1%
Excellent	29%	28%	11%	17%
Good	27%	34%	20%	28%
Fair	27%	15%	33%	25%
Poor	7%	22%	24%	27%
Worse	2%	0	9%	1%

Table 4: Clinical Signs: Mean Improvements Over Baseline

	CUTIVATE Cream		Vehicle	
	Study 1	Study 2	Study 1	Study 2
Erythema	1.19	1.07	0.55	0.84
Thickening	1.22	1.17	0.81	0.97
Scaling	1.53	1.39	0.95	1.21

Table 5: Physician's Assessment of Clinical Response

	CUTIVATE Cream Once Daily		CUTIVATE Cream Twice Daily	
	Study 1 (n = 64)	Study 2 (n = 106)	Study 1 (n = 65)	Study 2 (n = 100)
Cleared	30%	20%	48%	21%
Excellent	42%	32%	32%	50%
Good	17%	26%	5%	12%
Fair	3%	14%	6%	10%
Poor	5%	3%	8%	4%
Worse	3%	6%	2%	3%

This product information is based on labeling in effect on June 23, 2000. For further information, contact via direct mail, phone, or web site. Medical Information, Glaxo Wellcome Inc., PO Box 13398, Research Triangle Park, NC 27709. Healthcare Professionals (Medical Information): 800-334-0089. Patients (Customer Response Center): 1-888-825-5249. Glaxo Wellcome Corporate Web Site: www.glaxowellcome.com

Cutivate—Cont.

area of 64% (range, 35% to 95%). The mean morning cortisol levels with standard deviations before treatment (prestimulation mean value = 13.76 ± 6.94 mcg/dL, poststimulation mean value = 30.53 ± 7.23 mcg/dL) and at end treatment (prestimulation mean value = 12.32 ± 6.92 mcg/dL, poststimulation mean value = 28.84 ± 7.16 mcg/dL) showed little change. In 2 of 43 (4.7%) patients with end-treatment results, peak cortisol levels following cosyntropin stimulation testing were ≤18 μg/dL, indicating adrenal suppression. Follow-up testing after treatment discontinuation, available for 1 of the 2 subjects, demonstrated a normally responsive HPA axis. Local drug-related adverse events were transient burning, resolving the same day it was reported; transient urticaria, resolving the same day it was reported; erythematous rash; dusky erythema, resolving within 1 month after cessation of CUTIVATE Cream; and telangiectasia, resolving within 3 months after stopping CUTIVATE Cream.

[See table 1 at top of previous page]
[See table 2 on previous page]

The following local adverse reactions have been reported infrequently with topical corticosteroids, and they may occur more frequently with the use of occlusive dressings and higher potency corticosteroids. These reactions are listed in an approximately decreasing order of occurrence: irritation, folliculitis, acneiform eruptions, hypopigmentation, perioral dermatitis, allergic contact dermatitis, secondary infection, skin atrophy, striae, and miliaria. Also, there are reports of the development of pustular psoriasis from chronic plaque psoriasis following reduction or discontinuation of potent topical corticosteroid products.

OVERDOSAGE

Topically applied CUTIVATE Cream can be absorbed in sufficient amounts to produce systemic effects (see PRECAUTIONS).

DOSAGE AND ADMINISTRATION

CUTIVATE Cream may be used in adult and pediatric patients 3 months of age or older. Safety and efficacy of CUTIVATE Cream in pediatric patients for more than 4 weeks of use have not been established (see PRECAUTIONS: Pediatric Use). The safety and efficacy of CUTIVATE Cream in pediatric patients below 3 months of age have not been established.

Atopic Dermatitis: Apply a thin film of CUTIVATE Cream to the affected skin areas once or twice daily. Rub in gently.

Other Corticosteroid-Responsive Dermatoses: Apply a thin film of CUTIVATE Cream to the affected skin areas twice daily. Rub in gently.

As with other corticosteroids, therapy should be discontinued when control is achieved. If no improvement is seen within 2 weeks, reassessment of diagnosis may be necessary.

CUTIVATE Cream should not be used with occlusive dressings. CUTIVATE Cream should not be applied in the diaper area, as diapers or plastic pants may constitute occlusive dressings.

CLINICAL STUDIES

Psoriasis Studies: In 2 vehicle-controlled studies, CUTIVATE Cream applied twice daily was significantly more effective than the vehicle in the treatment of moderate to severe psoriasis. The investigator's global evaluation after 28 days of treatment is shown in Table 3.

[See table 3 on previous page]

The clinical signs of psoriasis were scored on a scale of 0 = absent, 1 = mild, 2 = moderate, and 3 = severe. The mean improvements over baseline in the clinical signs at the end of treatment are shown in Table 4.

[See table 4 on previous page]

Atopic Dermatitis Studies: In 2 controlled 28-day studies, CUTIVATE Cream once daily was equivalent to CUTIVATE Cream twice daily in the treatment of moderate to severe eczema. The investigator's global evaluation after 28 days of treatment is shown in Table 5.

[See table 5 on previous page]

The clinical signs and symptoms of atopic dermatitis were scored on a scale of 0 = absent, 1 = mild, 2 = moderate, and 3 = severe. The mean improvements over baseline at the end of treatment are shown in Table 6.

[See table 6 below]

HOW SUPPLIED

CUTIVATE Cream is supplied in:
15-g tubes (NDC 0173-0430-00)
30-g tubes (NDC 0173-0430-01)
60-g tubes (NDC 0173-0430-02)

Store between 2° and 30°C (36° and 86°F).
Glaxo Wellcome Inc., Research Triangle Park, NC 27709
August 1999/RL-734
Shown in Product Identification Guide, page 314

Table 6: Clinical Signs and Symptoms: Mean Improvements Over Baseline

	CUTIVATE Cream Once Daily		CUTIVATE Cream Twice Daily	
	Study 1	Study 2	Study 1	Study 2
Erythema	1.7	1.5	1.8	1.7
Pruritus	2.1	1.6	2.1	1.7
Thickening	1.6	1.3	1.6	1.5
Lichenification	1.2	1.2	1.2	1.3
Vesiculation	0.5	0.4	0.5	0.5
Crusting	0.6	0.7	0.8	0.8

CUTIVATE® ℞

[*kyoot 'ə-vāt "*]
(fluticasone propionate ointment)
Ointment, 0.005%

For Dermatologic Use Only—
Not for Ophthalmic Use.

DESCRIPTION

CUTIVATE Ointment, 0.005% contains fluticasone propionate [(6α,11β,16α,17α)-6,9,-difluoro-11-hydroxy-16-methyl-3-oxo-17-(1-oxopropoxy) androsta-1,4-diene-17-carbothioic acid, S-fluoromethyl ester], a synthetic fluorinated corticosteroid, for topical dermatologic use. The topical corticosteroids constitute a class of primarily synthetic steroids used as anti-inflammatory and antipruritic agents.

Chemically, fluticasone propionate is $C_{25}H_{31}F_3O_5S$.

Fluticasone propionate has a molecular weight of 500.6. It is a white to off-white powder and is insoluble in water.

Each gram of CUTIVATE Ointment contains fluticasone propionate 0.05 mg in a base of propylene glycol, sorbitan sesquioleate, microcrystalline wax, and liquid paraffin.

CLINICAL PHARMACOLOGY

Like other topical corticosteroids, fluticasone propionate has anti-inflammatory, antipruritic, and vasoconstrictive properties. The mechanism of the anti-inflammatory activity of the topical steroids, in general, is unclear. However, corticosteroids are thought to act by the induction of phospholipase A_2 inhibitory proteins, collectively called lipocortins. It is postulated that these proteins control the biosynthesis of potent mediators of inflammation such as prostaglandins and leukotrienes by inhibiting the release of their common precursor, arachidonic acid. Archidonic acid is released from membrane phospholipids by phospholipase A_2.

Pharmacokinetics: The extent of percutaneous absorption of topical corticosteroids is determined by many factors, including the vehicle and the integrity of the epidermal barrier. Occlusive dressing with hydrocortisone for up to 24 hours has not been demonstrated to increase penetration; however, occlusion of hydrocortisone for 96 hours markedly enhances penetration. Topical corticosteroids can be absorbed from normal intact skin. Inflammation and/or other disease processes in the skin increase percutaneous absorption.

Studies performed with CUTIVATE Ointment indicate that it is in the medium range of potency as compared with other topical corticosteroids.

INDICATIONS AND USAGE

CUTIVATE Ointment is a medium potency corticosteroid indicated for the relief of the inflammatory and pruritic manifestations of corticosteroid-responsive dermatoses.

CONTRAINDICATIONS

CUTIVATE Ointment is contraindicated in those patients with a history of hypersensitivity to any of the components of the preparation.

PRECAUTIONS

General: Systemic absorption of topical corticosteroids can produce reversible hypothalamic-pituitary-adrenal (HPA) axis suppression with the potential for glucocorticosteroid insufficiency after withdrawal from treatment. Manifestations of Cushing's syndrome, hyperglycemia, and glucosuria can also be produced in some patients by systemic absorption of topical corticosteroids while on treatment.

Patients applying a topical steroid to a large surface area or to areas under occlusion should be evaluated periodically for evidence of HPA axis suppression. This may be done by using the ACTH stimulation, A.M. plasma cortisol, and urinary free cortisol tests.

Fluticasone propionate ointment, 0.05% (a concentration 10 times that of fluticasone propionate ointment, 0.005%) suppressed 24-hour urinary free cortisol levels in 2 of 6 patients when used at a dose of 30 g/day for a week in patients with psoriasis or atopic eczema. In a second study, fluticasone propionate ointment, 0.05% caused depression of A.M. plasma cortisol levels in 3 of 12 normal volunteers when applied at doses of 50 g/day for 21 days. Morning plasma levels returned to normal levels within the first week upon discontinuation of fluticasone propionate. In this study there was no corresponding decrease in 24-hour urinary free cortisol levels.

If HPA axis suppression is noted, an attempt should be made to withdraw the drug, to reduce the frequency of application, or to substitute a less potent corticosteroid. Recovery of HPA axis function is generally prompt upon discontinuation of topical corticosteroids. Infrequently, signs and symptoms of glucocorticosteroid insufficiency may occur, requiring supplemental systemic corticosteroids. For information on systemic supplementation, see prescribing information for those products.

Children may be more susceptible to systemic toxicity from equivalent doses due to their larger skin surface to body mass ratios (see PRECAUTIONS: Pediatric Use).

If irritation develops, CUTIVATE Ointment should be discontinued and appropriate therapy instituted. Allergic contact dermatitis with corticosteroids is usually diagnosed by observing failure to heal rather than noting a clinical exacerbation as with most topical products not containing corticosteroids. Such an observation should be corroborated with appropriate diagnostic patch testing.

If concomitant skin infections are present or develop, an appropriate antifungal or antibacterial agent should be used. If a favorable response does not occur promptly, use of CUTIVATE Ointment should be discontinued until the infection has been adequately controlled.

CUTIVATE Ointment should not be used in the treatment of preexisting skin atrophy and should not be used where infection is present at the treatment site. CUTIVATE Ointment should not be used in the treatment of rosacea and perioral dermatitis.

Information for Patients: Patients using topical corticosteroids should receive the following information and instructions:

1. This medication is to be used as directed by the physician. It is for external use only. Avoid contact with the eyes.
2. This medication should not be used for any disorder other than that for which it was prescribed.
3. The treated skin area should not be bandaged or otherwise covered or wrapped so as to be occlusive unless directed by the physician.
4. Patients should report to their physician any signs of local adverse reactions.

Laboratory Tests: The following tests may be helpful in evaluating patients for HPA axis suppression:
ACTH stimulation test
A.M. plasma cortisol test
Urinary free cortisol test

Carcinogenesis, Mutagenesis, and Impairment of Fertility: Two 18-month studies were performed in mice to evaluate the carcinogenic potential of fluticasone propionate when given topically (as an 0.05% ointment) and orally. No evidence of carcinogenicity was found in either study.

Fluticasone propionate was not mutagenic in the standard Ames test, *E. coli* fluctuation test, *S. cerevisiae* gene conversion test, or Chinese Hamster ovarian cell assay. It was not clastogenic in mouse micronucleus or cultured human lymphocyte tests.

In a fertility and general reproductive performance study in rats, fluticasone propionate administered subcutaneously to females at up to 50 mcg/kg per day and to males at up to 100 mcg/kg per day (later reduced to 50 mcg/kg per day) had no effect upon mating performance or fertility. These doses are approximately 150 and 300 times, respectively, the human systemic exposure following use of the recommended human topical dose of fluticasone propionate ointment, 0.005%, assuming human percutaneous absorption of approximately 3% and the use in a 70-kg person of 15 g/day.

Pregnancy: ***Teratogenic Effects:*** Pregnancy Category C. Corticosteroids have been shown to be teratogenic in laboratory animals when administered systemically at relatively low dosage levels. Some corticosteroids have been shown to be teratogenic after dermal application in laboratory animals. Teratology studies in the mouse demonstrated fluticasone propionate to be teratogenic (cleft palate) when administered subcutaneously in doses of 45 mcg/kg per day and 150 mcg/kg per day. This dose is approximately 140 and 450 times, respectively, the human topical dose of fluticasone propionate ointment, 0.005%. There are no adequate and well-controlled studies in pregnant women. CUTIVATE Ointment should be used during pregnancy only if the potential benefit justifies the potential risk to the fetus.

Nursing Mothers: Systemically administered corticosteroids appear in human milk and could suppress growth, interfere with endogenous corticosteroid production, or cause other untoward effects. It is not known whether topical administration of corticosteroids could result in sufficient systemic absorption to produce detectable quantities in human milk. Because many drugs are excreted in human milk, caution should be exercised when CUTIVATE Ointment is administered to a nursing woman.

Pediatric Use: Safety and effectiveness in pediatric patients have not been established. Because of a higher ratio of skin surface area to body mass, pediatric patients are at a greater risk than adults of HPA axis suppression and Cushing's syndrome when they are treated with topical corticosteroids. They are therefore also at greater risk of adrenal insufficiency during or after withdrawal of treatment. Adverse effects including striae have been reported with inappropriate use of topical corticosteroids in pediatric patients.

HPA axis suppression, Cushing's syndrome, linear growth retardation, delayed weight gain, and intracranial hypertension have been reported in pediatric patients receiving topical corticosteroids. Manifestations of adrenal suppression in pediatric patients include low plasma cortisol levels and an absence of response to ACTH stimulation. Manifestations of intracranial hypertension include bulging fontanelles, headaches, and bilateral papilledema.

ADVERSE REACTIONS

In controlled clinical trials, the total incidence of adverse reactions associated with the use of CUTIVATE Ointment was approximately 4%. These adverse reactions were usually mild, self-limiting, and consisted primarily of pruritus, burning, hypertrichosis, increased erythema, hives, irritation, and lightheadedness. Each of these events occurred individually in less than 1% of patients.

The following additional local adverse reactions have been reported infrequently with topical corticosteroids, including fluticasone propionate, and they may occur more frequently with the use of occlusive dressings and higher potency corticosteroids. These reactions are listed in an approximately decreasing order of occurrence: dryness, folliculitis, acneiform eruptions, hypopigmentation, perioral dermatitis, allergic contact dermatitis, secondary infection, skin atrophy, striae, and miliaria. Also, there are reports of the development of pustular psoriasis from chronic plaque psoriasis following reduction or discontinuation of potent topical corticosteroid products.

OVERDOSAGE

Topically applied CUTIVATE Ointment can be absorbed in sufficient amounts to produce systemic effects (see PRECAUTIONS).

DOSAGE AND ADMINISTRATION

Apply a thin film of CUTIVATE Ointment to the affected skin areas twice daily. Rub in gently.

HOW SUPPLIED

CUTIVATE Ointment, 0.005% is supplied in 15-g (NDC 0173-0431-00), 30-g (NDC 0173-0431-01), and 60-g (NDC 0173-0431-02) tubes.

Store between 2° and 30°C (36° and 86°F).

Glaxo Wellcome Inc., Research Triangle Park, NC 27709

April 1999/RL-706

Shown in Product Identification Guide, page 314

DARAPRIM® ℞

[*dair 'ah-prĭm "*]

(pyrimethamine)

25 mg Scored Tablets

DESCRIPTION

DARAPRIM (pyrimethamine) is an antiparasitic compound available in tablet form for oral administration. Each scored tablet contains 25 mg pyrimethamine and the inactive ingredients corn and potato starch, lactose, and magnesium stearate.

Pyrimethamine is known chemically as 5-(4-chlorophenyl)-6-ethyl-2,4-pyrimidinediamine.

$C_{12}H_{13}ClN_4$

Mol. Wt 248.71

CLINICAL PHARMACOLOGY

Pyrimethamine is well absorbed with peak levels occurring between 2 to 6 hours following administration. It is eliminated slowly and has a plasma half-life of approximately 96 hours. Pyrimethamine is 87% bound to human plasma proteins.

Microbiology: Pyrimethamine is a folic acid antagonist and the rationale for its therapeutic action is based on the differential requirement between host and parasite for nucleic acid precursors involved in growth. This activity is highly selective against plasmodia and *Toxoplasma gondii*.

Pyrimethamine possesses blood schizonticidal and some tissue schizonticidal activity against malaria parasites of humans. However, the 4-amino-quinoline compounds are more effective against the erythrocytic schizonts. It does not destroy gametocytes, but arrests sporogony in the mosquito.

The action of pyrimethamine against *Toxoplasma gondii* is greatly enhanced when used in conjunction with sulfonamides. This was demonstrated by Eyles and Coleman[1] in the treatment of experimental toxoplasmosis in the mouse. Jacobs et al[2] demonstrated that combination of the two drugs effectively prevented the development of severe uveitis in most rabbits following the inoculation of the anterior chamber of the eye with toxoplasma.

INDICATIONS AND USAGE

Treatment of Toxoplasmosis: DARAPRIM is indicated for the treatment of toxoplasmosis when used conjointly with a sulfonamide, since synergism exists with this combination.

Treatment of Acute Malaria: DARAPRIM is also indicated for the treatment of acute malaria. It should not be used alone to treat acute malaria. Fast-acting schizonticides such as chloroquine or quinine are indicated and preferable for the treatment of acute malaria. However, conjoint use of DARAPRIM with a sulfonamide (e.g., sulfadoxine) will initiate transmission control and suppression of susceptible strains of plasmodia.

Chemoprophylaxis of Malaria: DARAPRIM is indicated for the chemoprophylaxis of malaria due to susceptible strains of plasmodia. However, resistance to pyrimethamine is prevalent worldwide. It is not suitable as a prophylactic agent for travelers to most areas.

CONTRAINDICATIONS

Use of DARAPRIM is contraindicated in patients with known hypersensitivity to pyrimethamine. Use of the drug is also contraindicated in patients with documented megaloblastic anemia due to folate deficiency.

WARNINGS

The dosage of pyrimethamine required for the treatment of toxoplasmosis is 10 to 20 times the recommended antimalaria dosage and approaches the toxic level. If signs of folate deficiency develop (see ADVERSE REACTIONS), reduce the dosage or discontinue the drug according to the response of the patient. Folinic acid (leucovorin) should be administered in a dosage of 5 to 15 mg daily (orally, IV, or IM) until normal hematopoiesis is restored.

Data in two humans indicate that pyrimethamine may be carcinogenic: a 51-year-old female who developed chronic granulocytic leukemia after taking pyrimethamine for 2 years for toxoplasmosis,[3] and a 56-year-old patient who developed reticulum cell sarcoma after 14 months of pyrimethamine for toxoplasmosis.[4]

Pyrimethamine has been reported to produce a significant increase in the number of lung tumors in mice when given intraperitoneally at doses of 25 mg/kg.[5]

DARAPRIM should be kept out of the reach of infants and children as they are extremely susceptible to adverse effects from an overdose. Deaths in pediatric patients have been reported after accidental ingestion.

PRECAUTIONS

General: The recommended dosage for chemoprophylaxis of malaria should not be exceeded. A small "starting" dose for toxoplasmosis is recommended in patients with convulsive disorders to avoid the potential nervous system toxicity of pyrimethamine. DARAPRIM should be used with caution in patients with impaired renal or hepatic function or in patients with possible folate deficiency, such as individuals with malabsorption syndrome, alcoholism, or pregnancy, and those receiving therapy, such as phenytoin, affecting folate levels (see Pregnancy subsection).

Information for Patients: Patients should be warned that at the first appearance of a skin rash they should stop use of DARAPRIM and seek medical attention immediately. Patients should also be warned that the appearance of sore throat, pallor, purpura, or glossitis may be early indications of serious disorders which require treatment with DARAPRIM to be stopped and medical treatment to be sought.

Women of childbearing potential who are taking DARAPRIM should be warned against becoming pregnant. Patients should be warned to keep DARAPRIM out of the reach of children. Patients should be advised not to exceed recommended doses. Patients should be warned that if anorexia and vomiting occur, they may be minimized by taking the drug with meals.

Concurrent administration of folinic acid is strongly recommended when used for the treatment of toxoplasmosis in all patients.

Laboratory Tests: In patients receiving high dosage, as for the treatment of toxoplasmosis, semiweekly blood counts, including platelet counts, should be performed.

Drug Interactions: Pyrimethamine may be used with sulfonamides, quinine and other antimalarials, and with other antibiotics. However, the concomitant use of other antifolic drugs, such as sulfonamides or trimethoprim-sulfamethoxazole combinations, while the patient is receiving pyrimethamine, may increase the risk of bone marrow suppression. If signs of folate deficiency develop, pyrimethamine should be discontinued. Folinic acid (leucovorin) should be administered until normal hematopoiesis is restored (see WARNINGS). Mild hepatotoxicity has been reported in some patients when lorazepam and pyrimethamine were administered concomitantly.

Carcinogenesis, Mutagenesis, Impairment of Fertility: See WARNINGS section for information on carcinogenesis.

Mutagenesis: Pyrimethamine has been shown to be nonmutagenic in the following in vitro assays: the Ames point mutation assay, the Rec assay, and the *E. coli* WP2 assay. It was positive in the L5178Y/TK +/- mouse lymphoma assay in the absence of exogenous metabolic activation.[6] Human blood lymphocytes cultured in vitro had structural chromosome aberrations induced by pyrimethamine.

In vivo, chromosomes analyzed from the bone marrow of rats dosed with pyrimethamine showed an increased number of structural and numerical aberrations.

Pregnancy: ***Teratogenic Effects:*** Pregnancy Category C. Pyrimethamine has been shown to be teratogenic in rats when given in oral doses 7 times the human dose for chemoprophylaxis of malaria or 2.5 times the human dose for treatment of toxoplasmosis. At these doses in rats, there was a significant increase in abnormalities such as cleft palate, brachygnathia, oligodactyly, and microphthalmia. Pyrimethamine has also been shown to produce terata, such as meningocele in hamsters and cleft palate in miniature pigs, when given in oral doses 170 and 5 times the human dose, respectively, for chemoprophylaxis of malaria or for treatment of toxoplasmosis.

There are no adequate and well-controlled studies in pregnant women. DARAPRIM should be used during pregnancy only if the potential benefit justifies the potential risk to the fetus.

Concurrent administration of folinic acid is strongly recommended when used for the treatment of toxoplasmosis during pregnancy.

Nursing Mothers: Pyrimethamine is excreted in human milk. Because of the potential for serious adverse reactions in nursing infants from pyrimethamine, a decision should be made whether to discontinue nursing or to discontinue the drug, taking into account the importance of the drug to the mother (see WARNINGS and PRECAUTIONS: Pregnancy).

Pediatric Use: See DOSAGE AND ADMINISTRATION section.

ADVERSE REACTIONS

Hypersensitivity reactions, occasionally severe (such as Stevens-Johnson syndrome, toxic epidermal necrolysis, erythema multiforme, and anaphylaxis), and hyperphenylalaninemia can occur particularly when pyrimethamine is administered concomitantly with a sulfonamide. With doses of pyrimethamine used for the treatment of toxoplasmosis, anorexia and vomiting may occur. Vomiting may be minimized by giving the medication with meals; it usually disappears promptly upon reduction of dosage. Doses used in toxoplasmosis may produce megaloblastic anemia, leukopenia, thrombocytopenia, pancytopenia, atrophic glossitis, hematuria, and disorders of cardiac rhythm. Hematologic effects, however, may also occur at low doses in certain individuals (see PRECAUTIONS: General).

Pulmonary eosinophilia has been reported rarely.

OVERDOSAGE

Following the ingestion of 300 mg or more of pyrimethamine, gastrointestinal and/or central nervous system signs may be present, including convulsions. The initial symptoms are usually gastrointestinal and may include abdominal pain, nausea, severe and repeated vomiting, possibly including hematemesis. Central nervous system toxicity may be manifest by initial excitability, generalized and prolonged convulsions which may be followed by respiratory depression, circulatory collapse, and death within a few hours. Neurological symptoms appear rapidly (30 minutes to 2 hours after drug ingestion), suggesting that in gross overdosage pyrimethamine has a direct toxic effect on the central nervous system.

The fatal dose is variable, with the smallest reported fatal single dose being 375 mg. There are, however, reports of pediatric patients who have recovered after taking 375 to 625 mg.

There is no specific antidote to acute pyrimethamine poisoning. In the event of overdosage, symptomatic and supportive measures should be employed. Gastric lavage is recommended and is effective if carried out very soon after drug ingestion. Parenteral diazepam may be used to control convulsions. Folinic acid should also be administered within 2 hours of drug ingestion to be most effective in counteracting the effects on the hematopoietic system (see WARNINGS). Due to the long half-life of pyrimethamine, daily monitoring of peripheral blood counts is recommended for up to several weeks after the overdose until normal hematologic values are restored.

DOSAGE AND ADMINISTRATION

For Treatment of Toxoplasmosis: The dosage of DARAPRIM for the treatment of toxoplasmosis must be carefully adjusted so as to provide maximum therapeutic effect and a minimum of side effects. At the dosage required, there is a marked variation in the tolerance to the drug. Young patients may tolerate higher doses than older individuals. Concurrent administration of folinic acid is strongly recommended in all patients.

The adult *starting* dose is 50 to 75 mg of the drug daily, together with 1 to 4 g daily of a sulfonamide of the sulfapyrimidine type, e.g., sulfadoxine. This dosage is ordinarily continued for 1 to 3 weeks, depending on the response of the patient and tolerance to therapy. The dosage may then be reduced to about one-half that previously given for each drug and continued for an additional 4 to 5 weeks.

The pediatric dosage of DARAPRIM is 1 mg/kg per day divided into two equal daily doses; after 2 to 4 days this dose may be reduced to one-half and continued for approximately 1 month. The usual pediatric sulfonamide dosage is used in conjunction with DARAPRIM.

For Treatment of Acute Malaria: DARAPRIM is NOT recommended alone in the treatment of acute malaria. Fast-acting schizonticides, such as chloroquine or quinine, are indicated for treatment of acute malaria. However, DARAPRIM at a dosage of 25 mg daily for 2 days with a sulfonamide will initiate transmission control and suppression of non-*falciparum* malaria. DARAPRIM is only recommended for patients infected in areas where susceptible plasmodia exist. Should circumstances arise wherein DARAPRIM must be used alone in semi-immune persons, the adult dosage for acute malaria is 50 mg for 2 days; children 4 through 10 years old may be given 25 mg daily for 2 days. In any event, clinical cure should be followed by the once-weekly regimen described below for chemoprophylaxis. Regimens which include suppression should be extended

Continued on next page

This product information is based on labeling in effect on June 23, 2000. For further information, contact via direct mail, phone, or web site. Medical Information, Glaxo Wellcome Inc., PO Box 13398, Research Triangle Park, NC 27709. Healthcare Professionals (Medical Information): 800-334-0089. Patients (Customer Response Center): 1-888-825-5249. Glaxo Wellcome Corporate Web Site: www.glaxowellcome.com

Daraprim—Cont.

through any characteristic periods of early recrudescence and late relapse, i.e., for at least 10 weeks in each case.

For Chemoprophylaxis of Malaria:

Adults and pediatric patients over 10 years—25 mg (1 tablet) once weekly

Children 4 through 10 years—12.5 mg (½ tablet) once weekly

Infants and children under 4 years—6.25 mg (¼ tablet) once weekly

HOW SUPPLIED

White, scored tablets containing 25 mg pyrimethamine, imprinted with "DARAPRIM" and "A3A" in bottles of 100 (NDC 0173-0201-55).

Store at 15° to 25°C (59° to 77°F) in a dry place and protect from light.

REFERENCES

1. Eyles DE, Coleman N. Synergistic effect of sulfadiazine and Daraprim against experimental toxoplasmosis in the mouse. *Antibiot Chemother.* 1953;3:483-490.
2. Jacobs L, Melton ML, Kaufman HE. Treatment of experimental ocular toxoplasmosis. *Arch Ophthalmol.* 1964;71:111-118.
3. Jim RTS, Elizaga FV. Development of chronic granulocytic leukemia in a patient treated with pyrimethamine. *Hawaii Med J.* 1977;36:173-176.
4. Sadoff L. Antimalarial drugs and Burkitt's lymphoma. *Lancet.* 1973;2:1262-1263.
5. Bahna L. Pyrimethamine. *LARC Monogr Eval Carcinog Risk Chem.* 1977;13:233-242.
6. Clive D, Johnson KO, Spector JKS, et al. Validation and characterization of the L5178Y/TK +/- mouse lymphoma mutagen assay system. *Mut Res.* 1979;59:61-108.

Manufactured by Catalytica Pharmaceuticals, Inc.
Greenville, NC 27834
for Glaxo Wellcome Inc., Research Triangle Park, NC 27709

April 1998/RL-560

Shown in Product Identification Guide, page 314

DIGIBIND® ℞
[*dij 'ə-bīnd*]
DIGOXIN IMMUNE FAB (OVINE)

DESCRIPTION

DIGIBIND, Digoxin Immune Fab (Ovine), is a sterile lyophilized powder of antigen binding fragments (Fab) derived from specific antidigoxin antibodies raised in sheep. Production of antibodies specific for digoxin involves conjugation of digoxin as a hapten to human albumin. Sheep are immunized with this material to produce antibodies specific for the antigenic determinants of the digoxin molecule. The antibody is then papain-digested and digoxin-specific Fab fragments of the antibody are isolated and purified by affinity chromatography. These antibody fragments have a molecular weight of approximately 46,200.

Each vial, which will bind approximately 0.5 mg of digoxin (or digitoxin), contains 38 mg of digoxin-specific Fab fragments derived from sheep plus 75 mg of sorbitol as a stabilizer and 28 mg of sodium chloride. The vial contains no preservatives.

DIGIBIND is administered by intravenous injection after reconstitution with Sterile Water for Injection (4 mL per vial).

CLINICAL PHARMACOLOGY

After intravenous injection of Digoxin Immune Fab (Ovine) in the baboon, digoxin-specific Fab fragments are excreted in the urine with a biological half-life of about 9 to 13 hours.[1] In humans with normal renal function, the half-life appears to be 15 to 20 hours.[2] Experimental studies in animals indicate that these antibody fragments have a large volume of distribution in the extracellular space, unlike whole antibody which distributes in a space only about twice the plasma volume.[1] Ordinarily, following administration of DIGIBIND, improvement in signs and symptoms of digitalis intoxication begins within one-half hour or less.[2,3,4,5]

The affinity of DIGIBIND for digoxin is in the range of 10^9 to 10^{11} M^{-1}, which is greater than the affinity of digoxin for (sodium, potassium) ATPase, the presumed receptor for its toxic effects. The affinity of DIGIBIND for digitoxin is about 10^8 to 10^9 M^{-1}.

DIGIBIND binds molecules of digoxin, making them unavailable for binding at their site of action on cells in the body. The Fab fragment-digoxin complex accumulates in the blood, from which it is excreted by the kidney. The net effect is to shift the equilibrium away from binding of digoxin to its receptors in the body, thereby reversing its effects.

INDICATIONS AND USAGE

DIGIBIND, Digoxin Immune Fab (Ovine), is indicated for treatment of potentially life-threatening digoxin intoxication.[3] Although designed specifically to treat life-threatening digoxin overdose, it has also been used successfully to treat life-threatening digitoxin overdose.[3] Since human experience is limited and the consequences of repeated exposures are unknown, DIGIBIND is not indicated for milder cases of digitalis toxicity.

Manifestations of life-threatening toxicity include severe ventricular arrhythmias such as ventricular tachycardia or ventricular fibrillation, or progressive bradyarrhythmias such as severe sinus bradycardia or second or third degree heart block not responsive to atropine.

Ingestion of more than 10 mg of digoxin in previously healthy adults or 4 mg of digoxin in previously healthy children, or ingestion causing steady-state serum concentrations greater than 10 ng/mL, often results in cardiac arrest. Digitalis-induced progressive elevation of the serum potassium concentration also suggests imminent cardiac arrest. If the potassium concentration exceeds 5 mEq/L in the setting of severe digitalis intoxication, therapy with DIGIBIND is indicated.

CONTRAINDICATIONS

There are no known contraindications to the use of DIGIBIND.

WARNINGS

Suicidal ingestion often involves more than one drug; thus, toxicity from other drugs should not be overlooked.

One should consider the possibility of anaphylactic, hypersensitivity, or febrile reactions. If an anaphylactoid reaction occurs, the drug infusion should be discontinued and appropriate therapy initiated using aminophylline, oxygen, volume expansion, diphenhydramine, corticosteroids, and airway management as indicated. The need for epinephrine should be balanced against its potential risk in the setting of digitalis toxicity.

Since the Fab fragment of the antibody lacks the antigenic determinants of the Fc fragment, it should pose less of an immunogenic threat to patients than does an intact immunoglobulin molecule. Patients with known allergies would be particularly at risk, as would individuals who have previously received antibodies or Fab fragments raised in sheep. Papain is used to cleave the whole antibody into Fab and Fc fragments, and traces of papain or inactivated papain residues may be present in DIGIBIND. Patients with allergies to papain, chymopapain, or other papaya extracts also may be particularly at risk.

Skin testing for allergy was performed during the clinical investigation of DIGIBIND. Only one patient developed erythema at the site of skin testing, with no accompanying wheal reaction; this individual had no adverse reaction to systemic treatment with DIGIBIND. Since allergy testing can delay urgently needed therapy, it is not routinely required before treatment of life-threatening digitalis toxicity with DIGIBIND.

Skin testing may be appropriate for high risk individuals, especially patients with known allergies or those previously treated with Digoxin Immune Fab (Ovine). The intradermal skin test can be performed by:

1. Diluting 0.1 mL of reconstituted DIGIBIND (9.5 mg/mL) in 9.9 mL sterile isotonic saline (1:100 dilution, 95 mcg/mL).
2. Injecting 0.1 mL of the 1:100 dilution (95 mcg) intradermally and observing for an urticarial wheal surrounded by a zone of erythema. The test should be read at 20 minutes.

The scratch test procedure is performed by placing one drop of a 1:100 dilution of DIGIBIND on the skin and then making a ¼-inch scratch through the drop with a sterile needle. The scratch site is inspected at 20 minutes for an urticarial wheal surrounded by erythema.

If skin testing causes a systemic reaction, a tourniquet should be applied above the site of testing and measures to treat anaphylaxis should be instituted. Further administration of DIGIBIND should be avoided unless its use is absolutely essential, in which case the patient should be pretreated with corticosteroids and diphenhydramine. The physician should be prepared to treat anaphylaxis.

PRECAUTIONS

General: Standard therapy for digitalis intoxication includes withdrawal of the drug and correction of factors that may contribute to toxicity, such as electrolyte disturbances, hypoxia, acid-base disturbances, and agents such as catecholamines. Also, treatment of arrhythmias may include judicious potassium supplements, lidocaine, phenytoin, procainamide, and/or propranolol; treatment of sinus bradycardia or atrioventricular block may involve atropine or pacemaker insertion. Massive digitalis intoxication can cause hyperkalemia; administration of potassium supplements in the setting of massive intoxication may be hazardous (see Laboratory Tests). After treatment with DIGIBIND, the serum potassium concentration may drop rapidly[2] and must be monitored frequently, especially over the first several hours after DIGIBIND is given (see Laboratory Tests).

The elimination half-life in the setting of renal failure has not been clearly defined. Patients with renal dysfunction have been successfully treated with DIGIBIND.[4] There is no evidence to suggest the time-course of therapeutic effect is any different in these patients than in patients with normal renal function, but excretion of the Fab fragment-digoxin complex from the body is probably delayed. In patients who are functionally anephric, one would anticipate failure to clear the Fab fragment-digoxin complex from the blood by glomerular filtration and renal excretion. Whether failure to eliminate the Fab fragment-digoxin complex in severe renal failure can lead to reintoxication following release of newly unbound digoxin into the blood is uncertain. Such patients should be monitored for a prolonged period for possible recurrence of digitalis toxicity.

Patients with intrinsically poor cardiac function may deteriorate from withdrawal of the inotropic action of digoxin. Studies in animals have shown that the reversal of inotropic effect is relatively gradual, occurring over hours. When needed, additional support can be provided by use of intravenous inotropes, such as dopamine or dobutamine, or vasodilators. One must be careful in using catecholamines not to aggravate digitalis toxic rhythm disturbances. Clearly, other types of digitalis glycosides should not be used in this setting.

Redigitalization should be postponed, if possible, until the Fab fragments have been eliminated from the body, which may require several days. Patients with impaired renal function may require a week or longer.

Laboratory Tests: DIGIBIND will interfere with digitalis immunoassay measurements.[6] Thus, the standard serum digoxin concentration measurement can be clinically misleading until the Fab fragment is eliminated from the body. Serum digoxin or digitoxin concentration should be obtained before administration of DIGIBIND if at all possible. These measurements may be difficult to interpret if drawn soon after the last digitalis dose, since at least 6 to 8 hours are required for equilibration of digoxin between serum and tissue. Patients should be closely monitored, including temperature, blood pressure, electrocardiogram, and potassium concentration, during and after administration of DIGIBIND. The total serum digoxin concentration may rise precipitously following administration of DIGIBIND, but this will be almost entirely bound to the Fab fragment and therefore not able to react with receptors in the body.

Potassium concentrations should be followed carefully. Severe digitalis intoxication can cause life-threatening elevation in serum potassium concentration by shifting potassium from inside to outside the cell. The elevation in serum potassium concentration can lead to increased renal excretion of potassium. Thus, these patients may have hyperkalemia with a total body deficit of potassium. When the effect of digitalis is reversed by DIGIBIND, potassium shifts back inside the cell, with a resulting decline in serum potassium concentration.[4] Hypokalemia may thus develop rapidly. For these reasons, serum potassium concentration should be monitored repeatedly, especially over the first several hours after DIGIBIND is given, and cautiously treated when necessary.

Carcinogenesis, Mutagenesis, Impairment of Fertility: There have been no long-term studies performed in animals to evaluate carcinogenic potential.

Pregnancy: Pregnancy Category C. Animal reproduction studies have not been conducted with DIGIBIND. It is also not known whether DIGIBIND can cause fetal harm when administered to a pregnant woman or can affect reproduction capacity. DIGIBIND should be given to a pregnant woman only if clearly needed.

Nursing Mothers: It is not known whether this drug is excreted in human milk. Because many drugs are excreted in human milk, caution should be exercised when DIGIBIND is administered to a nursing woman.

Pediatric Use: DIGIBIND has been successfully used in infants with no apparent adverse sequelae. As in all other circumstances, use of this drug in infants should be based on careful consideration of the benefits of the drug balanced against the potential risk involved.

ADVERSE REACTIONS

Allergic reactions to DIGIBIND have been reported rarely. Patients with a history of allergy, especially to antibiotics, appear to be at particular risk (see WARNINGS). In a few instances, low cardiac output states and congestive heart failure could have been exacerbated by withdrawal of the inotropic effects of digitalis. Hypokalemia may occur from re-activation of (sodium, potassium) ATPase (see Laboratory Tests). Patients with atrial fibrillation may develop a rapid ventricular response from withdrawal of the effects of digitalis on the atrioventricular node.[4]

DOSAGE AND ADMINISTRATION

General Guidelines: The dosage of DIGIBIND varies according to the amount of digoxin (or digitoxin) to be neutralized. The average dose used during clinical testing was 10 vials.

Dosage for Acute Ingestion of Unknown Amount: Twenty (20) vials (760 mg) of DIGIBIND is adequate to treat most life-threatening ingestions in both **adults and children.** However, in children it is important to monitor for volume overload. In general, a large dose of DIGIBIND has a faster onset of effect but may enhance the possibility of a febrile reaction. The physician may consider administering 10 vials, observing the patient's response, and following with an additional 10 vials if clinically indicated.

Dosage for Toxicity During Chronic Therapy: For adults, six vials (228 mg) usually is adequate to reverse most cases of toxicity. This dose can be used in patients who are in acute distress or for whom a serum digoxin or digitoxin concentration is not available. In infants and small children ($\leq$ 20 kg) a single vial usually should suffice.

Methods for calculating the dose of DIGIBIND required to neutralize the known or estimated amount of digoxin or digitoxin in the body are given below (see DOSAGE CALCULATION section).

When determining the dose for DIGIBIND, the following guidelines should be considered:

— Erroneous calculations may result from inaccurate estimates of the amount of digitalis ingested or absorbed or from nonsteady-state serum digitalis concentrations. Inaccurate serum digitalis concentration measurements are a possible source of error. Most serum digoxin assay kits are designed to measure values less than 5 ng/mL. Dilution of samples is required to obtain accurate measures above 5 ng/mL.

— Dosage calculations are based on a steady-state volume of distribution of approximately 5 L/kg for digoxin (0.5

Table 2: Adult Dose Estimate of DIGIBIND (in # of vials) from Steady-State Serum Digoxin Concentration

Patient Weight (kg)	Serum Digoxin Concentration (ng/mL) 1	2	4	8	12	16	20
40	0.5 V	1 V	2 V	3 V	5 V	7 V	8 V
60	0.5 V	1 V	3 V	5 V	7 V	10 V	12 V
70	1 V	2 V	3 V	6 V	9 V	11 V	14 V
80	1 V	2 V	3 V	7 V	10 V	13 V	16 V
100	1 V	2 V	4 V	8 V	12 V	16 V	20 V

V = vials

Table 3: Infants and Small Children Dose Estimates of DIGIBIND (in mg) from Steady-State Serum Digoxin Concentration

Patient Weight (kg)	Serum Digoxin Concentration (ng/mL) 1	2	4	8	12	16	20
1	0.4* mg	1* mg	1.5* mg	3* mg	5 mg	6 mg	8 mg
3	1* mg	2* mg	5 mg	9 mg	14 mg	18 mg	23 mg
5	2* mg	4 mg	8 mg	15 mg	23 mg	30 mg	38 mg
10	4 mg	8 mg	15 mg	30 mg	46 mg	61 mg	76 mg
20	8 mg	15 mg	30 mg	61 mg	91 mg	122 mg	152 mg

* Dilution of reconstituted vial to 1 mg/mL may be desirable.

L/kg for digitoxin) to convert serum digitalis concentration to the amount of digitalis in the body. The conversion is based on the principle that body load equals drug steady-state serum concentration multiplied by volume of distribution. These volumes are population averages and vary widely among individuals. Many patients may require higher doses for complete neutralization. Doses should ordinarily be rounded up to the next whole vial.

— If toxicity has not adequately reversed after several hours or appears to recur, readministration of DIGIBIND at a dose guided by clinical judgment may be required.

— Failure to respond to DIGIBIND raises the possibility that the clinical problem is not caused by digitalis intoxication. If there is no response to an adequate dose of DIGIBIND, the diagnosis of digitalis toxicity should be questioned.

DOSAGE CALCULATION

Acute Ingestion of Known Amount: Each vial of DIGIBIND contains 38 mg of purified digoxin-specific Fab fragments which will bind approximately 0.5 mg of digoxin (or digitoxin). Thus one can calculate the total number of vials required by dividing the total digitalis body load in mg by 0.5 mg/vial (see Formula 1).

For toxicity from an acute ingestion, total body load in milligrams will be approximately equal to the amount ingested in milligrams for digoxin capsules and digitoxin, or the amount ingested in milligrams multiplied by 0.80 (to account for incomplete absorption) for digoxin tablets.

Table 1 gives dosage estimates in number of vials for **adults and children** who have ingested a single large dose of digoxin and for whom the approximate number of tablets or capsules is known. The dose of DIGIBIND (in number of vials) represented in Table 1 can be approximated using the following formula:

Formula 1

$$\text{Dose (in \# of vials)} = \frac{\text{Total digitalis body load in mg}}{\text{0.5 mg of digitalis bound/vial}}$$

Table 1: Approximate Dose of DIGIBIND for Reversal of a Single Large Digoxin Overdose

Number of Digoxin Tablets or Capsules Ingested*	Dose of DIGIBIND # of Vials
25	10
50	20
75	30
100	40
150	60
200	80

* 0.25 mg tablets with 80% bioavailability or 0.2 mg LANOXICAPS® Capsules with 100% bioavailability.

Calculations Based on Steady-State Serum Digoxin Concentrations: Table 2 gives dosage estimates in number of vials for **adult patients** for whom a steady-state serum digoxin concentration is known. The dose of DIGIBIND (in number of vials) represented in Table 2 can be approximated using the following formula:

Formula 2

$$\text{Dose (in \# of vials)} = \frac{\text{(Serum digoxin concentration in ng/mL) (weight in kg)}}{100}$$

[See table 2 above]

Table 3 gives dosage estimates in milligrams **for infants and small children** based on the steady-state serum digoxin concentration. The dose of DIGIBIND represented in Table 3 can be estimated by multiplying the dose (in number of vials) calculated from Formula 2 by the amount of DIGIBIND contained in a vial (38 mg/vial) (see Formula 3). Since infants and small children can have much smaller dosage requirements, it is recommended that the 38-mg vial be reconstituted as directed and administered with a tuberculin syringe. For very small doses, a reconstituted vial can be diluted with 34 mL of sterile isotonic saline to achieve a concentration of 1 mg/mL.

Formula 3

Dose (in mg) = (Dose [in # of vials]) (38 mg/vial)

[See table 3 above]

Calculation Based on Steady-State Digitoxin Concentration: The dose of DIGIBIND for digitoxin toxicity can be approximated using the following formula:

Formula 4

$$\text{Dose (in \# of vials)} = \frac{\text{(Serum digitoxin concentration in ng/mL) (weight in kg)}}{1000}$$

If the dose based on ingested amount differs substantially from that calculated from the serum digoxin or digitoxin concentration, it may be preferable to use the higher dose.

ADMINISTRATION: The contents in each vial to be used should be dissolved with 4 mL of Sterile Water for Injection, by gentle mixing, to give a clear, colorless, approximately isosmotic solution with a protein concentration of 9.5 mg/mL. Reconstituted product should be used promptly. If it is not used immediately, it may be stored under refrigeration at 2° to 8°C (36° to 46°F) for up to 4 hours. The reconstituted product may be diluted with sterile isotonic saline to a convenient volume. Parenteral drug products should be inspected visually for particulate matter and discoloration prior to administration, whenever solution and container permit.

DIGIBIND, Digoxin Immune Fab (Ovine), is administered by the intravenous route over 30 minutes. It is recommended that it be infused through a 0.22-micron membrane filter to ensure no undissolved particulate matter is administered. If cardiac arrest is imminent, it can be given as a bolus injection.

HOW SUPPLIED

Vials containing 38 mg of purified lyophilized digoxin-specific Fab fragments. Box of 1. (NDC 0173-0230-44).

STORAGE

Refrigerate at 2° to 8°C (36° to 46°F). Unreconstituted vials can be stored at up to 30°C (86°F) for a total of 30 days.

REFERENCES

1. Smith TW, Lloyd BL, Spicer N, Haber E. Immunogenicity and kinetics of distribution and elimination of sheep digoxin-specific IgG and Fab fragments in the rabbit and baboon. *Clin Exp Immunol.* 1979; 36:384-396.
2. Smith TW, Haber E, Yeatman L, Butler VP Jr. Reversal of advanced digoxin intoxication with Fab fragments of digoxin-specific antibodies. *N Engl J Med.* 1976; 294:797-800.
3. Smith TW, Butler VP Jr, Haber E, Fozzard H, Marcus FI, Bremner WF, Schulman IC, Phillips A. Treatment of life-threatening digitalis intoxication with digoxin-specific Fab antibody fragments: Experience in 26 cases. *N Engl J Med.* 1982; 307:1357-1362.
4. Wenger TL, Butler VP Jr, Haber E, Smith TW. Treatment of 63 severely digitalis-toxic patients with digoxin-specific antibody fragments. *J Am Coll Cardiol.* 1985; 5:118A-123A.
5. Spiegel A, Marchlinski FE. Time course for reversal of digoxin toxicity with digoxin-specific antibody fragments. *Am Heart J.* 1985:109:1397-1399.
6. Gibb I, Adams PC, Parnham AJ, Jennings K. Plasma digoxin: Assay anomalies in Fab-treated patients. *Br J Clin Pharmacol.* 1983; 16:445-447.

THE WELLCOME FOUNDATION LTD., Beckenham, Kent, England BR3 3BS
U.S. License No. 129

Distributed by: Glaxo Wellcome Inc.
Research Triangle Park, NC 27709
June 1996/RL-239

Shown in Product Identification Guide, page 314

EMGEL® ℞
(erythromycin) 2%
Topical Gel

For Dermatologic Use Only—
Not for Ophthalmic Use.

DESCRIPTION

EMGEL Topical Gel contains erythromycin. Erythromycin is a macrolide antibiotic obtained from cultures of *Streptomyces erythreus.*

Erythromycin has the empirical formula $C_{37}H_{67}NO_{13}$ and a molecular weight of 733.94.

EMGEL Topical Gel contains erythromycin, USP 2% (20 mg/g) with SD 40-2 alcohol 77%, propylene glycol, and hydroxypropyl cellulose.

CLINICAL PHARMACOLOGY

The exact mechanism by which erythromycin reduces lesions of acne vulgaris is not fully known; however, the effect appears to be due in part to the antibacterial activity of the drug.

Microbiology: Erythromycin appears to inhibit protein synthesis in susceptible organisms by reversibly binding to ribosomal subunits, thereby inhibiting translocation of aminoacyl transfer-RNA and inhibiting polypeptide synthesis. Antagonism has been demonstrated between erythromycin, lincomycin, chloramphenicol, and clindamycin.

INDICATIONS AND USAGE

EMGEL Topical Gel is indicated for the topical treatment of acne vulgaris.

CONTRAINDICATIONS

EMGEL Topical Gel is contraindicated in those individuals who have shown hypersensitivity to any of its components.

PRECAUTIONS

General: For topical use only; not for ophthalmic use. Concomitant topical acne therapy should be used with caution since a possible cumulative irritancy effect may occur, especially with the use of peeling, desquamating, or abrasive agents.

Avoid contact with eyes and all mucous membranes. The use of antibiotic agents may be associated with the overgrowth of antibiotic-resistant organisms. If this occurs, discontinue use and take appropriate measures.

Carcinogenesis, Mutagenesis, Impairment of Fertility: Animal studies to evaluate carcinogenic and mutagenic potential or effects on fertility have not been performed with erythromycin.

Pregnancy Category B: There was no evidence of teratogenicity or any other adverse effect on reproduction in female rats fed erythromycin base (up to 0.25% of diet) before and during mating, during gestation, and through weaning of two successive litters. There are, however, no adequate and well-controlled studies in pregnant women. Because animal reproduction studies are not always predictive of human response, this drug should be used in pregnancy only if clearly needed. Erythromycin has been reported to cross the placental barrier in humans, but fetal plasma levels are generally low.

Nursing Mothers: It is not known whether topically applied erythromycin is excreted in human milk. A decision should be made whether to discontinue nursing or to discontinue the drug, taking into account the importance of the drug to the mother.

Pediatric Use: Safety and effectiveness in children have not been established.

ADVERSE REACTIONS

The most common adverse reaction reported with EMGEL Topical Gel was burning. The following have been reported occasionally: peeling, dryness, itching, erythema, and oiliness. Irritation of the eyes and tenderness of the skin have also been reported with the topical use of erythromycin. A generalized urticarial reaction, which was possibly related to the use of erythromycin and required systemic steroid therapy, has been reported.

DOSAGE AND ADMINISTRATION

Apply sparingly as a thin layer to affected area(s) twice a day, in the morning and the evening, after the skin has been thoroughly washed with soap and water and patted dry. The hands should be washed after application. If there has been no improvement after 6 to 8 weeks, or if the condition becomes worse, treatment should be discontinued, and the physician should be reconsulted. Spread the medication lightly rather than rubbing it in.

Continued on next page

Emgel—Cont.

HOW SUPPLIED

EMGEL 2% Topical Gel is supplied in plastic bottles containing 27 g (NDC 0173-0440-01) and 50 g (NDC 0173-0440-02).

Note: FLAMMABLE: Keep away from heat and flame. Keep bottle tightly closed. Store at room temperature.

Manufactured for Glaxo Wellcome Inc.
Research Triangle Park, NC 27709
by DPT Laboratories, Inc., San Antonio, TX 78215
September 1996/RL-358

Shown in Product Identification Guide, page 314

EPIVIR® ℞
[ep' ə-vir]
(lamivudine tablets)
Tablets

EPIVIR® ℞
(lamivudine oral solution)
Oral Solution

WARNING: LACTIC ACIDOSIS AND SEVERE HEPATOMEGALY WITH STEATOSIS, INCLUDING FATAL CASES, HAVE BEEN REPORTED WITH THE USE OF NUCLEOSIDE ANALOGUES ALONE OR IN COMBINATION, INCLUDING LAMIVUDINE AND OTHER ANTIRETROVIRALS (SEE WARNINGS).

DESCRIPTION

EPIVIR (formerly known as 3TC) is the brand name for lamivudine, a synthetic nucleoside analogue with activity against HIV. The chemical name of lamivudine is (2R,cis)-4-amino-1-(2-hydroxymethyl-1,3-oxathiolan-5-yl)-(1H)-pyrimidin-2-one. Lamivudine is the (-)enantiomer of a dideoxy analogue of cytidine. Lamivudine has also been referred to as (-)2',3'-dideoxy, 3'-thiacytidine. It has a molecular formula of $C_8H_{11}N_3O_3S$ and a molecular weight of 229.3. Lamivudine is a white to off-white crystalline solid with a solubility of approximately 70 mg/mL in water at 20°C.

EPIVIR Tablets are for oral administration. Each tablet contains 150 mg of lamivudine and the inactive ingredients magnesium stearate, microcrystalline cellulose, and sodium starch glycolate. Opadry YS-1-7706-G White is the coloring agent in the tablet coating.

EPIVIR Oral Solution is for oral administration. One milliliter (1 mL) of EPIVIR Oral Solution contains 10 mg of lamivudine (10 mg/mL) in an aqueous solution and the inactive ingredients artificial strawberry and banana flavors, citric acid (anhydrous), methylparaben, propylene glycol, propylparaben, sodium citrate (dihydrate), and sucrose.

CLINICAL PHARMACOLOGY

Mechanism of Action: Lamivudine is a synthetic nucleoside analogue. Intracellularly, lamivudine is phosphorylated to its active 5'-triphosphate metabolite, lamivudine triphosphate (L-TP). The principal mode of action of L-TP is inhibition of reverse transcriptase (RT) via DNA chain termination after incorporation of the nucleoside analogue. L-TP is a weak inhibitor of mammalian DNA polymerases α and β, and mitochondrial DNA polymerase.

Microbiology: *Antiviral Activity In Vitro:* The relationship between *in vitro* susceptibility of HIV to lamivudine and the inhibition of HIV replication in humans has not been established. *In vitro* activity of lamivudine against HIV-1 was assessed in a number of cell lines (including monocytes and fresh human peripheral blood lymphocytes) using standard susceptibility assays. IC_{50} values (50% inhibitory concentrations) were in the range of 2 nM to 15 µM. Lamivudine had anti–HIV-1 activity in all acute virus-cell infections tested. In HIV-1–infected MT-4 cells, lamivudine in combination with zidovudine had synergistic antiretroviral activity. Synergistic activity of lamivudine/zidovudine was also shown in a variable-ratio study.

Drug Resistance: Lamivudine-resistant isolates of HIV-1 have been selected *in vitro*. The resistant isolates showed reduced susceptibility to lamivudine and genotypic analysis showed that the resistance was due to specific substitution mutations in the HIV-1 reverse transcriptase at codon 184 from methionine to either isoleucine or valine. HIV-1 strains resistant to both lamivudine and zidovudine have been isolated.

Susceptibility of clinical isolates to lamivudine and zidovudine was monitored in controlled clinical trials. In patients receiving lamivudine monotherapy or combination therapy with lamivudine plus zidovudine, HIV-1 isolates from most patients became phenotypically and genotypically resistant to lamivudine within 12 weeks. In some patients harboring zidovudine-resistant virus, phenotypic sensitivity to zidovudine by 12 weeks of treatment was restored. Combination therapy with lamivudine plus zidovudine delayed the emergence of mutations conferring resistance to zidovudine.

Cross-Resistance: Cross-resistance among certain reverse transcriptase inhibitors has been observed. Cross-resistance between lamivudine and zidovudine has not been reported. In some patients treated with lamivudine alone or in combination with zidovudine, isolates have emerged with a mutation at codon 184 which confers resistance to lamivudine. In the presence of the 184 mutation, cross-resistance to didanosine and zalcitabine has been seen in some patients; the clinical significance is unknown. In some patients treated with zidovudine plus didanosine or zalcitabine, isolates resistant to multiple reverse transcriptase inhibitors, including lamivudine, have emerged.

Table 1: Pharmacokinetic Parameters (Mean ± SD) After a Single 300-mg Oral Dose of Lamivudine in 3 Groups of Adults With Varying Degrees of Renal Function (CrCl>60 mL/min, CrCl = 10-30 mL/min, and CrCl<10 mL/min)

Number of subjects	6	4	6
Creatinine clearance criterion	>60 mL/min	10-30 mL/min	<10 mL/min
Creatinine clearance (mL/min)	111 ± 14	28 ± 8	6 ± 2
C_{max} (µg/mL)	2.6 ± 0.5	3.6 ± 0.8	5.8 ± 1.2
AUC∞ (µg•h/mL)	11.0 ± 1.7	48.0 ± 19	157 ± 74
Cl/F (mL/min)	464 ± 76	114 ± 34	36 ± 11

Table 2: Number of Patients (%) With At Least One HIV Disease Progression Event or Death

Endpoint	Current Therapy (n = 460)	EPIVIR plus Current Therapy (n = 896)	EPIVIR plus a NNRTI* plus Current Therapy (n = 460)
HIV progression or death	90 (19.6%)	86 (9.6%)	41 (8.9%)
Death	27 (5.9%)	23 (2.6%)	14 (3.0%)

*An investigational non-nucleoside reverse transcriptase inhibitor not approved in the United States.

Table 3: Number of Patients (%) Reaching a Primary Clinical Endpoint (Disease Progression or Death)

Endpoint	EPIVIR plus RETROVIR (n = 236)	Didanosine (n = 235)
HIV disease progression or death (total)	15 (6.4%)	37 (15.7%)
Physical growth failure	7 (3.0%)	6 (2.6%)
Central nervous system deterioration	4 (1.7%)	12 (5.1%)
CDC Clinical Category C	2 (0.8%)	8 (3.4%)
Death	2 (0.8%)	11 (4.7%)

Pharmacokinetics in Adults: The pharmacokinetic properties of lamivudine have been studied in asymptomatic, HIV-infected adult patients after administration of single intravenous (IV) doses ranging from 0.25 to 8 mg/kg, as well as single and multiple (b.i.d. regimen) oral doses ranging from 0.25 to 10 mg/kg.

Absorption and Bioavailability: Lamivudine was rapidly absorbed after oral administration in HIV-infected patients. Absolute bioavailability in 12 adult patients was 86% ± 16% (mean ± SD) for the tablet and 87% ± 13% for the oral solution. After oral administration of 2 mg/kg twice a day to 9 adults with HIV, the peak serum lamivudine concentration (C_{max}) was 1.5 ± 0.5 µg/mL (mean ± SD). The area under the plasma concentration versus time curve (AUC) and C_{max} increased in proportion to oral dose over the range from 0.25 to 10 mg/kg.

An investigational 25-mg dosage form of lamivudine was administered orally to 12 asymptomatic, HIV-infected patients on 2 occasions, once in the fasted state and once with food (1099 kcal; 75 grams fat, 34 grams protein, 72 grams carbohydrate). Absorption of lamivudine was slower in the fed state (T_{max}: 3.2 ± 1.3 hours) compared with the fasted state (T_{max}: 0.9 ± 0.3 hours); C_{max} in the fed state was 40% ± 23% (mean ± SD) lower than in the fasted state. There was no significant difference in systemic exposure (AUC∞) in the fed and fasted states; therefore, EPIVIR Tablets and Oral Solution may be administered with or without food.

The accumulation ratio of lamivudine in HIV-positive asymptomatic adults with normal renal function has been 1.50 following 15 days of oral administration of 2 mg/kg b.i.d.

Distribution: The apparent volume of distribution after IV administration of lamivudine to 20 patients was 1.3 ± 0.4 L/kg, suggesting that lamivudine distributes into extravascular spaces. Volume of distribution was independent of dose and did not correlate with body weight.

Binding of lamivudine to human plasma proteins is low (<36%). *In vitro* studies showed that, over the concentration range of 0.1 to 100 µg/mL, the amount of lamivudine associated with erythrocytes ranged from 53% to 57% and was independent of concentration.

Metabolism: Metabolism of lamivudine is a minor route of elimination. In man, the only known metabolite of lamivudine is the trans-sulfoxide metabolite. Within 12 hours after a single oral dose of lamivudine in 6 HIV-infected adults, 5.2% ± 1.4% (mean ± SD) of the dose was excreted as the trans-sulfoxide metabolite in the urine. Serum concentrations of this metabolite have not been determined.

Elimination: The majority of lamivudine is eliminated unchanged in urine. In 20 patients given a single IV dose, renal clearance was 0.22 ± 0.06 L/hr*kg (mean ± SD), representing 71% ± 16% (mean ± SD) of total clearance of lamivudine.

In most single-dose studies in HIV-infected patients with serum sampling for 24 hours after dosing, the observed mean elimination half-life ($t_{½}$) ranged from 5 to 7 hours. Oral clearance was 0.37 ± 0.05 L/hr*kg (mean ± SD). Oral clearance and elimination half-life were independent of dose and body weight over an oral dosing range from 0.25 to 10 mg/kg.

Special Populations: *Adults With Impaired Renal Function:* The pharmacokinetic properties of lamivudine have been determined in a small group of HIV-infected adults with impaired renal function, as summarized in Table 1.

[See table 1 above]

Exposure (AUC∞), C_{max}, and half-life increased with diminishing renal function (as expressed by creatinine clearance). Apparent total oral clearance (Cl/F) of lamivudine decreased as creatinine clearance decreased. T_{max} was not significantly affected by renal function. Based on these observations, it is recommended that the dosage of lamivudine be modified in patients with renal impairment (see DOSAGE AND ADMINISTRATION). The effects of renal impairment on lamivudine pharmacokinetics in pediatric patients are not known.

Pediatric Patients: For pharmacokinetic properties of lamivudine in pediatric patients, see PRECAUTIONS: Pediatric Use.

Geriatric Patients: Lamivudine pharmacokinetics have not been specifically studied in patients over 65 years of age.

Gender: There are no significant gender differences in lamivudine pharmacokinetics.

Race: There are no significant racial differences in lamivudine pharmacokinetics.

Drug Interactions: No clinically significant alterations in lamivudine or zidovudine pharmacokinetics were observed in 12 asymptomatic HIV-infected adult patients given a single dose of zidovudine (200 mg) in combination with multiple doses of lamivudine (300 mg q 12 h).

Lamivudine and trimethoprim/sulfamethoxazole (TMP/SMX) were coadministered to 14 HIV-positive patients in a single-center, open-label, randomized, crossover study. Each patient received treatment with a single 300-mg dose of lamivudine and TMP 160 mg/SMX 800 mg once a day for 5 days with concomitant administration of lamivudine 300 mg with the fifth dose in a crossover design. Coadministration of TMP/SMX with lamivudine resulted in an increase of 44% ± 23% (mean ± SD) in lamivudine AUC∞, a decrease of 29% ± 13% in lamivudine oral clearance, and a decrease of 30% ± 36% in lamivudine renal clearance. The pharmacokinetic properties of TMP and SMX were not altered by coadministration with lamivudine.

INDICATIONS AND USAGE

EPIVIR in combination with other antiretroviral agents is indicated for the treatment of HIV infection (see Description of Clinical Studies).

Description of Clinical Studies: *Clinical Endpoint Study in Adults:* B3007 (CAESAR) was a multicenter, double-blind, placebo-controlled study comparing continued current therapy [zidovudine alone (62% of patients) or zidovudine with didanosine or zalcitabine (38% of patients)] to the addition of EPIVIR or EPIVIR plus an investigational non-nucleoside reverse transcriptase inhibitor, randomized 1:2:1. A total of 1816 HIV-infected adults with 25 to 250 CD4 cells/mm³ (median = 122 cells/mm³) at baseline were enrolled: median age was 36 years, 87% were male, 84% were nucleoside-experienced, and 16% were therapy-naive. The median duration on study was 12 months. Results are summarized in Table 2.

[See table 2 above]

Clinical Endpoint Study in Pediatric Patients: ACTG300 was a multicenter, randomized, double-blind study that provided for comparison of EPIVIR plus RETROVIR to didanosine monotherapy. A total of 471 symptomatic, HIV-infected therapy-naive (≤56 days of antiretroviral therapy) pediatric patients were enrolled in these 2 treatment arms. The median age was 2.7 years (range 6 weeks to 14 years), 58% were female, and 86% were non-Caucasian. The mean baseline CD4 cell count was 868 cells/mm³ (mean: 1060 cells/mm³ and range: 0 to 4650 cells/mm³ for patients ≤5 years of age; mean 419 cells/mm³ and range: 0 to 1555 cells/mm³ for patients >5 years of age) and the mean baseline plasma HIV RNA was 5.0 $\log_{10}$ copies/mL. The median duration on study was 10.1 months for the patients receiving EPIVIR plus RETROVIR and 9.2 months for patients receiving didanosine monotherapy. Results are summarized in Table 3.

[See table 3 above]

Surrogate Endpoint Studies: Therapy-Naive Adults: A3001 was a randomized, double-blind study comparing EPIVIR 150 mg b.i.d. plus RETROVIR 200 mg t.i.d.; EPIVIR 300 mg b.i.d. plus RETROVIR; EPIVIR 300 mg b.i.d.; and RETROVIR. Three hundred sixty-six adults enrolled: male (87%), Caucasian (61%), median age of 34 years, asymptomatic HIV infection (80%), baseline CD4 cell counts of 200 to 500 cells/mm^3 (median = 352 cells/mm^3), and mean baseline plasma HIV RNA of 4.47 ($\log_{10}$ copies/mL). B3001 was a randomized, double-blind study comparing EPIVIR 300 mg b.i.d. plus RETROVIR 200 mg t.i.d. versus RETROVIR. One hundred twenty-nine adults enrolled: male (74%), Caucasian (82%), median age of 33 years, asymptomatic HIV infection (64%), and baseline CD4 cell counts of 100 to 400 cells/mm^3 (median = 260 cells/mm^3). Mean changes in CD4 cell count and HIV RNA through 24 weeks of treatment for study A3001 are summarized in Figures 1 and 2, respectively. Mean change in CD4 cell count through 24 weeks of treatment for study B3001 is summarized in Figure 3.

Figure 1: Mean Absolute CD4 Cell Count Change (cells/mm^3) From Baseline in Study A3001

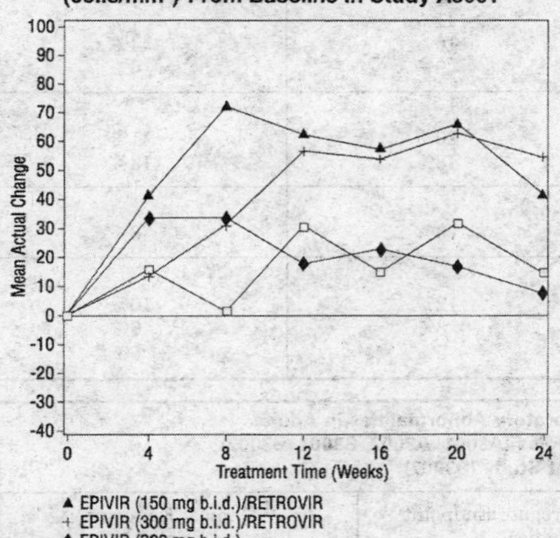

Figure 2: Mean Change From Baseline in Plasma HIV RNA ($\log_{10}$ copies/mL) in Study A3001

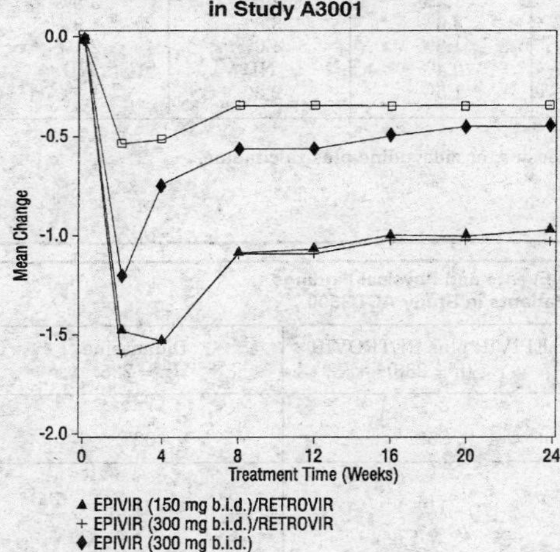

Figure 3: Mean Absolute CD4 Cell Count Change (cells/mm^3) From Baseline in Study B3001

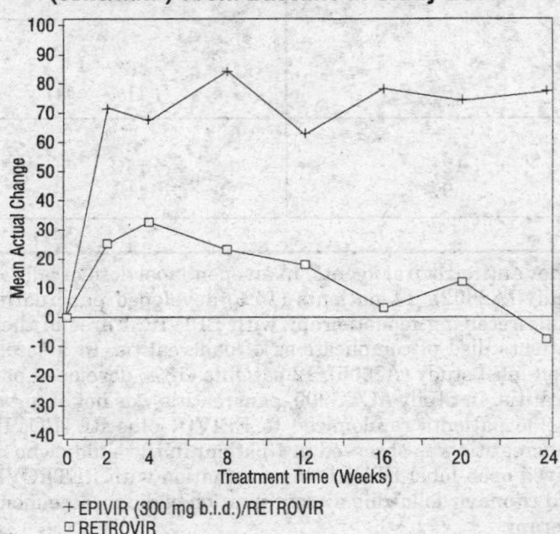

Therapy-Experienced Adults (≥24 Weeks of Prior Zidovudine Therapy): A3002 was a randomized, double-blind study comparing EPIVIR 150 mg b.i.d. plus RETROVIR 200 mg t.i.d.; EPIVIR 300 mg b.i.d. plus RETROVIR; and RETROVIR plus zalcitabine 0.75 mg t.i.d. Two hundred fifty-four adults enrolled: male (83%), Caucasian (63%), median age of 37 years, asymptomatic HIV infection (58%), median duration of prior zidovudine use of 24 months, baseline CD4 cell counts of 100 to 300 cells/mm^3 (median = 211 cells/mm^3), and mean baseline plasma HIV RNA of 4.60 ($\log_{10}$ copies/mL). B3002 was a randomized, double-blind study comparing EPIVIR 150 mg b.i.d. plus RETROVIR, EPIVIR 300 mg b.i.d. plus RETROVIR, and RETROVIR. Two hundred twenty-three adults enrolled: male (83%), Caucasian (96%), median age of 36 years, asymptomatic HIV infection (53%), median duration of prior zidovudine use of 23 months, and baseline CD4 cell counts of 100 to 400 cells/mm^3 (median = 241 cells/mm^3). Mean changes in CD4 cell count and HIV RNA through 24 weeks of treatment in study A3002 are summarized in Figures 4 and 5, respectively. Mean change in CD4 cell count through 24 weeks of treatment for study B3002 is summarized in Figure 6.

Figure 4: Mean Absolute CD4 Cell Count Change (cells/mm^3) From Baseline in Study A3002

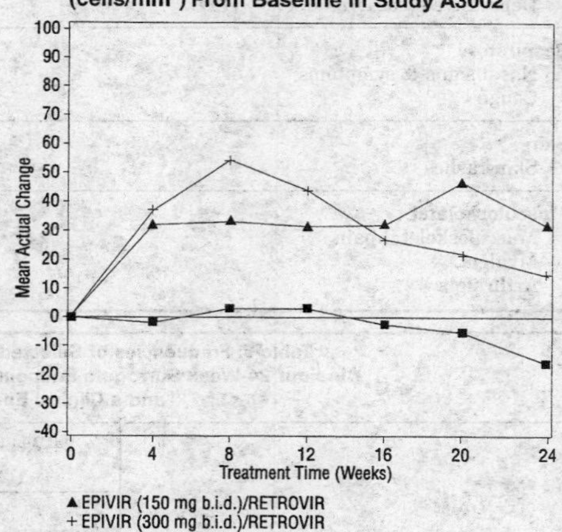

Figure 5: Mean Change From Baseline in Plasma HIV RNA ($\log_{10}$ copies/mL) in Study A3002

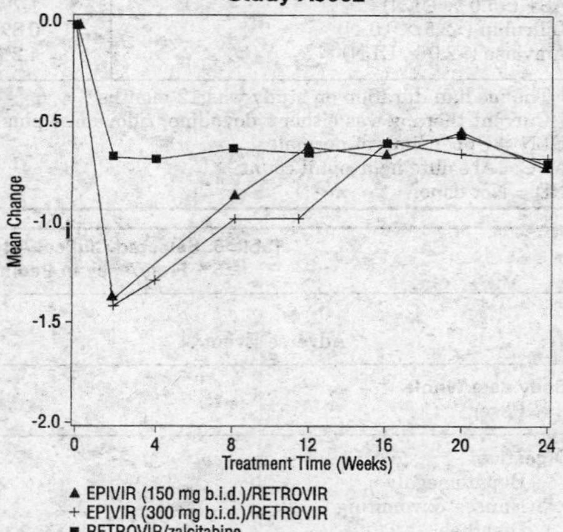

Figure 6: Mean Absolute CD4 Cell Count Change (cells/mm^3) From Baseline in Study B3002

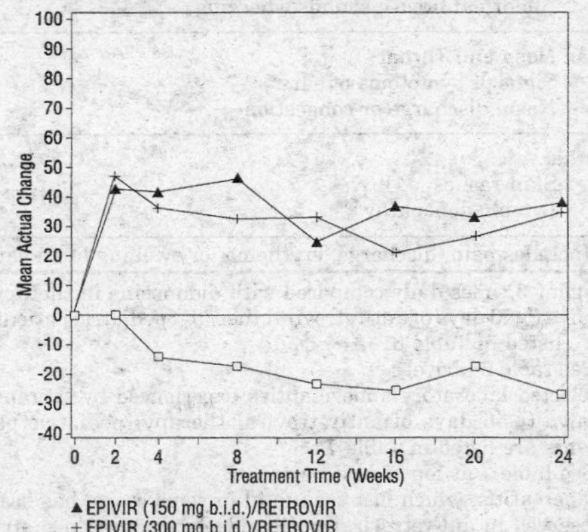

CONTRAINDICATIONS

EPIVIR Tablets and Oral Solution are contraindicated in patients with previously demonstrated clinically significant hypersensitivity to any of the components of the products.

WARNINGS

In pediatric patients with a history of prior antiretroviral nucleoside exposure, a history of pancreatitis, or other significant risk factors for the development of pancreatitis, EPIVIR should be used with caution. Treatment with EPIVIR should be stopped immediately if clinical signs, symptoms, or laboratory abnormalities suggestive of pancreatitis occur (see ADVERSE REACTIONS).

Lactic Acidosis/Severe Hepatomegaly with Steatosis: Lactic acidosis and severe hepatomegaly with steatosis, including fatal cases, have been reported with the use of nucleoside analogues alone or in combination, including lamivudine and other antiretrovirals. A majority of these cases have been in women. Obesity and prolonged nucleoside exposure may be risk factors. Particular caution should be exercised when administering EPIVIR to any patient with known risk factors for liver disease; however, cases have also been reported in patients with no known risk factors. Treatment with EPIVIR should be suspended in any patient who develops clinical or laboratory findings suggestive of lactic acidosis or pronounced hepatotoxicity (which may include hepatomegaly and steatosis even in the absence of marked transaminase elevations).

PRECAUTIONS

Patients With Impaired Renal Function: Reduction of the dosage of EPIVIR is recommended for patients with impaired renal function (see CLINICAL PHARMACOLOGY and DOSAGE AND ADMINISTRATION).

Patients With HIV and Hepatitis B Virus Coinfection: In clinical trials and postmarketing experience, some patients with HIV infection who have chronic liver disease due to hepatitis B virus infection experienced clinical or laboratory evidence of recurrent hepatitis upon discontinuation of lamivudine. Consequences may be more severe in patients with decompensated liver disease.

Information for Patients: EPIVIR is not a cure for HIV infection and patients may continue to experience illnesses associated with HIV infection, including opportunistic infections. Patients should remain under the care of a physician when using EPIVIR. Patients should be advised that the use of EPIVIR has not been shown to reduce the risk of transmission of HIV to others through sexual contact or blood contamination.

Patients should be advised that the long-term effects of EPIVIR are unknown at this time.

EPIVIR Tablets and Oral Solution are for oral ingestion only.

Patients should be advised of the importance of taking EPIVIR exactly as it is prescribed.

Parents or guardians should be advised to monitor pediatric patients for signs and symptoms of pancreatitis.

Drug Interaction: TMP 160 mg/SMX 800 mg once daily has been shown to increase lamivudine exposure (AUC). The effect of higher doses of TMP/SMX on lamivudine pharmacokinetics has not been investigated (see CLINICAL PHARMACOLOGY).

Carcinogenesis, Mutagenesis, and Impairment of Fertility: Lamivudine long-term carcinogenicity studies in mice and rats showed no evidence of carcinogenic potential at exposures up to 10 times (mice) and 58 times (rats) those observed in humans at the recommended therapeutic dose. Lamivudine was not active in a microbial mutagenicity screen or an *in vitro* cell transformation assay, but showed weak *in vitro* mutagenic activity in a cytogenetic assay using cultured human lymphocytes and in the mouse lymphoma assay. However, lamivudine showed no evidence of *in vivo* genotoxic activity in the rat at oral doses of up to 2000 mg/kg (approximately 65 times the recommended human dose based on body surface area comparisons). In a study of reproductive performance, lamivudine, administered to rats at doses up to 130 times the usual adult dose based on body surface area comparisons, revealed no evidence of impaired fertility and no effect on the survival, growth, and development to weaning of the offspring.

Pregnancy: Pregnancy Category C. Reproduction studies have been performed in rats and rabbits at orally administered doses up to approximately 130 and 60 times, respectively, the usual adult dose and have revealed no evidence of harm to the fetus due to lamivudine. Some evidence of early embryolethality was seen in the rabbit at doses similar to those produced by the usual adult dose and higher, but there was no indication of this effect in the rat at orally administered doses up to 130 times the usual adult dose. Studies in pregnant rats and rabbits showed that lamivudine is transferred to the fetus through the placenta. There are no

Continued on next page

This product information is based on labeling in effect on June 23, 2000. For further information, contact via direct mail, phone, or web site. Medical Information, Glaxo Wellcome Inc., PO Box 13398, Research Triangle Park, NC 27709. Healthcare Professionals (Medical Information): 800-334-0089. Patients (Customer Response Center): 1-888-825-5249. Glaxo Wellcome Corporate Web Site: www.glaxowellcome.com

Epivir—Cont.

adequate and well-controlled studies in pregnant women. Because animal reproductive toxicity studies are not always predictive of human response, lamivudine should be used during pregnancy only if the potential benefits outweigh the risks.

Antiretroviral Pregnancy Registry: To monitor maternal-fetal outcomes of pregnant women exposed to EPIVIR, an Antiretroviral Pregnancy Registry has been established. Physicians are encouraged to register patients by calling 1-800-258-4263.

Nursing Mothers: The Centers for Disease Control and Prevention recommend that HIV-infected mothers not breastfeed their infants to avoid risking postnatal transmission of HIV infection.

A study in which lactating rats were administered 45 mg/kg of lamivudine showed that lamivudine concentrations in milk were slightly greater than those in plasma. Although it is not known if lamivudine is excreted in human milk, there is the potential for adverse effects from lamivudine in nursing infants.

Mothers should be instructed not to breastfeed if they are receiving EPIVIR.

Pediatric Use: The safety and effectiveness of EPIVIR in combination with other antiretroviral agents have been established in pediatric patients 3 months of age and older.

In Study A2002, pharmacokinetic properties of lamivudine were assessed in a subset of 57 HIV-infected pediatric patients (age range: 4.8 months to 16 years, weight range: 5 to 66 kg) after oral and IV administration of 1, 2, 4, 8, 12, and 20 mg/kg per day. In the 9 infants and children (range: 5 months to 12 years of age) receiving oral solution 4 mg/kg twice daily (the usual recommended pediatric dose), absolute bioavailability was 66% ± 26% (mean ± SD), which was less than the 86% ± 16% (mean ± SD) observed in adults. The mechanism for the diminished absolute bioavailability of lamivudine in infants and children is unknown.

Systemic clearance decreased with increasing age in pediatric patients, as shown in Figure 7.

Figure 7: Systemic Clearance (L/hr∗kg) of Lamivudine in Relation to Age

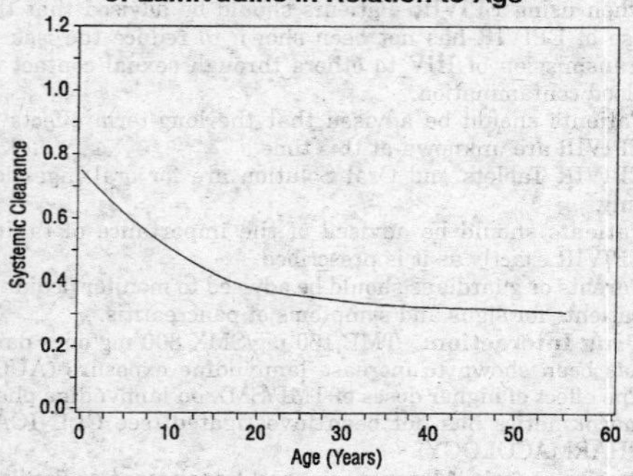

After oral administration of lamivudine 4 mg/kg twice daily to 11 pediatric patients ranging from 4 months to 14 years of age, C_{max} was 1.1 ± 0.6 µg/mL and half-life was 2.0 ± 0.6 hours. (In adults with similar blood sampling, the half-life was 3.7 ± 1 hours.) Total exposure to lamivudine, as reflected by mean AUC values, was comparable between pediatric patients receiving an 8-mg/kg-per-day dose and adults receiving a 4-mg/kg-per-day dose.

Distribution of lamivudine into cerebrospinal fluid (CSF) was assessed in 38 pediatric patients after multiple oral dosing with lamivudine. CSF samples were collected between 2 and 4 hours postdose. At the dose of 8 mg/kg per day, CSF lamivudine concentrations in 8 patients ranged from 5.6% to 30.9% (mean ± SD of 14.2% ± 7.9%) of the concentration in a simultaneous serum sample, with CSF lamivudine concentrations ranging from 0.04 to 0.3 µg/mL.

The safety and pharmacokinetic properties of EPIVIR in combination with other antiretroviral agents have not been established in pediatric patients less than 3 months of age.

See INDICATIONS AND USAGE: Description of Clinical Studies, CLINICAL PHARMACOLOGY, WARNINGS, ADVERSE REACTIONS, and DOSAGE AND ADMINISTRATION.

ADVERSE REACTIONS

Adults: Selected clinical adverse events with a ≥5% frequency during therapy with EPIVIR 150 mg b.i.d. plus RETROVIR 200 mg t.i.d. compared with zidovudine are listed in Table 4.

[See table 4 above]

Pancreatitis was observed in 3 of the 656 adult patients (<0.5%) who received EPIVIR in controlled clinical trials.

Selected laboratory abnormalities observed during therapy are summarized in Table 5.

[See table 5 above]

Pediatric Patients: Selected clinical adverse events and physical findings with a ≥5% frequency during therapy with EPIVIR 4 mg/kg twice daily plus RETROVIR 160 mg/m² 3 times daily compared with didanosine in therapy-naive (≤56 days of antiretroviral therapy) pediatric patients are listed in Table 6.

[See table 6 above]

Selected laboratory abnormalities experienced by therapy-naive (≤56 days of antiretroviral therapy) pediatric patients are listed in Table 7.

[See table 7 at top of next page]

Pancreatitis, which has been fatal in some cases, has been observed in antiretroviral nucleoside-experienced pediatric patients receiving EPIVIR alone or in combination with other antiretroviral agents. In an open-label dose-escalation study (A2002), 14 patients (14%) developed pancreatitis while receiving monotherapy with EPIVIR. Three of these patients died of complications of pancreatitis. In a second open-label study (A2005), 12 patients (18%) developed pancreatitis. In Study ACTG300, pancreatitis was not observed in 236 patients randomized to EPIVIR plus RETROVIR. Pancreatitis was observed in 1 patient in this study who received open-label EPIVIR in combination with RETROVIR and ritonavir following discontinuation of didanosine monotherapy.

Table 4: Selected Clinical Adverse Events (≥5% Frequency) In Four Controlled Clinical Trials (A3001, A3002, B3001, B3002)

Adverse Event	EPIVIR 150 mg b.i.d. plus RETROVIR (n = 251)	RETROVIR (n = 230)
Body as a whole		
Headache	35%	27%
Malaise & fatigue	27%	23%
Fever or chills	10%	12%
Digestive		
Nausea	33%	29%
Diarrhea	18%	22%
Nausea & vomiting	13%	12%
Anorexia and/or decreased appetite	10%	7%
Abdominal pain	9%	11%
Abdominal cramps	6%	3%
Dyspepsia	5%	5%
Nervous system		
Neuropathy	12%	10%
Insomnia & other sleep disorders	11%	7%
Dizziness	10%	4%
Depressive disorders	9%	4%
Respiratory		
Nasal signs & symptoms	20%	11%
Cough	18%	13%
Skin		
Skin rashes	9%	6%
Musculoskeletal		
Musculoskeletal pain	12%	10%
Myalgia	8%	6%
Arthralgia	5%	5%

Table 5: Frequencies of Selected Laboratory Abnormalities in Adults in Four 24-Week Surrogate Endpoint Studies (A3001, A3002, B3001, B3002) and a Clinical Endpoint Study (B3007)

Test (Abnormal Level)	24-Week Surrogate Endpoint Studies: EPIVIR plus RETROVIR	24-Week Surrogate Endpoint Studies: RETROVIR	Clinical Endpoint Study*: EPVIR plus Current Therapy	Clinical Endpoint Study*: Placebo plus Current Therapy†
Neutropenia (ANC<750/mm³)	7.2%	5.4%	15%	13%
Anemia (Hgb<8.0 g/dL)	2.9%	1.8%	2.2%	3.4%
Thrombocytopenia (platelets<50,000/mm³)	0.4%	1.3%	2.8%	3.8%
ALT (>5.0 × ULN)	3.7%	3.6%	3.8%	1.9%
AST (>5.0 × ULN)	1.7%	1.8%	4.0%	2.1%
Bilirubin (>2.5 × ULN)	0.8%	0.4%	ND	ND
Amylase (>2.0 × ULN)	4.2%	1.5%	2.2%	1.1%

* The median duration on study was 12 months.
† Current therapy was either zidovudine, zidovudine plus didanosine, or zidovudine plus zalcitabine.
ULN = Upper limit of normal.
ANC = Absolute neutrophil count.
ND = Not done.

Table 6: Selected Clinical Adverse Events and Physical Findings (≥5% Frequency in Pediatric Patients in Study ACTG300

Adverse Event	EPIVIR plus RETROVIR (n = 236)	Didanosine (n = 235)
Body as a whole		
Fever	25%	32%
Digestive		
Hepatomegaly	11%	11%
Nausea & vomiting	8%	7%
Diarrhea	8%	6%
Stomatitis	6%	12%
Splenomegaly	5%	8%
Respiratory		
Cough	15%	18%
Abnormal breath sounds/wheezing	7%	9%
Ear, Nose and Throat		
Signs or symptoms of ears*	7%	6%
Nasal discharge or congestion	8%	11%
Other		
Skin rashes	12%	14%
Lymphadenopathy	9%	11%

*Includes pain, discharge, erythema, or swelling of an ear.

Table 7: Frequencies of Selected Laboratory Abnormalities in Pediatric Patients in Study ACTG300

Test (Abnormal Level)	EPIVIR plus RETROVIR	Didanosine
Neutropenia (ANC<400/mm^3)	8%	3%
Anemia (Hgb<7.0 g/dL)	4%	2%
Thrombocytopenia (platelets<50,000/mm^3)	1%	3%
ALT (>10 × ULN)	1%	3%
AST (>10 × ULN)	2%	4%
Lipase (>2.5 × ULN)	3%	3%
Total Amylase (>2.5 × ULN)	3%	3%

ULN = Upper limit of normal.
ANC = Absolute neutrophil count.

Paresthesias and peripheral neuropathies were reported in 15 patients (15%) in Study A2002, 6 patients (9%) in Study A2005, and 2 patients (<1%) in Study ACTG300.

Observed During Clinical Practice: In addition to adverse events reported from clinical trials, the following events have been identified during post-approval use of EPIVIR. Because they are reported voluntarily from a population of unknown size, estimates of frequency cannot be made. These events have been chosen for inclusion due to a combination of their seriousness, frequency of reporting, or potential causal connection to EPIVIR.

Endocrine and Metabolic: Hyperglycemia.

General: Anaphylaxis, weakness.

Hepatobiliary Tract and Pancreas: Lactic acidosis and hepatic steatosis (see WARNINGS).

Musculoskeletal: Muscle weakness, CPK elevation, rhabdomyolysis.

Nervous: Peripheral neuropathy.

Skin: Alopecia, rash, pruritus, urticaria.

OVERDOSAGE

There is no known antidote for EPIVIR. One case of an adult ingesting 6 g of EPIVIR was reported; there were no clinical signs or symptoms noted and hematologic tests remained normal. Two cases of pediatric overdose were reported in ACTG300. One case was a single dose of 7 mg/kg of EPIVIR; the second case involved use of 5 mg/kg of EPIVIR twice daily for 30 days. There were no clinical signs or symptoms noted in either case. It is not known whether lamivudine can be removed by peritoneal dialysis or hemodialysis.

DOSAGE AND ADMINISTRATION

Adults: The recommended oral dose of EPIVIR for adults is 150 mg twice daily, administered in combination with other antiretroviral agents.

Pediatric Patients: The recommended oral dose of EPIVIR for pediatric patients 3 months up to 16 years of age is 4 mg/kg twice daily (up to a maximum of 150 mg twice a day), administered in combination with other antiretroviral agents.

Dose Adjustment: It is recommended that doses of EPIVIR be adjusted in accordance with renal function (see Table 8). (See CLINICAL PHARMACOLOGY section.)

Table 8: Adjustment of Dosage of EPIVIR in Adults and Adolescents in Accordance With Creatinine Clearance

Creatinine Clearance (mL/min)	Recommended Dosage of EPIVIR
≥50	150 mg twice daily
30-49	150 mg once daily
15-29	150 mg first dose, then 100 mg once daily
5-14	150 mg first dose, then 50 mg once daily
<5	50 mg first dose, then 25 mg once daily

Insufficient data are available to recommend a dosage of EPIVIR in patients undergoing dialysis. Although there are insufficient data to recommend a specific dose adjustment of EPIVIR in pediatric patients with renal impairment, a reduction in the dose and/or an increase in the dosing interval should be considered.

HOW SUPPLIED

EPIVIR Tablets, 150 mg, are white, modified diamond-shaped, film-coated tablets imprinted with "150" on one side and "GX CJ7" on the reverse side. They are available in bottles of 60 tablets (NDC 0173-0470-01) with child-resistant closures.

Store in tightly closed bottles at 25°C (77°F) (see USP Controlled Room Temperature).

EPIVIR Oral Solution, a clear, colorless to pale yellow, strawberry-banana flavored liquid, contains 10 mg of lamivudine in each 1 mL in plastic bottles of 240 mL (NDC 0173-0471-00) with child-resistant closures. This product does not require reconstitution.

Store in tightly closed bottles at 25°C (77°F) (see USP Controlled Room Temperature).

Glaxo Wellcome Inc., Research Triangle Park, NC 27709
Manufactured under agreement from
BioChem Pharma Inc., 275 Armand Frappier Blvd.
Laval, Quebec, Canada H7V 4A7
US Patent No. 5,047,407

December 1999/RL-784

Shown in Product Identification Guide, page 314

EPIVIR-HBV® Tablets ℞

[ep 'ə-vir]
(lamivudine)

EPIVIR-HBV® Oral Solution

(lamivudine)

WARNING: LACTIC ACIDOSIS AND SEVERE HEPATOMEGALY WITH STEATOSIS, INCLUDING FATAL CASES, HAVE BEEN REPORTED WITH THE USE OF NUCLEOSIDE ANALOGUES ALONE OR IN COMBINATION, INCLUDING LAMIVUDINE AND OTHER ANTIRETROVIRALS (SEE WARNINGS).

HUMAN IMMUNODEFICIENCY VIRUS (HIV) COUNSELING AND TESTING SHOULD BE OFFERED TO ALL PATIENTS BEFORE BEGINNING EPIVIR-HBV AND PERIODICALLY DURING TREATMENT (SEE WARNINGS), BECAUSE EPIVIR-HBV TABLETS AND ORAL SOLUTION CONTAIN A LOWER DOSE OF THE SAME ACTIVE INGREDIENT (LAMIVUDINE) AS EPIVIR® TABLETS AND ORAL SOLUTION USED TO TREAT HIV INFECTION. IF TREATMENT WITH EPIVIR-HBV IS PRESCRIBED FOR CHRONIC HEPATITIS B FOR A PATIENT WITH UNRECOGNIZED OR UNTREATED HIV INFECTION, RAPID EMERGENCE OF HIV RESISTANCE IS LIKELY BECAUSE OF SUBTHERAPEUTIC DOSE AND INAPPROPRIATE MONOTHERAPY.

DESCRIPTION

EPIVIR-HBV is a brand name for lamivudine, a synthetic nucleoside analogue with activity against HBV and HIV. Lamivudine was initially developed for the treatment of HIV infection as EPIVIR®. Please see the complete prescribing information for EPIVIR Tablets and Oral Solution for additional information. The chemical name of lamivudine is (2R,cis)-4-amino-1-(2-hydroxymethyl-1,3-oxathiolan-5-yl)-(1H)-pyrimidin-2-one. Lamivudine is the (-)enantiomer of a dideoxy analogue of cytidine. Lamivudine has also been referred to as (-)2′,3′-dideoxy, 3′-thiacytidine. It has a molecular formula of $C_8H_{11}N_3O_3S$ and a molecular weight of 229.3.

Lamivudine is a white to off-white crystalline solid with a solubility of approximately 70 mg/mL in water at 20°.

EPIVIR-HBV Tablets are for oral administration. Each tablet contains 100 mg of lamivudine and the inactive ingredients magnesium stearate, microcrystalline cellulose, and sodium starch glycolate. Opadry YS-1-17307-A Butterscotch is the coloring agent in the tablet coating.

EPIVIR-HBV Oral Solution is for oral administration. One milliliter (1 mL) of EPIVIR-HBV Oral Solution contains 5 mg of lamivudine (5 mg/mL) in an aqueous solution and the inactive ingredients artificial strawberry and banana flavors, citric acid (anhydrous), methylparaben, propylene glycol, propylparaben, sodium citrate (dihydrate), and sucrose.

MICROBIOLOGY

Mechanism of Action: Lamivudine is a synthetic nucleoside analogue. Lamivudine is phosphorylated intracellularly to lamivudine triphosphate, L-TP. Incorporation of the monophosphate form into viral DNA by hepatitis B virus (HBV) polymerase results in DNA chain termination. L-TP also inhibits the RNA- and DNA-dependent DNA polymerase activities of HIV-1 reverse transcriptase (RT). L-TP is a weak inhibitor of mammalian alpha-, beta-, and gamma-DNA polymerases.

Antiviral Activity: ***In Vitro:*** *In vitro* activity of lamivudine against HBV was assessed in HBV DNA-transfected 2.2.15 cells, HB611 cells, and infected human primary hepatocytes. IC_{50} values (the concentration of drug needed to reduce the level of extracellular HBV DNA by 50%) varied from 0.01 μM (2.3 ng/mL) to 5.6 μM (1.3 μg/mL) depending upon the duration of exposure of cells to lamivudine, the cell model system, and the protocol used. *In vitro* activity of lamivudine against HIV-1 has been previously demonstrated.

In Vivo: Activity of lamivudine against hepatitis B viruses was evaluated in two animal models. In ducklings chronically infected with duck hepatitis B virus (DHBV), lamivudine administration for 14 days resulted in a decrease of serum DHBV DNA. Increasing levels of serum DHBV DNA were observed within 4 days after cessation of treatment.

In two chimpanzees chronically infected with HBV, lamivudine administration for 28 days resulted in a decrease in serum HBV DNA in one animal and a modest decrease in e antigen (HBeAg) levels in both animals. Treatment of four chimpanzees with escalating doses of lamivudine from 0.1 to 6.0 mg/kg twice daily resulted in a decrease in serum HBV DNA. Within 14 days after cessation of therapy, three chimpanzees tested all showed an increase in HBV DNA serum levels.

Drug Resistance: ***Preclinical Studies: HBV:*** Genotypic analysis of viral isolates obtained from patients who show renewed evidence of replication of HBV while receiving lamivudine suggests that a reduction in sensitivity of HBV to lamivudine is associated with mutations resulting in a methionine to valine or isoleucine substitution in the YMDD motif of the catalytic domain of HBV polymerase (position 552) and a leucine to methionine substitution at position 528. HBV recombinants containing the YMDD mutations are less replication-competent than wild-type HBV *in vitro*. It is not known whether other HBV mutations may be associated with reduced lamivudine susceptibility *in vitro*.

HIV: Lamivudine-resistant isolates of HIV-1 have been selected *in vitro*.

Clinical Studies: HBV: In four controlled clinical trials, YMDD-mutant HBV were detected in 81 of 335 patients receiving lamivudine 100 mg once daily for 52 weeks. The prevalence of YMDD mutations was less than 10% in each of these trials for patients studied at 24 weeks and increased to an average of 24% (range in four studies: 16% to 32%) at 52 weeks. In limited data from a long-term follow-up trial in patients who continued 100 mg/day lamivudine after one of these studies, YMDD mutations further increased from 16% at 1 year to 42% at 2 years. Mutant viruses were associated with evidence of diminished treatment response at 52 weeks relative to lamivudine-treated patients without evidence of YMDD mutations (see PRECAUTIONS). The long-term clinical significance of YMDD-mutant HBV is not known.

HIV: In studies of HIV-1-infected patients who received lamivudine monotherapy or combination therapy with lamivudine plus zidovudine for at least 12 weeks, HIV-1 isolates with reduced *in vitro* susceptibility to lamivudine were detected in most patients (see WARNINGS).

CLINICAL PHARMACOLOGY

Pharmacokinetics in Adults: The pharmacokinetic properties of lamivudine have been studied as single and multiple oral doses ranging from 5 to 600 mg per day administered to HBV-infected patients.

The pharmacokinetic properties of lamivudine have also been studied in asymptomatic, HIV-infected adult patients after administration of single intravenous (IV) doses ranging from 0.25 to 8 mg/kg, as well as single and multiple (twice-daily regimen) oral doses ranging from 0.25 to 10 mg/kg.

Absorption and Bioavailability: Lamivudine was rapidly absorbed after oral administration in HBV-infected patients and in healthy subjects. Following single oral doses of 100 mg, the peak serum lamivudine concentration (C_{max}) in HBV-infected patients (steady state) and healthy subjects (single dose) was 1.28 ± 0.56 μg/mL and 1.05 ± 0.32 μg/mL (mean ± SD), respectively, which occurred between 0.5 and 2 hours after administration. The area under the plasma concentration versus time curve ($AUC_{[0-24\ h]}$) following 100 mg lamivudine oral single and repeated daily doses to steady state was 4.3 ± 1.4 (mean ± SD) and 4.7 ± 1.7 μg•h/mL, respectively. The relative bioavailability of the tablet and solution were then demonstrated in healthy subjects. Although the solution demonstrated a slightly higher peak serum concentration (C_{max}), there was no significant difference in systemic exposure (AUC_{∞}) between the solution and the tablet. Therefore, the solution and the tablet may be used interchangeably.

After oral administration of lamivudine once daily to HBV-infected adults, the AUC and peak serum levels (C_{max}) increased in proportion to dose over the range from 5 mg to 600 mg once daily.

The 100-mg tablet was administered orally to 24 healthy subjects on two occasions, once in the fasted state and once with food (standard meal: 967 kcal; 67 grams fat, 33 grams protein, 58 grams carbohydrate). There was no significant difference in systemic exposure (AUC_{∞}) in the fed and fasted states; therefore, EPIVIR-HBV Tablets and Oral Solution may be administered with or without food.

Lamivudine was rapidly absorbed after oral administration in HIV-infected patients. Absolute bioavailability in 12 adult patients was 86% ± 16% (mean ± SD) for the 150-mg tablet and 87% ± 13% for the 10-mg/mL oral solution.

Distribution: The apparent volume of distribution after IV administration of lamivudine to 20 asymptomatic HIV-infected patients was 1.3 ± 0.4 L/kg, suggesting that lamivudine distributes into extravascular spaces. Volume of distribution was independent of dose and did not correlate with body weight.

Binding of lamivudine to human plasma proteins is low (<36%) and independent of dose. *In vitro* studies showed that, over the concentration range of 0.1 to 100 μg/mL, the amount of lamivudine associated with erythrocytes ranged from 53% to 57% and was independent of concentration.

Continued on next page

This product information is based on labeling in effect on June 23, 2000. For further information, contact via direct mail, phone, or web site. Medical Information, Glaxo Wellcome Inc., PO Box 13398, Research Triangle Park, NC 27709. Healthcare Professionals (Medical Information): 800-334-0089. Patients (Customer Response Center): 1-888-825-5249. Glaxo Wellcome Corporate Web Site: www.glaxowellcome.com

Epivir-HBV—Cont.

Metabolism: Metabolism of lamivudine is a minor route of elimination. In man, the only known metabolite of lamivudine is the trans-sulfoxide metabolite. In nine healthy subjects receiving 300 mg of lamivudine as single oral doses, a total of 4.2% (range 1.5% to 7.5%) of the dose was excreted as the trans-sulfoxide metabolite in the urine, the majority of which was excreted in the first 12 hours.
Serum concentrations of the trans-sulfoxide metabolite have not been determined.
Elimination: The majority of lamivudine is eliminated unchanged in urine. In nine healthy subjects given a single 300-mg oral dose of lamivudine, renal clearance was 199.7 ± 56.9 mL/min (mean ± SD). In 20 HIV-infected patients given a single IV dose, renal clearance was 280.4 ± 75.2 mL/min (mean ± SD), representing 71% ± 16% (mean ± SD) of total clearance of lamivudine.
In most single-dose studies in HIV- or HBV-infected patients or healthy subjects with serum sampling for 24 hours after dosing, the observed mean elimination half-life ($t_{½}$) ranged from 5 to 7 hours. In HIV-infected patients, total clearance was 398.5 ± 69.1 mL/min (mean ± SD). Oral clearance and elimination half-life were independent of dose and body weight over an oral dosing range from 0.25 to 10 mg/kg.
Special Populations: ***Adults With Impaired Renal Function:*** The pharmacokinetic properties of lamivudine have been determined in healthy subjects and in subjects with impaired renal function, with and without hemodialysis (Table 1):
[See table 1 at right]
Exposure (AUC_∞), C_{max}, and half-life increased with diminishing renal function (as expressed by creatinine clearance). Apparent total oral clearance (Cl/F) of lamivudine decreased as creatinine clearance decreased. T_{max} was not significantly affected by renal function. Based on these observations, it is recommended that the dosage of lamivudine be modified in patients with renal impairment (see DOSAGE AND ADMINISTRATION).
Hemodialysis increases lamivudine clearance from a mean of 64 to 88 mL/min; however, the length of time of hemodialysis (4 hours) was insufficient to significantly alter mean lamivudine exposure after a single-dose administration. Therefore, it is recommended, following correction of dose for creatinine clearance, that no additional dose modification is made after routine hemodialysis.
It is not known whether lamivudine can be removed by peritoneal dialysis or continuous (24-hour) hemodialysis.
The effect of renal impairment on lamivudine pharmacokinetics in pediatric patients with chronic hepatitis B is not known.
Adults With Impaired Hepatic Function: The pharmacokinetic properties of lamivudine have been determined in adults with impaired hepatic function (Table 2). Patients were stratified by severity of hepatic functional impairment.
[See table 2 at right]
Pharmacokinetic parameters were not altered by diminishing hepatic function. Therefore, no dose adjustment for lamivudine is required for patients with impaired hepatic function. Safety and efficacy of EPIVIR-HBV have not been established in the presence of decompensated liver disease (see PRECAUTIONS)
Post-Hepatic Transplant: Fourteen HBV-infected patients received liver transplant following lamivudine therapy and completed pharmacokinetic assessments at enrollment, 2 weeks after 100-mg once-daily dosing (pre-transplant), and 3 months following transplant; there were no significant differences in pharmacokinetic parameters. The overall exposure of lamivudine is primarily affected by renal dysfunction; consequently, transplant patients with reduced renal function had generally higher exposure than patients with normal renal function. Safety and efficacy of EPIVIR-HBV have not been established in this population (see PRECAUTIONS).
Gender: There are no significant gender differences in lamivudine pharmacokinetics.
Race: There are no significant racial differences in lamivudine pharmacokinetics.
Drug Interactions: Multiple doses of lamivudine and a single dose of interferon were coadministered to 19 healthy male subjects in a pharmacokinetics study. Results indicated a small (10%) reduction in lamivudine AUC, but no change in interferon pharmacokinetic parameters when the two drugs were given in combination. All other pharmacokinetic parameters (C_{max}, T_{max}, and $t_{½}$) were unchanged. There was no significant pharmacokinetic interaction between lamivudine and interferon alfa in this study.
Lamivudine and zidovudine were coadministered to 12 asymptomatic HIV-positive adult patients in a single-center, open-label, randomized, crossover study. No significant differences were observed in AUC_∞ or total clearance for lamivudine or zidovudine when the two drugs were administered together. Coadministration of lamivudine with zidovudine resulted in an increase of 39% ± 62% (mean ± SD) in C_{max} of zidovudine.
Lamivudine and trimethoprim/sulfamethoxazole (TMP/SMX) were coadministered to 14 HIV-positive patients in a single-center, open-label, randomized, crossover study. Each patient received treatment with a single 300-mg dose of lamivudine and TMP 160 mg/SMX 800 mg once a day for 5 days with concomitant administration of lamivudine 300 mg with the fifth dose in a crossover design. Coadministration of TMP/SMX with lamivudine resulted in an increase of 44% ± 23% (mean ± SD) in lamivudine AUC_∞, a decrease of 29% ± 13% in lamivudine oral clearance, and a decrease of 30% ± 36% in lamivudine renal clearance. The pharmacokinetic properties of TMP and SMX were not altered by coadministration with lamivudine (see PRECAUTIONS: Drug Interactions).

Table 1: Pharmacokinetic Parameters (Mean ± SD) Dose-Normalized to a Single 100-mg Oral Dose of Lamivudine in Patients With Varying Degrees of Renal Function

Parameter	Creatinine Clearance Criterion (Number of Subjects) ≥80 mL/min (n = 9)	20–59 mL/min (n = 8)	<20 mL/min (n = 6)
Creatinine clearance (mL/min)	97 (range 82–117)	39 (range 25–49)	15 (range 13–19)
C_{max} (µg/mL)	1.31 ± 0.35	1.85 ± 0.40	1.55 ± 0.31
AUC_∞ (µg•h/mL)	5.28 ± 1.01	14.67 ± 3.74	27.33 ± 6.56
Cl/F (mL/min)	326.4 ± 63.8	120.1 ± 29.5	64.5 ± 18.3

Table 2: Pharmacokinetic Parameters (Mean ± SD) Dose-Normalized to a Single 100-mg Dose of Lamivudine in Three Groups of Subjects With Normal or Impaired Hepatic Function

Parameter	Normal (n = 8)	Impairment* Moderate (n = 8)	Severe (n = 8)
C_{max} (µg/mL)	0.92 ± 0.31	1.06 ± 0.58	1.08 ± 0.27
AUC_∞ (µg•h/mL)	3.96 ± 0.58	3.97 ± 1.36	4.30 ± 0.63
T_{max} (h)	1.3 ± 0.8	1.4 ± 0.8	1.4 ± 1.2
Cl/F (mL/min)	424.7 ± 61.9	456.9 ± 129.8	395.2 ± 51.8
Clr (mL/min)	279.2 ± 79.2	323.5 ± 100.9	216.1 ± 58.0

*Hepatic impairment assessed by aminopyrine breath test.

Table 3: Histologic Response at Week 52 Among Patients Receiving EPIVIR-HBV 100 mg Once Daily or Placebo

Assessment	Study 1 EPIVIR-HBV (n = 62)	Study 1 Placebo (n = 63)	Study 2 EPIVIR-HBV (n = 131)	Study 2 Placebo (n = 68)	Study 3 EPIVIR-HBV (n = 110)	Study 3 Placebo (n = 54)
Improvement*	55%	25%	56%	26%	56%	26%
No Improvement	27%	59%	36%	62%	25%	54%
Missing Data	18%	16%	8%	12%	19%	20%

*Improvement was defined as a ≥2-point decrease in the Knodell Histologic Activity Index (HAI)[1] at Week 52 compared with pretreatment HAI. Patients with missing data at baseline were excluded.

Table 4: HBeAg Seroconversion* at Week 52 Among Patients Receiving EPIVIR-HBV 100 mg Once Daily or Placebo

Seroconversion	Study 1 EPIVIR-HBV (n = 63)	Study 1 Placebo (n = 69)	Study 2 EPIVIR-HBV (n = 140)	Study 2 Placebo (n = 70)	Study 3 EPIVIR-HBV (n = 108)	Study 3 Placebo (n = 53)
Responder	17%	6%	16%	4%	15%	13%
Nonresponder	67%	78%	80%	91%	69%	68%
Missing Data	16%	16%	4%	4%	17%	19%

*Three-component seroconversion was defined as Week 52 values showing loss of HBeAg, gain of HBeAb, and reduction of HBV DNA to below the solution hybridization assay limit. Subjects with negative baseline HBeAg or HBV DNA assay were excluded from the analysis.

INDICATIONS AND USAGE

EPIVIR-HBV is indicated for the treatment of chronic hepatitis B associated with evidence of hepatitis B viral replication and active liver inflammation. This indication is based on 1-year histologic and serologic responses in patients with compensated chronic hepatitis B as described below.
Description of Clinical Studies: The safety and efficacy of EPIVIR-HBV were evaluated in four controlled studies in 967 patients with compensated chronic hepatitis B. All patients were 16 years of age or older and had chronic hepatitis B virus infection (serum HBsAg positive for at least 6 months) accompanied by evidence of HBV replication (serum HBeAg positive and positive for serum HBV DNA, as measured by a research solution-hybridization assay) and persistently elevated ALT levels and/or chronic inflammation on liver biopsy compatible with a diagnosis of chronic viral hepatitis. Three of these studies provided comparisons of EPIVIR-HBV 100 mg once daily versus placebo, and results of these comparisons are summarized below.

- Study 1 was a randomized, double-blind study of EPIVIR-HBV 100 mg once daily versus placebo for 52 weeks, followed by a 16-week no-treatment period, in treatment-naive US patients.
- Study 2 was a randomized, double-blind, three-arm study that compared EPIVIR-HBV 25 mg once daily versus EPIVIR-HBV 100 mg once daily versus placebo for 52 weeks in Asian patients.
- Study 3 was a randomized, partially-blind, three-arm study conducted primarily in North America and Europe in patients who had ongoing evidence of active chronic hepatitis B despite previous treatment with interferon alfa. The study compared EPIVIR-HBV 100 mg once daily for 52 weeks, followed by either EPIVIR-HBV 100 mg or matching placebo once daily for 16 weeks (Arm 1), versus placebo once daily for 68 weeks (Arm 2). (A third arm using a combination of interferon and lamivudine is not presented here because there was not sufficient information to evaluate this regimen.)

Principal endpoint comparisons for the histologic and serologic outcomes in lamivudine (100 mg daily) and placebo recipients in placebo-controlled studies are shown in the following tables.
[See table 3 above]
[See table 4 above]
Normalization of serum ALT levels was more frequent with lamivudine treatment compared with placebo in Studies 1-3.
The majority of lamivudine-treated patients showed a decrease of HBV DNA to below the assay limit early in the course of therapy. However, reappearance of assay-detectable HBV DNA during lamivudine treatment was observed in approximately one third of patients after this initial response.

CONTRAINDICATIONS

EPIVIR-HBV Tablets and EPIVIR-HBV Oral Solution are contraindicated in patients with previously demonstrated clinically significant hypersensitivity to any of the components of the products.

WARNINGS

Lactic Acidosis/Severe Hepatomegaly with Steatosis: Lactic acidosis and severe hepatomegaly with steatosis, including fatal cases, have been reported with the use of nucleoside analogues alone or in combination, including lamivudine and other antiretrovirals. A majority of these cases have been in women. Obesity and prolonged nucleoside exposure may be risk factors. Most of these reports have described patients receiving nucleoside analogues for treatment of HIV infection, but there have been reports of lactic acidosis in patients receiving lamivudine for hepatitis B. Particular caution should be exercised when administering EPIVIR or EPIVIR-HBV to any patient with known risk factors for liver disease; however, cases have also been reported in patients with no known risk factors. Treatment with EPIVIR or EPIVIR-HBV should be suspended in any patient who develops clinical or laboratory findings suggestive of lactic acidosis or pronounced hepatotoxicity (which may include hepatomegaly and steatosis even in the absence of marked transaminase elevations).

Important Differences Between Lamivudine-Containing Products, HIV Testing, and Risk of Emergence of Resistant HIV: EPIVIR-HBV Tablets and Oral Solution contain a lower dose of the same active ingredient (lamivudine) as EPIVIR Tablets and Oral Solution (and COMBIVIR® [lamivudine/zidovudine] Tablets) used to treat HIV infection. The formulation and dosage of lamivudine in EPIVIR-HBV are not appropriate for patients dually infected with HBV and HIV. If a decision is made to administer lamivudine to such patients, the higher dosage indicated for HIV therapy should be used as part of an appropriate combination regimen, and the prescribing information for EPIVIR or COMBIVIR as well as for EPIVIR-HBV should be consulted. HIV counseling and testing should be offered to all patients before beginning EPIVIR-HBV and periodically during treatment because of the risk of rapid emergence of resistant HIV and limitation of treatment options if EPIVIR-HBV is prescribed to treat chronic hepatitis B in a patient who has unrecognized or untreated HIV infection or acquires HIV infection during treatment.

Posttreatment Exacerbations of Hepatitis: Clinical and laboratory evidence of exacerbations of hepatitis have occurred after discontinuation of EPIVIR-HBV (these have been primarily detected by serum ALT elevations, in addition to the re-emergence of HBV DNA commonly observed after stopping treatment; see Table 7 for more information regarding frequency of posttreatment ALT elevations). Although most events appear to have been self-limited, fatalities have been reported in some cases. The causal relationship to discontinuation of lamivudine treatment is unknown. Patients should be closely monitored with both clinical and laboratory follow-up for at least several months after stopping treatment. There is insufficient evidence to determine whether re-initiation of therapy alters the course of posttreatment exacerbations of hepatitis.

Pancreatitis: Pancreatitis has been reported in patients receiving lamivudine, particularly in HIV-infected pediatric patients with prior nucleoside exposure.

PRECAUTIONS

General: Patients should be assessed before beginning treatment with EPIVIR-HBV by a physician experienced in the management of chronic hepatitis B.

Emergence of Resistance-Associated HBV Mutations: In controlled clinical trials, YMDD-mutant HBV were detected in patients with on-lamivudine re-appearance of HBV DNA after an initial decline below the solution hybridization assay limit (see MICROBIOLOGY: Drug Resistance). These mutations can be detected by a research assay and have been associated with reduced susceptibility to lamivudine *in vitro*. Lamivudine-treated patients with YMDD-mutant HBV at 52 weeks showed diminished treatment responses in comparison to lamivudine-treated patients without evidence of YMDD mutations, including lower rates of HBeAg seroconversion and HBeAg loss (no greater than placebo recipients), more frequent return of positive HBV DNA by solution hybridization assay, and more frequent ALT elevations. In the controlled trials, when patients developed YMDD-mutant HBV, they had a rise in HBV DNA and ALT from their own previous on-treatment levels. Progression of hepatitis B, including death, has been reported in some patients with YMDD-mutant HBV, including patients from the liver transplant setting and from other clinical trials. The long-term clinical significance of YMDD-mutant HBV is not known. Increased clinical and laboratory monitoring may aid in treatment decisions if emergence of viral mutants is suspected.

Limitations of Populations Studied: Safety and efficacy of EPIVIR-HBV have not been established in patients with decompensated liver disease or organ transplants; pediatric patients; patients dually infected with HBV and HCV, hepatitis delta, or HIV; or other populations not included in the principal phase III controlled studies. There are no studies in pregnant women and no data regarding effect on vertical transmission, and appropriate infant immunization should be used to prevent neonatal acquisition of HBV.

Assessing Patients During Treatment: Patients should be monitored regularly during treatment by a physician experienced in the management of chronic hepatitis B. The safety and effectiveness of treatment with EPIVIR-HBV beyond 1 year have not been established. During treatment, combinations of such events such as return of persistently elevated ALT, increasing levels of HBV DNA over time after an initial decline below assay limit, progression of clinical signs or symptoms of hepatic disease, and/or worsening of hepatic necroinflammatory findings may be considered as potentially reflecting loss of therapeutic response. Such observations should be taken into consideration when determining the advisability of continuing therapy with EPIVIR-HBV.

Table 5: Selected Clinical Adverse Events (≥5% Frequency) in Three Placebo-Controlled Clinical Trials During Treatment* (Studies 1–3)

Adverse Event	EPIVIR-HBV (n = 332)	Placebo (n = 200)
Non-site specific		
Malaise and fatigue	24%	28%
Fever or chills	7%	9%
Ear, nose, and throat		
Ear, nose, and throat infections	25%	21%
Sore throat	13%	8%
Gastrointestinal		
Nausea and vomiting	15%	17%
Abdominal discomfort and pain	16%	17%
Diarrhea	14%	12%
Musculoskeletal		
Myalgia	14%	17%
Arthralgia	7%	5%
Neurological		
Headache	21%	21%
Skin		
Skin rashes	5%	5%

*Includes patients treated for 52 to 68 weeks.

Table 6: Frequencies of Specified Laboratory Abnormalities in Three Placebo-Controlled Trials During Treatment* (Studies 1–3)

Test (Abnormal Level)	Patients with Abnormality/Patients with Observations	
	EPIVIR-HBV	Placebo
ALT >3 × baseline†	37/331 (11%)	26/199 (13%)
Albumin <2.5 g/dL	0/331 (0%)	2/199 (1%)
Amylase >3 × baseline	2/259 (<1%)	4/167 (2%)
Serum Lipase ≥2.5 × ULN‡	19/189 (10%)	9/127 (7%)
CPK ≥7 × baseline	31/329 (9%)	9/198 (5%)
Neutrophils <750/mm^3	0/331 (0%)	1/199 (<1%)
Platelets <50,000/mm^3	10/272 (4%)	5/168 (3%)

*Includes patients treated for 52 to 68 weeks
†See Table 7 for posttreatment ALT values.
‡Includes observations during and after treatment in the two placebo-controlled trials that collected this information.
ULN = Upper limit of normal.

Table 7: Posttreatment ALT Elevations in Two Placebo-Controlled Studies With No-Active-Treatment Follow-up (Studies 1 and 3)

Abnormal Value	Patients with ALT Elevation/ Patients with Observations*	
	EPIVIR-HBV	Placebo
ALT ≥2 × baseline value	37/137 (27%)	22/116 (19%)
ALT ≥3 × baseline value†	29/137 (21%)	9/116 (8%)
ALT ≥2 × baseline value and absolute ALT >500 IU/L	21/137 (15%)	8/116 (7%)
ALT ≥2 × baseline value; and bilirubin >2 × ULN and ≥2 × baseline value	1/137 (0.7%)	1/116 (0.9%)

*Each patient may be represented in one or more category.
†Comparable to a Grade 3 toxicity in accordance with modified WHO criteria.
ULN = Upper limit of normal.

The optimal duration of treatment, the durability of HBeAg seroconversions occurring during treatment, and the relationship between treatment response and long-term outcomes such as hepatocellular carcinoma or decompensated cirrhosis are not known.

Patients with Impaired Renal Function: Reduction of the dosage of EPIVIR-HBV is recommended for patients with impaired renal function (see CLINICAL PHARMACOLOGY and DOSAGE AND ADMINISTRATION).

Information for Patients: A Patient Package Insert (PPI) for EPIVIR-HBV is available for patient information.

Patients should remain under the care of a physician while taking EPIVIR-HBV. They should discuss any new symptoms or concurrent medications with their physician.

Patients should be advised that EPIVIR-HBV is not a cure for hepatitis B, that the long-term treatment benefits of EPIVIR-HBV are unknown at this time, and, in particular, that the relationship of initial treatment response to outcomes such as hepatocellular carcinoma and decompensated cirrhosis is unknown. Patients should be informed that deterioration of liver disease has occurred in some cases if treatment was discontinued, and that they should discuss any change in regimen with their physician. Patients should be informed that emergence of resistant hepatitis B virus and worsening of disease can occur during treatment, and they should promptly report any new symptoms to their physician.

Patients should be counseled on the importance of testing for HIV to avoid inappropriate therapy and development of resistant HIV, and HIV counseling and testing should be offered before starting EPIVIR-HBV and periodically during therapy. Patients should be advised that EPIVIR-HBV Tablets and EPIVIR-HBV Oral Solution contain a lower dose of the same active ingredient (lamivudine) as EPIVIR Tablets, EPIVIR Oral Solution, and COMBIVIR Tablets. EPIVIR-HBV should not be taken concurrently with EPIVIR or COMBIVIR (see WARNINGS). Patients infected with both HBV and HIV who are planning to change their HIV treat-

Continued on next page

This product information is based on labeling in effect on June 23, 2000. For further information, contact via direct mail, phone, or web site. Medical Information, Glaxo Wellcome Inc., PO Box 13398, Research Triangle Park, NC 27709. Healthcare Professionals (Medical Information): 800-334-0089. Patients (Customer Response Center): 1-888-825-5249. Glaxo Wellcome Corporate Web Site: www.glaxowellcome.com

Epivir-HBV—Cont.

ment regimen to a regimen that does not include EPIVIR or COMBIVIR should discuss continued therapy for hepatitis B with their physician.

Patients should be advised that treatment with EPIVIR-HBV has not been shown to reduce the risk of transmission of HBV to others through sexual contact or blood contamination (see Pregnancy section).

Drug Interaction: TMP 160 mg/SMX 800 mg once daily has been shown to increase lamivudine exposure (AUC). The effect of higher doses of TMP/SMX on lamivudine pharmacokinetics has not been investigated (see CLINICAL PHARMACOLOGY).

Carcinogenesis, Mutagenesis, and Impairment of Fertility: Lamivudine long-term carcinogenicity studies in mice and rats showed no evidence of carcinogenic potential at exposures up to 34 times (mice) and 200 times (rats) those observed in humans at the recommended therapeutic dose for chronic hepatitis B. Lamivudine was not active in a microbial mutagenicity screen or an *in vitro* cell transformation assay, but showed weak *in vitro* mutagenic activity in a cytogenetic assay using cultured human lymphocytes and in the mouse lymphoma assay. However, lamivudine showed no evidence of *in vivo* genotoxic activity in the rat at oral doses of up to 2000 mg/kg producing plasma levels of 60 to 70 times those in humans at the recommended dose for chronic hepatitis B. In a study of reproductive performance, lamivudine administered to rats at doses up to 4000 mg/kg per day, producing plasma levels 80 to 120 times those in humans, revealed no evidence of impaired fertility and no effect on the survival, growth, and development to weaning of the offspring.

Pregnancy: Pregnancy Category C. Reproduction studies have been performed in rats and rabbits at orally administered doses up to 4000 mg/kg per day and 1000 mg/kg per day, respectively, producing plasma levels up to approximately 60 times that for the adult HBV dose. No evidence of teratogenicity due to lamivudine was observed. Evidence of early embryolethality was seen in the rabbit at exposure levels similar to those observed in humans, but there was no indication of this effect in the rat at exposures up to 60 times that in humans. Studies in pregnant rats and rabbits showed that lamivudine is transferred to the fetus through the placenta. There are no adequate and well-controlled studies in pregnant women. Because animal reproductive toxicity studies are not always predictive of human response, lamivudine should be used during pregnancy only if the potential benefits outweigh the risks.

Lamivudine has not been shown to affect the transmission of HBV from mother to infant, and appropriate infant immunizations should be used to prevent neonatal acquisition of HBV.

Pregnancy Registry: To monitor maternal-fetal outcomes of pregnant women exposed to lamivudine, a Pregnancy Registry has been established. Physicians are encouraged to register patients by calling 1-800-258-4263.

Nursing Mothers: A study in lactating rats showed that lamivudine concentrations in milk were similar to those in plasma. Although it is not known if lamivudine is excreted in human milk, there is the potential for adverse effects from lamivudine in nursing infants. Mothers should be instructed not to breastfeed if they are receiving lamivudine.

Pediatric Use: ***HBV:*** Safety and efficacy of lamivudine for treatment of chronic hepatitis B in children have not been established. Lamivudine pharmacokinetics were evaluated in a 28-day dose-ranging study in 53 pediatric patients with chronic hepatitis B. Patients aged 2 to 12 years were randomized to receive lamivudine 0.35 mg/kg twice daily, 3 mg/kg once daily, 1.5 mg/kg twice daily, or 4 mg/kg twice daily. Patients aged 13 to 17 years received lamivudine 100 mg once daily. Lamivudine was rapidly absorbed (T_{max} 0.5 to 1 hour). In general, both C_{max} and exposure (AUC) showed dose proportionality in the dosing range studied. In children, weight-corrected oral clearances were higher, resulting in lower AUCs compared with adults. Age-stratified oral clearance was highest at age 2 and declined from 2 to 12 years, where values were then similar to those seen in adults. A dose of 3 mg/kg given once daily produced a steady-state lamivudine AUC (mean 5953 ng•hr/mL ± 1562 SD) similar to that associated with a dose of 100 mg/day in adults.

HIV: See the complete prescribing information for EPIVIR Tablets and Oral Solution for additional information on pharmacokinetics of lamivudine in HIV-infected children.

Geriatric Use: Clinical studies of EPIVIR-HBV did not include sufficient numbers of subjects aged 65 and over to determine whether they respond differently from younger subjects. Because elderly patients are more likely to have decreased renal function, care should be taken in dose selection, and it may be useful to monitor renal function (see DOSAGE AND ADMINISTRATION).

ADVERSE REACTIONS

Several serious adverse events reported with lamivudine (lactic acidosis and severe hepatomegaly with steatosis, posttreatment exacerbations of hepatitis B, pancreatitis, and emergence of viral mutants associated with reduced drug susceptibility and diminished treatment response) are also described in WARNINGS and PRECAUTIONS.

Clinical Trials In Chronic Hepatitis B: ***Adults:*** Selected clinical adverse events observed with a ≥5% frequency during therapy with EPIVIR-HBV compared with placebo are listed in Table 5. Frequencies of specified laboratory abnormalities during therapy with EPIVIR-HBV compared with placebo are listed in Table 6.

[See table 5 at top of previous page]

[See table 6 on previous page]

In patients followed for up to 16 weeks after discontinuation of treatment, posttreatment ALT elevations were observed more frequently in patients who had received EPIVIR-HBV than in patients who had received placebo. A comparison of ALT elevations between weeks 52 and 68 in patients who discontinued EPIVIR-HBV at week 52 and patients in the same studies who received placebo throughout the treatment course is shown in Table 7.

[See table 7 on previous page]

Lamivudine in Patients with HIV: In HIV-infected patients, safety information reflects a higher dose of lamivudine (150 mg b.i.d.) than the dose used to treat chronic hepatitis B in HIV-negative patients. In clinical trials using lamivudine as part of a combination regimen for treatment of HIV infection, several clinical adverse events occurred more often in lamivudine-containing treatment arms than in comparator arms. These included nasal signs and symptoms (20% vs 11%), dizziness (10% vs 4%), and depressive disorders (9% vs 4%). Pancreatitis was observed in three of the 656 adult patients (<0.5%) who received EPIVIR in controlled clinical trials. Laboratory abnormalities reported more often in lamivudine-containing arms included neutropenia and elevations of liver function tests (also more frequent in lamivudine-containing arms for a retrospective analysis of HIV/HBV dually infected patients in one study), and amylase elevations. Please see the complete prescribing information for EPIVIR Tablets and Oral Solution for more information.

Pediatric Patients with Hepatitis B: Limited information on the incidence of adverse events in children (2 to 12 years) and adolescents (13 to 17 years) receiving EPIVIR-HBV Oral Solution or Tablets is available from a 1-month pharmacokinetic study of lamivudine in children and adolescents with chronic hepatitis B. Malaise and fatigue; cough; fever; diarrhea, headache, and viral respiratory infections were the most commonly observed adverse events in lamivudine-treated pediatric patients.

Pediatric Patients with HIV Infection: In early open-label studies of lamivudine in children with HIV, peripheral neuropathy and neutropenia were reported, and pancreatitis was observed in 14% to 15% of patients.

Observed During Clinical Practice: The following events have been identified during post-approval use of lamivudine in clinical practice. Because they are reported voluntarily from a population of unknown size, estimates of frequency cannot be made. These events have been chosen for inclusion due to either their seriousness, frequency of reporting, potential causal connection to lamivudine, or a combination of these factors. Post-marketing experience with lamivudine at this time is largely limited to use in HIV-infected patients.

Digestive: Stomatitis.

Endocrine and Metabolic: Hyperglycemia.

General: Weakness.

Hemic and Lymphatic: Anemia, lymphadenopathy, splenomegaly.

Hepatic and Pancreatic: Lactic acidosis and steatosis, pancreatitis, posttreatment exacerbation of hepatitis (see WARNINGS and PRECAUTIONS).

Hypersensitivity: Anaphylaxis, urticaria.

Musculoskeletal: Rhabdomyolysis

Nervous: Paresthesia, peripheral neuropathy.

Respiratory: Abnormal breath sounds/wheezing.

Skin: Alopecia, pruritus, rash.

OVERDOSAGE

There is no known antidote for EPIVIR-HBV. One case of an adult ingesting 6 g of EPIVIR was reported; there were no clinical signs or symptoms noted and hematologic tests remained normal. It is not known whether lamivudine can be removed by peritoneal dialysis or hemodialysis.

DOSAGE AND ADMINISTRATION

The recommended oral dose of EPIVIR-HBV for treatment of chronic hepatitis B in adults is 100 mg once daily (see paragraph below and WARNINGS). Safety and effectiveness of treatment beyond 1 year have not been established and the optimum duration of treatment is not known (see PRECAUTIONS).

The formulation and dosage of lamivudine in EPIVIR-HBV are not appropriate for patients dually infected with HBV and HIV. If lamivudine is administered to such patients, the higher dosage indicated for HIV therapy should be used as part of an appropriate combination regimen, and the prescribing information for EPIVIR as well as EPIVIR-HBV should be consulted.

Pediatric Patients: See PRECAUTIONS: Pediatric Use.

Dose Adjustment: It is recommended that doses of EPIVIR-HBV be adjusted in accordance with renal function (Table 8) (see CLINICAL PHARMACOLOGY: Special Populations).

[See table 8 below]

Table 8: Adjustment of Adult Dosage of EPIVIR-HBV in Accordance With Creatinine Clearance

Creatinine Clearance (mL/min)	Recommended Dosage of EPIVIR-HBV
≥50	100 mg once daily
30–49	100 mg first dose, then 50 mg once daily
15–29	100 mg first dose, then 25 mg once daily
5–14	35 mg first dose, then 15 mg once daily
<5	35 mg first dose, then 10 mg once daily

No additional dosing of EPIVIR-HBV is required after routine (4-hour) hemodialysis. Insufficient data are available to recommend a dosage of EPIVIR-HBV in patients undergoing peritoneal dialysis (see CLINICAL PHARMACOLOGY: Special Populations).

HOW SUPPLIED

EPIVIR-HBV Tablets, 100 mg, are butterscotch-colored, film-coated, biconvex, capsule-shaped tablets imprinted with "GX CG5" on one side.

Bottles of 60 tablets (NDC 0173-0662-00) with child-resistant closures.

Store at controlled room temperature of 20° to 25°C (68° to 77°F) (see USP) in tightly closed bottles.

EPIVIR-HBV Oral Solution, a clear, colorless to pale yellow, strawberry-banana flavored liquid, contains 5 mg of lamivudine in each 1 mL in plastic bottles of 240 mL.

Bottles of 240 mL (NDC 0173-0663-00) with child-resistant closures. This product does not require reconstitution.

Store at controlled room temperature of 20° to 25°C (68° to 77°F) (see USP) in tightly closed bottles.

REFERENCES

1. Knodell RG, Ishak KG, Black WC, et al. Formulation and application of a numerical scoring system for assessing histological activity in asymptomatic chronic active hepatitis. *Hepatology.* 1982;1:431-435.

Glaxo Wellcome Inc., Research Triangle Park, NC 27709
Manufactured under agreement from
BioChem Pharma Inc.
275 Armand Frappier Blvd., Laval, Quebec, Canada
H7V 4A7

US Patent Nos. 5,047,407; 6,004,968; 5,905,082; and 5,532,246

April 2000/RL-808

Shown in Product Identification Guide, page 314

EXOSURF NEONATAL® ℞

[*ĕx 'ō-sŭrf nē-ə-năd' əl*]
(colfosceril palmitate, cetyl alcohol, tyloxapol)
for Intratracheal Suspension

DESCRIPTION

EXOSURF NEONATAL (colfosceril palmitate, cetyl alcohol, tyloxapol) for Intratracheal Suspension is a protein-free synthetic lung surfactant stored under vacuum as a sterile lyophilized powder. EXOSURF NEONATAL is reconstituted with preservative-free Sterile Water for Injection prior to administration by intratracheal instillation. Each 10-mL vial contains 108 mg colfosceril palmitate, commonly known as dipalmitoylphosphatidylcholine (DPPC), 12 mg cetyl alcohol, 8 mg tyloxapol, and 47 mg sodium chloride. Sodium hydroxide or hydrochloric acid may have been added to adjust pH. When reconstituted with 8 mL Sterile Water for Injection, the EXOSURF NEONATAL suspension contains 13.5 mg/mL colfosceril palmitate, 1.5 mg/mL cetyl alcohol, and 1 mg/mL tyloxapol in 0.1 N NaCl. The suspension appears milky white with a pH of 5 to 7 and an osmolality of 185 mOsm/kg.

The chemical names of the compounds of EXOSURF NEONATAL are as follows:

colfosceril palmitate: (*R*)-4-hydroxy-*N,N,N*-trimethyl-10-oxo-7-[(1-oxohexadecyl)oxy]-3,5,9-trioxa-4-phosphapentacosan-1-aminium hydroxide inner salt, 4-oxide; **cetyl alcohol:** (1-hexadecanol); and **tyloxapol:** 4-(1,1,3,3-tetramethylbutyl)phenol polymer with formaldehyde and oxirane.

CLINICAL PHARMACOLOGY

Surfactant deficiency is an important factor in the development of the neonatal respiratory distress syndrome (RDS). Thus, surfactant replacement therapy early in the course of RDS should ameliorate the disease and improve symptoms. Natural surfactant, a combination of lipids and apoproteins, exhibits not only surface tension reducing properties (conferred by the lipids), but also rapid spreading and adsorption (conferred by the apoproteins). The major fraction of the lipid component of natural surfactant is DPPC, which comprises up to 70% of natural surfactant by weight.

Although DPPC reduces surface tension, DPPC alone is ineffective in RDS because DPPC spreads and adsorbs poorly. In EXOSURF NEONATAL, which is protein free, cetyl alcohol acts as the spreading agent for the DPPC on the air-fluid interface. Tyloxapol, a polymeric long-chain repeating alcohol, is a nonionic surfactant which acts to disperse both DPPC and cetyl alcohol. Sodium chloride is added to adjust osmolality.

Pharmacokinetics: EXOSURF NEONATAL is administered directly into the trachea. Human pharmacokinetic

Table 1: Efficacy Assessments—Prophylactic Treatment

Number of Doses: Birth Weight Range:	Single Dose 500 to 700 g		Single Dose 700 to 1350 g		Single Dose 700 to 1100 g		1 vs 3 Doses 700 to 1100 g	
Treatment Group: Number of Infants:	Placebo (Air) n = 106	EXOSURF n = 109	Placebo (Air) n = 185	EXOSURF n = 176	Placebo (Air) n = 222	EXOSURF n = 224	EXOSURF 1 Dose n = 356	EXOSURF 3 Doses n = 360
	% of Infants		% of Infants		% of Infants		% of Infants	
Death ≤ day 28*	53	50	11	6	21	15	16	9[†]
Death through 1 year*	59	60	14	11	30	20[#]	17	12[†]
Death from RDS[§]	25	13[†]	4	3	10	5[‖]	3	2
Intact cardiopulmonary survival*,[¶]	29	25	69	78[†]	65	68	74	78
Bronchopulmonary dysplasia*, [#]	43	44	23	18	19	21	8	12
RDS incidence[§]	73	81	46	42	55	55	63	68

* "Intent-to-treat" analyses (as randomized) except for the 700 to 1350-g, single-dose study in which infants with congenital infections and anomalies were excluded.
[†] $P<0.05$.
[‡] $P<0.01$.
[§] "As-treated" analyses.
[‖] $P=0.051$.
[¶] Defined by survival through 28 days of life without bronchopulmonary dysplasia.
[#] Defined by a combination of clinical and radiographic criteria.

studies of the absorption, biotransformation, and excretion of the components of EXOSURF NEONATAL have not been performed. Nonclinical studies, however, have shown that DPPC can be absorbed from the alveolus into lung tissue where it can be catabolized extensively and reutilized for further phospholipid synthesis and secretion. In the developing rabbit, 90% of alveolar phospholipids are recycled. In premature rabbits, the alveolar half-life of intratracheally administered H^3-labeled phosphatidylcholine is approximately 12 hours.

Animal Studies: In animal models of RDS, treatment with EXOSURF NEONATAL significantly improved lung volume, compliance, and gas exchange in premature rabbits and lambs. The amount and distribution of lung water were not affected by treatment with EXOSURF NEONATAL of premature rabbit pups. The extent of lung injury in premature rabbit pups undergoing mechanical ventilation was reduced significantly by treatment with EXOSURF NEONATAL. In premature lambs, neither systemic blood flow nor flow through the ductus arteriosus were affected by treatment with EXOSURF NEONATAL. Survival was significantly better in both premature rabbits and premature lambs treated with EXOSURF NEONATAL.

Clinical Studies: EXOSURF NEONATAL has been studied in the United States and Canada in controlled clinical trials involving more than 4400 infants. Over 10 000 infants have received EXOSURF NEONATAL through an open, uncontrolled, North American study designed to provide the drug to premature infants who might benefit and to obtain additional safety information (EXOSURF NEONATAL Treatment IND).

Prophylactic Treatment: The efficacy of a single dose of EXOSURF NEONATAL in prophylactic treatment of infants at risk of developing RDS was examined in three double-blind, placebo-controlled studies, one involving 215 infants weighing 500 to 700 g, one involving 385 infants weighing 700 to 1350 g, and one involving 446 infants weighing 700 to 1100 g. The infants were intubated and placed on mechanical ventilation, and received 5 mL/kg of EXOSURF NEONATAL or placebo (air) within 30 minutes of birth.

The efficacy of one versus three doses of EXOSURF NEONATAL in prophylactic treatment of infants at risk of developing RDS was examined in a double-blind, placebo-controlled study of 823 infants weighing 700 to 1100 g. The infants were intubated and placed on mechanical ventilation, and received a first 5-mL/kg dose of EXOSURF NEONATAL within 30 minutes. Repeat 5-mL/kg doses of EXOSURF NEONATAL or placebo (air) were given to all infants who remained on mechanical ventilation at approximately 12 and 24 hours of age. An initial analysis of 716 infants is available.

The major efficacy parameters from these studies are presented in Table 1.

[See table 1 above]

Rescue Treatment: The efficacy of EXOSURF NEONATAL in the rescue treatment of infants with RDS was examined in two double-blind, placebo-controlled studies. One study enrolled 419 infants weighing 700 to 1350 g; the second enrolled 1237 infants weighing 1250 g and above. In the rescue treatment studies, infants received an initial dose (5 mL/kg) of EXOSURF NEONATAL or placebo (air) between 2 and 24 hours of life followed by a second dose (5 mL/kg) approximately 12 hours later to infants who remained on mechanical ventilation. The major efficacy parameters from these studies are presented in Table 2.

[See table 2 at top of next page]

Clinical Results: In these six controlled clinical studies, infants in the group receiving EXOSURF NEONATAL showed significant improvements in FiO_2 and ventilator settings that persisted for at least 7 days. Pulmonary air leaks were significantly reduced in each study. Five of these studies also showed a significant reduction in death from RDS. Further, overall mortality was reduced for all infants weighing >700 g. The one- versus three-dose prophylactic treatment study in 700 to 1100-g infants showed a further reduction in overall mortality with two additional doses.

Safety information is presented in Tables 3 and 4 (see ADVERSE REACTIONS). Beneficial effects in the group receiving EXOSURF NEONATAL were observed for some safety assessments. Various forms of pulmonary air leak and use of pancuronium were reduced in infants receiving EXOSURF NEONATAL in all six studies.

Follow-up data at 1 year adjusted age are available on 1094 of 2470 surviving infants. Growth and development of infants who received EXOSURF NEONATAL in this sample were comparable to infants who received placebo.

INDICATIONS AND USAGE

EXOSURF NEONATAL is indicated for:

1. **Prophylactic** treatment of infants with birth weights of less than 1350 g who are at risk of developing RDS (see PRECAUTIONS),
2. **Prophylactic** treatment of infants with birth weights greater than 1350 g who have evidence of pulmonary immaturity, and
3. **Rescue** treatment of infants who have developed RDS.

For **prophylactic** treatment, the first dose of EXOSURF NEONATAL should be administered as soon as possible after birth (see DOSAGE AND ADMINISTRATION: General Guidelines for Administration).

Infants considered as candidates for **rescue** treatment with EXOSURF NEONATAL should be on mechanical ventilation and have a diagnosis of RDS by both of the following criteria:

1. Respiratory distress not attributable to causes other than RDS, based on clinical and laboratory assessments.
2. Chest radiographic findings consistent with the diagnosis of RDS.

During the clinical development of EXOSURF NEONATAL, all infants who received the drug were intubated and on mechanical ventilation. For three-dose prophylactic treatment with EXOSURF NEONATAL, the first dose of drug was administered as soon as possible after birth and repeat doses were given at approximately 12 and 24 hours after birth if infants remained on mechanical ventilation at those times. For rescue treatment, two doses were given; one between 2 and 24 hours of life, and a second approximately 12 hours later if infants remained on mechanical ventilation. Infants who received rescue treatment with EXOSURF NEONATAL had a documented arterial to alveolar oxygen tension ratio (a/A) <0.22.

CONTRAINDICATIONS

There are no known contraindications to treatment with EXOSURF NEONATAL.

WARNINGS

Intratracheal Administration Only: EXOSURF NEONATAL should be administered only by instillation into the trachea (see DOSAGE AND ADMINISTRATION).

General: The use of EXOSURF NEONATAL requires expert clinical care by experienced neonatologists and other clinicians who are accomplished at neonatal intubation and ventilatory management. Adequate personnel, facilities, equipment, and medications are required to optimize perinatal outcome in premature infants.

Instillation of EXOSURF NEONATAL should be performed **only** by trained medical personnel experienced in airway and clinical management of unstable premature infants. Vigilant clinical attention should be given to all infants prior to, during, and after administration of EXOSURF NEONATAL.

Acute Effects: EXOSURF NEONATAL can rapidly affect oxygenation and lung compliance.

Lung Compliance: If chest expansion improves substantially after dosing, peak ventilator inspiratory pressures should be reduced immediately, without waiting for confirmation of respiratory improvement by blood gas assessment. Failure to reduce inspiratory ventilator pressures rapidly in such instances can result in lung overdistention and fatal pulmonary air leak.

Hyperoxia: If the infant becomes pink and transcutaneous oxygen saturation is in excess of 95%, FiO_2 should be reduced in small but repeated steps (until saturation is 90% to 95%) without waiting for confirmation of elevated arterial pO_2 by blood gas assessment. Failure to reduce FiO_2 in such instances can result in hyperoxia.

Hypocarbia: If arterial or transcutaneous CO_2 measurements are <30 torr, the ventilator rate should be reduced at once. Failure to reduce ventilator rates in such instances can result in marked hypocarbia, which is known to reduce brain blood flow.

Pulmonary Hemorrhage: In the single study conducted in infants weighing <700 g at birth, the incidence of pulmonary hemorrhage (10% vs 2% in the placebo group) was significantly increased in the group receiving EXOSURF NEONATAL. None of the five studies involving infants with birth weights >700 g showed a significant increase in pulmonary hemorrhage in the group receiving EXOSURF NEONATAL. In a cross-study analysis of these five studies, pulmonary hemorrhage was reported for 1% (14/1420) of infants in the placebo group and 2% (27/1411) of infants in the group receiving EXOSURF NEONATAL. Fatal pulmonary hemorrhage occurred in three infants; two in the group receiving EXOSURF NEONATAL and one in the placebo group. Mortality from all causes among infants who developed pulmonary hemorrhage was 43% in the placebo group and 37% in the group receiving EXOSURF NEONATAL.

Pulmonary hemorrhage in infants treated with either EXOSURF NEONATAL or placebo was more frequent in infants who were younger, smaller, male, or who had a patent ductus arteriosus. Pulmonary hemorrhage typically occurred in the first 2 days of life in both treatment groups.

In more than 7700 infants in the open, uncontrolled study, pulmonary hemorrhage was reported in 4%, but fatal pulmonary hemorrhage was reported rarely (0.4%).

In the controlled clinical studies, infants treated with EXOSURF NEONATAL who received steroids more than 24 hours prior to delivery or indomethacin postnatally had a lower rate of pulmonary hemorrhage than other infants treated with EXOSURF NEONATAL. Attention should be paid to early and aggressive diagnosis and treatment (unless contraindicated) of patent ductus arteriosus during the first 2 days of life (while the ductus arteriosus is often clinically silent). Other potentially protective measures include attempting to decrease FiO_2 preferentially over ventilator pressures during the first 24 to 48 hours after dosing, and attempting to decrease PEEP minimally for at least 48 hours after dosing.

Mucous Plugs: Infants whose ventilation becomes markedly impaired during or shortly after dosing may have mucous plugging of the endotracheal tube, particularly if pulmonary secretions were prominent prior to drug administration. Suctioning of all infants prior to dosing may lessen the chance of mucous plugs obstructing the endotracheal tube. If endotracheal tube obstruction from such plugs is suspected, and suctioning is unsuccessful in removing the obstruction, the blocked endotracheal tube should be replaced immediately.

PRECAUTIONS

General: In the controlled clinical studies, infants known prenatally or postnatally to have major congenital anomalies or who were suspected of having congenital infection were excluded from entry. However, these disorders cannot be recognized early in life in all cases, and a few infants with these conditions were entered. The benefits of EXOSURF NEONATAL in the affected infants who received drug appeared to be similar to the benefits observed in infants without anomalies or occult infection.

Prophylactic Treatment—Infants <700 g: In infants weighing 500 to 700 g, a single prophylactic dose of EXOSURF NEONATAL significantly improved FiO_2 and ventilator settings, reduced pneumothorax, and reduced death from RDS, but increased pulmonary hemorrhage (see WARNINGS).

Continued on next page

This product information is based on labeling in effect on June 23, 2000. For further information, contact via direct mail, phone, or web site. Medical Information, Glaxo Wellcome Inc., PO Box 13398, Research Triangle Park, NC 27709. Healthcare Professionals (Medical Information): 800-334-0089. Patients (Customer Response Center): 1-888-825-5249. Glaxo Wellcome Corporate Web Site: www.glaxowellcome.com

Exosurf—Cont.

Overall mortality did not differ significantly between the group receiving placebo and the group receiving EXOSURF NEONATAL (see Table 1). Data on multiple doses in infants in this weight class are not yet available. Accordingly, clinicians should carefully evaluate the potential risks and benefits of administration of EXOSURF NEONATAL in these infants.

Rescue Treatment—Number of Doses: A small number of infants with RDS have received more than two doses of EXOSURF NEONATAL as rescue treatment. Definitive data on the safety and efficacy of these additional doses are not available.

Carcinogenesis, Mutagenesis, Impairment of Fertility: EXOSURF NEONATAL at concentrations up to 10 000 mcg/plate was not mutagenic in the Ames Salmonella assay. Long-term studies have not been performed in animals to evaluate the carcinogenic potential of EXOSURF NEONATAL.

The effects of EXOSURF NEONATAL on fertility have not been studied.

ADVERSE REACTIONS

General: Premature birth is associated with a high incidence of morbidity and mortality. Despite significant reductions in overall mortality associated with EXOSURF NEONATAL, some infants who received EXOSURF NEONATAL developed severe complications and either survived with permanent handicaps or died.

In controlled clinical studies evaluating the safety and efficacy of EXOSURF NEONATAL, numerous safety assessments were made. In infants receiving EXOSURF NEONATAL, pulmonary hemorrhage, apnea, and use of methylxanthines were increased. A number of other adverse events were significantly reduced in the group receiving EXOSURF NEONATAL, particularly various forms of pulmonary air leak and use of pancuronium (see CLINICAL PHARMACOLOGY: Clinical Results). Tables 3 and 4 summarize the results of the major safety evaluations from the controlled clinical studies.

[See table 3 below]

[See table 4 on next page]

Pulmonary Hemorrhage: See WARNINGS.

Abnormal Laboratory Values: Abnormal laboratory values are common in critically ill, mechanically ventilated, premature infants. A higher incidence of abnormal laboratory values in the group receiving EXOSURF NEONATAL was not reported.

Table 2: Efficacy Assessments—Rescue Treatment

Number of Doses: / Birth Weight Range:	2 Doses 700 to 1350 g		2 Doses 1250 g and above	
Treatment Group: / Number of Infants:	Placebo (Air) n = 213	EXOSURF n = 206	Placebo (Air) n = 623	EXOSURF n = 614
	% of Infants		% of Infants	
Death ≤ day 28*	23	11†	7	4‡
Death through 1 Year*	27	15†	9	6§
Death from RDS‖	10	3¶	3	1‡
Intact cardiopulmonary survival*,#	62	75¶	88	93¶
Bronchopulmonary dysplasia *,**	18	15	6	3‡

* "Intent-to-treat" analyses (as randomized).
† $P<0.001$.
‡ $P<0.05$.
§ $P=0.067$.
‖ "As-treated" analyses.
¶ $P<0.01$.
\# Defined by survival through 28 days of life without bronchopulmonary dysplasia.
** Defined by a combination of clinical and radiographic criteria.

Events During Dosing: Data on events during dosing are available from more than 8800 infants in the open, uncontrolled clinical study (Table 5).

[See table 5 on next page]

Reflux: Reflux of EXOSURF NEONATAL into the endotracheal tube during dosing has been observed and may be associated with rapid drug administration. If reflux occurs, drug administration should be halted and, if necessary, peak inspiratory pressure on the ventilator should be increased by 4 to 5 cm H_2O until the endotracheal tube clears.

Greater than Twenty Percent Drop in Transcutaneous Oxygen Saturation: If transcutaneous oxygen saturation declines during dosing, drug administration should be halted and, if necessary, peak inspiratory pressure on the ventilator should be increased by 4 to 5 cm H_2O for 1 to 2 minutes. In addition, increases of FiO_2 may be required for 1 to 2 minutes.

Mucous Plugs: See WARNINGS.

OVERDOSAGE

There have been no reports of massive overdosage with EXOSURF NEONATAL.

DOSAGE AND ADMINISTRATION

Preparation of Suspension: EXOSURF NEONATAL is best reconstituted immediately before use because it does not contain antibacterial preservatives. However, the reconstituted suspension is chemically and physically stable and remains sterile (when reconstituted using aseptic techniques) when stored at 2° to 30°C (36° to 86°F) for up to 12 hours following reconstitution.

Solutions containing buffers or preservatives should not be used for reconstitution. **Do Not Use Bacteriostatic Water for Injection, USP.** Each vial of EXOSURF NEONATAL should be reconstituted only with **8 mL** of the accompanying diluent (preservative-free Sterile Water for Injection) as follows:

1. Fill a 10- or 12-mL syringe with 8 mL of preservative-free Sterile Water for Injection using an 18- or 19-gauge needle;
2. Allow the vacuum in the vial to draw the Sterile Water into the vial;
3. Aspirate as much as possible of the 8 mL out of the vial into the syringe (while maintaining the vacuum), then SUDDENLY release the syringe plunger.

Step 3 should be repeated three or four times to assure adequate mixing of the vial contents. If vacuum is not present, the vial of EXOSURF NEONATAL should not be used.

The appropriate dosage volume for the entire dose (5 mL/kg) should then be drawn into the syringe from **below** the froth in the vial (again maintaining the vacuum). If the infant weighs less than 1600 g, unused EXOSURF

Table 3: Safety Assessments*—Prophylactic Treatment

Number of Doses: / Birth Weight Range:	Single Dose 500 to 700 g		Single Dose 700 to 1350 g		Single Dose 700 to 1100 g		1 vs 3 Doses 700 to 1100 g	
Treatment Group: / Number of Infants:	Placebo (Air) n = 108	EXOSURF n = 107	Placebo (Air) n = 193	EXOSURF n = 192	Placebo (Air) n = 222	EXOSURF n = 224	EXOSURF 1 Dose n = 356	EXOSURF 3 Doses n = 360
	% of Infants		% of Infants		% of Infants		% of Infants	
Intraventricular hemorrhage (IVH)								
Overall	51	57	31	27	36	36	38	35
Severe IVH	26	25	10	8	13	14	9	9
Pulmonary air leak (PAL)								
Overall	52	48	16	11	32	25	29	27
Pneumothorax	23	10†	5	6	19	11†	14	12
Pneumopericardium	1	4	2	0	<1	1	1	1
Pneumomediastinum	2	1	2	3	7	1‡	3	2
Pulmonary interstitial emphysema	43	44	13	7†	26	20	23	22
Death from PAL	4	6	<1	<1	2	1	2	1
Patent ductus arteriosus	49	53	66	70	50	55	59	57
Necrotizing enterocolitis	2	4	11	13	3	4	6	2†
Pulmonary hemorrhage	2	10‡	2	4	1	4	4	6
Congenital pneumonia	4	4	2	4	2	2	1	1
Nosocomial pneumonia	10	10	2	4	4	7	14	15
Nonpulmonary infections	33	35	34	39	28	29	35	34
Sepsis	30	34	30	34	23	24	30	27
Death from sepsis	4	4	3	3	1	2	3	2
Meningitis	4	6	3	1	2	3	1	2
Other infections	7	4	5	3	6	10	10	11
Major anomalies	3	1	2	4	7	4	4	4
Hypotension	70	77	52	47	59	62	54	50
Hyperbilirubinemia	22	21	63	61	27	31	20	21
Exchange transfusion	4	3	1	2	2	2	3	1
Thrombocytopenia§	21	25	not available		9	8	12	10
Persistent fetal circulation	0	1	1	1	0	2†	1	<1
Seizures	11	8	2	2	11	9	6	5
Apnea	34	33	76	73	55	65†	62	68
Drug therapy								
Antibiotics	96	99	98	96	98	99	>99	99
Diuretics	55	60	39	37	59	63	64	65
Anticonvulsants	14	18	23	24	20	16	9	8
Inotropes	46	40	20	20	26	20	28	27
Sedatives	62	71	65	64	63	57	52	52
Pancuronium	19	11	22	14†	19	13†	15	11
Methylxanthines	38	43	77	77	61	72†	75	82†

* All parameters were examined with "as-treated" analyses.
† $P<0.05$.
‡ $P<0.01$.
§ Thrombocytopenia requiring platelet transfusion.

NEONATAL suspension will remain in the vial after the entire dose is drawn into the syringe. If the infant weighs more than 1600 g, at least two vials will be required for each dose.

Reconstituted EXOSURF NEONATAL is a milky white suspension with a total volume of 8 mL per vial. Each milliliter of reconstituted EXOSURF NEONATAL contains 13.5 mg colfosceril palmitate, 1.5 mg cetyl alcohol, 1 mg tyloxapol, and sodium chloride to provide a 0.1 N concentration. If the suspension appears to separate, gently shake or swirl the vial to resuspend the preparation. The reconstituted product should be inspected visually for homogeneity immediately before administration; if persistent large flakes or particulates are present, the vial should not be used.

Dosage: Accurate determination of weight at birth is the key to accurate dosing.

Prophylactic Treatment: The first dose of EXOSURF NEONATAL should be administered as a single 5-mL/kg dose as soon as possible after birth. Second and third doses should be administered approximately 12 and 24 hours later to all infants who remain on mechanical ventilation at those times.

Rescue Treatment: EXOSURF NEONATAL should be administered in two 5-mL/kg doses. The initial dose should be administered as soon as possible after the diagnosis of RDS is confirmed. The second dose should be administered approximately 12 hours following the first dose, provided the infant remains on mechanical ventilation. A small number of infants with RDS have received more than two doses of EXOSURF NEONATAL as rescue treatment. Definitive data on the safety and efficacy of these additional doses are not available (see PRECAUTIONS).

Use of Special Endotracheal Tube Adapter: With each vial of EXOSURF NEONATAL for Intratracheal Suspension, five different sized endotracheal tube adapters each with a special right angle Luer®-lock sideport are supplied. The adapters are clean but not sterile. The adapters should be used as follows:

1. Select an adapter size that corresponds to the inside diameter of the endotracheal tube.
2. Insert the adapter into the endotracheal tube with a firm push-twist motion.
3. Connect the breathing circuit wye to the adapter.
4. Remove the cap from the sideport on the adapter. Attach the syringe containing drug to the sideport.
5. After completion of dosing, remove the syringe and RECAP THE SIDEPORT.

Administration: The infant should be suctioned prior to administration of EXOSURF NEONATAL.

EXOSURF NEONATAL suspension is administered via the sideport on the special endotracheal tube adapter **WITHOUT INTERRUPTING MECHANICAL VENTILATION.**

Each dose of EXOSURF NEONATAL is administered in two 2.5-mL/kg half-doses. Each half-dose is instilled slowly over 1 to 2 minutes (30 to 50 mechanical breaths) in small bursts timed with inspiration. After the first 2.5-mL/kg half-dose is administered in the midline position, the infant's head and torso are turned 45° to the **right** for 30 seconds while mechanical ventilation is continued. After the infant is returned to the midline position, the second 2.5-mL/kg half-dose is given in an identical fashion over another 1 to 2 minutes. The infant's head and torso are then turned 45° to the **left** for 30 seconds while mechanical ventilation is continued, and the infant is then turned back to the midline position. These maneuvers allow gravity to assist in the distribution of EXOSURF NEONATAL in the lungs.

During dosing, heart rate, color, chest expansion, facial expressions, the oximeter, and the endotracheal tube patency and position should be monitored. If heart rate slows, the infant becomes dusky or agitated, transcutaneous oxygen saturation falls more than 15%, or EXOSURF NEONATAL backs up in the endotracheal tube, dosing should be slowed or halted and, if necessary, the peak inspiratory pressure, ventilator rate, and/or FiO_2 turned up. On the other hand, rapid improvements in lung function may require immediate reductions in peak inspiratory pressure, ventilator rate, and/or FiO_2. (See WARNINGS and see below for additional information concerning administration.)

Suctioning should not be performed for two hours after EXOSURF NEONATAL is administered, except when dictated by clinical necessity.

General Guidelines for Administration: Administration of EXOSURF NEONATAL should not take precedence over clinical assessment and stabilization of critically ill infants.

Intubation: Prior to dosing with EXOSURF NEONATAL, it is important to ensure that the endotracheal tube tip is in the trachea and not in the esophagus or right or left mainstem bronchus. Brisk and symmetrical chest movement with each mechanical inspiration should be confirmed prior to dosing, as should equal breath sounds in the two axillae. In prophylactic treatment, dosing with EXOSURF NEONATAL need not be delayed for radiographic confirmation of the endotracheal tube tip position. In rescue treatment, bedside confirmation of endotracheal tube tip position is usually sufficient, if at least one chest radiograph subsequent to the last intubation confirmed proper position of the endotracheal tube tip. Some lung areas will remain undosed if the endotracheal tube tip is too low.

Monitoring: Continuous electrocardiogram and transcutaneous oxygen saturation monitoring during dosing are essential. In most infants treated prophylactically, it should be possible to initiate such monitoring prior to administration of the first dose of EXOSURF NEONATAL. For subsequent prophylactic and all rescue doses, arterial blood pressure monitoring during dosing is also highly desirable. After both prophylactic and rescue dosing, frequent arterial blood gas sampling is required to prevent postdosing hyperoxia and hypocarbia (see WARNINGS).

Ventilatory Support During Dosing: The 5-mL/kg dosage volume may cause transient impairment of gas exchange by physical blockage of the airway, particularly in infants on low ventilator settings. As a result, infants may exhibit a drop in oxygen saturation during dosing, especially if they are on low ventilator settings prior to dosing. These transient effects are easily overcome by increasing peak inspiratory pressure on the ventilator by 4 to 5 cm H_2O for 1 to 2 minutes during dosing. FiO_2 can also be increased if necessary. In infants who are particularly fragile or reactive to external stimuli, increasing peak inspiratory pressure by 4 to 5 cm H_2O and/or FiO_2 20% just prior to dosing may minimize any transient deterioration in oxygenation. However, in virtually all cases it should be possible to return the infant to predose settings within a very short time of dose completion.

Postdosing: At the end of dosing, position of the endotracheal tube should be confirmed by listening for equal breath sounds in the two axillae. Attention should be paid to chest expansion, color, transcutaneous saturation, and arterial blood gases. Some infants who receive EXOSURF NEONATAL and other surfactants respond with rapid improvements in pulmonary compliance, minute ventilation, and gas exchange (see WARNINGS). Constant bedside attention of an experienced clinician for at least 30 minutes after dosing is essential. Frequent blood gas sampling also is absolutely essential. Rapid changes in lung function require immediate changes in peak inspiratory pressure, ventilator rate, and/or FiO_2.

Table 4: Safety Assessments*—Rescue Treatment

Number of Doses: Birth Weight Range:	2 Doses 700 to 1350 g		2 Doses 1250 g and above	
Treatment Group: Number of Infants:	Placebo (Air) n = 213	EXOSURF n = 206	Placebo (Air) n = 622	EXOSURF n = 615
	% of Infants		% of Infants	
Intraventricular hemorrhage (IVH)				
Overall	48	52	23	18[†]
Severe IVH	13	9	5	4
Pulmonary air leak (PAL)				
Overall	54	34[‡]	30	18[‡]
Pneumothorax	29	20[†]	20	10[‡]
Pneumopericardium	4	1	1	2
Pneumomediastinum	8	4	5	2[§]
Pulmonary interstitial emphysema	48	25[‡]	24	13[‡]
Death from PAL	7	3	<1	1
Patent ductus arteriosus	66	57	54	45[†]
Necrotizing enterocolitis	3	3	1	2
Pulmonary hemorrhage	3	1	<1	1
Congenital pneumonia	2	3	2	2
Nosocomial pneumonia	5	7	2	2
Nonpulmonary infections	19	22	13	13
Sepsis	15	17	8	8
Death from sepsis	<1	<1	1	<1
Meningitis	1	<1	1	<1[†]
Other infections	5	8	5	6
Major anomalies	3	3	4	4
Hypotension	62	57	50	39[§]
Hyperbilirubinemia	17	19	12	10
Exchange transfusion	3	4	1	2
Thrombocytopenia[‖]	10	11	4	<1[§]
Persistent fetal circulation	1	1	6	2[§]
Seizures	10	10	6	3[†]
Apnea	48	65[§]	37	44[†]
Drug therapy				
Antibiotics	100	99	98	98
Diuretics	60	65	45	34[‡]
Anticonvulsants	17	17	10	5[§]
Inotropes	36	31	27	16[‡]
Sedatives	72	68	76	64[‡]
Pancuronium	34	17[§]	33	15[‡]
Methylxanthines	62	74[§]	49	53

* All parameters were examined with "as-treated" analyses.
[†] $P<0.05$.
[‡] $P<0.001$.
[§] $P<0.01$.
[‖] Thrombocytopenia requiring platelet transfusion.

Table 5: Events During Dosing in the Open, Uncontrolled Study*

Treatment Type: Number of Infants:	Prophylactic Treatment n = 1127	Rescue Treatment n = 7711
	% of Infants	% of Infants
Reflux of EXOSURF NEONATAL	20	31
Drop in O_2 saturation (≥20%)	6	22
Rise in O_2 saturation (≥10%)	5	6
Drop in transcutaneous pO_2 (≥20 mm Hg)	1	8
Rise in transcutaneous pO_2 (≥20 mm Hg)	2	5
Drop in transcutaneous pCO_2 (≥20 mm Hg)	<1	1
Rise in transcutaneous pCO_2 (≥20 mm Hg)	1	3
Bradycardia (<60 beats/min)	1	3
Tachycardia (>200 beats/min)	<1	<1
Gagging	1	5
Mucous plugs	<1	<1

* Infants may have experienced more than one event. Investigators were prohibited from adjusting FiO_2 and/or ventilator settings during dosing unless significant clinical deterioration occurred.

HOW SUPPLIED

EXOSURF NEONATAL for Intratracheal Suspension is supplied in a carton containing one 10-mL vial of EXOSURF NEONATAL for Intratracheal Suspension, one 10-mL vial of Sterile Water for Injection, and five endotracheal tube adapters (2.5, 3.0, 3.5, 4.0, and 4.5 mm I.D.) (NDC 0173-0207-01).

Store EXOSURF NEONATAL for Intratracheal Suspension at 15° to 30°C (59° to 86°F) in a dry place.

Licensed under US Patent Nos. 4,312,860; 4,826,821; and 5,110,806.

Manufactured by Catalytica Pharmaceuticals, Inc.
Greenville, NC 27834

Continued on next page

This product information is based on labeling in effect on June 23, 2000. For further information, contact via direct mail, phone, or web site. Medical Information, Glaxo Wellcome Inc., PO Box 13398, Research Triangle Park, NC 27709. Healthcare Professionals (Medical Information): 800-334-0089. Patients (Customer Response Center): 1-888-825-5249. Glaxo Wellcome Corporate Web Site: www.glaxowellcome.com

Exosurf—Cont.

for Glaxo Wellcome Inc., Research Triangle Park, NC 27709

January 1998/RL-524
Shown in Product Identification Guide, page 314

FLOLAN® ℞
[flō 'lan]
(epoprostenol sodium)
for Injection

DESCRIPTION

FLOLAN (epoprostenol sodium) for Injection is a sterile sodium salt formulated for intravenous (IV) administration. Each vial of FLOLAN contains epoprostenol sodium equivalent to either 0.5 mg (500,000 ng) or 1.5 mg (1,500,000 ng) epoprostenol, 3.76 mg glycine, 2.93 mg sodium chloride, and 50 mg mannitol. Sodium hydroxide may have been added to adjust pH.

Epoprostenol (PGI_2, PGX, prostacyclin), a metabolite of arachidonic acid, is a naturally occurring prostaglandin with potent vasodilatory activity and inhibitory activity of platelet aggregation.

Epoprostenol is (5Z,9α,11α,13*E*,15*S*)-6,9-epoxy-11,15-dihydroxyprosta-5,13-dien-1-oic acid.

Epoprostenol sodium has a molecular weight of 374.45 and a molecular formula of $C_{20}H_{31}NaO_5$. The structural formula is:

FLOLAN is a white to off-white powder that must be reconstituted with STERILE DILUENT for FLOLAN. STERILE DILUENT for FLOLAN is supplied in 50-mL glass vials containing 94 mg glycine, 73.5 mg sodium chloride, sodium hydroxide (added to adjust pH), and Water for Injection, USP.

The reconstituted solution of FLOLAN has a pH of 10.2 to 10.8 and is increasingly unstable at a lower pH.

CLINICAL PHARMACOLOGY

General: Epoprostenol has two major pharmacological actions: (1) direct vasodilation of pulmonary and systemic arterial vascular beds, and (2) inhibition of platelet aggregation. In animals, the vasodilatory effects reduce right and left ventricular afterload and increase cardiac output and stroke volume. The effect of epoprostenol on heart rate in animals varies with dose. At low doses, there is vagally mediated bradycardia, but at higher doses, epoprostenol causes reflex tachycardia in response to direct vasodilation and hypotension. No major effects on cardiac conduction have been observed. Additional pharmacologic effects of epoprostenol in animals include bronchodilation, inhibition of gastric acid secretion, and decreased gastric emptying.

Pharmacokinetics: Epoprostenol is rapidly hydrolyzed at neutral pH in blood and is also subject to enzymatic degradation. Animal studies using tritium-labelled epoprostenol have indicated a high clearance (93 mL/min per kg), small volume of distribution (357 mL/kg), and a short half-life (2.7 minutes). During infusions in animals, steady-state plasma concentrations of tritium-labelled epoprostenol were reached within 15 minutes and were proportional to infusion rates.

No available chemical assay is sufficiently sensitive and specific to assess the in vivo human pharmacokinetics of epoprostenol. The in vitro half-life of epoprostenol in human blood at 37°C and pH 7.4 is approximately 6 minutes; the in vivo half-life of epoprostenol in humans is therefore expected to be no greater than 6 minutes. The in vitro pharmacologic half-life of epoprostenol in human plasma, based on inhibition of platelet aggregation, was similar for males (n = 954) and females (n = 1024).

Tritium-labelled epoprostenol has been administered to humans in order to identify the metabolic products of epoprostenol. Epoprostenol is metabolized to two primary metabolites: 6-keto-$PGF_{1\alpha}$ (formed by spontaneous degradation) and 6,15-diketo-13,14-dihydro-$PGF_{1\alpha}$ (enzymatically formed), both of which have pharmacological activity orders of magnitude less than epoprostenol in animal test systems. The recovery of radioactivity in urine and feces over a 1-week period was 82% and 4% of the administered dose, respectively. Fourteen additional minor metabolites have been isolated from urine, indicating that epoprostenol is extensively metabolized in humans.

CLINICAL TRIALS IN PULMONARY HYPERTENSION

Acute Hemodynamic Effects: Acute intravenous infusions of FLOLAN for up to 15 minutes in patients with secondary and primary pulmonary hypertension produce dose-related increases in cardiac index (CI) and stroke volume (SV), and dose-related decreases in pulmonary vascular resistance (PVR), total pulmonary resistance (TPR), and mean systemic arterial pressure (SAPm). The effects of FLOLAN on mean pulmonary artery pressure (PAPm) were variable and minor.

Table 1: Hemodynamics During Chronic Administration of FLOLAN in Patients with PPH

Hemodynamic Parameter	Baseline		Mean change from baseline at end of treatment period*	
	FLOLAN (N = 52)	Standard Therapy (N = 54)	FLOLAN (N = 48)	Standard Therapy (N = 41)
CI (L/min/m²)	2.0	2.0	0.3**	-0.1
PAPm (mm Hg)	60	60	-5**	1
PVR (Wood U)	16	17	-4**	1
SAPm (mm Hg)	89	91	-4	-3
SV (mL/beat)	44	43	6**	-1
TPR (Wood U)	20	21	-5**	1

* At 8 weeks: FLOLAN N = 10; Conventional Therapy N = 11 (N is the number of patients with hemodynamic data).
At 12 weeks: FLOLAN N = 38; Conventional Therapy N = 30 (N is the number of patients with hemodynamic data).
**Denotes statistically significant difference between FLOLAN and Conventional Therapy groups. CI = cardiac index; PAPm = mean pulmonary arterial pressure; PVR = pulmonary vascular resistance; SAPm = mean systemic arterial pressure; SV = stroke volume; TPR = total pulmonary resistance.

Table 2: Hemodynamics During Chronic Administration of FLOLAN in Patients with PH/SSD

Hemodynamic Parameter	Baseline		Mean change from baseline at 12 weeks	
	FLOLAN (N = 56)	Conventional Therapy (N = 55)	FLOLAN (N = 50)	Conventional Therapy (N = 48)
CI (L/min/m²)	1.9	2.2	0.5*	-0.1
PAPm (mm Hg)	51	49	-5*	1
RAPm (mm Hg)	13	11	-1*	1
PVR (Wood U)	14	11	-5*	1
SAPm (mm Hg)	93	89	-8*	-1

*Denotes statistically significant difference between FLOLAN and Conventional Therapy groups (N is the number of patients with hemodynamic data).
CI = cardiac index; PAPm = mean pulmonary arterial pressure; RAPm = mean right arterial pressure; PVR = pulmonary vascular resistance; SAPm = mean systemic arterial pressure.

Chronic Infusion in Primary Pulmonary Hypertension (PPH): ***Hemodynamic Effects:*** Chronic continuous infusions of FLOLAN in patients with PPH were studied in two prospective, open, randomized trials of 8 and 12 weeks' duration comparing FLOLAN plus conventional therapy to conventional therapy alone. Dosage of FLOLAN was determined as described in DOSAGE AND ADMINISTRATION and averaged 9.2 ng/kg per minute at study end. Conventional therapy varied among patients and included some or all of the following: anticoagulants in essentially all patients; oral vasodilators, diuretics, and digoxin in one half to two thirds of patients; and supplemental oxygen in about half the patients. Except for two New York Heart Association (NYHA) functional Class II patients, all patients were either functional Class III or Class IV. As results were similar in the two studies, the pooled results are described. Chronic hemodynamic effects were generally similar to acute effects. Increases in CI, SV, and arterial oxygen saturation and decreases in PAPm, mean right atrial pressure (RAPm), TPR, and systemic vascular resistance (SVR) were observed in patients who received FLOLAN chronically compared to those who did not. Table 1 illustrates the treatment-related hemodynamic changes in these patients after 8 or 12 weeks of treatment.

[See table 1 above]

These hemodynamic improvements appeared to persist when FLOLAN was administered for at least 36 months in an open, nonrandomized study.

Clinical Effects: Statistically significant improvement was observed in exercise capacity, as measured by the 6-minute walk test in patients receiving continuous intravenous FLOLAN plus conventional therapy (N = 52) for 8 or 12 weeks compared to those receiving conventional therapy alone (N = 54). Improvements were apparent as early as the first week of therapy. Increases in exercise capacity were accompanied by statistically significant improvement in dyspnea and fatigue, as measured by the Chronic Heart Failure Questionnaire and the Dyspnea Fatigue Index.

Survival was improved in NYHA functional Class III and Class IV PPH patients treated with FLOLAN for 12 weeks in a multicenter, open, randomized, parallel study. At the end of the treatment period, 8 of 40 (20%) patients receiving conventional therapy alone died, whereas none of the 41 patients receiving FLOLAN died ($P = 0.003$).

Chronic Infusion in Pulmonary Hypertension Associated with the Scleroderma Spectrum of Diseases (PH/SSD): ***Hemodynamic Effects:*** Chronic continuous infusions of FLOLAN in patients with PH/SSD were studied in a prospective, open, randomized trial of 12 weeks' duration comparing FLOLAN plus conventional therapy (N = 56) to conventional therapy alone (N = 55). Except for five New York Heart Association (NYHA) functional Class II patients, all patients were either functional Class III or Class IV. Dosage of FLOLAN was determined as described in DOSAGE AND ADMINISTRATION and averaged 11.2 ng/kg per minute at study end. Conventional therapy varied among patients and included some or all of the following: anticoagulants in essentially all patients, supplemental oxygen and diuretics in two-thirds of the patients, oral vasodilators in 40% of the patients, and digoxin in a third of the patients. A statistically significant increase in CI, and statistically significant decreases in PAPm, RAPm, PVR, and SAPm after 12 weeks of treatment were observed in patients who received FLOLAN chronically compared to those who did not. Table 2 illustrates the treatment-related hemodynamic changes in these patients after 12 weeks of treatment.

[See table 2 above]

Clinical Effects: Statistically significant improvement was observed in exercise capacity, as measured by the 6-minute walk, in patients receiving continuous intravenous FLOLAN plus conventional therapy for 12 weeks compared to those receiving conventional therapy alone. Improvements were apparent in some patients at the end of the first week of therapy. Increases in exercise capacity were accompanied by statistically significant improvements in dyspnea and fatigue, as measured by the Borg Dyspnea Index and Dyspnea Fatigue Index. At week 12, NYHA functional class improved in 21 of 51 (41%) patients treated with FLOLAN compared to none of the 48 patients treated with conventional therapy alone. However, more patients in both treatment groups (28/51 [55%] with FLOLAN and 35/48 [73%] with conventional therapy alone) showed no change in functional class and 2/51 (4%) with FLOLAN and 13/48 (27%) with conventional therapy alone worsened. Of the patients randomized, NYHA functional class data at 12 weeks were not available for 5 patients treated with FLOLAN and 7 patients treated with conventional therapy alone.

No statistical difference in survival over 12 weeks was observed in PH/SSD patients treated with FLOLAN as compared to those receiving conventional therapy alone. At the

Table 4: Adverse Events Regardless of Attribution Occurring in Patients with PPH with ≥10% Difference Between FLOLAN and Conventional Therapy Alone

Adverse Event	FLOLAN (n = 52)	Conventional Therapy (n = 54)
Occurrence More Common with FLOLAN		
GENERAL		
Chills/Fever/Sepsis/Flu-like symptoms	25%	11%
CARDIOVASCULAR		
Tachycardia	35%	24%
Flushing	42%	2%
GASTROINTESTINAL		
Diarrhea	37%	6%
Nausea/Vomiting	67%	48%
MUSCULOSKELETAL		
Jaw Pain	54%	0%
Myalgia	44%	31%
Nonspecific musculoskeletal pain	35%	15%
NEUROLOGICAL		
Anxiety/nervousness/tremor	21%	9%
Dizziness	83%	70%
Headache	83%	33%
Hypesthesia, Hyperesthesia, Paresthesia	12%	2%
Occurrence More Common with Standard Therapy		
CARDIOVASCULAR		
Heart Failure	31%	52%
Syncope	13%	24%
Shock	0%	13%
RESPIRATORY		
Hypoxia	25%	37%

end of the treatment period, 4 of 56 (7%) patients receiving FLOLAN died, whereas 5 of 55 (9%) patients receiving conventional therapy alone died.

No controlled clinical trials with FLOLAN have been performed in patients with pulmonary hypertension associated with other diseases.

INDICATIONS AND USAGE

FLOLAN is indicated for the long-term intravenous treatment of primary pulmonary hypertension and pulmonary hypertension associated with the scleroderma spectrum of disease in NYHA Class III and Class IV patients who do not respond adequately to conventional therapy (see CLINICAL TRIALS IN PULMONARY HYPERTENSION).

CONTRAINDICATIONS

A large study evaluating the effect of FLOLAN on survival in NYHA Class III and IV patients with CHF due to severe left ventricular systolic dysfunction was terminated after an interim analysis of 471 patients revealed a higher mortality in patients receiving FLOLAN plus conventional therapy than in those receiving conventional therapy alone. The chronic use of FLOLAN in patients with CHF due to severe left ventricular systolic dysfunction is therefore contraindicated.

Some patients with pulmonary hypertension have developed pulmonary edema during dose initiation, which may be associated with pulmonary veno-occlusive disease. FLOLAN should not be used chronically in patients who develop pulmonary edema during dose initiation.

FLOLAN is also contraindicated in patients with known hypersensitivity to the drug or to structurally-related compounds.

WARNINGS

FLOLAN must be reconstituted only as directed using STERILE DILUENT for FLOLAN. FLOLAN must not be reconstituted or mixed with any other parenteral medications or solutions prior to or during administration.

Abrupt Withdrawal: Abrupt withdrawal (including interruptions in drug delivery) or sudden large reductions in dosage of FLOLAN may result in symptoms associated with rebound pulmonary hypertension, including dyspnea, dizziness, and asthenia. In clinical trials, one Class III PPH patient's death was judged attributable to the interruption of FLOLAN. Abrupt withdrawal should be avoided.

Sepsis: See ADVERSE REACTIONS: Adverse Events Attributable to the Drug Delivery System.

PRECAUTIONS

General: FLOLAN should be used only by clinicians experienced in the diagnosis and treatment of pulmonary hypertension. The diagnosis of PPH or PH/SSD should be carefully established.

FLOLAN is a potent pulmonary and systemic vasodilator. Dose initiation with FLOLAN must be performed in a setting with adequate personnel and equipment for physiologic monitoring and emergency care. Dose initiation in controlled PPH clinical trials was performed during right heart catheterization. In uncontrolled PPH and controlled PH/SSD clinical trials, dose initiation was performed without cardiac catheterization. The risk of cardiac catheterization in patients with pulmonary hypertension should be carefully weighed against the potential benefits. During dose initiation, asymptomatic increases in pulmonary artery pressure coincident with increases in cardiac output occurred rarely. In such cases, dose reduction should be considered, but such an increase does not imply that chronic treatment is contraindicated.

During chronic use, FLOLAN is delivered continuously on an ambulatory basis through a permanent indwelling central venous catheter. Unless contraindicated, anticoagulant therapy should be administered to PPH and PH/SSD patients receiving FLOLAN to reduce the risk of pulmonary thromboembolism or systemic embolism through a patent foramen ovale. In order to reduce the risk of infection, aseptic technique must be used in the reconstitution and administration of FLOLAN as well as in routine catheter care. Because FLOLAN is metabolized rapidly, even brief interruptions in the delivery of FLOLAN may result in symptoms associated with rebound pulmonary hypertension including dyspnea, dizziness, and asthenia. The decision to initiate therapy with FLOLAN should be based upon the understanding that there is a high likelihood that intravenous therapy with FLOLAN will be needed for prolonged periods, possibly years, and the patient's ability to accept and care for a permanent intravenous catheter and infusion pump should be carefully considered.

Based on clinical trials, the acute hemodynamic response to FLOLAN did not correlate well with improvement in exercise tolerance or survival during chronic use of FLOLAN. Dosage of FLOLAN during chronic use should be adjusted at the first sign of recurrence or worsening of symptoms attributable to pulmonary hypertension or the occurrence of adverse events associated with FLOLAN (see DOSAGE AND ADMINISTRATION). Following dosage adjustments, standing and supine blood pressure and heart rate should be monitored closely for several hours.

Information for Patients: Patients receiving FLOLAN should receive the following information: **FLOLAN must be reconstituted only with STERILE DILUENT for FLOLAN.** FLOLAN is infused continuously through a permanent indwelling central venous catheter via a small, portable infusion pump. Thus, therapy with FLOLAN requires commitment by the patient to drug reconstitution, drug administration, and care of the permanent central venous catheter. Sterile technique must be adhered to in preparing the drug and in the care of the catheter, and even brief interruptions in the delivery of FLOLAN may result in rapid symptomatic deterioration. A patient's decision to receive FLOLAN should be based upon the understanding that there is a high likelihood that therapy with FLOLAN will be needed for prolonged periods, possibly years. The patient's ability to accept and care for a permanent intravenous catheter and infusion pump should also be carefully considered.

Drug Interactions: Additional reductions in blood pressure may occur when FLOLAN is administered with diuretics, antihypertensive agents, or other vasodilators. When other antiplatelet agents or anticoagulants are used concomitantly, there is the potential for FLOLAN to increase the risk of bleeding. However, patients receiving infusions of FLOLAN in clinical trials were maintained on anticoagulants without evidence of increased bleeding. In clinical trials, FLOLAN was used with digoxin, diuretics, anticoagulants, oral vasodilators, and supplemental oxygen.

In a pharmacokinetic substudy in patients with congestive heart failure receiving furosemide or digoxin in whom FLOLAN therapy was initiated, apparent oral clearance values for furosemide (n = 23) and digoxin (n = 30) were decreased by 13% and 15%, respectively, on the second day of therapy and had returned to baseline values by day 87. These changes are not likely to be clinically significant; however, clinicians should be aware of the potential for short-term elevations of digoxin concentrations after initiation of FLOLAN therapy, especially for patients prone to digoxin toxicity.

Carcinogenesis, Mutagenesis, Impairment of Fertility: Long-term studies in animals have not been performed to evaluate carcinogenic potential. A micronucleus test in rats revealed no evidence of mutagenicity. The Ames test and DNA elution tests were also negative, although the instability of epoprostenol makes the significance of these tests uncertain. Fertility was not impaired in rats given FLOLAN by subcutaneous injection at doses up to 100 mcg/kg per day [600 mcg/m^2 per day, 2.5 times the recommended human dose (4.6 ng/kg per minute or 245.1 mcg/m^2 per day, IV) based on body surface area].

Pregnancy: Pregnancy Category B. Reproductive studies have been performed in pregnant rats and rabbits at doses up to 100 mcg/kg per day (600 mcg/m^2 per day in rats, 2.5 times the recommended human dose, and 1180 mcg/m^2 per day in rabbits, 4.8 times the recommended human dose based on body surface area) and have revealed no evidence of impaired fertility or harm to the fetus due to FLOLAN. There are, however, no adequate and well-controlled studies in pregnant women. Because animal reproduction studies are not always predictive of human response, this drug should be used during pregnancy only if clearly needed.

Labor and Delivery: The use of FLOLAN during labor, vaginal delivery, or caesarean section has not been adequately studied in humans.

Nursing Mothers: It is not known whether this drug is excreted in human milk. Because many drugs are excreted in human milk, caution should be exercised when FLOLAN is administered to a nursing woman.

Pediatric Use: Safety and effectiveness in pediatric patients have not been established.

Geriatric Use: Clinical studies of FLOLAN in pulmonary hypertension did not include sufficient numbers of subjects aged 65 and over to determine whether they respond differently from younger patients. Other reported clinical experience has not identified differences in responses between the elderly and younger patients. In general, dose selection for an elderly patient should be cautious, usually starting at the low end of the dosing range, reflecting the greater frequency of decreased hepatic, renal, or cardiac function and of concomitant disease or other drug therapy.

ADVERSE REACTIONS

During clinical trials, adverse events were classified as follows: (1) adverse events during dose initiation and escalation, (2) adverse events during chronic dosing, and (3) adverse events associated with the drug delivery system.

Adverse Events During Dose Initiation and Escalation: During early clinical trials, FLOLAN was increased in 2-ng/kg-per-minute increments until the patients developed symptomatic intolerance. The most common adverse events and the adverse events that limited further increases in dose were generally related to the major pharmacologic effect of FLOLAN, vasodilation. The most common dose-limiting adverse events (occurring in ≥1% of patients) were nausea, vomiting, headache, hypotension, and flushing, but also include chest pain, anxiety, dizziness, bradycardia, dyspnea, abdominal pain, musculoskeletal pain, and tachycardia. Table 3 lists the adverse events reported during dose initiation and escalation in decreasing order of frequency.

Table 3: Adverse Events During Dose Initiation and Escalation

Adverse Events Occurring in ≥1% of Patients	FLOLAN (n = 391)
Flushing	58%
Headache	49%
Nausea/Vomiting	32%
Hypotension	16%
Anxiety, nervousness, agitation	11%
Chest pain	11%
Dizziness	8%
Bradycardia	5%
Abdominal pain	5%
Musculoskeletal pain	3%
Dyspnea	2%
Back pain	2%
Sweating	1%
Dyspepsia	1%
Hypesthesia/Paresthesia	1%
Tachycardia	1%

Adverse Events During Chronic Administration: Interpretation of adverse events is complicated by the clinical fea-

Continued on next page

This product information is based on labeling in effect on June 23, 2000. For further information, contact via direct mail, phone, or web site. Medical Information, Glaxo Wellcome Inc., PO Box 13398, Research Triangle Park, NC 27709. Healthcare Professionals (Medical Information): 800-334-0089. Patients (Customer Response Center): 1-888-825-5249. Glaxo Wellcome Corporate Web Site: www.glaxowellcome.com

Flolan—Cont.

tures of PPH and PH/SSD, which are similar to some of the pharmacologic effects of FLOLAN (e.g., dizziness, syncope). Adverse events probably related to the underlying disease include dyspnea, fatigue, chest pain, edema, hypoxia, right ventricular failure, and pallor. Several adverse events, on the other hand, can clearly be attributed to FLOLAN. These include headache, jaw pain, flushing, diarrhea, nausea and vomiting, flu-like symptoms, and anxiety/nervousness.

Adverse Events During Chronic Administration for PPH: In an effort to separate the adverse effects of the drug from the adverse effects of the underlying disease, Table 4 lists adverse events that occurred at a rate of at least 10% different in the two groups in controlled trials for PPH.

[See table 4 at top of previous page]

Thrombocytopenia has been reported during uncontrolled clinical trials in patients receiving FLOLAN.

Table 5 lists additional adverse events reported in PPH patients receiving FLOLAN plus conventional therapy or conventional therapy alone during controlled clinical trials.

[See table 5 at right]

Adverse Events During Chronic Administration for PH/SSD: In an effort to separate the adverse effects of the drug from the adverse effects of the underlying disease, Table 6 lists adverse events that occurred at a rate at least 10% different in the two groups in the controlled trial for patients with PH/SSD.

[See table 6 at right]

Table 7 lists additional adverse events reported in PH/SSD patients receiving FLOLAN plus conventional therapy or conventional therapy alone during controlled clinical trials.

Although the relationship to FLOLAN administration has not been established, pulmonary embolism has been reported in several patients taking FLOLAN and there have been reports of hepatic failure and pancytopenia.

Adverse Events Attributable to the Drug Delivery System: Chronic infusions of FLOLAN are delivered using a small, portable infusion pump through an indwelling central venous catheter. During controlled PPH trials of up to 12 weeks' duration, up to 21% of patients reported a local infection and up to 13% of patients reported pain at the injection site. During controlled PH/SSD trial of 12 weeks' duration, 14% of patients reported a local infection and 9% of patients reported pain at the injection site. During long-term follow-up in the clinical trial of PPH, sepsis was reported at least once in 14% of patients and occurred at a rate of 0.32 infections per patient per year in patients treated with FLOLAN. This rate was higher than reported in patients using chronic indwelling central venous catheters to administer parenteral nutrition, but lower than reported in oncology patients using theses catheters. Malfunctions in the delivery system resulting in an inadvertent bolus of or a reduction in FLOLAN were associated with symptoms related to excess or insufficient FLOLAN, respectively (see ADVERSE REACTIONS: Adverse Events During Chronic Administration).

[See table 7 at top of next page]

Observed During Clinical Practice: In addition to adverse reactions reported from clinical trials, the following events have been identified during post-approval use of FLOLAN. Because they are reported voluntarily from a population of unknown size, estimates of frequency cannot be made. These events have been chosen for inclusion due to a combination of their seriousness, frequency of reporting, or potential causal connection to FLOLAN.

Blood and Lymphatic: anemia, splenomegaly.

Endocrine and Metabolic: hyperthyroidism.

OVERDOSAGE

Signs and symptoms of excessive doses of FLOLAN during clinical trials are the expected dose-limiting pharmacologic effects of FLOLAN, including flushing, headache, hypotension, tachycardia, nausea, vomiting, and diarrhea. Treatment will ordinarily require dose reduction of FLOLAN.

One patient with secondary pulmonary hypertension accidentally received 50 mL of an unspecified concentration of FLOLAN. The patient vomited and become unconscious with an initially unrecordable blood pressure. FLOLAN was discontinued and the patient regained consciousness within seconds. In clinical practice, fatal events have been reported following overdosage of FLOLAN.

Single intravenous doses of FLOLAN at 10 and 50 mg/kg (2703 and 27,027 times the recommended acute phase human dose based on body surface area) were lethal to mice and rats, respectively. Symptoms of acute toxicity were hypoactivity, ataxia, loss of righting reflex, deep slow breathing, and hypothermia.

DOSAGE AND ADMINISTRATION

Important Note: FLOLAN must be reconstituted only with STERILE DILUENT for FLOLAN. Reconstituted solutions of FLOLAN must not be diluted or administered with other parenteral solutions or medications (see WARNINGS).

Dosage: Continuous chronic infusion of FLOLAN should be administered through a central venous catheter. Temporary peripheral intravenous infusion may be used until central access is established. Chronic infusion of FLOLAN should be initiated at 2 ng/kg/min and increased in increments of 2 ng/kg per minute every 15 minutes or longer until dose-limiting pharmacologic effects are elicited or until a tolerance limit to the drug is established and further increases in the infusion rate are not clinically warranted (see Dosage Adjustments). If dose-limiting pharmacologic effects occur, then the infusion rate should be decreased to an appropriate chronic infusion rate whereby the pharmacologic effects of FLOLAN are tolerated. In clinical trials, the most common dose-limiting adverse events were nausea, vomiting, hypotension, sepsis, headache, abdominal pain, or respiratory disorder (most treatment limiting adverse events were not serious). If the initial infusion rate of 2 ng/kg per minute is not tolerated, a lower dose which is tolerated by the patient should be identified.

In the controlled 12-week trial in PH/SSD, for example, the dose increased from a mean starting dose of 2.2 ng/kg per minute. During the first seven days of treatment, the dose was increased daily to a mean dose of 4.1 mg/kg per minute on Day 7 of treatment. At the end of week 12, the mean dose was 11.2 ng/kg per minute. The mean incremental increase was 2 to 3 ng/kg per minute every 3 weeks.

Dosage Adjustments: Changes in the chronic infusion rate should be based on persistence, recurrence, or worsening of the patient's symptoms of pulmonary hypertension

Table 5: Adverse Events Regardless of Attribution Occurring in Patients with PPH with <10% Difference Between FLOLAN and Conventional Therapy Alone

Adverse Event	FLOLAN (n = 52)	Conventional Therapy (n = 54)
GENERAL		
Asthenia	87%	81%
CARDIOVASCULAR		
Angina pectoris	19%	20%
Arrhythmia	27%	20%
Bradycardia	15%	9%
Supraventricular tachycardia	8%	0%
Pallor	21%	30%
Cyanosis	31%	39%
Palpitation	63%	61%
Cerebrovascular accident	4%	0%
Hemorrhage	19%	11%
Hypotension	27%	31%
Myocardial ischemia	2%	6%
GASTROINTESTINAL		
Abdominal pain	27%	31%
Anorexia	25%	30%
Ascites	12%	17%
Constipation	6%	2%
METABOLIC		
Edema	60%	63%
Hypokalemia	6%	4%
Weight reduction	27%	24%
Weight gain	6%	4%
MUSCULOSKELETAL		
Arthralgia	6%	0%
Bone pain	0%	4%
Chest pain	67%	65%
NEUROLOGICAL		
Confusion	6%	11%
Convulsion	4%	0%
Depression	37%	44%
Insomnia	4%	4%
RESPIRATORY		
Cough increase	38%	46%
Dyspnea	90%	85%
Epistaxis	4%	2%
Pleural effusion	4%	2%
SKIN AND APPENDAGES		
Pruritus	4%	0%
Rash	10%	13%
Sweating	15%	20%
SPECIAL SENSES		
Amblyopia	8%	4%
Vision abnormality	4%	0%

Table 6: Adverse Events Regardless of Attribution Occurring in Patients with PH/SSD with ≥10% Difference Between FLOLAN and Conventional Therapy Alone

Adverse Event	FLOLAN (n = 56)	Conventional Therapy (n = 55)
Occurrence More Common with FLOLAN		
CARDIOVASCULAR		
Flushing	23%	0%
Hypotension	13%	0%
GASTROINTESTINAL		
Anorexia	66%	47%
Nausea/Vomiting	41%	16%
Diarrhea	50%	5%
MUSCULOSKELETAL		
Jaw Pain	75%	0%
Pain/neck pain/arthralgia	84%	65%
NEUROLOGICAL		
Headache	46%	5%
SKIN AND APPENDAGES		
Skin ulcer	39%	24%
Eczema/rash/urticaria	25%	4%
Occurrence More Common with Conventional Therapy		
CARDIOVASCULAR		
Cyanosis	54%	80%
Pallor	32%	53%
Syncope	7%	20%
GASTROINTESTINAL		
Ascites	23%	33%
Esophageal reflux/gastritis	61%	73%
METABOLIC		
Weight decrease	45%	56%
NEUROLOGICAL		
Dizziness	59%	76%
RESPIRATORY		
Hypoxia	55%	65%

Table 7: Adverse Events Regardless of Attribution Occurring in Patients with PH/SSD With <10% Difference Between FLOLAN and Conventional Therapy Alone

Adverse Event*	FLOLAN (n = 56)	Conventional Therapy (n = 55)
GENERAL		
Asthenia	100%	98%
Hemorrhage/hemorrhage injection site/ hemorrhage rectal	11%	2%
Infection/rhinitis	21%	20%
Chills/fever/sepsis/flu-like symptoms	13%	11%
BLOOD AND LYMPHATIC		
Thrombocytopenia	4%	0%
CARDIOVASCULAR		
Heart failure/heart failure right	11%	13%
Myocardial Infarction	4%	0%
Palpitation	63%	71%
Shock	5%	5%
Tachycardia	43%	42%
Vascular disorder peripheral	96%	100%
Vascular disorder	95%	89%
GASTROINTESTINAL		
Abdominal enlargement	4%	0%
Abdominal pain	14%	7%
Constipation	4%	2%
Flatulence	5%	4%
METABOLIC		
Edema/edema peripheral/edema genital	79%	87%
Hypercalcemia	48%	51%
Hyperkalemia	4%	0%
Thirst	0%	4%
MUSCULOSKELETAL		
Arthritis	52%	45%
Back pain	13%	5%
Chest pain	52%	45%
Cramps leg	5%	7%
RESPIRATORY		
Cough increase	82%	82%
Dyspnea	100%	100%
Epistaxis	9%	7%
Pharyngitis	5%	2%
Pleural effusion	7%	0%
Pneumonia	5%	0%
Pneumothorax	4%	0%
Pulmonary edema	4%	2%
Respiratory disorder	7%	4%
Sinusitis	4%	4%
NEUROLOGICAL		
Anxiety/hyperkinesia/nervousness/tremor	7%	5%
Depression/depression psychotic	13%	4%
Hyperesthesia/hypesthesia/paresthesia	5%	0%
Insomnia	9%	0%
Somnolence	4%	2%
SKIN AND APPENDAGES		
Collagen disease	82%	84%
Pruritus	4%	2%
Sweat	41%	36%
UROGENITAL		
Hematuria	5%	0%
Urinary tract infection	7%	0%

*Table lists adverse events which occurred in at least 2 patients in either treatment group.

Table 8: Reconstitution and Dilution Instructions

To make 100 mL of solution with final concentration (ng/mL) of:	Directions:
3000 ng/mL	Dissolve contents of one 0.5-mg vial with 5 mL of STERILE DILUENT for FLOLAN. Withdraw 3 mL and add to sufficient STERILE DILUENT for FLOLAN to make a total of 100 mL.
5000 ng/mL	Dissolve contents of one 0.5-mg vial with 5 mL of STERILE DILUENT for FLOLAN. Withdraw entire vial contents and add sufficient STERILE DILUENT for FLOLAN to make a total of 100 mL.
10,000 ng/mL	Dissolve contents of two 0.5-mg vials each with 5 mL of STERILE DILUENT for FLOLAN. Withdraw entire vial contents and add sufficient STERILE DILUENT for FLOLAN to make a total of 100 mL.
15,000 ng/mL*	Dissolve contents of one 1.5-mg vial with 5 mL of STERILE DILUENT for FLOLAN. Withdraw entire vial contents and add sufficient STERILE DILUENT for FLOLAN to make a total of 100 mL.

* Higher concentrations may be required for patients who receive FLOLAN long-term.

and the occurrence of adverse events due to excessive doses of FLOLAN. In general, increases in dose from the initial chronic dose should be expected.

Increments in dose should be considered if symptoms of pulmonary hypertension persist or recur after improving. The infusion should be increased by 1- to 2-ng/kg-per-minute increments at intervals sufficient to allow assessment of clinical response; these intervals should be at least 15 minutes. In clinical trials, incremental increases in dose occurred at intervals of 24 to 48 hours or longer. Following establishment of a new chronic infusion rate, the patient should be observed, and standing and supine blood pressure and heart rate monitored for several hours to ensure that the new dose is tolerated.

During chronic infusion, the occurrence of dose-limiting pharmacological events may necessitate a decrease in infusion rate, but the adverse event may occasionally resolve without dosage adjustment. Dosage decreases should be made gradually in 2-ng/kg-per-minute decrements every 15 minutes or longer until the dose-limiting effects resolve. Abrupt withdrawal of FLOLAN or sudden large reductions in infusion rates should be avoided. Except in life-threatening situations (e.g., unconsciousness, collapse, etc.), infusion rates of FLOLAN should be adjusted only under the direction of a physician.

In patients receiving lung transplants, doses of FLOLAN were tapered after the initiation of cardiopulmonary bypass.

Administration: FLOLAN is administered by continuous intravenous infusion via a central venous catheter using an ambulatory infusion pump. During initiation of treatment, FLOLAN may be administered peripherally.

The ambulatory infusion pump used to administer FLOLAN should: (1) be small and lightweight, (2) be able to adjust infusion rates in 2-ng/kg-per-minute increments, (3) have occlusion, end of infusion, and low battery alarms, (4) be accurate to ±6% of the programmed rate, and (5) be positive pressure-driven (continuous or pulsatile) with intervals between pulses not exceeding 3 minutes at infusion rates used to deliver FLOLAN. The reservoir should be made of polyvinyl chloride, polypropylene, or glass. The infusion pump used in the most recent clinical trials was the CADD-1 HFX 5100 (SIMS Deltec). A 60" microbore non-DEHP extension set with proximal antisyphon valve, low priming volume (0.9 mL), and inline 0.22 micron filter was used during clinical trials.

To avoid potential interruptions in drug delivery, the patient should have access to a backup infusion pump and intravenous infusion sets. A multi-lumen catheter should be considered if other intravenous therapies are routinely administered.

To facilitate extended use at ambient temperatures exceeding 25°C (77°F), a cold pouch with frozen gel packs was used in clinical trials (see DOSAGE AND ADMINISTRATION: Storage and Stability). The cold pouches and gel packs used in clinical trials were obtained from Palco Labs, Palo Alto, California. Any cold pouch used must be capable of maintaining the temperature of reconstituted FLOLAN between 2° and 8°C for 12 hours.

Reconstitution: FLOLAN is stable only when reconstituted with STERILE DILUENT for FLOLAN. FLOLAN must not be reconstituted or mixed with any other parenteral medications or solutions prior to or during administration.

A concentration for the solution of FLOLAN should be selected which is compatible with the infusion pump being used with respect to minimum and maximum flow rates, reservoir capacity, and the infusion pump criteria listed above. FLOLAN, when administered chronically, should be prepared in a drug delivery reservoir appropriate for the infusion pump with a total reservoir volume of at least 100 mL. FLOLAN should be prepared using 2 vials of STERILE DILUENT for FLOLAN for use during a 24-hour period. Table 8 gives directions for preparing several different concentrations of FLOLAN:

[See table 8 at left]

Generally, 3000 ng/mL and 10,000 ng/mL are satisfactory concentrations to deliver between 2 to 16 ng/kg per minute in adults. Infusion rates may be calculated using the following formula:

Infusion Rate (mL/hr) =

$$\frac{\text{[Dose (ng/kg/min)} \times \text{Weight (kg)} \times \text{60 min/hr]}}{\text{Final Concentration (ng/mL)}}$$

Table 9 through 12 provide infusion delivery rates for doses up to 16 ng/kg per minute based upon patient weight, drug delivery rate, and concentration of the solution of FLOLAN to be used. These tables may be used to select the most appropriate concentration of FLOLAN that will result in an infusion rate between the minimum and maximum flow rates of the infusion pump and which will allow the desired duration of infusion from a given reservoir volume. Higher infusion rates, and therefore, more concentrated solutions may be necessary with long-term administration of FLOLAN.

Table 9: Infusion Rates for FLOLAN at a Concentration of 3000 ng/mL

Patient Weight (kg)	Dose or Drug Delivery Rate (ng/kg per minute) 2	4	6	8	10	12	14	16
	Infusion Delivery Rate (mL/hr)							
10	—	—	1.2	1.6	2.0	2.4	2.8	3.2
20	—	1.6	2.4	3.2	4.0	4.8	5.6	6.4
30	1.2	2.4	3.6	4.8	6.0	7.2	8.4	9.6
40	1.6	3.2	4.8	6.4	8.0	9.6	11.2	12.8
50	2.0	4.0	6.0	8.0	10.0	12.0	14.0	16.0
60	2.4	4.8	7.2	9.6	12.0	14.4	16.8	19.2
70	2.8	5.6	8.4	11.2	14.0	16.8	19.6	22.4
80	3.2	6.4	9.6	12.8	16.0	19.2	22.4	25.6
90	3.6	7.2	10.8	14.4	18.0	21.6	25.2	28.8
100	4.0	8.0	12.0	16.0	20.0	24.0	28.0	32.0

Table 10: Infusion Rates for FLOLAN at a Concentration of 5000 ng/mL

Patient Weight (kg)	Dose or Drug Delivery Rate (ng/kg per minute) 2	4	6	8	10	12	14	16
	Infusion Delivery Rate (mL/hr)							
10	—	—	—	1.0	1.2	1.4	1.7	1.9
20	—	1.0	1.4	1.9	2.4	2.9	3.4	3.8
30	—	1.4	2.2	2.9	3.6	4.3	5.0	5.8
40	1.0	1.9	2.9	3.8	4.8	5.8	6.7	7.7
50	1.2	2.4	3.6	4.8	6.0	7.2	8.4	9.6
60	1.4	2.9	4.3	5.8	7.2	8.6	10.1	11.5
70	1.7	3.4	5.0	6.7	8.4	10.1	11.8	13.4
80	1.9	3.8	5.8	7.7	9.6	11.5	13.4	15.4
90	2.2	4.3	6.5	8.6	10.8	13.0	15.1	17.3
100	2.4	4.8	7.2	9.6	12.0	14.4	16.8	19.2

Continued on next page

This product information is based on labeling in effect on June 23, 2000. For further information, contact via direct mail, phone, or web site. Medical Information, Glaxo Wellcome Inc., PO Box 13398, Research Triangle Park, NC 27709. Healthcare Professionals (Medical Information): 800-334-0089. Patients (Customer Response Center): 1-888-825-5249. Glaxo Wellcome Corporate Web Site: www.glaxowellcome.com

Flolan—Cont.

Table 11: Infusion Rates for FLOLAN at a Concentration of 10,000 ng/mL

Patient Weight (kg)	Dose or Drug Delivery Rate (ng/kg per minute)						
	4	6	8	10	12	14	16
	Infusion Delivery Rate (mL/hr)						
20	—	—	1.0	1.2	1.4	1.7	1.9
30	—	1.1	1.4	1.8	2.2	2.5	2.9
40	1.0	1.4	1.9	2.4	2.9	3.4	3.8
50	1.2	1.8	2.4	3.0	3.6	4.2	4.8
60	1.4	2.2	2.9	3.6	4.3	5.0	5.8
70	1.7	2.5	3.4	4.2	5.0	5.9	6.7
80	1.9	2.9	3.8	4.8	5.8	6.7	7.7
90	2.2	3.2	4.3	5.4	6.5	7.6	8.6
100	2.4	3.6	4.8	6.0	7.2	8.4	9.6

Table 12: Infusion Rates for FLOLAN at a Concentration of 15,000 ng/mL

Patient Weight (kg)	Dose or Drug Delivery Rate (ng/kg per minute)						
	4	6	8	10	12	14	16
	Infusion Delivery Rate (mL/hr)						
30	—	—	1.0	1.2	1.4	1.7	1.9
40	—	1.0	1.3	1.6	1.9	2.2	2.6
50	—	1.2	1.6	2.0	2.4	2.8	3.2
60	1.0	1.4	1.9	2.4	2.9	3.4	3.8
70	1.1	1.7	2.2	2.8	3.4	3.9	4.5
80	1.3	1.9	2.6	3.2	3.8	4.5	5.1
90	1.4	2.2	2.9	3.6	4.3	5.0	5.8
100	1.6	2.4	3.2	4.0	4.8	5.6	6.4

Storage and Stability: Unopened vials of FLOLAN are stable until the date indicated on the package when stored at 15° to 25°C (59° to 77°F) and protected from light in the carton. Unopened vials of STERILE DILUENT for FLOLAN are stable until the date indicated on the package when stored at 15° to 25°C (59° to 77°F).

Prior to use, reconstituted solutions of FLOLAN must be protected from light and must be refrigerated at 2° to 8°C (36° to 46°F) if not used immediately. **Do not freeze reconstituted solutions of FLOLAN. Discard any reconstituted solution that has been frozen. Discard any reconstituted solution if it has been refrigerated for more than 48 hours.** During use, a single reservoir of reconstituted solution of FLOLAN can be administered at room temperature for a total duration of 8 hours, or it can be used with a cold pouch and administered up to 24 hours with the use of two frozen 6-oz gel packs in a cold pouch. When stored or in use, reconstituted FLOLAN must be insulated from temperatures greater than 25°C (77°F) and less than 0°C (32°F), and must not be exposed to direct sunlight.

Use at Room Temperature: Prior to use at room temperature, 15° to 25°C (59° to 77°F), reconstituted solutions of FLOLAN may be stored refrigerated at 2° to 8°C (36° to 46°F) for no longer than 40 hours. When administered at room temperature, reconstituted solutions may be used for no longer than 8 hours. This 48-hour period allows the patient to reconstitute a 2-day supply (200 mL) of FLOLAN. Each 100-mL daily supply may be divided into three equal portions. Two of the portions are stored refrigerated at 2° to 8°C (36° to 46°F) until they are used.

Use with a Cold Pouch: Prior to infusion with the use of a cold pouch, solutions may be stored refrigerated at 2° to 8°C (36° to 46°F) for up to 24 hours. When a cold pouch is employed during the infusion, reconstituted solutions of FLOLAN may be used for no longer than 24 hours. The gel packs should be changed every 12 hours. Reconstituted solutions may be kept at 2° to 8°C (36° to 46°F), either in refrigerated storage or in a cold pouch or a combination of the two, for no more than 48 hours.

Parenteral drug products should be inspected visually for particular matter and discoloration prior to administration whenever solution and container permit. If either occurs, FLOLAN should not be administered.

HOW SUPPLIED

FLOLAN for Injection is supplied as a sterile freeze-dried powder in 17-mL flint glass vials with gray butyl rubber closures, individually packaged in a carton.

17-mL vial containing epoprostenol sodium equivalent to 0.5 mg (500,000 ng), carton of 1 (NDC 0173-0517-00).

17-mL vial containing epoprostenol sodium equivalent to 1.5 mg (1,500,000 ng), carton of 1 (NDC 0173-0519-00).

Store the vials of FLOLAN at 15° to 25°C (59° to 77°F) Protect from light.

The STERILE DILUENT for FLOLAN is supplied in 50-mL flint glass vials with fluororesin-faced butyl rubber closures.

50-mL vial of STERILE DILUENT for FLOLAN, tray of 4 (NDC 0173-0518-00).

Store the vials of STERILE DILUENT for FLOLAN at 15° to 25°C (59° to 77°F). DO NOT FREEZE.

Glaxo Wellcome Inc., Research Triangle Park, NC 27709

US Patent Nos. 4,539,333 and 4,883,812 (Use Patent)

Sterile Diluent for FLOLAN manufactured by
Catalytica Pharmaceuticals, Inc.
Greenville, NC 27834
for Glaxo Wellcome Inc., Research Triangle Park, NC 27709
April 2000 RL-809

Shown in Product Identification Guide, page 315

FLONASE® ℞

[*flō'nāz*]

(fluticasone propionate)
Nasal Spray, 50 mcg

For Intranasal Use Only.
SHAKE GENTLY BEFORE USE.

DESCRIPTION

Fluticasone propionate, the active ingredient of FLONASE Nasal Spray, is a synthetic corticosteroid with the chemical name of S-fluoromethyl 6α,9α-difluoro-11β-hydroxy-16α-methyl-3-oxo-17α-propionyloxyandrosta-1,4-diene-17β-carbothioate.

Fluticasone propionate is a white to off-white powder with a molecular weight of 500.6. It is practically insoluble in water, freely soluble in dimethyl sulfoxide and dimethylformamide, and slightly soluble in methanol and 95% ethanol.

FLONASE Nasal Spray 50 mcg is an aqueous suspension of microfine fluticasone propionate for topical administration to the nasal mucosa by means of a metering, atomizing spray pump. FLONASE Nasal Spray also contains microcrystalline cellulose and carboxymethylcellulose sodium, dextrose, 0.02% w/w benzalkonium chloride, polysorbate 80, and 0.25% w/w phenylethyl alcohol, and has a pH between 5 and 7.

It is necessary to prime the pump before first use or after a period of non-use (1 week or more). After initial priming (six actuations), each actuation delivers 50 mcg of fluticasone propionate in 100 mg of formulation through the nasal adapter. Each bottle of FLONASE Nasal Spray provides 120 metered sprays. After 120 metered sprays, the amount of fluticasone propionate delivered per actuation may not be consistent and the unit should be discarded.

CLINICAL PHARMACOLOGY

Fluticasone propionate is a synthetic, trifluorinated corticosteroid with anti-inflammatory activity. In vitro dose response studies on a cloned human glucocorticoid receptor system involving binding and gene expression afforded 50% responses at 1.25 and 0.17 nM concentrations, respectively. Fluticasone propionate was threefold to fivefold more potent than dexamethasone in these assays. Data from the McKenzie vasoconstrictor assay in man also support its potent glucocorticoid activity.

In preclinical studies, fluticasone propionate revealed progesterone-like activity similar to the natural hormone. However, the clinical significance of these findings in relation to the low plasma levels (see Pharmacokinetics) is not known.

The precise mechanism through which fluticasone propionate affects allergic rhinitis symptoms is not known. Corticosteroids have been shown to have a wide range of effects on multiple cell types (e.g., mast cells, eosinophils, neutrophils, macrophages, and lymphocytes) and mediators (e.g., histamine, eicosanoids, leukotrienes, and cytokines) involved in inflammation. In seven trials in adults, FLONASE Nasal Spray has decreased nasal mucosal eosinophils in 66% (35% for placebo) of patients and basophils in 39% (28% for placebo) of patients. The direct relationship of these findings to long-term symptom relief is not known.

FLONASE Nasal Spray, like other corticosteroids, is an agent that does not have an immediate effect on allergic symptoms. A decrease in nasal symptoms has been noted in some patients 12 hours after initial treatment with FLONASE Nasal Spray. Maximum benefit may not be reached for several days. Similarly, when corticosteroids are discontinued, symptoms may not return for several days.

Pharmacokinetics: ***Absorption:*** The activity of FLONASE Nasal Spray is due to the parent drug, fluticasone propionate. Indirect calculations indicate that fluticasone propionate delivered by the intranasal route has an absolute bioavailability averaging less than 2%. After intranasal treatment of patients with allergic rhinitis for 3 weeks, fluticasone propionate plasma concentrations were above the level of detection (50 pg/mL) only when recommended doses were exceeded and then only in occasional samples at low plasma levels. Due to the low bioavailability by the intranasal route, the majority of the pharmacokinetic data was obtained via other routes of administration. Studies using oral dosing of radiolabeled drug have demonstrated that fluticasone propionate is highly extracted from plasma and absorption is low. Oral bioavailability is negligible, and the majority of the circulating radioactivity is due to an inactive metabolite.

Distribution: Following intravenous administration, the initial disposition phase for fluticasone propionate was rapid and consistent with its high lipid solubility and tissue binding. The volume of distribution averaged 4.2 L/kg. The percentage of fluticasone propionate bound to human plasma proteins averaged 91% with no obvious concentration relationship. Fluticasone propionate is weakly and reversibly bound to erythrocytes and freely equilibrates between erythrocytes and plasma. Fluticasone propionate is not significantly bound to human transcortin.

Metabolism: The total blood clearance of fluticasone propionate is high (average, 1093 mL/min), with renal clearance accounting for less than 0.02% of the total. The only circulating metabolite detected in man is the 17β-carboxylic acid derivative of fluticasone propionate, which is formed through the cytochrome P450 3A4 pathway. This inactive metabolite had approximately 2000 times less affinity than the parent drug for the glucocorticoid receptor of human lung cytosol in vitro and negligible pharmacological activity in animal studies. Other metabolites detected in vitro using cultured human hepatoma cells have not been detected in man.

In a multiple-dose drug interaction study, coadministration of orally inhaled fluticasone propionate (500 mcg twice daily) and erythromycin (333 mg three times daily) did not affect fluticasone propionate pharmacokinetics.

In a drug interaction study, coadministration of orally inhaled fluticasone propionate (1000 mcg, 5 times the maximum daily intranasal dose) and ketoconazole (200 mg once daily) resulted in increased fluticasone propionate concentrations, a reduction in plasma cortisol AUC, and no effect on urinary excretion of cortisol.

Excretion: Following intravenous dosing, fluticasone propionate showed polyexponential kinetics and had a terminal elimination half-life of approximately 7.8 hours. Less than 5% of a radiolabeled oral dose was excreted in the urine as metabolites, with the remainder excreted in the feces as parent drug and metabolites.

Special Populations: Fluticasone propionate was not studied in any special populations, and no gender-specific pharmacokinetic data have been obtained.

Pharmacodynamics: In a trial to evaluate the potential systemic and topical effects of FLONASE Nasal Spray on allergic rhinitis symptoms, the benefits of comparable drug blood levels produced by FLONASE Nasal Spray and oral fluticasone propionate were compared. The doses used were 200 mcg of FLONASE Nasal Spray, the nasal spray vehicle (plus oral placebo), and 5 and 10 mg of oral fluticasone propionate (plus nasal spray vehicle) per day for 14 days. Plasma levels were undetectable in the majority of patients after intranasal dosing, but present at low levels in the majority after oral dosing. FLONASE Nasal Spray was significantly more effective in reducing symptoms of allergic rhinitis than either the oral fluticasone propionate or the nasal vehicle. This trial demonstrated that the therapeutic effect of FLONASE Nasal Spray can be attributed to the topical effects of fluticasone propionate.

In another trial, the potential systemic effects of FLONASE Nasal Spray on the hypothalamic-pituitary-adrenal (HPA) axis were also studied in allergic patients. FLONASE Nasal Spray given as 200 mcg once daily or 400 mcg twice daily was compared with placebo or oral prednisone 7.5 or 15 mg given in the morning. FLONASE Nasal Spray at either dose for 4 weeks did not affect the adrenal response to 6-hour cosyntropin stimulation, while both doses of oral prednisone significantly reduced the response to cosyntropin.

Clinical Trials: A total of 13 randomized, double-blind, parallel, multicenter, vehicle-controlled clinical trials were conducted in the United States in adults and pediatric patients (4 years of age and older) with seasonal or perennial allergic rhinitis. The trials included 2633 adults (1439 men and 1194 women) with a mean age of 37 years (range, 18 to 79). A total of 440 adolescents (405 boys and 35 girls), mean age of 14 (range, 12 to 17), and 500 children (325 boys and 175 girls), mean age of 9 (range, 4 to 11) were also studied. The overall racial distribution was 89% white, 4% black, and 7% other. These trials evaluated the total nasal symptom scores (TNSS) that included rhinorrhea, nasal obstruction, sneezing, and nasal itching in known allergic patients who were treated for 2 to 24 weeks. Subjects treated with FLONASE Nasal Spray exhibited significantly greater decreases in TNSS than vehicle placebo-treated patients. Nasal mucosal basophils and eosinophils were also reduced at the end of treatment in adult studies; however, the clinical significance of this decrease is not known.

There were no significant differences between fluticasone propionate regimens whether administered as a single daily dose of 200 mcg (two 50-mcg sprays in each nostril) or as 100 mcg (one 50-mcg spray in each nostril) twice daily in six clinical trials. A clear dose response could not be identified in clinical trials. In one trial, 200 mcg/day was slightly more effective than 50 mcg/day during the first few days of treatment; thereafter, no difference was seen.

Three randomized, double-blind, parallel, vehicle-controlled trials were conducted in 1191 patients with perennial nonallergic rhinitis. These trials evaluated the patient-rated total nasal symptom scores (nasal obstruction, postnasal drip, rhinorrhea) in patients treated for 28 days of double-blind therapy and in one of the 3 trials for 6 months of open-label treatment. Two of these trials demonstrated that patients treated with FLONASE Nasal Spray at a dose of 100 mcg twice daily exhibited statistically significant decreases in total nasal symptom scores compared with patients treated with vehicle.

Individualization of Dosage: Adult patients may be started on a 200-mcg once-a-day regimen (two 50-mcg sprays in each nostril once-a-day). An alternative 200-mcg/day dosage regimen can be given as 100 mcg twice daily (one 50-mcg spray in each nostril twice-a-day).

Individual patients will experience a variable time to onset and different degree of symptom relief. In 4 randomized, double-blind, placebo-controlled, parallel group allergic rhinitis studies and 2 studies of patients in an outdoor "park" setting (park studies), a decrease in nasal symptoms in treated subjects compared to placebo was shown to occur as soon as 12 hours after treatment with a 200-mcg dose of FLONASE Nasal Spray. Maximum effect may take several days. Patients who have responded may be able to be maintained (after 4 to 7 days) on 100 mcg/day (one spray in each nostril once daily).

Pediatric patients (4 years of age and older) should be started with 100 mcg (one spray in each nostril once-a-day). Treatment with 200 mcg (two sprays in each nostril once daily or one spray in each nostril twice daily) should be reserved for pediatric patients not adequately responding to 100 mcg daily. Once adequate control is achieved, the dosage should be decreased to 100 mcg (one spray in each nostril) daily.

Maximum total daily doses should not exceed two sprays in each nostril (total dose, 200 mcg/day). There is no evidence that exceeding the recommended dose is more effective.

INDICATIONS AND USAGE

FLONASE Nasal Spray is indicated for the management of the nasal symptoms of seasonal and perennial allergic and nonallergic rhinitis in adults and pediatric patients 4 years of age and older.

Safety and effectiveness of FLONASE Nasal Spray in children below 4 years of age have not been adequately established.

CONTRAINDICATIONS

FLONASE Nasal Spray is contraindicated in patients with a hypersensitivity to any of its ingredients.

WARNINGS

The replacement of a systemic corticosteroid with a topical corticosteroid can be accompanied by signs of adrenal insufficiency, and in addition some patients may experience symptoms of withdrawal, e.g., joint and/or muscular pain, lassitude, and depression. Patients previously treated for prolonged periods with systemic corticosteroids and transferred to topical corticosteroids should be carefully monitored for acute adrenal insufficiency in response to stress. In those patients who have asthma or other clinical conditions requiring long-term systemic corticosteroid treatment, too rapid a decrease in systemic corticosteroids may cause a severe exacerbation of their symptoms.

The concomitant use of intranasal corticosteroids with other inhaled corticosteroids could increase the risk of signs or symptoms of hypercorticism and/or suppression of the HPA axis.

Patients who are on immunosuppressant drugs are more susceptible to infections than healthy individuals. Chickenpox and measles, for example, can have a more serious or even fatal course in patients on immunosuppressant doses of corticosteroids. In such patients who have not had these diseases, particular care should be taken to avoid exposure. How the dose, route, and duration of corticosteroid administration affects the risk of developing a disseminated infection is not known. The contribution of the underlying disease and/or prior corticosteroid treatment to the risk is also not known. If exposed to chickenpox, prophylaxis with varicella zoster immune globulin (VZIG) may be indicated. If exposed to measles, prophylaxis with pooled intramuscular immunoglobulin (IG) may be indicated. (See the respective package inserts for complete VZIG and IG prescribing information). If chickenpox develops, treatment with antiviral agents may be considered.

PRECAUTIONS

General: Rarely, immediate hypersensitivity reactions or contact dermatitis may occur after the administration of FLONASE Nasal Spray. Rare instances of wheezing, nasal septum perforation, cataracts, glaucoma, and increased intraocular pressure have been reported following the intranasal application of corticosteroids, including fluticasone propionate.

Use of excessive doses of corticosteroids may lead to signs or symptoms of hypercorticism, suppression of HPA function, and/or reduction of growth velocity in children or teenagers. Physicians should closely follow the growth of children and adolescents taking corticosteroids, by any route, and weigh the benefits of corticosteroid therapy against the possibility of growth suppression if growth appears slowed.

Although systemic effects have been minimal with recommended doses of FLONASE Nasal Spray, potential risk increases with larger doses. Therefore, larger than recommended doses of FLONASE Nasal Spray should be avoided.

When used at higher than recommended doses, or in rare individuals at recommended doses, systemic corticosteroid effects such as hypercorticism and adrenal suppression may appear. If such changes occur, the dosage of FLONASE Nasal Spray should be discontinued slowly consistent with accepted procedures for discontinuing oral corticosteroid therapy.

In clinical studies with fluticasone propionate administered intranasally, the development of localized infections of the nose and pharynx with *Candida albicans* has occurred only rarely. When such an infection develops, it may require treatment with appropriate local therapy and discontinuation of treatment with FLONASE Nasal Spray. Patients using FLONASE Nasal Spray over several months or longer should be examined periodically for evidence of *Candida* infection or other signs of adverse effects on the nasal mucosa.

FLONASE Nasal Spray should be used with caution, if at all, in patients with active or quiescent tuberculous infection; untreated local or systemic fungal or bacterial, or systemic viral infections or parasitic infection; or ocular herpes simplex.

Because of the inhibitory effect of corticosteroids on wound healing, patients who have experienced recent nasal septal ulcers, nasal surgery, or nasal trauma should not use a nasal corticosteroid until healing has occurred.

Information for Patients: Patients being treated with FLONASE Nasal Spray should receive the following information and instructions. This information is intended to aid them in the safe and effective use of this medication. It is not a disclosure of all possible adverse or intended effects. Patients should be warned to avoid exposure to chickenpox or measles and, if exposed, to consult their physician without delay.

Patients should use FLONASE Nasal Spray at regular intervals as directed since its effectiveness depends on its regular use. A decrease in nasal symptoms may occur as soon as 12 hours after starting therapy with FLONASE Nasal Spray. Results in several clinical trials indicate statistically significant improvement within the first day or two of treatment; however, the full benefit of FLONASE Nasal Spray may not be achieved until treatment has been administered for several days. The patient should not increase the prescribed dosage but should contact the physician if symptoms do not improve or if the condition worsens. For the proper use of the nasal spray and to attain maximum improvement, the patient should read and follow carefully the patient's instructions accompanying the product.

Drug Interactions: In a placebo-controlled, crossover study in eight healthy volunteers, coadministration of a single dose of orally inhaled fluticasone propionate (1000 mcg, 5 times the maximum daily intranasal dose) with multiple doses of ketoconazole (200 mg) to steady state resulted in increased mean fluticasone propionate concentrations, a reduction in plasma cortisol AUC, and no effect on urinary excretion of cortisol. This interaction may be due to an inhibition of the cytochrome P450 3A4 isoenzyme system by ketoconazole, which is also the route of metabolism of fluticasone propionate. No drug interaction studies have been conducted with FLONASE Nasal Spray; however, care should be exercised when fluticasone propionate is coadministered with long-term ketoconazole and other known cytochrome P450 3A4 inhibitors.

Carcinogenesis, Mutagenesis, Impairment of Fertility: Fluticasone propionate demonstrated no tumorigenic potential in mice at oral doses up to 1000 mcg/kg (approximately 20 times the maximum recommended daily intranasal dose in adults and approximately 10 times the maximum recommended daily intranasal dose in children on a mcg/m^2 basis) for 78 weeks or in rats at inhalation doses up to 57 mcg/kg (approximately 2 times the maximum recommended daily intranasal dose in adults and approximately equivalent to the maximum recommended daily intranasal dose in children on a mcg/m^2 basis) for 104 weeks.

Fluticasone propionate did not induce gene mutation in prokaryotic or eukaryotic cells in vitro. No significant clastogenic effect was seen in cultured human peripheral lymphocytes in vitro or in the mouse micronucleus test when administered at high doses by the oral or subcutaneous routes. Furthermore, the compound did not delay erythroblast division in bone marrow.

No evidence of impairment of fertility was observed in reproductive studies conducted in male and female rats at subcutaneous doses up to 50 mcg/kg (approximately 2 times the maximum recommended daily intranasal dose in adults on a mcg/m^2 basis). Prostate weight was significantly reduced at a subcutaneous dose of 50 mcg/kg.

Pregnancy: *Teratogenic Effects:* Pregnancy Category C. Subcutaneous studies in the mouse and rat at 45 and 100 mcg/kg, respectively (approximately equivalent to and 4 times the maximum recommended daily intranasal dose in adults on a mcg/m^2 basis, respectively) revealed fetal toxicity characteristic of potent corticosteroid compounds, including embryonic growth retardation, omphalocele, cleft palate, and retarded cranial ossification.

In the rabbit, fetal weight reduction and cleft palate were observed at a subcutaneous dose of 4 mcg/kg (less than the maximum recommended daily intranasal dose in adults on a mcg/m^2 basis).

However, no teratogenic effects were reported at oral doses up to 300 mcg/kg (approximately 25 times the maximum recommended daily intranasal dose in adults on a mcg/m^2 basis) of fluticasone propionate to the rabbit. No fluticasone propionate was detected in the plasma in this study, consistent with the established low bioavailability following oral administration (see CLINICAL PHARMACOLOGY).

Fluticasone propionate crossed the placenta following oral administration of 100 mcg/kg to rats or 300 mcg/kg to rabbits (approximately 4 and 25 times, respectively, the maximum recommended daily intranasal dose in adults on a mcg/m^2 basis).

There are no adequate and well-controlled studies in pregnant women. Fluticasone propionate should be used during pregnancy only if the potential benefit justifies the potential risk to the fetus.

Experience with oral corticosteroids since their introduction in pharmacologic, as opposed to physiologic, doses suggests that rodents are more prone to teratogenic effects from corticosteroids than humans. In addition, because there is a natural increase in corticosteroid production during pregnancy, most women will require a lower exogenous corticosteroid dose and many will not need corticosteroid treatment during pregnancy.

Nursing Mothers: It is not known whether fluticasone propionate is excreted in human breast milk. When tritiated fluticasone propionate was administered to rats at a subcutaneous dose of 10 mcg/kg (less than the maximum recommended daily intranasal dose in adults on a mcg/m^2 basis), radioactivity was excreted in the milk. Because other corticosteroids are excreted in human milk, caution should be exercised when FLONASE Nasal Spray is administered to a nursing woman.

Pediatric Use: Five hundred (500) patients aged 4 to 11 years of age and 440 patients aged 12 to 17 years were studied in US clinical trials with fluticasone propionate nasal spray. The safety and effectiveness of FLONASE Nasal Spray in children below 4 years of age have not been established.

Oral and, to a less clear extent, inhaled and intranasal corticosteroids have been shown to have the potential to cause a reduction in growth velocity in children and adolescents with extended use. If a child or adolescent on any corticosteroid appears to have growth suppression, the possibility that they are particularly sensitive to this effect of corticosteroids should be considered (see PRECAUTIONS).

Geriatric Use: A limited number of patients above 60 years of age (n = 275) have been treated with FLONASE Nasal Spray in US and non-US clinical trials. While the number of patients is too small to permit separate analysis of efficacy and safety, the adverse reactions reported in this population were similar to those reported by younger patients.

ADVERSE REACTIONS

In controlled US studies, more than 3300 patients with seasonal allergic, perennial allergic, or perennial nonallergic rhinitis received treatment with intranasal fluticasone propionate. In general, adverse reactions in clinical studies have been primarily associated with irritation of the nasal mucous membranes, and the adverse reactions were reported with approximately the same frequency by patients treated with the vehicle itself. The complaints did not usually interfere with treatment. Less than 2% of patients in clinical trials discontinued because of adverse events; this rate was similar for vehicle placebo and active comparators.

Systemic corticosteroid side effects were not reported during controlled clinical studies up to 6 months' duration with FLONASE Nasal Spray. If recommended doses are exceeded, however, or if individuals are particularly sensitive, or taking FLONASE Nasal Spray in conjunction with administration of other corticosteroids, symptoms of hypercorticism, e.g., Cushing's syndrome, could occur.

The following incidence of common adverse reactions (>3%, where incidence in fluticasone propionate-treated subjects exceeded placebo) is based upon seven controlled clinical trials in which 536 patients (57 girls and 108 boys aged 4 to 11 years, 137 female and 234 male adolescents and adults) were treated with FLONASE Nasal Spray 200 mcg once daily over 2 to 4 weeks and two controlled clinical trials in which 246 patients (119 female and 127 male adolescents and adults) were treated with FLONASE Nasal Spray 200 mcg once daily over 6 months. Also included in the table are adverse events from two studies in which 167 children (45

Continued on next page

Overall Adverse Experiences With >3% Incidence on Fluticasone Propionate in Controlled Clinical Trials With FLONASE Nasal Spray in Patients ≥4 Years With Seasonal or Perennial Allergic Rhinitis

	Vehicle Placebo (n = 758) %	FLONASE 100 mcg Once Daily (n = 167) %	FLONASE 200 mcg Once Daily (n = 782) %
Headache	14.6	6.6	16.1
Pharyngitis	7.2	6.0	7.8
Epistaxis	5.4	6.0	6.9
Nasal burning/irritation	2.6	2.4	3.2
Nausea/vomiting	2.0	4.8	2.6
Asthma symptoms	2.9	7.2	3.3
Cough	2.8	3.6	3.8

This product information is based on labeling in effect on June 23, 2000. For further information, contact via direct mail, phone, or web site. Medical Information, Glaxo Wellcome Inc., PO Box 13398, Research Triangle Park, NC 27709. Healthcare Professionals (Medical Information): 800-334-0089. Patients (Customer Response Center): 1-888-825-5249. Glaxo Wellcome Corporate Web Site: www.glaxowellcome.com

Flonase—Cont.

girls and 122 boys aged 4 to 11 years) were treated with FLONASE Nasal Spray 100 mcg once daily for 2 to 4 weeks.
[See table at top of previous page]
Other adverse events that occurred in ≤3% but ≥1% of patients and that were more common with fluticasone propionate (with uncertain relationship to treatment) included: blood in nasal mucus, runny nose, abdominal pain, diarrhea, fever, flu-like symptoms, aches and pains, dizziness, bronchitis.

Observed During Clinical Practice: In addition to adverse events reported from clinical trials, the following events have been identified during postapproval use of fluticasone propionate in clinical practice. Because they are reported voluntarily from a population of unknown size, estimates of frequency cannot be made. These events have been chosen for inclusion due to either their seriousness, frequency of reporting, causal connection to fluticasone propionate, occurrence during clinical trials, or a combination of these factors.

General: Hypersensitivity reactions, including angioedema, skin rash, edema of the face and tongue, pruritus, urticaria, bronchospasm, wheezing, dyspnea, and anaphylaxis/anaphylactoid reactions, which in rare instances were severe.

Ear, Nose, and Throat: Alteration or loss of sense of taste and/or smell and, rarely, nasal septal perforation, nasal ulcer, sore throat, throat irritation and dryness, cough, hoarseness, and voice changes.

Eye: Dryness and irritation, conjunctivitis, blurred vision, glaucoma, increased intraocular pressure, and cataracts.

OVERDOSAGE

Chronic overdosage with FLONASE Nasal Spray may result in signs/symptoms of hypercorticism (see PRECAUTIONS). Intranasal administration of 2 mg (10 times the recommended dose) of fluticasone propionate twice daily for 7 days to healthy human volunteers was well tolerated. Single oral doses up to 16 mg have been studied in human volunteers with no acute toxic effects reported. Repeat oral doses up to 80 mg daily for 10 days in volunteers and repeat oral doses up to 10 mg daily for 14 days in patients were well tolerated. Adverse reactions were of mild or moderate severity, and incidences were similar in active and placebo treatment groups. Acute overdosage with this dosage form is unlikely since one bottle of FLONASE Nasal Spray contains approximately 8 mg of fluticasone propionate.

The oral and subcutaneous median lethal doses in mice and rats were >1000 mg/kg (>20000 and >41000 times, respectively, the maximum recommended daily intranasal dose in adults and >10000 and >20000 times, respectively, the maximum recommended daily intranasal dose in children on a mg/m^2 basis).

DOSAGE AND ADMINISTRATION

Patients should use FLONASE Nasal Spray at regular intervals as directed since its effectiveness depends on its regular use.

Adults: The recommended starting dosage in **adults** is two sprays (50 mcg of fluticasone propionate each) in each nostril once-a-day (total daily dose, 200 mcg). The same dosage divided into 100 mcg given twice-a-day (e.g., 8 a.m. and 8 p.m.) is also effective. After the first few days, patients may be able to reduce their dosage to 100 mcg (one spray in each nostril) once daily for maintenance therapy.

Adolescents and Children (4 Years of Age and Older): Patients should be started with 100 mcg (one spray in each nostril once-a-day). Patients not adequately responding to 100 mcg may use 200 mcg (two sprays in each nostril). Once adequate control is achieved, the dosage should be decreased to 100 mcg (one spray in each nostril) daily.

The maximum total daily dosage should not exceed two sprays in each nostril (200 mcg/day). (See Individualization of Dosage and Clinical Trials sections.)

FLONASE Nasal Spray is not recommended for children under 4 years of age.

Directions for Use: Illustrated patient's instructions for proper use accompany each package of FLONASE Nasal Spray.

HOW SUPPLIED

FLONASE Nasal Spray 50 mcg is supplied in an amber glass bottle providing 120 actuations, net fill weight 16 g (NDC 0173-0453-01). Each actuation delivers 50 mcg of fluticasone propionate in 100 mg of formulation through the nasal adapter. The bottle should be discarded when the labeled number of actuations has been reached even though the bottle is not completely empty. Each bottle is fitted with a white metering atomizing pump, white nasal adapter, and green dust cover in a box of one with patient's instructions for use.

Store between 4° and 30°C (39° and 86°F).

Glaxo Wellcome Inc., Research Triangle Park, NC 27709

U.S. Patent 4,335,121
December 1998/RL-645

Shown in Product Identification Guide, page 315

FLOVENT® 44 mcg ℞
(fluticasone propionate, 44 mcg)
Inhalation Aerosol

FLOVENT® 110 mcg
(fluticasone propionate, 110 mcg)
Inhalation Aerosol

FLOVENT® 220 mcg
(fluticasone propionate, 220 mcg)
Inhalation Aerosol

For Oral Inhalation Only

DESCRIPTION

The active component of FLOVENT 44 mcg Inhalation Aerosol, FLOVENT 110 mcg Inhalation Aerosol, and FLOVENT 220 mcg Inhalation Aerosol is fluticasone propionate, a glucocorticoid having the chemical name S-(fluoromethyl)6α,9-difluoro-11β, 17-dihydroxy-16α-methyl-3-oxoandrosta-1,4-diene-17β-carbothioate, 17-propionate.

Fluticasone propionate is a white to off-white powder with a molecular weight of 500.6. It is practically insoluble in water, freely soluble in dimethyl sulfoxide and dimethylformamide, and slightly soluble in methanol and 95% ethanol.

FLOVENT 44 mcg Inhalation Aerosol, FLOVENT 110 mcg Inhalation Aerosol, and FLOVENT 220 mcg Inhalation Aerosol are pressurized, metered-dose aerosol units intended for oral inhalation only. Each unit contains a microcrystalline suspension of fluticasone propionate (micronized) in a mixture of two chlorofluorocarbon propellants (trichlorofluoromethane and dichlorodifluoromethane) with lecithin. Each actuation of the inhaler delivers 50, 125, or 250 mcg of fluticasone propionate from the valve, and 44, 110, or 220 mcg, respectively, of fluticasone propionate from the actuator.

CLINICAL PHARMACOLOGY

Fluticasone propionate is a synthetic, trifluorinated glucocorticoid with potent anti-inflammatory activity. In vitro assays using human lung cytosol preparations have established fluticasone propionate as a human glucocorticoid receptor agonist with an affinity 18 times greater than dexamethasone, almost twice that of beclomethasone-17-monopropionate (BMP), the active metabolite of beclomethasone dipropionate, and over 3 times that of budesonide. Data from the McKenzie vasoconstrictor assay in man are consistent with these results.

The precise mechanisms of glucocorticoid action in asthma are unknown. Inflammation is recognized as an important component in the pathogenesis of asthma. Glucocorticoids have been shown to inhibit multiple cell types (e.g., mast cells, eosinophils, basophils, lymphocytes, macrophages, and neutrophils) and mediator production or secretion (e.g., histamine, eicosanoids, leukotrienes, and cytokines) involved in the asthmatic response. These anti-inflammatory actions of glucocorticoids may contribute to their efficacy in asthma.

Though highly effective for the treatment of asthma, glucocorticoids do not affect asthma symptoms immediately. However, improvement following inhaled administration of fluticasone propionate can occur within 24 hours of beginning treatment, although maximum benefit may not be achieved for 1 to 2 weeks or longer after starting treatment. When glucocorticoids are discontinued, asthma stability may persist for several days or longer.

Pharmacokinetics: ***Absorption:*** The activity of FLOVENT Inhalation Aerosol is due to the parent drug, fluticasone propionate. Studies using oral dosing of labeled and unlabeled drug have demonstrated that the oral systemic bioavailability of fluticasone propionate is negligible (<1%), primarily due to incomplete absorption and pre-systemic metabolism in the gut and liver. In contrast, the majority of the fluticasone propionate delivered to the lung is systemically absorbed. The systemic bioavailability of fluticasone propionate inhalation aerosol in healthy volunteers averaged about 30% of the dose delivered from the actuator.

Peak plasma concentrations after an 800-mcg inhaled dose ranged from 0.1 to 1.0 ng/mL.

Distribution: Following intravenous administration, the initial disposition phase for fluticasone propionate was rapid and consistent with its high lipid solubility and tissue binding. The volume of distribution averaged 4.2 L/kg. The percentage of fluticasone propionate bound to human plasma proteins averaged 91%. Fluticasone propionate is weakly and reversibly bound to erythrocytes. Fluticasone propionate is not significantly bound to human transcortin.

Metabolism: The total clearance of fluticasone propionate is high (average, 1093 mL/min), with renal clearance accounting for less than 0.02% of the total. The only circulating metabolite detected in man is the 17β-carboxylic acid derivative of fluticasone propionate, which is formed through the cytochrome P450 3A4 pathway. This metabolite had approximately 2000 times less affinity than the parent drug for the glucocorticoid receptor of human lung cytosol in vitro and negligible pharmacological activity in animal studies. Other metabolites detected in vitro using cultured human hepatoma cells have not been detected in man.

Excretion: Following intravenous dosing, fluticasone propionate showed polyexponential kinetics and had a terminal elimination half-life of approximately 7.8 hours. Less than 5% of a radiolabeled oral dose was excreted in the urine as metabolites, with the remainder excreted in the feces as parent drug and metabolites.

Special Populations: Formal pharmacokinetic studies using fluticasone propionate were not carried out in any special populations. In a clinical study using fluticasone propionate inhalation powder, trough fluticasone propionate plasma concentrations were collected in 76 males and 74 females after inhaled administration of 100 and 500 mcg twice daily. Full pharmacokinetic profiles were obtained from 7 female patients and 13 male patients at these doses, and no overall differences in pharmacokinetic behavior were found.

Pharmacodynamics: To confirm that systemic absorption does not play a role in the clinical response to inhaled fluticasone propionate, a double-blind clinical study comparing inhaled and oral fluticasone propionate was conducted. Doses of 100 and 500 mcg twice daily of fluticasone propionate inhalation powder were compared to oral fluticasone propionate, 20,000 mcg given once daily, and placebo for 6 weeks. Plasma levels of fluticasone propionate were detectable in all three active groups, but the mean values were highest in the oral group. Both doses of inhaled fluticasone propionate were effective in maintaining asthma stability and improving lung function while oral fluticasone propionate and placebo were ineffective. This demonstrates that the clinical effectiveness of inhaled fluticasone propionate is due to its direct local effect and not to an indirect effect through systemic absorption.

The potential systemic effects of inhaled fluticasone propionate on the hypothalamic-pituitary-adrenal (HPA) axis were also studied in asthma patients. Fluticasone propionate given by inhalation aerosol at doses of 220, 440, 660, or 880 mcg twice daily was compared with placebo or oral prednisone 10 mg given once daily for 4 weeks. For most patients, the ability to increase cortisol production in response to stress, as assessed by 6-hour cosyntropin stimulation, remained intact with inhaled fluticasone propionate treatment. No patient had an abnormal response (peak less than 18 mcg/dL) after dosing with placebo or 220 mcg twice daily. Ten percent (10%) to 16% of patients treated with fluticasone propionate at doses of 440 mcg or more twice daily had an abnormal response as compared to 29% of patients treated with prednisone.

Clinical Trials: Double-blind, parallel, placebo-controlled, US clinical trials were conducted in 1818 adolescent and adult patients with asthma to assess the efficacy and/or safety of FLOVENT Inhalation Aerosol in the treatment of asthma. Fixed doses ranging from 22 to 880 mcg twice daily were compared to placebo to provide information about appropriate dosing to cover a range of asthma severity. Patients with asthma included in these studies were those not adequately controlled with beta-agonists alone, those already maintained on daily inhaled corticosteroids, and those requiring oral corticosteroid therapy. In all efficacy trials, at all doses, measures of pulmonary function (forced expiratory volume in 1 second [FEV_1] and morning peak expiratory flow rate [AM PEFR]) were statistically significantly improved as compared with placebo.

In 2 clinical trials of 660 patients with asthma inadequately controlled on bronchodilators alone, fluticasone propionate administered by inhalation aerosol was evaluated at doses of 44 and 88 mcg twice daily. Both doses of fluticasone propionate improved asthma control significantly as compared with placebo.

Displayed in the figure below are results of pulmonary function tests for the recommended starting dosage of fluticasone propionate inhalation aerosol (88 mcg twice daily) and placebo from a 12-week trial in patients with asthma inadequately controlled on bronchodilators alone. Because this trial used predetermined criteria for lack of efficacy, which caused more patients in the placebo group to be withdrawn, pulmonary function results at endpoint, which is the last evaluable FEV_1 result and includes most patients' lung function data, are also provided. Pulmonary function improved significantly with fluticasone propionate compared with placebo by the second week of treatment, and this improvement was maintained over the duration of the trial.

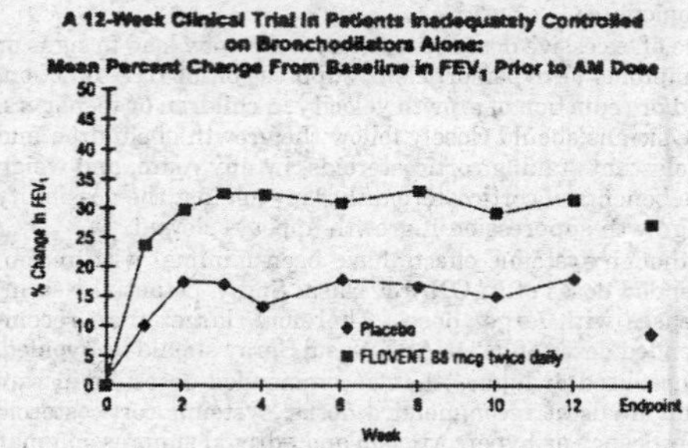

In clinical trials of 924 patients with asthma already receiving daily inhaled corticosteroid therapy (doses of at least 336 mcg/day of beclomethasone dipropionate) in addition to as-needed albuterol and theophylline (46% of all patients), fluticasone propionate inhalation aerosol doses of 22 to 440 mcg twice daily were also evaluated. All doses of fluticasone propionate were efficacious when compared to placebo on major endpoints including lung function and symptom scores. Patients treated with fluticasone propionate were also less likely to discontinue study participation due to asthma deterioration (as defined by predetermined criteria for lack of efficacy including lung function and patient-recorded variables such as AM PEFR, albuterol use, and nighttime awakenings due to asthma).

Displayed in the figure below are results of pulmonary function from a 12-week clinical trial in patients with asthma already receiving daily inhaled corticosteroid therapy (beclomethasone dipropionate 336 to 672 mcg/day). The mean percent change from baseline in lung function results for fluticasone propionate inhalation aerosol dosages of 88, 220, and 440 mcg twice daily and placebo are shown over the 12-week trial. Because this trial also used predetermined criteria for lack of efficacy, which caused more patients in the placebo group to be withdrawn, pulmonary function results at endpoint are included. Pulmonary function improved significantly with fluticasone propionate compared with placebo by the first week of treatment, and the improvement was maintained over the duration of the trial. Analysis of the endpoint results that adjusted for differential withdrawal rates indicated that pulmonary function significantly improved with fluticasone propionate compared with placebo treatment. Similar improvements in lung function were seen in the other two trials in patients treated with inhaled corticosteroids at baseline.

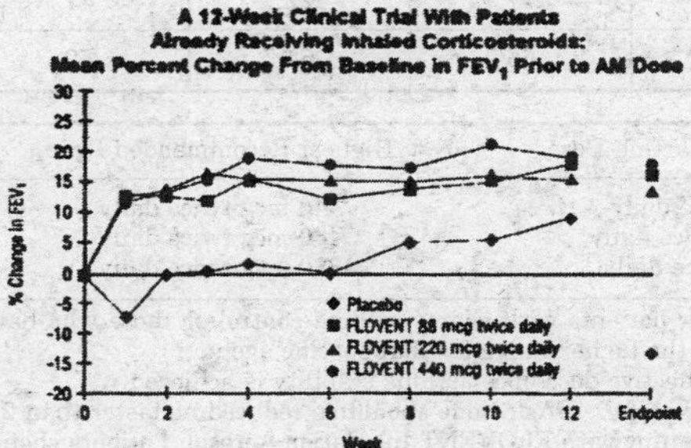

In a clinical trial of 96 patients with severe asthma requiring chronic oral prednisone therapy (average baseline daily prednisone dose was 10 mg), twice-daily doses of 660 and 880 mcg of FLOVENT Inhalation Aerosol doses were evaluated. Both doses enabled a statistically significantly larger percentage of patients to wean successfully from oral prednisone as compared with placebo (69% of the patients on 660 mcg twice daily and 88% of the patients on 880 mcg twice daily as compared with 3% of patients on placebo). Accompanying the reduction in oral corticosteroid use, patients treated with FLOVENT Inhalation Aerosol had significantly improved lung function and fewer asthma symptoms as compared with the placebo group.

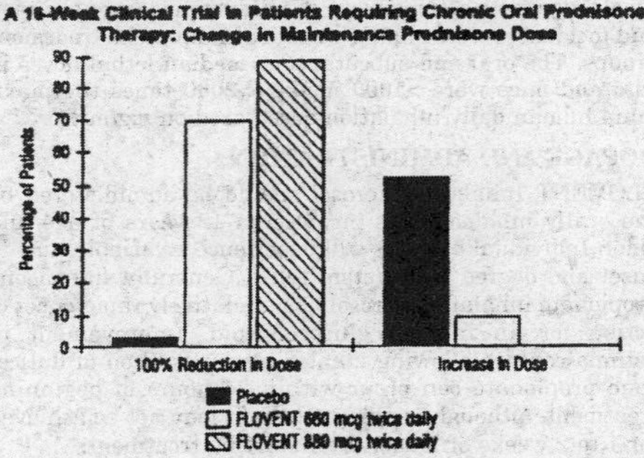

INDICATIONS AND USAGE

FLOVENT Inhalation Aerosol is indicated for the maintenance treatment of asthma as prophylactic therapy. It is also indicated for patients requiring oral corticosteroid therapy for asthma. Many of these patients may be able to reduce or eliminate their requirement for oral corticosteroids over time.

FLOVENT Inhalation Aerosol is NOT indicated for the relief of acute bronchospasm.

CONTRAINDICATIONS

FLOVENT Inhalation Aerosol is contraindicated in the primary treatment of status asthmaticus or other acute episodes of asthma where intensive measures are required.

Hypersensitivity to any of the ingredients of these preparations contraindicates their use.

WARNINGS

Particular care is needed for patients who are transferred from systemically active corticosteroids to FLOVENT Inhalation Aerosol because deaths due to adrenal insufficiency have occurred in patients with asthma during and after transfer from systemic corticosteroids to less systemically available inhaled corticosteroids. After withdrawal from systemic corticosteroids, a number of months are required for recovery of HPA function.

Patients who have been previously maintained on 20 mg or more per day of prednisone (or its equivalent) may be most susceptible, particularly when their systemic corticosteroids have been almost completely withdrawn. During this period of HPA suppression, patients may exhibit signs and symptoms of adrenal insufficiency when exposed to trauma, surgery, or infection (particularly gastroenteritis) or other conditions associated with severe electrolyte loss. Although fluticasone propionate inhalation aerosol may provide control of asthma symptoms during these episodes, in recommended doses it supplies less than normal physiological amounts of glucocorticoid systemically and does NOT provide the mineralocorticoid activity that is necessary for coping with these emergencies.

During periods of stress or a severe asthma attack, patients who have been withdrawn from systemic corticosteroids should be instructed to resume oral corticosteroids (in large doses) immediately and to contact their physicians for further instruction. These patients should also be instructed to carry a warning card indicating that they may need supplementary systemic corticosteroids during periods of stress or a severe asthma attack.

Patients requiring oral corticosteroids should be weaned slowly from systemic corticosteroid use after transferring to fluticasone propionate inhalation aerosol. In a trial of 96 patients, prednisone reduction was successfully accomplished by reducing the daily prednisone dose by 2.5 mg on a weekly basis during transfer to inhaled fluticasone propionate. Successive reduction of prednisone dose was allowed only when lung function, symptoms, and as-needed beta-agonist use were better than or comparable to that seen before initiation of prednisone dose reduction. Lung function (FEV_1 or AM PEFR), beta-agonist use, and asthma symptoms should be carefully monitored during withdrawal of oral corticosteroids. In addition to monitoring asthma signs and symptoms, patients should be observed for signs and symptoms of adrenal insufficiency such as fatigue, lassitude, weakness, nausea and vomiting, and hypotension.

Transfer of patients from systemic corticosteroid therapy to fluticasone propionate inhalation aerosol may unmask conditions previously suppressed by the systemic corticosteroid therapy, e.g., rhinitis, conjunctivitis, eczema, and arthritis.

Persons who are on drugs that suppress the immune system are more susceptible to infections than healthy individuals. Chickenpox and measles, for example, can have a more serious or even fatal course in susceptible children or adults on corticosteroids. In such children or adults who have not had these diseases, particular care should be taken to avoid exposure. How the dose, route, and duration of corticosteroid administration affects the risk of developing a disseminated infection is not known. The contribution of the underlying disease and/or prior corticosteroid treatment to the risk is also not known. If exposed to chickenpox, prophylaxis with varicella zoster immune globulin (VZIG) may be indicated. If exposed to measles, prophylaxis with pooled intramuscular immunoglobulin (IG) may be indicated. (See the respective package inserts for complete VZIG and IG prescribing information.) If chickenpox develops, treatment with antiviral agents may be considered.

Fluticasone propionate inhalation aerosol is not to be regarded as a bronchodilator and is not indicated for rapid relief of bronchospasm.

As with other inhaled asthma medications, bronchospasm may occur with an immediate increase in wheezing after dosing. If bronchospasm occurs following dosing with FLOVENT Inhalation Aerosol, it should be treated immediately with a fast-acting inhaled bronchodilator. Treatment with FLOVENT Inhalation Aerosol should be discontinued and alternative therapy instituted.

Patients should be instructed to contact their physicians immediately when episodes of asthma that are not responsive to bronchodilators occur during the course of treatment with fluticasone propionate inhalation aerosol. During such episodes, patients may require therapy with oral corticosteroids.

PRECAUTIONS

General: During withdrawal from oral corticosteroids, some patients may experience symptoms of systemically active corticosteroid withdrawal, e.g., joint and/or muscular pain, lassitude, and depression, despite maintenance or even improvement of respiratory function.

Fluticasone propionate will often permit control of asthma symptoms with less suppression of HPA function than therapeutically equivalent oral doses of prednisone. Since fluticasone propionate is absorbed into the circulation and can be systemically active at higher doses, the beneficial effects of fluticasone propionate inhalation aerosol in minimizing HPA dysfunction may be expected only when recommended dosages are not exceeded and individual patients are titrated to the lowest effective dose. A relationship between plasma levels of fluticasone propionate and inhibitory effects on stimulated cortisol production has been shown after 4 weeks of treatment with fluticasone propionate inhalation aerosol. Since individual sensitivity to effects on cortisol production exists, physicians should consider this information when prescribing fluticasone propionate inhalation aerosol.

Because of the possibility of systemic absorption of inhaled corticosteroids, patients treated with these drugs should be observed carefully for any evidence of systemic corticosteroid effects. Particular care should be taken in observing patients postoperatively or during periods of stress for evidence of inadequate adrenal response.

It is possible that systemic corticosteroid effects such as hypercorticism and adrenal suppression may appear in a small number of patients, particularly at higher doses. If such changes occur, fluticasone propionate inhalation aerosol should be reduced slowly, consistent with accepted procedures for reducing systemic corticosteroids and for management of asthma symptoms.

A reduction of growth velocity in children or teenagers may occur as a result of inadequate control of chronic diseases such as asthma or from use of corticosteroids for treatment. Physicians should closely follow the growth of adolescents taking corticosteroids by any route and weigh the benefits of corticosteroid therapy and asthma control against the possibility of growth suppression if an adolescent's growth appears slowed.

The long-term effects of fluticasone propionate in human subjects are not fully known. In particular, the effects resulting from chronic use of fluticasone propionate on developmental or immunologic processes in the mouth, pharynx, trachea, and lung are unknown. Some patients have received fluticasone propionate inhalation aerosol on a continuous basis for periods of 3 years or longer. In clinical studies with patients treated for nearly 2 years with inhaled fluticasone propionate, no apparent differences in the type or severity of adverse reactions were observed after long- versus short-term treatment.

Rare instances of glaucoma, increased intraocular pressure, and cataracts have been reported following the inhaled administration of corticosteroids, including fluticasone propionate.

In clinical studies with inhaled fluticasone propionate, the development of localized infections of the pharynx with *Candida albicans* has occurred. When such an infection develops, it should be treated with appropriate local or systemic (i.e., oral antifungal) therapy while remaining on treatment with fluticasone propionate inhalation aerosol, but at times therapy with fluticasone propionate may need to be interrupted.

Inhaled corticosteroids should be used with caution, if at all, in patients with active or quiescent tuberculosis infection of the respiratory tract; untreated systemic fungal, bacterial, viral or parasitic infections; or ocular herpes simplex.

Eosinophilic Conditions: In rare cases, patients on inhaled fluticasone propionate may present with systemic eosinophilic conditions, with some patients presenting with clinical features of vasculitis consistent with Churg-Strauss syndrome, a condition that is often treated with systemic corticosteroid therapy. These events usually, but not always, have been associated with the reduction and/or withdrawal of oral costicosteroid therapy following the introduction of fluticasone propionate. Cases of serious eosinophilic conditions have also been reported with other inhaled corticosteroids in this clinical setting. Physicians should be alert to eosinophilia, vasculitic rash, worsening pulmonary symptoms, cardiac complications, and/or neuropathy presenting in their patients. A causal relationship between fluticasone propionate and these underlying conditions has not been established (see ADVERSE REACTIONS).

Information for Patients: Patients being treated with FLOVENT Inhalation Aerosol should receive the following information and instructions. This information is intended to aid them in the safe and effective use of this medication. It is not a disclosure of all possible adverse or intended effects.

Patients should use FLOVENT Inhalation Aerosol at regular intervals as directed. Results of clinical trials indicated significant improvement may occur within the first day or two of treatment; however, the full benefit may not be achieved until treatment has been administered for 1 to 2 weeks or longer. The patient should not increase the prescribed dosage but should contact the physician if symptoms do not improve or if the condition worsens.

Patients should be warned to avoid exposure to chickenpox or measles and, if they are exposed, to consult their physicians without delay.

For the proper use of FLOVENT Inhalation Aerosol and to attain maximum improvement, the patient should read and follow carefully the Patient's Instructions for Use accompanying the product.

Carcinogenesis, Mutagenesis, Impairment of Fertility: Fluticasone propionate demonstrated no tumorigenic potential in studies of oral doses up to 1000 mcg/kg (approximately 2 times the maximum human daily inhalation dose based on mcg/m^2) for 78 weeks in the mouse or inhalation of up to 57 mcg/kg (approximately $^1/_4$ the maximum human daily inhalation dose based on mcg/m^2) for 104 weeks in the rat.

Fluticasone propionate did not induce gene mutation in prokaryotic or eukaryotic cells in vitro. No significant clastogenic effect was seen in cultured human peripheral lymphocytes in vitro or in the mouse micronucleus test when administered at high doses by the oral or subcutaneous routes. Furthermore, the compound did not delay erythroblast division in bone marrow.

No evidence of impairment of fertilty was observed in reproductive studies conducted in rats dosed subcutaneously with doses up to 50 mcg/kg (approximately $^1/_4$ the maximum

Continued on next page

This product information is based on labeling in effect on June 23, 2000. For further information, contact via direct mail, phone, or web site. Medical Information, Glaxo Wellcome Inc., PO Box 13398, Research Triangle Park, NC 27709. Healthcare Professionals (Medical Information): 800-334-0089. Patients (Customer Response Center): 1-888-825-5249. Glaxo Wellcome Corporate Web Site: www.glaxowellcome.com

Flovent—Cont.

human daily inhalation dose based on mcg/m^2) in males and females. However, prostate weight was significantly reduced in rats.

Pregnancy: ***Teratogenic Effects:*** Pregnancy Category C. Subcutaneous studies in the mouse and rat at 45 and 100 mcg/kg, respectively (approximately $^1/_{10}$ and $^1/_2$ the maximum human daily inhalation dose based on mcg/m^2, respectively), revealed fetal toxicity characteristic of potent glucocorticoid compounds, including embryonic growth retardation, omphalocele, cleft palate, and retarded cranial ossification.

In the rabbit, fetal weight reduction and cleft palate were observed following subcutaneous doses of 4 mcg/kg (approximately $^1/_{25}$ the maximum human daily inhalation dose based on mcg/m^2). However, following oral administration of up to 300 mcg/kg (approximately 3 times the maximum human daily inhalation dose based on mcg/m^2) of fluticasone propionate to the rabbit, there were no maternal effects nor increased incidence of external, visceral, or skeletal fetal defects. No fluticasone propionate was detected in the plasma in this study, consistent with the established low bioavailability following oral administration (see CLINICAL PHARMACOLOGY).

Less than 0.008% of the administered dose crossed the placenta following oral administration of 100 mcg/kg to rats or 300 mcg/kg to rabbits (approximately $^1/_2$ and 3 times the maximum human daily inhalation dose based on mcg/m^2, respectively).

There are no adequate and well-controlled studies in pregnant women. Fluticasone propionate should be used during pregnancy only if the potential benefit justifies the potential risk to the fetus.

Experience with oral glucocorticoids since their introduction in pharmacologic, as opposed to physiologic, doses suggests that rodents are more prone to teratogenic effects from glucocorticoids than humans. In addition, because there is a natural increase in glucocorticoid production during pregnancy, most women will require a lower exogenous glucocorticoid dose and many will not need glucocorticoid treatment during pregnancy.

Nursing Mothers: It is not known whether fluticasone propionate is excreted in human breast milk. Subcutaneous administration of 10 mcg/kg tritiated drug to lactating rats (approximately $^1/_{20}$ the maximum human daily inhalation dose based on mcg/m^2) resulted in measurable radioactivity in both plasma and milk. Because glucocorticoids are excreted in human milk, caution should be exercised when fluticasone propionate inhalation aerosol is administered to a nursing woman.

Pediatric Use: One hundred thirty-seven (137) patients between the ages of 12 and 16 years were treated with fluticasone propionate inhalation aerosol in the US pivotal clinical trials. The safety and effectiveness of FLOVENT Inhalation Aerosol in children below 12 years of age have not been established. Oral corticosteroids have been shown to cause a reduction in growth velocity in children and teenagers with extended use. If a child or teenager on any corticosteroid appears to have growth suppression, the possibility that they are particularly sensitive to this effect of corticosteroids should be considered (see PRECAUTIONS).

Geriatric Use: Five hundred seventy-four (574) patients 65 years of age or older have been treated with fluticasone propionate inhalation aerosol in US and non-US clinical trials. There were no differences in adverse reactions compared to those reported by younger patients.

ADVERSE REACTIONS

The following incidence of common adverse experiences is based upon 7 placebo-controlled US clinical trials in which 1243 patients (509 female and 734 male adolescents and adults previously treated with as-needed bronchodilators and/or inhaled corticosteroids) were treated with fluticasone propionate inhalation aerosol (doses of 88 to 440 mcg twice daily for up to 12 weeks) or placebo.

[See first table above]

Overall Adverse Experiences With >3% Incidence on Fluticasone Propionate in US Contolled Clinical Trials With MDI in Patients Previously Receiving Bronchodilators and/or Inhaled Corticosteroids

Adverse Event	Placebo (n = 475) %	FLOVENT 88 mcg twice daily (n = 488) %	FLOVENT 220 mcg twice daily (n = 95) %	FLOVENT 440 mcg twice daily (n = 185) %
Ear, nose, and throat				
Pharyngitis	7	10	14	14
Nasal congestion	8	8	16	10
Sinusitis	4	3	6	5
Nasal discharge	3	5	4	4
Dysphonia	1	4	3	8
Allergic rhinitis	4	5	3	3
Oral candidiasis	1	2	3	5
Respiratory				
Upper respiratory infection	12	15	22	16
Influenza	2	3	8	5
Neurological				
Headache	14	17	22	17
Average duration of exposure (days)	44	66	64	59

The table above includes all events (whether considered drug-related or nondrug-related by the investigator) that occurred at a rate of over 3% in the combined fluticasone propionate inhalation aerosol groups and were more common than in the placebo group. In considering these data, differences in average duration of exposure should be taken into account.

These adverse reactions were mostly mild to moderate in severity, with ≤2% of patients discontinuing the studies because of adverse events. Rare cases of immediate and delayed hypersensitivity reactions, including urticaria and rash and other rare events of angioedema and bronchospasm, have been reported.

Systemic glucocorticoid side effects were not reported during controlled clinical trials with fluticasone propionate inhalation aerosol. If recommended doses are exceeded, however, or if individuals are particularly sensitive, symptoms of hypercorticism, e.g., Cushing's syndrome, could occur.

Other adverse events that occurred in these clinical trials using fluticasone propionate inhalation aerosol with an incidence of 1% to 3% and which occurred at a greater incidence than with placebo were:

Ear, Nose, and Throat: Pain in nasal sinus(es), rhinitis.
Eye: Irritation of the eye(s).
Gastrointestinal: Nausea and vomiting, diarrhea, dyspepsia and stomach disorder.
Miscellaneous: Fever.
Mouth and Teeth: Dental problem.
Musculoskeletal: Pain in joint, sprain/strain, aches and pains, pain in limb.
Neurological: Dizziness/giddiness.
Respiratory: Bronchitis, chest congestion.
Skin: Dermatitis, rash/skin eruption.
Urogenital: Dysmenorrhea.

In a 16-week study in patients with asthma requiring oral corticosteroids, the effects of fluticasone propionate inhalation aerosol, 660 mcg twice daily (n = 32) and 880 mcg twice daily (n = 32), were compared with placebo. Adverse events (whether considered drug-related or nondrug-related by the investigator) reported by more than 3 patients in either fluticasone propionate group and which were more common with fluticasone propionate than placebo are shown below:

Ear, Nose, and Throat: Pharyngitis (9% and 25%), nasal congestion (19% and 22%), sinusitis (19% and 22%), nasal discharge (16% and 16%), dysphonia (19% and 9%), pain in nasal sinus(es) (13% and 0%), Candida-like oral lesions (16% and 9%), oropharyngeal candidiasis (25% and 19%).
Respiratory: Upper respiratory infection (31% and 19%), influenza (0% and 13%).
Other: Headache (28% and 34%), pain in joint (19% and 13%), nausea and vomiting (22% and 16%), muscular soreness (22% and 13%), malaise/fatigue (22% and 28%), insomnia (3% and 13%).

Observed During Clinical Practice: In addition to adverse events reported from clinical trials, the following events have been identified during postapproval use of fluticasone propionate in clinical practice. Because they are reported voluntarily from a population of unknown size, estimates of frequency cannot be made. These events have been chosen for inclusion due to either their seriousness, frequency of reporting, causal connection to fluticasone propionate, or a combination of these factors.

Ear, Nose, and Throat: Throat soreness and irritation, hoarseness, laryngitis, aphonia.
Endocrine and Metabolic: Cushingoid features, growth velocity reduction in children/adolescents, weight gain, hyperglycemia.
Psychiatry: Restlessness, agitation, aggression, depression.
Respiratory: Immediate bronchospasm, asthma exacerbation, dyspnea, wheeze, chest tightness, bronchospasm, cough.
Skin: Pruritus, contusions, ecchymoses.
Eosinophilic Conditions: In rare cases, patients on inhaled fluticasone propionate may present with systemic eosinophilic conditions, with some patients presenting with clinical features of vasculitis consistent with Churg-Strauss syndrome, a condition that is often treated with systemic corticosteroid therapy. These events usually, but not always, have been associated with the reduction and/or withdrawal of oral costicosteroid therapy following the introduction of fluticasone propionate. Cases of serious eosinophilic conditions have also been reported with other inhaled corticosteroids in this clinical setting. Physicians should be alert to eosinophilia, vasculitic rash, worsening pulmonary symptoms, cardiac complications, and/or neuropathy presenting in their patients. A causal relationship between fluticasone propionate and these underlying conditions has not been established (see PRECAUTIONS: Eosinophilic Conditions).

OVERDOSAGE

Chronic overdosage may result in signs/symptoms of hypercorticism (see PRECAUTIONS). Inhalation by healthy volunteers of a single dose of 1760 or 3520 mcg of fluticasone propionate inhalation aerosol was well tolerated. Fluticasone propionate given by inhalation aerosol at doses of 1320 mcg twice daily for 7 to 15 days to healthy human volunteers was also well tolerated. Repeat oral doses up to 80 mg daily for 10 days in healthy volunteers and repeat oral doses up to 20 mg daily for 42 days in patients were well tolerated. Adverse reactions were of mild or moderate severity, and incidences were similar in active and placebo treatment groups. The oral and subcutaneous median lethal doses in rats and mice were >1000 mg/kg (>2000 times the maximum human daily inhalation dose based on mg/m^2).

DOSAGE AND ADMINISTRATION

FLOVENT Inhalation Aerosol should be administered by the orally inhaled route in patients 12 years of age and older. Individual patients will experience a variable time to onset and degree of symptom relief. Generally, fluticasone propionate inhalation aerosol has a relatively rapid onset of action for an inhaled glucocorticoid. Improvement in asthma control following inhaled administration of fluticasone propionate can occur within 24 hours of beginning treatment, although maximum benefit may not be achieved for 1 to 2 weeks or longer after starting treatment.

After asthma stability has been achieved (see below), it is always desirable to titrate to the lowest effective dose to reduce the possibility of side effects. For patients who do not respond adequately to the starting dose after 2 weeks of therapy, higher doses may provide additional asthma control. The safety and efficacy of FLOVENT Inhalation Aerosol when administered in excess of recommended doses has not been established.

Rinsing the mouth after inhalation is advised.

The recommended starting dose and the highest recommended dose of fluticasone propionate inhalation aerosol, based on prior antiasthma therapy, are listed in the following table.

[See second table above]

Previous Therapy	Recommended Starting Dose	Highest Recommended Dose
Bronchodilators alone	88 mcg twice daily	440 mcg twice daily
Inhaled corticosteroids	88-220 mcg twice daily*	440 mcg twice daily
Oral corticosteroids†	880 mcg twice daily	880 mcg twice daily

*Starting doses above 88 mcg twice daily may be considered for patients with poorer asthma control or those who have previously required doses of inhaled corticosteroids that are in the higher range for that specific agent.

NOTE: In all patients, it is desirable to titrate to the lowest effective dose once asthma stability is achieved.

†**For Patients Currently Receiving Chronic Oral Corticosteroid Therapy:** Prednisone should be reduced no faster than 2.5 mg/day on a weekly basis, beginning after at least 1 week of therapy with FLOVENT Inhalation Aerosol. Patients should be carefully monitored for signs of asthma instability, including serial objective measures of airflow, and for signs of adrenal insufficiency (see WARNINGS). Once prednisone reduction is complete, the dosage of fluticasone propionate should be reduced to the lowest effective dosage.

Geriatric Use: In studies where geriatric patients (65 years of age or older, see PRECAUTIONS) have been treated with fluticasone propionate inhalation aerosol, efficacy and safety did not differ from that in younger patients. Consequently, no dosage adjustment is recommended.

Directions for Use: Illustrated Patient's Instructions for Use accompany each package of FLOVENT Inhalation Aerosol.

HOW SUPPLIED

FLOVENT 44 mcg Inhalation Aerosol is supplied in 7.9-g canisters containing 60 metered inhalations in boxes of one (NDC 0173-0497-00) and in 13-g canisters containing 120 metered inhalations in boxes of one (NDC 0173-0491-00). Each canister is supplied with a dark orange-colored oral actuator with a peach-colored strapcap and patient's instructions. Each actuation of the inhaler delivers 44 mcg of fluticasone propionate from the actuator.

FLOVENT 110 mcg Inhalation Aerosol is supplied in 7.9-g canisters containing 60 metered inhalations in boxes of one (NDC 0173-0498-00) and in 13-g canisters containing 120 metered inhalations in boxes of one (NDC 0173-0494-00).

Each canister is supplied with a dark orange-colored oral actuator with a peach-colored strapcap and patient's instructions. Each actuation of the inhaler delivers 110 mcg of fluticasone propionate from the actuator.

FLOVENT 220 mcg Inhalation Aerosol is supplied in 7.9-g canisters containing 60 metered inhalations in boxes of one (NDC 0173-0499-00) and in 13-g canisters containing 120 metered inhalations in boxes of one (NDC 0173-0495-00). Each canister is supplied with a dark orange-colored oral actuator with a peach-colored strapcap and patient's instructions. Each actuation of the inhaler delivers 220 mcg of fluticasone propionate from the actuator.

FLOVENT canisters are for use with FLOVENT Inhalation Aerosol actuators only. The actuators should not be used with other aerosol medications.

The correct amount of medication in each inhalation cannot be assured after 60 inhalations from the 7.9-g canister or 120 inhalations from the 13-g canister even though the canister is not completely empty. The canister should be discarded when the labeled number of actuations has been used.

Store between 2° and 30°C (36° and 86°F). Store canister with nozzle end down. Protect from freezing temperatures and direct sunlight.

Avoid spraying in eyes. Contents under pressure. Do not puncture or incinerate. Do not store at temperatures above 120°F. Keep out of reach of children. For best results, the canister should be at room temperature before use. Shake well before using.

Glaxo Wellcome Inc., Research Triangle Park, NC 27709

US Patent No. 4,335,121

April 1999/RL-687

Shown in Product Identification Guide, page 315

FLOVENT® ROTADISK® 50 mcg ℞

[*flō'vĕnt rōt 'ə -dĭsk*]

(fluticasone propionate inhalation powder, 50 mcg)

FLOVENT® ROTADISK® 100 mcg

(fluticasone propionate inhalation powder, 100 mcg)

FLOVENT® ROTADISK® 250 mcg

(fluticasone propionate inhalation powder, 250 mcg)

For Oral Inhalation Only

For Use With the DISKHALER® Inhalation Device

DESCRIPTION

The active component of FLOVENT ROTADISK 50 mcg, FLOVENT ROTADISK 100 mcg, and FLOVENT ROTADISK 250 mcg is fluticasone propionate, a corticosteroid having the chemical name S-(fluoromethyl)6α,9-difluoro-11β,17-dihydroxy-16α-methyl-3-oxoandrosta-1,4-diene-17β-carbothioate, 17-propionate.

Fluticasone propionate is a white to off-white powder with a molecular weight of 500.6, and the empirical formula is $C_{25}H_{31}F_3O_5S$. It is practically insoluble in water, freely soluble in dimethyl sulfoxide and dimethylformamide, and slightly soluble in methanol and 95% ethanol.

FLOVENT ROTADISK 50 mcg, FLOVENT ROTADISK 100 mcg, and FLOVENT ROTADISK 250 mcg contain a dry powder presentation of fluticasone propionate intended for oral inhalation only. Each double-foil ROTADISK contains 4 blisters. Each blister contains a mixture of 50, 100, or 250 mcg of microfine fluticasone propionate blended with lactose to a total weight of 25 mg. The contents of each blister are inhaled using a specially designed plastic device for inhaling powder called the DISKHALER. After a fluticasone propionate ROTADISK is loaded into the DISKHALER, a blister containing medication is pierced and the fluticasone propionate is dispersed into the air stream created when the patient inhales through the mouthpiece.

The amount of drug delivered to the lung will depend on patient factors such as inspiratory flow. Under standardized in vitro testing, FLOVENT ROTADISK delivers 44, 88, or 220 mcg of fluticasone propionate from FLOVENT ROTADISK 50 mcg, FLOVENT ROTADISK 100 mcg, or FLOVENT ROTADISK 250 mcg, respectively, when tested at a flow rate of 60 L/min for 3 seconds. In adult and adolescent patients with asthma, mean peak inspiratory flow (PIF) through the DISKHALER was 123 L/min (range, 88 to 159 L/min), and in pediatric patients 4 to 11 years of age with asthma, mean PIF was 110 L/min (range, 43 to 175 L/min).

CLINICAL PHARMACOLOGY

Fluticasone propionate is a synthetic, trifluorinated corticosteroid with potent anti-inflammatory activity. In vitro assays using human lung cytosol preparations have established fluticasone propionate as a human glucocorticoid receptor agonist with an affinity 18 times greater than dexamethasone, almost twice that of beclomethasone-17-monopropionate (BMP), the active metabolite of beclomethasone dipropionate, and over 3 times that of budesonide. Data from the McKenzie vasoconstrictor assay in man are consistent with these results.

The precise mechanisms of fluticasone propionate action in asthma are unknown. Inflammation is recognized as an important component in the pathogenesis of asthma. Corticosteroids have been shown to inhibit multiple cell types (e.g., mast cells, eosinophils, basophils, lymphocytes, macrophages, and neutrophils) and mediator production or secretion (e.g., histamine, eicosanoids, leukotrienes, and cytokines) involved in the asthmatic response. These anti-inflammatory actions of corticosteroids may contribute to their efficacy in asthma.

Though highly effective for the treatment of asthma, corticosteroids do not affect asthma symptoms immediately. However, improvement following inhaled administration of fluticasone propionate can occur within 24 hours of beginning treatment, although maximum benefit may not be achieved for 1 to 2 weeks or longer after starting treatment. When corticosteroids are discontinued, asthma stability may persist for several days or longer.

Pharmacokinetics: ***Absorption:*** The activity of FLOVENT ROTADISK Inhalation Powder is due to the parent drug, fluticasone propionate. Studies using oral dosing of labeled and unlabeled drug have demonstrated that the oral systemic bioavailability of fluticasone propionate is negligible (<1%), primarily due to incomplete absorption and presystemic metabolism in the gut and liver. In contrast, the majority of the fluticasone propionate delivered to the lung is systemically absorbed. The systemic bioavailability of fluticasone propionate inhalation powder in healthy volunteers averaged about 13.5% of the nominal dose.

Peak plasma concentrations after a 1000-mcg dose of fluticasone propionate inhalation powder ranged from 0.1 to 1.0 ng/mL.

Distribution: Following intravenous administration, the initial disposition phase for fluticasone propionate was rapid and consistent with its high lipid solubility and tissue binding. The volume of distribution averaged 4.2 L/kg. The percentage of fluticasone propionate bound to human plasma proteins averaged 91%.

Fluticasone propionate is weakly and reversibly bound to erythrocytes. Fluticasone propionate is not significantly bound to human transcortin.

Metabolism: The total clearance of fluticasone propionate is high (average, 1093 mL/min), with renal clearance accounting for less than 0.02% of the total. The only circulating metabolite detected in man is the 17β-carboxylic acid derivative of fluticasone propionate, which is formed through the cytochrome P450 3A4 pathway. This metabolite had approximately 2000 times less affinity than the parent drug for the glucocorticoid receptor of human lung cytosol in vitro and negligible pharmacological activity in animal studies. Other metabolites detected in vitro using cultured human hepatoma cells have not been detected in man.

In a multiple-dose drug interaction study, coadministration of fluticasone propionate (500 mcg twice daily) and erythromycin (333 mg 3 times daily) did not affect fluticasone propionate pharmacokinetics.

In a drug interaction study, coadministration of fluticasone propionate (1000 mcg) and ketoconazole (200 mg once daily) resulted in increased fluticasone propionate concentrations, a reduction in plasma cortisol AUC, and no effect on urinary excretion of cortisol.

Excretion: Following intravenous dosing, fluticasone propionate showed polyexponential kinetics and had a terminal elimination half-life of approximately 7.8 hours. Less than 5% of a radiolabeled oral dose was excreted in the urine as metabolites, with the remainder excreted in the feces as parent drug and metabolites.

Special Populations: Formal pharmacokinetic studies using fluticasone propionate were not carried out in any special populations. In a clinical study using fluticasone propionate inhalation powder, trough fluticasone propionate plasma concentrations were collected in 76 males and 74 females after inhaled administration of 100 and 500 mcg twice daily. Full pharmacokinetic profiles were obtained from 7 female patients and 13 male patients at these doses, and no overall differences in pharmacokinetic behavior were found.

Plasma concentrations of fluticasone propionate were measured 20 and 40 minutes after dosing from 29 children aged 4 to 11 years who were taking either 50 or 100 mcg twice daily of fluticasone propionate inhalation powder. Plasma concentration values ranged from below the limit of quantitation (25 pg/mL) to 117 pg/mL (50-mcg dose) or 154 pg/mL (100-mcg dose). In a study with adults taking the 100-mcg twice-daily dose, the plasma concentrations observed ranged from below the limit of quantitation to 73.1 pg/mL. The median fluticasone propionate plasma concentrations for the 100-mcg dose in children was 58.7 pg/mL; in adults the median plasma concentration was 39.5 pg/mL.

Pharmacodynamics: To confirm that systemic absorption does not play a role in the clinical response to inhaled fluticasone propionate, a double-blind clinical study comparing inhaled and oral fluticasone propionate was conducted. Doses of 100 and 500 mcg twice daily of fluticasone propionate inhalation powder were compared to oral fluticasone propionate, 20,000 mcg given once daily, and placebo for 6 weeks. Plasma levels of fluticasone propionate were detectable in all 3 active groups, but the mean values were highest in the oral group. Both doses of inhaled fluticasone propionate were effective in maintaining asthma stability and improving lung function while oral fluticasone propionate and placebo were ineffective. This demonstrates that the clinical effectiveness of inhaled fluticasone propionate is due to its direct local effect and not to an indirect effect through systemic absorption.

The potential systemic effects of inhaled fluticasone propionate on the hypothalamic-pituitary-adrenal (HPA) axis were also studied in asthma patients. Fluticasone propionate given by inhalation aerosol at doses of 220, 440, 660, or 880 mcg twice daily was compared with placebo or oral prednisone 10 mg given once daily for 4 weeks. For most patients, the ability to increase cortisol production in response to stress, as assessed by 6-hour cosyntropin stimulation, remained intact with inhaled fluticasone propionate treatment. No patient had an abnormal response (peak serum cortisol <18 mcg/dL) after dosing with placebo or fluticasone propionate 220 mcg twice daily. For patients treated with 440, 660, and 880 mcg twice daily, 10%, 16%, and 12%, respectively, had an abnormal response as compared to 29% of patients treated with prednisone.

In clinical trials with fluticasone propionate inhalation powder, using doses up to and including 250 mcg twice daily, occasional abnormal short cosyntropin tests (peak serum cortisol <18 mcg/dL) were noted in patients receiving fluticasone propionate or placebo. The incidence of abnormal tests at 500 mcg twice daily was greater than placebo. In a 2-year study carried out in 64 patients randomized to fluticasone propionate 500 mcg twice daily or placebo, 1 patient receiving fluticasone propionate (4%) had an abnormal response to 6-hour cosyntropin infusion at 1 year; repeat testing at 18 months and 2 years was normal. Another patient receiving fluticasone propionate (5%) had an abnormal response at 2 years. No patient on placebo had an abnormal response at 1 or 2 years.

Clinical Trials: Double-blind, parallel, placebo-controlled, US clinical trials were conducted in 1197 adolescent and adult asthma patients to assess the efficacy and safety of FLOVENT ROTADISK in the treatment of asthma. Fixed doses of 50, 100, 250, and 500 mcg twice daily were compared to placebo to provide information about appropriate dosing to cover a range of asthma severity. Asthmatic patients included in these studies were those not adequately controlled with beta-agonists alone, and those already maintained on daily inhaled corticosteroids. In these efficacy trials, at all doses, measures of pulmonary function (forced expiratory volume in 1 second [FEV_1] and morning peak expiratory flow rate [AM PEFR]) were statistically significantly improved as compared with placebo. All doses were delivered by inhalation of the contents of 1 or 2 blisters from the DISKHALER twice daily.

Displayed in the figure below are results of pulmonary function tests for 2 recommended dosages of fluticasone propionate inhalation powder (100 and 250 mcg twice daily) and placebo from a 12-week trial in 331 adolescent and adult asthma patients (baseline FEV_1 = 2.63 L/sec) inadequately controlled on bronchodilators alone. Because this trial used predetermined criteria for lack of efficacy, which caused more patients in the placebo group to be withdrawn, pulmonary function results at Endpoint, which is the last evaluable FEV_1 result and includes most patients' lung function data, are also provided. Pulmonary function at both fluticasone propionate dosages improved significantly compared with placebo by the first week of treatment, and this improvement was maintained over the duration of the trial.

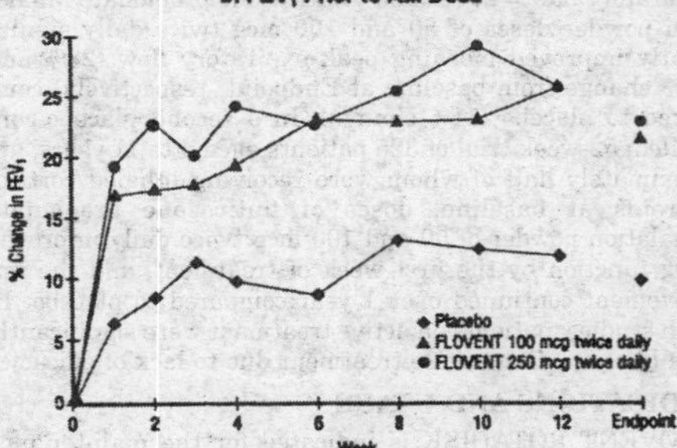

In a second clinical study of 75 patients, 500 mcg twice daily was evaluated in a similar population. In this trial fluticasone propionate significantly improved pulmonary function as compared with placebo.

Displayed in the figure below are results of pulmonary function tests for 2 recommended dosages of fluticasone propionate inhalation powder (100 and 250 mcg twice daily) and placebo from a 12-week trial in 342 adolescent and adult asthma patients (baseline FEV_1 = 2.49 L/sec) already receiving daily inhaled corticosteroid therapy (≥336 mcg/day of beclomethasone dipropionate or ≥800 mcg/day of triamcinolone acetonide) in addition to as-needed albuterol and theophylline (38% of all patients). Because this trial also used predetermined criteria for lack of efficacy, which caused more patients in the placebo group to be withdrawn, pulmonary function results at Endpoint are included. Pulmonary function at both fluticasone propionate dosages improved significantly compared with placebo by the first

Continued on next page

This product information is based on labeling in effect on June 23, 2000. For further information, contact via direct mail, phone, or web site. Medical Information, Glaxo Wellcome Inc., PO Box 13398, Research Triangle Park, NC 27709. Healthcare Professionals (Medical Information): 800-334-0089. Patients (Customer Response Center): 1-888-825-5249. Glaxo Wellcome Corporate Web Site: www.glaxowellcome.com

Flovent Rotadisk—Cont.

week of treatment and the improvement was maintained over the duration of the trial.

A 12-Week Clinical Trial in Patients Already Receiving Inhaled Corticosteroids: Mean Percent Change From Baseline in FEV_1 Prior to AM Dose

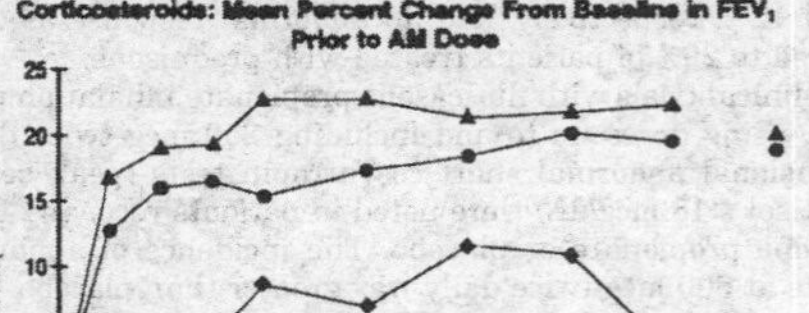
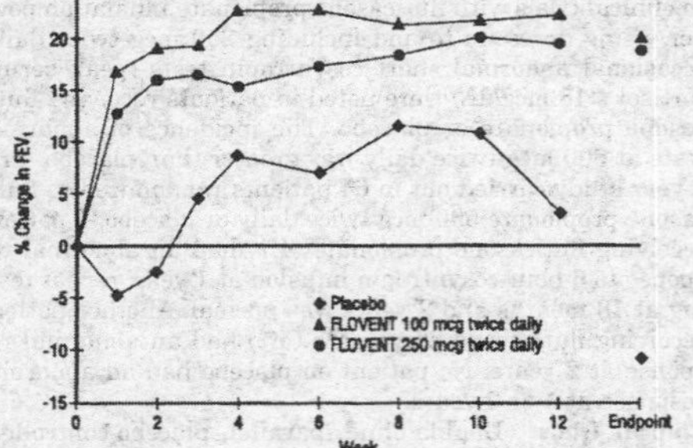

In a second clinical study of 139 patients, treatment with 500 mcg twice daily was evaluated in a similar patient population. In this trial fluticasone propionate significantly improved pulmonary function as compared with placebo.

In the 4 trials described above, all dosages of fluticasone propionate were efficacious; however, at higher dosages, patients were less likely to discontinue study participation due to asthma deterioration (as defined by predetermined criteria for lack of efficacy including lung function and patient-recorded variables such as AM PEFR, albuterol use, and nighttime awakenings due to asthma).

In a clinical trial of 96 severe asthmatic patients requiring chronic oral prednisone therapy (average baseline daily prednisone dose was 10 mg), fluticasone propionate given by inhalation aerosol at doses of 660 and 880 mcg twice daily was evaluated. Both doses enabled a statistically significantly larger percentage of patients to wean successfully from oral prednisone as compared with placebo (69% of the patients on 660 mcg twice daily and 88% of the patients on 880 mcg twice daily as compared with 3% of patients on placebo). Accompanying the reduction in oral corticosteroid use, patients treated with fluticasone propionate had significantly improved lung function and fewer asthma symptoms as compared with the placebo group. These data were obtained from a clinical study using fluticasone propionate inhalation aerosol; no direct assessment of the clinical comparability of equal nominal doses for the FLOVENT ROTADISK and FLOVENT Inhalation Aerosol formulations in this population has been conducted.

Pediatric Experience: In a 12-week, placebo-controlled clinical trial of 263 patients aged 4 to 11 years inadequately controlled on bronchodilators alone (baseline morning peak expiratory flow = 200 L/min), fluticasone propionate inhalation powder doses of 50 and 100 mcg twice daily significantly improved morning peak expiratory flow (28% and 34% change from baseline at Endpoint, respectively) compared to placebo (11% change). In a second placebo-controlled, 52-week trial of 325 patients aged 4 to 11 years, approximately half of whom were receiving inhaled corticosteroids at baseline, doses of fluticasone propionate inhalation powder of 50 and 100 mcg twice daily improved lung function by the first week of treatment, and the improvement continued over 1 year compared to placebo. In both studies, patients on active treatment were significantly less likely to discontinue treatment due to lack of efficacy.

INDICATIONS AND USAGE

FLOVENT ROTADISK is indicated for the maintenance treatment of asthma as prophylactic therapy in patients 4 years of age and older. It is also indicated for patients requiring oral corticosteroid therapy for asthma. Many of these patients may be able to reduce or eliminate their requirement for oral corticosteroids over time.

FLOVENT ROTADISK is NOT indicated for the relief of acute bronchospasm.

CONTRAINDICATIONS

FLOVENT ROTADISK is contraindicated in the primary treatment of status asthmaticus or other acute episodes of asthma where intensive measures are required.

Hypersensitivity to any of the ingredients of these preparations contraindicates their use.

WARNINGS

Particular care is needed for patients who are transferred from systemically active corticosteroids to FLOVENT ROTADISK because deaths due to adrenal insufficiency have occurred in asthmatic patients during and after transfer from systemic corticosteroids to less systemically available inhaled corticosteroids. After withdrawal from systemic corticosteroids, a number of months are required for recovery of HPA function.

Patients who have been previously maintained on 20 mg or more per day of prednisone (or its equivalent) may be most susceptible, particularly when their systemic corticosteroids have been almost completely withdrawn. During this period of HPA suppression, patients may exhibit signs and symptoms of adrenal insufficiency when exposed to trauma, surgery, or infection (particularly gastroenteritis) or other conditions associated with severe electrolyte loss. Although fluticasone propionate inhalation powder may provide control of asthma symptoms during these episodes, in recommended doses it supplies less than normal physiological amounts of corticosteroid systemically and does NOT provide the mineralocorticoid activity that is necessary for coping with these emergencies.

During periods of stress or a severe asthma attack, patients who have been withdrawn from systemic corticosteroids should be instructed to resume oral corticosteroids (in large doses) immediately and to contact their physicians for further instruction. These patients should also be instructed to carry a warning card indicating that they may need supplementary systemic corticosteroids during periods of stress or a severe asthma attack.

Patients requiring oral corticosteroids should be weaned slowly from systemic corticosteroid use after transferring to fluticasone propionate inhalation powder. In a clinical trial of 96 patients, prednisone reduction was successfully accomplished by reducing the daily prednisone dose by 2.5 mg on a weekly basis during transfer to inhaled fluticasone propionate. Successive reduction of prednisone dose was allowed only when lung function, symptoms, and as-needed beta-agonist use were better than or comparable to that seen before initiation of prednisone dose reduction. Lung function (FEV_1 or AM PEFR), beta-agonist use, and asthma symptoms should be carefully monitored during withdrawal of oral corticosteroids. In addition to monitoring asthma signs and symptoms, patients should be observed for signs and symptoms of adrenal insufficiency such as fatigue, lassitude, weakness, nausea and vomiting, and hypotension.

Transfer of patients from systemic corticosteroid therapy to fluticasone propionate inhalation powder may unmask conditions previously suppressed by the systemic corticosteroid therapy, e.g., rhinitis, conjunctivitis, eczema, and arthritis.

Persons who are on drugs that suppress the immune system are more susceptible to infections than healthy individuals. Chickenpox and measles, for example, can have a more serious or even fatal course in susceptible children or adults on corticosteroids. In such children or adults who have not had these diseases, particular care should be taken to avoid exposure. How the dose, route, and duration of corticosteroid administration affect the risk of developing a disseminated infection is not known. The contribution of the underlying disease and/or prior corticosteroid treatment to the risk is also not known. If exposed to chickenpox, prophylaxis with varicella zoster immune globulin (VZIG) may be indicated. If exposed to measles, prophylaxis with pooled intramuscular immunoglobulin (IG) may be indicated. (See the respective package inserts for complete VZIG and IG prescribing information.) If chickenpox develops, treatment with antiviral agents may be considered.

Fluticasone propionate inhalation powder is not to be regarded as a bronchodilator and is not indicated for rapid relief of bronchospasm.

As with other inhaled asthma medications, bronchospasm may occur with an immediate increase in wheezing after dosing. If bronchospasm occurs following dosing with FLOVENT ROTADISK, it should be treated immediately with a fast-acting inhaled bronchodilator. Treatment with inhaled fluticasone propionate should be discontinued and alternative therapy instituted.

Patients should be instructed to contact their physicians immediately when episodes of asthma that are not responsive to bronchodilators occur during the course of treatment with fluticasone propionate inhalation powder. During such episodes, patients may require therapy with oral corticosteroids.

PRECAUTIONS

General: During withdrawal from oral corticosteroids, some patients may experience symptoms of systemically active corticosteroid withdrawal, e.g., joint and/or muscular pain, lassitude, and depression, despite maintenance or even improvement of respiratory function.

Fluticasone propionate will often permit control of asthma symptoms with less suppression of HPA function than therapeutically equivalent oral doses of prednisone. Since fluticasone propionate is absorbed into the circulation and can be systemically active at higher doses, the beneficial effects of fluticasone propionate inhalation powder in minimizing HPA dysfunction may be expected only when recommended dosages are not exceeded and individual patients are titrated to the lowest effective dose. A relationship between plasma levels of fluticasone propionate and inhibitory effects on stimulated cortisol production has been shown after 4 weeks of treatment with fluticasone propionate inhalation aerosol. Since individual sensitivity to effects on cortisol production exists, physicians should consider this information when prescribing fluticasone propionate inhalation powder.

Because of the possibility of systemic absorption of inhaled corticosteroids, patients treated with these drugs should be observed carefully for any evidence of systemic corticosteroid effects. Particular care should be taken in observing patients postoperatively or during periods of stress for evidence of inadequate adrenal response.

It is possible that systemic corticosteroid effects such as hypercorticism and adrenal suppression may appear in a small number of patients, particularly at higher doses. If such changes occur, fluticasone propionate inhalation powder should be reduced slowly, consistent with accepted procedures for reducing systemic corticosteroids and for management of asthma symptoms.

A reduction of growth velocity in children or adolescents may occur as a result of poorly controlled asthma or from the therapeutic use of corticosteroids, including inhaled corticosteroids. A 52-week placebo-controlled study to assess the potential growth effects of fluticasone propionate inhalation powder at 50 and 100 mcg twice daily was conducted in the US in 325 prepubescent children (244 males and 81 females) 4 to 11 years of age. The mean growth velocities at 52 weeks observed in the intent-to-treat population were 6.32 cm/year in the placebo group (n = 76), 6.07 cm/year in the 50-mcg group (n = 98), and 5.66 cm/year in the 100-mcg group (n = 89). An imbalance in the proportion of children entering puberty between groups and a higher dropout rate in the placebo group due to poorly controlled asthma may be confounding factors in interpreting these data. A separate subset analysis of children who remained prepubertal during the study revealed growth rates at 52 weeks of 6.10 cm/year in the placebo group (n = 57), 5.91 cm/year in the 50-mcg group (n = 74), and 5.67 cm/year in the 100-mcg group (n = 79). The clinical significance of these growth data is not certain. In children 8.5 years of age, the mean age of children in this study, the range for expected growth velocity is: boys – 3rd percentile = 3.8 cm/year, 50th percentile = 5.4 cm/year, and 97th percentile = 7.0 cm/year; girls – 3rd percentile = 4.2 cm/year, 50th percentile = 5.7 cm/year, and 97th percentile = 7.3 cm/year. The effects of long-term treatment of children with inhaled corticosteroids, including fluticasone propionate, on final adult height are not known. Physicians should closely follow the growth of children and adolescents taking corticosteroids by any route, and weigh the benefits of corticosteroid therapy against the possibility of growth suppression if growth appears slowed. Patients should be maintained on the lowest dose of inhaled corticosteroid that effectively controls their asthma.

The long-term effects of fluticasone propionate in human subjects are not fully known. In particular, the effects resulting from chronic use of fluticasone propionate on developmental or immunologic processes in the mouth, pharynx, trachea, and lung are unknown. Some patients have received inhaled fluticasone propionate on a continuous basis for periods of 3 years or longer. In clinical studies with patients treated for 2 years with inhaled fluticasone propionate, no apparent differences in the type or severity of adverse reactions were observed after long- versus short-term treatment.

Rare instances of glaucoma, increased intraocular pressure, and cataracts have been reported following the inhaled administration of corticosteroids, including fluticasone propionate.

In clinical studies with inhaled fluticasone propionate, the development of localized infections of the pharynx with *Candida albicans* has occurred. When such an infection develops, it should be treated with appropriate local or systemic (i.e., oral antifungal) therapy while remaining on treatment with fluticasone propionate inhalation powder, but at times therapy with fluticasone propionate may need to be interrupted.

Inhaled corticosteroids should be used with caution, if at all, in patients with active or quiescent tuberculous infections of the respiratory tract; untreated systemic fungal, bacterial, viral, or parasitic infections; or ocular herpes simplex.

Eosinophilic Conditions: In rare cases, patients on inhaled fluticasone propionate may present with systemic eosinophilic conditions, with some patients presenting with clinical features of vasculitis consistent with Churg-Strauss syndrome, a condition that is often treated with systemic corticosteroid therapy. These events usually, but not always, have been associated with the reduction and/or withdrawal of oral corticosteroid therapy following the introduction of fluticasone propionate. Cases of serious eosinophilic conditions have also been reported with other inhaled corticosteroids in this clinical setting. Physicians should be alert to eosinophilia, vasculitic rash, worsening pulmonary symptoms, cardiac complications, and/or neuropathy presenting in their patients. A causal relationship between fluticasone propionate and these underlying conditions has not been established (see ADVERSE REACTIONS).

Information for Patients: Patients being treated with FLOVENT ROTADISK should receive the following information and instructions. This information is intended to aid them in the safe and effective use of this medication. It is not a disclosure of all possible adverse or intended effects.

Patients should use FLOVENT ROTADISK at regular intervals as directed. Results of clinical trials indicated significant improvement may occur within the first day or two of treatment; however, the full benefit may not be achieved until treatment has been administered for 1 to 2 weeks or longer. The patient should not increase the prescribed dosage but should contact the physician if symptoms do not improve or if the condition worsens.

Patients should be warned to avoid exposure to chickenpox or measles and, if they are exposed, to consult their physicians without delay.

For the proper use of FLOVENT ROTADISK Inhalation Powder and to attain maximum improvement, the patient should read and follow carefully the Patient's Instructions for Use accompanying the product.

Drug Interactions: In a placebo-controlled, crossover study in 8 healthy volunteers, coadministration of a single dose of fluticasone propionate (1000 mcg) with multiple doses of ketoconazole (200 mg) to steady state resulted in increased mean fluticasone propionate concentrations, a reduction in plasma cortisol AUC, and no effect on urinary excretion of cortisol. This interaction may be due to an inhibition of the cytochrome P450 3A4 isoenzyme system by ketoconazole, which is also the route of metabolism of fluticasone propionate. Care should be exercised when FLOVENT is coadministered with long-term ketoconazole and other known cytochrome P450 3A4 inhibitors.

Carcinogenesis, Mutagenesis, Impairment of Fertility: Fluticasone propionate demonstrated no tumorigenic potential in mice at oral doses up to 1000 mcg/kg (approximately 2 times the maximum recommended daily inhalation dose in adults and approximately 10 times the maximum recommended daily inhalation dose in children on a mcg/m^2 basis) for 78 weeks or in rats at inhalation doses up to 57 mcg/kg (approximately 1/4 the maximum recommended daily inhalation dose in adults and comparable to the maximum recommended daily inhalation dose in children on a mcg/m^2 basis) for 104 weeks.

Fluticasone propionate did not induce gene mutation in prokaryotic or eukaryotic cells in vitro. No significant clastogenic effect was seen in cultured human peripheral lymphocytes in vitro or in the mouse micronucleus test when administered at high doses by the oral or subcutaneous routes. Furthermore, the compound did not delay erythroblast division in bone marrow.

No evidence of impairment of fertility was observed in reproductive studies conducted in male and female rats at subcutaneous doses up to 50 mcg/kg (approximately 1/5 the maximum recommended daily inhalation dose in adults on a mcg/m^2 basis). Prostate weight was significantly reduced at a subcutaneous dose of 50 mcg/kg.

Pregnancy: ***Teratogenic Effects:*** Pregnancy Category C. Subcutaneous studies in the mouse and rat at 45 and 100 mcg/kg, respectively, (approximately 1/10 and 1/3, respectively, the maximum recommended daily inhalation dose in adults on a mcg/m^2 basis) revealed fetal toxicity characteristic of potent corticosteroid compounds, including embryonic growth retardation, omphalocele, cleft palate, and retarded cranial ossification.

In the rabbit, fetal weight reduction and cleft palate were observed at a subcutaneous dose of 4 mcg/kg (approximately 1/30 the maximum recommended daily inhalation dose in adults on a mcg/m^2 basis). However, no teratogenic effects were reported at oral doses up to 300 mcg/kg (approximately 2 times the maximum recommended daily inhalation dose in adults on a mcg/m^2 basis) of fluticasone propionate. No fluticasone propionate was detected in the plasma in this study, consistent with the established low bioavailability following oral administration (see CLINICAL PHARMACOLOGY).

Fluticasone propionate crossed the placenta following oral administration of 100 mcg/kg to rats or 300 mcg/kg to rabbits (approximately 1/3 and 2 times, respectively, the maximum recommended daily inhalation dose in adults on a mcg/m^2 basis).

There are no adequate and well-controlled studies in pregnant women. Fluticasone propionate should be used during pregnancy only if the potential benefit justifies the potential risk to the fetus.

Experience with oral corticosteroids since their introduction in pharmacologic, as opposed to physiologic, doses suggests that rodents are more prone to teratogenic effects from corticosteroids than humans. In addition, because there is a natural increase in corticosteroid production during pregnancy, most women will require a lower exogenous corticosteroid dose and many will not need corticosteroid treatment during pregnancy.

Nursing Mothers: It is not known whether fluticasone propionate is excreted in human breast milk. Subcutaneous administration to lactating rats of 10 mcg/kg tritiated fluticasone propionate (approximately 1/25 the maximum recommended daily inhalation dose in adults on a mcg/m^2 basis) resulted in measurable radioactivity in milk. Because other corticosteroids are excreted in human milk, caution should be exercised when fluticasone propionate inhalation powder is administered to a nursing woman.

Pediatric Use: Two hundred fourteen (214) patients 4 to 11 years of age and 142 patients 12 to 16 years of age were treated with fluticasone propionate inhalation powder in US clinical trials. The safety and effectiveness of FLOVENT ROTADISK Inhalation Powder in children below 4 years of age have not been established.

Inhaled corticosteroids, including fluticasone propionate, may cause a reduction in growth in children and adolescents (see PRECAUTIONS). If a child or adolescent on any corticosteroid appears to have growth suppression, the possibility that they are particularly sensitive to this effect of corticosteroids should be considered. Patients should be maintained on the lowest dose of inhaled corticosteroid that effectively controls their asthma.

Geriatric Use: One hundred seventy-three (173) patients 65 years of age or older have been treated with fluticasone propionate inhalation powder in US and non-US clinical trials. There were no differences in adverse reactions compared to those reported by younger patients.

ADVERSE REACTIONS

The following incidence of common adverse experiences is based upon 6 placebo-controlled clinical trials in which 1384 patients ≥4 years of age (520 females and 864 males) previously treated with as-needed bronchodilators and/or inhaled corticosteroids were treated with fluticasone propionate inhalation powder (doses of 50 to 500 mcg twice daily for up to 12 weeks) or placebo.

Overall Adverse Experiences With >3% Incidence on Fluticasone Propionate in Controlled Clinical Trials With FLOVENT ROTADISK in Patients ≥4 Years Previously Receiving Bronchodilators and/or Inhaled Corticosteroids

Adverse Event	Placebo (n = 438) %	FLOVENT 50 mcg Twice Daily (n = 255) %	FLOVENT 100 mcg Twice Daily (n = 331) %	FLOVENT 250 mcg Twice Daily (n = 176) %	FLOVENT 500 mcg Twice Daily (n = 184) %
Ear, nose, and throat					
Pharyngitis	7	6	8	8	13
Nasal congestion	5	4	4	7	7
Sinusitis	4	5	4	6	4
Rhinitis	4	4	9	2	3
Dysphonia	0	<1	4	6	4
Oral candidiasis	1	3	3	4	11
Respiratory					
Upper respiratory infection	13	16	17	22	16
Influenza	2	3	3	3	4
Bronchitis	2	4	2	1	2
Other					
Headache	11	11	9	14	15
Diarrhea	1	2	2	0	4
Back problems	<1	<1	1	1	4
Fever	3	4	4	2	2
Average duration of exposure (days)	53	77	68	78	60

Previous Therapy	Recommended Starting Dose	Highest Recommended Dose
Adults and Adolescents		
Bronchodilators alone	100 mcg twice daily	500 mcg twice daily
Inhaled corticosteroids	100-250 mcg twice daily*	500 mcg twice daily
Oral corticosteroids†	1000 mcg twice daily‡	1000 mcg twice daily‡
Children 4 to 11 Years		
Bronchodilators alone	50 mcg twice daily	100 mcg twice daily
Inhaled corticosteroids	50 mcg twice daily	100 mcg twice daily

* Starting doses above 100 mcg twice daily for adults and adolescents and 50 mcg twice daily for children 4 to 11 years of age may be considered for patients with poorer asthma control or those who have previously required doses of inhaled corticosteroids that are in the higher range for that specific agent.

NOTE: In all patients, it is desirable to titrate to the lowest effective dose once asthma stability is achieved.

† **For Patients Currently Receiving Chronic Oral Corticosteroid Therapy:** Prednisone should be reduced no faster than 2.5 mg/day on a weekly basis, beginning after at least 1 week of therapy with FLOVENT. Patients should be carefully monitored for signs of asthma instability, including serial objective measures of airflow, and for signs of adrenal insufficiency (see WARNINGS). Once prednisone reduction is complete, the dosage of fluticasone propionate should be reduced to the lowest effective dosage.

‡ This dosing recommendation is based on clinical data from a study conducted using FLOVENT Inhalation Aerosol. No clinical trials have been conducted in patients on oral corticosteroids using the ROTADISK formulation; no direct assessment of the clinical comparability of equal nominal doses for the FLOVENT ROTADISK and FLOVENT Inhalation Aerosol formulations in this population has been conducted.

[See first table above]

The table above includes all events (whether considered drug-related or nondrug-related by the investigator) that occurred at a rate of over 3% in any of the fluticasone propionate inhalation powder groups and were more common than in the placebo group. In considering these data, differences in average duration of exposure should be taken into account.

These adverse reactions were mostly mild to moderate in severity, with <2% of patients discontinuing the studies because of adverse events. Rare cases of immediate and delayed hypersensitivity reactions, including rash and other rare events of angioedema and bronchospasm, have been reported.

Other adverse events that occurred in these clinical trials using fluticasone propionate inhalation powder with an incidence of 1% to 3% and which occurred at a greater incidence than with placebo were:

Ear, Nose, and Throat: Otitis media, tonsillitis, nasal discharge, earache, laryngitis, epistaxis, sneezing.

Eye: Conjunctivitis.

Gastrointestinal: Abdominal pain, viral gastroenteritis, gastroenteritis/colitis, abdominal discomfort.

Miscellaneous: Injury.

Mouth and Teeth: Mouth irritation.

Musculoskeletal: Sprain/strain, pain in joint, disorder/symptoms of neck, muscular soreness, aches and pains.

Neurological: Migraine, nervousness.

Respiratory: Chest congestion, acute nasopharyngitis, dyspnea, irritation due to inhalant.

Skin: Dermatitis, urticaria.

Urogenital: Dysmenorrhea, candidiasis of vagina, pelvic inflammatory disease, vaginitis/vulvovaginitis, irregular menstrual cycle.

There were no clinically relevant differences in the pattern or severity of adverse events in children compared with those reported in adults.

Fluticasone propionate inhalation aerosol (660 or 880 mcg twice daily) was administered for 16 weeks to asthmatics requiring oral corticosteroids. Adverse events reported more frequently in these patients compared to patients not on oral corticosteroids included sinusitis, nasal discharge, oropharyngeal candidiasis, headache, joint pain, nausea and vomiting, muscular soreness, malaise/fatigue, and insomnia.

Observed During Clinical Practice: The following events have been identified during postapproval use of fluticasone propionate in clinical practice. Because they are reported voluntarily from a population of unknown size, estimates of frequency cannot be made. These events have been chosen for inclusion due to either their seriousness, frequency of reporting, causal connection to fluticasone propionate, or a combination of these factors.

Ear, Nose, and Throat: Aphonia, cough, hoarseness, laryngitis, and throat soreness and irritation.

Endocrine and Metabolic: Cushingoid features, growth velocity reduction in children/adolescents, hyperglycemia, and weight gain.

Psychiatry: Agitation, aggression, depression, and restlessness.

Respiratory: Asthma exacerbation, bronchospasm, chest tightness, dyspnea, paradoxical bronchospasm, and wheezing.

Skin: Contusions, ecchymoses, and pruritus.

Eosinophilic Conditions: In rare cases, patients on inhaled fluticasone propionate may present with systemic eosinophilic conditions, with some patients presenting with clinical features of vasculitis consistent with Churg-Strauss syndrome, a condition that is often treated with systemic corticosteroid therapy. These events usually, but not always, have been associated with the reduction and/or withdrawal of oral corticosteroid therapy following the introduction of fluticasone propionate. Cases of serious eosinophilic conditions have also been reported with other inhaled corticosteroids in this clinical setting. Physicians should be alert to eosinophilia, vasculitic rash, worsening pulmonary symptoms, cardiac complications, and/or neuropathy presenting in their patients. A causal relationship between fluticasone propionate and these underlying conditions has not been established (see PRECAUTIONS: Eosinophilic Conditions).

OVERDOSAGE

Chronic overdosage may result in signs/symptoms of hypercorticism (see PRECAUTIONS). Inhalation by healthy vol-

Continued on next page

This product information is based on labeling in effect on June 23, 2000. For further information, contact via direct mail, phone, or web site. Medical Information, Glaxo Wellcome Inc., PO Box 13398, Research Triangle Park, NC 27709. Healthcare Professionals (Medical Information): 800-334-0089. Patients (Customer Response Center): 1-888-825-5249. Glaxo Wellcome Corporate Web Site: www.glaxowellcome.com

Flovent Rotadisk—Cont.

unteers of a single dose of 4000 mcg of fluticasone propionate inhalation powder or single doses of 1760 or 3520 mcg of fluticasone propionate inhalation aerosol was well tolerated. Fluticasone propionate given by inhalation aerosol at doses of 1320 mcg twice daily for 7 to 15 days to healthy human volunteers was also well tolerated. Repeat oral doses up to 80 mg daily for 10 days in healthy volunteers and repeat oral doses up to 20 mg daily for 42 days in patients were well tolerated. Adverse reactions were of mild or moderate severity, and incidences were similar in active and placebo treatment groups. The oral and subcutaneous median lethal doses in mice and rats were >1000 mg/kg (>2000 and >4100 times, respectively, the maximum recommended daily inhalation dose in adults and >9600 and >19,000 times, respectively, the maximum recommended daily inhalation dose in children on a mg/m^2 basis).

DOSAGE AND ADMINISTRATION

FLOVENT ROTADISK should be administered by the orally inhaled route in patients 4 years of age and older. Individual patients will experience a variable time to onset and degree of symptom relief. Generally, fluticasone propionate inhalation powder has a relatively rapid onset of action for an inhaled corticosteroid. Improvement in asthma control following inhaled administration of fluticasone propionate can occur within 24 hours of beginning treatment, although maximum benefit may not be achieved for 1 to 2 weeks or longer after starting treatment.

After asthma stability has been achieved, it is always desirable to titrate to the lowest effective dose to reduce the possibility of side effects. Doses as low as 50 mcg twice daily have been shown to be effective in some patients. For patients who do not respond adequately to the starting dose after 2 weeks of therapy, higher doses may provide additional asthma control. The safety and efficacy of FLOVENT ROTADISK when administered in excess of recommended doses have not been established.

Rinsing the mouth after inhalation is advised.

The recommended starting dose and the highest recommended dose of fluticasone propionate inhalation powder, based on prior anti-asthma therapy, are listed in the following table.

[See second table on previous page]

Geriatric Use: In studies where geriatric patients (65 years of age or older, see PRECAUTIONS) have been treated with fluticasone propionate inhalation powder, efficacy and safety did not differ from that in younger patients. Consequently, no dosage adjustment is recommended.

Directions for Use: Illustrated Patient's Instructions for Use accompany each package of FLOVENT ROTADISK.

HOW SUPPLIED

FLOVENT ROTADISK 50 mcg is a circular double-foil pack containing 4 blisters of the drug. Fifteen (15) ROTADISKS are packaged in a white polypropylene tube, and the tube is packaged in a plastic-coated, moisture-protective foil pouch. A carton contains the foil pouch of 15 ROTADISKS and 1 dark orange- and peach-colored DISKHALER inhalation device (NDC 0173-0511-00).

FLOVENT ROTADISK 100 mcg is a circular double-foil pack containing 4 blisters of the drug. Fifteen (15) ROTADISKS are packaged in a white polypropylene tube, and the tube is packaged in a plastic-coated, moisture-protective foil pouch. A carton contains the foil pouch of 15 ROTADISKS and 1 dark orange- and peach-colored DISKHALER inhalation device (NDC 0173-0509-00).

FLOVENT ROTADISK 250 mcg is a circular double-foil pack containing 4 blisters of the drug. Fifteen (15) ROTADISKS are packaged in a white polypropylene tube, and the tube is packaged in a plastic-coated, moisture-protective foil pouch. A carton contains the foil pouch of 15 ROTADISKS and 1 dark orange- and peach-colored DISKHALER inhalation device (NDC 0173-0504-00).

Store at controlled room temperature (see USP), 20° to 25°C (68° to 77°F) in a dry place. Keep out of reach of children. Do not puncture any fluticasone propionate ROTADISK blister until taking a dose using the DISKHALER.

Use the ROTADISK blisters within 2 months after opening of the moisture-protective foil overwrap or before the expiration date, whichever comes first. Place the sticker provided with the product on the tube and enter the date the foil overwrap is opened and the 2-month use date.

Glaxo Wellcome Inc., Research Triangle Park, NC 27709
October 1999/RL-772

Shown in Product Identification Guide, page 315

FORTAZ® ℞

[for ' taz]
(ceftazidime for injection)

FORTAZ® ℞

(ceftazidime sodium injection)

For Intravenous or Intramuscular Use

DESCRIPTION

Ceftazidime is a semisynthetic, broad-spectrum, beta- lactam antibiotic for parenteral administration. It is the pentahydrate of pyridinium, 1-[[7-[[(2-amino-4-thiazolyl)[(1-carboxy-1-methylethoxy) imino]acetyl] amino]-2-carboxy-8-oxo-5-thia-1-azabicyclo[4.2.0]oct-2-en-3-yl]methyl]-, hydroxide, inner salt, [6R-[6α,7β(Z)]].

The empirical formula is $C_{22}H_{32}N_6O_{12}S_2$, representing a molecular weight of 636.6.

FORTAZ is a sterile, dry powdered mixture of ceftazidime pentahydrate and sodium carbonate. The sodium carbonate at a concentration of 118 mg/g of ceftazidime activity has been admixed to facilitate dissolution. The total sodium content of the mixture is approximately 54 mg (2.3 mEq)/g of ceftazidime activity.

FORTAZ in sterile crystalline form is supplied in vials equivalent to 500 mg, 1 g, 2 g, or 6 g of anhydrous ceftazidime and in ADD-Vantage® vials equivalent to 1 or 2 g of anhydrous ceftazidime. Solutions of FORTAZ range in color from light yellow to amber, depending on the diluent and volume used. The pH of freshly constituted solutions usually ranges from 5 to 8.

FORTAZ is available as a frozen, iso-osmotic, sterile, nonpyrogenic solution with 1 or 2 g of ceftazidime as ceftazidime sodium premixed with approximately 2.2 or 1.6 g, respectively, of dextrose hydrous, USP. Dextrose has been added to adjust the osmolality. Sodium hydroxide is used to adjust pH and neutralize ceftazidime pentahydrate free acid to the sodium salt. The pH may have been adjusted with hydrochloric acid. Solutions of premixed FORTAZ range in color from light yellow to amber. The solution is intended for intravenous (IV) use after thawing to room temperature. The osmolality of the solution is approximately 300 mOsmol/kg, and the pH of thawed solutions ranges from 5 to 7.5.

The plastic container for the frozen solution is fabricated from a specially designed multilayer plastic, PL 2040. Solutions are in contact with the polyethylene layer of this container and can leach out certain chemical components of the plastic in very small amounts within the expiration period. The suitability of the plastic has been confirmed in tests in animals according to USP biological tests for plastic containers as well as by tissue culture toxicity studies.

CLINICAL PHARMACOLOGY

After IV administration of 500-mg and 1-g doses of ceftazidime over 5 minutes to normal adult male volunteers, mean peak serum concentrations of 45 and 90 mcg/mL, respectively, were achieved. After IV infusion of 500-mg, 1-g, and 2-g doses of ceftazidime over 20 to 30 minutes to normal adult male volunteers, mean peak serum concentrations of 42, 69, and 170 mcg/mL, respectively, were achieved. The average serum concentrations following IV infusion of 500-mg, 1-g, and 2-g doses to these volunteers over an 8-hour interval are given in Table 1.

Table 1

Ceftazidime IV Dose	Serum Concentrations (mcg/mL)				
	0.5 h	1 h	2 h	4 h	8 h
500 mg	42	25	12	6	2
1 g	60	39	23	11	3
2 g	129	75	42	13	5

The absorption and elimination of ceftazidime were directly proportional to the size of the dose. The half-life following IV administration was approximately 1.9 hours. Less than 10% of ceftazidime was protein bound. The degree of protein binding was independent of concentration. There was no evidence of accumulation of ceftazidime in the serum in individuals with normal renal function following multiple IV doses of 1 and 2 g every 8 hours for 10 days.

Following intramuscular (IM) administration of 500-mg and 1-g doses of ceftazidime to normal adult volunteers, the mean peak serum concentrations were 17 and 39 mcg/mL, respectively, at approximately 1 hour. Serum concentrations remained above 4 mcg/mL for 6 and 8 hours after the IM administration of 500-mg and 1-g doses, respectively. The half-life of ceftazidime in these volunteers was approximately 2 hours.

The presence of hepatic dysfunction had no effect on the pharmacokinetics of ceftazidime in individuals administered 2 g intravenously every 8 hours for 5 days. Therefore, a dosage adjustment from the normal recommended dosage is not required for patients with hepatic dysfunction, provided renal function is not impaired.

Approximately 80% to 90% of an IM or IV dose of ceftazidime is excreted unchanged by the kidneys over a 24-hour period. After the IV administration of single 500-mg or 1-g doses, approximately 50% of the dose appeared in the urine in the first 2 hours. An additional 20% was excreted between 2 and 4 hours after dosing, and approximately another 12% of the dose appeared in the urine between 4 and 8 hours later. The elimination of ceftazidime by the kidneys resulted in high therapeutic concentrations in the urine.

The mean renal clearance of ceftazidime was approximately 100 mL/min. The calculated plasma clearance of approximately 115 mL/min indicated nearly complete elimination of ceftazidime by the renal route. Administration of probenecid before dosing had no effect on the elimination kinetics of ceftazidime. This suggested that ceftazidime is eliminated by glomerular filtration and is not actively secreted by renal tubular mechanisms.

Since ceftazidime is eliminated almost solely by the kidneys, its serum half-life is significantly prolonged in patients with impaired renal function. Consequently, dosage adjustments in such patients as described in the DOSAGE AND ADMINISTRATION section are suggested.

Therapeutic concentrations of ceftazidime are achieved in the following body tissues and fluids.

[See table 2 below]

Microbiology: Ceftazidime is bactericidal in action, exerting its effect by inhibition of enzymes responsible for cell-wall synthesis. A wide range of gram-negative organisms is susceptible to ceftazidime *in vitro*, including strains resistant to gentamicin and other aminoglycosides. In addition, ceftazidime has been shown to be active against gram-positive organisms. It is highly stable to most clinically important beta-lactamases, plasmid or chromosomal, which are produced by both gram-negative and gram-positive organisms and, consequently, is active against many strains resistant to ampicillin and other cephalosporins.

Ceftazidime has been shown to be active against the following organisms both *in vitro* and in clinical infections (see INDICATIONS AND USAGE).

Aerobes, Gram-negative: *Citrobacter* spp., including *Citrobacter freundii* and *Citrobacter diversus; Enterobacter* spp., including *Enterobacter cloacae* and *Enterobacter aerogenes; Escherichia coli; Haemophilus influenzae,* including ampicillin-resistant strains; *Klebsiella* spp. (including *Klebsiella pneumoniae*); *Neisseria meningitidis; Proteus mirabilis; Proteus vulgaris; Pseudomonas* spp. (including *Pseudomonas aeruginosa*); and *Serratia* spp.

Aerobes, Gram-positive: *Staphylococcus aureus,* including penicillinase- and non–penicillinase-producing strains; *Streptococcus agalactiae* (group B streptococci); *Streptococcus pneumoniae;* and *Streptococcus pyogenes* (group A beta-hemolytic streptococci).

Anaerobes: *Bacteroides* spp. (NOTE: many strains of *Bacteroides fragilis* are resistant).

Ceftazidime has been shown to be active *in vitro* against most strains of the following organisms; however, the clinical significance of these data is unknown: *Acinetobacter* spp., *Clostridium* spp. (not including *Clostridium difficile*), *Haemophilus parainfluenzae, Morganella morganii* (formerly *Proteus morganii*), *Neisseria gonorrhoeae, Peptococcus* spp., *Peptostreptococcus* spp., *Providencia* spp. (including *Providencia rettgeri,* formerly *Proteus rettgeri*), *Salmonella* spp., *Shigella* spp., *Staphylococcus epidermidis,* and *Yersinia enterocolitica.*

Ceftazidime and the aminoglycosides have been shown to be synergistic *in vitro* against *Pseudomonas aeruginosa* and

Table 2: Ceftazidime Concentrations in Body Tissues and Fluids

Tissue or Fluid	Dose/ Route	No. of Patients	Time of Sample Postdose	Average Tissue or Fluid Level (mcg/mL or mcg/g)
Urine	500 mg IM	6	0–2 h	2,100.0
	2 g IV	6	0–2 h	12,000.0
Bile	2 g IV	3	90 min	36.4
Synovial fluid	2 g IV	13	2 h	25.6
Peritoneal fluid	2 g IV	8	2 h	48.6
Sputum	1 g IV	8	1 h	9.0
Cerebrospinal fluid	2 g q8h IV	5	120 min	9.8
(inflamed meninges)	2 g q8h IV	6	180 min	9.4
Aqueous humor	2 g IV	13	1–3 h	11.0
Blister fluid	1 g IV	7	2–3 h	19.7
Lymphatic fluid	1 g IV	7	2–3 h	23.4
Bone	2 g IV	8	0.67 h	31.1
Heart muscle	2 g IV	35	30–280 min	12.7
Skin	2 g IV	22	30–180 min	6.6
Skeletal muscle	2 g IV	35	30–280 min	9.4
Myometrium	2 g IV	31	1–2 h	18.7

the enterobacteriaceae. Ceftazidime and carbenicillin have also been shown to be synergistic *in vitro* against *Pseudomonas aeruginosa.*

Ceftazidime is not active *in vitro* against methicillin-resistant staphylococci, *Streptococcus faecalis* and many other enterococci, *Listeria monocytogenes, Campylobacter* spp., or *Clostridium difficile.*

Susceptibility Tests: ***Diffusion Techniques:*** Quantitative methods that require measurement of zone diameters give an estimate of antibiotic susceptibility. One such procedure[1–3] has been recommended for use with disks to test susceptibility to ceftazidime.

Reports from the laboratory giving results of the standard single-disk susceptibility test with a 30-mcg ceftazidime disk should be interpreted according to the following criteria:

Susceptible organisms produce zones of 18 mm or greater, indicating that the test organism is likely to respond to therapy.

Organisms that produce zones of 15 to 17 mm are expected to be susceptible if high dosage is used or if the infection is confined to tissues and fluids (e.g., urine) in which high antibiotic levels are attained.

Resistant organisms produce zones of 14 mm or less, indicating that other therapy should be selected.

Organisms should be tested with the ceftazidime disk since ceftazidime has been shown by *in vitro* tests to be active against certain strains found resistant when other beta-lactam disks are used.

Standardized procedures require the use of laboratory control organisms. The 30-mcg ceftazidime disk should give zone diameters between 25 and 32 mm for *Escherichia coli* ATCC 25922. For *Pseudomonas aeruginosa* ATCC 27853, the zone diameters should be between 22 and 29 mm. For *Staphylococcus aureus* ATCC 25923, the zone diameters should be between 16 and 20 mm.

Dilution Techniques: In other susceptibility testing procedures, e.g., ICS agar dilution or the equivalent, a bacterial isolate may be considered susceptible if the minimum inhibitory concentration (MIC) value for ceftazidime is not more than 16 mcg/mL. Organisms are considered resistant to ceftazidime if the MIC is ≥ 64 mcg/mL. Organisms having an MIC value of < 64 mcg/mL but > 16 mcg/mL are expected to be susceptible if high dosage is used or if the infection is confined to tissues and fluids (e.g., urine) in which high antibiotic levels are attained.

As with standard diffusion methods, dilution procedures require the use of laboratory control organisms. Standard ceftazidime powder should give MIC values in the range of 4 to 16 mcg/mL for *Staphylococcus aureus* ATCC 25923. For *Escherichia coli* ATCC 25922, the MIC range should be between 0.125 and 0.5 mcg/mL. For *Pseudomonas aeruginosa* ATCC 27853, the MIC range should be between 0.5 and 2 mcg/mL.

INDICATIONS AND USAGE

FORTAZ is indicated for the treatment of patients with infections caused by susceptible strains of the designated organisms in the following diseases:

1. **Lower Respiratory Tract Infections,** including pneumonia, caused by *Pseudomonas aeruginosa* and other *Pseudomonas* spp.; *Haemophilus influenzae,* including ampicillin-resistant strains; *Klebsiella* spp.; *Enterobacter* spp.; *Proteus mirabilis; Escherichia coli; Serratia* spp.; *Citrobacter* spp.; *Streptococcus pneumoniae;* and *Staphylococcus aureus* (methicillin-susceptible strains).
2. **Skin and Skin-Structure Infections** caused by *Pseudomonas aeruginosa; Klebsiella* spp.; *Escherichia coli; Proteus* spp., including *Proteus mirabilis* and indole-positive *Proteus; Enterobacter* spp.; *Serratia* spp.; *Staphylococcus aureus* (methicillin-susceptible strains); and *Streptococcus pyogenes* (group A beta-hemolytic streptococci).
3. **Urinary Tract Infections,** both complicated and uncomplicated, caused by *Pseudomonas aeruginosa; Enterobacter* spp.; *Proteus* spp., including *Proteus mirabilis* and indole-positive *Proteus; Klebsiella* spp.; and *Escherichia coli.*
4. **Bacterial Septicemia** caused by *Pseudomonas aeruginosa, Klebsiella* spp., *Haemophilus influenzae, Escherichia coli, Serratia* spp., *Streptococcus pneumoniae,* and *Staphylococcus aureus* (methicillin-susceptible strains).
5. **Bone and Joint Infections** caused by *Pseudomonas aeruginosa, Klebsiella* spp., *Enterobacter* spp., and *Staphylococcus aureus* (methicillin-susceptible strains).
6. **Gynecologic Infections,** including endometritis, pelvic cellulitis, and other infections of the female genital tract caused by *Escherichia coli.*
7. **Intra-abdominal Infections,** including peritonitis caused by *Escherichia coli, Klebsiella* spp., and *Staphylococcus aureus* (methicillin-susceptible strains) and polymicrobial infections caused by aerobic and anaerobic organisms and *Bacteroides* spp. (many strains of *Bacteroides fragilis* are resistant).
8. **Central Nervous System Infections,** including meningitis, caused by *Haemophilus influenzae* and *Neisseria meningitidis.* Ceftazidime has also been used successfully in a limited number of cases of meningitis due to *Pseudomonas aeruginosa* and *Streptococcus pneumoniae.*

Specimens for bacterial cultures should be obtained before therapy in order to isolate and identify causative organisms and to determine their susceptibility to ceftazidime. Therapy may be instituted before results of susceptibility studies are known; however, once these results become available, the antibiotic treatment should be adjusted accordingly.

Table 3: Recommended Dosage Schedule

	Dose	Frequency
Adults		
Usual recommended dosage	**1 gram IV or IM**	**q8–12h**
Uncomplicated urinary tract infections	250 mg IV or IM	q12h
Bone and joint infections	2 grams IV	q12h
Complicated urinary tract infections	500 mg IV or IM	q8–12h
Uncomplicated pneumonia; mild skin and skin-structure infections	500 mg–1 gram IV or IM	q8h
Serious gynecologic and intra-abdominal infections	2 grams IV	q8h
Meningitis	2 grams IV	q8h
Very severe life-threatening infections, especially in immunocompromised patients	2 grams IV	q8h
Lung infections caused by *Pseudomonas* spp. in patients with cystic fibrosis with normal renal function*	30–50 mg/kg IV to a maximum of 6 grams per day	q8h
Neonates (0–4 weeks)	30 mg/kg IV	q12h
Infants and Children (1 month–12 years)	30–50 mg/kg IV to a maximum of 6 grams per day†	q8h

* Although clinical improvement has been shown, bacteriologic cures cannot be expected in patients with chronic respiratory disease and cystic fibrosis.

† The higher dose should be reserved for immunocompromised pediatric patients or pediatric patients with cystic fibrosis or meningitis.

FORTAZ may be used alone in cases of confirmed or suspected sepsis. Ceftazidime has been used successfully in clinical trials as empiric therapy in cases where various concomitant therapies with other antibiotics have been used.

FORTAZ may also be used concomitantly with other antibiotics, such as aminoglycosides, vancomycin, and clindamycin; in severe and life-threatening infections; and in the immunocompromised patient. When such concomitant treatment is appropriate, prescribing information in the labeling for the other antibiotics should be followed. The dose depends on the severity of the infection and the patient's condition.

CONTRAINDICATIONS

FORTAZ is contraindicated in patients who have shown hypersensitivity to ceftazidime or the cephalosporin group of antibiotics.

WARNINGS

BEFORE THERAPY WITH FORTAZ IS INSTITUTED, CAREFUL INQUIRY SHOULD BE MADE TO DETERMINE WHETHER THE PATIENT HAS HAD PREVIOUS HYPERSENSITIVITY REACTIONS TO CEFTAZIDIME, CEPHALOSPORINS, PENICILLINS, OR OTHER DRUGS. IF THIS PRODUCT IS TO BE GIVEN TO PENICILLIN-SENSITIVE PATIENTS, CAUTION SHOULD BE EXERCISED BECAUSE CROSS-HYPERSENSITIVITY AMONG BETA-LACTAM ANTIBIOTICS HAS BEEN CLEARLY DOCUMENTED AND MAY OCCUR IN UP TO 10% OF PATIENTS WITH A HISTORY OF PENICILLIN ALLERGY. IF AN ALLERGIC REACTION TO FORTAZ OCCURS, DISCONTINUE THE DRUG. SERIOUS ACUTE HYPERSENSITIVITY REACTIONS MAY REQUIRE TREATMENT WITH EPINEPHRINE AND OTHER EMERGENCY MEASURES, INCLUDING OXYGEN, IV FLUIDS, IV ANTIHISTAMINES, CORTICOSTEROIDS, PRESSOR AMINES, AND AIRWAY MANAGEMENT, AS CLINICALLY INDICATED.

Pseudomembranous colitis has been reported with nearly all antibacterial agents, including ceftazidime, and may range in severity from mild to life threatening. Therefore, it is important to consider this diagnosis in patients who present with diarrhea subsequent to the administration of antibacterial agents.

Treatment with antibacterial agents alters the normal flora of the colon and may permit overgrowth of clostridia. Studies indicate that a toxin produced by *Clostridium difficile* is one primary cause of "antibiotic-associated colitis."

After the diagnosis of pseudomembranous colitis has been established, appropriate therapeutic measures should be initiated. Mild cases of pseudomembranous colitis usually respond to drug discontinuation alone. In moderate to severe cases, consideration should be given to management with fluids and electrolytes, protein supplementation, and treatment with an antibacterial drug clinically effective against *Clostridium difficile* colitis.

Elevated levels of ceftazidime in patients with renal insufficiency can lead to seizures, encephalopathy, asterixis, neuromuscular excitability, and myoclonia (see PRECAUTIONS).

PRECAUTIONS

General: High and prolonged serum ceftazidime concentrations can occur from usual dosages in patients with transient or persistent reduction of urinary output because of renal insufficiency. The total daily dosage should be reduced when ceftazidime is administered to patients with renal insufficiency (see DOSAGE AND ADMINISTRATION). Elevated levels of ceftazidime in these patients can lead to seizures, encephalopathy, asterixis, neuromuscular excitability, and myoclonia. Continued dosage should be determined by degree of renal impairment, severity of infection, and susceptibility of the causative organisms.

As with other antibiotics, prolonged use of FORTAZ may result in overgrowth of nonsusceptible organisms. Repeated evaluation of the patient's condition is essential. If superinfection occurs during therapy, appropriate measures should be taken.

Inducible type I beta-lactamase resistance has been noted with some organisms (e.g., *Enterobacter* spp., *Pseudomonas* spp., and *Serratia* spp.). As with other extended-spectrum beta-lactam antibiotics, resistance can develop during therapy, leading to clinical failure in some cases. When treating infections caused by these organisms, periodic susceptibility testing should be performed when clinically appropriate. If patients fail to respond to monotherapy, an aminoglycoside or similar agent should be considered.

Cephalosporins may be associated with a fall in prothrombin activity. Those at risk include patients with renal and hepatic impairment, or poor nutritional state, as well as patients receiving a protracted course of antimicrobial therapy. Prothrombin time should be monitored in patients at risk and exogenous vitamin K administered as indicated.

FORTAZ should be prescribed with caution in individuals with a history of gastrointestinal disease, particularly colitis.

Distal necrosis can occur after inadvertent intra-arterial administration of ceftazidime.

Drug Interactions: Nephrotoxicity has been reported following concomitant administration of cephalosporins with aminoglycoside antibiotics or potent diuretics such as furosemide. Renal function should be carefully monitored, especially if higher dosages of the aminoglycosides are to be administered or if therapy is prolonged, because of the potential nephrotoxicity and ototoxicity of aminoglycosidic antibiotics. Nephrotoxicity and ototoxicity were not noted when ceftazidime was given alone in clinical trials.

Chloramphenicol has been shown to be antagonistic to beta-lactam antibiotics, including ceftazidime, based on *in vitro* studies and time kill curves with enteric gram-negative bacilli. Due to the possibility of antagonism *in vivo,* particularly when bactericidal activity is desired, this drug combination should be avoided.

Drug/Laboratory Test Interactions: The administration of ceftazidime may result in a false-positive reaction for glucose in the urine using CLINITEST® tablets, Benedict's solution, or Fehling's solution. It is recommended that glucose tests based on enzymatic glucose oxidase reactions (such as CLINISTIX® or TES-TAPE®) be used.

Carcinogenesis, Mutagenesis, Impairment of Fertility: Long-term studies in animals have not been performed to evaluate carcinogenic potential. However, a mouse Micronucleus test and an Ames test were both negative for mutagenic effects.

Pregnancy: ***Teratogenic Effects:*** Pregnancy Category B. Reproduction studies have been performed in mice and rats at doses up to 40 times the human dose and have revealed no evidence of impaired fertility or harm to the fetus due to FORTAZ. There are, however, no adequate and well-controlled studies in pregnant women. Because animal reproduction studies are not always predictive of human response, this drug should be used during pregnancy only if clearly needed.

Continued on next page

This product information is based on labeling in effect on June 23, 2000. For further information, contact via direct mail, phone, or web site. Medical Information, Glaxo Wellcome Inc., PO Box 13398, Research Triangle Park, NC 27709. Healthcare Professionals (Medical Information): 800-334-0089. Patients (Customer Response Center): 1-888-825-5249. Glaxo Wellcome Corporate Web Site: www.glaxowellcome.com

Fortaz—Cont.

Nursing Mothers: Ceftazidime is excreted in human milk in low concentrations. Caution should be exercised when FORTAZ is administered to a nursing woman.
Pediatric Use: (see DOSAGE AND ADMINISTRATION).

ADVERSE REACTIONS

Ceftazidime is generally well tolerated. The incidence of adverse reactions associated with the administration of ceftazidime was low in clinical trials. The most common were local reactions following IV injection and allergic and gastrointestinal reactions. Other adverse reactions were encountered infrequently. No disulfiramlike reactions were reported.
The following adverse effects from clinical trials were considered to be either related to ceftazidime therapy or were of uncertain etiology:
Local Effects, reported in fewer than 2% of patients, were phlebitis and inflammation at the site of injection (1 in 69 patients).
Hypersensitivity Reactions, reported in 2% of patients, were pruritus, rash, and fever. Immediate reactions, generally manifested by rash and/or pruritus, occurred in 1 in 285 patients. Toxic epidermal necrolysis, Stevens-Johnson syndrome, and erythema multiforme have also been reported with cephalosporin antibiotics, including ceftazidime. Angioedema and anaphylaxis (bronchospasm and/or hypotension) have been reported very rarely.
Gastrointestinal Symptoms, reported in fewer than 2% of patients, were diarrhea (1 in 78), nausea (1 in 156), vomiting (1 in 500), and abdominal pain (1 in 416). The onset of pseudomembranous colitis symptoms may occur during or after treatment (see WARNINGS).
Central Nervous System Reactions (fewer than 1%) included headache, dizziness, and paresthesia. Seizures have been reported with several cephalosporins, including ceftazidime. In addition, encephalopathy, asterixis, neuromuscular excitability, and myoclonia have been reported in renally impaired patients treated with unadjusted dosing regimens of ceftazidime (see PRECAUTIONS: General).
Less Frequent Adverse Events (fewer than 1%) were candidiasis (including oral thrush) and vaginitis.
Hematologic: Rare cases of hemolytic anemia have been reported.
Laboratory Test Changes noted during FORTAZ clinical trials were transient and included: eosinophilia (1 in 13), positive Coombs' test without hemolysis (1 in 23), thrombocytosis (1 in 45), and slight elevations in one or more of the hepatic enzymes, aspartate aminotransferase (AST, SGOT) (1 in 16), alanine aminotransferase (ALT, SGPT) (1 in 15), LDH (1 in 18), GGT (1 in 19), and alkaline phosphatase (1 in 23). As with some other cephalosporins, transient elevations of blood urea, blood urea nitrogen, and/or serum creatinine were observed occasionally. Transient leukopenia, neutropenia, agranulocytosis, thrombocytopenia, and lymphocytosis were seen very rarely.
Observed During Clinical Practice: In addition to the adverse events reported from clinical trials, the following events have been identified during post-approval use of FORTAZ. Because they are reported voluntarily from a population of unknown size, estimates of frequency cannot be made. These events have been chosen for inclusion due to a combination of their seriousness, frequency of reporting, or potential causal connection to FORTAZ.
General: Anaphylactic or anaphylactoid reactions, which, in rare instances, were severe (e.g., cardiopulmonary arrest), including laryngeal edema, stridor, and urticaria; pain at injection site.
Hepatobiliary Tract and Pancreas: Hyperbilirubinemia.
Renal and Genitourinary: Renal impairment.
Cephalosporin-Class Adverse Reactions: In addition to the adverse reactions listed above that have been observed in patients treated with ceftazidime, the following adverse reactions and altered laboratory tests have been reported for cephalosporin-class antibiotics:
Adverse Reactions: Colitis, toxic nephropathy, hepatic dysfunction including cholestasis, aplastic anemia, hemorrhage.
Altered Laboratory Tests: Prolonged prothrombin time, false-positive test for urinary glucose, pancytopenia.

OVERDOSAGE

Ceftazidime overdosage has occurred in patients with renal failure. Reactions have included seizure activity, encephalopathy, asterixis, neuromuscular excitability, and coma. Patients who receive an acute overdosage should be carefully observed and given supportive treatment. In the presence of renal insufficiency, hemodialysis or peritoneal dialysis may aid in the removal of ceftazidime from the body.

DOSAGE AND ADMINISTRATION

Dosage: The usual adult dosage is 1 gram administered intravenously or intramuscularly every 8 to 12 hours. The dosage and route should be determined by the susceptibility of the causative organisms, the severity of infection, and the condition and renal function of the patient.
The guidelines for dosage of FORTAZ are listed in Table 3. The following dosage schedule is recommended.
[See table 3 at top of previous page]
Impaired Hepatic Function: No adjustment in dosage is required for patients with hepatic dysfunction.
Impaired Renal Function: Ceftazidime is excreted by the kidneys, almost exclusively by glomerular filtration. Therefore, in patients with impaired renal function (glomerular filtration rate [GFR] <50 mL/min), it is recommended that the dosage of ceftazidime be reduced to compensate for its slower excretion. In patients with suspected renal insufficiency, an initial loading dose of 1 gram of FORTAZ may be given. An estimate of GFR should be made to determine the appropriate maintenance dosage. The recommended dosage is presented in Table 4.

Table 4: Recommended Maintenance Dosages of FORTAZ in Renal Insufficiency
NOTE: IF THE DOSE RECOMMENDED IN TABLE 3 ABOVE IS LOWER THAN THAT RECOMMENDED FOR PATIENTS WITH RENAL INSUFFICIENCY AS OUTLINED IN TABLE 4, THE LOWER DOSE SHOULD BE USED.

Creatinine Clearance (mL/min)	Recommended Unit Dose of FORTAZ	Frequency of Dosing
50–31	1 gram	q12h
30–16	1 gram	q24h
15–6	500 mg	q24h
<5	500 mg	q48h

When only serum creatinine is available, the following formula (Cockcroft's equation)[4] may be used to estimate creatinine clearance. The serum creatinine should represent a steady state of renal function:
Males:

$$\text{Creatinine clearance (mL/min)} = \frac{\text{Weight (kg)} \times (140 - \text{age})}{72 \times \text{serum creatinine (mg/dL)}}$$

Females: 0.85 × male value
In patients with severe infections who would normally receive 6 grams of FORTAZ daily were it not for renal insufficiency, the unit dose given in the table above may be increased by 50% or the dosing frequency may be increased appropriately. Further dosing should be determined by therapeutic monitoring, severity of the infection, and susceptibility of the causative organism.
In pediatric patients as for adults, the creatinine clearance should be adjusted for body surface area or lean body mass, and the dosing frequency should be reduced in cases of renal insufficiency.
In patients undergoing hemodialysis, a loading dose of 1 gram is recommended, followed by 1 gram after each hemodialysis period.
FORTAZ can also be used in patients undergoing intraperitoneal dialysis and continuous ambulatory peritoneal dialysis. In such patients, a loading dose of 1 gram of FORTAZ may be given, followed by 500 mg every 24 hours. In addition to IV use, FORTAZ can be incorporated in the dialysis fluid at a concentration of 250 mg for 2 L of dialysis fluid.
Note: Generally FORTAZ should be continued for 2 days after the signs and symptoms of infection have disappeared, but in complicated infections longer therapy may be required.
Administration: FORTAZ may be given intravenously or by deep IM injection into a large muscle mass such as the upper outer quadrant of the gluteus maximus or lateral part of the thigh. Intra-arterial administration should be avoided (see PRECAUTIONS).
Intramuscular Administration: For IM administration, FORTAZ should be constituted with one of the following diluents: Sterile Water for Injection, Bacteriostatic Water for Injection, or 0.5% or 1% Lidocaine Hydrochloride Injection. Refer to Table 5.
Intravenous Administration: The IV route is preferable for patients with bacterial septicemia, bacterial meningitis, peritonitis, or other severe or life-threatening infections, or for patients who may be poor risks because of lowered resistance resulting from such debilitating conditions as malnutrition, trauma, surgery, diabetes, heart failure, or malignancy, particularly if shock is present or pending.
For direct intermittent IV administration, constitute FORTAZ as directed in Table 5 with Sterile Water for Injection. Slowly inject directly into the vein over a period of 3 to 5 minutes or give through the tubing of an administration set while the patient is also receiving one of the compatible IV fluids (see COMPATIBILITY AND STABILITY).
For IV infusion, constitute the 1- or 2-gram infusion pack with 100 mL of Sterile Water for Injection or one of the compatible IV fluids listed under the COMPATIBILITY AND STABILITY section. Alternatively, constitute the 500-mg, 1-gram, or 2-gram vial and add an appropriate quantity of the resulting solution to an IV container with one of the compatible IV fluids.
Intermittent IV infusion with a Y-type administration set can be accomplished with compatible solutions. However, during infusion of a solution containing ceftazidime, it is desirable to discontinue the other solution.
ADD-Vantage vials are to be constituted only with 50 or 100 mL of 5% Dextrose Injection, 0.9% Sodium Chloride Injection, or 0.45% Sodium Chloride Injection in Abbott ADD-Vantage flexible diluent containers (see Instructions for Constitution section of the product package insert). ADD-Vantage vials that have been joined to Abbott ADD-Vantage diluent containers and activated to dissolve the drug are stable for 24 hours at room temperature or for 7 days under refrigeration. Joined vials that have not been activated may be used within a 14-day period; this period corresponds to that for use of Abbott ADD-Vantage containers following removal of the outer packaging (overwrap).
Freezing solutions of FORTAZ in the ADD-Vantage system is not recommended.
[See table 5 below]
All vials of FORTAZ as supplied are under reduced pressure. When FORTAZ is dissolved, carbon dioxide is released and a positive pressure develops. For ease of use please follow the recommended techniques of constitution described on the detachable Instructions for Constitution section of the product package insert.
Solutions of FORTAZ, like those of most beta-lactam antibiotics, should not be added to solutions of aminoglycoside antibiotics because of potential interaction.
However, if concurrent therapy with FORTAZ and an aminoglycoside is indicated, each of these antibiotics can be administered separately to the same patient.
Directions for Use of FORTAZ Frozen in GALAXY® Plastic Containers: FORTAZ supplied as a frozen, sterile, iso-osmotic, nonpyrogenic solution in plastic containers is to be administered after thawing either as a continuous or intermittent IV infusion. The thawed solution is stable for 24 hours at room temperature or for 7 days if stored under refrigeration. **Do not Refreeze.**
Thaw container at room temperature (25°C) or under refrigeration (5°C). Do not force thaw by immersion in water baths or by microwave irradiation. Components of the solution may precipitate in the frozen state and will dissolve upon reaching room temperature with little or no agitation. Potency is not affected. Mix after solution has reached room temperature. Check for minute leaks by squeezing bag firmly. Discard bag if leaks are found as sterility may be impaired. Do not add supplementary medication. Do not use unless solution is clear and seal is intact.
Use sterile equipment.
Caution: Do not use plastic containers in series connections. Such use could result in air embolism due to residual air being drawn from the primary container before administration of the fluid from the secondary container is complete.
Preparation for Administration:
1. Suspend container from eyelet support.
2. Remove protector from outlet port at bottom of container.
3. Attach administration set. Refer to complete directions accompanying set.

COMPATIBILITY AND STABILITY

Intramuscular: FORTAZ, when constituted as directed with Sterile Water for Injection, Bacteriostatic Water for Injection, or 0.5% or 1% Lidocaine Hydrochloride Injection, maintains satisfactory potency for 24 hours at room temperature or for 7 days under refrigeration. Solutions in Sterile Water for Injection that are frozen immediately after constitution in the original container are stable for 3 months when stored at −20°C. Once thawed, solutions should not be refrozen. Thawed solutions may be stored for up to 8 hours at room temperature or for 4 days in a refrigerator.
Intravenous: FORTAZ, when constituted as directed with Sterile Water for Injection, maintains satisfactory potency for 24 hours at room temperature or for 7 days under refrigeration. Solutions in Sterile Water for Injection in the infu-

Table 5: Preparation of Solutions of FORTAZ

Size	Amount of Diluent to be Added (mL)	Approximate Available Volume (mL)	Approximate Ceftazidime Concentration (mg/mL)
Intramuscular			
500-mg vial	1.5	1.8	280
1-gram vial	3.0	3.6	280
Intravenous			
500-mg vial	5.0	5.3	100
1-gram vial	10.0	10.6	100
2-gram vial	10.0	11.5	170
Infusion pack			
1-gram vial	100 *	100	10
2-gram vial	100 *	100	20
Pharmacy bulk package			
6-gram vial	26	30	200

* **Note:** Addition should be in two stages (see Instructions for Constitution accompanying the product package insert).

sion vial or in 0.9% Sodium Chloride Injection in VIAFLEX® small-volume containers that are frozen immediately after constitution are stable for 6 months when stored at −20°C. Do not force thaw by immersion in water baths or by microwave irradiation. Once thawed, solutions should not be refrozen. Thawed solutions may be stored for up to 24 hours at room temperature or for 7 days in a refrigerator. More concentrated solutions in Sterile Water for Injection in the original container that are frozen immediately after constitution are stable for 3 months when stored at −20°C. Once thawed, solutions should not be refrozen. Thawed solutions may be stored for up to 8 hours at room temperature or for 4 days in a refrigerator.

FORTAZ is compatible with the more commonly used IV infusion fluids. Solutions at concentrations between 1 and 40 mg/mL in 0.9% Sodium Chloride Injection; 1/6 M Sodium Lactate Injection; 5% Dextrose Injection; 5% Dextrose and 0.225% Sodium Chloride Injection; 5% Dextrose and 0.45% Sodium Chloride Injection; 5% Dextrose and 0.9% Sodium Chloride Injection; 10% Dextrose Injection; Ringer's Injection, USP; Lactated Ringer's Injection, USP; 10% Invert Sugar in Water for Injection; and NORMOSOL®-M in 5% Dextrose Injection may be stored for up to 24 hours at room temperature or for 7 days if refrigerated.

The 1- and 2-g FORTAZ ADD-Vantage vials, when diluted in 50 or 100 mL of 5% Dextrose Injection, 0.9% Sodium Chloride Injection, or 0.45% Sodium Chloride Injection, may be stored for up to 24 hours at room temperature or for 7 days under refrigeration.

FORTAZ is less stable in Sodium Bicarbonate Injection than in other IV fluids. It is not recommended as a diluent. Solutions of FORTAZ in 5% Dextrose Injection and 0.9% Sodium Chloride Injection are stable for at least 6 hours at room temperature in plastic tubing, drip chambers, and volume control devices of common IV infusion sets.

Ceftazidime at a concentration of 4 mg/mL has been found compatible for 24 hours at room temperature or for 7 days under refrigeration in 0.9% Sodium Chloride Injection or 5% Dextrose Injection when admixed with: cefuroxime sodium (ZINACEF®) 3 mg/mL; heparin 10 or 50 U/mL; or potassium chloride 10 or 40 mEq/L.

Vancomycin solution exhibits a physical incompatibility when mixed with a number of drugs, including ceftazidime. The likelihood of precipitation with ceftazidime is dependent on the concentrations of vancomycin and ceftazidime present. It is therefore recommended, when both drugs are to be administered by intermittent IV infusion, that they be given separately, flushing the IV lines (with one of the compatible IV fluids) between the administration of these two agents.

Note: Parenteral drug products should be inspected visually for particulate matter before administration whenever solution and container permit.

As with other cephalosporins, FORTAZ powder as well as solutions tend to darken, depending on storage conditions; within the stated recommendations, however, product potency is not adversely affected.

HOW SUPPLIED

FORTAZ in the dry state should be stored between 15° and 30°C (59° and 86°F) and protected from light. FORTAZ is a dry, white to off-white powder supplied in vials and infusion packs as follows:

NDC 0173-0377-31 500-mg* Vial (Tray of 25)
NDC 0173-0378-35 1-g* Vial (Tray of 25)
NDC 0173-0379-34 2-g* Vial (Tray of 10)
NDC 0173-0380-32 1-g* Infusion Pack (Tray of 10)
NDC 0173-0381-32 2-g* Infusion Pack (Tray of 10)
NDC 0173-0382-37 6-g* Pharmacy Bulk Package (Tray of 6)
NDC 0173-0434-00 1-g ADD-Vantage® Vial (Tray of 25)
NDC 0173-0435-00 2-g ADD-Vantage® Vial (Tray of 10)
(The above ADD-Vantage vials are to be used only with Abbott ADD-Vantage diluent containers.)

FORTAZ frozen as a premixed solution of ceftazidime sodium should not be stored above −20° C. FORTAZ is supplied frozen in 50-mL, single-dose, plastic containers as follows:

NDC 0173-0412-00 1-g* Plastic Container (Carton of 24)
NDC 0173-0413-00 2-g* Plastic Container (Carton of 24)
*Equivalent to anhydrous ceftazidime.

REFERENCES

1. Bauer AW, Kirby WMM, Sherris JC, Turck M. Antibiotic susceptibility testing by a standardized single disk method. *Am J Clin Pathol.* 1966;45:493–496.
2. National Committee for Clinical Laboratory Standards. *Approved Standard: Performance Standards for Antimicrobial Disc Susceptibility Tests.* (M2-A3). December 1984.
3. Certification procedure for antibiotic sensitivity discs (21 CFR 460.1). *Federal Register.* May 30, 1974;39:19182-19184.
4. Cockcroft DW, Gault MH. Prediction of creatinine clearance from serum creatinine. *Nephron.* 1976;16:31-41.

FORTAZ® (ceftazidime for injection):
Glaxo Wellcome Inc., Research Triangle Park, NC 27709
FORTAZ® (ceftazidime sodium injection):
Manufactured for Glaxo Wellcome Inc.
Research Triangle Park, NC 27709
by Baxter Healthcare Corporation, Deerfield, IL 60015
FORTAZ and ZINACEF are registered trademarks of Glaxo Wellcome.
ADD-Vantage is a registered trademark of Abbott Laboratories.
CLINITEST and CLINISTIX are registered trademarks of Ames Division, Miles Laboratories, Inc.
TES-TAPE is a registered trademark of Eli Lilly and Company.
GALAXY and VIAFLEX are registered trademarks of Baxter International Inc.
US Patent Nos. 4,329,453 and 4,582,830
June 1999/RL-722

Shown in Product Identification Guide, page 315

IMITREX® ℞
[*ĭm ′-ĭ-trĕx ″*]
(sumatriptan succinate)
Injection

For Subcutaneous Use Only.

DESCRIPTION

IMITREX (sumatriptan succinate) Injection is a selective 5-hydroxytryptamine$_1$ receptor subtype agonist. Sumatriptan succinate is chemically designated as 3-[2-(dimethylamino)ethyl]-N-methyl-indole-5-methanesulfonamide succinate (1:1).

The empirical formula is $C_{14}H_{21}N_3O_2S{\bullet}C_4H_6O_4$, representing a molecular weight of 413.5.

Sumatriptan succinate is a white to off-white powder that is readily soluble in water and in saline.

IMITREX Injection is a clear, colorless to pale yellow, sterile, nonpyrogenic solution for subcutaneous injection. Each 0.5 mL of solution contains 6 mg of sumatriptan (base) as the succinate salt and 3.5 mg of sodium chloride, USP in water for injection, USP. The pH range of the solution is approximately 4.2 to 5.3. The osmolality of the injection is 291 mOsmol.

CLINICAL PHARMACOLOGY

Mechanism of Action: Sumatriptan has been demonstrated to be a selective agonist for a vascular 5-hydroxytryptamine$_1$ receptor subtype (probably a member of the 5-HT$_{1D}$ family) with no significant affinity (as measured using standard radioligand binding assays) or pharmacological activity at 5-HT$_2$, 5-HT$_3$ receptor subtypes or at alpha$_1$-, alpha$_2$-, or beta-adrenergic; dopamine$_1$; dopamine$_2$; muscarinic; or benzodiazepine receptors.

The vascular 5-HT$_1$ receptor subtype to which sumatriptan binds selectively, and through which it presumably exerts its antimigrainous effect, has been shown to be present on cranial arteries in both dog and primate, on the human basilar artery, and in the vasculature of the isolated dura mater of humans. In these tissues, sumatriptan activates this receptor to cause vasoconstriction, an action in humans correlating with the relief of migraine and cluster headache. In the anesthetized dog, sumatriptan selectively reduces the carotid arterial blood flow with little or no effect on arterial blood pressure or total peripheral resistance. In the cat, sumatriptan selectively constricts the carotid arteriovenous anastomoses while having little effect on blood flow or resistance in cerebral or extracerebral tissues.

Corneal Opacities: Dogs receiving oral sumatriptan developed corneal opacities and defects in the corneal epithelium. Corneal opacities were seen at the lowest dosage tested, 2 mg/kg per day, and were present after 1 month of treatment. Defects in the corneal epithelium were noted in a 60-week study. Earlier examinations for these toxicities were not conducted and no-effect doses were not established; however, the relative exposure at the lowest dose tested was approximately 5 times the human exposure after a 100-mg oral dose or 3 times the human exposure after a 6-mg subcutaneous dose.

Melanin Binding: In rats with a single subcutaneous dose (0.5 mg/kg) of radiolabeled sumatriptan, the elimination half-life of radioactivity from the eye was 15 days, suggesting that sumatriptan and its metabolites bind to the melanin of the eye. The clinical significance of this binding is unknown.

Pharmacokinetics: Pharmacokinetic parameters following a 6-mg subcutaneous injection into the deltoid area of the arm in 9 males (*mean age, 33 years; mean weight, 77 kg*) were systemic clearance: 1194 ± 149 mL/min (*mean ± S.D.*), distribution half-life: 15 ± 2 minutes, terminal half-life: 115 ± 19 minutes, and volume of distribution central compartment: 50 ± 8 liters. Of this dose, 22% ± 4% was excreted in the urine as unchanged sumatriptan and 38% ± 7% as the indole acetic acid metabolite.

After a single 6-mg subcutaneous manual injection into the deltoid area of the arm in 18 healthy males (*age, 24 ± 6 years; weight, 70 kg*), the maximum serum concentration (C_{max}) was (*mean ± standard deviation*) 74 ± 15 ng/mL and the time to peak concentration (t_{max}) was 12 minutes after injection (*range, 5 to 20 minutes*). In this study, the same dose injected subcutaneously in the thigh gave a C_{max} of 61 ± 15 ng/mL by manual injection versus 52 ± 15 ng/mL by autoinjector techniques. The t_{max} or amount absorbed was not significantly altered by either the site or technique of injection.

The bioavailability of sumatriptan via subcutaneous site injection to 18 healthy male subjects was 97% ± 16% of that obtained following intravenous injection. Protein binding, determined by equilibrium dialysis over the concentration range of 10 to 1000 ng/mL, is low, approximately 14% to 21%. The effect of sumatriptan on the protein binding of other drugs has not been evaluated.

Special Populations: ***Renal Impairment:*** The effect of renal impairment on the pharmacokinetics of sumatriptan has not been examined, but little clinical effect would be expected as sumatriptan is largely metabolized to an inactive substance.

Hepatic Impairment: The effect of hepatic disease on the pharmacokinetics of subcutaneously and orally administered sumatriptan has been evaluated. There were no statistically significant differences in the pharmacokinetics of subcutaneously administered sumatriptan in hepatically impaired patients compared to healthy controls. However, the liver plays an important role in the presystemic clearance of orally administered sumatriptan. Accordingly, the bioavailability of sumatriptan following oral administration may be markedly increased in patients with liver disease. In 1 small study of hepatically impaired patients (n = 8) matched for sex, age, and weight with healthy subjects, the hepatically impaired patients had an approximately 70% increase in AUC and C_{max} and a t_{max} 40 minutes earlier compared to the healthy subjects.

Age: The pharmacokinetics of sumatriptan in the elderly (*mean age, 72 years, 2 males and 4 females*) and in patients with migraine (*mean age, 38 years, 25 male and 155 females*) were similar to that in healthy male subjects (*mean age, 30 years*) (see PRECAUTIONS: Geriatric Use).

Race: The systemic clearance and C_{max} of sumatriptan were similar in black (n = 34) and Caucasian (n = 38) healthy male subjects.

Drug Interactions: ***MAO Inhibitors:*** In vitro studies with human microsomes suggest that sumatriptan is metabolized by monoamine oxidase (MAO), predominantly the A isoenzyme. In a study of 14 healthy females, pretreatment with MAO-A inhibitor decreased the clearance of sumatriptan. Under the conditions of this experiment, the result was a 2-fold increase in the area under the sumatriptan plasma concentration × time curve (AUC), corresponding to a 40% increase in elimination half-life. No significant effect was seen with an MAO-B inhibitor.

Pharmacodynamics:

Typical Physiologic Responses:

Blood Pressure: (see WARNINGS)

Peripheral (small) Arteries: In healthy volunteers (n = 18), a study evaluating the effects of sumatriptan on peripheral (small vessel) arterial reactivity failed to detect a clinically significant increase in peripheral resistance.

Heart Rate: Transient increases in blood pressure observed in some patients in clinical studies carried out during sumatriptan's development as a treatment for migraine were not accompanied by any clinically significant changes in heart rate.

Respiratory Rate: Experience gained during the clinical development of sumatriptan as a treatment for migraine failed to detect an effect of the drug on respiratory rate.

Clinical Studies: ***Migraine:*** In US controlled clinical trials enrolling more than 1000 patients during migraine attacks who were experiencing moderate or severe pain and 1 or more of the symptoms enumerated in Table 2 below, onset of relief began as early as 10 minutes following a 6-mg IMITREX Injection. Smaller doses of sumatriptan may also prove effective, although the proportion of patients obtaining adequate relief is decreased and the latency to that relief is greater.

In 1 well-controlled study where placebo (n = 62) was compared to 6 different doses of IMITREX Injection (n = 30 each group) in a single-attack, parallel-group design, the dose response relationship was found to be as shown in the following Table 1.

[See table 1 at top of next page]

In 2 US well-controlled clinical trials in 1104 migraine patients with moderate and severe migraine pain, the onset of relief was rapid (less than 10 minutes). Headache relief, as evidenced by a reduction in pain from severe or moderately severe to mild or no headache, was achieved in 70% of the patients within 1 hour of a single 6-mg subcutaneous dose of IMITREX Injection. Headache relief was achieved in approximately 82% of patients within 2 hours, and 65% of all patients were pain free within 2 hours.

The following table shows the 1- and 2-hour efficacy results.

[See table 2 on next page]

IMITREX Injection also relieved photophobia, phonophobia (sound sensitivity), nausea, and vomiting associated with migraine attacks. Similar efficacy was seen when patients self-administered IMITREX Injection using an autoinjector. The efficacy of IMITREX Injection is unaffected by whether or not migraine is associated with aura, duration of attack, gender or age of the patient, or concomitant use of common migraine prophylactic drugs (e.g., beta-blockers).

Cluster Headache: The efficacy of IMITREX Injection in the acute treatment of cluster headache was demonstrated in 2 randomized, double-blind, placebo-controlled, 2-period crossover trials. Patients age 21 to 65 were enrolled and were instructed to treat a moderate to very severe headache within 10 minutes of onset. Headache relief was defined as a reduction in headache severity to mild or no pain. In both

Continued on next page

This product information is based on labeling in effect on June 23, 2000. For further information, contact via direct mail, phone, or web site. Medical Information, Glaxo Wellcome Inc., PO Box 13398, Research Triangle Park, NC 27709. Healthcare Professionals (Medical Information): 800-334-0089. Patients (Customer Response Center): 1-888-825-5249. Glaxo Wellcome Corporate Web Site: www.glaxowellcome.com

Imitrex Injection—Cont.

trials, the proportion of individuals gaining relief at 10 or 15 minutes was significantly greater among patients receiving 6 mg of IMITREX Injection compared to those who received placebo (see Table 3, below). One study evaluated a 12-mg dose; there was no statistically significant difference in outcome between patients randomized to the 6- and 12-mg doses.
[See table 3 at right]
The Kaplan-Meier (product limit) Survivorship Plot below (Figure 1) provides an estimate of the cumulative probability of a patient with a cluster headache obtaining relief after being treated with either sumatriptan or placebo.

Figure 1: Time to Relief From Time of Injection*

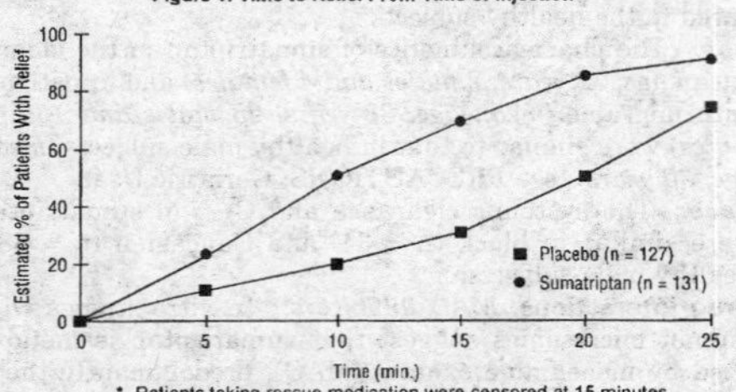

* Patients taking rescue medication were censored at 15 minutes.

The plot was constructed with data from patients who either experienced relief or did not require (request) rescue medication within a period of 2 hours following treatment. As a consequence, the data in the plot are derived from only a subset of the 258 headaches treated (rescue medication was required in 52 of the 127 placebo-treated headaches and 18 of the 131 sumatriptan-treated headaches).
Other data suggest that sumatriptan treatment is not associated with an increase in early recurrence of headache, and that treatment with sumatriptan has little effect on the incidence of latter occurring headaches (i.e., those occurring after 2, but before 18 or 24 hours).

INDICATIONS AND USAGE

IMITREX Injection is indicated for 1) the acute treatment of migraine attacks with or without aura and 2) the acute treatment of cluster headache episodes.
IMITREX Injection is not for use in the management of hemiplegic or basilar migraine (see CONTRAINDICATIONS).

CONTRAINDICATIONS

IMITREX Injection should not be given intravenously because of its potential to cause coronary vasospasm.
IMITREX Injection should not be given to patients with history, symptoms, or signs of ischemic cardiac, cerebrovascular, or peripheral vascular syndromes. In addition, patients with other significant underlying cardiovascular diseases should not receive IMITREX Injection. Ischemic cardiac syndromes include, but are not limited to, angina pectoris of any type (e.g., stable angina of effort and vasospastic forms of angina such as the Prinzmetal variant), all forms of myocardial infarction, and silent myocardial ischemia. Cerebrovascular syndromes include, but are not limited to, strokes of any type as well as transient ischemic attacks. Peripheral vascular disease includes, but is not limited to, ischemic bowel disease (see WARNINGS).
Because IMITREX Injection may increase blood pressure, it should not be given to patients with uncontrolled hypertension.
IMITREX Injection and any ergotamine-containing or ergot-type medication (like dihydroergotamine or methysergide) should not be used within 24 hours of each other, nor should IMITREX Injection and another 5-HT_1 agonist.
IMITREX Injection should not be administered to patients with hemiplegic or basilar migraine.
IMITREX Injection is contraindicated in patients with hypersensitivity to sumatriptan or any of its components.
IMITREX Injection is contraindicated in patients with severe hepatic impairment.

WARNINGS

IMITREX Injection should only be used where a clear diagnosis of migraine or cluster headache has been established. The prescriber should be aware that cluster headache patients often possess one or more predictive risk factors for coronary artery disease (CAD).
Risk of Myocardial Ischemia and/or Infarction and Other Adverse Cardiac Events: Sumatriptan should not be given to patients with documented ischemic or vasospastic CAD (see CONTRAINDICATIONS). It is strongly recommended that sumatriptan not be given to patients in whom unrecognized CAD is predicted by the presence of risk factors (e.g., hypertension, hypercholesterolemia, smoker, obesity, diabetes, strong family history of CAD, female with surgical or physiological menopause, or male over 40 years of age) unless a cardiovascular evaluation provides satisfactory clinical evidence that the patient is reasonably free of coronary artery and ischemic myocardial disease or other significant underlying cardiovascular disease. The sensitivity of cardiac diagnostic procedures to detect cardiovascular disease or predisposition to coronary artery vasospasm is modest, at best. If, during the cardiovascular evaluation, the patient's medical history or electrocardiographic investigations reveal findings indicative of or consistent with coronary artery vasospasm or myocardial ischemia, sumatriptan should not be administered (see CONTRAINDICATIONS).
For patients with risk factors predictive of CAD who are determined to have a satisfactory cardiovascular evaluation, it is strongly recommended that administration of the first dose of sumatriptan injection take place in the setting of a physician's office or similar medically staffed and equipped facility. Because cardiac ischemia can occur in the absence of clinical symptoms, consideration should be given to obtaining on the first occasion of use an electrocardiogram (ECG) during the interval immediately following IMITREX Injection, in these patients with risk factors.
It is recommended that patients who are intermittent long-term users of sumatriptan and who have or acquire risk factors predictive of CAD, as described above, undergo periodic interval cardiovascular evaluation as they continue to use sumatriptan. In considering this recommendation for periodic cardiovascular evaluation, it is noted that patients with cluster headache are predominantly male and over 40 years of age, which are risk factors for CAD.
The systematic approach described above is intended to reduce the likelihood that patients with unrecognized cardiovascular disease will be inadvertently exposed to sumatriptan.
Drug-Associated Cardiac Events and Fatalities: Serious adverse cardiac events, including acute myocardial infarction, life-threatening disturbances of cardiac rhythm, and death have been reported within a few hours following the administration of IMITREX Injection or IMITREX® (sumatriptan succinate) Tablets. Considering the extent of use of sumatriptan in patients with migraine, the incidence of these events is extremely low.
The fact that sumatriptan can cause coronary vasospasm, that some of these events have occurred in patients with no prior cardiac disease history and with documented absence of CAD, and the close proximity of the events to sumatriptan use support the conclusion that some of these cases were caused by the drug. In many cases, however, where there has been known underlying CAD, the relationship is uncertain.
Premarketing Experience With Sumatriptan: Among the more than 1900 patients with migraine who participated in premarketing controlled clinical trials of subcutaneous sumatriptan, there were 8 patients who sustained clinical events during or shortly after receiving sumatriptan that may have reflected coronary artery vasospasm. Six of these 8 patients had ECG changes consistent with transient ischemia, but without accompanying clinical symptoms or signs. Of these 8 patients, 4 had either findings suggestive of CAD or risk factors predictive of CAD prior to study enrollment.
Of 6348 patients with migraine who participated in premarketing controlled and uncontrolled clinical trials of oral sumatriptan, 2 experienced clinical adverse events shortly after receiving oral sumatriptan that may have reflected coronary vasospasm. Neither of these adverse events was associated with a serious clinical outcome.
Among approximately 4000 patients with migraine who participated in premarketing controlled and uncontrolled clinical trials of sumatriptan nasal spray, 1 patient experienced an asymptomatic subendocardial infarction possibly subsequent to a coronary vasospastic event.
Postmarketing Experience With Sumatriptan: Serious cardiovascular events, some resulting in death, have been reported in association with the use of IMITREX Injection or IMITREX Tablets. The uncontrolled nature of postmarketing surveillance, however, makes it impossible to determine definitively the proportion of the reported cases that were actually caused by sumatriptan or to reliably assess causation in individual cases. On clinical grounds, the longer the latency between the administration of IMITREX and the onset of the clinical event, the less likely the association is

Table 1: Dose Response Relationship For Efficacy

IMITREX Dose (mg)	% Patients With Relief* at 10 Minutes	% Patients With Relief* at 30 Minutes	% Patients With Relief* at 1 Hour	% Patients With Relief* at 2 Hours	Adverse Events Incidence (%)
placebo	5	15	24	21	55
1	10	40	43	40	63
2	7	23	57	43	63
3	17	47	57	60	77
4	13	37	50	57	80
6	10	63	73	70	83
8	23	57	80	83	93

*Relief is defined as the reduction of moderate or severe pain to no or mild pain after dosing without use of rescue medication.

Table 2: Efficacy Data From US Phase III Trials

	Study 1		Study 2	
1-Hour Data	Placebo (n = 190)	IMITREX 6 mg (n = 384)	Placebo (n = 180)	IMITREX 6 mg (n = 350)
Patients with pain relief (grade 0/1)	18%	70%*	26%	70%*
Patients with no pain	5%	48%*	13%	49%*
Patients without nausea	48%	73%*	50%	73%*
Patients without photophobia	23%	56%*	25%	58%*
Patients with little or no clinical disability§	34%	76%*	34%	76%*
	Study 1		Study 2	
2-Hour Data	Placebo†	IMITREX 6 mg‡	Placebo†	IMITREX 6 mg‡
Patients with pain relief (grade 0/1)	31%	81%*	39%	82%*
Patients with no pain	11%	63%*	19%	65%*
Patients without nausea	56%	82%*	63%	81%*
Patients without photophobia	31%	72%*	35%	71%*
Patients with little or no clinical disability§	42%	85%*	49%	84%*

* $P<0.05$ versus placebo.
† Includes patients that may have received an additional placebo injection 1 hour after the initial injection.
‡ Includes patients that may have received an additional 6 mg of IMITREX Injection 1 hour after the initial injection.
§ A successful outcome in terms of clinical disability was defined prospectively as ability to work mildly impaired or ability to work and function normally.

Table 3: Efficacy Data From the Pivotal Cluster Headache Studies

	Study 1		Study 2	
	Placebo (n = 39)	IMITREX 6 mg (n = 39)	Placebo (n = 88)	IMITREX 6 mg (n = 92)
Patients with pain relief (no/mild)				
5 minutes postinjection	8%	21%	7%	23%*
10 minutes postinjection	10%	49%*	25%	49%*
15 minutes postinjection	26%	74%*	35%	75%*

* $P<0.05$.
(n = Number of headaches treated.)

to be causative. Accordingly, interest has focused on events beginning within 1 hour of the administration of IMITREX. Cardiac events that have been observed to have onset within 1 hour of sumatriptan administration include: coronary artery vasospasm, transient ischemia, myocardial infarction, ventricular tachycardia and ventricular fibrillation, cardiac arrest, and death.

Some of these events occurred in patients who had no findings of CAD and appear to represent consequences of coronary artery vasospasm. However, among domestic reports of serious cardiac events within 1 hour of sumatriptan administration, the majority had risk factors predictive of CAD and the presence of significant underlying CAD was established in most cases (see CONTRAINDICATIONS).

Drug-Associated Cerebrovascular Events and Fatalities: Cerebral hemorrhage, subarachnoid hemorrhage, stroke, and other cerebrovascular events have been reported in patients treated with oral or subcutaneous sumatriptan, and some have resulted in fatalities. The relationship of sumatriptan to these events is uncertain. In a number of cases, it appears possible that the cerebrovascular events were primary, sumatriptan having been administered in the incorrect belief the symptoms experienced were a consequence of migraine when they were not. As with other acute migraine therapies, before treating headaches in patients not previously diagnosed as migraineurs, and in migraineurs who present with atypical symptoms, care should be taken to exclude other potentially serious neurological conditions. It should also be noted that patients with migraine may be at increased risk of certain cerebrovascular events (e.g., cerebrovascular accident, transient ischemic attack).

Other Vasospasm-Related Events: Sumatriptan may cause vasospastic reactions other than coronary artery vasospasm. Both peripheral vascular ischemia and colonic ischemia with abdominal pain and bloody diarrhea have been reported.

Increase in Blood Pressure: Significant elevation in blood pressure, including hypertensive crisis, has been reported on rare occasions in patients with and without a history of hypertension. Sumatriptan is contraindicated in patients with uncontrolled hypertension (see CONTRAINDICATIONS). Sumatriptan should be administered with caution to patients with controlled hypertension as transient increases in blood pressure and peripheral vascular resistance have been observed in a small proportion of patients.

Concomitant Drug Use: In patients taking MAO-A inhibitors, sumatriptan plasma levels attained after treatment with recommended doses are nearly double those obtained under other conditions. Accordingly, the coadministration of sumatriptan and an MAO-A inhibitor is not generally recommended. If such therapy is clinically warranted, however, suitable dose adjustment and appropriate observation of the patient is advised (see CLINICAL PHARMACOLOGY).

Use in Women of Childbearing Potential: (see PRECAUTIONS).

Hypersensitivity: Hypersensitivity (anaphylaxis/anaphylactoid) reactions have occurred on rare occasions in patients receiving sumatriptan. Such reactions can be life threatening or fatal. In general, hypersensitivity reactions to drugs are more likely to occur in individuals with a history of sensitivity to multiple allergens (see CONTRAINDICATIONS).

PRECAUTIONS

General: Chest, jaw, or neck tightness is relatively common after administration of IMITREX Injection. Chest discomfort and jaw or neck tightness has been reported following use of IMITREX Tablets and has also been reported infrequently following the administration of IMITREX® (sumatriptan) Nasal Spray. Only rarely have these symptoms been associated with ischemic ECG changes. However, because sumatriptan may cause coronary artery vasospasm, patients who experience signs or symptoms suggestive of angina following sumatriptan should be evaluated for the presence of CAD or a predisposition to Prinzmetal variant angina before receiving additional doses of sumatriptan and should be monitored electrocardiographically if dosing is resumed and similar symptoms recur. Similarly, patients who experience other symptoms or signs suggestive of decreased arterial flow, such as ischemic bowel syndrome or Raynaud syndrome, following sumatriptan should be evaluated for atherosclerosis or predisposition to vasospasm (see WARNINGS).

IMITREX should also be administered with caution to patients with diseases that may alter the absorption, metabolism, or excretion of drugs, such as impaired hepatic or renal function.

There have been rare reports of seizure following administration of sumatriptan. Sumatriptan should be used with caution in patients with a history of epilepsy or structural brain lesions that lower their seizure threshold.

Care should be taken to exclude other potentially serious neurologic conditions before treating headache in patients not previously diagnosed with migraine or cluster headache or who experience a headache that is atypical for them. There have been rare reports where patients received sumatriptan for severe headaches that were subsequently shown to have been secondary to an evolving neurologic lesion (see WARNINGS). For a given attack, if a patient does not respond to the first dose of sumatriptan, the diagnosis of migraine or cluster headache should be reconsidered before administration of a second dose.

Binding to Melanin-Containing Tissues: Because sumatriptan binds to melanin, it could accumulate in melanin-rich tissues (such as the eye) over time. This raises the possibility that sumatriptan could cause toxicity in these tissues after extended use. However, no effects on the retina related to treatment with sumatriptan were noted in any of the toxicity studies. Although no systematic monitoring of ophthalmologic function was undertaken in clinical trials, and no specific recommendations for ophthalmologic function was undertaken in clinical trials, and no specific recommendations for ophthalmologic monitoring are offered, prescribers should be aware of the possibility of long-term ophthalmologic effects (see CLINICAL PHARMACOLOGY).

Corneal Opacities: Sumatriptan causes corneal opacities and defects in the corneal epithelium in dogs; this raises the possibility that these changes may occur in humans. While patients were not systematically evaluated for these changes in clinical trials, and no specific recommendations for monitoring are being offered, prescribers should be aware of the possibility of these changes (see CLINICAL PHARMACOLOGY).

Patients who are advised to self-administer IMITREX Injection in medically unsupervised situations should receive instruction on the proper use of the product from the physician or other suitably qualified health care professional prior to doing so for the first time.

Information for Patients: With the autoinjector, the needle penetrates approximately 1/4 of an inch (5 to 6 mm). Since the injection is intended to be given subcutaneously, intramuscular or intravascular delivery should be avoided. Patients should be directed to use injection sites with an adequate skin and subcutaneous thickness to accommodate the length of the needle. See PATIENT INFORMATION at the end of this labeling for the text of the separate leaflet provided for patients.

Laboratory Tests: No specific laboratory tests are recommended for monitoring patients prior to and/or after treatment with sumatriptan.

Drug Interactions: There is no evidence that concomitant use of migraine prophylactic medications has any effect on the efficacy of sumatriptan. In 2 Phase III trials in the US, a retrospective analysis of 282 patients who had been using prophylactic drugs (verapamil n = 63, amitriptyline n = 57, propranolol n = 94, for 45 other drugs n = 123) were compared to those who had not used prophylaxis (n = 452). There were no differences in relief rates at 60 minutes postdose for IMITREX Injection, whether or not prophylactic medications were used.

Ergot-containing drugs have been reported to cause prolonged vasospastic reactions. Because there is a theoretical basis that these effects may be additive, use of ergotamine-containing or ergot-type medications (like dihydroergotamine or methysergide) and sumatriptan within 24 hours of each other should be avoided (see CONTRAINDICATIONS).

MAO-A inhibitors reduce sumatriptan clearance, significantly increasing systemic exposure. Therefore, the use of sumatriptan in patients receiving MAO-A inhibitors is not ordinarily recommended. If the clinical situation warrants the combined use of sumatriptan and an MAOI, the dose of sumatriptan employed should be reduced (see CLINICAL PHARMACOLOGY and WARNINGS).

Selective serotonin reuptake inhibitors (SSRIs) (e.g., fluoxetine, fluvoxamine, paroxetine, sertraline) have been reported, rarely, to cause weakness, hyperreflexia, and incoordination when coadministered with sumatriptan. If concomitant treatment with sumatriptan and an SSRI is clinically warranted, appropriate observation of the patient is advised.

Drug/Laboratory Test Interactions: IMITREX is not known to interfere with commonly employed clinical laboratory tests.

Carcinogenesis, Mutagenesis, Impairment of Fertility: In carcinogenicity studies, rats and mice were given sumatriptan by oral gavage (rats, 104 weeks) or drinking water (mice, 78 weeks). Average exposures achieved in mice receiving the highest dose were approximately 110 times the exposure attained in humans after the maximum recommended single dose of 6 mg. The highest dose to rats was approximately 260 times the maximum single dose of 6 mg on a mg/m^2 basis. There was no evidence of an increase in tumors in either species related to sumatriptan administration.

Sumatriptan was not mutagenic in the presence or absence of metabolic activation when tested in 2 gene mutation assays (the Ames test and the in vitro mammalian Chinese hamster V79/HGPRT assay). In 2 cytogenetics assays (the in vitro human lymphocyte assay and the in vivo rat micronucleus assay) sumatriptan was not associated with clastogenic activity.

A fertility study (Segment I) by the subcutaneous route, during which male and female rats were dosed daily with sumatriptan prior to and throughout the mating period, has shown no evidence of impaired fertility at doses equivalent to approximately 100 times the maximum recommended single human dose of 6 mg on a mg/m^2 basis. However, following oral administration, a treatment-related decrease in fertility, secondary to a decrease in mating, was seen for rats treated with 50 and 500 mg/kg per day. The no-effect dose for this finding was approximately 8 times the maximum recommended single human dose of 6 mg on a mg/m^2 basis. It is not clear whether the problem is associated with the treatment of males or females or both.

Pregnancy: Pregnancy Category C. Sumatriptan has been shown to be embryolethal in rabbits when given daily at a dose approximately equivalent to the maximum recommended single human subcutaneous dose of 6 mg on a mg/m^2 basis. There is no evidence that establishes that sumatriptan is a human teratogen; however, there are no adequate and well-controlled studies in pregnant women. IMITREX Injection should be used during pregnancy only if the potential benefit justifies the potential risk to the fetus. In assessing this information, the following additional findings should be considered.

Embryolethality: When given intravenously to pregnant rabbits daily throughout the period of organogenesis, sumatriptan caused embryolethality at doses at or close to those producing maternal toxicity. The mechanism of the embryolethality is not known. These doses were approximately equivalent to the maximum single human dose of 6 mg on a mg/m^2 basis.

The intravenous administration of sumatriptan to pregnant rats throughout organogenesis at doses that are approximately 20 times a human dose of 6 mg on a mg/m^2 basis, did not cause embryolethality. Additionally, in a study of pregnant rats given subcutaneous sumatriptan daily prior to and throughout pregnancy, there was no evidence of increased embryo/fetal lethality.

Teratogenicity: Term fetuses from Dutch Stride rabbits treated during organogenesis with oral sumatriptan exhibited an increased incidence of cervicothoracic vascular and skeletal abnormalities. The functional significance of these abnormalities is not known. The highest no-effect dose for these effects was 15 mg/kg per day, approximately 50 times the maximum single dose of 6 mg on a mg/m^2 basis.

In a study in rats dosed daily with subcutaneous sumatriptan prior to and throughout pregnancy, there was no evidence of teratogenicity.

To monitor fetal outcomes of pregnant women exposed to IMITREX, Glaxo Wellcome Inc. maintains a Sumatriptan Pregnancy Registry. Physicians are encouraged to register patients by calling (800) 336-2176.

Nursing Mothers: Sumatriptan is excreted in human breast milk. Therefore, caution should be exercised when considering the administration of IMITREX Injection to a nursing woman.

Pediatric Use: Safety and effectiveness of IMITREX Injection in pediatric patients have not been established.

Completed placebo-controlled clinical trials evaluating oral sumatriptan (25 to 100 mg) in pediatric patients aged 12 to 17 years enrolled a total of 701 adolescent migraineurs. These studies did not establish the efficacy of oral sumatriptan compared to placebo in the treatment of migraine in adolescents. Adverse events observed in these clinical trials were similar in nature to those reported in clinical trials in adults. The frequency of all adverse events in these patients appeared to be both dose- and age-dependent, with younger patients reporting events more commonly than older adolescents. Postmarketing experience includes a limited number of reports that describe pediatric patients who have experienced adverse events, some clinically serious, after use of subcutaneous sumatriptan and/or oral sumatriptan. These reports include events similar in nature to those reported rarely in adults. A myocardial infarct has been reported in a 14-year-old male following the use of oral sumatriptan; clinical signs occurred within 1 day of drug administration. Since clinical data to determine the frequency of serious adverse events in pediatric patients who might receive injectable, oral, or intranasal sumatriptan are not presently available, the use of sumatriptan in patients aged younger than 18 years is not recommended.

Geriatric Use: The use of sumatriptan in elderly patients is not recommended because elderly patients are more likely to have decreased hepatic function, they are at higher risk for CAD, and blood pressure increases may be more pronounced in the elderly (see WARNINGS).

ADVERSE REACTIONS

Serious cardiac events, including some that have been fatal, have occurred following the use of IMITREX Injection or Tablets. These events are extremely rare and most have been reported in patients with risk factors predictive of CAD. Events reported have included coronary artery vasospasm, transient myocardial ischemia, myocardial infarction, ventricular tachycardia, and ventricular fibrillation (see CONTRAINDICATIONS, WARNINGS, and PRECAUTIONS).

Significant hypertensive episodes, including hypertensive crises, have been reported on rare occasions in patients with or without a history of hypertension (see WARNINGS).

Among patients in clinical trials of subcutaneous IMITREX Injection (n = 6218), up to 3.5% of patients withdrew for reasons related to adverse events.

Incidence in Controlled Clinical Trials of Migraine Headache: The following Table 4 lists adverse events that occurred in 2 large US, Phase III, placebo-controlled clinical

Continued on next page

This product information is based on labeling in effect on June 23, 2000. For further information, contact via direct mail, phone, or web site. Medical Information, Glaxo Wellcome Inc., PO Box 13398, Research Triangle Park, NC 27709. Healthcare Professionals (Medical Information): 800-334-0089. Patients (Customer Response Center): 1-888-825-5249. Glaxo Wellcome Corporate Web Site: www.glaxowellcome.com

Imitrex Injection—Cont.

trials in migraine patients following either a single dose of IMITREX Injection or placebo. Only events that occurred at a frequency of 1% or more in groups treated with IMITREX Injection and were at least as frequent as in the placebo group are included in Table 4.

[See table 4 below]

The incidence of adverse events in controlled clinical trials was not affected by gender or age of the patients. There were insufficient data to assess the impact of race on the incidence of adverse events.

Incidence in Controlled Trials of Cluster Headache: In the controlled clinical trials assessing sumatriptan's efficacy as a treatment for cluster headache, no new significant adverse events associated with the use of sumatriptan were detected that had not already been identified in association with the drug's use in migraine.

Overall, the frequency of adverse events reported in the studies of cluster headache were generally lower. Exceptions include reports of paresthesia (5% IMITREX, 0% placebo), nausea and vomiting (4% IMITREX, 0% placebo), and bronchospasm (1% IMITREX, 0% placebo).

Other Events Observed in Association With the Administration of IMITREX Injection: In the paragraphs that follow, the frequencies of less commonly reported adverse clinical events are presented. Because the reports include events observed in open and uncontrolled studies, the role of IMITREX Injection in their causation cannot be reliably determined. Furthermore, variability associated with adverse event reporting, the terminology used to describe adverse events, etc., limit the value of the quantitative frequency estimates provided.

Event frequencies are calculated as the number of patients reporting an event divided by the total number of patients (n = 6218) exposed to subcutaneous IMITREX Injection. All reported events are included except those already listed in the previous table, those too general to be informative, and those not reasonably associated with the use of the drug. Events are further classified within body system categories and enumerated in order of decreasing frequency using the following definitions: frequent adverse events are defined as those occurring in at least 1/100 patients, infrequent adverse events are those occurring in 1/100 to 1/1000 patients, and rare adverse events are those occurring in fewer than 1/1000 patients.

Cardiovascular: Infrequent were hypertension, hypotension, bradycardia, tachycardia, palpitations, pulsating sensations, various transient ECG changes (nonspecific ST or T wave changes, prolongation of PR or QTc intervals, sinus arrhythmia, nonsustained ventricular premature beats, isolated junctional ectopic beats, atrial ectopic beats, delayed activation of the right ventricle), and syncope. Rare were pallor, arrhythmia, abnormal pulse, vasodilatation, and Raynaud syndrome.

Endocrine and Metabolic: Infrequent was thirst. Rare were polydipsia and dehydration.

Eye: Infrequent was irritation of the eye.

Gastrointestinal: Infrequent were gastroesophageal reflux, diarrhea, and disturbances of liver function tests. Rare were peptic ulcer, retching, flatulence/eructation, and gallstones.

Musculoskeletal: Infrequent were various joint disturbances (pain, stiffness, swelling, ache). Rare were muscle stiffness, need to flex calf muscles, backache, muscle tiredness, and swelling of the extremities.

Neurological: Infrequent were mental confusion, euphoria, agitation, relaxation, chills, sensation of lightness, tremor, shivering, disturbances of taste, prickling sensations, paresthesia, stinging sensations, facial pain, photophobia, and lacrimation. Rare were transient hemiplegia, hysteria, globus hystericus, intoxication, depression, myoclonia, monoplegia/diplegia, sleep disturbance, difficulties in concentration, disturbances of smell, hyperesthesia, dysesthesia, simultaneous hot and cold sensations, tickling sensations, dysarthria, yawning, reduced appetite, hunger, and dystonia.

Respiratory: Infrequent was dyspnea. Rare were influenza, diseases of the lower respiratory tract, and hiccoughs.

Skin: Infrequent were erythema, pruritus, and skin rashes and eruptions. Rare was skin tenderness.

Urogenital: Rare were dysuria, frequency, dysmenorrhea, and renal calculus.

Miscellaneous: Infrequent were miscellaneous laboratory abnormalities, including minor disturbances in liver function tests, "serotonin agonist effect", and hypersensitivity to various agents. Rare was fever.

Other Events Observed in the Clinical Development of IMITREX: The following adverse events occurred in clinical trials with IMITREX Tablets and IMITREX Nasal Spray. Because the reports include events observed in open and uncontrolled studies, the role of IMITREX in their causation cannot be reliably determined. All reported events are included except those already listed, those too general to be informative, and those not reasonably associated with the use of the drug.

Breasts: Breast swelling, cysts, disorder of breasts, lumps, masses of breasts, nipple discharge, primary malignant breast neoplasm, and tenderness.

Cardiovascular: Abdominal aortic aneurysm, angina, atherosclerosis, cerebral ischemia, cerebrovascular lesion, heart block, peripheral cyanosis, phlebitis, thrombosis, and transient myocardial ischemia.

Ear, Nose, and Throat: Allergic rhinitis; disorder of nasal cavity/sinuses; ear, nose, and throat hemorrhage; ear infection; external otitis; feeling of fullness in the ear(s); hearing disturbances; hearing loss; Meniere disease; nasal inflammation; otalgia; sensitivity to noise; sinusitis; tinnitus; and upper respiratory inflammation.

Endocrine and Metabolic: Elevated thyrotropin stimulating hormone (TSH) levels; endocrine cysts, lumps, and masses; fluid disturbances; galactorrhea; hyperglycemia; hypoglycemia; hypothyroidism; weight gain; and weight loss.

Eye: Accommodation disorders, blindness and low vision, conjunctivitis, disorders of sclera, external ocular muscle disorders, eye edema and swelling, eye hemorrhage, eye itching, eye pain, keratitis, mydriasis, and visual disturbances.

Gastrointestinal: Abdominal distention, colitis, constipation, dental pain, dyspeptic symptoms, feelings of gastrointestinal pressure, gastric symptoms, gastritis, gastroenteritis, gastrointestinal bleeding, gastrointestinal pain, hematemesis, hypersalivation, hyposalivation, intestinal obstruction, melena, nausea and/or vomiting, oral itching and irritation, pancreatitis, salivary gland swelling, and swallowing disorders.

Hematological Disorders: Anemia.

Mouth and Teeth: Disorder of mouth and tongue (e.g., burning of tongue, numbness of tongue, dry mouth).

Musculoskeletal: Acquired musculoskeletal deformity, arthralgia and articular rheumatitis, arthritis, intervertebral disc disorder, muscle atrophy, muscle tightness and rigidity, musculoskeletal inflammation, and tetany.

Neurological: Apathy, aggressiveness, bad/unusual taste, bradylogia, cluster headache, convulsions, depressive disorders, detachment, disturbance of emotions, drug abuse, facial paralysis, hallucinations, heat sensitivity, incoordination, increased alertness, memory disturbance, migraine, motor dysfunction, neoplasm or pituitary, neuralgia, neurotic disorders, paralysis, personality change, phobia, phonophobia, psychomotor disorders, radiculopathy, raised intracranial pressure, rigidity, stress, syncopy, suicide, and twitching.

Respiratory: Asthma, breathing disorders, bronchitis, cough, and lower respiratory tract infection.

Skin: Dry/scaly skin, eczema, herpes, seborrheic dermatitis, skin nodules, tightness of skin, and wrinkling of skin.

Urogenital: Abnormal menstrual cycle, abortion, bladder inflammation, endometriosis, hematuria, increased urination, inflammation of fallopian tubes, intermenstrual bleeding, menstruation symptoms, micturition disorders, urethritis, and urinary infections.

Miscellaneous: Contusions, difficulty in walking, edema, hematoma, hypersensitivity, fever, fluid retention, lymphadenopathy, overdose, speech disturbance, swelling of extremities, swelling of face, and voice disturbances.

Pain and Other Pressure Sensations: Chest pain and/or heaviness, neck/throat/jaw pain/tightness/pressure, and pain (location specified).

Postmarketing Experience (Reports for Subcutaneous or Oral Sumatriptan): The following section enumerates potentially important adverse events that have occurred in clinical practice and that have been reported spontaneously to various surveillance systems. The events enumerated represent reports arising from both domestic and nondomestic use of oral or subcutaneous dosage forms of sumatriptan. The events enumerated include all except those already listed in the ADVERSE REACTIONS section above or those too general to be informative. Because the reports cite events reported spontaneously from worldwide postmarketing experience, frequency of events and the role of IMITREX Injection in their causation cannot be reliably determined. It is assumed, however, that systemic reactions following sumatriptan use are likely to be similar regardless of route of administration.

Blood: Hemolytic anemia, pancytopenia, thrombocytopenia.

Cardiovascular: Atrial fibrillation, cardiomyopathy, colonic ischemia, (see WARNINGS), Prinzmetal variant angina, pulmonary embolism, shock, thrombophlebitis.

Ear, Nose, and Throat: Deafness.

Eye: Ischemic optic neuropathy, retinal artery occlusion, retinal vein thrombosis.

Gastrointestinal: Ischemic colitis with rectal bleeding (see WARNINGS), xerostomia.

Hepatic: Elevated liver function tests.

Neurological: Central nervous system vasculitis, cerebrovascular accident, dysphasia, subarachnoid hemorrhage.

Table 4: Treatment-Emergent Adverse Experience Incidence in 2 Large Placebo-Controlled Migraine Clinical Trials: Events Reported by at Least 1% of IMITREX Injection Patients

	Percent of Patients Reporting	
Adverse Event Type	IMITREX Injection 6 mg Subcutaneous n = 547	Placebo n = 370
Atypical sensations	42.0	9.2
Tingling	13.5	3.0
Warm/hot sensation	10.8	3.5
Burning sensation	7.5	0.3
Feeling of heaviness	7.3	1.1
Pressure sensation	7.1	1.6
Feeling of tightness	5.1	0.3
Numbness	4.6	2.2
Feeling strange	2.2	0.3
Tight feeling in head	2.2	0.3
Cold sensation	1.1	0.5
Cardiovascular		
Flushing	6.6	2.4
Chest discomfort	4.5	1.4
Tightness in chest	2.7	0.5
Pressure in chest	1.8	0.3
Ear, nose, and throat		
Throat discomfort	3.3	0.5
Discomfort: nasal cavity/sinuses	2.2	0.3
Eye		
Vision alterations	1.1	0.0
Gastrointestinal		
Abdominal discomfort	1.3	0.8
Dysphagia	1.1	0.0
Injection site reaction	58.7	23.8
Miscellaneous		
Jaw discomfort	1.8	0.0
Mouth and teeth		
Discomfort of mouth/tongue	4.9	4.6
Musculoskeletal		
Weakness	4.9	0.3
Neck pain/stiffness	4.8	0.5
Myalgia	1.8	0.5
Muscle cramp(s)	1.1	0.0
Neurological		
Dizziness/vertigo	11.9	4.3
Drowsiness/sedation	2.7	2.2
Headache	2.2	0.3
Anxiety	1.1	0.5
Malaise/fatigue	1.1	0.8
Skin		
Sweating	1.6	1.1

The sum of the percentages cited is greater than 100% because patients may experience more than 1 type of adverse event. Only events that occurred at a frequency of 1% or more in groups treated with IMITREX Injection and were at least as frequent in the placebo groups are included.

Non-Site Specific: Angioneurotic edema, cyanosis, death (see WARNINGS), temporal arteritis.
Psychiatry: Panic disorder.
Respiratory: Bronchospasm in patients with and without a history of asthma.
Skin: Exacerbation of sunburn, hypersensitivity reactions (allergic vasculitis, erythema, pruritus, rash, shortness of breath, urticaria; in addition, severe anaphylaxis/anaphylactoid reactions have been reported [see WARNINGS]), photosensitivity. Following subcutaneous administration of sumatriptan, pain, redness, stinging, induration, swelling, contusion, subcutaneous bleeding, and, on rare occasions, lipoatrophy (depression in the skin) or lipohypertrophy (enlargement or thickening of tissue) have been reported.
Urogenital: Acute renal failure.

DRUG ABUSE AND DEPENDENCE

The abuse potential of IMITREX Injection cannot be fully delineated in advance of extensive marketing experience. One clinical study enrolling 12 patients with a history of substance abuse failed to induce subjective behavior and/or physiologic response ordinarily associated with drugs that have an established potential for abuse.

OVERDOSAGE

Patients (n = 269) have received single injections of 8 to 12 mg without significant adverse effects. Volunteers (n = 47) have received single subcutaneous doses of up to 16 mg without serious adverse events.
No gross overdoses in clinical practice have been reported. Coronary vasospasm was observed after intravenous administration of IMITREX Injection (see CONTRAINDICATIONS). Overdoses would be expected from animal data (dogs at 0.1 g/kg, rats at 2 g/kg) to possibly cause convulsions, tremor, inactivity, erythema of the extremities, reduced respiratory rate, cyanosis, ataxia, mydriasis, injection site reactions (desquamation, hair loss, and scab formation), and paralysis. The half-life of elimination of sumatriptan is about 2 hours (see CLINICAL PHARMACOLOGY), and therefore monitoring of patients after overdose with IMITREX Injection should continue while symptoms or signs persist, and for at least 10 hours.
It is unknown what effect hemodialysis or peritoneal dialysis has on the serum concentrations of sumatriptan.

DOSAGE AND ADMINISTRATION

The maximum single recommended adult dose of IMITREX Injection is 6 mg injected subcutaneously. Controlled clinical trials have failed to show that clear benefit is associated with the administration of a second 6-mg dose in patients who have failed to respond to a first injection.
The maximum recommended dose that may be given in 24 hours is two 6-mg injections separated by at least 1 hour. Although the recommended dose is 6 mg, if side effects are dose limiting, then lower doses may be used (see CLINICAL PHARMACOLOGY). In patients receiving MAO inhibitors, decreased doses of sumatriptan should be considered (see WARNINGS and CLINICAL PHARMACOLOGY). In patients receiving doses lower than 6 mg, only the single-dose vial dosage form should be used. An autoinjection device is available for use with 6-mg prefilled syringe cartridges to facilitate self-administration in patients in whom this dose is deemed necessary. With this device, the needle penetrates approximately 1/4 of an inch (5 to 6 mm). Since the injection is intended to be given subcutaneously, intramuscular or intravascular delivery should be avoided. Patients should be directed to use injection sites with an adequate skin and subcutaneous thickness to accommodate the length of the needle.
Parenteral drug products should be inspected visually for particulate matter and discoloration before administration whenever solution and container permit.

HOW SUPPLIED

IMITREX Injection 6 mg (12 mg/mL) containing sumatriptan (base) as the succinate salt is supplied as a clear, colorless to pale yellow, sterile, nonpyrogenic solution as follows:
(NDC 0173-0479-00) IMITREX STATdose System® containing 2 prefilled single-dose syringe cartridges, 1 IMITREX STATdose Pen®, and instructions for use
(NDC 0173-0478-00) IMITREX Injection cartridge pack containing 2 prefilled syringe cartridges for refill of IMITREX STATdose System only.
(NDC 0173-0449-01) Unit-of-use syringe (0.5 mL in 1 mL) in cartons of 2 syringes. Not for use with IMITREX STATdose System.
(NDC 0173-0449-02) 6-mg Single-dose vials (0.5 mL in 2 mL) in cartons of 5 vials.
Store between 2° and 30°C (36° and 86°F). Protect from light.

PATIENT INFORMATION

The following wording is contained in a separate leaflet provided for patients.

Information for the Patient
IMITREX® (sumatriptan succinate) Injection

Please read this leaflet carefully before you take IMITREX Injection. This provides a summary of the information available on your medicine. Please do not throw away this leaflet until you have finished your medicine. You may need to read this leaflet again. This leaflet does not contain all the information on IMITREX Injection. For further information or advice, ask your doctor or pharmacist.
Information About Your Medicine:
The name of your medicine is IMITREX (sumatriptan succinate) Injection. It can be obtained only by prescription from your doctor. The decision to use IMITREX Injection is one that you and your doctor should make jointly, taking into account your individual preferences and medical circumstances. If you have risk factors for heart disease (such as high blood pressure, high cholesterol, obesity, diabetes, smoking, strong family history of heart disease, or you are postmenopausal or a male over 40), you should tell your doctor, who should evaluate you for heart disease in order to determine if IMITREX is appropriate for you. Although the vast majority of those who have taken IMITREX have not experienced any significant side effects, some individuals have experienced serious heart problems and, rarely, considering the extensiveness of IMITREX use worldwide, deaths have been reported. In all but a few instances, however, serious problems occurred in people with known heart diseases and it was not clear whether IMITREX was a contributory factor in these deaths.
1. The Purpose of Your Medicine:
IMITREX Injection is intended to relieve your migraine or cluster headache, but not to prevent or reduce the number of attacks you experience. Use IMITREX Injection only to treat an actual migraine or cluster headache attack.
2. Important Questions to Consider Before Taking IMITREX Injection:
If the answer to any of the following questions is **YES** or if you do not know the answer, then please discuss with your doctor before you use IMITREX Injection.

- Are you pregnant? Do you think you might be pregnant? Are you trying to become pregnant? Are you using inadequate contraception? Are you breastfeeding?
- Do you have any chest pain, heart disease, shortness of breath, or irregular heartbeats? Have you had a heart attack?
- Do you have risk factors for heart disease (such as high blood pressure, high cholesterol, obesity, diabetes, smoking, strong family history of heart disease, or you are postmenopausal or a male over 40)?
- Have you had a stroke, transient ischemic attacks (TIAs), or Raynaud syndrome?
- Do you have high blood pressure?
- Have you ever had to stop taking this or any other medication because of an allergy or other problems?
- Are you taking any other migraine medications, including other 5–HT_1 agonists or any other medications containing ergotamine, dihydroergotamine, or methysergide?
- Are you taking any medication for depression (monoamine oxidase inhibitors or selective serotonin reuptake inhibitors [SSRIs])?
- Have you had, or do you have, any disease of the liver or kidney?
- Have you had, or do you have, epilepsy or seizures?
- Is this headache different from your usual migraine attacks?

Remember, if you answered **YES** to any of the above questions, then discuss it with your doctor.
3. The Use of IMITREX Injection During Pregnancy:
Do not use IMITREX Injection if you are pregnant, think you might be pregnant, are trying to become pregnant, or are not using adequate contraception, unless you have discussed this with your doctor.
4. How to Use IMITREX Injection:
Before injecting IMITREX, check with your doctor on acceptable injection sites and see the instructions (on or inside the carton) on discarding empty syringes and loading an autoinjector device.
Never reuse a syringe.
For adults, the usual dose is a single injection given just below the skin. It should be given as soon as the symptoms of your migraine appear, but it may be given at any time during an attack. A second injection may be given if your symptoms of migraine come back. If your symptoms do not improve following the first injection, do not give a second injection for the same attack without first consulting with your doctor. Do not have more than 2 injections in any 24 hours and allow at least 1 hour between each dose.
5. Side Effects to Watch for:

- Some patients experience pain or tightness in the chest or throat when using IMITREX Injection. If this happens to you, then discuss it with your doctor before using any more IMITREX Injection. If the chest pain is severe or does not go away, call your doctor immediately.
- If you have sudden and/or severe abdominal pain following IMITREX Injection, call your doctor immediately.
- Shortness of breath; wheeziness; heart throbbing; swelling of eyelids, face, or lips; or a skin rash, skin lumps, or hives happens rarely. If it happens to you, then tell your doctor immediately. Do not take any more IMITREX Injection unless your doctor tells you to do so.
- Some people may have feelings of tingling, heat, flushing (redness of face lasting a short time), heaviness or pressure after treatment with IMITREX Injection. A few people may feel drowsy, dizzy, tired, or sick. Tell your doctor of these symptoms at your next visit.
- You may experience pain or redness at the site of injection, but this usually lasts less than an hour.
- If you feel unwell in any other way or have any symptoms that you do not understand, you should contact your doctor immediately.

6. What to Do If an Overdose Is Taken:
If you have taken more medication than you have been told, contact either your doctor, hospital emergency department, or nearest poison control center immediately.
7. Storing Your Medicine:
Keep your medicine in a safe place where children cannot reach it. It may be harmful to children.
Store your medication away from heat and light. Keep your medication in the case provided and do not store at temperatures above 86°F (30°C).
If your medication has expired (the expiration date is printed on the treatment pack), throw it away as instructed. Do not throw away your autoinjector.
If your doctor decides to stop your treatment, do not keep any leftover medicine unless your doctor tells you to. Throw away your medicine as instructed.
Glaxo Wellcome Inc., Research Triangle Park, NC 27709
US Patent Nos. 4,816,470 and 5,037,845

September 1999/RL-759
Shown in Product Identification Guide, page 315

IMITREX® ℞
[*ĭm′ ĭ-trĕx″*]
(sumatriptan)
Nasal Spray

DESCRIPTION

IMITREX (sumatriptan) Nasal Spray contains sumatriptan, a selective 5-hydroxytryptamine$_1$ receptor subtype agonist. Sumatriptan is chemically designated as 3-[2-(dimethylamino) ethyl] -N-methyl-1H-indole-5-methanesulfonamide.
The empirical formula is $C_{14}H_{21}N_3O_2S$, representing a molecular weight of 295.4. Sumatriptan is a white to off-white powder that is readily soluble in water and in saline. Each IMITREX Nasal Spray contains 5 or 20 mg of sumatriptan in a 100-μL unit dose aqueous buffered solution containing monobasic potassium phosphate NF, anhydrous dibasic sodium phosphate USP, sulfuric acid NF, sodium hydroxide NF, and purified water USP. The pH of the solution is approximately 5.5. The osmolality of the solution is 372 or 742 mOsmol for the 5- and 20-mg IMITREX Nasal Spray, respectively.

CLINICAL PHARMACOLOGY

Mechanism of Action: Sumatriptan is an agonist for a vascular 5-hydroxytryptamine$_1$ receptor subtype (probably a member of the 5-HT_{1D} family) having only a weak affinity for 5-HT_{1A}, 5-HT_{5A}, and 5-HT_7 receptors and no significant affinity (as measured using standard radioligand binding assays) or pharmacological activity at 5-HT_2, 5-HT_3, or 5-HT_4 receptor subtypes or at alpha$_1$-, alpha$_2$-, or beta-adrenergic; dopamine$_1$; dopamine$_2$; muscarinic; or benzodiazepine receptors.
The vascular 5-HT_1 receptor subtype that sumatriptan activates is present on cranial arteries in both dog and primate, on the human basilar artery, and in the vasculature of human dura mater and mediates vasoconstriction. This action in humans correlates with the relief of migraine headache. In addition to causing vasoconstriction, experimental data from animal studies show that sumatriptan also activates 5-HT_1 receptors on peripheral terminals of the trigeminal nerve innervating cranial blood vessels. Such an action may contribute to the antimigrainous effect of sumatriptan in humans.
In the anesthetized dog, sumatriptan selectively reduces the carotid arterial blood flow with little or no effect on arterial blood pressure or total peripheral resistance. In the cat, sumatriptan selectively constricts the carotid arteriovenous anastomoses while having little effect on blood flow or resistance in cerebral or extracerebral tissues.
Pharmacokinetics: In a study of 20 female volunteers, the mean maximum concentration following a 5- and 20-mg intranasal dose was 5 and 16 ng/mL, respectively. The mean C_{max} following a 6-mg subcutaneous injection is 71 ng/mL (range, 49 to 110 ng/mL). The mean C_{max} is 18 ng/mL (range, 7 to 47 ng/mL) following oral dosing with 25 mg and 51 mg/mL (range, 28 to 100 ng/mL) following oral dosing with 100 mg of sumatriptan. In a study of 24 male volunteers, the bioavailability relative to subcutaneous injection was low, approximately 17%, primarily due to presystemic metabolism and partly due to incomplete absorption.
Protein binding, determined by equilibrium dialysis over the concentration range of 10 to 1000 ng/mL, is low, approximately 14% to 21%. The effect of sumatriptan on the protein binding of other drugs has not been evaluated, but would be expected to be minor, given the low rate of protein binding. The mean volume of distribution after subcutaneous dosing is 2.7 L/kg and the total plasma clearance is approximately 1200 mL/min.
The elimination half-life of sumatriptan administered as a nasal spray is approximately 2 hours, similar to the half-life seen after subcutaneous injection. Only 3% of the dose is

Continued on next page

This product information is based on labeling in effect on June 23, 2000. For further information, contact via direct mail, phone, or web site. Medical Information, Glaxo Wellcome Inc., PO Box 13398, Research Triangle Park, NC 27709. Healthcare Professionals (Medical Information): 800-334-0089. Patients (Customer Response Center): 1-888-825-5249. Glaxo Wellcome Corporate Web Site: www.glaxowellcome.com

Imitrex Nasal Spray—Cont.

excreted in the urine as unchanged sumatriptan; 42% of the dose is excreted as the major metabolite, the indole acetic acid analogue of sumatriptan.

Clinical and pharmacokinetic data indicate that administration of two 5-mg doses, 1 dose in each nostril, is equivalent to administration of a single 10-mg dose in 1 nostril.

Special Populations: *Renal Impairment:* The effect of renal impairment on the pharmacokinetics of sumatriptan has not been examined, but little clinical effect would be expected as sumatriptan is largely metabolized to an inactive substance.

Hepatic Impairment: The effect of hepatic disease on the pharmacokinetics of subcutaneously and orally administered sumatriptan has been evaluated, but the intranasal dosage form has not been studied in hepatic impairment. There were no statistically significant differences in the pharmacokinetics of subcutaneously administered sumatriptan in hepatically impaired patients compared to healthy controls. However, the liver plays an important role in the presystemic clearance of orally administered sumatriptan. In 1 small study involving oral sumatriptan in hepatically impaired patients (n = 8) matched for sex, age, and weight with healthy subjects, the hepatically impaired patients had an approximately 70% increase in AUC and C_{max} and a t_{max} 40 minutes earlier compared to the healthy subjects. The bioavailability of nasally absorbed sumatriptan following intranasal administration, which would not undergo first-pass metabolism, should not be altered in hepatically impaired patients. The bioavailability of the swallowed portion of the intranasal sumatriptan dose has not been determined, but would be increased in these patients. The swallowed intranasal dose is small, however, compared to the usual oral dose, so that its impact should be minimal.

Age: The pharmacokinetics of oral sumatriptan in the elderly (mean age; 72 years, 2 males and 4 females) and in patients with migraine (mean age; 38 years, 25 males and 155 females) were similar to that in healthy male subjects (mean age, 30 years). Intranasal sumatriptan has not been evaluated for age differences (see PRECAUTIONS: Geriatric Use).

Race: The systemic clearance and C_{max} of sumatriptan were similar in black (n = 34) and Caucasian (n = 38) healthy male subjects. Intranasal sumatriptan has not been evaluated for race differences.

Drug Interactions: *Monoamine Oxidase Inhibitors (MAOIs):* Treatment with MAOIs generally leads to an increase of sumatriptan plasma levels (see CONTRAINDICATIONS and PRECAUTIONS).

MAOI interaction studies have not been performed with intranasal sumatriptan. Due to gut and hepatic metabolic first-pass effects, the increase of systemic exposure after coadministration of an MAO-A inhibitor with oral sumatriptan is greater than after coadministration of the MAOI with subcutaneous sumatriptan. The effects of an MAOI on systemic exposure after intranasal sumatriptan would be expected to be greater than the effect after subcutaneous sumatriptan but smaller than the effect after oral sumatriptan because only swallowed drug would be subject to first-pass effects.

In a study of 14 healthy females, pretreatment with an MAO-A inhibitor decreased the clearance of subcutaneous sumatriptan. Under the conditions of this experiment, the result was a 2-fold increase in the area under the sumatriptan plasma concentration x time curve (AUC), corresponding to a 40% increase in elimination half-life. This interaction was not evident with an MAO-B inhibitor.

A small study evaluating the effect of pretreatment with an MAO-A inhibitor on the bioavailability from a 25-mg oral sumatriptan tablet resulted in an approximately 7-fold increase in systemic exposure.

Xylometazoline: An in vivo drug interaction study indicated that 3 drops of xylometazoline (0.1% w/v), a decongestant, administered 15 minutes prior to a 20-mg nasal dose of sumatriptan did not alter the pharmacokinetics of sumatriptan.

CLINICAL TRIALS

The efficacy of IMITREX Nasal Spray in the acute treatment of migraine headaches was demonstrated in 8, randomized, double-blind, placebo-controlled studies, of which 5 used the recommended dosing regimen and used the marketed formulation. Patients enrolled in these 5 studies were predominately female (86%) and Caucasian (95%), with a mean age of 41 (range of 18 to 65). Patients were instructed to treat a moderate to severe headache. Headache response, defined as a reduction in headache severity from moderate or severe pain to mild or no pain, was assessed up to 2 hours after dosing. Associated symptoms such as nausea, photophobia, and phonophobia were also assessed. Maintenance of response was assessed for up to 24 hours postdose. A second dose of IMITREX Nasal Spray or other medication was allowed 2 to 24 hours after the initial treatment for recurrent headache. The frequency and time to use of these additional treatments were also determined. In all studies, doses of 10 and 20 mg were compared to placebo in the treatment of 1 to 3 migraine attacks. Patients received doses as a single spray into 1 nostril. In 2 studies, a 5-mg dose was also evaluated.

In all 5 trials utilizing the market formulation and recommended dosage regimen, the percentage of patients achieving headache response 2 hours after treatment was significantly greater among patients receiving IMITREX Nasal Spray at all doses (with one exception) compared to those who received placebo. In 4 of the 5 studies, there was a statistically significant greater percentage of patients with headache response at 2 hours in the 20-mg group when compared to the lower dose groups (5 and 10 mg). There were no statistically significant differences between the 5- and 10-mg dose groups in any study. The results from the 5 controlled clinical trials are summarized in Table 1. Note that, in general, comparisons of results obtained in studies conducted under different conditions by different investigators with different samples of patients are ordinarily unreliable for purposes of quantitative comparison.

[See table 1 below]

The estimated probability of achieving an initial headache response over the 2 hours following treatment is depicted in Figure 1.

Figure 1: Estimated Probability of Achieving Initial Headache Response Within 120 Minutes*

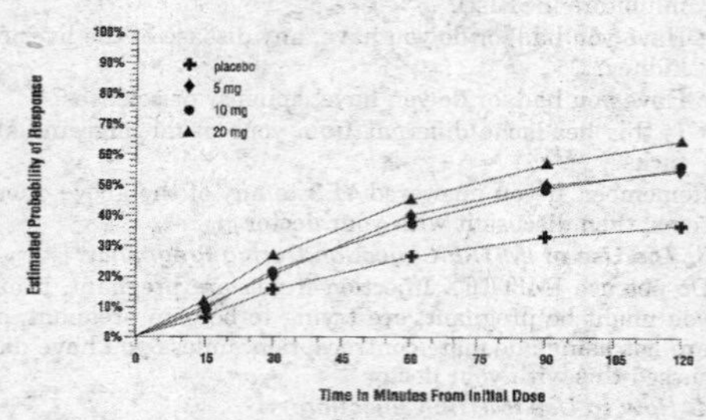

* The figure shows the probability over time of obtaining headache response (no or mild pain) following treatment with intranasal sumatriptan. The averages displayed are based on pooled data from the 5 clinical controlled trials providing evidence of efficacy. Kaplan-Meier plot with patients not achieving response within 120 minutes censored to 120 minutes.

For patients with migraine-associated nausea, photophobia, and phonophobia at baseline, there was a lower incidence of these symptoms at 2 hours following administration of IMITREX Nasal Spray compared to placebo.

Two to 24 hours following the initial dose of study treatment, patients were allowed to use additional treatment for pain relief in the form of a second dose of study treatment or other medication. The estimated probability of patients taking a second dose or other medication for migraine over the 24 hours following the initial dose of study treatment is summarized in Figure 2.

Figure 2: The Estimated Probability of Patients Taking a Second Dose or Other Medication for Migraine Over the 24 Hours Following the Initial Dose of Study Treatment*

Estimated Probability of Remedication or Rescue

placebo / 5 mg / 10 mg / 20 mg

Time in Hours From Initial Dose

* Kaplan-Meier plot based on data obtained in the 3 clinical controlled trials providing evidence of efficacy with patients not using additional treatments censored to 24 hours. Plot also includes patients who had no response to the initial dose. No remedication was allowed within 2 hours postdose.

There is evidence that doses above 20 mg do not provide a greater effect than 20 mg. There was no evidence to suggest that treatment with sumatriptan was associated with an increase in the severity of recurrent headaches. The efficacy of IMITREX Nasal Spray was unaffected by presence of aura; duration of headache prior to treatment; gender, age, or weight of the patient; or concomitant use of common migraine prophylactic drugs (e.g., beta-blockers, calcium channel blockers, tricyclic antidepressants). There were insufficient data to assess the impact of race on efficacy.

INDICATIONS AND USAGE

IMITREX Nasal Spray is indicated for the acute treatment of migraine attacks with or without aura in adults.

IMITREX Nasal Spray is not intended for the prophylactic therapy of migraine or for use in the management of hemiplegic or basilar migraine (see CONTRAINDICATIONS). Safety and effectiveness of IMITREX Nasal Spray have not been established for cluster headache, which is present in an older, predominantly male population.

CONTRAINDICATIONS

IMITREX Nasal Spray should not be given to patients with history, symptoms, or signs of ischemic cardiac, cerebrovascular, or peripheral vascular syndromes. In addition, patients with other significant underlying cardiovascular diseases should not receive IMITREX Nasal Spray. Ischemic cardiac syndromes include, but are not limited to, angina pectoris of any type (e.g., stable angina of effort and vasospastic forms of angina such as the Prinzmetal variant), all forms of myocardial infarction, and silent myocardial ischemia. Cerebrovascular syndromes include, but are not limited to, strokes of any type as well as transient ischemic attacks. Peripheral vascular disease includes, but is not limited to, ischemic bowel disease (see WARNINGS).

Because IMITREX Nasal Spray may increase blood pressure, it should not be given to patients with uncontrolled hypertension.

Concurrent administration of MAO-A inhibitors or use within 2 weeks of discontinuation of MAO-A inhibitor therapy is contraindicated (see CLINICAL PHARMACOLOGY: Drug Interactions and PRECAUTIONS: Drug Interactions).

IMITREX Nasal Spray and any ergotamine-containing or ergot-type medication (like dihydroergotamine or methysergide) should not be used within 24 hours of each other, nor should IMITREX Nasal Spray and another 5-HT_1 agonist.

IMITREX Nasal Spray should not be administered to patients with hemiplegic or basilar migraine.

IMITREX Nasal Spray is contraindicated in patients with hypersensitivity to sumatriptan or any of its components.

IMITREX Nasal Spray is contraindicated in patients with severe hepatic impairment.

WARNINGS

IMITREX Nasal Spray should only be used where a clear diagnosis of migraine headache has been established.

Risk of Myocardial Ischemia and/or Infarction and Other Adverse Cardiac Events: Sumatriptan should not be given to patients with documented ischemic or vasospastic coronary artery disease (CAD) (see CONTRAINDICATIONS). It is strongly recommended that sumatriptan not be given to patients in whom unrecognized CAD is predicted by the presence of risk factors (e.g., hypertension, hypercholesterolemia, smoker, obesity, diabetes, strong family history of CAD, female with surgical or physiological menopause, or male over 40 years of age) unless a cardiovascular evaluation provides satisfactory clinical evidence that the patient is reasonably free of coronary artery and ischemic myocardial disease or other significant underlying cardiovascular disease. The sensitivity of cardiac diagnostic procedures to detect cardiovascular disease or predisposition to coronary artery vasospasm is modest, at best. If, during the cardiovascular evaluation, the patient's medical history or electrocardiographic investigations reveal findings indicative of, or consistent with, coronary artery vasospasm or myocardial ischemia, sumatriptan should not be administered (see CONTRAINDICATIONS).

For patients with risk factors predictive of CAD, who are determined to have a satisfactory cardiovascular evalua-

Table 1: Percentage of Patients With Headache Response (No or Mild Pain) 2 Hours Following Treatment

	Placebo	IMITREX Nasal Spray 5 mg	IMITREX Nasal Spray 10 mg	IMITREX Nasal Spray 20 mg
Study 1	25% (n = 63)	49%* (n = 121)	46%* (n = 112)	64%*†‡ (n = 118)
Study 2	25% (n = 138)	Not applicable	44%* (n = 273)	55%*† (n = 277)
Study 3	35% (n = 100)	Not applicable	54%* (n = 106)	63%* (n = 202)
Study 4	29% (n = 112)	Not applicable	43% (n = 106)	62%*† (n = 215)
Study 5§	36% (n = 198)	45%* (n = 296)	53%* (n = 291)	60%*‡ (n = 286)

* $P<0.05$ in comparison with placebo.
† $P<0.05$ in comparison with 10 mg.
‡ $P<0.05$ in comparison with 5 mg.
§ Data are for attack 1 only of multiattack study for comparison.

tion, it is strongly recommended that administration of the first dose of sumatriptan nasal spray take place in the setting of a physician's office or similar medically staffed and equipped facility unless the patient has previously received sumatriptan. Because cardiac ischemia can occur in the absence of clinical symptoms, consideration should be given to obtaining on the first occasion of use an electrocardiogram (ECG) during the interval immediately following IMITREX Nasal Spray, in these patients with risk factors.

It is recommended that patients who are intermittent long-term users of sumatriptan and who have or acquire risk factors predictive of CAD, as described above, undergo periodic interval cardiovascular evaluation as they continue to use sumatriptan.

The systematic approach described above is intended to reduce the likelihood that patients with unrecognized cardiovascular disease will be inadvertently exposed to sumatriptan.

Drug-Associated Cardiac Events and Fatalities: Serious adverse cardiac events, including acute myocardial infarction, life-threatening disturbances of cardiac rhythm, and death have been reported within a few hours following the administration of IMITREX® (sumatriptan succinate) Injection or IMITREX® (sumatriptan succinate) Tablets. Considering the extent of use of sumatriptan in patients with migraine, the incidence of these events is extremely low.

The fact that sumatriptan can cause coronary vasospasm, that some of these events have occurred in patients with no prior cardiac disease history and with documented absence of CAD, and the close proximity of the events to sumatriptan use support the conclusion that some of these cases were caused by the drug. In many cases, however, where there has been known underlying coronary artery disease, the relationship is uncertain.

Premarketing Experience With Sumatriptan: Among approximately 4000 patients with migraine who participated in premarketing controlled and uncontrolled clinical trials of sumatriptan nasal spray, 1 patient experienced an asymptomatic subendocardial infarction possibly subsequent to a coronary vasospastic event.

Of 6348 patients with migraine who participated in premarketing controlled and uncontrolled clinical trials of oral sumatriptan, 2 experienced clinical adverse events shortly after receiving oral sumatriptan that may have reflected coronary vasospasm. Neither of these adverse events was associated with a serious clinical outcome.

Among the more than 1900 patients with migraine who participated in premarketing controlled clinical trials of subcutaneous sumatriptan, there were 8 patients who sustained clinical events during or shortly after receiving sumatriptan that may have reflected coronary artery vasospasm. Six of these 8 patients had ECG changes consistent with transient ischemia, but without accompanying clinical symptoms or signs. Of these 8 patients, 4 had either findings suggestive of CAD or risk factors predictive of CAD prior to study enrollment.

Postmarketing Experience With Sumatriptan: Serious cardiovascular events, some resulting in death, have been reported in association with the use of IMITREX Injection or IMITREX Tablets. The uncontrolled nature of postmarketing surveillance, however, makes it impossible to determine definitively the proportion of the reported cases that were actually caused by sumatriptan or to reliably assess causation in individual cases. On clinical grounds, the longer the latency between the administration of IMITREX and the onset of the clinical event, the less likely the association is to be causative. Accordingly, interest has focused on events beginning within 1 hour of the administration of IMITREX.

Cardiac events that have been observed to have onset within 1 hour of sumatriptan administration include: coronary artery vasospasm, transient ischemia, myocardial infarction, ventricular tachycardia and ventricular fibrillation, cardiac arrest, and death.

Some of these events occurred in patients who had no findings of CAD and appear to represent consequences of coronary artery vasospasm. However, among domestic reports of serious cardiac events within 1 hour of sumatriptan administration, almost all of the patients had risk factors predictive of CAD and the presence of significant underlying CAD was established in most cases (see CONTRAINDICATIONS).

Drug-Associated Cerebrovascular Events and Fatalities: Cerebral hemorrhage, subarachnoid hemorrhage, stroke, and other cerebrovascular events have been reported in patients treated with oral or subcutaneous sumatriptan, and some have resulted in fatalities. The relationship of sumatriptan to these events is uncertain. In a number of cases, it appears possible that the cerebrovascular events were primary, sumatriptan having been administered in the incorrect belief that the symptoms experienced were a consequence of migraine when they were not. As with other acute migraine therapies, before treating headaches in patients not previously diagnosed as migraineurs, and in migraineurs who present with atypical symptoms, care should be taken to exclude other potentially serious neurological conditions. It should also be noted that patients with migraine may be at increased risk of certain cerebrovascular events (e.g., cerebrovascular accident, transient ischemic attack).

Other Vasospasm-Related Events: Sumatriptan may cause vasospastic reactions other than coronary artery vasospasm. Both peripheral vascular ischemia and colonic ischemia with abdominal pain and bloody diarrhea have been reported.

Increase in Blood Pressure: Significant elevation in blood pressure, including hypertensive crisis, has been reported on rare occasions in patients with and without a history of hypertension. Sumatriptan is contraindicated in patients with uncontrolled hypertension (see CONTRAINDICATIONS). Sumatriptan should be administered with caution to patients with controlled hypertension as transient increases in blood pressure and peripheral vascular resistance have been observed in a small proportion of patients.

Local Irritation: Of the 3378 patients using the nasal spray (5-, 10-, or 20-mg doses) on 1 or 2 occasions in controlled clinical studies, approximately 5% noted irritation in the nose and throat. Irritative symptoms such as burning, numbness, paresthesia, discharge, pain or soreness were noted to be severe in about 1% of patients treated. The symptoms were transient and in approximately 60% of the cases, the symptoms resolved in less than 2 hours. Limited examinations of the nose and throat did not reveal any clinically noticeable injury in these patients. The consequences of extended and repeated use of IMITREX Nasal Spray on the nasal and/or respiratory mucosa have not been systematically evaluated in patients.

No increase in the incidence of local irritation was observed in patients using IMITREX Nasal Spray repeatedly for up to 1 year.

In inhalation studies in rats dosed daily for up to 1 month at exposures as low as one half the maximum daily human exposure (based on dose per surface area of nasal cavity), epithelial hyperplasia (with and without keratinization) and squamous metaplasia were observed in the larynx at all doses tested. These changes were partially reversible after a 2-week drug-free period. When dogs were dosed daily with various formulations by intranasal instillation for up to 13 weeks at exposures of 2 to 4 times the maximum daily human exposure (based on dose per surface area of nasal cavity), respiratory and nasal mucosa exhibited evidence of epithelial hyperplasia, focal squamous metaplasia, granulomata, bronchitis, and fibrosing alveolitis. A no-effect dose was not established. The changes observed in both species are not considered to be signs of either preneoplastic or neoplastic transformation.

Local effects on nasal and respiratory tissues after chronic intranasal dosing in animals have not been studied.

Concomitant Drug Use: In patients taking MAO-A inhibitors, sumatriptan plasma levels attained after treatment with recommended doses are 2-fold (following subcutaneous administration) to 7-fold (following oral administration) higher than those obtained under other conditions. Accordingly, the coadministration of IMITREX Nasal Spray and an MAO-A inhibitor is contraindicated (see CLINICAL PHARMACOLOGY and CONTRAINDICATIONS).

Hypersensitivity: Hypersensitivity (anaphylaxis/anaphylactoid) reactions have occurred on rare occasions in patients receiving sumatriptan. Such reactions can be life threatening or fatal. In general, hypersensitivity reactions to drugs are more likely to occur in individuals with a history of sensitivity to multiple allergens (see CONTRAINDICATIONS).

PRECAUTIONS

General: Chest discomfort and jaw or neck tightness have been reported infrequently following the administration of IMITREX Nasal Spray and have also been reported following use of IMITREX Tablets. Chest, jaw, or neck tightness is relatively common after administration of IMITREX Injection. Only rarely have these symptoms been associated with ischemic ECG changes. However, because sumatriptan may cause coronary artery vasospasm, patients who experience signs or symptoms suggestive of angina following sumatriptan should be evaluated for the presence of CAD or a predisposition to Prinzmetal variant angina before receiving additional doses of sumatriptan, and should be monitored electrocardiographically if dosing is resumed and similar symptoms recur. Similarly, patients who experience other symptoms or signs suggestive of decreased arterial flow, such as ischemic bowel syndrome or Raynaud syndrome following sumatriptan should be evaluated for atherosclerosis or predisposition to vasospasm (see WARNINGS).

IMITREX Nasal Spray should also be administered with caution to patients with diseases that may alter the absorption, metabolism, or excretion of drugs, such as impaired hepatic or renal function.

There have been rare reports of seizure following administration of sumatriptan. Sumatriptan should be used with caution in patients with a history of epilepsy or structural brain lesions that lower their seizure threshold.

Care should be taken to exclude other potentially serious neurologic conditions before treating headache in patients not previously diagnosed with migraine headache or who experience a headache that is atypical for them. There have been rare reports where patients received sumatriptan for severe headaches that were subsequently shown to have been secondary to an evolving neurologic lesion (see WARNINGS).

For a given attack, if a patient does not respond to the first dose of sumatriptan, the diagnosis of migraine headache should be reconsidered before administration of a second dose

Binding to Melanin-Containing Tissues: In rats treated with a single subcutaneous dose (0.5 mg/kg) or oral dose (2 mg/kg) of radiolabeled sumatriptan, the elimination half-life of radioactivity from the eye was 15 and 23 days, respectively, suggesting that sumatriptan and/or its metabolites bind to the melanin of the eye. Comparable studies were not performed by the intranasal route. Because there could be an accumulation in melanin-rich tissues over time, this raises the possibility that sumatriptan could cause toxicity in these tissues after extended use. However, no effects on the retina related to treatment with sumatriptan were noted in any of the oral or subcutaneous toxicity studies. Although no systematic monitoring of ophthalmologic function was undertaken in clinical trials, and no specific recommendations for ophthalmologic monitoring are offered, prescribers should be aware of the possibility of long-term ophthalmologic effects.

Corneal Opacities: Sumatriptan causes corneal opacities and defects in the corneal epithelium in dogs; this raises the possibility that these changes may occur in humans. While patients were not systematically evaluated for these changes in clinical trials, and no specific recommendations for monitoring are being offered, prescribers should be aware of the possibility of these changes (see ANIMAL TOXICOLOGY).

Information for Patients: See PATIENT INFORMATION at the end of this labeling for the text of the separate leaflet provided for patients.

Laboratory Tests: No specific laboratory tests are recommended for monitoring patients prior to and/or after treatment with sumatriptan.

Drug Interactions: Ergot-containing drugs have been reported to cause prolonged vasospastic reactions. Because there is a theoretical basis that these effects may be additive, use of ergotamine-containing or ergot-type medications (like dihydroergotamine or methysergide) and sumatriptan within 24 hours of each other should be avoided (see CONTRAINDICATIONS).

MAO-A inhibitors reduce sumatriptan clearance, significantly increasing systemic exposure. Therefore, the use of IMITREX Nasal Spray in patients receiving MAO-A inhibitors is contraindicated (see CLINICAL PHARMACOLOGY and CONTRAINDICATIONS).

Selective serotonin reuptake inhibitors (SSRIs) (e.g., fluoxetine, fluvoxamine, paroxetine, sertraline) have been reported, rarely, to cause weakness, hyperreflexia, and incoordination when coadministered with sumatriptan. If concomitant treatment with sumatriptan and an SSRI is clinically warranted, appropriate observation of the patient is advised.

Drug/Laboratory Test Interactions: IMITREX Nasal Spray is not known to interfere with commonly employed clinical laboratory tests.

Carcinogenesis, Mutagenesis, Impairment of Fertility: ***Carcinogenesis:*** In carcinogenicity studies, rats and mice were given sumatriptan by oral gavage (rats, 104 weeks) or drinking water (mice, 78 weeks). Average exposures, achieved in mice receiving the highest dose (target dose of 160 mg/kg per day) were approximately 184 times the exposure attained in humans after the maximum recommended single intranasal dose of 20 mg. The highest dose administered to rats (160 mg/kg per day, reduced from 360 mg/kg per day during week 21) was approximately 78 times the maximum recommended single intranasal dose of 20 mg on a mg/m^2 basis. There was no evidence of an increase in tumors in either species related to sumatriptan administration. Local effects on nasal and respiratory tissue after chronic intranasal dosing in animals have not been evaluated (see WARNINGS).

Mutagenesis: Sumatriptan was not mutagenic in the presence or absence of metabolic activation when tested in 2 gene mutation assays (the Ames test and the in vitro mammalian Chinese hamster V79/HGPRT assay). In 2 cytogenetics assays (the in vitro human lymphocyte assay and the in vivo rat micronucleus assay) sumatriptan was not associated with clastogenic activity.

Impairment of Fertility: In a study in which male and female rats were dosed daily with oral sumatriptan prior to and throughout the mating period, there was a treatment-related decrease in fertility secondary to a decrease in mating in animals treated with 50 and 500 mg/kg per day. The highest no-effect dose for this finding was 5 mg/kg per day, or approximately twice the maximum recommended single human intranasal dose of 20 mg on a mg/m^2 basis. It is not clear whether the problem is associated with treatment of the males or females or both combined. In a similar study by the subcutaneous route there was no evidence of impaired fertility at 60 mg/kg per day, the maximum dose tested, which is equivalent to approximately 29 times the maximum recommended single human intranasal dose of 20 mg on a mg/m^2 basis. Fertility studies, in which sumatriptan was administered by the intranasal route, were not conducted.

Pregnancy: Pregnancy Category C. In reproductive toxicity studies in rats and rabbits, oral treatment with sumatriptan was associated with embryolethality, fetal abnormalities, and pup mortality. When administered by the intravenous route to rabbits, sumatriptan has been shown

Continued on next page

This product information is based on labeling in effect on June 23, 2000. For further information, contact via direct mail, phone, or web site. Medical Information, Glaxo Wellcome Inc., PO Box 13398, Research Triangle Park, NC 27709. Healthcare Professionals (Medical Information): 800-334-0089. Patients (Customer Response Center): 1-888-825-5249. Glaxo Wellcome Corporate Web Site: www.glaxowellcome.com

Imitrex Nasal Spray—Cont.

to be embryolethal. Reproductive toxicity studies for sumatriptan by the intranasal route have not been conducted.

There are no adequate and well-controlled studies in pregnant women. Therefore, IMITREX Nasal Spray should be used during pregnancy only if the potential benefit justifies the potential risk to the fetus. In assessing this information, the following findings should be considered.

Embryolethality: When given orally or intravenously to pregnant rabbits daily throughout the period of organogenesis, sumatriptan caused embryolethality at doses at or close to those producing maternal toxicity. In the oral studies this dose was 100 mg/kg per day, and in the intravenous studies this dose was 2.0 mg/kg per day. The mechanism of the embryolethality is not known. The highest no-effect dose for embryolethality by the oral route was 50 mg/kg per day, which is approximately 48 times the maximum single recommended human intranasal dose of 20 mg on a mg/m^2 basis. By the intravenous route, the highest no-effect dose was 0.75 mg/kg per day, or approximately 0.7 times the maximum single recommended human intranasal dose of 20 mg on a mg/m^2 basis.

The intravenous administration of sumatriptan to pregnant rats throughout organogenesis at 12.5 mg/kg per day, the maximum dose tested, did not cause embryolethality. This dose is approximately 6 times the maximum single recommended human intranasal dose of 20 mg on a mg/m^2 basis. Additionally, in a study in rats given subcutaneous sumatriptan daily, prior to and throughout pregnancy, at 60 mg/kg per day, the maximum dose tested, there was no evidence of increased embryo/fetal lethality. This dose is equivalent to approximately 29 times the maximum recommended single human intranasal dose of 20 mg on a mg/m^2 basis.

Teratogenicity: Oral treatment of pregnant rats with sumatriptan during the period of organogenesis resulted in an increased incidence of blood vessel abnormalities (cervicothoracic and umbilical) at doses of approximately 250 mg/kg per day or higher. The highest no-effect dose was approximately 60 mg/kg per day, which is approximately 29 times the maximum single recommended human intranasal dose of 20 mg on a mg/m^2 basis. Oral treatment of pregnant rabbits with sumatriptan during the period of organogenesis resulted in an increased incidence of cervicothoracic vascular and skeletal abnormalities. The highest no-effect dose for these effects was 15 mg/kg per day, or approximately 14 times the maximum single recommended human intranasal dose of 20 mg on a mg/m^2 basis.

A study in which rats were dosed daily with oral sumatriptan prior to and throughout gestation demonstrated embryo/fetal toxicity (decreased body weight, decreased ossification, increased incidence of rib variations) and an increased incidence of a syndrome of malformations (short tail/short body and vertebral disorganization) at 500 mg/kg per day. The highest no-effect dose was 50 mg/kg per day, or approximately 24 times the maximum single recommended human intranasal dose of 20 mg on a mg/m^2 basis. In a study in rats dosed daily with subcutaneous sumatriptan prior to and throughout pregnancy, at a dose of 60 mg/kg per day, the maximum dose tested, there was no evidence of teratogenicity. This dose is equivalent to approximately 29 times the maximum recommended single human intranasal dose of 20 mg on a mg/m^2 basis.

Pup Deaths: Oral treatment of pregnant rats with sumatriptan during the period of organogenesis resulted in a decrease in pup survival between birth and postnatal day 4 at doses of approximately 250 mg/kg per day or higher. The highest no-effect dose for this effect was approximately 60 mg/kg per day, or 29 times the maximum single recommended human intranasal dose of 20 mg on a mg/m^2 basis.

Oral treatment of pregnant rats with sumatriptan from gestational day 17 through postnatal day 21 demonstrated a decrease in pup survival measured at postnatal days 2, 4, and 20 at the dose of 1000 mg/kg per day. The highest no-effect dose for this finding was 100 mg/kg per day, approximately 49 times the maximum single recommended human intranasal dose of 20 mg on a mg/m^2 basis. In a similar study in rats by the subcutaneous route there was no increase in pup death at 81 mg/kg per day, the highest dose tested, which is equivalent to 40 times the maximum single recommended human intranasal dose of 20 mg on a mg/m^2 basis.

To monitor fetal outcomes of pregnant women exposed to IMITREX, Glaxo Wellcome Inc. maintains a Sumatriptan Pregnancy Registry. Physicians are encouraged to register patients by calling (800) 336-2176.

Nursing Mothers: Sumatriptan is excreted in human breast milk. Therefore, caution should be exercised when considering the administration of IMITREX Nasal Spray to a nursing woman.

Pediatric Use: Safety and effectiveness of IMITREX Nasal Spray in pediatric patients have not been established.

Completed placebo-controlled clinical trials evaluating oral sumatriptan (25 to 100 mg) in pediatric patients aged 12 to 17 years enrolled a total of 701 adolescent migraineurs. These studies did not establish the efficacy of oral sumatriptan compared to placebo in the treatment of migraine in adolescents. Adverse events observed in these clinical trials were similar in nature to those reported in clinical trials in adults. The frequency of all adverse events in these patients appeared to be both dose- and age-dependent, with younger patients reporting events more commonly than older adolescents. Postmarketing experience includes a limited number of reports that describe pediatric patients who have experienced adverse events, some clinically serious, after use of subcutaneous sumatriptan and/or oral sumatriptan. These reports include events similar in nature to those reported rarely in adults. A myocardial infarct has been reported in a 14-year-old male following the use of oral sumatriptan; clinical signs occurred within 1 day of drug administration. Since clinical data to determine the frequency of serious adverse events in pediatric patients who might receive injectable, oral, or intranasal sumatriptan are not presently available, the use of sumatriptan in patients aged younger than 18 years is not recommended.

Geriatric Use: The use of sumatriptan in elderly patients is not recommended because elderly patients are more likely to have decreased hepatic function, they are at higher risk for CAD, and blood pressure increases may be more pronounced in the elderly (see WARNINGS).

ADVERSE REACTIONS

Serious cardiac events, including some that have been fatal, have occurred following the use of IMITREX Injection or Tablets. These events are extremely rare and most have been reported in patients with risk factors predictive of CAD. Events reported have included coronary artery vasospasm, transient myocardial ischemia, myocardial infarction, ventricular tachycardia, and ventricular fibrillation (see CONTRAINDICATIONS, WARNINGS, and PRECAUTIONS).

Significant hypertensive episodes, including hypertensive crises, have been reported on rare occasions in patients with or without a history of hypertension (see WARNINGS).

Incidence in Controlled Clinical Trials: Among 3653 patients treated with IMITREX Nasal Spray in active- and placebo-controlled clinical trials, less than 0.4% of patients withdrew for reasons related to adverse events. Table 2 lists adverse events that occurred in worldwide placebo-controlled clinical trials in 3419 migraineurs. The events cited reflect experience gained under closely monitored conditions of clinical trials in a highly selected patient population. In actual clinical practice or in other clinical trials, these frequency estimates may not apply, as the conditions of use, reporting behavior, and the kinds of patients treated may differ.

Only events that occurred at a frequency of 1% or more in the IMITREX Nasal Spray 20-mg treatment group and were more frequent in that group than in the placebo group are included in Table 2.

[See table 2 below]

Phonophobia also occurred in more than 1% of patients but was more frequent on placebo.

IMITREX Nasal Spray is generally well tolerated. Across all doses, most adverse reactions were mild and transient and did not lead to long-lasting effects. The incidence of adverse events in controlled clinical trials was not affected by gender, weight, or age of the patients; use of prophylactic medications; or presence of aura. There was insufficient data to assess the impact of race on the incidence of adverse events.

Other Events Observed in Association With the Administration of IMITREX Nasal Spray: In the paragraphs that follow, the frequencies of less commonly reported adverse clinical events are presented. Because the reports include events observed in open and uncontrolled studies, the role of IMITREX Nasal Spray in their causation cannot be reliably determined. Furthermore, variability associated with adverse event reporting, the terminology used to describe adverse events, etc., limit the value of the quantitative frequency estimates provided. Event frequencies are calculated as the number of patients who used IMITREX Nasal Spray (5, 10, or 20 mg in controlled and uncontrolled trials) and reported an event divided by the total number of patients (n = 3711) exposed to IMITREX Nasal Spray. All reported events are included except those already listed in the previous table, those too general to be informative, and those not reasonably associated with the use of the drug. Events are further classified within body system categories and enumerated in order of decreasing frequency using the following definitions: infrequent adverse events are those occurring in 1/100 to 1/1000 patients and rare adverse events are those occurring in fewer than 1/1000 patients.

Atypical Sensations: Infrequent were tingling, warm/hot sensation, numbness, pressure sensation, feeling strange, feeling of heaviness, feeling of tightness, paresthesia, cold sensation, and tight feeling in head. Rare were dysesthesia and prickling sensation.

Cardiovascular: Infrequent were flushing and hypertension (see WARNINGS), palpitations, tachycardia, changes in ECG, and arrhythmia (see WARNINGS and PRECAUTIONS). Rare were abdominal aortic aneurysm, hypotension, bradycardia, pallor, and phlebitis.

Chest Symptoms: Infrequent were chest tightness, chest discomfort, and chest pressure/heaviness (see PRECAUTIONS: General).

Ear, Nose, and Throat: Infrequent were disturbance of hearing and ear infection. Rare were otalgia and Meniere disease.

Endocrine and Metabolic: Infrequent was thirst. Rare were galactorrhea, hypothyroidism, and weight loss.

Eye: Infrequent were irritation of eyes and visual disturbance.

Gastrointestinal: Infrequent were abdominal discomfort, diarrhea, dysphagia, and gastroesophageal reflux. Rare were constipation, flatulence/eructation, hematemesis, intestinal obstruction, melena, gastroenteritis, colitis, hemorrhage of gastrointestinal tract, and pancreatitis.

Mouth and Teeth: Infrequent was disorder of mouth and tongue (e.g., burning of tongue, numbness of tongue, dry mouth).

Musculoskeletal: Infrequent were neck pain/stiffness, backache, weakness, joint symptoms, arthritis, and myalgia. Rare were muscle cramps, tetany, intervertebral disc disorder, and muscle stiffness.

Neurological: Infrequent were drowsiness/sedation, anxiety, sleep disturbances, tremors, syncope, shivers, chills, depression, agitation, sensation of lightness, and mental confusion. Rare were difficulty concentrating, hunger, lacrimation, memory disturbances, monoplegia/diplegia, apathy, disturbance of smell, disturbance of emotions, dysarthria, facial pain, intoxication, stress, decreased appetite, difficulty coordinating, euphoria, and neoplasm of pituitary.

Respiratory: Infrequent were dyspnea and lower respiratory tract infection. Rare was asthma.

Skin: Infrequent were rash/skin eruption, pruritus, and erythema. Rare were herpes, swelling of face, sweating, and peeling of skin.

Urogenital: Infrequent were dysuria, disorder of breasts, and dysmenorrhea. Rare were endometriosis and increased urination.

Miscellaneous: Infrequent were cough, edema, and fever. Rare were hypersensitivity, swelling of extremities, voice disturbances, difficulty in walking, and lymphadenopathy.

Other Events Observed in the Clinical Development of IMITREX: The following adverse events occurred in clinical trials with IMITREX Injection and IMITREX Tablets. Because the reports include events observed in open and uncontrolled studies, the role of IMITREX in their causation cannot be reliably determined. All reported events are included except those already listed, those too general to be informative, and those not reasonably associated with the use of the drug.

Breasts: Breast swelling; cysts, lumps, and masses of breasts; nipple discharge; primary malignant breast neoplasm; and tenderness.

Cardiovascular: Abnormal pulse, angina, atherosclerosis, cerebral ischemia, cerebrovascular lesion, heart block, peripheral cyanosis, pulsating sensations, Raynaud syndrome, thrombosis, transient myocardial ischemia, various transient ECG changes (nonspecific ST or T wave changes, prolongation of PR or QTc intervals, sinus arrhythmia, nonsustained ventricular premature beats, isolated junctional ectopic beats, atrial ectopic beats, delayed activation of the right ventricle), and vasodilation.

Ear, Nose, and Throat: Allergic rhinitis; ear, nose, and throat hemorrhage; external otitis; feeling of fullness in the ear(s); hearing disturbances; hearing loss; nasal inflammation; sensitivity to noise; sinusitis; tinnitus; and upper respiratory inflammation.

Endocrine and Metabolic: Dehydration; endocrine cysts, lumps, and masses; elevated thyrotropin stimulating hor-

Table 2: Treatment-Emergent Adverse Events Reported by at Least 1% of Patients in Controlled Migraine Trials

	Percent of Patients Reporting			
Adverse Event Type	Placebo (n = 704)	IMITREX 5 mg (n = 496)	IMITREX 10 mg (n = 1007)	IMITREX 20 mg (n = 1212)
Atypical sensations				
Burning sensation	0.1%	0.4%	0.6%	1.4%
Ear, nose, and throat				
Disorder/discomfort of nasal cavity/sinuses	2.4%	2.8%	2.5%	3.8%
Throat discomfort	0.9%	0.8%	1.8%	2.4%
Gastrointestinal				
Nausea and/or vomiting	11.3%	12.2%	11.0%	13.5%
Neurological				
Bad/unusual taste	1.7%	13.5%	19.3%	24.5%
Dizziness/vertigo	0.9%	1.0%	1.7%	1.4%

mone (TSH) levels; fluid disturbances; hyperglycemia; hypoglycemia; polydipsia; and weight gain.
Eye: Accommodation disorders, blindness and low vision, conjunctivitis, disorders of sclera, external ocular muscle disorders, eye edema and swelling, eye itching, eye hemorrhage, eye pain, keratitis, mydriasis, and vision alterations
Gastrointestinal: Abdominal distention, dental pain, disturbances of liver function tests, dyspeptic symptoms, feelings of gastrointestinal pressure, gallstones, gastric symptoms, gastritis, gastrointestinal pain, hypersalivation, hyposalivation, oral itching and irritation, peptic ulcer, retching, salivary gland swelling, and swallowing disorders.
Hematological Disorders: Anemia.
Injection Site Reaction
Miscellaneous: Contusions, fluid retention, hematoma, hypersensitivity to various agents, jaw discomfort, miscellaneous laboratory abnormalities, overdose, "serotonin agonist effect", and speech disturbance.
Musculoskeletal: Acquired musculoskeletal deformity, arthralgia and articular rheumatitis, muscle atrophy, muscle tiredness, musculoskeletal inflammation, need to flex calf muscles, rigidity, tightness, and various joint disturbances (pain, stiffness, swelling, ache).
Neurological: Aggressiveness, bradylogia, cluster headache, convulsions, detachment, disturbances of taste, drug abuse, dystonia, facial paralysis, globus hystericus, hallucinations, headache, heat sensitivity, hyperesthesia, hysteria, increased alertness, malaise/fatigue, migraine, motor dysfunction, myoclonia, neuralgia, neurotic disorders, paralysis, personality change, phobia, photophobia, psychomotor disorders, radiculopathy, raised intracranial pressure, relaxation, stinging sensations, transient hemiplegia, simultaneous hot and cold sensations, suicide, tickling sensations, twitching, and yawning.
Pain and Other Pressure Sensations: Chest pain, neck tightness/pressure, throat/jaw pain/tightness/pressure, and pain (location specified).
Respiratory: Breathing disorders, bronchitis, diseases of the lower respiratory tract, hiccoughs, and influenza.
Skin: Dry/scaly skin, eczema, seborrheic dermatitis, skin nodules, skin tenderness, tightness of skin, and wrinkling of skin.
Urogenital: Abortion, abnormal menstrual cycle, bladder inflammation, hematuria, inflammation of fallopian tubes, intermenstrual bleeding, menstruation symptoms, micturition disorders, renal calculus, urethritis, urinary frequency, and urinary infections.

Postmarketing Experience (Reports for Subcutaneous or Oral Sumatriptan): The following section enumerates potentially important adverse events that have occurred in clinical practice and that have been reported spontaneously to various surveillance systems. The events enumerated represent reports arising from both domestic and nondomestic use of oral or subcutaneous dosage forms of sumatriptan. The events enumerated include all except those already listed in the ADVERSE REACTIONS section above or those too general to be informative. Because the reports cite events reported spontaneously from worldwide postmarketing experience, frequency of events and the role of sumatriptan in their causation cannot be reliably determined. It is assumed, however, that systemic reactions following sumatriptan use are likely to be similar regardless of route of administration.
Blood: Hemolytic anemia, pancytopenia, thrombocytopenia.
Cardiovascular Atrial fibrillation, cardiomyopathy, colonic ischemia (see WARNINGS), Prinzmetal variant angina, pulmonary embolism, shock, thrombophlebitis.
Ear, Nose, and Throat: Deafness.
Eye: Ischemic optic neuropathy, retinal artery occlusion, retinal vein thrombosis.
Gastrointestinal: Ischemic colitis with rectal bleeding (see WARNINGS), xerostomia.
Hepatic: Elevated liver function tests.
Neurological: Central nervous system vasculitis, cerebrovascular accident, dysphasia, subarachnoid hemorrhage.
Non-Site Specific: Angioneurotic edema, cyanosis, death (see WARNINGS), temporal arteritis.
Psychiatry: Panic disorder.
Respiratory: Bronchospasm in patients with and without a history of asthma.
Skin: Exacerbation of sunburn, hypersensitivity reactions (allergic vasculitis, erythema, pruritus, rash, shortness of breath, urticaria; in addition, severe anaphylaxis/anaphylactoid reactions have been reported [see WARNINGS]), photosensitivity.
Urogenital: Acute renal failure.

DRUG ABUSE AND DEPENDENCE

One clinical study with IMITREX (sumatriptan succinate) Injection enrolling 12 patients with a history of substance abuse failed to induce subjective behavior and/or physiologic response ordinarily associated with drugs that have an established potential for abuse.

OVERDOSAGE

In clinical trials, the highest single doses of IMITREX Nasal Spray administered without significant adverse effects were 40 mg to 12 volunteers and 40 mg to 85 migraine patients, which is twice the highest single recommended dose. In addition, 12 volunteers were administered a total daily dose of 60 mg (20 mg 3 times daily) for 3.5 days without significant adverse events.

Overdose in animals has been fatal and has been heralded by convulsions, tremor, paralysis, inactivity, ptosis, erythema of the extremities, abnormal respiration, cyanosis, ataxia, mydriasis, salivation, and lacrimation. The elimination half-life of sumatriptan is about 2 hours (see CLINICAL PHARMACOLOGY), and therefore monitoring of patients after overdose with IMITREX Nasal Spray should continue for at least 10 hours or while symptoms or signs persist. It is unknown what effect hemodialysis or peritoneal dialysis has on the serum concentrations of sumatriptan.

DOSAGE AND ADMINISTRATION

In controlled clinical trials, single doses of 5, 10, or 20 mg of IMITREX Nasal Spray administered into one nostril were effective for the acute treatment of migraine in adults. A greater proportion of patients had headache response following a 20-mg dose than following a 5- or 10-mg dose (see CLINICAL TRIALS). Individuals may vary in response to doses of IMITREX Nasal Spray. The choice of dose should therefore be made on an individual basis, weighing the possible benefit of the 20-mg dose with the potential for a greater risk of adverse events. A 10-mg dose may be achieved by the administration of a single 5-mg dose in each nostril. There is evidence that doses above 20 mg do not provide a greater effect than 20 mg.

If the headache returns, the dose may be repeated once after 2 hours, not to exceed a total daily dose of 40 mg. The safety of treating an average of more than four headaches in a 30-day period has not been established.

HOW SUPPLIED

IMITREX Nasal Spray 5 mg (NDC 0173-0524-00) and 20 mg (NDC 0173-0523-00) are each supplied in boxes of 6 nasal spray devices. Each unit dose spray supplies 5 and 20 mg, respectively, of sumatriptan.

Store between 36° and 86°F (2° and 30°C). Protect from light.

ANIMAL TOXICOLOGY

Corneal Opacities: Dogs receiving oral sumatriptan developed corneal opacities and defects in the corneal epithelium. Corneal opacities were seen at the lowest dosage tested, 2 mg/kg per day, and were present after 1 month of treatment. Defects in the corneal epithelium were noted in a 60-week study. Earlier examinations for these toxicities were not conducted and no-effect doses were not established; however, the relative exposure at the lowest dose tested was approximately 5 times the human exposure after a 100-mg oral dose or 3 times the human exposure after a 6-mg subcutaneous dose or 22 times the human exposure after a single 20-mg intranasal dose. There is evidence of alterations in corneal appearance on the first day of intranasal dosing to dogs. Changes were noted at the lowest dose tested, which was approximately 2 times the maximum single human intranasal dose of 20 mg on a mg/m^2 basis.

PATIENT INFORMATION

The following wording is contained in a separate leaflet provided for patients.

Information for the Patient
IMITREX® (sumatriptan) Nasal Spray

Please read this leaflet carefully before you administer IMITREX Nasal Spray. This provides a summary of the information available on your medicine. Please do not throw away this leaflet until you have finished your medicine. You may need to read this leaflet again. This leaflet does not contain all the information on IMITREX Nasal Spray. For further information or advice, ask your doctor or pharmacist.

Information About Your Medicine:
The name of your medicine is IMITREX (sumatriptan) Nasal Spray. It can be obtained only by prescription from your doctor. The decision to use IMITREX Nasal Spray is one that you and your doctor should make jointly, taking into account your individual preferences and medical circumstances. If you have risk factors for heart disease (such as high blood pressure, high cholesterol, obesity, diabetes, smoking, strong family history of heart disease, or you are postmenopausal or a male over 40), you should tell your doctor, who should evaluate you for heart disease in order to determine if IMITREX is appropriate for you. Although the vast majority of those who have taken IMITREX have not experienced any significant side effects, some individuals have experienced serious heart problems and, rarely, considering the extensiveness of IMITREX use worldwide, deaths have been reported. In all but a few instances, however, serious problems occurred in people with known heart disease and it was not clear whether IMITREX was a contributory factor in these deaths.

1. The Purpose of Your Medicine:
IMITREX Nasal Spray is intended to relieve your migraine, but not to prevent or reduce the number of attacks you experience. Use IMITREX Nasal Spray only to treat an actual migraine attack.

2. Important Questions to Consider Before Using IMITREX Nasal Spray:
If the answer to any of the following questions is **YES** or if you do not know the answer, then please discuss it with your doctor before you use IMITREX Nasal Spray.

- Are you pregnant? Do you think you might be pregnant? Are you trying to become pregnant? Are you using inadequate contraception? Are you breastfeeding?
- Do you have any chest pain, heart disease, shortness of breath or irregular heartbeats? Have you had a heart attack?
- Do you have risk factors for heart disease (such as high blood pressure, high cholesterol, obesity, diabetes, smoking, strong family history of heart disease, or you are postmenopausal or a male over 40)?
- Have you had a stroke, transient ischemic attacks (TIAs), or Raynaud syndrome?
- Do you have high blood pressure?
- Have you ever had to stop taking this or any other medication because of an allergy or other problems?
- Are you taking any other migraine medications, including other 5-HT$_1$ agonists or any other medications containing ergotamine, dihydroergotamine, or methysergide?
- Are you taking any medication for depression (monoamine oxidase inhibitors or selective serotonin reuptake inhibitors [SSRIs])?
- Have you had, or do you have, any disease of the liver or kidney?
- Have you had, or do you have, epilepsy or seizures?
- Is this headache different from your usual migraine attacks?

Remember, if you answered **YES** to any of the above questions, then discuss it with your doctor.

3. The Use of IMITREX Nasal Spray During Pregnancy:
Do not use IMITREX Nasal Spray if you are pregnant, think you might be pregnant, are trying to become pregnant, or are not using adequate contraception, unless you have discussed this with your doctor.

4. How to Use IMITREX Nasal Spray:
Before using IMITREX Nasal Spray, see the enclosed instruction pamphlet. For adults, the usual dose is a single nasal spray administered into 1 nostril. If your headache comes back, a second nasal spray may be administered anytime after 2 hours of administering the first spray. For any attack where you have no response to the first nasal spray, do not take a second nasal spray without first consulting with your doctor. Do not administer more than a total of 40 mg of IMITREX Nasal Spray in any 24-hour period. The effects of long-term repeated use of IMITREX Nasal Spray on the surfaces of the nose and throat have not been specifically studied. The safety of treating an average of more than 4 headaches in a 30-day period has not been established.

5. Side Effects to Watch for:

- Some patients experience pain or tightness in the chest or throat when using IMITREX Nasal Spray. If this happens to you, then discuss it with your doctor before using any more IMITREX Nasal Spray. If the chest pain is severe or does not go away, call your doctor immediately.
- If you have sudden and/or severe abdominal pain following IMITREX Nasal Spray, call your doctor immediately.
- Shortness of breath; wheeziness; heart throbbing; swelling of eyelids, face, or lips; or a skin rash, skin lumps, or hives happens rarely. If it happens to you, then tell your doctor immediately. Do not take any more IMITREX Nasal Spray unless your doctor tells you to do so.
- Some people may have feelings of tingling, heat, flushing (redness of face lasting a short time), heaviness or pressure after treatment with IMITREX Nasal Spray. A few people may feel drowsy, dizzy, tired, sick, or may experience nasal irritation. Tell your doctor of these symptoms at your next visit.
- If you feel unwell in any other way or have any symptoms that you do not understand, you should contact your doctor immediately.

6. What to Do if an Overdose Is Taken:
If you have taken more medication than you have been told, contact either your doctor, hospital emergency department, or nearest poison control center immediately.

7. Storing Your Medicine:
Keep your medicine in a safe place where children cannot reach it. It may be harmful to children. Store your medication away from heat and light. Do not store at temperatures above 86°F (30°C), or below 36°F (2°C). If your medication has expired (the expiration date is printed on the treatment pack), throw it away as instructed. If your doctor decides to stop your treatment, do not keep any leftover medicine unless your doctor tells you to. Throw away your medicine as instructed.

Glaxo Wellcome Inc., Research Triangle Park, NC 27709
US Patent Nos. 4,816,470; 5,037,845; and 5,554,639

September 1999/RL-757

Shown in Product Identification Guide, page 315

IMITREX® ℞
[*ĭm ′-ĭ-trĕx ″*]
(sumatriptan succinate)
Tablets

DESCRIPTION

IMITREX Tablets contain sumatriptan (as the succinate), a selective 5-hydroxytryptamine$_1$ receptor subtype agonist.

Continued on next page

This product information is based on labeling in effect on June 23, 2000. For further information, contact via direct mail, phone, or web site. Medical Information, Glaxo Wellcome Inc., PO Box 13398, Research Triangle Park, NC 27709. Healthcare Professionals (Medical Information): 800-334-0089. Patients (Customer Response Center): 1-888-825-5249. Glaxo Wellcome Corporate Web Site: www.glaxowellcome.com

Imitrex Tablets—Cont.

Sumatriptan succinate is chemically designated as 3-[2-(dimethylamino)ethyl]-N-methyl-indole-5-methanesulfonamide succinate (1:1).

The empirical formula is $C_{14}H_{21}N_3O_2S{\bullet}C_4H_6O_4$, representing a molecular weight of 413.5. Sumatriptan succinate is a white to off-white powder that is readily soluble in water and in saline. Each IMITREX Tablet for oral administration contains 35 or 70 mg of sumatriptan succinate equivalent to 25 or 50 mg of sumatriptan, respectively. Each tablet also contains the inactive ingredients croscarmellose sodium, lactose, magnesium stearate, microcrystalline cellulose, and titanium dioxide dye.

CLINICAL PHARMACOLOGY

Mechanism of Action: Sumatriptan is an agonist for a vascular 5-hydroxytryptamine$_1$ receptor subtype (probably a member of the 5-HT_{1D} family) having only a weak affinity for 5-HT_{1A}, 5-HT_{5A}, and 5-HT_7 receptors and no significant affinity (as measured using standard radioligand binding assays) or pharmacological activity at 5-HT_2, 5-HT_3, or 5-HT_4 receptor subtypes or at alpha$_1$-, alpha$_2$-, or beta-adrenergic, dopamine$_1$, dopamine$_2$, muscarinic, or benzodiazepine receptors.

The vascular 5-HT_1 receptor subtype that sumatriptan activates is present on cranial arteries in both dog and primate, on the human basilar artery, and in the vasculature of human dura mater and mediates vasoconstriction. This action in humans correlates with the relief of migraine headache. In addition to causing vasoconstriction, experimental data from animal studies show that sumatriptan also activates 5-HT_1 receptors on peripheral terminals of the trigeminal nerve innervating cranial blood vessels. Such an action may also contribute to the antimigrainous effect of sumatriptan in humans.

In the anesthetized dog, sumatriptan selectively reduces the carotid arterial blood flow with little or no effect on arterial blood pressure or total peripheral resistance. In the cat, sumatriptan selectively constricts the carotid arteriovenous anastomoses while having little effect on blood flow or resistance in cerebral or extracerebral tissues.

Pharmacokinetics: The mean maximum concentration following oral dosing with 25 mg is 18 ng/mL (range, 7 to 47 ng/mL) and 51 ng/mL (range, 28 to 100 ng/mL) following oral dosing with 100 mg of sumatriptan. This compares with a C_{max} of 5 and 16 ng/mL following dosing with a 5- and 20-mg intranasal dose, respectively. The mean C_{max} following a 6-mg subcutaneous injection is 71 ng/mL (range, 49 to 110 ng/mL). The bioavailability is approximately 15%, primarily due to presystemic metabolism and partly due to incomplete absorption. The C_{max} is similar during a migraine attack and during a migraine-free period, but the t_{max} is slightly later during the attack, approximately 2.5 hours compared to 2.0 hours. When given as a single dose, sumatriptan displays dose proportionality in its extent of absorption (area under the curve [AUC]) over the dose range of 25 to 200 mg, but the C_{max} after 100 mg is approximately 25% less than expected (based on the 25-mg dose). Food has no significant effect on the bioavailability of sumatriptan, but delays the t_{max} slightly (by about 0.5 hours).

Plasma protein binding is low (14% to 21%). The effect of sumatriptan on the protein binding of other drugs has not been evaluated, but would be expected to be minor, given the low rate of protein binding. The apparent volume of distribution is 2.4 L/kg.

The elimination half-life of sumatriptan is approximately 2.5 hours. Radiolabeled ^{14}C-sumatriptan administered orally is largely renally excreted (about 60%) with about 40% found in the feces. Most of the radiolabeled compound excreted in the urine is the major metabolite, indole acetic acid (IAA), which is inactive, or the IAA glucuronide. Only 3% of the dose can be recovered as unchanged sumatriptan. In vitro studies with human microsomes suggest that sumatriptan is metabolized by monoamine oxidase (MAO), predominantly the A isoenzyme, and inhibitors of that enzyme may alter sumatriptan pharmacokinetics to increase systemic exposure. No significant effect was seen with an MAO-B inhibitor (see CONTRAINDICATIONS, WARNINGS, and PRECAUTIONS: Drug Interactions).

Special Populations: ***Renal Impairment:*** The effect of renal impairment on the pharmacokinetics of sumatriptan has not been examined, but little clinical effect would be expected as sumatriptan is largely metabolized to an inactive substance.

Hepatic Impairment: The liver plays an important role in the presystemic clearance of orally administered sumatriptan. Accordingly, the bioavailability of sumatriptan following oral administration may be markedly increased in patients with liver disease. In 1 small study of hepatically impaired patients (n = 8) matched for sex, age, and weight with healthy subjects, the hepatically impaired patients had an approximately 70% increase in AUC and C_{max} and a t_{max} 40 minutes earlier compared to the healthy subjects (see DOSAGE AND ADMINISTRATION).

Age: The pharmacokinetics of oral sumatriptan in the elderly (mean age; 72 years, 2 males and 4 females) and in patients with migraine (mean age; 38 years, 25 males and 155 females) were similar to that in healthy male subjects (mean age, 30 years) (see PRECAUTIONS: Geriatric Use).

Gender: In a study comparing females to males, no pharmacokinetic differences were observed between genders for AUC, C_{max}, t_{max}, and half-life.

Race: The systemic clearance and C_{max} of sumatriptan were similar in black (n = 34) and Caucasian (n = 38) healthy male subjects.

Drug Interactions: ***Monoamine Oxidase Inhibitors (MAOI):*** Treatment with MAO-A inhibitors generally leads to an increase of sumatriptan plasma levels (see CONTRAINDICATIONS and PRECAUTIONS).

Due to gut and hepatic metabolic first-pass effects, the increase of systemic exposure after coadministration of an MAO-A inhibitor with oral sumatriptan is greater than after coadministration of the MAOI with subcutaneous sumatriptan. In a study of 14 healthy females, pretreatment with an MAO-A inhibitor decreased the clearance of subcutaneous sumatriptan. Under the conditions of this experiment, the result was a 2-fold increase in the area under the sumatriptan plasma concentration x time curve (AUC), corresponding to a 40% increase in elimination half-life. This interaction was not evident with an MAO-B inhibitor.

A small study evaluating the effect of pretreatment with an MAO-A inhibitor on the bioavailability from a 25-mg oral sumatriptan tablet resulted in an approximately 7-fold increase in systemic exposure.

Alcohol: Alcohol consumed 30 minutes prior to sumatriptan ingestion had no effect on the pharmacokinetics of sumatriptan.

CLINICAL STUDIES

The efficacy of IMITREX Tablets in the acute treatment of migraine headaches was demonstrated in 3, randomized, double-blind, placebo-controlled studies. Patients enrolled in these 3 studies were predominately female (87%) and Caucasian (97%), with a mean age of 40 (range of 18 to 65). Patients were instructed to treat a moderate to severe headache. Headache response, defined as a reduction in headache severity from moderate or severe pain to mild or no pain, was assessed up to 4 hours after dosing. Associated symptoms such as nausea, photophobia, and phonophobia were also assessed. Maintenance of response was assessed for up to 24 hours postdose. A second dose of IMITREX Tablets or other medication was allowed 4 to 24 hours after the initial treatment for recurrent headache. Acetaminophen was offered to patients in Studies 2 and 3 beginning at 2 hours after initial treatment if the migraine pain had not improved or worsened. Additional medications were allowed 4 to 24 hours after the initial treatment for recurrent headache or as rescue in all 3 studies. The frequency and time to use of these additional treatments were also determined. In all studies, doses of 25, 50, and 100 mg were compared to placebo in the treatment of migraine attacks. In 1 study, doses of 25, 50, and 100 mg were also compared to each other.

In all 3 trials, the percentage of patients achieving headache response 2 and 4 hours after treatment was significantly greater among patients receiving IMITREX Tablets at all doses compared to those who received placebo. In 1 of the 3 studies, there was a statistically significant greater percentage of patients with headache response at 2 and 4 hours in the 50- or 100-mg group when compared to the 25-mg dose groups. There were no statistically significant differences between the 50- and 100-mg dose groups in any study. The results from the 3 controlled clinical trials are summarized in Table 1.

Comparisons of drug performance based upon results obtained in different clinical trials are never reliable. Because studies are conducted at different times, with different samples of patients, by different investigators, employing different criteria and/or different interpretations of the same criteria, under different conditions (dose, dosing regimen, etc.), quantitative estimates of treatment response and the timing of response may be expected to vary considerably from study to study.

[See table 1 below]

The estimated probability of achieving an initial headache response over the 4 hours following treatment is depicted in Figure 1.

Figure 1: Estimated Probability of Achieving Initial Headache Response Within 240 Minutes*

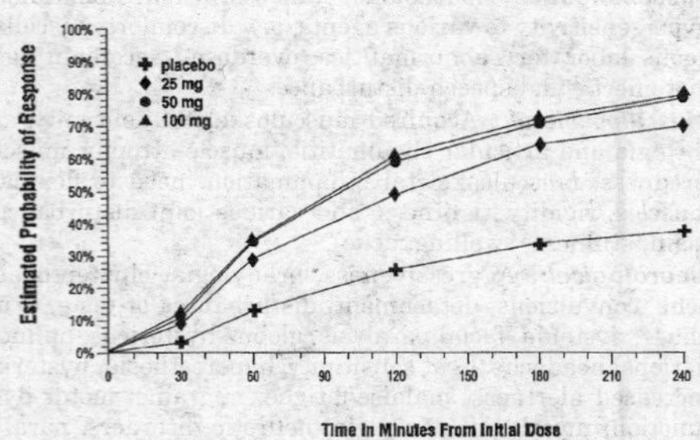

* The figure shows the probability over time of obtaining headache response (no or mild pain) following treatment with sumatriptan. The averages displayed are based on pooled data from the 3 clinical controlled trials providing evidence of efficacy. Kaplan-Meier plot with patients not achieving response and/or taking rescue within 240 minutes censored to 240 minutes.

For patients with migraine-associated nausea, photophobia, and/or phonophobia at baseline, there was a lower incidence of these symptoms at 2 hours (Study 1) and at 4 hours (Studies 1, 2, and 3) following administration of IMITREX Tablets compared to placebo.

As early as 2 hours in Studies 2 and 3 or 4 hours in Study 1, through 24 hours following the initial dose of study treatment, patients were allowed to use additional treatment for pain relief in the form of a second dose of study treatment or other medication. The estimated probability of patients taking a second dose or other medication for migraine over the 24 hours following the initial dose of study treatment is summarized in Figure 2.

Figure 2: The Estimated Probability of Patients Taking a Second Dose or Other Medication for Migraine Over the 24 Hours Following the Initial Dose of Study Treatment*

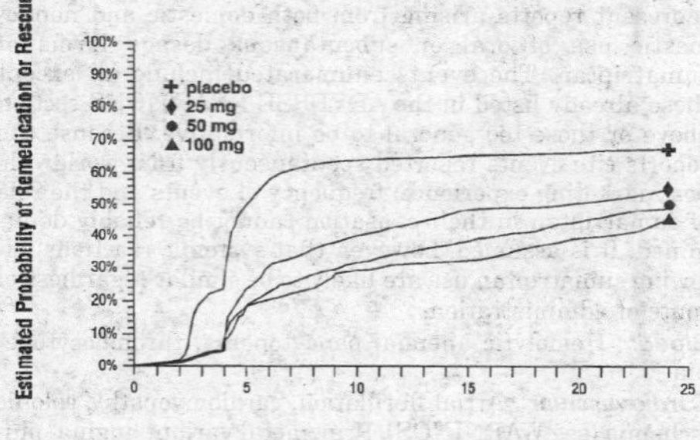

* Kaplan-Meier plot based on data obtained in the 3 clinical controlled trials providing evidence of efficacy with patients not using additional treatments censored to 24 hours. Plot also includes patients who had no response to the initial dose. No remedication was allowed within 2 hours postdose.

There is evidence that doses above 50 mg do not provide a greater effect than 50 mg. There was no evidence to suggest that treatment with sumatriptan was associated with an increase in the severity of recurrent headaches. The efficacy of IMITREX Tablets was unaffected by presence of aura; duration of headache prior to treatment; gender, age, or weight of the patient; relationship to menses; or concomitant use of common migraine prophylactic drugs (e.g., beta-blockers, calcium channel blockers, tricyclic antidepressants). There were insufficient data to assess the impact of race on efficacy.

INDICATIONS AND USAGE

IMITREX Tablets are indicated for the acute treatment of migraine attacks with or without aura in adults.

IMITREX Tablets are not intended for the prophylactic therapy of migraine or for use in the management of hemiplegic or basilar migraine (see CONTRAINDICATIONS). Safety and effectiveness of IMITREX Tablets have not been established for cluster headache, which is present in an older, predominantly male population.

CONTRAINDICATIONS

IMITREX Tablets should not be given to patients with history, symptoms, or signs of ischemic cardiac, cerebrovascular, or peripheral vascular syndromes. In addition, patients with other significant underlying cardiovascular diseases should not receive IMITREX Tablets. Ischemic cardiac syndromes include, but are not limited to, angina pectoris of any type (e.g., stable angina of effort and vasospastic forms of angina such as the Prinzmetal variant), all forms of myocardial infarction, and silent myocardial ischemia.

Table 1: Percentage of Patients With Headache Response (No or Mild Pain) 2 and 4 Hours Following Treatment

	Placebo		IMITREX Tablets 25 mg		IMITREX Tablets 50 mg		IMITREX Tablets 100 mg	
	2 hr	4 hr	2 hr	4 hr	2 hr	4 hr	2 hr	4 hr
Study 1	27%	38%	52%*	67%*	61%*†	78%*†	62%*†	79%*†
	(n = 94)		(n = 298)		(n = 296)		(n = 296)	
Study 2	26%	38%	52%*	70%*	50%*	68%*	56%*	71%*
	(n = 65)		(n = 66)		(n = 62)		(n = 66)	
Study 3	17%	19%	52%*	65%*	54%*	72%*	57%*	78%*
	(n = 47)		(n = 48)		(n = 46)		(n = 46)	

* $P<0.05$ in comparison with placebo.
† $P<0.05$ in comparison with 25 mg.

Cerebrovascular sydromes include, but are not limited to, strokes of any type as well as transient ischemic attacks. Peripheral vascular disease includes, but is not limited to, ischemic bowel disease (see WARNINGS).

Because IMITREX Tablets may increase blood pressure, they should not be given to patients with uncontrolled hypertension.

Concurrent administration of MAO-A inhibitors or use within 2 weeks of discontinuation of MAO-A inhibitor therapy is contraindicated (see CLINICAL PHARMACOLOGY: Drug Interactions and PRECAUTIONS: Drug Interactions).

IMITREX Tablets should not be administered to patients with hemiplegic or basilar migraine.

IMITREX Tablets and any ergotamine-containing or ergot-type medication (like dihydroergotamine or methysergide) should not be used within 24 hours of each other, nor should IMITREX and another 5-HT_1 agonist.

IMITREX Tablets are contraindicated in patients with hypersensitivity to sumatriptan or any of their components.

IMITREX Tablets are contraindicated in patients with severe hepatic impairment.

WARNINGS

IMITREX Tablets should only be used where a clear diagnosis of migraine headache has been established.

Risk of Myocardial Ischemia and/or Infarction and Other Adverse Cardiac Events: Sumatriptan should not be given to patients with documented ischemic or vasospastic coronary artery disease (CAD) (see CONTRAINDICATIONS). It is strongly recommended that sumatriptan not be given to patients in whom unrecognized CAD is predicted by the presence of risk factors (e.g., hypertension, hypercholesterolemia, smoker, obesity, diabetes, strong family history of CAD, female with surgical or physiological menopause, or male over 40 years of age) unless a cardiovascular evaluation provides satisfactory clinical evidence that the patient is reasonably free of coronary artery and ischemic myocardial disease or other significant underlying cardiovascular disease. The sensitivity of cardiac diagnostic procedures to detect cardiovascular disease or predisposition to coronary artery vasospasm is modest, at best. If, during the cardiovascular evaluation, the patient's medical history or electrocardiographic investigations reveal findings indicative of, or consistent with, coronary artery vasospasm or myocardial ischemia, sumatriptan should not be administered (see CONTRAINDICATIONS).

For patients with risk factors predictive of CAD, who are determined to have a satisfactory cardiovascular evaluation, it is strongly recommended that administration of the first dose of sumatriptan tablets take place in the setting of a physician's office or similar medically staffed and equipped facility unless the patient has previously received sumatriptan. Because cardiac ischemia can occur in the absence of clinical symptoms, consideration should be given to obtaining on the first occasion of use an electrocardiogram (ECG) during the interval immediately following IMITREX Tablets, in these patients with risk factors.

It is recommended that patients who are intermittent long-term users of sumatriptan and who have or acquire risk factors predictive of CAD, as described above, undergo periodic interval cardiovascular evaluation as they continue to use sumatriptan.

The systematic approach described above is intended to reduce the likelihood that patients with unrecognized cardiovascular disease will be inadvertently exposed to sumatriptan.

Drug-Associated Cardiac Events and Fatalities: Serious adverse cardiac events, including acute myocardial infarction, life-threatening disturbances of cardiac rhythm, and death have been reported within a few hours following the administration of IMITREX® (sumatriptan succinate) Injection or IMITREX Tablets. Considering the extent of use of sumatriptan in patients with migraine, the incidence of these events is extremely low.

The fact that sumatriptan can cause coronary vasospasm, that some of these events have occurred in patients with no prior cardiac disease history and with documented absence of CAD, and the close proximity of the events to sumatriptan use support the conclusion that some of these cases were caused by the drug. In many cases, however, where there has been known underlying coronary artery disease, the relationship is uncertain.

Premarketing Experience With Sumatriptan: Of 6348 patients with migraine who participated in premarketing controlled and uncontrolled clinical trials of oral sumatriptan, 2 experienced clinical adverse events shortly after receiving oral sumatriptan that may have reflected coronary vasospasm. Neither of these adverse events was associated with a serious clinical outcome.

Among the more than 1900 patients with migraine who participated in premarketing controlled clinical trials of subcutaneous sumatriptan, there were 8 patients who sustained clinical events during or shortly after receiving sumatriptan that may have reflected coronary artery vasospasm. Six of these 8 patients had ECG changes consistent with transient ischemia, but without accompanying clinical symptoms or signs. Of these 8 patients, 4 had either findings suggestive of CAD or risk factors predictive of CAD prior to study enrollment.

Among approximately 4000 patients with migraine who participated in premarketing controlled and uncontrolled clinical trials of sumatriptan nasal spray, 1 patient experienced an asymptomatic subendocardial infarction possibly subsequent to a coronary vasospastic event.

Postmarketing Experience With Sumatriptan: Serious cardiovascular events, some resulting in death, have been reported in association with the use of IMITREX Injection or IMITREX Tablets. The uncontrolled nature of postmarketing surveillance, however, makes it impossible to determine definitively the proportion of the reported cases that were actually caused by sumatriptan or to reliably assess causation in individual cases. On clinical grounds, the longer the latency between the administration of IMITREX and the onset of the clinical event, the less likely the association is to be causative. Accordingly, interest has focused on events begining within 1 hour of the administration of IMITREX. Cardiac events that have been observed to have onset within 1 hour of sumatriptan administration include: coronary artery vasospasm, transient ischemia, myocardial infarction, ventricular tachycardia and ventricular fibrillation, cardiac arrest, and death.

Some of these events occurred in patients who had no findings of CAD and appear to represent consequences of coronary artery vasospasm. However, among domestic reports of serious cardiac events within 1 hour of sumatriptan administration, almost all of the patients had risk factors predictive of CAD and the presence of significant underlying CAD was established in most cases (see CONTRAINDICATIONS).

Drug-Associated Cerebrovascular Events and Fatalities: Cerebral hemorrhage, subarachnoid hemorrhage, stroke, and other cerebrovascular events have been reported in patients treated with oral or subcutaneous sumatriptan, and some have resulted in fatalities. The relationship of sumatriptan to these events is uncertain. In a number of cases, it appears possible that the cerebrovascular events were primary, sumatriptan having been administered in the incorrect belief that the symptoms experienced were a consequence of migraine when they were not. As with other acute migraine therapies, before treating headaches in patients not previously diagnosed as migraineurs, and in migraineurs who present with atypical symptoms, care should be taken to exclude other potentially serious neurological conditions. It should also be noted that patients with migraine may be at increased risk of certain cerebrovascular events (e.g., cerebrovascular accident, transient ischemic attack).

Other Vasospasm-Related Events: Sumatriptan may cause vasospastic reactions other than coronary artery vasospasm. Both peripheral vascular ischemia and colonic ischemia with abdominal pain and bloody diarrhea have been reported.

Increase in Blood Pressure: Significant elevation in blood pressure, including hypertensive crisis, have been reported on rare occasions in patients with and without a history of hypertension. Sumatriptan is contraindicated in patients with uncontrolled hypertension (see CONTRAINDICATIONS). Sumatriptan should be administered with caution to patients with controlled hypertension as transient increases in blood pressure and peripheral vascular resistance have been observed in a small proportion of patients.

Concomitant Drug Use: In patients taking MAO-A inhibitors, sumatriptan plasma levels attained after treatment with recommended doses are 7-fold higher following oral administration than those obtained under other conditions. Accordingly, the coadministration of IMITREX Tablets and an MAO-A inhibitor is contraindicated (see CLINICAL PHARMACOLOGY and CONTRAINDICATIONS).

Hypersensitivity: Hypersensitivity (anaphylaxis/anaphylactoid) reactions have occurred on rare occasions in patients receiving sumatriptan. Such reactions can be life threatening or fatal. In general, hypersensitivity reactions to drugs are more likely to occur in individuals with a history of sensitivity to multiple allergens (see CONTRAINDICATIONS).

PRECAUTIONS

General: Chest discomfort and jaw or neck tightness have been reported following use of IMITREX Tablets and have also been reported infrequently following administration of IMITREX Nasal Spray. Chest, jaw, or neck tightness is relatively common after administration of IMITREX Injection. Only rarely have these symptoms been associated with ischemic ECG changes. However, because sumatriptan may cause coronary artery vasospasm, patients who experience signs or symptoms suggestive of angina following sumatriptan should be evaluated for the presence of CAD or a predisposition to Prinzmetal variant angina before receiving additional doses of sumatriptan, and should be monitored electrocardiographically if dosing is resumed and similar symptoms recur. Similarly, patients who experience other symptoms or signs suggestive of decreased arterial flow, such as ischemic bowel syndrome or Raynaud syndrome following sumatriptan should be evaluated for atherosclerosis or predisposition to vasospasm (see WARNINGS).

IMITREX should also be administered with caution to patients with diseases that may alter the absorption, metabolism, or excretion of drugs, such as impaired hepatic or renal function.

There have been rare reports of seizure following administration of sumatriptan. Sumatriptan should be used with caution in patients with a history of epilepsy or structural brain lesions that lower their seizure threshold.

Care should be taken to exclude other potentially serious neurologic conditions before treating headache in patients not previously diagnosed with migraine headache or who experience a headache that is atypical for them. There have been rare reports where patients received sumatriptan for severe headaches that were subsequently shown to have been secondary to an evolving neurologic lesion (see WARNINGS).

For a given attack, if a patient does not respond to the first dose of sumatriptan, the diagnosis of migraine should be reconsidered before administration of a second dose.

Binding to Melanin-Containing Tissues: In rats treated with a single subcutaneous dose (0.5 mg/kg) or oral dose (2 mg/kg) of radiolabeled sumatriptan, the elimination half-life of radioactivity from the eye was 15 and 23 days, respectively, suggesting that sumatriptan and/or its metabolites bind to the melanin of the eye. Because there could be an accumulation in melanin-rich tissues over time, this raises the possibility that sumatriptan could cause toxicity in these tissues after extended use. However, no effects on the retina related to treatment with sumatriptan were noted in any of the oral or subcutaneous toxicity studies. Although no systematic monitoring of ophthalmologic function was undertaken in clinical trials, and no specific recommendations for ophthalmologic monitoring are offered, prescribers should be aware of the possibility of long-term ophthalmologic effects.

Corneal Opacities: Sumatriptan causes corneal opacities and defects in the corneal epithelium in dogs; this raises the possibility that these changes may occur in humans. While patients were not systematically evaluated for these changes in clinical trials, and no specific recommendations for monitoring are being offered, prescribers should be aware of the possibility of these changes (see ANIMAL TOXICOLOGY).

Information for Patients: See PATIENT INFORMATION at the end of this labeling for the text of the separate leaflet provided for patients.

Laboratory Tests: No specific laboratory tests are recommended for monitoring patients prior to and/or after treatment with sumatriptan.

Drug Interactions: Ergot-containing drugs have been reported to cause prolonged vasospastic reactions. Because there is a theoretical basis that these effects may be additive, use of ergotamine-containing or ergot-type medications (like dihydroergotamine or methysergide) and sumatriptan within 24 hours of each other should be avoided (see CONTRAINDICATIONS).

MAO-A inhibitors reduce sumatriptan clearance, significantly increasing systemic exposure. Therefore, the use of IMITREX Tablets in patients receiving MAO-A inhibitors is contraindicated (see CLINICAL PHARMACOLOGY and CONTRAINDICATIONS).

Selective serotonin reuptake inhibitors (SSRIs) (e.g., fluoxetine, fluvoxamine, paroxetine, sertraline) have been reported, rarely, to cause weakness, hyperreflexia, and incoordination when coadministered with sumatriptan. If concomitant treatment with sumatriptan and an SSRI is clinically warranted, appropriate observation of the patient is advised.

Drug/Laboratory Test Interactions: IMITREX Tablets are not known to interfere with commonly employed clinical laboratory tests.

Carcinogenesis, Mutagenesis, Impairment of Fertility: ***Carcinogenesis:*** In carcinogenicity studies, rats and mice were given sumatriptan by oral gavage (rats, 104 weeks) or drinking water (mice, 78 weeks). Average exposures achieved in mice receiving the highest dose (target dose of 160 mg/kg per day) were approximately 40 times the exposure attained in humans after the maximum recommended single oral dose of 100 mg. The highest dose administered to rats (160 mg/kg per day, reduced from 360 mg/kg per day during week 21) was approximately 15 times the maximum recommended single human oral dose of 100 mg on a mg/m^2 basis. There was no evidence of an increase in tumors in either species related to sumatriptan administration.

Mutagenesis: Sumatriptan was not mutagenic in the presence or absence of metabolic activation when tested in 2 gene mutation assays (the Ames test and the in vitro mammalian Chinese hamster V79/HGPRT assay). In 2 cytogenetics assays (the in vitro human lymphocyte assay and the in vivo rat micronucleus assay) sumatriptan was not associated with clastogenic activity.

Impairment of Fertility: In a study in which male and female rats were dosed daily with oral sumatriptan prior to and throughout the mating period, there was a treatment-related decrease in fertility secondary to a decrease in mating in animals treated with 50 and 500 mg/kg per day. The highest no-effect dose for this finding was 5 mg/kg per day, or approximately one half of the maximum recommended single human oral dose of 100 mg on a mg/m^2 basis. It is not clear whether the problem is associated with treatment of the males or females or both combined. In a similar study by the subcutaneous route there was no evidence of impaired

Continued on next page

This product information is based on labeling in effect on June 23, 2000. For further information, contact via direct mail, phone, or web site. Medical Information, Glaxo Wellcome Inc., PO Box 13398, Research Triangle Park, NC 27709. Healthcare Professionals (Medical Information): 800-334-0089. Patients (Customer Response Center): 1-888-825-5249. Glaxo Wellcome Corporate Web Site: www.glaxowellcome.com

Imitrex Tablets—Cont.

fertility at 60 mg/kg per day, the maximum dose tested, which is equivalent to approximately 6 times the maximum recommended single human oral dose of 100 mg on a mg/m^2 basis.

Pregnancy: Pregnancy Category C. In reproductive toxicity studies in rats and rabbits, oral treatment with sumatriptan was associated with embryolethality, fetal abnormalities, and pup mortality. When administered by the intravenous route to rabbits, sumatriptan has been shown to be embryolethal. There are no adequate and well-controlled studies in pregnant women. Therefore, IMITREX should be used during pregnancy only if the potential benefit justifies the potential risk to the fetus. In assessing this information, the following findings should be considered.

Embryolethality: When given orally or intravenously to pregnant rabbits daily throughout the period of organogenesis, sumatriptan caused embryolethality at doses at or close to those producing maternal toxicity. In the oral studies this dose was 100 mg/kg per day and in the intravenous studies this dose was 2.0 mg/kg per day. The mechanism of the embryolethality is not known. The highest no-effect dose for embryolethality by the oral route was 50 mg/kg per day, which is approximately 9 times the maximum single recommended human oral dose of 100 mg on a mg/m^2 basis. By the intravenous route, the highest no-effect dose was 0.75 mg/kg per day, or approximately one tenth of the maximum single recommended human oral dose of 100 mg on a mg/m^2 basis.

The intravenous administration of sumatriptan to pregnant rats throughout organogenesis at 12.5 mg/kg per day, the maximum dose tested, did not cause embryolethality. This dose is equivalent to the maximum single recommended human oral dose of 100 mg on a mg/m^2 basis. Additionally, in a study in rats given subcutaneous sumatriptan daily prior to and throughout pregnancy at 60 mg/kg per day, the maximum dose tested, there was no evidence of increased embryo/fetal lethality. This dose is equivalent to approximately 6 times the maximum recommended single human oral dose of 100 mg on a mg/m^2 basis.

Teratogenicity: Oral treatment of pregnant rats with sumatriptan during the period of organogenesis resulted in an increased incidence of blood vessel abnormalities (cervicothoracic and umbilical) at doses of approximately 250 mg/kg per day or higher. The highest no-effect dose was approximately 60 mg/kg per day, which is approximately 6 times the maximum single recommended human oral dose of 100 mg on a mg/m^2 basis. Oral treatment of pregnant rabbits with sumatriptan during the period of organogenesis resulted in an increased incidence of cervicothoracic vascular and skeletal abnormalities. The highest no-effect dose for these effects was 15 mg/kg per day, or approximately 3 times the maximum single recommended human oral dose of 100 mg on a mg/m^2 basis.

A study in which rats were dosed daily with oral sumatriptan prior to and throughout gestation demonstrated embryo/fetal toxicity (decreased body weight, decreased ossification, increased incidence of rib variations) and an increased incidence of a syndrome of malformations (short tail/short body and vertebral disorganization) at 500 mg/kg per day. The highest no-effect dose was 50 mg/kg per day, or approximately 5 times the maximum single recommended human oral dose of 100 mg on a mg/m^2 basis. In a study in rats dosed daily with subcutaneous sumatriptan prior to and throughout pregnancy, at a dose of 60 mg/kg per day, the maximum dose tested, there was no evidence of teratogenicity. This dose is equivalent to approximately 6 times the maximum recommended single human oral dose of 100 mg on a mg/m^2 basis.

Pup Deaths: Oral treatment of pregnant rats with sumatriptan during the period of organogenesis resulted in a decrease in pup survival between birth and postnatal day 4 at doses of approximately 250 mg/kg per day or higher. The highest no-effect dose for this effect was approximately 60 mg/kg per day, or 6 times the maximum single recommended human oral dose of 100 mg on a mg/m^2 basis.

Oral treatment of pregnant rats with sumatriptan from gestational day 17 through postnatal day 21 demonstrated a decrease in pup survival measured at postnatal days 2, 4, and 20 at the dose of 1000 mg/kg per day. The highest no-effect dose for this finding was 100 mg/kg per day, approximately 10 times the maximum single recommended human oral dose of 100 mg on a mg/m^2 basis. In a similar study in rats by the subcutaneous route there was no increase in pup death at 81 mg/kg per day, the highest dose tested, which is equivalent to 8 times the maximum single recommended human oral dose of 100 mg on a mg/m^2 basis.

To monitor fetal outcomes of pregnant women exposed to IMITREX, Glaxo Wellcome Inc. maintains a Sumatriptan Pregnancy Registry. Physicians are encouraged to register patients by calling (800) 336-2176.

Nursing Mothers: Sumatriptan is excreted in human breast milk. Therefore, caution should be exercised when considering the administration of IMITREX Tablets to a nursing woman.

Pediatric Use: Safety and effectiveness of IMITREX Tablets in pediatric patients have not been established.

Completed placebo-controlled clinical trials evaluating oral sumatriptan (25 to 100 mg) in pediatric patients aged 12 to 17 years enrolled a total of 701 adolescent migraineurs. These studies did not establish the efficacy of oral sumatriptan compared to placebo in the treatment of migraine in adolescents. Adverse events observed in these clinical trials were similar in nature to those reported in clinical trials in adults. The frequency of all adverse events in these patients appeared to be both dose- and age-dependent, with younger patients reporting events more commonly than older adolescents. Postmarketing experience includes a limited number of reports that describe pediatric patients who have experienced adverse events, some clinically serious, after use of subcutaneous sumatriptan and/or oral sumatriptan. These reports include events similar in nature to those reported rarely in adults. A myocardial infarct has been reported in a 14-year-old male following the use of oral sumatriptan; clinical signs occurred within 1 day of drug administration. Since clinical data to determine the frequency of serious adverse events in pediatric patients who might receive injectable, oral, or intranasal sumatriptan are not presently available, the use of sumatriptan in patients aged younger than 18 years is not recommended.

Geriatric Use: The use of sumatriptan in elderly patients is not recommended because elderly patients are more likely to have decreased hepatic function, they are at higher risk for CAD, and blood pressure increases may be more pronounced in the elderly (see WARNINGS).

ADVERSE REACTIONS

Serious cardiac events, including some that have been fatal, have occurred following the use of IMITREX Injection or Tablets. These events are extremely rare and most have been reported in patients with risk factors predictive of CAD. Events reported have included coronary artery vasospasm, transient myocardial ischemia, myocardial infarction, ventricular tachycardia, and ventricular fibrillation (see CONTRAINDICATIONS, WARNINGS, and PRECAUTIONS).

Significant hypertensive episodes, including hypertensive crises, have been reported on rare occasions in patients with or without a history of hypertension (see WARNINGS).

Incidence in Controlled Clinical Trials: Table 2 lists adverse events that occurred in placebo-controlled clinical trials in patients who took at least 1 dose of study drug. Only events that occurred at a frequency of 2% or more in any group treated with IMITREX Tablets and were more frequent in that group than in the placebo group are included in Table 2. The events cited reflect experience gained under closely monitored conditions of clinical trials in a highly selected patient population. In actual clinical practice or in other clinical trials, these frequency estimates may not apply, as the conditions of use, reporting behavior, and the kinds of patients treated may differ.

[See table 2 below]

Table 2: Treatment-Emergent Adverse Events Reported by at Least 2% of Patients in Controlled Migraine Trials *

	Percent of Patients Reporting			
Adverse Event Type	Placebo (n = 309)	IMITREX 25 mg (n = 417)	IMITREX 50 mg (n = 771)	IMITREX 100 mg (n = 437)
Atypical sensations	4%	5%	6%	6%
Paresthesia (all types)	2%	3%	5%	3%
Sensation warm/cold	2%	3%	2%	3%
Pain and other pressure sensations	4%	6%	6%	8%
Chest - pain/tightness/ pressure and/or heaviness	1%	1%	2%	2%
Neck/throat/jaw - pain/tightness/pressure	<1%	<1%	2%	3%
Pain -location specified	1%	2%	1%	1%
Other - pressure/tightness/ heaviness	2%	1%	1%	3%
Neurological				
Vertigo	<1%	<1%	<1%	2%
Other				
Malaise/fatigue	<1%	2%	2%	3%

* Events that occurred at a frequency of 2% or more in the group treated with IMITREX Tablets and that occurred more frequently in that group than the placebo group.

Other events that occurred in more than 1% of patients receiving IMITREX Tablets and at least as often on placebo included nausea and/or vomiting, migraine, headache, hyposalivation, dizziness, and drowsiness/sleepiness.

IMITREX Tablets are generally well tolerated. Across all doses, most adverse reactions were mild and transient and did not lead to long-lasting effects. The incidence of adverse events in controlled clinical trials was not affected by gender or age of the patients. There were insufficient data to assess the impact of race on the incidence of adverse events.

Other Events Observed in Association With the Administration of IMITREX Tablets: In the paragraphs that follow, the frequencies of less commonly reported adverse clinical events are presented. Because the reports include events observed in open and uncontrolled studies, the role of IMITREX Tablets in their causation cannot be reliably determined. Furthermore, variability associated with adverse event reporting, the terminology used to describe adverse events, etc., limit the value of quantitative frequency estimates provided. Event frequencies are calculated as the number of patients who used IMITREX Tablets (25, 50, or 100 mg) and reported an event divided by the total number of patients (n = 6348) exposed to IMITREX Tablets. All reported events are included except those already listed in the previous table, those too general to be informative, and those not reasonably associated with the use of the drug. Events are further classified within body system categories and enumerated in order of decreasing frequency using the following definitions: frequent adverse events are defined as those occurring in at least 1/100 patients, infrequent adverse events are those occurring in 1/100 to 1/1000 patients, and rare adverse events are those occurring in fewer than 1/1000 patients.

Atypical Sensations: Frequent were burning sensation and numbness. Infrequent was tight feeling in head. Rare were dysesthesia.

Cardiovascular: Frequent were palpitations, syncope, decreased blood pressure, and increased blood pressure. Infrequent were arrhythmia, changes in ECG, hypertension, hypotension, pallor, pulsating sensations, and tachycardia. Rare were angina, atherosclerosis, bradycardia, cerebral ischemia, cerebrovascular lesion, heart block, peripheral cyanosis, thrombosis, transient myocardial ischemia, and vasodilation.

Ear, Nose, and Throat: Frequent were sinusitis, tinnitus; allergic rhinitis; upper respiratory inflammation; ear, nose, and throat hemorrhage; external otitis; hearing loss; nasal inflammation; and sensitivity to noise. Infrequent were hearing disturbances and otalgia. Rare was feeling of fullness in the ear(s).

Endocrine and Metabolic: Infrequent was thirst. Rare were elevated thyrotropin stimulating hormone (TSH) levels; galactorrhea; hyperglycemia; hypoglycemia; hypothyroidism; polydipsia; weight gain; weight loss; endocrine cysts, lumps, and masses; and fluid disturbances.

Eye: Rare were disorders of sclera, mydriasis, blindness and low vision, visual disturbances, eye edema and swelling, eye irritation and itching, accommodation disorders, external ocular muscle disorders, eye hemorrhage, eye pain, and keratitis and conjunctivitis.

Gastrointestinal: Frequent were diarrhea and gastric symptoms. Infrequent were constipation, dysphagia, and gastroesophageal reflux. Rare were gastrointestinal bleeding, hematemesis, melena, peptic ulcer, gastrointestinal pain, dyspeptic symptoms, dental pain, feelings of gastrointestinal pressure, gastroesophageal reflux, gastritis, gastroenteritis, hypersalivation, abdominal distention, oral itching and irritation, salivary gland swelling, and swallowing disorders.

Hematological Disorders: Rare was anemia.

Musculoskeletal: Frequent was myalgia. Infrequent was muscle cramps. Rare were tetany; muscle atrophy, weakness, and tiredness; arthralgia and articular rheumatitis; acquired musculoskeletal deformity; muscle stiffness, tightness, and rigidity; and musculoskeletal inflammation.

Neurological: Frequent were phonophobia and photophobia. Infrequent were confusion, depression, difficulty concentrating, disturbance of smell, dysarthria, euphoria, facial pain, heat sensitivity, incoordination, lacrimation, monoplegia, sleep disturbance, shivering, syncope, and tremor. Rare were aggressiveness, apathy, bradylogia, cluster headache, convulsions, decreased appetite, drug abuse, dystonic reaction, facial paralysis, hallucinations, hunger, hyperesthesia, hysteria, increased alertness, memory disturbance, neuralgia, paralysis, personality change, phobia, radiculopathy, rigidity, suicide, twitching, agitation, anxiety, depressive disorders, detachment, motor dysfunction, neurotic disorders, psychomotor disorders, taste disturbances, and raised intracranial pressure.

Respiratory: Frequent was dyspnea. Infrequent was asthma. Rare were hiccoughs, breathing disorders, cough, and bronchitis.

Skin: Frequent was sweating. Infrequent were erythema, pruritus, rash, and skin tenderness. Rare were dry/scaly skin, tightness of skin, wrinkling of skin, eczema, seborrheic dermatitis, and skin nodules.
Breasts: Infrequent was tenderness. Rare were nipple discharge; breast swelling; cysts, lumps, and masses of breasts; and primary malignant breast neoplasm.
Urogenital: Infrequent were dysmenorrhea, increased urination, and intermenstrual bleeding. Rare were abortion and hematuria, urinary frequency, bladder inflammation, micturition disorders, urethritis, urinary infections, menstruation symptoms, abnormal menstrual cycle, inflammation of fallopian tubes, and menstrual cycle symptoms.
Miscellaneous: Frequent was hypersensitivity. Infrequent were fever, fluid retention, and overdose. Rare were edema, hematoma, lymphadenopathy, speech disturbance, voice disturbances, contusions.
Other Events Observed in the Clinical Development of IMITREX: The following adverse events occurred in clinical trials with IMITREX Injection and IMITREX Nasal Spray. Because the reports include events observed in open and uncontrolled studies, the role of IMITREX in their causation cannot be reliably determined. All reported events are included except those already listed, those too general to be informative, and those not reasonably associated with the use of the drug.
Atypical Sensations: Feeling strange, prickling sensation, tingling, and hot sensation.
Cardiovascular: Abdominal aortic aneurysm, abnormal pulse, flushing, phlebitis, Raynaud syndrome, and various transient ECG changes (nonspecific ST or T wave changes, prolongation of PR or QTc intervals, sinus arrhythmia, nonsustained ventricular premature beats, isolated junctional ectopic beats, atrial ectopic beats, delayed activation of the right ventricle).
Chest Symptoms: Chest discomfort.
Endocrine and Metabolic: Dehydration.
Ear, Nose, and Throat: Disorder/discomfort nasal cavity and sinuses, ear infection, Meniere disease, and throat discomfort.
Eye: Vision alterations.
Gastrointestinal: Abdominal discomfort, colitis, disturbance of liver function tests, flatulence/eructation, gallstones, intestinal obstruction, pancreatitis, and retching.
Injection Site Reaction
Miscellaneous: Difficulty in walking, hypersensitivity to various agents, jaw discomfort, miscellaneous laboratory abnormalities, "serotonin agonist effect", swelling of the extremities, and swelling of the face.
Mouth and Teeth: Disorder of mouth and tongue (e.g., burning of tongue, numbness of tongue, dry mouth).
Musculoskeletal: Arthritis, backache, intervertebral disc disorder, neck pain/stiffness, need to flex calf muscles, and various joint disturbances (pain, stiffness, swelling, ache).
Neurological: Bad/unusual taste, chills, diplegia, disturbance of emotions, sedation, globus hystericus, intoxication, myoclonia, neoplasm of pituitary, relaxation, sensation of lightness, simultaneous hot and cold sensations, stinging sensations, stress, tickling sensations, transient hemiplegia, and yawning.
Respiratory: Influenza and diseases of the lower respiratory tract and lower respiratory tract infection.
Skin: Skin eruption, herpes, and peeling of the skin.
Urogenital: Disorder of breasts, endometriosis, and renal calculus.
Postmarketing Experience (Reports for Subcutaneous or Oral Sumatriptan): The following section enumerates potentially important adverse events that have occurred in clinical practice and that have been reported spontaneously to various surveillance systems. The events enumerated represent reports arising from both domestic and nondomestic use of oral or subcutaneous dosage forms of sumatriptan. The events enumerated include all except those already listed in the ADVERSE REACTIONS section above or those too general to be informative. Because the reports cite events reported spontaneously from worldwide postmarketing experience, frequency of events and the role of sumatriptan in their causation cannot be reliably determined. It is assumed, however, that systemic reactions following sumatriptan use are likely to be similar regardless of route of administration.
Blood: Hemolytic anemia, pancytopenia, thrombocytopenia.
Cardiovascular: Atrial fibrillation, cardiomyopathy, colonic ischemia (see WARNINGS), Prinzmetal variant angina, pulmonary embolism, shock, thrombophlebitis.
Ear, Nose, and Throat: Deafness.
Eye: Ischemic optic neuropathy, retinal artery occlusion, retinal vein thrombosis.
Gastrointestinal: Ischemic colitis with rectal bleeding (see WARNINGS), xerostomia.
Hepatic: Elevated liver function tests.
Neurological: Central nervous system vasculitis, cerebrovascular accident, dysphasia, subarachnoid hemorrhage.
Non-Site Specific: Angioneurotic edema, cyanosis, death (see WARNINGS), temporal arteritis.
Psychiatry: Panic disorder.
Respiratory: Bronchospasm in patients with and without a history of asthma.
Skin: Exacerbation of sunburn, hypersensitivity reactions (allergic vasculitis, erythema, pruritus, rash, shortness of breath, urticaria; in addition, severe anaphylaxis/anaphylactoid reactions have been reported [see WARNINGS]), photosensitivity.
Urogenital: Acute renal failure.

DRUG ABUSE AND DEPENDENCE

One clinical study with IMITREX® (sumatriptan succinate) Injection enrolling 12 patients with a history of substance abuse failed to induce subjective behavior and/or physiologic response ordinarily associated with drugs that have an established potential for abuse.

OVERDOSAGE

Patients (n = 670) have received single oral doses of 140 to 300 mg without significant adverse effects. Volunteers (n = 174) have received single oral doses of 140 to 400 mg without serious adverse events.
Overdose in animals has been fatal and has been heralded by convulsions, tremor, paralysis, inactivity, ptosis, erythema of the extremities, abnormal respiration, cyanosis, ataxia, mydriasis, salivation, and lacrimation. The elimination half-life of sumatriptan is approximately 2.5 hours (see CLINICAL PHARMACOLOGY), and therefore monitoring of patients after overdose with IMITREX Tablets should continue for at least 12 hours or while symptoms or signs persist.
It is unknown what effect hemodialysis or peritoneal dialysis has on the serum concentrations of sumatriptan.

DOSAGE AND ADMINISTRATION

In controlled clinical trials, single doses of 25, 50, or 100 mg of IMITREX TABLETS were effective for the acute treatment of migraine in adults. There is evidence that doses 50 and 100 mg may provide a greater effect than 25 mg (see CLINICAL TRIALS). There is also evidence that doses of 100 mg do not provide a greater effect than 50 mg. Individuals may vary in response to doses of IMITREX TABLETS. The choice of dose should therefore be made on an individual basis, weighing the possible benefit of a higher dose with the potential for a greater risk of adverse events.
If the headache returns or the patient has a partial response to the initial dose, the dose may be repeated after 2 hours, not to exceed a total daily dose of 200 mg. If a headache returns following an initial treatment with IMITREX Injection, additional single IMITREX Tablets (up to 100 mg/day) may be given with an interval of at least 2 hours between tablet doses. The safety of treating an average of more than 4 headaches in a 30-day period has not been established.
Because of the potential of MAO-A inhibitors to cause unpredictable elevations in the bioavailability of oral sumatriptan, their combined use is contraindicated (see CONTRAINDICATIONS).
Hepatic disease/functional impairment may also cause unpredictable elevations in the bioavailability of orally administered sumatriptan. Consequently, if treatment is deemed advisable in the presence of liver disease, the maximum single dose should in general not exceed 50 mg (see CLINICAL PHARMACOLOGY for the basis of this recommendation).

HOW SUPPLIED

IMITREX Tablets, 25 and 50 mg of sumatriptan (base) as the succinate. IMITREX Tablets, 25 mg are white, round, film-coated tablets embossed with "I" on one side and "25" on the other in blister packs of 9 tablets (NDC 0173-0460-02). IMITREX Tablets, 50 mg are white, capsule-shaped, film-coated tablets embossed with "Imitrex" on one side and "50" on the other in blister packs of 9 tablets (NDC 0173-0459-00).
Store between 36° and 86°F (2° and 30°C).

ANIMAL TOXICOLOGY

Corneal Opacities: Dogs receiving oral sumatriptan developed corneal opacities and defects in the corneal epithelium. Corneal opacities were seen at the lowest dosage tested, 2 mg/kg per day, and were present after 1 month of treatment. Defects in the corneal epithelium were noted in a 60-week study. Earlier examinations for these toxicities were not conducted and no-effect doses were not established; however, the relative exposure at the lowest dose tested was approximately 5 times the human exposure after a 100-mg oral dose. There is evidence of alterations in corneal appearance on the first day of intranasal dosing to dogs. Changes were noted at the lowest dose tested, which was approximately one half the maximum single human oral dose of 100 mg on a mg/m^2 basis.

PATIENT INFORMATION

The following wording is contained in a separate leaflet provided for patients.

Information for the Patient
IMITREX® (sumatriptan succinate) Tablets

Please read this leaflet carefully before you take IMITREX Tablets. This provides a summary of the information available on your medicine. Please do not throw away this leaflet until you have finished your medicine. You may need to read this leaflet again. This leaflet does not contain all the information on IMITREX Tablets. For further information or advice, ask your doctor or pharmacist.
Information About Your Medicine:
The name of your medicine is IMITREX (sumatriptan succinate) Tablets. It can be obtained only by prescription from your doctor. The decision to use IMITREX Tablets is one that you and your doctor should make jointly, taking into account your individual preferences and medical circumstances. If you have risk factors for heart disease (such as high blood pressure, high cholesterol, obesity, diabetes, smoking, strong family history of heart disease, or you are postmenopausal or a male over 40), you should tell your doctor, who should evaluate you for heart disease in order to determine if IMITREX is appropriate for you. Although the vast majority of those who have taken IMITREX have not experienced any significant side effects, some individuals have experienced serious heart problems and, rarely, considering the extensiveness of IMITREX use worldwide, deaths have been reported. In all but a few instances, however, serious problems occurred in people with known heart disease and it was not clear whether IMITREX was a contributory factor in these deaths.
1. The Purpose of Your Medicine:
IMITREX Tablets are intended to relieve your migraine, but not to prevent or reduce the number of attacks you experience. Use IMITREX Tablets only to treat an actual migraine attack.
2. Important Questions to Consider Before Taking IMITREX Tablets:
If the answer to any of the following questions is **YES** or if you do not know the answer, then please discuss it with your doctor before you use IMITREX Tablets.

- Are you pregnant? Do you think you might be pregnant? Are you trying to become pregnant? Are you using inadequate contraception? Are you breastfeeding?
- Do you have any chest pain, heart disease, shortness of breath, or irregular heartbeats? Have you had a heart attack?
- Do you have risk factors for heart disease (such as high blood pressure, high cholesterol, obesity, diabetes, smoking, strong family history of heart disease, or you are postmenopausal or a male over 40)?
- Have you had a stroke, transient ischemic attacks (TIAs), or Raynaud syndrome?
- Do you have high blood pressure?
- Have you ever had to stop taking this or any other medication because of an allergy or other problems?
- Are you taking any other migraine medications, including other 5-HT$_1$ agonists or any other medications containing ergotamine, dihydroergotamine, or methysergide?
- Are you taking any medication for depression (monoamine oxidase inhibitors or selective serotonin reuptake inhibitors [SSRIs])?
- Have you had, or do you have, any disease of the liver or kidney?
- Have you had, or do you have, epilepsy or seizures?
- Is this headache different from your usual migraine attacks?

Remember, if you answered **YES** to any of the above questions, then discuss it with your doctor.
3. The Use of IMITREX Tablets During Pregnancy:
Do not use IMITREX Tablets if you are pregnant, think you might be pregnant, are trying to become pregnant, or are not using adequate contraception, unless you have discussed this with your doctor.
4. How to Use IMITREX Tablets:
For adults, the usual dose is a single tablet taken whole with fluids. A second tablet may be taken if your symptoms of migraine come back or if you have a partial response to the initial dose, but not sooner than 2 hours following the first tablet. For a given attack, if you have no response to the first tablet, do not take a second tablet without first consulting with your doctor. Do not take more than a total of 200 mg of IMITREX Tablets in any 24-hour period. The safety of treating an average of more than 4 headaches in a 30-day period has not been established.
5. Side Effects to Watch for:

- Some patients experience pain or tightness in the chest or throat when using IMITREX Tablets. If this happens to you, then discuss it with your doctor before using any more IMITREX Tablets. If the chest pain is severe or does not go away, call your doctor immediately.
- If you have sudden and/or severe abdominal pain following IMITREX Tablets, call your doctor immediately.
- Shortness of breath; wheeziness; heart throbbing; swelling of eyelids, face, or lips; or a skin rash, skin lumps, or hives happens rarely. If it happens to you, then tell your doctor immediately. Do not take any more IMITREX Tablets unless your doctor tells you to do so.
- Some people may have feelings of tingling, heat, flushing (redness of face lasting a short time), heaviness or pressure after treatment with IMITREX Tablets. A few people may feel drowsy, dizzy, tired, or sick. Tell your doctor of these symptoms at your next visit.
- If you feel unwell in any other way or have any symptoms that you do not understand, you should contact your doctor immediately.

6. What to Do if an Overdose is Taken:
If you have taken more medication than you have been told, contact either your doctor, hospital emergency department, or nearest poison control center immediately.
7. Storing Your Medicine:
Keep your medicine in a safe place where children cannot reach it. It may be harmful to children. Store your medica-

Continued on next page

This product information is based on labeling in effect on June 23, 2000. For further information, contact via direct mail, phone, or web site. Medical Information, Glaxo Wellcome Inc., PO Box 13398, Research Triangle Park, NC 27709. Healthcare Professionals (Medical Information): 800-334-0089. Patients (Customer Response Center): 1-888-825-5249. Glaxo Wellcome Corporate Web Site: www.glaxowellcome.com

Imitrex Tablets—Cont.

tion away from heat and light. Do not store at temperatures above 86°F (30°C), or below 36°F (2°C). If your medication has expired (the expiration date is printed on the treatment pack), throw it away as instructed. If your doctor decides to stop your treatment, do not keep any leftover medicine unless your doctor tells you to. Throw away your medicine as instructed.

Glaxo Wellcome Inc., Research Triangle Park, NC 27709
US Patent Nos. 4,816,470 and 5,037,845

September 1999/RL-758

Shown in Product Identification Guide, page 315

LAMICTAL® ℞
[la-mik' tal]
(lamotrigine)
Tablets

LAMICTAL®
(lamotrigine)
Chewable Dispersible Tablets

SERIOUS RASHES REQUIRING HOSPITALIZATION AND DISCONTINUATION OF TREATMENT HAVE BEEN REPORTED IN ASSOCIATION WITH THE USE OF LAMICTAL. THE INCIDENCE OF THESE RASHES, WHICH HAVE INCLUDED STEVENS-JOHNSON SYNDROME, IS APPROXIMATELY 1% (1/100) IN PEDIATRIC PATIENTS (AGE <16 YEARS) AND 0.3% (3/1000) IN ADULTS. IN WORLDWIDE POSTMARKETING EXPERIENCE, RARE CASES OF TOXIC EPIDERMAL NECROLYSIS AND/OR RASH-RELATED DEATH HAVE BEEN REPORTED, BUT THEIR NUMBERS ARE TOO FEW TO PERMIT A PRECISE ESTIMATE OF THE RATE.

BECAUSE THE RATE OF SERIOUS RASH IS GREATER IN PEDIATRIC PATIENTS THAN IN ADULTS, IT BEARS EMPHASIS THAT LAMICTAL IS APPROVED ONLY FOR USE IN PEDIATRIC PATIENTS BELOW THE AGE OF 16 YEARS WHO HAVE SEIZURES ASSOCIATED WITH THE LENNOX-GASTAUT SYNDROME (SEE INDICATIONS).

OTHER THAN AGE, THERE ARE AS YET NO FACTORS IDENTIFIED THAT ARE KNOWN TO PREDICT THE RISK OF OCCURRENCE OR THE SEVERITY OF RASH ASSOCIATED WITH LAMICTAL. THERE ARE SUGGESTIONS, YET TO BE PROVEN, THAT THE RISK OF RASH MAY ALSO BE INCREASED BY 1) COADMINISTRATION OF LAMICTAL WITH VALPROIC ACID (VPA), 2) EXCEEDING THE RECOMMENDED INITIAL DOSE OF LAMICTAL, OR 3) EXCEEDING THE RECOMMENDED DOSE ESCALATION FOR LAMICTAL. HOWEVER, CASES HAVE BEEN REPORTED IN THE ABSENCE OF THESE FACTORS.

NEARLY ALL CASES OF LIFE-THREATENING RASHES ASSOCIATED WITH LAMICTAL HAVE OCCURRED WITHIN 2 TO 8 WEEKS OF TREATMENT INITIATION. HOWEVER, ISOLATED CASES HAVE BEEN REPORTED AFTER PROLONGED TREATMENT (e.g., 6 MONTHS). ACCORDINGLY, DURATION OF THERAPY CANNOT BE RELIED UPON AS A MEANS TO PREDICT THE POTENTIAL RISK HERALDED BY THE FIRST APPEARANCE OF A RASH.

ALTHOUGH BENIGN RASHES ALSO OCCUR WITH LAMICTAL, IT IS NOT POSSIBLE TO PREDICT RELIABLY WHICH RASHES WILL PROVE TO BE SERIOUS OR LIFE THREATENING. ACCORDINGLY, LAMICTAL SHOULD ORDINARILY BE DISCONTINUED AT THE FIRST SIGN OF RASH, UNLESS THE RASH IS CLEARLY NOT DRUG RELATED. DISCONTINUATION OF TREATMENT MAY NOT PREVENT A RASH FROM BECOMING LIFE THREATENING OR PERMANENTLY DISABLING OR DISFIGURING.

DESCRIPTION

LAMICTAL (lamotrigine), an antiepileptic drug (AED) of the phenyltriazine class, is chemically unrelated to existing antiepileptic drugs. Its chemical name is 3,5-diamino-6-(2,3-dichlorophenyl)-*as*-triazine, its molecular formula is $C_9H_7N_5Cl_2$, and its molecular weight is 256.09. Lamotrigine is a white to pale cream-colored powder and has a pK_a of 5.7. Lamotrigine is very slightly soluble in water (0.17 mg/mL at 25°C) and slightly soluble in 0.1 M HCl (4.1 mg/mL at 25°C).

LAMICTAL Tablets are supplied for oral administration as 25-mg (white), 100-mg (peach), 150-mg (cream), and 200-mg (blue) tablets. Each tablet contains the labeled amount of lamotrigine and the following inactive ingredients: lactose; magnesium stearate; microcrystalline cellulose; povidone; sodium starch glycolate; FD&C Yellow No. 6 Lake (100-mg tablet only); ferric oxide, yellow (150-mg tablet only); and FD&C Blue No. 2 Lake (200-mg tablet only).

LAMICTAL Chewable Dispersible Tablets are supplied for oral administration. The tablets contain 5 mg (white) or 25 mg (white) of lamotrigine and the following inactive ingredients: blackcurrant flavor, calcium carbonate, low-substituted hydroxypropylcellulose, magnesium aluminum silicate, magnesium stearate, povidone, saccharin sodium, and sodium starch glycolate.

Table 1: Mean* Pharmacokinetic Parameters in Adult Patients With Epilepsy or Healthy Volunteers

Adult Study Population	Number of Subjects	t_{max}: Time of Maximum Plasma Concentration (h)	$t_{½}$: Elimination Half-life (h)	Cl/F: Apparent Plasma Clearance (mL/min/kg)
Patients taking enzyme-inducing antiepileptic drugs (EIAEDs)†:				
Single-dose LAMICTAL	24	2.3 (0.5-5.0)	14.4 (6.4-30.4)	1.10 (0.51-2.22)
Multiple-dose LAMICTAL	17	2.0 (0.75-5.93)	12.6 (7.5-23.1)	1.21 (0.66-1.82)
Patients taking EIAEDs + VPA:				
Single-dose LAMICTAL	25	3.8 (1.0-10.0)	27.2 (11.2-51.6)	0.53 (0.27-1.04)
Patients taking VPA only:				
Single-dose LAMICTAL	4	4.8 (1.8-8.4)	58.8 (30.5-88.8)	0.28 (0.16-0.40)
Healthy volunteers taking VPA:				
Single-dose LAMICTAL	6	1.8 (1.0-4.0)	48.3 (31.5-88.6)	0.30 (0.14-0.42)
Multiple-dose LAMICTAL	18	1.9 (0.5-3.5)	70.3 (41.9-113.5)	0.18 (0.12-0.33)
Healthy volunteers taking no other medications:				
Single-dose LAMICTAL	179	2.2 (0.25-12.0)	32.8 (14.0-103.0)	0.44 (0.12-1.10)
Multiple-dose LAMICTAL	36	1.7 (0.5-4.0)	25.4 (11.6-61.6)	0.58 (0.24-1.15)

*The majority of parameter means determined in each study had coefficients of variation between 20% and 40% for half-life and Cl/F and between 30% and 70% for t_{max}. The overall mean values were calculated from individual study means that were weighted based on the number of volunteers/patients in each study. The numbers in parentheses below each parameter mean represent the range of individual volunteer/patient values across studies.

† Examples of EIAEDs are carbamazepine, phenobarbital, phenytoin, and primidone.

CLINICAL PHARMACOLOGY

Mechanism of Action: The precise mechanism(s) by which lamotrigine exerts its anticonvulsant action are unknown. In animal models designed to detect anticonvulsant activity, lamotrigine was effective in preventing seizure spread in the maximum electroshock (MES) and pentylenetetrazol (scMet) tests, and prevented seizures in the visually and electrically evoked after-discharge (EEAD) tests for antiepileptic activity. The relevance of these models to human epilepsy, however, is not known.

One proposed mechanism of action of LAMICTAL, the relevance of which remains to be established in humans, involves an effect on sodium channels. In vitro pharmacological studies suggest that lamotrigine inhibits voltage-sensitive sodium channels, thereby stabilizing neuronal membranes and consequently modulating presynaptic transmitter release of excitatory amino acids (e.g., glutamate and aspartate).

Pharmacological Properties: Although the relevance for human use is unknown, the following data characterize the performance of LAMICTAL in receptor binding assays. Lamotrigine had a weak inhibitory effect on the serotonin $5\text{-}HT_3$ receptor (IC_{50} = 18 μM). It does not exhibit high affinity binding (IC_{50}>100 μM) to the following neurotransmitter receptors: adenosine A_1 and A_2; adrenergic α_1, α_2, and β; dopamine D_1 and D_2; γ-aminobutyric acid (GABA) A and B; histamine H_1; kappa opioid; muscarinic acetylcholine; and serotonin $5\text{-}HT_2$. Studies have failed to detect an effect of lamotrigine on dihydropyridine-sensitive calcium channels. It had weak effects at sigma opioid receptors (IC_{50} = 145 μM). Lamotrigine did not inhibit the uptake of norepinephrine, dopamine, serotonin, or aspartic acid (IC_{50}>100 μM).

Effect of Lamotrigine on N-Methyl d-Aspartate (NMDA)-Mediated Activity: Lamotrigine did not inhibit NMDA-induced depolarizations in rat cortical slices or NMDA-induced cyclic GMP formation in immature rat cerebellum, nor did lamotrigine displace compounds that are either competitive or noncompetitive ligands at this glutamate receptor complex (CNQX, CGS, TCHP). The IC_{50} for lamotrigine effects on NMDA-induced currents (in the presence of 3 μM of glycine) in cultured hippocampal neurons exceeded 100 μM.

Folate Metabolism: In vitro, lamotrigine was shown to be an inhibitor of dihydrofolate reductase, the enzyme that catalyzes the reduction of dihydrofolate to tetrahydrofolate. Inhibition of this enzyme may interfere with the biosynthesis of nucleic acids and proteins. When oral daily doses of lamotrigine were given to pregnant rats during organogenesis, fetal, placental, and maternal folate concentrations were reduced. Significantly reduced concentrations of folate are associated with teratogenesis (see PRECAUTIONS: Pregnancy). Folate concentrations were also reduced in male rats given repeated oral doses of lamotrigine. Reduced concentrations were partially returned to normal when supplemented with folinic acid.

Accumulation in Kidneys: Lamotrigine was found to accumulate in the kidney of the male rat, causing chronic progressive nephrosis, necrosis, and mineralization. These findings are attributed to α-2 microglobulin, a species- and sex-specific protein that has not been detected in humans or other animal species.

Melanin Binding: Lamotrigine binds to melanin-containing tissues, e.g., in the eye and pigmented skin. It has been found in the uveal tract up to 52 weeks after a single dose in rodents.

Cardiovascular: In dogs, lamotrigine is extensively metabolized to a 2-N-methyl metabolite. This metabolite causes dose-dependent prolongations of the PR interval, widening of the QRS complex, and, at higher doses, complete AV conduction block. Similar cardiovascular effects are not anticipated in humans because only trace amounts of the 2-N-methyl metabolite (<0.6% of lamotrigine dose) have been found in human urine (see Drug Disposition below). However, it is conceivable that plasma concentrations of this metabolite could be increased in patients with a reduced capacity to glucuronidate lamotrigine (e.g., in patients with liver disease).

Pharmacokinetics and Drug Metabolism: The pharmacokinetics of lamotrigine have been studied in patients with epilepsy, healthy young and elderly volunteers, and volunteers with chronic renal failure. Lamotrigine pharmacokinetic parameters for adult and pediatric patients and healthy normal volunteers are summarized in Tables 1 and 2.

[See table 1 above]

The apparent clearance of lamotrigine is affected by the coadministration of AEDs. Lamotrigine is eliminated more rapidly in patients who have been taking hepatic EIAEDs, including carbamazepine, phenytoin, phenobarbital, and primidone. Most clinical experience is derived from this population.

VPA, however, actually decreases the apparent clearance of lamotrigine (i.e., more than doubles the elimination half-life of lamotrigine), whether given with or without EIAEDs. Accordingly, if lamotrigine is to be administered to a patient receiving VPA, lamotrigine must be given at a reduced dosage, less than half the dose used in patients not receiving VPA (see DOSAGE AND ADMINISTRATION and PRECAUTIONS: Drug Interactions).

Absorption: Lamotrigine is rapidly and completely absorbed after oral administration with negligible first-pass metabolism (absolute bioavailability is 98%). The bioavailability is not affected by food. Peak plasma concentrations occur anywhere from 1.4 to 4.8 hours following drug administration. The lamotrigine chewable/dispersible tablets were found to be equivalent, whether they were administered as dispersed in water, chewed and swallowed, or swallowed as whole, to the lamotrigine compressed tablets in terms of rate and extent of absorption.

Distribution: Estimates of the mean apparent volume of distribution (Vd/F) of lamotrigine following oral administration ranged from 0.9 to 1.3 L/kg. Vd/F is independent of dose and is similar following single and multiple doses in both patients with epilepsy and in healthy volunteers.

Protein Binding: Data from in vitro studies indicate that lamotrigine is approximately 55% bound to human plasma proteins at plasma lamotrigine concentrations from 1 to 10 mcg/mL (10 mcg/mL is four to six times the trough plasma concentration observed in the controlled efficacy trials). Because lamotrigine is not highly bound to plasma proteins, clinically significant interactions with other drugs through competition for protein binding sites are unlikely. The binding of lamotrigine to plasma proteins did not change in the presence of therapeutic concentrations of phenytoin, phenobarbital, or VPA. Lamotrigine did not displace other AEDs (carbamazepine, phenytoin, phenobarbital) from protein binding sites.

Drug Disposition: Lamotrigine is metabolized predominantly by glucuronic acid conjugation; the major metabolite is an inactive 2-N-glucuronide conjugate. After oral administration of 240 mg of ^{14}C-lamotrigine (15 µCi) to six healthy volunteers, 94% was recovered in the urine and 2% was recovered in the feces. The radioactivity in the urine consisted of unchanged lamotrigine (10%), the 2-N-glucuronide (76%), a 5-N-glucuronide (10%), a 2-N-methyl metabolite (0.14%), and other unidentified minor metabolites (4%).

Enzyme Induction: The effects of lamotrigine on specific families of mixed-function oxidase isozymes have not been systematically evaluated.

Following multiple administrations (150 mg twice daily) to normal volunteers taking no other medications, lamotrigine induced its own metabolism, resulting in a 25% decrease in $T_{½}$ and a 37% increase in Cl/F at steady state compared to values obtained in the same volunteers following a single dose. Evidence gathered from other sources suggests that self-induction by LAMICTAL may not occur when LAMICTAL is given as adjunctive therapy in patients receiving EIAEDs.

Dose Proportionality: In healthy volunteers not receiving any other medications and given single doses, the plasma concentrations of lamotrigine increased in direct proportion to the dose administered over the range of 50 to 400 mg. In two small studies (n = 7 and 8) of patients with epilepsy who were maintained on other AEDs, there also was a linear relationship between dose and lamotrigine plasma concentrations at steady state following doses of 50 to 350 mg twice daily.

Elimination: (See Table 1)

Special Populations: Patients With Renal Insufficiency: Twelve volunteers with chronic renal failure (mean creatinine clearance = 13 mL/min; range = 6 to 23) and another six individuals undergoing hemodialysis were each given a single 100-mg dose of LAMICTAL. The mean plasma half-lives determined in the study were 42.9 hours (chronic renal failure), 13.0 hours (during hemodialysis), and 57.4 hours (between hemodialysis) compared to 26.2 hours in healthy volunteers. On average, approximately 20% (range = 5.6 to 35.1) of the amount of lamotrigine present in the body was eliminated by hemodialysis during a 4-hour session.

Hepatic Disease: The pharmacokinetics of lamotrigine following a single 100-mg dose of LAMICTAL were evaluated in 24 subjects with moderate to severe hepatic dysfunction and compared with 12 subjects without hepatic impairment. The median apparent clearance of lamotrigine was 0.31, 0.24, or 0.10 mL/kg/min in patients with Grade A, B, or C (Child-Pugh Classification) hepatic impairment, respectively, compared to 0.34 mL/kg/min in the healthy controls. Median half-life of lamotrigine was 36, 60, or 110 hours in patients with Grade A, B, or C hepatic impairment, respectively, versus 32 hours in healthy controls.

Age: Pediatric Patients: The pharmacokinetics of LAMICTAL following a single 2-mg/kg dose were evaluated in two studies of pediatric patients with epilepsy (n = 25 for patients aged 10 months to 5.3 years and n = 19 for patients aged 5 to 11 years). All patients were receiving concomitant therapy with other AEDs. Lamotrigine pharmacokinetic parameters for pediatric patients are summarized in Table 2. As with adults, the elimination of lamotrigine in pediatric patients was similarly affected by concomitant AEDs. Weight normalized oral clearance (Cl/F) was higher (onefold to threefold) in infants and children (age 10 months to 11 years) than in the adolescents and adults, while adolescents and adults had similar mean values of Cl/F.

[See table 2 above]

Elderly: In a single-dose study (150 mg of LAMICTAL), the pharmacokinetics of lamotrigine in 12 elderly volunteers between the ages of 65 and 76 years (mean creatinine clearance = 61 mL/min, range = 33 to 108) were similar to those of young, healthy volunteers in other studies.

Gender: The clearance of lamotrigine is not affected by gender.

Race: The apparent oral clearance of lamotrigine was 25% lower in non-Caucasians than Caucasians.

Table 2: Mean Pharmacokinetic Parameters in Pediatric Patients With Epilepsy

Pediatric Study Population	Number of Subjects	t_{max} (h)	$t_{½}$ (h)	Cl/F (mL/min/kg)
Ages 10 months-5.3 years				
Patients taking EIAEDs	10	3.0 (1.0-5.9)	7.7 (5.7-11.4)	3.62 (2.44-5.28)
Patients taking AEDs with no known effect on drug-metabolizing enzymes	7	5.2 (2.9-6.1)	19.0 (12.9-27.1)	1.2 (0.75-2.42)
Patients taking VPA only	8	2.9 (1.0-6.0)	44.9 (29.5-52.5)	0.47 (0.23-0.77)
Ages 5-11 years				
Patients taking EIAEDs	7	1.6 (1.0-3.0)	7.0 (3.8-9.8)	2.54 (1.35-5.58)
Patients taking EIAEDs plus VPA	8	3.3 (1.0-6.4)	19.1 (7.0-31.2)	0.89 (0.39-1.93)
Patients taking VPA only*	3	4.5 (3.0-6.0)	65.8 (50.7-73.7)	0.24 (0.21-0.26)
Ages 13-18 years				
Patients taking EIAEDs	11	†	†	1.3
Patients taking EIAEDs plus VPA	8	†	†	0.5
Patients taking VPA only	4	†	†	0.3

*Two subjects were included in the calculation for mean t_{max}.

† Parameter not estimated.

CLINICAL STUDIES

The results of controlled clinical trials established the efficacy of LAMICTAL as monotherapy in adults with partial onset seizures already receiving treatment with a single enzyme-inducing antiepileptic drug (EIAED), as adjunctive therapy in adults with partial seizures, and as adjunctive therapy in the generalized seizures of Lennox-Gastaut syndrome in pediatric and adult patients.

Monotherapy With LAMICTAL in Adults With Partial Seizures Already Receiving Treatment With a Single EIAED: The effectiveness of monotherapy with LAMICTAL was established in a multicenter, double-blind clinical trial enrolling 156 adult outpatients with partial seizures. The patients experienced at least four simple partial, complex partial, and/or secondarily generalized seizures during each of two consecutive 4-week periods while receiving carbamazepine or phenytoin monotherapy during baseline. LAMICTAL (target dose of 500 mg/day) or VPA (1000 mg/day) was added to either carbamazepine or phenytoin monotherapy over a 4-week period. Patients were then converted to monotherapy with LAMICTAL or VPA during the next 4 weeks, then continued on monotherapy for an additional 12-week period.

Study endpoints were completion of all weeks of study treatment or meeting an escape criterion. Criteria for escape relative to baseline were: (1) doubling of average monthly seizure count, (2) doubling of highest consecutive 2-day seizure frequency, (3) emergence of a new seizure type (defined as a seizure that did not occur during the 8-week baseline) that is more severe than seizure types that occur during study treatment, or (4) clinically significant prolongation of generalized-tonic-clonic (GTC) seizures. The primary efficacy variable was the proportion of patients in each treatment group who met escape criteria.

The percentage of patients who met escape criteria was 42% (32/76) in the LAMICTAL group and 69% (55/80) in the VPA group. The difference in the percentage of patients meeting escape criteria was statistically significant (P = 0.0012) in favor of LAMICTAL. No differences in efficacy based on age, sex, or race were detected.

Patients in the control group were intentionally treated with a relatively low dose of valproate; as such, the sole objective of this study was to demonstrate the effectiveness and safety of monotherapy with LAMICTAL, and cannot be interpreted to imply the superiority of LAMICTAL to an adequate dose of valproate.

Adjunctive Therapy With LAMICTAL in Adults: The effectiveness of LAMICTAL as adjunctive therapy (added to other AEDs) was established in three multicenter, placebo-controlled, double-blind clinical trials in 355 adults with refractory partial seizures. The patients had a history of at least 4 partial seizures per month in spite of receiving one or more AEDs at therapeutic concentrations and, in 2 of the studies, were observed on their established AED regimen during baselines that varied between 8 to 12 weeks. In the third, patients were not observed in a prospective baseline. In patients continuing to have at least 4 seizures per month during the baseline, LAMICTAL or placebo was then added to the existing therapy. In all three studies, change from baseline in seizure frequency was the primary measure of effectiveness. The results given below are for all partial seizures in the intent-to-treat population (all patients who received at least one dose of treatment) in each study, unless otherwise indicated. The median seizure frequency at baseline was 3 per week while the mean at baseline was 6.6 per week for all patients enrolled in efficacy studies.

One study (n = 216) was a double-blind, placebo-controlled, parallel trial consisting of a 24-week treatment period. Patients could not be on more than two other anticonvulsants and VPA was not allowed. Patients were randomized to receive placebo, a target dose of 300 mg/day of LAMICTAL, or a target dose of 500 mg/day of LAMICTAL. The median reductions in the frequency of all partial seizures relative to baseline were 8% in patients receiving placebo, 20% in patients receiving 300 mg/day of LAMICTAL, and 36% in patients receiving 500 mg/day of LAMICTAL. The seizure frequency reduction was statistically significant in the 500-mg/day group compared to the placebo group, but not in the 300-mg/day group.

A second study (n = 98) was a double-blind, placebo-controlled, randomized, crossover trial consisting of two 14-week treatment periods (the last 2 weeks of which consisted of dose tapering) separated by a 4-week washout period. Patients could not be on more than two other anticonvulsants and VPA was not allowed. The target dose of LAMICTAL was 400 mg/day. When the first 12 weeks of the treatment periods were analyzed, the median change in seizure frequency was a 25% reduction on LAMICTAL compared to placebo (P<0.001).

The third study (n = 41) was a double-blind, placebo-controlled, crossover trial consisting of two 12-week treatment periods separated by a 4-week washout period. Patients could not be on more than two other anticonvulsants. Thirteen patients were on concomitant VPA; these patients received 150 mg/day of LAMICTAL. The 28 other patients had a target dose of 300 mg/day of LAMICTAL. The median change in seizure frequency was a 26% reduction on LAMICTAL compared to placebo (P<0.01).

No differences in efficacy based on age, sex, or race, as measured by change in seizure frequency, were detected.

Adjunctive Therapy With LAMICTAL in Pediatric and Adult Patients With Lennox-Gastaut Syndrome: The effectiveness of LAMICTAL as adjunctive therapy in patients with Lennox-Gastaut syndrome was established in a multicenter, double-blind, placebo-controlled trial in 169 patients aged 3 to 25 years (n = 79 on LAMICTAL, n = 90 on placebo). Following a 4-week single-blind, placebo phase, patients were randomized to 16 weeks of treatment with LAMICTAL or placebo added to their current AED regimen of up to three drugs. Patients were dosed on a fixed-dose regimen based on body weight and VPA use. Target doses were designed to approximate 5 mg/kg per day for patients taking VPA (maximum dose, 200 mg/day) and 15 mg/kg per day for patients not taking VPA (maximum dose, 400 mg/day). The primary efficacy endpoint was median reduction from baseline in major motor seizures (atonic, tonic, major myoclonic, and tonic-clonic seizures). For the intent-to-treat population, the median reduction of major motor seizures was 32% in patients treated with LAMICTAL and 9% on placebo, a difference that was statistically significant (P<0.05). Drop attacks were significantly reduced by LAMICTAL (34%) compared to placebo (9%), as were tonic-clonic seizures (36% reduction versus 10% increase for LAMICTAL and placebo, respectively).

INDICATIONS AND USAGE

Adjunctive Use: LAMICTAL is indicated as adjunctive therapy in adults with partial seizures and as adjunctive therapy in the generalized seizures of Lennox-Gastaut syndrome in pediatric and adult patients.

Monotherapy Use: LAMICTAL is indicated for conversion to monotherapy in adults with partial seizures who are receiving treatment with a single EIAED.

Safety and effectiveness of LAMICTAL have not been established 1) as initial monotherapy, 2) for conversion to monotherapy from non–enzyme-inducing AEDs (e.g., valproate), or 3) for simultaneous conversion to monotherapy from two or more concomitant AEDs (see DOSAGE AND ADMINISTRATION).

Safety and effectiveness in patients below the age of 16 other than those with Lennox-Gastaut syndrome have not been established (see BOX WARNING).

CONTRAINDICATIONS

LAMICTAL is contraindicated in patients who have demonstrated hypersensitivity to the drug or its ingredients.

WARNINGS

SEE BOX WARNING REGARDING THE RISK OF SERIOUS RASHES REQUIRING HOSPITALIZATION AND DISCONTINUATION OF LAMICTAL.

ALTHOUGH BENIGN RASHES ALSO OCCUR WITH LAMICTAL, IT IS NOT POSSIBLE TO PREDICT RELIABLY WHICH RASHES WILL PROVE TO BE SERIOUS OR LIFE THREATENING. ACCORDINGLY, LAMICTAL SHOULD ORDINARILY BE DISCONTINUED AT THE FIRST SIGN OF RASH, UNLESS THE RASH IS CLEARLY NOT DRUG RELATED. DISCONTINUATION OF TREATMENT MAY NOT PREVENT A RASH FROM BECOMING LIFE THREATENING OR PERMANENTLY DISABLING OR DISFIGURING.

Continued on next page

This product information is based on labeling in effect on June 23, 2000. For further information, contact via direct mail, phone, or web site. Medical Information, Glaxo Wellcome Inc., PO Box 13398, Research Triangle Park, NC 27709. Healthcare Professionals (Medical Information): 800-334-0089. Patients (Customer Response Center): 1-888-825-5249. Glaxo Wellcome Corporate Web Site: www.glaxowellcome.com

Lamictal—Cont.

Serious Rash: ***Pediatric Population:*** The incidence of serious rash associated with hospitalization and discontinuation of LAMICTAL in a prospectively followed cohort of pediatric patients was approximately 1.1% (14/1233). When these 14 cases were reviewed by 3 expert dermatologists, there was considerable disagreement as to their proper classification. To illustrate, one dermatologist considered none of the cases to be Stevens-Johnson syndrome; another assigned 7 of the 14 to this diagnosis. There were no deaths or permanent sequelae in these patients. Additionally, there have been rare cases of toxic epidermal necrolysis with and without permanent sequelae and/or death in US and foreign postmarketing experience. It bears emphasis, accordingly, that LAMICTAL is only approved for use in those patients below the age of 16 who have seizures associated with the Lennox-Gastaut syndrome (see INDICATIONS).

Because foreign postmarketing reports suggested that the rate of serious rash was greater with concomitant VPA use and because metabolism of LAMICTAL is inhibited by VPA, resulting in increased LAMICTAL plasma levels, the drug development database was examined for concomitant VPA use. In pediatric patients who used VPA concomitantly, 1.1% (5/443) experienced a serious rash compared to 1% (6/628) patients not taking VPA. Although the numbers are small, 1.7% (5/294) patients taking either VPA alone or VPA + non-EIAEDs experienced a serious rash compared to 0% (0/149) patients taking VPA + EIAEDs.

Adult Population: Serious rash associated with hospitalization and discontinuation of LAMICTAL occurred in 0.3% (11/3348) of patients who received LAMICTAL in premarketing clinical trials. No fatalities occurred among these individuals. However, in worldwide postmarketing experience, rare cases of rash-related death have been reported, but their numbers are too few to permit a precise estimate of the rate.

Among the rashes leading to hospitalization were Stevens-Johnson syndrome, toxic epidermal necrolysis, angioedema, and a rash associated with a variable number of the following systemic manifestations: fever, lymphadenopathy, facial swelling, hematologic, and hepatologic abnormalities.

There is evidence that the inclusion of VPA in a multidrug regimen increases the risk of serious, potentially life-threatening rash in adults. Specifically, of 584 patients administered LAMICTAL with VPA in clinical trials, 6 (1%) were hospitalized in association with rash; in contrast, 4 (0.16%) of 2398 clinical trial patients and volunteers administered LAMICTAL in the absence of VPA were hospitalized.

Other examples of serious and potentially life-threatening rash that did not lead to hospitalization also occurred in premarketing development. Among these, one case was reported to be Stevens-Johnson-like.

Hypersensitivity Reactions: Hypersensitivity reactions, some fatal or life threatening, have also occurred. Some of these reactions have included clinical features of multiorgan failure/dysfunction, including hepatic abnormalities and evidence of disseminated intravascular coagulation. It is important to note that early manifestations of hypersensitivity (e.g., fever, lymphadenopathy) may be present even though a rash is not evident. If such signs or symptoms are present, the patient should be evaluated immediately. LAMICTAL should be discontinued if an alternative etiology for the signs or symptoms cannot be established.

Prior to initiation of treatment with LAMICTAL, the patient should be instructed that a rash or other signs or symptoms of hypersensitivity (e.g., fever, lymphadenopathy) may herald a serious medical event and that the patient should report any such occurrence to a physician immediately.

Acute Multiorgan Failure: Multiorgan failure, which in some cases has been fatal or irreversible, has been observed in patients receiving LAMICTAL. Fatalities associated with multiorgan failure and various degrees of hepatic failure have been reported in 2/3796 adult patients and 3/1136 pediatric patients who received LAMICTAL during premarketing clinical trials. Rare fatalities from multiorgan failure have also been reported in compassionate plea and postmarketing use. The majority of these deaths occurred in association with other serious medical events, including status epilepticus and overwhelming sepsis, making it difficult to identify the initial cause.

Additionally, three patients (a 45-year-old woman, a 3.5-year-old boy, and an 11-year-old girl) developed multiorgan dysfunction and disseminated intravascular coagulation 9 to 14 days after LAMICTAL was added to their AED regimens. Rash and elevated transaminases were also present in all patients and rhabdomyolysis was noted in two patients. Both pediatric patients were receiving concomitant therapy with VPA, while the adult patient was being treated with carbamazepine and clonazepam. All patients subsequently recovered with supportive care after treatment with LAMICTAL was discontinued.

Pure Red Cell Aplasia (PRCA): A case of PRCA was reported in a 32-year-old male with a history of β-thalassemia. The patient had a microcytic anemia (hemoglobin 11 g/dL) that was stable while the patient received carbamazepine but became more severe in the 3 months after LAMICTAL was added. A bone marrow aspirate revealed markedly decreased erythropoiesis but normal granulopoiesis and thrombopoiesis. Erythropoiesis resumed after discontinuation of LAMICTAL and transfusions of packed red cells. Although PRCA is known to occur in patients with hemoglobinopathies, it is not known if β-thalassemia is a specific risk factor for the development of PRCA.

Withdrawal Seizures: As a rule, AEDs should not be abruptly discontinued because of the possibility of increasing seizure frequency. Unless safety concerns require a more rapid withdrawal, the dose of LAMICTAL should be tapered over a period of at least 2 weeks (see DOSAGE and ADMINISTRATION).

Special Dosing Considerations for Pediatric Patients: The lowest available strength of LAMICTAL Chewable Dispersible Tablets is 5 mg, and only whole tablets should be administered. Since the dosing of LAMICTAL in pediatric patients is based on body weight and the lowest tablet strength is 5 mg, some low-weight pediatric patients should not receive LAMICTAL. Specifically, pediatric patients who weigh less than 17 kg (37 lb) should not receive LAMICTAL because therapy cannot be initiated using the dosing guidelines and the currently available tablet strengths (see DOSAGE AND ADMINISTRATION).

PRECAUTIONS

Dermatological Events (see BOX WARNING, WARNINGS): Serious rashes associated with hospitalization and discontinuation of LAMICTAL have been reported. Rare deaths have been reported, but their numbers are too few to permit a precise estimate of the rate. There are suggestions, yet to be proven, that the risk of rash may also be increased by 1) coadministration of LAMICTAL with VPA, 2) exceeding the recommended initial dose of LAMICTAL, or 3) exceeding the recommended dose escalation for LAMICTAL. However, cases have been reported in the absence of these factors.

In clinical trials, approximately 10% of all patients exposed to LAMICTAL developed a rash. Rashes associated with LAMICTAL do not appear to have unique identifying features. Typically, rash occurs in the first 2 to 8 weeks following treatment initiation. However, isolated cases have been reported after prolonged treatment (e.g., 6 months). Accordingly, duration of therapy cannot be relied upon as a means to predict the potential risk heralded by the first appearance of a rash.

Although most rashes resolved even with continuation of treatment with LAMICTAL, it is not possible to predict reliably which rashes will prove to be serious or life threatening. **ACCORDINGLY, LAMICTAL SHOULD ORDINARILY BE DISCONTINUED AT THE FIRST SIGN OF RASH, UNLESS THE RASH IS CLEARLY NOT DRUG RELATED. DISCONTINUATION OF TREATMENT MAY NOT PREVENT A RASH FROM BECOMING LIFE THREATENING OR PERMANENTLY DISABLING OR DISFIGURING.**

Sudden Unexplained Death in Epilepsy (SUDEP): During the premarketing development of LAMICTAL, 20 sudden and unexplained deaths were recorded among a cohort of 4700 patients with epilepsy (5747 patient-years of exposure).

Some of these could represent seizure-related deaths in which the seizure was not observed, e.g., at night. This represents an incidence of 0.0035 deaths per patient-year. Although this rate exceeds that expected in a healthy population matched for age and sex, it is within the range of estimates for the incidence of sudden unexplained deaths in patients with epilepsy not receiving LAMICTAL (ranging from 0.0005 for the general population of patients with epilepsy, to 0.004 for a recently studied clinical trial population similar to that in the clinical development program for LAMICTAL, to 0.005 for patients with refractory epilepsy). Consequently, whether these figures are reassuring or suggest concern depends on the comparability of the populations reported upon to the cohort receiving LAMICTAL and the accuracy of the estimates provided. Probably most reassuring is the similarity of estimated SUDEP rates in patients receiving LAMICTAL and those receiving another antiepileptic drug that underwent clinical testing in a similar population at about the same time. Importantly, that drug is chemically unrelated to LAMICTAL. This evidence suggests, although it certainly does not prove, that the high SUDEP rates reflect population rates, not a drug effect.

Status Epilepticus: Valid estimates of the incidence of treatment emergent status epilepticus among patients treated with LAMICTAL are difficult to obtain because reporters participating in clinical trials did not all employ identical rules for identifying cases. At a minimum, 7 of 2343 adult patients had episodes that could unequivocally be described as status. In addition, a number of reports of variably defined episodes of seizure exacerbation (e.g., seizure clusters, seizure flurries, etc.) were made.

Addition of LAMICTAL to a Multidrug Regimen That Includes VPA (Dosage Reduction): Because VPA reduces the clearance of lamotrigine, the dosage of lamotrigine in the presence of VPA is less than half of that required in its absence (see DOSAGE AND ADMINISTRATION).

Use in Patients With Concomitant Illness: Clinical experience with LAMICTAL in patients with concomitant illness is limited. Caution is advised when using LAMICTAL in patients with diseases or conditions that could affect metabolism or elimination of the drug, such as renal, hepatic, or cardiac functional impairment.

Hepatic metabolism to the glucuronide followed by renal excretion is the principal route of elimination of lamotrigine (see CLINICAL PHARMACOLOGY).

A study in individuals with severe chronic renal failure (mean creatinine clearance = 13 mL/min) not receiving other AEDs indicated that the elimination half-life of unchanged lamotrigine is prolonged relative to individuals with normal renal function. Until adequate numbers of patients with severe renal impairment have been evaluated during chronic treatment with LAMICTAL, it should be used with caution in these patients, generally using a reduced maintenance dose for patients with significant impairment.

Because there is limited experience with the use of LAMICTAL in patients with impaired liver function, the use in such patients may be associated with as yet unrecognized risks (see CLINICAL PHARMACOLOGY and DOSAGE AND ADMINISTRATION).

Binding in the Eye and Other Melanin-Containing Tissues: Because lamotrigine binds to melanin, it could accumulate in melanin-rich tissues over time. This raises the possibility that lamotrigine may cause toxicity in these tissues after extended use. Although ophthalmological testing was performed in one controlled clinical trial, the testing was inadequate to exclude subtle effects or injury occurring after long-term exposure. Moreover, the capacity of available tests to detect potentially adverse consequences, if any, of lamotrigine's binding to melanin is unknown.

Accordingly, although there are no specific recommendations for periodic ophthalmological monitoring, prescribers should be aware of the possibility of long-term ophthalmologic effects.

Information for Patients: Prior to initiation of treatment with LAMICTAL, the patient should be instructed that a rash or other signs or symptoms of hypersensitivity (e.g., fever, lymphadenopathy) may herald a serious medical event and that the patient should report any such occurrence to a physician immediately. In addition, the patient should notify his physician if worsening of seizure control occurs.

Patients should be advised that LAMICTAL may cause dizziness, somnolence, and other symptoms and signs of central nervous system (CNS) depression. Accordingly, they should be advised neither to drive a car nor to operate other complex machinery until they have gained sufficient experience on LAMICTAL to gauge whether or not it adversely affects their mental and/or motor performance.

Patients should be advised to notify their physicians if they become pregnant or intend to become pregnant during therapy. Patients should be advised to notify their physicians if they intend to breast-feed or are breast-feeding an infant.

Patients should be informed of the availability of a patient information leaflet, and they should be instructed to read the leaflet prior to taking LAMICTAL. See PATIENT INFORMATION at the end of this labeling for the text of the leaflet provided for patients.

Laboratory Tests: The value of monitoring plasma concentrations of LAMICTAL has not been established. Because of the possible pharmacokinetic interactions between LAMICTAL and other AEDs being taken concomitantly (see Table 3), monitoring of the plasma levels of LAMICTAL and concomitant AEDs may be indicated, particularly during dosage adjustments. In general, clinical judgment should be exercised regarding monitoring of plasma levels of LAMICTAL and other anti-seizure drugs and whether or not dosage adjustments are necessary.

Drug Interactions: ***Antiepileptic Drugs:*** The use of AEDs in combination is complicated by the potential for pharmacokinetic interactions.

The interaction of lamotrigine with phenytoin, carbamazepine, and VPA has been studied. The net effects of these various AED combinations on individual AED plasma concentrations are summarized in Table 3.

Table 3: Summary of AED Interactions With LAMICTAL

AED	AED Plasma Concentration With Adjunctive LAMICTAL*	Lamotrigine Plasma Concentration With Adjunctive AEDs†
Phenytoin (PHT)	↔	↓
Carbamazepine (CBZ)	↔	↓
CBZ epoxide‡	?	
Valproic acid (VPA)	↓	↑
VPA + PHT and/or CBZ	NE	↔

* From adjunctive clinical trials and volunteer studies.
† Net effects were estimated by comparing the mean clearance values obtained in adjunctive clinical trials and volunteers studies.
‡ Not administered, but an active metabolite of carbamazepine.
↔ = No significant effect.
? = Conflicting data.
NE = not evaluated.

Specific Effects of Lamotrigine on the Pharmacokinetics of Other AED Products: LAMICTAL Added to Phenytoin: LAMICTAL has no appreciable effect on steady-state phenytoin plasma concentration.

LAMICTAL Added to Carbamazepine: LAMICTAL has no appreciable effect on steady-state carbamazepine plasma concentration. Limited clinical data suggest there is a higher incidence of dizziness, diplopia, ataxia, and blurred vision in patients receiving carbamazepine with LAMICTAL than in patients receiving other EIAEDs with LAMICTAL (see ADVERSE REACTIONS). The mechanism of this interaction is unclear. The effect of lamotrigine on plasma concentrations of carbamazepine-epoxide is unclear.

In a small subset of patients (n = 7) studied in a placebo-controlled trial, lamotrigine had no effect on carbamazepine-epoxide plasma concentrations, but in a small, uncontrolled study (n = 9), carbamazepine-epoxide levels were seen to increase.

LAMICTAL Added to VPA: When LAMICTAL was administered to 18 healthy volunteers receiving VPA in a pharmacokinetic study, the trough steady-state VPA concentrations in plasma decreased by an average of 25% over a 3-week period, and then stabilized. However, adding LAMICTAL to the existing therapy did not cause a change in plasma VPA concentrations in either adult or pediatric patients in controlled clinical trials.

Specific Effects of Other AED Products on the Pharmacokinetics of Lamotrigine: Phenytoin Added to LAMICTAL: The addition of phenytoin decreases lamotrigine steady-state concentrations by approximately 45% to 54% depending upon the total daily dose of phenytoin (i.e., from 100 to 400 mg).

Carbamazepine Added to LAMICTAL: The addition of carbamazepine decreases lamotrigine steady-state concentrations by approximately 40%.

Phenobarbital or Primidone Added to LAMICTAL: The addition of phenobarbital or primidone decreases lamotrigine steady-state concentrations by approximately 40%.

VPA Added to LAMICTAL: The addition of VPA increases lamotrigine steady-state concentrations in normal volunteers by slightly more than twofold.

Interactions With Drug Products Other Than AEDs: Folate Inhibitors: Lamotrigine is an inhibitor of dihydrofolate reductase. Prescribers should be aware of this action when prescribing other medications that inhibit folate metabolism.

Drug/Laboratory Test Interactions: None known.

Carcinogenesis, Mutagenesis, Impairment of Fertility: No evidence of carcinogenicity was seen in one mouse study or two rat studies following oral administration of lamotrigine for up to 2 years at maximum tolerated doses (30 mg/kg per day for mice and 10 to 15 mg/kg per day for rats, doses that are equivalent to 90 mg/m^2 and 60 to 90 mg/m^2, respectively). Steady-state plasma concentrations ranged from 1 to 4 mcg/mL in the mouse study and 1 to 10 mcg/mL in the rat study. Plasma concentrations associated with the recommended human doses of 300 to 500 mg/day are generally in the range of 2 to 5 mcg/mL, but concentrations as high as 19 mcg/mL have been recorded.

Lamotrigine was not mutagenic in the presence or absence of metabolic activation when tested in two gene mutation assays (the Ames test and the in vitro mammalian mouse lymphoma assay). In two cytogenetic assays (the in vitro human lymphocyte assay and the in vivo rat bone marrow assay), lamotrigine did not increase the incidence of structural or numerical chromosomal abnormalities.

No evidence of impairment of fertility was detected in rats given oral doses of lamotrigine up to 2.4 times the highest usual human maintenance dose of 8.33 mg/kg per day or 0.4 times the human dose on a mg/m^2 basis. The effect of lamotrigine on human fertility is unknown.

Pregnancy: Pregnancy Category C. No evidence of teratogenicity was found in mice, rats, or rabbits when lamotrigine was orally administered to pregnant animals during the period of organogenesis at doses up to 1.2, 0.5, and 1.1 times, respectively, on a mg/m^2 basis, the highest usual human maintenance dose (i.e., 500 mg/day). However, maternal toxicity and secondary fetal toxicity producing reduced fetal weight and/or delayed ossification were seen in mice and rats, but not in rabbits at these doses. Teratology studies were also conducted using bolus intravenous administration of the isethionate salt of lamotrigine in rats and rabbits. In rat dams administered an intravenous dose at 0.6 times the highest usual human maintenance dose, the incidence of intrauterine death without signs of teratogenicity was increased.

A behavioral teratology study was conducted in rats dosed during the period of organogenesis. At day 21 postpartum, offspring of dams receiving 5 mg/kg per day or higher displayed a significantly longer latent period for open field exploration and a lower frequency of rearing. In a swimming maze test performed on days 39 to 44 postpartum, time to completion was increased in offspring of dams receiving 25 mg/kg per day. These doses represent 0.1 and 0.5 times the clinical dose on a mg/m^2 basis, respectively.

Lamotrigine did not affect fertility, teratogenesis, or postnatal development when rats were dosed prior to and during mating, and throughout gestation and lactation at doses equivalent to 0.4 times the highest usual human maintenance dose on a mg/m^2 basis.

When pregnant rats were orally dosed at 0.1, 0.14, or 0.3 times the highest human maintenance dose (on a mg/m^2 basis) during the latter part of gestation (days 15 to 20), maternal toxicity and fetal death were seen. In dams, food consumption and weight gain were reduced, and the gestation period was slightly prolonged (22.6 vs. 22.0 days in the control group). Stillborn pups were found in all three drug-treated groups with the highest number in the high-dose group. Postnatal death was also seen, but only in the two highest doses, and occurred between day 1 and 20. Some of these deaths appear to be drug-related and not secondary to the maternal toxicity. A no-observed-effect level (NOEL) could not be determined for this study.

Although LAMICTAL was not found to be teratogenic in the above studies, lamotrigine decreases fetal folate concentrations in rats, an effect known to be associated with teratogenesis in animals and humans. There are no adequate and well-controlled studies in pregnant women. Because animal reproduction studies are not always predictive of human response, this drug should be used during pregnancy only if the potential benefit justifies the potential risk to the fetus.

Pregnancy Exposure Registry: To facilitate monitoring fetal outcomes of pregnant women exposed to lamotrigine, physicians are encouraged to register patients, **before fetal outcome (e.g., ultrasound, results of amniocentesis, birth, etc.) is known,** and can obtain information by calling the Lamotrigine Pregnancy Registry at (800) 336-2176 (toll-free). Patients can enroll themselves in the North American Antiepileptic Drug Pregnancy Registry by calling (888) 233-2334 (toll free).

Labor and Delivery: The effect of LAMICTAL on labor and delivery in humans is unknown.

Use in Nursing Mothers: Preliminary data indicate that lamotrigine passes into human milk. Because the effects on the infant exposed to LAMICTAL by this route are unknown, breast-feeding while taking LAMICTAL is not recommended.

Pediatric Use: In pediatric patients, LAMICTAL is only indicated as adjunctive therapy for the generalized seizures of Lennox-Gastaut syndrome. Safety and effectiveness for other uses in patients below the age of 16 years have not been established (see BOX WARNING).

Geriatric Use: Because few patients over the age of 65 (approximately 20) were exposed to LAMICTAL during its premarket evaluation, no specific statements about the safety or effectiveness of LAMICTAL in this age-group can be made.

Table 4: Treatment-Emergent Adverse Event Incidence in Placebo-Controlled Adjunctive Trials*
(Events in at least 2% of patients treated with LAMICTAL and numerically more frequent than in the placebo group.)

Body System/Adverse Experience†	Percent of Patients Receiving Adjunctive LAMICTAL (n = 711)	Percent of Patients Receiving Adjunctive Placebo (n = 419)
Body as a whole		
Headache	29	19
Flu syndrome	7	6
Fever	6	4
Abdominal pain	5	4
Neck pain	2	1
Reaction aggravated (seizure exacerbation)	2	1
Digestive		
Nausea	19	10
Vomiting	9	4
Diarrhea	6	4
Dyspepsia	5	2
Constipation	4	3
Tooth disorder	3	2
Anorexia	2	1
Musculoskeletal		
Arthralgia	2	0
Nervous		
Dizziness	38	13
Ataxia	22	6
Somnolence	14	7
Incoordination	6	2
Insomnia	6	2
Tremor	4	1
Depression	4	3
Anxiety	4	3
Convulsion	3	1
Irritability	3	2
Speech disorder	3	0
Concentration disturbance	2	1
Respiratory		
Rhinitis	14	9
Pharyngitis	10	9
Cough Increased	8	6
Skin and appendages		
Rash	10	5
Pruritus	3	2
Special Senses		
Diplopia	28	7
Blurred vision	16	5
Vision abnormality	3	1
Urogenital		
Female patients only	(n = 365)	(n = 207)
Dysmenorrhea	7	6
Vaginitis	4	1
Amenorrhea	2	1

*Patients in these adjunctive studies were receiving one to three concomitant EIAEDs in addition to LAMICTAL or placebo. Patients may have reported multiple adverse experiences during the study or at discontinuation; thus, patients may be included in more than one category.

† Adverse experiences reported by at least 2% of patients treated with LAMICTAL are included.

Table 5: Dose-Related Adverse Events From a Randomized, Placebo-Controlled Trial in Adults

Adverse Experience	Percent of Patients Experiencing Adverse Experiences		
	Placebo (n = 73)	LAMICTAL 300 mg (n = 71)	LAMICTAL 500 mg (n = 72)
Ataxia	10	10	28*†
Blurred vision	10	11	25*†
Diplopia	8	24*	49*†
Dizziness	27	31	54*†
Nausea	11	18	25*
Vomiting	4	11	18*

*Significantly greater than placebo group (P<0.05).

† Significantly greater than group receiving LAMICTAL 300 mg (P<0.05).

ADVERSE REACTIONS

SERIOUS RASH REQUIRING HOSPITALIZATION AND DISCONTINUATION OF LAMICTAL, INCLUDING STEVENS-JOHNSON SYNDROME AND TOXIC EPIDERMAL NECROLYSIS, HAVE OCCURRED IN ASSOCIATION WITH THERAPY WITH LAMICTAL. RARE DEATHS HAVE BEEN REPORTED, BUT THEIR NUMBERS ARE TOO FEW TO PERMIT A PRECISE ESTIMATE OF THE RATE (see BOX WARNING).

Continued on next page

This product information is based on labeling in effect on June 23, 2000. For further information, contact via direct mail, phone, or web site. Medical Information, Glaxo Wellcome Inc., PO Box 13398, Research Triangle Park, NC 27709. Healthcare Professionals (Medical Information): 800-334-0089. Patients (Customer Response Center): 1-888-825-5249. Glaxo Wellcome Corporate Web Site: www.glaxowellcome.com

Lamictal—Cont.

Most Common Adverse Events in All Clinical Studies:
Adjunctive Therapy in Adults: The most commonly observed (≥5%) adverse experiences seen in association with LAMICTAL during adjunctive therapy in adults and not seen at an equivalent frequency among placebo-treated patients were: dizziness, ataxia, somnolence, headache, diplopia, blurred vision, nausea, vomiting, and rash. Dizziness, diplopia, ataxia, blurred vision, nausea, and vomiting were dose related. Dizziness, diplopia, ataxia, and blurred vision occurred more commonly in patients receiving carbamazepine with LAMICTAL than in patients receiving other EIAEDs with LAMICTAL. Clinical data suggest a higher incidence of rash, including serious rash, in patients receiving concomitant VPA than in patients not receiving VPA (see WARNINGS).

Approximately 11% of the 3378 adult patients who received LAMICTAL as adjunctive therapy in premarketing clinical trials discontinued treatment because of an adverse experience. The adverse events most commonly associated with discontinuation were rash (3.0%), dizziness (2.8%), and headache (2.5%).

In a dose response study in adults, the rate of discontinuation of LAMICTAL for dizziness, ataxia, diplopia, blurred vision, nausea, and vomiting was dose related.

Monotherapy in Adults: The most commonly observed (≥ 5%) adverse experiences seen in association with the use of LAMICTAL during the monotherapy phase of the controlled trial in adults not seen at an equivalent rate in the control group were vomiting, coordination abnormality, dyspepsia, nausea, dizziness, rhinitis, anxiety, insomnia, infection, pain, weight decrease, chest pain, and dysmenorrhea. The most commonly observed (≥ 5%) adverse experiences associated with the use of LAMICTAL during the conversion to monotherapy (add-on) period, not seen at an equivalent frequency among low-dose valproate-treated patients, were dizziness, headache, nausea, asthenia, coordination abnormality, vomiting, rash, somnolence, diplopia, ataxia, accidental injury, tremor, blurred vision, insomnia, nystagmus, diarrhea, lymphadenopathy, pruritus, and sinusitis.

Approximately 10% of the 420 adult patients who received LAMICTAL as monotherapy in premarketing clinical trials discontinued treatment because of an adverse experience. The adverse events most commonly associated with discontinuation were rash (4.5%), headache (3.1%), and asthenia (2.4%).

Adjunctive Therapy in Pediatric Patients With Lennox-Gastaut Syndrome: The most commonly observed (≥ 5%) adverse experiences seen in association with the use of LAMICTAL as adjunctive treatment in pediatric patients with Lennox-Gastaut syndrome and not seen at an equivalent rate in the control group were pharyngitis, infection, rash, vomiting, bronchitis, accidental injury, constipation, and flu syndrome.

In 169 patients with Lennox-Gastaut syndrome (26 patients were between the ages of 16 and 25), 3.8% of patients on LAMICTAL and 7.8% of patients on placebo discontinued due to adverse experiences. The most commonly reported adverse experiences that led to discontinuation were rash for patients treated with LAMICTAL and deterioration of seizure control for patients treated with placebo.

Approximately 10% of the 1136 pediatric patients who received LAMICTAL as adjunctive therapy in premarketing clinical trials discontinued treatment because of an adverse experience. The adverse events most commonly associated with discontinuation were rash (3.9%), reaction aggravated (1.7%), and ataxia (0.9%).

Incidence in Controlled Clinical Studies: The prescriber should be aware that the figures in Tables 4, 5, 6, and 7 cannot be used to predict the frequency of adverse experiences in the course of usual medical practice where patient characteristics and other factors may differ from those prevailing during clinical studies. Similarly, the cited frequencies cannot be directly compared with figures obtained from other clinical investigations involving different treatments, uses, or investigators. An inspection of these frequencies, however, does provide the prescriber with one basis to estimate the relative contribution of drug and nondrug factors to the adverse event incidences in the population studied.

Incidence in Controlled Adjunctive Clinical Studies in Adults: Table 4 lists treatment-emergent signs and symptoms that occurred in at least 2% of adult patients with epilepsy treated with LAMICTAL in placebo-controlled trials and were numerically more common in the patients treated with LAMICTAL. In these studies, either LAMICTAL or placebo was added to the patient's current AED therapy. Adverse events were usually mild to moderate in intensity.

[See table 4 on previous page]

In a randomized, parallel study comparing placebo and 300 and 500 mg/day of LAMICTAL, some of the more common drug-related adverse events were dose related (see Table 5).

[See table 5 on previous page]

Other events that occurred in more than 1% of patients but equally or more frequently in the placebo group included: asthenia, back pain, chest pain, flatulence, menstrual disorder, myalgia, paresthesia, respiratory disorder, and urinary tract infection.

The overall adverse experience profile for LAMICTAL was similar between females and males, and was independent of age. Because the largest non-Caucasian racial subgroup was only 6% of patients exposed to LAMICTAL in placebo-controlled trials, there are insufficient data to support a statement regarding the distribution of adverse experience reports by race. Generally, females receiving either adjunctive LAMICTAL or placebo were more likely to report adverse experiences than males. The only adverse experience for which the reports on LAMICTAL were greater than 10% more frequent in females than males (without a corresponding difference by gender on placebo) was dizziness (difference = 16.5%). There was little difference between females and males in the rates of discontinuation of LAMICTAL for individual adverse experiences.

Table 6: Treatment-Emergent Adverse Event Incidence in Adults in a Controlled Monotherapy Trial*
(Events in at least 2% of patients treated with LAMICTAL and numerically more frequent than in the valproate [VPA] group.)

Body System/Adverse Experience†	Percent of Patients Receiving LAMICTAL Monotherapy‡ (n = 43)	Percent of Patients Receiving Low-Dose VPA§ Monotherapy (n = 44)
Body as a whole		
Pain	5	0
Infection	5	2
Chest pain	5	2
Asthenia	2	0
Fever	2	0
Digestive		
Vomiting	9	0
Dyspepsia	7	2
Nausea	7	2
Anorexia	2	0
Dry mouth	2	0
Rectal hemorrhage	2	0
Peptic ulcer	2	0
Metabolic and nutritional		
Weight decrease	5	2
Peripheral edema	2	0
Nervous		
Coordination abnormality	7	0
Dizziness	7	0
Anxiety	5	0
Insomnia	5	2
Amnesia	2	0
Ataxia	2	0
Depression	2	0
Hypesthesia	2	0
Libido increase	2	0
Decreased reflexes	2	0
Increased reflexes	2	0
Nystagmus	2	0
Irritability	2	0
Suicidal ideation	2	0
Respiratory		
Rhinitis	7	2
Epistaxis	2	0
Bronchitis	2	0
Dyspnea	2	0
Skin and appendages		
Contact dermatitis	2	0
Dry skin	2	0
Sweating	2	0
Special senses		
Vision abnormality	2	0
Urogenital (female patients only)	(n = 21)	(n = 28)
Dysmenorrhea	5	0

*Patients in these studies were converted to LAMICTAL or VPA monotherapy from adjunctive therapy with carbamazepine or phenytoin. Patients may have reported multiple adverse experiences during the study; thus, patients may be included in more than one category.
† Adverse experiences reported by at least 2% of patients are included.
‡ Up to 500 mg/day.
§ 1000 mg/day.

Table 7: Treatment-Emergent Adverse Event Incidence in Placebo-Controlled Adjunctive Trial in Adult and Pediatric Patients With Lennox-Gastaut Syndrome
(Events in at least 2% of patients treated with LAMICTAL and numerically more frequent than in the placebo group.)

Body System/Adverse Experience	Percent of Patients Receiving LAMICTAL (n = 79)	Percent of Patients Receiving Placebo (n = 90)
Body as a whole		
Infection	13	8
Accidental injury	9	7
Flu syndrome	5	0
Asthenia	3	1
Abdominal pain	3	0
Cardiovascular		
Hemorrhage	3	0
Digestive		
Vomiting	9	7
Constipation	5	2
Diarrhea	4	2
Nausea	4	1
Anorexia	3	1
Nervous system		
Ataxia	4	1
Convulsions	4	1
Tremor	3	0
Respiratory		
Pharyngitis	14	10
Bronchitis	9	7
Pneumonia	3	0
Skin		
Rash	9	7
Eczema	4	0
Urogenital		
Urinary tract infection	3	0
Balanitis	2	0
Penis disorder	2	0

Incidence in a Controlled Monotherapy Trial in Adults With Partial Seizures: Table 6 lists treatment-emergent signs and symptoms that occurred in at least 2% of patients with epilepsy treated with monotherapy with LAMICTAL in a double-blind trial following discontinuation of either concomitant carbamazepine or phenytoin not seen at an equivalent frequency in the control group.

[See table 6 on previous page]

Incidence in a Controlled Adjunctive Trial in Adult and Pediatric Patients With Lennox-Gastaut Syndrome: Table 7 lists adverse events that occurred in at least 2% of 79 adult and pediatric patients who received LAMICTAL up to 15 mg/kg per day or a maximum of 400 mg per day. Reported adverse events were classified using COSTART terminology.

[See table 7 on previous page]

Other Adverse Events Observed During All Clinical Trials For Adult and Pediatric Patients: LAMICTAL has been administered to 3923 individuals for whom complete adverse event data was captured during all clinical trials, only some of which were placebo controlled. During these trials, all adverse events were recorded by the clinical investigators using terminology of their own choosing. To provide a meaningful estimate of the proportion of individuals having adverse events, similar types of events were grouped into a smaller number of standardized categories using modified COSTART dictionary terminology. The frequencies presented represent the proportion of the 3923 individuals exposed to LAMICTAL who experienced an event of the type cited on at least one occasion while receiving LAMICTAL. All reported events are included except those already listed in the previous table, those too general to be informative, and those not reasonably associated with the use of the drug.

Events are further classified within body system categories and enumerated in order of decreasing frequency using the following definitions: *frequent* adverse events are defined as those occurring in at least 1/100 patients; *infrequent* adverse events are those occurring in 1/100 to 1/1000 patients; *rare* adverse events are those occurring in fewer than 1/1000 patients.

Body as a Whole: Frequent: Pain. ***Infrequent:*** Accidental injury, allergic reaction, back pain, chills, face edema, halitosis, infection, and malaise. ***Rare:*** Abdomen enlarged, abscess, photosensitivity, and suicide attempt.

Cardiovascular System: Infrequent: Flushing, hot flashes, migraine, palpitations, postural hypotension, syncope, tachycardia, and vasodilation. ***Rare:*** Angina pectoris, atrial fibrillation, deep thrombophlebitis, hemorrhage, hypertension, and myocardial infarction.

Dermatological: Infrequent: Acne, alopecia, dry skin, erythema, hirsutism, maculopapular rash, skin discoloration, Stevens-Johnson syndrome, sweating, urticaria, and vesiculobullous rash. ***Rare:*** Angioedema, erythema multiforme, fungal dermatitis, herpes zoster, leukoderma, petechial rash, pustular rash, and seborrhea.

Digestive System: Infrequent: Dry mouth, dysphagia, gingivitis, glossitis, gum hyperplasia, increased appetite, increased salivation, liver function tests abnormal, mouth ulceration, stomatitis, thirst, and tooth disorder. ***Rare:*** Eructation, gastritis, gastrointestinal hemorrhage, gum hemorrhage, hematemesis, hemorrhagic colitis, hepatitis, melena, stomach ulcer, and tongue edema.

Endocrine System: Rare: Goiter and hypothyroidism.

Hematologic and Lymphatic System: Infrequent: Anemia, ecchymosis, leukocytosis, leukopenia, lymphadenopathy, and petechia. ***Rare:*** Eosinophilia, fibrin decrease, fibrinogen decrease, iron deficiency anemia, lymphocytosis, macrocytic anemia, and thrombocytopenia.

Metabolic and Nutritional Disorders: Infrequent: Peripheral edema, weight gain, and weight loss. ***Rare:*** Alcohol intolerance, alkaline phosphatase increase, bilirubinemia, general edema, and hyperglycemia.

Musculoskeletal System: Infrequent: Joint disorder, myasthenia, and twitching. ***Rare:*** Arthritis, bursitis, leg cramps, pathological fracture, and tendinous contracture.

Nervous System: Frequent: Amnesia, confusion, hostility, memory decrease, nervousness, nystagmus, thinking abnormality, and vertigo. ***Infrequent:*** Abnormal dreams, abnormal gait, agitation, akathisia, apathy, aphasia, CNS depression, depersonalization, dysarthria, dyskinesia, dysphoria, emotional lability, euphoria, faintness, grand mal convulsions, hallucinations, hyperkinesia, hypertonia, hypesthesia, libido increased, mind racing, muscle spasm, myoclonus, panic attack, paranoid reaction, personality disorder, psychosis, sleep disorder, and stupor. ***Rare:*** Cerebrovascular accident, cerebellar syndrome, cerebral sinus thrombosis, choreoathetosis, CNS stimulation, delirium, delusions, dystonia, hemiplegia, hyperalgesia, hyperesthesia, hypoesthesia, hypokinesia, hypomania, hypotonia, libido decreased, manic depression reaction, movement disorder, neuralgia, neurosis, paralysis, and suicidal ideation.

Respiratory System: Infrequent: Dyspnea, epistaxis, and hyperventilation. ***Rare:*** Bronchospasm, hiccup, and sinusitis.

Special Senses: Infrequent: Abnormality of accommodation, conjunctivitis, ear pain, oscillopsia, photophobia, taste perversion, and tinnitus. ***Rare:*** Deafness, dry eyes, lacrimation disorder, parosmia, ptosis, strabismus, taste loss, and uveitis.

Urogenital System: Infrequent: Female lactation, hematuria, polyuria, urinary frequency, urinary incontinence, urinary retention, and vaginal moniliasis. ***Rare:*** Abnormal ejaculation, acute kidney failure, breast abscess, breast neoplasm, breast pain, creatinine increase, cystitis, dysuria, epididymitis, impotence, kidney failure, kidney pain, menorrhagia, and urine abnormality.

Postmarketing and Other Experience: In addition to the adverse experiences reported during clinical testing of LAMICTAL, the following adverse experiences have been reported in patients receiving marketed LAMICTAL and from worldwide noncontrolled investigational use. These adverse experiences have not been listed above, and data are insufficient to support an estimate of their incidence or to establish causation.

Blood and Lymphatic: Agranulocytosis, aplastic anemia, disseminated intravascular coagulation, hemolytic anemia, neutropenia, pancytopenia, red cell aplasia.

Gastrointestinal: Esophagitis.

Hepatobiliary Tract and Pancreas: Pancreatitis.

Immunologic: Lupus-like reaction, vasculitis.

Lower Respiratory: Apnea.

Musculoskeletal: Rhabdomyolysis has been observed in patients experiencing hypersensitivity reactions.

Neurology: Exacerbation of parkinsonian symptoms in patients with pre-existing Parkinson's disease, tics.

Non-site Specific: Hypersensitivity reaction, multiorgan failure, progressive immunosuppression.

DRUG ABUSE AND DEPENDENCE

The abuse and dependence potential of LAMICTAL have not been evaluated in human studies.

OVERDOSAGE

Human Overdose Experience: Overdoses involving quantities up to 15 g have been reported for LAMICTAL, some of which have been fatal. Overdose has resulted in ataxia, nystagmus, increased seizures, decreased level of consciousness, coma, and intraventricular conduction delay.

Management of Overdose: There are no specific antidotes for LAMICTAL. Following a suspected overdose, hospitalization of the patient is advised. General supportive care is indicated, including frequent monitoring of vital signs and close observation of the patient. If indicated, emesis should be induced or gastric lavage should be performed; usual precautions should be taken to protect the airway. It should be kept in mind that lamotrigine is rapidly absorbed (see CLINICAL PHARMACOLOGY). It is uncertain whether hemodialysis is an effective means of removing lamotrigine from the blood. In six renal failure patients, about 20% of the amount of lamotrigine in the body was removed by hemodialysis during a 4-hour session. A Poison Control Center should be contacted for information on the management of overdosage of LAMICTAL.

DOSAGE AND ADMINISTRATION

Adjunctive Use: LAMICTAL is indicated as adjunctive therapy in adults with partial seizures and as adjunctive therapy in the generalized seizures of Lennox-Gastaut syndrome in pediatric and adult patients.

Monotherapy Use: LAMICTAL is indicated for conversion to monotherapy in adults with partial seizures who are receiving treatment with a single EIAED (e.g., carbamazepine, phenytoin, phenobarbital, etc.).

Safety and effectiveness of LAMICTAL have not been established 1) as initial monotherapy, 2) for conversion to monotherapy from non–enzyme-inducing AEDs (e.g., valproate), or 3) for simultaneous conversion to monotherapy from two or more concomitant AEDs.

Safety and effectiveness in pediatric patients below the age of 16 years other than those with Lennox-Gastaut syndrome have not been established (see BOX WARNING).

General Dosing Considerations: The risk of nonserious rash is increased when the recommended initial dose and/or the rate of dose escalation of LAMICTAL is exceeded. There are suggestions, yet to be proven, that the risk of severe, potentially life-threatening rash may be increased by 1) coadministration of LAMICTAL with valproic acid (VPA), 2) exceeding the recommended initial dose of LAMICTAL, or 3) exceeding the recommended dose escalation for LAMICTAL. However, cases have been reported in the absence of these factors (see BOX WARNING). Therefore, it is important that the dosing recommendations be followed closely.

Adjunctive Therapy With LAMICTAL: This section provides specific dosing recommendations for patients 2 to 12 years of age and patients greater than 12 years of age. Within each of these age-groups, specific dosing recommendations are provided depending upon whether or not the patient is receiving VPA (Tables 8 and 9 for patients 2 to 12 years of age, Tables 10 and 11 for patients greater than 12 years of age). In addition, the section provides a discussion of dosing for those patients receiving concomitant AEDs that have not been systematically evaluated in combination with LAMICTAL.

For dosing guidelines for LAMICTAL below, enzyme-inducing antiepileptic drugs (EIAEDs) include phenytoin, carbamazepine, phenobarbital, and primidone.

Patients 2 to 12 Years of Age: Recommended dosing guidelines for LAMICTAL added to an antiepileptic drug (AED) regimen containing VPA are summarized in Table 8. Recommended dosing guidelines for LAMICTAL added to EIAEDs are summarized in Table 9. Note that the starting doses and dose escalations listed below are different than those used in clinical trials; however, the maintenance doses are the same as in clinical trials. Smaller starting doses and slower dose escalations than those used in clinical trials are recommended because of the suggestions that the risk of rash may be decreased by smaller starting doses and slower dose escalations. Therefore, maintenance doses will take longer to reach in clinical practice than in clinical trials. It may take several weeks to months to achieve an individualized maintenance dose. It is likely that patients aged 2 to 6 years will require a maintenance dose at the higher end of the maintenance dose range.

The smallest available strength of LAMICTAL Chewable Dispersible Tablets is 5 mg, and only whole tablets should be administered. If the calculated dose cannot be achieved using whole tablets, the dose should be rounded down to the nearest whole tablet.

Pediatric patients who weigh less than 17 kg (37 lb) should not receive LAMICTAL because therapy cannot be initiated

Continued on next page

Table 8: LAMICTAL Added to an AED Regimen Containing VPA in Patients 2 to 12 Years of Age

Weeks 1 and 2	0.15 mg/kg/day in one or two divided doses, rounded down to the nearest 5 mg. If the initial calculated daily dose of LAMICTAL is 2.5 to 5 mg, then 5 mg of LAMICTAL should be taken on alternate days for the first 2 weeks.
Weeks 3 and 4	0.3 mg/kg/day in one or two divided doses, rounded down to the nearest 5 mg.

Usual maintenance dose: 1 to 5 mg/kg/day (maximum 200 mg/day in one or two divided doses). To achieve the usual maintenance dose, subsequent doses should be increased every 1 to 2 weeks as follows: calculate 0.3 mg/kg/day, round this amount down to the nearest 5 mg, and add this amount to the previously administered daily dose.

Table 9: LAMICTAL Added to EIAEDs (Without VPA) in Patients 2 to 12 Years of Age

Weeks 1 and 2	0.6 mg/kg/day in two divided doses, rounded down to the nearest 5 mg.
Weeks 3 and 4	1.2 mg/kg/day in two divided doses, rounded down to the nearest 5 mg.

Usual maintenance dose: 5 to 15 mg/kg/day (maximum 400 mg/day in two divided doses). To achieve the usual maintenance dose, subsequent doses should be increased every 1 to 2 weeks as follows: calculate 1.2 mg/kg/day, round this amount down to the nearest 5 mg, and add this amount to the previously administered daily dose.

Table 10: LAMICTAL Added to an AED Regimen Containing VPA in Patients Over 12 Years of Age

Weeks 1 and 2	25 mg every *other* day
Weeks 3 and 4	25 mg every day

Usual maintenance dose: 100 to 400 mg/day (1 or 2 divided doses). To achieve maintenance, doses may be increased by 25 to 50 mg/day every 1 to 2 weeks. The usual maintenance dose in patients adding LAMICTAL to VPA alone ranges from 100 to 200 mg/day.

This product information is based on labeling in effect on June 23, 2000. For further information, contact via direct mail, phone, or web site. Medical Information, Glaxo Wellcome Inc., PO Box 13398, Research Triangle Park, NC 27709. Healthcare Professionals (Medical Information): 800-334-0089. Patients (Customer Response Center): 1-888-825-5249. Glaxo Wellcome Corporate Web Site: www.glaxowellcome.com

Lamictal—Cont.

using the dosing guidelines (see Table 8 and Table 9) and the currently available tablet strengths (see WARNINGS).
[See table 8 on previous page]
[See table 9 on previous page]
Patients Over 12 Years of Age: Recommended dosing guidelines for LAMICTAL added to VPA are summarized in Table 10. Recommended dosing guidelines for LAMICTAL added to EIAEDs are summarized in Table 11.
[See table 10 on previous page]
[See table 11 at right]
Conversion From a Single EIAED to Monotherapy With LAMICTAL in Patients ≥16 Years of Age: The goal of the transition regimen is to effect the conversion to monotherapy with LAMICTAL under conditions that ensure adequate seizure control while mitigating the risk of serious rash associated with the rapid titration of LAMICTAL.
The conversion regimen involves two steps. In the first, LAMICTAL is titrated to the targeted dose while maintaining the dose of the EIAED at a fixed level; in the second step, the EIAED is gradually withdrawn over a period of 4 weeks.
The recommended maintenance dose of LAMICTAL as monotherapy is 500 mg/day given in two divided doses.
LAMICTAL should be added to an EIAED to achieve a dose of 500 mg/day according to the guidelines in Table 11 above. The regimen for the withdrawal of the concomitant EIAED is based on experience gained in the controlled monotherapy clinical trial. In that trial, the concomitant EIAED was withdrawn by 20% decrements each week over a 4-week period.
Because of an increased risk of rash, the recommended initial dose and subsequent dose escalations of LAMICTAL should not be exceeded (see BOX WARNING).
Usual Maintenance Dose: The usual maintenance doses identified in the tables above are derived from dosing regimens employed in the placebo-controlled adjunctive studies in which the efficacy of LAMICTAL was established. In patients receiving multidrug regimens employing EIAEDs **without VPA**, maintenance doses of adjunctive LAMICTAL as high as 700 mg/day have been used. In patients receiving **VPA alone**, maintenance doses of adjunctive LAMICTAL as high as 200 mg/day have been used. The advantage of using doses above those recommended in the tables above has not been established in controlled trials.
LAMICTAL Added to AEDs Other Than EIAEDs and VPA: The effect of AEDs other than EIAEDs and VPA on the metabolism of LAMICTAL cannot be predicted. Therefore, no specific dosing guidelines can be provided in that situation. Conservative starting doses and dose escalations (as with concomitant VPA) would be prudent; maintenance dosing would be expected to fall between the maintenance dose with VPA and the maintenance dose without VPA, but with an EIAED.
Patients With Hepatic Impairment: Experience in patients with hepatic impairment is limited. Based on a clinical pharmacology study in 24 patients with moderate to severe liver dysfunction (see CLINICAL PHARMACOLOGY), the following general recommendations can be made. Initial, escalation, and maintenance doses should generally be reduced by approximately 50% in patients with moderate (Child-Pugh Grade B) and 75% in patients with severe (Child-Pugh Grade C) hepatic impairment. Escalation and maintenance doses should be adjusted according to clinical response.
Patients With Renal Functional Impairment: Initial doses of LAMICTAL should be based on patients' AED regimen (see above); reduced maintenance doses may be effective for patients with significant renal functional impairment (see CLINICAL PHARMACOLOGY). Few patients with severe renal impairment have been evaluated during chronic treatment with LAMICTAL. Because there is inadequate experience in this population, LAMICTAL should be used with caution in these patients.
Discontinuation Strategy: For patients receiving LAMICTAL in combination with other AEDs, a reevaluation of all AEDs in the regimen should be considered if a change in seizure control or an appearance or worsening of adverse experiences is observed.
If a decision is made to discontinue therapy with LAMICTAL, a step-wise reduction of dose over at least 2 weeks (approximately 50% per week) is recommended unless safety concerns require a more rapid withdrawal (see PRECAUTIONS).
Discontinuing an EIAED should prolong the half-life of lamotrigine; discontinuing VPA should shorten the half-life of lamotrigine.
Target Plasma Levels: A therapeutic plasma concentration range has not been established for lamotrigine. Dosing of LAMICTAL should be based on therapeutic response.
Administration of LAMICTAL Chewable Dispersible Tablets: LAMICTAL Chewable Dispersible Tablets may be swallowed whole, chewed, or dispersed in water or diluted fruit juice. If the tablets are chewed, consume a small amount of water or diluted fruit juice to aid in swallowing.
To disperse LAMICTAL Chewable Dispersible Tablets, add the tablets to a small amount of liquid (1 teaspoon, or enough to cover the medication). Approximately 1 minute later, when the tablets are completely dispersed, swirl the solution and consume the entire quantity immediately. *No attempt should be made to administer partial quantities of the dispersed tablets.*

Table 11: LAMICTAL Added to EIAEDs (Without VPA) in Patients Over 12 Years of Age

Weeks 1 and 2	50 mg/day
Weeks 3 and 4	100 mg/day in two divided doses

Usual maintenance dose: 300 to 500 mg/day (in two divided doses). To achieve maintenance, doses may be increased by 100 mg/day every 1 to 2 weeks.

LAMICTAL® (lamotrigine) Tablets

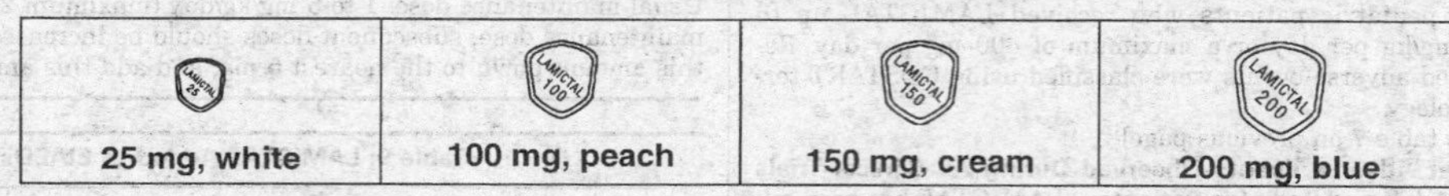

LAMICTAL® (lamotrigine) Chewable Dispersible Tablets

GX CL2
5 mg, white
GX CL5
25 mg, white

HOW SUPPLIED

LAMICTAL Tablets, 25 mg, white, scored, shield-shaped tablets engraved with "LAMICTAL" and "25", bottle of 100 (NDC 0173-0633-02).
Store at 15° to 25°C (59° to 77°F) in a dry place.
LAMICTAL Tablets, 100 mg, peach, scored, shield-shaped tablets engraved with "LAMICTAL" and "100", bottle of 100 (NDC 0173-0642-55).
LAMICTAL Tablets, 150 mg, cream, scored, shield-shaped tablets engraved with "LAMICTAL" and "150", bottle of 60 (NDC 0173-0643-60).
LAMICTAL Tablets, 200 mg, blue, scored, shield-shaped tablets engraved with "LAMICTAL" and "200", bottle of 60 (NDC 0173-0644-60).
Store at 15° to 25°C (59° to 77°F) in a dry place and protect from light.
LAMICTAL Chewable Dispersible Tablets, 5 mg, white, caplet-shaped tablets engraved with "GX CL2", bottle of 100 (NDC 0173-0526-00).
LAMICTAL Chewable Dispersible Tablets, 25 mg, white, super elliptical-shaped tablets engraved with "GX CL5", bottle of 100 (NDC 0173-0527-00).
Store at controlled room temperature, 20° to 25°C (68° to 77°F) (see USP) in a dry place.

PATIENT INFORMATION

The following wording is contained in a separate leaflet provided for patients.

Information for the Patient

[See tablet graphic above]
Please read this leaflet carefully before you take LAMICTAL and read the leaflet provided with any refill, in case any information has changed. This leaflet provides a summary of the information about your medicine. Please do not throw away this leaflet until you have finished your medicine. This leaflet does not contain all the information about LAMICTAL and is not meant to take the place of talking with your doctor. If you have any questions about LAMICTAL, ask your doctor or pharmacist.
Information About Your Medicine:
The name of your medicine is LAMICTAL (lamotrigine). The decision to use LAMICTAL is one that you and your doctor should make together.
1. The Purpose of Your Medicine:
Lamotrigine is intended to be used either alone or in combination with other medicines to treat seizures in people age 16 years or older and/or only those patients below the age of 16 years who have seizures associated with the Lennox-Gastaut syndrome. When taking lamotrigine, it is important to follow your doctor's instructions.
2. Who Should Not Take LAMICTAL:
You should not take LAMICTAL if you had an allergic reaction to it in the past.
3. Side Effects to Watch for:
- Most people who take LAMICTAL tolerate it well. The most common side effects with LAMICTAL are dizziness, headache, blurred or double vision, lack of coordination, sleepiness, nausea, vomiting, and rash.
- Although most patients who develop rash while receiving LAMICTAL have mild to moderate symptoms, some individuals may develop a serious skin reaction that requires hospitalization. Rarely, deaths have been reported. These serious skin reactions are most likely to happen within the first 8 weeks of treatment with LAMICTAL. Serious skin reactions occur more often in children than in adults.
- Rashes may be more likely to occur if you: 1) take LAMICTAL in combination with valproic acid (DEPAKENE® or DEPAKOTE®), 2) take a higher starting dose of LAMICTAL than your doctor prescribed, or 3) increase your dose of LAMICTAL faster than prescribed.
- It is not possible to predict whether a mild rash will develop into a more serious reaction. **Therefore, if you experience a skin rash, hives, fever, swollen lymph glands, painful sores in the mouth or around the eyes, or swelling of lips or tongue, tell a doctor immediately, since these symptoms may be the first signs of a serious reaction. A doctor should evaluate your condition and decide if you should continue taking LAMICTAL.**

4. The Use of LAMICTAL During Pregnancy and Breast-feeding:
The effects of LAMICTAL during pregnancy are not known at this time. If you are pregnant or are planning to become pregnant, talk to your doctor. Some LAMICTAL passes into breast milk and the effects of this on infants are unknown. Therefore, if you are breast-feeding, you should discuss this with your doctor to determine if you should continue to take LAMICTAL.
5. How to Use LAMICTAL:
- It is important to take LAMICTAL exactly as instructed by your doctor. The dose of LAMICTAL must be increased slowly. It may take several weeks or months before your final dosage can be determined by your doctor, based on your response.
- Do not increase your dose of LAMICTAL or take more frequent doses than those indicated by your doctor.
- If you miss a dose of LAMICTAL, do not double your next dose.
- Do NOT stop taking LAMICTAL or any of your other seizure medicines unless instructed by your doctor.
- Use caution before driving a car or operating complex, hazardous machinery until you know if LAMICTAL affects your ability to perform these tasks.
- Tell your doctor if your seizures get worse or if you have any new types of seizures.
- Always tell your doctor and pharmacist if you are taking or plan to take any other prescription or over-the-counter medicines.

6. How to Take LAMICTAL:
LAMICTAL Tablets should be swallowed whole. Chewing the tablets may leave a bitter taste.
LAMICTAL Chewable Dispersible Tablets may be swallowed whole, chewed, or mixed in water or diluted fruit juice. If the tablets are chewed, consume a small amount of water or diluted fruit juice to aid in swallowing.
To disperse LAMICTAL Chewable Dispersible Tablets, add the tablets to a small amount of liquid (1 teaspoon, or enough to cover the medication) in a glass or spoon. Approximately 1 minute later, when the tablets are completely dispersed, mix the solution and take the entire amount immediately.
7. Storing Your Medicine:
Store LAMICTAL at room temperature away from heat and light. Always keep your medicines out of the reach of children.
This medicine was prescribed for your use only to treat seizures. Do not give the drug to others.
If your doctor decides to stop your treatment, do not keep any leftover medicine unless your doctor tells you to. Throw away your medicine as instructed.
Glaxo Wellcome Inc., Research Triangle Park, NC 27709
DEPAKENE and DEPAKOTE are registered trademarks of Abbott Laboratories.
US Patent No. 4,602,017

June 2000/RL-832
Shown in Product Identification Guide, page 315

LANOXICAPS® ℞

[*lă-nŏx 'ĭ-kăps*"]
(digoxin solution in capsules)
50 mcg (0.05 mg) I.D. Imprint A2C (red)
100 mcg (0.1 mg) I.D. Imprint B2C (yellow)
200 mcg (0.2 mg) I.D. Imprint C2C (green)

DESCRIPTION

LANOXIN (digoxin) is one of the cardiac (or digitalis) glycosides, a closely related group of drugs having in common specific effects on the myocardium. These drugs are found in a number of plants. Digoxin is extracted from the leaves of *Digitalis lanata*. The term "digitalis" is used to designate the whole group of glycosides. The glycosides are composed of two portions: a sugar and a cardenolide (hence "glycosides").
Digoxin is described chemically as (3β,5β,12β)-3-[(*O*-2,6-dideoxy-β-*D*-*ribo*-hexopyranosyl-(1→4)-*O*-2,6-dideoxy-β-*D*-*ribo*-hexopyranosyl-(1→4)-2,6-dideoxy-β-*D*-*ribo*-hexopy-

Table 1: Comparisons of the Systemic Availability and Equivalent Doses for Preparations of LANOXIN

Product	Absolute Bioavailability	Equivalent Doses (mcg)* Among Dosage Forms			
LANOXIN Tablets	60–80%	62.5	125	250	500
LANOXIN Elixir Pediatric	70–85%	62.5	125	250	500
LANOXICAPS®	90–100%	50	100	200	400
LANOXIN Injection/IV	100%	50	100	200	400

* For example, 125 mcg LANOXIN Tablets equivalent to 125 mcg LANOXIN Elixir Pediatric equivalent to 100 mcg LANOXICAPS equivalent to 100 mcg LANOXIN Injection/IV.

ranosyl)oxy]-12,14-dihydroxy-card-20(22)-enolide. Its molecular formula is $C_{41}H_{64}O_{14}$, its molecular weight is 780.95. Digoxin exists as odorless white crystals that melt with decomposition above 230°C. The drug is practically insoluble in water and in ether; slightly soluble in diluted (50%) alcohol and in chloroform; and freely soluble in pyridine.

LANOXICAPS is a stable solution of digoxin enclosed within a soft gelatin capsule for oral use. Each capsule contains the labeled amount of digoxin USP dissolved in a solvent comprised of polyethylene glycol 400 USP, 8 percent ethyl alcohol, propylene glycol USP, and purified water USP. Inactive ingredients in the capsule shell include FD&C Red No. 40 (0.05-mg Capsule), D&C Yellow No. 10 (0.1-mg and 0.2-mg Capsules), FD&C Blue No. 1 (0.2-mg Capsule), gelatin, glycerin, methylparaben and propylparaben (added as preservatives), purified water, and sorbitol. Capsules are printed with edible ink.

CLINICAL PHARMACOLOGY

Mechanism of Action: Digoxin inhibits sodium-potassium ATPase, an enzyme that regulates the quantity of sodium and potassium inside cells. Inhibition of the enzyme leads to an increase in the intracellular concentration of sodium and thus (by stimulation of sodium-calcium exchange) an increase in the intracellular concentration of calcium. The beneficial effects of digoxin result from direct actions on cardiac muscle, as well as indirect actions on the cardiovascular system mediated by effects on the autonomic nervous system. The autonomic effects include: (1) a vagomimetic action, which is responsible for the effects of digoxin on the sinoatrial and atrioventricular (AV) nodes; and (2) baroreceptor sensitization, which results in increased afferent inhibitory activity and reduced activity of the sympathetic nervous system and renin-angiotensin system for any given increment in mean arterial pressure. The pharmacologic consequences of these direct and indirect effects are: (1) an increase in the force and velocity of myocardial systolic contraction (positive inotropic action); (2) a decrease in the degree of activation of the sympathetic nervous system and renin-angiotensin system (neurohormonal deactivating effect); and (3) slowing of the heart rate and decreased conduction velocity through the AV node (vagomimetic effect). The effects of digoxin in heart failure are mediated by its positive inotropic and neurohormonal deactivating effects, whereas the effects of the drug in atrial arrhythmias are related to its vagomimetic actions. In high doses, digoxin increases sympathetic outflow from the central nervous system (CNS). This increase in sympathetic activity may be an important factor in digitalis toxicity.

Pharmacokinetics: *Absorption:* Absorption of digoxin from LANOXICAPS Capsules has been demonstrated to be 90% to 100% complete compared to an identical intravenous dose of digoxin (absolute bioavailability). In comparison, the absolute bioavailability of conventional digoxin tablets has been demonstrated to be 60% to 80%. The enhanced absorption from LANOXICAPS compared to digoxin tablets and elixir is associated with reduced between-patient and within-patient variability in steady-state serum concentrations. The peak serum concentrations are higher than those observed after tablets. When digoxin tablets or capsules are taken after meals, the rate of absorption is slowed, but the total amount of digoxin absorbed is usually unchanged. When taken with meals high in bran fiber, however, the amount absorbed from an oral dose may be reduced. Comparisons of the systemic availability and equivalent doses for preparations of LANOXIN are shown in Table 1:

[See table 1 above]

In some patients, orally administered digoxin is converted to inactive reduction products (e.g., dihydrodigoxin) by colonic bacteria in the gut. Data suggest that one in ten patients treated with digoxin tablets will degrade 40% or more of the ingested dose. As a result, certain antibiotics may increase the absorption of digoxin in such patients. Although inactivation of these bacteria by antibiotics is rapid, the serum digoxin concentration will rise at a rate consistent with the elimination half-life of digoxin. The magnitude of rise in serum digoxin concentration relates to the extent of bacterial inactivation, and may be as much as two-fold in some cases. This phenomenon is minimized with LANOXICAPS because they are rapidly absorbed in the upper gastrointestinal tract.

Distribution: Following drug administration, a 6- to 8-hour tissue distribution phase is observed. This is followed by a much more gradual decline in the serum concentration of the drug, which is dependent on the elimination of digoxin from the body. The peak height and slope of the early portion (absorption/distribution phases) of the serum concentration-time curve are dependent upon the route of administration and the absorption characteristics of the formulation. Clinical evidence indicates that the early high serum concentrations (particularly high for digoxin capsules) do not reflect the concentration of digoxin at its site of action, but that with chronic use, the steady-state post-distribution serum levels are in equilibrium with tissue concentrations and correlate with pharmacologic effects. In individual patients, these post-distribution serum concentrations may be useful in evaluating therapeutic and toxic effects (see DOSAGE AND ADMINISTRATION: Serum Digoxin Concentrations).

Digoxin is concentrated in tissues and therefore has a large apparent volume of distribution. Digoxin crosses both the blood-brain barrier and the placenta. At delivery, the serum digoxin concentration in the newborn is similar to the serum concentration in the mother. Approximately 25% of digoxin in the plasma is bound to protein. Serum digoxin concentrations are not significantly altered by large changes in fat tissue weight, so that its distribution space correlates best with lean (i.e., ideal) body weight, not total body weight.

Metabolism: Only a small percentage (16%) of a dose of digoxin is metabolized. The end metabolites, which include 3 β-digoxigenin, 3-keto-digoxigenin, and their glucuronide and sulfate conjugates, are polar in nature and are postulated to be formed via hydrolysis, oxidation, and conjugation. The metabolism of digoxin is not dependent upon the cytochrome P-450 system, and digoxin is not known to induce or inhibit the cytochrome P-450 system.

Excretion: Elimination of digoxin follows first-order kinetics (that is, the quantity of digoxin eliminated at any time is proportional to the total body content). Following intravenous administration to healthy volunteers, 50% to 70% of a digoxin dose is excreted unchanged in the urine. Renal excretion of digoxin is proportional to glomerular filtration rate and is largely independent of urine flow. In healthy volunteers with normal renal function, digoxin has a half-life of 1.5 to 2.0 days. The half-life in anuric patients is prolonged to 3.5 to 5 days. Digoxin is not effectively removed from the body by dialysis, exchange transfusion, or during cardiopulmonary bypass because most of the drug is bound to tissue and does not circulate in the blood.

Special Populations: Race differences in digoxin pharmacokinetics have not been formally studied. Because digoxin is primarily eliminated as unchanged drug via the kidney and because there are no important differences in creatinine clearance among races, pharmacokinetic differences due to race are not expected.

The clearance of digoxin can be primarily correlated with renal function as indicated by creatinine clearance. The Cockcroft and Gault formula for estimation of creatinine clearance includes age, body weight, and gender. A table that provides the usual daily maintenance dose requirements of LANOXICAPS Capsules based on creatinine clearance (per 70-kg) is presented in the DOSAGE AND ADMINISTRATION section.

Plasma digoxin concentration profiles in patients with acute hepatitis generally fell within the range of profiles in a group of healthy subjects.

Pharmacodynamic and Clinical Effects: The times to onset of pharmacologic effect and to peak effect of preparations of LANOXIN are shown in Table 2:

[See table 2 at top of next page]

Hemodynamic Effects: Digoxin produces hemodynamic improvement in patients with heart failure. Short- and long-term therapy with the drug increases cardiac output and lowers pulmonary artery pressure, pulmonary capillary wedge pressure, and systemic vascular resistance. These hemodynamic effects are accompanied by an increase in the left ventricular ejection fraction and a decrease in end-systolic and end-diastolic dimensions.

Chronic Heart Failure: Two 12-week, double-blind, placebo-controlled studies enrolled 178 (RADIANCE trial) and 88 (PROVED trial) patients with NYHA class II or III heart failure previously treated with digoxin, a diuretic, and an ACE inhibitor (RADIANCE only) and randomized them to placebo or treatment with LANOXIN Tablets. Both trials demonstrated better preservation of exercise capacity in patients randomized to LANOXIN. Continued treatment with LANOXIN reduced the risk of developing worsening heart failure, as evidenced by heart failure-related hospitalizations and emergency care and the need for concomitant heart failure therapy. The larger study also showed treatment-related benefits in NYHA class and patients' global assessment. In the smaller trial, these trended in favor of a treatment benefit.

The Digitalis Investigation Group (DIG) main trial was a multicenter, randomized, double-blind, placebo-controlled mortality study of 6801 patients with heart failure and left ventricular ejection fraction ≤0.45. At randomization, 67% were NYHA class I or II, 71% had heart failure of ischemic etiology, 44% had been receiving digoxin, and most were receiving concomitant ACE inhibitor (94%) and diuretic (82%). Patients were randomized to placebo or LANOXIN Tablets, the dose of which was adjusted for the patient's age, sex, lean body weight, and serum creatinine (see DOSAGE AND ADMINISTRATION), and followed for up to 58 months (median 37 months). The median daily dose prescribed was 0.25 mg. Overall all-cause mortality was 35% with no difference between groups (95% confidence limits for relative risk of 0.91 to 1.07). LANOXIN was associated with a 25% reduction in the number of hospitalizations for heart failure, a 28% reduction in the risk of a patient having at least one hospitalization for heart failure, and a 6.5% reduction in total hospitalizations (for any cause).

Use of LANOXIN was associated with a trend to increase time to all-cause death or hospitalization. The trend was evident in subgroups of patients with mild heart failure as well as more severe disease, as shown in Table 3. Although the effect on all-cause death or hospitalization was not statistically significant, much of the apparent benefit derived from effects on mortality and hospitalization attributed to heart failure.

[See table 3 on next page]

In situations where there is no statistically significant benefit of treatment evident from a trial's primary endpoint, results pertaining to a secondary endpoint should be interpreted cautiously.

Chronic Atrial Fibrillation: In patients with chronic atrial fibrillation, digoxin slows rapid ventricular response rate in a linear dose-response fashion from 0.25 to 0.75 mg/day. Digoxin should not be used for the treatment of multifocal atrial tachycardia.

INDICATIONS AND USAGE

Heart Failure: LANOXIN is indicated for the treatment of mild to moderate heart failure. LANOXIN increases left ventricular ejection fraction and improves heart failure symptoms as evidenced by exercise capacity and heart failure-related hospitalizations and emergency care, while having no effect on mortality. Where possible, LANOXIN should be used with a diuretic and an angiotensin-converting enzyme inhibitor, but an optimal order for starting these three drugs cannot be specified.

Atrial Fibrillation: LANOXIN is indicated for the control of ventricular response rate in patients with chronic atrial fibrillation.

CONTRAINDICATIONS

Digitalis glycosides are contraindicated in patients with ventricular fibrillation or in patients with a known hypersensitivity to digoxin. A hypersensitivity reaction to other digitalis preparations usually constitutes a contraindication to digoxin.

WARNINGS

Sinus Node Disease and AV Block: Because digoxin slows sinoatrial and AV conduction, the drug commonly prolongs the PR interval. The drug may cause severe sinus bradycardia or sinoatrial block in patients with pre-existing sinus node disease and may cause advanced or complete heart block in patients with pre-existing incomplete AV block. In such patients consideration should be given to the insertion of a pacemaker before treatment with digoxin.

Accessory AV Pathway (Wolff-Parkinson-White Syndrome): After intravenous digoxin therapy, some patients with paroxysmal atrial fibrillation or flutter and a coexisting accessory AV pathway have developed increased antegrade conduction across the accessory pathway bypassing the AV node, leading to a very rapid ventricular response or ventricular fibrillation. Unless conduction down the accessory pathway has been blocked (either pharmacologically or by surgery), digoxin should not be used in such patients. The treatment of paroxysmal supraventricular tachycardia in such patients is usually direct-current cardioversion.

Use in Patients with Preserved Left Ventricular Systolic Function: Patients with certain disorders involving heart failure associated with preserved left ventricular ejection fraction may be particularly susceptible to toxicity of the drug. Such disorders include restrictive cardiomyopathy, constrictive pericarditis, amyloid heart disease, and acute cor pulmonale. Patients with idiopathic hypertrophic subaortic stenosis may have worsening of the outflow obstruction due to the inotropic effects of digoxin.

PRECAUTIONS

Use in Patients with Impaired Renal Function: Digoxin is primarily excreted by the kidneys; therefore, patients with impaired renal function require smaller than usual maintenance doses of digoxin (see DOSAGE AND ADMINISTRATION). Because of the prolonged elimination half-life, a longer period of time is required to achieve an initial or new steady-state serum concentration in patients with renal impairment than in patients with normal renal function. If appropriate care is not taken to reduce the dose of digoxin, such patients are at high risk for toxicity, and toxic effects will last longer in such patients than in patients with normal renal function.

Use in Patients with Electrolyte Disorders: In patients with hypokalemia or hypomagnesemia, toxicity may occur despite serum digoxin concentrations below 2.0 ng/mL, be-

Continued on next page

This product information is based on labeling in effect on June 23, 2000. For further information, contact via direct mail, phone, or web site. Medical Information, Glaxo Wellcome Inc., PO Box 13398, Research Triangle Park, NC 27709. Healthcare Professionals (Medical Information): 800-334-0089. Patients (Customer Response Center): 1-888-825-5249. Glaxo Wellcome Corporate Web Site: www.glaxowellcome.com

Lanoxicaps—Cont.

cause potassium or magnesium depletion sensitizes the myocardium to digoxin. Therefore, it is desirable to maintain normal serum potassium and magnesium concentrations in patients being treated with digoxin. Deficiencies of these electrolytes may result from malnutrition, diarrhea, or prolonged vomiting, as well as the use of the following drugs or procedures: diuretics, amphotericin B, corticosteroids, antacids, dialysis, and mechanical suction of gastrointestinal secretions.

Hypercalcemia from any cause predisposes the patient to digitalis toxicity. Calcium, particularly when administered rapidly by the intravenous route, may produce serious arrhythmias in digitalized patients. On the other hand, hypocalcemia can nullify the effects of digoxin in humans; thus, digoxin may be ineffective until serum calcium is restored to normal. These interactions are related to the fact that digoxin affects contractility and excitability of the heart in a manner similar to that of calcium.

Use in Thyroid Disorders and Hypermetabolic States: Hypothyroidism may reduce the requirements for digoxin. Heart failure and/or atrial arrhythmias resulting from hypermetabolic or hyperdynamic states (e.g., hyperthyroidism, hypoxia, or arteriovenous shunt) are best treated by addressing the underlying condition. Atrial arrhythmias associated with hypermetabolic states are particularly resistant to digoxin treatment. Care must be taken to avoid toxicity if digoxin is used.

Use in Patients with Acute Myocardial Infarction: Digoxin should be used with caution in patients with acute myocardial infarction. The use of inotropic drugs in some patients in this setting may result in undesirable increases in myocardial oxygen demand and ischemia.

Use During Electrical Cardioversion: It may be desirable to reduce the dose of digoxin for 1 to 2 days prior to electrical cardioversion of atrial fibrillation to avoid the induction of ventricular arrhythmias, but physicians must consider the consequences of increasing the ventricular response if digoxin is withdrawn. If digitalis toxicity is suspected, elective cardioversion should be delayed. If it is not prudent to delay cardioversion, the lowest possible energy level should be selected to avoid provoking ventricular arrhythmias.

Laboratory Test Monitoring: Patients receiving digoxin should have their serum electrolytes and renal function (serum creatinine concentrations) assessed periodically; the frequency of assessments will depend on the clinical setting. For discussion of serum digoxin concentrations, see DOSAGE AND ADMINISTRATION.

Drug Interactions: Potassium-depleting *diuretics* are a major contributing factor to digitalis toxicity. *Calcium*, particularly if administered rapidly by the intravenous route, may produce serious arrhythmias in digitalized patients. *Quinidine, verapamil, amiodarone, propafenone, indomethacin, itraconazole, alprazolam,* and *spironolactoneraise* the serum digoxin concentration due to a reduction in clearance and/or in volume of distribution of the drug, with the implication that digitalis intoxication may result. *Erythromycin* and *clarithromycin* (and possibly other *macrolide antibiotics*) and *tetracycline* may increase digoxin absorption in patients who inactivate digoxin by bacterial metabolism in the lower intestine, so that digitalis intoxication may result. The risk of this interaction may be reduced if digoxin is given as LANOXICAPS (see CLINICAL PHARMACOLOGY: Absorption). *Propantheline* and *diphenoxylate*, by decreasing gut motility, may increase digoxin absorption. *Antacids, kaolin-pectin, sulfasalazine, neomycin, cholestyramine,* certain *anticancer drugs,* and *metoclopramide* may interfere with intestinal digoxin absorption, resulting in unexpectedly low serum concentrations. *Rifampin* may decrease serum digoxin concentration, especially in patients with renal dysfunction, by increasing the non-renal clearance of digoxin. There have been inconsistent reports regarding the effects of other drugs [e.g., *quinine, penicillamine*] on serum digoxin concentration. *Thyroid* administration to a digitalized, hypothyroid patient may increase the dose requirement of digoxin. Concomitant use of digoxin and *sympathomimetics* increases the risk of cardiac arrhythmias. *Succinylcholine* may cause a sudden extrusion of potassium from muscle cells, and may thereby cause arrhythmias in digitalized patients. Although beta-adrenergic blockers or calcium channel blockers and digoxin may be useful in combination to control atrial fibrillation, their additive effects on AV node conduction can result in advanced or complete heart block.

Due to the considerable variability of these interactions, the dosage of digoxin should be individualized when patients receive these medications concurrently. Furthermore, caution should be exercised when combining digoxin with any drug that may cause a significant deterioration in renal function, since a decline in glomerular filtration or tubular secretion may impair the excretion of digoxin.

Drug/Laboratory Test Interactions: The use of therapeutic doses of digoxin may cause prolongation of the PR interval and depression of the ST segment on the electrocardiogram. Digoxin may produce false positive ST-T changes on the electrocardiogram during exercise testing. These electrophysiologic effects reflect an expected effect of the drug and are not indicative of toxicity.

Carcinogenesis, Mutagenesis, Impairment of Fertility: There have been no long-term studies performed in animals to evaluate carcinogenic potential, nor have studies

Table 2: Times to Onset of Pharmacologic Effect and to Peak Effect of Preparations of LANOXIN

Product	Time to Onset of Effect*	Time to Peak Effect*
LANOXIN Tablets	0.5–2 hours	2–6 hours
LANOXIN Elixir Pediatric	0.5–2 hours	2–6 hours
LANOXICAPS	0.5–2 hours	2–6 hours
LANOXIN Injection/IV	5–30 minutes†	1–4 hours

* Documented for ventricular response rate in atrial fibrillation, inotropic effects and electrocardiographic changes.
† Depending upon rate of infusion.

Table 3: Subgroup Analyses of Mortality and Hospitalization During the First Two Years Following Randomization

		Risk of All-Cause Mortality or All-Cause Hospitalization*			Risk of HF-Related Mortality or HF-Related Hospitalization*		
	n	Placebo	LANOXIN	Relative risk†	Placebo	LANOXIN	Relative risk†
All patients (EF ≤0.45)	6801	604	593	0.94 (0.88–1.00)	294	217	0.69 (0.63–0.76)
NYHA I/II	4571	549	541	0.96 (0.89–1.04)	242	178	0.70 (0.62–0.80)
EF 0.25–0.45	4543	568	571	0.99 (0.91–1.07)	244	190	0.74 (0.66–0.84)
CTR ≤0.55	4455	561	563	0.98 (0.91–1.06)	239	180	0.71 (0.63–0.81)
NYHA III/IV	2224	719	696	0.88 (0.80–0.97)	402	295	0.65 (0.57–0.75)
EF <0.25	2258	677	637	0.84 (0.76–0.93)	394	270	0.61 (0.53–0.71)
CTR >0.55	2346	687	650	0.85 (0.77–0.94)	398	287	0.65 (0.57–0.75)
EF >0.45‡	987	571	585	1.04 (0.88–1.23)	179	136	0.72 (0.53–0.99)

* Number of patients with an event during the first 2 years per 1000 randomized patients.
† Relative risk (95% confidence interval).
‡ DIG Ancillary Study.

been conducted to assess the mutagenic potential of digoxin or its potential to affect fertility.

Pregnancy: ***Teratogenic Effects:*** Pregnancy Category C. Animal reproduction studies have not been conducted with digoxin. It is also not known whether digoxin can cause fetal harm when administered to a pregnant woman or can affect reproduction capacity. Digoxin should be given to a pregnant woman only if clearly needed.

Nursing Mothers: Studies have shown that digoxin concentrations in the mother's serum and milk are similar. However, the estimated exposure of a nursing infant to digoxin via breast feeding will be far below the usual infant maintenance dose. Therefore, this amount should have no pharmacologic effect upon the infant. Nevertheless, caution should be exercised when digoxin is administered to a nursing woman.

Pediatric Use: Newborn infants display considerable variability in their tolerance to digoxin. Premature and immature infants are particularly sensitive to the effects of digoxin, and the dosage of the drug must not only be reduced but must be individualized according to their degree of maturity. Digitalis glycosides can cause poisoning in children due to accidental ingestion.

Geriatric Use: The majority of clinical experience gained with digoxin has been in the elderly population. This experience has not identified differences in response or adverse effects between the elderly and younger patients. However, this drug is known to be substantially excreted by the kidney, and the risk of toxic reactions to this drug may be greater in patients with impaired renal function. Because elderly patients are more likely to have decreased renal function, care should be taken in dose selection, which should be based on renal function, and it may be useful to monitor renal function (see DOSAGE AND ADMINISTRATION).

ADVERSE REACTIONS

In general, the adverse reactions of digoxin are dose-dependent and occur at doses higher than those needed to achieve a therapeutic effect. Hence, adverse reactions are less common when digoxin is used within the recommended dose range or therapeutic serum concentration range and when there is careful attention to concurrent medications and conditions.

Because some patients may be particularly susceptible to side effects with digoxin, the dosage of the drug should always be selected carefully and adjusted as the clinical condition of the patient warrants. In the past, when high doses of digoxin were used and little attention was paid to clinical status or concurrent medications, adverse reactions to digoxin were more frequent and severe. Cardiac adverse reactions accounted for about one-half, gastrointestinal disturbances for about one-fourth, and CNS and other toxicity for about one-fourth of these adverse reactions. However, available evidence suggests that the incidence and severity of digoxin toxicity has decreased substantially in recent years. In recent controlled clinical trials, in patients with predominantly mild to moderate heart failure, the incidence of adverse experiences was comparable in patients taking digoxin and in those taking placebo. In a large mortality trial, the incidence of hospitalization for suspected digoxin toxicity was 2% in patients taking LANOXIN Tablets compared to 0.9% in patients taking placebo. In this trial, the most common manifestations of digoxin toxicity included gastrointestinal and cardiac disturbances; CNS manifestations were less common.

Adults: ***Cardiac:*** Therapeutic doses of digoxin may cause heart block in patients with pre-existing sinoatrial or AV conduction disorders; heart block can be avoided by adjusting the dose of digoxin. Prophylactic use of a cardiac pacemaker may be considered if the risk of heart block is considered unacceptable. High doses of digoxin may produce a variety of rhythm disturbances, such as first-degree, second-degree (Wenckebach), or third-degree heart block (including asystole); atrial tachycardia with block; AV dissociation; accelerated junctional (nodal) rhythm; unifocal or multiform ventricular premature contractions (especially bigeminy or trigeminy); ventricular tachycardia; and ventricular fibrillation. Digoxin produces PR prolongation and ST segment depression which should not by themselves be considered digoxin toxicity. Cardiac toxicity can also occur at therapeutic doses in patients who have conditions which may alter their sensitivity to digoxin (see WARNINGS and PRECAUTIONS).

Gastrointestinal: Digoxin may cause anorexia, nausea, vomiting, and diarrhea. Rarely, the use of digoxin has been associated with abdominal pain, intestinal ischemia, and hemorrhagic necrosis of the intestines.

CNS: Digoxin can produce visual disturbances (blurred or yellow vision), headache, weakness, dizziness, apathy, confusion, and mental disturbances (such as anxiety, depression, delirium, and hallucination).

Other: Gynecomastia has been occasionally observed following the prolonged use of digoxin. Thrombocytopenia and maculopapular rash and other skin reactions have been rarely observed.

The following table summarizes the incidence of those adverse experiences listed above for patients treated with LANOXIN Tablets or placebo from two randomized, double-blind, placebo-controlled withdrawal trials. Patients in these trials were also receiving diuretics with or without angiotensin-converting enzyme inhibitors. These patients had been stable on digoxin, and were randomized to digoxin or placebo. The results shown in Table 4 reflect the experience in patients following dosage titration with the use of serum digoxin concentrations and careful follow-up. These adverse experiences are consistent with results from a large, placebo-controlled mortality trial (DIG trial) wherein over half the patients were not receiving digoxin prior to enrollment.

[See table 4 at top of next page]

Infants and Children: The side effects of digoxin in infants and children differ from those seen in adults in several respects. Although digoxin may produce anorexia, nausea, vomiting, diarrhea, and CNS disturbances in young patients, these are rarely the initial symptoms of overdosage. Rather, the earliest and most frequent manifestation of excessive dosing with digoxin in infants and children is the appearance of cardiac arrhythmias, including sinus bradycardia. In children, the use of digoxin may produce any arrhythmia. The most common are conduction disturbances or supraventricular tachyarrhythmias, such as atrial tachycardia (with or without block) and junctional (nodal) tachycardia. Ventricular arrhythmias are less common. Sinus bradycardia may be a sign of impending digoxin intoxication, especially in infants, even in the absence of first-degree heart block. Any arrhythmia or alteration in cardiac conduction that develops in a child taking digoxin should be assumed to be caused by digoxin, until further evaluation proves otherwise.

OVERDOSAGE

Treatment of Adverse Reactions Produced by Overdosage: Digoxin should be temporarily discontinued until the adverse reaction resolves. Every effort should also be made to correct factors that may contribute to the adverse reaction (such as electrolyte disturbances or concurrent medications). Once the adverse reaction has resolved, therapy with digoxin may be reinstituted, following a careful reassessment of dose.

Withdrawal of digoxin may be all that is required to treat the adverse reaction. However, when the primary manifestation of digoxin overdosage is a cardiac arrhythmia, additional therapy may be needed.

If the rhythm disturbance is a symptomatic bradyarrhythmia or heart block, consideration should be given to the reversal of toxicity with DIGIBIND® [Digoxin Immune Fab (Ovine)] (see below), the use of atropine, or the insertion of a temporary cardiac pacemaker. However, asymptomatic bradycardia or heart block related to digoxin may require only temporary withdrawal of the drug and cardiac monitoring of the patient.

If the rhythm disturbance is a ventricular arrhythmia, consideration should be given to the correction of electrolyte disorders, particularly if hypokalemia (see below) or hypomagnesemia is present. DIGIBIND is a specific antidote for digoxin and may be used to reverse potentially life-threatening ventricular arrhythmias due to digoxin overdosage.

Administration of Potassium: Every effort should be made to maintain the serum potassium concentration between 4.0 and 5.5 mmol/L. Potassium is usually administered orally, but when correction of the arrhythmia is urgent and the serum potassium concentration is low, potassium may be administered cautiously by the intravenous route. The electrocardiogram should be monitored for any evidence of potassium toxicity (e.g., peaking of T waves) and to observe the effect on the arrhythmia. Potassium salts may be dangerous in patients who manifest bradycardia or heart block due to digoxin (unless primarily related to supraventricular tachycardia) and in the setting of massive digitalis overdosage (see Massive Digitalis Overdosage subsection).

Massive Digitalis Overdosage: Manifestations of life-threatening toxicity include ventricular tachycardia or ventricular fibrillation, or progressive bradyarrhythmias, or heart block. The administration of more than 10 mg of digoxin in a previously healthy adult, or more than 4 mg in a previously healthy child, or a steady-state serum concentration greater than 10 ng/mL, often results in cardiac arrest. DIGIBIND should be used to reverse the toxic effects of ingestion of a massive overdose. The decision to administer DIGIBIND to a patient who has ingested a massive dose of digoxin but who has not yet manifested life-threatening toxicity should depend on the likelihood that life-threatening toxicity will occur (see above).

Patients with massive digitalis ingestion should receive large doses of activated charcoal to prevent absorption and bind digoxin in the gut during enteroenteric recirculation. Emesis or gastric lavage may be indicated especially if ingestion has occurred within 30 minutes of the patient's presentation at the hospital. Emesis should not be induced in patients who are obtunded. If a patient presents more than 2 hours after ingestion or already has toxic manifestations, it may be unsafe to induce vomiting or attempt passage of a gastric tube, because such maneuvers may induce an acute vagal episode that can worsen digitalis-related arrhythmias.

Severe digitalis intoxication can cause a massive shift of potassium from inside to outside the cell, leading to life-threatening hyperkalemia. The administration of potassium supplements in the setting of massive intoxication may be hazardous and should be avoided. Hyperkalemia caused by massive digitalis toxicity is best treated with DIGIBIND; initial treatment with glucose and insulin may also be required if hyperkalemia itself is acutely life-threatening.

DOSAGE AND ADMINISTRATION

General: Recommended dosages of digoxin may require considerable modification because of individual sensitivity of the patient to the drug, the presence of associated conditions, or the use of concurrent medications. Due to the more complete absorption of digoxin from soft capsules, recommended oral doses are only 80 percent of those for Tablets and Elixir.

Because the significance of the higher peak serum concentrations associated with once daily capsules is not established, divided daily dosing is presently recommended for:

1. Infants and children under 10 years of age;
2. Patients requiring a daily dose of 300 mcg (0.3 mg) or greater;
3. Patients with a previous history of digitalis toxicity;
4. Patients considered likely to become toxic;
5. Patients in whom compliance is not a problem.

Where compliance is considered a problem, single daily dosing may be appropriate.

In selecting a dose of digoxin, the following factors must be considered:

1. The body weight of the patient. Doses should be calculated based upon lean (i.e., ideal) body weight.
2. The patient's renal function, preferably evaluated on the basis of estimated creatinine clearance.
3. The patient's age. Infants and children require different doses of digoxin than adults. Also, advanced age may be indicative of diminished renal function even in patients with normal serum creatinine concentration (i.e., below 1.5 mg/dL).
4. Concomitant disease states, concurrent medications, or other factors likely to alter the pharmacokinetic or pharmacodynamic profile of digoxin (see PRECAUTIONS).

Serum Digoxin Concentrations: In general, the dose of digoxin used should be determined on clinical grounds. However, measurement of serum digoxin concentrations can be helpful to the clinician in determining the adequacy of digoxin therapy and in assigning certain probabilities to the likelihood of digoxin intoxication. About two-thirds of adults considered adequately digitalized (without evidence of toxicity) have serum digoxin concentrations ranging from 0.8 to 2.0 ng/mL. However, digoxin may produce clinical benefits even at serum concentrations below this range. About two-thirds of adult patients with clinical toxicity have serum digoxin concentrations greater than 2.0 ng/mL. However, since one-third of patients with clinical toxicity have concentrations less than 2.0 ng/mL, values below 2.0 ng/mL do not rule out the possibility that a certain sign or symptom is related to digoxin therapy. Rarely, there are patients who are unable to tolerate digoxin at serum concentrations below 0.8 ng/mL. Consequently, the serum concentration of digoxin should always be interpreted in the overall clinical context, and an isolated measurement should not be used alone as the basis for increasing or decreasing the dose of the drug.

To allow adequate time for equilibration of digoxin between serum and tissue, sampling of serum concentrations should be done just before the next scheduled dose of the drug. If this is not possible, sampling should be done at least 6 to 8 hours after the last dose, regardless of the route of administration or the formulation used. On a once-daily dosing schedule, the concentration of digoxin will be 10% to 25% lower when sampled at 24 versus 8 hours, depending upon the patient's renal function. On a twice-daily dosing schedule, there will be only minor differences in serum digoxin concentrations whether sampling is done at 8 or 12 hours after a dose.

If a discrepancy exists between the reported serum concentration and the observed clinical response, the clinician should consider the following possibilities:

1. Analytical problems in the assay procedure.
2. Inappropriate serum sampling time.
3. Administration of a digitalis glycoside other than digoxin.
4. Conditions (described in WARNINGS and PRECAUTIONS) causing an alteration in the sensitivity of the patient to digoxin.

Table 4: Adverse Experiences in Two Parallel, Double-Blind, Placebo-Controlled Withdrawal Trials (Number of Patients Reporting)

Adverse Experience	Digoxin Patients (n = 123)	Placebo Patients (n = 125)
Cardiac		
Palpitation	1	4
Ventricular extrasystole	1	1
Tachycardia	2	1
Heart arrest	1	1
Gastrointestinal		
Anorexia	1	4
Nausea	4	2
Vomiting	2	1
Diarrhea	4	1
Abdominal pain	0	6
CNS		
Headache	4	4
Dizziness	6	5
Mental disturbances	5	1
Other		
Rash	2	1
Death	4	3

Table 5: Usual Daily Maintenance Dose Requirements (mcg) of LANOXICAPS Capsules for Estimated Peak Body Stores of 10 mcg/kg

Corrected Ccr	Lean Body Weight							Number of Days Before Steady State Achieved†
	kg	50	60	70	80	90	100	
(mL/min per 70 kg)*	lb	110	132	154	176	198	220	
0		50‡	100	100	100	150	150	22
10		100	100	100	150	150	150	19
20		100	100	150	150	150	200	16
30		100	150	150	150	200	200	14
40		100	150	150	200	200	250	13
50		150	150	200	200	250	250	12
60		150	150	200	200	250	300	11
70		150	200	200	250	250	300	10
80		150	200	200	250	300	300	9
90		150	200	250	250	300	350	8
100		200	200	250	300	300	350	7

* Ccr is creatinine clearance, corrected to 70 kg body weight or 1.73 m^2 body surface area. *For adults,* if only serum creatinine concentrations (Scr) are available, a Ccr (corrected to 70 kg body weight) may be estimated in men as (140 - Age)/Scr. For women, this result should be multiplied by 0.85. *Note: This equation cannot be used for estimating creatinine clearance in infants or children.*

† If no loading dose administered.

‡ 50 mcg= 0.05 mg

Table 6: Usual Digitalizing and Maintenance Dosages for LANOXICAPS in Children with Normal Renal Function Based on Lean Body Weight

Age	Digitalizing* Dose (mcg/kg)	Daily Maintenance Dose† (mcg/kg)
2 to 5 Years	25 to 35	25% to 35% of
5 to 10 Years	15 to 30	the oral or I.V.
Over 10 Years	8 to 12	digitalizing dose‡

* IV digitalizing doses are the same as digitalizing doses of LANOXICAPS.

† Divided daily dosing is recommended for children under 10 years of age.

‡ Projected or actual digitalizing dose providing desired clinical response.

Continued on next page

This product information is based on labeling in effect on June 23, 2000. For further information, contact via direct mail, phone, or web site. Medical Information, Glaxo Wellcome Inc., PO Box 13398, Research Triangle Park, NC 27709. Healthcare Professionals (Medical Information): 800-334-0089. Patients (Customer Response Center): 1-888-825-5249. Glaxo Wellcome Corporate Web Site: www.glaxowellcome.com

Lanoxicaps—Cont.

5. Serum digoxin concentration may decrease acutely during periods of exercise without any associated change in clinical efficacy due to increased binding of digoxin to skeletal muscle.

Heart Failure: ***Adults:*** Digitalization may be accomplished by either of two general approaches that vary in dosage and frequency of administration, but reach the same endpoint in terms of total amount of digoxin accumulated in the body.

1. If rapid digitalization is considered medically appropriate, it may be achieved by administering a loading dose based upon projected peak digoxin body stores. Maintenance dose can be calculated as a percentage of the loading dose.
2. More gradual digitalization may be obtained by beginning an appropriate maintenance dose, thus allowing digoxin body stores to accumulate slowly. Steady-state serum digoxin concentrations will be achieved in approximately five half-lives of the drug for the individual patient. Depending upon the patient's renal function, this will take between 1 and 3 weeks.

Rapid Digitalization with a Loading Dose: Peak digoxin body stores of 8 to 12 mcg/kg should provide therapeutic effect with minimum risk of toxicity in most patients with heart failure and normal sinus rhythm. Because of altered digoxin distribution and elimination, projected peak body stores for patients with renal insufficiency should be conservative (i.e., 6 to 10 mcg/kg) [see PRECAUTIONS].

The loading dose should be administered in several portions, with roughly half the total given as the first dose. Additional fractions of this planned total dose may be given at 6- to 8-hour intervals, **with careful assessment of clinical response before each additional dose.**

If the patient's clinical response necessitates a change from the calculated loading dose of digoxin, then calculation of the maintenance dose should be based upon the amount actually given.

A single initial dose of 400 to 600 mcg (0.4 to 0.6 mg) of LANOXICAPS usually produces a detectable effect in 0.5 to 2 hours that becomes maximal in 2 to 6 hours. Additional doses of 100 to 300 mcg (0.1 to 0.3 mg) may be given cautiously at 6- to 8-hour intervals until clinical evidence of an adequate effect is noted. The usual amount of LANOXICAPS that a 70-kg patient requires to achieve 8 to 12 mcg/kg peak body stores is 600 to 1000 mcg (0.6 to 1.0 mg).

LANOXIN Injection is frequently used to achieve rapid digitalization, with conversion to LANOXIN Tablets or LANOXICAPS for maintenance therapy. If patients are switched from intravenous to oral digoxin formulations, allowances must be made for differences in bioavailability when calculating maintenance dosages (see Table 1, CLINICAL PHARMACOLOGY).

Maintenance Dosing: The doses of digoxin tablets used in controlled trials in patients with heart failure have ranged from 125 to 500 mcg (0.125 to 0.5 mg) once daily. In these studies, the digoxin dose has been generally titrated according to the patient's age, lean body weight, and renal function. Therapy is generally initiated at a dose of 250 mcg (0.25 mg) once daily in patients under age 70 with good renal function, at a dose of 125 mcg (0.125 mg) once daily in patients over age 70 or with impaired renal function, and at a dose of 62.5 mcg (0.0625 mg) in patients with marked renal impairment. Doses may be increased every 2 weeks according to clinical response.

In a subset of approximately 1800 patients enrolled in the DIG trial (wherein dosing was based on an algorithm similar to that in Table 5) the mean (±SD) serum digoxin concentrations at 1 month and 12 months were 1.01±0.47 ng/mL and 0.97±0.43 ng/mL, respectively.

The maintenance dose should be based upon the percentage of the peak body stores lost each day through elimination. The following formula has had wide clinical use:

Maintenance Dose = Peak Body Stores (i.e., Loading Dose) x % Daily Loss/100

Where: % Daily Loss = 14 + Ccr/5

(Ccr is creatinine clearance, corrected to 70 kg body weight or 1.73 m^2 body surface area)

Table 5 provides average daily maintenance dose requirements of LANOXICAPS Capsules for patients with heart failure based upon lean body weight and renal function:

[See table 5 on previous page]

Example: Based on the above table, a patient in heart failure with an estimated lean body weight of 70 kg and a Ccr of 60 mL/min, should be given a dose of 200 mcg (0.2 mg) daily of LANOXICAPS, usually taken as a divided dose of one 100-mcg (0.1-mg) capsule after the morning and evening meals. If no loading dose is administered, steady-state serum concentrations in this patient should be anticipated at approximately 11 days.

Infants and Children: In general, divided daily dosing is recommended for infants and young children (under age 10). In these patients, where dosage adjustment is frequent and outside the fixed dosages available, LANOXICAPS may not be the formulation of choice. In the newborn period, renal clearance of digoxin is diminished and suitable dosage adjustments must be observed. This is especially pronounced in the premature infant. Beyond the immediate newborn period, children generally require proportionally larger doses than adults on the basis of body weight or body surface area. Children over 10 years of age require adult dosages in proportion to their body weight. Some researchers have suggested that infants and young children tolerate slightly higher serum concentrations than do adults.

Daily maintenance doses for each age group are given in Table 6 and should provide therapeutic effects with minimum risk of toxicity in most patients with heart failure and normal sinus rhythm. These recommendations assume the presence of normal renal function:

[See table 6 on previous page]

In children with renal disease, digoxin must be carefully titrated based upon clinical response.

It cannot be overemphasized that both the adult and pediatric dosage guidelines provided are based upon average patient response and substantial individual variation can be expected. Accordingly, ultimate dosage selection must be based upon clinical assessment of the patient.

Atrial Fibrillation: Peak digoxin body stores larger than the 8 to 12 mcg/kg required for most patients with heart failure and normal sinus rhythm have been used for control of ventricular rate in patients with atrial fibrillation. Doses of digoxin used for the treatment of chronic atrial fibrillation should be titrated to the minimum dose that achieves the desired ventricular rate control without causing undesirable side effects. Data are not available to establish the appropriate resting or exercise target rates that should be achieved.

Dosage Adjustment When Changing Preparations: The absolute bioavailability of the capsule formulation is greater than that of the standard tablets and very near that of the intravenous dosage form. As a result, the doses recommended for LANOXICAPS Capsules are the same as those for LANOXIN Injection (see Table 1 in CLINICAL PHARMACOLOGY: Pharmacokinetics). Adjustments in dosage will seldom be necessary when converting a patient from the intravenous formulation to LANOXICAPS. The difference in bioavailability between LANOXIN Injection or LANOXICAPS and LANOXIN Elixir Pediatric or LANOXIN Tablets must be considered when changing patients from one dosage form to another.

Doses of 100 mcg (0.1 mg) and 200 mcg (0.2 mg) of LANOXICAPS are approximately equivalent to 125-mcg (0.125-mg) and 250-mcg (0.25-mg) doses of LANOXIN Tablets and Elixir Pediatric, respectively (see Table 1 in CLINICAL PHARMACOLOGY: Pharmacokinetics).

HOW SUPPLIED

LANOXICAPS (digoxin solution in capsules), 50 mcg (0.05 mg): Bottle of 100 (NDC 0173-0270-55). Imprint A2C (red).

LANOXICAPS (digoxin solution in capsules), 100 mcg (0.1 mg): Bottle of 100 (NDC 0173-0272-55). Imprint B2C (yellow).

LANOXICAPS (digoxin solution in capsules), 200 mcg (0.2 mg): Bottle of 100 (NDC 0173-0274-55). Imprint C2C (green).

Store at 25°C (77°F); excursions permitted to 15 to 30°C (59 to 86°F) [see USP Controlled Room Temperature] in a dry place and protect from light.

Manufactured by R. P. Scherer North America
St. Petersburg, FL 33702
for Glaxo Wellcome Inc.
Research Triangle Park, NC 27709

September 1998/RL-620

Shown in Product Identification Guide, page 315

LANOXIN® ℞

[*lă-nŏx'ĭn"*]
(digoxin)
Elixir Pediatric
50 mcg (0.05 mg) per mL

DESCRIPTION

LANOXIN (digoxin) is one of the cardiac (or digitalis) glycosides, a closely related group of drugs having in common specific effects on the myocardium. These drugs are found in a number of plants. Digoxin is extracted from the leaves of *Digitalis lanata.* The term "digitalis" is used to designate the whole group of glycosides. The glycosides are composed of two portions: a sugar and a cardenolide (hence "glycosides").

Digoxin is described chemically as (3β,5β, 12β)-3-[(*O*-2,6-dideoxy-β-*D*-*ribo*-hexopyranosyl-(1→4)-*O*-2,6-dideoxy-β-*D*-*ribo*-hexopyranosyl-(1→4)-2,6-dideoxy-β-*D*-*ribo*-hexopyranosyl)oxy]-12,14-dihydroxy-card-20(22)-enolide. Its molecular formula is $C_{41}H_{64}O_{14}$, and its molecular weight is 780.95.

Digoxin exists as odorless white crystals that melt with decomposition above 230°C. The drug is practically insoluble in water and in ether; slightly soluble in diluted (50%) alcohol and in chloroform; and freely soluble in pyridine.

LANOXIN Elixir Pediatric is a stable solution of digoxin specially formulated for oral use in infants and children. Each mL contains 50 mcg (0.05 mg) digoxin, USP. The lime-flavored elixir contains the inactive ingredients alcohol 10%, methylparaben 0.1% (added as a preservative), citric acid, D&C Green No. 5 and Yellow No. 10, flavor, propylene glycol, sodium phosphate, and sucrose. Each package is supplied with a specially calibrated dropper to facilitate the administration of accurate dosage even in premature infants. Starting at 0.2 mL, this 1-mL dropper is marked in divisions of 0.1 mL, each corresponding to 5 mcg (0.005 mg) digoxin.

CLINICAL PHARMACOLOGY

Mechanism of Action: Digoxin inhibits sodium-potassium ATPase, an enzyme that regulates the quantity of sodium and potassium inside cells. Inhibition of the enzyme leads to an increase in the intracellular concentration of sodium and thus (by stimulation of sodium-calcium exchange) an increase in the intracellular concentration of calcium. The beneficial effects of digoxin result from direct actions on cardiac muscle, as well as indirect actions on the cardiovascular system mediated by effects on the autonomic nervous system. The autonomic effects include: (1) a vagomimetic action, which is responsible for the effects of digoxin on the sinoatrial and atrioventricular (AV) nodes; and (2) baroreceptor sensitization, which results in increased afferent inhibitory activity and reduced activity of the sympathetic nervous system and renin-angiotensin system for any given increment in mean arterial pressure. The pharmacologic consequences of these direct and indirect effects are: (1) an increase in the force and velocity of myocardial systolic contraction (positive inotropic action); (2) a decrease in the degree of activation of the sympathetic nervous system and renin-angiotensin system (neurohormonal deactivating effect); and (3) slowing of the heart rate and decreased conduction velocity through the AV node (vagomimetic effect). The effects of digoxin in heart failure are mediated by its positive inotropic and neurohormonal deactivating effects, whereas the effects of the drug in atrial arrhythmias are related to its vagomimetic actions. In high doses, digoxin increases sympathetic outflow from the central nervous system (CNS). This increase in sympathetic activity may be an important factor in digitalis toxicity.

Pharmacokinetics: Note: The following data are from studies performed in adults, unless otherwise stated.

Absorption: Absorption of digoxin from LANOXIN Elixir Pediatric formulation has been demonstrated to be 70% to 85% complete compared to an identical intravenous dose of digoxin (absolute bioavailability). When the elixir is taken after meals, the rate of absorption is slowed, but the total amount of digoxin absorbed is usually unchanged. When taken with meals high in bran fiber, however, the amount absorbed from an oral dose may be reduced. Comparisons of the systemic availability and equivalent doses for preparations of LANOXIN are shown in Table 1:

[See table 1 below]

In some patients, orally administered digoxin is converted to inactive reduction products (e.g., dihydrodigoxin) by colonic bacteria in the gut. Data suggest that one in ten patients treated with digoxin tablets will degrade 40% or more of the ingested dose. As a result, certain antibiotics may increase the absorption of digoxin in such patients. Although inactivation of these bacteria by antibiotics is rapid, the serum digoxin concentration will rise at a rate consistent with the elimination half-life of digoxin. The magnitude of rise in serum digoxin concentration relates to the extent of bacterial inactivation, and may be as much as two-fold in some cases.

Distribution: Following drug administration, a 6- to 8-hour tissue distribution phase is observed. This is followed by a much more gradual decline in the serum concentration of the drug, which is dependent on the elimination of digoxin from the body. The peak height and slope of the early portion (absorption/distribution phases) of the serum concentration-time curve are dependent upon the route of administration and the absorption characteristics of the formulation. Clinical evidence indicates that the early high serum concentrations do not reflect the concentration of digoxin at its site of action, but that with chronic use, the steady-state post-distribution serum concentrations are in equilibrium with tissue concentrations and correlate with pharmacologic effects. In individual patients, these post-distribution serum concentrations may be useful in evaluating therapeutic and toxic effects (see DOSAGE AND ADMINISTRATION: Serum Digoxin Concentrations).

Digoxin is concentrated in tissues and therefore has a large apparent volume of distribution. Digoxin crosses both the

Table 1: Comparisons of the Systemic Availability and Equivalent Doses for Preparations of LANOXIN

Product	Absolute Bioavailability	Equivalent Doses (mcg)* Among Dosage Forms			
LANOXIN Tablets	60 – 80%	62.5	125	250	500
LANOXIN Elixir Pediatric	70 – 85%	62.5	125	250	500
LANOXICAPS®	90 – 100%	50	100	200	400
LANOXIN Injection/IV	100%	50	100	200	400

*For example, 125 mcg LANOXIN Tablets equivalent to 125 mcg LANOXIN Elixir Pediatric equivalent to 100 mcg LANOXICAPS equivalent to 100 mcg LANOXIN Injection/IV.

blood-brain barrier and the placenta. At delivery, the serum digoxin concentration in the newborn is similar to the serum concentration in the mother. Approximately 25% of digoxin in the plasma is bound to protein. Serum digoxin concentrations are not significantly altered by large changes in fat tissue weight, so that its distribution space correlates best with lean (i.e., ideal) body weight, not total body weight.

Metabolism: Only a small percentage (16%) of a dose of digoxin is metabolized. The end metabolites, which include 3 β-digoxigenin, 3-keto-digoxigenin, and their glucuronide and sulfate conjugates, are polar in nature and are postulated to be formed via hydrolysis, oxidation, and conjugation. The metabolism of digoxin is not dependent upon the cytochrome P-450 system, and digoxin is not known to induce or inhibit the cytochrome P-450 system.

Excretion: Elimination of digoxin follows first-order kinetics (that is, the quantity of digoxin eliminated at any time is proportional to the total body content). Following intravenous administration to healthy volunteers, 50% to 70% of a digoxin dose is excreted unchanged in the urine. Renal excretion of digoxin is proportional to glomerular filtration rate and is largely independent of urine flow. In healthy volunteers with normal renal function, digoxin has a half-life of 1.5 to 2.0 days. The half-life in anuric patients is prolonged to 3.5 to 5 days. Digoxin is not effectively removed from the body by dialysis, exchange transfusion, or during cardiopulmonary bypass because most of the drug is bound to tissue and does not circulate in the blood.

Special Populations: Race differences in digoxin pharmacokinetics have not been formally studied. Because digoxin is primarily eliminated as unchanged drug via the kidney and because there are no important differences in creatinine clearance among races, pharmacokinetic differences due to race are not expected.

The clearance of digoxin can be primarily correlated with renal function as indicated by creatinine clearance. In children with renal disease, digoxin must be carefully titrated based on clinical response.

Plasma digoxin concentration profiles in patients with acute hepatitis generally fell within the range of profiles in a group of healthy subjects.

Pharmacodynamic and Clinical Effects: The times to onset of pharmacologic effect and to peak effect of preparations of LANOXIN are shown in Table 2:

[See table 2 above]

Hemodynamic Effects: Digoxin produces hemodynamic improvement in patients with heart failure. Short- and long-term therapy with the drug increases cardiac output and lowers pulmonary artery pressure, pulmonary capillary wedge pressure, and systemic vascular resistance. These hemodynamic effects are accompanied by an increase in the left ventricular ejection fraction and a decrease in end-systolic and end-diastolic dimensions.

Chronic Heart Failure: Two 12-week, double-blind, placebo-controlled studies enrolled 178 (RADIANCE trial) and 88 (PROVED trial) adult patients with NYHA class II or III heart failure previously treated with digoxin, a diuretic, and an ACE inhibitor (RADIANCE only) and randomized them to placebo or treatment with LANOXIN. Both trials demonstrated better preservation of exercise capacity in patients randomized to LANOXIN Tablets. Continued treatment with LANOXIN reduced the risk of developing worsening heart failure, as evidenced by heart failure-related hospitalizations and emergency care and the need for concomitant heart failure therapy. The larger study also showed treatment-related benefits in NYHA class and patients' global assessment. In the smaller trial, these trended in favor of a treatment benefit.

The Digitalis Investigation Group (DIG) main trial was a multicenter, randomized, double-blind, placebo-controlled mortality study of 6801 adult patients with heart failure and left ventricular ejection fraction ≤0.45. At randomization, 67% were NYHA class I or II, 71% had heart failure of ischemic etiology, 44% had been receiving digoxin, and most were receiving concomitant ACE inhibitor (94%) and diuretic (82%). Patients were randomized to placebo or LANOXIN Tablets, the dose of which was adjusted for the patient's age, sex, lean body weight, and serum creatinine (see DOSAGE AND ADMINISTRATION), and followed for up to 58 months (median 37 months). The median daily dose prescribed was 0.25 mg. Overall all-cause mortality was 35% with no difference between groups (95% confidence limits for relative risk of 0.91 to 1.07). LANOXIN was associated with a 25% reduction in the number of hospitalizations for heart failure, a 28% reduction in the risk of a patient having at least one hospitalization for heart failure, and a 6.5% reduction in total hospitalizations (for any cause).

Use of LANOXIN was associated with a trend to increase time to all-cause death or hospitalization. The trend was evident in subgroups of patients with mild heart failure as well as more severe disease, as shown in Table 3. Although the effect on all-cause death or hospitalization was not statistically significant, much of the apparent benefit derived from effects on mortality and hospitalization attributed to heart failure.

[See table 3 above]

In situations where there is no statistically significant benefit of treatment evident from a trial's primary endpoint, results pertaining to a secondary endpoint should be interpreted cautiously.

Chronic Atrial Fibrillation: In adult patients with chronic atrial fibrillation, digoxin slows rapid ventricular response rate in a linear dose-response fashion from 0.25 to 0.75 mg/day. Digoxin should not be used for the treatment of multifocal atrial tachycardia.

Table 2: Times to Onset of Pharmacologic Effect and to Peak Effect of Preparations of LANOXIN

Product	Time to Onset of Effect*	Time to Peak Effect*
LANOXIN Tablets	0.5 – 2 hours	2 – 6 hours
LANOXIN Elixir Pediatric	0.5 – 2 hours	2 – 6 hours
LANOXICAPS	0.5 – 2 hours	2 – 6 hours
LANOXIN Injection/IV	5 – 30 minutes†	1 – 4 hours

* Documented for ventricular response rate in atrial fibrillation, inotropic effects and electrocardiographic changes.
† Depending upon rate of infusion.

Table 3: Subgroup Analyses of Mortality and Hospitalization During the First Two Years Following Randomization

		Risk of All-Cause Mortality or All-Cause Hospitalization*			Risk of HF-Related Mortality or HF-Related Hospitalization*		
	n	Placebo	LANOXIN	Relative risk†	Placebo	LANOXIN	Relative risk†
All patients (EF ≤0.45)	6801	604	593	0.94 (0.88–1.00)	294	217	0.69 (0.63–0.76)
NYHA I/II	4571	549	541	0.96 (0.89–1.04)	242	178	0.70 (0.62–0.80)
EF 0.25–0.45	4543	568	571	0.99 (0.91–1.07)	244	190	0.74 (0.66–0.84)
CTR ≤0.55	4455	561	563	0.98 (0.91–1.06)	239	180	0.71 (0.63–0.81)
NYHA III/IV	2224	719	696	0.88 (0.80–0.97)	402	295	0.65 (0.57–0.75)
EF <0.25	2258	677	637	0.84 (0.76–0.93)	394	270	0.61 (0.53–0.71)
CTR >0.55	2346	687	650	0.85 (0.77–0.94)	398	287	0.65 (0.57–0.75)
EF >0.45‡	987	571	585	1.04 (0.88–1.23)	179	136	0.72 (0.53–0.99)

*Number of patients with an event during the first 2 years per 1000 randomized patients.
†Relative risk (95% confidence interval).
‡DIG Ancillary Study.

INDICATIONS AND USAGE

Heart Failure: LANOXIN is indicated for the treatment of mild to moderate heart failure. LANOXIN increases left ventricular ejection fraction and improves heart failure symptoms as evidenced by exercise capacity and heart failure-related hospitalizations and emergency care, while having no effect on mortality. Where possible, LANOXIN should be used with a diuretic and an angiotensin-converting enzyme inhibitor, but an optimal order for starting these three drugs cannot be specified.

Atrial Fibrillation: LANOXIN is indicated for the control of ventricular response rate in patients with chronic atrial fibrillation.

CONTRAINDICATIONS

Digitalis glycosides are contraindicated in patients with ventricular fibrillation or in patients with a known hypersensitivity to digoxin. A hypersensitivity reaction to other digitalis preparations usually constitutes a contraindication to digoxin.

WARNINGS

Sinus Node Disease and AV Block: Because digoxin slows sinoatrial and AV conduction, the drug commonly prolongs the PR interval. The drug may cause severe sinus bradycardia or sinoatrial block in patients with pre-existing sinus node disease and may cause advanced or complete heart block in patients with pre-existing incomplete AV block. In such patients consideration should be given to the insertion of a pacemaker before treatment with digoxin.

Accessory AV Pathway (Wolff-Parkinson-White Syndrome): After intravenous digoxin therapy, some patients with paroxysmal atrial fibrillation or flutter and a coexisting accessory AV pathway have developed increased antegrade conduction across the accessory pathway bypassing the AV node, leading to a very rapid ventricular response or ventricular fibrillation. Unless conduction down the accessory pathway has been blocked (either pharmacologically or by surgery), digoxin should not be used in such patients. The treatment of paroxysmal supraventricular tachycardia in such patients is usually direct-current cardioversion.

Use in Patients with Preserved Left Ventricular Systolic Function: Patients with certain disorders involving heart failure associated with preserved left ventricular ejection fraction may be particularly susceptible to toxicity of the drug. Such disorders include restrictive cardiomyopathy, constrictive pericarditis, amyloid heart disease, and acute cor pulmonale. Patients with idiopathic hypertrophic subaortic stenosis may have worsening of the outflow obstruction due to the inotropic effects of digoxin.

PRECAUTIONS

Use in Patients with Impaired Renal Function: Digoxin is primarily excreted by the kidneys; therefore, patients with impaired renal function require smaller than usual maintenance doses of digoxin (see DOSAGE AND ADMINISTRATION). Because of the prolonged elimination half-life, a longer period of time is required to achieve an initial or new steady-state serum concentration in patients with renal impairment than in patients with normal renal function. If appropriate care is not taken to reduce the dose of digoxin, such patients are at high risk for toxicity, and toxic effects will last longer in such patients than in patients with normal renal function.

Use in Patients with Electrolyte Disorders: In patients with hypokalemia or hypomagnesemia, toxicity may occur despite serum digoxin concentrations below 2.0 ng/mL, because potassium or magnesium depletion sensitizes the myocardium to digoxin. Therefore, it is desirable to maintain normal serum potassium and magnesium concentrations in patients being treated with digoxin. Deficiencies of these electrolytes may result from malnutrition, diarrhea, or prolonged vomiting, as well as the use of the following drugs or procedures: diuretics, amphotericin B, corticosteroids, antacids, dialysis, and mechanical suction of gastrointestinal secretions.

Hypercalcemia from any cause predisposes the patient to digitalis toxicity. Calcium, particularly when administered rapidly by the intravenous route, may produce serious arrhythmias in digitalized patients. On the other hand, hypocalcemia can nullify the effects of digoxin in humans; thus, digoxin may be ineffective until serum calcium is restored to normal. These interactions are related to the fact that digoxin affects contractility and excitability of the heart in a manner similar to that of calcium.

Use in Thyroid Disorders and Hypermetabolic States: Hypothyroidism may reduce the requirements for digoxin. Heart failure and/or atrial arrhythmias resulting from hypermetabolic or hyperdynamic states (e.g., hyperthyroidism, hypoxia, or arteriovenous shunt) are best treated by addressing the underlying condition. Atrial arrhythmias associated with hypermetabolic states are particularly resistant to digoxin treatment. Care must be taken to avoid toxicity if digoxin is used.

Use in Patients with Acute Myocardial Infarction: Digoxin should be used with caution in patients with acute myocardial infarction. The use of inotropic drugs in some patients in this setting may result in undesirable increases in myocardial oxygen demand and ischemia.

Use During Electrical Cardioversion: It may be desirable to reduce the dose of digoxin for 1 to 2 days prior to electrical cardioversion of atrial fibrillation to avoid the induction of ventricular arrhythmias, but physicians must consider the consequences of increasing the ventricular response if digoxin is withdrawn. If digitalis toxicity is suspected, elective cardioversion should be delayed. If it is not prudent to delay cardioversion, the lowest possible energy level should be selected to avoid provoking ventricular arrhythmias.

Laboratory Test Monitoring: Patients receiving digoxin should have their serum electrolytes and renal function

Continued on next page

This product information is based on labeling in effect on June 23, 2000. For further information, contact via direct mail, phone, or web site. Medical Information, Glaxo Wellcome Inc., PO Box 13398, Research Triangle Park, NC 27709. Healthcare Professionals (Medical Information): 800-334-0089. Patients (Customer Response Center): 1-888-825-5249. Glaxo Wellcome Corporate Web Site: www.glaxowellcome.com

Lanoxin Elixir Pediatric—Cont.

(serum creatinine concentrations) assessed periodically; the frequency of assessments will depend on the clinical setting. For discussion of serum digoxin concentrations, see DOSAGE AND ADMINISTRATION.

Drug Interactions: Potassium-depleting *diuretics* are a major contributing factor to digitalis toxicity. *Calcium*, particularly if administered rapidly by the intravenous route, may produce serious arrhythmias in digitalized patients. *Quinidine, verapamil, amiodarone, propafenone, indomethacin, itraconazole, alprazolam*, and *spironolactone* raise the serum digoxin concentration due to a reduction in clearance and/or in volume of distribution of the drug, with the implication that digitalis intoxication may result. *Erythromycin* and *clarithromycin* (and possibly other *macrolide antibiotics*) and *tetracycline* may increase digoxin absorption in patients who inactivate digoxin by bacterial metabolism in the lower intestine, so that digitalis intoxication may result (see CLINICAL PHARMACOLOGY: Absorption). *Propantheline* and *diphenoxylate*, by decreasing gut motility, may increase digoxin absorption. *Antacids, kaolin-pectin, sulfasalazine, neomycin, cholestyramine, certain anticancer drugs*, and *metoclopramide* may interfere with intestinal digoxin absorption, resulting in unexpectedly low serum concentrations. *Rifampin* may decrease serum digoxin concentration, especially in patients with renal dysfunction, by increasing the non-renal clearance of digoxin. There have been inconsistent reports regarding the effects of other drugs [e.g., *quinine, penicillamine*] on serum digoxin concentration. *Thyroid* administration to a digitalized, hypothyroid patient may increase the dose requirement of digoxin. Concomitant use of digoxin and *sympathomimetics* increases the risk of cardiac arrhythmias. *Succinylcholine* may cause a sudden extrusion of potassium from muscle cells, and may thereby cause arrhythmias in digitalized patients. Although beta-adrenergic blockers or calcium channel blockers and digoxin may be useful in combination to control atrial fibrillation, their additive effects on AV node conduction can result in advanced or complete heart block.

Due to the considerable variability of these interactions, the dosage of digoxin should be individualized when patients receive these medications concurrently. Furthermore, caution should be exercised when combining digoxin with any drug that may cause a significant deterioration in renal function, since a decline in glomerular filtration or tubular secretion may impair the excretion of digoxin.

Drug/Laboratory Test Interactions: The use of therapeutic doses of digoxin may cause prolongation of the PR interval and depression of the ST segment on the electrocardiogram. Digoxin may produce false positive ST-T changes on the electrocardiogram during exercise testing. These electrophysiologic effects reflect an expected effect of the drug and are not indicative of toxicity.

Carcinogenesis, Mutagenesis, Impairment of Fertility: There have been no long-term studies performed in animals to evaluate carcinogenic potential, nor have studies been conducted to assess the mutagenic potential of digoxin or its potential to affect fertility.

Pregnancy: ***Teratogenic Effects:*** Pregnancy Category C. Animal reproduction studies have not been conducted with digoxin. It is also not known whether digoxin can cause fetal harm when administered to a pregnant woman or can affect reproduction capacity. Digoxin should be given to a pregnant woman only if clearly needed.

Nursing Mothers: Studies have shown that digoxin concentrations in the mother's serum and milk are similar. However, the estimated exposure of a nursing infant to digoxin via breast feeding will be far below the usual infant maintenance dose. Therefore, this amount should have no pharmacologic effect upon the infant. Nevertheless, caution should be exercised when digoxin is administered to a nursing woman.

Pediatric Use: Newborn infants display considerable variability in their tolerance to digoxin. Premature and immature infants are particularly sensitive to the effects of digoxin, and the dosage of the drug must not only be reduced but must be individualized according to their degree of maturity. Digitalis glycosides can cause poisoning in children due to accidental ingestion.

Geriatric Use: The majority of clinical experience gained with digoxin has been in the elderly population. This experience has not identified differences in response or adverse effects between the elderly and younger patients. However, this drug is known to be substantially excreted by the kidney, and the risk of toxic reactions to this drug may be greater in patients with impaired renal function. Because elderly patients are more likely to have decreased renal function, care should be taken in dose selection, which should be based on renal function, and it may be useful to monitor renal function.

ADVERSE REACTIONS

In general, the adverse reactions of digoxin are dose-dependent and occur at doses higher than those needed to achieve a therapeutic effect. Hence, adverse reactions are less common when digoxin is used within the recommended dose range or therapeutic serum concentration range and when there is careful attention to concurrent medications and conditions.

Because some patients may be particularly susceptible to side effects with digoxin, the dosage of the drug should always be selected carefully and adjusted as the clinical condition of the patient warrants. In the past, when high doses of digoxin were used and little attention was paid to clinical status or concurrent medications, adverse reactions to digoxin were more frequent and severe. Cardiac adverse reactions accounted for about one-half, gastrointestinal disturbances for about one-fourth, and CNS and other toxicity for about one-fourth of these adverse reactions. However, available evidence suggests that the incidence and severity of digoxin toxicity has decreased substantially in recent years. In recent controlled clinical trials, in patients with predominantly mild to moderate heart failure, the incidence of adverse experiences was comparable in patients taking digoxin and in those taking placebo. In a large mortality trial, the incidence of hospitalization for suspected digoxin toxicity was 2% in patients taking LANOXIN Tablets compared to 0.9% in patients taking placebo. In this trial, the most common manifestations of digoxin toxicity included gastrointestinal and cardiac disturbances; CNS manifestations were less common.

Adults: ***Cardiac:*** Therapeutic doses of digoxin may cause heart block in patients with pre-existing sinoatrial or AV conduction disorders; heart block can be avoided by adjusting the dose of digoxin. Prophylactic use of a cardiac pacemaker may be considered if the risk of heart block is considered unacceptable. High doses of digoxin may produce a variety of rhythm disturbances, such as first-degree, second-degree (Wenckebach), or third-degree heart block (including asystole); atrial tachycardia with block; AV dissociation; accelerated junctional (nodal) rhythm; unifocal or multiform ventricular premature contractions (especially bigeminy or trigeminy); ventricular tachycardia; and ventricular fibrillation. Digoxin produces PR prolongation and ST segment depression which should not by themselves be considered digoxin toxicity. Cardiac toxicity can also occur at therapeutic doses in patients who have conditions which may alter their sensitivity to digoxin (see WARNINGS and PRECAUTIONS).

Gastrointestinal: Digoxin may cause anorexia, nausea, vomiting, and diarrhea. Rarely, the use of digoxin has been associated with abdominal pain, intestinal ischemia, and hemorrhagic necrosis of the intestines.

CNS: Digoxin can produce visual disturbances (blurred or yellow vision), headache, weakness, dizziness, apathy, confusion, and mental disturbances (such as anxiety, depression, delirium, and hallucination).

Other: Gynecomastia has been occasionally observed following the prolonged use of digoxin. Thrombocytopenia and maculopapular rash and other skin reactions have been rarely observed.

Table 4 summarizes the incidence of those adverse experiences listed above for patients treated with LANOXIN Tablets or placebo from two randomized, double-blind, placebo-controlled withdrawal trials. Patients in these trials were also receiving diuretics with or without angiotensin-converting enzyme inhibitors. These patients had been stable on digoxin, and were randomized to digoxin or placebo. The results shown in Table 4 reflect the experience in patients following dosage titration with the use of serum digoxin concentrations and careful follow-up. These adverse experiences are consistent with results from a large, placebo-controlled mortality trial (DIG trial) wherein over half the patients were not receiving digoxin prior to enrollment.

[See table 4 above]

Table 4: Adverse Experiences In Two Parallel, Double-Blind, Placebo-Controlled Withdrawal Trials (Number of Patients Reporting)

Adverse Experience	Digoxin Patients (n = 123)	Placebo Patients (n = 125)
Cardiac		
Palpitation	1	4
Ventricular extrasystole	1	1
Tachycardia	2	1
Heart arrest	1	1
Gastrointestinal		
Anorexia	1	4
Nausea	4	2
Vomiting	2	1
Diarrhea	4	1
Abdominal pain	0	6
CNS		
Headache	4	4
Dizziness	6	5
Mental disturbances	5	1
Other		
Rash	2	1
Death	4	3

Infants and Children: The side effects of digoxin in infants and children differ from those seen in adults in several respects. Although digoxin may produce anorexia, nausea, vomiting, diarrhea, and CNS disturbances in young patients, these are rarely the initial symptoms of overdosage. Rather, the earliest and most frequent manifestation of excessive dosing with digoxin in infants and children is the appearance of cardiac arrhythmias, including sinus bradycardia. In children, the use of digoxin may produce any arrhythmia. The most common are conduction disturbances or supraventricular tachyarrhythmias, such as atrial tachycardia (with or without block) and junctional (nodal) tachycardia. Ventricular arrhythmias are less common. Sinus bradycardia may be a sign of impending digoxin intoxication, especially in infants, even in the absence of first-degree heart block. Any arrhythmia or alteration in cardiac conduction that develops in a child taking digoxin should be assumed to be caused by digoxin, until further evaluation proves otherwise.

OVERDOSAGE

Treatment of Adverse Reactions Produced by Overdosage: Digoxin should be temporarily discontinued until the adverse reaction resolves. Every effort should also be made to correct factors that may contribute to the adverse reaction (such as electrolyte disturbances or concurrent medications). Once the adverse reaction has resolved, therapy with digoxin may be reinstituted, following a careful reassessment of dose.

Withdrawal of digoxin may be all that is required to treat the adverse reaction. However, when the primary manifestation of digoxin overdosage is a cardiac arrhythmia, additional therapy may be needed.

If the rhythm disturbance is a symptomatic bradyarrhythmia or heart block, consideration should be given to the reversal of toxicity with DIGIBIND® [Digoxin Immune Fab (Ovine)] (see below), the use of atropine, or the insertion of a temporary cardiac pacemaker. However, asymptomatic bradycardia or heart block related to digoxin may require only temporary withdrawal of the drug and cardiac monitoring of the patient.

If the rhythm disturbance is a ventricular arrhythmia, consideration should be given to the correction of electrolyte disorders, particularly if hypokalemia (see below) or hypomagnesemia is present. DIGIBIND is a specific antidote for digoxin and may be used to reverse potentially life-threatening ventricular arrhythmias due to digoxin overdosage.

Administration of Potassium: Every effort should be made to maintain the serum potassium concentration between 4.0 and 5.5 mmol/L. Potassium is usually administered orally, but when correction of the arrhythmia is urgent and the serum potassium concentration is low, potassium may be administered cautiously by the intravenous route. The electrocardiogram should be monitored for any evidence of potassium toxicity (e.g., peaking of T waves) and to observe the effect on the arrhythmia. Potassium salts may be dangerous in patients who manifest bradycardia or heart block due to digoxin (unless primarily related to supraventricular tachycardia) and in the setting of massive digitalis overdosage (see Massive Digitalis Overdosage subsection).

Massive Digitalis Overdosage: Manifestations of life-threatening toxicity include ventricular tachycardia or ventricular fibrillation, or progressive bradyarrhythmias, or heart block. The administration of more than 10 mg of digoxin in a previously healthy adult or more than 4 mg in a previously healthy child, or a steady-state serum concentration greater than 10 ng/mL often results in cardiac arrest. DIGIBIND should be used to reverse the toxic effects of ingestion of a massive overdose. The decision to administer DIGIBIND to a patient who has ingested a massive dose of digoxin but who has not yet manifested life-threatening toxicity should depend on the likelihood that life-threatening toxicity will occur (see above).

Patients with massive digitalis ingestion should receive large doses of activated charcoal to prevent absorption and bind digoxin in the gut during enteroenteric recirculation. Emesis or gastric lavage may be indicated especially if ingestion has occurred within 30 minutes of the patient's presentation at the hospital. Emesis should not be induced in patients who are obtunded. If a patient presents more than 2 hours after ingestion or already has toxic manifestations, it may be unsafe to induce vomiting or attempt passage of a gastric tube, because such maneuvers may induce an acute vagal episode that can worsen digitalis-related arrhythmias.

Severe digitalis intoxication can cause a massive shift of potassium from inside to outside the cell, leading to life-threatening hyperkalemia. The administration of potassium supplements in the setting of massive intoxication may be hazardous and should be avoided. Hyperkalemia

Table 5: Usual Digitalizing and Maintenance Dosages for LANOXIN Elixir Pediatric in Children with Normal Renal Function Based on Lean Body Weight

Age	Oral Digitalizing* Dose (mcg/kg)	**Daily** Maintenance Dose† (mcg/kg)
Premature	20 to 30	20% to 30% of *oral* digitalizing dose‡
Full-Term	25 to 35	
1 to 24 Months	35 to 60	
2 to 5 Years	30 to 40	25% to 35% of *oral* digitalizing dose‡
5 to 10 Years	20 to 35	
Over 10 Years	10 to 15	

*IV digitalizing doses are 80% of oral digitalizing doses.
†Divided daily dosing is recommended for children under 10 years of age.
‡Projected or actual digitalizing dose providing clinical response.

caused by massive digitalis toxicity is best treated with DIGIBIND; initial treatment with glucose and insulin may also be required if hyperkalemia itself is acutely life-threatening.

DOSAGE AND ADMINISTRATION

General: Recommended dosages of digoxin may require considerable modification because of individual sensitivity of the patient to the drug, the presence of associated conditions, or the use of concurrent medications. In selecting a dose of digoxin, the following factors must be considered:

1. The body weight of the patient. Doses should be calculated based upon lean (i.e., ideal) body weight.
2. The patient's renal function, preferably evaluated on the basis of estimated creatinine clearance.
3. The patient's age. Infants and children require different doses of digoxin than adults. Also, advanced age may be indicative of diminished renal function even in patients with normal serum creatinine concentration (i.e., below 1.5 mg/dL).
4. Concomitant disease states, concurrent medications, or other factors likely to alter the pharmacokinetic or pharmacodynamic profile of digoxin (see PRECAUTIONS).

Serum Digoxin Concentrations: In general, the dose of digoxin used should be determined on clinical grounds. However, measurement of serum digoxin concentrations can be helpful to the clinician in determining the adequacy of digoxin therapy and in assigning certain probabilities to the likelihood of digoxin intoxication. About two-thirds of adults considered adequately digitalized (without evidence of toxicity) have serum digoxin concentrations ranging from 0.8 to 2.0 ng/mL. However, digoxin may produce clinical benefits even at serum concentrations below this range. About two-thirds of adult patients with clinical toxicity have serum digoxin concentrations greater than 2.0 ng/mL. However, since one-third of patients with clinical toxicity have concentrations less than 2.0 ng/mL, values below 2.0 ng/mL do not rule out the possibility that a certain sign or symptom is related to digoxin therapy. Rarely, there are patients who are unable to tolerate digoxin at serum concentrations below 0.8 ng/mL. Consequently, the serum concentration of digoxin should always be interpreted in the overall clinical context, and an isolated measurement should not be used alone as the basis for increasing or decreasing the dose of the drug.

To allow adequate time for equilibration of digoxin between serum and tissue, sampling of serum concentrations should be done just before the next scheduled dose of the drug. If this is not possible, sampling should be done at least 6 to 8 hours after the last dose, regardless of the route of administration or the formulation used. On a once-daily dosing schedule, the concentration of digoxin will be 10% to 25% lower when sampled at 24 versus 8 hours, depending upon the patient's renal function. On a twice-daily dosing schedule, there will be only minor differences in serum digoxin concentrations whether sampling is done at 8 or 12 hours after a dose.

If a discrepancy exists between the reported serum concentration and the observed clinical response, the clinician should consider the following possibilities:

1. Analytical problems in the assay procedure.
2. Inappropriate serum sampling time.
3. Administration of a digitalis glycoside other than digoxin.
4. Conditions (described in WARNINGS and PRECAUTIONS) causing an alteration in the sensitivity of the patient to digoxin.
5. Serum digoxin concentration may decrease acutely during periods of exercise without any associated change in clinical efficacy due to increased binding of digoxin to skeletal muscle.

Heart Failure: Adults: See the LANOXIN Tablets or LANOXICAPS Capsules package insert for specific recommendations.

Infants and Children: In general, divided daily dosing is recommended for infants and young children (under age 10). In the newborn period, renal clearance of digoxin is diminished and suitable dosage adjustments must be observed. This is especially pronounced in the premature infant. Beyond the immediate newborn period, children generally require proportionally larger doses than adults on the basis of body weight or body surface area. Children over 10 years of age require adult dosages in proportion to their body weight. Some researchers have suggested that infants and young children tolerate slightly higher serum concentrations than do adults.

Digitalization may be accomplished by either of two general approaches that vary in dosage and frequency of administration, but reach the same endpoint in terms of total amount of digoxin accumulated in the body.

1. If rapid digitalization is considered medically appropriate, it may be achieved by administering a loading dose based upon projected peak digoxin body stores. Maintenance dose can be calculated as a percentage of the loading dose.
2. More gradual digitalization may be obtained by beginning an appropriate maintenance dose, thus allowing digoxin body stores to accumulate slowly. Steady-state serum digoxin concentrations will be achieved in approximately five half-lives of the drug for the individual patient. Depending upon the patient's renal function, this will take between 1 and 3 weeks.

Rapid Digitalization with a Loading Dose: LANOXIN Injection Pediatric can be used to achieve rapid digitalization, with conversion to an oral formulation of LANOXIN for maintenance therapy. If patients are switched from intravenous to oral digoxin formulations, allowances must be made for differences in bioavailability when calculating maintenance dosages (see Table 1 in CLINICAL PHARMACOLOGY: Pharmacokinetics and dosing Table 5 below).

Peak digoxin body stores of 8 to 12 mcg/kg should provide therapeutic effect with minimum risk of toxicity in most patients with heart failure and normal sinus rhythm. Because of altered digoxin distribution and elimination, projected peak body stores for patients with renal insufficiency should be conservative (i.e., 6 to 10 mcg/kg [see PRECAUTIONS]).

Digitalizing and daily maintenance doses for each age group are given in Table 5 and should provide therapeutic effect with minimum risk of toxicity in most patients with heart failure and normal sinus rhythm. These recommendations assume the presence of normal renal function.

The loading dose should be administered in several portions, with roughly half the total given as the first dose. Additional fractions of this planned total dose may be given at 6- to 8-hour intervals, **with careful assessment of clinical response before each additional dose.** If the patient's clinical response necessitates a change from the calculated loading dose of digoxin, then calculation of the maintenance dose should be based upon the amount actually given.

[See table 5 above]

In children with renal disease, digoxin dosing must be carefully titrated based upon desired clinical response.

Gradual Digitalization With A Maintenance Dose: More gradual digitalization can also be accomplished by beginning an appropriate maintenance dose. The range of percentages provided in Table 5 can be used in calculating this dose for patients with normal renal function.

It cannot be overemphasized that these pediatric dosage guidelines are based upon average patient response and substantial individual variation can be expected. Accordingly, ultimate dosage selection must be based upon clinical assessment of the patient.

Atrial Fibrillation: Peak digoxin body stores larger than the 8 to 12 mcg/kg required for most patients with heart failure and normal sinus rhythm have been used for control of ventricular rate in patients with atrial fibrillation. Doses of digoxin used for the treatment of chronic atrial fibrillation should be titrated to the minimum dose that achieves the desired ventricular rate control without causing undesirable side effects. Data are not available to establish the appropriate resting or exercise target rates that should be achieved.

Dosage Adjustment When Changing Preparations: The difference in bioavailability between LANOXIN Injection or LANOXICAPS and LANOXIN Elixir Pediatric or LANOXIN Tablets must be considered when changing patients from one dosage form to another.

Doses of 100 mcg (0.1 mg) and 200 mcg (0.2 mg) of LANOXICAPS are approximately equivalent to 125-mcg (0.125-mg) and 250-mcg (0.25-mg) doses of LANOXIN Tablets and Elixir Pediatric, respectively (see Table 1 in CLINICAL PHARMACOLOGY: Pharmacokinetics).

HOW SUPPLIED

LANOXIN (digoxin) Elixir Pediatric, 50 mcg (0.05 mg) per mL; Bottle of 60 mL with calibrated dropper (NDC 0173-0264-27).

Store at 25°C (77°F); excursions permitted to 15° to 30°C (59° to 86°F) [see USP Controlled Room Temperature] and protect from light.

Glaxo Wellcome Inc., Research Triangle Park, NC 27709

October 1998/RL-619

Shown in Product Identification Guide, page 315

LANOXIN® ℞
[*lă-nŏx'ĭn"*]
(digoxin)
Injection
500 mcg (0.5 mg) in 2 mL (250 mcg [0.25 mg] per mL)

DESCRIPTION

LANOXIN (digoxin) is one of the cardiac (or digitalis) glycosides, a closely related group of drugs having in common specific effects on the myocardium. These drugs are found in a number of plants. Digoxin is extracted from the leaves of *Digitalis lanata*. The term "digitalis" is used to designate the whole group of glycosides. The glycosides are composed of two portions: a sugar and a cardenolide (hence "glycosides").

Digoxin is described chemically as (3β,5β,12β)-3-[(*O*-2,6-dideoxy-β-*D*-*ribo*-hexopyranosyl-(1→4)-*O*-2,6-dideoxy-β-*D*-*ribo*-hexopyranosyl-(1→4)-2,6-dideoxy-β-*D*-*ribo*-hexopyranosyl)oxy]-12,14-dihydroxy-card-20(22)-enolide. Its molecular formula is $C_{41}H_{64}O_{14}$, and its molecular weight is 780.95.

Digoxin exists as odorless white crystals that melt with decomposition above 230°C. The drug is practically insoluble in water and in ether; slightly soluble in diluted (50%) alcohol and in chloroform; and freely soluble in pyridine.

LANOXIN Injection is a sterile solution of digoxin for intravenous injection. The vehicle contains 40% propylene glycol and 10% alcohol. The injection is buffered to a pH of 6.8 to 7.2 with 0.17% sodium phosphate and 0.08% anhydrous citric acid. Each 2-mL ampul contains 500 mcg (0.5 mg) digoxin (250 mcg [0.25 mg] per mL). Dilution is not required.

CLINICAL PHARMACOLOGY

Mechanism of Action: Digoxin inhibits sodium-potassium ATPase, an enzyme that regulates the quantity of sodium and potassium inside cells. Inhibition of the enzyme leads to an increase in the intracellular concentration of sodium and thus (by stimulation of sodium-calcium exchange) an increase in the intracellular concentration of calcium. The beneficial effects of digoxin result from direct actions on cardiac muscle, as well as indirect actions on the cardiovascular system mediated by effects on the autonomic nervous system. The autonomic effects include: (1) a vagomimetic action, which is responsible for the effects of digoxin on the sinoatrial and atrioventricular (AV) nodes; and (2) baroreceptor sensitization, which results in increased afferent inhibitory activity and reduced activity of the sympathetic nervous system and renin-angiotensin system for any given increment in mean arterial pressure. The pharmacologic consequences of these direct and indirect effects are: (1) an increase in the force and velocity of myocardial systolic contraction (positive inotropic action); (2) a decrease in the degree of activation of the sympathetic nervous system and renin-angiotensin system (neurohormonal deactivating effect); and (3) slowing of the heart rate and decreased conduction velocity through the AV node (vagomimetic effect). The effects of digoxin in heart failure are mediated by its positive inotropic and neurohormonal deactivating effects, whereas the effects of the drug in atrial arrhythmias are related to its vagomimetic actions. In high doses, digoxin increases sympathetic outflow from the central nervous system (CNS). This increase in sympathetic activity may be an important factor in digitalis toxicity.

Pharmacokinetics: Note: the following data are from studies performed in adults, unless otherwise stated.

Absorption: Comparisons of the systemic availability and equivalent doses for preparations of LANOXIN are shown in Table 1:

[See table 1 at top of next page]

Distribution: Following drug administration, a 6- to 8-hour tissue distribution phase is observed. This is followed by a much more gradual decline in the serum concentration of the drug, which is dependent on the elimination of digoxin from the body. The peak height and slope of the early portion (absorption/distribution phases) of the serum concentration-time curve are dependent upon the route of administration and the absorption characteristics of the formulation. Clinical evidence indicates that the early high serum concentrations do not reflect the concentration of digoxin at its site of action, but that with chronic use, the steady-state post-distribution serum concentrations are in equilibrium with tissue concentrations and correlate with pharmacologic effects. In individual patients, these post-distribution serum concentrations may be useful in evaluating therapeutic and toxic effects (see DOSAGE AND ADMINISTRATION: Serum Digoxin Concentrations).

Continued on next page

This product information is based on labeling in effect on June 23, 2000. For further information, contact via direct mail, phone, or web site. Medical Information, Glaxo Wellcome Inc., PO Box 13398, Research Triangle Park, NC 27709. Healthcare Professionals (Medical Information): 800-334-0089. Patients (Customer Response Center): 1-888-825-5249. Glaxo Wellcome Corporate Web Site: www.glaxowellcome.com

Lanoxin Injection—Cont.

Digoxin is concentrated in tissues and therefore has a large apparent volume of distribution. Digoxin crosses both the blood-brain barrier and the placenta. At delivery, the serum digoxin concentration in the newborn is similar to the serum concentration in the mother. Approximately 25% of digoxin in the plasma is bound to protein. Serum digoxin concentrations are not significantly altered by large changes in fat tissue weight, so that its distribution space correlates best with lean (i.e., ideal) body weight, not total body weight.

Metabolism: Only a small percentage (16%) of a dose of digoxin is metabolized. The end metabolites, which include 3 β-digoxigenin, 3-keto-digoxigenin, and their glucuronide and sulfate conjugates, are polar in nature and are postulated to be formed via hydrolysis, oxidation, and conjugation. The metabolism of digoxin is not dependent upon the cytochrome P-450 system, and digoxin is not known to induce or inhibit the cytochrome P-450 system.

Excretion: Elimination of digoxin follows first-order kinetics (that is, the quantity of digoxin eliminated at any time is proportional to the total body content). Following intravenous administration to healthy volunteers, 50% to 70% of a digoxin dose is excreted unchanged in the urine. Renal excretion of digoxin is proportional to glomerular filtration rate and is largely independent of urine flow. In healthy volunteers with normal renal function, digoxin has a half-life of 1.5 to 2.0 days. The half-life in anuric patients is prolonged to 3.5 to 5 days. Digoxin is not effectively removed from the body by dialysis, exchange transfusion, or during cardiopulmonary bypass because most of the drug is bound to tissue and does not circulate in the blood.

Special Populations: Race differences in digoxin pharmacokinetics have not been formally studied. Because digoxin is primarily eliminated as unchanged drug via the kidney and because there are no important differences in creatinine clearance among races, pharmacokinetic differences due to race are not expected.

The clearance of digoxin can be primarily correlated with renal function as indicated by creatinine clearance. The Cockcroft and Gault formula for estimation of creatinine clearance includes age, body weight, and gender. A table that provides the usual daily maintenance dose requirements of LANOXIN Tablets based on creatinine clearance (per 70 kg) is presented in the DOSAGE AND ADMINISTRATION section.

Plasma digoxin concentration profiles in patients with acute hepatitis generally fell within the range of profiles in a group of healthy subjects.

Pharmacodynamic and Clinical Effects: The times to onset of pharmacologic effect and to peak effect of preparations of LANOXIN are shown in Table 2:

[See table 2 above]

Hemodynamic Effects: Digoxin produces hemodynamic improvement in patients with heart failure. Short- and long-term therapy with the drug increases cardiac output and lowers pulmonary artery pressure, pulmonary capillary wedge pressure, and systemic vascular resistance. These hemodynamic effects are accompanied by an increase in the left ventricular ejection fraction and a decrease in end-systolic and end-diastolic dimensions.

Chronic Heart Failure: Two 12-week, double-blind, placebo-controlled studies enrolled 178 (RADIANCE trial) and 88 (PROVED trial) patients with NYHA class II or III heart failure previously treated with oral digoxin, a diuretic, and an ACE inhibitor (RADIANCE only) and randomized them to placebo or treatment with LANOXIN Tablets. Both trials demonstrated better preservation of exercise capacity in patients randomized to LANOXIN. Continued treatment with LANOXIN reduced the risk of developing worsening heart failure, as evidenced by heart failure-related hospitalizations and emergency care and the need for concomitant heart failure therapy. The larger study also showed treatment-related benefits in NYHA class and patients' global assessment. In the smaller trial, these trended in favor of a treatment benefit.

The Digitalis Investigation Group (DIG) main trial was a multicenter, randomized, double-blind, placebo-controlled mortality study of 6801 patients with heart failure and left ventricular ejection fraction ≤0.45. At randomization, 67% were NYHA class I or II, 71% had heart failure of ischemic etiology, 44% had been receiving digoxin, and most were receiving concomitant ACE inhibitor (94%) and diuretic (82%). Patients were randomized to placebo or LANOXIN Tablets, the dose of which was adjusted for the patient's age, sex, lean body weight, and serum creatinine (see DOSAGE AND ADMINISTRATION), and followed for up to 58 months (median 37 months). The median daily dose prescribed was 0.25 mg. Overall all-cause mortality was 35% with no difference between groups (95% confidence limits for relative risk of 0.91 to 1.07). LANOXIN was associated with a 25% reduction in the number of hospitalizations for heart failure, a 28% reduction in the risk of a patient having at least one hospitalization for heart failure, and a 6.5% reduction in total hospitalizations (for any cause).

Use of LANOXIN was associated with a trend to increase time to all-cause death or hospitalization. The trend was evident in subgroups of patients with mild heart failure as well as more severe disease, as shown in Table 3. Although the effect on all-cause death or hospitalization was not statistically significant, much of the apparent benefit derived from effects on mortality and hospitalization attributed to heart failure.

[See table 3 at top of next page]

Table 1: Comparisons of the Systemic Availability and Equivalent Doses for Preparations of LANOXIN

Product	Absolute Bioavailability	Equivalent Doses (mcg)* Among Dosage Forms			
LANOXIN Tablets	60 - 80%	62.5	125	250	500
LANOXIN Elixir Pediatric	70 - 85%	62.5	125	250	500
LANOXICAPS®	90 - 100%	50	100	200	400
LANOXIN Injection/IV	100%	50	100	200	400

*For example, 125 mcg LANOXIN Tablets equivalent to 125 mcg LANOXIN Elixir Pediatric equivalent to 100 mcg LANOXICAPS equivalent to 100 mcg LANOXIN Injection/IV.

Table 2: Times to Onset of Pharmacologic Effect and to Peak Effect of Preparations of LANOXIN

Product	Time to Onset of Effect*	Time to Peak Effect*
LANOXIN Tablets	0.5 - 2 hours	2 - 6 hours
LANOXIN Elixir Pediatric	0.5 - 2 hours	2 - 6 hours
LANOXICAPS	0.5 - 2 hours	2 - 6 hours
LANOXIN Injection/IV	5 - 30 minutes†	1 - 4 hours

*Documented for ventricular response rate in atrial fibrillation, inotropic effects and electrocardiographic changes.
†Depending upon rate of infusion.

In situations where there is no statistically significant benefit of treatment evident from a trial's primary endpoint, results pertaining to a secondary endpoint should be interpreted cautiously.

Chronic Atrial Fibrillation: In patients with chronic atrial fibrillation, digoxin slows rapid ventricular response rate in a linear dose-response fashion from 0.25 to 0.75 mg/day. Digoxin should not be used for the treatment of multifocal atrial tachycardia.

INDICATIONS AND USAGE

Heart Failure: LANOXIN is indicated for the treatment of mild to moderate heart failure. LANOXIN increases left ventricular ejection fraction and improves heart failure symptoms as evidenced by exercise capacity and heart failure-related hospitalizations and emergency care, while having no effect on mortality. Where possible, LANOXIN should be used with a diuretic and an angiotensin-converting enzyme inhibitor, but an optimal order for starting these three drugs cannot be specified.

Atrial Fibrillation: LANOXIN is indicated for the control of ventricular response rate in patients with chronic atrial fibrillation.

CONTRAINDICATIONS

Digitalis glycosides are contraindicated in patients with ventricular fibrillation or in patients with a known hypersensitivity to digoxin. A hypersensitivity reaction to other digitalis preparations usually constitutes a contraindication to digoxin.

WARNINGS

Sinus Node Disease and AV Block: Because digoxin slows sinoatrial and AV conduction, the drug commonly prolongs the PR interval. The drug may cause severe sinus bradycardia or sinoatrial block in patients with pre-existing sinus node disease and may cause advanced or complete heart block in patients with pre-existing incomplete AV block. In such patients consideration should be given to the insertion of a pacemaker before treatment with digoxin.

Accessory AV Pathway (Wolff-Parkinson-White Syndrome): After intravenous digoxin therapy, some patients with paroxysmal atrial fibrillation or flutter and a coexisting accessory AV pathway have developed increased antegrade conduction across the accessory pathway bypassing the AV node, leading to a very rapid ventricular response or ventricular fibrillation. Unless conduction down the accessory pathway has been blocked (either pharmacologically or by surgery), digoxin should not be used in such patients. The treatment of paroxysmal supraventricular tachycardia in such patients is usually direct-current cardioversion.

Use in Patients with Preserved Left Ventricular Systolic Function: Patients with certain disorders involving heart failure associated with preserved left ventricular ejection fraction may be particularly susceptible to toxicity of the drug. Such disorders include restrictive cardiomyopathy, constrictive pericarditis, amyloid heart disease, and acute cor pulmonale. Patients with idiopathic hypertrophic subaortic stenosis may have worsening of the outflow obstruction due to the inotropic effects of digoxin.

PRECAUTIONS

Use in Patients with Impaired Renal Function: Digoxin is primarily excreted by the kidneys; therefore, patients with impaired renal function require smaller than usual maintenance doses of digoxin (see DOSAGE AND ADMINISTRATION). Because of the prolonged elimination half-life, a longer period of time is required to achieve an initial or new steady-state serum concentration in patients with renal impairment than in patients with normal renal function. If appropriate care is not taken to reduce the dose of digoxin, such patients are at high risk for toxicity, and toxic effects will last longer in such patients than in patients with normal renal function.

Use in Patients with Electrolyte Disorders: In patients with hypokalemia or hypomagnesemia, toxicity may occur despite serum digoxin concentrations below 2.0 ng/mL, because potassium or magnesium depletion sensitizes the myocardium to digoxin. Therefore, it is desirable to maintain normal serum potassium and magnesium concentrations in patients being treated with digoxin. Deficiencies of these electrolytes may result from malnutrition, diarrhea, or prolonged vomiting, as well as the use of the following drugs or procedures: diuretics, amphotericin B, corticosteroids, antacids, dialysis, and mechanical suction of gastrointestinal secretions.

Hypercalcemia from any cause predisposes the patient to digitalis toxicity. Calcium, particularly when administered rapidly by the intravenous route, may produce serious arrhythmias in digitalized patients. On the other hand, hypocalcemia can nullify the effects of digoxin in humans; thus, digoxin may be ineffective until serum calcium is restored to normal. These interactions are related to the fact that digoxin affects contractility and excitability of the heart in a manner similar to that of calcium.

Use in Thyroid Disorders and Hypermetabolic States: Hypothyroidism may reduce the requirements for digoxin. Heart failure and/or atrial arrhythmias resulting from hypermetabolic or hyperdynamic states (e.g., hyperthyroidism, hypoxia, or arteriovenous shunt) are best treated by addressing the underlying condition. Atrial arrhythmias associated with hypermetabolic states are particularly resistant to digoxin treatment. Care must be taken to avoid toxicity if digoxin is used.

Use in Patients with Acute Myocardial Infarction: Digoxin should be used with caution in patients with acute myocardial infarction. The use of inotropic drugs in some patients in this setting may result in undesirable increases in myocardial oxygen demand and ischemia.

Use During Electrical Cardioversion: It may be desirable to reduce the dose of digoxin for 1 to 2 days prior to electrical cardioversion of atrial fibrillation to avoid the induction of ventricular arrhythmias, but physicians must consider the consequences of increasing the ventricular response if digoxin is withdrawn. If digitalis toxicity is suspected, elective cardioversion should be delayed. If it is not prudent to delay cardioversion, the lowest possible energy level should be selected to avoid provoking ventricular arrhythmias.

Laboratory Test Monitoring: Patients receiving digoxin should have their serum electrolytes and renal function (serum creatinine concentrations) assessed periodically; the frequency of assessments will depend on the clinical setting. For discussion of serum digoxin concentrations, see DOSAGE AND ADMINISTRATION.

Drug Interactions: Potassium-depleting *diuretics* are a major contributing factor to digitalis toxicity. *Calcium*, particularly if administered rapidly by the intravenous route, may produce serious arrhythmias in digitalized patients. *Quinidine, verapamil, amiodarone, propafenone, indomethacin, itraconazole, alprazolam,* and *spironolactone* raise the serum digoxin concentration due to a reduction in clearance and/or in volume of distribution of the drug, with the implication that digitalis intoxication may result. *Erythromycin* and *clarithromycin* (and possibly other *macrolide antibiotics*) and *tetracycline* may increase digoxin absorption in patients who inactivate digoxin by bacterial metabolism in the lower intestine, so that digitalis intoxication may result. *Propantheline* and *diphenoxylate*, by decreasing gut motility, may increase digoxin absorption. *Antacids, kaolin-pectin, sulfasalazine, neomycin, cholestyramine,* certain *anticancer drugs*, and *metoclopramide* may interfere with intestinal digoxin absorption, resulting in unexpectedly low serum concentrations. *Rifampin* may decrease serum digoxin concentration, especially in patients with renal dysfunction, by increasing the non-renal clearance of digoxin. There have been inconsistent reports regarding the effects of other drugs (e.g., *quinine, penicillamine*) on serum digoxin concentration. *Thyroid* administration to a digitalized, hypothyroid patient may increase the dose requirement of digoxin. Concomitant use of digoxin and *sympathomimetics* increases the risk of cardiac arrhythmias. *Succinylcholine* may cause a sudden extrusion of potassium from muscle cells, and may thereby cause arrhythmias in digitalized patients. Although beta-adrenergic blockers or calcium channel blockers and digoxin may be useful in combination to control atrial fibrillation, their additive effects on AV node conduction can result in advanced or complete heart block.

Due to the considerable variability of these interactions, the dosage of digoxin should be individualized when patients re-

Table 3: Subgroup Analyses of Mortality and Hospitalization During the First Two Years Following Randomization

	n	Risk of All-Cause Mortality or All-Cause Hospitalization*			Risk of HF-Related Mortality or HF-Related Hospitalization*		
		Placebo	LANOXIN	Relative risk†	Placebo	LANOXIN	Relative risk†
All patients (EF ≤0.45)	6801	604	593	0.94 (0.88-1.00)	294	217	0.69 (0.63-0.76)
NYHA I/II	4571	549	541	0.96 (0.89-1.04)	242	178	0.70 (0.62-0.80)
EF 0.25–0.45	4543	568	571	0.99 (0.91-1.07)	244	190	0.74 (0.66-0.84)
CTR ≤0.55	4455	561	563	0.98 (0.91-1.06)	239	180	0.71 (0.63-0.81)
NYHA III/IV	2224	719	696	0.88 (0.80-0.97)	402	295	0.65 (0.57-0.75)
EF <0.25	2258	677	637	0.84 (0.76-0.93)	394	270	0.61 (0.53-0.71)
CTR >0.55	2346	687	650	0.85 (0.77-0.94)	398	287	0.65 (0.57-0.75)
EF >0.45‡	987	571	585	1.04 (0.88-1.23)	179	136	0.72 (0.53-0.99)

*Number of patients with an event during the first 2 years per 1000 randomized patients.
†Relative risk (95% confidence interval).
‡DIG Ancillary Study.

ceive these medications concurrently. Furthermore, caution should be exercised when combining digoxin with any drug that may cause a significant deterioration in renal function, since a decline in glomerular filtration or tubular secretion may impair the excretion of digoxin.

Drug/Laboratory Test Interactions: The use of therapeutic doses of digoxin may cause prolongation of the PR interval and depression of the ST segment on the electrocardiogram. Digoxin may produce false positive ST-T changes on the electrocardiogram during exercise testing. These electrophysiologic effects reflect an expected effect of the drug and are not indicative of toxicity.

Carcinogenesis, Mutagenesis, Impairment of Fertility: There have been no long-term studies performed in animals to evaluate carcinogenic potential, nor have studies been conducted to assess the mutagenic potential of digoxin or its potential to affect fertility.

Pregnancy: ***Teratogenic Effects:*** Pregnancy Category C. Animal reproduction studies have not been conducted with digoxin. It is also not known whether digoxin can cause fetal harm when administered to a pregnant woman or can affect reproduction capacity. Digoxin should be given to a pregnant woman only if clearly needed.

Nursing Mothers: Studies have shown that digoxin concentrations in the mother's serum and milk are similar. However, the estimated exposure of a nursing infant to digoxin via breast feeding will be far below the usual infant maintenance dose. Therefore, this amount should have no pharmacologic effect upon the infant. Nevertheless, caution should be exercised when digoxin is administered to a nursing woman.

Pediatric Use: Newborn infants display considerable variability in their tolerance to digoxin. Premature and immature infants are particularly sensitive to the effects of digoxin, and the dosage of the drug must not only be reduced but must be individualized according to their degree of maturity. Digitalis glycosides can cause poisoning in children due to accidental ingestion.

Geriatric Use: The majority of clinical experience gained with digoxin has been in the elderly population. This experience has not identified differences in response or adverse effects between the elderly and younger patients. However, this drug is known to be substantially excreted by the kidney, and the risk of toxic reactions to this drug may be greater in patients with impaired renal function. Because elderly patients are more likely to have decreased renal function, care should be taken in dose selection, which should be based on renal function, and it may be useful to monitor renal function (see DOSAGE AND ADMINISTRATION).

ADVERSE REACTIONS

In general, the adverse reactions of digoxin are dose-dependent and occur at doses higher than those needed to achieve a therapeutic effect. Hence, adverse reactions are less common when digoxin is used within the recommended dose range or therapeutic serum concentration range and when there is careful attention to concurrent medications and conditions.

Because some patients may be particularly susceptible to side effects with digoxin, the dosage of the drug should always be selected carefully and adjusted as the clinical condition of the patient warrants. In the past, when high doses of digoxin were used and little attention was paid to clinical status or concurrent medications, adverse reactions to digoxin were more frequent and severe. Cardiac adverse reactions accounted for about one-half, gastrointestinal disturbances for about one-fourth, and CNS and other toxicity for about one-fourth of these adverse reactions. However, available evidence suggests that the incidence and severity of digoxin toxicity has decreased substantially in recent years. In recent controlled clinical trials, in patients with predominantly mild to moderate heart failure, the incidence of adverse experiences was comparable in patients taking digoxin and in those taking placebo. In a large mortality trial, the incidence of hospitalization for suspected digoxin toxicity was 2% in patients taking LANOXIN Tablets compared to 0.9% in patients taking placebo. In this trial, the most common manifestations of digoxin toxicity included gastrointestinal and cardiac disturbances; CNS manifestations were less common.

Adults: ***Cardiac:*** Therapeutic doses of digoxin may cause heart block in patients with pre-existing sinoatrial or AV conduction disorders; heart block can be avoided by adjusting the dose of digoxin. Prophylactic use of a cardiac pacemaker may be considered if the risk of heart block is considered unacceptable. High doses of digoxin may produce a variety of rhythm disturbances, such as first-degree, second-degree (Wenckebach), or third-degree heart block (including asystole); atrial tachycardia with block; AV dissociation; accelerated junctional (nodal) rhythm; unifocal or multiform ventricular premature contractions (especially bigeminy or trigeminy); ventricular tachycardia; and ventricular fibrillation. Digoxin produces PR prolongation and ST segment depression which should not by themselves be considered digoxin toxicity. Cardiac toxicity can also occur at therapeutic doses in patients who have conditions which may alter their sensitivity to digoxin (see WARNINGS and PRECAUTIONS).

Gastrointestinal: Digoxin may cause anorexia, nausea, vomiting, and diarrhea. Rarely, the use of digoxin has been associated with abdominal pain, intestinal ischemia, and hemorrhagic necrosis of the intestines.

CNS: Digoxin can produce visual disturbances (blurred or yellow vision), headache, weakness, dizziness, apathy, confusion, and mental disturbances (such as anxiety, depression, delirium, and hallucination).

Other: Gynecomastia has been occasionally observed following the prolonged use of digoxin. Thrombocytopenia and maculopapular rash and other skin reactions have been rarely observed.

The following table summarizes the incidence of those adverse experiences listed above for patients treated with LANOXIN Tablets or placebo from two randomized, double-blind, placebo-controlled withdrawal trials. Patients in these trials were also receiving diuretics with or without angiotensin-converting enzyme inhibitors. These patients had been stable on digoxin, and were randomized to digoxin or placebo. The results shown in Table 4 reflect the experience in patients following dosage titration with the use of serum digoxin concentrations and careful follow-up. These adverse experiences are consistent with results from a large, placebo-controlled mortality trial (DIG trial) wherein over half the patients were not receiving digoxin prior to enrollment.

[See table 4 at top of next page]

Infants and Children: The side effects of digoxin in infants and children differ from those seen in adults in several respects. Although digoxin may produce anorexia, nausea, vomiting, diarrhea, and CNS disturbances in young patients, these are rarely the initial symptoms of overdosage. Rather, the earliest and most frequent manifestation of excessive dosing with digoxin in infants and children is the appearance of cardiac arrhythmias, including sinus bradycardia. In children, the use of digoxin may produce any arrhythmia. The most common are conduction disturbances or supraventricular tachyarrhythmias, such as atrial tachycardia (with or without block) and junctional (nodal) tachycardia. Ventricular arrhythmias are less common. Sinus bradycardia may be a sign of impending digoxin intoxication, especially in infants, even in the absence of first-degree heart block. Any arrhythmia or alteration in cardiac conduction that develops in a child taking digoxin should be assumed to be caused by digoxin, until further evaluation proves otherwise.

OVERDOSAGE

Treatment of Adverse Reactions Produced by Overdosage: Digoxin should be temporarily discontinued until the adverse reaction resolves. Every effort should also be made to correct factors that may contribute to the adverse reaction (such as electrolyte disturbances or concurrent medications). Once the adverse reaction has resolved, therapy with digoxin may be reinstituted, following a careful reassessment of dose.

Withdrawal of digoxin may be all that is required to treat the adverse reaction. However, when the primary manifestation of digoxin overdosage is a cardiac arrhythmia, additional therapy may be needed.

If the rhythm disturbance is a symptomatic bradyarrhythmia or heart block, consideration should be given to the reversal of toxicity with DIGIBIND® [Digoxin Immune Fab (Ovine)] (see below), the use of atropine, or the insertion of a temporary cardiac pacemaker. However, asymptomatic bradycardia or heart block related to digoxin may require only temporary withdrawal of the drug and cardiac monitoring of the patient.

If the rhythm disturbance is a ventricular arrhythmia, consideration should be given to the correction of electrolyte disorders, particularly if hypokalemia (see below) or hypomagnesemia is present. DIGIBIND is a specific antidote for digoxin and may be used to reverse potentially life-threatening ventricular arrhythmias due to digoxin overdosage.

Administration of Potassium: Every effort should be made to maintain the serum potassium concentration between 4.0 and 5.5 mmol/L. Potassium is usually administered orally, but when correction of the arrhythmia is urgent and the serum potassium concentration is low, potassium may be administered cautiously by the intravenous route. The electrocardiogram should be monitored for any evidence of potassium toxicity (e.g., peaking of T waves) and to observe the effect on the arrhythmia. Potassium salts may be dangerous in patients who manifest bradycardia or heart block due to digoxin (unless primarily related to supraventricular tachycardia) and in the setting of massive digitalis overdosage (see Massive Digitalis Overdosage subsection).

Massive Digitalis Overdosage: Manifestations of life-threatening toxicity include ventricular tachycardia or ventricular fibrillation, or progressive bradyarrhythmias, or heart block. The administration of more than 10 mg of digoxin in a previously healthy adult, or more than 4 mg in a previously healthy child, or a steady-state serum concentration greater than 10 ng/mL often results in cardiac arrest. DIGIBIND should be used to reverse the toxic effects of ingestion of a massive overdose. The decision to administer DIGIBIND to a patient who has ingested a massive dose of digoxin but who has not yet manifested life-threatening toxicity should depend on the likelihood that life-threatening toxicity will occur (see above).

Patients with massive digitalis ingestion should receive large doses of activated charcoal to prevent absorption and bind digoxin in the gut during enteroenteric recirculation. Emesis or gastric lavage may be indicated especially if ingestion has occurred within 30 minutes of the patient's presentation at the hospital. Emesis should not be induced in patients who are obtunded. If a patient presents more than 2 hours after ingestion or already has toxic manifestations, it may be unsafe to induce vomiting or attempt passage of a gastric tube, because such maneuvers may induce an acute vagal episode that can worsen digitalis-related arrhythmias.

Continued on next page

This product information is based on labeling in effect on June 23, 2000. For further information, contact via direct mail, phone, or web site. Medical Information, Glaxo Wellcome Inc., PO Box 13398, Research Triangle Park, NC 27709. Healthcare Professionals (Medical Information): 800-334-0089. Patients (Customer Response Center): 1-888-825-5249. Glaxo Wellcome Corporate Web Site: www.glaxowellcome.com

Lanoxin Injection—Cont.

Severe digitalis intoxication can cause a massive shift of potassium from inside to outside the cell, leading to life-threatening hyperkalemia. The administration of potassium supplements in the setting of massive intoxication may be hazardous and should be avoided. Hyperkalemia caused by massive digitalis toxicity is best treated with DIGIBIND; initial treatment with glucose and insulin may also be required if hyperkalemia itself is acutely life-threatening.

DOSAGE AND ADMINISTRATION

General: Recommended dosages of digoxin may require considerable modification because of individual sensitivity of the patient to the drug, the presence of associated conditions, or the use of concurrent medications.

Parenteral administration of digoxin should be used only when the need for rapid digitalization is urgent or when the drug cannot be taken orally. Intramuscular injection can lead to severe pain at the injection site, thus intravenous administration is preferred. If the drug must be administered by the intramuscular route, it should be injected deep into the muscle followed by massage. No more than 500 mcg (2 mL) should be injected into a single site.

LANOXIN Injection can be administered undiluted or diluted with a 4-fold or greater volume of Sterile Water for Injection, 0.9% Sodium Chloride Injection, or 5% Dextrose Injection. The use of less than a 4-fold volume of diluent could lead to precipitation of the digoxin. Immediate use of the diluted product is recommended.

If tuberculin syringes are used to measure very small doses, one must be aware of the problem of inadvertent overadministration of digoxin. The syringe should *not* be flushed with the parenteral solution after its contents are expelled into an indwelling vascular catheter.

Slow infusion of LANOXIN Injection is preferable to bolus administration. Rapid infusion of digitalis glycosides has been shown to cause systemic and coronary arteriolar constriction, which may be clinically undesirable. Caution is thus advised and LANOXIN Injection should probably be administered over a period of 5 minutes or longer. Mixing of LANOXIN Injection with other drugs in the same container or simultaneous administration in the same intravenous line is not recommended.

In selecting a dose of digoxin, the following factors must be considered:

1. The body weight of the patient. Doses should be calculated based upon lean (i.e., ideal) body weight.
2. The patient's renal function, preferably evaluated on the basis of estimated creatinine clearance.
3. The patient's age. Infants and children require different doses of digoxin than adults. Also, advanced age may be indicative of diminished renal function even in patients with normal serum creatinine concentration (i.e., below 1.5 mg/dL).
4. Concomitant disease states, concurrent medications, or other factors likely to alter the pharmacokinetic or pharmacodynamic profile of digoxin (see PRECAUTIONS).

Serum Digoxin Concentrations: In general, the dose of digoxin used should be determined on clinical grounds. However, measurement of serum digoxin concentrations can be helpful to the clinician in determining the adequacy of digoxin therapy and in assigning certain probabilities to the likelihood of digoxin intoxication. About two-thirds of adults considered adequately digitalized (without evidence of toxicity) have serum digoxin concentrations ranging from 0.8 to 2.0 ng/mL. However, digoxin may produce clinical benefits even at serum concentrations below this range. About two-thirds of adult patients with clinical toxicity have serum digoxin concentrations greater than 2.0 ng/mL. However, since one-third of patients with clinical toxicity have concentrations less than 2.0 ng/mL, values below 2.0 ng/mL do not rule out the possibility that a certain sign or symptom is related to digoxin therapy. Rarely, there are patients who are unable to tolerate digoxin at serum concentrations below 0.8 ng/mL. Consequently, the serum concentration of digoxin should always be interpreted in the overall clinical context, and an isolated measurement should not be used alone as the basis for increasing or decreasing the dose of the drug.

To allow adequate time for equilibration of digoxin between serum and tissue, sampling of serum concentrations should be done just before the next scheduled dose of the drug. If this is not possible, sampling should be done at least 6 to 8 hours after the last dose, regardless of the route of administration or the formulation used. On a once-daily dosing schedule, the concentration of digoxin will be 10% to 25% lower when sampled at 24 versus 8 hours, depending upon the patient's renal function. On a twice-daily dosing schedule, there will be only minor differences in serum digoxin concentrations whether sampling is done at 8 or 12 hours after a dose.

If a discrepancy exists between the reported serum concentration and the observed clinical response, the clinician should consider the following possibilities:

1. Analytical problems in the assay procedure.
2. Inappropriate serum sampling time.
3. Administration of a digitalis glycoside other than digoxin.
4. Conditions (described in WARNINGS and PRECAUTIONS) causing an alteration in the sensitivity of the patient to digoxin.

Table 4: Adverse Experiences In Two Parallel, Double-Blind, Placebo-Controlled Withdrawal Trials (Number of Patients Reporting)

Adverse Experience	Digoxin Patients (n = 123)	Placebo Patients (n = 125)
Cardiac		
Palpitation	1	4
Ventricular extrasystole	1	1
Tachycardia	2	1
Heart arrest	1	1
Gastrointestinal		
Anorexia	1	4
Nausea	4	2
Vomiting	2	1
Diarrhea	4	1
Abdominal pain	0	6
CNS		
Headache	4	4
Dizziness	6	5
Mental disturbances	5	1
Other		
Rash	2	1
Death	4	3

Table 5: Usual Daily Maintenance Dose Requirements (mcg) of LANOXIN Injection for Estimated Peak Body Stores of 10 mcg/kg*

Corrected Ccr (mL/min per 70 kg)†	Lean Body Weight kg / lb	50 / 110	60 / 132	70 / 154	80 / 176	90 / 198	100 / 220	Number of Days Before Steady State Achieved‡
0		75§	75	100	100	125	150	22
10		75	100	100	125	150	150	19
20		100	100	125	150	150	175	16
30		100	125	150	150	175	200	14
40		100	125	150	175	200	225	13
50		125	150	175	200	225	250	12
60		125	150	175	200	225	250	11
70		150	175	200	225	250	275	10
80		150	175	200	250	275	300	9
90		150	200	225	250	300	325	8
100		175	200	250	275	300	350	7

*Daily maintenance doses have been rounded to the nearest 25-mcg increment.

†Ccr is creatinine clearance, corrected to 70 mg body weight or 1.73 m^2 body surface area. *For adults,* if only serum creatinine concentrations (Scr) are available, a Ccr (corrected to 70 kg body weight) may be estimated in men as (140 - Age)/Scr. For women, this result should be multiplied by 0.85. *Note: This equation cannot be used for estimating creatinine clearance in infants or children.*

‡If no loading dose administered.

§75 mcg = 0.075 mg

5. Serum digoxin concentration may decrease acutely during periods of exercise without any associated change in clinical efficacy due to increased binding of digoxin to skeletal muscle.

Heart Failure: ***Adults:*** Digitalization may be accomplished by either of two general approaches that vary in dosage and frequency of administration, but reach the same endpoint in terms of total amount of digoxin accumulated in the body.

1. If rapid digitalization is considered medically appropriate, it may be achieved by administering a loading dose based upon projected peak digoxin body stores. Maintenance dose can be calculated as a percentage of the loading dose.
2. More gradual digitalization may be obtained by beginning an appropriate maintenance dose, thus allowing digoxin body stores to accumulate slowly. Steady-state serum digoxin concentrations will be achieved in approximately five half-lives of the drug for the individual patient. Depending upon the patient's renal function, this will take between 1 and 3 weeks.

Rapid Digitalization with a Loading Dose: LANOXIN Injection is frequently used to achieve rapid digitalization, with conversion to LANOXIN Tablets or LANOXICAPS for maintenance therapy. If patients are switched from intravenous to oral digoxin formulations, allowances must be made for differences in bioavailability when calculating maintenance dosages (see Table 1, CLINICAL PHARMACOLOGY: Pharmacokinetics and dosing Table 5 below).

Intramuscular injection of digoxin is extremely painful and offers no advantages unless other routes of administration are contraindicated.

Peak digoxin body stores of 8 to 12 mcg/kg should provide therapeutic effect with minimum risk of toxicity in most patients with heart failure and normal sinus rhythm. Because of altered digoxin distribution and elimination, projected peak body stores for patients with renal insufficiency should be conservative (i.e., 6 to 10 mcg/kg) [see PRECAUTIONS].

The loading dose should be administered in several portions, with roughly half the total given as the first dose. Additional fractions of this planned total dose may be given at 6- to 8-hour intervals, **with careful assessment of clinical response before each additional dose.** If the patient's clinical response necessitates a change from the calculated loading dose of digoxin, then calculation of the maintenance dose should be based upon the amount actually given.

A single initial intravenous dose of 400 to 600 mcg (0.4 to 0.6 mg) of LANOXIN Injection usually produces a detectable effect in 5 to 30 minutes that becomes maximal in 1 to 4 hours. Additional doses of 100 to 300 mcg (0.1 to 0.3 mg) may be given cautiously at 6- to 8-hour intervals until clinical evidence of an adequate effect is noted. The usual amount of LANOXIN Injection that a 70-kg patient requires to achieve 8- to 12-mcg/kg peak body stores is 600 to 1,000 mcg (0.6 to 1.0 mg).

Maintenance Dosing: The doses of oral digoxin used in controlled trials in patients with heart failure have ranged from 125 to 500 mcg (0.125 to 0.5 mg) once daily. In these studies, the digoxin dose has been generally titrated according to the patient's age, lean body weight, and renal function. Therapy is generally initiated at a dose of 250 mcg (0.25 mg) once daily in patients under age 70 with good renal function, at a dose of 125 mcg (0.125 mg) once daily in patients over age 70 or with impaired renal function, and at a dose of 62.5 mcg (0.0625 mg) in patients with marked renal impairment. Doses may be increased every 2 weeks according to clinical response.

In a subset of approximately 1,800 patients enrolled in the DIG trial (wherein dosing was based on an algorithm similar to that in Table 5) the mean (± SD) serum digoxin concentrations at 1 month and 12 months were 1.01 ± 0.47 ng/mL and 0.97 ± 0.43 ng/mL, respectively.

The maintenance dose should be based upon the percentage of the peak body stores lost each day through elimination. The following formula has had wide clinical use:

Maintenance Dose = Peak Body Stores (i.e., Loading Dose) × % Daily Loss/100

Where: % Daily Loss = 14 + Ccr/5

(Ccr is creatinine clearance, corrected to 70 kg body weight or 1.73 m^2 body surface area.)

Table 5 provides average daily maintenance dose requirements of LANOXIN Injection for patients with heart failure based upon lean body weight and renal function:

[See table 5 above]

Example: Based on the above table, a patient in heart failure with an estimated lean body weight of 70 kg and a Ccr of 60 mL/min should be given a dose of 175 mcg (0.175 mg) daily of LANOXIN Injection. If no loading dose is administered, steady-state serum concentrations in this patient should be anticipated at approximately 11 days.

Infants and Children: See the full prescribing information for LANOXIN Injection Pediatric for specific recommendations.

It cannot be overemphasized that dosage guidelines provided are based upon average patient response and substantial individual variation can be expected. Accordingly, ultimate dosage selection must be based upon clinical assessment of the patient.

Atrial Fibrillation: Peak digoxin body stores larger than the 8 to 12 mcg/kg required for most patients with heart failure and normal sinus rhythm have been used for control of ventricular rate in patients with atrial fibrillation. Doses of digoxin used for the treatment of chronic atrial fibrillation should be titrated to the minimum dose that achieves the desired ventricular rate control without causing undesirable side effects. Data are not available to establish the appropriate resting or exercise target rates that should be achieved.

Dosage Adjustment When Changing Preparations: The difference in bioavailability between LANOXIN Injection or LANOXICAPS and LANOXIN Elixir Pediatric or LANOXIN Tablets must be considered when changing patients from one dosage form to another.

Doses of 100 mcg (0.1 mg) and 200 mcg (0.2 mg) of LANOXICAPS are approximately equivalent to 125-mcg (0.125-mg) and 250-mcg (0.25-mg) doses of LANOXIN Tablets and Elixir Pediatric, respectively (see Table 1 in CLINICAL PHARMACOLOGY: Pharmacokinetics).

HOW SUPPLIED

LANOXIN (digoxin) Injection, 500 mcg (0.5 mg) in 2 mL (250 mcg [0.25 mg] per mL); Boxes of 10 (NDC 0173-0260-10) and 50 ampuls (NDC 0173-0260-35).

Store at 25°C (77°F); excursions permitted to 15 to 30°C (59 to 86°F) [see USP Controlled Room Temperature] and protect from light.

Manufactured by Catalytica Pharmaceuticals, Inc.
Greenville, NC 27834
for Glaxo Wellcome Inc.
Research Triangle Park, NC 27709

November 1998/RL-622

Shown in Product Identification Guide, page 315

LANOXIN® ℞

[lă-nŏx ʹĭn ʺ]
(digoxin)
Injection Pediatric
100 mcg (0.1 mg) in 1 mL

DESCRIPTION

LANOXIN (digoxin) is one of the cardiac (or digitalis) glycosides, a closely related group of drugs having in common specific effects on the myocardium. These drugs are found in a number of plants. Digoxin is extracted from the leaves of *Digitalis lanata*. The term "digitalis" is used to designate the whole group of glycosides. The glycosides are composed of two portions: a sugar and a cardenolide (hence "glycosides").

Digoxin is described chemically as (3β,5β,12β)-3-[(*O*-2,6-dideoxy-β-*D*-*ribo*-hexopyranosyl-(1→4)-*O*-2,6-di-deoxy-β-*D*-*ribo*-hexopyranosyl-(1→4)-2,6-dideoxy-β-*D*-*ribo*-hexopyranosyl)oxy]-12,14-dihydroxy-card-20(22)-enolide. Its molecular formula is $C_{41}H_{64}O_{14}$, and its molecular weight is 780.95.

Digoxin exists as odorless white crystals that melt with decomposition above 230°C. The drug is practically insoluble in water and in ether; slightly soluble in diluted (50%) alcohol and in chloroform; and freely soluble in pyridine.

LANOXIN Injection Pediatric is a sterile solution of digoxin for intravenous injection. The vehicle contains 40% propylene glycol and 10% alcohol. The injection is buffered to a pH of 6.8 to 7.2 with 0.17% sodium phosphate and 0.08% anhydrous citric acid. Each 1-mL ampul contains 100 mcg (0.1 mg) digoxin. Dilution is not required.

CLINICAL PHARMACOLOGY

Mechanism of Action: Digoxin inhibits sodium-potassium ATPase, an enzyme that regulates the quantity of sodium and potassium inside cells. Inhibition of the enzyme leads to an increase in the intracellular concentration of sodium and thus (by stimulation of sodium-calcium exchange) an increase in the intracellular concentration of calcium. The beneficial effects of digoxin result from direct actions on cardiac muscle, as well as indirect actions on the cardiovascular system mediated by effects on the autonomic nervous system. The autonomic effects include: (1) a vagomimetic action, which is responsible for the effects of digoxin on the sinoatrial and atrioventricular (AV) nodes; and (2) baroreceptor sensitization, which results in increased afferent inhibitory activity and reduced activity of the sympathetic nervous system and renin-angiotensin system for any given increment in mean arterial pressure. The pharmacologic consequences of these direct and indirect effects are: (1) an increase in the force and velocity of myocardial systolic contraction (positive inotropic action); (2) a decrease in the degree of activation of the sympathetic nervous system and renin-angiotensin system (neurohormonal deactivating effect); and (3) slowing of the heart rate and decreased conduction velocity through the AV node (vagomimetic effect).

The effects of digoxin in heart failure are mediated by its positive inotropic and neurohormonal deactivating effects, whereas the effects of the drug in atrial arrhythmias are related to its vagomimetic actions. In high doses, digoxin increases sympathetic outflow from the central nervous system (CNS). This increase in sympathetic activity may be an important factor in digitalis toxicity.

Pharmacokinetics: Note: The following data are from studies performed in adults, unless otherwise stated.

Absorption: Comparisons of the systemic availability and equivalent doses for preparations of digoxin are shown in Table 1:

Table 1: Comparisons of the Systemic Availability and Equivalent Doses for Preparations of LANOXIN

Product	Absolute Bioavailability	Equivalent Doses (mcg)* Among Dosage Forms			
LANOXIN Tablets	60 - 80%	62.5	125	250	500
LANOXIN Elixir Pediatric	70 - 85%	62.5	125	250	500
LANOXICAPS®	90 - 100%	50	100	200	400
LANOXIN Injection/IV	100%	50	100	200	400

*For example, 125 mcg LANOXIN Tablets equivalent to 125 mcg LANOXIN Elixir Pediatric equivalent to 100 mcg LANOXICAPS equivalent to 100 mcg LANOXIN Injection/IV.

Table 2: Times to Onset of Pharmacologic Effect and to Peak Effect of Preparations of LANOXIN

Product	Time to Onset of Effect*	Time to Peak Effect*
LANOXIN Tablets	0.5 - 2 hours	2 - 6 hours
LANOXIN Elixir Pediatric	0.5 - 2 hours	2 - 6 hours
LANOXICAPS	0.5 - 2 hours	2 - 6 hours
LANOXIN Injection/IV	5 - 30 minutes†	1 - 4 hours

*Documented for ventricular response rate in atrial fibrillation, inotropic effects and electrocardiographic changes.
†Depending upon rate of infusion.

Table 3: Subgroup Analyses of Mortality and Hospitalization During the First Two Years Following Randomization

		Risk of All-Cause Mortality or All-Cause Hospitalization*			Risk of HF-Related Mortality or HF-Related Hospitalization*		
	n	Placebo	LANOXIN	Relative risk†	Placebo	LANOXIN	Relative risk†
All patients (EF ≤0.45)	6801	604	593	0.94 (0.88-1.00)	294	217	0.69 (0.63-0.76)
NYHA I/II	4571	549	541	0.96 (0.89-1.04)	242	178	0.70 (0.62-0.80)
EF 0.25-0.45	4543	568	571	0.99 (0.91-1.07)	244	190	0.74 (0.66-0.84)
CTR ≤0.55	4455	561	563	0.98 (0.91-1.06)	239	180	0.71 (0.63-0.81)
NYHA III/IV	2224	719	696	0.88 (0.80-0.97)	402	295	0.65 (0.57-0.75)
EF <0.25	2258	677	637	0.84 (0.76-0.93)	394	270	0.61 (0.53-0.71)
CTR >0.55	2346	687	650	0.85 (0.77-0.94)	398	287	0.65 (0.57-0.75)
EF >0.45‡	987	571	585	1.04 (0.88-1.23)	179	136	0.72 (0.53-0.99)

*Number of patients with an event during the first 2 years per 1000 randomized patients.
†Relative risk (95% confidence interval).
‡DIG Ancillary Study.

[See table 1 above]

Distribution: Following drug administration, a 6- to 8-hour tissue distribution phase is observed. This is followed by a much more gradual decline in the serum concentration of the drug, which is dependent on the elimination of digoxin from the body. The peak height and slope of the early portion (absorption/distribution phases) of the serum concentration-time curve are dependent upon the route of administration and the absorption characteristics of the formulation. Clinical evidence indicates that the early high serum concentrations do not reflect the concentration of digoxin at its site of action, but that with chronic use, the steady-state post-distribution serum concentrations are in equilibrium with tissue concentrations and correlate with pharmacologic effects. In individual patients, these post-distribution serum concentrations may be useful in evaluating therapeutic and toxic effects (see DOSAGE AND ADMINISTRATION: Serum Digoxin Concentrations).

Digoxin is concentrated in tissues and therefore has a large apparent volume of distribution. Digoxin crosses both the blood-brain barrier and the placenta. At delivery, the serum digoxin concentration in the newborn is similar to the serum concentration in the mother. Approximately 25% of digoxin in the plasma is bound to protein. Serum digoxin concentrations are not significantly altered by large changes in fat tissue weight, so that its distribution space correlates best with lean (i.e., ideal) body weight, not total body weight.

Metabolism: Only a small percentage (16%) of a dose of digoxin is metabolized. The end metabolites, which include 3 β-digoxigenin, 3-keto-digoxigenin, and their glucuronide and sulfate conjugates, are polar in nature and are postulated to be formed via hydrolysis, oxidation, and conjugation. The metabolism of digoxin is not dependent upon the cytochrome P-450 system, and digoxin is not known to induce or inhibit the cytochrome P-450 system.

Excretion: Elimination of digoxin follows first-order kinetics (that is, the quantity of digoxin eliminated at any time is proportional to the total body content). Following intravenous administration to healthy volunteers, 50% to 70% of a digoxin dose is excreted unchanged in the urine. Renal excretion of digoxin is proportional to glomerular filtration rate and is largely independent of urine flow. In healthy volunteers with normal renal function, digoxin has a half-life of 1.5 to 2.0 days. The half-life in anuric patients is prolonged to 3.5 to 5 days. Digoxin is not effectively removed from the body by dialysis, exchange transfusion, or during cardiopulmonary bypass because most of the drug is bound to tissue and does not circulate in the blood.

Special Populations: Race differences in digoxin pharmacokinetics have not been formally studied. Because digoxin is primarily eliminated as unchanged drug via the kidney and because there are no important differences in creatinine clearance among races, pharmacokinetic differences due to race are not expected.

The clearance of digoxin can be primarily correlated with renal function as indicated by creatinine clearance. In children with renal disease, digoxin must be carefully titrated based upon clinical response. Plasma digoxin concentration profiles in patients with acute hepatitis generally fell within the range of profiles in a group of healthy subjects.

Pharmacodynamic and Clinical Effects:
The times to onset of pharmacologic effect and to peak effect of preparations of LANOXIN are shown in Table 2:
[See table 2 above]

Hemodynamic Effects: Digoxin produces hemodynamic improvement in patients with heart failure. Short- and long-term therapy with the drug increases cardiac output and lowers pulmonary artery pressure, pulmonary capillary wedge pressure, and systemic vascular resistance. These hemodynamic effects are accompanied by an increase in the left ventricular ejection fraction and a decrease in end-systolic and end-diastolic dimensions.

Chronic Heart Failure: Two 12-week, double-blind, placebo-controlled studies enrolled 178 (RADIANCE trial) and 88 (PROVED trial) adult patients with NYHA class II or III heart failure previously treated with oral digoxin, a diuretic, and an ACE inhibitor (RADIANCE only) and randomized them to placebo or treatment with LANOXIN Tablets. Both trials demonstrated better preservation of exercise capacity in patients randomized to LANOXIN. Continued treatment with LANOXIN reduced the risk of

Continued on next page

This product information is based on labeling in effect on June 23, 2000. For further information, contact via direct mail, phone, or web site. Medical Information, Glaxo Wellcome Inc., PO Box 13398, Research Triangle Park, NC 27709. Healthcare Professionals (Medical Information): 800-334-0089. Patients (Customer Response Center): 1-888-825-5249. Glaxo Wellcome Corporate Web Site: www.glaxowellcome.com

Lanoxin Inj.—Cont.

developing worsening heart failure, as evidenced by heart failure-related hospitalizations and emergency care and the need for concomitant heart failure therapy. The larger study also showed treatment-related benefits in NYHA class and patients' global assessment. In the smaller trial, these trended in favor of a treatment benefit.

The Digitalis Investigation Group (DIG) main trial was a multicenter, randomized, double-blind, placebo-controlled mortality study of 6801 adult patients with heart failure and left ventricular ejection fraction ≤0.45. At randomization, 67% were NYHA class I or II, 71% had heart failure of ischemic etiology, 44% had been receiving digoxin, and most were receiving concomitant ACE inhibitor (94%) and diuretic (82%). Patients were randomized to placebo or LANOXIN Tablets, the dose of which was adjusted for the patient's age, sex, lean body weight, and serum creatinine (see DOSAGE AND ADMINISTRATION), and followed for up to 58 months (median 37 months). The median daily dose prescribed was 0.25 mg. Overall all-cause mortality was 35% with no difference between groups (95% confidence limits for relative risk of 0.91 to 1.07). LANOXIN was associated with a 25% reduction in the number of hospitalizations for heart failure, a 28% reduction in the risk of a patient having at least one hospitalization for heart failure, and a 6.5% reduction in total hospitalizations (for any cause).

Use of LANOXIN was associated with a trend to increase time to all-cause death or hospitalization. The trend was evident in subgroups of patients with mild heart failure as well as more severe disease, as shown in Table 3. Although the effect on all-cause death or hospitalization was not statistically significant, much of the apparent benefit derived from effects on mortality and hospitalization attributed to heart failure.

[See table 3 on previous page]

In situations where there is no statistically significant benefit of treatment evident from a trial's primary endpoint, results pertaining to a secondary endpoint should be interpreted cautiously.

Chronic Atrial Fibrillation: In adult patients with chronic atrial fibrillation, digoxin slows rapid ventricular response rate in a linear dose-response fashion from 0.25 to 0.75 mg/day. Digoxin should not be used for the treatment of multifocal atrial tachycardia.

INDICATIONS AND USAGE

Heart Failure: LANOXIN is indicated for the treatment of mild to moderate heart failure. LANOXIN increases left ventricular ejection fraction and improves heart failure symptoms as evidenced by exercise capacity and heart failure-related hospitalizations and emergency care, while having no effect on mortality. Where possible, LANOXIN should be used with a diuretic and an angiotensin-converting enzyme inhibitor, but an optimal order for starting these three drugs cannot be specified.

Atrial Fibrillation: LANOXIN is indicated for the control of ventricular response rate in patients with chronic atrial fibrillation.

CONTRAINDICATIONS

Digitalis glycosides are contraindicated in patients with ventricular fibrillation or in patients with a known hypersensitivity to digoxin. A hypersensitivity reaction to other digitalis preparations usually constitutes a contraindication to digoxin.

WARNINGS

Sinus Node Disease and AV Block: Because digoxin slows sinoatrial and AV conduction, the drug commonly prolongs the PR interval. The drug may cause severe sinus bradycardia or sinoatrial block in patients with pre-existing sinus node disease and may cause advanced or complete heart block in patients with pre-existing incomplete AV block. In such patients consideration should be given to the insertion of a pacemaker before treatment with digoxin.

Accessory AV Pathway (Wolff-Parkinson-White Syndrome): After intravenous digoxin therapy, some patients with paroxysmal atrial fibrillation or flutter and a coexisting accessory AV pathway have developed increased antegrade conduction across the accessory pathway bypassing the AV node, leading to a very rapid ventricular response or ventricular fibrillation. Unless conduction down the accessory pathway has been blocked (either pharmacologically or by surgery), digoxin should not be used in such patients. The treatment of paroxysmal supraventricular tachycardia in such patients is usually direct-current cardioversion.

Use in Patients with Preserved Left Ventricular Systolic Function: Patients with certain disorders involving heart failure associated with preserved left ventricular ejection fraction may be particularly susceptible to toxicity of the drug. Such disorders include restrictive cardiomyopathy, constrictive pericarditis, amyloid heart disease, and acute cor pulmonale. Patients with idiopathic hypertrophic subaortic stenosis may have worsening of the outflow obstruction due to the inotropic effects of digoxin.

PRECAUTIONS

Use in Patients with Impaired Renal Function: Digoxin is primarily excreted by the kidneys; therefore, patients with impaired renal function require smaller than usual maintenance doses of digoxin (see DOSAGE AND ADMINISTRATION). Because of the prolonged elimination half-life, a longer period of time is required to achieve an initial or new steady-state serum concentration in patients with renal impairment than in patients with normal renal function. If appropriate care is not taken to reduce the dose of digoxin, such patients are at high risk for toxicity, and toxic effects will last longer in such patients than in patients with normal renal function.

Use in Patients with Electrolyte Disorders: In patients with hypokalemia or hypomagnesemia, toxicity may occur despite serum digoxin concentrations below 2.0 ng/mL, because potassium or magnesium depletion sensitizes the myocardium to digoxin. Therefore, it is desirable to maintain normal serum potassium and magnesium concentrations in patients being treated with digoxin. Deficiencies of these electrolytes may result from malnutrition, diarrhea, or prolonged vomiting, as well as the use of the following drugs or procedures: diuretics, amphotericin B, corticosteroids, antacids, dialysis, and mechanical suction of gastrointestinal secretions.

Hypercalcemia from any cause predisposes the patient to digitalis toxicity. Calcium, particularly when administered rapidly by the intravenous route, may produce serious arrhythmias in digitalized patients. On the other hand, hypocalcemia can nullify the effects of digoxin in humans; thus, digoxin may be ineffective until serum calcium is restored to normal. These interactions are related to the fact that digoxin affects contractility and excitability of the heart in a manner similar to that of calcium.

Use in Thyroid Disorders and Hypermetabolic States: Hypothyroidism may reduce the requirements for digoxin. Heart failure and/or atrial arrhythmias resulting from hypermetabolic or hyperdynamic states (e.g., hyperthyroidism, hypoxia, or arteriovenous shunt) are best treated by addressing the underlying condition. Atrial arrhythmias associated with hypermetabolic states are particularly resistant to digoxin treatment. Care must be taken to avoid toxicity if digoxin is used.

Use in Patients with Acute Myocardial Infarction: Digoxin should be used with caution in patients with acute myocardial infarction. The use of inotropic drugs in some patients in this setting may result in undesirable increases in myocardial oxygen demand and ischemia.

Use During Electrical Cardioversion: It may be desirable to reduce the dose of digoxin for 1 to 2 days prior to electrical cardioversion of atrial fibrillation to avoid the induction of ventricular arrhythmias, but physicians must consider the consequences of increasing the ventricular response if digoxin is withdrawn. If digitalis toxicity is suspected, elective cardioversion should be delayed. If it is not prudent to delay cardioversion, the lowest possible energy level should be selected to avoid provoking ventricular arrhythmias.

Laboratory Test Monitoring: Patients receiving digoxin should have their serum electrolytes and renal function (serum creatinine concentrations) assessed periodically; the frequency of assessments will depend on the clinical setting. For discussion of serum digoxin concentrations, see DOSAGE AND ADMINISTRATION.

Drug Interactions: Potassium-depleting *diuretics* are a major contributing factor to digitalis toxicity. *Calcium*, particularly if administered rapidly by the intravenous route, may produce serious arrhythmias in digitalized patients. *Quinidine, verapamil, amiodarone, propafenone, indomethacin, itraconazole, alprazolam,* and *spironolactone* raise the serum digoxin concentration due to a reduction in clearance and/or volume of distribution of the drug, with the implication that digitalis intoxication may result. *Erythromycin* and *clarithromycin* (and possibly other *macrolide antibiotics*) and *tetracycline* may increase digoxin absorption in patients who inactivate digoxin by bacterial metabolism in the lower intestine, so that digitalis intoxication may result. *Propantheline* and *diphenoxylate*, by decreasing gut motility, may increase digoxin absorption. *Antacids, kaolin-pectin, sulfasalazine, neomycin, cholestyramine*, certain *anticancer drugs*, and *metoclopramide* may interfere with intestinal digoxin absorption, resulting in unexpectedly low serum concentrations. *Rifampin* may decrease serum digoxin concentration, especially in patients with renal dysfunction, by increasing the non-renal clearance of digoxin. There have been inconsistent reports regarding the effects of other drugs [e.g., *quinine, penicillamine*] on serum digoxin concentration. *Thyroid* administration to a digitalized, hypothyroid patient may increase the dose requirement of digoxin. Concomitant use of digoxin and *sympathomimetics* increases the risk of cardiac arrhythmias. *Succinylcholine* may cause a sudden extrusion of potassium from muscle cells, and may thereby cause arrhythmias in digitalized patients. Although beta-adrenergic blockers or calcium channel blockers and digoxin may be useful in combination to control atrial fibrillation, their additive effects on AV node conduction can result in advanced or complete heart block.

Due to the considerable variability of these interactions, dosage of digoxin should be individualized when patients receive these medications concurrently. Furthermore, caution should be exercised when combining digoxin with any drug that may cause a significant deterioration in renal function, since a decline in glomerular filtration or tubular secretion may impair the excretion of digoxin.

Drug/Laboratory Test Interactions: The use of therapeutic doses of digoxin may cause prolongation of the PR interval and depression of the ST segment on the electrocardiogram. Digoxin may produce false positive ST-T changes on the electrocardiogram during exercise testing. These electrophysiologic effects reflect an expected effect of the drug and are not indicative of toxicity.

Carcinogenesis, Mutagenesis, Impairment of Fertility: There have been no long-term studies performed in animals to evaluate carcinogenic potential, nor have studies been conducted to assess the mutagenic potential of digoxin or its potential to affect fertility.

Pregnancy: *Teratogenic Effects:* Pregnancy Category C. Animal reproduction studies have not been conducted with digoxin. It is also not known whether digoxin can cause fetal harm when administered to a pregnant woman or can affect reproductive capacity. Digoxin should be given to a pregnant woman only if clearly needed.

Nursing Mothers: Studies have shown that digoxin concentrations in the mother's serum and milk are similar. However, the estimated exposure of a nursing infant to digoxin via breast feeding will be far below the usual infant maintenance dose. Therefore, this amount should have no pharmacologic effect upon the infant. Nevertheless, caution should be exercised when digoxin is administered to a nursing woman.

Pediatric Use: Newborn infants display considerable variability in their tolerance to digoxin. Premature and immature infants are particularly sensitive to the effects of digoxin, and the dosage of the drug must not only be reduced but must be individualized according to their degree of maturity. Digitalis glycosides can cause poisoning in children due to accidental ingestion.

Geriatric Use: The majority of clinical experience gained with digoxin has been in the elderly population. This experience has not identified differences in response or adverse effects between the elderly and younger patients. However, this drug is known to be substantially excreted by the kidney, and the risk of toxic reactions to this drug may be greater in patients with impaired renal function. Because elderly patients are more likely to have decreased renal function, care should be taken in dose selection, which should be based on renal function, and it may be useful to monitor renal function.

ADVERSE REACTIONS

In general, the adverse reactions of digoxin are dose-dependent and occur at doses higher than those needed to achieve a therapeutic effect. Hence, adverse reactions are less common when digoxin is used within the recommended dose range or therapeutic serum concentration range and when there is careful attention to concurrent medications and conditions.

Because some patients may be particularly susceptible to side effects with digoxin, the dosage of the drug should always be selected carefully and adjusted as the clinical condition of the patient warrants. In the past, when high doses of digoxin were used and little attention was paid to clinical status or concurrent medications, adverse reactions to digoxin were more frequent and severe. Cardiac adverse reactions accounted for about one-half, gastrointestinal disturbances for about one-fourth, and CNS and other toxicity for about one-fourth of these adverse reactions. However, available evidence suggests that the incidence and severity of digoxin toxicity has decreased substantially in recent years. In recent controlled clinical trials, in patients with predominantly mild to moderate heart failure, the incidence of adverse experiences was comparable in patients taking digoxin and in those taking placebo. In a large mortality trial, the incidence of hospitalization for suspected digoxin toxicity was 2% in patients taking LANOXIN Tablets compared to 0.9% in patients taking placebo. In this trial, the most common manifestations of digoxin toxicity included gastrointestinal and cardiac disturbances; CNS manifestations were less common.

Adults: *Cardiac:* Therapeutic doses of digoxin may cause heart block in patients with pre-existing sinoatrial or AV conduction disorders; heart block can be avoided by adjusting the dose of digoxin. Prophylactic use of a cardiac pacemaker may be considered if the risk of heart block is considered unacceptable. High doses of digoxin may produce a variety of rhythm disturbances, such as first-degree, second-degree (Wenckebach), or third-degree heart block (including asystole); atrial tachycardia with block; AV dissociation; accelerated junctional (nodal) rhythm; unifocal or multiform ventricular premature contractions (especially bigeminy or trigeminy); ventricular tachycardia; and ventricular fibrillation. Digoxin produces PR prolongation and ST segment depression which should not by themselves be considered digoxin toxicity. Cardiac toxicity can also occur at therapeutic doses in patients who have conditions which may alter their sensitivity to digoxin (see WARNINGS and PRECAUTIONS).

Gastrointestinal: Digoxin may cause anorexia, nausea, vomiting, and diarrhea. Rarely, the use of digoxin has been associated with abdominal pain, intestinal ischemia, and hemorrhagic necrosis of the intestines.

CNS: Digoxin can produce visual disturbances (blurred or yellow vision), headache, weakness, dizziness, apathy, confusion, and mental disturbances (such as anxiety, depression, delirium, and hallucination).

Other: Gynecomastia has been occasionally observed following the prolonged use of digoxin. Thrombocytopenia and maculopapular rash and other skin reactions have been rarely observed.

The following table summarizes the incidence of those adverse experiences listed above for patients treated with LANOXIN Tablets or placebo from two randomized, double-blind, placebo-controlled withdrawal trials. Patients in these trials were also receiving diuretics with or without angiotensin-converting enzyme inhibitors. These patients had been stable on digoxin, and were randomized to digoxin or placebo. The results shown in Table 4 reflect the experience in patients following dosage titration with the use of serum digoxin concentrations and careful follow-up. These adverse experiences are consistent with results from a large, placebo-controlled mortality trial (DIG trial) wherein over half the patients were not receiving digoxin prior to enrollment. [See table 4 at right]

Infants and Children: The side effects of digoxin in infants and children differ from those seen in adults in several respects. Although digoxin may produce anorexia, nausea, vomiting, diarrhea, and CNS disturbances in young patients, these are rarely the initial symptoms of overdosage. Rather, the earliest and most frequent manifestation of excessive dosing with digoxin in infants and children is the appearance of cardiac arrhythmias, including sinus bradycardia. In children, the use of digoxin may produce any arrhythmia. The most common are conduction disturbances or supraventricular tachyarrhythmias, such as atrial tachycardia (with or without block) and junctional (nodal) tachycardia. Ventricular arrhythmias are less common. Sinus bradycardia may be a sign of impending digoxin intoxication, especially in infants, even in the absence of first-degree heart block. Any arrhythmia or alteration in cardiac conduction that develops in a child taking digoxin should be assumed to be caused by digoxin, until further evaluation proves otherwise.

Table 4: Adverse Experiences in Two Parallel, Double-Blind, Placebo-Controlled Withdrawal Trials (Number of Patients Reporting)

Adverse Experience	Digoxin Patients (n = 123)	Placebo Patients (n = 125)
Cardiac		
Palpitation	1	4
Ventricular extrasystole	1	1
Tachycardia	2	1
Heart arrest	1	1
Gastrointestinal		
Anorexia	1	4
Nausea	4	2
Vomiting	2	1
Diarrhea	4	1
Abdominal pain	0	6
CNS		
Headache	4	4
Dizziness	6	5
Mental disturbances	5	1
Other		
Rash	2	1
Death	4	3

OVERDOSAGE

Treatment of Adverse Reactions Produced by Overdosage: Digoxin should be temporarily discontinued until the adverse reaction resolves. Every effort should also be made to correct factors that may contribute to the adverse reaction (such as electrolyte disturbances or concurrent medications). Once the adverse reaction has resolved, therapy with digoxin may be reinstituted, following a careful reassessment of dose.

Withdrawal of digoxin may be all that is required to treat the adverse reaction. However, when the primary manifestation of digoxin overdosage is a cardiac arrhythmia, additional therapy may be needed.

If the rhythm disturbance is a symptomatic bradyarrhythmia or heart block, consideration should be given to the reversal of toxicity with DIGIBIND® [Digoxin Immune Fab (Ovine)] (see below), the use of atropine, or the insertion of a temporary cardiac pacemaker. However, asymptomatic bradycardia or heart block related to digoxin may require only temporary withdrawal of the drug and cardiac monitoring of the patient.

If the rhythm disturbance is a ventricular arrhythmia, consideration should be given to the correction of electrolyte disorders, particularly if hypokalemia (see below) or hypomagnesemia is present. DIGIBIND is a specific antidote for digoxin and may be used to reverse potentially life-threatening ventricular arrhythmias due to digoxin overdosage.

Administration of Potassium: Every effort should be made to maintain the serum potassium concentration between 4.0 and 5.5 mmol/L. Potassium is usually administered orally, but when correction of the arrhythmia is urgent and the serum potassium concentration is low, potassium may be administered cautiously by the intravenous route. The electrocardiogram should be monitored for any evidence of potassium toxicity (e.g., peaking of T waves) and to observe the effect on the arrhythmia. Potassium salts may be dangerous in patients who manifest bradycardia or heart block due to digoxin (unless primarily related to supraventricular tachycardia) and in the setting of massive digitalis overdosage (see Massive Digitalis Overdosage subsection).

Massive Digitalis Overdosage: Manifestations of life-threatening toxicity include ventricular tachycardia or ventricular fibrillation, or progressive bradyarrhythmias or heart block. The administration of more than 10 mg of digoxin in a previously healthy adult, or more than 4 mg in a previously healthy child, or a steady-state serum concentration greater than 10 ng/mL often results in cardiac arrest. DIGIBIND should be used to reverse the toxic effects of ingestion of a massive overdose. The decision to administer DIGIBIND to a patient who has ingested a massive dose of digoxin but who has not yet manifested life-threatening toxicity should depend on the likelihood that life-threatening toxicity will occur (see above).

Patients with massive digitalis ingestion should receive large doses of activated charcoal to prevent absorption and bind digoxin in the gut during enteroenteric recirculation. Emesis or gastric lavage may be indicated especially if ingestion has occurred within 30 minutes of the patient's presentation at the hospital. Emesis should not be induced in patients who are obtunded. If a patient presents more than 2 hours after ingestion or already has toxic manifestations, it may be unsafe to induce vomiting or attempt passage of a gastric tube, because such maneuvers may induce an acute vagal episode that can worsen digitalis-related arrhythmias.

Severe digitalis intoxication can cause a massive shift of potassium from inside to outside the cell, leading to life-threatening hyperkalemia. The administration of potassium supplements in the setting of massive intoxication may be hazardous and should be avoided. Hyperkalemia caused by massive digitalis toxicity is best treated with DIGIBIND; initial treatment with glucose and insulin may also be required if hyperkalemia itself is acutely life-threatening.

DOSAGE AND ADMINISTRATION

General: Recommended dosages of digoxin may require considerable modification because of individual sensitivity of the patient to the drug, the presence of associated conditions, or the use of concurrent medications.

Table 5: Usual Digitalizing and Maintenance Dosages for LANOXIN® Injection Pediatric in Children with Normal Renal Function Based on Lean Body Weight

Age	IV Digitalizing* Dose (mcg/kg)	Daily IV Maintenance Dose† (mcg/kg)
Premature	15 to 25	20% to 30% of the IV digitalizing dose‡
Full-Term	20 to 30	
1 to 24 Months	30 to 50	
2 to 5 Years	25 to 35	25% to 35% of the IV digitalizing dose‡
5 to 10 Years	15 to 30	
Over 10 Years	8 to 12	

* IV digitalizing doses are 80% of oral digitalizing doses.
† Divided daily dosing is recommended for children under 10 years of age.
‡ Projected or actual digitalizing dose providing clinical response.

Parenteral administration of digoxin should be used only when the need for rapid digitalization is urgent or when the drug cannot be taken orally. Intramuscular injection can lead to severe pain at the injection site, thus intravenous administration is preferred. If the drug must be administered by the intramuscular route, it should be injected deep into the muscle followed by massage. No more than 200 mcg (2 mL) should be injected into a single site.

LANOXIN Injection Pediatric can be administered undiluted or diluted with a 4-fold or greater volume of Sterile Water for Injection, 0.9% Sodium Chloride Injection, or 5% Dextrose Injection. The use of less than a 4-fold volume of diluent could lead to precipitation of the digoxin. Immediate use of the diluted product is recommended.

If tuberculin syringes are used to measure very small doses, one must be aware of the problem of inadvertent overadministration of digoxin. The syringe should *not* be flushed with the parenteral solution after its contents are expelled into an indwelling vascular catheter.

Slow infusion of LANOXIN Injection Pediatric is preferable to bolus administration. Rapid infusion of digitalis glycosides has been shown to cause systemic and coronary arteriolar constriction, which may be clinically undesirable. Caution is thus advised and LANOXIN Injection Pediatric should probably be administered over a period of 5 minutes or longer. Mixing of LANOXIN Injection Pediatric with other drugs in the same container or simultaneous administration in the same intravenous line is not recommended.

In selecting a dose of digoxin, the following factors must be considered:

1. The body weight of the patient. Doses should be calculated based upon lean (i.e., ideal) body weight.
2. The patient's renal function, preferably evaluated on the basis of estimated creatinine clearance.
3. The patient's age. Infants and children require different doses of digoxin than adults. Also, advanced age may be indicative of diminished renal function even in patients with normal serum creatinine concentration (i.e., below 1.5 mg/dL).
4. Concomitant disease states, concurrent medications, or other factors likely to alter the pharmacokinetic or pharmacodynamic profile of digoxin (see PRECAUTIONS).

Serum Digoxin Concentrations: In general, the dose of digoxin used should be determined on clinical grounds. However, measurement of serum digoxin concentrations can be helpful to the clinician in determining the adequacy of digoxin therapy and in assigning certain probabilities to the likelihood of digoxin intoxication. About two-thirds of adults considered adequately digitalized (without evidence of toxicity) have serum digoxin concentrations ranging from 0.8 to 2.0 ng/mL. However, digoxin may produce clinical benefits even at serum concentrations below this range. About two-thirds of adult patients with clinical toxicity have serum digoxin concentrations greater than 2.0 ng/mL. However, since one-third of patients with clinical toxicity have concentrations less than 2.0 ng/mL, values below 2.0 ng/mL do not rule out the possibility that a certain sign or symptom is related to digoxin therapy. Rarely, there are patients who are unable to tolerate digoxin at serum concentrations below 0.8 ng/mL. Consequently, the serum concentration of digoxin should always be interpreted in the overall clinical context, and an isolated measurement should not be used alone as the basis for increasing or decreasing the dose of the drug.

To allow adequate time for equilibration of digoxin between serum and tissue, sampling of serum concentrations should be done just before the next scheduled dose of the drug. If this is not possible, sampling should be done at least 6 to 8 hours after the last dose, regardless of the route of administration or the formulation used. On a once-daily dosing schedule, the concentration of digoxin will be 10% to 25% lower when sampled at 24 versus 8 hours, depending upon the patient's renal function. On a twice-daily dosing schedule, there will be only minor differences in serum digoxin concentrations whether sampling is done at 8 or 12 hours after a dose.

If a discrepancy exists between the reported serum concentration and the observed clinical response, the clinician should consider the following possibilities:

1. Analytical problems in the assay procedure.
2. Inappropriate serum sampling time.
3. Administration of a digitalis glycoside other than digoxin.
4. Conditions (described in WARNINGS and PRECAUTIONS) causing an alteration in the sensitivity of the patient to digoxin.
5. Serum digoxin concentration may decrease acutely during periods of exercise without any associated change in clinical efficacy due to increased binding of digoxin to skeletal muscle.

Heart Failure: Adults: See the full prescribing information for LANOXIN Injection for specific recommendations.

Infants and Children: In general, divided daily dosing is recommended for infants and young children (under age 10). In the newborn period, renal clearance of digoxin is diminished and suitable dosage adjustments must be observed. This is especially pronounced in the premature infant. Beyond the immediate newborn period, children generally require proportionally larger doses than adults on the basis of body weight or body surface area. Children over 10 years of age require adult dosages in proportion to their body weight. Some researchers have suggested that infants and young children tolerate slightly higher serum concentrations than do adults.

Continued on next page

This product information is based on labeling in effect on June 23, 2000. For further information, contact via direct mail, phone, or web site. Medical Information, Glaxo Wellcome Inc., PO Box 13398, Research Triangle Park, NC 27709. Healthcare Professionals (Medical Information): 800-334-0089. Patients (Customer Response Center): 1-888-825-5249. Glaxo Wellcome Corporate Web Site: www.glaxowellcome.com

Lanoxin Inj.—Cont.

Digitalization may be accomplished by either of two general approaches that vary in dosage and frequency of administration, but reach the same endpoint in terms of total amount of digoxin accumulated in the body.

1. If rapid digitalization is considered medically appropriate, it may be achieved by administering a loading dose based upon projected peak digoxin body stores. Maintenance dose can be calculated as a percentage of the loading dose.
2. More gradual digitalization may be obtained by beginning an appropriate maintenance dose, thus allowing digoxin body stores to accumulate slowly. Steady-state serum digoxin concentrations will be achieved in approximately five half-lives of the drug for the individual patient. Depending upon the patient's renal function, this will take between 1 and 3 weeks.

Rapid Digitalization with a Loading Dose: LANOXIN Injection Pediatric can be used to achieve rapid digitalization, with conversion to an oral formulation of LANOXIN for maintenance therapy. If patients are switched from intravenous to oral digoxin formulations, allowances must be made for differences in bioavailability when calculating maintenance dosages (see Table 1 in CLINICAL PHARMACOLOGY: Pharmacokinetics and dosing Table 5 below).

Intramuscular injection of digoxin is extremely painful and offers no advantages unless other routes of administration are contraindicated.

Peak digoxin body stores of 8 to 12 mcg/kg should provide therapeutic effect with minimum risk of toxicity in most patients with heart failure and normal sinus rhythm. Because of altered digoxin distribution and elimination, projected peak body stores for patients with renal insufficiency should be conservative (i.e., 6 to 10 mcg/kg) [see PRECAUTIONS].

Digitalizing and daily maintenance doses for each age group are given in Table 5 and should provide therapeutic effect with minimum risk of toxicity in most patients with heart failure and normal sinus rhythm. These recommendations assume the presence of normal renal function.

The loading dose should be administered in several portions, with roughly half the total given as the first dose. Additional fractions of this planned total dose may be given at 4- to 8-hour intervals, **with careful assessment of clinical response before each additional dose.** If the patient's clinical response necessitates a change from the calculated loading dose of digoxin, then calculation of the maintenance dose should be based upon the amount actually given.

[See table 5 on previous page]

In children with renal disease, digoxin dosing must be carefully titrated based on clinical response.

Gradual Digitalization With A Maintenance Dose: More gradual digitalization can also be accomplished by beginning an appropriate maintenance dose. The range of percentages provided in Table 5 can be used in calculating this dose for patients with normal renal function.

It cannot be overemphasized that these pediatric dosage guidelines are based upon average patient response and substantial individual variation can be expected. Accordingly, ultimate dosage selection must be based upon clinical assessment of the patient.

Atrial Fibrillation: Peak digoxin body stores larger than the 8 to 12 mcg/kg required for most patients with heart failure and normal sinus rhythm have been used for control of ventricular rate in patients with atrial fibrillation. Doses of digoxin used for the treatment of chronic atrial fibrillation should be titrated to the minimum dose that achieves the desired ventricular rate control without causing undesirable side effects. Data are not available to establish the appropriate resting or exercise target rates that should be achieved.

Dosage Adjustment When Changing Preparations: The differences in bioavailability between injectable LANOXIN or LANOXICAPS and LANOXIN Elixir Pediatric or LANOXIN Tablets must be considered when changing patients from one dosage form to another.

Doses of 100 mcg (0.1 mg) and 200 mcg (0.2 mg) of LANOXICAPS are approximately equivalent to 125 mcg (0.125 mg) and 250 mcg (0.25 mg) doses of LANOXIN Tablets and Elixir Pediatric, respectively (see Table 1 in CLINICAL PHARMACOLOGY: Pharmacokinetics).

HOW SUPPLIED

LANOXIN (digoxin) Injection Pediatric, 100 mcg (0.1 mg) in 1 mL; box of 10 ampuls (NDC 0173-0262-10).

Store at 25°C (77°F); excursions permitted to 15° to 30°C (59° to 86°F) [see USP Controlled Room Temperature] and protect from light.

Manufactured by Catalytica Pharmaceuticals, Inc.
Greenville, NC 27834
for Glaxo Wellcome Inc.
Research Triangle Park, NC 27709

December 1998/RL-623

Shown in Product Identification Guide, page 315

LANOXIN® ℞

[*lă-nŏx ' in*]
(digoxin)
Tablets, USP
125 mcg (0.125 mg) Scored I.D. Imprint Y3B (yellow)
250 mcg (0.25 mg) Scored I.D. Imprint X3A (white)

DESCRIPTION

LANOXIN (digoxin) is one of the cardiac (or digitalis) glycosides, a closely related group of drugs having in common specific effects on the myocardium. These drugs are found in a number of plants. Digoxin is extracted from the leaves of *Digitalis lanata*. The term "digitalis" is used to designate the whole group of glycosides. The glycosides are composed of two portions: a sugar and a cardenolide (hence "glycosides").

Digoxin is described chemically as (3β,5β,12β)-3-[(*O*-2,6-dideoxy-β-*D-ribo*-hexopyranosyl-(1→4)-*O*-2,6-dideoxy-β-*D-ribo*-hexopyranosyl-(1→4)-2,6-dideoxy-β-*D-ribo*-hexopyranosyl)oxy]-12,14-dihydroxy-card-20(22)-enolide. Its molecular formula is $C_{41}H_{64}O_{14}$, and its molecular weight is 780.95.

Digoxin exists as odorless white crystals that melt with decomposition above 230°C. The drug is practically insoluble in water and in ether; slightly soluble in diluted (50%) alcohol and in chloroform; and freely soluble in pyridine.

LANOXIN is supplied as 125-mcg (0.125-mg) or 250-mcg (0.25-mg) tablets for oral administration. Each tablet contains the labeled amount of digoxin USP and the following inactive ingredients: corn and potato starches, lactose, and magnesium stearate. In addition, the dyes used in the 125-mcg (0.125-mg) tablets are D&C Yellow No. 10 and FD&C Yellow No. 6.

CLINICAL PHARMACOLOGY

Mechanism of Action: Digoxin inhibits sodium-potassium ATPase, an enzyme that regulates the quantity of sodium and potassium inside cells. Inhibition of the enzyme leads to an increase in the intracellular concentration of sodium and thus (by stimulation of sodium-calcium exchange) an increase in the intracellular concentration of calcium. The beneficial effects of digoxin result from direct actions on cardiac muscle, as well as indirect actions on the cardiovascular system mediated by effects on the autonomic nervous system. The autonomic effects include: (1) a vagomimetic action, which is responsible for the effects of digoxin on the sinoatrial and atrioventricular (AV) nodes; and (2) baroreceptor sensitization, which results in increased afferent inhibitory activity and reduced activity of the sympathetic nervous system and renin-angiotensin system for any given increment in mean arterial pressure. The pharmacologic consequences of these direct and indirect effects are: (1) an increase in the force and velocity of myocardial systolic contraction (positive inotropic action); (2) a decrease in the degree of activation of the sympathetic nervous system and renin-angiotensin system (neurohormonal deactivating effect); and (3) slowing of the heart rate and decreased conduction velocity through the AV node (vagomimetic effect). The effects of digoxin in heart failure are mediated by its positive inotropic and neurohormonal deactivating effects, whereas the effects of the drug in atrial arrhythmias are related to its vagomimetic actions. In high doses, digoxin increases sympathetic outflow from the central nervous system (CNS). This increase in sympathetic activity may be an important factor in digitalis toxicity.

Pharmacokinetics: ***Absorption:*** Following oral administration, peak serum concentrations of digoxin occur at 1 to 3 hours. Absorption of digoxin from LANOXIN Tablets has been demonstrated to be 60% to 80% complete compared to an identical intravenous dose of digoxin (absolute bioavailability) or LANOXICAPS® (relative bioavailability). When LANOXIN Tablets are taken after meals, the rate of absorption is slowed, but the total amount of digoxin absorbed is usually unchanged. When taken with meals high in bran fiber, however, the amount absorbed from an oral dose may be reduced. Comparisons of the systemic availability and equivalent doses for oral preparations of LANOXIN are shown in Table 1:

[See table 1 below]

In some patients, orally administered digoxin is converted to inactive reduction products (e.g., dihydrodigoxin) by colonic bacteria in the gut. Data suggest that one in ten patients treated with digoxin tablets will degrade 40% or more of the ingested dose. As a result, certain antibiotics may increase the absorption of digoxin in such patients. Although inactivation of these bacteria by antibiotics is rapid, the serum digoxin concentration will rise at a rate consistent with the elimination half-life of digoxin. The magnitude of rise in serum digoxin concentration relates to the extent of bacterial inactivation, and may be as much as two-fold in some cases.

Distribution: Following drug administration, a 6- to 8-hour tissue distribution phase is observed. This is followed by a much more gradual decline in the serum concentration of the drug, which is dependent on the elimination of digoxin from the body. The peak height and slope of the early portion (absorption/distribution phases) of the serum concentration-time curve are dependent upon the route of administration and the absorption characteristics of the formulation. Clinical evidence indicates that the early high serum concentrations do not reflect the concentration of digoxin at its site of action, but that with chronic use, the steady-state post-distribution serum concentrations are in equilibrium with tissue concentrations and correlate with pharmacologic effects. In individual patients, these post-distribution serum concentrations may be useful in evaluating therapeutic and toxic effects (see DOSAGE AND ADMINISTRATION: Serum Digoxin Concentrations).

Digoxin is concentrated in tissues and therefore has a large apparent volume of distribution. Digoxin crosses both the blood-brain barrier and the placenta. At delivery, the serum digoxin concentration in the newborn is similar to the serum concentration in the mother. Approximately 25% of digoxin in the plasma is bound to protein. Serum digoxin concentrations are not significantly altered by large changes in fat tissue weight, so that its distribution space correlates best with lean (i.e., ideal) body weight, not total body weight.

Metabolism: Only a small percentage (16%) of a dose of digoxin is metabolized. The end metabolites, which include 3 β-digoxigenin, 3-keto-digoxigenin, and their glucuronide and sulfate conjugates, are polar in nature and are postulated to be formed via hydrolysis, oxidation, and conjugation. The metabolism of digoxin is not dependent upon the cytochrome P-450 system, and digoxin is not known to induce or inhibit the cytochrome P-450 system.

Excretion: Elimination of digoxin follows first-order kinetics (that is, the quantity of digoxin eliminated at any time is proportional to the total body content). Following intravenous administration to healthy volunteers, 50% to 70% of a digoxin dose is excreted unchanged in the urine. Renal excretion of digoxin is proportional to glomerular filtration rate and is largely independent of urine flow. In healthy volunteers with normal renal function, digoxin has a half-life of 1.5 to 2.0 days. The half-life in anuric patients is prolonged to 3.5 to 5 days. Digoxin is not effectively removed from the body by dialysis, exchange transfusion, or during cardiopulmonary bypass because most of the drug is bound to tissue and does not circulate in the blood.

Special Populations: Race differences in digoxin pharmacokinetics have not been formally studied. Because digoxin is primarily eliminated as unchanged drug via the kidney and because there are no important differences in creatinine clearance among races, pharmacokinetic differences due to race are not expected.

The clearance of digoxin can be primarily correlated with renal function as indicated by creatinine clearance. The Cockcroft and Gault formula for estimation of creatinine clearance includes age, body weight, and gender. A table that provides the usual daily maintenance dose requirements of LANOXIN Tablets based on creatinine clearance (per 70 kg) is presented in the DOSAGE AND ADMINISTRATION section.

Plasma digoxin concentration profiles in patients with acute hepatitis generally fell within the range of profiles in a group of healthy subjects.

Pharmacodynamic and Clinical Effects: The times to onset of pharmacologic effect and to peak effect of preparations of LANOXIN are shown in Table 2:

[See table 2 at top of next page]

Hemodynamic Effects: Digoxin produces hemodynamic improvement in patients with heart failure. Short- and long-term therapy with the drug increases cardiac output and lowers pulmonary artery pressure, pulmonary capillary wedge pressure, and systemic vascular resistance. These hemodynamic effects are accompanied by an increase in the left ventricular ejection fraction and a decrease in end-systolic and end-diastolic dimensions.

Chronic Heart Failure: Two 12-week, double-blind, placebo-controlled studies enrolled 178 (RADIANCE trial) and 88 (PROVED trial) patients with NYHA class II or III heart failure previously treated with digoxin, a diuretic, and an ACE inhibitor (RADIANCE only) and randomized them to placebo or treatment with LANOXIN. Both trials demonstrated better preservation of exercise capacity in patients randomized to LANOXIN. Continued treatment with LANOXIN reduced the risk of developing worsening heart failure, as evidenced by heart failure-related hospitalizations and emergency care and the need for concomitant heart failure therapy. The larger study also showed treatment-related benefits in NYHA class and patients' global assessment. In the smaller trial, these trended in favor of a treatment benefit.

The Digitalis Investigation Group (DIG) main trial was a multicenter, randomized, double-blind, placebo-controlled mortality study of 6801 patients with heart failure and left ventricular ejection fraction ≤0.45. At randomization, 67% were NYHA class I or II, 71% had heart failure of ischemic etiology, 44% had been receiving digoxin, and most were receiving concomitant ACE inhibitor (94%) and diuretic (82%). Patients were randomized to placebo or LANOXIN, the dose of which was adjusted for the patient's age, sex, lean body weight, and serum creatinine (see DOSAGE AND ADMIN-

Table 1: Comparisons of the Systemic Availability and Equivalent Doses for Oral Preparations of LANOXIN

Product	Absolute Bioavailability	Equivalent Doses (mcg)* Among Dosage Forms			
LANOXIN Tablets	60 – 80%	62.5	125	250	500
LANOXIN Elixir Pediatric	70 – 85%	62.5	125	250	500
LANOXICAPS®	90 – 100%	50	100	200	400
LANOXIN Injection/IV	100%	50	100	200	400

*For example, 125-mcg LANOXIN Tablets equivalent to 125-mcg LANOXIN Elixir Pediatric equivalent to 100-mcg LANOXICAPS equivalent to 100-mcg LANOXIN Injection/IV.

ISTRATION), and followed for up to 58 months (median 37 months). The median daily dose prescribed was 0.25 mg. Overall all-cause mortality was 35% with no difference between groups (95% confidence limits for relative risk of 0.91 to 1.07). LANOXIN was associated with a 25% reduction in the number of hospitalizations for heart failure, a 28% reduction in the risk of a patient having at least one hospitalization for heart failure, and a 6.5% reduction in total hospitalizations (for any cause).

Use of LANOXIN was associated with a trend to increase time to all-cause death or hospitalization. The trend was evident in subgroups of patients with mild heart failure as well as more severe disease, as shown in Table 3. Although the effect on all-cause death or hospitalization was not statistically significant, much of the apparent benefit derived from effects on mortality and hospitalization attributed to heart failure.

[See table 3 at right]

In situations where there is no statistically significant benefit of treatment evident from a trial's primary endpoint, results pertaining to a secondary endpoint should be interpreted cautiously.

Chronic Atrial Fibrillation: In patients with chronic atrial fibrillation, digoxin slows rapid ventricular response rate in a linear dose-response fashion from 0.25 to 0.75 mg/day. Digoxin should not be used for the treatment of multifocal atrial tachycardia.

Table 2: Times to Onset of Pharmacologic Effect and to Peak Effect of Preparations of LANOXIN

Product	Time to Onset of Effect*	Time to Peak Effect*
LANOXIN Tablets	0.5 – 2 hours	2 – 6 hours
LANOXIN Elixir Pediatric	0.5 – 2 hours	2 – 6 hours
LANOXICAPS	0.5 – 2 hours	2 – 6 hours
LANOXIN Injection/IV	5 – 30 minutes†	1 – 4 hours

* Documented for ventricular response rate in atrial fibrillation, inotropic effects and electrocardiographic changes.
† Depending upon rate of infusion.

Table 3: Subgroup Analyses of Mortality and Hospitalization During the First Two Years Following Randomization

	n	Risk of All-Cause Mortality or All-Cause Hospitalization*			Risk of HF-Related Mortality or HF-Related Hospitalization*		
		Placebo	LANOXIN	Relative risk†	Placebo	LANOXIN	Relative risk†
All patients (EF ≤0.45)	6801	604	593	0.94 (0.88-1.00)	294	217	0.69 (0.63-0.76)
NYHA I / II	4571	549	541	0.96 (0.89-1.04)	242	178	0.70 (0.62-0.80)
EF 0.25-0.45	4543	568	571	0.99 (0.91-1.07)	244	190	0.74 (0.66-0.84)
CTR ≤0.55	4455	561	563	0.98 (0.91-1.06)	239	180	0.71 (0.63-0.81)
NYHA III / IV	2224	719	696	0.88 (0.80-0.97)	402	295	0.65 (0.57-0.75)
EF <0.25	2258	677	637	0.84 (0.76-0.93)	394	270	0.61 (0.53-0.71)
CTR >0.55	2346	687	650	0.85 (0.77-0.94)	398	287	0.65 (0.57-0.75)
EF >0.45‡	987	571	585	1.04 (0.88-1.23)	179	136	0.72 (0.53-0.99)

* Number of patients with an event during the first 2 years per 1000 randomized patients.
† Relative risk (95% confidence interval).
‡ DIG Ancillary Study.

INDICATIONS AND USAGE

Heart Failure: LANOXIN is indicated for the treatment of mild to moderate heart failure. LANOXIN increases left ventricular ejection fraction and improves heart failure symptoms as evidenced by exercise capacity and heart failure-related hospitalizations and emergency care, while having no effect on mortality. Where possible, LANOXIN should be used with a diuretic and an angiotensin-converting enzyme inhibitor, but an optimal order for starting these three drugs cannot be specified.

Atrial Fibrillation: LANOXIN is indicated for the control of ventricular response rate in patients with chronic atrial fibrillation.

CONTRAINDICATIONS

Digitalis glycosides are contraindicated in patients with ventricular fibrillation or in patients with a known hypersensitivity to digoxin. A hypersensitivity reaction to other digitalis preparations usually constitutes a contraindication to digoxin.

WARNINGS

Sinus Node Disease and AV Block: Because digoxin slows sinoatrial and AV conduction, the drug commonly prolongs the PR interval. The drug may cause severe sinus bradycardia or sinoatrial block in patients with pre-existing sinus node disease and may cause advanced or complete heart block in patients with pre-existing incomplete AV block. In such patients consideration should be given to the insertion of a pacemaker before treatment with digoxin.

Accessory AV Pathway (Wolff-Parkinson-White Syndrome): After intravenous digoxin therapy, some patients with paroxysmal atrial fibrillation or flutter and a coexisting accessory AV pathway have developed increased antegrade conduction across the accessory pathway bypassing the AV node, leading to a very rapid ventricular response or ventricular fibrillation. Unless conduction down the accessory pathway has been blocked (either pharmacologically or by surgery), digoxin should not be used in such patients. The treatment of paroxysmal supraventricular tachycardia in such patients is usually direct-current cardioversion.

Use in Patients with Preserved Left Ventricular Systolic Function: Patients with certain disorders involving heart failure associated with preserved left ventricular ejection fraction may be particularly susceptible to toxicity of the drug. Such disorders include restrictive cardiomyopathy, constrictive pericarditis, amyloid heart disease, and acute cor pulmonale. Patients with idiopathic hypertrophic subaortic stenosis may have worsening of the outflow obstruction due to the inotropic effects of digoxin.

PRECAUTIONS

Use in Patients with Impaired Renal Function: Digoxin is primarily excreted by the kidneys; therefore, patients with impaired renal function require smaller than usual maintenance doses of digoxin (see DOSAGE AND ADMINISTRATION). Because of the prolonged elimination half-life, a longer period of time is required to achieve an initial or new steady-state serum concentration in patients with renal impairment than in patients with normal renal function. If appropriate care is not taken to reduce the dose of digoxin, such patients are at high risk for toxicity, and toxic effects will last longer in such patients than in patients with normal renal function.

Use in Patients with Electrolyte Disorders: In patients with hypokalemia or hypomagnesemia, toxicity may occur despite serum digoxin concentrations below 2.0 ng/mL, because potassium or magnesium depletion sensitizes the myocardium to digoxin. Therefore, it is desirable to maintain normal serum potassium and magnesium concentrations in patients being treated with digoxin. Deficiencies of these electrolytes may result from malnutrition, diarrhea, or prolonged vomiting, as well as the use of the following drugs or procedures: diuretics, amphotericin B, corticosteroids, antacids, dialysis, and mechanical suction of gastrointestinal secretions.

Hypercalcemia from any cause predisposes the patient to digitalis toxicity. Calcium, particularly when administered rapidly by the intravenous route, may produce serious arrhythmias in digitalized patients. On the other hand, hypocalcemia can nullify the effects of digoxin in humans; thus, digoxin may be ineffective until serum calcium is restored to normal. These interactions are related to the fact that digoxin affects contractility and excitability of the heart in a manner similar to that of calcium.

Use in Thyroid Disorders and Hypermetabolic States: Hypothyroidism may reduce the requirements for digoxin. Heart failure and/or atrial arrhythmias resulting from hypermetabolic or hyperdynamic states (e.g., hyperthyroidism, hypoxia, or arteriovenous shunt) are best treated by addressing the underlying condition. Atrial arrhythmias associated with hypermetabolic states are particularly resistant to digoxin treatment. Care must be taken to avoid toxicity if digoxin is used.

Use in Patients with Acute Myocardial Infarction: Digoxin should be used with caution in patients with acute myocardial infarction. The use of inotropic drugs in some patients in this setting may result in undesirable increases in myocardial oxygen demand and ischemia.

Use During Electrical Cardioversion: It may be desirable to reduce the dose of digoxin for 1 to 2 days prior to electrical cardioversion of atrial fibrillation to avoid the induction of ventricular arrhythmias, but physicians must consider the consequences of increasing the ventricular response if digoxin is withdrawn. If digitalis toxicity is suspected, elective cardioversion should be delayed. If it is not prudent to delay cardioversion, the lowest possible energy level should be selected to avoid provoking ventricular arrhythmias.

Laboratory Test Monitoring: Patients receiving digoxin should have their serum electrolytes and renal function (serum creatinine concentrations) assessed periodically; the frequency of assessments will depend on the clinical setting. For discussion of serum digoxin concentrations, see DOSAGE AND ADMINISTRATION section.

Drug Interactions: Potassium-depleting *diuretics* are a major contributing factor to digitalis toxicity. *Calcium*, particularly if administered rapidly by the intravenous route, may produce serious arrhythmias in digitalized patients. *Quinidine, verapamil, amiodarone, propafenone, indomethacin, itraconazole, alprazolam*, and *spironolactone* raise the serum digoxin concentration due to a reduction in clearance and/or in volume of distribution of the drug, with the implication that digitalis intoxication may result. *Erythromycin* and *clarithromycin* (and possibly other *macrolide antibiotics*) and *tetracycline* may increase digoxin absorption in patients who inactivate digoxin by bacterial metabolism in the lower intestine, so that digitalis intoxication may result (see CLINICAL PHARMACOLOGY: Absorption). *Propantheline* and *diphenoxylate*, by decreasing gut motility, may increase digoxin absorption. *Antacids, kaolin-pectin, sulfasalazine, neomycin, cholestyramine*, certain *anticancer drugs*, and *metoclopramide* may interfere with intestinal digoxin absorption, resulting in unexpectedly low serum concentrations. *Rifampin* may decrease serum digoxin concentration, especially in patients with renal dysfunction, by increasing the non-renal clearance of digoxin. There have been inconsistent reports regarding the effects of other drugs [e.g., *quinine, penicillamine*] on serum digoxin concentration. *Thyroid* administration to a digitalized, hypothyroid patient may increase the dose requirement of digoxin. Concomitant use of digoxin and *sympathomimetics* increases the risk of cardiac arrhythmias. *Succinylcholine* may cause a sudden extrusion of potassium from muscle cells, and may thereby cause arrhythmias in digitalized patients. Although beta-adrenergic blockers or calcium channel blockers and digoxin may be useful in combination to control atrial fibrillation, their additive effects on AV node conduction can result in advanced or complete heart block.

Due to the considerable variability of these interactions, the dosage of digoxin should be individualized when patients receive these medications concurrently. Furthermore, caution should be exercised when combining digoxin with any drug that may cause a significant deterioration in renal function, since a decline in glomerular filtration or tubular secretion may impair the excretion of digoxin.

Drug/Laboratory Test Interactions: The use of therapeutic doses of digoxin may cause prolongation of the PR interval and depression of the ST segment on the electrocardiogram. Digoxin may produce false positive ST-T changes on the electrocardiogram during exercise testing. These electrophysiologic effects reflect an expected effect of the drug and are not indicative of toxicity.

Carcinogenesis, Mutagenesis, Impairment of Fertility: There have been no long-term studies performed in animals to evaluate carcinogenic potential, nor have studies been conducted to assess the mutagenic potential of digoxin or its potential to affect fertility.

Pregnancy: ***Teratogenic Effects:*** Pregnancy Category C. Animal reproduction studies have not been conducted with digoxin. It is also not known whether digoxin can cause fetal harm when administered to a pregnant woman or can affect reproductive capacity. Digoxin should be given to a pregnant woman only if clearly needed.

Nursing Mothers: Studies have shown that digoxin concentrations in the mother's serum and milk are similar. However, the estimated exposure of a nursing infant to digoxin via breast feeding will be far below the usual infant maintenance dose. Therefore, this amount should have no pharmacologic effect upon the infant. Nevertheless, caution should be exercised when digoxin is administered to a nursing woman.

Pediatric Use: Newborn infants display considerable variability in their tolerance to digoxin. Premature and immature infants are particularly sensitive to the effects of digoxin, and the dosage of the drug must not only be reduced but must be individualized according to their degree of maturity. Digitalis glycosides can cause poisoning in children due to accidental ingestion.

Continued on next page

This product information is based on labeling in effect on June 23, 2000. For further information, contact via direct mail, phone, or web site. Medical Information, Glaxo Wellcome Inc., PO Box 13398, Research Triangle Park, NC 27709. Healthcare Professionals (Medical Information): 800-334-0089. Patients (Customer Response Center): 1-888-825-5249. Glaxo Wellcome Corporate Web Site: www.glaxowellcome.com

Lanoxin Tablets—Cont.

Table 5: Usual Daily Maintenance Dose Requirements (mcg) of LANOXIN for Estimated Peak Body Stores of 10 mcg/kg

Corrected Ccr (mL/min per 70 kg)*	kg / lb	Lean Body Weight 50 / 110	60 / 132	70 / 154	80 / 176	90 / 198	100 / 220	Number of Days Before Steady State Achieved†
0		62.5‡	125	125	125	187.5	187.5	22
10		125	125	125	187.5	187.5	187.5	19
20		125	125	187.5	187.5	187.5	250	16
30		125	187.5	187.5	187.5	250	250	14
40		125	187.5	187.5	250	250	250	13
50		187.5	187.5	250	250	250	250	12
60		187.5	187.5	250	250	250	375	11
70		187.5	250	250	250	250	375	10
80		187.5	250	250	250	375	375	9
90		187.5	250	250	250	375	500	8
100		250	250	250	375	375	500	7

* Ccr is creatinine clearance, corrected to 70 kg body weight or 1.73 m^2 body surface area. *For adults*, if only serum creatinine concentrations (Scr) are available, a Ccr (corrected to 70 kg body weight) may be estimated in men as (140 - Age)/Scr. For women, this result should be multiplied by 0.85. *Note*: This equation cannot be used for estimating creatinine clearance in infants or children.
† If no loading dose administered.
‡ 62.5 mcg = 0.0625 mg

Geriatric Use: The majority of clinical experience gained with digoxin has been in the elderly population. This experience has not identified differences in response or adverse effects between the elderly and younger patients. However, this drug is known to be substantially excreted by the kidney, and the risk of toxic reactions to this drug may be greater in patients with impaired renal function. Because elderly patients are more likely to have decreased renal function, care should be taken in dose selection, which should be based on renal function, and it may be useful to monitor renal function (see DOSAGE AND ADMINISTRATION).

ADVERSE REACTIONS

In general, the adverse reactions of digoxin are dose-dependent and occur at doses higher than those needed to achieve a therapeutic effect. Hence, adverse reactions are less common when digoxin is used within the recommended dose range or therapeutic serum concentration range and when there is careful attention to concurrent medications and conditions.

Because some patients may be particularly susceptible to side effects with digoxin, the dosage of the drug should always be selected carefully and adjusted as the clinical condition of the patient warrants. In the past, when high doses of digoxin were used and little attention was paid to clinical status or concurrent medications, adverse reactions to digoxin were more frequent and severe. Cardiac adverse reactions accounted for about one-half, gastrointestinal disturbances for about one-fourth, and CNS and other toxicity for about one-fourth of these adverse reactions. However, available evidence suggests that the incidence and severity of digoxin toxicity has decreased substantially in recent years. In recent controlled clinical trials, in patients with predominantly mild to moderate heart failure, the incidence of adverse experiences was comparable in patients taking digoxin and in those taking placebo. In a large mortality trial, the incidence of hospitalization for suspected digoxin toxicity was 2% in patients taking LANOXIN compared to 0.9% in patients taking placebo. In this trial, the most common manifestations of digoxin toxicity included gastrointestinal and cardiac disturbances; CNS manifestations were less common.

Adults: *Cardiac*: Therapeutic doses of digoxin may cause heart block in patients with pre-existing sinoatrial or AV conduction disorders; heart block can be avoided by adjusting the dose of digoxin. Prophylactic use of a cardiac pacemaker may be considered if the risk of heart block is considered unacceptable. High doses of digoxin may produce a variety of rhythm disturbances, such as first-degree, second-degree (Wenckebach), or third-degree heart block (including asystole); atrial tachycardia with block; AV dissociation; accelerated junctional (nodal) rhythm; unifocal or multiform ventricular premature contractions (especially bigeminy or trigeminy); ventricular tachycardia; and ventricular fibrillation. Digoxin produces PR prolongation and ST segment depression which should not by themselves be considered digoxin toxicity. Cardiac toxicity can also occur at therapeutic doses in patients who have conditions which may alter their sensitivity to digoxin (see WARNINGS and PRECAUTIONS).

Gastrointestinal: Digoxin may cause anorexia, nausea, vomiting, and diarrhea. Rarely, the use of digoxin has been associated with abdominal pain, intestinal ischemia, and hemorrhagic necrosis of the intestines.

CNS: Digoxin can produce visual disturbances (blurred or yellow vision), headache, weakness, dizziness, apathy, confusion, and mental disturbances (such as anxiety, depression, delirium, and hallucination).

Other: Gynecomastia has been occasionally observed following the prolonged use of digoxin. Thrombocytopenia and maculopapular rash and other skin reactions have been rarely observed.

The following table summarizes the incidence of those adverse experiences listed above for patients treated with LANOXIN Tablets or placebo from two randomized, double-blind, placebo-controlled withdrawal trials. Patients in these trials were also receiving diuretics with or without angiotensin-converting enzyme inhibitors. These patients had been stable on digoxin, and were randomized to digoxin or placebo. The results shown in Table 4 reflect the experience in patients following dosage titration with the use of serum digoxin concentrations and careful follow-up. These adverse experiences are consistent with results from a large, placebo-controlled mortality trial (DIG trial) wherein over half the patients were not receiving digoxin prior to enrollment.

Table 4: Adverse Experiences In Two Parallel, Double-Blind, Placebo-Controlled Withdrawal Trials (Number of Patients Reporting)

Adverse Experience	Digoxin Patients (n = 123)	Placebo Patients (n = 125)
Cardiac		
Palpitation	1	4
Ventricular extrasystole	1	1
Tachycardia	2	1
Heart arrest	1	1
Gastrointestinal		
Anorexia	1	4
Nausea	4	2
Vomiting	2	1
Diarrhea	4	1
Abdominal pain	0	6
CNS		
Headache	4	4
Dizziness	6	5
Mental disturbances	5	1
Other		
Rash	2	1
Death	4	3

Infants and Children: The side effects of digoxin in infants and children differ from those seen in adults in several respects. Although digoxin may produce anorexia, nausea, vomiting, diarrhea, and CNS disturbances in young patients, these are rarely the initial symptoms of overdosage. Rather, the earliest and most frequent manifestation of excessive dosing with digoxin in infants and children is the appearance of cardiac arrhythmias, including sinus bradycardia. In children, the use of digoxin may produce any arrhythmia. The most common are conduction disturbances or supraventricular tachyarrhythmias, such as atrial tachycardia (with or without block) and junctional (nodal) tachycardia. Ventricular arrhythmias are less common. Sinus bradycardia may be a sign of impending digoxin intoxication, especially in infants, even in the absence of first-degree heart block. Any arrhythmia or alteration in cardiac conduction that develops in a child taking digoxin should be assumed to be caused by digoxin, until further evaluation proves otherwise.

OVERDOSAGE

Treatment of Adverse Reactions Produced by Overdosage: Digoxin should be temporarily discontinued until the adverse reaction resolves. Every effort should also be made to correct factors that may contribute to the adverse reaction (such as electrolyte disturbances or concurrent medications). Once the adverse reaction has resolved, therapy with digoxin may be reinstituted, following a careful reassessment of dose.

Withdrawal of digoxin may be all that is required to treat the adverse reaction. However, when the primary manifestation of digoxin overdosage is a cardiac arrhythmia, additional therapy may be needed.

If the rhythm disturbance is a symptomatic bradyarrhythmia or heart block, consideration should be given to the reversal of toxicity with DIGIBIND® [Digoxin Immune Fab (Ovine)] (see below), the use of atropine, or the insertion of a temporary cardiac pacemaker. However, asymptomatic bradycardia or heart block related to digoxin may require only temporary withdrawal of the drug and cardiac monitoring of the patient.

If the rhythm disturbance is a ventricular arrhythmia, consideration should be given to the correction of electrolyte disorders, particularly if hypokalemia (see below) or hypomagnesemia is present. DIGIBIND is a specific antidote for digoxin and may be used to reverse potentially life-threatening ventricular arrhythmias due to digoxin overdosage.

Administration of Potassium: Every effort should be made to maintain the serum potassium concentration between 4.0 and 5.5 mmol/L. Potassium is usually administered orally, but when correction of the arrhythmia is urgent and the serum potassium concentration is low, potassium may be administered cautiously by the intravenous route. The electrocardiogram should be monitored for any evidence of potassium toxicity (e.g., peaking of T waves) and to observe the effect on the arrhythmia. Potassium salts may be dangerous in patients who manifest bradycardia or heart block due to digoxin (unless primarily related to supraventricular tachycardia) and in the setting of massive digitalis overdosage (see Massive Digitalis Overdosage subsection).

Massive Digitalis Overdosage: Manifestations of life-threatening toxicity include ventricular tachycardia or ventricular fibrillation, or progressive bradyarrhythmias, or heart block. The administration of more than 10 mg of digoxin in a previously healthy adult, or more than 4 mg in a previously healthy child, or a steady-state serum concentration greater than 10 ng/mL often results in cardiac arrest.

DIGIBIND should be used to reverse the toxic effects of ingestion of a massive overdose. The decision to administer DIGIBIND to a patient who has ingested a massive dose of digoxin but who has not yet manifested life-threatening toxicity should depend on the likelihood that life-threatening toxicity will occur (see above).

Patients with massive digitalis ingestion should receive large doses of activated charcoal to prevent absorption and bind digoxin in the gut during enteroenteric recirculation. Emesis or gastric lavage may be indicated especially if ingestion has occurred within 30 minutes of the patient's presentation at the hospital. Emesis should not be induced in patients who are obtunded. If a patient presents more than 2 hours after ingestion or already has toxic manifestations, it may be unsafe to induce vomiting or attempt passage of a gastric tube, because such maneuvers may induce an acute vagal episode that can worsen digitalis-related arrhythmias.

Severe digitalis intoxication can cause a massive shift of potassium from inside to outside the cell, leading to life-threatening hyperkalemia. The administration of potassium supplements in the setting of massive intoxication may be hazardous and should be avoided. Hyperkalemia caused by massive digitalis toxicity is best treated with DIGIBIND; initial treatment with glucose and insulin may also be required if hyperkalemia itself is acutely life-threatening.

DOSAGE AND ADMINISTRATION

General: Recommended dosages of digoxin may require considerable modification because of individual sensitivity of the patient to the drug, the presence of associated conditions, or the use of concurrent medications. In selecting a dose of digoxin, the following factors must be considered:

1. The body weight of the patient. Doses should be calculated based upon lean (i.e., ideal) body weight.
2. The patient's renal function, preferably evaluated on the basis of estimated creatinine clearance.
3. The patient's age. Infants and children require different doses of digoxin than adults. Also, advanced age may be indicative of diminished renal function even in patients with normal serum creatinine concentration (i.e., below 1.5 mg/dL).
4. Concomitant disease states, concurrent medications, or other factors likely to alter the pharmacokinetic or pharmacodynamic profile of digoxin (see PRECAUTIONS).

Serum Digoxin Concentrations: In general, the dose of digoxin used should be determined on clinical grounds. However, measurement of serum digoxin concentrations can be helpful to the clinician in determining the adequacy of digoxin therapy and in assigning certain probabilities to the likelihood of digoxin intoxication. About two-thirds of adults considered adequately digitalized (without evidence of toxicity) have serum digoxin concentrations ranging from 0.8 to 2.0 ng/mL. However, digoxin may produce clinical benefits even at serum concentrations below this range. About two-thirds of adult patients with clinical toxicity have serum digoxin concentrations greater than 2.0 ng/mL. However, since one-third of patients with clinical toxicity have concentrations less than 2.0 ng/mL, values below 2.0 ng/mL do not rule out the possibility that a certain sign or symptom is related to digoxin therapy. Rarely, there are patients who are unable to tolerate digoxin at serum concentrations below 0.8 ng/mL. Consequently, the serum concentration of digoxin should always be interpreted in the overall clinical context, and an isolated measurement should not be used alone as the basis for increasing or decreasing the dose of the drug.

To allow adequate time for equilibration of digoxin between serum and tissue, sampling of serum concentrations should be done just before the next scheduled dose of the drug. If this is not possible, sampling should be done at least 6 to 8 hours after the last dose, regardless of the route of administration or the formulation used. On a once-daily dosing schedule, the concentration of digoxin will be 10% to 25% lower when sampled at 24 versus 8 hours, depending upon the patient's renal function. On a twice-daily dosing schedule, there will be only minor differences in serum digoxin concentrations whether sampling is done at 8 or 12 hours after a dose.

If a discrepancy exists between the reported serum concentration and the observed clinical response, the clinician should consider the following possibilities:

1. Analytical problems in the assay procedure.
2. Inappropriate serum sampling time.
3. Administration of a digitalis glycoside other than digoxin.
4. Conditions (described in WARNINGS and PRECAUTIONS) causing an alteration in the sensitivity of the patient to digoxin.
5. Serum digoxin concentration may decrease acutely during periods of exercise without any associated change in clinical efficacy due to increased binding of digoxin to skeletal muscle.

Heart Failure: *Adults*: Digitalization may be accomplished by either of two general approaches that vary in dosage and frequency of administration, but reach the same endpoint in terms of total amount of digoxin accumulated in the body.

1. If rapid digitalization is considered medically appropriate, it may be achieved by administering a loading dose based upon projected peak digoxin body stores. Maintenance dose can be calculated as a percentage of the loading dose.
2. More gradual digitalization may be obtained by beginning an appropriate maintenance dose, thus allowing digoxin body stores to accumulate slowly. Steady-state serum digoxin concentrations will be achieved in approximately five half-lives of the drug for the individual patient. Depending upon the patient's renal function, this will take between 1 and 3 weeks.

***Rapid Digitalization with a Loading Dose*:** Peak digoxin body stores of 8 to 12 mcg/kg should provide therapeutic effect with minimum risk of toxicity in most patients with heart failure and normal sinus rhythm. Because of altered digoxin distribution and elimination, projected peak body stores for patients with renal insufficiency should be conservative (i.e., 6 to 10 mcg/kg) [see PRECAUTIONS].

The loading dose should be administered in several portions, with roughly half the total given as the first dose. Additional fractions of this planned total dose may be given at 6- to 8-hour intervals, **with careful assessment of clinical response before each additional dose.** If the patient's clinical response necessitates a change from the calculated loading dose of digoxin, then calculation of the maintenance dose should be based upon the amount actually given.

A single initial dose of 500 to 750 mcg (0.5 to 0.75 mg) of LANOXIN Tablets usually produces a detectable effect in 0.5 to 2 hours that becomes maximal in 2 to 6 hours. Additional doses of 125 to 375 mcg (0.125 to 0.375 mg) may be given cautiously at 6- to 8-hour intervals until clinical evidence of an adequate effect is noted. The usual amount of LANOXIN Tablets that a 70-kg patient requires to achieve 8 to 12 mcg/kg peak body stores is 750 to 1250 mcg (0.75 to 1.25 mg).

LANOXIN Injection is frequently used to achieve rapid digitalization, with conversion to LANOXIN Tablets or LANOXICAPS for maintenance therapy. If patients are switched from intravenous to oral digoxin formulations, allowances must be made for differences in bioavailability when calculating maintenance dosages (see table, CLINICAL PHARMACOLOGY).

***Maintenance Dosing*:** The doses of digoxin used in controlled trials in patients with heart failure have ranged from 125 to 500 mcg (0.125 to 0.5 mg) once daily. In these studies, the digoxin dose has been generally titrated according to the patient's age, lean body weight, and renal function. Therapy is generally initiated at a dose of 250 mcg (0.25 mg) once daily in patients under age 70 with good renal function, at a dose of 125 mcg (0.125 mg) once daily in patients over age 70 or with impaired renal function, and at a dose of 62.5 mcg (0.0625 mg) in patients with marked renal impairment. Doses may be increased every 2 weeks according to clinical response.

In a subset of approximately 1800 patients enrolled in the DIG trial (wherein dosing was based on an algorithm similar to that in Table 5) the mean (± SD) serum digoxin concentrations at 1 month and 12 months were 1.01 ± 0.47 ng/mL and 0.97 ± 0.43 ng/mL, respectively.

The maintenance dose should be based upon the percentage of the peak body stores lost each day through elimination. The following formula has had wide clinical use:

Maintenance Dose = Peak Body Stores
(i.e., Loading Dose) × % Daily Loss/100

Where: % Daily Loss = 14 + Ccr/5

(Ccr is creatinine clearance, corrected to 70 kg body weight or 1.73 m^2 body surface area.)

Table 5 provides average daily maintenance dose requirements of LANOXIN Tablets for patients with heart failure based upon lean body weight and renal function:

[See table 5 at top of previous page]

Example: Based on Table 5, a patient in heart failure with an estimated lean body weight of 70 kg and a Ccr of 60 mL/min should be given a dose of 250 mcg (0.25 mg) daily of LANOXIN Tablets, usually taken after the morning meal. If no loading dose is administered, steady-state serum concentrations in this patient should be anticipated at approximately 11 days.

Infants and Children: In general, divided daily dosing is recommended for infants and young children (under age 10). In the newborn period, renal clearance of digoxin is diminished and suitable dosage adjustments must be observed. This is especially pronounced in the premature infant. Beyond the immediate newborn period, children generally require proportionally larger doses than adults on the basis of body weight or body surface area. Children over 10 years of age require adult dosages in proportion to their body weight. Some researchers have suggested that infants and young children tolerate slightly higher serum concentrations than do adults.

Daily maintenance doses for each age group are given in Table 6 and should provide therapeutic effects with minimum risk of toxicity in most patients with heart failure and normal sinus rhythm. These recommendations assume the presence of normal renal function:

Table 6: Daily Maintenance Doses in Children with Normal Renal Function

Age	Daily Maintenance Dose (mcg/kg)
2 to 5 Years	10 to 15
5 to 10 Years	7 to 10
Over 10 Years	3 to 5

In children with renal disease, digoxin must be carefully titrated based upon clinical response.

It cannot be overemphasized that both the adult and pediatric dosage guidelines provided are based upon average patient response and substantial individual variation can be expected. Accordingly, ultimate dosage selection must be based upon clinical assessment of the patient.

Atrial Fibrillation: Peak digoxin body stores larger than the 8 to 12 mcg/kg required for most patients with heart failure and normal sinus rhythm have been used for control of ventricular rate in patients with atrial fibrillation. Doses of digoxin used for the treatment of chronic atrial fibrillation should be titrated to the minimum dose that achieves the desired ventricular rate control without causing undesirable side effects. Data are not available to establish the appropriate resting or exercise target rates that should be achieved.

Dosage Adjustment When Changing Preparations: The difference in bioavailability between LANOXIN Injection or LANOXICAPS and LANOXIN Elixir Pediatric or LANOXIN Tablets must be considered when changing patients from one dosage form to another.

Doses of 100 mcg (0.1 mg) and 200 mcg (0.2 mg) of LANOXICAPS are approximately equivalent to 125-mcg (0.125-mg) and 250-mcg (0.25-mg) doses of LANOXIN Tablets and Elixir Pediatric, respectively (see table in CLINICAL PHARMACOLOGY: Pharmacokinetics).

HOW SUPPLIED

LANOXIN (digoxin) Tablets, Scored 125 mcg (0.125 mg): Bottles of 100 with child-resistant cap (NDC 0173-0242-55) and 1000 (NDC 0173-0242-75); unit dose pack of 100 (NDC 0173-0242-56). Imprinted with LANOXIN and Y3B (yellow).

Store at 25°C (77°F); excursions permitted to 15° to 30°C (59° to 86°F) [see USP Controlled Room Temperature] in a dry place and protect from light.

LANOXIN (digoxin) Tablets, Scored 250 mcg (0.25 mg): Bottles of 100 with child-resistant cap (NDC 0173-0249-55), 1000 (NDC 0173-0249-75), and 5000 (NDC 0173-0249-80); carton of 12 bottles of 100 (NDC 0173-0249-01); unit dose pack of 100 (NDC 0173-0249-56). Imprinted with LANOXIN and X3A (white).

Store at 25°C (77°F); excursions permitted to 15° to 30°C (59° to 86°F) [see USP Controlled Room Temperature] in a dry place.

Glaxo Wellcome Inc., Research Triangle Park, NC 27709

November 1998/RL-621

Shown in Product Identification Guide, page 315

LEUKERAN® ℞

[lū 'kŭh-răn]
(chlorambucil)
2-mg Sugar-coated Tablets

WARNING: LEUKERAN (chlorambucil) can severely suppress bone marrow function. Chlorambucil is a carcinogen in humans. Chlorambucil is probably mutagenic and teratogenic in humans. Chlorambucil produces human infertility (see WARNINGS and PRECAUTIONS).

DESCRIPTION

LEUKERAN (chlorambucil) was first synthesized by Everett et al.[1] It is a bifunctional alkylating agent of the nitrogen mustard type that has been found active against selected human neoplastic diseases. Chlorambucil is known chemically as 4-[bis(2-chlorethyl)amino]benzenebutanoic acid.

Chlorambucil hydrolyzes in water and has a pKa of 5.8.

LEUKERAN (chlorambucil) is available in tablet form for oral administration. Each sugar-coated tablet contains 2 mg chlorambucil and the inactive ingredients acacia, corn and wheat starch, lactose, magnesium stearate, pharmaceutical glaze, polysorbate 60, sucrose, and talc. Printed with edible black ink.

CLINICAL PHARMACOLOGY

Chlorambucil is rapidly and completely absorbed from the gastrointestinal tract. After single oral doses of 0.6 to 1.2 mg/kg, peak plasma chlorambucil levels are reached within 1 hour and the terminal half-life of the parent drug is estimated at 1.5 hours. Chlorambucil undergoes rapid metabolism to phenylacetic acid mustard, the major metabolite, and the combined chlorambucil and phenylacetic acid mustard urinary excretion is extremely low—less than 1% in 24 hours. The peak plasma levels of chlorambucil and phenylacetic acid mustard are similar, approximating 1 mcg/mL; however, the metabolite's half-life is 1.6 times greater than that of the parent drug.[2,3]

Chlorambucil and its metabolites are extensively bound to plasma and tissue proteins. In vitro, chlorambucil is 99% bound to plasma proteins, specifically albumin.[4] Cerebrospinal fluid levels of chlorambucil have not been determined. Evidence of human teratogenicity suggests that the drug crosses the placenta.[5,6]

Chlorambucil is extensively metabolized in the liver primarily to phenylacetic acid mustard which has antineoplastic activity.[2,3] Chlorambucil and its major metabolite spontaneously degrade in vivo forming monohydroxy and dihydroxy derivatives.[2] After a single dose of radiolabeled chlorambucil (^{14}C), approximately 15% to 60% of the radioactivity appears in the urine after 24 hours. Again, less than 1% of the urinary radioactivity is in the form of chlorambucil or phenylacetic acid mustard.[2] In summary, the pharmacokinetic data suggest that oral chlorambucil undergoes rapid gastrointestinal absorption and plasma clearance and that it is almost completely metabolized, having extremely low urinary excretion.

INDICATIONS AND USAGE

LEUKERAN (chlorambucil) is indicated in the treatment of chronic lymphatic (lymphocytic) leukemia, malignant lymphomas including lymphosarcoma, giant follicular lymphoma, and Hodgkin's disease. It is not curative in any of these disorders but may produce clinically useful palliation.

CONTRAINDICATIONS

Chlorambucil should not be used in patients whose disease has demonstrated a prior resistance to the agent. Patients who have demonstrated hypersensitivity to chlorambucil should not be given the drug.[7–9] There may be cross-hypersensitivity (skin rash) between chlorambucil and other alkylating agents.[10]

WARNINGS

Because of its carcinogenic properties, chlorambucil should not be given to patients with conditions other than chronic lymphatic leukemia or malignant lymphomas. Convulsions,[11] infertility,[12] leukemia[13,14] and secondary malignancies[15] have been observed when chlorambucil was employed in the therapy of malignant and non-malignant diseases.

There are many reports of acute leukemia arising in patients with both malignant[16] and non-malignant[17] diseases following chlorambucil treatment. In many instances, these patients also received other chemotherapeutic agents or some form of radiation therapy. The quantitation of the risk of chlorambucil-induction of leukemia or carcinoma in humans is not possible. Evaluation of published reports of leukemia developing in patients who have received chlorambucil (and other alkylating agents) suggests that the risk of leukemogenesis increases with both chronicity of treatment and large cumulative doses. However, it has proved impossible to define a cumulative dose below which there is no risk of the induction of secondary malignancy. The potential benefits from chlorambucil therapy must be weighed on an individual basis against the possible risk of the induction of a secondary malignancy.

Chlorambucil has been shown to cause chromatid or chromosome damage in humans.[18,19] Both reversible and permanent sterility have been observed in both sexes receiving chlorambucil.

A high incidence of sterility has been documented when chlorambucil is administered to prepubertal and pubertal males.[20] Prolonged or permanent azoospermia has also been observed in adult males.[21] While most reports of gonadal dysfunction secondary to chlorambucil have related to males, the induction of amenorrhea in females with alkylating agents is well documented, and chlorambucil is capable of producing amenorrhea. Autopsy studies of the ovaries from women with malignant lymphoma treated with combination chemotherapy including chlorambucil have shown varying degrees of fibrosis, vasculitis, and depletion of primordial follicles.[22,23]

Rare instances of skin rash progressing to erythema multiforme, toxic epidermal necrolysis, or Stevens-Johnson syn-

Continued on next page

Leukeran—Cont.

drome have been reported.[8,9] Chlorambucil should be discontinued promptly in patients who develop skin reactions.

Pregnancy: Pregnancy Category D. Chlorambucil can cause fetal harm when administered to a pregnant woman. Unilateral renal agenesis has been observed in two offspring whose mothers received chlorambucil during the first trimester.[5,6] Urogenital malformations, including absence of a kidney, were found in fetuses of rats given chlorambucil.[24] There are no adequate and well-controlled studies in pregnant women. If this drug is used during pregnancy, or if the patient becomes pregnant while taking this drug, the patient should be apprised of the potential hazard to the fetus. Women of childbearing potential should be advised to avoid becoming pregnant.

PRECAUTIONS

General: Many patients develop a slowly progressive lymphopenia during treatment. The lymphocyte count usually rapidly returns to normal levels upon completion of drug therapy. Most patients have some neutropenia after the third week of treatment and this may continue for up to 10 days after the last dose. Subsequently, the neutrophil count usually rapidly returns to normal. Severe neutropenia appears to be related to dosage and usually occurs only in patients who have received a total dosage of 6.5 mg/kg or more in one course of therapy with continuous dosing. About one quarter of all patients receiving the continuous-dose schedule, and one third of those receiving this dosage in 8 weeks or less may be expected to develop severe neutropenia.[25]

While it is not necessary to discontinue chlorambucil at the first evidence of a fall in neutrophil count, it must be remembered that the fall may continue for 10 days after the last dose, and that as the total dose approaches 6.5 mg/kg, there is a risk of causing irreversible bone marrow damage. The dose of chlorambucil should be decreased if leukocyte or platelet counts fall below normal values and should be discontinued for more severe depression.

Chlorambucil should **not** be given at full dosages before 4 weeks after a full course of radiation therapy or chemotherapy because of the vulnerability of the bone marrow to damage under these conditions. If the pretherapy leukocyte or platelet counts are depressed from bone marrow disease process prior to institution of therapy, the treatment should be instituted at a reduced dosage.

Persistently low neutrophil and platelet counts or peripheral lymphocytosis suggest bone marrow infiltration. If confirmed by bone marrow examination, the daily dosage of chlorambucil should not exceed 0.1 mg/kg. Chlorambucil appears to be relatively free from gastrointestinal side effects or other evidence of toxicity apart from the bone marrow depressant action. In humans, single oral doses of 20 mg or more may produce nausea and vomiting.

Children with nephrotic syndrome[11] and patients receiving high pulse doses of chlorambucil[26] may have an increased risk of seizures. As with any potentially epileptogenic drug, caution should be exercised when administering chlorambucil to patients with a history of seizure disorder, or head trauma, or who are receiving other potentially epileptogenic drugs.

Information for Patients: Patients should be informed that the major toxicities of chlorambucil are related to hypersensitivity, drug fever, myelosuppression, hepatotoxicity, infertility, seizures, gastrointestinal toxicity, and secondary malignancies. Patients should never be allowed to take the drug without medical supervision and should consult their physician if they experience skin rash, bleeding, fever, jaundice, persistent cough, seizures, nausea, vomiting, amenorrhea, or unusual lumps/masses. Women of childbearing potential should be advised to avoid becoming pregnant.

Laboratory Tests: Patients must be followed carefully to avoid life-endangering damage to the bone marrow during treatment. Weekly examination of the blood should be made to determine hemoglobin levels, total and differential leukocyte counts, and quantitative platelet counts. Also, during the first 3 to 6 weeks of therapy, it is recommended that white blood cell counts be made 3 or 4 days after each of the weekly complete blood counts. Galton et al[25] have suggested that in following patients it is helpful to plot the blood counts on a chart at the same time that body weight, temperature, spleen size, etc., are recorded. It is considered dangerous to allow a patient to go more than 2 weeks without hematological and clinical examination during treatment.

Drug Interactions: There are no known drug/drug interactions with chlorambucil.

Carcinogenesis, Mutagenesis, Impairment of Fertility: See WARNINGS section for information on carcinogenesis, mutagenesis, and impairment of fertility.

Pregnancy: ***Teratogenic Effects:*** Pregnancy Category D: See WARNINGS section.

Nursing Mothers: It is not known whether this drug is excreted in human milk. Because many drugs are excreted in human milk and because of the potential for serious adverse reactions in nursing infants from chlorambucil, a decision should be made whether to discontinue nursing or to discontinue the drug, taking into account the importance of the drug to the mother.

Pediatric Use: The safety and effectiveness in pediatric patients have not been established.

ADVERSE REACTIONS

Hematologic: The most common side effect is bone marrow suppression.[27] Although bone marrow suppression frequently occurs, it is usually reversible if the chlorambucil is withdrawn early enough. However, irreversible bone marrow failure has been reported.[28,29]

Gastrointestinal: Gastrointestinal disturbances such as nausea and vomiting, diarrhea, and oral ulceration occur infrequently.

CNS: Tremors, muscular twitching, confusion, agitation, ataxia, flaccid paresis, and hallucinations have been reported as rare adverse experiences to chlorambucil which resolve upon discontinuation of drug. Rare, focal and/or generalized seizures have been reported to occur in both children[11,30,31] and adults[26,32–35] at both therapeutic daily doses and pulse-dosing regimens, and in acute overdose (see PRECAUTIONS: General).

Dermatologic: Skin hypersensitivity (including rare reports of skin rash progressing to erythema multiforme,[9] toxic epidermal necrolysis,[8] and Stevens-Johnson syndrome) has been reported (see WARNINGS).

Miscellaneous: Other reported adverse reactions include: pulmonary fibrosis, hepatotoxicity and jaundice, drug fever, peripheral neuropathy, interstitial pneumonia, sterile cystitis, infertility, leukemia, and secondary malignancies (see WARNINGS).

OVERDOSAGE

Reversible pancytopenia was the main finding of inadvertent overdoses of chlorambucil.[36,37] Neurological toxicity ranging from agitated behavior and ataxia to multiple grand mal seizures has also occurred.[30,36] As there is no known antidote, the blood picture should be closely monitored and general supportive measures should be instituted, together with appropriate blood transfusions, if necessary. Chlorambucil is not dialyzable.

Oral LD_{50} single doses in mice are 123 mg/kg. In rats, a single intraperitoneal dose of 12.5 mg/kg of chlorambucil produces typical nitrogen-mustard effects; these include atrophy of the intestinal mucous membrane and lymphoid tissues, severe lymphopenia becoming maximal in 4 days, anemia, and thrombocytopenia. After this dose, the animals begin to recover within 3 days and appear normal in about a week, although the bone marrow may not become completely normal for about 3 weeks. An intraperitoneal dose of 18.5 mg/kg kills about 50% of the rats with development of convulsions. As much as 50 mg/kg has been given orally to rats as a single dose, with recovery. Such a dose causes bradycardia, excessive salivation, hematuria, convulsions, and respiratory dysfunction.

DOSAGE AND ADMINISTRATION

The usual oral dosage is 0.1 to 0.2 mg/kg body weight daily for 3 to 6 weeks as required. This usually amounts to 4 to 10 mg per day for the average patient. The entire daily dose may be given at one time. These dosages are for initiation of therapy or for short courses of treatment. The dosage must be carefully adjusted according to the response of the patient and must be reduced as soon as there is an abrupt fall in the white blood cell count. Patients with Hodgkin's disease usually require 0.2 mg/kg daily, whereas patients with other lymphomas or chronic lymphocytic leukemia usually require only 0.1 mg/kg daily. When lymphocytic infiltration of the bone marrow is present, or when the bone marrow is hypoplastic, the daily dose should not exceed 0.1 mg/kg (about 6 mg for the average patient).

Alternate schedules for the treatment of chronic lymphocytic leukemia employing intermittent, biweekly, or once-monthly pulse doses of chlorambucil have been reported.[38,39] Intermittent schedules of chlorambucil begin with an initial single dose of 0.4 mg/kg. Doses are generally increased by 0.1 mg/kg until control of lymphocytosis or toxicity is observed. Subsequent doses are modified to produce mild hematologic toxicity. It is felt that the response rate of chronic lymphocytic leukemia to the biweekly or once-monthly schedule of chlorambucil administration is similar or better to that previously reported with daily administration and that hematologic toxicity was less than or equal to that encountered in studies using daily chlorambucil.

Radiation and cytotoxic drugs render the bone marrow more vulnerable to damage, and chlorambucil should be used with particular caution within 4 weeks of a full course of radiation therapy or chemotherapy. However, small doses of palliative radiation over isolated foci remote from the bone marrow will not usually depress the neutrophil and platelet count. In these cases chlorambucil may be given in the customary dosage.

It is presently felt that short courses of treatment are safer than continuous maintenance therapy, although both methods have been effective. It must be recognized that continuous therapy may give the appearance of "maintenance" in patients who are actually in remission and have no immediate need for further drug. If maintenance dosage is used, it should not exceed 0.1 mg/kg daily and may well be as low as 0.03 mg/kg daily. A typical maintenance dose is 2 mg to 4 mg daily, or less, depending on the status of the blood counts. It may, therefore, be desirable to withdraw the drug after maximal control has been achieved, since intermittent therapy reinstituted at time of relapse may be as effective as continuous treatment.

Procedures for proper handling and disposal of anticancer drugs should be considered. Several guidelines on this subject have been published.[40–46]

There is no general agreement that all of the procedures recommended in the guidelines are necessary or appropriate.

HOW SUPPLIED

White sugar-coated tablet containing 2 mg chlorambucil and printed with "635"; bottle of 50 (NDC 0173-0635-35).
Store at 15° to 25°C (59° to 77°F) in a dry place.

REFERENCES

1. Everett JL, Roberts JJ, Ross WCJ. Aryl-2-halogenoalkylamines. Pt. XII. Some carboxylic derivatives of NN-Di-2-chloroethylaniline. *J Chem Soc.* 1953;3:2386–2392.
2. Alberts DS, Chang SY, Chen H-SG, Larcom BJ, Jones SE. Pharmacokinetics and metabolism of chlorambucil in man. *Cancer Treat Rev.* 1979;6 (suppl):9–17.
3. McLean A, Woods RL, Catovsky D, Farmer P. Pharmacokinetics and metabolism of chlorambucil in patients with malignant disease. *Cancer Treat Rev.* 1979;6(suppl):33–42.
4. Ehrsson H, Lönroth U, Wallin I, Ehrnebo M, Nilsson SO. Degradation of chlorambucil in aqueous solution: influence of human albumin binding. *J Pharm Pharmacol.* 1981;33:313–315. Communications.
5. Shotton D, Monie IW. Possible teratogenic effect of chlorambucil on a human fetus. *JAMA.* 1963;186:74–75.
6. Steege JF, Caldwell DS. Renal agenesis after first trimester exposure to chlorambucil. *South Med J.* 1980;73:1414–1415.
7. Knisley RE, Settipane GA, Albala MM. Unusual reaction to chlorambucil in a patient with chronic lymphocytic leukemia. *Arch Dermatol.* 1971;104:77–79.
8. Pietrantonio F, Moriconi L, Torino F, Romano A, Gangovich A. Unusual reaction to chlorambucil: a case report. *Cancer Lett.* 1990;54:109–111.
9. Hitchins RN, Hocker GA, Thomson DB. Chlorambucil allergy—a series of three cases. *Aust NZ J Med.* 1987;17:600–602.
10. Weiss RB, Bruno S. Hypersensitivity reactions to cancer chemotherapeutic agents. *Ann Intern Med.* 1981; 94:66–72.
11. Williams SA, Makker SP, Grupe WE. Seizures: a significant side effect of chlorambucil therapy in children. *J Pediatr.* 1978;93:516–518.
12. Freckman HA, Fry HL, Mendez FL, Maurer ER. Chlorambucil-prednisolone therapy for disseminated breast carcinoma. *JAMA.* 1964;189:23–26.
13. Aymard JP, Frustin J, Witz F, Colomb JN, Lederlin P, Herbeuval R. Acute leukemia after prolonged chlorambucil treatment for non-malignant disease: a report of a new case and literature survey. *Acta Haematol (Basel).* 1980;63:283–285.
14. Berk PD, Goldberg JD, Silverstein MN, et al. Increased incidence of acute leukemia in polycythemia vera associated with chlorambucil therapy. *N Engl J Med.* 1981;304:441–447.
15. Lerner HJ. Acute myelogenous leukemia in patients receiving chlorambucil as long-term adjuvant chemotherapy for stage II breast cancer. *Cancer Treat Rep.* 1978;62:1135–1138.
16. Zarrabi MH, Grünwald HW, Rosner F. Chronic lymphocytic leukemia terminating in acute leukemia. *Arch Intern Med.* 1977;137:1059–1064.
17. Cameron S. Chlorambucil and leukemia. *N Eng J Med.* 1977;296:1065.
18. Lawler SD, Lele KP. Chromosomal damage induced by chlorambucil in chronic lymphocytic leukemia. *Scand J Haematol.* 1972;9:603–612.
19. Stevenson AC, Patel C. Effects of chlorambucil on human chromosomes. *Mutat Res.* 1973;18:333–351.
20. Guesry P, Lenoir G, Broyer M. Gonadal effects of chlorambucil given to prepubertal and pubertal boys for nephrotic syndrome. *J Pediatr.* 1978;92:299–303.
21. Richter P, Calamera JC, Morgenfeld MC, Kierszenbaum AL, Lavieri JC, Mancini RE. Effect of chlorambucil on spermatogenesis in the human with malignant lymphoma. *Cancer.* 1970;25:1026–1030.
22. Morgenfeld MC, Goldberg V, Parisier H, Bugnard SC, Bur GE. Ovarian lesions due to cytostatic agents during the treatment of Hodgkin's disease. *Surg Gynecol Obstet.* 1972;134:826–828.
23. Sobrinho LG, Levine RA, DeConti RC. Amenorrhea in patients with Hodgkin's disease treated with antineoplastic agents. *Am J Obstet Gynecol.* 1971;109:135–139.
24. Monie IW. Chlorambucil-induced abnormalities of the urogenital system of rat fetuses. *Anat Rec.* 1961;139:145–153.
25. Galton DAG, Israels LG, Nabarro JDN, Till M. Clinical trials of p-(DI-2-chloroethylamino)-phenylbutyric acid (CB 1348) in malignant lymphoma. *Br Med J.* 1955;2:1172–1176.
26. Ciobanu N, Runowicz C, Gucalp R, et al. Reversible central nervous system toxicity associated with high-dose chlorambucil in autologous bone marrow transplantation for ovarian carcinoma. *Cancer Treat Rep.* 1987;71:1324–1325.
27. Moore GE, Bross ID, Ausman R, et al. Effects of chlorambucil (NSC-3088) in 374 patients with advanced cancer. Eastern Clinical Drug Evaluation Program. *Cancer Chemother Rep.* 1968;52(pt 1):661–666.
28. Galton DA, Wiltshaw E, Szur L, Dacie JV. The use of chlorambucil and steroids in the treatment of chronic lymphocytic leukemia. *Br J Haematol.* 1961;7:73–98.

29. Rudd P, Fries JF, Epstein WV. Irreversible bone marrow failure with chlorambucil. *J Rheumatol.* 1975;2:421–429.
30. Wolfson S, Olney MB. Accidental ingestion of a toxic dose of chlorambucil: report of a case in a child. *JAMA.* 1957;165:239–240.
31. Byrne TN, Moseley TAE, Finer MA. Myoclonic seizures following chlorambucil overdose. *Ann Neurol.* 1981;9: 191–194.
32. LaDelfa I, Bayer N, Myers R, Hoffstein V. Chlorambucil-induced myoclonic seizures in an adult. *J Clin Oncol.* 1985;3:1691–1692.
33. Naysmith A, Robson RH: Focal fits during chlorambucil therapy. *Postgrad Med J.* 1979;55:806–807.
34. Blank DW, Nanji AA, Schreiber DH, Hudman C, Sanders HD. Acute renal failure and seizures associated with chlorambucil overdose. *J Toxicol Clin Toxicol.* 1983;20: 361–365.
35. Ammenti A, Reitter B, Muller-Wiefel DE. Chlorambucil neurotoxicity: report of two cases. *Helv Paediatr Acta.* 1980;35:281–287.
36. Green AA, Naiman JL. Chlorambucil poisoning. *Am J Dis Child.* 1968;116:190–191.
37. Enck RE, Bennett JM. Inadvertent chlorambucil overdose in adults. *NY State J Med.* 1977;77:1480–1481.
38. Knospe WH, Loeb V Jr, Huguley CM. Bi-weekly chlorambucil treatment of chronic lymphocytic leukemia. *Cancer.* 1974;33:555–562.
39. Sawitsky A, Rai KR, Glidewell O, et al. Comparison of daily versus intermittent chlorambucil and prednisone therapy in the treatment of patients with chronic lymphocytic leukemia. *Blood.* 1977;50:1049–1059.
40. Recommendations for the safe handling of parenteral antineoplastic drugs. Washington, DC: Division of Safety; National Institutes of Health; 1983. US Dept of Health and Human Services, Public Health Service publication NIH 83-2621.
41. AMA Council on Scientific Affairs. Guidelines for handling parenteral antineoplastics. *JAMA.* 1985;253:1590–1591.
42. National Study Commission on Cytotoxic Exposure. Recommendations for handling cytotoxic agents. 1987. Available from Louis P. Jeffrey, Chairman, National Study Commission on Cytotoxic Exposure. Massachusetts College of Pharmacy and Allied Health Sciences, 179 Longwood Avenue, Boston, MA, 02115.
43. Clinical Oncological Society of Australia. Guidelines and recommendations for safe handling of antineoplastic agents. *Med J Australia.* 1983;1:426–428.
44. Jones RB, Frank R, Mass T. Safe handling of chemotherapeutic agents: a report from the Mount Sinai Medical Center. *CA-A Cancer J for Clin.* 1983;33:258–263.
45. American Society of Hospital Pharmacists. ASHP technical assistance bulletin on handling cytotoxic and hazardous drugs. *Am J Hosp Pharm.* 1990;47:1033–1049.
46. Yodaiken RE, Bennett D. OSHA work-practice guidelines for personnel dealing with cytotoxic (antineoplastic) drugs. *Am J Hosp Pharm.* 1986;43:1193–1204.

Manufactured by Catalytica Pharmaceuticals, Inc.
Greenville, NC 27834
for Glaxo Wellcome Inc., Research Triangle Park, NC 27709

September 1997/RL-468

Shown in Product Identification Guide, page 315

LOTRONEX® ℞
[*lō' trə-nex*]
(alosetron hydrochloride)
Tablets

DESCRIPTION

The active ingredient in LOTRONEX Tablets is alosetron hydrochloride (HCl), a potent and selective antagonist of the serotonin 5-HT3 receptor type. Chemically, alosetron is designated as 2,3,4,5-tetrahydro-5-methyl-2-[(5-methyl-1H-imidazol-4-yl)methyl]-1H-pyrido[4,3-b]indol-1-one, monohydrochloride. Alosetron is achiral and has the empirical formula: $C_{17}H_{18}N_4O \bullet HCl$, representing a molecular weight of 330.8. Alosetron is a white to beige solid that has a solubility of 61 mg/mL in water, 42 mg/mL in 0.1M hydrochloric acid, 0.3 mg/mL in pH 6 phosphate buffer, and <0.1 mg/mL in pH 8 phosphate buffer. The chemical structure of alosetron is:

LOTRONEX Tablets for oral administration contain 1.124 mg alosetron HCl equivalent to 1 mg of alosetron. Each tablet also contains the inactive ingredients, lactose (anhydrous), magnesium stearate, microcrystalline cellulose, and pregelatinized starch. The blue film-coat contains hydroxypropyl methylcellulose, titanium dioxide, triacetin, and indigo carmine.

CLINICAL PHARMACOLOGY

Pharmacodynamics: ***Mechanism of Action:*** Alosetron is a potent and selective 5-HT3 receptor antagonist. 5-HT3 receptors are nonselective cation channels that are extensively distributed on enteric neurons in the human gastrointestinal tract, as well as other peripheral and central locations. Activation of these channels and the resulting neuronal depolarization affect the regulation of visceral pain, colonic transit and gastrointestinal secretions, processes that relate to the pathophysiology of irritable bowel syndrome (IBS). 5-HT3 receptor antagonists such as alosetron inhibit activation of non-selective cation channels which results in the modulation of the enteric nervous system.

The cause of IBS is unknown. IBS is characterized by visceral hypersensitivity and hyperactivity of the gastrointestinal tract, which lead to abnormal sensations of pain and motor activity. Following distention of the rectum, IBS patients exhibit pain and discomfort at lower volumes than healthy volunteers. Following such distention, alosetron reduced pain and exaggerated motor responses, possibly due to blockade of 5-HT3 receptors.

In healthy volunteers and IBS patients, alosetron (2 mg orally, twice daily for 8 days) increased colonic transit time without affecting orocecal transit time. In healthy volunteers, alosetron also increased basal jejunal water and sodium absorption after a single 4-mg dose. In IBS patients, multiple oral doses of alosetron (4 mg twice daily for 6.5 days) significantly increased colonic compliance.

Single oral doses of alosetron administered to healthy men produced a dose-dependent reduction in the flare response seen after intradermal injection of serotonin. Urinary 6-β-hydroxycortisol excretion decreased by 52% in elderly subjects after 27.5 days of alosetron 2 mg orally twice daily. This decrease was not statistically significant. In another study utilizing alosetron 1 mg orally twice daily for 4 days, there was a significant decrease in urinary 6-β-hydroxycortisol excretion. However, there was no change in the ratio of 6-β-hydroxycortisol to cortisol, indicating a possible decrease in cortisol production. The clinical significance of these findings is unknown.

Pharmacokinetics: The pharmacokinetics of alosetron have been studied after single oral doses ranging from 0.05 mg to 16 mg in healthy men. The pharmacokinetics of alosetron have also been evaluated in healthy women and men and in patients with IBS after repeated oral doses ranging from 1 mg twice daily to 8 mg twice daily.

Absorption: Alosetron is rapidly absorbed after oral administration with a mean absolute bioavailability of approximately 50 to 60% (approximate range 30 to >90%). After administration of radiolabeled alosetron, only 1% of the dose was recovered in the feces as unchanged drug. Following oral administration of a 1 mg alosetron dose to young men, a peak plasma concentration of approximately 5 ng/mL occurs at 1 hour. In young women, the mean peak plasma concentration is approximately 9 ng/mL, with a similar time to peak.

Food Effects: Alosetron absorption is decreased by approximately 25% by co-administration with food, with a mean delay in time to peak concentration of 15 minutes (see DOSAGE AND ADMINISTRATION).

Distribution: Alosetron demonstrates a volume of distribution of approximately 65 to 95 L. Plasma protein binding is 82% over a concentration range of 20 to 4000 ng/mL.

Metabolism and Elimination: Plasma concentrations of alosetron increase proportionately with increasing single oral doses up to 8 mg and more than proportionately at a single oral dose of 16 mg. Twice-daily oral dosing of alosetron does not result in accumulation. The terminal elimination half-life of alosetron is approximately 1.5 hours (plasma clearance is approximately 600 mL/min). Population pharmacokinetic analysis in IBS patients confirmed that alosetron clearance is minimally influenced by doses up to 8 mg.

Renal elimination of unchanged alosetron accounts for only 6% of the dose. Renal clearance is approximately 94 mL/min.

Alosetron is extensively metabolized in humans. The biological activity of these metabolites is unknown. A mass balance study was performed utilizing an orally administered dose of unlabeled and ^{14}C-labeled alosetron. This study indicates that on a molar basis, alosetron metabolites reach additive peak plasma concentrations 9-fold greater than alosetron and that the additive metabolite AUCs are 13-fold greater than alosetron's AUC. Plasma radioactivity declined with a half-life 2-fold longer than that of alosetron, indicating the presence of circulating metabolites. Approximately 73% of the radiolabeled dose was recovered in urine with another 24% of the dose recovered in feces. Only 7% of the dose was recovered as unchanged drug. At least 13 metabolites have been detected in urine. The predominant product in urine was a 6-hydroxy metabolite (15% of the dose). This metabolite was secondarily metabolized to a glucuronide that was also present in urine (14% of the dose). Smaller amounts of the 6-hydroxy metabolite and the 6-O-glucuronide also appear to be present in feces. A bis-oxidized dicarbonyl accounted for 14% of the dose and its monocarbonyl precursor accounted for another 4% in urine and 6% in feces. No other urinary metabolite accounted for more than 4% of the dose. Glucuronide or sulfate conjugates of unchanged alosetron were not detected in urine.

In studies of Japanese men, an N-desmethyl metabolite was found circulating in plasma in all subjects and accounted for up to 30% of the dose in one subject when alosetron was administered with food. The clinical significance of this finding is unknown.

Alosetron is metabolized by human microsomal cytochrome P450 (CYP), shown in vitro to involve enzymes 2C9 (30%), 3A4 (18%), and 1A2 (10%). Non-CYP mediated Phase I metabolic conversion also contributes to an extent of about 11% (see PRECAUTIONS: Drug Interactions).

Population Subgroups: ***Age:*** In some studies in healthy men or women, plasma concentrations were elevated by approximately 40% in individuals 65 years and older compared to young adults. However, this effect was not consistently observed in men (see PRECAUTIONS: Geriatric Use and DOSAGE AND ADMINISTRATION: Geriatric Patients).

Gender: Plasma concentrations are 30% to 50% lower and less variable in men compared to women given the same oral doses. Population pharmacokinetic analysis in IBS patients confirmed that alosetron concentrations were influenced by gender (27% lower in men).

Reduced Hepatic Function: No pharmacokinetic data are available in this patient group (see PRECAUTIONS: Hepatic Insufficiency and DOSAGE AND ADMINISTRATION: Patients with Hepatic Impairment).

Reduced Renal Function: Renal impairment (creatinine clearance 4 to 56 mL/min) has no effect on the renal elimination of alosetron due to the minor contribution of this pathway to elimination. The effect of renal impairment on metabolite kinetics and the effect of end-stage renal disease have not been assessed (see DOSAGE AND ADMINISTRATION: Patients with Renal Impairment).

CLINICAL TRIALS

Two 12-week treatment, multi-center, double-blind, placebo-controlled, dose-ranging studies were conducted to determine the dosage of oral LOTRONEX for subsequent evaluation in efficacy studies.

In women, of the doses studied, 1 mg of LOTRONEX twice daily was significantly more effective than placebo in providing relief of IBS pain and discomfort, decreasing the proportion of days with urgency, decreasing stool frequency, and producing firmer stools. Efficacy in men, as assessed by producing adequate relief of IBS pain and discomfort, was not demonstrated at any dose of LOTRONEX.

The efficacy and safety of 1 mg of oral LOTRONEX twice daily for 12 weeks was studied in two US multi-center, double-blind, placebo-controlled trials of identical design (Studies 1 and 2) in non-constipated women with IBS meeting the Rome Criteria (see Appendix) for at least 6 months. For enrollment into the studies, patients were required to meet entry pain and stool consistency criteria. An average pain score of at least mild pain, as collected during a 2-week screening period, was required. Women with severe pain were excluded. An entry stool consistency requirement was also incorporated to target women whose predominant bowel symptom was diarrhea or in which diarrhea was a prominent feature in their alternating pattern. Women with a history of severe constipation were excluded. Men were not studied.

The primary efficacy measure in these studies was the woman's weekly assessment of adequate relief of IBS pain and discomfort. Key secondary measures included percentage of days with urgency and daily assessment of stool frequency and consistency. Study 1 enrolled 647 women (71% diarrhea-predominant, 28% alternating between diarrhea and constipation, and 1% constipation-predominant) while Study 2 enrolled 626 women (71% diarrhea-predominant, 27% alternating between diarrhea and constipation, and 2% constipation-predominant). At entry into the studies, most women reported mild to moderate pain intensity and stool consistency of formed to loose.

In both trials, LOTRONEX 1 mg administered twice daily was significantly more effective than placebo in providing relief of IBS pain and discomfort.

In both Study 1 and Study 2, the beneficial effect on IBS pain and discomfort was demonstrated only in women with diarrhea-predominant IBS. Data in Figures 1 and 2 are presented for this subgroup. In Study 1, significantly more women reported relief of their abdominal pain and discomfort within 1 week of starting alosetron therapy than those who received placebo (Figure 1). In Study 2, this treatment effect was observed within 4 weeks (Figure 2). Once attained, significant treatment effect persisted throughout the remainder of the treatment period. Upon discontinuing LOTRONEX, symptoms returned. Within one week after discontinuing therapy, there was no difference between placebo and alosetron-treated women.

[See figures 1 & 2 at top of next column]

In each study, women who received LOTRONEX reported a significant decrease in the percentage of days with urgency as compared to those who received placebo. Treatment with LOTRONEX also resulted in firmer stools and a significant decrease in stool frequency. Significant improvement of these symptoms occurred within the first week of treatment and persisted throughout the 12 weeks of therapy. Upon dis-

Continued on next page

This product information is based on labeling in effect on June 23, 2000. For further information, contact via direct mail, phone, or web site. Medical Information, Glaxo Wellcome Inc., PO Box 13398, Research Triangle Park, NC 27709. Healthcare Professionals (Medical Information): 800-334-0089. Patients (Customer Response Center): 1-888-825-5249. Glaxo Wellcome Corporate Web Site: www.glaxowellcome.com

Lotronex—Cont.

Figure 1: Percentage of Women (Diarrhea-Predominant) Reporting Relief of IBS Pain and Discomfort in Study 1

*p<0.05

Figure 2: Percentage of Women (Diarrhea-Predominant) Reporting Relief of IBS Pain and Discomfort in Study 2

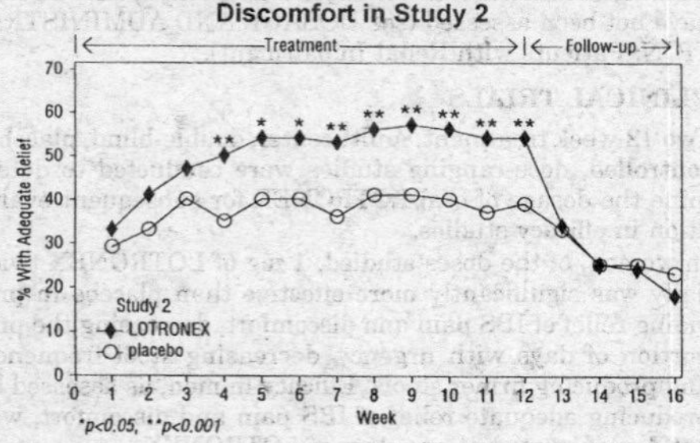

*p<0.05, **p<0.001

continuance of treatment these symptoms returned. Within one week after discontinuing therapy, there was no difference between placebo and alosetron-treated patients. The efficacy of LOTRONEX for treatment longer than 12 weeks has not been established.

INDICATIONS AND USAGE

LOTRONEX is indicated for the treatment of irritable bowel syndrome (IBS) in women whose predominant bowel symptom is diarrhea.

The safety and effectiveness of LOTRONEX in men have not been established.

CONTRAINDICATIONS

LOTRONEX is contraindicated in patients known to have hypersensitivity to any component of the product.

WARNINGS

Acute ischemic colitis was infrequently* reported in patients receiving LOTRONEX in 3-month clinical trials. The reported cases resolved over several days to weeks without sequelae or complications following supportive management. A causal association between treatment with LOTRONEX and acute colitis has not been established, nor have risk factors been identified. LOTRONEX should be discontinued in patients experiencing rectal bleeding and a sudden worsening of abdominal pain. These patients should be promptly evaluated and appropriate diagnostic testing considered.

Constipation is a frequent and dose-related side effect of treatment with LOTRONEX. LOTRONEX should not be used in IBS patients who are currently constipated or whose predominant bowel symptom is constipation. In clinical studies, 25% to 30% of patients receiving alosetron experienced constipation. For the majority of these patients, constipation was mild to moderate in intensity and self-limited; however, approximately 9% of patients studied required interruption of treatment for a few days and approximately 10% could not tolerate twice daily dosing on a continuous basis and discontinued therapy. Patients experiencing constipation who completed the 12-week treatment period had similar relief of abdominal pain as patients not experiencing constipation who completed the study. Management of constipation with usual care including laxatives, fiber, or with a brief interruption of therapy may be considered (see DOSAGE AND ADMINISTRATION).

*Infrequent is defined as occurring in 1/100 to 1/1000 patients.

PRECAUTIONS

Information for Patients: See the tear-off leaflet at the end of the labeling for Information for the Patient.

Drug Interactions: In vitro human liver microsome studies and an in vivo metabolic probe study demonstrated that alosetron did not inhibit CYP enzymes 2D6, 3A4, 2C9, or 2C19. In vitro, at total drug concentrations 27-fold higher than peak plasma concentrations observed with the 1-mg dosage, alosetron inhibited CYP enzymes 1A2 (60%) and 2E1 (50%). In an in vivo metabolic probe study, alosetron did not inhibit CYP2E1 but did produce 30% inhibition of both CYP1A2 and N-acetyltransferase. Although not studied with alosetron, inhibition of N-acetyltransferase may have clinically relevant consequences for drugs such as isoniazid, procainamide, and hydralazine. The effect on CYP1A2 was explored further in a clinical interaction study with theophylline and no effect on metabolism was observed. Another study showed that alosetron had no clinically significant effect on plasma concentrations of the oral contraceptive agents ethinyl estradiol and levonorgestrel (CYP3A4 substrates). A clinical interaction study was also conducted with alosetron and the CYP3A4 substrate cisapride. No significant effects on cisapride metabolism or QT interval were noted. The effect of alosetron on monoamine oxidases and on intestinal first pass secondary to high intraluminal concentrations have not been examined. Based on the above data from in vitro and in vivo studies, it is unlikely that alosetron will inhibit the hepatic metabolic clearance of drugs metabolized by the major CYP enzyme 3A4, as well as the CYP enzymes 2D6, 2C9, 2C19, 2E1, or 1A2.

Alosetron does not appear to induce the major cytochrome P450 (CYP) drug metabolizing enzyme 3A. Alosetron also does not appear in induce CYP enzymes 2E1 or 2C19. It is not known whether alosetron might induce other enzymes. Because alosetron is metabolized by a variety of hepatic CYP drug-metabolizing enzymes, inducers or inhibitors of these enzymes may change the clearance of alosetron. The effect of induction or inhibition of individual pathways on metabolite kinetics and pharmacodynamic consequences has not been examined.

Hepatic Insufficiency: Due to the extensive hepatic metabolism and first pass metabolism of alosetron and metabolites, increased exposure to alosetron is likely to occur in patients with hepatic insufficiency.

Carcinogenesis, Mutagenesis, Impairment of Fertility: In 2-year oral studies, alosetron was not carcinogenic in mice at doses up to 30 mg/kg/day or in rats at doses up to 40 mg/kg/day. These doses are, respectively, about 60 to 160 times the recommended human dose of alosetron of 2 mg/day (1 mg twice daily) based on body surface area. Alosetron was not genotoxic in the Ames tests, the mouse lymphoma cell (L5178Y/TK$^{\pm}$) forward gene mutation test, the human lymphocyte chromosome aberration test, the ex vivo rat hepatocyte unscheduled DNA synthesis (UDS) test, or the in vivo rat micronucleus test for mutagenicity. Alosetron at oral doses up to 40 mg/kg/day (about 160 times the recommended daily human dose based on body surface area) was found to have no effect on fertility and reproductive performance of male or female rats.

Pregnancy: ***Teratogenic Effects:*** Pregnancy Category B. Reproduction studies have been performed in rats at doses up to 40 mg/kg/day (about 160 times the recommended human dose based on body surface area) and rabbits at oral doses up to 30 mg/kg/day (about 240 times the recommended daily human dose based on body surface area). These studies have revealed no evidence of impaired fertility or harm to the fetus due to alosetron. There are, however, no adequate and well-controlled studies in pregnant women. Because animal reproduction studies are not always predictive of human response, LOTRONEX should be used during pregnancy only if clearly needed.

Nursing Mothers: Alosetron and/or metabolites of alosetron are excreted in the breast milk of lactating rats. It is not known whether alosetron is excreted in human milk. Because many drugs are excreted in human milk, caution should be exercised when LOTRONEX is administered to a nursing woman.

Pediatric Use: Safety and effectiveness in pediatric patients have not been established.

Geriatric Use: Of all patients who received at least one dose of alosetron in premarketing studies, 211 were 65 years of age and over and 39 were 75 years of age and over. The safety profile of LOTRONEX was similar in older and younger patients.

In 2 placebo-controlled IBS safety and efficacy trials (Studies 1 and 2), 60 patients 65 years of age and over and 14 patients 75 years of age and over received 1-mg oral doses of LOTRONEX twice daily for up to 12 weeks. In both studies, subgroup analyses showed no evidence of differential treatment effects across the age categories assessed. Other reported clinical experience has not identified differences in responses between elderly and younger patients, but greater sensitivity of some older individuals cannot be ruled out (see CLINICAL PHARMACOLOGY: Population Subgroups: Age).

ADVERSE REACTIONS

In two large, placebo-controlled clinical trials conducted in the US (Studies 1 and 2), women (18 years of age and older) were treated with 1 mg of LOTRONEX twice-daily for up to 12 weeks. The adverse events in Table 1 were reported in 1% or more of patients who received LOTRONEX and occurred more frequently on LOTRONEX than on placebo. A statistically significant difference was observed for constipation in patients treated with LOTRONEX compared to placebo (p<0.0001).

[See table 1 below]

Table 1: Adverse Events Reported in ≥1% of Female Patients and More Frequently on LOTRONEX 1 mg B.I.D. than Placebo (Studies 1 and 2)

Body System Adverse Event	LOTRONEX (N = 632)	Placebo (N = 637)
Cardiovascular		
Hypertension	2%	<1%
Ear, Nose, and Throat		
Allergic rhinitis	2%	<1%
Throat and tonsil discomfort and pain	1%	<1%
Bacterial ear, nose, and throat infections	1%	<1%
Gastrointestinal		
Constipation	28%	5%
Nausea	7%	6%
Gastrointestinal discomfort and pain	5%	4%
Abdominal discomfort and pain	5%	3%
Gastrointestinal gaseous symptoms	3%	2%
Viral gastrointestinal infections	3%	2%
Dyspeptic symptoms	3%	1%
Abdominal distention	2%	<1%
Hemorrhoids	2%	<1%
Neurology		
Sleep disorders	3%	2%
Psychiatry		
Depressive disorders	2%	1%

Gastrointestinal: The most frequent adverse event reported by patients treated with LOTRONEX was constipation (see WARNINGS). In clinical studies, constipation was reported in 25% to 30% of patients treated with LOTRONEX 1 mg twice daily for up to 12 weeks (n = 702). This effect was statistically significant compared to placebo (p<0.0001). Ten percent (10%) of patients treated with LOTRONEX withdrew from the studies due to constipation. Of the patients reporting constipation, 75% reported a single episode with the mean time to constipation onset of about 3 weeks. Occurrences of constipation were generally mild to moderate in intensity and transient in nature. Most constipation events resolved spontaneously with continued treatment. In studies 1 and 2, 9% of patients treated with LOTRONEX reported constipation and 4 consecutive days with no bowel movement; by protocol, therapy was withheld for 1 to 4 days. Following interruption of treatment, 88% of the affected patients resumed bowel movements within the 4-day period and were able to re-initiate treatment with LOTRONEX.

Hepatic: A similar incidence in elevation of ALT (>3-fold) was seen in patients receiving LOTRONEX or placebo (0.5% vs 0.4%) in studies of 12 weeks' and 12 months' duration. A single case of hepatitis (elevated ALT, AST, alkaline phosphatase, and bilirubin) without jaundice was reported in a 12-week study. A causal association with LOTRONEX has not been established.

Long-Term Safety: The pattern and frequency of adverse events in a long-term, placebo-controlled safety study in which women with IBS (n = 473) were treated with LOTRONEX 1 mg twice daily for up to 12 months were essentially the same as observed in 12-week safety and effectiveness trials. There were no reports of acute colitis in these alosetron-treated women.

Other Events Observed During the Premarketing Evaluation of LOTRONEX: During its premarketing assessment, multiple and single doses of LOTRONEX were administered resulting in 2574 patient exposures in 46 completed clinical studies. The conditions, dosages, and duration of exposure to LOTRONEX varied between trials, and the studies included healthy male and female volunteers as well as male and female patients with IBS.

In the listing that follows, reported adverse events were classified using a standardized coding dictionary. Only those events that an investigator believed were possibly related to alosetron, occurred in at least 2 patients, and occurred at a greater frequency during treatment with LOTRONEX than during placebo administration are presented. Serious adverse events occurring in at least 1 patient for which an in-

APPENDIX

Diagnostic Criteria: Irritable Bowel Syndrome (IBS)*

At least three months continuous or recurrent symptoms of:
1. abdominal pain or discomfort which is:
   (a) relieved with defecation,
   (b) and/or associated with a change in frequency of stool,
   (c) and/or associated with a change in consistency of stool;

and

2. two or more of the following, at least a quarter of occasions or days;
   (a) altered stool frequency,
   (b) altered stool form (lumpy/hard or loose/watery stool),
   (c) altered stool passage (straining, urgency, or feeling of incomplete evacuation),
   (d) passage of mucus,
   (e) bloating or feeling of abdominal distention.

*Thompson WG, Creed F, Drossman DA, et al. Functional bowel disease and functional abdominal pain. *Gastroenterol Int.* 1992;5:75-91.

vestigator believed there was reasonable possibility that the event was related to alosetron treatment and which occurred at a greater frequency in LOTRONEX than placebo-treated patients are also presented.

In the following listing, events are categorized by body system. Within each body system, events are presented in descending order of frequency. The following definitions are used: *Infrequent* adverse events are those occurring on one or more occasion in 1/100 to 1/1000 patients; *Rare* adverse events are those occurring on one or more occasion in fewer than 1/1000 patients.

Although the events reported occurred during treatment with LOTRONEX, they were not necessarily caused by it.

Cardiovascular—Infrequent: Arrhythmias.

Drug Interaction, Overdose and Trauma—Rare: Contusions and hematomas.

Ear, Nose, and Throat—Infrequent: Nasal signs and symptoms. ***Rare:*** Ear signs and symptoms.

Eyes—Rare: Photophobia.

Gastrointestinal—Infrequent: Ischemic colitis. ***Rare:*** proctitis.

Hepatobiliary Tract and Pancreas—Infrequent: Abnormal bilirubin levels.

Lower Respiratory—Infrequent: Breathing disorders. ***Rare:*** Cough.

Neurological—Rare: Sedation and abnormal dreams.

Non-site Specific—Rare: Allergies, allergic reactions, unusual odors and taste.

Psychiatry—Infrequent: Anxiety.

Reproduction—Infrequent: Menstrual disorders. ***Rare:*** Sexual function disorders.

Skin—Rare: Acne and folliculitis.

Urology—Rare: Urinary infections, polyuria, and diuresis.

DRUG ABUSE AND DEPENDENCE

LOTRONEX has no known potential for abuse or dependence.

OVERDOSAGE

There is no specific antidote for overdose of LOTRONEX. Patients should be managed with appropriate supportive therapy. Individual oral doses as large as 16 mg have been administered in clinical studies without significant adverse events. This dose is 8 times higher than the recommended total daily dose. Inhibition of the metabolic elimination and reduced first pass of other drugs might occur with overdoses of alosetron (see PRECAUTIONS: Drug Interactions). Single oral doses of LOTRONEX at 15 mg/kg in female mice and 60 mg/kg in female rats (30 and 240 times, respectively, the recommended human dose based on body surface area) were lethal. Symptoms of acute toxicity were labored respiration, subdued behavior, ataxia, tremors, and convulsions.

DOSAGE AND ADMINISTRATION

Usual Dose in Adults: The recommended adult dosage of LOTRONEX is 1 mg taken orally twice daily with or without food. Individual patients who experience constipation may need to interrupt treatment (see WARNINGS and ADVERSE REACTIONS: Gastrointestinal).

Pediatric Patients: No studies have been conducted in patients less than 18 years of age (see PRECAUTIONS: Pediatric Use).

Geriatric Patients: No dosage adjustment is recommended for elderly patients (65 years of age and older) (see CLINICAL PHARMACOLOGY: Population Subgroups: Age and PRECAUTIONS: Geriatric Use).

Patients with Renal Impairment: No dosage adjustment is recommended for patients with renal impairment (creatinine clearance 4 to 56 mL/min) (see CLINICAL PHARMACOLOGY: Reduced Renal Function).

Patients with Hepatic Impairment: No studies have been conducted in patients with hepatic impairment (see PRECAUTIONS: Hepatic Insufficiency and CLINICAL PHARMACOLOGY: Population Subgroups: Reduced Hepatic Function).

HOW SUPPLIED

LOTRONEX Tablets, 1 mg (1.124 mg alosetron HCl equivalent to 1 mg alosetron), are blue, oval, film-coated tablets debossed with GX CT1 on one face in bottles of 60 (NDC 0173-0690-00) with child-resistant closure.

Store at 25°C (77°F); excursions permitted to 15–30°C (59–86°F) [see USP Controlled Room Temperature].

[See table above]

Glaxo Wellcome Inc., Research Triangle Park, NC 27709
US Patent No. 5,360,800

April 2000/RL-812

Information for the Patient

LOTRONEX® (alosetron hydrochloride) Tablets

Read this information carefully before you start taking LOTRONEX (pronounced LOW-trah-nex) Tablets. Read the information included with LOTRONEX each time you refill your prescription, in case something has changed. This information does not take the place of discussions with your doctor.

What is LOTRONEX?

LOTRONEX is a prescription medicine used to treat irritable bowel syndrome (IBS) in women who have diarrhea as their main symptom. LOTRONEX has not been shown to work in men with IBS. IBS has been called by many names including irritable colon and spastic colon. IBS is a medical condition causing cramping abdominal pain, abdominal discomfort, urgency (a sudden need to have a bowel movement), and irregular bowel habits such as diarrhea or constipation.

It is not clear why some people develop IBS. It may be caused by your body's overreaction to a body chemical called serotonin. This overreaction may cause your intestinal system to be overactive. LOTRONEX works by blocking the action of serotonin on the intestinal system. This reduces the cramping abdominal pain, abdominal discomfort, urgency, and diarrhea caused by IBS.

LOTRONEX may not work for every patient who takes it. For women who are helped by LOTRONEX, the medicine works faster in some and slower in others. Some women taking LOTRONEX will have relief from their IBS pain and discomfort within the first week of use. Other women have relief of abdominal pain and discomfort within four weeks of starting LOTRONEX. Within one week, urgency and diarrhea occur less often for some patients. When you stop taking LOTRONEX, IBS symptoms will likely return within one week.

Who should not take LOTRONEX?

You should not start taking LOTRONEX when you are constipated or constipated most of the time.

Do not take LOTRONEX if you are allergic to LOTRONEX or any of its ingredients. The active ingredient in LOTRONEX is alosetron hydrochloride. The inactive ingredients are listed at the end of this leaflet.

LOTRONEX may not be right for you. Tell your doctor if you are:

- constipated most of the time.
- pregnant or plan to become pregnant.
- breast feeding.
- taking or planning to take any other medicines, including those you can get without a prescription.

How should LOTRONEX be taken?

Take LOTRONEX exactly as your doctor prescribes it. You can take LOTRONEX with or without food. If you miss a dose of LOTRONEX, do not double the next dose. Instead, simply go to the next regularly scheduled dosing time and take your normal prescribed dose of LOTRONEX.

What are the possible side effects of LOTRONEX?

If you have a sudden worsening of abdominal pain or if you see blood in your stool (bowel movement), call your doctor right away. These symptoms may be a sign of a serious medical condition.

Constipation is a common side effect of treatment with LOTRONEX. If you become constipated while taking LOTRONEX, call your doctor. Your doctor may tell you to stop taking LOTRONEX or suggest other ways to manage your constipation.

This description of side effects is not complete. Your doctor or pharmacist can give you a more complete list of side effects with LOTRONEX. Talk to your doctor right away about any side effects you have.

Medicines are sometimes prescribed for purposes not listed in patient information leaflets. Do not use LOTRONEX for a condition for which it was not prescribed. Do not share LOTRONEX with other people. As with any medicine, LOTRONEX may be harmful without appropriate medical supervision.

If you have questions about LOTRONEX, ask your doctor or pharmacist. They can show you detailed information about LOTRONEX that was written for health professionals.

Inactive Ingredients: lactose (anhydrous), magnesium stearate, microcrystalline cellulose, and pregelatinized starch. The blue film-coat contains hydroxypropyl methylcellulose, titanium dioxide, triacetin, and indigo carmine.

Glaxo Wellcome Inc., Research Triangle Park, NC 27709
US Patent No. 5,360,800

April 2000/RL-812

Shown in Product Identification Guide, page 315

MALARONE™ ℞

[*mă lă-rone*]
(atovaquone and proguanil hydrochloride) Tablets

MALARONE™ ℞

(atovaquone and proguanil hydrochloride) Pediatric Tablets

DESCRIPTION

MALARONE (atovaquone and proguanil hydrochloride) is a fixed-dose combination of the antimalarial agents atovaquone and proguanil hydrochloride. The chemical name of atovaquone is *trans*-2-[4-(4-chlorophenyl)cyclohexyl]-3-hydroxy-1,4-naphthalenedione. Atovaquone is a yellow crystalline solid that is practically insoluble in water. It has a molecular weight of 366.84 and the molecular formula $C_{22}H_{19}ClO_3$. The compound has the following structural formula:

The chemical name of proguanil hydrochloride is 1-(4-chlorophenyl)-5-isopropyl-biguanide hydrochloride. Proguanil hydrochloride is a white crystalline solid that is sparingly soluble in water. It has a molecular weight of 290.22 and the molecular formula $C_{11}H_{16}ClN_5$•HCl. The compound has the following structural formula:

MALARONE Tablets and MALARONE Pediatric Tablets are for oral administration. Each MALARONE Tablet contains 250 mg of atovaquone and 100 mg of proguanil hydrochloride and each MALARONE Pediatric Tablet contains 62.5 mg of atovaquone and 25 mg of proguanil hydrochloride. The inactive ingredients in both tablets are low-substituted hydroxypropyl cellulose, magnesium stearate, microcrystalline cellulose, poloxamer 188, povidone K30, and sodium starch glycolate. The tablet coating contains red iron oxide, polyethylene glycol 400, hydroxypropyl methylcellulose, polyethylene glycol 8000, and titanium dioxide.

CLINICAL PHARMACOLOGY

Microbiology:

Mechanism of Action: The constituents of MALARONE, atovaquone and proguanil hydrochloride, interfere with 2 different pathways involved in the biosynthesis of pyrimidines required for nucleic acid replication. Atovaquone is a selective inhibitor of parasite mitochondrial electron transport. Proguanil hydrochloride primarily exerts its effect by means of the metabolite cycloguanil, a dihydrofolate reductase inhibitor. Inhibition of dihydrofolate reductase in the malaria parasite disrupts deoxythymidylate synthesis.

Activity In Vitro and In Vivo: Atovaquone and cycloguanil (an active metabolite of proguanil) are active against the erythrocytic and exoerythrocytic stages of *Plasmodium* spp. Enhanced efficacy of the combination compared to either atovaquone or proguanil hydrochloride alone was demonstrated in clinical studies in both immune and nonimmune patients (see CLINICAL STUDIES).

Drug Resistance: Strains of *P. falciparum* with decreased susceptibility to atovaquone or proguanil/cycloguanil alone can be selected in vitro or in vivo. The combination of atovaquone and proguanil hydrochloride may not be effective for treatment of recrudescent malaria that develops after prior therapy with the combination.

Pharmacokinetics:

Absorption: Atovaquone is a highly lipophilic compound with low aqueous solubility. The bioavailability of atovaquone shows considerable inter-individual variability.

Continued on next page

This product information is based on labeling in effect on June 23, 2000. For further information, contact via direct mail, phone, or web site. Medical Information, Glaxo Wellcome Inc., PO Box 13398, Research Triangle Park, NC 27709. Healthcare Professionals (Medical Information): 800-334-0089. Patients (Customer Response Center): 1-888-825-5249. Glaxo Wellcome Corporate Web Site: www.glaxowellcome.com

Malarone—Cont.

Dietary fat taken with atovaquone increases the rate and extent of absorption, increasing AUC 2 to 3 times and C_{max} 5 times over fasting. The absolute bioavailability of the tablet formulation of atovaquone when taken with food is 23%. MALARONE Tablets should be taken with food or a milky drink.
Proguanil hydrochloride is extensively absorbed regardless of food intake.
Distribution: Atovaquone is highly protein bound (>99%) over the concentration range of 1 to 90 mcg/mL. The apparent volume of distribution of atovaquone after oral administration is approximately 3.5 L/kg.
Proguanil is 75% protein bound. The apparent volume of distribution is approximately 42 L/kg.
In human plasma, the binding of atovaquone and proguanil was unaffected by the presence of the other.
Metabolism: In a study where ^{14}C-labelled atovaquone was administered to healthy volunteers, greater than 94% of the dose was recovered as unchanged atovaquone in the feces over 21 days. There was little or no excretion of atovaquone in the urine (less than 0.6%). There is indirect evidence that atovaquone may undergo limited metabolism; however, a specific metabolite has not been identified. Between 40% to 60% of proguanil is excreted by the kidneys. Proguanil is metabolized to cycloguanil (primarily via CYP2C19) and 4-chlorophenylbiguanide. The main routes of elimination are hepatic biotransformation and renal excretion.
Elimination: The elimination half-life of atovaquone is about 2 to 3 days in adult patients.
The mean oral clearance of atovaquone is approximately 0.04 L/h per kg.
The mean oral clearance of proguanil is 3.22 L/h per kg. The elimination half-life of proguanil is 12 to 21 hours in both adult patients and pediatric patients, but may be longer in individuals who are slow metabolizers.
Special Populations:
Pediatrics: The pharmacokinetics of proguanil and cycloguanil are similar in adult patients and pediatric patients. However, the elimination half-life of atovaquone is shorter in pediatric patients (1 to 2 days) than in adult patients (2 to 3 days).
Geriatrics: No studies have been carried out in geriatric patients to assess the pharmacokinetics in this patient population. Since geriatric patients may have reduced renal function, caution should be taken when treating geriatric patients with MALARONE (see Special Populations: Renal Impairment and PRECAUTIONS).
Hepatic Impairment: The pharmacokinetics of MALARONE have not been studied in patients with hepatic impairment. The effect of hepatic dysfunction on the conversion of proguanil to cycloguanil is unknown.
Renal Impairment: The pharmacokinetics of MALARONE have not been studied in patients with renal impairment. Since proguanil and cycloguanil are eliminated primarily via the renal route, the clinical implication of treating patients with severe renal dysfunction with MALARONE is unknown (see PRECAUTIONS: General).
Drug Interactions: There are no pharmacokinetic interactions between atovaquone and proguanil at the recommended dose.
Concomitant treatment with **tetracycline** has been associated with approximately a 40% reduction in plasma concentrations of atovaquone.
Concomitant treatment with **metoclopramide** has also been associated with decreased bioavailability of atovaquone.
Concomitant administration of **rifampin** is known to reduce atovaquone levels by approximately 50% (see PRECAUTIONS: Drug Interactions). The mechanism of this interaction is unknown.
Atovaquone is highly protein bound (>99%) but does not displace other highly protein-bound drugs in vitro, indicating significant drug interactions arising from displacement are unlikely (see PRECAUTIONS: Drug Interactions). Proguanil is metabolized primarily by CYP2C19. Potential pharmacokinetic interactions with other substrates or inhibitors of this pathway are unknown.

INDICATIONS AND USAGE

Prevention of Malaria: MALARONE is indicated for the prophylaxis of *P. falciparum* malaria, including in areas where chloroquine resistance has been reported (see CLINICAL STUDIES).
Treatment of Malaria: MALARONE is indicated for the treatment of acute, uncomplicated *P. falciparum* malaria. MALARONE has been shown to be effective in regions where the drugs chloroquine, halofantrine, mefloquine, and amodiaquine may have unacceptable failure rates, presumably due to drug resistance.

CONTRAINDICATIONS

MALARONE is contraindicated in individuals with known hypersensitivity to atovaquone or proguanil hydrochloride or any component of the formulation. During clinical trials, one case of anaphylaxis following treatment with atovaquone/proguanil was observed.

PRECAUTIONS

General: MALARONE has not been evaluated for the treatment of cerebral malaria or other severe manifestations of complicated malaria, including hyperparasitemia, pulmonary edema, or renal failure. Patients with severe malaria are not candidates for oral therapy.
Absorption of atovaquone may be reduced in patients with diarrhea or vomiting. If MALARONE is used in patients who are vomiting (see DOSAGE AND ADMINISTRATION), parasitemia should be closely monitored and the use of an antiemetic considered. Vomiting occurred in up to 19% of pediatric patients given treatment doses of MALARONE. In the controlled clinical trials of MALARONE, 15.3% of adults who were treated with atovaquone/proguanil received an antiemetic drug during that part of the trial when they received atovaquone/proguanil. Of these patients, 98.3% were successfully treated. In patients with severe or persistent diarrhea or vomiting, alternative antimalarial therapy may be required.
Parasite relapse occurred commonly when *P. vivax* malaria was treated with MALARONE alone.
In the event of recrudescent *P. falciparum* infections after treatment with MALARONE or failure of chemoprophylaxis with MALARONE, patients should be treated with a different blood schizonticide.
The concomitant administration of MALARONE and any other medication containing proguanil hydrochloride should be avoided. Because proguanil is eliminated by renal excretion, proguanil hydrochloride, and hence MALARONE, should be administered with caution to patients with severe pre-existing renal failure.
Information for Patients: Patients should be instructed:
- to take MALARONE tablets at the same time each day with food or a milky drink.
- to take a repeat dose of MALARONE if vomiting occurs within 1 hour after dosing.
- to consult a healthcare professional regarding alternative forms of prophylaxis if prophylaxis with MALARONE is prematurely discontinued for any reason.
- that protective clothing, insect repellents, and bednets are important components of malaria prophylaxis.
- that no chemoprophylactic regimen is 100% effective; therefore, patients should seek medical attention for any febrile illness that occurs during or after return from a malaria-endemic area and inform their healthcare professional that they may have been exposed to malaria.
- that falciparum malaria carries a higher risk of death and serious complications in pregnant women than in the general population. Pregnant women anticipating travel to malarious areas should discuss the risks and benefits of such travel with their physicians (see Pregnancy section).

Drug Interactions: Concomitant treatment with **tetracycline** has been associated with approximately a 40% reduction in plasma concentrations of atovaquone. Parasitemia should be closely monitored in patients receiving tetracycline. While antiemetics may be indicated for patients receiving MALARONE, **metoclopramide** may reduce the bioavailability of atovaquone and should be used only if other antiemetics are not available.
Concomitant administration of rifampin is known to reduce atovaquone levels by approximately 50%. The concomitant administration of MALARONE and rifampin is not recommended.
Atovaquone is highly protein bound (>99%) but does not displace other highly protein-bound drugs in vitro, indicating significant drug interactions arising from displacement are unlikely.
Potential interactions between proguanil or cycloguanil and other drugs that are CYP2C19 substrates or inhibitors are unknown.

Table 1: Adverse Experiences in Clinical Trials of MALARONE for Prophylaxis of Malaria

Adverse Event	Percent of Subjects With Adverse Experiences (Percent of Subjects With Adverse Experiences Attributable to Therapy)				
	Adults			Children and Adolescents	
	Placebo (n = 206)	MALARONE* (n = 206)	MALRONE† (n = 381)	Placebo (n = 140)	MALARONE (n = 125)
Headache	27 (7)	22 (3)	17 (5)	21 (14)	19 (14)
Fever	13 (1)	5 (0)	3 (0)	11 (<1)	6 (0)
Myalgia	11 (0)	12 (0)	7 (0)	0 (0)	0 (0)
Abdominal pain	10 (5)	9 (4)	6 (3)	29 (29)	33 (31)
Cough	8 (<1)	6 (<1)	4 (1)	9 (0)	9 (0)
Diarrhea	8 (3)	6 (2)	4 (1)	3 (1)	2 (0)
Upper respiratory infection	7 (0)	8 (0)	5 (0)	0 (0)	<1 (0)
Dyspepsia	5 (4)	3 (2)	2 (1)	0 (0)	0 (0)
Back Pain	4 (0)	8 (0)	4 (0)	0 (0)	0 (0)
Gastritis	3 (2)	3 (3)	2 (2)	0 (0)	0 (0)
Vomiting	2 (<1)	1 (<1)	<1 (<1)	6 (6)	7 (7)
Flu syndrome	1 (0)	2 (0)	4 (0)	6 (0)	9 (0)
Any adverse event	65 (32)	54 (17)	49 (17)	62 (41)	60 (42)

*Subjects receiving the recommended dose of atovaquone and proguanil hydrochloride in placebo-controlled trials.
†Subjects receiving the recommended dose of atovaquone and proguanil hydrochloride in any trial.

Carcinogenesis, Mutagenesis, Impairment of Fertility:
Atovaquone: Carcinogenicity studies in rats were negative; 24-month studies in mice showed treatment-related increases in incidence of hepatocellular adenoma and hepatocellular carcinoma at all doses tested which ranged from approximately 5 to 8 times the average steady-state plasma concentrations in humans during prophylaxis of malaria. Atovaquone alone was negative with or without metabolic activation in the Ames *Salmonella* mutagenicity assay, the Mouse Lymphoma mutagenesis assay, and the Cultured Human Lymphocyte cytogenetic assay. No evidence of genotoxicity was observed in the in vivo Mouse Micronucleus assay.
Proguanil: Carcinogenicity studies with proguanil have not been completed. Proguanil was not genotoxic in in vitro or in vivo studies.
Proguanil alone was negative with or without metabolic activation in the Ames *Salmonella* mutagenicity assay and the Mouse Lymphoma mutagenesis assay. No evidence of genotoxicity was observed in the in vivo Mouse Micronucleus assay.
Genotoxicity studies have not been performed with atovaquone in combination with proguanil. Effects of MALARONE on male and female reproductive performance are unknown.
Pregnancy: Pregnancy Category C. Falciparum malaria carries a higher risk of morbidity and mortality in pregnant women than in the general population. Maternal death and fetal loss are both known complications of falciparum malaria in pregnancy. In pregnant women who must travel to malaria-endemic areas, personal protection against mosquito bites should always be employed (see Information for Patients) in addition to antimalarials.
Atovaquone was not teratogenic and did not cause reproductive toxicity in rats at maternal plasma concentrations up to 5 to 6.5 times the estimated human exposure during treatment of malaria. Following single-dose administration of ^{14}C-labeled atovaquone to pregnant rats, concentrations of radiolabel in rat fetuses were 18% (mid-gestation) and 60% (late gestation) of concurrent maternal plasma concentrations. In rabbits, atovaquone caused maternal toxicity at plasma concentrations that were approximately 0.6 to 1.3 times the estimated human exposure during treatment of malaria. Adverse fetal effects in rabbits, including decreased fetal body lengths and increased early resorptions and post-implantation losses, were observed only in the presence of maternal toxicity. Concentrations of atovaquone in rabbit fetuses averaged 30% of the concurrent maternal plasma concentrations.
The combination of atovaquone and proguanil hydrochloride was not teratogenic in rats at plasma concentrations up to 1.7 and 0.10 times, respectively, the estimated human exposure during treatment of malaria. In rabbits, the combination of atovaquone and proguanil hydrochloride was not teratogenic or embryotoxic to rabbit fetuses at plasma concentrations up to 0.34 and 0.82 times, respectively, the estimated human exposure during treatment of malaria.
While there are no adequate and well-controlled studies of atovaquone and/or proguanil hydrochloride in pregnant women, MALARONE may be used if the potential benefit justifies the potential risk to the fetus. The proguanil component of MALARONE acts by inhibiting the parasitic dihydrofolate reductase (see CLINICAL PHARMACOLOGY: Microbiology: Mechanism of Action). However, there are no clinical data indicating that folate supplementation diminishes drug efficacy, and for women of childbearing age re-

ceiving folate supplements to prevent neural tube birth defects, such supplements may be continued while taking MALARONE.

Nursing Mothers: It is not known whether atovaquone is excreted into human milk. In a rat study, atovaquone concentrations in the milk were 30% of the concurrent atovaquone concentrations in the maternal plasma.

Proguanil is excreted into human milk in small quantities. Caution should be exercised when MALARONE is administered to a nursing woman.

Pediatric Use: Safety and effectiveness for the treatment and prophylaxis of malaria in pediatric patients who weigh less than 11 kg have not been established.

Geriatric Use: Clinical studies of MALARONE did not include sufficient numbers of subjects aged 65 and over to determine whether they respond differently from younger subjects. In general, dose selection for an elderly patient should be cautious, reflecting the greater frequency of decreased hepatic, renal, or cardiac function, and of concomitant disease or other drug therapy (see CLINICAL PHARMACOLOGY: Special Populations: Geriatrics).

ADVERSE REACTIONS

Because MALARONE contains atovaquone and proguanil hydrochloride, the type and severity of adverse reactions associated with each of the compounds may be expected. The higher treatment doses of MALARONE were less well tolerated than the lower prophylactic doses.

Among adults who received MALARONE for treatment of malaria, attributable adverse experiences that occurred in ≥5% of patients were abdominal pain (17%), nausea (12%), vomiting (12%), headache (10%), diarrhea (8%), asthenia (8%), anorexia (5%), and dizziness (5%). Treatment was discontinued prematurely due to an adverse experience in 4 of 436 adults treated with MALARONE.

Among pediatric patients who received MALARONE for the treatment of malaria, attributable adverse experiences that occurred in ≥5% of patients were vomiting (10%) and pruritus (6%). Vomiting occurred in 43 of 319 (13%) pediatric patients who did not have symptomatic malaria but were given treatment doses of MALARONE for 3 days in a clinical trial. The design of this clinical trial required that any patient who vomited be withdrawn from the trial. Among pediatric patients with symptomatic malaria treated with MALARONE, treatment was discontinued prematurely due to an adverse experience in 1 of 116 (0.9%).

Abnormalities in laboratory tests reported in clinical trials were limited to elevations of transaminases in malaria patients being treated with MALARONE. The frequency of these abnormalities varied substantially across studies of treatment and were not observed in the randomized portions of the prophylaxis trials.

In one phase III trial of malaria treatment in Thai adults, early elevations of ALT and AST were observed to occur more frequently in patients treated with MALARONE compared to patients treated with an active control drug. Rates for patients who had normal baseline levels of these clinical laboratory parameters were: Day 7: ALT 26.7% versus 15.6%; AST 16.9% vs. 8.6%. By day 14 of this 28-day study, the frequency of transaminase elevations equalized across the two groups.

In this and other studies in which transaminase elevations occurred, they were noted to persist for up to 4 weeks following treatment with MALARONE for malaria. None were associated with untoward clinical events.

Among subjects who received MALARONE for prophylaxis of malaria, adverse experiences occurred in similar proportions of subjects receiving MALARONE or placebo (Table 1). The most commonly reported adverse experiences possibly attributable to MALARONE or placebo were headache and abdominal pain. Prophylaxis with MALARONE was discontinued prematurely due to a treatment-related adverse experience in 3 of 381 adults and 0 of 125 pediatric patients.
[See table 1 at top of previous page]

OVERDOSAGE

There have been no reports of overdosage from the administration of MALARONE.

There is no known antidote for atovaquone, and it is currently unknown if atovaquone is dialyzable. The median lethal dose is higher than the maximum oral dose tested in mice and rats (1825 mg/kg per day). Overdoses up to 31,500 mg of atovaquone have been reported. In one such patient who also took an unspecified dose of dapsone, methemoglobinemia occurred. Rash has also been reported after overdose.

Overdoses of proguanil hydrochloride as large as 1500 mg have been followed by complete recovery, and doses as high as 700 mg twice daily have been taken for over 2 weeks without serious toxicity. Adverse events occasionally associated with proguanil hydrochloride doses of 100 to 200 mg/day, such as epigastric discomfort and vomiting, would be likely to occur with overdose. There are also reports of reversible hair loss and scaling of the skin on the palms and/or soles, reversible aphthous ulceration, and hematologic side effects.

DOSAGE AND ADMINISTRATION

The daily dose should be taken at the same time each day with food or a milky drink. In the event of vomiting within 1 hour after dosing, a repeat dose should be taken.

Prevention of Malaria: Prophylactic treatment with MALARONE should be started 1 or 2 days before entering a malaria-endemic area and continued daily during the stay and for 7 days after return.

Table 2: Dosage for Prevention of Malaria in Pediatric Patients

Weight (kg)	Atovaquone/Proguanil HCl Total Daily Dose	Dosage Regimen
11–20	62.5 mg/25 mg	1 MALARONE Pediatric Tablet daily
21–30	125 mg/50 mg	2 MALARONE Pediatric Tablets as a single dose daily
31–40	187.5 mg/75 mg	3 MALARONE Pediatric Tablets as a single dose daily
>40	250 mg/100 mg	1 MALARONE Tablet (adult strength) as a single dose daily

Table 3: Dosage for Treatment of Acute Malaria in Pediatric Patients

Weight (kg)	Atovaquone/Proguanil HCl Total Daily Dose	Dosage Regimen
11–20	250 mg/100 mg	1 MALARONE Tablet (adult strength) daily for 3 consecutive days
21–30	500 mg/200 mg	2 MALARONE Tablets (adult strength) as a single dose daily for 3 consecutive days
31–40	750 mg/300 mg	3 MALARONE Tablets (adult strength) as a single dose daily for 3 consecutive days
>40	1 g/400 mg	4 MALARONE Tablets (adult strength) as a single dose daily for 3 consecutive days

Table 4: Parasitological Response in Clinical Trials of MALARONE for Treatment of *P. falciparum* Malaria

Study Site	MALARONE* Evaluable Patients (n)	MALARONE* % Sensitive Response**	Comparator Drug(s)	Comparator Evaluable Patients (n)	Comparator % Sensitive Response**
Brazil	74	98.6%	Quinine and tetracycline	76	100.0%
Thailand	79	100.0%	Mefloquine	79	86.1%
France†	21	100.0%	Halofantrine	18	100.0%
Kenya†‡	81	93.8%	Halofantrine	83	90.4%
Zambia	80	100.0%	Pyrimethamine/sulfadoxine (P/S)	80	98.8%
Gabon†	63	98.4%	Amodiaquine	63	81.0%
Philippines	54	100.0%	Chloroquine (Cq) Cq and P/S	23 32	30.4% 87.5%
Peru	19	100.0%	Chloroquine P/S	13 7	7.7% 100.0%

*MALARONE = 1000 mg atovaquone and 400 mg proguanil hydrochloride (or equivalent based on body weight for patients weighing ≤40 kg) once daily for 3 days.
**Elimination of parasitemia with no recurrent parasitemia during follow-up for 28 days.
†Patients hospitalized only for acute care. Follow-up conducted in outpatients.
‡Study in pediatric patients 3 to 12 years of age.

Adults: One MALARONE Tablet (adult strength = 250 mg atovaquone/100 mg proguanil hydrochloride) per day.

Pediatric Patients: The dosage for prevention of malaria in pediatric patients is based upon body weight (Table 2).
[See table 2 above]

Treatment of Acute Malaria:

Adults: Four MALARONE Tablets (adult strength; total daily dose 1 g atovaquone/400 mg proguanil hydrochloride) as a single dose daily for 3 consecutive days.

Pediatric Patients: The dosage for treatment of acute malaria in pediatric patients is based upon body weight (Table 3).
[See table 3 above]

HOW SUPPLIED

MALARONE Tablets, containing 250 mg atovaquone and 100 mg proguanil hydrochloride, are pink, film-coated, round, biconvex tablets engraved with "GX CM3" on one side.

Bottle of 100 tablets with child-resistant closure (NDC 0173-0675-01).

MALARONE Pediatric Tablets, containing 62.5 mg atovaquone and 25 mg proguanil hydrochloride, are pink, film-coated, round, biconvex tablets engraved with "GX CG7" on one side.

Bottle of 100 tablets with child-resistant closure (NDC 0173-0676-01).

Store at 25°C (77°F); excursions permitted to 15° to 30°C (59° to 86°F) (see USP Controlled Room Temperature).

ANIMAL TOXICOLOGY

Fibrovascular proliferation in the right atrium, pyelonephritis, bone marrow hypocellularity, lymphoid atrophy, and gastritis/enteritis were observed in dogs treated with proguanil hydrochloride for 6 months at a dose of 12 mg/kg per day (approximately 3.9 times the recommended daily human dose for malaria prophylaxis on a mg/m^2 basis). Bile duct hyperplasia, gall bladder mucosal atrophy, and interstitial pneumonia were observed in dogs treated with proguanil hydrochloride for 6 months at a dose of 4 mg/kg per day (approximately 1.3 times the recommended daily human dose for malaria prophylaxis on a mg/m^2 basis). Mucosal hyperplasia of the cecum and renal tubular basophilia were observed in rats treated with proguanil hydrochloride for 6 months at a dose of 20 mg/kg per day (approximately 1.6 times the recommended daily human dose for malaria prophylaxis on a mg/m^2 basis). Adverse heart, lung, liver, and gall bladder effects observed in dogs and kidney effects observed in rats were not shown to be reversible.

CLINICAL STUDIES

Treatment of Acute Malarial Infections: In 3 phase II clinical trials, atovaquone alone, proguanil hydrochloride alone, and the combination of atovaquone and proguanil hydrochloride were evaluated for the treatment of acute, uncomplicated malaria caused by *P. falciparum*. Among 156 evaluable patients, the parasitological cure rate was 59/89 (66%) with atovaquone alone, 1/17 (6%) with proguanil hydrochloride alone, and 50/50 (100%) with the combination of atovaquone and proguanil hydrochloride.

MALARONE was evaluated for treatment of acute, uncomplicated malaria caused by *P. falciparum* in 8 phase III controlled clinical trials. Among 471 evaluable patients treated with the equivalent of 4 MALARONE Tablets once daily for 3 days, 464 had a sensitive response (elimination of parasitemia with no recurrent parasitemia during follow-up for 28 days) (see Table 4). Seven patients had a response of R1 resistance (elimination of parasitemia but with recurrent parasitemia between 7 and 28 days after starting treatment).

Continued on next page

This product information is based on labeling in effect on June 23, 2000. For further information, contact via direct mail, phone, or web site. Medical Information, Glaxo Wellcome Inc., PO Box 13398, Research Triangle Park, NC 27709. Healthcare Professionals (Medical Information): 800-334-0089. Patients (Customer Response Center): 1-888-825-5249. Glaxo Wellcome Corporate Web Site: www.glaxowellcome.com

Malarone—Cont.

In these trials, the response to treatment with MALARONE was similar to treatment with the comparator drug in 4 trials, and better than the response to treatment with the comparator drug in the other 4 trials.
The overall efficacy in 521 evaluable patients was 98.7% (see Table 4).
[See table at top of previous page]
Eighteen of 521 (3.5%) evaluable patients with acute falciparum malaria presented with a pretreatment serum creatinine greater than 2.0 mg/dL (range 2.1 to 4.3 mg/dL). All were successfully treated with MALARONE and 17 of 18 (94.4%) had normal serum creatinine levels by day 7.
Data from a phase II trial of atovaquone conducted in Zambia suggested that approximately 40% of the study population in this country were HIV-infected patients. The enrollment criteria were similar for the phase III trial of MALARONE conducted in Zambia and the results are presented in Table 4. Efficacy rates for MALARONE in this study population were high and comparable to other populations studied.
The efficacy of MALARONE in the treatment of the erythrocytic phase of nonfalciparum malaria was assessed in a small number of patients. Of the 23 patients in Thailand infected with *P. vivax* and treated with atovaquone/proguanil hydrochloride 1000 mg/400 mg daily for 3 days, parasitemia cleared in 21 (91.3%) at 7 days. Parasite relapse occurred commonly when *P. vivax* malaria was treated with MALARONE alone. Seven patients in Gabon with malaria due to *P. ovale* or *P. malariae* were treated with atovaquone/proguanil hydrochloride 1000 mg/400 mg daily for 3 days. All 6 evaluable patients (3 with *P. malariae*, 2 with *P. ovale*, and 1 with mixed *P. falciparum* and *P. ovale*) were cured at 28 days. Relapsing malarias including *P. vivax* and *P. ovale* require additional treatment to prevent relapse.
Prevention of Malaria: MALARONE was evaluated for prophylaxis of malaria in 4 clinical trials in malaria-endemic areas.
Three placebo-controlled studies of 10 to 12 weeks' duration were conducted among residents of malaria-endemic areas in Kenya, Zambia, and Gabon. Of a total of 669 randomized patients (including 264 pediatric patients 5 to 16 years of age), 103 were withdrawn for reasons other than falciparum malaria or drug-related adverse events. (Fifty-five percent of these were lost to follow-up and 45% were withdrawn for protocol violations.) The results are listed in Table 5.

Table 5: Prevention of Parasitemia in Controlled Clinical Trials of MALARONE for Prophylaxis of *P. falciparum* Malaria

	MALARONE	Placebo
Total number of patients randomized	326	341
Failed to complete study	57	44
Developed parasitemia (*P. falciparum*)	2	92

In a 10-week study in 175 South African subjects who moved into malaria-endemic areas and were given prophylaxis with 1 MALARONE Tablet daily, parasitemia developed in 1 subject who missed several doses of medication. Since no placebo control was included, the incidence of malaria in this study was not known. In a malaria challenge study conducted in healthy US volunteers, atovaquone alone prevented malaria in 6/6 individuals, whereas 4/4 placebo-treated volunteers developed malaria. Although these data suggest that MALARONE prophylaxis is effective in both malaria-immune and nonimmune subjects, differences in the response rates may occur.
Causal Prophylaxis: In separate studies with small numbers of volunteers, atovaquone and proguanil hydrochloride were independently shown to have causal prophylactic activity directed against liver-stage parasites of *P. falciparum*. Six patients given a single dose of atovaquone 250 mg 24 hours prior to malaria challenge were protected from developing malaria, whereas all 4 placebo-treated patients developed malaria.
During the 4 weeks following cessation of prophylaxis in clinical trial participants who remained in malaria-endemic areas and were available for evaluation, malaria developed in 24/211 (11.4%) subjects who took placebo and 9/328 (2.7%) who took MALARONE. While new infections could not be distinguished from recrudescent infections, all but 1 of the infections in patients treated with MALARONE occurred more than 15 days after stopping therapy, probably representing new infections. The single case occurring on day 8 following cessation of therapy with MALARONE probably represents a failure of prophylaxis with MALARONE.
The possibility that delayed cases of *P. falciparum* malaria may occur some time after stopping prophylaxis with MALARONE cannot be ruled out. Hence, returning travelers developing febrile illnesses should be investigated for malaria.
Glaxo Wellcome Inc., Research Triangle Park, NC 27709
US Patent Nos. 5,053,432 and 5,998,449

July 2000/RL-843

MEPRON® ℞

[mĕ ′prŏn]
(atovaquone)
Suspension

DESCRIPTION

MEPRON (atovaquone) is an antiprotozoal agent. The chemical name of atovaquone is *trans*-2-[4-(4-chlorophenyl) cyclohexyl]-3-hydroxy-1,4-naphthalenedione. Atovaquone is a yellow crystalline solid that is practically insoluble in water. It has a molecular weight of 366.84 and the molecular formula $C_{22}H_{19}ClO_3$.
MEPRON Suspension is a formulation of micro-fine particles of atovaquone. The atovaquone particles, reduced in size to facilitate absorption, are significantly smaller than those in the previously marketed tablet formulation. MEPRON Suspension is for oral administration and is bright yellow with a citrus flavor. Each teaspoonful (5 mL) contains 750 mg of atovaquone and the inactive ingredients benzyl alcohol, flavor, poloxamer 188, purified water, saccharin sodium, and xanthan gum.

MICROBIOLOGY

Mechanism of Action: Atovaquone is a hydroxy-1,4-naphthoquinone, an analog of ubiquinone, with antipneumocystis activity. The mechanism of action against *Pneumocystis carinii* has not been fully elucidated. In *Plasmodium* species, the site of action appears to be the cytochrome bc_1 complex (Complex III). Several metabolic enzymes are linked to the mitochondrial electron transport chain via ubiquinone. Inhibition of electron transport by atovaquone will result in indirect inhibition of these enzymes. The ultimate metabolic effects of such blockade may include inhibition of nucleic acid and ATP synthesis.
Activity In Vitro: Several laboratories, using different in vitro methodologies, have shown the IC_{50} (50% Inhibitory Concentration) of atovaquone against rat *P. carinii* to be in the range of 0.1 to 3.0 mcg/mL.
Drug Resistance: Phenotypic resistance to atovaquone in vitro has not been demonstrated for *P. carinii*. However, in two patients who developed *P. carinii* pneumonia (PCP) after prophylaxis with atovaquone, DNA sequence analysis identified mutations in the predicted amino acid sequence of *P. carinii* cytochrome b (a likely target site for atovaquone). The clinical significance of this is unknown.

CLINICAL PHARMACOLOGY

Pharmacokinetics: ***Absorption:*** Atovaquone is a highly lipophilic compound with low aqueous solubility. The bioavailability of atovaquone is highly dependent on formulation and diet. The suspension formulation provides an approximately twofold increase in atovaquone bioavailability in the fasting or fed state compared to the previously marketed tablet formulation. The absolute bioavailability of a 750-mg dose of MEPRON Suspension administered under fed conditions in nine HIV-infected (CD4 >100 cells/mm^3) volunteers was 47% ± 15%. In the same study, the bioavailability of a 750-mg dose of the previously marketed tablet formulation was 23% ± 11%.
Administering atovaquone with food enhances its absorption by approximately two-fold. In one study, 16 healthy volunteers received a single dose of 750 mg MEPRON Suspension after an overnight fast and following a standard breakfast (23 g fat: 610 kCal). The mean (±SD) area under the concentration-time curve (AUC) values were 324 ± 115 and 801 ± 320 hr•mcg/mL under fasting and fed conditions, respectively, representing a 2.6 ± 1.0-fold increase. The effect of food (23 g fat: 400 kCal) on plasma atovaquone concentrations was also evaluated in a multiple-dose, randomized, crossover study in 19 HIV-infected volunteers (CD4 <200 cells/mm^3) receiving daily doses of 500 mg MEPRON Suspension. AUC was 280 ± 114 hr•mcg/mL when atovaquone was administered with food as compared to 169 ± 77 hr•mcg/mL under fasting conditions. Maximum plasma atovaquone concentration (C_{max}) was 15.1 ± 6.1 and 8.8 ± 3.7 mcg/mL when atovaquone was administered with food and under fasting conditions, respectively.
Dose Proportionality: Plasma atovaquone concentrations do not increase proportionally with dose. When MEPRON Suspension was administered with food at dosage regimens of 500 mg once daily, 750 mg once daily, and 1000 mg once daily, average steady-state plasma atovaquone concentrations were 11.7 ± 4.8, 12.5 ± 5.8, and 13.5 ± 5.1 mcg/mL, respectively. The corresponding C_{max} concentrations were 15.1 ± 6.1, 15.3 ± 7.6, and 16.8 ± 6.4 mcg/mL. When MEPRON Suspension was administered to five HIV-infected volunteers at a dose of 750 mg twice daily, the average steady-state plasma atovaquone concentration was 21.0 ± 4.9 mcg/mL and C_{max} was 24.0 ± 5.7 mcg/mL. The minimum plasma atovaquone concentration (C_{min}) associated with the 750-mg twice-daily regimen was 16.7 ± 4.6 mcg/mL.
Distribution: Following the intravenous administration of atovaquone, the volume of distribution at steady state (Vd_{ss}) was 0.60 ± 0.17 L/kg (n = 9). Atovaquone is extensively bound to plasma proteins (99.9%) over the concentration range of 1 to 90 mcg/mL. In three HIV-infected children who received 750 mg atovaquone as the tablet formulation four times daily for 2 weeks, the cerebrospinal fluid concentrations of atovaquone were 0.04, 0.14, and 0.26 mcg/mL, representing less than 1% of the plasma concentration.
Elimination: The plasma clearance of atovaquone following intravenous (IV) administration in nine HIV-infected volunteers was 10.4 ± 5.5 mL/min (0.15 ± 0.09 mL/min per kg). The half-life of atovaquone was 62.5 ± 35.3 hours after IV administration and ranged from 67.0 ± 33.4 to 77.6 ± 23.1 hours across studies following administration of MEPRON Suspension. The half-life of atovaquone is long due to presumed enterohepatic cycling and eventual fecal elimination. In a study where ^{14}C-labelled atovaquone was administered to healthy volunteers, greater than 94% of the dose was recovered as unchanged atovaquone in the feces over 21 days. There was little or no excretion of atovaquone in the urine (less than 0.6%). There is indirect evidence that atovaquone may undergo limited metabolism; however, a specific metabolite has not been identified.
Special Populations: ***Pediatrics:*** In a study of MEPRON Suspension in 27 HIV-infected, asymptomatic infants and children between 1 month and 13 years of age, the pharmacokinetics of atovaquone were age-dependent. These patients were dosed once daily with food for 12 days. The average steady-state plasma atovaquone concentrations in the 24 patients with available concentration data are shown in Table 1.
[See table 1 below]
Hepatic/Renal Impairment: The pharmacokinetics of atovaquone have not been studied in patients with hepatic or renal impairment.
Drug Interactions: ***Rifampin:*** In a study with 13 HIV-infected volunteers, the oral administration of rifampin 600 mg every 24 hours with MEPRON Suspension 750 mg every 12 hours resulted in a 52% ± 13% decrease in the average steady-state plasma atovaquone concentration and a 37% ± 42% increase in the average steady-state plasma rifampin concentration. The half-life of atovaquone decreased from

Table 1: Average Steady-State Plasma Atovaquone Concentrations in Pediatric Patients

Age	Dose of MEPRON Suspension: 10 mg/kg	30 mg/kg	45 mg/kg
	Average C_{ss} in mcg/mL (mean ±SD)		
1–3 months	5.9 (n = 1)	27.8 ± 5.8 (n = 4)	—
>3–24 months	5.7 ± 5.1 (n = 4)	9.8 ± 3.2 (n = 4)	15.4 ± 6.6 (n = 4)
>2–13 years	16.8 ± 6.4 (n = 4)	37.1 ± 10.9 (n = 3)	—

Table 2: Relationship Between Plasma Atovaquone Concentration and Successful Treatment

Steady-State Plasma Atovaquone Concentrations (mcg/mL)	Successful Treatment* (No. Successes/No. in Group) (%): Observed		Predicted†	
0 to <5	0/6	(0%)	1.5/6	(25%)
5 to <10	18/26	(69%)	14.7/26	(57%)
10 to <15	30/38	(79%)	31.9/38	(84%)
15 to <20	18/19	(95%)	18.1/19	(95%)
20 to <25	18/18	(100%)	17.8/18	(99%)
25+	6/6	(100%)	6/6	(100%)

*Successful treatment was defined as improvement in clinical and respiratory measures persisting at least 4 weeks after cessation of therapy. This was based on data from patients for which both outcome and steady-state plasma atovaquone concentration data are available.
†Based on logistic regression analysis.

82 ± 36 hours when administered without rifampin to 50 ± 16 hours with rifampin.
Rifabutin, another rifamycin, is structurally similar to rifampin and may possibly have some of the same drug interactions as rifampin. No interaction trials have been conducted with MEPRON and rifabutin.
Trimethoprim/Sulfamethoxazole (TMP-SMX): The possible interaction between atovaquone and TMP-SMX was evaluated in six HIV-infected adult volunteers as part of a larger multiple-dose, dose-escalation, and chronic dosing study of MEPRON Suspension. In this crossover study, MEPRON Suspension 500 mg once daily, or TMP-SMX tablets (160 mg trimethoprim and 800 mg sulfamethoxazole) twice daily, or the combination were administered with food to achieve steady state. No difference was observed in the average steady-state plasma atovaquone concentration after coadministration with TMP-SMX. Coadministration of MEPRON with TMP-SMX resulted in a 17% and 8% decrease in average steady-state concentrations of trimethoprim and sulfamethoxazole in plasma, respectively. This effect is minor and would not be expected to produce clinically significant events.
Zidovudine: Data from 14 HIV-infected volunteers who were given atovaquone tablets 750 mg every 12 hours with zidovudine 200 mg every 8 hours showed a 24% ± 12% decrease in zidovudine apparent oral clearance, leading to a 35% ± 23% increase in plasma zidovudine AUC. The glucuronide metabolite:parent ratio decreased from a mean of 4.5 when zidovudine was administered alone to 3.1 when zidovudine was administered with atovaquone tablets. This effect is minor and would not be expected to produce clinically significant events. Zidovudine had no effect on atovaquone pharmacokinetics.
Relationship Between Plasma Atovaquone Concentration and Clinical Outcome: In a comparative study of atovaquone tablets with TMP-SMX for oral treatment of mild-to-moderate *Pneumocystis carinii* pneumonia (PCP) (see INDICATIONS AND USAGE), where AIDS patients received 750 mg atovaquone tablets three times daily for 21 days, the mean steady-state atovaquone concentration was 13.9 ± 6.9 mcg/mL (n = 133). Analysis of these data established a relationship between plasma atovaquone concentration and successful treatment. This is shown in Table 2.
[See table 2 on previous page]
A dosing regimen of MEPRON Suspension for the treatment of mild-to-moderate PCP has been selected to achieve average plasma atovaquone concentrations of approximately 20 mcg/mL, because this plasma concentration was previously shown to be well tolerated and associated with the highest treatment success rates (Table 2). In an open-label PCP treatment study with MEPRON Suspension, dosing regimens of 1000 mg once daily, 750 mg twice daily, 1500 mg once daily, and 1000 mg twice daily were explored. The average steady-state plasma atovaquone concentration achieved at the 750-mg twice-daily dose given with meals was 22.0 ± 10.1 mcg/mL (n = 18).

INDICATIONS AND USAGE: MEPRON Suspension is indicated for the prevention of *Pneumocystis carinii* pneumonia in patients who are intolerant to trimethoprim-sulfamethoxazole (TMP-SMX).

MEPRON Suspension is also indicated for the acute oral treatment of mild-to-moderate PCP in patients who are intolerant to TMP-SMX.
Prevention of PCP: The indication for prevention of PCP is based on the results of two clinical trials comparing MEPRON Suspension to dapsone or aerosolized pentamidine in HIV-infected adult and adolescent patients at risk of PCP (CD4 count <200 cells/mm^3 or a prior episode of PCP) and intolerant to TMP-SMX.
Dapsone Comparative Study: This randomized, open-label trial enrolled a total of 1057 patients at 48 study centers. Patients were randomized to receive 1500 mg MEPRON Suspension once daily (n = 536) or 100 mg dapsone once daily (n = 521). Median follow-up was 24 months. Patients randomized to the dapsone arm who were seropositive for *Toxoplasma gondii* and had a CD4 count <100 cells/mm^3 also received pyrimethamine and folinic acid. PCP event rates are shown in Table 3. There was no significant difference in mortality rates between the groups.
Aerosolized Pentamidine Comparative Study: This randomized, open-label trial enrolled a total of 549 patients at 35 study centers. Patients were randomized to receive 1500 mg MEPRON Suspension once daily (n = 175), 750 mg MEPRON Suspension once daily (n = 188), or 300 mg aerosolized pentamidine once monthly (n = 186). Median follow-up was 11.3 months. The results of the PCP event rates appear in Table 3. There were no significant differences in mortality rates among the groups.
[See table 3 above]
An analysis of all PCP events (intent-to-treat analysis) showed results similar to those above.
Treatment of PCP: The indication for treatment of mild-to-moderate PCP is based on the results of comparative pharmacokinetic studies of the suspension and tablet formulations (see CLINICAL PHARMACOLOGY) and clinical efficacy studies of the tablet formulation which established a relationship between plasma atovaquone concentration and successful treatment. The results of a randomized, double-blind trial comparing MEPRON to TMP-SMX in AIDS patients with mild-to-moderate PCP (defined in the study protocol as an alveolar-arterial oxygen diffusion gradient [(A-a)DO_2][1] ≤45 mm Hg and PaO_2 ≥60 mm Hg on room air) and a randomized trial comparing MEPRON to IV pentamidine isethionate in patients with mild-to-moderate PCP intolerant to trimethoprim or sulfa-antimicrobials are summarized below:
TMP-SMX Comparative Study: This double-blind, randomized trial initiated in 1990 was designed to compare the safety and efficacy of MEPRON to that of TMP-SMX for the treatment of AIDS patients with histologically confirmed PCP. Only patients with mild-to-moderate PCP were eligible for enrollment.
A total of 408 patients were enrolled into the trial at 37 study centers. Eighty-six patients without histologic confirmation of PCP were excluded from the efficacy analyses. Of the 322 patients with histologically confirmed PCP, 160 were randomized to receive MEPRON and 162 to TMP-SMX.
Study participants randomized to treatment with MEPRON were to receive 750 mg MEPRON (three 250-mg tablets) three times daily for 21 days and those randomized to TMP-SMX were to receive 320 mg TMP plus 1600 mg SMX three times daily for 21 days.
Therapy success was defined as improvement in clinical and respiratory measures persisting at least 4 weeks after cessation of therapy. Therapy failures included lack of response, treatment discontinuation due to an adverse experience, and unevaluable.
There was a significant difference (P = 0.03) in mortality rates between the treatment groups. Among the 322 patients with confirmed PCP, 13 of 160 (8%) patients treated with MEPRON and four of 162 (2.5%) patients receiving

Continued on next page

Table 3: Confirmed or Presumed/Probable PCP Events (As-Treated Analysis)*

	Study 115-211		Study 115-213		
Assessment	Atovaquone 1500 mg/day (n = 527)	Dapsone 100 mg/day (n = 510)	Atovaquone 750 mg/day (n = 188)	Atovaquone 1500 mg/day (n = 172)	Aerosolized Pentamidine 300 mg/month (n = 169)
%	15%	19%	23%	18%	17%
Relative Risk† (CI)‡	0.77 (0.57, 1.04)		1.47 (0.86, 2.50)	1.14 (0.63, 2.06)	

*Those events occurring during or within 30 days of stopping assigned treatment.
†Relative risk <1 favors atovaquone and values >1 favor comparator. These trials were designed to show superiority of atovaquone to the comparator. This was not shown.
‡The confidence level of the interval for the dapsone comparative study was 95% and for the pentamidine comparative study was 97.5%.

Table 4: Outcome of Treatment for PCP-Positive Patients Enrolled in the TMP-SMX Comparative Study

Outcome of Therapy*	Number of Patients (% of Total) MEPRON (n = 160)		TMP-SMX (n = 162)		P Value
Therapy Success	99	(62%)	103	(64%)	0.75
Therapy Failure					
–Lack of Response	28	(17%)	10	(6%)	<0.01
–Adverse Experience	11	(7%)	33	(20%)	<0.01
–Unevaluable	22	(14%)	16	(10%)	0.28
Required Alternate PCP Therapy During Study	55	(34%)	55	(34%)	0.95

*As defined by the protocol and described in study description above.

Table 5: Outcome of Treatment for PCP-Positive Patients Enrolled in the Pentamidine Comparative Study

	Primary Treatment					Salvage Treatment				
Outcome of Therapy	MEPRON (n = 56)		Pentamidine (n = 53)		P Value	MEPRON (n = 14)		Pentamidine (n = 11)		P Value
Therapy Success	32	(57%)	21	(40%)	0.09	13	(93%)	7	(64%)	0.14
Therapy Failure										
–Lack of Response	16	(29%)	9	(17%)	0.18	0		0		—
–Adverse Experience	2	(3.6%)	19	(36%)	<0.01	0		3	(27%)	0.07
–Unevaluable	6	(11%)	4	(8%)	0.75	1	(7%)	1	(9%)	1.00
Required Alternate PCP Therapy During Study	19	(34%)	29	(55%)	0.04	0		4	(36%)	0.03

Table 6: Treatment-Limiting Adverse Experiences in the Dapsone Comparative PCP Prevention Study

	Percentage of Patients with Treatment-Limiting Adverse Experience			
	All Patients		Patients Not Taking Either Drug at Enrollment	
Treatment-Limiting Adverse Experience	MEPRON 1500 mg/day (n = 536)	Dapsone 100 mg/day (n = 521)	MEPRON 1500 mg/day (n = 238)	Dapsone 100 mg/day (n = 249)
Any event	24.4%	25.9%	20.2%	43.4%
Rash	6.3%	8.8%	7.6%	16.1%
Nausea	4.1%	0.6%	2.5%	0.8%
Diarrhea	3.2%	0.2%	2.1%	0.4%
Vomiting	2.2%	0.6%	1.3%	0.8%
Allergic reaction	1.1%	2.9%	0.8%	4.8%
Fever	0.6%	2.9%	0%	5.6%
Anemia	0%	1.5%	0%	2.0%

This product information is based on labeling in effect on June 23, 2000. For further information, contact via direct mail, phone, or web site. Medical Information, Glaxo Wellcome Inc., PO Box 13398, Research Triangle Park, NC 27709. Healthcare Professionals (Medical Information): 800-334-0089. Patients (Customer Response Center): 1-888-825-5249. Glaxo Wellcome Corporate Web Site: www.glaxowellcome.com

Mepron—Cont.

TMP-SMX died during the 21-day treatment course or 8-week follow-up period. In the intent-to-treat analysis for all 408 randomized patients, there were 16 (8%) deaths in the arm treated with MEPRON and seven (3.4%) deaths in the TMP-SMX arm ($P = 0.051$). Of the 13 patients treated with MEPRON who died, four died of PCP and five died with a combination of bacterial infections and PCP; bacterial infections did not appear to be a factor in any of the four deaths among TMP-SMX-treated patients.

A correlation between plasma atovaquone concentrations and death was demonstrated; in general, patients with lower plasma concentrations were more likely to die. For those patients for whom day 4 plasma atovaquone concentration data are available, five (63%) of the eight patients with concentrations <5 mcg/mL died during participation in the study. However, only one (2.0%) of the 49 patients with day 4 plasma atovaquone concentrations ≥5 mcg/mL died. Sixty-two percent of patients on MEPRON and 64% of patients on TMP-SMX were classified as protocol-defined therapy successes (Table 4).

[See table 4 on previous page]

The failure rate due to lack of response was significantly larger for patients receiving MEPRON while the failure rate due to adverse experiences was significantly larger for patients receiving TMP-SMX.

There were no significant differences in the effect of either treatment on additional indicators of response (i.e., arterial blood gas measurements, vital signs, serum LDH levels, clinical symptoms, and chest radiographs).

Pentamidine Comparative Study: This unblinded, randomized trial initiated in 1991 was designed to compare the safety and efficacy of MEPRON to that of pentamidine for the treatment of histologically confirmed mild or moderate PCP in AIDS patients. Approximately 80% of the patients either had a history of intolerance to trimethoprim or sulfa-antimicrobials (the primary therapy group) or were experiencing intolerance to TMP-SMX with treatment of an episode of PCP at the time of enrollment in the study (the salvage treatment group).

Patients randomized to MEPRON were to receive 750 mg atovaquone (three 250-mg tablets) three times daily for 21 days and those randomized to pentamidine isethionate were to receive a 3- to 4-mg/kg single IV infusion daily for 21 days.

A total of 174 patients were enrolled into the trial at 22 study centers. Thirty-nine patients without histologic confirmation of PCP were excluded from the efficacy analyses. Of the 135 patients with histologically confirmed PCP, 70 were randomized to receive MEPRON and 65 to pentamidine. One hundred and ten (110) of these were in the primary therapy group and 25 were in the salvage therapy group. One patient in the primary therapy group randomized to receive pentamidine did not receive study medication.

There was no difference in mortality rates between the treatment groups. Among the 135 patients with confirmed PCP, 10 of 70 (14%) patients randomized to MEPRON and nine of 65 (14%) patients randomized to pentamidine died during the 21-day treatment course or 8-week follow-up period. In the intent-to-treat analysis for all randomized patients, there were 11 (12.5%) deaths in the arm treated with MEPRON and 12 (14%) deaths in the pentamidine arm. For those patients for whom day 4 plasma atovaquone concentrations are available, three of five (60%) patients with concentrations <5 mcg/mL died during participation in the study. However, only two of 21 (9%) patients with day 4 plasma concentrations ≥5 mcg/mL died.

The therapeutic outcomes for the 134 patients who received study medication in this trial are presented in Table 5.

[See table 5 on previous page]

CONTRAINDICATIONS

MEPRON Suspension is contraindicated for patients who develop or have a history of potentially life-threatening allergic reactions to any of the components of the formulation.

WARNINGS

Clinical experience with MEPRON for the treatment of PCP has been limited to patients with mild-to-moderate PCP [(A-a)DO_2 ≤45 mm Hg]. Treatment of more severe episodes of PCP has not been systematically studied with this agent. Also, the efficacy of MEPRON in patients who are failing therapy with TMP-SMX has not been systematically studied.

PRECAUTIONS

General: Absorption of orally administered MEPRON is limited but can be significantly increased when the drug is taken with food. Plasma atovaquone concentrations have been shown to correlate with the likelihood of successful treatment and survival. Therefore, parenteral therapy with other agents should be considered for patients who have difficulty taking MEPRON with food (see CLINICAL PHARMACOLOGY). Gastrointestinal disorders may limit absorption of orally administered drugs. Patients with these disorders also may not achieve plasma concentrations of atovaquone associated with response to therapy in controlled trials.

Based upon the spectrum of in vitro antimicrobial activity, atovaquone is not effective therapy for concurrent pulmonary conditions such as bacterial, viral, or fungal pneumonia or mycobacterial diseases. Clinical deterioration in patients may be due to infections with other pathogens, as well as progressive PCP. All patients with acute PCP should be carefully evaluated for other possible causes of pulmonary disease and treated with additional agents as appropriate.

If it is necessary to treat patients with severe hepatic impairment, caution is advised and administration should be closely monitored.

Information for Patients: The importance of taking the prescribed dose of MEPRON should be stressed. Patients should be instructed to take their daily doses of MEPRON with meals, as the presence of food will significantly improve the absorption of the drug.

Drug Interactions: Atovaquone is highly bound to plasma protein (>99.9%). Therefore, caution should be used when administering MEPRON concurrently with other highly plasma protein-bound drugs with narrow therapeutic indices, as competition for binding sites may occur. The extent of plasma protein binding of atovaquone in human plasma is not affected by the presence of therapeutic concentrations of phenytoin (15 mcg/mL), nor is the binding of phenytoin affected by the presence of atovaquone.

Rifampin: Coadministration of rifampin and MEPRON Suspension results in a significant decrease in average steady-state plasma atovaquone concentrations (see CLINICAL PHARMACOLOGY: Drug Interactions). Alternatives to rifampin should be considered during the course of PCP treatment with MEPRON.

Rifabutin, another rifamycin, is structurally similar to rifampin and may possibly have some of the same drug interactions as rifampin. No interaction trials have been conducted with MEPRON and rifabutin.

Drug/Laboratory Test Interactions: It is not known if MEPRON interferes with clinical laboratory test or assay results.

Carcinogenesis, Mutagenesis, Impairment of Fertility: Carcinogenicity studies in rats were negative; 24-month studies in mice showed treatment-related increases in incidence of hepatocellular adenoma and hepatocellular carcinoma at all doses tested which ranged from 1.4 to 3.6 times the average steady-state plasma concentrations in humans during acute treatment of *Pneumocystis carinii* pneumonia. Atovaquone was negative with or without metabolic activation in the Ames *Salmonella* mutagenicity assay, the Mouse Lymphoma mutagenesis assay, and the Cultured Human Lymphocyte cytogenetic assay. No evidence of genotoxicity was observed in the in vivo Mouse Micronucleus assay.

Pregnancy: Pregnancy Category C. Atovaquone was not teratogenic and did not cause reproductive toxicity in rats at plasma concentrations up to two to three times the estimated human exposure. Atovaquone caused maternal toxicity in rabbits at plasma concentrations that were approxi-

Table 7: Treatment-Emergent Adverse Experiences in the Aerosolized Pentamidine Comparative PCP Prevention Study

Treatment-Emergent Adverse Experience	Percentage of Patients with Treatment-Emergent Adverse Experience		
	MEPRON 1500 mg/day (n = 175)	MEPRON 750 mg/day (n = 188)	Aerosolized Pentamidine (n = 186)
Diarrhea	42%	42%	35%
Rash	39%	46%	28%
Headache	28%	31%	22%
Nausea	26%	32%	23%
Cough increased	25%	25%	31%
Fever	25%	31%	18%
Rhinitis	24%	18%	17%
Asthenia	22%	31%	31%
Infection	22%	18%	19%
Abdominal pain	20%	21%	20%
Dyspnea	15%	21%	16%
Vomiting	15%	22%	11%
Patients Discontinuing Therapy Due to an Adverse Experience	25%	16%	7%
Patients Reporting At Least One Adverse Experience	98%	96%	89%

Table 8: Treatment-Emergent Adverse Experiences in the TMP-SMX Comparative PCP Treatment Study

Treatment-Emergent Adverse Experience	Percentage of Patients with Treatment-Emergent Adverse Experience	
	MEPRON (n = 203)	TMP-SMX (n = 205)
Rash (including maculopapular)	23%	34%
Nausea	21%	44%
Diarrhea	19%	7%
Headache	16%	22%
Vomiting	14%	35%
Fever	14%	25%
Insomnia	10%	9%
Asthenia	8%	8%
Pruritus	5%	9%
Monilia, Oral	5%	10%
Abdominal Pain	4%	7%
Constipation	3%	17%
Dizziness	3%	8%
No. Patients Discontinuing Therapy Due to an Adverse Experience	9%	24%
No. Patients Reporting At Least One Adverse Experience	63%	65%

Table 9: Treatment-Emergent Laboratory Test Abnormalities in the TMP-SMX Comparative PCP Treatment Study

Laboratory Test Abnormality	Percentage of Patients Developing a Laboratory Test Abnormality	
	MEPRON	TMP-SMX
Anemia (Hgb<8.0 g/dL)	6%	7%
Neutropenia (ANC<750 cells/mm^3)	3%	9%
Elevated ALT (>5 × ULN)	6%	16%
Elevated AST (>5 × ULN)	4%	14%
Elevated Alkaline Phosphatase (>2.5 × ULN)	8%	6%
Elevated Amylase (>1.5 × ULN)	7%	12%
Hyponatremia (<0.96 × LLN)	7%	26%

ULN = upper limit of normal range.
LLN = lower limit of normal range.

Table 10: Treatment-Emergent Adverse Experiences in the Pentamidine Comparative PCP Treatment Study (Primary Therapy Group)

Treatment-Emergent Adverse Experience	Percentage of Patients with Treatment-Emergent Adverse Experience	
	MEPRON (n = 73)	Pentamidine (n = 71)
Fever	40%	25%
Nausea	22%	37%
Rash	22%	13%
Diarrhea	21%	31%
Insomnia	19%	14%
Headache	18%	28%
Vomiting	14%	17%
Cough	14%	1%
Abdominal Pain	10%	11%
Pain	10%	10%
Sweat	10%	3%
Monilia, Oral	10%	3%
Asthenia	8%	14%
Dizziness	8%	14%
Anxiety	7%	10%
Anorexia	7%	10%
Sinusitis	7%	6%
Dyspepsia	5%	10%
Rhinitis	5%	7%
Taste Perversion	3%	13%
Hypoglycemia	1%	15%
Hypotension	1%	10%
No. Patients Discontinuing Therapy Due to an Adverse Experience	7%	41%
No. Patients Reporting At Least One Adverse Experience	63%	72%

mately one-half the estimated human exposure. Mean fetal body lengths and weights were decreased and there were higher numbers of early resorption and post-implantation loss per dam. It is not clear whether these effects were caused by atovaquone directly or were secondary to maternal toxicity. Concentrations of atovaquone in rabbit fetuses averaged 30% of the concurrent maternal plasma concentrations. In a separate study in rats given a single ^{14}C-radiolabelled dose, concentrations of radiocarbon in rat fetuses were 18% (middle gestation) and 60% (late gestation) of concurrent maternal plasma concentrations. There are no adequate and well-controlled studies in pregnant women. MEPRON should be used during pregnancy only if the potential benefit justifies the potential risk to the fetus.

Nursing Mothers: It is not known whether atovaquone is excreted into human milk. Because many drugs are excreted into human milk, caution should be exercised when MEPRON is administered to a nursing woman. In a rat study, atovaquone concentrations in the milk were 30% of the concurrent atovaquone concentrations in the maternal plasma.

Pediatric Use: Evidence of safety and effectiveness in pediatric patients has not been established. A relationship between plasma atovaquone concentrations and successful treatment of PCP has been established in adults (see Table 2). In a study of MEPRON Suspension in 27 HIV-infected, asymptomatic infants and children between 1 month and 13 years of age, the pharmacokinetics of atovaquone were age-dependent (see CLINICAL PHARMACOLOGY: Special Populations). No drug-related treatment-limiting adverse events were observed in the pharmacokinetic study.

Geriatric Use: Clinical studies of MEPRON did not include sufficient numbers of subjects aged 65 and over to determine whether they respond differently from younger subjects. Other reported clinical experience has not identified differences in responses between the elderly and younger patients. In general, dose selection for an elderly patient should be cautious, reflecting the greater frequency of decreased hepatic, renal, or cardiac function, and of concomitant disease or other drug therapy.

ADVERSE REACTIONS

Because many patients who participated in clinical trials with MEPRON had complications of advanced HIV disease, it was often difficult to distinguish adverse events caused by MEPRON from those caused by underlying medical conditions. There were no life-threatening or fatal adverse experiences caused by MEPRON.

PCP Prevention Studies: In the dapsone comparative study of MEPRON Suspension, adverse experience data were collected only for treatment-limiting events. Among the entire population (n = 1057), treatment-limiting events occurred at similar frequencies in patients treated with MEPRON Suspension or dapsone (Table 6). Among patients who were taking neither dapsone nor atovaquone at enrollment (n = 487), treatment-limiting events occurred in 43% of patients treated with dapsone and 20% of patients treated with MEPRON Suspension ($P < 0.001$). In both populations, the type of treatment-limiting events differed between the two treatment arms. Hypersensitivity reactions (rash, fever, allergic reaction) and anemia were more common in patients treated with dapsone, while gastrointestinal events (nausea, diarrhea, and vomiting) were more common in patients treated with MEPRON Suspension.

[See table 6 on page 1443]

Table 7 summarizes the clinical adverse experiences reported by ≥20% of patients in any group in the aerosolized pentamidine comparative study of MEPRON Suspension (n = 549), regardless of attribution. The incidence of adverse experiences at the recommended dose was similar to that seen with aerosolized pentamidine. Rash was the only individual adverse experience that occurred significantly more commonly in patients treated with both dosages of MEPRON Suspension (39% to 46%) than in patients treated with aerosolized pentamidine (28%). Among patients treated with MEPRON Suspension, there was no evidence of a dose-related increase in the incidence of adverse experiences. Treatment-limiting adverse experiences occurred less often in patients treated with aerosolized pentamidine (7%) than in patients treated with 1500 mg MEPRON Suspension once daily (25%, $P \leq 0.001$) or 750 mg MEPRON Suspension once daily (16%, $P = 0.004$). The most common adverse experiences requiring discontinuation of dosing in the group receiving 1500 mg MEPRON Suspension once daily were rash (6%), diarrhea (4%), and nausea (3%). The most common adverse experience requiring discontinuation of dosing in the group receiving aerosolized pentamidine was bronchospasm (2%).

[See table 7 at top of previous page]

Other events occurring in ≥10% of the patients receiving the recommended dose of MEPRON included sweating, flu syndrome, pain, sinusitis, pruritus, insomnia, depression, and myalgia. Bronchospasm occurred more frequently in patients receiving aerosolized pentamidine (11%) than in patients receiving MEPRON 1500 mg/day (4%) and MEPRON 750 mg/day (2%).

Neither MEPRON nor aerosolized pentamidine was associated with a substantial change from baseline values in any measured laboratory parameter, nor were there any significant differences in any measured laboratory parameter between MEPRON and aerosolized pentamidine. Some patients had laboratory abnormalities considered serious by the investigator or that contributed to discontinuation of therapy.

PCP Treatment Studies: Table 8 summarizes all the clinical adverse experiences reported by ≥5% of the study population during the TMP-SMX comparative study of MEPRON (n = 408), regardless of attribution. The incidence of adverse experiences with MEPRON Suspension at the recommended dose was similar to that seen with the tablet formulation of atovaquone.

[See table 8 on previous page]

Although an equal percentage of patients receiving MEPRON and TMP-SMX reported at least one adverse experience, more patients receiving TMP-SMX required discontinuation of therapy due to an adverse event. Twenty-four percent of patients receiving TMP-SMX were prematurely discontinued from therapy due to an adverse experience versus 9% of patients receiving MEPRON. Four percent of patients receiving MEPRON had therapy discontinued due to development of rash. The majority of cases of rash among patients receiving MEPRON were mild and did not require the discontinuation of dosing. The only other clinical adverse experience that led to premature discontinuation of dosing of MEPRON by more than one patient was vomiting (<1%). The most common adverse experience requiring discontinuation of dosing in the TMP-SMX group was rash (8%).

Laboratory test abnormalities reported for ≥5% of the study population during the treatment period are summarized in Table 9. Two percent of patients treated with MEPRON and 7% of patients treated with TMP-SMX had therapy prematurely discontinued due to elevations in ALT/AST. In general, patients treated with MEPRON developed fewer abnormalities in measures of hepatocellular function (ALT, AST, alkaline phosphatase) or amylase values than patients treated with TMP-SMX.

[See table 9 above]

Table 10 summarizes the clinical adverse experiences reported by ≥5% of the primary therapy study population (n = 144) during the comparative trial of MEPRON and intravenous pentamidine, regardless of attribution. A slightly lower

Continued on next page

This product information is based on labeling in effect on June 23, 2000. For further information, contact via direct mail, phone, or web site. Medical Information, Glaxo Wellcome Inc., PO Box 13398, Research Triangle Park, NC 27709. Healthcare Professionals (Medical Information): 800-334-0089. Patients (Customer Response Center): 1-888-825-5249. Glaxo Wellcome Corporate Web Site: www.glaxowellcome.com

Mepron—Cont.

percentage of patients who received MEPRON reported occurrence of adverse events than did those who received pentamidine (63% vs 72%). However, only 7% of patients discontinued treatment with MEPRON due to adverse events, while 41% of patients who received pentamidine discontinued treatment for this reason ($P<0.001$). Of the five patients who discontinued therapy with MEPRON, three reported rash (4%). Rash was not severe in any patient. No other reason for discontinuation of MEPRON was cited more than once. The most frequently cited reasons for discontinuation of pentamidine therapy were hypoglycemia (11%) and vomiting (9%).

[See table 10 on previous page]

Laboratory test abnormalities reported in ≥5% of patients in the pentamidine comparative study are presented in Table 11. Laboratory abnormality was reported as the reason for discontinuation of treatment in two of 73 patients who received MEPRON. One patient (1%) had elevated creatinine and BUN levels and one patient (1%) had elevated amylase levels. Laboratory abnormalities were the sole or contributing factor in 14 patients who prematurely discontinued pentamidine therapy. In the 71 patients who received pentamidine, laboratory parameters most frequently reported as reasons for discontinuation were hypoglycemia (11%), elevated creatinine levels (6%), and leukopenia (4%).

[See table 11 below]

Observed During Clinical Practice: In addition to adverse events reported from clinical trials, the following events have been identified during post-approval use of MEPRON. Because they are reported voluntarily from a population of unknown size, estimates of frequency cannot be made. These events have been chosen for inclusion due to a combination of their seriousness, frequency of reporting, or potential causal connection to MEPRON.

Blood and Lymphatic: Methemoglobinemia, thrombocytopenia.

Eye: Vortex keratopathy.

Hepatobiliary Tract and Pancreas: Pancreatitis.

Skin: Allergic reactions including erythema multiforme.

Urology: Acute renal impairment.

OVERDOSAGE

There is no known antidote for atovaquone, and it is currently unknown if atovaquone is dialyzable. The median lethal dose is higher than the maximum oral dose tested in mice and rats (1825 mg/kg per day). Overdoses up to 31,500 mg of atovaquone have been reported. In one such patient who also took an unspecified dose of dapsone, methemoglobinemia occurred. Rash has also been reported after overdose.

DOSAGE AND ADMINISTRATION

Dosage: ***Prevention of PCP: Adults and Adolescents (13 to 16 Years):*** The recommended oral dose is 1500 mg (10 mL) once daily administered with a meal.

Treatment of Mild-to-Moderate PCP: Adults and Adolescents (13 to 16 Years): The recommended oral dose is 750 mg (5 mL) administered with meals twice daily for 21 days (total daily dose 1500 mg).

Note: Failure to administer MEPRON Suspension with meals may result in lower plasma atovaquone concentrations and may limit response to therapy (see CLINICAL PHARMACOLOGY and PRECAUTIONS).

Administration: ***Foil Pouch:*** Open pouch by removing tab at perforation and tear at notch. Take entire contents by mouth. Can be discharged into a dosing spoon or cup or directly into the mouth.

Bottle: SHAKE BOTTLE GENTLY BEFORE USING.

HOW SUPPLIED

MEPRON Suspension (bright yellow, citrus flavored) containing 750 mg atovaquone in each teaspoonful (5 mL).

Bottle of 210 mL with child-resistant cap (NDC 0173-0665-18).

Store at 15° to 25°C (59° to 77°F). DO NOT FREEZE. Dispense in tight container as defined in USP.

5-mL child-resistant foil pouch—unit dose pack of 42 (NDC 0173-0547-00).

Store at 15° to 25°C (59° to 77°F). DO NOT FREEZE.

[1](A-a)DO_2 = [(713 × FiO_2) − ($PaCO_2$/0.8)] − PaO_2 (mm Hg)

US Patent No. 5,053,432

US Patent No. 4,981,874 (Use Patent)

Glaxo Wellcome Inc., Research Triangle Park, NC 27709

January 1999/RL-655

Shown in Product Identification Guide, page 315

MYLERAN® ℞

[mī 'lə-răn"]

(busulfan)

2-mg Scored Tablets

> **WARNING:** *MYLERAN is a potent drug. It should not be used unless a diagnosis of chronic myelogenous leukemia has been adequately established and the responsible physician is knowledgeable in assessing response to chemotherapy.*
>
> *MYLERAN can induce severe bone marrow hypoplasia. Reduce or discontinue the dosage immediately at the first sign of any unusual depression of bone marrow function as reflected by an abnormal decrease in any of the formed elements of the blood. A bone marrow examination should be performed if the bone marrow status is uncertain.*
>
> *SEE WARNINGS FOR INFORMATION REGARDING BUSULFAN-INDUCED LEUKEMOGENESIS IN HUMANS.*

DESCRIPTION

MYLERAN (busulfan) is a bifunctional alkylating agent. Busulfan is known chemically as 1,4-butanediol dimethanesulfonate.

Busulfan is *not* a structural analog of the nitrogen mustards. MYLERAN is available in tablet form for oral administration. Each scored tablet contains 2 mg busulfan and the inactive ingredients magnesium stearate and sodium chloride.

The activity of busulfan in chronic myelogenous leukemia was first reported by D.A.G. Galton in 1953.

CLINICAL PHARMACOLOGY

No analytical method has been found which permits the quantitation of nonradiolabeled busulfan or its metabolites in biological tissues or plasma. All studies of the pharmacokinetics of busulfan in humans have employed radiolabeled drug using either sulfur-35 (labeling the "carrier" portion of the molecule) or carbon-14 or tritium in the alkane portion of the 4-carbon chain (labels in the "alkylating" portion of the molecule).

Studies with ^{35}S-busulfan: Following the intravenous administration of a single therapeutic dose of ^{35}S-busulfan, there was rapid disappearance of radioactivity from the blood; 90% to 95% of the ^{35}S-label disappeared within 3 to 5 minutes after injection. Thereafter, a constant, low level of radioactivity (1% to 3% of the injected dose) was maintained during the subsequent 48-hour period of observation. Following the oral administration of ^{35}S-busulfan, there was a lag period of ½ to 2 hours prior to the detection of radioactivity in the blood. However, at 4 hours the (low) level of circulating radioactivity was comparable to that obtained following intravenous administration.

After either oral or intravenous administration of ^{35}S-busulfan to humans, 45% to 60% of the radioactivity was recovered in the urine in the 48 hours after administration; the majority of the total urinary excretion occurred in the first 24 hours. In humans, over 95% of the urinary sulfur-35 occurs as ^{35}S-methanesulfonic acid.

The fact that urinary recovery of sulfur-35 was equivalent, irrespective of whether the drug was given intravenously or orally, suggests virtually complete absorption by the oral route.

Studies with ^{14}C-busulfan: Oral and intravenous administration of 1,4-^{14}C-busulfan showed the same rapid initial disappearance of plasma radioactivity with a subsequent low-level plateau as observed following the administration of ^{35}S-labeled drug. Cumulative radioactivity in the urine after 48 hours was 25% to 30% of the administered dose (contrasting with 45% to 60% for ^{35}S-busulfan) and suggests a slower excretion of the alkylating portion of the molecule and its metabolites than for the sulfonoxymethyl moieties. Regardless of the route of administration, 1,4-^{14}C-busulfan yielded a complex mixture of at least 12 radiolabeled metabolites in urine; the main metabolite being 3-hydroxytetrahydrothiophene-1,1-dioxide.

Studies with ^{3}H-busulfan: Human pharmacokinetic studies have been conducted employing busulfan labeled with tritium on the tetramethylene chain. These experiments confirmed a rapid initial clearance of the radioactivity from plasma, irrespective of whether the drug was given orally or intravenously, and showed a gradual accumulation of radioactivity in the plasma after repeated doses. Urinary excretion of less than 50% of the total dose given suggested a slow elimination of the metabolic products from the body.

There is no experience with the use of dialysis in an attempt to modify the clinical toxicity of busulfan. One technical difficulty would derive from the extremely poor water solubility of busulfan. Additionally, all studies of the metabolism of busulfan employing radiolabeled materials indicate rapid chemical reactivity of the parent compound with prolonged retention of some of the metabolites (particularly the metabolites arising from the "alkylating" portion of the molecule). The effectiveness of dialysis at removing significant quantities of unreacted drug would be expected to be minimal in such a situation.

No information is available regarding the penetration of busulfan into brain or cerebrospinal fluid.

Biochemical Pharmacology: In aqueous media, busulfan undergoes a wide range of nucleophilic substitution reactions. While this chemical reactivity is relatively non-specific, alkylation of the DNA is felt to be an important biological mechanism for its cytotoxic effect. Coliphage T7 exposed to busulfan was found to have the DNA crosslinked by intrastrand crosslinkages, but no interstrand linkages were found.

The metabolic fate of busulfan has been studied in rats and humans using ^{14}C- and ^{35}S-labeled materials. In humans, as in the rat, almost all of the radioactivity in ^{35}S-labeled busulfan is excreted in the urine in the form of ^{35}S-methanesulfonic acid. No unchanged drug was found in human urine, although a small amount has been reported in rat urine. Roberts and Warwick demonstrated that the formation of methanesulfonic acid in vivo in the rat is not due to a simple hydrolysis of busulfan to 1,4-butanediol, since only about 4% of 2,3-^{14}C-busulfan was excreted as carbon dioxide whereas 2,3-^{14}C-1,4-butanediol was converted almost exclusively to carbon dioxide. The predominant reaction of busulfan in the rat is the alkylation of sulfhydryl groups (particularly cysteine and cysteine-containing compounds) to produce a cyclic sulfonium compound which is the precursor of the major urinary metabolite of the 4-carbon portion of the molecule, 3-hydroxytetrahydrothiophene-1,1-dioxide. This has been termed a "sulfur-stripping" action of busulfan and it may modify the function of certain sulfur-containing amino acids, polypeptides, and proteins; whether this action makes an important contribution to the cytotoxicity of busulfan is unknown.

The biochemical basis for acquired resistance to busulfan is largely a matter of speculation. Although altered transport of busulfan into the cell is one possibility, increased intracellular inactivation of the drug before it reaches the DNA is also possible. Experiments with other alkylating agents have shown that resistance to this class of compounds may reflect an acquired ability of the resistant cell to repair alkylation damage more effectively.

Clinical Studies: Although not curative, busulfan reduces the total granulocyte mass, relieves symptoms of the disease, and improves the clinical state of the patient. Approximately 90% of adults with previously untreated chronic myelogenous leukemia will obtain hematologic remission with regression or stabilization of organomegaly following the use of busulfan. It has been shown to be superior to splenic irradiation with respect to survival times and maintenance of hemoglobin levels, and to be equivalent to irradiation at controlling splenomegaly.

It is not clear whether busulfan unequivocally prolongs the survival of responding patients beyond the 31 months experienced by an untreated group of historical controls. Median survival figures of 31 to 42 months have been reported for several groups of patients treated with busulfan, but concurrent control groups of comparable, untreated patients are not available. The median survival figures reported from different studies will be influenced by the percentage of "poor risk" patients initially entered into the particular study. Patients who are alive 2 years following the diagnosis of chronic myelogenous leukemia, and who have been treated during that period with busulfan, are estimated to have a mean annual mortality rate during the second to fifth year which is approximately two thirds that of patients

Table 11: Treatment-Emergent Laboratory Test Abnormalities in the Pentamidine Comparative PCP Treatment Study

Laboratory Test Abnormality	Percentage of Patients Developing a Laboratory Test Abnormality	
	MEPRON	Pentamidine
Anemia (Hgb<8.0 g/dL)	4%	9%
Neutropenia (ANC<750 cells/mm^3)	5%	9%
Hyponatremia (<0.96 × LLN)	10%	10%
Hyperkalemia (>1.18 × ULN)	0%	5%
Alkaline Phosphatase (>2.5 ×ULN)	5%	2%
Hyperglycemia (>1.8 × ULN)	9%	13%
Elevated AST (>5 × ULN)	0%	5%
Elevated Amylase (>1.5 × ULN)	8%	4%
Elevated Creatinine (>1.5 × ULN)	0%	7%

ULN = upper limit of normal range.
LLN = lower limit of normal range.

who received either no treatment, conventional x-ray or ^{32}P-irradiation, or chemotherapy with minimally active drugs.

Busulfan is clearly less effective in patients with chronic myelogenous leukemia who lack the Philadelphia (Ph^1) chromosome. Also, the so-called "juvenile" type of chronic myelogenous leukemia, typically occurring in young children and associated with the absence of a Philadelphia chromosome, responds poorly to busulfan. The drug is of no benefit in patients whose chronic myelogenous leukemia has entered a "blastic" phase.

MYLERAN should not be used in patients whose chronic myelogenous leukemia has demonstrated prior resistance to this drug.

MYLERAN is of no value in chronic lymphocytic leukemia, acute leukemia, or in the "blastic crisis" of chronic myelogenous leukemia.

INDICATIONS AND USAGE

MYLERAN (busulfan) is indicated for the palliative treatment of chronic myelogenous (myeloid, myelocytic, granulocytic) leukemia.

CONTRAINDICATIONS

MYLERAN is contraindicated in patients in whom a definitive diagnosis of chronic myelogenous leukemia has not been firmly established.

MYLERAN is contraindicated in patients who have previously suffered a hypersensitivity reaction to busulfan or any other component of the preparation.

WARNINGS

The most frequent, serious side effect of treatment with busulfan is the induction of bone marrow failure (which may or may not be anatomically hypoplastic) resulting in severe pancytopenia. The pancytopenia caused by busulfan may be more prolonged than that induced with other alkylating agents. It is generally felt that the usual cause of busulfan-induced pancytopenia is the failure to stop administration of the drug soon enough; individual idiosyncrasy to the drug does not seem to be an important factor. *MYLERAN should be used with extreme caution and exceptional vigilance in patients whose bone marrow reserve may have been compromised by prior irradiation or chemotherapy, or whose marrow function is recovering from previous cytotoxic therapy.* Although recovery from busulfan-induced pancytopenia may take from 1 month to 2 years, this complication is potentially reversible, and the patient should be vigorously supported through any period of severe pancytopenia.

A rare, important complication of busulfan therapy is the development of bronchopulmonary dysplasia with pulmonary fibrosis. Symptoms have been reported to occur within 8 months to 10 years after initiation of therapy—the average duration of therapy being 4 years. The histologic findings associated with "busulfan lung" mimic those seen following pulmonary irradiation. Clinically, patients have reported the insidious onset of cough, dyspnea, and low-grade fever. In some cases, however, onset of symptoms may be acute. Pulmonary function studies have revealed diminished diffusion capacity and decreased pulmonary compliance. It is important to exclude more common conditions (such as opportunistic infections or leukemic infiltration of the lungs) with appropriate diagnostic techniques. If measures such as sputum cultures, virologic studies, and exfoliative cytology fail to establish an etiology for the pulmonary infiltrates, lung biopsy may be necessary to establish the diagnosis. Treatment of established busulfan-induced pulmonary fibrosis is unsatisfactory; in most cases the patients have died within 6 months after the diagnosis was established. There is no specific therapy for this complication. MYLERAN should be discontinued if this lung toxicity develops. The administration of corticosteroids has been suggested, but the results have not been impressive or uniformly successful.

Busulfan may cause cellular dysplasia in many organs in addition to the lung. Cytologic abnormalities characterized by giant, hyperchromatic nuclei have been reported in lymph nodes, pancreas, thyroid, adrenal glands, liver, and bone marrow. This cytologic dysplasia may be severe enough to cause difficulty in interpretation of exfoliative cytologic examinations from the lung, bladder, breast, and the uterine cervix.

In addition to the widespread epithelial dysplasia that has been observed during busulfan therapy, chromosome aberrations have been reported in cells from patients receiving busulfan.

Busulfan is mutagenic in mice and, possibly, in humans.

Malignant tumors and acute leukemias have been reported in patients who have received busulfan therapy, and this drug may be a human carcinogen. The World Health Organization has concluded that there is a causal relationship between busulfan exposure and the development of secondary malignancies. Four cases of acute leukemia occurred among 243 patients treated with busulfan as adjuvant chemotherapy following surgical resection of bronchogenic carcinoma. All four cases were from a subgroup of 19 of these 243 patients who developed pancytopenia while taking busulfan 5 to 8 years before leukemia became clinically apparent. These findings suggest that busulfan is leukemogenic, although its mode of action is uncertain.

Ovarian suppression and amenorrhea with menopausal symptoms commonly occur during busulfan therapy in premenopausal patients. Busulfan has been associated with ovarian failure including failure to achieve puberty in females. Busulfan interferes with spermatogenesis in experimental animals, and there have been clinical reports of sterility, azoospermia, and testicular atrophy in male patients.

Hepatic veno-occlusive disease, which may be life-threatening, has been reported in patients receiving busulfan, usually in combination with cyclophosphamide or other chemotherapeutic agents prior to bone marrow transplantation. Possible risk factors for the development of hepatic veno-occlusive disease include: total busulfan dose exceeding 16 mg/kg based on ideal body weight, and concurrent use of multiple alkylating agents. A clear cause-and-effect relationship with busulfan has not been demonstrated. Periodic measurement of serum transaminases, alkaline phosphatase, and bilirubin is indicated for early detection of hepatotoxicity.

Cardiac tamponade has been reported in a small number of patients with thalassemia (2% in one series) who received busulfan and cyclophosphamide as the preparatory regimen for bone marrow transplantation. In this series, the cardiac tamponade was often fatal. Abdominal pain and vomiting preceded the tamponade in most patients.

Pregnancy: Pregnancy Category D. Busulfan may cause fetal harm when administered to a pregnant woman. Although there have been a number of cases reported where apparently normal children have been born after busulfan treatment during pregnancy, one case has been cited where a malformed baby was delivered by a mother treated with busulfan. During the pregnancy that resulted in the malformed infant, the mother received x-ray therapy early in the first trimester, mercaptopurine until the third month, then busulfan until delivery. In pregnant rats, busulfan produces sterility in both male and female offspring due to the absence of germinal cells in testes and ovaries. Germinal cell aplasia or sterility in offspring of mothers receiving busulfan during pregnancy has not been reported in humans. There are no adequate and well-controlled studies in pregnant women. If this drug is used during pregnancy, or if the patient becomes pregnant while taking this drug, the patient should be apprised of the potential hazard to the fetus. Women of childbearing potential should be advised to avoid becoming pregnant.

PRECAUTIONS

General: The most consistent, dose-related toxicity is bone marrow suppression. This may be manifest by anemia, leukopenia, thrombocytopenia, or any combination of these. It is imperative that patients be instructed to report promptly the development of fever, sore throat, signs of local infection, bleeding from any site, or symptoms suggestive of anemia. Any one of these findings may indicate busulfan toxicity; however, they may also indicate transformation of the disease to an acute "blastic" form. Since busulfan may have a delayed effect, it is important to withdraw the medication temporarily at the first sign of an abnormally large or exceptionally rapid fall in any of the formed elements of the blood. *Patients should never be allowed to take the drug without close medical supervision.*

Seizures have been reported in patients receiving busulfan. As with any potentially epileptogenic drug, caution should be exercised when administering busulfan to patients with a history of seizure disorder, head trauma, or receiving other potentially epileptogenic drugs. Some investigators have used prophylactic anticonvulsant therapy in this setting.

Information for Patients: Patients beginning therapy with busulfan should be informed of the importance of having periodic blood counts and to immediately report any unusual fever or bleeding. Aside from the major toxicity of myelosuppression, patients should be instructed to report any difficulty in breathing, persistent cough, or congestion. They should be told that diffuse pulmonary fibrosis is an infrequent, but serious and potentially life-threatening, complication of long-term busulfan therapy. Patients should be alerted to report any signs of abrupt weakness, unusual fatigue, anorexia, weight loss, nausea and vomiting, and melanoderma that could be associated with a syndrome resembling adrenal insufficiency. Patients should never be allowed to take the drug without medical supervision and they should be informed that other encountered toxicities to busulfan include infertility, amenorrhea, skin hyperpigmentation, drug hypersensitivity, dryness of the mucous membranes, and rarely, cataract formation. Women of childbearing potential should be advised to avoid becoming pregnant. The increased risk of a second malignancy should be explained to the patient.

Laboratory Tests: It is recommended that evaluation of the hemoglobin or hematocrit, total white blood cell count and differential count, and quantitative platelet count be obtained weekly while the patient is on busulfan therapy. In cases where the cause of fluctuation in the formed elements of the peripheral blood is obscure, bone marrow examination may be useful for evaluation of marrow status. A decision to increase, decrease, continue, or discontinue a given dose of busulfan must be based not only on the absolute hematologic values, but also on the rapidity with which changes are occurring. The dosage of busulfan may need to be reduced if this agent is combined with other drugs whose primary toxicity is myelosuppression. Occasional patients may be unusually sensitive to busulfan administered at standard dosage and suffer neutropenia or thrombocytopenia after a relatively short exposure to the drug. Busulfan should not be used where facilities for complete blood counts, including quantitative platelet counts, are not available at weekly (or more frequent) intervals.

Drug Interactions: Busulfan may cause additive myelosuppression when used with other myelosuppressive drugs.

In one study, 12 of approximately 330 patients receiving continuous busulfan and thioguanine therapy for treatment of chronic myelogenous leukemia were found to have portal hypertension and esophageal varices associated with abnormal liver function tests. Subsequent liver biopsies were performed in four of these patients, all of which showed evidence of nodular regenerative hyperplasia. Duration of combination therapy prior to the appearance of esophageal varices ranged from 6 to 45 months. With the present analysis of the data, no cases of hepatotoxicity have appeared in the busulfan-alone arm of the study. Long-term continuous therapy with thioguanine and busulfan should be used with caution.

Busulfan-induced pulmonary toxicity may be additive to the effects produced by other cytotoxic agents. Patients should be monitored for signs of busulfan toxicity when itraconazole is used concomitantly with MYLERAN.

Carcinogenesis, Mutagenesis, Impairment of Fertility: See WARNINGS section. The World Health Organization has concluded that there is a causal relationship between busulfan exposure and the development of secondary malignancies.

Pregnancy: ***Teratogenic Effects:*** Pregnancy Category D. See WARNINGS section.

Nonteratogenic Effects: There have been reports in the literature of small infants being born after the mothers received busulfan during pregnancy, in particular, during the third trimester. One case was reported where an infant had mild anemia and neutropenia at birth after busulfan was administered to the mother from the eighth week of pregnancy to term.

Nursing Mothers: It is not known whether this drug is excreted in human milk. Because of the potential for tumorigenicity shown for busulfan in animal and human studies, a decision should be made whether to discontinue nursing or to discontinue the drug, taking into account the importance of the drug to the mother.

Pediatric Use: See INDICATIONS AND USAGE and DOSAGE AND ADMINISTRATION sections.

ADVERSE REACTIONS

Hematological Effects: The most frequent, serious, toxic effect of busulfan is myelosuppression resulting in leukopenia, thrombocytopenia, and anemia. Myelosuppression is most frequently the result of a failure to discontinue dosage in the face of an undetected decrease in leukocyte or platelet counts.

Pulmonary: Interstitial pulmonary fibrosis has been reported rarely, but it is a clinically significant adverse effect when observed and calls for immediate discontinuation of further administration of the drug. The role of corticosteroids in arresting or reversing the fibrosis has been reported to be beneficial in some cases and without effect in others.

Cardiac: Cardiac tamponade has been reported in a small number of patients with thalassemia who received busulfan and cyclophosphamide as the preparatory regimen for bone marrow transplantation (see WARNINGS).

One case of endocardial fibrosis has been reported in a 79-year-old woman who received a total dose of 7200 mg of busulfan over a period of 9 years for the management of chronic myelogenous leukemia. At autopsy, she was found to have endocardial fibrosis of the left ventricle in addition to interstitial pulmonary fibrosis.

Ocular: Busulfan is capable of inducing cataracts in rats and there have been several reports indicating that this is a rare complication in humans.

Dermatologic: Hyperpigmentation is the most common adverse skin reaction and occurs in 5% to 10% of patients, particularly those with a dark complexion.

Metabolic: In a few cases, a clinical syndrome closely resembling adrenal insufficiency and characterized by weakness, severe fatigue, anorexia, weight loss, nausea and vomiting, and melanoderma has developed after prolonged busulfan therapy. The symptoms have sometimes been reversible when busulfan was withdrawn. Adrenal responsiveness to exogenously administered ACTH has usually been normal. However, pituitary function testing with metyrapone revealed a blunted urinary 17-hydroxycorticosteroid excretion in two patients. Following the discontinuation of busulfan (which was associated with clinical improvement), rechallenge with metyrapone revealed normal pituitary-adrenal function.

Hyperuricemia and/or hyperuricosuria are not uncommon in patients with chronic myelogenous leukemia. Additional rapid destruction of granulocytes may accompany the initiation of chemotherapy and increase the urate pool. Adverse effects can be minimized by increased hydration, urine alkalinization, and the prophylactic administration of a xanthine oxidase inhibitor such as allopurinol.

Hepatic Effects: Esophageal varices have been reported in patients receiving continuous busulfan and thioguanine therapy for treatment of chronic myelogenous leukemia (see PRECAUTIONS: Drug Interactions). Hepatic veno-occlu-

Continued on next page

This product information is based on labeling in effect on June 23, 2000. For further information, contact via direct mail, phone, or web site. Medical Information, Glaxo Wellcome Inc., PO Box 13398, Research Triangle Park, NC 27709. Healthcare Professionals (Medical Information): 800-334-0089. Patients (Customer Response Center): 1-888-825-5249. Glaxo Wellcome Corporate Web Site: www.glaxowellcome.com

Myleran—Cont.

sive disease has been observed in patients receiving busulfan (see WARNINGS).

Miscellaneous: Other reported adverse reactions include: urticaria, erythema multiforme, erythema nodosum, alopecia, porphyria cutanea tarda, excessive dryness and fragility of the skin with anhidrosis, dryness of the oral mucous membranes and cheilosis, gynecomastia, cholestatic jaundice, and myasthenia gravis. Most of these are single case reports, and in many, a clear cause-and-effect relationship with busulfan has not been demonstrated.

Seizures (see PRECAUTIONS: General) have been observed in patients receiving higher than recommended doses of busulfan.

Observed During Clinical Practice: The following events have been identified during post-approval use of busulfan. Because they are reported voluntarily from a population of unknown size, estimates of frequency cannot be made. These events have been chosen for inclusion due to a combination of their seriousness, frequency of reporting, or potential causal connection to busulfan.

Blood and Lymphatic: Aplastic anemia.

Eye: Cataracts, corneal thinning, and lens changes.

Hepatobiliary Tract and Pancreas: Centrilobular sinusoidal fibrosis, hepatic veno-occlusive disease, hepatocellular atrophy, hepatocellular necrosis, and hyperbilirubinemia (see WARNINGS).

Non-site Specific: Infection, mucositis, and sepsis.

Respiratory: Pneumonia.

Skin: Rash. An increased local cutaneous reaction has been observed in patients receiving radiotherapy soon after busulfan.

OVERDOSAGE

There is no known antidote to busulfan. The principal toxic effect is on the bone marrow. The hematologic status should be closely monitored and vigorous supportive measures instituted if necessary. Induction of vomiting or gastric lavage followed by administration of charcoal would be indicated if ingestion were recent. It is not known whether busulfan is dialyzable (see CLINICAL PHARMACOLOGY).

Gastrointestinal toxicity with mucositis, nausea, vomiting, and diarrhea has been observed when MYLERAN was used in association with bone marrow transplantation.

Oral LD_{50} single doses in mice are 120 mg/kg. Two distinct types of toxic response are seen at median lethal doses given intraperitoneally. Within a matter of hours there are signs of stimulation of the central nervous system with convulsions and death on the first day. Mice are more sensitive to this effect than are rats. With doses at the LD_{50} there is also delayed death due to damage to the bone marrow. At three times the LD_{50}, atrophy of the mucosa of the large intestine is found after a week, whereas that of the small intestine is little affected. After doses in the order of 10 times those used therapeutically were added to the diet of rats, irreversible cataracts were produced after several weeks. Small doses had no such effect.

DOSAGE AND ADMINISTRATION

Busulfan is administered orally. The usual adult dose range for *remission induction* is 4 to 8 mg, total dose, daily. Dosing on a weight basis is the same for both pediatric patients and adults, approximately 60 mcg/kg of body weight or 1.8 mg/m^2 of body surface, daily. Since the rate of fall of the leukocyte count is dose related, daily doses exceeding 4 mg per day should be reserved for patients with the most compelling symptoms; the greater the total daily dose, the greater is the possibility of inducing bone marrow aplasia.

A decrease in the leukocyte count is not usually seen during the first 10 to 15 days of treatment; the leukocyte count may actually increase during this period and it should not be interpreted as resistance to the drug, nor should the dose be increased. Since the leukocyte count may continue to fall for more than 1 month after discontinuing the drug, it is important that busulfan be discontinued *prior* to the total leukocyte count falling into the normal range. When the total leukocyte count has declined to approximately 15,000/mcL, the drug should be withheld.

With a constant dose of busulfan, the total leukocyte count declines exponentially; a weekly plot of the leukocyte count on semi-logarithmic graph paper aids in predicting the time when therapy should be discontinued. With the recommended dose of busulfan, a normal leukocyte count is usually achieved in 12 to 20 weeks.

During remission, the patient is examined at monthly intervals and treatment resumed with the induction dosage when the total leukocyte count reaches approximately 50,000/mcL. When remission is shorter than 3 months, maintenance therapy of 1 to 3 mg daily may be advisable in order to keep the hematological status under control and prevent rapid relapse.

Procedures for proper handling and disposal of anticancer drugs should be considered. Several guidelines on this subject have been published.[1-7]

There is no general agreement that all of the procedures recommended in the guidelines are necessary or appropriate.

HOW SUPPLIED

White, scored tablets containing 2 mg busulfan, imprinted with "MYLERAN" and "K2A" on each tablet; bottle of 25 (NDC 0173-0713-25).

Store at 15° to 25°C (59° to 77°F) in a dry place.

REFERENCES:

1. Recommendations for the safe handling of parenteral antineoplastic drugs. Washington, DC: Division of Safety, National Institutes of Health; 1983. US Dept of Health and Human Services, Public Health Service publication NIH 83-2621.
2. AMA Council on Scientific Affairs. Guidelines for handling parenteral antineoplastics. *JAMA*. 1985;253:1590-1591.
3. National Study Commission on Cytotoxic Exposure. Recommendations for handling cytotoxic agents. 1987. Available from Louis P. Jeffrey, Chairman, National Study Commission on Cytotoxic Exposure. Massachusetts College of Pharmacy and Allied Health Sciences, 179 Longwood Avenue, Boston, MA 02115.
4. Clinical Oncological Society of Australia. Guidelines and recommendations for safe handling of antineoplastic agents. *Med J Australia*. 1983;1:426-428.
5. Jones RB, Frank R, Mass T. Safe handling of chemotherapeutic agents: a report from the Mount Sinai Medical Center. *CA-A Cancer J for Clin*. 1983;33:258-263.
6. American Society of Hospital Pharmacists. ASHP technical assistance bulletin on handling cytotoxic and hazardous drugs. *Am J Hosp Pharm*. 1990;47:1033-1049.
7. Controlling Occupational Exposure to Hazardous Drugs. (OSHA Work-Practice Guidelines.) *Am J. Health-Syst Pharm*. 1996:53:1669-1685.

Manufactured by Catalytica Pharmaceuticals, Inc.
Greenville, NC 27834
for Glaxo Wellcome Inc., Research Triangle Park, NC 27709

May 2000/RL-822

Shown in Product Identification Guide, page 316

NAVELBINE® ℞

[na 'vəl-bēn]
(vinorelbine tartrate)
Injection

> **WARNING:** NAVELBINE (vinorelbine tartrate) Injection should be administered under the supervision of a physician experienced in the use of cancer chemotherapeutic agents. This product is for intravenous (IV) use only. Intrathecal administration of other vinca alkaloids has resulted in death. Syringes containing this product should be labeled "WARNING—FOR IV USE ONLY. FATAL if given intrathecally."
>
> Severe granulocytopenia resulting in increased susceptibility to infection may occur. Granulocyte counts should be ≥1000 cells/mm^3 prior to the administration of NAVELBINE. The dosage should be adjusted according to complete blood counts with differentials obtained on the day of treatment.
>
> Caution—It is extremely important that the intravenous needle or catheter be properly positioned before NAVELBINE is injected. Administration of NAVELBINE may result in extravasation causing local tissue necrosis and/or thrombophlebitis (see DOSAGE AND ADMINISTRATION: Administration Precautions).

DESCRIPTION

NAVELBINE (vinorelbine tartrate) Injection is for intravenous administration. Each vial contains vinorelbine tartrate equivalent to 10 mg (1-mL vial) or 50 mg (5-mL vial) vinorelbine in Water for Injection. No preservatives or other additives are present. The aqueous solution is sterile and nonpyrogenic.

Vinorelbine tartrate is a semi-synthetic vinca alkaloid with antitumor activity. The chemical name is 3′,4′-didehydro-4′-deoxy-*C*′-norvincaleukoblastine [*R*-(*R**,*R**)-2,3-dihydroxybutanedioate (1:2)(salt)].

Vinorelbine tartrate is a white to yellow or light brown amorphous powder with the molecular formula $C_{45}H_{54}N_4O_8 \cdot 2C_4H_6O_6$ and molecular weight of 1079.12. The aqueous solubility is >1000 mg/mL in distilled water. The pH of NAVELBINE Injection is approximately 3.5.

CLINICAL PHARMACOLOGY

Vinorelbine is a vinca alkaloid that interferes with microtubule assembly. The vinca alkaloids are structurally similar compounds comprised of 2 multiringed units, vindoline and catharanthine. Unlike other vinca alkaloids, the catharanthine unit is the site of structural modification for vinorelbine. The antitumor activity of vinorelbine is thought to be due primarily to inhibition of mitosis at metaphase through its interaction with tubulin. Like other vinca alkaloids, vinorelbine may also interfere with: 1) amino acid, cyclic AMP, and glutathione metabolism, 2) calmodulin-dependent Ca^{++}-transport ATPase activity, 3) cellular respiration, and 4) nucleic acid and lipid biosynthesis. In intact tectal plates from mouse embryos, vinorelbine, vincristine, and vinblastine inhibited mitotic microtubule formation at the same concentration (2 μM), inducing a blockade of cells at metaphase. Vincristine produced depolymerization of axonal microtubules at 5 μM, but vinblastine and vinorelbine did not have this effect until concentrations of 30 μM and 40 μM, respectively. These data suggest relative selectivity of vinorelbine for mitotic microtubules.

Pharmacokinetics: The pharmacokinetics of vinorelbine were studied in 49 patients who received doses of 30 mg/m^2 in 4 clinical trials. Doses were administered by 15- to 20-minute constant-rate infusions. Following intravenous administration, vinorelbine concentration in plasma decays in a triphasic manner. The initial rapid decline primarily represents distribution of drug to peripheral compartments followed by metabolism and excretion of the drug during subsequent phases. The prolonged terminal phase is due to relatively slow efflux of vinorelbine from peripheral compartments. The terminal phase half-life averages 27.7 to 43.6 hours and the mean plasma clearance ranges from 0.97 to 1.26 L/h per kg. Steady-state volume of distribution (V_{SS}) values range from 25.4 to 40.1 L/kg.

Vinorelbine demonstrated high binding to human platelets and lymphocytes. The free fraction was approximately 0.11 in pooled human plasma over a concentration range of 234 to 1169 ng/mL. The binding to plasma constituents in cancer patients ranged from 79.6% to 91.2%. Vinorelbine binding was not altered in the presence of cisplatin, 5-fluorouracil, or doxorubicin.

Vinorelbine undergoes substantial hepatic elimination in humans, with large amounts recovered in feces after intravenous administration to humans. Two metabolites of vinorelbine have been identified in human blood, plasma, and urine; vinorelbine N-oxide and deacetylvinorelbine. Deacetylvinorelbine has been demonstrated to be the primary metabolite of vinorelbine in humans, and has been shown to possess antitumor activity similar to vinorelbine. Therapeutic doses of NAVELBINE (30 mg/m^2) yield very small, if any, quantifiable levels of either metabolite in blood or urine. The metabolism of vinca alkaloids has been shown to be mediated by hepatic cytochrome P450 isoenzymes in the CYP3A subfamily. This metabolic pathway may be impaired in patients with hepatic dysfunction or who are taking concomitant potent inhibitors of these isoenzymes (see PRECAUTIONS). The effects of renal or hepatic dysfunction on the disposition of vinorelbine have not been assessed, but based on experience with other anticancer vinca alkaloids, dose adjustments are recommended for patients with impaired hepatic function (see DOSAGE AND ADMINISTRATION).

The disposition of radiolabeled vinorelbine given intravenously was studied in a limited number of patients. Approximately 18% and 46% of the administered dose was recovered in the urine and in the feces, respectively. Incomplete recovery in humans is consistent with results in animals where recovery is incomplete, even after prolonged sampling times. A separate study of the urinary excretion of vinorelbine using specific chromatographic analytical methodology showed that 10.9% ± 0.7% of a 30-mg/m^2 intravenous dose was excreted unchanged in the urine.

The influence of age on the pharmacokinetics of vinorelbine was examined using data from 44 cancer patients (average age, 56.7 ± 7.8 years; range, 41 to 74 years; with 12 patients ≥60 years and 6 patients ≥65 years) in 3 studies. CL (the mean plasma clearance), $t_{1/2}$ (the terminal phase half-life), and V_Z (the volume of distribution during terminal phase) were independent of age. A separate pharmacokinetic study was conducted in 10 elderly patients with metastatic breast cancer (age range, 66 to 81 years; 3 patients >75 years; normal liver function tests) receiving vinorelbine 30 mg/m^2 intravenously. CL, V_{ss}, and $t_{1/2}$ were similar to those reported for younger adult patients in previous studies. No relationship between age, systemic exposure ($AUC_{0-\infty}$) and hematological toxicity was observed.

The pharmacokinetics of vinorelbine are not influenced by the concurrent administration of cisplatin with NAVELBINE (see PRECAUTIONS: Drug Interactions).

Clinical Trials: Data from 2 controlled clinical studies (823 patients), as well as additional data from more than 100 patients enrolled in 2 uncontrolled clinical trials, support the use of NAVELBINE in patients with advanced nonsmall cell lung cancer (NSCLC). In a large European clinical trial, 612 patients with Stage III or IV NSCLC, no prior chemotherapy, and WHO Performance Status of 0, 1, or 2 were randomized to treatment with single-agent NAVELBINE (30 mg/m^2 per week), NAVELBINE (30 mg/m^2 per week) plus cisplatin (120 mg/m^2 days 1 and 29, then every 6 weeks), and vindesine (3 mg/m^2 per week for 7 weeks, then every other week) plus cisplatin (120 mg/m^2 days 1 and 29, then every 6 weeks). NAVELBINE plus cisplatin produced longer survival times than vindesine plus cisplatin (median survival 40 weeks versus 32 weeks, *P* = 0.03). The median survival time for patients receiving single-agent NAVELBINE was similar to that observed with vindesine plus cisplatin (31 weeks versus 32 weeks). The 1-year survival rates were 35% for NAVELBINE plus cisplatin, 27% for vindesine plus cisplatin, and 30% for single-agent NAVELBINE. The overall objective response rate (all partial responses) was significantly higher in the patients treated with NAVELBINE plus cisplatin (28%) than in those treated with vindesine plus cisplatin (19%, *P* = 0.03) and in those treated with single-agent NAVELBINE (14%, *P* <0.001). The response rates reported for vindesine plus cisplatin and single-agent NAVELBINE were not significantly different. Significantly less nausea, vomiting, alopecia, and neurotoxicity were observed in patients receiving single-agent NAVELBINE compared to those receiving the combination of vindesine and cisplatin.

Single-agent NAVELBINE was studied in a North American, randomized clinical trial in which patients with Stage IV NSCLC, no prior chemotherapy, and Karnofsky Performance Status ≥70 were treated with NAVELBINE (30 mg/

m²) weekly or 5-fluorouracil (5-FU) (425 mg/m² IV bolus) plus leucovorin (LV) (20 mg/m² IV bolus) daily for 5 days every 4 weeks. A total of 211 patients were randomized at a 2:1 ratio to NAVELBINE (143) or 5-FU/LV (68). NAVELBINE showed improved survival time compared to 5-FU/LV. In an intent-to-treat analysis, the median survival time for patients receiving NAVELBINE was 30 weeks and for those receiving 5-FU/LV was 22 weeks ($P = 0.06$). The 1-year survival rates were 24% (±4% SE) for NAVELBINE and 16% (±5% SE) for the 5-FU/LV group, using the Kaplan-Meier product-limit estimates. The median survival time with 5-FU/LV was similar to, or slightly better than, that usually observed in untreated patients with advanced NSCLC, suggesting that the difference was not related to some unknown detrimental effect of 5-FU/LV therapy. The response rates (all partial responses) for NAVELBINE and 5-FU/LV were 12% and 3%, respectively. Quality of life (QOL) was also an endpoint in this study. Patients completed a modified Southwest Oncology Group QOL questionnaire which assessed the domains of role functioning, physical functioning, symptom distress, and global QOL. Quality of life was not adversely affected by NAVELBINE when compared to control.

A dose-ranging study of NAVELBINE (20, 25, or 30 mg/m² per week) plus cisplatin (120 mg/m² days 1 and 29, then every 6 weeks) in 32 patients with NSCLC demonstrated a median survival of 44 weeks. There were no responses at the lowest dose level; the response rate was 33% in the 21 patients treated at the 2 highest dose levels.

INDICATIONS AND USAGE

NAVELBINE is indicated as a single agent or in combination with cisplatin for the first-line treatment of ambulatory patients with unresectable, advanced nonsmall cell lung cancer (NSCLC). In patients with Stage IV NSCLC, NAVELBINE is indicated as a single agent or in combination with cisplatin. In Stage III NSCLC, NAVELBINE is indicated in combination with cisplatin.

CONTRAINDICATIONS

Administration of NAVELBINE is contraindicated in patients with pretreatment granulocyte counts <1000 cells/mm³ (see WARNINGS).

WARNINGS

NAVELBINE should be administered in carefully adjusted doses by or under the supervision of a physician experienced in the use of cancer chemotherapeutic agents.

Patients treated with NAVELBINE should be frequently monitored for myelosuppression both during and after therapy. Granulocytopenia is dose-limiting. Granulocyte nadirs occur between 7 and 10 days after dosing with granulocyte count recovery usually within the following 7 to 14 days. Complete blood counts with differentials should be performed and results reviewed prior to administering each dose of NAVELBINE. NAVELBINE should not be administered to patients with granulocyte counts <1000 cells/mm³. Patients developing severe granulocytopenia should be monitored carefully for evidence of infection and/or fever. See DOSAGE AND ADMINISTRATION for recommended dose adjustments for granulocytopenia.

Acute shortness of breath and severe bronchospasm have been reported frequently, following the administration of NAVELBINE and other vinca alkaloids, most commonly when the vinca alkaloid was used in combination with mitomycin. These adverse events may require treatment with supplemental oxygen, bronchodilators, and/or corticosteroids, particularly when there is pre-existing pulmonary dysfunction. Interstitial pulmonary changes and/or acute respiratory distress syndrome, which in some cases was fatal, have been observed in patients receiving single-agent NAVELBINE. These symptoms generally occurred within a week of treatment. Patients with alterations in their baseline pulmonary symptoms or with new onset of dyspnea, cough, hypoxia, or other symptoms should be evaluated promptly.

NAVELBINE has been reported to cause severe constipation (e.g., grade 3-4), paralytic ileus, intestinal obstruction, necrosis, and/or perforation. Some events have been fatal.

Pregnancy: Pregnancy Category D. NAVELBINE may cause fetal harm if administered to a pregnant woman. A single dose of vinorelbine has been shown to be embryo- and/or fetotoxic in mice and rabbits at doses of 9 mg/m² and 5.5 mg/m², respectively (one third and one sixth the human dose). At nonmaternotoxic doses, fetal weight was reduced and ossification was delayed. There are no studies in pregnant women. If NAVELBINE is used during pregnancy, or if the patient becomes pregnant while receiving this drug, the patient should be apprised of the potential hazard to the fetus. Women of childbearing potential should be advised to avoid becoming pregnant during therapy with NAVELBINE.

PRECAUTIONS

General: Most drug-related adverse events of NAVELBINE are reversible. If severe adverse events occur, NAVELBINE should be reduced in dosage or discontinued and appropriate corrective measures taken. Reinstitution of therapy with NAVELBINE should be carried out with caution and alertness as to possible recurrence of toxicity.

NAVELBINE should be used with extreme caution in patients whose bone marrow reserve may have been compromised by prior irradiation or chemotherapy, or whose marrow function is recovering from the effects of previous chemotherapy (see DOSAGE AND ADMINISTRATION).

Table 1: Summary of Adverse Events in 365 Patients Receiving Single-Agent NAVELBINE*†

Adverse Event		All Patients (n = 365) (% Incidence)	NSCLC (n = 143) (% Incidence)
Bone Marrow			
Granulocytopenia	<2000 cells/mm³	90	80
	<500 cells/mm³	36	29
Leukopenia	<4000 cells/mm³	92	81
	<1000 cells/mm³	15	12
Thrombocytopenia	<100,000 cells/mm³	5	4
	<50,000 cells/mm³	1	1
Anemia	<11 g/dL	83	77
	<8 g/dL	9	1
Hospitalizations due to granulocytopenic complications		9	8

Adverse Event	All Grades (% Incidence) All Patients	All Grades NSCLC	Grade 3 (% Incidence) All Patients	Grade 3 NSCLC	Grade 4 (% Incidence) All Patients	Grade 4 NSCLC
Clinical Chemistry Elevations						
Total Bilirubin (n = 351)	13	9	4	3	3	2
SGOT (n = 346)	67	54	5	2	1	1
General						
Asthenia	36	27	7	5	0	0
Injection Site Reactions	28	38	2	5	0	0
Injection Site Pain	16	13	2	1	0	0
Phlebitis	7	10	<1	1	0	0
Digestive						
Nausea	44	34	2	1	0	0
Vomiting	20	15	2	1	0	0
Constipation	35	29	3	2	0	0
Diarrhea	17	13	1	1	0	0
Peripheral Neuropathy‡	25	20	1	1	<1	0
Dyspnea	7	3	2	2	1	0
Alopecia	12	12	≤1	1	0	0

* None of the reported toxicities were influenced by age. Grade based on modified criteria from the National Cancer Institute.

† Patients with NSCLC had not received prior chemotherapy. The majority of the remaining patients had received prior chemotherapy.

‡ Incidence of paresthesia plus hypesthesia.

Administration of NAVELBINE to patients with prior radiation therapy may result in radiation recall reactions (see ADVERSE REACTIONS and Drug Interactions).

Patients with a prior history or pre-existing neuropathy, regardless of etiology, should be monitored for new or worsening signs and symptoms of neuropathy while receiving NAVELBINE.

Care must be taken to avoid contamination of the eye with concentrations of NAVELBINE used clinically. Severe irritation of the eye has been reported with accidental exposure to another vinca alkaloid. If exposure occurs, the eye should immediately be thoroughly flushed with water.

Information for Patients: Patients should be informed that the major acute toxicities of NAVELBINE are related to bone marrow toxicity, specifically granulocytopenia with increased susceptibility to infection. They should be advised to report fever or chills immediately. Women of childbearing potential should be advised to avoid becoming pregnant during treatment. Patients should be advised to contact their physician if they experience increased shortness of breath, cough, or other new pulmonary symptoms, or if they experience symptoms of abdominal pain or constipation.

Laboratory Tests: Since dose-limiting clinical toxicity is the result of depression of the white blood cell count, it is imperative that complete blood counts with differentials be obtained and reviewed on the day of treatment prior to each dose of NAVELBINE (see ADVERSE REACTIONS: Hematologic).

Hepatic: There is no evidence that the toxicity of NAVELBINE is enhanced in patients with elevated liver enzymes. No data are available for patients with severe baseline cholestasis, but the liver plays an important role in the metabolism of NAVELBINE. Because clinical experience in patients with severe liver disease is limited, caution should be exercised when administering NAVELBINE to patients with severe hepatic injury or impairment (see DOSAGE AND ADMINISTRATION).

Drug Interactions: Acute pulmonary reactions have been reported with NAVELBINE and other anticancer vinca alkaloids used in conjunction with mitomycin. Although the pharmacokinetics of vinorelbine are not influenced by the concurrent administration of cisplatin, the incidence of granulocytopenia with NAVELBINE used in combination with cisplatin is significantly higher than with single-agent NAVELBINE. Patients who receive NAVELBINE and paclitaxel, either concomitantly or sequentially, should be monitored for signs and symptoms of neuropathy. Administration of NAVELBINE to patients with prior or concomitant radiation therapy may result in radiosensitizing effects.

Caution should be exercised in patients concurrently taking drugs known to inhibit drug metabolism by hepatic cytochrome P450 isoenzymes in the CYP3A subfamily, or in patients with hepatic dysfunction. Concurrent administration of vinorelbine tartrate with an inhibitor of this metabolic pathway may cause an earlier onset and/or an increased severity of side effects.

Carcinogenesis, Mutagenesis, Impairment of Fertility: The carcinogenic potential of NAVELBINE has not been studied. Vinorelbine has been shown to affect chromosome number and possibly structure in vivo (polyploidy in bone marrow cells from Chinese hamsters and a positive micronucleus test in mice). It was not mutagenic in the Ames test and gave inconclusive results in the mouse lymphoma TK Locus assay. The significance of these or other short-term test results for human risk is unknown. Vinorelbine did not affect fertility to a statistically significant extent when administered to rats on either a once-weekly (9 mg/m², approximately one third the human dose) or alternate-day schedule (4.2 mg/m², approximately one seventh the human dose) prior to and during mating. However, biweekly administration for 13 or 26 weeks in the rat at 2.1 and 7.2 mg/m² (approximately one fifteenth and one fourth the human dose) resulted in decreased spermatogenesis and prostate/seminal vesicle secretion.

Pregnancy: Pregnancy Category D. See WARNINGS section.

Nursing Mothers: It is not known whether the drug is excreted in human milk. Because many drugs are excreted in human milk and because of the potential for serious adverse reactions in nursing infants from NAVELBINE, it is recommended that nursing be discontinued in women who are receiving therapy with NAVELBINE.

Pediatric Use: Safety and effectiveness in pediatric patients have not been established.

Geriatric Use: Of the total number of patients in North American clinical studies of IV NAVELBINE, approximately one third were 65 years of age or greater. No overall differences in effectiveness or safety were observed between these patients and younger patients. Other reported clinical experience has not identified differences in responses between the elderly and younger adult patients, but greater sensitivity of some older individuals cannot be ruled out. The pharmacokinetics of vinorelbine in elderly and younger adult patients are similar (see CLINICAL PHARMACOLOGY).

ADVERSE REACTIONS

Granulocytopenia is the major dose-limiting toxicity with NAVELBINE. Dose adjustments are required for hematologic toxicity and hepatic insufficiency (see DOSAGE AND ADMINISTRATION).

Continued on next page

This product information is based on labeling in effect on June 23, 2000. For further information, contact via direct mail, phone, or web site. Medical Information, Glaxo Wellcome Inc., PO Box 13398, Research Triangle Park, NC 27709. Healthcare Professionals (Medical Information): 800-334-0089. Patients (Customer Response Center): 1-888-825-5249. Glaxo Wellcome Corporate Web Site: www.glaxowellcome.com

Navelbine—Cont.

Data in the following table are based on the experience of 365 patients (143 patients with NSCLC; 222 patients with advanced breast cancer) treated with IV NAVELBINE as a single agent in 3 clinical studies. The dosing schedule in each study was 30 mg/m^2 NAVELBINE on a weekly basis. [See table 1 at top of previous page]

Hematologic: Granulocytopenia was the major dose-limiting toxicity with NAVELBINE; it was generally reversible and not cumulative over time. Granulocyte nadirs occurred 7 to 10 days after the dose, with granulocyte recovery usually within the following 7 to 14 days. Granulocytopenia resulted in hospitalizations for fever and/or sepsis in 8% of patients. Septic deaths occurred in approximately 1% of patients. Prophylactic hematologic growth factors have not been routinely used with NAVELBINE. If medically necessary, growth factors may be administered at recommended doses no earlier than 24 hours after the administration of cytotoxic chemotherapy. Growth factors should not be administered in the period 24 hours before the administration of chemotherapy.

Grade 3 or 4 anemia occurred in 1% of patients, although blood products were administered to 18% of patients who received NAVELBINE. Grade 3 or 4 thrombocytopenia was reported in 1% of patients.

Neurologic: Mild to moderate peripheral neuropathy manifested by paresthesia and hypesthesia were the most frequently reported neurologic toxicities. Loss of deep tendon reflexes occurred in less than 5% of patients. The development of severe peripheral neuropathy was infrequent (1%) and generally reversible.

Skin: Alopecia was reported in 12% of patients and was usually mild.

Like other anticancer vinca alkaloids, NAVELBINE is a moderate vesicant. Injection site reactions, including erythema, pain at injection site, and vein discoloration occurred in approximately one third of patients; 5% were severe. Chemical phlebitis along the vein proximal to the site of injection was reported in 10% of patients.

Gastrointestinal: Mild or moderate nausea occurred in 34% of patients treated with NAVELBINE; severe nausea was infrequent (<2%). Prophylactic administration of antiemetics was not routine in patients treated with single-agent NAVELBINE. Due to the low incidence of severe nausea and vomiting with single-agent NAVELBINE, the use of serotonin antagonists is generally not required. Constipation occurred in 29% of patients, with paralytic ileus occurring in 1%. Vomiting, diarrhea, anorexia, and stomatitis were usually mild or moderate and each occurred in less than 20% of patients.

Hepatic: Transient elevations of liver enzymes were reported without clinical symptoms.

Cardiovascular: Chest pain was reported in 5% of patients. Most reports of chest pain were in patients who had either a history of cardiovascular disease or tumor within the chest. There have been rare reports of myocardial infarction.

Pulmonary: Shortness of breath was reported in 3% of patients; it was severe in 2% (see WARNINGS). Interstitial pulmonary changes were documented.

Other: Fatigue occurred in 27% of patients. It was usually mild or moderate but tended to increase with cumulative dosing.

Other toxicities that have been reported in less than 5% of patients include jaw pain, myalgia, arthralgia, and rash. Hemorrhagic cystitis and the syndrome of inappropriate ADH secretion were each reported in <1% of patients.

Combination Use: In a randomized study, 206 patients received treatment with NAVELBINE plus cisplatin and 206 patients received single-agent NAVELBINE. The toxicity profile of cisplatin is known (see full prescribing information for cisplatin). The incidence of severe nausea and vomiting was 30% for NAVELBINE/cisplatin compared to <2% for single-agent NAVELBINE. Cisplatin did not appear to increase the incidence of neurotoxicity observed with single-agent NAVELBINE. However, myelosuppression, specifically Grade 3 and 4 granulocytopenia, was greater with the combination of NAVELBINE/cisplatin (79%) than with single-agent NAVELBINE (53%). The incidence of fever and infection may be increased with the combination.

Observed During Clinical Practice: In addition to the adverse events reported from clinical trials, the following events have been identified during post-approval use of NAVELBINE. Because they are reported voluntarily from a population of unknown size, estimates of frequency cannot be made. These events have been chosen for inclusion due to a combination of their seriousness, frequency of reporting, or potential causal connection to NAVELBINE.

Body As A Whole: Systemic allergic reactions reported as anaphylaxis, pruritus, urticaria, and angioedema; flushing; and radiation recall events such as dermatitis and esophagitis (see PRECAUTIONS) have been reported.

Hematologic: Thromboembolic events including pulmonary embolus and deep venous thrombosis have been reported primarily in seriously ill and debilitated patients with known predisposing risk factors for these events.

Neurologic: Peripheral neurotoxicities such as, but not limited to, muscle weakness and disturbance of gait, have been observed in patients with and without prior symptoms. There may be increased potential for neurotoxicity in patients with pre-existing neuropathy, regardless of etiology, who receive NAVELBINE. Vestibular and auditory deficits have been observed with NAVELBINE, usually when used in combination with cisplatin.

Skin: Injection site reactions, including localized rash and urticaria, blister formation, and skin sloughing have been observed in clinical practice. Some of these reactions may be delayed in appearance.

Gastrointestinal: Dysphagia and mucositis have been reported.

Cardiovascular: Hypertension, hypotension, vasodilation, tachycardia, and pulmonary edema have been reported.

Pulmonary: Pneumonia has been reported.

Musculoskeletal: Headache has been reported, with and without other musculoskeletal aches and pains.

Other: Pain in tumor-containing tissue, back pain, and abdominal pain have been reported. Electrolyte abnormalities, including hyponatremia with or without the syndrome of inappropriate ADH secretion, have been reported in seriously ill and debilitated patients.

Combination Use: Patients with prior exposure to paclitaxel and who have demonstrated neuropathy should be monitored closely for new or worsening neuropathy. Patients who have experienced neuropathy with previous drug regimens should be monitored for symptoms of neuropathy while receiving NAVELBINE. NAVELBINE may result in radiosensitizing effects with prior or concomitant radiation therapy (see PRECAUTIONS).

OVERDOSAGE

There is no known antidote for overdoses of NAVELBINE. Overdoses involving quantities up to 10 times the recommended dose (30 mg/m^2) have been reported. The toxicities described were consistent with those listed in the ADVERSE REACTIONS section including paralytic ileus, stomatitis, and esophagitis. Bone marrow aplasia, sepsis, and paresis have also been reported. Fatalities have occurred following overdose of NAVELBINE. If overdosage occurs, general supportive measures together with appropriate blood transfusions, growth factors, and antibiotics should be instituted as deemed necessary by the physician.

DOSAGE AND ADMINISTRATION

The usual initial dose of NAVELBINE is 30 mg/m^2 administered weekly. The recommended method of administration is an intravenous injection over 6 to 10 minutes. In controlled trials, single-agent NAVELBINE was given weekly until progression or dose-limiting toxicity. NAVELBINE was used at the same dose in combination with 120 mg/m^2 of cisplatin, given on days 1 and 29, then every 6 weeks.

No dose adjustments are required for renal insufficiency. If moderate or severe neurotoxicity develops, NAVELBINE should be discontinued. The dosage should be adjusted according to hematologic toxicity or hepatic insufficiency, whichever results in the lower dose.

Dose Modifications for Hematologic Toxicity: Granulocyte counts should be $\geq$1000 cells/mm^3 prior to the administration of NAVELBINE. Adjustments in the dosage of NAVELBINE should be based on granulocyte counts obtained on the day of treatment according to Table 2.

Table 2: Dose Adjustments Based on Granulocyte Counts

Granulocytes (cells/mm^3) on Days of Treatment	Dose of NAVELBINE (mg/m^2)
$\geq$1500	30
1000 to 1499	15
<1000	Do not administer. Repeat granulocyte count in 1 week. If 3 consecutive weekly doses are held because granulocyte count is $<$1000 cells/mm^3, discontinue NAVELBINE.

Note: For patients who, during treatment with NAVELBINE, have experienced fever and/or sepsis while granulocytopenic or had 2 consecutive weekly doses held due to granulocytopenia, subsequent doses of NAVELBINE should be:

22.5 mg/m^2 for granulocytes $\geq$1500 cells/mm^3
11.25 mg/m^2 for granulocytes 1000 to 1499 cells/mm^3

Dose Modification for Hepatic Insufficiency: NAVELBINE should be administered with caution to patients with hepatic insufficiency. In patients who develop hyperbilirubinemia during treatment with NAVELBINE, the dose should be adjusted for total bilirubin according to Table 3.

Table 3: Dose Modification Based on Total Bilirubin

Total Bilirubin (mg/dL)	Dose of NAVELBINE (mg/m^2)
$\leq$2.0	30
2.1 to 3.0	15
>3.0	7.5

Dose Modification for Concurrent Hematologic Toxicity and Hepatic Insufficiency: In patients with both hematologic toxicity and hepatic insufficiency, the lower of the doses determined from Table 2 and Table 3 should be administered.

Administration Precautions: Caution—NAVELBINE must be administered intravenously. It is extremely important that the intravenous needle or catheter be properly positioned before any NAVELBINE is injected. Leakage into surrounding tissue during intravenous administration of NAVELBINE may cause considerable irritation, local tissue necrosis, and/or thrombophlebitis. If extravasation occurs, the injection should be discontinued immediately, and any remaining portion of the dose should then be introduced into another vein. Since there are no established guidelines for the treatment of extravasation injuries with NAVELBINE, institutional guidelines may be used. The *ONS Chemotherapy Guidelines* provide additional recommendations for the prevention of extravasation injuries.[1]

As with other toxic compounds, caution should be exercised in handling and preparing the solution of NAVELBINE. Skin reactions may occur with accidental exposure. The use of gloves is recommended. If the solution of NAVELBINE contacts the skin or mucosa, immediately wash the skin or mucosa thoroughly with soap and water. Severe irritation of the eye has been reported with accidental contamination of the eye with another vinca alkaloid. If this happens with NAVELBINE, the eye should be flushed with water immediately and thoroughly.

Procedures for proper handling and disposal of anticancer drugs should be used. Several guidelines on this subject have been published.[2-8] There is no general agreement that all of the procedures recommended in the guidelines are necessary or appropriate.

NAVELBINE Injection is a clear, colorless to pale yellow solution. Parenteral drug products should be visually inspected for particulate matter and discoloration prior to administration whenever solution and container permit. If particulate matter is seen, NAVELBINE should not be administered.

Preparation for Administration: NAVELBINE Injection must be diluted in either a syringe or IV bag using one of the recommended solutions. The diluted NAVELBINE should be administered over 6 to 10 minutes into the side port of a free-flowing IV **closest to the IV bag** followed by flushing with at least 75 to 125 mL of one of the solutions. Diluted NAVELBINE may be used for up to 24 hours under normal room light when stored in polypropylene syringes or polyvinyl chloride bags at 5° to 30°C (41° to 86°F).

Syringe: The calculated dose of NAVELBINE should be diluted to a concentration between 1.5 and 3.0 mg/mL. The following solutions may be used for dilution:

5% Dextrose Injection, USP
0.9% Sodium Chloride Injection, USP

IV Bag: The calculated dose of NAVELBINE should be diluted to a concentration between 0.5 and 2 mg/mL. The following solutions may be used for dilution:

5% Dextrose Injection, USP
0.9% Sodium Chloride Injection, USP
0.45% Sodium Chloride Injection, USP
5% Dextrose and 0.45% Sodium Chloride Injection, USP
Ringer's Injection, USP
Lactated Ringer's Injection, USP

Stability: Unopened vials of NAVELBINE are stable until the date indicated on the package when stored under refrigeration at 2° to 8°C (36° to 46°F) and protected from light in the carton. Unopened vials of NAVELBINE are stable at temperatures up to 25°C (77°F) for up to 72 hours. This product should not be frozen.

HOW SUPPLIED

NAVELBINE Injection is a clear, colorless to pale yellow solution in Water for Injection, containing 10 mg vinorelbine per mL. NAVELBINE Injection is available in single-use, clear glass vials with elastomeric stoppers and royal blue caps, individually packaged in a carton in the following vial sizes:

10 mg/1 mL Single-Use Vial, Carton of 1 (NDC 0173-0656-01).

50 mg/5 mL Single-Use Vial, Carton of 1 (NDC 0173-0656-44).

Store the vials under refrigeration at 2° to 8°C (36° to 46°F) in the carton. Protect from light. DO NOT FREEZE.

REFERENCES

1. ONS Clinical Practice Committee. Cancer Chemotherapy Guidelines: Recommendations for the management of vesicant extravasation, hypersensitivity, and anaphylaxis. Pittsburgh, Pa: Oncology Nursing Society; 1992: 1-4.
2. Recommendations for the safe handling of parenteral antineoplastic drugs. Washington, DC: Division of Safety, National Institutes of Health; 1983. US Dept of Health and Human Services, Public Health Service publication NIH 83-2621.
3. AMA Council on Scientific Affairs. Guidelines for handling parenteral antineoplastics. *JAMA.* 1985;253:1590-1591.
4. National Study Commission on Cytotoxic Exposure. Recommendations for handling cytotoxic agents. 1987. Available from Louis P. Jeffrey, Chairman, National Study Commission on Cytotoxic Exposure. Massachusetts College of Pharmacy and Allied Health Sciences, 179 Longwood Avenue, Boston, MA 02115.
5. Clinical Oncological Society of Australia. Guidelines and recommendations for safe handling of antineoplastic agents. *Med J Australia.* 1983;1:426-428.

6. Jones RB, Frank R, Mass T. Safe handling of chemotherapeutic agents: a report from the Mount Sinai Medical Center. *CA-A Cancer J for Clin.* 1983;33:258-263.
7. American Society of Hospital Pharmacists. ASHP technical assistance bulletin on handling cytotoxic and hazardous drugs. *Am J Hosp Pharm.* 1990;47:1033-1049.
8. Yodaiken RE, Bennet D. OSHA work-practice guidelines for personnel dealing with cytotoxic (antineoplastic) drugs. *Am J Hosp Pharm.* 1986;43:1193-1204.

Manufactured by Pierre Fabre Medicament Production
64320 Idron, FRANCE
for Glaxo Wellcome Inc., Research Triangle Park, NC 27709
Under license of Pierre Fabre Médicament–Centre National de la Recherche Scientifique-France
US Patent No. 4,307,100

June 2000/RL-836
Shown in Product Identification Guide, page 316

OXISTAT® ℞

[*äx 'ē-stat"*]
(oxiconazole nitrate cream)
Cream, 1%*

OXISTAT®

(oxiconazole nitrate lotion)
Lotion, 1%*

***Potency expressed as oxiconazole**
FOR TOPICAL DERMATOLOGIC USE ONLY—
NOT FOR OPHTHALMIC OR INTRAVAGINAL USE

DESCRIPTION

OXISTAT Cream and Lotion formulations contain the antifungal active compound oxiconazole nitrate. Both formulations are for topical dermatologic use only.
Chemically, oxiconazole nitrate is 2′,4′-dichloro-2-imidazol-1-ylacetophenone (*Z*)-[*0*-(2,4-dichlorobenzyl)oxime], mononitrate. The compound has the empirical formula $C_{18}H_{13}ON_3Cl_4 \cdot HNO_3$, and a molecular weight of 492.15.
Oxiconazole nitrate is a nearly white crystalline powder, soluble in methanol; sparingly soluble in ethanol, chloroform, and acetone; and very slightly soluble in water.
OXISTAT Cream contains 10 mg of oxiconazole per gram of cream in a white to off-white, opaque cream base of purified water USP, white petrolatum USP, stearyl alcohol NF, propylene glycol USP, polysorbate 60 NF, cetyl alcohol NF, and benzoic acid USP 0.2% as a preservative.
OXISTAT Lotion contains 10 mg of oxiconazole per gram of lotion in a white to off-white, opaque lotion base of purified water USP, white petrolatum USP, stearyl alcohol NF, propylene glycol USP, polysorbate 60 NF, cetyl alcohol NF, and benzoic acid USP 0.2% as a preservative.

CLINICAL PHARMACOLOGY

Pharmacokinetics: The penetration of oxiconazole nitrate into different layers of the skin was assessed using an in vitro permeation technique with human skin. Five hours after application of 2.5 mg/cm^2 of oxiconazole nitrate cream onto human skin, the concentration of oxiconazole nitrate was demonstrated to be 16.2 μmol in the epidermis, 3.64 μmol in the upper corium, and 1.29 μmol in the deeper corium. Systemic absorption of oxiconazole nitrate is low. Using radiolabeled drug, less than 0.3% of the applied dose of oxiconazole nitrate was recovered in the urine of volunteer subjects up to 5 days after application of the cream formulation.
Neither in vitro nor in vivo studies have been conducted to establish relative activity between the lotion and cream formulations.
Microbiology: Oxiconazole nitrate is an imidazole derivative whose antifungal activity is derived primarily from the inhibition of ergosterol biosynthesis, which is critical for cellular membrane integrity. It has in vitro activity against a wide range of pathogenic fungi.
Oxiconazole has been shown to be active against most strains of the following organisms both in vitro and in clinical infections at indicated body sites (see INDICATIONS AND USAGE):
Epidermophyton floccosum
Trichophyton mentagrophytes
Trichophyton rubrum
Malassezia furfur
The following in vitro data are available; **however, their clinical significance is unknown**. Oxiconazole exhibits satisfactory in vitro minimum inhibitory concentrations (MICs) against most strains of the following organisms; however, the safety and efficacy of oxiconazole in treating clinical infections due to these organisms have not been established in adequate and well-controlled clinical trials:
Candida albicans
Microsporum audouini
Microsporum canis
Microsporum gypseum
Trichophyton tonsurans
Trichophyton violaceum

INDICATIONS AND USAGE

OXISTAT Cream and Lotion are indicated for the topical treatment of the following dermal infections: tinea pedis, tinea cruris, and tinea corporis due to *Trichophyton rubrum, Trichophyton mentagrophytes,* or *Epidermophyton floccosum.* OXISTAT Cream is indicated for the topical treatment of tinea (pityriasis) versicolor due to *Malassezia furfur* (see DOSAGE AND ADMINISTRATION and CLINICAL STUDIES).
OXISTAT Cream may be used in pediatric patients for tinea corporis, tinea cruris, tinea pedis, and tinea (pityriasis) versicolor; however, these indications for which OXISTAT Cream has been shown to be effective rarely occur in children below the age of 12.

CONTRAINDICATIONS

OXISTAT Cream and Lotion are contraindicated in individuals who have shown hypersensitivity to any of their components.

WARNINGS

OXISTAT Cream and Lotion are not for ophthalmic or intravaginal use.

PRECAUTIONS

General: OXISTAT Cream and Lotion are for external dermal use only. Avoid introduction of OXISTAT Cream or Lotion into the eyes or vagina. If a reaction suggesting sensitivity or chemical irritation should occur with the use of OXISTAT Cream or Lotion, treatment should be discontinued and appropriate therapy instituted. If signs of epidermal irritation should occur, the drug should be discontinued.
Information for Patients: The patient should be instructed to:

1. Use OXISTAT as directed by the physician. The hands should be washed after applying the medication to the affected area(s). Avoid contact with the eyes, nose, mouth, and other mucous membranes. OXISTAT is for external use only.
2. Use the medication for the **full** treatment time recommended by the physician, even though symptoms may have improved. Notify the physician if there is no improvement after 2 to 4 weeks, or sooner if the condition worsens (see below).
3. Inform the physician if the area of application shows signs of increased irritation, itching, burning, blistering, swelling, or oozing.
4. Avoid the use of occlusive dressings unless otherwise directed by the physician.
5. Do not use this medication for any disorder other than that for which it was prescribed.

Drug Interactions: Potential drug interactions between OXISTAT and other drugs have not been systematically evaluated.
Carcinogenesis, Mutagenesis, Impairment of Fertility: Although no long-term studies in animals have been performed to evaluate carcinogenic potential, no evidence of mutagenic effect was found in 2 mutation assays (Ames test and Chinese hamster V79 in vitro cell mutation assay) or in 2 cytogenetic assays (human peripheral blood lymphocyte in vitro chromosome aberration assay and in vivo micronucleus assay in mice).
Reproductive studies revealed no impairment of fertility in rats at oral doses of 3 mg/kg per day in females (one time the human dose based on mg/m^2) and 15 mg/kg per day in males (4 times the human dose based on mg/m^2). However, at doses above this level, the following effects were observed: a reduction in the fertility parameters of males and females, a reduction in the number of sperm in vaginal smears, extended estrous cycle, and a decrease in mating frequency.
Pregnancy: Teratogenic Effects: Pregnancy Category B. Reproduction studies have been performed in rabbits, rats, and mice at oral doses up to 100, 150, and 200 mg/kg per day (57, 40, and 27 times the human dose based on mg/m^2), respectively, and revealed no evidence of harm to the fetus due to oxiconazole nitrate. There are, however, no adequate and well-controlled studies in pregnant women. Because animal reproduction studies are not always predictive of human response, this drug should be used during pregnancy only if clearly needed.
Nursing Mothers: Because oxiconazole is excreted in human milk, caution should be exercised when the drug is administered to a nursing woman.
Pediatric Use: OXISTAT Cream may be used in pediatric patients for tinea corporis, tinea cruris, tinea pedis, and tinea (pityriasis) versicolor; however, these indications for which OXISTAT Cream has been shown to be effective rarely occur in children below the age of 12.

ADVERSE REACTIONS

During clinical trials, of 955 patients treated with oxiconazole nitrate cream, 1%, 41 (4.3%) reported adverse reactions thought to be related to drug therapy. These reactions included pruritus (1.6%); burning (1.4%); irritation and allergic contact dermatitis (0.4% each); folliculitis (0.3%); erythema (0.2%); and papules, fissure, maceration, rash, stinging, and nodules (0.1% each).
In a controlled, multicenter clinical trial of 269 patients treated with oxiconazole nitrate lotion, 1%, 7 (2.6%) reported adverse reactions thought to be related to drug therapy. These reactions included burning and stinging (0.7% each) and pruritus, scaling, tingling, pain, and dyshidrotic eczema (0.4% each).

OVERDOSAGE

When 5% oxiconazole cream (5 times the concentration of the marketed product) was applied at a rate of 1 g/kg to approximately 10% of body surface area of a group of 40 male and female rats for 35 days, 3 deaths and severe dermal inflammation were reported. No overdoses in humans have been reported with use of oxiconazole nitrate cream or lotion.

DOSAGE AND ADMINISTRATION

OXISTAT Cream or Lotion should be applied to affected and immediately surrounding areas once to twice daily in patients with tinea pedis, tinea corporis, or tinea cruris. OXISTAT Cream should be applied once daily in the treatment of tinea (pityriasis) versicolor. Tinea corporis, tinea cruris, and tinea (pityriasis) versicolor should be treated for 2 weeks and tinea pedis for 1 month to reduce the possibility of recurrence. If a patient shows no clinical improvement after the treatment period, the diagnosis should be reviewed.
Note: Tinea (pityriasis) versicolor may give rise to hyperpigmented or hypopigmented patches on the trunk that may extend to the neck, arms, and upper thighs. Treatment of the infection may not immediately result in restoration of pigment to the affected sites. Normalization of pigment following successful therapy is variable and may take months, depending on individual skin type and incidental sun exposure. Although tinea (pityriasis) versicolor is not contagious, it may recur because the organism that causes the disease is part of the normal skin flora.

HOW SUPPLIED

OXISTAT Cream, 1% is supplied in 15-g tubes (NDC 0173-0423-00), 30-g tubes (NDC 0173-0423-01), and 60-g tubes (NDC 0173-0423-04). **Store between 15° and 30°C (59° and 86°F).**
OXISTAT Lotion, 1% is supplied in a 30-mL bottle (NDC 0173-0448-01). **Store between 15° and 30°C (59° and 86°F). Shake well before using.**

CLINICAL STUDIES

The following definitions were applied to the clinical and microbiological outcomes in patients enrolled in the clinical trials that form the basis for the approvals of OXISTAT Lotion and OXISTAT Cream.
Definitions:

1. Mycological Cure: No evidence (culture and KOH preparation) of the baseline (original) pathogen in a specimen from the affected area taken at the 2-week post-treatment visit (for tinea [pityriasis] versicolor, mycological cure was limited to KOH only).
2. Treatment Success: Both a global evaluation of ≥90% clinical improvement and a microbiologic eradication (see above) at the 2-week post-treatment visit.

Tinea Pedis: THERE ARE NO HEAD-TO-HEAD COMPARISON TRIALS OF THE OXISTAT CREAM AND LOTION FORMULATIONS IN THE TREATMENT OF TINEA PEDIS.
Lotion Formulation: The clinical trial for the lotion formulation line extension involved 332 evaluable patients with clinically and microbiologically established tinea pedis. Of these evaluable patients, 64% were diagnosed with hyperkeratotic plantar tinea pedis and 28% with interdigital tinea pedis. Seventy-seven percent (77%) had disease secondary to infection with *Trichophyton rubrum*, 18% had disease secondary to infection with *Trichophyton mentagrophytes*, and 4% had disease secondary to infection with *Epidermophyton floccosum*.
The results of this clinical trial at the 2-week post-treatment follow-up visit are shown in the following table:

Patient Outcome	OXISTAT Lotion b.i.d.	OXISTAT Lotion q.d.	Vehicle
Mycological cure	67%	64%	28%
Treatment success	41%	34%	10%

In this study, the improvement and cure rates of the b.i.d.- and q.d.-treated groups did not differ significantly (95% confidence interval) from each other but were statistically (95% confidence interval) superior to the vehicle-treated group.
Cream Formulation: The two pivotal trials for the cream formulation involved 281 evaluable patients (total from both trials) with clinically and microbiologically established tinea pedis.
The combined results of these two clinical trials at the 2-week post-treatment follow-up visit are shown in the following table:

Patient Outcome	OXISTAT Cream b.i.d.	OXISTAT Cream q.d	Vehicle
Mycological cure	77%	79%	33%
Treatment success	52%	43%	14%

Continued on next page

This product information is based on labeling in effect on June 23, 2000. For further information, contact via direct mail, phone, or web site. Medical Information, Glaxo Wellcome Inc., PO Box 13398, Research Triangle Park, NC 27709. Healthcare Professionals (Medical Information): 800-334-0089. Patients (Customer Response Center): 1-888-825-5249. Glaxo Wellcome Corporate Web Site: www.glaxowellcome.com

Oxistat—Cont.

All the improvement and cure rates of the b.i.d.- and q.d.-treated groups did not differ significantly (95% confidence interval) from each other but were statistically (95% confidence interval) superior to the vehicle-treated group.
In addition, pediatric data (95 children ages 10 and under) available with the cream formulation indicate that it is safe and effective for use in children when used as directed. Adverse events were reported in 2 children; 1 child was reported to have reddening of the skin and 1 child was reported to have eczema-like skin alterations.
Tinea (pityriasis) Versicolor: Two pivotal clinical trials of OXISTAT Cream in tinea (pityriasis) versicolor involved 219 evaluable patients in the q day OXISTAT and vehicle arms of the trial with clinical and mycological evidence of tinea (pityriasis) versicolor. Patients were treated for 2 weeks with OXISTAT Cream once daily, or with cream vehicle. The combined results of these clinical trials at the 2-week post-treatment follow-up visit are shown in the following table. These results are based on 207 patients (110 in the OXISTAT group and 97 in the vehicle group) with efficacy evaluations at this visit.

	OXISTAT Cream	
Patient Outcome	q.d.	Vehicle
Mycological cure	88%	67%
Treatment success	83%	62%

Only once a day was shown in both studies to be statistically superior to vehicle for all efficacy parameters at 2 weeks and follow-up.
Glaxo Wellcome Inc., Research Triangle Park, NC 27709
January 1999/RL-679

Shown in Product Identification Guide, page 316

PURINETHOL® ℞

[pur 'ĭn-thawl]
(mercaptopurine)
50-mg Scored Tablets

CAUTION: PURINETHOL (mercaptopurine) is a potent drug. It should not be used unless a diagnosis of acute lymphatic leukemia has been adequately established and the responsible physician is knowledgeable in assessing response to chemotherapy.

DESCRIPTION

PURINETHOL (mercaptopurine) was synthesized and developed by Hitchings, Elion, and associates at the Wellcome Research Laboratories.[1] It is one of a large series of purine analogues which interfere with nucleic acid biosynthesis and has been found active against human leukemias.
Mercaptopurine, known chemically as 1,7-dihydro-6*H*-purine-6-thione monohydrate, is an analogue of the purine bases adenine and hypoxanthine.
PURINETHOL is available in tablet form for oral administration. Each scored tablet contains 50 mg mercaptopurine and the inactive ingredients corn and potato starch, lactose, magnesium stearate, and stearic acid.

CLINICAL PHARMACOLOGY

Clinical studies have shown that the absorption of an oral dose of mercaptopurine in humans is incomplete and variable, averaging approximately 50% of the administered dose.[2] The factors influencing absorption are unknown. Intravenous administration of an investigational preparation of mercaptopurine revealed a plasma half-disappearance time of 21 minutes in pediatric patients and 47 minutes in adults. The volume of distribution usually exceeded that of the total body water.[2]
Following the oral administration of ^{35}S-6-mercaptopurine in one subject, a total of 46% of the dose could be accounted for in the urine (as parent drug and metabolites) in the first 24 hours. Metabolites of mercaptopurine were found in urine within the first 2 hours after administration. Radioactivity (in the form of sulfate) could be found in the urine for weeks afterwards.[3]
There is negligible entry of mercaptopurine into cerebrospinal fluid.
Plasma protein binding averages 19% over the concentration range 10 to 50 mcg/mL (a concentration only achieved by intravenous administration of mercaptopurine at doses exceeding 5 to 10 mg/kg).[2]
Monitoring of plasma levels of mercaptopurine during therapy is of questionable value.[3] There is technical difficulty in determining plasma concentrations which are seldom greater than 1 to 2 mcg/mL after a therapeutic oral dose. More significantly, mercaptopurine enters rapidly into the anabolic and catabolic pathways for purines, and the active intracellular metabolites have appreciably longer half-lives than the parent drug. The biochemical effects of a single dose of mercaptopurine are evident long after the parent drug has disappeared from plasma. Because of this rapid metabolism of mercaptopurine to active intracellular derivatives, hemodialysis would not be expected to appreciably reduce toxicity of the drug. There is no known pharmacologic antagonist to the biochemical actions of mercaptopurine in vivo.
Mercaptopurine competes with hypoxanthine and guanine for the enzyme hypoxanthine-guanine phosphoribosyltransferase (HGPRTase) and is itself converted to thioinosinic acid (TIMP). This intracellular nucleotide inhibits several reactions involving inosinic acid (IMP), including the conversion of IMP to xanthylic acid (XMP) and the conversion of IMP to adenylic acid (AMP) via adenylosuccinate (SAMP). In addition, 6-methylthioinosinate (MTIMP) is formed by the methylation of TIMP. Both TIMP and MTIMP have been reported to inhibit glutamine-5-phosphoribosylpyrophosphate amidotransferase, the first enzyme unique to the de novo pathway for purine ribonucleotide synthesis.[3]
Experiments indicate that radiolabeled mercaptopurine may be recovered from the DNA in the form of deoxythioguanosine.[4] Some mercaptopurine is converted to nucleotide derivatives of 6-thioguanine (6-TG) by the sequential actions of inosinate (IMP) dehydrogenase and xanthylate (XMP) aminase, converting TIMP to thioguanylic acid (TGMP).
Animal tumors that are resistant to mercaptopurine often have lost the ability to convert mercaptopurine to TIMP. However, it is clear that resistance to mercaptopurine may be acquired by other means as well, particularly in human leukemias.
It is not known exactly which of any one or more of the biochemical effects of mercaptopurine and its metabolites are directly or predominantly responsible for cell death.[5]
The catabolism of mercaptopurine and its metabolites is complex. In humans, after oral administration of ^{35}S-6-mercaptopurine, urine contains intact mercaptopurine, thiouric acid (formed by direct oxidation by xanthine oxidase, probably via 6-mercapto-8-hydroxypurine), and a number of 6-methylated thiopurines. The methylthiopurines yield appreciable amounts of inorganic sulfate.[3] The importance of the metabolism by xanthine oxidase relates to the fact that ZYLOPRIM® (allopurinol) inhibits this enzyme and retards the catabolism of mercaptopurine and its active metabolites. A significant reduction in mercaptopurine dosage is mandatory if a potent xanthine oxidase inhibitor and mercaptopurine are used simultaneously in a patient (see PRECAUTIONS).

INDICATIONS AND USAGE

PURINETHOL (mercaptopurine) is indicated for remission induction and maintenance therapy of acute lymphatic leukemia. The response to this agent depends upon the particular subclassification of acute lymphatic leukemia and the age of the patient (pediatric patient or adult).
Acute Lymphatic (Lymphocytic, Lymphoblastic) Leukemia: Given as a single agent for remission induction, PURINETHOL induces complete remission in approximately 25% of pediatric patients and 10% of adults. However, reliance upon PURINETHOL alone is not justified for initial remission induction of acute lymphatic leukemia since combination chemotherapy with vincristine, prednisone, and L-asparaginase results in more frequent complete remission induction than with PURINETHOL alone or in combination. The duration of complete remission induced in acute lymphatic leukemia is so brief without the use of maintenance therapy that some form of drug therapy is considered essential. PURINETHOL, as a single agent, is capable of significantly prolonging complete remission duration; however, combination therapy has produced remission duration longer than that achieved with PURINETHOL alone.
Acute Myelogenous (and Acute Myelomonocytic) Leukemia: As a single agent, PURINETHOL will induce complete remission in approximately 10% of pediatric patients and adults with acute myelogenous leukemia or its subclassifications. These results are inferior to those achieved with combination chemotherapy employing optimum treatment schedules.
Central Nervous System Leukemia: PURINETHOL is not effective for prophylaxis or treatment of central nervous system leukemia.
Other Neoplasms: PURINETHOL is not effective in chronic lymphatic leukemia, the lymphomas (including Hodgkin's Disease), or solid tumors.

CONTRAINDICATIONS

PURINETHOL should not be used unless a diagnosis of acute lymphatic leukemia has been adequately established and the responsible physician is knowledgeable in assessing response to chemotherapy.
PURINETHOL should not be used in patients whose disease has demonstrated prior resistance to this drug. In animals and humans, there is usually complete cross-resistance between mercaptopurine and thioguanine.

WARNINGS

SINCE DRUGS USED IN CANCER CHEMOTHERAPY ARE POTENTIALLY HAZARDOUS, IT IS RECOMMENDED THAT ONLY PHYSICIANS EXPERIENCED WITH THE RISKS OF PURINETHOL AND KNOWLEDGEABLE IN THE NATURAL HISTORY OF ACUTE LEUKEMIAS ADMINISTER THIS DRUG.
Bone Marrow Toxicity: The most consistent, dose-related toxicity is bone marrow suppression. This may be manifest by anemia, leukopenia, thrombocytopenia, or any combination of these. Any of these findings may also reflect progression of the underlying disease. Since mercaptopurine may have a delayed effect, it is important to withdraw the medication temporarily at the first sign of an abnormally large fall in any of the formed elements of the blood.
There are rare individuals with an inherited deficiency of the enzyme thiopurine methyltransferase (TPMT) who may be unusually sensitive to the myelosuppressive effects of mercaptopurine and prone to developing rapid bone marrow suppression following the initiation of treatment.[6,7] Substantial dosage reductions may be required to avoid the development of life-threatening bone marrow suppression in these patients. This toxicity may be more profound in patients treated with concomitant allopurinol (see PRECAUTIONS: Drug Interactions).
Hepatotoxicity: Mercaptopurine is hepatotoxic in animals and humans. A small number of deaths have been reported which may have been attributed to hepatic necrosis due to administration of mercaptopurine. Hepatic injury can occur with any dosage, but seems to occur with more frequency when doses of 2.5 mg/kg/day are exceeded. The histologic pattern of mercaptopurine hepatotoxicity includes features of both intrahepatic cholestasis and parenchymal cell necrosis, either of which may predominate. It is not clear how much of the hepatic damage is due to direct toxicity from the drug and how much may be due to a hypersensitivity reaction. In some patients jaundice has cleared following withdrawal of mercaptopurine and reappeared with its reintroduction.[8]
Published reports have cited widely varying incidences of overt hepatotoxicity. In a large series of patients with various neoplastic diseases, mercaptopurine was administered orally in doses ranging from 2.5 mg/kg to 5.0 mg/kg without any evidence of hepatotoxicity. It was noted by the authors that no definite clinical evidence of liver damage could be ascribed to the drug, although an occasional case of serum hepatitis did occur in patients receiving 6-MP who previously had transfusions.[8] In reports of smaller cohorts of adult and pediatric leukemic patients, the incidence of hepatotoxicity ranged from 0% to 6%.[9-11] In an isolated report by Einhorn and Davidsohn, jaundice was observed more frequently (40%), especially when doses exceeded 2.5 mg/kg.[12]
Usually, clinically detectable jaundice appears early in the course of treatment (1 to 2 months). However, jaundice has been reported as early as 1 week and as late as 8 years after the start of treatment with mercaptopurine.[13]
Monitoring of serum transaminase levels, alkaline phosphatase, and bilirubin levels may allow early detection of hepatotoxicity. It is advisable to monitor these liver function tests at weekly intervals when first beginning therapy and at monthly intervals thereafter. Liver function tests may be advisable more frequently in patients who are receiving mercaptopurine with other hepatotoxic drugs or with known pre-existing liver disease.
The concomitant administration of mercaptopurine with other hepatotoxic agents requires especially careful clinical and biochemical monitoring of hepatic function. Combination therapy involving mercaptopurine with other drugs not felt to be hepatotoxic should nevertheless be approached with caution. The combination of mercaptopurine with doxorubicin was reported to be hepatotoxic in 19 of 20 patients undergoing remission-induction therapy for leukemia resistant to previous therapy.[14]
The hepatotoxicity has been associated in some cases with anorexia, diarrhea, jaundice, and ascites. Hepatic encephalopathy has occurred.
The onset of clinical jaundice, hepatomegaly, or anorexia with tenderness in the right hypochondrium are immediate indications for withholding mercaptopurine until the exact etiology can be identified. Likewise, any evidence of deterioration in liver function studies, toxic hepatitis, or biliary stasis should prompt discontinuation of the drug and a search for an etiology of the hepatotoxicity.
Immunosuppression: Mercaptopurine recipients may manifest decreased cellular hypersensitivities and impaired allograft rejection. Induction of immunity to infectious agents or vaccines will be subnormal in these patients; the degree of immunosuppression will depend on antigen dose and temporal relationship to drug. This immunosuppressive effect should be carefully considered with regard to intercurrent infections and risk of subsequent neoplasia.
Pregnancy: Pregnancy Category D. Mercaptopurine can cause fetal harm when administered to a pregnant woman. Women receiving mercaptopurine in the first trimester of pregnancy have an increased incidence of abortion; the risk of malformation in offspring surviving first trimester exposure is not accurately known.[15] In a series of 28 women receiving mercaptopurine after the first trimester of pregnancy, three mothers died undelivered, one delivered a stillborn child, and one aborted; there were no cases of macroscopically abnormal fetuses.[16] Since such experience cannot exclude the possibility of fetal damage, mercaptopurine should be used during pregnancy only if the benefit clearly justifies the possible risk to the fetus, and particular caution should be given to the use of mercaptopurine in the first trimester of pregnancy.
There are no adequate and well-controlled studies in pregnant women. If this drug is used during pregnancy or if the patient becomes pregnant while taking the drug, the patient should be apprised of the potential hazard to the fetus. Women of childbearing potential should be advised to avoid becoming pregnant.

PRECAUTIONS

General: The safe and effective use of PURINETHOL demands a thorough knowledge of the natural history of the condition being treated. After selection of an initial dosage schedule, therapy will frequently need to be modified depending upon the patient's response and manifestations of toxicity.

The most frequent, serious, toxic effect of PURINETHOL is myelosuppression resulting in leukopenia, thrombocytopenia, and anemia. These toxic effects are often unavoidable during the induction phase of adult acute leukemia if remission induction is to be successful. Whether or not these manifestations demand modification or cessation of dosage depends both upon the response of the underlying disease and a careful consideration of supportive facilities (granulocyte and platelet transfusions) which may be available. Life-threatening infections and bleeding have been observed as a consequence of mercaptopurine-induced granulocytopenia and thrombocytopenia. Severe hematologic toxicity may require supportive therapy with platelet transfusions for bleeding, and antibiotics and granulocyte transfusions if sepsis is documented.

If it is not the intent to deliberately induce bone marrow hypoplasia, it is important to discontinue the drug temporarily at the first evidence of an abnormally large fall in white blood cell count, platelet count, or hemoglobin concentration. In many patients with severe depression of the formed elements of the blood due to PURINETHOL, the bone marrow appears hypoplastic on aspiration or biopsy, whereas in other cases it may appear normocellular. The qualitative changes in the erythroid elements toward the megaloblastic series, characteristically seen with the folic acid antagonists and some other antimetabolites, are not seen with this drug.

It is probably advisable to start with smaller dosages in patients with impaired renal function, since the latter might result in slower elimination of the drug and metabolites and a greater cumulative effect.

Information for Patients: Patients should be informed that the major toxicities of PURINETHOL are related to myelosuppression, hepatotoxicity, and gastrointestinal toxicity. Patients should never be allowed to take the drug without medical supervision and should be advised to consult their physician if they experience fever, sore throat, jaundice, nausea, vomiting, signs of local infection, bleeding from any site, or symptoms suggestive of anemia. Women of childbearing potential should be advised to avoid becoming pregnant.

Laboratory Tests: It is recommended that evaluation of the hemoglobin or hematocrit, total white blood cell count and differential count, and quantitative platelet count be obtained weekly while the patient is on therapy with PURINETHOL. In cases where the cause of fluctuations in the formed elements in the peripheral blood is obscure, bone marrow examination may be useful for the evaluation of marrow status. The decision to increase, decrease, continue, or discontinue a given dosage of PURINETHOL must be based not only on the absolute hematologic values, but also upon the rapidity with which changes are occurring. In many instances, particularly during the induction phase of acute leukemia, complete blood counts will need to be done more frequently than once weekly in order to evaluate the effect of the therapy.

Drug Interactions: ***Interaction with Allopurinol:*** When allopurinol and mercaptopurine are administered concomitantly, it is imperative that the dose of mercaptopurine be reduced to one third to one quarter of the usual dose. Failure to observe this dosage reduction will result in a delayed catabolism of mercaptopurine and the strong likelihood of inducing severe toxicity.

There is usually complete cross-resistance between mercaptopurine and thioguanine.

The dosage of mercaptopurine may need to be reduced when this agent is combined with other drugs whose primary or secondary toxicity is myelosuppression. Enhanced marrow suppression has been noted in some patients also receiving trimethoprim-sulfamethoxazole.[17,18]

Carcinogenesis, Mutagenesis, Impairment of Fertility: Mercaptopurine causes chromosomal aberrations in animals and humans and induces dominant-lethal mutations in male mice. In mice, surviving female offspring of mothers who received chronic low doses of mercaptopurine during pregnancy were found sterile, or if they became pregnant, had smaller litters and more dead fetuses as compared to control animals.[19] Carcinogenic potential exists in humans, but the extent of the risk is unknown.

The effect of mercaptopurine on human fertility is unknown for either males or females.

Pregnancy: ***Teratogenic Effects:*** Pregnancy Category D. See WARNINGS section.

Nursing Mothers: It is not known whether this drug is excreted in human milk. Because many drugs are excreted in human milk, and because of the potential for serious adverse reactions in nursing infants from mercaptopurine, a decision should be made whether to discontinue nursing or to discontinue the drug, taking into account the importance of the drug to the mother.

Pediatric Use: See DOSAGE AND ADMINISTRATION section.

ADVERSE REACTIONS

The principal and potentially serious toxic effects of PURINETHOL are bone marrow toxicity and hepatotoxicity (see WARNINGS).

Hematologic: The most frequent adverse reaction to PURINETHOL is myelosuppression. The induction of complete remission of acute lymphatic leukemia frequently is associated with marrow hypoplasia. Maintenance of remission generally involves multiple-drug regimens whose component agents cause myelosuppression. Anemia, leukopenia, and thrombocytopenia are frequently observed. Dosages and schedules are adjusted to prevent life-threatening cytopenias.

Renal: Hyperuricemia may occur in patients receiving PURINETHOL as a consequence of rapid cell lysis accompanying the antineoplastic effect. Adverse effects can be minimized by increased hydration, urine alkalinization, and the prophylactic administration of a xanthine oxidase inhibitor such as allopurinol. The dosage of PURINETHOL should be reduced to one third to one quarter of the usual dose if allopurinol is given concurrently.

Gastrointestinal: Intestinal ulceration has been reported.[20] Nausea, vomiting, and anorexia are uncommon during initial administration. Mild diarrhea and sprue-like symptoms have been noted occasionally, but it is difficult at present to attribute these to the medication. Oral lesions are rarely seen, and when they occur they resemble thrush rather than antifolic ulcerations.

An increased risk of pancreatitis may be associated with the investigational use of PURINETHOL in inflammatory bowel disease.[21-23]

Miscellaneous: While dermatologic reactions can occur as a consequence of disease, the administration of PURINETHOL has been associated with skin rashes and hyperpigmentation.[24]

Drug fever has been very rarely reported with PURINETHOL. Before attributing fever to PURINETHOL, every attempt should be made to exclude more common causes of pyrexia, such as sepsis, in patients with acute leukemia.

OVERDOSAGE

Signs and symptoms of overdosage may be immediate such as anorexia, nausea, vomiting and diarrhea; or delayed such as myelosuppression, liver dysfunction, and gastroenteritis. Dialysis cannot be expected to clear mercaptopurine. Hemodialysis is thought to be of marginal use due to the rapid intracellular incorporation of mercaptopurine into active metabolites with long persistence. The oral LD_{50} of mercaptopurine was determined to be 480 mg/kg in the mouse and 425 mg/kg in the rat.[25]

There is no known pharmacologic antagonist of mercaptopurine. The drug should be discontinued immediately if unintended toxicity occurs during treatment. If a patient is seen immediately following an accidental overdosage of the drug, it may be useful to induce emesis.

DOSAGE AND ADMINISTRATION

Induction Therapy: PURINETHOL is administered orally. The dosage which will be tolerated and be effective varies from patient to patient, and therefore careful titration is necessary to obtain the optimum therapeutic effect without incurring excessive, unintended toxicity. The usual initial dosage for pediatric patients and adults is 2.5 mg/kg of body weight per day (100 to 200 mg in the average adult and 50 mg in an average 5-year-old child). Pediatric patients with acute leukemia have tolerated this dose without difficulty in most cases; it may be continued daily for several weeks or more in some patients. If, after 4 weeks at this dosage, there is no clinical improvement and no definite evidence of leukocyte or platelet depression, the dosage may be increased up to 5 mg/kg daily. A dosage of 2.5 mg/kg per day may result in a rapid fall in leukocyte count within 1 to 2 weeks in some adults with acute lymphatic leukemia and high total leukocyte counts.

The total daily dosage may be given at one time. It is calculated to the nearest multiple of 25 mg. The dosage of PURINETHOL should be reduced to one third to one quarter of the usual dose if allopurinol is given concurrently. Because the drug may have a delayed action, it should be discontinued at the first sign of an abnormally large or rapid fall in the leukocyte or platelet count. If subsequently the leukocyte count or platelet count remains constant for 2 or 3 days, or rises, treatment may be resumed.

Maintenance Therapy: Once a complete hematologic remission is obtained, maintenance therapy is considered essential. Maintenance doses will vary from patient to patient. A usual daily maintenance dose of PURINETHOL is 1.5 to 2.5 mg/kg per day as a single dose. It is to be emphasized that in pediatric patients with acute lymphatic leukemia in remission, superior results have been obtained when PURINETHOL has been combined with other agents (most frequently with methotrexate) for remission maintenance. PURINETHOL should rarely be relied upon as a single agent for the maintenance of remissions induced in acute leukemia.

Procedures for proper handling and disposal of anticancer drugs should be considered. Several guidelines on this subject have been published.[26-32]

There is no general agreement that all of the procedures recommended in the guidelines are necessary or appropriate.

HOW SUPPLIED

Pale yellow to buff, scored tablets containing 50 mg mercaptopurine, imprinted with "PURINETHOL" and "04A"; bottles of 25 (NDC 0173-0807-25) and 250 (NDC 0173-0807-65).

Store at 15° to 25°C (59°to 77°F) in a dry place.

REFERENCES

1. Hitchings GH, Elion GB. The chemistry and biochemistry of purine analogs. *Ann NY Acad Sci.* 1954; 60:195-199.
2. Loo TL, Luce JK, Sullivan MP, Frei E III. Clinical pharmacologic observations on 6-mercaptopurine and 6-methylthiopurine ribonucleoside. *Clin Pharmacol Ther.* 1968; 9:180-194.
3. Elion GB. Biochemistry and pharmacology of purine analogs. *Fed Proc.* 1967;26:898-904.
4. Scannell JP, Hitchings GH. Thioguanine in deoxyribonucleic acid from tumors of 6-mercaptopurine-treated mice. *Proc Soc Exp Biol Med.* 1966;122:627-629.
5. Paterson ARP, Tidd DM. 6-thiopurines. In Sartorelli AC, Johns DG (eds). *Antineoplastic and Immunosuppressive Agents,* Part II. Berlin, Springer-Verlag; 1975;384-403.
6. Lennard L, Gibson BES, Nicole T, Lilleyman JS. Congenital thiopurine methyltransferase deficiency and 6-mercaptopurine toxicity during treatment for acute lymphoblastic leukemia. *Arch Dis Child.* 1993:69:577-579.
7. Evans WE, Horner M, Chu YQ, Kalwinsky D, Roberts WM. Altered mercaptopurine metabolism, toxic effects, and dosage requirement in a thiopurine methyltransferase-deficient child with acute lymphocytic leukemia. *J Pediatr.* 1991;119:985-989.
8. Burchenal JH, Ellison RR, Murphy ML, et al. Clinical studies on 6-mercaptopurine. *Ann NY Acad Sci.* 1954; 60:359-368.
9. Farber S. Summary of experience with 6-mercaptopurine. *Ann NY Acad Sci.* 1954;60:412-414.
10. Fountain JR. Clinical observations of the treatment of leukemia and allied disorders with 6-mercaptopurine. *Ann NY Acad Sci.* 1954;60:439-446.
11. Hyman GA, Gellhorn A, Wolff JA. The therapeutic effect of mercaptopurine in a variety of human neoplastic diseases. *Ann NY Acad Sci.* 1954;60:430-435.
12. Einhorn M, Davidsohn I. Hepatotoxicity of mercaptopurine. *JAMA.* 1964;188:802-806.
13. Schein PS, Winokur SH. Immunosuppressive and cytotoxic chemotherapy: long-term complications. *Ann Intern Med.* 1975;82:84-95.
14. Stern MH, Minow RA, Casey JH, Luna MA. Hepatotoxicity in patients treated with adriamycin and 6-mercaptopurine for refractory leukemia. *Am J Clin Pathol.* 1975;63:758-759. Abstract.
15. Blatt J, Mulvihill JJ, Ziegler JL, Young RC, Poplack DG. Pregnancy outcome following cancer chemotherapy. *Am J Med.* 1980;69:828-832.
16. Nicholson HO. Cytotoxic drugs in pregnancy: review of reported cases. *J Obstet Gynaecol Br Commonw.* 1968; 75:307-312.
17. Woods WG, Daigle AE, Hutchinson RJ, Robison LL. Myelosuppression associated with cotrimoxazole as a prophylactic antibiotic in the maintenance phase of childhood acute lymphocytic leukemia. *J Pediatr.* 1984; 105: 639-644.
18. Rees CA, Lennard L, Lilleyman JS, Maddocks JL. Disturbance of 6-mercaptopurine metabolism by cotrimoxazole in childhood lymphoblastic leukemia. *Cancer Chemother Pharmacol.* 1984;12:87-89.
19. Reimers TJ, Sluss PM. 6-mercaptopurine treatment of pregnant mice: effects on second and third generations. *Science.* 1978;201:65-67.
20. Clark PA, Hsia YE, Huntsman RG. Toxic complications of treatment with 6-mercaptopurine. *Br Med J. [Clin Res].* 1960;1:393-395.
21. Present DH, Meltzer SJ, Wolke A, Korelitz BI. Short and long term toxicity to 6-mercaptopurine in the management of inflammatory bowel disease. *Gastroenterology.* 1985;88:1545. Abstract.
22. Bank L, Wright JP. 6-mercaptopurine-related pancreatitis in 2 patients with inflammatory bowel disease. *Dig Dis Sci.* 1984;29:357-359.
23. Singleton JW, Law DH, Kelley ML Jr, Mekhjian HS, Sturdevant RAL. National cooperative Crohn's disease study: adverse reactions to study drugs. *Gastroenterology.* 1979;77:870-882.
24. Dreizen S, Bodey GP, Rodriguez V, McCredie KB. Cutaneous complications of cancer chemotherapy. *Postgrad Med.* 1975;58:150-158.
25. Unpublished data on file with Glaxo Wellcome Inc.
26. Recommendations for the safe handling of parenteral antineoplastic drugs. Washington, DC: Division of Safety; National Institutes of Health; 1983. US Dept of Health and Human Services. Public Health Service publication NIH 83-2621.
27. AMA Council on Scientific Affairs. Guidelines for handling parenteral antineoplastics. *JAMA.* 1985; 253: 1590-1591.
28. National Study Commission on Cytotoxic Exposure. Recommendations for handling cytotoxic agents. 1987.

Continued on next page

This product information is based on labeling in effect on June 23, 2000. For further information, contact via direct mail, phone, or web site. Medical Information, Glaxo Wellcome Inc., PO Box 13398, Research Triangle Park, NC 27709. Healthcare Professionals (Medical Information): 800-334-0089. Patients (Customer Response Center): 1-888-825-5249. Glaxo Wellcome Corporate Web Site: www.glaxowellcome.com

Purinethol—Cont.

Available from Louis P. Jeffrey, Chairman, National Study Commission on Cytotoxic Exposure. Massachusetts College of Pharmacy and Allied Health Sciences, 179 Longwood Avenue, Boston, MA 02115.

29. Clinical Oncological Society of Australia. Guidelines and recommendations for safe handling of antineoplastic agents. *Med J Australia.* 1983;1:426-428.
30. Jones RB, Frank R, Mass T. Safe handling of chemotherapeutic agents: a report from the Mount Sinai Medical Center. *CA-A Cancer J for Clinicians.* 1983;33:258-263.
31. American Society of Hospital Pharmacists. ASHP technical assistance bulletin on handling cytotoxic and hazardous drugs. *Am J Hosp Pharm.* 1990;47:1033-1049.
32. Yodaiken RE, Bennett D. OSHA work-practice guidelines for personnel dealing with cytotoxic (antineoplastic) drugs. *Am J Hosp Pharm.* 1986;43:1193-1204.

Manufactured by Catalytica Pharmaceuticals, Inc.
Greenville, NC 27834
for Glaxo Wellcome Inc., Research Triangle Park, NC 27709

November 1997/RL-497

Shown in Product Identification Guide, page 316

RELENZA® ℞

[ra-lin' za]
(zanamivir for inhalation)

For Oral Inhalation Only
For Use with the DISKHALER® Inhalation Device

DESCRIPTION

The active component of RELENZA is zanamivir. The chemical name of zanamivir is 5-(acetylamino)-4-[(aminoiminomethyl)-amino]-2,6-anhydro-3,4,5-trideoxy-D-glycero-D-galacto-non-2-enonic acid. It has a molecular formula of $C_{12}H_{20}N_4O_7$ and a molecular weight of 332.3. It has the following structural formula:

Zanamivir is a white to off-white powder with a solubility of approximately 18 mg/mL in water at 20°C.

RELENZA is for administration to the respiratory tract by oral inhalation only. Each RELENZA ROTADISK® contains 4 regularly spaced double-foil blisters with each blister containing a powder mixture of 5 mg of zanamivir and 20 mg of lactose. The contents of each blister are inhaled using a specially designed breath-activated plastic device for inhaling powder called the DISKHALER. After a RELENZA ROTADISK is loaded into the DISKHALER, a blister that contains medication is pierced and the zanamivir is dispersed into the air stream created when the patient inhales through the mouthpiece. The amount of drug delivered to the respiratory tract will depend on patient factors such as inspiratory flow. Under standardized in vitro testing, RELENZA ROTADISK delivers 4 mg of zanamivir from the DISKHALER device when tested at a pressure drop of 3 kPa (corresponding to a flow rate of about 62 to 65 L/min) for 3 seconds. In a study of 5 adult and 5 adolescent patients with obstructive airway diseases, the combined peak inspiratory flow rates (PIFR) ranged from 66 to 140 L/min. In a separate study of 16 pediatric patients, PIFR results were more variable; 4 did not achieve measurable flow rates, and PIFR for measurable inhalations by 12 children ranged from 30.5 to 122.4 L/min. Only 1 of 4 children under age 8 had a measurable flow rate (see CLINICAL PHARMACOLOGY: Pediatric Patients, INDICATIONS AND USAGE: Description of Clinical Studies, and PRECAUTIONS: Pediatric Use).

MICROBIOLOGY

Mechanism of Action: The proposed mechanism of action of zanamivir is via inhibition of influenza virus neuraminidase with the possibility of alteration of virus particle aggregation and release.

Antiviral Activity In Vitro: The antiviral activity of zanamivir against laboratory and clinical isolates of influenza virus was determined in cell culture assays. The concentrations of zanamivir required for inhibition of influenza virus were highly variable depending on the assay method used and virus isolate tested. The 50% and 90% inhibitory concentrations (IC_{50} and IC_{90}) of zanamivir were in the range of 0.005 to 16.0 µM and 0.05 to >100 µM, respectively (1 µM = 0.33 µg/mL). The relationship between the in vitro inhibition of influenza virus by zanamivir and the inhibition of influenza virus replication in humans has not been established.

Drug Resistance: Influenza viruses with reduced susceptibility to zanamivir have been recovered in vitro by passage of the virus in the presence of increasing concentrations of the drug. Genetic analysis of these viruses showed that the reduced susceptibility in vitro to zanamivir is associated with mutations that result in amino acid changes in the viral neuraminidase or viral hemagglutinin or both.

In an immunocompromised patient infected with influenza B virus, a variant virus emerged after treatment with an investigational nebulized solution of zanamivir for 2 weeks. Analysis of this variant showed a hemagglutinin mutation (Thr 198 lle) which resulted in a reduced affinity for human cell receptors, and a mutation in the neuraminidase active site (Arg 152 Lys) which reduced the enzyme's activity to zanamivir by 1000-fold.

Insufficient information is available to characterize the risk of emergence of zanamivir resistance in clinical use.

Cross-Resistance: Cross-resistance has been observed between zanamivir-resistant and oseltamivir-resistant influenza virus mutants generated in vitro. No studies have been performed to assess risk of emergence of cross-resistance during clinical use.

Influenza Vaccine Interaction Study: An interaction study (n = 138) was conducted to evaluate the effects of zanamivir (10 mg once daily) on the serological response to a single dose of trivalent inactivated influenza vaccine, as measured by hemagglutination inhibition titers. There was no clear difference in hemagglutination inhibition antibody titers at 2 weeks and 4 weeks after vaccine administration between zanamivir and placebo recipients.

Influenza Challenge Studies: Antiviral activity of zanamivir was supported for influenza A, and to a more limited extent for influenza B, by Phase 1 studies in volunteers who received intranasal inoculations of challenge strains of influenza virus, and received an intranasal formulation of zanamivir or placebo starting before or shortly after viral inoculation.

CLINICAL PHARMACOLOGY

Pharmacokinetics: ***Absorption and Bioavailability:*** Pharmacokinetic studies of orally inhaled zanamivir indicate that approximately 4% to 17% of the inhaled dose is systemically absorbed. The peak serum concentrations ranged from 17 to 142 ng/mL within 1 to 2 hours following a 10-mg dose. The area under the serum concentration versus time curve (AUC_∞) ranged from 111 to 1364 ng•h/mL.

Distribution: Zanamivir has limited plasma protein binding (<10%).

Metabolism: Zanamivir is renally excreted as unchanged drug. No metabolites have been detected in humans.

Elimination: The serum half-life of zanamivir following administration by oral inhalation ranges from 2.5 to 5.1 hours. It is excreted unchanged in the urine with excretion of a single dose completed within 24 hours. Total clearance ranges from 2.5 to 10.9 L/h. Unabsorbed drug is excreted in the feces.

Special Populations: Impaired Hepatic Function: The pharmacokinetics of zanamivir have not been studied in patients with impaired hepatic function.

Impaired Renal Function: Systemic exposure is limited after inhalation (see Absorption and Bioavailability). After a single intravenous dose of 4 mg or 2 mg of zanamivir in volunteers with mild/moderate or severe renal impairment, respectively, significant decreases in renal clearance (and hence total clearance: normals 5.3 L/h, mild/moderate 2.7 L/h, and severe 0.8 L/h; median values) and significant increases in half-life (normals 3.1 h, mild/moderate 4.7 h, and severe 18.5 h; median values) and systemic exposure were observed. Safety and efficacy have not been documented in the presence of severe renal insufficiency.

Pediatric Patients: The pharmacokinetics of zanamivir were evaluated in pediatric patients with signs and symptoms of respiratory illness. Sixteen patients, 6 to 12 years of age, received a single dose of 10-mg zanamivir dry powder via DISKHALER. Five patients had either undetectable zanamivir serum concentrations or had low drug concentrations (8.32 to 10.38 ng/mL) that were not detectable after 1.5 hours. Eleven patients had C_{max} median values of 43 ng/mL (range 15 to 74) and AUC_∞ median values of 167 ng•h/mL (range 58 to 279). Low or undetectable serum concentrations were related to lack of measurable PIFR in individual patients (see DESCRIPTION, INDICATIONS AND USAGE: Description of Clinical Studies, and PRECAUTIONS: Pediatric Use).

Geriatric Patients: The pharmacokinetics of zanamivir have not been studied in patients over 65 years of age (see PRECAUTIONS: Geriatric Use).

Gender, Race, and Weight: In a population pharmacokinetic analysis in patient studies, no clinically significant differences in serum concentrations and/or pharmacokinetic parameters (V/F, CL/F, ka, AUC_{0-3}, C_{max}, T_{max}, CLr, and % excreted in urine) were observed when demographic variables (gender, age, race, and weight) and indices of infection (laboratory evidence of infection, overall symptoms, symptoms of upper respiratory illness, and viral titers) were considered. There were no significant correlations between measures of systemic exposure and safety parameters.

Drug Interactions: No clinically significant pharmacokinetic drug interactions are predicted based on data from in vitro studies.

Zanamivir is not a substrate nor does it affect cytochrome P450 (CYP) isoenzymes (CYP1A1/2, 2A6, 2C9, 2C18, 2D6, 2E1, and 3A4) in human liver microsomes.

INDICATIONS AND USAGE

RELENZA is indicated for treatment of uncomplicated acute illness due to influenza A and B virus in adults and pediatric patients 7 years and older who have been symptomatic for no more than 2 days (see Description of Clinical Studies and PRECAUTIONS).

Description of Clinical Studies: ***Adults and Adolescents:*** The efficacy of RELENZA 10 mg inhaled twice daily for 5 days in the treatment of influenza has been evaluated in placebo-controlled studies conducted in North America, the Southern Hemisphere, and Europe during their respective influenza seasons. The magnitude of treatment effect varied between studies, with possible relationships to population-related factors including amount of symptomatic relief medication used.

Populations Studied: The principal Phase 3 studies enrolled 1588 patients ages 12 years and older (median age 34 years, 49% male, 91% Caucasian), with uncomplicated influenza-like illness within 2 days of symptom onset. Influenza was confirmed by culture, hemagglutination inhibition antibodies, or investigational direct tests. Of 1164 patients with confirmed influenza, 89% had influenza A and 11% had influenza B. These studies served as the principal basis for efficacy evaluation, with more limited Phase 2 studies providing supporting information where necessary. Following randomization to either zanamivir or placebo (inhaled lactose vehicle), all patients received instruction and supervision by a healthcare professional for the initial dose.

Principal Results: The definition of time to improvement in major symptoms of influenza included no fever and self-assessment of "none" or "mild" for headache, myalgia, cough, and sore throat. A Phase 2 and a Phase 3 study conducted in North America (total of over 600 influenza-positive patients) suggested up to one day of shortening of median time to this defined improvement in symptoms in patients receiving zanamivir compared to placebo, although statistical significance was not reached in either of these studies. In a study conducted in the Southern Hemisphere (321 influenza-positive patients), a 1.5-day difference in median time to symptom improvement was observed. Additional evidence of efficacy was provided by the European study.

Other Findings:

- There was no consistent difference in treatment effect in patients with influenza A compared to influenza B; however, these trials enrolled smaller numbers of patients with influenza B and thus provided less evidence in support of efficacy in influenza B.
- In general, patients with lower temperature (e.g., 38.2°C or less) or investigator-rated as having less severe symptoms at entry derived less benefit from therapy.
- No consistent treatment effect was demonstrated in patients with underlying chronic medical conditions, including respiratory or cardiovascular disease (see WARNINGS and PRECAUTIONS).
- No consistent differences in rate of development of complications were observed between treatment groups.
- Some fluctuation of symptoms was observed after the primary study endpoint in both treatment groups.

Pediatric Patients: The efficacy of RELENZA 10 mg inhaled twice daily for 5 days in the treatment of influenza in pediatric patients has been evaluated in a placebo-controlled study conducted in North America and Europe, enrolling 471 patients, ages 5 to 12 years (55% male, 90% Caucasian), within 36 hours of symptom onset. Of 346 patients with confirmed influenza, 65% had influenza A and 35% had influenza B. The definition of time to improvement included no fever and parental assessment of no or mild cough and absent/minimal muscle and joint aches or pains, sore throat, chills/feverishness, and headache. Median time to symptom improvement was one day shorter in patients receiving zanamivir compared with placebo. No consistent differences in rate of development of complications were observed between treatment groups. Some fluctuation of symptoms was observed after the primary study endpoint in both treatment groups.

Although this study was designed to enroll children ages 5 to 12 years, the product is indicated only for children ages 7 years and older. This evaluation is based on the combination of lower estimates of treatment effect in 5 and 6 year olds compared with the overall study population, and evidence of inadequate inhalation through the DISKHALER in a pharmacokinetic study (see DESCRIPTION, CLINICAL PHARMACOLOGY: Pediatric Patients, and PRECAUTIONS: Pediatric Use).

CONTRAINDICATIONS

RELENZA is contraindicated in patients with a known hypersensitivity to any component of the formulation.

WARNINGS

BRONCHOSPASM AND DECLINE IN LUNG FUNCTION HAVE BEEN REPORTED IN SOME PATIENTS RECEIVING RELENZA. MANY BUT NOT ALL OF THESE PATIENTS HAD UNDERLYING AIRWAYS DISEASE SUCH AS ASTHMA OR CHRONIC OBSTRUCTIVE PULMONARY DISEASE. BECAUSE OF THE RISK OF SERIOUS ADVERSE EVENTS AND BECAUSE EFFICACY HAS NOT BEEN DEMONSTRATED IN THIS POPULATION, RELENZA IS NOT GENERALLY RECOMMENDED FOR TREATMENT OF PATIENTS WITH UNDERLYING AIRWAYS DISEASE (SEE PRECAUTIONS). Some patients with serious adverse events during treatment with RELENZA have had fatal outcomes, although causality was difficult to assess.

RELENZA SHOULD BE DISCONTINUED IN ANY PATIENT WHO DEVELOPS BRONCHOSPASM OR DECLINE IN RESPIRATORY FUNCTION; immediate treatment and hospitalization may be required. Some patients without prior pulmonary disease may also have respiratory abnormalities from acute respiratory infection that could resemble adverse drug reactions or increase patient vulnerability to adverse drug reactions.

PRECAUTIONS

General: Patients should be instructed in the use of the delivery system. Instructions should include a demonstration whenever possible. Patients should read and follow carefully the Patient Instructions for Use accompanying the product. Effective and safe use of RELENZA requires proper use of the DISKHALER to inhale the drug.

There is no evidence for efficacy of zanamivir in any illness caused by agents other than influenza virus A and B.

No data are available to support safety or efficacy in patients who begin treatment after 48 hours of symptoms.

Safety and efficacy of repeated treatment courses have not been studied.

Patients with Respiratory Disease: SAFETY AND EFFICACY OF RELENZA HAVE NOT BEEN DEMONSTRATED IN PATIENTS WITH UNDERLYING CHRONIC PULMONARY DISEASE (SEE WARNINGS). IN PARTICULAR, RELENZA HAS NOT BEEN SHOWN TO BE EFFECTIVE IN PATIENTS WITH SEVERE OR DECOMPENSATED CHRONIC OBSTRUCTIVE PULMONARY DISEASE OR ASTHMA, AND SERIOUS ADVERSE EVENTS HAVE BEEN REPORTED IN SUCH PATIENTS. THEREFORE, RELENZA IS NOT GENERALLY RECOMMENDED FOR TREATMENT OF PATIENTS WITH UNDERLYING AIRWAYS DISEASE SUCH AS ASTHMA OR CHRONIC OBSTRUCTIVE PULMONARY DISEASE (SEE WARNINGS).

Bronchospasm was documented following administration of zanamivir in 1 of 13 patients with mild or moderate asthma (but without acute influenza-like illness) in a Phase 1 study. In interim results from an ongoing treatment study in patients with acute influenza-like illness superimposed on underlying asthma or chronic obstructive pulmonary disease, more patients on zanamivir than on placebo experienced greater than 20% decline in FEV_1 or peak expiratory flow rate.

If treatment with RELENZA is considered for a patient with underlying airways disease, the potential risks and benefits should be carefully weighed. If a decision is made to prescribe RELENZA for such a patient, this should be done only under conditions of careful monitoring of respiratory function, close observation, and appropriate supportive care including availability of fast-acting bronchodilators.

Allergic Reactions: Allergic-like reactions, including oropharyngeal edema and serious skin rashes, have been reported in post-marketing experience with RELENZA. RELENZA should be stopped and appropriate treatment instituted if an allergic reaction occurs or is suspected.

Bacterial Infections: Serious bacterial infections may begin with influenza-like symptoms or may coexist with or occur as complications during the course of influenza. RELENZA has not been shown to prevent such complications.

Prevention of Influenza: Use of zanamivir should not affect the evaluation of individuals for annual influenza vaccination in accordance with guidelines of the Centers for Disease Control and Prevention Advisory Committee on Immunization Practices. Safety and efficacy of zanamivir have not been established for prophylactic use of zanamivir to prevent influenza.

Limitations of Populations Studied: Safety and efficacy have not been demonstrated in patients with high-risk underlying medical conditions (see INDICATIONS AND USAGE: Description of Clinical Studies, and WARNINGS). No information is available regarding treatment of influenza in patients with any medical condition sufficiently severe or unstable to be considered at imminent risk of requiring inpatient management.

Information for Patients: Patients should be instructed in use of the delivery system. Instructions should include a demonstration whenever possible.

For the proper use of RELENZA, the patient should read and follow carefully the accompanying Patient Instructions for Use.

Patients should be advised that the use of RELENZA for treatment of influenza has not been shown to reduce the risk of transmission of influenza to others.

Patients should be advised of the risk of bronchospasm, especially in the setting of underlying airways disease, and should stop RELENZA and contact their physician if they experience increased respiratory symptoms during treatment such as worsening wheezing, shortness of breath, or other signs or symptoms of bronchospasm (see WARNINGS). If a decision is made to prescribe RELENZA for a patient with asthma or chronic obstructive pulmonary disease, the patient should be made aware of the risks and should have a fast-acting bronchodilator available. Patients scheduled to take inhaled bronchodilators at the same time as RELENZA should be advised to use their bronchodilators before taking RELENZA.

Drug Interactions: No clinically significant pharmacokinetic drug interactions are predicted based on data from in vitro studies.

Carcinogenesis, Mutagenesis, and Impairment of Fertility:
Carcinogenesis: In 2-year carcinogenicity studies conducted in rats and mice using a powder formulation administered through inhalation, zanamivir induced no statistically significant increases in tumors over controls. The maximum daily exposures in rats and mice were approximately 23 to 25 and 20 to 22 times, respectively, greater than those in humans at the proposed clinical dose based on AUC comparisons.

Table 1: Summary of Adverse Events ≥1.5% Incidence During Treatment in Adults and Adolescents

Adverse Event	RELENZA 10 mg b.i.d. **Inhaled** (n = 1132)	RELENZA All Dosing Regimens* (n = 2289)	Placebo (Lactose Vehicle†) (n = 1520)
Body as a whole			
Headaches	2%	2%	3%
Digestive			
Diarrhea	3%	3%	4%
Nausea	3%	3%	3%
Vomiting	1%	1%	2%
Respiratory			
Nasal signs and symptoms	2%	3%	3%
Bronchitis	2%	2%	3%
Cough	2%	2%	3%
Sinusitis	3%	2%	2%
Ear, nose, & throat infections	2%	1%	2%
Nervous system			
Dizziness	2%	1%	<1%

*Includes studies where RELENZA was administered intranasally (6.4 mg 2 to 4 times per day in addition to inhaled preparation) and/or inhaled more frequently (q.i.d.) than the currently recommended dose.

†Because the placebo consisted of inhaled lactose powder, which is also the vehicle for the active drug, some adverse events occurring at similar frequencies in different treatment groups could be related to lactose vehicle inhalation.

Table 2: Summary of Adverse Events ≥1.5% Incidence During Treatment in Pediatric Patients*

Adverse Event	RELENZA 10 mg b.i.d. Inhaled (n = 291)	Placebo (Lactose Vehicle†) (n = 318)
Respiratory		
Ear, nose, & throat infections	5%	5%
Ear, nose, & throat hemorrhage	<1%	2%
Asthma	<1%	2%
Cough	<1%	2%
Digestive		
Vomiting	2%	3%
Diarrhea	2%	2%
Nausea	<1%	2%

* Includes a subset of patients receiving RELENZA for treatment of influenza in a prophylaxis study.

† Because the placebo consisted of inhaled lactose powder which is also the vehicle for the active drug, some adverse events occurring at similar frequencies in different treatment groups could be related to lactose vehicle inhalation.

Mutagenesis: Zanamivir was not mutagenic in in vitro and in vivo genotoxicity assays which included bacterial mutation assays in *S. typhimurium* and *E. coli*, mammalian mutation assays in mouse lymphoma, chromosomal aberration assays in human peripheral blood lymphocytes, and the in vivo mouse bone marrow micronucleus assay.

Impairment of Fertility: The effects of zanamivir on fertility and general reproductive performance were investigated in male (dosed for 10 weeks prior to mating, and throughout mating, gestation/lactation, and shortly after weaning) and female rats (dosed for 3 weeks prior to mating through day 19 of pregnancy, or day 21 post partum) at IV doses 1, 9, and 90 mg/kg per day. Zanamivir did not impair mating or fertility of male or female rats, and did not affect the sperm of treated male rats. The reproductive performance of the F1 generation born to female rats given zanamivir was not affected. Based on a subchronic study in rats at a 90 mg/kg-per-day IV dose, AUC values ranged between 142 and 199 μg•h/mL (>300 times the human exposure at the proposed clinical dose).

Pregnancy: Pregnancy Category C. Embryo/fetal development studies were conducted in rats (dosed from days 6 to 15 of pregnancy) and rabbits (dosed from days 7 to 19 of pregnancy) using the same IV doses. Pre- and post-natal developmental studies were performed in rats (dosed from day 16 of pregnancy until litter day 21 to 23). In all studies, intravenous (1, 9, and 90 mg/kg per day) instead of the inhalational route of drug administration was used. No malformations, maternal toxicity, or embryotoxicity were observed in pregnant rats or rabbits and their fetuses. Because of insufficient blood sampling timepoints in both rat and rabbit reproductive toxicity studies, AUC values were not available. However, in a subchronic study in rats at the 90 mg/kg-per-day IV dose, the AUC values were greater than 300 times the human exposure at the proposed clinical dose.

An additional embryo/fetal study, in a different strain of rat, was conducted using subcutaneous administration of zanamivir, 3 times daily, at doses of 1, 9, or 80 mg/kg during days 7 to 17 of pregnancy. There was an increase in the incidence rates of a variety of minor skeleton alterations and variants in the exposed offspring in this study. Based on AUC measurements, the high dose in the study produced an exposure greater than 1000 times the human exposure at the proposed clinical dose. However, the individual incidence rate of each skeletal alteration or variant, in most instances, remained within the background rates of the historical occurrence in the strain studied.

Zanamivir has been shown to cross the placenta in rats and rabbits. In these animals, fetal blood concentrations of zanamivir were significantly lower than zanamivir concentrations in the maternal blood.

There are no adequate and well-controlled studies of zanamivir in pregnant women. Zanamivir should be used during pregnancy only if the potential benefit justifies the potential risk to the fetus.

Nursing Mothers: Studies in rats have demonstrated that zanamivir is excreted in milk. However, nursing mothers should be instructed that it is not known whether zanamivir is excreted in human milk. Because many drugs are excreted in human milk, caution should be exercised when RELENZA is administered to a nursing mother.

Pediatric Use: Safety and effectiveness of RELENZA have not been established in pediatric patients under 7 years of age.

The safety and effectiveness of RELENZA have been studied in a Phase 3 treatment study in pediatric patients, where 471 children 5 to 12 years of age received zanamivir or placebo (see INDICATIONS AND USAGE: Description of Clinical Studies, ADVERSE REACTIONS, and DOSAGE AND ADMINISTRATION). In a Phase 1 study of 16 children ages 6 to 12 years with signs and symptoms of respiratory disease, 4 did not produce a measurable peak inspiratory flow rate (PIFR) through the DISKHALER (3 with no adequate inhalation on request, 1 with missing data), 9 had measurable PIFR on each of 2 inhalations, and 3 achieved measurable PIFR on only 1 of 2 inhalations. Neither of two 6-year-olds and one of two 7-year-olds produced measurable PIFR. Overall, 8 of the 16 children (including all those under 8 years old) either did not produce measurable inspiratory flow through the DISKHALER or produced peak inspiratory flow rates below the 60 L/min considered optimal for the device under standardized in vitro testing; lack of measurable flow rate was related to low or undetectable serum concentrations (see DESCRIPTION, CLINICAL PHARMACOLOGY: Pediatric Patients, and INDICATIONS AND USAGE: Description of Clinical Studies). Prescribers should carefully evaluate the ability of young children to use the delivery system if prescription of RELENZA is considered. When RELENZA is prescribed for children, it should be used only under adult supervision and with attention to proper use of the delivery system.

Adolescents were included in the 3 principal Phase 3 adult treatment studies. In these studies, 67 patients were 12 to 16 years of age. No definite differences in safety and efficacy were observed between these adolescent patients and young adults.

Geriatric Use: Of the total number of patients in 6 clinical treatment studies of RELENZA, 59 were 65 and over, while 24 were 75 and over. No overall differences in safety or effectiveness were observed between these subjects and youn-

Continued on next page

This product information is based on labeling in effect on June 23, 2000. For further information, contact via direct mail, phone, or web site. Medical Information, Glaxo Wellcome Inc., PO Box 13398, Research Triangle Park, NC 27709. Healthcare Professionals (Medical Information): 800-334-0089. Patients (Customer Response Center): 1-888-825-5249. Glaxo Wellcome Corporate Web Site: www.glaxowellcome.com

Relenza—Cont.

ger patients, and other reported clinical experience has not identified differences in responses between the elderly and younger patients, but greater sensitivity of some older individuals cannot be ruled out.

ADVERSE REACTIONS

See WARNINGS and PRECAUTIONS for information about risk of serious adverse events such as bronchospasm and allergic-like reactions, and for safety information in patients with underlying respiratory disease.

Clinical Trials in Adults and Adolescents: Adverse events that occurred with an incidence ≥1.5% in treatment studies are listed in Table 1. This table shows adverse events occurring in patients ≥ 12 years of age receiving RELENZA 10 mg inhaled twice daily, RELENZA in all inhalation regimens, and placebo inhaled twice daily (where placebo consisted of the same lactose vehicle used in RELENZA).

[See table 1 at top of previous page]

Additional adverse reactions occurring in less than 1.5% of patients receiving RELENZA included malaise, fatigue, fever, abdominal pain, myalgia, arthralgia, and urticaria.

The most frequent laboratory abnormalities in Phase 3 treatment studies included elevations of liver enzymes and CPK, lymphopenia, and neutropenia. These were reported in similar proportions of zanamivir and lactose vehicle placebo recipients with acute influenza-like illness.

Clinical Trials in Pediatric Patients: Adverse events that occurred with an incidence ≥1.5% in children receiving treatment doses of RELENZA in 2 Phase 3 studies are listed in Table 2. This table shows adverse events occurring in pediatric patients 5 to 12 years old receiving RELENZA 10 mg inhaled twice daily, and placebo inhaled twice daily (where placebo consisted of the same lactose vehicle used in RELENZA).

[See table 2 on previous page]

In 1 of the 2 studies described in Table 2, some additional information is available from children (5 to 12 years old) without acute influenza-like illness who received an investigational prophylaxis regimen of RELENZA; 132 children received RELENZA and 145 children received placebo. Among these children, nasal signs and symptoms (zanamivir 20%, placebo 9%), cough (zanamivir 16%, placebo 8%), and throat/tonsil discomfort and pain (zanamivir 11%, placebo 6%) were reported more frequently with RELENZA than placebo. In a subset with chronic respiratory disease, lower respiratory adverse events (described as asthma, cough, or viral respiratory infections which could include influenza-like symptoms) were reported in 7 of 7 zanamivir recipients and 5 of 12 placebo recipients.

Observed During Clinical Practice: In addition to adverse events reported from clinical trials, the following events have been identified during post-marketing use of zanamivir (RELENZA). Because they are reported voluntarily from a population of unknown size, estimates of frequency cannot be made. These events have been chosen for inclusion due to a combination of their seriousness, frequency of reporting, or potential causal connection to zanamivir (RELENZA).

General: Allergic or allergic-like reaction, including oropharyngeal edema (see PRECAUTIONS).

Cardiac: Arrhythmias, syncope.

Neurologic: Seizures.

Respiratory: Bronchospasm, dyspnea (see WARNINGS and PRECAUTIONS).

Skin: Rash, including serious cutaneous reactions (see PRECAUTIONS).

OVERDOSAGE

There have been no reports of overdosage from administration of RELENZA. Doses of zanamivir up to 64 mg/day have been administered by nebulizer. Additionally, doses of up to 1200 mg/day for 5 days have been administered intravenously. Adverse effects were similar to those seen in clinical studies at the recommended dose.

DOSAGE AND ADMINISTRATION

RELENZA is for administration to the respiratory tract by oral inhalation only, using the DISKHALER device provided. **Patients should be instructed in the use of the delivery system. Instructions should include a demonstration whenever possible. If RELENZA is prescribed for children, it should be used only under adult supervision and instruction, and the supervising adult should first be instructed by a healthcare professional (see PRECAUTIONS).**

The recommended dose of RELENZA for treatment of influenza in adults and pediatric patients ages 7 years and older is 2 inhalations (one 5-mg blister per inhalation for a total dose of 10 mg) twice daily (approximately 12 hours apart) for 5 days. Two doses should be taken on the first day of treatment whenever possible provided there is at least 2 hours between doses. On subsequent days, doses should be about 12 hours apart (e.g., morning and evening) at approximately the same time each day. There are no data on the effectiveness of treatment with RELENZA when initiated more than 2 days after the onset of signs or symptoms.

Patients scheduled to use an inhaled bronchodilator at the same time as RELENZA should use their bronchodilator before taking RELENZA. (See WARNINGS and PRECAUTIONS regarding patients with chronic respiratory disease and other medical conditions.)

HOW SUPPLIED

RELENZA is supplied in a circular double-foil pack (a ROTADISK) containing 4 blisters of the drug. Five ROTADISKS are packaged in a white polypropylene tube. The tube is packaged in a carton with 1 blue and gray DISKHALER inhalation device (NDC 0173-0681-01).

Store at 25°C (77°F); excursions permitted to 15° to 30°C (59° to 86°F) (see USP Controlled Room Temperature). Keep out of reach of children. Do not puncture any RELENZA ROTADISK blister until taking a dose using the DISKHALER.

Glaxo Wellcome Inc., Research Triangle Park, NC 27709
US Patent Nos. 4,627,432; 4,778,054; 4,811,731; 5,360,817; 5,648,379; 5,035,237; Des. 379,506

April 2000/RL-817

Shown in Product Identification Guide, page 316

RETROVIR® ℞
[re 'trō-vir]
(zidovudine)
Tablets

RETROVIR® ℞
(zidovudine)
Capsules

RETROVIR® ℞
(zidovudine)
Syrup

WARNING: RETROVIR (ZIDOVUDINE) MAY BE ASSOCIATED WITH HEMATOLOGIC TOXICITY INCLUDING GRANULOCYTOPENIA AND SEVERE ANEMIA PARTICULARLY IN PATIENTS WITH ADVANCED HIV DISEASE (SEE WARNINGS). PROLONGED USE OF RETROVIR HAS BEEN ASSOCIATED WITH SYMPTOMATIC MYOPATHY SIMILAR TO THAT PRODUCED BY HUMAN IMMUNODEFICIENCY VIRUS.
RARE OCCURRENCES OF POTENTIALLY FATAL LACTIC ACIDOSIS IN THE ABSENCE OF HYPOXEMIA, AND SEVERE HEPATOMEGALY WITH STEATOSIS HAVE BEEN REPORTED WITH THE USE OF CERTAIN ANTIRETROVIRAL NUCLEOSIDE ANALOGUES (SEE WARNINGS).

DESCRIPTION

RETROVIR is the brand name for zidovudine (formerly called azidothymidine [AZT]), a pyrimidine nucleoside analogue active against human immunodeficiency virus (HIV).

Tablets: RETROVIR Tablets are for oral administration. Each film-coated tablet contains 300 mg of zidovudine and the inactive ingredients hydroxypropyl methylcellulose, magnesium stearate, microcrystalline cellulose, polyethylene glycol, sodium starch glycolate, and titanium dioxide.

Capsules: RETROVIR Capsules are for oral administration. Each capsule contains 100 mg of zidovudine and the inactive ingredients corn starch, magnesium stearate, microcrystalline cellulose, and sodium starch glycolate. The 100-mg empty hard gelatin capsule, printed with edible black ink, consists of black iron oxide, dimethylpolysiloxane, gelatin, pharmaceutical shellac, soya lecithin, and titanium dioxide. The blue band around the capsule consists of gelatin and FD&C Blue No. 2.

Syrup: RETROVIR Syrup is for oral administration. Each teaspoonful (5 mL) of RETROVIR Syrup contains 50 mg of zidovudine and the inactive ingredients sodium benzoate 0.2% (added as a preservative), citric acid, flavors, glycerin, and liquid sucrose. Sodium hydroxide may be added to adjust pH.

The chemical name of zidovudine is 3′-azido-3′-deoxythymidine.

Zidovudine is a white to beige, odorless, crystalline solid with a molecular weight of 267.24 and a solubility of 20.1 mg/mL in water at 25°C. The molecular formula is $C_{10}H_{13}N_5O_4$.

MICROBIOLOGY

Mechanism of Action: Zidovudine is a synthetic nucleoside analogue of the naturally occurring nucleoside, thymidine, in which the 3′-hydroxy (-OH) group is replaced by an azido (-N_3) group. Within cells, zidovudine is converted to the active metabolite, zidovudine 5′-triphosphate (AztTP), by the sequential action of the cellular enzymes. Zidovudine 5′-triphosphate inhibits the activity of the HIV reverse transcriptase both by competing for utilization with the natural substrate, deoxythymidine 5′-triphosphate (dTTP), and by its incorporation into viral DNA. The lack of a 3′-OH group in the incorporated nucleoside analogue prevents the formation of the 5′ to 3′ phosphodiester linkage essential for DNA chain elongation and, therefore, the viral DNA growth is terminated. The active metabolite AztTP is also a weak inhibitor of the cellular DNA polymerase-alpha and mitochondrial polymerase-gamma and has been reported to be incorporated into the DNA of cells in culture.

In Vitro HIV Susceptibility: The in vitro anti-HIV activity of zidovudine was assessed by infecting cell lines of lymphoblastic and monocytic origin and peripheral blood lymphocytes with laboratory and clinical isolates of HIV. The IC_{50} and IC_{90} values (50% and 90% inhibitory concentrations) were 0.003 to 0.013 and 0.03 to 0.13 mcg/mL, respectively (1 nM = 0.27 ng/mL). The IC_{50} and IC_{90} values of HIV isolates recovered from 18 untreated AIDS/ARC patients were in the range of 0.003 to 0.013 mcg/mL and 0.03 to 0.3 mcg/mL, respectively. Zidovudine showed antiviral activity in all acutely infected cell lines; however, activity was substantially less in chronically infected cell lines. In drug combination studies with zalcitabine, didanosine, lamivudine, saquinavir, indinavir, ritonavir, nevirapine, delavirdine, or interferon-alpha, zidovudine showed additive to synergistic activity in cell culture. The relationship between the in vitro susceptibility of HIV to reverse transcriptase inhibitors and the inhibition of HIV replication in humans has not been established.

Drug Resistance: HIV isolates with reduced sensitivity to zidovudine have been selected in vitro and were also recovered from patients treated with RETROVIR. Genetic analysis of the isolates showed mutations which result in five amino acid substitutions (Met41→Leu, A67→Asn, Lys70→Arg, Thr215→Tyr or Phe, and Lys219→Gln) in the viral reverse transcriptase. In general, higher levels of resistance were associated with greater number of mutations with 215 mutation being the most significant.

Cross-Resistance: The potential for cross-resistance between HIV reverse transcriptase inhibitors and protease inhibitors is low because of the different enzyme targets involved. Combination therapy with zidovudine plus zalcitabine or didanosine does not appear to prevent the emergence of zidovudine-resistant isolates. Combination therapy with RETROVIR plus EPIVIR® delayed the emergence of mutations conferring resistance to zidovudine. In some patients harboring zidovudine-resistant virus, combination therapy with RETROVIR plus EPIVIR restored phenotypic sensitivity to zidovudine by 12 weeks of treatment. HIV isolates with multidrug resistance to zidovudine, didanosine, zalcitabine, stavudine, and lamivudine were recovered from a small number of patients treated for ≥1 year with the combination of zidovudine and didanosine or zalcitabine. The pattern of resistant mutations in the combination therapy was different (Ala62→Val, Val75→Ile, Phe77→116Tyr, and Gln→151Met) from monotherapy, with mutation 151 being most significant for multidrug resistance. Site-directed mutagenesis studies showed that these mutations could also result in resistance to zalcitabine, lamivudine, and stavudine.

CLINICAL PHARMACOLOGY

Pharmacokinetics: ***Adults:*** The pharmacokinetics of zidovudine has been evaluated in 22 adult HIV-infected patients in a Phase 1 dose-escalation study. After oral dosing (capsules), zidovudine was rapidly absorbed from the gastrointestinal tract with peak serum concentrations occurring within 0.5 to 1.5 hours. Dose-independent kinetics was observed over the range of 2 mg/kg every 8 hours to 10 mg/kg every 4 hours. The mean zidovudine half-life was approximately 1 hour and ranged from 0.78 to 1.93 hours following oral dosing.

Zidovudine is rapidly metabolized to 3′-azido-3′-deoxy-5′-*O*-β-*D*-glucopyranuronosylthymidine (GZDV) which has an apparent elimination half-life of 1 hour (range 0.61 to 1.73 hours). Following oral administration, urinary recovery of zidovudine and GZDV accounted for 14% and 74% of the dose, respectively, and the total urinary recovery averaged 90% (range 63% to 95%), indicating a high degree of absorption. However, as a result of first-pass metabolism, the average oral capsule bioavailability of zidovudine is 65% (range 52% to 75%). A second metabolite, 3′-amino-3′-deoxythymidine (AMT), has been identified in the plasma following single-dose intravenous (IV) administration of zidovudine. AMT area-under-the-curve (AUC) was one fifth of the AUC of zidovudine and had a half-life of 2.7 ± 0.7 hours. In comparison, GZDV AUC was about threefold greater than the AUC of zidovudine.

Additional pharmacokinetic data following intravenous dosing indicated dose-independent kinetics over the range of 1 to 5 mg/kg with a mean zidovudine half-life of 1.1 hours (range 0.48 to 2.86 hours). Total body clearance averaged 1900 mL/min per 70 kg and the apparent volume of distribution was 1.6 L/kg. Renal clearance is estimated to be 400 mL/min per 70 kg, indicating glomerular filtration and active tubular secretion by the kidneys. Zidovudine plasma protein binding is 34% to 38%, indicating that drug interactions involving binding site displacement are not anticipated.

The zidovudine cerebrospinal fluid (CSF)/plasma concentration ratio was determined in 39 patients receiving chronic therapy with RETROVIR. The median ratio measured in 50 paired samples drawn 1 to 8 hours after the last dose of RETROVIR was 0.6.

Adults with Impaired Renal Function: The pharmacokinetics of zidovudine has been evaluated in patients with impaired renal function following a single 200-mg oral dose. In 14 patients (mean creatinine clearance 18 ± 2 mL/min) the half-life of zidovudine was 1.4 hours compared to 1.0 hour for control subjects with normal renal function; AUC values were approximately twice those of controls. Additionally, GZDV half-life in these patients was 8.0 hours (vs 0.9 hours for control) and AUC was 17 times higher than for control subjects. The pharmacokinetics and tolerance were evaluated in a multiple-dose study in patients undergoing hemodialysis (n = 5) or peritoneal dialysis (n = 6). Patients received escalating doses of zidovudine up to 200 mg five times daily for 8 weeks. Daily doses of 500 mg or less were well tolerated despite significantly elevated plasma levels of GZDV. Apparent oral clearance of zidovudine was approximately 50% of that reported in patients with normal renal function. The plasma concentrations of AMT are not known in patients with renal insufficiency. Daily doses of 300 to 400 mg should be appropriate in HIV-infected patients with severe renal dysfunction (see DOSAGE AND ADMINISTRATION: Dose Adjustment). Hemodialysis and peritoneal dialysis appear to have a negligible effect on the removal of zidovudine, whereas GZDV elimination is enhanced.

Pediatrics: The pharmacokinetics and bioavailability of zidovudine have been evaluated in 21 HIV-infected pediatric patients, aged 6 months through 12 years, following intravenous doses administered over the range of 80 to 160 mg/m^2 every 6 hours, and following oral doses of the IV solution administered over the range of 90 to 240 mg/m^2 every 6 hours. After discontinuation of the IV infusion, zidovudine plasma concentrations decayed biexponentially, consistent with two-compartment pharmacokinetics. Proportional increases in AUC and in zidovudine concentrations were observed with increasing dose, consistent with dose-independent kinetics over the dose range studied. The mean terminal half-life and total body clearance across all dose levels administered were 1.5 hours and 30.9 mL/min per kg, respectively. These values compare to mean half-life and total body clearance in adults of 1.1 hours and 27.1 mL/min per kg.

The mean oral bioavailability of 65% was independent of dose. This value is the same as the bioavailability in adults. Doses of 180 mg/m^2 four times daily in pediatric patients produced similar systemic exposure (24-hour AUC 10.7 hr•mcg/mL) as doses of 200 mg six times daily in adult patients (10.9 hr•mcg/mL).

The pharmacokinetics of zidovudine have been studied in pediatric patients from birth to 3 months of life. In one study of the pharmacokinetics of zidovudine in women during the last trimester of pregnancy, zidovudine elimination was determined immediately after birth in eight neonates who were exposed to zidovudine in utero. The half-life was 13.0 ± 5.8 hours. In another study, the pharmacokinetics of zidovudine was evaluated in pediatric patients (ranging in age of 1 day to 3 months) of normal birth weight for gestational age and with normal renal and hepatic function. In neonates less than or equal to 14 days old, mean ± SD total body clearance was 10.9 ± 4.8 mL/min per kg (n = 18) and half-life was 3.1 ± 1.2 hours (n = 21). In neonates and infants greater than 14 days old, total body clearance was 19.0 ± 4.0 mL/min per kg (n = 16) and half-life was 1.9 ± 0.7 hours (n = 18). Bioavailability was 89% ± 19% (n = 15) in the younger age group and decreased to 61% ± 19% (n = 17) in patients older than 14 days.

Concentrations of zidovudine in cerebrospinal fluid were measured after both intermittent oral and IV drug administration in 21 pediatric patients during Phase 1 and Phase 2 studies. The mean zidovudine CSF/plasma concentration ratio measured at an average time of 2.2 hours postdose at oral doses of 120 to 240 mg/m^2 was 0.52 ± 0.44 (n = 28); after an IV infusion of doses of 80 to 160 mg/m^2 over 1 hour, the mean CSF/plasma concentration ratio was 0.87 ± 0.66 (n = 23) at 3.2 hours after the start of the infusion. During continuous IV infusion, mean steady-state CSF/plasma ratio was 0.26 ± 0.17 (n = 28).

As in adult patients, the major route of elimination in pediatric patients was by metabolism to GZDV. After IV dosing, about 29% of the dose was excreted in the urine unchanged and about 45% of the dose was excreted as GZDV. Overall, the pharmacokinetics of zidovudine in pediatric patients greater than 3 months of age are similar to that of zidovudine in adult patients.

Pregnancy: The pharmacokinetics of zidovudine have been studied in a Phase 1 study of eight women during the last trimester of pregnancy. As pregnancy progressed, there was no evidence of drug accumulation. The pharmacokinetics of zidovudine were similar to that of nonpregnant adults. Consistent with passive transmission of the drug across the placenta, zidovudine concentrations in infant plasma at birth were essentially equal to those in maternal plasma at delivery. Although data are limited, methadone maintenance therapy in five pregnant women did not appear to alter zidovudine pharmacokinetics. However, in another patient population, a potential for interaction has been identified (see PRECAUTIONS).

Nursing Mothers: The U.S. Public Health Service Centers for Disease Control and Prevention advises HIV-infected women not to breastfeed to avoid postnatal transmission of HIV to a child who may not yet be infected. After administration of a single dose of 200 mg zidovudine to 13 HIV-infected women, the mean concentration of zidovudine was similar in human milk and serum (see PRECAUTIONS: Nursing Mothers).

Effect of Food on Absorption: Administration of RETROVIR Capsules with food decreased peak plasma concentrations by greater than 50%; however, bioavailability as determined by AUC may not be affected.

The effect of food on the absorption of zidovudine from the tablet formulation is not known.

Tablets: In a single-dose study of 23 healthy volunteers, the mean ± SD relative bioavailability of the RETROVIR 300-mg Tablet relative to three 100-mg RETROVIR Capsules was 110 ± 18%. After administration of the 300-mg RETROVIR Tablet or three 100-mg RETROVIR Capsules, the mean ± SD C_{max} values were 1.81 ± 0.52 and 1.50 ± 0.46 mcg/mL, respectively.

Syrup: In a multiple-dose bioavailability study conducted in 12 HIV-infected adults receiving doses of 100 or 200 mg every 4 hours, RETROVIR Syrup was demonstrated to be bioequivalent to RETROVIR Capsules with respect to area under the zidovudine plasma concentration-time curve (AUC). The rate of absorption of RETROVIR Syrup was greater than that of RETROVIR Capsules, as indicated by mean times to peak concentration of 0.5 and 0.8 hours, respectively. Mean values for steady-state peak concentration (dose-normalized to 200 mg) were 1.5 and 1.2 mcg/mL for syrup and capsules, respectively.

Table 1
First AIDS-Defining Event or Death and Death Only by Study Arm and Antiretroviral Experience

Treatment Antiretroviral Experience	Event	RETROVIR	Didanosine	RETROVIR plus Didanosine	RETROVIR plus Zalcitabine
Overall	No. of Patients	619	620	613	615
	AIDS/Death	96 (16%)	71 (11%)	66 (11%)	76 (12%)
	Death Only	54 (9%)	29 (5%)	31 (5%)	40 (7%)
Naive	No. of Patients	269	268	263	267
	AIDS/Death	32 (12%)	23 (9%)	20 (8%)	16 (6%)
	Death Only	18 (7%)	11 (4%)	11 (4%)	9 (3%)
Experienced	No. of Patients	350	352	350	348
	AIDS/Death	64 (18%)	48 (14%)	45 (13%)	60 (17%)
	Death Only	36 (10%)	18 (5%)	20 (6%)	31 (9%)

INDICATIONS AND USAGE

RETROVIR is indicated for the treatment of HIV infection when antiretroviral therapy is warranted (see Description of Clinical Studies).

The duration of clinical benefit from antiretroviral therapy may be limited. Alterations in antiretroviral therapy should be considered if disease progression occurs during treatment.

Maternal-Fetal HIV Transmission: RETROVIR is also indicated for the prevention of maternal-fetal HIV transmission as part of a regimen that includes oral RETROVIR beginning between 14 and 34 weeks of gestation, intravenous RETROVIR during labor, and administration of RETROVIR Syrup to the neonate after birth. The efficacy of this regimen for preventing HIV transmission in women who have received RETROVIR for a prolonged period before pregnancy has not been evaluated. The safety of RETROVIR for the mother or fetus during the first trimester of pregnancy has not been assessed (see Description of Clinical Studies).

Description of Clinical Studies: Therapy with RETROVIR has been shown to prolong survival and decrease the incidence of opportunistic infections in patients with advanced HIV disease at the initiation of therapy and to delay disease progression in asymptomatic HIV-infected patients.

Other randomized studies suggest that the duration of the clinical benefit of monotherapy with RETROVIR is time-limited.

Combination Therapy-Adults: ACTG175 was a randomized, double-blind, controlled trial that compared RETROVIR 200 mg t.i.d.; didanosine 200 mg b.i.d.; RETROVIR plus didanosine; and RETROVIR plus zalcitabine 0.75 mg t.i.d. A total of 2467 HIV-infected adults with baseline CD4 counts of 200 to 500 cells/mm^3 (mean = 352) and no prior AIDS-defining event enrolled with the following demographics: male (82%), Caucasian (70%), mean age of 35 years, asymptomatic HIV infection (81%), and prior antiretroviral use (57%, mean duration = 89.5 weeks). The overall median duration of study treatment was 118 weeks. The incidence of AIDS-defining events or death is shown in Table 1.

[See table 1 above]

RETROVIR in combination with certain antiretroviral agents has been shown to be superior to monotherapy in one or more of the following: delaying death, delaying development of AIDS, increasing CD4 cell counts, and decreasing plasma HIV RNA. Use of RETROVIR in some combinations is based on surrogate marker data. The complete prescribing information for each drug should be consulted before combination therapy which includes RETROVIR is initiated.

Pregnant Women and Their Neonates: The utility of RETROVIR for the prevention of maternal-fetal HIV transmission was demonstrated in a randomized, double-blind, placebo-controlled trial (ACTG 076) conducted in HIV-infected pregnant women with CD4 cell counts of 200 to 1818 cells/mm^3 (median in the treated group: 560 cells/mm^3) who had little or no previous exposure to RETROVIR. Oral RETROVIR was initiated between 14 and 34 weeks of gestation (median 11 weeks of therapy) followed by IV administration of RETROVIR during labor and delivery. After birth, neonates received oral RETROVIR Syrup for 6 weeks. The study showed a statistically significant difference in the incidence of HIV infection in the neonates (based on viral culture from peripheral blood) between the group receiving RETROVIR and the group receiving placebo. Of 363 neonates evaluated in the study, the estimated risk of HIV infection was 7.8% in the group receiving RETROVIR and 24.9% in the placebo group, a relative reduction in transmission risk of 68.7%. RETROVIR was well tolerated by mothers and infants. There was no difference in pregnancy-related adverse events between the treatment groups.

Dose-Frequency Study: A randomized, double-blind, dose-frequency study of RETROVIR in 320 patients with AIDS or advanced ARC was conducted to assess the safety and tolerability of 600 mg RETROVIR per day given as either 100 mg every 4 hours or as 300 mg every 12 hours for 48 weeks. No significant difference was detected between the two dose frequencies with regard to adverse experiences or hematologic abnormalities. Although this study was not designed to determine efficacy, no differences in the frequency of or time to opportunistic infections, neoplasms, or death were noted between treatment groups. Changes in CD4 cell counts and β_2-microglobulin levels were similar between treatment groups.

CONTRAINDICATIONS

RETROVIR Tablets, Capsules, and Syrup are contraindicated for patients who have potentially life-threatening allergic reactions to any of the components of the formulations.

WARNINGS

Before combination therapy with RETROVIR is initiated, consult the complete prescribing information for each drug. The safety profile of RETROVIR plus other antiretroviral agents reflects the individual safety profiles of each component.

The incidence of adverse reactions appears to increase with disease progression, and patients should be monitored carefully, especially as disease progression occurs.

Bone Marrow Suppression: RETROVIR should be used with caution in patients who have bone marrow compromise evidenced by granulocyte count <1000 cells/mm^3 or hemoglobin <9.5 g/dL. In patients with advanced symptomatic HIV disease, anemia and neutropenia were the most significant adverse events observed (see ADVERSE REACTIONS). There have been reports of pancytopenia associated with the use of RETROVIR, which was reversible in most instances after discontinuance of the drug. However, significant anemia, in many cases requiring dose adjustment, discontinuation of RETROVIR, and/or blood transfusions has occurred during treatment with RETROVIR alone or in combination with other antiretrovirals.

Frequent blood counts are strongly recommended in patients with advanced HIV disease who are treated with RETROVIR. For HIV-infected individuals and patients with asymptomatic or early HIV disease, periodic blood counts are recommended. If anemia or neutropenia develops, dosage adjustments may be necessary (see DOSAGE AND ADMINISTRATION).

Myopathy: Myopathy and myositis with pathological changes, similar to that produced by HIV disease, have been associated with prolonged use of RETROVIR.

Lactic Acidosis/Severe Hepatomegaly with Steatosis: Rare occurrences of potentially fatal lactic acidosis in the absence of hypoxemia, and severe hepatomegaly with steatosis have been reported with the use of certain antiretroviral nucleoside analogues. Lactic acidosis should be considered whenever a patient receiving therapy with RETROVIR develops unexplained tachypnea, dyspnea, or fall in serum bicarbonate level. Under these circumstances, therapy with RETROVIR should be suspended until the diagnosis of lactic acidosis has been excluded. Caution should be exercised when administering RETROVIR to any patient, particularly obese women, with hepatomegaly, hepatitis, or other known risk factor for liver disease. These patients should be followed closely while on therapy with RETROVIR. The significance of elevated aminotransferase levels suggesting hepatic injury in HIV-infected patients prior to starting RETROVIR or while on RETROVIR is unclear. Treatment with RETROVIR should be suspended in the setting of rap-

Continued on next page

This product information is based on labeling in effect on June 23, 2000. For further information, contact via direct mail, phone, or web site. Medical Information, Glaxo Wellcome Inc., PO Box 13398, Research Triangle Park, NC 27709. Healthcare Professionals (Medical Information): 800-334-0089. Patients (Customer Response Center): 1-888-825-5249. Glaxo Wellcome Corporate Web Site: www.glaxowellcome.com

Retrovir Capsules/Syrup—Cont.

idly elevating aminotransferase levels, progressive hepatomegaly, or metabolic/lactic acidosis of unknown etiology.

Other Serious Adverse Reactions: Several serious adverse events have been reported with use of RETROVIR in clinical practice. Reports of pancreatitis, sensitization reactions (including anaphylaxis in one patient), vasculitis, and seizures have been rare. These adverse events, except for sensitization, have also been associated with HIV disease. Changes in skin and nail pigmentation have been associated with the use of RETROVIR.

PRECAUTIONS

General: Zidovudine is eliminated from the body primarily by renal excretion following metabolism in the liver (glucuronidation). In patients with severely impaired renal function, dosage reduction is recommended (see CLINICAL PHARMACOLOGY: Pharmacokinetics and DOSAGE AND ADMINISTRATION). Although very little data are available, patients with severely impaired hepatic function may be at greater risk of toxicity.

Information for Patients: RETROVIR is not a cure for HIV infection, and patients may continue to acquire illnesses associated with HIV infection, including opportunistic infections. Therefore, patients should be advised to seek medical care for any significant change in their health status.

The safety and efficacy of RETROVIR in women, intravenous drug users, and racial minorities is not significantly different than that observed in white males.

Patients should be informed that the major toxicities of RETROVIR are neutropenia and/or anemia. The frequency and severity of these toxicities are greater in patients with more advanced disease and in those who initiate therapy later in the course of their infection. They should be told that if toxicity develops, they may require transfusions or dose modifications including possible discontinuation. They should be told of the extreme importance of having their blood counts followed closely while on therapy, especially for patients with advanced symptomatic HIV disease. They should be cautioned about the use of other medications, including ganciclovir and interferon-alpha, that may exacerbate the toxicity of RETROVIR (see PRECAUTIONS: Drug Interactions). Patients should be informed that other adverse effects of RETROVIR include nausea and vomiting. Patients should also be encouraged to contact their physician if they experience muscle weakness, shortness of breath, symptoms of hepatitis or pancreatitis, or any other unexpected adverse events while being treated with RETROVIR.

RETROVIR Tablets, Capsules, and Syrup are for oral ingestion only. Patients should be told of the importance of taking RETROVIR exactly as prescribed. They should be told not to share medication and not to exceed the recommended dose. Patients should be told that the long-term effects of RETROVIR are unknown at this time.

Pregnant women considering the use of RETROVIR during pregnancy for prevention of HIV-transmission to their infants should be advised that transmission may still occur in some cases despite therapy. The long-term consequences of in utero and infant exposure to RETROVIR are unknown, including the possible risk of cancer.

HIV-infected pregnant women should be advised not to breastfeed to avoid postnatal transmission of HIV to a child who may not yet be infected.

Patients should be advised that therapy with RETROVIR has not been shown to reduce the risk of transmission of HIV to others through sexual contact or blood contamination.

Drug Interactions: ***Ganciclovir:*** Use of RETROVIR in combination with ganciclovir increases the risk of hematologic toxicities in some patients with advanced HIV disease. Should the use of this combination become necessary in the treatment of patients with HIV disease, dose reduction or interruption of one or both agents may be necessary to minimize hematologic toxicity. Hematologic parameters, including hemoglobin, hematocrit, and white blood cell count with differential, should be monitored frequently in all patients receiving this combination.

Interferon-alpha: Hematologic toxicities have also been seen when RETROVIR is used concomitantly with interferon-alpha. As with the concomitant use of RETROVIR and ganciclovir, dose reduction or interruption of one or both agents may be necessary, and hematologic parameters should be monitored frequently.

Bone Marrow Suppressive Agents/Cytotoxic Agents: Coadministration of RETROVIR with drugs that are cytotoxic or which interfere with RBC/WBC number or function (e.g., dapsone, flucytosine, vincristine, vinblastine, or adriamycin) may increase the risk of hematologic toxicity.

Probenecid: Limited data suggest that probenecid may increase zidovudine levels by inhibiting glucuronidation and/or by reducing renal excretion of zidovudine. Some patients who have used RETROVIR concomitantly with probenecid have developed flu-like symptoms consisting of myalgia, malaise, and/or fever and maculopapular rash.

Phenytoin: Phenytoin plasma levels have been reported to be low in some patients receiving RETROVIR, while in one case a high level was documented. However, in a pharmacokinetic interaction study in which 12 HIV-positive volunteers received a single 300-mg phenytoin dose alone and during steady-state zidovudine conditions (200 mg every 4 hours), no change in phenytoin kinetics was observed. Although not designed to optimally assess the effect of phenytoin on zidovudine kinetics, a 30% decrease in oral zidovudine clearance was observed with phenytoin.

Table 2

Stage of Disease	RETROVIR Daily Dose* (mg)	Granulocytopenia (<750 cells/mm^3)	Anemia (Hgb <8.0 g/dL)
Asymptomatic			
ACTG 019	500	1.8%†	1.1%†
Early HIV Disease (CD4 >200 cells/mm^3)			
ACTG 016	1200	4%	4%
Advanced HIV Disease (CD4 > 200 cells/mm^3)			
BW 02	1500	10%†	3%†‡
(CD4 ≤200 cells/mm^3)			
ACTG 002	600	37%	29%
BW 02	1500	47%	29%‡

*The currently recommended dose is 500 to 600 mg daily.
†Not statistically significant compared to placebo.
‡Anemia = Hgb <7.5 g/dL.

Methadone: In a pharmacokinetic study of nine HIV-positive patients receiving methadone-maintenance (30 to 90 mg daily) concurrent with 200 mg of RETROVIR every 4 hours, no changes were observed in the pharmacokinetics of methadone upon initiation of therapy with RETROVIR and after 14 days of treatment with RETROVIR. No adjustments in methadone-maintenance requirements were reported. For four patients, the mean zidovudine AUC was elevated twofold, while for five patients, the value was equal to that of control patients. The exact mechanism and clinical significance of these data are unknown.

Fluconazole: The coadministration of fluconazole with RETROVIR has been reported to interfere with the oral clearance and metabolism of RETROVIR. In a pharmacokinetic interaction study in which 12 HIV-positive men received RETROVIR 200 mg every 8 hours alone and in combination with fluconazole 400 mg daily, fluconazole increased the zidovudine AUC (74%; range 28% to 173%) and the zidovudine half-life (128%; range -4% to 189%) at steady state. The clinical significance of this interaction is unknown.

Atovaquone: Data from 14 HIV-infected volunteers who were given atovaquone tablets 750 mg every 12 hours with zidovudine 200 mg every 8 hours showed a 24% ± 12% decrease in zidovudine oral clearance, leading to a 35% ± 23% increase in plasma zidovudine AUC. The glucuronide metabolite:parent ratio decreased from a mean of 4.5 when zidovudine was administered alone to 3.1 when zidovudine was administered with atovaquone tablets. Zidovudine had no effect on atovaquone pharmacokinetics.

Valproic Acid: The concomitant administration of valproic acid 250 mg (n = 5) or 500 mg (n = 1) every 8 hours and zidovudine 100 mg orally every 8 hours for 4 days to six HIV-infected, asymptomatic male volunteers resulted in a 79% ± 61% (mean ± SD) increase in the plasma zidovudine AUC and a 22% ± 10% decrease in the plasma GZDV AUC as compared to the administration of zidovudine in the absence of valproic acid. The GZDV/zidovudine urinary excretion ratio decreased 58% ± 12%. Because no change in the zidovudine plasma half-life occurred, these results suggest that valproic acid may increase the oral bioavailability of zidovudine through inhibition of first-pass metabolism. Although the clinical significance of this interaction is unknown, patients should be monitored more closely for a possible increase in zidovudine-related adverse effects. The effect of zidovudine on the pharmacokinetics of valproic acid was not evaluated.

Lamivudine: RETROVIR and lamivudine were coadministered to 12 asymptomatic HIV-positive patients in a single-center, open-label, randomized, crossover study. No significant differences were observed in AUC∞ or total clearance for lamivudine or zidovudine when the two drugs were administered together.

Coadministration of RETROVIR with lamivudine resulted in an increase of 39% ± 62% (mean ± SD) in C_{max} of zidovudine.

Other Agents: Preliminary data from a drug interaction study (n = 10) suggest that coadministration of 200 mg RETROVIR and 600 mg rifampin decreases the area under the plasma concentration curve by an average of 48% ± 34%. However, the effect of once-daily dosing of rifampin on multiple daily doses of RETROVIR is unknown. Some nucleoside analogues affecting DNA replication, such as ribavirin, antagonize the in vitro antiviral activity of RETROVIR against HIV; concomitant use of such drugs should be avoided.

Carcinogenesis, Mutagenesis, Impairment of Fertility: Zidovudine was administered orally at three dosage levels to separate groups of mice and rats (60 females and 60 males in each group). Initial single daily doses were 30, 60, and 120 mg/kg per day in mice and 80, 220, and 600 mg/kg per day in rats. The doses in mice were reduced to 20, 30, and 40 mg/kg per day after day 90 because of treatment-related anemia, whereas in rats only the high dose was reduced to 450 mg/kg per day on day 91 and then to 300 mg/kg per day on day 279.

In mice, seven late-appearing (after 19 months) vaginal neoplasms (five nonmetastasizing squamous cell carcinomas, one squamous cell papilloma, and one squamous polyp) occurred in animals given the highest dose. One late-appearing squamous cell papilloma occurred in the vagina of a middle-dose animal. No vaginal tumors were found at the lowest dose.

In rats, two late-appearing (after 20 months), nonmetastasizing vaginal squamous cell carcinomas occurred in animals given the highest dose. No vaginal tumors occurred at the low or middle dose in rats. No other drug-related tumors were observed in either sex of either species.

At doses that produced tumors in mice and rats, the estimated drug exposure (as measured by AUC) was approximately three times (mouse) and 24 times (rat) the estimated human exposure at the recommended therapeutic dose of 100 mg every 4 hours.

Two transplacental carcinogenicity studies were conducted in mice. One study administered zidovudine at doses of 20 mg/kg per day or 40 mg/kg per day from gestation day 10 through parturition and lactation with dosing continuing in offspring for 24 months postnatally. The doses of zidovudine employed in this study produced zidovudine exposures approximately three times the estimated human exposure at recommended doses. After 24 months, an increase in incidence of vaginal tumors was noted with no increase in tumors in the liver or lung or any other organ in either gender. These findings are consistent with results of the standard oral carcinogenicity study in mice, as described earlier. A second study administered zidovudine at maximum tolerated doses of 12.5 mg/day or 25 mg/day (~1000 mg/kg nonpregnant body weight or ~450 mg/kg of term body weight) to pregnant mice from days 12 through 18 of gestation. There was an increase in the number of tumors in the lung, liver, and female reproductive tracts in the offspring of mice receiving the higher dose level of zidovudine.

It is not known how predictive the results of rodent carcinogenicity studies may be for humans.

Zidovudine was mutagenic in a 5178Y/TK$^{+/-}$ mouse lymphoma assay, positive in an in vitro cell transformation assay, clastogenic in a cytogenetic assay using cultured human lymphocytes, and positive in mouse and rat micronucleus tests after repeated doses. It was negative in a cytogenetic study in rats given a single dose.

Zidovudine, administered to male and female rats at doses up to seven times the usual adult dose based on body surface area considerations, had no effect on fertility judged by conception rates.

Pregnancy: Pregnancy Category C. Oral teratology studies in the rat and in the rabbit at doses up to 500 mg/kg per day revealed no evidence of teratogenicity with zidovudine. Zidovudine treatment resulted in embryo/fetal toxicity as evidenced by an increase in the incidence of fetal resorptions in rats given 150 or 450 mg/kg per day and rabbits given 500 mg/kg per day. The doses used in the teratology studies resulted in peak zidovudine plasma concentrations (after one half of the daily dose) in rats 66 to 226 times, and in rabbits 12 to 87 times, mean steady-state peak human plasma concentrations (after one sixth of the daily dose) achieved with the recommended daily dose (100 mg every 4 hours). In an in vitro experiment with fertilized mouse oocytes, zidovudine exposure resulted in a dose-dependent reduction in blastocyst formation. In an additional teratology study in rats, a dose of 3000 mg/kg per day (very near the oral median lethal dose in rats of 3683 mg/kg) caused marked maternal toxicity and an increase in the incidence of fetal malformations. This dose resulted in peak zidovudine plasma concentrations 350 times peak human plasma concentrations. (Estimated area-under-the-curve [AUC] in rats at this dose level was 300 times the daily AUC in humans given 600 mg per day.) No evidence of teratogenicity was seen in this experiment at doses of 600 mg/kg per day or less.

Two rodent transplacental carcinogenicity studies were conducted (see Carcinogenesis, Mutagenesis, Impairment of Fertility).

A randomized, double-blind, placebo-controlled trial was conducted in HIV-infected pregnant women to determine the utility of RETROVIR for the prevention of maternal-fetal HIV-transmission (see INDICATIONS AND USAGE: Description of Clinical Studies). Congenital abnormalities occurred with similar frequency between neonates born to mothers who received RETROVIR and neonates born to mothers who received placebo. Abnormalities were either problems in embryogenesis (prior to 14 weeks) or were recognized on ultrasound before or immediately after initiation of study drug.

Antiretroviral Pregnancy Registry: To monitor maternal-fetal outcomes of pregnant women exposed to RETROVIR, an Antiretroviral Pregnancy Registry has been established. Physicians are encouraged to register patients by calling 1-800-258-4263.

Nursing Mothers: The U.S. Public Health Service Centers for Disease Control and Prevention advises HIV-infected women not to breastfeed to avoid postnatal transmission of HIV to a child who may not yet be infected. Zidovudine is excreted in human milk (see Pharmacokinetics).

Pediatric Use: RETROVIR has been studied in HIV-infected pediatric patients over 3 months of age who have HIV-related symptoms or who are asymptomatic with abnormal laboratory values indicating significant HIV-related immunosuppression (see ADVERSE REACTIONS, DOSAGE AND ADMINISTRATION, and INDICATIONS AND USAGE: Description of Clinical Studies, and Pharmacokinetics).

ADVERSE REACTIONS

Monotherapy: ***Adults:*** The frequency and severity of adverse events associated with the use of RETROVIR in adults are greater in patients with more advanced infection at the time of initiation of therapy. The following table summarizes the relative incidence of hematologic adverse events observed in clinical studies by severity of HIV disease present at the start of treatment:

[See table 2 on previous page]

The anemia reported in patients with advanced HIV disease receiving RETROVIR appeared to be the result of impaired erythrocyte maturation as evidenced by macrocytosis while on drug. Although mean platelet counts in patients receiving RETROVIR were significantly increased compared to mean baseline values, thrombocytopenia did occur in some of these patients with advanced disease. Twelve percent of patients receiving RETROVIR compared to 5% of patients receiving placebo had >50% decreases from baseline platelet count. Mild drug-associated elevations in total bilirubin levels have been reported as an uncommon occurrence in patients treated for asymptomatic HIV infection.

The HIV-infected adults participating in these clinical trials often had baseline symptoms and signs of HIV disease and/or experienced adverse events at some time during study. It was often difficult to distinguish adverse events possibly associated with administration of RETROVIR from underlying signs of HIV disease or intercurrent illnesses. The following table summarizes clinical adverse events or symptoms which occurred in at least 5% of all patients with advanced HIV disease treated with 1500 mg/day of RETROVIR in the original placebo-controlled study. Of the items listed in the table, only severe headache, nausea, insomnia, and myalgia were reported at a significantly greater rate in patients receiving RETROVIR.

[See table 3 at right]

All events of a severe or life-threatening nature were monitored for adults in the placebo-controlled studies in early HIV disease and asymptomatic HIV infection. Data concerning the occurrence of additional signs or symptoms were also collected. No distinction was made in reporting events between those possibly associated with the administration of the study medication and those due to the underlying disease. The following tables summarize all those events reported at a statistically significant greater incidence for patients receiving RETROVIR in these studies:

[See table 4 at right]
[See table 5 at right]

Several serious adverse events have been reported with the use of RETROVIR in clinical practice. Myopathy and myositis with pathological changes, similar to that produced by HIV disease, have been associated with prolonged use of RETROVIR. Reports of hepatomegaly with steatosis, hepatitis, pancreatitis, lactic acidosis, sensitization reactions (including anaphylaxis in one patient), hyperbilirubinemia, vasculitis, and seizures have been rare. These adverse events, except for sensitization, have also been associated with HIV disease. A single case of macular edema has been reported with the use of RETROVIR.

Additional adverse events reported in clinical trials at a rate not significantly different from placebo are listed below. Selected events from post-marketing clinical experience with RETROVIR are also included. Many of these events may also occur as part of HIV disease. The clinical significance of the association between treatment with RETROVIR and these events is unknown.

Body as a Whole: Abdominal pain, back pain, body odor, chest pain, chills, edema of the lip, fever, flu syndrome, hyperalgesia.

Cardiovascular: Syncope, vasodilation.

Gastrointestinal: Bleeding gums, constipation, diarrhea, dysphagia, edema of the tongue, eructation, flatulence, mouth ulcer, rectal hemorrhage.

Hemic and Lymphatic: Lymphadenopathy.

Musculoskeletal: Arthralgia, muscle spasm, tremor, twitch.

Nervous: Anxiety, confusion, depression, dizziness, emotional lability, loss of mental acuity, nervousness, paresthesia, somnolence, vertigo.

Respiratory: Cough, dyspnea, epistaxis, hoarseness, pharyngitis, rhinitis, sinusitis.

Skin: Acne, changes in skin and nail pigmentation, pruritus, rash, sweat, urticaria.

Special senses: Amblyopia, hearing loss, photophobia, taste perversion.

Table 3
Percentage (%) of Patients with Clinical Events in Advanced HIV Disease (BW 02)

Adverse Event	RETROVIR 1500 mg/day* (n = 144) %	Placebo (n = 137) %
BODY AS A WHOLE		
Asthenia	19	18
Diaphoresis	5	4
Fever	16	12
Headache	42	37
Malaise	8	7
GASTROINTESTINAL		
Anorexia	11	8
Diarrhea	12	18
Dyspepsia	5	4
GI Pain	20	19
Nausea	46	18
Vomiting	6	3
MUSCULOSKELETAL		
Myalgia	8	2
NERVOUS		
Dizziness	6	4
Insomnia	5	1
Paresthesia	6	3
Somnolence	8	9
RESPIRATORY		
Dyspnea	5	3
SKIN		
Rash	17	15
SPECIAL SENSES		
Taste Perversion	5	8

*The currently recommended dose is 500 to 600 mg daily.

Table 4
Percentage (%) of Patients with Adverse Events in Early HIV Disease (ACTG 016)

Adverse Event	RETROVIR 1200 mg/day* (n = 361) %	Placebo (n = 352) %
BODY AS A WHOLE		
Asthenia	69	62
GASTROINTESTINAL		
Dyspepsia	6	1
Nausea	61	41
Vomiting	25	13

*The currently recommended dose is 500 to 600 mg daily.

Table 5
Percentage (%) of Patients with Adverse Events* in Asymptomatic HIV Infection (ACTG 019)

Adverse Event	RETROVIR 500 mg/day (n = 453) %	Placebo (n = 428) %
BODY AS A WHOLE		
Asthenia	8.6†	5.8
Headache	62.5	52.6
Malaise	53.2	44.9
GASTROINTESTINAL		
Anorexia	20.1	10.5
Constipation	6.4†	3.5
Nausea	51.4	29.9
Vomiting	17.2	9.8
NERVOUS		
Dizziness	17.9†	15.2

*Reported in ≥5% of study population.
†Not statistically significant versus placebo.

Urogenital: Dysuria, polyuria, urinary frequency, urinary hesitancy.

Pediatrics: Anemia and granulocytopenia among pediatric patients with advanced HIV disease receiving RETROVIR occurred with similar incidence to that reported for adults with AIDS or advanced ARC (see above). Management of neutropenia and anemia included, in some cases, dose modification and/or blood product transfusions. In the open-label studies, 17% had their dose modified (generally a reduction in dose by 30%) due to anemia and 25% had their dose modified (temporary discontinuation or dose reduction by 30%) for neutropenia. Four pediatric patients had RETROVIR permanently discontinued for neutropenia. The following table summarizes the occurrence of anemia (Hgb <7.5 g/dL) and granulocytopenia (<750 cells/mm^3) among 124 pediatric patients receiving RETROVIR for a mean of 267 days (range 3 to 855 days):

Table 6

Advanced Pediatric HIV Disease (n=124)	Granulocytopenia (<750 cells/mm^3)		Anemia (Hgb <7.5 g/dL)	
	n	%	n	%
	48	39	28*	23

* Twenty-two pediatric patients received one or more transfusions due to a decline in hemoglobin to <7.5 g/dL; an additional 15 pediatric patients were transfused for hemoglobin levels >7.5 g/dL. Fifty-nine percent of the patients transfused had a prestudy history of anemia or transfusion requirement.

Macrocytosis was observed among the majority of pediatric patients enrolled in the studies.

In the open-label studies involving 124 pediatric patients, 16 clinical adverse events were reported by 24 pediatric patients. No event was reported by more than 5.6% of the study populations. Due to the open-label design of the studies, it was difficult to determine possible events related to the use of RETROVIR versus disease-related events. Therefore, all clinical events reported as associated with therapy with RETROVIR or of unknown relationship to therapy with RETROVIR are presented in the following table:

[See table 7 at bottom of next page]

The clinical adverse events reported among adult recipients of RETROVIR may also occur in pediatric patients.

Use for the Prevention of Maternal-Fetal Transmission of HIV: In a randomized, double-blind, placebo-controlled

Continued on next page

This product information is based on labeling in effect on June 23, 2000. For further information, contact via direct mail, phone, or web site. Medical Information, Glaxo Wellcome Inc., PO Box 13398, Research Triangle Park, NC 27709. Healthcare Professionals (Medical Information): 800-334-0089. Patients (Customer Response Center): 1-888-825-5249. Glaxo Wellcome Corporate Web Site: www.glaxowellcome.com

Retrovir Capsules/Syrup—Cont.

trial in HIV-infected women and their neonates conducted to determine the utility of RETROVIR for the prevention of maternal-fetal HIV transmission, RETROVIR Syrup at 2 mg/kg was administered every 6 hours for 6 weeks to neonates beginning within 12 hours after birth. The most commonly reported adverse experiences were anemia (hemoglobin <9.0 g/dL) and neutropenia (<1000 cells/mm^3). Anemia occurred in 22% of the neonates who received RETROVIR and in 12% of the neonates who received placebo. The mean difference in hemoglobin values was less than 1.0 g/dL for neonates receiving RETROVIR compared to neonates receiving placebo. No neonates with anemia required transfusion and all hemoglobin values spontaneously returned to normal within 6 weeks after completion of therapy with RETROVIR. Neutropenia was reported with similar frequency in the group that received RETROVIR (21%) and in the group that received placebo (27%). The long-term consequences of in utero and infant exposure to RETROVIR are unknown.

OVERDOSAGE

Cases of acute overdoses in both pediatric patients and adults have been reported with doses up to 50 grams. None were fatal. The only consistent finding in these cases of overdose was spontaneous or induced nausea and vomiting. Hematologic changes were transient and not severe. Some patients experienced nonspecific CNS symptoms such as headache, dizziness, drowsiness, lethargy, and confusion. One report of a grand mal seizure possibly attributable to RETROVIR occurred in a 35-year-old male 3 hours after ingesting 36 grams of RETROVIR. No other cause could be identified. All patients recovered without permanent sequelae. Hemodialysis and peritoneal dialysis appear to have a negligible effect on the removal of zidovudine while elimination of its primary metabolite, GZDV, is enhanced.

DOSAGE AND ADMINISTRATION

Adults: The recommended total oral daily dose of RETROVIR is 600 mg per day in divided doses in combination with other antiretroviral agents and 500 mg (100 mg every 4 hours while awake) or 600 mg per day in divided doses for monotherapy. The effectiveness of this dose compared to higher dosing regimens in improving the neurologic dysfunction associated with HIV disease is unknown. A small randomized study found a greater effect of higher doses of RETROVIR on improvement of neurological symptoms in patients with pre-existing neurological disease.

Pediatrics: The recommended dose in pediatric patients 3 months to 12 years of age is 180 mg/m^2 every 6 hours (720 mg/m^2 per day), not to exceed 200 mg every 6 hours.

Maternal-Fetal HIV Transmission: The recommended dosing regimen for administration to pregnant women (>14 weeks of pregnancy) and their neonates is:

Maternal Dosing: 100 mg orally five times per day until the start of labor (see INDICATIONS AND USAGE: Description of Clinical Studies). During labor and delivery, intravenous RETROVIR should be administered at 2 mg/kg (total body weight) over 1 hour followed by a continuous intravenous infusion of 1 mg/kg per hour (total body weight) until clamping of the umbilical cord.

Neonatal Dosing: 2 mg/kg orally every 6 hours starting within 12 hours after birth and continuing through 6 weeks of age. Neonates unable to receive oral dosing may be administered RETROVIR intravenously at 1.5 mg/kg, infused over 30 minutes, every 6 hours. (See PRECAUTIONS if hepatic disease or renal insufficiency is present.)

Monitoring of Patients: Hematologic toxicities appear to be related to pretreatment bone marrow reserve and to dose and duration of therapy. In patients with poor bone marrow reserve, particularly in patients with advanced symptomatic HIV disease, frequent monitoring of hematologic indices is recommended to detect serious anemia or neutropenia (see WARNINGS). In patients who experience hematologic toxicity, reduction in hemoglobin may occur as early as 2 to 4 weeks, and neutropenia usually occurs after 6 to 8 weeks.

Dose Adjustment: Significant anemia (hemoglobin of <7.5 g/dL or reduction of >25% of baseline) and/or significant neutropenia (granulocyte count of <750 cells/mm^3 or reduction of >50% from baseline) may require a dose interruption until evidence of marrow recovery is observed (see WARNINGS). For less severe anemia or neutropenia, a reduction in daily dose may be adequate. In patients who develop significant anemia, dose modification does not necessarily eliminate the need for transfusion. If marrow recovery occurs following dose modification, gradual increases in dose may be appropriate depending on hematologic indices and patient tolerance.

In end-stage renal disease patients maintained on hemodialysis or peritoneal dialysis, recommended dosing is 100 mg every 6 to 8 hours (see CLINICAL PHARMACOLOGY: Pharmacokinetics).

There are insufficient data to recommend dose adjustment of RETROVIR in patients with impaired hepatic function.

HOW SUPPLIED

RETROVIR Tablets 300 mg (biconvex, white, round, film-coated) containing 300 mg zidovudine, one side engraved "GX CW3" and "300" on the other side. Bottle of 60 (NDC 0173-0501-00).

Store at 15° to 25°C (59° to 77°F).

RETROVIR Capsules 100 mg (white, opaque cap and body with a dark blue band) containing 100 mg zidovudine and printed with "Wellcome" and unicorn logo on cap and "Y9C" and "100" on body. Bottles of 100 (NDC 0173-0108-55) and Unit Dose Pack of 100 (NDC 0173-0108-56).

Store at 15° to 25°C (59° to 77°F) and protect from moisture.

RETROVIR Syrup (colorless to pale yellow, strawberry-flavored) containing 50 mg zidovudine in each teaspoonful (5 mL). Bottle of 240 mL (NDC 0173-0113-18) with child-resistant cap.

Store at 15° to 25°C (59° to 77°F).

US Patent Nos. 4,818,538 and 4,828,838 (Product Patents); 4,724,232; 4,833,130; and 4,837,208 (Use Patents)

Glaxo Wellcome Inc., Research Triangle Park, NC 27709

May 1998/RL-581

Shown in Product Identification Guide, page 316

RETROVIR® ℞

[re 'trō-vir]

(zidovudine)

IV Infusion

FOR INTRAVENOUS INFUSION ONLY

WARNING: RETROVIR (ZIDOVUDINE) MAY BE ASSOCIATED WITH HEMATOLOGIC TOXICITY INCLUDING NEUTROPENIA AND SEVERE ANEMIA PARTICULARLY IN PATIENTS WITH ADVANCED HIV DISEASE (SEE WARNINGS). PROLONGED USE OF RETROVIR HAS BEEN ASSOCIATED WITH SYMPTOMATIC MYOPATHY SIMILAR TO THAT PRODUCED BY HUMAN IMMUNODEFICIENCY VIRUS. RARE OCCURRENCES OF POTENTIALLY FATAL LACTIC ACIDOSIS IN THE ABSENCE OF HYPOXEMIA, AND SEVERE HEPATOMEGALY WITH STEATOSIS HAVE BEEN REPORTED WITH THE USE OF CERTAIN ANTIRETROVIRAL NUCLEOSIDE ANALOGUES (SEE WARNINGS).

DESCRIPTION

RETROVIR is the brand name for zidovudine (formerly called azidothymidine [AZT]), a pyrimidine nucleoside analogue active against human immunodeficiency virus (HIV). RETROVIR IV Infusion is a sterile solution for intravenous infusion only. Each mL contains 10 mg zidovudine in Water for Injection. Hydrochloric acid and/or sodium hydroxide may have been added to adjust the pH to approximately 5.5. RETROVIR IV Infusion contains no preservatives.

The chemical name of zidovudine is 3′-azido-3′-deoxythymidine.

Zidovudine is a white to beige, odorless, crystalline solid with a molecular weight of 267.24 and a solubility of 20.1 mg/mL in water at 25°C. The molecular formula is $C_{10}H_{13}N_5O_4$.

MICROBIOLOGY

Mechanism of Action: Zidovudine is a synthetic nucleoside analogue of the naturally occurring nucleoside, thymidine, in which the 3′-hydroxy (-OH) group is replaced by an azido (-N_3) group. Within cells, zidovudine is converted to the active metabolite, zidovudine 5′-triphosphate (AztTP), by the sequential action of the cellular enzymes. Zidovudine 5′-triphosphate inhibits the activity of the HIV reverse transcriptase both by competing for utilization with the natural substrate, deoxythymidine 5′-triphosphate (dTTP), and by its incorporation into viral DNA. The lack of a 3′- OH group in the incorporated nucleoside analogue prevents the formation of the 5′ to 3′ phosphodiester linkage essential for DNA chain elongation and, therefore, the viral DNA growth is terminated. The active metabolite AztTP is also a weak inhibitor of the cellular DNA polymerase-alpha and mitochondrial polymerase-gamma and has been reported to be incorporated into the DNA of cells in culture.

In Vitro HIV Susceptibility: The in vitro anti-HIV activity of zidovudine was assessed by infecting cell lines of lymphoblastic and monocytic origin and peripheral blood lymphocytes with laboratory and clinical isolates of HIV. The IC_{50} and IC_{90} values (50% and 90% inhibitory concentrations) were 0.003 to 0.013 and 0.03 to 0.13 mcg/mL, respectively (1 nM = 0.27 ng/mL). The IC_{50} and IC_{90} values of HIV isolates recovered from 18 untreated AIDS/ARC patients were in the range of 0.003 to 0.013 mcg/mL and 0.03 to 0.3 mcg/mL, respectively. Zidovudine showed antiviral activity in all acutely infected cell lines; however, activity was substantially less in chronically infected cell lines. In drug combination studies with zalcitabine, didanosine, lamivudine, saquinavir, indinavir, ritonavir, nevirapine, delavirdine, or interferon-alpha, zidovudine showed additive to synergistic activity in cell culture. The relationship between the in vitro susceptibility of HIV to reverse transcriptase inhibitors and the inhibition of HIV replication in humans has not been established.

Drug Resistance: HIV isolates with reduced sensitivity to zidovudine have been selected in vitro and were also recovered from patients treated with RETROVIR. Genetic analysis of the isolates showed mutations which result in five amino acid substitutions (Met41→Leu, A67→Asn, Lys70→Arg, Thr215→Tyr or Phe, and Lys219→Gln) in the viral reverse transcriptase. In general, higher levels of resistance were associated with greater number of mutations with 215 mutation being the most significant.

Cross-Resistance: The potential for cross-resistance between HIV reverse transcriptase inhibitors and protease inhibitors is low because of the different enzyme targets involved. Combination therapy with zidovudine plus zalcitabine or didanosine does not appear to prevent the emergence of zidovudine-resistant isolates. Combination therapy with RETROVIR plus EPIVIR® delayed the emergence of mutations conferring resistance to zidovudine. In some patients harboring zidovudine-resistant virus, combination therapy with RETROVIR plus EPIVIR restored phenotypic sensitivity to zidovudine by 12 weeks of treatment. HIV isolates with multidrug resistance to zidovudine, didanosine, zalcitabine, stavudine, and lamivudine were recovered from a small number of patients treated for ≥1 year with the combination of zidovudine and didanosine or zalcitabine. The pattern of resistant mutations in the combination therapy was different (Ala62→Val, Val75→Ile, Phe77→116Tyr, and Gln→151Met) from monotherapy, with mutation 151 being most significant for multidrug resistance. Site-directed mutagenesis studies showed that these mutations could also result in resistance to zalcitabine, lamivudine, and stavudine.

CLINICAL PHARMACOLOGY

Pharmacokinetics: ***Adults:*** The pharmacokinetics of zidovudine has been evaluated in 22 adult HIV-infected patients in a Phase 1 dose-escalation study. Following intravenous dosing, dose-independent kinetics was observed over the range of 1 to 5 mg/kg with a mean zidovudine half-life of 1.1 hours (range 0.48 to 2.86 hours). Total body clearance averaged 1900 mL/min per 70 kg, and the apparent volume of distribution was 1.6 L/kg. At a dose of 7.5 mg/kg every 4 hours, total body clearance was calculated to be about 1200 mL/min per 70 kg, with no change in half-life. Renal clearance is estimated to be 400 mL/min per 70 kg, indicating glomerular filtration and active tubular secretion by the kidneys. Zidovudine plasma protein binding is 34% to 38%, indicating that drug interactions involving binding site displacement are not anticipated.

The mean steady-state peak and trough concentrations of zidovudine at 2.5 mg/kg every 4 hours were 1.06 and 0.12 mcg/mL, respectively.

Table 7
Percentage (%) of Pediatric Patients with Clinical Events in Open-Label Studies

Adverse Event	n	%
BODY AS A WHOLE		
Fever	4	3.2
Phlebitis*/Bacteremia	2	1.6
Headache	2	1.6
GASTROINTESTINAL		
Nausea	1	0.8
Vomiting	6	4.8
Abdominal Pain	4	3.2
Diarrhea	1	0.8
Weight Loss	1	0.8
NERVOUS		
Insomnia	3	2.4
Nervousness/Irritability	2	1.6
Decreased Reflexes	7	5.6
Seizure	1	0.8
CARDIOVASCULAR		
Left Ventricular Dilation	1	0.8
Cardiomyopathy	1	0.8
S_3 Gallop	1	0.8
Congestive Heart Failure	1	0.8
Generalized Edema	1	0.8
ECG Abnormality	3	2.4
UROGENITAL		
Hematuria/Viral Cystitis	1	0.8

*Peripheral vein IV catheter site.

The zidovudine cerebrospinal fluid (CSF)/plasma concentration ratio was determined in 39 patients receiving chronic therapy with RETROVIR. The median ratio measured in 50 paired samples drawn 1 to 8 hours after the last dose of RETROVIR was 0.6.

Zidovudine is rapidly metabolized to GZDV which has an apparent elimination half-life of 1 hour (range 0.61 to 1.73 hours). A second metabolite, 3′-amino-3′-deoxythymidine (AMT), has been identified in the plasma following single-dose intravenous administration of zidovudine. AMT area-under-the-curve (AUC) was one fifth of the AUC of zidovudine and had a half-life of 2.7 ± 0.7 hours. In comparison, GZDV AUC was about threefold greater than the AUC of zidovudine. Following intravenous administration, urinary recoveries of zidovudine and GZDV accounted for 18% and 60% of the dose, respectively, and the total urinary recovery averaged 77% (range 64% to 98%).

Adults with Impaired Renal Function: The pharmacokinetics of zidovudine has been evaluated in patients with impaired renal function following a single 200-mg oral dose. In 14 patients (mean creatinine clearance 18 ± 2 mL/min) the half-life of zidovudine was 1.4 hours compared to 1.0 hour for control subjects with normal renal function; AUC values were approximately twice those of controls. Additionally, GZDV half-life in these patients was 8.0 hours (versus 0.9 hours for control) and AUC was 17 times higher than for control subjects. The pharmacokinetics and tolerance were evaluated in a multiple-dose study in patients undergoing hemodialysis (n = 5) or peritoneal dialysis (n = 6). Patients received escalating oral doses of zidovudine up to 200 mg five times daily for 8 weeks. Daily oral doses of 500 mg or less were well tolerated despite significantly elevated plasma levels of GZDV. Apparent oral clearance of zidovudine was approximately 50% of that reported in patients with normal renal function. The plasma concentrations of AMT are not known in patients with renal insufficiency. Daily doses of 300 to 400 mg should be appropriate in HIV-infected patients with severe renal dysfunction (see DOSAGE AND ADMINISTRATION: Dose Adjustment). Hemodialysis and peritoneal dialysis appear to have a negligible effect on the removal of zidovudine, whereas GZDV elimination is enhanced.

Pediatrics: The pharmacokinetics and bioavailability of zidovudine have been evaluated in 21 HIV-infected pediatric patients, aged 6 months through 12 years, following intravenous doses administered over the range of 80 to 160 mg/m^2 every 6 hours, and following oral doses of the intravenous solution administered over the range of 90 to 240 mg/m^2 every 6 hours. After discontinuation of the IV infusion, zidovudine plasma concentrations decayed biexponentially, consistent with two-compartment pharmacokinetics. Proportional increases in AUC and in zidovudine concentrations were observed with increasing dose, consistent with dose-independent kinetics over the dose range studied. The mean terminal half-life and total body clearance across all dose levels administered were 1.5 hours and 30.9 mL/min per kg, respectively. These values compare to mean half-life and total body clearance in adults of 1.1 hours and 27.1 mL/min per kg.

The pharmacokinetics of zidovudine has been studied in pediatric patients from birth to 3 months of life. In one study of the pharmacokinetics of zidovudine in women during the last trimester of pregnancy, zidovudine elimination was determined immediately after birth in eight neonates who were exposed to zidovudine in utero. The half-life was 13.0 ± 5.8 hours. In another study, the pharmacokinetics of zidovudine was evaluated in pediatric patients (ranging in age of 1 day to 3 months) of normal birth weight for gestational age and with normal renal and hepatic function. In neonates less than or equal to 14 days old, mean ± SD total body clearance was 10.9 ± 4.8 mL/min per kg (n = 18) and half-life was 3.1 ± 1.2 hours (n = 21). In neonates and infants greater than 14 days old, total body clearance was 19.0 ± 4.0 mL/min per kg (n = 16) and half-life was 1.9 ± 0.7 hours (n = 18).

Concentrations of zidovudine in cerebrospinal fluid were measured after both intermittent oral and IV drug administration in 21 pediatric patients during Phase 1 and Phase 2 studies. The mean zidovudine CSF/plasma concentration ratio measured at an average time of 2.2 hours postdose at oral doses of 120 to 240 mg/m^2 was 0.52 ± 0.44 (n = 28); after an IV infusion of doses of 80 to 160 mg/m^2 over 1 hour, the mean CSF/plasma concentration ratio was 0.87 ± 0.66 (n = 23) at 3.2 hours after the start of the infusion. During continuous IV infusion, mean steady-state CSF/plasma ratio was 0.26 ± 0.17 (n = 28).

As in adult patients, the major route of elimination in pediatric patients was by metabolism to GZDV. After IV dosing, about 29% of the dose was excreted in the urine unchanged and about 45% of the dose was excreted as GZDV. Overall, the pharmacokinetics of zidovudine in pediatric patients greater than 3 months of age is similar to that of zidovudine in adult patients.

Pregnancy: The pharmacokinetics of zidovudine has been studied in a Phase 1 study of eight women during the last trimester of pregnancy. As pregnancy progressed, there was no evidence of drug accumulation. The pharmacokinetics of zidovudine was similar to that of nonpregnant adults. Consistent with passive transmission of the drug across the placenta, zidovudine concentrations in infant plasma at birth were essentially equal to those in maternal plasma at delivery. Although data are limited, methadone maintenance therapy in five pregnant women did not appear to alter zidovudine pharmacokinetics. However, in another patient population, a potential for interaction has been identified (see PRECAUTIONS).

Nursing Mothers: The US Public Health Service Centers for Disease Control and Prevention advises HIV-infected women not to breastfeed to avoid postnatal transmission of HIV to a child who may not yet be infected. After administration of a single dose of 200 mg zidovudine to 13 HIV-infected women, the mean concentration of zidovudine was similar in human milk and serum (see PRECAUTIONS: Nursing Mothers).

INDICATIONS AND USAGE

RETROVIR IV Infusion is indicated for the treatment of HIV infection when antiretroviral therapy is warranted (see Description of Clinical Studies).

The duration of clinical benefit from antiretroviral therapy may be limited. Alterations in antiretroviral therapy should be considered if disease progression occurs during treatment.

Maternal-Fetal HIV Transmission: RETROVIR is also indicated for the prevention of maternal-fetal HIV transmission as part of a regimen that includes oral RETROVIR beginning between 14 and 34 weeks of gestation, intravenous RETROVIR during labor, and administration of RETROVIR Syrup to the neonate after birth. The efficacy of this regimen for preventing HIV transmission in women who have received RETROVIR for a prolonged period before pregnancy has not been evaluated. The safety of RETROVIR for the mother or fetus during the first trimester of pregnancy has not been assessed (see Description of Clinical Studies).

Description of Clinical Studies: RETROVIR has been shown to prolong survival and decrease the incidence of opportunistic infections in patients with advanced HIV disease at the initiation of therapy and to delay disease progression in asymptomatic HIV-infected patients.

Other randomized studies suggest that the duration of the clinical benefit of monotherapy with RETROVIR is time-limited.

Pregnant Women and Their Neonates: The utility of RETROVIR for the prevention of maternal-fetal HIV transmission was demonstrated in a randomized, double-blind, placebo-controlled trial (ACTG 076) conducted in HIV-infected pregnant women with CD4 cell counts of 200 to 1818 $cells/mm^3$ (median in the treated group: 560 $cells/mm^3$) who had little or no previous exposure to RETROVIR. Oral RETROVIR was initiated between 14 and 34 weeks of gestation (median 11 weeks of therapy) followed by intravenous administration of RETROVIR during labor and delivery. After birth, neonates received oral RETROVIR Syrup for 6 weeks. The study showed a statistically significant difference in the incidence of HIV infection in the neonates (based on viral culture from peripheral blood) between the group receiving RETROVIR and the group receiving placebo. Of 363 neonates evaluated in the study, the estimated risk of HIV infection was 7.8% in the group receiving RETROVIR and 24.9% in the placebo group, a relative reduction in transmission risk of 68.7%. RETROVIR was well tolerated by mothers and infants. There was no difference in pregnancy-related adverse events between the treatment groups.

CONTRAINDICATIONS

RETROVIR IV Infusion is contraindicated for patients who have potentially life-threatening allergic reactions to any of the components of the formulation.

WARNINGS

The incidence of adverse reactions appears to increase with disease progression, and patients should be monitored carefully, especially as disease progression occurs.

Bone Marrow Suppression: RETROVIR should be used with caution in patients who have bone marrow compromise evidenced by granulocyte count <1000 $cells/mm^3$ or hemoglobin <9.5 g/dL. In patients with advanced symptomatic HIV disease, anemia and neutropenia were the most significant adverse events observed (see ADVERSE REACTIONS). There have been reports of pancytopenia associated with the use of RETROVIR, which was reversible in most instances after discontinuance of the drug. However, significant anemia, in many cases requiring dose adjustment, discontinuation of RETROVIR, and/or blood transfusions has occurred during treatment with RETROVIR alone or in combination with other antiretrovirals.

Frequent blood counts are strongly recommended in patients with advanced HIV disease who are treated with RETROVIR. For HIV-infected individuals and patients with asymptomatic or early HIV disease, periodic blood counts are recommended. If anemia or neutropenia develops, dosage adjustments may be necessary (see DOSAGE AND ADMINISTRATION).

Myopathy: Myopathy and myositis with pathological changes, similar to that produced by HIV disease, have been associated with prolonged use of RETROVIR.

Lactic Acidosis/Severe Hepatomegaly with Steatosis: Rare occurrences of potentially fatal lactic acidosis in the absence of hypoxemia, and severe hepatomegaly with steatosis have been reported with the use of certain antiretroviral nucleoside analogues. Lactic acidosis should be considered whenever a patient receiving therapy with RETROVIR develops unexplained tachypnea, dyspnea, or fall in serum bicarbonate level. Under these circumstances, therapy with RETROVIR should be suspended until the diagnosis of lactic acidosis has been excluded. Caution should be exercised when administering RETROVIR to any patient, particularly obese women, with hepatomegaly, hepatitis, or other known risk factor for liver disease. These patients should be followed closely while on therapy with RETROVIR. The significance of elevated aminotransferase levels suggesting hepatic injury in HIV-infected patients prior to starting RETROVIR or while on RETROVIR is unclear. Treatment with RETROVIR should be suspended in the setting of rapidly elevating aminotransferase levels, progressive hepatomegaly, or metabolic/lactic acidosis of unknown etiology.

Other Serious Adverse Reactions: Several serious adverse events have been reported with use of RETROVIR in clinical practice. Reports of pancreatitis, sensitization reactions (including anaphylaxis in one patient), vasculitis, and seizures have been rare. These adverse events, except for sensitization, have also been associated with HIV disease. Changes in skin and nail pigmentation have been associated with the use of RETROVIR.

PRECAUTIONS

General: Zidovudine is eliminated from the body primarily by renal excretion following metabolism in the liver (glucuronidation). In patients with severely impaired renal function, dosage reduction is recommended (see CLINICAL PHARMACOLOGY: Pharmacokinetics and DOSAGE AND ADMINISTRATION). Although very little data are available, patients with severely impaired hepatic function may be at greater risk of toxicity.

Information for Patients: RETROVIR is not a cure for HIV infection, and patients may continue to acquire illnesses associated with HIV infection, including opportunistic infections. Therefore, patients should be advised to seek medical care for any significant change in their health status.

The safety and efficacy of RETROVIR in treating women, intravenous drug users, and racial minorities is not significantly different than that observed in white males.

Patients should be informed that the major toxicities of RETROVIR are neutropenia and/or anemia. The frequency and severity of these toxicities are greater in patients with more advanced disease and in those who initiate therapy later in the course of their infection. They should be told that if toxicity develops, they may require transfusions or dose modifications including possible discontinuation. They should be told of the extreme importance of having their blood counts followed closely while on therapy, especially for patients with advanced symptomatic HIV disease. They should be cautioned about the use of other medications, including ganciclovir and interferon-alpha, that may exacerbate the toxicity of RETROVIR (see PRECAUTIONS: Drug Interactions). Patients should be informed that other adverse effects of RETROVIR include nausea and vomiting. Patients should also be encouraged to contact their physician if they experience muscle weakness, shortness of breath, symptoms of hepatitis or pancreatitis, or any other unexpected adverse events while being treated with RETROVIR.

Pregnant women considering the use of RETROVIR during pregnancy for prevention of HIV-transmission to their infants should be advised that transmission may still occur in some cases despite therapy. The long-term consequences of in utero and neonatal exposure to RETROVIR are unknown, including the possible risk of cancer.

HIV-infected pregnant women should be advised not to breastfeed to avoid postnatal transmission of HIV to a child who may not yet be infected.

Patients should be advised that therapy with RETROVIR has not been shown to reduce the risk of transmission of HIV to others through sexual contact or blood contamination.

Drug Interactions: *Ganciclovir:* Use of RETROVIR in combination with ganciclovir increases the risk of hematologic toxicities in some patients with advanced HIV disease. Should the use of this combination become necessary in the treatment of patients with HIV disease, dose reduction or interruption of one or both agents may be necessary to minimize hematologic toxicity. Hematologic parameters, including hemoglobin, hematocrit, and white blood cell count with differential, should be monitored frequently in all patients receiving this combination.

Interferon-alpha: Hematologic toxicities have also been seen when RETROVIR is used concomitantly with interferon-alpha. As with the concomitant use of RETROVIR and ganciclovir, dose reduction or interruption of one or both agents may be necessary, and hematologic parameters should be monitored frequently.

Bone Marrow Suppressive Agents/Cytotoxic Agents: Coadministration of RETROVIR with drugs that are cytotoxic or which interfere with RBC/WBC number or function (e.g., dapsone, flucytosine, vincristine, vinblastine, or adriamycin) may increase the risk of hematologic toxicity.

Probenecid: Limited data suggest that probenecid may increase zidovudine levels by inhibiting glucuronidation and/or by reducing renal excretion of zidovudine. Some patients who have used RETROVIR concomitantly with pro-

Continued on next page

This product information is based on labeling in effect on June 23, 2000. For further information, contact via direct mail, phone, or web site. Medical Information, Glaxo Wellcome Inc., PO Box 13398, Research Triangle Park, NC 27709. Healthcare Professionals (Medical Information): 800-334-0089. Patients (Customer Response Center): 1-888-825-5249. Glaxo Wellcome Corporate Web Site: www.glaxowellcome.com

Retrovir I.V.—Cont.

benecid have developed flu-like symptoms consisting of myalgia, malaise, and/or fever and maculopapular rash.

Phenytoin: Phenytoin plasma levels have been reported to be low in some patients receiving RETROVIR, while in one case a high level was documented. However, in a pharmacokinetic interaction study in which 12 HIV-positive volunteers received a single 300-mg phenytoin dose alone and during steady-state zidovudine conditions (200 mg every 4 hours), no change in phenytoin kinetics was observed. Although not designed to optimally assess the effect of phenytoin on zidovudine kinetics, a 30% decrease in oral zidovudine clearance was observed with phenytoin.

Methadone: In a pharmacokinetic study of nine HIV-positive patients receiving methadone-maintenance (30 to 90 mg daily) concurrent with 200 mg of RETROVIR every 4 hours, no changes were observed in the pharmacokinetics of methadone upon initiation of therapy with RETROVIR and after 14 days of treatment with RETROVIR. No adjustments in methadone-maintenance requirements were reported. For four patients, the mean zidovudine AUC was elevated twofold, while for five patients, the value was equal to that of control patients. The exact mechanism and clinical significance of these data are unknown.

Fluconazole: The coadministration of fluconazole with RETROVIR has been reported to interfere with the oral clearance and metabolism of RETROVIR. In a pharmacokinetic interaction study in which 12 HIV-positive men received RETROVIR 200 mg every 8 hours alone and in combination with fluconazole 400 mg daily, fluconazole increased the zidovudine AUC (74%; range 28% to 173%) and the zidovudine half-life (128%; range -4% to 189%) at steady state. The clinical significance of this interaction is unknown.

Atovaquone: Data from 14 HIV-infected volunteers who were given atovaquone tablets 750 mg every 12 hours with zidovudine 200 mg every 8 hours showed a 24% ± 12% decrease in zidovudine oral clearance, leading to a 35% ± 23% increase in plasma zidovudine AUC. The glucuronide metabolite:parent ratio decreased from a mean of 4.5 when zidovudine was administered alone to 3.1 when zidovudine was administered with atovaquone tablets. Zidovudine had no effect on atovaquone pharmacokinetics.

Valproic Acid: The concomitant administration of valproic acid 250 mg (n = 5) or 500 mg (n = 1) every 8 hours and zidovudine 100 mg orally every 8 hours for 4 days to six HIV-infected, asymptomatic male volunteers resulted in a 79% ± 61% (mean ± SD) increase in the plasma zidovudine AUC and a 22% ± 10% decrease in the plasma GZDV AUC as compared to the administration of zidovudine in the absence of valproic acid. The GZDV/zidovudine urinary excretion ratio decreased 58% ± 12%. Because no change in the zidovudine plasma half-life occurred, these results suggest that valproic acid may increase the oral bioavailability of zidovudine through inhibition of first-pass metabolism. Although the clinical significance of this interaction is unknown, patients should be monitored more closely for a possible increase in zidovudine-related adverse effects. The effect of zidovudine on the pharmacokinetics of valproic acid was not evaluated.

Lamivudine: RETROVIR and lamivudine were coadministered to 12 asymptomatic HIV-positive patients in a single-center, open-label, randomized, crossover study. No significant differences were observed in AUC∞ or total clearance for lamivudine or zidovudine when the two drugs were administered together. Coadministration of RETROVIR with lamivudine resulted in an increase of 39% ± 62% (mean ± SD) in C_{max} of zidovudine.

Other Agents: Preliminary data from a drug interaction study (n = 10) suggest that coadministration of 200 mg RETROVIR and 600 mg rifampin decreases the area under the plasma concentration curve by an average of 48% ± 34%. However, the effect of once daily dosing of rifampin on multiple daily doses of RETROVIR is unknown. Some nucleoside analogues affecting DNA replication, such as ribavirin, antagonize the in vitro antiviral activity of RETROVIR against HIV; concomitant use of such drugs should be avoided.

Carcinogenesis, Mutagenesis, Impairment of Fertility: Zidovudine was administered orally at three dosage levels to separate groups of mice and rats (60 females and 60 males in each group). Initial single daily doses were 30, 60, and 120 mg/kg per day in mice and 80, 220, and 600 mg/kg per day in rats. The doses in mice were reduced to 20, 30, and 40 mg/kg per day after day 90 because of treatment-related anemia, whereas in rats only the high dose was reduced to 450 mg/kg per day on day 91, and then to 300 mg/kg per day on day 279.

In mice, seven late-appearing (after 19 months) vaginal neoplasms (five nonmetastasizing squamous cell carcinomas, one squamous cell papilloma, and one squamous polyp) occurred in animals given the highest dose. One late-appearing squamous cell papilloma occurred in the vagina of a middle-dose animal. No vaginal tumors were found at the lowest dose.

In rats, two late-appearing (after 20 months), nonmetastasizing vaginal squamous cell carcinomas occurred in animals given the highest dose. No vaginal tumors occurred at the low or middle dose in rats. No other drug-related tumors were observed in either sex of either species.

At doses that produced tumors in mice and rats, the estimated drug exposure (as measured by AUC) was approximately three times (mouse) and 24 times (rat) the estimated human exposure at the recommended therapeutic dose of 100 mg every 4 hours.

Table 1

Stage of Disease	RETROVIR Daily Dose* (mg)	Neutropenia (<750 cells/mm^3)	Anemia (Hgb <8.0 g/dL)
Asymptomatic			
ACTG 019	500	1.8%†	1.1%†
Early HIV Disease (CD4 >200 cells/mm^3)			
ACTG 016	1200	4%	4%
Advanced HIV Disease (CD4 >200 cells/mm^3)			
BW 02	1500	10%†	3%†‡
(CD4 ≤200 cells/mm^3)			
ACTG 002	600	37%	29%
BW 02	1500	47%	29%‡

* The currently recommended oral dose is 500 to 600 mg daily.
† Not statistically significant compared to placebo.
‡ Anemia = Hgb <7.5 g/dL.

Table 2: Percentage (%) of Patients with Adverse Events in Advanced HIV Disease (BW 02)

Adverse Event	RETROVIR 1500 mg/day* (n = 144) %	Placebo (n = 137) %
BODY AS A WHOLE		
Asthenia	19	18
Diaphoresis	5	4
Fever	16	12
Headache	42	37
Malaise	8	7
GASTROINTESTINAL		
Anorexia	11	8
Diarrhea	12	18
Dyspepsia	5	4
GI Pain	20	19
Nausea	46	18
Vomiting	6	3
MUSCULOSKELETAL		
Myalgia	8	2
NERVOUS		
Dizziness	6	4
Insomnia	5	1
Paresthesia	6	3
Somnolence	8	9
RESPIRATORY		
Dyspnea	5	3
SKIN		
Rash	17	15
SPECIAL SENSES		
Taste Perversion	5	8

*The currently recommended oral dose is 500 to 600 mg daily.

Table 3: Percentage (%) of Patients with Adverse Events in Early HIV Disease (ACTG 016)

Adverse Event	RETROVIR 1200 mg/day* (n = 361) %	Placebo (n = 352) %
BODY AS A WHOLE		
Asthenia	69	62
GASTROINTESTINAL		
Dyspepsia	6	1
Nausea	61	41
Vomiting	25	13

*The currently recommended oral dose is 500 to 600 mg daily.

Two transplacental carcinogenicity studies were conducted in mice. One study administered zidovudine at doses of 20 mg/kg per day or 40 mg/kg per day from gestation day 10 through parturition and lactation with dosing continuing in offspring for 24 months postnatally. The doses of zidovudine employed in this study produced zidovudine exposures approximately three times the estimated human exposure at recommended doses. After 24 months, an increase in incidence of vaginal tumors was noted with no increase in tumors in the liver or lung or any other organ in either gender. These findings are consistent with results of the standard oral carcinogenicity study in mice, as described earlier. A second study administered zidovudine at maximum tolerated doses of 12.5 mg/day or 25 mg/day (~1,000 mg/kg nonpregnant body weight or ~450 mg/kg of term body weight) to pregnant mice from days 12 through 18 of gestation. There was an increase in the number of tumors in the lung, liver, and female reproductive tracts in the offspring of mice receiving the higher dose level of zidovudine. It is not known how predictive the results of rodent carcinogenicity studies may be for humans.

Zidovudine was mutagenic in a 5178Y/TK$^{+/-}$ mouse lymphoma assay, positive in an in vitro cell transformation assay, clastogenic in a cytogenetic assay using cultured human lymphocytes, and positive in mouse and rat micronucleus tests after repeated doses. It was negative in a cytogenetic study in rats given a single dose.

Zidovudine, administered to male and female rats at doses up to seven times the usual adult dose based on body surface area considerations, had no effect on fertility judged by conception rates.

Pregnancy: Pregnancy Category C. Oral teratology studies in the rat and in the rabbit at doses up to 500 mg/kg per day revealed no evidence of teratogenicity with zidovudine. Zidovudine treatment resulted in embryo/fetal toxicity as evidenced by an increase in the incidence of fetal resorptions in rats given 150 or 450 mg/kg per day and rabbits given 500 mg/kg per day. The doses used in the teratology studies resulted in peak zidovudine plasma concentrations (after one-half of the daily dose) in rats 66 to 226 times, and in rabbits 12 to 87 times, mean steady-state peak human plasma concentrations (after one-sixth of the daily dose) achieved with the recommended daily dose (100 mg every 4 hours). In an in vitro experiment with fertilized mouse oocytes, zidovudine exposure resulted in a dose-dependent reduction in blastocyst formation. In an additional teratology study in rats, a dose of 3000 mg/kg per day (very near the oral median lethal dose in rats of 3683 mg/kg) caused marked maternal toxicity and an increase in the incidence of fetal malformations. This dose resulted in peak zidovudine plasma concentrations 350 times peak human plasma concentrations. (Estimated area-under-the-curve [AUC] in rats at this dose level was 300 times the daily AUC in humans given 600 mg per day.) No evidence of teratogenicity was seen in this experiment at doses of 600 mg/kg per day or less.

Two rodent transplacental carcinogenicity studies were conducted (see Carcinogenesis, Mutagenesis, Impairment of Fertility).

A randomized, double-blind, placebo-controlled trial was conducted in HIV-infected pregnant women to determine the utility of RETROVIR for the prevention of maternal-fetal HIV-transmission (see INDICATIONS AND USAGE: Description of Clinical Studies). Congenital abnormalities occurred with similar frequency between neonates born to mothers who received RETROVIR and neonates born to mothers who received placebo. Abnormalities were either problems in embryogenesis (prior to 14 weeks) or were recognized on ultrasound before or immediately after initiation of study drug.

Antiretroviral Pregnancy Registry: To monitor maternal-fetal outcomes of pregnant women exposed to RETROVIR, an Antiretroviral Pregnancy Registry has been established. Physicians are encouraged to register patients by calling 1-800-258-4263.

Nursing Mothers: The US Public Health Service Centers for Disease Control and Prevention advises HIV-infected women not to breastfeed to avoid postnatal transmission of HIV to a child who may not yet be infected.

Zidovudine is excreted in human milk (see Pharmacokinetics).

Pediatric Use: RETROVIR has been studied in HIV-infected pediatric patients over 3 months of age who have HIV-related symptoms or who are asymptomatic with abnormal laboratory values indicating significant HIV-related immunosuppression (see ADVERSE REACTIONS, DOSAGE AND ADMINISTRATION, and INDICATIONS AND USAGE: Description of Clinical Studies, and Pharmacokinetics).

ADVERSE REACTIONS

The adverse events reported during intravenous administration of RETROVIR IV Infusion are similar to those reported with oral administration; neutropenia and anemia were reported most frequently. Long-term intravenous administration beyond 2 to 4 weeks has not been studied in adults and may enhance hematologic adverse events. Local reaction, pain, and slight irritation during intravenous administration occur infrequently.

Adults: The frequency and severity of adverse events associated with the use of oral RETROVIR in adults are greater in patients with more advanced infection at the time of initiation of therapy. Table 1 summarizes the relative incidence of hematologic adverse events observed in clinical studies by severity of HIV disease present at the start of treatment with oral RETROVIR:

[See table 1 at top of previous page]

The anemia reported in patients with advanced HIV disease receiving RETROVIR appeared to be the result of impaired erythrocyte maturation as evidenced by macrocytosis while on drug. Although mean platelet counts in patients receiving RETROVIR were significantly increased compared to mean baseline values, thrombocytopenia did occur in some of these patients with advanced disease. Twelve percent of patients receiving RETROVIR compared to 5% of patients receiving placebo had >50% decreases from baseline platelet count. Mild drug-associated elevations in total bilirubin levels have been reported as an uncommon occurrence in patients treated for asymptomatic HIV infection.

The HIV-infected adults participating in these clinical trials often had baseline symptoms and signs of HIV disease and/or experienced adverse events at some time during study. It was often difficult to distinguish adverse events possibly associated with administration of RETROVIR from underlying signs of HIV disease or intercurrent illnesses. Table 2 summarizes clinical adverse events or symptoms which occurred in at least 5% of all patients with advanced HIV disease treated with 1500 mg/day of oral RETROVIR in the original placebo-controlled study. Of the items listed in the table, only severe headache, nausea, insomnia, and myalgia were reported at a significantly greater rate in patients receiving RETROVIR.

[See table 2 on previous page]

All events of a severe or life-threatening nature were monitored for adults in the placebo-controlled studies in early HIV disease and asymptomatic HIV infection. Data concerning the occurrence of additional signs or symptoms were also collected. No distinction was made in reporting events between those possibly associated with the administration of the study medication and those due to the underlying disease. Tables 3 and 4 summarize all those events reported at a statistically significant greater incidence for patients receiving RETROVIR in these studies:

[See table 3 on previous page]

[See table 4 above]

Several serious adverse events have been reported with the use of RETROVIR in clinical practice. Myopathy and myositis with pathological changes, similar to that produced by HIV disease, have been associated with prolonged use of RETROVIR. Reports of hepatomegaly with steatosis, hepatitis, pancreatitis, lactic acidosis, sensitization reactions (including anaphylaxis in one patient), hyperbilirubinemia, vasculitis, and seizures have been rare. These adverse events, except for sensitization, have also been associated with HIV disease. A single case of macular edema has been reported with the use of RETROVIR.

Additional adverse events reported in clinical trials at a rate not significantly different from placebo are listed below. Selected events from post-marketing clinical experience with RETROVIR are also included. Many of these events may also occur as part of HIV disease. The clinical significance of the association between treatment with RETROVIR and these events is unknown.

Body as a Whole: Abdominal pain, back pain, body odor, chest pain, chills, edema of the lip, fever, flu syndrome, hyperalgesia.

Cardiovascular: Syncope, vasodilation.

Table 4: Percentage (%) of Patients with Adverse Events* in Asymptomatic HIV Infection (ACTG 019)

Adverse Event	RETROVIR 500 mg/day (n = 453) %	Placebo (n = 428) %
BODY AS A WHOLE		
Asthenia	8.6†	5.8
Headache	62.5	52.6
Malaise	53.2	44.9
GASTROINTESTINAL		
Anorexia	20.1	10.5
Constipation	6.4†	3.5
Nausea	51.4	29.9
Vomiting	17.2	9.8
NERVOUS		
Dizziness	17.9†	15.2

* Reported in ≥5% of study population.
† Not statistically significant versus placebo.

Table 5

Advanced Pediatric HIV Disease (n = 124)	Neutropenia (<750 cells/mm³)		Anemia (Hgb <7.5 g/dL)	
	n	%	n	%
	48	39	28*	23

*Twenty-two pediatric patients received one or more transfusions due to a decline in hemoglobin to <7.5 g/dL; an additional 15 pediatric patients were transfused for hemoglobin levels >7.5 g/dL. Fifty-nine percent of the patients transfused had a prestudy history of anemia or transfusion requirement.

Table 6: Percentage (%) of Pediatric Patients with Clinical Events in Open-Label Studies

Adverse Event	n	%
BODY AS A WHOLE		
Fever	4	3.2
Phlebitis*/Bacteremia	2	1.6
Headache	2	1.6
GASTROINTESTINAL		
Nausea	1	0.8
Vomiting	6	4.8
Abdominal Pain	4	3.2
Diarrhea	1	0.8
Weight Loss	1	0.8
NERVOUS		
Insomnia	3	2.4
Nervousness/Irritability	2	1.6
Decreased Reflexes	7	5.6
Seizure	1	0.8
CARDIOVASCULAR		
Left Ventricular Dilation	1	0.8
Cardiomyopathy	1	0.8
S_3 Gallop	1	0.8
Congestive Heart Failure	1	0.8
Generalized Edema	1	0.8
ECG Abnormality	3	2.4
UROGENITAL		
Hematuria/Viral Cystitis	1	0.8

*Peripheral vein IV catheter site.

Gastrointestinal: Bleeding gums, constipation, diarrhea, dysphagia, edema of the tongue, eructation, flatulence, mouth ulcer, rectal hemorrhage.

Hemic and Lymphatic: Lymphadenopathy.

Musculoskeletal: Arthralgia, muscle spasm, tremor, twitch.

Nervous: Anxiety, confusion, depression, dizziness, emotional lability, loss of mental acuity, nervousness, paresthesia, somnolence, vertigo.

Respiratory: Cough, dyspnea, epistaxis, hoarseness, pharyngitis, rhinitis, sinusitis.

Skin: Acne, changes in skin and nail pigmentation, pruritus, rash, sweat, urticaria.

Special Senses: Amblyopia, hearing loss, photophobia, taste perversion.

Urogenital: Dysuria, polyuria, urinary frequency, urinary hesitancy.

Pediatrics: Anemia and neutropenia among pediatric patients with advanced HIV disease receiving RETROVIR occurred with similar incidence to that reported for adults with AIDS or advanced ARC (see above). Management of neutropenia and anemia included, in some cases, dose modification and/or blood product transfusions. In the open-label studies, 17% had their dose modified (generally a reduction in dose by 30%) due to anemia and 25% had their dose modified (temporary discontinuation or dose reduction by 30%) for neutropenia. Four pediatric patients had RETROVIR permanently discontinued for neutropenia. Table 5 summarizes the occurrence of anemia (Hgb <7.5 g/dL) and neutropenia (<750 cells/mm³) among 124 pediatric patients receiving oral RETROVIR for a mean of 267 days (range 3 to 855 days):

[See table 5 above]

Macrocytosis was observed among the majority of pediatric patients enrolled in the studies.

In the open-label studies involving 124 pediatric patients, 16 clinical adverse events were reported by 24 pediatric patients. No event was reported by more than 5.6% of the study populations. Due to the open-label design of the studies, it was difficult to determine possible events related to the use of RETROVIR versus disease-related events. Therefore, all clinical events reported as associated with therapy with RETROVIR or of unknown relationship to therapy with RETROVIR are presented in Table 6:

[See table 6 above]

The clinical adverse events reported among adult recipients of RETROVIR may also occur in pediatric patients.

Use for the Prevention of Maternal-Fetal Transmission of HIV: In a randomized, double-blind, placebo-controlled trial in HIV-infected women and their neonates conducted to determine the utility of RETROVIR for the prevention of maternal-fetal HIV transmission, RETROVIR Syrup at 2 mg/kg was administered every 6 hours for 6 weeks to neonates beginning within 12 hours after birth. The most commonly reported adverse experiences were anemia (hemoglobin <9.0 g/dL) and neutropenia (<1000 cells/mm³). Anemia occurred in 22% of the neonates who received RETROVIR and in 12% of the neonates who received placebo. The mean difference in hemoglobin values was less than 1.0 g/dL for

Continued on next page

This product information is based on labeling in effect on June 23, 2000. For further information, contact via direct mail, phone, or web site. Medical Information, Glaxo Wellcome Inc., PO Box 13398, Research Triangle Park, NC 27709. Healthcare Professionals (Medical Information): 800-334-0089. Patients (Customer Response Center): 1-888-825-5249. Glaxo Wellcome Corporate Web Site: www.glaxowellcome.com

Retrovir I.V.—Cont.

neonates receiving RETROVIR compared to neonates receiving placebo. No neonates with anemia required transfusion, and all hemoglobin values spontaneously returned to normal within 6 weeks after completion of therapy with RETROVIR. Neutropenia was reported with similar frequency in the group that received RETROVIR (21%) and in the group that received placebo (27%). The long-term consequences of in utero and neonatal exposure to RETROVIR are unknown.

OVERDOSAGE

Cases of acute overdoses in both pediatric patients and adults have been reported with doses up to 50 grams. None were fatal. The only consistent finding in these cases of overdose was spontaneous or induced nausea and vomiting. Hematologic changes were transient and not severe. Some patients experienced nonspecific CNS symptoms such as headache, dizziness, drowsiness, lethargy, and confusion. One report of a grand mal seizure possibly attributable to RETROVIR occurred in a 35-year-old male 3 hours after ingesting 36 grams of RETROVIR. No other cause could be identified. All patients recovered without permanent sequelae. Hemodialysis appears to have a negligible effect on the removal of zidovudine while elimination of its primary metabolite, GZDV, is enhanced.

DOSAGE AND ADMINISTRATION

Adults: The recommended intravenous dose is 1 mg/kg infused over 1 hour. This dose should be administered five to six times daily (5 to 6 mg/kg daily). The effectiveness of this dose compared to higher dosing regimens in improving the neurologic dysfunction associated with HIV disease is unknown. A small randomized study found a greater effect of higher doses of RETROVIR on improvement of neurological symptoms in patients with pre-existing neurological disease.

Patients should receive RETROVIR IV Infusion only until oral therapy can be administered. The intravenous dosing regimen equivalent to the oral administration of 100 mg every 4 hours is approximately 1 mg/kg intravenously every 4 hours.

Maternal-Fetal HIV Transmission: The recommended dosing regimen for administration to pregnant women (>14 weeks of pregnancy) and their neonates is:

Maternal Dosing: 100 mg orally five times per day until the start of labor. During labor and delivery, intravenous RETROVIR should be administered at 2 mg/kg (total body weight) over 1 hour followed by a continuous intravenous infusion of 1 mg/kg per hour (total body weight) until clamping of the umbilical cord.

Neonatal Dosing: 2 mg/kg orally every 6 hours starting within 12 hours after birth and continuing through 6 weeks of age. Neonates unable to receive oral dosing may be administered RETROVIR intravenously at 1.5 mg/kg, infused over 30 minutes, every 6 hours. (See PRECAUTIONS if hepatic disease or renal insufficiency is present.)

Monitoring of Patients: Hematologic toxicities appear to be related to pretreatment bone marrow reserve and to dose and duration of therapy. In patients with poor bone marrow reserve, particularly in patients with advanced symptomatic HIV disease, frequent monitoring of hematologic indices is recommended to detect serious anemia or neutropenia (see WARNINGS). In patients who experience hematologic toxicity, reduction in hemoglobin may occur as early as 2 to 4 weeks, and neutropenia usually occurs after 6 to 8 weeks.

Dose Adjustment: Significant anemia (hemoglobin of <7.5 g/dL or reduction of >25% of baseline) and/or significant neutropenia (granulocyte count of <750 cells/mm^3 or reduction of >50% from baseline) may require a dose interruption until some evidence of marrow recovery is observed. For less severe anemia or neutropenia, a reduction in daily dose may be adequate. In patients who develop significant anemia, dose modification does not necessarily eliminate the need for transfusion. If marrow recovery occurs following dose modification, gradual increases in dose may be appropriate depending on hematologic indices and patient tolerance.

In end-stage renal disease patients maintained on hemodialysis or peritoneal dialysis, recommended dosing is 1 mg/kg every 6 to 8 hours (see CLINICAL PHARMACOLOGY: Pharmacokinetics).

There are insufficient data to recommend dose adjustment of zidovudine in patients with impaired hepatic function.

Method of Preparation: RETROVIR IV Infusion must be diluted prior to administration. The calculated dose should be removed from the 20-mL vial and added to 5% Dextrose Injection solution to achieve a concentration no greater than 4 mg/mL. Admixture in biologic or colloidal fluids (e.g., blood products, protein solutions, etc.) is not recommended.

After dilution, the solution is physically and chemically stable for 24 hours at room temperature and 48 hours if refrigerated at 2° to 8°C (36° to 46°F). Care should be taken during admixture to prevent inadvertent contamination. As an additional precaution, the diluted solution should be administered within 8 hours if stored at 25°C (77°F) or 24 hours if refrigerated at 2° to 8°C to minimize potential administration of a microbially contaminated solution.

Parenteral drug products should be inspected visually for particulate matter and discoloration prior to administration whenever solution and container permit. Should either be observed, the solution should be discarded and fresh solution prepared.

Administration: RETROVIR IV Infusion is administered intravenously at a constant rate over one hour. Rapid infusion or bolus injection should be avoided. RETROVIR IV Infusion should not be given intramuscularly.

HOW SUPPLIED

RETROVIR IV Infusion, 10 mg zidovudine in each mL. 20-mL Single-Use Vial, Tray of 10 (NDC 0173-0107-93).

Store vials at 15° to 25°C (59° to 77°F) and protect from light.

US Patent Nos. 4,818,538 (Product Patent)
4,724,232; 4,833,130; and 4,837,208 (Use Patents)
Manufactured by Catalytica Pharmaceuticals, Inc.
Greenville, NC 27834
for Glaxo Wellcome Inc., Research Triangle Park, NC 27709

April 1998/RL-559

Shown in Product Identification Guide, page 316

SEREVENT® ℞

[ser' a-vent"]
(salmeterol xinafoate)
Inhalation Aerosol

Bronchodilator Aerosol
For Oral Inhalation Only

DESCRIPTION

SEREVENT (salmeterol xinafoate) Inhalation Aerosol contains salmeterol xinafoate as the racemic form of the 1-hydroxy-2-naphthoic acid salt of salmeterol. The active component of the formulation is salmeterol base, a highly selective beta$_2$-adrenergic bronchodilator. The chemical name of salmeterol xinafoate is 4-hydroxy-α^1-[[[6-(4-phenylbutoxy) hexyl]amino]methyl]-1,3-benzenedimethanol, 1-hydroxy-2-naphthalenecarboxylate.

The molecular weight of salmeterol xinafoate is 603.8, and the empirical formula is $C_{25}H_{37}NO_4 \bullet C_{11}H_8O_3$. Salmeterol xinafoate is a white to off-white powder. It is freely soluble in methanol; slightly soluble in ethanol, chloroform, and isopropanol; and sparingly soluble in water.

SEREVENT Inhalation Aerosol is a pressurized, metered-dose aerosol unit for oral inhalation. It contains a microcrystalline suspension of salmeterol xinafoate in a mixture of 2 chlorofluorocarbon propellants (trichlorofluoromethane and dichlorodifluoromethane) with lecithin. 36.25 mcg of salmeterol xinafoate is equivalent to 25 mcg of salmeterol base. Each actuation delivers 25 mcg of salmeterol base (as salmeterol xinafoate) from the valve and 21 mcg of salmeterol base (as salmeterol xinafoate) from the actuator. Each 6.5-g canister provides 60 inhalations and each 13-g canister provides 120 inhalations.

CLINICAL PHARMACOLOGY

Mechanism of Action: Salmeterol is a long-acting beta-adrenergic agonist. In vitro studies and in vivo pharmacologic studies demonstrate that salmeterol is selective for beta$_2$-adrenoceptors compared with isoproterenol, which has approximately equal agonist activity on beta$_1$- and beta$_2$-adrenoceptors. In vitro studies show salmeterol to be at least 50 times more selective for beta$_2$-adrenoceptors than albuterol. Although beta$_2$-adrenoceptors are the predominant adrenergic receptors in bronchial smooth muscle and beta$_1$-adrenoceptors are the predominant receptors in the heart, there are also beta$_2$-adrenoceptors in the human heart comprising 10% to 50% of the total beta-adrenoceptors. The precise function of these is not yet established, but they raise the possibility that even highly selective beta$_2$-agonists may have cardiac effects.

The pharmacologic effects of beta$_2$-adrenoceptor agonist drugs, including salmeterol, are at least in part attributable to stimulation of intracellular adenyl cyclase, the enzyme that catalyzes the conversion of adenosine triphosphate (ATP) to cyclic-3',5'-adenosine monophosphate (cyclic AMP). Increased cyclic AMP levels cause relaxation of bronchial smooth muscle and inhibition of release of mediators of immediate hypersensitivity from cells, especially from mast cells.

In vitro tests show that salmeterol is a potent and long-lasting inhibitor of the release of mast cell mediators, such as histamine, leukotrienes, and prostaglandin D_2, from human lung. Salmeterol inhibits histamine-induced plasma protein extravasation and inhibits platelet activating factor-induced eosinophil accumulation in the lungs of guinea pigs when administered by the inhaled route. In humans, single doses of salmeterol attenuate allergen-induced bronchial hyper-responsiveness.

Pharmacokinetics: Salmeterol acts locally in the lung; plasma levels therefore do not predict therapeutic effect. Because of the low therapeutic dose, systemic levels of salmeterol are low or undetectable after inhalation of recommended doses (42 mcg twice daily). Following chronic administration of an inhaled dose of 42 mcg twice daily, salmeterol was detected in plasma within 5 to 10 minutes in 6 asthmatic patients; plasma concentrations were very low, with peak concentrations of 150 pg/mL and no accumulation with repeated doses. Larger inhaled doses gave approximately proportionally increased blood levels. In these patients, a second peak concentration of 115 pg/mL occurred at about 45 minutes, probably due to absorption of the swallowed portion of the dose (most of the dose delivered by a metered-dose inhaler is swallowed). Oral administration of 1 mg of radiolabeled salmeterol (as salmeterol xinafoate) to 2 healthy subjects gave peak plasma salmeterol concentrations of about 650 pg/mL at about 45 minutes; the terminal elimination half-life was about 5.5 hours (1 volunteer only).

Salmeterol xinafoate, an ionic salt, dissociates in solution so that the salmeterol and 1-hydroxy-2-naphthoic acid (xinafoate) moieties are absorbed, distributed, metabolized, and excreted independently. Salmeterol base is extensively metabolized by hydroxylation, with subsequent elimination predominantly in the feces. In 2 healthy subjects who received 1 mg of radiolabeled salmeterol (as salmeterol xinafoate) orally, approximately 25% and 60% of the radiolabeled salmeterol was eliminated in urine and feces, respectively, over a period of 7 days. No significant amount of unchanged salmeterol base was detected in either urine or feces.

Salmeterol is 94% to 98% bound to human plasma proteins in vitro over the concentration range of 8 to 7722 ng of base per milliliter, much higher concentrations than those achieved following therapeutic doses of salmeterol.

The xinafoate moiety has no apparent pharmacologic activity, is highly protein bound (>99%), and has a long elimination half-life of 11 days.

The pharmacokinetics of salmeterol base has not been studied in elderly patients nor in patients with hepatic or renal impairment. Since salmeterol is predominantly cleared by hepatic metabolism, liver function impairment may lead to accumulation of salmeterol in plasma. Therefore, patients with hepatic disease should be closely monitored.

Pharmacodynamics: Inhaled salmeterol, like other beta-adrenergic agonist drugs, can in some patients produce cardiovascular effects (see PRECAUTIONS). The cardiovascular effects (heart rate, blood pressure) associated with salmeterol occur with similar frequency, and are of similar type and severity, as those noted following albuterol administration.

The effects of rising inhaled doses of salmeterol and standard inhaled doses of albuterol were studied in volunteers and in patients with asthma. Salmeterol doses up to 84 mcg resulted in heart rate increases of 3 to 16 beats/min, about the same as albuterol dosed at 180 mcg by inhalation aerosol (4 to 10 beats/min). In 2 double-blind asthma studies, patients receiving either 42 mcg of salmeterol inhalation aerosol twice daily (n = 81) or 180 mcg of albuterol inhalation aerosol 4 times daily (n = 80) underwent continuous electrocardiographic monitoring during four 24-hour periods; no clinically significant dysrhythmias were noted. Continuous electrocardiographic monitoring was also performed in 2 double-blind studies in COPD patients (see ADVERSE REACTIONS).

Studies in laboratory animals (minipigs, rodents, and dogs) have demonstrated the occurrence of cardiac arrhythmias and sudden death (with histologic evidence of myocardial necrosis) when beta-agonists and methylxanthines are administered concurrently. The clinical significance of these findings is unknown.

Clinical Trials: ***Asthma:*** In placebo- and albuterol-controlled, single-dose clinical trials with SEREVENT Inhalation Aerosol, the time to onset of effective bronchodilatation (>15% improvement in forced expiratory volume in 1 second [FEV_1]) was 10 to 20 minutes after a 42-mcg dose. Maximum improvement in FEV_1 generally occurred within 180

Table 1: Daily Efficacy Measurements in 2 Large 12-Week Clinical Trials (Combined Data)

Parameter	Time	Placebo	SEREVENT Inhalation Aerosol	Albuterol Inhalation Aerosol
No. of randomized subjects		187	184	185
Mean AM peak expiratory flow rate (L/min)	baseline	412	409	398
	12 weeks	414	438*	390
Mean % days with no asthma symptoms	baseline	11	11	14
	12 weeks	17	35*	24
Mean % nights with no awakenings	baseline	67	67	65
	12 weeks	74	87*	74
Rescue medications (mean no. of inhalations per day)	baseline	4.4	4.1	4.0
	12 weeks	3.3	1.3†‡	1.9
Asthma exacerbations		17%	11%	14%

* P<0.001 versus albuterol and placebo.
† P<0.05 versus albuterol.
‡ P<0.001 versus placebo.

minutes, and clinically significant improvement continued for 12 hours in most patients.

In 2 large, randomized, double-blind studies, SEREVENT Inhalation Aerosol was compared with albuterol and placebo in patients with mild-to-moderate asthma, including both patients who did and who did not receive concomitant inhaled corticosteroids. The efficacy of SEREVENT Inhalation Aerosol was demonstrated over the 12-week period with no change in effectiveness over this period of time. There were no gender-related differences in safety or efficacy. No development of tachyphylaxis to the bronchodilator effect has been noted in these studies. FEV_1 measurements (percent of predicted) from these two 12-week trials are shown below for both the first and last treatment days.

Figure 1: FEV_1, as Percent of Predicted, From 2 Large 12-Week Clinical Trials

First Treatment Day

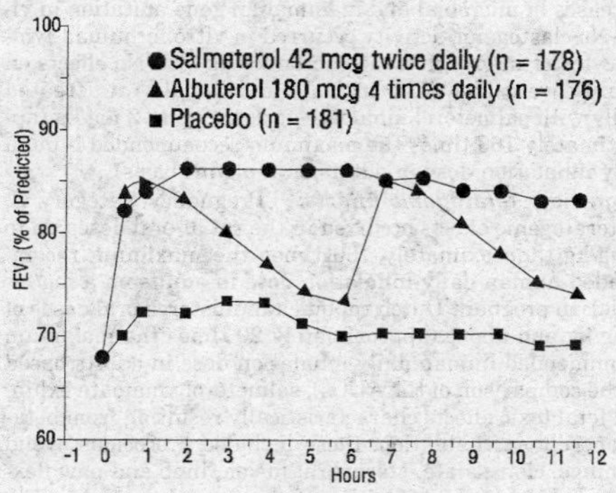

Last Treatment Day (Week 12)

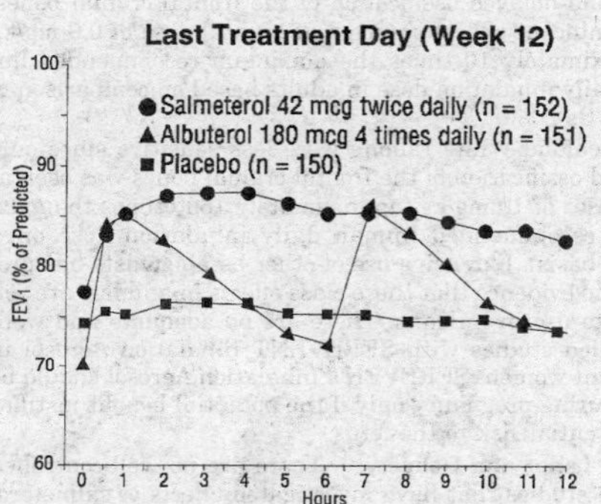

During daily treatment with SEREVENT Inhalation Aerosol for 12 weeks in patients with asthma, the following treatment effects were seen:

[See table 1 at bottom of previous page]

Safe usage with maintenance of efficacy for periods up to 1 year has been documented.

Exercise-Induced Bronchospasm: Protection against exercise-induced bronchospasm was examined in 3 controlled studies. Based on median values, patients who received SEREVENT Inhalation Aerosol had consistently less exercise-induced fall in FEV_1 than patients who received placebo, and they were protected for a longer period of time than patients who received albuterol (see table below). There were, however, some patients who were not protected from exercise-induced bronchospasm after SEREVENT administration and others in whom protection against exercise-induced bronchospasm decreased with continued administration over a period of 4 weeks.

[See table 2 above]

Chronic Obstructive Pulmonary Disease (COPD): In 2 large randomized, double-blind studies, SEREVENT Inhalation Aerosol administered twice daily was compared with placebo and ipratropium bromide inhalation aerosol administered 4 times daily in patients with COPD (emphysema and chronic bronchitis), including patients who were reversible (≥12% and ≥200 mL increase in baseline FEV_1 after albuterol treatment) and nonreversible to albuterol. After a single 42-mcg dose of SEREVENT, significant improvement in pulmonary function (mean FEV_1 increase of 12% or more) occurred within 30 minutes, reached a peak within 4 hours on average, and persisted for 12 hours with no loss in effectiveness observed over a 12-week treatment period. Serial 12-hour measurements of FEV_1 from these two 12-week trials are shown below for both the first and last treatment days.

[See figure 2 in next column]

Table 2: Exercise-Induced Bronchospasm Mean Percentage Fall in Postexercise FEV_1

Clinical Trials/Time After Dose	Treatment		
	Placebo	SEREVENT Inhalation Aerosol	Albuterol Inhalation Aerosol
Study A: 1st Dose			
6 hours	37	9*	
12 hours	27	16*	
Study A: 4th Week			
6 hours	30	19	
12 hours	24	12	
Study B:			
1 hour	37	0*	2*
6 hours	37	5*†	27
12 hours	34	6*†	33
Study C:			
0.5 hour	43	16*	8*
2.5 hours	33	12*†	30
4.5 hours	—	12†	36
6.0 hours	—	19†	41

* Statistically superior to placebo ($P \leq 0.05$).
† Statistically superior to albuterol ($P \leq 0.05$).

Figure 2: FEV_1 From 2 Large 12-Week Clinical Trials

First Treatment Day

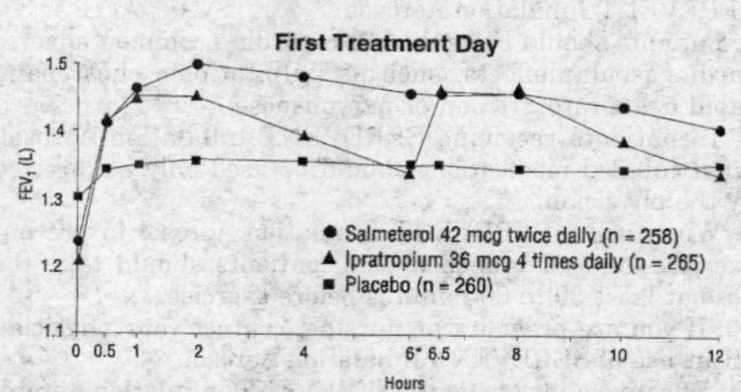

*Ipratropium Inhalation Aerosol (or matching placebo) administered immediately following hour 6 assessment.

Last Treatment Day (Week 12)

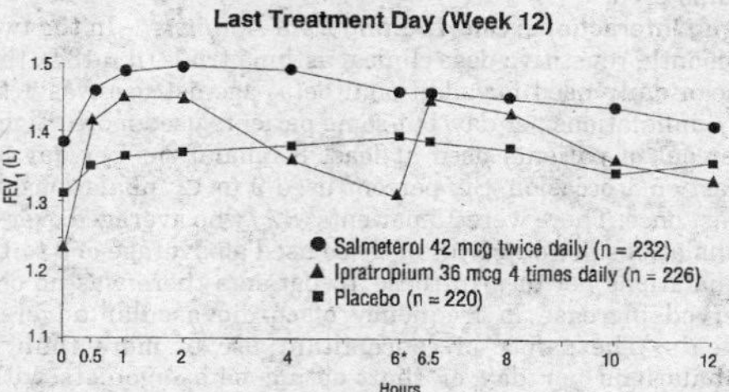

*Ipratropium inhalation aerosol (or matching placebo) administered immediately following hour 6 assessment.

INDICATIONS AND USAGE

Asthma: SEREVENT Inhalation Aerosol is indicated for long-term, twice-daily (morning and evening) administration in the maintenance treatment of asthma and in the prevention of bronchospasm in patients 12 years of age and older with reversible obstructive airway disease, including patients with symptoms of nocturnal asthma, who require regular treatment with inhaled, short-acting $beta_2$-agonists. It should not be used in patients whose asthma can be managed by occasional use of inhaled, short-acting $beta_2$-agonists.

SEREVENT Inhalation Aerosol may be used with or without concurrent inhaled or systemic corticosteroid therapy.

SEREVENT Inhalation Aerosol is also indicated for prevention of exercise-induced bronchospasm in patients 12 years of age and older.

COPD: SEREVENT Inhalation Aerosol is indicated for long-term, twice daily (morning and evening) administration in the maintenance treatment of bronchospasm associated with COPD (including emphysema and chronic bronchitis).

CONTRAINDICATIONS

SEREVENT Inhalation Aerosol is contraindicated in patients with a history of hypersensitivity to salmeterol or any of its components.

WARNINGS

IMPORTANT INFORMATION: SEREVENT INHALATION AEROSOL SHOULD NOT BE INITIATED IN PATIENTS WITH SIGNIFICANTLY WORSENING OR ACUTELY DETERIORATING ASTHMA, WHICH MAY BE A LIFE-THREATENING CONDITION. Serious acute respiratory events, including fatalities, have been reported, both in the United States and worldwide, when SEREVENT Inhalation Aerosol has been initiated in this situation.

Although it is not possible from these reports to determine whether SEREVENT Inhalation Aerosol contributed to these adverse events or simply failed to relieve the deteriorating asthma, the use of SEREVENT Inhalation Aerosol in this setting is inappropriate.

SEREVENT INHALATION AEROSOL SHOULD NOT BE USED TO TREAT ACUTE SYMPTOMS. It is crucial to inform patients of this and prescribe an inhaled, short-acting $beta_2$-agonist for this purpose as well as warn them that increasing inhaled $beta_2$-agonist use is a signal of deteriorating asthma.

SEREVENT INHALATION AEROSOL IS NOT A SUBSTITUTE FOR INHALED OR ORAL CORTICOSTEROIDS. Corticosteroids should not be stopped or reduced when SEREVENT Inhalation Aerosol is initiated.

(See PRECAUTIONS: Information for Patients below and the PATIENT'S INSTRUCTIONS FOR USE leaflet.)

1. Do Not Introduce SEREVENT Inhalation Aerosol as a Treatment for Acutely Deteriorating Asthma: SEREVENT Inhalation Aerosol is intended for the maintenance treatment of asthma (see INDICATIONS AND USAGE) and should not be introduced in acutely deteriorating asthma, which is a potentially life-threatening condition. There are no data demonstrating that SEREVENT Inhalation Aerosol provides greater efficacy than or additional efficacy to inhaled, short-acting $beta_2$-agonists in patients with worsening asthma. Serious acute respiratory events, including fatalities, have been reported, both in the United States and worldwide, in patients receiving SEREVENT Inhalation Aerosol. In most cases, these have occurred in patients with severe asthma (e.g., patients with a history of corticosteroid dependence, low pulmonary function, intubation, mechanical ventilation, frequent hospitalizations, or previous life-threatening acute asthma exacerbations) and/or in some patients in whom asthma has been acutely deteriorating (e.g., unresponsive to usual medications; increasing need for inhaled, short-acting $beta_2$-agonists; increasing need for systemic corticosteroids; significant increase in symptoms; recent emergency room visits; sudden or progressive deterioration in pulmonary function). However, they have occurred in a few patients with less severe asthma as well. It was not possible from these reports to determine whether SEREVENT Inhalation Aerosol contributed to these events or simply failed to relieve the deteriorating asthma.

2. Do Not Use SEREVENT Inhalation Aerosol to Treat Acute Symptoms: An inhaled, short-acting $beta_2$-agonist, not SEREVENT Inhalation Aerosol, should be used to relieve acute asthma or COPD symptoms. When prescribing SEREVENT Inhalation Aerosol, the physician must also provide the patient with an inhaled, short-acting $beta_2$-agonist (e.g., albuterol) for treatment of symptoms that occur acutely, despite regular twice-daily (morning and evening) use of SEREVENT Inhalation Aerosol.

When beginning treatment with SEREVENT Inhalation Aerosol, patients who have been taking inhaled, short-acting $beta_2$-agonists on a regular basis (e.g., 4 times a day) should be instructed to discontinue the regular use of these drugs and use them only for symptomatic relief of acute asthma or COPD symptoms (see PRECAUTIONS: Information for Patients).

3. Watch for Increasing Use of Inhaled, Short-Acting $Beta_2$-Agonists, Which Is a Marker of Deteriorating Asthma: Asthma may deteriorate acutely over a period of hours or chronically over several days or longer. If the patient's inhaled, short-acting $beta_2$-agonist becomes less effective or the patient needs more inhalations than usual, this may be a marker of destabilization of asthma. In this setting, the patient requires immediate reevaluation with reassessment of the treatment regimen, giving special consideration to the possible need for corticosteroids. If the patient uses 4 or more inhalations per day of an inhaled, short-acting $beta_2$-agonist for 2 or more consecutive days, or if more than 1 canister (200 inhalations per canister) of inhaled, short-acting $beta_2$-agonist is used in an 8-week period in conjunction with SEREVENT Inhalation Aerosol, then the patient should consult the physician for reevaluation. **Increasing the daily dosage of SEREVENT Inhalation Aerosol in this situation is not appropriate. SEREVENT Inhalation Aerosol should not be used more frequently than twice daily (morning and evening) at the recommended dose of 2 inhalations.**

4. Do Not Use SEREVENT Inhalation Aerosol as a Substitute for Oral or Inhaled Corticosteroids: The use of beta-

Continued on next page

This product information is based on labeling in effect on June 23, 2000. For further information, contact via direct mail, phone, or web site. Medical Information, Glaxo Wellcome Inc., PO Box 13398, Research Triangle Park, NC 27709. Healthcare Professionals (Medical Information): 800-334-0089. Patients (Customer Response Center): 1-888-825-5249. Glaxo Wellcome Corporate Web Site: www.glaxowellcome.com

Serevent—Cont.

adrenergic agonist bronchodilators alone may not be adequate to control asthma in many patients. Early consideration should be given to adding anti-inflammatory agents, e.g., corticosteroids. There are no data demonstrating that SEREVENT Inhalation Aerosol has a clinical anti-inflammatory effect and could be expected to take the place of, or reduce the dose of, corticosteroids. Patients who already require oral or inhaled corticosteroids for treatment of asthma should be continued on this type of treatment even if they feel better as a result of initiating SEREVENT Inhalation Aerosol. Any change in corticosteroid dosage should be made ONLY after clinical evaluation (see PRECAUTIONS: Information for Patients).

5. Do Not Exceed Recommended Dosage: As with other inhaled $beta_2$-adrenergic drugs, SEREVENT Inhalation Aerosol should not be used more often or at higher doses than recommended. Fatalities have been reported in association with excessive use of inhaled sympathomimetic drugs. Large doses of inhaled or oral salmeterol (12 to 20 times the recommended dose) have been associated with clinically significant prolongation of the QT_c interval, which has the potential for producing ventricular arrhythmias.

6. Paradoxical Bronchospasm: SEREVENT Inhalation Aerosol can produce paradoxical bronchospasm, which may be life threatening. If paradoxical bronchospasm occurs, SEREVENT Inhalation Aerosol should be discontinued immediately and alternative therapy instituted. It should be recognized that paradoxical bronchospasm, when associated with inhaled formulations, frequently occurs with the first use of a new canister or vial.

7. Immediate Hypersensitivity Reactions: Immediate hypersensitivity reactions may occur after administration of SEREVENT Inhalation Aerosol, as demonstrated by rare cases of urticaria, angioedema, rash, and bronchospasm.

8. Upper Airway Symptoms: Symptoms of laryngeal spasm, irritation, or swelling, such as stridor and choking, have been reported rarely in patients receiving SEREVENT Inhalation Aerosol.

SEREVENT Inhalation Aerosol, like all other beta-adrenergic agonists, can produce a clinically significant cardiovascular effect in some patients as measured by pulse rate, blood pressure, and/or symptoms. Although such effects are uncommon after administration of SEREVENT Inhalation Aerosol at recommended doses, if they occur, the drug may need to be discontinued. In addition, beta-agonists have been reported to produce electrocardiogram (ECG) changes, such as flattening of the T wave, prolongation of the QTc interval, and ST segment depression. The clinical significance of these findings is unknown. Therefore, SEREVENT Inhalation Aerosol, like all sympathomimetic amines, should be used with caution in patients with cardiovascular disorders, especially coronary insufficiency, cardiac arrhythmias, and hypertension.

PRECAUTIONS

General: 1. Use With Spacer or Other Devices: The safety and effectiveness of SEREVENT Inhalation Aerosol when used with a spacer or other devices have not been adequately studied.

2. Cardiovascular and Other Effects: No effect on the cardiovascular system is usually seen after the administration of inhaled salmeterol in recommended doses, but the cardiovascular and central nervous system effects seen with all sympathomimetic drugs (e.g., increased blood pressure, heart rate, excitement) can occur after use of salmeterol and may require discontinuation of the drug. Salmeterol, like all sympathomimetic amines, should be used with caution in patients with cardiovascular disorders, especially coronary insufficiency, cardiac arrhythmias, and hypertension; in patients with convulsive disorders or thyrotoxicosis; and in patients who are unusually responsive to sympathomimetic amines.

As has been described with other beta-adrenergic agonist bronchodilators, clinically significant changes in systolic and/or diastolic blood pressure, pulse rate, and electrocardiograms have been seen infrequently in individual patients in controlled clinical studies with salmeterol.

3. Metabolic Effects: Doses of the related $beta_2$-adrenoceptor agonist albuterol, when administered intravenously, have been reported to aggravate preexisting diabetes mellitus and ketoacidosis. No effects on glucose have been seen with SEREVENT Inhalation Aerosol at recommended doses. Beta-adrenergic agonist medications may produce significant hypokalemia in some patients, possibly through intracellular shunting, which has the potential to produce adverse cardiovascular effects. The decrease is usually transient, not requiring supplementation.

Clinically significant changes in blood glucose and/or serum potassium were seen rarely during clinical studies with long-term administration of SEREVENT Inhalation Aerosol at recommended doses.

Information for Patients: See illustrated PATIENT'S INSTRUCTIONS FOR USE. **SHAKE WELL BEFORE USING.**

It is important that patients understand how to use SEREVENT Inhalation Aerosol appropriately and how it should be used in relation to other asthma or COPD medications they are taking. Patients should be given the following information:

1. Shake well before using.
2. The action of SEREVENT Inhalation Aerosol may last up to 12 hours or longer. The recommended dosage (2 inhalations twice daily, morning and evening) should not be exceeded.
3. SEREVENT Inhalation Aerosol is not meant to relieve acute asthma or COPD symptoms and extra doses should not be used for that purpose. Acute symptoms should be treated with an inhaled, short-acting $beta_2$-agonist such as albuterol (the physician should provide the patient with such medication and instruct the patient in how it should be used).
4. Patients should not stop SEREVENT therapy for COPD without physician/provider guidance since symptoms may recur after discontinuation.
5. The physician should be notified immediately if any of the following situations occur, which may be a sign of seriously worsening asthma.
   - Decreasing effectiveness of inhaled, short-acting $beta_2$-agonists
   - Need for more inhalations than usual of inhaled, short-acting $beta_2$-agonists
   - Use of 4 or more inhalations per day of a short-acting $beta_2$-agonist for 2 or more days consecutively
   - Use of more than one 200-inhalation canister of an inhaled, short-acting $beta_2$-agonist (e.g., albuterol) in an 8-week period
6. SEREVENT Inhalation Aerosol should not be used as a substitute for oral or inhaled corticosteroids. The dosage of these medications should not be changed and they should not be stopped without consulting the physician, even if the patient feels better after initiating treatment with SEREVENT Inhalation Aerosol.
7. Patients should be cautioned regarding common adverse cardiovascular effects, such as palpitations, chest pain, rapid heart rate, tremor, or nervousness.
8. In patients receiving SEREVENT Inhalation Aerosol, other inhaled medications should be used only as directed by the physician.
9. When using SEREVENT Inhalation Aerosol to prevent exercise-induced bronchospasm, patients should take the dose at least 30 to 60 minutes before exercise.
10. If you are pregnant or nursing, contact your physician about use of SEREVENT Inhalation Aerosol.
11. Effective and safe use of SEREVENT Inhalation Aerosol includes an understanding of the way that it should be administered.

Drug Interactions: ***Short-Acting Beta-Agonists:*** In the two 3-month, repetitive-dose clinical asthma trials (n = 184), the mean daily need for additional $beta_2$-agonist use was 1 to $1^1/_2$ inhalations per day, but some patients used more. Eight percent of patients used at least 8 inhalations per day at least on 1 occasion. Six percent used 9 to 12 inhalations at least once. There were 15 patients (8%) who averaged over 4 inhalations per day. Four of these used an average of 8 to 11 inhalations per day. In these 15 patients there was no observed increase in frequency of cardiovascular adverse events. The safety of concomitant use of more than 8 inhalations per day of short-acting $beta_2$-agonists with SEREVENT Inhalation Aerosol has not been established. In 15 patients who experienced worsening of asthma while receiving SEREVENT Inhalation Aerosol, nebulized albuterol (1 dose in most) led to improvement in FEV_1 and no increase in occurrence of cardiovascular adverse events.

Monoamine Oxidase Inhibitors and Tricyclic Antidepressants: Salmeterol should be administered with extreme caution to patients being treated with monoamine oxidase inhibitors or tricyclic antidepressants, or within 2 weeks of discontinuation of such agents, because the action of salmeterol on the vascular system may be potentiated by these agents.

Corticosteroids and Cromoglycate: In clinical trials, inhaled corticosteroids and/or inhaled cromolyn sodium did not alter the safety profile of SEREVENT Inhalation Aerosol when administered concurrently.

Methylxanthines: The concurrent use of intravenously or orally administered methylxanthines (e.g., aminophylline, theophylline) by patients receiving SEREVENT Inhalation Aerosol has not been completely evaluated. In 1 clinical asthma trial, 87 patients receiving SEREVENT Inhalation Aerosol 42 mcg twice daily concurrently with a theophylline product had adverse event rates similar to those in 71 patients receiving SEREVENT Inhalation Aerosol without theophylline. Resting heart rates were slightly higher in the patients on theophylline but were little affected by SEREVENT Inhalation Aerosol therapy.

Beta-adrenergic receptor blocking agents not only block the pulmonary effect of beta-agonists, such as SEREVENT Inhalation Aerosol, but may also produce severe bronchospasm in asthmatic patients. Therefore, patients with asthma should not normally be treated with beta-blockers. However, under certain circumstances, e.g., as prophylaxis after myocardial infarction, there may be no acceptable alternatives to the use of beta-adrenergic blocking agents in patients with asthma. In this setting, cardioselective beta-blockers could be considered, although they should be administered with caution.

The ECG changes and/or hypokalemia that may result from the administration of nonpotassium-sparing diuretics (such as loop or thiazide diuretics) can be acutely worsened by beta-agonists, especially when the recommended dose of the beta-agonist is exceeded. Although the clinical significance of these effects is not known, caution is advised in the coadministration of beta-agonists with nonpotassium-sparing diuretics.

Carcinogenesis, Mutagenesis, Impairment of Fertility: In an 18-month oral carcinogenicity study in CD-mice, salmeterol xinafoate at oral doses of 1.4 mg/kg and above (approximately 9 times the maximum recommended daily inhalation dose in adults based on comparison of the areas under the plasma concentration versus time curves [AUCs]) caused dose-related increases in the incidence of smooth muscle hyperplasia, cystic glandular hyperplasia, leiomyomas of the uterus, and cysts in the ovaries. The incidence of leiomyosarcomas was not statistically significant. No tumors were seen at 0.2 mg/kg (comparable to the maximum recommended human daily inhalation dose in adults based on comparison of the AUCs).

In a 24-month inhalation and oral carcinogenicity study in Sprague Dawley rats, salmeterol caused dose-related increases in the incidence of mesovarian leiomyomas and ovarian cysts at inhalation and oral doses of 0.68 mg/kg per day and above (approximately 55 times the maximum recommended human daily inhalation dose in adults on a mg/m^2 basis). No tumors were seen at 0.21 mg/kg per day (approximately 15 times the maximum recommended human daily inhalation dose in adults on a mg/m^2 basis). These findings in rodents are similar to those reported previously for other beta-adrenergic agonist drugs. The relevance of these findings to human use is unknown.

Salmeterol xinafoate produced no detectable or reproducible increases in microbial and mammalian gene mutation in vitro. No clastogenic activity occurred in vitro in human lymphocytes or in vivo in a rat micronucleus test. No effects on fertility were identified in male and female rats treated orally with salmeterol xinafoate at doses up to 2 mg/kg (approximately 160 times the maximum recommended human daily inhalation dose in adults on a mg/m^2 basis).

Pregnancy: ***Teratogenic Effects:*** Pregnancy Category C. No teratogenic effects occurred in the rat at oral doses up to 2 mg/kg (approximately 160 times the maximum recommended human daily inhalation dose in adults on a mg/m^2 basis). In pregnant Dutch rabbits administered oral doses of 1 mg/kg and above (approximately 20 times the maximum recommended human daily inhalation dose in adults based on the comparison of the AUCs), salmeterol xinafoate exhibited fetal toxic effects characteristically resulting from beta-adrenoceptor stimulation; these included precocious eyelid openings, cleft palate, sternebral fusion, limb and paw flexures, and delayed ossification of the frontal cranial bones. No significant effects occurred at an oral dose of 0.6 mg/kg (approximately 10 times the maximum recommended human daily inhalation dose in adults based on comparison of the AUCs).

New Zealand White rabbits were less sensitive since only delayed ossification of the frontal cranial bones was seen at oral doses of 10 mg/kg (approximately 1600 times the maximum recommended human daily inhalation dose on a mg/m^2 basis). Extensive use of other beta-agonists has provided no evidence that these class effects in animals are relevant to use in humans. There are no adequate and well-controlled studies with SEREVENT Inhalation Aerosol in pregnant women. SEREVENT Inhalation Aerosol should be used during pregnancy only if the potential benefit justifies the potential risk to the fetus.

Use in Labor and Delivery: There are no well-controlled human studies that have investigated effects of salmeterol on preterm labor or labor at term. Because of the potential for beta-agonist interference with uterine contractility, use of SEREVENT Inhalation Aerosol for prevention of bronchospasm during labor should be restricted to those patients in whom the benefits clearly outweigh the risks.

Nursing Mothers: Plasma levels of salmeterol after inhaled therapeutic doses are very low. In rats, salmeterol xinafoate is excreted in milk. However, since there is no experience with use of SEREVENT Inhalation Aerosol by nursing mothers, a decision should be made whether to discontinue nursing or to discontinue the drug, taking into account the importance of the drug to the mother. Caution should be exercised when salmeterol xinafoate is administered to a nursing woman.

Pediatric Use: The safety and effectiveness of SEREVENT Inhalation Aerosol in children younger than 12 years of age have not been established.

Geriatric Use: Of the total number of patients who received SEREVENT Inhalation Aerosol in all asthma clinical studies, 241 were 65 years of age and older. Geriatric patients (65 years and older) with reversible obstructive airway disease were evaluated in 4 well-controlled studies of 3 weeks' to 3 months' duration. Two placebo-controlled, crossover studies evaluated twice-daily dosing with salmeterol for 21 to 28 days in 45 patients. An additional 75 geriatric patients were treated with salmeterol for 3 months in 2 large parallel-group, multicenter studies. These 120 patients experienced increases in AM and PM peak expiratory flow rate and decreases in diurnal variation in peak expiratory flow rate similar to responses seen in the total populations of the 2 latter studies. The adverse event type and frequency in geriatric patients were not different from those of the total populations studied.

In 2 large, randomized, double-blind, placebo-controlled 3-month studies involving patients with COPD, 133 patients using SEREVENT Inhalation Aerosol were 65 years and older. These patients experienced similar improvements in FEV_1 as observed for patients younger than 65.

No apparent differences in the efficacy and safety of SEREVENT Inhalation Aerosol were observed when geriatric patients were compared with younger patients in asthma and COPD clinical trials. As with other $beta_2$-agonists, however, special caution should be observed when using SEREVENT Inhalation Aerosol in geriatric patients who have concomitant cardiovascular disease that could be adversely affected by this class of drug. Based on available data, no adjustment of salmeterol dosage in geriatric patients is warranted.

ADVERSE REACTIONS

Adverse reactions to salmeterol are similar in nature to reactions to other selective $beta_2$-adrenoceptor agonists, i.e., tachycardia; palpitations; immediate hypersensitivity reactions, including urticaria, angioedema, rash, bronchospasm (see WARNINGS); headache; tremor; nervousness; and paradoxical bronchospasm (see WARNINGS).

Asthma: Two multicenter, 12-week, controlled studies have evaluated twice-daily doses of SEREVENT Inhalation Aerosol in patients 12 years of age and older with asthma. The following table reports the incidence of adverse events in these 2 studies.

[See table 3 at right]

Table 3: Adverse Experience Incidence in 2 Large 12-Week Asthma Clinical Trials*

Adverse Event Type	Percent of Patients		
	Placebo n = 187	SEREVENT Inhalation Aerosol 42 mcg twice daily n = 184	Albuterol Inhalation Aerosol 180 mcg 4 times daily n = 185
Ear, nose, and throat			
Upper respiratory tract infection	13	14	16*
Nasopharyngitis	12	14	11
Disease of nasal cavity/sinus	4	6	1
Sinus headache	2	4	<1
Gastrointestinal			
Stomachache	0	4	0
Neurological			
Headache	23	28	27
Tremor	2	4	3
Respiratory			
Cough	6	7	3
Lower respiratory infection	2	4	2

* The only adverse experience classified as serious was 1 case of upper respiratory tract infection in a patient treated with albuterol.

The table above includes all events (whether considered drug-related or nondrug-related by the investigator) that occurred at a rate of over 3% in the SEREVENT Inhalation Aerosol treatment group and were more common in the SEREVENT Inhalation Aerosol group than in the placebo group.

Pharyngitis, allergic rhinitis, dizziness/giddiness, and influenza occurred at 3% or more but were equally common on placebo. Other events occurring in the SEREVENT Inhalation Aerosol treatment group at a frequency of 1% to 3% were as follows:

Cardiovascular: Tachycardia, palpitations.
Ear, Nose, and Throat: Rhinitis, laryngitis.
Gastrointestinal: Nausea, viral gastroenteritis, nausea and vomiting, diarrhea, abdominal pain.
Hypersensitivity: Urticaria.
Mouth and Teeth: Dental pain.
Musculoskeletal: Pain in joint, back pain, muscle cramp/contraction, myalgia/myositis, muscular soreness.
Neurological: Nervousness, malaise/fatigue.
Respiratory: Tracheitis/bronchitis.
Skin: Rash/skin eruption.
Urogenital: Dysmenorrhea.

In small dose-response studies, tremor, nervousness, and palpitations appeared to be dose related.

COPD: Two multicenter, 12-week, controlled studies have evaluated twice-daily doses of SEREVENT Inhalation Aerosol in patients with COPD. The following table reports the incidence of adverse events in these 2 studies.

[See table 4 at right]

Table 4: Adverse Experience Incidence in 2 Large 12-Week COPD Clinical Trials

Adverse Event Type	Percent of Patients		
	Placebo n = 278	SEREVENT Inhalation Aerosol 42 mcg twice daily n = 267	Ipratropium Inhalation Aerosol 36 mcg 4 times daily n = 271
Ear, nose, and throat			
Upper respiratory tract infection	7	9	9
Sore throat	3	8	6
Nasal sinus infection	1	4	2
Gastrointestinal			
Diarrhea	3	5	4
Musculoskeletal			
Back pain	3	4	3
Neurological			
Headache	10	12	8
Respiratory			
Chest congestion	3	4	3

The table above includes all events (whether considered drug-related or nondrug-related by the investigator) that occurred at a rate of over 3% in the SEREVENT Inhalation Aerosol treatment group and were more common in the SEREVENT Inhalation Aerosol group than in the placebo group.

Common cold, rhinorrhea, bronchitis, cough, exacerbation of chest congestion, chest pain, and dizziness occurred at 3% or more but were equally common on placebo. Other events occurring in the SEREVENT Inhalation Aerosol treatment group at a frequency of 1% to 3% were as follows:

Ear, Nose, and Throat: Cold symptoms, earache, epistaxis, nasal congestion, nasal sinus congestion, sneezing.
Gastrointestinal: Nausea, dyspepsia, gastric pain, gastric upset, abdominal pain, constipation, heartburn, oral candidiasis, xerostomia, vomiting, surgical removal of tooth.
Musculoskeletal: Leg cramps, myalgia, neck pain, pain in arm, shoulder pain, muscle injury of neck.
Neurological: Insomnia, sinus headache.
Non-Site Specific: Fatigue, fever, pain in body, discomfort in chest.
Respiratory: Acute bronchitis, dyspnea, influenza, lower respiratory tract infection, pneumonia, respiratory tract infection, shortness of breath, wheezing.
Urogenital: Urinary tract infection.

Electrocardiographic Monitoring in Patients With COPD: Continuous electrocardiographic (Holter) monitoring was performed on 284 patients in 2 large COPD clinical trials during five 24-hour periods. No cases of sustained ventricular tachycardia were observed. At baseline, non-sustained, asymptomatic ventricular tachycardia was recorded for 7 (7.1%), 8 (9.4%), and 3 (3.0%) patients in the placebo, SEREVENT, and ipratropium groups, respectively. During treatment, nonsustained, asymptomatic ventricular tachycardia that represented a clinically significant change from baseline was reported for 11 (11.6%), 15 (18.3%), and 20 (20.8%) patients receiving placebo, SEREVENT, and ipratropium, respectively. Four of these cases of ventricular tachycardia were reported as adverse events (1 placebo, 3 SEREVENT) by 1 investigator based upon review of Holter data. One case of ventricular tachycardia was observed during ECG evaluation of chest pain (ipratropium) and reported as an adverse event.

Observed During Clinical Practice: In extensive US and worldwide postmarketing experience, serious exacerbations of asthma, including some that have been fatal, have been reported. In most cases, these have occurred in patients with severe asthma and/or in some patients in whom asthma has been acutely deteriorating (see WARNINGS no. 1), but they have occurred in a few patients with less severe asthma as well. It was not possible from these reports to determine whether SEREVENT Inhalation Aerosol contributed to these events or simply failed to relieve the deteriorating asthma.

The following events have also been identified during post-approval use of SEREVENT in clinical practice. Because they are reported voluntarily from a population of unknown size, estimates of frequency cannot be made. These events have been chosen for inclusion due to a combination of their seriousness, frequency of reporting, or potential causal connection to SEREVENT.

Respiratory: Rare reports of upper airway symptoms of laryngeal spasm, irritation, or swelling such as stridor or choking.

Cardiovascular: Hypertension, arrhythmias, (including atrial fibrillation, supraventricular tachycardia, extrasystoles).

OVERDOSAGE

The expected signs and symptoms with overdosage are those of excessive beta-adrenergic stimulation and/or occurrence or exaggeration of any of the symptoms listed under ADVERSE REACTIONS, e.g., seizures, angina, hypertension or hypotension, tachycardia with rates up to 200 beats/min, arrhythmias, nervousness, headache, tremor, muscle cramps, dry mouth, palpitation, nausea, dizziness, fatigue, malaise, and insomnia. Overdosage with salmeterol may be expected to result in exaggeration of the pharmacologic adverse effects associated with beta-adrenoceptor agonists, including tachycardia and/or arrhythmia, tremor, headache, and muscle cramps. Overdosage with salmeterol can lead to clinically significant prolongation of the QT_c interval, which can produce ventricular arrhythmias. Other signs of overdosage may include hypokalemia and hyperglycemia.

As with all sympathomimetic aerosol medications, cardiac arrest and even death may be associated with abuse of SEREVENT Inhalation Aerosol.

Treatment consists of discontinuation of SEREVENT Inhalation Aerosol together with appropriate symptomatic therapy. The judicious use of a cardioselective beta-receptor blocker may be considered, bearing in mind that such medication can produce bronchospasm. There is insufficient evidence to determine if dialysis is beneficial for overdosage of SEREVENT Inhalation Aerosol. Cardiac monitoring is recommended in cases of overdosage.

No deaths were seen in rats at inhalation doses of 2.9 mg/kg (approximately 240 times the maximum recommended human daily inhalation dose on a mg/m^2 basis) and in dogs at 0.7 mg/kg (approximately 190 times the maximum recommended human daily inhalation dose on a mg/m^2 basis). By the oral route, no deaths occurred in mice at 150 mg/kg (approximately 6100 times the maximum recommended human daily inhalation dose on a mg/m^2 basis) and in rats at 1000 mg/kg (approximately 81,000 times the maximum recommended human daily inhalation dose on a mg/m^2 basis).

DOSAGE AND ADMINISTRATION

SEREVENT Inhalation Aerosol should be administered by the orally inhaled route only (see PATIENT'S INSTRUCTIONS FOR USE). It is recommended to "test spray" SEREVENT Inhalation Aerosol into the air 4 times before using for the first time and in cases where the aerosol has not been used for a prolonged period of time (i.e., more than 4 weeks).

Asthma: For maintenance of bronchodilatation and prevention of symptoms of asthma, including the symptoms of nocturnal asthma, the usual dosage for patients 12 years of age and older is 2 inhalations (42 mcg) twice daily (morning and evening, approximately 12 hours apart). Adverse effects are more likely to occur with higher doses of salmeterol, and more frequent administration or administration of a larger number of inhalations is not recommended.

To gain full therapeutic benefit, SEREVENT Inhalation Aerosol should be administered twice daily (morning and evening) in the treatment of reversible airway obstruction. If a previously effective dosage regimen fails to provide the usual response, medical advice should be sought immediately as this is often a sign of destabilization of asthma. Under these circumstances, the therapeutic regimen should be re-evaluated and additional therapeutic options, such as inhaled or systemic corticosteroids, should be considered. If symptoms arise in the period between doses, an inhaled, short-acting $beta_2$-agonist should be taken for immediate relief.

COPD: For maintenance treatment of bronchospasm associated with COPD (including chronic bronchitis and emphysema), the usual dosage for adults is 2 inhalations (42 mcg) twice daily (morning and evening, approximately 12 hours apart).

Prevention of Exercise-Induced Bronchospasm: Two inhalations at least 30 to 60 minutes before exercise have been shown to protect against exercise-induced bronchospasm in many patients for up to 12 hours. Additional doses of SEREVENT Inhalation Aerosol should not be used for 12 hours after the administration of this drug. Patients who are receiving SEREVENT Inhalation Aerosol twice daily (morning and evening) should not use additional SEREVENT Inhalation Aerosol for prevention of exercise-induced bronchospasm. If this dose is not effective, other appropriate therapy for exercise-induced bronchospasm should be considered.

Geriatric Use: In studies where geriatric patients (65 years of age or older, see PRECAUTIONS) have been

Continued on next page

This product information is based on labeling in effect on June 23, 2000. For further information, contact via direct mail, phone, or web site. Medical Information, Glaxo Wellcome Inc., PO Box 13398, Research Triangle Park, NC 27709. Healthcare Professionals (Medical Information): 800-334-0089. Patients (Customer Response Center): 1-888-825-5249. Glaxo Wellcome Corporate Web Site: www.glaxowellcome.com

Serevent—Cont.

treated with SEREVENT Inhalation Aerosol, efficacy and safety of 42 mcg given twice daily (morning and evening) did not differ from that in younger patients. Consequently, no dosage adjustment is recommended.

HOW SUPPLIED

SEREVENT Inhalation Aerosol is supplied in 13-g canisters containing 120 metered actuations in boxes of 1. Each actuation delivers 25 mcg of salmeterol base (as salmeterol xinafoate) from the valve and 21 mcg of salmeterol base (as salmeterol xinafoate) from the actuator. Each canister is supplied with a green plastic actuator with a teal-colored strapcap and patient's instructions (NDC 0173-0464-00). Also available, SEREVENT Inhalation Aerosol Refill (NDC 0173-0465-00), a 13-g canister only with patient's instructions.

SEREVENT Inhalation Aerosol is also supplied in a pack that consists of a 6.5-g canister containing 60 metered actuations in boxes of 1. Each actuation delivers 25 mcg of salmeterol base (as salmeterol xinafoate) from the valve and 21 mcg of salmeterol base from the actuator (as salmeterol xinafoate). Each canister is supplied with a green plastic actuator with a teal-colored strapcap and patient's instructions (NDC 0173-0467-00).

For use with SEREVENT Inhalation Aerosol actuator only. The green actuator with SEREVENT Inhalation Aerosol should not be used with other aerosol medications, and actuators from other aerosol medications should not be used with a SEREVENT Inhalation Aerosol canister.

The correct amount of medication in each inhalation cannot be assured after 120 actuations from the 13-g canister or 60 actuations from the 6.5-g canister even though the canister is not completely empty. The canister should be discarded when the labeled number of actuations has been used.

Store between 15° and 30°C (59° and 86°F). Store canister with nozzle end down. Protect from freezing temperatures and direct sunlight.

Avoid spraying in eyes. Contents under pressure. Do not puncture or incinerate. Do not store at temperatures above 120°F. Keep out of reach of children. As with most inhaled medications in aerosol canisters, the therapeutic effect of this medication may decrease when the canister is cold; for best results, the canister should be at room temperature before use. Shake well before using.

Glaxo Wellcome Inc., Research Triangle Park, NC 27709
US Patent Nos. 4,992,474; 5,225,445; and 5,380,922

May 2000/RL-826

Shown in Product Identification Guide, page 316

SEREVENT® DISKUS® ℞

[*sĕr' ə-vent dĭsk' us*]
(salmeterol xinafoate inhalation powder)

For Oral Inhalation Only

DESCRIPTION

SEREVENT DISKUS (salmeterol xinafoate inhalation powder) contains salmeterol xinafoate as the racemic form of the 1-hydroxy-2-naphthoic acid salt of salmeterol. The active component of the formulation is salmeterol base, a highly selective beta$_2$-adrenergic bronchodilator. The chemical name of salmeterol xinafoate is 4-hydroxy-α^1-[[[6-(4-phenylbutoxy)hexyl]amino]methyl]-1,3-benzenedimethanol, 1-hydroxy-2-naphthalenecarboxylate.

The molecular weight of salmeterol xinafoate is 603.8, and the empirical formula is $C_{25}H_{37}NO_4 \bullet C_{11}H_8O_3$. Salmeterol xinafoate is a white to off-white powder. It is freely soluble in methanol; slightly soluble in ethanol, chloroform, and isopropanol; and sparingly soluble in water.

SEREVENT DISKUS is a specially designed plastic device containing a double-foil blister strip of a powder formulation of salmeterol xinafoate intended for oral inhalation only. Each blister on the double-foil strip within the device contains 50 mcg of salmeterol administered as the salmeterol xinafoate salt in 12.5 mg of formulation containing lactose. When a blister containing medication is opened by activating the device, the medication is dispersed into the air stream created when the patient inhales through the mouthpiece.

The amount of drug delivered to the lung will depend on patient factors such as inspiratory flow. Under standardized in vitro testing, SEREVENT DISKUS delivers 47 mcg when tested at 60 L/min flow rate for 3 seconds. In adult patients with obstructive lung disease and severely compromised lung function (mean forced expiratory volume in 1 second [FEV$_1$] 0.65 L [range, 0.35 to 0.92 L], 20% to 30% predicted FEV$_1$), mean peak inspiratory flow (PIF) through SEREVENT DISKUS was 82.4 L/min (range, 46.1 to 115.3 L/min). The emitted dose of salmeterol xinafoate determined in an in vitro experiment modeling these patient-generated flow rates was 46 mcg (range, 45 to 51 mcg).

CLINICAL PHARMACOLOGY

Mechanism of Action: Salmeterol is a long-acting beta-adrenergic agonist. In vitro studies and in vivo pharmacologic studies demonstrate that salmeterol is selective for beta$_2$-adrenoceptors compared with isoproterenol, which has approximately equal agonist activity on beta$_1$- and beta$_2$-adrenoceptors. In vitro studies show salmeterol to be at least 50 times more selective for beta$_2$-adrenoceptors than albuterol. Although beta$_2$-adrenoceptors are the predominant adrenergic receptors in bronchial smooth muscle and beta$_1$-adrenoceptors are the predominant receptors in the heart, there are also beta$_2$-adrenoceptors in the human heart comprising 10% to 50% of the total beta-adrenoceptors. The precise function of these receptors has not been established, but they raise the possibility that even highly selective beta$_2$-agonists may have cardiac effects.

The pharmacologic effects of beta$_2$-adrenoceptor agonist drugs, including salmeterol, are at least in part attributable to stimulation of intracellular adenyl cyclase, the enzyme that catalyzes the conversion of adenosine triphosphate (ATP) to cyclic-3′,5′-adenosine monophosphate (cyclic AMP). Increased cyclic AMP levels cause relaxation of bronchial smooth muscle and inhibition of release of mediators of immediate hypersensitivity from cells, especially from mast cells.

In vitro tests show that salmeterol is a potent and long-lasting inhibitor of the release of mast cell mediators, such as histamine, leukotrienes, and prostaglandin D$_2$, from human lung. Salmeterol inhibits histamine-induced plasma protein extravasation and inhibits platelet activating factor-induced eosinophil accumulation in the lungs of guinea pigs when administered by the inhaled route. In humans, single doses of salmeterol administered via inhalation aerosol attenuate allergen-induced bronchial hyper-responsiveness.

Pharmacokinetics: Salmeterol acts locally in the lung; plasma levels therefore do not predict therapeutic effect. Because of the low therapeutic dose, systemic levels of salmeterol inhalation powder are low or undetectable after inhalation of recommended doses (50 mcg twice daily). Following chronic administration of an inhaled dose of 50 mcg of salmeterol inhalation powder twice daily, salmeterol was detected in plasma within 5 to 45 minutes in seven asthmatic patients; plasma concentrations were very low, with mean peak concentrations of 167 ± 75 pg/mL and no accumulation with repeated doses. Oral administration of 1 mg of radiolabeled salmeterol (as salmeterol xinafoate) to two healthy subjects gave peak plasma salmeterol concentrations of about 650 pg/mL at about 45 minutes; the terminal elimination half-life was about 5.5 hours (one volunteer only).

Salmeterol xinafoate, an ionic salt, dissociates in solution so that the salmeterol and 1-hydroxy-2-naphthoic acid (xinafoate) moieties are absorbed, distributed, metabolized, and excreted independently. Salmeterol base is extensively metabolized by hydroxylation, with subsequent elimination predominantly in the feces. In two healthy subjects who received 1 mg of radiolabeled salmeterol (as salmeterol xinafoate) orally, approximately 25% and 60% of the radiolabeled salmeterol was eliminated in urine and feces, respectively, over a period of 7 days. No significant amount of unchanged salmeterol base was detected in either urine or feces.

Salmeterol is 94% to 98% bound to human plasma proteins in vitro over the concentration range of 8 to 7722 ng of base per milliliter, much higher concentrations than those achieved following therapeutic doses of salmeterol.

The xinafoate moiety has no apparent pharmacologic activity, is highly protein bound (>99%), and has a long elimination half-life of 11 days.

The pharmacokinetics of salmeterol base has not been studied in elderly patients nor in patients with hepatic or renal impairment. Since salmeterol is predominantly cleared by hepatic metabolism, liver function impairment may lead to accumulation of salmeterol in plasma. Therefore, patients with hepatic disease should be closely monitored.

Pharmacodynamics: Inhaled salmeterol, like other beta-adrenergic agonist drugs, can in some patients produce cardiovascular effects (see PRECAUTIONS). The cardiovascular effects (heart rate, blood pressure) associated with salmeterol inhalation powder occur with similar frequency, and are of similar type and severity, as those noted following albuterol administration.

The effects of rising doses of salmeterol and standard inhaled doses of albuterol were studied in volunteers and in patients with asthma. Salmeterol doses up to 84 mcg administered as inhalation aerosol resulted in heart rate increases of 3 to 16 beats/min, about the same as albuterol dosed at 180 mcg by inhalation aerosol (4 to 10 beats/min). Adolescent and adult patients receiving 50-mcg doses of salmeterol inhalation powder (n = 60) underwent continuous electrocardiographic monitoring during two 12-hour periods after the first dose and after 1 month of therapy, and no clinically significant dysrhythmias were noted. Also, pediatric patients receiving 50-mcg doses of salmeterol inhalation powder (n = 67) underwent continuous electrocardiographic monitoring during two 12-hour periods after the first dose and after 3 months of therapy, and no clinically significant dysrhythmias were noted.

Studies in laboratory animals (minipigs, rodents, and dogs) have demonstrated the occurrence of cardiac arrhythmias and sudden death (with histologic evidence of myocardial necrosis) when beta-agonists and methylxanthines are administered concurrently. The clinical significance of these findings is unknown.

Clinical Trials: During the initial treatment day in several multiple-dose clinical trials with salmeterol inhalation powder in patients with asthma, the median time to onset of clinically significant bronchodilatation (≥15% improvement in FEV$_1$) ranged from 30 to 48 minutes after a 50-mcg dose. One hour after a single dose of 50 mcg of salmeterol inhalation powder, the majority of patients had ≥15% improvement in FEV$_1$. Maximum improvement in FEV$_1$ generally occurred within 180 minutes, and clinically significant improvement continued for 12 hours in most patients.

In two large, randomized, double-blind studies, salmeterol inhalation powder was compared with albuterol inhalation aerosol and placebo in adolescent and adult patients with mild-to-moderate asthma (protocol defined as 50% to 80% predicted FEV$_1$, actual mean of 67.7% at baseline), including patients who did and who did not receive concurrent inhaled corticosteroids. The efficacy of salmeterol inhalation powder was demonstrated over the 12-week period with no change in effectiveness over this time period. There were no gender- or age-related differences in safety or efficacy. No development of tachyphylaxis to the bronchodilator effect has been noted in these studies. FEV$_1$ measurements (mean change from baseline) from these two 12-week studies are shown below for both the first and last treatment days.

FEV$_1$, As Percent of Predicted, From Two Large 12-Week Clinical Trials
First Treatment Day

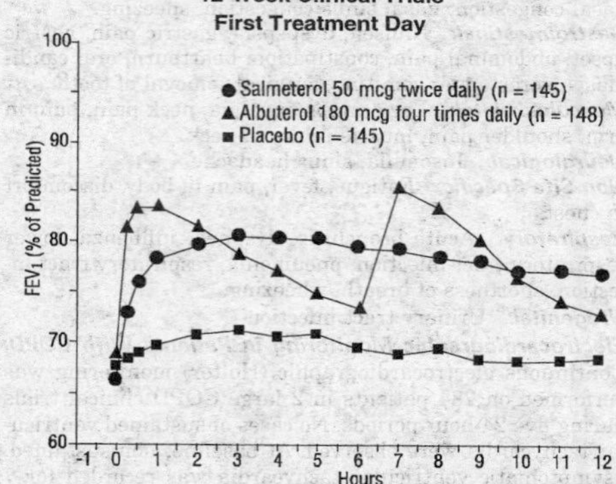

Last Treatment Day (Week 12)

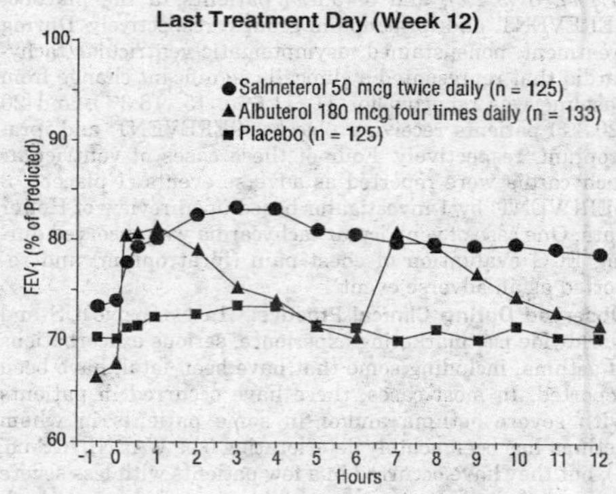

During daily treatment with salmeterol inhalation powder for 12 weeks in adolescent and adult patients with mild-to-moderate asthma, the following treatment effects were seen:

[See table 1 above]

Table 1: Daily Efficacy Measurements in Two Large 12-Week Clinical Trials (Combined Data)

Parameter	Time	Placebo	SEREVENT	Albuterol
No. of randomized subjects		152	149	148
Mean AM peak expiratory flow rate (L/min)	baseline	394	395	394
	12 weeks	396	427*	394
Mean % days with no asthma symptoms	baseline	14	13	12
	12 weeks	20	33	21
Mean % nights with no awakenings	baseline	70	63	68
	12 weeks	73	85*	71
Rescue medications (mean no. of inhalations per day)	baseline	4.2	4.3	4.3
	12 weeks	3.3	1.6†	2.2
Asthma exacerbations		14%	15%	16%

* Statistically superior to placebo and albuterol ($P<0.001$).
† Statistically superior to placebo ($P<0.001$).

Safe usage with maintenance of efficacy for periods up to 1 year has been documented.

Salmeterol inhalation powder and salmeterol aerosol were compared to placebo in two additional randomized, double-blind clinical trials in adolescent and adult patients with mild-to-moderate asthma. Salmeterol inhalation powder 50 mcg administered via the DISKUS and salmeterol inhalation aerosol 42 mcg, both administered twice daily, produced significant improvements in pulmonary function compared with placebo over the 12-week period. While no statistically significant differences were observed between the active treatments for any of the efficacy assessments or safety evaluations performed, there were some efficacy measures on which the metered-dose inhaler appeared to provide better results. Similar findings were noted in two randomized, single-dose, crossover comparisons of salmeterol inhalation powder and salmeterol aerosol for the prevention of exercise-induced bronchospasm. Therefore, while SEREVENT DISKUS was comparable to SEREVENT® (salmeterol xinafoate) Inhalation Aerosol in clinical trials in mild-to-moderate asthmatics, it should not be assumed that the SEREVENT Inhalation Aerosol and SEREVENT DISKUS drug products will produce clinically equivalent outcomes in all patients.

In a large, randomized, double-blind, controlled study (n = 449), 50 mcg of salmeterol inhalation powder, via the SEREVENT DISKUS, was administered twice daily to pediatric asthma patients who did and who did not receive concurrent inhaled corticosteroids. The efficacy of salmeterol inhalation powder was demonstrated over the 12-week treatment period with respect to periodic serial peak expiratory flow (36% to 39% postdose increase from baseline) and FEV_1 (32% to 33% postdose increase from baseline). Salmeterol was effective in demographic subgroup analyses (gender and age) and was effective when coadministered with other inhaled asthma medications such as short-acting bronchodilators and inhaled corticosteroids. A second large, randomized, double-blind, placebo-controlled study (n = 207) with 50 mcg of salmeterol inhalation powder via an alternate device supported the findings of the trial with SEREVENT DISKUS.

In two randomized, single-dose, crossover studies in adolescents and adults with exercise-induced bronchospasm (EIB) (n = 53), 50 mcg of salmeterol inhalation powder prevented EIB when dosed 30 minutes prior to exercise. For many patients, this protective effect against EIB was still apparent up to 8.5 hours following a single dose.

[See table 2 above]

Table 2: Results of Two Exercise-Induced Bronchospasm Studies in Adolescents and Adults

		Placebo (n = 52)		SEREVENT DISKUS (n = 52)	
		n	% Total	n	% Total
0.5 Hour postdose exercise challenge	% Fall in FEV_1				
	<10%	15	29	31	60
	≥10%,<20%	3	6	11	21
	≥20%	34	65	10	19
Mean maximal % fall in FEV_1 (SE)		−25% (1.8)		−11% (1.9)	
8.5 Hour postdose exercise challenge	% Fall in FEV_1				
	<10%	12	23	26	50
	≥10%,<20%	7	13	12	23
	≥20%	33	63	14	27
Mean maximal % fall in FEV_1 (SE)		−27% (1.5)		−16% (2.0)	

In two randomized studies in children 4 to 11 years old with asthma and EIB (n = 50), a single 50-mcg dose of salmeterol inhalation powder prevented EIB when dosed 30 minutes prior to exercise, with protection lasting up to 11.5 hours in repeat testing following this single dose in many patients.

INDICATIONS AND USAGE

SEREVENT DISKUS inhalation powder is indicated for long-term, twice-daily (morning and evening) administration in the maintenance treatment of asthma and in the prevention of bronchospasm in patients 4 years of age and older with reversible obstructive airway disease, including patients with symptoms of nocturnal asthma, who require regular treatment with inhaled, short-acting $beta_2$-agonists. It is not indicated for patients whose asthma can be managed by occasional use of inhaled, short-acting $beta_2$-agonists.

SEREVENT DISKUS is also indicated for prevention of exercise-induced bronchospasm in patients 4 years of age and older.

SEREVENT DISKUS may be used with or without concurrent inhaled or systemic corticosteroid therapy.

CONTRAINDICATIONS

SEREVENT DISKUS is contraindicated in patients with a history of hypersensitivity to salmeterol or any of its components.

WARNINGS

IMPORTANT INFORMATION: SEREVENT DISKUS SHOULD NOT BE INITIATED IN PATIENTS WITH SIGNIFICANTLY WORSENING OR ACUTELY DETERIORATING ASTHMA, WHICH MAY BE A LIFE-THREATENING CONDITION. Serious acute respiratory events, including fatalities, have been reported, both in the United States and worldwide, when SEREVENT has been initiated in this situation. Although it is not possible from these reports to determine whether SEREVENT contributed to these adverse events or simply failed to relieve the deteriorating asthma, the use of SEREVENT DISKUS in this setting is inappropriate.

SEREVENT DISKUS SHOULD NOT BE USED TO TREAT ACUTE SYMPTOMS. It is crucial to inform patients of this and prescribe an inhaled, short-acting $beta_2$-agonist for this purpose as well as warn them that increasing inhaled $beta_2$-agonist use is a signal of deteriorating asthma.

SEREVENT DISKUS IS NOT A SUBSTITUTE FOR INHALED OR ORAL CORTICOSTEROIDS. Corticosteroids should not be stopped or reduced when SEREVENT DISKUS is initiated.

(See PRECAUTIONS: Information for Patients and the accompanying PATIENT'S INSTRUCTIONS FOR USE.)

1. Do Not Introduce SEREVENT DISKUS as a Treatment for Acutely Deteriorating Asthma: SEREVENT DISKUS is intended for the maintenance treatment of asthma (see INDICATIONS AND USAGE) and should not be introduced in acutely deteriorating asthma, which is a potentially life-threatening condition. There are no data demonstrating that SEREVENT DISKUS provides greater efficacy than or additional efficacy to inhaled, short-acting $beta_2$-agonists in patients with worsening asthma. Serious acute respiratory events, including fatalities, have been reported, both in the United States and worldwide, in patients receiving SEREVENT. In most cases, these have occurred in patients with severe asthma (e.g., patients with a history of corticosteroid dependence, low pulmonary function, intubation, mechanical ventilation, frequent hospitalizations, or previous life-threatening acute asthma exacerbations) and/or in some patients in whom asthma has been acutely deteriorating (e.g., unresponsive to usual medications; increasing need for inhaled, short-acting $beta_2$-agonists; increasing need for systemic corticosteroids; significant increase in symptoms; recent emergency room visits; sudden or progressive deterioration in pulmonary function). However, they have occurred in a few patients with less severe asthma as well. It was not possible from these reports to determine whether SEREVENT contributed to these events or simply failed to relieve the deteriorating asthma.

2. Do Not Use SEREVENT DISKUS to Treat Acute Symptoms: An inhaled, short-acting $beta_2$-agonist, not SEREVENT DISKUS, should be used to relieve acute asthma symptoms. When prescribing SEREVENT DISKUS, the physician must also provide the patient with an inhaled, short-acting $beta_2$-agonist (e.g., albuterol) for treatment of symptoms that occur acutely, despite regular twice-daily (morning and evening) use of SEREVENT DISKUS.

When beginning treatment with SEREVENT DISKUS, patients who have been taking inhaled, short-acting $beta_2$-agonists on a regular basis (e.g., four times a day) should be instructed to discontinue the regular use of these drugs and use them only for symptomatic relief of acute asthma symptoms (see PRECAUTIONS: Information for Patients).

3. Watch for Increasing Use of Inhaled, Short-Acting $Beta_2$-Agonists, Which Is a Marker of Deteriorating Asthma: Asthma may deteriorate acutely over a period of hours or chronically over several days or longer. If the patient's inhaled, short-acting $beta_2$-agonist becomes less effective or the patient needs more inhalations than usual, this may be a marker of destabilization of asthma. In this setting, the patient requires immediate reevaluation with reassessment of the treatment regimen, giving special consideration to the possible need for corticosteroids. If the patient uses four or more inhalations per day of an inhaled, short-acting $beta_2$-agonist for 2 or more consecutive days, or if more than one canister (200 inhalations per canister) of inhaled, short-acting $beta_2$-agonist is used in an 8-week period in conjunction with SEREVENT DISKUS, then the patient should consult the physician for reevaluation. **Increasing the daily dosage of SEREVENT DISKUS in this situation is not appropriate. SEREVENT DISKUS should not be used more frequently than twice daily (morning and evening) at the recommended dose of one inhalation.**

4. Do Not Use SEREVENT DISKUS as a Substitute for Oral or Inhaled Corticosteroids: The use of beta-adrenergic agonist bronchodilators alone may not be adequate to control asthma in many patients. Early consideration should be given to adding anti-inflammatory agents, e.g., corticosteroids. There are no data demonstrating that SEREVENT DISKUS has a clinical anti-inflammatory effect and could be expected to take the place of, or reduce the dose of, corticosteroids. Patients who already require oral or inhaled corticosteroids for treatment of asthma should be continued on a suitable dose to maintain clinical stability even if they feel better as a result of initiating SEREVENT DISKUS. Any change in corticosteroid dosage should be made ONLY after clinical evaluation (see PRECAUTIONS: Information for Patients).

5. Do Not Exceed Recommended Dosage: As with other inhaled $beta_2$-adrenergic drugs, SEREVENT DISKUS should not be used more often or at higher doses than recommended. Fatalities have been reported in association with excessive use of inhaled sympathomimetic drugs. Large doses of inhaled or oral salmeterol (12 to 20 times the recommended dose) have been associated with clinically significant prolongation of the QT_c interval, which has the potential for producing ventricular arrhythmias.

6. Paradoxical Bronchospasm: Inhalation of salmeterol xinafoate can produce paradoxical bronchospasm, which may be life threatening. If paradoxical bronchospasm occurs, SEREVENT DISKUS should be discontinued immediately and alternative therapy instituted.

7. Immediate Hypersensitivity Reactions: Immediate hypersensitivity reactions may occur after administration of SEREVENT DISKUS, as demonstrated by cases of urticaria, angioedema, rash, and bronchospasm.

8. Upper Airway Symptoms: Symptoms of laryngeal spasm, irritation, or swelling, such as stridor and choking, have been reported in patients receiving SEREVENT DISKUS.

SEREVENT DISKUS, like all other beta-adrenergic agonists, can produce a clinically significant cardiovascular effect in some patients as measured by pulse rate, blood pressure, and/or symptoms. Although such effects are uncommon after administration of SEREVENT DISKUS at recommended doses, if they occur, the drug may need to be discontinued. In addition, beta-agonists have been reported to produce electrocardiogram (ECG) changes, such as flattening of the T wave, prolongation of the QT_c interval, and ST segment depression. The clinical significance of these findings is unknown. Therefore, SEREVENT DISKUS, like all sympathomimetic amines, should be used with caution in patients with cardiovascular disorders, especially coronary insufficiency, cardiac arrhythmias, and hypertension.

PRECAUTIONS

General: 1. Cardiovascular and Other Effects: No effect on the cardiovascular system is usually seen after the administration of inhaled salmeterol at recommended doses, but the cardiovascular and central nervous system effects seen with all sympathomimetic drugs (e.g., increased blood pressure, heart rate, excitement) can occur after use of salmeterol and may require discontinuation of the drug. Salmeterol, like all sympathomimetic amines, should be used with caution in patients with cardiovascular disorders, especially coronary insufficiency, cardiac arrhythmias, and hypertension; in patients with convulsive disorders or thyrotoxicosis; and in patients who are unusually responsive to sympathomimetic amines.

As has been described with other beta-adrenergic agonist bronchodilators, clinically significant changes in systolic and/or diastolic blood pressure, pulse rate, and electrocardiograms have been seen infrequently in individual patients in controlled clinical studies with salmeterol.

2. Metabolic Effects: Doses of the related $beta_2$-adrenoceptor agonist albuterol, when administered intravenously, have been reported to aggravate preexisting diabetes mellitus and ketoacidosis. No effects on glucose have been seen with SEREVENT DISKUS at recommended doses. Beta-adrenergic agonist medications may produce significant hypokalemia in some patients, possibly through intracellular shunting, which has the potential to produce adverse cardiovascular effects. The decrease in serum potassium is usually transient, not requiring supplementation.

Clinically significant changes in blood glucose and/or serum potassium were seen rarely during clinical studies with long-term administration of SEREVENT DISKUS at recommended doses.

Information for Patients: See illustrated PATIENT'S INSTRUCTIONS FOR USE.

It is important that patients understand how to use the DISKUS inhalation device appropriately and how it should be used in relation to other asthma medications they are taking. Patients should be given the following information:

1. The action of SEREVENT DISKUS may last up to 12 hours or longer. The recommended dosage (one inhalation twice daily, morning and evening) should not be exceeded.

2. SEREVENT DISKUS is not meant to relieve acute asthma symptoms and extra doses should not be used for that purpose. Acute symptoms should be treated with an inhaled, short-acting $beta_2$-agonist such as albuterol (the physician should provide the patient with such medication and instruct the patient in how it should be used).

Continued on next page

This product information is based on labeling in effect on June 23, 2000. For further information, contact via direct mail, phone, or web site. Medical Information, Glaxo Wellcome Inc., PO Box 13398, Research Triangle Park, NC 27709. Healthcare Professionals (Medical Information): 800-334-0089. Patients (Customer Response Center): 1-888-825-5249. Glaxo Wellcome Corporate Web Site: www.glaxowellcome.com

Serevent Diskus—Cont.

3. • When used for the treatment of EIB, one inhalation of SEREVENT DISKUS inhalation powder should be taken 30 minutes before exercise.
- Additional doses of SEREVENT should not be used for 12 hours.
- Patients who are receiving SEREVENT DISKUS inhalation powder twice daily should not use additional SEREVENT for prevention of EIB.

4. The physician should be notified immediately if any of the following situations occur, which may be a sign of seriously worsening asthma:
- Decreasing effectiveness of inhaled, short-acting $beta_2$-agonists
- Need for more inhalations than usual of inhaled, short-acting $beta_2$-agonists
- Use of four or more inhalations per day of a short-acting $beta_2$-agonist for 2 or more days consecutively
- Use of more than one canister of an inhaled, short-acting $beta_2$-agonist in an 8-week period (i.e., canister with 200 inhalations)

5. SEREVENT DISKUS should not be used as a substitute for oral or inhaled corticosteroids. The dosage of these medications should not be changed and they should not be stopped without consulting the physician, even if the patient feels better after initiating treatment with SEREVENT DISKUS.
6. Patients should be cautioned regarding common adverse cardiovascular effects, such as palpitations, chest pain, rapid heart rate, tremor, or nervousness.
7. In patients receiving SEREVENT DISKUS, other inhaled medications should be used only as directed by the physician.
8. SEREVENT DISKUS should not be used with a spacer.
9. If you are pregnant or nursing, contact your physician about use of SEREVENT DISKUS.
10. Effective and safe use of the DISKUS device includes an understanding of the way that it should be used:
- Never exhale into the DISKUS device.
- Always activate and use the DISKUS device in a level, horizontal position.
- Never wash the mouthpiece or any part of the DISKUS device. KEEP IT DRY.

Drug Interactions: ***Short-Acting Beta-Agonists:*** In the two 12-week, repetitive-dose adolescent and adult clinical trials (n = 149), the mean daily need for additional $beta_2$-agonist use in patients using salmeterol inhalation powder was approximately $1^1/_2$ inhalations per day. Twenty-six percent of the patients in these trials used between 8 and 24 inhalations of short-acting beta-agonist per day on one or more occasions. Nine percent of the patients in these trials averaged over 4 inhalations per day over the course of the 12-week trials. No observed increase in frequency of cardiovascular events was noted among the 3 patients who used an average of 8 to 11 inhalations per day; however, the safety of concomitant use of more than 8 inhalations per day of short-acting $beta_2$-agonist with salmeterol inhalation powder has not been established. In 29 patients who experienced worsening of asthma while receiving salmeterol inhalation powder during these trials, albuterol therapy administered via either nebulizer or inhalation aerosol (one dose in most cases) led to improvement in FEV_1 and no increase in occurrence of cardiovascular adverse events.

Monoamine Oxidase Inhibitors and Tricyclic Antidepressants: Salmeterol should be administered with extreme caution to patients being treated with monoamine oxidase inhibitors or tricyclic antidepressants, or within 2 weeks of discontinuation of such agents, because the action of salmeterol on the vascular system may be potentiated by these agents.

Corticosteroids and Cromoglycate: In clinical trials, inhaled corticosteroids and/or inhaled cromolyn sodium did not alter the safety profile of SEREVENT when administered concurrently.

Methylxanthines: The concurrent use of intravenously or orally administered methylxanthines (e.g., aminophylline, theophylline) by patients receiving SEREVENT has not been completely evaluated. In one clinical asthma trial, 87 patients receiving SEREVENT Inhalation Aerosol 42 mcg twice daily concurrently with a theophylline product had adverse event rates similar to those in 71 patients receiving SEREVENT Inhalation Aerosol without theophylline. Resting heart rates were slightly higher in the patients on theophylline but were little affected by therapy with SEREVENT Inhalation Aerosol.

Beta-adrenergic receptor blocking agents not only block the pulmonary effect of beta-agonists, such as SEREVENT DISKUS, but may produce severe bronchospasm in asthmatic patients. Therefore, patients with asthma should not normally be treated with beta-blockers. However, under certain circumstances, e.g., as prophylaxis after myocardial infarction, there may be no acceptable alternatives to the use of beta-adrenergic blocking agents in patients with asthma. In this setting, cardioselective beta-blockers could be considered, although they should be administered with caution.

The ECG changes and/or hypokalemia that may result from the administration of nonpotassium-sparing diuretics (such as loop or thiazide diuretics) can be acutely worsened by beta-agonists, especially when the recommended dose of the beta-agonist is exceeded. Although the clinical significance of these effects is not known, caution is advised in the coadministration of beta-agonists with nonpotassium-sparing diuretics.

Table 3: Adverse Experience Incidence in Two Large 12-Week Adolescent and Adult Clinical Trials

Adverse Event Type	Percent of Patients		
	Placebo n = 152	SEREVENT Inhalation Powder 50 mcg twice daily n = 149	Albuterol Inhalation Aerosol 180 mcg four times daily n = 150
Ear, nose, and throat			
Nasal/sinus congestion, pallor	6	9	8
Rhinitis	4	5	4
Neurological			
Headache	9	13	12
Respiratory			
Asthma	1	3	<1
Tracheitis/bronchitis	4	7	3
Influenza	2	5	5

Table 4: Adverse Experience Incidence in Two Large 12-Week Pediatric Clinical Trials

Adverse Event Type	Percent of Patients		
	Placebo n = 215	SEREVENT Inhalation Powder 50 mcg twice daily n = 211	Albuterol Powder 200 mcg four times daily n = 115
Ear, nose, and throat			
Ear signs and symptoms	3	4	9
Pharyngitis	3	6	3
Neurological			
Headache	14	17	20
Respiratory			
Asthma	2	4	<1
Skin			
Skin rashes	3	4	2
Urticaria	0	3	2

Carcinogenesis, Mutagenesis, Impairment of Fertility: In an 18-month carcinogenicity study in CD-mice, salmeterol xinafoate at oral doses of 1.4 mg/kg and above (approximately 20 times the maximum recommended daily inhalation dose in adults and children based on comparison of the area under the plasma concentration versus time curves [AUCs]) caused a dose-related increase in the incidence of smooth muscle hyperplasia, cystic glandular hyperplasia, leiomyomas of the uterus, and cysts in the ovaries. The incidence of leiomyosarcomas was not statistically significant. No tumors were seen at 0.2 mg/kg (approximately 3 times the maximum recommended daily inhalation doses in adults and children based on comparison of the AUCs).

In a 24-month oral and inhalation carcinogenicity study in Sprague Dawley rats, salmeterol caused a dose-related increase in the incidence of mesovarian leiomyomas and ovarian cysts at doses of 0.68 mg/kg and above (approximately 60 times the maximum recommended daily inhalation dose in adults and approximately 30 times the maximum recommended daily inhalation dose in children on a mg/m^2 basis). No tumors were seen at 0.21 mg/kg (approximately 20 times the maximum recommended daily inhalation dose in adults and approximately 9 times the maximum recommended daily inhalation dose in children on a mg/m^2 basis). These findings in rodents are similar to those reported previously for other beta-adrenergic agonist drugs. The relevance of these findings to human use is unknown.

Salmeterol produced no detectable or reproducible increases in microbial and mammalian gene mutation in vitro. No clastogenic activity occurred in vitro in human lymphocytes or in vivo in a rat micronucleus test. No effects on fertility were identified in male and female rats treated with salmeterol at oral doses up to 2 mg/kg (approximately 170 times the maximum recommended daily inhalation dose in adults on a mg/m^2 basis).

Pregnancy: ***Teratogenic Effects:*** Pregnancy Category C. No teratogenic effects occurred in rats at oral doses up to 2 mg/kg (approximately 170 times the maximum recommended daily inhalation dose in adults on a mg/m^2 basis). In pregnant Dutch rabbits administered oral doses of 1 mg/kg and above (approximately 50 times the maximum recommended daily inhalation dose in adults based on comparison of the AUCs), salmeterol exhibited fetal toxic effects characteristically resulting from beta-adrenoceptor stimulation. These included precocious eyelid openings, cleft palate, sternebral fusion, limb and paw flexures, and delayed ossification of the frontal cranial bones. No significant effects occurred at an oral dose of 0.6 mg/kg (approximately 20 times the maximum recommended daily inhalation dose in adults based on comparison of the AUCs).

New Zealand White rabbits were less sensitive since only delayed ossification of the frontal bones was seen at an oral dose of 10 mg/kg (approximately 1700 times the maximum recommended daily inhalation dose in adults on a mg/m^2 basis). Extensive use of other beta-agonists has provided no evidence that these class effects in animals are relevant to their use in humans. There are no adequate and well-controlled studies with SEREVENT DISKUS in pregnant women. SEREVENT DISKUS should be used during pregnancy only if the potential benefit justifies the potential risk to the fetus.

Use in Labor and Delivery: There are no well-controlled human studies that have investigated effects of salmeterol on preterm labor or labor at term. Because of the potential for beta-agonist interference with uterine contractility, use of SEREVENT DISKUS for relief of bronchospasm during labor should be restricted to those patients in whom the benefits clearly outweigh the risks.

Nursing Mothers: Plasma levels of salmeterol after inhaled therapeutic doses are very low. In rats, salmeterol xinafoate is excreted in the milk. However, since there are no data from controlled trials on the use of SEREVENT by nursing mothers, a decision should be made whether to discontinue nursing or to discontinue the drug, taking into account the importance of the drug to the mother. Caution should be exercised when salmeterol xinafoate is administered to a nursing woman.

Pediatric Use: The safety and efficacy of salmeterol inhalation powder has been evaluated in over 2500 patients aged 4 to 11 years with asthma, 346 of whom were administered salmeterol inhalation powder for 1 year. Based on available data, no adjustment of salmeterol dosage in pediatric patients is warranted for either asthma or EIB (see DOSAGE AND ADMINISTRATION).

In two randomized, double-blind, controlled clinical trials of 12 weeks' duration, salmeterol 50-mcg powder was administered to 211 pediatric asthma patients who did and who did not receive concurrent inhaled corticosteroids. The efficacy of salmeterol inhalation powder was demonstrated over the 12-week treatment period with respect to peak expiratory flow and FEV_1. Salmeterol inhalation powder was effective in demographic subgroups (gender and age) of the population. Salmeterol was effective when coadministered with other inhaled asthma medications, such as short-acting bronchodilators and inhaled corticosteroids. Salmeterol inhalation powder was well tolerated in the pediatric population, and there were no safety issues identified specific to the administration of salmeterol inhalation powder to pediatric patients.

In two randomized studies in children 4 to 11 years old with asthma and EIB, a single 50-mcg dose of salmeterol inhalation powder prevented EIB when dosed 30 minutes prior to exercise, with protection lasting up to 11.5 hours in repeat testing following this single dose in many patients.

Geriatric Use: Of the total number of patients who received salmeterol inhalation powder in adolescent and adult chronic dosing clinical trials, 209 were 65 years of age and older. No apparent differences in the efficacy and safety of SEREVENT inhalation powder were observed when geriatric patients were compared with younger patients in clinical trials. As with other $beta_2$-agonists, however, special caution should be observed when using SEREVENT inhalation powder in geriatric patients who have concomitant cardiovascular disease that could be adversely affected by this class of drug. Based on available data, no adjustment of salmeterol dosage in geriatric patients is warranted.

ADVERSE REACTIONS

Adverse reactions to salmeterol are similar in nature to reactions to other selective $beta_2$-adrenoceptor agonists, i.e., tachycardia; palpitations; immediate hypersensitivity reactions, including urticaria, angioedema, rash, bronchospasm (see WARNINGS); headache; tremor; nervousness; and paradoxical bronchospasm (see WARNINGS).

Two multicenter, 12-week, controlled studies have evaluated twice-daily doses of SEREVENT inhalation powder in patients 12 years of age and older with asthma. The following table reports the incidence of adverse events in these two studies.

[See table 3 at top of previous page]

The table above includes all events (whether considered drug-related or nondrug-related by the investigator) that occurred at a rate of ≥3% in the SEREVENT inhalation powder treatment group and were more common in the SEREVENT inhalation powder group than in the placebo group.

Pharyngitis, sinusitis, upper respiratory tract infection, and cough occurred at ≥3% but were more common in the placebo group. However, throat irritation has been described at rates exceeding that of placebo in other controlled clinical trials. Other events occurring in the SEREVENT inhalation powder group at a frequency of 1% to 3% and at a greater rate than in placebo were as follows:

Ear, Nose, and Throat: Sinus headache.
Gastrointestinal: Nausea.
Mouth and Teeth: Oral mucosal abnormality.
Musculoskeletal: Pain in joint.
Neurological: Sleep disturbance, paresthesia.
Skin: Contact dermatitis, eczema.
Miscellaneous: Localized aches and pains, pyrexia of unknown origin.

Two multicenter, 12-week, controlled studies have evaluated twice-daily doses of salmeterol inhalation powder in patients aged 4 to 11 years with asthma. The following table includes all events (whether considered drug-related or nondrug-related by the investigator) that occurred at a rate of ≥3% in the SEREVENT inhalation powder treatment group and were more common in the SEREVENT inhalation powder group than in the placebo group.

[See table 4 on previous page]

The following events were reported at an incidence of 1% to 2% (3 to 4 patients) in the salmeterol group and with a higher incidence than in the albuterol and placebo groups: gastrointestinal signs and symptoms, lower respiratory signs and symptoms, photodermatitis, and arthralgia and articular rheumatism.

Observed During Clinical Practice: In extensive United States and worldwide postmarketing experience with SEREVENT, serious exacerbations of asthma, including some that have been fatal, have been reported. In most cases, these have occurred in patients with severe asthma and/or in some patients in whom asthma has been acutely deteriorating (see WARNINGS no. 1), but they have also occurred in a few patients with less severe asthma as well. It was not possible from these reports to determine whether SEREVENT contributed to these events or simply failed to relieve the deteriorating asthma.

The following events have also been identified during post-approval use of SEREVENT in clinical practice. Because they are reported voluntarily from a population of unknown size, estimates of frequency cannot be made. These events have been chosen for inclusion due to a combination of their seriousness, frequency of reporting, or potential causal connection to SEREVENT.

Respiratory: Reports of upper airway symptoms of laryngeal spasm, irritation, or swelling such as stridor or choking.

Cardiovascular: Cases of hypertension, arrhythmias (including atrial fibrillation, supraventricular tachycardia, extrasystoles), and anaphylaxis.

OVERDOSAGE

The expected signs and symptoms with overdosage of SEREVENT DISKUS are those of excessive beta-adrenergic stimulation and/or occurrence or exaggeration of any of the signs and symptoms listed under ADVERSE REACTIONS, e.g., seizures, angina, hypertension or hypotension, tachycardia with rates up to 200 beats/min, arrhythmias, nervousness, headache, tremor, muscle cramps, dry mouth, palpitation, nausea, dizziness, fatigue, malaise, and insomnia. Overdosage with salmeterol may be expected to result in exaggeration of the pharmacologic adverse effects associated with beta-adrenoceptor agonists, including tachycardia and/or arrhythmia, tremor, headache, and muscle cramps. Overdosage with salmeterol can lead to clinically significant prolongation of the QT_c interval, which can produce ventricular arrhythmias. Other signs of overdosage may include hypokalemia and hyperglycemia.

As with all sympathomimetic medications, cardiac arrest and even death may be associated with abuse of SEREVENT DISKUS.

Treatment consists of discontinuation of SEREVENT DISKUS together with appropriate symptomatic therapy. The judicious use of a cardioselective beta-receptor blocker may be considered, bearing in mind that such medication can produce bronchospasm. There is insufficient evidence to determine if dialysis is beneficial for overdosage of SEREVENT DISKUS. Cardiac monitoring is recommended in cases of overdosage.

No deaths were seen in rats at an inhalation dose of 2.9 mg/kg (approximately 250 times the maximum recommended daily inhalation dose in adults and approximately 120 times the maximum recommended daily inhalation dose in children on a mg/m^2 basis) and in dogs at an inhalation dose of 0.7 mg/kg (approximately 200 times the maximum recommended daily inhalation dose in adults and approximately 95 times the maximum recommended daily inhalation dose in children on a mg/m^2 basis). By the oral route, no deaths occurred in mice at 150 mg/kg (approximately 6500 times the maximum recommended daily inhalation dose in adults and approximately 3100 times the maximum recommended daily inhalation dose in children on a mg/m^2 basis) and in rats at 1000 mg/kg (approximately 86,000 times the maximum recommended daily inhalation dose in adults and approximately 41,000 times the maximum recommended daily inhalation dose in children on a mg/m^2 basis).

DOSAGE AND ADMINISTRATION

SEREVENT DISKUS inhalation powder should be administered by the orally inhaled route only (see PATIENT'S INSTRUCTIONS FOR USE). For maintenance of bronchodilatation and prevention of symptoms of asthma, including the symptoms of nocturnal asthma, the usual dosage for adults and children 4 years of age and older is one inhalation (50 mcg) twice daily (morning and evening, approximately 12 hours apart). Adverse effects are more likely to occur with higher doses of salmeterol, and more frequent administration or administration of a larger number of inhalations is not recommended.

To gain full therapeutic benefit, SEREVENT DISKUS should be administered twice daily (morning and evening) in the treatment of reversible airway obstruction. The patient must not exhale into the device and the device should only be activated and used in a level, horizontal position.

If a previously effective dosage regimen fails to provide the usual response, medical advice should be sought immediately as this is often a sign of destabilization of asthma. Under these circumstances, the therapeutic regimen should be reevaluated and additional therapeutic options, such as inhaled or systemic corticosteroids, should be considered. If symptoms arise in the period between doses, an inhaled, short-acting beta$_2$-agonist should be taken for immediate relief.

Geriatric Use: In studies where geriatric patients (65 years of age or older, see PRECAUTIONS) have been treated with SEREVENT inhalation powder, efficacy and safety of 50 mcg given twice daily (morning and evening) did not differ from that in younger patients. Consequently, no dosage adjustment is recommended.

Prevention of Exercise-Induced Bronchospasm (EIB): One inhalation of SEREVENT DISKUS inhalation powder at least 30 minutes before exercise has been shown to protect patients against EIB. When used intermittently as needed for prevention of EIB, this protection may last up to 9 hours in adolescents and adults and up to 12 hours in patients 4 to 11 years of age. Additional doses of SEREVENT should not be used for 12 hours after the administration of this drug. Patients who are receiving SEREVENT DISKUS inhalation powder twice daily should not use additional SEREVENT for prevention of EIB. If regular, twice-daily dosing is not effective in preventing EIB, other appropriate therapy for EIB should be considered.

HOW SUPPLIED

SEREVENT DISKUS inhalation powder is supplied as a disposable, teal green colored device containing 60 blisters. The DISKUS inhalation device is packaged within a teal green colored, plastic-coated foil pouch (NDC 0173-0521-00).

SEREVENT DISKUS is also supplied in an institutional pack of one teal green colored, disposable DISKUS inhalation device containing 28 blisters. The DISKUS inhalation device is packaged within a teal green colored, plastic-coated foil pouch (NDC 0173-0520-00).

Store at controlled room temperature, 20° to 25°C (68° to 77°F) in a dry place away from direct heat or sunlight. Keep out of reach of children. The DISKUS inhalation device is not reusable and should be discarded after every blister has been used (when the dose indicator reads "0") or 6 weeks after removal from the moisture-protective foil overwrap pouch, whichever comes first. Do not attempt to take the device apart.

Glaxo Wellcome Inc., Research Triangle Park, NC 27709
US Patent Nos. 4,992,474; 5,225,445; 5,380,922; 5,590,645; and Des. 342,994

September 1998/RL-628

Shown in Product Identification Guide, page 316

TABLOID® brand Thioguanine ℞

[tab 'loid]

40-mg Scored Tablets

CAUTION: TABLOID brand Thioguanine is a potent drug. It should not be used unless a diagnosis of acute nonlymphocytic leukemia has been adequately established and the responsible physician is knowledgeable in assessing response to chemotherapy.

DESCRIPTION

TABLOID brand Thioguanine was synthesized and developed by Hitchings, Elion, and associates at the Wellcome Research Laboratories. It is one of a large series of purine analogues which interfere with nucleic acid biosynthesis, and has been found active against selected human neoplastic diseases.[1]

Thioguanine, known chemically as 2-amino-1,7-dihydro-6*H*-purine-6-thione, is an analogue of the nucleic acid constituent guanine, and is closely related structurally and functionally to PURINETHOL® (mercaptopurine).

TABLOID brand Thioguanine is available in tablets for oral administration. Each scored tablet contains 40 mg thioguanine and the inactive ingredients gum acacia, lactose, magnesium stearate, potato starch, and stearic acid.

CLINICAL PHARMACOLOGY

Clinical studies have shown that the absorption of an oral dose of thioguanine in humans is incomplete and variable, averaging approximately 30% of the administered dose (range: 14% to 46%).[2,3] Following oral administration of ^{35}S-6-thioguanine, total plasma radioactivity reached a maximum at 8 hours and declined slowly thereafter. Parent drug represented only a very small fraction of the total plasma radioactivity at any time, being virtually undetectable throughout the period of measurements.

The oral administration of radiolabeled thioguanine revealed only trace quantities of parent drug in the urine. However, a methylated metabolite, 2-amino-6-methylthiopurine (MTG), appeared very early, rose to a maximum 6 to 8 hours after drug administration, and was still being excreted after 12 to 22 hours. Radiolabeled sulfate appeared somewhat later than MTG but was the principal metabolite after 8 hours. Thiouric acid and some unidentified products were found in the urine in small amounts.[3] Intravenous administration of ^{35}S-6-thioguanine disclosed a median plasma half-disappearance time of 80 minutes (range: 25 to 240 minutes) when the compound was given in single doses of 65 to 300 mg/m^2. Although initial plasma levels of thioguanine did correlate with the dose level, there was no correlation between the plasma half-disappearance time and the dose.[2]

Thioguanine is incorporated into the DNA and the RNA of human bone marrow cells. Studies with intravenous ^{35}S-6-thioguanine have shown that the amount of thioguanine incorporated into nucleic acids is more than 100 times higher after five daily doses than after a single dose. With the five-dose schedule, from one-half to virtually all of the guanine in the residual DNA was replaced by thioguanine.[2] Tissue distribution studies of ^{35}S-6-thioguanine in mice showed only traces of radioactivity in brain after oral administration. No measurements have been made of thioguanine concentrations in human cerebrospinal fluid (CSF), but observations on tissue distribution in animals, together with the lack of CNS penetration by the closely related compound, mercaptopurine, suggest that thioguanine does not reach therapeutic concentrations in the CSF.

Monitoring of plasma levels of thioguanine during therapy is of questionable value.[3] There is technical difficulty in determining plasma concentrations, which are seldom greater than 1 to 2 mcg/mL after a therapeutic oral dose. More significantly, thioguanine enters rapidly into the anabolic and catabolic pathways for purines, and the active intracellular metabolites have appreciably longer half-lives than the parent drug. The biochemical effects of a single dose of thioguanine are evident long after the parent drug has disappeared from plasma. Because of this rapid metabolism of thioguanine to active intracellular derivatives, hemodialysis would not be expected to appreciably reduce toxicity of the drug.

Thioguanine competes with hypoxanthine and guanine for the enzyme hypoxanthine-guanine phosphoribosyltransferase (HGPRTase) and is itself converted to 6-thioguanylic acid (TGMP). This nucleotide reaches high intracellular concentrations at therapeutic doses. TGMP interferes at several points with the synthesis of guanine nucleotides. It inhibits de novo purine biosynthesis by pseudo-feedback inhibition of glutamine-5-phosphoribosylpyrophosphate amidotransferase—the first enzyme unique to the de novo pathway for purine ribonucleotide synthesis. TGMP also inhibits the conversion of inosinic acid (IMP) to xanthylic acid (XMP) by competition for the enzyme IMP dehydrogenase. At one time TGMP was felt to be a significant inhibitor of ATP:GMP phosphotransferase (guanylate kinase),[4] but recent results have shown this not to be so.[5]

Thioguanylic acid is further converted to the di- and triphosphates, thioguanosine diphosphate (TGDP) and thioguanosine triphosphate (TGTP) (as well as their 2'-deoxyribosyl analogues) by the same enzymes which metabolize guanine nucleotides.[6] Thioguanine nucleotides are incorporated into both the RNA and the DNA by phosphodiester linkages[2] and it has been argued that incorporation of such fraudulent bases contributes to the cytotoxicity of thioguanine.

Thus, thioguanine has multiple metabolic effects and at present it is not possible to designate one major site of action. Its tumor inhibitory properties may be due to one or more of its effects on (a) feedback inhibition of de novo purine synthesis; (b) inhibition of purine nucleotide interconversions; or (c) incorporation into the DNA and the RNA. The net consequence of its actions is a sequential blockade of the synthesis and utilization of the purine nucleotides.[4,6,7]

The catabolism of thioguanine and its metabolites is complex and shows significant differences between humans and the mouse.[2,3] In both humans and mice, after oral adminis-

Continued on next page

This product information is based on labeling in effect on June 23, 2000. For further information, contact via direct mail, phone, or web site. Medical Information, Glaxo Wellcome Inc., PO Box 13398, Research Triangle Park, NC 27709. Healthcare Professionals (Medical Information): 800-334-0089. Patients (Customer Response Center): 1-888-825-5249. Glaxo Wellcome Corporate Web Site: www.glaxowellcome.com.

Thioguanine, Tabloid Brand—Cont.

tration of ^{35}S-6-thioguanine, urine contains virtually no detectable intact thioguanine. While deamination and subsequent oxidation to thiouric acid occurs only to a small extent in humans, it is the main pathway in mice. The product of deamination by guanase, 6-thioxanthine is inactive, having negligible antitumor activity. This pathway of thioguanine inactivation is not dependent on the action of xanthine oxidase, and an inhibitor of that enzyme (such as allopurinol) will not block the detoxification of thioguanine even though the inactive 6-thioxanthine is normally further oxidized by xanthine oxidase to thiouric acid before it is eliminated. In humans, methylation of thioguanine is much more extensive than in the mouse. The product of methylation, 2-amino-6-methylthiopurine, is also substantially less active and less toxic than thioguanine and its formation is likewise unaffected by the presence of allopurinol. Appreciable amounts of inorganic sulfate are also found in both murine and human urine, presumably arising from further metabolism of the methylated derivatives.

In some animal tumors, resistance to the effect of thioguanine correlates with the loss of HGPRTase activity and the resulting inability to convert thioguanine to thioguanylic acid. However, other resistance mechanisms, such as increased catabolism of TGMP by a nonspecific phosphatase, may be operative. Although not invariable, it is usual to find cross-resistance between thioguanine and its close analogue, PURINETHOL (mercaptopurine).

INDICATIONS AND USAGE

a) Acute Nonlymphocytic Leukemias: TABLOID brand Thioguanine is indicated for remission induction, remission consolidation, and maintenance therapy of acute nonlymphocytic leukemias.[8,9] The response to this agent depends upon the age of the patient (younger patients faring better than older) and whether thioguanine is used in previously treated or previously untreated patients. Reliance upon thioguanine alone is seldom justified for initial remission induction of acute nonlymphocytic leukemias because combination chemotherapy including thioguanine results in more frequent remission induction and longer duration of remission than thioguanine alone.

b) Other Neoplasms: TABLOID brand Thioguanine is not effective in chronic lymphocytic leukemia, Hodgkin's lymphoma, multiple myeloma, or solid tumors. Although thioguanine is one of several agents with activity in the treatment of the chronic phase of chronic myelogenous leukemia, more objective responses are observed with MYLERAN® (busulfan), and therefore busulfan is usually regarded as the preferred drug.

CONTRAINDICATIONS

Thioguanine should not be used in patients whose disease has demonstrated prior resistance to this drug. In animals and humans, there is usually complete cross-resistance between PURINETHOL (mercaptopurine) and TABLOID brand Thioguanine.

WARNINGS

SINCE DRUGS USED IN CANCER CHEMOTHERAPY ARE POTENTIALLY HAZARDOUS, IT IS RECOMMENDED THAT ONLY PHYSICIANS EXPERIENCED WITH THE RISKS OF THIOGUANINE AND KNOWLEDGEABLE IN THE NATURAL HISTORY OF ACUTE NONLYMPHOCYTIC LEUKEMIAS ADMINISTER THIS DRUG.

The most consistent, dose-related toxicity is bone marrow suppression. This may be manifested by anemia, leukopenia, thrombocytopenia, or any combination of these. Any one of these findings may also reflect progression of the underlying disease. Since thioguanine may have a delayed effect, it is important to withdraw the medication temporarily at the first sign of an abnormally large fall in any of the formed elements of the blood.

It is recommended that evaluation of the hemoglobin concentration or hematocrit, total white blood cell count and differential count, and quantitative platelet count be obtained frequently while the patient is on thioguanine therapy. In cases where the cause of fluctuations in the formed elements in the peripheral blood is obscure, bone marrow examination may be useful for the evaluation of marrow status. The decision to increase, decrease, continue, or discontinue a given dosage of thioguanine must be based not only on the absolute hematologic values, but also upon the rapidity with which changes are occurring. In many instances, particularly during the induction phase of acute leukemia, complete blood counts will need to be done more frequently in order to evaluate the effect of the therapy. The dosage of thioguanine may need to be reduced when this agent is combined with other drugs whose primary toxicity is myelosuppression.

Myelosuppression is often unavoidable during the induction phase of adult acute nonlymphocytic leukemias if remission induction is to be successful. Whether or not this demands modification or cessation of dosage depends both upon the response of the underlying disease and a careful consideration of supportive facilities (granulocyte and platelet transfusions) which may be available. Life-threatening infections and bleeding have been observed as consequences of thioguanine-induced granulocytopenia and thrombocytopenia.

The effect of thioguanine on the immunocompetence of patients is unknown.

Pregnancy: Pregnancy Category D. Drugs such as thioguanine are potential mutagens and teratogens. Thioguanine may cause fetal harm when administered to a pregnant woman. Thioguanine has been shown to be teratogenic in rats when given in doses five times the human dose. When given to the rat on the 4th and 5th days of gestation, 13% of surviving placentas did not contain fetuses, and 19% of offspring were malformed or stunted. The malformations noted included generalized edema, cranial defects, and general skeletal hypoplasia, hydrocephalus, ventral hernia, situs inversus, and incomplete development of the limbs.[10] There are no adequate and well-controlled studies in pregnant women. If this drug is used during pregnancy, or if the patient becomes pregnant while taking the drug, the patient should be apprised of the potential hazard to the fetus. Women of childbearing potential should be advised to avoid becoming pregnant.

PRECAUTIONS

General: Although the primary toxicity of thioguanine is myelosuppression, other toxicities have occasionally been observed, particularly when thioguanine is used in combination with other cancer chemotherapeutic agents.

A few cases of jaundice have been reported in patients with leukemia receiving thioguanine. Among these were two adult male patients and four pediatric patients with acute myelogenous leukemia and an adult male with acute lymphocytic leukemia who developed veno-occlusive hepatic disease while receiving chemotherapy for their leukemia.[11,12] Six patients had received cytarabine prior to treatment with thioguanine, and some were receiving other chemotherapy in addition to thioguanine when they became symptomatic. While veno-occlusive hepatic disease has not been reported in patients treated with thioguanine alone, it is recommended that thioguanine be withheld if there is evidence of toxic hepatitis or biliary stasis, and that appropriate clinical and laboratory investigations be initiated to establish the etiology of the hepatic dysfunction. Deterioration in liver function studies during thioguanine therapy should prompt discontinuation of treatment and a search for an explanation of the hepatotoxicity.

Information for Patients: Patients should be informed that the major toxicities of thioguanine are related to myelosuppression, hepatotoxicity, and gastrointestinal toxicity. Patients should never be allowed to take the drug without medical supervision and should be advised to consult their physician if they experience fever, sore throat, jaundice, nausea, vomiting, signs of local infection, bleeding from any site, or symptoms suggestive of anemia. Women of childbearing potential should be advised to avoid becoming pregnant.

Laboratory Tests: It is advisable to monitor liver function tests (serum transaminases, alkaline phosphatase, bilirubin) at weekly intervals when first beginning therapy and at monthly intervals thereafter. It may be advisable to perform liver function tests more frequently in patients with known pre-existing liver disease or in patients who are receiving thioguanine and other hepatotoxic drugs. Patients should be instructed to discontinue thioguanine immediately if clinical jaundice is detected (see WARNINGS).

Drug Interactions: There is usually complete cross-resistance between PURINETHOL (mercaptopurine) and TABLOID brand Thioguanine.

In one study, 12 of approximately 330 patients receiving continuous busulfan and thioguanine therapy for treatment of chronic myelogenous leukemia were found to have esophageal varices associated with abnormal liver function tests.[13] Subsequent liver biopsies were performed in four of these patients, all of which showed evidence of nodular regenerative hyperplasia. Duration of combination therapy prior to the appearance of esophageal varices ranged from 6 to 45 months. With the present analysis of the data, no cases of hepatotoxicity have appeared in the busulfan-alone arm of the study. Long-term continuous therapy with thioguanine and busulfan should be used with caution.

Carcinogenesis, Mutagenesis, Impairment of Fertility: In view of its action on cellular DNA, thioguanine is potentially mutagenic and carcinogenic, and consideration should be given to the theoretical risk of carcinogenesis when thioguanine is administered (see WARNINGS).

Pregnancy: ***Teratogenic Effects:*** Pregnancy Category D. See WARNINGS section.

Nursing Mothers: It is not known whether this drug is excreted in human milk. Because of the potential for tumorigenicity shown for thioguanine, a decision should be made whether to discontinue nursing or to discontinue the drug, taking into account the importance of the drug to the mother.

Pediatric Use: See DOSAGE AND ADMINISTRATION section.

ADVERSE REACTIONS

The most frequent adverse reaction to thioguanine is myelosuppression. The induction of complete remission of acute myelogenous leukemia usually requires combination chemotherapy in dosages which produce marrow hypoplasia.[14] Since consolidation and maintenance of remission are also effected by multiple-drug regimens whose component agents cause myelosuppression, pancytopenia is observed in nearly all patients. Dosages and schedules must be adjusted to prevent life-threatening cytopenias whenever these adverse reactions are observed.

Hyperuricemia frequently occurs in patients receiving thioguanine as a consequence of rapid cell lysis accompanying the antineoplastic effect. Adverse effects can be minimized by increased hydration, urine alkalinization, and the prophylactic administration of a xanthine oxidase inhibitor such as ZYLOPRIM® (allopurinol). Unlike PURINETHOL (mercaptopurine) and IMURAN® (azathioprine), thioguanine may be continued in the usual dosage when allopurinol is used conjointly to inhibit uric acid formation.

Less frequent adverse reactions include nausea, vomiting, anorexia, and stomatitis. Intestinal necrosis and perforation have been reported in patients who received multiple-drug chemotherapy including thioguanine.

Hepatic Effects: Liver enzyme and other liver function studies are occasionally abnormal. If jaundice, hepatomegaly, or anorexia with tenderness in the right hypochondrium occurs, thioguanine should be withheld until the exact etiology can be determined. There have been reports of veno-occlusive liver disease occurring in patients who received combination chemotherapy including thioguanine.[11,12] Esophageal varices have been reported in patients receiving continuous busulfan and thioguanine therapy for treatment of chronic myelogenous leukemia (see PRECAUTIONS: Drug Interactions).

OVERDOSAGE

Signs and symptoms of overdosage may be immediate, such as nausea, vomiting, malaise, hypertension, and diaphoresis; or delayed, such as myelosuppression and azotemia.[15] It is not known whether thioguanine is dialyzable. Hemodialysis is thought to be of marginal use due to the rapid intracellular incorporation of thioguanine into active metabolites with long persistence. The oral LD_{50} of thioguanine was determined to be 823 mg/kg ± 50.73 mg/kg and 740 mg/kg ± 45.24 mg/kg for male and female rats, respectively.[16] Symptoms of overdosage may occur after a single dose of as little as 2.0 to 3.0 mg/kg thioguanine. As much as 35 mg/kg has been given in a single oral dose with reversible myelosuppression observed. There is no known pharmacologic antagonist of thioguanine. The drug should be discontinued immediately if unintended toxicity occurs during treatment. Severe hematologic toxicity may require supportive therapy with platelet transfusions for bleeding, and granulocyte transfusions and antibiotics if sepsis is documented. If a patient is seen immediately following an accidental overdosage of the drug, it may be useful to induce emesis.

DOSAGE AND ADMINISTRATION

TABLOID brand Thioguanine is administered orally. The dosage which will be tolerated and effective varies according to the stage and type of neoplastic process being treated. Because the usual therapies for adult and pediatric acute nonlymphocytic leukemias involve the use of thioguanine with other agents in combination, physicians responsible for administering these therapies should be experienced in the use of cancer chemotherapy and in the chosen protocol.

Ninety-six (59%) of 163 pediatric patients with previously untreated acute nonlymphocytic leukemia obtained complete remission with a multiple-drug protocol including thioguanine, prednisone, cytarabine, cyclophosphamide, and vincristine. Remission was maintained with daily thioguanine, 4-day pulses of cytarabine and cyclophosphamide, and a single dose of vincristine every 28 days. The median duration of remission was 11.5 months.[8]

Fifty-three percent of previously untreated adults with acute nonlymphocytic leukemias attained remission following use of the combination of thioguanine and cytarabine according to a protocol developed at The Memorial Sloan-Kettering Cancer Center. A median duration of remission of 8.8 months was achieved with the multiple-drug maintenance regimen which included thioguanine.[9]

On those occasions when single-agent chemotherapy with thioguanine may be appropriate, the usual initial dosage for pediatric patients and adults is approximately 2 mg/kg of body weight per day. If, after 4 weeks on this dosage, there is no clinical improvement and no leukocyte or platelet depression, the dosage may be cautiously increased to 3 mg/kg per day. The total daily dose may be given at one time.

The dosage of thioguanine used does not depend on whether or not the patient is receiving ZYLOPRIM (allopurinol); **this is in contradistinction to the dosage reduction which is mandatory when PURINETHOL (mercaptopurine) or IMURAN (azathioprine) is given simultaneously with allopurinol.**

Procedures for proper handling and disposal of anticancer drugs should be considered. Several guidelines on this subject have been published.[17-23]

There is no general agreement that all of the procedures recommended in the guidelines are necessary or appropriate.

HOW SUPPLIED

Greenish-yellow, scored tablets containing 40 mg thioguanine, imprinted with "WELLCOME" and "U3B" on each tablet; in bottle of 25 (NDC 0173-0880-25).

Store at 15° to 25°C (59° to 77°F) in a dry place.

REFERENCES

1. Hitchings GH, Elion GB. The chemistry and biochemistry of purine analogs. *Ann NY Acad Sci.* 1954;60:195-199.
2. LePage GA, Whitecar JP Jr. Pharmacology of 6-thioguanine in man. *Cancer Res.* 1971;31:1627-1631.
3. Elion GB. Biochemistry and pharmacology of purine analogues. *Fed Proc.* 1967;26:898-904.
4. Miech RP, Parks RE Jr, Anderson JH Jr, Sartorelli AC. An hypothesis on the mechanism of action of 6-thioguanine. *Biochem Pharmacol.* 1967;16:2222-2227.

5. Miller RL, Adamczyk DL, Spector T, Agarwal KC, Miech RP, Panks RE Jr. Reassessment of the interactions of guanylate kinase and 6-thioguanine 5′-phosphate. *Biochem Pharmacol.* 1977;26:1573-1576.
6. Paterson ARP, Tidd DN. 6-Thiopurines. In: Sartorelli AC, Johns DG, eds. *Antineoplastic and Immunosuppressive Agents,* Part II. Berlin: Springer Verlag; 1975:384-403.
7. Nelson JA, Carpenter JW, Rose LM, Adamson DJ. Mechanisms of action of 6-thioguanine, 6-mercaptopurine, and 8-azaguanine. *Cancer Res.* 1975;35:2872-2878.
8. Chard RL Jr, Finklestein JZ, Sonley MJ, et al. Increased survival in childhood acute nonlymphocytic leukemia after treatment with prednisone, cytosine arabinoside, 6-thioguanine, cyclophosphamide, and oncovin (PATCO) combination therapy. *Med Ped Oncol.* 1978;4:263-273.
9. Mertelsmann R, Drapkin RL, Gee TS, et al. Treatment of acute nonlymphocytic leukemia in adults: response to 2,2-anhydro-1-B-D-arabinofuranosyl-5-fluorocytosine and thioguanine on the L-12 protocol. *Cancer.* 1981;48: 2136-2142.
10. Thiersch JB. Effect of 2-6 diaminopurine (2-6DP): 6 chlorpurine (CIP) and thioguanine (ThG) on rat litter *in utero. Proc Soc Exp Biol Med.* 1957;94:40-43.
11. Griner PF, Elbadawi A, Packman CH. Veno-occlusive disease of the liver after chemotherapy of acute leukemia: report of two cases. *Ann Intern Med.* 1976;85:578-582.
12. Gill RA, Onstad GR, Cardamone JM, Maneval DC, Sumner HW. Hepatic veno-occlusive disease caused by 6-thioguanine. *Ann Intern Med.* 1982;96:58-60.
13. Key NS, Kelly PMA, Emerson PM, Chapman RWG, Allan NC, McGee JO'D. Oesophageal varices associated with busulfan-thioguanine combination therapy for chronic myeloid leukaemia. *Lancet.* 1987;2:1050-1052.
14. Clarkson BD, Dowling MD, Gee TS, Cunningham IB, Burchenal JH. Treatment of acute leukemia in adults. *Cancer.* 1975;36:775-795.
15. Presant CA, Denes AE, Klein L, Garrett S, Metter GE. Phase I and preliminary phase II observations of high-dose intermittent 6-thioguanine. *Cancer Treat Rep.* 1980;64:1109-1113.
16. Unpublished data on file with Glaxo Wellcome Inc.
17. Recommendations for the safe handling of parenteral antineoplastic drugs. Washington, DC: Division of Safety, National Institutes of Health; 1983. US Dept of Health and Human Services, Public Health Service publication NIH 83-2621.
18. AMA Council on Scientific Affairs. Guidelines for handling parenteral antineoplastics. *JAMA.* 1985;253: 1590-1591.
19. National Study Commission on Cytotoxic Exposure. Recommendations for handling cytotoxic agents. 1987. Available from Louis P. Jeffrey, Chairman, National Study Commission on Cytotoxic Exposure. Massachusetts College of Pharmacy and Allied Health Sciences, 179 Longwood Avenue, Boston, MA 02115.
20. Clinical Oncological Society of Australia. Guidelines and recommendations for safe handling of antineoplastic agents. *Med J Australia.* 1983;1:426-428.
21. Jones RB, Frank R, Mass T. Safe handling of chemotherapeutic agents: a report from the Mount Sinai Medical Center. *CA-A Cancer J for Clin.* 1983;33:258-263.
22. American Society of Hospital Pharmacists. ASHP technical assistance bulletin on handling cytotoxic and hazardous drugs. *Am J Hosp Pharm.* 1990;47:1033-1049.
23. Yodaiken RE, Bennett D. OSHA work-practice guidelines for personnel dealing with cytotoxic (antineoplastic) drugs. *Am J Hosp Pharm.* 1986;43:1193-1204.

Manufactured by Catalytica Pharmaceuticals, Inc.
Greenville, NC 27834
for Glaxo Wellcome Inc., Research Triangle Park, NC 27709

October 1997/RL-490

Shown in Product Identification Guide, page 316

TEMOVATE® ℞
[*tim 'ō-vāt*]
(clobetasol propionate cream)
Cream, 0.05%

TEMOVATE® ℞
(clobetasol propionate ointment)
Ointment, 0.05%

For Dermatologic Use Only—
Not for Ophthalmic Use.

DESCRIPTION

TEMOVATE (clobetasol propionate cream and ointment) Cream and Ointment contain the active compound clobetasol propionate, a synthetic corticosteroid, for topical dermatologic use. Clobetasol, an analog of prednisolone, has a high degree of glucocorticoid activity and a slight degree of mineralocorticoid activity.

Chemically, clobetasol propionate is (11β,16β)-21-chloro-9-fluoro-11-hydroxy-16-methyl -17- (1-oxopropoxy)-pregna-1,4-diene-3,20-dione.

Clobetasol propionate has the empirical formula $C_{25}H_{32}ClFO_5$ and a molecular weight of 467. It is a white to cream-colored crystalline powder insoluble in water.

TEMOVATE Cream contains clobetasol propionate 0.5 mg/g in a cream base of propylene glycol, glyceryl monostearate, cetostearyl alcohol, glyceryl stearate, PEG 100 stearate, white wax, chlorocresol, sodium citrate, citric acid monohydrate, and purified water.

TEMOVATE Ointment contains clobetasol propionate 0.5 mg/g in a base of propylene glycol, sorbitan sesquioleate, and white petrolatum.

CLINICAL PHARMACOLOGY

Like other topical corticosteroids, clobetasol propionate has anti-inflammatory, antipruritic, and vasoconstrictive properties. The mechanism of the anti-inflammatory activity of the topical steroids, in general, is unclear. However, corticosteroids are thought to act by the induction of phospholipase A_2 inhibitory proteins, collectively called lipocortins. It is postulated that these proteins control the biosynthesis of potent mediators of inflammation such as prostaglandins and leukotrienes by inhibiting the release of their common precursor, arachidonic acid. Arachidonic acid is released from membrane phospholipids by phospholipase A_2.

Pharmacokinetics: The extent of percutaneous absorption of topical corticosteroids is determined by many factors, including the vehicle and the integrity of the epidermal barrier. Occlusive dressing with hydrocortisone for up to 24 hours has not been demonstrated to increase penetration; however, occlusion of hydrocortisone for 96 hours markedly enhances penetration. Topical corticosteroids can be absorbed from normal intact skin. Inflammation and/or other disease processes in the skin may increase percutaneous absorption.

Studies performed with TEMOVATE Cream and Ointment indicate that they are in the super-high range of potency as compared with other topical corticosteroids.

INDICATIONS AND USAGE

TEMOVATE Cream and Ointment are super-high potency corticosteroid formulations indicated for the relief of the inflammatory and pruritic manifestations of corticosteroid-responsive dermatoses. Treatment beyond 2 consecutive weeks is not recommended, and the total dosage should not exceed 50 g/week because of the potential for the drug to suppress the hypothalamic-pituitary-adrenal (HPA) axis. Use in children under 12 years of age is not recommended. As with other highly active corticosteroids, therapy should be discontinued when control has been achieved. If no improvement is seen within 2 weeks, reassessment of the diagnosis may be necessary.

CONTRAINDICATIONS

TEMOVATE Cream and Ointment are contraindicated in those patients with a history of hypersensitivity to any of the components of the preparations.

PRECAUTIONS

General: TEMOVATE Cream and Ointment should not be used in the treatment of rosacea or perioral dermatitis, and should not be used on the face, groin, or axillae.

Systemic absorption of topical corticosteroids can produce reversible HPA axis suppression with the potential for glucocorticosteroid insufficiency after withdrawal from treatment. Manifestations of Cushing's syndrome, hyperglycemia, and glucosuria can also be produced in some patients by systemic absorption of topical corticosteroids while on therapy.

Patients applying a topical steroid to a large surface area or to areas under occlusion should be evaluated periodically for evidence of HPA axis suppression. This may be done by using the ACTH stimulation, A.M. plasma cortisol, and urinary free cortisol tests. Patients receiving super-potent corticosteroids should not be treated for more than 2 weeks at a time, and only small areas should be treated at any one time due to the increased risk of HPA suppression.

TEMOVATE Cream and Ointment produced HPA axis suppression when used at doses as low as 2 g/day for 1 week in patients with eczema.

If HPA axis suppression is noted, an attempt should be made to withdraw the drug, to reduce the frequency of application, or to substitute a less potent corticosteroid. Recovery of HPA axis function is generally prompt upon discontinuation of topical corticosteroids. Infrequently, signs and symptoms of glucocorticosteroid insufficiency may occur, requiring supplemental systemic corticosteroids. For information on systemic supplementation, see prescribing information for those products.

Pediatric patients may be more susceptible to systemic toxicity from equivalent doses due to their larger skin surface to body mass ratios (see PRECAUTIONS: Pediatric Use).

If irritation develops, TEMOVATE Cream and Ointment should be discontinued and appropriate therapy instituted. Allergic contact dermatitis with corticosteroids is usually diagnosed by observing *failure to heal* rather than noting a clinical exacerbation as with most topical products not containing corticosteroids. Such an observation should be corroborated with appropriate diagnostic patch testing.

If concomitant skin infections are present or develop, an appropriate antifungal or antibacterial agent should be used. If a favorable response does not occur promptly, use of TEMOVATE Cream and Ointment should be discontinued until the infection has been adequately controlled.

Information for Patients: Patients using topical corticosteroids should receive the following information and instructions:

1. This medication is to be used as directed by the physician. It is for external use only. Avoid contact with the eyes.
2. This medication should not be used for any disorder other than that for which it was prescribed.
3. The treated skin area should not be bandaged, otherwise covered, or wrapped so as to be occlusive unless directed by the physician.
4. Patients should report any signs of local adverse reactions to the physician.

Laboratory Tests: The following tests may be helpful in evaluating patients for HPA axis suppression:
ACTH stimulation test
A.M. plasma cortisol test
Urinary free cortisol test

Carcinogenesis, Mutagenesis, Impairment of Fertility: Long-term animal studies have not been performed to evaluate the carcinogenic potential of clobetasol propionate.

Studies in the rat following oral administration at dosage levels up to 50 mg/kg per day revealed that the females exhibited an increase in the number of resorbed embryos and a decrease in the number of living fetuses at the highest dose.

Clobetasol propionate was nonmutagenic in three different test systems: the Ames test, the *Saccharomyces cerevisiae* gene conversion assay, and the *E. coli* B WP2 fluctuation test.

Pregnancy: ***Teratogenic Effects:*** Pregnancy Category C. Corticosteroids have been shown to be teratogenic in laboratory animals when administered systemically at relatively low dosage levels. Some corticosteroids have been shown to be teratogenic after dermal application to laboratory animals.

Clobetasol propionate has not been tested for teratogenicity when applied topically; however, it is absorbed percutaneously, and when administered subcutaneously it was a significant teratogen in both the rabbit and mouse. Clobetasol propionate has greater teratogenic potential than steroids that are less potent.

Teratogenicity studies in mice using the subcutaneous route resulted in fetotoxicity at the highest dose tested (1 mg/kg) and teratogenicity at all dose levels tested down to 0.03 mg/kg. These doses are approximately 0.33 and 0.01 times, respectively, the human topical dose of TEMOVATE Cream and Ointment. Abnormalities seen included cleft palate and skeletal abnormalities.

In rabbits, clobetasol propionate was teratogenic at doses of 3 and 10 mcg/kg. These doses are approximately 0.001 and 0.003 times, respectively, the human topical dose of TEMOVATE Cream and Ointment. Abnormalities seen included cleft palate, cranioschisis, and other skeletal abnormalities.

There are no adequate and well-controlled studies of the teratogenic potential of clobetasol propionate in pregnant women. TEMOVATE Cream and Ointment should be used during pregnancy only if the potential benefit justifies the potential risk to the fetus.

Nursing Mothers: Systemically administered corticosteroids appear in human milk and could suppress growth, interfere with endogenous corticosteroid production, or cause other untoward effects. It is not known whether topical administration of corticosteroids could result in sufficient systemic absorption to produce detectable quantities in human milk. Because many drugs are excreted in human milk, caution should be exercised when TEMOVATE Cream or Ointment is administered to a nursing woman.

Pediatric Use: Safety and effectiveness of TEMOVATE in pediatric patients have not been established. Use in children under 12 years of age is not recommended. Because of a higher ratio of skin surface area to body mass, pediatric patients are at a greater risk than adults of HPA axis suppression and Cushing's syndrome when they are treated with topical corticosteroids. They are therefore also at greater risk of adrenal insufficiency during or after withdrawal of treatment. Adverse effects including striae have been reported with inappropriate use of topical corticosteroids in infants and children.

HPA axis suppression, Cushing's syndrome, linear growth retardation, delayed weight gain, and intracranial hypertension have been reported in children receiving topical corticosteroids. Manifestations of adrenal suppression in children include low plasma cortisol levels and an absence of response to ACTH stimulation. Manifestations of intracranial hypertension include bulging fontanelles, headaches, and bilateral papilledema.

ADVERSE REACTIONS

In controlled clinical trials, the most frequent adverse reactions reported for TEMOVATE Cream were burning and stinging sensation in 1% of treated patients. Less frequent adverse reactions were itching, skin atrophy, and cracking and fissuring of the skin.

In controlled clinical trials, the most frequent adverse events reported for TEMOVATE Ointment were burning sensation, irritation, and itching in 0.5% of treated patients. Less frequent adverse reactions were stinging, cracking, erythema, folliculitis, numbness of fingers, skin atrophy, and telangiectasia.

Continued on next page

This product information is based on labeling in effect on June 23, 2000. For further information, contact via direct mail, phone, or web site. Medical Information, Glaxo Wellcome Inc., PO Box 13398, Research Triangle Park, NC 27709. Healthcare Professionals (Medical Information): 800-334-0089. Patients (Customer Response Center): 1-888-825-5249. Glaxo Wellcome Corporate Web Site: www.glaxowellcome.com

Temovate Cream/Ointment—Cont.

Cushing's syndrome has been reported in infants and adults as a result of prolonged use of topical clobetasol propionate formulations.
The following additional local adverse reactions have been reported with topical corticosteroids, and they may occur more frequently with the use of occlusive dressings and higher potency corticosteroids. These reactions are listed in an approximately decreasing order of occurrence: dryness, acneiform eruptions, hypopigmentation, perioral dermatitis, allergic contact dermatitis, secondary infection, irritation, striae, and miliaria.

OVERDOSAGE

Topically applied TEMOVATE Cream and Ointment can be absorbed in sufficient amounts to produce systemic effects (see PRECAUTIONS).

DOSAGE AND ADMINISTRATION

Apply a thin layer of TEMOVATE Cream or Ointment to the affected skin areas twice daily and rub in gently and completely.
TEMOVATE Cream and Ointment are super-high potency topical corticosteroids; therefore, **treatment should be limited to 2 consecutive weeks, and amounts greater than 50 g/week should not be used.**
As with other highly active corticosteroids, therapy should be discontinued when control has been achieved. If no improvement is seen within 2 weeks, reassessment of diagnosis may be necessary.
TEMOVATE Cream and Ointment should not be used with occlusive dressings.

HOW SUPPLIED

TEMOVATE Cream, 0.05% is supplied in 15-g (NDC 0173-0375-73), 30-g (NDC 0173-0375-72), 45-g (NDC 0173-0375-01), and 60-g (NDC 0173-0375-02) tubes.
TEMOVATE Ointment, 0.05% is supplied in 15-g (NDC 0173-0376-73), 30-g (NDC 0173-0376-72), 45-g (NDC 0173-0376-01), and 60-g (NDC 0173-0376-02) tubes.
Store between 15° and 30°C (59° and 86°F). TEMOVATE Cream should not be refrigerated.
Glaxo Wellcome Inc., Research Triangle Park, NC 27709
March 1999/RL-705

Shown in Product Identification Guide, page 316

TEMOVATE® ℞

[tim 'ō-vāt]
(clobetasol propionate gel)
Gel, 0.05%

FOR TOPICAL DERMATOLOGIC USE ONLY—NOT FOR OPHTHALMIC, ORAL, OR INTRAVAGINAL USE

DESCRIPTION

TEMOVATE Gel contains the active compound clobetasol propionate, a synthetic corticosteroid, for topical dermatologic use. Clobetasol, an analog of prednisolone, has a high degree of glucocorticoid activity and a slight degree of mineralocorticoid activity.
Chemically, clobetasol propionate is (11β,16β)-21-chloro-9-fluoro-11-hydroxy-16-methyl-17- (1-oxopropoxy)-pregna-1,4-diene-3,20-dione.
Clobetasol propionate has the empirical formula $C_{25}H_{32}ClFO_5$ and a molecular weight of 467. It is a white to cream-colored crystalline powder insoluble in water.
TEMOVATE Gel contains clobetasol propionate 0.5 mg/g in a base of propylene glycol, carbomer 934P, sodium hydroxide, and purified water.

CLINICAL PHARMACOLOGY

Like other topical corticosteroids, clobetasol propionate has anti-inflammatory, antipruritic, and vasoconstrictive properties. The mechanism of the anti-inflammatory activity of the topical steroids, in general, is unclear. However, corticosteroids are thought to act by the induction of phospholipase A_2 inhibitory proteins, collectively called lipocortins. It is postulated that these proteins control the biosynthesis of potent mediators of inflammation such as prostaglandins and leukotrienes by inhibiting the release of their common precursor, arachidonic acid. Arachidonic acid is released from membrane phospholipids by phospholipase A_2.
Pharmacokinetics: The extent of percutaneous absorption of topical corticosteroids is determined by many factors, including the vehicle and the integrity of the epidermal barrier. Occlusive dressing with hydrocortisone for up to 24 hours has not been demonstrated to increase penetration; however, occlusion of hydrocortisone for 96 hours markedly enhances penetration. Topical corticosteroids can be absorbed from normal intact skin, while inflammation and/or other disease processes in the skin may increase percutaneous absorption. Greater absorption was observed for the TEMOVATE gel formulation as compared to the cream formulation in in vitro human skin penetration studies.
Studies performed with TEMOVATE Gel indicate that it is in the super-high range of potency as compared with other topical corticosteroids.

INDICATIONS AND USAGE

TEMOVATE Gel is a super-high potency corticosteroid formulation indicated for the relief of the inflammatory and pruritic manifestations of corticosteroid-responsive dermatoses. Treatment beyond 2 consecutive weeks is not recommended, and the total dosage should not exceed 50 g/week because of the potential for the drug to suppress the hypothalamic-pituitary- adrenal (HPA) axis. Use in children under 12 years of age is not recommended.

CONTRAINDICATIONS

TEMOVATE Gel is contraindicated in those patients with a history of hypersensitivity to any of the components of the preparation.

PRECAUTIONS

General: Clobetasol propionate is a highly potent topical corticosteroid that has been shown to suppress the HPA axis at doses as low as 2 g/day.
Systemic absorption of topical corticosteroids can produce reversible HPA axis suppression with the potential for glucocorticosteroid insufficiency after withdrawal from treatment. Manifestations of Cushing's syndrome, hyperglycemia, and glucosuria can also be produced in some patients by systemic absorption of topical corticosteroids while on therapy.
Patients receiving a large dose applied to a large surface area should be evaluated periodically for evidence of HPA axis suppression. This may be done by using the ACTH stimulation, A.M. plasma cortisol, and urinary free cortisol tests. Patients receiving super-potent corticosteroids should not be treated for more than 2 weeks at a time, and only small areas should be treated at any one time due to the increased risk of HPA suppression.
If HPA axis suppression is noted, an attempt should be made to withdraw the drug, to reduce the frequency of application, or to substitute a less potent corticosteroid. Recovery of HPA axis function is generally prompt and complete upon discontinuation of topical corticosteroids. Infrequently, signs and symptoms of glucocorticosteroid insufficiency may occur that require supplemental systemic corticosteroids. For information on systemic supplementation, see prescribing information for those products.
Children may be more susceptible to systemic toxicity from equivalent doses due to their larger skin surface to body mass ratios (see PRECAUTIONS: Pediatric Use).
If irritation develops, TEMOVATE Gel should be discontinued and appropriate therapy instituted. Allergic contact dermatitis with corticosteroids is usually diagnosed by observing *failure to heal* rather than noting a clinical exacerbation as with most topical products not containing corticosteroids. Such an observation should be corroborated with appropriate diagnostic patch testing.
If concomitant skin infections are present or develop, an appropriate antifungal or antibacterial agent should be used. If a favorable response does not occur promptly, use of TEMOVATE Gel should be discontinued until the infection has been adequately controlled.
TEMOVATE Gel should not be used in the treatment of rosacea or perioral dermatitis, and should not be used on the face, groin, or axillae.
Information for Patients: Patients using topical corticosteroids should receive the following information and instructions:
1. This medication is to be used as directed by the physician. It is for external use only. Avoid contact with the eyes.
2. This medication should not be used for any disorder other than that for which it was prescribed.
3. The treated skin area should not be bandaged or otherwise covered or wrapped so as to be occlusive unless directed by the physician.
4. Patients should report any signs of local adverse reactions to the physician.
5. Patients should inform their physicians that they are using TEMOVATE if surgery is contemplated.

Laboratory Tests: The following tests may be helpful in evaluating patients for HPA axis suppression:
ACTH stimulation test
A.M. plasma cortisol test
Urinary free cortisol test
Carcinogenesis, Mutagenesis, Impairment of Fertility: Long-term animal studies have not been performed to evaluate the carcinogenic potential of clobetasol propionate.
Studies in the rat following oral administration at dosage levels up to 50 mg/kg per day revealed no significant effect on the males. The females exhibited an increase in the number of resorbed embryos and a decrease in the number of living fetuses at the highest dose.
Clobetasol propionate was nonmutagenic in 3 different test systems: the Ames test, the *Saccharomyces cerevisiae* gene conversion assay, and the *E. coli* B WP2 fluctuation test.
Pregnancy: *Teratogenic Effects:* Pregnancy Category C. Corticosteroids have been shown to be teratogenic in laboratory animals when administered systemically at relatively low dosage levels. Some corticosteroids have been shown to be teratogenic after dermal application to laboratory animals.
Clobetasol propionate has not been tested for teratogenicity by this route; however, it is absorbed percutaneously, and when administered subcutaneously it was a significant teratogen in both the rabbit and mouse. Clobetasol propionate has greater teratogenic potential than steroids that are less potent.
Teratogenicity studies in mice using the subcutaneous route resulted in fetotoxicity at the highest dose tested (1 mg/kg) and teratogenicity at all dose levels tested down to 0.03 mg/kg. These doses are approximately 0.33 and 0.01 times, respectively, the human topical dose of TEMOVATE Gel. Abnormalities seen included cleft palate and skeletal abnormalities.
In rabbits, clobetasol propionate given by the same route was teratogenic at doses of 3 and 10 mcg/kg. These doses are approximately 0.001 and 0.003 times, respectively, the human topical dose of TEMOVATE Gel. Abnormalities seen included cleft palate, cranioschisis, and other skeletal abnormalities.
There are no adequate and well-controlled studies of the teratogenic potential of clobetasol propionate in pregnant women. TEMOVATE Gel should be used during pregnancy only if the potential benefit justifies the potential risk to the fetus.
Nursing Mothers: Systemically administered corticosteroids appear in human milk and could suppress growth, interfere with endogenous corticosteroid production, or cause other untoward effects. It is not known whether topical administration of corticosteroids could result in sufficient systemic absorption to produce detectable quantities in human milk. Because many drugs are excreted in human milk, caution should be exercised when TEMOVATE Gel is administered to a nursing woman.
Pediatric Use: Safety and effectiveness of TEMOVATE Gel in children and infants have not been established; therefore, use in children under 12 years of age is not recommended. Because of a higher ratio of skin surface area to body mass, children are at a greater risk than adults of HPA axis suppression when they are treated with topical corticosteroids. They are therefore also at greater risk of glucocorticosteroid insufficiency after withdrawal of treatment and of Cushing's syndrome while on treatment. Adverse effects including striae have been reported with inappropriate use of topical corticosteroids in infants and children (see PRECAUTIONS).
HPA axis suppression, Cushing's syndrome, and intracranial hypertension have been reported in children receiving topical corticosteroids. Manifestations of adrenal suppression in children include linear growth retardation, delayed weight gain, low plasma cortisol levels, and absence of response to ACTH stimulation. Manifestations of intracranial hypertension include bulging fontanelles, headaches, and bilateral papilledema.

ADVERSE REACTIONS

In a controlled trial with TEMOVATE Gel, the only reported adverse reaction that was considered to be drug related was a report of burning sensation (1.8% of treated patients).
In larger controlled clinical trials with other clobetasol propionate formulations, the most frequently reported adverse reactions have included burning, stinging, irritation, pruritus, erythema, folliculitis, cracking and fissuring of the skin, numbness of fingers, skin atrophy, and telangiectasia (all less than 2%).
Cushing's syndrome has been reported in infants and adults as a result of prolonged use of topical clobetasol propionate formulations.
The following additional local adverse reactions are reported infrequently with topical corticosteroids, but may occur more frequently with super-high potency corticosteroids such as TEMOVATE Gel. These reactions are listed in approximate decreasing order of occurrence: dryness, hypertrichosis, acneiform eruptions, hypopigmentation, perioral dermatitis, allergic contact dermatitis, secondary infection, irritation, striae, and miliaria.

OVERDOSAGE

Topically applied TEMOVATE Gel can be absorbed in sufficient amounts to produce systemic effects (see PRECAUTIONS).

DOSAGE AND ADMINISTRATION

Apply a thin layer of TEMOVATE Gel to the affected skin areas twice daily and rub in gently and completely (see INDICATIONS AND USAGE).
TEMOVATE Gel is a super-high potency topical corticosteroid; therefore, **treatment should be limited to 2 consecutive weeks, and amounts greater than 50 g/week should not be used.**
As with other highly active corticosteroids, therapy should be discontinued when control has been achieved. If no improvement is seen within 2 weeks, reassessment of diagnosis may be necessary.
TEMOVATE Gel should not be used with occlusive dressings.

HOW SUPPLIED

TEMOVATE Gel, 0.05% is supplied in 15-g (NDC 0173-0455-01), 30-g (NDC 0173-0455-02), and 60-g (NDC 0173-0455-03) tubes.
Store between 2° and 30°C (36° and 86°F).
Glaxo Wellcome Inc., Research Triangle Park, NC 27709
March 1999/RL-704

Shown in Product Identification Guide, page 316

TEMOVATE® ℞

[tim 'ō-vāt]
(clobetasol propionate scalp application)
Scalp Application, 0.05%

For Dermatologic Use Only—
Not for Ophthalmic Use.

DESCRIPTION

TEMOVATE Scalp Application contains the active compound clobetasol propionate, a synthetic corticosteroid, for topical dermatologic use. Clobetasol, an analog of prednisolone, has a high degree of glucocorticoid activity and a slight degree of mineralocorticoid activity.

Chemically, clobetasol propionate is (11β,16β)-21-chloro-9-fluoro-11-hydroxy-16-methyl-17-(1-oxopropoxy)pregna-1,4-diene-3,20-dione.

Clobetasol propionate has the empirical formula $C_{25}H_{32}ClFO_5$ and a molecular weight of 467. It is a white to cream-colored crystalline powder insoluble in water.

TEMOVATE Scalp Application contains clobetasol propionate 0.5 mg/g in a base composed of purified water, isopropyl alcohol (39.3%), carbomer 934P, and sodium hydroxide.

CLINICAL PHARMACOLOGY

The corticosteroids are a class of compounds comprising steroid hormones secreted by the adrenal cortex and their synthetic analogs. In pharmacologic doses, corticosteroids are used primarily for their anti-inflammatory and/or immunosuppressive effects. Topical corticosteroids such as clobetasol propionate are effective in the treatment of corticosteroid-responsive dermatoses primarily because of their anti-inflammatory, antipruritic, and vasoconstrictive actions. However, while the physiologic, pharmacologic, and clinical effects of the corticosteroids are well known, the exact mechanisms of their actions in each disease are uncertain. Clobetasol propionate, a corticosteroid, has been shown to have topical (dermatologic) and systemic pharmacologic and metabolic effects characteristic of this class of drugs.

Pharmacokinetics: The extent of percutaneous absorption of topical corticosteroids, including clobetasol propionate, is determined by many factors, including the vehicle, the integrity of the epidermal barrier, and the use of occlusive dressings (see DOSAGE AND ADMINISTRATION).

As with all topical corticosteroids, clobetasol propionate can be absorbed from normal intact skin. Inflammation and/or other disease processes in the skin may increase percutaneous absorption. Occlusive dressings substantially increase the percutaneous absorption of topical corticosteroids (see DOSAGE AND ADMINISTRATION).

Once absorbed through the skin, topical corticosteroids enter pharmacokinetic pathways similarly to systemically administered corticosteroids. Corticosteroids are bound to plasma proteins in varying degrees. Corticosteroids are metabolized primarily in the liver and are then excreted by the kidneys. Some of the topical corticosteroids, including clobetasol propionate and its metabolites, are also excreted into the bile.

Following repeated nonocclusive application in the treatment of scalp psoriasis, there is some evidence that TEMOVATE Scalp Application has the potential to depress plasma cortisol levels in some patients. However, hypothalamic-pituitary-adrenal (HPA) axis effects produced by systemically absorbed clobetasol propionate have been shown to be transient and reversible upon completion of a 2-week course of treatment.

INDICATIONS AND USAGE

TEMOVATE Scalp Application is indicated for short-term topical treatment of inflammatory and pruritic manifestations of moderate to severe corticosteroid-responsive dermatoses of the scalp. Treatment beyond 2 consecutive weeks is not recommended, and the total dosage should not exceed 50 mL/week because of the potential for the drug to suppress the HPA axis.

This product is not recommended for use in children under 12 years of age.

CONTRAINDICATIONS

TEMOVATE Scalp Application is contraindicated in patients with primary infections of the scalp, or in patients who are hypersensitive to clobetasol propionate, other corticosteroids, or any ingredient in this preparation.

PRECAUTIONS

General: Clobetasol propionate is a highly potent topical corticosteroid that has been shown to suppress the HPA axis at doses as low as 2 g (of ointment) per day. Systemic absorption of topical corticosteroids has resulted in reversible HPA axis suppression, manifestations of Cushing's syndrome, hyperglycemia, and glucosuria in some patients.

Conditions that augment systemic absorption include the application of the more potent corticosteroids, use over large surface areas, prolonged use, and the addition of occlusive dressings. Therefore, patients receiving a large dose of a potent topical steroid applied to a large surface area should be evaluated periodically for evidence of HPA axis suppression by using the urinary free cortisol and ACTH stimulation tests. If HPA axis suppression is noted, an attempt should be made to withdraw the drug, to reduce the frequency of application, or to substitute a less potent steroid.

Recovery of HPA axis function is generally prompt and complete upon discontinuation of the drug. Infrequently, signs and symptoms of steroid withdrawal may occur, requiring supplemental systemic corticosteroids.

Children may absorb proportionally larger amounts of topical corticosteroids and thus be more susceptible to systemic toxicity (see PRECAUTIONS: Pediatric Use).

If irritation develops, topical corticosteroids should be discontinued and appropriate therapy instituted. Irritation is possible if TEMOVATE Scalp Application contacts the eye. If that should occur, immediate flushing of the eye with a large volume of water is recommended.

If the inflammatory lesion becomes infected, the use of an appropriate antifungal or antibacterial agent should be instituted. If a favorable response does not occur promptly, the corticosteroid should be discontinued until the infection has been adequately controlled.

Although TEMOVATE Scalp Application is intended for the treatment of inflammatory conditions of the scalp, it should be noted that certain areas of the body, such as the face, groin, and axillae, are more prone to atrophic changes than other areas of the body following treatment with corticosteroids. Frequent observation of the patient is important if these areas are to be treated.

As with other potent topical corticosteroids, TEMOVATE Scalp Application should not be used in the treatment of rosacea and perioral dermatitis. Topical corticosteroids in general should not be used in the treatment of acne or as sole therapy in widespread plaque psoriasis.

Information For Patients: Patients using TEMOVATE Scalp Application should receive the following information and instructions:

1. This medication is to be used as directed by the physician and should not be used longer than the prescribed time period. It is for external use only. Avoid contact with the eyes.
2. This medication should not be used for any disorder other than that for which it was prescribed.
3. The treated skin area should not be bandaged or otherwise covered or wrapped so as to be occlusive.
4. Patients should report any signs of local adverse reactions to the physician.

Laboratory Tests: The following tests may be helpful in evaluating HPA axis suppression:

Urinary free cortisol test

ACTH stimulation test

Carcinogenesis, Mutagenesis, Impairment of Fertility: Long-term animal studies have not been performed to evaluate the carcinogenic potential or the effect on fertility of topical corticosteroids.

Studies to determine mutagenicity with prednisolone have revealed negative results.

Pregnancy: ***Teratogenic Effects: Pregnancy Category C:*** The more potent corticosteroids have been shown to be teratogenic in animals after dermal application. Clobetasol propionate has not been tested for teratogenicity by this route; however, it is absorbed percutaneously, and when administered subcutaneously it was a significant teratogen in both the rabbit and the mouse. Clobetasol propionate has greater teratogenic potential than steroids that are less potent.

There are no adequate and well-controlled studies of the teratogenic effects of topically applied corticosteroids, including clobetasol, in pregnant women. Therefore, clobetasol and other topical corticosteroids should be used during pregnancy only if the potential benefit justifies the potential risk to the fetus, and they should not be used extensively on pregnant patients, in large amounts, or for prolonged periods of time.

Nursing Mothers: It is not known whether topical administration of corticosteroids could result in sufficient systemic absorption to produce detectable quantities in breast milk. Systemically administered corticosteroids are secreted into breast milk in quantities not likely to have a deleterious effect on the infant. Nevertheless, caution should be exercised when topical corticosteroids are prescribed for a nursing woman.

Pediatric Use: Use of TEMOVATE Scalp Application in children under 12 years of age is not recommended.

Pediatric patients may demonstrate greater susceptibility to topical corticosteroid-induced HPA axis suppression and Cushing's syndrome than mature patients because of a larger skin surface area to body weight ratio.

HPA axis suppression, Cushing's syndrome, and intracranial hypertension have been reported in children receiving topical corticosteroids. Manifestations of adrenal suppression in children include linear growth retardation, delayed weight gain, low plasma cortisol levels, and absence of response to ACTH stimulation. Manifestations of intracranial hypertension include bulging fontanelles, headaches, and bilateral papilledema.

ADVERSE REACTIONS

TEMOVATE Scalp Application is generally well tolerated when used for 2-week treatment periods.

The most frequent adverse events reported for TEMOVATE Scalp Application have been local and have included burning and/or stinging sensation, which occurred in 29 of 294 patients; scalp pustules, which occurred in 3 of 294 patients; and tingling and folliculitis, each of which occurred in 2 of 294 patients. Less frequent adverse events were itching and tightness of the scalp, dermatitis, tenderness, headache, hair loss, and eye irritation, each of which occurred in 1 of 294 patients.

The following local adverse reactions are reported infrequently when topical corticosteroids are used as recommended. These reactions are listed in an approximately decreasing order of occurrence: burning, itching, irritation, dryness, folliculitis, hypertrichosis, acneiform eruptions, hypopigmentation, perioral dermatitis, allergic contact dermatitis, maceration of the skin, secondary infection, skin atrophy, striae, and miliaria. Systemic absorption of topical corticosteroids has produced reversible HPA axis suppression, manifestations of Cushing's syndrome, hyperglycemia, and glucosuria in some patients. In rare instances, treatment (or withdrawal of treatment) of psoriasis with corticosteroids is thought to have exacerbated the disease or provoked the pustular form of the disease, so careful patient supervision is recommended.

OVERDOSAGE

Topically applied TEMOVATE Scalp Application can be absorbed in sufficient amounts to produce systemic effects (see PRECAUTIONS).

DOSAGE AND ADMINISTRATION

TEMOVATE Scalp Application should be applied to the affected scalp areas twice daily, once in the morning and once at night.

TEMOVATE Scalp Application is potent; therefore, **treatment must be limited to 2 consecutive weeks, and amounts greater than 50 mL/week should not be used. TEMOVATE Scalp Application is not to be used with occlusive dressings.**

HOW SUPPLIED

TEMOVATE Scalp Application, 0.05% is supplied in plastic squeeze bottles, 25 mL (NDC 0173-0432-00) and 50 mL (NDC 0173-0432-01).

Store between 4° and 25°C (39° and 77°F). Do not use near an open flame.

Glaxo Wellcome Inc., Research Triangle Park, NC 27709

March 1999/RL-702

Shown in Product Identification Guide, page 316

TEMOVATE E® ℞

[*tim 'ō-vāt"*]

(clobetasol propionate emollient cream)

Emollient, 0.05%

FOR TOPICAL DERMATOLOGIC USE ONLY—NOT FOR OPHTHALMIC, ORAL, OR INTRAVAGINAL USE

DESCRIPTION

TEMOVATE E Emollient contains the active compound clobetasol propionate, a synthetic corticosteroid, for topical dermatologic use. Clobetasol, an analog of prednisolone, has a high degree of glucocorticoid activity and a slight degree of mineralocorticoid activity.

Chemically, clobetasol propionate is (11β,16β)-21-chloro-9-fluoro-11-hydroxy-16-methyl-17-(1-oxopropoxy)-pregna-1,4-diene-3,20-dione.

Clobetasol propionate has the empirical formula $C_{25}H_{32}ClFO_5$ and a molecular weight of 467. It is a white to cream-colored crystalline powder insoluble in water.

TEMOVATE E Emollient contains clobetasol propionate 0.5 mg/g in an emollient base of cetostearyl alcohol, isopropyl myristate, propylene glycol, cetomacrogol 1000, dimethicone 360, citric acid, sodium citrate, purified water, and imidurea as a preservative.

CLINICAL PHARMACOLOGY

Like other topical corticosteroids, clobetasol propionate has anti-inflammatory, antipruritic, and vasoconstrictive properties. The mechanism of the anti-inflammatory activity of the topical steroids, in general, is unclear. However, corticosteroids are thought to act by the induction of phospholipase A_2 inhibitory proteins, collectively called lipocortins. It is postulated that these proteins control the biosynthesis of potent mediators of inflammation such as prostaglandins and leukotrienes by inhibiting the release of their common precursor, arachidonic acid. Arachidonic acid is released from membrane phospholipids by phospholipase A_2.

Pharmacokinetics: The extent of percutaneous absorption of topical corticosteroids is determined by many factors, including the vehicle and the integrity of the epidermal barrier. Occlusive dressing with hydrocortisone for up to 24 hours has not been demonstrated to increase penetration; however, occlusion of hydrocortisone for 96 hours markedly enhances penetration. Topical corticosteroids can be absorbed from normal intact skin. Inflammation and/or other disease processes in the skin may increase percutaneous absorption.

Studies performed with TEMOVATE E Emollient indicate that it is in the super-high range of potency as compared with other topical corticosteroids.

INDICATIONS AND USAGE

TEMOVATE E Emollient is a super-high potency corticosteroid formulation indicated for the relief of the inflammatory and pruritic manifestations of corticosteroid-responsive dermatoses. Treatment beyond 2 consecutive weeks is not recommended, and the total dosage should not exceed 50 g/week because of the potential for the drug to suppress the hypothalamic-pituitary-adrenal (HPA) axis. Use in children under 12 years of age is not recommended.

In the treatment of moderate to severe plaque-type psoriasis, TEMOVATE E Emollient applied to 5% to 10% of body

Continued on next page

This product information is based on labeling in effect on June 23, 2000. For further information, contact via direct mail, phone, or web site. Medical Information, Glaxo Wellcome Inc., PO Box 13398, Research Triangle Park, NC 27709. Healthcare Professionals (Medical Information): 800-334-0089. Patients (Customer Response Center): 1-888-825-5249. Glaxo Wellcome Corporate Web Site: www.glaxowellcome.com

Temovate E—Cont.

surface area can be used up to 4 consecutive weeks. The total dosage should not exceed 50 g/week. When dosing for more than 2 weeks, any additional benefits of extending treatment should be weighed against the risk of HPA suppression. Treatment beyond 4 consecutive weeks is not recommended. Patients should be instructed to use TEMOVATE E Emollient for the minimum amount of time necessary to achieve the desired results (see PRECAUTIONS and INDICATIONS AND USAGE). Use in pediatric patients under 16 years of age has not been studied.

CONTRAINDICATIONS

TEMOVATE E Emollient is contraindicated in those patients with a history of hypersensitivity to any of the components of the preparation.

PRECAUTIONS

General: Clobetasol propionate is a highly potent topical corticosteroid that has been shown to suppress the HPA axis at doses as low as 2 g/day.

Systemic absorption of topical corticosteroids can produce reversible HPA axis suppression with the potential for glucocorticosteroid insufficiency after withdrawal from treatment. Manifestations of Cushing's syndrome, hyperglycemia, and glucosuria can also be produced in some patients by systemic absorption of topical corticosteroids while on therapy.

Patients applying a dose to a large surface area or to areas under occlusion should be evaluated periodically for evidence of HPA axis suppression. This may be done by using the ACTH stimulation, A.M. plasma cortisol, and urinary free cortisol tests. Patients receiving super-potent corticosteroids should not be treated for more than 2 weeks at a time, and only small areas should be treated at any one time due to the increased risk of HPA suppression.

In a controlled clinical trial involving patients with moderate to severe plaque-type psoriasis, TEMOVATE E Emollient applied to 5% to 10% of body surface area resulted in additional benefits in the treatment of patients for 4 consecutive weeks. In this trial, there were no clobetasol-treated patients with clinically significant decreases in morning cortisol levels after 4 weeks of treatment; however, morning cortisol levels may not identify patients with adrenal dysfunction. Therefore, the additional benefits of extending treatment beyond 2 weeks should be weighed against the potential for HPA suppression. Therapy should be discontinued when control has been achieved. Treatment beyond 4 consecutive weeks is not recommended.

If HPA axis suppression is noted, an attempt should be made to withdraw the drug, to reduce the frequency of application, or to substitute a less potent corticosteroid. Recovery of HPA axis function is generally prompt upon discontinuation of topical corticosteroids. Infrequently, signs and symptoms of glucocorticosteroid insufficiency may occur that require supplemental systemic corticosteroids. For information on systemic supplementation, see prescribing information for those products.

Pediatric patients may be more susceptible to systemic toxicity from equivalent doses due to their larger skin surface to body mass ratios (see PRECAUTIONS: Pediatric Use). The use of TEMOVATE E Emollient for 4 consecutive weeks has not been studied in pediatric patients under 16 years of age.

If irritation develops, TEMOVATE E Emollient should be discontinued and appropriate therapy instituted. Allergic contact dermatitis with corticosteroids is usually diagnosed by observing a *failure to heal* rather than noting a clinical exacerbation as with most topical products not containing corticosteroids. Such an observation should be corroborated with appropriate diagnostic patch testing.

If concomitant skin infections are present or develop, an appropriate antifungal or antibacterial agent should be used. If a favorable response does not occur promptly, use of TEMOVATE E Emollient should be discontinued until the infection has been adequately controlled.

TEMOVATE E Emollient should not be used in the treatment of rosacea or perioral dermatitis, and should not be used on the face, groin, or axillae.

Information for Patients: Patients using topical corticosteroids should receive the following information and instructions:

1. This medication is to be used as directed by the physician. It is for external use only. Avoid contact with the eyes.
2. This medication should not be used for any disorder other than that for which it was prescribed.
3. The treated skin area should not be bandaged, otherwise covered, or wrapped so as to be occlusive unless directed by the physician.
4. Patients should report any signs of local adverse reactions to the physician.
5. Patients should inform their physicians that they are using TEMOVATE if surgery is contemplated.
6. This medication should not be used on the face, underarms, or groin areas.
7. As with other corticosteroids, therapy should be discontinued when control has been achieved. If no improvement is seen within 2 weeks, contact the physician.

Laboratory Tests: The following tests may be helpful in evaluating patients for HPA axis suppression:
ACTH stimulation test
A.M. plasma cortisol test
Urinary free cortisol test

Carcinogenesis, Mutagenesis, Impairment of Fertility: Long-term animal studies have not been performed to evaluate the carcinogenic potential of clobetasol propionate.

Studies in the rat following oral administration at dosage levels up to 50 mg/kg per day revealed no significant effect on the males. The females exhibited an increase in the number of resorbed embryos and a decrease in the number of living fetuses at the highest dose.

Clobetasol propionate was nonmutagenic in three different test systems: the Ames test, the *Saccharomyces cerevisiae* gene conversion assay, and the *E. coli* B WP2 fluctuation test.

Pregnancy: *Teratogenic Effects:* Pregnancy Category C. Corticosteroids have been shown to be teratogenic in laboratory animals when administered systemically at relatively low dosage levels. Some corticosteroids have been shown to be teratogenic after dermal application to laboratory animals.

Clobetasol propionate has not been tested for teratogenicity by this route; however, it is absorbed percutaneously, and when administered subcutaneously it was a significant teratogen in both the rabbit and mouse. Clobetasol propionate has greater teratogenic potential than steroids that are less potent.

Teratogenicity studies in mice using the subcutaneous route resulted in fetotoxicity at the highest dose tested (1 mg/kg) and teratogenicity at all dose levels tested down to 0.03 mg/kg. These doses are approximately 0.33 and 0.01 times, respectively, the human topical dose of TEMOVATE E Emollient. Abnormalities seen included cleft palate and skeletal abnormalities.

In rabbits, clobetasol propionate was teratogenic at doses of 3 and 10 mcg/kg. These doses are approximately 0.001 and 0.003 times, respectively, the human topical dose of TEMOVATE E Emollient. Abnormalities seen included cleft palate, cranioschisis, and other skeletal abnormalities.

There are no adequate and well-controlled studies of the teratogenic potential of clobetasol propionate in pregnant women. TEMOVATE E Emollient should be used during pregnancy only if the potential benefit justifies the potential risk to the fetus.

Nursing Mothers: Systemically administered corticosteroids appear in human milk and could suppress growth, interfere with endogenous corticosteroid production, or cause other untoward effects. It is not known whether topical administration of corticosteroids could result in sufficient systemic absorption to produce detectable quantities in human milk. Because many drugs are excreted in human milk, caution should be exercised when TEMOVATE E Emollient is administered to a nursing woman.

Pediatric Use: Safety and effectiveness of TEMOVATE E Emollient in pediatric patients have not been established, and its use in pediatric patients under 12 years of age is not recommended. For continued use beyond 2 consecutive weeks, the safety of TEMOVATE E Emollient has not been studied. Because of a higher ratio of skin surface area to body mass, pediatric patients are at a greater risk than adults of HPA axis suppression and Cushing's syndrome when they are treated with topical corticosteroids. They are therefore also at greater risk of glucocorticosteroid insufficiency during or after withdrawal of treatment. Adverse effects including striae have been reported with inappropriate use of topical corticosteroids in infants and children.

HPA axis suppression, Cushing's syndrome, linear growth retardation, delayed weight gain, and intracranial hypertension have been reported in children receiving topical corticosteroids. Manifestations of adrenal suppression in children include low plasma cortisol levels and absence of response to ACTH stimulation. Manifestations of intracranial hypertension include bulging fontanelles, headaches, and bilateral papilledema.

ADVERSE REACTIONS

In controlled trials with all clobetasol propionate formulations, the following adverse reactions have been reported: burning/stinging, pruritus, irritation, erythema, folliculitis, cracking and fissuring of the skin, numbness of the fingers, tenderness in the elbow, skin atrophy, and telangiectasia. The incidence of local adverse reactions reported in the trials with TEMOVATE E Emollient was <2% of patients treated with the exception of burning/stinging, which occured in 5% of treated patients.

Cushing's syndrome has been reported in infants and adults as a result of prolonged use of other topical clobetasol propionate formulations.

The following additional local adverse reactions are reported infrequently with topical corticosteroids, but may occur more frequently with super-high potency corticosteroids such as TEMOVATE E Emollient. These reactions are listed in an approximately decreasing order of occurrence: dryness, hypertrichosis, acneiform eruptions, hypopigmentation, perioral dermatitis, allergic contact dermatitis, secondary infection, striae, and miliaria.

OVERDOSAGE

Topically applied TEMOVATE E Emollient can be absorbed in sufficient amounts to produce systemic effects.

DOSAGE AND ADMINISTRATION

Apply a thin layer of TEMOVATE E Emollient to the affected skin areas twice daily and rub in gently and completely (see INDICATIONS AND USAGE).

TEMOVATE E Emollient is a super-high potency topical corticosteroid; therefore, **treatment should be limited to 2 consecutive weeks and amounts greater than 50 g/week should not be used.** Use in children under 12 years of age is not recommended.

In moderate to severe plaque-type psoriasis, TEMOVATE E Emollient applied to 5% to 10% of body surface area can be used up to 4 weeks. The total dosage should not exceed 50 g/week. When dosing for more than 2 weeks, any additional benefits of extending treatment should be weighed against the risk of HPA suppression. Therapy should be discontinued when control has been achieved. If no improvement is seen within 2 weeks, reassessment of diagnosis may be necessary. Treatment beyond 4 consecutive weeks is not recommended. Use in pediatric patients under 16 years of age has not been studied.

TEMOVATE E Emollient should not be used with occlusive dressings.

HOW SUPPLIED

TEMOVATE E Emollient, 0.05% is supplied in 15-g (NDC 0173-0454-01), 30-g (NDC 0173-0454-02), and 60-g (NDC 0173-0454-03) tubes.

Store between 15° and 30°C (59° and 86°F). TEMOVATE E Emollient should not be refrigerated.

Glaxo Wellcome Inc., Research Triangle Park, NC 27709
March 1999/RL-703

Shown in Product Identification Guide, page 316

VALTREX® ℞

[*val'trĕx*]
(valacyclovir hydrochloride)
Caplets

DESCRIPTION

VALTREX (valacyclovir hydrochloride) is the hydrochloride salt of L-valyl ester of the antiviral drug acyclovir (ZOVIRAX® Brand, Glaxo Wellcome Inc.).

VALTREX Caplets are for oral administration. Each caplet contains valacyclovir hydrochloride equivalent to 500 mg or 1 gram valacyclovir and the inactive ingredients carnauba wax, colloidal silicon dioxide, crospovidone, FD&C Blue No. 2 Lake, hydroxypropyl methylcellulose, magnesium stearate, microcrystalline cellulose, polyethylene glycol, polysorbate 80, povidone, and titanium dioxide. The blue, film-coated caplets are printed with edible white ink.

The chemical name of valacyclovir hydrochloride is L-valine, 2-[(2-amino-1,6-dihydro-6-oxo-9*H*-purin-9-yl)methoxy]ethyl ester, monohydrochloride.

Valacyclovir hydrochloride is a white to off-white powder with the molecular formula $C_{13}H_{20}N_6O_4 \bullet HCl$ and a molecular weight of 360.80. The maximum solubility in water at 25°C is 174 mg/mL. The pk_a's for valacyclovir hydrochloride are 1.90, 7.47, and 9.43.

MICROBIOLOGY

Mechanism of Antiviral Action: Valacyclovir hydrochloride is rapidly converted to acyclovir which has demonstrated antiviral activity against herpes simplex virus types 1 (HSV-1) and 2 (HSV-2) and varicella-zoster virus (VZV) both in vitro and in vivo. In cell culture, acyclovir's highest antiviral activity is against HSV-1, followed in decreasing order of potency against HSV-2 and VZV.

The inhibitory activity of acyclovir is highly selective due to its affinity for the enzyme thymidine kinase (TK) encoded by HSV, VZV, and EBV. This viral enzyme converts acyclovir into acyclovir monophosphate, a nucleotide analogue. The monophosphate is further converted into diphosphate by cellular guanylate kinase and into triphosphate by a number of cellular enzymes. In vitro, acyclovir triphosphate stops replication of herpes viral DNA. This is accomplished in 3 ways: 1) competitive inhibition of viral DNA polymerase, 2) incorporation and termination of the growing viral DNA chain, and 3) inactivation of the viral DNA polymerase. The greater antiviral activity of acyclovir against HSV compared to VZV is due to its more efficient phosphorylation by the viral TK.

Antiviral Activities: The quantitative relationship between the in vitro susceptibility of herpesviruses to antivirals and the clinical response to therapy has not been established in humans, and virus sensitivity testing has not been standardized. Sensitivity testing results, expressed as the concentration of drug required to inhibit by 50% the growth of virus in cell culture (IC_{50}), vary greatly depending upon a number of factors. Using plaque-reduction assays, the IC_{50} against herpes simplex virus isolates ranges from 0.02 to 13.5 mcg/mL for HSV-1 and from 0.01 to 9.9 mcg/mL for HSV-2. The IC_{50} for acyclovir against most laboratory strains and clinical isolates of VZV ranges from 0.12 to 10.8 mcg/mL. Acyclovir also demonstrates activity against the Oka vaccine strain of VZV with a mean IC_{50} of 1.35 mcg/mL.

Drug Resistance: Resistance of VZV to antiviral nucleoside analogues can result from qualitative or quantitative changes in the viral TK or DNA polymerase. Clinical isolates of VZV with reduced susceptibility to acyclovir have been recovered from patients with AIDS. In these cases, TK-deficient mutants of VZV have been recovered.

Resistance of HSV to antiviral nucleoside analogues occurs by the same mechanisms as resistance to VZV. While most of the acyclovir-resistant mutants isolated thus far from immunocompromised patients have been found to be TK-deficient mutants, other mutants involving the viral TK gene (TK partial and TK altered) and DNA polymerase have also been isolated. TK-negative mutants may cause severe disease in immunocompromised patients. The possibility of viral resistance to valacyclovir (and therefore, to acyclovir) should be considered in patients who show poor clinical response during therapy.

CLINICAL PHARMACOLOGY

After oral administration, valacyclovir hydrochloride is rapidly absorbed from the gastrointestinal tract and nearly completely converted to acyclovir and L-valine by first-pass intestinal and/or hepatic metabolism.

Pharmacokinetics: The pharmacokinetics of valacyclovir and acyclovir after oral administration of VALTREX have been investigated in 14 volunteer studies involving 283 adults.

Absorption and Bioavailability: The absolute bioavailability of acyclovir after administration of VALTREX is 54.5% ± 9.1% as determined following a 1-gram oral dose of VALTREX and a 350-mg intravenous acyclovir dose to 12 healthy volunteers. Acyclovir bioavailability from the administration of VALTREX is not altered by administration with food (30 minutes after an 873 Kcal breakfast, which included 51 grams of fat).

There was a lack of dose proportionality in acyclovir maximum concentration (C_{max}) and area under the acyclovir concentration-time curve (AUC) after single-dose administration of 100 mg, 250 mg, 500 mg, 750 mg, and 1 gram of VALTREX to 8 healthy volunteers. The mean C_{max} (±SD) was 0.83 (± 0.14), 2.15 (± 0.50), 3.28 (± 0.83), 4.17 (± 1.14), and 5.65 (± 2.37) mcg/mL, respectively; and the mean AUC (± SD) was 2.28 (± 0.40), 5.76 (± 0.60), 11.59 (± 1.79), 14.11 (± 3.54), and 19.52 (± 6.04) hr•mcg/mL, respectively.

There was also a lack of dose proportionality in acyclovir C_{max} and AUC after the multiple-dose administration of 250 mg, 500 mg, and 1 gram of VALTREX administered 4 times daily for 11 days in parallel groups of 8 healthy volunteers. The mean C_{max} (± SD) was 2.11 (± 0.33), 3.69 (± 0.87), and 4.96 (± 0.64) mcg/mL, respectively, and the mean AUC (± SD) was 5.66 (± 1.09), 9.88 (± 2.01), and 15.70 (± 2.27) hr•mcg/mL, respectively.

There is no accumulation of acyclovir after the administration of valacyclovir at the recommended dosage regimens in healthy volunteers with normal renal function.

Distribution: The binding of valacyclovir to human plasma proteins ranged from 13.5% to 17.9%.

Metabolism: After oral administration, valacyclovir hydrochloride is rapidly absorbed from the gastrointestinal tract. Valacyclovir is converted to acyclovir and L-valine by first-pass intestinal and/or hepatic metabolism. Acyclovir is converted to a small extent to inactive metabolites by aldehyde oxidase and by alcohol and aldehyde dehydrogenase. Neither valacyclovir nor acyclovir metabolism is associated with liver microsomal enzymes. Plasma concentrations of unconverted valacyclovir are low and transient, generally becoming non-quantifiable by 3 hours after administration. Peak plasma valacyclovir concentrations are generally less than 0.5 mcg/mL at all doses. After single-dose administration of 1 gram of VALTREX, average plasma valacyclovir concentrations observed were 0.5, 0.4, and 0.8 mcg/mL in patients with hepatic dysfunction, renal insufficiency, and in healthy volunteers who received concomitant cimetidine and probenecid, respectively.

Elimination: The pharmacokinetic disposition of acyclovir delivered by valacyclovir is consistent with previous experience from intravenous and oral acyclovir. Following the oral administration of a single 1-gram dose of radiolabeled valacyclovir to 4 healthy subjects, 45.60% and 47.12% of administered radioactivity was recovered in urine and feces over 96 hours, respectively. Acyclovir accounted for 88.60% of the radioactivity excreted in the urine. Renal clearance of acyclovir following the administration of a single 1-gram dose of VALTREX to 12 healthy volunteers was approximately 255 ± 86 mL/min which represents 41.9% of total acyclovir apparent plasma clearance.

The plasma elimination half-life of acyclovir typically averaged 2.5 to 3.3 hours in all studies of VALTREX in volunteers with normal renal function.

End-Stage Renal Disease (ESRD): Following administration of VALTREX to volunteers with ESRD, the average acyclovir half-life is approximately 14 hours. During hemodialysis, the acyclovir half-life is approximately 4 hours. Approximately one-third of acyclovir in the body is removed by dialysis during a 4-hour hemodialysis session. Apparent plasma clearance of acyclovir in dialysis patients was 86.3 ± 21.3 mL/min/1.73 m^2, compared to 679.16 ± 162.76 mL/min/1.73 m^2 in healthy volunteers.

Reduction in dosage is recommended in patients with renal impairment (see DOSAGE AND ADMINISTRATION).

Geriatrics: After single-dose administration of 1 gram of VALTREX in healthy geriatric volunteers (n = 9, mean age ± SD = 74.0 ± 5.4 years), the half-life of acyclovir was 3.11 ± 0.51 hours, compared to 2.91 ± 0.63 hours in healthy volunteers (n = 33, mean age ± SD = 41.2 ± 10.1 years). Dosage modification may be necessary in geriatric patients with reduced renal function (see DOSAGE AND ADMINISTRATION).

Pediatrics: Valacyclovir pharmacokinetics have not been evaluated in pediatric patients.

Liver Disease: Administration of VALTREX to patients with moderate (biopsy-proven cirrhosis) or severe (with and without ascites and biopsy-proven cirrhosis) liver disease indicated that the rate but not the extent of conversion of valacyclovir to acyclovir is reduced, and the acyclovir half-life is not affected. Dosage modification is not recommended for patients with cirrhosis.

Table 1: Proportions of Patients Recurrence-free at 6 and 12 Months

	6 Months			12 Months		
Treatment Arm	VALTREX 1 gram q.d. (n = 269)	ZOVIRAX 400 mg b.i.d. (n = 267)	Placebo (n = 134)	VALTREX 1 gram q.d. (n = 269)	ZOVIRAX 400 mg b.i.d. (n = 267)	Placebo (n = 134)
Recurrence-free (%)	55	54	7	34	34	4
Recurrences (%)	35	36	83	46	46	85
Unknowns (%)	10	10	10	19	19	10

Table 2: Incidence (%) of Adverse Events in Herpes Zoster and Genital Herpes Study Populations

	Herpes Zoster		Genital Herpes Treatment			Genital Herpes Suppression		
Adverse Event	VALTREX 1 gram t.i.d. (n = 967)	Placebo (n = 195)	VALTREX 1 gram b.i.d. (n = 1194)	VALTREX 500 mg b.i.d. (n = 359)	Placebo (n = 439)	VALTREX 1 gram q.d. (n = 269)	VALTREX 500 mg q.d. (n = 266)	Placebo (n = 134)
Nausea	15	8	6	6	8	11	11	8
Headache	14	12	16	17	14	35	38	34
Vomiting	6	3	1	1	<1	3	3	2
Dizziness	3	2	3	2	3	4	2	1
Abdominal Pain	3	2	2	3	3	11	9	6
Dysmenorrhea	0	0	<1	1	1	8	5	4
Arthralgia	1	0	<1	1	<1	6	5	4
Depression	1	1	1	0	<1	7	5	5

HIV Disease: In 9 patients with advanced HIV disease (CD4 cell counts <150 cells/mm^3) who received VALTREX at a dosage of 1 gram 4 times daily for 30 days, the pharmacokinetics of valacyclovir and acyclovir were not different from that observed in healthy volunteers (see WARNINGS).

Drug Interactions: The pharmacokinetics of digoxin was not affected by coadministration of VALTREX 1 gram 3 times daily, and the pharmacokinetics of acyclovir after a single dose of VALTREX (1 gram) was unchanged by coadministration of digoxin (2 doses of 0.75 mg), single doses of antacids (Al^{3+} or Mg^{++}), or multiple doses of thiazide diuretics. Acyclovir C_{max} and AUC following a single dose of VALTREX (1 gram) increased by 8% and 32%, respectively, after a single dose of cimetidine (800 mg), or by 22% and 49%, respectively, after probenecid (1 gram), or by 30% and 78%, respectively, after a combination of cimetidine and probenecid, primarily due to a reduction in renal clearance of acyclovir. These effects are not considered to be of clinical significance in subjects with normal renal function. Therefore, no dosage adjustment is recommended when VALTREX is coadministered with digoxin, antacids, thiazide diuretics, cimetidine, or probenecid in subjects with normal renal function.

Clinical Trials: *Herpes Zoster Infections:* Two randomized double-blind clinical trials in immunocompetent adults with localized herpes zoster were conducted. VALTREX was compared to placebo in patients less than 50 years of age, and to ZOVIRAX in patients greater than 50 years of age. All patients were treated within 72 hours of appearance of zoster rash. In patients less than 50 years of age, the median time to cessation of new lesion formation was 2 days for those treated with VALTREX compared to 3 days for those treated with placebo. In patients greater than 50 years of age, the median time to cessation of new lesions was 3 days in patients treated with either VALTREX or ZOVIRAX. In patients less than 50 years of age, no difference was found with respect to the duration of pain after rash healing (post-herpetic neuralgia) between the recipients of VALTREX and placebo. In patients greater than 50 years of age, among the 83% who reported pain after healing (post-herpetic neuralgia), the median duration of pain after healing [95% confidence interval] in days was: 40 [31, 51], 43 [36, 55], and 59 [41, 77] for 7-day VALTREX, 14-day VALTREX, and 7-day ZOVIRAX, respectively.

Genital Herpes Infections: Initial Episode: Six hundred and forty-three immunocompetent adults with first episode genital herpes who presented within 72 hours of symptom onset were randomized in a double-blind trial to receive 10 days of VALTREX 1 gram b.i.d. (n = 323) or ZOVIRAX 200 mg 5 times a day (n = 320). For both treatment groups: the median time to lesion healing was 9 days, the median time to cessation of pain was 5 days, the median time to cessation of viral shedding was 3 days.

Recurrent Episodes: Two double-blind placebo-controlled trials in immunocompetent adults with recurrent genital herpes were conducted. Patients self-initiated therapy within 24 hours of the first sign or symptom of a recurrent genital herpes episode.

In 1 study, patients were randomized to receive 5 days of treatment with either VALTREX 500 mg b.i.d. (n = 360) or placebo (n = 259). The median time to lesion healing was 4 days in the group receiving VALTREX 500 mg versus 6 days in the placebo group, and the median time to cessation of viral shedding in patients with at least 1 positive culture (42% of the overall study population) was 2 days in the group receiving VALTREX 500 mg versus 4 days in the placebo group. The median time to cessation of pain was 3 days in the group receiving VALTREX 500 mg versus 4 days in the placebo group. Results supporting efficacy were replicated in a second trial.

Suppressive Therapy: One thousand four hundred seventy-nine (1479) immunocompetent adults with a history of 6 or more recurrences per year were randomized into a double-blind, placebo-controlled study. Outcomes for the overall study population are shown in Table 1.

[See table 1 above]

Subjects with 9 or fewer recurrences per year showed comparable results with VALTREX 500 mg once daily.

INDICATIONS AND USAGE

Herpes Zoster: VALTREX is indicated for the treatment of herpes zoster (shingles).

Genital Herpes: VALTREX is indicated for the treatment or suppression of genital herpes.

CONTRAINDICATIONS

VALTREX is contraindicated in patients with a known hypersensitivity or intolerance to valacyclovir, acyclovir, or any component of the formulation.

WARNINGS

Thrombotic thrombocytopenic purpura/hemolytic uremic syndrome (TTP/HUS), in some cases resulting in death, has occurred in patients with advanced HIV disease and also in allogeneic bone marrow transplant and renal transplant recipients participating in clinical trials of VALTREX at doses of 8 grams per day.

PRECAUTIONS

Dosage reduction is recommended when administering VALTREX to patients with renal impairment (see DOSAGE AND ADMINISTRATION). Acute renal failure and central nervous system symptoms have been reported in patients with underlying renal disease who have received inappropriately high doses of VALTREX for their level of renal function. Similar caution should be exercised when administering VALTREX to geriatric patients (see Geriatric Use) and patients receiving potentially nephrotoxic agents.

Precipitation of acyclovir in renal tubules may occur when the solubility (2.5 mg/mL) is exceeded in the intratubular fluid. In the event of acute renal failure and anuria, the patient may benefit from hemodialysis until renal function is restored (see DOSAGE AND ADMINISTRATION).

The efficacy of VALTREX has not been established for the treatment of disseminated herpes zoster or in immunocompromised patients.

Information for Patients: *Herpes Zoster:* There are no data on treatment initiated more than 72 hours after onset of the zoster rash. Patients should be advised to initiate treatment as soon as possible after a diagnosis of herpes zoster.

Genital Herpes: Patients should be informed that VALTREX is not a cure for genital herpes. There are no data evaluating whether VALTREX will prevent transmission of infection to others. Because genital herpes is a sexually transmitted disease, patients should avoid contact with lesions or intercourse when lesions and/or symptoms are present to avoid infecting partners. Genital herpes can also be transmitted in the absence of symptoms through asymptomatic viral shedding. If medical management of a genital herpes recurrence is indicated, patients should be advised to initiate therapy at the first sign or symptom of an episode.

There are no data on the effectiveness of treatment initiated more than 72 hours after the onset of signs and symptoms of a first episode of genital herpes or more than 24 hours of the onset of signs and symptoms of a recurrent episode.

Continued on next page

This product information is based on labeling in effect on June 23, 2000. For further information, contact via direct mail, phone, or web site. Medical Information, Glaxo Wellcome Inc., PO Box 13398, Research Triangle Park, NC 27709. Healthcare Professionals (Medical Information): 800-334-0089. Patients (Customer Response Center): 1-888-825-5249. Glaxo Wellcome Corporate Web Site: www.glaxowellcome.com

Valtrex—Cont.

There are no data on the safety or effectiveness of chronic suppressive therapy of more than 1 year's duration.
Drug Interactions: See CLINICAL PHARMACOLOGY: Pharmacokinetics.
Carcinogenesis, Mutagenesis, Impairment of Fertility: The data presented below include references to the steady-state acyclovir AUC observed in humans treated with 1 gram VALTREX given orally 3 times a day to treat herpes zoster. Plasma drug concentrations in animal studies are expressed as multiples of human exposure to acyclovir (see CLINICAL PHARMACOLOGY: Pharmacokinetics).
Valacyclovir was noncarcinogenic in lifetime carcinogenicity bioassays at single daily doses (gavage) of up to 120 mg/kg per day for mice and 100 mg/kg per day for rats. There was no significant difference in the incidence of tumors between treated and control animals, nor did valacyclovir shorten the latency of tumors. Plasma concentrations of acyclovir were equivalent to human levels in the mouse bioassay and 1.4 to 2.3 times human levels in the rat bioassay.
Valacyclovir was tested in 5 genetic toxicity assays. An Ames assay was negative in the absence or presence of metabolic activation. Also negative were an in vitro cytogenetic study with human lymphocytes and a rat cytogenetic study at a single oral dose of 3000 mg/kg (8 to 9 times human plasma levels).
In the mouse lymphoma assay, valacyclovir was negative in the absence of metabolic activation. In the presence of metabolic activation (76% to 88% conversion to acyclovir), valacyclovir was weakly mutagenic.
A mouse micronucleus assay was negative at 250 mg/kg but weakly positive at 500 mg/kg (acyclovir concentrations 26 to 51 times human plasma levels).
Valacyclovir did not impair fertility or reproduction in rats at 200 mg/kg per day (6 times human plasma levels).
Pregnancy: *Teratogenic Effects:* Pregnancy Category B. Valacyclovir was not teratogenic in rats or rabbits given 400 mg/kg (which results in exposures of 10 and 7 times human plasma levels, respectively) during the period of major organogenesis.
There are no adequate and well-controlled studies of VALTREX or ZOVIRAX in pregnant women. A prospective epidemiologic registry of acyclovir use during pregnancy was established in 1984 and completed in April 1999. There were 756 pregnancies followed in women exposed to systemic acyclovir during the first trimester of pregnancy. The occurrence rate of birth defects approximates that found in the general population. However, the small size of the registry is insufficient to evaluate the risk for less common defects or to permit reliable or definitive conclusions regarding the safety of acyclovir in pregnant women and their developing fetuses. VALTREX should be used during pregnancy only if the potential benefit justifies the potential risk to the fetus.
Nursing Mothers: There is no experience with VALTREX. However, acyclovir concentrations have been documented in breast milk in 2 women following oral administration of ZOVIRAX and ranged from 0.6 to 4.1 times corresponding plasma levels. These concentrations would potentially expose the nursing infant to a dose of acyclovir as high as 0.3 mg/kg per day. VALTREX should be administered to a nursing mother with caution and only when indicated.
Pediatric Use: Safety and effectiveness of VALTREX in pediatric patients have not been established.
Geriatric Use: Of the total number of patients included in clinical studies of VALTREX, 861 were age 65 or older, and 344 were age 75 or older. A total of 34 volunteers age 65 or older completed a pharmacokinetic trial of VALTREX. The pharmacokinetics of acyclovir following single- and multiple-dose oral administration of VALTREX in geriatric volunteers varied with renal function. Dosage reduction may be required in geriatric patients, depending on the underlying renal status of the patient (see CLINICAL PHARMACOLOGY and DOSAGE AND ADMINISTRATION).

ADVERSE REACTIONS

Frequently reported adverse events in clinical trials of VALTREX are listed in Table 2.
[See table 2 on previous page]
Laboratory abnormalities reported in clinical trials of VALTREX are listed in Table 3.
[See table 3 above]
Observed During Clinical Practice: The following events have been identified during post-approval use of VALTREX in clinical practice. Because they are reported voluntarily from a population of unknown size, estimates of frequency cannot be made. These events have been chosen for inclusion due to either their seriousness, frequency of reporting, causal connection to VALTREX, or a combination of these factors.
General: Facial edema, hypertension, tachycardia.
Allergic: Acute hypersensitivity reactions including anaphylaxis, angioedema, dyspnea, pruritus, rash, and urticaria.
CNS Symptoms: Confusion, agitation, hallucinations (auditory and visual), aggressive behavior, mania.
Gastrointestinal: Diarrhea.
Hepatobiliary Tract and Pancreas: Liver enzyme abnormalities, hepatitis.
Renal: Elevated creatinine, renal failure.
Hemic: Thrombocytopenia, aplastic anemia.

Table 3: Incidence (%) of Laboratory Abnormalities in Herpes Zoster and Genital Herpes Study Populations

Laboratory Abnormality	Herpes Zoster: VALTREX 1 gram t.i.d.	Herpes Zoster: Placebo	Genital Herpes Treatment: VALTREX 1 gram b.i.d.	Genital Herpes Treatment: VALTREX 500 mg b.i.d.	Genital Herpes Treatment: Placebo	Genital Herpes Suppression: VALTREX 1 gram q.d.	Genital Herpes Suppression: VALTREX 500 mg q.d.	Genital Herpes Suppression: Placebo
Anemia	0.8	0	0.3	0.3	0	0	0.8	0.8
Leukopenia	1.3	0.6	0.7	0.8	0.2	0.7	0.8	1.5
Thrombocytopenia	1.0	1.2	0.3	0.6	0.7	0.4	1.1	1.5
AST (SGOT)	1.0	0	1.0	*	0.5	4.1	3.8	3.0
Serum Creatinine	0.2	0	0.7	0	0	0	0	0

* Data were not collected prospectively in this study.

Table 4: Dosages for Patients with Renal Impairment

Indications	Normal Dosage Regimen (Creatinine Clearance ≥50)	Creatinine Clearance (mL/min): 30–49	10–29	<10
Herpes zoster	1 gram every 8 hours	1 gram every 12 hours	1 gram every 24 hours	500 mg every 24 hours
Genital herpes				
Initial treatment	1 gram every 12 hours	no reduction	1 gram every 24 hours	500 mg every 24 hours
Recurrent episodes	500 mg every 12 hours	no reduction	500 mg every 24 hours	500 mg every 24 hours
Suppressive therapy	1 gram every 24 hours	no reduction	500 mg every 24 hours	500 mg every 24 hours
Suppressive therapy	500 mg every 24 hours	no reduction	500 mg every 48 hours	500 mg every 48 hours

Skin: Erythema multiforme, rashes including photosensitivity.
Renal Impairment: Renal failure and CNS symptoms have been reported in patients with renal impairment who received VALTREX or acyclovir at greater than the recommended dose. **Dosage adjustment is recommended in this patient population (see DOSAGE AND ADMINISTRATION).**

OVERDOSAGE

Caution should be exercised to prevent inadvertent overdose (see PRECAUTIONS). Precipitation of acyclovir in renal tubules may occur when the solubility (2.5 mg/mL) is exceeded in the intratubular fluid. In the event of acute renal failure and anuria, the patient may benefit from hemodialysis until renal function is restored (see DOSAGE AND ADMINISTRATION).

DOSAGE AND ADMINISTRATION

VALTREX Caplets may be given without regard to meals.
Herpes Zoster: The recommended dosage of VALTREX for the treatment of herpes zoster is 1 gram orally 3 times daily for 7 days. Therapy should be initiated at the earliest sign or symptom of herpes zoster and is most effective when started within 48 hours of the onset of zoster rash. No data are available on efficacy of treatment started greater than 72 hours after rash onset.
Genital Herpes: *Initial Episodes:* The recommended dosage of VALTREX for treatment of initial genital herpes is 1 gram twice daily for 10 days.
There are no data on the effectiveness of treatment with VALTREX when initiated more than 72 hours after the onset of signs and symptoms. Therapy was most effective when administered within 48 hours of the onset of signs and symptoms.
Recurrent Episodes: The recommended dosage of VALTREX for the treatment of recurrent genital herpes is 500 mg twice daily for 5 days. If medical management of a genital herpes recurrence is indicated, patients should be advised to initiate therapy at the first sign or symptom of an episode. There are no data on the effectiveness of treatment with VALTREX when initiated more than 24 hours after the onset of signs or symptoms.
Suppressive Therapy: The recommended dosage of VALTREX for chronic suppressive therapy of recurrent genital herpes is 1 gram once daily. In patients with a history of 9 or fewer recurrences per year, an alternative dose is 500 mg once daily. The safety and efficacy of therapy with VALTREX beyond 1 year have not been established.
Patients with Acute or Chronic Renal Impairment: In patients with reduced renal function, reduction in dosage is recommended (see Table 4).
[See table 4 above]
Hemodialysis: During hemodialysis, the half-life of acyclovir after administration of VALTREX is approximately 4 hours. About one third of acyclovir in the body is removed by dialysis during a 4-hour hemodialysis session. Patients requiring hemodialysis should receive the recommended dose of VALTREX after hemodialysis.
Peritoneal Dialysis: There is no information specific to administration of VALTREX in patients receiving peritoneal dialysis. The effect of chronic ambulatory peritoneal dialysis (CAPD) and continuous arteriovenous hemofiltration/dialysis (CAVHD) on acyclovir pharmacokinetics has been studied. The removal of acyclovir after CAPD and CAVHD is less pronounced than with hemodialysis, and the pharmacokinetic parameters closely resemble those observed in patients with ESRD not receiving hemodialysis. Therefore, supplemental doses of VALTREX should not be required following CAPD or CAVHD.

HOW SUPPLIED

VALTREX Caplets (blue, film-coated, capsule-shaped tablets) containing valacyclovir hydrochloride equivalent to 500 mg valacyclovir and printed with "VALTREX 500 mg" - Bottle of 42 (NDC 0173-0933-03) and unit dose pack of 100 (NDC 0173-0933-56).
VALTREX Caplets (blue, film-coated, capsule-shaped tablets) containing valacyclovir hydrochloride equivalent to 1 gram valacyclovir and printed with "VALTREX 1 gram" - Bottle of 20 (NDC 0173-0565-00).
Store at 15° to 25°C (59° to 77°F).

Manufactured by Catalytica Pharmaceuticals, Inc.
Greenville, NC 27834
for Glaxo Wellcome Inc.
Research Triangle Park, NC 27709
U.S. Patent No. 4,957,924

January 2000/RL-790
Shown in Product Identification Guide, page 316

VENTOLIN® ℞

[*vent 'ō-lin*]
(albuterol, USP)
Inhalation Aerosol

Bronchodilator Aerosol
For Oral Inhalation Only

DESCRIPTION

The active component of VENTOLIN Inhalation Aerosol is albuterol, USP, racemic (α^1-[(*tert*-butylamino)methyl]-4-hydroxy-*m*-xylene-α,α'-diol) and a relatively selective beta$_2$-adrenergic bronchodilator.
Albuterol is the official generic name in the United States. The World Health Organization recommended name for the drug is salbutamol. The molecular weight of albuterol is 239.3, and the empirical formula is $C_{13}H_{21}NO_3$. Albuterol is a white to off-white crystalline solid. It is soluble in ethanol, sparingly soluble in water, and very soluble in chloroform.
VENTOLIN Inhalation Aerosol is a pressurized metered-dose aerosol unit for oral inhalation. It contains a microcrystalline (95%≤10 µm) suspension of albuterol in propellants (trichloromonofluoromethane and dichlorodifluoromethane) with oleic acid. Each actuation delivers 100 mcg of albuterol from the valve and 90 mcg of albuterol from the mouthpiece. Each 6.8-g canister provides 80 inhalations and each 17-g canister provides 200 inhalations.

CLINICAL PHARMACOLOGY

In vitro studies and in vivo pharmacologic studies have demonstrated that albuterol has a preferential effect on beta$_2$-adrenergic receptors compared with isoproterenol. While it is recognized that beta$_2$-adrenergic receptors are the predominant receptors in bronchial smooth muscle, data indicate that there is a population of beta$_2$-receptors in the human heart existing in a concentration between 10% and 50%. The precise function of these receptors has not been established.

The pharmacologic effects of beta-adrenergic agonist drugs, including albuterol, are at least in part attributable to stimulation through beta-adrenergic receptors of intracellular adenyl cyclase, the enzyme that catalyzes the conversion of adenosine triphosphate (ATP) to cyclic-3′,5′-adenosine monophosphate (cyclic AMP). Increased cyclic AMP levels are associated with relaxation of bronchial smooth muscle and inhibition of release of mediators of immediate hypersensitivity from cells, especially from mast cells.

Albuterol has been shown in most controlled clinical trials to have more effect on the respiratory tract, in the form of bronchial smooth muscle relaxation, than isoproterenol at comparable doses while producing fewer cardiovascular effects. Controlled clinical studies and other clinical experience have shown that inhaled albuterol, like other beta-adrenergic agonist drugs, can produce a significant cardiovascular effect in some patients, as measured by pulse rate, blood pressure, symptoms, and/or electrocardiographic changes.

Albuterol is longer acting than isoproterenol in most patients by any route of administration because it is not a substrate for the cellular uptake processes for catecholamines nor for catechol-*O*-methyl transferase.

The effects of rising doses of albuterol and isoproterenol aerosols were studied in volunteers and asthmatic patients. Results in normal volunteers indicated that albuterol is one half to one quarter as active as isoproterenol in producing increases in heart rate. In asthmatic patients similar cardiovascular differentiation between the two drugs was also seen.

Preclinical: Intravenous studies in rats with albuterol sulfate have demonstrated that albuterol crosses the blood-brain barrier and reaches brain concentrations amounting to approximately 5.0% of the plasma concentrations. In structures outside the brain barrier (pineal and pituitary glands), albuterol concentrations were found to be 100 times those in the whole brain.

Studies in laboratory animals (minipigs, rodents, and dogs) have demonstrated the occurrence of cardiac arrhythmias and sudden death (with histologic evidence of myocardial necrosis) when beta-agonists and methylxanthines are administered concurrently. The clinical significance of these findings is unknown.

Pharmacokinetics: Because of its gradual absorption from the bronchi, systemic levels of albuterol are low after inhalation of recommended doses. Studies undertaken with four subjects administered tritiated albuterol resulted in maximum plasma concentrations occurring within 2 to 4 hours. Due to the sensitivity of the assay method, the metabolic rate and half-life of elimination of albuterol in plasma could not be determined. However, urinary excretion provided data indicating that albuterol has an elimination half-life of 3.8 hours. Approximately 72% of the inhaled dose is excreted within 24 hours in the urine, and consists of 28% as unchanged drug and 44% as metabolite.

Clinical Trials: In controlled clinical trials involving adults with asthma, the onset of improvement in pulmonary function was within 15 minutes, as determined by both MMEF (maximum midexpiratory flow rate) and FEV_1 (forced expiratory volume in 1 second). MMEF measurements also showed that near maximum improvement in pulmonary function generally occurs within 60 to 90 minutes following two inhalations of albuterol and that clinically significant improvement generally continues for 3 to 4 hours in most patients. Some patients showed a therapeutic response (defined by maintaining FEV_1 values 15% or more above baseline) that was still apparent at 6 hours. Continued effectiveness of albuterol was demonstrated over a 13-week period in these same trials.

In controlled clinical trials involving children 4 to 12 years of age, FEV_1 measurements showed that maximum improvement in pulmonary function occurs within 30 to 60 minutes. The onset of clinically significant (≥15%) improvement in FEV_1 was observed as soon as 5 minutes following 180 mcg of albuterol in 18 of 30 (60%) children in a controlled dose-ranging study. Clinically significant improvement in FEV_1 continued in the majority of patients for 2 hours and in 33% to 47% for 4 hours among 56 patients receiving inhalation aerosol in one pediatric study. In a second study among 48 patients receiving inhalation aerosol, clinically significant improvement continued in the majority for up to 1 hour and in 23% to 40% for 4 hours. In addition, at least 50% of the patients in both studies achieved an improvement in $FEF_{25\%-75\%}$ (forced expiratory flow rate between 25% and 75% of the forced vital capacity) of at least 20% for 2 to 5 hours. Continued effectiveness of albuterol was demonstrated over the 12-week study period.

In other clinical studies in adults and children, two inhalations of VENTOLIN Inhalation Aerosol taken approximately 15 minutes before exercise prevented exercise-induced bronchospasm, as demonstrated by the maintenance of FEV_1 within 80% of baseline values in the majority of patients. One study in adults also evaluated the duration of the prophylactic effect to repeated exercise challenges, which was evident at 4 hours in the majority of patients and at 6 hours in approximately one third of the patients.

INDICATIONS AND USAGE

VENTOLIN Inhalation Aerosol is indicated for the prevention and relief of bronchospasm in patients 4 years of age and older with reversible obstructive airway disease and for the prevention of exercise-induced bronchospasm in patients 4 years of age and older.

VENTOLIN Inhalation Aerosol can be used with or without concomitant steroid therapy.

CONTRAINDICATIONS

VENTOLIN Inhalation Aerosol is contraindicated in patients with a history of hypersensitivity to albuterol or any of its components.

WARNINGS

Paradoxical Bronchospasm: VENTOLIN Inhalation Aerosol can produce paradoxical bronchospasm, which may be life threatening. If paradoxical bronchospasm occurs, VENTOLIN Inhalation Aerosol should be discontinued immediately and alternative therapy instituted. It should be recognized that paradoxical bronchospasm, when associated with inhaled formulations, frequently occurs with the first use of a new canister or vial.

Cardiovascular Effects: VENTOLIN Inhalation Aerosol, like all other beta-adrenergic agonists, can produce a clinically significant cardiovascular effect in some patients as measured by pulse rate, blood pressure, and/or symptoms. Although such effects are uncommon after administration of VENTOLIN Inhalation Aerosol at recommended doses, if they occur, the drug may need to be discontinued. In addition, beta-agonists have been reported to produce electrocardiogram (ECG) changes, such as flattening of the T wave, prolongation of the QT_c interval, and ST segment depression. The clinical significance of these findings is unknown. Therefore, VENTOLIN Inhalation Aerosol, like all sympathomimetic amines, should be used with caution in patients with cardiovascular disorders, especially coronary insufficiency, cardiac arrhythmias, and hypertension.

Deterioration of Asthma: Asthma may deteriorate acutely over a period of hours or chronically over several days or longer. If the patient needs more doses of VENTOLIN Inhalation Aerosol than usual, this may be a marker of destabilization of asthma and requires reevaluation of the patient and treatment regimen, giving special consideration to the possible need for anti-inflammatory treatment, e.g., corticosteroids.

Use of Anti-Inflammatory Agents: The use of beta-adrenergic agonist bronchodilators alone may not be adequate to control asthma in many patients. Early consideration should be given to adding anti-inflammatory agents, e.g., corticosteroids.

Immediate Hypersensitivity Reactions: Immediate hypersensitivity reactions may occur after administration of albuterol inhalation aerosol, as demonstrated by rare cases of urticaria, angioedema, rash, bronchospasm, anaphylaxis, and oropharyngeal edema.

The contents of VENTOLIN Inhalation Aerosol are under pressure. Do not puncture. Do not use or store near heat or open flame. Exposure to temperatures above 120°F may cause bursting. Never throw container into fire or incinerator. Keep out of reach of children.

PRECAUTIONS

General: Albuterol, as with all sympathomimetic amines, should be used with caution in patients with cardiovascular disorders, especially coronary insufficiency, cardiac arrhythmias, and hypertension; in patients with convulsive disorders, hyperthyroidism, or diabetes mellitus; and in patients who are unusually responsive to sympathomimetic amines. Clinically significant changes in systolic and diastolic blood pressure have been seen in individual patients and could be expected to occur in some patients after use of any beta-adrenergic bronchodilator.

Large doses of intravenous albuterol have been reported to aggravate preexisting diabetes mellitus and ketoacidosis. As with other beta-agonists, albuterol may produce significant hypokalemia in some patients, possibly through intracellular shunting, which has the potential to produce adverse cardiovascular effects. The decrease is usually transient, not requiring supplementation.

Although there have been no reports concerning the use of VENTOLIN Inhalation Aerosol during labor and delivery, it has been reported that high doses of albuterol administered intravenously inhibit uterine contractions. Although this effect is extremely unlikely as a consequence of aerosol use, it should be kept in mind.

Information for Patients: The action of VENTOLIN Inhalation Aerosol may last up to 6 hours or longer. VENTOLIN Inhalation Aerosol should not be used more frequently than recommended. Do not increase the dose or frequency of VENTOLIN Inhalation Aerosol without consulting your physician. If you find that treatment with VENTOLIN Inhalation Aerosol becomes less effective for symptomatic relief, your symptoms become worse, and/or you need to use the product more frequently than usual, you should seek medical attention immediately. While you are using VENTOLIN Inhalation Aerosol, other inhaled drugs and asthma medications should be taken only as directed by your physician. Common adverse effects include palpitations, chest pain, rapid heart rate, and tremor or nervousness. If you are pregnant or nursing, contact your physician about use of VENTOLIN Inhalation Aerosol. Effective and safe use of VENTOLIN Inhalation Aerosol includes an understanding of the way that it should be administered.

In general, the technique for administering VENTOLIN Inhalation Aerosol to children is similar to that for adults, since children's smaller ventilatory exchange capacity automatically provides proportionally smaller aerosol intake. Children should use VENTOLIN Inhalation Aerosol under adult supervision, as instructed by the patient's physician. See illustrated Patient's Instructions for Use section of the full prescribing information.

Drug Interactions: Other short-acting sympathomimetic aerosol bronchodilators should not be used concomitantly with albuterol. If additional adrenergic drugs are to be administered by any route, they should be used with caution to avoid deleterious cardiovascular effects.

Monoamine Oxidase Inhibitors or Tricyclic Antidepressants: Albuterol should be administered with extreme caution to patients being treated with monoamine oxidase inhibitors or tricyclic antidepressants, or within 2 weeks of discontinuation of such agents, because the action of albuterol on the vascular system may be potentiated.

Beta-Blockers: Beta-adrenergic receptor blocking agents not only block the pulmonary effect of beta-agonists, such as VENTOLIN Inhalation Aerosol, but may produce severe bronchospasm in asthmatic patients. Therefore, patients with asthma should not normally be treated with beta-blockers. However, under certain circumstances, e.g., as prophylaxis after myocardial infarction, there may be no acceptable alternatives to the use of beta-adrenergic blocking agents in patients with asthma. In this setting, cardioselective beta-blockers should be considered, although they should be administered with caution.

Diuretics: The ECG changes and/or hypokalemia that may result from the administration of nonpotassium-sparing diuretics (such as loop or thiazide diuretics) can be acutely worsened by beta-agonists, especially when the recommended dose of the beta-agonist is exceeded. Although the clinical significance of these effects is not known, caution is advised in the coadministration of beta-agonists with nonpotassium-sparing diuretics.

Digoxin: Mean decreases of 16% to 22% in serum digoxin levels were demonstrated after single-dose intravenous and oral administration of albuterol, respectively, to normal volunteers who had received digoxin for 10 days. The clinical significance of these findings for patients with obstructive airway disease who are receiving albuterol and digoxin on a chronic basis is unclear. Nevertheless, it would be prudent to carefully evaluate the serum digoxin levels in patients who are currently receiving digoxin and albuterol.

Carcinogenesis, Mutagenesis, Impairment of Fertility: In a 2-year study in Sprague-Dawley rats, albuterol sulfate caused a significant dose-related increase in the incidence of benign leiomyomas of the mesovarium at dietary doses of 2.0, 10, and 50 mg/kg (approximately 15, 70, and 340 times, respectively, the maximum recommended daily inhalation dose for adults on a mg/m^2 basis or approximately 6, 30, and 160 times, respectively, the maximum recommended daily inhalation dose for children on a mg/m^2basis). In another study this effect was blocked by the coadministration of propranolol, a non-selective beta-adrenergic antagonist. In an 18-month study in CD-1 mice albuterol sulfate showed no evidence of tumorigenicity at dietary doses of up to 500 mg/kg (approximately 1700 times the maximum recommended daily inhalation dose for adults on a mg/m^2 basis or approximately 800 times the maximum recommended daily inhalation dose for children on a mg/m^2 basis). In a 22-month study in the Golden hamster albuterol sulfate showed no evidence of tumorigenicity at dietary doses of up to 50 mg/kg (approximately 225 times the maximum recommended daily inhalation dose for adults on a mg/m^2 basis or approximately 110 times the maximum recommended daily inhalation dose for children on a mg/m^2 basis).

Albuterol sulfate was not mutagenic in the Ames test with or without metabolic activation using tester strains *S. typhimurium* TA1537, TA1538, and TA98 or *E. coli* WP2, WP2uvrA, and WP67. No forward mutation was seen in yeast strain *S. cerevisiae* S9 nor any mitotic gene conversion in yeast strain *S. cerevisiae* JD1 with or without metabolic activation. Fluctuation assays in *S. typhimurium* TA98 and *E. coli* WP2, both with metabolic activation, were negative. Albuterol sulfate was not clastogenic in a human peripheral lymphocyte assay or in an AH1 strain mouse micronucleus assay at intraperitoneal doses of up to 200 mg/kg.

Reproduction studies in rats demonstrated no evidence of impaired fertility at oral doses up to 50 mg/kg (approximately 340 times the maximum recommended daily inhalation dose for adults on a mg/m^2 basis).

Pregnancy: ***Teratogenic Effects:*** Pregnancy Category C. Albuterol sulfate has been shown to be teratogenic in mice. A study in CD-1 mice at subcutaneous doses of 0.025, 0.25, and 2.5 mg/kg (approximately 2/25, 1.0, and 8.0 times, respectively, the maximum recommended daily inhalation dose for adults on a mg/m^2 basis), showed cleft palate formation in 5 of 111 (4.5%) fetuses at 0.25 mg/kg and in 10 of 108 (9.3%) fetuses at 2.5 mg/kg. The drug did not induce cleft palate formation at the lowest dose, 0.025 mg/kg. Cleft palate also occurred in 22 of 72 (30.5%) fetuses from females treated with 2.5 mg/kg of isoproterenol (positive control) subcutaneously (approximately 8 times the maximum recommended daily inhalation dose for adults on a mg/m^2 basis).

A reproduction study in Stride Dutch rabbits revealed cranioschisis in 7 of 19 (37%) fetuses when albuterol sulfate

Continued on next page

This product information is based on labeling in effect on June 23, 2000. For further information, contact via direct mail, phone, or web site. Medical Information, Glaxo Wellcome Inc., PO Box 13398, Research Triangle Park, NC 27709. Healthcare Professionals (Medical Information): 800-334-0089. Patients (Customer Response Center): 1-888-825-5249. Glaxo Wellcome Corporate Web Site: www.glaxowellcome.com

Ventolin Inh. Aero.—Cont.

was administered orally at a 50 mg/kg dose (approximately 680 times the maximum recommended daily inhalation dose for adults on a mg/m^2 basis).
There are no adequate and well-controlled studies in pregnant women. Albuterol should be used during pregnancy only if the potential benefit justifies the potential risk to the fetus.
During worldwide marketing experience, various congenital anomalies, including cleft palate and limb defects, have been rarely reported in the offspring of patients being treated with albuterol. Some of the mothers were taking multiple medications during their pregnancies. No consistent pattern of defects can be discerned, and a relationship between albuterol use and congenital anomalies has not been established.
Use in Labor and Delivery: Because of the potential for beta-agonist interference with uterine contractility, use of VENTOLIN Inhalation Aerosol for relief of bronchospasm during labor should be restricted to those patients in whom the benefits clearly outweigh the risk.
Tocolysis: Albuterol has not been approved for the management of preterm labor. The benefit:risk ratio when albuterol is administered for tocolysis has not been established. Serious adverse reactions, including maternal pulmonary edema, have been reported during or following treatment of premature labor with beta$_2$-agonists, including albuterol.
Nursing Mothers: It is not known whether this drug is excreted in human milk. Because of the potential for tumorigenicity shown for albuterol in some animal studies, a decision should be made whether to discontinue nursing or to discontinue the drug, taking into account the importance of the drug to the mother.
Pediatric Use: Safety and effectiveness in children below 4 years of age have not been established.

ADVERSE REACTIONS

The adverse reactions to albuterol are similar in nature to reactions to other sympathomimetic agents, although the incidence of certain cardiovascular effects is lower with albuterol.

Percent Incidence of Adverse Reactions in Patients ≥12 Years of Age in a 13-Week Clinical Trial*

Reaction	Percent Incidence	
	Albuterol	Isoproterenol
Tremor	<15%	<15%
Nausea	<15%	<15%
Tachycardia	10%	10%
Palpitations	<10%	<15%
Nervousness	<10%	<15%
Increased blood pressure	<5%	<5%
Dizziness	<5%	<5%
Heartburn	<5%	<5%

* A 13-week double-blind study compared albuterol and isoproterenol inhalation aerosols in 147 asthmatic patients.

Percent Incidence of Adverse Reactions in Children 4 to 11 Years of Age in a 12-Week Trial*

Reaction	Percent Incidence
Central nervous system	
Headache	3%
Nervousness	1%
Lightheadedness	<1%
Tremor	<1%
Agitation	1%
Nightmares	1%
Hyperactivity	1%
Aggressive behavior	1%
Gastrointestinal	
Nausea and/or vomiting	6%
Stomachache	3%
Diarrhea	1%
Oropharyngeal	
Throat irritation	6%
Discoloration of teeth	1%
Respiratory	
Epistaxis	3%
Cough	2%
Musculoskeletal	
Muscle cramp	1%

* A 12-week double-blind trial in 104 patients aged 4 to 11 years.

Cases of urticaria, angioedema, rash, bronchospasm, hoarseness, oropharyngeal edema, and arrhythmias (including atrial fibrillation, supraventricular tachycardia, extrasystoles) have been reported after the use of VENTOLIN Inhalation Aerosol.
In addition, albuterol, like other sympathomimetic agents, can cause adverse reactions such as hypertension, angina, vertigo, central nervous system stimulation, sleeplessness, and unusual taste.

OVERDOSAGE

The expected symptoms with overdosage are those of excessive beta-adrenergic stimulation and/or occurrence or exaggeration of any of the symptoms listed under ADVERSE REACTIONS, e.g., seizures, angina, hypertension or hypotension, tachycardia with rates up to 200 beats/min, arrhythmias, nervousness, headache, tremor, dry mouth, palpitation, nausea, dizziness, fatigue, malaise, and sleeplessness. Hypokalemia may also occur.
As with all sympathomimetic aerosol medications, cardiac arrest and even death may be associated with abuse of VENTOLIN Inhalation Aerosol. Treatment consists of discontinuation of VENTOLIN Inhalation Aerosol together with appropriate symptomatic therapy. The judicious use of a cardioselective beta-receptor blocker may be considered, bearing in mind that such medication can produce bronchospasm. There is insufficient evidence to determine if dialysis is beneficial for overdosage of VENTOLIN Inhalation Aerosol.
The oral median lethal dose of albuterol sulfate in mice is greater than 2000 mg/kg (approximately 6800 times the maximum recommended daily inhalation dose for adults on a mg/m^2 basis or approximately 3200 times the maximum recommended daily inhalation dose for children on a mg/m^2 basis). In mature rats, the subcutaneous median lethal dose of albuterol sulfate is approximately 450 mg/kg (approximately 3000 times the maximum recommended daily inhalation dose for adults on a mg/m^2 basis or approximately 1400 times the maximum recommended daily inhalation dose for children on a mg/m^2 basis). In small young rats, the subcutaneous median lethal dose is approximately 2000 mg/kg (approximately 14,000 times the maximum recommended daily inhalation dose for adults on a mg/m^2 basis or approximately 6400 times the maximum recommended daily inhalation dose for children on a mg/m^2 basis). The inhalation median lethal dose has not been determined in animals.

DOSAGE AND ADMINISTRATION

For treatment of acute episodes of bronchospasm or prevention of asthmatic symptoms, the usual dosage for adults and children 4 years of age and older is two inhalations repeated every 4 to 6 hours; in some patients, one inhalation every 4 hours may be sufficient. More frequent administration or a larger number of inhalations are not recommended. It is recommended to "test spray" VENTOLIN Inhalation Aerosol. Do this by spraying four times into the air before using for the first time and when the inhaler has not been used for a prolonged period of time (i.e., more than 4 weeks).
The use of VENTOLIN Inhalation Aerosol can be continued as medically indicated to control recurring bouts of bronchospasm. During this time most patients gain optimal benefit from regular use of the inhaler. Safe usage for periods extending over several years has been documented.
If a previously effective dosage regimen fails to provide the usual response, this may be a marker of destabilization of asthma and requires reevaluation of the patient and the treatment regimen, giving special consideration to the possible need for anti-inflammatory treatment, e.g., corticosteroids.
Exercise-Induced Bronchospasm Prevention: The usual dosage for adults and children 4 years and older is two inhalations 15 minutes before exercise.
For treatment, see above.

HOW SUPPLIED

VENTOLIN Inhalation Aerosol is supplied in 6.8-g canisters containing 80 metered inhalations (NDC 0173-0463-00) and in 17-g canisters containing 200 metered inhalations (NDC 0173-0321-88), each in boxes of one. Each actuation delivers 100 mcg of albuterol from the valve and 90 mcg of albuterol from the mouthpiece. Each canister is supplied with a blue oral adapter and patient's instructions. Also available, VENTOLIN Inhalation Aerosol Refill 17-g canister only with patient's instructions (NDC 0173-0321-98).
The blue adapter supplied with VENTOLIN Inhalation Aerosol should not be used with any other product canisters, and adapters from other products should not be used with a VENTOLIN Inhalation Aerosol canister. The correct amount of medication in each canister cannot be assured after 80 actuations from the 6.8-g canister and 200 actuations from the 17.0-g canister, even though the canister is not completely empty. The canister should be discarded when the labeled number of actuations have been used. Store between 15° and 30°C (59° and 86°F). As with most inhaled medications in aerosol canisters, the therapeutic effect of this medication may decrease when the canister is cold; for best results, the canister should be at room temperature before use. Shake well before using.
Glaxo Wellcome Inc., Research Triangle Park, NC 27709
August 1998/RL-627

Shown in Product Identification Guide, page 316

VENTOLIN® ℞

[vent' ō-lin]
(albuterol sulfate, USP)
Inhalation Solution, 0.5%*
***Potency expressed as albuterol.**

DESCRIPTION

The active component of VENTOLIN Inhalation Solution is albuterol sulfate, USP, the racemic form of albuterol and a relatively selective beta$_2$-adrenergic bronchodilator (see CLINICAL PHARMACOLOGY). It has the chemical name α^1-[(*tert*-butylamino)methyl]-4-hydroxy-*m*-xylene-α, α'-diol sulfate (2:1)(salt).
Albuterol sulfate has a molecular weight of 576.7, and the empirical formula is $(C_{13}H_{21}NO_3)_2 \cdot H_2SO_4$. Albuterol sulfate is a white crystalline powder, soluble in water and slightly soluble in ethanol.
The World Health Organization recommended name for albuterol base is salbutamol.
VENTOLIN Inhalation Solution, 0.5% is in concentrated form. Dilute the appropriate volume of the solution (see DOSAGE AND ADMINISTRATION) with sterile normal saline solution to a total volume of 3 mL and administer by nebulization.
Each milliliter of VENTOLIN Inhalation Solution contains 5 mg of albuterol (as 6 mg of albuterol sulfate) in an aqueous solution containing benzalkonium chloride; sulfuric acid is used to adjust the pH to between 3 and 5. VENTOLIN Inhalation Solution contains no sulfiting agents. It is supplied in a 20-mL amber glass bottle.
VENTOLIN Inhalation Solution is a clear, colorless to light yellow solution.

CLINICAL PHARMACOLOGY

In vitro studies and in vivo pharmacologic studies have demonstrated that albuterol has a preferential effect on beta$_2$-adrenergic receptors compared with isoproterenol. While it is recognized that beta$_2$-adrenergic receptors are the predominant receptors in bronchial smooth muscle, data indicate that there is a population of beta$_2$-receptors in the human heart existing in a concentration between 10% and 50%. The precise function of these receptors has not been established (see WARNINGS).
The pharmacologic effects of beta-adrenergic agonist drugs, including albuterol, are at least in part attributable to stimulation through beta-adrenergic receptors of intracellular adenyl cyclase, the enzyme that catalyzes the conversion of adenosine triphosphate (ATP) to cyclic-3',5'-adenosine monophosphate (cyclic AMP). Increased cyclic AMP levels are associated with relaxation of bronchial smooth muscle and inhibition of release of mediators of immediate hypersensitivity from cells, especially from mast cells.
Albuterol has been shown in most controlled clinical trials to have more effect on the respiratory tract, in the form of bronchial smooth muscle relaxation, than isoproterenol at comparable doses while producing fewer cardiovascular effects.
Controlled clinical studies and other clinical experience have shown that inhaled albuterol, like other beta-adrenergic agonist drugs, can produce a significant cardiovascular effect in some patients, as measured by pulse rate, blood pressure, symptoms, and/or electrocardiographic changes.
Albuterol is longer acting than isoproterenol in most patients by any route of administration because it is not a substrate for the cellular uptake processes for catecholamines nor for catechol-*O*-methyl transferase.
Pharmacokinetics: Studies in asthmatic patients have shown that less than 20% of a single albuterol dose was absorbed following either intermittent positive-pressure breathing (IPPB) or nebulizer administration; the remaining amount was recovered from the nebulizer and apparatus and expired air. Most of the absorbed dose was recovered in the urine within 24 hours after drug administration. Following a 3-mg dose of nebulized albuterol in adults, the maximum albuterol plasma levels at 0.5 hours were 2.1 ng/mL (range, 1.4 to 3.2 ng/mL). There was a significant dose-related response in FEV$_1$ (forced expiratory volume in 1 second) and peak flow rate. It has been demonstrated that following oral administration of 4 mg of albuterol, the elimination half-life was 5 to 6 hours.
Preclinical: Intravenous studies in rats with albuterol sulfate have demonstrated that albuterol crosses the blood-brain barrier and reaches brain concentrations amounting to approximately 5.0% of the plasma concentrations. In structures outside the brain barrier (pineal and pituitary glands), albuterol concentrations were found to be 100 times those in the whole brain.
Studies in laboratory animals (minipigs, rodents, and dogs) have demonstrated the occurrence of cardiac arrhythmias and sudden death (with histologic evidence of myocardial necrosis) when beta-agonists and methylxanthines are administered concurrently. The clinical significance of these findings is unknown.
Clinical Trials: In controlled clinical trials in adults, most patients exhibited an onset of improvement in pulmonary function within 5 minutes as determined by FEV$_1$. FEV$_1$ measurements also showed that the maximum average improvement in pulmonary function usually occurred at approximately 1 hour following inhalation of 2.5 mg of albuterol by compressor-nebulizer and remained close to peak for 2 hours. Clinically significant improvement in pulmonary function (defined as maintenance of a 15% or more increase in FEV$_1$ over baseline values) continued for 3 to 4

hours in most patients, with some patients continuing up to 6 hours.

Published reports of trials in asthmatic children aged 3 years or older have demonstrated significant improvement in either FEV_1 or PEFR within 2 to 20 minutes following single doses of albuterol inhalation solution. An increase of 15% or more in baseline FEV_1 has been observed in children aged 5 to 11 years up to 6 hours after treatment with doses of 0.10 mg/kg or higher of albuterol inhalation solution. Single doses of 3, 4, or 10 mg resulted in improvement in baseline PEFR that was comparable in extent and duration to a 2-mg dose, but doses above 3 mg were associated with heart rate increases of more than 10%.

INDICATIONS AND USAGE

VENTOLIN Inhalation Solution is indicated for the relief of bronchospasm in patients 2 years of age and older with reversible obstructive airway disease and acute attacks of bronchospasm.

CONTRAINDICATIONS

VENTOLIN Inhalation Solution is contraindicated in patients with a history of hypersensitivity to albuterol or any of its components.

WARNINGS

Paradoxical Bronchospasm: VENTOLIN Inhalation Solution can produce paradoxical bronchospasm, which may be life threatening. If paradoxical bronchospasm occurs, VENTOLIN Inhalation Solution should be discontinued immediately and alternative therapy instituted. It should be recognized that paradoxical bronchospasm, when associated with inhaled formulations, frequently occurs with the first use of a new canister or vial.

Fatalities have been reported in association with excessive use of inhaled sympathomimetic drugs and with the home use of nebulizers. It is therefore essential that the physician instruct the patient in the need for further evaluation if his/her asthma becomes worse.

Cardiovascular Effects: VENTOLIN Inhalation Solution, like all other beta-adrenergic agonists, can produce a clinically significant cardiovascular effect in some patients as measured by pulse rate, blood pressure, and/or symptoms. Although such effects are uncommon after administration of VENTOLIN Inhalation Solution at recommended doses, if they occur, the drug may need to be discontinued. In addition, beta-agonists have been reported to produce electrocardiogram (ECG) changes, such as flattening of the T wave, prolongation of the QT_c interval, and ST segment depression. The clinical significance of these findings is unknown. Therefore, VENTOLIN Inhalation Solution, like all sympathomimetic amines, should be used with caution in patients with cardiovascular disorders, especially coronary insufficiency, cardiac arrhythmias, and hypertension.

Deterioration of Asthma: Asthma may deteriorate acutely over a period of hours or chronically over several days or longer. If the patient needs more doses of VENTOLIN Inhalation Solution than usual, this may be a marker of destabilization of asthma and requires reevaluation of the patient and treatment regimen, giving special consideration to the possible need for anti-inflammatory treatment, e.g., corticosteroids.

Immediate Hypersensitivity Reactions: Immediate hypersensitivity reactions may occur after administration of albuterol, as demonstrated by rare cases of urticaria, angioedema, rash, bronchospasm, and oropharyngeal edema.

Use of Anti-Inflammatory Agents: The use of beta-adrenergic agonist bronchodilators alone may not be adequate to control asthma in many patients. Early consideration should be given to adding anti-inflammatory agents, e.g., corticosteroids.

Microbial Contamination: To avoid microbial contamination, proper aseptic technique should be used each time the bottle is opened. Precautions should be taken to prevent contact of the dropper tip of the bottle with any surface, including the nebulizer reservoir and associated ventilatory equipment. In addition, if the solution changes color or becomes cloudy, it should not be used.

PRECAUTIONS

General: Albuterol, as with all sympathomimetic amines, should be used with caution in patients with cardiovascular disorders, especially coronary insufficiency, hypertension, and cardiac arrhythmia; in patients with convulsive disorders, hyperthyroidism, or diabetes mellitus; and in patients who are unusually responsive to sympathomimetic amines. Clinically significant changes in systolic and diastolic blood pressure have been seen in individual patients and could be expected to occur in some patients after use of any beta-adrenergic bronchodilator.

Large doses of intravenous albuterol have been reported to aggravate preexisting diabetes mellitus and ketoacidosis. As with other beta-agonists, albuterol may produce significant hypokalemia in some patients, possibly through intracellular shunting, which has the potential to produce adverse cardiovascular effects. The decrease is usually transient, not requiring supplementation.

Repeated dosing with 0.15 mg/kg of albuterol inhalation solution in children aged 5 to 17 years who were initially normokalemic has been associated with an asymptomatic decline of 20% to 25% in serum potassium levels.

Information for Patients: The action of VENTOLIN Inhalation Solution may last up to 6 hours or longer. VENTOLIN Inhalation Solution should not be used more frequently than recommended. Do not increase the dose or frequency of VENTOLIN Inhalation Solution without consulting your

Approximate Weight (kg)	Approximate Weight (lb)	Dose (mg)	Volume of Inhalation Solution
10–15	22–33	1.25	0.25 mL
>15	>33	2.5	0.5 mL

physician. If you find that treatment with VENTOLIN Inhalation Solution becomes less effective for symptomatic relief, your symptoms become worse, and/or you need to use the product more frequently than usual, you should seek medical attention immediately. While you are using VENTOLIN Inhalation Solution, other inhaled drugs and asthma medications should be taken only as directed by your physician. Common adverse effects include palpitations, chest pain, rapid heart rate, and tremor or nervousness. If you are pregnant or nursing, contact your physician about use of VENTOLIN Inhalation Solution. Effective and safe use of VENTOLIN Inhalation Solution includes an understanding of the way that it should be administered.

To avoid microbial contamination, proper aseptic techniques should be used each time the bottle is opened. Precautions should be taken to prevent contact of the dropper tip of the bottle with any surface, including the nebulizer reservoir and associated ventilatory equipment. In addition, if the solution changes color or becomes cloudy, it should not be used.

Drug compatibility (physical and chemical), efficacy, and safety of VENTOLIN Inhalation Solution when mixed with other drugs in a nebulizer have not been established.

See illustrated Patient's Instructions for Use section of the full prescribing information.

Drug Interactions: Other short-acting sympathomimetic aerosol bronchodilators or epinephrine should not be used concomitantly with albuterol. If additional adrenergic drugs are to be administered by any route, they should be used with caution to avoid deleterious cardiovascular effects.

Monoamine Oxidase Inhibitors or Tricyclic Antidepressants: Albuterol should be administered with extreme caution to patients being treated with monoamine oxidase inhibitors or tricyclic antidepressants, or within 2 weeks of discontinuation of such agents, because the action of albuterol on the vascular system may be potentiated.

Beta-Blockers: Beta-adrenergic receptor blocking agents not only block the pulmonary effect of beta-agonists, such as VENTOLIN Inhalation Solution, but may produce severe bronchospasm in asthmatic patients. Therefore, patients with asthma should not normally be treated with beta-blockers. However, under certain circumstances, e.g., as prophylaxis after myocardial infarction, there may be no acceptable alternatives to the use of beta-adrenergic blocking agents in patients with asthma. In this setting, cardioselective beta-blockers could be considered, although they should be administered with caution.

Diuretics: The ECG changes and/or hypokalemia that may result from the administration of nonpotassium-sparing diuretics (such as loop or thiazide diuretics) can be acutely worsened by beta-agonists, especially when the recommended dose of the beta-agonist is exceeded. Although the clinical significance of these effects is not known, caution is advised in the coadministration of beta-agonists with nonpotassium-sparing diuretics.

Digoxin: Mean decreases of 16% to 22% in serum digoxin levels were demonstrated after single-dose intravenous and oral administration of albuterol, respectively, to normal volunteers who had received digoxin for 10 days. The clinical significance of these findings for patients with obstructive airway disease who are receiving albuterol and digoxin on a chronic basis is unclear. Nevertheless, it would be prudent to carefully evaluate the serum digoxin levels in patients who are currently receiving digoxin and albuterol.

Carcinogenesis, Mutagenesis, Impairment of Fertility: In a 2-year study in Sprague-Dawley rats, albuterol sulfate caused a significant dose-related increase in the incidence of benign leiomyomas of the mesovarium at dietary doses of 2.0, 10, and 50 mg/kg (approximately 2, 8, and 40 times, respectively, the maximum recommended daily inhalation dose for adults on a mg/m^2 basis or approximately 3/5, 3, and 15 times, respectively, the maximum recommended daily inhalation dose in children on a mg/m^2 basis). In another study this effect was blocked by the coadministration of propranolol, a non-selective beta-adrenergic antagonist. In an 18-month study in CD-1 mice, albuterol sulfate showed no evidence of tumorigenicity at dietary doses of up to 500 mg/kg (approximately 200 times the maximum recommended daily inhalation dose for adults on a mg/m^2 basis or approximately 75 times the maximum recommended daily inhalation dose for children on a mg/m^2 basis). In a 22-month study in the Golden hamster, albuterol sulfate showed no evidence of tumorigenicity at dietary doses of up to 50 mg/kg (approximately 25 times the maximum recommended daily inhalation dose for adults on a mg/m^2 basis or approximately 10 times the maximum recommended daily inhalation dose for children on a mg/m^2 basis).

Albuterol sulfate was not mutagenic in the Ames test with or without metabolic activation using tester strains *S. typhimurium* TA1537, TA1538, and TA98 or *E. coli* WP2, WP2uvrA, and WP67. No forward mutation was seen in yeast strain *S. cerevisiae* S9 nor any mitotic gene conversion in yeast strain *S. cerevisiae* JD1 with or without metabolic activation. Fluctuation assays in *S. typhimurium* TA98 and *E. coli* WP2, both with metabolic activation, were negative. Albuterol sulfate was not clastogenic in a human peripheral lymphocyte assay or in an AH1 strain mouse micronucleus assay at intraperitoneal doses of up to 200 mg/kg.

Reproduction studies in rats demonstrated no evidence of impaired fertility at oral doses up to 50 mg/kg (approximately 40 times the maximum recommended daily inhalation dose for adults on a mg/m^2 basis).

Pregnancy: ***Teratogenic Effects:*** Pregnancy Category C. Albuterol has been shown to be teratogenic in mice. A study in CD-1 mice at subcutaneous doses of 0.025, 0.25, and 2.5 mg/kg (approximately 1/100, 1/10, and 1.0 times, respectively, the maximum recommended daily inhalation dose for adults on a mg/m^2 basis) showed cleft palate formation in 5 of 111 (4.5%) fetuses at 0.25 mg/kg and in 10 of 108 (9.3%) fetuses at 2.5 mg/kg. The drug did not induce cleft palate formation at the lowest dose, 0.025 mg/kg. Cleft palate also occurred in 22 of 72 (30.5%) fetuses from females treated with 2.5 mg/kg of isoproterenol (positive control) subcutaneously (approximately 1.0 time the maximum recommended daily inhalation dose for adults on a mg/m^2 basis).

A reproduction study in Stride Dutch rabbits revealed cranioschisis in 7 of 19 (37%) fetuses when albuterol was administered orally at a 50-mg/kg dose (approximately 80 times the maximum recommended daily inhalation dose for adults on a mg/m^2 basis).

There are no adequate and well-controlled studies in pregnant women. Albuterol should be used during pregnancy only if the potential benefit justifies the potential risk to the fetus.

During worldwide marketing experience, various congenital anomalies, including cleft palate and limb defects, have been rarely reported in the offspring of patients being treated with albuterol. Some of the mothers were taking multiple medications during their pregnancies. No consistent pattern of defects can be discerned, and a relationship between albuterol use and congenital anomalies has not been established.

Use in Labor and Delivery: Because of the potential for beta-agonist interference with uterine contractility, use of VENTOLIN Inhalation Solution for relief of bronchospasm during labor should be restricted to those patients in whom the benefits clearly outweigh the risk.

Tocolysis: Albuterol has not been approved for the management of preterm labor. The benefit:risk ratio when albuterol is administered for tocolysis has not been established. Serious adverse reactions, including maternal pulmonary edema, have been reported during or following treatment of premature labor with $beta_2$-agonists, including albuterol.

Nursing Mothers: It is not known whether this drug is excreted in human milk. Because of the potential for tumorigenicity shown for albuterol in some animal studies, a decision should be made whether to discontinue nursing or to discontinue the drug, taking into account the importance of the drug to the mother.

Pediatric Use: The safety and effectiveness of VENTOLIN Inhalation Solution have been established in children 2 years of age and older. Use of VENTOLIN Inhalation Solution in these age-groups is supported by evidence from adequate and well-controlled studies of VENTOLIN Inhalation Solution in adults; the likelihood that the disease course, pathophysiology, and the drug's effect in pediatric and adult patients are substantially similar; and published reports of trials in pediatric patients 3 years of age or older. The recommended dose for the pediatric population is based upon three published dose comparison studies of efficacy and safety in children 5 to 17 years, and on the safety profile in both adults and pediatric patients at doses equal to or higher than the recommended doses. The safety and effectiveness of VENTOLIN Inhalation Solution in children below 2 years of age have not been established.

ADVERSE REACTIONS

The results of clinical trials with VENTOLIN Inhalation Solution in 135 patients showed the following side effects that were considered probably or possibly drug related:

Percent Incidence of Adverse Reactions

Reaction	Percent Incidence n = 135
Central nervous system	
Tremors	20%
Dizziness	7%
Nervousness	4%
Headache	3%
Sleeplessness	1%
Gastrointestinal	
Nausea	4%
Dyspepsia	1%

Continued on next page

This product information is based on labeling in effect on June 23, 2000. For further information, contact via direct mail, phone, or web site. Medical Information, Glaxo Wellcome Inc., PO Box 13398, Research Triangle Park, NC 27709. Healthcare Professionals (Medical Information): 800-334-0089. Patients (Customer Response Center): 1-888-825-5249. Glaxo Wellcome Corporate Web Site: www.glaxowellcome.com

Ventolin Inh. Soln—Cont.

Ear, nose, and throat	
Nasal congestion	1%
Pharyngitis	<1%
Cardiovascular	
Tachycardia	1%
Hypertension	1%
Respiratory	
Bronchospasm	8%
Cough	4%
Bronchitis	4%
Wheezing	1%

No clinically relevant laboratory abnormalities related to VENTOLIN Inhalation Solution administration were determined in these studies.
Cases of urticaria, angioedema, rash, bronchospasm, hoarseness, oropharyngeal edema, and arrhythmias (including atrial fibrillation, supraventricular tachycardia, extrasystoles) have been reported after the use of VENTOLIN Inhalation Solution.

OVERDOSAGE

The expected symptoms with overdosage are those of excessive beta-adrenergic stimulation and/or occurrence or exaggeration of any of the symptoms listed under ADVERSE REACTIONS, e.g., seizures, angina, hypertension or hypotension, tachycardia with rates up to 200 beats/min, arrhythmias, nervousness, headache, tremor, dry mouth, palpitation, nausea, dizziness, fatigue, malaise, and sleeplessness. Hypokalemia may also occur. In isolated cases in children 2 to 12 years of age, tachycardia with rates >200 beats/min has been observed.
As with all sympathomimetic medications, cardiac arrest and even death may be associated with abuse of VENTOLIN Inhalation Solution. Treatment consists of discontinuation of VENTOLIN Inhalation Solution together with appropriate symptomatic therapy. The judicious use of a cardioselective beta-receptor blocker may be considered, bearing in mind that such medication can produce bronchospasm. There is insufficient evidence to determine if dialysis is beneficial for overdosage of VENTOLIN Inhalation Solution.
The oral median lethal dose of albuterol sulfate in mice is greater than 2000 mg/kg (approximately 810 times the maximum recommended daily inhalation dose for adults on a mg/m^2 basis or approximately 300 times the maximum recommended daily dose for children on a mg/m^2 basis). In mature rats, the subcutaneous (SC) median lethal dose of albuterol sulfate is approximately 450 mg/kg (approximately 365 times the maximum recommended daily inhalation dose for adults on a mg/m^2 basis or approximately 135 times the maximum recommended daily inhalation dose for children on a mg/m^2 basis). In small young rats, the SC median lethal dose is approximately 2000 mg/kg (approximately 1600 times the maximum recommended daily inhalation dose for adults on a mg/m^2 basis or approximately 600 times the maximum recommended daily inhalation dose for children on a mg/m^2 basis). The inhalational median lethal dose has not been determined in animals.

DOSAGE AND ADMINISTRATION

To avoid microbial contamination, proper aseptic techniques should be used each time the bottle is opened. Precautions should be taken to prevent contact of the dropper tip of the bottle with any surface, including the nebulizer reservoir and associated ventilatory equipment. In addition, if the solution changes color or becomes cloudy, it should not be used.
Children 2 to 12 Years of Age: For children 2 to 12 years of age, initial dosing should be based upon body weight (0.1 to 0.15 mg/kg per dose), with subsequent dosing titrated to achieve the desired clinical response. Dosing should not exceed 2.5 mg three to four times daily by nebulization. The following table outlines approximate dosing according to body weight.
[See table at top of previous page]
The appropriate volume of the 0.5% inhalation solution should be diluted in sterile normal saline solution to a total volume of 3 mL prior to administration via nebulization.
Adults and Children Over 12 Years of Age: The usual dosage for adults and children over 12 years of age is 2.5 mg of albuterol administered three to four times daily by nebulization. More frequent administration or higher doses are not recommended. To administer 2.5 mg of albuterol, dilute 0.5 mL of the 0.5% inhalation solution with 2.5 mL of sterile normal saline solution. The flow rate is regulated to suit the particular nebulizer so that VENTOLIN Inhalation Solution will be delivered over approximately 5 to 15 minutes.
The use of VENTOLIN Inhalation Solution can be continued as medically indicated to control recurring bouts of bronchospasm. During this time most patients gain optimal benefit from regular use of the inhalation solution.
If a previously effective dosage regimen fails to provide the usual relief, medical advice should be sought immediately as this is often a sign of seriously worsening asthma that would require reassessment of therapy.
Drug compatibility (physical and chemical), efficacy, and safety of VENTOLIN Inhalation Solution when mixed with other drugs in a nebulizer have not been established.

HOW SUPPLIED

VENTOLIN Inhalation Solution, 0.5% is supplied in amber glass bottles of 20 mL (NDC 0173-0385-58) with accompanying calibrated dropper in boxes of one.
Store between 2° and 25°C (36° and 77°F).
Glaxo Wellcome Inc., Research Triangle Park, NC 27709
September 1998/RL-634
Shown in Product Identification Guide, page 316

VENTOLIN ROTACAPS® ℞

[vent'ō-lin]
(albuterol sulfate, USP)
for Inhalation

FOR ORAL INHALATION ONLY
For Use with the ROTAHALER®
Inhalation Device

DESCRIPTION

VENTOLIN ROTACAPS for Inhalation contain a dry powder presentation of albuterol sulfate intended for oral inhalation only. Each light blue and clear, hard gelatin capsule contains a mixture of 200 mcg of microfine (95%≤10 µm) albuterol (as the sulfate) with 25 mg of lactose.
The contents of each capsule are inhaled using a specially designed plastic device for inhaling powder called the ROTAHALER®. When turned, this device opens the capsule and facilitates dispersion of the albuterol sulfate into the airstream created when the patient inhales through the mouthpiece.
VENTOLIN ROTACAPS for Inhalation are an alternative inhalation form of albuterol to the metered-dose pressurized inhaler.
The active component of VENTOLIN ROTACAPS for Inhalation is albuterol sulfate, USP, the racemic form of albuterol and a relatively selective beta$_2$-adrenergic bronchodilator. It has the chemical name α^1-[(*tert*-butylamino)methyl]-4-hydroxy-*m*-xylene-α,α'-diol sulfate (2:1)(salt).
Albuterol sulfate has a molecular weight of 576.7, and the empirical formula is $(C_{13}H_{21}NO_3)_2 \cdot H_2SO_4$. Albuterol sulfate is a white crystalline powder, soluble in water and slightly soluble in ethanol.
The World Health Organization recommended name for albuterol base is salbutamol.

CLINICAL PHARMACOLOGY

In vitro studies and in vivo pharmacologic studies have demonstrated that albuterol has a preferential effect on beta$_2$-adrenergic receptors compared with isoproterenol. While it is recognized that beta$_2$-adrenergic receptors are the predominant receptors in bronchial smooth muscle, data indicate that there is a population of beta$_2$-receptors in the human heart existing in a concentration between 10% and 50%. The precise function of these receptors has not been established (see WARNINGS).
The pharmacologic effects of beta-adrenergic agonist drugs, including albuterol, are at least in part attributable to stimulation through beta-adrenergic receptors of intracellular adenyl cyclase, the enzyme that catalyzes the conversion of adenosine triphosphate (ATP) to cyclic-3',5'-adenosine monophosphate (cyclic AMP). Increased cyclic AMP levels are associated with relaxation of bronchial smooth muscle and inhibition of release of mediators of immediate hypersensitivity from cells, especially from mast cells.
Albuterol has been shown in most controlled clinical trials to have more effect on the respiratory tract, in the form of bronchial smooth muscle relaxation, than isoproterenol at comparable doses while producing fewer cardiovascular effects. Controlled clinical studies and other clinical experience have shown that inhaled albuterol, like other beta-adrenergic agonist drugs, can produce a significant cardiovascular effect in some patients, as measured by pulse rate, blood pressure, symptoms, and/or electrocardiographic changes.
Albuterol is longer acting than isoproterenol in most patients by any route of administration because it is not a substrate for the normal cellular uptake processes for catecholamines nor for catechol-*O*-methyl transferase.
Pharmacokinetics: Studies undertaken with four subjects administered tritiated albuterol from a metered-dose aerosol inhaler resulted in maximum plasma concentrations occurring within 2 to 4 hours. Due to the sensitivity of the assay method, the metabolic rate and half-life elimination of albuterol in plasma could not be determined. However, urinary excretion provided data indicating that albuterol has an elimination half-life of 3.8 hours. Approximately 72% of the inhaled dose is excreted within 24 hours in the urine, and consists of 28% as unchanged drug and 44% as metabolite.
Preclinical: Intravenous studies in rats with albuterol sulfate have demonstrated that albuterol crosses the blood-brain barrier and reaches brain concentrations amounting to approximately 5.0% of the plasma concentrations. In structures outside the brain barrier (pineal and pituitary glands), albuterol concentrations were found to be 100 times those in the whole brain.
Studies in laboratory animals (minipigs, rodents, and dogs) have demonstrated the occurrence of cardiac arrhythmias and sudden death (with histologic evidence of myocardial necrosis) when beta-agonists and methylxanthines are administered concurrently. The clinical significance of these findings is unknown.
Clinical Trials: In single, dose-range, crossover trials with VENTOLIN ROTACAPS for Inhalation in patients 12 years of age and older, the onset of improvement in pulmonary function was within 5 minutes as determined by a 15% increase in forced expiratory volume in 1 second (FEV$_1$) following administration of either a 200- or 400-mcg dose. Maximum increases in FEV$_1$ occurred within 60 minutes following inhalation of either dose. The duration of effect (defined as an increase in FEV$_1$ of 15% or greater in a single-dose study) was 1 to 2 hours after the 200-mcg dose and 3 to 4 hours after the 400-mcg dose. In a single-dose study, an increase in forced expiratory flow rate between 25% and 75% of the forced vital capacity (FEF$_{25\%-75\%}$) of 20% or greater continued for 3 to 4 hours after the 200-mcg dose and for 3 to 6 hours following the 400-mcg dose. A therapeutic response continued for 4 hours in the majority of patients and for 6 hours in 38% of the patients following the 400-mcg dose. Twenty-two percent of the patients receiving the 200-mcg dose had a duration of effect of 8 hours.
In 12-week, double-blind, comparative evaluations in patients 12 years of age and older of one 200-mcg VENTOLIN ROTACAPS for Inhalation capsule versus two inhalations of VENTOLIN® (albuterol, USP) Inhalation Aerosol, the two dosage regimens were found to be clinically comparable. Based on a 15% or more increase in FEV$_1$ determinations, both provided a therapeutic response that persisted for 2 or 3 hours in 50% of 231 patients aged 12 years and older. Similar results were found in two controlled, 12-week clinical trials involving 204 children aged 4 to 11 years. Both formulations produced a therapeutic response (defined as maintenance of mean increase over baseline of at least 15% in FEV$_1$, or 20% in FEF$_{25\%-75\%}$). Therapeutic improvement of FEF$_{25\%-75\%}$ persisted for 3 to 5 hours in over 50% of the children throughout the study. Continued effectiveness and safety of VENTOLIN ROTACAPS for Inhalation were demonstrated over the 12-week study periods in both adults and children.
In other clinical studies in adults and children, one 200-mcg VENTOLIN ROTACAPS for Inhalation capsule taken approximately 15 minutes before exercise prevented exercise-induced bronchospasm, as demonstrated by the maintenance of FEV$_1$ within 80% of baseline values in the majority of patients. One study in adults also evaluated the duration of the prophylactic effect to repeated exercise challenges, which was evident at 4 hours in the majority of patients and at 6 hours in approximately one third of the patients.

INDICATIONS AND USAGE

VENTOLIN ROTACAPS for Inhalation are indicated for the prevention and relief of bronchospasm in patients 4 years of age and older with reversible obstructive airway disease and for the prevention of exercise-induced bronchospasm in patients 4 years of age and older. The VENTOLIN ROTACAPS for Inhalation formulation is particularly useful in patients who are unable to properly use the pressurized aerosol form of albuterol or who prefer an alternative formulation. VENTOLIN ROTACAPS for Inhalation can be used with or without concomitant steroid therapy.

CONTRAINDICATIONS

VENTOLIN ROTACAPS for Inhalation are contraindicated in patients with a history of hypersensitivity to albuterol or any of its components.

WARNINGS

Paradoxical Bronchospasm: VENTOLIN ROTACAPS for Inhalation can produce paradoxical bronchospasm, which may be life threatening. If paradoxical bronchospasm occurs, VENTOLIN ROTACAPS for Inhalation should be discontinued immediately and alternative therapy instituted.
Cardiovascular Effects: VENTOLIN ROTACAPS for Inhalation, like all other beta-adrenergic agonists, can produce a clinically significant cardiovascular effect in some patients as measured by pulse rate, blood pressure, and/or symptoms. Although such effects are uncommon after administration of VENTOLIN ROTACAPS for Inhalation at recommended doses, if they occur, the drug may need to be discontinued. In addition, beta-agonists have been reported to produce electrocardiogram (ECG) changes, such as flattening of the T wave, prolongation of the QT$_c$ interval, and ST segment depression. The clinical significance of these findings is unknown. Therefore, VENTOLIN ROTACAPS for Inhalation, like all sympathomimetic amines, should be used with caution in patients with cardiovascular disorders, especially coronary insufficiency, cardiac arrhythmias, and hypertension.
Deterioration of Asthma: Asthma may deteriorate acutely over a period of hours or chronically over several days or longer. If the patient needs more doses of VENTOLIN ROTACAPS for Inhalation than usual, this may be a marker of destabilization of asthma and requires reevaluation of the patient and treatment regimen, giving special consideration to the possible need for anti-inflammatory treatment, e.g., corticosteroids.
Immediate Hypersensitivity Reactions: Immediate hypersensitivity reactions may occur after administration of albuterol, as demonstrated by rare cases of urticaria, angioedema, rash, bronchospasm, anaphylaxis, and oropharyngeal edema.
Use of Anti-Inflammatory Agents: The use of beta-adrenergic agonist bronchodilators alone may not be adequate to control asthma in many patients. Early consideration

should be given to adding anti-inflammatory agents, e.g., corticosteroids.

Inhalation of capsule particles may result if damage to the capsule has occurred from handling by the patient.

PRECAUTIONS

General: Albuterol, as with all sympathomimetic amines, should be used with caution in patients with cardiovascular disorders, especially coronary insufficiency, hypertension, and cardiac arrhythmia; in patients with convulsive disorders, hyperthyroidism, or diabetes mellitus; and in patients who are unusually responsive to sympathomimetic amines. Clinically significant changes in systolic and diastolic blood pressure have been seen in individual patients and could be expected to occur in some patients after use of any beta-adrenergic bronchodilator. As with other beta-agonists, albuterol may produce significant hypokalemia in some patients, possibly through intracellular shunting, which has the potential to produce adverse cardiovascular effects. The decrease is usually transient, not requiring supplementation.

Information for Patients: The action of VENTOLIN ROTACAPS for Inhalation may last for up to 6 hours or longer. VENTOLIN ROTACAPS for Inhalation should not be used more frequently than recommended. Do not increase the dose or frequency of VENTOLIN ROTACAPS for Inhalation without consulting your physician. If you find that treatment with VENTOLIN ROTACAPS for Inhalation becomes less effective for symptomatic relief, your symptoms become worse, and/or you need to use the product more frequently than usual, you should seek medical attention immediately. While you are using VENTOLIN ROTACAPS for Inhalation, other inhaled drugs and asthma medications should be taken only as directed by your physician. Common adverse effects include palpitations, chest pain, rapid heart rate, and tremor or nervousness. If you are pregnant or nursing, contact your physician about use of VENTOLIN ROTACAPS for Inhalation. Effective and safe use of VENTOLIN ROTACAPS for Inhalation includes an understanding of the way that it should be administered. Children should use VENTOLIN ROTACAPS for Inhalation under adult supervision, as instructed by the patient's physician.

See illustrated Patient's Instructions for Use section of the full prescribing information.

Drug Interactions: Other short-acting sympathomimetic aerosol bronchodilators should not be used concomitantly with albuterol. If additional adrenergic drugs are to be administered by any route, they should be used with caution to avoid deleterious cardiovascular effects.

Monoamine Oxidase Inhibitors or Tricyclic Antidepressants: Albuterol should be administered with extreme caution to patients being treated with monoamine oxidase inhibitors or tricyclic antidepressants, or within 2 weeks of discontinuation of such agents, because the action of albuterol on the vascular system may be potentiated.

Beta-Blockers: Beta-adrenergic receptor blocking agents not only block the pulmonary effect of beta-agonists, such as VENTOLIN ROTACAPS for Inhalation, but may produce severe bronchospasm in asthmatic patients. Therefore, patients with asthma should not normally be treated with beta-blockers. However, under certain circumstances, e.g., as prophylaxis after myocardial infarction, there may be no acceptable alternatives to the use of beta-adrenergic blocking agents in patients with asthma. In this setting, cardioselective beta-blockers should be considered, although they could be administered with caution.

Diuretics: The ECG changes and/or hypokalemia that may result from the administration of nonpotassium-sparing diuretics (such as loop or thiazide diuretics) can be acutely worsened by beta-agonists, especially when the recommended dose of the beta-agonist is exceeded. Although the clinical significance of these effects is not known, caution is advised in the coadministration of beta-agonists with nonpotassium-sparing diuretics.

Digoxin: Mean decreases of 16% to 22% in serum digoxin levels were demonstrated after single-dose intravenous and oral administration of albuterol, respectively, to normal volunteers who had received digoxin for 10 days. The clinical significance of these findings for patients with obstructive airway disease who are receiving albuterol and digoxin on a chronic basis is unclear. Nevertheless, it would be prudent to carefully evaluate the serum digoxin levels in patients who are currently receiving digoxin and albuterol.

Carcinogenesis, Mutagenesis, Impairment of Fertility: In a 2-year study in Sprague-Dawley rats, albuterol sulfate caused a significant dose-related increase in the incidence of benign leiomyomas of the mesovarium at dietary doses of 2.0, 10, and 50 mg/kg (approximately 7, 35, and 170 times, respectively, the maximum recommended daily inhalation dose for adults on a mg/m^2 basis or approximately 3, 15, and 80 times, respectively, the maximum recommended daily inhalation dose in children on a mg/m^2 basis). In another study this effect was blocked by the coadministration of propranolol, a non-selective beta-adrenergic antagonist. In an 18-month study in CD-1 mice, albuterol sulfate showed no evidence of tumorigenicity at dietary doses of up to 500 mg/kg (approximately 850 times the maximum recommended daily inhalation dose for adults on a mg/m^2 basis or approximately 400 times the maximum recommended daily inhalation dose for children on a mg/m^2 basis). In a 22-month study in the Golden hamster, albuterol sulfate showed no evidence of tumorigenicity at dietary doses of up to 50 mg/kg (approximately 120 times the maximum recommended daily inhalation dose for adults on a mg/m^2 basis or approximately 55 times the maximum recommended daily inhalation dose for children on a mg/m^2 basis).

Albuterol sulfate was not mutagenic in the Ames test with or without metabolic activation using tester strains *S. typhimurium* TA1537, TA1538, and TA98 or *E. coli* WP2, WP2uvrA, and WP67. No forward mutation was seen in yeast strain *S. cerevisiae* S9 nor any mitotic gene conversion in yeast strain *S. cerevisiae* JD1 with or without metabolic activation. Fluctuation assays in *S. typhimurium* TA98 and *E. coli* WP2, both with metabolic activation, were negative. Albuterol sulfate was not clastogenic in a human peripheral lymphocyte assay or in an AH1 strain mouse micronucleus assay at intraperitoneal doses of up to 200 mg/kg.

Reproduction studies in rats demonstrated no evidence of impaired fertility at oral doses up to 50 mg/kg (approximately 170 times the maximum recommended daily inhalation dose for adults on a mg/m^2 basis).

Pregnancy: *Teratogenic Effects:* Pregnancy Category C. Albuterol has been shown to be teratogenic in mice. A study in CD-1 mice at subcutaneous doses of 0.025, 0.25, and 2.5 mg/kg (approximately 1/25, 2/5, and 4 times, respectively, the maximum recommended daily inhalation dose for adults on a mg/m^2 basis) showed cleft palate formation in 5 of 111 (4.5%) fetuses at 0.25 mg/kg and in 10 of 108 (9.3%) fetuses at 2.5 mg/kg. The drug did not induce cleft palate formation at the lowest dose, 0.025 mg/kg. Cleft palate also occurred in 22 of 72 (30.5%) fetuses from females treated with 2.5 mg/kg of isoproterenol (positive control) subcutaneously, approximately four times the maximum recommended daily inhalation dose for adults on a mg/m^2 basis.

A reproduction study in Stride Dutch rabbits revealed cranioschisis in 7 of 19 (37%) fetuses when albuterol was administered orally at a 50-mg/kg dose (approximately 340 times the maximum recommended daily inhalation dose for adults on a mg/m^2 basis).

There are no adequate and well-controlled studies in pregnant women. Albuterol should be used during pregnancy only if the potential benefit justifies the potential risk to the fetus.

During worldwide marketing experience, various congenital anomalies, including cleft palate and limb defects, have been rarely reported in the offspring of patients being treated with albuterol. Some of the mothers were taking multiple medications during their pregnancies. No consistent pattern of defects can be discerned, and a relationship between albuterol use and congenital anomalies has not been established.

Use in Labor and Delivery: Because of the potential for beta-agonist interference with uterine contractility, use of VENTOLIN ROTACAPS for Inhalation for relief of bronchospasm during labor should be restricted to those patients in whom the benefits clearly outweigh the risk.

Tocolysis: Albuterol has not been approved for the management of preterm labor. The benefit:risk ratio when albuterol is administered for tocolysis has not been established. Serious adverse reactions, including maternal pulmonary edema, have been reported during or following treatment of premature labor with beta$_2$-agonists, including albuterol.

Nursing Mothers: It is not known whether this drug is excreted in human milk after inhalation of recommended doses. Because of the potential for tumorigenicity shown for albuterol in some animal studies, a decision should be made whether to discontinue nursing or to discontinue the drug, taking into account the importance of the drug to the mother.

Pediatric Use: Safety and effectiveness in children below 4 years of age have not been established.

ADVERSE REACTIONS

The adverse reactions to albuterol are similar in nature to reactions to other sympathomimetic agents, although the incidence of certain cardiovascular effects is lower with albuterol. Results of clinical trials with VENTOLIN ROTACAPS® for Inhalation 200 mcg in 172 patients aged 12 years and older (adults) and 129 patients aged 4 to 12 years (children) are shown in the following tables:

Percent Incidence of Adverse Reactions in Patients ≥12 Years of Age

Reaction	Percent Incidence
Central nervous system	
Headache	2%
Nervousness	1%
Tremor	1%
Sleeplessness	<1%
Dizziness	<1%
Lightheadedness	<1%
Digestive system	
Throat irritation	2%
Burning in the stomach	<1%
Dry mouth	<1%
Bad taste	<1%
Respiratory system	
Coughing	5%
Bronchospasm	1%

Percent Incidence of Adverse Reactions in Children 4 to 12 Years of Age

Reaction	Percent Incidence
Central nervous system	
Headache	5%
Dizziness	<1%
Hyperactivity	<1%
Gastrointestinal	
Nausea and/or vomiting	4%
Stomachache	2%
Diarrhea	<1%
Respiratory system	
Epistaxis	2%
Hoarseness	2%
Nasal congestion	2%
Cough	2%
Oropharyngeal	
Throat irritation	2%
Unusual taste	2%

Cases of urticaria, angioedema, rash, bronchospasm, hoarseness, oropharyngeal edema, and arrhythmias (including atrial fibrillation, supraventricular tachycardia, extrasystoles) have been reported after the use of VENTOLIN ROTACAPS for Inhalation.

In addition, albuterol, like other sympathomimetic agents, can cause adverse reactions such as hypertension, angina, vertigo, and CNS stimulation.

OVERDOSAGE

The expected symptoms with overdosage are those of excessive beta-adrenergic stimulation and/or occurrence or exaggeration of any of the symptoms listed under ADVERSE REACTIONS, e.g., seizures, angina, hypertension or hypotension, tachycardia with rates up to 200 beats/min, arrhythmias, nervousness, headache, tremor, dry mouth, palpitation, nausea, dizziness, fatigue, malaise, and sleeplessness. Hypokalemia may also occur. As with all sympathomimetic medications, cardiac arrest and even death may be associated with abuse of VENTOLIN ROTACAPS for Inhalation. Treatment consists of discontinuation of VENTOLIN ROTACAPS for Inhalation together with appropriate symptomatic therapy. The judicious use of a cardioselective beta-receptor blocker may be considered, bearing in mind that such medication can produce bronchospasm. There is insufficient evidence to determine if dialysis is beneficial for overdosage of VENTOLIN ROTACAPS for Inhalation.

The oral median lethal dose of albuterol sulfate in mice is greater than 2000 mg/kg (approximately 3400 times the maximum recommended daily inhalation dose for adults on a mg/m^2 basis or approximately 1600 times the maximum recommended daily dose for children on a mg/m^2 basis). In mature rats, the subcutaneous median lethal dose of albuterol sulfate is approximately 450 mg/kg (approximately 1500 times the maximum recommended daily inhalation dose for adults on a mg/m^2 basis or approximately 700 times the maximum recommended daily dose for children on a mg/m^2 basis). In small young rats, the subcutaneous median lethal dose is approximately 2000 mg/kg (approximately 6800 times the maximum recommended daily inhalation dose for adults on a mg/m^2 basis or approximately 3200 times the maximum recommended daily inhalation dose for children on a mg/m^2 basis). The inhalational median lethal dose has not been determined in animals.

Dialysis is not appropriate treatment for overdosage of VENTOLIN ROTACAPS for Inhalation.

DOSAGE AND ADMINISTRATION

The usual dosage of VENTOLIN ROTACAPS for Inhalation for adults and children 4 years of age and older is the contents of one 200-mcg capsule inhaled every 4 to 6 hours using a ROTAHALER inhalation device. In some patients, the contents of two 200-mcg capsules inhaled every 4 to 6 hours may be required. Larger doses or more frequent administration is not recommended.

The use of VENTOLIN ROTACAPS for Inhalation can be continued as medically indicated to control recurring bouts of bronchospasm. During this time most patients gain optimal benefit from regular use of the VENTOLIN ROTACAPS for Inhalation formulation.

If a previously effective dosage regimen fails to provide the usual relief, medical advice should be sought immediately as this is often a sign of seriously worsening asthma that would require reassessment of therapy.

Exercise-Induced Bronchospasm Prevention: The usual dosage of VENTOLIN ROTACAPS for Inhalation for adults

Continued on next page

This product information is based on labeling in effect on June 23, 2000. For further information, contact via direct mail, phone, or web site. Medical Information, Glaxo Wellcome Inc., PO Box 13398, Research Triangle Park, NC 27709. Healthcare Professionals (Medical Information): 800-334-0089. Patients (Customer Response Center): 1-888-825-5249. Glaxo Wellcome Corporate Web Site: www.glaxowellcome.com

Ventolin Rotacaps—Cont.

and children 4 years of age and older is the contents of one 200-mcg capsule inhaled using a ROTAHALER 15 minutes before exercise.

HOW SUPPLIED

VENTOLIN ROTACAPS for Inhalation, 200 mcg, are light blue and clear, with "VENTOLIN 200" printed on the blue cap and "GLAXO" printed on the clear body.
VENTOLIN ROTACAPS for Inhalation are supplied in a kit containing one white plastic HDPE bottle of 100 capsules and one ROTAHALER inhalation device with patient's instructions (NDC 0173-0389-01). Also available, VENTOLIN ROTACAPS for Inhalation Refill in white plastic HDPE bottle of 100 capsules with patient's instructions (NDC 0173-0389-02).
Store between 2° and 30°C (36° and 86°F). Replace cap securely after each opening.

Glaxo Wellcome Inc., Research Triangle Park, NC 27709
November 1998/RL-648

Shown in Product Identification Guide, page 316

VENTOLIN® ℞
[*vent' ō-lin*]
(albuterol sulfate, USP)
Syrup

DESCRIPTION

VENTOLIN Syrup contains albuterol sulfate, USP, the racemic form of albuterol, a relatively selective beta$_2$-adrenergic bronchodilator. Albuterol sulfate has the chemical name α^1-[(*tert*-Butylamino)methyl]-4-hydroxy-*m*-xylene-α,α'-diol sulfate (2:1)(salt).
The molecular weight of albuterol sulfate is 576.7, and the empirical formula is $(C_{13}H_{21}NO_3)_2 \bullet H_2SO_4$. Albuterol sulfate is a white crystalline powder, soluble in water and slightly soluble in ethanol. The World Health Organization's recommended name for albuterol base is salbutamol.
VENTOLIN Syrup for oral administration contains 2 mg of albuterol as 2.4 mg of albuterol sulfate in each teaspoonful (5 mL). The inactive ingredients for VENTOLIN Syrup include: citric acid, USP anhydrous; FD&C Yellow No. 6; flavor strawberry artificial F-8636; hydroxypropyl methylcellulose 2906 or 2910, USP; saccharin, NF; sodium benzoate, NF; sodium citrate, USP dihydrate; and water purified, USP. The pH of the syrup is between 3.0 and 4.5.

CLINICAL PHARMACOLOGY

The primary action of beta-adrenergic drugs, including albuterol, is to stimulate adenyl cyclase, the enzyme which catalyzes the formation of cyclic-3',5'-adenosine monophosphate (cyclic AMP) from adenosine triphosphate (ATP) in beta-adrenergic cells. The cyclic AMP thus formed mediates the cellular responses. Increased cyclic AMP levels are associated with relaxation of bronchial smooth muscle and inhibition of release of mediators of immediate hypersensitivity from cells, especially from mast cells.
In vitro studies and *in vivo* pharmacologic studies have demonstrated that albuterol has a preferential effect on beta$_2$-adrenergic receptors compared with isoproterenol. While it is recognized that beta$_2$-adrenergic receptors are the predominant receptors in bronchial smooth muscle, data indicate that there is a population of beta$_2$-receptors in the human heart existing in a concentration between 10% and 50%. The precise function of these receptors has not been established.
In controlled clinical trials, albuterol has been shown to have more effect on the respiratory tract, in the form of bronchial smooth muscle relaxation, than isoproterenol at comparable doses, while producing fewer cardiovascular effects. Controlled clinical studies and other clinical experience have shown that inhaled albuterol, like other beta-adrenergic agonist drugs, can produce a significant cardiovascular effect in some patients, as measured by pulse rate, blood pressure, symptoms, and/or ECG changes.
Albuterol is longer acting than isoproterenol in most patients by any route of administration because it is not a substrate for the cellular uptake processes for catecholamines nor for catechol-*O*-methyl transferase.
Preclinical: Intravenous studies in rats with albuterol sulfate have demonstrated that albuterol crosses the blood-brain barrier and reaches brain concentrations that are amounting to approximately 5.0% of the plasma concentrations. In structures outside the blood-brain barrier (pineal and pituitary glands), albuterol concentrations were found to be 100 times those in the whole brain.
Studies in laboratory animals (minipigs, rodents, and dogs) have demonstrated the occurrence of cardiac arrhythmias and sudden death (with histologic evidence of myocardial necrosis) when beta-agonists and methylxanthines are administered concurrently. The clinical significance of these findings is unknown.
Pharmacokinetics: Albuterol is rapidly and well absorbed following oral administration. After oral administration of 10 mL of VENTOLIN Syrup (4 mg of albuterol) in normal volunteers, maximum plasma albuterol concentrations of about 18 ng/mL are achieved within 2 hours, and the drug is eliminated with a half-life of about 5 to 6 hours.
In other studies, the analysis of urine samples of patients given 8 mg of tritiated albuterol orally showed that 76% of the dose was excreted over 3 days, with the majority of the dose being excreted within the first 24 hours. Sixty percent of this radioactivity was shown to be the metabolite. Feces collected over this period contained 4% of the administered dose.
Clinical Trials: In controlled clinical trials in patients with asthma, the onset of improvement in pulmonary function, as measured by maximal midexpiratory flow rate (MMEF) and forced expiratory volume in 1 second (FEV$_1$), was within 30 minutes after a dose of VENTOLIN Syrup. Peak improvement of pulmonary function occurred between 2 and 3 hours. In a controlled clinical trial involving 55 children, clinically significant improvement (defined as maintenance of mean values over baseline of 15% or 20% or more in the FEV$_1$ and MMEF, respectively) continued to be recorded up to 6 hours. No decrease in the effectiveness was reported in one uncontrolled study of 32 children who took VENTOLIN Syrup for a 3-month period.

INDICATIONS AND USAGE

VENTOLIN Syrup is indicated for the relief of bronchospasm in adults and children 2 years of age and older with reversible obstructive airway disease.

CONTRAINDICATIONS

VENTOLIN Syrup is contraindicated in patients with a history of hypersensitivity to albuterol or any of its components.

WARNINGS

Deterioration of Asthma: Asthma may deteriorate acutely over a period of hours, or chronically over several days or longer. If the patient needs more doses of VENTOLIN Syrup than usual, this may be a marker of destabilization of asthma and requires re-evaluation of the patient and the treatment regimen, giving special consideration to the possible need for anti-inflammatory treatment, eg, corticosteroids.
Use of Anti-Inflammatory Agents: The use of beta-adrenergic agonist bronchodilators alone may not be adequate to control asthma in many patients. Early consideration should be given to adding anti-inflammatory agents, eg, corticosteroids.
Cardiovascular Effects: VENTOLIN Syrup, like all other beta-adrenergic agonists, can produce a clinically significant cardiovascular effect in some patients as measured by pulse rate, blood pressure, and/or symptoms. Although such effects are uncommon after administration of VENTOLIN Syrup at recommended doses, if they occur, the drug may need to be discontinued. In addition, beta-agonists have been reported to produce electrocardiogram (ECG) changes, such as flattening of the T wave, prolongation of the QTc interval, and ST segment depression. The clinical significance of these findings is unknown. Therefore, VENTOLIN Syrup, like all sympathomimetic amines, should be used with caution in patients with cardiovascular disorders, especially coronary insufficiency, cardiac arrhythmias, and hypertension.
Paradoxical Bronchospasm: VENTOLIN Syrup can produce paradoxical bronchospasm, which may be life threatening. If paradoxical bronchospasm occurs, VENTOLIN Syrup should be discontinued immediately and alternative therapy instituted.
Immediate Hypersensitivity Reactions: Immediate hypersensitivity reactions may occur after administration of albuterol, as demonstrated by rare cases of urticaria, angioedema, rash, bronchospasm, anaphylaxis, and oropharyngeal edema,.
Rarely, erythema multiforme and Stevens-Johnson syndrome have been associated with the administration of oral albuterol sulfate in children.

PRECAUTIONS

General: Albuterol, as with all sympathomimetic amines, should be used with caution in patients with cardiovascular disorders, especially coronary insufficiency, cardiac arrhythmias, and hypertension; in patients with convulsive disorders, hyperthyroidism, or diabetes mellitus; and in patients who are unusually responsive to sympathomimetic amines. Clinically significant changes in systolic and diastolic blood pressure have been seen and could be expected to occur in some patients after use of any beta-adrenergic bronchodilator.
Large doses of intravenous albuterol have been reported to aggravate preexisting diabetes and ketoacidosis. As with other beta-agonists, albuterol may produce significant hypokalemia in some patients, possibly through intracellular shunting, which has the potential to produce adverse cardiovascular effects. The decrease is usually transient, not requiring supplementation.
Information for Patients: The action of VENTOLIN Syrup may last up to 6 hours or longer. VENTOLIN Syrup should not be taken more frequently than recommended. Do not increase the dose or frequency of doses of VENTOLIN Syrup without consulting your physician. If you find that treatment with VENTOLIN Syrup becomes less effective for symptomatic relief, your symptoms become worse, and/or you need to take the product more frequently than usual, you should seek medical attention immediately. While you are taking VENTOLIN Syrup, other inhaled drugs and asthma medications should be taken only as directed by your physician. Common adverse effects include palpitations, chest pain, rapid heart rate, tremor, or nervousness. If you are pregnant or nursing, contact your physician about the use of VENTOLIN Syrup. Effective use of VENTOLIN Syrup includes an understanding of the way that it should be administered.
Drug Interactions: The concomitant use of VENTOLIN Syrup and other oral sympathomimetic agents is not recommended since such combined use may lead to deleterious cardiovascular effects. This recommendation does not preclude the judicious use of an aerosol bronchodilator of the adrenergic stimulant type in patients receiving VENTOLIN Syrup. Such concomitant use, however, should be individualized and not given on a routine basis. If regular coadministration is required, then alternative therapy should be considered.
Beta-Blockers: Beta-adrenergic receptor blocking agents not only block the pulmonary effect of beta-agonists, such as VENTOLIN Syrup, but may produce severe bronchospasm in asthmatic patients. Therefore, patients with asthma should not normally be treated with beta-blockers. However, under certain circumstances, eg, as prophylaxis after myocardial infarction, there may be no acceptable alternatives to the use of beta-adrenergic blocking agents in patients with asthma. In this setting, cardioselective beta-blockers could be considered, although they should be administered with caution.
Diuretics: The ECG changes and/or hypokalemia that may result from the administration of nonpotassium-sparing diuretics (such as loop or thiazide diuretics) can be acutely worsened by beta-agonists, especially when the recommended dose of the beta-agonist is exceeded. Although the clinical significance of these effects is not known, caution is advised in the coadministration of beta-agonists with nonpotassium-sparing diuretics.
Digoxin: Mean decreases of 16% to 22% in serum digoxin levels were demonstrated after single dose intravenous and oral administration of albuterol, respectively, to normal volunteers who had received digoxin for 10 days. The clinical significance of these findings for patients with obstructive airway disease who are receiving albuterol and digoxin on a chronic basis is unclear. Nevertheless, it would be prudent to carefully evaluate the serum digoxin levels in patients who are currently receiving digoxin and albuterol.
Monoamine Oxidase Inhibitors or Tricyclic Antidepressants: Albuterol should be administered with extreme caution to patients being treated with monoamine oxidase inhibitors or tricyclic antidepressants, or within 2 weeks of discontinuation of such agents, because the action of albuterol on the vascular system may be potentiated.
Carcinogenesis, Mutagenesis, and Impairment of Fertility: In a 2-year study in Sprague-Dawley rats, albuterol sulfate caused a significant dose-related increase in the incidence of benign leiomyomas of the mesovarium at and above dietary doses of 2 mg/kg (corresponding to less than the maximum recommended daily oral dose for adults and children on a mg/m^2 basis). In another study, this effect was blocked by the coadministration of propranolol, a nonselective beta-adrenergic antagonist.
In an 18-month study in CD-1 mice, albuterol sulfate showed no evidence of tumorigenicity at dietary doses up to 500 mg/kg (approximately 65 times the maximum recommended daily oral dose for adults on a mg/m^2 basis and approximately 50 times the maximum recommended daily oral dose for children on a mg/m^2 basis). In a 22-month study in the Golden hamster, albuterol sulfate showed no evidence of tumorigenicity at dietary doses up to 50 mg/kg (approximately 8 times the maximum recommended daily oral dose for adults and children on an mg/m^2 basis).
Albuterol sulfate was not mutagenic in the Ames test with or without metabolic activation using tester strains *S. typhimurium* TA1537, TA1538, and TA98 or *E. coli* WP2, WP2uvrA, and WP67. No forward mutation was seen in yeast strain *S. cerevisiae* S9 nor any mitotic gene conversion in yeast strain *S. cerevisiae* JD1 with or without metabolic activation. Fluctuation assays in *S. typhimurium* TA98 and *E. coli* WP2, both with metabolic activation, were negative. Albuterol sulfate was not clastogenic in a human peripheral lymphocyte assay or in an AH1 strain mouse micronucleus assay.
Reproduction studies in rats demonstrated no evidence of impaired fertility at oral doses of albuterol sulfate up to 50 mg/kg (approximately 15 times the maximum recommended daily oral dose for adults on a mg/m^2 basis).
Teratogenic Effects—Pregnancy Category C: Albuterol sulfate has been shown to be teratogenic in mice. A study in CD-1 mice at subcutaneous (sc) doses at and above 0.25 mg/kg (corresponding to less than the maximum recommended daily oral dose for adults on an mg/m^2 basis), induced cleft palate formation in 5 of 111 (4.5%) fetuses. At an sc dose of 2.5 mg/kg (corresponding to less than the maximum recommended daily oral dose for adults on an mg/m^2 basis), albuterol sulfate induced cleft palate formation in 10 of 108 (9.3%) fetuses. The drug did not induce cleft palate formation when administered at an sc dose of 0.025 mg/kg (significantly less than the maximum recommended daily oral dose for adults on an mg/m^2 basis). Cleft palate also occurred in 22 of 72 (30.5%) fetuses from females treated with 2.5 mg/kg of isoproterenol (positive control) administered subcutaneously.
A reproduction study in Stride Dutch rabbits revealed cranioschisis in 7 of 19 (37%) fetuses when albuterol was administered orally at a dose of 50 mg/kg (approximately 25 times the maximum recommended daily oral dose for adults on an mg/m^2 basis).
Studies in pregnant rats with tritiated albuterol demonstrated that approximately 10% of the circulating maternal

drug is transferred to the fetus. Disposition in the fetal lungs is comparable to maternal lungs, but fetal liver disposition is 1% of the maternal liver levels.

There are no adequate and well-controlled studies in pregnant women. Because animal reproduction studies are not always predictive of human response, albuterol should be used during pregnancy only if the potential benefit justifies the potential risk to the fetus.

During worldwide marketing experience, various congenital anomalies, including cleft palate and limb defects, have been reported in the offspring of patients being treated with albuterol. Some of the mothers were taking multiple medications during their pregnancies. Because no consistent pattern of defects can be discerned, a relationship between albuterol use and congenital anomalies has not been established.

Use in Labor and Delivery—Use in Labor: Because of the potential for beta-agonist interference with uterine contractility, use of VENTOLIN Syrup for relief of bronchospasm during labor should be restricted to those patients in whom the benefits clearly outweigh the risk.

Tocolysis: Albuterol has not been approved for the management of preterm labor. The benefit:risk ratio when albuterol is administered for tocolysis has not been established. Serious adverse reactions, including maternal pulmonary edema, have been reported during or following treatment of premature labor with beta$_2$-agonists, including albuterol.

Nursing Mothers: It is not known whether this drug is excreted in human milk. Because of the potential for tumorigenicity shown for albuterol in some animal studies, a decision should be made whether to discontinue nursing or to discontinue the drug, taking into account the importance of the drug to the mother.

Pediatric Use: Safety and effectiveness in children below the age of 2 years have not been established.

ADVERSE REACTIONS

The adverse reactions to albuterol are similar in nature to those of other sympathomimetic agents. In clinical trials, the most frequent adverse reactions to VENTOLIN Syrup in adults and older children were:

Percent Incidence of Adverse Reactions in Adults and Children (6–12 Years of Age)

Adverse Event	Percent Incidence
Central Nervous System	
Tremor	10
Nervousness	9
Shakiness	9
Headache	4
Dizziness	3
Excitement	2
Hyperactivity	2
Sleeplessness	1
Disturbed sleep	<1
Irritable behavior	<1
Dilated pupils	<1
Weakness	1
Cardiovascular	
Tachycardia	1
Palpitations	<1
Sweating	<1
Chest Pain	<1
Ear, Nose, and Throat	
Epistaxis	1
Gastrointestinal	
Increased appetite	3
Epigastric pain	<1
Stomachache	<1
Musculoskeletal	
Muscle spasm	<1
Respiratory	
Cough	<1

In clinical trials, the following adverse reactions to VENTOLIN Syrup were noted more frequently in young children 2 to 6 years of age than in adults and older children:

Percent Incidence of Adverse Reactions Noted More Frequently in Children 2 to 6 Years of Age Than in Older Children and Adults

Adverse Event	Percent Incidence
Central Nervous System	
Excitement	20
Nervousness	15
Hypokinesia	4
Sleeplessness	2
Emotional lability	1
Fatigue	1
Cardiovascular	
Tachycardia	2
Pallor	1
Gastrointestinal	
Gastrointestinal symptoms	2
Loss of appetite	1
Ophthalmologic	
Conjunctivitis	1

Cases of urticaria, angioedema, rash, bronchospasm, oropharyngeal edema, and arrhythmias (including atrial fibrillation, supraventricular tachycardia, and extrasystoles) have been reported after the use of VENTOLIN Syrup.

In addition, albuterol, like other sympathomimetic agents, can cause adverse reactions such as angina, central nervous system stimulation, drying or irritation of the oropharynx, hypertension, nausea, unusual taste, vertigo, and vomiting. The reactions are generally transient in nature, and it is usually not necessary to discontinue treatment with VENTOLIN Syrup. In selected cases, however, dosage may be reduced temporarily; after the reaction has subsided, dosage should be increased in small increments to the optimal dosage.

OVERDOSAGE

The expected symptoms with overdosage are those of excessive beta-adrenergic stimulation and/or occurrence or exaggeration of any of the symptoms listed under **ADVERSE REACTIONS**, eg, angina, hypertension, tachycardia with rates up to 200 beats per minute, nervousness, headache, tremor, dry mouth, palpitation, nausea, dizziness, fatigue, and insomnia. In addition, seizures, hypotension, arrhythmias, malaise, and hypokalemia may also occur. As with all sympathomimetic medications, cardiac arrest and even death may be associated with abuse of VENTOLIN Syrup. Treatment consists of discontinuation of VENTOLIN Syrup together with appropriate symptomatic therapy. The judicious use of a cardioselective beta-receptor blocker may be considered, bearing in mind that such medication can produce bronchospasm. There is insufficient evidence to determine if dialysis is beneficial for overdosage of VENTOLIN Syrup.

The oral median lethal dose of albuterol sulfate in mice is greater than 2000 mg/kg (approximately 250 times the maximum recommended daily oral dose for adults on an mg/m^2 basis and approximately 200 times the maximum recommended daily oral dose for children on an mg/m^2 basis). In mature rats, the subcutaneous (sc) median lethal dose of albuterol sulfate is approximately 450 mg/kg (approximately 110 times the maximum recommended daily oral dose for adults on an mg/m^2 basis and approximately 90 times the maximum recommended daily oral dose for children on an mg/m^2 basis). In small young rats, the sc median lethal dose is approximately 2000 mg/kg (approximately 510 times the maximum recommended daily oral dose for adults on an mg/m^2 basis and approximately 400 times the maximum recommended daily oral dose for children on an mg/m^2 basis).

DOSAGE AND ADMINISTRATION

The following dosages of VENTOLIN Syrup are expressed in terms of albuterol base:

Usual Dose

Adults and pediatric patients over 12 years of age: The usual starting dosage for adults and children over 12 years of age is 2 mg (1 teaspoonful) or 4 mg (2 teaspoonfuls) three or four times a day.

Pediatric patients 6 to 12 years of age: The usual starting dosage for children 6 to 12 years of age is 2 mg (1 teaspoonful) three or four times a day.

Pediatric patients 2 to 6 years of age: Dosing in children 2 to 6 years of age should be initiated at 0.1 mg/kg of body weight three times a day. The starting dosage should not exceed 2 mg (1 teaspoonful) three times a day.

Dosage Adjustment

Adults and pediatric patients over 12 years of age: For adults and children over 12 years of age, a dosage above 4 mg four times a day should be used *only* when the patient fails to respond to this dosage. If a favorable response does not occur with the 4 mg initial dosage, it may be cautiously increased stepwise as tolerated, but not to exceed 8 mg four times a day (total daily dose should not exceed 32 mg).

Pediatric patients 6 to 12 years of age who fail to respond to the initial starting dosage of 2 mg four times a day: For children 6 to 12 years of age who fail to respond to the initial starting dosage of 2 mg four times a day, the dosage may be cautiously increased stepwise as tolerated but not to exceed 6 mg four times a day (total daily dose should not exceed 24 mg).

Pediatric patients 2 to 6 years of age who do not respond satisfactorily to the initial dosage: For children 2 to 6 years of age who do not respond satisfactorily to the initial starting dosage, the dosage may be increased stepwise to 0.2 mg/kg of body weight three times a day as tolerated, but not to exceed a maximum of 4 mg (2 teaspoonfuls) given three times a day (total daily dose should not exceed 12 mg).

Elderly patients and those sensitive to beta-adrenergic stimulators: The initial dosage should be restricted to 2 mg three or four times a day. If adequate bronchodilation is not obtained, dosage may be increased gradually as tolerated to as much as 8 mg three or four times per day (total daily dose should not exceed 32 mg).

HOW SUPPLIED

VENTOLIN Syrup, a clear orange-yellow liquid with a strawberry flavor, contains 2 mg albuterol as the sulfate per 5 mL; amber glass bottles of 16 fluid ounces (NDC 0173-0351-54).

Store between 2° and 30°C (36° and 86°F). Dispense in tight, light-resistant containers as defined in the USP/NF.

Manufactured for Glaxo Wellcome Inc.,
Research Triangle Park, NC 27709
by Schering Corporation, Kenilworth, NJ 07033 USA
November 1998/RL-788

Shown in Product Identification Guide, page 316

WELLBUTRIN® ℞

[*wel 'byü-trin*]
(bupropion hydrochloride)
Tablets

DESCRIPTION

WELLBUTRIN (bupropion hydrochloride), an antidepressant of the aminoketone class, is chemically unrelated to tricyclic, tetracyclic, or other known antidepressant agents. Its structure closely resembles that of diethylpropion; it is related to phenylethylamines. It is designated as (±)-1-(3-chlorophenyl)-2-[(1,1-dimethylethyl)amino]-1-propanone hydrochloride. The molecular weight is 276.2. The empirical formula is $C_{13}H_{18}ClNO \bullet HCl$. Bupropion hydrochloride powder is white, crystalline, and highly soluble in water. It has a bitter taste and produces the sensation of local anesthesia on the oral mucosa.

WELLBUTRIN is supplied for oral administration as 75-mg (yellow-gold) and 100-mg (red) film-coated tablets. Each tablet contains the labeled amount of bupropion hydrochloride and the inactive ingredients: 75-mg tablet—D&C Yellow No. 10 Lake, FD&C Yellow No. 6 Lake, hydroxypropyl cellulose, hydroxypropyl methylcellulose, microcrystalline cellulose, polyethylene glycol, talc, and titanium dioxide; 100-mg tablet—FD&C Red No. 40 Lake, FD&C Yellow No. 6 Lake, hydroxypropyl cellulose, hydroxypropyl methylcellulose, microcrystalline cellulose, polyethylene glycol, talc, and titanium dioxide.

CLINICAL PHARMACOLOGY

Pharmacodynamics: The neurochemical mechanism of the antidepressant effect of bupropion is not known. Bupropion does not inhibit monoamine oxidase. Compared to classical tricyclic antidepressants, it is a weak blocker of the neuronal uptake of serotonin and norepinephrine; it also inhibits the neuronal re-uptake of dopamine to some extent.

Bupropion produces dose-related central nervous system (CNS) stimulant effects in animals, as evidenced by increased locomotor activity, increased rates of responding in various schedule-controlled operant behavior tasks, and, at high doses, induction of mild stereotyped behavior.

Bupropion causes convulsions in rodents and dogs at doses approximately tenfold the dose recommended as the human antidepressant dose.

Pharmacokinetics: In humans, following oral administration of WELLBUTRIN, peak plasma bupropion concentrations are usually achieved within 2 hours, followed by a biphasic decline. The average half-life of the second (postdistributional) phase is approximately 14 hours, with a range of 8 to 24 hours. Six hours after a single dose, plasma bupropion concentrations are approximately 30% of peak concentrations. Plasma bupropion concentrations are dose-proportional following single doses of 100 to 250 mg; however, it is not known if the proportionality between dose and plasma level is maintained in chronic use.

In vitro tests show that bupropion is 80% or more bound to human albumin at plasma concentrations up to 800 µmol/L (200 mcg/mL).

The absolute bioavailability of WELLBUTRIN Tablets in humans has not been determined because an intravenous formulation for human use is not available.

However, it appears likely that only a small proportion of any orally administered dose reaches the systemic circulation intact. For example, the absolute bioavailability of bupropion in animals (rats and dogs) ranges from 5% to 20%.

Metabolism: Following oral administration of 200 mg of ^{14}C-bupropion, 87% and 10% of the radioactive dose were recovered in the urine and feces, respectively. However, the fraction of the oral dose of WELLBUTRIN excreted unchanged was only 0.5%, a finding documenting the extensive metabolism of bupropion.

Several of the known metabolites of bupropion are pharmacologically active, but their potency and toxicity relative to bupropion have not been fully characterized. However, because of their longer elimination half-lives, the plasma concentrations of at least two of the known metabolites can be expected, especially in chronic use, to be very much higher than the plasma concentration of bupropion. This is of potential clinical importance because factors or conditions altering metabolic capacity (e.g., liver disease, congestive heart failure, age, concomitant medications, etc.) or elimination may be expected to influence the degree and extent of accumulation of these active metabolites.

Furthermore, bupropion has been shown to induce its own metabolism in three animal species (mice, rats, and dogs) following subchronic administration. If induction also occurs in humans, the relative contribution of bupropion and its metabolites to the clinical effects of WELLBUTRIN may be changed in chronic use.

Plasma and urinary metabolites so far identified include biotransformation products formed via reduction of the carbonyl group and/or hydroxylation of the *tert*-butyl group of bupropion. Four basic metabolites have been identified.

They are the *erythro-* and *threo-*amino alcohols of bupropion, the *erythro-*amino diol of bupropion, and hydroxybupropion.

Hydroxybupropion appears in the systemic circulation almost as rapidly as the parent drug following a single oral dose. Its peak level is three times the peak level of the parent drug; it has a half-life on the order of 24 hours; and its AUC 0 to 60 hours is about 15 times that of bupropion.

Continued on next page

This product information is based on labeling in effect on June 23, 2000. For further information, contact via direct mail, phone, or web site. Medical Information, Glaxo Wellcome Inc., PO Box 13398, Research Triangle Park, NC 27709. Healthcare Professionals (Medical Information): 800-334-0089. Patients (Customer Response Center): 1-888-825-5249. Glaxo Wellcome Corporate Web Site: www.glaxowellcome.com.

Wellbutrin—Cont.

The *threo*-amino alcohol metabolite has a plasma concentration-time profile similar to that of hydroxybupropion. The *erythro*-amino alcohol and the *erythro*-amino diol metabolites generally cannot be detected in the systemic circulation following a single oral dose of the parent drug. Hydroxybupropion and the *threo*-amino alcohol metabolites have been found to be half as potent as bupropion in animal screening tests for antidepressant drugs.

In vitro findings suggest that cytochrome P450IIB6 (CYP2B6) is the principal isoenzyme involved in the formation of hydroxybupropion, while cytochrome P450 isoenzymes are not involved in the formation of the *threo*-amino alcohol metabolite.

Because bupropion is extensively metabolized, there is the potential for drug-drug interactions, particularly with those agents that are metabolized by the cytochrome P450IIB6 (CYP2B6) isoenzyme. Although bupropion is not metablized by cytochrome P450IID6 (CYP2D6), there is the potential for drug-drug interactions when bupropion is co-administered with drugs metabolized by this isoenzyme (see PRECAUTIONS: Drug Interactions).

Populations Subgroups: Factors or conditions altering metabolic capacity (e.g., liver disease, congestive heart failure [CHF], age, concomitant medications, etc.) or elimination may be expected to influence the degree and extent of accumulation of the active metabolites of bupropion. The elimination of the major metabolites of bupropion may be affected by reduced renal or hepatic function because they are moderately polar compounds and are likely to undergo further metabolism or conjugation in the liver prior to urinary excretion.

Hepatic: The effect of hepatic impairment on the pharmacokinetics of bupropion was characterized in two single-dose studies, one in patients with alcoholic liver disease and one in patients with mild to severe cirrhosis. The first study showed that the half-life of hydroxybupropion was significantly longer in 8 patients with alcoholic liver disease than in 8 healthy volunteers (32±14 hours versus 21±5 hours, respectively). Although not statistically significant, the AUCs for bupropion and hydroxybupropion were more variable and tended to be greater (by 53% to 57%) in volunteers with alcoholic liver disease. The differences in half-life for bupropion and the other metabolites in the two patient groups were minimal.

The second study showed that there were no statistically significant differences in the pharmacokinetics of bupropion and its active metabolites in 9 patients with mild to moderate hepatic cirrhosis compared to 8 healthy volunteers. There was, however, more variability observed in some of the pharmacokinetic parameters for bupropion (AUC, C_{max}, and T_{max}) and its active metabolites ($t_{1/2}$) in patients with mild to moderate hepatic cirrhosis. In addition, in patients with severe hepatic cirrhosis, the bupropion C_{max} and AUC were substantially increased (mean difference: by approximately 70% and 3-fold, respectively) and more variable when compared to values in healthy volunteers; the mean bupropion half-life was also longer (by approximately 40%). For the metabolites, the mean C_{max} was lower (by approximately 30% to 70%), the mean AUC tended to be higher (by approximately 30% to 50%), the median T_{max} was later (by approximately 20 hours), and the mean half-lives were longer (by approximately 2- to 4-fold) in patients with severe hepatic cirrhosis than in healthy volunteers (see WARNINGS, PRECAUTIONS, and DOSAGE AND ADMINISTRATION).

Renal: The effect of renal disease on the pharmacokinetics of bupropion has not been studied. The elimination of the major metabolites of bupropion may be affected by reduced renal function.

Left Ventricular Dysfunction: During a chronic dosing study in 14 depressed patients with left ventricular dysfunction, it was found that there was substantial interpatient variability (twofold to fivefold) in the trough steady-state concentrations of bupropion, hydroxybupropion, and *threo*-amino alcohol metabolites. In addition, the steady-state plasma concentrations of these metabolites were 10 to 100 times the steady-state concentrations of the parent drug.

Age: The effects of age on the pharmacokinetics of bupropion and its metabolites have not been fully characterized, but an exploration of steady-state bupropion concentrations from several depression efficacy studies involving patients dosed in a range of 300 to 750 mg/day, on a three times daily schedule, revealed no relationship between age (18 to 83 years) and plasma concentration of bupropion. A single-dose pharmacokinetic study demonstrated that the disposition of bupropion and its metabolites in elderly subjects was similar to that of younger subjects. These data suggest there is no prominent effect of age on bupropion concentration; however, another pharmacokinetic study, single and multiple dose, has suggested that the elderly are at increased risk for accumulation of bupropion and its metabolites (see PRECAUTIONS: Geriatric Use).

INDICATIONS AND USAGE

WELLBUTRIN is indicated for the treatment of depression.

A physician considering WELLBUTRIN for the management of a patient's first episode of depression should be aware that the drug may cause generalized seizures in a dose-dependent manner with an approximate incidence of 0.4% (4/1000). This incidence of seizures may exceed that of other marketed antidepressants by as much as fourfold. This relative risk is only an approximate estimate because no direct comparative studies have been conducted (see WARNINGS).

The efficacy of WELLBUTRIN has been established in three placebo-controlled trials, including two of approximately 3 weeks' duration in depressed inpatients and one of approximately 6 weeks' duration in depressed outpatients. The depressive disorder of the patients studied corresponds most closely to the Major Depression category of the APA Diagnostic and Statistical Manual III.

Major Depression implies a prominent and relatively persistent depressed or dysphoric mood that usually interferes with daily functioning (nearly every day for at least 2 weeks); it should include at least four of the following eight symptoms: change in appetite, change in sleep, psychomotor agitation or retardation, loss of interest in usual activities or decrease in sexual drive, increased fatigability, feelings of guilt or worthlessness, slowed thinking or impaired concentration, and suicidal ideation or attempts.

Effectiveness of WELLBUTRIN in long-term use, that is, for more than 6 weeks, has not been systematically evaluated in controlled trials. Therefore, the physician who elects to use WELLBUTRIN for extended periods should periodically reevaluate the long-term usefulness of the drug for the individual patient.

CONTRAINDICATIONS

WELLBUTRIN is contraindicated in patients with a seizure disorder.

WELLBUTRIN is contraindicated in patients treated with ZYBAN® (bupropion hydrochloride) Sustained-Release Tablets, or any other medications that contain bupropion because the incidence of seizure is dose dependent.

WELLBUTRIN is also contraindicated in patients with a current or prior diagnosis of bulimia or anorexia nervosa because of a higher incidence of seizures noted in such patients treated with WELLBUTRIN.

The concurrent administration of WELLBUTRIN and a monoamine oxidase (MAO) inhibitor is contraindicated. At least 14 days should elapse between discontinuation of an MAO inhibitor and initiation of treatment with WELLBUTRIN.

WELLBUTRIN is contraindicated in patients who have shown an allergic response to bupropion or the other ingredients that make up WELLBUTRIN Tablets.

WARNINGS

Patients should be made aware that WELLBUTRIN contains the same active ingredient found in ZYBAN, used as an aid to smoking cessation treatment, and that WELLBUTRIN should not be used in combination with ZYBAN, or any other medications that contain bupropion.

Seizures: Bupropion is associated with seizures in approximately 0.4% (4/1000) of patients treated at doses up to 450 mg/day. This incidence of seizures may exceed that of other marketed antidepressants by as much as fourfold. This relative risk is only an approximate estimate because no direct comparative studies have been conducted. The estimated seizure incidence for WELLBUTRIN increases almost tenfold between 450 and 600 mg/day, which is twice the usually required daily dose (300 mg) and one and one-third the maximum recommended daily dose (450 mg). Given the wide variability among individuals and their capacity to metabolize and eliminate drugs this disproportionate increase in seizure incidence with dose incrementation calls for caution in dosing.

During the initial development, 25 among approximately 2400 patients treated with WELLBUTRIN experienced seizures. At the time of seizure, seven patients were receiving daily doses of 450 mg or below for an incidence of 0.33% (3/1000) within the recommended dose range. Twelve patients experienced seizures at 600 mg/day (2.3% incidence); six additional patients had seizures at daily doses between 600 and 900 mg (2.8% incidence).

A separate, prospective study was conducted to determine the incidence of seizure during an 8-week treatment exposure in approximately 3200 additional patients who received daily doses of up to 450 mg. Patients were permitted to continue treatment beyond 8 weeks if clinically indicated. Eight seizures occurred during the initial 8-week treatment period and five seizures were reported in patients continuing treatment beyond 8 weeks, resulting in a total seizure incidence of 0.4%.

The risk of seizure appears to be strongly associated with dose. Sudden and large increments in dose may contribute to increased risk. While many seizures occurred early in the course of treatment, some seizures did occur after several weeks at fixed dose.

The risk of seizure is also related to patient factors, clinical situations, and concomitant medications, which must be considered in selection of patients for therapy with WELLBUTRIN.

- **Patient factors: Predisposing factors that may increase the risk of seizure with bupropion use include history of head trauma or prior seizure, CNS tumor, the presence of severe hepatic cirrhosis, and concomitant medications that lower seizure threshold.**
- **Clinical situations: Circumstances associated with an increased seizure risk include, among others, excessive use of alcohol; abrupt withdrawal from alcohol or other sedatives; addiction to opiates, cocaine, or stimulants; use of over-the-counter stimulants and anorectics; and diabetes treated with oral hypoglycemics or insulin.**
- **Concomitant medications: Many medications (e.g., antipsychotics, antidepressants, theophylline, systemic steroids) and treatment regimens (e.g., abrupt discontinuation of benzodiazepines) are known to lower seizure threshold.**

Recommendations for Reducing the Risk of Seizure: **Retrospective analysis of clinical experience gained during the development of WELLBUTRIN suggests that the risk of seizure may be minimized if**

- **the total daily dose of WELLBUTRIN does *not* exceed 450 mg,**
- **the daily dose is administered three times daily, with each single dose *not* to exceed 150 mg to avoid high peak concentrations of bupropion and/or its metabolites, and**
- **the rate of incrementation of dose is very gradual.**

Extreme caution should be used when WELLBUTRIN is administered to patients with a history of seizure, cranial trauma, or other predisposition(s) toward seizure, or prescribed with other agents (e.g., antipsychotics, other antidepressants, theophylline, systemic steroids, etc.) or treatment regimens (e.g., abrupt discontinuation of a benzodiazepine) that lower seizure threshold.

Hepatic Impairment: WELLBUTRIN should be used with extreme caution in patients with severe hepatic cirrhosis. In these patients a reduced dose and frequency is required, as peak bupropion levels are substantially increased and accumulation is likely to occur in such patients to a greater extent than usual. The dose should not exceed 75 mg once a day in these patients (see CLINICAL PHARMACOLOGY, PRECAUTIONS, and DOSAGE AND ADMINISTRATION).

Potential for Hepatotoxicity: In rats receiving large doses of bupropion chronically, there was an increase in incidence of hepatic hyperplastic nodules and hepatocellular hypertrophy. In dogs receiving large doses of bupropion chronically, various histologic changes were seen in the liver, and laboratory tests suggesting mild hepatocellular injury were noted.

PRECAUTIONS

General: ***Agitation and Insomnia:*** A substantial proportion of patients treated with WELLBUTRIN experience some degree of increased restlessness, agitation, anxiety, and insomnia, especially shortly after initiation of treatment. In clinical studies, these symptoms were sometimes of sufficient magnitude to require treatment with sedative/hypnotic drugs. In approximately 2% of patients, symptoms were sufficiently severe to require discontinuation of treatment with WELLBUTRIN.

Psychosis, Confusion, and Other Neuropsychiatric Phenomena: Patients treated with WELLBUTRIN have been reported to show a variety of neuropsychiatric signs and symptoms including delusions, hallucinations, psychotic episodes, confusion, and paranoia. Because of the uncontrolled nature of many studies, it is impossible to provide a precise estimate of the extent of risk imposed by treatment with WELLBUTRIN. In several cases, neuropsychiatric phenomena abated upon dose reduction and/or withdrawal of treatment.

Activation of Psychosis and/or Mania: Antidepressants can precipitate manic episodes in Bipolar Manic Depressive patients during the depressed phase of their illness and may activate latent psychosis in other susceptible patients. WELLBUTRIN is expected to pose similar risks.

Altered Appetite and Weight: A weight loss of greater than 5 lbs occurred in 28% of patients receiving WELLBUTRIN. This incidence is approximately double that seen in comparable patients treated with tricyclics or placebo. Furthermore, while 34.5% of patients receiving tricyclic antidepressants gained weight, only 9.4% of patients treated with WELLBUTRIN did. Consequently, if weight loss is a major presenting sign of a patient's depressive illness, the anorectic and/or weight reducing potential of WELLBUTRIN should be considered.

Suicide: The possibility of a suicide attempt is inherent in depression and may persist until significant remission occurs. Accordingly, prescriptions for WELLBUTRIN should be written for the smallest number of tablets consistent with good patient management.

Allergic Reactions: Anaphylactoid/anaphylactic reactions characterized by symptoms such as pruritus, urticaria, angioedema, and dyspnea requiring medical treatment have been reported in clinical trials with bupropion. In addition, there have been rare spontaneous postmarketing reports of erythema multiforme, Stevens-Johnson syndrome, and anaphylactic shock associated with bupropion. A patient should stop taking WELLBUTRIN and consult a doctor if experiencing allergic or anaphylactoid/anaphylactic reactions (e.g., skin rash, pruritus, hives, chest pain, edema, and shortness of breath) during treatment.

Arthralgia, myalgia, and fever with rash and other symptoms suggestive of delayed hypersensitivity have been reported in association with bupropion. These symptoms may resemble serum sickness.

Cardiovascular Effects: In clinical practice, hypertension, in some cases severe, requiring acute treatment, has been reported in patients receiving bupropion alone and in combination with nicotine replacement therapy. These events have been observed in both patients with and without evidence of preexisting hypertension.

Data from a comparative study of the sustained-release formulation of bupropion (ZYBAN® Sustained-Release Tablets), nicotine transdermal system (NTS), the combination of sustained-release buproprion plus NTS, and placebo as an aid to smoking cessation suggest a higher incidence of treatment-emergent hypertension in patients treated with the combination of sustained-release bupropion and NTS. In this study, 6.1% of patients treated with the combination of sustained-release bupropion and NTS had treatment-emergent hypertension compared to 2.5%, 1.6%, and 3.1% of patients treated with sustained-release bupropion, NTS, and placebo, respectively. The majority of these patients had evidence of preexisting hypertension. Three patients (1.2%) treated with the combination of ZYBAN and NTS and one patient (0.4%) treated with NTS had study medication discontinued due to hypertension compared to none of the patients treated with ZYBAN or placebo. Monitoring of blood pressure is recommended in patients who receive the combination of bupropion and nicotine replacement.

There is no clinical experience establishing the safety of WELLBUTRIN in patients with a recent history of myocardial infarction or unstable heart disease. Therefore, care should be exercised if it is used in these groups. Bupropion was well tolerated in depressed patients who had previously developed orthostatic hypotension while receiving tricyclic antidepressants and was also generally well tolerated in a group of 36 depressed inpatients with stable congestive heart failure (CHF). However, bupropion was associated with a rise in supine blood pressure in the study of patients with CHF, resulting in discontinuation of treatment in two patients for exacerbation of baseline hypertension.

Hepatic Impairment: WELLBUTRIN should be used with extreme caution in patients with severe hepatic cirrhosis. In these patients, a reduced dose and frequency is required. WELLBUTRIN should be used with caution in patients with hepatic impairment (including mild to moderate hepatic cirrhosis) and a reduced frequency and/or dose should be considered in patients with mild to moderate hepatic cirrhosis.

All patients with hepatic impairment should be closely monitored for possible adverse effects that could indicate high drug and metabolite levels (see CLINICAL PHARMACOLOGY, WARNINGS, and DOSAGE AND ADMINISTRATION).

Renal Impairment: No studies have been conducted in patients with renal impairment. Bupropion is extensively metabolized in the liver to active metabolites, which are further metabolized and excreted by the kidneys. WELLBUTRIN should be used with caution in patients with renal impairment and a reduced frequency and/or dose should be considered as bupropion and its metabolites may accumulate in such patients to a greater extent than usual. The patient should be closely monitored for possible adverse effects that could indicate high drug or metabolite levels.

Information for Patients: Patients should be made aware that WELLBUTRIN contains the same active ingredient found in ZYBAN, used as an aid to smoking cessation, and that WELLBUTRIN should not be used in combination with ZYBAN or any other medications that contain bupropion hydrochloride.

Physicians are advised to discuss the following issues with patients:

Patients should be instructed to take WELLBUTRIN in equally divided doses three or four times a day to minimize the risk of seizure.

Patients should be told that any CNS-active drug like WELLBUTRIN may impair their ability to perform tasks requiring judgment or motor and cognitive skills. Consequently, until they are reasonably certain that WELLBUTRIN does not adversely affect their performance, they should refrain from driving an automobile or operating complex, hazardous machinery.

Patients should be told that the use and cessation of use of alcohol may alter the seizure threshold, and, therefore, that the consumption of alcohol should be minimized, and, if possible, avoided completely.

Patients should be advised to inform their physicians if they are taking or plan to take any prescription or over-the-counter drugs. Concern is warranted because WELLBUTRIN and other drugs may affect each other's metabolism.

Patients should be advised to notify their physicians if they become pregnant or intend to become pregnant during therapy.

Laboratory Tests: There are no specific laboratory tests recommended.

Drug Interactions: In vitro studies indate that bupropion is primarily metabolized to hydroxybupropion by the cytochrome P450IIB6 (CYP2B6) isoenzyme. Therefore, the potential exists for a drug interaction between WELLBUTRIN and drugs that affect the CYP2B6 isoenzyme (e.g., orphenadrine and cyclophosphamide). The *threo*-amino alcohol metabolite of bupropion does not appear to be produced by the cytochrome P450IID6 (CYP2D6) isoenzymes. Few systemic data have been collected on the metabolism of WELLBUTRIN following concomitant administration with other drugs or, alternatively, the effect of concomitant administration of WELLBUTRIN on the metabolism of other drugs.

However, animal data suggest that WELLBUTRIN may be an inducer of drug metabolizing enzymes. This may be of potential clinical importance because the blood levels of coadministered drugs may be altered. Alternatively, because bupropion is extensively metabolized, the coadministration of other drugs may affect its clinical activity. In particular, care should be exercised when administering drugs known to affect hepatic drug-metabolizing enzyme systems (e.g., carbamazepine, cimetidine, phenobarbital, phenytoin).

Drugs Metabolized by Cytochrome P450IID6 (CYP2D6): Many drugs, including most antidepressants (SSRIs, many tricyclics), beta-blockers, antiarrhythmics, and antipsychotics are metabolized by the CYP2D6 isoenzyme. Although bupropion is not metabolized by this isoenzyme, bupropion and hydroxybupropion are inhibitors of the CYP2D6 isoenzyme in vitro. In a study of 15 male subjects (ages 19 to 35 years) who were extensive metabolizers of the CYP2D6 isoenzyme, daily doses of bupropion given as 150 mg twice daily followed by a single dose of 50 mg desipramine increased the C_{max}, AUC, and $t_{1/2}$ of desipramine by an average of approximately two-, five- and two-fold, respectively. The effect was present for at least 7 days after the last dose of bupropion. Concomitant use of bupropion with other drugs metabolized by CYP2D6 has not been formally studied.

Therefore, co-administration of bupropion with drugs that are metabolized by CYP2D6 isoenzyme including certain antidepressants (e.g., nortriptyline, imipramine, desipramine, paroxetine, fluoxetine, sertraline), antipsychotics (e.g., haloperidol, risperidone, thioridazine), beta-blockers (e.g., metoprolol), and Type 1C antiarrhythmics (e.g., propafenone, flecainide), should be approached with caution and should be initiated at the lower end of the dose range of the concomitant medication. If bupropion is added to the treatment regimen of a patient already receiving a drug metabolized by CYP2D6, the need to decrease the dose of the original medication should be considered, particularly for those concomitant medications with a narrow therapeutic index.

MAO Inhibitors: Studies in animals demonstrate that the acute toxicity of bupropion is enhanced by the MAO inhibitor phenelzine (see CONTRAINDICATIONS).

Levodopa: Limited clinical data suggest a higher incidence of adverse experiences in patients receiving concurrent administration of WELLBUTRIN and L-dopa. Administration of WELLBUTRIN to patients receiving L-dopa concurrently should be undertaken with caution, using small initial doses and small gradual dose increases.

Drugs that Lower Seizure Threshold: Concurrent administration of WELLBUTRIN and agents (e.g., antipsychotics, other antidepressants, theophylline, systemic steroids, etc.) or treatment regimens (e.g., abrupt discontinuation of benzodiazepines) that lower seizure threshold should be undertaken only with extreme caution (see WARNINGS). Low initial dosing and small gradual dose increases should be employed.

Nicotine Transdermal System: (see PRECAUTIONS: Cardiovascular Effects).

Carcinogenesis, Mutagenesis, Impairment of Fertility: Lifetime carcinogenicity studies were performed in rats and mice at doses up to 300 and 150 mg/kg per day, respectively. In the rat study there was an increase in nodular proliferative lesions of the liver at doses of 100 to 300 mg/kg per day; lower doses were not tested. The question of whether or not such lesions may be precursors of neoplasms of the liver is currently unresolved. Similar liver lesions were not seen in the mouse study, and no increase in malignant tumors of the liver and other organs was seen in either study.

Bupropion produced a borderline positive response (two to three times control mutation rate) in some strains in the Ames bacterial mutagenicity test, and a high oral dose (300 mg/kg, but not 100 or 200 mg/kg) produced a low incidence of chromosomal aberrations in rats. The relevance of these results in estimating the risk of human exposure to therapeutic doses is unknown.

A fertility study was performed in rats; no evidence of impairment of fertility was encountered at oral doses up to 300 mg/kg per day.

Pregnancy: *Teratogenic Effects:* Pregnancy Category B. Reproduction studies have been performed in rabbits and rats at doses up to 15 to 45 times the human daily dose and have revealed no definitive evidence of impaired fertility or harm to the fetus due to bupropion. (In rabbits, a slightly increased incidence of fetal abnormalities was seen in two studies, but there was no increase in any specific abnormality). There are no adequate and well-controlled studies in pregnant women. Because animal reproduction studies are not always predictive of human response, this drug should be used during pregnancy only if clearly needed.

To monitor fetal outcomes of pregnant women exposed to WELLBUTRIN, Glaxo Wellcome Inc. maintains a Bupropion Pregnancy Registry. Health care providers are encouraged to register patients by calling (800) 336-2176.

Labor and Delivery: The effect of WELLBUTRIN on labor and delivery in humans is unknown.

Nursing Mothers: Like many other drugs, bupropion and its metabolites are secreted in human milk. Because of the potential for serious adverse reactions in nursing infants from WELLBUTRIN, a decision should be made whether to discontinue nursing or to discontinue the drug, taking into account the importance of the drug to the mother.

Pediatric Use: The safety and effectiveness of WELLBUTRIN in pediatric patients under 18 years old have not been established. The immediate-release formulation of bupropion was studied in 104 pediatric patients (age range, 6 to 16) in clinical trials of the drug for other indications. Although generally well tolerated, the limited exposure is insufficient to assess the safety of bupropion in pediatric patients.

Geriatric Use: Of the approximately 6000 patients who participated in clinical trials with bupropion sustained-release tablets (depression and smoking cessation studies), 275 were 65 and over and 47 were 75 and over. In addition, several hundred patients 65 and over participated in clinical trials using the immediate-release formulation of bupropion (depression studies). No overall differences in safety or effectiveness were observed between these subjects and younger subjects, and other reported clinical experience has not identified differences in responses between the elderly and younger patients, but greater sensitivity of some older individuals cannot be ruled out.

A single-dose pharmacokinetic study demonstrated that the disposition of bupropion and its metabolites in elderly subjects was similar to that of younger subjects; however, another pharmacokinetic study, single and multiple dose, has suggested that the elderly are at increased risk for accumulation of bupropion and its metabolites (see CLINICAL PHARMACOLOGY).

Bupropion is extensively metabolized in the liver to active metabolites, which are further metabolized and excreted by the kidneys. The risk of toxic reaction to this drug may be greater in patients with impaired renal function. Because elderly patients are more likely to have decreased renal function, care should be taken in dose selection, and it may be useful to monitor renal function (see PRECAUTIONS: Renal Impairment and DOSAGE AND ADMINISTRATION).

ADVERSE REACTIONS

(see also WARNINGS and PRECAUTIONS) Adverse events commonly encountered in patients treated with WELLBUTRIN are agitation, dry mouth, insomnia, headache/migraine, nausea/vomiting, constipation, and tremor.

Adverse events were sufficiently troublesome to cause discontinuation of treatment with WELLBUTRIN in approximately 10% of the 2400 patients and volunteers who participated in clinical trials during the product's initial development. The more common events causing discontinuation include neuropsychiatric disturbances (3.0%), primarily agitation and abnormalities in mental status; gastrointestinal disturbances (2.1%), primarily nausea and vomiting; neurological disturbances (1.7%), primarily seizures, headaches, and sleep disturbances; and dermatologic problems (1.4%), primarily rashes. It is important to note, however, that many of these events occurred at doses that exceed the recommended daily dose.

Accurate estimates of the incidence of adverse events associated with the use of any drug are difficult to obtain. Estimates are influenced by drug dose, detection technique, setting, physician judgments, etc. Consequently, the table below is presented solely to indicate the relative frequency of adverse events reported in representative controlled clinical studies conducted to evaluate the safety and efficacy of WELLBUTRIN under relatively similar conditions of daily dosage (300 to 600 mg), setting, and duration (3 to 4 weeks). The figures cited cannot be used to predict precisely the incidence of untoward events in the course of usual medical practice where patient characteristics and other factors must differ from those which prevailed in the clinical trials. These incidence figures also cannot be compared with those obtained from other clinical studies involving related drug products as each group of drug trials is conducted under a different set of conditions.

Finally, it is important to emphasize that the tabulation does not reflect the relative severity and/or clinical importance of the events. A better perspective on the serious adverse events associated with the use of WELLBUTRIN is provided in WARNINGS and PRECAUTIONS.

[See first table at top of next page]

Other Events Observed During the Development of WELLBUTRIN: The conditions and duration of exposure to WELLBUTRIN varied greatly, and a substantial proportion of the experience was gained in open and uncontrolled clinical settings. During this experience, numerous adverse events were reported; however, without appropriate controls, it is impossible to determine with certainty which events were or were not caused by WELLBUTRIN. The following enumeration is organized by organ system and describes events in terms of their relative frequency of reporting in the data base. Events of major clinical importance are also described in WARNINGS and PRECAUTIONS.

The following definitions of frequency are used: Frequent adverse events are defined as those occurring in at least 1/100 patients. Infrequent adverse events are those occurring in 1/100 to 1/1000 patients, while rare events are those occurring in less than 1/1000 patients.

Cardiovascular: Frequent was edema; infrequent were chest pain, electrocardiogram (ECG) abnormalities (premature beats and nonspecific ST-T changes), and shortness of breath/dyspnea; rare were flushing, pallor, phlebitis, and myocardial infarction.

Dermatologic: Frequent were nonspecific rashes; infrequent were alopecia and dry skin; rare were change in hair color, hirsutism, and acne.

Continued on next page

This product information is based on labeling in effect on June 23, 2000. For further information, contact via direct mail, phone, or web site. Medical Information, Glaxo Wellcome Inc., PO Box 13398, Research Triangle Park, NC 27709. Healthcare Professionals (Medical Information): 800-334-0089. Patients (Customer Response Center): 1-888-825-5249. Glaxo Wellcome Corporate Web Site: www.glaxowellcome.com

Wellbutrin—Cont.

Endocrine: Infrequent was gynecomastia; rare were glycosuria and hormone level change.
Gastrointestinal: Infrequent were dysphagia, thirst disturbance, and liver damage/jaundice; rare were rectal complaints, colitis, gastrointestinal bleeding, intestinal perforation, and stomach ulcer.
Genitourinary: Frequent was nocturia; infrequent were vaginal irritation, testicular swelling, urinary tract infection, painful erection, and retarded ejaculation; rare were dysuria, enuresis, urinary incontinence, menopause, ovarian disorder, pelvic infection, cystitis, dyspareunia, and painful ejaculation.
Hematologic/Oncologic: Rare were lymphadenopathy, anemia, and pancytopenia.
Musculoskeletal: Rare was musculosketetal chest pain.
Neurological: (see WARNINGS) Frequent were ataxia/incoordination, seizure, myoclonus, dyskinesia, and dystonia; infrequent were mydriasis, vertigo, and dysarthria; rare were electroencephalogram (EEG) abnormality, abnormal neurological exam, impaired attention, sciatica, and aphasia.
Neuropsychiatric: (see PRECAUTIONS) Frequent were mania/hypomania, increased libido, hallucinations, decrease in sexual function, and depression; infrequent were memory impairment, depersonalization, psychosis, dysphoria, mood instability, paranoia, formal thought disorder, and frigidity; rare was suicidal ideation.
Oral Complaints: Frequent was stomatitis; infrequent were toothache, bruxism, gum irritation, and oral edema; rare was glossitis.
Respiratory: Infrequent were bronchitis and shortness of breath/dyspnea; rare were epistaxis, rate or rhythm disorder, pneumonia, and pulmonary embolism.
Special Senses: Infrequent was visual disturbance; rare was diplopia.
Nonspecific: Frequent were flu-like symptoms; infrequent was nonspecific pain; rare were body odor, surgically related pain, infection, medication reaction, and overdose.
Postintroduction Reports: Voluntary reports of adverse events temporally associated with bupropion that have been received since market introduction and which may have no causal relationship with the drug include the following:
Body (General): arthralgia, myalgia, and fever with rash and other symptoms suggestive of delayed hypersensitivity. These symptoms may resemble serum sickness (see PRECAUTIONS).
Cardiovascular: hypertension (in some cases severe, see PRECAUTIONS), orthostatic hypotension, third degree heart block.
Endocrine: syndrome of inappropriate antidiuretic hormone secretion, hyperglycemia, hypoglycemia
Gastrointestinal: esophagitis, hepatitis, liver damage
Hemic and Lymphatic: ecchymosis, leukocytosis, leukopenia, thrombocytopenia
Musculoskeletal: arthralgia, myalgia, muscle rigidity/fever/rhabdomyolysis, muscle weakness
Nervous: coma, delirium, dream abnormalities, paresthesia, unmasking of tardive dyskinesia
Skin and Appendages: Stevens-Johnson syndrome, angioedema, exfoliative dermatitis, urticaria
Special Senses: tinnitus

DRUG ABUSE AND DEPENDENCE

Humans: Controlled clinical studies conducted in normal volunteers, in subjects with a history of multiple drug abuse, and in depressed patients showed some increase in motor activity and agitation/excitement.
In a population of individuals experienced with drugs of abuse, a single dose of 400 mg WELLBUTRIN produced mild amphetamine-like activity as compared to placebo on the Morphine-Benzedrine Subscale of the Addiction Research Center Inventories (ARCI) and a score intermediate between placebo and amphetamine on the Liking Scale of the ARCI. These scales measure general feelings of euphoria and drug desirability.
Findings in clinical trials, however, are not known to predict the abuse potential of drugs reliably. Nonetheless, evidence from single-dose studies does suggest that the recommended daily dosage of bupropion when administered in divided doses is not likely to be especially reinforcing to amphetamine or stimulant abusers. However, higher doses, which could not be tested because of the risk of seizure, might be modestly attractive to those who abuse stimulant drugs.
Animals: Studies in rodents have shown that bupropion exhibits some pharmacologic actions common to psychostimulants, including increases in locomotor activity and the production of a mild stereotyped behavior and increases in rates of responding in several schedule-controlled behavior paradigms. Drug discrimination studies in rats showed stimulus generalization between bupropion and amphetamine and other psychostimulants. Rhesus monkeys have been shown to self-administer bupropion intravenously.

OVERDOSAGE

Human Overdose Experience: There has been extensive clinical experience with overdosage of WELLBUTRIN Tablets. Thirteen overdoses occurred during clinical trials. Twelve patients ingested 850 to 4200 mg and recovered without significant sequelae. Another patient who ingested 9000 mg of WELLBUTRIN and 300 mg of tranylcypromine experienced a grand mal seizure and recovered without further sequelae.
Since introduction, overdoses of WELLBUTRIN Tablets up to 17,500 mg have been reported. Seizure was reported in approximately one third of all cases. Other serious reactions reported with overdoses of WELLBUTRIN Tablets alone included hallucinations, loss of consciousness, and sinus tachycardia. Fever, muscle rigidity, rhabdomyolysis, hypotension, stupor, coma, and respiratory failure have been reported when WELLBUTRIN Tablets was part of multiple drug overdoses.
Although most patients recovered without sequelae, deaths associated with overdoses of WELLBUTRIN Tablets alone have been reported rarely in patients ingesting massive doses of WELLBUTRIN Tablets. Multiple uncontrolled seizures, bradycardia, cardiac failure, and cardiac arrest prior to death were reported in these patients.
Overdosage Management: Ensure an adequate airway, oxygenation, and ventilation. Monitor cardiac rhythm and vital signs. EEG monitoring is also recommended for the first 48 hours post-ingestion. General supportive and symptomatic measures are also recommended. Induction of emesis is not recommended. Gastric lavage with a large-bore orogastric tube with appropriate airway protection, if needed, may be indicated if performed soon after ingestion or in symptomatic patients.
Activated charcoal should be administered. There is no experience with the use of forced diuresis, dialysis, hemoperfusion, or exchange transfusion in the management of bupropion overdoses. No specific antidotes for bupropion are known.
Due to the dose-related risk of seizures with WELLBUTRIN, hospitalization following suspected overdose should be considered. Based on studies in animals, it is recommended that seizures be treated with intravenous benzodiazepine administration and other supportive measures, as appropriate.
In managing overdosage, consider the possibility of multiple drug involvement. The physician should consider contacting a poison control center for additional information on the treatment of any overdose. Telephone numbers for certified poison control centers are listed in the *Physicians' Desk Reference* (PDR).

DOSAGE AND ADMINISTRATION

General Dosing Considerations: It is particularly important to administer WELLBUTRIN in a manner most likely to minimize the risk of seizure (see WARNINGS). Increases in dose should not exceed 100 mg/day in a 3-day period. Gradual escalation in dosage is also important if agitation, motor restlessness, and insomnia, often seen during the initial days of treatment, are to be minimized. If necessary, these effects may be managed by temporary reduction of dose or the short-term administration of an intermediate to long-acting sedative hypnotic. A sedative hypnotic usually is not required beyond the first week of treatment. Insomnia may also be minimized by avoiding bedtime doses. If distressing, untoward effects supervene, dose escalation should be stopped.
No single dose of WELLBUTRIN should exceed 150 mg. WELLBUTRIN should be administered three times daily, preferably with at least 6 hours between successive doses.
Usual Dosage for Adults: The usual adult dose is 300 mg/day, given three times daily. Dosing should begin at 200 mg/day, given as 100 mg twice daily. Based on clinical response, this dose may be increased to 300 mg/day, given as 100 mg three times daily, no sooner than 3 days after beginning therapy (see table below).
[See second table above]
Increasing the Dosage Above 300 mg/Day: As with other antidepressants, the full antidepressant effect of WELLBUTRIN may not be evident until 4 weeks of treatment or longer. An increase in dosage, up to a maximum of 450 mg/day, given in divided doses of not more than 150 mg each, may be considered for patients in whom no clinical improvement is noted after several weeks of treatment at 300 mg/day. Dosing above 300 mg/day may be accomplished using the 75- or 100-mg tablets. The 100-mg tablet must be administered four times daily with at least 4 hours between successive doses, in order not to exceed the limit of 150 mg in a single dose. WELLBUTRIN should be discontinued in patients who do not demonstrate an adequate response after an appropriate period of treatment at 450 mg/day.
Maintenance: The lowest dose that maintains remission is recommended. Although it is not known how long the patient should remain on WELLBUTRIN, it is generally recognized that acute episodes of depression require several months or longer of antidepressant drug treatment.
Dosage Adjustment for Patients with Impaired Hepatic Function: WELLBUTRIN should be used with extreme caution in patients with severe hepatic cirrhosis. The dose should not exceed 75 mg once a day in these patients. WELLBUTRIN should be used with caution in patients with hepatic impairment (including mild to moderate hepatic cirrhosis) and a reduced frequency and/or dose should be considered in patients with mild to moderate hepatic cirrhosis (see CLINICAL PHARMACOLOGY and PRECAUTIONS).
Dosage Adjustment for Patients with Impaired Renal Function: WELLBUTRIN should be used with caution in pa-

Treatment Emergent Adverse Experience Incidence in Placebo-Controlled Clinical Trials*
(Percent of Patients Reporting)

Adverse Experience	WELLBUTRIN Patients (n = 323)	Placebo Patients (n = 185)	Adverse Experience	WELLBUTRIN Patients (n = 323)	Placebo Patients (n = 185)
Cardiovascular			Dry mouth	27.6	18.4
Cardiac arrhythmias	5.3	4.3	Excessive sweating	22.3	14.6
Dizziness	22.3	16.2	Headache/migraine	25.7	22.2
Hypertension	4.3	1.6	Impaired sleep quality	4.0	1.6
Hypotension	2.5	2.2	Increased salivary flow	3.4	3.8
Palpitations	3.7	2.2	Insomnia	18.6	15.7
Syncope	1.2	0.5	Muscle spasms	1.9	3.2
Tachycardia	10.8	8.6	Pseudoparkinsonism	1.5	1.6
Dermatologic			Sedation	19.8	19.5
Pruritus	2.2	0.0	Sensory disturbance	4.0	3.2
Rash	8.0	6.5	Tremor	21.1	7.6
Gastrointestinal			Neuropsychiatric		
Anorexia	18.3	18.4	Agitation	31.9	22.2
Appetite increase	3.7	2.2	Anxiety	3.1	1.1
Constipation	26.0	17.3	Confusion	8.4	4.9
Diarrhea	6.8	8.6	Decreased libido	3.1	1.6
Dyspepsia	3.1	2.2	Delusions	1.2	1.1
Nausea/vomiting	22.9	18.9	Disturbed concentration	3.1	3.8
Weight gain	13.6	22.7	Euphoria	1.2	0.5
Weight loss	23.2	23.2	Hostility	5.6	3.8
Genitourinary			Nonspecific		
Impotence	3.4	3.1	Fatigue	5.0	8.6
Menstrual complaints	4.7	1.1	Fever/chills	1.2	0.5
Urinary frequency	2.5	2.2	Respiratory		
Urinary retention	1.9	2.2	Upper respiratory complaints	5.0	11.4
Musculoskeletal			Special Senses		
Arthritis	3.1	2.7	Auditory disturbance	5.3	3.2
Neurological			Blurred vision	14.6	10.3
Akathisia	1.5	1.1	Gustatory disturbance	3.1	1.1
Akinesia/bradykinesia	8.0	8.6			
Cutaneous temperature disturbance	1.9	1.6			

* Events reported by at least 1% of patients receiving WELLBUTRIN are included.

Dosing Regimen

Treatment Day	Total Daily Dose	Tablet Strength	Number of Tablets: Morning	Midday	Evening
1	200 mg	100 mg	1	0	1
4	300 mg	100 mg	1	1	1

tients with renal impairment and a reduced frequency and/or dose should be considered (see CLINICAL PHARMACOLOGY and PRECAUTIONS).

HOW SUPPLIED

WELLBUTRIN Tablets, 75 mg of bupropion hydrochloride, are yellow-gold, round, biconvex tablets printed with "WELLBUTRIN 75" in bottles of 100 (NDC 0173-0177-55).
WELLBUTRIN Tablets, 100 mg of bupropion hydrochloride, are red, round, biconvex tablets printed with "WELLBUTRIN 100" in bottles of 100 (NDC 0173-0178-55).
Store at 15° to 25°C (59° to 77°F). Protect from light and moisture.
Manufactured by Catalytica Pharmaceuticals, Inc.
Greenville, NC 27834
for Glaxo Wellcome Inc., Research Triangle Park, NC 27709

May 2000/RL-816
Shown in Product Identification Guide, page 316

WELLBUTRIN SR® ℞
(bupropion hydrochloride)
Sustained-Release Tablets

DESCRIPTION

WELLBUTRIN SR (bupropion hydrochloride), an antidepressant of the aminoketone class, is chemically unrelated to tricyclic, tetracyclic, selective serotonin re-uptake inhibitor, or other known antidepressant agents. Its structure closely resembles that of diethylpropion; it is related to phenylethylamines. It is designated as (±)-1-(3-chlorophenyl)-2-[(1,1-dimethylethyl)amino]-1-propanone hydrochloride. The molecular weight is 276.2. The molecular formula is $C_{13}H_{18}ClNO \bullet HCl$. Bupropion hydrochloride powder is white, crystalline, and highly soluble in water. It has a bitter taste and produces the sensation of local anesthesia on the oral mucosa.

WELLBUTRIN SR Tablets are supplied for oral administration as 100-mg (blue) and 150-mg (purple), film-coated, sustained-release tablets. Each tablet contains the labeled amount of bupropion hydrochloride and the inactive ingredients: carnauba wax, cysteine hydrochloride, hydroxypropyl methylcellulose, magnesium stearate, microcrystalline cellulose, polyethylene glycol, and titanium dioxide and is printed with edible black ink. In addition, the 100-mg tablet contains FD&C Blue No. 1 Lake and polysorbate 80, and the 150-mg tablet contains FD&C Blue No. 2 Lake, FD&C Red No. 40 Lake, and polysorbate 80.

CLINICAL PHARMACOLOGY

Pharmacodynamics: Bupropion is a relatively weak inhibitor of the neuronal uptake of norepinephrine, serotonin, and dopamine, and does not inhibit monoamine oxidase. While the mechanism of action of bupropion, as with other antidepressants, is unknown, it is presumed that this action is mediated by noradrenergic and/or dopaminergic mechanisms.

Pharmacokinetics: Bupropion is a racemic mixture. The pharmacologic activity and pharmacokinetics of the individual enantiomers have not been studied.

Following oral administration of WELLBUTRIN SR Tablets to healthy volunteers, peak plasma concentrations of bupropion are achieved within 3 hours. Food increased C_{max} and AUC of bupropion by 11% and 17%, respectively, indicating that there is no clinically significant food effect.

In vitro tests show that bupropion is 84% bound to human plasma proteins at concentrations up to 200 mcg/mL. The extent of protein binding of the hydroxybupropion metabolite is similar to that for bupropion, whereas the extent of protein binding of the threohydrobupropion metabolite is about half that seen with bupropion.

Following oral administration of 200 mg of ^{14}C-bupropion in humans, 87% and 10% of the radioactive dose were recovered in the urine and feces, respectively. The fraction of the oral dose of bupropion excreted unchanged was only 0.5%, a finding consistent with the extensive metabolism of bupropion.

The mean elimination half-life (±SD) of bupropion after chronic dosing is 21 (±9) hours, and steady-state plasma concentrations of bupropion are reached within 8 days.

Bupropion is extensively metabolized in humans. Three metabolites have been shown to be active: hydroxybupropion, which is formed via hydroxylation of the *tert*-butyl group of bupropion, and the amino-alcohol isomers threohydrobupropion and erythrohydrobupropion, which are formed via reduction of the carbonyl group. In vitro findings suggest that cytochrome P450IIB6 (CYP2B6) is the principal isoenzyme involved in the formation of hydroxybupropion, while cytochrome P450 isoenzymes are not involved in the formation of threohydrobupropion. Oxidation of the bupropion side chain results in the formation of a glycine conjugate of meta-chlorobenzoic acid, which is then excreted as the major urinary metabolite. The potency and toxicity of the metabolites relative to bupropion have not been fully characterized. Nevertheless, they may be clinically important because their plasma concentrations are higher than those of bupropion.

Because bupropion is extensively metabolized, there is the potential for drug-drug interactions, particularly with those agents that are metabolized by the cytochrome P450IIB6 (CYP2B6) isoenzyme. Although bupropion is not metabolized by cytochrome P450IID6 (CYP2D6), there is the potential for drug-drug interactions when bupropion is co-administered with drugs metabolized by this isoenzyme (see PRECAUTIONS: Drug Interactions).

Following a single dose in humans, peak plasma concentrations of hydroxybupropion occur approximately 6 hours after administration of WELLBUTRIN SR Tablets. Peak plasma concentrations of hydroxybupropion are approximately 10 times the peak level of the parent drug at steady state. The elimination half-life of hydroxybupropion is approximately 20 (±5) hours, and its AUC at steady state is about 17 times that of bupropion. The times to peak concentrations for the erythrohydrobupropion and threohydrobupropion metabolites are similar to that of the hydroxybupropion metabolite. However, their elimination half-lives are longer, 33 (±10) and 37 (±13) hours, respectively, and steady-state AUCs are 1.5 and 7 times that of bupropion, respectively.

In a study comparing chronic dosing with WELLBUTRIN SR Tablets 150 mg twice daily to the immediate-release formulation of bupropion at 100 mg three times daily, peak plasma concentrations of bupropion at steady state for WELLBUTRIN SR Tablets were approximately 85% of those achieved with the immediate-release formulation. There was equivalence for bupropion AUCs, as well as equivalence for both peak plasma concentration and AUCs for all three of the detectable bupropion metabolites. Thus, at steady state, WELLBUTRIN SR Tablets, given twice daily, and the immediate-release formulation of bupropion, given three times daily, are essentially bioequivalent for both bupropion and the three quantitatively important metabolites.

Bupropion and its metabolites exhibit linear kinetics following chronic administration of 300 to 450 mg/day.

Population Subgroups: Factors or conditions altering metabolic capacity (e.g., liver disease, congestive heart failure [CHF], age, concomitant medications, etc.) or elimination may be expected to influence the degree and extent of accumulation of the active metabolites of bupropion. The elimination of the major metabolites of bupropion may be affected by reduced renal or hepatic function because they are moderately polar compounds and are likely to undergo further metabolism or conjugation in the liver prior to urinary excretion.

Hepatic: The effect of hepatic impairment on the pharmacokinetics of bupropion was characterized in two single-dose studies, one in patients with alcoholic liver disease and one in patients with mild to severe cirrhosis. The first study showed that the half-life of hydroxybupropion was significantly longer in 8 patients with alcoholic liver disease than in 8 healthy volunteers (32±14 hours versus 21±5 hours, respectively). Although not statistically significant, the AUCs for bupropion and hydroxybupropion were more variable and tended to be greater (by 53% to 57%) in patients with alcoholic liver disease. The differences in half-life for bupropion and the other metabolites in the two patient groups were minimal.

The second study showed that there were no statistically significant differences in the pharmacokinetics of bupropion and its active metabolites in 9 patients with mild to moderate hepatic cirrhosis compared to 8 healthy volunteers. There was, however, more variability observed in some of the pharmacokinetic parameters for bupropion (AUC, C_{max}, and T_{max}) and its active metabolites ($t^{1}/_{2}$) in patients with mild to moderate hepatic cirrhosis. In addition, in patients with severe hepatic cirrhosis, the bupropion C_{max} and AUC were substantially increased (mean difference: by approximately 70% and 3-fold, respectively) and more variable when compared to values in healthy volunteers; the mean bupropion half-life was also longer (by approximately 40%). For the metabolites, the mean C_{max} was lower (by approximately 30% to 70%), the mean AUC tended to be higher (by approximately 30% to 50%), the median T_{max} was later (by approximately 20 hours), and the mean half-lives were longer (by approximately 2- to 4-fold) in patients with severe hepatic cirrhosis than in healthy volunteers (see WARNINGS, PRECAUTIONS, and DOSAGE AND ADMINISTRATION).

Renal: The effect of renal disease on the pharmacokinetics of bupropion has not been studied. The elimination of the major metabolites of bupropion may be affected by reduced renal function.

Left Ventricular Dysfunction: During a chronic dosing study with bupropion in 14 depressed patients with left ventricular dysfunction (history of CHF or an enlarged heart on x-ray), no apparent effect on the pharmacokinetics of bupropion or its metabolites, compared to healthy normal volunteers, was revealed.

Age: The effects of age on the pharmacokinetics of bupropion and its metabolites have not been fully characterized, but an exploration of steady-state bupropion concentrations from several depression efficacy studies involving patients dosed in a range of 300 to 750 mg/day, on a three times daily schedule, revealed no relationship between age (18 to 83 years) and plasma concentration of bupropion. A single-dose pharmacokinetic study demonstrated that the disposition of bupropion and its metabolites in elderly subjects was similar to that of younger subjects. These data suggest there is no prominent effect of age on bupropion concentration; however, another pharmacokinetic study, single and multiple dose, has suggested that the elderly are at increased risk for accumulation of bupropion and its metabolites (see PRECAUTIONS: Geriatric Use).

Gender: A single-dose study involving 12 healthy male and 12 healthy female volunteers revealed no sex-related differences in the pharmacokinetic parameters of bupropion.

Smokers: The effects of cigarette smoking on the pharmacokinetics of bupropion were studied in 34 healthy male and female volunteers; 17 were chronic cigarette smokers and 17 were nonsmokers. Following oral administration of a single 150-mg dose of bupropion, there was no statistically significant difference in C_{max}, half-life, t_{max}, AUC, or clearance of bupropion or its active metabolites between smokers and nonsmokers.

CLINICAL TRIALS

The efficacy of the immediate-release formulation of bupropion as a treatment for depression was established in two 4-week, placebo-controlled trials in adult inpatients with depression and in one 6-week, placebo-controlled trial in adult outpatients with depression. In the first study, patients were titrated in a bupropion dose range of 300 to 600 mg/day on a three times daily schedule; 78% of patients received maximum doses of 450 mg/day or less. This trial demonstrated the effectiveness of the immediate-release formulation of bupropion on the Hamilton Depression Rating Scale (HDRS) total score, the depressed mood item (item 1) from that scale, and the Clinical Global Impressions (CGI) severity score. A second study included two fixed doses of the immediate-release formulation of bupropion (300 and 450 mg/day) and placebo. This trial demonstrated the effectiveness of the immediate-release formulation of bupropion, but only at the 450-mg/day dose; the results were positive for the HDRS total score and the CGI severity score, but not for HDRS item 1. In the third study, outpatients received 300 mg/day of the immediate-release formulation of bupropion. This study demonstrated the effectiveness of the immediate-release formulation of bupropion on the HDRS total score, HDRS item 1, the Montgomery-Asberg Depression Rating Scale, the CGI severity score, and the CGI improvement score.

Although there are not as yet independent trials demonstrating the antidepressant effectiveness of the sustained-release formulation of bupropion, studies have demonstrated the bioequivalence of the immediate-release and sustained-release forms of bupropion under steady-state conditions, i.e., bupropion sustained-release 150 mg twice daily was shown to be bioequivalent to 100 mg three times daily of the immediate-release formulation of bupropion, with regard to both rate and extent of absorption, for parent drug and metabolites.

INDICATIONS AND USAGE

WELLBUTRIN SR is indicated for the treatment of depression.

The efficacy of bupropion in the treatment of depression was established in two 4-week controlled trials of depressed inpatients and in one 6-week controlled trial of depressed outpatients whose diagnoses corresponded most closely to the Major Depression category of the APA Diagnostic and Statistical Manual (DSM) (see CLINICAL PHARMACOLOGY).

A major depressive episode (DSM-IV) implies the presence of 1) depressed mood or 2) loss of interest or pleasure; in addition, at least five of the following symptoms have been present during the same 2-week period and represent a change from previous functioning: depressed mood, markedly diminished interest or pleasure in usual activities, significant change in weight and/or appetite, insomnia or hypersomnia, psychomotor agitation or retardation, increased fatigue, feelings of guilt or worthlessness, slowed thinking or impaired concentration, a suicide attempt or suicidal ideation.

Effectiveness of bupropion in long-term use (more than 6 weeks) has not been systematically evaluated in controlled trials. Therefore, the physician who elects to use WELLBUTRIN SR Tablets for extended periods should periodically reevaluate the long-term usefulness of the drug for the individual patient.

CONTRAINDICATIONS

WELLBUTRIN SR is contraindicated in patients with a seizure disorder.

WELLBUTRIN SR is contraindicated in patients treated with ZYBAN® (bupropion hydrochloride) Sustained-Release Tablets, or any other medications that contain bupropion because the incidence of seizure is dose dependent.

WELLBUTRIN SR is contraindicated in patients with a current or prior diagnosis of bulimia or anorexia nervosa because of a higher incidence of seizures noted in patients treated for bulimia with the immediate-release formulation of bupropion.

The concurrent administration of WELLBUTRIN SR Tablets and a monoamine oxidase (MAO) inhibitor is contraindicated. At least 14 days should elapse between discontinuation of an MAO inhibitor and initiation of treatment with WELLBUTRIN SR Tablets.

Continued on next page

This product information is based on labeling in effect on June 23, 2000. For further information, contact via direct mail, phone, or web site. Medical Information, Glaxo Wellcome Inc., PO Box 13398, Research Triangle Park, NC 27709. Healthcare Professionals (Medical Information): 800-334-0089. Patients (Customer Response Center): 1-888-825-5249. Glaxo Wellcome Corporate Web Site: www.glaxowellcome.com

Wellbutrin SR—Cont.

WELLBUTRIN SR is contraindicated in patients who have shown an allergic response to bupropion or the other ingredients that make up WELLBUTRIN SR Tablets.

WARNINGS

Patients should be made aware that WELLBUTRIN SR contains the same active ingredient found in ZYBAN, used as an aid to smoking cessation treatment, and that WELLBUTRIN SR should not be used in combination with ZYBAN, or any other medications that contain bupropion.

Seizures: Bupropion is associated with a dose-related risk of seizures. The risk of seizures is also related to patient factors, clinical situations, and concomitant medications, which must be considered in selection of patients for therapy with WELLBUTRIN SR.

- **Dose: At doses of WELLBUTRIN SR up to a dose of 300 mg/day, the incidence of seizure is approximately 0.1% (1/1000) and increases to approximately 0.4% (4/1000) at the maximum recommended dose of 400 mg/day.**
  Data for the immediate-release formulation of bupropion revealed a seizure incidence of approximately 0.4% (i.e., 13 of 3200 patients followed prospectively) in patients treated at doses in a range of 300 to 450 mg/day. The 450-mg/day upper limit of this dose range is close to the currently recommended maximum dose of 400 mg/day for WELLBUTRIN SR Tablets. This seizure incidence (0.4%) may exceed that of other marketed antidepressants and WELLBUTRIN SR Tablets up to 300 mg/day by as much as fourfold. This relative risk is only an approximate estimate because no direct comparative studies have been conducted.
  Additional data accumulated for the immediate-release formulation of bupropion suggested that the estimated seizure incidence increases almost tenfold between 450 and 600 mg/day, which is twice the usual adult dose and one and one-half the maximum recommended daily dose (400 mg) of WELLBUTRIN SR Tablets. This disproportionate increase in seizure incidence with dose incrementation calls for caution in dosing.
  Data for WELLBUTRIN SR Tablets revealed a seizure incidence of approximately 0.1% (i.e., 3 of 3100 patients followed prospectively) in patients treated at doses in a range of 100 to 300 mg/day. It is not possible to know if the lower seizure incidence observed in this study involving the sustained-release formulation of bupropion resulted from the different formulation or the lower dose used. However, as noted above, the immediate-release and sustained-release formulations are bioequivalent with regard to both rate and extent of absorption during steady state (the most pertinent condition to estimating seizure incidence), since most observed seizures occur under steady-state conditions.
- **Patient factors: Predisposing factors that may increase the risk of seizure with bupropion use include history of head trauma or prior seizure, central nervous system (CNS) tumor, the presence of severe hepatic cirrhosis, and concomitant medications that lower seizure threshold.**
- **Clinical situations: Circumstances associated with an increased seizure risk include, among others, excessive use of alcohol; abrupt withdrawal from alcohol or other sedatives; addiction to opiates, cocaine, or stimulants; use of over-the-counter stimulants and anorectics; and diabetes treated with oral hypoglycemics or insulin.**
- **Concomitant medications: Many medications (e.g., antipsychotics, antidepressants, theophylline, systemic steroids) and treatment regimens (e.g., abrupt discontinuation of benzodiazepines) are known to lower seizure threshold.**

Recommendations for Reducing the Risk of Seizure: **Retrospective analysis of clinical experience gained during the development of bupropion suggests that the risk of seizure may be minimized if**

- **the total daily dose of WELLBUTRIN SR Tablets does *not* exceed 400 mg,**
- **the daily dose is administered twice daily, and**
- **the rate of incrementation of dose is gradual.**
- **No single dose should exceed 200 mg to avoid high peak concentrations of bupropion and/or its metabolites.**

WELLBUTRIN SR should be administered with extreme caution to patients with a history of seizure, cranial trauma, or other predisposition(s) toward seizure, or patients treated with other agents (e.g., antipsychotics, other antidepressants, theophylline, systemic steroids, etc.) or treatment regimens (e.g., abrupt discontinuation of a benzodiazepine) that lower seizure threshold.

Hepatic Impairment: WELLBUTRIN SR should be used with extreme caution in patients with severe hepatic cirrhosis. In these patients a reduced frequency and/or dose is required, as peak bupropion levels are substantially increased and accumulation is likely to occur in such patients to a greater extent than usual. The dose should not exceed 100 mg every day or 150 mg every other day in these patients (see CLINICAL PHARMACOLOGY, PRECAUTIONS, and DOSAGE AND ADMINISTRATION).

Potential for Hepatotoxicity: In rats receiving large doses of bupropion chronically, there was an increase in incidence of hepatic hyperplastic nodules and hepatocellular hypertrophy. In dogs receiving large doses of bupropion chronically, various histologic changes were seen in the liver, and laboratory tests suggesting mild hepatocellular injury were noted.

PRECAUTIONS

General: ***Agitation and Insomnia:*** Patients in placebo-controlled trials with WELLBUTRIN SR Tablets experienced agitation, anxiety, and insomnia as shown in Table 1.

Table 1: Incidence of Agitation, Anxiety, and Insomnia in Placebo-Controlled Trials

Adverse Event Term	WELLBUTRIN SR 300 mg/day (n = 376)	WELLBUTRIN SR 400 mg/day (n = 114)	Placebo (n = 385)
Agitation	3%	9%	2%
Anxiety	5%	6%	3%
Insomnia	11%	16%	6%

In clinical studies, these symptoms were sometimes of sufficient magnitude to require treatment with sedative/hypnotic drugs.

Symptoms were sufficiently severe to require discontinuation of treatment in 1% and 2.6% of patients treated with 300 and 400 mg/day, respectively, of WELLBUTRIN SR Tablets and 0.8% of patients treated with placebo.

Psychosis, Confusion, and Other Neuropsychiatric Phenomena: Depressed patients treated with an immediate-release formulation of bupropion or with WELLBUTRIN SR Tablets have been reported to show a variety of neuropsychiatric signs and symptoms, including delusions, hallucinations, psychosis, concentration disturbance, paranoia, and confusion. In some cases, these symptoms abated upon dose reduction and/or withdrawal of treatment.

Activation of Psychosis and/or Mania: Antidepressants can precipitate manic episodes in bipolar disorder patients during the depressed phase of their illness and may activate latent psychosis in other susceptible patients. WELLBUTRIN SR is expected to pose similar risks.

Altered Appetite and Weight: In placebo-controlled studies, patients experienced weight gain or weight loss as shown in Table 2.

Table 2: Incidence of Weight Gain and Weight Loss in Placebo-Controlled Trials

Weight Change	WELLBUTRIN SR 300 mg/day (n = 339)	WELLBUTRIN SR 400 mg/day (n = 112)	Placebo (n = 347)
Gained >5 lbs	3%	2%	4%
Lost >5 lbs	14%	19%	6%

In studies conducted with the immediate-release formulation of bupropion, 35% of patients receiving tricyclic antidepressants gained weight, compared to 9% of patients treated with the immediate-release formulation of bupropion. If weight loss is a major presenting sign of a patient's depressive illness, the anorectic and/or weight-reducing potential of WELLBUTRIN SR Tablets should be considered.

Suicide: The possibility of a suicide attempt is inherent in depression and may persist until significant remission occurs. Accordingly, prescriptions for WELLBUTRIN SR Tablets should be written for the smallest number of tablets consistent with good patient management.

Allergic Reactions: Anaphylactoid/anaphylactic reactions characterized by symptoms such as pruritus, urticaria, angioedema, and dyspnea requiring medical treatment have been reported in clinical trials with bupropion. In addition, there have been rare spontaneous postmarketing reports of erythema multiforme, Stevens-Johnson syndrome, and anaphylactic shock associated with bupropion. A patient should stop taking WELLBUTRIN SR and consult a doctor if experiencing allergic or anaphylactoid/anaphylactic reactions (e.g., skin rash, pruritus, hives, chest pain, edema, and shortness of breath) during treatment.

Arthralgia, myalgia, and fever with rash and other symptoms suggestive of delayed hypersensitivity have been reported in association with bupropion. These symptoms may resemble serum sickness.

Cardiovascular Effects: In clinical practice, hypertension, in some cases severe, requiring acute treatment, has been reported in patients receiving bupropion alone and in combination with nicotine replacement therapy. These events have been observed in both patients with and without evidence of preexisting hypertension.

Data from a comparative study of the sustained-release formulation of bupropion (ZYBAN® Sustained-Release Tablets), nicotine transdermal system (NTS), the combination of sustained-release bupropion plus NTS, and placebo as an aid to smoking cessation suggest a higher incidence of treatment-emergent hypertension in patients treated with the combination of sustained-release bupropion and NTS. In this study, 6.1% of patients treated with the combination of sustained-release bupropion and NTS had treatment-emergent hypertension compared to 2.5%, 1.6%, and 3.1% of patients treated with sustained-release bupropion, NTS, and placebo, respectively. The majority of these patients had evidence of preexisting hypertension. Three patients (1.2%) treated with the combination of ZYBAN and NTS and one patient (0.4%) treated with NTS had study medication discontinued due to hypertension compared to none of the patients treated with ZYBAN or placebo. Monitoring of blood pressure is recommended in patients who receive the combination of bupropion and nicotine replacement.

There is no clinical experience establishing the safety of WELLBUTRIN SR Tablets in patients with a recent history of myocardial infarction or unstable heart disease. Therefore, care should be exercised if it is used in these groups. Bupropion was well tolerated in depressed patients who had previously developed orthostatic hypotension while receiving tricyclic antidepressants, and was also generally well tolerated in a group of 36 depressed inpatients with stable congestive heart failure (CHF). However, bupropion was associated with a rise in supine blood pressure in the study of patients with CHF, resulting in discontinuation of treatment in two patients for exacerbation of baseline hypertension.

Hepatic Impairment: WELLBUTRIN SR should be used with extreme caution in patients with severe hepatic cirrhosis. In these patients, a reduced frequency and/or dose is required. WELLBUTRIN SR should be used with caution in patients with hepatic impairment (including mild to moderate hepatic cirrhosis) and reduced frequency and/or dose should be considered in patients with mild to moderate hepatic cirrhosis.

All patients with hepatic impairment should be closely monitored for possible adverse effects that could indicate high drug and metabolite levels (see CLINICAL PHARMACOLOGY, WARNINGS, and DOSAGE AND ADMINISTRATION).

Renal Impairment: No studies have been conducted in patients with renal impairment. Bupropion is extensively metabolized in the liver to active metabolites, which are further metabolized and excreted by the kidneys. WELLBUTRIN SR should be used with caution in patients with renal impairment and a reduced frequency and/or dose should be considered as bupropion and its metabolites may accumulate in such patients to a greater extent than usual. The patient should be closely monitored for possible adverse effects that could indicate high drug or metabolite levels.

Information for Patients: See the text of the tear-off leaflet at the end of this labeling for Information for the Patient.

Patients should be made aware that WELLBUTRIN SR contains the same active ingredient found in ZYBAN, used as an aid to smoking cessation treatment, and that WELLBUTRIN SR should not be used in combination with ZYBAN or any other medications that contain bupropion hydrochloride.

Physicians are advised to discuss the following issues with patients:

As dose is increased during initial titration to doses above 150 mg/day, patients should be instructed to take WELLBUTRIN SR Tablets in two divided doses, preferably with at least 8 hours between successive doses, to minimize the risk of seizures.

Patients should be told that any CNS-active drug like WELLBUTRIN SR Tablets may impair their ability to perform tasks requiring judgment or motor and cognitive skills. Consequently, until they are reasonably certain that WELLBUTRIN SR Tablets do not adversely affect their performance, they should refrain from driving an automobile or operating complex, hazardous machinery.

Patients should be told that the use and cessation of use of alcohol may alter the seizure threshold, and, therefore, that the consumption of alcohol should be minimized, and, if possible, avoided completely.

Patients should be advised to inform their physicians if they are taking or plan to take any prescription or over-the-counter drugs. Concern is warranted because WELLBUTRIN SR Tablets and other drugs may affect each other's metabolism.

Patients should be advised to notify their physicians if they become pregnant or intend to become pregnant during therapy.

Patients should be advised to swallow WELLBUTRIN SR Tablets whole so that the release rate is not altered. Do not chew, divide, or crush tablets.

Laboratory Tests: There are no specific laboratory tests recommended.

Drug Interactions: Few systemic data have been collected on the metabolism of WELLBUTRIN SR following concomitant administration with other drugs or, alternatively, the effect of concomitant administration of WELLBUTRIN SR on the metabolism of other drugs.

Because bupropion is extensively metabolized, the coadministration of other drugs may affect its clinical activity. In vitro studies indicate that bupropion is primarily metabolized to hydroxybupropion by the CYP2B6 isoenzyme. Therefore, the potential exists for a drug interaction between WELLBUTRIN SR and drugs that affect the CYP2B6 isoenzyme (e.g., orphenadrine and cyclophosphamide). The threohydrobupropion metabolite of bupropion does not appear to be produced by the cytochrome P450 isoenzymes.

The effects of concomitant administration of cimetidine on the pharmacokinetics of bupropion and its active metabolites were studied in 24 healthy young male volunteers. Following oral administration of two 150-mg WELLBUTRIN SR Tablets with and without 800 mg of cimetidine, the pharmacokinetics of bupropion and hydroxybupropion were unaffected. However, there were 16% and 32% increases in the AUC and C_{max}, respectively, of the combined moieties of threohydrobupropion and erythrohydrobupropion.

While not systematically studied, certain drugs may induce the metabolism of bupropion (e.g., carbamazepine, phenobarbital, phenytoin).

Animal data indicated that bupropion may be an inducer of drug-metabolizing enzymes in humans. In one study, following chronic administration of bupropion, 100 mg three times daily to eight healthy male volunteers for 14 days, there was no evidence of induction of its own metabolism. Nevertheless, there may be the potential for clinically important alterations of blood levels of coadministered drugs.

Drugs Metabolized By Cytochrome P450IID6 (CYP2D6): Many drugs, including most antidepressants (SSRIs, many tricyclics), beta-blockers, antiarrhythmics, and antipsychotics are metabolized by the CYP2D6 isoenzyme. Although bupropion is not metabolized by this isoenzyme, bupropion and hydroxybupropion are inhibitors of CYP2D6 isoenzyme in vitro. In a study of 15 male subjects (ages 19 to 35 years) who were extensive metabolizers of the CYP2D6 isoenzyme, daily doses of bupropion given as 150 mg twice daily followed by a single dose of 50 mg desipramine increased the C_{max}, AUC, and $t_{½}$ of desipramine by an average of approximately two-, five-, and two-fold, respectively. The effect was present for at least 7 days after the last dose of bupropion. Concomitant use of bupropion with other drugs metabolized by CYP2D6 has not been formally studied.

Therefore, co-administration of bupropion with drugs that are metabolized by CYP2D6 isoenzyme including certain antidepressants (e.g., nortriptyline, imipramine, desipramine, paroxetine, fluoxetine, sertraline), antipsychotics (e.g., haloperidol, risperidone, thioridazine), beta-blockers (e.g., metoprolol), and Type 1C antiarrhythmics (e.g., propafenone, flecainide), should be approached with caution and should be initiated at the lower end of the dose range of the concomitant medication. If bupropion is added to the treatment regimen of a patient already receiving a drug metabolized by CYP2D6, the need to decrease the dose of the original medication should be considered, particularly for those concomitant medications with a narrow therapeutic index.

MAO Inhibitors: Studies in animals demonstrate that the acute toxicity of bupropion is enhanced by the MAO inhibitor phenelzine (see CONTRAINDICATIONS).

Levodopa: Limited clinical data suggest a higher incidence of adverse experiences in patients receiving concurrent administration of bupropion and levodopa. Administration of WELLBUTRIN SR Tablets to patients receiving levodopa concurrently should be undertaken with caution, using small initial doses and gradual dose increases.

Drugs That Lower Seizure Threshold: Concurrent administration of WELLBUTRIN SR Tablets and agents (e.g., antipsychotics, other antidepressants, theophylline, systemic steroids, etc.) or treatment regimens (e.g., abrupt discontinuation of benzodiazepines) that lower seizure threshold should be undertaken only with extreme caution (see WARNINGS). Low initial dosing and gradual dose increases should be employed.

Nicotine Transdermal System: (see PRECAUTIONS: Cardiovascular Effects).

Carcinogenesis, Mutagenesis, Impairment of Fertility: Lifetime carcinogenicity studies were performed in rats and mice at doses up to 300 and 150 mg/kg per day, respectively. These doses are approximately seven and two times the maximum recommended human dose (MRHD), respectively, on a mg/m^2 basis. In the rat study there was an increase in nodular proliferative lesions of the liver at doses of 100 to 300 mg/kg per day (approximately two to seven times the MRHD on a mg/m^2 basis); lower doses were not tested. The question of whether or not such lesions may be precursors of neoplasms of the liver is currently unresolved. Similar liver lesions were not seen in the mouse study, and no increase in malignant tumors of the liver and other organs was seen in either study.

Bupropion produced a positive response (two to three times control mutation rate) in two of five strains in the Ames bacterial mutagenicity test and an increase in chromosomal aberrations in one of three in vivo rat bone marrow cytogenetic studies.

A fertility study in rats at doses up to 300 mg/kg revealed no evidence of impaired fertility.

Pregnancy: ***Teratogenic Effects:*** Pregnancy Category B. Teratology studies have been performed at doses up to 450 mg/kg in rats, and at doses up to 150 mg/kg in rabbits (approximately 7 to 11 and 7 times the MRHD, respectively, on a mg/m^2 basis), and have revealed no evidence of harm to the fetus due to bupropion. There are no adequate and well-controlled studies in pregnant women. Because animal reproduction studies are not always predictive of human response, this drug should be used during pregnancy only if clearly needed.

To monitor fetal outcomes of pregnant women exposed to WELLBUTRIN SR, Glaxo Wellcome Inc. maintains a Bupropion Pregnancy Registry. Health care providers are encouraged to register patients by calling (800) 336-2176.

Labor and Delivery: The effect of WELLBUTRIN SR Tablets on labor and delivery in humans is unknown.

Nursing Mothers: Like many other drugs, bupropion and its metabolites are secreted in human milk. Because of the potential for serious adverse reactions in nursing infants from WELLBUTRIN SR Tablets, a decision should be made whether to discontinue nursing or to discontinue the drug, taking into account the importance of the drug to the mother.

Pediatric Use: The safety and effectiveness of WELLBUTRIN SR Tablets in pediatric patients below 18 years old have not been established. The immediate-release formulation of bupropion was studied in 104 pediatric patients (age range, 6 to 16) in clinical trials of the drug for other indications. Although generally well tolerated, the limited exposure is insufficient to assess the safety of bupropion in pediatric patients.

Geriatric Use: Of the approximately 6000 patients who participated in clinical trials with bupropion sustained-release tablets (depression and smoking cessation studies), 275 were 65 and over and 47 were 75 and over. In addition, several hundred patients 65 and over participated in clinical trials using the immediate-release formulation of bupropion (depression studies). No overall differences in safety or effectiveness were observed between these subjects and younger subjects, and other reported clinical experience has not identified differences in responses between the elderly and younger patients, but greater sensitivity of some older individuals cannot be ruled out.

A single-dose pharmacokinetic study demonstrated that the disposition of bupropion and its metabolites in elderly subjects was similar to that of younger subjects; however, another pharmacokinetic study, single and multiple dose, has suggested that the elderly are at increased risk for accumulation of bupropion and its metabolites (see CLINICAL PHARMACOLOGY).

Bupropion is extensively metabolized in the liver to active metabolites, which are further metabolized and excreted by the kidneys. The risk of toxic reaction to this drug may be greater in patients with impaired renal function. Because elderly patients are more likely to have decreased renal function, care should be taken in dose selection, and it may be useful to monitor renal function (see PRECAUTIONS: Renal Impairment and DOSAGE AND ADMINISTRATION).

ADVERSE REACTIONS: (See also WARNINGS and PRECAUTIONS)

The information included under the Incidence in Controlled Trials subsection of ADVERSE REACTIONS is based primarily on data from controlled clinical trials with WELLBUTRIN SR Tablets. Information on additional adverse events associated with the sustained-release formulation of bupropion in smoking cessation trials, as well as the immediate-release formulation of bupropion, is included in a separate section (see Other Events Observed During the Clinical Development and Postmarketing Experience of Bupropion).

Incidence in Controlled Trials With WELLBUTRIN SR: ***Adverse Events Associated With Discontinuation of Treatment Among Patients Treated With WELLBUTRIN SR Tablets:*** In placebo-controlled clinical trials, 9% and 11% of patients treated with 300 and 400 mg/day, respectively, of WELLBUTRIN SR Tablets and 4% of patients treated with placebo discontinued treatment due to adverse events. The specific adverse events in these trials that led to discontinuation in at least 1% of patients treated with either 300 or 400 mg/day of WELLBUTRIN SR Tablets and at a rate at least twice the placebo rate are listed in Table 3.

Table 3: Treatment Discontinuations Due to Adverse Events in Placebo-Controlled Trials

Adverse Event Term	WELLBUTRIN SR 300 mg/day (n = 376)	WELLBUTRIN SR 400 mg/day (n = 114)	Placebo (n = 385)
Rash	2.4%	0.9%	0.0%
Nausea	0.8%	1.8%	0.3%
Agitation	0.3%	1.8%	0.3%
Migraine	0.0%	1.8%	0.3%

Adverse Events Occurring at an Incidence of 1% or More Among Patients Treated With WELLBUTRIN SR Tablets: Table 4 enumerates treatment-emergent adverse events that occurred among patients treated with 300 and 400 mg/day of WELLBUTRIN SR Tablets and with placebo in placebo-controlled trials. Events that occurred in either the 300- or 400-mg/day group at an incidence of 1% or more and were more frequent than in the placebo group are included. Reported adverse events were classified using a COSTART-based Dictionary.

Accurate estimates of the incidence of adverse events associated with the use of any drug are difficult to obtain. Estimates are influenced by drug dose, detection technique, setting, physician judgments, etc. The figures cited cannot be used to predict precisely the incidence of untoward events in the course of usual medical practice where patient characteristics and other factors differ from those that prevailed in the clinical trials. These incidence figures also cannot be compared with those obtained from other clinical studies involving related drug products as each group of drug trials is conducted under a different set of conditions.

Finally, it is important to emphasize that the tabulation does not reflect the relative severity and/or clinical importance of the events. A better perspective on the serious adverse events associated with the use of WELLBUTRIN SR Tablets is provided in the WARNINGS and PRECAUTIONS sections.

Table 4: Treatment-Emergent Adverse Events in Placebo-Controlled Trials*

Body System/ Adverse Event	WELLBUTRIN SR 300 mg/day (n = 376)	WELLBUTRIN SR 400 mg/day (n = 114)	Placebo (n = 385)
Body (General)			
Headache	26%	25%	23%
Infection	8%	9%	6%
Abdominal pain	3%	9%	2%
Asthenia	2%	4%	2%
Chest pain	3%	4%	1%
Pain	2%	3%	2%
Fever	1%	2%	—
Cardiovascular			
Palpitation	2%	6%	2%
Flushing	1%	4%	—
Migraine	1%	4%	1%
Hot flashes	1%	3%	1%
Digestive			
Dry mouth	17%	24%	7%
Nausea	13%	18%	8%
Constipation	10%	5%	7%
Diarrhea	5%	7%	6%
Anorexia	5%	3%	2%
Vomiting	4%	2%	2%
Dysphagia	0%	2%	0%
Musculoskeletal			
Myalgia	2%	6%	3%
Arthralgia	1%	4%	1%
Arthritis	0%	2%	0%
Twitch	1%	2%	—
Nervous system			
Insomnia	11%	16%	6%
Dizziness	7%	11%	5%
Agitation	3%	9%	2%
Anxiety	5%	6%	3%
Tremor	6%	3%	1%
Nervousness	5%	3%	3%
Somnolence	2%	3%	2%
Irritability	3%	2%	2%
Memory decreased	—	3%	1%
Paresthesia	1%	2%	1%
Central nervous system stimulation	2%	1%	1%
Respiratory			
Pharyngitis	3%	11%	2%
Sinusitis	3%	1%	2%
Increased cough	1%	2%	1%
Skin			
Sweating	6%	5%	2%
Rash	5%	4%	1%
Pruritus	2%	4%	2%
Urticaria	2%	1%	0%
Special senses			
Tinnitus	6%	6%	2%
Taste perversion	2%	4%	—
Amblyopia	3%	2%	2%
Urogenital			
Urinary frequency	2%	5%	2%
Urinary urgency	—	2%	0%
Vaginal hemorrhage†	0%	2%	—
Urinary tract infection	1%	0%	—

* Adverse events that occurred in at least 1% of patients treated with either 300 or 400 mg/day of WELLBUTRIN SR Tablets, but equally or more frequently in the placebo group, were: abnormal dreams, accidental injury, acne, appetite increased, back pain, bronchitis, dysmenorrhea, dyspepsia, flatulence, flu syndrome, hypertension, neck pain, respiratory disorder, rhinitis, and tooth disorder.

Continued on next page

This product information is based on labeling in effect on June 23, 2000. For further information, contact via direct mail, phone, or web site. Medical Information, Glaxo Wellcome Inc., PO Box 13398, Research Triangle Park, NC 27709. Healthcare Professionals (Medical Information): 800-334-0089. Patients (Customer Response Center): 1-888-825-5249. Glaxo Wellcome Corporate Web Site: www.glaxowellcome.com

Wellbutrin SR—Cont.

† Incidence based on the number of female patients.
—Hyphen denotes adverse events occurring in greater than 0 but less than 0.5% of patients.

Incidence of Commonly Observed Adverse Events in Controlled Clinical Trials: Adverse events from Table 4 occurring in at least 5% of patients treated with WELLBUTRIN SR Tablets and at a rate at least twice the placebo rate are listed below for the 300- and 400-mg/day dose groups.

WELLBUTRIN SR 300 mg/day: Anorexia, dry mouth, rash, sweating, tinnitus, and tremor.

WELLBUTRIN SR 400 mg/day: Abdominal pain, agitation, anxiety, dizziness, dry mouth, insomnia, myalgia, nausea, palpitation, pharyngitis, sweating, tinnitus, and urinary frequency.

Other Events Observed During the Clinical Development and Postmarketing Experience of Bupropion: In addition to the adverse events noted above, the following events have been reported in clinical trials and postmarketing experience with the sustained-release formulation of bupropion in depressed patients and in nondepressed smokers, as well as in clinical trials and postmarketing clinical experience with the immediate-release formulation of bupropion.

Adverse events for which frequencies are provided below occurred in clinical trials with the sustained-release formulation of bupropion. The frequencies represent the proportion of patients who experienced a treatment-emergent adverse event on at least one occasion in placebo-controlled studies for depression (n = 987) or smoking cessation (n = 1013), or patients who experienced an adverse event requiring discontinuation of treatment in an open-label surveillance study with WELLBUTRIN SR Tablets (n = 3100). All treatment-emergent adverse events are included except those listed in Tables 1 through 4, those events listed in other safety-related sections, those adverse events subsumed under COSTART terms that are either overly general or excessively specific so as to be uninformative, those events not reasonably associated with the use of the drug, and those events that were not serious and occurred in fewer than two patients. Events of major clinical importance are described in the WARNINGS and PRECAUTIONS sections of the labeling. Events are further categorized by body system and listed in order of decreasing frequency according to the following definitions of frequency: Frequent adverse events are defined as those occurring in at least 1/100 patients. Infrequent adverse events are those occurring in 1/100 to 1/1000 patients, while rare events are those occurring in less than 1/1000 patients.

Adverse events for which frequencies are not provided occurred in clinical trials or postmarketing experience with bupropion. Only those adverse events not previously listed for sustained-release bupropion are included. The extent to which these events may be associated with WELLBUTRIN SR is unknown.

Body (General): Infrequent were chills, facial edema, musculoskeletal chest pain, and photosensitivity. Rare was malaise. Also observed were arthralgia, myalgia, and fever with rash and other symptoms suggestive of delayed hypersensitivity. These symptoms may resemble serum sickness (see PRECAUTIONS).

Cardiovascular: Infrequent were postural hypotension, stroke, tachycardia, and vasodilation. Rare was syncope. Also observed were complete atrioventricular block, extrasystoles, hypotension, hypertension (in come cases severe, see PRECAUTIONS), myocardial infarction, phlebitis, and pulmonary embolism.

Digestive: Infrequent were abnormal liver function, bruxism, gastric reflux, gingivitis, glossitis, increased salivation, jaundice, mouth ulcers, stomatitis, and thirst. Rare was edema of tongue. Also observed were colitis, esophagitis, gastrointestinal hemorrhage, gum hemorrhage, hepatitis, intestinal perforation, liver damage, pancreatitis, and stomach ulcer.

Endocrine: Also observed were hyperglycemia, hypoglycemia, and syndrome of inappropriate antidiuretic hormone.

Hemic and Lymphatic: Infrequent was ecchymosis. Also observed were anemia, leukocytosis, leukopenia, lymphadenopathy, pancytopenia, and thrombocytopenia.

Metabolic and Nutritional: Infrequent were edema and peripheral edema. Also observed was glycosuria.

Musculoskeletal: Infrequent were leg cramps. Also observed were muscle rigidity/fever/rhabdomyolysis and muscle weakness.

Nervous System: Infrequent were abnormal coordination, decreased libido, depersonalization, dysphoria, emotional lability, hostility, hyperkinesia, hypertonia, hypesthesia, suicidal ideation, and vertigo. Rare were amnesia, ataxia, derealization, and hypomania. Also observed were abnormal electroencephalogram (EEG), akinesia, aphasia, coma, delirium, dysarthria, dyskinesia, dystonia, euphoria, extrapyramidal syndrome, hypokinesia, increased libido, manic reaction, neuralgia, neuropathy, paranoid reaction, and unmasking tardive dyskinesia.

Respiratory: Rare was bronchospasm. Also observed was pneumonia.

Skin: Rare was maculopapular rash. Also observed were alopecia, angioedema, exfoliative dermatitis, and hirsutism.

Special Senses: Infrequent were accommodation abnormality and dry eye. Also observed were deafness, diplopia, and mydriasis.

Urogenital: Infrequent were impotence, polyuria, and prostate disorder. Also observed were abnormal ejaculation, cystitis, dyspareunia, dysuria, gynecomastia, menopause, painful erection, salpingitis, urinary incontinence, urinary retention, and vaginitis.

DRUG ABUSE AND DEPENDENCE

Controlled Substance Class: Bupropion is not a controlled substance.

Humans: Controlled clinical studies of bupropion conducted in normal volunteers, in subjects with a history of multiple drug abuse, and in depressed patients showed some increase in motor activity and agitation/excitement.

In a population of individuals experienced with drugs of abuse, a single dose of 400 mg of bupropion produced mild amphetamine-like activity as compared to placebo on the Morphine-Benzedrine Subscale of the Addiction Research Center Inventories (ARCI), and a score intermediate between placebo and amphetamine on the Liking Scale of the ARCI. These scales measure general feelings of euphoria and drug desirability.

Findings in clinical trials, however, are not known to reliably predict the abuse potential of drugs. Nonetheless, evidence from single-dose studies does suggest that the recommended daily dosage of bupropion when administered in divided doses is not likely to be especially reinforcing to amphetamine or stimulant abusers. However, higher doses that could not be tested because of the risk of seizure might be modestly attractive to those who abuse stimulant drugs.

Animals: Studies in rodents and primates have shown that bupropion exhibits some pharmacologic actions common to psychostimulants. In rodents, it has been shown to increase locomotor activity, elicit a mild stereotyped behavioral response, and increase rates of responding in several schedule-controlled behavior paradigms. In primate models to assess the positive reinforcing effects of psychoactive drugs, bupropion was self-administered intravenously. In rats, bupropion produced amphetamine-like and cocaine-like discriminative stimulus effects in drug discrimination paradigms used to characterize the subjective effects of psychoactive drugs.

OVERDOSAGE

Human Overdose Experience: There has been very limited experience with overdosage of WELLBUTRIN SR Tablets; three cases were reported during clinical trials. One patient ingested 3000 mg of WELLBUTRIN SR Tablets and vomited quickly after the overdose; the patient experienced blurred vision and lightheadedness. A second patient ingested a "handful" of WELLBUTRIN SR Tablets and experienced confusion, lethargy, nausea, jitteriness, and seizure. A third patient ingested 3600 mg of WELLBUTRIN SR Tablets and a bottle of wine; the patient experienced nausea, visual hallucinations, and "grogginess." None of the patients experienced further sequelae.

There has been extensive experience with overdosage of the immediate-release formulation of bupropion. Thirteen overdoses occurred during clinical trials. Twelve patients ingested 850 to 4200 mg and recovered without significant sequelae. Another patient who ingested 9000 mg of the immediate-release formulation of bupropion and 300 mg of tranylcypromine experienced a grand mal seizure and recovered without further sequelae.

Since introduction, overdoses of up to 17,500 mg of the immediate-release formulation of bupropion have been reported. Seizure was reported in approximately one third of all cases. Other serious reactions reported with overdoses of the immediate-release formulation of bupropion alone included hallucinations, loss of consciousness, and sinus tachycardia. Fever, muscle rigidity, rhabdomyolysis, hypotension, stupor, coma, and respiratory failure have been reported when the immediate-release formulation of bupropion was part of multiple drug overdoses.

Although most patients recovered without sequelae, deaths associated with overdoses of the immediate-release formulation of bupropion alone have been reported rarely in patients ingesting massive doses of the drug. Multiple uncontrolled seizures, bradycardia, cardiac failure, and cardiac arrest prior to death were reported in these patients.

Overdosage Management: Ensure an adequate airway, oxygenation, and ventilation. Monitor cardiac rhythm and vital signs. EEG monitoring is also recommended for the first 48 hours post-ingestion. General supportive and symptomatic measures are also recommended. Induction of emesis is not recommended. Gastric lavage with a large-bore orogastric tube with appropriate airway protection, if needed, may be indicated if performed soon after ingestion or in symptomatic patients.

Activated charcoal should be administered. There is no experience with the use of forced diuresis, dialysis, hemoperfusion, or exchange transfusion in the management of bupropion overdoses. No specific antidotes for bupropion are known.

Due to the dose-related risk of seizures with WELLBUTRIN SR, hospitalization following suspected overdose should be considered. Based on studies in animals, it is recommended that seizures be treated with intravenous benzodiazepine administration and other supportive measures, as appropriate.

In managing overdosage, consider the possibility of multiple drug involvement. The physician should consider contacting a poison control center for additional information on the treatment of any overdose. Telephone numbers for certified poison control centers are listed in the *Physicians' Desk Reference* (PDR).

DOSAGE AND ADMINISTRATION

General Dosing Considerations: It is particularly important to administer WELLBUTRIN SR Tablets in a manner most likely to minimize the risk of seizure (see WARNINGS). Gradual escalation in dosage is also important if agitation, motor restlessness, and insomnia, often seen during the initial days of treatment, are to be minimized. If necessary, these effects may be managed by temporary reduction of dose or the short-term administration of an intermediate to long-acting sedative hypnotic. A sedative hypnotic usually is not required beyond the first week of treatment. Insomnia may also be minimized by avoiding bedtime doses. If distressing, untoward effects supervene, dose escalation should be stopped.

Initial Treatment: The usual adult target dose for WELLBUTRIN SR Tablets is 300 mg/day, given as 150 mg twice daily. Dosing with WELLBUTRIN SR Tablets should begin at 150 mg/day given as a single daily dose in the morning. If the 150-mg initial dose is adequately tolerated, an increase to the 300-mg/day target dose, given as 150 mg twice daily, may be made as early as day 4 of dosing. There should be an interval of at least 8 hours between successive doses.

Increasing the Dosage Above 300 mg/day: As with other antidepressants, the full antidepressant effect of WELLBUTRIN SR Tablets may not be evident until 4 weeks of treatment or longer. An increase in dosage to the maximum of 400 mg/day, given as 200 mg twice daily, may be considered for patients in whom no clinical improvement is noted after several weeks of treatment at 300 mg/day.

Maintenance: The lowest dose that maintains remission is recommended. Although it is not known how long the patient should remain on WELLBUTRIN SR Tablets, it is generally recognized that acute episodes of depression require several months or longer of antidepressant drug treatment.

Dosage Adjustment for Patients with Impaired Hepatic Function: WELLBUTRIN SR should be used with extreme caution in patients with severe hepatic cirrhosis. The dose should not exceed 100 mg every day or 150 mg every other day in these patients. WELLBUTRIN SR should be used with caution in patients with hepatic impairment (including mild to moderate hepatic cirrhosis) and a reduced frequency and/or dose should be considered in patients with mild to moderate hepatic cirrhosis (see CLINICAL PHARMACOLOGY, WARNINGS, and PRECAUTIONS)

Dosage Adjustment for Patients with Impaired Renal Function: WELLBUTRIN SR should be used with caution in patients with renal impairment and a reduced frequency and/or dose should be considered (see CLINICAL PHARMACOLOGY and PRECAUTIONS).

HOW SUPPLIED

WELLBUTRIN SR Sustained-Release Tablets, 100 mg of bupropion hydrochloride, are blue, round, biconvex, film-coated tablets printed with "WELLBUTRIN SR 100" in bottles of 60 (NDC 0173-0947-55) tablets.

WELLBUTRIN SR Sustained-Release Tablets, 150 mg of bupropion hydrochloride, are purple, round, biconvex, film-coated tablets printed with "WELLBUTRIN SR 150" in bottles of 60 (NDC 0173-0135-55) tablets.

Store at controlled room temperature, 20° to 25°C (68° to 77°F) [see USP]. Dispense in a tight, light-resistant container as defined in the USP.

Information for the Patient
WELLBUTRIN SR® (bupropion hydrochloride)
Sustained-Release Tablets

Please read this information before you start taking WELLBUTRIN SR. Also read this leaflet each time you renew your prescription, in case anything has changed. This information is not intended to take the place of discussions between you and your doctor. You and your doctor should discuss WELLBUTRIN SR as it relates to the treatment of your depression. Do not let anyone else use your WELLBUTRIN SR.

IMPORTANT WARNING:

At a dose of 300 mg each day, there is a chance that approximately 1 out of every 1000 people taking bupropion hydrochloride, the active ingredient in WELLBUTRIN SR, will have a seizure. At a dose of 400 mg each day, there is a chance that approximately 4 out of every 1000 people will have a seizure. The chance of this happening increases if you:

- have a seizure disorder (for example, epilepsy);
- have or have had an eating disorder (for example, bulimia or anorexia nervosa);
- take more than the recommended amount of WELLBUTRIN SR; or
- take other medicines with the same active ingredient that is in WELLBUTRIN SR, such as ZYBAN® (bupropion hydrochloride) Sustained-Release Tablets (used to help people quit smoking).

You can reduce the chance of experiencing a seizure by following your doctor's directions on how to take WELLBUTRIN SR. You should also discuss with your doctor whether WELLBUTRIN SR is right for you.

1. What is WELLBUTRIN SR?

WELLBUTRIN SR is a prescription medicine used to treat depression.

2. Who should not take WELLBUTRIN SR:

You should not take WELLBUTRIN SR if you:

- have a seizure disorder (for example, epilepsy);
- are already taking ZYBAN or any other medicines that contain bupropion hydrochloride;
- have or have had an eating disorder (for example, bulimia or anorexia nervosa);
- are currently taking or have recently taken a monoamine oxidase inhibitor (MAOI); or
- are allergic to bupropion.

3. Are there special concerns for women?
WELLBUTRIN SR is not recommended for women who are pregnant or breast-feeding. Women should notify their doctor if they become pregnant or intend to become pregnant while taking WELLBUTRIN SR.

4. Are there any concerns for patients with liver or kidney disease?
If you have liver or kidney disease, tell your doctor before taking WELLBUTRIN SR. Depending on the severity of your condition, your doctor may need to adjust your dosage.

5. How should I take WELLBUTRIN SR?
- You should take WELLBUTRIN SR as directed by your doctor. The usual recommended dosing is to begin treatment with WELLBUTRIN SR by taking one 150-mg tablet in the morning. As early as day 4 of treatment, your doctor may increase your dose to one 150-mg tablet in the morning and one 150-mg tablet in the early evening (for a total of 300 mg each day).
  If your depression does not improve after several weeks, your doctor may increase the dose of WELLBUTRIN SR to a total of 400 mg each day (taken as 200 mg in the morning and 200 mg in the early evening). Doses should be taken at least 8 hours apart.
- **Never take an "extra" dose of WELLBUTRIN SR tablets for any reason, even if you miss a dose.** If you forget to take a dose, do not take an extra tablet to "catch up" for the dose you forgot. Wait and take your next tablet at the regular time. Do not take more tablets than your doctor prescribed. This is important so you do not increase your chance of having a seizure.
- It is important to swallow WELLBUTRIN SR tablets whole. Do not chew, divide, or crush tablets.

6. How long should I take WELLBUTRIN SR?
Only you and your doctor can determine how long you should take WELLBUTRIN SR. You and your doctor should discuss your signs and symptoms of depression regularly to determine how long you should take WELLBUTRIN SR. Do not stop taking your medicine or decrease the amount of medicine you are taking without talking to your doctor first.

7. What are possible side effects of WELLBUTRIN SR?
Like all medicines, WELLBUTRIN SR may cause side effects.
- The most common side effects of WELLBUTRIN SR in clinical studies were:
  At 300 mg/day: Loss of appetite, dry mouth, skin rash, sweating, ringing in the ears, and shakiness.
  At 400 mg/day: Abdominal (stomach) pain, agitation, anxiety, dizziness, dry mouth, difficulty sleeping, muscle pain, nausea, rapid heart beat, sore throat, sweating, ringing in the ears, and urinating more often.
- The side effects of WELLBUTRIN SR are generally mild and often disappear after a few weeks. If you have nausea, you may want to take your medicine with food. If you have difficulty sleeping, avoid taking your medicine too close to bedtime.
- The most common side effects that caused people to stop taking WELLBUTRIN SR during clinical studies were skin rash, nausea, agitation, and migraine (a severe type of headache).
- Stop taking WELLBUTRIN SR and contact your doctor or health care professional if you have signs of an allergic reaction such as a skin rash, or difficulty in breathing. Discuss any other troublesome side effects with your doctor.
- Use caution before driving a car or operating complex, hazardous machinery until you know if WELLBUTRIN SR affects your ability to perform these tasks.

8. Will taking WELLBUTRIN SR change my body weight?
In clinical studies with WELLBUTRIN SR, some people lost weight and other people gained weight.
For people who lost weight, 14 out of 100 people taking 300 mg/day of WELLBUTRIN SR lost more than 5 lbs, 19 out of 100 people taking 400 mg/day lost more than 5 lbs, and 6 out of 100 people taking placebo (a sugar pill) lost more than 5 lbs.
For people who gained weight, 3 out of 100 people taking 300 mg/day of WELLBUTRIN SR gained more than 5 lbs, 2 out of 100 people taking 400 mg/day gained more than 5 lbs, and 4 out of 100 people taking placebo (a sugar pill) gained more than 5 lbs.
Since weight change (loss or gain) also can be a symptom of depression, you should discuss with your doctor whether WELLBUTRIN SR is right for you.

9. Should I drink alcohol while I am taking WELLBUTRIN SR?
It is best to not drink alcohol at all or to drink very little while taking WELLBUTRIN SR. If you usually drink a lot of alcohol, or if you drink a lot of alcohol and suddenly stop, you may increase your chance of having a seizure. Therefore, it is important to discuss your use of alcohol with your doctor before you begin taking WELLBUTRIN SR.

10. Will WELLBUTRIN SR affect other medicines I am taking?
WELLBUTRIN SR may affect other medicines you're taking. It is important not to take medicines that may increase the chance for you to have a seizure. Therefore, you should make sure that your doctor knows about all medicines—prescription and over-the-counter—you are taking or plan to take.

11. Do WELLBUTRIN SR tablets have a characteristic odor?
WELLBUTRIN SR tablets may have a characteristic odor. If present, this odor is normal.

12. How should I store WELLBUTRIN SR?
- Store WELLBUTRIN SR at room temperature, out of direct sunlight.
- Keep WELLBUTRIN SR in a tightly closed container.
- Keep WELLBUTRIN SR out of the reach of children.

This summary provides important information about WELLBUTRIN SR. This summary cannot replace the more detailed information that you need from your doctor. If you have any questions or concerns about either WELLBUTRIN SR or depression, talk to your doctor or other health care professional.
Distributed by:
Glaxo Wellcome Inc., Research Triangle Park, NC 27709
Manufactured by:
Glaxo Wellcome Inc., Research Triangle Park, NC 27709
or Catalytica Pharmaceuticals, Inc., Greenville, NC 27834
US Patent Nos. 5,358,970; 5,427,798; 5,731,000; 5,763,493; and Re. 33,994

May 2000/RL-815
Shown in Product Identification Guide, page 316

ZANTAC® ℞
[zan 'tak]
(ranitidine hydrochloride)
Injection
ZANTAC® ℞
(ranitidine hydrochloride)
Injection Premixed

DESCRIPTION

The active ingredient in ZANTAC Injection and ZANTAC Injection Premixed is ranitidine hydrochloride (HCl), a histamine H_2-receptor antagonist. Chemically it is N[2-[[[5-[(dimethylamino)methyl]-2-furanyl]methyl]thio]ethyl]-N′-methyl-2-nitro-1,1-ethenediamine, hydrochloride.
The empirical formula is $C_{13}H_{22}N_4O_3S \bullet HCl$, representing a molecular weight of 350.87.
Ranitidine HCl is a white to pale yellow, granular substance that is soluble in water.
ZANTAC Injection is a clear, colorless to yellow, nonpyrogenic liquid. The yellow color of the liquid tends to intensify without adversely affecting potency. The pH of the injection solution is 6.7 to 7.3.
Sterile Injection for Intramuscular or Intravenous Administration: Each 1 mL of aqueous solution contains ranitidine 25 mg (as the hydrochloride); phenol 5 mg as preservative; and 0.96 mg of monobasic potassium phosphate and 2.4 mg of dibasic sodium phosphate as buffers.
A pharmacy bulk package is a container of a sterile preparation for parenteral use that contains many single doses. The contents are intended for use in a pharmacy admixture program and are restricted to the preparation of admixtures for intravenous (IV) infusion.
Sterile, Premixed Solution for Intravenous Administration in Single-Dose, Flexible Plastic Containers: Each 50 mL contains ranitidine HCl equivalent to 50 mg of ranitidine, sodium chloride 225 mg, and citric acid 15 mg and dibasic sodium phosphate 90 mg as buffers in water for injection. It contains no preservatives. The osmolarity of this solution is 180 mOsm/L (approx.), and the pH is 6.7 to 7.3.
The flexible plastic container is fabricated from a specially formulated, nonplasticized, thermoplastic co-polyester (CR3). Water can permeate from inside the container into the overwrap but not in amounts sufficient to affect the solution significantly. Solutions inside the plastic container also can leach out certain of the chemical components in very small amounts before the expiration period is attained. However, the safety of the plastic has been confirmed by tests in animals according to USP biological standards for plastic containers.

CLINICAL PHARMACOLOGY

ZANTAC is a competitive, reversible inhibitor of the action of histamine at the histamine H_2-receptors, including receptors on the gastric cells. ZANTAC does not lower serum Ca^{++} in hypercalcemic states. ZANTAC is not an anticholinergic agent.
Pharmacokinetics: ***Absorption:*** ZANTAC is absorbed very rapidly after intramuscular (IM) injection. Mean peak levels of 576 ng/mL occur within 15 minutes or less following a 50-mg IM dose. Absorption from IM sites is virtually complete, with a bioavailability of 90% to 100% compared with intravenous (IV) administration. Following oral administration, the bioavailability of ZANTAC Tablets is 50%.
Distribution: The volume of distribution is about 1.4 L/kg. Serum protein binding averages 15%.
Metabolism: In humans, the N-oxide is the principal metabolite in the urine; however, this amounts to <4% of the dose. Other metabolites are the S-oxide (1%) and the desmethyl ranitidine (1%). The remainder of the administered dose is found in the stool. Studies in patients with hepatic dysfunction (compensated cirrhosis) indicate that there are minor, but clinically insignificant, alterations in ranitidine half-life, distribution, clearance, and bioavailability.
Excretion: Following IV injection, approximately 70% of the dose is recovered in the urine as unchanged drug. Renal clearance averages 530 mL/min, with a total clearance of 760 mL/min. The elimination half-life is 2.0 to 2.5 hours. Four patients with clinically significant renal function impairment (creatinine clearance 25 to 35 mL/min) administered 50 mg of ranitidine intravenously had an average plasma half-life of 4.8 hours, a ranitidine clearance of 29 mL/min, and a volume of distribution of 1.76 L/kg. In general, these parameters appear to be altered in proportion to creatinine clearance (see DOSAGE AND ADMINISTRATION).
Pediatrics: There are no significant differences in the pharmacokinetic parameter values for ranitidine in pediatric patients (from 1 month up to 16 years of age) and healthy adults when correction is made for body weight. The pharmacokinetics of ZANTAC in pediatric patients are summarized in Table 1.
[See table 1 at top of next page]
Plasma clearance in neonatal patients (less than 1 month of age) receiving ECMO was considerably lower (3 to 4 mL/min/kg) than observed in children or adults. The elimination half-life in neonates averages 6.6 hours as compared to approximately 2 hours in adults and pediatric patients.
Pharmacodynamics: Serum concentrations necessary to inhibit 50% of stimulated gastric acid secretion are estimated to be 36 to 94 ng/mL. Following single IV or IM 50-mg doses, serum concentrations of ZANTAC are in this range for 6 to 8 hours.
Antisecretory Activity: ***1. Effects on Acid Secretion:*** ZANTAC Injection inhibits basal gastric acid secretion as well as gastric acid secretion stimulated by betazole and pentagastrin, as shown in Table 2:
[See table 2 at top of next page]
In a group of 10 known hypersecretors, ranitidine plasma levels of 71, 180, and 376 ng/mL inhibited basal acid secretion by 76%, 90%, and 99.5%, respectively.
It appears that basal- and betazole-stimulated secretions are most sensitive to inhibition by ZANTAC, while pentagastrin-stimulated secretion is more difficult to suppress.
2. Effects on Other Gastrointestinal Secretions:
Pepsin: ZANTAC does not affect pepsin secretion. Total pepsin output is reduced in proportion to the decrease in volume of gastric juice.
Intrinsic Factor: ZANTAC has no significant effect on pentagastrin-stimulated intrinsic factor secretion.
Serum Gastrin: ZANTAC has little or no effect on fasting or postprandial serum gastrin.
Other Pharmacologic Actions:
a. Gastric bacterial flora—increase in nitrate-reducing organisms, significance not known.
b. Prolactin levels—no effect in recommended oral or intravenous (IV) dosage, but small, transient, dose-related increases in serum prolactin have been reported after IV bolus injections of 100 mg or more.
c. Other pituitary hormones—no effect on serum gonadotropins, TSH, or GH. Possible impairment of vasopressin release.
d. No change in cortisol, aldosterone, androgen, or estrogen levels.
e. No antiandrogenic action.
f. No effect on count, motility, or morphology of sperm.
Pediatrics: The ranitidine concentration necessary to suppress basal acid secretion by at least 90% has been reported to be 40 to 60 ng/mL in pediatric patients with duodenal or gastric ulcers.
In a study of 20 critically ill pediatric patients receiving ranitidine IV at 1 mg/kg every 6 hours, 10 patients with a baseline pH≥4 maintained this baseline throughout the study. Eight of the remaining 10 patients with a baseline of pH≤2 achieved pH≥4 throughout varying periods after dosing. It should be noted, however, that because these pharmacodynamic parameters were assessed in critically ill pediatric patients, the data should be interpreted with caution when dosing recommendations are made for a less seriously ill pediatric population.
In another small study of neonatal patients (n=5) receiving ECMO, gastric pH<4 pretreatment increased to >4 after a 2 mg/kg dose and remained above 4 for at least 15 hours.
Clinical Trials: ***Active Duodenal Ulcer:*** In a multicenter, double-blind, controlled, US study of endoscopically diagnosed duodenal ulcers, earlier healing was seen in the patients treated with oral ZANTAC as shown in Table 3:
[See table 3 at top of next page]
In these studies, patients treated with oral ZANTAC reported a reduction in both daytime and nocturnal pain, and they also consumed less antacid than the placebo-treated patients.
[See table 4 at top of next page]
Pathological Hypersecretory Conditions (such as Zollinger-Ellison syndrome): ZANTAC inhibits gastric acid secretion and reduces occurrence of diarrhea, anorexia, and pain in patients with pathological hypersecretion associated with Zollinger-Ellison syndrome, systemic mastocytosis, and other pathological hypersecretory conditions (e.g., postoperative, "short-gut" syndrome, idiopathic). Use of oral ZANTAC was followed by healing of ulcers in 8 of 19 (42%) patients who were intractable to previous therapy.

Continued on next page

This product information is based on labeling in effect on June 23, 2000. For further information, contact via direct mail, phone, or web site. Medical Information, Glaxo Wellcome Inc., PO Box 13398, Research Triangle Park, NC 27709. Healthcare Professionals (Medical Information): 800-334-0089. Patients (Customer Response Center): 1-888-825-5249. Glaxo Wellcome Corporate Web Site: www.glaxowellcome.com

Zantac Injection—Cont.

In a retrospective review of 52 Zollinger-Ellison patients given ZANTAC as a continuous IV infusion for up to 15 days, no patients developed complications of acid-peptic disease such as bleeding or perforation. Acid output was controlled to ≤10 mEq/h.

INDICATIONS AND USAGE

ZANTAC Injection and ZANTAC Injection Premixed are indicated in some hospitalized patients with pathological hypersecretory conditions or intractable duodenal ulcers, or as an alternative to the oral dosage form for short-term use in patients who are unable to take oral medication.

CONTRAINDICATIONS

ZANTAC Injection and ZANTAC Injection Premixed are contraindicated for patients known to have hypersensitivity to the drug.

PRECAUTIONS

General: 1. Symptomatic response to therapy with ZANTAC does not preclude the presence of gastric malignancy.
2. Since ZANTAC is excreted primarily by the kidney, dosage should be adjusted in patients with impaired renal function (see DOSAGE AND ADMINISTRATION). Caution should be observed in patients with hepatic dysfunction since ZANTAC is metabolized in the liver.
3. In controlled studies in normal volunteers, elevations in SGPT have been observed when H_2-antagonists have been administered intravenously at greater than recommended dosages for 5 days or longer. Therefore, it seems prudent in patients receiving IV ranitidine at dosages ≥100 mg q.i.d. for periods of 5 days or longer to monitor SGPT daily (from day 5) for the remainder of IV therapy.
4. Bradycardia in association with rapid administration of ZANTAC Injection has been reported rarely, usually in patients with factors predisposing to cardiac rhythm disturbances. Recommended rates of administration should not be exceeded (see DOSAGE AND ADMINISTRATION).
5. Rare reports suggest that ZANTAC may precipitate acute porphyric attacks in patients with acute porphyria. ZANTAC should therefore be avoided in patients with a history of acute porphyria.

Laboratory Tests: False-positive tests for urine protein with MULTISTIX® may occur during therapy with ZANTAC and therefore testing with sulfosalicylic acid is recommended.

Drug Interactions: Although ZANTAC has been reported to bind weakly to cytochrome P-450 *in vitro,* recommended doses of the drug do not inhibit the action of the cytochrome P-450–linked oxygenase enzymes in the liver. However, there have been isolated reports of drug interactions that suggest that ZANTAC may affect the bioavailability of certain drugs by some mechanism as yet unidentified (e.g., a pH-dependent effect on absorption or a change in volume of distribution).
Increased or decreased prothrombin times have been reported during concurrent use of ranitidine and warfarin. However, in human pharmacokinetic studies with dosages of ranitidine up to 400 mg/day, no interaction occurred; ranitidine had no effect on warfarin clearance or prothrombin time. The possibility of an interaction with warfarin at dosages of ranitidine higher than 400 mg/day has not been investigated.
In a ranitidine-triazolam drug-drug interaction study, triazolam plasma concentrations were higher during b.i.d. dosing of ranitidine than triazolam given alone. The mean area under the triazolam concentration-time curve (AUC) values, in 18- to 60-year-old subjects were 10% and 28% higher following administration of 75-mg and 150-mg ranitidine tablets, respectively, than triazolam given alone. In subjects older than 60 years of age, the mean AUC values were approximately 30% higher following administration of 75-mg and 150-mg ranitidine tablets. It appears that there were no changes in pharmacokinetics of triazolam and α-hydroxytriazolam, a major metabolite, and in their elimination. Reduced gastric acidity due to ranitidine may have resulted in an increase in the availability of triazolam. The clinical significance of this triazolam and ranitidine pharmacokinetic interaction is unknown.

Carcinogenesis, Mutagenesis, Impairment of Fertility: There was no indication of tumorigenic or carcinogenic effects in life-span studies in mice and rats at oral dosages up to 2000 mg/kg per day.
Ranitidine was not mutagenic in standard bacterial tests *(Salmonella, Escherichia coli)* for mutagenicity at concentrations up to the maximum recommended for these assays. In a dominant lethal assay, a single oral dose of 1000 mg/kg to male rats was without effect on the outcome of two matings per week for the next 9 weeks.

Pregnancy: ***Teratogenic Effects: Pregnancy Category B:*** Reproduction studies have been performed in rats and rabbits at oral doses up to 160 times the human oral dose and have revealed no evidence of impaired fertility or harm to the fetus due to ZANTAC. There are, however, no adequate and well-controlled studies in pregnant women. Because animal reproduction studies are not always predictive of human response, this drug should be used during pregnancy only if clearly needed.

Nursing Mothers: ZANTAC is secreted in human milk. Caution should be exercised when ZANTAC is administered to a nursing mother.

Table 1: Ranitidine Pharmacokinetics in Pediatric Patients Following IV Dosing

Population (age)	n	Dose (mg/kg)	$T_{1/2}$ (hours)	Vd (L/kg)	CLp (mL/min/kg)
Peptic ulcer disease					
(<6 years)	6	1.25 or 2.5	2.2	1.29	11.41
(6–11.9 years)	11	1.25 or 2.5	2.1	1.14	8.96
(>12 years)	6	1.25 or 2.5	1.7	0.98	9.89
Adults	6	2.5	1.9	1.04	8.77
Peptic ulcer disease (3.5–16 years)	12	0.13–0.80	1.8	2.3	795 mL/min/1.73/m²
Children in intensive care (1 day–12.6 years)	17	1.0	2.4	2	11.7
Neonates receiving ECMO	12	2	6.6	1.8	4.3

$T_{1/2}$ = Terminal half-life; CLp = Plasma clearance of ranitidine.
ECMO = extracorporeal membrane oxygenation.

Table 2: Effect of Intravenous ZANTAC on Gastric Acid Secretion

	Time After Dose, h	% Inhibition of Gastric Acid Output by Intravenous Dose, mg		
		20 mg	60 mg	100 mg
Betazole	Up to 2	93	99	99
Pentagastrin	Up to 3	47	66	77

Table 3: Duodenal Ulcer Patient Healing Rates

	Oral ZANTAC*		Oral Placebo*	
	Number Entered	Healed/ Evaluable	Number Entered	Healed/ Evaluable
Outpatients				
Week 2	195	69/182 (38%)†	188	31/164 (19%)
Week 4		137/187 (73%)†		76/168 (45%)

*All patients were permitted p.r.n. antacids for relief of pain.
†P<0.0001.

Table 4: Mean Daily Doses of Antacid

	Ulcer Healed	Ulcer Not Healed
Oral ZANTAC	0.06	0.71
Oral placebo	0.71	1.43

Pediatric Use: The safety and effectiveness of ZANTAC Injection have been established in the age-group of 1 month to 16 years for the treatment of duodenal ulcer. Use of ZANTAC in this age-group is supported by adequate and well-controlled studies in adults, as well as additional pharmacokinetic data in pediatric patients, and an analysis of the published literature.
Safety and effectiveness in pediatric patients for the treatment of pathological hypersecretory conditions have not been established.
Limited data in neonatal patients (less than one month of age) receiving ECMO suggest that ZANTAC may be useful and safe for increasing gastric pH for patients at risk of gastrointestinal hemorrhage.

Use in Elderly Patients: Ulcer healing rates in elderly patients (65 to 82 years of age) treated with oral ZANTAC were no different from those in younger age-groups. The incidence rates for adverse events and laboratory abnormalities were also not different from those seen in other age-groups.

ADVERSE REACTIONS

Transient pain at the site of IM injection has been reported. Transient local burning or itching has been reported with IV administration of ZANTAC.
The following have been reported as events in clinical trials or in the routine management of patients treated with oral or parenteral ZANTAC. The relationship to therapy with ZANTAC has been unclear in many cases. Headache, sometimes severe, seems to be related to administration of ZANTAC.

Central Nervous System: Rarely, malaise, dizziness, somnolence, insomnia, and vertigo. Rare cases of reversible mental confusion, agitation, depression, and hallucinations have been reported, predominantly in severely ill elderly patients. Rare cases of reversible blurred vision suggestive of a change in accommodation have been reported. Rare reports of reversible involuntary motor disturbances have been received.

Cardiovascular: As with other H_2-blockers, rare reports of arrhythmias such as tachycardia, bradycardia, asystole, atrioventricular block, and premature ventricular beats.

Gastrointestinal: Constipation, diarrhea, nausea/vomiting, abdominal discomfort/pain, and rare reports of pancreatitis.

Hepatic: In normal volunteers, SGPT values were increased to at least twice the pretreatment levels in 6 of 12 subjects receiving 100 mg q.i.d. intravenously for 7 days, and in 4 of 24 subjects receiving 50 mg q.i.d. intravenously for 5 days. There have been occasional reports of hepatocellular, cholestatic, or mixed hepatitis, with or without jaundice. In such circumstances, ranitidine should be immediately discontinued. These events are usually reversible, but in rare circumstances death has occurred. Rare cases of hepatic failure have also been reported.

Musculoskeletal: Rare reports of arthralgias and myalgias.

Hematologic: Blood count changes (leukopenia, granulocytopenia, and thrombocytopenia) have occurred in a few patients. These were usually reversible. Rare cases of agranulocytosis, pancytopenia, sometimes with marrow hypoplasia, and aplastic anemia and exceedingly rare cases of acquired immune hemolytic anemia have been reported.

Endocrine: Controlled studies in animals and humans have shown no stimulation of any pituitary hormone by ZANTAC and no antiandrogenic activity, and cimetidine-induced gynecomastia and impotence in hypersecretory patients have resolved when ZANTAC has been substituted. However, occasional cases of gynecomastia, impotence, and loss of libido have been reported in male patients receiving ZANTAC, but the incidence did not differ from that in the general population.

Integumentary: Rash, including rare cases of erythema multiforme, and, rarely, alopecia.

Other: Rare cases of hypersensitivity reactions (e.g., bronchospasm, fever, rash, eosinophilia), anaphylaxis, angioneurotic edema, and small increases in serum creatinine.

OVERDOSAGE

There has been virtually no experience with overdosage with ZANTAC Injection and limited experience with oral doses of ranitidine. Reported acute ingestions of up to 18 g orally have been associated with transient adverse effects similar to those encountered in normal clinical experience (see ADVERSE REACTIONS). In addition, abnormalities of gait and hypotension have been reported.
When overdosage occurs, clinical monitoring and supportive therapy should be employed.
Studies in dogs receiving dosages of ZANTAC in excess of 225 mg/kg per day have shown muscular tremors, vomiting, and rapid respiration. Single oral doses of 1000 mg/kg in mice and rats were not lethal. Intravenous LD_{50} values in mice and rats were 77 and 83 mg/kg, respectively.

DOSAGE AND ADMINISTRATION

Parenteral Administration: In some hospitalized patients with pathological hypersecretory conditions or intractable duodenal ulcers, or in patients who are unable to take oral medication, ZANTAC may be administered parenterally according to the following recommendations:

Intramuscular Injection: 50 mg (2 mL) every 6 to 8 hours. (No dilution necessary.)

Intermittent Intravenous Injection:

a. Intermittent Bolus: 50 mg (2 mL) every 6 to 8 hours. Dilute ZANTAC Injection, 50 mg, in 0.9% sodium chloride injection or other compatible IV solution (see Stability) to a concentration no greater than 2.5 mg/mL (20 mL). Inject at a rate no greater than 4 mL/min (5 minutes).

b. Intermittent Infusion: 50 mg (2 mL) every 6 to 8 hours. Dilute ZANTAC Injection, 50 mg, in 5% dextrose injection or other compatible IV solution (see Stability) to a concentration no greater than 0.5 mg/mL (100 mL). Infuse at a rate no greater than 5 to 7 mL/min (15 to 20 minutes).

ZANTAC Injection Premixed solution, 50 mg, in 0.45% sodium chloride, 50 mL, requires no dilution and should be infused over 15 to 20 minutes.

In some patients it may be necessary to increase dosage. When this is necessary, the increases should be made by more frequent administration of the dose, but generally should not exceed 400 mg/day.

Continuous Intravenous Infusion: Add ZANTAC Injection to 5% dextrose injection or other compatible IV solution (see Stability). Deliver at a rate of 6.25 mg/h (e.g., 150 mg [6 mL] of ZANTAC Injection in 250 mL of 5% dextrose injection at 10.7 mL/h).

For Zollinger-Ellison patients, dilute ZANTAC Injection in 5% dextrose injection or other compatible IV solution (see Stability) to a concentration no greater than 2.5 mg/mL. Start the infusion at a rate of 1.0 mg/kg per hour. If after 4 hours either a measured gastric acid output is >10 mEq/h or the patient becomes symptomatic, the dose should be adjusted upward in 0.5-mg/kg per hour increments, and the acid output should be remeasured. Dosages up to 2.5 mg/kg per hour and infusion rates as high as 220 mg/h have been used.

Pediatric Use: While limited data exist on the administration of IV ranitidine to children, the recommended dose in pediatric patients is for a total daily dose of 2 to 4 mg/kg, to be divided and administered every 6 to 8 hours, up to a maximum of 50 mg given every 6 to 8 hours. This recommendation is derived from adult clinical studies and pharmacokinetic data in pediatric patients. Limited data in neonatal patients (less than one month of age) receiving ECMO have shown that a dose of 2 mg/kg is usually sufficient to increase gastric pH to >4 for at least 15 hours. Therefore, doses of 2 mg/kg given every 12 to 24 hours or as a continuous infusion should be considered.

ZANTAC Injection Premixed in Flexible Plastic Containers: Instructions for Use: ***To Open:*** Tear outer wrap at notch and remove solution container. Check for minute leaks by squeezing container firmly. If leaks are found, discard unit as sterility may be impaired.

Preparation for Administration: Use aseptic technique.

1. Close flow control clamp of administration set.
2. Remove cover from outlet port at bottom of container.
3. Insert piercing pin of administration set into port with a twisting motion until the pin is firmly seated. NOTE: See full directions on administration set carton.
4. Suspend container from hanger.
5. Squeeze and release drip chamber to establish proper fluid level in chamber during infusion of ZANTAC Injection Premixed.
6. Open flow control clamp to expel air from set. Close clamp.
7. Attach set to venipuncture device. If device is not indwelling, prime and make venipuncture.
8. Perform venipuncture.
9. Regulate rate of administration with flow control clamp.

Caution: ZANTAC Injection Premixed in flexible plastic containers is to be administered by slow IV drip infusion only. **Additives should not be introduced into this solution.** If used with a primary IV fluid system, the primary solution should be discontinued during ZANTAC Injection Premixed infusion.

Do not administer unless solution is clear and container is undamaged.

Warning: Do not use flexible plastic container in series connections.

Dosage Adjustment for Patients With Impaired Renal Function: The administration of ranitidine as a continuous infusion has not been evaluated in patients with impaired renal function. On the basis of experience with a group of subjects with severely impaired renal function treated with ZANTAC, the recommended dosage in patients with a creatinine clearance <50 mL/min is 50 mg every 18 to 24 hours. Should the patient's condition require, the frequency of dosing may be increased to every 12 hours or even further with caution. Hemodialysis reduces the level of circulating ranitidine. Ideally, the dosing schedule should be adjusted so that the timing of a scheduled dose coincides with the end of hemodialysis.

Stability: Undiluted, ZANTAC Injection tends to exhibit a yellow color that may intensify over time without adversely affecting potency. ZANTAC Injection is stable for 48 hours at room temperature when added to or diluted with most commonly used IV solutions, e.g., 0.9% sodium chloride injection, 5% dextrose injection, 10% dextrose injection, lactated ringer's injection, or 5% sodium bicarbonate injection. ZANTAC Injection Premixed in flexible plastic containers is sterile through the expiration date on the label when stored under recommended conditions.

Note: Parenteral drug products should be inspected visually for particulate matter and discoloration before administration whenever solution and container permit.

Directions for Dispensing: ***Pharmacy Bulk Package—Not for Direct Infusion:*** The pharmacy bulk package is for use in a pharmacy admixture service only under a laminar flow hood. The closure should be penetrated only once with a sterile transfer set or other sterile dispensing device, which allows measured distribution of the contents, and the contents dispensed in aliquots using aseptic technique. CONTENTS SHOULD BE USED AS SOON AS POSSIBLE FOLLOWING INITIAL CLOSURE PUNCTURE. DISCARD ANY UNUSED PORTION WITHIN 24 HOURS OF FIRST ENTRY. Following closure puncture, container should be maintained below 30°C (86°F) under a laminar flow hood until contents are dispensed.

HOW SUPPLIED

ZANTAC Injection, 25 mg/mL, containing phenol 0.5% as preservative, is available as follows:

NDC 0173-0362-38 2-mL single-dose vials (Tray of 10)
NDC 0173-0363-01 6-mL multidose vials (Singles)
NDC 0173-0363-00 40-mL pharmacy bulk packages (Singles)

Store between 4° and 30°C (39° and 86°F). Protect from light. Store the 40-mL pharmacy bulk vial in carton until time of use.

ZANTAC Injection Premixed, 50 mg/50 mL, in 0.45% sodium chloride, is available as a sterile, premixed solution for IV administration in single-dose, flexible plastic containers (NDC 0173-0441-00) (case of 24). It contains no preservatives.

Store between 2° and 25°C (36° and 77°F). Protect from light.

Exposure of pharmaceutical products to heat should be minimized. Avoid excessive heat; however, brief exposure up to 40°C does not adversely affect the product. Protect from freezing.

ZANTAC® Injection:
Glaxo Wellcome Inc., Research Triangle Park, NC 27709
ZANTAC® Injection Premixed:
Manufactured for Glaxo Wellcome Inc.
Research Triangle Park, NC 27709
by Abbott Laboratories, North Chicago, IL 60064
US Patent No. 4,585,790

November 1999/RL-774
Shown in Product Identification Guide, page 316 and 317

ZANTAC® 150 ℞
[zan 'tak]
(ranitidine hydrochloride)
Tablets, USP

ZANTAC® 300 ℞
(ranitidine hydrochloride)
Tablets, USP

ZANTAC® 150 ℞
(ranitidine hydrochloride effervescent)
EFFERdose® Tablets

ZANTAC® 150 ℞
(ranitidine hydrochloride effervescent)
EFFERdose® Granules

ZANTAC® ℞
(ranitidine hydrochloride)
Syrup, USP

DESCRIPTION

The active ingredient in ZANTAC 150 Tablets, ZANTAC 300 Tablets, ZANTAC 150 EFFERdose Tablets, ZANTAC 150 EFFERdose Granules, and ZANTAC Syrup is ranitidine hydrochloride (HCl), USP, a histamine H_2-receptor antagonist. Chemically it is N[2-[[[5-[(dimethylamino) methyl]-2-furanyl]methyl]thio]ethyl]-N'-methyl-2-nitro-1,1-ethenediamine, HCl.

The empirical formula is $C_{13}H_{22}N_4O_3S \bullet HCl$, representing a molecular weight of 350.87.

Ranitidine HCl is a white to pale yellow, granular substance that is soluble in water. It has a slightly bitter taste and sulfurlike odor.

Each ZANTAC 150 Tablet for oral administration contains 168 mg of ranitidine HCl equivalent to 150 mg of ranitidine. Each tablet also contains the inactive ingredients FD&C Yellow No. 6 Aluminum Lake, hydroxypropyl methylcellulose, magnesium stearate, microcrystalline cellulose, titanium dioxide, triacetin, and yellow iron oxide.

Each ZANTAC 300 Tablet for oral administration contains 336 mg of ranitidine HCl equivalent to 300 mg of ranitidine. Each tablet also contains the inactive ingredients croscarmellose sodium, D&C Yellow No. 10 Aluminum Lake, hydroxypropyl methylcellulose, magnesium stearate, microcrystalline cellulose, titanium dioxide, and triacetin.

ZANTAC 150 EFFERdose Tablets and ZANTAC 150 EFFERdose Granules for oral administration are effervescent formulations of ranitidine that must be dissolved in water before use. Each individual tablet or the contents of a packet contain 168 mg of ranitidine HCl equivalent to 150 mg of ranitidine and the following inactive ingredients: aspartame, monosodium citrate anhydrous, povidone, and sodium bicarbonate. Each tablet also contains sodium benzoate. The total sodium content of each tablet is 183.12 mg (7.96 mEq) per 150 mg of ranitidine, and the total sodium content of each packet of granules is 173.54 mg (7.55 mEq) per 150 mg of ranitidine.

Each 1 mL of ZANTAC Syrup contains 16.8 mg of ranitidine HCl equivalent to 15 mg of ranitidine. ZANTAC Syrup also contains the inactive ingredients alcohol (7.5%), butylparaben, dibasic sodium phosphate, hydroxypropyl methylcellulose, peppermint flavor, monobasic potassium phosphate, propylparaben, purified water, saccharin sodium, sodium chloride, and sorbitol.

CLINICAL PHARMACOLOGY

ZANTAC is a competitive, reversible inhibitor of the action of histamine at the histamine H_2-receptors, including receptors on the gastric cells. ZANTAC does not lower serum Ca^{++} in hypercalcemic states. ZANTAC is not an anticholinergic agent.

Pharmacokinetics:

Absorption: ZANTAC is 50% absorbed after oral administration, compared to an intravenous (IV) injection with mean peak levels of 440 to 545 ng/mL occurring 2 to 3 hours after a 150-mg dose. The syrup and EFFERdose formulations are bioequivalent to the tablets. Absorption is not significantly impaired by the administration of food or antacids. Propantheline slightly delays and increases peak blood levels of ZANTAC, probably by delaying gastric emptying and transit time. In one study, simultaneous administration of high-potency antacid (150 mmol) in fasting subjects has been reported to decrease the absorption of ZANTAC.

Distribution: The volume of distribution is about 1.4 L/kg. Serum protein binding averages 15%.

Metabolism: In humans, the N-oxide is the principal metabolite in the urine; however, this amounts to <4% of the dose. Other metabolites are the S-oxide (1%) and the desmethyl ranitidine (1%). The remainder of the administered dose is found in the stool. Studies in patients with hepatic dysfunction (compensated cirrhosis) indicate that there are minor, but clinically insignificant, alterations in ranitidine half-life, distribution, clearance, and bioavailability.

Excretion: The principal route of excretion is the urine, with approximately 30% of the orally administered dose collected in the urine as unchanged drug in 24 hours. Renal clearance is about 410 mL/min, indicating active tubular excretion. The elimination half-life is 2.5 to 3 hours. Four patients with clinically significant renal function impairment (creatinine clearance 25 to 35 mL/min) administered 50 mg of ranitidine intravenously had an average plasma half-life of 4.8 hours, a ranitidine clearance of 29 mL/min, and a volume of distribution of 1.76 L/kg. In general, these parameters appear to be altered in proportion to creatinine clearance (see DOSAGE AND ADMINISTRATION).

Pediatrics: There are no significant differences in the pharmacokinetic parameter values for ranitidine in pediatric patients (from 1 month up to 16 years of age) and healthy adults when correction is made for body weight. The average bioavailability of ranitidine given orally to pediatric patients is 48% which is comparable to the bioavailability of ranitidine in the adult population. All other pharmacokinetic parameter values ($t_{1/2}$, Vd, and CL) are similar to those observed with intravenous ranitidine use in pediatric patients. Estimates of C_{max} and T_{max} are displayed in Table 1.

[See table 1 at top of next page]

Plasma clearance measured in two neonatal patients (less than 1 month of age) was considerably lower (3 mL/min/kg) than children or adults and is likely due to reduced renal function observed in this population.

Pharmacodynamics: Serum concentrations necessary to inhibit 50% of stimulated gastric acid secretion are estimated to be 36 to 94 ng/mL. Following a single oral dose of 150 mg, serum concentrations of ZANTAC are in this range up to 12 hours. However, blood levels bear no consistent relationship to dose or degree of acid inhibition.

In a pharmacodynamic comparison of the EFFERdose with the ZANTAC Tablets, during the first hour after administration, the EFFERdose tablet formulation gave a significantly higher intragastric pH, by approximately 1 pH unit, compared to the ZANTAC tablets.

Antisecretory Activity: ***1. Effects on Acid Secretion:*** ZANTAC inhibits both daytime and nocturnal basal gastric acid secretions as well as gastric acid secretion stimulated by food, betazole, and pentagastrin, as shown in Table 2:

[See table 2 on next page]

It appears that basal-, nocturnal-, and betazole-stimulated secretions are most sensitive to inhibition by ZANTAC, responding almost completely to doses of 100 mg or less, while pentagastrin- and food-stimulated secretions are more difficult to suppress.

2. Effects on Other Gastrointestinal Secretions:

Pepsin: Oral ZANTAC does not affect pepsin secretion. Total pepsin output is reduced in proportion to the decrease in volume of gastric juice.

Intrinsic Factor: Oral ZANTAC has no significant effect on pentagastrin-stimulated intrinsic factor secretion.

Serum Gastrin: ZANTAC has little or no effect on fasting or postprandial serum gastrin.

Continued on next page

This product information is based on labeling in effect on June 23, 2000. For further information, contact via direct mail, phone, or web site. Medical Information, Glaxo Wellcome Inc., PO Box 13398, Research Triangle Park, NC 27709. Healthcare Professionals (Medical Information): 800-334-0089. Patients (Customer Response Center): 1-888-825-5249. Glaxo Wellcome Corporate Web Site: www.glaxowellcome.com

Zantac—Cont.

Other Pharmacologic Actions:
a. Gastric bacterial flora—increase in nitrate-reducing organisms, significance not known.
b. Prolactin levels—no effect in recommended oral or intravenous (IV) dosage, but small, transient, dose-related increases in serum prolactin have been reported after IV bolus injections of 100 mg or more.
c. Other pituitary hormones—no effect on serum gonadotropins, TSH, or GH. Possible impairment of vasopressin release.
d. No change in cortisol, aldosterone, androgen, or estrogen levels.
e. No antiandrogenic action.
f. No effect on count, motility, or morphology of sperm.

Pediatrics: Oral doses of 6 to 10 mg/kg per day in two or three divided doses maintain gastric pH >4 throughout most of the dosing interval.

Clinical Trials: ***Active Duodenal Ulcer:*** In a multicenter, double-blind, controlled, US study of endoscopically diagnosed duodenal ulcers, earlier healing was seen in the patients treated with ZANTAC as shown in Table 3:

[See table 3 at right]

In these studies, patients treated with ZANTAC reported a reduction in both daytime and nocturnal pain, and they also consumed less antacid than the placebo-treated patients.

[See table 4 at right]

Foreign studies have shown that patients heal equally well with 150 mg b.i.d. and 300 mg h.s. (85% versus 84%, respectively) during a usual 4-week course of therapy. If patients require extended therapy of 8 weeks, the healing rate may be higher for 150 mg b.i.d. as compared to 300 mg h.s. (92% versus 87%, respectively).

Studies have been limited to short-term treatment of acute duodenal ulcer. Patients whose ulcers healed during therapy had recurrences of ulcers at the usual rates.

Maintenance Therapy in Duodenal Ulcer: Ranitidine has been found to be effective as maintenance therapy for patients following healing of acute duodenal ulcers. In two independent, double-blind, multicenter, controlled trials, the number of duodenal ulcers observed was significantly less in patients treated with ZANTAC (150 mg h.s.) than in patients treated with placebo over a 12-month period.

Table 5: Duodenal Ulcer Prevalence

Double-blind, Multicenter, Placebo-Controlled Trials

Multicenter Trial	Drug	Duodenal Ulcer Prevalence			No. of Patients
		0-4 Months	0-8 Months	0-12 Months	
USA	RAN	20%*	24%*	35%*	138
	PLC	44%	54%	59%	139
Foreign	RAN	12%*	21%*	28%*	174
	PLC	56%	64%	68%	165

% = Life table estimate.
* = $P<0.05$ (ZANTAC versus comparator).
RAN = ranitidine (ZANTAC).
PLC = placebo.

As with other H_2-antagonists, the factors responsible for the significant reduction in the prevalence of duodenal ulcers include prevention of recurrence of ulcers, more rapid healing of ulcers that may occur during maintenance therapy, or both.

Gastric Ulcer: In a multicenter, double-blind, controlled, US study of endoscopically diagnosed gastric ulcers, earlier healing was seen in the patients treated with ZANTAC as shown in Table 6:

Table 6: Gastric Ulcer Patient Healing Rates

	ZANTAC*		Placebo*	
	Number Entered	Healed/ Evaluable	Number Entered	Healed/ Evaluable
Outpatients				
Week 2	92	16/83 (19%)	94	10/83 (12%)
Week 6		50/73 (68%)†		35/69 (51%)

* All patients were permitted p.r.n. antacids for relief of pain.
† $P= 0.009$.

In this multicenter trial, significantly more patients treated with ZANTAC became pain free during therapy.

Maintenance of Healing of Gastric Ulcers: In two multicenter, double-blind, randomized, placebo-controlled, 12-month trials conducted in patients whose gastric ulcers had been previously healed, ZANTAC 150 mg h.s. was significantly more effective than placebo in maintaining healing of gastric ulcers.

Pathological Hypersecretory Conditions (such as Zollinger-Ellison syndrome): ZANTAC inhibits gastric acid secretion and reduces occurrence of diarrhea, anorexia, and pain in patients with pathological hypersecretion associated with Zollinger-Ellison syndrome, systemic mastocytosis, and other pathological hypersecretory conditions (e.g., postoperative, "short-gut" syndrome, idiopathic). Use of ZANTAC was followed by healing of ulcers in 8 of 19 (42%) patients who were intractable to previous therapy.

Gastroesophageal Reflux Disease (GERD): In two multicenter, double-blind, placebo-controlled, 6-week trials performed in the United States and Europe, ZANTIC 150 mg b.i.d. was more effective than placebo for the relief of heartburn and other symptoms associated with GERD. Ranitidine-treated patients consumed significantly less antacid than did placebo-treated patients.

The US trial indicated that ZANTAC 150 mg b.i.d. significantly reduced the frequency of heartburn attacks and severity of heartburn pain within 1 to 2 weeks after starting therapy. The improvement was maintained throughout the 6-week trial period. Moreover, patient response rates demonstrated that the effect on heartburn extends through both the day and night time periods.

In two additional US multicenter, double-blind, placebo-controlled, 2-week trials, ZANTAC 150 mg b.i.d. was shown to provide relief of heartburn pain within 24 hours of initiating therapy and a reduction in the frequency of severity of heartburn. In these trials, ZANTAC EFFERdose Tablets were shown to provide heartburn relief within 45 minutes of dosing.

Erosive Esophagitis: In two multicenter, double-blind, randomized, placebo-controlled, 12-week trials performed in the United States, ZANTAC 150 mg q.i.d. was significantly more effective than placebo in healing endoscopically diagnosed erosive esophagitis and in relieving associated heartburn. The erosive esophagitis healing rates were as follows:

Table 7: Erosive Esophagitis Patient Healing Rates

	Healed/Evaluable	
	Placebo* n = 229	ZANTAC 150 mg q.i.d.* n = 215
Week 4	43/198 (22%)	96/206 (47%)†
Week 8	63/176 (36%)	142/200 (71%)†
Week 12	92/159 (58%)	162/192 (84%)†

* All patients were permitted p.r.n. antacids for relief of pain.
† $P<0.001$ versus placebo.

No additional benefit in healing of esophagitis or in relief of heartburn was seen with a ranitidine dose of 300 mg q.i.d.

Maintenance of Healing of Erosive Esophagitis: In two multicenter, double-blind, randomized, placebo-controlled, 48-week trials conducted in patients whose erosive esophagitis had been previously healed, ZANTAC 150 mg b.i.d. was significantly more effective than placebo in maintaining healing of erosive esophagitis.

Table 1: Ranitidine Pharmacokinetics in Pediatric Patients Following Oral Dosing

Population (age)	n	Dosage Form (dose)	C_{max} (ng/mL)	T_{max} (hours)
Gastric or duodenal ulcer (3.5 to 16 years)	12	Tablets (1 to 2 mg/kg)	54 to 492	2.0
Otherwise healthy requiring ZANTAC (0.7 to 14 years, Single dose)	10	Syrup (2 mg/kg)	244	1.61
Otherwise healthy requiring ZANTAC (0.7 to 14 years, Multiple dose)	10	Syrup (2 mg/kg)	320	1.66

Table 2: Effect of Oral ZANTAC on Gastric Acid Secretion

	Time After Dose, h	% Inhibition of Gastric Acid Output by Dose, mg			
		75–80	100	150	200
Basal	Up to 4		99	95	
Nocturnal	Up to 13	95	96	92	
Betazole	Up to 3		97	99	
Pentagastrin	Up to 5	58	72	72	80
Meal	Up to 3		73	79	95

Table 3: Duodenal Ulcer Patient Healing Rates

	ZANTAC*		Placebo*	
	Number Entered	Healed/ Evaluable	Number Entered	Healed/ Evaluable
Outpatients				
Week 2	195	69/182 (38%)†	188	31/164 (19%)
Week 4		137/187 (73%)†		76/168 (45%)

*All patients were permitted p.r.n. antacids for relief of pain.
†$P<0.0001$.

Table 4: Mean Daily Doses of Antacid

	Ulcer Healed	Ulcer Not Healed
ZANTAC	0.06	0.71
Placebo	0.71	1.43

INDICATIONS AND USAGE

ZANTAC is indicated in:

1. Short-term treatment of active duodenal ulcer. Most patients heal within 4 weeks. Studies available to date have not assessed the safety of ranitidine in uncomplicated duodenal ulcer for periods of more than 8 weeks.
2. Maintenance therapy for duodenal ulcer patients at reduced dosage after healing of acute ulcers. No placebo-controlled comparative studies have been carried out for periods of longer than 1 year.
3. The treatment of pathological hypersecretory conditions (e.g., Zollinger-Ellison syndrome and systemic mastocytosis).
4. Short-term treatment of active, benign gastric ulcer. Most patients heal within 6 weeks and the usefulness of further treatment has not been demonstrated. Studies available to date have not assessed the safety of ranitidine in uncomplicated, benign gastric ulcer for periods of more than 6 weeks.
5. Maintenance therapy for gastric ulcer patients at reduced dosage after healing of acute ulcers. Placebo-controlled studies have been carried out for 1 year.
6. Treatment of GERD. Symptomatic relief commonly occurs within 24 hours after starting therapy with ZANTAC 150 mg b.i.d.
7. Treatment of endoscopically diagnosed erosive esophagitis. Symptomatic relief of heartburn commonly occurs within 24 hours of therapy initiation with ZANTAC 150 mg q.i.d.
8. Maintenance of healing of erosive esophagitis. Placebo-controlled trials have been carried out for 48 weeks.

Concomitant antacids should be given as needed for pain relief to patients with active duodenal ulcer; active, benign gastric ulcer; hypersecretory states; GERD; and erosive esophagitis.

CONTRAINDICATIONS

ZANTAC is contraindicated for patients known to have hypersensitivity to the drug or any of the ingredients (see PRECAUTIONS).

PRECAUTIONS

General: 1. Symptomatic response to therapy with ZANTAC does not preclude the presence of gastric malignancy.
2. Since ZANTAC is excreted primarily by the kidney, dosage should be adjusted in patients with impaired renal function (see DOSAGE AND ADMINISTRATION). Caution should be observed in patients with hepatic dysfunction since ZANTAC is metabolized in the liver.
3. Rare reports suggest that ZANTAC may precipitate acute porphyric attacks in patients with acute porphyria. ZANTAC should therefore be avoided in patients with a history of acute porphyria.

Information for Patients: ***Phenylketonurics:*** ZANTAC 150 EFFERdose Tablets and ZANTAC 150 EFFERdose Granules contain phenylalanine 16.84 mg per 150 mg of ranitidine.

Laboratory Tests: False-positive tests for urine protein with MULTISTIX® may occur during ZANTAC therapy, and therefore testing with sulfosalicylic acid is recommended.

Drug Interactions: Although ZANTAC has been reported to bind weakly to cytochrome P-450 in vitro, recommended doses of the drug do not inhibit the action of the cytochrome P-450–linked oxygenase enzymes in the liver. However, there have been isolated reports of drug interactions that suggest that ZANTAC may affect the bioavailability of certain drugs by some mechanism as yet unidentified (e.g., a pH-dependent effect on absorption or a change in volume of distribution).

Increased or decreased prothrombin times have been reported during concurrent use of ranitidine and warfarin. However, in human pharmacokinetic studies with dosages of ranitidine up to 400 mg/day, no interaction occurred; ranitidine had no effect on warfarin clearance or prothrombin time. The possibility of an interaction with warfarin at dosages of ranitidine higher than 400 mg/day has not been investigated.

In a ranitidine-triazolam drug-drug interaction study, triazolam plasma concentrations were higher during b.i.d. dosing of ranitidine than triazolam given alone. The mean area under the triazolam concentration-time curve (AUC) values in 18- to 60-year old subjects were 10% and and 28% higher following administration of 75-mg and 150-mg ranitidine tablets, respectively, than triazolam given alone. In subjects older than 60 years of age, the mean AUC values were approximately 30% higher following administraiton of 75-mg and 150-mg ranitidine tablets. It appears that there were no changes in pharmacokinetics of triazolam and α-hydroxytriazolam, a major metabolite, and in their elimination. Reduced gastric acidity due to ranitidine may have resulted in an increase in the availability of triazolam. The clinical significance of this triazolam and ranitidine pharmacokinetic interaction is unknown.

Carcinogenesis, Mutagenesis, Impairment of Fertility: There was no indication of tumorigenic or carcinogenic effects in life-span studies in mice and rats at dosages up to 2000 mg/kg per day.

Ranitidine was not mutagenic in standard bacterial tests *(Salmonella, Escherichia coli)* for mutagenicity at concentrations up to the maximum recommended for these assays.

In a dominant lethal assay, a single oral dose of 1000 mg/kg to male rats was without effect on the outcome of two matings per week for the next 9 weeks.

Pregnancy: ***Teratogenic Effects: Pregnancy Category B:*** Reproduction studies have been performed in rats and rabbits at doses up to 160 times the human dose and have revealed no evidence of impaired fertility or harm to the fetus due to ZANTAC. There are, however, no adequate and well-controlled studies in pregnant women. Because animal reproduction studies are not always predictive of human response, this drug should be used during pregnancy only if clearly needed.

Nursing Mothers: ZANTAC is secreted in human milk. Caution should be exercised when ZANTAC is administered to a nursing mother.

Pediatric Use: The safety and effectiveness of ZANTAC have been established in the age-group of 1 month to 16 years for the treatment of duodenal and gastric ulcers, gastroesophageal reflux disease and erosive esophagitis, and the maintenance of healed duodenal and gastric ulcer. Use of ZANTAC in this age-group is supported by adequate and well-controlled studies in adults, as well as additional pharmacokinetic data in pediatric patients and an analysis of the published literature.

Safety and effectiveness in pediatric patients for the treatment of pathological hypersecretory conditions or the maintenance of healing of erosive esophagitis have not been established.

Safety and effectiveness in neonates (less than one month of age) have not been established (see CLINICAL PHARMACOLOGY: Pediatrics).

Use in Elderly Patients: Ulcer healing rates in elderly patients (65 to 82 years of age) were no different from those in younger age-groups. The incidence rates for adverse events and laboratory abnormalities were also not different from those seen in other age-groups.

ADVERSE REACTIONS

The following have been reported as events in clinical trials or in the routine management of patients treated with ZANTAC. The relationship to therapy with ZANTAC has been unclear in many cases. Headache, sometimes severe, seems to be related to administration of ZANTAC.

Central Nervous System: Rarely, malaise, dizziness, somnolence, insomnia, and vertigo. Rare cases of reversible mental confusion, agitation, depression, and hallucinations have been reported, predominantly in severely ill elderly patients. Rare cases of reversible blurred vision suggestive of a change in accommodation have been reported. Rare reports of reversible involuntary motor disturbances have been received.

Cardiovascular: As with other H_2-blockers, rare reports of arrhythmias such as tachycardia, bradycardia, atrioventricular block, and premature ventricular beats.

Gastrointestinal: Constipation, diarrhea, nausea/vomiting, abdominal discomfort/pain, and rare reports of pancreatitis.

Hepatic: There have been occasional reports of hepatocellular, cholestatic, or mixed hepatitis, with or without jaundice. In such circumstances, ranitidine should be immediately discontinued. These events are usually reversible, but in rare circumstances death has occurred. Rare cases of hepatic failure have also been reported. In normal volunteers, SGPT values were increased to at least twice the pretreatment levels in 6 of 12 subjects receiving 100 mg q.i.d. intravenously for 7 days, and in 4 of 24 subjects receiving 50 mg q.i.d. intravenously for 5 days.

Musculoskeletal: Rare reports of arthralgias and myalgias.

Hematologic: Blood count changes (leukopenia, granulocytopenia, and thrombocytopenia) have occurred in a few patients. These were usually reversible. Rare cases of agranulocytosis, pancytopenia, sometimes with marrow hypoplasia, and aplastic anemia and exceedingly rare cases of acquired immune hemolytic anemia have been reported.

Endocrine: Controlled studies in animals and man have shown no stimulation of any pituitary hormone by ZANTAC and no antiandrogenic activity, and cimetidine-induced gynecomastia and impotence in hypersecretory patients have resolved when ZANTAC has been substituted. However, occasional cases of gynecomastia, impotence, and loss of libido have been reported in male patients receiving ZANTAC, but the incidence did not differ from that in the general population.

Integumentary: Rash, including rare cases of erythema multiforme, and, rarely, alopecia.

Other: Rare cases of hypersensitivity reactions (e.g., bronchospasm, fever, rash, eosinophilia), anaphylaxis, angioneurotic edema, and small increases in serum creatinine.

OVERDOSAGE

There has been limited experience with overdosage. Reported acute ingestions of up to 18 g orally have been associated with transient adverse effects similar to those encountered in normal clinical experience (see ADVERSE REACTIONS). In addition, abnormalities of gait and hypotension have been reported.

When overdosage occurs, the usual measures to remove unabsorbed material from the gastrointestinal tract, clinical monitoring, and supportive therapy should be employed.

Studies in dogs receiving dosages of ZANTAC in excess of 225 mg/kg per day have shown muscular tremors, vomiting, and rapid respiration. Single oral doses of 1,000 mg/kg in mice and rats were not lethal. Intravenous LD_{50} values in mice and rats were 77 and 83 mg/kg, respectively.

DOSAGE AND ADMINISTRATION

Active Duodenal Ulcer: The current recommended adult oral dosage of ZANTAC for duodenal ulcer is 150 mg or 10 mL (2 teaspoonfuls equivalent to 150 mg of ranitidine) twice daily. An alternative dosage of 300 mg or 20 mL (4 teaspoonfuls equivalent to 300 mg of ranitidine) once daily after the evening meal or at bedtime can be used for patients in whom dosing convenience is important. The advantages of one treatment regimen compared to the other in a particular patient population have yet to be demonstrated (see Clinical Trials: *Active Duodenal Ulcer*). Smaller doses have been shown to be equally effective in inhibiting gastric acid secretion in US studies, and several foreign trials have shown that 100 mg b.i.d. is as effective as the 150-mg dose.

Antacid should be given as needed for relief of pain (see CLINICAL PHARMACOLOGY: Pharmacokinetics).

Maintenance of Healing of Duodenal Ulcers: The current recommended adult oral dosage is 150 mg or 10 mL (2 teaspoonfuls equivalent to 150 mg of ranitidine) at bedtime.

Pathological Hypersecretory Conditions (such as Zollinger-Ellison syndrome): The current recommended adult oral dosage is 150 mg or 10 mL (2 teaspoonfuls equivalent to 150 mg of ranitidine) twice a day. In some patients it may be necessary to administer ZANTAC 150-mg doses more frequently. Dosages should be adjusted to individual patient needs, and should continue as long as clinically indicated. Dosages up to 6 g/day have been employed in patients with severe disease.

Benign Gastric Ulcer: The current recommended adult oral dosage is 150 mg or 10 mL (2 teaspoonfuls equivalent to 150 mg of ranitidine) twice a day.

Maintenance of Healing of Gastric Ulcers: The current recommended adult oral dosage is 150 mg or 10 mL (2 teaspoonfuls equivalent to 150 mg of ranitidine) at bedtime.

GERD: The current recommended adult oral dosage is 150 mg or 10 mL (2 teaspoonfuls equivalent to 150 mg of ranitidine) twice a day.

Erosive Esophagitis: The current recommended adult oral dosage is 150 mg or 10 mL (2 teaspoonfuls equivalent to 150 mg of ranitidine) four times a day.

Maintenance of Healing of Erosive Esophagitis: The current recommended adult oral dosage is 150 mg or 10 mL (2 teaspoonfuls equivalent to 150 mg of ranitidine) twice a day.

Pediatric Use: The safety and effectiveness of ZANTAC have been established in the age-group of 1 month to 16 years. There is insufficient information about the pharmacokinetics of ZANTAC in neonatal patients (less than 1 month of age) to make dosing recommendations.

Treatment of Duodenal and Gastric Ulcers: The recommended oral dose for the treatment of active duodenal and gastric ulcers is 2 to 4 mg/kg per day twice daily to a maximum of 300 mg/day. This recommendation is derived from adult clinical studies and pharmacokinetic data in pediatric patients.

Maintenance of Healing of Duodenal and Gastric Ulcers: The recommended oral dose for the maintenance of healing of duodenal and gastric ulcers is 2 to 4 mg/kg once daily to a maximum of 150 mg/day. This recommendation is derived from adult clinical studies and pharmacokinetic data in pediatric patients.

Treatment of GERD and Erosive Esophagitis: Although limited data exist for these conditions in pediatric patients, published literature supports a dosage of 5 to 10 mg/kg per day, usually given as two divided doses.

Dosage Adjustment for Patients With Impaired Renal Function: On the basis of experience with a group of subjects with severely impaired renal function treated with ZANTAC, the recommended dosage in patients with a creatinine clearance <50 mL/min is 150 mg or 10 mL (2 teaspoonfuls equivalent to 150 mg of ranitidine) every 24 hours. Should the patient's condition require, the frequency of dosing may be increased to every 12 hours or even further with caution. Hemodialysis reduces the level of circulating ranitidine. Ideally, the dosing schedule should be adjusted so that the timing of a scheduled dose coincides with the end of hemodialysis.

Preparation of ZANTAC 150 EFFERdose Tablets and ZANTAC 150 EFFERdose Granules: Dissolve each dose in approximately 6 to 8 oz of water before drinking.

HOW SUPPLIED

ZANTAC 150 Tablets (ranitidine HCl equivalent to 150 mg of ranitidine) are peach, film-coated, five-sided tablets embossed with "ZANTAC 150" on one side and "Glaxo" on the other. They are available in bottles of 60 (NDC 0173-0344-42), 180 (NDC 0173-0344-17), 500 (NDC 0173-0344-14), and 1000 (NDC 0173-0344-12) tablets and unit dose packs of 100 (NDC 0173-0344-47) tablets.

ZANTAC 300 Tablets (ranitidine HCl equivalent to 300 mg of ranitidine) are yellow, film-coated, capsule-shaped tablets embossed with "ZANTAC 300" on one side and "Glaxo" on the other. They are available in bottles of 30 (NDC 0173-0393-40) and 250 (NDC 0173-0393-06) tablets and unit dose packs of 100 (NDC 0173-0393-47) tablets.

Store between 15° and 30°C (59° and 86°F) in a dry place. Protect from light. Replace cap securely after each opening.

ZANTAC 150 EFFERdose Tablets (ranitidine HCl equivalent to 150 mg of ranitidine) are white to pale yellow, round, flat-faced, bevel-edged tablets embossed with "ZANTAC 150" on one side and "427" on the other. They are packaged individually in foil and are available in cartons of 30 (NDC 0173-0427-00) and 60 (NDC 0173-0427-02) tablets.

ZANTAC 150 EFFERdose Granules (ranitidine HCl equivalent to 150 mg of ranitidine) are white to pale yellow granules. Each 150-mg dose of granules (approximately 1.44 g) is packaged in individual foil packets and is available in cartons of 30 (NDC 0173-0451-00) and 60 (NDC 0173-0451-01) packets.

Store between 2° and 30°C (36° and 86°F).

ZANTAC Syrup, a clear, peppermint-flavored liquid, contains 16.8 mg of ranitidine HCl equivalent to 15 mg of ranitidine per 1 mL in bottles of 16 fluid ounces (one pint) (NDC 0173-0383-54).

Store between 4° and 25°C (39° and 77°F). Dispense in tight, light-resistant containers as defined in the USP/NF.

ZANTAC® 150 Tablets/ZANTAC® 300 Tablets/
ZANTAC® 150 EFFERdose® Tablets/ZANTAC® 150 EFFERdose® Granules:
Glaxo Wellcome Inc., Research Triangle Park, NC 27709
US Patent Nos. 4,521,431; 4,880,636; and 5,102,665
ZANTAC® Syrup:
Manufactured for Glaxo Wellcome Inc.
Research Triangle Park, NC 27709
by Roxane Laboratories, Inc., Columbus, OH 43216
US Patent Nos. 4,585,790 and 5,068,249

November 1999/RL-773

Shown in Product Identification Guide, page 316

ZIAGEN® ℞
[zī'ə-jin]
(abacavir sulfate)
Tablets

ZIAGEN® ℞
(abacavir sulfate)
Oral Solution

> **WARNING: FATAL HYPERSENSITIVITY REACTIONS HAVE BEEN ASSOCIATED WITH THERAPY WITH ZIAGEN. PATIENTS DEVELOPING SIGNS OR SYMPTOMS OF HYPERSENSITIVITY (WHICH INCLUDE FEVER; SKIN RASH; FATIGUE; GASTROINTESTINAL SYMPTOMS SUCH AS NAUSEA, VOMITING, DIARRHEA, OR ABDOMINAL PAIN; AND RESPIRATORY SYMPTOMS SUCH AS PHARYNGITIS, DYSPNEA, OR COUGH) SHOULD DISCONTINUE ZIAGEN AS SOON**

Continued on next page

This product information is based on labeling in effect on June 23, 2000. For further information, contact via direct mail, phone, or web site. Medical Information, Glaxo Wellcome Inc., PO Box 13398, Research Triangle Park, NC 27709. Healthcare Professionals (Medical Information): 800-334-0089. Patients (Customer Response Center): 1-888-825-5249. Glaxo Wellcome Corporate Web Site: www.glaxowellcome.com.

Ziagen—Cont.

AS A HYPERSENSITIVITY REACTION IS SUSPECTED. ZIAGEN SHOULD NOT BE RESTARTED FOLLOWING A HYPERSENSITIVITY REACTION BECAUSE MORE SEVERE SYMPTOMS WILL RECUR WITHIN HOURS AND MAY INCLUDE LIFE-THREATENING HYPOTENSION AND DEATH (see WARNINGS, PRECAUTIONS: Information for Patients, and ADVERSE REACTIONS). LACTIC ACIDOSIS AND SEVERE HEPATOMEGALY WITH STEATOSIS, INCLUDING FATAL CASES, HAVE BEEN REPORTED WITH THE USE OF NUCLEOSIDE ANALOGUES ALONE OR IN COMBINATION, INCLUDING ZIAGEN AND OTHER ANTIRETROVIRALS (SEE WARNINGS).

ZIAGEN in combination with other antiretroviral agents is indicated for the treatment of HIV-1 infection. This indication is based on analyses of surrogate markers in controlled studies of up to 24 weeks in duration. At present, there are no results from controlled trials evaluating long-term suppression of HIV RNA or disease progression with ZIAGEN.

DESCRIPTION

ZIAGEN is the brand name for abacavir sulfate, a synthetic carbocyclic nucleoside analogue with inhibitory activity against HIV. The chemical name of abacavir sulfate is (1*S*,*cis*)-4-[2-amino-6-(cyclopropylamino)-9*H*-purin-9-yl]-2-cyclopentene-1-methanol sulfate (salt) (2:1). Abacavir sulfate is the enantiomer with *1S, 4R* absolute configuration on the cyclopentene ring. It has a molecular formula of $(C_{14}H_{18}N_6O)_2 \bullet H_2SO_4$ and a molecular weight of 670.76 daltons.

Abacavir sulfate is a white to off-white solid with a solubility of approximately 77 mg/mL in distilled water at 25°C. It has an octanol/water (pH 7.1 to 7.3) partition coefficient (log *P*) of approximately 1.20 at 25°C.

ZIAGEN Tablets are for oral administration. Each tablet contains abacavir sulfate equivalent to 300 mg of abacavir and the inactive ingredients colloidal silicon dioxide, magnesium stearate, microcrystalline cellulose, and sodium starch glycolate. The tablets are coated with a film that is made of hydroxypropyl methylcellulose, polysorbate 80, synthetic yellow iron oxide, titanium dioxide, and triacetin.

ZIAGEN Oral Solution is for oral administration. One milliliter (1 mL) of ZIAGEN Oral Solution contains abacavir sulfate equivalent to 20 mg of abacavir (20 mg/mL) in an aqueous solution and the inactive ingredients artificial strawberry and banana flavors, citric acid (anhydrous), methylparaben and propylparaben (added as preservatives), propylene glycol, saccharin sodium, sodium citrate (dihydrate), and sorbitol solution.

In vivo, abacavir sulfate dissociates to its free base, abacavir. In this insert, all dosages for ZIAGEN are expressed in terms of abacavir.

MICROBIOLOGY

Mechanism of Action: Abacavir is a carbocyclic synthetic nucleoside analogue. Intracellularly, abacavir is converted by cellular enzymes to the active metabolite carbovir triphosphate. Carbovir triphosphate is an analogue of deoxyguanosine-5′-triphosphate (dGTP). Carbovir triphosphate inhibits the activity of HIV-1 reverse transcriptase (RT) both by competing with the natural substrate dGTP and by its incorporation into viral DNA. The lack of a 3′-OH group in the incorporated nucleoside analogue prevents the formation of the 5′ to 3′ phosphodiester linkage essential for DNA chain elongation, and therefore, the viral DNA growth is terminated.

Antiviral Activity *In Vitro*: The *in vitro* anti-HIV-1 activity of abacavir was evaluated against a T-cell tropic laboratory strain HIV-1 IIIB in lymphoblastic cell lines, a monocyte/macrophage tropic laboratory strain HIV-1 BaL in primary monocytes/macrophages, and clinical isolates in peripheral blood mononuclear cells. The concentration of drug necessary to inhibit viral replication by 50 percent (IC_{50}) ranged from 3.7 to 5.8 μM against HIV-1 IIIB, and was 0.26 ± 0.18 μM (1 μM = 0.28 mcg/mL) against 8 clinical isolates. The IC_{50} of abacavir against HIV-1 BaL varied from 0.07 to 1.0 μM. Abacavir had synergistic activity in combination with amprenavir, nevirapine, and zidovudine, and additive activity in combination with didanosine, lamivudine, stavudine, and zalcitabine *in vitro*. These drug combinations have not been adequately studied in humans. The relationship between *in vitro* susceptibility of HIV to abacavir and the inhibition of HIV replication in humans has not been established.

Drug Resistance: HIV-1 isolates with reduced sensitivity to abacavir have been selected *in vitro* and were also obtained from patients treated with abacavir. Genetic analysis of isolates from abacavir-treated patients showed point mutations in the reverse transcriptase gene that resulted in amino acid substitutions at positions K65R, L74V, Y115F, and M184V. Mutations M184V and L74V were most frequently observed in clinical isolates. Phenotypic analysis of HIV-1 isolates that harbor abacavir-associated mutations from 17 patients after 12 weeks of abacavir monotherapy exhibited a 3-fold decrease in susceptibility to abacavir *in vitro*. The clinical relevance of genotypic and phenotypic changes associated with abacavir therapy has not been established.

Cross-Resistance: Recombinant laboratory strains of HIV-1 (HXB2) containing multiple reverse transcriptase mutations conferring abacavir resistance exhibited cross-resistance to lamivudine, didanosine, and zalcitabine *in vitro*. For clinical information in treatment-experienced patients, see INDICATIONS AND USAGE: Description of Clinical Studies and PRECAUTIONS.

Cross-resistance between abacavir and HIV protease inhibitors is unlikely because of the different enzyme targets involved. Cross-resistance between abacavir and non-nucleoside reverse transcriptase inhibitors is unlikely because of different binding sites on reverse transcriptase.

CLINICAL PHARMACOLOGY

Pharmacokinetics in Adults: The pharmacokinetic properties of abacavir have been studied in asymptomatic, HIV-infected adult patients after administration of a single intravenous (IV) dose of 150 mg and after single and multiple oral doses. The pharmacokinetic properties of abacavir were independent of dose over the range of 300 to 1200 mg/day.

Absorption and Bioavailability: Abacavir was rapidly and extensively absorbed after oral administration. The geometric mean absolute bioavailability of the tablet was 83%. After oral administration of 300 mg twice daily in 20 patients, the steady-state peak serum abacavir concentration (C_{max}) was 3.0 ± 0.89 mcg/mL (mean ± SD) and $AUC_{(0-12\ h)}$ was 6.02 ± 1.73 mcg•h/mL. Bioavailability of abacavir tablets was assessed in the fasting and fed states. There was no significant difference in systemic exposure (AUC∞) in the fed and fasting states; therefore, ZIAGEN Tablets may be administered with or without food. Systemic exposure to abacavir was comparable after administration of ZIAGEN Oral Solution and ZIAGEN Tablets. Therefore, these products may be used interchangeably.

Distribution: The apparent volume of distribution after IV administration of abacavir was 0.86 ± 0.15 L/kg, suggesting that abacavir distributes into extravascular space. In 3 subjects, the CSF $AUC_{(0-6\ h)}$ to plasma abacavir $AUC_{(0-6\ h)}$ ratio ranged from 27% to 33%.

Binding of abacavir to human plasma proteins is approximately 50%. Binding of abacavir to plasma proteins was independent of concentration. Total blood and plasma drug-related radioactivity concentrations are identical, demonstrating that abacavir readily distributes into erythrocytes.

Metabolism: In humans, abacavir is not significantly metabolized by cytochrome P450 enzymes. The primary routes of elimination of abacavir are metabolism by alcohol dehydrogenase (to form the 5′-carboxylic acid) and glucuronyl transferase (to form the 5′-glucuronide). The metabolites do not have antiviral activity. *In vitro* experiments reveal that abacavir does not inhibit human CYP3A4, CYP2D6, or CYP2C9 activity at clinically relevant concentrations.

Elimination: Elimination of abacavir was quantified in a mass balance study following administration of a 600-mg dose of ^{14}C-abacavir: 99% of the radioactivity was recovered, 1.2% was excreted in the urine as abacavir, 30% as the 5′-carboxylic acid metabolite, 36% as the 5′-glucuronide metabolite, and 15% as unidentified minor metabolites in the urine. Fecal elimination accounted for 16% of the dose.

In single-dose studies, the observed elimination half-life ($t_{1/2}$) was 1.54 ± 0.63 hours. After intravenous administration, total clearance was 0.80 ± 0.24 L/hr per kg (mean ± SD).

Special Populations: *Adults With Impaired Renal Function:* The pharmacokinetic properties of ZIAGEN have not been determined in patients with impaired renal function. Renal excretion of unchanged abacavir is a minor route of elimination in humans.

Pediatric Patients: The pharmacokinetics of abacavir have been studied after either single or repeat doses of ZIAGEN in 68 pediatric patients. Following multiple-dose administration of ZIAGEN 8 mg/kg twice daily, steady-state $AUC_{(0-12\ h)}$ and C_{max} were 9.8 ± 4.56 mcg•h/mL and 3.71 ± 1.36 mcg/mL (mean ± SD), respectively (see PRECAUTIONS: Pediatric Use).

Geriatric Patients: The pharmacokinetics of ZIAGEN have not been studied in patients over 65 years of age.

Gender: The pharmacokinetics of ZIAGEN with respect to gender have not been determined.

Race: The pharmacokinetics of ZIAGEN with respect to race have not been determined.

Drug Interactions: In human liver microsomes, abacavir did not inhibit cytochrome P450 isoforms (2C9, 2D6, 3A4). Based on these data, it is unlikely that clinically significant drug interactions will occur between abacavir and drugs metabolized through these pathways.

Due to their common metabolic pathways via glucuronyl transferase with zidovudine, 15 HIV-infected patients were enrolled in a crossover study evaluating single doses of abacavir (600 mg), lamivudine (150 mg), and zidovudine (300 mg) alone or in combination. Analysis showed no clinically relevant changes in the pharmacokinetics of abacavir with the addition of lamivudine or zidovudine or the combination of lamivudine and zidovudine. Lamivudine exposure (AUC decreased 15%) and zidovudine exposure (AUC increased 10%) did not show clinically relevant changes with concurrent abacavir.

Due to their common metabolic pathways via alcohol dehydrogenase, the pharmacokinetic interaction between abacavir and ethanol was studied in 24 HIV-infected male patients. Each patient received the following treatments on separate occasions: a single 600-mg dose of abacavir, 0.7 g/kg ethanol (equivalent to five alcoholic drinks), and abacavir 600 mg plus 0.7 g/kg ethanol. Coadministration of ethanol and abacavir resulted in a 41% increase in abacavir AUC∞ and a 26% increase in abacavir $t_{1/2}$. In males, abacavir had no effect on the pharmacokinetic properties of ethanol, so no clinically significant interaction is expected in men. This interaction has not been studied in females.

INDICATIONS AND USAGE

ZIAGEN Tablets and Oral Solution, in combination with other antiretroviral agents, are indicated for the treatment of HIV-1 infection. This indication is based on analyses of surrogate markers in controlled studies up to 24 weeks in duration. At present there are no results from controlled trials evaluating long-term suppression of HIV RNA or disease progression with therapy with ZIAGEN (see Description of Clinical Studies).

Description of Clinical Studies: *Therapy-Naive Adults:* CNAAB3003 is an ongoing, multicenter, double-blind, placebo-controlled study in which 173 HIV-infected, therapy-naive adults were randomized to receive either ZIAGEN (300 mg twice daily), lamivudine (150 mg twice daily), and zidovudine (300 mg twice daily) or lamivudine (150 mg twice daily) and zidovudine (300 mg twice daily). The duration of double-blind treatment was 16 weeks. Study participants were: male (76%), Caucasian (54%), African-American (28%), and Hispanic (16%). The median age was 34 years, the median pretreatment CD4 cell count was 450 cells/mm^3, and median plasma HIV-1 RNA was 4.5 log_{10} copies/mL. Proportions of patients with plasma HIV-1 RNA ≤400 copies/mL (using Roche Amplicor HIV-1 MONITOR® Test) through 16 weeks of treatment are summarized in Figure 1.

Figure 1: Proportions of Patients with HIV-1 RNA ≤400 copies/mL in Study CNAAB3003[1]

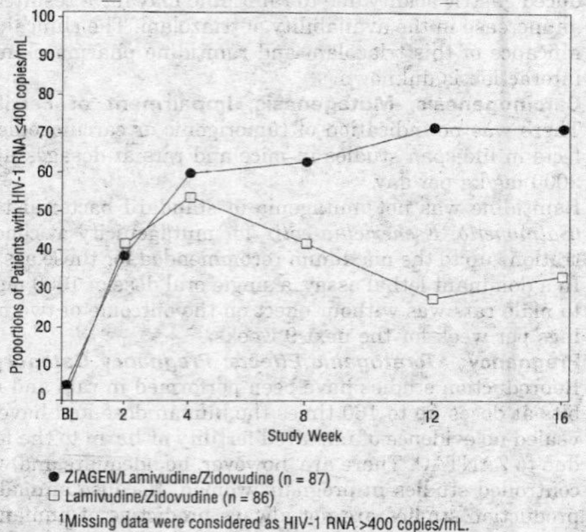

After 16 weeks of therapy, the median CD4 increases from baseline were 47 cells/mm^3 in the group receiving ZIAGEN and 112 cells/mm^3 in the placebo group.

Preliminary findings from a second controlled study in therapy-naive adults were supportive of the efficacy of abacavir through 16 weeks of treatment.

Therapy-Experienced Pediatric Patients: CNAA3006 is an ongoing, randomized, double-blind study comparing ZIAGEN 8 mg/kg twice daily and lamivudine 4 mg/kg twice daily and zidovudine 180 mg/m^2 twice daily versus lamivudine 4 mg/kg twice daily and zidovudine 180 mg/m^2 twice daily. Two hundred and five pediatric patients were enrolled: female (56%), Caucasian (17%), African-American (50%), Hispanic (30%), median age of 5.4 years, baseline CD4 cell percent >15% (median = 27%), and median baseline plasma HIV-1 RNA of 4.6 log_{10} copies/mL. Eighty percent and 55% of patients had prior therapy with zidovudine and lamivudine, respectively, most often in combination. The median duration of prior nucleoside analogue therapy was 2 years. Proportions of patients with plasma HIV-1 RNA levels ≤10,000 and ≤400 copies/mL, respectively, through 24 weeks of treatment are summarized in Figure 2.

Figure 2: Proportions of Patients with Plasma HIV-1 RNA ≤10,000 copies/mL or ≤400 copies/mL Through Week 24 in Study CNAA3006[1,2]

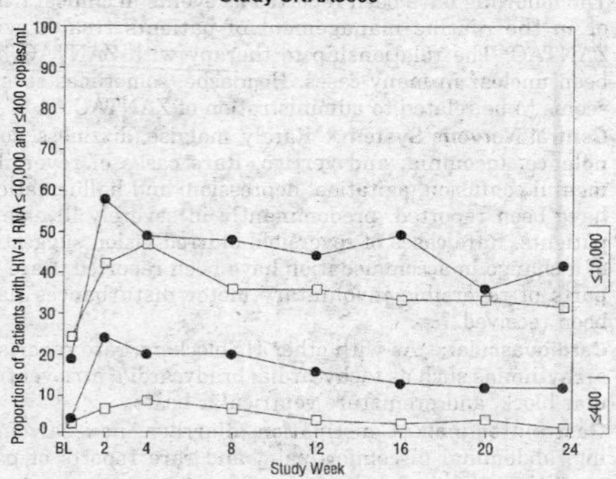

After 16 weeks of therapy, the median CD4 increases from baseline were 69 cells/mm^3 in the group receiving ZIAGEN and 9 cells/mm^3 in the control group.

CONTRAINDICATIONS

ZIAGEN Tablets and Oral Solution are contraindicated in patients with previously demonstrated hypersensitivity to any of the components of the products (see WARNINGS).

WARNINGS

Hypersensitivity Reaction: Fatal hypersensitivity reactions have been associated with therapy with ZIAGEN. Patients developing signs or symptoms of hypersensitivity (which include fever; skin rash; fatigue; gastrointestinal symptoms such as nausea, vomiting, diarrhea, or abdominal pain; and respiratory symptoms such as pharyngitis, dyspnea, or cough) should discontinue ZIAGEN as soon as a hypersensitivity reaction is first suspected, and should seek medical evaluation immediately. The diagnosis of hypersensitivity reaction should be carefully considered for patients presenting with symptoms of acute onset respiratory diseases, even if alternative respiratory diagnoses (pneumonia, bronchitis, pharyngitis, or flu-like illness) are possible. ZIAGEN SHOULD NOT be restarted following a hypersensitivity reaction because more severe symptoms will recur within hours and may include life-threatening hypotension and death (see PRECAUTIONS: Information for Patients and ADVERSE REACTIONS).

In ongoing clinical trials, hypersensitivity reactions have been reported in approximately 5% of adult and pediatric patients receiving abacavir. Symptoms usually appear within the first 6 weeks of treatment with ZIAGEN although these reactions may occur at any time during therapy (see PRECAUTIONS: Information for Patients and ADVERSE REACTIONS).

Abacavir Hypersensitivity Reaction Registry: To facilitate reporting of hypersensitivity reactions and collection of information on each case, an Abacavir Hypersensitivity Registry has been established. Physicians should register patients by calling 1-800-270-0425.

Lactic Acidosis/Severe Hepatomegaly with Steatosis: Lactic acidosis and severe hepatomegaly with steatosis, including fatal cases, have been reported with the use of nucleoside analogues alone or in combination, including abacavir and other antiretrovirals. A majority of these cases have been in women. Obesity and prolonged nucleoside exposure may be risk factors. Particular caution should be exercised when administering ZIAGEN to any patient with known risk factors for liver disease; however, cases have also been reported in patients with no known risk factors. Treatment with ZIAGEN should be suspended in any patient who develops clinical or laboratory findings suggestive of lactic acidosis or pronounced hepatotoxicity (which may include hepatomegaly and steatosis even in the absence of marked transaminase elevations).

PRECAUTIONS

General: Abacavir should always be used in combination with other antiretroviral agents. Abacavir should not be added as a single agent when antiretroviral regimens are changed due to loss of virologic response.

Therapy-Experienced Patients: In clinical trials, patients with prolonged prior nucleoside reverse transcriptase inhibitor (NRTI) exposure or who had HIV-1 isolates that contained multiple mutations conferring resistance to NRTIs had limited response to abacavir. The potential for cross-resistance between abacavir and other NRTIs should be considered when choosing new therapeutic regimens in therapy-experienced patients (see MICROBIOLOGY: Cross-Resistance).

Information for Patients: Patients should be advised of the possibility of hypersensitivity reaction to ZIAGEN that may result in death. Patients developing signs or symptoms of hypersensitivity (which include fever; skin rash; fatigue; gastrointestinal symptoms such as nausea, vomiting, diarrhea, or abdominal pain; and respiratory symptoms such as sore throat, shortness of breath, or cough) should discontinue treatment with ZIAGEN and seek medical evaluation immediately. **ZIAGEN SHOULD NOT be restarted following a hypersensitivity reaction because more severe symptoms will recur within hours and may include life-threatening hypotension and death (see ADVERSE REACTIONS and WARNINGS).**

The Medication Guide provides written information for the patient, and should be dispensed with each new prescription and refill. The complete text of the Medication Guide is reprinted at the end of this document. A Warning Card summarizing the symptoms of the abacavir hypersensitivity reaction should be provided to the patient by the pharmacist with each prescription. Patients should be instructed to carry this card with them.

ZIAGEN is not a cure for HIV infection and patients may continue to experience illnesses associated with HIV infection, including opportunistic infections. Patients should remain under the care of a physician when using ZIAGEN.

Patients should be advised that the use of ZIAGEN has not been shown to reduce the risk of transmission of HIV to others through sexual contact or blood contamination.

Patients should be advised that the long-term effects of ZIAGEN are unknown at this time.

ZIAGEN Tablets and Oral Solution are for oral ingestion only.

Patients should be advised of the importance of taking ZIAGEN exactly as it is prescribed.

Table 1: Selected Clinical Adverse Events Grades 1-4 (≥5% Frequency) in Therapy-Naive Adults (CNAAB3003) Through 16 Weeks of Treatment

Adverse Event	ZIAGEN/Lamivudine/ Zidovudine (n = 83)	Lamivudine/Zidovudine (n = 81)
Nausea	47%	41%
Nausea and vomiting	16%	11%
Diarrhea	12%	11%
Loss of appetite/anorexia	11%	10%
Insomnia and other sleep disorders	7%	5%

Table 2: Selected Clinical Adverse Events Grades 1-4 (≥5% Frequency) in Therapy-Experienced Pediatric Patients (CNAAB3006) Through 24 Weeks of Treatment

Adverse Event	ZIAGEN/Lamivudine/ Zidovudine (n = 102)	Lamivudine/Zidovudine (n = 103)
Nausea and vomiting	38%	18%
Fever	19%	12%
Headache	16%	12%
Diarrhea	16%	15%
Skin rashes	11%	8%
Loss of appetite/anorexia	9%	2%

Drug Interactions: Pharmacokinetic properties of abacavir were not altered by the addition of either lamivudine or zidovudine or the combination of lamivudine and zidovudine. No clinically significant changes to lamivudine or zidovudine pharmacokinetics were observed following concomitant administration of abacavir.

Abacavir has no effect on the pharmacokinetic properties of ethanol. Ethanol decreases the elimination of abacavir causing an increase in overall exposure (see CLINICAL PHARMACOLOGY: Drug Interactions).

Carcinogenesis, Mutagenesis, and Impairment of Fertility: Abacavir induced chromosomal aberrations both in the presence and absence of metabolic activation in an *in vitro* cytogenetic study in human lymphocytes. Abacavir was mutagenic in the absence of metabolic activation, although it was not mutagenic in the presence of metabolic activation in an L5178Y mouse lymphoma assay. At systemic exposures approximately 9 times higher than that in humans at the therapeutic dose, abacavir was clastogenic in males and not clastogenic in females in an *in vivo* mouse bone marrow micronucleus assay.

Abacavir was not mutagenic in bacterial mutagenicity assays in the presence and absence of metabolic activation.

Abacavir had no adverse effects on the mating performance or fertility of male and female rats at doses of up to 500 mg/kg per day, a dose expected to produce exposures approximately 8 fold higher than that in humans at the therapeutic dose based on body surface area comparisons.

Pregnancy: Pregnancy Category C. Studies in pregnant rats showed that abacavir is transferred to the fetus through the placenta. Developmental toxicity (depressed fetal body weight and reduced crown-rump length) and increased incidences of fetal anasarca and skeletal malformations were observed when rats were treated with abacavir at doses of 1000 mg/kg during organogenesis. This dose produced 35 times the human exposure, based on AUC. In a fertility study, evidence of toxicity to the developing embryo and fetuses (increased resorptions, decreased fetal body weights) occurred only at 500 mg/kg per day. The offspring of female rats treated with abacavir at 500 mg/kg per day (beginning at embryo implantation and ending at weaning) showed increased incidence of stillbirth and lower body weights throughout life. In the rabbit, there was no evidence of drug-related developmental toxicity and no increases in fetal malformations at doses up to 700 mg/kg (8.5 times the human exposure at the recommended dose, based on AUC).

There are no adequate and well-controlled studies in pregnant women. ZIAGEN should be used during pregnancy only if the potential benefits outweigh the risk.

Antiretroviral Pregnancy Registry: To monitor maternal-fetal outcomes of pregnant women exposed to ZIAGEN, an Antiretroviral Pregnancy Registry has been established. Physicians are encouraged to register patients by calling 1-800-258-4263.

Nursing Mothers: The Centers for Disease Control and Prevention recommend that HIV-infected mothers not breastfeed their infants to avoid risking postnatal transmission of HIV infection.

Although it is not known if abacavir is excreted in human milk, abacavir is present in the milk of lactating rats dosed with abacavir. Because of both the potential for HIV transmission and any possible adverse effects of abacavir, **mothers should be instructed not to breastfeed if they are receiving ZIAGEN.**

Pediatric Use: The safety and effectiveness of ZIAGEN have been established in pediatric patients aged 3 months to 13 years. Use of ZIAGEN in these age groups is supported by pharmacokinetic studies and evidence from adequate and well-controlled studies of ZIAGEN in adults and pediatric patients (see CLINICAL PHARMACOLOGY: Pharmacokinetics: Special Populations: Pediatric Patients; INDICATIONS AND USAGE: Description of Clinical Studies; WARNINGS; ADVERSE REACTIONS; and DOSAGE AND ADMINISTRATION).

Geriatric Use: Clinical studies of ZIAGEN did not include sufficient numbers of patients aged 65 and over to determine whether they respond differently from younger patients. Other reported clinical experience has not identified differences in response between elderly and younger patients. In general, dose selection for an elderly patient should be cautious, reflecting the greater frequency of decreased hepatic, renal, or cardiac function, and of concomitant disease or other drug therapy.

ADVERSE REACTIONS

Hypersensitivity Reaction: Fatal hypersensitivity reactions have been associated with therapy with ZIAGEN. Therapy with ZIAGEN SHOULD NOT be restarted following a hypersensitivity reaction because more severe symptoms will recur within hours and may include life-threatening hypotension and death. Patients developing signs or symptoms of hypersensitivity should discontinue treatment as soon as a hypersensitivity reaction is first suspected, and should seek medical evaluation immediately (see WARNINGS, PRECAUTIONS, and Information for Patients).

In ongoing clinical studies, approximately 5% of adult and pediatric patients receiving ZIAGEN developed a hypersensitivity reaction. This reaction is characterized by the appearance of symptoms indicating multi-organ/body system involvement. Symptoms usually appear within the first 6 weeks of treatment with ZIAGEN, although these reactions may occur at any time during therapy. Frequently observed signs and symptoms include fever; skin rash; fatigue; and gastrointestinal symptoms such as nausea, vomiting, diarrhea, or abdominal pain. Other signs and symptoms include malaise, lethargy, myalgia, myolysis, arthralgia, edema, pharyngitis, cough, dyspnea, headache, and paresthesia. Some patients who experienced a hypersensitivity reaction were initially thought to have acute onset or worsening respiratory disease. The diagnosis of hypersensitivity reaction should be carefully considered for patients presenting with symptoms of acute onset respiratory diseases, even if alternative respiratory diagnoses (pneumonia, bronchitis, pharyngitis, or flu-like illness) are possible. Physical findings include lymphadenopathy, mucous membrane lesions (conjunctivitis and mouth ulcerations), and rash. The rash usually appears maculopapular or urticarial but may be variable in appearance. Hypersensitivity reactions have occurred without rash. Laboratory abnormalities include elevated liver function tests, increased creatine phosphokinase or creatinine, and lymphopenia. Anaphylaxis, liver failure, renal failure, hypotension, and death have occurred in association with hypersensitivity reactions. Symptoms worsen with continued therapy but often resolve upon discontinuation of ZIAGEN.

Risk factors that may predict the occurrence or severity of hypersensitivity to abacavir have not been identified.

Adults: Selected clinical adverse events with a ≥5% frequency during therapy with ZIAGEN 300 mg twice daily and lamivudine 150 mg twice daily and zidovudine 300 mg twice daily compared with lamivudine 150 mg twice daily and zidovudine 300 mg twice daily from CNAAB3003 are listed in Table 1.

[See table 1 above]

Pediatric Patients: Selected clinical adverse events with a ≥5% frequency during therapy with ZIAGEN 8 mg/kg twice daily and lamivudine 4 mg/kg twice daily and zidovudine 180 mg/m^2 twice daily compared with lamivudine 4 mg/kg

Continued on next page

This product information is based on labeling in effect on June 23, 2000. For further information, contact via direct mail, phone, or web site. Medical Information, Glaxo Wellcome Inc., PO Box 13398, Research Triangle Park, NC 27709. Healthcare Professionals (Medical Information): 800-334-0089. Patients (Customer Response Center): 1-888-825-5249. Glaxo Wellcome Corporate Web Site: www.glaxowellcome.com

Ziagen—Cont.

twice daily and zidovudine 180 mg/m^2 twice daily from CNAA3006 are listed in Table 2.

[See table 2 on previous page]

Laboratory Abnormalities: Laboratory abnormalities (anemia, neutropenia, liver function test abnormalities, and CPK elevations) were observed with similar frequencies in the 2 treatment groups in studies CNAAB3003 and CNAA3006. Mild elevations of blood glucose were more frequent in subjects receiving abacavir. In study CNAAB3003, triglyceride elevations (all grades) were more common on the abacavir arm (25%) than on the placebo arm (11%).

Other Adverse Events: In addition to adverse events in Tables 1 and 2, other adverse events observed in the expanded access program were pancreatitis and increased GGT.

OVERDOSAGE

There is no known antidote for ZIAGEN. It is not known whether abacavir can be removed by peritoneal dialysis or hemodialysis.

DOSAGE AND ADMINISTRATION

A Medication Guide and Warning Card that provide information about recognition of hypersensitivity reactions should be dispensed with each new prescription and refill. To facilitate reporting of hypersensitivity reactions and collection of information on each case, an Abacavir Hypersensitivity Registry has been established. Physicians should register patients by calling 1-800-270-0425.

ZIAGEN may be taken with or without food.

Adults: The recommended oral dose of ZIAGEN for adults is 300 mg twice daily in combination with other antiretroviral agents.

Adolescents and Pediatric Patients: The recommended oral dose of ZIAGEN for adolescents and pediatric patients 3 months to up to 16 years of age is 8 mg/kg twice daily (up to a maximum of 300 mg twice daily) in combination with other antiretroviral agents.

Dose Adjustment in Hepatic Impairment: Insufficient data are available to recommend a dosage of ZIAGEN in patients with hepatic impairment.

HOW SUPPLIED

ZIAGEN is available as tablets and oral solution.

ZIAGEN Tablets: Each tablet contains abacavir sulfate equivalent to 300 mg abacavir. The tablets are yellow, biconvex, capsule-shaped, film-coated, and imprinted with "GX 623" on one side with no marking on the reverse side. They are packaged as follows:

Bottles of 60 tablets (NDC 0173-0661-01).

Unit dose blister packs of 60 tablets (NDC 0173-0661-00). Each pack contains 6 blister cards of 10 tablets each.

Store at controlled room temperature of 20° to 25°C (68° to 77°F) (see USP).

ZIAGEN Oral Solution: It is a clear to opalescent, yellowish, strawberry-banana-flavored liquid. Each mL of the solution contains abacavir sulfate equivalent to 20 mg of abacavir. It is packaged in plastic bottles as follows:

Bottles of 240 mL (NDC 0173-0664-00) with child-resistant closure. This product does not require reconstitution.

Store at controlled room temperature of 20° to 25°C (68° to 77°F) (see USP). DO NOT FREEZE. May be refrigerated.

Glaxo Wellcome Inc., Research Triangle Park, NC 27709
US Patent Nos. 5,034,394 and 5,089,500

January 2000/RL-791

MEDICATION GUIDE

ZIAGEN® (z-EYE-uh-jen) (abacavir sulfate) Tablets and Oral Solution

Established name: abacavir (uh-BACK-ah-veer) sulfate tablets and oral solution

In order to take Ziagen safely, you should read all of the information in this Medication Guide each time you fill your prescription for Ziagen.

What is the most important information I should know about Ziagen?

About 5% of patients (5 in 100) who take Ziagen have a hypersensitivity reaction (a serious allergic reaction) **that may result in death.** If you have **skin rash** or 2 or more of the following sets of symptoms, you may be having this kind of reaction:

- **fever**
- **nausea, vomiting, diarrhea, or abdominal pain**
- **severe tiredness, achiness, or generally ill feeling**
- **sore throat, shortness of breath, or cough**

A written list of these symptoms is on the Warning Card provided by your pharmacist. You should carry this Warning Card with you. **IF YOU NOTICE THESE SYMPTOMS WHILE TAKING ZIAGEN, STOP TAKING ZIAGEN AND CALL YOUR DOCTOR IMMEDIATELY.**

If you must stop treatment with Ziagen because you have had this serious reaction, **NEVER TAKE ZIAGEN AGAIN.** If you take Ziagen again after you have had this serious reaction, **WITHIN HOURS** you may experience **LIFE-THREATENING** symptoms that may include **LOWERING OF YOUR BLOOD PRESSURE OR DEATH.**

Ziagen can have other serious side effects. Be sure to read "What are the possible side effects of Ziagen?" in the section below.

What is Ziagen?

Ziagen is a medication used to treat HIV infection. Ziagen is taken by mouth as a tablet or a strawberry-banana flavored liquid. It belongs to a class of anti-HIV medicines called nucleoside analogue reverse transcriptase inhibitors (NRTIs). Ziagen is only proven to work when taken in combination with other anti-HIV medications. When used in combination with these other medications, Ziagen helps lower the amount of HIV found in your blood and keep your immune system as healthy as possible so that it can help fight infection. However, Ziagen does not have these effects in all patients.

Ziagen does not cure HIV infection or AIDS. At this time, there is no evidence that Ziagen will help you live longer or have fewer of the medical problems that are associated with HIV infection or AIDS. Because of this, you must be sure to be seen regularly by your health care provider.

Who should not take Ziagen?

Do not take Ziagen if you have ever had a hypersensitivity reaction (a serious allergic reaction) to Ziagen. In such cases, you should return all of your unused Ziagen to your doctor or pharmacist for proper disposal.

How should I take Ziagen?

Take Ziagen exactly as your doctor prescribes it.

The usual dosage for adults (at least 16 years of age) is one 300-mg tablet twice a day.

Adolescents and children from 3 months to 16 years of age can also take Ziagen. Your doctor will tell you if the oral solution or tablet is best for your child. Also, your child's doctor will decide the right dose based on your child's weight and age. Ziagen has not been studied in children under 3 months of age.

Ziagen can be taken with food or on an empty stomach.

To help make sure that your anti-HIV therapy is as effective as it can be, be very careful to take all of your medication exactly as your doctor prescribed it and do not skip any doses.

If you miss a dose of Ziagen, take the missed dose immediately. Then, take the next dose at the regularly scheduled time.

When your supply of Ziagen and other anti-HIV drugs starts to run low, get more from your doctor or pharmacy. It is very important that you take anti-HIV drugs as prescribed by your doctor because the amount of virus in your blood may increase if one or more of the drugs is stopped, even for a short time.

What should I avoid while taking Ziagen?

Ziagen has not been shown to reduce the risk of passing HIV to others through sexual contact or blood contamination. Continue to practice safe sex while using Ziagen. Do not use or share dirty needles.

Talk to your doctor if you are pregnant or if you become pregnant while taking Ziagen. Ziagen has not been studied in pregnant women and the risk to the unborn child is not known.

Mothers with HIV should not breastfeed their infants because HIV in the breast milk can be passed to the infant.

What are the possible side effects of Ziagen?

Some people have had a hypersensitivity reaction (a serious allergic reaction) to Ziagen, which can be fatal. Instructions on how to recognize a possible reaction, as well as what to do if such a reaction is suspected, are discussed in the section "What is the most important information I should know about Ziagen?"

The class of medicines to which Ziagen belongs (NRTIs) can cause a condition called lactic acidosis, together with an enlarged liver. In some cases, this condition can be fatal. Women are more likely than men to experience this rare but serious side effect.

Ziagen can cause other side effects. In studies, the most common side effects with Ziagen were nausea, vomiting, malaise or fatigue, headache, diarrhea, and loss of appetite. Most of these side effects did not cause people to stop taking Ziagen. This listing of side effects is not complete. Your doctor or pharmacist can discuss with you a more complete list of side effects with Ziagen. Talk to your doctor promptly about any side effects you have.

Medicines are sometimes prescribed for purposes other than those listed in a Medication Guide. Ask a health care professional about any concerns about Ziagen. Professional labeling is available to your doctor and other health care professionals. If you want more information, ask your doctor or pharmacist to let you read the professional labeling.

Glaxo Wellcome Inc., Research Triangle Park, NC 27709
January 2000/MG-005

This Medication Guide has been approved by the US Food and Drug Administration.

Shown in Product Identification Guide, page 317

ZINACEF® ℞
[*zin 'ah-sef*]
(cefuroxime for injection)

ZINACEF® ℞
(cefuroxime injection)

DESCRIPTION

Cefuroxime is a semisynthetic, broad-spectrum, cephalosporin antibiotic for parenteral administration. It is the sodium salt of (6R, 7R)-3-carbamoyloxymethyl-7-[Z-2-methoxyimino-2-(fur-2-yl) acetamido]ceph-3-em-4-carboxylate.

The empirical formula is $C_{16}H_{15}N_4NaO_8S$, representing a molecular weight of 446.4.

ZINACEF contains approximately 54.2 mg (2.4 mEq) of sodium per gram of cefuroxime activity.

ZINACEF in sterile crystalline form is supplied in vials equivalent to 750 mg, 1.5 g, or 7.5 g of cefuroxime as cefuroxime sodium and in ADD-Vantage® vials equivalent to 750 mg or 1.5 g of cefuroxime as cefuroxime sodium. Solutions of ZINACEF range in color from light yellow to amber, depending on the concentration and diluent used. The pH of freshly constituted solutions usually ranges from 6 to 8.5.

ZINACEF is available as a frozen, iso-osmotic, sterile, nonpyrogenic solution with 750 mg or 1.5 g of cefuroxime as cefuroxime sodium. Approximately 1.4 g of Dextrose Hydrous, USP has been added to the 750-mg dose to adjust the osmolality. Sodium Citrate Hydrous, USP has been added as a buffer (300 mg and 600 mg to the 750-mg and 1.5-g doses, respectively). ZINACEF contains approximately 111 mg (4.8 mEq) and 222 mg (9.7 mEq) of sodium in the 750-mg and 1.5-g doses, respectively. The pH has been adjusted with hydrochloric acid and may have been adjusted with sodium hydroxide. Solutions of premixed ZINACEF range in color from light yellow to amber. The solution is intended for intravenous (IV) use after thawing to room temperature. The osmolality of the solution is approximately 300 mOsmol/kg, and the pH of thawed solutions ranges from 5 to 7.5.

The plastic container for the frozen solution is fabricated from a specially designed multilayer plastic, PL 2040. Solutions are in contact with the polyethylene layer of this container and can leach out certain chemical components of the plastic in very small amounts within the expiration period. The suitability of the plastic has been confirmed in tests in animals according to USP biological tests for plastic containers as well as by tissue culture toxicity studies.

CLINICAL PHARMACOLOGY

After intramuscular (IM) injection of a 750-mg dose of cefuroxime to normal volunteers, the mean peak serum concentration was 27 mcg/mL. The peak occurred at approximately 45 minutes (range, 15 to 60 minutes). Following IV doses of 750 mg and 1.5 g, serum concentrations were approximately 50 and 100 mcg/mL, respectively, at 15 minutes. Therapeutic serum concentrations of approximately 2 mcg/mL or more were maintained for 5.3 hours and 8 hours or more, respectively. There was no evidence of accumulation of cefuroxime in the serum following IV administration of 1.5-g doses every 8 hours to normal volunteers. The serum half-life after either IM or IV injections is approximately 80 minutes.

Approximately 89% of a dose of cefuroxime is excreted by the kidneys over an 8-hour period, resulting in high urinary concentrations.

Following the IM administration of a 750-mg single dose, urinary concentrations averaged 1300 mcg/mL during the first 8 hours. Intravenous doses of 750 mg and 1.5 g produced urinary levels averaging 1150 and 2500 mcg/mL, respectively, during the first 8-hour period.

The concomitant oral administration of probenecid with cefuroxime slows tubular secretion, decreases renal clearance by approximately 40%, increases the peak serum level by approximately 30%, and increases the serum half-life by approximately 30%. Cefuroxime is detectable in therapeutic concentrations in pleural fluid, joint fluid, bile, sputum, bone, and aqueous humor.

Cefuroxime is detectable in therapeutic concentrations in cerebrospinal fluid (CSF) of adults and pediatric patients with meningitis. The following table shows the concentrations of cefuroxime achieved in cerebrospinal fluid during multiple dosing of patients with meningitis.

[See table at top of next page]

Cefuroxime is approximately 50% bound to serum protein.

Microbiology: Cefuroxime has *in vitro* activity against a wide range of gram-positive and gram-negative organisms, and it is highly stable in the presence of beta-lactamases of certain gram-negative bacteria. The bactericidal action of cefuroxime results from inhibition of cell-wall synthesis.

Cefuroxime is usually active against the following organisms *in vitro.*

Aerobes, Gram-positive: *Staphylococcus aureus, Staphylococcus epidermidis, Streptococcus pneumoniae,* and *Streptococcus pyogenes* (and other streptococci).

NOTE: Most strains of enterococci, e.g., *Enterococcus faecalis* (formerly *Streptococcus faecalis*), are resistant to cefuroxime. Methicillin-resistant staphylococci and *Listeria monocytogenes* are resistant to cefuroxime.

Aerobes, Gram-negative: *Citrobacter* spp., *Enterobacter* spp., *Escherichia coli, Haemophilus influenzae* (including ampicillin-resistant strains), *Haemophilus parainfluenzae, Klebsiella* spp. (including *Klebsiella pneumoniae*), *Moraxella (Branhamella) catarrhalis* (including ampicillin- and cephalothin-resistant strains), *Morganella morganii* (formerly *Proteus morganii*), *Neisseria gonorrhoeae* (including penicillinase- and non–penicillinase-producing strains), *Neisseria meningitidis, Proteus mirabilis, Providencia rettgeri* (formerly *Proteus rettgeri*), *Salmonella* spp., and *Shigella* spp.

NOTE: Some strains of *Morganella morganii, Enterobacter cloacae,* and *Citrobacter* spp. have been shown by *in vitro* tests to be resistant to cefuroxime and other cephalosporins. *Pseudomonas* and *Campylobacter* spp., *Acinetobacter calcoaceticus,* and most strains of *Serratia* spp. and *Proteus vulgaris* are resistant to most first- and second-generation cephalosporins.

Anaerobes: Gram-positive and gram-negative cocci (including *Peptococcus* and *Peptostreptococcus* spp.), gram-positive bacilli (including *Clostridium* spp.), and gram-negative bacilli (including *Bacteroides* and *Fusobacterium* spp.).

NOTE: *Clostridium difficile* and most strains of *Bacteroides fragilis* are resistant to cefuroxime.

Susceptibility Tests: *Diffusion Techniques:* Quantitative methods that require measurement of zone diameters give an estimate of antibiotic susceptibility. One such standard procedure[1] that has been recommended for use with disks to test susceptibility of organisms to cefuroxime uses the 30-mcg cefuroxime disk. Interpretation involves the correlation of the diameters obtained in the disk test with the minimum inhibitory concentration (MIC) for cefuroxime.

A report of "Susceptible" indicates that the pathogen is likely to be inhibited by generally achievable blood levels. A report of "Moderately Susceptible" suggests that the organism would be susceptible if high dosage is used or if the infection is confined to tissues and fluids in which high antibiotic levels are attained. A report of "Intermediate" suggests an equivocable or indeterminate result. A report of "Resistant" indicates that achievable concentrations of the antibiotic are unlikely to be inhibitory and other therapy should be selected.

Reports from the laboratory giving results of the standard single-disk susceptibility test for organisms other than *Haemophilus* spp. and *Neisseria gonorrhoeae* with a 30-mcg cefuroxime disk should be interpreted according to the following criteria:

Zone Diameter (mm)	Interpretation
≥18	(S) Susceptible
15-17	(MS) Moderately Susceptible
≤14	(R) Resistant

Results for *Haemophilus* spp. should be interpreted according to the following criteria:

Zone Diameter (mm)	Interpretation
≥24	(S) Susceptible
21-23	(I) Intermediate
≤20	(R) Resistant

Results for *Neisseria gonorrhoeae* should be interpreted according to the following criteria:

Zone Diameter (mm)	Interpretation
≥31	(S) Susceptible
26-30	(MS) Moderately Susceptible
≤25	(R) Resistant

Organisms should be tested with the cefuroxime disk since cefuroxime has been shown by *in vitro* tests to be active against certain strains found resistant when other beta-lactam disks are used. The cefuroxime disk should not be used for testing susceptibility to other cephalosporins.

Standardized procedures require the use of laboratory control organisms. The 30-mcg cefuroxime disk should give the following zone diameters.

1. Testing for organisms other than *Haemophilus* spp. and *Neisseria gonorrhoeae:*

Organism	Zone Diameter (mm)
Staphylococcus aureus ATCC 25923	27-35
Escherichia coli ATCC 25922	20-26

2. Testing for *Haemophilus* spp.:

Organism	Zone Diameter (mm)
Haemophilus influenzae ATCC 49766	28-36

3. Testing for *Neisseria gonorrhoeae:*

Organism	Zone Diameter (mm)
Neisseria gonorrhoeae ATCC 49226	33-41
Staphylococcus aureus ATCC 25923	29-33

Dilution Techniques: Use a standardized dilution method[1] (broth, agar, microdilution) or equivalent with cefuroxime powder. The MIC values obtained for bacterial isolates other than *Haemophilus* spp. and *Neisseria gonorrhoeae* should be interpreted according to the following criteria:

MIC (mcg/mL)	Interpretation
≤8	(S) Susceptible
16	(MS) Moderately Susceptible
≥32	(R) Resistant

MIC values obtained for *Haemophilus* spp. should be interpreted according to the following criteria:

MIC (mcg/mL)	Interpretation
≤4	(S) Susceptible
8	(I) Intermediate
≥16	(R) Resistant

MIC values obtained for *Neisseria gonorrhoeae* should be interpreted according to the following criteria:

MIC (mcg/mL)	Interpretation
≤1	(S) Susceptible
2	(MS) Moderately Susceptible
≥4	(R) Resistant

As with standard diffusion techniques, dilution methods require the use of laboratory control organisms. Standard cefuroxime powder should provide the following MIC values.

1. For organisms other than *Haemophilus* spp. and *Neisseria gonorrhoeae:*

Organism	MIC (mcg/mL)
Staphylococcus aureus ATCC 29213	0.5-2.0
Escherichia coli ATCC 25922	2.0-8.0

2. For *Haemophilus* spp.:

Organism	MIC (mcg/mL)
Haemophilus influenzae ATCC 49766	0.25-1.0

3. For *Neisseria gonorrhoeae:*

Organism	MIC (mcg/mL)
Neisseria gonorrhoeae ATCC 49226	0.25-1.0
Staphylococcus aureus ATCC 29213	0.25-1.0

Patients	Dose	Number of Patients	Mean (Range) CSF Cefuroxime Concentrations (mcg/mL) Achieved Within 8 Hours Post Dose
Pediatric patients (4 weeks to 6.5 years)	200 mg/kg/day, divided q 6 hours	5	6.6 (0.9-17.3)
Pediatric patients (7 months to 9 years)	200 to 230 mg/kg/day, divided q 8 hours	6	8.3 (<2-22.5)
Adults	1.5 grams q 8 hours	2	5.2 (2.7-8.9)
Adults	1.5 grams q 6 hours	10	6.0 (1.5-13.5)

INDICATIONS AND USAGE

ZINACEF is indicated for the treatment of patients with infections caused by susceptible strains of the designated organisms in the following diseases:

1. **Lower Respiratory Tract Infections**, including pneumonia, caused by *Streptococcus pneumoniae, Haemophilus influenzae* (including ampicillin-resistant strains), *Klebsiella* spp., *Staphylococcus aureus* (penicillinase- and non–penicillinase-producing strains), *Streptococcus pyogenes,* and *Escherichia coli.*
2. **Urinary Tract Infections** caused by *Escherichia coli* and *Klebsiella* spp.
3. **Skin and Skin-Structure Infections** caused by *Staphylococcus aureus* (penicillinase- and non–penicillinase-producing strains), *Streptococcus pyogenes, Escherichia coli, Klebsiella* spp., and *Enterobacter* spp.
4. **Septicemia** caused by *Staphylococcus aureus* (penicillinase- and non–penicillinase-producing strains), *Streptococcus pneumoniae, Escherichia coli, Haemophilus influenzae* (including ampicillin-resistant strains), and *Klebsiella* spp.
5. **Meningitis** caused by *Streptococcus pneumoniae, Haemophilus influenzae* (including ampicillin-resistant strains), *Neisseria meningitidis,* and *Staphylococcus aureus* (penicillinase- and non–penicillinase-producing strains).
6. **Gonorrhea**: Uncomplicated and disseminated gonococcal infections due to *Neisseria gonorrhoeae* (penicillinase- and non–penicillinase-producing strains) in both males and females.
7. **Bone and Joint Infections** caused by *Staphylococcus aureus* (penicillinase- and non–penicillinase-producing strains).

Clinical microbiological studies in skin and skin-structure infections frequently reveal the growth of susceptible strains of both aerobic and anaerobic organisms. ZINACEF has been used successfully in these mixed infections in which several organisms have been isolated. Appropriate cultures and susceptibility studies should be performed to determine the susceptibility of the causative organisms to ZINACEF.

Therapy may be started while awaiting the results of these studies; however, once these results become available, the antibiotic treatment should be adjusted accordingly. In certain cases of confirmed or suspected gram-positive or gram-negative sepsis or in patients with other serious infections in which the causative organism has not been identified, ZINACEF may be used concomitantly with an aminoglycoside (see PRECAUTIONS). The recommended doses of both antibiotics may be given depending on the severity of the infection and the patient's condition.

Prevention: The preoperative prophylactic administration of ZINACEF may prevent the growth of susceptible disease-causing bacteria and thereby may reduce the incidence of certain postoperative infections in patients undergoing surgical procedures (e.g., vaginal hysterectomy) that are classified as clean-contaminated or potentially contaminated procedures. Effective prophylactic use of antibiotics in surgery depends on the time of administration. ZINACEF should usually be given one-half to 1 hour before the operation to allow sufficient time to achieve effective antibiotic concentrations in the wound tissues during the procedure. The dose should be repeated intraoperatively if the surgical procedure is lengthy.

Prophylactic administration is usually not required after the surgical procedure ends and should be stopped within 24 hours. In the majority of surgical procedures, continuing prophylactic administration of any antibiotic does not reduce the incidence of subsequent infections but will increase the possibility of adverse reactions and the development of bacterial resistance.

The perioperative use of ZINACEF has also been effective during open heart surgery for surgical patients in whom infections at the operative site would present a serious risk. For these patients it is recommended that therapy with ZINACEF be continued for at least 48 hours after the surgical procedure ends. If an infection is present, specimens for culture should be obtained for the identification of the causative organism, and appropriate antimicrobial therapy should be instituted.

CONTRAINDICATIONS

ZINACEF is contraindicated in patients with known allergy to the cephalosporin group of antibiotics.

WARNINGS

BEFORE THERAPY WITH ZINACEF IS INSTITUTED, CAREFUL INQUIRY SHOULD BE MADE TO DETERMINE WHETHER THE PATIENT HAS HAD PREVIOUS HYPERSENSITIVITY REACTIONS TO CEPHALOSPORINS, PENICILLINS, OR OTHER DRUGS. THIS PRODUCT SHOULD BE GIVEN CAUTIOUSLY TO PENICILLIN-SENSITIVE PATIENTS. ANTIBIOTICS SHOULD BE ADMINISTERED WITH CAUTION TO ANY PATIENT WHO HAS DEMONSTRATED SOME FORM OF ALLERGY, PARTICULARLY TO DRUGS. IF AN ALLERGIC REACTION TO ZINACEF OCCURS, DISCONTINUE THE DRUG. SERIOUS ACUTE HYPERSENSITIVITY REACTIONS MAY REQUIRE EPINEPHRINE AND OTHER EMERGENCY MEASURES.

Pseudomembranous colitis has been reported with nearly all antibacterial agents, including cefuroxime, and may range in severity from mild to life threatening. Therefore, it is important to consider this diagnosis in patients who present with diarrhea subsequent to the administration of antibacterial agents.

Treatment with antibacterial agents alters the normal flora of the colon and may permit overgrowth of clostridia. Studies indicate that a toxin produced by *Clostridium difficile* is one primary cause of "antibiotic-associated colitis."

After the diagnosis of pseudomembranous colitis has been established, appropriate therapeutic measures should be initiated. Mild cases of pseudomembranous colitis usually respond to drug discontinuation alone. In moderate to severe cases, consideration should be given to management with fluids and electrolytes, protein supplementation, and treatment with an antibacterial drug clinically effective against *Clostridium difficile* colitis.

When the colitis is not relieved by drug discontinuation or when it is severe, oral vancomycin is the treatment of choice for antibiotic-associated pseudomembranous colitis produced by *Clostridium difficile.* Other causes of colitis should also be considered.

PRECAUTIONS

Although ZINACEF rarely produces alterations in kidney function, evaluation of renal status during therapy is recommended, especially in seriously ill patients receiving the maximum doses. Cephalosporins should be given with caution to patients receiving concurrent treatment with potent diuretics as these regimens are suspected of adversely affecting renal function.

The total daily dose of ZINACEF should be reduced in patients with transient or persistent renal insufficiency (see DOSAGE AND ADMINISTRATION), because high and prolonged serum antibiotic concentrations can occur in such individuals from usual doses.

As with other antibiotics, prolonged use of ZINACEF may result in overgrowth of nonsusceptible organisms. Careful observation of the patient is essential. If superinfection occurs during therapy, appropriate measures should be taken.

Broad-spectrum antibiotics should be prescribed with caution in individuals with a history of gastrointestinal disease, particularly colitis.

Nephrotoxicity has been reported following concomitant administration of aminoglycoside antibiotics and cephalosporins.

As with other therapeutic regimens used in the treatment of meningitis, mild-to-moderate hearing loss has been reported in a few pediatric patients treated with cefuroxime. Persistence of positive CSF (cerebrospinal fluid) cultures at 18 to 36 hours has also been noted with cefuroxime injection, as well as with other antibiotic therapies; however, the clinical relevance of this is unknown.

Drug/Laboratory Test Interactions: A false-positive reaction for glucose in the urine may occur with copper reduction tests (Benedict's or Fehling's solution or with CLINITEST® tablets) but not with enzyme-based tests for glycosuria (e.g., TES-TAPE®). As a false-negative result may occur in the ferricyanide test, it is recommended that either the glucose oxidase or hexokinase method be used to determine blood plasma glucose levels in patients receiving ZINACEF.

Cefuroxime does not interfere with the assay of serum and urine creatinine by the alkaline picrate method.

Carcinogenesis, Mutagenesis, Impairment of Fertility: Although no long-term studies in animals have been performed to evaluate carcinogenic potential, no mutagenic potential of cefuroxime was found in standard laboratory tests.

Continued on next page

This product information is based on labeling in effect on June 23, 2000. For further information, contact via direct mail, phone, or web site. Medical Information, Glaxo Wellcome Inc., PO Box 13398, Research Triangle Park, NC 27709. Healthcare Professionals (Medical Information): 800-334-0089. Patients (Customer Response Center): 1-888-825-5249. Glaxo Wellcome Corporate Web Site: www.glaxowellcome.com

Zinacef—Cont.

Reproductive studies revealed no impairment of fertility in animals.

Pregnancy: ***Teratogenic Effects:*** Pregnancy Category B. Reproduction studies have been performed in mice and rabbits at doses up to 60 times the human dose and have revealed no evidence of impaired fertility or harm to the fetus due to cefuroxime. There are, however, no adequate and well-controlled studies in pregnant women. Because animal reproduction studies are not always predictive of human response, this drug should be used during pregnancy only if clearly needed.

Nursing Mothers: Since cefuroxime is excreted in human milk, caution should be exercised when ZINACEF is administered to a nursing woman.

Pediatric Use: Safety and effectiveness in pediatric patients below 3 months of age have not been established. Accumulation of other members of the cephalosporin class in newborn infants (with resulting prolongation of drug half-life) has been reported.

ADVERSE REACTIONS

ZINACEF is generally well tolerated. The most common adverse effects have been local reactions following IV administration. Other adverse reactions have been encountered only rarely.

Local Reactions: Thrombophlebitis has occurred with IV administration in 1 in 60 patients.

Gastrointestinal: Gastrointestinal symptoms occurred in 1 in 150 patients and included diarrhea (1 in 220 patients) and nausea (1 in 440 patients). The onset of pseudomembranous colitis may occur during or after antibacterial treatment (see WARNINGS).

Hypersensitivity Reactions: Hypersensitivity reactions have been reported in fewer than 1% of the patients treated with ZINACEF and include rash (1 in 125). Pruritus, urticaria, and positive Coombs' test each occurred in fewer than 1 in 250 patients, and, as with other cephalosporins, rare cases of anaphylaxis, drug fever, erythema multiforme, interstitial nephritis, toxic epidermal necrolysis, and Stevens-Johnson syndrome have occurred.

Blood: A decrease in hemoglobin and hematocrit has been observed in 1 in 10 patients and transient eosinophilia in 1 in 14 patients. Less common reactions seen were transient neutropenia (fewer than 1 in 100 patients) and leukopenia (1 in 750 patients). A similar pattern and incidence were seen with other cephalosporins used in controlled studies. As with other cephalosporins, there have been rare reports of thrombocytopenia.

Hepatic: Transient rise in SGOT and SGPT (1 in 25 patients), alkaline phosphatase (1 in 50 patients), LDH (1 in 75 patients), and bilirubin (1 in 500 patients) levels has been noted.

Kidney: Elevations in serum creatinine and/or blood urea nitrogen and a decreased creatinine clearance have been observed, but their relationship to cefuroxime is unknown.

Observed During Clinical Practice: In addition to adverse events reported from clinical trials, the following events have been identified during post-approval use of ZINACEF. Because they are reported voluntarily from a population of unknown size, estimates of frequency cannot be made. These events have been chosen for inclusion due to a combination of their seriousness, frequency of reporting, or potential causal connection to ZINACEF.

Neurologic: Seizure.

Non-site specific: Angioedema.

Cephalosporin-class Adverse Reactions: In addition to the adverse reactions listed above that have been observed in patients treated with cefuroxime, the following adverse reactions and altered laboratory tests have been reported for cephalosporin-class antibiotics:

Adverse Reactions: Vomiting, abdominal pain, colitis, vaginitis including vaginal candidiasis, toxic nephropathy, hepatic dysfunction including cholestasis, aplastic anemia, hemolytic anemia, hemorrhage.

Several cephalosporins have been implicated in triggering seizures, particularly in patients with renal impairment when the dosage was not reduced (see DOSAGE AND ADMINISTRATION). If seizures associated with drug therapy should occur, the drug should be discontinued. Anticonvulsant therapy can be given if clinically indicated.

Altered Laboratory Tests: Prolonged prothrombin time, pancytopenia, agranulocytosis.

OVERDOSAGE

Overdosage of cephalosporins can cause cerebral irritation leading to convulsions. Serum levels of cefuroxime can be reduced by hemodialysis and peritoneal dialysis.

DOSAGE AND ADMINISTRATION

Dosage: ***Adults:*** The usual adult dosage range for ZINACEF is 750 mg to 1.5 grams every 8 hours, usually for 5 to 10 days. In uncomplicated urinary tract infections, skin and skin-structure infections, disseminated gonococcal infections, and uncomplicated pneumonia, a 750-mg dose every 8 hours is recommended. In severe or complicated infections, a 1.5-gram dose every 8 hours is recommended.

In bone and joint infections, a 1.5-gram dose every 8 hours is recommended. In clinical trials, surgical intervention was performed when indicated as an adjunct to therapy with ZINACEF. A course of oral antibiotics was administered when appropriate following the completion of parenteral administration of ZINACEF.

In life-threatening infections or infections due to less susceptible organisms, 1.5 grams every 6 hours may be required. In bacterial meningitis, the dosage should not exceed 3 grams every 8 hours. The recommended dosage for uncomplicated gonococcal infection is 1.5 grams given intramuscularly as a single dose at two different sites together with 1 gram of oral probenecid. For preventive use for clean-contaminated or potentially contaminated surgical procedures, a 1.5-gram dose administered intravenously just before surgery (approximately one-half to 1 hour before the initial incision) is recommended. Thereafter, give 750 mg intravenously or intramuscularly every 8 hours when the procedure is prolonged.

For preventive use during open heart surgery, a 1.5-gram dose administered intravenously at the induction of anesthesia and every 12 hours thereafter for a total of 6 grams is recommended.

Impaired Renal Function: A reduced dosage must be employed when renal function is impaired. Dosage should be determined by the degree of renal impairment and the susceptibility of the causative organism (see Table 1).

Table 1: Dosage of ZINACEF in Adults With Reduced Renal Function

Creatinine Clearance (mL/min)	Dose	Frequency
>20	750 mg-1.5 grams	q8h
10–20	750 mg	q12h
<10	750 mg	q24h*

* Since ZINACEF is dialyzable, patients on hemodialysis should be given a further dose at the end of the dialysis.

When only serum creatinine is available, the following formula[2] (based on sex, weight, and age of the patient) may be used to convert this value into creatinine clearance. The serum creatinine should represent a steady state of renal function.

Males: $\text{Creatinine clearance (mL/min)} = \dfrac{\text{Weight (kg)} \times (140-\text{age})}{72 \times \text{serum creatinine (mg/dL)}}$

Females: $0.85 \times$ male value

Note: As with antibiotic therapy in general, administration of ZINACEF should be continued for a minimum of 48 to 72 hours after the patient becomes asymptomatic or after evidence of bacterial eradication has been obtained; a minimum of 10 days of treatment is recommended in infections caused by *Streptococcus pyogenes* in order to guard against the risk of rheumatic fever or glomerulonephritis; frequent bacteriologic and clinical appraisal is necessary during therapy of chronic urinary tract infection and may be required for several months after therapy has been completed; persistent infections may require treatment for several weeks; and doses smaller than those indicated above should not be used. In staphylococcal and other infections involving a collection of pus, surgical drainage should be carried out where indicated.

Pediatric Patients Above 3 Months of Age: Administration of 50 to 100 mg/kg per day in equally divided doses every 6 to 8 hours has been successful for most infections susceptible to cefuroxime. The higher dosage of 100 mg/kg per day (not to exceed the maximum adult dosage) should be used for the more severe or serious infections.

In bone and joint infections, 150 mg/kg per day (not to exceed the maximum adult dosage) is recommended in equally divided doses every 8 hours. In clinical trials, a course of oral antibiotics was administered to pediatric patients following the completion of parenteral administration of ZINACEF.

In cases of bacterial meningitis, a larger dosage of ZINACEF is recommended, 200 to 240 mg/kg per day intravenously in divided doses every 6 to 8 hours.

In pediatric patients with renal insufficiency, the frequency of dosing should be modified consistent with the recommendations for adults.

Preparation of Solution and Suspension: The directions for preparing ZINACEF for both IV and IM use are summarized in Table 2.

For Intramuscular Use: Each 750-mg vial of ZINACEF should be constituted with 3.0 mL of Sterile Water for Injection. Shake gently to disperse and withdraw completely the resulting suspension for injection.

For Intravenous Use: Each 750-mg vial should be constituted with 8.0 mL of Sterile Water for Injection. Withdraw completely the resulting solution for injection.

Each 1.5-gram vial should be constituted with 16.0 mL of Sterile Water for Injection, and the solution should be completely withdrawn for injection.

The 7.5-gram pharmacy bulk vial should be constituted with 77 mL of Sterile Water for Injection; each 8 mL of the resulting solution contains 750 mg of cefuroxime.

Each 750-mg and 1.5-gram infusion pack should be constituted with 100 mL of Sterile Water for Injection, 5% Dextrose Injection, 0.9% Sodium Chloride Injection, or any of the solutions listed under the Intravenous portion of the COMPATIBILITY AND STABILITY section.

[See table 2 below]

Administration: After constitution, ZINACEF may be given intravenously or by deep IM injection into a large muscle mass (such as the gluteus or lateral part of the thigh). Before injecting intramuscularly, aspiration is necessary to avoid inadvertent injection into a blood vessel.

Intravenous Administration: The IV route may be preferable for patients with bacterial septicemia or other severe or life-threatening infections or for patients who may be poor risks because of lowered resistance, particularly if shock is present or impending.

For direct intermittent IV administration, slowly inject the solution into a vein over a period of 3 to 5 minutes or give it through the tubing system by which the patient is also receiving other IV solutions.

For intermittent IV infusion with a Y-type administration set, dosing can be accomplished through the tubing system by which the patient may be receiving other IV solutions. However, during infusion of the solution containing ZINACEF, it is advisable to temporarily discontinue administration of any other solutions at the same site.

ADD-Vantage vials are to be constituted only with 50 or 100 mL of 5% Dextrose Injection, 0.9% Sodium Chloride Injection, or 0.45% Sodium Chloride Injection in Abbott ADD-Vantage flexible diluent containers (see Instructions for Constitution section of the product package insert). ADD-Vantage vials that have been joined to Abbott ADD-Vantage diluent containers and activated to dissolve the drug are stable for 24 hours at room temperature or for 7 days under refrigeration. Joined vials that have not been activated may be used within a 14-day period; this period corresponds to that for use of Abbott ADD-Vantage containers following removal of the outer packaging (overwrap). Freezing solutions of ZINACEF in the ADD-Vantage system is not recommended.

For continuous IV infusion, a solution of ZINACEF may be added to an IV infusion pack containing one of the following fluids: 0.9% Sodium Chloride Injection; 5% Dextrose Injection; 10% Dextrose Injection; 5% Dextrose and 0.9% Sodium Chloride Injection; 5% Dextrose and 0.45% Sodium Chloride Injection; or 1/6 M Sodium Lactate Injection.

Solutions of ZINACEF, like those of most beta-lactam antibiotics, should not be added to solutions of aminoglycoside antibiotics because of potential interaction.

However, if concurrent therapy with ZINACEF and an aminoglycoside is indicated, each of these antibiotics can be administered separately to the same patient.

Directions for Use of ZINACEF Frozen in GALAXY® Plastic Containers: ZINACEF supplied as a frozen, sterile, iso-osmotic, nonpyrogenic solution in plastic containers is to be administered after thawing either as a continuous or intermittent IV infusion. The thawed solution of the premixed product is stable for 28 days if stored under refrigeration (5° C) or for 24 hours if stored at room temperature (25° C). **Do not Refreeze.**

Thaw container at room temperature (25°C) or under refrigeration (5°C). Do not force thaw by immersion in water baths or by microwave irradiation. Components of the solution may precipitate in the frozen state and will dissolve upon reaching room temperature with little or no agitation. Potency is not affected. Mix after solution has reached room temperature. Check for minute leaks by squeezing bag firmly. Discard bag if leaks are found as sterility may be impaired. Do not add supplementary medication. Do not use unless solution is clear and seal is intact.

Use sterile equipment.

Caution: Do not use plastic containers in series connections. Such use could result in air embolism due to residual air being drawn from the primary container before administration of the fluid from the secondary container is complete.

Table 2: Preparation of Solution and Suspension

Strength	Amount of Diluent to Be Added (mL)	Volume to Be Withdrawn	Approximate Cefuroxime Concentration (mg/mL)
750-mg Vial	3.0 (IM)	Total*	220
750-mg Vial	8.0 (IV)	Total	90
1.5-gram Vial	16.0 (IV)	Total	90
750-mg Infusion pack	100 (IV)	—	7.5
1.5-gram Infusion pack	100 (IV)	—	15
7.5-gram Pharmacy bulk package	77 (IV)	Amount Needed†	95

***Note:** ZINACEF is a suspension at IM concentrations.

†8 mL of solution contains 750 mg of cefuroxime; 16 mL of solution contains 1.5 grams of cefuroxime.

Preparation for Administration:
1. Suspend container from eyelet support.
2. Remove protector from outlet port at bottom of container.
3. Attach administration set. Refer to complete directions accompanying set.

COMPATIBILITY AND STABILITY

Intramuscular: When constituted as directed with Sterile Water for Injection, suspensions of ZINACEF for IM injection maintain satisfactory potency for 24 hours at room temperature and for 48 hours under refrigeration (5°C).
After the periods mentioned above any unused suspensions should be discarded.

Intravenous: When the 750-mg, 1.5-g, and 7.5-g pharmacy bulk vials are constituted as directed with Sterile Water for Injection, the solutions of ZINACEF for IV administration maintain satisfactory potency for 24 hours at room temperature and for 48 hours (750-mg and 1.5-g vials) or for 7 days (7.5-g pharmacy bulk vial) under refrigeration (5°C). More dilute solutions, such as 750 mg or 1.5 g plus 100 mL of Sterile Water for Injection, 5% Dextrose Injection, or 0.9% Sodium Chloride Injection, also maintain satisfactory potency for 24 hours at room temperature and for 7 days under refrigeration.
These solutions may be further diluted to concentrations of between 1 and 30 mg/mL in the following solutions and will lose not more than 10% activity for 24 hours at room temperature or for at least 7 days under refrigeration: 0.9% Sodium Chloride Injection; 1/6 M Sodium Lactate Injection; Ringer's Injection, USP; Lactated Ringer's Injection, USP; 5% Dextrose and 0.9% Sodium Chloride Injection; 5% Dextrose Injection; 5% Dextrose and 0.45% Sodium Chloride Injection; 5% Dextrose and 0.225% Sodium Chloride Injection; 10% Dextrose Injection; and 10% Invert Sugar in Water for Injection.
Unused solutions should be discarded after the time periods mentioned above.
ZINACEF has also been found compatible for 24 hours at room temperature when admixed in IV infusion with heparin (10 and 50 U/mL) in 0.9% Sodium Chloride Injection and Potassium Chloride (10 and 40 mEq/L) in 0.9% Sodium Chloride Injection. Sodium Bicarbonate Injection, USP is not recommended for the dilution of ZINACEF.
The 750-mg and 1.5-g ZINACEF ADD-Vantage vials, when diluted in 50 or 100 mL of 5% Dextrose Injection, 0.9% Sodium Chloride Injection, or 0.45% Sodium Chloride Injection, may be stored for up to 24 hours at room temperature or for 7 days under refrigeration.

Frozen Stability: Constitute the 750-mg, 1.5-g, or 7.5-g vial as directed for IV administration in Table 2. Immediately withdraw the total contents of the 750-mg or 1.5-g vial or 8 or 16 mL from the 7.5-g bulk vial and add to a Baxter VIAFLEX® MINI-BAG™ containing 50 or 100 mL of 0.9% Sodium Chloride Injection or 5% Dextrose Injection and freeze. Frozen solutions are stable for 6 months when stored at −20°C. Frozen solutions should be thawed at room temperature and not refrozen. Do not force thaw by immersion in water baths or by microwave irradiation. Thawed solutions may be stored for up to 24 hours at room temperature or for 7 days in a refrigerator.

Note: Parenteral drug products should be inspected visually for particulate matter and discoloration before administration whenever solution and container permit.
As with other cephalosporins, ZINACEF powder as well as solutions and suspensions tend to darken, depending on storage conditions, without adversely affecting product potency.

Directions for Dispensing: *Pharmacy Bulk Package —Not for Direct Infusion:* The pharmacy bulk package is for use in a pharmacy admixture service only under a laminar flow hood. Entry into the vial must be made with a sterile transfer set or other sterile dispensing device, and the contents dispensed in aliquots using aseptic technique. The use of syringe and needle is not recommended as it may cause leakage (see DOSAGE AND ADMINISTRATION). AFTER INITIAL WITHDRAWAL USE ENTIRE CONTENTS OF VIAL PROMPTLY. ANY UNUSED PORTION MUST BE DISCARDED WITHIN 24 HOURS.

HOW SUPPLIED

ZINACEF in the dry state should be stored between 15° and 30°C (59° and 86°F) and protected from light. ZINACEF is a dry, white to off-white powder supplied in vials and infusion packs as follows:
NDC 0173-0352-31 750-mg* Vial (Tray of 25)
NDC 0173-0354-35 1.5-g* Vial (Tray of 25)
NDC 0173-0353-32 750-mg* Infusion Pack (Tray of 10)
NDC 0173-0356-32 1.5-g* Infusion Pack (Tray of 10)
NDC 0173-0400-00 7.5-g* Pharmacy Bulk Package (Tray of 6)
NDC 0173-0436-00 750-mg ADD-Vantage Vial (Tray of 25)
NDC 0173-0437-00 1.5-g ADD-Vantage Vial (Tray of 10)
(The above ADD-Vantage vials are to be used only with Abbott ADD-Vantage diluent containers.)
ZINACEF frozen as a premixed solution of cefuroxime injection should not be stored above −20° C. ZINACEF is supplied frozen in 50-mL, single-dose, plastic containers as follows:
NDC 0173-0424-00 750-mg* Plastic Container (Carton of 24)
NDC 0173-0425-00 1.5-g* Plastic Container (Carton of 24)
*Equivalent to cefuroxime.

REFERENCES

1. National Committee for Clinical Laboratory Standards. *Performance Standards for Antimicrobial Susceptibility Testing.* Third Informational Supplement. NCCLS Document M100-S3, Vol. 11, No. 17. Villanova, Pa: NCCLS; 1991.
2. Cockcroft DW, Gault MH. Prediction of creatinine clearance from serum creatinine. *Nephron.* 1976;16:31-41.

ZINACEF® (cefuroxime for injection):
Glaxo Wellcome Inc., Research Triangle Park, NC 27709
ZINACEF® (cefuroxime injection):
Manufactured for Glaxo Wellcome Inc.
Research Triangle Park, NC 27709
by Baxter Healthcare Corporation, Deerfield, IL 60015
ZINACEF is a registered trademark of Glaxo Wellcome.
ADD-Vantage is a registered trademark of Abbott Laboratories.
CLINITEST is a registered trademark of Ames Division, Miles Laboratories, Inc.
TES-TAPE is a registered trademark of Eli Lilly and Company.
GALAXY and VIAFLEX are registered trademarks of Baxter International Inc.
November 1998/RL-642

Shown in Product Identification Guide, page 317

ZOFRAN® ℞
[zō' fran]
(ondansetron hydrochloride)
Injection

ZOFRAN® ℞
(ondansetron hydrochloride)
Injection Premixed

DESCRIPTION

The active ingredient in ZOFRAN Injection and ZOFRAN Injection Premixed is ondansetron hydrochloride (HCl), the racemic form of ondansetron and a selective blocking agent of the serotonin 5-HT_3 receptor type. Chemically it is (±) 1, 2, 3, 9-tetrahydro-9-methyl-3-[(2-methyl-1H-imidazol-1-yl) methyl]-4H-carbazol-4-one, monohydrochloride, dihydrate.
The empirical formula is $C_{18}H_{19}N_3O \bullet HCl \bullet 2H_2O$, representing a molecular weight of 365.9.
Ondansetron HCl is a white to off-white powder that is soluble in water and normal saline.

Sterile Injection for Intravenous (I.V.) or Intramuscular (I.M.) Administration: Each 1 mL of aqueous solution in the 2-mL single-dose vial contains 2 mg of ondansetron as the hydrochloride dihydrate; 9.0 mg of sodium chloride, USP; and 0.5 mg of citric acid monohydrate, USP and 0.25 mg of sodium citrate dihydrate, USP as buffers in Water for Injection, USP.
Each 1 mL of aqueous solution in the 20-mL multidose vial contains 2 mg of ondansetron as the hydrochloride dihydrate; 8.3 mg of sodium chloride, USP; 0.5 mg of citric acid monohydrate, USP and 0.25 mg of sodium citrate dihydrate, USP as buffers; and 1.2 mg of methylparaben, NF and 0.15 mg of propylparaben, NF as preservatives in Water for Injection, USP.
ZOFRAN Injection is a clear, colorless, nonpyrogenic, sterile solution. The pH of the injection solution is 3.3 to 4.0.

Sterile, Premixed Solution for Intravenous Administration in Single-Dose, Flexible Plastic Containers: Each 50 mL contains ondansetron 32 mg (as the hydrochloride dihydrate); dextrose 2500 mg; and citric acid 26 mg and sodium citrate 11.5 mg as buffers in Water for Injection, USP. It contains no preservatives. The osmolarity of this solution is 270 mOsm/L (approx.), and the pH is 3.0 to 4.0.
The flexible plastic container is fabricated from a specially formulated, nonplasticized, thermoplastic co-polyester (CR3). Water can permeate from inside the container into the overwrap but not in amounts sufficient to affect the solution significantly. Solutions inside the plastic container also can leach out certain of the chemical components in very small amounts before the expiration period is attained. However, the safety of the plastic has been confirmed by tests in animals according to USP biological standards for plastic containers.

CLINICAL PHARMACOLOGY

Pharmacodynamics: Ondansetron is a selective 5-HT_3 receptor antagonist. While ondansetron's mechanism of action has not been fully characterized, it is not a dopamine-receptor antagonist. Serotonin receptors of the 5-HT_3 type are present both peripherally on vagal nerve terminals and centrally in the chemoreceptor trigger zone of the area postrema. It is not certain whether ondansetron's antiemetic action in chemotherapy-induced emesis is mediated centrally, peripherally, or in both sites. However, cytotoxic chemotherapy appears to be associated with release of serotonin from the enterochromaffin cells of the small intestine. In humans, urinary 5-HIAA (5-hydroxyindoleacetic acid) excretion increases after cisplatin administration in parallel with the onset of emesis. The released serotonin may stimulate the vagal afferents through the 5-HT_3 receptors and initiate the vomiting reflex.
In animals, the emetic response to cisplatin can be prevented by pretreatment with an inhibitor of serotonin synthesis, bilateral abdominal vagotomy and greater splanchnic nerve section, or pretreatment with a serotonin 5-HT_3 receptor antagonist.
In normal volunteers, single I.V. doses of 0.15 mg/kg of ondansetron had no effect on esophageal motility, gastric motility, lower esophageal sphincter pressure, or small intestinal transit time. In another study in six normal male volunteers, a 16-mg dose infused over 5 minutes showed no effect of the drug on cardiac output, heart rate, stroke volume, blood pressure, or electrocardiogram (ECG). Multiday administration of ondansetron has been shown to slow colonic transit in normal volunteers. Ondansetron has no effect on plasma prolactin concentrations.
In a gender-balanced pharmacodynamic study (n = 56), ondansetron 4 mg administered intravenously or intramuscularly was dynamically similar in the prevention of emesis and nausea using the ipecacuanha model of emesis. Both treatments were well tolerated.
Ondansetron does not alter the respiratory depressant effects produced by alfentanil or the degree of neuromuscular blockade produced by atracurium. Interactions with general or local anesthetics have not been studied.

Pharmacokinetics: Ondansetron is extensively metabolized in humans, with approximately 5% of a radiolabeled dose recovered as the parent compound from the urine. The primary metabolic pathway is hydroxylation on the indole ring followed by glucuronide or sulfate conjugation.
Although some nonconjugated metabolites have pharmacologic activity, these are not found in plasma at concentrations likely to significantly contribute to the biological activity of ondansetron.
Ondansetron is a substrate for human hepatic cytochrome P-450 enzymes, including CYP1A2, CYP2D6, and CYP3A4. Because of the multiplicity of metabolic enzymes capable of metabolizing ondansetron, inhibition or loss of one enzyme (e.g., CYP2D6 genetic deficiency) results in little change in overall rates of ondansetron elimination.
In normal volunteers, the following mean pharmacokinetic data have been determined following a single 0.15-mg/kg I.V. dose.

Table 1: Pharmacokinetics in Normal Volunteers

Age-group	n	Peak Plasma Concentration (ng/mL)	Mean Elimination Half-life (h)	Plasma Clearance (L/h/kg)
19-40	11	102	3.5	0.381
61-74	12	106	4.7	0.319
≥75	11	170	5.5	0.262

A reduction in clearance and increase in elimination half-life are seen in patients over 75 years of age. In clinical trials with cancer patients, safety and efficacy were similar in patients over 65 years of age and those under 65 years of age; there was an insufficient number of patients over 75 years of age to permit conclusions in that age-group. No dosage adjustment is recommended in the elderly.
In patients with mild-to-moderate hepatic impairment, clearance is reduced twofold and mean half-life is increased to 11.6 hours compared to 5.7 hours in normals. In patients with severe hepatic impairment (Child-Pugh score[1] of 10 or greater), clearance is reduced twofold to threefold and apparent volume of distribution is increased with a resultant increase in half-life to 20 hours and bioavailability approaching 100%. In such patients, a total daily dose of 8 mg should not be exceeded.
Ondansetron plasma clearance was reduced by 41% (95% Cl 20% to 57%) in patients with severe renal impairment (creatinine clearance <30 mL/min). This reduction in clearance is variable and was not consistent with an increase in half-life. No reduction in dose or dosing frequency in these patients is warranted.
In adult cancer patients, the mean elimination half-life was 4.0 hours, and there was no difference in the multidose pharmacokinetics over a 4-day period. In a study of 21 pediatric cancer patients (aged 4 to 18 years) who received three I.V. doses of 0.15 mg/kg of ondansetron at 4-hour intervals, patients older than 15 years of age exhibited ondansetron pharmacokinetic parameters similar to those of adults. Patients aged 4 to 12 years generally showed higher clearance and somewhat larger volume of distribution than adults. Most pediatric patients younger than 15 years of age with cancer had a shorter (2.4 hours) ondansetron plasma half-life than patients older than 15 years of age. It is not known whether these differences in ondansetron plasma half-life may result in differences in efficacy between adults and some young pediatric patients (see CLINICAL TRIALS: Pediatric Studies).
In a study of 21 pediatric patients (aged 3 to 12 years) who were undergoing surgery requiring anesthesia for a duration of 45 minutes to 2 hours, a single I.V. dose of ondansetron, 2 mg (3 to 7 years) or 4 mg (8 to 12 years), was administered immediately prior to anesthesia induction. Mean weight-normalized clearance and volume of distribution values in these pediatric surgical patients were similar to those previously reported for young adults. Mean termi-

Continued on next page

This product information is based on labeling in effect on June 23, 2000. For further information, contact via direct mail, phone, or web site. Medical Information, Glaxo Wellcome Inc., PO Box 13398, Research Triangle Park, NC 27709. Healthcare Professionals (Medical Information): 800-334-0089. Patients (Customer Response Center): 1-888-825-5249. Glaxo Wellcome Corporate Web Site: www.glaxowellcome.com

Zofran Inj.—Cont.

nal half-life was slightly reduced in pediatric patients (range, 2.5 to 3 hours) in comparison with adults (range, 3 to 3.5 hours).

In normal volunteers (19 to 39 years old, n = 23), the peak plasma concentration was 264 ng/mL following a single 32-mg dose administered as a 15-minute I.V. infusion. The mean elimination half-life was 4.1 hours. Systemic exposure to 32 mg of ondansetron was not proportional to dose as measured by comparing dose-normalized AUC values to an 8-mg dose. This is consistent with a small decrease in systemic clearance with increasing plasma concentrations.

A study was performed in normal volunteers (n = 56) to evaluate the pharmacokinetics of a single 4-mg dose administered as a 5-minute infusion compared to a single intramuscular injection. Systemic exposure as measured by mean AUC was equivalent, with values of 156 [95% CI 136, 180] and 161 [95% CI 137, 190] ng•h/mL for I.V. and I.M. groups, respectively. Mean peak plasma concentrations were 42.9 [95% CI 33.8, 54.4] ng/mL at 10 minutes after I.V. infusion and 31.9 [95% CI 26.3, 38.6] ng/mL at 41 minutes after I.M. injection. The mean elimination half-life was not affected by route of administration.

Plasma protein binding of ondansetron as measured in vitro was 70% to 76%, with binding constant over the pharmacologic concentration range (10 to 500 ng/mL). Circulating drug also distributes into erythrocytes.

A positive lymphoblast transformation test to ondansetron has been reported, which suggests immunologic sensitivity to ondansetron.

CLINICAL TRIALS

Chemotherapy-Induced Nausea and Vomiting: In a double-blind study of three different dosing regimens of ZOFRAN Injection, 0.015 mg/kg, 0.15 mg/kg, and 0.30 mg/kg, each given three times during the course of cancer chemotherapy, the 0.15-mg/kg dosing regimen was more effective than the 0.015-mg/kg dosing regimen. The 0.30-mg/kg dosing regimen was not shown to be more effective than the 0.15-mg/kg dosing regimen.

Cisplatin-Based Chemotherapy: In a double-blind study in 28 patients, ZOFRAN Injection (three 0.15-mg/kg doses) was significantly more effective than placebo in preventing nausea and vomiting induced by cisplatin-based chemotherapy. Treatment response was as follows:

[See table 2 below]

Ondansetron was compared with metoclopramide in a single-blind trial in 307 patients receiving cisplatin ≥100 mg/m^2 with or without other chemotherapeutic agents. Patients received the first dose of ondansetron or metoclopramide 30 minutes before cisplatin. Two additional ondansetron doses were administered 4 and 8 hours later, or five additional metoclopramide doses were administered 2, 4, 7, 10, and 13 hours later. Cisplatin was administered over a period of 3 hours or less. Episodes of vomiting and retching were tabulated over the period of 24 hours after cisplatin. The results of this study are summarized below:

[See table 3 on next page]

In a stratified, randomized, double-blind, parallel-group, multicenter study, a single 32-mg dose of ondansetron was compared with three 0.15-mg/kg doses in patients receiving cisplatin doses of either 50 to 70 mg/m^2 or ≥100 mg/m^2. Patients received the first ondansetron dose 30 minutes before cisplatin. Two additional ondansetron doses were administered 4 and 8 hours later to the group receiving three 0.15-mg/kg doses. In both strata, significantly fewer patients on the single 32-mg dose than those receiving the three-dose regimen failed.

[See table 4 on next page]

Cyclophosphamide-Based Chemotherapy: In a double-blind, placebo-controlled study of ZOFRAN Injection (three 0.15-mg/kg doses) in 20 patients receiving cyclophosphamide (500 to 600 mg/m^2) chemotherapy, ZOFRAN Injection was significantly more effective than placebo in preventing nausea and vomiting. The results are summarized below:

[See table 5 on next page]

Re-treatment: In uncontrolled trials, 127 patients receiving cisplatin (median dose, 100 mg/m^2) and ondansetron who had two or fewer emetic episodes were re-treated with ondansetron and chemotherapy, mainly cisplatin, for a total of 269 re-treatment courses (median, 2; range, 1 to 10). No emetic episodes occurred in 160 (59%), and two or fewer emetic episodes occurred in 217 (81%) re-treatment courses.

Pediatric Studies: Four open-label, noncomparative (one US, three foreign) trials have been performed with 209 pediatric cancer patients aged 4 to 18 years given a variety of cisplatin or noncisplatin regimens. In the three foreign trials, the initial ZOFRAN Injection dose ranged from 0.04 to 0.87 mg/kg for a total dose of 2.16 to 12 mg. This was followed by the oral administration of ondansetron ranging from 4 to 24 mg daily for 3 days. In the US trial, ZOFRAN was administered intravenously (only) in three doses of 0.15 mg/kg each for a total daily dose of 7.2 to 39 mg. In these studies, 58% of the 196 evaluable patients had a complete response (no emetic episodes) on day 1. Thus, prevention of emesis in these pediatric patients was essentially the same as for patients older than 18 years of age. Overall, ZOFRAN Injection was well tolerated in these pediatric patients.

Postoperative Nausea and Vomiting: ***Prevention of Postoperative Nausea and Vomiting:*** Adult surgical patients who received ondansetron immediately before the induction of general balanced anesthesia (barbiturate: thiopental, methohexital, or thiamylal; opioid: alfentanil or fentanyl; nitrous oxide; neuromuscular blockade: succinylcholine/curare and/or vecuronium or atracurium; and supplemental isoflurane) were evaluated in two double-blind US studies involving 554 patients. ZOFRAN Injection (4 mg) I.V. given over 2 to 5 minutes was significantly more effective than placebo. The results of these studies are summarized below:

[See table 6 at top of page 1506]

The study populations in Table 6 consisted mainly of females undergoing laparoscopic procedures.

In a placebo-controlled study conducted in 468 males undergoing outpatient procedures, a single 4 mg I.V. ondansetron dose prevented postoperative vomiting over a 24-hour study period in 79% of males receiving drug compared to 63% of males receiving placebo (P<0.001).

Two other placebo-controlled studies were conducted in 2792 patients undergoing major abdominal or gynecological surgeries to evaluate a single 4-mg or 8-mg I.V. ondansetron dose for prevention of postoperative nausea and vomiting over a 24-hour study period. At the 4-mg dosage, 59% of patients receiving ondansetron versus 45% receiving placebo in the first study (P<0.001) and 41% of patients receiving ondansetron versus 30% receiving placebo in the second study (P=0.001) experienced no emetic episodes. No additional benefit was observed in patients who received I.V. ondansetron 8 mg compared to patients who received I.V. ondansetron 4 mg.

Pediatric Studies: Three double-blind, placebo-controlled studies have been performed (one US, two foreign) in 1049 male and female patients (2 to 12 years of age) undergoing general anesthesia with nitrous oxide. The surgical procedures included tonsillectomy with or without adenoidectomy, strabismus surgery, herniorrhaphy, and orchidopexy. Patients were randomized to either single I.V. doses of ondansetron (0.1 mg/kg for pediatric patients weighing 40 kg or less, 4 mg for pediatric patients weighing more than 40 kg) or placebo. Study drug was administered over at least 30 seconds, immediately prior to or following anesthesia induction. Ondansetron was significantly more effective than placebo in preventing nausea and vomiting. The results of these studies are summarized below:

[See table 7 on page 1506]

Prevention of Further Postoperative Nausea and Vomiting: Adult surgical patients receiving general balanced anesthesia (barbiturate: thiopental, methohexital, or thiamylal; opioid: alfentanil or fentanyl; nitrous oxide; neuromuscular blockade: succinylcholine/curare and/or vecuronium or atracurium; and supplemental isoflurane) who received no prophylactic antiemetics and who experienced nausea and/or vomiting within 2 hours postoperatively were evaluated in two double-blind US studies involving 441 patients. Patients who experienced an episode of postoperative nausea and/or vomiting were given ZOFRAN Injection (4 mg) I.V. over 2 to 5 minutes, and this was significantly more effective than placebo. The results of these studies are summarized below:

[See table 8 on page 1506]

The study populations in Table 8 consisted mainly of women undergoing laparoscopic procedures.

Pediatric Studies: One double-blind, placebo-controlled, US study was performed in 351 male and female outpatients (2 to 12 years of age) who received general anesthesia with nitrous oxide and no prophylactic antiemetics. Surgical procedures were unrestricted. Patients who experienced two or more emetic episodes within 2 hours following discontinuation of nitrous oxide were randomized to either single I.V. doses of ondansetron (0.1 mg/kg for pediatric patients weighing 40 kg or less, 4 mg for pediatric patients weighing more than 40 kg) or placebo administered over at least 30 seconds. Ondansetron was significantly more effective than placebo in preventing further episodes of nausea and vomiting. The results of the study are summarized below:

[See table 9 at top of page 1507]

Repeat Dosing in Adults: In patients who do not achieve adequate control of postoperative nausea and vomiting following a single, prophylactic, preinduction, I.V. dose of ondansetron 4 mg, administration of a second I.V. dose of ondansetron 4 mg postoperatively does not provide additional control of nausea and vomiting.

INDICATIONS AND USAGE

1. Prevention of nausea and vomiting associated with initial and repeat courses of emetogenic cancer chemotherapy, including high-dose cisplatin. Efficacy of the 32-mg single dose beyond 24 hours in these patients has not been established.
2. Prevention of postoperative nausea and/or vomiting. As with other antiemetics, routine prophylaxis is not recommended for patients in whom there is little expectation that nausea and/or vomiting will occur postoperatively. In patients where nausea and/or vomiting must be avoided postoperatively, ZOFRAN Injection is recommended even where the incidence of postoperative nausea and/or vomiting is low. For patients who do not receive prophylactic ZOFRAN Injection and experience nausea and/or vomiting postoperatively, ZOFRAN Injection may be given to prevent further episodes (see CLINICAL TRIALS).

CONTRAINDICATIONS

ZOFRAN Injection and ZOFRAN Injection Premixed are contraindicated for patients known to have hypersensitivity to the drug.

WARNINGS

Hypersensitivity reactions have been reported in patients who have exhibited hypersensitivity to other selective 5-HT_3 receptor antagonists.

PRECAUTIONS

Ondansetron is not a drug that stimulates gastric or intestinal peristalsis. It should not be used instead of nasogastric suction. The use of ondansetron in patients following abdominal surgery or in patients with chemotherapy-induced nausea and vomiting may mask a progressive ileus and/or gastric distention.

Drug Interactions: Ondansetron does not itself appear to induce or inhibit the cytochrome P-450 drug-metabolizing enzyme system of the liver. Because ondansetron is metabolized by hepatic cytochrome P-450 drug-metabolizing enzymes, inducers or inhibitors of these enzymes may change the clearance and, hence, the half-life of ondansetron. On the basis of limited available data, no dosage adjustment is recommended for patients on these drugs. Tumor response to chemotherapy in the P 388 mouse leukemia model is not affected by ondansetron. In humans, carmustine, etoposide, and cisplatin do not affect the pharmacokinetics of ondansetron.

Ondansetron has no effect on the pharmacokinetics of high-dose methotrexate.

Carcinogenesis, Mutagenesis, Impairment of Fertility: Carcinogenic effects were not seen in 2-year studies in rats and mice with oral ondansetron doses up to 10 and 30 mg/kg per day, respectively. Ondansetron was not mutagenic in standard tests for mutagenicity. Oral administration of ondansetron up to 15 mg/kg per day did not affect fertility or general reproductive performance of male and female rats.

Pregnancy: ***Teratogenic Effects:*** Pregnancy Category B. Reproduction studies have been performed in pregnant rats and rabbits at I.V. doses up to 4 mg/kg per day and have revealed no evidence of impaired fertility or harm to the fetus due to ondansetron. There are, however, no adequate and well-controlled studies in pregnant women. Because animal reproduction studies are not always predictive of human response, this drug should be used during pregnancy only if clearly needed.

Table 2: Prevention of Chemotherapy-Induced Nausea and Emesis in Single-Day Cisplatin Therapy*

	ZOFRAN Injection	Placebo	P Value†
Number of patients	14	14	
Treatment response			
0 Emetic episodes	2 (14%)	0 (0%)	
1–2 Emetic episodes	8 (57%)	0 (0%)	
3–5 Emetic episodes	2 (14%)	1 (7%)	
More than 5 emetic episodes/rescued	2 (14%)	13 (93%)	0.001
Median number of emetic episodes	1.5	Undefined‡	
Median time to first emetic episode (h)	11.6	2.8	0.001
Median nausea scores (0–100)§	3	59	0.034
Global satisfaction with control of nausea and vomiting (0–100)ǁ	96	10.5	0.009

* Chemotherapy was high dose (100 and 120 mg/m^2; ZOFRAN Injection n = 6, placebo n = 5) or moderate dose (50 and 80 mg/m^2; ZOFRAN Injection n = 8, placebo n = 9). Other chemotherapeutic agents included fluorouracil, doxorubicin, and cyclophosphamide. There was no difference between treatments in the types of chemotherapy that would account for differences in response.

† Efficacy based on "all patients treated" analysis.

‡ Median undefined since at least 50% of the patients were rescued or had more than five emetic episodes.

§ Visual analog scale assessment of nausea: 0 = no nausea, 100 = nausea as bad as it can be.

ǁ Visual analog scale assessment of satisfaction: 0 = not at all satisfied, 100 = totally satisfied.

Nursing Mothers: Ondansetron is excreted in the breast milk of rats. It is not known whether ondansetron is excreted in human milk. Because many drugs are excreted in human milk, caution should be exercised when ondansetron is administered to a nursing woman.

Pediatric Use: Little information is available about dosage in pediatric patients under 2 years of age (see DOSAGE AND ADMINISTRATION section for use in pediatric patients 4 to 18 years of age receiving cancer chemotherapy or for use in pediatric patients 2 to 12 years of age receiving general anesthesia).

Geriatric Use: Of the total number of subjects enrolled in cancer chemotherapy-induced and postoperative nausea and vomiting in US- and foreign-controlled clinical trials, 862 were 65 years of age and over. No overall differences in safety or effectiveness were observed between these subjects and younger subjects, and other reported clinical experience has not identified differences in responses between the elderly and younger patients, but greater sensitivity of some older individuals cannot be ruled out. Dosage adjustment is not needed in patients over the age of 65 (see CLINICAL PHARMACOLOGY).

Table 3: Prevention of Emesis Induced by Cisplatin (≥100 mg/m²) Single-Day Therapy*

	ZOFRAN Injection	Metoclopramide	*P* Value
Dose	0.15 mg/kg × 3	2 mg/kg × 6	
Number of patients in efficacy population	136	138	
Treatment response			
0 Emetic episodes	54 (40%)	41 (30%)	
1–2 Emetic episodes	34 (25%)	30 (22%)	
3–5 Emetic episodes	19 (14%)	18 (13%)	
More than 5 emetic episodes/rescued	29 (21%)	49 (36%)	
Comparison of treatments with respect to			
0 Emetic episodes	54/136	41/138	0.083
More than 5 emetic episodes/rescued	29/136	49/138	0.009
Median number of emetic episodes	1	2	0.005
Median time to first emetic episode (h)	20.5	4.3	<0.001
Global satisfaction with control of nausea and vomiting (0–100)†	85	63	0.001
Acute dystonic reactions	0	8	0.005
Akathisia	0	10	0.002

*In addition to cisplatin, 68% of patients received other chemotherapeutic agents, including cyclophosphamide, etoposide, and fluorouracil. There was no difference between treatments in the types of chemotherapy that would account for differences in response.
†Visual analog scale assessment: 0 = not at all satisfied, 100 = totally satisfied.

Table 4: Prevention of Chemotherapy-Induced Nausea and Emesis in Single-Dose Therapy

	Ondansetron Dose		
	0.15 mg/kg x 3	32 mg x 1	*P* Value
High-dose cisplatin (≥100 mg/m²)			
Number of patients	100	102	
Treatment response			
0 Emetic episodes	41 (41%)	49 (48%)	0.315
1–2 Emetic episodes	19 (19%)	25 (25%)	
3–5 Emetic episodes	4 (4%)	8 (8%)	
More than 5 emetic episodes/rescued	36 (36%)	20 (20%)	0.009
Median time to first emetic episode (h)	21.7	23	0.173
Median nausea scores (0–100)*	28	13	0.004
Medium-dose cisplatin (50–70 mg/m²)			
Number of patients	101	93	
Treatment response			
0 Emetic episodes	62 (61%)	68 (73%)	0.083
1–2 Emetic episodes	11 (11%)	14 (15%)	
3–5 Emetic episodes	6 (6%)	3 (3%)	
More than 5 emetic episodes/rescued	22 (22%)	8 (9%)	0.011
Median time to first emetic episode (h)	Undefined†	Undefined	
Median nausea scores (0–100)*	9	3	0.131

*Visual analog scale assessment: 0 = no nausea, 100 = nausea as bad as it can be.
†Median undefined since at least 50% of patients did not have any emetic episodes.

Table 5: Prevention of Chemotherapy-Induced Nausea and Emesis in Single-Day Cyclophosphamide Therapy*

	ZOFRAN Injection	Placebo	*P* Value†
Number of patients	10	10	
Treatment response			
0 Emetic episodes	7 (70%)	0 (0%)	0.001
1–2 Emetic episodes	0 (0%)	2 (20%)	
3–5 Emetic episodes	2 (20%)	4 (40%)	
More than 5 emetic episodes/rescued	1 (10%)	4 (40%)	0.131
Median number of emetic episodes	0	4	0.008
Median time to first emetic episode (h)	Undefined‡	8.79	
Median nausea scores (0–100)§	0	60	0.001
Global satisfaction with control of nausea and vomiting (0–100)‖	100	52	0.008

*Chemotherapy consisted of cyclophosphamide in all patients, plus other agents, including fluorouracil, doxorubicin, methotrexate, and vincristine. There was no difference between treatments in the type of chemotherapy that would account for differences in response.
†Efficacy based on "all patients treated" analysis.
‡Median undefined since at least 50% of patients did not have any emetic episodes.
§Visual analog scale assessment of nausea: 0 = no nausea, 100 = nausea as bad as it can be.
‖Visual analog scale assessment of satisfaction: 0 = not at all satisfied, 100 = totally satisfied.

ADVERSE REACTIONS

Chemotherapy-Induced Nausea and Vomiting: The following adverse events have been reported in individuals receiving ondansetron at a dosage of three 0.15-mg/kg doses or as a single 32-mg dose in clinical trials. These patients were receiving concomitant chemotherapy, primarily cisplatin, and I.V. fluids. Most were receiving a diuretic.
[See table 10 on page 1507]
The following have been reported during controlled clinical trials:

Cardiovascular: Rare cases of angina (chest pain), electrocardiographic alterations, hypotension, and tachycardia have been reported. In many cases, the relationship to ZOFRAN Injection was unclear.

Gastrointestinal: Constipation has been reported in 11% of chemotherapy patients receiving multiday ondansetron.

Hepatic: In comparative trials in cisplatin chemotherapy patients with normal baseline values of aspartate transaminase (AST) and alanine transaminase (ALT), these enzymes have been reported to exceed twice the upper limit of normal in approximately 5% of patients. The increases were transient and did not appear to be related to dose or duration of therapy. On repeat exposure, similar transient elevations in transaminase values occurred in some courses, but symptomatic hepatic disease did not occur.

Integumentary: Rash has occurred in approximately 1% of patients receiving ondansetron.

Neurological: There have been rare reports consistent with, but not diagnostic of, extrapyramidal reactions in patients receiving ZOFRAN Injection, and rare cases of grand mal seizure. The relationship to ZOFRAN was unclear.

Other: Rare cases of hypokalemia have been reported. The relationship to ZOFRAN Injection was unclear.

Postoperative Nausea and Vomiting: The following adverse events have been reported in ≥2% of adults receiving ondansetron at a dosage of 4 mg I.V. over 2 to 5 minutes in clinical trials. Rates of these events were not significantly different in the ondansetron and placebo groups. These patients were receiving multiple concomitant perioperative and postoperative medications.
[See table 11 on page 1507]

Pediatric Use: The following were the most commonly reported adverse events in pediatric patients receiving ondansetron (a single 0.1-mg/kg dose for pediatric patients weighing 40 kg or less, or 4 mg for pediatric patients weighing more than 40 kg) administered intravenously over at least 30 seconds. Rates of these events were not significantly different in the ondansetron and placebo groups. These patients were receiving multiple concomitant perioperative and postoperative medications.
[See table 12 on page 1507]

Observed During Clinical Practice: In addition to adverse events reported from clinical trials, the following events have been identified during post-approval use of intravenous formulations of ZOFRAN. Because they are reported voluntarily from a population of unknown size, estimates of frequency cannot be made. The events have been chosen for inclusion due to a combination of their seriousness, frequency of reporting, or potential causal connection to ZOFRAN.

Cardiovascular: Arrhythmias (including ventricular and supraventricular tachycardia, premature ventricular contractions, and atrial fibrillation), bradycardia, electrocardiographic alterations (including second degree heart block and ST segment depression), palpitations, and syncope.

General: Flushing. Rare cases of hypersensitivity reactions, sometimes severe (e.g., anaphylaxis/anaphylactoid reactions, angioedema, bronchospasm, cardiopulmonary arrest, hypotension, laryngeal edema, laryngospasm, shock, shortness of breath, stridor) have also been reported.

Hepatobiliary: Liver enzyme abnormalities have been reported. Liver failure and death have been reported in patients with cancer receiving concurrent medications including potentially hepatotoxic cytotoxic chemotherapy and antibiotics. The etiology of the liver failure is unclear.

Local Reactions: Pain, redness, and burning at site of injection.

Lower Respiratory: Hiccups

Neurological: Oculogyric crisis, appearing alone, as well as with other dystonic reactions.

Continued on next page

This product information is based on labeling in effect on June 23, 2000. For further information, contact via direct mail, phone, or web site. Medical Information, Glaxo Wellcome Inc., PO Box 13398, Research Triangle Park, NC 27709. Healthcare Professionals (Medical Information): 800-334-0089. Patients (Customer Response Center): 1-888-825-5249. Glaxo Wellcome Corporate Web Site: www.glaxowellcome.com

Zofran Inj.—Cont.

Skin: Urticaria
Special Senses: Transient blurred vision, in some cases associated with abnormalities of accommodation, and transient dizziness during or shortly after I.V. infusion.

DRUG ABUSE AND DEPENDENCE

Animal studies have shown that ondansetron is not discriminated as a benzodiazepine nor does it substitute for benzodiazepines in direct addiction studies.

OVERDOSAGE

There is no specific antidote for ondansetron overdose. Patients should be managed with appropriate supportive therapy. Individual doses as large as 150 mg and total daily dosages (three doses) as large as 252 mg have been administered intravenously without significant adverse events. These doses are more than 10 times the recommended daily dose.

In addition to the adverse events listed above, the following events have been described in the setting of ondansetron overdose: "Sudden blindness" (amaurosis) of 2 to 3 minutes' duration plus severe constipation occurred in one patient that was administered 72 mg of ondansetron intravenously as a single dose. Hypotension (and faintness) occurred in another patient that took 48 mg of oral ondansetron. Following infusion of 32 mg over only a 4-minute period, a vasovagal episode with transient second-degree heart block was observed. In all instances, the events resolved completely.

DOSAGE AND ADMINISTRATION

Prevention of Chemotherapy-Induced Nausea and Vomiting: The recommended I.V. dosage of ZOFRAN is a single 32-mg dose or three 0.15-mg/kg doses. A single 32-mg dose is infused over 15 minutes beginning 30 minutes before the start of emetogenic chemotherapy. The recommended infusion rate should not be exceeded (see OVERDOSAGE). With the three-dose (0.15-mg/kg) regimen, the first dose is infused over 15 minutes beginning 30 minutes before the start of emetogenic chemotherapy. Subsequent doses (0.15 mg/kg) are administered 4 and 8 hours after the first dose of ZOFRAN.

ZOFRAN Injection should not be mixed with solutions for which physical and chemical compatibility have not been established. In particular, this applies to alkaline solutions as a precipitate may form.

Vial: **DILUTE BEFORE USE.** ZOFRAN Injection should be diluted in 50 mL of 5% Dextrose Injection or 0.9% Sodium Chloride Injection before administration.

Flexible Plastic Container: ZOFRAN Injection Premixed, 32 mg in 5% Dextrose, 50 mL, **REQUIRES NO DILUTION.**

Pediatric Use: On the basis of the limited available information (see CLINICAL TRIALS: Pediatric Studies and CLINICAL PHARMACOLOGY: Pharmacokinetics), the dosage in pediatric patients 4 to 18 years of age should be three 0.15-mg/kg doses (see above). Little information is available about dosage in pediatric patients 3 years of age and younger.

Geriatric Use: The dosage recommendation is the same as for the general population.

Prevention of Postoperative Nausea and Vomiting: The recommended I.V. dosage of ZOFRAN for adults is 4 mg **undiluted** administered intravenously in not less than 30 seconds, preferably over 2 to 5 minutes, immediately before induction of anesthesia, or postoperatively if the patient experiences nausea and/or vomiting occurring shortly after surgery. Alternatively, 4 mg **undiluted** may be administered intramuscularly as a single injection for adults. While recommended as a fixed dose for patients weighing more than 40 kg, few patients above 80 kg have been studied. In patients who do not achieve adequate control of postoperative nausea and vomiting following a single, prophylactic, preinduction, I.V. dose of ondansetron 4 mg, administration of a second I.V. dose of 4 mg ondansetron postoperatively does not provide additional control of nausea and vomiting.

Vial: ZOFRAN Injection **REQUIRES NO DILUTION FOR ADMINISTRATION FOR POSTOPERATIVE NAUSEA AND VOMITING.**

Pediatric Use: The recommended I.V. dosage of ZOFRAN for pediatric patients (2 to 12 years of age) is a single 0.1-mg/kg dose for pediatric patients weighing 40 kg or less, or a single 4-mg dose for pediatric patients weighing more than 40 kg. The rate of administration should not be less than 30 seconds, preferably over 2 to 5 minutes. Little information is available about dosage in pediatric patients younger than 2 years of age.

Geriatric Use: The dosage recommendation is the same as for the general population.

Dosage Adjustment for Patients With Impaired Renal Function: The dosage recommendation is the same as for the general population. There is no experience beyond first-day administration of ondansetron.

Dosage Adjustment for Patients With Impaired Hepatic Function: In patients with severe hepatic impairment according to Child-Pugh[1] criteria, a single maximal daily dose of 8 mg to be infused over 15 minutes beginning 30 minutes before the start of the emetogenic chemotherapy is recommended. There is no experience beyond first-day administration of ondansetron.

ZOFRAN Injection Premixed in Flexible Plastic Containers: Instructions for Use: ***To Open:*** Tear outer wrap at notch and remove solution container. Check for minute leaks by squeezing container firmly. If leaks are found, discard unit as sterility may be impaired.

Preparation for Administration: Use aseptic technique.

1. Close flow control clamp of administration set.
2. Remove cover from outlet port at bottom of container.
3. Insert piercing pin of administration set into port with a twisting motion until the pin is firmly seated. NOTE: See full directions on administration set carton.
4. Suspend container from hanger.
5. Squeeze and release drip chamber to establish proper fluid level in chamber during infusion of ZOFRAN Injection Premixed.
6. Open flow control clamp to expel air from set. Close clamp.
7. Attach set to venipuncture device. If device is not indwelling, prime and make venipuncture.
8. Perform venipuncture.
9. Regulate rate of administration with flow control clamp.

Caution: ZOFRAN Injection Premixed in flexible plastic containers is to be administered by I.V. drip infusion only. ZOFRAN Injection Premixed should not be mixed with solutions for which physical and chemical compatibility have not been established. In particular, this applies to alkaline solutions as a precipitate may form. If used with a primary

Table 6: Prevention of Postoperative Nausea and Vomiting in Adult Patients

	Ondansetron 4 mg I.V.	Placebo	*P* Value
Study 1			
Emetic episodes:			
Number of patients	136	139	
Treatment response over 24-h postoperative period			
0 Emetic episodes	103 (76%)	64 (46%)	<0.001
1 Emetic episode	13 (10%)	17 (12%)	
More than 1 emetic episode/rescued	20 (15%)	58 (42%)	
Nausea assessments:			
Number of patients	134	136	
No nausea over 24-h postoperative period	56 (42%)	39 (29%)	
Study 2			
Emetic episodes:			
Number of patients	136	143	
Treatment response over 24-h postoperative period			
0 Emetic episodes	85 (63%)	63 (44%)	0.002
1 Emetic episode	16 (12%)	29 (20%)	
More than 1 emetic episode/rescued	35 (26%)	51 (36%)	
Nausea assessments:			
Number of patients	125	133	
No nausea over 24-h postoperative period	48 (38%)	42 (32%)	

Table 7: Prevention of Postoperative Nausea and Vomiting in Pediatric Patients

Treatment Response Over 24 Hours	Ondansetron n (%)	Placebo n (%)	*P* Value
Study 1			
Number of patients	205	210	
0 Emetic episodes	140 (68%)	82 (39%)	≤0.001
Failure*	65 (32%)	128 (61%)	
Study 2			
Number of patients	112	110	
0 Emetic episodes	68 (61%)	38 (35%)	≤0.001
Failure*	44 (39%)	72 (65%)	
Study 3			
Number of patients	206	206	
0 Emetic episodes	123 (60%)	96 (47%)	≤0.01
Failure*	83 (40%)	110 (53%)	
Nausea assessments:†			
Number of patients	185	191	
None	119 (64%)	99 (52%)	≤0.01

*Failure was one or more emetic episodes, rescued, or withdrawn.
†Nausea measured as none, mild, or severe.

Table 8: Prevention of Further Postoperative Nausea and Vomiting in Adult Patients

	Ondansetron 4 mg I.V.	Placebo	*P* Value
Study 1			
Emetic episodes:			
Number of patients	104	117	
Treatment response 24 h after study drug			
0 Emetic episodes	49 (47%)	19 (16%)	<0.001
1 Emetic episode	12 (12%)	9 (8%)	
More than 1 emetic episode/rescued	43 (41%)	89 (76%)	
Median time to first emetic episode (min)*	55.0	43.0	
Nausea assessments:			
Number of patients	98	102	
Mean nausea score over 24-h postoperative period†	1.7	3.1	
Study 2			
Emetic episodes:			
Number of patients	112	108	
Treatment response 24 h after study drug			
0 Emetic episodes	49 (44%)	28 (26%)	0.006
1 Emetic episode	14 (13%)	3 (3%)	
More than 1 emetic episode/rescued	49 (44%)	77 (71%)	
Median time to first emetic episode (min)*	60.5	34.0	
Nausea assessments:			
Number of patients	105	85	
Mean nausea score over 24-h postoperative period†	1.9	2.9	

*After administration of study drug.
†Nausea measured on a scale of 0-10 with 0 = no nausea, 10 = nausea as bad as it can be.

Table 9: Prevention of Further Postoperative Nausea and Vomiting in Pediatric Patients

Treatment Response Over 24 Hours	Ondansetron n (%)	Placebo n (%)	*P* Value
Number of patients	180	171	
0 Emetic episodes	96 (53%)	29 (17%)	≤0.001
Failure*	84 (47%)	142 (83%)	

*Failure was one or more emetic episodes, rescued, or withdrawn.

Table 10: Principal Adverse Events in Comparative Trials

	Number of Patients With Event			
	ZOFRAN Injection 0.15 mg/kg × 3 n = 419	ZOFRAN Injection 32 mg × 1 n = 220	Metoclopramide n = 156	Placebo n = 34
Diarrhea	16%	8%	44%	18%
Headache	17%	25%	7%	15%
Fever	8%	7%	5%	3%
Akathisia	0%	0%	6%	0%
Acute dystonic reactions*	0%	0%	5%	0%

*See Neurological.

Table 11: Adverse Events in ≥2% of Adults Receiving Ondansetron at a Dosage of 4 mg I.V. over 2 to 5 Minutes in Clinical Trials

	ZOFRAN Injection 4 mg I.V. n = 547 patients	Placebo n = 547 patients
Headache	92 (17%)	77 (14%)
Dizziness	67 (12%)	88 (16%)
Musculoskeletal pain	57 (10%)	59 (11%)
Drowsiness/sedation	44 (8%)	37 (7%)
Shivers	38 (7%)	39 (7%)
Malaise/fatigue	25 (5%)	30 (5%)
Injection site reaction	21 (4%)	18 (3%)
Urinary retention	17 (3%)	15 (3%)
Postoperative CO_2-related pain*	12 (2%)	16 (3%)
Chest pain (unspecified)	12 (2%)	15 (3%)
Anxiety/agitation	11 (2%)	16 (3%)
Dysuria	11 (2%)	9 (2%)
Hypotension	10 (2%)	12 (2%)
Fever	10 (2%)	6 (1%)
Cold sensation	9 (2%)	8 (1%)
Pruritus	9 (2%)	3 (<1%)
Paresthesia	9 (2%)	2 (<1%)

* Sites of pain included abdomen, stomach, joints, rib cage, shoulder.

Table 12: Frequency of Adverse Events From Controlled Studies in Pediatric Patients

Adverse Event	Ondansetron n = 755 Patients	Placebo n = 731 Patients
Wound problem	80 (11%)	86 (12%)
Anxiety/agitation	49 (6%)	47 (6%)
Headache	44 (6%)	43 (6%)
Drowsiness/sedation	41 (5%)	56 (8%)
Pyrexia	32 (4%)	41 (6%)

I.V. fluid system, the primary solution should be discontinued during ZOFRAN Injection Premixed infusion.

Do not administer unless solution is clear and container is undamaged.

Warning: Do not use flexible plastic container in series connections.

Stability: ZOFRAN Injection is stable at room temperature under normal lighting conditions for 48 hours after dilution with the following I.V. fluids: 0.9% Sodium Chloride Injection, 5% Dextrose Injection, 5% Dextrose and 0.9% Sodium Chloride Injection, 5% Dextrose and 0.45% Sodium Chloride Injection, and 3% Sodium Chloride Injection.

Although ZOFRAN Injection is chemically and physically stable when diluted as recommended, sterile precautions should be observed because diluents generally do not contain preservative. After dilution, do not use beyond 24 hours.

Note: Parenteral drug products should be inspected visually for particulate matter and discoloration before administration whenever solution and container permit.

Precaution: Occasionally, ondansetron precipitates at the stopper/vial interface in vials stored upright. Potency and safety are not affected. If a precipitate is observed, resolubilize by shaking the vial vigorously.

HOW SUPPLIED

ZOFRAN Injection, 2 mg/mL, is supplied as follows:
NDC 0173-0442-02 2-mL single-dose vials (Carton of 5)
NDC 0173-0442-00 20-mL multidose vials (Singles)

Store between 2° and 30°C (36° and 86°F). Protect from light.

ZOFRAN Injection Premixed, 32 mg/50 mL, in 5% Dextrose, contains no preservatives and is supplied as a sterile, premixed solution for I.V. administration in single-dose, flexible plastic containers (NDC 0173-0461-00) (case of 6).

Store between 2° and 30°C (36° and 86°F). Protect from light. Avoid excessive heat. Protect from freezing.

REFERENCE:

1. Pugh RNH, Murray-Lyon IM, Dawson JL, Pietroni MC, Williams R. Transection of the oesophagus for bleeding oesophageal varices. *Brit J Surg.* 1973;60:646–649.

Glaxo Wellcome Inc., Research Triangle Park, NC 27709
ZOFRAN® Injection Premixed:
Manufactured for Glaxo Wellcome Inc.
Research Triangle Park, NC 27709
by Abbott Laboratories, North Chicago, IL 60064
US Patent Nos. 4,695,578; 4,753,789; and 5,578,628

May 2000/RL-811

Shown in Product Identification Guide, page 317

ZOFRAN® ℞
[zō′fran]
(ondansetron hydrochloride)
Tablets

ZOFRAN® ODT® ℞
(ondansetron)
Orally Disintegrating Tablets

ZOFRAN® ℞
(ondansetron hydrochloride)
Oral Solution

DESCRIPTION

The active ingredient in ZOFRAN Tablets and ZOFRAN Oral Solution is ondansetron hydrochloride (HCl) as the dihydrate, the racemic form of ondansetron and a selective blocking agent of the serotonin 5-HT_3 receptor type. Chemically it is (±) 1, 2, 3, 9-tetrahydro-9-methyl-3-[(2-methyl-1H-imidazol-1-yl)methyl]-4H-carbazol-4-one, monohydrochloride, dihydrate.

The empirical formula is $C_{18}H_{19}N_3O \bullet HCl \bullet 2H_2O$, representing a molecular weight of 365.9.

Ondansetron HCl dihydrate is a white to off-white powder that is soluble in water and normal saline.

The active ingredient in ZOFRAN ODT Orally Disintegrating Tablets is ondansetron base, the racemic form of ondansetron, and a selective blocking agent of the serotonin 5-HT_3 receptor type. Chemically it is (±) 1, 2, 3, 9-tetrahydro-9-methyl-3-[(2-methyl-1H-imidazol-1-yl)methyl]-4H-carbazol-4-one.

The empirical formula is $C_{18}H_{19}N_3O$ representing a molecular weight of 293.4.

Each 4-mg ZOFRAN Tablet for oral administration contains ondansetron HCl dihydrate equivalent to 4 mg of ondansetron. Each 8-mg ZOFRAN Tablet for oral administration contains ondansetron HCl dihydrate equivalent to 8 mg of ondansetron. Each 24-mg ZOFRAN Tablet for oral administration contains ondansetron HCl dihydrate equivalent to 24 mg of ondansetron. Each tablet also contains the inactive ingredients lactose, microcrystalline cellulose, pregelatinized starch, hydroxypropyl methylcellulose, magnesium stearate, titanium dioxide, triacetin, iron oxide yellow (8-mg tablet only), and iron oxide red (24-mg tablet only).

Each 4-mg ZOFRAN ODT Orally Disintegrating Tablet for oral administration contains 4 mg ondansetron base. Each 8-mg ZOFRAN ODT Orally Disintegrating Tablet for oral administration contains 8 mg ondansetron base. Each ZOFRAN ODT Tablet also contains the inactive ingredients aspartame, gelatin, mannitol, methylparaben sodium, propylparaben sodium, and strawberry flavor. ZOFRAN ODT Tablets are a freeze-dried, orally administered formulation of ondansetron which rapidly disintegrates on the tongue and does not require water to aid dissolution or swallowing.

Each 5 mL of ZOFRAN Oral Solution contains 5 mg of ondansetron HCl dihydrate equivalent to 4 mg of ondansetron. ZOFRAN Oral Solution contains the inactive ingredients citric acid anhydrous, purified water, sodium benzoate, sodium citrate, sorbitol, and strawberry flavor.

CLINICAL PHARMACOLOGY

Pharmacodynamics: Ondansetron is a selective 5-HT_3 receptor antagonist. While its mechanism of action has not been fully characterized, ondansetron is not a dopamine-receptor antagonist. Serotonin receptors of the 5-HT_3 type are present both peripherally on vagal nerve terminals and centrally in the chemoreceptor trigger zone of the area postrema. It is not certain whether ondansetron's antiemetic action is mediated centrally, peripherally, or in both sites. However, cytotoxic chemotherapy appears to be associated with release of serotonin from the enterochromaffin cells of the small intestine. In humans, urinary 5-HIAA (5-hydroxyindoleacetic acid) excretion increases after cisplatin administration in parallel with the onset of emesis. The released serotonin may stimulate the vagal afferents through the 5-HT_3 receptors and initiate the vomiting reflex.

In animals, the emetic response to cisplatin can be prevented by pretreatment with an inhibitor of serotonin synthesis, bilateral abdominal vagotomy and greater splanchnic nerve section, or pretreatment with a serotonin 5-HT_3 receptor antagonist.

In normal volunteers, single intravenous doses of 0.15 mg/kg of ondansetron had no effect on esophageal motility, gastric motility, lower esophageal sphincter pressure, or small intestinal transit time. Multiday administration of ondansetron has been shown to slow colonic transit in normal volunteers. Ondansetron has no effect on plasma prolactin concentrations.

Ondansetron does not alter the respiratory depressant effects produced by alfentanil or the degree of neuromuscular blockade produced by atracurium. Interactions with general or local anesthetics have not been studied.

Pharmacokinetics: Ondansetron is extensively metabolized in humans, with approximately 5% of a radiolabeled dose recovered from the urine as the parent compound. The primary metabolic pathway is hydroxylation on the indole ring followed by subsequent glucuronide or sulfate conjugation. Although some nonconjugated metabolites have pharmacologic activity, these are not found in plasma at concentrations likely to significantly contribute to the biological activity of ondansetron.

Ondansetron is a substrate for human hepatic cytochrome P-450 enzymes, including CYP1A2, CYP2D6, and CYP3A4. Because of the multiplicity of metabolic enzymes capable of metabolizing ondansetron, inhibition or loss of one enzyme (e.g., CYP2D6 genetic deficiency) results in little change in overall rates of ondansetron elimination.

Ondansetron is passively and completely absorbed from the gastrointestinal tract and undergoes some first-pass metabolism. Mean bioavailability in healthy subjects has ranged from 48% to 75%.

Gender differences were shown in the disposition of ondansetron given as a single dose. The extent and rate of ondansetron's absorption is greater in women than men. Slower clearance in women, a smaller apparent volume of distribution (adjusted for weight), and higher absolute bioavailability resulted in higher plasma ondansetron levels. These higher plasma levels may in part be explained by dif-

Continued on next page

This product information is based on labeling in effect on June 23, 2000. For further information, contact via direct mail, phone, or web site. Medical Information, Glaxo Wellcome Inc., PO Box 13398, Research Triangle Park, NC 27709. Healthcare Professionals (Medical Information): 800-334-0089. Patients (Customer Response Center): 1-888-825-5249. Glaxo Wellcome Corporate Web Site: www.glaxowellcome.com

Zofran—Cont.

ferences in body weight between men and women. It is not known whether these gender-related differences were clinically important. More detailed pharmacokinetic information is contained in Tables 1 and 2 taken from two studies.
[See table 1 at right]
[See table 2 at right]
A reduction in clearance and increase in elimination half-life are seen in patients over 75 years of age. In clinical trials with cancer patients, safety and efficacy was similar in patients over 65 years of age and those under 65 years of age; there was an insufficient number of patients over 75 years of age to permit conclusions in that age-group. No dosage adjustment is recommended in the elderly.
Ondansetron systemic exposure does not increase proportionately to dose. AUC from a 16-mg tablet was 24% greater than predicted from an 8-mg tablet dose. This may reflect some reduction of first-pass metabolism at higher oral doses. Bioavailability is also slightly enhanced by the presence of food but unaffected by antacids.
In patients with severe hepatic impairment (Child-Pugh[1] score of 10 or greater), clearance is reduced twofold to threefold and apparent volume of distribution is increased with a resultant increase in half-life to 20 hours and bioavailability approaching 100%. In such patients, a total daily dose of 8 mg should not be exceeded.
Ondansetron oral plasma clearance was reduced 50% (95% CI 22% to 68%) in patients with severe renal impairment (creatinine clearance <30 mL/min). This reduction in clearance is variable and was not consistent with an increase in half-life. No reduction in dose or dosing frequency in these patients is warranted.
Plasma protein binding of ondansetron as measured in vitro was 70% to 76% over the concentration range of 10 to 500 ng/mL. Circulating drug also distributes into erythrocytes.
Four- and 8-mg doses of either ZOFRAN Oral Solution or ZOFRAN ODT Orally Disintegrating Tablets are bioequivalent to corresponding doses of ZOFRAN Tablets and may be used interchangeably. One 24-mg ZOFRAN Tablet is bioequivalent to and interchangeable with three 8-mg ZOFRAN Tablets.

CLINICAL TRIALS

Chemotherapy-Induced Nausea and Vomiting: ***Highly Emetogenic Chemotherapy:*** In two randomized, double-blind, monotherapy trials, a single 24-mg ZOFRAN Tablet was superior to a relevant historical placebo control in the prevention of nausea and vomiting associated with highly emetogenic cancer chemotherapy, including cisplatin ≥50 mg/m². Steroid administration was excluded from these clinical trials. More than 90% of patients receiving a cisplatin dose ≥50 mg/m² in the historical placebo comparator experienced vomiting in the absence of antiemetic therapy.
The first trial compared oral doses of ondansetron 24 mg once a day, 8 mg twice a day, and 32 mg once a day in 357 adult cancer patients receiving chemotherapy regimens containing cisplatin ≥50 mg/m². A total of 66% of patients in the ondansetron 24 mg once a day group, 55% in the ondansetron 8 mg twice a day group, and 55% in the ondansetron 32 mg once a day group completed the 24-hour study period with zero emetic episodes and no rescue antiemetic medications, the primary endpoint of efficacy. Each of the three treatment groups was shown to be statistically significantly superior to a historical placebo control.
In the same trial, 56% of patients receiving oral ondansetron 24 mg once a day experienced no nausea during the 24-hour study period, compared with 36% of patients in the oral ondansetron 8 mg twice a day group (p = 0.001) and 50% in the oral ondansetron 32 mg once a day group.
In a second trial, efficacy of the oral ondansetron 24 mg once a day regimen in the prevention of nausea and vomiting associated with highly emetogenic cancer chemotherapy, including cisplatin ≥50 mg/m², was confirmed.
Moderately Emetogenic Chemotherapy: In one double-blind US study in 67 patients, ZOFRAN Tablets 8 mg administered twice a day were significantly more effective than placebo in preventing vomiting induced by cyclophosphamide-based chemotherapy containing doxorubicin. Treatment response is based on the total number of emetic episodes over the 3-day study period. The results of this study are summarized below in Table 3.
[See table 3 above]
In one double-blind US study in 336 patients, ZOFRAN Tablets 8 mg administered twice a day were as effective as ZOFRAN Tablets 8 mg administered three times a day in preventing nausea and vomiting induced by cyclophosphamide-based chemotherapy containing either methotrexate or doxorubicin. Treatment response is based on the total number of emetic episodes over the 3-day study period. The results of this study are summarized below in Table 4.
[See table 4 above]
Re-treatment: In uncontrolled trials, 148 patients receiving cyclophosphamide-based chemotherapy were re-treated with ZOFRAN Tablets 8 mg t.i.d. of oral ondansetron during subsequent chemotherapy for a total of 396 re-treatment courses. No emetic episodes occurred in 314 (79%) of the re-treatment courses, and only one to two emetic episodes occurred in 43 (11%) of the re-treatment courses.
Pediatric Studies: Three open-label, uncontrolled, foreign trials have been performed with 182 patients 4 to 18 years old with cancer who were given a variety of cisplatin or noncisplatin regimens. In these foreign trials, the initial dose of ZOFRAN® (ondansetron HCl) Injection ranged from 0.04 to 0.87 mg/kg for a total dose of 2.16 to 12 mg. This was followed by the administration of ZOFRAN Tablets ranging from 4 to 24 mg daily for 3 days. In these studies, 58% of the 170 evaluable patients had a complete response (no emetic episodes) on day 1. Two studies showed the response rates for patients less than 12 years of age who received ZOFRAN Tablets 4 mg three times a day to be similar to those in patients 12 to 18 years of age who received ZOFRAN Tablets 8 mg three times daily. Thus, prevention of emesis in these children was essentially the same as for patients older than 18 years of age. Overall, ZOFRAN Tablets were well tolerated in these pediatric patients.

Table 1: Pharmacokinetics in Normal Volunteers: Single 8-mg ZOFRAN Tablet Dose

Age-group (years)	Mean Weight (kg)	n	Peak Plasma Concentration (ng/mL)	Time of Peak Plasma Concentration (h)	Mean Elimination Half-life (h)	Systemic Plasma Clearance L/h/kg	Absolute Bioavailability
18–40 M	69.0	6	26.2	2.0	3.1	0.403	0.483
F	62.7	5	42.7	1.7	3.5	0.354	0.663
61–74 M	77.5	6	24.1	2.1	4.1	0.384	0.585
F	60.2	6	52.4	1.9	4.9	0.255	0.643
≥75 M	78.0	5	37.0	2.2	4.5	0.277	0.619
F	67.6	6	46.1	2.1	6.2	0.249	0.747

Table 2: Pharmacokinetics in Normal Volunteers: Single 24-mg ZOFRAN Tablet Dose

Age-group (years)	Mean Weight (kg)	n	Peak Plasma Concentration (ng/mL)	Time of Peak Plasma Concentration (h)	Mean Elimination Half-life (h)
18–43 M	84.1	8	125.8	1.9	4.7
F	71.8	8	194.4	1.6	5.8

Table 3: Emetic Episodes: Treatment Response

	Ondansetron 8-mg b.i.d. ZOFRAN Tablets*	Placebo	*P* Value
Number of patients	33	34	
Treatment response			
0 Emetic episodes	20 (61%)	2 (6%)	<0.001
1–2 Emetic episodes	6 (18%)	8 (24%)	
More than 2 emetic episodes/withdrawn	7 (21%)	24 (71%)	<0.001
Median number of emetic episodes	0.0	Undefined†	
Median time to first emetic episode (h)	Undefined‡	6.5	

*The first dose was administered 30 minutes before the start of emetogenic chemotherapy, with a subsequent dose 8 hours after the first dose. An 8-mg ZOFRAN Tablet was administered twice a day for 2 days after completion of chemotherapy.
†Median undefined since at least 50% of the patients were withdrawn or had more than two emetic episodes.
‡Median undefined since at least 50% of patients did not have any emetic episodes.

Table 4: Emetic Episodes: Treatment Response

	Ondansetron	
	8-mg b.i.d. ZOFRAN Tablets*	8-mg t.i.d. ZOFRAN Tablets†
Number of patients	165	171
Treatment response		
0 Emetic episodes	101 (61%)	99 (58%)
1–2 Emetic episodes	16 (10%)	17 (10%)
More than 2 emetic episodes/withdrawn	48 (29%)	55 (32%)
Median number of emetic episodes	0.0	0.0
Median time to first emetic episode (h)	Undefined‡	Undefined‡
Median nausea scores (0–100)§	6	6

*The first dose was administered 30 minutes before the start of emetogenic chemotherapy, with a subsequent dose 8 hours after the first dose. An 8-mg ZOFRAN Tablet was administered twice a day for 2 days after completion of chemotherapy.
† The first dose was administered 30 minutes before the start of emetogenic chemotherapy, with subsequent doses 4 and 8 hours after the first dose. An 8-mg ZOFRAN Tablet was administered three times a day for 2 days after completion of chemotherapy.
‡ Median undefined since at least 50% of patients did not have any emetic episodes.
§ Visual analog scale assessment: 0 = no nausea, 100 = nausea as bad as it can be.

Radiation-Induced Nausea and Vomiting: ***Total Body Irradiation:*** In a randomized, double-blind study in 20 patients, ZOFRAN Tablets (8 mg given 1.5 hours before each fraction of radiotherapy for 4 days) were significantly more effective than placebo in preventing vomiting induced by total body irradiation. Total body irradiation consisted of 11 fractions (120 cGy per fraction) over 4 days for a total of 1320 cGy. Patients received three fractions for 3 days, then two fractions on day 4.
Single High-Dose Fraction Radiotherapy: Ondansetron was significantly more effective than metoclopramide with respect to complete control of emesis (0 emetic episodes) in a double-blind trial in 105 patients receiving single high-dose radiotherapy (800 to 1000 cGy) over an anterior or posterior field size of ≥80 cm² to the abdomen. Patients received the first dose of ZOFRAN Tablets (8 mg) or metoclopramide (10 mg) 1 to 2 hours before radiotherapy. If radiotherapy was given in the morning, two additional doses of study treatment were given (one tablet late afternoon and one tablet before bedtime). If radiotherapy was given in the afternoon, patients took only one further tablet that day before bedtime. Patients continued the oral medication on a t.i.d. basis for 3 days.
Daily Fractionated Radiotherapy: Ondansetron was significantly more effective than prochlorperazine with respect to complete control of emesis (0 emetic episodes) in a double-blind trial in 135 patients receiving a 1- to 4-week course of fractionated radiotherapy (180 cGy doses) over a field size of ≥100 cm² to the abdomen. Patients received the first dose of ZOFRAN Tablets (8 mg) or prochlorperazine (10 mg) 1 to 2 hours before the patient received the first daily radiotherapy fraction, with two subsequent doses on a t.i.d. basis. Patients continued the oral medication on a t.i.d. basis on each day of radiotherapy.
Postoperative Nausea and Vomiting: Surgical patients who received ondansetron 1 hour before the induction of general balanced anesthesia (barbiturate: thiopental, methohexital, or thiamylal; opioid: alfentanil, sufentanil, morphine, or fentanyl; nitrous oxide; neuromuscular blockade: succinylcholine/curare or gallamine and/or vecuronium, pancuronium, or atracurium; and supplemental isoflurane or enflurane) were evaluated in two double-blind studies (one US study, one foreign) involving 865 patients. ZOFRAN Tablets (16 mg) were significantly more effective than placebo in preventing postoperative nausea and vomiting.
The study populations in all trials thus far consisted of women undergoing inpatient surgical procedures. No studies have been performed in males. No controlled clinical study comparing ZOFRAN Tablets to ZOFRAN Injection has been performed.

INDICATIONS AND USAGE

1. Prevention of nausea and vomiting associated with highly emetogenic cancer chemotherapy, including cisplatin ≥50 mg/m².
2. Prevention of nausea and vomiting associated with initial and repeat courses of moderately emetogenic cancer chemotherapy.

3. Prevention of nausea and vomiting associated with radiotherapy in patients receiving either total body irradiation, single high-dose fraction to the abdomen, or daily fractions to the abdomen.
4. Prevention of postoperative nausea and/or vomiting. As with other antiemetics, routine prophylaxis is not recommended for patients in whom there is little expectation that nausea and/or vomiting will occur postoperatively. In patients where nausea and/or vomiting must be avoided postoperatively, ZOFRAN Tablets, ZOFRAN ODT Orally Disintegrating Tablets, and ZOFRAN Oral Solution are recommended even where the incidence of postoperative nausea and/or vomiting is low.

CONTRAINDICATIONS

ZOFRAN Tablets, ZOFRAN ODT Orally Disintegrating Tablets, and ZOFRAN Oral Solution are contraindicated for patients known to have hypersensitivity to the drug.

WARNINGS

Hypersensitivity reactions have been reported in patients who have exhibited hypersensitivity to other selective 5-HT_3 receptor antagonists.

PRECAUTIONS

Ondansetron is not a drug that stimulates gastric or intestinal peristalsis. It should not be used instead of nasogastric suction. The use of ondansetron in patients following abdominal surgery or in patients with chemotherapy-induced nausea and vomiting may mask a progressive ileus and/or gastric distension.

Information for Patients: ***Phenylketonurics:*** Phenylketonuric patients should be informed that ZOFRAN ODT Orally Disintegrating Tablets contain phenylalanine (a component of aspartame). Each 4-mg and 8-mg orally disintegrating tablet contains <0.03 mg phenylalanine.

Patients should be instructed not to remove ZOFRAN ODT Tablets from the blister until just prior to dosing. The tablet should not be pushed through the foil. With dry hands, the blister backing should be peeled completely off the blister. The tablet should be gently removed and immediately placed on the tongue to dissolve and be swallowed with the saliva. Peelable illustrated stickers are affixed to the product carton that can be provided with the prescription to ensure proper use and handling of the product.

Drug Interactions: Ondansetron does not itself appear to induce or inhibit the cytochrome P-450 drug-metabolizing enzyme system of the liver. Because ondansetron is metabolized by hepatic cytochrome P-450 drug-metabolizing enzymes, inducers or inhibitors of these enzymes may change the clearance and, hence, the half-life of ondansetron. On the basis of available data, no dosage adjustment is recommended for patients on these drugs. Tumor response to chemotherapy in the P 388 mouse leukemia model is not affected by ondansetron. In humans, carmustine, etoposide, and cisplatin do not affect the pharmacokinetics of ondansetron.

Ondansetron has no effect on the pharmacokinetics of high-dose methotrexate.

Use in Surgical Patients: The coadministration of ondansetron had no effect on the pharmacokinetics and pharmacodynamics of temazepam.

Carcinogenesis, Mutagenesis, Impairment of Fertility: Carcinogenic effects were not seen in 2-year studies in rats and mice with oral ondansetron doses up to 10 and 30 mg/kg per day, respectively. Ondansetron was not mutagenic in standard tests for mutagenicity. Oral administration of ondansetron up to 15 mg/kg per day did not affect fertility or general reproductive performance of male and female rats.

Pregnancy: ***Teratogenic Effects: Pregnancy Category B:*** Reproduction studies have been performed in pregnant rats and rabbits at daily oral doses up to 15 and 30 mg/kg per day, respectively, and have revealed no evidence of impaired fertility or harm to the fetus due to ondansetron. There are, however, no adequate and well-controlled studies in pregnant women. Because animal reproduction studies are not always predictive of human response, this drug should be used during pregnancy only if clearly needed.

Nursing Mothers: Ondansetron is excreted in the breast milk of rats. It is not known whether ondansetron is excreted in human milk. Because many drugs are excreted in human milk, caution should be exercised when ondansetron is administered to a nursing woman.

Pediatric Use: Little information is available about dosage in children 4 years of age or younger (see CLINICAL PHARMACOLOGY and DOSAGE AND ADMINISTRATION sections for use in children 4 to 18 years of age).

Geriatric Use: Of the total number of subjects enrolled in cancer chemotherapy-induced and post-operative nausea and vomiting in US- and foreign-controlled clinical trials, for which there were subgroup analyses, 938 were 65 years of age and over. No overall differences in safety or effectiveness were observed between these subjects and younger subjects, and other reported clinical experience has not identified differences in responses between the elderly and younger patients, but greater sensitivity of some older individuals cannot be ruled out. Dosage adjustment is not needed in patients over the age of 65 (see CLINICAL PHARMACOLOGY).

ADVERSE REACTIONS

The following have been reported as adverse events in clinical trials of patients treated with ondansetron, the active ingredient of ZOFRAN. A causal relationship to therapy with ZOFRAN has been unclear in many cases.

Table 5: Principal Adverse Events in US Trials: Single Day Therapy With 24-mg ZOFRAN Tablets (Highly Emetogenic Chemotherapy)

Event	Ondansetron 24 mg q.d. n = 300	Ondansetron 8 mg b.i.d. n = 124	Ondansetron 32 mg q.d. n = 117
Headache	33 (11%)	16 (13%)	17 (15%)
Diarrhea	13 (4%)	9 (7%)	3 (3%)

Table 6: Principal Adverse Events in US Trials: 3 Days of Therapy With 8 mg ZOFRAN Tablets (Moderately Emetogenic Chemotherapy)

Event	Ondansetron 8 mg b.i.d. n = 242	Ondansetron 8 mg t.i.d. n = 415	Placebo n = 262
Headache	58 (24%)	113 (27%)	34 (13%)
Malaise/fatigue	32 (13%)	37 (9%)	6 (2%)
Constipation	22 (9%)	26 (6%)	1 (<1%)
Diarrhea	15 (6%)	16 (4%)	10 (4%)
Dizziness	13 (5%)	18 (4%)	12 (5%)

Table 7: Frequency of Adverse Events From Controlled Studies With ZOFRAN Tablets (Postoperative Nausea and Vomiting)

Adverse Event	Ondansetron 16 mg (n = 550)	Placebo (n = 531)
Wound problem	152 (28%)	162 (31%)
Drowsiness/sedation	112 (20%)	122 (23%)
Headache	49 (9%)	27 (5%)
Hypoxia	49 (9%)	35 (7%)
Pyrexia	45 (8%)	34 (6%)
Dizziness	36 (7%)	34 (6%)
Gynecological disorder	36 (7%)	33 (6%)
Anxiety/agitation	33 (6%)	29 (5%)
Bradycardia	32 (6%)	30 (6%)
Shiver(s)	28 (5%)	30 (6%)
Urinary retention	28 (5%)	18 (3%)
Hypotension	27 (5%)	32 (6%)
Pruritus	27 (5%)	20 (4%)

Chemotherapy-Induced Nausea and Vomiting: The following adverse events have been reported in ≥5% of adult patients receiving a single 24-mg ZOFRAN Tablet in two trials. These patients were receiving concurrent highly emetogenic cisplatin-based chemotherapy regimens (cisplatin dose ≥50 mg/m^2).

[See table 5 above]

The following adverse events have been reported in ≥5% of adults receiving either 8 mg of ZOFRAN Tablets two or three times a day for 3 days or placebo in four trials. These patients were receiving concurrent moderately-emetogenic chemotherapy, primarily cyclophosphamide-based regimens.

[See table 6 above]

Central Nervous System: There have been rare reports consistent with, but not diagnostic of, extrapyramidal reactions in patients receiving ondansetron.

Hepatic: In 723 patients receiving cyclophosphamide-based chemotherapy in US clinical trials, AST and/or ALT values have been reported to exceed twice the upper limit of normal in approximately 1% to 2% of patients receiving ZOFRAN Tablets. The increases were transient and did not appear to be related to dose or duration of therapy. On repeat exposure, similar transient elevations in transaminase values occurred in some courses, but symptomatic hepatic disease did not occur. The role of cancer chemotherapy in these biochemical changes cannot be clearly determined.

There have been reports of liver failure and death in patients with cancer receiving concurrent medications including potentially hepatotoxic cytotoxic chemotherapy and antibiotics. The etiology of the liver failure is unclear.

Integumentary: Rash has occurred in approximately 1% of patients receiving ondansetron.

Other: Rare cases of anaphylaxis, bronchospasm, tachycardia, angina (chest pain), hypokalemia, electrocardiographic alterations, vascular occlusive events, and grand mal seizures have been reported. Except for bronchospasm and anaphylaxis, the relationship to ZOFRAN was unclear.

Radiation-Induced Nausea and Vomiting: The adverse events reported in patients receiving ZOFRAN Tablets and concurrent radiotherapy were similar to those reported in patients receiving ZOFRAN Tablets and concurrent chemotherapy. The most frequently reported adverse events were headache, constipation, and diarrhea.

Postoperative Nausea and Vomiting: The following adverse events have been reported in ≥5% of patients receiving ZOFRAN Tablets at a dosage of 16 mg orally in clinical trials. With the exception of headache, rates of these events were not significantly different in the ondansetron and placebo groups. These patients were receiving multiple concomitant perioperative and postoperative medications.

[See table 7 above]

Preliminary observations in a small number of subjects suggest a higher incidence of headache when ZOFRAN ODT Orally Disintegrating Tablets are taken with water, when compared to without water.

Observed During Clinical Practice: In addition to adverse events reported from clinical trials, the following events have been identified during post-approval use of oral formulations of ZOFRAN. Because they are reported voluntarily from a population of unknown size, estimates of frequency cannot be made. The events have been chosen for inclusion due to a combination of their seriousness, frequency of reporting, or potential causal connection to ZOFRAN.

General: Flushing. Rare cases of hypersensitivity reactions, sometimes severe (e.g., anaphylaxis/anaphylactoid reactions, angioedema, bronchospasm, shortness of breath, hypotension, laryngeal edema, stridor) have also been reported. Laryngospasm, shock, and cardiopulmonary arrest have occurred during allergic reactions in patients receiving injectable ondansetron.

Hepatobiliary: Liver enzyme abnormalities

Lower Respiratory: Hiccups

Neurology: Oculogyric crisis, appearing alone, as well as with other dystonic reactions

Skin: Urticaria

DRUG ABUSE AND DEPENDENCE

Animal studies have shown that ondansetron is not discriminated as a benzodiazepine nor does it substitute for benzodiazepines in direct addiction studies.

OVERDOSAGE

There is no specific antidote for ondansetron overdose. Patients should be managed with appropriate supportive therapy. Individual intravenous doses as large as 150 mg and total daily intravenous doses as large as 252 mg have been inadvertently administered without significant adverse events. These doses are more than 10 times the recommended daily dose.

In addition to the adverse events listed above, the following events have been described in the setting of ondansetron overdose: "Sudden blindness" (amaurosis) of 2 to 3 minutes duration plus severe constipation occurred in one patient that was administered 72 mg of ondansetron intravenously as a single dose. Hypotension (and faintness) occurred in a patient that took 48 mg of ZOFRAN Tablets. Following infusion of 32 mg over only a 4-minute period, a vasovagal episode with transient second degree heart block was observed. In all instances, the events resolved completely.

DOSAGE AND ADMINISTRATION

Instructions for Use/Handling ZOFRAN ODT Orally Disintegrating Tablets: Do not attempt to push ZOFRAN ODT Tablets through the foil backing. With dry hands, PEEL BACK the foil backing of one blister and GENTLY remove the tablet. IMMEDIATELY place the ZOFRAN ODT Tablet on top of the tongue where it will dissolve in seconds, then swallow with saliva. Administration with liquid is not necessary.

Continued on next page

This product information is based on labeling in effect on June 23, 2000. For further information, contact via direct mail, phone, or web site. Medical Information, Glaxo Wellcome Inc., PO Box 13398, Research Triangle Park, NC 27709. Healthcare Professionals (Medical Information): 800-334-0089. Patients (Customer Response Center): 1-888-825-5249. Glaxo Wellcome Corporate Web Site: www.glaxowellcome.com

Zofran—Cont.

Prevention of Nausea and Vomiting Associated With Highly Emetogenic Cancer Chemotherapy: The recommended adult oral dosage of ZOFRAN is a single 24-mg tablet administered 30 minutes before the start of single-day highly emetogenic chemotherapy, including cisplatin ≥50 mg/m². Multi-day, single-dose administration of ZOFRAN 24-mg Tablets has not been studied.

Pediatric Use: There is no experience with the use of 24-mg ZOFRAN Tablets in children.

Geriatric Use: The dosage recommendation is the same as for the general population.

Prevention of Nausea and Vomiting Associated With Moderately Emetogenic Cancer Chemotherapy: The recommended adult oral dosage is one 8-mg ZOFRAN Tablet or one 8-mg ZOFRAN ODT Tablet or 10 mL (2 teaspoonfuls equivalent to 8 mg of ondansetron) of ZOFRAN Oral Solution given twice a day. The first dose should be administered 30 minutes before the start of emetogenic chemotherapy, with a subsequent dose 8 hours after the first dose. One 8-mg ZOFRAN Tablet or one 8-mg ZOFRAN ODT Tablet or 10 mL (2 teaspoonfuls equivalent to 8 mg of ondansetron) of ZOFRAN Oral Solution should be administered twice a day (every 12 hours) for 1 to 2 days after completion of chemotherapy.

Pediatric Use: For patients 12 years of age and older, the dosage is the same as for adults. For patients 4 through 11 years of age, the dosage is one 4-mg ZOFRAN Tablet or one 4-mg ZOFRAN ODT Tablet or 5 mL (1 teaspoonful equivalent to 4 mg of ondansetron) of ZOFRAN Oral Solution given three times a day. The first dose should be administered 30 minutes before the start of emetogenic chemotherapy, with subsequent doses 4 and 8 hours after the first dose. One 4-mg ZOFRAN Tablet or one 4-mg ZOFRAN ODT Tablet or 5 mL (1 teaspoonful equivalent to 4 mg of ondansetron) of ZOFRAN Oral Solution should be administered three times a day (every 8 hours) for 1 to 2 days after completion of chemotherapy.

Geriatric Use: The dosage is the same as for the general population.

Prevention of Nausea and Vomiting Associated With Radiotherapy, Either Total Body Irradiation, or Single High-Dose Fraction or Daily Fractions to the Abdomen: The recommended oral dosage is one 8-mg ZOFRAN Tablet or one 8-mg ZOFRAN ODT Tablet or 10 mL (2 teaspoonfuls equivalent to 8 mg of ondansetron) of ZOFRAN Oral Solution given three times a day.

For total body irradiation, one 8-mg ZOFRAN Tablet or one 8-mg ZOFRAN ODT Tablet or 10 mL (2 teaspoonfuls equivalent to 8 mg of ondansetron) of ZOFRAN Oral Solution should be administered 1 to 2 hours before each fraction of radiotherapy administered each day.

For single high-dose fraction radiotherapy to the abdomen, one 8-mg ZOFRAN Tablet or one 8-mg ZOFRAN ODT Tablet or 10 mL (2 teaspoonfuls equivalent to 8 mg of ondansetron) of ZOFRAN Oral Solution should be administered 1 to 2 hours before radiotherapy, with subsequent doses every 8 hours after the first dose for 1 to 2 days after completion of radiotherapy.

For daily fractionated radiotherapy to the abdomen, one 8-mg ZOFRAN Tablet or one 8-mg ZOFRAN ODT Tablet or 10 mL (2 teaspoonfuls equivalent to 8 mg of ondansetron) of ZOFRAN Oral Solution should be administered 1 to 2 hours before radiotherapy, with subsequent doses every 8 hours after the first dose for each day radiotherapy is given.

Pediatric Use: There is no experience with the use of ZOFRAN Tablets, ZOFRAN ODT Tablets, or ZOFRAN Oral Solution in the prevention of radiation-induced nausea and vomiting in children.

Geriatric Use: The dosage recommendation is the same as for the general population.

Postoperative Nausea and Vomiting: The recommended dosage is 16 mg given as two 8-mg ZOFRAN Tablets or two 8-mg ZOFRAN ODT Tablets or 20 mL (4 teaspoonfuls equivalent to 16 mg of ondansetron) of ZOFRAN Oral Solution 1 hour before induction of anesthesia.

Pediatric Use: There is no experience with the use of ZOFRAN Tablets, ZOFRAN ODT Tablets, or ZOFRAN Oral Solution in the prevention of postoperative nausea and vomiting in children.

Geriatric Use: The dosage is the same as for the general population.

Dosage Adjustment for Patients With Impaired Renal Function: The dosage recommendation is the same as for the general population. There is no experience beyond first-day administration of ondansetron.

Dosage Adjustment for Patients With Impaired Hepatic Function: In patients with severe hepatic impairment according to Child-Pugh[1] criteria, clearance is reduced, apparent volume of distribution is increased with a resultant increase in plasma half-life, and bioavailability approaches 100%. In such patients, a total daily dose of 8 mg should not be exceeded.

HOW SUPPLIED

ZOFRAN Tablets, 4 mg (ondansetron HCl dihydrate equivalent to 4 mg of ondansetron), are white, oval, film-coated tablets engraved with "Zofran" on one side and "4" on the other in daily unit dose packs of 3 tablets (NDC 0173-0446-04), bottles of 30 tablets (NDC 0173-0446-00), and unit dose packs of 100 tablets (NDC 0173-0446-02).

ZOFRAN Tablets, 8 mg (ondansetron HCl dihydrate equivalent to 8 mg of ondansetron), are yellow, oval, film-coated tablets engraved with "Zofran" on one side and "8" on the other in daily unit dose packs of 3 tablets (NDC 0173-0447-04), bottles of 30 tablets (NDC 0173-0447-00), and unit dose packs of 100 tablets (NDC 0173-0447-02).

Store between 2° and 30°C (36° and 86°F). Protect from light. Store blisters and bottles in cartons.

ZOFRAN Tablets, 24 mg (ondansetron HCl dihydrate equivalent to 24 mg of ondansetron), are pink, oval, film-coated tablets engraved with "GX CF7" on one side and "24" on the other in daily unit dose packs of 1 tablet (NDC 0173-0680-00).

Store between 2° and 30°C (36° and 86°F).

ZOFRAN ODT Orally Disintegrating Tablets, 4 mg (as 4 mg ondansetron base) are white, round and plano-convex tablets with no marking on either side in unit dose packs of 30 tablets (NDC 0173-0569-00).

ZOFRAN ODT Orally Disintegrating Tablets, 8 mg (as 8 mg ondansetron base) are white, round and plano-convex tablets with no marking on either side in unit dose packs of 30 tablets (NDC 0173-0570-00).

Store between 2° and 30°C (36° and 86°F).

ZOFRAN Oral Solution, a clear, colorless to light yellow liquid with a characteristic strawberry odor, contains 5 mg of ondansetron HCl dihydrate equivalent to 4 mg of ondansetron per 5 mL in amber glass bottles of 50 mL with child-resistant closures (NDC 0173-0489-00).

Store upright between 15° and 30°C (59° and 86°F). Protect from light. Store bottles upright in cartons.

REFERENCE

1. Pugh RNH, Murray-Lyon IM, Dawson JL, Pietroni MC, Williams R. Transection of the oesophagus for bleeding oesophageal varices. *Brit J Surg.* 1973;60:646-649.

ZOFRAN Tablets and Oral Solution:
Glaxo Wellcome Inc., Research Triangle Park, NC 27709
ZOFRAN ODT Orally Disintegrating Tablets:
Manufactured for Glaxo Wellcome Inc.
Research Triangle Park, NC 27709
by Scherer DDS, Blagrove, Swindon, Wiltshire, UK SN5 8RU
US Patent Nos. 4,695,578; 4,753,789; 5,344,658; and 5,578,628

February 2000/RL-798

Shown in Product Identification Guide, page 317

ZOVIRAX® ℞
[*zō vī′rax*]
(acyclovir)
Capsules

ZOVIRAX® ℞
(acyclovir)
Tablets

ZOVIRAX® ℞
(acyclovir)
Suspension

DESCRIPTION

ZOVIRAX is the brand name for acyclovir, a synthetic nucleoside analogue active against herpesviruses. ZOVIRAX Capsules, Tablets, and Suspension are formulations for oral administration. Each capsule of ZOVIRAX contains 200 mg of acyclovir and the inactive ingredients corn starch, lactose, magnesium stearate, and sodium lauryl sulfate. The capsule shell consists of gelatin, FD&C Blue No. 2, and titanium dioxide. May contain one or more parabens. Printed with edible black ink.

Each 800-mg tablet of ZOVIRAX contains 800 mg of acyclovir and the inactive ingredients FD&C Blue No. 2, magnesium stearate, microcrystalline cellulose, povidone, and sodium starch glycolate.

Each 400-mg tablet of ZOVIRAX contains 400 mg of acyclovir and the inactive ingredients magnesium stearate, microcrystalline cellulose, povidone, and sodium starch glycolate.

Each teaspoonful (5 mL) of ZOVIRAX Suspension contains 200 mg of acyclovir and the inactive ingredients methylparaben 0.1% and propylparaben 0.02% (added as preservatives), carboxymethylcellulose sodium, flavor, glycerin, microcrystalline cellulose, and sorbitol.

Acyclovir is a white, crystalline powder with the molecular formula $C_8H_{11}N_5O_3$ and a molecular weight of 225. The maximum solubility in water at 37°C is 2.5 mg/mL. The pka's of acyclovir are 2.27 and 9.25.

The chemical name of acyclovir is 2-amino-1,9-dihydro-9-[(2-hydroxyethoxy)methyl]-6*H*-purin-6-one.

VIROLOGY

Mechanism of Antiviral Action: Acyclovir is a synthetic purine nucleoside analogue with in vitro and in vivo inhibitory activity against herpes simplex virus types 1 (HSV-1), 2 (HSV-2), and varicella-zoster virus (VZV). In cell culture, acyclovir's highest antiviral activity is against HSV-1, followed in decreasing order of potency against HSV-2 and VZV.

The inhibitory activity of acyclovir is highly selective due to its affinity for the enzyme thymidine kinase (TK) encoded by HSV and VZV. This viral enzyme converts acyclovir into acyclovir monophosphate, a nucleotide analogue. The monophosphate is further converted into diphosphate by cellular guanylate kinase and into triphosphate by a number of cellular enzymes. In vitro, acyclovir triphosphate stops replication of herpes viral DNA. This is accomplished in 3 ways: 1) competitive inhibition of viral DNA polymerase, 2) incorporation into and termination of the growing viral DNA chain, and 3) inactivation of the viral DNA polymerase. The greater antiviral activity of acyclovir against HSV compared to VZV is due to its more efficient phosphorylation by the viral TK.

Antiviral Activities: The quantitative relationship between the in vitro susceptibility of herpes viruses to antivirals and the clinical response to therapy has not been established in humans, and virus sensitivity testing has not been standardized. Sensitivity testing results, expressed as the concentration of drug required to inhibit by 50% the growth of virus in cell culture (IC_{50}), vary greatly depending upon a number of factors. Using plaque-reduction assays, the IC_{50} against herpes simplex virus isolates ranges from 0.02 to 13.5 mcg/mL for HSV-1 and from 0.01 to 9.9 mcg/mL for HSV-2. The IC_{50} for acyclovir against most laboratory strains and clinical isolates of VZV ranges from 0.12 to 10.8 mcg/mL. Acyclovir also demonstrates activity against the Oka vaccine strain of VZV with a mean IC_{50} of 1.35 mcg/mL.

Drug Resistance: Resistance of HSV and VZV to antiviral nucleoside analogues can result from qualitative or quantitative changes in the viral TK or DNA polymerase. Clinical isolates of HSV and VZV with reduced susceptibility to acyclovir have been recovered from immunocompromised patients, especially with advanced HIV infection.

While most of the acyclovir-resistant mutants isolated thus far from immunocompromised patients have been found to be TK-deficient mutants, other mutants involving the viral TK gene (TK partial and TK altered) and DNA polymerase have been isolated. TK-negative mutants may cause severe disease in infants and immunocompromised adults. The possibility of viral resistance to acyclovir should be considered in patients who show poor clinical response during therapy.

CLINICAL PHARMACOLOGY

Pharmacokinetics: The pharmacokinetics of acyclovir after oral administration have been evaluated in healthy volunteers and in immunocompromised patients with herpes simplex or varicella-zoster virus infection. Acyclovir pharmacokinetic parameters are summarized in Table 1.

Table 1: Acyclovir Pharmacokinetic Characteristics (Range)

Parameter	Range
Plasma protein binding	9% to 33%
Plasma elimination half-life	2.5 to 3.3 hr
Average oral bioavailability	10% to 20%*

* Bioavailability decreases with increasing dose.

In one multiple-dose, cross-over study in healthy subjects (n = 23), it was shown that increases in plasma acyclovir concentrations were less than dose proportional with increasing dose, as shown in Table 2. The decrease in bioavailability is a function of the dose and not the dosage form.

Table 2: Acyclovir Peak and Trough Concentrations at Steady State

Parameter	200 mg	400 mg	800 mg
C^{ss}_{max}	0.83 mcg/mL	1.21 mcg/mL	1.61 mcg/mL
C^{ss}_{trough}	0.46 mcg/mL	0.63 mcg/mL	0.83 mcg/mL

There was no effect of food on the absorption of acyclovir (n = 6); therefore ZOVIRAX Capsules, Tablets, and Suspension may be administered with or without food.

The only known urinary metabolite is 9-[(carboxymethoxy)methyl]guanine.

Special Populations: ***Adults with Impaired Renal Function:*** The half-life and total body clearance of acyclovir are dependent on renal function. A dosage adjustment is recommended for patients with reduced renal function (see DOSAGE AND ADMINISTRATION).

Pediatrics: In general, the pharmacokinetics of acyclovir in pediatric patients is similar to that of adults. Mean half-life after oral doses of 300 mg/m² and 600 mg/m² in pediatric patients ages 7 months to 7 years was 2.6 hours (range 1.59 to 3.74 hours).

Drug Interactions: Coadministration of probenecid with intravenous acyclovir has been shown to increase the mean acyclovir half-life and the area under the concentration-time curve. Urinary excretion and renal clearance were correspondingly reduced.

Clinical Trials: ***Initial Genital Herpes:*** Double-blind, placebo-controlled studies have demonstrated that orally administered ZOVIRAX significantly reduced the duration of acute infection and duration of lesion healing. The duration of pain and new lesion formation was decreased in some patient groups.

Recurrent Genital Herpes: Double-blind, placebo-controlled studies in patients with frequent recurrences (6 or more episodes per year) have shown that orally administered ZOVIRAX given daily for 4 months to 10 years prevented or reduced the frequency and/or severity of recurrences in greater than 95% of patients.

In a study of patients who received ZOVIRAX 400 mg twice daily for 3 years, 45%, 52%, and 63% of patients remained free of recurrences in the first, second, and third years, respectively. Serial analyses of the 3-month recurrence rates for the patients showed that 71% to 87% were recurrence-free in each quarter.

Herpes Zoster Infections: In a double-blind, placebo-controlled study of immunocompetent patients with localized cutaneous zoster infection, ZOVIRAX (800 mg 5 times daily for 10 days) shortened the times to lesion scabbing, healing, and complete cessation of pain, and reduced the duration of viral shedding and the duration of new lesion formation.

In a similar double-blind, placebo-controlled study, ZOVIRAX (800 mg 5 times daily for 7 days) shortened the times to complete lesion scabbing, healing, and cessation of pain, reduced the duration of new lesion formation, and reduced the prevalence of localized zoster-associated neurologic symptoms (paresthesia, dysesthesia, or hyperesthesia).

Treatment was begun within 72 hours of rash onset and was most effective if started within the first 48 hours.

Adults greater than 50 years of age showed greater benefit.

Chickenpox: Three randomized, double-blind, placebo-controlled trials were conducted in 993 pediatric patients ages 2 to 18 years with chickenpox. All patients were treated within 24 hours after the onset of rash. In 2 trials, ZOVIRAX was administered at 20 mg/kg 4 times daily (up to 3200 mg per day) for 5 days. In the third trial, doses of 10, 15, or 20 mg/kg were administered 4 times daily for 5 to 7 days. Treatment with ZOVIRAX shortened the time to 50% healing, reduced the maximum number of lesions, reduced the median number of vesicles, decreased the median number of residual lesions on day 28, and decreased the proportion of patients with fever, anorexia, and lethargy by day 2. Treatment with ZOVIRAX did not affect varicella-zoster virus-specific humoral or cellular immune responses at 1 month or 1 year following treatment.

INDICATIONS AND USAGE

Herpes Zoster Infections: ZOVIRAX is indicated for the acute treatment of herpes zoster (shingles).

Genital Herpes: ZOVIRAX is indicated for the treatment of initial episodes and the management of recurrent episodes of genital herpes.

Chickenpox: ZOVIRAX is indicated for the treatment of chickenpox (varicella).

CONTRAINDICATIONS

ZOVIRAX is contraindicated for patients who develop hypersensitivity to acyclovir or valacyclovir.

WARNINGS

ZOVIRAX Capsules, Tablets, and Suspension are intended for oral ingestion only. Renal failure, in some cases resulting in death, has been observed with acyclovir therapy (see ADVERSE REACTIONS: Observed During Clinical Practice and OVERDOSAGE). Thrombotic thrombocytopenic purpura/hemolytic uremic syndrome (TTP/HUS), which has resulted in death, has occurred in immunocompromised patients receiving acyclovir therapy.

PRECAUTIONS

Dosage adjustment is recommended when administering ZOVIRAX to patients with renal impairment (see DOSAGE AND ADMINISTRATION). Caution should also be exercised when administering ZOVIRAX to patients receiving potentially nephrotoxic agents since this may increase the risk of renal dysfunction and/or the risk of reversible central nervous system symptoms such as those that have been reported in patients treated with intravenous acyclovir.

Information for Patients: Patients are instructed to consult with their physician if they experience severe or troublesome adverse reactions, they become pregnant or intend to become pregnant, they intend to breastfeed while taking orally administered ZOVIRAX, or they have any other questions.

Herpes Zoster: There are no data on treatment initiated more than 72 hours after onset of the zoster rash. Patients should be advised to initiate treatment as soon as possible after a diagnosis of herpes zoster.

Genital Herpes Infections: Patients should be informed that ZOVIRAX is not a cure for genital herpes. There are no data evaluating whether ZOVIRAX will prevent transmission of infection to others. Because genital herpes is a sexually transmitted disease, patients should avoid contact with lesions or intercourse when lesions and/or symptoms are present to avoid infecting partners. Genital herpes can also be transmitted in the absence of symptoms through asymptomatic viral shedding. If medical management of a genital herpes recurrence is indicated, patients should be advised to initiate therapy at the first sign or symptom of an episode.

Chickenpox: Chickenpox in otherwise healthy children is usually a self-limited disease of mild to moderate severity. Adolescents and adults tend to have more severe disease. Treatment was initiated within 24 hours of the typical chickenpox rash in the controlled studies, and there is no information regarding the effects of treatment begun later in the disease course.

Drug Interactions: See CLINICAL PHARMACOLOGY: Pharmacokinetics.

Carcinogenesis, Mutagenesis, Impairment of Fertility: The data presented below include references to peak steady-state plasma acyclovir concentrations observed in humans treated with 800 mg given orally 6 times a day (dosing appropriate for treatment of herpes zoster) or 200 mg given orally 6 times a day (dosing appropriate for treatment of genital herpes). Plasma drug concentrations in animal studies are expressed as multiples of human exposure to acyclovir at the higher and lower dosing schedules (see CLINICAL PHARMACOLOGY: Pharmacokinetics).

Table 3: Dosage Modification for Renal Impairment

Normal Dosage Regimen	Creatinine Clearance (mL/min/1.73 m^2)	Adjusted Dosage Regimen: Dose (mg)	Adjusted Dosage Regimen: Dosing Interval
200 mg every 4 hours	>10	200	every 4 hours, 5x daily
	0-10	200	every 12 hours
400 mg every 12 hours	>10	400	every 12 hours
	0–10	200	every 12 hours
800 mg every 4 hours	>25	800	every 4 hours, 5x daily
	10–25	800	every 8 hours
	0–10	800	every 12 hours

Acyclovir was tested in lifetime bioassays in rats and mice at single daily doses of up to 450 mg/kg administered by gavage. There was no statistically significant difference in the incidence of tumors between treated and control animals, nor did acyclovir shorten the latency of tumors. Maximum plasma concentrations were 3 to 6 times human levels in the mouse bioassay and 1 to 2 times human levels in the rat bioassay.

Acyclovir was tested in 16 genetic toxicity assays. No evidence of mutagenicity was observed in 4 microbial assays. Acyclovir demonstrated mutagenic activity in 2 in vitro cytogenetic assays (1 mouse lymphoma cell line and human lymphocytes). No mutagenic activity was observed in 5 in vitro cytogenetic assays (3 Chinese hamster ovary cell lines and 2 mouse lymphoma cell lines).

A positive result was demonstrated in 1 of 2 in vitro cell transformation assays, and morphologically transformed cells obtained in this assay formed tumors when inoculated into immunosuppressed, syngeneic, weanling mice. No activity was demonstrated in another, possibly less sensitive, in vitro cell transformation assay.

Acyclovir caused chromosomal damage in Chinese hamsters at 380 to 760 times human dose levels. In rats, acyclovir produced a nonsignificant increase in chromosomal damage at 62 to 125 times human levels. No activity was observed in a dominant lethal study in mice at 36 to 73 times human levels.

Acyclovir did not impair fertility or reproduction in mice (450 mg/kg per day, PO) or in rats (25 mg/kg per day, SC). In the mouse study, plasma levels were 9 to 18 times human levels, while in the rat study, they were 8 to 15 times human levels. At higher doses (50 mg/kg per day, SC) in rats and rabbits (11 to 22 and 16 to 31 times human levels, respectively) implantation efficacy, but not litter size, was decreased. In a rat peri- and post-natal study at 50 mg/kg per day, SC, there was a statistically significant decrease in group mean numbers of corpora lutea, total implantation sites, and live fetuses.

No testicular abnormalities were seen in dogs given 50 mg/kg per day, IV for 1 month (21 to 41 times human levels) or in dogs given 60 mg/kg per day orally for 1 year (6 to 12 times human levels). Testicular atrophy and aspermatogenesis were observed in rats and dogs at higher dose levels.

Pregnancy: ***Teratogenic Effects:*** Pregnancy Category B. Acyclovir was not teratogenic in the mouse (450 mg/kg per day, PO), rabbit (50 mg/kg per day, SC and IV), or rat (50 mg/kg per day, SC). These exposures resulted in plasma levels 9 and 18, 16 and 106, and 11 and 22 times, respectively, human levels.

There are no adequate and well-controlled studies in pregnant women. A prospective epidemiologic registry of acyclovir use during pregnancy was established in 1984 and completed in April 1999. There were 756 pregnancies followed in women exposed to systemic acyclovir during the first trimester of pregnancy. The occurrence rate of birth defects approximates that found in the general population. However, the small size of the registry is insufficient to evaluate the risk for less common defects or to permit reliable or definitive conclusions regarding the safety of acyclovir in pregnant women and their developing fetuses. Acyclovir should be used during pregnancy only if the potential benefit justifies the potential risk to the fetus.

Nursing Mothers: Acyclovir concentrations have been documented in breast milk in 2 women following oral administration of ZOVIRAX and ranged from 0.6 to 4.1 times corresponding plasma levels. These concentrations would potentially expose the nursing infant to a dose of acyclovir up to 0.3 mg/kg per day. ZOVIRAX should be administered to a nursing mother with caution and only when indicated.

Geriatric Use: Clinical studies of ZOVIRAX did not include sufficient numbers of patients aged 65 and over to determine whether they respond differently than younger patients. Other reported clinical experience has not identified differences in responses between elderly and younger patients. In general, dose selection for an elderly patient should be cautious, usually starting at the low end of the dosing range, reflecting the greater frequency of decreased renal function, and of concomitant disease or other drug therapy.

Pediatric Use: Safety and effectiveness in pediatric patients less than 2 years of age have not been adequately studied.

ADVERSE REACTIONS

Herpes Simplex: ***Short-Term Administration:*** The most frequent adverse events reported during clinical trials of treatment of genital herpes with ZOVIRAX 200 mg administered orally 5 times daily every 4 hours for 10 days were nausea and/or vomiting in 8 of 298 patient treatments (2.7%). Nausea and/or vomiting occurred in 2 of 287 (0.7%) patients who received placebo.

Long-Term Administration: The most frequent adverse events reported in a clinical trial for the prevention of recurrences with continuous administration of 400 mg (two 200-mg capsules) 2 times daily for 1 year in 586 patients treated with ZOVIRAX were nausea (4.8%) and diarrhea (2.4%). The 589 control patients receiving intermittent treatment of recurrences with ZOVIRAX for 1 year reported diarrhea (2.7%), nausea (2.4%), and headache (2.2%).

Herpes Zoster: The most frequent adverse event reported during 3 clinical trials of treatment of herpes zoster (shingles) with 800 mg of oral ZOVIRAX 5 times daily for 7 to 10 days in 323 patients was malaise (11.5%). The 323 placebo recipients reported malaise (11.1%).

Chickenpox: The most frequent adverse event reported during 3 clinical trials of treatment of chickenpox with oral ZOVIRAX at doses of 10 to 20 mg/kg 4 times daily for 5 to 7 days or 800 mg 4 times daily for 5 days in 495 patients was diarrhea (3.2%). The 498 patients receiving placebo reported diarrhea (2.2%).

Observed During Clinical Practice: In addition to adverse events reported from clinical trials, the following events have been identified during post-approval use of ZOVIRAX. Because they are reported voluntarily from a population of unknown size, estimates of frequency cannot be made. These events have been chosen for inclusion due to either their seriousness, frequency of reporting, potential causal connection to ZOVIRAX, or a combination of these factors.

General: Anaphylaxis, fever, headache, pain, peripheral edema.

Nervous: Agitation, coma, confusion, delirium, dizziness, hallucinations, paresthesia, psychosis, seizure, somnolence. These symptoms may be marked, particularly in older adults (see PRECAUTIONS).

Digestive: Diarrhea, gastrointestinal distress, nausea.

Hemic and Lymphatic: Leukopenia, lymphadenopathy, thrombocytopenia.

Hepatobiliary Tract and Pancreas: Elevated liver function tests, hepatitis, jaundice.

Musculoskeletal: Myalgia.

Skin: Alopecia, erythema multiforme, photosensitive rash, pruritus, rash, Stevens-Johnson syndrome, toxic epidermal necrolysis, urticaria.

Special Senses: Visual abnormalities.

Urogenital: Renal failure, elevated blood urea nitrogen, elevated creatinine, hematuria (see WARNINGS).

OVERDOSAGE

Overdoses involving ingestion of up to 100 capsules (20 g) have been reported. Adverse events that have been reported only in association with overdosage include convulsions and lethargy. Precipitation of acyclovir in renal tubules may occur when the solubility (2.5 mg/mL) is exceeded in the intratubular fluid. Overdosage has been reported following bolus injections or inappropriately high doses and in patients whose fluid and electrolyte balance were not properly monitored. This has resulted in elevated BUN and serum creatinine and subsequent renal failure. In the event of acute renal failure and anuria, the patient may benefit from hemodialysis until renal function is restored (see DOSAGE AND ADMINISTRATION).

DOSAGE AND ADMINISTRATION

Acute Treatment of Herpes Zoster: 800 mg every 4 hours orally, 5 times daily for 7 to 10 days.

Genital Herpes: ***Treatment of Initial Genital Herpes:*** 200 mg every 4 hours, 5 times daily for 10 days.

Continued on next page

This product information is based on labeling in effect on June 23, 2000. For further information, contact via direct mail, phone, or web site. Medical Information, Glaxo Wellcome Inc., PO Box 13398, Research Triangle Park, NC 27709. Healthcare Professionals (Medical Information): 800-334-0089. Patients (Customer Response Center): 1-888-825-5249. Glaxo Wellcome Corporate Web Site: www.glaxowellcome.com

Zovirax Caps/Tabs/Susp.—Cont.

Chronic Suppressive Therapy for Recurrent Disease: 400 mg 2 times daily for up to 12 months, followed by re-evaluation. Alternative regimens have included doses ranging from 200 mg 3 times daily to 200 mg 5 times daily.
The frequency and severity of episodes of untreated genital herpes may change over time. After 1 year of therapy, the frequency and severity of the patient's genital herpes infection should be re-evaluated to assess the need for continuation of therapy with ZOVIRAX.
Intermittent Therapy: 200 mg every 4 hours, 5 times daily for 5 days. Therapy should be initiated at the earliest sign or symptom (prodrome) of recurrence.
Treatment of Chickenpox: ***Children (2 years of age and older):*** 20 mg/kg **per dose** orally 4 times daily (80 mg/kg per day) for 5 days. Children over 40 kg should receive the adult dose for chickenpox.
Adults and Children over 40 kg: 800 mg 4 times daily for 5 days.
Intravenous ZOVIRAX is indicated for the treatment of varicella-zoster infections in immunocompromised patients.
When therapy is indicated, it should be initiated at the earliest sign or symptom of chickenpox. There is no information about the efficacy of therapy initiated more than 24 hours after onset of signs and symptoms.
Patients With Acute or Chronic Renal Impairment: In patients with renal impairment, the dose of ZOVIRAX Capsules, Tablets, or Suspension should be modified as shown in Table 3:
[See table 3 at top of previous page]
Hemodialysis: For patients who require hemodialysis, the mean plasma half-life of acyclovir during hemodialysis is approximately 5 hours. This results in a 60% decrease in plasma concentrations following a 6-hour dialysis period. Therefore, the patient's dosing schedule should be adjusted so that an additional dose is administered after each dialysis.
Peritoneal Dialysis: No supplemental dose appears to be necessary after adjustment of the dosing interval.
Bioequivalence of Dosage Forms: ZOVIRAX Suspension was shown to be bioequivalent to ZOVIRAX Capsules (n = 20) and 1 ZOVIRAX 800-mg tablet was shown to be bioequivalent to 4 ZOVIRAX 200-mg capsules (n = 24).

HOW SUPPLIED

ZOVIRAX Capsules (blue, opaque cap and body) containing 200 mg acyclovir and printed with "Wellcome ZOVIRAX 200"—Bottle of 100 (NDC 0173-0991-55) and unit dose pack of 100 (NDC 0173-0991-56).
Store at 15° to 25°C (59° to 77°F) and protect from moisture.
ZOVIRAX Tablets (light blue, oval) containing 800 mg acyclovir and engraved with "ZOVIRAX 800"—Bottle of 100 (NDC 0173-0945-55) and unit dose pack of 100 (NDC 0173-0945-56).
Store at 15° to 25°C (59° to 77°F) and protect from moisture.
ZOVIRAX Tablets (white, shield-shaped) containing 400 mg acyclovir and engraved with "ZOVIRAX" on one side and a triangle on the other side—Bottle of 100 (NDC 0173-0949-55).
Store at 15° to 25°C (59° to 77°F) and protect from moisture.
ZOVIRAX Suspension (off-white, banana-flavored) containing 200 mg acyclovir in each teaspoonful (5 mL)—Bottle of 1 pint (473 mL) (NDC 0173-0953-96).
Store at 15° to 25°C (59° to 77°F).
Glaxo Wellcome Inc., Research Triangle Park, NC 27709

March 2000/RL-804
Shown in Product Identification Guide, page 317

ZOVIRAX® ℞
[zō-vī ′răx]
(acyclovir)
Ointment 5%

DESCRIPTION

ZOVIRAX is the brand name for acyclovir, an antiviral drug active against herpes viruses. ZOVIRAX Ointment 5% is a formulation for topical administration. Each gram of ZOVIRAX Ointment 5% contains 50 mg of acyclovir in a polyethylene glycol (PEG) base.
The chemical name of acyclovir is 2-amino-1,9-dihydro-9-[(2-hydroxyethoxy)methyl]-6*H*-purin-6-one.
Acyclovir is a white, crystalline powder with a molecular weight of 225 daltons, and a maximum solubility in water of 1.3 mg/mL.

CLINICAL PHARMACOLOGY

Acyclovir is a synthetic acyclic purine nucleoside analogue with in vitro inhibitory activity against Herpes simplex types 1 and 2 (HSV-1 and HSV-2), varicella-zoster, Epstein-Barr, and cytomegalovirus. In cell cultures, the inhibitory activity of acyclovir for Herpes simplex virus is highly selective. Cellular thymidine kinase does not effectively utilize acyclovir as a substrate. Herpes simplex virus-coded thymidine kinase, however, converts acyclovir into acyclovir monophosphate, a nucleotide. The monophosphate is further converted into diphosphate by cellular guanylate kinase and into triphosphate by a number of cellular enzymes.[1] Acyclovir triphosphate interferes with Herpes simplex virus DNA polymerase and inhibits viral DNA replication. Acyclovir triphosphate also inhibits cellular α-DNA polymerase but to a lesser degree. In vitro, acyclovir triphosphate can be incorporated into growing chains of DNA by viral DNA polymerase and to a much smaller extent by cellular α-DNA polymerase.[2] When incorporation occurs, the DNA chain is terminated.[3] Acyclovir is preferentially taken up and selectively converted to the active triphosphate form by herpes-virus-infected cells. Thus, acyclovir is much less toxic in vitro for normal uninfected cells because: 1) less is taken up; 2) less is converted to the active form; 3) cellular α-DNA polymerase is less sensitive to the effects of the active form.
The relationship between in vitro susceptibility of Herpes simplex virus to antiviral drugs and clinical response has not been established. The techniques and cell culture types used for determining in vitro susceptibility may influence the results obtained. Using a quantitative assay to determine the acyclovir concentration producing 50% inhibition of viral cytopathic effect (ID_{50}), 28 HSV-1 clinical isolates had a mean ID_{50} of 0.17 mcg/mL and 32 HSV-2 clinical isolates had a mean ID_{50} of 0.46 mcg/mL.* Results from other studies using different assays have yielded mean ID_{50} values for clinical HSV-1 isolates of 0.018, 0.03, and 0.043 mcg/mL and for clinical HSV-2 isolates of 0.027, 0.36, and 0.03 mcg/mL, respectively.[4,5,6]
Two clinical pharmacology studies were performed with ZOVIRAX Ointment 5% in adult immunocompromised patients at risk of developing mucocutaneous Herpes simplex virus infections or with localized varicella-zoster infections. These studies were designed to evaluate the dermal tolerance, systemic toxicity, and percutaneous absorption of acyclovir.
In one of these studies, which included 16 inpatients, the complete ointment or its vehicle were randomly administered in a dose of 1-cm strips (25 mg acyclovir) four times a day for 7 days to an intact skin surface area of 4.5 square inches. No local intolerance, systemic toxicity, or contact dermatitis were observed. In addition, no drug was detected in blood and urine by radioimmunoassay (sensitivity, 0.01 mcg/mL).
The other study included 11 patients with localized varicella-zoster. In this uncontrolled study, acyclovir was detected in the blood of nine patients and in the urine of all patients tested. Acyclovir levels in plasma ranged from <0.01 to 0.28 mcg/mL in eight patients with normal renal function, and from <0.01 to 0.78 mcg/mL in one patient with impaired renal function. Acyclovir excreted in the urine ranged from <0.02% to 9.4% of the daily dose. Therefore, systemic absorption of acyclovir after topical application is minimal.

INDICATIONS AND USAGE

ZOVIRAX (acyclovir) Ointment 5% is indicated in the management of initial herpes genitalis and in limited nonlife-threatening mucocutaneous Herpes simplex virus infections in immunocompromised patients. In clinical trials of initial herpes genitalis, ZOVIRAX Ointment 5% has shown a decrease in healing time and, in some cases, a decrease in duration of viral shedding and duration of pain. In studies in immunocompromised patients with mainly herpes labialis, there was a decrease in duration of viral shedding and a slight decrease in duration of pain.
By contrast, in studies of recurrent herpes genitalis and of herpes labialis in nonimmunocompromised patients, there was no evidence of clinical benefit; there was some decrease in duration of viral shedding.
Diagnosis: Whereas cutaneous lesions associated with Herpes simplex infections are often characteristic, the finding of multinucleated giant cells in smears prepared from lesion exudate or scrapings may assist in the diagnosis.[7] Positive cultures for Herpes simplex virus offer a reliable means for confirmation of the diagnosis. In genital herpes, appropriate examinations should be performed to rule out other sexually transmitted diseases.

CONTRAINDICATIONS

ZOVIRAX Ointment 5% is contraindicated for patients who develop hypersensitivity or chemical intolerance to the components of the formulation.

WARNINGS

ZOVIRAX Ointment 5% is intended for cutaneous use only and should not be used in the eye.

PRECAUTIONS

General: The recommended dosage, frequency of applications, and length of treatment should not be exceeded (see DOSAGE AND ADMINISTRATION). There exist no data which demonstrate that the use of ZOVIRAX Ointment 5% will either prevent transmission of infection to other persons or prevent recurrent infections when applied in the absence of signs and symptoms. ZOVIRAX Ointment 5% should not be used for the prevention of recurrent HSV infections. Although clinically significant viral resistance associated with the use of ZOVIRAX Ointment 5% has not been observed, this possibility exists.
Drug Interactions: Clinical experience has identified no interactions resulting from topical or systemic administration of other drugs concomitantly with ZOVIRAX Ointment 5%.
Carcinogenesis, Mutagenesis, Impairment of Fertility: Acyclovir was tested in lifetime bioassays in rats and mice at single daily doses of 50, 150, and 450 mg/kg per day given by gavage. These studies showed no statistically significant difference in the incidence of benign and malignant tumors produced in drug-treated as compared to control animals, nor did acyclovir induce the occurrence of tumors earlier in drug-treated animals as compared to controls. In two in vitro cell transformation assays, used to provide preliminary assessment of potential oncogenicity in advance of these more definitive lifetime bioassays in rodents, conflicting results were obtained. Acyclovir was positive at the highest dose used in one system and the resulting morphologically transformed cells formed tumors when inoculated into immunosuppressed, syngeneic, weanling mice. Acyclovir was negative in another transformation system.
No chromosome damage was observed at maximum tolerated parenteral doses of 100 mg/kg acyclovir in rats or Chinese hamsters; higher doses of 500 and 1000 mg/kg were clastogenic in Chinese hamsters. In addition, no activity was found in a dominant lethal study in mice. In nine of 11 microbial and mammalian cell assays, no evidence of mutagenicity was observed. In two mammalian cell assays (human lymphocytes and L5178Y mouse lymphoma cells in vitro), positive response for mutagenicity and chromosomal damage occurred, but only at concentrations at least 1000 times the plasma levels achieved in humans following topical application.
Acyclovir does not impair fertility or reproduction in mice at oral doses up to 450 mg/kg per day or in rats at subcutaneous doses up to 25 mg/kg per day. In rabbits given a high dose of acyclovir (50 mg/kg per day, SC), there was a statistically significant decrease in implantation efficiency.
Pregnancy: ***Teratogenic Effects:*** Pregnancy Category C. Acyclovir was not teratogenic in the mouse (450 mg/kg per day, PO), rabbit (50 mg/kg per day, SC and IV) or in standard tests in the rat (50 mg/kg per day, SC). In a nonstandard test in rats, fetal abnormalities, such as head and tail anomalies, were observed following subcutaneous administration of acyclovir at very high doses associated with toxicity to the maternal rat. The clinical relevance of these findings is uncertain.[8] There are no adequate and well-controlled studies in pregnant women. Acyclovir should not be used during pregnancy unless the potential benefit justifies the potential risk to the fetus.
Nursing Mothers: It is not known whether topically applied acyclovir is excreted in breast milk. After oral administration of ZOVIRAX, acyclovir concentrations have been documented in breast milk in two women and ranged from 0.6 to 4.1 times the corresponding plasma levels.[9,10] Caution should be exercised when ZOVIRAX Ointment is administered to a nursing woman.
Pediatric Use: Safety and effectiveness in pediatric patients have not been established.

ADVERSE REACTIONS

Because ulcerated genital lesions are characteristically tender and sensitive to any contact or manipulation, patients may experience discomfort upon application of ointment. In the controlled clinical trials, mild pain (including transient burning and stinging) was reported by 103 (28.3%) of 364 patients treated with acyclovir and by 115 (31.1%) of 370 patients treated with placebo; treatment was discontinued in two of these patients. Other local reactions among acyclovir-treated patients included pruritus in 15 (4.1%), rash in one (0.3%), and vulvitis in one (0.3%). Among the placebo-treated patients, pruritus was reported by 17 (4.6%) and rash by one (0.3%).
In all studies, there was no significant difference between the drug and placebo group in the rate or type of reported adverse reactions nor were there any differences in abnormal clinical laboratory findings.
Observed During Clinical Practice: Based on clinical practice experience in patients treated with ZOVIRAX Ointment in the US, spontaneously reported adverse events are uncommon. Data are insufficient to support an estimate of their incidence or to establish causation. These events may also occur as part of the underlying disease process. Voluntary reports of adverse events which have been received since market introduction include:
General: Edema and/or pain at the application site
Skin: Pruritus, rash

OVERDOSAGE

Overdosage by topical application of ZOVIRAX Ointment 5% is unlikely because of limited transcutaneous absorption (see CLINICAL PHARMACOLOGY).

DOSAGE AND ADMINISTRATION

Apply sufficient quantity to adequately cover all lesions every 3 hours, six times per day for 7 days. The dose size per application will vary depending upon the total lesion area but should approximate a one-half inch ribbon of ointment per 4 square inches of surface area. A finger cot or rubber glove should be used when applying ZOVIRAX to prevent autoinoculation of other body sites and transmission of infection to other persons. **Therapy should be initiated as early as possible following onset of signs and symptoms.**

HOW SUPPLIED

ZOVIRAX Ointment 5% is supplied in 15-g tubes (NDC 0173-0993-94) and 3-g tubes (NDC 0173-0993-41). Each gram contains 50 mg acyclovir in a polyethylene glycol base.
Store at 15° to 25°C (59° to 77°F) in a dry place.

ANIMAL PHARMACOLOGY AND ANIMAL TOXICOLOGY

Topical treatment of guinea pigs with 10% acyclovir in polyethylene glycol ointment for 3 weeks did not result in cu-

taneous irritation or systemic toxicity. Also, a wide variety of animal tests by parenteral routes demonstrated that acyclovir has a low order of toxicity.
Acyclovir did not cause dermal sensitization in guinea pigs.

REFERENCES

1. Miller WH, Miller RL. Phosphorylation of acyclovir (acycloguanosine) monophosphate by GMP kinase. *J Biol Chem.* 1980;255:7204-7207.
2. Furman PA, St. Clair MH, Fyfe JA, et al. Inhibition of herpes simplex virus-induced DNA polymerase activity and viral DNA replication by 9-(2-hydroxyethoxymethyl)guanine and its triphosphate. *J Virol.* 1979; 32:72-77.
3. Derse D, Cheng YC, Furman PA, et al. Inhibition of purified human and herpes simplex virus-induced DNA polymerases by 9-(2-hydroxyethoxymethyl)guanine triphosphate: effects on primer-template function. *J Biol Chem.* 1981;256:11447-11451.
4. Collins P, Bauer DJ. The activity in vitro against herpes virus of 9-(2-hydroxyethoxymethyl)guanine (acycloguanosine), a new antiviral agent. *J Antimicrob Chemother.* 1979;5:431-436.
5. Crumpacker CS, Schnipper LE, Zaia JA, et al. Growth inhibition of acycloguanosine of herpesviruses isolated from human infections. *Antimicrob Agents Chemother.* 1979;15:642-645.
6. DeClercq E, Descamps J, Verhelst G, et al. Comparative efficacy of antiherpes drugs against different strains of herpes simplex virus. *J Infect Dis.* 1980;141:563-574.
7. Naib ZM, Nahmias AJ, Josey WE, et al. Relation of cytohistopathology of genital herpesvirus infection to cervical anaplasia. *Cancer Res.* 1973;33:1452-1463.
8. Stahlmann R, Klug S, Lewandowski C, et al. Teratogenicity of acyclovir in rats. *Infection.* 1987;15:261-262.
9. Lau RJ, Emery MG, Galinsky RE, et al. Unexpected accumulation of acyclovir in breast milk with estimate of infant exposure. *Obstet Gynecol.* 1987;69:468-471.
10. Meyer LJ, deMiranda P, Sheth N, et al. Acyclovir in human breast milk. *Am J Obstet Gynecol.* 1988;158: 586-588.

*Data on file at Glaxo Wellcome Inc.
Glaxo Wellcome Inc., Research Triangle Park, NC 27709

March 1998/RL-552

Shown in Product Identification Guide, page 317

ZOVIRAX® ℞
[*zō vī′răx*]
(acyclovir sodium)
for Injection
FOR INTRAVENOUS INFUSION ONLY

DESCRIPTION

ZOVIRAX is the brand name for acyclovir, a synthetic nucleoside analog active against herpesviruses. Acyclovir sodium for injection is a sterile lyophilized powder for intravenous administration only. Each 500-mg vial contains 500 mg of acyclovir and 49 mg of sodium, and each 1000-mg vial contains 1000 mg acyclovir and 98 mg of sodium. Reconstitution of the 500-mg or 1000-mg vials with 10 mL or 20 mL, respectively, of Sterile Water for Injection, USP results in a solution containing 50 mg/mL of acyclovir. The pH of the reconstituted solution is approximately 11. Further dilution in any appropriate intravenous solution must be performed before infusion (see DOSAGE AND ADMINISTRATION: Method of Preparation and Administration).
Acyclovir sodium is a white, crystalline powder with the molecular formula $C_8H_{10}N_5NaO_3$ and a molecular weight of 247.19. The maximum solubility in water at 25°C exceeds 100 mg/mL. At physiologic pH, acyclovir sodium exists as the un-ionized form with a molecular weight of 225 and a maximum solubility in water at 37°C of 2.5 mg/mL. The pka's of acyclovir are 2.27 and 9.25.
The chemical name of acyclovir sodium is 2-amino-1,9-dihydro-9-[(2-hydroxyethoxy)methyl]-6*H*-purin-6-one monosodium salt.

VIROLOGY

Mechanism of Antiviral Action: Acyclovir is a synthetic purine nucleoside analogue with in vitro and in vivo inhibitory activity against herpes simplex virus types 1 (HSV-1), 2 (HSV-2), and varicella-zoster virus (VZV). In cell culture, acyclovir's highest antiviral activity is against HSV-1, followed in decreasing order of potency against HSV-2 and VZV.
The inhibitory activity of acyclovir is highly selective due to its affinity for the enzyme thymidine kinase (TK) encoded by HSV and VZV. This viral enzyme converts acyclovir into acyclovir monophosphate, a nucleotide analogue. The monophosphate is further converted into diphosphate by cellular guanylate kinase and into triphosphate by a number of cellular enzymes. In vitro, acyclovir triphosphate stops replication of herpes viral DNA. This is accomplished in 3 ways: 1) competitive inhibition of viral DNA polymerase, 2) incorporation into and termination of the growing viral DNA chain, and 3) inactivation of the viral DNA polymerase. The greater antiviral activity of acyclovir against HSV compared to VZV is due to its more efficient phosphorylation by the viral TK.
Antiviral Activities: The quantitative relationship between the in vitro susceptibility of herpes viruses to antivirals and the clinical response to therapy has not been established in humans, and virus sensitivity testing has not been standardized. Sensitivity testing results, expressed as the concentration of drug required to inhibit by 50% the growth of virus in cell culture (IC_{50}), vary greatly depending upon a number of factors. Using plaque-reduction assays, the IC_{50} against herpes simplex virus isolates ranges from 0.02 to 13.5 mcg/mL for HSV-1 and from 0.01 to 9.9 mcg/mL for HSV-2. The IC_{50} for acyclovir against most laboratory strains and clinical isolates of VZV ranges from 0.12 to 10.8 mcg/mL. Acyclovir also demonstrates activity against the Oka vaccine strain of VZV with a mean IC_{50} of 1.35 mcg/mL.
Drug Resistance: Resistance of HSV and VZV to antiviral nucleoside analogues can result from qualitative or quantitative changes in the viral TK or DNA polymerase. Clinical isolates of HSV and VZV with reduced susceptibility to acyclovir have been recovered from immunocompromised patients, especially with advanced HIV infection. While most of the acyclovir-resistant mutants isolated thus far from such patients have been found to be TK-deficient mutants, other mutants involving the viral TK gene (TK partial and TK altered) and DNA polymerase have been isolated. TK-negative mutants may cause severe disease in infants and immunocompromised adults. The possibility of viral resistance to acyclovir should be considered in patients who show poor clinical response during therapy.

CLINICAL PHARMACOLOGY

Pharmacokinetics: The pharmacokinetics of acyclovir after intravenous administration have been evaluated in adult patients with normal renal function during Phase 1/2 studies after single doses ranging from 0.5 to 15 mg/kg and after multiple doses ranging from 2.5 to 15 mg/kg every 8 hours. Proportionality between dose and plasma levels is seen after single doses or at steady state after multiple dosing. Average steady-state peak and trough concentrations from 1-hour infusions administered every 8 hours are given in Table 1.

Table 1: Acyclovir Peak and Trough Concentrations at Steady State

Dosage Regimen	C^{ss}_{max}	C^{ss}_{trough}
5 mg/kg q 8 h (n = 8)	9.8 mcg/mL range: 5.5 to 13.8	0.7 mcg/mL range: 0.2 to 1.0
10 mg/kg q 8 h (n = 7)	22.9 mcg/mL range: 14.1 to 44.1	1.9 mcg/mL range: 0.5 to 2.9

Concentrations achieved in the cerebrospinal fluid are approximately 50% of plasma values. Plasma protein binding is relatively low (9% to 33%) and drug interactions involving binding site displacement are not anticipated.
Renal excretion of unchanged drug is the major route of acyclovir elimination accounting for 62% to 91% of the dose. The only major urinary metabolite detected is 9-carboxymethoxymethylguanine accounting for up to 14.1% of the dose in patients with normal renal function.
The half-life and total body clearance of acyclovir are dependent on renal function as shown in Table 2.
[See table 2 above]

Table 2: Acyclovir Half-life and Total Body Clearance

Creatinine Clearance (mL/min per 1.73 m²)	Half-life (h)	Total Body Clearance	
		(mL/min per 1.73 m²)	(mL/min per kg)
>80	2.5	327	5.1
50 – 80	3.0	248	3.9
15 – 50	3.5	190	3.4
0 (Anuric)	19.5	29	0.5

Special Populations: ***Adults With Impaired Renal Function:*** ZOVIRAX was administered at a dose of 2.5 mg/kg to 6 adult patients with severe renal failure. The peak and trough plasma levels during the 47 hours preceding hemodialysis were 8.5 mcg/mL and 0.7 mcg/mL, respectively.
Consult DOSAGE AND ADMINISTRATION section for recommended adjustments in dosing based upon creatinine clearance.
Pediatrics: Acyclovir pharmacokinetics were determined in 16 pediatric patients with normal renal function ranging in age from 3 months to 16 years at doses of approximately 10 mg/kg and 20 mg/kg every 8 hours (Table 3). Concentrations achieved at these regimens are similar to those in adults receiving 5 mg/kg and 10 mg/kg every 8 hours, respectively (Table 1). Acyclovir pharmacokinetics were determined in 12 patients ranging in age from birth to 3 months at doses of 5 mg/kg, 10 mg/kg, and 15 mg/kg every 8 hours (Table 3).
[See table 3 above]

Table 3: Acyclovir Pharmacokinetics in Pediatric Patients (Mean ± SD)

Parameter	Birth to 3 Months of Age (n = 12)	3 Months to 12 Years of Age (n = 16)
CL (mL/min per kg)	4.46 ± 1.61	8.44 ± 2.92
VDSS (L/kg)	1.08 ± 0.35	1.01 ± 0.28
Elimination Half-life (h)	3.80 ± 1.19	2.36 ± 0.97

Drug Interactions: Coadministration of probenecid with acyclovir has been shown to increase the mean acyclovir half-life and the area under the concentration-time curve. Urinary excretion and renal clearance were correspondingly reduced.
Clinical Trials: ***Herpes Simplex Infections in Immunocompromised Patients:*** A multicenter trial of ZOVIRAX for Injection at a dose of 250 mg/m² every 8 hours (750 mg/m² per day) for 7 days was conducted in 98 immunocompromised patients (73 adults and 25 children) with orofacial, esophageal, genital, and other localized infections (52 treated with ZOVIRAX and 46 with placebo). ZOVIRAX decreased virus excretion, reduced pain, and promoted healing of lesions.
Initial Episodes of Herpes Genitalis: In placebo-controlled trials, 58 patients with initial genital herpes were treated with intravenous ZOVIRAX 5 mg/kg or placebo (27 patients treated with ZOVIRAX and 31 treated with placebo) every 8 hours for 5 days. ZOVIRAX decreased the duration of viral excretion, new lesion formation, and duration of vesicles, and promoted healing of lesions.
Herpes Simplex Encephalitis: Sixty-two patients ages 6 months to 79 years with brain biopsy-proven herpes simplex encephalitis were randomized to receive either ZOVIRAX (10 mg/kg every 8 hours) or vidarabine (15 mg/kg per day) for 10 days (28 were treated with ZOVIRAX and 34 with vidarabine). Overall mortality at 12 months for patients treated with ZOVIRAX was 25% compared to 59% for patients treated with vidarabine. The proportion of patients treated with ZOVIRAX functioning normally or with only mild sequelae (e.g., decreased attention span) was 32% compared to 12% of patients treated with vidarabine.
Patients less than 30 years of age and those who had the least severe neurologic involvement at time of entry into study had the best outcome with treatment with ZOVIRAX. An additional controlled study performed in Europe demonstrated similar findings.
Neonatal Herpes Simplex Virus Infection: Two hundred and two infants with neonatal herpes simplex infections were randomized to receive either ZOVIRAX 10 mg/kg every 8 hours (n = 107) or vidarabine 30 mg/kg per day (n = 95) for 10 days. Outcomes are presented in Table 4.

Table 4: Mortality at 1 Year

HSV Disease Classification	Treatment Group	
	Acyclovir (n = 107)	Vidarabine (n = 95)
SEM* (n = 85)	0/54	0/31
CNS† (n = 71)	5/35	5/36
DISS‡ (n = 46)	11/18	14/28

*SEM refers to localized infection with disease limited to skin, eye, and/or mouth.
†CNS refers to infection of the central nervous system with compatible neurologic and CSF findings.
‡DISS refers to visceral organ involvement such as hepatitis or pneumonitis with or without CNS involvement.

Rates of neurologic sequelae at 1 year were comparable between the treatment groups.
Varicella-Zoster Infections in Immunocompromised Patients: A multicenter trial of ZOVIRAX for Injection at a

Continued on next page

This product information is based on labeling in effect on June 23, 2000. For further information, contact via direct mail, phone, or web site. Medical Information, Glaxo Wellcome Inc., PO Box 13398, Research Triangle Park, NC 27709. Healthcare Professionals (Medical Information): 800-334-0089. Patients (Customer Response Center): 1-888-825-5249. Glaxo Wellcome Corporate Web Site: www.glaxowellcome.com

Zovirax for Injection—Cont.

dose of 500 mg/m^2 every 8 hours for 7 days was conducted in immunocompromised patients with zoster infections (shingles). Ninety-four (94) patients were evaluated (52 patients were treated with ZOVIRAX and 42 with placebo). ZOVIRAX was superior to placebo as measured by reductions in cutaneous dissemination and visceral dissemination.

INDICATIONS AND USAGE

Herpes Simplex Infections in Immunocompromised Patients: ZOVIRAX for Injection is indicated for the treatment of initial and recurrent mucosal and cutaneous herpes simplex (HSV-1 and HSV-2) in immunocompromised patients.

Initial Episodes of Herpes Genitalis: ZOVIRAX for Injection is indicated for the treatment of severe initial clinical episodes of herpes genitalis in immunocompetent patients.

Herpes Simplex Encephalitis: ZOVIRAX for Injection is indicated for the treatment of herpes simplex encephalitis.

Neonatal Herpes Simplex Virus Infection: ZOVIRAX for Injection is indicated for the treatment of neonatal herpes infections.

Varicella-Zoster Infections in Immunocompromised Patients: ZOVIRAX for Injection is indicated for the treatment of varicella-zoster (shingles) infections in immunocompromised patients.

CONTRAINDICATIONS

ZOVIRAX for Injection is contraindicated for patients who develop hypersensitivity to acyclovir or valacyclovir.

WARNINGS

ZOVIRAX for Injection is intended for intravenous infusion only, and should not be administered topically, intramuscularly, orally, subcutaneously, or in the eye. Intravenous infusions must be given over a period of at least 1 hour to reduce the risk of renal tubular damage (see PRECAUTIONS and DOSAGE AND ADMINISTRATION).

Renal failure, in some cases resulting in death, has been observed with acyclovir therapy (see ADVERSE REACTIONS: Observed During Clinical Practice and OVERDOSAGE).

Thrombotic thrombocytopenic purpura/hemolytic uremic syndrome (TTP/HUS), which has resulted in death, has occurred in immunocompromised patients receiving acyclovir therapy.

PRECAUTIONS

General: Precipitation of acyclovir crystals in renal tubules can occur if the maximum solubility of free acyclovir (2.5 mg/mL at 37°C in water) is exceeded or if the drug is administered by bolus injection. Ensuing renal tubular damage can produce acute renal failure.

Abnormal renal function (decreased creatinine clearance) can occur as a result of acyclovir administration and depends on the state of the patient's hydration, other treatments, and the rate of drug administration. Concomitant use of other nephrotoxic drugs, pre-existing renal disease, and dehydration make further renal impairment with acyclovir more likely.

Administration of ZOVIRAX by intravenous infusion must be accompanied by adequate hydration.

When dosage adjustments are required, they should be based on estimated creatinine clearance (see DOSAGE AND ADMINISTRATION).

Approximately 1% of patients receiving intravenous acyclovir have manifested encephalopathic changes characterized by either lethargy, obtundation, tremors, confusion, hallucinations, agitation, seizures, or coma. ZOVIRAX should be used with caution in those patients who have underlying neurologic abnormalities and those with serious renal, hepatic, or electrolyte abnormalities, or significant hypoxia.

Drug Interactions: See CLINICAL PHARMACOLOGY: Pharmacokinetics.

Carcinogenesis, Mutagenesis, Impairment of Fertility: The data presented below include references to peak steady-state plasma acyclovir concentrations observed in humans treated with 30 mg/kg per day (10 mg/kg every 8 hours, dosing appropriate for treatment of herpes zoster or herpes encephalitis), or 15 mg/kg per day (5 mg/kg every 8 hours, dosing appropriate for treatment of primary genital herpes or herpes simplex infections in immunocompromised patients). Plasma drug concentrations in animal studies are expressed as multiples of human exposure to acyclovir at the higher and lower dosing schedules (see CLINICAL PHARMACOLOGY: Pharmacokinetics).

Acyclovir was tested in lifetime bioassays in rats and mice at single daily doses of up to 450 mg/kg administered by gavage. There was no statistically significant difference in the incidence of tumors between treated and control animals, nor did acyclovir shorten the latency of tumors. At 450 mg/kg per day, plasma concentrations in both the mouse and rat bioassay were lower than concentrations in humans.

Acyclovir was tested in 16 genetic toxicity assays. No evidence of mutagenicity was observed in 4 microbial assays. Acyclovir demonstrated mutagenic activity in 2 in vitro cytogenetic assays (1 mouse lymphoma cell line and human lymphocytes). No mutagenic activity was observed in 5 in vitro cytogenetic assays (3 Chinese hamster ovary cell lines and 2 mouse lymphoma cell lines).

A positive result was demonstrated in 1 of 2 in vitro cell transformation assays, and morphologically transformed cells obtained in this assay formed tumors when inoculated into immunosuppressed, syngeneic, weanling mice. No activity was demonstrated in another, possibly less sensitive, in vitro cell transformation assay.

Acyclovir caused chromosomal damage in Chinese hamsters at 31 to 61 times human dose levels. In rats, acyclovir produced a nonsignificant increase in chromosomal damage at 5 to 10 times human levels. No activity was observed in a dominant lethal study in mice at 3 to 6 times human levels.

Acyclovir did not impair fertility or reproduction in mice (450 mg/kg per day, PO) or in rats (25 mg/kg per day, SC). In the mouse study, plasma levels were the same as human levels, while in the rat study, they were 1 to 2 times human levels. At higher doses (50 mg/kg per day, SC) in rats and rabbits (1 to 2 and 1 to 3 times human levels, respectively) implantation efficacy, but not litter size, was decreased. In a rat peri- and post-natal study at 50 mg/kg per day, SC, there was a statistically significant decrease in group mean numbers of corpora lutea, total implantation sites, and live fetuses.

No testicular abnormalities were seen in dogs given 50 mg/kg per day, IV for 1 month (1 to 3 times human levels) or in dogs given 60 mg/kg per day orally for 1 year (the same as human levels). Testicular atrophy and aspermatogenesis were observed in rats and dogs at higher dose levels.

Pregnancy: ***Teratogenic Effects:*** Pregnancy Category B. Acyclovir was not teratogenic in the mouse (450 mg/kg per day, PO), rabbit (50 mg/kg per day, SC and IV), or rat (50 mg/kg per day, SC). These exposures resulted in plasma levels the same as, 4 and 9, and 1 and 2 times, respectively, human levels.

There are no adequate and well-controlled studies in pregnant women. A prospective epidemiologic registry of acyclovir use during pregnancy was established in 1984 and completed in April 1999. There were 756 pregnancies followed in women exposed to systemic acyclovir during the first trimester of pregnancy. The occurrence rate of birth defects approximates that found in the general population. However, the small size of the registry is insufficient to evaluate the risk for less common defects or to permit reliable or definitive conclusions regarding the safety of acyclovir in pregnant women and their developing fetuses. Acyclovir should be used during pregnancy only if the potential benefit justifies the potential risk to the fetus.

Nursing Mothers: Acyclovir concentrations have been documented in breast milk in 2 women following oral administration of ZOVIRAX and ranged from 0.6 to 4.1 times corresponding plasma levels. These concentrations would potentially expose the nursing infant to a dose of acyclovir up to 0.3 mg/kg per day. ZOVIRAX should be administered to a nursing mother with caution and only when indicated.

Geriatric Use: Clinical studies of ZOVIRAX did not include sufficient numbers of patients aged 65 and over to determine whether they respond differently than younger patients. In general, dose selection for an elderly patient should be cautious, usually starting at the low end of the dosing range, reflecting the greater frequency of decreased renal function, and of concomitant disease or other drug therapy.

Pediatric Use: See DOSAGE AND ADMINISTRATION.

ADVERSE REACTIONS

The adverse reactions listed below have been observed in controlled and uncontrolled clinical trials in approximately 700 patients who received ZOVIRAX at ~5 mg/kg (250 mg/m^2) 3 times daily, and approximately 300 patients who received ~10 mg/kg (500 mg/m^2) 3 times daily.

The most frequent adverse reactions reported during administration of ZOVIRAX were inflammation or phlebitis at the injection site in approximately 9% of the patients, and transient elevations of serum creatinine or BUN in 5% to 10% (the higher incidence occurred usually following rapid [less than 10 minutes] intravenous infusion). Nausea and/or vomiting occurred in approximately 7% of the patients (the majority occurring in nonhospitalized patients who received 10 mg/kg). Itching, rash, or hives occurred in approximately 2% of patients. Elevation of transaminases occurred in 1% to 2% of patients.

The following hematologic abnormalities occurred at a frequency of less than 1%: anemia, neutropenia, thrombocytopenia, thrombocytosis, leukocytosis, and neutrophilia. In addition, anorexia and hematuria were observed.

Observed During Clinical Practice: In addition to adverse events reported from clinical trials, the following events have been identified during post-approval use of ZOVIRAX for Injection in clinical practice. Because they are reported voluntarily from a population of unknown size, estimates of frequency cannot be made. These events have been chosen for inclusion due to either their seriousness, frequency of reporting, potential causal connection to ZOVIRAX, or a combination of these factors.

General: Anaphylaxis, fever, headache, pain, peripheral edema.

Digestive: Diarrhea, gastrointestinal distress, nausea.

Cardiovascular: Hypotension.

Hemic and Lymphatic: Disseminated intravascular coagulation, hemolysis, leukopenia, lymphadenopathy.

Hepatobiliary Tract and Pancreas: Elevated liver function tests, hepatitis, jaundice.

Musculoskeletal: Myalgia.

Nervous: Agitation, coma, confusion, delirium, dizziness, hallucinations, obtundation, psychosis, seizure, somnolence. These symptoms may be marked, particularly in older adults (see PRECAUTIONS).

Skin: Alopecia, erythema multiforme, photosensitive rash, pruritus, rash, Stevens-Johnson syndrome, toxic epidermal necrolysis, urticaria.

Special Senses: Visual abnormalities.

Urogenital: Renal failure, elevated blood urea nitrogen, elevated creatinine (see WARNINGS).

OVERDOSAGE

Overdoses involving ingestions of up to 20 g have been reported. Adverse events that have been reported only in association with overdosage include convulsions and lethargy. Precipitation of acyclovir in renal tubules may occur when the solubility (2.5 mg/mL) is exceeded in the intratubular fluid. Overdosage has been reported following bolus injections or inappropriately high doses, and in patients whose fluid and electrolyte balance were not properly monitored. This has resulted in elevated BUN and serum creatinine, and subsequent renal failure. In the event of acute renal failure and anuria, the patient may benefit from hemodialysis until renal function is restored (see DOSAGE AND ADMINISTRATION).

DOSAGE AND ADMINISTRATION

CAUTION—RAPID OR BOLUS INTRAVENOUS INJECTION MUST BE AVOIDED (see WARNINGS and PRECAUTIONS).

INTRAMUSCULAR OR SUBCUTANEOUS INJECTION MUST BE AVOIDED (see WARNINGS).

Therapy should be initiated as early as possible following onset of signs and symptoms of herpes infections.

A maximum dose equivalent to 20 mg/kg every 8 hours should not be exceeded for any patient.

Dosage: ***Herpes Simplex Infections: Mucosal and Cutaneous Herpes Simplex (HSV-1 and HSV-2) Infections in Immunocompromised Patients:***

Adults and Adolescents (12 years of age and older): 5 mg/kg infused at a constant rate over 1 hour, every 8 hours for 7 days.

Pediatrics (Under 12 years of age): 10 mg/kg infused at a constant rate over 1 hour, every 8 hours for 7 days.

Severe Initial Clinical Episodes of Herpes Genitalis:

Adults and Adolescents (12 years of age and older): 5 mg/kg infused at a constant rate over 1 hour, every 8 hours for 5 days.

Herpes Simplex Encephalitis:

Adults and Adolescents (12 years of age and older): 10 mg/kg infused at a constant rate over 1 hour, every 8 hours for 10 days.

Pediatrics (3 months to 12 years of age): 20 mg/kg infused at a constant rate over 1 hour, every 8 hours for 10 days.

Neonatal Herpes Simplex Virus Infections (Birth to 3 months): 10 mg/kg infused at a constant rate over 1 hour, every 8 hours for 10 days. In neonatal herpes simplex infections, doses of 15 mg/kg or 20 mg/kg (infused at a constant rate over 1 hour every 8 hours) have been used; the safety and efficacy of these doses are not known.

Varicella Zoster Infections: Zoster in Immunocompromised Patients:

Adults and Adolescents (12 years of age and older): 10 mg/kg infused at a constant rate over 1 hour, every 8 hours for 7 days.

Pediatrics (Under 12 years of age): 20 mg/kg infused at a constant rate over 1 hour, every 8 hours for 7 days.

Obese Patients: Obese patients should be dosed at the recommended adult dose using Ideal Body Weight.

Patients with Acute or Chronic Renal Impairment: Refer to DOSAGE AND ADMINISTRATION section for recommended doses, and adjust the dosing interval as indicated in Table 5.

Table 5: Dosage Adjustments for Patients with Renal Impairment

Creatinine Clearance (mL/min per 1.73 m^2)	Percent of Recommended Dose	Dosing Interval (h)
>50	100%	8
25 – 50	100%	12
10 – 25	100%	24
0 – 10	50%	24

Hemodialysis: For patients who require dialysis, the mean plasma half-life of acyclovir during hemodialysis is approximately 5 hours. This results in a 60% decrease in plasma concentrations following a 6-hour dialysis period. Therefore, the patient's dosing schedule should be adjusted so that an additional dose is administered after each dialysis.

Peritoneal Dialysis: No supplemental dose appears to be necessary after adjustment of the dosing interval.

Method of Preparation: Each 10-mL vial contains acyclovir sodium equivalent to 500 mg of acyclovir. Each 20-mL vial contains acyclovir sodium equivalent to 1000 mg of acyclovir. The contents of the vial should be dissolved in Sterile Water for Injection as follows:

Contents of Vial	Amount of Diluent
500 mg	10 mL
1000 mg	20 mL

The resulting solution in each case contains 50 mg acyclovir per mL (pH approximately 11). Shake the vial well to assure complete dissolution before measuring and transferring each individual dose. The reconstituted solution should be used within 12 hours. Refrigeration of reconstituted solution may result in the formation of a precipitate which will redissolve at room temperature.

DO NOT USE BACTERIOSTATIC WATER FOR INJECTION CONTAINING BENZYL ALCOHOL OR PARABENS.

Administration: The calculated dose should then be removed and added to any appropriate intravenous solution at a volume selected for administration during each 1-hour infusion. Infusion concentrations of approximately 7 mg/mL or lower are recommended. In clinical studies, the average 70-kg adult received between 60 and 150 mL of fluid per dose. Higher concentrations (e.g., 10 mg/mL) may produce phlebitis or inflammation at the injection site upon inadvertent extravasation. Standard, commercially available electrolyte and glucose solutions are suitable for intravenous administration; biologic or colloidal fluids (e.g., blood products, protein solutions, etc.) are not recommended.

Once diluted for administration, each dose should be used within 24 hours.

HOW SUPPLIED

10-mL sterile vials, each containing acyclovir sodium equivalent to 500 mg of acyclovir, tray of 10 (NDC 0173-0995-01).

20-mL sterile vials, each containing acyclovir sodium equivalent to 1000 mg of acyclovir, tray of 10 (NDC 0173-0952-01).

Store at 15° to 25°C (59° to 77°F).

Manufactured by Catalytica Pharmaceuticals, Inc.
Greenville, NC 27834
for Glaxo Wellcome Inc.
Research Triangle Park, NC 27709

April 2000/RL-806

Shown in Product Identification Guide, page 317

ZYBAN® ℞

[*zī′ ban*]
(bupropion hydrochloride)
Sustained-Release Tablets

DESCRIPTION

ZYBAN (bupropion hydrochloride) Sustained-Release Tablets are a non-nicotine aid to smoking cessation. ZYBAN is chemically unrelated to nicotine or other agents currently used in the treatment of nicotine addiction. Initially developed and marketed as an antidepressant (WELLBUTRIN® [bupropion hydrochloride] Tablets and WELLBUTRIN SR® [bupropion hydrochloride] Sustained-Release Tablets), ZYBAN is also chemically unrelated to tricyclic, tetracyclic, selective serotonin re-uptake inhibitor, or other known antidepressant agents. Its structure closely resembles that of diethylpropion; it is related to phenylethylamines. It is (±)-1-(3-chlorophenyl)-2-[(1,1-dimethylethyl)amino]-1-propanone hydrochloride. The molecular weight is 276.2. The molecular formula is $C_{13}H_{18}ClNO \cdot HCl$. Bupropion hydrochloride powder is white, crystalline, and highly soluble in water. It has a bitter taste and produces the sensation of local anesthesia on the oral mucosa.

ZYBAN is supplied for oral administration as 150-mg (purple), film-coated, sustained-release tablets. Each tablet contains the labeled amount of bupropion hydrochloride and the inactive ingredients carnauba wax, cysteine hydrochloride, hydroxypropyl methylcellulose, magnesium stearate, microcrystalline cellulose, polyethylene glycol, polysorbate 80 and titanium dioxide and is printed with edible black ink. In addition, the 150-mg tablet contains FD&C Blue No. 2 Lake and FD&C Red No. 40 Lake.

CLINICAL PHARMACOLOGY

Pharmacodynamics: Bupropion is a relatively weak inhibitor of the neuronal uptake of norepinephrine, serotonin, and dopamine, and does not inhibit monoamine oxidase. The mechanism by which ZYBAN enhances the ability of patients to abstain from smoking is unknown. However, it is presumed that this action is mediated by noradrenergic and/or dopaminergic mechanisms.

Pharmacokinetics: Bupropion is a racemic mixture. The pharmacologic activity and pharmacokinetics of the individual enantiomers have not been studied. Bupropion follows biphasic pharmacokinetics best described by a two-compartment model. The terminal phase has a mean half-life (±% CV) of about 21 hours (±20%), while the distribution phase has a mean half-life of 3 to 4 hours.

Absorption: Bupropion has not been administered intravenously to humans; therefore, the absolute bioavailability of ZYBAN Sustained-Release Tablets in humans has not been determined. In rat and dog studies, the bioavailability of bupropion ranged from 5% to 20%.

Following oral administration of ZYBAN to healthy volunteers, peak plasma concentrations of bupropion are achieved within 3 hours. The mean peak concentration (C_{max}) values were 91 and 143 ng/mL from two single-dose (150-mg) studies. At steady state, the mean C_{max} following a 150-mg dose every 12 hours is 136 ng/mL.

In a single-dose study, food increased the C_{max} of bupropion by 11% and the extent of absorption as defined by area under the plasma concentration-time curve (AUC) by 17%. The mean time to peak concentration (t_{max}) was prolonged by 1 hour. This effect was of no clinical significance.

Distribution: In vitro tests show that bupropion is 84% bound to human plasma proteins at concentrations up to 200 mcg/mL. The extent of protein binding of the hydroxybupropion metabolite is similar to that for bupropion, whereas the extent of protein binding of the threohydrobupropion metabolite is about half that seen with bupropion. The volume of distribution (V_{ss}/F) estimated from a single 150-mg dose given to 17 subjects is 1950 L (20% CV).

Metabolism: Bupropion is extensively metabolized in humans. There are three active metabolites: hydroxybupropion and the amino-alcohol isomers threohydrobupropion and erythrohydrobupropion, which are formed via hydroxylation of the *tert*-butyl group of bupropion and/or reduction of the carbonyl group. Oxidation of the bupropion side chain results in the formation of a glycine conjugate of meta-chlorobenzoic acid, which is then excreted as the major urinary metabolite. The potency and toxicity of the metabolites relative to bupropion have not been fully characterized; however, it has been demonstrated in mice that hydroxybupropion is comparable in potency to bupropion, while the other metabolites are one tenth to one half as potent. This may be of clinical importance because the plasma concentrations of the metabolites are higher than those of bupropion. In vitro findings suggest that cytochrome P450IIB6 (CYP2B6) is the principal isoenzyme involved in the formation of hydroxybupropion, while cytochrome P450 isoenzymes are not involved in the formation of threohydrobupropion.

Because bupropion is extensively metabolized, there is the potential for drug-drug interactions, particularly with those agents that are metabolized by the cytochrome P450IIB6 (CYP2B6) isoenzyme. Although bupropion is not metabolized by cytochrome P450IID6 (CYP2D6), there is the potential for drug-drug interactions when bupropion is co-administered with drugs metabolized by this isoenzyme (see PRECAUTIONS: Drug Interactions).

Following a single dose in humans, peak plasma concentrations of hydroxybupropion occur approximately 6 hours after administration. Peak plasma concentrations of hydroxybupropion are approximately 10 times the peak level of the parent drug at steady state. The AUC at steady state is about 17 times that of bupropion. The times to peak concentrations for the erythrohydrobupropion and threohydrobupropion metabolites are similar to that of the hydroxybupropion metabolite, and steady-state AUCs are 1.5 and 7 times that of bupropion, respectively.

Elimination: The mean (±% CV) apparent clearance (Cl/F) estimated from two single-dose (150-mg) studies are 135 (±20%) and 209 L/hr (±21%). Following chronic dosing of 150 mg of ZYBAN every 12 hours for 14 days (n = 34), the mean Cl/F at steady state was 160 L/hr (±23%). The mean elimination half-life of bupropion estimated from a series of studies is approximately 21 hours. Estimates of the half-lives of the metabolites determined from a multiple-dose study were 20 hours (±25%) for hydroxybupropion, 37 hours (±35%) for threohydrobupropion, and 33 hours (±30%) for erythrohydrobupropion. Steady-state plasma concentrations of bupropion and metabolites are reached within 5 and 8 days, respectively.

Following oral administration of 200 mg of ^{14}C-bupropion in humans, 87% and 10% of the radioactive dose were recovered in the urine and feces, respectively. The fraction of the oral dose of bupropion excreted unchanged was only 0.5%.

The effects of cigarette smoking on the pharmacokinetics of bupropion were studied in 34 healthy male and female volunteers; 17 were chronic cigarette smokers and 17 were nonsmokers. Following oral administration of a single 150-mg dose of ZYBAN, there was no statistically significant difference in C_{max}, half-life, t_{max}, AUC, or clearance of bupropion or its major metabolites between smokers and nonsmokers.

In a study comparing the treatment combination of ZYBAN and nicotine transdermal system (NTS) versus ZYBAN alone, no statistically significant differences were observed between the two treatment groups of combination ZYBAN and NTS (n = 197) and ZYBAN alone (n = 193) in the plasma concentrations of bupropion or its active metabolites at weeks 3 and 6.

Bupropion and its metabolites exhibit linear kinetics following chronic administration of 150 to 300 mg/day.

Population Subgroups: Factors or conditions altering metabolic capacity (e.g., liver disease, congestive heart failure, age, concomitant medications, etc.) or elimination may be expected to influence the degree and extent of accumulation of the active metabolites of bupropion. The elimination of the major metabolites of bupropion may be affected by reduced renal or hepatic function because they are moderately polar compounds and are likely to undergo further metabolism or conjugation in the liver prior to urinary excretion.

Hepatic: The disposition of bupropion following a single 200-mg oral dose was compared in eight healthy volunteers and eight weight- and age-matched volunteers with alcoholic liver disease. The half-life of hydroxybupropion was significantly prolonged in subjects with alcoholic liver disease (32 hours [±41%] versus 21 hours [±23%]). The differences in half-life for bupropion and the other metabolites in the two patient groups were minimal.

Renal: The effect of renal disease on the pharmacokinetics of bupropion has not been studied. The elimination of the major metabolites of bupropion may be affected by reduced renal function.

Left Ventricular Dysfunction: During a chronic dosing study with bupropion in 14 depressed patients with left ventricular dysfunction (history of congestive heart failure [CHF] or an enlarged heart on x-ray), no apparent effect on the pharmacokinetics of bupropion or its metabolites, compared to healthy normal volunteers, was revealed.

Age: The effects of age on the pharmacokinetics of bupropion and its metabolites have not been fully characterized, but an exploration of steady-state bupropion concentrations from several depression efficacy studies involving patients dosed in a range of 300 to 750 mg/day, on a three times a day schedule, revealed no relationship between age (18 to 83 years) and plasma concentration of bupropion. A single-dose pharmacokinetic study demonstrated that the disposition of bupropion and its metabolites in elderly subjects was similar to that of younger subjects. These data suggest there is no prominent effect of age on bupropion concentration; however, another pharmacokinetic study, single and multiple dose, has suggested that the elderly are at increased risk for accumulation of bupropion and its metabolites (see PRECAUTIONS: Geriatric Use).

Gender: A single-dose study involving 12 healthy male and 12 healthy female volunteers revealed no sex-related differences in the pharmacokinetic parameters of bupropion.

CLINICAL TRIALS

The efficacy of ZYBAN as an aid to smoking cessation was demonstrated in three placebo-controlled, double-blind trials in nondepressed chronic cigarette smokers (n = 1940, ≥15 cigarettes per day). In these studies, ZYBAN was used in conjunction with individual smoking cessation counseling.

The first study was a dose-response trial conducted at three clinical centers. Patients in this study were treated for 7 weeks with one of three doses of ZYBAN (100, 150, or 300 mg/day) or placebo; quitting was defined as total abstinence during the last 4 weeks of treatment (weeks 4 through 7). Abstinence was determined by patient daily diaries and verified by carbon monoxide levels in expired air.

Results of this dose-response trial with ZYBAN demonstrated a dose-dependent increase in the percentage of patients able to achieve 4-week abstinence (weeks 4 through 7). Treatment with ZYBAN at both 150 and 300 mg/day was significantly more effective than placebo in this study.

Table 1 presents quit rates over time in the multicenter trial by treatment group. The quit rates are the proportions of all persons initially enrolled (i.e., intent to treat analysis) who abstained from week 4 of the study through the specified week. Treatment with ZYBAN (150 or 300 mg/day) was more effective than placebo in helping patients achieve 4-week abstinence. In addition, treatment with ZYBAN (7 weeks at 300 mg/day) was more effective than placebo in helping patients maintain continuous abstinence through week 26 (6 months) of the study.

[See table 1 at top of next page]

The second study was a comparative trial conducted at four clinical centers. Four treatments were evaluated: ZYBAN 300 mg/day, nicotine transdermal system (NTS) 21 mg/day, combination of ZYBAN 300 mg/day plus NTS 21 mg/day, and placebo. Patients were treated for 9 weeks. Treatment with ZYBAN was initiated at 150 mg/day while the patient was still smoking and was increased after 3 days to 300 mg/day given as 150 mg twice daily. NTS 21 mg/day was added to treatment with ZYBAN after approximately 1 week when the patient reached the target quit date. During weeks 8 and 9 of the study, NTS was tapered to 14 and 7 mg/day, respectively. Quitting, defined as total abstinence during weeks 4 through 7, was determined by patient daily diaries and verified by expired air carbon monoxide levels. In this study, patients treated with any of the three treatments achieved greater 4-week abstinence rates than patients treated with placebo.

Table 2 presents quit rates over time by treatment group for the comparative trial.

[See table 2 on next page]

When patients in this study were followed out to one year, the superiority of ZYBAN and the combination of ZYBAN and NTS over placebo in helping patients to achieve abstinence from smoking was maintained. The continuous abstinence rate was 30% (95% Cl 24-35) in the ZYBAN treated patients, and 33% (95% Cl 27-39) for patients treated with the combination at 26 weeks compared with 13% (95% Cl 7-18) in the placebo group. At 52 weeks, the continuous abstinence rate was 23% (95% Cl 18-28) in the ZYBAN treated patients, and 28% (95% Cl 23-34) for patients treated with the combination, compared with 8% (95% Cl 3-12) in the

Continued on next page

This product information is based on labeling in effect on June 23, 2000. For further information, contact via direct mail, phone, or web site. Medical Information, Glaxo Wellcome Inc., PO Box 13398, Research Triangle Park, NC 27709. Healthcare Professionals (Medical Information): 800-334-0089. Patients (Customer Response Center): 1-888-825-5249. Glaxo Wellcome Corporate Web Site: www.glaxowellcome.com

Zyban—Cont.

placebo group. Although the treatment combination of ZYBAN and NTS displayed the highest rates of continuous abstinence throughout the study, the quit rates for the combination were not significantly higher (P>0.05) than for ZYBAN alone.
The comparisons between ZYBAN, NTS, and combination treatment in this study have not been replicated, and, therefore should not be interpreted as demonstrating the superiority of any of the active treatment arms over any other.
The third study was a long-term maintenance trial conducted at five clinical centers. Patients in this study received open-label ZYBAN 300 mg/day for 7 weeks. Patients who quit smoking while receiving ZYBAN (n = 432) were then randomized to ZYBAN 300 mg/day or placebo for a total study duration of 1 year. Abstinence from smoking was determined by patient self-report and verified by expired air carbon monoxide levels. This trial demonstrated that at 6 months, continuous abstinence rates were significantly higher for patients continuing to receive ZYBAN than for those switched to placebo (P<0.05; 55% versus 44%).
Quit rates in clinical trials are influenced by the population selected. Quit rates in an unselected population may be lower than the above rates. Quit rates for ZYBAN were similar in patients with and without prior quit attempts using nicotine replacement therapy.
Treatment with ZYBAN reduced withdrawal symptoms compared to placebo. Reductions on the following withdrawal symptoms were most pronounced: irritability, frustration, or anger; anxiety; difficulty concentrating; restlessness; and depressed mood or negative affect. Depending on the study and the measure used, treatment with ZYBAN showed evidence of reduction in craving for cigarettes or urge to smoke compared to placebo.

Table 1: Dose-Response Trial: Quit Rates by Treatment Group

Abstinence From Week 4 Through Specified Week	Treatment Groups			
	Placebo (n = 151) % (95% CI)	ZYBAN 100 mg/day (n = 153) % (95% CI)	ZYBAN 150 mg/day (n = 153) % (95% CI)	ZYBAN 300 mg/day (n = 156) % (95% CI)
Week 7 (4-week quit)	17% (11–23)	22% (15–28)	27%* (20–35)	36%* (28–43)
Week 12	14% (8–19)	20% (13–26)	20% (14–27)	25%* (18–32)
Week 26	11% (6–16)	16% (11–22)	18% (12–24)	19%* (13–25)

* Significantly different from placebo (P≤0.05).

Table 2: Comparative Trial: Quit Rates by Treatment Group

Abstinence From Week 4 Through Specified Week	Treatment Groups			
	Placebo (n = 160) % (95% CI)	Nicotine Transdermal System (NTS) 21 mg/day (n = 244) % (95% CI)	ZYBAN 300 mg/day (n = 244) % (95% CI)	ZYBAN 300 mg/day and NTS 21 mg/day (n = 245) % (95% CI)
Week 7 (4-week quit)	23% (17–30)	36% (30–42)	49% (43–56)	58% (51–64)
Week 10	20% (14–26)	32% (26–37)	46% (39–52)	51% (45–58)

INDICATIONS AND USAGE

ZYBAN is indicated as an aid to smoking cessation treatment.

CONTRAINDICATIONS

ZYBAN is contraindicated in patients with a seizure disorder.
ZYBAN is contraindicated in patients treated with WELLBUTRIN, WELLBUTRIN SR, or any other medications that contain bupropion because the incidence of seizure is dose dependent.
ZYBAN is contraindicated in patients with a current or prior diagnosis of bulimia or anorexia nervosa because of a higher incidence of seizures noted in patients treated for bulimia with the immediate-release formulation of bupropion.
The concurrent administration of ZYBAN and a monoamine oxidase (MAO) inhibitor is contraindicated. At least 14 days should elapse between discontinuation of an MAO inhibitor and initiation of treatment with ZYBAN.
ZYBAN is contraindicated in patients who have shown an allergic response to bupropion or the other ingredients that make up ZYBAN.

WARNINGS

Patients should be made aware that ZYBAN contains the same active ingredient found in WELLBUTRIN and WELLBUTRIN SR used to treat depression, and that ZYBAN should not be used in combination with WELLBUTRIN, WELLBUTRIN SR, or any other medications that contain bupropion.
Because the use of bupropion is associated with a dose-dependent risk of seizures, *clinicians should not prescribe doses over 300 mg/day for smoking cessation.* The risk of seizures is also related to patient factors, clinical situation, and concurrent medications, which must be considered in selection of patients for therapy with ZYBAN.

- **Dose: *For smoking cessation, doses above 300 mg/day should not be used.* The seizure rate associated with doses of sustained-release bupropion up to 300 mg/day is approximately 0.1% (1/1000). This incidence was prospectively determined during an 8-week treatment exposure in approximately 3100 depressed patients. Data for the immediate-release formulation of bupropion revealed a seizure incidence of approximately 0.4% (4/1000) in depressed patients treated at doses in a range of 300 to 450 mg/day. In addition, the estimated seizure incidence increases almost tenfold between 450 and 600 mg/day.**
- **Patient factors: Predisposing factors that may increase the risk of seizure with bupropion use include history of head trauma or prior seizure, central nervous system (CNS) tumor, and concomitant medications that lower seizure threshold.**
- **Clinical situations: Circumstances associated with an increased seizure risk include, among others, excessive use of alcohol; abrupt withdrawal from alcohol or other sedatives; addiction to opiates, cocaine, or stimulants; use of over-the-counter stimulants and anorectics; and diabetes treated with oral hypoglycemics or insulin.**
- **Concomitant medications: Many medications (e.g., antipsychotics, antidepressants, theophylline, systemic steroids) and treatment regimens (e.g., abrupt discontinuation of benzodiazepines) are known to lower seizure threshold.**

Recommendations for Reducing the Risk of Seizure: Retrospective analysis of clinical experience gained during the development of bupropion suggests that the risk of seizure may be minimized if

- **the total daily dose of ZYBAN does *not* exceed 300 mg (the maximum recommended dose for smoking cessation), and**
- **the recommended daily dose for most patients (300 mg/day) is administered in divided doses (150 mg twice daily).**
- **No single dose should exceed 150 mg to avoid high peak concentrations of bupropion and/or its metabolites.**
- **ZYBAN should be administered with extreme caution to patients with a history of seizure, cranial trauma, or other predisposition(s) toward seizure, or patients treated with other agents (e.g., antipsychotics, antidepressants, theophylline, systemic steroids, etc.) or treatment regimens (e.g., abrupt discontinuation of a benzodiazepine) that lower seizure threshold.**

Potential for Hepatotoxicity: In rats receiving large doses of bupropion chronically, there was an increase in incidence of hepatic hyperplastic nodules and hepatocellular hypertrophy. In dogs receiving large doses of bupropion chronically, various histologic changes were seen in the liver, and laboratory tests suggesting mild hepatocellular injury were noted.

PRECAUTIONS

General: ***Allergic Reactions:*** Anaphylactoid/anaphylactic reactions characterized by symptoms such as pruritus, urticaria, angioedema, and dyspnea requiring medical treatment have been reported at a rate of about 1 to 3 per thousand in clinical trials of ZYBAN. In addition, there have been rare spontaneous postmarketing reports of erythema multiforme, Stevens-Johnson syndrome, and anaphylactic shock associated with bupropion. A patient should stop taking ZYBAN and consult a doctor if experiencing allergic or anaphylactoid/anaphylactic reactions (e.g., skin rash, pruritus, hives, chest pain, edema, and shortness of breath) during treatment.
Arthralgia, myalgia, and fever with rash and other symptoms suggestive of delayed hypersensitivity have been reported in association with bupropion. These symptoms may resemble serum sickness.
Insomnia: In the dose-response smoking cessation trial, 29% of patients treated with 150 mg/day of ZYBAN and 35% of patients treated with 300 mg/day of ZYBAN experienced insomnia, compared to 21% of placebo-treated patients. Symptoms were sufficiently severe to require discontinuation of treatment in 0.6% of patients treated with ZYBAN and none of the patients treated with placebo.
In the comparative trial, 40% of the patients treated with 300 mg/day of ZYBAN, 28% of the patients treated with 21 mg/day of NTS, and 45% of the patients treated with the combination of ZYBAN and NTS experienced insomnia compared to 18% of placebo-treated patients. Symptoms were sufficiently severe to require discontinuation of treatment in 0.8% of patients treated with ZYBAN and none of the patients in the other three treatment groups.
Insomnia may be minimized by avoiding bedtime doses and, if necessary, reduction in dose.
Psychosis, Confusion, and Other Neuropsychiatric Phenomena: In clinical trials with ZYBAN conducted in nondepressed smokers, the incidence of neuropsychiatric side effects was generally comparable to placebo. Depressed patients treated with bupropion in depression trials have been reported to show a variety of neuropsychiatric signs and symptoms including delusions, hallucinations, psychosis, concentration disturbance, paranoia, and confusion. In some cases, these symptoms abated upon dose reduction and/or withdrawal of treatment.
Activation of Psychosis and/or Mania: Antidepressants can precipitate manic episodes in bipolar disorder patients during the depressed phase of their illness and may activate latent psychosis in other susceptible individuals. The sustained-release formulation of bupropion is expected to pose similar risks. There were no reports of activation of psychosis or mania in clinical trials with ZYBAN conducted in nondepressed smokers.
Cardiovascular Effects: In clinical practice, hypertension, in some cases severe, requiring acute treatment, has been reported in patients receiving bupropion alone and in combination with nicotine replacement therapy. These events have been observed in both patients with and without evidence of preexisting hypertension.
Data from a comparative study of ZYBAN, nicotine transdermal system (NTS), the combination of sustained-release bupropion plus NTS, and placebo as an aid to smoking cessation suggest a higher incidence of treatment-emergent hypertension in patients treated with the combination of ZYBAN and NTS. In this study, 6.1% of patients treated with the combination of ZYBAN and NTS had treatment-emergent hypertension compared to 2.5%, 1.6%, and 3.1% of patients treated with ZYBAN, NTS, and placebo, respectively. The majority of these patients had evidence of preexisting hypertension. Three patients (1.2%) treated with the combination of ZYBAN and NTS and one patient (0.4%) treated with NTS had study medication discontinued due to hypertension compared to none of the patients treated with ZYBAN or placebo. Monitoring of blood pressure is recommended in patients who receive the combination of bupropion and nicotine replacement.
There is no clinical experience establishing the safety of ZYBAN in patients with a recent history of myocardial infarction or unstable heart disease. Therefore, care should be exercised if it is used in these groups. Bupropion was well tolerated in depressed patients who had previously developed orthostatic hypotension while receiving tricyclic antidepressants, and was also generally well tolerated in a group of 36 depressed inpatients with stable congestive heart failure (CHF). However, bupropion was associated with a rise in supine blood pressure in the study of patients with CHF, resulting in discontinuation of treatment in two patients for exacerbation of baseline hypertension.
Renal or Hepatic Impairment: Because bupropion hydrochloride and its metabolites are almost completely excreted through the kidney and metabolites are likely to undergo conjugation in the liver prior to urinary excretion, treatment of patients with renal or hepatic impairment should be initiated at reduced dosage as bupropion and its metabolites may accumulate in such patients to a greater extent than usual. The patient should be closely monitored for possible toxic effects of elevated blood and tissue levels of drug and metabolites.
Information for Patients: See PATIENT INFORMATION at the end of this labeling for the text of the separate leaflet provided for patients. Physicians are advised to review the leaflet with their patients and to emphasize that ZYBAN contains the same active ingredient found in WELLBUTRIN and WELLBUTRIN SR used to treat depression and that ZYBAN should not be used in conjunction with WELLBUTRIN, WELLBUTRIN SR, or any other medications that contain bupropion hydrochloride.
Laboratory Tests: There are no specific laboratory tests recommended.
Drug Interactions: In vitro studies indicate that bupropion is primarily metabolized to hydroxybupropion by the cytochrome P450IIB6 (CYP2B6) isoenzyme. Therefore, the potential exists for a drug interaction between ZYBAN and

drugs that affect the CYP2B6 isoenzyme (e.g., orphenadrine and cyclophosphamide). The threohydrobupropion metabolite of bupropion does not appear to be produced by the cytochrome P450 isoenzymes. Few systemic data have been collected on the metabolism of ZYBAN following concomitant administration with other drugs or, alternatively, the effect of concomitant administration of ZYBAN on the metabolism of other drugs.

Animal data indicated that bupropion may be an inducer of drug-metabolizing enzymes in humans. However, following chronic administration of bupropion, 100 mg t.i.d. to 8 healthy male volunteers for 14 days, there was no evidence of induction of its own metabolism. Because bupropion is extensively metabolized, the coadministration of other drugs may affect its clinical activity. In particular, certain drugs may induce the metabolism of bupropion (e.g., carbamazepine, phenobarbital, phenytoin), while other drugs may inhibit the metabolism of bupropion (e.g., cimetidine). The effects of concomitant administration of cimetidine on the pharmacokinetics of bupropion and its active metabolites were studied in 24 healthy young male volunteers. Following oral administration of two 150-mg ZYBAN tablets with and without 800 mg of cimetidine, the pharmacokinetics of bupropion and its hydroxy metabolite were unaffected. However, there were 16% and 32% increases, respectively, in the AUC and C_{max} of the combined moieties of theohydro- and erythrohydro bupropion.

Drugs Metabolized by Cytochrome P450IID6 (CYP2D6): Many drugs, including most antidepressants (SSRIs, many tricyclics), beta-blockers, antiarrhythmics, and antipsychotics are metabolized by the CYP2D6 isoenzyme. Although bupropion is not metabolized by this isoenzyme, bupropion and hydroxybupropion are inhibitors of the CYP2D6 isoenzyme in vitro. In a study of 15 male subjects (ages 19 to 35 years) who were extensive metabolizers of the CYP2D6 isoenzyme, daily doses of bupropion given as 150 mg twice daily followed by a single dose of 50 mg desipramine increased the C_{max}, AUC, and $t_{1/2}$ of desipramine by an average of approximately two-, five- and two-fold, respectively. The effect was present for at least 7 days after the last dose of bupropion. Concomitant use of bupropion with other drugs metabolized by CYP2D6 has not been formally studied.

Therefore, co-administration of bupropion with drugs that are metabolized by CYP2D6 isoenzyme including certain antidepressants (e.g., nortriptyline, imipramine, desipramine, paroxetine, fluoxetine, sertraline), antipsychotics (e.g., haloperidol, risperidone, thioridazine), beta-blockers (e.g., metoprolol), and Type 1C antiarrhythmics (e.g., propafenone, flecainide), should be approached with caution and should be initiated at the lower end of the dose range of the concomitant medication. If bupropion is added to the treatment regimen of a patient already receiving a drug metabolized by CYP2D6, the need to decrease the dose of the original medication should be considered, particularly for those concomitant medications with a narrow therapeutic index.

MAO Inhibitors: Studies in animals demonstrate that the acute toxicity of bupropion is enhanced by the MAO inhibitor phenelzine (see CONTRAINDICATIONS).

Levodopa: Limited clinical data suggest a higher incidence of adverse experiences in patients receiving concurrent administration of bupropion and levodopa. Administration of ZYBAN to patients receiving levodopa concurrently should be undertaken with caution, using small initial doses and gradual dose increases.

Drugs that Lower Seizure Threshold: Concurrent administration of ZYBAN and agents (e.g., antipsychotics, antidepressants, theophylline, systemic steroids, etc.) or treatment regimens (e.g., abrupt discontinuation of benzodiazepines) that lower seizure threshold should be undertaken only with extreme caution (see WARNINGS).

Nicotine Transdermal System: (see PRECAUTIONS: Cardiovascular Effects).

Smoking Cessation: Physiological changes resulting from smoking cessation itself, with or without treatment with ZYBAN, may alter the pharmacokinetics of some concomitant medications, which may require dosage adjustment.

Carcinogenesis, Mutagenesis, Impairment of Fertility: Lifetime carcinogenicity studies were performed in rats and mice at doses up to 300 and 150 mg/kg per day, respectively. These doses are approximately ten and two times the maximum recommended human dose (MRHD), respectively, on a mg/m^2 basis. In the rat study, there was an increase in nodular proliferative lesions of the liver at doses of 100 to 300 mg/kg per day (approximately three to ten times the MRHD on a mg/m^2 basis); lower doses were not tested. The question of whether or not such lesions may be precursors of neoplasms of the liver is currently unresolved. Similar liver lesions were not seen in the mouse study, and no increase in malignant tumors of the liver and other organs was seen in either study.

Bupropion produced a positive response (two to three times control mutation rate) in two of five strains in the Ames bacterial mutagenicity test and an increase in chromosomal aberrations in one of three in vivo rat bone marrow cytogenic studies.

A fertility study in rats at doses up to 300 mg/kg revealed no evidence of impaired fertility.

Pregnancy: *Teratogenic Effects: Pregnancy Category B:* Teratology studies have been performed at doses up to 450 mg/kg in rats (approximately 14 times the MRHD on a mg/m^2 basis), and at doses up to 150 mg/kg in rabbits (approximately 10 times the MRHD on a mg/m^2 basis). There is no evidence of impaired fertility or harm to the fetus due to bupropion. There are no adequate and well-controlled studies in pregnant women. Because animal reproduction studies are not always predictive of human response, this drug should be used during pregnancy only if clearly needed. Pregnant smokers should be encouraged to attempt cessation using educational and behavioral interventions before pharmacological approaches are used.

To monitor fetal outcomes of pregnant women exposed to ZYBAN, Glaxo Wellcome Inc. maintains a Bupropion Pregnancy Registry. Health care providers are encouraged to register patients by calling (800) 336-2176.

Labor and Delivery: The effect of ZYBAN on labor and delivery in humans is unknown.

Nursing Mothers: Bupropion and its metabolites are secreted in human milk. Because of the potential for serious adverse reactions in nursing infants from ZYBAN, a decision should be made whether to discontinue nursing or to discontinue the drug, taking into account the importance of the drug to the mother.

Pediatric Use: Clinical trials with ZYBAN did not include individuals under the age of 18. Therefore, the safety and efficacy in a pediatric smoking population have not been established. The immediate-release formulation of bupropion was studied in 104 pediatric patients (age range, 6 to 16) in clinical trials of the drug for other indications. Although generally well tolerated, the limited exposure is insufficient to assess the safety of bupropion in pediatric patients.

Geriatric Use: Of the approximately 6000 patients who participated in clinical trials with bupropion sustained-release tablets (depression and smoking cessation studies), 275 were 65 and over and 47 were 75 and over. In addition, several hundred patients 65 and over participated in clinical trials using the immediate-release formulation of bupropion (depression studies). No overall differences in safety or effectiveness were observed between these subjects and younger subjects, and other reported clinical experience has not identified differences in responses between the elderly and younger patients, but greater sensitivity of some older individuals cannot be ruled out.

A single-dose pharmacokinetic study demonstrated that the disposition of bupropion and its metabolites in elderly subjects was similar to that of younger subjects; however, another pharmacokinetic study, single and multiple dose, has suggested that the elderly are at increased risk for accumulation of bupropion and its metabolites (see CLINICAL PHARMACOLOGY).

Bupropion hydrochloride and its metabolites are almost completely excreted through the kidney and metabolites are likely to undergo conjugation in the liver prior to urinary excretion. The risk of toxic reaction to this drug may be greater in patients with impaired renal function. Because elderly patients are more likely to have decreased renal function, care should be taken in dose selection, and it may be useful to monitor renal function (see Use in Patients with Systemic Illness).

ADVERSE REACTIONS (see also WARNINGS and PRECAUTIONS)

The information included under ADVERSE REACTIONS is based primarily on data from the dose-response trial and the comparative trial that evaluated ZYBAN for smoking cessation (see CLINICAL TRIALS). Information on additional adverse events associated with the sustained-release formulation of bupropion in depression trials, as well as the immediate-release formulation of bupropion, is included in a separate section (see Other Events Observed During the Clinical Development and Postmarketing Experience of Bupropion).

Adverse Events Associated With the Discontinuation of Treatment: Adverse events were sufficiently troublesome to cause discontinuation of treatment in 8% of the 706 patients treated with ZYBAN and 5% of the 313 patients treated with placebo. The more common events leading to discontinuation of treatment with ZYBAN included nervous system disturbances (3.4%), primarily tremors, and skin disorders (2.4%), primarily rashes.

Incidence of Commonly Observed Adverse Events: The most commonly observed adverse events consistently associated with the use of ZYBAN were dry mouth and insomnia. The most commonly observed adverse events were defined as those that consistently occurred at a rate of five percentage points greater than that for placebo across clinical studies.

Dose Dependency of Adverse Events: The incidence of dry mouth and insomnia may be related to the dose of ZYBAN. The occurrence of these adverse events may be minimized by reducing the dose of ZYBAN. In addition, insomnia may be minimized by avoiding bedtime doses.

Adverse Events Occurring at an Incidence of 1% or More Among Patients Treated With ZYBAN: Table 3 enumerates selected treatment-emergent adverse events from the dose-response trial that occurred at an incidence of 1% or more and were more common in patients treated with ZYBAN compared to those treated with placebo. Table 4 enumerates selected treatment-emergent adverse events from the comparative trial that occurred at an incidence of 1% or more and were more common in patients treated with ZYBAN, NTS, or the combination of ZYBAN and NTS compared to those treated with placebo. Reported adverse events were classified using a COSTART-based dictionary.

[See table 3 above]

Table 3: Treatment-Emergent Adverse Event Incidence in the Dose-Response Trial*

Body System/ Adverse Experience	ZYBAN 100 to 300 mg/day (n = 461) %	Placebo (n = 150) %
Body (General)		
Neck pain	2	<1
Allergic reaction	1	0
Cardiovascular		
Hot flashes	1	0
Hypertension	1	<1
Digestive		
Dry mouth	11	5
Increased appetite	2	<1
Anorexia	1	<1
Musculoskeletal		
Arthralgia	4	3
Myalgia	2	1
Nervous system		
Insomnia	31	21
Dizziness	8	7
Tremor	2	1
Somnolence	2	1
Thinking abnormality	1	0
Respiratory		
Bronchitis	2	0
Skin		
Pruritus	3	<1
Rash	3	<1
Dry skin	2	0
Urticaria	1	0
Special senses		
Taste perversion	2	<1

*Selected adverse events with an incidence of at least 1% of patients treated with ZYBAN and more frequent than in the placebo group.

[See table 4 at top of next page]

In the long-term maintenance trial, which evaluated chronic administration of ZYBAN for up to 1 year, ZYBAN was well tolerated. Adverse events were quantitatively and qualitatively similar to those observed in the dose-response and comparative trials.

Other Events Observed During the Clinical Development and Postmarketing Experience of Bupropion: In addition to the adverse events noted above, the following events have been reported in clinical trials and postmarketing experience with the sustained-release formulation of bupropion in depressed patients and in nondepressed smokers, as well as in clinical trials and postmarketing clinical experience with the immediate-release formulation of bupropion.

Adverse events for which frequencies are provided below occurred in clinical trials with bupropion sustained-release. The frequencies represent the proportion of patients who experienced a treatment-emergent adverse event on at least

Continued on next page

This product information is based on labeling in effect on June 23, 2000. For further information, contact via direct mail, phone, or web site. Medical Information, Glaxo Wellcome Inc., PO Box 13398, Research Triangle Park, NC 27709. Healthcare Professionals (Medical Information): 800-334-0089. Patients (Customer Response Center): 1-888-825-5249. Glaxo Wellcome Corporate Web Site: www.glaxowellcome.com

Zyban—Cont.

one occasion in placebo-controlled studies for depression (n = 987) or smoking cessation (n = 1013), or patients who experienced an adverse event requiring discontinuation of treatment in an open-label surveillance study with bupropion sustained-release tablets (n = 3100). All treatment-emergent adverse events are included except those listed in Tables 3 and 4, those events listed in other safety-related sections of the insert, those adverse events subsumed under COSTART terms that are either overly general or excessively specified so as to be uninformative, those events not reasonably associated with the use of the drug, and those events that were not serious and occurred in fewer than two patients.

Events are further categorized by body system and listed in order of decreasing frequency according to the following definitions of frequency: Frequent adverse events are defined as those occurring in at least 1/100 patients. Infrequent adverse events are those occurring in 1/100 to 1/1000 patients, while rare events are those occurring in less than 1/1000 patients.

Adverse events for which frequencies are not provided occurred in clinical trials or postmarketing experience with bupropion. Only those adverse events not previously listed for sustained-release bupropion are included. The extent to which these events may be associated with ZYBAN is unknown.

Body (General): Frequent were asthenia, fever, and headache. Infrequent were back pain, chills, inguinal hernia, musculoskeletal chest pain, pain, and photosensitivity. Rare was malaise. Also observed were arthralgia, myalgia, and fever with rash and other symptoms suggestive of delayed hypersensitivity. These symptoms may resemble serum sickness (see PRECAUTIONS).

Cardiovascular: Infrequent were flushing, migraine, postural hypotension, stroke, tachycardia, and vasodilation. Rare was syncope. Also observed were cardiovascular disorder, complete AV block, extrasystoles, hypotension, hypertension (in some cases severe, see PRECAUTIONS), myocardial infarction, phlebitis, and pulmonary embolism.

Digestive: Frequent were dyspepsia, flatulence, and vomiting. Infrequent were abnormal liver function, bruxism, dysphagia, gastric reflux, gingivitis, glossitis, jaundice, and stomatitis. Rare was edema of tongue. Also observed were colitis, esophagitis, gastrointestinal hemorrhage, gum hemorrhage, hepatitis, increased salivation, intestinal perforation, liver damage, pancreatitis, stomach ulcer, and stool abnormality.

Endocrine: Also observed were hyperglycemia, hypoglycemia, and syndrome of inappropriate antidiuretic hormone.

Hemic and Lymphatic: Infrequent was ecchymosis. Also observed were anemia, leukocytosis, leukopenia, lymphadenopathy, pancytopenia, and thrombocytopenia.

Metabolic and Nutritional: Infrequent were edema, increased weight, and peripheral edema. Also observed was glycosuria.

Musculoskeletal: Infrequent were leg cramps and twitching. Also observed were arthritis and muscle rigidity/fever/rhabdomyolysis, and muscle weakness.

Nervous System: Frequent were agitation, depression, and irritability. Infrequent were abnormal coordination, CNS stimulation, confusion, decreased libido, decreased memory, depersonalization, emotional lability, hostility, hyperkinesia, hypertonia, hypesthesia, paresthesia, suicidal ideation, and vertigo. Rare were amnesia, ataxia, derealization, and hypomania. Also observed were abnormal electroencephalogram (EEG), akinesia, aphasia, coma, delirium, delusions, dysarthria, dyskinesia, dystonia, euphoria, extrapyramidal syndrome, hypokinesia, increased libido, manic reaction, neuralgia, neuropathy, paranoid reaction, and unmasking tardive dyskinesia.

Respiratory: Rare was bronchospasm. Also observed was pneumonia.

Skin: Frequent was sweating. Infrequent was acne and dry skin. Rare was maculopapular rash. Also observed were alopecia, angioedema, exfoliative dermatitis, and hirsutism.

Special Senses: Frequent was amblyopia. Infrequent were accommodation abnormality and dry eye. Also observed were deafness, diplopia, and mydriasis.

Urogenital: Frequent was urinary frequency. Infrequent were impotence, polyuria, and urinary urgency. Also observed were abnormal ejaculation, cystitis, dyspareunia, dysuria, gynecomastia, menopause, painful erection, prostate disorder, salpingitis, urinary incontinence, urinary retention, urinary tract disorder, and vaginitis.

Table 4: Treatment-Emergent Adverse Event Incidence in the Comparative Trial*

Adverse Experience (COSTART Term)	ZYBAN 300 mg/day (n = 243) %	Nicotine Transdermal System (NTS) 21 mg/day (n = 243) %	ZYBAN and NTS (n = 244) %	Placebo (n = 159) %
Body				
Abdominal pain	3	4	1	1
Accidental injury	2	2	1	1
Chest pain	<1	1	3	1
Neck pain	2	1	<1	0
Facial edema	<1	0	1	0
Cardiovascular				
Hypertension	1	<1	2	0
Palpitations	2	0	1	0
Digestive				
Nausea	9	7	11	4
Dry mouth	10	4	9	4
Constipation	8	4	9	3
Diarrhea	4	4	3	1
Anorexia	3	1	5	1
Mouth ulcer	2	1	1	1
Thirst	<1	<1	2	0
Musculoskeletal				
Myalgia	4	3	5	3
Arthralgia	5	3	3	2
Nervous system				
Insomnia	40	28	45	18
Dream abnormality	5	18	13	3
Anxiety	8	6	9	6
Disturbed concentration	9	3	9	4
Dizziness	10	2	8	6
Nervousness	4	<1	2	2
Tremor	1	<1	2	0
Dysphoria	<1	1	2	1
Respiratory				
Rhinitis	12	11	9	8
Increased cough	3	5	<1	1
Pharyngitis	3	2	3	0
Sinusitis	2	2	2	1
Dyspnea	1	0	2	1
Epistaxis	2	1	1	0
Skin				
Application site reaction†	11	17	15	7
Rash	4	3	3	2
Pruritus	3	1	5	1
Urticaria	2	0	2	0
Special senses				
Taste perversion	3	1	3	2
Tinnitus	1	0	<1	0

*Selected adverse events with an incidence of at least 1% of patients treated with either ZYBAN, NTS, or the combination of ZYBAN and NTS and more frequent than in the placebo group.

†Patients randomized to ZYBAN or placebo received placebo patches.

DRUG ABUSE AND DEPENDENCE

ZYBAN is likely to have a low abuse potential.

Humans: There have been few reported cases of drug dependence and withdrawal symptoms associated with the immediate-release formulation of bupropion. In human studies of abuse liability, individuals experienced with drugs of abuse reported that bupropion produced a feeling of euphoria and desirability. In these subjects, a single dose of 400 mg (1.33 times the recommended daily dose) of bupropion produced mild amphetamine-like effects compared to placebo on the Morphine-Benzedrine Subscale of the Addiction Research Center Inventories (ARCI), which is indicative of euphorigenic properties and a score intermediate between placebo and amphetamine on the Liking Scale of the ARCI.

Animals: Studies in rodents and primates have shown that bupropion exhibits some pharmacologic actions common to psychostimulants. In rodents, it has been shown to increase locomotor activity, elicit a mild stereotyped behavioral response, and increase rates of responding in several schedule-controlled behavior paradigms. In primate models to assess the positive reinforcing effects of psychoactive drugs, bupropion was self-administered intravenously. In rats, bupropion produced amphetamine- and cocaine-like discriminative stimulus effects in drug discrimination paradigms used to characterize the subjective effects of psychoactive drugs.

The possibility that bupropion may induce dependence should be kept in mind when evaluating the desirability of including the drug in smoking cessation programs of individual patients.

OVERDOSAGE

Human Overdose Experience: There has been very limited experience with overdosage of the sustained-release formulation of bupropion; three such cases were reported during clinical trials in depressed patients. One patient ingested 3000 mg of bupropion sustained-release tablets and vomited quickly after the overdose; the patient experienced blurred vision and lightheadedness. A second patient ingested a "handful" of bupropion sustained-release tablets and experienced confusion, lethargy, nausea, jitteriness, and seizure. A third patient ingested 3600 mg of bupropion sustained-release tablets and a bottle of wine; the patient experienced nausea, visual hallucinations, and "grogginess." None of the patients experienced further sequelae.

There has been extensive experience with overdosages of the immediate-release formulation of bupropion. Thirteen overdoses occurred during clinical trials in depressed patients. Twelve patients ingested 850 to 4200 mg and recovered without significant sequelae. Another patient who ingested 9000 mg of the immediate-release formulation of bupropion and 300 mg of tranylcypromine experienced a grand mal seizure and recovered without further sequelae.

Since introduction, overdoses of up to 17,500 mg of the immediate-release formulation of bupropion have been reported. Seizure was reported in approximately one third of all cases. Other serious reactions reported with overdoses of the immediate-release formulation of bupropion alone included hallucinations, loss of consciousness, and sinus tachycardia. Fever, muscle rigidity, rhabdomyolysis, hypotension, stupor, coma, and respiratory failure have been reported when the immediate-release formulation of bupropion was part of multiple drug overdoses.

Although most patients recovered without sequelae, deaths associated with overdoses of the immediate-release formulation of bupropion alone have been reported rarely in patients ingesting massive doses of the drug. Multiple uncontrolled seizures, bradycardia, cardiac failure, and cardiac arrest prior to death were reported in these patients.

Overdosage Management: Ensure an adequate airway, oxygenation, and ventilation. Monitor cardiac rhythm and vital signs. EEG monitoring is also recommended for the first 48 hours post-ingestion. General supportive and symptomatic measures are also recommended. Induction of emesis is not recommended. Gastric lavage with a large-bore orogastric tube with appropriate airway protection, if needed, may be indicated if performed soon after ingestion or in symptomatic patients.

Activated charcoal should be administered. There is no experience with the use of forced diuresis, dialysis, hemoperfusion, or exchange transfusion in the management of bupropion overdoses. No specific antidotes for bupropion are known.

Due to the dose-related risk of seizures with ZYBAN, hospitalization following suspected overdose should be considered. Based on studies in animals, it is recommended that seizures be treated with intravenous benzodiazepine administration and other supportive measures, as appropriate.

In managing overdosage, consider the possibility of multiple drug involvement. The physician should consider contacting a poison control center for additional information on the treatment of any overdose. Telephone numbers for certified poison control centers are listed in the *Physicians' Desk Reference* (PDR).

DOSAGE AND ADMINISTRATION

ZYBAN: *Usual Dosage for Adults:* The recommended and maximum dose of ZYBAN is 300 mg/day, given as 150 mg twice daily. Dosing should begin at 150 mg/day given every day for the first 3 days, followed by a dose increase for most patients to the recommended usual dose of 300 mg/day.

There should be an interval of at least 8 hours between successive doses. Doses above 300 mg/day should not be used (see WARNINGS). Treatment with ZYBAN should be initiated **while the patient is still smoking**, since approximately 1 week of treatment is required to achieve steady-state blood levels of bupropion. Patients should set a "target quit date" within the first 2 weeks of treatment with ZYBAN, generally in the second week. Treatment with ZYBAN should be continued for 7 to 12 weeks; longer treatment should be guided by the relative benefits and risks for individual patients. If a patient has not made significant progress towards abstinence by the seventh week of therapy with ZYBAN, it is unlikely that he or she will quit during that attempt, and treatment should probably be discontinued. Conversely, a patient who successfully quits after 7 to 12 weeks of treatment should be considered for ongoing therapy with ZYBAN. Dose tapering of ZYBAN is not required when discontinuing treatment. It is important that patients continue to receive counseling and support throughout treatment with ZYBAN, and for a period of time thereafter.

Individualization of Therapy: Patients are more likely to quit smoking and remain abstinent if they are seen frequently and receive support from their physicians or other health care professionals. It is important to ensure that patients read the instructions provided to them and have their questions answered. Physicians should review the patient's overall smoking cessation program that includes treatment with ZYBAN. Patients should be advised of the importance of participating in the behavioral interventions, counseling, and/or support services to be used in conjunction with ZYBAN. See information for patients at the end of the package insert.

The goal of therapy with ZYBAN is complete abstinence. If a patient has not made significant progress towards abstinence by the seventh week of therapy with ZYBAN, it is unlikely that he or she will quit during that attempt, and treatment should probably be discontinued.

Patients who fail to quit smoking during an attempt may benefit from interventions to improve their chances for success on subsequent attempts. Patients who are unsuccessful should be evaluated to determine why they failed. A new quit attempt should be encouraged when factors that contributed to failure can be eliminated or reduced, and conditions are more favorable.

Maintenance: Nicotine dependence is a chronic condition. Some patients may need continuous treatment. Systematic evaluation of ZYBAN 300 mg/day for maintenance therapy demonstrated that treatment for up to 6 months was efficacious. Whether to continue treatment with ZYBAN for periods longer than 12 weeks for smoking cessation must be determined for individual patients.

Combination Treatment With ZYBAN and a Nicotine Transdermal System (NTS): Combination treatment with ZYBAN and NTS may be prescribed for smoking cessation. The prescriber should review the complete prescribing information for both ZYBAN and NTS before using combination treatment. See also CLINICAL TRIALS for methods and dosing used in the ZYBAN and NTS combination trial. Monitoring for treatment-emergent hypertension in patients treated with the combination of ZYBAN and NTS is recommended.

HOW SUPPLIED

ZYBAN Sustained-Release Tablets, 150 mg of bupropion hydrochloride, are purple, round, biconvex, film-coated tablets printed with "ZYBAN 150" in bottles of 60 (NDC 0173-0556-02) tablets and the ZYBAN Advantage Pack™ containing 1 bottle of 60 (NDC 0173-0556-01) tablets.

Store at controlled room temperature, 20° to 25°C (68° to 77°F) (see USP). Dispense in tight, light-resistant containers as defined in the USP.

PATIENT INFORMATION: The following wording is contained in a separate leaflet provided for patients.

Information for the Patient

ZYBAN® (bupropion hydrochloride) Sustained-Release Tablets

Please read this information before you start taking ZYBAN. Also read this leaflet each time you renew your prescription, in case anything has changed. This information is not intended to take the place of discussions between you and your doctor. You and your doctor should discuss ZYBAN as part of your plan to stop smoking. Your doctor has prescribed ZYBAN for your use only. Do not let anyone else use your ZYBAN.

IMPORTANT WARNING:

There is a chance that approximately 1 out of every 1000 people taking bupropion hydrochloride, the active ingredient in ZYBAN, will have a seizure. The chance of this happening increases if you:

- have a seizure disorder (for example, epilepsy);
- have or have had an eating disorder (for example, bulimia or anorexia nervosa);
- take more than the recommended amount of ZYBAN; or
- take other medicines with the same active ingredient that is in ZYBAN, such as WELLBUTRIN® (bupropion hydrochloride) Tablets and WELLBUTRIN SR® (bupropion hydrochloride) Sustained-Release Tablets. (Both of these medicines are used to treat depression.)

You can reduce the chance of experiencing a seizure by following your doctor's directions on how to take ZYBAN. You should also discuss with your doctor whether ZYBAN is right for you.

1. What is ZYBAN?

ZYBAN is a prescription medicine to help people quit smoking. Studies have shown that more than one third of people quit smoking for at least 1 month while taking ZYBAN and participating in a patient support program. For many patients, ZYBAN reduces withdrawal symptoms and the urge to smoke. ZYBAN should be used with a patient support program. It is important to participate in the behavioral program, counseling, or other support program your health care professional recommends.

2. Who should not take ZYBAN?

You should not take ZYBAN if you:

- have a seizure disorder (for example, epilepsy).
- are already taking WELLBUTRIN, WELLBUTRIN SR, or any other medicines that contain bupropion hydrochloride.
- have or have had an eating disorder (for example, bulimia or anorexia nervosa).
- are currently taking or have recently taken a monoamine oxidase inhibitor (MAOI).
- are allergic to bupropion.

3. Are there special concerns for women?

ZYBAN is not recommended for women who are pregnant or breast-feeding. Women should notify their doctor if they become pregnant or intend to become pregnant while taking ZYBAN.

4. How should I take ZYBAN?

- You should take ZYBAN as directed by your doctor. The usual recommended dosing is to take one 150-mg tablet in the morning for the first 3 days. On the fourth day, begin taking one 150-mg tablet in the morning and one 150-mg tablet in the early evening. Doses should be taken at least 8 hours apart.
- **Never take an "extra" dose of ZYBAN.** If you forget to take a dose, do not take an extra tablet to "catch up" for the dose you forgot. Wait and take your next tablet at the regular time. Do not take more tablets than your doctor prescribed. This is important so you do not increase your chance of having a seizure.
- It is important to swallow ZYBAN Tablets whole. Do not chew, divide, or crush tablets.

5. How long should I take ZYBAN?

Most people should take ZYBAN for at least 7 to 12 weeks. Some people may need to take ZYBAN for a longer period of time to assist in their smoking cessation efforts. Follow your doctor's instructions.

6. When should I stop smoking?

It takes about 1 week for ZYBAN to reach the right levels in your body to be effective. So, to maximize your chance of quitting, you should not stop smoking until you have been taking ZYBAN for 1 week. You should set a date to stop smoking during the second week you're taking ZYBAN.

7. Can I smoke while taking ZYBAN?

It is not physically dangerous to smoke and use ZYBAN at the same time. However, continuing to smoke after the date you set to stop smoking will seriously reduce your chance of breaking your smoking habit.

8. Can ZYBAN be used at the same time as nicotine patches?

Yes, ZYBAN and nicotine patches can be used at the same time but should only be used together under the supervision of your doctor. Using ZYBAN and nicotine patches together may raise your blood pressure. Your doctor will probably want to check your blood pressure regularly to make sure that it stays within acceptable levels.

DO NOT SMOKE AT ANY TIME if you are using a nicotine patch or any other nicotine product along with ZYBAN. It is possible to get too much nicotine and have serious side effects.

9. What are possible side effects of ZYBAN?

Like all medicines, ZYBAN may cause side effects.

- The most common side effects include dry mouth and difficulty sleeping. These side effects are generally mild and often disappear after a few weeks. If you have difficulty sleeping, avoid taking your medicine too close to bedtime.
- The most common side effects that caused people to stop taking ZYBAN during clinical studies were shakiness and skin rash.
- Stop taking ZYBAN and contact your doctor or health care professional if you have signs of an allergic reaction such as a rash, hives, or difficulty in breathing. Discuss any other troublesome side effects with your doctor.
- Use caution before driving a car or operating complex, hazardous machinery until you know if ZYBAN affects your ability to perform these tasks.

10. Can I drink alcohol while I am taking ZYBAN?

It is best to not drink alcohol at all or to drink very little while taking ZYBAN. If you drink a lot of alcohol and suddenly stop, you may increase your chance of having a seizure. Therefore, it is important to discuss your use of alcohol with your doctor before you begin taking ZYBAN.

11. Will ZYBAN affect other medicines I am taking?

ZYBAN may affect other medicines you're taking. It is important not to take medicines that may increase the chance for you to have a seizure. Therefore, you should make sure that your doctor knows about all medicines—prescription or over-the-counter—you are taking or plan to take.

12. Do ZYBAN Tablets have a characteristic odor?

ZYBAN Tablets may have a characteristic odor. If present, this odor is normal.

13. How should I store ZYBAN?

- Store ZYBAN at room temperature, out of direct sunlight.
- Keep ZYBAN in a tightly closed container.
- Keep ZYBAN out of the reach of children.

This summary provides important information about ZYBAN. This summary cannot replace the more detailed information that you need from your doctor. If you have any questions or concerns about either ZYBAN or smoking cessation, talk to your doctor or other health care professional.

Manufactured by Catalytica Pharmaceuticals, Inc., Greenville, NC 27834
for Glaxo Wellcome Inc., Research Triangle Park, NC 27709
US Patent Nos. 5,358,970; 5,427,798; 5,731,000; and 5,763,493

September 1999/RL-754

Shown in Product Identification Guide, page 317

Glenwood

82 N. SUMMIT STREET
TENAFLY, NJ 07670

Direct Inquiries to:
Professional Services Department
201 569-0050
800 542-0772

For Medical Information Contact:
In Emergencies:
Professional Services Department
201 569-0050
800 542-0772

POTABA® ℞
Systemic ANTIFIBROSIS THERAPY

PRODUCT OVERVIEW

KEY FACTS

Potaba® (Aminobenzoate Potassium) is considered a member of the vitamin B complex. It has been suggested that the antifibrotic action of Potaba® is due to its mediation of increased oxygen uptake at the tissue level.

MAJOR USES

Potaba® offers a means of treatment of serious and often chronic entities, such as scleroderma and Peyronie's Disease.

SAFETY INFORMATION

Contraindicated in patients taking sulfonamides. Anorexia, nausea, fever and rash have occurred infrequently and subside with omission of the drug. Often, desensitization can be accomplished and treatment resumed.

PRESCRIBING INFORMATION

POTABA® ℞
Systemic ANTIFIBROSIS THERAPY

FORMULA

POTABA is chemically pure potassium p-aminobenzoate

INDICATIONS

Based on a review of this drug by the National Academy of Sciences-National Research Council and/or other information, FDA has classified the indications as follows:

"Possibly" effective: Potassium aminobenzoate is possibly effective in the treatment of scleroderma, dermatomyositis, morphea, linear scleroderma, pemphigus, and Peyronie's disease.

Final classification of the less-than-effective indications requires further investigation.

ADVANTAGES

POTABA offers a means of treatment of serious and often chronic entities involving fibrosis and nonsuppurative inflammation.

PHARMACOLOGY

p-Aminobenzoate is considered a member of the vitamin B complex. Small amounts are found in cereal, eggs, milk and meats. Detectable amounts are normally present in human blood, spinal fluid, urine, and sweat. PABA is a component of several biologically important systems, and it participates in a number of fundamental biological processes.

It has been suggested that the antifibrosis action of POTABA is due to its mediation of increased oxygen uptake at the tissue level. Fibrosis is believed to occur from either too much serotonin or too little monoamine oxidase (MAO) activity over a period of time. Monoamine oxidase requires an adequate supply of oxygen to function properly. By increasing oxygen supply at the tissue level POTABA may enhance MAO activity and prevent or bring about regression of fibrosis.

Continued on next page

Potaba—Cont.

CLINICAL USES

PEYRONIE'S DISEASE: 21 patients with Peyronie's disease were placed on POTABA therapy for periods ranging from 3 months to 2 years. Pain disappeared from 16 of 16 cases in which it had been present. There was objective improvement in penile deformity in 10 of 17 patients, and decrease in plaque size in 16 of 21. The authors suggest that this medication offers no hazard of further local injury as may result from other therapy. There were no significant untoward effects encountered on long term POTABA therapy.

SCLERODERMA: Of 135 patients with diffuse systemic sclerosis treated with POTABA every patient but one has shown softening of the involved skin if treatment has been continued for 3 months or longer. The responses have been reported in a number of publications. The treatment program consists of systemic antifibrosis therapy with POTABA, physical therapy, including deep breathing exercises and dynamic traction splints where indicated, and bethanechol chloride for relief of dysphagia as well as small doses of reserpine for amelioration of Raynaud's phenomena.

DERMATOMYOSITIS: Five patients with scleroderma and 2 with dermatomyositis were treated with POTABA. There was striking clinical improvement in each patient. Doses of 15-20 grams per day were well tolerated, and patients were easily able to take these doses.

MORPHEA and LINEAR SCLERODERMA: All 14 patients with localized forms of scleroderma placed on long-term POTABA treatment showed softening of the sclerotic component of their disorder. Treatment is particularly indicated in patients where persistent compressive sclerosis may contribute even greater disfigurement or functional embarrassment from secondary pressure atrophy.

DOSAGE AND ADMINISTRATION

The average adult daily dose of POTABA is 12 grams, usually given in four to six divided doses. Tablets and capsules 0.5 gram are given at the rate of 4 tablets or capsules 6 times daily, or 6 given four times daily, usually with meals, and at bed-time with a snack. Tablets must be dissolved in an adequate amount of liquid to prevent gastrointestinal upset.

POTABA Envules contain 2 grams pure drug each. 6 Envules are given for a total of 12 grams POTABA daily.

Children are given 1 gram POTABA daily in divided doses for each 10 lbs. of body weight.

SIDE EFFECTS

Anorexia, nausea, fever and rash have occurred infrequently and subside with omission of the drug. Desensitization can be accomplished and treatment resumed.

USAGE IN PREGNANCY

Safety for use in pregnancy or during lactation has not been established.

PRECAUTIONS

Should anorexia or nausea occur, therapy is interrupted until the patient is eating normally again. This permits prompt subsidence of symptoms and also avoids the possible development of hypoglycemia. Give cautiously to patients with renal disease. If a hypersensitivity reaction should occur, POTABA should be stopped.

CONTRAINDICATIONS

POTABA should not be administered to patients taking sulfonamides.

HOW SUPPLIED

POTABA Capsules—0.5 gm.
NDC 0516-0051-25 Bottle of 250
NDC 0516-0051-10 Bottle of 1000
POTABA Tablets—0.5 gm.
NDC 0516-0054-01 Bottle of 100
NDC 0516-0054-10 Bottle of 1000
POTABA Powder—2.0 gm Envule
NDC 0516-0052-50 Box of 50 × 2.0 gm

Shown in Product Identification Guide, page 317

YODOXIN® ℞

210 mg. & 650 mg. Tablets
(IODOQUINOL TABLETS U.S.P.)

PRODUCT OVERVIEW

KEY FACTS

Yodoxin (Iodoquinol) is amebicidal against the cyst and trophozoite forms of Entamoeba histolytica. Yodoxin® contains 64% organically bound iodine.

MAJOR USES

Yodoxin® is used in the treatment of intestinal amebiasis.

SAFETY INFORMATION

Contraindicated in patients with hepatic damage and in patients with known hypersensitivity to iodine and 8-hydroxyquinolines. Long term use of this drug should be avoided as optic neuritis, optic atrophy and peripheral neuropathy have been reported following prolonged high dosage with halogenated 8-hydroxyquinolines.

PRESCRIBING INFORMATION

YODOXIN® ℞

210 mg. & 650 mg. Tablets
(IODOQUINOL TABLETS U.S.P.)

DESCRIPTION

Iodoquinol is a light yellowish to tan color, nearly odorless and stable in air. The compound is practically insoluble in water, and sparingly soluble in most other solvents. It contains 64 per cent organically bound iodine.

ACTION

Iodoquinol is amebicidal against Entamoeba histolytica and is considered effective against the trophozoite and cyst forms.

INDICATIONS

Iodoquinol is used in the treatment of intestinal amebiasis. Iodoquinol is not recommended for the treatment of nonspecific diarrhea.

CONTRAINDICATIONS

Known hypersensitivity to iodine and 8-hydroxyquinolines. Contraindicated in patients with hepatic damage.

WARNINGS

Optic neuritis, optic atrophy, and peripheral neuropathy have been reported following prolonged high dosage therapy with halogenated 8-hydroxyquinolines. Long term use of this drug should be avoided.

USE IN PREGNANCY

Safety for use in pregnancy or during lactation has not been established.

PRECAUTIONS

Iodoquinol should be used with caution in patients with thyroid disease.

Protein-bound serum iodine levels may be increased during treatment with iodoquinol and therefore interfere with certain thyroid function tests. These effects may persist for as long as six months after discontinuation of therapy. Discontinue the drug if hypersensitivity reactions occur.

ADVERSE REACTIONS

Skin: various forms of skin eruptions (acneiform papular and pustular; bullae; vegetating or tuberous iododerma), urticaria and pruritus. Gastrointestinal: nausea, vomiting, abdominal cramps, diarrhea, and pruritus ani.

Fever, chills, headache, vertigo and enlargement of thyroid have been reported. Optic neuritis, optic atrophy and peripheral neuropathy have been reported in association with prolonged high-dosage 8-hydroxyquinoline therapy.

DOSAGE AND ADMINISTRATION

Usual adult dose: (210 mg tablet) 3 tablets three times a day, to be taken after meals for twenty days. Usual adult dose: (650 mg tablet) 1 tablet three times a day, to be taken after meals for twenty days. Usual pediatric dose: 10 to 13.3 mg per kg of body weight, three times a day for 20 days. Dose should not exceed 1.95 grams in twenty-four hours.

HOW SUPPLIED

YODOXIN Tablets—210 mg.
NDC-0516-0092-01 Bottle of 100
YODOXIN Tablets—650 mg.
NDC-0516-0093-01 Bottle of 100

STORAGE

Store at Controlled Room Temperature 15–30°C. (59–86°F.)
Rx only

Gordon Laboratories

6801 LUDLOW STREET
UPPER DARBY, PA 19082

Direct inquiries to:
Customer Service
(610) 734-2011
Fax (610) 734-2049
Website: http://www.gordonlabs.com
E-mail: gordonlabs@worldnet.att.net
For medical emergencies contact:
David Dercher (610) 734-2011
Fax (610) 734-2049

GORDOCHOM™ Solution OTC

[gōrdō'kōm]

DESCRIPTION

Gordochom is an antifungal solution for topical use containing 25% Undecylenic Acid and 3% Chloroxylenol as its active ingredients in a penetrating oil base. Undecylenic Acid is chemically 10 hendecenoic acid having the empirical formula $C_{11}H_{20}O_2$ and the chemical bond structure CH_2=CH $(CH_2)8$ CO_2H.

Undecylenic Acid is a colorless to pale yellow liquid. It is insoluble in water and soluble in alcohol, chloroform and ether.

Chloroxylenol is chemically 2-chloro-5-hydroxy-1,3-dimethylbenzene having the empirical formula C_8H_9 ClO.

CLINICAL PHARMACOLOGY

Undecylenic Acid is a fungistatic agent employed in the treatment of tinea pedis, ringworm and dermatophytosis. Chloroxylenol is a topical antiseptic germicide and antifungal agent effective against a wide variety of causative fungi and yeast organisms. Among those affected by chloroxylenol are candida albicans, aspergillus niger, aspergillus flavus, trichophyton rubrum, trichophyton mentagrophytes, penicillum luteum and epidermophyton floccosum.

The penetrating oil base vehicle serves as a delivery system, enhancing the impregnation of Undecylenic Acid and Chloroxylenol as antimicrobial agents.

INDICATIONS

Cures athlete's foot (tinea pedis), and ringworm (tinea corporis).

CONTRAINDICATIONS

Gordochom is contraindicated in patients who are sensitive to Undecylenic Acid or Chloroxylenol.

WARNINGS

FOR EXTERNAL USE ONLY. Not for opthalmic or optic use. Avoid inhaling and contact with eyes or other mucous membranes. Not to be applied over blistered, raw or oozing areas of skin or over deep puncture wounds.

PRECAUTIONS

If a reaction suggesting sensitivity or chemical irritation should occur with the use of Gordochom, treatment should be discontinued. Use of Gordochom in pregnancy has not been established.

ADVERSE REACTIONS

No significant adverse reactions have been reported. However, attention should be paid to localized hypersensitivity.

DOSAGE AND ADMINISTRATION

Cleanse and dry affected areas. Apply a thin application twice a day (morning and night) to the affected area, or as recommended by your physician. Supervise children in the use of this product. For athlete's foot, pay special attention to the spaces between the toes; wear well-fitting, ventilated shoes, and change shoes and socks at least once daily. For athlete's foot and ringworm, use daily for 4 weeks. If condition persists longer, consult a physician. This product has not been proven effective on the scalp or nails.

HOW SUPPLIED

Gordochom is available in 1 oz. bottles with special brush applicator. (NDC 104818010-2)
Store at controlled room temperatures (59°–86°F).
For external use only.
Keep out of reach of children.

A.C. Grace Co.

1100 QUITMAN ROAD
P.O. BOX 570
BIG SANDY, TX 75755

Direct Inquiries to:
Inquiries: (903) 636-4368
Orders Only: 800-833-4368

UNIQUE E® OTC

NATURAL VITAMIN E COMPLEX
MIXED TOCOPHEROLS CONCENTRATE

DESCRIPTION

OUR SOLE PRODUCT! Established 1962. WHY UNIQUE? ALL NATURAL UNESTERIFIED HIGH ANTI*THROMBIC*, d-Alpha TOCOPHEROL FUNCTION, FULL ANTI*OXIDANT* d-Beta, d-GAMMA, d-Delta PROTECTION against harmful free radical damage *PLUS* the total biological activity and synergistic benefit of the complete natural Vitamin E Complex.

NOT the dl synthetic chemical form, not ESTERified tocopher(y)l acetate, (or succinate) nor ordinary soy oil diluted Mixed Tocopherols or any adulterated mixture.

NO SOY, or other oil fillers to turn RANCID and cause harmful free radical pathology.

NO allergy causing additives, preservatives, colors or flavorings.

400 I.U. d-alpha tocopherol in MIXED TOCOPHEROLS COMPLEX (Certified by Assay) in pure Bovine gelatin Softgel capsules.

DOSAGE

Up to 6 capsules daily as directed by your physician according to individual weight or need, usually 1 capsule for each 40 lbs. of total body weight. Best results when entire daily dose is taken just before or with the morning meal.

HOW SUPPLIED

Bottles of 180 and 90 Softgel Capsules is safety-sealed, light protected plastic bottles.

Grifols America, Inc.

8880 N.W. 18TH. TERRACE
MIAMI, FLORIDA 33172

Direct Inquiries to:
Ph: (305) 593 8366
Fax: (305) 593 8166
(305) 594 4090
E-mail: grifamer@bellsouth.net

HUMAN ALBUMIN GRIFOLS® 20% ℞
Albumin (Human), USP, 20% Solution

DESCRIPTION

Albumin (Human), Human Albumin Grifols® 20% is a sterile aqueous solution for single dose intravenous administration containing 20% human albumin (weight/volume). Human Albumin Grifols® 20% is prepared by a cold alcohol fractionation method from pooled human plasma obtained from venous blood. The product is stabilized with 0.08 millimole sodium caprylate and 0.08 millimole sodium acetyltryptophanate per gram of protein. Human Albumin Grifols® 20% is osmotically equivalent to four times its volume of normal citrated plasma.

A liter of Human Albumin Grifols® 20% solution contains 130–160 milliequivalents of sodium ion. The product contains no preservatives.

Human Albumin Grifols® 20% is heated at 60°C for ten hours. No positive assertion can be made, however, that this heat treatment completely destroys the causative agents of viral hepatitis. There are no known cases of viral hepatitis, which have resulted from the administration of Human Albumin Grifols® 20%.

HOW SUPPLIED

Albumin (Human), Human Albumin Grifols® 20% is supplied in 50 ml vial.
NDC 61953-0001-1 May 1998

Guardian Laboratories

a division of United-Guardian, Inc.
P.O. Box 18050
HAUPPAUGE, N.Y. 11788

For Medical Information Contact:
Director of Medical Research
(516) 273-0900
(800) 645-5566

CLORPACTIN® WCS-90 OTC
[*klor-pak 'tin*]
(brand of sodium oxychlorosene)

COMPOSITION

Stabilized organic derivative of hypochlorous acid. A white, water soluble powder with a characteristic smell of hypochlorous acid. Active chlorine derived from calcium hypochlorite: 3–4%.

ACTION AND USES

For use as a topical antiseptic for treating localized infections, particularly when resistant organisms are present. Complete spectrum (bacteria, fungi, viruses, mold, yeast and spores); effective in cases of antibiotic resistance; nontoxic and non-allergenic in use concentrations.

ADMINISTRATION AND DOSAGE

Applied by irrigation, instillations, spray, soaks or wet compresses, preferably thoroughly cleansing with gravity flow irrigation or syringe to provide copious quantities of fresh solution to remove the organic wastes and debris from the site of the involvement. Also for preoperative skin preparation and postoperative protection. Generally applied as the 0.4% solution in water, or isotonic saline, but as the 0.1% to 0.2% in Urology and Ophthalmology.

CONTRAINDICATIONS

The use of this product is contraindicated where the site of the infection is not exposed to the direct contact with the solution. Not for systemic use.

HOW SUPPLIED

In boxes containing 5 x 2 gram bottles. NDC: 0327-0001-10
Store under refrigeration.

RENACIDIN® ℞
(Citric Acid, Glucono-delta-lactone, and Magnesium Carbonate)
Irrigation

DESCRIPTION

Renacidin® (Citric Acid, Glucono-delta-lactone, and Magnesium Carbonate) Irrigation is a sterile, non-pyrogenic irrigation for use within the urinary tract in the prevention and dissolution of calculi.

Each 100 ml. of Renacidin Irrigation contains:
Active ingredients:

Citric Acid (anhydrous), U.S.P. $C_6H_8O_7$	6.602 grams
Glucono-delta-lactone $C_6H_{10}O_6$	0.198 grams
Magnesium Carbonate, U.S.P. $(MgCO_3)_4{\cdot}Mg(OH)_2{\cdot}3H_2O$	3.177 grams

Citric Acid **Glucono-delta-lactone**

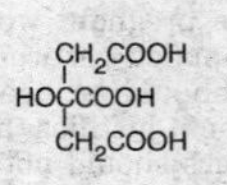

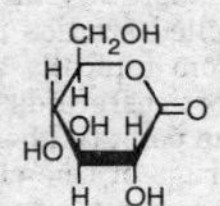

Magnesium Carbonate
$(MgCO_3)_4{\cdot}Mg(OH)_2{\cdot}3H_2O$

Inert ingredients:

Benzoic Acid, U.S.P.	0.023 grams

Solution pH: 3.85 (3.50–4.20)

HOW SUPPLIED

Renacidin Irrigation is available as a sterile, non-pyrogenic solution in 500 ml containers, packaged in cartons of six. Exposure of Renacidin Irrigation to heat or cold should be minimized. Renacidin Irrigation should be stored at controlled room temperature, 59° to 86°F (15° to 30°C). Avoid excessive heat or cold (keep from freezing). Brief exposure to temperatures of up to 40°C or temperatures down to 5°C does not adversely affect the product.
NDC: 0327-0011-05
PRODUCT CODE: RN500

Healthpoint

2600 AIRPORT FWY
FORT WORTH, TX 76111

Direct Inquiries to:
800-441-8227

ACCUZYME® ℞
PAPAIN-UREA DEBRIDING OINTMENT

DESCRIPTION

Each gram of ACCUZYME enzymatic debriding ointment contains papain (8.3×10^5 USP units of activity) and 100mg urea in a hydrophilic ointment base composed of purified water, emulsifying wax, glycerin, isopropyl palmitate, potassium phosphate monobasic, fragrance, methylparaben and propylparaben.

CLINICAL PHARMACOLOGY

Papain, the proteolytic enzyme from the fruit of carica papaya, is a potent digestant of nonviable protein matter but is harmless to viable tissue. It is active over a pH range of 3 to 12. Papain is relatively ineffective when used alone as a debriding agent and requires the presence of activators to stimulate its digestive potency. In ACCUZYME, papain is combined with urea, a denaturant of proteins, to bring about two supplemental chemical actions: (1) to expose by solvent action the activators of papain, and (2) to denature the nonviable protein matter in lesions and thereby render it more susceptible to enzymatic digestion. Pharmacologic studies have shown that the combination of papain and urea result in twice as much digestive activity as papain alone.

INDICATIONS AND USAGE

ACCUZYME is indicated for debridement of necrotic tissue and liquefication of slough in acute and chronic lesions such as pressure ulcers, varicose and diabetic ulcers, burns, postoperative wounds, pilonidal cyst wounds, carbuncles and miscellaneous traumatic or infected wounds.

CONTRAINDICATIONS

ACCUZYME is contraindicated in patients who have shown sensitivity to papain or any other components of this preparation.

PRECAUTIONS

See Dosage and Administration. Not to be used in eyes.

ADVERSE REACTIONS

ACCUZYME is generally well-tolerated and non-irritating. A transient "burning" sensation may be experienced by a small percentage of patients upon applying ACCUZYME. Occasionally, the profuse exudate from enzymatic digestion may irritate the skin. In such cases, more frequent dressing changes will alleviate discomfort until exudate decreases.

DOSAGE AND ADMINISTRATION

Cleanse the wound with ALLCLENZ® Wound Cleanser or saline. Avoid cleansing with hydrogen peroxide solution as it may inactivate the papain. Apply ACCUZYME directly to the wound, cover with appropriate dressing, secure into place. Daily or twice daily applications are preferred. Irrigate the wound at each redressing to remove any accumulation of liquefied necrotic material. NOTE: Papain may also be inactivated by the salts of heavy metals such as lead, silver and mercury. Contact with medications containing these metals should be avoided.

HOW SUPPLIED

30g tubes. Store in a cool place.
CAUTION: Avoid freezing or extreme heat.
Rx only
NDC–0064-1000-01
HEALTHPOINT®
HEALTHPOINT, San Antonio, Texas 78215
1-800-441-8227
REORDER NO. 1000-01 126959-1195
Shown in Product Identification Guide, page 317

AKNE-MYCIN® ℞
[*ak-nē-mīcin*]
(Erythromycin)
2% TOPICAL OINTMENT FOR ACNE

DESCRIPTION

Akne-mycin (erythromycin) topical ointment contains erythromycin which is produced from a strain of *Streptomyces erythraeus*. Each gram of Akne-mycin topical ointment contains 20 mg of erythromycin base in a vehicle consisting of mineral oil, petrolatum, paraffin, talc, titanium dioxide, tri-laureth 4 phosphate, oleyl oleate, trilaneth 4 phosphate, cetostearyl alcohol, sorbitol and fragrance. Akne-mycin marketed in the United States is not of the same composition as Akne-mycin marketed in Europe.

CLINICAL PHARMACOLOGY

Although the mechanism by which Akne-mycin acts in reducing the inflammatory lesions of acne vulgaris is unknown, it is presumably due to the antibiotic action of the drug.

INDICATIONS AND USAGE

Akne-mycin is indicated for topical control of acne vulgaris.

CONTRAINDICATIONS

Akne-mycin is contraindicated in persons who have shown hypersensitivity to erythromycin or to any of the other listed ingredients.

WARNINGS

The safe use of Akne-mycin during pregnancy or lactation has not been established.

PRECAUTIONS

Akne-mycin is for topical use only and should be kept out of the eyes, nose and mouth.

The use of antibiotic agents may be associated with the overgrowth of antibiotic resistant organisms. If this occurs, administration of the drug should be discontinued and appropriate measures taken.

ADVERSE REACTIONS

In clinical trials there was one report of a possible contact sensitization which could not be confirmed. There were isolated reports of skin irritation, such as erythema and peeling.

DOSAGE AND ADMINISTRATION

Akne-mycin should be applied to the affected area twice daily, morning and evening.

HOW SUPPLIED

Akne-mycin is supplied in a 25 gram sealed tube. NDC 0064-3000-25. Store below 27°C (80°F).
Distributed by:
HEALTHPOINT®
Healthpoint, Ltd.
San Antonio, Texas 78215
1-800-441-8227
Reorder No. 0064-3000-25
127553-1098
Manufactured in:
Republic of Germany
by HERMAL KURT HERRMANN
GmbH & Co
41002708
Shown in Product Identification Guide, page 317

CLODERM® CREAM, 0.1% ℞
[*clō - dĕrm*]
(clocortolone pivalate)
For Topical Use Only

DESCRIPTION

Cloderm Cream 0.1% contains the medium potency topical corticosteroid, clocortolone pivalate, in a specially formulated water-washable emollient cream base consisting of purified water, white petrolatum, mineral oil, stearyl alcohol, polyoxyl 40 stearate, carbomer 934P, edetate disodium, sodium hydroxide, with methylparaben and propylparaben as preservatives.

Chemically, clocortolone pivalate is 9-chloro-6α-fluoro-11β, 21-dihydroxy-16α-methylpregna-1, 4-diene-3, 20-dione 21-pivalate.

Continued on next page

Cloderm—Cont.

Its structure is as follows:

CLINICAL PHARMACOLOGY

Topical corticosteroids share anti-inflammatory, anti-pruritic and vasoconstrictive actions.
The mechanism of anti-inflammatory activity of the topical corticosteroids is unclear. Various laboratory methods, including vasoconstrictor assays, are used to compare and predict potencies and/or clinical efficacies of the topical corticosteroids. There is some evidence to suggest that a recognizable correlation exists between vasoconstrictor potency and therapeutic efficacy in man.
Pharmacokinetics: The extent of percutaneous absorption of topical corticosteroids is determined by many factors including the vehicle, the integrity of the epidermal barrier, and the use of occlusive dressings.
Topical corticosteroids can be absorbed from normal intact skin. Inflammation and/or other disease processes in the skin increase percutaneous absorption. Occlusive dressings substantially increase the percutaneous absorption of topical corticosteroids. Thus, occlusive dressings may be a valuable therapeutic adjunct for treatment of resistant dermatoses. (See **DOSAGE AND ADMINISTRATION**).
Once absorbed through the skin, topical corticosteroids are handled through pharmacokinetic pathways similar to systemically administered corticosteroids. Corticosteroids are bound to plasma proteins in varying degrees. Corticosteroids are metabolized primarily in the liver and are then excreted by the kidneys. Some of the topical corticosteroids and their metabolites are also excreted into the bile.

INDICATIONS AND USAGE

Topical corticosteroids are indicated for the relief of the inflammatory and pruritic manifestations of corticosteroid-responsive dermatoses.

CONTRAINDICATIONS

Topical corticosteroids are contraindicated in those patients with a history of hypersensitivity to any of the components of the preparation.

PRECAUTIONS

General: Systemic absorption of topical corticosteroids has produced reversible hypothalamic-pituitary-adrenal (HPA) axis suppression, manifestations of Cushing's syndrome, hyperglycemia, and glucosuria in some patients.
Conditions which augment systemic absorption include the application of the more potent steroids, use over large surface areas, prolonged use, and the addition of occlusive dressings.
Therefore, patients receiving a large dose of a potent topical steroid applied to a large surface area or under an occlusive dressing should be evaluated periodically for evidence of HPA axis suppression by using the urinary free cortisol and ACTH stimulation tests. If HPA axis suppression is noted, an attempt should be made to withdraw the drug, to reduce the frequency of application, or to substitute a less potent steroid.
Recovery of HPA axis function is generally prompt and complete upon discontinuation of the drug. Infrequently, signs and symptoms of steroid withdrawal may occur, requiring supplemental systemic corticosteroids.
Children may absorb proportionally larger amounts of topical corticosteroids and thus be more susceptible to systemic toxicity (See **PRECAUTIONS**–*Pediatric Use*).
If irritation develops, topical corticosteroids should be discontinued and appropriate therapy instituted.
In the presence of dermatological infections, the use of an appropriate antifungal or antibacterial agent should be instituted. If a favorable response does not occur promptly, the corticosteroid should be discontinued until the infection has been adequately controlled.
Information for the Patient: Patients using topical corticosteroids should receive the following information and instructions:

1. This medication is to be used as directed by the physician. It is for external use only. Avoid contact with the eyes.
2. Patients should be advised not to use this medication for any disorder other than for which it was prescribed.
3. The treated skin area should not be bandaged or otherwise covered or wrapped as to be occlusive unless directed by the physician.
4. Patients should report any signs of local adverse reactions especially under occlusive dressing.
5. Parents of pediatric patients should be advised not to use tight-fitting diapers or plastic pants on a child being treated in the diaper area, as these garments may constitute occlusive dressings.

Laboratory Tests: The following tests may be helpful in evaluating the HPA axis suppression:
Urinary free cortisol test
ACTH stimulation test

Carcinogenesis, Mutagenesis, and Impairment of Fertility: Long-term animal studies have not been performed to evaluate the carcinogenic potential or the effect on fertility of topical corticosteroids.
Studies to determine mutagenicity with prednisolone and hydrocortisone have revealed negative results.
Pregnancy Category C: Corticosteroids are generally teratogenic in laboratory animals when administered systemically at relatively low dosage levels. The more potent corticosteroids have been shown to be teratogenic after dermal application in laboratory animals. There are no adequate and well-controlled studies in pregnant women on teratogenic effects from topically applied corticosteroids. Therefore, topical corticosteroids should be used during pregnancy only if the potential benefit justifies the potential risk to the fetus. Drugs of this class should not be used extensively on pregnant patients, in large amounts, or for prolonged periods of time.
Nursing Mothers: It is not known whether topical administration of corticosteroids could result in sufficient systemic absorption to produce detectable quantities in breast milk. Systemically administered corticosteroids are secreted into breast milk in quantities *not* likely to have a deleterious effect on the infant. Nevertheless, caution should be exercised when topical corticosteroids are administered to a nursing woman.
Pediatric Use: Pediatric patients may demonstrate greater susceptibility to topical corticosteroid-induced HPA axis suppression and Cushing's syndrome than mature patients because of a larger skin surface area to body weight ratio.
Hypothalamic-pituitary-adrenal (HPA) axis suppression, Cushing's syndrome, and intracranial hypertension have been reported in children receiving topical corticosteroids. Manifestations of adrenal suppression in children include linear growth retardation, delayed weight gain, low plasma cortisol levels, and absence of response to ACTH stimulation. Manifestations of intracranial hypertension include bulging fontanelles, headaches, and bilateral papilledema.
Administration of topical corticosteroids to children should be limited to the least amount compatible with an effective therapeutic regimen. Chronic corticosteroid therapy may interfere with the growth and development of children.

ADVERSE REACTIONS

The following local adverse reactions are reported infrequently with topical corticosteroids, but may occur more frequently with the use of occlusive dressings. These reactions are listed in an approximate decreasing order of occurrence:
Burning
Itching
Irritation
Dryness
Folliculitis
Hypertrichosis
Acneform eruptions
Hypopigmentation
Perioral dermatitis
Allergic contact dermatitis
Maceration of the skin
Secondary infection
Skin atrophy
Striae
Miliaria

OVERDOSAGE

Topically applied corticosteroids can be absorbed in sufficient amounts to produce systemic effects (see **PRECAUTIONS**).

DOSAGE AND ADMINISTRATION

Apply Cloderm (clocortolone pivalate) Cream 0.1% sparingly to the affected areas three times a day and rub in gently.
Occlusive dressings may be used for the management of psoriasis or recalcitrant conditions.
If an infection develops, the use of occlusive dressings should be discontinued and appropriate anti–microbial therapy instituted.

HOW SUPPLIED

Cloderm (clocortolone pivalate) Cream 0.1% is supplied in tubes containing 15 grams and 45 grams.
Store Cloderm Cream between 15° and 30° C (59° and 86° F). Avoid freezing.
Distributed by:
HEALTHPOINT®
Healthpoint, Ltd.
San Antonio, Texas 78215
1-800-441-8227
Manufactured by:
DPT Laboratories, Ltd.
San Antonio, Texas 78215
Reorder No. 0064-3100-45 (45 g)
Reorder No. 0064-3100-15 (15 g)
127351-0198
Shown in Product Identification Guide, page 317

EMBELINE™ E ℞

[*ĕm-bĕlīne E*]
Emollient, 0.05%*
****potency expressed as clobetasol propionate (clobetasol propionate cream-emollient)***

FOR TOPICAL DERMATOLOGIC USE ONLY—NOT FOR OPHTHALMIC, ORAL, OR INTRAVAGINAL USE

DESCRIPTION

Embeline E (Clobetasol Propionate Cream—Emollient) Emollient contains the active compound clobetasol propionate, a synthetic corticosteroid, for topical dermatologic use. Clobetasol, an analog of prednisolone, has a high degree of glucocorticoid activity and a slight degree of mineralocorticoid activity.
Chemically, clobetasol propionate is 21-chloro-9-fluoro-11β, 17-dihydroxy-16β-methylpregna-1,4 diene-3,20-dione 17-propionate, and it has the following structural formula:

Clobetasol propionate has the molecular formula $C_{25}H_{32}ClFO_5$ and a molecular weight of 466.96. It is a white to cream-colored crystalline powder insoluble in water.
Each gram of Embeline E Emollient contains 0.5 mg clobetasol propionate in an emollient base of cetostearyl alcohol, isopropyl myristate, propylene glycol, cetomacrogol 1000, dimethicone 360, citric acid, sodium citrate, purified water, and imidurea as a preservative.

CLINICAL PHARMACOLOGY

Like other topical corticosteroids, clobetasol propionate has anti-inflammatory, antipruritic, and vasoconstrictive properties. The mechanism of the anti-inflammatory activity of the topical steroids, in general, is unclear. However, corticosteroids are thought to act by the induction of phospholipase A_2 inhibitory proteins, collectively called lipocortins. It is postulated that these proteins control the biosynthesis of potent mediators of inflammation such as prostaglandins and leukotrienes by inhibiting the release of their common precursor, arachidonic acid. Arachidonic acid is released from membrane phospholipids by phospholipase A_2.
Pharmacokinetics: The extent of percutaneous absorption of topical corticosteroids is determined by many factors, including the vehicle and integrity of the epidermal barrier. Occlusive dressing with hydrocortisone for up to 24 hours has not been demonstrated to increase penetration; however, occlusion of hydrocortisone for 96 hours markedly enhances penetration. Topical corticosteroids can be absorbed from normal intact skin. Inflammation and/or other disease processes in the skin may increase percutaneous absorption.
Studies performed with Clobetasol Propionate Cream—Emollient indicate that it is in the super-high range of potency as compared with other topical corticosteroids.

INDICATIONS AND USAGE

Embeline E (Clobetasol Propionate Cream—Emollient) Emollient is a super-high potency corticosteroid formulation indicated for the relief of the inflammatory and pruritic manifestations of corticosteroid-responsive dermatoses. Treatment beyond 2 consecutive weeks is not recommended, and the total dosage should not exceed 50 g/week because of the potential for the drug to suppress the hypothalamic-pituitary-adrenal (HPA) axis. Use in children under 12 years of age is not recommended.
In the treatment of moderate to severe plaque-type psoriasis, Embeline E Emollient applied to 5% to 10% of body surface area can be used up to 4 consecutive weeks. The total dosage should not exceed 50 g/week. When dosing for more than 2 weeks, any additional benefits of extending treatment should be weighed against the risk of HPA suppression. Treatment beyond 4 consecutive weeks is not recommended. Patients should be instructed to use Embeline E Emollient for the minimum amount of time necessary to achieve the desired results (see PRECAUTIONS and INDICATIONS AND USAGE). Use in pediatric patients under 16 years of age has not been studied.

CONTRAINDICATIONS

Embeline E (Clobetasol Propionate Cream—Emollient) Emollient is contraindicated in those patients with a history of hypersensitivity to any of the components of this preparation.

PRECAUTIONS

General: Clobetasol propionate is a highly potent topical corticosteroid that has been shown to suppress the HPA axis at doses as low as 2 g/day.
Systemic absorption of topical corticosteroids can produce reversible HPA axis suppression with the potential for glucocorticosteroid insufficiency after withdrawal from treatment. Manifestations of Cushing's syndrome, hyperglycemia, and glucosuria can also be produced in some patients by systemic absorption of topical corticosteroids while on therapy.
Patients applying a dose to a large surface area or to areas under occlusion should be evaluated periodically for evidence of HPA axis suppression. This may be done by using the ACTH stimulation, A.M. plasma cortisol, and urinary free cortisol tests. Patients receiving super-potent corticosteroids should not be treated for more than 2 weeks at a time, and only small areas should be treated at any one time due to the increased risk of HPA suppression.
If HPA axis suppression is noted, an attempt should be made to withdraw the drug, to reduce the frequency of ap-

plication, or to substitute a less potent corticosteroid. Recovery of HPA axis function is generally prompt upon discontinuation of topical corticosteroids. Infrequently, signs and symptoms of glucocorticosteroid insufficiency may occur that require supplemental systemic corticosteroids. For information on systemic supplementation, see prescribing information for those products.

Pediatric patients may be more susceptible to systemic toxicity from equivalent doses due to their larger skin surface to body mass ratios (see PRECAUTIONS: Pediatric Use).

If irritation develops, Embeline E (Clobetasol Propionate Cream—Emollient) Emollient should be discontinued and appropriate therapy instituted. Allergic contact dermatitis with corticosteroids is usually diagnosed by observing *failure to heal* rather than noting a clinical exacerbation as with most topical products not containing corticosteroids. Such an observation should be corroborated with appropriate diagnostic patch testing.

If concomitant skin infections are present or develop, an appropriate antifungal or antibacterial agent should be used. If a favorable response does not occur promptly, use of Embeline E Emollient should be discontinued until the infection has been adequately controlled.

Embeline E Emollient should not be used in the treatment of rosacea or perioral dermatitis, and should not be used on the face, groin, or axillae.

Information for Patients: Patients using topical corticosteroids should receive the following information and instructions:

1. This medication is to be used as directed by the physician. It is for external use only. Avoid contact with the eyes.
2. This medication should not be used for any disorder other than that for which it was prescribed.
3. The treated skin area should not be bandaged, otherwise covered, or wrapped so as to be occlusive unless directed by the physician.
4. Patients should report any signs of local adverse reactions to the physician.
5. Patients should inform their physicians that they are using Embeline E Emollient if surgery is contemplated.
6. This medication should not be used on the face, underarms, or groin area.
7. As with other corticosteroids, therapy should be discontinued when control has been achieved. If no improvement is seen within 2 weeks, contact the physician.

Laboratory Tests: The following tests may be helpful in evaluating patients for HPA axis suppression:

ACTH stimulation test
A.M. plasma cortisol test
Urinary free cortisol test

Carcinogenesis, Mutagenesis, Impairment of Fertility: Long-term animal studies have not been performed to evaluate the carcinogenic potential of clobetasol propionate.

Studies in the rat following oral administration at dosage levels up to 50 mg/kg per day revealed no significant effect on the males. The females exhibited an increase in the number of resorbed embryos and a decrease in the number of living fetuses at the highest dose.

Clobetasol propionate was nonmutagenic in three different test systems: the Ames test, the *Saccharomyces cerevisiae* gene conversion assay, and the *E. coli* B WP2 fluctuation test.

Pregnancy: *Teratogenic Effects: Pregnancy Category C:* Corticosteroids have been shown to be teratogenic in laboratory animals when administered systemically at relatively low dosage levels. Some corticosteroids have been shown to be teratogenic after dermal application to laboratory animals.

Clobetasol propionate has not been tested for teratogenicity by this route; however, it is absorbed percutaneously, and when administered subcutaneously it was a significant teratogen in both the rabbit and mouse. Clobetasol propionate has greater teratogenic potential than steroids that are less potent.

Teratogenicity studies in mice using the subcutaneous route resulted in fetotoxicity at the highest dose tested (1mg/kg) and teratogenicity at all dose levels tested down to 0.03 mg/kg. These doses are approximately 0.33 and 0.01 times, respectively, the human topical dose of Embeline E Emollient. Abnormalities seen included cleft palate and skeletal abnormalities.

In rabbits, clobetasol propionate was teratogenic at doses of 3 and 10 mcg/kg. These doses are approximately 0.001 and 0.003 times, respectively, the human topical dose of Embeline E Emollient. Abnormalities seen included cleft palate, cranioschisis, and other skeletal abnormalities.

There are no adequate and well-controlled studies of the teratogenic potential of clobetasol propionate in pregnant women. Embeline E Emollient should be used during pregnancy only if the potential benefit justifies the potential risk to the fetus.

Nursing Mothers: Systemically administered corticosteroids appear in human milk and could suppress growth, interfere with endogenous corticosteroid production, or cause other untoward effects. It is not known whether topical administration of corticosteroids could result in sufficient systemic absorption to produce detectable quantities in human milk. Because many drugs are excreted in human milk, caution should be exercised when Embeline E Emollient is administered to a nursing woman.

Pediatric Use: Safety and effectiveness of Embeline E Emollient in pediatric patients have not been established, and its use in pediatric patients under 12 years of age is not recommended. Because of a higher ratio of skin surface area to body mass, pediatric patients are at a greater risk than adults of HPA axis suppression and Cushing's syndrome when they are treated with topical corticosteroids. They are therefore also at greater risk of glucocorticosteroid insufficiency during or after withdrawal of treatment. Adverse effects including striae have been reported with inappropriate use of topical corticosteroids in pediatric patients.

HPA axis suppression, Cushing's syndrome, linear growth retardation, delayed weight gain, and intracranial hypertension have been reported in pediatric patients receiving topical corticosteroids. Manifestations of adrenal suppression in children include low plasma cortisol levels and absence of response to ACTH stimulation. Manifestations of intracranial hypertension include bulging fontanelles, headaches, and bilateral papilledema.

ADVERSE REACTIONS

In controlled trials with all clobetasol propionate formulations, the following adverse reactions have been reported: burning/stinging, pruritus, irritation, erythema, folliculitis, cracking and fissuring of the skin, numbness of the fingers, tenderness in the elbow, skin atrophy, and telangiectasia. The incidence of local adverse reactions reported in the trials with Clobetasol Propionate Cream—Emollient was less than 2% of patients treated with the exception of burning/stinging, which occurred in 5% of treated patients.

Cushing's syndrome has been reported in infants and adults as a result of prolonged use of topical clobetasol propionate formulations.

The following additional local adverse reactions are reported infrequently with topical corticosteroids, but may occur more frequently with super-high potency corticosteroids such as Embeline E (Clobetasol Propionate Cream—Emollient) Emollient. These reactions are listed in an approximately decreasing order of occurrence: dryness, hypertrichosis, acneiform eruptions, hypopigmentation, perioral dermatitis, allergic contact dermatitis, secondary infection, striae, and miliaria.

OVERDOSAGE

Topically applied Embeline E (Clobetasol Propionate Cream—Emollient) Emollient can be absorbed in sufficient amounts to produce systemic effects.

DOSAGE AND ADMINISTRATION

Apply a thin layer of Embeline E (Clobetasol Propionate Cream—Emollient) Emollient to the affected skin areas twice daily and rub in gently and completely (see INDICATIONS AND USAGE).

Embeline E Emollient is a super-high potency topical corticosteroid; therefore, **treatment should be limited to 2 consecutive weeks, and amounts greater than 50 g/week should not be used.** Use in children under 12 years of age is not recommended.

In moderate to severe plaque-type psoriasis, Embeline E Emollient applied to 5% to 10% of body surface area can be used up to 4 weeks. The total dosage should not exceed 50 g/week. When dosing for more than 2 weeks, any additional benefits of extending treatment should be weighed against the risk of HPA suppression. They should be discontinued when control has been achieved. If no improvement is seen within 2 weeks, reassessment of diagnosis may be necessary. Treatment beyond 4 consecutive weeks is not recommended. Use in pediatric patients under 16 years of age has not been studied.

Embeline E Emollient should not be used with occlusive dressings.

HOW SUPPLIED

Embeline E (Clobetasol Propionate Cream—Emollient) Emollient, 0.05% is supplied in 15 g (NDC 0064-0440-15), 30 g (NDC 0064-0440-30), and 60 g (NDC 0064-0440-60) tubes.

Store between 15° and 30°C (59°–86°F). Embeline E Emollient should not be refrigerated.

Rx Only

Marketed by:
HEALTHPOINT®
Healthpoint, Ltd.
San Antonio, Texas 78215
1-800-441-8227
Manufactured by:
DPT Laboratories, Ltd.
San Antonio, Texas 78215
127467-0998

Shown in Product Identification Guide, page 317

NUTRACORT® ℞

[nutră-cŏrt]
(hydrocortisone)
lotion 1% & 2.5%

DESCRIPTION

NUTRACORT® lotion is a topical hydrocortisone preparation. Hydrocortisone is therapeutically classed as an anti-inflammatory and anti-pruritic agent. Hydrocortisone is a white crystalline powder that is very slightly soluble in water and in ether and sparingly soluble in acetone and in alcohol. It is represented by the structural formula:

[See chemical structure at top of next column]

Chemical Name: Pregn-4-ene-3, 20-dione, 11, 17, 21-trihydroxy-, (11β)-.

Molecular Formula: $C_{21}H_{30}O_5$

Molecular Weight: 362.47

NUTRACORT® Lotion 1% contains: Hydrocortisone 1.0% (10 mg/mL) in a lotion base containing **Inactive:** purified water, light mineral oil, sorbitan monostearate, stearyl alcohol, cetyl alcohol, glyceryl stearate SE, sodium lauryl sulfate, edetate sodium, methylparaben, propylparaben, and certified color. May contain citric acid and/or sodium hydroxide for pH adjustment.

NUTRACTORT® Lotion 2.5% contains: Hydrocortisone 2.5% (25 mg/mL) in a lotion base containing **Inactive:** purified water, light mineral oil, sorbitan monostearate, stearyl alcohol, glyceryl stearate SE, sodium lauryl sulfate, cetyl alcohol, edetate disodium, methylparaben, propylparaben, and certified colors. May contain citric acid and/or sodium hydroxide for pH adjustment.

CLINICAL PHARMACOLOGY

Topical corticosteroids share anti-inflammatory, anti-pruritic and vasoconstrictive actions.

The mechanism of anti-inflammatory activity of the topical corticosteroids is unclear. Various laboratory methods, including vasoconstrictor assays, are used to compare and predict potencies and/or clinical efficacies of the topical corticosteroids. There is some evidence to suggest that a recognizable correlation exists between vasoconstrictor potency and therapeutic efficacy in man.

Pharmacokinetics: The extent of percutaneous absorption of topical corticosteroids is determined by many factors including the vehicle, the integrity of the epidermal barrier, and the use of occlusive dressings.

Topical corticosteroids can be absorbed from normal intact skin. Inflammation and/or other disease processes in the skin increase percutaneous absorption. Occlusive dressings substantially increase the percutaneous absorption of topical corticosteroids. Thus, occlusive dressings may be a valuable therapeutic adjunct for treatment of resistant dermatoses. (See DOSAGE AND ADMINISTRATION).

Once absorbed through the skin, topical corticosteroids are handled through pharmacokinetic pathways similar to systemically administered corticosteroids. Corticosteroids are bound to plasma proteins in varying degrees. Corticosteroids are metabolized primarily in the liver and are then excreted by the kidneys. Some of the topical corticosteroids and their metabolites are also excreted into the bile.

INDICATIONS AND USAGE

Topical corticosteroids are indicated for the relief of the inflammatory and pruritic manifestations of corticosteroid-responsive dermatoses.

CONTRAINDICATIONS

Topical corticosteroids are contraindicated in those patients with a history of hypersensitivity to any of the components of the preparation.

PRECAUTIONS

General: Systemic absorption of topical corticosteroids has produced reversible hypothalmic-pituitary-adrenal (HPA) axis suppression, manifestations of Cushing's syndrome, hyperglycemia, and glucosuria in some patients.

Conditions which augment systemic absorption include the application of the more potent steroids, use over large surface areas, prolonged use, and the addition of occlusive dressings. Therefore, patients receiving a large dose of a potent topical steroid applied to a large surface area or under an occlusive dressing should be evaluated periodically for evidence of HPA axis suppression by using the urinary free cortisol and ACTH stimulation tests. If HPA axis suppression is noted, an attempt should be made to withdraw the drug, to reduce the frequency of application, or to substitute a less potent steroid.

Recovery of HPA axis function is generally prompt and complete upon discontinuation of the drug. Infrequently, signs and symptoms of steroid withdrawal may occur, requiring supplemental systemic corticosteroids.

Children may absorb proportionally larger amounts of topical corticosteroids and thus be more susceptible to systemic toxicity. (See PRECAUTIONS—Pediatric Use).

If irritation develops, topical corticosteroids should be discontinued and appropriate therapy instituted.

In the presence of dermatological infections, the use of an appropriate antifungal or antibacterial agent should be instituted. If a favorable response does not occur promptly, the corticosteroid should be discontinued until the infection has been adequately controlled.

Information for the Patient: Patients using topical corticosteroids should receive the following information and instructions:

1. This medication is to be used as directed by the physician. It is for external use only. Avoid contact with the eyes.
2. Patients should be advised not to use this medication for any disorder other than for which it was prescribed.

Continued on next page

Nutracort—Cont.

3. The treated skin area should not be bandaged or otherwise covered or wrapped as to be occlusive unless directed by the physician.
4. Patients should report any signs of local adverse reactions especially under occlusive dressing.
5. Parents of pediatric patients should be advised not to use tight-fitting diapers or plastic pants on a child being treated in the diaper area, as these garments may constitute occlusive dressings.

Laboratory Tests: The following tests may be helpful in evaluating the HPA axis suppression:
Urinary free cortisol test
ACTH stimulation test

Carcinogenesis, Mutagenesis, and Impairment of Fertility: Long-term animal studies have not been performed to evaluate the carcinogenic potential or the effect on fertility of topical corticosteroids. Studies to determine mutagenicity with prednisolone and hydrocortisone have revealed negative results.

Pregnancy Category C: Corticosteroids are generally teratogenic in laboratory animals when administered systemically at relatively low dosage levels. The more potent corticosteroids have been shown to be teratogenic after dermal application in laboratory animals. There are no adequate and well-controlled studies in pregnant women on teratogenic effects from topically applied corticosteroids. Therefore, topical corticosteroids should be used during pregnancy only if the potential benefit justifies the potential risk to the fetus. Drugs of this class should not be used extensively on pregnant patients, in large amounts, or for prolonged periods of time.

Nursing Mothers: It is not known whether topical administration of corticosteroids could result in sufficient systemic absorption to produce detectable quantities in breast milk. Systemically administered corticosteroids are secreted into breast milk in quantities *not* likely to have a deleterious effect on the infant. Nevertheless, caution should be exercised when topical corticosteroids are administered to a nursing woman.

Pediatric Use: *Pediatric patients may demonstrate greater susceptibility to topical corticosteroid-induced HPA axis suppression and Cushing's syndrome than mature patients because of a larger skin surface area to body weight ratio.*
Hypothalmic-pituitary-adrenal (HPA) axis suppression. Cushing's syndrome, and intracranial hypertension have been reported in children receiving topical corticosteroids. Manifestations of adrenal suppression in children include linear growth retardation, delayed weight gain, low plasma cortisol levels, and absence of response to ACTH stimulation. Manifestations of intracranial hypertension include bulging fontanelles, headaches, and bilateral papilledema. Administration of topical corticosteroids to children should be limited to the least amount compatible with an effective therapeutic regimen. Chronic corticosteroid therapy may interfere with the growth and development of children.

ADVERSE REACTIONS

The following local adverse reactions are reported infrequently with topical corticosteroids, but may occur more frequently with the use of occlusive dressings. These reactions are listed in an approximate decreasing order of occurrence:

1. Burning
2. Itching
3. Irritation
4. Dryness
5. Folliculitis
6. Hypertrichosis
7. Acneiform eruptions
8. Hypopigmentation
9. Perioral dermatitis
10. Allergic contact dermatitis
11. Maceration of the skin
12. Secondary infection
13. Skin atrophy
14. Striae
15. Miliaria

OVERDOSAGE

Topically applied corticosteroids can be absorbed in sufficient amounts to produce systemic effects (See PRECAUTIONS).

DOSAGE AND ADMINISTRATION

Topical corticosteroids are generally applied to the affected area as a thin film three or four times daily depending on the severity of the condition.
Occlusive dressings may be used for the management of psoriasis or recalcitrant conditions.
If an infection develops, the use of occlusive dressings should be discontinued and appropriate antimicrobial therapy instituted.

HOW SUPPLIED

NUTRACORT® Lotion 1% is supplied in HDPE bottles:
2 fl. oz. **NDC** 0064-2200-02
4 fl. oz. **NDC** 0064-2200-04
NUTRACORT® Lotion 2.5% is supplied in HDPE bottles:
2 fl. oz. **NDC** 0064-2210-02
4 fl. oz. **NDC** 0064-2210-04
Store at room temperature.
CAUTION: Federal law prohibits dispensing without prescription.

HEALTHPOINT®
San Antonio, Texas 78215
1-800-441-8227
127118-1196
Shown in Product Identification Guide, page 317

PANAFIL® ℞
DEBRIDING, DEODORIZING AND HEALING OINTMENT
NDC 0064-3410-30 (30g tube)
Papain-Urea-Chlorophyllin Copper Complex Sodium

DESCRIPTION

PANAFIL Ointment is an enzymatic debriding-healing ointment which contains standardized Papain, USP (not less than 521,700 USP units per gram of ointment), Urea USP 10% and Chlorophyllin Copper Complex Sodium 0.5% in a hydrophilic base composed of Purified Water, USP; Propylene Glycol, USP, White Petrolatum, USP; Stearyl Alcohol, NF; Polyoxyl 40 Stearate, NF; Sorbitan Monostearate, NF; Boric Acid, NF; Chlorobutanol (Anhydrous), NF as a preservative; Sodium Borate, NF.

CLINICAL PHARMACOLOGY

Papain, the proteolytic enzyme derived from the fruit of carica papaya, is a potent digestant of nonviable protein matter, but is harmless to viable tissue. It has the unique advantage of being active over a wide pH range, 3 to 12. Despite its recognized value as a digestive agent, papain is relatively ineffective when used alone as a debriding agent, primarily because it requires the presence of activators to exert its digestive function. Urea is combined with papain to provide two supplementary chemical actions: 1) to expose by solvent action the activators of papain (sulfhydryl groups) which are always present, but not necessarily accessible, in the nonviable tissue or debris of lesions, and 2) to denature the nonviable protein matter in lesions and thereby render it more susceptible to enzymatic digestion. In pharmacologic studies involving digestion of beef powder, Miller[1] showed that the combination of papain and urea produced twice as much digestion as papain alone.
Chlorophyllin Copper Complex Sodium adds healing action to the cleansing action of the proteolytic papain-urea combination. The basic wound-healing properties of Chlorophyllin Copper Complex Sodium are promotion of healthy granulations, control of local inflammation and reduction of wound odors.[2] Specifically, Chlorophyllin Copper Complex Sodium inhibits the hemagglutinating and inflammatory properties of protein degradation products in the wound, including the products of enzymatic digestion, thus providing an additional protective factor.[1,3] The incorporation of Chlorophyllin Copper Complex Sodium in PANAFIL Ointment permits its continuous use for as long as desired to help produce and then maintain a clean wound base and to promote healing.

INDICATIONS AND USES

PANAFIL Ointment is suggested for treatment of acute and chronic lesions such as varicose, diabetic and decubitus ulcers, burns, postoperative wounds, pilonidal cyst wounds, carbuncles and miscellaneous traumatic or infected wounds.
PANAFIL Ointment is applied continuously throughout treatment of these conditions (1) for enzymatic debridement of necrotic tissue and liquefaction of fibrinous, purulent debris, (2) to keep the wound clean, and simultaneously (3) to promote normal healing.

CONTRAINDICATIONS

None known.

PRECAUTIONS

See Dosage and Administration. Not to be used in eyes.

ADVERSE REACTIONS

PANAFIL Ointment is generally well tolerated and nonirritating. A small percentage of patients may experience a transient "burning" sensation on application of the ointment. Occasionally, the profuse exudate resulting from enzymatic digestion may cause irritation. In such cases, more frequent changes of dressings until exudate diminishes will alleviate discomfort.

DOSAGE AND ADMINISTRATION

Cleanse the wound with ALLCLENZ® Wound Cleanser or saline. Avoid cleansing with hydrogen peroxide solution as it may inactivate the papain. Apply PANAFIL directly to the wound, cover with appropriate dressing, and secure into place. Note: Papain may also be inactivated by the salts of heavy metals such as lead, silver and mercury. Contact with medications containing these metals should be avoided. When practicable, daily or twice daily changes of dressings are preferred. Longer intervals between redressings (two or three days) have proved satisfactory, and PANAFIL Ointment may be applied under pressure dressings.

HOW SUPPLIED

30g tube
Store at controlled room temperature (59°–86°F, 15°–30°C).
Rx only

REFERENCES

1. Miller, J.M.: The Interaction of Papain, Urea and Water-Soluble Chlorophyll in a Proteolytic Ointment for Infected Wounds, Surgery 43:939, 1958.
2. Smith, L.W.: The Present Status of Topical Chlorophyll Therapy, New York, J. Med. 55:2041, 1955.
3. Barnard, R.D.: Elucidation of Chemically Defined Haptens For Competitive Inhibition of Aggressin Activity. Immunol. 8:78, 1954.

HEALTHPOINT®
1-800-441-8227
www.healthpoint.com
Shown in Product Identification Guide, page 317

PRUDOXIN™ ℞
[prū 'dock-cĭn]
DOXEPIN HYDROCHLORIDE CREAM, 5%
NDC 0064-3600-45
For Topical Dermatologic Use Only—
Not For Ophthalmic, Oral, or Intravaginal Use.

DESCRIPTION

PRUDOXIN Cream (doxepin hydrochloride cream) is a topical antipuritic cream. Each gram contains: 50 mg of doxepin hydrochloride (equivalent to 44.3 mg of doxepin). Doxepin hydrochloride is one of a class of agents known as dibenzoxepine tricyclic compounds. It is an isomeric mixture of N,N-Dimethyldibenz [*b,e*] oxepin-$\Delta^{11,6H,\gamma}$-propylamine hydrochloride. Doxepin hydrochloride has an empirical formula of $C_{19}H_{21}NO \bullet HCl$ and a molecular weight of 316. The base is a cream of pH 3.5 to 5.5 that includes the inactive ingredients: sorbitol, cetyl alcohol, isopropyl myristate, glyceryl stearate, PEG-100 stearate, petrolatum, benzyl alcohol, titanium dioxide and purified water.

CLINICAL PHARMACOLOGY

The exact mechanism by which doxepin exerts its antipuritic effect is unknown. Doxepin HCl does have potent H1 and potent H2 receptor blocking actions. Histamine-blocking drugs appear to compete at histamine receptor sites and inhibit the biological activation of histamine receptors. In addition, doxepin drowsiness in significant numbers of patients. Sedation may have an effect on certain pruritic symptoms. In 19 pruritic eczema patients treated with Doxepin HCl Cream 5%, plasma doxepin concentrations ranged from nondetectable to 47 ng/mL from percutaneous absorption. Target therapeutic plasma levels of ORAL doxepin HCl for the treatment of depression range from 30 to 150 ng/mL. Once absorbed into the systemic circulation, doxepin undergoes hepatic metabolism that results in conversion to pharmacologically-active desmethyldoxepin. Further glucuronidation results in urinary excretion of the parent drug and its metabolites. Desmethyldoxepin has a half life reportedly that ranges from 28 to 52 hours and is not affected by multiple dosing. Plasma levels of both doxepin and desmethyldoxepin are highly variable and are poorly correlated with dosage. Wide distribution occurs in body tissues including lungs, heart, brain, and liver. Renal disease, genetic factors, age, and other medications affect the metabolism and subsequent elimination of doxepin. (See **PRECAUTIONS: Drug Interactions.**)

INDICATIONS AND USAGE

PRUDOXIN Cream is indicated for the short-term (up to 8 days) management of moderate pruritus in adult patients with the following forms of eczematous dermatitis: atopic dermatitis and lichen simplex chronicus. (See **DOSAGE AND ADMINISTRATION.**)

CONTRAINDICATIONS

Because doxepin HCl has an anticholinergic effect and because significant plasma levels of doxepin are detectable after topical PRUDOXIN Cream application, the use of PRUDOXIN Cream is contraindicated in patients with untreated narrow angle glaucoma or a tendency to urinary retention.
PRUDOXIN Cream is contraindicated in individuals who have shown previous sensitivity to any of its components.

WARNINGS

Drowsiness occurs in over 20% of patients treated with PRUDOXIN Cream, especially in patients receiving treatment to greater than 10% of their body surface area. Patients should be warned of this possibility and cautioned against driving a motor vehicle or operating hazardous machinery while being treated with PRUDOXIN Cream. Patients should also be warned that the effects of alcoholic beverages can be potentiated when using PRUDOXIN Cream. If excessive drowsiness occurs it may be necessary to reduce the number of applications, the amount of cream applied, and/or the percentage of body surface area treated, or discontinue the drug.
Keep this product away from the eyes.

PRECAUTIONS

Drug Interactions: Studies have not been performed examining drug interactions with PRUDOXIN Cream. However, data are available regarding potentially significant drug interactions regarding doxepin. As plasma levels of doxepin similar to therapeutic ranges for antidepressant therapy can be obtained following topical application of PRUDOXIN Cream, it would not be unexpected for the following drug interactions to be possible following topical PRUDOXIN Cream application.

MAO Inhibitors: Serious side effects and even death have been reported following the concomitant use of certain orally administered drugs chemically related to doxepin and MAO inhibitors. Therefore, MAO inhibitors should be discontinued at least two weeks prior to the initiation of treatment with PRUDOXIN Cream.

Cimetidine: Cimetidine has been reported to produce clinically significant fluctuations in steady-state serum concentrations of various tricyclic antidepressants. Serious anticholinergic symptoms have been associated with elevations in the serum levels of tricyclic antidepressants when cimetidine therapy is initiated. Additionally, higher than expected tricyclic antidepressant levels have been observed in patients already taking cimetidine. In patients who have been reported to be well-controlled on tricyclic antidepressants receiving concurrent cimetidine therapy, discontinuation of cimetidine has been reported to decrease steady-state serum tricyclic antidepressant levels and compromise their therapeutic effects.
Alcohol: Alcohol ingestion may exacerbate the potential sedative effects of PRUDOXIN Cream.
Drugs Metabolized by P_{450}IID6: A subset (3% to 10%) of the population has reduced activity of certain drug metabolizing enzymes such as the cytochrome P_{450} isozyme P_{450}IID6. Such individuals are referred to as "poor metabolizers" of drugs such as debrisoquin, dextromethorphan, and the tricyclic antidepressants. These individuals may have higher than expected plasma concentrations of tricyclic antidepressant when given usual doses. In addition, certain drugs that are metabolized by this isozyme, including many antidepressants (tricyclic antidepressants, selective serotonin reuptake inhibitors, and others), may inhibit the activity of this isozyme, and thus may make normal metabolizers resemble poor metabolizers with regard to concomitant therapy with other drugs metabolized by this enzyme system, leading to drug interaction.
Concomitant use of tricyclic antidepressants with other drugs metabolized by cytochrome P_{450}IID6 may require lower doses than usually prescribed for either the tricyclic antidepressant or the other drug. Therefore, co-administration of tricyclic antidepressants with other drugs that are metabolized by this isoenzyme, including other antidepressants, phenothiazines, carbamazepine, and Type IC antiarrhythmics (e.g., propafenone, flecainide and encainide), or that inhibit this enzyme (e.g., quinidine), should be approached with caution. Concomitant use of PRUDOXIN Cream with drugs metabolized by cytochrome P_{450}IID6 has not been formally studied.
Carcinogenesis, Mutagenesis, Impairment of Fertility: Carcinogenesis, mutagenesis, impairment of fertility studies have not been conducted with doxepin hydrochloride.
Pregnancy: Pregnancy Category B: Teratology studies have been performed in rats and rabbits at oral doses up to 8 times the topical human dose (based on a mg/kg basis) and have revealed no evidence of impaired fertility or harm to the fetus due to doxepin. There are however, no adequate and well-controlled studies in pregnant women. Because animal reproduction studies are not always predictive of human response, this drug should be used during pregnancy only if clearly needed.
Nursing Mothers: Doxepin is excreted in human milk after oral administration. There have been no studies conducted to date to determine if doxepin is excreted in human milk after topical administration; however, it is known that significant systemic levels of doxepin are obtained after topical administration. It is therefore possible that doxepin could be secreted in human milk following topical administration. One case has been reported of apnea and drowsiness in a nursing infant whose mother was taking an oral dosage form of doxepin HCl.
Because of the potential for serious adverse reactions in nursing infants from doxepin, a decision should be made whether to discontinue nursing or to discontinue the drug, taking into account the importance of the drug to the mother.
Pediatric Use: Safety and effectiveness of PRUDOXIN Cream in children have not been established.

ADVERSE REACTIONS

CONTROLLED CLINICAL TRIALS:
Systemic Adverse Effects: In controlled clinical trials of patients treated with PRUDOXIN Cream, the most common systemic adverse effect reported was drowsiness. Drowsiness occurred in 22% of patients treated with PRUDOXIN Cream (and 2% of patients treated with placebo cream) and resulted in the premature discontinuation of the drug in approximately 5% of patients treated.
Other systemic adverse effects reported in approximately 1 to 10% of these patients included: Dry mouth, dry lips, thirst, headache, fatigue, dizziness, emotional changes, and taste changes.
Other systemic adverse effects reported in less than 1% of these patients included: Nausea, anxiety, and fever.
Local Site Adverse Effects: In controlled clinical trials of patients treated with PRUDOXIN Cream, the most common local site adverse effect reported was burning and/or stinging at the site of application. These occurred in approximately 21% of these patients. Most of these reactions were categorized as "mild": however, approximately 25% of patients who reported burning and/or stinging reported the reaction as "severe." Four patients treated with PRUDOXIN Cream withdrew from the study because of the burning and/or stinging.
Other local site adverse effects reported in approximately 1 to 10% of these patients included: Pruritus exacerbation, eczema exacerbation, dryness and tightness to skin, paresthesias, and edema.
Other local site adverse effects reported in less than 1% of these patients included: Irritation, tingling, scaling, and cracking.

POST MARKETING EXPERIENCE
PRUDOXIN Cream has been associated with allergic contact dermatitis.

OVERDOSAGE

Overdosage with a topical product is unlikely; should it occur, the signs and symptoms include: Mild: Drowsiness, stupor, blurred vision, excessive dryness of mouth. Severe: Respiratory depression, hypotension, coma, convulsions, cardiac arrhythmias and tachycardias. Also, urinary retention (bladder atony), decreased gastrointestinal motility (paralytic ileus), hyperthermia (or hypothermia), hypertension, dilated pupils, hyperactive reflexes.
Management and Treatment:
Mild: Observation and supportive therapy is all that is usually necessary. It may be necessary to reduce the percent of body surface area treated or the frequency of application or apply a thinner layer of cream. Severe: Medical management of severe doxepin overdosage consists of aggressive supportive therapy. The area covered with doxepin HCl cream should be thoroughly washed. An adequate airway should be established in comatose patients and assisted ventilation used if necessary. EKG monitoring may be required for several days, because relapse after apparent recovery has been reported with oral doxepin HCl. Arrhythmias should be treated with the appropriate antiarrhythmic agent. It has been reported that many of the cardiovascular and CNS symptoms of tricyclic antidepressant poisoning in adults may be reversed by the slow intravenous administration of 1 mg to 3 mg of physostigmine salicylate. Because physostigmine is rapidly metabolized, the dosage should be repeated as required. Convulsions may respond to standard anticonvulsant therapy; however, barbiturates may potentiate any respiratory depression. Dialysis and forced diuresis generally are not of value in the management of overdosage due to high tissue and protein binding of doxepin HCl.

DOSAGE AND ADMINISTRATION

A thin film of PRUDOXIN Cream should be applied four times each day with at least a 3 to 4 hour interval between applications. There are no data to establish the safety and effectiveness of PRUDOXIN Cream when used for greater than 8 days. Chronic use beyond 8 days may result in higher systemic levels.
Clinical experience has shown that drowsiness is significantly more common in patients applying PRUDOXIN Cream to over 10% of body surface area; therefore, patients with greater than 10% of body surface area affected should be particularly cautioned concerning possible drowsiness and other systemic adverse effects of doxepin. If excessive drowsiness occurs it may be necessary to do one or more of the following: reduce the body surface area treated, reduce the number of applications per day, reduce the amount of cream applied, or discontinue the drug.
Occlusive dressings may increase the absorption of most topical drugs; therefore, occlusive dressings with PRUDOXIN Cream should not be utilized.

HOW SUPPLIED

PRUDOXIN Cream is available in a 45 g (NDC 0064-3600-45) aluminum tube. Store at or below 27°C (80°F).
Rx ONLY
Distributed by:
HEALTHPOINT®
Healthpoint, Ltd.
San Antonio, Texas 78215
1-800-441-8227
Manufactured by:
DPT Laboratories, Ltd.
San Antonio, Texas 78215

REFERENCES

1. Breneman DL, Dunlap FE, Monroe EW, Schupbach CW, Shmunes E, Phillips SB. Doxepin cream relieves eczema-associated pruritus within 15 minutes and is not accompanied by a risk of rebound upon discontinuation. *J Dermatol Treat.* 1997, 8:161–168.
2. Drake LA, Fallon JD, Sober A, and The Doxepin Study Group. Relief of pruritus in patients with atopic dermatitis after treatment with topical doxepin cream. *J Am Acad Dermatol.* 1994: 31: 613–616.
3. Berberian BJ, Breneman DL, Drake LA, Gratton D, Raimir SS, Phillips S, Sulica VI, Bernstein JE. The addition of topical doxepin to corticosteroid therapy: an improved treatment regimen for atopic dermatitis. *Intl J Dermatol.* 1999: 38: 145–148.

Shown in Product Identification Guide, page 317

For information on over-the-counter drugs,
consult **PDR For Nonprescription Drugs.**

Heel Inc.

11600 COCHITI SE
ALBUQUERQUE, NM 87123

Direct Inquiries to:
Medical Department
800–621–7644
(505) 293–3843
Fax: (505) 275–1672
www.heelbhi.com

TRAUMEEL® Gel OTC
Anti-inflammatory/Analgesic

TRAUMEEL® Tablets OTC
Anti-inflammatory/Analgesic

TRAUMEEL® Ointment OTC
Anti-inflammatory/Analgesic

TRAUMEEL® Oral Drops OTC
Anti-inflammatory/Analgesic

TRAUMEEL® Oral Liquid in Vials OTC
Anti-inflammatory/Analgesic

TRAUMEEL® Injection Solution ℞

DESCRIPTION

TRAUMEEL® Injection Solution is an anti-inflammatory, analgesic, anti-edematous, anti-exudative combination formulation of 12 botanical substances and 1 mineral substance. TRAUMEEL® Injection Solution is officially classified as a homeopathic combination remedy (1).
1. Botanical ingredients:
Arnica montana, radix (mountain arnica)
Calendula officinalis (marigold)
Hamamelis virginiana (witch hazel)
Millefolium (milfoil)
Belladonna (deadly nightshade)
Aconitum napellus (monkshood)
Chamomilla (chamomile)
Symphytum officinale (comfrey)
Bellis perennis (daisy)
Echinacea angustifolia (narrow-leafed cone flower)
Echinacea purpurea (purple cone flower)
Hypericum perforatum (St. John's wort)
2. Mineral ingredients:
Hepar sulphuris calcareum (calcium sulfide)
Injection Solution: Each 2.0 ml ampule contains as active ingredients: Hepar sulphuris calcareum 8X 200.0 µl; Belladonna 3X 20.0 µl; Calendula officinalis 3X 20.0 µl; Chamomilla 4X 20.0 µl; Millefolium 4X 20.0 µl; Aconitum napellus 3X 12.0 µl; Bellis perennis 3X 10.0 µl; Hypericum perforatum 3X 6.0 µl; Echinacea angustifolia 3X 5.0 µl; Echinacea purpurea 3X 5.0 µl; Arnica montana, radix 2X 2.0 µl; Hamamelis virginiana 2X 2.0 µl; Symphytum officinale 6X 2.0 µl. Each 2.0 ml ampule contains as an inactive ingredient: Sterile isotonic sodium chloride solution.

CLINICAL PHARMACOLOGY

The exact mechanism of action of TRAUMEEL® Injection Solution is not fully understood. Various cellular and biochemical pathways appear to be modulated by the product ingredients. The mechanism of action of TRAUMEEL® Injection Solution does not appear to be the result of cyclooxygenase or lipoxygenase enzyme inhibition, as is the case with nonsteroidal anti-inflammatory drugs (NSAIDs). TRAUMEEL® Injection Solution does not inhibit the arachidonic acid pathway of prostaglandin synthesis. Instead, the mechanism of action of TRAUMEEL® Injection Solution appears to be the result of modulation of the release of oxygen radicals from activated neutrophils, and inhibition of the release of inflammatory mediators (possibly interleukin-1 from activated macrophages) and neuropeptides (2).
In vitro studies show that the ingredients in TRAUMEEL® Injection Solution are noncytotoxic to granulocytes, lymphocytes, platelets, and endothelia, which indicates that the defensive functions of these cells are preserved during treatment with TRAUMEEL® Injection Solution (3).
The anti-inflammatory, analgesic, anti-edematous, and anti-exudative effects of TRAUMEEL® Injection Solution have been demonstrated in clinical trials as well as in *in vivo* experimental models including the carrageenin-induced edema test and the adjuvant arthritis test (3).

INDICATIONS AND USAGE

TRAUMEEL® Injection Solution is indicated for the treatment of symptoms associated with inflammatory, exudative, and degenerative processes due to acute trauma (such as contusions, lacerations, fractures, sprains, post-operative wounds, etc.), repetitive or overuse injuries (such as tendonitis, bursitis, epicondylitis, etc.), and for minor aches and pains associated with such conditions. TRAUMEEL® Injection Solution is also indicated for the treatment of minor aches and pains associated with backache, muscular aches, and the minor pain from rheumatoid arthritis, osteoarthritis, gouty arthritis, and ankylosing spondylitis.

Continued on next page

Traumeel Injection—Cont.

CONTRAINDICATIONS

TRAUMEEL® Injection Solution is contraindicated in patients with a known hypersensitivity to TRAUMEEL® Injection Solution or any of its ingredients (see **ADVERSE REACTIONS**).

WARNINGS

If pain persists or worsens, if new symptoms occur, or if redness or swelling is present, the patient should be carefully re-evaluated because these could be signs of a serious condition.

PRECAUTIONS

General:
Adverse effects with TRAUMEEL® Injection Solution are extremely rare. TRAUMEEL® Injection Solution exhibits no known adverse renal, hepatic, cardiovascular, gastrointestinal or central nervous system effects.

Information for Patients:
No harmful or potentially hazardous side effects such as central nervous system depression are known. TRAUMEEL® Injection Solution is generally well-tolerated. However, if symptoms persist or worsen, a physician should be consulted (see **WARNINGS**).

Drug Interactions:
TRAUMEEL® Injection Solution is not known to interact with other medications. Furthermore, the administration of TRAUMEEL® Injection Solution can be safely augmented by the application of a topical dosage form of TRAUMEEL®.

Drug/Laboratory Test Interactions:
TRAUMEEL® Injection Solution is not known to interact with any laboratory tests.

Carcinogenesis:
No studies have been performed to evaluate the carcinogenicity of TRAUMEEL® Injection Solution. In world-wide post-marketing surveillance studies no evidence of carcinogenicity has been found (2).

Pregnancy:
Pregnancy Category C. In general, medications such as TRAUMEEL® Injection Solution that are classified as homeopathic are not known to cause direct or indirect harm to the fetus. However, animal reproduction studies have not been performed and there are no well-controlled studies in pregnant women. In cases of pregnancy or suspected pregnancy, TRAUMEEL® Injection Solution should be used only if potential benefits justify potential risks to the fetus.

Nursing Mothers:
It is not known whether any of the ingredients in TRAUMEEL® Injection Solution are excreted in human milk. However, because many drugs are excreted in human milk, TRAUMEEL® Injection Solution should be administered with caution to nursing mothers.

Pediatric Use:
TRAUMEEL® Injection Solution can be safely administered to children as young as 2 years (see **DOSAGE AND ADMINISTRATION**).

ADVERSE REACTIONS

In rare cases, patients with hypersensitivity to botanicals of the Compositae family may experience an allergic reaction after the administration of TRAUMEEL® Injection Solution including anaphylactic reaction. TRAUMEEL® Injection Solution ingredients of the Compositae family are:

- Arnica montana, radix (mountain arnica)
- Calendula officinalis (marigold)
- Millefolium (milfoil)
- Chamomilla (chamomile)
- Bellis perennis (daisy)
- Echinacea angustifolia (narrow-leafed cone flower)
- Echinacea purpurea (purple cone flower)

OVERDOSAGE

Due to the low concentration of active ingredients in homeopathic preparations such as TRAUMEEL® Injection Solution, adverse reactions following overdosage are extremely unlikely. However, care must be taken not to exceed the recommended dosage.

DOSAGE AND ADMINISTRATION

The dosage schedules listed below can be used as a general guide for the administration of TRAUMEEL® Injection Solution. TRAUMEEL® Injection Solution shows individual differences in clinical response. Therefore, the dosage for each patient should be individualized according to the patient's response to therapy. For best results, treatment with TRAUMEEL® Injection Solution should be initiated immediately following injury or at the first sign of symptoms. TRAUMEEL® Injection Solution may be administered until symptoms disappear.

TRAUMEEL® Injection Solution:

Adults and children above 6 years: 1 ampule daily for acute disorders, or 1 to 2 ampules 1 to 3 times weekly.
Children (2 to 6 years): Half the adult dosage. Discard unused solution.

TRAUMEEL® Injection Solution may be administered intravenously, intramuscularly, subcutaneously or intradermally. TRAUMEEL® Injection Solution is indicated for peri-articular administration. However, TRAUMEEL® Injection Solution is not indicated for intra-articular use. If coadministration with a local anesthetic is desired, TRAUMEEL® Injection Solution may be mixed in a 1:1 ratio with 1% or 2% lidocaine hydrochloride. Similar local anesthetics may also be used. The required dose of TRAUMEEL® Injection Solution is first withdrawn from the ampule into the syringe. The local anesthetic is then withdrawn into the syringe, and the syringe is then shaken briefly. Normally, about 0.5 to 1.0 milliliters of each drug is withdrawn into the syringe.

TRAUMEEL® Injection Solution should be administered using a narrow gauge needle (e.g., 22 to 30 gauge). **Note:** Parenteral drug products like TRAUMEEL® Injection Solution should be inspected visually for particulate matter and discoloration prior to administration whenever solution and container permit. TRAUMEEL® Injection Solution is a clear, colorless solution. Discolored solutions should be discarded.

HOW SUPPLIED

TRAUMEEL® Injection Solution in 2.0 ml ampules:
Packs of 10: NDC 50114-7000-1.
Avoid freezing and excessive heat. Store at controlled room temperature. Protect from light.
CAUTION: Rx only.

REFERENCES

(1) The Homeopathic Pharmacopoeia of the United States (HPUS), 8th edition, Falls Church, Virginia, 1979; and the Homeopathic Pharmacopoeia of the United States Revision Service (HPRS), 1988.
(2) Data on file, Heel GmbH, Baden-Baden, Germany.
(3) Conforti A, *et al.* Experimental Studies on the Anti-inflammatory Activity of a Homeopathic Preparation. *Biomedical Therapy XV* No.1:28-31, 1997.

This full prescribing information has been compiled in accordance with the Code of Federal Regulations (CFR), 21 sections 201.56 and 201.57.

VERTIGOHEEL® Tablets ℞
VERTIGOHEEL® Oral Drops ℞
VERTIGOHEEL® Oral Liquid in Vials ℞

DESCRIPTION

VERTIGOHEEL® is a homeopathic combination formulation for the treatment of vertigo consisting of 2 botanical substances, 1 zoological substance, and 1 mineral substance (1, 2). VERTIGOHEEL® is officially classified as a homeopathic combination remedy.

1. Botanical ingredients:
   Conium maculatum (umbelliferae)
   Cocculus indicus (menispermaceae)
2. Zoological ingredient:
   Ambra grisea (ambergris)
3. Mineral ingredient:
   Petroleum (purified mineral oil)

Tablets: Each 300 mg tablet contains as active ingredients: Cocculus indicus 4X 210 mg; Conium maculatum 3X 30 mg; Ambra grisea 6X 30 mg; Petroleum 8X 30 mg; in a lactose base. Each 300 mg tablet contains as an inactive ingredient: Magnesium stearate.

Oral Drops: Each 100 ml of solution contains as active ingredients: Cocculus indicus 4X 70 ml; Conium maculatum 3X 10 ml; Ambra grisea 6X 10 ml; Petroleum 8X 10 ml. Contains ethyl alcohol 35% by volume.

Oral Liquid in Vials: Each 100 ml of solution contains as active ingredients: Cocculus indicus 3X 0.7 ml; Conium maculatum 2X 0.1 ml; Ambra grisea 5X 0.1 ml; Petroleum 7X 0.1 ml. Each 100 ml of solution contains as an inactive ingredient: Isotonic sodium chloride solution.

CLINICAL PHARMACOLOGY

The exact mechanism of action of VERTIGOHEEL® is not fully understood. Pharmacologic studies suggest that the effectiveness of VERTIGOHEEL® for the treatment of vertigo and nausea, and for improving vestibulo-ocular and proprioceptive symptoms, is due in part to central nervous system stimulation. Studies have confirmed that VERTIGOHEEL® activates the vestibular regulatory systems located in the brainstem area. Computer-processed brain mapping recordings indicate an increase in activity in the neuropathways, which connect the vestibulo-pathways with the corpora quadrigemina (3, 4).

Clinical Studies: In a randomized, double blind, controlled clinical study (119 patients) Vertigoheel® reduced the frequency, duration, and intensity of the vertigo attacks during a 6-week treatment period; effectiveness and tolerability was good compared to betahistine (5).

INDICATIONS AND USAGE

VERTIGOHEEL® is indicated for the treatment of vertigo (3,4,5) and other related imbalance disorders, and related symptoms such as nausea. VERTIGOHEEL® is also indicated for the prevention and treatment of motion sickness (6).

CONTRAINDICATIONS

VERTIGOHEEL® is contraindicated in patients with a known hypersensitivity to VERTIGOHEEL® or any of its ingredients.

WARNINGS

VERTIGOHEEL® should not be administered for more than 10 days for adults or 5 days for children without follow-up assessment by a physician. If during the course of treatment symptoms persist or worsen, or if new symptoms occur, the patient should consult a physician because these could be signs of a serious condition requiring more aggressive therapy.

PRECAUTIONS

General:
Adverse effects with VERTIGOHEEL® are extremely rare. VERTIGOHEEL® exhibits no known adverse renal, hepatic, cardiovascular, gastrointestinal, or central nervous system effects.

Information for Patients:
No harmful or potentially hazardous side effects such as central nervous system depression are known. VERTIGOHEEL® is generally well-tolerated even during long term administration.

Drug Interactions:
VERTIGOHEEL® is not known to interact with other medications.

Drug/Laboratory Test Interactions:
VERTIGOHEEL® is not known to interact with any laboratory tests.

Carcinogenesis:
No studies have been performed to evaluate the carcinogenicity of VERTIGOHEEL®. In world-wide post-marketing surveillance no evidence of carcinogenicity has been found (5).

Pregnancy:
Pregnancy Category C. In general, medications such as VERTIGOHEEL® which are classified as homeopathic are not known to cause direct or indirect harm to the fetus. However, animal reproduction studies have not been performed and there are no well-controlled studies in pregnant women. In cases of pregnancy or suspected pregnancy, a physician should be consulted before administering VERTIGOHEEL®.

Nursing Mothers:
It is not known whether any of the ingredients in VERTIGOHEEL® are excreted in human milk. However, because many drugs are excreted in human milk, VERTIGOHEEL® should be administered with caution to nursing mothers.

Pediatric Use:
VERTIGOHEEL® Tablets and VERTIGOHEEL® Oral Liquid in Vials can be safely administered to children as young as 2 years (see **DOSAGE AND ADMINISTRATION**). However, due to its alcohol content (ethyl alcohol 35% by volume), VERTIGOHEEL® Oral Drops should be administered with caution to children below the age of 12 years.

ADVERSE REACTIONS

VERTIGOHEEL® exhibits no known adverse reactions.

OVERDOSAGE

Due to the low concentrations of active ingredients in homeopathic preparations such as VERTIGOHEEL®, adverse reactions following overdosage are extremely unlikely. However, care must be taken not to exceed the recommended dosage.

DOSAGE AND ADMINISTRATION

The dosage schedules listed below can be used as a general guide for the administration of VERTIGOHEEL®. The dosage for each patient should be individualized according to the patient's response to therapy. For the treatment or prevention of vertigo or motion sickness, the onset of action of VERTIGOHEEL® may not be immediate. Patients responding to VERTIGOHEEL® therapy will normally show benefit within one week (5,6). The frequency of administration of the 3 dosage forms may be increased to every 15 minutes over a 2-hour period for acute exacerbations of the symptoms of vertigo, in both children and adults, unless otherwise directed by a physician. VERTIGOHEEL® Tablets, Oral Drops, and Oral Liquid in Vials should be administered at least 30 minutes after meals and when the oral cavity is free of food material. For best results, treatment with VERTIGOHEEL® should be initiated at the first sign of symptoms and continued for a physician-specified period. If symptoms persist or worsen, the patient should contact a physician (see **WARNINGS**).

VERTIGOHEEL® Tablets:

Adults and Children above 6 years: 2 to 3 tablets sublingually or dissolved completely in the mouth 3 times daily.
Children 2 to 6 years: 1 to 2 tablets sublingually or dissolved completely in the mouth 3 times daily.
For best results, VERTIGOHEEL® Tablets should be dissolved under the tongue or in the mouth since the absorption is via the buccal lining. For small children tablets may be divided or crushed for easier administration.

VERTIGOHEEL® Oral Drops:

Adults and Children above 11 years: 15 to 20 drops taken sublingually 3 times daily.
Children 2 to 11 years: Half the adult dosage. Due to its alcohol content (ethyl alcohol 35% by volume), VERTIGOHEEL® Oral Drops should be administered with caution to children below the age of 12 years.
VERTIGOHEEL® Oral Drops may be added to clear, non-sparkling water prior to administration.

VERTIGOHEEL® Oral Liquid in Vials:

Adults and Children above 6 years: The contents of 1 vial taken orally 1 to 3 times daily.
Children 2 to 6 years: Half the contents of 1 vial taken orally 1 to 3 times daily.
VERTIGOHEEL® Oral Liquid in Vials may be added to clear, non-sparkling water prior to administration. **Note:** The unused portion of the open vials should be discarded. **NOT FOR INJECTION.**

HOW SUPPLIED

VERTIGOHEEL® Tablets (white, unscored with "Heel" impressed on one side) in bottles of 100: NDC 50114-6155-2. Avoid freezing and excessive heat. Store at room temperature. Keep container tightly closed. Protect from light and moisture.

VERTIGOHEEL® Oral Drops in 50 ml (1.6 fluid oz) bottles: NDC 50114-1170-4. Avoid freezing and excessive heat. Store at controlled room temperature. Keep container tightly closed. Protect from light.

VERTIGOHEEL® Oral Liquid in Vials, 1.1 ml packs of 10: NDC 50114-1122-4. Avoid freezing and excessive heat. Store at controlled room temperature. Protect from light.

CAUTION: Rx only.

REFERENCES

(1) The Homeopathic Pharmacopoeia of the United States (HPUS), 5th Edition, Falls Church, Virginia, 1979.
(2) The Homeopathic Pharmacopoeia of the United States Revision Service (HPRS), 1988.
(3) Claussen, CF. Treatment of the Syndrome of the Slowed Down Brainstem with Vertigoheel. *Biological Therapy*, Vol. V, No. 1, 1-24, 1987, and Vol. V, No. 2, 25-49, 1987.
(4) Claussen CF, Bergmann J, Bertora G, Claussen E. Clinico-experimental Study and Equilibrimetric Measurements Assessing the Therapeutic Efficacy of a Homeopathic Drug with the Ingredients Ambra, Cocculus, Conium, and Mineral Oil in Vertigo and Nausea Cases, *Arzneimittel-Forschung* (Drug Research) 34(ll), 12, 1791-1798, 1984.
(5) Data on file, Heel GmbH, Baden-Baden, Germany. Weiser M, Strosser W, Klein P, Homeopathic vs Conventional Treatment of Vertigo. *Arch Otolaryngol Head Neck Surg*. 124:879–885, 1998.
(6) Bruckner G. Vertigoheel in an Internal Medicine Practice, *Biomedical Therapy*, Vol. IV, No. 1, 2-5, 1986.

High Chemical Co.

3901-A NEBRASKA ST.
LEVITTOWN, PA 19056

Direct Inquiries to:
800-447-8792
877–SARAPIN

SARAPIN® ℞

DESCRIPTION

A sterile aqueous solution of soluble salts of the volatile bases from Sarraceniaceae (Pitcher Plant). Benzyl Alcohol 0.75%.

ACTIONS

The painful syndromes most commonly encountered in general practice which are relieved by SARAPIN® treatment are as follows:
Sciatic Pain
Intercostal Neuralgia
Alcoholic Neuritis
Occipital Neuritis
Brachial Plexus Neuralgia
Meralgia Paresthetica
Lumbar Neuralgia
Trigeminal Neuralgia

ADMINISTRATION

These and allied conditions may be treated with success in a majority of cases by nerve block or local infiltration:
Paravertebral—Careful localization of the zone of tenderness permits a determination of the corresponding trunk levels to be injected.
Perineural—In some instances, as in sciatica, the affected nerve can be injected at a site distant from its origin.
Local Infiltration—Multiple injections throughout an area of tenderness provide for diffusion into all the affected parts.

DOSAGE

Paravertebral Injections

Cervical	2–3 ml
Dorsal	5–10 ml
Lumbar	5–10 ml
Sacral	3–5 ml
Caudal Canal	10 ml
Sciatic Nerve	10 ml
Local Infiltration	5–10 ml

WARNINGS

Withdraw plunger of syringe to make sure the needle point is not in a blood vessel.

PRECAUTIONS

Procedure should be gentle and unhurried.
SARAPIN® is intended only for professional use. Its successful employment depends upon a thorough knowledge of the anatomy involved.

ADVERSE REACTIONS

Patients should be maintained in a recumbent position for 10 to 15 minutes following injection. A local sensation is to be expected, limited to the distribution of the nerve injected, and usually appearing as a temporary feeling of heaviness, although some cases will feel heat or a transitory aggravation of symptoms.

CONTRAINDICATIONS

SARAPIN® is non-toxic, has no side effects other than above and is contraindicated only in areas of local infection.

HOW SUPPLIED

50 ml Multiple Dose Vial.
NDC-10541-492-50
CAUTION: Federal law prohibits dispensing without prescription.

HIGH CHEMICAL COMPANY
3901-A Nebraska Street
Levittown, PA 19056-3333
800-447-8792

Hill Dermaceuticals, Inc.

2650 SO. MELLONVILLE AVE.
SANFORD, FL 32773

Direct Inquiries to:
Rosario G. Ramirez
(407) 323-1887
FAX: (407) 649-9213/323-1871

DERMA-SMOOTHE/FS TOPICAL OIL ℞
Fluocinolone acetonide, 0.01%, Topical Oil

FS SHAMPOO, 0.01% ℞
Fluocinolone acetonide, 0.01%, Shampoo

Hoechst Marion Roussel

Due to the merger of Hoechst Marion Roussel and Rhône-Poulenc Rorer, please refer to Aventis Pharmaceuticals for product information.

ICN Pharmaceuticals, Inc.

ICN PLAZA
3300 HYLAND AVENUE
COSTA MESA, CA 92626

Direct Inquiries to:
Medical Emergency Contact
Boanerges Rubalcava, M.D., Ph.D.
(800) 548-5100, ext. 3531
FAX: (714) 641-7287

8-MOP® CAPSULES ℞
(Methoxsalen Capsules, USP, 10 mg)
℞ Only

CAUTION: METHOXSALEN IS A POTENT DRUG. READ ENTIRE BROCHURE PRIOR TO PRESCRIBING OR DISPENSING THIS MEDICATION.

Methoxsalen with UV radiation should be used only by physicians who have special competence in the diagnosis and treatment of psoriasis and vitiligo and who have special training and experience in photochemotherapy. Psoralen and ultraviolet radiation therapy should be under constant supervision of such a physician. For the treatment of patients with psoriasis, photochemotherapy should be restricted to patients with severe, recalcitrant, disabling psoriasis which is not adequately responsive to other forms of therapy, and only when the diagnosis has been supported by biopsy. Because of the possibilities of ocular damage, aging of the skin, and skin cancer (including melanoma), the patient should be fully informed by the physician of the risks inherent in this therapy. When methoxsalen is used in combination with photopheresis, refer to the UVAR* System Operator's Manual for specific warnings, cautions, indications, and instructions related to photopheresis.

CAUTION: 8-MOP® Capsules (Methoxsalen Hard Gelatin Capsules) may not be interchanged with Oxsoralen-Ultra® Capsules (Methoxsalen Soft Gelatin Capsules) without retitration of the patient.

I. DESCRIPTION

8-MOP (Methoxsalen, 8-Methoxypsoralen) Capsules, 10mg. Methoxsalen is a naturally occurring photoactive substance found in the seeds of the **Ammi majus** (Umbelliferae) plant and in the roots of **Heracleum Candicans**. It belongs to a group of compounds known as psoralens, or furocoumarins. The chemical name of methoxsalen is 9-methoxy-7 H-furo[3,2-g][1]-benzopyran-7-one; it has the following structure:

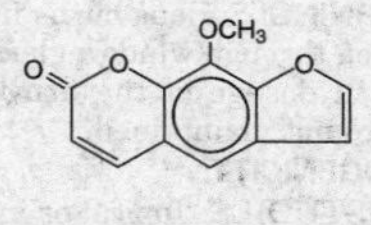

II. CLINICAL PHARMACOLOGY

The combination treatment regimen of psoralen (P) and ultraviolet radiation of 320–400 nm wavelength commonly referred to as UVA is known by the acronym, PUVA. Skin reactivity to UVA (320–400 nm) radiation is markedly enhanced by the ingestion of methoxsalen. The drug reaches its maximum bioavailability $1\frac{1}{2}$–3 hours after oral administration and may last for up to 8 hours (Pathak et al., 1974)[1]. Methoxsalen is reversibly bound to serum albumin and is also preferentially taken up by epidermal cells (Artuc et al. 1979)[2]. At a dose which is six times larger than that used in humans, it induces mixed function oxidases in the liver of mice (Mandula et al. 1978)[3]. In both mice and man, methoxsalen is rapidly metabolized. Approximately 95% of the drug is excreted as a series of metabolites in the urine within 24 hours (Pathak et al. 1977)[4].

The exact mechanism of action of methoxsalen with the epidermal melanocyctes and keratinocytes is not known. The best known biochemical reaction of methoxsalen is with DNA. Methoxsalen, upon photoactivation, conjugates and forms covalent bonds with DNA which leads to the formation of both monofunctional (addition to a single strand of DNA) and bifunctional adducts (crosslinking of psoralen to both strands of DNA) (Dall' Acqua et al., 1971[5]; Cole, 1970[6]; Musajo et al., 1974[7]; Dall'Acqua et al., 1979[8]). Reactions with proteins have also been described (Yoshikawa, et al., 1979[9]).

Methoxsalen acts as a photosensitizer. Administration of the drug and subsequent exposure to UVA can lead to cell injury. Orally administered methoxsalen reaches the skin via the blood and UVA penetrates well into the skin. If sufficient cell injury occurs in the skin, an inflammatory reaction occurs. The most obvious manifestation of this reaction is delayed erythema, which may not begin for several hours and peaks at 48–72 hours. The inflammation is followed, over several days to weeks, by repair which is manifested by increased melanization of the epidermis and thickening of the stratum corneum. The mechanisms of therapy are not known. In the treatment of vitiligo, it has been suggested that melanocytes in the hair follicle are stimulated to move up the follicle and to repopulate the epidermis (Ortonne et al, 1979[10]). In the treatment of psoriasis, the mechanism is most often assumed to be DNA photodamage and resulting decrease in cell proliferation but other vascular, leukocyte, or cell regulatory mechanisms may also be playing some role. Psoriasis is a hyperproliferative disorder and other agents known to be therapeutic for psoriasis are known to inhibit DNA synthesis.

III. INDICATIONS AND USAGE

A. Photochemotherapy (methoxsalen with long wave UVA radiation) is indicated for the symptomatic control of severe, recalcitrant, disabling psoriasis not adequately responsive to other forms of therapy and when the diagnosis has been supported by biopsy. Photochemotherapy is intended to be administered only in conjunction with a schedule of controlled doses of long wave ultraviolet radiation.

B. Photochemotherapy (methoxsalen with long wave ultraviolet radiation) is indicated for the repigmentation of idiopathic vitiligo.

C. Photopheresis (methoxsalen with long wave ultraviolet radiation of white blood cells) is indicated for use with the UVAR* System in the palliative treatment of the skin manifestations of cutaneous T-cell lymphoma (CTCL) in persons who have not been responsive to other forms of treatment. While this dosage form of methoxsalen has been approved for use in combination with photopheresis, Oxsoralen Ultra® Capsules have not been approved for that use.

IV. CONTRAINDICATIONS

A. Patients exhibiting idiosyncratic reactions to psoralen compounds.

B. Patients possessing a specific history of light sensitive disease states should not initiate methoxsalen therapy. Diseases associated with photosensitivity include lupus erythematosus, porphyria cutanea tarda, erythropoietic protoporphyria, variegate porphyria, xeroderma pigmentosum, and albinism.

C. Patients exhibiting melanoma or possessing a history of melanoma.

D. Patients exhibiting invasive squamous cell carcinomas.

Continued on next page

8-Mop—Cont.

E. Patients with aphakia, because of the significantly increased risk of retinal damage due to the absence of lenses.

V. WARNINGS—GENERAL

A. SKIN BURNING: Serious burns from either UVA or sunlight (even through window glass) can result if the recommended dosage of the drug and/or exposure schedules are not maintained.

B. CARCINOGENICITY:

1. ANIMAL STUDIES: Topical or intraperitoneal methoxsalen has been reported to be a potent photocarcinogen in albino mice and hairless mice. However, methoxsalen given by the oral route to albino mice or by any route in pigmented mice is considerably less phototoxic or carcinogenic (Hakim et al. 1960[11]; Pathak et al. 1959[12]).

2. HUMAN STUDIES: A prospective study of 1380 patients over 5 years revealed an approximately ninefold increase in risks of squamous cell carcinoma among PUVA treated patients (Stern et al. 1979[13] and Stern et al. 1980[14]). This increase in risk appears greatest among patients who are fair skinned or had pre-PUVA exposure to 1) prolonged tar and UVB treatment, 2) ionizing radiation, or 3) arsenic.

In addition, an approximately two-fold increase in the risk of basal cell carcinoma was noted in this study. Roenigk et al. 1980[15] studied 690 patients for up to 4 years and found no increase in the risk of non-melanoma skin cancer. However, patients in this cohort had significantly less exposure to PUVA than in the Stern et al study. After 5 years, two of 1380 patients in the Stern et al PUVA study have developed malignant melanoma. In addition, more than 1/5 of patients in this cohort have developed macular pigmented lesions on the buttocks. While there is no evidence that an increased risk of melanoma exists in PUVA treated patients, these observations indicate the need for continued evaluation of melanoma risk in PUVA treated patients.

In a study in Indian patients treated for 4 years for vitiligo, 12 percent developed keratoses, but not cancer, in the depigmented, vitiliginous areas (Mosher, 1980[16]). Clinically, the keratoses were keratotic papules, actinic keratosis-like macules, nonscaling dome-shaped papules, and lichenoid porokeratotic-like papules.

C. CATARACTOGENICITY:

1. ANIMAL STUDIES: Exposure to large doses of UVA causes cataracts in animals, and this effect is enhanced by the administration of methoxsalen (Cloud et al. 1960[17]; Cloud et al. 1961[18]; Freeman et al. 1969[19]).

2. HUMAN STUDIES: It has been found that the concentration of methoxsalen in the lens is proportional to the serum level. If the lens is exposed to UVA during the time methoxsalen is present in the lens, photochemical action may lead to irreversible binding of methoxsalen to proteins and the DNA components of the lens (Lerman et al. 1980[20]). However, if the lens is shielded from UVA, the methoxsalen will diffuse out of the lens in a 24 hour period[20]. Patients should be told emphatically to wear UVA-absorbing, wrap-around sunglasses for the twenty-four (24) hour period following ingestion of methoxsalen, whether exposed to direct or indirect sunlight in the open or through a window glass.

Among patients using proper eye protection, there is no evidence for a significantly increased risk of cataracts in association with PUVA therapy.[13] Thirty-five of 1380 patients have developed cataracts in the five years since their first PUVA treatment. This incidence is comparable to that expected in a population of this size and age distribution. No relationship between PUVA dose and cataract risk in this group has been noted.

D. ACTINIC DEGENERATION: Exposure to sunlight and/or ultraviolet radiation may result in "premature aging" of the skin.

E. BASAL CELL CARCINOMAS: Patients exhibiting multiple basal cell carcinomas or having a history of basal cell carcinomas should be diligently observed and treated.

F. RADIATION THERAPY: Patients having a history of previous x-ray therapy or grenz ray therapy should be diligently observed for signs of carcinoma.

G. ARSENIC THERAPY: Patients having a history of previous arsenic therapy should be diligently observed for signs of carcinoma.

H. HEPATIC DISEASES: Patients with hepatic insufficiency should be treated with caution since hepatic biotransformation is necessary for drug urinary excretion.

I. CARDIAC DISEASES: Patients with cardiac diseases or others who may be unable to tolerate prolonged standing or exposure to heat stress should not be treated in a vertical UVA chamber.

J. TOTAL DOSAGE: The total cumulative dose of UVA that can be given over long periods of time with safety has not as yet been established.

K. CONCOMITANT THERAPY: Special care should be exercised in treating patients who are receiving concomitant therapy (either topically or systemically) with known photosensitizing agents such as anthralin, coal tar or coal tar derivatives, griseofulvin, phenothiazines, nalidixic acid, halogenated salicylanilides (bacteriostatic soaps), sulfonamides, tetracyclines, thiazides, and certain organic staining dyes such as methylene blue, toluidine blue, rose bengal, and methyl orange.

VI. PRECAUTIONS

A. GENERAL—APPLICABLE TO BOTH VITILIGO AND PSORIASIS TREATMENT:

1. BEFORE METHOXSALEN INGESTION

Patients must not sunbathe during the 24 hours prior to methoxsalen ingestion and UV exposure. The presence of a sunburn may prevent an accurate evaluation of the patient's response to photochemotherapy.

2. AFTER METHOXSALEN INGESTION

a. UVA-absorbing wrap-around sunglasses should be worn during daylight for 24 hours after methoxsalen ingestion. The protective eyewear must be designed to prevent entry of stray radiation to the eyes, including that which may enter from the sides of the eyewear. The protective eyewear is used to prevent the irreversible binding of methoxsalen to the proteins and DNA components of the lens. Cataracts form when enough of the binding occurs. Visual discrimination should be permitted by the eyewear for patient well-being and comfort.

b. Patients must avoid sun exposure, even through window glass or cloud cover, for at least 8 hours after methoxsalen ingestion. If sun exposure cannot be avoided, the patient should wear protective devices such as a hat and gloves, and/or apply sunscreens which contain ingredients that filter out UVA radiation (e.g., sunscreens containing benzophenone and/or PABA esters which exhibit a sun protective factor equal to or greater than 15). These chemical sunscreens should be applied to all areas that might be exposed to the sun (including lips). Sunscreens should not be applied to areas affected by psoriasis until after the patient has been treated in the UVA chamber.

3. DURING PUVA THERAPY

a. Total UVA-absorbing/blocking goggles mechanically designed to give maximal ocular protection must be worn. Failure to do so may increase the risk of cataract formation. A reliable radiometer can be used to verify elimination of UVA transmission through the goggles.

b. Abdominal skin, breasts, genitalia, and other sensitive areas should be protected for approximately $^1/_3$ of the initial exposure time until tanning occurs.

c. Unless affected by disease, male genitalia should be shielded.

4. AFTER COMBINED METHOXSALEN/UVA THERAPY

a. UVA-absorbing wrap-around sunglasses should be worn during the daylight for 24 hours after combined methoxsalen/UVA therapy.

b. Patients should not sunbathe for 48 hours after therapy. Erythema and/or burning due to photochemotherapy and sunburn due to sun exposure are additive.

5. VITILIGO THERAPY

a. The dosage of methoxsalen should not be increased above 0.6 mg/kg since overdosage may result in serious burning of the skin.

b. Eye and skin sun protection as described in the Precautions—General section should be observed.

B. INFORMATION FOR PATIENTS: See accompanying Patient Package Insert.

C. LABORATORY TESTS:

1. Patients should have an ophthalmologic examination prior to the start of therapy, and thence yearly.

2. Patients should have the following tests prior to the start of therapy and should be retested 6–12 months subsequently. Additional tests at more extended time periods should be conducted as clinically indicated.

a. Complete Blood Count (Hemoglobin or Hematocrit; White Blood Count—if abnormal, a differential count).

b. Anti-nuclear Antibodies.

c. Liver Function Tests.

d. Renal Function Tests (Creatinine or Blood Urea Nitrogen).

D. DRUG INTERACTIONS: See Warnings Section.

E. CARCINOGENESIS: See Warnings Section.

F. PREGNANCY:

Pregnancy Category C. Animal reproduction studies have not been conducted with methoxsalen. It is also not known whether methoxsalen can cause fetal harm when administered to a pregnant woman or can affect reproduction capacity. Methoxsalen should be given to a woman only if clearly needed.

G. NURSING MOTHERS:

It is not known whether this drug is excreted in human milk. Because many drugs are excreted in human milk, caution should be exercised when methoxsalen is administered to a nursing woman.

H. PEDIATRIC USE:

Safety in children has not been established. Potential hazards of long-term therapy include the possibilities of carcinogenicity and cataractogenicity as described in the Warnings Section as well as the probability of actinic degeneration which is also described in the Warnings Section.

VII. ADVERSE REACTIONS

A. METHOXSALEN:

The most commonly reported side effect of methoxsalen alone is nausea, which occurs with approximately 10% of all patients. This effect may be minimized or avoided by instructing the patient to take methoxsalen with milk or food, or to divide the dose into two portions, taken approximately one-half hour apart. Other effects include nervousness, insomnia, and psychological depression.

B. COMBINED METHOXSALEN/UVA THERAPY:

1. PRURITUS: This adverse reaction occurs with approximately 10% of all patients. In most cases, pruritus can be alleviated with frequent application of bland emollients or other topical agents; severe pruritus may require systemic treatment. If pruritus is unresponsive to these measures, shield pruritic areas from further UVA exposure until the condition resolves. If intractable pruritus is generalized, UVA treatment should be discontinued until the pruritus disappears.

2. ERYTHEMA: Mild, transient erythema at 24–48 hours after PUVA therapy is an expected reaction and indicates that a therapeutic interaction between methoxsalen and UVA occurred. Any area showing moderate erythema (greater than Grade 2—See Table 1 for grades of erythema) should be shielded during subsequent UVA exposures until the erythema has resolved. Erythema greater than Grade 2 which appears within 24 hours after UVA treatment may signal a potentially severe burn. Erythema may become progressively worse over the next 24 hours, since the peak erythemal reaction characteristically occurs 48 hours or later after methoxsalen ingestion. The patient should be protected from further UVA exposures and sunlight, and should be monitored closely.

3. IMPORTANT DIFFERENCES BETWEEN PUVA ERYTHEMA AND SUNBURN: PUVA-induced inflammation differs from sunburn or UVB phototherapy in several ways. The **in situ** depth of photochemistry is deeper within the tissue because UVA is transmitted further into the skin. The DNA lesions induced by PUVA are very different from UV-induced thymine dimers and may lead to a DNA crosslink. This DNA lesion may be more problematic to the cell because crosslinks are more lethal and psoralen-DNA photoproducts may be "new" or unfamiliar substrates for DNA repair enzymes. DNA synthesis is also suppressed longer after PUVA. The time course of delayed erythema is different with PUVA and may not involve the usual mediators seen in sunburn. PUVA-induced redness may be just beginning at 24 hours, when UVB erythema has already passed its peak. The erythema dose-response curve is also steeper for PUVA. Compared to equally erythemogenic doses of UVB, the histologic alterations induced by PUVA show more dermal vessel damage and longer duration of epidermal and dermal abnormalities.

4. OTHER ADVERSE REACTIONS: Those reported include edema, dizziness, headache, malaise, depression, hypopigmentation, vesiculation and bullae formation, non-specific rash, herpes simplex, miliaria, urticaria, folliculitis, gastrointestinal disturbances, cutaneous tenderness, leg cramps, hypotension, and extension of psoriasis.

VIII. OVERDOSAGE

In the event of methoxsalen overdosage, induce emesis and keep the patient in a darkened room for at least 24 hours. Emesis is beneficial only within the first 2 to 3 hours after ingestion of methoxsalen, since maximum blood levels are reached by this time.

IX. DRUG DOSAGE & ADMINISTRATION

A. VITILIGO THERAPY

1. DRUG DOSAGE: Two capsules (10 mg each) in one dose taken with milk or in food two to four hours before ultraviolet light exposure.

2. LIGHT EXPOSURE: The exposure time to sunlight should comply with the following guide:

	Basic Skin Color		
	Light	**Medium**	**Dark**
Initial Exposure	15 min.	20 min.	25 min.
Second Exposure	20 min.	25 min.	30 min.
Third Exposure	25 min.	30 min.	35 min.
Fourth Exposure	30 min.	35 min.	40 min.

Subsequent Exposure: Gradually increase exposure based on erythema and tenderness of the amelanotic skin.

Therapy should be on alternate days and never two consecutive days.

B. PSORIASIS THERAPY

1. DRUG DOSAGE—INITIAL THERAPY: The methoxsalen capsules should be taken 2 hours before UVA exposure with some food or milk according to the following table:

Patient's Weight (kg)	(lbs)	Dose (mg)
<30	<66	10
30–50	66–110	20
51–65	112–143	30
66–80	146–176	40
81–90	179–198	50
91–115	201–254	60
>115	>254	70

Additional drug dosage directions are as follows:
a. Weight Change: In the event that the weight of a patient changes during treatment such that he/she falls into an adjacent weight range/dose category, no change in the dose of methoxsalen is usually required. If, in the physician's opinion, however, a weight change is sufficiently great to modify the drug dose, then an adjustment in the time of exposure to UVA should be made.
b. Dose/Week: The number of doses per week of methoxsalen capsules will be determined by the patient's schedule of UVA exposures. In no case should treatments be given more often than once every other day because the full extent of phototoxic reactions may not be evident until 48 hours after each exposure.
c. Dosage Increase: Dosage may be increased by 10 mg. after the fifteenth treatment under the conditions outlined in section XI.B.4.b.

X. UVA RADIATION SOURCE SPECIFICATIONS & INFORMATION

A. IRRADIANCE UNIFORMITY: (For photopheresis, refer to the UVAR* System Operator's Manual.)
The following specifications should be met with the window of the detector held in a vertical plane:
1. Vertical variation: For readings taken at any point along the vertical center axis of the chamber (to within 15 cm from the top and bottom), the lowest reading should not be less than 70 percent of the highest reading.
2. Horizontal variation: Throughout any specific horizontal plane, the lowest reading must be at least 80 percent of the highest reading, excluding the peripheral 3 cm of the patient treatment space:

B. PATIENT SAFETY FEATURES:
The following safety features should be present: (1) Protection from electrical hazard: All units should be grounded and conform to applicable electrical codes. The patient or operator should not be able to touch any live electrical parts. There should be ground fault protection. (2) Protective shielding of lamps: The patient should not be able to come in contact with the bare lamps. In the event of lamp breakage, the patient should not be exposed to broken lamp components. (3) Hand rails and hand holds: Appropriate supports should be available to the patient. (4) Patient viewing window: A window which blocks UV should be provided for viewing the patient during treatment. (5) Door and latches: Patients should be able to open the door from the inside with only slight pressure to the door. (6) Non-skid floor: The floor should be of a non-skid nature. (7) Thermoregulation: Sufficient air flow should be provided for patient safety and comfort, limiting temperature within the UVA radiator cabinet to approximately less than 100° F. (8) Timer: The irradiator should be equipped with an automatic timer which terminates the exposure at the conclusion of a pre-set time interval. (9) Patient alarm device: An alarm device within the UVA irradiator chamber should be accessible to the patient for emergency activation. (10) Danger label: The unit should have a label prominently displayed which reads as follows:
DANGER—Ultraviolet Radiation—Follow your physician's instructions—Failure to use protective eyewear may result in eye injury.

C. UVA EXPOSURE DOSIMETRY MEASUREMENTS:
The maximum radiant exposure or irradiance (within ± 15 percent) of UVA (320–400 nm) delivered to the patient should be determined by using an appropriate radiometer calibrated to be read in Joules/cm^2 or mW/cm^2. In the absence of a standard measuring technique approved by the National Bureau of Standards, the system should use a detector corrected to a cosine spatial response. The use and recalibration frequency of such a radiometer for a specific UVA irradiator chamber should be specified by the manufacturer because the UVA dose (exposure) is determined by the design of the irradiator, the number of lamps, and the age of the lamps. If irradiance is measured, the radiometer reading in mW/cm^2 is used to calculate the exposure time in minutes to deliver the required UVA dose in Joules/cm^2 to a patient in the UVA irradiator cabinet. The equation is:

$$\text{Exposure Time in minutes} = \frac{\text{Desired UVA Dose (J/cm}^2\text{)}}{0.06 \times \text{Irradiance (mW/cm}^2\text{)}}$$

Overexposure due to human error should be minimized by using an accurate automatic timing device, which is set by the operator and controlled by energizing and de-energizing the UVA irradiator lamp.

Skin Type	History	Recommended Joules/cm ^{2}
I	Always burn, never tan (Patients with Erythrodermic psoriasis are to be classed as Type I for determination of UVA dosage.)	0.5 J/cm^2
II	Always burn, but sometimes tan	1.0 J/cm^2
III	Sometimes burn, but always tan	1.5 J/cm^2
IV	Never burn, always tan	2.0 J/cm ^{2}
	Physician Examination	
V*	Moderately pigmented	2.5 J/cm ^{2}
VI*	Blacks	3.0 J/cm^2

[*Patients with natural pigmentation of these types should be classified into a lower skin type category if the sunburning history so indicates.]

The timing device calibration interval should be specified by the manufacturer. Safety systems should be included to minimize the possibility of delivering a UVA exposure which exceeds the prescribed dose, in the event the timer or radiometer should malfunction.

D. UVA SPECTRAL OUTPUT DISTRIBUTION:
The spectral distributions of the lamps should meet the following specifications:

Wavelength Band (Nanometers)	Output [1]
<310	<1
310 to 320	1 to 3
320 to 330	4 to 8
330 to 340	11 to 17
340 to 350	18 to 25
350 to 360	19 to 28
360 to 370	15 to 23
370 to 380	8 to 12
380 to 390	3 to 7
390 to 400	1 to 3

[1]As a percentage of total irradiance between 320 and 400 nanometers.

XI. PUVA TREATMENT PROTOCOL

A. INITIAL EXPOSURE: The initial UVA exposure should be conducted according to the guidelines presented previously under IX.B.1 and 2, Psoriasis therapy, Drug dosage-initial Therapy and Exposure.
[See table at top of page]

B. CLEARING PHASE: Specific recommendations for patient treatment are as follows:
1. SKIN TYPES I, II & III. Patients with skin types I, II and III may be treated 2 or 3 times per week. UVA exposure may be held constant or increased by up to 1.0 Joule/cm^2 at each treatment, according to the patient's response. If erythema occurs, however, do not increase exposure time until erythema resolves. The severity and extent of the patient's erythema may be used to determine whether the next exposure should be shortened, omitted, or maintained at the previous dosage. See Adverse Reactions section for additional information.
2. SKIN TYPES IV, V & VI. Patients with skin types IV, V and VI may be treated 2 or 3 times per week. UVA exposure may be held constant or increased by up to 1.5 Joules/cm^2 at each treatment unless erythema occurs. If erythema occurs, follow instructions outlined above in the procedures for patients with skin types I, II and III.
3. ERYTHRODERMIC PSORIASIS. Patients with erythrodermic psoriasis should be treated with special attention because pre-existing erythema may obscure observations of possible treatment-related phototoxic erythema. These patients may be treated 2 or 3 times per week, as a Type I patient.
4. MISCELLANEOUS SITUATIONS:
a. If there is no response after a total of 10 treatments, the exposure of UVA energy may be increased by an additional 0.5–1.0 Joules/cm^2 above the prior incremental increases for each treatment. (Example: a patient whose exposure dosage is being increased by 1.0 Joule/cm^2 may now have all subsequent doses increased by 1.5–2.0 Joules/cm^2.)
b. If there is no response, or only minimal response, after 15 treatments, the dosage of methoxsalen may be increased by 10 mg. (a one-time increase in dosage). This increased dosage may be continued for the remainder of the course of treatment but should not be exceeded.
c. If a patient misses a treatment, the UVA exposure time of the next treatment should not be increased. If more than one treatment is missed, reduce the exposure by 0.5 Joules/cm^2 for each treatment missed.
d. If the lower extremities are not responding as well as the rest of the body and do not show erythema, cover all other body area and give 25 percent of the present exposure dose as an additional exposure to the lower extremities. This additional exposure to the lower extremities should be terminated if erythema develops on these areas.
e. Non-responsive psoriasis: If a patient's generalized psoriasis is not responding, or if the condition appears to be worsening during treatment, the possibility of a generalized phototoxic reaction should be considered. This may be confirmed by the improvement of the condition following temporary discontinuance of this therapy for two weeks. If no improvement occurs during the interruption of treatment, this patient may be considered a treatment failure.

C. ALTERNATIVE EXPOSURE SCHEDULE:
As an alternative to increasing the UVA exposure at each treatment, the following schedule may be followed; this schedule may reduce the total number of Joules/cm^2 received by the patient over the entire course of therapy.
1. Incremental increases in UVA exposure for all patients may range from 0.5 to 1.5 Joules/cm^2, according to the patient's response to therapy.
2. Once Grade 2 clearing (see Table 2) has been reached and the patient is progressing adequately, UVA dosage is held constant. This dosage is maintained until Grade 4 clearing is reached.
3. If the rate of clearing significantly decreases, exposure dosage may be increased at each treatment (0.1–1.5 Joules/cm^2) until Grade 3 clearing and a satisfactory progress rate is attained. The UVA exposure will be held constant again until Grade 4 clearing is attained. These increases may be used also if the rate of clearing significantly decreases between Grade 3 and Grade 4 response. However, the possibility of a phototoxic reaction should be considered; see Non-responsive Psoriasis, above.
4. In summary, this schedule raises slightly the increments (Joules/cm^2) of UVA dosage, but limits these increases to those periods when the patient is not responding adequately. Otherwise, the UVA exposure is held at the lowest effective dose.

D. MAINTENANCE PHASE:
The goal of maintenance treatment is to keep the patient as symptom-free as possible with the least amount of UVA exposure.
1. SCHEDULE OF EXPOSURES: When patients have achieved 95 percent clearing, or Grade 4 response (Table 2), they may be placed on the following maintenance schedules (M_1–M_4), in sequence. It is recommended that each maintenance schedule be adhered to for at least 2 treatments (unless erythema or psoriatic flare occurs, in which case see (2a) and (2b) below).

Maintenance Schedules
M_1–once/week
M_2–once/2 week
M_3–once/3 weeks
M_4–p.r.n. (i.e., for flares)

2. LENGTH OF EXPOSURE: The UVA exposure for the first maintenance treatment of any schedule (ex-

Continued on next page

Table 2. Response to Therapy

Grade	Criteria	Percent Improvement (compared to original extent of disease)
−1	Psoriasis worse	0
0	No change	0
1	Minimal improvement—slightly less scale and/or erythema	5–20
2	Definite improvement—partial flattening of all plaques—less scaling and less erythema	20–50
3	Considerable improvement—nearly complete flattening of all plaques but borders of plaques still palpable	50–95
4	Clearing; complete flattening of plaques including borders; plaques may be outlined by pigmentation	95

8-Mop—Cont.

cept M_4 as noted below) is the same as that of the patient's last treatment under the previous schedule. For skin types I-IV, however, it is recommended that the maximum UVA dosage during maintenance treatments not exceed the following:

Skin Types	Joules/cm²/treatment
I	12
II	14
III	18
IV	22

If the patient develops erythema or new lesions of psoriasis, proceed as follows:
a. Erythema: During maintenance therapy, the patient's tan and threshold dose for erythema may gradually decrease. If maintenance treatments produce significant erythema, the exposure to UVA should be decreased by 25 percent until further treatments no longer produce erythema.
b. Psoriasis: If the patient develops new areas of psoriasis during maintenance therapy (but still is classified as having a Grade 4 response), the exposure to UVA may be increased by 0.5–1.5 Joules/cm² at each treatment; this is appropriate for all types of patients. These increases are continued until the psoriasis is brought under control and the patient is again clear. The exposure being administered when this clearing is reached should be used for further maintenance treatment.
3. FLARES DURING MAINTENANCE: If the patient flares during maintenance treatment (i.e., develops psoriasis on more than 5 percent of the originally involved areas of the body) his maintenance treatment schedule may be changed to the preceding maintenance or clearing schedule. The patient may be kept on his schedule until again 95 percent clear. If the original maintenance treatment schedule is unable to control the psoriasis, the schedule may be changed to a more frequent regimen. If a flare occurs less than 6 weeks after the last treatment, 25 percent of the maximum exposure received during the clearing phase, may be used and then proceed with the clearing schedule previously followed for this patient. (At 95 percent clearing follow regular maintenance until the optimum maintenance schedule is determined for the patient.) If more than 6 weeks have elapsed since the last treatment was given, treat patients as if they were beginning therapy insofar as exposure dosages are concerned, since their threshold for erythema may have decreased.

Table 1. Grades of Erythema

Grade	Erythema Level
0	No erythema
1	Minimally perceptible erythema—faint pink
2	Marked erythema but with no edema
3	Fiery erythema with edema
4	Fiery erythema with edema and blistering

[See table 2 at bottom of previous page]

XII. HOW SUPPLIED

8-MOP Capsules, each containing 10 mg. of methoxsalen (8-methoxypsoralen) packaged in amber glass bottles of 50 (NDC 0187-0651-42).
Store at 25°C (77°F); excursions permitted to 15°C–30°C (59°F–86°F).

BIBLIOGRAPHY

1. Pathak, M.A., Kramer, D.M., Fitzpatrick, T.B.: Photobiology and Photochemistry of Furocoumarins (Psoralens), SUNLIGHT AND MAN: Normal and Abnormal Photobiologic Responses. Edited by M.A. Pathak, L.C. Harbor, M. Seiji et al. University of Tokyo Press. 1974, pp. 335–368.
2. Artuc, M., Stuettgen, G., Schalla, W., Schaefer, H., and Gazith, J.: Reversible binding of 5- and 8-methoxypsoralen to human serum proteins (albumin) and to epidermis in vitro: Brit. J. Dermat. 101, pp. 669–677 (1979).
3. Mandula, B.B., Pathak, M.A., Nakayama, Y., and Davidson, S.J.: Induction of mixed-function oxidases in mouse liver by psoralens., Ibid, 99, pp. 687–692 (1978).
4. Pathak, M.A., Fitzpatrick, T.B., Parrish, J.A.: PSORIASIS, Proceedings of the Second International Symposium. Edited by E.M. Farber, A.J. Cox, Yorke Medical Books, pp. 262–265 (1977).
5. Dall'Acqua, F., Marciani, S., Ciavatta, L, Rodighiero, G.: Formation of interstrand cross-linkings in the photoreactions between furocoumarins and DNA; Z Naturforsch (B), 26, pp. 561–569 (1971).
6. Cole, R.S.: Light-induced cross-linkings of DNA in the presence of a furocoumarin (psoralen), Biochem. Biophys. Acta, 217, pp. 30–39 (1970).
7. Musajo, L., Rodighiero, G., Caporale, G., Dall'Acqua, F., Marciani, S., Bordin, F., Baccichetti, F., Bevilacqua, R.: Photoreactions between Skin-Photosensitizing Furocoumarins and Nucleic Acids, SUNLIGHT AND MAN; Normal and Abnormal Photobiologic Responses. Edited by M.A. Pathak, L.C. Harber, M. Seiji et al. University of Tokyo Press, pp. 369–387 (1974).
8. Dall'Acqua, F., Vedaldi, D., Bordin, F., and Rodighiero, G.: New studies in the interaction between 8-methoxypsoralen and DNA in vitro; J. Investigative Dermat., 73, pp. 191–197 (1979).
9. Yoshikawa, K., Mori, N., Sakakibara, S., Mizuno, N., Song, P.: Photo-Conjugation of 8-methoxypsoralen with Proteins; Photochem. & Photobiol. 29, pp. 1127–1133 (1979).
10. Ortonne, J. P., MacDonald, D.M., Micoud, A., Thivolet, J.: PUVA-induced repigmentation of vitiligo: a histochemical (split-DOPA) and ultra-structural study: Brit. J. of Dermat., 101, pp. 1–12 (1979).
11. Hakim, R.E., Griffin, A.C., Knox, J.M.: Erythema and tumor formation in methoxsalen treated mice exposed to fluorescent light; Arch. Dermatol. 82, 572–577 (1960).
12. Pathak, M.A., Daniels, F., Hopkins, C.E., Fitzpatrick, T.B.: Ultraviolet carcinogenesis in albino and pigmented mice receiving furocoumarins: psoralens and 8-methoxypsoralen, Nature 183, pp. 728–730 (1959).
13. Stern, R.S., Thibodeau, L.A., Kleinerman, R.A., Parrish, J.A., Fitzpatrick, T.B., and 22 Participating Investigators: Risk of Cutaneous Carcinoma in Patients Treated with Oral Methoxsalen Photochemotherapy for Psoriasis: NEJM, 300. No. 15, pp. 809–813 (1979).
14. Stern, R.S., Parrish, J.A., Zierler, S.: Skin Carcinoma in Patients with Psoriasis Treated with Topical Tar and Artificial Ultraviolet Radiation. Lancet, 1, pp. 732–735 (1980).
15. Roenigk, Jr., H.H., and 12 Cooperating Investigators: Skin Cancer in the PUVA-48 Cooperative Study of Psoriasis. Program for Forty-First Annual Meeting for The Society of Investigative Dermatology, Inc., Sheraton Washington Hotel, Washington, D.C., May 12, 13, and 14, 1980. Abstracts JID, 74, No. 4, p. 250 (April, 1980).
16. Mosher, D.B., Pathak, M.A., Harris, T.J., Fitzpatrick, T.B.: Development of Cutaneous Lesions in Vitiligo During Long-Term PUVA Therapy. Program for Forty-First Annual Meeting for The Society for Investigative Dermatology, Inc., Sheraton Washington Hotel, Washington, D.C., May 12, 13, and 14, 1980. Abstracts JID, 74, No. 4, p. 259 (April, 1980).
17. Cloud, T.M., Hakim, R., Griffin, A.C.: Photosensitization of the eye with methoxsalen. I. Acute effects; Arch. Ophthalmol. 64, pp. 346–352 (1960).
18. Cloud, T.M., Hakim, R., Griffen, A.C.: Photosensitization of the eye with methoxsalen. II. Chronic effects, Ibid, 66, pp. 689–694 (1961).
19. Freeman, R.G., Troll, D.: Photosensitization of the eye by 8-methoxypsoralen, JID, 53, pp. 449–453 (1969).
20. Lerman, S., Megaw, J., Willis, I.: Potential ocular complications from PUVA therapy and their prevention; J. Invest. Dermat., 74, pp. 197–199 (1980).

2579-01A EL ICN Pharmaceuticals, Inc. Rev. 2-00
3300 Hyland Ave.
Costa Mesa, CA 92626

Shown in Product Identification Guide, page 317

ANCOBON® ℞

[an 'co-bon]
brand of flucytosine
CAPSULES

> **WARNING**
> **Use with extreme caution in patients with impaired renal function. Close monitoring of hematologic, renal and hepatic status of all patients is essential. These instructions should be thoroughly reviewed before administration of Ancobon.**

DESCRIPTION

Ancobon (flucytosine), an antifungal agent, is available as 250-mg and 500-mg capsules for oral administration. Each capsule also contains corn starch, lactose and talc. Gelatin capsule shells contain parabens (butyl, methyl, propyl) and sodium propionate, with the following dye systems: 250-mg capsules—black iron oxide, FD&C Blue No. 1, FD&C Yellow No. 6, D&C Yellow No. 10 and titanium dioxide; 500-mg capsules—black iron oxide and titanium dioxide. Chemically, flucytosine is 5-fluorocytosine, a fluorinated pyrimidine which is related to fluorouracil and floxuridine. It is a white to off-white crystalline powder with a molecular weight of 129.09 and the following structural formula:

CLINICAL PHARMACOLOGY

Flucytosine is rapidly and virtually completely absorbed following oral administration. Bioavailability estimated by comparing the area under the curve of serum concentrations after oral and intravenous administration showed 78% to 89% absorption of the oral dose. Peak blood concentrations of 30 to 40 mcg/mL were reached within 2 hours of administration of a 2-gm oral dose to normal subjects. The mean blood concentrations were approximately 70 to 80 mcg/mL 1 to 2 hours after a dose in patients with normal renal function who received a 6-week regimen of flucytosine (150 mg/kg/day given in divided doses every 6 hours) in combination with amphotericin B. The half-life in the majority of normal subjects ranged between 2.4 and 4.8 hours. Flucytosine is excreted via the kidneys by means of glomerular filtration without significant tubular reabsorption. More than 90% of the total radioactivity after oral administration was recovered in the urine as intact drug. Approximately 1% of the dose is present in the urine as the α-fluoro-β-ureido-propionic acid metabolite. A small portion of the dose is excreted in the feces.
The half-life of flucytosine is prolonged in patients with renal insufficiency; the average half-life in nephrectomized or anuric patients was 85 hours (range: 29.9 to 250 hours). A linear correlation was found between the elimination rate constant of flucytosine and creatinine clearance.
In vitro studies have shown that 2.9% to 4% of flucytosine is protein-bound over the range of therapeutic concentrations found in the blood. Flucytosine readily penetrates the blood-brain barrier, achieving clinically significant concentrations in cerebrospinal fluid. Studies in pregnant rats have shown that flucytosine injected intraperitoneally crosses the placental barrier (see PRECAUTIONS).

Microbiology
Flucytosine has in vitro and in vivo activity against Candida and Cryptococcus. Although the exact mode of action is unknown, it has been proposed that flucytosine acts directly on fungal organisms by competitive inhibition of purine and pyrimidine uptake and indirectly by intracellular metabolism to 5-fluorouracil. Flucytosine enters the fungal cell via cytosine permease; thus, flucytosine is metabolized to 5-fluorouracil within fungal organisms. The 5-fluorouracil is extensively incorporated into fungal RNA and inhibits synthesis of both DNA and RNA. The result is unbalanced growth and death of the fungal organism. Antifungal synergism between Ancobon and polyene antibiotics, particularly amphotericin B, has been reported.

Actions
Flucytosine has in vitro and in vivo activity against Candida and Cryptococcus. The exact mode of action against these fungi is not known. Ancobon is not metabolized significantly when given orally to man.

Susceptibility
Cryptococcus: Most strains initially isolated from clinical material have shown flucytosine minimal inhibitory concentrations (MIC's) ranging from .46 to 7.8 mcg/mL. Any isolate with an MIC greater than 12.5 mcg/mL is considered resistant. In vitro resistance has developed in originally susceptible strains during therapy. It is recommended that clinical cultures for susceptibility testing be taken initially and at weekly intervals during therapy. The initial culture should be reserved as a reference in susceptibility testing of subsequent isolates.
Candida: As high as 40% to 50% of the pretreatment clinical isolates of Candida have been reported to be resistant to flucytosine. It is recommended that susceptibility studies be performed as early as possible and be repeated during therapy. An MIC value greater than 100 mcg/mL is considered resistant.
Interference with in vitro activity of flucytosine occurs in complex or semisynthetic media. In order to rely upon the recommended in vitro interpretations of susceptibility, it is essential that the broth medium and the testing procedure used be that described by Shadomy.[1]

INDICATIONS AND USAGE

Ancobon is indicated only in the treatment of serious infections caused by susceptible strains of Candida and/or Cryptococcus. *Candida:* Septicemia, endocarditis and urinary system infections have been effectively treated with flucytosine. Limited trials in pulmonary infections justify the use of flucytosine. *Cryptococcus:* Meningitis and pulmonary infections have been treated effectively. Studies in septicemias and urinary tract infections are limited, but good responses have been reported.

CONTRAINDICATIONS

Ancobon should not be used in patients with a known hypersensitivity to the drug.

WARNINGS

Ancobon must be given with extreme caution to patients with impaired renal function. Since Ancobon is excreted primarily by the kidneys, renal impairment may lead to accumulation of the drug. Ancobon blood concentrations should be monitored to determine the adequacy of renal excretion in such patients.[1] Dosage adjustments should be made in patients with renal insufficiency to prevent progressive accumulation of active drug.
Ancobon must be given with extreme caution to patients with bone marrow depression. Patients may be more prone to depression of bone marrow function if they: 1) have a hematologic disease, 2) are being treated with radiation or drugs which depress bone marrow, or 3) have a history of treatment with such drugs or radiation. Bone marrow toxicity can be irreversible and may lead to death in immunosuppressed patients. Frequent monitoring of hepatic function and of the hematopoietic system is indicated during therapy.

PRECAUTIONS

General: Before therapy with Ancobon is instituted, electrolytes (because of hypokalemia) and the hematologic and renal status of the patient should be determined (see WARNINGS). Close monitoring of the patient during therapy is essential.
Laboratory Tests: Since renal impairment can cause progressive accumulation of the drug, blood concentrations and kidney function should be monitored during therapy. Hematologic status (leucocyte and thrombocyte count) and liver

function (alkaline phosphatase, SGOT and SGPT) should be determined at frequent intervals during treatment as indicated.

Drug Interactions: Cytosine arabinoside, a cytostatic agent, has been reported to inactivate the antifungal activity of Ancobon by competitive inhibition. Drugs which impair glomerular filtration may prolong the biological half-life of flucytosine. Antifungal synergism between Ancobon and polyene antibiotics, particularly amphotericin B, has been reported.

Drug/Laboratory Test Interactions: Measurement of serum creatinine levels should be determined by the Jaffe method, since Ancobon does not interfere with the determination of creatinine values by this method, as it does when the dry-slide enzymatic method with the Kodak Ektachem analyzer is used.

Carcinogenesis, Mutagenesis, Impairment of Fertility: Flucytosine has not undergone adequate animal testing to evaluate carcinogenic potential. The mutagenic potential of flucytosine was evaluated in Ames-type studies with five different mutants of *S. typhimurium* and no mutagenicity was detected in the presence or absence of activating enzymes. Flucytosine was nonmutagenic in three different repair assay systems.

There have been no adequate trials in animals on the effects of flucytosine on fertility or reproductive performance. The fertility and reproductive performance of the offspring (F_1 generation) of mice treated with 100, 200 or 400 mg/kg/day of flucytosine on days 7 to 13 of gestation was studied; the *in utero* treatment had no adverse effect on the fertility or reproductive performance of the offspring.

Pregnancy: Teratogenic Effects. Pregnancy Category C. Although standard segment II studies have not been done, flucytosine was shown to be teratogenic (vertebral fusions) in the rat at doses of 40 mg/kg/day (0.27 times the maximum human dose, based on nominal dose). At higher doses (700 mg/kg/day, 4.7 times the maximum human dose, based on nominal dose), cleft lip and palate and micrognathia were reported. Flucytosine was not teratogenic in rabbits up to a dose of 100 mg/kg/day (0.68 times the maximum human dose, based on nominal dose). In mice, 400 mg/kg/day of flucytosine (2.7 times the maximum human dose, based on nominal dose) was associated with a low incidence of cleft palate that was not statistically significant. There are no adequate and well-controlled studies in pregnant women. Ancobon should be used during pregnancy only if the potential benefits justifies the potential risk to the fetus.

Nursing Mothers: It is not known whether this drug is excreted in human milk. Because many drugs are excreted in human milk and because of the potential for serious adverse reactions in nursing infants from Ancobon, a decision should be made whether to discontinue nursing or to discontinue the drug, taking into account the importance of the drug to the mother.

Pediatric Use: Safety and effectiveness in children have not been established.

ADVERSE REACTIONS

The adverse reactions which have occurred during treatment with Ancobon are grouped according to organ system affected.

Cardiovascular: Cardiac arrest, myocardial toxicity, ventricular dysfunction.

Respiratory: Respiratory arrest, chest pain, dyspnea.

Dermatologic: Rash, pruritus, urticaria, photosensitivity.

Gastrointestinal: Nausea, emesis, abdominal pain, diarrhea, anorexia, dry mouth, duodenal ulcer, gastrointestinal hemorrhage, acute hepatic injury with possible fatal outcome in debilitated patients, hepatic dysfunction, jaundice, ulcerative colitis, bilirubin elevation.

Genitourinary: Azotemia, creatinine and BUN elevation, crystalluria, renal failure.

Hematologic: Anemia, agranulocytosis, aplastic anemia, eosinophilia, leukopenia, pancytopenia, thrombocytopenia.

Neurologic: Ataxia, hearing loss, headache, paresthesia, parkinsonism, peripheral neuropathy, pyrexia, vertigo, sedation, convulsions.

Psychiatric: Confusion, hallucinations, psychosis.

Miscellaneous: Fatigue, hypoglycemia, hypokalemia, weakness, allergic reactions, Lyell's syndrome.

OVERDOSAGE

There is no experience with intentional overdosage. It is reasonable to expect that overdosage may produce pronounced manifestations of the known clinical adverse reactions. Prolonged serum concentrations in excess of 100 mcg/mL may be associated with an increased incidence of toxicity, especially gastrointestinal (diarrhea, nausea, vomiting), hematologic (leukopenia, thrombocytopenia) and hepatic (hepatitis).

In the management of overdosage, prompt gastric lavage or the use of an emetic is recommended. Adequate fluid intake should be maintained, by the intravenous route if necessary, since Ancobon is excreted unchanged via the renal tract. The hematologic parameters should be monitored frequently; liver and kidney function should be carefully monitored. Should any abnormalities appear in any of these parameters, appropriate therapeutic measures should be instituted. Since hemodialysis has been shown to rapidly reduce serum concentrations in anuric patients, this method may be considered in the management of overdosage.

DOSAGE AND ADMINISTRATION

The usual dosage of Ancobon is 50 to 150 mg/kg/day administered in divided doses at 6-hour intervals. Nausea or vomiting may be reduced or avoided if the capsules are given a few at a time over a 15-minute period. If the BUN or the serum creatinine is elevated, or if there are other signs of renal impairment, the initial dose should be at the lower level (see WARNINGS).

HOW SUPPLIED

Capsules, 250 mg (gray and green), imprinted ANCOBON® 250 ROCHE; bottles of 100 (NDC 0004-0077-01). *Capsules,* 500 mg (gray and white), imprinted ANCOBON® 500 ROCHE, bottles of 100 (NDC 0004-0079-01).

REFERENCE

1. Shadomy S: *Appl Microbiol.* June 1969, 17: 871–877.

Revised: December 1996

ANDROID® Ⓒ℞

Brand of
Methyltestosterone
Capsules USP, 10 mg

Rx Only

DESCRIPTION

The androgens are steroids that develop and maintain primary and secondary male sex characteristics.

Androgens are derivatives of cyclopentanoperhydrophenanthrene. Endogenous androgens are C-19 steroids with a side chain at C-17, and with two angular methyl groups. Testosterone is the primary endogenous androgen. In their active form, all drugs in the class have a 17-beta hydroxy group. 17-alpha alkylation (methyltestosterone) increases the pharmacologic activity per unit weight compared to testosterone when given orally.

Methyltestosterone, a synthetic derivative of testosterone, is an androgenic preparation given by the oral route in a capsule form. Each capsule contains 10 mg of Methyltestosterone USP. It has the following structural formula:

$C_{20}H_{30}O_2$ M.W. 302.46
17-β-hydroxy-17-methylandrost-4-en-3-one

Methyltestosterone occurs as white or creamy white crystals or powder, which is soluble in various organic solvents but is practically insoluble in water.

Each capsule, for oral administration, contains 10 mg of Methyltestosterone. In addition, each capsule contains the following inactive ingredients: Corn starch NF, Gelatin NF, FD&C Blue #1, FD&C Red #40.

CLINICAL PHARMACOLOGY

Endogenous androgens are responsible for the normal growth and development of the male sex organs and for maintenance of secondary sex characteristics. These effects include the growth and maturation of prostate, seminal vesicles, penis, and scrotum. The development of male hair distribution, such as beard, pubic, chest, and axillary hair; laryngeal enlargement, vocal chord thickening, alterations in body musculature, and fat distribution. Drugs in this class also cause retention of nitrogen, sodium, potassium, phosphorus, and decreased urinary excretion of calcium. Androgens have been reported to increase protein anabolism and decrease protein catabolism. Nitrogen balance is improved only when there is sufficient intake of calories and protein.

Androgens are responsible for the growth spurt of adolescence and for the eventual termination of linear growth which is brought about by fusion of the epiphyseal growth centers. In children, exogenous androgens accelerate linear growth rates, but may cause a disproportionate advancement in bone maturation. Use over long periods may result in fusion of the epiphyseal growth centers and termination of growth process. Androgens have been reported to stimulate the production of red blood cells by enhancing the production of erythropoietic stimulating factor.

During exogenous administration of androgens, endogenous testosterone release is inhibited through feedback inhibition of pituitary luteinizing hormone (LH). At large doses of exogenous androgens, spermatogenesis may also be suppressed through feedback inhibition of pituitary follicle stimulating hormone (FSH).

There is a lack of substantial evidence that androgens are effective in fractures, surgery, convalescence and functional uterine bleeding.

Pharmacokinetics

Testosterone given orally is metabolized by the gut and 44 percent is cleared by the liver of the first pass. Oral doses as high as 400 mg per day are needed to achieve clinically effective blood levels for full replacement therapy. The synthetic androgen, methyltestosterone, is less extensively metabolized by the liver and has a longer half-life. It is more suitable than testosterone for oral administration.

Testosterone in plasma is 98 percent bound to a specific testosterone-estradiol binding globulin, and about 2 percent is free. Generally, the amount of this sex-hormone binding globulin in the plasma will determine the distribution of testosterone between free and bound forms, and the free testosterone concentration will determine its half-life.

About 90 percent of a dose of testosterone is excreted in the urine as glucuronic and sulfuric acid conjugates of testosterone and its metabolites: and 6 percent of a dose is excreted in the feces, mostly in the unconjugated form. Inactivation of testosterone occurs primarily in the liver. Testosterone is metabolized to various 17-keto steroids through two different pathways. There are considerable variations of the half-life of testosterone as reported in the literature, ranging from 10 to 100 minutes.

In many tissues the activity of testosterone appears to depend on reduction to dihydrotestosterone, which binds to cytosol receptor proteins. The steroid-receptor complex is transported to the nucleus where it initiates transcription events and cellular changes related to androgen action.

INDICATIONS AND USAGE

1. Males

Androgens are indicated for replacement therapy in conditions associated with a deficiency or absence of endogenous testosterone.

a. Primary hipogonadism (congenital or acquired) — testicular failure due to cryptorchidism, bilateral torsions, orchitis, vanishing testis syndrome; or orchidectomy.
b. Hypogonadotropic hypogonadism (congenital or acquired) — idiopathic gonadotropin or LHRH deficiency, or pituitary hypothalamic injury from tumors, trauma, or radiation. If the above conditions occur prior to puberty, androgen replacement therapy will be needed during the adolescent years for development of secondary sexual characteristics. Prolonged androgen treatment will be required to maintain sexual characteristics in these and other males who develop testosterone deficiency after puberty.
c. Androgens may be used to stimulate puberty in carefully selected males with clearly delayed puberty. These patients usually have a familial pattern of delayed puberty that is not secondary to a pathological disorder; puberty is expected to occur spontaneously at a relatively late date. Brief treatment with conservative doses may occasionally be justified in these patients if they do not respond to psychological support. The potential adverse effect on bone maturation should be discussed with the patient and parents prior to androgen administration. An X-ray of the hand and wrist to determine bone age should be obtained every 6 months to assess the effect of treatment on the epiphyseal centers (see WARNINGS).

2. Females

Androgens may be used secondarily in women with advancing inoperable metastatic (skeletal) mammary cancer who are 1 to 5 years postmenopausal. Primary goals of therapy in these women include ablation of the ovaries. Other methods of counteracting estrogen activity are adrenalectomy, hypophysectomy, and/or antiestrogen therapy. This treatment has also been used in premenopausal women with breast cancer who have benefited from oophorectomy and are considered to have a hormone-responsive tumor. Judgment concerning androgen therapy should be made by an oncologist with expertise in this field.

CONTRAINDICATIONS

Androgens are contraindicated in men with carcinomas of the breast or with known or suspected carcinomas of the prostate, and in women who are or may become pregnant. When administered to pregnant woman, androgens cause virilization of the external genitalia of the female fetus. This virilization includes clitoromegaly, abnormal vaginal development, and fusion of genital folds to form a scrotal-like structure. The degree of masculinization is related to the amount of drug given and the age of the fetus, and is most likely to occur in the female fetus when the drugs are given in the first trimester. If the patient becomes pregnant while taking these drugs, she should be apprised of the potential hazard to the fetus.

WARNINGS

In patients with breast cancer, androgen therapy may cause hypercalcemia by stimulating osteolysis. In this case, the drug should be discontinued.

Prolonged use of high doses of androgens has been associated with the development of peliosis hepatis and hepatic neoplasms including hepatocellular carcinoma. (See PRECAUTIONS—Carcinogenesis). Peliosis hepatis can be a life-threatening or fatal complication.

Cholestatic hepatitis and jaundice occur with 17-alpha-alkylandrogens at a relatively low dose. If cholestatic hepatitis with jaundice appears or if liver function tests become abnormal, the androgen should be discontinued and the etiology should be determined. Drug-induced jaundice is reversible when the medication is discontinued.

Geriatric patients treated with androgens may be at an increased risk for the development of prostatic hypertrophy and prostatic carcinoma.

Edema with or without congestive heart failure may be a serious complication in patients with preexisting cardiac, renal, or hepatic disease. In addition to discontinuation of the drug, diuretic therapy may be required.

Gynecomastia frequently develops and occasionally persists in patients being treated for hypogonadism.

Androgen therapy should be used cautiously in healthy males with delayed puberty. The effect on bone maturation should be monitored by assessing bone age of the wrist and hand every 6 months. In children, androgen treatment may accelerate bone maturation without producing compensa-

Continued on next page

Android—Cont.

tory gain in linear growth. This adverse effect may result in compromised adult stature. The younger the child the greater the risk of compromising final mature height.
This drug has not been shown to be safe and effective for the enhancement of athletic performance. Because of the potential risk of serious adverse health effects, this drug should not be used for such purpose.

PRECAUTIONS

General

Women should be observed for signs of virilization (deepening of the voice, hirsutism, acne, clitoromegaly and menstrual irregularities). Discontinuation of drug therapy at the time of evidence of mild virilism is necessary to prevent irreversible virilization. Such virilization is usual following androgen use at high doses. A decision may be made by the patient and the physician that some virilization will be tolerated during treatment for breast carcinoma.

Information for the Patient

The physician should instruct patients to report any of the following side effects of androgens:

Adult or Adolescent Males:	Too frequent or persistent erections of the penis. Any male adolescent patient receiving androgens for delayed puberty should have bone development checked every six months.
Women:	Hoarseness, acne, changes in menstrual periods or more hair on the face.
All Patients:	Any nausea, vomiting, changes in skin color or ankle swelling.

Laboratory Tests

1. Women with disseminated breast carcinoma should have frequent determination of urine and serum calcium levels during the course of androgen therapy (See WARNINGS).
2. Because of the hepatotoxicity associated with the use of 17-alpha-alkylated androgens, liver function tests should be obtained periodically.
3. Periodic (every 6 months) X-ray examinations of bone age should be made during treatment of prepubertal males to determine the rate of bone maturation and the effects of androgen therapy on the epiphyseal centers.
4. Hemoglobin and hematocrit should be checked periodically for polycythemia in patients who are receiving high doses of androgens.

Drug Interactions

1. Anticoagulants: C-17 substituted derivatives of testosterone, such as methandrostenolone, have been reported to decrease the anticoagulant requirements of patients receiving oral anticoagulants. Patients receiving oral anticoagulant therapy require close monitoring, especially when androgens are started or stopped.

2. Oxyphenbutazone: Concurrent administration of oxyphenbutazone and androgens may result in elevated serum levels of oxyphenbutazone.

3. Insulin: In diabetic patients the metabolic effects of androgens may decrease blood glucose and insulin requirements.

Drug/Laboratory Test Interferences

Androgens may decrease levels of thyroxine-binding globulin, resulting in decreased total T4 serum levels and increased resin uptake of T3 and T4. Free thyroid hormone levels remain unchanged, however, and there is no clinical evidence of thyroid dysfunction.

Carcinogenesis

Animal Data

Testosterone has been tested by subcutaneous injection and implantation in mice and rats. The implant induced cervical-uterine tumors in mice, which metastasized in some cases. There is suggestive evidence that injection of testosterone into some strains of female mice increases their susceptibility to hepatoma. Testosterone is also known to increase the number of tumors and decrease the degree of differentiation of chemically induced carcinomas of the liver in rats.

Human Data

There are rare reports of hepatocellular carcinoma in patients receiving long-term therapy with androgens in high doses. Withdrawal of the drugs did not lead to regression of the tumors in all cases.
Geriatric patients treated with androgens may be at an increased risk for the development of prostatic hypertrophy and prostatic carcinoma.

Pregnancy

Teratogenic effects. Pregnancy Category X (See CONTRAINDICATIONS).

Nursing Mothers

It is not known whether androgens are excreted in human milk. Because many drugs are excreted in human milk and because of the potential for serious adverse reactions in nursing infants from androgens, a decision should be made whether to discontinue nursing or to discontinue the drug, taking into account the importance of the drug to the mother.

Pediatric Use

Androgen therapy should be used very cautiously in children and only by specialists who are aware of the adverse effects on bone maturation. Skeletal maturation must be monitored every six months by an X-ray of hand and wrist (See INDICATIONS AND USAGE and WARNINGS).

ADVERSE REACTIONS

Endocrine and Urogenital

Female: The most common side effects of androgen therapy are amenorrhea and other menstrual irregularities, inhibition of gonadotropin secretion and virilization, including deepening of the voice and clitoral enlargement. The latter usually is not reversible after androgens are discontinued. When administered to a pregnant woman androgens cause virilization of external genitalia of the female fetus.
Male: Gynecomastia, and excessive frequency and duration of penile erections. Oligospermia may occur at high dosages (see CLINICAL PHARMACOLOGY).
Skin and appendages: Hirsutism, male pattern of baldness, and acne.
Fluid and Electrolyte Disturbances: Retention of sodium, chloride, water, potassium, calcium and inorganic phosphates.
Gastrointestinal: Nausea, cholestatic jaundice, alterations in liver function tests, rarely hepatocellular neoplasms and peliosis hepatitis (see WARNINGS).
Hematologic: Suppression of clotting factors II, V, VII, and X, bleeding in patients on concomitant anticoagulant therapy and polycythemia.
Nervous System: Increased or decreased libido, headache, anxiety, depression, and generalized paresthesia.
Metabolic: Increased serum cholesterol.
Miscellaneous: Rarely anaphylactoid reactions.

DRUG ABUSE AND DEPENDENCE

Methyltestosterone Capsules are classified as a schedule III Controlled Substance under the Anabolic Steroids Act of 1990.

OVERDOSAGE

There have been no reports of acute overdosage with the androgens.

DOSAGE AND ADMINISTRATION

Methyltestosterone capsules are administered orally. The suggested dosage for androgens varies depending on the age, sex, and diagnosis of the individual patient. Dosage is adjusted according to the patient's response and the appearance of adverse reactions.
Replacement therapy in androgen-deficient males is 10 to 50 mg of methyltestosterone daily. Various dosage regimens have been used to induce pubertal changes in hypogonadal males, some experts have advocated lower dosages initially, gradually increasing the dose as puberty progresses with or without a decrease to maintenance levels. Other experts emphasize that higher dosages are needed to induce pubertal changes and lower dosages can be used for maintenance after puberty. The chronological and skeletal ages must be taken into consideration both in determining the initial dose and in adjusting the dose.
Doses used in delayed puberty generally are in the lower range of that given above, and for a limited duration, for example 4 to 6 months.
Women with metastatic breast carcinoma must be followed closely because androgen therapy occasionally appears to accelerate the disease. Thus, many experts prefer to use the shorter acting androgen preparations rather than those with prolonged activity for treating breast carcinoma, particularly during the early stages of androgen therapy. The dosage of methyltestosterone for androgen therapy in breast carcinoma in females is from 50–200 mg daily.

HOW SUPPLIED

Methyltestosterone capsules USP 10 mg are red capsules imprinted "ICN 0901" on both sections. They are available in bottles of 100 (NDC 0187-0902-01).
Store at 25°C (77°F); excursion permitted to 15°C–30°C (59°F–86°F).

ICN Pharmaceuticals, Inc.
ICN Plaza
3300 Hyland Avenue
Costa Mesa, CA 92626
(714)545-0100
7004821 Revision May 1999

BENOQUIN® CREAM 20% ℞

(Monobenzone, Cream, USP)

Rx Only.

FOR EXTERNAL USE ONLY

DESCRIPTION

Monobenzone is the monobenzyl ether of hydroquinone. Monobenzone occurs as a white, almost tasteless crystalline powder, soluble in alcohol and practically insoluble in water. Chemically, monobenzone is designated as p-(benzyloxy)phenol; the empirical formula is $C_{13}H_{12}O_2$; molecular weight 200.24. The structural formula is:
[See chemical structure at top of next column]
Each gram of Benoquin Cream contains 200 mg of monobenzone USP, in a water-washable base consisting of purified water USP, cetyl alcohol NF, propylene glycol USP, sodium lauryl sulfate NF and white wax NF.

CLINICAL PHARMACOLOGY

Benoquin Cream 20% is a depigmenting agent whose mechanism of action is not fully understood.

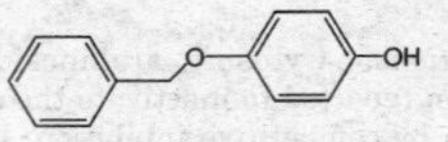

OH

$C_{13}H_{12}O_2$ 200.24

The topical application of monobenzone in animals, increases the excretion of melanin from the melanocytes. The same action is thought to be responsible for the depigmenting effect of the drug in humans. Monobenzone may cause destruction of melanocytes and permanent depigmentation. This effect is erratic and may take one to four months to occur while existing melanin is lost with normal sloughing of the stratum corneum. Hyperpigmented skin appears to fade more rapidly than does normal skin, and exposure to sunlight reduces the depigmenting effect of the drug. The histology of the skin after depigmentation with topical monobenzone is the same as that seen in vitiligo; the epidermis is normal except for the absence of identifiable melanocytes.

INDICATIONS AND USAGE

Benoquin Cream 20% is indicated for final depigmentation in extensive Vitiligo.
Benoquin Cream 20% is applied topically to permanently depigment normal skin surrounding vitiliginous lesions in patients with disseminated (greater than 50 percent of body surface area) idiopathic vitiligo.
Benoquin Cream 20% is not recommended in freckling; hyperpigmentation caused by photosensitization following the use of certain perfumes (berlock dermatitis); melasma (chloasma) of pregnancy; or hyperpigmentation resulting from inflammation of the skin. Benoquin Cream 20% is not effective for the treatment of cafe-au-lait spots, pigmented nevi, malignant melanoma or pigmentation resulting from pigments other than melanin (e.g.: bile, silver, or artificial pigments).

CONTRAINDICATIONS

Benoquin Cream 20% contains a potent depigmenting agent and is not a cosmetic skin bleach. Use of Benoquin Cream 20% is contraindicated in any conditions other than disseminated vitiligo. Benoquin Cream 20% frequently produces irreversible depigmentation, and it must not be used as a substitute for hydroquinone.
Benoquin Cream 20% is also contraindicated in individuals with a history of sensitivity or allergic reactions to this product, or any of its ingredients.

WARNINGS

Benoquin Cream 20% is a potent depigmenting agent, not a mild cosmetic bleach. Do not use except for final depigmentation in extensive vitiligo.
Keep this, and all medications out of the reach of children. In case of accidental ingestion, call a physician or a Poison Control Center immediately.

PRECAUTIONS (See Warnings)

General. Benoquin Cream 20% is for External Use Only. Following therapy with Benoquin Cream 20%, the skin will be sensitive for the rest of the patient's life. He/she must use sunscreens during exposure to the sun.
Information for the Patient. Benoquin Cream 20% contains a potent depigmenting agent and is not a cosmetic skin bleach. Use of Benoquin Cream 20% is contraindicated in any conditions other than disseminated vitiligo. Use only for final depigmentation in extensive vitiligo. Areas of normal skin distant to the site of Benoquin Cream 20% application may become depigmented, and irregular, excessive, unsightly, and frequently permanent depigmentation may occur.
Carcinogenesis, mutagenesis, impairment of fertility. No long term studies have been performed to evaluate carcinogenic potential.
Pregnancy: Category C. Animal reproduction studies have not been conducted with Benoquin Cream 20%. It is also not known whether Benoquin Cream 20% can cause fetal harm when administered to a pregnant woman, or can affect reproduction capacity. Benoquin Cream 20% should be given to a pregnant woman only if clearly needed.
Nursing Mothers. It is not known whether this drug is excreted in human milk. Because many drugs are excreted in human milk, caution should be exercised when Benoquin Cream 20% is administered to a nursing woman.
Pediatric Use. The safety and effectiveness of Benoquin Cream 20% in pediatric patients below the age of 12 years have not been established.

ADVERSE REACTIONS

Mild, transient skin irritation and sensitization, including erythematous and eczematous reactions have occurred following topical application of Benoquin Cream 20%. Although those reactions are usually transient, treatment with Benoquin Cream 20% should be discontinued if irritation, a burning sensation, or dermatitis occur. Areas of normal skin distant to the site of Benoquin Cream 20% application frequently have become depigmented, and irregular, excessive, unsightly, and frequently permanent depigmentation has occurred.

DOSAGE AND ADMINISTRATION

A thin layer of Benoquin Cream 20% should be applied and rubbed into the pigmented area two or three times daily, or

as directed by a physician. Prolonged exposure to sunlight should be avoided during treatment with Benoquin Cream 20%, or a sunscreen should be used.
Depigmentation is usually accomplished after one to four months of Benoquin Cream 20% treatment. If satisfactory results are not obtained after four months of Benoquin Cream 20% treatment, the drug should be discontinued. When the desired degree of depigmentation is obtained, Benoquin Cream 20% should be applied only as often as needed to maintain depigmentation (usually only two times weekly).

HOW SUPPLIED

Benoquin Cream 20% in $1^1/_4$ oz. tubes (35.4 g) (NDC 0187-0380-34).
Benoquin Cream 20% should be stored at 25°C (77°F); excursions permitted to 15–30°C (59–86°F).
ICN Pharmaceuticals, Inc.
3300 Hyland Ave.
Costa Mesa, CA 92626
(714) 545–0100
2393-04 EL
Rev. 6-98

EFUDEX ® ℞

[ef 'u-dex]
brand of fluorouracil
TOPICAL SOLUTIONS AND CREAM

For Topical Dermatological Use Only — Not for Ophthalmic Use

DESCRIPTION

Efudex Solutions and Cream are topical preparations containing the fluorinated pyrimidine 5-fluorouracil, an antineoplastic antimetabolite.
Efudex Solution consists of 2% or 5% fluorouracil on a weight/weight basis, compounded with propylene glycol, tris(hydroxymethyl)aminomethane, hydroxypropylcellulose, parabens (methyl and propyl) and disodium edetate.
Efudex Cream contains 5% fluorouracil in a vanishing cream base consisting of white petrolatum, stearyl alcohol, propylene glycol, polysorbate 60 and parabens (methyl and propyl).
Chemically, fluorouracil is 5-fluoro-2,4(*1H,3H*)-pyrimidinedione. It is a white to practically white, crystalline powder which is sparingly soluble in water and slightly soluble in alcohol. One gram of fluorouracil is soluble in 100 mL of propylene glycol. The molecular weight of 5-fluorouracil is 130.08 and the structural formula is:

H N O NH F O

CLINICAL PHARMACOLOGY

There is evidence that the metabolism of fluorouracil in the anabolic pathway blocks the methylation reaction of deoxyuridylic acid to thymidylic acid. In this manner fluorouracil interferes with the synthesis of deoxyribonucleic acid (DNA) and to a lesser extent inhibits the formation of ribonucleic acid (RNA). Since DNA and RNA are essential for cell division and growth, the effect of fluorouracil may be to create a thymine deficiency which provokes unbalanced growth and death of the cell. The effects of DNA and RNA deprivation are most marked on those cells which grow more rapidly and take up fluorouracil at a more rapid rate.
The catabolic metabolism of fluorouracil results in degradation products (eg, CO_2, urea, α-fluoro-β-alanine) which are inactive.
Systemic absorption studies of topically applied fluorouracil have been performed on patients with actinic keratoses using tracer amounts of ^{14}C-labeled fluorouracil added to a 5% preparation. All patients had been receiving nonlabeled fluorouracil until the peak of the inflammatory reaction occurred (2 to 3 weeks), ensuring that the time of maximum absorption was used for measurement. One gram of labeled preparation was applied to the entire face and neck and left in place for 12 hours. Urine samples were collected. At the end of 3 days, the total recovery ranged between 0.48% and 0.94% with an average of 0.76%, indicating that approximately 5.98% of the topical dose was absorbed systematically. If applied twice daily, this would indicate systemic absorption of topical fluorouracil to be in the range of 5 to 6 mg per daily dose of 100 mg. In an additional study, negligible amounts of labeled material were found in plasma, urine and expired CO_2 after 3 days of treatment with topically applied ^{14}C-labeled fluorouracil.

INDICATIONS AND USAGE

Efudex is recommended for the topical treatment of actinic or solar keratoses. In the 5% strength it is also useful in the treatment of superficial basal cell carcinomas when conventional methods are impractical, such as with multiple lesions or difficult treatment sites. Safety and efficacy in other indications have not been established.
The diagnosis should be established prior to treatment, since this method has not been proven effective in other types of basal cell carcinomas. With isolated, easily accessible basal cell carcinomas, surgery is preferred since success with such lesions is almost 100%. The success rate with Efudex Cream and Solution is approximately 93%, based on 113 lesions in 54 patients.Twenty-five lesions treated with the solution produced 1 failure and 88 lesions treated with the cream produced 7 failures.

CONTRAINDICATIONS

Efudex may cause fetal harm when administered to a pregnant woman.
There are no adequate and well-controlled studies in pregnant women with either the topical or parenteral forms of fluorouracil. One birth defect (cleft lip and palate) has been reported in the newborn of a patient using Efudex as recommended. One birth defect (ventricular septal defect) and cases of miscarriage have been reported when Efudex was applied to mucous membrane areas. Multiple birth defects have been reported in a fetus of a patient treated with intravenous fluorouracil.
Animal reproduction studies have not been conducted with Efudex. Fluorouracil administered parenterally has been shown to be teratogenic in mice, rats, and hamsters when given at doses equivalent to the usual human intravenous dose; however, the amount of fluorouracil absorbed systemically after topical administration to actinic keratoses is minimal (see CLINICAL PHARMACOLOGY). Fluorouracil exhibited maximum teratogenicity when given to mice as single intraperitoneal injections of 10 to 40 mg/kg on Day 10 or 12 of gestation. Similarly, intraperitoneal doses of 12 to 37 mg/kg given to rats between Days 9 and 12 of gestation and intramuscular doses of 3 to 9 mg/kg given to hamsters between Days 8 and 11 of gestation were teratogenic and/or embryotoxic (ie, resulted in increased resorptions or embryolethality). In monkeys, divided doses of 40 mg/kg given between Days 20 and 24 of gestation were not teratogenic. Doses higher than 40 mg/kg resulted in abortion.
Efudex is contraindicated in women who are or may become pregnant during therapy. If this drug is used during pregnancy, or if the patient becomes pregnant while using this drug, the patient should be apprised of the potential hazard to the fetus.
Efudex is also contraindicated in patients with known hypersensitivity to any of its components.

WARNINGS

Application to mucous membranes should be avoided due to the possibility of local inflammation and ulceration. Additionally, cases of miscarriage and a birth defect (ventricular septal defect) have been reported when Efudex was applied to mucous membrane areas during pregnancy.
Occlusion of the skin with resultant hydration has been shown to increase precutaneous penetration of several topical preparations. If any occlusive dressing is used in treatment of basal cell carcinoma, there may be an increase in the severity of inflammatory reactions in the adjacent normal skin. A porous gauze dressing may be applied for cosmetic reasons without increase in reaction.
Exposure to ultraviolet rays should be minimized during and immediately following treatment with Efudex because the intensity of the reaction may be increased.

PRECAUTIONS

General: There is a possibility of increased absorption through ulcerated or inflamed skin.
Information for Patients: Patients should be forewarned that the reaction in the treated areas may be unsightly during therapy and, usually, for several weeks following cessation of therapy. Patients should be instructed to avoid exposure to ultraviolet rays during and immediately following treatment with Efudex because the intensity of the reaction may be increased. If Efudex is applied with the fingers, the hands should be washed immediately afterward. Efudex should not be applied on the eyelids or directly into the eyes, nose or mouth because irritation may occur.
Laboratory Tests: Solar keratoses which do not respond should be biopsied to confirm the diagnosis. Follow-up biopsies should be performed as indicated in the management of superficial basal cell carcinoma.
Carcinogenesis, Mutagenesis, Impairment of Fertility: Adequate long-term studies in animals to evaluate carcinogenic potential have not been conducted with fluorouracil. Studies with the active ingredient of Efudex, 5-fluorouracil, have shown positive effects in in vitro tests for mutagenicity and on impairment of fertility.
5-Fluorouracil was positive in three in vitro cell neoplastic transformation assays. In the C3H/10T½ clone 8 mouse embryo cell system, the resulting morphologically transformed cells formed tumors when inoculated into immunosuppressed syngeneic mice.
While no evidence for mutagenic activity was observed in the Ames test (3 studies), fluorouracil has been shown to be mutagenic in the survival count rec-assay with *Bacillus subtilis* and in the Drosophilia wing-hair spot test. Fluorouracil produced petite mutations in *Saccharomyces cerevisiae* and was positive in the mironucleus test (bone marrow cells of male mice).
Fluorouracil was clastogenic in vitro (ie, chromatid gaps, breaks and exchanges) in Chinese hamster fibroblasts at concentrations of 1.0 and 2.0 μg/mL and has been shown to increase sister chromatid exchange in vitro in human lymphocytes. In addition, 5-fluorouracil has been reported to produce an increase in numerical and structural chromosome aberrations in peripheral lymphocytes of patients with this product.
Doses of 125 to 250 mg/kg, administered intraperitoneally, have been shown to induce chromosomal aberrations and changes in chromosome organization of spermatogonia in rats. Spermatogonial differentiation was also inhibited by fluorouracil, resulting in transient infertility. However, in studies with a strain of mouse which is sensitive to the induction of sperm head abnormalities after exposure to a range of chemical mutagens and carcinogens, fluorouracil was inactive at oral doses of 5 to 80 mg/kg/day. In female rats, fluorouracil administered intraperitoneally at doses of 25 and 50 mg/kg during the preovulatory phase of oogenesis significantly reduced the incidence of fertile matings, delayed the development of preimplantation and postimplantation embryos, increased the incidence of preimplantation lethality and induced chromosomal anomalies in these embryos. Single dose intravenous and intraperitoneal injections of 5-fluorouracil have been reported to kill differentiated spermatogonia and spermatocytes (at 500 mg/kg) and to produce abnormalities in spermatids (at 50 mg/kg) in mice.
Pregnancy: Pregnancy: **Teratogenic Effects: Pregnancy Category X:** See CONTRAINDICATIONS section.
Nursing Mothers: It is not known whether Efudex is excreted in human milk. Because there is some systemic absorption of fluorouracil after topical administration (see CLINICAL PHARMACOLOGY), because many drugs are excreted in human milk, and because of the potential for serious adverse reactions in nursing infants, a decision should be made whether to discontinue nursing or to discontinue use of the drug, taking into account the importance of the drug to the mother.
Pediatric Use: Safety and effectiveness in children have not been established.

ADVERSE REACTIONS

The most frequent adverse reactions to Efudex occur locally and are often related to an extension of the pharmacological activity of the drug. These include burning, crusting, allergic contact dermatitis, erosions, erythema, hyperpigmentation, irritation, pain, photosensitivity, pruritus, scarring, rash, soreness and ulceration. Ulcerations, other local reactions, cases of miscarriage and a birth defect (ventricular septal defect) have been reported when Efudex was applied to mucous membrane areas. Leukocytosis is the most frequent hematological side effect.
Although a causal relationship is remote, other adverse reactions which have been reported infrequently are:
Central Nervous System: Emotional upset, insomnia, irritability.
Gastrointestinal: Medicinal taste, stomatitis.
Hematological: Eosinophilia, thrombocytopenia, toxic granulation.
Integumentary: Alopecia, blistering, bullous pemphigoid, discomfort, ichthyosis, scaling, suppuration, swelling, telangiectasia, tenderness, urticaria, skin rash.
Special Senses: Conjunctival reaction, corneal reaction, lacrimation, nasal irritaiton.
Miscellaneous: Herpes simplex.

OVERDOSAGE

There have been no reports of overdosage with Efudex.
The oral LD_{50} for the 5% topical cream was 234 mg/kg in rats and 39 mg/kg in dogs. These doses represented 11.7 and 1.95 mg/kg of fluorouracil, respectively. Studies with a 5% topical solution yielded an oral LD_{50} of 214 mg/kg in rats and 28.5 in dogs, corresponding to 10.7 and 14.3 mg/kg of fluorouracil, respectively. The topical application of the 5% cream to rats yielded an LD_{50} of greater than 500 mg/kg.

DOSAGE AND ADMINISTRATION

When Efudex is applied to a lesion, a response occurs with the following sequence; erythema, usually followed by vesiculation, desquamation, erosion and reepithelialization.
Efudex should be applied preferably with a nonmetal applicator or suitable glove. If Efudex is applied with the fingers, the hands should be washed immediately afterward.
Actinic or Solar Keratosis: Apply cream or solution twice daily in an amount sufficient to cover the lesions. Medication should be continued until the inflammatory response reaches the erosion state, at which time use of the drug should be terminated. The usual duraton of therapy is from 2 to 4 weeks. Complete healing of the lesions may not be evident for 1 to 2 months following cessation of Efudex therapy.
Superficial Basal Cell Carcinomas: **Only the 5% strength is recommended.** Apply cream or solution twice daily in an amount sufficient to cover the lesions. Treatment should be continued for at least 3 to 6 weeks. Therapy may be required for as long as 10 to 12 weeks before the lesions are obliterated. As in any neoplastic condition, the patient should be followed for a reasonable period of time to determine if a cure has been obtained.

HOW SUPPLIED

Efudex Solution is available in 10-mL drop dispensers containing either 2% (NDC 0187-3202-10) or 5% (NDC 0187-3203-10) fluorouracil on a weight/weight basis compounded with propylene glycol, tris(hydroxymethyl)aminomethane, hyroxypropyl cellulose, parabens (methyl and propyl) and disodium edetate.
Efudex Cream is available in 25-gm tubes containing 5% fluorouracil (NDC 0187-3204-26) in a vanishing cream base consisting of white petrolatum, stearyl alcohol, propylene glycol, polysorbate 60 and parabens (methyl and propyl).

Continued on next page

Efudex—Cont.

Store at 25°C (77°F); excursion permitted to 15°C–30°C (59°F–86°F).
Manufactured for ICN Pharmaceuticals Inc.
Costa Mesa, CA 92626
by Hoffman-La Roche Inc.
Nutley, N.J. 07110
ICN Pharmaceuticals, Inc.
ICN Plaza
3300 Hyland Avenue
Costa Mesa, California 92626
714-545-0100
Revised: February 1998

ELDOQUIN FORTE® 4% Cream ℞
(Hydroquinone USP, 4%)
(Skin Bleaching Cream)
ELDOPAQUE FORTE® 4% Cream
(Hydroquinone USP, 4%)
(Skin Bleaching Cream with Sunblock)
SOLAQUIN FORTE® 4% Cream
(Hydroquinone USP, 4%)
(Skin Bleaching Cream with Sunscreens, SPF 17)
SOLAQUIN FORTE® 4% Gel
(Hydroquinone USP, 4%)
(Skin Bleaching Gel with Sunscreens)

FOR EXTERNAL USE ONLY

DESCRIPTION

Hydroquinone is 1,4-benzenediol. Hydroquinone is structurally related to monobenzone. Hydroquinone occurs as fine, white needles. The drug is freely soluble in water and in alcohol and has a pK_a of 9.96. Chemically, hydroquinone is designated as p-dihydroxybenzene; the empirical formula is $C_6H_6O_2$; molecular weight 110.0.
The structural formula is:

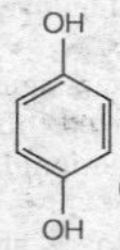

OH / OH — $C_6H_6O_2$

Each gram of Eldoquin Forte 4% Cream contains 40 mg of Hydroquinone USP in a vanishing cream base of purified water USP, stearic acid NF, propylene glycol USP, polyoxyl 40 stearate NF, polyoxyethylene (25) propylene glycol stearate, glycerol monostearate, light mineral oil NF, squalane NF, propylparaben NF and sodium metabisulfite NF.
Each gram of Eldopaque Forte 4% Cream contains 40 mg of Hydroquinone USP in a tinted sunblocking cream base of purified water USP, stearic acid NF, talc USP, polyoxyl 40 stearate NF, polyoxyethylene (25) propylene glycol stearate, propylene glycol USP, glycerol monostearate, iron oxides, light mineral oil NF, squalane NF, edetate disodium USP, sodium metabisulfite NF and potassium sorbate NF.
Each gram of Solaquin Forte 4% Cream contains 40 mg of Hydroquinone USP, 80 mg Padimate O USP, 30 mg Dioxybenzone USP and 20 mg Oxybenzone USP in a vanishing cream base of purified water USP, glycerol monostearate and polyoxyethylene stearate, ootyldodecyl stearoyl stearate, glyceryl dilaurate, quaternium-26, cetearyl alcohol and ceteareth-20, stearyl alcohol NF, propylene glycol USP, diethylaminoethyl stearate, polydimethylsiloxane, polysorbate 80 NF, lactic acid USP, ascorbic acid USP, hydroxyethyl cellulose, quaternium-14 and myristalkonium chloride, edetate disodium USP and sodium metabisulfite NF.
Each gram of Solaquin Forte 4% Gel contains 40 mg of Hydroquinone USP, 50 mg of Padimate O USP and 30 mg Dioxybenzone USP, in a hydro-alcoholic base of alcohol USP, purified water USP, propylene glycol USP, entprol, carbomer 940, edetate disodium USP and sodium metabisulfite NF.

CLINICAL PHARMACOLOGY

Topical application of hydroquinone produces a reversible depigmentation of the skin by inhibition of the enzymatic oxidation of tyrosine to 3,4-dihydroxyphenylalanine (dopa) (Denton, C. et al., 1952)[1] and suppression of other melanocyte metabolic processes (Jimbow, K. et al., 1974).[2] Exposure to sunlight or ultraviolet light will cause repigmentation of bleached areas which may be prevented by the sunblocking agents contained in Eldopaque Forte 4% Cream and by the broad spectrum sunscreen agents contained in Solaquin Forte 4% Cream and Solaquin Forte 4% Gel (Parrish, J.A. et al., 1978).[3]

INDICATIONS AND USAGE

For the gradual bleaching of hyperpigmented skin conditions such as chloasma, melasma, freckles, senile lentigines and other unwanted areas of melanin hyperpigmentation.

CONTRAINDICATIONS

Prior history of sensitivity or allergic reaction to these products or any of the ingredients. The safety of topical hydroquinone use during pregnancy or in children (12 years and under) has not been established.

WARNINGS

Caution: Hydroquinone is a skin bleaching agent which may produce unwanted cosmetic effects if not used as directed. The physician should be familiar with the contents of the package insert before prescribing or dispensing these medications.
Test for skin sensitivity before using by applying a small amount to an unbroken patch of skin and check in 24 hours. Minor redness is not a contraindication, but where there is itching or vesicle formation or excessive inflammatory response, further treatment is not advised. Close patient supervision is recommended. Contact with the eyes should be avoided. If no bleaching or lightening effect is noted after 2 months of treatment use, the medication should be discontinued. Eldoquin Forte 4% Cream, Eldopaque Forte 4% Cream, Solaquin Forte 4% Cream and Solaquin Forte 4% Gel are formulated for use as skin bleaching agents and should not be used for the prevention of sunburn.
Sunscreen use is an essential aspect of hydroquinone therapy because even minimal sunlight sustains melanocytic activity. The sunblock in Eldopaque Forte 4% Cream and the sunscreens in Solaquin Forte 4% Cream, and Solaquin Forte 4% Gel provide the necessary sun protection during skin bleaching therapy.
After clearing and during maintenance therapy, sun exposure should be avoided on bleached skin by application of a sunscreen or sunblock agent or protective clothing to prevent repigmentation
Keep this and all medication out of the reach of children. In case of accidental ingestion, call a physician or a poison control center immediately.
Warning: Contains sodium metabisulfite, a sulfite that may cause serious allergic type reactions (e.g., hives, itching, wheezing, anaphylaxis, severe asthma attack) in certain susceptible persons.

PRECAUTIONS (SEE WARNINGS)

General. Treatment should be limited to relatively small areas of the body at one time since some patients experience a transient skin reddening and a mild burning sensation which does not preclude treatment.
Pregnancy Category C. Animal reproduction studies have not been conducted with topical hydroquinone. It is also not known whether hydroquinone can cause fetal harm when used topically on a pregnant woman or affect reproductive capacity. It is not known to what degree, if any, topical hydroquinone is absorbed systemically. Topical hydroquinone should be used in pregnant women only when clearly indicated.
Nursing mothers. It is not known whether topical hydroquinone is absorbed or excreted in human milk. Caution is advised when topical hydroquinone is used by a nursing mother.
Pediatric usage. Safety and effectiveness in pediatric patients below the age of 12 years have not been established.

ADVERSE REACTIONS

No systemic adverse reactions have been reported. Occasional hypersensitivity (localized contact dermatitis) may occur, in which case the medication should be discontinued and the physician notified immediately.

DOSAGE AND ADMINISTRATION

Solaquin Forte 4% Cream and Solaquin Forte 4% Gel should be applied to the affected area and rubbed in well twice daily or as directed by a physician.
Eldopaque Forte 4% Cream should be applied to the affected area twice daily or as directed by a physician. Do not rub in.
Eldoquin Forte 4% Cream should be applied to the affected area and rubbed in well twice daily or as directed by a physician. During the day, an effective broad spectrum sunscreen should be used and unnecessary solar exposure avoided, or protective clothing should be worn to cover bleached skin in order to prevent repigmentation from occurring.

HOW SUPPLIED

ELDOQUIN FORTE 4% CREAM is available as follows:

SIZE	NDC NUMBER
1.0 ounce tube (28.4 grams)	0187-0394-31

ELDOPAQUE FORTE 4% CREAM is available as follows:

SIZE	NDC NUMBER
1.0 ounce tube (28.4 grams)	0187-0395-31

SOLAQUIN FORTE 4% CREAM is available as follows:

SIZE	NDC NUMBER
1.0 ounce tube (28.4 grams)	0187-0396-31

SOLAQUIN FORTE 4% GEL is available as follows:

SIZE	NDC NUMBER
1.0 ounce tube (28.4 grams)	0187-0523-31

Store at 25°C (77°F); excursion permitted to 15°C–30°C (59°–86°F)
Rx only

REFERENCES

1. Denton, C., A.B. Lerner and T.B. Fitzpatrick, "Inhibition of Melanin Formation by Chemical Agents," *Journal of Investigative Dermatology*, 18:119–135, 1952.
2. Jimbow, K., H. Obata, M. Pathak and T.B. Fitzpatrick, "Mechanism of Depigmentation by Hydroquinone," *Journal of Investigative Dermatology*, 62:436–449, 1974.
3. Parrish, J.A., R.R. Anderson, F. Urbach, D. Pitts, "UVA, Biological Effects of Ultraviolet Radiation with Emphasis on Human Responses to Longwave Ultraviolet," *Plenum Press*, New York and London, 1978, p. 151.

2614-00 EL Orig. 8/97
ICN PHARMACEUTICALS, INC.
3300 Hyland Avenue
Costa Mesa, CA 92626, U.S.A.
(714) 545-0100

LEVO-DROMORAN® Ⓒ ℞
[lee "vo dro 'mo-ran]
brand of
levorphanol tartrate
AMPULS, VIALS, TABLETS
Potent Synthetic Opioid
For Parenteral or Oral Administration

WARNING: May be habit forming

DESCRIPTION

Levo-Dromoran (levorphanol tartrate) is a potent opioid analgesic with empirical formula $C_{17}H_{23}NO{\cdot}C_4H_6O_6{\cdot}2H_2O$ and molecular weight 443.5. Each mg of levorphanol tartrate is equivalent to 0.58 mg levorphanol base. Chemically levorphanol is levo-3-hydroxy-N-methylmorphinan. The USP nomenclature is 17-methylmorphinan 3-ol tartrate (1:1)(Salt) dihydrate. The material has 3 asymmetric carbon atoms. The chemical structure is:

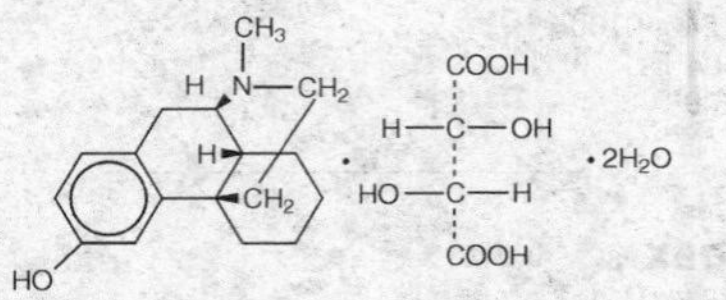

CH_3, H, N, CH_2, H, CH_2, HO · COOH, H—C—OH, HO—C—H, COOH · $2H_2O$

Levorphanol tartrate is a white crystalline powder, soluble in water and ether but insoluble in chloroform.
Each 1-mL ampul contains 2 mg levorphanol tartrate, 1.8 mg methyl paraben preservative, 0.2 mg propyl paraben preservative, sodium hydroxide to adjust pH to approximately 4.3 and Water for Injection.
Each milliliter in the 10 mL vials contains 2 mg levorphanol tartrate, 4.5 mg phenol preservative, sodium hydroxide to adjust pH to approximately 4.3 and Water for Injection.
Each tablet contains 2 mg levorphanol tartrate, lactose, corn starch, stearic acid and talc.

CLINICAL PHARMACOLOGY

Pharmacodynamics: Levo-Dromoran is a potent synthetic opioid similar to morphine in its actions. Like other mu-agonist opioids it is believed to act at receptors in the periventricular and periaqueductal gray matter in both the brain and spinal cord to alter the transmission and perception of pain. Onset of analgesia and peak analgesic effect following administration of levorphanol are similar to morphine when administered at equianalgesic doses.
Levorphanol produces a degree of respiratory depression similar to that produced by morphine at equianalgesic doses, and like many mu-opioid drugs, levorphanol produces euphoria or has a positive effect on mood in many individuals. Two mg of intramuscular levorphanol tartrate depresses respiration to a degree approximately equivalent to that produced by 10 to 15 mg of intramuscular morphine in man. The hemodynamic changes after intravenous administration of levorphanol have not been studied in man but are expected to clinically resemble those seen after morphine.
As with other opioids, the blood levels required for analgesia are determined by the opioid tolerance of the patient and are likely to rise with chronic use. The rate of development of tolerance is highly variable and is determined by the dose, dosing interval, age, use of concomitant drugs and physical status of the patient. While blood levels of opioid drugs may be helpful in assessing individual cases, dosage is usually adjusted by careful clinical observation of the patient.
Pharmacokinetics: The pharmacokinetics of levorphanol have been studied in a limited number of cancer patients following intravenous (IV), intramuscular (IM) and oral (PO) administration. Following IV administration, plasma concentrations of levorphanol decline in a triexponential manner with a terminal half-life of approximately 11 to 16 hours and a clearance of 0.78 to 1.1 L/kg/hr. Based on terminal half-life, steady-state plasma concentrations should be achieved by the third day of dosing. Levorphanol is rapidly distributed (<1 hr) and redistributed (1 to 2 hours) following IV administration and has a steady-state volume of distribution of 10 to 13 L/kg. In vitro studies of protein binding indicate that levorphanol is only 40% bound to plasma proteins.
No pharmacokinetic studies of the absorption of IM levorphanol are available, but clinical data suggests that absorption is rapid with onset of effects within 15 to 30 minutes of administration.
Levorphanol is well absorbed after PO administration with peak plasma concentrations occurring approximately 1 hour after dosing. The bioavailability of levorphanol tablets compared to IM or IV administration is not known.
Plasma concentrations of levorphanol following chronic administration in patients with cancer increased with the dose, but the analgesic effect was dependent on the degree of opioid tolerance of the patient. Expected steady-state plasma concentrations for a 6-hour dosing interval can reach 2 to 5 times those following a single dose, depending on the patient's individual clearance of the drug. Very high plasma concentrations of levorphanol can be reached in patients on chronic therapy due to the long half-life of the drug. One study in 11 patients using the drug for control of cancer pain reported plasma concentrations from 5 to 10 ng/mL after a single 2-mg dose up to 50 to 100 ng/mL after repeated oral doses of 20 to 50 mg/day.

Animal studies suggest that levorphanol is extensively metabolized in the liver and is eliminated as the glucuronide metabolite. This renally excreted inactive glucuronide metabolite accumulates with chronic dosing in plasma at concentrations that reach fivefold that of the parent compound.

The effects of age, gender, hepatic and renal disease on the pharmacokinetics of levorphanol are not known. As with all drugs of this class, patients at the extremes of age are expected to be more susceptible to adverse effects because of a greater pharmacodynamic sensitivity and probable increased variability in pharmacokinetics due to age or disease.

CLINICAL TRIALS

Clinical trials have been reported in the medical literature that investigated the use of Levo-Dromoran as a preoperative medication, as a postoperative analgesic and in the management of chronic pain due primarily to malignancy. In each of these clinical settings Levo-Dromoran has been shown to be an effective analgesic of the mu-opioid type and similar to morphine, meperidine or fentanyl.
A single 2 mg intramuscular dose of Levo-Dromoran was studied as a routine preoperative medication in 100 patients as part of a blinded 1500 patient trial of a number of synthetic opioids and was found to provide sedation similar to that observed with 100 mg meperidine or 10 mg of methadone.
Levo-Dromoran has been studied in chronic cancer patients. Dosages were individualized to each patient's level of opioid tolerance. In one study, starting doses of 2 mg twice a day often had to be advanced by 50% or more within a few weeks of starting therapy. A study of levorphanol indicates that the relative potency is approximately 4 to 8 times that of morphine, depending on the specific circumstances of use. In postoperative patients, intramuscular levorphanol was determined to be about 8 times as potent as intramuscular morphine, whereas in cancer patients with chronic pain, it was found to be only about 4 times as potent.

INDIVIDUALIZATION OF DOSAGE

Accepted medical practice dictates that the dose of any opioid analgesic be appropriate to the degree of pain to be relieved, the clinical setting, the physical condition of the patient, and the kind and dose of concurrent medication. This is especially important during recovery from anesthesia because of the residual CNS-depressant effects of anesthetic agents and the adverse effects of surgery on respiratory reserve. In consequence, the dose of Levo-Dromoran should be reduced under circumstances likely to increase the patient's sensitivity to the adverse effects of opioids. As there is substantial redistribution involved in the kinetics of levorphanol, the duration of effect of a single dose may vary and physicians must judge the need for a repeat dose based on the clinical response of the patient. Clinicians are advised to remember that while the long terminal half-life of levorphanol may reduce the need for postoperative analgesics, the administration of an excessive dose preoperatively may cause a delay in the return of spontaneous respirations or prolonged hypoventilation in the postoperative period. In addition, accumulation of the drug following excessive dosage postoperatively may prolong or result in hypoventilation.
Levo-Dromoran has a long half-life similar to methadone or other slowly excreted opioids, rather than quickly excreted agents such as morphine or meperidine. Slowly excreted drugs may have some advantages in the management of chronic pain. Unfortunately, the duration of pain relief after a single dose of a slowly excreted opioid cannot always be predicted from pharmacokinetic principles, and the interdose interval may have to be adjusted to suit the patient's individual pharmacodynamic response.
Levo-Dromoran is 4 to 8 times as potent as morphine and has a longer half-life. Because there is incomplete cross-tolerance among opioids, when converting a patient from morphine to Levo-Dromoran, the total *daily* dose of oral Levo-Dromoran should begin at approximately $^1/_{15}$ to $^1/_{12}$ of the total *daily* dose of oral morphine that such patients had previously required and then the dose should be adjusted to the patient's clinical response. If a patient is to be placed on fixed-schedule dosing (round-the-clock) with this drug, care should be taken to allow adequate time after each dose change (approximately 72 hours) for the patient to reach a new steady-state before a subsequent dose adjustment to avoid excessive sedation due to drug accumulation.

INDICATIONS

Levo-Dromoran is indicated for the management of moderate to severe pain or as a preoperative medication where an opioid analgesic is appropriate.

CONTRAINDICATIONS

Levo-Dromoran is contraindicated in patients hypersensitive to levorphanol tartrate.

WARNINGS

Respiratory Depression: Levo-Dromoran, like morphine, may be expected to produce serious or potentially fatal respiratory depression if given in an excessive dose, too frequently, or if given in full dosage to compromised or vulnerable patients. This is because the doses required to produce analgesia in the general clinical population may cause serious respiratory depression in vulnerable patients. Safe usage of this potent opioid requires that the dose and dosage interval be individualized to each patient based on the severity of the pain, weight, age, diagnosis and physical status of the patient, and the kind and dose of concurrently administered medication.
The initial dose of Levo-Dromoran should be reduced by 50% or more when the drug is given to patients with any condition affecting respiratory reserve or in conjunction with other drugs affecting the respiratory center. Subsequent doses should then be individually titrated according to the patient's response. Respiratory depression produced by levorphanol tartrate can be reversed by naloxone, a specific antagonist (see OVERDOSAGE).
Preexisting Pulmonary Disease: Because Levo-Dromoran causes respiratory depression, it should be administered with caution to patients with impaired respiratory reserve or respiratory depression from some other cause (eg, from other medication, uremia, severe infection, obstructive respiratory conditions, restrictive respiratory diseases, intrapulmonary shunting or chronic bronchial asthma). As with other strong opioids, use of Levo-Dromoran in acute or severe bronchial asthma is not recommended (see *Respiratory Depression*).
Head Injury and Increased Intracranial Pressure: The respiratory depressant effects of Levo-Dromoran with carbon dioxide retention and secondary elevation of cerebral spinal fluid pressure may be markedly exaggerated in the presence of head injury, other intracranial lesions or pre-existing increase in intracranial pressure. Opioids, including Levo-Dromoran, produce effects that may obscure neurological signs of further increase in pressure in patients with head injuries. In addition, Levo-Dromoran may affect level of consciousness that may complicate neurological evaluation.
Cardiovascular Effects: The use of Levo-Dromoran in acute myocardial infarction or in cardiac patients with myocardial dysfunction or coronary insufficiency should be limited because the effects of levorphanol on the work of the heart are unknown.
Hypotensive Effect: The administration of Levo-Dromoran may result in severe hypotension in the postoperative patient or in any individual whose ability to maintain blood pressure has been compromised by a depleted blood volume or by administration of drugs, such as phenothiazines or general anesthetics. Opioids may produce orthostatic hypotension in ambulatory patients.
Use in Liver Disease: Levo-Dromoran should be administered with caution to patients with extensive liver disease who may be vulnerable to excessive sedation due to increased pharmacodynamic sensitivity or impaired metabolism of the drug.
Biliary Surgery: Levo-Dromoran has been shown to cause moderate to marked rises in pressure in the common bile duct when given in analgesic doses. It is not recommended for use in biliary surgery.
Use in Alcoholism or Drug Dependence: Levo-Dromoran has an abuse potential as great as morphine, and the prescription of this drug must always balance the prospective benefits against the risk of abuse and dependence. The use of levorphanol in patients with a history of alcohol or other drug dependence, either active or in remission, has not been specifically studied (see DRUG ABUSE AND DEPENDENCE).

PRECAUTIONS

General: As with other opioids, the administration of Levo-Dromoran may obscure the diagnosis or clinical course in patients with acute abdominal conditions. Levo-Dromoran should be administered with caution and the initial dose should be reduced in patients who are elderly or debilitated and in those patients with severe impairment of hepatic or renal function, hypothyroidism, Addison's disease, toxic psychosis, prostatic hypertrophy or urethral stricture, acute alcoholism, or delirium tremens.
Information for Patients: If Levo-Dromoran is administered to ambulatory patients, they should be cautioned against engaging in hazardous occupations requiring complete mental alertness such as operating machinery or driving a motor vehicle. They should also be warned that concurrent use of Levo-Dromoran with central nervous system depressants (eg, alcohol, sedatives, hypnotics, other opioids, barbiturates, tricyclic antidepressants, phenothiazines, tranquilizers, skeletal muscle relaxants and antihistamines) may result in additive central nervous system depressant effects. Patients should be made aware of the risk of orthostatic hypotension, dizziness and syncope in ambulatory patients taking Levo-Dromoran.
Drug Interactions: *Interactions with Other CNS Agents:* Concurrent use of Levo-Dromoran with all central nervous system depressants (eg, alcohol, sedatives, hypnotics, other opioids, general anesthetics, barbiturates, tricyclic antidepressants, phenothiazines, tranquilizers, skeletal muscle relaxants and antihistamines) may result in additive central nervous system depressant effects. Respiratory depression, hypotension, and profound sedation or coma may occur. When such combined therapy is contemplated, the dose of one or both agents should be reduced. Although no interaction between MAO inhibitors and Levo-Dromoran has been observed, it is not recommended for use with MAO inhibitors.
Most cases of serious or fatal adverse events involving Levo-Dromoran reported to the manufacturer or the FDA have involved either the administration of large initial doses or too frequent doses of the drug to nonopioid tolerant patients, or the simultaneous administration of levorphanol with other drugs affecting respiration (see INDIVIDUALIZATION OF DOSAGE and WARNINGS). The initial dose of levorphanol should be reduced by approximately 50% or more when it is given to patients along with another drug affecting respiration.
Interactions with Mixed Agonist/Antagonist Opioid Analgesics: Agonist/antagonist analgesics (eg, pentazocine, nalbuphine, butorphanol, dezocine and buprenorphine) should NOT be administered to a patient who has received or is receiving a course of therapy with a pure agonist opioid analgesic such as Levo-Dromoran. In opioid-dependent patients, mixed agonist/antagonist analgesics may precipitate withdrawal symptoms.
Use in Ambulatory Patients: Levo-Dromoran has been used in both inpatient and outpatient settings, but both physicians and patients must be aware of the risk of orthostatic hypotension, dizziness and syncope in ambulatory patients.

As with other opioids, the use of Levo-Dromoran may impair mental and/or physical abilities required for the performance of potentially hazardous tasks or for the exercise of normal good judgement and patients and staff should be advised accordingly.
Concurrent use of Levo-Dromoran with central nervous system depressants (eg, alcohol, sedatives, hypnotics, other opioids, barbiturates, tricyclic antidepressants, phenothiazines, tranquilizers, skeletal muscle relaxants and antihistamines) may result in additive central nervous system depressant effects.
Carcinogenesis, Mutagenesis, Impairment of Fertility: No information about the effects of Levo-Dromoran on carcinogenesis, mutagenesis, or fertility is available.
Pregnancy: Teratogenic Effects: Pregnancy Category C. Levo-Dromoran has been shown to be teratogenic in mice when given at a single oral dose of 25 mg/kg. The tested dose caused a near 50% mortality of the mouse embryos. There are no adequate and well-controlled studies in pregnant women. Levo-Dromoran should be used in pregnancy only if the potential benefit justifies the potential risk to the fetus.

Nonteratogenic Effects: Babies born to mothers who have been taking opioids regularly prior to delivery may be physically dependent.
A study in rabbits has demonstrated that at doses of 1.5 to 20 mg/kg, Levo-Dromoran administered intravenously crosses the placental barrier and depresses fetal respiration.
Labor and Delivery: The use of Levo-Dromoran in labor and delivery in humans has not been studied. However, as with other opioids, administration of Levo-Dromoran to the mother during labor and delivery may result in respiratory depression in the newborn. Therefore, its use during labor and delivery is not recommended.
Nursing Mothers: Studies of levorphanol concentrations in breast milk have not been performed. However, morphine, which is structurally similar to levorphanol, is excreted in human milk. Because of the potential for serious adverse reactions from Levo-Dromoran in nursing infants, a decision should be made whether to discontinue nursing or to discontinue the drug, taking into account the importance of the drug to the mother.
Pediatric Use: Levo-Dromoran is not recommended in children under the age of 18 years as the safety and efficacy of the drug in this population has not been established.
Geriatric Use: The initial dose of Levo-Dromoran should be reduced by 50% or more in the infirm elderly patient, even though there have been no reports of unexpected adverse events in older populations. All drugs of this class may be associated with a profound or prolonged effect in elderly patients for both pharmacokinetic and pharmacodynamic reasons and caution is indicated.

ADVERSE REACTIONS

In approximately 1400 patients treated with Levo-Dromoran in controlled clinical trials, the type and incidence of side effects were those expected of an opioid analgesic, and no unforeseen or unusual toxicity was reported.
Drugs of this type are expected to produce a cluster of typical opioid effects in addition to analgesia, consisting of nausea, vomiting, altered mood and mentation, pruritus, flushing, difficulties in urination, constipation and biliary spasm. The frequency and intensity of these effects appears to be dose related. Although listed as adverse events these are expected pharmacologic actions of these drugs and should be interpreted as such by the clinician.
The following adverse events have been reported with the use of Levo-Dromoran:
Body as a Whole: abdominal pain, dry mouth, sweating
Cardiovascular System: cardiac arrest, shock, hypotension, arrhythmias including bradycardia and tachycardia, palpitations, extra-systoles
Digestive System: nausea, vomiting, dyspepsia, biliary tract spasm
Nervous System: coma, suicide attempt, convulsions, depression, dizziness, confusion, lethargy, abnormal dreams, abnormal thinking, nervousness, drug withdrawal, hypokinesia, dyskinesia, hyperkinesia, CNS stimulation, personality disorder, amnesia, insomnia
Respiratory System: apnea, cyanosis, hypoventilation
Skin & Appendages: pruritus, urticaria, rash, injection site reaction
Special Senses: abnormal vision, pupillary disorder, diplopia

Continued on next page

Levo-Dromoran—Cont.

Urogenital System: kidney failure, urinary retention, difficulty urinating

DRUG ABUSE AND DEPENDENCE

Warning: May be Habit Forming

Levo-Dromoran is a Schedule II Controlled Substance. All drugs of this class (mu-opioids of the morphine type) are habit forming and should be stored, prescribed, used and disposed of accordingly. Psychological/physical dependence and tolerance may develop upon repeated administration of Levo-Dromoran.

Discontinuation of Levo-Dromoran after chronic use has been reported to result in withdrawal syndromes, and some reports of overuse and self-reported addiction have been received. Neither withdrawal nor withdrawal symptoms are usually expected in postoperative patients who used the drug for less than a week or in patients who are gradually tapered off the drug after longer use.

OVERDOSAGE

Most reports of overdosage known to the manufacturer and to the FDA involve three clinical situations. These are: 1. the use of larger than recommended doses or too frequent doses, 2. administration of the drug to children or small adults without any reduction in dosage, and 3. the use of the drug in ordinary dosage in patients compromised by concurrent illness.

As with all opioids, overdose can occur due to accidental or intentional misuse of this product, especially in infants and children who may gain access to the drug in the home. Based on its pharmacology, levorphanol overdosage would be expected to produce signs of respiratory depression, cardiovascular failure (especially in predisposed patients) and/or central nervous system depression. Serious overdosage with Levo-Dromoran is characterized by respiratory depression (a decrease in respiratory rate and/or tidal volume, periodic breathing, cyanosis), extreme somnolence progressing to stupor or coma, skeletal muscle flaccidity, cold and clammy skin, constricted pupils, and sometimes bradycardia and hypotension. In severe overdosage, apnea, circulatory collapse, cardiac arrest and death may occur.

Treatment: The specific treatment of suspected levorphanol tartrate overdosage is immediate establishment of an adequate airway and ventilation, followed (if necessary) by intravenous naloxone. The respiratory and cardiac status of the patient should be continuously monitored and appropriate supportive measures instituted, such as oxygen, intravenous fluids and/or vasopressors, if required. Physicians are reminded that the duration of levorphanol action far exceeds the duration of action of naloxone, and repeated dosing with naloxone may be required. Naloxone should be administered cautiously to persons known or suspected to be physically dependent on Levo-Dromoran. In such cases an abrupt and complete reversal of opioid effects may precipitate an acute abstinence syndrome. If necessary to administer naloxone to the physically dependent patient, the antagonist should be administered with extreme care and by titration with smaller than usual doses of the antagonist.

DOSAGE AND ADMINISTRATION

Intravenous: The usual recommended starting dose for IV administration is up to 1 mg, given in divided doses, by slow injection. This may be repeated in 3 to 6 hours as needed, provided the patient is assessed for signs of hypoventilation or excessive sedation. Dosage should be adjusted according to the severity of the pain; age, weight and physical status of the patient; the patient's underlying diseases; use of concomitant medications; and other factors (see INDIVIDUALIZATION OF DOSAGE, WARNINGS and PRECAUTIONS). Total *daily* doses or more than 4 to 8 mg IV in 24 hours are generally not recommended as starting doses in nonopioid tolerant patients; lower total *daily* doses may be appropriate.

Intramuscular or Subcutaneous: The usual recommended starting dose for IM or SC administration is 1 to 2 mg. This may be repeated in 6 to 8 hours as needed, provided the patient is assessed for signs of hypoventilation or excessive sedation. Dosage should be adjusted according to the severity of the pain; age, weight and physical status of the patient; the patient's underlying diseases; use of concomitant medications; and other factors (see INDIVIDUALIZATION OF DOSAGE, WARNINGS and PRECAUTIONS). Total *daily* doses of more than 3 to 8 mg IM in 24 hours are generally not recommended as starting doses in nonopioid tolerant patients; lower total *daily* doses may be appropriate.

Oral: The usual recommended starting dose for oral administration is 2 mg. This may be repeated in 6 to 8 hours as needed, provided the patient is assessed for signs of hypoventilation and excessive sedation. If necessary, the dose may be increased to up to 3 mg every 6 to 8 hours, after adequate evaluation of the patient's response. Higher doses may be appropriate in opioid tolerant patients. Dosage should be adjusted according to the severity of the pain; age, weight and physical status of the patient; the patient's underlying diseases; use of concomitant medications; and other factors (see INDIVIDUALIZATION OF DOSAGE, WARNINGS and PRECAUTIONS). Total oral *daily* doses of more than 6 to 12 mg in 24 hours are generally not recommended as starting doses in nonopioid tolerant patients; lower total *daily* doses may be appropriate.

Use in Chronic Pain: The dosage of Levo-Dromoran in patients with cancer or with other conditions for which chronic opioid therapy is indicated must be individualized (see INDIVIDUALIZATION OF DOSAGE). Levo-Dromoran is 4 to 8 times as potent as morphine and has a longer half-life. Because there is incomplete cross-tolerance among opioids, when converting a patient from morphine to Levo-Dromoran, the total *daily* dose of oral Levo-Dromoran should begin at approximately $1/15$ to $1/12$ of the total *daily* dose of oral morphine that such patients had previously required and then the dose should be adjusted to the patient's clinical response. If a patient is to be placed on fixed-schedule dosing (round-the-clock) with this drug, care should be taken to allow adequate time after each dose change (approximately 72 hours) for the patient to reach a new steady-state before a subsequent dose adjustment to avoid excessive sedation due to drug accumulation.

Use in The Perioperative Period: Levo-Dromoran has been used for analgesic action during premedication and the postoperative period. Factors to be considered in determining the dosage include age, body weight, physical status, underlying pathological condition, use of other drugs, type of anesthesia used, the surgical procedure involved and the severity of pain (see INDIVIDUALIZATION OF DOSAGE, WARNINGS and PRECAUTIONS).

Premedication: The preoperative medication dose of Levo-Dromoran should be individualized (see INDIVIDUALIZATION OF DOSAGE, WARNINGS and PRECAUTIONS). The usual dose for healthy young adults is 1 to 2 mg intramuscularly or subcutaneously, administered 60 to 90 minutes before surgery. Older or debilitated patients usually require less drug. Two mg of Levo-Dromoran is approximately equivalent to 10 to 15 mg of morphine or 100 mg of meperidine.

NOTE: Parenteral drug products should be inspected visually for particulate matter and discoloration prior to administration, whenever solution and container permit.

Pharmaceutical Incompatibilities of Levo-Dromoran: Levorphanol tartrate injection has been reported to be physically incompatible with solutions containing aminophylline, ammonium chloride, amobarbital sodium, chlorothiazide sodium, heparin sodium, methicillin sodium, nitrofurantoin sodium, novobiocin sodium, pentobarbital sodium, perphenazine, phenobarbital sodium, phenytoin sodium, secobarbital sodium, sodium bicarbonate, sodium iodide, sulfadiazine sodium, sulfisoxazole diethanolamine and thiopental sodium.

Safety and Handling: Levo-Dromoran is packaged in sealed systems that have a low risk of accidental exposure to health care workers. Ordinary care should be taken to avoid aerosol generation while preparing a syringe for use. Significant absorption from accidental dermal exposure is unlikely, and spilled Levo-Dromoran should be washed from the skin by rinsing with cool water. As with all controlled substances, abuse by health care personnel is possible and the drug should be handled accordingly.

HOW SUPPLIED

Ampuls: 1 mL, 2 mg/mL levorphanol tartrate—boxes of 10 (NDC 0187-3072-10).

Multiple-Dose Vials: 10 mL, 2 mg/mL levorphanol tartrate—boxes of 1 (NDC 0187-3074-20).

Scored Oral Tablets: 2 mg levorphanol tartrate—bottles of 100 (NDC 0187-3251-10).

Storage: Tablets should be stored at 59° to 86°F (15° to 30°C).

Dispense in tight containers as defined in USP/NF.

Parenteral dosage forms should be stored at 59° to 86° F (15° to 30°C).

WARNING: May be habit forming.

DEA Order Form Required.

Revised: November 1998

LIBRIUM® Ⓒ ℞

[lib 'ree-um]

brand of chlordiazepoxide HCl
CAPSULES

DESCRIPTION

Librium, the original chlordiazepoxide HCl and prototype for the benzodiazepine compounds, was synthesized and developed at Hoffmann-La Roche Inc. It is a versatile therapeutic agent of proven value for the relief of anxiety. Librium is among the safer of the effective psychopharmacologic compounds available, as demonstrated by extensive clinical evidence.

Librium is available as capsules containing 5 mg, 10 mg or 25 mg chlordiazepoxide HCl. Each capsule also contains corn starch, lactose and talc. Gelatin capsule shells may contain methyl and propyl parabens and potassium sorbate, with the following dye systems: 5-mg capsules—FD&C Yellow No. 6 plus D&C Yellow No. 10 and either FD&C Blue No. 1 or FD&C Green No. 3. 10-mg capsules—FD&C Yellow No. 6 plus D&C Yellow No. 10 and either FD&C Blue No. 1 plus FD&C Red No. 3 or FD&C Green No. 3 plus FD&C Red No. 40. 25-mg capsules—D&C Yellow No. 10 and either FD&C Green No. 3 or FD&C Blue No. 1.

Chlordiazepoxide hydrochloride is 7-chloro-2-(methylamino)-5-phenyl-3H-1,4-benzodiazepine 4-oxide hydrochloride. A white to practically white crystalline substance, it is soluble in water. It is unstable in solution and the powder must be protected from light. The molecular weight is 336.22. The structural formula of chlordiazepoxide hydrochloride is as follows:

NHCH₃ … CH₂ … Cl … • HCl … C₆H₅

ACTIONS

Librium (chlordiazepoxide HCl) has antianxiety, sedative, appetite-stimulating and weak analgesic actions. The precise mechanism of action is not known. The drug blocks EEG arousal from stimulation of the brain stem reticular formation. It takes several hours for peak blood levels to be reached and the half-life of the drug is between 24 and 48 hours. After the drug is discontinued plasma levels decline slowly over a period of several days. Chlordiazepoxide is excreted in the urine, with 1% to 2% unchanged and 3% to 6% as a conjugate.

Animal Pharmacology: The drug has been studied extensively in many species of animals and these studies are suggestive of action on the limbic system of the brain, which recent evidence indicates is involved in emotional responses.

Hostile monkeys were made tame by oral drug doses which did not cause sedation. Chlordiazepoxide HCl revealed a "taming" action with the elimination of fear and aggression. The taming effect of chlordiazepoxide HCl was further demonstrated in rats made vicious by lesions in the septal area of the brain. The drug dosage which effectively blocked the vicious reaction was well below the dose which caused sedation in these animals.

The LD_{50} of parenterally administered chlordiazepoxide HCl was determined in mice (72 hours) and rats (5 days), and calculated according to the method of Miller and Tainter, with the following results: mice, IV, 123 ±12 mg/kg; mice, IM, 366 ±7 mg/kg; rats, IV, 120 ±7 mg/kg; rats, IM, >160 mg/kg.

Effects on Reproduction: Reproduction studies in rats fed 10, 20 and 80 mg/kg daily and bred through one or two matings showed no congenital anomalies, nor were there adverse effects on lactation of the dams or growth of the newborn. However, in another study at 100 mg/kg daily there was noted a significant decrease in the fertilization rate and a marked decrease in the viability and body weight of offspring which may be attributable to sedative activity, thus resulting in lack of interest in mating and lessened maternal nursing and care of the young. One neonate in each of the first and second matings in the rat reproduction study at the 100 mg/kg dose exhibited major skeletal defects. Further studies are in progress to determine the significance of these findings.

INDICATIONS

Librium is indicated for the management of anxiety disorders or for the short-term relief of symptoms of anxiety, withdrawal symptoms of acute alcoholism, and preoperative apprehension and anxiety. Anxiety or tension associated with the stress of everyday life usually does not require treatment with an anxiolytic.

The effectiveness of Librium in long-term use, that is, more than 4 months, has not been assessed by systematic clinical studies. The physician should periodically reassess the usefulness of the drug for the individual patient.

CONTRAINDICATIONS

Librium is contraindicated in patients with known hypersensitivity to the drug.

WARNINGS

Chlordiazepoxide HCl may impair the mental and/or physical abilities required for the performance of potentially hazardous tasks such as driving a vehicle or operating machinery. Similarly, it may impair mental alertness in children. The concomitant use of alcohol or other central nervous system depressants may have an additive effect. PATIENTS SHOULD BE WARNED ACCORDINGLY.

Usage in Pregnancy: An increased risk of congenital malformations associated with the use of minor tranquilizers (chlordiazepoxide, diazepam and meprobamate) during the first trimester of pregnancy has been suggested in several studies. Because use of these drugs is rarely a matter of urgency, their use during this period should almost always be avoided. The possibility that a woman of childbearing potential may be pregnant at the time of institution of therapy should be considered. Patients should be advised that if they become pregnant during therapy or intend to become pregnant they should communicate with their physicians about the desirability of discontinuing the drug.

Withdrawal symptoms of the barbiturate type have occurred after the discontinuation of benzodiazepines. (See DRUG ABUSE AND DEPENDENCE section.)

PRECAUTIONS

In elderly and debilitated patients, it is recommended that the dosage be limited to the smallest effective amount to preclude the development of ataxia or oversedation (10 mg or less per day initially, to be increased gradually as needed and tolerated). In general, the concomitant administration of Librium and other psychotropic agents is not recommended. If such combination therapy seems indicated, careful consideration should be given to the pharmacology of the agents to be employed — particularly when the known potentiating compounds such as the MAO inhibitors and phenothiazines are to be used. The usual precautions in treating patients with impaired renal or hepatic function should be observed.

Paradoxical reactions, eg, excitement, stimulation and acute rage, have been reported in psychiatric patients and in hyperactive aggressive pediatric patients, and should be watched for during Librium therapy. The usual precautions are indicated when Librium is used in the treatment of anxiety states where there is any evidence of impending depression; it should be borne in mind that suicidal tendencies may be present and protective measures may be necessary.

Although clinical studies have not established a cause and effect relationship, physicians should be aware that variable effects on blood coagulation have been reported very rarely in patients receiving oral anticoagulants and Librium. In view of isolated reports associating chlordiazepoxide with exacerbation of porphyria, caution should be exercised in prescribing chlordiazepoxide to patients suffering from this disease.

Pediatric Use: Because of the varied response of pediatric patients to CNS-acting drugs, therapy should be initiated with the lowest dose and increased as required (see DOSAGE AND ADMINISTRATION). Since clinical experience with Librium in pediatric patients under 6 years of age is limited, use in this age group is not recommended. Hyperactive aggressive pediatric patients should be monitored for paradoxical reactions to Librium (see PRECAUTIONS).

Information for Patients: To assure the safe and effective use of benzodiazepines, patients should be informed that, since benzodiazepines may produce psychological and physical dependence it is advisable that they consult with their physician before either increasing the dose or abruptly discontinuing this drug.

ADVERSE REACTIONS

The necessity of discontinuing therapy because of undesirable effects has been rare. Drowsiness, ataxia and confusion have been reported in some patients — particularly the elderly and debilitated. While these effects can be avoided in almost all instances by proper dosage adjustment, they have occasionally been observed at the lower dosage ranges. In a few instances syncope has been reported.

Other adverse reactions reported during therapy include isolated instances of skin eruptions, edema, minor menstrual irregularities, nausea and constipation, extrapyramidal symptoms, as well as increased and decreased libido. Such side effects have been infrequent and are generally controlled with reduction of dosage. Changes in EEG patterns (low-voltage fast activity) have been observed in patients during and after Librium treatment.

Blood dyscrasias (including agranulocytosis), jaundice and hepatic dysfunction have occasionally been reported during therapy. When Librium treatment is protracted, periodic blood counts and liver function tests are advisable.

DRUG ABUSE AND DEPENDENCE

Chlordiazepoxide hydrochloride capsules are classified by the Drug Enforcement Administration as a Schedule IV controlled substance.

Withdrawal symptoms, similar in character to those noted with barbiturates and alcohol (convulsions, tremor, abdominal and muscle cramps, vomiting and sweating), have occurred following abrupt discontinuance of chlordiazepoxide. The more severe withdrawal symptoms have usually been limited to those patients who had received excessive doses over an extended period of time. Generally milder withdrawal symptoms (eg, dysphoria and insomnia) have been reported following abrupt discontinuance of benzodiazepines taken continuously at therapeutic levels for several months. Consequently, after extended therapy, abrupt discontinuation should generally be avoided and a gradual dosage tapering schedule followed. Addiction-prone individuals (such as drug addicts or alcoholics) should be under careful surveillance when receiving chlordiazepoxide or other psychotropic agents because of the predisposition of such patients to habituation and dependence.

OVERDOSAGE

Manifestations of Librium overdosage include somnolence, confusion, coma and diminished reflexes. Respiration, pulse and blood pressure should be monitored, as in all cases of drug overdosage, although, in general, these effects have been minimal following Librium overdosage. General supportive measures should be employed, along with immediate gastric lavage. Intravenous fluids should be administered and an adequate airway maintained. Hypotension may be combated by the use of Levophed® (norepinephrine) or Aramine (metaraminol). Dialysis is of limited value. There have been occasional reports of excitation in patients following chlordiazepoxide HCl overdosage; if this occurs barbiturates should not be used. As with the management of intentional overdosage with any drug, it should be borne in mind that multiple agents may have been ingested.

Flumazenil, a specific benzodiazepine-receptor antagonist, is indicated for the complete or partial reversal of the sedative effects of benzodiazepines and may be used in situations when an overdose with a benzodiazepine is known or suspected. Prior to the administration of flumazenil, necessary measures should be instituted to secure airway, ventilation and intravenous access. Flumazenil is intended as an adjunct to, not as a substitute for, proper management of benzodiazepine overdose. Patients treated with flumazenil should be monitored for resedation, respiratory depression and other residual benzodiazepine effects for an appropriate period after treatment. **The prescriber should be aware of a risk of seizure in association with flumazenil treatment, particularly in long-term benzodiazepine users and in cyclic antidepressant overdose.** The complete flumazenil package insert, including CONTRAINDICATIONS, WARNINGS and PRECAUTIONS, should be consulted prior to use.

DOSAGE AND ADMINISTRATION

Because of the wide range of clinical indications for Librium, the optimum dosage varies with the diagnosis and response of the individual patient. The dosage, therefore, should be individualized for maximum beneficial effects.

ADULTS	*USUAL DAILY DOSE*
Relief of Mild and Moderate Anxiety Disorders and Symptoms of Anxiety	5 mg or 10 mg, 3 or 4 times daily
Relief of Severe Anxiety Disorders and Symptoms of Anxiety	20 mg or 25 mg, 3 or 4 times daily
Geriatric Patients, or in the presence of debilitating disease	5 mg, 2 to 4 times daily

Preoperative Apprehension and Anxiety:
On days preceding surgery, 5 to 10 mg orally, 3 or 4 times daily. If used as preoperative medication, 50 to 100 mg IM* 1 hour prior to surgery.

PEDIATRIC PATIENTS	*USUAL DAILY DOSE*
Because of the varied response of pediatric patients to CNS-acting drugs, therapy should be initiated with the lowest dose and increased as required. Since clinical experience in pediatric patients under 6 years of age is limited, the use of the drug in this age group is not recommended.	5 mg, 2 to 4 times daily (may be increased in some pediatric patients to 10 mg, 2 to 3 times daily)

For the relief of withdrawal symptoms of acute alcoholism, the parenteral form* is usually used initially. If the drug is administered orally, the suggested initial dose is 50 to 100 mg, to be followed by repeated doses as needed until agitation is controlled — up to 300 mg per day. Dosage should then be reduced to maintenance levels.

* See package insert for Injectable Librium (chlordiazepoxide HCl).

HOW SUPPLIED

Librium (chlordiazepoxide HCl) capsules — 5 mg, green and yellow — bottles of 100 (NDC 0140-0001-01) and 500 (NDC 0140-0001-14); 10 mg, green and black — bottles of 100 (NDC 0140-0002-01) and 500 (NDC 0140-0002-14); 25 mg. green and white — bottles of 100 (NDC 0140–0003–01) and 500 (NDC 0140–0003–14).

Revised: December 1996

Shown in Product Identification Guide, page 317

LIBRIUM® FOR INJECTION ℂ℞

[lib 'ree-um]

brand of chlordiazepoxide HCl

for the relief of acute anxiety when rapid action is required

DESCRIPTION

Librium is a versatile therapeutic agent of proven value for the relief of anxiety and tension.

Librium is the first of a new class, unrelated chemically and pharmacologically to other types of tranquilizers. Librium promptly relieves anxiety and is among the safer of the effective psychopharmacologic compounds available.

Chlordiazepoxide HCl is 7-chloro-2-methylamino-5-phenyl-3H-1,4-benzodiazepine 4-oxide hydrochloride. A colorless, crystalline substance, it is soluble in water. It is unstable in solution and the powder must be protected from light. The molecular weight is 336.22. The structural formula of chlordiazepoxide HCl is as follows:

ANIMAL PHARMACOLOGY

The drug has been studied extensively in many species of animals and these studies are suggestive of action on the limbic system of the brain, which recent evidence indicates is involved in emotional responses.

Hostile monkeys were made tame by oral drug doses which did not cause sedation. Librium revealed a "taming" action with the elimination of fear and aggression. The taming effect of Librium was further demonstrated in rats made vicious by lesions in the septal area of the brain. The drug dosage which effectively blocked the vicious reaction was well below the dose which caused sedation in these animals.

The LD_{50} of parenterally administered chlordiazepoxide HCl was determined in mice (72 hours) and rats (5 days), and calculated according to the method of Miller and Tainter, with the following results: mice, IV, 123 ± 12 mg/kg; mice, IM, 366 ± 7 mg/kg; rats, IV, 120 ± 7 mg/kg; rats, IM, >160 mg/kg.

Effects on Reproduction: Reproduction studies in rats fed 10, 20 and 80 mg/kg daily and bred through one or two matings showed no congenital anomalies, nor were there adverse effects on lactation of the dams or growth of the newborn. However, in another study at 100 mg/kg daily there was noted a significant decrease in the fertilization rate and a marked decrease in the viability and body weight of offspring which may be attributable to sedative activity, thus resulting in lack of interest in mating and lessened maternal nursing and care of the young. One neonate in each of the first and second matings in the rat reproduction study at the 100 mg/kg dose exhibited major skeletal defects. Further studies are in progress to determine the significance of these findings.

INDICATIONS

Injectable Librium is indicated for the management of anxiety disorders or for the short-term relief of symptoms of anxiety, withdrawal symptoms of acute alcoholism, and preoperative apprehension and anxiety. Anxiety or tension associated with the stress of everyday life usually does not require treatment with an anxiolytic.

CONTRAINDICATIONS

Librium is contraindicated in patients with known hypersensitivity to the drug.

WARNINGS

As in the case of other CNS-acting drugs, patients receiving Librium should be cautioned about possible combined effects with alcohol and other CNS depressants.

As is true of all preparations containing CNS-acting drugs, patients receiving Librium should be cautioned against hazardous occupations requiring complete mental alertness such as operating machinery or driving a motor vehicle.

***Usage in Pregnancy:* An increased risk of congenital malformations associated with the use of minor tranquilizers (chlordiazepoxide, diazepam and meprobamate) during the first trimester of pregnancy has been suggested in several studies. Because use of these drugs is rarely a matter of urgency, their use during this period should almost always be avoided. The possibility that a woman of childbearing potential may be pregnant at the time of institution of therapy should be considered. Patients should be advised that if they become pregnant during therapy or intend to become pregnant they should communicate with their physicians about the desirability of discontinuing the drug.**

Management of Overdosage: Manifestations of Librium overdosage include somnolence, confusion, coma and diminished reflexes. Respiration, pulse and blood pressure should be monitored, as in all cases of drug overdosage, although, in general, these effects have been minimal following Librium overdosage. General supportive measures should be employed, along with immediate gastric lavage.

Intravenous fluids should be administered and an adequate airway maintained. Hypotension may be combated by the use of Levophed® (levarterenol) or Aramine (metaraminol). Dialysis is of limited value. There have been occasional reports of excitation in patients following Librium overdosage; if this occurs barbiturates should not be used. As with the management of intentional overdosage with any drug, it should be borne in mind that multiple agents may have been ingested.

Flumazenil, a specific benzodiazepine-receptor antagonist, is indicated for the complete or partial reversal of the sedative effects of benzodiazepines and may be used in situations when an overdose with a benzodiazepine is known or suspected. Prior to the administration of flumazenil, necessary measures should be instituted to secure airway, ventilation and intravenous access. Flumazenil is intended as an adjunct to, not as a substitute for, proper management of benzodiazepine overdose. Patients treated with flumazenil should be monitored for resedation, respiratory depression and other residual benzodiazepine effects for an appropriate period after treatment. **The prescriber should be aware of a risk of seizure in association with flumazenil treatment, particularly in long-term benzodiazepine users and in cyclic antidepressant overdose.** The complete flumazenil package insert, including CONTRAINDICATIONS, WARNINGS and PRECAUTIONS, should be consulted prior to use.

Withdrawal symptoms of the barbiturate type have occurred after the discontinuation of benzodiazepines. (See DRUG ABUSE AND DEPENDENCE section.)

PRECAUTIONS

Injectable Librium (intramuscular or intravenous) is indicated primarily in acute states, and patients receiving this form of therapy should be kept under observation, preferably in bed, for a period of up to 3 hours. Ambulatory patients should not be permitted to operate a vehicle following an injection. Injectable Librium should not be given to patients in shock or comatose states. Reduced dosage (usually 25 to 50 mg) should be used for elderly or debilitated pa-

Continued on next page

Librium Injectable—Cont.

tients. In general, the concomitant administration of Librium and other psychotropic agents is not recommended. If such combination therapy seems indicated, careful consideration should be given to the pharmacology of the agents to be employed—particularly when the known potentiating compounds such as the MAO inhibitors and phenothiazines are to be used. The usual precautions in treating patients with impaired renal or hepatic function should be observed. Paradoxical reactions, eg, excitement, stimulation and acute rage, have been reported in psychiatric patients and in hyperactive aggressive pediatric patients, and should be watched for during Librium therapy. The usual precautions are indicated when Librium is used in the treatment of anxiety states where there is any evidence of impending depression; it should be borne in mind that suicidal tendencies may be present and protective measures may be necessary. Although clinical studies have not established a cause and effect relationship, physicians should be aware that variable effects on blood coagulation have been reported very rarely in patients receiving oral anticoagulants and Librium. In view of isolated reports associating chlordiazepoxide with exacerbation of porphyria, caution should be exercised in prescribing chlordiazepoxide to patients suffering from this disease.

Pediatric Use: Reduced dosage (usually 25 to 50 mg) should be used for pediatric patients age 12 years and older (see DOSAGE AND ADMINISTRATION). Since clinical experience in pediatric patients under 12 years of age is limited, the use of the drug in this age group is not recommended. Hyperactive aggressive pediatric patients should be monitored for paradoxical reactions to Librium (see PRECAUTIONS).

ADVERSE REACTIONS

The necessity of discontinuing therapy because of undesirable effects has been rare. Drowsiness, ataxia and confusion are more commonly seen in the elderly and debilitated.

Other adverse reactions reported during therapy include isolated instances of syncope, hypotension, tachycardia, skin eruptions, edema, minor menstrual irregularities, nausea and constipation, extrapyramidal symptoms, blurred vision, as well as increased and decreased libido. Such side effects have been infrequent and are generally controlled with reduction of dosage. Similarly, hypotension associated with spinal anesthesia has occurred. Pain following intramuscular injection has been reported. Changes in EEG patterns (low-voltage fast activity) have been observed in patients during and after Librium treatment.

Blood dyscrasias (including agranulocytosis), jaundice and hepatic dysfunction, have occasionally been reported during therapy. When Librium treatment is protracted, periodic blood counts and liver function tests are advisable.

DRUG ABUSE AND DEPENDENCE

Withdrawal symptoms, similar in character to those noted with barbiturates and alcohol (convulsions, tremor, abdominal and muscle cramps, vomiting and sweating), have occurred following abrupt discontinuance of chlordiazepoxide. The more severe withdrawal symptoms have usually been limited to those patients who had received excessive doses over an extended period of time. Generally milder withdrawal symptoms (eg, dysphoria and insomnia) have been reported following abrupt discontinuance of benzodiazepines taken continuously at therapeutic levels for several months. Consequently, after extended therapy, abrupt discontinuation should generally be avoided and a gradual dosage tapering schedule followed. Addiction-prone individuals (such as drug addicts or alcoholics) should be under careful surveillance when receiving chlordiazepoxide or other psychotropic agents because of the predisposition of such patients to habituation and dependence.

PREPARATION AND ADMINISTRATION OF SOLUTIONS

Solutions of Librium for intramuscular or intravenous use should be prepared aseptically. Sterilization by heating should not be attempted.

Intramuscular: Add 2 mL of *Special Intramuscular Diluent* to contents of 5-mL dry-filled amber ampul of Librium Sterile Powder (100 mg). Avoid excessive pressure in injecting this special diluent into the ampul containing the powder since bubbles will form on the surface of the solution. Agitate gently until completely dissolved. Solution should be prepared immediately before administration. Any unused solution should be discarded. Deep intramuscular injection should be given *slowly* into the upper outer quadrant of the gluteus muscle.

Caution: Librium solution made with the Special Intramuscular Diluent should not be given intravenously because of the air bubbles which form when the intramuscular diluent is added to the Librium powder. Do not use diluent solution if it is opalescent or hazy.

Intravenous: In most cases, intramuscular injection is the preferred route of administration of Injectable Librium since beneficial effects are usually seen within 15 to 30 minutes. When, in the judgment of the physician, even more rapid action is mandatory, Injectable Librium may be administered intravenously. A suitable solution for intravenous administration may be prepared as follows: Add 5 mL of *sterile physiological saline* or *sterile water for injection* to contents of 5-mL dry-filled amber ampul of Librium Sterile Powder (100 mg). Agitate gently until thoroughly dissolved. Solution should be prepared immediately before administration. Any unused portion should be discarded. *Intravenous injection should be given slowly over a 1-minute period. Caution: Librium solution made with physiological saline or sterile water for injection should not be given intramuscularly because of pain on injection.*

DOSAGE

Dosage should be individualized according to the diagnosis and the response of the patient. While 300 mg may be given during a 6-hour period, this dose should not be exceeded in any 24-hour period.

INDICATION	*ADULT DOSAGE**
Withdrawal Symptoms of Acute Alcoholism	50 to 100 mg IM or IV initially; repeat in 2 to 4 hours, if necessary
Acute or Severe Anxiety Disorders or Symptoms of Anxiety	50 to 100 mg IM or IV initially; then 25 to 50 mg 3 or 4 times daily, if necessary
Preoperative Apprehension and Anxiety	50 to 100 mg IM 1 hour prior to surgery

* Lower doses (usually 25 to 50 mg) should be used for elderly or debilitated patients, and for pediatric patients age 12 years and older. Because of limited clinical experience in pediatric patients under 12 years of age, the use of the drug in this age group is not recommended.

In most cases, acute symptoms may be rapidly controlled by parenteral administration so that subsequent treatment, if necessary, may be given orally. (See package insert for Oral Librium.)

HOW SUPPLIED

For Parenteral Administration: Ampuls—Duplex package consisting of a 5-mL dry-filled ampul containing 100 mg chlordiazepoxide HCl in dry crystalline form, and a 2-mL ampul of Special Intramuscular Diluent (for intramuscular administration) compounded with 1.5% benzyl alcohol, 4% polysorbate 80, 20% propylene glycol, 1.6% maleic acid and sodium hydroxide to adjust pH to approximately 3. Boxes of 10 (NDC 0187-3755-74).

CAUTION

Before preparing solution for intramuscular or intravenous administration, please read instructions for PREPARATION AND ADMINISTRATION OF SOLUTIONS.

Manufactured for ICN Pharmaceuticals, Inc, Costa Mesa, CA 92626 by Hoffmann-La Roche Inc., Nutley, NJ 07110

Revised: March 1999

LIMBITROL® Ⓒ℞

[*lim 'bit-roll*]

(chlordiazepoxide and amitriptyline HCl)
DS (double strength) TABLETS
TABLETS
Tranquilizer—Antidepressant

DESCRIPTION

Limbitrol combines for oral administration, chlordiazepoxide, an agent for the relief of anxiety and tension, and amitriptyline, an antidepressant. It is available in DS (double strength) white, film-coated tablets, each containing 10 mg chlordiazepoxide and 25 mg amitriptyline (as the hydrochloride salt); and in blue, film-coated tablets, each containing 5 mg chlordiazepoxide and 12.5 mg amitriptyline (as the hydrochloride salt). Each tablet also contains corn starch, hydroxypropyl cellulose, hydroxypropyl methylcellulose, lactose, magnesium stearate, polyethylene glycol, povidone and propylene glycol; Limbitrol tablets contain the following colorant system—FD&C Blue No. 1 aluminum lake and titanium dioxide; Limbitrol DS tablets contain titanium dioxide.

Chlordiazepoxide is a benzodiazepine with the formula 7-chloro-2-(methylamino)-5-phenyl-*3H*-1,4-benzodiazepine 4-oxide. It is a slightly yellow crystalline material and is insoluble in water. The molecular weight is 299.76.

Amitriptyline is a dibenzocycloheptadiene derivative. The formula is 10,11-dihydro-*N,N*-dimethyl-5H-dibenzo [a,d] cycloheptene-$\Delta^{5,\gamma}$-propylamine hydrochloride. It is a white or practically white crystalline compound that is freely soluble in water. The molecular weight is 313.87.

ACTIONS

Both components of Limbitrol exert their action in the central nervous system. Extensive studies with chlordiazepoxide in many animal species suggest action in the limbic system. Recent evidence indicates that the limbic system is involved in emotional response. Taming action was observed in some species. The mechanism of action of amitriptyline in man is not known, but the drug appears to interfere with the reuptake of norepinephrine into adrenergic nerve endings. This action may prolong the sympathetic activity of biogenic amines.

INDICATIONS

Limbitrol is indicated for the treatment of patients with moderate to severe depression associated with moderate to severe anxiety.

The therapeutic response to Limbitrol occurs earlier and with fewer treatment failures than when either amitriptyline or chlordiazepoxide is used alone.

Symptoms likely to respond in the first week of treatment include: insomnia, feelings of guilt or worthlessness, agitation, psychic and somatic anxiety, suicidal ideation and anorexia.

CONTRAINDICATIONS

Limbitrol is contraindicated in patients with hypersensitivity to either benzodiazepines or tricyclic antidepressants. It should not be given concomitantly with a monoamine oxidase inhibitor. Hyperpyretic crises, severe convulsions and deaths have occurred in patients receiving a tricyclic antidepressant and a monoamine oxidase inhibitor simultaneously. When it is desired to replace a monoamine oxidase inhibitor with Limbitrol, a minimum of 14 days should be allowed to elapse after the former is discontinued. Limbitrol should then be initiated cautiously with gradual increase in dosage until optimum response is achieved.

This drug is contraindicated during the acute recovery phase following myocardial infarction.

WARNINGS

Because of the atropine-like action of the amitriptyline component, great care should be used in treating patients with a history of urinary retention or angle-closure glaucoma. In patients with glaucoma, even average doses may precipitate an attack. Severe constipation may occur in patients taking tricyclic antidepressants in combination with anticholinergic-type drugs.

Patients with cardiovascular disorders should be watched closely. Tricyclic antidepressant drugs, particularly when given in high doses, have been reported to produce arrhythmias, sinus tachycardia and prolongation of conduction time. Myocardial infarction and stroke have been reported in patients receiving drugs of this class.

Because of the sedative effects of Limbitrol, patients should be cautioned about combined effects with alcohol or other CNS depressants. The additive effects may produce a harmful level of sedation and CNS depression.

Patients receiving Limbitrol should be cautioned against engaging in hazardous occupations requiring complete mental alertness, such as operating machinery or driving a motor vehicle.

Usage in Pregnancy: Safe use of Limbitrol during pregnancy and lactation has not been established. Because of the chlordiazepoxide component, please note the following:

An increased risk of congenital malformations associated with the use of minor tranquilizers (chlordiazepoxide, diazepam and meprobamate) during the first trimester of pregnancy has been suggested in several studies. Because use of these drugs is rarely a matter of urgency, their use during this period should almost always be avoided. The possibility that a woman of childbearing potential may be pregnant at the time of institution of therapy should be considered. Patients should be advised that if they become pregnant during therapy or intend to become pregnant they should communicate with their physicians about the desirability of discontinuing the drug.

Withdrawal symptoms of the barbiturate type have occurred after the discontinuation of benzodiazepines. (See DRUG ABUSE AND DEPENDENCE section.)

PRECAUTIONS

General: Use with caution in patients with a history of seizures.

Close supervision is required when Limbitrol is given to hyperthyroid patients or those on thyroid medication.

The usual precautions should be observed when treating patients with impaired renal or hepatic function.

Patients with suicidal ideation should not have easy access to large quantities of the drug. The possibility of suicide in depressed patients remains until significant remission occurs.

Essential Laboratory Tests: Patients on prolonged treatment should have periodic liver function tests and blood counts.

Drug and Treatment Interactions: Because of its amitriptyline component, Limbitrol may block the antihypertensive action of guanethidine or compounds with a similar mechanism of action.

Drugs Metabolized by P450 2D6: The biochemical activity of the drug metabolizing isozyme cytochrome P450 2D6 (debrisoquin hydroxylase) is reduced in a subset of the caucasian population (about 7% to 10% of caucasians are so called "poor metabolizers"); reliable estimates of the prevalence of reduced P450 2D6 isozyme activity among Asian, African and other populations are not yet available. Poor metabolizers have higher than expected plasma concentrations of tricyclic antidepressants (TCAs) when given usual doses. Depending on the fraction of drug metabolized by P450 2D6, the increase in plasma concentration may be small or quite large (8-fold increase in plasma AUC of the TCA).

In addition, certain drugs inhibit the activity of this isozyme and make normal metabolizers resemble poor metabolizers. An individual who is stable on a given dose of TCA may become abruptly toxic when given one of these inhibiting drugs as concomitant therapy. The drugs that inhibit cytochrome P450 2D6 include some that are not metabolized by the enzyme (quinidine; cimetidine) and many that are substrates for P450 2D6 (many other antidepressants, phenothiazines, and the type 1c antiarrhythmics propafenone and flecainide). While all the selective serotonin reuptake in-

hibitors (SSRIs), eg, fluoxetine, sertraline and paroxetine, inhibit P450 2D6, they may vary in the extent of inhibition. The extent to which SSRI TCA interactions may pose clinical problems will depend on the degree of inhibition and the pharmacokinetics of the SSRI involved. Nevertheless, caution is indicated in the coadministration of TCAs with any of the SSRIs and also in switching from one class to the other. Of particular importance, sufficient time must elapse before initiating TCA treatment in a patient being withdrawn from fluoxetine, given the long half-life of the parent and active metabolite (at least 5 weeks may be necessary). Concomitant use of tricyclic antidepressants with drugs that can inhibit cytochrome P450 2D6 may require lower doses than usually prescribed for either the tricyclic antidepressant or the other drug. Furthermore, whenever one of these other drugs is withdrawn from cotherapy, an increased dose of tricyclic antidepressant may be required. It is desirable to monitor TCA plasma levels whenever a TCA is going to be coadministered with another drug known to be an inhibitor of P450 2D6.
The effects of concomitant administration of Limbitrol and other psychotropic drugs have not been evaluated. Sedative effects may be additive.
Cimetidine is reported to reduce hepatic metabolism of certain tricyclic antidepressants and benzodiazepines, thereby delaying elimination and increasing steady-state concentrations of these drugs. Clinically significant effects have been reported with the tricyclic antidepressants when used concomitantly with cimetidine (Tagamet).
The drug should be discontinued several days before elective surgery.
Concurrent administration of ECT and Limbitrol should be limited to those patients for whom it is essential.
Pregnancy: See WARNINGS section.
Nursing Mothers: It is not known whether this drug is excreted in human milk. As a general rule, nursing should not be undertaken while a patient is on a drug, since many drugs are excreted in human milk.
Pediatric Use: Safety and effectiveness in children below the age of 12 years have not been established.
Elderly Patients: In elderly and debilitated patients it is recommended that dosage be limited to the smallest effective amount to preclude the development of ataxia, oversedation, confusion or anticholinergic effects.
Information for Patients: To assure the safe and effective use of benzodiazepines, patients should be informed that, since benzodiazepines may produce psychological and physical dependence, it is advisable that they consult with their physician before either increasing the dose or abruptly discontinuing this drug.

ADVERSE REACTIONS

Adverse reactions to Limbitrol are those associated with the use of either component alone. Most frequently reported were drowsiness, dry mouth, constipation, blurred vision, dizziness and bloating. Other side effects occurring less commonly included vivid dreams, impotence, tremor, confusion and nasal congestion. Many symptoms common to the depressive state, such as anorexia, fatigue, weakness, restlessness and lethargy, have been reported as side effects of treatment with both Limbitrol and amitriptyline.
Granulocytopenia, jaundice and hepatic dysfunction of uncertain etiology have also been observed rarely with Limbitrol. When treatment with Limbitrol is prolonged, periodic blood counts and liver function tests are advisable.
Note: Included in the listing which follows are adverse reactions which have not been reported with Limbitrol. However, they are included because they have been reported during therapy with one or both of the components or closely related drugs.
Cardiovascular: Hypotension, hypertension, tachycardia, palpitations, myocardial infarction, arrhythmias, heart block, stroke.
Psychiatric: Euphoria, apprehension, poor concentration, delusions, hallucinations, hypomania and increased or decreased libido.
Neurologic: Incoordination, ataxia, numbness, tingling and paresthesias of the extremities, extrapyramidal symptoms, syncope, changes in EEG patterns.
Anticholinergic: Disturbance of accommodation, paralytic ileus, urinary retention, dilatation of urinary tract.
Allergic: Skin rash, urticaria, photosensitization, edema of face and tongue, pruritus.
Hematologic: Bone marrow depression including agranulocytosis, eosinophilia, purpura, thrombocytopenia.
Gastrointestinal: Nausea, epigastric distress, vomiting, anorexia, stomatitis, peculiar taste, diarrhea, black tongue.
Endocrine: Testicular swelling and gynecomastia in the male, breast enlargement, galactorrhea and minor menstrual irregularities in the female, elevation and lowering of blood sugar levels, and syndrome of inappropriate ADH (antidiuretic hormone) secretion.
Other: Headache, weight gain or loss, increased perspiration, urinary frequency, mydriasis, jaundice, alopecia, parotid swelling.

DRUG ABUSE AND DEPENDENCE

Withdrawal symptoms, similar in character to those noted with barbiturates and alcohol (convulsions, tremor, abdominal and muscle cramps, vomiting and sweating), have occurred following abrupt discontinuance of chlordiazepoxide. The more severe withdrawal symptoms have usually been limited to those patients who had received excessive doses over an extended period of time. Generally milder withdrawal symptoms (eg, dysphoria and insomnia) have been reported following abrupt discontinuance of benzodiazepines taken continuously at therapeutic levels for several months. Withdrawal symptoms (eg, nausea, headache and malaise) have also been reported in association with abrupt amitriptyline discontinuation. Consequently, after extended therapy, abrupt discontinuation should generally be avoided and a gradual dosage tapering schedule followed. Addiction-prone individuals (such as drug addicts or alcoholics) should be under careful surveillance when receiving chlordiazepoxide or other psychotropic agents because of the predisposition of such patients to habituation and dependence.

OVERDOSAGE*

Deaths may occur from overdosage with this class of drugs. Multiple drug ingestion (including alcohol) is common in deliberate tricyclic antidepressant overdose. As the management is complex and changing, it is recommended that the physician contact a poison control center for current information on treatment. Signs and symptoms of toxicity develop rapidly after tricyclic antidepressant overdose; therefore, hospital monitoring is required as soon as possible.
Manifestations: Critical manifestations of overdose include: cardiac dysrhythmias, severe hypotension, convulsions and CNS depression, including coma. Changes in the electrocardiogram, particularly in QRS axis or width, are clinically significant indicators of tricyclic antidepressant toxicity.
Other signs of overdose may include: confusion, disturbed concentration, transient visual hallucinations, dilated pupils, agitation, hyperactive reflexes, stupor, drowsiness, muscle rigidity, vomiting, hypothermia, hyperpyrexia or any of the symptoms listed under ADVERSE REACTIONS.
Management: *General:* Obtain an ECG and immediately initiate cardiac monitoring. Protect the patient's airway, establish an intravenous line and initiate gastric decontamination. A minimum of 6 hours of observation with cardiac monitoring and observation for signs of CNS or respiratory depression, hypotension, cardiac dysrhythmias and/or conduction blocks, and seizures is necessary. If signs of toxicity occur at any time during this period, extended monitoring is required. *There are case reports of patients succumbing to fatal dysrhythmias late after overdose; these patients had clinical evidence of significant poisoning prior to death and most received inadequate gastrointestinal decontamination.* Monitoring of plasma drug levels should not guide management of the patient.
Gastrointestinal Decontamination: All patients suspected of tricyclic antidepressant overdose should receive gastrointestinal decontamination. This should include large volume gastric lavage followed by activated charcoal. If consciousness is impaired, the airway should be secured prior to lavage. Emesis is contraindicated.
Cardiovascular: A maximal limb-lead QRS duration of ≥ 0.10 seconds may be the best indication of the severity of the overdose. Serum alkalinization, to a pH of 7.45 to 7.56, using intravenous sodium bicarbonate and hyperventilation (as needed) should be instituted for patients with dysrhythmias and/or QRS widening. A pH > 7.60 or a $pCO_2 < 20$ mm Hg is undesirable. Dysrhythmias unresponsive to sodium bicarbonate therapy/hyperventilation may respond to lidocaine, bretylium or phenytoin. Type *1A and 1C* antiarrhythmics are generally contraindicated (eg, quinidine, disopyramide and procainamide).
In rare instances, hemoperfusion may be beneficial in acute refractory cardiovascular instability in patients with acute toxicity. However, hemodialysis, peritoneal dialysis, exchange transfusions and forced diuresis generally have been reported as ineffective in tricyclic antidepressant poisoning.
CNS: In patients with CNS depression, early intubation is advised because of the potential for abrupt deterioration. Seizures should be controlled with benzodiazepines, or if these are ineffective, other anticonvulsants (eg, phenobarbital, phenytoin). *Physostigmine is not recommended except to treat life-threatening symptoms that have been unresponsive to other therapies,* and then only in consultation with a poison control center.
Psychiatric Follow-up: Since overdosage is often deliberate, patients may attempt suicide by other means during the recovery phase. Psychiatric referral may be appropriate.
Pediatric Management: The principles of management of child and adult overdosages are similar. It is strongly recommended that the physician contact the local poison control center for specific pediatric treatment.
*Poisindex® Toxicologic Management. Topic: Antidepressants, Tricyclic. *Micromedex Inc.* Vol. 85.
Chlordiazepoxide Overdosage: Manifestations of benzodiazepine overdosage include somnolence, confusion, coma and diminished reflexes. Dialysis is of limited value. There have been occasional reports of excitation in patients following benzodiazepine overdosage; if this occurs, barbiturates should not be used. Withdrawal symptoms of the barbiturate type have occurred after the discontinuation of benzodiazepines (see DRUG ABUSE AND DEPENDENCE section). Since Limbitrol contains amitriptyline, it is important to note that use of the benzodiazepine antagonist flumazenil is contraindicated in patients who are showing signs of serious cyclic antidepressant overdose.

DOSAGE AND ADMINISTRATION

Optimum dosage varies with the severity of the symptoms and the response of the individual patient. When a satisfactory response is obtained, dosage should be reduced to the smallest amount needed to maintain the remission. The larger portion of the total daily dose may be taken at bedtime. In some patients, a single dose at bedtime may be sufficient. In general, lower dosages are recommended for elderly patients.
Limbitrol DS (double strength) Tablets are recommended in an initial dosage of 3 or 4 tablets daily in divided doses; this may be increased to 6 tablets daily as required. Some patients respond to smaller doses and can be maintained on 2 tablets daily.
Limbitrol Tablets in an initial dosage of 3 or 4 tablets daily in divided doses may be satisfactory in patients who do not tolerate higher doses.

HOW SUPPLIED

DS (double strength) Tablets, containing 10 mg chlordiazepoxide and 25 mg amitriptyline (as the hydrochloride salt)—bottles of 100 (NDC 0140-0071-01) and 500 (NDC 0140-0071-14).
Tablets, containing 5 mg chlordiazepoxide and 12.5 mg amitriptyline (as the hydrochloride salt)—bottles of 100 (NDC 0140-0070-01) and 500 (NDC 0140-0070-14).

Revised: June 1996

Shown in Product Identification Guide, page 317

MESTINON® ℞

[mes 'tin-on]
(pyridostigmine bromide)
SYRUP, TABLETS, and TIMESPAN® TABLETS

DESCRIPTION

Mestinon (pyridostigmine bromide) is an orally active cholinesterase inhibitor. Chemically, pyridostigmine bromide is 3-hydroxy-1-methylpyridinium bromide dimethylcarbamate. Its structural formula is:

Mestinon is available in the following forms: *Syrup* containing 60 mg pyridostigmine bromide per teaspoonful in a vehicle containing 5% alcohol, glycerin, lactic acid, sodium benzoate, sorbitol, sucrose, FD&C Red No. 40, FD&C Blue No. 1, flavors and water. *Tablets* containing 60 mg pyridostigmine bromide; each tablet also contains lactose, silicon dioxide and stearic acid. *Timespan Tablets* containing 180 mg pyridostigmine bromide; each tablet also contains carnauba wax, corn-derived proteins, magnesium stearate, silica gel and tribasic calcium phosphate.

ACTIONS

Mestinon inhibits the destruction of acetylcholine by cholinesterase and thereby permits freer transmission of nerve impulses across the neuromuscular junction. Pyridostigmine is an analog of neostigmine (Prostigmin®), but differs from it in certain clinically significant respects; for example, pyridostigmine is characterized by a longer duration of action and fewer gastrointestinal side effects.

INDICATION

Mestinon is useful in the treatment of myasthenia gravis.

CONTRAINDICATIONS

Mestinon is contraindicated in mechanical intestinal or urinary obstruction, and particular caution should be used in its administration to patients with bronchial asthma. Care should be observed in the use of atropine for counteracting side effects, as discussed below.

WARNINGS

Although failure of patients to show clinical improvement may reflect underdosage, it can also be indicative of overdosage. As is true of all cholinergic drugs, overdosage of Mestinon may result in cholinergic crisis, a state characterized by increasing muscle weakness which, through involvement of the muscles of respiration, may lead to death. Myasthenic crisis due to an increase in the severity of the disease is also accompanied by extreme muscle weakness, and thus may be difficult to distinguish from cholinergic crisis on a symptomatic basis. Such differentiation is extremely important, since increases in doses of Mestinon or other drugs of this class in the presence of cholinergic crisis or of a refractory or "insensitive" state could have grave consequences. Osserman and Genkins[1] indicate that the differential diagnosis of the two types of crisis may require the use of Tensilon® (edrophonium chloride) as well as clinical judgment. The treatment of the two conditions obviously differs radically. Whereas the presence of myasthenic crisis suggests the need for more intensive anticholinesterase therapy, the diagnosis of cholinergic crisis, according to Osserman and Genkins,[1] calls for the prompt *withdrawal* of all drugs of this type. The immediate use of atropine in cholinergic crisis is also recommended.

Continued on next page

Mestinon—Cont.

Atropine may also be used to abolish or obtund gastrointestinal side effects or other muscarinic reactions; but such use, by masking signs of overdosage, can lead to inadvertent induction of cholinergic crisis.
For detailed information on the management of patients with myasthenia gravis, the physician is referred to one of the excellent reviews such as those by Osserman and Genkins,[2] Grob[3] or Schwab.[4,5]
Usage in Pregnancy: The safety of Mestinon during pregnancy or lactation in humans has not been established. Therefore, use of Mestinon in women who may become pregnant requires weighing the drug's potential benefits against its possible hazards to mother and child.

PRECAUTION

Pyridostigmine is mainly excreted unchanged by the kidney.[6,7,8] Therefore, lower doses may be required in patients with renal disease, and treatment should be based on titration of drug dosage to effect.[6,7]
Pediatric Use: Safety and effectiveness in pediatric patients have not been established.

ADVERSE REACTIONS

The side effects of Mestinon are most commonly related to overdosage and generally are of two varieties, muscarinic and nicotinic. Among those in the former group are nausea, vomiting, diarrhea, abdominal cramps, increased peristalsis, increased salivation, increased bronchial secretions, miosis and diaphoresis. Nicotinic side effects are comprised chiefly of muscle cramps, fasciculation and weakness. Muscarinic side effects can usually be counteracted by atropine, but for reasons shown in the preceding section the expedient is not without danger. As with any compound containing the bromide radical, a skin rash may be seen in an occasional patient. Such reactions usually subside promptly upon discontinuance of the medication.

DOSAGE AND ADMINISTRATION

Mestinon is available in three dosage forms:
Syrup —raspberry-flavored, containing 60 mg pyridostigmine bromide per teaspoonful (5 mL). This form permits accurate dosage adjustment for children and "brittle" myasthenic patients who require fractions of 60-mg doses. It is more easily swallowed, especially in the morning, by patients with bulbar involvement.
Conventional Tablets —each containing 60 mg pyridostigmine bromide.
Timespan Tablets —each containing 180 mg pyridostigmine bromide. This form provides uniformly slow release, hence prolonged duration of drug action; it facilitates control of myasthenic symptoms with fewer individual doses daily. The immediate effect of a 180-mg Timespan Tablet is about equal to that of a 60-mg Conventional Tablet; however, its duration of effectiveness, although varying in individual patients, averages $2^1/_2$ times that of a 60-mg dose.
Dosage: The size and frequency of the dosage must be adjusted to the needs of the individual patient.
Syrup and Conventional Tablets —The average dose is ten 60-mg tablets or ten 5-mL teaspoonfuls daily, spaced to provide maximum relief when maximum strength is needed. In severe cases as many as 25 tablets or teaspoonfuls a day may be required, while in mild cases one to six tablets or teaspoonfuls a day may suffice.
Timespan Tablets —One to three 180-mg tablets, once or twice daily, will usually be sufficient to control symptoms; however, the needs of certain individuals may vary markedly from this average. The interval between doses should be at least 6 hours. For optimum control, it may be necessary to use the more rapidly acting regular tablets or syrup in conjunction with Timespan therapy.
Note: For information on a diagnostic test for myasthenia gravis, and for the evaluation and stabilization of therapy, please see product literature on Tensilon® (edrophonium chloride).

HOW SUPPLIED

Syrup, 60 mg pyridostigmine bromide per teaspoonful (5 mL) and 5% alcohol—bottles of 16 fluid ounces (1 pint) (NDC 0187-3012-20).
Tablets, scored, 60 mg pyridostigmine bromide each—bottles of 100 (NDC 0187-3010-30) and 500 (NDC 0187-3010-40).
Timespan Tablets, scored, 180 mg pyridostigmine bromide each—bottles of 30 (NDC 0187-3013-30).
Note: Because of the hygroscopic nature of the Timespan Tablets, mottling may occur. This does not affect their efficacy.

REFERENCES

1. Osserman KE, Genkins G. Studies in myasthenia gravis: Reduction in mortality rate after crisis. *JAMA.* Jan 1963; 183:97–101.
2. Osserman KE, Genkins G. Studies in myasthenia gravis. *NY State J. Med.* June 1961; 61:2076–2085.
3. Grob D. Myasthenia gravis. A review of pathogenesis and treatment. *Arch Intern Med.* Oct 1961; 108:615–638.
4. Schwab RS. Management of myasthenia gravis. *New Eng J Med.* Mar 1963; 268:596–597.
5. Schwab RS.Management of myasthenia gravis. *New Eng J Med.* Mar 1963; 268:717–719.
6. Cronnelly R, Stanski DR, Miller RD, Sheiner LB. Pyridostigmine kinetics with and without renal function. *Clin Pharmacol Ther.* 1980; 28:No. 1, 78–81.
7. Miller RD. Pharmacodynamics and pharmacokinetics of anticholinesterase. In: Ruegheimer E, Zindler M, ed. *Anaesthesiology.* (Hamburg, Germany: Congress; Sep 14–21, 1980; 222–223.) (Int Congr. No. 538), Amsterdam, Netherlands: Excerpta Medica; 1981.
8. Breyer-Pfaff U, Maier U, Brinkmann AM, Schumm F. Pyridostigmine kinetics in healthy subjects and patients with myasthenia gravis. *Clin Pharmacol Ther.* 1985;5: 495–501.

ICN Pharmaceuticals, Inc.
ICN Plaza
3300 Hyland Avenue
Costa Mesa, CA 92626
(714) 545-0100

Rev. 11/98
Shown in Product Identification Guide, page 317

OXSORALEN® LOTION 1% ℞

[ox 'sore "a-len]
(methoxsalen USP, 1%)
Rx only

CAUTION: METHOXSALEN LOTION IS A POTENT TOPICAL DRUG. READ ENTIRE BROCHURE BEFORE PRESCRIBING OR USING THIS MEDICATION.

WARNING: METHOXSALEN LOTION IS A POTENT DRUG CAPABLE OF PRODUCING SEVERE BURNS IF IMPROPERLY USED. IT SHOULD BE APPLIED ONLY BY A PHYSICIAN UNDER CONTROLLED CONDITIONS FOR LIGHT EXPOSURE AND SUBSEQUENT LIGHT SHIELDING.

THIS PREPARATION SHOULD NEVER BE DISPENSED TO A PATIENT.

I. DESCRIPTION

Each ml. of Oxsoralen Lotion contains 10 mg methoxsalen in an inert vehicle containing alcohol (71% v/v), propylene glycol, acetone, and purified water.
Methoxsalen is a naturally occurring substance found in the seeds of the **Ammi majus** (Umbelliferae) plant and in the roots of **Heracleum Candicans.** It belongs to a group of compounds known as psoralens or furocoumarins. The chemical name of methoxsalen is 9-methoxy-7H-furo(3, 2g) (1)-benzopyran-7-one. It has the following structure:

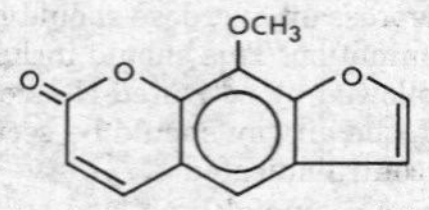

OCH_3

II. CLINICAL PHARMACOLOGY

The exact mechanism of action of methoxsalen with the epidermal melanocytes and keratinocytes is not known. Psoralens given orally are preferentially taken up by epidermal cells (Artuc et al, 1979).[1] The best known biochemical reaction of methoxsalen is with DNA. Methoxsalen, upon photoactivation, conjugates and forms covalent bonds with DNA which leads to the formation of both monofunctional (addition to a single strand of DNA) and bifunctional adducts (crosslinking of psoralen to both strands of DNA) (Dall'Acqua et al, 1971).[2] Reactions with proteins have also been described (Yoshikawa et al, 1979).[3]
Methoxsalen acts as a photosensitizer. Topical application of this drug and subsequent exposure to UVA, whether artificial or sunlight, can cause cell injury. If sufficient cell injury occurs in the skin an inflammatory reaction will result. The most obvious manifestation of this reaction is delayed erythema which may not begin for several hours and may not peak for 2 to 3 days or longer. It is crucial to realize that the length of time the skin remains sensitized or when the maximum erythema will occur is quite variable from person to person. The erythematous reaction is followed over several days or weeks by repair which is manifested by increased melanization of the epidermis and thickening of the stratum corneum. The exact mechanics are unknown but it has been suggested melanocytes in the hair follicles are stimulated to move up the follicle and to repopulate the epidermis. (Ortonne, et al, 1979).[4]

III. INDICATIONS AND USAGE

As a topical repigmenting agent in vitiligo in conjunction with controlled doses of ultraviolet A (320–400 nm) or sunlight.

IV. CONTRAINDICATIONS

A. Patients exhibiting idiosyncratic reactions to psoralen compounds or a history of sensitivity reactions to them.
B. Patients exhibiting melanoma or with a history of melanoma.
C. Patients exhibiting invasive skin carcinoma generally.
D. Patients with photosensitivity diseases such as porphyria, acute lupus erythematosus, xeroderma pigmentosum, etc.
E. Children under 12 since clinical studies to determine the efficacy and safety of treatment in this age group have not been done.

V. WARNINGS

A. **Skin Burns**
Serious skin burns from either UVA or sunlight (even through window glass) can result if recommended exposure schedule is exceeded and/or protective covering or sunscreens are not used. The blistering of the skin sometimes encountered after UVA exposure generally heals without complication or scarring. (Farrington Daniels, Jr, M.D., personal communication). Suitable covering of the area of application or a topical sunblock should follow the therapeutic UVA exposure.
B. **Carcinogenicity**
1. Animal Studies. Topical methoxsalen has been reported to be a potent photocarcinogen in certain strains of mice. (Pathak et al 1959).[5]
2. Human Studies. None of our clinical investigators reported skin cancer as a complication of topical treatment for vitiligo. However, it is recommended that caution be exercised when the patient is fair-skinned or has a history of prior coal tar UVA treatment, or has had ionizing radiation or taken arsenical compounds. Such patients who subsequently have **oral** psoralen—UVA treatment (PUVA) are at increased risk for developing skin cancer.
C. **Concomitant Therapy**
Special care should be exercised in treating patients who are receiving concomitant therapy (either topically or systemically) with known photosensitizing agents such as anthralin, coal tar or coal tar derivatives, griseofulvin, phenothiazines, nalidixic acid, halogenated salicylanilides (bacteriostatic soaps), sulfonamides, tetracyclines, thiazides, and certain organic staining dyes such as methylene blue, toluidine blue, rose bengal, and methyl orange.

VI. PRECAUTIONS

A. This product should be applied only in small well defined lesions and preferably on lesions which can be protected by clothing or a sunscreen from subsequent exposure to radiant UVA. If this product is used to treat vitiligo of face or hands, be very emphatic when instructing patient to keep the treated areas protected from light by use of protective clothing or sunscreening agents. The area of application may be highly photosensitive for several days and may result in severe burn injury if exposed to additional UV or sunlight.
B. CARCINOGENESIS: See Warning Section
C. Pregnancy Category C. Animal reproduction studies have not been conducted with topical methoxsalen. It is also not known whether methoxsalen can cause fetal harm when used topically on a pregnant woman or affect reproductive capacity. It is not known to what degree, if any, topical methoxsalen is absorbed systemically. Topical methoxsalen should be used in pregnant women only when clearly indicated.
D. Nursing Mothers. It is not known whether topical methoxsalen is absorbed or excreted in human milk. Caution is advised when topical methoxsalen is used in a nursing mother.
E. Pediatric Usage. Safety and effectiveness in children below the age of 12 years have not been established.

VII. ADVERSE REACTIONS

Systemic adverse reactions have not been reported. The most common adverse reaction is severe burns of the treated area from overexposure to UVA, including sunlight. TREATMENT MUST BE INDIVIDUALIZED. Minor blistering of the skin is not a contraindication to further treatment and generally heals without incident. Treatment would be the standard for burn therapy. Since 1953, many studies have demonstrated the safety and effectiveness of topical methoxsalen and UVA for the treatment of vitiligo when used as directed. (Lerner, A.B., et al, 1953)[6] (Fitzpatrick, T.B., et al, 1966)[7] (Fulton, James F. et al, 1969)[8].

VIII. OVERDOSAGE

This does not apply to topical usage. In the unlikely event that the lotion is ingested, standard procedures for poisoning should be followed, including gastric lavage. Protection from UVA or daylight for hours or days would also be necessary. The patient should be kept in a darkened room.

IX. ADMINISTRATION

OXSORALEN Lotion is applied to a well-defined area of vitiligo by the physician and the area is then exposed to a suitable source of UVA. Initial exposure time should be conservative and not exceed that which is predicted to be one-half the minimal erythema dose. Treatment intervals should be regulated by the erythema response; generally once a week is recommended or less often depending on the results. The hands and fingers of the person applying the medication should be protected by gloves or finger cots to avoid photosensitization and possible burns.
Pigmentation may begin after a few weeks but significant repigmentation may require up to 6 to 9 months of treatment. Periodic re-treatment may be necessary to retain all of the new pigment. Idiopathic vitiligo is reversible but not equally reversible in every patient. Treatment must be individualized. Repigmentation will vary in completeness, time of onset, and duration. Repigmentation occurs more rapidly in fleshy areas such as face, abdomen, and buttocks and less rapidly over less fleshy areas such as the dorsum of the hands or feet.

X. HOW SUPPLIED

Oxsoralen Lotion containing 1% methoxsalen (8-methoxypsoralen) packaged in 1 ounce (29.57 ml) amber glass bottles (NDC 0187-0402-31).
Store at 25°C (77°F); excursion permitted to 15°C–30°C (59°F–86°F).

REFERENCES

1. Artuc, M.; Stuettgen, G.; Schalla, W.; Schaefer, H.; Gazith, J.: Reversible binding of 5- and 8-methoxypsor-

alen to human serum proteins (albumin) and to epidermis **in vitro; Brit. J. Dermat., 101**, pp. 669–677 (1979).
2. Dall'Acqua, F.; Marciani, S.; Ciavatta, L.; Rodighiero, G.: formation of interstrand cross-linkings in the photoreactions between furocoumarins and DNA.; **Z Naturforsch** (B), **26,** pp. 561–569 (1971).
3. Yoshikawa, K; Mori, N.; Sakakibara, S.; Mizuno, N.; Song, P.: Photo-Conjugation of 8-methoxypsoralen with Proteins; **Photochem & Photobiol, 29,** pp. 1127–1133 (1979).
4. Ortonne, J.P.; MacDonald, D.M.; Micoud, A.; Thivolet, J.: PUVA-induced repigmentation of vitiligo: a histochemical (split-DOPA) and ultra-structural study; **Brit. J. Dermat., 101,** pp. 1–12 (1979).
5. Pathak, M.A.; Daniels, F.; Hopkins, C.E.; Fitzpatrick, T.B.: Ultraviolet carcinogenesis in albino and pigmented mice receiving furocoumarins: psoralens and 8-methoxypsoralen, **Nature, 183,** pp. 728–730 (1959).
6. Lerner, A.B.; Denton, C.R.; Fitzpatrick, T.B.: Clinical and experimental studies with 8-methoxypsoralen in vitiligo; **J. Invest. Derm., 20,** pp. 299–314 (April, 1953).
7. Fitzpatrick, T.B.; Arndt, K.A.; El Mofty, A.M.: Hydroquinone and psoralens in the therapy of hypermelanosis and vitiligo; **Arch Derm., 93,** pp. 589–599 (May, 1966).
8. Fulton, James F.; Leyden, James; Papa, Christopher: Treatment of vitiligo with topical methoxsalen and blacklite; **Arch. Derm., 101,** pp. 224–229 (1969).

2398-03 EL
Rev. 5-98

OXSORALEN–ULTRA® CAPSULES ℞

[ox '-sore "a-len]
(Methoxsalen Capsules, USP, 10 mg)

Rx only

CAUTION: METHOXSALEN IS A POTENT DRUG. READ ENTIRE BROCHURE PRIOR TO PRESCRIBING OR DISPENSING THIS MEDICATION.

Methoxsalen with UV radiation should be used only by physicians who have special competence in the diagnosis and treatment of psoriasis and who have special training and experience in photochemotherapy. The use of Psoralen and ultraviolet radiation therapy should be under constant supervision of such a physician. For the treatment of patients with psoriasis, photochemotherapy should be restricted to patients with severe, recalcitrant, disabling psoriasis which is not adequately responsive to other forms of therapy, and only when the diagnosis has been supported by biopsy. Because of the possibilities of ocular damage, aging of the skin, and skin cancer (including melanoma), the patient should be fully informed by the physician of the risks inherent in this therapy.

CAUTION: Oxsoralen-Ultra® (Methoxsalen Soft Gelatin Capsules) should not be used interchangeably with regular Oxsoralen® or 8-MOP® (Methoxsalen Hard Gelatin Capsules). This new dosage form of methoxsalen exhibits significantly greater bioavailability and earlier photosensitization onset time than previous methoxsalen dosage forms. Patients should be treated in accordance with the dosimetry specifically recommended for this product. The minimum phototoxic dose (MPD) and phototoxic peak time after drug administration prior to onset of photochemotherapy with this dosage form should be determined.

I. DESCRIPTION

Oxsoralen-Ultra (methoxsalen, 8-methoxypsoralen) Capsules, 10 mg. Methoxsalen is a naturally occurring photoactive substance found in the seeds of the **Ammi majus** (Umbelliferae) plant and in the roots of **Heracleum Candicans**. It belongs to a group of compounds known as psoralens, or furocoumarins. The chemical name of methoxsalen is 9-methoxy-7H-furo [3,2-g] [1]benzopyran-7-one; it has the following structure:

II. CLINICAL PHARMACOLOGY

The combination treatment regimen of psoralen (P) and ultraviolet radiation of 320–400 nm wavelength commonly referred to as UVA is known by the acronym, PUVA. Skin reactivity to UVA (320–400 nm) radiation is markedly enhanced by the ingestion of methoxsalen. In a well controlled bioavailability study, Oxsoralen-Ultra Capsules reached peak drug levels in the blood of test subjects between 0.5 and 4 hours (Mean = 1.8 hours) as compared to between 1.5 and 6 hours (Mean = 3.0 hours) for regular Oxsoralen when administered with 8 ounces of milk. Peak drug levels were 2 to 3 fold greater when the overall extent of drug absorption was approximately two fold greater for Oxsoralen-Ultra Capsules as compared to regular Oxsoralen Capsules. Detectable methoxsalen levels were observed up to 12 hours post dose. The drug half-life is approximately 2 hours. Photosensitivity studies demonstrate a shorter time of peak photosensitivity of 1.5 to 2.1 hours vs. 3.9 to 4.25 hours for regular Oxsoralen capsules. In addition, the mean minimal erythema dose (MED), J/cm^2, for the Oxsoralen-Ultra Capsules is substantially less than that required for regular Oxsoralen Capsules (Levins et al., 1984 and private communication[1]).

Methoxsalen is reversibly bound to serum albumin and is also preferentially taken up by epidermal cells (Artuc et al., 1979[2]). At a dose which is six times larger than that used in humans, it induces mixed function oxidases in the liver of mice (Mandula et al., 1978[3]). In both mice and man, methoxsalen is rapidly metabolized. Approximately 95% of the drug is excreted as a series of metabolites in the urine within 24 hours (Pathak et al., 1977[4]). The exact mechanism of action of methoxsalen with the epidermal melanocytes and keratinocytes is not known. The best known biochemical reaction of methoxsalen is with DNA. Methoxsalen, upon photoactivation, conjugates and forms covalent bonds with DNA which leads to the formation of both monofunctional (addition to a single strand of DNA) and bifunctional (crosslinking of psoralen to both strands of DNA) adducts (Dall' Acqua et al., 1971[5]; Cole, 1970[6]; Musajo et al., 1974[7]; Dall' Acqua et al., 1979[8]). Reactions with proteins have also been described (Yoshikawa, et al., 1979[9]).

Methoxsalen acts as a photosensitizer. Administration of the drug and subsequent exposure to UVA can lead to cell injury. Orally administered methoxsalen reaches the skin via the blood and UVA penetrates well into the skin. If sufficient cell injury occurs in the skin, an inflammatory reaction occurs. The most obvious manifestation of this reaction is delayed erythema, which may not begin for several hours and peaks at 48–72 hours. The inflammation is followed, over several days to weeks, by repair which is manifested by increased melanization of the epidermis and thickening of the stratum corneum. The mechanisms of therapy are not known. In the treatment of psoriasis, the mechanism is most often assumed to be DNA photodamage and resulting decrease in cell proliferation but other vascular, leukocyte, or cell regulatory mechanisms may also be playing some role. Psoriasis is a hyper-proliferative disorder and other agents known to be therapeutic for psoriasis are known to inhibit DNA synthesis.

III. INDICATIONS AND USAGE

Photochemotherapy (Methoxsalen with long wave UVA radiation) is indicated for the symptomatic control of severe, recalcitrant, disabling psoriasis not adequately responsive to other forms of therapy and when the diagnosis has been supported by biopsy. Methoxsalen is intended to be administered only in conjunction with a schedule of controlled doses of long wave ultraviolet radiation.

IV. CONTRAINDICATIONS

A. Patients exhibiting idiosyncratic reactions to psoralen compounds.
B. Patients possessing a specific history of light sensitive disease states should not initiate methoxsalen therapy except under special circumstances. Diseases associated with photosensitivity include lupus erythematosus, porphyria cutanea tarda, erythropoietic protoporphyria, variegate porphyria, xeroderma pigmentosum, and albinism.
C. Patients with melanoma or with a history of melanoma.
D. Patients with invasive squamous cell carcinomas.
E. Patients with aphakia, because of the significantly increased risk of retinal damage due to the absence of lenses.

V. WARNINGS—GENERAL

A. SKIN BURNING: Serious burns from either UVA or sunlight (even through window glass) can result if the recommended dosage of the drug and/or exposure schedules are exceeded.

B. CARCINOGENICITY:

1. ANIMAL STUDIES: Topical or intraperitoneal methoxsalen has been reported to be a potent photocarcinogen in albino mice and hairless mice (Hakim et al., 1960[10]). However, methoxsalen given by the oral route to Swiss albino mice suggests this agent exerts a protective effect against ultraviolet carcinogenesis; mice given 8-methoxypsoralen in their diet showed 38% ear tumors 180 days after the start of ultraviolet therapy compared to 62% for controls (O'Neal et al., 1957[11]).

2. HUMAN STUDIES: A 5.7 year prospective study of 1380 psoriasis patients treated with oral methoxsalen and ultraviolet A photochemotherapy (PUVA) demonstrated that the risk of cutaneous squamous-cell carcinoma developing at least 22 months following the first PUVA exposure was approximately 12.8 times higher in the high dose patients than in the low dose patients (Stern et al., 1979[12], Stern et al., 1980[13], and Stern et al., 1984[14]). The substantial dose-dependent increase was observed in patients with neither a prior history of skin cancer nor significant exposure to cutaneous carcinogens. Reduction in PUVA dosage significantly reduces the risk. No substantial dose related increase was noted for basal cell carcinoma according to Stern et al., 1984[14]. Increases appear greatest in patients who have pre-PUVA exposure to 1) prolonged tar and UVB treatment, 2) ionizing radiation, or 3) arsenic.

Roenigk et al., 1980[15], studied 690 patients for up to 4 years and found no increase in the risk of non-melanoma skin cancer, although patients in this cohort had significantly less exposure to PUVA than in the Stern et al. study. After 5 years, two of 1380 patients in the Stern et al. PUVA study have developed malignant melanoma. In addition, more than $^1/_5$ of the patients in this cohort have developed macular pigmented lesions on the buttocks. While there is no evidence that an increased risk of melanoma exists in PUVA treated patients, these observations indicate the need for continued evaluation of melanoma risk of PUVA treated patients.

In a study in Indian patients treated for 4 years for vitiligo, 12 percent developed keratoses, but not cancer, in the depigmented, vitiliginous areas (Mosher, 1980[16]). Clinically, the keratoses were keratotic papules, actinic keratosis-like macules, nonscaling dome-shaped papules, and lichenoid porokeratotic-like papules.

C. CATARACTOGENICITY:

1. ANIMAL STUDIES: Exposure to large doses of UVA causes cataracts in animals, and this effect is enhanced by the administration of methoxsalen (Cloud et al, 1960[17]; Cloud et al, 1961[18]; Freeman et al, 1969[19]).

2. HUMAN STUDIES: It has been found that the concentration of methoxsalen in the lens is proportional to the serum level. If the lens is exposed to UVA during the time methoxsalen is present in the lens, photochemical action may lead to irreversible binding of methoxsalen to proteins and the DNA components of the lens (Lerman et al, 1980[20]). However, if the lens is shielded from UVA, the methoxsalen will diffuse out of the lens in a 24 hour period (Lerman et al., 1980[20]). Patients should be told emphatically to wear UVA-absorbing, wrap-around sunglasses for the twenty-four (24) hour period following ingestion of methoxsalen, whether exposed to direct or indirect sunlight in the open or through a window glass. Among patients using proper eye protection, there is no evidence for a significantly increased risk of cataracts in association with PUVA therapy. (Stern et al., 1979[12]). Thirty-five of 1380 patients have developed cataracts in the five years since their first PUVA treatment. This incidence is comparable to that expected in a population of this size and age distribution. No relationship between PUVA dose and cataract risk in this group has been noted.

D. ACTINIC DEGENERATION: Exposure to sunlight and/or ultraviolet radiation may result in "premature aging" of the skin.

E. BASAL CELL CARCINOMAS: Patients exhibiting multiple basal cell carcinomas or having a history of basal cell carcinomas should be diligently observed and treated.

F. RADIATION THERAPY: Patients having a history of previous x-ray therapy or grenz ray therapy should be diligently observed for signs of carcinoma.

G. ARSENIC THERAPY: Patients having a history of previous arsenic therapy should be diligently observed for signs of carcinoma.

H. HEPATIC DISEASES: Patients with hepatic insufficiency should be treated with caution since hepatic biotransformation is necessary for drug urinary excretion.

I. CARDIAC DISEASES: Patients with cardiac diseases or others who may be unable to tolerate prolonged standing or exposure to heat stress should not be treated in a vertical UVA chamber.

J. TOTAL DOSAGE: The total cumulative dose of UVA that can be given over long periods of time with safety has not as yet been established.

K. CONCOMITANT THERAPY: Special care should be exercised in treating patients who are receiving concomitant therapy (either topically or systemically) with known photosensitizing agents such as anthralin, coal tar or coal tar derivatives, griseofulvin, phenothiazines, nalidixic acid, halogenated salicylanilides (bacteriostatic soaps), sulfonamides, tetracyclines, thiazides and certain organic staining dyes such as methylene blue, toluidine blue, rose bengal, and methyl orange.

VI. PRECAUTIONS

A. GENERAL—APPLICABLE TO PSORIASIS TREATMENT:

1. BEFORE METHOXSALEN INGESTION

Patients must not sunbathe during the 24 hours prior to methoxsalen ingestion and UV exposure. The presence of a sunburn may prevent an accurate evaluation of the patient's response to photochemotherapy.

2. AFTER METHOXSALEN INGESTION

a. UVA-absorbing wrap-around sunglasses should be worn during daylight for 24 hours after methoxsalen ingestion. The protective eyewear must be designed to prevent entry of stray radiation to the eyes, including that which may enter from the sides of the eyewear. The protective eyewear is used to prevent the irreversible binding of methoxsalen to the proteins and DNA components of the lens. Cataracts form when enough of the binding occurs. Visual discrimination should be permitted by the eyewear for patient well-being and comfort.

b. Patients must avoid sun exposure, even through window glass or cloud cover, for at least 8 hours after methoxsalen ingestion. If sun exposure cannot be avoided, the patient should wear protective devices such as a hat and gloves, and/or apply sunscreens which contain ingredients that filter out UVA radiation (e.g. sunscreens containing benzophenone and/or PABA esters which exhibit a sun protective factor

Continued on next page

Oxsoralen Ultra—Cont.

equal to or greater than 15). These chemical sunscreens should be applied to all areas that might be exposed to the sun (including lips). Sunscreens should not be applied to areas affected by psoriasis until after the patient has been treated in the UVA chamber.

3. DURING PUVA THERAPY

a. Total UVA-absorbing/blocking goggles mechanically designed to give maximal ocular protection must be worn. Failure to do so may increase the risk of cataract formation. A reliable radiometer can be used to verify elimination of UVA transmission through the goggles.

b. Abdominal skin, breasts, genitalia, and other sensitive areas should be protected for approximately $^1/_3$ of the initial exposure time until tanning occurs.

c. Unless affected by disease, male genitalia should be shielded.

4. AFTER COMBINED METHOXSALEN/UVA THERAPY

a. UVA-absorbing wrap-around sunglasses should be worn during daylight for 24 hours after combined methoxsalen/UVA therapy.

b. Patients should not sunbathe for 48 hours after therapy. Erythema and/or burning due to photochemotherapy and sunburn due to sun exposure are additive.

B. INFORMATION FOR PATIENTS: See accompanying Patient Package Insert.

C. LABORATORY TESTS:

1. Patients should have an ophthalmologic examination prior to start of therapy, and thence yearly.
2. Patients should have routine laboratory tests prior to the start of therapy and at regular periods thereafter if patients are on extended treatments.

D. DRUG INTERACTIONS: See Warnings Section.

E. CARCINOGENESIS: See Warnings Section.

F. PREGNANCY:

Pregnancy Category C. Animal reproduction studies have not been conducted with methoxsalen. It is also not known whether methoxsalen can cause fetal harm when administered to a pregnant woman or can affect reproduction capacity. Methoxsalen should be given to a woman with reproductive capacity only if clearly needed.

G. NURSING MOTHERS:

It is not known whether this drug is excreted in human milk. Because many drugs are excreted in human milk, either methoxsalen ingestion or nursing should be discontinued.

H. PEDIATRIC USE:

Safety in children has not been established. Potential hazards of long-term therapy include the possibilities of carcinogenicity and cataractogenicity as described in the Warnings Section as well as the probability of actinic degeneration which is also described in the Warnings Section.

VII. ADVERSE REACTIONS

A. METHOXSALEN:

The most commonly reported side effect of methoxsalen alone is nausea, which occurs with approximately 10% of all patients. This effect may be minimized or avoided by instructing the patient to take methoxsalen in milk or food, or to divide the dose into two portions, taken approximately one-half hour apart. Other effects include nervousness, insomnia, and depression.

B. COMBINED METHOXSALEN/UVA THERAPY:

1. PRURITUS: This adverse reaction occurs with approximately 10% of all patients. In most cases, pruritus can be alleviated with frequent application of bland emollients or other topical agents; severe pruritus may require systemic treatment. If pruritus is unresponsive to these measures, shield pruritic areas from further UVA exposure until the condition resolves. If intractable pruritus is generalized, UVA treatment should be discontinued until the pruritus disappears.

2. ERYTHEMA: Mild, transient erythema at 24–48 hours after PUVA therapy is an expected reaction and indicates that a therapeutic interaction between methoxsalen and UVA occurred. Any area showing moderate erythema (greater than Grade 2—See Table 1 for grades of erythema) should be shielded during subsequent UVA exposures until the erythema has resolved. Erythema greater than Grade 2 which appears within 24 hours after UVA treatment may signal a potentially severe burn. Erythema may become progressively worse over the next 24 hours, since the peak erythemal reaction characteristically occurs 48 hours or later after methoxsalen ingestion. The patient should be protected from further UVA exposures and sunlight, and should be monitored closely.

3. IMPORTANT DIFFERENCES BETWEEN PUVA ERYTHEMA AND SUNBURN: PUVA-induced inflammation differs from sunburn or UVB phototherapy in several ways. The percent transmission of UVB varies between 0% to 34% through skin whereas UVA varies between 1% to 80% transmission; thus, UVA is transmitted to a larger percent through the skin. (Diffey, 1982[21]). The DNA lesions induced by PUVA are very different from UV-induced thymine dimers and may lead to a DNA crosslink. This DNA lesion may be more problematic to the cell because crosslinks are more lethal and psoralen-DNA photoproducts may be "new" or unfamiliar substrates for DNA repair enzymes. DNA synthesis is also suppressed longer after PUVA. The time course of delayed erythema is different with PUVA and may not involve the usual mediators seen in sunburn. PUVA-induced redness may be just beginning at 24 hours, when UVB erythema has already passed its peak. The erythema dose-response curve is also steeper for PUVA. Compared to equally erythemogenic doses of UVB, the histologic alterations induced by PUVA show more dermal vessel damage and longer duration of epidermal and dermal abnormalities.

4. OTHER ADVERSE REACTIONS: Those reported include edema, dizziness, headache, malaise, depression, hypopigmentation, vesiculation and bullae formation, non-specific rash, herpes simplex, miliaria, urticaria, folliculitis, gastrointestinal disturbances, cutaneous tenderness, leg cramps, hypotension, and extension of psoriasis.

VIII. OVERDOSAGE

In the event of methoxsalen overdosage, induce emesis and keep the patient in a darkened room for at least 24 hours. Emesis is most beneficial within the first 2 to 3 hours after ingestion of methoxsalen, since maximum blood levels are reached by this time.

IX. DRUG DOSAGE AND ADMINISTRATION

CAUTION: Oxsoralen-Ultra represents a new dose form of methoxsalen. This new dosage form of methoxsalen exhibits significantly greater bioavailability and earlier photosensitization onset time than previous methoxsalen dosage forms. Each patient should be evaluated by determining the minimum phototoxic dose (MPD) and phototoxic peak time after drug administration prior to onset of photochemotherapy with this dosage form. Human bioavailability studies have indicated the following drug dosage and administration directions are to be used as a guideline only.

PSORIASIS THERAPY

1. DRUG DOSAGE-INITIAL THERAPY: The methoxsalen capsules should be taken $1^1/_2$ to 2 hours before UVA exposure with some low fat food or milk according to the following table:

Patient's Weight (kg)	(lbs)	Dose (mg)
<30	<66	10
30–50	66–110	20
51–65	112–143	30
66–80	146–176	40
81–90	179–198	50
91–115	201–254	60
>115	>254	70

2. INITIAL EXPOSURE: The initial UVA exposure energy level and corresponding time of exposure is determined by the patient's skin characteristics for sunburning and tanning as follows:

Skin Type	History	Recommended Joules/cm²
I	Always burn, never tan (patients with erythrodermic psoriasis are to be classed as Type I for determination of UVA dosage.)	0.5 J/cm²
II	Always burn, but sometimes tan	1.0 J/cm²
III	Sometimes burn, but always tan	1.5 J/cm²
IV	Never burn, always tan	2.0 J/cm²
Skin Type	**Physician Examination**	**Joules/cm²**
V*	Moderately pigmented	2.5 J/cm²
VI*	Blacks	3.0 J/cm²

(*Patients with natural pigmentation of these types should be classified into a lower skin type category if the sunburning history so indicates.)

If the MPD is done, start at $^1/_2$ MPD.

Additional drug dosage directions are as follows:

a. Weight Change: In the event that the weight of a patient changes during treatment such that he/she falls into an adjacent weight range/dose category, no change in the dose of methoxsalen is usually required. If, in the physician's opinion, however, a weight change is sufficiently great to modify the drug dose, then an adjustment in the time of exposure to UVA should be made.

b. Dose/Week: The number of doses per week of methoxsalen capsules will be determined by the patient's schedule of UVA exposures. In no case should treatments be given more often than once every other day because the full extent of phototoxic reactions may not be evident until 48 hours after each exposure.

c. Dosage Increase: Dosage may be increased by 10 mg after the fifteenth treatment under the conditions outlined in section XI.B.4b.

X. UVA RADIATION SOURCE SPECIFICATIONS & INFORMATION

A. IRRADIANCE UNIFORMITY:

The following specifications should be met with the window of the detector held in a vertical plane:

1. Vertical variation: For readings taken at any point along the vertical center axis of the chamber (to within 15 cm from the top and bottom), the lowest reading should not be less than 70 percent of the highest reading.

2. Horizontal variation: Throughout any specific horizontal plane, the lowest reading must be at least 80 percent of the highest reading, excluding the peripheral 3 cm of the patient treatment space.

B. PATIENT SAFETY FEATURES:

The following safety features should be present: (1) Protection from electrical hazard: All units should be grounded and conform to applicable electrical codes. The patient or operator should not be able to touch any live electrical parts. There should be ground fault protection. (2) Protective shielding of lamps: The patient should not be able to come in contact with the bare lamps. In the event of lamp breakage, the patient should not be exposed to broken lamp components. (3) Hand rails and hand holds: Appropriate supports should be available to the patient. (4) Patient viewing window: A window which blocks UV should be provided for viewing the patient during treatment. (5) Door and latches: Patients should be able to open the door from the inside with only slight pressure to the door. (6) Non-skid floor: The floor should be of a non-skid nature. (7) Thermoregulation: Sufficient air flow should be provided for patient safety and comfort, limiting temperature within the UVA radiator cabinet to approximately less than 100°F. (8) Timer: The irradiator should be equipped with an automatic timer which terminates the exposure at the conclusion of a preset time interval. (9) Patient alarm device: An alarm device within the UVA irradiator chamber should be accessible to the patient for emergency activation. (10) Danger label: The unit should have a label prominently displayed which reads as follows:

DANGER—Ultraviolet Radiation—Follow your physician's instructions—Failure to use protective eyewear may result in eye injury.

C. UVA EXPOSURE DOSIMETRY MEASUREMENTS:

The maximum radiant exposure or irradiance (within ± 15 percent) of UVA (320–400 nm) delivered to the patient should be determined by using an appropriate radiometer calibrated to be read in Joules/cm² or mW/cm². In the absence of a standard measuring technique approved by the National Bureau of Standards, the system should use a detector corrected to a cosine spatial response. The use and recalibration frequency of such a radiometer for a specific UVA irradiator chamber should be specified by the manufacturer because the UVA dose (exposure) is determined by the design of the irradiator, the number of lamps, and the age of the lamp. If irradiance is measured, the radiometer reading in mW/cm² is used to calculate the exposure time in minutes to deliver the required UVA in Joules/cm² to a patient in the UVA irradiator cabinet. The equation is:

$$\text{Exposure Time (minutes)} = \frac{\text{Desired UVA Dose (J/cm}^2\text{)}}{0.06 \times \text{Irradiance (mW/cm}^2\text{)}}.$$

Overexposure due to human error should be minimized by using an accurate automatic timing device, which is set by the operator and controlled by energizing and de-energizing the UVA irradiator lamp. The timing device calibration interval should be specified by the manufacturer. Safety systems should be included to minimize the possibility of delivering a UVA exposure which exceeds the prescribed dose, in the event the timer or radiometer should malfunction.

D. UVA SPECTRAL OUTPUT DISTRIBUTION:

The spectral distributions of the lamps should meet the following specifications:

Wavelength band (nanometers)	Output[1]
<310	<1
310 to 320	1 to 3
320 to 330	4 to 8
330 to 340	11 to 17
340 to 350	18 to 25
350 to 360	19 to 28
360 to 370	15 to 23
370 to 380	8 to 12
380 to 390	3 to 7
390 to 400	1 to 3

[1] As a percentage of total irradiance between 320 and 400 nanometers.

XI. PUVA TREATMENT PROTOCOL

INTRODUCTION:

The Oxsoralen-Ultra® Capsules reach their maximum bioavailability in $1^1/_2$ to 2 hours after ingestion.

On average, the serum level achieved with Oxsoralen-Ultra is twice that obtained with 8-MOP (formerly Oxsoralen) and reach their peak concentration in less than $^1/_2$ the time of the 8-MOP capsules.

As a result the mean MED J/cm² for the Oxsoralen-Ultra Capsules is substantially less than that required for 8-MOP (Levins et al., 1984 and private communication[1]).

Photosensitivity studies demonstrate a shorter time of peak photosensitivity of 1.5 to 2.1 hours vs. 3.9 to 4.25 hours for regular methoxsalen capsules.

A. INITIAL EXPOSURE: The initial UVA exposures should be conducted according to the guidelines presented previously under IX.B.1 and 2, Psoriasis therapy, Drug dosage-initial Therapy and Exposure.

B. CLEARING PHASE: Specific recommendations for patient treatment are as follows:

1. SKIN TYPES I, II, & III. Patients with skin types I, II, and III may be treated 2 or 3 times per week. UVA exposure may be held constant or increased by up to 1.0 Joule/cm² at each treatment, according to the patient's response. If erythema occurs, however, do not increase

exposure time until erythema resolves. The severity and extent of the patient's erythema may be used to determine whether the next exposure should be shortened, omitted, or maintained at the previous dosage. See Adverse Reactions section for additional information.

2. SKIN TYPES IV, V, & VI. Patients with skin types IV, V, and VI may be treated 2 or 3 times per week. UVA exposure may be held constant or increased by up to 1.5 Joules/cm^2 at each treatment unless erythema occurs. If erythema occurs, follow instructions outlined above in the procedures for patients with skin types I, II, and III.

3. ERYTHRODERMIC PSORIASIS. Patients with erythrodermic psoriasis should be treated with special attention because pre-existing erythema may obscure observations of possible treatment-related phototoxic erythema. These patients may be treated 2 or 3 times per week, as a Type I patient.

4. MISCELLANEOUS SITUATIONS:

a. If there is no response after a total of 10 treatments, the exposure of UVA energy may be increased by an additional 0.5-1.0 Joules/cm^2 above the prior incremental increases for each treatment. (Example: a patient whose exposure dose is being increased by 1.0 Joule/cm^2 may now have all subsequent doses increased by 1.5-2.0 Joules/cm^2.)

b. If there is no response, or only minimal response, after 15 treatments, the dosage of methoxsalen may be increased by 10 mg (a one-time increase in dosage). This increased dosage may be continued for the remainder of the course of treatment but should not be exceeded.

c. If a patient misses a treatment, the UVA exposure time of the next treatment should not be increased. If more than one treatment is missed, reduce the exposure by 0.5 Joules/cm^2 for each treatment missed.

d. If the lower extremities are not responding as well as the rest of the body and do not show erythema, cover all other body areas and give 25 percent of the present exposure dose as an additional exposure to the lower extremities. This additional exposure to the lower extremities should be terminated if erythema develops on these areas.

e. Non-responsive psoriasis: If a patient's generalized psoriasis is not responding, or if the condition appears to be worsening during treatment, the possibility of a generalized phototoxic reaction should be considered. This may be confirmed by the improvement of the condition following temporary discontinuance of this therapy for two weeks. If no improvement occurs during the interruption of treatment, this patient may be considered a treatment failure.

C. ALTERNATIVE EXPOSURE SCHEDULE:

As an alternative to increasing the UVA exposure at each treatment, the following schedule may be followed; this schedule may reduce the total number of Joules/cm^2 received by the patient over the entire course of therapy.

1. Incremental increases in UVA exposure for all patients may range from 0.5 to 1.5 Joules/cm^2, according to the patient's response to therapy.

2. Once Grade 2 clearing (see Table 2) has been reached and the patient is progressing adequately, UVA dosage is held constant. The dosage is maintained until Grade 4 clearing is reached.

3. If the rate of clearing significantly decreases, exposure dosage may be increased at each treatment (0.1–1.5 Joules/cm^2) until Grade 3 clearing and a satisfactory progress rate is attained. The UVA exposure will be held constant again until Grade 4 clearing is attained. These increases may be used also if the rate of clearing significantly decreases between Grade 3 and Grade 4 response. However, the possibility of a phototoxic reaction should be considered; see Non-responsive Psoriasis, above.

4. In summary, this schedule raises slightly the increments (Joules/cm^2) of UVA dosage, but limits these increases to those periods when the patient is not responding adequately. Otherwise, the UVA exposure is held at the lowest effective dose.

D. MAINTENANCE PHASE:

The goal of maintenance treatment is to keep the patient as symptom-free as possible with the least amount of UVA exposure.

1. SCHEDULE OF EXPOSURES: When patients have achieved 95 percent clearing, or Grade 4 response (Table 2), they may be placed on the following maintenance schedules (M_1–M_4), in sequence. It is recommended that each maintenance schedule be adhered to for at least 2 treatments (unless erythema or psoriatic flare occurs, in which case see (2a) and (2b) below).

Maintenance Schedules
M_1—once/week
M_2—once/2 weeks
M_3—once/3 weeks
M_4—p.r.n. (i.e., for flares)

2. LENGTH OF EXPOSURE: The UVA exposure for the first maintenance treatment of any schedule (except M_4 as noted below) is the same as that of the patient's last treatment under the previous schedule. For skin types I–IV, however, it is recommended that the maximum UVA dosage during maintenance treatments not exceed the following:

Skin Types	Joules/cm^2/treatment
I	12
II	14
III	18
IV	22

If the patient develops erythema or new lesions of psoriasis, proceed as follows:

a. Erythema: During maintenance therapy, the patient's tan and threshold dose for erythema may gradually decrease. If maintenance treatments produce significant erythema, the exposure to UVA should be decreased by 25 percent until further treatments no longer produce erythema.

b. Psoriasis: If the patient develops new areas of psoriasis during maintenance therapy (but still is classified as having a Grade 4 response), the exposure to UVA may be increased by 0.5–1.5 Joules/cm^2 at each treatment; this is appropriate for all types of patients. These increases are continued until the psoriasis is brought under control and the patient is again clear. The exposure being administered when this clearing is reached should be used for further maintenance treatment.

3. FLARES DURING MAINTENANCE: If the patient flares during maintenance treatment (i.e., develops psoriasis on more than 5 percent of the originally involved areas of the body) his maintenance treatment schedule may be changed to the preceding maintenance or clearing schedule. The patient may be kept on his schedule until again 95 percent clear. If the original maintenance treatment schedule is unable to control the psoriasis, the schedule may be changed to a more frequent regimen. If a flare occurs less than 6 weeks after the last treatment, 25 percent of the maximum exposure received during the clearing phase, with the clearing schedule received during the clearing phase, may be used and then proceed with the clearing schedule previously followed for this patient. (At 95 percent clearing, follow regular maintenance until the optimum maintenance schedule is determined for the patient.) If more than 6 weeks have elapsed since the last treatment was given, treat patients as if they were beginning therapy insofar as exposure dosages are concerned, since their threshold for erythema may have decreased.

Table 1. Grades of Erythema

Grades	Erythema
0	No erythema
1	Minimally perceptible erythema—faint pink
2	Marked erythema but with no edema
3	Fiery erythema with edema
4	Fiery erythema with edema and blistering

Table 2. Response to Therapy

Grade	Criteria	Percent Improvement (compared to original extent of disease)
−1	Psoriasis worse	0
0	No change	0
1	Minimal improvement— slightly less scale and/or erythema	5–20
2	Definite improvement— partial flattening of all plaques— less scaling and less erythema	20–50
3	Considerable improvement— nearly complete flattening of all plaques but borders of plaques still palpable	50–95
4	Clearing; complete flattening of plaques including borders; plaques may be outlined by pigmentation	95

XII. HOW SUPPLIED

Oxsoralen-Ultra Capsules, each containing 10 mg of methoxsalen (8-methoxypsoralen) in a soft gelatin capsule packaged in amber glass bottles are available as follows:

Unit Count	NDC Number
50	NDC 0187-0650-42

Store at 25°C (77°F); excursion permitted to 15°C–30°C (59°F–86°F).

ICN Pharmaceuticals, Inc. Rev. 4-98
3300 Hyland Ave.
Costa Mesa, Ca 92626, U.S.A. 2400–02 EL

BIBLIOGRAPHY

1. Levins, P.C., Gange, R.W., Momtaz-T.K., Parrish, J.A., and Fitzpatrick, T.B.: A New Liquid Formulation of 8-Methoxypsoralen: Bioactivity and Effect of Diet: JID, *82,* No. 2, pp. 185–187 (1984) and private communication.
2. Artuc, M., Stuettgen, G. Schalla, W., Schaefer, H., and Gazith, J.: Reversible binding of 5- and 8-methoxypsoralen to human serum proteins (albumin) and to epidermis in vitro: Brit. J. Dermat. *101,* pp. 669–677 (1979).
3. Mandula, B.B., Pathak, M.A., Nakayama, T., and Davidson, S.J.: Induction of mixed-function oxidases in mouse liver by psoralens., Ibid, *99,* pp. 687–692 (1978).
4. Pathak, M.A., Fitzpatrick, T.B., Parrish, J.A.: PSORIASIS, Proceedings of the Second International Symposium. Edited by E.M. Farber, A.J. Cox, Yorke Medical Books, pp. 262–265 (1977).
5. Dall'Acqua, F., Marciani, S., Ciavatta, L., Rodighiero, G.: Formation of interstrand cross-linkings in the photoreactions between furocoumarins and DNA; Z Naturforsch (B), *26,* pp. 561–569 (1971).
6. Cole, R.S.: Light-induced cross-linkings of DNA in the presence of a furocoumarin (psoralen), Biochem. Biophys. Acta, *217,* pp. 30–39 (1970).
7. Musajo, L, Rodighiero, G., Caporale, G., Dall'Acqua, F, Marciani, S., Bordin, F., Bacchichetti, F., Bevilacqua, R.: Photoreactions between Skin-Photosensitizing Furocoumarins and Nucleic Acids, *Sunlight and Man;* Normal and Abnormal Photobiologic Responses. Edited by M.A. Pathak, LC. Harber, M. Seiji et al. University of Tokyo Press, pp. 369–387 (1974).
8. Dall'Acqua, F., Vedaldi, D., Bordin, F., and Rodighiero, G.: New studies in the interaction between 8-methoxypsoralen and DNA *in vitro:* JID, *73,* pp. 191–197 (1979).
9. Yoshikawa, K., Mori, N., Sakakibara, S., Mizuno, N. Song, P.: Photo Conjugation of 8-methoxypsoralen with Proteins; Photochem. & Photobiol. *29,* pp. 1127–1133 (1979).
10. Hakim, R.E., Griffin, A.C.: Knox, J.M.: Erythema and tumor formation in methoxsalen treated mice exposed to fluorescent light; Arch. Dermatol. *82,* pp. 572–577 (1960).
11. O'Neal, M.A., Griffin, A.C.: The Effect of Oxypsoralen upon Ultraviolet Carcinogenesis in Albino Mice, Cancer Res., *17,* pp. 911–916 (1957).
12. Stern, R.S., Unpublished personal communication.
13. Stern, R.S., Parrish, J.A., Zierler, S.: Skin Carcinoma in Patients with Psoriasis Treated with Topical Tar and Artificial Ultraviolet Radiation. Lancet, *1,* pp. 732–735 (1980).
14. Stern, R.S., Laird, N., Melski, J. Parrish, J.A., Fitzpatrick, T.B., Bleich, H.L.: Cutaneous Squamous-Cell Carcinoma in Patients Treated with PUVA: NEJM, *310,* No. 18, pp. 1156–1161 (1984).
15. Roenigk, Jr., H.H., and 12 Cooperating Investigators: Skin Cancer in the PUVA-48 Cooperative Study of Psoriasis. Program for Forty-First Annual Meeting for The Society of Investigative Dermatology, Inc., Sheraton Washington Hotel, Washington, D.C., May 12, 13, and 14, 1980. Abstracts JID, *74,* No. 4, p. 250 (April, 1980).
16. Mosher, D.B., Pathak, M.A., Harris, T.J., Fitzpatrick, T.B.: Development of Cutaneous Lesions in Vitiligo During Long-Term PUVA Therapy. Program for Forty-First Annual Meeting for the Society for Investigative Dermatology, Inc., Sheraton Washington Hotel, Washington, D.C., May 12, 13, and 14, 1980. Abstracts JID, *74,* No. 4, p 259 (April, 1980).
17. Cloud, T.M. Hakim, R., Griffin, A.C.: Photosensitization of the eye with methoxsalen. I. Acute effects; Arch. Ophthalmol. *64,* pp. 346–352 (1960).
18. Cloud, T.M. Hakim, R., Griffin, A.C.: Photosensitization of the eye with methoxsalen. II. Chronic effects, Ibid, *66,* pp. 689–694 (1961).
19. Freeman, R.G., Troll, D.: Photosensitization of the eye by 8-methoxypsoralen, JID, *53,* pp. 449–453 (1969).
20. Lerman, S., Megaw, J., Willis, I.:Potential ocular complications from PUVA therapy and their prevention; JID, *74,* pp. 197–199 (1980).
21. Diffey, B.L., Medical Physics Handbook 11, Ultraviolet Radiation in Medicine, Adam Hilger, Ltd., Bristol, p. 86 (1982).

Shown in Product Identification Guide, page 317

PROSTIGMIN® ℞
[*pro-stig 'min*]
(neostigmine methylsulfate)
INJECTABLE

DESCRIPTION

Prostigmin (neostigmine methylsulfate) Injectable, an anticholinesterase agent, is a sterile aqueous solution intended for intramuscular, intravenous or subcutaneous administration.

Prostigmin Injectable is available in the following concentrations:

Prostigmin 1:2000 Ampuls — each mL contains 0.5 mg neostigmine methylsulfate compounded with 0.2% parabens (methyl and propyl) as preservatives and sodium hydroxide to adjust pH to approximately 5.9.

Prostigmin 1:4000 Ampuls— each mL contains 0.25 mg neostigmine methylsulfate compounded with 0.2% parabens (methyl and propyl) as preservatives and sodium hydroxide to adjust pH to approximately 5.9.

Prostigmin 1:1000 Multiple Dose Vials — each mL contains 1 mg neostigmine methylsulfate compounded with 0.45% phenol as preservative, 0.2 mg sodium acetate, and acetic acid and sodium hydroxide to adjust pH to approximately 5.9.

Prostigmin 1:2000 Multiple Dose Vials — each mL contains 0.5 mg neostigmine methylsulfate compounded with 0.45% phenol as preservative, 0.2 mg sodium acetate, and acetic acid and sodium hydroxide to adjust pH to approximately 5.9.

Chemically, neostigmine methylsulfate is (*m*-hydroxyphenyl)trimethylammonium methylsulfate dimethylcarbam-

Continued on next page

Prostigmin Injectable—Cont.

ate. It has a molecular weight of 334.39 and the following structural formula:

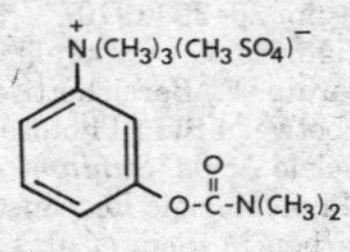

CLINICAL PHARMACOLOGY

Neostigmine inhibits the hydrolysis of acetylcholine by competing with acetylcholine for attachment to acetylcholinesterase at sites of cholinergic transmission. It enhances cholinergic action by facilitating the transmission of impulses across neuromuscular junctions. It also has a direct cholinomimetic effect on skeletal muscle and possibly on autonomic ganglion cells and neurons of the central nervous system. Neostigmine undergoes hydrolysis by cholinesterase and is also metabolized by microsomal enzymes in the liver. Protein binding to human serum albumin ranges from 15 to 25 percent.

Following intramuscular administration, neostigmine is rapidly absorbed and eliminated. In a study of five patients with myasthenia gravis, peak plasma levels were observed at 30 minutes, and the half-life ranged from 51 to 90 minutes. Approximately 80 percent of the drug was eliminated in urine within 24 hours; approximately 50% as the unchanged drug, and 30 percent as metabolites. Following intravenous administration, plasma half-life ranges from 47 to 60 minutes have been reported with a mean half-life of 53 minutes.

The clinical effects of neostigmine usually begin within 20 to 30 minutes after intramuscular injection and last from 2.5 to 4 hours.

INDICATIONS AND USAGE

Prostigmin is indicated for:

— the symptomatic control of myasthenia gravis when oral therapy is impractical.

— the prevention and treatment of postoperative distention and urinary retention after mechanical obstruction has been excluded.

— reversal of effects of nondepolarizing neuromuscular blocking agents (*e.g.*, tubocurarine, metocurine, gallamine, or pancuronium) after surgery.

CONTRAINDICATIONS

Prostigmin is contraindicated in patients with known hypersensitivity to the drug. It is also contraindicated in patients with peritonitis or mechanical obstruction of the intestinal or urinary tract.

WARNINGS

Prostigmin should be used with caution in patients with epilepsy, bronchial asthma, bradycardia, recent coronary occlusion, vagotonia, hyperthyroidism, cardiac arrhythmias or peptic ulcer. When large doses of Prostigmin are administered, the prior or simultaneous injection of atropine sulfate may be advisable. Separate syringes should be used for the Prostigmin and atropine. Because of the possibility of hypersensitivity in an occasional patient, atropine and antishock medication should always be readily available.

PRECAUTIONS

General: It is important to differentiate between myasthenic crisis and cholinergic crisis caused by overdosage of Prostigmin. Both conditions result in extreme muscle weakness but require radically different treatment. (See OVERDOSAGE section.)

Drug Interactions: Prostigmin does not antagonize, and may in fact prolong, the Phase I block of *depolarizing* muscle relaxants such as succinylcholine or decamethonium. Certain antibiotics, especially neomycin, streptomycin and kanamycin, have a mild but definite nondepolarizing blocking action which may accentuate neuromuscular block. These antibiotics should be used in the myasthenic patient only where definitely indicated, and then careful adjustment should be made of the anticholinesterase dosage. Local and some general anesthetics, antiarrhythmic agents and other drugs that interfere with neuromuscular transmission should be used cautiously, if at all, in patients with myasthenia gravis; the dose of Prostigmin may have to be increased accordingly.

Carcinogenesis, Mutagenesis and Impairment of Fertility: There have been no studies with Prostigmin which would permit an evaluation of its carcinogenic or mutagenic potential. Studies on the effect of Prostigmin on fertility and reproduction have not been performed.

Pregnancy:

Teratogenic Effects: Pregnancy Category C. There are no adequate or well-controlled studies of Prostigmin in either laboratory animals or in pregnant women. It is not known whether Prostigmin can cause fetal harm when administered to a pregnant woman or can affect reproductive capacity. Prostigmin should be given to a pregnant woman only if clearly needed.

Nonteratogenic Effects: Anticholinesterase drugs may cause uterine irritability and induce premature labor when given intravenously to pregnant women near term.

Nursing Mothers: It is not known whether Prostigmin is excreted in human milk. Because many drugs are excreted in human milk and because of the potential for serious adverse reactions from Prostigmin in nursing infants, a decision should be made whether to discontinue nursing or to discontinue the drug, taking into account the importance of the drug to the mother.

Pediatric Use: Safety and effectiveness in children have not been established.

ADVERSE REACTIONS

Side effects are generally due to an exaggeration of pharmacological effects of which salivation and fasciculation are the most common. Bowel cramps and diarrhea may also occur. The following additional adverse reactions have been reported following the use of either neostigmine bromide or neostigmine methylsulfate:

Allergic: Allergic reactions and anaphylaxis.

Neurologic: Dizziness, convulsions, loss of consciousness, drowsiness, headache, dysarthria, miosis and visual changes.

Cardiovascular: Cardiac arrhythmias (including bradycardia, tachycardia, A-V block and nodal rhythm) and nonspecific EKG changes have been reported, as well as cardiac arrest, syncope and hypotension. These have been predominantly noted following the use of the injectable form of Prostigmin.

Respiratory: Increased oral, pharyngeal and bronchial secretions, dyspnea, respiratory depression, respiratory arrest and bronchospasm.

Dermatologic: Rash and urticaria.

Gastrointestinal: Nausea, emesis, flatulence and increased peristalsis.

Genitourinary: Urinary frequency.

Musculoskeletal: Muscle cramps and spasms, arthralgia.

Miscellaneous: Diaphoresis, flushing and weakness.

OVERDOSAGE

Overdosage of Prostigmin can cause cholinergic crisis, which is characterized by increasing muscle weakness, and through involvement of the muscles of respiration, may result in death. Myasthenic crisis, due to an increase in the severity of the disease, is also accompanied by extreme muscle weakness and may be difficult to distinguish from cholinergic crisis on a symptomatic basis. However, such differentiation is extremely important because increases in the dose of Prostigmin or other drugs in this class, in the presence of cholinergic crisis or of a refractory or "insensitive" state, could have grave consequences. The two types of crises may be differentiated by the use of Tensilon® (edrophonium chloride) as well as by clinical judgment.

Treatment of the two conditions differs radically. Whereas the presence of *myasthenic crisis* requires more intensive anticholinesterase therapy, *cholinergic crisis* calls for the prompt withdrawal of all drugs of this type. The immediate use of atropine in cholinergic crisis is also recommended.

Atropine may also be used to abolish or minimize gastrointestinal side effects or other muscarinic reactions; but such use, by masking signs of overdosage, can lead to inadvertent induction of cholinergic crisis.

The LD_{50} of neostigmine methylsulfate in mice is 0.3 ± 0.02 mg/kg intravenously, 0.54 ± 0.03 mg/kg subcutaneously, and 0.395 ± 0.025 mg/kg intramuscularly; in rats the LD_{50} is 0.315 ± 0.019 mg/kg intravenously, 0.445 ± 0.032 mg/kg subcutaneously, and 0.423 ± 0.032 mg/kg intramuscularly.

DOSAGE AND ADMINISTRATION

Symptomatic control of myasthenia gravis: One mL of the 1:2000 solution (0.5 mg) subcutaneously or intramuscularly. Subsequent doses should be based on the individual patient's response. In most patients, however, oral treatment with Prostigmin (neostigmine bromide) tablets, 15 mg each, is adequate for control of symptoms.

Prevention of postoperative distention and urinary retention: One mL of the 1:4000 solution (0.25 mg) subcutaneously or intramuscularly as soon as possible after operation; repeat every 4 to 6 hours for two or three days.

Treatment of postoperative distention: One mL of the 1:2000 solution (0.5 mg) subcutaneously or intramuscularly, as required.

Treatment of urinary retention: One mL of the 1:2000 solution (0.5 mg) subcutaneously or intramuscularly. If urination does not occur within an hour, the patient should be catheterized. After the patient has voided, or the bladder has been emptied, continue the 0.5 mg injections every three hours for at least 5 injections.

Reversal of Effects of Nondepolarizing Neuromuscular Blocking Agents: When Prostigmin is administered intravenously, it is recommended that atropine sulfate (0.6 to 1.2 mg) also be given intravenously using separate syringes. Some authorities have recommended that the atropine be injected several minutes before the Prostigmin rather than concomitantly. The usual dose is 0.5 to 2 mg Prostigmin given by *slow* intravenous injection, repeated as required. Only in exceptional cases should the total dose of Prostigmin exceed 5 mg. It is recommended that the patient be well ventilated and a patent airway maintained until complete recovery of normal respiration is assured. The optimum time for administration of the drug is during hyperventilation when the carbon dioxide level of the blood is low. It should never be administered in the presence of high concentrations of halothane or cyclopropane. In cardiac cases and severely ill patients, it is advisable to titrate the exact dose of Prostigmin required, using a peripheral nerve stimulator device. In the presence of bradycardia, the pulse rate should be increased to about 80/minute with atropine before administering Prostigmin.

Parenteral drug products should be inspected visually for particulate matter and discoloration prior to administration, whenever solution and container permit.

HOW SUPPLIED

Prostigmin 1:2000 (0.5 mg neostigmine methylsulfate/mL), 1-mL ampuls — boxes of 10 (NDC 0187-3101-30).

Prostigmin 1:4000 (0.25 mg neostigmine methylsulfate/mL), 1-mL ampuls — boxes of 10 (NDC 0187-3102-40).

Prostigmin 1:1000 (1 mg neostigmine methylsulfate/mL), 10-mL multiple dose vials — boxes of 10 (NDC 0187-3103-50).

Prostigmin 1:2000 (0.5 mg neostigmine methylsulfate/mL), 10-mL multiple dose vials — boxes of 10 (NDC 0187-3104-60).

Manufactured for ICN Pharmaceuticals, Inc.
Costa Mesa, CA 92626
by Hoffmann-La Roche Inc.
Nutley, N.J. 07110
Rev. 7/90

PROSTIGMIN® ℞

[*pro-stig 'min*]
(neostigmine bromide)
TABLETS

DESCRIPTION

Prostigmin (neostigmine bromide), an anticholinesterase agent, is available for oral administration in 15-mg tablets. Each tablet also contains gelatin, lactose, corn starch, stearic acid, sugar and talc.

Chemically, neostigmine bromide is (*m* -hydroxyphenyl)trimethylammonium bromide dimethylcarbamate. It is a white, crystalline, bitter powder, soluble 1:1 in water, with a molecular weight of 303.20 and the following structural formula:

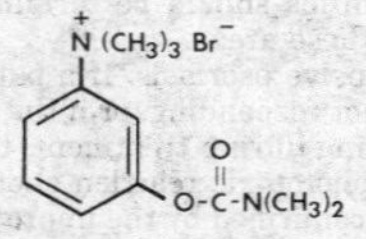

CLINICAL PHARMACOLOGY

Neostigmine inhibits the hydrolysis of acetylcholine by competing with acetylcholine for attachment to acetylcholinesterase at sites of cholinergic transmission. It enhances cholinergic action by facilitating the transmission of impulses across neuromuscular junctions. It also has a direct cholinomimetic effect on skeletal muscle and possibly on autonomic ganglion cells and neurons of the central nervous system. Neostigmine undergoes hydrolysis by cholinesterase and is also metabolized by microsomal enzymes in the liver. Protein binding to human serum albumin ranges from 15 to 25 percent.

Neostigmine bromide is poorly absorbed from the gastrointestinal tract following oral administration. As a rule, 15 mg of neostigmine bromide orally is equivalent to 0.5 mg of neostigmine methylsulfate parenterally, due to poor absorption of the tablet from the intestinal tract. In a study in fasting myasthenic patients, the extent of absorption was estimated to be 1 to 2 percent of the ingested 30-mg single oral dose. Peak concentrations in plasma occurred 1 to 2 hours following drug ingestion, with considerable individual variations. The half-life ranged from 42 to 60 minutes with a mean half-life of 52 minutes.

INDICATIONS AND USAGE

Prostigmin is indicated for the symptomatic treatment of myasthenia gravis. Its greatest usefulness is in prolonged therapy where no difficulty in swallowing is present. In acute myasthenic crisis where difficulty in breathing and swallowing is present, the parenteral form (neostigmine methylsulfate) should be used. The patient can be transferred to the oral form as soon as it can be tolerated.

CONTRAINDICATIONS

Prostigmin is contraindicated in patients with known hypersensitivity to the drug. Because of the presence of the bromide ion, it should not be used in patients with a previous history of reaction to bromides. It is contraindicated in patients with peritonitis or mechanical obstruction of the intestinal or urinary tract.

WARNINGS

Prostigmin should be used with caution in patients with epilepsy, bronchial asthma, bradycardia, recent coronary occlusion, vagotonia, hyperthyroidism, cardiac arrhythmias or peptic ulcer. As a rule, 15 mg of neostigmine bromide orally is equivalent to 0.5 mg of neostigmine methylsulfate parenterally, due to poor absorption of the tablet from the intestinal tract. Large doses should be avoided in situations where there might be an increased absorption rate from the intestinal tract. It should be used with caution when coadministered with anticholinergic drugs, in order to avoid reduction of intestinal motility.

PRECAUTIONS

General: It is important to differentiate between myasthenic crisis and cholinergic crisis caused by overdosage of Prostigmin. Both conditions result in extreme muscle weakness but require radically different treatment. (See OVERDOSAGE section.)

Drug Interactions: Certain antibiotics, especially neomycin, streptomycin and kanamycin, have a mild but definite nondepolarizing blocking action which may accentuate neuromuscular block. These antibiotics should be used in the myasthenic patient only where definitely indicated, and then careful adjustment should be made of adjunctive anticholinesterase dosage.
Local and some general anesthetics, antiarrhythmic agents and other drugs that interfere with neuromuscular transmission should be used cautiously, if at all, in patients with myasthenia gravis; the dose of Prostigmin may have to be increased accordingly.
Carcinogenesis, Mutagenesis and Impairment of Fertility: There have been no studies with Prostigmin which would permit an evaluation of its carcinogenic or mutagenic potential. Studies on the effect of Prostigmin on fertility and reproduction have not been performed.
Pregnancy:
Teratogenic Effects: Pregnancy Category C. There are no adequate or well-controlled studies of Prostigmin in either laboratory animals or in pregnant women. It is not known whether Prostigmin can cause fetal harm when administered to a pregnant woman or can affect reproductive capacity. Prostigmin should be given to a pregnant woman only if clearly needed.
Nonteratogenic Effects: Anticholinesterase drugs may cause uterine irritability and induce premature labor when given intravenously to pregnant women near term.
Nursing Mothers: It is not known whether Prostigmin is excreted in human milk. Because many drugs are excreted in human milk and because of the potential for serious adverse reactions from Prostigmin in nursing infants, a decision should be made whether to discontinue nursing or to discontinue the drug, taking into account the importance of the drug to the mother.
Pediatric Use: Safety and effectiveness in children have not been established.

ADVERSE REACTIONS

Side effects are generally due to an exaggeration of pharmacological effects of which salivation and fasciculation are the most common. Bowel cramps and diarrhea may also occur. The following additional adverse reactions have been reported following the use of either neostigmine bromide or neostigmine methylsulfate:
Allergic: Allergic reactions and anaphylaxis.
Neurologic: Dizziness, convulsions, loss of consciousness, drowsiness, headache, dysarthria, miosis and visual changes.
Cardiovascular: Cardiac arrhythmias (including bradycardia, tachycardia, A-V block and nodal rhythm) and nonspecific EKG changes have been reported, as well as cardiac arrest, syncope and hypotension. These have been predominantly noted following the use of the injectable form of Prostigmin.
Respiratory: Increased oral, pharyngeal and bronchial secretions, and dyspnea. Respiratory depression, respiratory arrest and bronchospasm have been reported following the use of the injectable form of Prostigmin.
Dermatologic: Rash and urticaria.
Gastrointestinal: Nausea, emesis, flatulence and increased peristalsis.
Genitourinary: Urinary frequency.
Musculoskeletal: Muscle cramps and spasms, arthralgia.
Miscellaneous: Diaphoresis, flushing and weakness.

OVERDOSAGE

Overdosage of Prostigmin can cause cholinergic crisis, which is characterized by increasing muscle weakness, and through involvement of the muscles of respiration, may result in death. Myasthenic crisis, due to an increase in the severity of the disease, is also accompanied by extreme muscle weakness and may be difficult to distinguish from cholinergic crisis on a symptomatic basis. However, such differentiation is extremely important because increases in the dose of Prostigmin or other drugs in this class, in the presence of cholinergic crisis or of a refractory or "insensitive" state, could have grave consequences. The two types of crises may be differentiated by the use of Tensilon® (edrophonium chloride) as well as by clinical judgment.
Treatment of the two conditions differs radically. Whereas the presence of *myasthenic crisis* requires more intensive anticholinesterase therapy, *cholinergic crisis* calls for the prompt withdrawal of all drugs of this type. The immediate use of atropine in cholinergic crisis is also recommended.
Atropine may also be used to abolish or minimize gastrointestinal side effects or other muscarinic reactions; but such use, by masking signs of overdosage, can lead to inadvertent induction of cholinergic crisis.
The LD_{50} of neostigmine methylsulfate in mice is 0.3 ± 0.02 mg/kg intravenously, 0.54 ± 0.03 mg/kg subcutaneously, and 0.395 ± 0.025 mg/kg intramuscularly; in rats the LD_{50} is 0.315 ± 0.019 mg/kg intravenously, 0.445 ± 0.032 mg/kg subcutaneously, and 0.423 ± 0.032 mg/kg intramuscularly.

DOSAGE AND ADMINISTRATION

The onset of action of Prostigmin given orally is slower than when given parenterally, but the duration of action is longer and the intensity of action more uniform. Dosage requirements for optimal results vary from 15 mg to 375 mg per day. In some instances it may be necessary to exceed these dosages, but the possibility of cholinergic crisis must be recognized. The average dose is 10 tablets (150 mg) administered over a 24-hour period. The interval between doses is of paramount importance. The dosage schedule should be adjusted for each patient and changed as the need arises. Frequently, therapy is required day and night. Larger portions of the total daily dose may be given at times when the patient is more prone to fatigue (afternoon, mealtimes, etc.). The patient should be encouraged to keep a daily record of his or her condition to assist the physician in determining an optimal therapeutic regimen.

HOW SUPPLIED

Scored, white tablets containing 15 mg neostigmine bromide — bottles of 100 (NDC 0187-3100-10). Imprint on tablets: (front) PROSTIGMIN 15: (back) ICN.
Manufactured for ICN Pharmaceuticals, Inc.
Costa Mesa, CA 92626
by Hoffmann-La Roche Inc.
Nutley, N.J. 07110
Rev. 9/97

Shown in Product Identification Guide, page 318

TENSILON® ℞

[*ten 'sil-on*]
(edrophonium chloride)
Injectable Solution
ampuls • vials

DESCRIPTION

Tensilon is a short and rapid-acting cholinergic drug. Chemically, edrophonium chloride is ethyl (*m*- hydroxyphenyl)dimethylammonium chloride.
10-ml vials: Each ml contains, in a sterile solution, 10 mg edrophonium chloride compounded with 0.45% phenol and 0.2% sodium sulfite as preservatives, buffered with sodium citrate and citric acid, and pH adjusted to approximately 5.4.
1-ml ampuls: Each ml contains, in a sterile solution, 10 mg edrophonium chloride compounded with 0.2% sodium sulfite, buffered with sodium citrate and citric acid, and pH adjusted to approximately 5.4.

ACTIONS

Tensilon is an anticholinesterase drug. Its pharmacological action is due primarily to the inhibition of acetylcholinesterase at sites of cholinergic transmission. Its effect is manifest within 30 to 60 seconds after injection and lasts an average of 10 minutes.

INDICATIONS

Tensilon is recommended for the differential diagnosis of myasthenia gravis and as an adjunct in the evaluation of treatment requirements in this disease. It may also be used for evaluating emergency treatment in myasthenic crises. Because of its brief duration of action, it is not recommended for maintenance therapy in myasthenia gravis.
Tensilon is also useful whenever a curare antagonist is needed to reverse the neuromuscular block produced by curare, tubocurarine, gallamine triethiodide or dimethyl-tubocurarine. It is *not* effective against decamethonium bromide and succinylcholine chloride. It may be used adjunctively in the treatment of respiratory depression caused by curare overdosage.

CONTRAINDICATIONS

Known hypersensitivity to anticholinesterase agents; intestinal and urinary obstructions of mechanical type.

WARNINGS

Whenever anticholinesterase drugs are used for testing, a syringe containing 1 mg of atropine sulfate should be immediately available to be given in aliquots intravenously to counteract severe cholinergic reactions which may occur in the hypersensitive individual, whether he is normal or myasthenic. Tensilon should be used with caution in patients with bronchial asthma or cardiac dysrhythmias. The transient bradycardia which sometimes occurs can be relieved by atropine sulfate. Isolated instances of cardiac and respiratory arrest following administration of Tensilon have been reported. It is postulated that these are vagotonic effects.
Tensilon solution contains sodium sulfite, a sulfite that may cause allergic-type reactions, including anaphylactic symptoms and life-threatening or less severe asthmatic episodes in certain susceptible people. The overall prevalence of sulfite sensitivity in the general population is unknown and probably low. Sulfite sensitivity is seen more frequently in asthmatic than in nonasthmatic people.
Usage in Pregnancy: The safety of Tensilon during pregnancy or lactation in humans has not been established. Therefore, use of Tensilon in women who may become pregnant requires weighing the drug's potential benefits against its possible hazards to mother and child.

PRECAUTIONS

Patients may develop "anticholinesterase insensitivity" for brief or prolonged periods. During these periods the patients should be carefully monitored and may need respiratory assistance. Dosages of anticholinesterase drugs should be reduced or withheld until patients again become sensitive to them.

ADVERSE REACTIONS

Careful observation should be made for severe cholinergic reactions in the hyperreactive individual. The myasthenic patient in crisis who is being tested with Tensilon should be observed for bradycardia or cardiac standstill and cholinergic reactions if an overdose is given. The following reactions common to anticholinesterase agents may occur, although not all of these reactions have been reported with the administration of Tensilon, probably because of its short duration of action and limited indications: **Eye:** Increased lacrimation, pupillary constriction, spasm of accommodation, diplopia, conjunctival hyperemia. **CNS:** Convulsions, dysarthria, dysphonia, dysphagia. **Respiratory:** Increased tracheobronchial secretions, laryngospasm, bronchiolar constriction, paralysis of muscles of respiration, central respiratory paralysis. **Cardiac:** Arrhythmias (especially bradycardia), fall in cardiac output leading to hypotension. **G.I.:** Increased salivary, gastric and intestinal secretion, nausea, vomiting, increased peristalsis, diarrhea, abdominal cramps. **Skeletal Muscle:** Weakness, fasciculations. **Miscellaneous:** Increased urinary frequency and incontinence, diaphoresis.

DOSAGE AND ADMINISTRATION

Tensilon Test in the Differential Diagnosis of Myasthenia Gravis:[1–8]
Intravenous Dosage (Adults): A tuberculin syringe containing 1 mL (10 mg) of Tensilon is prepared with an intravenous needle, and 0.2 mL (2 mg) is injected intravenously within 15 to 30 seconds. The needle is left *in situ. Only* if no reaction occurs after 45 seconds is the remaining 0.8 mL (8 mg) injected. If a cholinergic reaction (muscarinic side effects, skeletal muscle fasciculations and increased muscle weakness) occurs after injection of 0.2 mL (2 mg), the test is discontinued and atropine sulfate 0.4 mg to 0.5 mg is administered intravenously. After one-half hour the test may be repeated.
Intramuscular Dosage (Adults): In adults with inaccessible veins, dosage for intramuscular injection is 1 mL (10 mg) of Tensilon. Subjects who demonstrate hyperreactivity to this injection (cholinergic reaction), should be retested after one-half hour with 0.2 mL (2 mg) of Tensilon intramuscularly to rule out false-negative reactions.
Dosage (Children): The intravenous testing dose of Tensilon in children weighing up to 75 lbs is 0.1 mL (1 mg); above this weight, the dose is 0.2 mL (2 mg). If there is no response after 45 seconds, it may be titrated up to 0.5 mL (5 mg) in children under 75 lbs, given in increments of 0.1 mL (1 mg) every 30 to 45 seconds and up to 1 mL (10 mg) in heavier children. In infants, the recommended dose is 0.05 mL (0.5 mg). Because of technical difficulty with intravenous injection in children, the intramuscular route may be used. In children weighing up to 75 lbs, 0.2 mL (2 mg) is injected intramuscularly. In children weighing more than 75 lbs, 0.5 mL (5 mg) is injected intramuscularly. All signs which would appear with the intravenous test appear with the intramuscular test except that there is a delay of two to ten minutes before a reaction is noted.
Tensilon Test for Evaluation of Treatment Requirements in Myasthenia Gravis: The recommended dose is 0.1 mL to 0.2 mL (1 mg to 2 mg) of Tensilon, administered intravenously one hour after oral intake of the drug being used in treatment.[1–5] Response will be myasthenic in the undertreated patient, adequate in the controlled patient, and cholinergic in the overtreated patient. Responses to Tensilon in myasthenic and nonmyasthenic individuals are summarized in the following chart:[2]
[See table below]
Tensilon Test in Crisis: The term *crisis* is applied to the myasthenic whenever severe respiratory distress with ob-

Continued on next page

	Myasthenic*	**Adequate†**	**Cholinergic‡**
Muscle Strength (ptosis, diplopia, dysphonia, dysphagia, dysarthria, respiration, limb strength)	Increased	No change	Decreased
Fasciculations (orbicularis oculi, facial muscles, limb muscles)	Absent	Present or absent	Present or absent
Side reactions (lacrimation, diaphoresis, salivation, abdominal cramps, nausea, vomiting, diarrhea)	Absent	Minimal	Severe

* Myasthenic Response—occurs in untreated myasthenics and may serve to establish diagnosis; in patients under treatment, indicates that therapy is inadequate.
† Adequate Response—observed in treated patients when therapy is stabilized; a typical response in normal individuals. In addition to this response in nonmyasthenics, the phenomenon of forced lid closure is often observed in psychoneurotics.[1]
‡ Cholinergic Response—seen in myasthenics who have been overtreated with anticholinesterase drugs.

Tensilon—Cont.

jective ventilatory inadequacy occurs and the response to medication is not predictable. This state may be secondary to a sudden increase in severity of myasthenia gravis (myasthenic crisis), or to overtreatment with anticholinesterase drugs (cholinergic crisis).

When a patient is apneic, controlled ventilation must be secured immediately in order to avoid cardiac arrest and irreversible central nervous system damage. No attempt is made to test with Tensilon until respiratory exchange is adequate. *Dosage used at this time is most important:* If the patient is cholinergic, Tensilon will cause increased oropharyngeal secretions and further weakness in the muscles of respiration. If the crisis is myasthenic, the test clearly improves respiration and the patient can be treated with longer-acting intravenous anticholinesterase medication. When the test is performed, there should not be more than 0.2 mL (2 mg) Tensilon in the syringe. An intravenous dose of 0.1 mL (1 mg) is given initially. The patient's heart action is carefully observed. If, after an interval of one minute, this dose does not further impair the patient, the remaining 0.1 mL (1 mg) can be injected. If no clear improvement of respiration occurs after 0.2 mL (2 mg) dose, it is usually wisest to discontinue all anticholinesterase drug therapy and secure controlled ventilation by tracheostomy with assisted respiration.[5]

For Use as a Curare Antagonist: Tensilon should be administered by intravenous injection in 1 mL (10 mg) doses given slowly over a period of 30 to 45 seconds so that the onset of cholinergic reaction can be detected. This dosage may be repeated whenever necessary. The maximal dose for any one patient should be 4 mL (40 mg). Because of its brief effect, Tensilon should not be given prior to the administration of curare, tubocurarine, gallamine triethiodide or dimethyl-tubocurarine; it should be used at the time when its effect is needed. When given to counteract curare overdosage, the effect of each dose on the respiration should be carefully observed before it is repeated, and assisted ventilation should always be employed.

DRUG INTERACTIONS

Care should be given when administering this drug to patients with symptoms of myasthenic weakness who are also on anticholinesterase drugs. Since symptoms of anticholinesterase overdose (cholinergic crisis) may mimic underdosage (myasthenic weakness), their condition may be worsened by the use of this drug. (See OVERDOSAGE section for treatment.)

OVERDOSAGE

With drugs of this type, muscarine-like symptoms (nausea, vomiting, diarrhea, sweating, increased bronchial and salivary secretions and bradycardia) often appear with overdosage (cholinergic crisis). An important complication that can arise is obstruction of the airway by bronchial secretions. These may be managed with suction (especially if tracheostomy has been performed) and by the use of atropine. Many experts have advocated a wide range of dosages of atropine *(for Tensilon, see atropine dosage below),* but if there are copious secretions, up to 1.2 mg intravenously may be given initially and repeated every 20 minutes until secretions are controlled. Signs of atropine overdosage such as dry mouth, flush and tachycardia should be avoided as tenacious secretions and bronchial plugs may form. A total dose of atropine of 5 to 10 mg or even more may be required. The following steps should be taken in the management of overdosage of Tensilon:

1. Adequate respiratory exchange should be maintained by assuring an open airway, and the use of assisted respiration augmented by oxygen.
2. Cardiac function should be monitored until complete stabilization has been achieved.
3. Atropine sulfate in doses of 0.4 to 0.5 mg should be administered intravenously. This may be repeated every 3 to 10 minutes. Because of the short duration of action of Tensilon the total dose required will seldom exceed 2 mg.
4. If convulsions or shock is present, appropriate measures should be instituted.

HOW SUPPLIED

Multiple Dose Vials, 10 ml, boxes of 10 (NDC 0187-3200-20).
Ampuls, 1 ml, boxes of 10 (NDC 0187-3200-10).

REFERENCES

1. Osserman, K.E. and Kaplan, L.I., *J.A.M.A., 150:* 265, 1952.
2. Osserman, K.E., Kaplan, L.I. and Besson, G., *J. Mt. Sinai Hosp., 20:* 165, 1953.
3. Osserman, K.E. and Kaplan, L.I., *Arch. Neurol. & Psychiat., 70:* 385, 1953.
4. Osserman, K.E. and Teng, P., *J.A.M.A., 160:* 153, 1956.
5. Osserman, K.E. and Genkins, G., *Ann. N.Y. Acad. Sci., 135:* 312, 1966.
6. Tether, J.E., Second International Symposium Proceedings, Myasthenia Gravis, 1961, p. 444.
7. Tether, J.E., in H.F. Conn: *Current Therapy 1960,* Philadelphia, W. B. Saunders Company, p. 551.
8. Tether, J.E., in H.F. Conn: *Current Therapy 1965,* Philadelphia, W. B. Saunders Company, p. 556.

Manufactured for ICN Pharmaceuticals, Inc.
Costa Mesa, CA 92626
by Hoffmann-La Roche Inc.
Nutley, NJ 07110
Rev. 11/93

TESTRED® Ⓒ℞
Brand of
Methyltestosterone Capsules, USP 10 mg
Rx only

DESCRIPTION

The androgens are steroids that develop and maintain primary and secondary male sex characteristics.

Androgens are derivatives of cyclopentanoperhydrophenanthrene. Endogenous androgens are C-19 steroids with a side chain at C-17, and with two angular methyl groups. Testosterone is the primary endogenous androgen. In their active form, all drugs in the class have a 17-beta-hydroxy group. 17-alpha alkylation (methyltestosterone) increases the pharmacologic activity per unit weight compared to testosterone when given orally.

Methyltestosterone, a synthetic derivative of testosterone, is an androgenic preparation given by the oral route in a capsule form. Each capsule contains 10 mg of Methyltestosterone USP. It has the following structural formula:

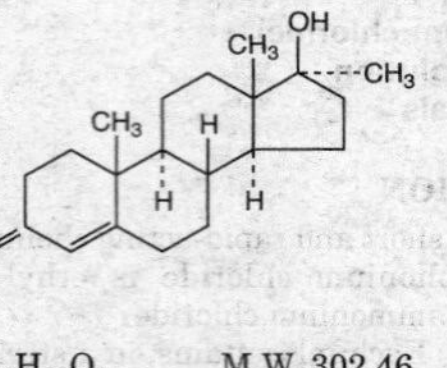

$C_{20}H_{30}O_2$ M.W. 302.46
17β-hydroxy-17-methylandrost-4-en-3-one

Methyltestosterone occurs as white or creamy white crystals or powder, which is soluble in various organic solvents but is practically insoluble in water.

Each capsule, for oral administration, contains 10 mg of Methyltestosterone. In addition, each capsule contains the following inactive ingredients: Corn starch NF, Gelatin NF, FD&C Blue #1, FD&C Red #40.

CLINICAL PHARMACOLOGY

Endogenous androgens are responsible for the normal growth and development of the male sex organs and for maintenance of secondary sex characteristics. These effects include the growth and maturation of prostate, seminal vesicles, penis, and scrotum. The development of male hair distribution, such as beard, pubic, chest, and axillary hair; laryngeal enlargement, vocal chord thickening, alterations in body musculature and fat distribution. Drugs in this class also cause retention of nitrogen, sodium, potassium, phosphorus, and decreased urinary excretion of calcium. Androgens have been reported to increase protein anabolism and decrease protein catabolism. Nitrogen balance is improved only when there is sufficient intake of calories and protein.

Androgens are responsible for the growth spurt of adolescence and for the eventual termination of linear growth which is brought about by fusion of the epiphyseal growth centers. In children, exogenous androgens accelerate linear growth rates, but may cause a disproportionate advancement in bone maturation. Use over long periods may result in fusion of the epiphyseal growth centers and termination of growth process. Androgens have been reported to stimulate the production of red blood cells by enhancing the production of erythropoietic stimulating factor.

During exogenous administration of androgens, endogenous testosterone release is inhibited through feedback inhibition of pituitary luteinizing hormone (LH). At large doses of exogenous androgens, spermatogenesis may also be suppressed through feedback inhibition of pituitary follicle stimulating hormone (FSH).

There is a lack of substantial evidence that androgens are effective in fractures, surgery, convalescence and functional uterine bleeding.

Pharmacokinetics

Testosterone given orally is metabolized by the gut and 44 percent is cleared by the liver of the first pass. Oral doses as high as 400 mg per day are needed to achieve clinically effective blood levels for full replacement therapy. The synthetic androgen, methyltestosterone, is less extensively metabolized by the liver and has a longer half-life. It is more suitable than testosterone for oral administration.

Testosterone in plasma is 98 percent bound to a specific testosterone-estradiol binding globulin, and about 2 percent is free. Generally, the amount of this sex-hormone binding globulin in the plasma will determine the distribution of testosterone between free and bound forms, and the free testosterone concentration will determine its half-life.

About 90 percent of a dose of testosterone is excreted in the urine as glucuronic and sulfuric acid conjugates of testosterone and its metabolites; about 6 percent of a dose is excreted in the feces, mostly in the unconjugated form. Inactivation of testosterone occurs primarily in the liver. Testosterone is metabolized to various 17-keto steroids through two different pathways. There are considerable variations of the half-life of testosterone as reported in the literature, ranging from 10 to 100 minutes.

In many tissues the activity of testosterone appears to depend on reduction to dihydrotestosterone, which binds to cytosol receptor proteins. The steroid-receptor complex is transported to the nucleus where it initiates transcription events and cellular changes related to androgen action.

INDICATIONS AND USAGE

1. Males

Androgens are indicated for replacement therapy in conditions associated with a deficiency or absence of endogenous testosterone;

a. Primary hypogonadism (congenital or acquired)—testicular failure due to cryptorchidism, bilateral torsions, orchitis, vanishing testis syndrome; or orchidectomy.
b. Hypogonadotropic hypogonadism (congenital or acquired)—idiopathic gonadotropin or LHRH deficiency, or pituitary-hypothalamic injury from tumors, trauma or radiation.
   If the above conditions occur prior to puberty, androgen replacement therapy will be needed during the adolescent years for development of secondary sexual characteristics. Prolonged androgen treatment will be required to maintain sexual characteristics in these and other males who develop testosterone deficiency after puberty.
c. Androgens may be used to stimulate puberty in carefully selected males with clearly delayed puberty. These patients usually have a familial pattern of delayed puberty that is not secondary to a pathological disorder; puberty is expected to occur spontaneously at a relatively late date. Brief treatment with conservative doses may occasionally be justified in these patients if they do not respond to psychological support. The potential adverse effect on bone maturation should be discussed with the patient and parents prior to androgen adminstration. An X-ray of the hand and wrist to determine bone age should be obtained every 6 months to assess the effect of treatment on the epiphyseal centers (see WARNINGS).

2. Females

Androgens may be used secondarily in women with advancing inoperable metastatic (skeletal) mammary cancer who are 1 to 5 years postmenopausal. Primary goals of therapy in these women include ablation of the ovaries. Other methods of counteracting estrogen activity are adrenalectomy, hypophysectomy, and/or antiestrogen therapy. This treatment has also been used in premenopausal women with breast cancer who have benefited from oophorectomy and are considered to have a hormone-responsive tumor. Judgment concerning androgen therapy should be made by an oncologist with expertise in this field.

CONTRAINDICATIONS

Androgens are contraindicated in men with carcinomas of the breast or with known or suspected carcinomas of the prostate, and in women who are or may become pregnant. When administered to pregnant women, androgens cause virilization of the external genitalia of the female fetus. This virilization includes clitoromegaly, abnormal vaginal development, and fusion of genital folds to form a scrotal-like structure. The degree of masculinization is related to the amount of drug given and the age of the fetus, and is most likely to occur in the female fetus when the drugs are given in the first trimester. If the patient becomes pregnant while taking these drugs, she should be apprised of the potential hazard to the fetus.

WARNINGS

In patients with breast cancer, androgen therapy may cause hypercalcemia by stimulating osteolysis. In this case, the drug should be discontinued.

Prolonged use of high doses of androgens has been associated with the development of peliosis hepatis and hepatic neoplasms including hepatocellular carcinoma. (See PRECAUTIONS-Carcinogenesis). Peliosis hepatis can be a life-threatening or fatal complication.

Cholestatic hepatitis and jaundice occur with 17-alphaalkylandrogens at a relatively low dose. If cholestatic hepatitis with jaundice appears or if liver function tests become abnormal, the androgen should be discontinued and the etiology should be determined. Drug-induced jaundice is reversible when the medication is discontinued.

Geriatric patients treated with androgens may be at an increased risk for the development of prostatic hypertrophy and prostatic carcinoma.

Edema with or without congestive heart failure may be a serious complication in patients with preexisting cardiac, renal, or hepatic disease. In addition to discontinuation of the drug, diuretic therapy may be required.

Gynecomastia frequently develops and occasionally persists in patients being treated for hypogonadism.

Androgen therapy should be used cautiously in healthy males with delayed puberty. The effect on bone maturation should be monitored by assessing bone age of the wrist and hand every 6 months. In children, androgen treatment may accelerate bone maturation without producing compensatory gain in linear growth. This adverse effect may result in compromised adult stature. The younger the child the greater the risk of compromising final mature height.

This drug has not been shown to be safe and effective for the enhancement of athletic performance. Because of the potential risk of serious adverse health effects, this drug should not be used for such purpose.

PRECAUTIONS

General

Women should be observed for signs of virilization (deepening of the voice, hirsutism, acne, clitoromegaly and menstrual irregularities). Discontinuation of drug therapy at the time of evidence of mild virilism is necessary to prevent irreversible virilization. Such virilization is usual following androgen use at high doses. A decision may be made by the patient and the physician that some virilization will be tolerated during treatment for breast carcinoma.

Information for the Patient

The physician should instruct patients to report any of the following side effects of androgens:

Adult or Adolescent Males:	Too frequent or persistent erections of the penis. Any male adolescent patient receiving androgens for delayed puberty should have bone development checked every six months.
Women:	Hoarseness, acne, changes in menstrual periods, or more hair on the face.
All Patients:	Any nausea, vomiting, changes in skin color or ankle swelling.

Laboratory Tests

1. Women with disseminated breast carcinoma should have frequent determination of urine and serum calcium levels during the course of androgen therapy. (See WARNINGS).
2. Because of the hepatotoxicity associated with the use of 17-alpha-alkylated androgens, liver function tests should be obtained periodically.
3. Periodic (every 6 months) x-ray examinations of bone age should be made during treatment of prepubertal males to determine the rate of bone maturation and the effects of androgen therapy on the epiphyseal centers.
4. Hemoglobin and hematocrit should be checked periodically for polycythemia in patients who are receiving high doses of androgens.

Drug Interactions

1. **Anticoagulants:** C-17 substituted derivatives of testosterone, such as methandrostenolone, have been reported to decrease the anticoagulant requirements of patients receiving oral anticoagulants. Patients receiving oral anticoagulant therapy require close monitoring, especially when androgens are started or stopped.
2. **Oxyphenbutazone:** Concurrent administration of oxyphenbutazone and androgens may result in elevated serum levels of oxyphenbutazone.
3. **Insulin:** In diabetic patients the metabolic effects of androgens may decrease blood glucose and insulin requirements.

Drug/Laboratory Test Interferences

Androgens may decrease levels of thyroxine-binding globulin, resulting in decreased total T4 serum levels and increased resin uptake of T3 and T4. Free thyroid hormone levels remain unchanged, however, and there is no clinical evidence of thyroid dysfunction.

Carcinogenesis

Animal Data

Testosterone has been tested by subcutaneous injection and implantation in mice and rats. The implant induced cervical-uterine tumors in mice, which metastasized in some cases. There is suggestive evidence that injection of testosterone into some strains of female mice increases their susceptibility to hepatoma. Testosterone is also known to increase the number of tumors and decrease the degree of differentiation of chemically induced carcinomas of the liver in rats.

Human Data

There are rare reports of hepatocellular carcinoma in patients receiving long-term therapy with androgens in high doses. Withdrawal of the drugs did not lead to regression of the tumors in all cases.

Geriatric patients treated with androgens may be at an increased risk for the development of prostatic hypertrophy and prostatic carcinoma.

Pregnancy

Teratogenic effects. Pregnancy Category X (See CONTRAINDICATIONS).

Nursing Mothers

It is not known whether androgens are excreted in human milk. Because many drugs are excreted in human milk and because of the potential for serious adverse reactions in nursing infants from androgens, a decision should be made whether to discontinue nursing or to discontinue the drug, taking into account the importance of the drug to the mother.

Pediatric Use

Androgen therapy should be used very cautiously in children and only by specialists who are aware of the adverse effects on bone maturation. Skeletal maturation must be monitored every six months by an x-ray of hand and wrist (See INDICATIONS AND USAGE and WARNINGS).

ADVERSE REACTIONS

Endocrine and Urogenital

Female: The most common side effects of androgen therapy are amenorrhea and other menstrual irregularities, inhibition of gonadotropin secretion, and virilization, including deepening of the voice and clitoral enlargement. The latter usually is not reversible after androgens are discontinued. When administered to a pregnant woman androgens cause virilization of external genitalia of the female fetus.

Male: Gynecomastia, and excessive frequency and duration of penile erections. Oligospermia may occur at high dosages (see CLINICAL PHARMACOLOGY).

Skin and appendages: Hirsutism, male pattern of baldness, and acne.

Fluid and Electrolyte Disturbances: Retention of sodium, chloride, water, potassium, calcium, and inorganic phosphates.

Gastrointestinal: Nausea, cholestatic jaundice, alterations in liver function tests, rarely hepatocellular neoplasms and peliosis hepatis (see WARNINGS).

Hematologic: Suppression of clotting factors II, V, VII, and X, bleeding in patients on concomitant anticoagulant therapy, and polycythemia.

Nervous System: Increased or decreased libido, headache, anxiety, depression, and generalized paresthesia.

Metabolic: Increased serum cholesterol.

Miscellaneous: Rarely anaphylactoid reactions.

DRUG ABUSE AND DEPENDENCE

Testred Capsules are classified as a schedule III Controlled Substance under the Anabolic Steroids Act of 1990.

OVERDOSAGE

There have been no reports of acute overdosage with the androgens.

DOSAGE AND ADMINISTRATION

Methyltestosterone capsules are administered orally. The suggested dosage for androgens varies depending on the age, sex, and diagnosis of the individual patient. Dosage is adjusted according to the patient's response and the appearance of adverse reactions.

Replacement therapy in androgen-deficient males is 10 to 50 mg of methyltestosterone daily. Various dosage regimens have been used to induce pubertal changes in hypogonadal males; some experts have advocated lower dosages initially, gradually increasing the dose as puberty progresses with or without a decrease to maintenance levels. Other experts emphasize that higher dosages are needed to induce pubertal changes and lower dosages can be used for maintenance after puberty. The chronological and skeletal ages must be taken into consideration, both in determining the initial dose and in adjusting the dose.

Doses used in delayed puberty generally are in the lower range of that given above, and for a limited duration, for example 4 to 6 months.

Women with metastatic breast carcinoma must be followed closely because androgen therapy occasionally appears to accelerate the disease. Thus, many experts prefer to use the shorter acting androgen preparations rather than those with prolonged activity for treating breast carcinoma, particularly during the early stages of androgen therapy. The dosage of methyltestosterone for androgen therapy in breast carcinoma in females is from 50–200 mg daily.

HOW SUPPLIED

Methyltestosterone capsules USP 10 mg are red capsules imprinted "ICN 0901" on both sections. They are available in bottles of 100 (NDC 0187-0901-01).

Store at 25°C (77°F); excursion permitted to 15°C–30°C (59°F–86°F).

Revision May 1999

ICN Pharmaceuticals, Inc.
ICN Plaza
3300 Hyland Avenue
Costa Mesa, CA 92626
(714) 545-0100

Shown in Product Identification Guide, page 318

VIRAZOLE® ℞

[*vira 'zahl '*]

(Ribavirin for Inhalation Solution)

WARNINGS:

USE OF AEROSOLIZED VIRAZOLE IN PATIENTS REQUIRING MECHANICAL VENTILATOR ASSISTANCE SHOULD BE UNDERTAKEN ONLY BY PHYSICIANS AND SUPPORT STAFF FAMILIAR WITH THE SPECIFIC VENTILATOR BEING USED AND THIS MODE OF ADMINISTRATION OF THE DRUG. STRICT ATTENTION MUST BE PAID TO PROCEDURES THAT HAVE BEEN SHOWN TO MINIMIZE THE ACCUMULATION OF DRUG PRECIPITATE, WHICH CAN RESULT IN MECHANICAL VENTILATOR DYSFUNCTION AND ASSOCIATED INCREASED PULMONARY PRESSURES (SEE WARNINGS).

SUDDEN DETERIORATION OF RESPIRATORY FUNCTION HAS BEEN ASSOCIATED WITH INITIATION OF AEROSOLIZED VIRAZOLE USE IN INFANTS. RESPIRATORY FUNCTION SHOULD BE CAREFULLY MONITORED DURING TREATMENT. IF INITIATION OF AEROSOLIZED VIRAZOLE TREATMENT APPEARS TO PRODUCE SUDDEN DETERIORATION OF RESPIRATORY FUNCTION, TREATMENT SHOULD BE STOPPED AND REINSTITUTED ONLY WITH EXTREME CAUTION, CONTINUOUS MONITORING AND CONSIDERATION OF CONCOMITANT ADMINISTRATION OF BRONCHODILATORS (SEE WARNINGS).

VIRAZOLE IS NOT INDICATED FOR USE IN ADULTS. PHYSICIANS AND PATIENTS SHOULD BE AWARE THAT RIBAVIRIN HAS BEEN SHOWN TO PRODUCE TESTICULAR LESIONS IN RODENTS AND TO BE TERATOGENIC IN ALL ANIMAL SPECIES IN WHICH ADEQUATE STUDIES HAVE BEEN CONDUCTED (RODENTS AND RABBITS); (SEE CONTRAINDICATIONS).

DESCRIPTION

Virazole® is a brand name for ribavirin, a synthetic nucleoside with antiviral activity. VIRAZOLE for inhalation solution is a sterile, lyophilized powder to be reconstituted for aerosol administration. Each 100 ml glass vial contains 6 grams of ribavirin, and when reconstituted to the recommended volume of 300 ml with sterile water for injection or sterile water for inhalation (no preservatives added), will contain 20 mg of ribavirin per ml, pH approximately 5.5. Aerosolization is to be carried out in a Small Particle Aerosol Generator (SPAG-2) nebulizer only.

Ribavirin is 1-beta-D-ribofuranosyl-1H-1,2,4-triazole-3-carboxamide, with the following structural formula:

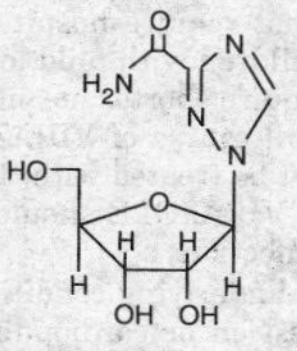

Ribavirin is a stable, white crystalline compound with a maximum solubility in water of 142 mg/ml at 25°C and with only a slight solubility in ethanol. The empirical formula is $C_8H_{12}N_4O_5$ and the molecular weight is 244.21.

CLINICAL PHARMACOLOGY

Mechanism of Action

In cell cultures the inhibitory activity of ribavirin for respiratory syncytial virus (RSV) is selective. The mechanism of action is unknown. Reversal of the *in vitro* antiviral activity by guanosine or xanthosine suggests ribavirin may act as an analogue of these cellular metabolites.

Microbiology

Ribavirin has demonstrated antiviral activity against RSV *in vitro*[1] and in experimentally infected cotton rats.[2] Several clinical isolates of RSV were evaluated for ribavirin susceptibility by plaque reduction in tissue culture. Plaques were reduced 85–98% by 16 µg/ml; however, results may vary with the test system. The development of resistance has not been evaluated *in vitro* or in clinical trials.

In addition to the above, ribavirin has been shown to have *in vitro* activity against influenza A and B viruses and herpes simplex virus, but the clinical significance of these data is unknown.

Immunologic Effects

Neutralizing antibody responses to RSV were decreased in aerosolized VIRAZOLE treated infants compared to placebo treated infants.[3] One study also showed that RSV-specific IgE antibody in bronchial secretions was decreased in patients treated with aerosolized VIRAZOLE. In rats, ribavirin administration resulted in lymphoid atrophy of the thymus, spleen, and lymph nodes. Humoral immunity was reduced in guinea pigs and ferrets. Cellular immunity was also mildly depressed in animal studies. The clinical significance of these observations is unknown.

Pharmacokinetics

Assay for VIRAZOLE in human materials is by a radioimmunoassay which detects ribavirin and at least one metabolite.

VIRAZOLE brand of ribavirin, when administered by aerosol, is absorbed systemically. Four pediatric patients inhaling VIRAZOLE aerosol administered by face mask for 2.5 hours each day for 3 days had plasma concentrations ranging from 0.44 to 1.55 µM, with a mean concentration of 0.76 µM. The plasma half-life was reported to be 9.5 hours. Three pediatric patients inhaling aerosolized VIRAZOLE administered by face mask or mist tent for 20 hours each day for 5 days had plasma concentrations ranging from 1.5 to 14.3 µM, with a mean concentration of 6.8 µM.

The bioavailability of aerosolized VIRAZOLE is unknown and may depend on the mode of aerosol delivery. After aerosol treatment, peak plasma concentrations of ribavirin are 85% to 98% less than the concentration that reduced RSV plaque formation in tissue culture. After aerosol treatment, respiratory tract secretions are likely to contain ribavirin in concentrations many fold higher than those required to reduce plaque formation. However, RSV is an intracellular virus and it is unknown whether plasma concentrations or respiratory secretion concentrations of the drug better reflect intracellular concentrations in the respiratory tract.

In man, rats, and rhesus monkeys, accumulation of ribavirin and/or metabolites in the red blood cells has been noted, plateauing in red cells in man in about 4 days and gradually declining with an apparent half-life of 40 days (the half-life of erythrocytes). The extent of accumulation of ribavirin following inhalation therapy is not well defined.

Animal Toxicology

Ribavirin, when administered orally or as an aerosol, produced cardiac lesions in mice, rats, and monkeys, when given at doses of 30, 36 and 120 mg/kg or greater for 4 weeks or more (estimated human equivalent doses of 4.8, 12.3 and 111.4 mg/kg for a 5 kg child, or 2.5, 5.1 and 40

Continued on next page

Virazole—Cont.

mg/kg for a 60 kg adult, based on body surface area adjustment). Aerosolized ribavirin administered to developing ferrets at 60 mg/kg for 10 or 30 days resulted in inflammatory and possibly emphysematous changes in the lungs. Proliferative changes were seen in the lungs following exposure at 131 mg/kg for 30 days. The significance of these findings to human administration is unknown.

INDICATIONS AND USAGE

VIRAZOLE is indicated for the treatment of hospitalized infants and young children with severe lower respiratory tract infections due to respiratory syncytial virus. Treatment early in the course of severe lower respiratory tract infection may be necessary to achieve efficacy.

Only severe RSV lower respiratory tract infection should be treated with VIRAZOLE. The vast majority of infants and children with RSV infection have disease that is mild, self-limited, and does not require hospitalization or antiviral treatment. Many children with mild lower respiratory tract involvement will require shorter hospitalization than would be required for a full course of VIRAZOLE aerosol (3 to 7 days) and should not be treated with the drug. Thus the decision to treat with VIRAZOLE should be based on the severity of the RSV infection.

The presence of an underlying condition such as prematurity, immunosuppression or cardiopulmonary disease may increase the severity of clinical manifestations and complications of RSV infection.

Use of aerosolized VIRAZOLE in patients requiring mechanical ventilator assistance should be undertaken only by physicians and support staff familiar with this mode of administration and the specific ventilator being used (see Warnings, and Dosage and Administration).

Diagnosis

RSV infection should be documented by a rapid diagnostic method such as demonstration of viral antigen in respiratory tract secretions by immunofluorescence[3,4] or ELISA[5] before or during the first 24 hours of treatment. Treatment may be initiated while awaiting rapid diagnostic test results. However, treatment should not be continued without documentation of RSV infection.

Non-culture antigen detection techniques may have false positive or false negative results. Assessment of the clinical situation, the time of year and other parameters may warrant reevaluation of the laboratory diagnosis.

Description of Studies

Non-Mechanically-Ventilated Infants: In two placebo controlled trials in infants hospitalized with RSV lower respiratory tract infection, aerosolized VIRAZOLE treatment had a therapeutic effect, as judged by the reduction in severity of clinical manifestations of disease by treatment day 3.[3,4] Treatment was most effective when instituted within the first 3 days of clinical illness. Virus titers in respiratory secretions were also significantly reduced with VIRAZOLE in one of these original studies.[4] Additional controlled studies conducted since these initial trials of aerosolized VIRAZOLE in the treatment of RSV infection have supported these data.

Mechanically-Ventilated Infants: A randomized, double-blind, placebo controlled evaluation of aerosolized VIRAZOLE at the recommended dose was conducted in 28 infants requiring mechanical ventilation for respiratory failure caused by documented RSV infection.[6] Mean age was 1.4 months (SD, 1.7 months). Seven patients had underlying diseases predisposing them to severe infection and 21 were previously normal. Aerosolized VIRAZOLE treatment significantly decreased the duration of mechanical ventilation required (4.9 vs. 9.9 days, p=0.01) and duration of required supplemental oxygen (8.7 vs 13.5 days, p=0.01). Intensive patient management and monitoring techniques were employed in this study. These included endotracheal tube suctioning every 1 to 2 hours; recording of proximal airway pressure, ventilatory rate, and F_1O_2 every hour; and arterial blood gas monitoring every 2 to 6 hours. To reduce the risk of VIRAZOLE precipitation and ventilator malfunction, heated wire tubing, two bacterial filters connected in series in the expiratory limb of the ventilator (with filter changes every 4 hours), and water column pressure release valves to monitor internal ventilator pressures were used in connecting ventilator circuits to the SPAG-2.

Employing these techniques, no technical difficulties with VIRAZOLE administration were encountered during the study. Adverse events consisted of bacterial pneumonia in one case, staphyloccus bacteremia in one case and two cases of post-extubation stridor. None were felt to be related to VIRAZOLE administration.

CONTRAINDICATIONS

VIRAZOLE is contraindicated in individuals who have shown hypersensitivity to the drug or its components, and in women who are or may become pregnant during exposure to the drug. Ribavirin has demonstrated significant teratogenic and/or embryocidal potential in all animal species in which adequate studies have been conducted (rodents and rabbits). Therefore, although clinical studies have not been performed, it should be assumed that VIRAZOLE may cause fetal harm in humans. Studies in which the drug has been administered systemically demonstrate that ribavirin is concentrated in the red blood cells and persists for the life of the erythrocyte.

WARNINGS

SUDDEN DETERIORATION OF RESPIRATORY FUNCTION HAS BEEN ASSOCIATED WITH INITIATION OF AEROSOLIZED VIRAZOLE USE IN INFANTS. Respiratory function should be carefully monitored during treatment. If initiation of aerosolized VIRAZOLE treatment appears to produce sudden deterioration of respiratory function, treatment should be stopped and reinstituted only with extreme caution, continuous monitoring, and consideration of concomitant administration of bronchodilators.

Use with Mechanical Ventilators

USE OF AEROSOLIZED VIRAZOLE IN PATIENTS REQUIRING MECHANICAL VENTILATOR ASSISTANCE SHOULD BE UNDERTAKEN ONLY BY PHYSICIANS AND SUPPORT STAFF FAMILIAR WITH THIS MODE OF ADMINISTRATION AND THE SPECIFIC VENTILATOR BEING USED. Strict attention must be paid to procedures that have been shown to minimize the accumulation of drug precipitate, which can result in mechanical ventilator dysfunction and associated increased pulmonary pressures. These procedures include the use of bacteria filters in series in the expiratory limb of the ventilator circuit with frequent changes (every 4 hours), water column pressure release valves to indicate elevated ventilator pressures, frequent monitoring of these devices and verification that ribavirin crystals have not accumulated within the ventilator circuitry, and frequent suctioning and monitoring of the patient (see Clinical Studies).

Those administering aersolized VIRAZOLE in conjunction with mechanical ventilator use should be thoroughly familiar with detailed descriptions of these procedures as outlined in the SPAG-2 manual.

PRECAUTIONS

General: Patients with severe lower respiratory tract infection due to respiratory syncytial virus require optimum monitoring and attention to respiratory and fluid status (see SPAG-2 manual).

Drug Interactions

Clinical studies of interactions of VIRAZOLE with other drugs commonly used to treat infants with RSV infections, such as digoxin, bronchodilators, other antiviral agents, antibiotics, or anti-metabolites have not been conducted. Interference by VIRAZOLE with laboratory tests has not been evaluated.

Carcinogenesis and Mutagenesis

Ribavirin increased the incidence of cell transformations and mutations in mouse Balb/c 3T3 (fibroblasts) and L5178Y (lymphoma) cells at concentrations of 0.015 and 0.03–5.0 mg/ml, respectively (without metabolic activation.) Modest increases in mutation rates (3–4x) were observed at concentrations between 3.75–10.0 mg/ml in L5178Y cells *in vitro* with the addition of a metabolic activation fraction. In the mouse micronucleus assay, ribavirin was clastogenic at intravenous doses of 20–200 mg/kg, (estimated human equivalent of 1.67–16.7 mg/kg, based on body surface area adjustment for a 60 kg adult). Ribavirin was not mutagenic in a dominant lethal assay in rats at intraperitoneal doses between 50–200 mg/kg when administered for 5 days (estimated human equivalent of 7.14–28.6 mg/kg, based on body surface area adjustment; see Pharmacokinetics).

In vivo carcinogenicity studies with ribavirin are incomplete. However, results of a chronic feeding study with ribavirin in rats, at doses of 16–100 mg/kg/day (estimated human equivalent of 2.3–14.3 mg/kg/day, based on body surface area adjustment for the adult), suggest that ribavirin may induce benign mammary, pancreatic, pituitary and adrenal tumors. Preliminary results of 2 oral gavage oncogenicity studies in the mouse and rat (18–24 months; doses of 20–75 and 10–40 mg/kg/day, respectively [estimated human equivalent of 1.67–6.25 and 1.43–5.71 mg/kg/day, respectively, based on body surface area adjustment for the adult]) are inconclusive as to the carcinogenic potential of ribavirin (see Pharmacokinetics). However, these studies have demonstrated a relationship between chronic ribavirin exposure and increased incidences of vascular lesions (microscopic hemorrhages in mice) and retinal degeneration (in rats).

Impairment of Fertility

The fertility of ribavirin-treated animals (male or female) has not been fully investigated. However, in the mouse, administration of ribavirin at doses between 35–150 mg/kg/day (estimated human equivalent of 2.92–12.5 mg/kg/day, based on body surface area adjustment for the adult) resulted in significant seminiferous tubule atrophy, decreased sperm concentrations, and increased numbers of sperm with abnormal morphology. Partial recovery of sperm production was apparent 3–6 months following dose cessation. In several additional toxicology studies, ribavirin has been shown to cause testicular lesions (tubular atrophy), in adult rats at oral dose levels as low as 16 mg/kg/day (estimated human equivalent of 2.29 mg/kg/day, based on body surface area adjustment; see Pharmacokinetics). Lower doses were not tested. The reproductive capacity of treated male animals has not been studied.

Pregnancy: Category X

Ribavirin has demonstrated significant teratogenic and/or embryocidal potential in all animal species in which adequate studies have been conducted. Teratogenic effects were evident after single oral doses of 2.5 mg/kg or greater in the hamster, and after daily oral doses of 0.3 and 1.0 mg/kg in the rabbit and rat, respectively (estimated human equivalent doses of 0.12 and 0.14 mg/kg, based on body surface area adjustment for the adult). Malformations of the skull, palate, eye, jaw, limbs, skeleton, and gastrointestinal tract were noted. The incidence and severity of teratogenic effects increased with escalation of the drug dose. Survival of fetuses and offspring was reduced. Ribavirin caused embryolethality in the rabbit at daily oral dose levels as low as 1 mg/kg. No teratogenic effects were evident in the rabbit and rat administered daily oral doses of 0.1 and 0.3 mg/kg, respectively with estimated human equivalent doses of 0.01 and 0.04 mg/kg, based on body surface area adjustment (see Pharmacokinetics). These doses are considered to define the "No Observable Teratogenic Effects Level" (NOTEL) for ribavirin in the rabbit and rat.

Following oral administration of ribavirin in the pregnant rat (1.0 mg/kg) and rabbit (0.3 mg/kg), mean plasma levels of drug ranged from 0.10–0.20 μM [0.024–0.049 μg/ml] at 1 hour after dosing, to undetectable levels at 24 hours. At 1 hour following the administration of 0.3 or 0.1 mg/kg in the rat and rabbit (NOTEL), respectively, mean plasma levels of drug in both species were near or below the limit of detection (0.05 μM; see Pharmacokinetics),

Although clinical studies have not been performed, VIRAZOLE may cause fetal harm in humans. As noted previously, ribavirin is concentrated in red blood cells and persists for the life of the cell. Thus the terminal half-life for the systemic elimination of ribavirin is essentially that of the half-life of circulating erythrocytes. The minimum interval following exposure to VIRAZOLE before pregnancy may be safely initiated is unknown (see Contraindications, Warnings, and Information for Health Care Personnel).

Nursing Mothers

VIRAZOLE has been shown to be toxic to lactating animals and their offspring. It is not known if VIRAZOLE is excreted in human milk.

Information for Health Care Personnel

Health care workers directly providing care to patients receiving aerosolized VIRAZOLE should be aware that ribavirin has been shown to be teratogenic in all animal species in which adequate studies have been conducted (rodents and rabbits). Although no reports of teratogenesis in offspring of mothers who were exposed to aerosolized VIRAZOLE during pregnancy have been confirmed, no controlled studies have been conducted in pregnant women. Studies of environmental exposure in treatment settings have shown that the drug can disperse into the immediate bedside area during routine patient care activities with highest ambient levels closest to the patient and extremely low levels outside of the immediate bedside area. Adverse reactions resulting from actual occupational exposure in adults are described below (see Adverse Events in Health Care Workers). Some studies have documented ambient drug concentrations at the bedside that could potentially lead to systemic exposures above those considered safe for exposure during pregnancy (1/1000 of the NOTEL dose in the most sensitive animal species).[7,8,9]

A 1992 study conducted by the National Institute of Occupational Safety and Health (NIOSH) demonstrated measurable urine levels of ribavirin in health care workers exposed to aerosol in the course of direct patient care.[7] Levels were lowest in workers caring for infants receiving aerosolized VIRAZOLE with mechanical ventilation and highest in those caring for patients being administered the drug via an oxygen tent or hood. This study employed a more sensitive assay to evaluate ribavirin levels in urine than was available for several previous studies of environmental exposure that failed to detect measurable ribavirin levels in exposed workers. Creatinine adjusted urine levels in the NIOSH study ranged from less than 0.001 to 0.140 μM of ribavirin per gram of creatinine in exposed workers. However, the relationship between urinary ribavirin levels in exposed workers, plasma levels in animal studies, and the specific risk of teratogenesis in exposed pregnant women is unknown.

It is good practice to avoid unnecessary occupational exposure to chemicals wherever possible. Hospitals are encouraged to conduct training programs to minimize potential occupational exposure to VIRAZOLE. Health care workers who are pregnant should consider avoiding direct care of patients receiving aerosolized VIRAZOLE. If close patient contact cannot be avoided, precautions to limit exposure should be taken. These include administration of VIRAZOLE in negative pressure rooms; adequate room ventilation (at least six air exchanges per hour); the use of VIRAZOLE aerosol scavenging devices; turning off the SPAG-2 device for 5 to 10 minutes prior to prolonged patient contact, and wearing appropriately fitted respirator masks. Surgical masks do not provide adequate filtration of VIRAZOLE particles. Further information is available from NIOSH's Hazard Evaluation and Technical Assistance Branch and additional recommendations have been published in an Aerosol Consensus Statement by the American Respiratory Care Foundation and the American Association for Respiratory Care.[10]

ADVERSE REACTIONS

The description of adverse reactions is based on events from clinical studies (approximately 200 patients) conducted prior to 1986, and the controlled trial of aerosolized VIRAZOLE conducted in 1989–1990. Additional data from spontaneous post-marketing reports of adverse events in individual patients have been available since 1986.

Deaths

Deaths during or shortly after treatment with aerosolized VIRAZOLE have been reported in 20 cases of patients treated with VIRAZOLE (12 of these patients were being treated for RSV infections). Several cases have been characterized as "possibly related" to VIRAZOLE by the treating physician; these were in infants who experienced worsening respiratory status related to bronchospasm while being treated with the drug. Several other cases have been attributed to mechanical ventilator malfunction in which VIRAZOLE precipitation within the ventilator apparatus led to excessively high pulmonary pressures and diminished oxygenation. In these cases the monitoring procedures described in the current package insert were not employed (see Description of Studies, Warnings, and Dosage and Administration).

Pulmonary and Cardiovascular

Pulmonary function significantly deteriorated during aerosolized VIRAZOLE treatment in six of six adults with chronic obstructive lung disease and in four of six asthmatic adults. Dyspnea and chest soreness were also reported in the latter group. Minor abnormalities in pulmonary function were also seen in healthy adult volunteers.

In the original study population of approximately 200 infants who received aerosolized VIRAZOLE, several serious adverse events occurred in severely ill infants with life-threatening underlying diseases, many of whom required assisted ventilation. The role of VIRAZOLE in these events is indeterminate. Since the drug's approval in 1986, additional reports of similar serious, though non-fatal, events have been filed infrequently. Events associated with aerosolized VIRAZOLE use have included the following:

Pulmonary: Worsening of respiratory status, bronchospasm, pulmonary edema, hypoventilation, cyanosis, dyspnea, bacterial pneumonia, pneumothorax, apnea, atelectasis and ventilator dependence.

Cardiovascular: Cardiac arrest, hypotension, bradycardia and digitalis toxicity. Bigeminy, bradycardia and tachycardia have been described in patients with underlying congenital heart disease.

Some subjects requiring assisted ventilation experienced serious difficulties, due to inadequate ventilation and gas exchange. Precipitation of drug within the ventilatory apparatus, including the endotracheal tube, has resulted in increased positive end expiratory pressure and increased positive inspiratory pressure. Accumulation of fluid in tubing ("rain out") has also been noted. Measures to avoid these complications should be followed carefully (see Dosage and Administration).

Hematologic

Although anemia was not reported with use of aerosolized VIRAZOLE in controlled clinical trials, most infants treated with the aerosol have not been evaluated 1 to 2 weeks post-treatment when anemia is likely to occur. Anemia has been shown to occur frequently with experimental oral and intravenous VIRAZOLE in humans. Also, cases of anemia (type unspecified), reticulocytosis and hemolytic anemia associated with aerosolized VIRAZOLE use have been reported through post-marketing reporting systems. All have been reversible with discontinuation of the drug.

Other

Rash and conjunctivitis have been associated with the use of aerosolized VIRAZOLE. These usually resolve within hours of discontinuing therapy. Seizures and asthenia associated with experimental intravenous VIRAZOLE therapy have also been reported.

Adverse Events in Health Care Workers

Studies of environmental exposure to aerosolized VIRAZOLE in health care workers administering care to patients receiving the drug have not detected adverse signs or symptoms related to exposure. However, 152 health care workers have reported experiencing adverse events through post-marketing surveillance. Nearly all were in individuals providing direct care to infants receiving aerosolized VIRAZOLE. Of 358 events from these 152 individual health care worker reports, the most common signs and symptoms were headache (51% of reports), conjunctivitis (32%), and rhinitis, nausea, rash, dizziness, pharyngitis, or lacrimation (10–20% each). Several cases of bronchospasm and/or chest pain were also reported, usually in individuals with known underlying reactive airway disease. Several case reports of damage to contact lenses after prolonged close exposure to aerosolized VIRAZOLE have also been reported. Most signs and symptoms reported as having occurred in exposed health care workers resolved within minutes to hours of discontinuing close exposure to aerosolized VIRAZOLE (also see Information for Health Care Personnel).

The symptoms of RSV in adults can include headache, conjunctivitis, sore throat and/or cough, fever, hoarseness, nasal congestion and wheezing, although RSV infections in adults are typically mild and transient. Such infections represent a potential hazard to uninfected hospital patients. It is unknown whether certain symptoms cited in reports from health care workers were due to exposure to the drug or infection with RSV. Hospitals should implement appropriate infection control procedures.

Overdosage

No overdosage with VIRAZOLE by aerosol administration has been reported in humans. The LD_{50} in mice is 2 gm orally and is associated with hypoactivity and gastrointestinal symptoms (estimated human equivalent dose of 0.17gm/kg, based on body surface area conversion). The mean plasma half-life after administration of aerosolized VIRAZOLE for pediatric patients is 9.5 hours. VIRAZOLE is concentrated and persists in red blood cells for the life of the erythrocyte (see Pharmacokinetics).

DOSAGE AND ADMINISTRATION

BEFORE USE, READ THOROUGHLY THE ICN SMALL PARTICLE AEROSOL GENERATOR MODEL SPAG-2 OPERATOR'S MANUAL FOR SMALL PARTICLE AEROSOL GENERATOR OPERATING INSTRUCTIONS. AEROSOLIZED VIRAZOLE SHOULD NOT BE ADMINISTERED WITH ANY OTHER AEROSOL GENERATING DEVICE.

The recommended treatment regimen is 20 mg/ml VIRAZOLE as the starting solution in the drug reservoir of the SPAG-2 unit, with continuous aerosol administration for 12–18 hours per day for 3 to 7 days. Using the recommended drug concentration of 20 mg/ml the average aerosol concentration for a 12 hour delivery period would be 190 micrograms/liter of air. Aerosolized VIRAZOLE should not be administered in a mixture for combined aerosolization or simultaneously with other aerosolized medications.

Non-mechanically ventilated infants

VIRAZOLE should be delivered to an infant oxygen hood from the SPAG-2 aerosol generator. Administration by face mask or oxygen tent may be necessary if a hood cannot be employed (see SPAG-2 manual). However, the volume and condensation area are larger in a tent and this may alter delivery dynamics of the drug.

Mechanically ventilated infants

The recommended dose and administration schedule for infants who require mechanical ventilation is the same as for those who do not. Either a pressure or volume cycle ventilator may be used in conjunction with the SPAG-2. In either case, patients should have their endotracheal tubes suctioned every 1–2 hours, and their pulmonary pressures monitored frequently (every 2–4 hours). For both pressure and volume ventilators, heated wire connective tubing and bacteria filters in series in the expiratory limb of the system (which must be changed frequently, i.e., every 4 hours) must be used to minimize the risk of VIRAZOLE precipitation in the system and the subsequent risk of ventilator dysfunction. Water column pressure release valves should be used in the ventilator circuit for pressure cycled ventilators, and may be utilized with volume cycled ventilators (SEE SPAG-2 MANUAL FOR DETAILED INSTRUCTIONS).

Method of Preparation

VIRAZOLE brand of ribavirin is supplied as 6 grams of lyophilized powder per 100 ml vial for aerosol administration only. By sterile technique, reconstitute drug with a minimum of 75 ml of **sterile USP water for injection or inhalation** in the original 100 ml glass vial. Shake well. Transfer to the clean, sterilized 500 ml SPAG-2 reservoir and further dilute to a final volume of 300 ml with Sterile Water for Injection, USP, or Inhalation. The final concentration should be 20 mg/ml. **Important:** This water should NOT have had any antimicrobial agent or other substance added. The solution should be inspected visually for particulate matter and discoloration prior to administration. Solutions that have been placed in the SPAG-2 unit should be discarded at least every 24 hours and when the liquid level is low before adding newly reconstituted solution.

HOW SUPPLIED

VIRAZOLE (ribavirin for inhalation solution) is supplied in 100 ml glass vials with 6 grams of sterile, lyophilized drug which is to be reconstituted with 300 ml Sterile Water for Injection or Sterile Water for Inhalation (no preservatives added) and administered only by a small particle aerosol generator (SPAG-2). Vials containing the lyophilized drug powder should be stored in a dry place at 15–25°C (59–78°F). Reconstituted solutions may be stored, under sterile conditions, at room temperature (20–30°C, 68–86°F) for 24 hours. Solutions which have been placed in the SPAG-2 unit should be discarded at least every 24 hours.

VIRAZOLE is available as follows:

Package Size	NDC Number
4 × 6 g vials	NDC 0187-0007-14

REFERENCES

1. Hruska JF, Bernstein JM, Douglas Jr., RG, and Hall CB. Effects of Virazole on respiratory syncytial virus in vitro. Antimicrob Agents Chemother 17:770–775, 1 1980.
2. Hruska JF, Morrow PE, Suffin SC, and Douglas Jr., RG. In vivo inhibition of respiratory syncytial virus by Virazole. Antimicrob Agents Chemother 21:125–130, 1982.
3. Taber LH, Knight V, Gilbert BE, McClung HW et al. Virazole aerosol treatment of bronchiolitis associated with respiratory tract infection in infants. Pediatrics 72:613–618, 1983.
4. Hall CB, McBride JT, Walsh EE, Bell DM et al. Aerosolized Virazole treatment of infants with respiratory syncytial viral infection. N Engl J Med 308:1443–7, 1983.
5. Hendry RM, McIntosh K, Fahnestock ML, and Pierik LT. Enzyme-linked immunosorbent assay for detection of respiratory syncytial virus infection. J Clin Microbiol 16:329–33, 1982.
6. Smith, David W., Frankel, Lorry R., Mather, Larry H., Tang, Allen T.S., Ariagno, Ronald L., Prober, Charles G. A Controlled Trial of Aerosolized Ribavirin in Infants Receiving Mechanical Ventilation for Severe Respiratory Syncytial Virus Infection. The New England Journal of Medicine 1991; 325:24–29.
7. Decker, John, Shultz, Ruth A., Health Hazard Evaluation Report: Florida Hospital, Orlando, Florida, Cincinnati OH: U.S. Department of Health and Human Services, Public Health Service, Centers for NIOSH Report No. HETA 91-104-2229.*
8. Barnes, D.J. and Doursew, M. Reference dose: Description and use in health risk assessments. Regul Tox. and Pharm. Vol. 8; p. 471–486, 1988.
9. Federal Register Vol. 53 No. 126 Thurs. June 30, 1988 p. 24834–24847.
10. American Association for Respirtory Care [1991]. Aerosol Consensus Statement-1991. Respiratory Care 36(9): 916–921.

*Copies of the Report may be purchased from National Technical Information Service, 5285 Port Royal Road, Springfield, VA 22161; Ask for Publication PB 93119-345.

1957-06 EL
Rev. 5-96

ICN PHARMACEUTICALS, INC.
ICN Plaza
3300 Hyland Avenue
Costa Mesa, California 92626
714-545-0100

IDEC Pharmaceuticals Corporation

3030 CALLAN ROAD
SAN DIEGO, CA 92121

Direct Inquiries to:
(858) 431-8500

RITUXAN®
Rituximab ℞

WARNINGS

Infusion-related reactions: Infusion-related deaths (death within 24 hours of infusion) have been reported at a rate of approximately 0.04–0.07% (4–7 per 10,000 patients treated). These events appear as manifestations of an infusion-related complex and include hypoxia, pulmonary infiltrates, adult respiratory distress syndrome, myocardial infarction, ventricular fibrillation or cardiogenic shock. Nearly all fatal infusion-related events occurred in association with the first infusion. In the reported cases, the following factors were more frequently associated with fatal outcomes: women, patients with pulmonary infiltrates, and patients with CLL or mantle cell lymphoma (see WARNINGS).

Regarding the management of infusion-related reactions:

- Patients who develop clinically significant cardiopulmonary events should have RITUXAN infusion discontinued and receive medical treatment.
- Patients with pre-existing cardiac and pulmonary conditions or those with prior clinically significant cardiopulmonary adverse events should be monitored during and after subsequent infusions of RITUXAN.
- Patients with high numbers of circulating malignant cells (≥25,000/mm^3) with or without other evidence of high tumor burden should be more closely monitored for infusion reactions and tumor lysis syndrome.

Tumor Lysis Syndrome (TLS): Acute renal failure requiring dialysis with instances of fatal outcome has been reported in the setting of TLS. Assessment of serum electrolytes and renal function is indicated in patients with rapid decreases in tumor volume (see WARNINGS).

DESCRIPTION

The RITUXAN (Rituximab) antibody is a genetically engineered chimeric murine/human monoclonal antibody directed against the CD20 antigen found on the surface of normal and malignant B lymphocytes. The antibody is an IgG_1 kappa immunoglobulin containing murine light- and heavy-chain variable region sequences and human constant region sequences. Rituximab is composed of two heavy chains of 451 amino acids and two light chains of 213 amino acids (based on cDNA analysis) and has an approximate molecular weight of 145 kD. Rituximab has a binding affinity for the CD20 antigen of approximately 8.0 nM.

The chimeric anti-CD20 antibody is produced by mammalian cell (Chinese Hamster Ovary) suspension culture in a nutrient medium containing the antibiotic gentamicin. Gentamicin is not detectable in the final product. The anti-CD20 antibody is purified by affinity and ion exchange chromatography. The purification process includes specific viral inactivation and removal procedures. Rituximab drug product is manufactured from either bulk drug substance manufactured by Genentech, Inc. (US License No. 1048), or utilizing formulation bulk Rituximab supplied by IDEC Pharmaceuticals Corporation (US License No. 1235) under a shared manufacturing arrangement.

RITUXAN is a sterile, clear, colorless, preservative-free liquid concentrate for intravenous (IV) administration. RITUXAN is supplied at a concentration of 10 mg/mL in either 100 mg (10 mL) or 500 mg (50 mL) single-use vials. The product is formulated for IV administration in 9.0 mg/mL sodium chloride, 7.35 mg/mL sodium citrate dihydrate, 0.7 mg/mL polysorbate 80, and Sterile Water for Injection. The pH is adjusted to 6.5.

Continued on next page

Rituxan—Cont.

CLINICAL PHARMACOLOGY

General

Rituximab binds specifically to the antigen CD20 (human B-lymphocyte-restricted differentiation antigen, Bp35), a hydrophobic transmembrane protein with a molecular weight of approximately 35 kD located on pre-B and mature B lympocytes.[1,2] The antigen is also expressed on >90% of B-cell non-Hodgkin's lymphomas (NHL)[3] but is not found on hematopoietic stem cells, pro-B cells, normal plasma cells or other normal tissues.[4] CD20 regulates an early step(s) in the activation process for cell cycle initiation and differentiation,[4] and possibly functions as a calcium ion channel.[5] CD20 is not shed from the cell surface and does not internalize upon antibody binding.[6] Free CD20 antigen is not found in the circulation.[2]

Preclinical Pharmacology and Toxicology

Mechanism of Action: The Fab domain of Rituximab binds to thd CD20 antigen on B lymphocytes, and the Fc domain recruits immune effector functions to mediate B-cell lysis in vitro. Possible mechanisms of cell lysis include complement-dependent cytotoxicity (CDC)[7] and antibody-dependent cell mediated cytotoxicity (ADCC). The antibody has been shown to induce apoptosis in the DHL-4 human B-cell lymphoma line.[8]

Normal Tissue Cross-reactivity: Rituximab binding was observed on lymphoid cells in the thymus, the white pulp of the spleen, and a majority of B lymphocytes in peripheral blood and lymph nodes. Little or no binding was observed in the non-lymphoid tissues examined.

Human Pharmacokinetics/Pharmacodynamics

In patients given single doses at 10, 50, 100, 250 or 500 mg/m^2 as an IV infusion, serum levels and the half-life of Rituximab were proportional to dose. In nine patients given 375 mg/m^2 as an IV infusion for four doses, the mean serum half-life was 59.8 hours (range 11.1 to 104.6 hours) after the first infusion and 174 hours (range 26 to 442 hours) after the fourth infusion. The wide range of half-lives may reflect the variable tumor burden among patients and the changes in CD20 positive (normal and malignant) B-cell populations upon repeated administrations.

Rituximab at a dose of 375 mg/m^2 was administered as an IV infusion at weekly intervals for four doses to 166 patients. The peak and trough serum levels of Rituximab were inversely correlated with baseline values for the number of circulating CD20 positive B cells and measures of disease burden. Median steady-state serum levels were higher for responders compared to nonresponders; however, no difference was found in the rate of elimination as measured by serum half-life. Serum levels were higher in patients with International Working Formulation (IWF) subtypes B, C, and D as compared to those with subtype A. Rituximab was detectable in the serum of patients three to six months after completion of treatment.

The pharmacokinetic profile of Rituximab when administered as six infusions of 375 mg/m^2 in combination with six cycles of CHOP chemotherapy was similar to that seen with Rituximab alone.

Administration of RITUXAN resulted in a rapid and sustained depletion of circulating and tissue-based B cells. Lymph node biopsies performed 14 days after therapy showed a decrease in the percentage of B cells in seven of eight patients who had received single doses of Rituximab ≥100 mg/m^2.[9] Among the 166 patients in the pivotal study, circulating B cells (measured as CD19 positive cells) were depleted within the first three doses with sustained depletion for up to 6 to 9 months posttreatment in 83% of patients. One of the responding patients (1%), failed to show significant depletion of CD19 positive cells after the third infusion of Rituximab as compared to 19% of the nonresponding patients. B-cell recovery began at approximately six months following completion of treatment. Median B-cell levels returned to normal by twelve months following completion of treatment.

There were sustained and statistically significant reductions in both IgM and IgG serum levels observed from 5 through 11 months following Rituximab administration. However, only 14% of patients had reductions in IgM and/or IgG serum levels, resulting in values below the normal range.

CLINICAL STUDIES

A multicenter, open-label, single-arm study was conducted in 166 patients with relapsed or refractory low-grade or follicular B-cell NHL who received 375 mg/m^2 of RITUXAN given as an IV infusion weekly for four doses. Patients with tumor masses >10 cm or with >5,000 lymphocytes/μL in the peripheral blood were excluded from the study. The overall response rate (ORR) was 48% (80/166) with a 6% (10/166) complete response (CR) and a 42% (70/166) partial response (PR) rate. Disease-related signs and symptoms (including B-symptoms) were present in 23% (39/166) of patients at study entry and resolved in 64% (25/39) of those patients. The median time to onset of response was 50 days and the median duration of response is projected to be 10 to 12 months.

In a multivariate analysis, the ORR was higher in patients with IWF B, C, and D histologic subtypes as compared to IWF subtype A (58% vs. 12%), higher in patients whose largest lesion was <5 cm vs. >7 cm in greatest diameter (53% vs. 38%), and higher in patients with chemosensitive relapse as compared to chemoresistant (defined as duration of response <3 months) relapse (53% vs. 36%). ORR in patients previously treated with autologous bone marrow transplant was 78% (18/23). The following factors were not associated with a lower response rate: age ≥60 years, extranodal disease, prior anthracycline therapy, and bone marrow involvement.

In a second multicenter, multiple-dose study, 37 patients with relapsed or refractory B-cell NHL received 375 mg/m^2 of RITUXAN as an IV infusion once weekly for four doses.[10,11] The ORR was 46% with a median duration of response of 8.6 months (range 2.6 to 26.2+). Single doses of up to 500 mg/m^2 were well tolerated.[9]

Twenty patients have received two courses and one patient has received three courses of RITUXAN as four weekly infusions of 375 mg/m^2 per infusion. The percentage of patients reporting adverse events upon retreatment was similar to that reported following the first course, although the incidence of specific adverse events differed (see ADVERSE REACTIONS). All patients had obtained an objective clinical response (CR or PR) to the first course of RITUXAN; upon retreatment, 6 of 12 patients evaluable for response obtained a complete or partial remission.

Twenty-nine patients with relapsed or refractory, bulky (single lesion of >10 cm in diameter), low-grade NHL received 375 mg/m^2 of RITUXAN as four weekly infusions. The overall incidence of adverse events and the incidence of Grade 3 and 4 adverse events was higher in patients with bulky disease than in patients with non-bulky disease (see ADVERSE REACTIONS). Ten of 21 patients evaluable for response have obtained a complete or partial remission.

INDICATIONS AND USAGE

RITUXAN is indicated for the treatment of patients with relapsed or refractory low-grade or follicular, CD20 positive, B-cell non-Hodgkin's lymphoma.

CONTRAINDICATIONS

RITUXAN is contraindicated in patients with known Type I hypersensitivity or anaphylactic reactions to murine proteins or to any component of this product. (See WARNINGS.)

WARNINGS (see BOXED WARNINGS)

Infusion-Related Events (see BOXED WARNING): An infusion-related symptom complex consisting of fever and chills/rigors occurred in the majority of patients during the first RITUXAN infusion. Other frequent infusion-related symptoms included nausea, urticaria, fatigue, headache, pruritus, bronchospasm, dyspnea, sensation of tongue or throat swelling (angioedema), rhinitis, vomiting, hypotension, flushing, and pain at disease sites. These reactions generally occurred within 30 minutes to 2 hours of beginning the first infusion, and resolved with slowing or interruption of the RITUXAN infusion and with supportive care (diphenhydramine, acetaminophen, IV saline, and vasopressors). RITUXAN infusion should be interrupted for severe reactions. In most cases, the infusion can be resumed at a 50% reduction in rate (e.g., from 100 mg/hr to 50 mg/hr) when symptoms have completely resolved. In clinical studies, the incidence of infusion-related events decreased from 80% (7% Grade 3/4) during the first infusion to approximately 40% (5% to 10% Grade 3/4) with subsequent infusions. Mild to moderate hypotension requiring interruption of RITUXAN infusion with or without the administration of IV saline occurred in 32 (10%) patients. Angioedema was reported in 41 (13%) patients and was serious in one patient. Bronchospasm occurred in 24 (8%) patients; one-quarter of these patients were treated with bronchodilators.

Tumor Lysis Syndrome (see BOXED WARNING): TLS, characterized by rapid reduction in tumor volume, renal insufficiency, hyperkalemia, hypocalcemia, hyperuricemia, or hyperphosphatasemia, has been reported within 12 to 24 hours after the first RITUXAN infusion at a reported rate of 0.04%–0.05%. The risks of TLS appear to be higher in patients with high numbers of circulating malignant cells. Correction of electrolytes abnormalities, monitoring of renal function and fluid balance, and supportive care, including dialysis, should be initiated as indicated. Following complete resolution of the complications of TLS, RITUXAN has been tolerated when re-administered in conjunction with prophylactic therapy for TLS in a limited number of cases.

General

RITUXAN is associated with hypersensitivity reactions which may respond to adjustments in the infusion rate. Hypotension, bronchospasm, and angioedema have occurred in association with RITUXAN infusion as part of an infusion-related symptom complex. RITUXAN infusion should be interrupted for severe reactions and can be resumed at a 50% reduction in rate (e.g., from 100 mg/hr to 50 mg/hr) when symptoms have completely resolved. Treatment of these symptoms with diphenhydramine and acetaminophen is recommended; additional treatment with bronchodilators or IV saline may be indicated. In most cases, patients who have experienced non-life-threatening reactions have been able to complete the full course of therapy. (See DOSAGE and ADMINISTRATION.) Medications for the treatment of hypersensitivity reactions, e.g., epinephrine, antihistamines and corticosteroids, should be available for immediate use in the event of a reaction during administration.

Cardiovascular

Infusions should be discontinued in the event of serious or life-threatening cardiac arrhythmias. Patients who develop clinically significant arrhythmias should undergo cardiac monitoring during and after subsequent infusions of RITUXAN. Patients with preexisting cardiac conditions including arrhythmias and angina have had recurrences of these events during RITUXAN therapy and should be monitored throughout the infusion and immediate post-infusion period.

PRECAUTIONS

Laboratory Monitoring: Complete blood counts (CBC) and platelet counts should be obtained at regular intervals during RITUXAN therapy and more frequently in patients who develop cytopenias (see ADVERSE REACTIONS).

Drug/Laboratory Interactions: There have been no formal drug interaction studies performed with RITUXAN.

HAMA/HACA Formation: Human anti-murine antibody (HAMA) was not detected in 67 patients evaluated. Less than 1.0% (3/355) of patients evaluated for human anti-chimeric antibody (HACA) were positive. Patients who develop HAMA/HACA titers may have allergic or hypersensitivity reactions when treated with this or other murine or chimeric monoclonal antibodies.

Immunization: The safety of immunization with any vaccine, particularly live viral vaccines, following RITUXAN therapy has not been studied. The ability to generate a primary or anamnestic humoral response to any vaccine has also not been studied.

Carcinogenesis, Mutagenesis, Impairment of Fertility: No long-term animal studies have been performed to establish the carcinogenic or mutagenic potential of RITUXAN, or to determine its effects on fertility in males or females. Individuals of childbearing potential should use effective contraceptive methods during treatment and for up to 12 months following RITUXAN therapy.

Pregnancy Category C: Animal reproduction studies have not been conducted with RITUXAN. It is not known whether RITUXAN can cause fetal harm when administered to a pregnant woman or whether it can affect reproductive capacity. Human IgG is known to pass the placental barrier, and thus may potentially cause fetal B-cell depletion; therefore, RITUXAN should be given to a pregnant woman only if clearly needed.

Nursing Mothers: It is not known whether RITUXAN is excreted in human milk. Because human IgG is excreted in human milk and the potential for absorption and immunosuppression in the infant is unknown, women should be advised to discontinue nursing until circulating drug levels are no longer detectable. (See CLINICAL PHARMACOLOGY.)

Pediatric Use: The safety and effectiveness of RITUXAN in pediatric patients have not been established.

ADVERSE REACTIONS

Safety data, except where indicated, are based on 315 patients treated in five single-agent studies of RITUXAN. These include patients with bulky disease (lesions >10 cm), those who have received more than one course of RITUXAN, and patients receiving 375 mg/m^2 for eight doses.

Infusion-Related Events: (See BOXED WARNING and WARNINGS.)

Immunologic Events: RITUXAN induced B-cell depletion in 70 to 80% of patients was associated with decreased serum immunoglobulins in a minority of patients. The incidence of infection did not appear to be increased. During the treatment period, 50 out of 166 patients (30%) in the pivotal trial developed 68 infectious events; six (9%) were Grade 3 in severity and none were Grade 4 events. Of the six serious infections events, none were associated with neutropenia. The serious bacterial events included sepsis due to *Listeria* (n=1), *Staphylococcal* bacteremia (n=1), and polymicrobial sepsis (n=1). In the posttreatment period (30 days to 11 months following the last dose), bacterial infections included sepsis (n=1); significant viral infections included *Herpes simplex* infections (n=2) and *Herpes zoster* (n=3). Additional reports of focal bacterial infections, sepsis, and viral infections have been received in the postmarketing setting. Serious infections, including sepsis, have been reported in patients with and without neutropenia.

Retreatment Events: Twenty-one patients have received more than one course of RITUXAN. The percentage of patients reporting any adverse event upon retreatment was similar to the percentage of patients reporting adverse events upon initial exposure. The following adverse events were reported more frequently in retreated subjects: asthenia, throat irritation, flushing, tachycardia, anorexia, leukopenia, thrombocytopenia, anemia, peripheral edema, dizziness, depression, respiratory symptoms, night sweats, and pruritus.

Hematologic Events: Severe cytopenias were reported including thrombocytopenia (1.3%), neutropenia (1.9%), and anemia (1.0%). A single occurrence of transient aplastic anemia (pure red cell aplasia) and two occurrences of hemolytic anemia following RITUXAN therapy were reported. In addition, there have been rare postmarketing reports of prolonged pancytopenia and marrow hypoplasia.

Cardiac Events (see BOXED WARNING): Four patients developed ventricular or supraventricular arrhythmias and one patient developed angina in association with the RITUXAN infusion. Rare, fatal cardiac failure with symptomatic onset weeks after RITUXAN has also been reported. Patients who develop clinically significant cardiopulmonary events should have RITUXAN infusion discontinued.

Pulmonary Events (see BOXED WARNING): Three pulmonary events have been reported in temporal association with RITUXAN infusion as a single agent: acute, infusion-related bronchospasm, an acute pneumonitis presenting 1–4 weeks post-RITUXAN infusion, and bronchiolitis obliterans. The bronchiolitis obliterans was associated with pro-

Table 1
Adverse Events ≥5% of Patients (N=315)

	Incidence All Grades N	%
Any Adverse Event	**275**	**87**
Body As A Whole		
Fever	154	49
Chills	102	32
Asthenia	49	16
Headache	43	14
Throat Irritation	19	6
Abdominal Pain	18	6
Cardiovascular System		
Hypotension	32	10
Digestive System		
Nausea	55	18
Vomiting	23	7
Hemic and Lymphatic System		
Leukopenia	33	11
Thrombocytopenia	25	8
Neutropenia	21	7
Metabolic and Nutritional System		
Angioedema	41	13
Musculo-Skeletal System		
Myalgia	21	7
Nervous System		
Dizziness	23	7
Respiratory System		
Rhinitis	25	8
Bronchospasm	24	8
Skin and Appendages		
Pruritus	32	10
Rash	31	10
Urticaria	24	8

gressive pulmonary symptoms and culminated in death several months following the last RITUXAN infusion. The safety of resumption or continued administration of RITUXAN in patients with pneumonitis or bronchiolitis obliterans is unknown.

[See table above]

Severe and life-threatening (Grade 3 and 4) events were reported in 10% (32/315) of patients. The following Grade 3 and 4 adverse events were reported: neutropenia (1.9%), chills (1.6%), leukopenia and thrombocytopenia (1.3% for each), hypotension, anemia, bronchospasm, and urticaria (1.0% for each), headache, abdominal pain, and arrhythmia (0.6% for each), asthenia, hypertension, nausea, vomiting, coagulation disorder, angioedema, arthralgia, pain, rhinitis, increased cough, dyspnea, bronchiolitis obliterans, hypoxia, asthma, pruritus, and rash (one patient each, 0.3%).

The following adverse events occurred in ≥1.0% but <5.0% of patients, in order of decreasing incidence: flushing, arthralgia, diarrhea, anemia, cough increase, hypertension, lacrimation disorder, pain, hyperglycemia, back pain, peripheral edema, paresthesia, dyspepsia, chest pain, anorexia, anxiety, malaise, tachycardia, agitation, insomnia, sinusitis, conjunctivitis, abdominal enlargement, postural hypotension, LDH increase, hypocalcemia, hypesthesia, respiratory disorder, tumor pain, pain at injection site, bradycardia, hypertonia, nervousness, bronchitis, and taste perversion.

Multisystem adverse events—The following serious adverse reactions have been reported at a frequency of less than 0.1% in the postmarketing setting:

Body as a Whole: Lupus-like syndrome and serum sickness
Cardiovascular System: Systemic vasculitis
Musculoskeletal System: Polyarticular arthritis
Respiratory System: Pleuritis
Skin and Appendages: Severe bullous skin reactions (including toxic epidermal necrolysis) and pemphigus; some with fatal outcome
Special Senses: Optic neuritis and uveitis

Several of these events were reported as individual components of multisystem processes (e.g., optic neuritis in a patient with systemic vasculitis, pleuritis in association with lupus-like syndrome, etc.) and often in conjunction with rash and polyarthritis.

The proportion of patients reporting any adverse event was similar in patients with bulky disease and those with lesions <10 cm in diameter. However, the incidence of dizziness, neutropenia, thrombocytopenia, myalgia, anemia, and chest pain was higher in patients with lesions >10 cm. The incidence of any Grade 3 and 4 event was higher (31% vs. 13%) and the incidence of Grade 3 or 4 neutropenia, anemia, hypotension, and dyspnea was also higher in patients with bulky disease compared with patients with lesions <10 cm.

OVERDOSAGE

There has been no experience with overdosage in human clinical trials. Single doses higher than 500 mg/m^2 have not been tested.

DOSAGE AND ADMINISTRATION

Usual Dose:

The recommended dosage of RITUXAN is 375 mg/m^2 given as an IV infusion once weekly for four doses (Days 1, 8, 15, and 22). RITUXAN may be administered in an outpatient setting. **DO NOT ADMINISTER AS AN INTRAVENOUS PUSH OR BOLUS. (See Administration).**

Instructions for Administration

Preparation for Administration: Use appropriate aseptic technique. Withdraw the necessary amount of RITUXAN and dilute to a final concentration of 1 to 4 mg/mL into an infusion bag containing either 0.9% Sodium Chloride, USP, or 5% Dextrose in Water, USP. Gently invert the bag to mix the solution. Discard any unused portion left in the vial. Parenteral drug products should be inspected visually for particulate matter and discoloration prior to administration.

RITUXAN solutions for infusion are stable at 2–8°C (36–46°F) for 24 hours and at room temperature for an additional 12 hours. No incompatibilities between RITUXAN and polyvinylchloride or polyethylene bags have been observed.

Administration: DO NOT ADMINISTER AS AN INTRAVENOUS PUSH OR BOLUS. Hypersensitivity reactions may occur (see WARNINGS). Premedication consisting of acetaminophen and diphenhydramine should be considered before each infusion of RITUXAN. Premedication may attenuate infusion-related events. Since transient hypotension may occur during RITUXAN infusion, consideration should be given to withholding antihypertensive medications 12 hours prior to RITUXAN infusion.

First Infusion: The RITUXAN solution for infusion should be administered intravenously at an initial rate of 50 mg/hr. RITUXAN should not be mixed or diluted with other drugs. If hypersensitivity or infusion-related events do not occur, escalate the infusion rate in 50 mg/hr increments every 30 minutes, to a maximum of 400 mg/hr. If hypersensitivity or an infusion-related event develops, the infusion should be temporarily slowed or interrupted (see WARNINGS). The infusion can continue at one-half the previous rate upon improvement of patient symptoms.

Subsequent Infusions: Subsequent RITUXAN infusions can be administered at an initial rate of 100 mg/hr, and increased by 100 mg/hr increments at 30-minute intervals, to a maximum of 400 mg/hr as tolerated.

Stability and Storage: RITXUAN vials are stable at 2–8°C (36–46°F). Do not use beyond expiration date stamped on carton. RITUXAN vials should be protected from direct sunlight.

HOW SUPPLIED

RITUXAN is supplied as 100 mg and 500 mg of sterile, preservative-free, single-use vials.

Single unit 100 mg carton: Contains one 10 mL vial of RITUXAN (10 mg/mL).

NDC 50242-051-21

Single unit 500 mg carton: Contains one 50 mL vial of RITUXAN (10 mg/mL).

NDC 50242-053-06

REFERENCES

1. Valentine MA, Meier KE, Rossie S, et al. Phosphorylation of the CD20 phosphoprotein in resting B lymphocytes. *J Biol Chem* 1989 264(19): 11282–11287.
2. Einfeld DA, Brown JP, Valentine MA, et al. Molecular cloning of the human B cell CD20 receptor predicts a hydrophobic protein with multiple transmembrane domains. *EMBO J* 1988 7(3):711–717.
3. Anderson KC, Bates MP, Slaughenhoupt BL, et al. Expression of human B cell-associated antigens on leukemias and lymphomas: A model of human B cell differentiation. *Blood* 1984 63(6):1424–1433.
4. Tedder TF, Boyd AW, Freedman AS, et al. The B cell surface molecule B1 is functionally linked with B cell activation and differentiation. *J Immunol* 1985 135(2):973–979.
5. Tedder TF, Zhou LJ, Bell PD, et al. The CD20 surface molecule of B lympocytes functions as a calcium channel. *J Cell Biochem* 1990 14D:195.
6. Press OW, Applebaum F, Ledbetter JA, Martin PJ, Zarling J, Kidd P, et al. Monoclonal antibody 1F5 (anti-CD20) serotherapy of human B-cell lymphomas. *Blood* 1987 69(2):584–591.
7. Reff ME, Carner C, Chambers KS, Chinn PC, Leonard JE, Raab R, et al. Depletion of B cells in vivo by a chimeric mouse human monoclonal antibody to CD20. *Blood* 1994 83(2):435–445.
8. Demidem A, Lam T, Alas S, Hariharan K, Hanna N, and Bonavida B. Chimeric anti-CD20 (IDEC-C2B8) monoclonal antibody sensitizes a B cell lymphoma cell line to cell killing by cytotoxic drugs. *Cancer Biotherapy & Radiopharmaceuticals* 1997 12(3):177–186.
9. Maloney DG, Liles TM, Czerwinski C, Waldichuk J, Rosenberg J, Grillo-López A, et al. Phase I clinical trial using escalating single-dose infusion of chimeric anti-CD20 monoclonal antibody (IDEC-C2B8) in patients with recurrent B-cell lymphoma. *Blood* 1994 84(8):2457–2466.
10. Maloney DG, Grillo-López AJ, Bodkin D, White CA, Liles T-M, Royston I, et al. IDEC-C2B8: Results of a phase I multiple-dose trial in patients with relapsed non-Hodgkin's lympoma. *J Clin Oncol* 1997 15(10):3266–3274.
11. Maloney DG, Grillo-López AJ, White CA, Bodkin D, Schlider RJ, Neidhart JA, et al. IDEC-C2B8 (Rituximab) anti-CD20 monoclonal antibody therapy in patients with relapsed low-grade non-Hodgkin's lymphoma. *Blood* 1997 90(6):2188–2195.

Jointly Marketed by:
IDEC Pharmaceuticals Corporation
3030 Callan Road
San Diego, CA 92121
7202000 LJ0070
Genentech, Inc.
1 DNA Way
South San Francisco, CA 94080-4990
(4809703 Revised July 1999)

Shown in Product Identification Guide, page 318

Immunex Corporation

51 UNIVERSITY STREET
SEATTLE, WA 98101

For Medical Information Contact:
Generally:
Professional Services
(800) 466-8639
FAX: (800) 221-6820
FAX: (206) 223-5525
In Emergencies:
Professional Services
(800) 466-8639
FAX: (800) 221-6820
FAX: (206) 223-5525

ENBREL® ℞
[*ĕn-brĕl*]
(etanercept)

DESCRIPTION

ENBREL (etanercept) is a dimeric fusion protein consisting of the extracellular ligand-binding portion of the human 75 kilodalton (p75) tumor necrosis factor receptor (TNFR) linked to the Fc portion of human IgG1. The Fc component of etanercept contains the C_H2 domain, the C_H3 domain and hinge region, but not the C_H1 domain of IgG1. Etanercept is produced by recombinant DNA technology in a Chinese hamster ovary (CHO) mammalian cell expression system. It consists of 934 amino acids and has an apparent molecular weight of approximately 150 kilodaltons.

ENBREL is supplied as a sterile, white, preservative-free, lyophilized powder for parenteral administration after reconstitution with 1 mL of the supplied Sterile Bacteriostatic Water for Injection, USP (containing 0.9% benzyl alcohol). Following reconstitution, the solution of ENBREL is clear and colorless, with a pH of 7.4 ± 0.3. Each single-use vial of ENBREL contains 25 mg etanercept, 40 mg mannitol, 10 mg sucrose, and 1.2 mg tromethamine.

CLINICAL PHARMACOLOGY

General

Etanercept binds specifically to tumor necrosis factor (TNF) and blocks its interaction with cell surface TNF receptors. TNF is a naturally occurring cytokine that is involved in normal inflammatory and immune responses. It plays an important role in the inflammatory processes of rheumatoid arthritis (RA), polyarticular-course juvenile rheumatoid arthritis (JRA), and the resulting joint pathology.[1, 2] Elevated levels of TNF are found in the synovial fluid of RA patients.[3] Two distinct receptors for TNF (TNFRs), a 55 kilodalton protein (p55) and a 75 kilodalton protein (p75), exist natu-

Continued on next page

Enbrel—Cont.

rally as monomeric molecules on cell surfaces and in soluble forms.[4] Biological activity of TNF is dependent upon binding to either cell surface TNFR.

Etanercept is a dimeric soluble form of the p75 TNF receptor that can bind to two TNF molecules. It inhibits the activity of TNF in vitro and has been shown to affect several animal models of inflammation, including murine collagen-induced arthritis.[5, 6] Etanercept inhibits binding of both TNFα and TNFβ (lymphotoxin alpha [LTα]) to cell surface TNFRs, rendering TNF biologically inactive.[6] Cells expressing transmembrane TNF that bind ENBREL are not lysed in vitro in the presence or absence of complement.[6]

Etanercept can also modulate biological responses that are induced or regulated by TNF, including expression of adhesion molecules responsible for leukocyte migration (i.e., E-selectin and to a lesser extent intercellular adhesion molecule-1 [ICAM-1]), serum levels of cytokines (e.g., IL-6), and serum levels of matrix metalloproteinase-3 (MMP-3 or stromelysin).[6]

Pharmacokinetics

After administration of 25 mg of ENBREL by a single subcutaneous (SC) injection to three patients with RA, a median half-life of 115 hours (range 98 to 300 hours) was observed with a clearance of 89 mL/hr (52 mL/hr/m^2). A maximum serum concentration (Cmax) of 1.2 mcg/mL (range 0.6 to 1.5 mcg/mL) and time to Cmax of 72 hours (range 48 to 96 hours) was observed in these patients. After continued dosing of RA patients (N=25) with ENBREL for 6 months with 25 mg twice weekly, the median observed level was 3.0 mcg/mL (range 1.7 to 5.6 mcg/mL). Based on the available data, individual patients may undergo a two- to five-fold increase in serum levels with repeated dosing. Serum concentrations in patients with RA have not been measured for periods of dosing that exceed 6 months.

Pharmacokinetic parameters were not different between men and women and did not vary with age in adult patients. No formal pharmacokinetic studies have been conducted to examine the effects of renal or hepatic impairment or interactions with methotrexate.

Pediatric patients with JRA (ages 4 to 17 years) were administered 0.4 mg/kg of ENBREL for up to 18 weeks. The average serum concentration after repeated dosing was 2.1 mcg/mL, with a range of 0.7 to 4.3 mcg/mL. Preliminary data suggests that the clearance of ENBREL is reduced slightly in children ages 4 to 8 years. Children < 4 years of age have not been studied.

CLINICAL STUDIES

Adult Rheumatoid Arthritis

The safety and efficacy of ENBREL were assessed in three randomized, double-blind, controlled studies. Study I evaluated 234 patients with active RA who were ≥ 18 years old, had failed therapy with at least one but no more than four disease-modifying antirheumatic drugs (DMARDs; e.g., hydroxychloroquine, oral or injectable gold, methotrexate [MTX], azathioprine, D-penicillamine, sulfasalazine), and had ≥ 12 tender joints, ≥ 10 swollen joints, and either ESR ≥ 28 mm/hour, CRP > 20 mg/dL, or morning stiffness for ≥ 45 minutes. Doses of 10 mg or 25 mg ENBREL or placebo were administered SC twice a week for 6 consecutive months. Results from patients receiving 25 mg are presented below.

Study II evaluated 89 patients and had similar inclusion criteria to Study I except that subjects in Study II had additionally received MTX for at least 6 months with a stable dose (12.5 to 25 mg/wk) for at least 4 weeks and they had at least 6 tender or painful joints. Subjects in Study II received a dose of 25 mg ENBREL or placebo SC twice a week for 6 months in addition to their stable MTX dose.

Study III compared the efficacy of ENBREL to MTX in patients with active RA. This study evaluated 632 patients who were ≥18 years old with early (≤ 3 years disease duration) active RA; had never received treatment with MTX; and had ≥ 12 tender joints, ≥ 10 swollen joints, and either ESR ≥ 28 mm/hr, CRP > 2.0 mg/dL, or morning stiffness for ≥ 45 minutes. Doses of 10 mg or 25 mg ENBREL were administered SC twice a week for 12 consecutive months. Results from patients receiving 25 mg are presented below. MTX tablets (escalated from 7.5 mg/week to a maximum of 20 mg/week over the first 8 weeks of the trial) or placebo tablets were given once a week on the same day as the injection of placebo or ENBREL doses, respectively.

The results of all three trials were expressed in percentage of patients with improvement in RA using American College of Rheumatology (ACR) response criteria.[7]

Clinical Response

The percent of ENBREL-treated patients achieving ACR 20, 50, and 70 responses was consistent across all three trials. The results of the three trials are summarized in Table 1.

[See table 1 above]

Table 1: ACR Responses in Placebo- and Active-Controlled Trials (Percent of Patients)

	Placebo Controlled				Active Controlled	
	Study I		Study II		Study III	
Response	Placebo N = 80	ENBREL[a] N = 78	MTX/ Placebo N = 30	MTX/ ENBREL[a] N = 59	MTX N = 217	ENBREL[a] N = 207
ACR 20						
Month 3	23%	62%[b]	33%	66%[b]	56%	62%
Month 6	11%	59%[b]	27%	71%[b]	58%	65%
Month 12	NA	NA	NA	NA	65%	72%
ACR 50						
Month 3	8%	41%[b]	0%	42%[b]	24%	29%
Month 6	5%	40%[b]	3%	39%[b]	32%	40%
Month 12	NA	NA	NA	NA	43%	49%
ACR 70						
Month 3	4%	15%[b]	0	15%[b]	7%	13%[c]
Month 6	1%	15%[b]	0	15%[b]	14%	21%[c]
Month 12	NA	NA	NA	NA	22%	25%

a. 25 mg ENBREL SC twice weekly.
b. $p < 0.01$, ENBREL vs. placebo.
c. $p < 0.05$, ENBREL vs. MTX.

Table 2: Components of ACR Response in Study I

	Placebo N = 80		ENBREL[a] N = 78	
Parameter (median)	Baseline	3 Months	Baseline	3 Months*
Number of tender joints[b]	34.0	29.5	31.2	10.0[f]
Number of swollen joints[c]	24.0	22.0	23.5	12.6[f]
Physician global assessment[d]	7.0	6.5	7.0	3.0[f]
Patient global assessment[d]	7.0	7.0	7.0	3.0[f]
Pain[d]	6.9	6.6	6.9	2.4[f]
Disability index[e]	1.7	1.8	1.6	1.0[f]
ESR (mm/hour)	31.0	32.0	28.0	15.5[f]
CRP (mg/dL)	2.8	3.9	3.5	0.9[f]

** Results at 6 months showed similar improvement.*
a. 25 mg ENBREL SC twice weekly.
b. Scale 0–71.
c. Scale 0–68.
d. Visual analog scale; 0 = best, 10 = worst.
e. Health Assessment Questionnaire[8]; 0 = best, 3 = worst; includes eight categories: dressing and grooming, arising, eating, walking, hygiene, reach, grip, and activities.
f. $p < 0.01$, ENBREL vs. placebo, based on mean percent change from baseline.

Table 3: Mean Radiographic Change Over 6 and 12 Months In Study III

		MTX	25 mg ENBREL	MTX-ENBREL (95% Confidence Interval*)	P-value
12 Months	Total Sharp score	1.59	1.00	0.59 (−0.12, 1.30)	0.110
	Erosion score	1.03	0.47	0.56 (0.11, 1.00)	0.002
	JSN score	0.56	0.52	0.04 (−0.39, 0.46)	0.529
6 Months	Total Sharp score	1.06	0.57	0.49 (0.06, 0.91)	0.001
	Erosion score	0.68	0.30	0.38 (0.09, 0.66)	0.001
	JSN score	0.38	0.27	0.11 (−0.14, 0.35)	0.585

** 95% confidence intervals for the differences in change scores between MTX and ENBREL*

The time course for ACR 20 response rates for patients receiving placebo or 25 mg ENBREL in Studies I and II is summarized in Figure 1. The time course of responses to ENBREL in Study III was similar.

[See figure 1 in next column]

Among patients receiving ENBREL, the clinical responses generally appeared within 1 to 2 weeks after initiation of therapy and nearly always occurred by 3 months. A dose response was seen in Studies I and III: 25 mg ENBREL was more effective than 10 mg (10 mg was not evaluated in Study II). ENBREL was significantly better than placebo in

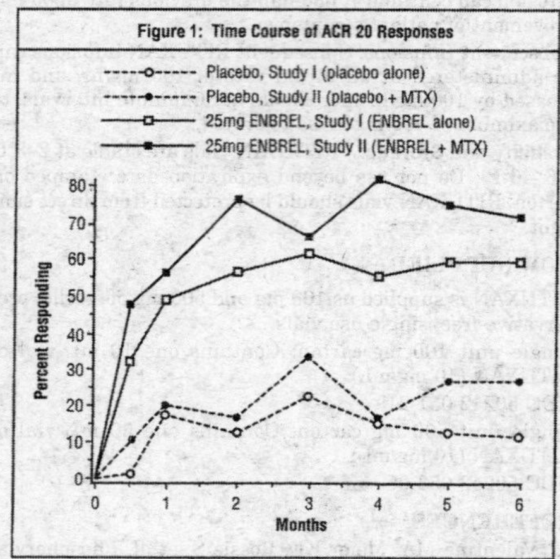

all components of the ACR criteria as well as other measures of RA disease activity not included in the ACR response criteria, such as morning stiffness.

In Study III, approximately 10% of patients treated with ENBREL achieved a major clinical response, defined as maintenance of an ACR 70 response over a 6-month period.

The results of the components of the ACR response criteria for Study I are shown in Table 2. Findings were similar in Studies II and III for patients treated with ENBREL.

[See table 2 above]

After discontinuation of ENBREL, symptoms of arthritis generally returned within a month. Reintroduction of treatment with ENBREL after discontinuations of up to 18 months resulted in the same magnitudes of response as patients who received ENBREL without interruption of therapy based on results of open-label studies. Continued durable responses have been seen for up to 36 months in open-label extension treatment trials when patients received ENBREL without interruption.

A Health Assessment Questionnaire (HAQ),[8] which included disability, vitality, mental health, general health status, and arthritis-associated health status subdomains, was administered every 3 months during Studies I and III. All subdomains of the HAQ were improved in patients treated with ENBREL.

In Study III, health outcome measures were assessed by the SF-36 questionnaire. The eight subscales of the SF-36 were combined into two summary scales, the physical component summary (PCS) and the mental component summary (MCS).[9] At 12 months, patients treated with 25 mg ENBREL showed significantly more improvement in the PCS compared to the 10 mg ENBREL group, but not in the MCS.

Radiographic Response

In Study III, structural joint damage was assessed radiographically and expressed as change in total Sharp score (TSS) and its components, the erosion score and joint space narrowing (JSN) score. Radiographs of hands/wrists and forefeet were read at baseline, 6 months, and 12 months. The results are shown in Table 3. A significant difference for change in erosion score was observed at 6 months and maintained at 12 months.

[See table 3 above]

Polyarticular-Course Juvenile Rheumatoid Arthritis (JRA)

The safety and efficacy of ENBREL were assessed in a two-part study in 69 children with polyarticular-course JRA who had a variety of JRA onset types. Patients ages 4 to 17 years with moderately to severely active polyarticular-course JRA refractory to or intolerant of methotrexate were enrolled; patients remained on a stable dose of a single nonsteroidal anti-inflammatory drug and/or prednisone (≤ 0.2 mg/kg/day or 10 mg maximum). In part 1, all patients received 0.4

mg/kg (maximum 25 mg per dose) ENBREL SC twice weekly. In part 2, patients with a clinical response at day 90 were randomized to remain on ENBREL or receive placebo for four months and assessed for disease flare. Responses were measured using the JRA Definition of Improvement (DOI),[10] defined as ≥ 30% improvement in at least three of six and ≥ 30% worsening in no more than one of six JRA core set criteria, including active joint count, limitation of motion, physician and patient/parent global assessments, functional assessment, and ESR. Disease flare was defined as a ≥ 30% worsening in three of the six JRA core set criteria and ≥ 30% improvement in not more than one of the six JRA core set criteria and a minimum of two active joints. In part 1 of the study, 51 of 69 (74%) patients demonstrated a clinical response and entered part 2.[11] In part 2, 6 of 25 (24%) patients remaining on ENBREL experienced a disease flare compared to 20 of 26 (77%) patients receiving placebo (p = 0.007). From the start of part 2, the median time to flare was ≥ 116 days for patients who received ENBREL and 28 days for patients who received placebo. Each component of the JRA core set criteria worsened in the arm that received placebo and remained stable or improved in the arm that continued on ENBREL. The data suggested the possibility of a higher flare rate among those patients with a higher baseline ESR. Of patients who demonstrated a clinical response at 90 days and entered part 2 of the study, some of the patients remaining on ENBREL continued to improve from month 3 through month 7, while those who received placebo did not improve.

The majority of JRA patients who developed a disease flare in part 2 and reintroduced ENBREL treatment up to 4 months after discontinuation re-responded to ENBREL therapy, in open-label studies. Most of the responding patients who continued ENBREL therapy without interruption have maintained responses for up to 18 months.

Studies have not been done in patients with polyarticular-course JRA to assess the effects of continued ENBREL therapy in patients who do not respond within 3 months of initiating ENBREL therapy, or to assess the combination of ENBREL with methotrexate.

Immunogenicity

Patients were tested at multiple timepoints for antibodies to ENBREL. Antibodies to ENBREL, all non-neutralizing, were detected at least once in sera of < 16% of adult rheumatoid arthritis patients. No apparent correlation of antibody development to clinical response or adverse events was observed. Results from JRA patients were similar to those seen in adult RA patients treated with ENBREL. The long-term immunogenicity of ENBREL is unknown.

The data reflect the percentage of patients whose test results were considered positive for antibodies to ENBREL in an ELISA assay, and are highly dependent on the sensitivity and specificity of the assay. Additionally, the observed incidence of antibody positivity in an assay may be influenced by several factors including sample handling, concomitant medications, and underlying disease. For these reasons, comparison of the incidence of antibodies to ENBREL with the incidence of antibodies to other products may be misleading.

INDICATIONS AND USAGE

ENBREL is indicated for reducing signs and symptoms and delaying structural damage in patients with moderately to severely active rheumatoid arthritis. ENBREL can be used in combination with methotrexate in patients who do not respond adequately to methotrexate alone.

ENBREL is indicated for reducing signs and symptoms of moderately to severely active polyarticular-course juvenile rheumatoid arthritis in patients who have had an inadequate response to one or more DMARDs.

CONTRAINDICATIONS

ENBREL should not be administered to patients with sepsis or with known hypersensitivitiy to ENBREL or any of its components.

WARNINGS

IN POST-MARKETING REPORTS, SERIOUS INFECTIONS AND SEPSIS, INCLUDING FATALITIES, HAVE BEEN REPORTED WITH THE USE OF ENBREL. MANY OF THESE SERIOUS EVENTS HAVE OCCURRED IN PATIENTS WITH UNDERLYING DISEASES THAT IN ADDITION TO THEIR RHEUMATOID ARTHRITIS COULD PREDISPOSE THEM TO INFECTIONS. PATIENTS WHO DEVELOP A NEW INFECTION WHILE UNDERGOING TREATMENT WITH ENBREL SHOULD BE MONITORED CLOSELY. ADMINISTRATION OF ENBREL SHOULD BE DISCONTINUED IF A PATIENT DEVELOPS A SERIOUS INFECTION OR SEPSIS. TREATMENT WITH ENBREL SHOULD NOT BE INITIATED IN PATIENTS WITH ACTIVE INFECTIONS INCLUDING CHRONIC OR LOCALIZED INFECTIONS. PHYSICIANS SHOULD EXERCISE CAUTION WHEN CONSIDERING THE USE OF ENBREL IN PATIENTS WITH A HISTORY OF RECURRING INFECTIONS OR WITH UNDERLYING CONDITIONS WHICH MAY PREDISPOSE PATIENTS TO INFECTIONS, SUCH AS ADVANCED OR POORLY CONTROLLED DIABETES (see PRECAUTIONS, ADVERSE REACTIONS, Infections).

PRECAUTIONS

General

Allergic reactions associated with administration of ENBREL during clinical trials have been reported in < 2% of patients. If an anaphylactic reaction or other serious allergic reaction occurs, administration of ENBREL should be discontinued immediately and appropriate therapy initiated.

Table 4: Percent of RA Patients Reporting Adverse Events In Controlled Clinical Trials*

	Placebo Controlled		Active Controlled (Study III)	
	Percent of patients		Precent of patients	
Event	Placebo† (n = 152)	ENBREL (n = 349)	MTX (n = 217)	ENBREL (n = 415)
Injection site reaction	10	37	7	34
Infection	32	35	72	64
Non-upper respiratory infection**	32	38	60	51
Upper respiratory infection**	16	29	39	31
Headache	13	17	27	24
Nausea	10	9	29	15
Rhinitis	8	12	14	16
Dizziness	5	7	11	8
Pharyngitis	5	7	9	6
Cough	3	6	6	5
Asthenia	3	5	12	11
Abdominal pain	3	5	10	10
Rash	3	5	23	14
Peripheral edema	3	2	4	8
Respiratory disorder	1	5	NA	NA
Dyspepsia	1	4	10	11
Sinusitis	2	3	3	5
Vomiting	–	3	8	5
Mouth ulcer	1	2	14	6
Alopecia	1	1	12	6
Pneumonitis ("MTX lung")	–	–	2	0

* *Includes data from the 6-month study in which patients received concurrent MTX therapy.*
† *The duration of exposure for patients receiving placebo was less than the ENBREL-treated patients.*
** *Includes data from two placebo-controlled trials.*

Information to Patients

If a patient or caregiver is to self-administer ENBREL, he/she should be instructed in injection techniques and how to measure the correct dose to help ensure the proper administration of ENBREL (see **How to Use ENBREL, Instructions for Preparing and Giving an Injection**). The first injection should be performed under the supervision of a qualified health care professional. The patient's or caregiver's ability to self-inject subcutaneously should be assessed. A puncture-resistant container for disposal of needles and syringes should be used. Patients and caregivers should be instructed in the technique as well as proper syringe and needle disposal, and be cautioned against reuse of these items.

Immunosuppression

The possibility exists for anti-TNF therapies, including ENBREL, to affect host defenses against infections and malignancies since TNF mediates inflammation and modulates cellular immune responses. In a study of 49 patients with RA treated with ENBREL, there was no evidence of depression of delayed-type hypersensitivity, depression of immunoglobulin levels, or change in enumeration of effector cell populations. The impact of treatment with ENBREL on the development and course of malignancies as well as active and/or chronic infections is not fully understood (see **WARNINGS, ADVERSE REACTIONS, Infections** and **Malignancies**). The safety and efficacy of ENBREL in patients with immunosuppression or chronic infections have not been evaluated.

Immunizations

No data are available on the effects of vaccination in patients receiving ENBREL. Live vaccines should not be given concurrently with ENBREL. No data are available on the secondary transmission of infection by live vaccines in patients receiving ENBREL (see **PRECAUTIONS, Immunosuppression**).

It is recommended that JRA patients, if possible, be brought up to date with all immunizations in agreement with current immunization guidelines prior to initiating ENBREL therapy. Two JRA patients developed varicella infection and signs and symptoms of aseptic meningitis, which resolved without sequelae. Patients with a significant exposure to varicella virus should temporarily discontinue ENBREL therapy and be considered for prophylactic treatment with Varicella Zoster Immune Globulin.

Autoantibody Formation

Treatment with ENBREL may result in the formation of autoimmune antibodies (see **ADVERSE REACTIONS, Autoantibodies**).

Drug Interactions

Specific drug interaction studies have not been conducted with ENBREL.

Carcinogenesis, Mutagenesis, and Impairment of Fertility

Long-term animal studies have not been conducted to evaluate the carcinogenic potential of ENBREL or its effect on fertility. Mutagenesis studies were conducted in vitro and in vivo, and no evidence of mutagenic activity was observed.

Pregnancy (Category B)

Developmental toxicity studies have been performed in rats and rabbits at doses ranging from 60- to 100-fold higher than the human dose and have revealed no evidence of harm to the fetus due to ENBREL. There are, however, no studies in pregnant women. Because animal reproduction studies are not always predictive of human response, this drug should be used during pregnancy only if clearly needed.

Nursing Mothers

It is not known whether ENBREL is excreted in human milk or absorbed systemically after ingestion. Because many drugs and immunoglobulins are excreted in human milk, and because of the potential for serious adverse reactions in nursing infants from ENBREL, a decision should be made whether to discontinue nursing or to discontinue the drug.

Geriatric Use

A total of 197 RA patients ages 65 years or older have been studied in clinical trials. No overall differences in safety or effectiveness were observed between these patients and younger patients. Because there is a higher incidence of infections in the elderly population in general, caution should be used in treating the elderly.

Pediatric Use

ENBREL is indicated for treatment of polyarticular-course juvenile rheumatoid arthritis in patients who have had an inadequate response to one or more DMARDs. For issues relevant to pediatric patients, in addition to other sections of the label, see also **PRECAUTIONS, Immunizations,** and **ADVERSE REACTIONS, Adverse Reactions in Pediatric Patients**. ENBREL has not been studied in children < 4 years of age.

ADVERSE REACTIONS

ENBREL has been studied in 1197 patients with RA, followed for up to 36 months. The proportion of patients who discontinued treatment due to adverse events was approximately 4% in both ENBREL and placebo-treated patients.

Injection Site Reactions

In controlled trials, 37% of patients treated with ENBREL developed injection site reactions. All injection site reactions were described as mild to moderate (erythema and/or itching, pain, or swelling) and generally did not necessitate drug discontinuation. Injection site reactions generally occurred in the first month and subsequently decreased in frequency. The mean duration of injection site reactions was 3 to 5 days. Seven percent of patients experienced redness at a previous injection site when subsequent injections were given.

Infections

In controlled trials, there were no differences in rates of infection among patients treated with ENBREL and those treated with placebo or MTX. The most common type of infection was upper respiratory infection, which occurred in 16% of placebo-treated patients and 29% of patients treated with ENBREL. When the longer observation of patients on ENBREL was accounted for, the event rate was similar in both groups.

In placebo-controlled trials in DMARD-refractory RA, no increase in the incidence of serious infections was observed (approximately 1% in both placebo and ENBREL-treated groups). The rates of infections for the ENBREL arm in Study III were similar. In all clinical trials in RA, 50 of 1197 subjects exposed to ENBREL for up to 36 months experienced serious infections, including pyelonephritis, bronchitis, septic arthritis, abdominal abscess, cellulitis, osteomyelitis, wound infection, pneumonia, foot abscess, leg ulcer, diarrhea, sinusitis, and sepsis. Serious infections, including sepsis and death, have also been reported during post-marketing use of ENBREL. Some have occurred within a few weeks after initiating treatment with ENBREL. Many of the patients had underlying conditions (e.g., diabetes, congestive heart failure, history of active or chronic infections) in addition to their rheumatoid arthritis. (See **WARNINGS**). Data from a sepsis clinical trial not specifically in patients with RA suggest that ENBREL treatment may increase mortality in patients with established sepsis.[12]

Continued on next page

Enbrel—Cont.

Malignancies
Seventeen malignancies of various types were observed in 1197 RA patients treated in clinical trials with ENBREL for up to 36 months. The observed rates and incidences were similar to those expected for the population studied.
Autoantibodies
Patients had serum samples tested for autoantibodies at multiple timepoints. In Studies I and II, the percentage of patients evaluated for antinuclear antibodies (ANA), the percentage of patients who developed new positive ANA (≥ 1:40) was higher in patients treated with ENBREL (11%) than in placebo-treated patients (5%). The percentage of patients who developed new positive anti-double-stranded DNA antibodies was also higher by radioimmunoassay (15% of patients treated with ENBREL compared to 4% of placebo-treated patients) and by crithidia lucilae assay (3% of patients treated with ENBREL compared to none of placebo-treated patients). The proportion of patients treated with ENBREL who developed anticardiolipin antibodies was similarly increased compared to placebo-treated patients. In Study III, no pattern of increased autoantibody development was seen in ENBREL patients compared to MTX patients. No patients in placebo- and active-controlled trials developed clinical signs suggestive of a lupus-like syndrome. The impact of long-term treatment with ENBREL on the development of autoimmune diseases is unknown.
Other Adverse Reactions
Table 4 summarizes events reported in at least 3% of all patients with higher incidence in patients treated with ENBREL compared to controls in placebo-controlled RA trials (including the combination methotrexate trial) and relevant events from Study III.
[See table 4 at top of previous page]
Among patients with rheumatoid arthritis treated in placebo-controlled trials, serious adverse events occurred at a frequency of 4% in 349 patients treated with ENBREL compared to 5% of 152 placebo-treated patients. In Study III, serious adverse events occurred at a frequency of 6% in 415 patients treated with ENBREL compared to 8% of 217 MTX-treated patients. Among patients with RA in placebo-controlled, active-controlled, and open-label trials of ENBREL, malignancies (see **ADVERSE REACTIONS, Malignancies**) and infections (see **ADVERSE REACTIONS, Infections**) were the most common serious adverse events observed. Other infrequent serious adverse events observed included heart failure, myocardial infarction, myocardial ischemia, cerebral ischemia, hypertension, hypotension, cholecystitis, pancreatitis, gastrointestinal hemorrhage, bursitis, depression, dyspnea, deep vein thrombosis, pulmonary embolism, membranous glomerulonephropathy, polymyositis, and thrombophlebitis.
Adverse Reactions in Pediatric Patients
In general, the adverse events in pediatric patients were similar in frequency and type as those seen in adult patients. Differences from adult and other special considerations are discussed in the following paragraphs.
Severe adverse reactions reported in 69 JRA patients ages 4 to 17 years included varicella (see also **PRECAUTIONS, Immunizations**), gastroenteritis, depression/personality disorder, cutaneous ulcer, esophagitis/gastritis, group A streptococcal septic shock, type I diabetes mellitus, and soft tissue and post-operative wound infection.
Forty-three of 69 (62%) children with JRA experienced an infection while receiving ENBREL during three months of study (part 1 open-label), and the frequency and severity of infections was similar in 58 patients completing 12 months of open-label extension therapy. The types of infections reported in JRA patients were generally mild and consistent with those commonly seen in outpatient pediatric populations.
The following adverse events were reported more commonly in 69 JRA patients receiving 3 months of ENBREL compared to the 349 adult RA patients in placebo-controlled trials. These included headache (19% of patients, 1.7 events per patient year), nausea (9%, 1.0 events per patient year), abdominal pain (19%, 0.74 events per patient year), and vomiting (13%, 0.74 events per patient year).

OVERDOSAGE
The maximum tolerated dose of ENBREL has not been established in humans. Toxicology studies have been performed in monkeys at doses up to 30 times the human dose with no evidence of dose-limiting toxicities. No dose-limiting toxicities have been observed during clinical trials of ENBREL. Single IV doses up to 60 mg/m^2 have been administered to healthy volunteers in an endotoxemia study without evidence of dose-limiting toxicities. The highest dose level evaluated in RA patients has been a single IV loading dose of 32 mg/m^2 followed by SC doses of 16 mg/m^2 (~25 mg) administered twice weekly. In one RA trial, one patient mistakenly self-administered 62 mg ENBREL SC twice weekly for 3 weeks without experiencing adverse effects.

DOSAGE AND ADMINISTRATION
The recommended dose of ENBREL for adult patients with rheumatoid arthritis is 25 mg given twice weekly as a subcutaneous injection 72–96 hours apart (see **Clinical Studies**). Methotrexate, glucocorticoids, salicylates, nonsteroidal anti-inflammatory drugs (NSAIDs) or analgesics may be continued during treatment with ENBREL. Higher doses of ENBREL have not been studied.
The recommended dose of ENBREL for pediatric patients ages 4 to 17 years with active polyarticular-course JRA is 0.4 mg/kg (up to a maximum 25 mg per dose) given twice weekly as a subcutaneous injection 72–96 hours apart. Glucocorticoids, nonsteroidal anti-inflamatory drugs (NSAIDs), or analgesics may be continued during treatment with ENBREL. Concurrent use with methotrexate and higher doses of ENBREL have not been studied in pediatric patients.
Preparation of ENBREL
ENBREL is intended for use under the guidance and supervision of a physician. Patients may self-inject only if their physician determines that it is appropriate and with medical follow-up, as necessary, after proper training in how to measure the correct dose and in injection technique.
Note: The needle cover of the diluent syringe contains dry natural rubber (latex), which should not be handled by persons sensitive to this substance.
ENBREL should be reconstituted aseptically with 1 mL of the supplied Sterile Bacteriostatic Water for Injection, USP (0.9% benzyl alcohol) giving a solution of 1.0 mL containing 25 mg of ENBREL. During reconstitution of ENBREL, the diluent should be injected very slowly into the vial. Some foaming will occur. This is normal. To avoid excessive foaming, **do not shake or vigorously agitate**. The contents should be swirled gently during dissolution. Generally, dissolution of ENBREL takes less than 10 minutes. The reconstituted solution should be clear and colorless and used within 6 hours (see **Storage and Stability**).
Visually inspect the solution for particulate matter and discoloration prior to administration. The solution should not be used if discolored or cloudy, or if particulate matter remains. Withdraw the solution into a syringe, removing only the dose to be given from the vial. Some foam or bubbles may remain in the vial.
No other medications should be added to solutions containing ENBREL, and do not reconstitute ENBREL with other diluents. Do not filter reconstituted solution during preparation or administration.
Rotate sites for injection (thigh, abdomen, or upper arm). New injections should be given at least one inch from an old site and never into areas where the skin is tender. bruised, red, or hard. (See **How to Use ENBREL, Instructions for Preparing and Giving an Injection** instruction sheet.)
Storage and Stability
Do not use a dose tray beyond the date stamped on the carton, dose tray label, vial label, or diluent syringe label. The dose tray containing ENBREL (sterile powder) must be refrigerated at 2–8°C (36–46°F). DO NOT FREEZE.
Administer reconstituted solutions of ENBREL as soon as possible after reconstitution. If not administered immediately after reconstitution, ENBREL may be stored in the vial at 2–8° (36–46°F) for up to 6 hours. **ANY ENBREL NOT USED WITHIN 6 HOURS OF RECONSTITUTION SHOULD BE DISCARDED. PRODUCT STABILITY AND STERILITY CANNOT BE ASSURED.**

HOW SUPPLIED
ENBREL is supplied in a carton containing four dose trays (NDC 58406-425-34). Each dose tray contains one 25 mg single-use vial of etanercept, one syringe (1 mL Sterile Bacteriostatic Water for Injection, USP, containing 0.9% benzyl alcohol), one plunger, and two alcohol swabs.
Rx only

REFERENCES

1. Feldman M, Brennan FM, Maini RN. The role of cytokines in rheumatoid arthritis. Ann Rev Immunol 1996;14: 397.
2. Grom A, Murray KF, Luyrink L, et al. Patterns of expression of tumor necrosis factor α, tumor necrosis factor β, and their receptors in synovia of patients with juvenile rheumatoid arthritis and juvenile spondyloarthropathy. Arthritis Rheum 1996;39:1703.
3. Saxne T, Palladino Jr MA, Heinegard D, et al. Detection of tumor necrosis factor alpha but not tumor necrosis factor beta in rheumatoid arthritis synovial fluid and serum. Arthritis Rheum 1988;31:1041.
4. Smith CA, Farrah T, Goodwin RG. The TNF receptor superfamily of cellular and viral proteins: activation, costimulation, and death. Cell 1994;75:959.
5. Wooley PH, Dutcher J, Widmer MB, et al. Influence of a recombinant human soluble tumor necrosis factor receptor FC fusion protein on type II collagen-induced arthritis in mice. J Immunol 1993;151:6602.
6. Data on file, Immunex Corporation.
7. Felson DT, Anderson JJ, Boers M, et al. American College of Rheumatology preliminary definition of improvement in rheumatoid arthritis. Arthritis Rheum 1995;6: 727.
8. Ramey DR, Fries JF, Singh G. The Health Assessment Questionnaire 1995 – Status and Review. In: Spilker B, ed. "Quality of Life and Pharmacoeconomics in Clinical Trials." 2nd ed. Philadelphia, PA. Lippincott-Raven;1996.
9. Ware JE, Gandek, B. Overview of the SF-36 Health Survey and the International Quality of Life Assessment (IQOLA) Project. J. Clin Epidemiol 1998;51(11):903–12.
10. Giannini EH, Ruperto N, Ravelli A, et al. Preliminary definition of improvement in juvenile arthritis. Arthr Rheum 1997;40(7):1202.
11. Lovell DJ, Giannini EH, Reiff A, et al. Etanercept in children with polyarticular juvenile rheumatoid arthritis. N Engl J Med 2000;342(11):763–9.
12. Fisher CJ Jr, Agosti JM, Opal SM, et al. Treatment of septic shock with the tumor necrosis factor receptor:Fc fusion protein. The Soluble TNF Receptor Sepsis Study Group. N Engl J Med 1996;334(26):1697.

0311-04 Issue Date 06/2000
Manufactured by:
Immunex Corporation
Seattle, Washington 98101
U.S. License Number 1132
Marketed by Immunex Corporation and Wyeth-Ayerst Pharmaceuticals

Immunex U.S. Patent Numbers:
5,605,690; 5,712,155; 5,395,760; 5,945,397

LEUKINE® ℞
SARGRAMOSTIM

Caution: Federal law prohibits dispensing without prescription.

DESCRIPTION
LEUKINE® (sargramostim) is a recombinant human granulocyte-macrophage colony stimulating factor (rhu GM-CSF) produced by recombinant DNA technology in a yeast *(S. cerevisiae)* expression system. GM-CSF is a hematopoietic growth factor which stimulates proliferation and differentiation of hematopoietic progenitor cells. LEUKINE is a glycoprotein of 127 amino acids characterized by 3 primary molecular species having molecular masses of 19,500, 16,800 and 15,500 daltons. The amino acid sequence of LEUKINE differs from the natural human GM-CSF by a substitution of leucine at position 23, and the carbohydrate moiety may be different from the native protein. Sargramostim has been selected as the proper name for yeast-derived rhu GM-CSF.
The LEUKINE Liquid presentation is formulated as a sterile, preserved (1.1% benzyl alcohol), injectable solution (500 mcg/mL) in a vial. Lyophilized LEUKINE is a sterile, white, preservative-free powder (250 mcg) that requires reconstitution with 1 mL Sterile Water for Injection, USP or 1 mL Bacteriostatic Water for Injection, USP.
LEUKINE Liquid and reconstituted lyophilized LEUKINE are clear, colorless liquids suitable for subcutaneous injection or intravenous infusion. LEUKINE Liquid contains 500 mcg (2.8×10^6 IU/mL) sargramostim and 1.1% benzyl alcohol in a 1 mL solution. The vial of lyophilized LEUKINE contains 250 mcg (1.4×10^6 IU/vial) sargramostim. The LEUKINE Liquid vial and reconstituted lyophilized LEUKINE vial also contain 40 mg/mL mannitol, USP; 10 mg/mL sucrose, NF; and 1.2 mg/mL tromethamine, USP, as excipients. Biological potency is expressed in International Units (IU) as tested against the WHO First International Reference Standard. The specific activity of LEUKINE is approximately 5.6×10^6 IU/mg.

CLINICAL PHARMACOLOGY
General GM-CSF belongs to a group of growth factors termed colony stimulating factors which support survival, clonal expansion, and differentiation of hematopoietic progenitor cells. GM-CSF induces partially committed progenitor cells to divide and differentiate in the granulocyte-macrophage pathways.
GM-CSF is also capable of activating mature granulocytes and macrophages. GM-CSF is a multilineage factor and, in addition to dose-dependent effects on the myelomonocytic lineage, can promote the proliferation of megakaryocytic and erythroid progenitors.[1] However, other factors are required to induce complete maturation in these two lineages. The various cellular responses (i.e., division, maturation, activation) are induced through GM-CSF binding to specific receptors expressed on the cell surface of target cells.[2]
***In vitro* Studies of LEUKINE in Human Cells** The biological activity of GM-CSF is species-specific. Consequently, *in vitro* studies have been performed on human cells to characterize the pharmacological activity of LEUKINE. *In vitro* exposure of human bone marrow cells to LEUKINE at concentrations ranging from 1–100 ng/mL results in the proliferation of hematopoietic progenitors and in the formation of pure granulocyte, pure macrophage and mixed granulocyte-macrophage colonies.[3] Chemotactic, anti-fungal and anti-parasitic[4] activities of granulocytes and monocytes are increased by exposure to LEUKINE *in vitro*. LEUKINE increases the cytotoxicity of monocytes toward certain neoplastic cell lines[3] and activates polymorphonuclear neutrophils to inhibit the growth of tumor cells.
***In vivo* Primate Studies of LEUKINE** Pharmacology/toxicology studies of LEUKINE were performed in cynomolgus monkeys. An acute toxicity study revealed an absence of treatment-related toxicity following a single IV bolus injection at a dose of 300 mcg/kg. Two subacute studies were performed using IV injection (maximum dose 200 mcg/kg/day × 14 days) and subcutaneous injection (maximum dose 200 mcg/kg/day × 28 days). No major visceral organ toxicity was documented. Notable histopathology findings included increased cellularity in hematologic organs and heart and lung tissues. A dose-dependent increase in leukocyte count, which consisted primarily of segmented neutrophils, occurred during the dosing period; increases in monocytes, basophils, eosinophils and lymphocytes were also noted. Leukocyte counts decreased to pretreatment values over a 1–2 week recovery period.
Pharmacokinetics Pharmacokinetic profiles have been analyzed in controlled studies of 24 normal male volunteers.

Liquid and lyophilized LEUKINE, at the recommended dose of 250 mcg/m^2, have been determined to be bioequivalent based on the statistical evaluation of AUC.[5]

When LEUKINE (either liquid or lyophilized) was administered IV over 2 hours to normal volunteers, the mean beta half-life was approximately 60 minutes. Peak concentrations of GM-CSF were observed in blood samples obtained during or immediately after completion of LEUKINE infusion. For LEUKINE Liquid, the mean maximum concentration (Cmax) was 5.0 ng/mL, the mean clearance rate was approximately 420 mL/min/m^2 and the mean AUC (0–inf) was 640 ng/mL·min. Corresponding results for lyophilized LEUKINE in the same subjects were mean Cmax of 5.4 ng/mL, mean clearance rate of 431 mL/min/m^2, and mean AUC (0–inf) of 677 ng/mL·min. GM-CSF was last detected in blood samples obtained at 3 or 6 hours.

When LEUKINE (either liquid or lyophilized) was administered SC to normal volunteers, GM-CSF was detected in the serum at 15 minutes, the first sample point. The mean beta half-life was approximately 162 minutes. Peak levels occurred at 1 to 3 hours post injection, and LEUKINE remained undetectable for up to 6 hours after injection. The mean Cmax was 1.5 ng/mL. For LEUKINE Liquid, the mean clearance was 549 mL/min/m^2 and the mean AUC (0–inf) was 549 ng/mL·min. For lyophilized LEUKINE, the mean clearance was 529 mL/min/m^2 and the mean AUC (0–inf) was 501 ng/mL·min.

Antibody Formation Serum samples collected before and after LEUKINE treatment from 214 patients with a variety of underlying diseases have been examined for the presence of antibodies. Neutralizing antibodies were detected in 5 of 214 patients (2.3%) after receiving LEUKINE by continuous IV infusion (3 patients) or subcutaneous injection (2 patients) for 28 to 84 days in multiple courses. All 5 patients had impaired hematopoiesis before the administration of LEUKINE and consequently the effect of the development of anti-GM-CSF antibodies on normal hematopoiesis could not be assessed. Drug-induced neutropenia, neutralization of endogenous GM-CSF activity and diminution of the therapeutic effect of LEUKINE secondary to formation of neutralizing antibody remain a theoretical possibility.

INDICATIONS AND USAGE

Use Following Induction Chemotherapy in Acute Myelogenous Leukemia LEUKINE is indicated for use following induction chemotherapy in older adult patients with acute myelogenous leukemia (AML) to shorten time to neutrophil recovery and to reduce the incidence of severe and life-threatening infections and infections resulting in death. The safety and efficacy of LEUKINE have not been assessed in patients with AML under 55 years of age.

The term acute myelogenous leukemia, also referred to as acute non-lymphocytic leukemia (ANLL), encompasses a heterogeneous group of leukemias arising from various nonlymphoid cell lines which have been defined morphologically by the French-American-British (FAB) system of classification.

Use in Mobilization and Following Transplantation of Autologous Peripheral Blood Progenitor Cells LEUKINE is indicated for the mobilization of hematopoietic progenitor cells into peripheral blood for collection by leukapheresis. Mobilization allows for the collection of increased numbers of progenitor cells capable of engraftment as compared with collection without mobilization. After myeloablative chemotherapy, the transplantation of an increased number of progenitor cells can lead to more rapid engraftment, which may result in a decreased need for supportive care. Myeloid reconstitution is further accelerated by administration of LEUKINE following peripheral blood progenitor cell transplantation.

Use in Myeloid Reconstitution After Autologous Bone Marrow Transplantation LEUKINE is indicated for acceleration of myeloid recovery in patients with non-Hodgkin's lymphoma (NHL), acute lymphoblastic leukemia (ALL) and Hodgkin's disease undergoing autologous bone marrow transplantation (BMT). After autologous BMT in patients with NHL, ALL, or Hodgkin's disease, LEUKINE has been found to be safe and effective in accelerating myeloid engraftment, decreasing median duration of antibiotic administration, reducing the median duration of infectious episodes and shortening the median duration of hospitalization. Hematologic response to LEUKINE can be detected by complete blood count (CBC) with differential performed twice per week.

Use in Myeloid Reconstitution After Allogeneic Bone Marrow Transplantation LEUKINE is indicated for acceleration of myeloid recovery in patients undergoing allogeneic BMT from HLA-matched related donors. LEUKINE has been found to be safe and effective in accelerating myeloid engraftment, reducing the incidence of bacteremia and other culture positive infections, and shortening the median duration of hospitalization.

Use in Bone Marrow Transplantation Failure or Engraftment Delay LEUKINE is indicated in patients who have undergone allogeneic or autologous bone marrow transplantation (BMT) in whom engraftment is delayed or has failed. LEUKINE has been found to be safe and effective in prolonging survival of patients who are experiencing graft failure or engraftment delay, in the presence or absence of infection, following autologous or allogeneic BMT. Survival benefit may be relatively greater in those patients who demonstrate one or more of the following characteristics: autologous BMT failure or engraftment delay, no previous total body irradiation, malignancy other than leukemia or a multiple organ failure (MOF) score ≤ 2 (See CLINICAL EXPERIENCE). Hematologic response to LEUKINE can be detected by complete blood count (CBC) with differential performed twice per week.

Hematological Recovery (in Days): Induction

Dataset	sargramostim n=52* Median (25%, 75%)	Placebo n=47 Median (25%, 75%)	p-value**
ANC>500/mm^3 [a]	13 (11, 16)	17 (13, 25)	0.009
ANC>1000/mm^3 [b]	14 (12, 18)	21 (13, 34)	0.003
PLT>20,000/mm^3 [c]	11 (7, 14)	12 (9, >42)	0.10
RBC[d]	12 (9, 24)	14 (9, 42)	0.53

** Patients with missing data censored.*
[a] 2 patients on sargramostim and 4 patients on placebo had missing values.
[b] 2 patients on sargramostim and 3 patients on placebo had missing values.
[c] 4 patients on placebo had missing values.
[d] 3 patients on sargramostim and 4 patients on placebo had missing values.
*** p=Generalized Wilcoxon*

ANC and Platelet Recovery after PBPC Transplant

	Route for Mobilization	Post-transplant LEUKINE	ENGRAFTMENT (median value in days) ANC>500/mm^3	Last platelet transfusion
No Mobilization	-	no	29	28
LEUKINE 250 mcg/m^2	IV	no	21	24
	IV	yes	12	19
	SC	yes	12	17

CLINICAL EXPERIENCE

Acute Myelogenous Leukemia The safety and efficacy of sargramostim in patients with AML who are younger than 55 years of age have not been determined. Based on Phase II data suggesting the best therapeutic effects could be achieved in patients at highest risk for severe infections and mortality while neutropenic, the Phase III clinical trial was conducted in older patients. The safety and efficacy of LEUKINE in the treatment of AML were evaluated in a multicenter, randomized, double-blind placebo-controlled trial of 99 newly diagnosed adult patients, 55–70 years of age, receiving induction with or without consolidation.[6] A combination of standard doses of daunorubicin (days 1–3) and ara-C (days 1–7) was administered during induction and high dose ara-C was administered days 1–6 as a single course of consolidation, if given. Bone marrow evaluation was performed on day 10 following induction chemotherapy. If hypoplasia with <5% blasts was not achieved, patients immediately received a second cycle of induction chemotherapy. If the bone marrow was hypoplastic with <5% blasts on day 10 or 4 days following the second cycle of induction chemotherapy, LEUKINE (250 mcg/m^2/day) or placebo was given IV over 4 hours each day, starting 4 days after the completion of chemotherapy. Study drug was continued until an ANC ≥1500/mm^3 for three consecutive days was attained or a maximum of 42 days. LEUKINE or placebo was also administered after the single course of consolidation chemotherapy if delivered (ara-C 3–6 weeks after induction following neutrophil recovery). Study drug was discontinued immediately if leukemic regrowth occurred.

[See first table above]

LEUKINE (sargramostim) significantly shortened the median duration of ANC <500/mm^3 by 4 days and <1000/mm^3 by 7 days following induction (see table at right). 75% of patients receiving LEUKINE achieved ANC >500/mm^3 by day 16, compared to day 25 for patients receiving placebo. The proportion of patients receiving 1 cycle (70%) or 2 cycles (30%) of induction was similar in both treatment groups; LEUKINE significantly shortened the median times to neutrophil recovery whether one cycle (12 versus 15 days) or two cycles (14 versus 23 days) of induction chemotherapy was administered. Median times to platelet (>20,000/mm^3) and RBC transfusion independence were not significantly different between treatment groups.

During the consolidation phase of treatment, LEUKINE did not shorten the median time to recovery of ANC to 500/mm^3 (13 days) or 1000/mm^3 (14.5 days) compared to placebo. There were no significant differences in time to platelet and RBC transfusion independence.

The incidence of severe infections and deaths associated with infections was significantly reduced in patients who received LEUKINE. During induction or consolidation, 27 of 52 patients receiving LEUKINE and 35 of 47 patients receiving placebo had at least one grade 3, 4 or 5 infection (p=0.02). Twenty-five patients receiving LEUKINE and 30 patients receiving placebo experienced severe and fatal infections during induction only. There were significantly fewer deaths from infectious causes in the sargramostim arm (3 versus 11, p=0.02). The majority of deaths in the placebo group were associated with fungal infections with pneumonia as the primary infection.

Disease outcomes were not adversely affected by the use of LEUKINE. The proportion of patients achieving complete remission (CR) was higher in the LEUKINE group (69% as compared to 55% for the placebo group), but the difference was not significant (p=0.21). There was no significant difference in relapse rates; 12 of 36 patients who received LEUKINE and 5 of 26 patients who received placebo relapsed within 180 days of documented CR (p=0.26). The overall median survival was 378 days for patients receiving LEUKINE and 268 days for those on placebo (p=0.17). The study was not sized to assess the impact of LEUKINE treatment on response or survival.

Mobilization and Engraftment of PBPC A retrospective review was conducted of data from patients with cancer undergoing collection of peripheral blood progenitor cells (PBPC) at a single transplant center. Mobilization of PBPC and myeloid reconstitution post-transplant were compared between four groups of patients (n=196) receiving LEUKINE for mobilization and a historical control group who did not receive any mobilization treatment [progenitor cells collected by leukapheresis without mobilization (n=100)]. Sequential cohorts received LEUKINE. The cohorts differed by dose (125 or 250 mcg/m^2/day), route (IV over 24 hours or SC) and use of LEUKINE post-transplant. Leukaphereses were initiated for all mobilization groups after the WBC reached 10,000/mm^3. Leukaphereses continued until both a minimum number of mononucleated cells (MNC) were collected (6.5 or 8.0 × 10^8/kg body weight) and a minimum number of phereses (5–8) were performed. Both minimum requirements varied by treatment cohort and planned conditioning regimen. If subjects failed to reach a WBC of 10,000 cells/mm^3 by day 5, another cytokine was substituted for LEUKINE; these subjects were all successfully leukapheresed and transplanted. The most marked mobilization and post-transplant effects were seen in patients administered the higher dose of LEUKINE (250 mcg/m^2) either IV (n=63) or SC (n=41).

PBPCs from patients treated at the 250 mcg/m^2/day dose had significantly higher number of granulocyte-macrophage colony-forming units (CFU-GM) than those collected without mobilization. The mean value after thawing was 11.41 × 10^4 CFU-GM/kg for all LEUKINE-mobilized patients, compared to 0.96 × 10^4/kg for the non-mobilized group. A similar difference was observed in the mean number of erythrocyte burst-forming units (BFU-E) collected (23.96 × 10^4/kg for patients mobilized with 250 mcg/m^2 doses of LEUKINE administered SC vs. 1.63 × 10^4/kg for non-mobilized patients).

[See second table above]

After transplantation, mobilized subjects had shorter times to myeloid engraftment and fewer days between transplantation and the last platelet transfusion compared to non-mobilized subjects. Neutrophil recovery (ANC >500/mm^3) was more rapid in patients administered LEUKINE following PBPC transplantation with LEUKINE-mobilized cells (see table at right). Mobilized patients also had fewer days to the last platelet transfusion and last RBC transfusion, and a shorter duration of hospitalization than did non-mobilized subjects.

A second retrospective review of data from patients undergoing PBPC at another single transplant center was also conducted. LEUKINE was given SC at 250 mcg/m^2/day once a day (n=10) or twice a day (n=21) until completion of the phereses. Phereses were begun on day 5 of LEUKINE administration and continued until the targeted MNC count of 9 × 10^8/kg or CD34+ cell count of 1 × 10^6/kg was reached. There was no difference in CD34+ cell count in patients receiving LEUKINE once or twice a day. The median time to ANC>500/mm^3 was 12 days and to platelet recovery (>25,000/mm^3) was 23 days.

Survival studies comparing mobilized study patients to the non-mobilized patients and to an autologous historical bone marrow transplant group showed no differences in median survival time.

Autologous Bone Marrow Transplantation[7] Following a dose-ranging Phase I/II trial in patients undergoing autologous BMT for lymphoid malignancies,[8, 9] three single center,

Continued on next page

Leukine—Cont.

randomized, placebo-controlled and double-blinded studies were conducted to evaluate the safety and efficacy of LEUKINE for promoting hematopoietic reconstitution following autologous BMT. A total of 128 patients (65 LEUKINE, 63 placebo) were enrolled in these 3 studies. The majority of the patients had lymphoid malignancy (87 NHL, 17 ALL), 23 patients had Hodgkin's disease, and 1 patient had acute myeloblastic leukemia (AML). In 72 patients with NHL or ALL, the bone marrow harvest was purged prior to storage with one of several monoclonal antibodies. No chemical agent was used for *in vitro* treatment of the bone marrow. Preparative regimens in the 3 studies included cyclophosphamide (total dose 120–150 mg/kg) and total body irradiation (total dose 1,200–1,575 rads). Other regimens used in patients with Hodgkin's disease and NHL without radiotherapy consisted of 3 or more of the following in combination (expressed as total dose): cytosine arabinoside (400 mg/m^2) and carmustine (300 mg/m^2), cyclophosphamide (140–150 mg/kg), hydroxyurea (4.5 grams/m^2) and etoposide (375–450 mg/m^2).

Compared to placebo, administration of LEUKINE in 2 studies (n=44 and 47) significantly improved the following hematologic and clinical endpoints: time to neutrophil engraftment, duration of hospitalization and infection experience or antibacterial usage. In the third study (n=37) there was a positive trend toward earlier myeloid engraftment in favor of LEUKINE. This latter study differed from the other 2 in having enrolled a large number of patients with Hodgkin's disease who had also received extensive radiation and chemotherapy prior to harvest of autologous bone marrow. A subgroup analysis of the data from all 3 studies revealed that the median time to engraftment for patients with Hodgkin's disease, regardless of treatment, was 6 days longer when compared to patients with NHL and ALL, but that the overall beneficial LEUKINE treatment effect was the same. In the following combined analysis of the 3 studies, these 2 subgroups (NHL and ALL vs. Hodgkin's disease) are presented separately.

Patients with Lymphoid Malignancy (Non-Hodgkin's Lymphoma and Acute Lymphoblastic Leukemia): Myeloid engraftment (absolute neutrophil count [ANC] ≥ 500 cells/mm^3) in 54 patients receiving LEUKINE was observed 6 days earlier than in 50 patients treated with placebo (see table at right).

[See first table above]

Autologous BMT: Combined Analysis from Placebo-Controlled Clinical Trials of Responses in Patients with NHL and ALL

	Median Value (days)				
	ANC ≥500/mm^3	ANC ≥1000/mm^3	Duration of Hospitalization	Duration of Infection	Duration of Antibacterial Therapy
LEUKINE (n=54)	18*#	24*#	25*	1*	21*
Placebo (n=50)	24	32	31	4	25

* $p<0.05$ *Wilcoxon or CMH ridit chi-squared*
\# $p<0.05$ *Log rank*
Note: The single AML patient was not included.

Accelerated myeloid engraftment was associated with significant clinical benefits. The median duration of hospitalization was 6 days shorter for the LEUKINE group than for the placebo group. Median duration of infectious episodes (defined as fever and neutropenia; or 2 positive cultures of the same organism; or fever >38°C and 1 positive blood culture; or clinical evidence of infection) was 3 days less in the group treated with LEUKINE. The median duration of antibacterial administration in the post-transplantation period was 4 days shorter for the patients treated with LEUKINE than for placebo-treated patients. The study was unable to detect a significant difference between the treatment groups in rate of disease relapse 24 months post-transplantation. As a group, leukemic subjects receiving LEUKINE derived less benefit than NHL subjects. However, both the leukemic and NHL groups receiving LEUKINE engrafted earlier than controls.

Patients with Hodgkin's Disease: If patients with Hodgkin's disease are analyzed separately, a trend toward earlier myeloid engraftment is noted. LEUKINE-treated patients engrafted earlier (by 5 days) than the placebo-treated patients (p=0.189, Wilcoxon) but the number of patients was small (n=22). Studies are in progress to confirm statistically the trend toward earlier engraftment with LEUKINE in patients with Hodgkin's disease.

Allogeneic Bone Marrow Transplantation A multi-center, randomized, placebo-controlled, and double-blinded study was conducted to evaluate the safety and efficacy of LEUKINE for promoting hematopoietic reconstitution following allogeneic BMT. A total of 109 patients (53 LEUKINE, 56 placebo) were enrolled in the study. Twenty-three patients (11 LEUKINE, 12 placebo) were 18 years old or younger. Sixty-seven patients had myeloid malignancies (33 AML, 34 CML), 17 had lymphoid malignancies (12 ALL, 5 NHL), 3 patients had Hodgkin's disease, 6 had multiple myeloma, 9 had myelodysplastic disease, and 7 patients had aplastic anemia. In 22 patients at one of the seven study sites, bone marrow harvests were depleted of T cells. Preparative regimens included cyclophosphamide, busulfan, cytosine arabinoside, etoposide, methotrexate, corticosteroids, and asparaginase. Some patients also received total body, splenic, or testicular irradiation. Primary graft-versus-host disease (GVHD) prophylaxis was cyclosporine A and a corticosteroid.

Accelerated myeloid engraftment was associated with significant laboratory and clinical benefits. Compared to placebo, administration of LEUKINE significantly improved the following: time to neutrophil engraftment, duration of hospitalization, number of patients with bacteremia and overall incidence of infection (see table at right).

[See second table above]

Allogeneic BMT: Analysis of Data from Placebo-Controlled Clinical Trial

	Median Values (days or number of patients)				
	ANC ≥ 500/mm^3	ANC ≥ 1000/mm^3	Number of Patients with Infections	Number of Patients with Bacteremia	Days of Hospitalization
LEUKINE (n=53)	13*	14*	30*	9**	25*
Placebo (n=56)	17	19	42	19	26

* $p<0.05$ *generalized Wilcoxon test*
** $p<0.05$ *simple chi-square test*

Median time to myeloid engraftment (ANC ≥500 cells/mm^3) in 53 patients receiving LEUKINE (sargramostim) was 4 days less than in 56 patients treated with placebo (see table at right). The number of patients with bacteremia and infection was significantly lower in the LEUKINE group compared to the placebo group (9/53 versus 19/56 and 30/53 versus 42/56, respectively). There were a number of secondary laboratory and clinical endpoints. Of these, only the incidence of severe (grade 3/4) mucositis was significantly improved in the LEUKINE group (4/53) compared to the placebo group (16/56) at p<0.05. LEUKINE-treated patients also had a shorter median duration of post-transplant IV antibiotic infusions, and shorter median number of days to last platelet and RBC transfusions compared to placebo patients, but none of these differences reached statistical significance.

Bone Marrow Transplantation Failure or Engraftment Delay A historically controlled study was conducted in patients experiencing graft failure following allogeneic or autologous BMT to determine whether LEUKINE improved survival after BMT failure.

Three categories of patients were eligible for this study:

1) patients displaying a delay in engraftment (ANC ≤ 100 cells/mm^3 by day 28 post-transplantation);
2) patients displaying a delay in engraftment (ANC ≤ 100 cells/mm^3 by day 21 post-transplantation) and who had evidence of an active infection, and
3) patients who lost their marrow graft after a transient engraftment (manifested by an average of ANC ≥ 500 cells/mm^3 for at least one week followed by loss of engraftment with ANC <500 cells/mm^3 for at least one week beyond day 21 post-transplantation).

A total of 140 eligible patients from 35 institutions were treated with LEUKINE and evaluated in comparison to 103 historical control patients from a single institution. One hundred sixty-three patients had lymphoid or myeloid leukemia, 24 patients had non-Hodgkin's lymphoma, 19 patients had Hodgkin's disease and 37 patients had other diseases, such as aplastic anemia, myelodysplasia or non-hematologic malignancy. The majority of patients (223 out of 243) had received prior chemotherapy with or without radiotherapy and/or immunotherapy prior to preparation for transplantation.

One hundred day survival was improved in favor of the patients treated with LEUKINE after graft failure following either autologous or allogeneic BMT. In addition, the median survival was improved by greater than 2-fold. The median survival of patients treated with LEUKINE after autologus failure was 474 days versus 161 days for the historical patients. Similarly, after allogeneic failure, the median survival was 97 days with LEUKINE treatment and 35 days for the historical controls. Improvement in survival was better in patients with fewer impaired organs.

The MOF score is a simple clinical and laboratory assessment of 7 major organ systems: cardiovascular, respiratory, gastrointestinal, hematologic, renal, hepatic and neurologic.[10] Assessment of the MOF score is recommended as an additional method of determining the need to initiate treatment with LEUKINE in patients with graft failure or delay in engraftment following autologous or allogeneic BMT.

[See third table above]

Median Survival by Multiple Organ Failure (MOF) Category

	Median Survival (days)		
	MOF ≤ 2 Organs	MOF > 2 Organs	MOF (Composite of Both Groups)
Autologous BMT			
LEUKINE	474 (n=58)	78.5 (n=10)	474 (n=68)
Historical	165 (n=14)	39 (n=3)	161 (n=17)
Allogeneic BMT			
LEUKINE	174 (n=50)	27 (n=22)	97 (n=72)
Historical	52.5 (n=60)	15.5 (n=26)	35 (n=86)

Factors that Contribute to Survival: The probability of survival was relatively greater for patients with any one of the following characteristics: autologous BMT failure or delay in engraftment, exclusion of total body irradiation from the preparative regimen, a non-leukemic malignancy or MOF score ≤ 2 (0, 1 or 2 dysfunctional organ systems). Leukemic subjects derived less benefit than other subjects.

CONTRAINDICATIONS

LEUKINE is contraindicated:

1) in patients with excessive leukemic myeloid blasts in the bone marrow or peripheral blood (≥ 10%);
2) in patients with known hypersensitivity to GM-CSF, yeast-derived products or any component of the product;
3) for concomitant use with chemotherapy and radiotherapy.

Due to the potential sensitivity of rapidly dividing hematopoietic progenitor cells, LEUKINE should not be administered simultaneously with cytotoxic chemotherapy or radiotherapy or within 24 hours preceding or following chemotherapy or radiotherapy. In one controlled study, patients with small cell lung cancer received LEUKINE and concurrent thoracic radiotherapy and chemotherapy or the identical radiotherapy and chemotherapy without LEUKINE. The patients randomized to LEUKINE had significantly higher incidence of adverse events, including higher mortality and a higher incidence of grade 3 and 4 infections and grade 3 and 4 thrombocytopenia.[11]

WARNINGS

Pediatric Use Benzyl alcohol is a constituent of LEUKINE Liquid and Bacteriostatic Water for Injection diluent. Benzyl alcohol has been reported to be associated with a fatal "Gasping Syndrome" in premature infants. **Liquid solutions containing benzyl alcohol (including LEUKINE Liquid) or lyophilized LEUKINE reconstituted with Bacteriostatic Water for Injection, USP (0.9% benzyl alcohol) should not be administered to neonates** (see PRECAUTIONS and DOSAGE AND ADMINISTRATION).

Fluid Retention Edema, capillary leak syndrome, pleural and/or pericardial effusion have been reported in patients after LEUKINE administration. In 156 patients enrolled in placebo-controlled studies using LEUKINE at a dose of 250 mcg/m^2/day by 2-hour IV infusion, the reported incidences of fluid retention (LEUKINE vs. placebo) were as follows: peripheral edema, 11% vs. 7%; pleural effusion, 1% vs. 0%; and pericardial effusion, 4% vs. 1%. Capillary leak syndrome was not observed in this limited number of studies; based on other uncontrolled studies and reports from users of marketed LEUKINE, the incidence is estimated to be less than 1%. In patients with preexisting pleural and pericardial effusions, administration of LEUKINE may aggravate fluid retention; however, fluid retention associated with or worsened by LEUKINE has been reversible after interruption or dose reduction of LEUKINE with or without diuretic therapy. LEUKINE should be used with caution in patients with preexisting fluid retention, pulmonary infiltrates or congestive heart failure.

Respiratory Symptoms Sequestration of granulocytes in the pulmonary circulation has been documented following LEUKINE infusion,[12] and dyspnea has been reported occasionally in patients treated with LEUKINE. Special attention should be given to respiratory symptoms during or immediately following LEUKINE infusion, especially in patients with preexisting lung disease. In patients displaying dyspnea during LEUKINE administration, the rate of infusion should be reduced by half. If respiratory symptoms worsen despite infusion rate reduction, the infusion should be discontinued. Subsequent IV infusions may be administered following the standard dose schedule with careful monitoring. LEUKINE should be administered with caution in patients with hypoxia.

Cardiovascular Symptoms Occasional transient supraventricular arrhythmia has been reported in uncontrolled studies during LEUKINE administration, particularly in patients with a previous history of cardiac arrhythmia. However, these arrhythmias have been reversible after discontinuation of LEUKINE. LEUKINE should be used with caution in patients with preexisting cardiac disease.

Renal and Hepatic Dysfunction In some patients with preexisting renal or hepatic dysfunction enrolled in uncontrolled clinical trials, administration of LEUKINE has induced elevation of serum creatinine or bilirubin and hepatic enzymes. Dose reduction or interruption of LEUKINE administration has resulted in a decrease to pretreatment values. However, in controlled clinical trials the incidences of renal and hepatic dysfunction were comparable between LEUKINE (250 mcg/m^2/day by 2-hour IV infusion) and placebo-treated patients. Monitoring of renal and hepatic function in patients displaying renal or hepatic dysfunction prior to initiation of treatment is recommended at least every other week during LEUKINE administration.

PRECAUTIONS

General Parenteral administration of recombinant proteins should be attended by appropriate precautions in case an allergic or untoward reaction occurs. Serious allergic or anaphylactic reactions have been reported. If any serious allergic or anaphylactic reaction occurs, LEUKINE therapy should immediately be discontinued and appropriate therapy initiated.

A syndrome characterized by respiratory distress, hypoxia, flushing, hypotension, syncope, and/or tachycardia has been reported following the first administration of LEUKINE (sargramostim) in a particular cycle. These signs have resolved with symptomatic treatment and usually do not recur with subsequent doses in the same cycle of treatment.

Stimulation of marrow precursors with LEUKINE may result in a rapid rise in white blood cell (WBC) count. If the ANC exceeds 20,000 cells/mm^3 or if the platelet count exceeds 500,000/mm^3, LEUKINE administration should be interrupted or the dose reduced by half. The decision to reduce the dose or interrupt treatment should be based on the clinical condition of the patient. Excessive blood counts have returned to normal or baseline levels within 3 to 7 days following cessation of LEUKINE therapy. Twice weekly monitoring of CBC with differential (including examination for the presence of blast cells) should be performed to preclude development of excessive counts.

Growth Factor Potential LEUKINE is a growth factor that primarily stimulates normal myeloid precursors. However, the possibility that LEUKINE can act as a growth factor for any tumor type, particularly myeloid malignancies, cannot be excluded. Because of the possibility of tumor growth potentiation, precaution should be exercised when using this drug in any malignancy with myeloid characteristics.

Should disease progression be detected during LEUKINE treatment, LEUKINE therapy should be discontinued.

LEUKINE has been administered to patients with myelodysplastic syndromes (MDS) in uncontrolled studies without evidence of increased relapse rates.[13, 14, 15] Controlled studies have not been performed in patients with MDS.

Use in Patients Receiving Purged Bone Marrow LEUKINE is effective in accelerating myeloid recovery in patients receiving bone marrow purged by anti-B lymphocyte monoclonal antibodies. Data obtained from uncontrolled studies suggest that if *in vitro* marrow purging with chemical agents causes a significant decrease in the number of responsive hematopoietic progenitors, the patient may not respond to LEUKINE. When the bone marrow purging process preserves a sufficient number of progenitors (>1.2 × 10^4/kg), a beneficial effect of LEUKINE on myeloid engraftment has been reported.[16]

Use in Patients Previously Exposed to Intensive Chemotherapy/Radiotherapy In patients who before autologous BMT, have received extensive radiotherapy to hematopoietic sites for the treatment of primary disease in the abdomen or chest, or have been exposed to multiple myelotoxic agents (alkylating agents, anthracycline antibiotics and antimetabolites), the effect of LEUKINE on myeloid reconstitution may be limited.

Use in Patients with Malignancy Undergoing LEUKINE-Mobilized PBPC Collection When using LEUKINE to mobilize PBPC, the limited *in vitro* data suggest that tumor cells may be released and reinfused into the patient in the leukapheresis product. The effect of reinfusion of tumor cells has not been well studied and the data are inconclusive.

Patient Monitoring LEUKINE can induce variable increases in WBC and/or platelet counts. In order to avoid potential complications of excessive leukocytosis (WBC >50,000 cells/mm^3; ANC >20,000 cells/mm^3), a CBC is recommended twice per week during LEUKINE therapy. Monitoring of renal and hepatic function in patients displaying renal or hepatic dysfunction prior to initiation of treatment is recommended at least biweekly during LEUKINE administration. Body weight and hydration status should be carefully monitored during LEUKINE administration.

Drug Interaction Interactions between LEUKINE and other drugs have not been fully evaluated. Drugs which may

Percent of AuBMT Patients Reporting Events

Events by Body System	LEUKINE (n=79)	Placebo (n=77)	Events by Body System	LEUKINE (n=79)	Placebo (n=77)
Body, General			**Metabolic/Nutritional Disorder**		
Fever	95	96	Edema	34	35
Mucous membrane disorder	75	78	Peripheral edema	11	7
Asthenia	66	51	**Respiratory System**		
Malaise	57	51	Dyspnea	28	31
Sepsis	11	14	Lung disorder	20	23
Digestive System			**Hemic and Lymphatic System**		
Nausea	90	96	Blood dyscrasia	25	27
Diarrhea	89	82	**Cardiovascular System**		
Vomiting	85	90	Hemorrhage	23	30
Anorexia	54	58	**Urogenital System**		
GI disorder	37	47	Urinary tract disorder	14	13
GI hemorrhage	27	33	Kidney function abnormal	8	10
Stomatitis	24	29	**Nervous System**		
Liver damage	13	14	CNS disorder	11	16
Skin and Appendages					
Alopecia	73	74			
Rash	44	38			

Percent of Allogeneic BMT Patients Reporting Events

Events by Body System	LEUKINE (n=53)	Placebo (n=56)	Events by Body System	LEUKINE (n=53)	Placebo (n=56)
Body, General			**Metabolic/Nutritional Disorders**		
Fever	77	80	Bilirubinemia	30	27
Abdominal pain	38	23	Hyperglycemia	25	23
Headache	36	36	Peripheral edema	15	21
Chills	25	20	Increased creatinine	15	14
Pain	17	36	Hypomagnesemia	15	9
Asthenia	17	20	Increased SGPT	13	16
Chest pain	15	9	Edema	13	11
Back pain	9	18	Increased alk. phosphatase	8	14
Digestive System			**Respiratory System**		
Diarrhea	81	66	Pharyngitis	23	13
Nausea	70	66	Epistaxis	17	16
Vomiting	70	57	Dyspnea	15	14
Stomatitis	62	63	Rhinitis	11	14
Anorexia	51	57	**Hemic and Lymphatic System**		
Dyspepsia	17	20	Thrombocytopenia	19	34
Hematemesis	13	7	Leukopenia	17	29
Dysphagia	11	7	Petechia	6	11
GI hemorrhage	11	5	Agranulocytosis	6	11
Constipation	8	11	**Urogenital System**		
Skin and Appendages			Hematuria	9	21
Rash	70	73	**Nervous System**		
Alopecia	45	45	Paresthesia	11	13
Pruritis	23	13	Insomnia	11	9
Musculo-skeletal System			Anxiety	11	2
Bone pain	21	5	**Laboratory Abnormalities***		
Arthralgia	11	4	High glucose	41	49
Special Senses			Low albumin	27	36
Eye hemorrhage	11	0	High BUN	23	17
Cardiovascular System			Low calcium	2	7
Hypertension	34	32	High cholesterol	17	8
Tachycardia	11	9			

** Grade 3 and 4 laboratory abnormalities only. Denominators may vary due to missing laboratory measurements.*

potentiate the myeloproliferative effects of LEUKINE, such as lithium and corticosteroids, should be used with caution.

Carcinogenesis, Mutagenesis, Impairment of Fertility Animal studies have not been conducted with LEUKINE to evaluate the carcinogenic potential or the effect on fertility.

Pregnancy (Category C) Animal reproduction studies have not been conducted with LEUKINE. It is not known whether LEUKINE can cause fetal harm when administered to a pregnant woman or can affect reproductive capability. LEUKINE should be given to a pregnant woman only if clearly needed.

Nursing Mothers It is not known whether LEUKINE is excreted in human milk. Because many drugs are excreted in human milk, LEUKINE should be administered to a nursing women only if clearly needed.

Pediatric Use Safety and effectiveness in pediatric patients have not been established; however, available safety data indicate that LEUKINE does not exhibit any greater toxicity in pediatric patients than in adults. A total of 124 pediatric subjects between the ages of 4 months and 18 years have been treated with LEUKINE in clinical trials at doses ranging from 60–1,000 mcg/m^2/day intravenously and 4–1,500 mcg/m^2/day subcutaneously. In 53 pediatric patients enrolled in controlled studies at a dose of 250 mcg/m^2/day by 2-hour IV infusion, the type and frequency of adverse events were comparable to those reported for the adult population. **Liquid solutions containing benzyl alcohol (including LEUKINE Liquid) or lyophilized LEUKINE reconstituted with Bacteriostatic Water for Injection, USP (0.9% benzyl alcohol) should not be administered to neonates (see WARNINGS).**

ADVERSE REACTIONS

Autologous and Allogeneic Bone Marrow Transplantation

LEUKINE is generally well tolerated. In 3 placebo-controlled studies enrolling a total of 156 patients after autologous BMT or peripheral blood progenitor cell transplantation, events reported in at least 10% of patients who received IV LEUKINE or placebo were as reported at right: [See first table above]

No significant differences were observed between LEUKINE and placebo-treated patients in the type or frequency of laboratory abnormalities, including renal and hepatic parameters. In some patients with preexisting renal or hepatic dysfunction enrolled in uncontrolled clinical trials, administration of LEUKINE has induced elevation of serum creatinine or bilirubin and hepatic enzymes (see WARNINGS). In addition, there was no significant difference in relapse rate and 24 month survival between the LEUKINE and placebo-treated patients.

In the placebo-controlled trial of 109 patients after allogeneic BMT, events reported in at least 10% of patients who received IV LEUKINE or placebo were as reported at right: [See second table above]

There were no significant differences in the incidence or severity of GVHD, relapse rates and survival between the LEUKINE and placebo-treated patients.

Adverse events observed for the patients treated with LEUKINE (sargramostim) in the historically controlled BMT failure study were similar to those reported in the placebo-controlled studies. In addition, headache (26%), pericardial effusion (25%), arthralgia (21%) and myalgia (18%) were also reported in patients treated with LEUKINE in the graft failure study.

In uncontrolled Phase I/II studies with LEUKINE in 215 patients, the most frequent adverse events were fever, asthenia, headache, bone pain, chills and myalgia. These systemic events were generally mild or moderate and were usually prevented or reversed by the administration of analgesics and antipyretics such as acetaminophen. In these uncontrolled trials, other infrequent events reported were dyspnea, peripheral edema, and rash.

Reports of events occurring with marketed LEUKINE include arrhythmia, fainting, eosinophilia, dizziness, hypotension, injection site reactions, pain (including abdominal, back, chest, and joint pain), tachycardia, thrombosis, and transient liver function abnormalities.

In patients with preexisting edema, capillary leak syndrome, pleural and/or pericardial effusion, administration of LEUKINE may aggravate fluid retention (see WARNINGS). Body weight and hydration status should be carefully monitored during LEUKINE administration.

Adverse events observed in pediatric patients in controlled studies were comparable to those observed in adult patients.

Continued on next page

Leukine—Cont.

Acute Myelogenous Leukemia Adverse events reported in at least 10% of patients who received LEUKINE or placebo were as reported at right:
[See table below]
Nearly all patients reported leukopenia, thrombocytopenia and anemia. The frequency and type of adverse events observed following induction were similar between LEUKINE and placebo groups. The only significant difference in the rates of these adverse events was an increase in skin associated events in the LEUKINE group (p=0.002). No significant differences were observed in laboratory results, renal or hepatic toxicity. No significant differences were observed between the LEUKINE- and placebo-treated patients for adverse events following consolidation. There was no significant difference in response rate or relapse rate.
In a historically controlled study of 86 patients with acute myelogenous leukemia (AML), the LEUKINE treated group exhibited an increased incidence of weight gain (p=0.007), low serum proteins and prolonged prothrombin time (p=0.02) when compared to the control group. Two LEUKINE treated patients had progressive increase in circulating monocytes and promonocytes and blasts in the marrow which reversed when LEUKINE was discontinued. The historical control group exhibited an increased incidence of cardiac events (p=0.018), liver function abnormalities (p=0.008), and neurocortical hemorrhagic events (p=0.025).[15]
Overdosage The maximum amount of LEUKINE that can be safely administered in single or multiple doses has not been determined. Doses up to 100 mcg/kg/day (4,000 mcg/m^2/day or 16 times the recommended dose) were administered to 4 patients in a Phase I uncontrolled clinical study by continuous IV infusion for 7 to 18 days. Increases in WBC up to 200,000 cells/mm^3 were observed. Adverse events reported were dyspnea, malaise, nausea, fever, rash, sinus tachycardia, headache and chills. All these events were reversible after discontinuation of LEUKINE.
In case of overdosage, LEUKINE therapy should be discontinued and the patient carefully monitored for WBC increase and respiratory symptoms.

DOSAGE AND ADMINISTRATION

Neutrophil Recovery Following Chemotherapy in Acute Myelogenous Leukemia The recommended dose is 250 mcg/m^2/day administered intravenously over a 4 hour period starting approximately on day 11 or 4 days following the completion of induction chemotherapy, if the day 10 bone marrow is hypoplastic with <5% blasts. If a second cycle of induction chemotherapy is necessary, LEUKINE should be administered approximately 4 days after the completion of chemotherapy if the bone marrow is hypoplastic with <5% blasts. LEUKINE should be continued until an ANC >1500 cells/mm^3 for 3 consecutive days or a maximum of 42 days. LEUKINE should be discontinued immediately if leukemic regrowth occurs. If a severe adverse reaction occurs, the dose can be reduced by 50% or temporarily discontinued until the reaction abates.
In order to avoid potential complications of excessive leukocytosis (WBC >50,000 cells/mm^3 or ANC >20,000 cells/mm^3) a CBC with differential is recommended twice per week during LEUKINE therapy. LEUKINE treatment should be interrupted or the dose reduced by half if the ANC exceeds 20,000 cells/mm^3.
Mobilization of Peripheral Blood Progenitor Cells The recommended dose is 250 mcg/m^2/day administered IV over 24 hours or SC once daily. Dosing should continue at the same dose through the period of PBPC collection. The optimal schedule for PBPC collection has not been established. In clinical studies, collection of PBPC was usually begun by day 5 and performed daily until protocol specified targets were achieved (see CLINICAL EXPERIENCE, Mobilization and Engraftment of PBPC). If WBC >50,000 cells/mm^3, the LEUKINE dose should be reduced by 50%. If adequate numbers of progenitor cells are not collected, other mobilization therapy should be considered.
Post Peripheral Blood Progenitor Cell Transplantation The recommended dose is 250 mcg/m^2/day administered IV over 24 hours or SC once daily beginning immediately following infusion of progenitor cells and continuing until an ANC>1500 cells/mm^3 for 3 consecutive days is attained.
Myeloid Reconstitution After Autologous or Allogeneic Bone Marrow Transplantation The recommended dose is 250 mcg/m^2/day administered IV over a 2-hour period beginning 2 to 4 hours after bone marrow infusion, and not less than 24 hours after the last dose of chemotherapy or radiotherapy. Patients should not receive LEUKINE until the post marrow infusion ANC is less than 500 cells/mm^3. LEUKINE should be continued until an ANC >1500 cells/mm^3 for 3 consecutive days is attained. If a severe adverse reaction occurs, the dose can be reduced by 50% or temporarily discontinued until the reaction abates. LEUKINE should be discontinued immediately if blast cells appear or disease progression occurs.
In order to avoid potential complications of excessive leukocytosis (WBC >50,000 cells/mm^3, ANC >20,000 cells/mm^3) a CBC with differential is recommended twice per week during LEUKINE therapy. LEUKINE treatment should be interrupted or the dose reduced by 50% if the ANC exceeds 20,000 cells/mm^3.
Bone Marrow Transplantation Failure or Engraftment Delay The recommended dose is 250 mcg/m^2/day for 14 days as a 2-hour IV infusion. The dose can be repeated after 7 days off therapy if engraftment has not occurred. If engraftment still has not occurred, a third course of 500 mcg/m^2/day for 14 days may be tried after another 7 days off therapy. If there is still no improvement, it is unlikely that further dose escalation will be beneficial. If a severe adverse reaction occurs, the dose can be reduced by 50% or temporarily discontinued until the reaction abates. LEUKINE should be discontinued immediately if blast cells appear or disease progression occurs.
In order to avoid potential complications of excessive leukocytosis (WBC >50,000 cells/mm^3, ANC >20,000 cells/mm^3) a CBC with differential is recommended twice per week during LEUKINE therapy. LEUKINE treatment should be interrupted or the dose reduced by half if the ANC exceeds 20,000 cells/mm^3.

Preparation of LEUKINE

1. LEUKINE Liquid is formulated as a sterile, preserved (1.1% benzyl alcohol), injectable solution (500 mcg/mL) in a vial. Lyophilized LEUKINE is a sterile, white, preservative-free powder (250 mcg) that requires reconstitution with 1 mL Sterile Water for Injection, USP, or 1 mL Bacteriostatic Water for Injection, USP.
2. LEUKINE Liquid may be stored for up to 20 days at 2–8°C once the vial has been entered. Discard any remaining solution after 20 days.
3. Lyophilized LEUKINE (250 mcg) should be reconstituted aseptically with 1.0 mL of diluent (see below). The contents of vials reconstituted with different diluents should not be mixed together.
   Sterile Water for Injection, USP (without preservative): Lyophilized LEUKINE vials contain no antibacterial preservative, and therefore solutions prepared with Sterile Water for Injection, USP should be administered as soon as possible, and within 6 hours following reconstitution and/or dilution for IV infusion. The vial should not be reentered or reused. Do not save any unused portion for administration more than 6 hours following reconstitution.
   Bacteriostatic Water for Injection, USP (0.9% benzyl alcohol): Reconstituted solutions prepared with Bacteriostatic Water for Injection, USP (0.9% benzyl alcohol) may be stored for up to 20 days at 2–8°C prior to use. Discard reconstituted solution after 20 days. Previously reconstituted solutions mixed with freshly reconstituted solutions must be administered within 6 hours following mixing. **Preparations containing benzyl alcohol (including LEUKINE Liquid and lyophilized LEUKINE reconstituted with Bacteriostatic Water for Injection) should not be used in neonates** (see WARNINGS).
4. During reconstitution of lyophilized LEUKINE the diluent should be directed at the side of the vial and the contents gently swirled to avoid foaming during dissolution. Avoid excessive or vigorous agitation; do not shake.
5. LEUKINE should be used for SC injection without further dilution. Dilution for IV infusion should be performed in 0.9% Sodium Chloride Injection, USP. If the final concentration of LEUKINE is below 10 mcg/mL, Albumin (Human) at a final concentration of 0.1% should be added to the saline prior to addition of LEUKINE to prevent adsorption to the components of the drug delivery system. To obtain a final concentration of 0.1% Albumin (Human), add 1 mg Albumin (Human) per 1 mL 0.9% Sodium Chloride Injection, USP (e.g., use 1 mL 5% Albumin [Human] in 50 mL 0.9% Sodium Chloride Injection, USP).
6. An in-line membrane filter should NOT be used for intravenous infusion of LEUKINE.
7. Store LEUKINE Liquid and reconstituted lyophilized LEUKINE solutions under refrigeration at 2–8°C (36–46°F); DO NOT FREEZE.
8. In the absence of compatibility and stability information, no other medication should be added to infusion solutions containing LEUKINE. Use only 0.9% Sodium Chloride Injection, USP to prepare IV infusion solutions.
9. Aseptic technique should be employed in the preparation of all LEUKINE solutions. To assure correct concentration following reconstitution, care should be exercised to eliminate any air bubbles from the needle hub of the syringe used to prepare the diluent. Parenteral drug products should be inspected visually for particulate matter and discoloration prior to administration whenever solution and container permit.

HOW SUPPLIED

LEUKINE Liquid is available in vials containing 500 mcg/mL (2.8 × 10^6 IU/mL) sargramostim. Lyophilized LEUKINE is available in vials containing 250 mcg (1.4 × 10^6 IU/vial) sargramostim.
Each dosage form is supplied as follows:
Carton of 5 vials of lyophilized LEUKINE 250 mcg (NDC 58406-002-33).
Carton of 5 multiple-dose vials; each vial contains 1 mL of preserved 500 mcg/mL LEUKINE Liquid (NDC 58406-050-30).

STORAGE

LEUKINE should be refrigerated at 2–8°C (36–46°F). Do not freeze or shake. Do not use beyond the expiration date printed on the vial.

REFERENCES

1. Metcalf D. The molecular biology and functions of the granulocyte-macrophage colony-stimulating factors. Blood 1986; 67(2):257–267.
2. Park LS, Friend D, Gillis S, Urdal DL. Characterization of the cell surface receptor for human granulocyte/macrophage colony stimulating factor. J Exp Med 1986; 164: 251–262.
3. Grabstein KH, Urdal DL, Tushinski RJ, *et al.* Induction of macrophage tumoricidal activity by granulocyte-macrophage colony-stimulating factors. Science 1986; 232: 506–508.
4. Reed SG, Nathan CF, Pihl DL, *et al.* Recombinant granulocyte/macrophage colony-stimulating factor activates macrophages to inhibit *Trypanosoma cruzi* and release hydrogen peroxide. J Exp Med 1987; 166:1734–1746.
5. Data on file Immunex Corporation; Seattle, WA.
6. Rowe JM, Andersen JW, Mazza JJ, *et al.* A randomized placebo-controlled phase III study of granulocyte-macrophage colony-stimulating factor in adult patients (>55 to 70 years of age) with acute myelogenous leukemia: a study of the Eastern Cooperative Oncology Group (E1490). Blood 1995; 86(2):457–462.
7. Nemunaitis J, Rabinowe SN, Singer JW, *et al.* Recombinant human granulocyte-macrophage colony-stimulating factor after autologous bone marrow transplantation for lymphoid malignancy: Pooled results of a randomized, double-blind, placebo controlled trial. NEJM 1991; 324(25):1773–1778.
8. Nemunaitis J, Singer JW, Buckner CD, *et al.* Use of recombinant human granulocyte-macrophage colony-stimulating factor in autologous bone marrow transplantation for lymphoid malignancies. Blood 1988; 72(2):834–836.
9. Nemunaitis J, Singer JW, Buckner CD, *et al.* Long-term follow-up of patients who received recombinant human granulocyte-macrophage colony-stimulating factor after autologous bone marrow transplantation for lymphoid malignancy. BMT 1991; 7:49–52.
10. Goris RJA, Boekhorst TPA, Nuytinck JKS, *et al.* Multiple organ failure: Generalized auto-destructive inflammation? Arch Surg 1985; 120:1109–1115.
11. Bunn P, Crowley J, Kelly J, *et al.* Chemoradiotherapy with or without granulocyte-macrophage colony-stimulating factor in the treatment of limited-state small-cell lung cancer: a prospective phase III randomized study of the southwest oncology group. JCO 1995; 13(7):1632–1641.
12. Herrmann F, Schultz G, Lindemann A, *et al.* Yeast-expressed granulocyte-macrophage colony-stimulating factor in cancer patients: A phase lb clinical study. In Behring Institute Research Communications, Colony Stimulating Factors-CSF. International Symposium, Garmisch-Partenkirchen, West Germany, 1988; 83:107–118.
13. Estey EH, Dixon D, Kantarjian H, *et al.* Treatment of poor-prognosis, newly diagnosed acute myeloid leukemia with Ara-C and recombinant human granulocyte-macrophage colony-stimulating factor. Blood 1990: 75(9):1766–1769.

Percent of AML Patients Reporting Events

Events by Body System	LEUKINE (n=52)	Placebo (n=47)	Events by Body System	LEUKINE (n=52)	Placebo (n=47)
Body, General			**Metabolic/Nutritional Disorder**		
Fever (no infection)	81	74	Metabolic	58	49
Infection	65	68	Edema	25	23
Weight loss	37	28	**Respiratory System**		
Weight gain	8	21	Pulmonary	48	64
Chills	19	26	**Hemic and Lymphatic System**		
Allergy	12	15	Coagulation	19	21
Sweats	6	13	**Cardiovascular System**		
Digestive System			Hemorrhage	29	43
Nausea	58	55	Hypertension	25	32
Liver	77	83	Cardiac	23	32
Diarrhea	52	53	Hypotension	13	26
Vomiting	46	34	**Urogenital System**		
Stomatitis	42	43	GU	50	57
Anorexia	13	11	**Nervous System**		
Abdominal distention	4	13	Neuro-clinical	42	53
Skin and Appendages			Neuro-motor	25	26
Skin	77	45	Neuro-psych	15	26
Alopecia	37	51	Neuro-sensory	6	11

14. Vadhan-Raj S, Keating M, LeMaistre A, *et al.* Effects of recombinant human granulocyte-macrophage colony-stimulating factor in patients with myelodysplastic syndromes. NEJM 1987; 317:1545–1552.
15. Buchner BR, Hiddemann W, Koenigsmann M, *et al.* Recombinant human granulocyte-macrophage colony stimulating factor after chemotherapy in patients with acute myeloid leukemia at higher age or after relapse. Blood 1991; 78(5):1190–1197.
16. Blazar BR, Kersey JH, McGlave, *et al. In vivo* administration of recombinant human granylocyte/macrophage colony-stimulating factor in acute lymphoblastic patients receiving purged autografts. Blood 1989; 73(3): 849–857.

IMMUNEX®
LEUKINE® is a registered trademark of Immunex Corporation, Seattle WA 98101

Rev 0230-02
Issued 02/98

NOVANTRONE® ℞
mitoxantrone for injection concentrate

WARNING
NOVANTRONE® (mitoxantrone for injection concentrate) should be administered under the supervision of a physician experienced in the use of cancer chemotherapeutic agents.
Except for the treatment of acute nonlymphocytic leukemia, NOVANTRONE® therapy generally should not be given to patients with baseline neutrophil counts of less than 1,500 cells/mm^3. In order to monitor the occurrence of bone marrow suppression, primarily neutropenia, which may be severe and result in infection, it is recommended that frequent peripheral blood cell counts be performed on all patients receiving NOVANTRONE®.

DESCRIPTION
NOVANTRONE® (mitoxantrone hydrochloride) is a synthetic antineoplastic anthracenedione for intravenous use. The molecular formula is $C_{22}H_{28}N_4O_6 \bullet 2HCl$ and the molecular weight is 517.41. It is supplied as a concentrate which MUST BE DILUTED PRIOR TO INJECTION. The concentrate is a sterile, nonpyrogenic, dark blue aqueous solution containing mitoxantrone hydrochloride equivalent to 2 mg/mL mitoxantrone free base, with sodium chloride (0.80% w/v), sodium acetate (0.005% w/v), and acetic acid (0.046% w/v) as inactive ingredients. The solution has a pH of 3.0 to 4.5 and contains 0.14 mEq of sodium per mL. The product does not contain preservatives. The chemical name is 1,4-dihydroxy-5,8-bis[[2-[(2-hydroxyethyl) amino]ethyl]amino]-9,10-anthracenedione dihydrochloride and the structural formula is:

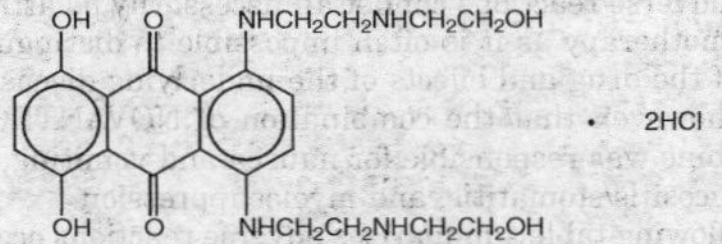

CLINICAL PHARMACOLOGY
Mechanism of Action
Although its mechanism of action is not fully elucidated, mitoxantrone is a DNA-reactive agent. It has a cytocidal effect on both proliferating and nonproliferating cultured human cells, suggesting lack of cell cycle phase specificity.
Pharmacokinetics
Pharmacokinetics of mitoxantrone in patients following a single intravenous administration of NOVANTRONE can be characterized by a three-compartment model. The mean alpha half-life of mitoxantrone is 6 to 12 minutes, the mean beta half-life is 1.1 to 3.1 hours and the mean gamma (terminal or elimination) half-life is 23 to 215 hours (median approximately 75 hours). Pharmacokinetic studies have not been performed in humans receiving multiple daily dosing. Distribution to tissues is extensive: steady-state volume of distribution exceeds 1,000 L/m2. Tissue concentrations of mitoxantrone appear to exceed those in the blood during the terminal elimination phase. In the monkey, distribution to brain, spinal cord, eye, and spinal fluid is low.
In patients administered 15-90 mg/m^2 of NOVANTRONE intravenously, there is a linear relationship between dose and the area under the concentration-time curve.
Mitoxantrone is 78% bound to plasma proteins in the observed concentration range of 26-455 ng/mL. This binding is independent of concentration and is not affected by the presence of phenytoin, doxorubicin, methotrexate, prednisone, prednisolone, heparin, or aspirin.
Metabolism and Elimination: Metabolism and elimination of mitoxantrone following NOVANTRONE administration are not well characterized. Eleven percent or less of mitoxantrone is recovered in the urine, and 25% or less is recovered in the feces, within five days after drug administration. Of the material recovered in the urine, 65% is unchanged drug. The remaining 35% is comprised primarily of a mono- and a dicarboxylic acid derivative and their glucuronide conjugates. These carboxylic acid metabolites are not DNA-reactive/cytocidal, and their route of formation is unknown.
Special Populations:
Gender: The effect of gender on mitoxantrone pharmacokinetics is unknown.
Geriatric: Mitoxantrone pharmacokinetics in the elderly are unknown.
Pediatric: Mitoxantrone pharmacokinetics in the pediatric population are unknown.
Race: The effect of race on mitoxantrone pharmacokinetics is unknown.
Renal Impairment: Mitoxantrone pharmacokinetics in patients with renal impairment are unknown.
Hepatic Impairment: Mitoxantrone clearance is reduced by hepatic impairment. Patients with severe hepatic dysfunction (bilirubin greater than 3.4 mg/dL) have an AUC more than 3-fold that of patients with normal hepatic function receiving the same dose. For patients with hepatic impairment, there is at present no laboratory measurement that allows for dose adjustment recommendations.
Drug Interactions: Pharmacokinetic studies of the interaction of NOVANTRONE with concomitantly administered medications have not been performed. The interaction of mitoxantrone with the human P450 system has not been investigated.
Clinical Trials
Advanced Hormone-Refractory Prostate Cancer
A multicenter phase 2 trial of NOVANTRONE and low-dose prednisone (N + P) was conducted in 27 symptomatic patients with hormone-refractory prostate cancer. Using NPCP (National Prostate Cancer Project) criteria for disease response, there was one partial responder and 12 patients with stable disease. However, nine patients or 33% achieved a palliative response defined on the basis of reduction in analgesic use or pain intensity.
These findings led to the initiation of a randomized multicenter trial (CCI-NOV22) comparing the effectiveness of (N + P) to low-dose prednisone alone (P). Eligible patients were required to have metastatic or locally advanced disease that had progressed on standard hormonal therapy, a castrate serum testosterone level, and at least mild pain at study entry. NOVANTRONE was administered at a dose of 12 mg/m^2 by short IV infusion every three weeks. Prednisone was administered orally at a dose of 5 mg twice a day. Patients randomized to the prednisone arm were crossed over to the N + P arm if they progressed or if they were not improved after a minimum of six weeks of therapy with prednisone alone.
A total of 161 patients were randomized, 80 to the N + P arm and 81 to the P arm. The median NOVANTRONE dose administered was 12 mg/m^2 per cycle. The median cumulative NOVANTRONE dose administered was 73 mg/m^2 (range of 12 to 212 mg/m^2).
A primary palliative response (defined as a 2-point decrease in pain intensity in a 6-point pain scale, associated with stable analgesic use, and lasting a minimum of 6 weeks) was achieved in 29% of patients randomized to N + P compared to 12% of patients randomized to P alone (p = 0.011). Two responders left the study after meeting primary response criterion for two consecutive cycles. For the purposes of this analysis, these two patients were assigned a response duration of zero days. A secondary palliative response was defined as a 50% or greater decrease in analgesic use, associated with stable pain intensity, and lasting a minimum of 6 weeks. An overall palliative response (defined as primary plus secondary responses) was achieved in 38% of patients randomized to N + P compared to 21% of patients randomized to P (p = 0.025).
The median duration of primary palliative response for patients randomized to N + P was 7.6 months compared to 2.1 months for patients randomized to P alone (p = 0.0009). The median duration of overall palliative response for patients randomized to N + P was 5.6 months compared to 1.9 months for patients randomized to P alone (p = 0.0004).
Time to progression was defined as a 1-point increase in pain intensity, or a >25% increase in analgesic use, or evidence of disease progression on radiographic studies, or requirement for radiotherapy. The median time to progression for all patients randomized to N + P was 4.4 months compared to 2.3 months for all patients randomized to P alone (p = 0.0001). Median time to death was 11.3 months for all patients on the N + P arm compared to 10.8 months for all patients on P alone (p = 0.2324).
Forty-eight patients on the P arm crossed over to receive N + P. Of these, thirty patients had progressed on P, while 18 had stable disease on P. The median cycle of crossover was 5 cycles (range of 2 to 16 cycles). Time trends for pain intensity prior to crossover were significantly worse for patients who crossed over than for those who remained on P alone (p = 0.012). Nine patients (19%) demonstrated a palliative response on N + P after crossover. The median time to death for patients who crossed over to N + P was 12.7 months.
The clinical significance of a fall in prostate specific antigen (PSA) concentrations after chemotherapy is unclear. On the CCI-NOV22 trial, a PSA fall of 50% or greater for two consecutive follow-up assessments after baseline was reported in 33% of all patients randomized to the N+P arm and 9% of all patients randomized to the P arm. These findings should be interpreted with caution since PSA responses were not defined prospectively. A number of patients were inevaluable for response, and there was an imbalance between treatment arms in the numbers of evaluable patients. In addition, PSA reduction did not correlate precisely with palliative response, the primary efficacy endpoint of this study. For example, among the 26 evaluable patients randomized to the N+P arm who had a ≥50% reduction in PSA, only 13 had a primary palliative response. Also, among 42 evaluable patients on this arm who did not have this reduction in PSA, 8 nonetheless had a primary palliative response.
Investigators at Cancer and Leukemia Group B (CALGB) conducted a phase III comparative trial of NOVANTRONE plus hydrocortisone (N + H) versus hydrocortisone alone (H) in patients with hormone-refractory prostate cancer (CALGB 9182). Eligible patients were required to have metastatic disease that had progressed despite at least one hormonal therapy. Progression at study entry was defined on the basis of progressive symptoms, increases in measurable or osseous disease, or rising PSA levels. NOVANTRONE was administered intravenously at a dose of 14 mg/m^2 every 21 days and hydrocortisone was administered orally at a daily dose of 40 mg. A total of 242 subjects were randomized, 119 to the N + H arm and 123 to the H arm. There were no differences in survival between the two arms, with a median of 11.1 months in the N + H arm, and 12 months in the H arm (p = 0.3298).
Using NPCP criteria for response, partial responses were achieved in 10 patients (8.4%) randomized to the N + H arm compared with 2 patients (1.6%) randomized to the H arm (p = 0.018). The median time to progression, defined by NPCP criteria, for patients randomized to the N + H arm was 7.3 months compared to 4.1 months for patients randomized to H alone (p = 0.0654).
Approximately 60% of patients on each arm required analgesics at baseline. Analgesic use was measured in this study using a 5-point scale. The best percent change from baseline in mean analgesic use was -17% for 61 patients with available data on the N + H arm, compared with +17% for 61 patients on H alone (p = 0.014). A time trend analysis for analgesic use in individual patients also showed a trend favoring the N + H arm over H alone but was not statistically significant.
Pain intensity was measured using the Symptom Distress Scale (SDS) Pain Item 2 (a 5-point scale). The best percent change from baseline in mean pain intensity was -14% for 37 patients with available data on the N + H arm, compared with +8% for 38 patients on H alone (p = 0.057). A time trend analysis for pain intensity in individual patients showed no difference between treatment arms.
Acute Nonlymphocytic Leukemia
In two large randomized multicenter trials, remission induction therapy for acute nonlymphocytic leukemia (ANLL) with NOVANTRONE 12 mg/m^2 daily for 3 days as a 10-minute intravenous infusion and cytarabine 100 mg/m^2 for 7 days given as a continuous 24-hour infusion was compared with daunorubicin 45 mg/m^2 daily by intravenous infusion for 3 days plus the same dose and schedule of cytarabine used with NOVANTRONE. Patients who had an incomplete antileukemic response received a second induction course in which NOVANTRONE or daunorubicin was administered for 2 days and cytarabine for 5 days using the same daily dosage schedule. Response rates and median survival information for both the U.S. and international multicenter trials are given in the following table:
[See table above]

Trial	% Complete Response (CR)		Median Time to CR (days)		Median Survival (days)	
	NOV	DAUN	NOV	DAUN	NOV	DAUN
U.S.	63 (62/98)	53 (54/102)	35	42	312	237
International	50 (56/112)	51 (62/123)	36	42	192	230

NOV = NOVANTRONE® + cytarabine
DAUN = daunorubicin + cytarabine

In these studies, two consolidation courses were administered to complete responders on each arm. Consolidation therapy consisted of the same drug and daily dosage used for remission induction, but only 5 days of cytarabine and 2 days of NOVANTRONE or daunorubicin were given. The first consolidation course was administered 6 weeks after the start of the final induction course if the patient achieved a complete remission. The second consolidation course was generally administered 4 weeks later. Full hematologic recovery was necessary for patients to receive consolidation therapy. For the U.S. trial, median granulocyte nadirs for patients receiving NOVANTRONE + cytarabine for consolidation courses 1 and 2 were 10/mm^3 for both courses, and for those patients receiving daunorubicin + cytarabine nadirs were 170/mm^3 and 260/mm^3, respectively. Median platelet nadirs for patients who received NOVANTRONE +

Continued on next page

Novantrone—Cont.

cytarabine for consolidation courses 1 and 2 were 17,000/mm^3 and 14,000/mm^3, respectively, and were 33,000/mm^3 and 22,000/mm^3 in courses 1 and 2 for those patients who received daunorubicin + cytarabine. The benefit of consolidation therapy in ANLL patients who achieve a complete remission remains controversial. However, in the only well-controlled prospective, randomized multicenter trials with NOVANTRONE in ANLL, consolidation therapy was given to all patients who achieved a complete remission. During consolidation in the U.S. study, two myelosuppression-related deaths occurred on the NOVANTRONE arm and one on the daunorubicin arm. However, in the international study there were eight deaths on the NOVANTRONE arm during consolidation which were related to the myelosuppression and none on the daunorubicin arm where less myelosuppression occurred.

INDICATIONS AND USAGE

NOVANTRONE in combination with corticosteroids is indicated as initial chemotherapy for the treatment of patients with pain related to advanced hormone-refractory prostate cancer.

NOVANTRONE in combination with other approved drug(s) is indicated in the initial therapy of acute nonlymphocytic leukemia (ANLL) in adults. This category includes myelogenous, promyelocytic, monocytic, and erythroid acute leukemias.

CONTRAINDICATIONS

NOVANTRONE is contraindicated in patients who have demonstrated prior hypersensitivity to it.

WARNINGS

WHEN NOVANTRONE IS USED IN DOSES INDICATED FOR THE TREATMENT OF LEUKEMIA, SEVERE MYELOSUPPRESSION WILL OCCUR. THEREFORE, IT IS RECOMMENDED THAT NOVANTRONE BE ADMINISTERED ONLY BY PHYSICIANS EXPERIENCED IN THE CHEMOTHERAPY OF THIS DISEASE. LABORATORY AND SUPPORTIVE SERVICES MUST BE AVAILABLE FOR HEMATOLOGIC AND CHEMISTRY MONITORING AND ADJUNCTIVE THERAPIES, INCLUDING ANTIBIOTICS. BLOOD AND BLOOD PRODUCTS MUST BE AVAILABLE TO SUPPORT PATIENTS DURING THE EXPECTED PERIOD OF MEDULLARY HYPOPLASIA AND SEVERE MYELOSUPPRESSION. PARTICULAR CARE SHOULD BE GIVEN TO ASSURING FULL HEMATOLOGIC RECOVERY BEFORE UNDERTAKING CONSOLIDATION THERAPY (IF THIS TREATMENT IS USED) AND PATIENTS SHOULD BE MONITORED CLOSELY DURING THIS PHASE.

Patients with preexisting myelosuppression as the result of prior drug therapy should not receive NOVANTRONE unless it is felt that the possible benefit from such treatment warrants the risk of further medullary suppression.

The safety of NOVANTRONE in patients with hepatic insufficiency is not established. (See **CLINICAL PHARMACOLOGY** section.)

Safety for use by routes other than intravenous administration has not been established.

Pregnancy - NOVANTRONE may cause fetal harm when administered to a pregnant woman. In treated rats, at doses of ≥0.1 mg/kg (0.05 fold the recommended human dose on a mg/m^2 basis) low fetal birth weight and retarded development of the fetal kidney were seen in greater frequency. In treated rabbits, an increased incidence of premature delivery was observed at doses ≥0.01 mg/kg (0.01 fold the recommended human dose on a mg/m^2 basis). NOVANTRONE was not teratogenic in rabbits. There are no adequate and well-controlled studies in pregnant women. If this drug is used during pregnancy, or if the patient becomes pregnant while taking this drug, the patient should be apprised of the potential hazard to the fetus. Women of childbearing potential should be advised to avoid becoming pregnant.

Topoisomerase II inhibitors, including NOVANTRONE, in combination with other antineoplastic agents, have been associated with the development of acute leukemia.

Cardiac Effects

Because of the possible danger of cardiac effects in patients previously treated with daunorubicin or doxorubicin, the benefit-to-risk ratio of NOVANTRONE therapy in such patients should be determined before starting therapy.

General - Functional cardiac changes including decreases in left ventricular ejection fraction (LVEF) and irreversible congestive heart failure can occur with NOVANTRONE. Cardiac toxicity may be more common in patients with prior treatment with anthracyclines, prior mediastinal radiotherapy, or with preexisting cardiovascular disease. Such patients should have regular cardiac monitoring of LVEF from the initiation of therapy. In investigational trials of intermittent single doses in other tumor types, patients who received up to the cumulative dose of 140 mg/m^2 had a cumulative 2.6% probability of clinical congestive heart failure. The overall cumulative probability rate of moderate or serious decreases in LVEF at this dose was 13% in comparative trials.

Leukemia - Acute congestive heart failure may occasionally occur in patients treated with NOVANTRONE for ANLL. In first-line comparative trials of NOVANTRONE + cytarabine *vs* daunorubicin + cytarabine in adult patients with previously untreated ANLL, therapy was associated with congestive heart failure in 6.5% of patients on each arm. A causal relationship between drug therapy and cardiac effects is difficult to establish in this setting since myocardial function is frequently depressed by the anemia, fever and infection, and hemorrhage which often accompany the underlying disease.

Hormone-Refractory Prostate Cancer- Functional cardiac changes such as decreases in LVEF and congestive heart failure may occur in patients with hormone-refractory prostate cancer treated with NOVANTRONE. In a randomized comparative trial of NOVANTRONE plus low-dose prednisone vs low-dose prednisone, 7 of 128 patients (5.5%) treated with NOVANTRONE had a cardiac event defined as any decrease in LVEF below the normal range, congestive heart failure (n = 3), or myocardial ischemia. Two patients had a prior history of cardiac disease. The total NOVANTRONE dose administered to patients with cardiac effects ranged from >48 to 212 mg/m^2.

Among 112 patients evaluable for safety on the NOVANTRONE + hydrocortisone arm of the CALGB trial, 18 patients (19%) had a reduction in cardiac function, 5 patients (5%) had cardiac ischemia, and 2 patients (2%) experienced pulmonary edema. The range of total NOVANTRONE doses administered to these patients is not available.

PRECAUTIONS

General: Therapy with NOVANTRONE should be accompanied by close and frequent monitoring of hematologic and chemical laboratory parameters, as well as frequent patient observation.

Systemic infections should be treated concomitantly with or just prior to commencing therapy with NOVANTRONE.

Information for Patients: NOVANTRONE may impart a blue-green color to the urine for 24 hours after administration, and patients should be advised to expect this during therapy. Bluish discoloration of the sclera may also occur. Patients should be advised of the signs and symptoms of myelosuppression.

Laboratory Tests: Serial complete blood counts and liver function tests are necessary for appropriate dose adjustments. (See **DOSAGE AND ADMINISTRATION** section.)

In leukemia treatment, hyperuricemia may occur as a result of rapid lysis of tumor cells by NOVANTRONE. Serum uric acid levels should be monitored and hypouricemic therapy instituted prior to the initiation of antileukemic therapy.

Carcinogenesis, Mutagenesis, Impairment of Fertility

Carcinogenesis: Intravenous treatment of rats and mice, once every 21 days for 24 months, with NOVANTRONE resulted in an increased incidence of fibroma and external auditory canal tumors in rats at a dose of 0.03 mg/kg (0.02 fold the recommended human dose, on a mg/m^2 basis), and hepatocellular adenoma in male mice at a dose of 0.1 mg/kg (0.03 fold the recommended human dose, on a mg/m^2 basis).

Mutagenesis: NOVANTRONE produced a clastogenic effect *in vivo* (rat bone marrow metaphase analysis) and *in vitro* (induced DNA damage in primary rat hepatocytes and SCE in CHO cells), and is mutagenic in bacterial (Ames/Salmonella and E.Coli) and mammalian (L5178Y TK+/-mouse lymphoma) test systems.

Impairment of Fertility: Daily treatment of male rats (71 days prior to, and during the mating period, and until confirmation of pregnancy in females) and female rats (15 days prior to, and during the mating period) with NOVANTRONE IV doses up to 0.03 mg/kg (0.02 fold the recommended human dose, on a mg/m^2 basis) had no effects on fertility.

Drug Interactions: There is no evidence for drug-drug interactions when NOVANTRONE is administered with corticosteroids.

Pregnancy: Pregnancy Category D: (See **WARNINGS** section.)

Nursing Mothers: NOVANTRONE is excreted in human milk and significant concentrations (18 ng/mL) have been reported for 28 days after the last administration. Because of the potential for serious adverse reactions in infants from NOVANTRONE, breast feeding should be discontinued before starting treatment.

Pediatric Use: Safety and effectiveness in pediatric patients have not been established.

ADVERSE REACTIONS

Leukemia - NOVANTRONE® has been studied in approximately 600 patients with ANLL. The table below represents the adverse reaction experience in the large U.S. comparative study of mitoxantrone + cytarabine *vs* daunorubicin + cytarabine. Experience in the large international study was similar. A much wider experience in a variety of other tumor types revealed no additional important reactions other than cardiomyopathy. (See WARNINGS section.) It should be appreciated that the listed adverse reaction categories include overlapping clinical symptoms related to the same condition, e.g., dyspnea, cough and pneumonia. In addition, the listed adverse reactions cannot all necessarily be attributed to chemotherapy as it is often impossible to distinguish effects of the drug and effects of the underlying disease. It is clear, however, that the combination of NOVANTRONE + cytarabine was responsible for nausea and vomiting, alopecia, mucositis/stomatitis, and myelosuppression.

The following table summarizes adverse reactions occurring in patients treated with NOVANTRONE + cytarabine in comparison with those who received daunorubicin + cytarabine for therapy of ANLL in a large multicenter randomized prospective U.S. trial. Adverse reactions are presented as major categories and selected examples of clinically significant subcategories.

[See table at left]

	ALL INDUCTION [percentage of pts entering induction]		ALL CONSOLIDATION [percentage of pts entering consolidation]	
	NOV N=102	DAUN N=102	NOV N=55	DAUN N=49
Cardiovascular	26	28	11	24
CHF	5	6	0	0
Arrhythmias	3	3	4	4
Bleeding	37	41	20	6
GI	16	12	2	2
Petechiae/Ecchymoses	7	9	11	2
Gastrointestinal	88	85	58	51
Nausea/Vomiting	72	67	31	31
Diarrhea	47	47	18	8
Abdominal Pain	15	9	9	4
Mucositis/Stomatitis	29	33	18	8
Hepatic	10	11	14	2
Jaundice	3	8	7	0
Infections	66	73	60	43
UTI	7	2	7	2
Pneumonia	9	7	9	0
Sepsis	34	36	31	18
Fungal Infections	15	13	9	6
Renal Failure	8	6	0	2
Fever	78	71	24	18
Alopecia	37	40	22	16
Pulmonary	43	43	24	14
Cough	13	9	9	2
Dyspnea	18	20	6	0
CNS	30	30	34	35
Seizures	4	4	2	8
Headache	10	9	13	8
Eye	7	6	2	4
Conjunctivitis	5	1	0	0

Hormone-Refractory Prostate Cancer - Detailed safety information is available for a total of 353 patients with hormone-refractory prostate cancer treated with NOVANTRONE, including 274 patients who received NOVANTRONE in combination with corticosteroids.

The following table summarizes adverse reactions of all grades occurring in ≥5% of patients in Trial CCI-NOV22.

Adverse Events of Any Intensity Occurring in ≥5% of Patients Trial CCI-NOV22

Event	N+P (n = 80) %	P (n = 81) %
Nausea	61	35
Fatigue	39	14
Alopecia	29	0
Anorexia	25	6
Constipation	16	14
Dyspnea	11	5
Nail bed changes	11	0
Edema	10	4
Systemic Infection	10	7
Mucositis	10	0
UTI	9	4
Emesis	9	5

Pain	8	9
Fever	6	3
Hemorrhage/bruise	6	1
Anemia	5	3
Cough	5	0
Decreased LVEF	5	0
Anxiety/depression	5	3
Dyspepsia	5	6
Skin infection	5	3
Blurred vision	3	5

No non-hematologic adverse events of Grade 3/4 were seen in >5% of patients.

The next table summarizes adverse events of all grades occurring in ≥5% of patients in Trial CALGB 9182.

Adverse Events of Any Intensity Occurring in ≥5% of Patients Trial CALGB 9182

	M+H (n = 112)		H (n = 113)	
Event	n	%	n	%
Decreased WBC	96	87	4	4
Granulocytes/bands	88	79	3	3
Decreased hemoglobin	83	75	42	39
Lymphocytes	78	72	27	25
Pain	45	41	44	39
Platelets	43	39	8	7
Alkaline Phosphatase	41	37	42	38
Malaise/fatigue	37	34	16	14
Hyperglycemia	33	31	32	30
Edema	31	30	15	14
Nausea	28	26	9	8
Anorexia	24	22	16	14
BUN	24	22	22	20
Transaminase	22	20	16	14
Alopecia	20	20	1	1
Cardiac function	19	18	0	0
Infection	18	17	4	4
Weight loss	18	17	13	12
Dyspnea	16	15	9	8
Diarrhea	16	14	4	4
Fever in absence of infection	15	14	7	6
Weight gain	15	14	16	15
Creatinine	14	13	11	10
Other gastrointestinal	13	14	11	11
Vomiting	12	11	6	5
Other neurologic	11	11	5	5
Hypocalcemia	10	10	5	5
Hematuria	9	11	5	6
Hyponatremia	9	9	3	3
Sweats	9	9	2	2
Other liver	8	8	8	8
Stomatitis	8	8	1	1
Cardiac dysrrhythmia	7	7	3	3
Hypokalemia	7	7	4	4
Neuro/constipation	7	7	2	2
Neuro/motor	7	7	3	3
Neuro/mood	6	6	2	2
Skin	6	6	4	4
Cardiac ischemia	5	5	1	1
Chills	5	5	0	0
Hemorrhage	5	5	3	3
Myalgias/arthralgias	5	5	3	3
Other kidney/bladder	5	5	3	3
Other endocrine	5	6	3	4
Other pulmonary	5	5	3	3
Hypertension	4	4	5	5
Impotence/libido	4	7	2	3
Proteinuria	4	6	2	3
Sterility	3	5	2	3

General

Allergic Reaction: Hypotension, urticaria, dyspnea, and rashes have been reported occasionally.

Cutaneous: Extravasation at the infusion site has been reported, which may result in erythema, swelling, pain, burning, and/or blue discoloration of the skin. Extravasation can result in tissue necrosis with resultant need for debridement and skin grafting. Phlebitis has also been reported at the site of infusion.

Hematologic: Topoisomerase II inhibitors, including NOVANTRONE in combination with other antineoplastic agents, have been associated with the development of acute leukemia.

Leukemia - Myelosuppression is rapid in onset and is consistent with the requirement to produce significant marrow hypoplasia in order to achieve a response in acute leukemia. The incidences of infection and bleeding seen in the U.S. trial are consistent with those reported for other standard induction regimens.

Hormone-refractory prostate cancer - In a randomized study where dose escalation was required for nadir neutrophil counts greater than 1000/mm^3, Grade 4 neutropenia (ANC < 500 /mm^3) was observed in 54% of patients treated with NOVANTRONE + low-dose prednisone. In a separate randomized trial where patients were treated with 14 mg/m^2, Grade 4 neutropenia in 23% of patients treated with NOVANTRONE + hydrocortisone was observed. Neutropenic fever/infection occurred in 11% and 10% of patients receiving NOVANTRONE + corticosteroids, respectively, on the two trials. Platelets < 50,000/mm^3 were noted in 4% and 3% of patients receiving NOVANTRONE + corticosteroids on these trials, and there was one patient death on NOVANTRONE + hydrocortisone due to intracranial hemorrhage after a fall.

Gastrointestinal: Nausea and vomiting occurred acutely in most patients and may have contributed to reports of dehydration, but were generally mild to moderate and could be controlled through the use of antiemetics. Stomatitis/mucositis occurred within 1 week of therapy.

Cardiovascular: Congestive heart failure, tachycardia, EKG changes including arrhythmias, chest pain, and asymptomatic decreases in left ventricular ejection fraction have occurred. (See **WARNINGS** section.)

Pulmonary: Interstitial pneumonitis has been reported in cancer patients receiving combination chemotherapy that included NOVANTRONE.

OVERDOSAGE

There is no known specific antidote for NOVANTRONE. Accidental overdoses have been reported. Four patients receiving 140 - 180 mg/m^2 as a single bolus injection died as a result of severe leukopenia with infection. Hematologic support and antimicrobial therapy may be required during prolonged periods of medullary hypoplasia.

Although patients with severe renal failure have not been studied, NOVANTRONE is extensively tissue bound and it is unlikely that the therapeutic effect or toxicity would be mitigated by peritoneal or hemodialysis.

DOSAGE AND ADMINISTRATION (See WARNINGS section.)

Hormone-Refractory Prostate Cancer: Based on data from two Phase III comparative trials of NOVANTRONE plus corticosteroids versus corticosteroids alone, the recommended dosage of NOVANTRONE is 12 to 14 mg/m^2 given as a short intravenous infusion every 21 days.

Combination Initial Therapy for ANLL in Adults: For induction, the recommended dosage is 12 mg/m^2 of NOVANTRONE daily on days 1-3 given as an intravenous infusion, and 100 mg/m^2 of cytarabine for 7 days given as a continuous 24-hour infusion on days 1-7.

Most complete remissions will occur following the initial course of induction therapy. In the event of an incomplete antileukemic response, a second induction course may be given. NOVANTRONE should be given for 2 days and cytarabine for 5 days using the same daily dosage levels.

If severe or life-threatening nonhematologic toxicity is observed during the first induction course, the second induction course should be withheld until toxicity clears.

Consolidation therapy which was used in 2 large randomized multicenter trials consisted of NOVANTRONE, 12 mg/m^2 given by intravenous infusion daily on days 1 and 2 and cytarabine, 100 mg/m^2 for 5 days given as a continuous 24-hour infusion on days 1-5. The first course was given approximately 6 weeks after the final induction course, the second was generally administered 4 weeks after the first. Severe myelosuppression occurred. (See **CLINICAL PHARMACOLOGY** section.)

Hepatic Impairment: For patients with hepatic impairment, there is at present no laboratory measurement that allows for dose adjustment recommendations. (See **CLINICAL PHARMACOLOGY**, Special Populations: *Hepatic Impairment*)

Preparation and Administration Precautions: NOVANTRONE CONCENTRATE MUST BE DILUTED PRIOR TO USE.

Parenteral drug products should be inspected visually for particulate matter and discoloration prior to administration whenever solution and container permit.

The dose of NOVANTRONE should be diluted to at least 50 mL with either 0.9% Sodium Chloride Injection (USP) or 5% Dextrose Injection (USP). NOVANTRONE may be further diluted into Dextrose 5% in Water, Normal Saline or Dextrose 5% with Normal Saline and used immediately. DO NOT FREEZE.

NOVANTRONE should not be mixed in the same infusion as heparin since a precipitate may form. Because specific compatibility data are not available, it is recommended that NOVANTRONE not be mixed in the same infusion with other drugs. The diluted solution should be introduced slowly into the tubing as a freely running intravenous infusion of 0.9% Sodium Chloride Injection (USP) or 5% Dextrose Injection (USP) over a period of not less than 3 minutes. Unused infusion solutions should be discarded immediately in an appropriate fashion. In the case of multidose use, after penetration of the stopper, the remaining portion of the undiluted NOVANTRONE concentrate should be stored not longer than 7 days between 15°-25° C (59°-77° F) or 14 days under refrigeration. DO NOT FREEZE. CONTAINS NO PRESERVATIVE.

If extravasation occurs, the administration should be stopped immediately and restarted in another vein. The nonvesicant properties of NOVANTRONE minimize the possibility of severe local reactions following extravasation. However, care should be taken to avoid extravasation at the infusion site and to avoid contact of NOVANTRONE with the skin, mucous membranes or eyes.

Skin accidentally exposed to NOVANTRONE should be rinsed copiously with warm water and if the eyes are involved, standard irrigation techniques should be used immediately. The use of goggles, gloves, and protective gowns is recommended during preparation and administration of the drug.

Procedures for proper handling and disposal of anticancer drugs should be considered. Several guidelines on this subject have been published.[1-7] There is no general agreement that all of the procedures recommended in the guidelines are necessary or appropriate.

REFERENCES

1. Recommendations for the Safe Handling of Parenteral Antineoplastic Drugs. NIH Publication No. 83-2621. For sale by the Superintendent of Documents, US Government Printing Office, Washington, DC 20402.

2. AMA Council Report. Guidelines for Handling Parenteral Antineoplastics. *JAMA*. 1985; 253 (11) :1590-1592.

3. National Study Commission on Cytotoxic Exposure - Recommendations for Handling Cytotoxic Agents. Available from Louis P. Jeffrey, Sc D, Chairman, National Study Commission on Cytotoxic Exposure, Massachusetts College of Pharmacy and Allied Health Sciences, 179 Longwood Avenue, Boston, Massachusetts 02115.

4. Clinical Oncological Society of Australia: Guidelines and recommendations for safe handling of antineoplastic agents. *Med J Australia.* 1983; 1:426-428.

5. Jones RB, et al. Safe handling of chemotherapeutic agents: A report from the Mount Sinai Medical Center. *Ca - A Cancer Journal for Clinicians*. Sept/Oct 1983; 258-263.

6. American Society of Hospital Pharmacists technical assistance bulletin on handling cytotoxic and hazardous drugs. *Am J Hosp Pharm*. 1990; 47:1033-1049.

7. OSHA Work-Practice guidelines for personnel dealing with cytotoxic (antineoplastic) drugs. *Am J Hosp Pharm* 1986; 43:1193-1204.

HOW SUPPLIED

NOVANTRONE® (mitoxantrone for injection concentrate) is a sterile aqueous solution containing mitoxantrone hydrochloride at a concentration equivalent to 2 mg mitoxantrone free base per mL supplied in vials for multidose use as follows:

NDC 58406-640-03 - 10 mL/multidose vial (20 mg)
NDC 58406-640-05 - 12.5 mL/multidose vial (25 mg)
NDC 58406-640-07 - 15 mL/multidose vial (30 mg)

NOVANTRONE® (mitoxantrone for injection concentrate) should be stored between 15°-25°C (59°-77°F). DO NOT FREEZE.

Manufactured for IMMUNEX CORPORATION, Seattle, WA 98101
by LEDERLE PARENTERALS, INC., Carolina, Puerto Rico 00987

Rev 0166-08 CI 6102-1
Revised 03/2000

THIOPLEX® ℞

(Thiotepa For Injection)
15 mg/Vial

DESCRIPTION

THIOPLEX® (thiotepa for injection) is an ethylenimine-type compound. It is supplied as a non-pyrogenic, sterile lyophilized powder for intravenous, intracavitary or intravesical administration, containing 15 mg of thiotepa. THIOPLEX is a synthetic product with antitumor activity. The chemical name for thiotepa is Aziridine, 1,1′,1″-phosphinothioylidynetris-, or Tris (1-aziridinyl) phosphine sulfide.

Thiotepa has the following structural formula:

Thiotepa has the empirical formula $C_6H_{12}N_3PS$ and a molecular weight of 189.22. When reconstituted with Sterile Water for Injection, the resulting solution has a pH of approximately 5.5 - 7.5. Thiotepa is stable in alkaline medium and unstable in acid medium.

CLINICAL PHARMACOLOGY

Thiotepa is a cytotoxic agent of the polyfunctional type, related chemically and pharmacologically to nitrogen mustard. The radiomimetic action of thiotepa is believed to occur through the release of ethylenimine radicals which, like irradiation, disrupt the bonds of DNA. One of the principal bond disruptions is initiated by alkylation of guanine at the N-7 position, which severs the linkage between the purine base and the sugar and liberates alkylated guanines.

The pharmacokinetics of thiotepa and TEPA in thirteen female patients (45 - 84 years) with advanced stage ovarian cancer receiving 60 mg and 80 mg thiotepa by intravenous infusion on subsequent courses given at 4-week intervals are presented in the following table:

[See first table at top of next page]

TEPA, which possesses cytotoxic activity, appears to be the major metabolite of thiotepa found in human serum and urine. Urinary excretion of ^{14}C-labeled thiotepa and metabolites in a 34-year old patient with metastatic carcinoma of the cecum who received a dose of 0.3 mg/kg intravenously was 63%. Thiotepa and TEPA in urine each accounts for less than 2% of the administered dose.

Continued on next page

Thioplex—Cont.

The pharmacokinetics of thiotepa in renal and hepatic dysfunction patients have not been evaluated. Possible pharmacokinetic interactions of thiotepa with any concomitantly administered medications have not been formally investigated.

INDICATIONS AND USAGE

Thiotepa has been tried with varying results in the palliation of a wide variety of neoplastic diseases. However, the most consistent results have been seen in the following tumors:

1. Adenocarcinoma of the breast.
2. Adenocarcinoma of the ovary.
3. For controlling intracavitary effusions secondary to diffuse or localized neoplastic diseases of various serosal cavities.
4. For the treatment of superficial papillary carcinoma of the urinary bladder.

While now largely superseded by other treatments, thiotepa has been effective against other lymphomas, such as lymphosarcoma and Hodgkin's disease.

CONTRAINDICATIONS

THIOPLEX is contraindicated in patients with a known hypersensitivity (allergy) to this preparation.

Therapy is probably contraindicated in cases of existing hepatic, renal, or bone-marrow damage. However, if the need outweighs the risk in such patients, thiotepa may be used in low dosage, and accompanied by hepatic, renal and hemopoietic function tests.

WARNINGS

Death has occurred after intravesical administration, caused by bone-marrow depression from systematically absorbed drug.

Death from septicemia and hemorrhage has occurred as a direct result of hematopoietic depression by thiotepa.

Thiotepa is highly toxic to the hematopoietic system. A rapidly falling white blood cell or platelet count indicates the necessity for discontinuing or reducing the dosage of thiotepa. Weekly blood and platelet counts are recommended during therapy and for at least 3 weeks after therapy has been discontinued.

Thiotepa can cause fetal harm when administered to a pregnant woman. Thiotepa given by the intraperitoneal (IP) route was teratogenic in mice at doses ≥1 mg/kg (3.2 mg/m^2), approximately 8-fold less than the maximum recommended human therapeutic dose (0.8 mg/kg, 27 mg/m^2), based on body-surface area. Thiotepa given by the IP route was teratogenic in rats at doses ≥3 mg/kg (21 mg/m^2), approximately equal to the maximum recommended human therapeutic dose, based on body-surface area. Thiotepa was lethal to rabbit fetuses at a dose of 3 mg/kg (41 mg/m^2), approximately two times the maximum recommended human therapeutic dose based on body-surface area.

Effective contraception should be used during thiotepa therapy if either the patient or partner is of childbearing potential. There are no adequate and well-controlled studies in pregnant women. If thiotepa is used during pregnancy, or if pregnancy occurs during thiotepa therapy, the patient and partner should be apprised of the potential hazard to the fetus.

Thiotepa is a polyfunctional alkylating agent, capable of cross-linking the DNA within a cell and changing its nature. The replication of the cell is, therefore, altered, and thiotepa may be described as mutagenic. An *in vitro* study has shown that it causes chromosomal aberrations of the chromatid type and that the frequency of induced aberrations increases with the age of the subject.

Like many alkylating agents, thiotepa has been reported to be carcinogenic when administered to laboratory animals. Carcinogenicity is shown most clearly in studies using mice, but there is some evidence of carcinogenicity in man. In patients treated with thiotepa, cases of myelodysplastic syndromes and acute non-lymphocytic leukemia have been reported.

PRECAUTIONS

General

The serious complication of excessive thiotepa therapy, or sensitivity to the effects of thiotepa, is bone-marrow depression. If proper precautions are not observed thiotepa may cause leukopenia, thrombocytopenia, and anemia.

Information for Patients

The patient should notify the physician in the case of any sign of bleeding (epistaxis, easy bruising, change in color of urine, black stool) or infection (fever, chills) or for possible pregnancy to patient or partner.

Effective contraception should be used during thiotepa therapy if either the patient or the partner is of childbearing potential.

Laboratory Tests

The most reliable guide to thiotepa toxicity is the white blood cell count. If this falls to 3000 or less, the dose should be discontinued. Another good index of thiotepa toxicity is the platelet count; if this falls to 150,000, therapy should be discontinued. Red blood cell count is a less accurate indicator of thiotepa toxicity. If the drug is used in patients with hepatic or renal damage (see **CONTRAINDICATIONS** section), regular assessment of hepatic and renal function tests are indicated.

Pharmacokinetic Parameters	Mean ± SEM			
	Thiotepa		TEPA	
(units)	60 mg	80 mg	60 mg	80 mg
Peak Serum concentration (ng/mL)	1331 ± 119	1828 ± 135	273 ± 46	353 ± 46
Elimination half-life (h)	2.4 ± 0.3	2.3 ± 0.3	17.6 ± 3.6	15.7 ± 2.7
Area under the curve (ng/h/mL)	2832 ± 412	4127 ± 668	4789 ± 1022	7452 ± 1667
Total body clearance (mL/min)	446 ± 63	419 ± 56		

Label Claim (mg/vial)	Actual Content (mg/vial)	Amount of Diluent to be Added (mL)	Approximate Withdrawable Volume (mL)	Approximate Withdrawable Amount (mg/vial)	Approximate Reconstituted Concentration (mg/mL)
15.0	15.6	1.5	1.4	14.7	10.4

Drug Interactions

It is not advisable to combine, simultaneously or sequentially, cancer chemotherapeutic agents or a cancer chemotherapeutic agent and a therapeutic modality having the same mechanism of action. Therefore, thiotepa combined with other alkylating agents such as nitrogen mustard or cyclophosphamide or thiotepa combined with irradiation would serve to intensify toxicity rather than to enhance therapeutic response. If these agents must follow each other, it is important that recovery from the first agent, as indicated by white blood cell count, be complete before therapy with the second agent is instituted.

Other drugs which are known to produce bone-marrow depression should be avoided.

Carcinogenesis, Mutagenesis and Impairment of Fertility

Also see **WARNINGS** section.

Carcinogenesis

In mice, repeated IP administration of thiotepa (1.15 or 2.3 mg/kg three times per week for 52 or 43 weeks, respectively) produced a significant increase in the combined incidence of squamous-cell carcinomas of the skin, preputial gland, and ear canal, and combined incidence of lymphoma and lymphocytic leukemia. In other studies in mice, repeated IP administration of thiotepa (4 or 8 mg/kg three times per week for 4 weeks followed by a 20-week observation period or 1.8 mg/kg three times per week for 4 weeks followed by a 35-week observation period) resulted in an increased incidence of lung tumors. In rats, repeated IP administration of thiotepa (0.7 or 1.4 mg/kg three times per week for 52 or 34 weeks, respectively) produced significant increases in the incidence of squamous-cell carcinomas of the skin or ear canal, combined hematopoietic neoplasms, and uterine adenocarcinomas. Thiotepa given intravenously (IV) to rats (1 mg/kg once per week for 52 weeks) produced an increased incidence of malignant tumors (abdominal cavity sarcoma, lymphosarcoma, myelosis, seminoma, fibrosarcoma, salivary gland hemangioendothelioma, mammary sarcoma, pheochromocytoma) and benign tumors.

The lowest reported carcinogenic dose in mice (1.15 mg/kg, 3.68 mg/m^2) is approximately 7-fold less than the maximum recommended human therapeutic dose based on body-surface area. The lowest reported carcinogenic dose in rats (0.7 mg/kg, 4.9 mg/m^2) is approximately 6-fold less than the maximum recommended human therapeutic dose based on body-surface area.

Mutagenesis

Thiotepa was mutagenic in *in vitro* assays in *Salmonella typhimurium, E. coli*, Chinese hamster lung and human lymphocytes. Chromosomal aberrations and sister chromatid exchanges were observed *in vitro* with thiotepa in bean root tips, human lymphocytes, Chinese hamster lung, and monkey lymphocytes. Mutations were observed with oral thiotepa in mice at doses >2.5 mg/kg (8 mg/m^2). The mouse micronucleus test was positive with IP administration of >1 mg/kg (3.2 mg/m^2). Other positive *in vivo* chromosomal aberration or mutation assays included *Drosophila melanogaster*, Chinese hamster marrow, murine marrow, monkey lymphocyte, and murine germ cell.

Impairment of Fertility

Thiotepa impaired fertility in male mice at PO or IP doses ≥0.7 mg/kg (2.24 mg/m^2), approximately 12-fold less than the maximum recommended human therapeutic dose based on body-surface area. Thiotepa (0.5 mg) inhibited implantation in female rats when instilled into the uterine cavity. Thiotepa interfered with spermatogenesis in mice at IP doses ≥0.5 mg/kg (1.6 mg/m^2), approximately 17-fold less than the maximum recommended human therapeutic dose based on body-surface area. Thiotepa interfered with spermatogenesis in hamsters at an IP dose of 1 mg/kg (4.1 mg/m^2), approximately 7-fold less than the maximum recommended human therapeutic dose based on body-surface area.

Pregnancy

Category D: See **WARNINGS** section.

Thiotepa can cause fetal harm when administered to a pregnant woman. Thiotepa given by the IP route was teratogenic in mice at doses ≥1 mg/kg (3.2 mg/m^2), approximately 8-fold less than the maximum recommended human therapeutic dose based on body-surface area. Thiotepa given by the IP route was teratogenic in rats at doses ≥3 mg/kg (21 mg/m^2), approximately equal to the maximum recommended human therapeutic dose based on body-surface area. Thiotepa was lethal to rabbit fetuses at a dose of 3 mg/kg (41 mg/m^2), approximately 2 times the maximum recommended human therapeutic dose based on body-surface area. Patients of childbearing potential should be advised to avoid pregnancy. There are no adequate and well-controlled studies in pregnant women. If thiotepa is used during pregnancy, or if pregnancy occurs during thiotepa therapy, the patient and partner should be apprised of the potential hazard to the fetus.

Nursing Mothers

It is not known whether thiotepa is excreted in human milk. Because many drugs are excreted in human milk and because of the potential for tumorigenicity shown for thiotepa in animal studies, a decision should be made whether to discontinue nursing or to discontinue the drug, taking into account the importance of the drug to the mother.

Pediatric Use

Safety and effectiveness in pediatric patients have not been established.

Geriatric Use

Clinical studies of thiotepa did not include sufficient numbers of subjects aged 65 and over to determine whether elderly subjects respond differently from younger subjects, and other reported clinical experience has not identified differences in responses between the elderly and younger patients. In general, dose selection for an elderly patient should be cautious, usually starting at the low end of the dosing range, reflecting the greater frequency of decreasing hepatic, renal or cardiac function, and of concomitant disease or other drug therapy.

ADVERSE REACTIONS

In addition to its effect on the blood-forming elements (see **WARNINGS** and **PRECAUTIONS** sections), thiotepa may cause other adverse reactions.

General: Fatigue, weakness. Febrile reaction and discharge from a subcutaneous lesion may occur as the result of breakdown of tumor tissue.

Hypersensitivity Reactions: Allergic reactions - rash, urticaria, laryngeal edema, asthma, anaphylactic shock, wheezing.

Local Reactions: Contact dermatitis, pain at the injection site.

Gastrointestinal: Nausea, vomiting, abdominal pain, anorexia.

Renal: Dysuria, urinary retention. There have been rare reports of chemical cystitis or hemorrhagic cystitis following intravesical, but not parenteral administration of thiotepa.

Respiratory: Prolonged apnea has been reported when succinylcholine was administered prior to surgery, following combined use of thiotepa and other anticancer agents. It was theorized that this was caused by decrease of pseudocholinesterase activity caused by the anticancer drugs.

Neurologic: Dizziness, headache, blurred vision.

Skin: Dermatitis, alopecia. Skin depigmentation has been reported following topical use.

Special Senses: Conjunctivitis.

Reproductive: Amenorrhea, interference with spermatogenesis.

OVERDOSAGE

Hematopoietic toxicity can occur following overdose, manifested by a decrease in the white cell count and/or platelets. Red blood cell count is a less accurate indicator of thiotepa toxicity. Bleeding manifestations may develop. The patient may become more vulnerable to infection, and less able to combat such infection.

Dosages within and minimally above the recommended therapeutic doses have been associated with potentially life-threatening hematopoietic toxicity. Thiotepa has a toxic effect on the hematopoietic system that is dose related.

Thiotepa is dialyzable.

There is no known antidote for overdosage with thiotepa. Transfusions of whole blood or platelets have proven beneficial to the patient in combating hematopoietic toxicity.

DOSAGE AND ADMINISTRATION

Since absorption from the gastrointestinal tract is variable, thiotepa should not be administered orally.

Dosage must be carefully individualized. A slow response to thiotepa does not necessarily indicate a lack of effect. Therefore, increasing the frequency of dosing may only increase toxicity. After maximum benefit is obtained by initial therapy, it is necessary to continue the patient on maintenance therapy (1 to 4 week intervals). In order to continue optimal effect, maintenance doses should not be administered more frequently than weekly in order to preserve correlation between dose and blood counts.

Preparation and Administration Precautions: Thiotepa is a cytotoxic anticancer drug and as with other potentially toxic compounds, caution should be exercised in handling and preparation of thiotepa. Skin reactions associated with accidental exposure to thiotepa may occur. The use of gloves is recommended. If thiotepa solution contacts the skin, immediately wash the skin thoroughly with soap and water. If thiotepa contacts mucous membranes, the membranes should be flushed thoroughly with water.

Preparation of Solution: THIOPLEX (thiotepa for injection) should be reconstituted with **1.5 mL** of Sterile Water for Injection resulting in a drug concentration of approximately **10 mg/mL**. The actual withdrawable quantities and concentration achieved are illustrated in the following table:

[See second table at top of previous page]

The reconstituted solution is hypotonic and should be further diluted with Sodium Chloride Injection (0.9% sodium chloride) before use.

When reconstituted with Sterile Water for Injection, solutions of THIOPLEX should be stored in a refrigerator and used within 8 hours. Reconstituted solutions further diluted with Sodium Chloride Injection should be used immediately. **In order to eliminate haze, filter solutions through a 0.22 micron filter* prior to administration. Filtering does not alter solution potency. Reconstituted solutions should be clear. Solutions that remain opaque or precipitate after filtration should not be used.**

* Polysulfone membrane (Gelman's Sterile Acrodisc®, Single Use) or triton-free mixed ester of cellulose/PVC (Millipore's MILLEX®-GS Filter Unit).

Parenteral drug products should be inspected visually for particulate matter and discoloration prior to administration, whenever solution and container permit.

Initial and Maintenance Doses: Initially the higher dose in the given range is commonly administered. The maintenance dose should be adjusted weekly on the basis of pretreatment control blood counts and subsequent blood counts.

Intravenous Administration: Thiotepa may be given by rapid intravenous administration in doses of 0.3 to 0.4 mg/kg. Doses should be given at 1 to 4 week intervals.

Intracavitary Administration: The dosage recommended is 0.6 - 0.8 mg/kg. Administration is usually effected through the same tubing which is used to remove the fluid from the cavity involved.

Intravesical Administration: Patients with papillary carcinoma of the bladder are dehydrated for 8 to 12 hours prior to treatment. Then 60 mg of thiotepa in 30 - 60 mL of Sodium Chloride Injection is instilled into the bladder by catheter. For maximum effect, the solution should be retained for 2 hours. If the patient finds it impossible to retain 60 mL for 2 hours, the dose may be given in a volume of 30 mL. If desired, the patient may be positioned every 15 minutes for maximum area contact. The usual course of treatment is once a week for 4 weeks. The course may be repeated if necessary, but second and third courses must be given with caution since bone-marrow depression may be increased. Deaths have occurred after intravesical administration, caused by bone-marrow depression from systemically absorbed drug.

Handling and Disposal: Follow safe cytotoxic agent handling procedures. Several guidelines on this subject have been published.[1–6] There is no general agreement that all of the procedures recommended in the guidelines are necessary or appropriate.

HOW SUPPLIED

THIOPLEX® (thiotepa for injection), for single use only, is available in vials containing 15 mg of non-pyrogenic, sterile lyophilized powder, supplied as follows:

NDC 58406-661-31 - 6 x 15 mg/vial

STORAGE

Store in refrigerator between 2-8°C (36-46°F). PROTECT FROM LIGHT AT ALL TIMES.

REFERENCES

1. Recommendations for the Safe Handling of Parenteral Antineoplastic Drugs. NIH Publication No. 83-2621. For sale by the Superintendent of Documents, US Government Printing Office, Washington, DC 20402.
2. AMA Council Report. Guidelines for Handling Parenteral Antineoplastics. *JAMA*. 1985; 253(11):1590-1592.
3. National Study Commission on Cytotoxic Exposure - Recommendations for Handling Cytotoxic Agents. Available from Louis P. Jeffrey, Sc D, Chairman, National Study Commission on Cytotoxic Exposure, Massachusetts College of Pharmacy and Allied Health Sciences, 179 Longwood Avenue, Boston, Massachusetts 02115.
4. Clinical Oncological Society of Australia: Guidelines and recommendations for safe handling of antineoplastic agents. *Med J Australia*. 1983; 1:426-428.
5. Jones RB, et al. Safe handling of chemotherapeutic agents: A report from the Mount Sinai Medical Center. Ca - *A Cancer Journal for Clinicians*. Sept/Oct 1983; 258-263.
6. American Society of Hospital Pharmacists technical assistance bulletin on handling cytotoxic and hazardous drugs. *Am J Hosp Pharm*. 1990; 47:1033-1049.

Manufactured for IMMUNEX CORPORATION, Seattle, WA 98101

by LEDERLE PARENTERALS, INC., Carolina, Puerto Rico 00987

CI 4506-2

Immuno

1200 PARKDALE ROAD
ROCHESTER, MI 48307 USA

(For product information, see BAXTER HEALTHCARE CORPORATION)

Immunotec Research Ltd.

292 ADRIEN PATENEAUDE
VAUDREUIL-DORION (QUEBEC)
CANADA J7V 5V5

For Direct Inquiries Contact:
450-424-9992

IMMUNOCAL® OTC

GLUTATHIONE PRECURSOR
(undenatured whey protein isolate)
Powder Sachets

DESCRIPTION

Immunocal® is a U.S. patented natural food protein concentrate which assists the body in maintaining an optimal concentration of glutathione (GSH) by supplying the precursors required for intracellular glutathione synthesis. These precursors are derived from a specially prepared bovine whey protein isolate. Glutathione (L-gamma-glutamyl-L-cysteinylglycine) is the major endogenous antioxidant produced by the cell. Glutathione participates directly in the neutralization of free radicals, reactive oxygen compounds, and maintains exogenous antioxidants such as vitamins C and E in their reduced (active) forms. In addition, through direct conjugation, glutathione plays a role in the detoxification of many xenobiotics (foreign compounds) both organic and inorganic. Glutathione is an essential component of the human immune response. Proposed mechanisms of immune enhancement include:

1) optimizing macrophage functions, 2) offsetting oxidative damage associated with lymphocyte monoclonal expansion and 3) stabilizing the mitochondrial membrane thereby, reducing apoptosis in lymphocytes.

CLINICAL PHARMACOLOGY

The systemic availability of oral glutathione is negligible; the vast majority of it must be manufactured intracellularly. Glutathione (GSH) is a tripeptide made up of the three amino acids: cysteine, glycine and glutamate. Glutamate and glycine are readily available in most North American diets, but the availability of cysteine makes it be the rate-limiting substrate for the synthesis of glutathione within the cell. It is the sulfhydryl (thiol) group (SH) of cysteine that serves as proton-donor and is responsible for the biochemical activity of glutathione. The free amino acid cysteine does not represent an ideal delivery system to the cell. It is potentially toxic and is spontaneously catabolized in the gastrointestinal tract and blood plasma. Conversely, cysteine absorbed during digestion as cystine (two cysteine molecules linked by a disulfide bond) in the gastrointestinal tract is more stable than the free amino acid, cysteine. The disulfide bond is pepsin- and trypsin-resistant, but may be split by heat, low pH, and mechanical stress. Cystine travels safely through the GI tract and blood plasma and is promptly reduced to the two cysteine molecules upon cell entry. Immunocal can thus be viewed as a cystine delivery vehicle.

Cystine is the preferred form of cysteine for the synthesis of glutathione in macrophages and astrocytes. Lymphocytes and neurons prefer cysteine for glutathione production. Optimizing glutathione levels in macrophages and astrocytes with cystine allow these cells to provide cysteine to lymphocytes and neurons directly upon demand.

This specially prepared whey protein isolate contains the thermolabile proteins serum albumin, alpha lactalbumin and lactoferrin. These proteins contain high levels of cystine residues that could be denatured by heat, low pH, or mechanical stress (inherent in most extraction processes). In serum albumin there are 17 cystine residues and 6 glutamylcystine (Glu-Cys) dipeptides; in lactoferrin 17 cystine residues and 4 Glu-Cys dipeptides; and in alpha-lactalbumin 4 cystine residues. In particular, the Glu-Cys dipeptides very readily enter the cell to be synthesized into GSH. Of interest, the Glu-Cys dipeptide is an exclusive feature of the only obligatory foods in the early life of mammals and oviparous species, those being milk and egg white respectively. When subject to heat or shearing forces, the fragile disulfide bonds within these peptides are broken and the bioavailability of the glutathione precursors is greatly diminished.

As an antioxidant, glutathione is essential for allowing lymphocytes to express their full potential, without being hampered by oxyradical accumulation during the oxygen-requiring development of the immune response. In a similar fashion, GSH delays the muscular fatigue induced by oxyradicals during the aerobic phase of strenuous muscular contraction.

As a detoxification agent, glutathione has been demonstrated to be effective against a number of xenobiotics, including chemical pollutants, various carcinogens and ultraviolet radiation.

Glutathione is a tightly regulated intracellular constituent and is limited in its production by negative feedback inhibition of its own synthesis through the enzyme gamma-glutamylcysteine synthetase, thus greatly minimizing any possibility of overdosage.

INDICATIONS AND USAGE

Immunocal® is a natural food supplement and as such is limited from stating medical claims per se. Statements have not been evaluated by the FDA. As such, this product is not intended to diagnose, cure, prevent or treat any disease.

Glutathione augmentation is a strategy developed to address states of glutathione deficiency, high oxidative stress, and xenobiotic overload in which glutathione plays a part in the detoxification of the xenobiotic in question. Glutathione deficiency states include, but are not limited to: AIDS and cancer cachexia, chemical and infectious hepatitis, radiation poisoning, malnutritive states, arduous physical stress, and has been associated with sub-optimal immune response. Many clinical pathologies are associated with oxidative stress and are elaborated upon in numerous medical references.

CONTRAINDICATIONS

Immunocal® is contraindicated in individuals who develop or have known hypersensitivity to specific milk proteins.

PRECAUTIONS

Each sachet of **Immunocal®** contains nine grams of protein. Patients on a protein-restricted diet need to take this into account when calculating their daily protein load. Although a bovine milk derivative, **Immunocal®** contains less than 1% lactose and therefore is generally well tolerated by lactose-intolerant individuals.

WARNINGS

Patients undergoing immunosuppressive therapy should discuss the use of this product with their health professional.

Heating or adding **Immunocal®** to a hot liquid, or use of a high-speed blender to reconstitute it will significantly decrease the effectiveness of the product.

ADVERSE REACTIONS

Gastrointestinal bloating and cramps if not sufficiently rehydrated. Transient urticarial-like rash in rare individuals undergoing severe detoxification reaction. Rash abates when product intake stopped or reduced.

OVERDOSAGE

Overdosing on **Immunocal®** has not been reported. Unless hypersensitive to the constituents, no toxicity of milk proteins has been described.

DOSAGE AND ADMINISTRATION

Maintenance dose is one sachet (10 grams) per day. For mild to moderate health challenges, higher doses are recommended. Clinical trials in patients with AIDS, cancer and chronic fatigue syndrome have used 30–50 grams per day without ill effect. **Immunocal®** is best administered on an empty stomach or with a light meal. Concomitant intake of another high protein load may adversely affect absorption.

RECONSTITUTION: **Immunocal®** is a dehydrated powdered protein isolate. It must be appropriately rehydrated before use. If left standing too long after rehydration, activity of the product may be reduced. Times vary depending on temperature and pH of the liquid used. It is generally recommended to ingest the product within 30 minutes of reconstitution. DO NOT heat or use a hot liquid to rehydrate the product or use a high-speed blender for reconstitution. These methods will decrease the activity of the product. Special low-speed blenders or mixing cups can be made available through NuMedTec distribution networks.

Proper mixing is imperative. Consult instructions included in packaging.

HOW SUPPLIED

10 grams of bovine milk protein isolate powder per sachet. 30 sachets per box.

STORAGE

Store in a cool dry environment. Refrigeration is not necessary.

Patent no.'s 5,230,902 - 5,290,571 - 5,456,924 - 5,451,412 - 5,888,552

REFERENCES

1. Meister A. **Glutathione.** *Ann Rev Biochem* 52:711-60, 1983.
2. Kaplowitz N, Aw T, Ookhtens M. **The regulation of hepatic glutathione.** *Ann Rev Pharmacol Toxicol* 25:715-44, 1985.
3. Witschi A, Reddy S, Stofer B, Lauterberg B. **The systemic availability of oral glutathione.** *Eur J Clin Pharmacol* 43:667-9, 1992.
4. Meister A. **New aspects of glutathione biochemistry and transport, selective alteration of glutathione metabolism.** *Nutr Rev* 42:397-410, 1984.

Continued on next page

Immunocal—Cont.

5. Bray T, Taylor C. **Enhancement of tissue glutathione for antioxidant and immune functions in malnutrition.** *Biochem Pharmacol* 47:2113-23, 1994.
6. Lomaestro B, Malone M. **Glutathione in health and disease: Pharmacotherapeutic Issues.** *Ann Pharmacother* 29:1263-73, 1995.
7. Bounous G, Gold P. **The biological activity of undenatured whey proteins: The role of glutathione.** *Clin Invest Med* 14:296–309, 1991.
8. Bounous G, Kongshavn P. **Influence of dietary whey proteins on the immune system of mice.** *J Nutr* 112: 1747-55, 1982.
9. Bounous G, Letourneau L, Kongshavn P. **Influence of dietary protein type on the immune system of mice.** *J Nutr* 113:1415-21, 1983.
10. Bounous G, Kongshavn P. **Influence of protein type in nutritionally adequate diets on the development of immunity.** *Absorption and utilization of amino acids* 2:219-32, 1989.
11. Bounous G, Batist G, Gold P. **Immuno-enhancing property of dietary whey protein in mice: Role of glutathione.** *Clin Invest Med* 12:154-61, 1989.
12. Bounous G, Shenouda N, Kongshavn P, Osmond D. **Mechanism of altered B-cell response induced by changes in dietary protein type in mice.** *J Nutr* 115: 1409-17, 1985.
13. Bounous G, Papenburg R, Kongshavn P, Gold P, et al. **Dietary whey protein inhibits the development of DMH-induced malignancy.** *Clin Invest Med.* 11:213-17, 1988.
14. Bounous G, Gervais F, Amer V, Batist G, et al. **The influence of dietary whey protein on tissue glutathione and the diseases of aging.** *Clin Invest Med* 12:343-9, 1989.
15. Baruchel S, Viau G, Olivier R, Bounous G, Wainberg MA. **Nutriceutical modulation of glutathione with a humanized native milk serum protein isolate Immunocal: Application in AIDS and cancer.** In: *Oxidative stress in Cancer AIDS and Neurodegenerative Diseases.* Ed.; Montagnier L, Olivier R, Pasquier C. Pub.; Marcel Dekker Inc. New York, 1996.
16. Kennedy R, Konok G, Bounous G, Baruchel S, Lee T. **The use of a whey protein concentrate in the treatment of patients with metastatic carcinoma: A phase I-II clinical study.** *Anticancer Research* 15:2643-50, 1995.
17. Baruchel S, Bounous G, Gold P. **Place for an antioxidant therapy in HIV infection.** *Oxidative stress, Cell activation and viral infection*, 311-21,1994.
18. Bounous G, Baruchel S, Falutz J, Gold P. **Whey proteins as a food supplement in HIV-seropositive individuals.** *Clin Invest Med.* 16:3; 204–209.
19. Baruchel S, Viau G. **In-vitro selective modulation of cellular glutathione by a humanized native milk protein isolate in normal cells and rat mammary carcinoma mode.** *Anticancer Research.* 16:1095–1100, 1996.
20. Bounous G, Batist G, Gold P. **Whey proteins in cancer prevention.** *Cancer Letters.* 57:91–94, 1991.
21. Watanabe A, Higuchi K, Yasumura S, Shimizu Y, Kondo Y, Kohri H. **Nutritional modulation of glutathione level and cellular immunity in chronic hepatitis B and C.** *Hepatology.* 24:597A, 1996.
22. Lothian B, Grey V, Kimoff RJ, Lands LC. **Treatment of obstructive airway disease with a cysteine donor protein supplement: A case report.** *Chest* 117:914–916, 2000.
23. Cross CE, Halliwell B, Borish ET, et al. **Oxygen radicals and human disease.** *Annals of Internal Medicine* 107: 526–545, 1987.
24. Lands LC, Grey VL, Smountas AA. **Effect of supplementation with a cysteine donor on muscular performance.** *J. Appl. Physiol.* 87:1381–1385, 1999.
25. Short S, Merkel BJ, Caffrey R, McCoy KL. **Defective antigen processing correlates with a low level of intracellular glutathione.** *Eur. J. Immunol. 26(12):3015–3020, 1996.*
26. Macho A, Hirsch T, Marzo I, Marchetti P, Dallaporta B, Susin SA, Zamzami N, Kroemer G. **Glutathione depletion is an early and calcium elevation is a late event of thymocyte apoptosis.** *J. Immunol. 158(10):4612–4619, 1997.*
27. Gmunder H, Eck HP, Benninghoff B, Roth S, Droge W. **Macrophages regulate intracellular glutathione levels of lymphocytes. Evidence for an immunoregulatory role of cysteine.** *Cell. Immunol. 129(1)32–46, 1990.*
28. Kranich O, Dringen R, Sandberg M, Hamprecht B. **Utilization of cysteine and cysteine precursors for the synthesis of glutathione in astroglial cultures: preference for cystine.** *Glia 22(1):11–18, 1998.*
29. Droge W, Holm E. **Role of cysteine and glutathione in HIV infection and other diseases associated with muscle wasting and immunological dysfunction.** *FASEB J. 11(13):1077–1089, 1997.*

Immunotec Research Ltd.
Manufactured by Immunotec Research Ltd. and Immunotec Medical Corp
Distributed by AmmunoMed, LLC and NuMedTec
Tel: (877-687-2277)
www.Immunocal.Com

Interferon Sciences, Inc.

783 JERSEY AVENUE
NEW BRUNSWICK, NJ 08901-3660

Direct Inquiries to:
J.R. Knill, M.D.
(732) 249-3250, ext. 565
FAX: (732) 249-0623
For Medical Information Contact:
In Emergencies:
J.R. Knill, M.D.
(732) 249-3250, ext. 565

Prescribing information for the product Alferon N Injection® is listed under Interferon Sciences, Inc.

ALFERON N INJECTION® ℞
Interferon alfa-n3
(human leukocyte derived)

DESCRIPTION

Alferon N Injection® [Interferon alfa-n3 (human leukocyte derived)] is a sterile aqueous formulation of purified, natural, human interferon alpha proteins for use by injection. Alferon N Injection® consists of interferon alpha proteins comprising approximately 166 amino acids ranging in molecular weights from 16,000 to 27,000 daltons. The specific activity of Interferon alfa-n3 is approximately equal to, or greater than, 2×10^8 IU/mg of protein.

Alferon N Injection® is manufactured from pooled units of human leukocytes which have been induced by incomplete infection with a murine virus (Sendai virus) to produce Interferon alfa-n3. The manufacturing process includes immunoaffinity chromatography with a murine monoclonal antibody, acidification (pH 2) for 5 days at 4°C, and gel filtration chromatography.

Since Alferon N Injection® is manufactured using source leukocytes, human donor screening is performed to minimize the risk that the leukocytes could contain infectious agents. In addition, the manufacturing process contains steps which have been shown to inactivate viruses. There has been no evidence of infection transmission to recipients in clinical trials. The laboratory and clinical data obtained support the conclusion that Alferon N Injection® is equivalent to other products derived from human blood or plasma which are free of risk of transmission of infectious agents, such as immunoglobulin and albumin (See WARNINGS).

The Alferon N Injection® manufacturing process was evaluated for quantitative removal or inactivation of model pathogenic viruses. The viruses were deliberately added to the leukocytes in amounts far exceeding those present in contaminated blood, i.e., $\geq 10^9$ infectious units per milliliter. The manufacturing process yielded a cumulative reduction of $\geq 10^{14}$ of infectious HIV-1, i.e., $\geq 10^{6.5}$ removal by acid inactivation and $\geq 10^{7.9}$ removal by the purification process. In the validation studies, there was 10^8 reduction in the titer of hepatitis B virus as determined by HBsAg assay, and a 10^9 reduction in the infectious titer of herpes simplex virus-1 (HSV-1). Cultivation of Alferon N Injection® [Interferon alfa-n3 (human leukocyte derived)] Purified Drug Concentrate with human indicator cells, i.e., MRC-5 cells, peripheral blood leukocytes in the presence of Cyclosporin A, and fetal cord blood cells, did not detect the presence of infectious viruses.

As part of a validation study, Alferon N Injection® was examined for the presence of the following viruses; Sendai virus (SV), HIV-1, HTLV-1, HBV, HSV-1, CMV, and EBV. Alferon N Injection® contained no detectable quantities of these viruses. In addition, other studies, i.e., Polymerase Chain Reaction (PCR) and Dot Blot Hybridization (DBH), have shown no detectable genetic material from these viruses in Alferon N Injection®. The sensitivity of the PCR was 10 copies for HIV-1 (env gene probe) and 10 copies for HBV (S/P gene probe). The sensitivity of the DBH was 1 pg for EBV, < 10 pg for CMV, < 10 pg for HSV-1, and < 2 pg for SV. Furthermore, sera from 105 patients treated with Alferon N Injection® (95 with condylomata acuminata and 10 with cancer) were tested for antibody to HIV-1 and HIV p24 antigen. There was no evidence to suggest transmission of HIV-1 by Alferon N Injection®. Sera from 135 patients with condylomata acuminata treated with Alferon N Injection® were tested to determine abnormal SGOT laboratory values. There was no evidence to suggest transmission of hepatitis by Alferon N Injection® based on both SGOT results and patient data collected during clinical trials.

Alferon N Injection® has been extensively purified using immunoaffinity chromatography with a murine monoclonal antibody, acidification (pH 2) for 5 days at 4°C, and gel filtration chromatography. Alferon N Injection® has been subjected to the acid treatment for five days during its manufacture in order to reduce the risk of viral transmission. Subsequent analyses of the Alferon N Injection® [Interferon alfa-n3 (human leukocyte derived)] Purified Drug Concentrate confirm the absence of detectable infectious or non-infectious viral particles.

The leukocyte nutrient medium contains the antibiotic neomycin sulfate at a concentration of 35 mg/L; however, neomycin sulfate is not detectable in the final product, i.e., < 0.64 μg/ml.

Murine immunoglobulin (IgG) is detected in the Alferon N Injection® Purified Drug Concentrate at levels below 0.15% of the Interferon alfa-n3 protein. This equates to levels less than 8 ng of murine IgG per million of IU Interferon alfa-n3 (range of 0.9 to 5.6 ng typically found).

Alferon N Injection® is available in an injectable solution containing 5 million IU Interferon alfa-n3 per vial for intralesional injection. The solution is clear and colorless. Each milliliter (ml) contains five million IU of Interferon alfa-n3 in phosphate-buffered saline (8.0 mg sodium chloride, 1.74 mg sodium phosphate dibasic, 0.20 mg potassium phosphate monobasic, and 0.20 mg potassium chloride) containing 3.3 mg phenol as a preservative and 1 mg Albumin (Human) as a stabilizer.

CLINICAL PHARMACOLOGY

General Interferons are naturally occurring proteins with antiviral, antiproliferative, and immunoregulatory properties. They are produced and secreted in response to viral infections and to a variety of other synthetic and biological inducers. Four major families of interferons have been identified: alpha, beta, gamma, and omega. The interferon alpha family contains 13 different non-allelic molecular species. Their molecular weights range from 16,000 to 27,000 daltons.

Interferons bind to specific membrane receptors on cell surfaces. Interferon alfa-n3 has been shown to bind to the same receptors as Interferon alfa-2b. The receptors have a high degree of selectivity for the binding of human but not mouse interferon. This correlates with the high species specificity found in laboratory studies.

Binding of interferon to membrane receptors initiates a series of events including induction of protein synthesis. These actions are followed by a variety of cellular responses, including inhibition of virus replication and suppression of cell proliferation. Immunomodulation, including enhancement of phagocytosis by macrophages, augmentation of the cytotoxicity of lymphocytes and enhancement of human leukocyte antigen expression occurs in response to exposure to interferons. One or more of these activities may contribute to the therapeutic effect of interferon.

Pharmacokinetics In a study of intralesional use of Alferon N Injection® [Interferon alfa-n3 (human leukocyte derived)] for the treatment of condylomata acuminata, plasma concentrations of interferon were below the detection limit of the assay, i.e., ≤ 3 IU/ml. Minor systemic effects (e.g., myalgias, fever, and headaches) were noted, indicating that some of the injected interferon entered the systemic circulation (See ADVERSE REACTIONS).

Condylomata Acuminata Condylomata acuminata (venereal or genital warts) are associated with infections of human papilloma virus (HPV), especially HPV type-6 and possibly type-11. Given the antiviral and antiproliferative activities of interferons and the viral etiology of condylomata, a placebo-controlled clinical trial was conducted to evaluate the safety and efficacy of intralesional injection of Alferon N Injection® in the treatment of condylomata acuminata.

In a multicenter, randomized, double-blind, placebo-controlled, clinical trial, intralesional administration of Alferon N Injection® was an effective treatment for condylomata acuminata.[1–4] One hundred fifty-six (156) patients were evaluable for efficacy (81 Alferon N Injection® patients and 75 placebo patients). Patients had a mean of five warts (range was 2-14) and all warts were treated. Patients were injected intralesionally with a mean of 225,000 IU of Alferon N Injection® per wart 2 times a week for up to 8 weeks.

Overall, 80% ($^{65}/_{81}$) of patients treated with Alferon N Injection® had a complete or partial resolution of warts compared with 44% ($^{33}/_{75}$) of placebo-treated patients ($p < 0.001$). Alferon N Injection® was significantly more effective than placebo in producing a complete resolution of warts ($p < 0.001$), as shown by Table 1.

[See table below]

Of the patients who had a complete resolution of warts, approximately half ($^{21}/_{44}$) the patients had complete resolution of warts by the end of treatment, and half ($^{23}/_{44}$) had complete resolution of warts during the three months after the

Table 1
Degree of Resolution as Measured By Total Wart Volume per Patient

	Percent of Patients with: Complete Resolution	Partial Resolution (≥50% resolution)	Minor Resolution (<50% resolution)	Progression/ No change
Alferon (n = 81)	54%	26%	15%	5%
Placebo (n = 75)	20%	24%	13%	43%

cessation of treatment. Patients with complete resolution of warts were followed for a median of 48 weeks. Overall, 76% ($^{31}/_{41}$) of Alferon N Injection® [Interferon alfa-n3 (human leukocyte derived)]-treated patients who achieved complete resolution of warts remained clear of all treated lesions during follow-up, while 79% ($^{11}/_{14}$) of the placebo-treated patients remained clear of all treated lesions during follow-up. A total of 762 evaluable warts were injected in this trial. Of the 407 Alferon N Injection®-treated warts, 73% ($^{297}/_{407}$) completely resolved, as compared to 35% ($^{125}/_{355}$) of the placebo-treated warts ($p < 0.0001$). Alferon N Injection® was effective in treating lesions of all sizes, and there was no difference in resolution for perianal, penile, or vulvar lesions.

There was no difference in resolution for patients who had received prior treatment of their warts and for those who had not. Among patients with recalcitrant warts (i.e., warts that were refractory to previous treatment or recurring), 82% ($^{58}/_{71}$) of the evaluable patients had complete or partial resolution of warts due to intralesional administration of Alferon N Injection® as compared to 43% ($^{29}/_{67}$) of placebo patients ($p < 0.001$). Fifty-four percent ($^{38}/_{71}$) of the evaluable Alferon N Injection® patients had complete resolution of warts as compared to 18% ($^{12}/_{67}$) of placebo patients ($p < 0.001$). Patients with primary occurrence of genital warts (i.e., no prior treatment of warts) had a similar resolution rate compared to the patients with recalcitrant warts: 70% ($^{7}/_{10}$) had complete or partial resolution of warts due to Alferon N Injection® [Interferon alfa-n3 (human leukocyte derived)] treatment and 60% ($^{6}/_{10}$) had complete resolution of warts, as compared to 50% ($^{4}/_{8}$) of placebo recipients who had complete or partial resolution of warts and 38% ($^{3}/_{8}$) who had complete resolution. Overall, 83% ($^{5}/_{6}$) of Alferon N Injection®-treated patients with primary occurrence, who achieved complete resolution of warts, remained clear of all treated lesions during a median follow-up of 52 weeks. Because the number of patients with primary occurrence of warts was small (10 Alferon N Injection® recipients and 8 placebo recipients), the difference between Alferon N Injection® and placebo treatment was not statistically significant. However, when the resolution of primary warts was examined, 75% ($^{33}/_{44}$) of the Alferon N Injection®-treated primary warts resolved completely as compared to 39% ($^{11}/_{28}$) of the placebo-treated primary warts ($p = 0.003$).

In an open clinical trial using a once-a-week treatment schedule for up to 16 weeks, 28 patients were evaluable for efficacy. Eighty-nine percent ($^{25}/_{28}$) of patients had a complete or partial resolution of warts following treatment with Alferon N Injection®. The condylomata acuminata resolved completely in 46% ($^{13}/_{28}$) of the patients. Of the 154 warts treated, 77% ($^{118}/_{154}$) resolved completely.

After injections of Alferon N Injection®, side effects were minor and transient. After 4 weeks of treatment, the frequency of adverse reactions was similar in Alferon N Injection® and placebo treatment groups. The most frequent side effects were myalgias, fever, and headache (See ADVERSE REACTIONS).

Antigenicity

1. Alferon N Injection®
   One hundred five (105) patients treated with Alferon N Injection® [Interferon alfa-n3 (human leukocyte derived)] during clinical trials were tested for the presence of anti-interferon antibodies using three different antibody assays: Immunoradiometric Assay (IRMA), Enzyme Linked Immunosorbent Assay (ELISA), and neutralization by the Cytopathic Effect Assay (CPE). To date, no antibodies to Interferon alfa-n3 have been detected in any of the patients.
2. Mouse Proteins
   No hypersensitivity reactions to the components in Alferon N Injection® have been observed. Alferon N Injection® uses a murine monoclonal antibody in one of the purification procedures. A possibility exists that patients treated with Alferon N Injection® may develop hypersensitivity to the mouse proteins. However, none of the patients receiving Alferon N Injection® during clinical trials developed antibodies or hypersensitivity to mouse proteins (See CONTRAINDICATIONS).
3. Egg Protein
   The initial stage in the manufacture of Alferon N Injection® uses Sendai virus which was grown in chicken-embryonated eggs as the specific Interferon alfa-n3 inducer. Although no egg protein (ovalbumin) has been detected in the initial stage of interferon manufacture using an ELISA (sensitivity of 16 ng/ml), a possibility exists that patients treated with Alferon N Injection® may develop hypersensitivity to egg protein (See CONTRAINDICATIONS).

INDICATIONS AND USAGE

Alferon N Injection® is indicated for the intralesional treatment of refractory or recurring external condylomata acuminata in patients 18 years of age or older (See DOSAGE AND ADMINISTRATION).

The physician should select patients for treatment with Alferon N Injection® after consideration of a number of factors: the locations and sizes of the lesions, past treatment and response thereto, and the patient's ability to comply with the treatment regimen. Alferon N Injection® is particularly useful for patients who have not responded satisfactorily to other treatment modalities, e.g., podophyllin resin, surgery, laser or cryotherapy.

There have been no studies with this product in adolescents. This product is not recommended for use in patients less than 18 years of age.

CONTRAINDICATIONS

Alferon N Injection® [Interferon alfa-n3 (human leukocyte derived)] is contraindicated in patients with known hypersensitivity to human interferon alpha proteins or any component of the product. The product is also contraindicated in patients who have anaphylactic sensitivity to mouse immunoglobulin (IgG), egg protein or neomycin.

WARNINGS

Because of the fever and other "flu-like" symptoms associated with Alferon N Injection® (See ADVERSE REACTIONS), it should be used cautiously in patients with debilitating medical conditions such as cardiovascular disease (e.g., unstable angina and uncontrolled congestive heart failure), severe pulmonary disease (e.g., chronic obstructive pulmonary disease), or diabetes mellitus with ketoacidosis. Alferon N Injection® should be used cautiously in patients with coagulation disorders (e.g., thrombophlebitis, pulmonary embolism and hemophilia), severe myelosuppression, or seizure disorders. Acute, serious hypersensitivity reactions (e.g., urticaria, angioedema, bronchoconstriction, and anaphylaxis) have not been observed in patients receiving Alferon N Injection®. However, if such reactions develop, drug administration should be discontinued immediately and appropriate medical therapy should be instituted. In addition, because this product is made from human blood, it may carry a risk of transmitting infectious agents, e.g., viruses, and theoretically, the Creutzfeldt Jakob disease (CJD) agent.

PRECAUTIONS

General Patients being treated with Alferon N Injection® should be informed of the benefits and risks associated with the treatment. Because the manufacturing process, strength, and type of interferon (e.g., natural, human leukocyte interferon versus single-species recombinant interferon) may vary for different interferon formulations, changing brands may require a change in dosage. Therefore, physicians are cautioned not to change from one interferon product to another without considering these factors.

Information for Patients Patients should be informed of the early signs of hypersensitivity reactions including hives, generalized urticaria, tightness of the chest, wheezing, hypotension, and anaphylaxis, and should be advised to contact their physician if these symptoms occur.

Patients being treated with Alferon N Injection® [Interferon alfa-n3 (human leukocyte derived)] should be informed of benefits and risks associated with treatment.

Patients should be cautioned not to change brands of interferon without medical consultation, as a change in dosage may occur.

Carcinogenesis, Mutagenesis, Impairment of Fertility Studies with Alferon N Injection® have not been performed to determine carcinogenicity, mutagenicity, or the effect on fertility. In studies with adult females, interferon alpha has been shown to affect the menstrual cycle and decrease serum estradiol and progesterone levels[5].

Alferon N Injection® should be used with caution in fertile men. Fertile women should be cautioned to use effective contraception while being treated with Alferon N Injection®.

Changes in the menstrual cycle and abortions have been reported to occur in non-human primates given extremely high doses of recombinant interferon alpha[6]. In these studies, Macaca mulatta (rhesus monkeys) were given interferon daily by intramuscular injection. When given at daily intramuscular doses 326 times the average intralesional dose of Alferon N Injection® (120 times the maximum recommended dose), this recombinant interferon formulation produced menstrual cycle changes in the monkeys.

In human clinical trials with Alferon N Injection®, menstrual cycle data were reported by 51 patients (36 Alferon N Injection® and 15 placebo). There was no significant difference between Alferon N Injection® and placebo treatment groups with regard to menstrual cycle changes.

PREGNANCY Pregnancy Category C Animal reproduction studies have not been conducted with Alferon N Injection®. It is also not known whether Alferon N Injection® [Interferon alfa-n3 (human leukocyte derived)] can cause fetal harm when administered to a pregnant woman or can affect reproductive capacity. Alferon N Injection® should be given to a pregnant woman only if clearly needed.

Changes in the menstrual cycle and abortions have been reported to occur in non-human primates given extremely high doses of recombinant interferon alpha. In these studies, Macaca mulatta (rhesus monkeys) were given interferon daily by intramuscular injection. Abortifacient effects were noted when the recombinant interferon alpha was given daily during early to mid-gestation at intramuscular doses of 978 times the average intralesional dose of Alferon N Injection® (360 times the maximum recommended dose).

Nursing Mothers It is not known whether Alferon N Injection® is excreted in human milk. Studies in mice have shown that mouse interferons are excreted in milk[7]. Because many drugs are excreted in human milk and because of the potential for serious adverse reactions in nursing infants, a decision should be made whether to discontinue nursing or to not initiate drug treatment, taking into account the importance of the drug to the mother and the potential risks to the infant.

Pediatric Use Safety and effectiveness have not been established in patients below the age of 18 years.

ADVERSE REACTIONS

Adverse reactions were evaluated in 202 patients with condylomata acuminata receiving Alferon N Injection® by intralesional administration and in 31 patients with cancer receiving Alferon N Injection® by systemic administration. In the double-blind efficacy trial for the treatment of condylomata acuminata, 104 patients were treated with doses of Alferon N Injection® of 0.05 million to 2.5 million IU per treatment session (average dose = 0.92 million IU per treatment session) by intralesional injection. In open trials, an additional 98 patients received a dose range of 0.05 to 4.6 million IU of Alferon N Injection® per treatment session (average dose = 1.12 million IU per treatment session). Patients with cancer were given doses of Alferon N Injection® [Interferon alfa-n3 (human leukocyte derived)] of 3 million, 9 million, or 15 million IU per day for ten days by intramuscular injection.

Adverse Reactions in Patients with Condylomata Acuminata

A total of 104 patients with condylomata acuminata was treated with Alferon N Injection® during the double-blind clinical trial. Adverse reactions were reported to be likely, unlikely, or not known to be related to Alferon N Injection®. Adverse reactions consisted primarily of "flu-like" symptoms (myalgias, fever, and/or headache) which were in most cases mild or moderate, and transient, and did not interfere with treatment.

The "flu-like" adverse reactions, consisting of fever, myalgias, and/or headache, occurred primarily after the first treatment session and were reported by 30% of the patients. The frequency of "flu-like" adverse reactions abated with repeated dosing of Alferon N Injection® so that the incidences due to Alferon N Injection® and placebo were similar after three to four weeks of treatment (after six to eight treatment sessions). "Flu-like" symptoms were relieved by administration of acetaminophen.

Adverse reactions were reported at least once during the course of treatment in the following percentages of patients in each treatment group:

Table 2
Percent of Patients with Adverse Reactions

Adverse Reactions:	Alferon (n = 104)	Placebo (n = 85)
Autonomic Nervous System		
Sweating	2%	1%
Vasovagal Reaction	2%	0%
Body as a Whole		
Fever	40%	19%
Chills	14%	2%
Fatigue	14%	6%
Malaise	9%	9%
Skin		
Generalized Pruritus	2%	0%
Central & Peripheral Nervous System		
Dizziness	9%	4%
Insomnia	2%	1%
Gastrointestinal System		
Nausea	4%	7%
Vomiting	3%	0%
Dyspepsia/Heartburn	3%	1%
Diarrhea	2%	2%
Musculoskeletal System		
Arthralgia	5%	1%
Back Pain	4%	1%
Myalgias	45%	15%
Headache	31%	15%
Psychiatric Disorders		
Depression	2%	1%
Nasopharyngeal		
Nose/sinus drainage	2%	2%

Most of the systemic adverse reactions were mild or moderate. Severe systemic adverse reactions were reported by 18% of Alferon N Injection® [Interferon alfa-n3 (human leukocyte derived)]-treated patients and 13% of placebo-treated patients (not a statistically significant difference). Most of the severe systemic adverse reactions reported were "flu-like". Other severe systemic adverse reactions included back pain, insomnia, and sensitivity to allergens. Those ad-

Continued on next page

Alferon N—Cont.

verse reactions which were reported by 1% of patients treated with Alferon N Injection® in the double-blind trial include: left groin lymph node swelling, tongue hyperaesthesia, thirst, tingling of legs/feet, hot sensation on bottom of feet, strange taste in mouth, increased salivation, heat intolerance, visual disturbances, pharyngitis, sensitivity to allergens, muscle cramps, nosebleed, throat tightness, and papular rash on neck. Additional adverse reactions which were reported by 1% of patients treated with placebo include: pharyngitis, oral pain, penile discharge, cold, knuckle stiffness, herpes outbreak, cough, disorientation, and weight/appetite loss.
Additional adverse reactions which occurred only in open clinical trials of intralesional use of Alferon N Injection® [Interferon alfa-n3 (human leukocyte derived)] for treatment of condylomata acuminata were herpes labialis, hot flashes, nervousness, decrease in concentration, dysuria, photosensitivity, and swollen lymph nodes. These reactions occurred in 1% of the patients. One patient with a history of epilepsy, who was not taking anticonvulsant medication, had a grand mal seizure while being treated with Alferon N Injection®; this seizure was judged to be unrelated to Alferon N Injection® administration.
Application Site Disorders The frequency of application site disorders (such as itching and pain) for patients treated with Alferon N Injection® was significantly less than that reported with placebo (12% versus 26%). No severe application site disorders were reported by patients treated with Alferon N Injection®, while 7% of placebo-treated patients reported severe disorders.
Laboratory Test Values Abnormalities were seen with statistically equivalent frequencies in both the Alferon N Injection® and placebo groups. None of the laboratory abnormalities were considered clinically significant. The abnormalities in the Alferon N Injection®-treated patients consisted primarily of decreased WBC (11%). Decreases also occurred in 4% of the placebo patients (not a statistically significant difference). The abnormalities in Alferon N Injection®-treated patients involved increases of only one WHO grade.
Adverse Reactions in Patients with Cancer Thirty-one (31) patients with cancer were treated with a maximum of ten intramuscular injections of Alferon N Injection® in doses of 3 million IU, 9 million IU, or 15 million IU per treatment session. The occurrence of adverse reactions was judged to be unrelated to the dose of Alferon N Injection®. The following adverse reactions were reported at least once (the percentage of patients experiencing the reaction is indicated in parentheses): chills (87%), fever (81%), anorexia (68%), malaise (65%), nausea (48%), vomiting (29%), myalgias (16%), arthralgia (10%), chest pains (10%), soreness at injection site (10%), sleepiness (10%), headache (10%), diarrhea (6%), fatigue (6%), low blood pressure (6%), sore mouth/stomatitis (6%), and blurred vision (6%). Those adverse reactions which were each reported by only one patient treated with Alferon N Injection® [Interferon alfa-n3 (human leukocyte derived)] include: stiff shoulders, flushed face, edema, dry mouth, mucositis, coughing, numbness, numbness in hands, numbness in fingers, pain on ocular rotation, shakes/shivers, ringing in ears, cramps, constipation, muscle soreness, confusion, light-headedness, depression, upset stomach, and sweating. The following adverse reactions were reported as severe by at least one patient (the percentage of patients experiencing the reaction is indicated in parentheses): fever (55%), malaise (54%), anorexia (45%), chills (45%), nausea (16%), myalgias (13%), vomiting (10%), fatigue (6%), low blood pressure (6%), chest pains (6%), sore mouth/stomatitis (6%), headache (3%), diarrhea (3%), sleepiness (3%), arthralgia (3%), blurred vision (3%), stiff shoulders (3%), numbness (3%), pain on ocular rotation (3%), muscle soreness (3%), confusion (3%), light-headedness (3%), depression (3%), and sweating (3%).
The number and percentage of patients with cancer who experienced a significant abnormal laboratory test value (values that changed from WHO Grades 0, 1, or 2 at baseline to WHO Grades 3 or 4 during or after treatment) at least once during the trials are shown in the following table:

Table 3
Abnormal Laboratory Test Values

	Cancer (n = 31)
Hemoglobin Level	2 (7%)
White Blood Cell Count	1 (3%)
Platelet Count	1 (3%)
GGT	1 (6%)
SGOT	1 (3%)
Alkaline Phosphatase	2 (8%)
Total Bilirubin	1 (4%)

DOSAGE AND ADMINISTRATION

The recommended dose of Alferon N Injection® for the treatment of condylomata acuminata is 0.05 ml (250,000 IU) per wart. Alferon N Injection® should be administered twice weekly for up to 8 weeks. The maximum recommended dose per treatment session is 0.5 ml (2.5 million IU). Alferon N Injection® [Interferon alfa-n3 (human leukocyte derived)] should be injected into the base of each wart, preferably using a 30 gauge needle. For large warts, Alferon N Injection® may be injected at several points around the periphery of the wart, using a total dose of 0.05 ml per wart. The minimum effective dose of Alferon N Injection® for the treatment of condylomata acuminata has not been established. Moderate to severe adverse experiences may require modification of the dosage regimen or, in some cases, termination of therapy with Alferon N Injection®.
Genital warts usually begin to disappear after several weeks of treatment with Alferon N Injection®. Treatment should continue for a maximum of 8 weeks. In clinical trials with Alferon N Injection®, many patients who had partial resolution of warts during treatment experienced further resolution of their warts after cessation of treatment. Of the patients who had complete resolution of warts due to treatment, half the patients had complete resolution of warts by the end of the treatment and half had complete resolution of warts during the 3 months after cessation of treatment. Thus, it is recommended that no further therapy (Alferon N Injection® or conventional therapy) be administered for 3 months after the initial 8-week course of treatment unless the warts enlarge or new warts appear. Studies to determine the safety and efficacy of a second course of treatment with Alferon N Injection® have not been conducted.
Parenteral drug products should be inspected visually for particulate matter and discoloration prior to administration, whenever solution and container permit.

HOW SUPPLIED

Injectable Solution: Each vial contains 1 ml of Alferon N Injection®. Each ml of Alferon N Injection® contains 5 million IU of Interferon alfa-n3, 3.3 mg of phenol, and 1 mg of Albumin (Human) in a pH 7.4 phosphate-buffered saline solution (8.0 mg/ml sodium chloride, 1.74 mg/ml sodium phosphate dibasic, 0.20 mg/ml potassium phosphate monobasic, and 0.20 mg/ml potassium chloride). One vial per box. (NDC 54746-001-01).

STORAGE

Alferon N Injection® [Interferon alfa-n3 (human leukocyte derived)] should be stored at 2° to 8°C (36° to 46°F). Do not freeze. Do not shake.
CAUTION: FEDERAL (U.S.A.) LAW PROHIBITS DISPENSING WITHOUT PRESCRIPTION.

REFERENCES

1. Friedman-Kien, AE; Eron, LJ; Conant, M; et al., *JAMA* 1988; *259:* 533–538.
2. Kirby, P; (editorial comment), *JAMA* 1988; *259:* 570–572.
3. Friedman-Kien, AE; Plasse, TF; et al., *Papilloma Viruses: Molecular and Clinical Aspects* [Howley, PM, Broker, TR (eds)], New York, Alan R. Liss, Inc.; 1986; 217–233.
4. Geffen, JR; Klein, RJ; Friedman-Kien, AE; *J. Infect. Dis.* 1984; *150:* 612–615.
5. Kauppila, A; et al., *Int. J. Cancer* 1982; *29:* 291–294.
6. Trown, PW; et al., *Cancer* 1986; *57 (Suppl):* 1648–1656.
7. Schafer, TW; et al., *Science* 1972; *176:* 1326–1327.

Manufactured and Distributed by:
Interferon Sciences, Inc.
783 Jersey Avenue
New Brunswick, NJ 08901-3660
U.S. Lic. No. 930

4/00
Shown in Product Identification Guide, page 318

InterMune Pharmaceuticals, Inc.

1710 GILBRETH ROAD
SUITE 301
BURLINGAME, CA 94010

For Direct Inquiries Contact:
InterMune Customer Service
(888) 696-8036
Fax: (615) 287-0420
Corporate Offices:
(650) 409-2020

ACTIMMUNE® ℞

[*act-ĭmmune*]
(Interferon gamma-1b)
Injection

DESCRIPTION

ACTIMMUNE® (Interferon gamma-1b), a biologic response modifier, is a single-chain polypeptide containing 140 amino acids. Production of ACTIMMUNE is achieved by fermentation of a genetically engineered Escherichia coli bacterium containing the DNA which encodes for the human protein. Purification of the product is achieved by conventional column chromatography. ACTIMMUNE is a highly purified sterile solution consisting of non-covalent dimers of two identical 16,465 dalton monomers; with a specific activity of 20 million International Units (IU)/mg (2×10^6 IU per 0.5 mL) which is equivalent to 30 million units/mg.
ACTIMMUNE is a sterile, clear, colorless solution filled in a single-dose vial for subcutaneous injection. Each 0.5 mL of ACTIMMUNE contains: 100 mcg (2 million IU) of Interferon gamma-1b formulated in 20 mg mannitol, 0.36 mg sodium succinate, 0.05 mg polysorbate 20 and Sterile Water for Injection. *Note that the above activity is expressed in International Units (1 million IU/50mcg). This is equivalent to what was previously expressed as units (1.5 million U/50mcg).*

CLINICAL PHARMACOLOGY

General

Interferons are a family of functionally related, species-specific, proteins synthesized by eukaryotic cells in response to viruses and a variety of natural and synthetic stimuli. The most striking differences between interferon-gamma and other classes of interferon concern the immunomodulatory properties of this molecule. While gamma, alpha and beta interferons share certain properties, interferon-gamma has potent phagocyte-activating effects not seen with other interferon preparations. These effects include the generation of toxic oxygen metabolites within phagocytes in vitro, which are capable of mediating the intracellular killing of selected microorganisms such as Staphylococcus aureus, Toxoplasma gondii, Leishmania donovani, Listeria monocytogenes, and Mycobacterium avium intracellulare.
Clinical studies in patients using interferon-gamma, have revealed a broad range of biological activities including the enhancement of the oxidative metabolism of tissue macrophages, enhancement of antibody-dependent cellular cytotoxicity (ADCC) and natural killer (NK) cell activity. Additionally, effects on Fc receptor expression on monocytes and major histocompatibility antigen expression have been noted.[1,2]
To the extent that interferon-gamma is produced by antigen-stimulated T lymphocytes and regulates the activity of immune cells, it is appropriate to characterize interferon-gamma as a lymphokine of the interleukin type. There is growing evidence that interferon-gamma interacts functionally with other interleukin molecules such as interleukin-2 and that all of the interleukins form part of a complex, lymphokine regulatory network.[3] For example, interferon-gamma and interleukin-4 appear to reciprocally interact to regulate murine IgE levels; interferon-gamma can suppress IgE levels in humans.[4,5] Interferon-gamma also inhibits the production of collagen at the transcription level in human systems.[6]
With respect to Chronic Granulomatous Disease (an inherited disorder characterized by deficient phagocyte oxidative metabolism), pilot clinical trials of the systemic administration of ACTIMMUNE® in patients with Chronic Granulomatous Disease provided evidence for a treatment-related enhancement of phagocyte function including elevation of superoxide levels and improved killing of Staphylococcus aureus.[7,8]
In severe, malignant osteopetrosis (another inherited disorder characterized by an osteoclast defect leading to bone overgrowth and deficient phagocyte oxidative metabolism),[9] a treatment-related enhancement of superoxide production by phagocytes was observed in situ.[10] ACTIMMUNE was found to enhance osteoclast function in vitro.[11,12]

Pharmacokinetics

The intravenous, intramuscular, and subcutaneous pharmacokinetics of ACTIMMUNE® have been investigated in 24 healthy male subjects following single-dose administration of 100 mcg/m^2. ACTIMMUNE is rapidly cleared after intravenous administration (1.4 liters/minute) and slowly absorbed after intramuscular or subcutaneous injection. After intramuscular or subcutaneous injection, the apparent fraction of dose absorbed was greater than 89%. The mean elimination half-life after intravenous administration of 100 mcg/m^2 in healthy male subjects was 38 minutes. The mean elimination half-lives for intramuscular and subcutaneous dosing with 100 mcg/m^2 were 2.9 and 5.9 hours, respectively. Peak plasma concentrations, determined by ELISA, occurred approximately 4 hours (1.5 ng/mL) after intramuscular dosing and 7 hours (0.6 ng/mL) after subcutaneous dosing. Multiple dose subcutaneous pharmacokinetic studies were conducted in 38 healthy male subjects. There was no accumulation of ACTIMMUNE after 12 consecutive daily injections of 100 mcg/m^2. Pharmacokinetic studies in patients with Chronic Granulomatous Disease have not been performed.
Trace amounts of interferon-gamma were detected in the urine of squirrel monkeys following intravenous administration of 500 mcg/kg. Interferon-gamma was not detected in the urine of healthy human volunteers following administration of 100 mcg/m^2 of ACTIMMUNE by the intravenous, intramuscular and subcutaneous routes. In vitro perfusion studies utilizing rabbit livers and kidneys demonstrate that these organs are capable of clearing interferon-gamma from perfusate. Studies of the administration of interferon-gamma to nephrectomized mice and squirrel monkeys demonstrate a reduction in clearance of interferon-gamma from blood; however, prior nephrectomy did not prevent elimination.

Effects in Chronic Granulomatous Disease

A randomized, double-blind, placebo-controlled study of ACTIMMUNE® (Interferon gamma-1b) in patients with Chronic Granulomatous Disease (CGD), was performed to determine whether ACTIMMUNE administered subcutaneously on a three times weekly schedule could decrease the incidence of serious infectious episodes and improve existing infectious and inflammatory conditions in patients with

Chronic Granulomatous Disease. One hundred twenty-eight eligible patients were enrolled on this study including patients with different patterns of inheritance. Most patients received prophylactic antibiotics. Patients ranged in age from 1 to 44 years with the mean age being 14.6 years. The study was terminated early following demonstration of a highly statistically significant benefit of ACTIMMUNE therapy compared to placebo with respect to time to serious infection (p=0.0036), the primary endpoint of the investigation. Serious infection was defined as a clinical event requiring hospitalization and the use of parenteral antibiotics. The final analysis provided further support for the primary endpoint. (p=0.0006). There was a 67 percent reduction in relative risk of serious infection in patients receiving ACTIMMUNE (n=63) compared to placebo (n=65). Additional supportive evidence of treatment benefit included a twofold reduction in the number of primary serious infections in the ACTIMMUNE group (30 on placebo versus 14 on ACTIMMUNE, p=0.002) and the total number and rate of serious infections including recurrent events (56 on placebo versus 20 on ACTIMMUNE, p=<0.0001). Moreover, the length of hospitalization for the treatment of all clinical events provided evidence highly supportive of an ACTIMMUNE treatment benefit. Placebo patients required three times as many inpatient hospitalization days for treatment of clinical events compared to patients receiving ACTIMMUNE (1493 versus 497 total days, p=0.02). An ACTIMMUNE treatment benefit with respect to time to serious infection was consistently demonstrated in all subgroup analyses according to stratification factors, including pattern of inheritance, use of prophylactic antibiotics, as well as age. There was a 67 percent reduction in relative risk of serious infection in patients receiving ACTIMMUNE compared to placebo across all groups. The beneficial effect of ACTIMMUNE therapy was observed throughout the entire study, in which the mean duration of ACTIMMUNE administration was 8.9 months/patient.

Effects in Osteopetrosis

A controlled, randomized study in patients with severe, malignant osteopetrosis was conducted with ACTIMMUNE® administered subcutaneously three times weekly. Sixteen patients were randomized to receive either ACTIMMUNE plus calcitriol (n=11), or calcitriol alone (n=5). Patients ranged in age from 1 month to 8 years, mean 1.5 years. Treatment failure was considered to be disease progression as defined by 1) death, 2) significant reduction in hemoglobin or platelet counts, 3) a serious bacterial infection requiring antibiotics, or 4) a 50 dB decrease in hearing or progressive optic atrophy. The median time to disease progression was significantly delayed in the ACTIMMUNE plus calcitriol arm versus calcitriol alone. In the treatment arm, the median was not reached. Based on the observed data, however, the median time to progression in this arm was at least 165 days versus a median of 65 days in the calcitriol alone arm. In an analysis which combined data from a second study, 19 of 24 patients treated with ACTIMMUNE plus or minus calcitriol for at least 6 months had reduced trabecular bone volume compared to baseline.

INDICATIONS AND USAGE

ACTIMMUNE is indicated for reducing the frequency and severity of serious infections associated with Chronic Granulomatous Disease.

ACTIMMUNE is indicated for delaying time to disease progression in patients with severe, malignant osteopetrosis.

CONTRAINDICATIONS

ACTIMMUNE is contraindicated in patients who develop or have known hypersensitivity to interferon-gamma, E. coli derived products, or any component of the product.

WARNINGS

ACTIMMUNE should be used with caution in patients with pre-existing cardiac disease, including symptoms of ischemia, congestive heart failure or arrhythmia. No direct cardiotoxic effect has been demonstrated but it is possible that acute and transient "flu-like" or constitutional symptoms such as fever and chills frequently associated with ACTIMMUNE administration at doses of 250 mcg/m^2/day or higher may exacerbate pre-existing cardiac conditions.

Caution should be exercised when treating patients with known seizure disorders and or compromised central nervous system function. Central nervous system adverse reactions including decreased mental status, gait disturbance and dizziness have been observed, particularly in patients receiving doses greater than 250 mcg/m^2/day. Most of these abnormalities were mild and reversible within a few days upon dose reduction or discontinuation of therapy.

Caution should be exercised when administering ACTIMMUNE to patients with myelosuppression. Reversible neutropenia and elevation of hepatic enzymes can be dose limiting above 250 mcg/m^2/day. Thrombocytopenia and proteinuria have also been seen rarely.

PRECAUTIONS

General

Acute serious hypersensitivity reactions have not been observed in patients receiving ACTIMMUNE, however, if such an acute reaction develops the drug should be discontinued immediately and appropriate medical therapy instituted. Transient cutaneous rashes have occurred in some patients following injection but have rarely necessitated treatment interruption.

Information for Patients

Patients being treated with ACTIMMUNE and/or their parents should be informed regarding the potential benefits and risks associated with treatment. If home use is determined to be desirable by the physician, instructions on appropriate use should be given, including review of the contents of the Patient Information Insert. This information is intended to aid in the safe and effective use of the medication. It is not a disclosure of all possible adverse or intended effects.

If home use is prescribed, a puncture resistant container for the disposal of used syringes and needles should be supplied to the patient. Patients should be thoroughly instructed in the importance of proper disposal and cautioned against any reuse of needles and syringes. The full container should be disposed of according to the directions provided by the physician (see Patient Information Insert).

The most common adverse experiences occurring with ACTIMMUNE therapy are "flu-like" or constitutional symptoms such as fever, headache, chills, myalgia or fatigue (see ADVERSE REACTIONS Section) which may decrease in severity as treatment continues. Some of the "flu-like" symptoms may be minimized by bedtime administration. Acetaminophen may be used to prevent or partially alleviate the fever and headache.

The long-term effects of ACTIMMUNE therapy on growth, development or other parameters are not known.

Laboratory Tests

In addition to those tests normally required for monitoring patients with Chronic Granulomatous Disease and osteopetrosis, the following laboratory tests are recommended for all patients on ACTIMMUNE (Interferon gamma-1b) therapy prior to the beginning of and at three month intervals during treatment.

- Hematologic tests—including complete blood counts, differential and platelet counts
- Blood chemistries—including renal and liver function tests
- Urinalysis

Drug Interactions

Interactions between ACTIMMUNE and other drugs have not been fully evaluated. Caution should be exercised when administering ACTIMMUNE in combination with other potentially myelosuppressive agents (see WARNINGS).

Preclinical studies in rodents using species-specific interferon-gamma have demonstrated a decrease in hepatic microsomal cytochrome P-450 concentrations. This could potentially lead to a depression of the hepatic metabolism of certain drugs that utilize this degradative pathway.

Carcinogenesis, Mutagenesis and Impairment of Fertility

Carcinogenesis: ACTIMMUNE has not been tested for its carcinogenic potential.

Mutagenesis: Ames tests using five different tester strains of bacteria with and without metabolic activation revealed no evidence of mutagenic potential. ACTIMMUNE was tested in a micronucleus assay for its ability to induce chromosomal damage in bone marrow cells of mice following two intravenous doses of 20 mg/kg. No evidence of chromosomal damage was noted.

Impairment of Fertility: Female cynomolgus monkeys treated with daily subcutaneous doses of 30 or 150 mcg/kg ACTIMMUNE (approximately 20 and 100 times the human dose) exhibited irregular menstrual cycles or absence of cyclicity during treatment. Similar findings were not observed in animals treated with 3 mcg/kg ACTIMMUNE. No studies have been performed assessing any potential effects of ACTIMMUNE on male fertility.

Pregnancy

Teratogenic Effects: Pregnancy Category C. ACTIMMUNE has shown an increased incidence of abortions in primates when given in doses approximately 100 × the human dose. A study in pregnant primates treated with intravenous doses, 2–100 × the human dose failed to demonstrate teratogenic activity for ACTIMMUNE. There are no adequate and well-controlled studies in pregnant women. ACTIMMUNE should be used during pregnancy only if the potential benefit justifies the potential risk to the fetus. In addition, studies evaluating recombinant murine interferon-gamma in pregnant mice, revealed increased incidences of uterine bleeding and abortifacient activity and decreased neonatal viability at maternally toxic doses. The clinical significance of this latter observation with recombinant murine interferon-gamma tested in a homologous system is uncertain.

Nursing Mothers

It is not known whether ACTIMMUNE is excreted in human milk. Because many drugs are excreted in human milk and because of the potential for serious adverse reactions in nursing infants from ACTIMMUNE, a decision should be made whether to discontinue nursing or to discontinue the drug, dependent upon the importance of the drug to the mother.

Pediatric Use

Safety and effectiveness in children under the age of 1 year has not been established in patients with CGD.

ADVERSE REACTIONS

The following data on adverse reactions are based on the subcutaneous administration of ACTIMMUNE at a dose of 50 mcg/m^2, three times weekly, in patients with Chronic Granulomatous Disease (CGD) during an investigational trial in the United States and Europe. The most common adverse events observed in patients with CGD are shown in the following table:

Clinical Toxicity	Percent of Patients ACTIMMUNE® CGD(n=63)	Placebo CGD(n=65)
Fever	52	28
Headache	33	9
Rash	17	6
Chills	14	0
Injection site erythema or tenderness	14	2
Fatigue	14	11
Diarrhea	14	12
Vomiting	13	5
Nausea	10	2
Myalgia	6	0
Arthralgia	2	0
Injection site pain	0	2

Miscellaneous adverse events which occurred infrequently in patients with CGD and may have been related to underlying disease included back pain (2 percent versus 0 percent), abdominal pain (8 percent versus 3 percent) and depression (3 percent versus 0 percent) for ACTIMMUNE and placebo treated patients, respectively.

Similar safety data were observed in 34 patients with severe malignant osteopetrosis.

ACTIMMUNE has also been evaluated in additional disease states in studies in which patients have generally received higher doses (>100 mcg/m^2/day) administered by intramuscular injection or intravenous infusion. All of the previously described adverse reactions which occurred in patients with Chronic Granulomatous Disease have also been observed in patients receiving higher doses. Adverse reactions not observed in patients with Chronic Granulomatous Disease receiving doses less than 100 mcg/m^2/day but seen rarely in patients receiving ACTIMMUNE (Interferon gamma-1b) in other studies include: Cardiovascular—hypotension, syncope, tachyarrhythmia, heart block, heart failure, and myocardial infarction. Central Nervous System—confusion, disorientation, gait disturbance, Parkinsonian symptoms, seizure, hallucinations, and transient ischemic attacks. Gastrointestinal—hepatic insufficiency, gastrointestinal bleeding, and pancreatitis. Renal—reversible renal insufficiency. Hematologic—deep venous thrombosis and pulmonary embolism. Pulmonary—tachypnea, bronchospasm, and interstitial pneumonitis. Metabolic—hyponatremia and hyperglycemia. Other—exacerbation of dermatomyositis.

Abnormal Laboratory Test Values: The incidence of abnormal hematologic, coagulation, hepatic and renal laboratory tests were similar between ACTIMMUNE and placebo treatment groups in the Chronic Granulomatous Disease trial.

No neutralizing antibodies to ACTIMMUNE have been detected in any Chronic Granulomatous Disease patients receiving ACTIMMUNE.

DOSAGE AND ADMINISTRATION

The recommended dosage of ACTIMMUNE for the treatment of patients with Chronic Granulomatous Disease and severe, malignant osteopetrosis is 50 mcg/m^2 (1 million IU/m^2) for patients whose body surface area is greater than 0.5 m^2 and 1.5 mcg/kg/dose for patients whose body surface area is equal to or less than 0.5 m^2. *Note that the above activity is expressed in International Units (1 million IU/50mcg). This is equivalent to what was previously expressed as units (1.5 million U/50mcg).* Injections should be administered subcutaneously three times weekly (for example, Monday, Wednesday, Friday). The optimum sites of injection are the right and left deltoid and anterior thigh. ACTIMMUNE can be administered by a physician, nurse, family member or patient when trained in the administration of subcutaneous injections. Parenteral drug products should be inspected visually for particulate matter and discoloration prior to administration, whenever solution and container permit.

The formulation does not contain a preservative. A vial of ACTIMMUNE is suitable for a single dose only. The unused portion of any vial should be discarded.

Higher doses are not recommended. Safety and efficacy has not been established for ACTIMMUNE given in doses greater or less than the recommended dose of 50 mcg/m^2. The minimum effective dose of ACTIMMUNE has not been established.

If severe reactions occur, the dosage should be modified (50 percent reduction) or therapy should be discontinued until the adverse reaction abates.

ACTIMMUNE may be administered using either sterilized glass or plastic disposable syringes.

HOW SUPPLIED

ACTIMMUNE (Interferon gamma-1b) is a sterile, clear, colorless solution filled in a single-dose vial for subcutaneous injection. Each 0.5 mL of ACTIMMUNE contains: **100 mcg (2 million IU)** of Interferon gamma-1b, formulated in 20 mg mannitol, 0.36 mg sodium succinate, 0.05 mg polysorbate 20 and Sterile Water for Injection.

Single vial (NDC 64116-011-01)

Cartons of 12 (NDC 64116-011-12)

Stability and Storage

Vials of ACTIMMUNE must be placed in a 2–8°C (36–46°F) refrigerator immediately upon receipt to insure optimal retention of physical and biochemical integrity. DO NOT

Continued on next page

Actimmune—Cont.

FREEZE. Avoid excessive or vigorous agitation. DO NOT SHAKE. An unentered vial of ACTIMMUNE should not be left at room temperature for a total time exceeding 12 hours prior to use. Vials exceeding this time period should not be returned to the refrigerator; such vials should be discarded. Do not use beyond the expiration date stamped on the vial.

REFERENCES

1. Maluish AE, Urba WJ, Longo DL, et al: The determination of an immunologically active dose of interferon gamma in patients with melanoma. J Clin Onc 6: 434–445, 1988.
2. Nathan CF, Kaplan G, Levis W, et al: Local and systemic effects of intradermal recombinant interferon gamma in patients with lepromatous leprosy. NEJM 315: 6–11, 1986.
3. Fauci AS, Rosenberg SA, Sherwin SA, et al: Immunomodulators in clinical medicine. Ann Internal Med 106: 421–433, 1987.
4. Snapper CM, Paul WE: Interferon-gamma and B cell stimulatory factor-1 reciprocally regulate Ig isotype production. Science 236: 944–947, 1987.
5. King CL, Gallin JI, Malech HL, et al: Regulation of immunoglobulin production in hyperimmunoglobulin E recurrent-infection syndrome by interferon gamma. PNAS USA 86: 10085–10089, 1989.
6. Rosenbloom J, Feldman G, Freundlich B, Jimenez SA: Inhibition of excessive scleroderma fibroblast collagen production by recombinant gamma-interferon. Arth Rheum 29: 851–856, 1986.
7. Ezekowitz RAB, Dinauer MC, Jaffe HS, et al: Partial correction of the phagocyte defect in patients with X-linked chronic granulomatous disease by subcutaneous interferon gamma. NEJM 319: 146–151, 1988.
8. Sechler JMG, Malech HL, White CJ, Gallin JI: Recombinant human interferon-gamma reconstitutes defective phagocyte function in patients with chronic granulomatous disease of childhood. PNAS USA 85:4874–4878, 1988.
9. Shapiro F: Osteopetrosis, current clinical considerations. Clin Orth & Rel Res 296: 34–44, 1993.
10. Beard CJ, Key L, Newburger PE, Ezekowitz RAB, et al: Neutrophil defect associated with malignant infantile osteopetrosis. J Lab Clin Med 108: 498–505, 1986.
11. Shankar L, Gerritsen EJA, and Key LL: Osteopetrosis: pathogenesis and rationale for the use of interferon-γ-1b. Biodrugs 1: 23–29, 1997.
12. Key LL, Rodriguiz RM, Willi SM: Long-term treatment of osteopetrosis with recombinant human interferon gamma. NEJM 24: 1594–1599, 1995.

Manufactured by:
InterMune Pharmaceuticals, Inc.
Burlingame, CA 94010
U.S. License No. 1267
Revised March, 2000

4817801

 LB-0163

Shown in Product Identification Guide, page 318

Jacobus Pharmaceutical Co., Inc.

37 CLEVELAND LANE
P.O. BOX 5290
PRINCETON, NJ 08540

Direct Inquiries to:
Professional Services
(609) 921-7447
FAX: (609) 799-1176

For Medical Information Contact:
In Emergencies:
Medical Department
(609) 921-7447
FAX: (609) 799-1176

DAPSONE TABLETS USP ℞

[*dap 'sōne*]
25 mg. & 100 mg.

PRODUCT OVERVIEW

KEY FACTS

Dapsone is a sulfone for the primary treatment of Dermatitis herpetiformis and an antibacterial drug for susceptible cases of leprosy.

MAJOR USES

Dapsone is used to control the dermatologic symptoms of Dermatitis herpetiformis. Dapsone is used alone or in combination with other anti-leprosy drugs for leprosy.

SAFETY INFORMATION

Dapsone is contraindicated in patients with Dapsone hypersensitivity. Complete blood counts and laboratory monitoring should be done frequently. See labeling.

PRODUCT INFORMATION

DAPSONE TABLETS USP ℞

[*dap 'sōne*]
25 mg. & 100 mg.

DESCRIPTION

Dapsone-USP, 4,4′-diaminodiphenylsulfone (DDS) is a primary treatment for Dermatitis herpetiformis. It is an antibacterial drug for susceptible cases of leprosy. It is a white, odorless crystalline powder, practically insoluble in water and insoluble in fixed and vegetable oils.
Dapsone is issued on prescription in tablets of 25 and 100 mg. for oral use.

NH_2 — SO_2 — NH_2

Inactive Ingredients: Colloidal silicone dioxide, magnesium stearate, microcrystalline cellulose, and corn starch.

CLINICAL PHARMACOLOGY

Actions: The mechanism of action in Dermatitis herpetiformis has not been established. By the kinetic method in mice, Dapsone is bactericidal as well as bacteriostatic against *Mycobacterium leprae.*
Absorption and Excretion: Dapsone, when given orally, is rapidly and almost completely absorbed. About 85 percent of the daily intake is recoverable from the urine mainly in the form of water-soluble metabolites. Excretion of the drug is slow and a constant blood level can be maintained with the usual dosage.
Blood Levels: Detected a few minutes after ingestion, the drug reaches peak concentration in 4–8 hours. Daily administration for at least eight days is necessary to achieve a plateau level. With doses of 200 mg. daily, this level averaged 2.3 μg/ml with a range of 0.1–7.0 μg/ml. The half-life in the plasma in different individuals varies from ten hours to fifty hours and averages twenty-eight hours. Repeat tests in the same individual are constant. Daily administration (50–100 mg.) in leprosy patients will provide blood levels in excess of the usual minimum inhibitory concentration even for patients with a short Dapsone half-life.

INDICATIONS AND USAGE

Dermatitis herpetiformis: (D.H.)
Leprosy: All forms of leprosy except for cases of proven Dapsone resistance.

CONTRAINDICATION

Hypersensitivity to Dapsone and/or its derivatives.

WARNINGS

The patient should be warned to respond to the presence of clinical signs such as sore throat, fever, pallor, purpura or jaundice. Deaths associated with the administration of Dapsone have been reported from agranulocytosis, aplastic anemia and other blood dyscrasias. Complete blood counts should be done frequently in patients receiving Dapsone. The FDA Dermatology Advisory Committee recommended that, when feasible counts should be done weekly for the first month, monthly for six months and semi-annually thereafter. If a significant reduction in leucocytes, platelets or hemopoiesis is noted, Dapsone should be discontinued and the patient followed intensively. Folic acid antagonists have similar effects and may increase the incidence of hematologic reactions; if co-administered with Dapsone the patient should be monitored more frequently. Patients on weekly Pyrimethamine and Dapsone have developed agranulocytosis during the second and third month of therapy.
Severe anemia should be treated prior to initiation of therapy and hemoglobin monitored. Hemolysis and methemoglobin may be poorly tolerated by patients with severe cardio-pulmonary disease.
Cutaneous reactions, especially bullous, include exfoliative dermatitis and are probably one of the most serious, though rare, complications of sulfone therapy. They are directly due to drug sensitization. Such reactions include toxic erythema, erythema multiforme, toxic epidermal necrolysis, morbilliform and scarlatiniform reactions, urticaria and erythema nodosum. If new or toxic dermatologic reactions occur, sulfone therapy must be promptly discontinued and appropriate therapy instituted.
Leprosy reactional states, including cutaneous, are not hypersensitivity reactions to Dapsone and do not require discontinuation. See special section.

PRECAUTIONS

General: Hemolysis and Heinz body formation may be exaggerated in individuals with a glucose-6-phosphate dehydrogenase (G6PD) deficiency, or methemoglobin reductase deficiency, or hemoglobin M. This reaction is frequently dose-related. Dapsone should be given with caution to these patients or if the patient is exposed to other agents or conditions such as infection or diabetic ketosis capable of producing hemolysis. Drugs or chemicals which have produced significant hemolysis in G6PD or methemoglobin reductase deficient patients include Dapsone, sulfanilamide, nitrite, aniline, phenylhydrazine, napthalene, niridazole, nitrofurantoin and 8-amino-antimalarials such as primaquine.
Toxic hepatitis and cholestatic jaundice have been reported early in therapy. Hyperbilirubinemia may occur more often in G6PD deficient patients. When feasible, baseline and subsequent monitoring of liver function is recommended. If abnormal, Dapsone should be discontinued until the source of the abnormality is established.
Drug Interactions: Rifampin lowers Dapsone levels 7 to 10-fold by accelerating plasma clearance; in leprosy this reduction has not required a change in dosage.
Folic acid antagonists such as pyrimethamine may increase the likelihood of hematologic reactions.
A modest interaction has been reported for patients receiving 100 mg Dapsone od in combination with trimethoprim 5 mg/kg q6h. On Day 7, the serum Dapsone levels averaged 2.1 ± 1.0 μg/mL in comparison to 1.5 ± 0.5 μg/mL for Dapsone alone. On Day 7, trimethoprim levels averaged 18.4 ± 5.2 μg/mL in comparison to 12.4 ± 4.5 μg/mL for patients not receiving Dapsone. Thus, there is a mutual interaction between Dapsone and trimethoprim in which each raises the level of the other about 1.5 times.
Carcinogenesis, mutagenesis: Dapsone has been found carcinogenic (sarcomagenic) for male rats and female mice causing mesenchymal tumors in the spleen and peritoneum, and thyroid carcinoma in female rats. Dapsone is not mutagenic with or without microsomal activation in *S. typhimurium* tester strains 1535, 1537, 1538, 98, or 100.
Pregnancy Category C: Animal reproduction studies have not been conducted with Dapsone. Extensive, but uncontrolled experience and two published surveys on the use of Dapsone in pregnant women have not shown that Dapsone increases the risk of fetal abnormalities if administered during all trimesters of pregnancy or can affect reproduction capacity. Because of the lack of animal studies or controlled human experience, Dapsone should be given to a pregnant woman only if clearly needed. In general, for leprosy, USPHS at Carville recommends maintenance of Dapsone. Dapsone has been important for the management of some pregnant D.H. patients.
Nursing Mothers: Dapsone is excreted in breast milk in substantial amounts. Hemolytic reactions can occur in neonates. See section on hemolysis. Because of the potential for tumorgenicity shown for Dapsone in animal studies a decision should be made whether to discontinue nursing or discontinue the drug taking into account the importance of the drug to the mother.
Pediatric Use: Children are treated on the same schedule as adults but with correspondingly smaller doses. Dapsone is generally not considered to have an effect on the later growth, development and functional development of the child.

ADVERSE REACTIONS

In addition to the warnings listed above, the following syndromes and serious reactions have been reported in patients on Dapsone.
Hematologic Effects: Dose-related hemolysis is the most common adverse effect and is seen in patients with or without G6PD deficiency. Almost all patients demonstrate the interrelated changes of a loss of 1–2g of HB, an increase in the reticulocytes (2–12%), a shortened red cell life span and a rise in methemoglobin. G6PD deficient patients have greater responses.
Nervous System Effects: Peripheral neuropathy is a definite but unusual complication of Dapsone therapy in non-leprosy patients. Motor loss is predominent. If muscle weakness appears, Dapsone should be withdrawn. Recovery on withdrawal is usually substantially complete. The mechanism of recovery is reportedly by axonal regeneration. Some recovered patients have tolerated retreatment at reduced dosage. In leprosy this complication may be difficult to distinguish from a leprosy reactional state.
Body As A Whole: In addition to the warnings and adverse effects reported above, additional adverse reactions include: nausea, vomiting, abdominal pains, pancreatitis, vertigo, blurred vision, tinnitus, insomnia, fever, headache, psychosis, phototoxicity, pulmonary eosinophilia, tachycardia, albuminuria, the nephrotic syndrome, hypoalbuminemia without proteinuria, renal papillary necrosis, male infertility, drug-induced Lupus erythematosus and an infectious mononucleosis-like syndrome. In general, with the exception of the complications of severe anoxia from overdosage (retinal and optic nerve damage, etc.) these adverse reactions have regressed off drug.

OVERDOSAGE

Nausea, vomiting, hyperexcitability can appear a few minutes up to 24 hours after ingestion of an overdose. Methemoglobin induced depression, convulsions and severe cyanosis requires prompt treatment. In normal and methemoglobin reductase deficient patients, methylene blue, 1–2 mg/kg of body weight, given slowly intravenously is the treatment of choice. The effect is complete in 30 minutes, but may have to be repeated if methemoglobin reaccumulates. For non-emergencies, if treatment is needed, methylene blue may be given orally in doses of 3–5 mg/kg every 4–6 hours.
Methylene blue reduction depends on G6PD and should not be given to fully expressed G6PD deficient patients.

DOSAGE AND ADMINISTRATION

Dermatitis herpetiformis: The dosage should be individually titrated starting in adults with 50 mg. daily and correspondingly smaller doses in children. If full control is not achieved within the range of 50–300 mg. daily, higher doses may be tried. Dosage should be reduced to a minimum maintenance level as soon as possible. In responsive patients there is a prompt reduction in pruritus followed by clearance of skin lesions. There is no effect on the gastrointestinal component of the disease.
Dapsone levels are influenced by acetylation rates. Patients with high acetylation rates, or who are receiving treatment affecting acetylation may require an adjustment in dosage.

A strict gluten free diet is an option for the patient to elect, permitting many to reduce or eliminate the need for Dapsone; the average time for dosage reduction is 8 months with a range of 4 months to $2^1/_2$ years and for dosage elimination 29 months with a range of 6 months to 9 years.

Leprosy: In order to reduce secondary Dapsone resistance, the WHO Expert Committee on Leprosy and the USPHS at Carville, LA, recommend that Dapsone should be commenced in combination with one or more anti-leprosy drugs. In the multi-drug program Dapsone should be maintained at the full dosage of 100 mg. daily without interruption (with correspondingly smaller doses for children) and provided to all patients who have sensitive organisms with new or recrudescent disease or who have not yet completed a two year course of Dapsone monotherapy. For advice and other drugs, the USPHS at Carville, LA, (1 800-642-2477) should be contacted. Before using other drugs consult appropriate product labeling.

In bacteriologically negative tuberculoid and indeterminate disease, the recommendation is the coadministration of Dapsone 100 mg. daily with six months of Rifampin 600 mg. daily. Under WHO, daily Rifampin may be replaced by 600 mg. Rifampin monthly, if supervised. The Dapsone is continued until all signs of clinical activity are controlled—usually after an additional six months. Then Dapsone should be continued for an additional three years for tuberculoid and indeterminate patients and for five years for borderline tuberculoid patients.

In lepromatous and borderline lepromatous patients, the recommendation is the coadministration of Dapsone 100 mg. daily with two years of Rifampin 600 mg. daily. Under WHO, daily Rifampin may be replaced by 600 mg. Rifampin monthly, if supervised. One may elect the concurrent administration of a third anti-leprosy drug, usually either Clofazamine 50–100mg. daily or Ethionamide 250–500 mg. daily. Dapsone 100 mg. daily is continued 3–10 years until all signs of clinical activity are controlled with skin scrapings and biopsies negative for one year. Dapsone should then be continued for an additional 10 years for borderline patients and for life for lepromatous patients.

Secondary Dapsone resistance should be suspected whenever a lepromatous or borderline lepromatous patient receiving Dapsone treatment relapses clinically and bacteriologically, solid staining bacilli being found in the smears taken from the new active lesions. If such cases show no response to regular and supervised Dapsone therapy within three to six months or good compliance for the past 3–6 months can be assured, Dapsone resistance should be considered confirmed clinically. Determination of drug sensitivity using the mouse footpad method is recommended and, after prior arrangement, is available without charge from the USPHS, Carville, LA. Patients with proven Dapsone resistance should be treated with other drugs.

LEPROSY REACTIONAL STATES

Abrupt changes in clinical activity occur in leprosy with any effective treatment and are known as reactional states. The majority can be classified into two groups.

The "Reversal" reaction (Type 1) may occur in borderline or tuberculoid leprosy patients often soon after chemotherapy is started. The mechanism is presumed to result from a reduction in the antigenic load: the patient is able to mount an enhanced delayed hypersensitivity response to residual infection leading to swelling ("Reversal") of existing skin and nerve lesions. If severe, or if neuritis is present, large doses of steroids should always be used. If severe, the patient should be hospitalized. In general anti-leprosy treatment is continued and therapy to suppress the reaction is indicated such as analgesics, steroids, or surgical decompression of swollen nerve trunks. USPHS at Carville, LA should be contacted for advice in management.

Erythema nodosum leprosum (ENL) (lepromatous reaction) (Type 2 reaction) occurs mainly in lepromatous patients and small numbers of borderline patients. Approximately 50% of treated patients show this reaction in the first year. The principal clinical features are fever and tender erythematous skin nodules sometimes associated with malaise, neuritis, orchitis, albuminuria, joint swelling, iritis, epistaxis or depression. Skin lesions can become pustular and/or ulcerate. Histologically there is a vasculitis with an intense polymorphonuclear infiltrate. Elevated circulating immune complexes are considered to be the mechanism of reaction. If severe, patients should be hospitalized. In general, anti-leprosy treatment is continued. Analgesics, steroids, and other agents available from USPHS, Carville, LA, are used to suppress the reaction.

HOW SUPPLIED

Rx: Dapsone 25 mg, round white scored tablet, debossed "25" above and "102" below the score and on the obverse "Jacobus" in light and child-resistant bottles, of 100, NDC 49938-102-01.

Dapsone 100 mg, round white scored tablet, debossed "100" above and "101" below the score and on the obverse "Jacobus" in light and child-resistant bottles of 100, NDC 49938-101-01.

Store at controlled room temperature, 20°–25°C (68°–77°F). Protect from light.

CAUTION: Federal law prohibits dispensing without prescription.

Dispense this product in a well-closed child-resistant container.

JACOBUS PHARMACEUTICAL CO., INC.
P.O. Box 5290
Princeton, NJ 08540

9J JUNE, 1997

PASER® GRANULES ℞
(aminosalicylic acid granules)

DESCRIPTION

PASER granules are a delayed release granule preparation of aminosalicylic acid (p-aminosalicylic acid: 4–aminosalicylic acid) for use with other anti-tuberculosis drugs for the treatment of all forms of active tuberculosis due to susceptible strains of tubercle bacilli. The granules are designed for gradual release to avoid high peak levels not useful (and perhaps toxic) with bacteriostatic drugs. Aminosalicylic acid is rapidly degraded in acid media; the protective acid-resistant outer coating is rapidly dissolved in neutral media so a mildly acidic food such as orange, apple or tomato juice, yogurt or apple sauce should be used.

Aminosalicylic acid (p-aminosalicylic acid) is 4–Amino-2-hydroxybenzoic acid. PASER granules are the free base of aminosalicylic acid and do NOT contain sodium or a sugar. The molecular formula is $C_7H_7NO_3$ with a molecular weight of 153.14. With heat p-aminosalicylic acid is decarboxylated to produce CO_2 and m-aminophenol. If the airtight packets are swollen, storage has been improper. DO NOT USE if packets are swollen or the granules have lost their tan color and are dark brown or purple.

The structural formula is:

OH
H_2N– –COOH

PASER granules are supplied as off-white tan colored granules with an average diameter of 1.5 mm and an average content of 60% aminosalicylic acid by weight. The acid resistant outer coating will be completely removed by a few minutes at a neutral pH. The inert ingredients are:

colloidal silicon dioxide
dibutyl sebacate
hydroxypropyl methyl cellulose
methacrylic acid copolymer
microcystalline cellulose
talc

The packets contain 4 grams of aminosalicylic acid for oral administration three times a day by sprinkling an apple sauce or yogurt to be eaten without chewing. Suspension in an acidic fruit drink such as orange juice or tomato juice will protect the coating for at least 2 hours. Swirling the juice in the glass will help resuspend the granules if they sink.

CLINICAL PHARMACOLOGY

Mechanism of Action: Aminosalicylic acid is bacteriostatic against Mycobacterium tuberculosis. It inhibits the onset of bacterial resistance to streptomycin and isoniazid. The mechanism of action has been postulated to be inhibition of folic acid synthesis (but without potentiation with antifolic compounds) and/or inhibition of synthesis of the cell wall component, mycobactin, thus reducing iron uptake by M. tuberculosis.

Characteristics: The two major considerations in the clinical pharmacology of aminosalicylic acid are the prompt production of a toxic inactive metabolite under acid conditions and the short serum half life of one hour for the free drug. Both are discussed below.

After two hours in simulated gastric fluid, 10% of unprotected aminosalicylic acid is decarboxylated to form meta-aminophenol, a known hepatotoxin. The acid-resistant coating of the PASER granules protects against degradation in the stomach. The small granules are designed to escape the usual restriction on gastric emptying of large particles. Under neutral conditions such as are found in the small intestine or in neutral foods, the acid-resistant coating is dissolved within one minute. Care must be taken in the administration of these granules to protect the acid-resistant coating by maintaining the granules in an acidic food during dosage administration. Patients who have neutralized gastric acid with antacids will not need to protect the acid resistant coating with an acidic food since no acid is present to spoil the drug. Antacids may influence the absorption of other medications and are not necessary for PASER consumed with an acidic food.

Because PASER granules are protected by an enteric coating absorption does not commence until they leave the stomach; the soft skeletons of the granules remain and may be seen in the stool.

Absorption and excretion: In a single 4 gram pharmacokinetic study with food in normal volunteers the initial time to a 2 µg/mL serum level of aminosalicylic acid was 2 hours with a range of 45 minutes to 24 hours; the median time to peak was 6 hours with a range of 1.5 to 24 hours; the mean peak level was 20 µg/mL with a range of 9 to 35 µg/mL; a level of 2 µg/mL was maintained for an average of 7.9 hours with a range of 5 to 9; a level of 1 µg/mL was maintained for an average of 8.8 hours with a range of 6 to 11.5 hours. The recommended schedule is 4 grams every 8 hours.

80% of aminosalicylic acid is excreted in the urine, with 50% or more of the dosage excreted in acetylated form. The acetylation process is not genetically determined as is the case for isoniazid. Aminosalicylic acid is excreted by glomerular filtration; although previously reported otherwise, probenecid, a tubular blocking agent, does not enhance plasma concentration. In a 1954 study thyroxine synthesis but not iodide uptake was reported reduced about 40% when the sodium salt (not PASER granules) of aminosalicylic acid was administered one hour before radio-iodine; the sodium salt typically produces a serum level over 120 µg/mL at one hour lasting one hour. Occasional goiter development can be prevented by the administration of thyroxine but not iodide. Penetration into the cerebrospinal fluid occurs only if the meninges are inflamed.

Approximately 50–60% of aminosalicylic acid is protein bound; binding is reported to be reduced 50% in kwashiorkor.

Microbiology: The aminosalicylic acid MIC for M. tuberculosis in 7H11 agar was less than 1.0 µg/mL for nine strains including three multidrug resistant strains, but 4 and 8 µg/mL for two other multidrug resistant strains. The 90% inhibition in 7H12 broth (Bactec) showed little dose response but was interpreted as being less than or equal to 0.12–0.25 µg/mL for eight strains of which three were multi-resistant, 0.50 µg/mL for one resistant strain, questionable for four nonresistant strains and greater than 1 µg/mL for one non-resistant and three resistant strains. Aminosalicylic acid is not active in vitro against M. avium.

INDICATIONS AND USAGE

PASER is indicated for the treatment of tuberculosis in combination with other active agents. It is most commonly used in patients with Multi-drug Resistant TB (MDR-TB) or in situations when therapy with isoniazid and rifampin is not possible due to a combination of resistance and/or intolerance. When PASER is added to the treatment regimen in patients with proven or suspected drug resistance, it should be accompanied by at least one and preferably two other new agents to which the patient's organism is known or expected to be susceptible.

CONTRAINDICATIONS

Hypersensitivity to any component of this medication.

Severe renal disease.

Patients with severe renal disease will accumulate aminosalicylic acid and its acetyl metabolite but will continue to acetylate, thus leading exclusively to the inactive acetylated form; deacetylation, if any, is not significant.

The half life of free aminosalicylic acid in renal disease is 30.8 minutes in comparison to 26.4 minutes in normal volunteers, but the half life of the inactive metabolite is 309 minutes in uremic patients in comparison to 51 minutes in normal volunteers. Although aminosalicylic acid passes dialysis membranes, the frequency of dialysis usually is not comparable to the half-life of 50 minutes for the free acid. Patients with end stage renal disease should not receive aminosalicylic acid.

WARNINGS

Liver Function

In one retrospective study of 7492 patients on rapidly absorbed aminosalicylic acid preparations, drug-induced hepatitis occurred in 38 patients (0.5%); in these 38 the first symptom usually appeared within three months of the start of therapy with a rash as the most common event followed by fever and much less frequently by GI disturbances of anorexia, nausea or diarrhea. Only one patient was diagnosed on routine biochemistry.

Premonitory symptoms in 90% of these 38 patients preceded jaundice by a few days to several weeks with the mean time of onset 33 days with a range of 7–90 days. Half of the adverse reactions occurred during the third, fourth or fifth weeks. When aminosalicylic acid-induced hepatitis was diagnosed, hepatomegaly was invariably present with lymphadenopathy in 46%, leucocytosis in 79%, and eosinophilia in 55%. Prompt recognition with discontinuation led to the recovery of all 38 patients. If recognized in the premonitory stage, the reaction is reported to "settle" in 24 hours and no jaundice ensues. From other reported studies failure to recognize the reaction can result in a mortality of up to 21%. The patient must be monitored carefully during the first three months of therapy and treatment must be discontinued immediately at the first sign of a rash, fever or other premonitory signs of intolerance.

PRECAUTIONS

(1) General:

All drugs should be stopped at the first sign suggesting a hypersensitivity reaction. They may be restarted one at a time in very small but gradually increasing doses to determine whether the manifestations are drug-induced and, if so, which drug is responsible.

Desensitization has been accomplished successfully in 15 of 17 patients starting with 10 mg aminosalicylic acid given as a single dose. The dosage is doubled every 2 days until reaching a total of 1 gram after which the dosage is divided to follow the regular schedule of administration. If a mild temperature rise or skin reaction develops, the increment is to be dropped back one level or the progression held for one cycle. Reactions are rare after a total dosage of 1.5 grams.

Patients with hepatic disease may not tolerate aminosalicylic acid as well as normal patients, even though the metabolism in patients with hepatic disease has been reported to be comparable to that in normal volunteers.

(2) Information for Patients:

The patient should be advised that the first signs of hypersensitivity include a rash, often followed by fever, and much less frequently, GI disturbances of anorexia, nausea or diar-

Continued on next page

Paser—Cont.

rhea. If such symptoms develop, the patient should immediately cease taking the medication and arrange for a prompt clinical visit.
Patients should be advised that poor compliance in taking anti-TB medication often leads to treatment failure, and, not infrequently, to the development of resistance of the organisms in the individual patient.
Patients should be advised that the skeleton of the granules may be seen in the stool.
The coating to protect the PASER granules dissolves promptly under neutral conditions; the granules therefore should be administered by sprinkling on acidic foods such as apple sauce or yogurt or by suspension in a fruit drink which will protect the coating, but the granules sink and will have to be swirled. The coating will last at least 2 hours in either system. All juices tested to date have been satisfactory; tested are: tomato, orange, grapefruit, grape, cranberry, apple, "fruit punch".
Patients should be advised to store PASER in a refrigerator or freezer. PASER packets may be stored at room temperature for short periods of time.
Patients should be advised NOT to use if the packets are swollen or the granules have lost their tan color and are dark brown or purple. The patient should inform the pharmacist or physician immediately and return the medication.
(3) Laboratory Tests:
Aminosalicylic acid has been reported to interfere technically with the serum determinations of albumin by dye-binding. SGOT by the azoene dye method and with qualitative urine tests for ketones, bilirubin, urobilinogen or porphobilinogen.
(4) Drug Interactions:
Aminosalicytic acid at a dosage of 12 grams in a rapidly available form has been reported to produce a 20 percent reduction in the acetylation of isoniazid, especially in patients who are rapid acetylators; INH serum levels, half lives and excretions in fast acetylators still remain half of the levels seen in slow acetylators with or without p-aminosalicylic acid. The effect is dose related and, while it has not been studied with the current delayed release preparation, the lower serum levels with this preparation will result in a reduced effect on the acetylation of INH.
Aminosalicylic acid has previously been reported to block the absorption of rifampin. A subsequent report has shown that this blockade was due to an excipient not included in PASER granules. Oral administration of a solution containing both aminosalicylic acid and rifampin showed full absorption of each product.
As a result of competition, Vitamin B_{12} absorption has been reduced 55% by 5 grams of aminosalicylic acid with clinically significant erythrocyte abnormalities developing after depletion; patients on therapy of more than one month should be considered for maintenance B_{12}.
A malabsorption syndrome can develop in patients on aminosalicylic acid but is usually not complete. The complete syndrome includes steatorrhea, an abnormal small bowel pattern on x-ray, villus atrophy, depressed cholesterol, reduced D-xylose and iron absorption. Triglyceride absorption always is normal.
In one literature report 8 hours after the last dosage of aminosalicylic acid at 2 gm qid serum digoxin levels were reduced 40% in two of ten patients but not changed in the remaining eight.
(5) Carcinogenesis, mutagenesis, impairment of fertility: Sodium aminosalicylate produced an occipital bone defect, probably with a dose response, when administered to ten pregnant Wistar rats at five doses from 3.85 to 385 mg/kg from days 6 to 14. There were no significant changes from controls in any group in corpora lutea, early resorptions, total resorptions, fetal death, litter size, or hematomas. For all except the 77 mg/kg group, fetal weights were significantly greater than controls. Chinchilla rabbits on 5 mg/kg from days 7 to 14 did not show any significant differences as compared to controls for the same parameters studied.
Sodium aminosalicylic acid was not mutagenic in Ames tester strain TA 100. In human lymphocyte cultures in-vitro clastogenic effects of achromatic, chromatid, isochromatic breaks or chromatid translocations were not seen at 153 or 600 µg/mL. At 1500 and 3000 µg/mL there was a dose related increase in chromatid aberrations.
Patients on isoniazid and aminosalicylic acid have been reported to have an increased number of chromosomal aberrations as compared to controls.
(6) Pregnancy: Pregnancy Category C:
Aminosalicylic acid has been reported to produce occipital malformations in rats when given at doses within the human dose range. Although there probably is a dose response, the frequency of abnormalities was comparable to controls at the highest level tested (two times the human dosage). When administered to rabbits at 5 mg/kg, throughout all three trimesters, no teratologic embryocidal effects were seen. Literature reports on aminosalicylic acid in pregnant women always report coadministration of other medications. Because there are no adequate and well controlled studies of aminosalicylic acid in humans, PASER granules should be given to a pregnant woman only if clearly needed.
(8) Nursing mothers:
After administration of a different preparation of aminosalicylic acid to one patient, the maximum concentration in the milk was 1 µg/mL at 3 hours with a half-life of 2.5 hours; the maximum maternal plasma concentration was 70 µg/mL at two hours.

ADVERSE EFFECTS

The most common side effect is gastrointestinal intolerance manifested by nausea, vomiting, diarrhea, and abdominal pain.
Hypersensitivity reactions: Fever, skin eruptions of various types, including exfoliative dermatitis, infectious mononucleosis-like, or lymphoma-like syndrome, leucopenia, agranulocytosis, thrombocytopenia, Coombs' positive hemolytic anemia, jaundice, hepatitis, pericarditis, hypoglycemia, optic neuritis, encephalopathy, Leoffler's syndrome, and vasculitis and a reduction in prothrombin.
Crystalluria may be prevented by the maintenance of urine at a neutral or an alkaline pH.

OVERDOSAGE

Overdosage has not been reported.

DOSAGE AND ADMINISTRATION

PASER granules should be administered with other drugs to which the organism is known or expected to be susceptible. It is most commonly administered to patients with Multi-drug Resistant TB (MDR-TB) or in other situations in which therapy with isoniazid or rifampin is not possible due to a combination of resistance and/or tolerance. The adult dosage of four grams (one packet) three times per day or correspondingly smaller doses in children should be given by sprinking on apple sauce or yogurt or by swirling in the glass to suspend the granules in an acidic drink such as tomato or orange juice.
DO NOT USE if the packet is swollen or the granules have lost their tan color, turning dark brown or purple.

HOW SUPPLIED

Carton of 30 PASER packets (NDC 49938-107-04).
Each packet contains four grams aminosalicylic acid.
PASER granules are supplied in packets containing 4 grams of aminosalicylic acid for administration three times a day by suspension in an acidic drink or food with a pH less than 5. Examples include apple sauce, yogurt, tomato or orange juice.
Distributors and Pharmacists: Store below 59°F (15°C) (in a refrigerator or freezer).
Patients are urged to store PASER in a refrigerator or freezer. PASER packets may be stored at room temperature for short periods of time.
AVOID EXCESSIVE HEAT. DO NOT USE if packet is swollen or the granules have lost their tan color, turning dark brown or purple.
Caution: Federal, law prohibits dispensing without prescription.

JACOBUS PHARMACEUTICAL CO. INC.
P.O. Box 5290
Princeton, NJ 08540

2A JULY, 1996

Janssen Pharmaceutica Products, L.P.

1125 TRENTON-HARBOURTON ROAD
P.O. BOX 200
TITUSVILLE, NJ 08560-0200

For Medical Information Monday through Friday 9 am-5 pm EST Contact:
(800) JANSSEN
FAX: (609) 730-2461
After Hours and Weekends:
(800) JANSSEN

ACIPHEX® ℞

['a-sə-feks]
(rabeprazole sodium)
Delayed-Release Tablets

DESCRIPTION

The active ingredient in ACIPHEX® Delayed-Release Tablets is rabeprazole sodium, a substituted benzimidazole that inhibits gastric acid secretion. Rabeprazole sodium is known chemically as 2-[[[4-(3-methyoxypropoxy)-3-methyl-2-pyridinyl]-methyl]sulfinyl]-1*H*-benz-imidazole sodium salt. It has an empirical formula of $C_{18}H_{20}N_3NaO_3S$ and a molecular weight of 381.43. Rabeprazole sodium is a white to slightly yellowish-white solid. It is very soluble in water and methanol, freely soluble in ethanol, chloroform and ethyl acetate and insoluble in ether and n-hexane. The stability of rabeprazole sodium is a function of pH; it is rapidly degraded in acid media, and is more stable under alkaline conditions. The structural formula is:

RABEPRAZOLE SODIUM

ACIPHEX® is available for oral administration as delayed-release, enteric-coated tablets containing 20 mg of rabeprazole sodium. Inactive ingredients are mannitol, hydroxypropyl cellulose, magnesium oxide, low-substituted hydroxypropyl cellulose, magnesium stearate, ethylcellulose, hydroxypropyl methylcellulose phthalate, diacetylated monoglycerides, talc, titanium dioxide, carnauba wax, and ferric oxide (yellow) as a coloring agent.

CLINICAL PHARMACOLOGY

Pharmacokinetics and Metabolism

ACIPHEX® delayed-release tablets are enteric-coated to allow rabeprazole sodium, which is acid labile, to pass through the stomach relatively intact. After oral administration of 20 mg ACIPHEX®, peak plasma concentrations (C_{max}) of rabeprazole occur over a range of 2.0 to 5.0 hours (T_{max}). The rabeprazole C_{max} and AUC are linear over an oral dose range of 10 mg to 40 mg. There is no appreciable accumulation when doses of 10 mg to 40 mg are administered every 24 hours; the pharmacokinetics of rabeprazole are not altered by multiple dosing. The plasma half-life ranges from 1 to 2 hours.

Absorption: Following oral administration of 20 mg, rabeprazole is absorbed and can be detected in plasma by 1 hour. Absolute bioavailability for a 20 mg oral tablet of rabeprazole (compared to intravenous administration) is approximately 52%.
The effects of food on the absorption of rabeprazole have not been evaluated.

Distribution: Rabeprazole is 96.3% bound to human plasma proteins.

Metabolism: Rabeprazole is extensively metabolized. The thioether and sulphone are the primary metabolites measured in human plasma. These metabolites were not observed to have significant anti-secretory activity. *In vitro* studies have demonstrated that rabeprazole is primarily metabolized in the liver by cytochromes P450 3A (sulphone metabolite) and 2C19 (desmethyl rabeprazole). The thioether metabolite is formed by reduction of rabeprazole.

Elimination: Following a single 20 mg oral dose of ^{14}C-labeled rabeprazole, approximately 90% of the drug was eliminated in the urine, primarily as thioether carboxylic acid; its glucuronide, and mercapturic acid metabolites. The remainder of the dose was recovered in the feces. Total recovery of radioactivity was 99.8%. No unchanged rabeprazole was recovered in the urine or feces.

Special Populations

Geriatric: In 20 healthy elderly subjects administered 20 mg rabeprazole once daily for seven days, AUC values approximately doubled and the C_{max} increased by 60% compared to values in a parallel younger control group. There was no evidence of drug accumulation after once daily administration. (see PRECAUTIONS).

Pediatric: The pharmacokinetics of rabeprazole in pediatric patients under the age of 18 years have not been studied.

Gender and Race: In analyses adjusted for body mass and height, rabeprazole pharmacokinetics showed no clinically significant differences between male and female subjects. In studies that used different formulations of rabeprazole, $AUC_{0-\infty}$ values for healthy Japanese men were approximately 50–60% greater than values derived from pooled data from healthy men in the United States.

Renal Disease: In 10 patients with stable end-stage renal disease requiring maintenance hemodialysis (creatinine clearance ≤5 mL/min/1.73 m^2), no clinically significant differences were observed in the pharmacokinetics of rabeprazole after a single 20 mg oral dose when compared to 10 healthy volunteers.

Hepatic Disease: In a single dose study of 10 patients with chronic mild to moderate compensated cirrhosis of the liver who were administered a 20 mg dose of rabeprazole, AUC_{0-24} was approximately doubled, the elimination half-life was 2- to 3-fold higher, and total body clearance was decreased to less than half compared to values in healthy men.
In a multiple dose study of 12 patients with mild to moderate hepatic impairment administered 20 mg rabeprazole once daily for eight days, $AUC_{0-\infty}$ and C_{max} values increased approximately 20% compared to values in healthy age- and gender-matched subjects. These increases were not statistically significant.
No information exists on rabeprazole disposition in patients with severe hepatic impairment. Please refer to the DOSAGE AND ADMINISTRATION section for information on dosage adjustment in patients with hepatic impairment.

PHARMACODYNAMICS

Mechanism of Action

Rabeprazole belongs to a class of antisecretory compounds (substituted benzimidazole proton-pump inhibitors) that do not exhibit anticholinergic or histamine H_2-receptor antagonist properties, but supress gastric acid secretion by inhibiting the gastric H^+, K^+ATPase at the secretory surface of the gastric parietal cell. Because this enzyme is regarded as the acid (proton) pump within the parietal cell, rabeprazole has been characterized as a gastric proton-pump inhibitor. Rabeprazole blocks the final step of gastric acid secretion.
In gastric parietal cells, rabeprazole is protonated, accumulates, and is transformed to an active sulfenamide. When studied *in vitro*, rabeprazole is chemically activated at pH 1.2 with a half-life of 78 seconds. It inhibits acid transport in porcine gastric vesicles with a half-life of 90 seconds.

Antisecretory Activity

The anti-secretory effect begins within one hour after oral administration of 20 mg ACIPHEX®. The median inhibitory effect of ACIPHEX® on 24-hour gastric acidity is 88% of maximal after the first dose. ACIPHEX® 20 mg inhibits basal and peptone meal-stimulated acid secretion versus placebo by 86% and 95%, respectively, and increases the percent of a 24-hour period that the gastric pH>3 from 10% to 65% (see table below). This relatively prolonged pharmacodynamic action compared to the short pharmacokinetic half-life (1–2 hours) reflects the sustained inactivation of the H^+, K^+ATPase.

[See first table at right]

Compared to placebo, ACIPHEX®, 10 mg, 20 mg, and 40 mg, administered once daily for 7 days significantly decreased intragastric acidity with all doses for each of four meal-related intervals and the 24-hour time period overall. In this study, there were no statistically significant differences between doses; however, there was a significant dose-related decrease in intragastric acidity. The ability of rabeprazole to cause a dose-related decrease in mean intragastric acidity is illustrated below.

[See second table at right]

After administration of 20 mg ACIPHEX® once daily for eight days, the mean percent of time that gastric pH>3 or gastric pH>4 after a single dose (Day 1) and multiple doses (Day 8) was significantly greater than placebo (see table below). The decrease in gastric acidity and the increase in gastric pH observed with 20 mg ACIPHEX® administered once daily for eight days were compared to the same parameters for placebo, as illustrated below:

[See third table at right]

Effects on Esophageal Acid Exposure

In patients with gastroesophageal reflux disease (GERD) and moderate to severe esophageal acid exposure, ACIPHEX® 20 mg and 40 mg per day decreased 24-hour esophageal acid exposure. After seven days of treatment, the percentage of time that esophageal pH<4 decreased from baselines of 24.7% for 20 mg and 23.7% for 40 mg, to 5.1% and 2.0%, respectively. Normalization of 24-hour intraesophageal acid exposure was correlated to gastric pH>4 for at least 35% of the 24-hour period; this level was achieved in 90% of subjects receiving ACIPHEX® 20 mg and in 100% of subjects receiving ACIPHEX® 40 mg. With ACIPHEX® 20 mg and 40 mg per day, effects on gastric and esophageal pH were significant and substantial after one day of treatment, and more pronounced after seven days of treatment.

Effects on Serum Gastrin

In patients given daily doses of ACIPHEX® for up to eight weeks to treat ulcerative or erosive esophagitis and in patients treated for up to 52 weeks to prevent recurrence of disease the median fasting gastrin level increased in a dose-related manner. The group median values stayed within the normal range.

Effects on Enterochromaffin-like (ECL) Cells

Increased serum gastrin secondary to antisecretory agents stimulates proliferation of gastric ECL cells which, over time, may result in ECL cell hyperplasia in rats and mice and gastric carcinoids in rats, especially in females (see Carcinogenesis, Mutagenesis, Impairment of Fertility).

In over 400 patients treated with ACIPHEX® (10 or 20 mg/day) for up to one year, the incidence of ECL cell hyperplasia increased with time and dose, which is consistent with the pharmacological action of the proton-pump inhibitor. No patient developed the adenomatoid, dysplastic or neoplastic changes of ECL cells in the gastric mucosa. No patient developed the carcinoid tumors observed in rats.

Endocrine Effects

Studies in humans for up to one year have not revealed clinically significant effects on the endocrine system. In healthy male volunteers treated with ACIPHEX® for 13 days, no clinically relevant changes have been detected in the following endocrine parameters examined: 17 β-estradiol, thyroid stimulating hormone, tri-iodothyronine, thyroxine, thyroxine-binding protein, parathyroid hormone, insulin, glucagon, renin, aldosterone, follicle-stimulating hormone, luteotrophic hormone, prolactin, somatotrophic hormone, dehydroepiandrosterone, cortisol-binding globulin, and urinary 6β-hydroxycortisol, serum testosterone and circadian cortisol profile.

Other Effects

In humans treated with ACIPHEX® for up to one year, no systemic effects have been observed on the central nervous, lymphoid, hematopoietic, renal, hepatic, cardiovascular, or respiratory systems. No data are available on long-term treatment with ACIPHEX® and ocular effects.

CLINICAL STUDIES

Healing of Erosive or Ulcerative Gastroesophageal Reflux Disease (GERD)

In a U.S., multicenter, randomized, double-blind, placebo-controlled study, 103 patients were treated for up to eight weeks with placebo, 10 mg, 20 mg or 40 mg ACIPHEX® QD. For this and all studies of GERD healing, only patients with GERD symptoms and at least grade 2 esophagitis (modified Hetzel-Dent grading scale) were eligible for entry. Endoscopic healing was defined as grade 0 or 1. Each rabeprazole dose was significantly superior to placebo in producing endoscopic healing after four and eight weeks of treatment. The percentage of patients demonstrating endoscopic healing was as follows:

[See fourth table above]

In addition, there was a statistically significant difference in favor of the ACIPHEX® 10 mg, 20 mg, and 40 mg doses compared to placebo at Weeks 4 and 8 regarding complete resolution of GERD heartburn frequency (p≤0.026). All ACIPHEX® groups reported significantly greater rates of

Gastric Acid Parameters
ACIPHEX® Versus Placebo After 7 Days of Once Daily Dosing

Parameter	ACIPHEX® (20 mg QD)	Placebo
Basal Acid Output (mmol/hr)	0.4*	2.8
Stimulated Acid Output (mmol/hr)	0.6*	13.3
% Time Gastric pH>3	65*	10

* (p<0.01 versus placebo)

AUC Acidity (mmol•hr/L)
ACIPHEX® Versus Placebo on Day 7
of Once Daily Dosing (mean±SD)

AUC interval (hrs)	Treatment: 10 mg RBP (N=24)	20 mg RBP (N=24)	40 mg RBP (N=24)	Placebo (N=24)
08:00–13:00	19.6±21.5*	12.9±23*	7.6±14.7*	91.1±39.7
13:00–19:00	5.6±9.7*	8.3±29.8*	1.3±5.2*	95.5±48.7
19:00–22:00	0.1±0.1*	0.1±0.06*	0.0±0.02*	11.9±12.5
22:00–08:00	129.2±84*	109.6±67.2*	76.9±58.4*	479.9±165
AUC 0–24 hours	155.5±90.6*	130.9±81*	85.8±64.3*	678.5±216

*(p<0.001 versus placebo)

Gastric Acid Parameters
ACIPHEX® Once Daily Dosing Versus Placebo on Day 1 and Day 8

Parameter	ACIPHEX® 20 mg QD		Placebo	
	Day 1	Day 8	Day 1	Day 8
Mean AUC_{0-24} Acidity	340.8*	176.9*	925.5	862.4
Median trough pH (23-hr)[a]	3.77	3.51	1.27	1.38
% Time Gastric pH>3[b]	54.6*	68.7*	19.1	21.7
% Time Gastric pH>4[b]	44.1*	60.3*	7.6	11.0

[a]No inferential statistics conducted for this parameter.
*(p<0.001) versus placebo
[b]Gastric pH was measured every hour over a 24-hour period.

Healing of Erosive or Ulcerative
Gastroesophageal Reflux Disease (GERD)
Percentage of Patients Healed

Week	10 mg ACIPHEX® QD N=27	20 mg ACIPHEX® QD N=25	40 mg ACIPHEX® QD N=26	Placebo N=25
4	63%*	56%*	54%*	0%
8	93%*	84%*	85%*	12%

*(p<0.001 versus placebo)

Healing of Erosive or Ulcerative
Gastroesophageal Reflux Disease (GERD)
Percentage of Patients Healed

Week	ACIPHEX® 20 mg QD N=167	Ranitidine 150 mg QID N=169
4	59%*	36%
8	87%*	66%

*(p<0.001 versus ranitidine)

complete resolution of GERD daytime heartburn severity compared to placebo at Weeks 4 and 8 (p≤0.036). Mean reductions from baseline in daily antacid dose were statistically significant for all ACIPHEX® groups when compared to placebo at both Weeks 4 and 8 (p≤0.007).

In a North American multicenter, randomized, double-blind, active-controlled study of 336 patients, ACIPHEX® was statistically superior to rantidine with respect to the percentage of patients healed at endoscopy after four and eight weeks of treatment (see table below):

[See fifth table above]

ACIPHEX® 20 mg once daily was significantly more effective than ranitidine 150 mg QID in the percentage of patients with complete resolution of heartburn at Weeks 4 and 8 (p<0.001). ACIPHEX® 20 mg once daily was also more effective in complete resolution of daytime heartburn (p≤0.025), and night time heartburn (p≤0.012) at both Weeks 4 and 8, with significant differences by the end of the first week of the study.

Long-term Maintenance of Healing of Erosive or Ulcerative Gastroesophageal Reflux Disease (GERD Maintenance)

The long-term maintenance of healing in patients with erosive or ulcerative GERD previously healed with gastric antisecretory therapy was assessed in two U.S., multicenter, randomized, double-blind, placebo-controlled studies of identical design of 52 weeks duration. The two studies randomized 209 and 285 patients, respectively, to receive either 10 mg or 20 mg of ACIPHEX® QD or placebo. As demonstrated in the tables below, ACIPHEX® was significantly superior to placebo in both studies with respect to the maintenance of healing of GERD and the proportions of patients remaining free of heartburn symptoms at 52 weeks:

[See first table at top of next page]

[See second table on next page]

Healing of Duodenal Ulcers

In a U.S., randomized, double-blind, multi-center study assessing the effectiveness of 20 mg and 40 mg of ACIPHEX® QD versus placebo for healing endoscopically defined duodenal ulcers, 100 patients were treated for up to four weeks. ACIPHEX® was significantly superior to placebo in producing healing of duodenal ulcers. The percentages of patients with endoscopic healing are presented below:

[See third table on next page]

At Weeks 2 and 4, significantly more patients in the ACIPHEX® 20 and 40 mg groups reported complete resolution of ulcer pain frequency (p≤0.018), daytime pain severity (p≤0.023), and nighttime pain severity (p≤0.035) compared with placebo patients. The only exception was the ACIPHEX® 40 mg group versus placebo at Week 2 for duodenal ulcer pain frequency (p=0.094). Significant differences

Continued on next page

Aciphex—Cont.

in resolution of daytime and nighttime pain were noted in both ACIPHEX® groups relative to placebo by the end of the first week of the study. Significant reductions in daily antacid use were also noted in both ACIPHEX® groups compared to placebo at Weeks 2 and 4 ($p \leq 0.001$).

An international randomized, double-blind, active-controlled trial was conducted in 205 patients comparing 20 mg ACIPHEX® QD with 20 mg omeprazole QD. The study was designed to provide at least 80% power to exclude a difference of at least 10% between ACIPHEX® and omeprazole, assuming four-week healing response rate of 93% for both groups. In patients with endoscopically defined duodenal ulcers treated for up to four weeks, ACIPHEX® was comparable to omeprazole in producing healing of duodenal ulcers. The percentages of patients with endoscopic healing at two and four weeks are presented below:

[See fourth table at right]

ACIPHEX® and omeprazole were comparable in providing complete resolution of symptoms.

Pathological Hypersecretory Conditions Including Zollinger-Ellison Syndrome

Twelve patients with idiopathic gastric hypersecretion or Zollinger-Ellison syndrome have been treated successfully with ACIPHEX® at doses from 20 to 120 mg for up to 12 months. ACIPHEX® produced satisfactory inhibition of gastric acid secretion in all patients and complete resolution of signs and symptoms of acid-peptic disease where present. ACIPHEX® also prevented recurrence of gastric hypersecretion and manifestations of acid-peptic disease in all patients. The high doses of ACIPHEX® used to treat this small cohort of patients with gastric hypersecretion were not associated with drug-related adverse effects.

INDICATIONS AND USAGE

Healing of Erosive or Ulcerative Gastroesophageal Reflux Disease (GERD)

ACIPHEX® is indicated for short-term (4 to 8 weeks) treatment in the healing and symptomatic relief of erosive or ulcerative gastroesophageal reflux disease (GERD). For those patients who have not healed after 8 weeks of treatment, an additional 8-week course of ACIPHEX® may be considered.

Maintenance of Healing of Erosive or Ulcerative Gastroesophageal Reflux Disease (GERD)

ACIPHEX® is indicated for maintaining healing and reduction in relapse rates of heartburn symptoms in patients with erosive or ulcerative gastroesophageal reflux disease (GERD Maintenance).

Healing of Duodenal Ulcers

ACIPHEX® is indicated for short-term (up to four weeks) treatment in the healing and symptomatic relief of duodenal ulcers. Most patients heal within four weeks.

Treatment of Pathological Hypersecretory Conditions, Including Zollinger-Ellison Syndrome

ACIPHEX® is indicated for the long-term treatment of pathological hypersecretory conditions including Zollinger-Ellison syndrome.

CONTRAINDICATIONS

Rabeprazole is contraindicated in patients with known hypersensitivity to rabeprazole, substituted benzimidazoles or to any component of the formulation.

PRECAUTIONS

General

Symptomatic response to therapy with rabeprazole does not preclude the presence of gastric malignancy.

Patients with healed GERD were treated for up to 40 months with rabeprazole and monitored with serial gastric biopsies. Patients without *H. pylori* infection (221 of 326 patients) had no clinically important pathologic changes in the gastric mucosa. Patients with *H. pylori* infection at baseline (105 of 326 patients) had mild or moderate inflammation in the gastric body or mild inflammation in the gastric antrum. Patients with mild grades of infection or inflammation in the gastric body tended to change to moderate, whereas those graded moderate at baseline tended to remain stable. Patients with mild grades of infection or inflammation in the gastric antrum tended to remain stable. At baseline 8% of patients had atrophy of glands in the gastric body and 15% had atrophy in the gastric antrum. At endpoint, 15% of patients had atrophy of glands in the gastric body and 11% had atrophy in the gastric antrum. Approximately 4% of patients had intestinal metaplasia at some point during follow-up, but no consistent changes were seen.

Information for Patients

Patients should be cautioned that ACIPHEX® delayed-release tablets should be swallowed whole. The tablets should not be chewed, crushed, or split.

Drug Interactions

Rabeprazole is metabolized by the cytochrome P450 (CYP450) drug metabolizing enzyme system. Studies in healthy subjects have shown that rabeprazole does not have clinically significant interactions with other drugs metabolized by the CYP450 system, such as warfarin and theophylline given as single oral doses, diazepam as a single intravenous dose, and phenytoin given as a single intravenous dose (with supplemental oral dosing). *In vitro* incubations employing human liver microsomes indicated that rabeprazole inhibited cyclosporine metabolism with an IC_{50} of 62 micromolar, a concentration that is over 50 times higher than the C_{max} in healthy volunteers following 14 days of dosing with 20 mg of rabeprazole. This degree of inhibition is similar to that by omeprazole at equivalent concentrations.

Rabeprazole produces sustained inhibition of gastric acid secretion. An interaction with compounds which are dependent on gastric pH for absorption may occur due to the magnitude of acid suppression observed with rabeprazole. For example, in normal subjects, co-administration of rabeprazole 20 mg QD resulted in an approximately 30% decrease in the bioavailability of ketoconazole and increases in the AUC and C_{max} for digoxin of 19% and 29%, respectively. Therefore, patients may need to be monitored when such drugs are taken concomitantly with rabeprazole. Co-administration of rabeprazole and antacids produced no clinically relevant changes in plasma rabeprazole concentrations.

Carcinogenesis, Mutagenesis, Impairment of Fertility

In a 88/104-week carcinogenicity study in CD-1 mice, rabeprazole at oral doses up to 100 mg/kg/day did not produce any increased tumor occurrence. The highest tested dose produced a systemic exposure to rabeprazole (AUC) of 1.40

Long-term Maintenance of Healing of Erosive or Ulcerative Gastroesophageal Reflux Disease (GERD Maintenance) Percent of Patients in Endoscopic Remission

	ACIPHEX® 10 mg	ACIPHEX® 20 mg	Placebo
Study 1	N=66	N=67	N=70
Week 4	83%*	96%*	44%
Week 13	79%*	93%*	39%
Week 26	77%*	93%*	31%
Week 39	76%*	91%*	30%
Week 52	73%*	90%*	29%
Study 2	N=93	N=93	N=99
Week 4	89%*	94%*	40%
Week 13	86%*	91%*	33%
Week 26	85%*	89%*	30%
Week 39	84%*	88%*	29%
Week 52	77%*	86%*	29%
COMBINED STUDIES	N=159	N=160	N=169
Week 4	87%*	94%*	42%
Week 13	83%*	92%*	36%
Week 26	82%*	91%*	31%
Week 39	81%*	89%*	30%
Week 52	75%*	87%*	29%

*($p<0.001$ versus placebo)

Long-term Maintenance of Healing of Erosive or Ulcerative Gastroesophageal Reflux Disease (GERD Maintenance): Percent of Patients Without Relapse in Heartburn Frequency and Daytime and Nighttime Heartburn Severity at Week 52

	ACIPHEX® 10 mg	ACIPHEX® 20 mg	Placebo
Heartburn Frequency			
Study 1	46/55 (84%)*	48/52 (92%)*	17/45 (38%)
Study 2	50/72 (69%)*	57/72 (79%)*	22/79 (28%)
Daytime Heartburn Severity			
Study 1	61/64 (95%)*	60/62 (97%)*	42/61 (69%)
Study 2	73/84 (87%)†	82/87 (94%)*	67/90 (74%)
Nighttime Heartburn Severity			
Study 1	57/61 (93%)*	60/61 (98%)*	37/56 (66%)
Study 2	67/80 (84%)	79/87 (91%)†	64/87 (74%)

*$p \leq 0.001$ versus placebo
†$0.001 < p < 0.05$ versus placebo

Healing of Duodenal Ulcers Percentage of Patients Healed

Week	ACIPHEX® 20 mg QD N=34	ACIPHEX® 40 mg QD N=33	Placebo N=33
2	44%	42%	21%
4	79%*	91%*	39%

*$p \leq 0.001$ versus placebo

Healing of Duodenal Ulcers Percentage of Patients Healed

Week	ACIPHEX® 20 mg QD N=102	Omeprazole 20 mg QD N=103	95% Confidence Interval for the Treatment Difference (ACHIPEX®-Omeprazole)
2	69%	61%	(−6%, 22%)
4	98%	93%	(−3%, 15%)

μg•hr/mL which is 1.6 times the human exposure (plasma $AUC_{0-\infty}$ = 0.88 μg•hr/mL) at the recommended dose for GERD (20 mg/day). In a 104-week carcinogenicity study in Sprague-Dawley rats, males were treated with oral doses of 5, 15, 30 and 60 mg/kg/day and females with 5, 15, 30, 60 and 120 mg/kg/day. Rabeprazole produced gastric enterochromaffin-like (ECL) cell hyperplasia in male and female rats and ECL cell carcinoid tumors in female rats at all doses including the lowest tested dose. The lowest dose (5 mg/kg/day) produced a systemic exposure to rabeprazole (AUC) of about 0.1 μg•hr/mL which is about 0.1 times the human exposure at the recommended dose for GERD. In male rats, no treatment related tumors were observed at doses up to 60 mg/kg/day producing a rabeprazole plasma exposure (AUC) of about 0.2 μg•hr/mL (0.2 times the human exposure at the recommended dose for GERD).

Rabeprazole was positive in the Ames test, the Chinese hamster ovary cell (CHO/HGPRT) forward gene mutation test and the mouse lymphoma cell (L5178Y/TK+/−) forward gene mutation test. Its demethylated-metabolite was also positive in the Ames test. Rabeprazole was negative in the *in vitro* Chinese hamster lung cell chromosome aberration test, the *in vivo* mouse micronucleus test, and the *in vivo* and *ex vivo* rat hepatocyte unscheduled DNA synthesis (UDS) tests.

Rabeprazole at intravenous doses up to 30 mg/kg/day (plasma AUC of 8.8 μg•hr/mL, about 10 times the human exposure at the recommended dose for GERD) was found to have no effect on fertility and reproductive performance of male and female rats.

Pregnancy

Teratogenic Effects. Pregnancy Category B: Teratology studies have been performed in rats at intravenous doses up to 50 mg/kg/day (plasma AUC of 11.8 μg•hr/mL, about 13 times the human exposure at the recommended dose for GERD) and rabbits at intravenous doses up to 30 mg/kg/day (plasma AUC of 7.3 μg•hr/mL, about 8 times the human exposure at the recommended dose for GERD) and have revealed no evidence of impaired fertility or harm to the fetus due to rabeprazole. There are, however, no adequate and well-controlled studies in pregnant women. Because animal reproduction studies are not always predictive of human response, this drug should be used during pregnancy only if clearly needed.

Nursing Mothers

Following intravenous administration of ^{14}C-labeled rabeprazole to lactating rats, radioactivity in milk reached levels that were 2- to 7-fold higher than levels in the blood. It is not known if unmetabolized rabeprazole is excreted in human breast milk. Administration of rabeprazole to rats in late gestation and during lactation at doses of 400 mg/kg/day (about 195-times the human dose based on mg/m^2) resulted in decreases in body weight gain of the pups. Since many drugs are excreted in milk, and because of the potential for adverse reactions to nursing infants from rabeprazole, a decision should be made to discontinue nursing or discontinue the drug, taking into account the importance of the drug to the mother.

Pediatric Use

The safety and effectiveness of rabeprazole in pediatric patients have not been established.

Use in Women

Duodenal ulcer and erosive esophagitis healing rates in women are similar to those in men. Adverse events and laboratory test abnormalities in women occurred at rates similar to those in men.

Geriatric Use

Of the total number of subjects in clinical studies of ACIPHEX®, 19% were 65 years and over, while 4% were 75 years and over. No overall differences in safety or effectiveness were observed between these subjects and younger subjects, and other reported clinical experience has not identified differences in responses between the elderly and younger patients, but greater sensitivity of some older individuals cannot be ruled out.

ADVERSE REACTIONS

Worldwide, over 2900 patients have been treated with rabeprazole in Phase II–III clinical trials involving various dosages and durations of treatment. In general, rabeprazole treatment has been well-tolerated in both short-term and long-term trials. The adverse events rates were generally similar between the 10 and 20 mg doses.

Incidence in Controlled North American and European Clinical Trials

In an analysis of adverse events assessed as possibly or probably related to treatment appearing in greater than 1% of ACIPHEX® patients and appearing with greater frequency than placebo in controlled North American and European trials, the incidence of headache was 2.4% (n=1552) for ACIPHEX® versus 1.6% (n=258) for placebo.

In short and long-term studies, the following adverse events, regardless of causality, were reported in ACIPHEX®-treated patients. Rare events are those reported in ≤1/1000 patients.

Body as a Whole: asthenia, fever, allergic reaction, chills, malaise, chest pain substernal, neck rigidity, photosensitivity reaction. Rare: abdomen enlarged, face edema, hangover effect. *Cardiovascular System:* hypertension, myocardial infarct, electrocardiogram abnormal, migraine, syncope, angina pectoris, bundle branch block, palpitation, sinus bradycardia, tachycardia. Rare: bradycardia, pulmonary embolus, supraventricular tachycardia, thrombophlebitis, vasodilation, QTC prolongation and ventricular tachycardia. *Digestive System:* diarrhea, nausea, abdominal pain, vomiting, dyspepsia, flatulence, constipation, dry mouth, eructation, gastroenteritis, rectal hemorrhage, melena, anorexia, cholelithiasis, mouth ulceration, stomatitis, dysphagia, gingivitis, cholecystitis, increased appetite, abnormal stools, colitis, esophagitis, glossitis, pancreatitis, proctitis. Rare: bloody diarrhea, cholangitis, duodenitis, gastrointestinal hemorrhage, hepatic encephalopathy, hepatitis, hepatoma, liver fatty deposit, salivary gland enlargement, thirst. *Endocrine System:* hyperthyroidism, hypothyroidism. *Hemic & Lymphatic System:* anemia, ecchymosis, lymphadenopathy, hypochromic anemia. *Metabolic & Nutritional Disorders:* peripheral edema, edema, weight gain, gout, dehydration, weight loss. *Musculo-Skeletal System:* myalgia, arthritis, leg cramps, bone pain, arthrosis, bursitis. Rare: twitching. *Nervous System:* insomnia, anxiety, dizziness, depression, nervousness, somnolence, hypertonia, neuralgia, vertigo, convulsion, abnormal dreams, libido decreased, neuropathy, paresthesia, tremor. Rare: agitation, amnesia, confusion, extrapyramidal syndrome, hyperkinesia. *Respiratory System:* dyspnea, asthma, epistaxis, laryngitis, hiccup, hyperventilation. Rare: apnea, hypoventilation. *Skin and Appendages:* rash, pruritus, sweating, urticaria, alopecia. Rare: dry skin, herpes zoster, psoriasis, skin discoloration. *Special Senses:* cataract, amblyopia, glaucoma, dry eyes, abnormal vision, tinnitus, otitis media. Rare: corneal opacity, blurry vision, diplopia, deafness, eye pain, retinal degeneration, strabismus. *Urogenital System:* cystitis, urinary frequency, dysmenorrhea, dysuria, kidney calculus, metorrhagia, polyuria. Rare: breast enlargement, hematuria, impotence, leukorrhea, menorrhagia, orchitis, urinary incontinence.

Laboratory Values: The following changes in laboratory parameters were reported as adverse events: abnormal platelets, albuminuria, creatine phosphokinase increased, erythrocytes abnormal, hypercholesteremia, hyperglycemia, hyperlipemia, hypokalemia, hyponatremia, leukocytosis, leukorrhea, liver function tests abnormal, prostatic specific antigen increase, SGPT increased, urine abnormality, WBC abnormal.

In controlled clinical studies, 3/1456 (0.2%) patients treated with rabeprazole and 2/237 (0.8%) patients treated with placebo developed treatment-emergent abnormalities (which were either new on study or present at study entry with an increase of 1.25 × baseline value) in SGOT (AST), SGPT (ALT), or both. None of the three rabeprazole patients experienced chills, fever, right upper quadrant pain, nausea or jaundice.

Post-Marketing Adverse Events: Additional adverse events reported from worldwide marketing experience with rabeprazole sodium are: sudden death, coma and hyperammonemia, jaundice, rhabdomyolysis, disorientation and delirium, bullous and other drug eruptions of the skin, interstitial pneumonia, and TSH elevations. In most instances, the relationship to rabeprazole sodium was unclear. In addition, agranulocytosis, hemolytic anemia, leukopenia, pancytopenia, and thrombocytopenia have been reported.

OVERDOSAGE

Because strategies for the management of overdose are continually evolving, it is advisable to contact a Poison Control Center to determine the latest recommendations for the management of an overdose of any drug. There has been no experience with large overdoses with rabeprazole. Seven reports of accidental overdosage with rabeprazole have been received. The maximum reported overdosage was 80 mg. There were no clinical signs or symptoms associated with any reported overdose. Patients with Zollinger-Ellison syndrome have been treated with up to 120 mg rabeprazole QD. No specific antidote for rabeprazole is known. Rabeprazole is extensively protein bound and is not readily dialyzable. In the event of overdosage, treatment should be symptomatic and supportive.

Single oral doses of rabeprazole at 786 mg/kg and 1024 mg/kg were lethal to mice and rats, respectively. The single oral dose of 2000 mg/kg was not lethal to dogs. The major symptoms of acute toxicity were hypoactivity, labored respiration, lateral or prone position and convulsion in mice and rats and watery diarrhea, tremor, convulsion and coma in dogs.

DOSAGE AND ADMINISTRATION

Healing of Erosive or Ulcerative Gastroesophageal Reflux Disease (GERD)

The recommended adult oral dose is one ACIPHEX® 20 mg delayed-release tablet to be taken once daily for four to eight weeks. (See INDICATIONS AND USAGE). For those patients who have not healed after 8 weeks of treatment, an additional 8-week course of ACIPHEX® may be considered.

Maintenance of Healing of Erosive or Ulcerative Gastroesophageal Reflux Disease (GERD Maintenance)

The recommended adult oral dose is one ACIPHEX® 20 mg delayed-release tablet to be taken once daily. (See INDICATIONS AND USAGE).

Healing of Duodenal Ulcers

The recommended adult oral dose is one ACIPHEX® 20 mg delayed-release tablet to be taken once daily after the morning meal for a period up to four weeks. (See INDICATIONS AND USAGE). Most patients with duodenal ulcer heal within four weeks. A few patients may require additional therapy to achieve healing.

Treatment of Pathological Hypersecretory Conditions Including Zollinger-Ellison Syndrome

The dosage of ACIPHEX® in patients with pathologic hypersecretory conditions varies with the individual patient. The recommended adult oral starting dose is 60 mg once a day. Doses should be adjusted to individual patient needs and should continue for as long as clinically indicated. Some patients may require divided doses. Doses up to 100 mg QD and 60 mg BID have been administered. Some patients with Zollinger-Ellison syndrome have been treated continuously with ACIPHEX® for up to one year.

No dosage adjustment is necessary in elderly patients, in patients with renal disease or in patients with mild to moderate hepatic impairment. Administration of rabeprazole to patients with mild to moderate liver impairment resulted in increased exposure and decreased elimination. Due to the lack of clinical data on rabeprazole in patients with severe hepatic impairment, caution should be exercised in those patients.

ACIPHEX® tablets should be swallowed whole. The tablets should not be chewed, crushed, or split.

HOW SUPPLIED

ACIPHEX® 20 mg is supplied as delayed-release light yellow enteric-coated tablets. The medication code number (E243) is imprinted on one side.

Bottles of 30 (NDC#62856-243-30)

Unit Dose Blisters Package of 100 (10 × 10) (NDC#62856-243-41)

Store at 25°C (77°F); excursions permitted to 15–30°C (59–86°F).

Protect from moisture.

Rx only.

ACIPHEX® is a trademark of Eisai Co., Ltd., Tokyo, Japan.

Manufactured by Eisai Co., Ltd.
Misato, Japan
Made in Japan

Marketed by Eisai Inc., Teaneck, NJ 07666
and
Janssen Pharmaceutica Inc., Titusville, NJ 08560-0200

Revised October 1999

200120 © 2000 Eisai Inc.

Shown in Product Identification Guide, page 318

DURAGESIC® ℂ ℞

[*dūr-a-jē 'sik*]

(fentanyl transdermal system)

Full Prescribing Information

> BECAUSE SERIOUS OR LIFE-THREATENING HYPOVENTILATION COULD OCCUR, DURAGESIC® IS CONTRAINDICATED:
> - In the management of acute or post-operative pain, including use in out-patient surgeries
> - In the management of mild or intermittent pain responsive to PRN or non–opioid therapy
> - In doses exceeding 25 μg/hour at the initiation of opioid therapy
>
> (See CONTRAINDICATIONS for further information.)
>
> DURAGESIC® SHOULD NOT BE ADMINISTERED TO CHILDREN UNDER 12 YEARS OF AGE OR PATIENTS UNDER 18 YEARS OF AGE WHO WEIGH LESS THAN 50 KG (110 LBS) EXCEPT IN AN AUTHORIZED INVESTIGATIONAL RESEARCH SETTING. (See PRECAUTIONS - Pediatric Use.)
>
> *DURAGESIC® is indicated for treatment of chronic pain (such as that of malignancy) that:*
> - cannot be managed by lesser means such as acetaminophen-opioid combinations, non-steroidal analgesics, or PRN dosing with short-acting opioids and
> - requires continuous opioid administration.
>
> The 50, 75, and 100 mcg/hour dosages should ONLY be used in patients who are already on and are tolerant to opioid therapy.

DESCRIPTION

DURAGESIC® is a transdermal system providing continuous systemic delivery of fentanyl, a potent opioid analgesic, for 72 hours. The chemical name is N-Phenyl-N-(1-2-phenylethyl-4-piperidyl) propanamide.

The molecular weight of fentanyl base is 336.5, and the empirical formula is $C_{22}H_{28}N_2O$. The n-octanol:water partition coefficient is 860:1. The pKa is 8.4.

System Components and Structure

The amount of fentanyl released from each system per hour is proportional to the surface area (25 μg/h per 10 cm^2). The composition per unit area of all system sizes is identical. Each system also contains 0.1 mL of alcohol USP per 10 cm^2

Dose* (μg/h)	Size (cm^2)	Fentanyl Content (mg)
25	10	2.5
50 **	20	5
75 **	30	7.5
100 **	40	10

* Nominal delivery rate per hour

** FOR USE ONLY IN OPIOID TOLERANT PATIENTS

DURAGESIC® is a rectangular transparent unit comprising a protective liner and four functional layers. Proceeding from the outer surface toward the surface adhering to skin, these layers are:

Continued on next page

Duragesic—Cont.

1) a backing layer of polyester film; 2) a drug reservoir of fentanyl and alcohol USP gelled with hydroxyethyl cellulose;3) an ethylene-vinyl acetate copolymer membrane that controls the rate of fentanyl delivery to the skin surface; and4) a fentanyl containing silicone adhesive. Before use, a protective liner covering the adhesive layer is removed and discarded.

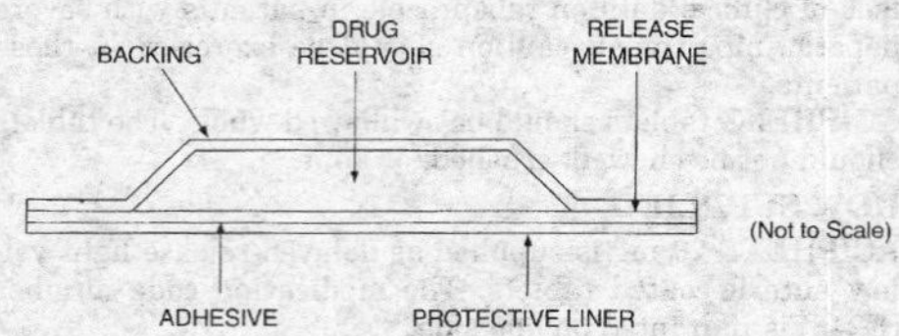

The active component of the system is fentanyl. The remaining components are pharmacologically inactive. Less than 0.2 mL of alcohol is also released from the system during use.

Do not cut or damage DURAGESIC®. If the DURAGESIC® system is cut or damaged, controlled drug delivery will not be possible.

CLINICAL PHARMACOLOGY

Pharmacology

Fentanyl is an opioid analgesic. Fentanyl interacts predominately with the opioid μ-receptor. These μ-binding sites are discretely distributed in the human brain, spinal cord, and other tissues.

In clinical settings, fentanyl exerts its principal pharmacologic effects on the central nervous system. Its primary actions of therapeutic value are analgesia and sedation. Fentanyl may increase the patient's tolerance for pain and decrease the perception of suffering, although the presence of the pain itself may still be recognized.

In addition to analgesia, alterations in mood, euphoria and dysphoria, and drowsiness commonly occur. Fentanyl depresses the respiratory centers, depresses the cough reflex, and constricts the pupils. Analgesic blood levels of fentanyl may cause nausea and vomiting directly by stimulating the chemoreceptor trigger zone, but nausea and vomiting are significantly more common in ambulatory than in recumbent patients, as is postural syncope.

Opioids increase the tone and decrease the propulsive contractions of the smooth muscle of the gastrointestinal tract. The resultant prolongation in gastrointestinal transit time may be responsible for the constipating effect of fentanyl. Because opioids may increase biliary tract pressure, some patients with biliary colic may experience worsening rather than relief of pain.

While opioids generally increase the tone of urinary tract smooth muscle, the net effect tends to be variable, in some cases producing urinary urgency, in others, difficulty in urination.

At therapeutic dosages, fentanyl usually does not exert major effects on the cardiovascular system. However, some patients may exhibit orthostatic hypotension and fainting.

Histamine assays and skin wheal testing in man indicate that clinically significant histamine release rarely occurs with fentanyl administration. Assays in man show no clinically significant histamine release in dosages up to 50 μg/kg.

Pharmacokinetics (see graph and tables)

DURAGESIC® releases fentanyl from the reservoir at a nearly constant amount per unit time. The concentration gradient existing between the saturated solution of drug in the reservoir and the lower concentration in the skin drives drug release. Fentanyl moves in the direction of the lower concentration at a rate determined by the copolymer release membrane and the diffusion of fentanyl through the skin layers. While the actual rate of fentanyl delivery to the skin varies over the 72 hour application period, each system is labeled with a nominal flux which represents the average amount of drug delivered to the systemic circulation per hour across average skin.

While there is variation in dose delivered among patients, the nominal flux of the systems (25, 50, 75, and 100 μg of fentanyl per hour) are sufficiently accurate as to allow individual titration of dosage for a given patient. The small amount of alcohol which has been incorporated into the system enhances the rate of drug flux through the rate-limiting copolymer membrane and increases the permeability of the skin to fentanyl.

Following DURAGESIC® application, the skin under the system absorbs fentanyl, and a depot of fentanyl concentrates in the upper skin layers. Fentanyl then becomes available to the systemic circulation. Serum fentanyl concentrations increase gradually following initial DURAGESIC® application, generally leveling off between 12 and 24 hours and remaining relatively constant, with some fluctuation, for the remainder of the 72 hour application period. Peak serum concentrations of fentanyl generally occurred between 24 and 72 hours after initial application (see Table A). Serum fentanyl concentrations achieved are proportional to the DURAGESIC® delivery rate. With continuous use, serum fentanyl concentrations continue to rise for the first few system applications. After several sequential 72-hour applications, patients reach and maintain a steady state serum concentration that is determined by individual variation in skin permeability and body clearance of fentanyl (see graph and Table B).

After system removal, serum fentanyl concentrations decline gradually, falling about 50% in approximately 17 (range 13–22) hours. Continued absorption of fentanyl from the skin accounts for a slower disappearance of the drug from the serum than is seen after an IV infusion, where the apparent half-life is approximately 7 (range 3–12) hours.

[See graphic at top of page]
[See table A above]
[See table B above]

Fentanyl plasma protein binding capacity decreases with increasing ionization of the drug. Alterations in pH may affect its distribution between plasma and the central nervous system. Fentanyl accumulates in the skeletal muscle and fat and is released slowly into the blood.

The average volume of distribution for fentanyl is 6 L/kg (range 3–8, N=8). The average clearance in patients undergoing various surgical procedures is 46 L/h (range 27–75, N=8). The kinetics of fentanyl in geriatric patients has not been well studied, but in geriatric patients the clearance of IV fentanyl may be reduced and the terminal half-life greatly prolonged (see PRECAUTIONS).

Fentanyl is metabolized primarily via human cytochrome P450 3A4 isoenzyme system. In humans the drug appears to be metabolized primarily by oxidative N-dealkylation to norfentanyl and other inactive metabolites that do not contribute materially to the observed activity of the drug. Within 72 hours of IV fentanyl administration, approximately 75% of the dose is excreted in urine, mostly as metabolites with less than 10% representing unchanged drug. Approximately 9% of the dose is recovered in the feces, primarily as metabolites. Mean values for unbound fractions of fentanyl in plasma are estimated to be between 13 and 21%. Skin does not appear to metabolize fentanyl delivered transdermally. This was determined in a human keratinocyte cell assay and in clinical studies in which 92% of the dose delivered from the system was accounted for as unchanged fentanyl that appeared in the systemic circulation.

Serum Fentanyl Concentrations Following Multiple Applications of DURAGESIC® 100 μg/h (n=10)

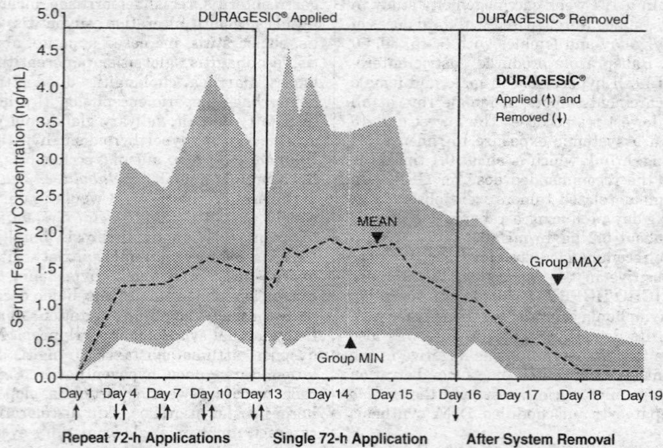

TABLE A
FENTANYL PHARMACOKINETIC PARAMETERS FOLLOWING FIRST 72-HOUR APPLICATION OF DURAGESIC®

Dose	Mean (SD) Time to Maximal Concentration T_{max} (h)	Mean (SD) Maximal Concentration C_{max} (ng/mL)
DURAGESIC® 25 μg/h	38.1 (18.0)	0.6 (0.3)
DURAGESIC® 50 μg/h	34.8 (15.4)	1.4 (0.5)
DURAGESIC® 75 μg/h	33.5 (14.5)	1.7 (0.7)
DURAGESIC® 100 μg/h	36.8 (15.7)	2.5 (1.2)

NOTE: After system removal there is continued systemic absorption from residual fentanyl in the skin so that serum concentrations fall 50%, on average, in 17 hours.

TABLE B
RANGE OF PHARMACOKINETIC PARAMETERS OF INTRAVENOUS FENTANYL IN PATIENTS

	Clearance (L/h) Range [70 kg]	Volume of Distribution V_{ss} (L/kg) Range	Half-Life t½ (h) Range
Surgical Patients	27–75	3–8	3–12
Hepatically Impaired Patients	3–80⁺	0.8–8⁺	4–12⁺
Renally Impaired Patients	30–78	—	—

⁺Estimated

NOTE: Information on volume of distribution and half-life not available for renally impaired patients.

Pharmacodynamics

Analgesia

DURAGESIC® is a strong opioid analgesic. In controlled clinical trials in non-opioid-tolerant patients, 60 mg/day IM morphine was considered to provide analgesia approximately equivalent to DURAGESIC® 100 μg/h in an acute pain model.

Minimum effective analgesic serum concentrations of fentanyl in opioid naive patients range from 0.2 to 1.2 ng/mL; side effects increase in frequency at serum levels above 2 ng/mL. Both the minimum effective concentration and the concentration at which toxicity occurs rise with increasing tolerance. The rate of development of tolerance varies widely among individuals.

Ventilatory Effects

At equivalent analgesic serum concentrations, fentanyl and morphine produce a similar degree of hypoventilation. A small number of patients have experienced clinically significant hypoventilation with DURAGESIC®. Hypoventilation was manifest by respiratory rates of less than 8 breaths/minute or a pCO_2 greater than 55 mm Hg. In clinical trials of 357 postoperative (acute pain) patients treated with DURAGESIC®, 13 patients experienced hypoventilation. In these studies the incidence of hypoventilation was higher in nontolerant women (10) than in men (3) and in patients weighing less than 63 kg (9 of 13). Although patients with impaired respiration were not common in the trials, they had higher rates of hypoventilation. In addition, post-marketing reports have been received of opioid-naive post-operative patients who have experienced clinically significant hypoventilation with DURAGESIC®. DURAGESIC® is contraindicated in the treatment of postoperative and acute pain.

While most patients using DURAGESIC® chronically develop tolerance to fentanyl induced hypoventilation, episodes of slowed respirations may occur at any time during therapy; medical intervention generally was not required in these instances.

Hypoventilation can occur throughout the therapeutic range of fentanyl serum concentrations. However, in non-opioid-tolerant patients the risk of hypoventilation increases at serum fentanyl concentrations greater than 2 ng/mL, especially for patients who have an underlying pulmonary condition or who receive usual doses of opioids or other CNS drugs associated with hypoventilation in addition to DURAGESIC®. The use of initial doses exceeding 25 µg/h is contraindicated in patients who are not tolerant to opioid therapy. The use of DURAGESIC® should be monitored by clinical evaluation. As with other drug level measurements, serum fentanyl concentrations may be useful clinically, although they do not reflect patient sensitivity to fentanyl and should not be used by physicians as a sole indicator of effectiveness or toxicity.

See BOX WARNING, CONTRAINDICATIONS, WARNINGS, PRECAUTIONS, ADVERSE REACTIONS, and OVERDOSAGE for additional information on hypoventilation.

Cardiovascular Effects

Fentanyl may infrequently produce bradycardia. The incidence of bradycardia in clinical trials with DURAGESIC® was less than 1%.

CNS Effects

In opioid naive patients, central nervous system effects increase when serum fentanyl concentrations are greater than 3 ng/mL.

CLINICAL TRIALS

DURAGESIC® (fentanyl transdermal system) was studied in patients with acute and chronic pain (postoperative and cancer pain models); however, DURAGESIC® is contraindicated for postoperative analgesia.

The analgesic efficacy of DURAGESIC® was demonstrated in an acute pain model with surgical procedures expected to produce various intensities of pain (eg hysterectomy, major orthopedic surgery). Clinical use and safety was evaluated in patients experiencing chronic pain due to malignancy. Based on the results of these trials, DURAGESIC® was determined to be effective in both populations, but safe only for use in patients with chronic pain. Because of the risk of hypoventilation (4% incidence) in postoperative patients with actue pain, DURAGESIC® is contraindicated for postoperative analgesia. (See BOX WARNING, CLINICAL PHARMACOLOGY–Ventilatory Effects, and CONTRAINDICATIONS.)

DURAGESIC® as therapy for pain due to cancer has been studied in 153 patients. In this patient population, DURAGESIC® has been administered in doses of 25 µg/h to 600 µg/h. Individual patients have used DURAGESIC® continuously for up to 866 days. At one month after initiation of DURAGESIC® therapy, patients generally reported lower pain intensity scores as compared to a prestudy analgesic regimen of oral morphine (see graph).

Visual Analogue Score of Pain Intensity Ratings at Entry in the Study and After One Month of DURAGESIC® Use

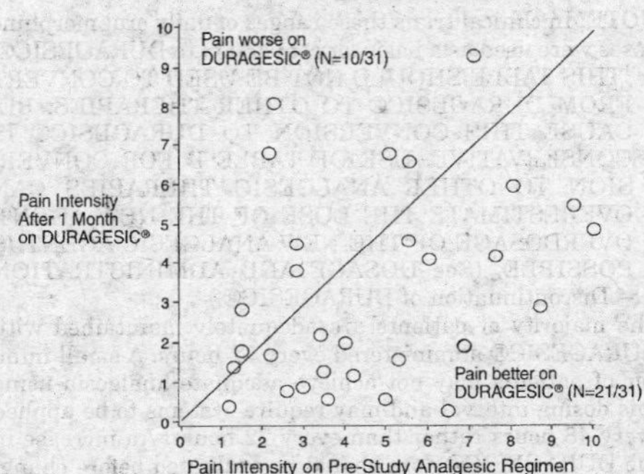

INDICATIONS AND USAGE

DURAGESIC® (fentanyl transdermal system) is indicated in the management of chronic pain in patients who require continuous opioid analgesia for pain that cannot be managed by lesser means such as acetaminophen-opioid combinations, non-steroidal analgesics, or PRN dosing with short-acting opioids.

DURAGESIC® should not be used in the management of acute or postoperative pain because serious or life-threatening hypoventilation could result. (See BOX WARNING and CONTRAINDICATIONS.)

In patients with chronic pain, it is possible to individually titrate the dose of the transdermal system to minimize the risk of adverse effects while providing analgesia. In properly selected patients, DURAGESIC® is a safe and effective alternative to other opioid regimens. (See DOSAGE AND ADMINISTRATION.)

CONTRAINDICATIONS

BECAUSE SERIOUS OR LIFE-THREATENING HYPOVENTILATION COULD OCCUR, DURAGESIC® (FENTANYL TRANSDERMAL SYSTEM) IS CONTRAINDICATED:

- **in the management of acute or post-operative pain, including use in out-patient surgeries because there is no opportunity for proper dose titration (See CLINICAL PHARMACOLOGY and DOSAGE AND ADMINISTRATION),**
- **in the management of mild or intermittent pain that can otherwise be managed by lesser means such as acetaminophen-opioid combinations, non-steriodal analgesics, or PRN dosing with short-acting opioids, and**
- **in doses exceeding 25 µg/hour at the initiation of opioid therapy because of the need to individualize dosing by titrating to the desired analgesic effect.**

DURAGESIC® is also contraindicated in patients with known hypersensitivity to fentanyl or adhesives.

WARNINGS

DURAGESIC® (FENTANYL TRANSDERMAL SYSTEM) SHOULD NOT BE ADMINISTERED TO CHILDREN UNDER 12 YEARS OF AGE OR PATIENTS UNDER 18 YEARS OF AGE WHO WEIGH LESS THAN 50 KG (110 LBS) EXCEPT IN AN AUTHORIZED INVESTIGATIONAL RESEARCH SETTING. (See PRECAUTIONS-Pediatric Use.)

PATIENTS WHO HAVE EXPERIENCED ADVERSE EVENTS SHOULD BE MONITORED FOR AT LEAST 12 HOURS AFTER DURAGESIC® REMOVAL SINCE SERUM FENTANYL CONCENTRATIONS DECLINE GRADUALLY AND REACH AN APPROXIMATE 50% REDUCTION IN SERUM CONCENTRATIONS 17 HOURS AFTER SYSTEM REMOVAL.

DURAGESIC® SHOULD BE PRESCRIBED ONLY BY PERSONS KNOWLEDGEABLE IN THE CONTINUOUS ADMINISTRATION OF POTENT OPIOIDS, IN THE MANAGEMENT OF PATIENTS RECEIVING POTENT OPIOIDS FOR TREATMENT OF PAIN, AND IN THE DETECTION AND MANAGEMENT OF HYPOVENTILATION INCLUDING THE USE OF OPIOID ANTAGONISTS.

THE CONCOMITANT USE OF OTHER CENTRAL NERVOUS SYSTEM DEPRESSANTS, INCLUDING OTHER OPIOIDS, SEDATIVES OR HYPNOTICS, GENERAL ANESTHETICS, PHENOTHIAZINES, TRANQUILIZERS, SKELETAL MUSCLE RELAXANTS, SEDATING ANTIHISTAMINES, AND ALCOHOLIC BEVERAGES MAY PRODUCE ADDITIVE DEPRESSANT EFFECTS. HYPOVENTILATION, HYPOTENSION AND PROFOUND SEDATION OR COMA MAY OCCUR. WHEN SUCH COMBINED THERAPY IS CONTEMPLATED, THE DOSE OF ONE OR BOTH AGENTS SHOULD BE REDUCED BY AT LEAST 50%.

ALL PATIENTS SHOULD BE ADVISED TO AVOID EXPOSING THE DURAGESIC® APPLICATION SITE TO DIRECT EXTERNAL HEAT SOURCES, SUCH AS HEATING PADS OR ELECTRIC BLANKETS, HEAT LAMPS, SAUNAS, HOT TUBS, AND HEATED WATER BEDS, ETC. WHILE WEARING THE SYSTEM. THERE IS A POTENTIAL FOR TEMPERATURE-DEPENDENT INCREASES IN FENTANYL RELEASE FROM THE SYSTEM. (See PRECAUTIONS, Patients with Fever/External Heat.)

PRECAUTIONS

General

DURAGESIC® (fentanyl transdermal system) doses greater than 25 µg/h are too high for initiation of therapy in non opioid-tolerant patients and should not be used to begin DURAGESIC® therapy in these patients. (See BOX WARNING.)

DURAGESIC® may impair mental and/or physical ability required for the performance of potentially hazardous tasks (eg driving, operating machinery). Patients who have been given DURAGESIC® should not drive or operate dangerous machinery unless they are tolerant to the side effects of the drug.

Patients should be instructed to keep both used and unused systems out of the reach of children. Used systems should be folded so that the adhesive side of the system adheres to itself and flushed down the toilet immediately upon removal. Patients should be advised to dispose of any systems remaining from a prescription as soon as they are no longer needed. Unused systems should be removed from their pouch and flushed down the toilet.

Hypoventilation (Respiratory Depression)

Hypoventilation may occur at any time during the use of DURAGESIC®.

Because significant amounts of fentanyl are absorbed from the skin for 17 hours or more after the system is removed, hypoventilation may persist beyond the removal of DURAGESIC®. Consequently, patients with hypoventilation should be carefully observed for degree of sedation and their respiratory rate monitored until respiration has stabilized.

The use of concomitant CNS active drugs requires special patient care and observation. (See WARNINGS.)

Chronic Pulmonary Disease

Because potent opioids can cause hypoventilation, DURAGESIC® (fentanyl transdermal system) should be administered with caution to patients with preexisting medical conditions predisposing them to hypoventilation. In such patients, normal analgesic doses of opioids may further decrease respiratory drive to the point of respiratory failure.

Head Injuries and Increased Intracranial Pressure

DURAGESIC® should not be used in patients who may be particularly susceptible to the intracranial effects of CO_2 retention such as those with evidence of increased intracranial pressure, impaired consciousness, or coma. Opioids may obscure the clinical course of patients with head injury. DURAGESIC® should be used with caution in patients with brain tumors.

Cardiac Disease

Intravenous fentanyl may produce bradycardia. Fentanyl should be administered with caution to patients with bradyarrhythmias.

Hepatic or Renal Disease

At the present time insufficient information exists to make recommendations regarding the use of DURAGESIC® in patients with impaired renal or hepatic function. If the drug is used in these patients, it should be used with caution because of the hepatic metabolism and renal excretion of fentanyl.

Patients with Fever/External Heat

Based on a pharmacokinetic model, serum fentanyl concentrations could theoretically increase by approximately one third for patients with a body temperature of 40°C (104°F) due to temperature-dependent increases in fentanyl release from the system and increased skin permeability. Therefore, patients wearing DURAGESIC® systems who develop fever should be monitored for opioid side effects and the DURAGESIC® dose should be adjusted if necessary.

ALL PATIENTS SHOULD BE ADVISED TO AVOID EXPOSING THE DURAGESIC® APPLICATION SITE TO DIRECT EXTERNAL HEAT SOURCES, SUCH AS HEATING PADS OR ELECTRIC BLANKETS, HEAT LAMPS, SAUNAS, HOT TUBS, AND HEATED WATER BEDS, ETC. WHILE WEARING THE SYSTEM. THERE IS A POTENTIAL FOR TEMPERATURE-DEPENDENT INCREASES IN FENTANYL RELEASE FROM THE SYSTEM.

Central Nervous System Depressants

When patients are receiving DURAGESIC®, the dose of additional opioids or other CNS depressant drugs (including benzodiazepines) should be reduced by at least 50%. With the concomitant use of CNS depressants, hypotension may occur.

Agents Affecting Cytochrome P450 3A4 Isoenzyme System

Fentanyl is metabolized mainly via the human cytochrome P450 3A4 isoenzyme system (CYP34A), therefore potential interactions may occur when DURAGESIC® is given concurrently with agents that affect CYP3A4 activity. It is therefore recommended to employ appropriate clinical monitoring when coadministering DURAGESIC® with agents that affect CYP3A4 activity.

Drug or Alcohol Dependence

Use of DURAGESIC® in combination with alcoholic beverages and/or other CNS depressants can result in increased risk to the patient. DURAGESIC® should be used with caution in individuals who have a history of drug or alcohol abuse, especially if they are outside a medically controlled environment.

Ambulatory Patients

Strong opioid analgesics impair the mental or physical abilities required for the performance of potentially dangerous tasks such as driving a car or operating machinery. Patients who have been given DURAGESIC® should not drive or operate dangerous machinery unless they are tolerant to the effects of the drug.

Carcinogenesis, Mutagenesis, and Impairment of Fertility

Because long-term animal studies have not been conducted, the potential carcinogenic effects of DURAGESIC® are unknown. There was no evidence of mutagenicity in the Ames *Salmonella typhimurium* mutagenicity assay, the primary rat hepatocyte unscheduled DNA synthesis assay, the BALB/c-3T3 transformation test, the mouse lymphoma assay, the human lymphocyte and CHO chromosomal aberration in-vitro assays or the in-vivo micronucleus test.

Pregnancy—Pregnancy Category C

Fentanyl has been shown to impair fertility and to have an embryocidal effect in rats when given in intravenous doses 0.3 times the human dose for a period of 12 days. No evidence of teratogenic effects has been observed after administration of fentanyl to rats. There are no adequate and well-controlled studies in pregnant women. DURAGESIC® should be used during pregnancy only if the potential benefit justifies the potential risk to the fetus.

Labor and Delivery

DURAGESIC® is not recommended for analgesia during labor and delivery.

Nursing Mothers

Fentanyl is excreted in human milk; therefore DURAGESIC® is not recommended for use in nursing women because of the possibility of effects in their infants.

Pediatric Use

The safety and efficacy of DURAGESIC® in pediatric patients has not been established. (See BOX WARNING and CONTRAINDICATIONS.)

DURAGESIC® SHOULD NOT BE ADMINISTERED TO CHILDREN UNDER 12 YEARS OF AGE OR PATIENTS UNDER 18 YEARS OF AGE WHO WEIGH LESS THAN 50 KG (110 LBS) EXCEPT IN AN AUTHORIZED INVESTIGATIONAL RESEARCH SETTING.

Geriatric Use

Information from a pilot study of the pharmacokinetics of IV fentanyl in geriatric patients indicates that the clearance of fentanyl may be greatly decreased in the population above the age of 60. The relevance of these findings to transdermal fentanyl is unknown at this time.

Since elderly, cachectic, or debilitated patients may have altered pharmacokinetics due to poor fat stores, muscle wasting, or altered clearance, they should not be started on DURAGESIC® doses higher than 25 µg/h unless they are already taking more than 135 mg of oral morphine a day or an equivalent dose of another opioid (see DOSAGE AND ADMINISTRATION).

Information for Patients

A patient instruction sheet is included in the package of DURAGESIC® systems dispensed to the patient.

Disposal of DURAGESIC®

DURAGESIC® should be kept out of the reach of children. DURAGESIC® systems should be folded so that the adhesive side of the system adheres to itself, then the system should be flushed down the toilet immediately upon removal. Patients should dispose of any systems remaining from a prescription as soon as they are no longer needed. Unused systems should be removed from their pouch and flushed down the toilet.

Continued on next page

Duragesic—Cont.

If the gel from the drug reservoir accidentally contacts the skin, the area should be washed with clear water.

ADVERSE REACTIONS

In post-marketing experience, deaths from hypoventilation due to inappropriate use of DURAGESIC® have been reported. (See BOX WARNING and CONTRAINDICATIONS.)

Pre-marketing Clinical Trial Experience:
The safety of DURAGESIC® has been evaluated in 357 postoperative patients and 153 cancer patients for a total of 510 patients. Patients with acute pain used DURAGESIC® for 1 to 3 days. The duration of DURAGESIC® use varied in cancer patients; 56% of patients used DURAGESIC® for over 30 days, 28% continued treatment for more than 4 months, and 10% used DURAGESIC® for more than 1 year.
Hypoventilation was the most serious adverse reaction observed in 13 (4%) postoperative patients and in 3 (2%) of the cancer patients. Hypotension and hypertension were observed in 11 (3%) and 4 (1%) of the opioid-naive patients.
Various adverse events were reported; a causal relationship to DURAGESIC® was not always determined. The frequencies presented here reflect the actual frequency of each adverse effect in patients who received DURAGESIC®. There has been no attempt to correct for a placebo effect, concomitant use of other opioids, or to subtract the frequencies reported by placebo-treated patients in controlled trials.
The following adverse reactions were reported in 153 cancer patients at a frequency of 1% or greater; similar reactions were seen in the 357 postoperative patients studied.
Body as a Whole: abdominal pain*, headache*
Cardiovascular: arrhythmia, chest pain
Digestive: nausea**, vomiting**, constipation**, dry mouth**, anorexia*, diarrhea*, dyspepsia*, flatulence
Nervous: somnolence**, confusion**, asthenia**, dizziness*, nervousness*, hallucinations*, anxiety*, depression*, euphoria*, tremor, abnormal coordination, speech disorder, abnormal thinking, abnormal gait, abnormal dreams, agitation, paresthesia, amnesia, syncope, paranoid reaction
Respiratory: dyspnea*, hypoventilation*, apnea*, hemoptysis, pharyngitis, hiccups
Skin and Appendages: sweating**, pruritus*, rash, application site reaction - erythema, papules, itching, edema
Urogenital: urinary retention*
*Reactions occurring in 3%–10% of DURAGESIC® patients
**Reactions occurring in 10% or more of DURAGESIC® patients

The following adverse effects have been reported in less than 1% of the 510 postoperative and cancer patients studied; the association between these events and DURAGESIC® administration is unknown. This information is listed to serve as alerting information for the physician.
Digestive: abdominal distention
Nervous: aphasia, hypertonia, vertigo, stupor, hypotonia, depersonalization, hostility
Respiratory: stertorous breathing, asthma, respiratory disorder
Skin and Appendages, General: exfoliative dermatitis, pustules
Special Senses: amblyopia
Urogenital: bladder pain, oliguria, urinary frequency

DRUG ABUSE AND DEPENDENCE

Fentanyl is a Schedule II controlled substance and can produce drug dependence similar to that produced by morphine. DURAGESIC® (fentanyl transdermal system) therefore has the potential for abuse. Tolerance, physical and psychological dependence may develop upon repeated administration of opioids. Iatrogenic addiction following opioid administration is relatively rare. Physicians should not let concerns of physical dependence deter them from using adequate amounts of opioids in the management of severe pain when such use is indicated.

OVERDOSAGE

Clinical Presentation
The manifestations of fentanyl overdosage are an extension of its pharmacologic actions with the most serious significant effect being hypoventilation.
Treatment
For the management of hypoventilation immediate countermeasures include removing the DURAGESIC® (fentanyl transdermal system) system and physically or verbally stimulating the patient. These actions can be followed by administration of a specific narcotic antagonist such as naloxone. The duration of hypoventilation following an overdose may be longer than the effects of the narcotic antagonist's action (the half-life of naloxone ranges from 30 to 81 minutes). The interval between IV antagonist doses should be carefully chosen because of the possibility of re-narcotization after system removal; repeated administration of naloxone may be necessary. Reversal of the narcotic effect may result in acute onset of pain and the release of catecholamines.
If the clinical situation warrants, ensure a patent airway is established and maintained, administer oxygen and assist or control respiration as indicated and use an oropharyngeal airway or endotracheal tube if necessary. Adequate body temperature and fluid intake should be maintained.
If severe or persistent hypotension occurs, the possibility of hypovolemia should be considered and managed with appropriate parenteral fluid therapy.

DOSAGE AND ADMINISTRATION

With all opioids, the safety of patients using the products is dependent on health care practitioners prescribing them in strict conformity with their approved labeling with respect to patient selection, dosing, and proper conditions for use.
As with all opioids, dosage should be individualized. The most important factor to be considered in determining the appropriate dose is the extent of preexisting opioid tolerance. (See BOX WARNING and CONTRAINDICATIONS.)
Initial doses should be reduced in elderly or debilitated patients (see PRECAUTIONS).
DURAGESIC® (fentanyl transdermal system) should be applied to non-irritated and non-irradiated skin on a flat surface such as chest, back, flank or upper arm. Hair at the application site should be clipped (not shaved) prior to system application. If the site of DURAGESIC® application must be cleansed prior to application of the system, do so with clear water. Do not use soaps, oils, lotions, alcohol, or any other agents that might irritate the skin or alter its characteristics. Allow the skin to dry completely prior to system application.
DURAGESIC® should be applied immediately upon removal from the sealed package. Do not alter the system, e.g., cut, in any way prior to application.
The transdermal system should be pressed firmly in place with the palm of the hand for 30 seconds, making sure the contact is complete, especially around the edges.
Each DURAGESIC® may be worn continuously for 72 hours. If analgesia for more than 72 hours is required, a new system should be applied to a different skin site after removal of the previous transdermal system.
DURAGESIC® should be kept out of the reach of children. Used systems should be folded so that the adhesive side of the system adheres to itself, then the system should be flushed down the toilet immediately upon removal. Patients should dispose of any systems remaining from a prescription as soon as they are no longer needed. Unused systems should be removed from their pouch and flushed down the toilet.
Dose Selection
DOSES MUST BE INDIVIDUALIZED BASED UPON THE STATUS OF EACH PATIENT AND SHOULD BE ASSESSED AT REGULAR INTERVALS AFTER DURAGESIC® APPLICATION. REDUCED DOSES OF DURAGESIC® ARE SUGGESTED FOR THE ELDERLY AND OTHER GROUPS DISCUSSED IN PRECAUTIONS.
DURAGESIC® DOSES GREATER THAN 25 µG/H SHOULD NOT BE USED FOR INITIATION OF DURAGESIC® THERAPY IN NON-OPIOID TOLERANT PATIENTS.
In selecting an initial DURAGESIC® dose, attention should be given to 1) the daily dose, potency, and characteristics of the opioid the patient has been taking previously (eg whether it is a pure agonist or mixed agonist-antagonist), 2) the reliability of the relative potency estimates used to calculate the DURAGESIC® dose needed (potency estimates may vary with the route of administration), 3) the degree of opioid tolerance, if any, and 4) the general condition and medical status of the patient. Each patient should be maintained at the lowest dose providing acceptable pain control.
Initial DURAGESIC® Dose Selection
There has been no systematic evaluation of DURAGESIC® as an initial opioid analgesic in the management of chronic pain, since most patients in the clinical trials were converted to DURAGESIC® from other narcotics. Therefore, unless the patient has pre-existing opioid tolerance, the lowest DURAGESIC® dose, 25 µg/h, should be used as the initial dose.
To convert patients from oral or parenteral opioids to DURAGESIC® use the following methodology:

1. Calculate the previous 24-hour analgesic requirement.
2. Convert this amount to the equianalgesic oral morphine dose using Table C.
3. Table D displays the range of 24-hour oral morphine doses that are recommended for conversion to each DURAGESIC® dose. Use this table to find the calculated 24-hour morphine dose and the corresponding DURAGESIC® dose. Initiate DURAGESIC® treatment using the recommended dose and titrate patients upwards (no more frequently than every 3 days after the initial dose or than every 6 days thereafter) until analgesic efficacy is attained. The recommended starting dose when converting from other opioids to DURAGESIC® is likely too low for 50% of patients. This starting dose is recommended to minimize the potential for overdosing patients with the first dose. For delivery rates in excess of 100 µg/h, multiple systems may be used.

TABLE C[a]
EQUIANALGESIC POTENCY CONVERSION

Name	Equianalgesic Dose (mg) IM[b,c]	PO
morphine	10	60 (30)[d]
hydromorphone (Dilaudid®)	1.5	7.5
methadone (Dolophine®)	10	20
oxycodone (Percocet®)	15	30
levorphanol (Levo-Dromoran®)	2	4
oxymorphone (Numorphan®)	1	10 (PR)
heroin	5	60
meperidine (Demerol®)	75	—
codeine	130	200

[a] All IM and PO doses in this chart are considered equivalent to 10 mg of IM morphine in analgesic effect. IM denotes intramuscular, PO oral, and PR rectal.
[b] Based on single-dose studies in which an intramuscular dose of each drug listed was compared with morphine to establish the relative potency. Oral doses are those recommended when changing from parenteral to an oral route. Reference: Foley, K.M. (1985) The treatment of cancer pain. NEJM 313(2): 84–95
[c] Although controlled studies are not available, in clinical practice it is customary to consider the doses of opioid given IM, IV or subcutaneously to be equivalent. There may be some differences in pharmacokinetic parameters such as C_{max} and T_{max}.
[d] The conversion ratio of 10 mg parenteral morphine = 30 mg oral morphine is based on clinical experience in patients with chronic pain. The conversion ratio of 10 mg parenteral morphine =60 mg oral morphine is based on a potency study in acute pain. Reference: Ashburn and Lipman (1993) Management of pain in the cancer patient. Anesth Analg 76: 402–416.

TABLE D
RECOMMENDED DURAGESIC® DOSE BASED UPON DAILY ORAL MORPHINE DOSE

Oral 24-hour Morphine (mg/day)	DURAGESIC® Dose (µg/hr)
45–134	25
135–224	50
225–314	75
315–404	100
405–494	125
495–584	150
585–674	175
675–764	200
765–854	225
855–944	250
945–1034	275
1035–1124	300

NOTE: In clinical trials these ranges of daily oral morphine doses were used as a basis for conversion to DURAGESIC®.
[1]THIS TABLE SHOULD NOT BE USED TO CONVERT FROM DURAGESIC® TO OTHER THERAPIES, BECAUSE THIS CONVERSION TO DURAGESIC® IS CONSERVATIVE. USE OF TABLE D FOR CONVERSION TO OTHER ANALGESIC THERAPIES CAN OVERESTIMATE THE DOSE OF THE NEW AGENT. OVERDOSAGE OF THE NEW ANALGESIC AGENT IS POSSIBLE. (See DOSAGE AND ADMINISTRATION—Discontinuation of DURAGESIC®.)
The majority of patients are adequately maintained with DURAGESIC® administered every 72 hours. A small number of patients may not achieve adequate analgesia using this dosing interval and may require systems to be applied every 48 hours rather than every 72 hours. An increase in the DURAGESIC® dose should be evaluated before changing dosing intervals in order to maintain patients on a 72-hour regimen.
Because of the increase in serum fentanyl concentration over the first 24 hours following initial system application, the initial evaluation of the maximum analgesic effect of DURAGESIC® cannot be made before 24 hours of wearing. The initial DURAGESIC® dosage may be increased after 3 days (see Dose Titration).
During the initial application of DURAGESIC®, patients should use short-acting analgesics as needed until analgesic efficacy with DURAGESIC® is attained. Thereafter, some patients still may require periodic supplemental doses of other short-acting analgesics for 'breakthrough' pain.
Dose Titration
The recommended initial DURAGESIC® dose based upon the daily oral morphine is conservative, and 50% of patients are likely to require a dose increase after initial application of DURAGESIC®. The initial DURAGESIC® dosage may be increased after 3 days, based on the daily dose of supplemental analgesics required by the patient in the second or third day of the initial application.
Physicians are advised that it may take up to 6 days after increasing the dose of DURAGESIC® for the patient to reach equilibrium on the new dose (see graph in CLINICAL PHARMACOLOGY). Therefore, patients should wear a higher dose through two applications before any further increase in dosage is made on the basis of the average daily use of a supplemental analgesic.
Appropriate dosage increments should be based on the daily dose of supplementary opioids, using the ratio of 90 mg/24 hours of oral morphine to a 25 µg/h increase in DURAGESIC® dose.

Discontinuation of DURAGESIC®

To convert patients to another opioid, remove DURAGESIC® and titrate the dose of the new analgesic based upon the patient's report of pain until adequate analgesia has been attained. Upon system removal, 17 hours or more are required for a 50% decrease in serum fentanyl concentrations. Opioid withdrawal symptoms (such as nausea, vomiting, diarrhea, anxiety, and shivering) are possible in some patients after conversion or dose adjustment. For patients requiring discontinuation of opioids, a gradual downward titration is recommended since it is not known what dose level the opioid may be discontinued without producing the signs and symptoms of abrupt withdrawal.

TABLE D SHOULD NOT BE USED TO CONVERT FROM DURAGESIC® TO OTHER THERAPIES. BECAUSE THE CONVERSION TO DURAGESIC® IS CONSERVATIVE, USE OF TABLE D FOR CONVERSION TO OTHER ANALGESIC THERAPIES CAN OVERESTIMATE THE DOSE OF THE NEW AGENT. OVERDOSAGE OF THE NEW ANALGESIC AGENT IS POSSIBLE.

HOW SUPPLIED

DURAGESIC® is supplied in cartons containing 5 individually packaged systems. See chart for information regarding individual systems.

DURAGESIC® Dose (µg/h)	System Size (cm^2)	Fentanyl Content (mg)	NDC Number
DURAGESIC®-25	10	2.5	50458-033-05
DURAGESIC®-50*	20	5	50458-034-05
DURAGESIC®-75*	30	7.5	50458-035-05
DURAGESIC®-100*	40	10	50458-036-05

* FOR USE ONLY IN OPIOID TOLERANT PATIENTS.

Safety and Handling

DURAGESIC® is supplied in sealed transdermal systems which pose little risk of exposure to health care workers. If the gel from the drug reservoir accidentally contacts the skin, the area should be washed with copious amounts of water. Do not use soap, alcohol, or other solvents to remove the gel because they may enhance the drug's ability to penetrate the skin. Do not cut or damage DURAGESIC®. If the DURAGESIC® system is cut or damaged, controlled drug delivery will not be possible.

Do not store above 77°F (25°C). Apply immediately after removal from individual sealed package. Do not use if the seal is broken. **For transdermal use only.**

CAUTION: Rx only

DEA order form required. A schedule CII narcotic.

Manufactured by:
ALZA Corporation
Mountain View, CA 94304
Distributed by:
JANSSEN PHARMACEUTICA
Titusville, NJ 08560

Revised November 1999, January 2000

Shown in Product Identification Guide, page 318

ERGAMISOL® ℞

[ər-gam 'ə-, sōl]
(levamisole hydrochloride)
Tablets

DESCRIPTION

ERGAMISOL® (levamisole hydrochloride) is an immunomodulator available in tablets for oral administration containing the equivalent of 50 mg as levamisole base. Fifty-nine (59) mg of levamisole HCl is equivalent to 50 mg of levamisole base. Inactive ingredients are colloidal silicon dioxide, hydrogenated vegetable oil, hydroxypropyl methylcellulose, lactose, microcystalline cellulose, polyethylene glycol 6000, polysorbate 80, and talc.

Levamisole hydrochloride is (-)-(S)-2,3,5,6-tetrahydro-6-phenylimidazo [2,1-b] thiazole monohydrochloride.

Levamisole hydrochloride is a white to almost white crystalline powder which is almost odorless and is freely soluble in water. It is quite stable in acid aqueous media but hydrolyzes in alkaline or neutral solutions. It has a molecular weight of 240.75.

CLINICAL PHARMACOLOGY

Two clinical trials having essentially the same design have demonstrated an increase in survival and a reduction in recurrence rate in the subset of patients with resected Dukes' C colon cancer treated with a regimen of ERGAMISOL® (levamisole hydrochloride) plus fluorouracil[1,2]. After surgery, patients were randomized to no further therapy, ERGAMISOL® alone, or ERGAMISOL® plus fluorouracil. In one clinical trial in which 408 Dukes' B and C colorectal cancer patients were studied, 262 Dukes' C patients were evaluated for a minimum follow-up of five years[1]. A subset analysis of these Dukes' C patients showed the estimated reduction in death rate was 27% for ERGAMISOL® plus fluorouracil (p = 0.11) and 28% for ERGAMISOL® alone (p = 0.11)[3]. The estimated reduction in recurrence rate was 36% for ERGAMISOL® plus fluorouracil (p = 0.025) and 28% for ERGAMISOL® alone (p = 0.11)[3]. In another clinical trial designed to confirm the above results, 929 Dukes' C colon cancer patients were evaluated for a minimum follow-up of 2 years[2]. The estimated reduction in death rate was 33% for ERGAMISOL® plus fluorouracil (p = 0.006). The estimated reduction in recurrence rate was 41% for ERGAMISOL® plus fluorouracil (p<0.0001). The ERGAMISOL® alone group did not show advantage over no treatment on improving recurrence or survival rates. There are presently insufficient data to evaluate the effect of the combination of ERGAMISOL® plus fluorouracil in Dukes' B patients. There are also insufficient data to evaluate the effect of ERGAMISOL® plus fluorouracil in patients with rectal cancer because only 12 patients with rectal cancer were treated with the combination in the first study and none in the second study.

The mechanism of action of ERGAMISOL® in combination with fluorouracil is unknown. The effects of levamisole on the immune system are complex. The drug appears to restore depressed immune function rather than to stimulate response to above-normal levels. Levamisole can stimulate formation of antibodies to various antigens, enhance T-cell responses by stimulating T-cell activation and proliferation, potentiate monocyte and macrophage functions including phagocytosis and chemotaxis, and increase neutrophil mobility, adherence, and chemotaxis. Other drugs have similar short-term effects and the clinical relevance is unclear.

Besides its immunomodulatory function, levamisole has other mammalian pharmacologic activities, including inhibition of alkaline phosphatase, and cholinergic activity.

The pharmacokinetics of ERGAMISOL® have not been studied in the dosage regimen recommended with fluorouracil. After administration of a single oral dose of 50 mg of a research formulation of ERGAMISOL®, it appears that levamisole is rapidly absorbed from the gastrointestinal tract. Mean peak plasma concentrations of 0.13 mcg/ml are attained within 1.5 to 2 hours. The plasma elimination half-life of levamisole is between 3–4 hours. Following a 150-mg radio-labeled dose, levamisole is extensively metabolized by the liver in humans and the metabolites excreted mainly by the kidneys (70% over 3 days). The elimination half-life of metabolite excretion is 16 hours. Approximately 5% is excreted in the feces. Less than 5% is excreted unchanged in the urine and less than 0.2% in the feces. Approximately 12% is recovered in the urine as the glucuronide of p-hydroxy-levamisole. The clinical significance of these data are unknown since a 150-mg dose may not be proportional to a 50-mg dose. In the presence of cirrhosis in twelve patients with alcoholic cirrhosis and hepatitis, the Cmax of ERGAMISOL® was not clearly increased, but the AUC was 1 to 20-fold increased compared to normal volunteers.

INDICATIONS AND USAGE

ERGAMISOL® (levamisole hydrochloride) is only indicated as adjuvant treatment in combination with fluorouracil after surgical resection in patients with Dukes' stage C colon cancer.

CONTRAINDICATIONS

ERGAMISOL® (levamisole hydrochloride) is contraindicated in patients with a known hypersensitivity to the drug or its components.

WARNINGS

Cases of an encephalopathy-like syndrome associated with demyelination have been reported in patients treated with ERGAMISOL® (levamisole hydrochloride). Worldwide post-marketing experience with the combination therapy of ERGAMISOL® and fluorouracil has also included reports of peripheral neuropathy and multifocal inflammatory leukoencephalopathy. The onset of symptoms and the clinical presentation in these cases are quite varied. Symptoms may include coma, confusion, lethargy, memory loss, muscle weakness, paresthesia, seizures, and speech disturbances. This condition has been associated with MRI and CT scan findings of demyelinating lesions in the white matter. If an acute neurological syndrome occurs, ERGAMISOL® and fluorouracil should be discontinued immediately. Patients have generally recovered/improved with drug discontinuation, but in some cases patients have not recovered/improved and deaths have been reported. Patients are generally treated with corticosteroids, but the efficacy of corticosteroids has not been proven.

ERGAMISOL® has been associated with agranulocytosis, sometimes fatal. The onset of agranulocytosis is frequently accompanied by a flu-like syndrome (fever, chills, etc.); however, in a small number of patients it is asymptomatic. A flu-like syndrome may also occur in the absence of agranulocytosis. It is essential that appropriate hematological monitoring be done routinely during therapy with ERGAMISOL® and fluorouracil. Neutropenia is usually reversible following discontinuation of therapy. Patients should be instructed to report immediately any flu-like symptoms.

Higher than recommended doses of ERGAMISOL® may be associated with an increased incidence of agranulocytosis, so the recommended dose should not be exceeded. The combination of ERGAMISOL® and fluorouracil has been associated with frequent neutropenia, anemia and thrombocytopenia.

In the presence of cirrhosis in twelve patients with alcoholic cirrhosis and hepatitis, the Cmax of ERGAMISOL® was not clearly increased, but the AUC was 1 to 20-fold increased compared to normal volunteers. Patients with hepatic impairment should be monitored for adverse events, including encephalopathy. Dose modification or discontinuation of ERGAMISOL® may be necessary if adverse experiences are observed.

PRECAUTIONS

Before beginning this combination adjuvant treatment, the physician should become familiar with the labeling for fluorouracil.

Information for Patients: The patient should be informed that if flu-like symptoms or malaise occurs, the physician should be notified immediately.

Drug Interactions: ERGAMISOL® (levamisole hydrochloride) has been reported to produce "ANTABUSE®"-like side effects when given concomitantly with alcohol. Concomitant administration of phenytoin and ERGAMISOL® plus fluorouracil has led to increased plasma levels of phenytoin. The physician is advised to monitor plasma levels of phenytoin and to decrease the dose if necessary.

Because of reports of prolongation of the prothrombin time beyond the therapeutic range in patients taking concurrent levamisole and warfarin sodium, it is suggested that the prothrombin time be monitored carefully, and the dose of warfarin sodium or other coumarin-like drugs should be adjusted accordingly, in patients taking both drugs.

Laboratory Tests: On the first day of therapy with ERGAMISOL®/fluorouracil, patients should have a CBC with differential and platelets, electrolytes and liver function tests performed. Thereafter, a CBC with differential and platelets should be performed weekly prior to each treatment with fluorouracil with electrolytes and liver function tests peformed every 3 months for a total of one year. Dosage modifications should be instituted as follows: If WBC is 2500-3500/mm^3 defer the fluorouracil dose until WBC is >3500/mm^3. If WBC is < 2500/mm^3, defer the fluorouracil dose until WBC is > 3500/mm^3; then resume the fluorouracil dose reduced by 20%. If WBC remains < 2500/mm^3 for over 10 days despite deferring fluorouracil, discontinue administration of ERGAMISOL®. Both drugs should be deferred unless enough platelets are present (≥ 100,000/mm^3).

Carcinogenesis, Mutagenesis, Impairment of Fertility: Adequate animal carcinogenicity studies have not been conducted with levamisole. Studies of levamisole administered in drinking water at 5, 20, and 80 mg/kg/day to mice for up to 18 months or adminstered to rats in the diet at 5, 20, and 80 mg/kg/day for 24 months showed no evidence of neoplastic effects. These studies were not conducted at the maximum tolerated dose, therefore the animals may not have been exposed to a reasonable drug challenge. No mutagenic effects were demonstrated in dominant lethal studies in male and female mice, in an Ames test, and in a study to detect chromosomal aberrations in cultured peripheral human lymphocytes.

Adverse effects were not observed on male or female fertility when levamisole was administered to rats in the diet at doses of 2.5, 10, 40, and 160 mg/kg. In a rat gavage study at doses of 20, 60, and 180 mg/kg, the copulation period was increased, the duration of pregnancy was slightly increased, and fertility, pup viability and weight, lactation index, and number of fetuses were decreased at 60 mg/kg. No negative reproductive effects were present when the offspring were allowed to mate and litter.

Pregnancy: Pregnancy Category C: Teratogenicity studies have been performed in rats and rabbits at oral doses up to 180 mg/kg. Fetal malformations were not observed. In rats, embryotoxicity was present at 160 mg/kg and in rabbits, significant embryotoxicity was observed at 180 mg/kg. There are no adequate and well-controlled studies in pregnant women and ERGAMISOL® should not be administered unless the potential benefits outweigh the risks. Women taking the combination of ERGAMISOL® and fluorouracil should be advised not to become pregnant.

Nursing Mothers: It is not known whether ERGAMISOL® is excreted in human milk; it is excreted in cows' milk. Because of the potential for serious adverse reactions in nursing infants from ERGAMISOL®, a decision should be made whether to discontinue nursing or to discontinue the drug, taking into account the importance of the drug to the mother.

Pediatric Use: Safety and effectiveness of ERGAMISOL® in children have not been established.

ADVERSE REACTIONS

Almost all patients receiving ERGAMISOL® (levamisole hydrochloride) and fluorouracil reported adverse experiences. Tabulated below is the incidence of adverse experiences that occurred in at least 1% of patients enrolled in two clinical trials who were adjuvantly treated with either ERGAMISOL® or ERGAMISOL® plus fluorouracil following colon surgery. In the larger clinical trial, 66 of 463 patients (14%) discontinued the combination of ERGAMISOL® plus fluorouracil because of adverse reactions. Forty-three of these patients (9%) developed isolated or a combination of gastrointestinal toxicities. (e.g., nausea, vomiting, diarrhea, stomatitis and anorexia). Ten patients developed rash and/or pruritus. Five patients discontinued therapy because of flu-like symptoms or fever with chills; ten patients developed central nervous system symptoms such as dizziness, ataxia, depression, confusion, memory loss, weakness, inability to concentrate, and headache; two patients developed reversible neutropenia and sepsis; one patient because of thrombocytopenia; one patient because of

Continued on next page

Ergamisol—Cont.

hyperbilirubinemia. One patient in the ERGAMISOL® plus fluorouracil group developed agranulocytosis and sepsis and died.

In the ERGAMISOL® alone arm of the trial, 15 of 310 patients (4.8%) discontinued therapy because of adverse experiences. Six of these (2%) discontinued because of rash, six because of arthralgia/myalgia, and one each for fever and neutropenia, urinary infection, and cough.

[See table below]

In worldwide experience with ERGAMISOL®, less frequent adverse experiences included exfoliative dermatitis, fixed drug eruptions, periorbital edema, vaginal bleeding, anaphylaxis, confusion, convulsions, hallucinations, impaired concentration, renal failure, pancreatitis, elevated serum creatinine, and increased alkaline phosphatase.

Reports of hyperlipidemia have been observed in patients receiving combination therapy of ERGAMISOL® and fluorouracil; elevations in triglyceride levels have been greater than increases in cholesterol levels. In worldwide postmarketing experience with the combination therapy, there have been rare cases of elevated hepatic enzymes and hepatosteatosis in patients. Isolated cases of Stevens-Johnson syndrome have also been reported.

The following additional adverse experiences have been reported for fluorouracil alone: esophagopharyngitis, pancytopenia, myocardial ischemia, angina, gastrointestinal ulceration and bleeding, anaphylaxis and generalized allergic reactions, acute cerebellar syndrome, nystagmus, dry skin, fissuring, photosensitivity, lacrimal duct stenosis, photophobia, euphoria, thrombophlebitis, and nail changes.

OVERDOSAGE

Fatalities have been reported in a three-year-old child who ingested 15 mg/kg and in an adult who ingested 32 mg/kg. No further clinical information is available. In cases of overdosage, gastric lavage is recommended together with symptomatic and supportive measures.

DOSAGE AND ADMINISTRATION

The adjuvant use of ERGAMISOL® (levamisole hydrochloride) and fluorouracil is limited to the following dosage schedule:

Initial Therapy:

ERGAMISOL®: 50 mg p.o. q8h for 3 days (starting 7–30 days post-surgery)

fluorouracil: 450 mg/m²/day IV for 5 days concomitant with a 3-day course of ERGAMISOL® (starting 21–34 days post-surgery)

Maintenance:

ERGAMISOL®: 50 mg p.o. q8h for 3 days every 2 weeks.

fluorouracil: 450 mg/m²/day IV once a week beginning 28 days after the initiation of the 5-day course.

Treatment: ERGAMISOL®, administered orally, should be initiated no earlier than 7 and no later than 30 days postsurgery at a dose of 50 mg q8h × 3 days repeated every 14 days for 1 year. Fluorouracil therapy should be initiated no earlier than 21 days and no later than 35 days after surgery providing the patient is out of the hospital, ambulatory, maintaining normal oral nutrition, has well-healed wounds, and is fully recovered from any postoperative complications. If ERGAMISOL® has been initiated from 7 to 20 days after surgery, initiation of fluorouracil therapy should be coincident with the second course of ERGAMISOL®, i.e., at 21 to 34 days. If ERGAMISOL® is initiated from 21 to 30 days after surgery, fluorouracil should be initiated simultaneously with the first course of ERGAMISOL®. Since the AUC of ERGAMISOL® is markedly increased in cirrhotic patients, such patients should be observed closely for adverse effects. Dose reduction or discontinuation of ERGAMISOL® may be warranted if adverse experiences are noted.

Fluorouracil should be administered by rapid IV push at a dosage of 450 mg/m²/day for 5 consecutive days. Dosage calculation is based on actual weight (estimated dry weight if there is evidence of fluid retention). *This course should be discontinued before the full 5 doses are administered if the patient develops any stomatitis or diarrhea* (5 or more loose stools). Twenty-eight days after initiation of this course, weekly fluorouracil should be instituted at a dosage of 450 mg/m²/week and continued for a total treatment time of 1 year. If stomatitis or diarrhea develop during weekly therapy, the next dose of fluorouracil should be deferred until these side effects have subsided. If these side effects are moderate to severe, the fluorouracil dose should be reduced 20% when it is resumed.

Dosage modifications should be instituted as follows: If WBC is 2500-3500/mm³ defer the fluorouracil dose until WBC is >3500/mm³. If WBC is <2500/mm³, defer the fluorouracil dose until WBC is >3500/mm³; then resume the fluorouracil dose reduced by 20%. If WBC remains <2500/mm³ for over 10 days despite deferring fluorouracil, discontinue administration of ERGAMISOL®. Both drugs should be deferred unless platelets are adequate (≥100,000/mm³).

ERGAMISOL® should not be used at doses exceeding the recommended dose or frequency. Clinical studies suggest a relationship between ERGAMISOL® adverse experiences and increasing dose, and since some of these, e.g. agranulocytosis, may be life-threatening, the recommended dosage regimen should not be exceeded (see **"WARNINGS"**).

Before beginning this combination adjuvant treatment, the physician should become familiar with the labeling for fluorouracil.

HOW SUPPLIED

ERGAMISOL® (levamisole hydrochloride) is available in white, coated tablets containing the equivalent of 50 mg of levamisole base, debossed "JANSSEN"and "L"/"50".

They are supplied in blister packages of 36 tablets (NDC 50458-270-36).

Store at controlled room temperature, (59°–77°F/15°–25°C). Protect from moisture.

REFERENCES

1. Laurie JA, Moertel CG, Fleming TR, et al. Surgical adjuvant therapy of large-bowel carcinoma: An evaluation of levamisole and the combination of levamisole and fluorouracil. *J Clin Oncol.* 1989; 7:1447–1456.
2. Moertel CG, Fleming TR, Macdonald JS, et al. Levamisole and fluorouracil for adjuvant therapy of resected colon carcinoma. *New Engl J Med.* 1990; 322:352–358.
3. Data on file, Janssen Pharmaceutica Inc.

Manufactured by:
Janssen Pharmaceutica, nv
Beerse, Belgium
Distributed by:
Janssen Pharmaceutica Inc.
Titusville, NJ 08560
Edition October 1998, August 1999
U.S. Patent Number 4,584,305

7500112

Shown in Product Identification Guide, page 318

Adverse experience	ERGAMISOL® N = 440 %	ERGAMISOL® plus fluorouracil N = 599 %
Gastrointestinal		
Nausea	22	65
Diarrhea	13	52
Stomatitis	3	39
Vomiting	6	20
Anorexia	2	6
Abdominal pain	2	5
Constipation	2	3
Flatulence	<1	2
Dyspepsia	<1	1
Hematological		
Leukopenia		
<2000/mm³	<1	1
≥2000 to <4000/mm³	4	19
≥4000/mm³	2	33
unscored category	0	<1
Thrombocytopenia		
<50,000/mm³	0	0
≥50,000 to <130,000/mm³	1	8
≥130,000/mm³	1	10
Anemia	0	6
Granulocytopenia	<1	2
Epistaxis	0	1
Skin and Appendages		
Dermatitis	8	23
Alopecia	3	22
Pruritus	1	2
Skin discoloration	0	2
Urticaria	<1	0
Body as a Whole		
Fatigue	6	11
Fever	3	5
Rigors	3	5
Chest pain	<1	1
Edema	1	1
Resistance Mechanisms		
Infection	5	12
Special Senses		
Taste Perversion	8	8
Altered sense of smell	1	1
Musculoskeletal System		
Arthralgia	5	4
Myalgia	3	2
Central and peripheral nervous system		
Dizziness	3	4
Headache	3	4
Paresthesia	2	3
Ataxia	0	2
Psychiatric		
Somnolence	3	2
Depression	1	2
Nervousness	1	2
Insomnia	1	1
Anxiety	1	1
Forgetfulness	0	1
Vision		
Abnormal tearing	0	4
Blurred vision	1	2
Conjunctivitis	<1	2
Liver and biliary system		
Hyperbilirubinemia	<1	1

IMODIUM (loperamide HCl) CAPSULES ℞

Please see full prescribing information for Imodium Capsules under McNeil Consumer.

NIZORAL (ketoconazole) 2% CREAM ℞

Please see full prescribing information for Nizoral 2% Cream under McNeil Consumer.

NIZORAL (ketoconazole) 2% SHAMPOO

Please see full prescribing information for Nizoral 2% Shampoo under McNeil Consumer.

NIZORAL® ℞

[nī 'zōr-ăl]
(ketoconazole)
Tablets

WARNING: When used orally, ketoconazole has been associated with hepatic toxicity, including some fatalities. Patients receiving this drug should be informed by the physician of the risk and should be closely monitored. See WARNINGS and PRECAUTIONS sections.
Coadministration of terfenadine with ketoconazole tablets is contraindicated. Rare cases of serious cardiovascular adverse events, including death, ventricular tachycardia and torsades de pointes have been observed in patients taking ketoconazole tablets concomitantly with terfenadine, due to increased terfenadine concentrations induced by ketoconazole tablets. See CONTRAINDICATIONS, WARNINGS, and PRECAUTIONS sections.

Pharmacokinetic data indicate that oral ketoconazole inhibits the metabolism of astemizole, resulting in elevated plasma levels of astemizole and its active metabolite desmethylastemizole which may prolong QT intervals. Coadministration of astemizole with ketoconazole tablets is therefore contraindicated. See CONTRAINDICATIONS, WARNINGS, and PRECAUTIONS sections.
Coadministration of cisapride with ketoconazole is contraindicated. Serious cardiovascular adverse events including ventricular tachycardia, ventricular fibrillation and torsades de pointes have occurred in patients taking ketoconazole concomitantly with cisapride. See CONTRAINDICATIONS, WARNINGS, and PRECAUTIONS sections.

DESCRIPTION

NIZORAL® (ketoconazole) is a synthetic broad-spectrum antifungal agent available in scored white tablets, each containing 200 mg ketoconazole base for oral administration. Inactive ingredients are colloidal silicon dioxide, corn starch, lactose, magnesium stearate, microcrystalline cellulose, and povidone. Ketoconazole is cis-1-acetyl-4-[4-[[2-(2,4-dichlorophenyl) -2- (1H-imidazol-1-ylmethyl)-1,3-dioxolan-4-yl] methoxyl]phenyl] piperazine.
Ketoconazole is a white to slightly beige, odorless powder, soluble in acids, with a molecular weight of 531.44.

CLINICAL PHARMACOLOGY

Mean peak plasma levels of approximately 3.5 µg/mL are reached within 1 to 2 hours, following oral administration of a single 200 mg dose taken with a meal. Subsequent plasma elimination is biphasic with a half-life of 2 hours during the first 10 hours and 8 hours thereafter. Following absorption from the gastrointestinal tract, NIZORAL® (ketoconazole) is converted into several inactive metabolites. The major identified metabolic pathways are oxidation and degradation of the imidazole and piperazine rings, oxidative O-dealkylation and aromatic hydroxylation. About 13% of the dose is excreted in the urine, of which 2 to 4% is unchanged drug. The major route of excretion is through the bile into the intestinal tract. *In vitro,* the plasma protein binding is about 99% mainly to the albumin fraction. Only a negligible proportion of ketoconazole reaches the cerebral-spinal fluid. Ketoconazole is a weak dibasic agent and thus requires acidity for dissolution and absorption.
NIZORAL® Tablets are active against clinical infections with *Blastomyces dermatitidis, Candida spp., Coccidioides immitis, Histoplasma capsulatum, Paracoccidioides brasiliensis,* and *Phialophora spp.* NIZORAL® Tablets are also active against *Trichophyton spp., Epidermophyton spp.,* and *Microsporum spp.* Ketoconazole is also active *in vitro* against a variety of fungi and yeast. In animal models, activity has been demonstrated against *Candida spp., Blastomyces dermatitidis, Histoplasma capsulatum, Malassezia furfur, Coccidioides immitis,* and *Cryptococcus neoformans.*
Mode of Action: In vitro studies suggest that ketoconazole impairs the synthesis of ergosterol, which is a vital component of fungal cell membranes.

INDICATIONS AND USAGE

NIZORAL® (ketoconazole) Tablets are indicated for the treatment of the following systemic fungal infections: candidiasis, chronic mucocutaneous candidiasis, oral thrush, candiduria, blastomycosis, coccidioidomycosis, histoplasmosis, chromomycosis, and paracoccidioidomycosis. NIZORAL® Tablets should not be used for fungal meningitis because it penetrates poorly into the cerebral-spinal fluid.
NIZORAL® Tablets are also indicated for the treatment of patients with severe recalcitrant cutaneous dermatophyte infections who have not responded to topical therapy or oral griseofulvin, or who are unable to take griseofulvin.

CONTRAINDICATIONS

Coadministration of terfenadine or astemizole with ketoconazole tablets is contraindicated. (See BOX WARNING, WARNINGS, and PRECAUTIONS sections.)
Concomitant administration of NIZORAL® Tablets with cisapride is contraindicated. (See BOX WARNING, WARNINGS, and PRECAUTIONS sections.)
Concomitant administration of NIZORAL® Tablets with oral triazolam is contraindicated. (See PRECAUTIONS section.)
NIZORAL® is contraindicated in patients who have shown hypersensitivity to the drug.

WARNINGS

Hepatotoxicity, primarily of the hepatocellular type, has been associated with the use of NIZORAL® (ketoconazole) Tablets, including rare fatalities. The reported incidence of hepatotoxicity has been about 1:10,000 exposed patients, but this probably represents some degree of under-reporting, as is the case for most reported adverse reactions to drugs. The median duration of NIZORAL® Tablet therapy in patients who developed symptomatic hepatotoxicity was about 28 days, although the range extended to as low as 3 days. The hepatic injury has usually, but not always, been reversible upon discontinuation of NIZORAL® Tablet treatment. Several cases of hepatitis have been reported in children.
Prompt recognition of liver injury is essential. Liver function tests (such as SGGT, alkaline phosphatase, SGPT, SGOT and bilirubin) should be measured before starting treatment and at frequent intervals during treatment. Patients receiving NIZORAL® Tablets concurrently with other potentially hepatotoxic drugs should be carefully monitored, particularly those patients requiring prolonged therapy or those who have had a history of liver disease.
Most of the reported cases of hepatic toxicity have to date been in patients treated for onychomycosis. Of 180 patients worldwide developing idiosyncratic liver dysfunction during NIZORAL® Tablet therapy, 61.3% had onychomycosis and 16.8% had chronic recalcitrant dermatophytoses.
Transient minor elevations in liver enzymes have occurred during treatment with NIZORAL® Tablets. The drug should be discontinued if these persist, if the abnormalities worsen, or if the abnormalities become accompanied by symptoms of possible liver injury.
In rare cases anaphylaxis has been reported after the first dose. Several cases of hypersensitivity reactions including urticaria have also been reported.
Coadministration of ketoconazole tablets and terfenadine has led to elevated plasma concentrations of terfenadine which may prolong QT intervals, sometimes resulting in life-threatening cardiac dysrhythmias. Cases of torsades de pointes and other serious ventricular dysrhythmias, in rare cases leading to fatality, have been reported among patients taking terfenadine concurrently with ketoconazole tablets. Coadministration of ketoconazole tablets and terfenadine is contraindicated.
Coadministration of astemizole with ketoconazole tablets is contraindicated. (See BOX WARNING, CONTRAINDICATIONS, and PRECAUTIONS sections.)
Concomitant administration of NIZORAL® Tablets with cisapride is contraindicated because it has resulted in markedly elevated cisapride plasma concentrations and prolonged QT interval, and has rarely been associated with ventricular arrhythmias and torsades de pointes. (See BOX WARNINGS, CONTRAINDICATIONS and PRECAUTIONS sections.)
In European clinical trials involving 350 patients with metastatic prostatic cancer, eleven deaths were reported within two weeks of starting treatment with high doses of ketoconazole tablets (1200 mg/day). It is not possible to ascertain from the information available whether death was related to ketoconazole therapy in these patients with serious underlying disease. However, high doses of ketoconazole tablets are known to suppress adrenal corticosteroid secretion.
In female rats treated three to six months with ketoconazole at dose levels of 80 mg/kg and higher, increased fragility of long bones, in some cases leading to fracture, was seen. The maximum "no-effect" dose level in these studies was 20 mg/kg (2.5 times the maximum recommended human dose). The mechanism responsible for this phenomenon is obscure. Limited studies in dogs failed to demonstrate such an effect on the metacarpals and ribs.

PRECAUTIONS

General: NIZORAL® (ketoconazole) Tablets have been demonstrated to lower serum testosterone. Once therapy with NIZORAL® Tablets has been discontinued, serum testosterone levels return to baseline values. Testosterone levels are impaired with doses of 800 mg per day and abolished by 1600 mg per day. NIZORAL® Tablets also decrease ACTH induced corticosteroid serum levels at similar high doses. The recommended dose of 200 mg–400 mg daily should be followed closely.
In four subjects with drug-induced achlorhydria, a marked reduction in ketoconazole absorption was observed. NIZORAL® Tablets require acidity for dissolution. If concomitant antacids, anticholinergics, and H_2-blockers are needed, they should be given at least two hours after administration of NIZORAL® Tablets. In cases of achlorhydria, the patients should be instructed to dissolve each tablet in 4 mL aqueous solution of 0.2 N HCl. For ingesting the resulting mixture, they should use a drinking straw so as to avoid contact with the teeth. This administration should be followed with a cup of tap water.
Information for Patients: Patients should be instructed to report any signs and symptoms which may suggest liver dysfunction so that appropriate biochemical testing can be done. Such signs and symptoms may include unusual fatigue, anorexia, nausea and/or vomiting, jaundice, dark urine or pale stools (see WARNINGS section).
Drug Interactions: Ketoconazole is a potent inhibitor of the cytochrome P450 3A4 enzyme system. Coadministration of NIZORAL® Tablets and drugs primarily metabolized by the cytochrome P450 3A4 enzyme system may result in increased plasma concentrations of the drugs that could increase or prolong both therapeutic and adverse effects. Therefore, unless otherwise specified, appropriate dosage adjustments may be necessary. The following drug interactions have been identified involving NIZORAL® Tablets and other drugs metabolized by the cytochrome P450 3A4 enzyme system.
Ketoconazole tablets inhibit the metabolism of terfenadine, resulting in an increased plasma concentration of terfenadine and a delay in the elimination of its acid metabolite. The increased plasma concentration of terfenadine or its metabolite may result in prolonged QT intervals. (See BOX WARNING, CONTRAINDICATIONS, and WARNINGS sections.)
Pharmacokinetic data indicate that oral ketoconazole inhibits the metabolism of astemizole, resulting in elevated plasma levels of astemizole and its active metabolite desmethylastemizole which may prolong QT intervals. Coadministration of astemizole with ketoconazole tablets is therefore contraindicated. (See BOX WARNING, CONTRAINDICATIONS, and WARNINGS sections.)
Human pharmacokinetics data indicate that oral ketoconazole potently inhibits the metabolism of cisapride resulting in a mean eight-fold increase in AUC of cisapride. Data suggest that coadministration of oral ketoconazole and cisapride can result in prolongation of the QT interval on the ECG. Therefore concomitant administration of ketoconazole tablets with cisapride is contraindicated. (See BOX WARNING, CONTRAINDICATIONS, and WARNINGS sections.)
Ketoconazole tablets may alter the metabolism of cyclosporine, tacrolimus, and methylprednisolone, resulting in elevated plasma concentrations of the latter drugs. Dosage adjustment may be required if cyclosporine, tacrolimus, or methylprednisolone are given concomitantly with NIZORAL® Tablets.
Coadministration of NIZORAL® Tablets with midazolam or triazolam has resulted in elevated plasma concentrations of the latter two drugs. This may potentiate and prolong hypnotic and sedative effects, especially with repeated dosing or chronic administration of these agents. These agents should not be used in patients treated with NIZORAL® Tablets. If midazolam is administered parenterally, special precaution is required since the sedative effect may be prolonged.
Rare cases of elevated plasma concentrations of digoxin have been reported. It is not clear whether this was due to the combination of therapy. It is, therefore, advisable to monitor digoxin concentrations in patients receiving ketoconazole.
When taken orally, imidazole compounds like ketoconazole may enhance the anticoagulant effect of coumarin-like drugs. In simultaneous treatment with imidazole drugs and coumarin drugs, the anticoagulant effect should be carefully titrated and monitored.
Because severe hypoglycemia has been reported in patients concomitantly receiving oral miconazole (an imidazole) and oral hypoglycemic agents, such a potential interaction involving the latter agents when used concomitantly with ketoconazole tablets (an imidazole) can not be ruled out.
Concomitant administration of ketoconazole tablets with phenytoin may alter the metabolism of one or both of the drugs. It is suggested to monitor both ketoconazole and phenytoin.
Concomitant administration of rifampin with ketoconazole tablets reduces the blood levels of the latter. INH (Isoniazid) is also reported to affect ketoconazole concentrations adversely. These drugs should not be given concomitantly.
After the coadministration of 200 mg oral ketoconazole twice daily and one 20 mg dose of loratadine to 11 subjects, the AUC and C_{max} of loratadine averaged 302% (± 142 S.D.) and 251% (± 68 S.D.), respectively, of those obtained after co-treatment with placebo. The AUC and C_{max} of descarboethoxyloratadine, an active metabolite, averaged 155% (± 27 S.D.) and 141% (± 35 S.D.), respectively. However, no related changes were noted in the QT_c on ECG taken at 2, 6, and 24 hours after the coadministration. Also, there were no clinically significant differences in adverse events when loratadine was administered with or without ketoconazole.
Rare cases of disulfiram-like reaction to alcohol have been reported. These experiences have been characterized by flushing, rash, peripheral edema, nausea, and headache. Symptoms resolved within a few hours.
Carcinogenesis, Mutagenesis, Impairment of Fertility: The dominant lethal mutation test in male and female mice revealed that single oral doses of ketoconazole as high as 80 mg/kg produced no mutation in any stage of germ cell development. The *Ames Salmonella* microsomal activator assay was also negative. A long term feeding study in Swiss Albino mice and in Wistar rats showed no evidence of oncogenic activity.
Pregnancy: Teratogenic effects: *Pregnancy Category C:* Ketoconazole has been shown to be teratogenic (syndactylia and oligodactylia) in the rat when given in the diet at 80 mg/kg/day (10 times the maximum recommended human dose). However, these effects may be related to maternal toxicity, evidence of which also was seen at this and higher dose levels.
There are no adequate and well controlled studies in pregnant women. NIZORAL® Tablets should be used during pregnancy only if the potential benefit justifies the potential risk to the fetus.
Nonteratogenic Effects: Ketoconazole has also been found to be embryotoxic in the rat when given in the diet at doses higher than 80 mg/kg during the first trimester of gestation.
In addition, dystocia (difficult labor) was noted in rats administered oral ketoconazole during the third trimester of gestation. This occurred when ketoconazole was administered at doses higher than 10 mg/kg (higher than 1.25 times the maximum human dose).
It is likely that both the malformations and the embryotoxicity resulting from the administration of oral ketoconazole during gestation are a reflection of the particular sensitivity of the female rat to this drug. For example, the oral LD_{50} of ketoconazole given by gavage to the female rat is 166 mg/kg whereas in the male rat the oral LD_{50} is 287 mg/kg.
Nursing Mothers: Since ketoconazole is probably excreted in the milk, mothers who are under treatment should not breast feed.

Continued on next page

Nizoral Tablets—Cont.

Pediatric Use: NIZORAL® (ketoconazole) Tablets have not been systematically studied in children of any age, and essentially no information is available on children under 2 years. NIZORAL® Tablets should not be used in pediatric patients unless the potential benefit outweighs the risks.

ADVERSE REACTIONS

In rare cases, anaphylaxis has been reported after the first dose. Several cases of hypersensitivity reactions including urticaria have also been reported. However, the most frequent adverse reactions were nausea and/or vomiting in approximately 3%, abdominal pain in 1.2%, pruritus in 1.5%, and the following in less than 1% of the patients: headache, dizziness, somnolence, fever and chills, photophobia, diarrhea, gynecomastia, impotence, thrombocytopenia, leukopenia, hemolytic anemia, and bulging fontanelles. Oligospermia has been reported in investigational studies with the drug at dosages above those currently approved. Oligospermia has not been reported at dosages up to 400 mg daily, however sperm counts have been obtained infrequently in patients treated with these dosages. Most of these reactions were mild and transient and rarely required discontinuation of NIZORAL® (ketoconazole) Tablets. In contrast, the rare occurrences of hepatic dysfunction require special attention (see WARNINGS section).

In worldwide postmarketing experience with NIZORAL® Tablets there have been rare reports of alopecia, paresthesia, and signs of increased intracranial pressure including bulging fontanelles and papilledema. Hypertriglyceridemia has also been reported but a causal association with NIZORAL® Tablets is uncertain.

Neuropsychiatric disturbances, including suicidal tendencies and severe depression, have occurred rarely in patients using NIZORAL® Tablets.

Ventricular dysrhythmias (prolonged QT intervals) have occurred with the concomitant use of terfenadine with ketoconazole tablets. (See BOX WARNING, CONTRAINDICATIONS, and WARNINGS sections.) Data suggest that coadministration of ketoconazole tablets and cisapride can result in prolongation of the QT interval and has rarely been associated with ventricular arrhythmias. (See CONTRAINDICATIONS, WARNINGS, and PRECAUTIONS sections.)

OVERDOSAGE

In the event of accidental overdosage, supportive measures, including gastric lavage with sodium bicarbonate, should be employed.

DOSAGE AND ADMINISTRATION

Adults: The recommended starting dose of NIZORAL® (ketoconazole) Tablets is a single daily administration of 200 mg (one tablet). In very serious infections or if clinical responsiveness is insufficient within the expected time, the dose of NIZORAL® Tablets may be increased to 400 mg (two tablets) once daily.

Children: In small numbers of children over 2 years of age, a single daily dose of 3.3 to 6.6 mg/kg has been used. NIZORAL® Tablets have not been studied in children under 2 years of age.

There should be laboratory as well as clinical documentation of infection prior to starting ketoconazole therapy. Treatment should be continued until tests indicate that active fungal infection has subsided. Inadequate periods of treatment may yield poor response and lead to early recurrence of clinical symptoms. Minimum treatment for candidiasis is one or two weeks. Patients with chronic mucocutaneous candidiasis usually require maintenance therapy. Minimum treatment for the other indicated systemic mycoses is six months.

Minimum treatment for recalcitrant dermatophyte infections is four weeks in cases involving glabrous skin. Palmar and plantar infections may respond more slowly. Apparent cures may subsequently recur after discontinuation of therapy in some cases.

HOW SUPPLIED

NIZORAL® (ketoconazole) is available as white, scored tablets containing 200 mg of ketoconazole debossed "JANSSEN" and on the reverse side debossed "NIZORAL". They are supplied in bottles of 100 tablets (NDC 50458-220-10).

Store at controlled room temperature
15°–25°C(59°–77°F). Protect from moisture.
U.S. Patent 4,335,125
Rev. March 1997, July 1998
JANSSEN PHARMACEUTICA
Titusville, NJ 08560-0200

Shown in Product Identification Guide, page 318

RISPERDAL® ℞

[*ris 'pər dăl*]
(risperidone) Tablets/Oral Solution

DESCRIPTION

RISPERDAL® (risperidone) is an antipsychotic agent belonging to a new chemical class, the benzisoxazole derivatives. The chemical designation is 3-[2-[4-(6-fluoro-1,2-benzisoxazol-3-yl)-1-piperidinyl]ethyl]-6,7,8,9-tetrahydro-2-methyl-4*H*-pyrido[1,2-a]pyrimidin-4-one. Its molecular formula is $C_{23}H_{27}FN_4O_2$ and its molecular weight is 410.49.

Risperidone is a white to slightly beige powder. It is practically insoluble in water, freely soluble in methylene chloride, and soluble in methanol and 0.1 N HCl.

RISPERDAL® tablets are available in 0.25 mg (dark yellow), 0.5 mg (red-brown), 1 mg (white), 2 mg (orange), 3 mg (yellow), and 4 mg (green) strengths. Inactive ingredients are colloidal silicon dioxide, hydroxypropyl methylcellulose, lactose, magnesium stearate, microcrystalline cellulose, propylene glycol, sodium lauryl sulfate, and starch (corn). Tablets of 0.25, 0.5, 2, 3, and 4 mg also contain talc and titanium dioxide. The 0.25 mg tablets contain yellow iron oxide; the 0.5 mg tablets contain red iron oxide, the 2 mg tablets contain FD&C Yellow No. 6 Aluminum Lake; the 3 mg and 4 mg tablets contain D&C Yellow No. 10; the 4 mg tablets contain FD&C Blue No. 2 Aluminum Lake.

RISPERDAL® is also available as a 1 mg/mL oral solution. The inactive ingredients for this solution are; tartaric acid, benzoic acid, sodium hydroxide and purified water.

CLINICAL PHARMACOLOGY

Pharmacodynamics

The mechanism of action of RISPERDAL® (risperidone), as with other antipsychotic drugs, is unknown. However, it has been proposed that this drug's antipsychotic activity is mediated through a combination of dopamine type 2 (D_2) and serotonin type 2 ($5HT_2$) antagonism. Antagonism at receptors other than D_2 and $5HT_2$ may explain some of the other effects of RISPERDAL®.

RISPERDAL® is a selective monoaminergic antagonist with high affinity (Ki of 0.12 to 7.3 nM) for the serotonin type 2 ($5HT_2$), dopamine type 2 (D_2), α_1 and α_2 adrenergic, and H_1 histaminergic receptors. RISPERDAL® antagonizes other receptors, but with lower potency. RISPERDAL® has low to moderate affinity (Ki of 47 to 253 nM) for the serotonin $5HT_{1C}$, $5HT_{1D}$, and $5HT_{1A}$ receptors, weak affinity (Ki of 620 to 800 nM) for the dopamine D_1 and haloperidol-sensitive sigma site, and no affinity (when tested at concentrations $>10^{-5}$ M) for cholinergic muscarinic or β_1 and β_2 adrenergic receptors.

Pharmacokinetics

Risperidone is well absorbed, as illustrated by a mass balance study involving a single 1 mg oral dose of ^{14}C-risperidone as a solution in three healthy male volunteers. Total recovery of radioactivity at one week was 85%, including 70% in the urine and 15% in the feces.

Risperidone is extensively metabolized in the liver by cytochrome $P_{450}IID_6$ to a major active metabolite, 9-hydroxyrisperidone, which is the predominant circulating specie, and appears approximately equi-effective with risperidone with respect to receptor binding activity and some effects in animals. (A second minor pathway is *N*-dealkylation). Consequently, the clinical effect of the drug likely results from the combined concentrations of risperidone plus 9-hydroxyrisperidone. Plasma concentrations of risperidone, 9-hydroxyrisperidone, and risperidone plus 9-hydroxyrisperidone are dose proportional over the dosing range of 1 to 16 mg daily (0.5 to 8 mg BID). The relative oral bioavailability of risperidone from a tablet was 94% (CV=10%) when compared to a solution. Food does not affect either the rate or extent of absorption of risperidone. Thus, risperidone can be given with or without meals. The absolute oral bioavailability of risperidone was 70% (CV=25%).

The enzyme catalyzing hydroxylation of risperidone to 9-hydroxyrisperidone is cytochrome $P_{450}IID_6$, also called debrisoquin hydroxylase, the enzyme responsible for metabolism of many neuroleptics, antidepressants, antiarrhythmics, and other drugs. Cytochrome $P_{450}IID_6$ is subject to genetic polymorphism (about 6-8% of Caucasians, and a very low percent of Asians have little or no activity and are "poor metabolizers") and to inhibition by a variety of substrates and some non-substrates, notably quinidine. Extensive metabolizers convert risperidone rapidly into 9-hydroxyrisperidone, while poor metabolizers convert it much more slowly. Extensive metabolizers, therefore, have lower risperidone and higher 9-hydroxyrisperidone concentrations than poor metabolizers. Following oral administration of solution or tablet, mean peak plasma concentrations occurred at about 1 hour. Peak 9-hydroxyrisperidone occurred at about 3 hours in extensive metabolizers, and 17 hours in poor metabolizers. The apparent half-life of risperidone was three hours (CV=30%) in extensive metabolizers and 20 hours (CV=40%) in poor metabolizers. The apparent half-life of 9-hydroxyrisperidone was about 21 hours (CV=20%) in extensive metabolizers and 30 hours (CV=25%) in poor metabolizers. Steady-state concentrations of risperidone are reached in 1 day in extensive metabolizers and would be expected to reach steady state in about 5 days in poor metabolizers. Steady-state concentrations of 9-hydroxyrisperidone are reached in 5-6 days (measured in extensive metabolizers).

Because risperidone and 9-hydroxyrisperidone are approximately equi-effective, the sum of their concentrations is pertinent. The pharmacokinetics of the sum of risperidone and 9-hydroxyrisperidone, after single and multiple doses, were similar in extensive and poor metabolizers, with an overall mean elimination half-life of about 20 hours. In analyses comparing adverse reaction rates in extensive and poor metabolizers in controlled and open studies, no important differences were seen.

Risperidone could be subject to two kinds of drug-drug interactions. First, inhibitors of cytochrome $P_{450}IID_6$ could interfere with conversion of risperidone to 9-hydroxyrisperidone. This in fact occurs with quinidine, giving essentially all recipients a risperidone pharmacokinetic profile typical of poor metabolizers. The favorable and adverse effects of risperidone in patients receiving quinidine have not been evaluated, but observations in a modest number (n is approximately equal to 70) of poor metabolizers given risperidone do not suggest important differences between poor and extensive metabolizers. It would also be possible for risperidone to interfere with metabolism of other drugs metabolized by cytochrome $P_{450}IID_6$. Relatively weak binding of risperidone to the enzyme suggests this is unlikely (See PRECAUTIONS and DRUG INTERACTIONS).

The plasma protein binding of risperidone was about 90% over the in vitro concentration range of 0.5 to 200 ng/mL and increased with increasing concentrations of α_1-acid glycoprotein. The plasma binding of 9-hydroxyrisperidone was 77%. Neither the parent nor the metabolite displaced each other from the plasma binding sites. High therapeutic concentrations of sulfamethazine (100 µg/mL), warfarin (10 µg/mL) and carbamazepine (10 µg/mL) caused only a slight increase in the free fraction of risperidone at 10 ng/mL and 9-hydroxyrisperidone at 50 ng/mL, changes of unknown clinical significance.

Special Populations

Renal Impairment: In patients with moderate to severe renal disease, clearance of the sum of risperidone and its active metabolite decreased by 60% compared to young healthy subjects. RISPERDAL® doses should be reduced in patients with renal disease (See PRECAUTIONS and DOSAGE AND ADMINISTRATION).

Hepatic Impairment: While the pharmacokinetics of risperidone in subjects with liver disease were comparable to those in young healthy subjects, the mean free fraction of risperidone in plasma was increased by about 35% because of the diminished concentration of both albumin and α_1-acid glycoprotein. RISPERDAL® doses should be reduced in patients with liver disease (See PRECAUTIONS and DOSAGE AND ADMINISTRATION).

Elderly: In healthy elderly subjects renal clearance of both risperidone and 9-hydroxyrisperidone was decreased, and elimination half-lives were prolonged compared to young healthy subjects. Dosing should be modified accordingly in the elderly patients (See DOSAGE AND ADMINISTRATION).

Race and Gender Effects: No specific pharmacokinetic study was conducted to investigate race and gender effects, but a population pharmacokinetic analysis did not identify important differences in the disposition of risperidone due to gender (whether corrected for body weight or not) or race.

Clinical Trials

The efficacy of RISPERDAL® in the management of the manifestations of psychotic disorders was established in four short-term (4- to 8-week) controlled trials of psychotic inpatients who met DSM-III-R criteria for schizophrenia.

Several instruments were used for assessing psychiatric signs and symptoms in these studies, among them the Brief Psychiatric Rating Scale (BPRS), a multi-item inventory of general psychopathology traditionally used to evaluate the effects of drug treatment in psychosis. The BPRS psychosis cluster (conceptual disorganization, hallucinatory behavior, suspiciousness, and unusual thought content) is considered a particularly useful subset for assessing actively psychotic schizophrenic patients. A second traditional assessment, the Clinical Global Impression (CGI), reflects the impression of a skilled observer, fully familiar with the manifestations of schizophrenia, about the overall clinical state of the patient. In addition, two more recently developed, but less well evaluated scales, were employed; these included the Positive and Negative Syndrome Scale (PANSS) and the Scale for Assessing Negative Symptoms (SANS).

The results of the trials follow:

(1) In a 6-week, placebo-controlled trial (n=160) involving titration of RISPERDAL® in doses up to 10 mg/day (BID schedule), RISPERDAL® was generally superior to placebo on the BPRS total score, on the BPRS psychosis cluster, and marginally superior to placebo on the SANS.

(2) In an 8-week, placebo-controlled trial (n=513) involving 4 fixed doses of RISPERDAL® (2, 6, 10, and 16 mg/day, on a BID schedule), all 4 RISPERDAL® groups were generally superior to placebo on the BPRS total score, BPRS psychosis cluster, and CGI severity score; the 3 highest RISPERDAL® dose groups were generally superior to placebo on the PANSS negative subscale. The most consistently positive responses on all measures were seen for the 6 mg dose group, and there was no suggestion of increased benefit from larger doses.

(3) In an 8-week, dose comparison trial (n=1356) involving 5 fixed doses of RISPERDAL® (1, 4, 8, 12, and 16 mg/day, on a BID schedule), the four highest RISPERDAL® dose groups were generally superior to the 1 mg RISPERDAL® dose group on BPRS total score, BPRS psychosis cluster, and CGI severity score. None of the dose groups were superior to the 1 mg group on the PANSS negative subscale. The most consistently positive responses were seen for the 4 mg dose group.

(4) In a 4-week, placebo-controlled dose comparison trial (n=246) involving 2 fixed doses of RISPERDAL® (4 and 8 mg/day on a QD schedule), both RISPERDAL® dose groups were generally superior to placebo on several PANSS measures, including a response measure (> 20% reduction in PANSS total score), PANSS total score, and the BPRS psychosis cluster (derived from PANSS). The results were generally stronger for the 8 mg than for the 4 mg dose group.

INDICATIONS AND USAGE

RISPERDAL® (risperidone) is indicated for the management of the manifestations of psychotic disorders.

The antipsychotic efficacy of RISPERDAL® was established in short-term (6 to 8-weeks) controlled trials of schizophrenic inpatients (See CLINICAL PHARMACOLOGY).

The effectiveness of RISPERDAL® in long-term use, that is, more than 6 to 8-weeks, has not been systematically evaluated in controlled trials. Therefore, the physician who elects to use RISPERDAL® for extended periods should periodically re-evaluate the long-term usefulness of the drug for the individual patient. (See DOSAGE AND ADMINISTRATION).

CONTRAINDICATIONS

RISPERDAL® (risperidone) is contraindicated in patients with a known hypersensitivity to the product.

WARNINGS

Neuroleptic Malignant Syndrome (NMS)

A potentially fatal symptom complex sometimes referred to as Neuroleptic Malignant Syndrome (NMS) has been reported in association with antipsychotic drugs. Clinical manifestations of NMS are hyperpyrexia, muscle rigidity, altered mental status and evidence of autonomic instability (irregular pulse or blood pressure, tachycardia, diaphoresis and cardiac dysrhythmia). Additional signs may include elevated creatine phosphokinase, myoglobinuria (rhabdomyolysis), and acute renal failure.

The diagnostic evaluation of patients with this syndrome is complicated. In arriving at a diagnosis, it is important to identify cases where the clinical presentation includes both serious medical illness (e.g., pneumonia, systemic infection, etc.) and untreated or inadequately treated extrapyramidal signs and symptoms (EPS). Other important considerations in the differential diagnosis include central anticholinergic toxicity, heat stroke, drug fever, and primary central nervous system pathology.

The management of NMS should include: 1) immediate discontinuation of antipsychotic drugs and other drugs not essential to concurrent therapy; 2) intensive symptomatic treatment and medical monitoring; and 3) treatment of any concomitant serious medical problems for which specific treatments are available. There is no general agreement about specific pharmacological treatment regimens for uncomplicated NMS.

If a patient requires antipsychotic drug treatment after recovery from NMS, the potential reintroduction of drug therapy should be carefully considered. The patient should be carefully monitored, since recurrences of NMS have been reported.

Tardive Dyskinesia

A syndrome of potentially irreversible, involuntary, dyskinetic movements may develop in patients treated with antipsychotic drugs. Although the prevalence of the syndrome appears to be highest among the elderly, especially elderly women, it is impossible to rely upon prevalence estimates to predict, at the inception of antipsychotic treatment, which patients are likely to develop the syndrome. Whether antipsychotic drug products differ in their potential to cause tardive dyskinesia is unknown.

The risk of developing tardive dyskinesia and the likelihood that it will become irreversible are believed to increase as the duration of treatment and the total cumulative dose of antipsychotic drugs administered to the patient increase. However, the syndrome can develop, although much less commonly, after relatively brief treatment periods at low doses.

There is no known treatment for established cases of tardive dyskinesia, although the syndrome may remit, partially or completely, if antipsychotic treatment is withdrawn. Antipsychotic treatment, itself, however, may suppress (or partially suppress) the signs and symptoms of the syndrome and thereby may possibly mask the underlying process. The effect that symptomatic suppression has upon the long-term course of the syndrome is unknown.

Given these considerations, RISPERDAL® (risperidone) should be prescribed in a manner that is most likely to minimize the occurrence of tardive dyskinesia. Chronic antipsychotic treatment should generally be reserved for patients who suffer from a chronic illness that (1) is known to respond to antipsychotic drugs, and (2) for whom alternative, equally effective, but potentially less harmful treatments are not available or appropriate. In patients who do require chronic treatment, the smallest dose and the shortest duration of treatment producing a satisfactory clinical response should be sought. The need for continued treatment should be reassessed periodically.

If signs and symptoms of tardive dyskinesia appear in a patient on RISPERDAL®, drug discontinuation should be considered. However, some patients may require treatment with RISPERDAL® despite the presence of the syndrome.

Potential for Proarrhythmic Effects: Risperidone and/or 9-hydroxyrisperidone appears to lengthen the QT interval in some patients, although there is no average increase in treated patients, even at 12–16 mg/day, well above the recommended dose. Other drugs that prolong the QT interval have been associated with the occurrence of torsades de pointes, a life-threatening arrhythmia. Bradycardia, electrolyte imbalance, concomitant use with other drugs that prolong QT, or the presence of congenital prolongation in QT can increase the risk for occurrence of this arrhythmia.

PRECAUTIONS

General

Orthostatic Hypotension: RISPERDAL® (risperidone) may induce orthostatic hypotension associated with dizziness, tachycardia, and in some patients, syncope, especially during the initial dose-titration period, probably reflecting its alpha-adrenergic antagonistic properties. Syncope was reported in 0.2% (6/2607) of RISPERDAL® treated patients in phase 2–3 studies. The risk of orthostatic hypotension and syncope may be minimized by limiting the initial dose to 2 mg total (either QD or 1 mg BID) in normal adults and 0.5 mg BID in the elderly and patients with renal or hepatic impairment (See DOSAGE AND ADMINISTRATION). Monitoring of orthostatic vital signs should be considered in patients for whom this is of concern. A dose reduction should be considered if hypotension occurs. RISPERDAL® should be used with particular caution in patients with known cardiovascular disease (history of myocardial infarction or ischemia, heart failure, or conduction abnormalities), cerebrovascular disease, and conditions which would predispose patients to hypotension e.g., dehydration and hypovolemia. Clinically significant hypotension has been observed with concomitant use of RISPERDAL® and antihypertensive medication.

Seizures: During premarketing testing, seizures occurred in 0.3% (9/2607) of RISPERDAL® treated patients, two in association with hyponatremia. RISPERDAL® should be used cautiously in patients with a history of seizures.

Dysphagia: Esophageal dysmotility and aspiration have been associated with antipsychotic drug use. Aspiration pneumonia is a common cause of morbidity and mortality in patients with advanced Alzheimer's dementia. RISPERDAL® and other antipsychotic drugs should be used cautiously in patients at risk for aspiration pneumonia.

Hyperprolactinemia: As with other drugs that antagonize dopamine D_2 receptors, risperidone elevates prolactin levels and the elevation persists during chronic administration. Tissue culture experiments indicate that approximately one-third of human breast cancers are prolactin dependent in vitro, a factor of potential importance if the prescription of these drugs is contemplated in a patient with previously detected breast cancer. Although disturbances such as galactorrhea, amenorrhea, gynecomastia, and impotence have been reported with prolactin-elevating compounds, the clinical significance of elevated serum prolactin levels is unknown for most patients. As is common with compounds which increase prolactin release, an increase in pituitary gland, mammary gland, and pancreatic islet cell hyperplasia and/or neoplasia was observed in the risperidone carcinogenicity studies conducted in mice and rats (See CARCINOGENESIS). However, neither clinical studies nor epidemiologic studies conducted to date have shown an association between chronic administration of this class of drugs and tumorigenesis in humans; the available evidence is considered too limited to be conclusive at this time.

Potential for Cognitive and Motor Impairment: Somnolence was a commonly reported adverse event associated with RISPERDAL® treatment, especially when ascertained by direct questioning of patients. This adverse event is dose related, and in a study utilizing a checklist to detect adverse events, 41% of the high dose patients (RISPERDAL® 16 mg/day) reported somnolence compared to 16% of placebo patients. Direct questioning is more sensitive for detecting adverse events than spontaneous reporting, by which 8% of RISPERDAL® 16 mg/day patients and 1% of placebo patients reported somnolence as an adverse event. Since RISPERDAL® has the potential to impair judgment, thinking, or motor skills, patients should be cautioned about operating hazardous machinery, including automobiles, until they are reasonably certain that RISPERDAL® therapy does not affect them adversely.

Priapism: Rare cases of priapism have been reported. While the relationship of the events to RISPERDAL® use has not been established, other drugs with alpha-adrenergic blocking effects have been reported to induce priapism, and it is possible that RISPERDAL® may share this capacity. Severe priapism may require surgical intervention.

Thrombotic Thrombocytopenic Purpura (TTP): A single case of TTP was reported in a 28 year-old female patient receiving RISPERDAL® in a large, open premarketing experience (approximately 1300 patients). She experienced jaundice, fever, and bruising, but eventually recovered after receiving plasmapheresis. The relationship to RISPERDAL® therapy is unknown.

Antiemetic effect: Risperidone has an antiemetic effect in animals; this effect may also occur in humans, and may mask signs and symptoms of overdosage with certain drugs or of conditions such as intestinal obstruction, Reye's syndrome, and brain tumor.

Body Temperature Regulation: Disruption of body temperature regulation has been attributed to antipsychotic agents. Both hyperthermia and hypothermia have been reported in association with RISPERDAL® use. Caution is advised when prescribing for patients who will be exposed to temperature extremes.

Suicide: The possibility of a suicide attempt is inherent in schizophrenia, and close supervision of high risk patients should accompany drug therapy. Prescriptions for RISPERDAL® should be written for the smallest quantity of tablets consistent with good patient management, in order to reduce the risk of overdose.

Use in Patients with Concomitant Illness: Clinical experience with RISPERDAL® in patients with certain concomitant systemic illnesses is limited. Caution is advisable in using RISPERDAL® in patients with diseases or conditions that could affect metabolism or hemodynamic responses. RISPERDAL® has not been evaluated or used to any appreciable extent in patients with a recent history of myocardial infarction or unstable heart disease. Patients with these diagnoses were excluded from clinical studies during the product's premarket testing. The electrocardiograms of approximately 380 patients who received RISPERDAL® and 120 patients who received placebo in two double-blind, placebo-controlled trials were evaluated and the data revealed one finding of potential concern, i.e., 8 patients taking RISPERDAL® whose baseline QTc interval was less than 450 msec were observed to have QTc intervals greater than 450 msec during treatment; no such prolongations were seen in the smaller placebo group. There were 3 such episodes in the approximately 125 patients who received haloperidol. Because of the risks of orthostatic hypotension and QT prolongation, caution should be observed in cardiac patients (See WARNINGS AND PRECAUTIONS).

Increased plasma concentrations of risperidone and 9-hydroxyrisperidone occur in patients with severe renal impairment (creatinine clearance <30 mL/min/1.73 m^2), and an increase in the free fraction of the risperidone is seen in patients with severe hepatic impairment. A lower starting dose should be used in such patients (See DOSAGE AND ADMINISTRATION).

Information for Patients

Physicians are advised to discuss the following issues with patients for whom they prescribe RISPERDAL®:

Orthostatic Hypotension: Patients should be advised of the risk of orthostatic hypotension, especially during the period of initial dose titration.

Interference With Cognitive and Motor Performance: Since RISPERDAL® has the potential to impair judgment, thinking, or motor skills, patients should be cautioned about operating hazardous machinery, including automobiles, until they are reasonably certain that RISPERDAL® therapy does not affect them adversely.

Pregnancy: Patients should be advised to notify their physician if they become pregnant or intend to become pregnant during therapy.

Nursing: Patients should be advised not to breast feed an infant if they are taking RISPERDAL®.

Concomitant Medication: Patients should be advised to inform their physicians if they are taking, or plan to take, any prescription or over-the-counter drugs, since there is a potential for interactions.

Alcohol: Patients should be advised to avoid alcohol while taking RISPERDAL®.

Laboratory Tests

No specific laboratory tests are recommended.

Drug Interactions

The interactions of RISPERDAL® and other drugs have not been systematically evaluated. Given the primary CNS effects of risperidone, caution should be used when RISPERDAL® is taken in combination with other centrally acting drugs and alcohol.

Because of its potential for inducing hypotension, RISPERDAL® may enhance the hypotensive effects of other therapeutic agents with this potential.

RISPERDAL® may antagonize the effects of levodopa and dopamine agonists.

Chronic administration of carbamazepine with risperidone may increase the clearance of risperidone.

Chronic administration of clozapine with risperidone may decrease the clearance of risperidone.

Fluoxetine may increase the plasma concentration of the anti-psychotic fraction (risperidone plus 9-hydroxyrisperidone) by raising the concentration of risperidone, although not the active metabolite, 9-hydroxyrisperidone).

Drugs that Inhibit Cytochrome $P_{450}IID_6$ and Other P_{450} Isozymes: Risperidone is metabolized to 9-hydroxyrisperidone by cytochrome $P_{450}IID_6$, an enzyme that is polymorphic in the population and that can be inhibited by a variety of psychotropic and other drugs (See CLINICAL PHARMACOLOGY). Drug interactions that reduce the metabolism of risperidone to 9-hydroxyrisperidone would increase the plasma concentrations of risperidone and lower the concentrations of 9-hydroxyrisperidone. Analysis of clinical studies involving a modest number of poor metabolizers (n is approximately equal to 70) does not suggest that poor and extensive metabolizers have different rates of adverse effects. No comparison of effectiveness in the two groups has been made.

In vitro studies showed that drugs metabolized by other P_{450} isozymes, including 1A1, 1A2, IIC9, MP, and IIIA4, are only weak inhibitors of risperidone metabolism.

Drugs Metabolized by Cytochrome $P_{450}IID_6$: In vitro studies indicate that risperidone is a relatively weak inhibitor of cytochrome $P_{450}IID_6$. Therefore, RISPERDAL® is not expected to substantially inhibit the clearance of drugs that are metabolized by this enzymatic pathway. However, clinical data to confirm this expectation are not available.

Carcinogenesis, Mutagenesis, Impairment of Fertility

Carcinogenesis: Carcinogenicity studies were conducted in Swiss albino mice and Wistar rats. Risperidone was administered in the diet at doses of 0.63, 2.5, and 10 mg/kg for 18 months to mice and for 25 months to rats. These doses are equivalent to 2.4, 9.4 and 37.5 times the maximum human dose (16 mg/day) on a mg/kg basis or 0.2, 0.75 and 3 times the maximum human dose (mice) or 0.4, 1.5, and 6 times the maximum human dose (rats) on a mg/m^2 basis. A maximum tolerated dose was not achieved in male mice. There were statistically significant increases in pituitary gland adenomas, endocrine pancreas adenomas and mam-

Continued on next page

Risperdal—Cont.

mary gland adenocarcinomas. The following table summarizes the multiples of the human dose on a mg/m^2 (mg/kg) basis at which these tumors occurred.

TUMOR TYPE	SPECIES	SEX	MULTIPLE OF MAXIMUM HUMAN DOSE in mg/m^2 (mg/kg) LOWEST EFFECT LEVEL	HIGHEST NO EFFECT LEVEL
Pituitary adenomas	mouse	female	0.75 (*9.4*)	0.2 (*2.4*)
Endocrine pancreas adenomas	rat	male	1.5 (*9.4*)	0.4 (*2.4*)
Mammary gland adeno-carcinomas	mouse	female	0.2 (*2.4*)	none
	rat	female	0.4 (*2.4*)	none
	rat	male	6 (*37.5*)	1.5 (*9.4*)
Mammary gland neoplasms, Total	rat	male	1.5 (*9.4*)	0.4 (*2.4*)

Antipsychotic drugs have been shown to chronically elevate prolactin levels in rodents. Serum prolactin levels were not measured during the risperidone carcinogenicity studies; however, measurements during subchronic toxicity studies showed that risperidone elevated serum prolactin levels 5 to 6 fold in mice and rats at the same doses used in the carcinogenicity studies. An increase in mammary, pituitary, and endocrine pancreas neoplasms has been found in rodents after chronic administration of other antipsychotic drugs and is considered to be prolactin mediated. The relevance for human risk of the findings of prolactin-mediated endocrine tumors in rodents is unknown (See Hyperprolactinemia under PRECAUTIONS, GENERAL).

Mutagenesis: No evidence of mutagenic potential for risperidone was found in the Ames reverse mutation test, mouse lymphoma assay, in vitro rat hepatocyte DNA-repair assay, in vivo micronucleus test in mice, the sex-linked recessive lethal test in Drosophila, or the chromosomal aberration test in human lymphocytes or Chinese hamster cells.

Impairment of Fertility: Risperidone (0.16 to 5 mg/kg) was shown to impair mating, but not fertility, in Wistar rats in three reproductive studies (two Segment I and a multigenerational study) at doses 0.1 to 3 times the maximum recommended human dose on a mg/m^2 basis. The effect appeared to be in females since impaired mating behavior was not noted in the Segment I study in which males only were treated. In a subchronic study in Beagle dogs in which risperidone was administered at doses of 0.31 to 5 mg/kg, sperm motility and concentration were decreased at doses 0.6 to 10 times the human dose on a mg/m^2 basis. Dose-related decreases were also noted in serum testosterone at the same doses. Serum testosterone and sperm parameters partially recovered but remained decreased after treatment was discontinued. No no-effect doses were noted in either rat or dog.

Pregnancy

Pregnancy Category C: The teratogenic potential of risperidone was studied in three Segment II studies in Sprague-Dawley and Wistar rats and in one Segment II study in New Zealand rabbits. The incidence of malformations was not increased compared to control in offspring of rats or rabbits given 0.4 to 6 times the human dose on a mg/m^2 basis. In three reproductive studies in rats (two Segment III and a multigenerational study), there was an increase in pup deaths during the first 4 days of lactation at doses 0.1 to 3 times the human dose on a mg/m^2 basis. It is not known whether these deaths were due to a direct effect on the fetuses or pups or to effects on the dams. There was no no-effect dose for increased rat pup mortality. In one Segment III study, there was an increase in stillborn rat pups at a dose 1.5 times higher than the human dose on a mg/m^2 basis.

Placental transfer of risperidone occurs in rat pups. There are no adequate and well-controlled studies in pregnant women. However, there was one report of a case of agenesis of the corpus callosum in an infant exposed to risperidone in utero. The causal relationship to RISPERDAL® therapy is unknown.

RISPERDAL® should be used during pregnancy only if the potential benefit justifies the potential risk to the fetus.

Labor and Delivery

The effect of RISPERDAL® on labor and delivery in humans is unknown.

Nursing Mothers

It is not known whether or not risperidone is excreted in human milk. In animal studies, risperidone and 9-hydroxyrisperidone were excreted in breast milk. Therefore, women receiving RISPERDAL® should not breast feed.

Pediatric Use

Safety and effectiveness in children have not been established.

Geriatric Use

Clinical studies of RISPERDAL® did not include sufficient numbers of patients aged 65 and over to determine whether they respond differently from younger patients. Other reported clinical experience has not identified differences in responses between elderly and younger patients. In general, a lower starting dose is recommended for an elderly patient, reflecting a decreased pharmacokinetic clearance in the elderly, as well as a greater frequency of decreased hepatic, renal, or cardiac function, and of concomitant disease or other drug therapy. (See CLINICAL PHARMACOLOGY and DOSAGE AND ADMINISTRATION). While elderly patients exhibit a greater tendency to orthostatic hypotension, its risk in the elderly may be minimized by limiting the initial dose to 0.5 mg BID followed by careful titration (See PRECAUTIONS). Monitoring of orthostatic vital signs should be considered in patients for whom this is of concern. This drug is known to be substantially excreted by the kidney, and the risk of toxic reactions to this drug may be greater in patients with impaired renal function. Because elderly patients are more likely to have decreased renal function, care should be taken in dose selection, and it may be useful to monitor renal function (See DOSAGE AND ADMINISTRATION).

ADVERSE REACTIONS

Associated with Discontinuation of Treatment

Approximately 9% percent (244/2607) of RISPERDAL® (risperidone)-treated patients in phase 2–3 studies discontinued treatment due to an adverse event, compared with about 7% on placebo and 10% on active control drugs. The more common events (≥0.3%) associated with discontinuation and considered to be possibly or probably drug-related included:

Adverse Event	RISPERDAL®	Placebo
Extrapyramidal symptoms	2.1%	0%
Dizziness	0.7%	0%
Hyperkinesia	0.6%	0%
Somnolence	0.5%	0%
Nausea	0.3%	0%

Suicide attempt was associated with discontinuation in 1.2% of RISPERDAL® treated patients compared to 0.6% of placebo patients, but, given the almost 40-fold greater exposure time in RISPERDAL® compared to placebo patients, it is unlikely that suicide attempt is a RISPERDAL® related adverse event (See PRECAUTIONS). Discontinuation for extrapyramidal symptoms was 0% in placebo patients but 3.8% in active-control patients in the phase 2–3 trials.

Incidence in Controlled Trials

Commonly Observed Adverse Events in Controlled Clinical Trials: In two 6- to 8-week placebo-controlled trials, spontaneously-reported, treatment-emergent adverse events with an incidence of 5% or greater in at least one of the RISPERDAL® groups and at least twice that of placebo were: anxiety, somnolence, extrapyramidal symptoms, dizziness, constipation, nausea, dyspepsia, rhinitis, rash, and tachycardia.

Adverse events were also elicited in one of these two trials (i.e., in the fixed-dose trial comparing RISPERDAL® at doses of 2, 6, 10, and 16 mg/day with placebo) utilizing a checklist for detecting adverse events, a method that is more sensitive than spontaneous reporting. By this method, the following additional common and drug-related adverse events were present at least 5% and twice the rate of placebo: increased dream activity, increased duration of sleep, accommodation disturbances, reduced salivation, micturition disturbances, diarrhea, weight gain, menorrhagia, diminished sexual desire, erectile dysfunction, ejaculatory dysfunction, and orgastic dysfunction.

Adverse Events Occurring at an Incidence of 1% or More Among RISPERDAL®-Treated Patients: The table that follows enumerates adverse events that occurred at an incidence of 1% or more, and were at least as frequent among RISPERDAL® treated patients treated at doses of ≤10 mg/day than among placebo-treated patients in the pooled results of two 6- to 8-week controlled trials. Patients received RISPERDAL® doses of 2, 6, 10, or 16 mg/day in the dose comparison trial, or up to a maximum dose of 10 mg/day in the titration study. This table shows the percentage of patients in each dose group (≤10 mg/day or 16 mg/day) who spontaneously reported at least one episode of an event at some time during their treatment. Patients given doses of 2, 6, or 10 mg did not differ materially in these rates. Reported adverse events were classified using the World Health Organization preferred terms.

The prescriber should be aware that these figures cannot be used to predict the incidence of side effects in the course of usual medical practice where patient characteristics and other factors differ from those which prevailed in this clinical trial. Similarly, the cited frequencies cannot be compared with figures obtained from other clinical investigations involving different treatments, uses and investigators. The cited figures, however, do provide the prescribing physician with some basis for estimating the relative contribution of drug and nondrug factors to the side effect incidence rate in the population studied.

Table 1: Treatment-Emergent Adverse Experience Incidence in 6- to 8-Week Controlled Clinical Trials[1]

Body System/ Preferred Term	RISPERDAL® ≤10 mg/day (N=324)	RISPERDAL® 16 mg/day (N=77)	Placebo (N=142)
Psychiatric Disorders			
Insomnia	26%	23%	19%
Agitation	22%	26%	20%
Anxiety	12%	20%	9%
Somnolence	3%	8%	1%
Aggressive reaction	1%	3%	1%
Nervous System			
Extrapyramidal symptoms[2]	17%	34%	16%
Headache	14%	12%	12%
Dizziness	4%	7%	1%
Gastrointestinal System			
Constipation	7%	13%	3%
Nausea	6%	4%	3%
Dyspepsia	5%	10%	4%
Vomiting	5%	7%	4%
Abdominal pain	4%	1%	0%
Saliva increased	2%	0%	1%
Toothache	2%	0%	0%
Respiratory System			
Rhinitis	10%	8%	4%
Coughing	3%	3%	1%
Sinusitis	2%	1%	1%
Pharyngitis	2%	3%	0%
Dyspnea	1%	0%	0%
Body as a Whole			
Back pain	2%	0%	1%
Chest pain	2%	3%	1%
Fever	2%	3%	0%
Dermatological			
Rash	2%	5%	1%
Dry skin	2%	4%	0%
Seborrhea	1%	0%	0%
Infections			
Upper respiratory	3%	3%	1%
Visual			
Abnormal vision	2%	1%	1%
Musculo-Skeletal			
Arthralgia	2%	3%	0%
Cardiovascular			
Tachycardia	3%	5%	0%

[1] Events reported by at least 1% of patients treated with RISPERDAL® ≤10 mg/day are included, and are rounded to the nearest %. Comparative rates for RISPERDAL® 16 mg/day and placebo are provided as well. Events for which the RISPERDAL® incidence (in both dose groups) was equal to or less than placebo are not listed in the table, but included the following: nervousness, injury, and fungal infection.

[2] Includes tremor, dystonia, hypokinesia, hypertonia, hyperkinesia, oculogyric crisis, ataxia, abnormal gait, involuntary muscle contractions, hyporeflexia, akathisia and extrapyramidal disorders. Although the incidence of 'extrapyramidal symptoms' does not appear to differ for the '≤10 mg/day' group and placebo, the data for individual dose groups in fixed dose trials do suggest a dose/response relationship (See DOSE DEPENDENCY OF ADVERSE EVENTS).

Dose Dependency of Adverse Events:

Extrapyramidal symptoms: Data from two fixed dose trials provided evidence of dose-relatedness for extrapyramidal symptoms associated with risperidone treatment.

Two methods were used to measure extrapyramidal symptoms (EPS) in an 8-week trial comparing four fixed doses of risperidone (2, 6, 10, and 16 mg/day), including (1) a parkinsonism score (mean change from baseline) from the Extrapyramidal Symptom Rating Scale and (2) incidence of spontaneous complaints of EPS:

Dose Groups	Placebo	Ris 2	Ris 6	Ris 10	Ris 16
Parkinsonism	1.2	0.9	1.8	2.4	2.6
EPS Incidence	13%	13%	16%	20%	31%

Similar methods were used to measure extrapyramidal symptoms (EPS) in an 8-week trial comparing five fixed doses of risperidone (1, 4, 8, 12, and 16 mg/day):

Dose Groups	Ris 1	Ris 4	Ris 8	Ris 12	Ris 16
Parkinsonism	0.6	1.7	2.4	2.9	4.1
EPS Incidence	7%	12%	18%	18%	21%

Other Adverse Events: Adverse event data elicited by a checklist for side effects from a large study comparing 5 fixed doses of RISPERDAL® (1, 4, 8, 12, and 16 mg/day) were explored for dose-relatedness of adverse events. A Cochran-Armitage Test for trend in these data revealed a positive trend ($p<0.05$) for the following adverse events: sleepiness, increased duration of sleep, accommodation disturbances, orthostatic dizziness, palpitations, weight gain, erectile dysfunction, ejaculatory dysfunction, orgastic dysfunction, asthenia/lassitude/increased fatiguability, and increased pigmentation.

Vital Sign Changes: RISPERDAL® is associated with orthostatic hypotension and tachycardia (See PRECAUTIONS).

Weight changes: The proportions of RISPERDAL® and placebo-treated patients meeting a weight gain criterion of ≥ 7% of body weight were compared in a pool of 6- to 8-week placebo-controlled trials, revealing a statistically significantly greater incidence of weight gain for RISPERDAL® (18%) compared to placebo (9%).

Laboratory Changes: A between group comparison for 6- to 8-week placebo-controlled trials revealed no statistically significant RISPERDAL®/placebo differences in the proportions of patients experiencing potentially important changes in routine serum chemistry, hematology, or urinalysis parameters. Similarly, there were no RISPERDAL®/placebo differences in the incidence of discontinuations for changes in serum chemistry, hematology, or urinalysis. However, RISPERDAL® administration was associated with increases in serum prolactin (See PRECAUTIONS).

ECG Changes: The electrocardiograms of approximately 380 patients who received RISPERDAL® and 120 patients who received placebo in two double-blind, placebo-controlled trials were evaluated and revealed one finding of potential concern; i.e., 8 patients taking RISPERDAL® whose baseline QTc interval was less than 450 msec were observed to have QTc intervals greater than 450 msec during treatment (See WARNINGS). Changes of this type were not seen among about 120 placebo patients, but were seen in patients receiving haloperidol (3/126).

Other Events Observed During the Pre-Marketing Evaluation of RISPERDAL®

During its premarketing assessment, multiple doses of RISPERDAL® (risperidone) were administered to 2607 patients in phase 2 and 3 studies. The conditions and duration of exposure to RISPERDAL® varied greatly, and included (in overlapping categories) open and double-blind studies, uncontrolled and controlled studies, inpatient and outpatient studies, fixed-dose and titration studies, and short-term or longer-term exposure. In most studies, untoward events associated with this exposure were obtained by spontaneous report and recorded by clinical investigators using terminology of their own choosing. Consequently, it is not possible to provide a meaningful estimate of the proportion of individuals experiencing adverse events without first grouping similar types of untoward events into a smaller number of standardized event categories. In two large studies, adverse events were also elicited utilizing the UKU (direct questioning) side effect rating scale, and these events were not further categorized using standard terminology (Note: These events are marked with an asterisk in the listings that follow).

In the listings that follow, spontaneously reported adverse events were classified using World Health Organization (WHO) preferred terms. The frequencies presented, therefore, represent the proportion of the 2607 patients exposed to multiple doses of RISPERDAL® who experienced an event of the type cited on at least one occasion while receiving RISPERDAL®. All reported events are included except those already listed in Table 1, those events for which a drug cause was remote, and those event terms which were so general as to be uninformative. It is important to emphasize that, although the events reported occurred during treatment with RISPERDAL®, they were not necessarily caused by it.

Events are further categorized by body system and listed in order of decreasing frequency according to the following definitions: frequent adverse events are those occurring in at least 1/100 patients (only those not already listed in the tabulated results from placebo controlled trials appear in this listing); infrequent adverse events are those occurring in 1/100 to 1/1000 patients; rare events are those occurring in fewer than 1/1000 patients.

Psychiatric Disorders: *Frequent:* increased dream activity*, diminished sexual desire*, nervousness. *Infrequent:* impaired concentration, depression, apathy, catatonic reaction, euphoria, increased libido, amnesia. *Rare:* emotional lability, nightmares, delirium, withdrawal syndrome, yawning.

Central and Peripheral Nervous System Disorders: *Frequent:* increased sleep duration*. *Infrequent:* dysarthria, vertigo, stupor, paraesthesia, confusion. *Rare:* aphasia, cholinergic syndrome, hypoesthesia, tongue paralysis, leg cramps, torticollis, hypotonia, coma, migraine, hyperreflexia, choreoathetosis.

Gastro-intestinal Disorders: *Frequent:* anorexia, reduced salivation*. *Infrequent:* flatulence, diarrhea, increased appetite, stomatitis, melena, dysphagia, hemorrhoids, gastritis. *Rare:* fecal incontinence, eructation, gastroesophageal reflux, gastroenteritis, esophagitis, tongue discoloration, cholelithiasis, tongue edema, diverticulitis, gingivitis, discolored feces, GI hemorrhage, hematemesis.

Body as a Whole/General Disorders: *Frequent:* fatigue. *Infrequent:* edema, rigors, malaise, influenza-like symptoms. *Rare:* pallor, enlarged abdomen, allergic reaction, ascites, sarcoidosis, flushing.

Respiratory System Disorders: *Infrequent:* hyperventilation, bronchospasm, pneumonia, stridor. *Rare:* asthma, increased sputum, aspiration.

Skin and Appendage Disorders: *Frequent:* increased pigmentation*, photosensitivity*. *Infrequent:* increased sweating, acne, decreased sweating, alopecia, hyperkeratosis, pruritus, skin exfoliation. *Rare:* bullous eruption, skin ulceration, aggravated psoriasis, furunculosis, verruca, dermatitis lichenoid, hypertrichosis, genital pruritus, urticaria.

Cardiovascular Disorders: *Infrequent:* palpitation, hypertension, hypotension, AV block, myocardial infarction. *Rare:* ventricular tachycardia, angina pectoris, premature atrial contractions, T wave inversions, ventricular extrasystoles, ST depression, myocarditis.

Vision Disorders: *Infrequent:* abnormal accommodation, xerophthalmia. *Rare:* diplopia, eye pain, blepharitis, photopsia, photophobia, abnormal lacrimation.

Metabolic and Nutritional Disorders: *Infrequent:* hyponatremia, weight increase, creatine phosphokinase increase, thirst, weight decrease, diabetes mellitus. *Rare:* decreased serum iron, cachexia, dehydration, hypokalemia, hypoproteinemia, hyperphosphatemia, hypertriglyceridemia, hyperuricemia, hypoglycemia.

Urinary System Disorders: *Frequent:* polyuria/polydipsia*. *Infrequent:* urinary incontinence, hematuria, dysuria. *Rare:* urinary retention, cystitis, renal insufficiency.

Musculo-skeletal System Disorders: *Infrequent:* myalgia. *Rare:* arthrosis, synostosis, bursitis, arthritis, skeletal pain.

Reproductive Disorders, Female: *Frequent:* menorrhagia*, orgastic dysfunction*, dry vagina*. *Infrequent:* nonpuerperal lactation, amenorrhea, female breast pain, leukorrhea, mastitis, dysmenorrhea, female perineal pain, intermenstrual bleeding, vaginal hemorrhage.

Liver and Biliary System Disorders: *Infrequent:* increased SGOT, increased SGPT. *Rare:* hepatic failure, cholestatic hepatitis, cholecystitis, cholelithiasis, hepatitis, hepatocellular damage.

Platelet, Bleeding and Clotting Disorders: *Infrequent:* epistaxis, purpura. *Rare:* hemorrhage, superficial phlebitis, thrombophlebitis, thrombocytopenia.

Hearing and Vestibular Disorders: *Rare:* tinnitus, hyperacusis, decreased hearing.

Red Blood Cell Disorders: *Infrequent:* anemia, hypochromic anemia. *Rare:* normocytic anemia.

Reproductive Disorders, Male: *Frequent:* erectile dysfunction*. *Infrequent:* ejaculation failure.

White Cell and Resistance Disorders: *Rare:* leukocytosis, lymphadenopathy, leucopenia, Pelger-Huet anomaly.

Endocrine Disorders: *Rare:* gynecomastia, male breast pain, antidiuretic hormone disorder.

Special Senses: *Rare:* bitter taste.

* Incidence based on elicited reports.

Post introduction Reports: Adverse events reported since market introduction which were temporally (but not necessarily causally) related to RISPERDAL® therapy, include the following: anaphylactic reaction, angioedema, apnea, atrial fibrillation, cerebrovascular disorder, diabetes mellitus aggravated, including diabetic ketoacidosis intestinal obstruction, jaundice, mania, pancreatitis, Parkinson's disease aggravated, pulmonary embolism. There have been rare reports of sudden death and/or cardiopulmonary arrest in patients receiving RISPERDAL®. A causal relationship with RISPERDAL® has not been established. It is important to note that sudden and unexpected death may occur in psychotic patients whether they remain untreated or whether they are treated with other antipsychotic drugs.

DRUG ABUSE AND DEPENDENCE

Controlled Substance Class: RISPERDAL® (risperidone) is not a controlled substance.

Physical and Psychologic Dependence: RISPERDAL® has not been systematically studied in animals or humans for its potential for abuse, tolerance or physical dependence. While the clinical trials did not reveal any tendency for any drug-seeking behavior, these observations were not systematic and it is not possible to predict on the basis of this limited experience the extent to which a CNS-active drug will be misused, diverted and/or abused once marketed. Consequently, patients should be evaluated carefully for a history of drug abuse, and such patients should be observed closely for signs of RISPERDAL® misuse or abuse (e.g., development of tolerance, increases in dose, drug-seeking behavior).

OVERDOSAGE

Human Experience: Premarketing experience included eight reports of acute RISPERDAL® overdosage with estimated doses ranging from 20 to 300 mg and no fatalities. In general, reported signs and symptoms were those resulting from an exaggeration of the drug's known pharmacological effects, i.e., drowsiness and sedation, tachycardia and hypotension, and extrapyramidal symptoms. One case, involving an estimated overdose of 240 mg, was associated with hyponatremia, hypokalemia, prolonged QT, and widened QRS. Another case, involving an estimated overdose of 36 mg, was associated with a seizure. Postmarketing experience includes reports of acute RISPERDAL® overdosage, with estimated doses of up to 360 mg. In general, the most frequently reported signs and symptoms are those resulting from an exaggeration of the drug's known pharmacological effects, i.e., drowsiness, sedation, tachycardia and hypotension. Other adverse events reported since market introduction which were temporally, (but not necessarily causally) related to RISPERDAL® overdose, include prolonged QT interval, convulsions, cardiopulmonary arrest, and rare fatality associated with multiple drug overdose.

Management of Overdosage: In case of acute overdosage, establish and maintain an airway and ensure adequate oxygenation and ventilation. Gastric lavage (after intubation, if patient is unconscious) and administration of activated charcoal together with a laxative should be considered. The possibility of obtundation, seizures or dystonic reaction of the head and neck following overdose may create a risk of aspiration with induced emesis. Cardiovascular monitoring should commence immediately and should include continuous electrocardiographic monitoring to detect possible arrhythmias. If antiarrhythmic therapy is administered, disopyramide, procainamide and quinidine carry a theoretical hazard of QT-prolonging effects that might be additive to those of risperidone. Similarly, it is reasonable to expect that the alpha-blocking properties of bretylium might be additive to those of risperidone, resulting in problematic hypotension.

There is no specific antidote to RISPERDAL®. Therefore appropriate supportive measures should be instituted. The possibility of multiple drug involvement should be considered. Hypotension and circulatory collapse should be treated with appropriate measures such as intravenous fluids and/or sympathomimetic agents (epinephrine and dopamine should not be used, since beta stimulation may worsen hypotension in the setting of risperidone-induced alpha blockade). In cases of severe extrapyramidal symptoms, anticholinergic medication should be administered. Close medical supervision and monitoring should continue until the patient recovers.

DOSAGE AND ADMINISTRATION

Usual Initial Dose: RISPERDAL® (risperidone) can be administered on either a BID or a QD schedule. In early clinical trials, RIPSERDAL® was generally administered at 1 mg BID initially, with increases in increments of 1 mg BID on the second and third day, as tolerated, to a target dose of 3 mg BID by the third day. Subsequent controlled trials have indicated that total daily risperidone doses of up to 8 mg on a QD regimen are also safe and effective. However, regardless of which regimen is employed, in some patients a slower titration may be medically appropriate. Further dosage adjustments, if indicated, should generally occur at intervals of not less than 1 week, since steady state for the active metabolite would not be achieved for approximately 1 week in the typical patient. When dosage adjustments are necessary, small increments/decrements of 1–2 mg are recommended.

Antipsychotic efficacy was demonstrated in a dose range of 4 to 16 mg/day in the clinical trials supporting effectiveness of RISPERDAL®, however, maximal effect was generally seen in a range of 4 to 8 mg/day. Doses above 6 mg/day for BID dosing were not demonstrated to be more efficacious than lower doses, were associated with more extrapyramidal symptoms and other adverse effects, and are not generally recommended. In a single study supporting QD dosing, the efficacy results were generally stronger for 8 mg than for 4 mg. The safety of doses above 16 mg/day has not been evaluated in clinical trials.

Pediatric Use: Safety and effectiveness in pediatric patients have not been established.

Dosage in Special Populations: The recommended initial dose is 0.5 mg BID in patients who are elderly or debilitated, patients with severe renal or hepatic impairment, and patients either predisposed to hypotension or for whom hypotension would pose a risk. Dosage increases in these patients should be in increments of no more than 0.5 mg BID. Increases to dosages above 1.5 mg BID should generally occur at intervals of at least 1 week. In some patients, slower titration may be medically appropriate.

Elderly or debilitated patients, and patients with renal impairment, may have less ability to eliminate RISPERDAL® than normal adults. Patients with impaired hepatic function may have increases in the free fraction of the risperidone, possibly resulting in an enhanced effect (See CLINICAL PHARMACOLOGY). Patients with a predisposition to hypotensive reactions or for whom such reactions would pose a particular risk likewise need to be titrated cautiously and carefully monitored (See PRECAUTIONS).

If a once-a-day dosing regimen in the elderly or debilitated patient is being considered, it is recommended that the patient be titrated on a twice-a-day regimen for 2–3 days at the target dose. Subsequent switches to a once-a-day dosing regimen can be done thereafter.

Maintenance Therapy: While there is no body of evidence available to answer the question of how long the patient treated with RISPERDAL® should remain on it, the effectiveness of maintenance treatment is well established for many other antipsychotic drugs. It is recommended that responding patients be continued on RISPERDAL®, but at the lowest dose needed to maintain remission. Patients should be periodically reassessed to determine the need for maintenance treatment.

Reinitiation of Treatment in Patients Previously Discontinued: Although there are no data to specifically address reinitiation of treatment, it is recommended that when restarting patients who have had an interval off RISPERDAL®, the initial titration schedule should be followed.

Switching from Other Antipsychotics: There are no systematically collected data to specifically address switching from other antipsychotics to RISPERDAL®, or concerning concomitant administration with other antipsychotics. While immediate discontinuation of the previous antipsy-

Continued on next page

Risperdal—Cont.

chotic treatment may be acceptable for some patients, more gradual discontinuation may be most appropriate for other patients. In all cases, the period of overlapping antipsychotic administration should be minimized. When switching patients from depot antipsychotics, if medically appropriate, initiate RISPERDAL® therapy in place of the next scheduled injection. The need for continuing existing EPS medication should be reevaluated periodically.

HOW SUPPLIED

RISPERDAL® (risperidone) tablets are imprinted "JANSSEN", and either "Ris" and the strength "0.25," "0.5" or "R" and the strength "1", "2", "3", or "4".

0.25 mg dark yellow tablet: bottles of 60 NDC 50458-301-04, bottles of 500 NDC 50458-301-50.

0.5 mg red-brown tablet: bottles of 60 NDC 50458-302-06, bottles of 500 NDC 50458-302-50.

1 mg white tablet: bottles of 60 NDC 50458-300-06, blister pack of 100 NDC 50458-300-01, bottles of 500 NDC 50458-300-50.

2 mg orange tablet: bottles of 60 NDC 50458-320-06, blister pack of 100 NDC 50458-320-01, bottles of 500 NDC 50458-320-50

3 mg yellow tablet: bottles of 60 NDC 50458-330-06, blister pack of 100 NDC 50458-330-01, bottles of 500 NDC 50458-330-50

4 mg green tablet: bottles of 60 NDC 50458-350-06, blister pack of 100 NDC 50458-350-01.

RISPERDAL® (risperidone) 1 mg/mL oral solution (NDC 50458-305-03) is supplied in 30mL bottles with a calibrated (in milligrams and milliliters) pipette. The minimum calibrated volume is 0.25 mL, while the maximum calibrated volume is 3 mL.

Patient Instructions (including illustrations) for using the RISPERDAL® (risperidone) calibrated dispensing-pipette are provided. Tests indicate that RISPERDAL® (risperidone) oral solution is compatible in the following beverages: water, coffee, orange juice and low-fat milk; it is NOT compatible with either cola or tea, however.

STORAGE AND HANDLING - RISPERDAL® tablets should be stored at controlled room temperature (59°–77°F/15°–25°C) away from children, and should be protected from light and moisture.

RISPERDAL® 1 mg/mL oral solution should be stored at controlled room temperature (59°–77°F/15°–25°C) away from children, and should be protected from light and freezing.

US Patent 4,804,663

July 1998, May 1999

JANSSEN
PHARMACEUTICA
Titusville, NJ 08560

Shown in Product Identification Guide, page 318

SPORANOX ℞

[*spər 'ah-näks"*]
(Itraconazole)
100 mg capsules

> **WARNING:** Coadministration of astemizole, cisapride, pimozide, or quinidine with SPORANOX® (itraconazole) Capsules, Injection or Oral Solution is contraindicated. SPORANOX®, a potent cytochrome P450 3A4 isoenzyme system (CYP3A4) inhibitor, may increase plasma concentrations of drugs metabolized by this pathway. Serious cardiovascular events, including QT prolongation, torsades de pointes, ventricular tachycardia, cardiac arrest, and/or sudden death have occurred in patients using astemizole, cisapride, pimozide, or quinidine, concomitantly with SPORANOX® and/or other CYP3A4 inhibitors. See CONTRAINDICATIONS, WARNINGS, and PRECAUTIONS: Drug Interactions for more information.

DESCRIPTION

SPORANOX® is the brand name for itraconazole, a synthetic triazole antifungal agent. Itraconazole is a 1:1:1:1 racemic mixture of four diastereomers (two enantiomeric pairs), each possessing three chiral centers. It may be represented by the following structural formula and nomenclature:

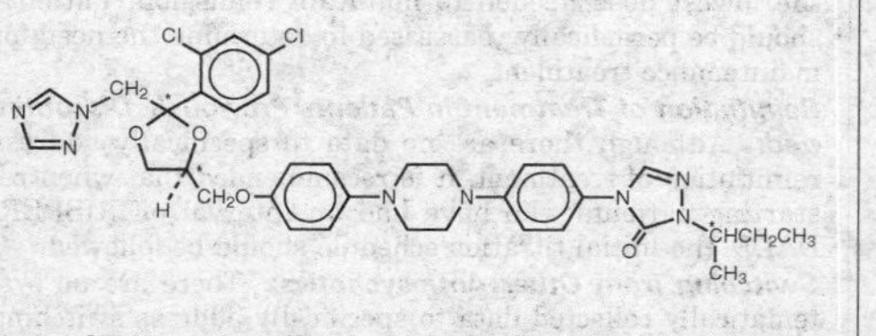

(±)-1-[(R*)-sec-butyl]-4-[p-[4-[p-[[(2R*,4S*)-2-(2,4-dichlorophenyl)-2-(1H-1,2,4-triazol-1-ylmethyl)-1,3-dioxolan-4-yl]methoxy]phenyl]-1-piperazinyl]phenyl]-Δ^2-1,2,4-triazolin-5-one mixture with (±)-1-[(R*)-sec-butyl]-4-[p-[4-[p-[[(2S*,4R*) -2-(2,4-dichlorophenyl) -2-(1H-1,2,4-triazol-1-ylmethyl)-1,3-dioxolan-4-yl]methoxy]phenyl]-1-piperazinyl]phenyl]-Δ^2-1,2,4-triazolin-5-one

or

(±)-1-[(RS)-sec-butyl]-4-[p-[4-[p-[[(2R,4S)-2-(2,4-dichlorophenyl)-2-(1H-1,2,4-triazol-1-ylmethyl)-1,3-dioxolan-4-yl]methoxy]phenyl]-1-piperazinyl]phenyl]-Δ^2-1,2,4-triazolin-5-one

Itraconazole has a molecular formula of $C_{35}H_{38}Cl_2N_8O_4$ and a molecular weight of 705.64. It is a white to slightly yellowish powder. It is insoluble in water, very slightly soluble in alcohols, and freely soluble in dichloromethane. It has a pKa of 3.70 (based on extrapolation of values obtained from methanolic solutions) and a log (n-octanol/water) partition coefficient of 5.66 at pH 8.1.

SPORANOX® Capsules contain 100 mg of itraconazole coated on sugar spheres. Inactive ingredients are gelatin, hydroxypropyl methylcellulose, polyethylene glycol (PEG) 20,000, starch, sucrose, titanium dioxide, FD&C Blue No. 1, FD&C Blue No. 2, D&C Red No. 22 and D&C Red No. 28.

CLINICAL PHARMACOLOGY

Pharmacokinetics and Metabolism: NOTE: The plasma concentrations reported below were measured by high-performance liquid chromatography (HPLC) specific for itraconazole. When itraconazole in plasma is measured by a bioassay, values reported are approximately 3.3 times higher than those obtained by HPLC due to the presence of the bioactive metabolite, hydroxyitraconazole. (See MICROBIOLOGY.)

The pharmacokinetics of itraconazole after intravenous administration and its absolute oral bioavailability from an oral solution were studied in a randomized crossover study in 6 healthy male volunteers. The observed absolute oral bioavailability of itraconazole was 55%.

The oral bioavailability of itraconazole is maximal when SPORANOX® (itraconazole) Capsules are taken with a full meal. The pharmacokinetics of itraconazole were studied in 6 healthy male volunteers who received, in a crossover design, single 100-mg doses of itraconazole as a polyethylene glycol capsule, with or without a full meal. The same 6 volunteers also received 50 mg or 200 mg with a full meal in a crossover design. In this study, only itraconazole plasma concentrations were measured. The respective pharmacokinetic parameters for itraconazole are presented in the table below:

[See first table at bottom of next page]

Doubling the SPORANOX® dose results in approximately a three-fold increase in the itraconazole plasma concentrations.

Values given in the table below represent data from a crossover pharmacokinetics study in which 27 healthy male volunteers each took a single 200-mg dose of SPORANOX® Capsules with or without a full meal:

[See second table at bottom of next page]

Absorption of itraconazole under fasted conditions in individuals with relative or absolute achlorhydria, such as patients with AIDS or volunteers taking gastric acid secretion suppressors (e.g., H_2 receptor antagonists), was increased when SPORANOX® Capsules were administered with a cola beverage. Eighteen men with AIDS received single 200-mg doses of SPORANOX® Capsules under fasted conditions with 8 ounces of water or 8 ounces of a cola beverage in a crossover design. The absorption of itraconazole was increased when SPORANOX® Capsules were coadministered with a cola beverage, with AUC_{0-24} and C_{max} increasing 75% ± 121% and 95% ± 128%, respectively.

Thirty healthy men received single 200-mg doses of SPORANOX® Capsules under fasted conditions either 1) with water; 2) with water, after ranitidine 150 mg b.i.d. for 3 days; or 3) with cola, after ranitidine 150 mg b.i.d. for 3 days. When SPORANOX® Capsules were administered after ranitidine pretreatment, itraconazole was absorbed to a lesser extent than when SPORANOX® Capsules were administered alone, with decreases in AUC_{0-24} and C_{max} of 39% ± 37% and 42% ± 39%, respectively. When SPORANOX® Capsules were administered with cola after ranitidine pretreatment, itraconazole absorption was comparable to that observed when SPORANOX® Capsules were administered alone. (See PRECAUTIONS: Drug Interactions.)

Steady-state concentrations were reached within 15 days following oral doses of 50 mg to 400 mg daily. Values given in the table below are data at steady-state from a pharmacokinetics study in which 27 healthy male volunteers took 200-mg SPORANOX® Capsules b.i.d. (with a full meal) for 15 days:

[See third table at bottom of next page]

The plasma protein binding of itraconazole is 99.8% and that of hydroxyitraconazole is 99.5%. Following intravenous administration, the volume of distribution of itraconazole averaged 796 ± 185 liters.

Itraconazole is metabolized predominately by the cytochrome P450 3A4 isoenzyme system (CYP3A4), resulting in the formation of several metabolites, including hydroxyitraconazole, the major metabolite. Results of a pharmacokinetics study suggest that itraconazole may undergo saturable metabolism with multiple dosing. Fecal excretion of the parent drug varies between 3–18% of the dose. Renal excretion of the parent drug is less than 0.03% of the dose. About 40% of the dose is excreted as inactive metabolites in the urine. No single excreted metabolite represents more than 5% of a dose. Itraconazole total plasma clearance averaged 381 ± 95 mL/minute following intravenous administration.

Special Populations:

Renal Insufficiency: A pharmacokinetic study using a single 200-mg dose of itraconazole (four 50-mg capsules) was conducted in three groups of patients with renal impairment (uremia: n=7; hemodialysis: n=7; and continuous ambulatory peritoneal dialysis: n=5). In uremic subjects with a mean creatinine clearance of 13 mL/min. × 1.73 m^2, the bioavailability was slightly reduced compared with normal population parameters. This study did not demonstrate any significant effect of hemodialysis or continuous ambulatory peritoneal dialysis on the pharmacokinetics of itraconazole (T_{max}, C_{max}, and AUC_{0-8}). Plasma concentration-versus-time profiles showed wide intersubject variation in all three groups.

Hepatic Insufficiency: A pharmacokinetic study using a single 100-mg dose of itraconazole (one 100-mg capsule) was conducted in 6 healthy and 12 cirrhotic subjects. No statistically significant differences in AUC were seen between these two groups. A statistically significant reduction in mean C_{max} (47%) and a two-fold increase in the elimination half-life (37 ± 17 hours) of itraconazole were noted in cirrhotic subjects compared with healthy subjects. Patients with impaired hepatic function should be carefully monitored when taking itraconazole. The prolonged elimination half-life of itraconazole observed in cirrhotic patients should be considered when deciding to initiate therapy with other medications metabolized by CYP3A4. (See BOXED WARNING, CONTRAINDICATIONS, and PRECAUTIONS: Drug Interactions.)

MICROBIOLOGY

Mechanism of Action: In vitro studies have demonstrated that itraconazole inhibits the cytochrome P-450-dependent synthesis of ergosterol, which is a vital component of fungal cell membranes.

Activity In Vitro and In Vivo: Itraconazole exhibits in vitro activity against *Blastomyces dermatitidis, Histoplasma capsulatum, Histoplasma duboisii, Aspergillus flavus, Aspergillus fumigatus, Candida albicans,* and *Cryptococcus neoformans.* Itraconazole also exhibits varying in vitro activity against *Sporothrix schenckii, Trichophyton* species, *Candida krusei*, and other *Candida* species. The bioactive metabolite, hydroxyitraconazole, has not been evaluated against *Histoplasma capsulatum* and *Blastomyces dermatitidis.* Correlation between minimum inhibitory concentration (MIC) results in vitro and clinical outcome has yet to be established for azole antifungal agents.

Itraconazole administered orally was active in a variety of animal models of fungal infection using standard laboratory strains of fungi. Fungistatic activity has been demonstrated against disseminated fungal infections caused by *Blastomyces dermatitidis, Histoplasma duboisii, Aspergillus fumigatus, Coccidioides immitis, Cryptococcus neoformans, Paracoccidioides brasiliensis, Sporothrix schenckii, Trichophyton rubrum,* and *Trichophyton mentagrophytes.*

Itraconazole administered at 2.5 mg/kg and 5 mg/kg via the oral and parenteral routes increased survival rates and sterilized organ systems in normal and immunosuppressed guinea pigs with disseminated *Aspergillus fumigatus* infections. Oral itraconazole administered daily at 40 mg/kg and 80 mg/kg increased survival rates in normal rabbits with disseminated disease and in immunosuppressed rats with pulmonary *Aspergillus fumigatus* infection, respectively. Itraconazole has demonstrated antifungal activity in a variety of animal models infected with *Candida albicans* and other *Candida* species.

Resistance: Isolates from several fungal species with decreased susceptibility to itraconazole have been isolated in vitro and from patients receiving prolonged therapy.

Several in vitro studies have reported that some fungal clinical isolates, including *Candida* species, with reduced susceptibility to one azole antifungal agent may also be less susceptible to other azole derivatives. The finding of cross-resistance is dependent on a number of factors, including the species evaluated, its clinical history, the particular azole compounds compared, and the type of susceptibility test that is performed. The relevance of these in vitro susceptibility data to clinical outcome remains to be elucidated.

Studies (both in vitro and in vivo) suggest that the activity of amphotericin B may be suppressed by prior azole antifungal therapy. As with other azoles, itraconazole inhibits the ^{14}C-demethylation step in the synthesis of ergosterol, a cell wall component of fungi. Ergosterol is the active site for amphotericin B. In one study the antifungal activity of amphotericin B against *Aspergillus fumigatus* infections in mice was inhibited by ketoconazole therapy. The clinical significance of test results obtained in this study is unknown.

INDICATIONS AND USAGE

SPORANOX® Capsules are indicated for the treatment of the following fungal infections in non-immunocompromised patients:

1. Onychomycosis of the toenail, with or without fingernail involvement, due to dermatophytes (tinea unguium), and
2. Onychomycosis of the fingernail due to dermatophytes (tinea unguium).

SPORANOX® (itraconazole) Capsules are indicated for the treatment of the following fungal infections in immunocompromised and non-immunocompromised patients:

1. Blastomycosis, pulmonary and extrapulmonary
2. Histoplasmosis, including chronic cavitary pulmonary disease and disseminated, non-meningeal histoplasmosis, and
3. Aspergillosis, pulmonary and extrapulmonary, in patients who are intolerant of or who are refractory to amphotericin B therapy.

Specimens for fungal cultures and other relevant laboratory studies (wet mount, histopathology, serology) should be obtained before therapy to isolate and identify causative organisms. Therapy may be instituted before the results of the cultures and other laboratory studies are known; however, once these results become available, anti-infective therapy should be adjusted accordingly.

Description of Clinical Studies:

Blastomycosis: Analyses were conducted on data from two open-label, non-concurrently controlled studies (N=73 combined) in patients with normal or abnormal immune status. The median dose was 200 mg/day. A response for most signs and symptoms was observed within the first 2 weeks, and all signs and symptoms cleared between 3 and 6 months. Results of these two studies demonstrated substantial evidence of the effectiveness of itraconazole for the treatment of blastomycosis compared with the natural history of untreated cases.

Histoplasmosis: Analyses were conducted on data from two open-label, non-concurrently controlled studies (N=34 combined) in patients with normal or abnormal immune status (not including HIV-infected patients). The median dose was 200 mg/day. A response for most signs and symptoms was observed within the first 2 weeks, and all signs and symptoms cleared between 3 and 12 months. Results of these two studies demonstrated substantial evidence of the effectiveness of itraconazole for the treatment of histoplasmosis, compared with the natural history of untreated cases.

Histoplasmosis in HIV-infected patients: Data from a small number of HIV-infected patients suggested that the response rate of histoplasmosis in HIV-infected patients is similar to that of non-HIV-infected patients. The clinical course of histoplasmosis in HIV-infected patients is more severe and usually requires maintenance therapy to prevent relapse.

Aspergillosis: Analyses were conducted on data from an open-label, "single-patient-use" protocol designed to make itraconazole available in the U.S. for patients who either failed or were intolerant of amphotericin B therapy (N=190). The findings were corroborated by two smaller open-label studies (N=31 combined) in the same patient population. Most adult patients were treated with a daily dose of 200 to 400 mg, with a median duration of 3 months. Results of these studies demonstrated substantial evidence of effectiveness of itraconazole as a second-line therapy for the treatment of aspergillosis compared with the natural history of the disease in patients who either failed or were intolerant of amphotericin B therapy.

Onychomycosis of the toenail: Analyses were conducted on data from three double-blind, placebo-controlled studies (N=214 total; 110 given SPORANOX® Capsules) in which patients with onychomycosis of the toenails received 200 mg of SPORANOX® Capsules once daily for 12 consecutive weeks. Results of these studies demonstrated mycologic cure, defined as simultaneous occurrence of negative KOH plus negative culture, in 54% of patients. Thirty-five percent (35%) of patients were considered an overall success (mycologic cure plus clear or minimal nail involvement with significantly decreased signs) and 14% of patients demonstrated mycologic cure plus clinical cure (clearance of all signs, with or without residual nail deformity). The mean time to overall success was approximately 10 months. Twenty-one percent (21%) of the overall success group had a relapse (worsening of the global score or conversion of KOH or culture from negative to positive).

Onychomycosis of the fingernail: Analyses were conducted on data from a double-blind, placebo-controlled study (N=73 total; 37 given SPORANOX® Capsules) in which patients with onychomycosis of the fingernails received a 1-week course (pulse) of 200 mg of SPORANOX® Capsules b.i.d., followed by a 3-week period without SPORANOX®, which was followed by a second 1-week pulse of 200 mg of SPORANOX® Capsules b.i.d. Results demonstrated mycologic cure in 61% of patients. Fifty-six percent (56%) of patients were considered an overall success and 47% of patients demonstrated mycologic cure plus clinical cure. The mean time to overall success was approximately 5 months. None of the patients who achieved overall success relapsed.

CONTRAINDICATIONS

Concomitant administration of SPORANOX® (itraconazole) Capsules, Injection, or Oral Solution and certain drugs metabolized by the cytochrome P450 3A4 isoenzyme system (CYP3A4) may result in increased plasma concentrations of those drugs, leading to potentially serious and/or life-threatening adverse events. Astemizole, cisapride, oral midazolam, pimozide, quinidine, and triazolam are contraindicated with SPORANOX®. HMG CoA-reductase inhibitors metabolized by CYP3A4, such as lovastatin and simvastatin, are also contraindicated with SPORANOX®. (See BOXED WARNING, and PRECAUTIONS: Drug Interactions.)

SPORANOX® should not be administered for the treatment of onychomycosis to pregnant patients or to women contemplating pregnancy.

SPORANOX® is contraindicated for patients who have shown hypersensitivity to itraconazole or its excipients. There is no information regarding cross-hypersensitivity between itraconazole and other azole antifungal agents. Caution should be used when prescribing SPORANOX® to patients with hypersensitivity to other azoles.

WARNINGS

SPORANOX® (itraconazole) Capsules and SPORANOX® Oral Solution should not be used interchangeably. This is because drug exposure is greater with the Oral Solution than with the Capsules when the same dose of drug is given. In addition, the topical effects of mucosal exposure may be different between the two formulations. Only the Oral Solution has been demonstrated effective for oral and/or esophageal candidiasis.

Hepatitis: Rare cases of reversible idiosyncratic hepatitis have been reported among patients taking SPORANOX® Capsules. SPORANOX® has been associated with rare cases of serious hepatotoxicity, including death, primarily in patients with serious underlying medical conditions who are taking multiple medications. The causal association with SPORANOX® is uncertain. If clinical signs and symptoms develop that are consistent with liver disease and may be attributable to itraconazole, SPORANOX® should be discontinued.

Cardiac Dysrhythmias: Life-threatening cardiac dysrhythmias and/or sudden death have occurred in patients using astemizole, cisapride, pimozide or quinidine concomitantly with SPORANOX® and/or other CYP3A4 inhibitors. Concomitant administration of these drugs with SPORANOX® is contraindicated. (See BOX WARNING, CONTRAINDICATIONS, and PRECAUTIONS: Drug Interactions.)

	50 mg (fed)	100 mg (fed)	100 mg (fasted)	200 mg (fed)
C_{max} (ng/mL)	45 ± 16*	132 ± 67	38 ± 20	289 ± 100
T_{max} (hours)	3.2 ± 1.3	4.0 ± 1.1	3.3 ± 1.0	4.7 ± 1.4
$AUC_{0-\infty}$ (ng•h/mL)	567 ± 264	1899 ± 838	722 ± 289	5211 ± 2116

*mean ± standard deviation

	Itraconazole		Hydroxyitraconazole	
	Fed	Fasted	Fed	Fasted
C_{max} (ng/mL)	239 ± 85*	140 ± 65	397 ± 103	286 ± 101
T_{max} (hours)	4.5 ± 1.1	3.9 ± 1.0	5.1 ± 1.6	4.5 ± 1.1
$AUC_{0-\infty}$ (ng•h/mL)	3423 ± 1154	2094 ± 905	7978 ± 2648	5191 ± 2489
$t_{1/2}$ (hours)	21 ± 5	21 ± 7	12 ± 3	12 ± 3

*mean ± standard deviation

	Itraconazole	Hydroxyitraconazole
C_{max} (ng/mL)	2282 ± 514*	3488 ± 742
C_{min} (ng/mL)	1855 ± 535	3349 ± 761
T_{max} (hours)	4.6 ± 1.8	3.4 ± 3.4
AUC_{0-12h} (ng•h/mL)	22569 ± 5375	38572 ± 8450
$t_{1/2}$ (hours)	64 ± 32	56 ± 24

*mean ± standard deviation

PRECAUTIONS

General: Hepatic enzyme test values should be monitored in patients with pre-existing hepatic function abnormalities or those who have experienced liver toxicity with other medications. Hepatic enzyme test values should be monitored periodically in all patients receiving continuous treatment for more than 1 month, or at any time a patient develops signs or symptoms suggestive of liver dysfunction.

SPORANOX® (itraconazole) Capsules should be administered after a full meal. (See CLINICAL PHARMACOLOGY: Pharmacokinetics and Metabolism.)

Under fasted conditions, itraconazole absorption was decreased in the presence of decreased gastric acidity. The absorption of itraconazole may be decreased with the concomitant administration of antacids or gastric acid secretion suppressors. Studies conducted under fasted conditions demonstrated that administration with 8 ounces of a cola beverage resulted in increased absorption of itraconazole in AIDS patients with relative or absolute achlorhydria. This increase relative to the effects of a full meal is unknown. (See CLINICAL PHARMACOLOGY: Pharmacokinetics and Metabolism.)

Information for Patients: The topical effects of mucosal exposure may be different between the SPORANOX® Capsules and Oral Solution. Only the Oral Solution has been demonstrated effective for oral and/or esophageal candidiasis.

Instruct patients to take SPORANOX® Capsules with a full meal.

Instruct patients to report any signs and symptoms that may suggest liver dysfunction so that the appropriate laboratory testing can be done. Such signs and symptoms may include unusual fatigue, anorexia, nausea and/or vomiting, jaundice, dark urine, or pale stools.

Instruct patients to contact their physician before taking any concomitant medications with itraconazole to ensure that there are no potential drug interactions.

Drug Interactions: Itraconazole and its major metabolite, hydroxyitraconazole, are inhibitors of CYP3A4. Therefore, the following drug interactions may occur (See Table 1 below and the following drug class subheadings that follow):

1. SPORANOX® may decrease the elimination of drugs metabolized by CYP3A4, resulting in increased plasma concentrations of these drugs when they are administered with SPORANOX®. These elevated plasma concentrations may increase or prolong both therapeutic and adverse effects of these drugs. Whenever possible, plasma concentrations of these drugs should be monitored, and dosage adjustments made after concomitant SPORANOX® therapy is initiated. When appropriate, clinical monitoring for signs or symptoms of increased or prolonged pharmacologic effects is advised. Upon discontinuation, depending on the dose and duration of treatment, itraconazole plasma concentrations decline gradually (especially in patients with hepatic cirrhosis or in those receiving CYP3A4 inhibitors). This is particularly important when initiating therapy with drugs whose metabolism is affected by itraconazole.
2. Inducers of CYP3A4 may decrease the plasma concentrations of itraconazole. SPORANOX® may not be effective in patients concomitantly taking SPORANOX® and one of these drugs. Therefore, administration of these drugs with SPORANOX® is not recommended.
3. Other inhibitors of CYP3A4 may increase the plasma concentrations of itraconazole. Patients who must take SPORANOX® concomitantly with one of these drugs should be monitored closely for signs or symptoms of increased or prolonged pharmacologic effects of SPORANOX®.

[See table 1 at top of next page]

Antiarrhythmics: The class IA antiarrhythmic quinidine is known to prolong the QT interval. Coadministration of quinidine with SPORANOX® increases plasma concentrations of quinidine which could result in serious cardiovascular events. Therefore, concomitant administration of SPORANOX® and quinidine is contraindicated. (See BOX WARNING, CONTRAINDICATIONS, and WARNINGS.)

Concomitant administration of digoxin and SPORANOX® has led to increased plasma concentrations of digoxin.

Anticonvulsants: Reduced plasma concentrations of itraconazole were reported when SPORANOX® was administered concomitantly with phenytoin. Carbamazepine, phenobarbital, and phenytoin are all inducers of CYP3A4. Although interactions with carbamazepine and phenobarbital have not been studied, concomitant administration of SPORANOX® and these drugs would be expected to result in decreased plasma concentrations of itraconazole. In addition, in vivo studies have demonstrated an increase in plasma carbamazepine concentrations in subjects concomitantly receiving ketoconazole. Although there are no data regarding the effect of itraconazole on carbamazepine metabolism, because of the similarities between ketoconazole and itraconazole, concomitant administration of SPORANOX® and carbamazepine may inhibit the metabolism of carbamazepine.

Antihistamines: Coadministration of astemizole with SPORANOX® has led to elevated plasma concentrations of astemizole and desmethylastemizole which could result in serious cardiovascular events. Therefore, concomitant administration of SPORANOX® with astemizole is contraindi-

Continued on next page

Sporanox Caps—Cont.

cated. (See BOX WARNING, CONTRAINDICATIONS, and WARNINGS.)

Antimycobacterials: Drug interaction studies have demonstrated that plasma concentrations of azole antifungal agents and their metabolites, including itraconazole and hydroxyitraconazole, were significantly decreased when these agents were given concomitantly with rifabutin or rifampin. In vivo data suggest that rifabutin is metabolized in part by CYP3A4. SPORANOX® may inhibit the metabolism of rifabutin. Although no formal study data are available for isoniazid, similar effects should be anticipated. Therefore, the efficacy of SPORANOX® could be substantially reduced if given concomitantly with one of these agents. Coadministration is not recommended.

Antineoplastics: SPORANOX® may inhibit the metabolism of busulfan, docetaxel, and vinca alkaloids.

Antipsychotics: Pimozide is known to prolong the QT interval and is partially metabolized by CYP3A4. Coadministration of pimozide with SPORANOX® could result in serious cardiovascular events. Therefore, concomitant administration of SPORANOX® and pimozide is contraindicated. (See BOX WARNING, CONTRAINDICATIONS, and WARNINGS.)

Benzodiazepines: Concomitant administration of SPORANOX® and alprazolam, diazepam, oral midazolam, or triazolam could lead to increased plasma concentrations of these benzodiazepines. Increased plasma concentrations could potentiate and prolong hypnotic and sedative effects. Concomitant administration of SPORANOX® and oral midazolam or triazolam is contraindicated. (See CONTRAINDICATIONS and WARNINGS.) If midazolam is administered parenterally, special precaution and patient monitoring is required since the sedative effect may be prolonged.

Calcium Channel Blockers: SPORANOX® may inhibit the metabolism of the dihydropyridines and verapamil.

Gastric Acid Suppressors/Neutralizers: Reduced plasma concentrations of itraconazole were reported when SPORANOX® Capsules were administered concomitantly with H_2-receptor antagonists. Studies have shown that absorption of itraconazole is impaired when gastric acid production is decreased. Therefore, SPORANOX® should be administered with a cola beverage if the patient has achlorhydria or is taking H_2-receptor antagonists or other gastric acid suppressors. Antacids should be administered at least 1 hour before or 2 hours after administration of SPORANOX® Capsules. In a clinical study, when SPORANOX® Capsules were administered with omeprazole (a proton pump inhibitor), the bioavailability of itraconazole was significantly reduced.

Gastrointestinal Motility Agents: Coadministration of SPORANOX® with cisapride can elevate plasma cisapride concentrations which could result in serious cardiovascular events. Therefore, concomitant administration of SPORANOX® with cisapride is contraindicated. (See BOX WARNING, CONTRAINDICATIONS, and WARNINGS.)

HMG CoA-Reductase Inhibitors: Human pharmacokinetic data suggest that SPORANOX® inhibits the metabolism of atorvastatin, cerivastatin, lovastatin, and simvastatin, which may increase the risk of skeletal muscle toxicity, including rhabdomyolysis. Concomitant administration of SPORANOX® and lovastatin or simvastatin is contraindicated. (See CONTRAINDICATIONS and WARNINGS.)

Immunosuppressants: Concomitant administration of SPORANOX® and cyclosporine or tacrolimus has led to increased plasma concentrations of these immunosuppressants. Concomitant administration of SPORANOX® and sirolimus could increase plasma concentrations of sirolimus.

Macrolide Antibiotics: Clarithromycin is a known inhibitor of CYP3A4 and may increase plasma concentrations of itraconazole.

Non-nucleoside Reverse Transcriptase Inhibitors: Nevirapine is an inducer of CYP3A4. In vivo studies have shown that nevirapine induces the metabolism of ketoconazole, significantly reducing the bioavailability of ketoconazole. Studies involving nevirapine and itraconazole have not been conducted. However, because of the similarities between ketoconazole and itraconazole, concomitant administration of SPORANOX® and nevirapine is not recommended.

In a clinical study, when 8 HIV-infected subjects were treated concomitantly with SPORANOX® Capsules 100 mg twice daily and the nucleoside reverse transcriptase inhibitor zidovudine 8 ± 0.4 mg/kg/day, the pharmacokinetics of zidovudine were not affected. Other nucleoside reverse transcriptase inhibitors have not been studied.

Oral Hypoglycemic Agents: Severe hypoglycemia has been reported in patients concomitantly receiving azole antifungal agents and oral hypoglycemic agents. Blood glucose concentrations should be carefully monitored when SPORANOX® and oral hypoglycemic agents are coadministered.

Polyenes: Prior treatment with itraconazole, like other azoles, may reduce or inhibit the activity of polyenes such as amphotericin B. However, the clinical significance of this drug effect has not been clearly defined.

Protease Inhibitors: Concomitant administration of SPORANOX® and protease inhibitors metabolized by CYP3A4, such as indinavir, ritonavir, and saquinavir, may increase plasma concentrations of these protease inhibitors. In addition, concomitant administration of SPORANOX® and indinavir and ritonavir (but not saquinavir) may increase plasma concentrations of itraconazole. Caution is advised when SPORANOX® and protease inhibitors must be given concomitantly.

Table 1. Selected Drugs that are predicted to alter the plasma concentration of Itraconazole or have their plasma concentration altered by SPORANOX®[1]

Drug plasma concentration increased by itraconazole	
Antiarrhythmics	digoxin, quinidine[2]
Anticonvulsants	carbamazepine
Antihistamines	astemizole[2]
Antimycobacterials	rifabutin
Antineoplastics	busulfan, docetaxel, vinca alkaloids
Antipsychotics	pimozide[2]
Benzodiazepines	alprazolam, diazepam, midazolam,[2,3] triazolam[2]
Calcium Channel Blockers	dihydropyridines, verapamil
Gastrointestinal Motility Agents	cisapride[2]
HMG CoA-Reductase Inhibitors	atorvastatin, cerivastatin, lovastatin,[2] simvastatin[2]
Immunosuppressants	cyclosporine, tacrolimus, sirolimus
Oral Hypoglycemics	oral hypoglycemics
Protease Inhibitors	indinavir, ritonavir, saquinavir
Other	alfentanil, buspirone, methylprednisolone, trimetrexate, warfarin
Decrease plasma concentration of itraconazole	
Anticonvulsants	carbamazepine, phenobarbital, phenytoin
Antimycobacterials	isoniazid, rifabutin, rifampin
Gastric Acid Suppressors/Neutralizers	antacids, H_2-receptor antagonists, proton pump inhibitors
Non-nucleoside Reverse Transcriptase Inhibitors	nevirapine
Increase plasma concentration of itraconazole	
Macrolide Antibiotics	clarithromycin
Protease Inhibitors	indinavir, ritonavir

[1] This list is not all-inclusive.
[2] Contraindicated with SPORANOX® based on clinical and/or pharmacokinetics studies. (See WARNINGS and below.)
[3] For information on parenterally administered midazolam, see the benzodiazepine paragraph below.

Other:

- In vitro data suggest that alfentanil is metabolized by CYP3A4. Administration with SPORANOX® may increase plasma concentrations of alfentanil.
- Human pharmacokinetic data suggest that concomitant administration of SPORANOX® and buspirone results in significant increases in plasma concentrations of buspirone.
- SPORANOX® may inhibit the metabolism of methylprednisolone.
- In vitro data suggest that trimetrexate is extensively metabolized by CYP3A4. In vitro animal models have demonstrated that ketoconazole potently inhibits the metabolism of trimetrexate. Although there are no data regarding the effect of itraconazole on trimetrexate metabolism, because of the similarities between ketoconazole and itraconazole, concomitant administration of SPORANOX® and trimetrexate may inhibit the metabolism of trimetrexate.
- SPORANOX® enhances the anticoagulant effect of coumarin-like drugs, such as warfarin.

Carcinogenesis, Mutagenesis, and Impairment of Fertility: Itraconazole showed no evidence of carcinogenicity potential in mice treated orally for 23 months at dosage levels up to 80 mg/kg/day (approximately 10× the maximum recommended human dose [MRHD]). Male rats treated with 25 mg/kg/day (3.1× MRHD) had a slightly increased incidence of soft tissue sarcoma. These sarcomas may have been a consequence of hypercholesterolemia, which is a response of rats, but not dogs or humans, to chronic itraconazole administration. Female rats treated with 50 mg/kg/day (6.25× MRHD) had an increased incidence of squamous cell carcinoma of the lung (2/50) as compared to the untreated group. Although the occurrence of squamous cell carcinoma in the lung is extremely uncommon in untreated rats, the increase in this study was not statistically significant.

Itraconazole produced no mutagenic effects when assayed in DNA repair test (unscheduled DNA synthesis) in primary rat hepatocytes, in Ames tests with *Salmonella typhimurium* (6 strains) and *Escherichia coli*, in the mouse lymphoma gene mutation tests, in a sex-linked recessive lethal mutation (*Drosophila melanogaster*) test, in chromosome aberration tests in human lymphocytes, in a cell transformation test with C3H/10T$^1/_2$ C18 mouse embryo fibroblasts cells, in a dominant lethal mutation test in male and female mice, and in micronucleus tests in mice and rats.

Itraconazole did not affect the fertility of male or female rats treated orally with dosage levels of up to 40 mg/kg/day (5× MRHD), even though parental toxicity was present at this dosage level. More severe signs of parental toxicity, including death, were present in the next higher dosage level, 160 mg/kg/day (20× MRHD).

Pregnancy: Teratogenic effects. Pregnancy Category C: Itraconazole was found to cause a dose-related increase in maternal toxicity, embryotoxicity, and teratogenicity in rats at dosage levels of approximately 40–160 mg/kg/day (5–20× MRHD), and in mice at dosage levels of approximately 80 mg/kg/day (10× MRHD). In rats, the teratogenicity consisted of major skeletal defects; in mice, it consisted of encephaloceles and/or macroglossia.

There are no studies in pregnant women. SPORANOX® should be used for the treatment of systemic fungal infections in pregnancy only if the benefit outweighs the potential risk. SPORANOX® should not be administered for the treatment of onychomycosis to pregnant patients or to women contemplating pregnancy. SPORANOX® should not be administered to women of childbearing potential for the treatment of onychomycosis unless they are using effective measures to prevent pregnancy and they begin therapy on the second or third day following the onset of menses. Effective contraception should be continued throughout SPORANOX® therapy and for 2 months following the end of treatment.

Nursing Mothers: Itraconazole is excreted in human milk; therefore, the expected benefits of SPORANOX® therapy for the mother should be weighed against the potential risk from exposure of itraconazole to the infant. The U.S. Public Health Service Centers for Disease Control and Prevention advises HIV-infected women not to breast-feed to avoid potential transmission of HIV to uninfected infants.

Pediatric Use: The efficacy and safety of SPORANOX® have not been established in pediatric patients. No pharmacokinetic data on SPORANOX® Capsules are available in children. A small number of patients ages 3 to 16 years have been treated with 100 mg/day of itraconazole capsules for systemic fungal infections, and no serious unexpected adverse effects have been reported. SPORANOX® Oral Solution (5 mg/kg/day) has been administered to pediatric patients (N=26; ages 6 months to 12 years) for 2 weeks and no serious unexpected adverse events were reported.

The long-term effects of itraconazole on bone growth in children are unknown. In three toxicology studies using rats, itraconazole induced bone defects at dosage levels as low as 20 mg/kg/day (2.5× MRHD). The induced defects included reduced bone plate activity, thinning of the zone compacta of the large bones, and increased bone fragility. At a dosage level of 80 mg/kg/day (10× MRHD) over 1 year or 160 mg/kg/day (20× MRHD) for 6 months, itraconazole induced small tooth pulp with hypocellular appearance in some rats. No such bone toxicity has been reported in adult patients.

HIV-Infected Patients: Because hypochlorhydria has been reported in HIV-infected individuals, the absorption of itraconazole in these patients may be decreased.

ADVERSE REACTIONS

Rare cases of reversible idiosyncratic hepatitis has been reported among patients taking SPORANOX® (itraconazole) Capsules. SPORANOX® has been associated with rare cases of serious hepatotoxicity, including fatalities, primarily in patients with serious underlying medical conditions who are taking multiple medications. The causal association with SPORANOX® is uncertain. If clinical signs and symptoms consistent with liver disease develop and could be attributed to itraconazole, SPORANOX® should be discontinued. (See WARNINGS.)

Adverse Events Reported in Toenail Onychomycosis Clinical Trials

Patients in these trials were on a continuous dosing regimen of 200 mg once daily for 12 consecutive weeks. The following adverse events led to temporary or permanent discontinuation of therapy.

[See table at right]

Clinical Trials of Onychomycosis of the Toenail: Adverse Events Leading to Temporary or Permanent Discontinuation of Therapy

Adverse Event	Incidence (%) Itraconazole (N=112)
Elevated Liver Enzymes (greater than twice the upper limit of normal)	4
Gastrointestinal Disorders	4
Rash	3
Hypertension	2
Orthostatic Hypotension	1
Headache	1
Malaise	1
Myalgia	1
Vasculitis	1
Vertigo	1

The following adverse events occurred with an incidence of greater than or equal to 1% (N=112): headache: 10%; rhinitis: 9%; upper respiratory tract infection: 8%; sinusitis, injury: 7%; diarrhea, dyspepsia, flatulence, abdominal pain, dizziness, rash, nausea: 4%; cystitis, urinary tract infection, liver function abnormality, myalgia: 3%; appetite increased, constipation, gastritis, gastroenteritis, pharyngitis, asthenia, fever, pain, tremor, herpes zoster, abnormal dreaming: 2%.

Adverse Events Reported in Fingernail Onychomycosis Clinical Trials

Patients in these trials were on a pulse regimen consisting of two 1-week treatment periods of 200 mg twice daily, separated by a 3-week period without drug.

The following adverse events led to temporary or permanent discontinuation of therapy.

For Onychomycosis of the Fingernail Clinical Trials: Adverse Events Leading to Temporary or Permanent Discontinuation of Therapy

Adverse Event	Incidence (%) Itraconazole (N=37)
Rash/Pruritus	3
Hypertriglyceridemia	3

The following adverse events occurred with an incidence of greater than or equal to 1% (N=37): headache: 8%; pruritus, nausea, rhinitis: 5%; rash, bursitis, anxiety, depression, constipation, abdominal pain, dyspepsia, ulcerative stomatitis, gingivitis, hypertriglyceridemia, sinusitis, fatigue, malaise, pain, injury: 3%.

Adverse Events in the Treatment of Systemic Fungal Infections

Adverse event data were derived from 602 patients treated for systemic fungal disease in U.S. clinical trials who were immunocompromised or receiving multiple concomitant medications. Treatment was discontinued in 10.5% of patients due to adverse events. The median duration before discontinuation of therapy was 81 days (range: 2 to 776 days). The table lists adverse events reported by at least 1% of patients.

Treatment of Systemic Fungal Infections: Adverse Events Occurring with an Incidence of Greater than or Equal to 1%

Body System/Adverse Event	Incidence (%) Itraconazole (N=602)
Gastrointestinal	
Nausea	11
Vomiting	5
Diarrhea	3
Abdominal Pain	2
Anorexia	1
Body as Whole	
Edema	4
Fatigue	3
Fever	3
Malaise	1
Skin and Appendages	
Rash*	9
Pruritus	3
Central/Peripheral Nervous System	
Headache	4
Dizziness	2
Psychiatric	
Libido Decreased	1
Somnolence	1
Cardiovascular	
Hypertension	3
Metabolic/Nutritional	
Hypokalemia	2
Urinary System	
Albuminuna	1
Liver and Biliary System	
Hepatic Function Abnormal	3
Reproductive System, Male	
Impotence	1

*Rash tends to occur more frequently in immunocompromised patients receiving immunosuppressive medications.

Adverse events infrequently reported in all studies included constipation, gastritis, depression, insomnia, tinnitus, menstrual disorder, adrenal insufficiency, gynecomastia, and male breast pain.

Post-marketing Experience

In worldwide post-marketing experience with SPORANOX® Capsules, allergic reactions, including rash, pruritus, urticaria, angioedema, and, in rare instances, anaphylaxis and Stevens-Johnson syndrome, have been reported. Post-marketing experiences have also included reports of elevated liver enzymes and rarely, hepatitis. Although the causal association with SPORANOX® is uncertain, rare cases of alopecia, hypertriglyceridemia, and neutropenia, and isolated cases of neuropathy have also been reported.

OVERDOSAGE

Itraconazole is not removed by dialysis. In the event of accidental overdosage, supportive measures, including gastric lavage with sodium bicarbonate, should be employed.

Limited data exist on the outcomes of patients ingesting high doses of itraconazole. In patients taking either 1000 mg of SPORANOX® (itraconazole) Oral Solution or up to 3000 mg of SPORANOX® (itraconazole) Capsules, the adverse event profile was similar to that observed at recommended doses.

DOSAGE AND ADMINISTRATION

SPORANOX® (itraconazole) Capsules should be taken with a full meal to ensure maximal absorption. For patients with achlorhydria, SPORANOX® Capsules should be taken with a cola beverage.

Treatment of Onychomycosis: Toenails with or without fingernail involvement: The recommended dose is 200 mg (2 capsules) once daily for 12 consecutive weeks.

Treatment of Onychomycosis: Fingernails only: The recommended dosing regimen is 2 treatment pulses, each consisting of 200 mg (2 capsules) b.i.d. (400 mg/day) for 1 week. The pulses are separated by a 3-week period without SPORANOX®.

Treatment of Blastomycosis and Histoplasmosis: The recommended dose is 200 mg once daily (2 capsules). If there is no obvious improvement, or there is evidence of progressive fungal disease, the dose should be increased in 100-mg increments to a maximum of 400 mg daily. Doses above 200 mg/day should be given in two divided doses.

Treatment of Aspergillosis: A daily dose of 200 to 400 mg is recommended.

Treatment in Life-Threatening Situations: In life-threatening situations, a loading dose should be used whether given as oral capsules or intravenously.

- IV Injection: the recommended intravenous dose is 200 mg b.i.d. for four consecutive doses, followed by 200 mg once daily thereafter. Each intravenous dose should be infused over 1 hour. The safety and efficacy of SPORANOX® Injection administered for greater than 14 days is not known. See complete prescribing information for SPORANOX® (itraconazole) Injection.
- Capsules: although clinical studies did not provide for a loading dose, it is recommended, based on pharmacokinetic data, that a loading dose of 200 mg (2 capsules) three times daily (600 mg/day) be given for the first 3 days of treatment.

Treatment should be continued for a minimum of three months and until clinical parameters and laboratory tests indicate that the active fungal infection has subsided. An inadequate period of treatment may lead to recurrence of active infection.

SPORANOX® Capsules and SPORANOX® Oral Solution should not be used interchangeably. Only the oral solution has been demonstrated effective for oral and/or esophageal candidiasis.

HOW SUPPLIED

SPORANOX® (itraconazole) Capsules are available containing 100 mg of itraconazole, with a blue opaque cap and pink transparent body, imprinted with "JANSSEN" and "SPORANOX 100." The capsules are supplied in unit-dose blister packs of 3 × 10 capsules (NDC 50458-290-01), bottles of 30 capsules (NDC 50458-290-04) and in the PulsePak® containing 7 blister packs × 4 capsules each (NDC 50458-290-28).

Store at controlled room temperature (59°–77°F/15°–25°C). Protect from light and moisture.

U.S. Patent Nos. 4,267,179; 4,791,111; 5,633,015

Rev. November 1999, January 2000

Distributed by:
JANSSEN PHARMACEUTICA INC.
Titusville, New Jersey 08560, USA

Capsule contents manufactured by:
JANSSEN PHARMACEUTICA N.V.
Beerse, Belgium

Shown in Product Identification Guide, page 318

SPORANOX® ℞

[*spŏr-a-nŏx*]

(ITRACONAZOLE) INJECTION

WARNING: Coadministration of astemizole, cisapride, pimozide, or quinidine with SPORANOX® (itraconazole) Capsules, Injection or Oral Solution is contraindicated. SPORANOX®, a potent cytochrome P450 3A4 isoenzyme system (CYP3A4) inhibitor, may increase plasma concentrations of drugs metabolized by this pathway. Serious cardiovascular events, including QT prolongation, torsades de pointes, ventricular tachycardia, cardiac arrest, and/or sudden death have occurred in patients using astemizole, cisapride, pimozide, or quinidine, concomitantly with SPORANOX® and/or other CYP3A4 inhibitors. See CONTRAINDICATIONS, WARNINGS and PRECAUTIONS: Drug Interactions for more information.

DESCRIPTION

For intravenous infusion (NOT FOR IV BOLUS INJECTION)

SPORANOX® is the brand name for itraconazole, a synthetic triazole antifungal agent. Itraconazole is a 1:1:1:1 racemic mixture of four diastereomers (two enantiomeric pairs), each possessing three chiral centers. It may be represented by the following structural formula and nomenclature:

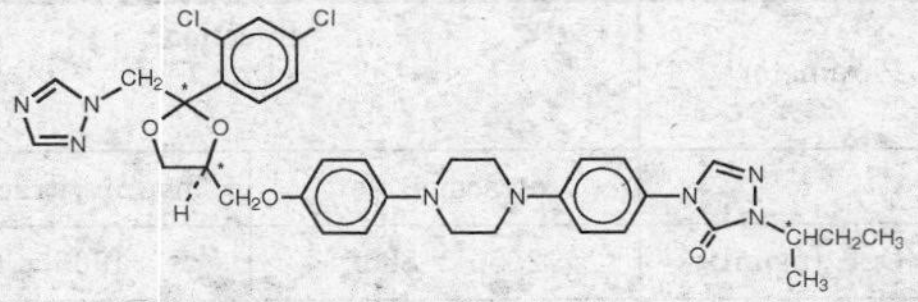

(±)-1-[(R*)-sec-butyl-4-[p-[4-[p-[[(2R*,4S*)-2-(2,4-dichlorophenyl)-2-(1H-1,2,4-triazol-1-ylmethyl)-1,3-dioxolan-4-yl]methoxy]phenyl]-1-piperazinyl]phenyl]-Δ^2-1,2,4-triazolin-5-one mixture with (±)-1-[(R*)-sec-butyl]-4-[p-[4-[p-[[2S*, 4R*)-2-(2,4-dichlorophenyl)-2-(1H-1,2,4-triazol-1-ylmethyl)-1,3-dioxolan-4-yl]methoxy] phenyl]-1-piperazinyl]phenyl]-Δ^2-1,2,4-triazolin-5-one

Continued on next page

Sporanox Inj.—Cont.

or

(±) -1- [(RS)-sec-butyl] -4- [p- [4- [p- [[(2R,4S) -2- (2,4-dichlorophenyl)-2-(1H-1,2,4-triazol-1-ylmethyl)-1,3-dioxolan-4-yl]methoxy]phenyl-1-piperazinyl]phenyl]-Δ^2-1,2,4-triazolin-5-one

Itraconazole has a molecular formula of $C_{35}H_{38}Cl_2N_8O_4$ and a molecular weight of 705.64. It is a white to slightly yellowish powder. It is insoluble in water, very slightly soluble in alcohols, and freely soluble in dichloromethane. It has a pKa of 3.70 (based on extrapolation of values obtained from methanolic solutions) and a log (n-octanol/water) partition coefficient of 5.66 at pH 8.1.

SPORANOX® (itraconazole) Injection is a sterile pyrogen-free clear, colorless to slightly yellow solution for intravenous infusion. Each mL contains 10 mg of itraconazole, solubilized by hydroxypropyl-β-cyclodextrin (400 mg) as a molecular inclusion complex, with 3.8 µL hydrochloric acid, 25 µL propylene glycol, and sodium hydroxide for pH adjustment to 4.5, in water for injection. SPORANOX® Injection is packaged in 25 mL colorless glass ampules, containing 250 mg of itraconazole, contents of which are diluted in 50 mL 0.9% Sodium Chloride Injection, USP (Normal Saline) prior to infusion. When properly administered, contents of one ampule will supply 200 mg of itraconazole.

CLINICAL PHARMACOLOGY

Pharmacokinetics and Metabolism: NOTE: The plasma concentrations reported below were measured by high-performance liquid chromatography (HPLC) specific for itraconazole. When itraconazole in plasma is measured by a bioassay, values reported may be higher than those obtained by HPLC due to the presence of the bioactive metabolite, hydroxyitraconazole. (See MICROBIOLOGY.)

The pharmacokinetics of SPORANOX® (itraconazole) Injection (200 mg b.i.d. for two days, then 200 mg q.d. for five days) followed by oral dosing of SPORANOX® Capsules were studied in patients with advanced HIV infection. Steady-state plasma concentrations were reached after the fourth dose for itraconazole and by the seventh dose for hydroxyitraconazole. Steady-state plasma concentrations were maintained by administration of SPORANOX® Capsules, 200 mg b.i.d. Pharmacokinetic parameters for itraconazole and hydroxyitraconazole are presented in the table below:

[See table below]

Parameter	Injection Day 7 n=29		Capsules, 200 mg b.i.d. Day 36 n=12	
	itraconazole	hydroxyitraconazole	itraconazole	hydroxyitraconazole
C_{max} (ng/mL)	2856 ± 866*	1906 ± 612	2010 ± 1420	2614 ± 1703
t_{max} (hr)	1.08 ± 0.14	8.53 ± 6.36	3.92 ± 1.83	5.92 ± 6.14
$AUC_{0\text{-}12h}$ (ng•h/mL)	—	—	18768 ± 13933	28516 ± 19149
$AUC_{0\text{-}24h}$ (ng•h/mL)	30605 ± 8961	42445 ± 13282	—	—

*mean ± standard deviation

The estimated mean ±SD half-life at steady-state of itraconazole after intravenous infusion was 35.4 ± 29.4 hours. In previous studies, the mean elimination half-life for itraconazole at steady-state after daily oral administration of 100 to 400 mg was 30–40 hours. Approximately 93–101% of hydroxypropyl-β-cyclodextrin was excreted unchanged in the urine within 12 hours after dosing.

The plasma protein binding of itraconazole is 99.8% and that of hydroxyitraconazole is 99.5%. Following intravenous administration, the volume of distribution of itraconazole averaged 796 ± 185 L.

Itraconazole is metabolized predominately by the cytochrome P450 3A4 isoenzyme system (CYP3A4), resulting in the formation of several metabolites, including hydroxyitraconazole, the major metabolite. Results of a pharmacokinetics study suggest that itraconazole may undergo saturable metabolism with multiple dosing. Fecal excretion of the parent drug varies between 3–18% of the dose. Renal excretion of the parent drug is less than 0.03% of the dose. About 40% of the dose is excreted as inactive metabolites in the urine. No single excreted metabolite represents more than 5% of a dose. Itraconazole total plasma clearance averaged 381 ± 95 mL/min following intravenous administration. Approximately 80–90% of hydroxypropyl-β-cyclodextrin is eliminated through the kidneys.

Special Populations

Renal Insufficiency: Plasma concentrations of itraconazole in patients with mild to moderate renal insufficiency were comparable to those obtained in healthy subjects. The majority of the 8-gram dose of hydroxypropyl-β-cyclodextrin was eliminated in the urine during the 120-hour collection period in normal subjects and in patients with mild to severe renal insufficiency. Following a single intravenous dose of 200 mg to subjects with severe renal impairment (creatinine clearance ≤ 19 mL/minute), clearance of hydroxypropyl-β-cyclodextrin was reduced six-fold compared with subjects with normal renal function. SPORANOX® Injection should not be used in patients with creatinine clearance < 30 mL/min.

Hepatic Insufficiency: Patients with impaired hepatic function should be carefully monitored when taking itraconazole. The prolonged elimination half-life of itraconazole observed in a clinical trial with itraconazole capsules in cirrhotic patients should be considered when deciding to initiate therapy with other medications metabolized by CYP3A4. (See BOX WARNING, CONTRAINDICATIONS, and PRECAUTIONS: Drug Interactions.)

MICROBIOLOGY

Mechanism of Action: In vitro studies have demonstrated that itraconazole inhibits the cytochrome P-450-dependent synthesis of ergosterol, which is a vital component of fungal cell membranes.

Activity In Vitro and In Vivo: Itraconazole exhibits in vitro activity against *Blastomyces dermatitidis, Histoplasma capsulatum, Histoplasma duboisii, Aspergillus flavus, Aspergillus fumigatus, Candida albicans,* and *Cryptococcus neoformans*. Itraconazole also exhibits varying in vitro activity against *Sporothrix schenckii, Trichophyton* species, *Candida krusei,* and other *Candida* species. The bioactive metabolite, hydroxyitraconazole, has not been evaluated against *Histoplasma capsulatum* and *Blastomyces dermatitidis*. Correlation between minimum inhibitory concentration (MIC) results in vitro and clinical outcome has yet to be established for azole antifungal agents.

Itraconazole administered orally was active in a variety of animal models of fungal infection using standard laboratory strains of fungi. Fungistatic activity has been demonstrated against disseminated fungal infections caused by *Blastomyces dermatitidis, Histoplasma duboisii, Aspergillus fumigatus, Coccidioides immitis, Cryptococcus neoformans, Paracoccidioides brasiliensis, Sporothix schenckii, Trichophyton rubrum,* and *Trichophyton mentagrophytes*.

Itraconazole administered at 2.5 mg/kg and 5 mg/kg via the oral and parenteral routes increased survival rates and sterilized organ systems in normal and immunosuppressed guinea pigs with disseminated *Aspergillus fumigatus* infections. Oral itraconazole administered daily at 40 mg/kg and 80 mg/kg increased survival rates in normal rabbits with disseminated disease and in immunosuppressed rats with pulmonary *Aspergillus fumigatus* infection, respectively. Itraconazole has demonstrated antifungal activity in a variety of animal models infected with *Candida albicans* and other *Candida* species.

Resistance: Isolates from several fungal species with decreased susceptibility to itraconazole have been isolated in vitro and from patients receiving prolonged therapy.

Several in vitro studies reported that some fungal clinical isolates, including *Candida* species, with reduced susceptibility to one azole antifungal agent may also be less susceptible to other azole derivatives. The finding of cross-resistance is dependent on a number of factors, including the species evaluated, its clinical history, the particular azole compounds compared, and the type of susceptibility test that is performed. The relevance of these in vitro susceptibility data to clinical outcome remains to be elucidated.

Studies (both in vitro and in vivo) suggest that the activity of amphotericin B may be suppressed by prior azole antifungal therapy. As with other azoles, itraconazole inhibits the ^{14}C-demethylation step in the synthesis of ergosterol, a cell wall component of fungi. Ergosterol is the active site for amphotericin B. In one study the antifungal activity of amphotericin B against *Aspergillus fumigatus* infections in mice was inhibited by ketoconazole therapy. The clinical significance of test results obtained in this study is unknown.

INDICATIONS AND USAGE

SPORANOX® (itraconazole) Injection is indicated for the treatment of the following fungal infections in immunocompromised and non-immunocompromised patients:

1. Blastomycosis, pulmonary and extrapulmonary;
2. Histoplasmosis, including chronic cavitary pulmonary disease and disseminated, non-meningeal histoplasmosis; and
3. Aspergillosis, pulmonary and extrapulmonary, in patients who are intolerant of or who are refractory to amphotericin B therapy.

Specimens for fungal cultures and other relevant laboratory studies (wet mount, histopathology, serology) should be obtained prior to therapy to isolate and identify causative organisms. Therapy may be instituted before the results of the cultures and other laboratory studies are known; however, once these results become available, anti-infective therapy should be adjusted accordingly.

CONTRAINDICATIONS

Concomitant administration of SPORANOX® (itraconazole) Capsules, Injection, or Oral Solution and certain drugs metabolized by the cytochrome P450 3A4 isoenzyme system (CYP3A4) may result in increased plasma concentrations of those drugs, leading to potentially serious and/or life-threatening adverse events. Astemizole, cisapride, oral midazolam, pimozide, quinidine, and triazolam are contraindicated with SPORANOX®, HMG CoA-reductase inhibitors metabolized by CYP3A4, such as lovastatin and simvastatin, are also contraindicated with SPORANOX®. (See BOX WARNING, and PRECAUTIONS: Drug Interactions.)

SPORANOX® is contraindicated in patients who have shown hypersensitivity to itraconazole or its excipients. There is no information regarding cross-hypersensitivity between itraconazole and other azole antifungal agents. Caution should be used when prescribing SPORANOX® to patients with hypersensitivity to other azoles.

WARNINGS

SPORANOX® (itraconazole) Injection contains the excipient hydroxypropyl-β-cyclodextrin which produced pancreatic adenocarcinomas in a rat carcinogenicity study. These findings were not observed in a similar mouse carcinogenicity study. The clinical relevance of these findings is unknown. (See PRECAUTIONS: Carcinogenesis, Mutagenesis, and Impairment of Fertility.)

Hepatitis: There have been rare cases of reversible idiosyncratic hepatitis reported among patients taking SPORANOX® Capsules. SPORANOX® has been associated with rare cases of serious hepatotoxicity, including fatalities, primarily in patients with serious underlying medical conditions taking multiple medications. The causal association with SPORANOX® is uncertain. If clinical signs and symptoms develop that are consistent with liver disease and may be attributable to itraconazole, SPORANOX® should be discontinued.

Cardiac Dysrhythmias: Life-threatening cardiac dysrhythmias and/or sudden death have occurred in patients using astemizole, cisapride, pimozide or quinidine concomitantly with SPORANOX® and/or other CYP3A4 inhibitors. Concomitant administration of these drugs with SPORANOX® is contraindicated. (See BOX WARNING, CONTRAINDICATIONS, and PRECAUTIONS: Drug Interactions.)

PRECAUTIONS

General: Hepatic enzyme test values should be monitored in patients with pre-existing hepatic function abnormalities or those who have experienced liver toxicity with other medications. Hepatic enzyme test values should be monitored periodically in all patients receiving continuous treatment for more than 1 month, or at any time a patient develops signs or symptoms suggestive of liver dysfunction.

As severe renal impairment prolongs the elimination rate of hydroxypropyl-β-cyclodextrin, SPORANOX® (itraconazole) Injection should not be used in patients with severe renal dysfunction (creatinine clearance ≤ 30 mL/min). (See CLINICAL PHARMACOLOGY: Special populations.)

Information for Patients: SPORANOX® Injection contains the excipient hydroxypropyl-β-cyclodextrin which produced pancreatic adenocarcinomas in a rat carcinogenicity study. These findings were not observed in a similar mouse carcinogenicity study. The clinical relevance of these findings is unknown. (See PRECAUTIONS: Carcinogenesis, Mutagenesis, and Impairment of Fertility.)

Drug Interactions: Itraconazole and its major metabolite, hydroxyitraconazole, are inhibitors of CYP3A4. Therefore, the following drug interactions may occur.

(See Table 1 below and the following drug class subheadings that follow):

1. SPORANOX® may decrease the elimination of drugs metabolized by CYP3A4, resulting in increased plasma concentrations of these drugs when they are administered with SPORANOX®. These elevated plasma concentrations may increase or prolong both therapeutic and adverse effects of these drugs. Whenever possible, plasma concentrations of these drugs should be monitored, and dosage adjustments made after concomitant SPORANOX® therapy is initiated. When appropriate, clinical monitoring for signs or symptoms of increased or prolonged pharmacologic effects is advised. Upon discontinuation, depending on the dose and duration of treatment, itraconazole plasma concentrations decline gradually (especially in patients with hepatic cirrhosis or in those receiving CYP3A4 inhibitors). This is particularly important when initiating therapy with drugs whose metabolism is affected by itraconazole.
2. Inducers of CYP3A4 may decrease the plasma concentrations of itraconazole. SPORANOX® may not be effective in patients concomitantly taking SPORANOX® and one of these drugs. Therefore, administration of these drugs with SPORANOX® is not recommended.
3. Other inhibitors of CYP3A4 may increase the plasma concentrations of itraconazole. Patients who must take SPORANOX® concomitantly with one of these drugs should be monitored closely for signs or symptoms of increased or prolonged pharmacologic effects of SPORANOX®.

[See table 1 at bottom of next page]

Antiarrhythmics: The class IA antiarrhythmic quinidine is known to prolong the QT interval. Coadministration of quinidine with SPORANOX® increases plasma concentrations of quinidine which could result in serious cardiovascular events. Therefore, concomitant administration of SPORANOX® and quinidine is contraindicated. (See BOX

WARNING, CONTRAINDICATIONS, and WARNINGS.)
Concomitant administration of digoxin and SPORANOX® has led to increased plasma concentrations of digoxin.

Anticonvulsants: Reduced plasma concentrations of itraconazole were reported when SPORANOX® was administered concomitantly with phenytoin. Carbamazepine, phenobarbital, and phenytoin are all inducers of CYP3A4. Although interactions with carbamazepine and phenobarbital have not been studied, concomitant administration of SPORANOX® and these drugs would be expected to result in decreased plasma concentrations of itraconazole. In addition, in vivo studies have demonstrated an increase in plasma carbamazepine concentrations in subjects concomitantly receiving ketoconazole. Although there are no data regarding the effect of itraconazole on carbamazepine metabolism, because of the similarities between ketoconazole and itraconazole, concomitant administration of SPORANOX® and carbamazepine may inhibit the metabolism of carbamazepine.

Antihistamines: Coadministration of astemizole with SPORANOX® has led to elevated plasma concentrations of astemizole and desmethylastemizole which could result in serious cardiovascular events. Therefore, concomitant administration of SPORANOX® with astemizole is contraindicated. (See BOX WARNING, CONTRAINDICATIONS, and WARNINGS.)

Antimycobacterials: Drug interaction studies have demonstrated that plasma concentrations of azole antifungal agents and their metabolites, including itraconazole and hydroxyitraconazole, were significantly decreased when these agents were given concomitantly with rifabutin or rifampin. In vivo data suggest that rifabutin is metabolized in part by CYP3A4. SPORANOX® may inhibit the metabolism of rifabutin. Although no formal study data are available for isoniazid, similar effects should be anticipated. Therefore, the efficacy of SPORANOX® could be substantially reduced if given concomitantly with one of these agents. Coadministration is not recommended.

Antineoplastics: SPORANOX® may inhibit the metabolism of busulfan, docetaxel, and vinca alkaloids.

Antipsychotics: Pimozide is known to prolong the QT interval and is partially metabolized by CYP3A4. Coadministration of pimozide with SPORANOX® could result in serious cardiovascular events. Therefore, concomitant administration of SPORANOX® and pimozide is contraindicated. (See BOX WARNING, CONTRAINDICATIONS, and WARNINGS.)

Benzodiazepines: Concomitant administration of SPORANOX® and alprazolam, diazepam, oral midazolam, or triazolam could lead to increased plasma concentrations of these benzodiazepines. Increased plasma concentrations could potentiate and prolong hypnotic and sedative effects. Concomitant administration of SPORANOX® and oral midazolam or triazolam is contraindicated. (See CONTRAINDICATIONS and WARNINGS.) If midazolam is administered parenterally, special precaution and patient monitoring is required since the sedative effect may be prolonged.

Calcium Channel Blockers: SPORANOX® may inhibit the metabolism of the dihydropyridines and verapamil.

Gastrointestinal Motility Agents: Coadministration of SPORANOX® with cisapride can elevate plasma cisapride concentrations which could result in serious cardiovascular events. Therefore, concomitant administration of SPORANOX® with cisapride is contraindicated. (See BOX WARNING, CONTRAINDICATIONS, and WARNINGS.)

HMG CoA-Reductase Inhibitors: Human pharmacokinetic data suggest that SPORANOX® inhibits the metabolism of atorvastatin, cerivastatin, lovastatin, and simvastatin, which may increase the risk of skeletal muscle toxicity, including rhabdomyolysis. Concomitant adminstration of SPORANOX® and lovastatin or simvastatin is contraindicated. (See CONTRAINDICATIONS and WARNINGS.)

Immunosuppressants: Concomitant administration of SPORANOX® and cyclosporine or tacrolimus has led to increased plasma concentrations of these immunosuppressants. Concomitant administration of SPORANOX® and sirolimus could increase plasma concentrations of sirolimus.

Macrolide Antibiotics: Clarithromycin is a known inhibitor of CYP3A4 and may increase plasma concentrations of itraconazole. There is no data regarding the pharmacokinetic effects of other macrolides on itraconazole.

Oral Hypoglycemic Agents: Severe hypoglycemia has been reported in patients concomitantly receiving azole antifungal agents and oral hypoglycemic agents. Blood glucose concentrations should be carefully monitored when SPORANOX® and oral hypoglycemic agents are coadministered.

Polyenes: Prior treatment with itraconazole, like other azoles, may reduce or inhibit the activity of polyenes such as amphoterecin B. However, the clinical significance of this drug effect has not been clearly defined.

Protease Inhibitors: Concomitant administration of SPORANOX® and protease inhibitors metabolized by CYP3A4, such as indinavir, ritonavir, and saquinavir, may increase plasma concentrations of these protease inhibitors. In addition, concomitant administration of SPORANOX® and indinavir and ritonavir (but not saquinavir) may increase plasma concentrations of itraconazole. Caution is advised when SPORANOX® and protease inhibitors must be given concomitantly.

Reverse Transcriptase Inhibitors: Nevirapine is an inducer of CYP3A4. In vivo studies have shown that nevirapine induces the metabolism of ketoconazole, significantly reducing the bioavailability of ketoconazole. Studies involving nevirapine and itraconazole have not been conducted. However, because of the similarities between ketoconazole and itraconazole, concomitant administration of SPORANOX® and nevirapine is not recommended. In a clinical study, when 8 HIV-infected subjects were treated concomitantly with SPORANOX® Capsules 100 mg twice daily and the nucleoside reverse transcriptase inhibitor zidovudine 8 ± 0.4 mg/kg/day, the pharmacokinetics of zidovudine were not affected. Other nucleoside reverse transcriptase inhibitors have not been studied.

Other:

- In vitro data suggest that alfentanil is metabolized by CYP3A4. Administration with SPORANOX® may increase plasma concentrations of alfentanil.
- Human pharmacokinetic data suggest that concomitant administration of SPORANOX® and buspirone results in significant increases in plasma concentrations of buspirone.
- SPORANOX® may inhibit the metabolism of methylprednisolone.
- In vitro data suggest that trimetrexate is extensively metabolized by CYP3A4. In vitro animal models have demonstrated that ketoconazaole potently inhibits the metabolism of trimetrexate. Although there are no data regarding the effect of itraconazole on trimetrexate metabolism, because of the similarities between ketoconazole and itraconazole, concomitant administration of SPORANOX® and trimetrexate may inhibit the metabolism of trimetrexate.
- SPORANOX® enhances the anticoagulant effect of coumarin-like drugs, such as warfarin.

Table 1. Selected Drugs that are predicted to alter the plasma concentration of itraconazole or have their plasma concentration altered by SPORANOX®[1]

Drug plasma concentration increased by itraconazole	
Antiarrhythmics	digoxin, quinidine[2]
Anticonvulsants	carbamazepine
Antihistamines	astemizole[2]
Antimycobacterials	rifabutin
Antineoplastics	busulfan, docetaxel, vinca alkaloids
Antipsychotics	pimozide[2]
Benzodiazepines	alprazolam, diazepam, midazolam,[2,3] triazolam[2]
Calcium Channel Blockers	dihydropyridines, verapamil
Gastrointestinal Motility Agents	cisapride[2]
HMG CoA-Reductase Inhibitors	atorvastatin, cerivastatin, lovastatin,[2] simvastatin[2]
Immunosuppressants	cyclosporine, tacrolimus, sirolimus
Oral Hypoglycemics	oral hypoglycemics
Protease Inhibitors	indinavir, ritonavir, saquinavir
Other	alfentanil, buspirone, methylprednisolone, trimetrexate, warfarin

Decrease plasma concentration of itraconazole	
Anticonvulsants	carbamazepine, phenobarbital, phenytoin
Antimycobacterials	isoniazid, rifabutin, rifampin
Reverse Transcriptase Inhibitors	nevirapine

Increase plasma concentration of itraconazole	
Macrolide Antibiotics	clarithromycin
Protease Inhibitors	indinavir, ritonavir

[1] This list is not all-inclusive.
[2] Contraindicated with SPORANOX® based on clinical and/or pharmacokinetics studies. (See WARNINGS and below.)
[3] For information on parenterally administered midazolam, see the benzodiazepine paragraph below.

Carcinogenesis, Mutagenesis and Impairment of Fertility: Itraconazole showed no evidence of carcinogenicity potential in mice treated orally for 23 months at dosage levels up to 80 mg/kg/day (approximately 10× the maximum recommended human dose [MRHD]). Male rats treated with 25 mg/kg/day (3.1× MRHD) had a slightly increased incidence of soft tissue sarcoma. These sarcomas may have been a consequence of hypercholesterolemia, which is a response of rats, but not dogs or humans, to chronic itraconazole administration. Female rats treated with 50 mg/kg/day (6.25× MRHD) had an increased incidence of squamous cell carcinoma of the lung (2/50) as compared to the untreated group. Although the occurrence of squamous cell carcinoma in the lung is extremely uncommon in untreated rats, the increase in this study was not statistically significant.

Hydroxypropyl-β-cyclodextrin (HP-β-CD), the solubilizing excipient used in SPORANOX® Injection and Oral Solution, was found to produce pancreatic exocrine hyperplasia and neoplasia when administered orally to rats at doses of 500, 2000 or 5000 mg/kg/day for 25 months. Adenocarcinomas of the exocrine pancreas produced in the treated animals were not seen in the untreated group and are not reported in the historical controls. Development of these tumors may be related to a mitogenic action of cholecystokinin. This finding was not observed in the mouse carcinogenicity study at doses of 500, 2000 or 5000 mg/kg/day for 22–23 months; however, the clinical relevance of these findings is unknown. Based on body surface area comparisons, the exposure to humans of HP-β-CD at the recommended clinical dose of SPORANOX® Oral Solution, is approximately equivalent to 1.7 times the exposure at the lowest dose in the rat study. The relevance of the findings with orally administered HP-β-CD to potential carcinogenic effects for SPORANOX® Injection is uncertain.

Itraconazole produced no mutagenic effects when assayed in DNA repair test (unscheduled DNA synthesis) in primary rat hepatocytes, in Ames tests with *Salmonella typhimurium* (6 strains) and *Escherichia coli*, in the mouse lymphoma gene mutation tests, in a sex-linked recessive lethal mutation (*Drosphila melanogaster*) test, in chromosome aberration tests in human lymphocytes, in a cell transformation test with C3H/10T$^{1}/_{2}$ C18 mouse embryo fibroblasts cells, in a dominant lethal mutation test in male and female mice, and in micronucleus tests in mice and rats.

Itraconazole did not affect the fertility of male or female rats treated orally with dosage levels of up to 40 mg/kg/day (5× MRHD), even though parental toxicity was present at this dosage level. More severe signs of parental toxicity, including death, were present in the next higher dosage level, 160 mg/kg/day (20× MRHD).

Pregnancy: Teratogenic Effects. Pregnancy Category C: Itraconazole was found to cause a dose-related increase in maternal toxicity, embryotoxicity, and teratogenicity in rats at dosage levels of approximately 40–160 mg/kg/day (5–20× MRHD), and in mice at dosage levels of approximately

Continued on next page

Sporanox Inj.—Cont.

80 mg/kg/day (10× MRHD). In rats, the teratogenicity consisted of major skeletal defects; in mice, it consisted of encephaloceles and/or macroglossia.

There are no studies in pregnant women, SPORANOX® should be used for the treatment of systemic fungal infections in pregnancy only if the benefit outweighs the potential risk.

Nursing Mothers: Itraconazole is excreted in human milk; therefore, the expected benefits of SPORANOX® therapy for the mother should be weighed against the potential risk from exposure of itraconazole to the infant. The U.S. Public Health Service Centers for Disease Control and Prevention advises HIV-infected women not to breast-feed to avoid potential transmission of HIV to uninfected infants.

Pediatric Use: The safety and efficacy of SPORANOX® have not been established in pediatric patients. No pharmacokinetic data on SPORANOX® Capsules or Injection are available in children. A small number of patients ages 3 to 16 years have been treated with 100 mg/day of itraconazole capsules for systemic fungal infections, and no serious unexpected adverse effects have been reported. SPORANOX® Oral Solution (5 mg/kg/day) has been administered to pediatric patients (N=26; ages 6 months to 12 years) for 2 weeks and no serious unexpected adverse events were reported.

The long-term effects of itraconazole on bone growth in children are unknown. In three toxicology studies using rats, itraconazole induced bone defects at dosage levels as low as 20 mg/kg/day (2.5× MRHD). The induced defects included reduced bone plate activity, thinning of the zona compacta of the large bones, and increased bone fragility. At a dosage level of 80 mg/kg/day (10× MRHD) over 1 year or 160 mg/kg/day (20× MRHD) for 6 months, itraconazole induced small tooth pulp with hypocellular appearance in some rats. No such bone toxicity has been reported in adult patients.

Geriatric Use: Clinical studies of SPORANOX® Injection did not include sufficient numbers of subjects aged 65 and over to determine whether they respond differently from younger subjects. Other reported clinical experience has not identified differences in responses between the elderly and younger patients. In general, dose selection for an elderly patient should be cautious reflecting the greater frequency of decreased hepatic, renal, or cardiac function, and of concomitant disease or other drug therapy.

ADVERSE REACTIONS

Rare cases of reversible idiosyncratic hepatitis have been reported among patients taking SPORANOX® (itraconazole) Capsules. SPORANOX® has been associated with rare cases of serious hepatotoxicity, including fatalities, primarily in patients with serious underlying medical conditions who are taking multiple medications. The causal association with SPORANOX® is uncertain. If clinical signs and symptoms consistent with liver disease develop and could be attributed to itraconazole, SPORANOX® should be discontinued. (See WARNINGS.)

Adverse events considered at least possibly drug related are listed below and are based on the experience of 360 patients treated with SPORANOX® Injection in four pharmacokinetic, one uncontrolled and four active controlled studies where the control was amphotericin B or fluconazole. Nearly all patients were neutropenic or were otherwise immunocompromised and were treated empirically for febrile episodes, for documented systemic fungal infections, or in trials to determine pharmacokinetics. The dose of SPORANOX® Injection was 200 mg twice daily for the first two days followed by a single daily dose of 200 mg for the remainder of the intravenous treatment period. The majority of patients received between 7 and 14 days of SPORANOX® Injection.

[See table below]

The following adverse events occurred in less than 1% of patients in clinical trials of SPORANOX® Injection: constipation, hyperglycemia, hepatitis, fever, rigors, dyspnea, and hypotension.

Post-marketing Experience

In worldwide post-marketing experience with SPORANOX® Capsules, allergic reactions, including rash, pruritus, urticaria, angioedema, and, in rare instances, anaphylaxis and Stevens-Johnson syndrome, have been reported. Post-marketing experiences have also included reports of elevated liver enzymes and rarely, hepatitis. Although the causal association with SPORANOX® is uncertain, rare cases of alopecia, hypertriglyceridemia, menstrual disorders, and neutropenia, and isolated cases of neuropathy have also been reported.

Summary of possibly or definitely drug-related adverse events reported by ≥1% of SPORANOX® Injection patients (TOTAL)

Adverse Event	Total SPORANOX® Injection (N=360) %	Comparative Studies		
		SPORANOX® Injection (N=234) %	Intravenous Fluconazole (N=32) %	Intravenous Amphotericin B (N=202) %
Gastrointestinal system disorders				
Nausea	8	9	0	15
Diarrhea	6	6	3	9
Vomiting	4	6	0	10
Abdominal pain	2	2	0	3
Metabolic and nutritional disorders				
Hypokalemia	5	8	0	29
Alkaline phosphatase increased	1	2	3	2
Serum creatinine increased	2	2	3	26
Hypomagnesemia	1	1	0	5
Liver and biliary system disorders				
Bilirubinemia	4	6	9	3
SGPT/ALT increased	2	3	3	1
Hepatic function abnormal	1	2	0	2
Jaundice	1	2	0	1
SGOT/AST increased	1	2	0	1
Body as a whole – General disorders				
Pain	1	2	0	1
Edema	1	1	0	1
Skin and appendages disorders				
Rash	3	3	3	3
Sweating increased	1	2	0	1
Central and peripheral nervous system disorders				
Dizziness	1	2	0	1
Headache	2	2	0	3
Urinary system disorders				
Renal function abnormal	1	1	0	11
Albuminuria	1	0	0	0
Application site disorder				
Application site reaction	4	0	0	0
Vascular (extracardiac) disorders				
Vein disorder	3	0	0	0

OVERDOSAGE

Itraconazole is not removed by dialysis.

There are limited data on the outcomes of patients ingesting high doses of itraconazole. In patients taking either 100 mg of SPORANOX® (itraconazole) Oral Solution or up to 3000 mg of SPORANOX® Capsules, the adverse event profile was similar to that observed at recommended doses.

DOSAGE AND ADMINISTRATION

Use only the components [SPORANOX® (itraconazole) Injection ampule, 0.9% Sodium Chloride Injection, USP (Normal Saline) bag and filtered infusion set] provided in the kit: **DO NOT SUBSTITUTE.**

SPORANOX® Injection should not be diluted with 5% Dextrose Injection, USP, or with Lactated Ringer's Injection, USP, alone or in combination with any other diluent. The compatibility of SPORANOX® Injection with diluents other than 0.9% Sodium Chloride Injection, USP (Normal Saline) is not known. **NOT FOR IV BOLUS INJECTION.**

NOTE: After reconstitution, the diluted SPORANOX® Injection may be stored refrigerated (2–8°C) or at room temperature (15–25°C) for up to 48 hours, when protected from direct light. During administration, exposure to normal room light is acceptable.

NOTE: Use only a dedicated infusion line for administration of SPORANOX® Injection. Do not introduce concomitant medication in the same bag nor through the same line as SPORANOX® Injection. Other medications may be administered after flushing the line/catheter with 0.9% Sodium Chloride Injection, USP, as described below, and removing and replacing the entire infusion line. Alternatively, utilize another lumen, in the case of a multi-lumen catheter.

Add the full contents (25 mL) of the SPORANOX® Injection ampule into the infusion bag provided, which contains 50 mL of 0.9% Sodium Chloride Injection, USP (Normal Saline). Mix gently after the solution is completely transferred. Using a flow control device, infuse 60 mL of the dilute solution (3.33 mg/mL = 200 mg itraconazole, pH apx. 48) intravenously over 60 minutes, using an extension line and the infusion set provided. After administration, flush the infusion set with 15–20 mL of 0.9% Sodium Chloride Injection, USP, over 30 seconds-15 minutes, via the two-way stopcock. Discard the entire infusion line.

Parenteral drug products should be inspected visually for particulate matter and discoloration prior to administration, whenever solution and container permit.

Treatment of Blastomycosis, Histoplasmosis and Aspergillosis: The recommended intravenous dose is 200 mg b.i.d. for four doses, followed by 200 mg q.d. Each intravenous dose should be infused over 1 hour.

For the treatment of blastomycosis, histoplasmosis and aspergillosis, SPORANOX® can be given as oral capsules or intravenously. The safety and efficacy of SPORANOX® Injection administered for greater than 14 days is not known. Total itraconazole therapy (SPORANOX® Injection followed by SPORANOX® Capsules) should be continued for a minimum of 3 months and until clinical parameters and laboratory tests indicate that the active fungal infection has subsided. An inadequate period of treatment may lead to recurrence of active infection.

SPORANOX® Injection should not be used in patients with creatinine clearance < 30 mL/min.

HOW SUPPLIED

SPORANOX® (itraconazole) Injection for intravenous infusion is supplied as a kit (NDC 50458-298-01), containing one 25 mL colorless glass ampule of itraconazole 10 mg/mL sterile, pyrogen-free solution (NDC 50458-297-10), one 50 mL bag (100 mL capacity) of 0.9% Sodium Chloride Injection, USP (Normal Saline) and one filtered infusion set. Store at or below 25°C (77°F). Protect from light and freezing.

Distributed by:
Ortho Biotech, Inc.
Raritan, NJ 08869
Manufactured by:
Abbott Laboratories, Inc.
North Chicago, IL 60064

631-10-938-2
U.S. Patents 4,267,179; 4,791,111
58-6011-R2
March 2000

SPORANOX® ℞
[*spŏr-a-nŏx*]
(ITRACONAZOLE)
ORAL SOLUTION

WARNING: Coadministration of astemizole, cisapride, pimozide, or quinidine with SPORANOX® (itraconazole) Capsules, Injection or Oral Solution is contraindicated. SPORANOX®, a potent cytochrome P450 3A4 isoenzyme system (CYP3A4) inhibitor, may increase plasma concentrations of drugs metabolized by this pathway. Serious cardiovascular events, including QT prolongation, torsades de pointes, ventricular tachycardia, cardiac arrest, and/or sudden death have occurred in patients using astemizole, cisapride, pimozide, or quinidine, concomitantly with SPORANOX® and/or other CYP3A4 inhibitors. See CONTRAINDICATIONS, WARNINGS, and PRECAUTIONS: Drug Interactions for more information.

DESCRIPTION
SPORANOX® is the brand name for itraconazole, a synthetic antifungal agent. Itraconazole is a 1:1:1:1 racemic mixture of four diastereomers (two enantiomeric pairs), each possessing three chiral centers. It may be represented by the following nomenclature:
(±)-1-[(R*)-sec-butyl]-4-[p-[4-[p-[[(2R*,4S*)-2-(2,4-dichlorophenyl)-2-(1H-1,2,4-triazol-1-ylmethyl)-1,3-dioxolan-4-yl-]methoxy]phenyl]-1-piperazinyl]phenyl]-Δ^2-1,2,4-triazolin-5-one mixture with (±)-1-[(R*)-sec-butyl]-4-[p-[4-[p-[[(2S*,4R*)-2-(2,4-dichlorophenyl)-2-(1H-1,2,4-triazol-1-ylmethyl)-1,3-dioxolan-4-yl]methoxy]phenyl]-1-piperazinyl]phenyl]-Δ^2-1,2,4-triazolin-5-one
or
(±)-1-[(RS)-sec-butyl]-4-[p-[4-[p-[[(2R,4S)-2-(2,4-dichlorophenyl)-2-(1H-1,2,4-triazol-1-ylmethyl)-1,3-dioxolan-4-yl-]methoxy]phenyl]-1-piperazinyl]phenyl]-Δ^2-1,2,4-triazolin-5-one.
Itraconazole has a molecular formula of $C_{35}H_{38}Cl_2N_8O_4$ and a molecular weight of 705.64. It is a white to slightly yellowish powder. It is insoluble in water, very slightly soluble in alcohols, and freely soluble in dichloromethane. It has a pKa of 3.70 (based on extrapolation of values obtained from methanolic solutions) and a log (n-octanol/water) partition coefficient of 5.66 at pH 8.1.
SPORANOX® (itraconazole) Oral Solution contains 10 mg of itraconazole per mL, solubilized by hydroxypropyl-β-cyclodextrin (400 mg/mL) as a molecular inclusion complex. SPORANOX® Oral Solution is clear and yellowish in color with a target pH of 2. Other ingredients are hydrochloric acid, propylene glycol, purified water, sodium hydroxide, sodium saccharin, sorbitol, cherry flavor 1, cherry flavor 2 and caramel flavor.

CLINICAL PHARMACOLOGY
Pharmacokinetics and Metabolism: NOTE: The plasma concentrations reported below were measured by high-performance liquid chromatography (HPLC) specific for itraconazole. When itraconazole in plasma is measured by a bioassay, values reported may be higher than those obtained by HPLC due to the presence of the bioactive metabolite, hydroxyitraconazole. (See MICROBIOLOGY.) The absolute bioavailability of itraconazole administered as a non-marketed solution formulation under fed conditions was 55% in 6 healthy male volunteers. However, the bioavailability of SPORANOX® (itraconazole) Oral Solution is increased under fasted conditions reaching higher maximum plasma concentrations (C_{max}) in a shorter period of time. In 27 healthy male volunteers, the steady-state area under the plasma concentration versus time curve (AUC_{0-24h}) of itraconazole (SPORANOX® Oral Solution, 200 mg daily for 15 days) under fasted conditions was 131 ± 30% of that obtained under fed conditions. Therefore, unlike SPORANOX® Capsules, it is recommended that SPORANOX® Oral Solution be administered without food.
Presented in the table below are the steady-state (Day 15) pharmacokinetic parameters for itraconazole and hydroxyitraconazole (SPORANOX® Oral Solution) under fasted and fed conditions:
[See table at top of page]

	Itraconazole		Hydroxyitraconazole	
	Fasted	Fed	Fasted	Fed
C_{max} (ng/mL)	1963 ± 601*	1435 ± 477	2055 ± 487	1781 ± 397
T_{max} (hours)	2.5 ± 0.8	4.4 ± 0.7	5.3 ± 4.3	4.3 ± 1.2
AUC_{0-24h} (ng·h/mL)	29271 ± 10285	22815 ± 7098	45184 ± 10981	38823 ± 8907
$t_{1/2}$ (hours)	39.7 ± 13	37.4 ± 13	27.3 ± 13	26.1 ± 10

*mean ± standard deviation

The bioavailability of SPORANOX® Oral Solution relative to SPORANOX® Capsules was studied in 30 healthy male volunteers who received 200 mg of itraconazole as the oral solution and capsules under fed conditions. The $AUC_{0-\infty}$ from SPORANOX® Oral Solution was 149 ± 68% of that obtained from SPORANOX® Capsules; a similar increase was observed for hydroxyitraconazole. In addition, a cross study comparison of itraconazole and hydroxyitraconazole pharmacokinetics following the administration of single 200 mg doses of SPORANOX® Oral Solution (under fasted conditions) or SPORANOX® Capsules (under fed conditions) indicates that when these two formulations are administered under conditions which optimize their systemic absorption, the bioavailability of the solution relative to capsules is expected to be increased further. Therefore, it is recommended that SPORANOX® Oral Solution and SPORANOX® Capsules not be used interchangeably. The following table contains pharmacokinetic parameters for itraconazole and hydroxyitraconazole following single 200 mg doses of SPORANOX® Oral Solution (n=27) or SPORANOX® Capsules (n=30) administered to healthy male volunteers under fasted and fed conditions, respectively:
[See first table at top of next page]
The plasma protein binding of itraconazole is 99.8% and that of hydroxyitraconazole is 99.5%. Following intravenous administration, the volume of distribution of itraconazole averaged 796 ± 185 L.
Itraconazole is metabolized predominately by the cytochrome P450 3A4 isoenzyme system (CYP3A4), resulting in the formation of several metabolites, including hydroxyitraconazole, the major metabolite. Results of a pharmacokinetics study suggest that itraconazole may undergo saturable metabolism with multiple dosing. Fecal excretion of the parent drug varies between 3–18% of the dose. Renal excretion of the parent drug is less than 0.03% of the dose. About 40% of the dose is excreted as inactive metabolites in the urine. No single excreted metabolite represents more than 5% of a dose. Itraconazole total plasma clearance averaged 381 ± 95 mL/minute following intravenous administration.
Special Populations:
Pediatrics: The pharmacokinetics of SPORANOX® Oral Solution were studied in 26 pediatric patients requiring systemic antifungal therapy. Patients were stratified by age: 6 months to 2 years (n=8), 2 to 5 years (n=7) and 5 to 12 years (n=11), and received itraconazole oral solution 5 mg/kg once daily for 14 days. Pharmacokinetic parameters at steady-state (Day 14) were not significantly different among the age strata and are summarized in the table below for all 26 patients:

	Itraconazole	Hydroxyitraconazole
C_{max} (ng/mL)	582.5 ± 382.4*	692.4 ± 355.0
C_{min} (ng/mL)	187.5 ± 161.4	403.8 ± 336.1
AUC_{0-24h} (ng·h/mL)	7706.7 ± 5245.2	13356.4 ± 8942.4
$t_{1/2}$ (hours)	35.8 ± 35.6	17.7 ± 13.0

*mean ± standard deviation

Renal Insufficiency: A pharmacokinetic study using a single 200-mg dose of itraconazole (four 50-mg capsules) was conducted in three groups of patients with renal impairment (uremia: n=7; hemodialysis: n=7; and continuous ambulatory peritoneal dialysis: n=5). In uremic subjects with a mean creatinine clearance of 13 mL/min. × 1.73 m^2, the bioavailability was slightly reduced compared with normal population parameters. This study did not demonstrate any significant effect of hemodialysis or continuous ambulatory peritoneal dialysis on the pharmacokinetics of itraconazole (T_{max}, C_{max}, and AUC_{0-8}). Plasma concentration-versus-time profiles showed wide intersubject variation in all three groups.
Hepatic Insufficiency: Patients with impaired hepatic function should be carefully monitored when taking itraconazole. The prolonged elimination half-life of itraconazole observed in cirrhotic patients should be considered when deciding to initiate therapy with other medications metabolized by CYP3A4. (See BOX WARNING, CONTRAINDICATIONS, and PRECAUTIONS: Drug Interactions.)

MICROBIOLOGY
Mechanism of Action: In vitro studies have demonstrated that itraconazole inhibits the cytochrome P-450-dependent synthesis of ergosterol, which is a vital component of fungal cell membranes.
Activity in Vitro and in Vivo: Itraconazole exhibits in vitro activity against *Blastomyces dermatitidis*, *Histoplasma capsulatum*, *Histoplasma duboisii*, *Aspergillus flavus*, *Aspergillus fumigatus*, *Candida albicans*, and *Cryptococcus neoformans*. Itraconazole also exhibits varying in vitro activity against *Sporothrix schenckii*, *Trichophyton* species, *Candida krusei*, and other *Candida* species. The bioactive metabolite, hydroxyitraconazole, has not been evaluated against *Histoplasma capsulatum* and *Blastomyces dermatitidis*. Correlation between minimum inhibitory concentration (MIC) results in vitro and clinical outcome has yet to be established for azole antifungal agents.
Itraconazole administered orally was active in a variety of animal models of fungal infection using standard laboratory strains of fungi. Fungistatic activity has been demonstrated against disseminated fungal infections caused by *Blastomyces dermatitidis*, *Histoplasma duboisii*, *Aspergillus fumigatus*, *Coccidioides immitis*, *Cryptococcus neoformans*, *Paracoccidioides brasiliensis*, *Sporothrix schenckii*, *Trichophyton rubrum*, and *Trichophyton mentagrophytes*.
Itraconazole administered at 2.5 mg/kg and 5 mg/kg via the oral and parenteral routes increased survival rates and sterilized organ systems in normal and immunosuppressed guinea pigs with disseminated *Aspergillus fumigatus* infections. Oral itraconazole administered daily at 40 mg/kg and 80 mg/kg increased survival rates in normal rabbits with disseminated disease and in immunosuppressed rats with pulmonary *Aspergillus fumigatus* infection, respectively. Itraconazole has demonstrated antifungal activity in a variety of animal models infected with *Candida albicans* and other *Candida* species.
Resistence: Isolates from several fungal species with decreased susceptibility to itraconazole have been isolated in vitro and from patients receiving prolonged therapy.
Several in vitro studies have reported that some fungal clinical isolates, including *Candida* species, with reduced susceptibility to one azole antifungal agent may also be less susceptible to other azole derivatives. The finding of cross-resistance is dependent on a number of factors, including the species evaluated, its clinical history, the particular azole compounds compared, and the type of susceptibility test that is performed. The relevance of these in vitro susceptibility data to clinical outcome remains to be elucidated.
Studies (both in vitro and in vivo) suggest that the activity of amphotericin B may be suppressed by prior azole antifungal therapy. As with other azoles, itraconazole inhibits the ^{14}C-demethylation step in the synthesis of ergosterol, a cell wall component of fungi. Ergosterol is the active site for amphotericin B. In one study the antifungal activity of amphotericin B against *Aspergillus fumigatus* infections in mice was inhibited by ketoconazole therapy. The clinical significance of test results obtained in this study is unknown.

INDICATIONS AND USAGE
SPORANOX® (itraconazole) Oral Solution is indicated for the treatment of oropharyngeal and esophageal candidiasis.
Description of Clinical Studies:
Oropharyngeal Candidiasis: Two randomized, controlled studies for the treatment of oropharyngeal candidiasis have been conducted (total n=344). In one trial, clinical response to either 7 or 14 days of itraconazole oral solution, 200 mg/day, was similar to fluconazole tablets and averaged 84% across all arms. Clinical response in this study was defined as cured or improved (only minimal signs and symptoms with no visible lesions). Approximately 5% of subjects were lost to follow-up before any evaluations could be performed. Response to 14 days therapy of itraconazole oral solution was associated with a lower relapse rate than 7 days of itraconazole therapy. In another trial, the clinical response rate (defined as cured or improved) for itraconazole oral solution was similar to clotrimazole troches and averaged approximately 71% across both arms, with approximately 3% of subjects lost to follow-up before any evaluations could be performed. Ninety-two percent of the patients in these studies were HIV seropositive.
In an uncontrolled, open-label study of selected patients clinically unresponsive to fluconazole tablets (n=74, all patients HIV seropositive), patients were treated with itraconazole oral solution 100 mg b.i.d. (Clinically unresponsive to fluconazole in this study was defined as having received a dose of fluconazole tablets at least 200 mg/day for a minimum of 14 days.) Treatment duration was 14–28 days based on response. Approximately 55% of patients had complete resolution of oral lesions. Of patients who responded and then entered a follow-up phase (n=22), all relapsed within 1 month (median 14 days) when treatment was discontinued. Although baseline endoscopies had not been performed, several patients in this study developed symptoms of esophageal candidiasis while receiving therapy with itraconazole oral solution. Itraconazole oral solution has not been directly compared to other agents in a controlled trial of similar patients.
Esophageal Candidiasis: A double-blind randomized study (n=119, 111 of whom were HIV seropositive) compared itraconazole oral solution (100 mg/day) to fluconazole tablets (100 mg/day). The dose of each was increased to 200 mg/day for patients not responding initially. Treatment continued for 2 weeks following resolution of symptoms, for a total duration of treatment of 3–8 weeks. Clinical response (a global assessment of cured or improved) was not significantly different between the two study arms, and averaged approximately 86% with 8% lost to follow-up. Six of 53 (11%) itraconazole-treated patients and 12/57 (21%) fluconazole-treated patients were escalated to the 200 mg dose in this trial. Of the subgroup of patients who responded and entered a follow-up phase (n=88), approximately 23% relapsed across both arms within 4 weeks.

CONTRAINDICATIONS
Concomitant administration of SPORANOX® (itraconazole) Capsules, Injection, or Oral Solution and certain drugs metabolized by the cytochrome P450 3A4 isoenzyme system (CYP3A4) may result in increased plasma concentrations of those drugs, leading to potentially serious and/or life-

Continued on next page

Sporanox Oral—Cont.

threatening adverse events. Astemizole, cisapride, oral midazolam, pimozide, quinidine, and triazolam are contraindicated with SPORANOX®. HMG CoA-reductase inhibitors metabolized by CYP3A4, such as lovastatin and simvastatin, are also contraindicated with SPORANOX®. (See BOX WARNING, and PRECAUTIONS: Drug Interactions.)

SPORANOX® is contraindicated for patients who have shown hypersensitivity to itraconazole or its excipients. There is no information regarding cross-hypersensitivity between itraconazole and other azole antifungal agents. Caution should be used when prescribing SPORANOX® to patients with hypersensitivity to other azoles.

WARNINGS

SPORANOX® (itraconazole) Oral Solution and SPORANOX® Capsules should not be used interchangeably. Only SPORANOX® Oral Solution has been demonstrated effective for oral and/or esophageal candidiasis. SPORANOX® Oral Solution contains the excipient hydroxypropyl-β-cyclodextrin which produced pancreatic adenocarcinomas in a rat carcinogenicity study. These findings were not observed in a similar mouse carcinogenicity study. The clinical relevance of these findings is unknown. (See Carcinogenesis, Mutagenesis, and Impairment of Fertility.)

Hepatitis: Rare cases of reversible idiosyncratic hepatitis have been reported among patients taking SPORANOX® Capsules. SPORANOX® has been associated with rare cases of serious hepatotoxicity, including death, primarily in patients with serious underlying medical conditions who are taking multiple medications. The causal association with SPORANOX® is uncertain. If clinical signs and symptoms develop that are consistent with liver disease and may be attributable to itraconazole, SPORANOX® should be discontinued.

Cardiac Dysrhythmias: Life-threatening cardiac dysrhythmias and/or sudden death have occurred in patients using astemizole, cisapride, pimozide or quinidine concomitantly with SPORANOX® and/or other CYP3A4 inhibitors. Concomitant administration of these drugs with SPORANOX® is contraindicated. (See BOX WARNING, CONTRAINDICATIONS, and PRECAUTIONS: Drug Interactions.)

PRECAUTIONS

General: Hepatic enzyme test values should be monitored in patients with pre-existing hepatic function abnormalities or those who have experienced liver toxicity with other medications. Hepatic enzyme test values should be monitored periodically in all patients receiving continuous treatment for more than 1 month, or at any time a patient develops signs or symptoms suggestive of liver dysfunction.

Information for Patients: Only SPORANOX® Oral Solution has been demonstrated effective for oral and/or esophageal candidiasis. SPORANOX® Oral Solution contains the excipient hydroxypropyl-β-cyclodextrin which produced pancreatic adenocarcinomas in a rat carcinogenicity study. These findings were not observed in a similar mouse carcinogenicity study. The clinical relevence of these findings is unknown. (See Carcinogenesis, Mutagenesis, and Impairment of Fertility.)

Taking SPORANOX® Oral Solution under fasted conditions improves the systemic availability of itraconazole. Instruct patients to take SPORANOX® Oral Solution without food, if possible.

Instruct patients to report any signs and symptoms that may suggest liver dysfunction so that the appropriate laboratory testing can be done. Such signs and symptoms may include unusual fatigue, anorexia, nausea and/or vomiting, jaundice, dark urine or pale stools.

Instruct patients to contact their physician before taking any concomitant medications with itraconazole to ensure there are no potential drug interactions.

Drug Interactions: Itraconazole and its major metabolite, hydroxyitraconazole, are inhibitors of CYP3A4. Therefore, the following drug interactions may occur (See Table 1 below and the following drug class subheadings that follow):

1. SPORANOX® may decrease the elimination of drugs metabolized by CYP3A4, resulting in increased plasma concentrations of these drugs when they are administered with SPORANOX®. These elevated plasma concentrations may increase or prolong both therapeutic and adverse effects of these drugs. Whenever possible, plasma concentrations of these drugs should be monitored, and dosage adjustments made after concomitant SPORANOX® therapy is initiated. When appropriate, clinical monitoring for signs or symptoms of increased or prolonged pharmacologic effects is advised. Upon discontinuation, depending on the dose and duration of treatment, itraconazole plasma concentrations decline gradually (especially in patients with hepatic cirrhosis or in those receiving CYP3A4 inhibitors). This is particularly important when initiating therapy with drugs whose metabolism is affected by intraconazole.
2. Inducers of CYP3A4 may decrease the plasma concentrations of itraconazole. SPORANOX® may not be effective in patients concomitantly taking SPORANOX® and one of these drugs. Therefore, administration of these drugs with SPORANOX® is not recommended.
3. Other inhibitors of CYP3A4 may increase the plasma concentrations of itraconazole. Patients who must take SPORANOX® concomitantly with one of these drugs should be monitored closely for signs or symptoms of increased or prolonged pharmacologic effects of SPORANOX®.

	Itraconazole		Hydroxyitraconazole	
	Oral Solution fasted	Capsules fed	Oral Solution fasted	Capsules fed
C_{max} (ng/mL)	544 ± 213*	302 ± 119	622 ± 116	504 ± 132
T_{max} (hours)	2.2 ± 0.8	5 ± 0.8	3.5 ± 1.2	5 ± 1
AUC_{0-24h} (ng·h/mL)	4505 ± 1670	2682 ± 1084	9552 ± 1835	7293 ± 2144

*mean ± standard deviation

Table 1. Selected Drugs that are predicted to alter the plasma concentration of itraconazole or have their plasma concentration altered by SPORANOX®[1]

Drug plasma concentration increased by itraconazole	
Antiarrhythmics	digoxin, quinidine[2]
Anticoagulants	warfarin
Anticonvulsants	carbamazepine
Antihistamines	astemizole[2]
Antimycobacterials	rifabutin
Antineoplastics	busulfan, docetaxel, vinca alkaloids
Antipsychotics	pimozide[2]
Benzodiazepines	alprazolam, diazepam, midazolam,[2,3] triazolam[2]
Calcium Channel Blockers	dihydropyridines, verapamil
Gastrointestinal Motility Agents	cisapride[2]
HMG CoA-Reductase Inhibitors	atorvastatin, cerivastatin, lovastatin,[2] simvastatin[2]
Immunosuppressants	cyclosporine, tacrolimus, sirolimus
Oral Hypoglycemics	oral hypoglycemics
Protease Inhibitors	indinavir, ritonavir, saquinavir
Other	alfentanil, buspirone, methylprednisolone, trimetrexate
Decrease plasma concentration of itraconazole	
Anticonvulsants	carbamazepine, phenobarbital, phenytoin
Antimycobacterials	isoniazid, rifabutin, rifampin
Gastric Acid Suppressors/Neutralizers	antacids, H_2-receptor antagonists, proton pump inhibitors
Reverse Transcriptase Inhibitors	nevirapine
Increase plasma concentration of itraconazole	
Macrolide Antibiotics	clarithromycin
Protease Inhibitors	indinavir, ritonavir

[1] This list is not all-inclusive.
[2] Contraindicated with SPORANOX® based on clinical and/or pharmacokinetics studies. (See WARNINGS and below.)
[3] For information on parenterally administered midazolam, see the Benzodiazepine paragraph below.

[See second table above]

Antiarrhythmics: The class IA antiarrhythmic quinidine is known to prolong the QT interval. Coadministration of quinidine with SPORANOX® increases plasma concentrations of quinidine which could result in serious cardiovascular events. Therefore, concomitant administration of SPORANOX® and quinidine is contraindicated. (See BOX WARNING, CONTRAINDICATIONS, and WARNINGS.) Concomitant administration of digoxin and SPORANOX® has led to increased plasma concentrations of digoxin.

Anticoagulants: SPORANOX® enhances the anticoagulant effect of coumarin-like drugs, such as warfarin.

Anticonvulsants: Reduced plasma concentrations of itraconazole were reported when SPORANOX® was administered concomitantly with phenytoin. Carbamazepine, phenobarbital, and phenytoin are all inducers of CYP3A4. Although interactions with carbamazepine and phenobarbital have not been studied, concomitant administration of SPORANOX® and these drugs would be expected to result in decreased plasma concentrations of itraconazole. In addition, in vivo studies have demonstrated an increase in plasma carbamazepine concentrations in subjects concomitantly receiving ketoconazole. Although there are no data regarding the effect of itraconazole on carbamazepine metabolism, because of the similarities between ketoconazole and itraconazole, concomitant administration of SPORANOX® and carbamazepine may inhibit the metabolism of carbamazepine.

Antihistamines: Coadministration of astemizole with SPORANOX® has led to elevated plasma concentrations of astemizole and desmethyl-astemizole which could result in serious cardiovascular events. Therefore, concomitant administration of SPORANOX® with astemizole is contraindicated. (See BOX WARNING, CONTRAINDICATIONS, and WARNINGS.)

Antimycobacterials: Drug interaction studies have demonstrated that plasma concentrations of azole antifungal agents and their metabolites, including itraconazole and hydroxyitraconazole, were significantly decreased when these agents were given concomitantly with rifabutin or rifampin. In vivo data suggest that rifabutin is metabolized in part by CYP3A4. SPORANOX® may inhibit the metabolism of rifabutin. Although no formal study data are available for isoniazid, similar effects should be anticipated. Therefore, the efficacy of SPORANOX® could be substantially reduced if given concomitantly with one of these agents. Coadministration is not recommended.

Antineoplastics: SPORANOX® may inhibit the metabolism of busulfan, docetaxel, and vinca alkaloids.

Antipsychotics: Pimozide is known to prolong the QT interval and is partially metabolized by CYP3A4. Coadministration of pimozide with SPORANOX® could result in serious cardiovascular events. Therefore, concomitant administration of SPORANOX® and pimozide is contraindicated. (See BOX WARNING, CONTRAINDICATIONS, and WARNINGS.)

Benzodiazepines: Concomitant administration of SPORANOX® and alprazolam, diazepam, oral midazolam, or triazolam could lead to increased plasma concentrations of these benzodiazepines. Increased plasma concentrations could potentiate and prolong hypnotic and sedative effects. Concomitant administration of SPORANOX® and oral midazolam or triazolam is contraindicated. (See CONTRAINDICATIONS and WARNINGS.) If midazolam is administered parenterally, special precaution and patient monitoring is required since the sedative effect may be prolonged.

Calcium Channel Blockers: SPORANOX® may inhibit the metabolism of the dihydropyridines and verapamil.

Gastric Acid Suppressors/Neutralizers: Reduced plasma concentrations of itraconazole were reported when SPORANOX® Capsules were administered concomitantly with H_2-receptor antagonists. Studies have shown that absorption of itraconazole is impaired when gastric acid production is decreased. Therefore, SPORANOX® should be administered with a cola beverage if the patient has achlorhydria or is taking H_2-receptor antagonists or other gastric acid suppressors. Antacids should be administered at least 1 hour before or 2 hours after administration of SPORANOX® Capsules. In a clinical study, when SPORANOX® Capsules were administered with omeprazole (a proton pump inhibitor), the bioavailability of itraconazole was significantly reduced. However, as itraconazole is already dissolved in SPORANOX® Oral Solution, the effect of H_2 antagonists is expected to be substantially less than with the capsules. Nevertheless, caution is advised when the two drugs are coadministered.

Gastrointestinal Motility Agents: Coadministration of SPORANOX® with cisapride can elevate plasma cisapride concentrations which could result in serious cardiovascular events. Therefore, concomitant administration of SPORANOX® with cisapride is contraindicated. (See BOX WARNING, CONTRAINDICATIONS, and WARNINGS.)

HMG CoA-Reductase Inhibitors: Human pharmacokinetic data suggest that SPORANOX® inhibits the metabolism of atorvastatin, cerivastatin, lovastatin, and simvastatin, which may increase the risk of skeletal muscle toxicity, including rhabdomyolysis. Concomitant administration of SPORANOX® and lovastatin or simvastatin is contraindicated. (See CONTRAINDICATIONS, and WARNINGS.)

Immunosuppressants: Concomitant administration of SPORANOX® and cyclosporine or tacrolimus has led to increased plasma concentrations of these immunosuppressants. Concomitant administration of SPORANOX® and sirolimus could increase plasma concentrations of sirolimus.

Macrolide Antibiotics: Clarithromycin is a known inhibitor of CYP3A4 and may increase plasma concentrations of itraconazole.

Oral Hypoglycemic Agents: Severe hypoglycemia has been reported in patients concomitantly receiving azole antifungal agents and oral hypoglycemic agents. Blood glucose concentrations should be carefully monitored when SPORANOX® and oral hypoglycemic agents are coadministered.

Polyenes: Prior treatment with itraconazole, like other azoles, may reduce or inhibit the activity of polyenes such as amphotericin B. However, the clinical significance of this drug effect has not been clearly defined.

Protease Inhibitors: Concomitant administration of SPORANOX® and protease inhibitors metabolized by CYP3A4, such as indinavir, ritonavir, and saquinavir, may increase plasma concentrations of these protease inhibitors. In addition, concomitant administration of SPORANOX® and indinavir and ritonavir (but not saquinavir) may increase plasma concentrations of itraconazole. Caution is advised when SPORANOX® and protease inhibitors must be given concomitantly.

Reverse Transcriptase Inhibitors: Nevirapine is an inducer of CYP3A4. In vivo studies have shown that nevirapine induces the metabolism of ketoconazole, significantly reducing the bioavailability of ketoconazole. Studies involving nevirapine and itraconazole have not been conducted. However, because of the similarities between ketoconazole and itraconazole, concomitant administration of SPORANOX® and nevirapine is not recommended. In a clinical study, when 8 HIV-infected subjects were treated concomitantly with SPORANOX® Capsules 100mg twice daily and the nucleoside reverse transcriptase inhibitor zidovudine 8 ± 0.4 mg/kg/day, the pharmacokinetics of zidovudine were not affected. Other nucleoside reverse transcriptase inhibitors have not been studied.

Other:

- In vitro data suggest that alfentanil is metabolized by CYP3A4. Administration with SPORANOX® may increase plasma concentrations of alfentanil.
- Human pharmacokinetic data suggest that concomitant administration of SPORANOX® and buspirone results in significant increases in plasma concentrations of buspirone.
- SPORANOX® may inhibit the metabolism of methylprednisolone.
- In vitro data suggest that trimetrexate is extensively metabolized by CYP3A4. In vitro animal models have demonstrated that ketoconazole potently inhibits the metabolism of trimetrexate. Although there are no data regarding the effect of itraconazole on trimetrexate metabolism, because of the similarities between ketoconazole and itraconazole, concomitant administration of SPORANOX® and trimetrexate may inhibit the metabolism of trimetrexate.

Carcinogenesis, Mutagenesis, and Impairment of Fertility: Itraconazole showed no evidence of carcinogenicity potential in mice treated orally for 23 months at dosage levels up to 80 mg/kg/day (approximately 10× the maximum recommended human dose [MRHD]). Male rats treated with 25 mg/kg/day (3.1× MRHD) had a slightly increased incidence of soft tissue sarcoma. These sarcomas may have been a consequence of hypercholesterolemia, which is a response of rats, but not dogs or humans, to chronic itraconazole administration. Female rats treated with 50 mg/kg/day (6.25× MRHD) had an increased incidence of squamous cell carcinoma of the lung (2/50) as compared to the untreated group. Although the occurrence of squamous cell carcinoma in the lung is extremely uncommon in untreated rats, the increase in this study was not statistically significant.

Hydroxypropyl-β-cyclodextrin (HP-β-CD), the solubilizing excipient used in SPORANOX® Oral Solution, was found to produce pancreatic exocrine hyperplasia and neoplasia when administered orally to rats at doses of 500, 2000 or 5000 mg/kg/day for 25 months. Adenocarcinomas of the exocrine pancreas produced in the treated animals were not seen in the untreated group and are not reported in the historical controls. Development of these tumors may be related to a mitogenic action of cholecystokinin. This finding was not observed in the mouse carcinogenicity study at doses of 500, 2000 or 5000 mg/kg/day for 22–23 months; however, the clinical relevance of these findings is unknown. Based on body surface area comparisons, the exposure to humans of HP-β-CD at the recommended clinical dose of SPORANOX® Oral Solution, is approximately equivalent to 1.7 times the exposure at the lowest dose in the rat study.

Itraconazole produced no mutagenic effects when assayed in a DNA repair test (unscheduled DNA synthesis) in primary rat hepatocytes, in Ames tests with *Salmonella typhimurium* (6 strains) and *Escherichia coli*, in the mouse lymphoma gene mutation tests, in a sex-linked recessive lethal mutation (*Drosophila melanogaster*) test, in chromosome aberration tests in human lymphocytes, in a cell transformation test with C3H/10T$^1/_2$ C18 mouse embryo fibroblasts cells, in a dominant lethal mutation test in male and female mice, and in micronucleus tests in mice and rats.

Itraconazole did not affect the fertility of male or female rats treated orally with dosage levels of up to 40 mg/kg/day (5× MRHD), even though parental toxicity was present at this dosage level. More severe signs of parental toxicity, including death, were present in the next higher dosage level, 160 mg/kg/day (20× MRHD).

Pregnancy: Teratogenic Effects. Pregnancy Category C: Itraconazole was found to cause a dose-related increase in maternal toxicity, embryotoxicity, and teratogenicity in rats at dosage levels of approximately 40–160 mg/kg/day (5–20× MRHD), and in mice at dosage levels of approximately 80 mg/kg/day (10× MRHD). In rats, the teratogenicity consisted of major skeletal defects; in mice, it consisted of encephaloceles and/or macroglossia.

There are no studies in pregnant women. SPORANOX® should be used in pregnancy only if the benefit outweighs the potential risk.

Nursing Mothers: Itraconazole is excreted in human milk; therefore, the expected benefits of SPORANOX® therapy for the mother should be weighed against the potential risk from exposure of itraconazole to the infant. The U.S. Public Health Service Centers for Disease Control and Prevention advises HIV-infected women not to breast-feed to avoid potential transmission of HIV to uninfected infants.

Pediatric Use: The efficacy and safety of SPORANOX® have not been established in pediatric patients. A pharmacokinetic study was conducted with SPORANOX® Oral Solution in 26 pediatric patients, ages 6 months to 12 years, requiring systemic antifungal treatment. Itraconazole was dosed at 5 mg/kg once daily for two weeks and no serious unexpected adverse events were reported. (See CLINICAL PHARMACOLOGY.)

The long-term effects of itraconazole on bone growth in children are unknown. In three toxicology studies using rats, itraconazole induced bone defects at dosage levels as low as 20 mg/kg/day (2.5× MRHD). The induced defects included reduced bone plate activity, thinning of the zona compacta of the large bones, and increased bone fragility. At a dosage level of 80 mg/kg/day (10× MRHD) over 1 year or 160 mg/kg/day (20× MRHD) for 6 months, itraconazole induced small tooth pulp with hypocellular appearance in some rats. No such bone toxicity has been reported in adult patients.

ADVERSE REACTIONS

Rare cases of reversible idiosyncratic hepatitis have been reported among patients taking SPORANOX® (itraconazole) Capsules. SPORANOX® has been associated with rare cases of serious hepatotoxicity, including fatalities, primarily in patients with serious underlying medical conditions who are taking multiple medications. The causal association with SPORANOX® is uncertain. If clinical signs and symptoms consistent with liver disease develop and could be attributed to itraconazole, SPORANOX® should be discontinued. (See WARNINGS.)

U.S. adverse experience data are derived from 350 immunocompromised patients (332 HIV seropositive/AIDS) treated for oropharyngeal or esophageal candidiasis. The table below lists adverse events reported by at least 2% of patients treated with SPORANOX® Oral Solution in U.S. clinical trials. Data on patients receiving comparator agents in these trials are included for comparison.

[See table above]

Body System/Adverse Event	Itraconazole		Fluconazole	Clotrimazole
	Total n=350*	All controlled studies n=272	n=125**	n=81***
Gastrointestinal disorders				
Nausea	11.1%	10.3%	11.2%	4.9%
Diarrhea	10.9%	10.3%	10.4%	3.7%
Vomiting	7.1%	5.5%	8.0%	1.2%
Abdominal Pain	5.7%	4.0%	7.2%	7.4%
Constipation	2.0%	2.2%	0.8%	0%
Body as a whole				
Fever	6.6%	6.3%	8.0%	4.9%
Chest pain	2.6%	2.9%	2.4%	0%
Pain	2.3%	1.8%	4.0%	0%
Fatigue	2.0%	1.1%	1.6%	0%
Respiratory disorders				
Coughing	4.0%	4.4%	9.6%	0%
Dyspnea	2.3%	2.6%	4.8%	1.2%
Pneumonia	2.0%	1.5%	0%	0%
Sinusitis	2.0%	1.8%	4.0%	0%
Sputum increased	2.0%	2.6%	3.2%	1.2%
Skin and appendages disorders				
Rash	4.0%	4.8%	4.0%	6.2%
Increased sweating	3.4%	3.7%	6.4%	1.2%
Skin disorder, unspecified	2.3%	2.2%	2.4%	1.2%
Central/peripheral nervous system				
Headache	4.3%	4.4%	5.6%	6.2%
Dizziness	2.0%	1.5%	4.0%	1.2%
Resistance mechanism disorders				
Pneumocystis carinii infection	2.3%	1.5%	1.6%	0%
Psychiatric disorders				
Depression	2.0%	1.1%	0%	1.2%

* Of the 350 patients, 209 were treated for oropharyngeal candidiasis in controlled studies, 63 were treated for esophageal candidiasis in controlled studies and 78 were treated for oropharyngeal candidiasis in an open study.
** Of the 125 patients, 62 were treated for oropharyngeal candidiasis and 63 were treated for esophageal candidiasis.
*** All 81 patients were treated for oropharyngeal candidiasis.

Adverse events reported by less than 2% of patients in U.S. clinical trials with SPORANOX® included: adrenal insufficiency, asthenia, back pain, dehydration, dyspepsia, dysphagia, flatulence, gynecomastia, hematuria, hemorrhoids, hot flushes, implantation complication, infection unspecified, injury, insomnia, male breast pain, myalgia, pharyngitis, pruritus, rhinitis, rigors, stomatitis ulcerative, taste perversion, tinnitus, upper respiratory tract infection, vision abnormal, and weight decrease. Edema, hypokalemia and menstrual disorders have been reported in clinical trials with itraconazole capsules.

Post-marketing Experience

In worldwide post-marketing experience with SPORANOX® Capsules, allergic reactions, including rash, pruritus, urticaria, angioedema, and, in rare instances, anaphylaxis and Stevens-Johnson syndrome, have been reported. Post-marketing experiences have also included reports of elevated liver enzymes and rarely, hepatitis. Although the causal association with SPORANOX® is uncertain, rare cases of alopecia, hypertriglyceridemia, menstrual disorders, neutropenia, and isolated cases of neuropathy have also been reported.

OVERDOSAGE

Itraconazole is not removed by dialysis. In the event of accidental overdosage, supportive measures, including gastric lavage with sodium bicarbonate, should be employed.

There are limited data on the outcomes of patients ingesting high doses of itraconazole. In patients taking either 1000

Continued on next page

Sporanox Oral—Cont.

mg of SPORANOX® (itraconazole) Oral Solution or up to 3000 mg of SPORANOX® Capsules, the adverse event profile was similar to that observed at recommended doses.

DOSAGE AND ADMINISTRATION

The solution should be vigorously swished in the mouth (10 mL at a time) for several seconds and swallowed.

The recommended dosage of SPORANOX® (itraconazole) Oral Solution for oropharyngeal candidiasis is 200 mg (20 mL) daily for 1 to 2 weeks. Clinical signs and symptoms of oropharyngeal candidiasis generally resolve within several days.

For patients with oropharyngeal candidiasis unresponsive/refractory to treatment with fluconazole tablets, the recommended dose is 100 mg (10 mL) b.i.d. For patients responding to therapy, clinical response will be seen in 2 to 4 weeks. Patients may be expected to relapse shortly after discontinuing therapy. Limited data on the safety of long-term use (>6 months) of SPORANOX® Oral Solution are available at this time.

The recommended dosage of SPORANOX® Oral Solution for esophageal candidiasis is 100 mg (10 mL) daily for a minimum treatment of three weeks. Treatment should continue for 2 weeks following resolution of symptoms. Doses up to 200 mg (20 mL) per day may be used based on medical judgement of the patient's response to therapy.

SPORANOX® Oral Solution and SPORANOX® Capsules should not be used interchangeably. Patients should be instructed to take SPORANOX® Oral Solution without food, if possible. Only SPORANOX® Oral Solution has been demonstrated effective for oral and/or esophageal candidiasis.

HOW SUPPLIED

SPORANOX® (itraconazole) Oral Solution is available in 150 mL amber glass bottles (NDC 50458-295-15) containing 10 mg of itraconazole per mL.

Store at or below 25°C (77°F). Do not freeze.

631-10-939-2

U.S. Patent Nos. 4,267,179; 4,791,111; 5,707,975; 4,727,064

February 1997, February 2000

Manufactured by:
Janssen Pharmaceutica N.V.
Beerse, Belgium
Distributed by:
Ortho Biotech Inc.
Raritan, NJ 08869

VERMOX (mebendazole) CHEWABLE TABLETS

Please see full prescribing information for Vermox Chewable Tablets under McNeil Consumer.

Johnson & Johnson • MERCK

Consumer Pharmaceuticals Co.
CAMP HILL ROAD
FORT WASHINGTON, PA 19034

Direct Inquiries to:
Consumer Affairs Department
Fort Washington, PA 19034
1-800-469-5268
For Medical Information Contact:
In Emergencies:
1-800-469-5268

CHILDREN'S MYLANTA® UPSET STOMACH RELIEF OTC
CALCIUM CARBONATE/ANTACID
LIQUID AND TABLETS

DESCRIPTION

Children's Mylanta is a specially formulated antacid to quickly and effectively relieve the upset stomach kids sometime experience.

ACTIVE INGREDIENTS

Each tablet or 5 ml teaspoonful contains 400 mg of calcium carbonate.

INACTIVE INGREDIENTS

Tablets: Citric acid, confectioner's sugar, D&C Red #27, flavors, magnesium stearate, sorbitol, starch.

Liquid: Butylparaben, cellulose, flavor propylparaben, purified water, D&C Red #22, D&C Red #28, simethicone, sodium saccharin, sorbitol, xanthan gum, may contain tartaric acid.

Acid Neutralizing Capacity:

Tablet	Liquid
8 mEq	8 mEq

INDICATIONS

For the relief of acid indigestion, sour stomach, or heartburn and upset stomach associated with these conditions, or overindulgence in food and drink.

DIRECTIONS

Find the right dose on the chart below. If possible use weight as your dosing guide; otherwise use age. Repeat dosing as needed. DO NOT USE MORE THAN THREE TIMES PER DAY.

WEIGHT (LB)	AGE (YR)	TABLET	LIQUID (TSP)
Under 24	Under 2	Consult Physician	
24–47	2–5	1	1
48–95	6–11	2	2

WARNINGS

Keep this and all drugs out of the reach of children. Do not take more than 3 tablets or 3 teaspoonfuls (2–5 years) or 6 tablets or 6 teaspoonfuls (6–11 years) in a 24-hour period, or use the maximum dosage of this product for more than two weeks, except under the advice and supervision of a physician.

DRUG INTERACTION PRECAUTION

Antacids may interact with certain prescription drugs. If your child is presently taking a prescription drug, do not give this product without checking with your physician or other health professional.

HOW SUPPLIED

Children's Mylanta Upset Stomach Relief is supplied as a liquid and chewable tablets in bubble gum flavor.

NDC 16837-810 Bubble Gum tablets
NDC 16837-820 Bubble Gum liquid

Shown in Product Identification Guide, page 318

INFANTS' MYLICON® Drops OTC
[*my 'li-con*]
Antiflatulent

INGREDIENTS

Each 0.6 mL of drops contains: Active: simethicone, 40 mg. Inactive: carboxymethylcellulose sodium, citric acid, manitol microcrystalline cellulose, natural flavor, purified water, Red 22, Red 28, sodium benzoate, sodium citrate, xanthan gum, non-staining formula contains no Red 22 or Red 20.

INDICATIONS

For relief of the symptoms of excess gas in the digestive tract. Such gas is frequently caused by excessive swallowing of air or by eating foods that disagree. The defoaming action of INFANTS' MYLICON® Drops relieves flatulence by dispersing and preventing the formation of mucus-surrounded gas pockets in the gastrointestinal tract. INFANTS' MYLICON® Drops act in the stomach and intestines to change the surface tension of gas bubbles enabling them to coalesce, thereby freeing and eliminating the gas more easily by belching or passing flatus.

DIRECTIONS

Infants (under 2 years): 0.3 ml four times daily after meals and at bedtime, or as directed by a physician. The dosage can also be mixed with 1 oz of cool water, infant formula or other suitable liquids to ease administration.

Adults and children: 0.6 ml four times daily, after meals and at bedtime, or as directed by a physician.

WARNINGS

Do not exceed 12 doses per day except under the advice and supervision of a physician. Keep this and all drugs out of the reach of children.

HOW SUPPLIED

INFANTS' MYLICON® Drops are available in bottles of 15 ml (0.5 fl oz) and 30 ml (1.0 fl oz) original pink, pleasant tasting liquid and non-staining formula. NDC 16837-630; 16837-911.

Shown in Product Identification Guide, page 318

FAST-ACTING MYLANTA® AND EXTRA STRENGTH FAST-ACTING MYLANTA® OTC
[*my-lan'ta*]
Aluminum, Magnesium and Simethicone
Liquid
Antacid/Anti-Gas

DESCRIPTION

Fast-acting MYLANTA® and Extra Strength Fast-Acting MYLANTA® are well-balanced, pleasant-tasting, antacid/anti-gas medications that provide consistent, effective relief of symptoms associated with gastric hyperacidity and excess gas. Non-constipating and very low sodium Fast-Acting MYLANTA® and Extra Strength Fast-Acting MYLANTA® contain two proven antacids, aluminum hydroxide and magnesium hydroxide, plus simethicone for gas relief.

ACTIVE INGREDIENTS

Each 5 mL teaspoon contains:

	MYLANTA®	MYLANTA® Extra Strength
Aluminum Hydroxide	200 mg	400 mg
Magnesium Hydroxide	200 mg	400 mg
Simethicone	20 mg	40 mg

INACTIVE INGREDIENTS

LIQUIDS:
Butylparaben, carboxymethylcellulose sodium, flavors, hydroxypropyl methylcellulose, microcrystalline cellulose, propylparaben, purified water, saccharin sodium, and sorbitol.

SODIUM CONTENT

Each 5 mL teaspoon contains the following amount of sodium:

	MYLANTA®	MYLANTA® Extra Strength
Liquid	0.6 mg (0.05 mEq)	0.9 mg (0.05 mEq)

ACID NEUTRALIZING CAPACITY

Two teaspoonfuls have the following acid neutralizing capacity:

	Fast Acting MYLANTA®	Extra Strength Fast Acting MYLANTA®
Liquid	25.4 mEq	50.8 mEq

INDICATIONS

Fast-Acting MYLANTA® and Extra Strength Fast-Acting MYLANTA® are indicated for the relief of acid indigestion, heartburn, sour stomach, and symptoms of gas and upset stomach associated with those conditions. Fast-Acting MYLANTA® and Extra Strength Fast-Acting MYLANTA® are also indicated as antacids for the symptomatic relief of hyperacidity associated with the diagnosis of peptic ulcer, gastritis, peptic esophagitis, heartburn and hiatal hernia and as antiflatulents to alleviate the symptoms of mucus-entrapped gas, including postoperative gas pain.

ADVANTAGES

Fast-Acting MYLANTA and Extra Strength Fast-Acting MYLANTA are homogenized for a smooth, creamy taste. The choice of three pleasant-tasting liquid flavors and the non-constipating formula encourage patient acceptance, thereby minimizing the skipping of prescribed doses. Fast-Acting MYLANTA and Extra Strength Fast-Acting MYLANTA are also available in tablets, and both the liquid and tablet forms are very low in sodium. Fast-Acting MYLANTA and Extra Strength Fast-Acting MYLANTA provide consistent relief in patients suffering from distress associated with hyperacidity, mucus-entrapped gas, or swallowed air.

DIRECTIONS

Liquid:
Shake well. 2-4 teaspoonfuls between meals and at bedtime, or as directed by a physician.

WARNINGS

Keep this and all drugs out of the reach of children. Do not take more than 24 tsps of Fast-Acting MYLANTA® or 12 tsps of Extra Strength Fast-Acting MYLANTA® in a 24-hour period or use the maximum dose of this product for more than two weeks, except under the advice and supervision of a physician. Do not use this product if you have kidney disease.

Prolonged use of aluminum-containing antacids in patients with renal failure may result in or worsen dialysis osteomalacia. Elevated tissue aluminum levels contribute to the development of the dialysis encephalopathy and osteomalacia syndromes. Small amounts of aluminum are absorbed from the gastrointestinal tract and renal excretion of aluminum is impaired in renal failure. Aluminum is not well removed by dialysis because it is bound to albumin and transferrin, which do not cross dialysis membranes. As a result, aluminum is deposited in bone, and dialysis osteomalacia may develop when large amounts of aluminum are ingested orally by patients with impaired renal function.

Aluminum forms insoluble complexes with phosphate in the gastrointestinal tract, thus decreasing phosphate absorption. Prolonged use of aluminum-containing antacids by normophosphatemic patients may result in hypophosphatemia if phosphate intake is not adequate. In its more severe forms, hypophosphatemia can lead to anorexia, malaise, muscle weakness, and osteomalacia.

DRUG INTERACTION PRECAUTION

Antacids may interact with certain prescription drugs. If you are presently taking a prescription drug, do not take this product without checking with your physician or other health professional.

HOW SUPPLIED

Fast-Acting MYLANTA® and Extra Strength Fast-Acting MYLANTA® are available as white liquid suspensions in pleasant-tasting flavors, Original, Cherry Creme and Cool Mint Creme. Liquids are supplied in bottles of 5 oz, 12 oz, and 24 oz. Also available for hospital use in liquid unit dose bottles of 1 oz and bottles of 5 oz.

MYLANTA®
NDC 16837-610 ORIGINAL LIQUID
NDC 16837-629 COOL MINT CREME LIQUID
NDC 16837-621 CHERRY CREME LIQUID
NDC 16837-817 Lemon Twist Liquid

MYLANTA® Extra Strength
NDC 16837-652 ORIGINAL LIQUID
NDC 16837-624 COOL MINT CREME LIQUID
NDC 16837-622 CHERRY CREME LIQUID
NDC 16837-818 Lemon Twist Liquid

Professional Labeling

INDICATIONS

Stress-induced upper gastrointestinal hemorrhage: Extra Strength Fast-Acting MYLANTA® is indicated for the prevention of stress-induced upper gastrointestinal hemorrhage. Hyperacidic conditions: As an antacid, for the symptomatic relief of hyperacidity associated with the diagnosis of peptic ulcer and other gastrointestinal conditions where a high degree of acid neutralization is desired.

DIRECTIONS

Prevention of stress-induced upper gastrointestinal hemorrhage: 1) Aspirate stomach via nasogastric tube* and record pH. 2) Instill 10 mL of Extra Strength Fast-Acting MYLANTA® followed by 30 mL of water via nasogastric tube. Clamp tube. 3) Wait one hour. Aspirate stomach and record pH. 4a) If pH equals or exceeds 4.0, apply drainage or intermittent suction for one hour, then repeat the cycle. 4b) If pH is less than 4.0, instill double (20 mL) Extra Strength Fast-Acting MYLANTA® followed by 30 mL of water. Clamp tube. 5) Wait one hour. If pH equals or exceeds 4.0, see number 7, if pH is still less than 4.0, instill double (40 mL) Extra Strength Fast-Acting MYLANTA® followed by 30 mL of water. Clamp tube. 6) Wait one hour. If pH equals or exceeds 4.0, see number 7. If pH is still less than 4.0, instill double (80 mL)† Extra Strength Fast-Acting MYLANTA® followed by 30 mL of water. 7) Drain for one hour and repeat cycle with the effective dosage of Extra Strength Fast-Acting MYLANTA®.

*If nasogastric tube is not in place, administer 20 mL of Extra Strength Fast-Acting MYLANTA® orally q2h.

† In a recent clinical study[1] 20 mL of Extra Strength Fast-Acting MYLANTA®, q2h, was sufficient in more than 85 percent of the patients. No patient studied required more than 80 mL of Extra Strength Fast-Acting MYLANTA® q2h.

In hyperacid states for symptomatic relief: One or two teaspoonfuls as needed between meals and at bedtime or as directed by a physician. Higher dosage regimens may be employed under the direct supervision of a physician in the treatment of active peptic ulcer disease.

PRECAUTIONS

Aluminum-magnesium hydroxide containing antacids should be used with caution in patients with renal impairment.

ADVERSE EFFECTS

Occasional regurgitation and mild diarrhea have been reported with the dosage recommended for the prevention of stress-induced upper gastrointestinal hemorrhage.

References: 1. Zinner MJ, Zuidema GD, Smigh PL, Mignosa M: The prevention of upper gastrointestinal tract bleeding in patients in an intensive care unit. *Surg Gynecol Obster* 153:214–220, 1981. 2. Lucas CE, Sugawa C, Riddle J, et al.: Natural history and surgical dilemma of "stress" gastric bleeding. *Arch Surg* 102:266–273, 1971. 3. Hastings PR, Skillman JJ, Bushnell LS, Silen W: Antacid titration in the prevention of acute gastrointestinal bleeding: a controlled, randomized trial in 100 critically ill patients. *N Engl J Med* 298:1042–1045, 1978. 4. Day SB, MacMillan BG, Altemeier WA: *Curling's Ulcer, An Experience of Nature.* Springfield, IL, Charles C Thomas Co., 1972, p. 205. 5. Skillman JJ, Bushnell LS, Goldman H, Silen W: Respiratory failure, hypotension, sepsis, and jaundice. A clinical syndrome associated with lethal hemorrhage from acute stress ulceration of the stomach. *Am J Surg* 117:523–530, 1969. 6. Priebe HJ, Skillman J, Bushnell LS, et al. Antacid versus cimetidine in preventing acute gastrointestinal bleeding. *N Engl J Med* 302:426–430, 1980. 7. Silen W: The prevention and management of stress ulcers. *Hosp Pract* 15:93–97, 1980. 8. Hermann V, Kaminski DL: Evaluation of intragastric pH in acutely ill patients. *Arch Surg* 114:511–514, 1979. 9. Martin LF, Staloch DK, Simonowitz DA, et al.: Failure of cimetidine prophylaxis in the critically ill. *Arch Surg* 114:492–496, 1979. 10. Zinner MJ, Turtinen L, Gurll NJ, Reynolds DG: The effect of metiamide on gastric mucosal injury in rat restraint. *Clin Res* 23:484A, 1975. 11. Zinner M, Turtinen BA, Gurll NJ: The role of acid and ischemia in production of stress ulcers during canine hemorrhagic shock. *Surgery* 77: 807–816, 1975. 12. Winans CS: Prevention and treatment of stress ulcer bleeding: Antacids or cimetidine? *Drug Ther Bull* (hospital) 12:37–45, 1981.

Shown in Product Identification Guide, page 318

FAST-ACTING MYLANTA ULTRA TABS AND FAST-ACTING MYLANTA ANTACID GELCAPS OTC

[*mylan 'ta*]

Calcium Carbonate and Magnesium Hydroxide Tablets/ Gelcaps Antacid

DESCRIPTION

Fast-Acting Mylanta Ultra Tabs and Fast-Acting Mylanta Antacid Gelcaps are well balanced, pleasant tasting antacid medications that provide consistent, effective relief of symptoms associated with gastric hyperacidity. Non-constipating and very low in sodium, Fast-Acting Mylanta Ultra Tabs and Fast-Acting Mylanta Antacid Gelcaps contain two proven antacids, calcium carbonate and magnesium hydroxide.

Active Ingredients

Each tablet/gelcap contains:

	Fast-Acting Mylanta Antacid Gelcaps	Fast-Acting Mylanta Ultra Tabs
Calcium Carbonate	500mg	700mg
Magnesium Hydroxide	125mg	300mg

Inactive Ingredients

Fast-Acting Mylanta Antacid Gelcaps: Benzyl alcohol, butylparaben, castor oil, crospovidone, D&C Red #28, D&C Yellow #10, disodium calcium edetate, FD&C Blue #1, FD&C Red #40, gelatin, hydroxypropyl methylcellulose, magnesium stearate, methylparaben microcrystalline cellulose, propylparaben, sodium lauryl sulfate, sodium propionate, starch, titanium dioxide. May also contain propylene glycol.

Fast-Acting Mylanta Ultra Tabs: Citric acid, confectioner's sugar, D&C Red #27, flavors, magnesium stearate, sodium lauryl sulfate, sorbitol, starch.

Sodium Content

Each tablet/gelcap contains the following amount of sodium:

Fast-Acting Mylanta Ultra Tabs	Fast-Acting Mylanta Antacid Gelcaps
0.6mg	.1087mEq

Acid Neutralizing Capacity

Two tablets/gelcaps have the following acid neutralizing capacity:

Fast-Acting Mylanta Ultra Tabs	Fast-Acting Mylanta Antacid Gelcaps
24.0mEq	23.0mEq

INDICATIONS

Fast-Acting Mylanta Ultra Tabs and Fast-Acting Mylanta Antacid Gelcaps are indicated for the relief of heartburn, acid indigestion, sour stomach and upset stomach associated with these conditions. Fast-Acting Mylanta Ultra Tabs and Fast-Acting Mylanta Antacid Gelcaps are also indicated as antacids for the symptomatic relief of hyperacidity associated with the diagnosis of peptic ulcer, gastritis, peptic esophagitis, heartburn and hiatal hernia.

DIRECTIONS

Thoroughly chew 2–4 tablets between meals, at bedtime or as directed by a physician.
Swallow 2–4 gelcaps as needed or directed by physician.

WARNINGS

Keep this and all drugs out of the reach of children. Do not take more than 10 Tablets of Fast-Acting Mylanta Ultra Tabs or 12 Gelcaps of Fast-Acting Mylanta Antacid Gelcaps in a 24-hour period, or use the maximum dosage for more than two weeks. Do not use this product if you have kidney disease, except under the advise and supervision of a physician.

DRUG INTERACTION PRECAUTION

Antacids may interact with certain prescription drugs. If you are presently taking a prescription drug, do not take this product without checking with your physician or other health professional.

HOW SUPPLIED

Fast-Acting Mylanta Antacid Gelcaps:
NDC: 16837-850-24 24 Gelcaps
NDC: 16837-850-50 50 Gelcaps
NDC: 16837-850-10 100 Gelcaps

Fast-Acting Mylanta Ultra Tabs:
NDC: 16837-849-36 3 Roll Mint Pack
NDC: 16837-849-35 35 Mint Tablets
NDC: 16837-849-70 70 Mint Tablets
NDC: 16837-869-35 35 Cherry Tablets
NDC: 16837-869-70 70 Cherry Tablets

FAST ACTING MYLANTA SUPREME ANTACID LIQUID OTC

DESCRIPTION

Fast acting Mylanta Supreme is a revolutionary liquid antacid that works fast and tastes great. It has a fresh smooth taste and texture that goes down easy and doesn't leave that chalky aftertaste. Plus, Mylanta Supreme is rich in calcium.

Active Ingredients: Each 5 ml teaspoon contains:
Calcium carbonate 400 mg
Magnesium hydroxide 135 mg

Inactive Ingredients: Flavors, hydroxyethyl cellulose, purified water, simethicone, sodium saccharin, sorbitol, xanthan gum, may also contain D&C Yellow #10 and FD&C Blue #1.

Sodium Content: Each 5 ml teaspoon contains 0.7 mg of sodium.

ACID NEUTRALIZING CAPACITY: Two teaspoonfuls provide 25.2 MEq of acid neutralizing capacity.

INDICATIONS

Mylanta Supreme is indicated for the relief of heartburn, acid indigestion, sour stomach, upset stomach associated with these conditions and overindulgence in food and drink.

DIRECTIONS

Shake Well. Take 2–4 teaspoonfuls between meals, at bedtime, or as directed by a physician.

WARNINGS

Keep this and all drugs out of the reach of children. Do not take more than 20 teaspoonfuls in a 24-hour period, or use the maximum dosage for more than two weeks, or use this product if you have kidney disease except under the advice and supervision of a physician.

DRUG INTERACTION PRECAUTION

Antacids may interact with certain prescription drugs. If you are presently taking a prescription drug, do not take this product without checking with your physician or other health professional.

HOW SUPPLIED

Fast Acting Mylanta Supreme is available as white liquid suspensions in cherry, and mint flavors.
NDC 16837-825 Cherry
NDC 16837-819 Mint

Shown in Product Identification Guide, page 318

MYLANTA® GAS Relief Tablets OTC
Maximum Strength MYLANTA® GAS Relief Tablets

[*My-lan '-ta*]

Maximum Strength MYLANTA® GAS Softgels

ACTIVE INGREDIENTS

Each tablet contains:

	Simethicone
MYLANTA® GAS Relief	80 mg
Maximum Strength MYLANTA® GAS Relief	125 mg
Maximum Strength MYLANTA® GAS Softgels	125 mg

INACTIVE INGREDIENTS

TABLETS: Dextrates, flavor, sorbitol, stearic acid, tricalcium phosphate. Cherry: Red 7.
SOFTGELS: FD&C blue #1, gelatin, glycerin, iron oxide black, peppermint oil, titanium dioxide.

INDICATIONS

For relief of the symptoms of excess gas in the digestive tract. Such gas is frequently caused by excessive swallowing of air or by eating foods that disagree. MYLANTA® GAS Softgels, MYLANTA® GAS Relief, and Maximum Strength MYLANTA® GAS Relief Tablets are high capacity antiflatulents for adjunctive treatment of many conditions in which the retention of gas may be a problem, such as the following: air swallowing, postoperative gaseous distention, peptic ulcer, spastic or irritable colon, diverticulosis. If condition persists, consult your physician.
MYLANTA® GAS Softgels, MYLANTA® GAS Relief, and Maximum Strength MYLANTA® GAS Relief Tablets have a defoaming action that relieves flatulence by dispersing and preventing the formation of mucus-surrounded gas pockets in the gastrointestinal tract. MYLANTA® GAS Softgels, MYLANTA® GAS Relief, and Maximum Strength MYLANTA® GAS Relief Tablets act in the stomach and intestines to change the surface tension of gas bubbles enabling them to coalesce, thereby freeing and eliminating the gas more easily by belching or passing flatus.

DIRECTIONS

MYLANTA® GAS Relief Tablets
One tablet four times daily after meals and at bedtime. May also be taken as needed up to six tablets daily or as directed by a physician.

Maximum Strength MYLANTA® GAS Relief Tablets
One tablet four times daily after meals and at bedtime or as directed by a physician.

Continued on next page

Mylanta Gas Relief—Cont.

Maximum Strength MYLANTA® GAS Softgels
Take 1–2 softgels as needed after meals and at bedtime. Do not exceed 4 softgels per day unless directed by a physician.

WARNINGS
Keep this and all drugs out of the reach of children.

HOW SUPPLIED
MYLANTA® GAS Relief Tablets are available as white (mint) or pink (cherry) scored, chewable tablets identified "MYL GAS 80." Mint NDC 16837-858. Cherry NDC 16837-859.
Maximum Strength MYLANTA® GAS Relief Tablets are available as white, scored, chewable tablets identified "MYL GAS 125." NDC 16837-455.
Maximum Strength MYLANTA® GAS Softgels are available as blue softgels. NDC 16837-611.
Shown in Product Identification Guide, page 318

MYLANTA NIGHT TIME STRENGTH OTC
Antacid

DESCRIPTION
Provides fast soothing relief of:
- heartburn
- acid indigestion
- sour stomach
- associated symptoms of upset stomach
- overindulgence in food and drink.

ACTIVE INGREDIENTS
Each 5 ml teaspoonful contains 500 mg aluminum hydroxide (equiv. to dried gel, USP) and 500 mg magnesium hydroxide.

INACTIVE INGREDIENTS
butylparaben, flavors, hydroxyethyl cellulose, propylparaben, purified water, simethicone, sodium saccharin, sorbitol.
Sodium Content: Each 5 ml teaspoon contains 1.0 mg of sodium.
Acid Neutralizing Capacity: Two Teaspoonfuls provide 63.8 mEq of acid neutralizing capacity.
DIRECTIONS
Liquid:
- Shake well
- Take 2–4 teaspoonfuls between meals, at bedtime, or as directed by a physician
- Do not take more than 9 teaspoonfuls in a 24-hour period, or use the maximum dosage for more than 2 weeks

Other Information:
This Product does not contain a Sleep Aid
While refrigeration is not necessary to maintain product quality, it can improve the flavor. Do not freeze.

WARNINGS
- **Ask a doctor before use if you have** kidney disease
- **Ask a doctor or pharmacist before use if you are** taking a prescription drug. Antacids may interact with certain prescription drugs.
- **Stop use and ask a doctor if** symptoms last for more than 2 weeks
- **Keep out of reach of children.** In case of overdose, get medical help or contact poison control center right away.

HOW SUPPLIED
Mylanta Night Time Strength is available as white liquid suspension in pleasant tasting flavors. Cherry and Mint supplied in bottles of 12 oz. and 24 oz.
NDC 16837-06212 Cherry 12 oz.
NDC 16837-06112 Mint 12 oz.
NDC 16837-06224 Cherry 24 oz.
Shown in Product Identification Guide, page 318

Ultra MYLANTA CALCI TABS OTC
Antacid/Calcium Supplement
Extra Strength MYLANTA CALCI TABS OTC
Antacid/Calcium Supplement

INDICATIONS
For fast relief of acid indigestion, heartburn, sour stomach and upset stomach associated with these symptoms. Can also be used as a daily source of extra calcium.

ACTIVE INGREDIENT
Ultra Mylanta Calci Tabs - Calcium Carbonate USP, 1,000 mg per tablet
Extra Strength Calci Tabs - Calcium Carbonate USP, 750 mg per tablet

ACTIONS
Mylanta Calci Tabs provide rapid neutralization of stomach acid. Each Ultra Mylanta Calci Tab tablet has an acid-neutralizing capacity (ANC) of 20 mEq and each Extra Strength Mylanta Calci Tab tablet has an ANC of 15 mEq per tablet.

WARNINGS
Ultra Mylanta Calci Tabs - Do not take more than 8 tablets in a 24-hour period or use the maximum dosage of this product for more than two weeks except under the advice and supervision of a physician. Keep this and all drugs out of the reach of children.

Serving Size	Ultra Mylanta Calci Tabs 2 Tablets		Extra Strength Mylanta Calci Tabs 2 Tablets	
Amount Per Serving		***% Daily Value***		***% Daily Value***
Calories	10		10	
Total Carbohydrates	2 g	less than 1%	2 g	less than 1%
Sugars	2 g		2 g	
Calcium	800 mg	80%	600	60%

Extra Strength Calci Tabs - Do not take more than 10 tablets in a 24-hour period or use the maximum dosage of this product for more than two weeks except under the advice and supervision of a physician. Keep this and all drugs out of the reach of children.

DRUG INTERACTION PRECAUTION
Antacids may interact with certain prescription drugs. If you are presently taking a prescription drug, do not take this product without checking with your physician or health professional.

INACTIVE INGREDIENTS
Ultra Mylanta Calci Tabs: Fruit Medley and Cool Mint: dextrose, maltodextrin, magnesium stearate, starch, cellulose, citric and fumaric acids, natural and artificial flavors, mineral oil, sucroseethylmaltol, crospovidone, hydroxypropyl methylcellulose and stearic acid and may contain (FD&C yellow #6, FD&C yellow #5, (tartrazine), FD&C blue #1, D&C red #27).
Extra Strength Calci Tabs: Fruit Medley and Cool Mint: dextrose, maltodextrin, microcrystalline cellulose, magnesium stearate, starch, cellulose, citric and fumaric acids, natural and artificial flavors, mineral oil, sucrose, ethylmaltol, crospovidone, hydroxypropyl methylcellulose and stearic acid and may contain (FD&C yellow #6, FD&C yellow #5, (tartrazine), FD&C blue #1, D&C red #27).

DIRECTIONS FOR ANTACID USE:
Ultra Mylanta Calci Tabs – Chew 2–3 tablets as symptoms occur. Repeat hourly if symptoms return or as directed by a physician.
Extra Strength Mylanta Calci Tabs – Chew 2–4 talbets as symptoms occur. Repeat hourly if symptoms return or as directed by a physician.

USE AS A DIETARY SUPPLEMENT:
IMPORTANT INFORMATION ON OSTEOPOROSIS:
Research shows that certain ethnic, age and other groups are at a higher risk for developing osteoporosis, including Caucasian and Asian teen and young adult women, menopausal women, older persons and those persons with a family history of fragile bones. **A balanced diet with enough calcium and regular exercise will help you to build and maintain healthy bones and may reduce your risk of developing osteoporosis later in life.** Adequate calcium is important, but daily intakes above 2,000 mg are not likely to provide any additional benefit.

Directions For Calcium Supplement Use:
Ultra Mylanta Calci Tabs – Chew 2 tablets twice daily. Average daily calcium intake should not exceed 6 tablets. ***Other Information:*** The 1,000 mg of calcium carbonate in each tablet provide 400 mg of elemental calcium.
Extra Strength Mylanta Calci Tabs – Chew 2 tablets twice daily. Average daily calcium intake should not exceed 8 tablets. ***Other Information:*** The 750 mg of calcium carbonate in each tablet provide 300 mg of elemental calcium.
SUPPLEMENT FACTS
[See table above]

HOW SUPPLIED
Ultra and Extra Strength Mylanta Calci Tab are provided in chewable tablets in Fruit Medley and Cool Mint Flavors.
NDC 16837-059-96 96 Chewable Tablets Fruit Medley
NDC 16837-057-96 96 Chewable Tablets Cool Mint
NDC 16837-058-72 72 Chewable Tablets Fruit Medley
NDC 16837-056-72 72 Chewable Tablets Cool Mint
Shown in Product Identification Guide, page 318

PEPCID AC® OTC
TABLETS, CHEWABLE TABLETS AND GELCAPS

DESCRIPTION
ACTIVE INGREDIENT: Famotidine 10 mg per tablet.
INACTIVE INGREDIENTS: TABLETS: Hydroxypropyl cellulose, hydroxypropyl methylcellulose, red iron oxide, magnesium stearate, microcrystalline cellulose, starch, talc, titanium dioxide.
CHEWABLE TABLETS: aspartame, cellulose acetate, flavors, hydroxypropyl cellulose, hydroxypropyl methylcellulose, lactose, magnesium stearate, mannitol, microcrystalline cellulose, red ferric oxide.
GELCAPS: benzyl alcohol, black iron oxide, butylparaben, castor oil, edetate calcium disodium, FD&C red #40, gelatin, hydroxypropyl methylcellulose, magnesium stearate, methylparaben, microcrystalline cellulose, pregelatinized corn starch, propylene glycol, propylparaben, sodium lauryl sulfate, sodium propionate, talc, titanium dioxide.

Product Benefits:
- **1 Tablet, Chewable Tablet or Gelcap** relieves heartburn and acid indigestion.
- Pepcid AC prevents heartburn and acid indigestion brought on by consuming food and beverages.

It contains famotidine, a prescription-proven medicine.
The ingredient in PEPCID AC, famotidine, has been prescribed by doctors for years to treat millions of patients safely and effectively. The active ingredient in PEPCID AC has been taken safely with many frequently prescribed medications.

ACTION
It is normal for the stomach to produce acid, especially after consuming food and beverages. However, acid in the wrong place (the esophagus), or too much acid, can cause burning pain and discomfort that interfere with everyday activities.
- **Heartburn—Caused by acid in the esophagus**

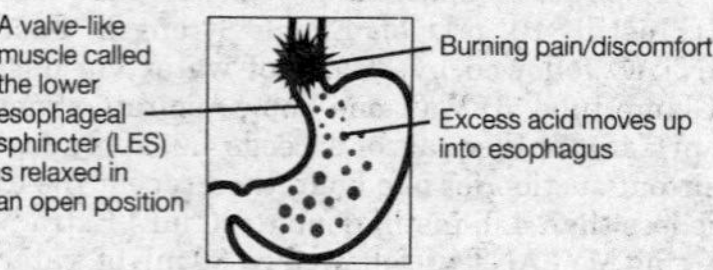

In clinical studies, PEPCID AC was significantly better than placebo pills in relieving and preventing heartburn.

Percent of heartburn episodes completely relieved

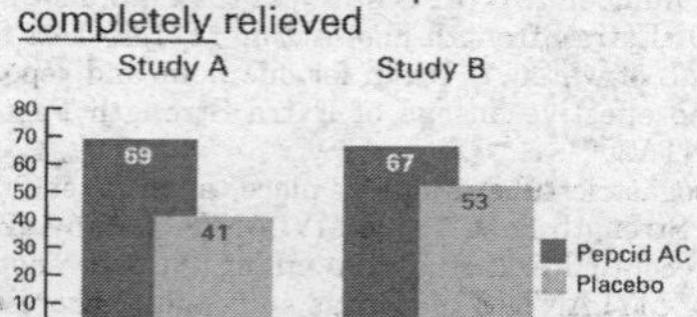

Percent of patients with prevention or reduction of heartburn symptoms

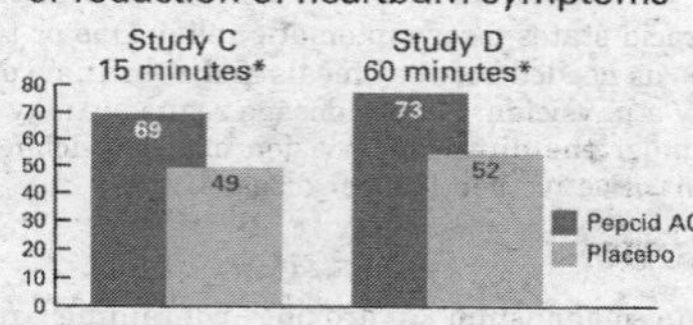

*Time taken before eating a meal that is expected to cause symptoms.

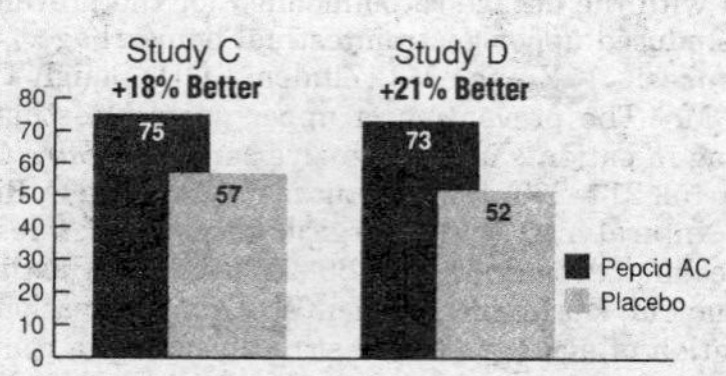

USES
- **For Relief of heartburn, associated with acid indigestion, and sour stomach;**
- **For Prevention of heartburn associated with acid indigestion and sour stomach brought on by consuming food and beverages.**

Tips for Managing Heartburn
- Do not lie flat or bend over soon after eating.
- Do not eat late at night, or just before bedtime.
- Avoid food or drinks that are more likely to cause heartburn, such as rich, spicy, fatty, and fried foods, chocolate, caffeine, alcohol, and even some fruits and vegetables.
- Eat slowly and do not eat big meals.
- If you are overweight, lose weight.
- If you smoke, quit smoking.
- Raise the head of your bed.
- Wear loose fitting clothing around your stomach.

WARNINGS
Allergy Warning: Do not use if you are allergic to Pepcid AC (famotidine) or other acid reducers.
- Do not take the maximum daily dosage for more than 2 weeks continuously except under the advice and supervision of a doctor.

- Do not use with other acid reducers.
- If you have trouble swallowing, or persistent abdominal pain, see your doctor promptly. You may have a serious condition that may need different treatment.
- As with any drug, if you are pregnant or nursing a baby, seek the advice of a health professional before using this product.
- Keep this and all drugs out of the reach of children.
- In case of accidental overdose, seek professional assistance or contact a poison control center immediately.

CAUTION

Heartburn and acid indigestion are common, but you should see your doctor promptly if:

- You have trouble swallowing or persistent abdominal pain. You may have a serious condition that may need different treatment.
- You have used the maximum dosage every day for two weeks continuously.

Important: As with any drug, if you are pregnant or nursing a baby, seek the advice of a health professional before using this product. This product should not be given to children under 12 years old, unless directed by a doctor. Keep this and all drugs out of the reach of children. In case of accidental overdose, seek professional assistance or contact a poison control center immediately.

DIRECTIONS

- Tablet: To relieve symptoms, swallow 1 tablet with a glass of water.
  Chewable Tablet: To relieve symptoms, Do not swallow tablet whole; chew one tablet completely
  Gelcap: To relieve symptoms, swallow one gelcap with a glass of water.
- To prevent symptoms, swallow 1 tablet with a glass of water at any time from 15 to 60 minutes before eating food or drinking beverages that cause heartburn.
- Can be used up to twice daily (up to 2 tablets in 24 hours).
- This product should not be given to children under 12 years old unless directed by a doctor.

HOW SUPPLIED

Pepcid AC Tablet is available as a rose-colored tablet identified as 'PEPCID AC'. NDC 16837-872

Pepcid AC Gelcap is available as a rose and white gelatin coated, capsule shaped tablet identified as 'PEPCID AC'. NDC 16837-856

Pepcid AC Chewable Tablet is available as a rose-colored chewable tablet identified as 'PEPCID AC'. NDC 16837-873

- Read the directions and warnings before use.
- Keep the carton. It contains important information.

Store between 25°–30°C (77–86°F).

Protect from moisture.

Shown in Product Identification Guide, page 318

Jones Pharma Incorporated

1945 CRAIG ROAD
PO BOX 46903
ST LOUIS, MO 63146

Direct Inquiries to:
Customer Service:
314-576-6100
Fax:
314-469-5749

BREVITAL® SODIUM Ⓒ℞
METHOHEXITAL SODIUM
FOR INJECTION, USP
For Intravenous Use

CYTOMEL® ℞
[*sigh "toe 'mel*]
brand of liothyronine sodium tablets

LEVOXYL® ℞
(Levothyroxine Sodium Tablets, USP)
FOR ORAL ADMINISTRATION
Shown in Product Identification Guide, page 318

TAPAZOLE® ℞
METHIMAZOLE TABLETS, USP

THROMBIN, TOPICAL U.S.P. (BOVINE ORIGIN)

THROMBIN-JMI™ ℞

TRIOSTAT™ ℞
[*try 'o-stat*]
brand of liothyronine sodium injection
(T_3)

Key Pharmaceuticals, Inc.

GALLOPING HILL ROAD
KENILWORTH, NJ 07033

For Medical Information Contact:
Generally:
Drug Information Services
(800) 526-4099
(9:00 AM to 5:00 PM EST)

After Hours and Weekends:
(908) 298-4000

Product Identification Codes

To provide quick and positive identification of Key Products, we have imprinted the product identification number of the National Drug Code on most tablets and capsules. In some cases, identification letters also appear.

Additionally: the following telephone numbers are provided for inquiries:

Drug Information Services
9:00 AM to 5:00 PM EST
1-800-526-4099

After regular hours and on weekends (908) 298-4000

IMDUR® ℞
(isosorbide mononitrate)
Extended Release Tablets
PRODUCT INFORMATION

DESCRIPTION

Isosorbide mononitrate (ISMN), an organic nitrate and the major biologically active metabolite of isosorbide dinitrate (ISDN), is a vasodilator with effects on both arteries and veins.

IMDUR® Tablets contain 30 mg, 60 mg, or 120 mg of isosorbide mononitrate in an extended-release formulation. The inactive ingredients are aluminum silicate, colloidal silicon dioxide, hydroxypropyl cellulose, hydroxypropyl methylcellulose, iron oxide, magnesium stearate, paraffin wax, polyethylene glycol, titanium dioxide, and trace amounts of ethanol.

The chemical name for ISMN is 1,4:3,6-dianhydro-, D-glucitol 5-nitrate; the compound has the following structural formula:

OH H … H ONO_2

ISMN is a white, crystalline, odorless compound which is stable in air and in solution, has a melting point of about 90°C, and an optical rotation of +144° (2% in water, 20°C). Isosorbide mononitrate is freely soluble in water, ethanol, methanol, chloroform, ethyl acetate, and dichloromethane.

CLINICAL PHARMACOLOGY

Mechanism of Action: The IMDUR product is an oral extended-release formulation of ISMN, the major active metabolite of isosorbide dinitrate; most of the clinical activity of the dinitrate is attributable to the mononitrate.

The principal pharmacological action of ISMN and all organic nitrates in general is relaxation of vascular smooth muscle, producing dilatation of peripheral arteries and veins, especially the latter. Dilatation of the veins promotes peripheral pooling of blood and decreases venous return to the heart, thereby reducing left ventricular end-diastolic pressure and pulmonary capillary wedge pressure (preload). Arteriolar relaxation reduces systemic vascular resistance, and systolic arterial pressure and mean arterial pressure (afterload). Dilatation of the coronary arteries also occurs. The relative importance of preload reduction, afterload reduction, and coronary dilatation remains undefined.

Pharmacodynamics: Dosing regimens for most chronically used drugs are designed to provide plasma concentrations that are continuously greater than a minimally effective concentration. This strategy is inappropriate for organic nitrates. Several well-controlled clinical trials have used exercise testing to assess the antianginal efficacy of continuously delivered nitrates. In the large majority of these trials, active agents were indistinguishable from placebo after 24 hours (or less) of continuous therapy. Attempts to overcome tolerance by dose escalation, even to doses far in excess of those used acutely, have consistently failed. Only after nitrates have been absent from the body for several hours has their antianginal efficacy been restored. IMDUR Tablets during long-term use over 42 days dosed at 120 mg once daily continued to improve exercise performance at 4 hours and at 12 hours after dosing, but its effects (although better than placebo) are less than or, at best, equal to the effects of the first dose of 60 mg.

Pharmacokinetics and Metabolism: After oral administration of ISMN as a solution or immediate-release tablets, maximum plasma concentrations of ISMN are achieved in 30 to 60 minutes, with an absolute bioavailability of approximately 100%. After intravenous administration, ISMN is distributed into total body water in about 9 minutes with a volume of distribution of approximately 0.6 to 0.7 L/kg. Isosorbide mononitrate is approximately 5% bound to human plasma proteins and is distributed into blood cells and saliva. Isosorbide mononitrate is primarily metabolized by the liver, but unlike oral isosorbide dinitrate, it is not subject to first-pass metabolism. Isosorbide mononitrate is cleared by denitration to isosorbide and glucuronidation as the mononitrate, with 96% of the administered dose excreted in the urine within 5 days and only about 1% eliminated in the feces. At least six different compounds have been detected in urine, with about 2% of the dose excreted as the unchanged drug and at least five metabolites. The metabolites are not pharmacologically active. Renal clearance accounts for only about 4% of total body clearance. The mean plasma elimination half-life of ISMN is approximately 5 hours.

The disposition of ISMN in patients with various degrees of renal insufficiency, liver cirrhosis, or cardiac dysfunction was evaluated and found to be similar to that observed in healthy subjects. The elimination half-life of ISMN was not prolonged, and there was no drug accumulation in patients with chronic renal failure after multiple oral dosing.

The pharmacokinetics and/or bioavailability of IMDUR Tablets have been studied in both normal volunteers and patients following single- and multiple-dose administration. Data from these studies suggest that the pharmacokinetics of ISMN administered as IMDUR Tablets are similar between normal healthy volunteers and patients with angina pectoris. In single- and multiple-dose studies, the pharmacokinetics of ISMN were dose proportional between 30 mg and 240 mg.

In a multiple-dose study, the effect of age on the pharmacokinetic profile of IMDUR 60 mg and 120 mg (2 × 60 mg) Tablets was evaluated in subjects ≥45 years. The results of that study indicate that there are no significant differences in any of the pharmacokinetic variables of ISMN between elderly (≥65 years) and younger individuals (45–64 years) for the IMDUR 60-mg dose. The administration of IMDUR Tablets 120 mg (2 × 60 mg tablets every 24 hours for 7 days) produced a dose-proportional increase in C_{max} and AUC, without changes in T_{max} or the terminal half-life. The older group (65–74 years) showed 30% lower apparent oral clearance (Cl/F) following the higher dose, ie, 120 mg, compared to the younger group (45–64 years); Cl/F was not different between the two groups following the 60-mg regimen. While Cl/F was independent of dose in the younger group, the older group showed slightly lower Cl/F following the 120-mg regimen compared to the 60-mg regimen. Differences between the two age groups, however, were not statistically significant. In the same study, females showed a slight (15%) reduction in clearance when the dose was increased. Females showed higher AUCs and C_{max} compared to males, but these differences were accounted for by differences in body weight between the two groups. When the data were analyzed using age as a variable, the results indicated that there were no significant differences in any of the pharmacokinetic variables of ISMN between older (≥65 years) and younger individuals (45–64 years). The results of this study, however, should be viewed with caution due to the small numbers of subjects in each age subgroup and consequently the lack of sufficient statistical power.

The following table summarizes key pharmacokinetic parameters of ISMN after single- and multiple-dose administration of ISMN as an oral solution or IMDUR Tablets:

[See table at top of next page]

Food Effects: The influence of food on the bioavailability of ISMN after single-dose administration of IMDUR Tablets 60 mg was evaluated in three different studies involving either a "light" breakfast or a high-calorie, high-fat breakfast. Results of these studies indicate that concomitant food intake may decrease the rate (increase in T_{max}) but not the extent (AUC) of absorption of ISMN.

CLINICAL TRIALS

Controlled trials with IMDUR Tablets have demonstrated antianginal activity following acute and chronic dosing. Administration of IMDUR Tablets once daily, taken early in the morning on arising, provided at least 12 hours of antianginal activity.

In a placebo-control parallel study, 30, 60, 120, and 240 mg of IMDUR Tablets were administered once daily for up to 6 weeks. Prior to randomization, all patients completed a 1- to 3-week single-blind placebo phase to demonstrate nitrate responsiveness and total exercise treadmill time reproducibility. Exercise tolerance tests using the Bruce Protocol were conducted prior to and at 4 and 12 hours after the morning dose on days 1, 7, 14, 28, and 42 of the double-blind period. IMDUR Tablets 30 and 60 mg (only doses evaluated acutely) demonstrated a significant increase from baseline in total treadmill time relative to placebo at 4 and 12 hours after the administration of the first dose. At day 42, the 120- and 240-mg dose of IMDUR Tablets demonstrated a significant increase in total treadmill time at 4 and 12 hours post-dosing, but by day 42, the 30- and 60-mg doses no longer

Continued on next page

Imdur—Cont.

were differentiable from placebo. Throughout chronic dosing, rebound was not observed in any IMDUR treatment group.

Pooled data from two other trials, comparing IMDUR Tablets 60 mg once daily, ISDN 30 mg QID, and placebo QID in patients with chronic stable angina using a randomized, double-blind, three-way crossover design found statistically significant increases in exercise tolerance times for IMDUR Tablets compared to placebo at hours 4, 8, and 12 and to ISDN at hour 4. The increases in exercise tolerance on day 14, although statistically significant compared to placebo, were about half of that seen on day 1 of the trial.

PARAMETER	SINGLE-DOSE STUDIES ISMN 60 mg	SINGLE-DOSE STUDIES IMDUR 60 mg	MULTIPLE-DOSE STUDIES IMDUR 60 mg	MULTIPLE-DOSE STUDIES IMDUR 120 mg
C_{max} (ng/mL)	1242–1534	424–541	557–572	1151–1180
T_{max} (hr)	0.6–0.7	3.1–4.5	2.9–4.2	3.1–3.2
AUC (ng•hr/mL)	8189–8313	5990–7452	6625–7555	14241–16800
$t_{1/2}$ (hr)	4.8–5.1	6.3–6.6	6.2–6.3	6.2–6.4
Cl/F (mL/min)	120–122	151–187	132–151	119–140

INDICATIONS AND USAGE

IMDUR Tablets are indicated for the prevention of angina pectoris due to coronary artery disease. The onset of action of oral isosorbide mononitrate is not sufficiently rapid for this product to be useful in aborting an acute anginal episode.

CONTRAINDICATIONS

IMDUR Tablets are contraindicated in patients who have shown hypersensitivity or idiosyncratic reactions to other nitrates or nitrites.

WARNINGS

Amplification of the vasodilatory effects of IMDUR by sildenafil can result in severe hypotension. The time course and dose dependence of this interaction have not been studied. Appropriate supportive care has not been studied, but it seems reasonable to treat this as a nitrate overdose, with elevation of the extremities and with central volume expansion.

The benefits of ISMN in patients with acute myocardial infarction or congestive heart failure have not been established. Because the effects of isosorbide mononitrate are difficult to terminate rapidly, this drug is not recommended in these settings.

If isosorbide mononitrate is used in these conditions, careful clinical or hemodynamic monitoring must be used to avoid the hazards of hypotension and tachycardia.

PRECAUTIONS

General: Severe hypotension, particularly with upright posture, may occur with even small doses of isosorbide mononitrate. This drug should therefore be used with caution in patients who may be volume depleted or who, for whatever reason, are already hypotensive. Hypotension induced by isosorbide mononitrate may be accompanied by paradoxical bradycardia and increased angina pectoris.

Nitrate therapy may aggravate the angina caused by hypertrophic cardiomyopathy.

In industrial workers who have had long-term exposure to unknown (presumably high) doses of organic nitrates, tolerance clearly occurs. Chest pain, acute myocardial infarction, and even sudden death have occurred during temporary withdrawal of nitrates from these workers, demonstrating the existence of true physical dependence. The importance of these observations to the routine, clinical use of oral isosorbide mononitrate is not known.

Information for Patients: Patients should be told that the antianginal efficacy of IMDUR Tablets can be maintained by carefully following the prescribed schedule of dosing. For most patients, this can be accomplished by taking the dose on arising.

As with other nitrates, daily headaches sometimes accompany treatment with isosorbide mononitrate. In patients who get these headaches, the headaches are a marker of the activity of the drug. Patients should resist the temptation to avoid headaches by altering the schedule of their treatment with isosorbide mononitrate, since loss of headache may be associated with simultaneous loss of antianginal efficacy. Aspirin or acetaminophen often successfully relieves isosorbide mononitrate-induced headaches with no deleterious effect on isosorbide mononitrate's antianginal efficacy.

Treatment with isosorbide mononitrate may be associated with light-headedness on standing, especially just after rising from a recumbent or seated position. This effect may be more frequent in patients who have also consumed alcohol.

Drug Interactions: The vasodilating effects of isosorbide mononitrate may be additive with those of other vasodilators. Alcohol, in particular, has been found to exhibit additive effects of this variety.

Marked symptomatic orthostatic hypotension has been reported when calcium channel blockers and organic nitrates were used in combination. Dose adjustments of either class of agents may be necessary.

Drug/Laboratory Test Interactions: Nitrates and nitrites may interfere with the Zlatkis-Zak color reaction, causing falsely low readings in serum cholesterol determinations.

Isosorbide mononitrate did not produce gene mutations (Ames test, mouse lymphoma test) or chromosome aberrations (human lymphocyte and mouse micronucleus tests) at biologically relevant concentrations.

No effects on fertility were observed in a study in which male and female rats were administered doses of up to 750 mg/kg/day beginning, in males, 9 weeks prior to mating, and in females, 2 weeks prior to mating.

PREGNANCY

Teratogenic Effects: *Pregnancy Category B* In studies designed to detect effects of isosorbide mononitrate on embryo-fetal development, doses of up to 240 or 248 mg/kg/day, administered to pregnant rats and rabbits, were unassociated with evidence of such effects. These animal doses are about 100 times the maximum recommended human dose (120 mg in a 50-kg woman) when comparison is based on body weight; when comparison is based on body surface area, the rat dose is about 17 times the human dose and the rabbit dose is about 38 times the human dose. There are, however, no adequate and well-controlled studies in pregnant women. Because animal reproduction studies are not always predictive of human response, IMDUR Tablets should be used during pregnancy only if clearly needed.

Nonteratogenic Effects: Neonatal survival and development and incidence of stillbirths were adversely affected when pregnant rats were administered oral doses of 750 (but not 300) mg isosorbide mononitrate/kg/day during late gestation and lactation. This dose (about 312 times the human dose when comparison is based on body weight and 54 times the human dose when comparison is based on body surface area) was associated with decreases in maternal weight gain and motor activity and evidence of impaired lactation.

Nursing Mothers: It is not known whether this drug is excreted in human milk. Because many drugs are excreted in human milk, caution should be exercised when ISMN is administered to a nursing mother.

Pediatric Use: The safety and effectiveness of ISMN in pediatric patients have not been established.

ADVERSE REACTIONS

The table below shows the frequencies of the adverse events that occurred in >5% of the subjects in three placebo-controlled North American studies in which patients in the active treatment arm received 30 mg, 60 mg, 120 mg, or 240 mg of isosorbide mononitrate as IMDUR Tablets once daily. In parentheses, the same table shows the frequencies with which these adverse events were associated with the discontinuation of treatment. Overall, 8% of the patients who received 30 mg, 60 mg, 120 mg, or 240 mg of isosorbide mononitrate in the three placebo-controlled North American studies discontinued treatment because of adverse events. Most of these discontinued because of headache. Dizziness was rarely associated with withdrawal from these studies. Since headache appears to be a dose-related adverse effect and tends to disappear with continued treatment, it is recommended that IMDUR treatment be initiated at low doses for several days before being increased to desired levels.

FREQUENCY AND ADVERSE EVENTS (DISCONTINUED)*

Three Controlled North American Studies

Dose	Placebo	30 mg	60 mg	120 mg**	240 mg**
Patients	96	60	102	65	65
Headache	15% (0%)	38% (5%)	51% (8%)	42% (5%)	57% (8%)
Dizziness	4% (0%)	8% (0%)	11% (1%)	9% (2%)	9% (2%)

* Some individuals discontinued for multiple reasons.
** Patients were started on 60 mg and titrated to their final dose.

In addition, the three North American trials were pooled with 11 controlled trials conducted in Europe. Among the 14 controlled trials, a total of 711 patients were randomized to IMDUR Tablets. When the pooled data were reviewed, headache and dizziness were the only adverse events that were reported by >5% of patients. Other adverse events, each reported by ≤5% of exposed patients, and in many cases of uncertain relation to drug treatment, were:

Autonomic Nervous System Disorders: Dry mouth, hot flushes.

Body as a Whole: Asthenia, back pain, chest pain, edema, fatigue, fever, flu-like symptoms, malaise, rigors.

Cardiovascular Disorders, General: Cardiac failure, hypertension, hypotension.

Central and Peripheral Nervous System Disorders: Dizziness, headache, hypoesthesia, migraine, neuritis, paresis, paresthesia, ptosis, tremor, vertigo.

Gastrointestinal System Disorders: Abdominal pain, constipation, diarrhea, dyspepsia, flatulence, gastric ulcer, gastritis, glossitis, hemorrhagic gastric ulcer, hemorrhoids, loose stools, melena, nausea, vomiting.

Hearing and Vestibular Disorders: Earache, tinnitus, tympanic membrane perforation.

Heart Rate and Rhythm Disorders: Arrhythmia, arrhythmia atrial, atrial fibrillation, bradycardia, bundle branch block, extrasystole, palpitation, tachycardia, ventricular tachycardia.

Liver and Biliary System Disorders: SGOT increase, SGPT increase.

Metabolic and Nutritional Disorders: Hyperuricemia, hypokalemia.

Musculoskeletal System Disorders: Arthralgia, frozen shoulder, muscle weakness, musculoskeletal pain, myalgia, myositis, tendon disorder, torticollis.

Myo-, Endo-, Pericardial, and Valve Disorders: Angina pectoris aggravated, heart murmur, heart sound abnormal, myocardial infarction, Q wave abnormality.

Platelet, Bleeding, and Clotting Disorders: Purpura, thrombocytopenia.

Psychiatric Disorders: Anxiety, concentration impaired, confusion, decreased libido, depression, impotence, insomnia, nervousness, paroniria, somnolence.

Red Blood Cell Disorder: Hypochromic anemia.

Reproductive Disorders, Female: Atrophic vaginitis, breast pain.

Resistance Mechanism Disorders: Bacterial infection, moniliasis, viral infection.

Respiratory System Disorders: Bronchitis, bronchospasm, coughing, dyspnea, increased sputum, nasal congestion, pharyngitis, pneumonia, pulmonary infiltration, rales, rhinitis, sinusitis.

Skin and Appendages Disorders: Acne, hair texture abnormal, increased sweating, pruritus, rash, skin nodule.

Urinary System Disorders: Polyuria, renal calculus, urinary tract infection.

Vascular (Extracardiac) Disorders: Flushing, intermittent claudication, leg ulcer, varicose vein.

Vision Disorders: Conjunctivitis, photophobia, vision abnormal.

In addition, the following spontaneous adverse event has been reported during the marketing of isosorbide mononitrate: syncope.

OVERDOSAGE

Hemodynamic Effects: The ill effects of isosorbide mononitrate overdose are generally the results of isosorbide mononitrate's capacity to induce vasodilatation, venous pooling, reduced cardiac output, and hypotension. These hemodynamic changes may have protean manifestations, including increased intracranial pressure, with any or all of persistent throbbing headache, confusion, and moderate fever; vertigo; palpitations; visual disturbances; nausea and vomiting (possibly with colic and even bloody diarrhea); syncope (especially in the upright posture); air hunger and dyspnea, later followed by reduced ventilatory effort; diaphoresis, with the skin either flushed or cold and clammy; heart block and bradycardia; paralysis; coma; seizures; and death.

Laboratory determinations of serum levels of isosorbide mononitrate and its metabolites are not widely available, and such determinations have, in any event, no established role in the management of isosorbide mononitrate overdose.

There are no data suggesting what dose of isosorbide mononitrate is likely to be life threatening in humans. In rats and mice, there is significant lethality at doses of 2000 mg/kg and 3000 mg/kg, respectively.

No data are available to suggest physiological maneuvers (eg, maneuvers to change the pH of the urine) that might accelerate elimination of isosorbide mononitrate. In particular, dialysis is known to be ineffective in removing isosorbide mononitrate from the body.

No specific antagonist to the vasodilator effects of isosorbide mononitrate is known, and no intervention has been subject to controlled study as a therapy of isosorbide mononitrate overdose. Because the hypotension associated with isosorbide mononitrate overdose is the result of venodilatation and arterial hypovolemia, prudent therapy in this situation should be directed toward an increase in central fluid volume. Passive elevation of the patient's legs may be sufficient, but intravenous infusion of normal saline or similar fluid may also be necessary.

The use of epinephrine or other arterial vasoconstrictors in this setting is likely to do more harm than good.

In patients with renal disease or congestive heart failure, therapy resulting in central volume expansion is not without hazard. Treatment of isosorbide mononitrate overdose in these patients may be subtle and difficult, and invasive monitoring may be required.

Methemoglobinemia: Methemoglobinemia has been reported in patients receiving other organic nitrates, and it probably could also occur as a side effect of isosorbide mononitrate. Certainly, nitrate ions liberated during metabolism of isosorbide mononitrate can oxidize hemoglobin into methemoglobin. Even in patients totally without cytochrome b_5 reductase activity, however, and even assuming that the nitrate moiety of isosorbide mononitrate is quantitatively applied to oxidation of hemoglobin, about 2 mg/kg of isosorbide mononitrate should be required before any of these patients manifest clinically significant (≥10%) methemoglobinemia. In patients with normal reductase function, significant production of methemoglobin should require even larger doses of isosorbide mononitrate. In one study in which 36 patients received 2 to 4 weeks of continuous nitroglycerin therapy at 3.1 to 4.4 mg/hr (equivalent, in total administered dose of nitrate ions, to 7.8–11.1 mg of isosorbide mononitrate per hour), the average methemoglobin level measured was 0.2%; this was comparable to that observed in parallel patients who received placebo.

Notwithstanding these observations, there are case reports of significant methemoglobinemia in association with moderate overdoses of organic nitrates. None of the affected patients had been thought to be unusually susceptible.

Methemoglobin levels are available from most clinical laboratories. The diagnosis should be suspected in patients who exhibit signs of impaired oxygen delivery despite adequate cardiac output and adequate arterial pO_2. Classically, methemoglobinemic blood is described as chocolate brown, without color change on exposure to air.

When methemoglobinemia is diagnosed, the treatment of choice is methylene blue, 1 to 2 mg/kg intravenously.

DOSAGE AND ADMINISTRATION

The recommended starting dose of IMDUR Tablets is 30 mg (given as a single 30-mg tablet or as $^1/_2$ of a 60-mg tablet) or 60 mg (given as a single tablet) once daily. After several days, the dosage may be increased to 120 mg (given as a single 120-mg tablet or as two 60-mg tablets) once daily. Rarely, 240 mg may be required. The daily dose of IMDUR Tablets should be taken in the morning on arising. IMDUR Extended Release Tablets should not be chewed or crushed and should be swallowed together with a half-glassful of fluid.

HOW SUPPLIED

IMDUR Extended Release Tablets

30 mg: rose-colored tablets, scored on both sides and branded with the tradename ("IMDUR") on one side and the strength on the other.

Bottles of 30	NDC 0085-3306-02
Bottles of 100	NDC 0085-3306-03
Unit Dose 100 (10 x 10 blister strips)	NDC 0085-3306-01
Unit Dose 90 (9 x 10 blister strips) Institutional Pack for Inpatient Use Only	NDC 0085-3306-04

60 mg: yellow-colored tablets, scored on both sides and branded with the tradename ("IMDUR") on one side and the strength on the other.

Bottles of 100	NDC 0085-4110-03
Unit Dose 100 (10 x 10 blister strips)	NDC 0085-4110-01
Unit Dose 90 (9 x 10 blister strips) Institutional Pack for Inpatient Use Only	NDC 0085-4110-05

120 mg: white-colored tablets, branded with the tradename ("IMDUR") on one side and the strength on the other.

Bottles of 100	NDC 0085-1153-03
Unit Dose 100 (10 x 10 blister strips)	NDC 0085-1153-04
Unit Dose 90 (9 x 10 blister strips) Institutional Pack for Inpatient Use Only	NDC 0085-1153-07

Store at controlled room temperature 20°–25°C (68°–77°F) [see USP].

Protect unit dose from excessive moisture.

Manufactured for Key Pharmaceuticals, Inc.,
Kenilworth, NJ 07033 by A.B. ASTRA, Sweden.

Rev. 10/99 B-17616978

18692937T

Shown in Product Identification Guide, page 319

INTEGRILIN® ℞

[*ĭn-tĕg-rĭl-in*]

(eptifibatide)

Injection

For Intravenous Administration

DESCRIPTION

Eptifibatide is a cyclic heptapeptide containing six amino acids and one mercaptopropionyl (des-amino cysteinyl) residue. An interchain disulfide bridge is formed between the cysteine amide and the mercaptopropionyl moieties. Chemically it is N^6-(aminoiminomethyl)-N^2-(3-mercapto-1-oxopropyl-L-lysylglycyl-L-α-aspartyl-L-tryptophyl-L-prolyl-L-cysteinamide, cyclic (1→6)-disulfide. Eptifibatide binds to the platelet receptor glycoprotein (GP) IIb/IIIa of human platelets and inhibits platelet aggregation.

The eptifibatide peptide is produced by solution-phase peptide synthesis, and is purified by preparative reverse-phase liquid chromatography and lyophilized. The structural formula is:

$C_{35}H_{49}N_{11}O_9S_2$ Mol wt: 831.96

INTEGRILIN (eptifibatide) Injection is a clear, colorless, sterile, non-pyrogenic solution for intravenous (IV) use. Each 10-mL vial contains 2 mg/mL of eptifibatide and each 100-mL vial contains 0.75 mg/mL of eptifibatide. Each vial of either size also contains 5.25 mg/mL citric acid and sodium hydroxide to adjust the pH to 5.25.

CLINICAL PHARMACOLOGY

Mechanism of Action. Eptifibatide reversibly inhibits platelet aggregation by preventing the binding of fibrinogen, von Willebrand factor, and other adhesive ligands to GP IIb/IIIa. When administered intravenously, eptifibatide inhibits *ex vivo* platelet aggregation in a dose- and concentration-dependent manner. Platelet aggregation inhibition is reversible following cessation of the eptifibatide infusion; this is thought to result from dissociation of eptifibatide from the platelet.

Pharmacodynamics. Infusion of eptifibatide into baboons caused a dose-dependent inhibition of *ex vivo* platelet aggregation, with complete inhibition of aggregation achieved at infusion rates greater than 5.0 µg/kg/min. In a baboon model that is refractory to aspirin and heparin, doses of eptifibatide that inhibit aggregation prevented acute thrombosis with only a modest prolongation (2- to 3-fold) of the bleeding time. Platelet aggregation in dogs was also inhibited by infusions of eptifibatide, with complete inhibition at 2.0 µg/kg/min. This infusion dose completely inhibited canine coronary thrombosis induced by coronary artery injury (Folts model).

Human pharmacodynamic data were obtained in healthy subjects and in patients presenting with unstable angina (UA) or non-Q-wave myocardial infarction (NQMI) and/or undergoing percutaneous coronary interventions. Studies in healthy subjects enrolled only males; patient studies enrolled approximately one third women. In these studies, eptifibatide inhibited *ex vivo* platelet aggregation induced by adenosine diphosphate (ADP) and other agonists in a dose- and concentration-dependent manner. The effect of eptifibatide was observed immediately after administration of a 180 µg/kg intravenous bolus. Table 1 shows the effects of the two doses of eptifibatide used in the two principal clinical studies on *ex vivo* platelet aggregation induced by 20 µM ADP in PPACK-anticoagulated platelet-rich plasma and on bleeding time.

Table 1
Platelet Inhibition and Bleeding Time

	IMPACT II 135/0.5*	PURSUIT 180/2.0**
Inhibition of platelet aggregation 15 min. after bolus	69%	84%
Inhibition of platelet aggregation at steady state	40–50%	>90%
Bleeding-time prolongation at steady state	<5×	<5×
Inhibition of platelet aggregation 4h after infusion discontinuation	<30%	<50%
Bleeding-time prolongation 6h after infusion discontinuation	1×	1.4×

*135 µg/kg bolus followed by a continuous infusion of 0.5 µg/kg/min

**180 µg/kg bolus followed by a continuous infusion of 2.0 µg/kg/min

When administered alone, eptifibatide has no measurable effect on prothrombin time (PT) or activated partial thromboplastin time (aPTT). (See also PRECAUTIONS: Drug Interactions.)

There were no important differences between men and women or between age groups in the pharmacodynamic properties of eptifibatide. Differences among ethnic groups have not been assessed.

Pharmacokinetics. The pharmacokinetics of eptifibatide are linear and dose-proportional for bolus doses ranging from 90 to 250 µg/kg and infusion rates from 0.5 to 3.0 µg/kg/min. Plasma elimination half-life is approximately 2.5 hours. The recommended regimens of a bolus followed by an infusion produce an early peak level, followed by a small decline with attainment of steady state within 4–6 hours. The extent of eptifibatide binding to human plasma protein is about 25%.

Excretion and Metabolism. Clearance in patients with coronary artery disease is 55–58 mL/kg/h. In healthy subjects, renal clearance accounts for approximately 50% of total body clearance, with the majority of the drug excreted in the urine as eptifibatide, deamidated eptifibatide, and other, more polar metabolites. No major metabolites have been detected in human plasma. Clinical studies have included 2418 patients with serum creatinine between 1.0 and 2.0 mg/dL (for the 180 µg/kg bolus and the 2.0 µg/kg/min infusion) and 7 patients with serum creatinine between 2.0 and 4.0 mg/dL (for the 135 µg/kg bolus and the 0.5 µg/kg/min infusion), without dose adjustment. No data are available in patients with more severe degrees of renal impairment, but plasma eptifibatide levels are expected to be higher in such patients (see CONTRAINDICATIONS).

Special Populations. Patients in clinical studies were older than the subjects in clinical pharmacology studies, and they had lower total body eptifibatide clearance and higher eptifibatide plasma levels. Clinical studies were conducted in patients aged 20 to 94 years with coronary artery disease without dose adjustment for age. Because patients over 75 years of age were enrolled into the PURSUIT clinical study only if their body weight exceeded 50 kg, minimal data are available on lighter-weight patients over 75 years of age. Men and women showed no important differences in the pharmacokinetics of eptifibatide.

CLINICAL STUDIES

Eptifibatide was studied in two placebo-controlled, randomized studies, one (PURSUIT) in patients with acute coronary syndrome (unstable angina (UA) or non-Q-wave myocardial infarction (NQMI)), the other (IMPACT II) in patients about to undergo a percutaneous cardiovascular intervention (PCI; balloon angioplasty in most cases, but sometimes directional atherectomy, transluminal extraction catheter atherectomy, rotational ablation atherectomy, or excimer-laser angioplasty).

Acute coronary syndrome is defined as prolonged (≥10 minutes) symptoms of cardiac ischemia within the previous 24 hours associated with either ST-segment changes (elevation between 0.6 mm and 1 mm or depression >0.5 mm), T-wave inversion (>1 mm), or positive CK-MB. This definition includes "unstable angina" and "non-Q-wave myocardial infarction" but excludes myocardial infarction that is associated with Q waves or greater degrees of ST-segment elevation.

PURSUIT was a 726-center, 27-country, double-blind, randomized, placebo-controlled study in 10,948 patients presenting with UA or NQMI. Patients could be enrolled only if they had experienced cardiac ischemia at rest (≥10 minutes) within the previous 24 hours and had either ST-segment changes (elevations between 0.6 mm and 1 mm or depression >0.5 mm), T-wave inversion (>1 mm), or increased CK-MB. Important exclusion criteria included a history of bleeding diathesis, evidence of abnormal bleeding within the previous 30 days, uncontrolled hypertension, major surgery within the previous 6 weeks, stroke within the previous 30 days, any history of hemorrhagic stroke, serum creatinine >2.0 mg/dL, dependency on renal dialysis, or platelet count <100,000/mm^3.

Patients were randomized to either placebo, eptifibatide 180 µg/kg bolus followed by a 2.0 µg/kg/min infusion (180/2.0), or eptifibatide 180 µg/kg bolus followed by a 1.3 µg/kg/min infusion (180/1.3). The infusion was continued for 72 hours, until hospital discharge, or until the time of coronary artery bypass grafting (CABG), whichever occurred first, except that if PCI was performed, the eptifibatide infusion was continued for 24 hours after the procedure, allowing for a duration of infusion up to 96 hours.

The lower-infusion-rate arm was stopped after the first interim analysis when the two active-treatment arms appeared to have the same incidence of bleeding.

Patient age ranged from 20 to 94 (mean 63) years, and 65% were male. The patients were 89% Caucasian, 6% Hispanic, and 5% Black, recruited in the United States and Canada (40%), Western Europe (39%), Eastern Europe (16%), and Latin America (5%).

This was a "real world" study; each patient was managed according to the usual standards of the investigational site; frequencies of angiography, PCI, and CABG therefore differed widely from site to site and from country to country. Of the patients in PURSUIT, 13% were managed with PCI during drug infusion, of whom 50% received intracoronary stents; 87% were managed medically (without PCI during drug infusion).

The majority of patients received aspirin (75–325 mg once daily). Heparin was administered intravenously or subcutaneously, at the physician's discretion, most commonly as an intravenous bolus of 5000 U followed by a continuous infusion of 1000 U/h. For patients weighing less than 70 kg, the recommended heparin bolus dose was 60 U/kg followed by a continuous infusion of 12 U/kg/h. A target aPTT of 50–70 seconds was recommended. A total of 1250 patients underwent PCI within 72 hours after randomization, in which case they received intravenous heparin to maintain an activated clotting time (ACT) of 300–350 seconds.

The primary endpoint of the study was the occurrence of death from any cause or new myocardial infarction (MI) (evaluated by a blinded Clinical Endpoints Committee) within 30 days of randomization.

Compared to placebo, eptifibatide administered as a 180 µg/kg bolus followed by a 2.0 µg/kg/min infusion significantly (p=0.042) reduced the incidence of endpoint events (see Table 2). The reduction in the incidence of endpoint events in patients receiving eptifibatide was evident early

Continued on next page

Integrilin—Cont.

during treatment, and this reduction was maintained through at least 30 days (see Figure 1). Table 2 also shows the incidence of the components of the primary endpoint, death (whether or not preceded by an MI) and new MI in surviving patients at 30 days.

[See table 2 at right]

Figure 1

Kaplan-Meier Plot of Time to Death or Myocardial Infarction Within 30 Days of Randomization

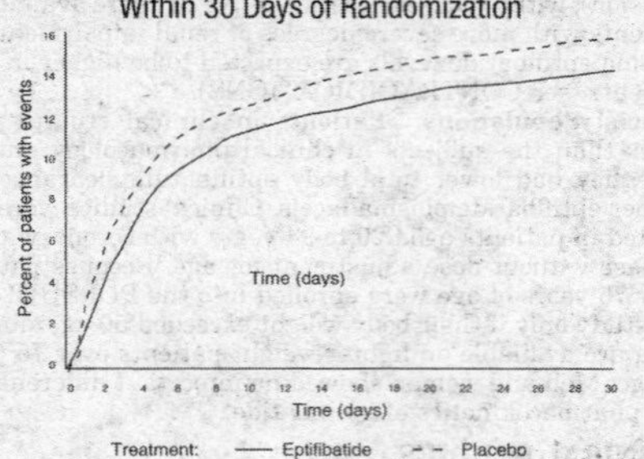

The effect of eptifibatide in PURSUIT did not appear to vary with patients' age. There were too few non-Caucasian patients to reach any conclusion as to possible differences related to race. Analysis of the PURSUIT results reveals a complex interaction of treatment, gender, and region. Throughout the world, eptifibatide was significantly less beneficial in women than in men, and in the overall study eptifibatide in women was nonsignificantly worse than placebo. These results were, however, strikingly heterogeneous across the several regions; eptifibatide appeared much worse than placebo in women in Latin America, while effects in men and women were scarcely distinguishable (relative risk reductions of 23% and 18%, respectively) in the U.S. and Canada. These results may reflect (a) genuine biological interactions between eptifibatide and gender, (b) interactions between eptifibatide and unknown international differences in concomitant therapy delivered to men and women, and (c) the play of chance, but the relative contributions of these possible factors are unknown.

Treatment with eptifibatide prior to determination of patient management strategy reduced clinical events regardless of whether patients ultimately underwent diagnostic catheterization, revascularization (i.e., PCI or CABG surgery) or continued to receive medical management alone. Table 3 shows the incidence of death or MI within 72 hours.

Table 3

Clinical Events (Death or MI) in the PURSUIT Study Within 72 Hours of Randomization

	Placebo	Eptifibatide 180/2.0
Overall Patient Population	n=4739	n=4722
- At 72 hours	7.6%	5.9%
Patients undergoing early PCI	n=631	n=619
- Pre-procedure (nonfatal MI only)	5.5%	1.8%
- At 72 hours	14.4%	9.0%
Patients not undergoing early PCI	n=4108	n=4103
- At 72 hours	6.5%	5.4%

All of the effect of eptifibatide was established within 72 hours (during the period of drug infusion), regardless of management strategy. Moreover, for patients undergoing early PCI, a reduction in events was evident prior to the procedure.

Follow-up data were available through 165 days for 10,611 patients enrolled in the PURSUIT trial (96.9 percent of the initial enrollment). This follow-up included 4,566 patients who received eptifibatide at the 180/2.0 dose. As reported by the investigators, the occurrence of death from any cause or new myocardial infarction for patients followed for at least 165 days was reduced from 13.6 percent with placebo to 12.1 percent with eptifibatide 180/2.0.

IMPACT II was a multi-center, double-blind, randomized, placebo-controlled study conducted in the United States in 4010 patients undergoing PCI. Major exclusion criteria included a history of bleeding diathesis, major surgery within 6 weeks of treatment, gastrointestinal bleeding within 30 days, any stroke or structural CNS abnormality, uncontrolled hypertension, PT >1.2 times control, hematocrit <30%, platelet count <100,000/mm^3, and pregnancy.

Patient age ranged from 24 to 89 (mean 60) years, and 75% were male. The patients were 92% Caucasian, 5% Black, and 3% Hispanic. Patients were randomly assigned to one of three treatment regimens, each incorporating a bolus dose initiated immediately prior to PCI followed by a continuous infusion lasting 20–24 hours: 1) 135 µg/kg bolus followed by a continuous infusion of 0.5 µg/kg/min of eptifibatide (135/0.5); 2) 135 µg/kg bolus followed by a continuous infusion of 0.75 µg/kg/min of eptifibatide (135/0.75); or 3) a matching placebo bolus followed by a matching placebo continuous infusion. Each patient received aspirin and an intravenous

Table 2

Clinical Events in The PURSUIT Study

Death or MI	Placebo (n = 4739) n (%)	Eptifibatide (180/2.0) (n = 4722) n (%)	p-value
3 days	359 (7.6%)	279 (5.9%)	0.001
7 days	552 (11.6%)	477 (10.1%)	0.016
30 days			
Death or MI (Primary Endpoint)	745 (15.7%)	672 (14.2%)	0.042
Death	177 (3.7%)	165 (3.5%)	
Nonfatal MI	568 (12.0%)	507 (10.7%)	

Table 4

Clinical Events in the IMPACT II Study

	Placebo n (%)	Eptifibatide (135/0.5) n (%)	Eptifibatide (135/0.75) n (%)
Patients	1285	1300	1286
Abrupt Closure	65 (5.1%)	36 (2.8%)	43 (3.3%)
p-value vs. placebo		0.003	0.030
Death, MI, or Urgent Intervention			
24 hours	123 (9.6%)	86 (6.6%)	89 (6.9%)
p-value vs. placebo		0.006	0.014
48 hours	131 (10.2%)	99 (7.6%)	102 (7.9%)
p-value vs. placebo		0.021	0.045
30 days (primary endpoint)	149 (11.6%)	118 (9.1%)	128 (10.0%)
p-value vs. placebo		0.035	0.179
Death or MI			
30 days	110 (8.6%)	89 (6.8%)	95 (7.4%)
p-value vs. placebo		0.102	0.272
6 months	151 (11.9%)*	136 (10.6%)*	130 (10.3%)*
p-value vs. placebo		0.297	0.182

*Kaplan-Meier estimate of event rate

Table 5

Clinical Events at 30 Days in the IMPACT II Study, Stratified by Acuity at Time of Randomization

Classification of Patients (%)	Placebo n (%)	Eptifibatide 135/0.5 n (%)	Eptifibatide 135/0.75 n (%)
Ongoing ACS, MI ongoing or within past 24h (41.3%)	538 (11.5%)	532 (10.0%)	527 (10.6%)
Others (58.7%)	747 (11.6%)	768 (8.5%)	759 (9.5%)

heparin bolus of 100 U/kg, with additional bolus infusions of up to 2000 additional units of heparin every 15 minutes to maintain an activated clotting time (ACT) of 300–350 seconds.

The primary endpoint was the composite of death, MI, or urgent revascularization, analyzed at 30 days after randomization in all patients who received at least one dose of study drug.

As shown in Table 4, each eptifibatide regimen reduced the rate of death, MI, or urgent intervention, although at 30 days, this finding was statistically significant only in the lower-dose eptifibatide group. As in the PURSUIT study, the effects of eptifibatide were seen early and persisted throughout the 30-day period.

[See table 4 above]

At the time of randomization, approximately 25% of the IMPACT II patients suffered from only chronic stable angina, or had had no angina at all since a remote (more than 14 days prior) myocardial infarction. At the other extreme, approximately 40% of the IMPACT II patients had ongoing acute coronary syndromes, including patients with rest angina, others with refractory recurrent angina, others with early post-infarction angina, and others about to receive percutaneous interventions during or immediately following acute myocardial infarction. The remaining patients had various histories of recent and remote acute coronary syndromes; data are not available to describe what fraction of these underwent PCI within only a day or two of an acute episode. The IMPACT II study was not powered to obtain stable estimates of efficacy in subpopulations defined by degree of acuity, but (as shown in Table 5) the data suggest that the benefit of eptifibatide was not limited to patients with ongoing acute coronary syndromes.

[See table 5 above]

INDICATIONS AND USAGE

INTEGRILIN is indicated:

- For the treatment of patients with acute coronary syndrome (UA/NQMI), including patients who are to be managed medically and those undergoing percutaneous coronary intervention (PCI). In this setting, INTEGRILIN has been shown to decrease the rate of a combined endpoint of death or new myocardial infarction.
- For the treatment of patients undergoing PCI. In this setting, INTEGRILIN has been shown to decrease the rate of a combined endpoint of death, new myocardial infarction, or need for urgent intervention.

In the clinical studies of eptifibatide, most patients received heparin and aspirin, as described in CLINICAL TRIALS.

CONTRAINDICATIONS

Treatment with eptifibatide is contraindicated in patients with:

- A history of bleeding diathesis, or evidence of active abnormal bleeding within the previous 30 days.
- Severe hypertension (systolic blood pressure >200 mm Hg or diastolic blood pressure >110 mm Hg) not adequately controlled on antihypertensive therapy.
- Major surgery within the preceding 6 weeks.
- History of stroke within 30 days or any history of hemorrhagic stroke.
- Current or planned administration of another parenteral GP IIb/IIIa inhibitor.
- Platelet count <100,000/mm^3.
- Serum creatinine ≥4.0 mg/dL. In patients with serum creatinine levels between 2.0 mg/dL and 4.0 mg/dL, the 135µg/kg bolus and 0.5 µg/kg/min infusion should be administered.
- Dependency on renal dialysis.
- Known hypersensitivity to any component of the product.

WARNINGS

Bleeding. Bleeding is the most common complication encountered during eptifibatide therapy. Administration of eptifibatide is associated with an increase in major and minor bleeding, as classified by the criteria of the Thrombolysis in Myocardial Infarction Study group (TIMI), (see ADVERSE REACTIONS). Most major bleeding associated with eptifibatide has been at the arterial access site for cardiac catheterization or from the gastrointestinal or genitourinary tract.

In patients undergoing percutaneous coronary interventions, patients receiving eptifibatide experience an increased incidence of major bleeding compared to those receiving placebo. Special care should be employed to minimize the risk of bleeding among these patients (see PRECAUTIONS).

If bleeding cannot be controlled with pressure, infusion of eptifibatide and concomitant heparin should be stopped immediately.

PRECAUTIONS

Bleeding Precautions

Care of the Femoral Artery Access Site in Patients Undergoing Percutaneous Coronary Intervention (PCI). In patients undergoing PCI, treatment with eptifibatide is associated with an increase in major and minor bleeding at the site of arterial sheath placement. After PCI, eptifibatide infusion should be continued for 20–24 hours. The femoral artery sheath may be removed during treatment with eptifibatide, but only after heparin has been discontinued and its effects largely reversed. In the IMPACT II study, heparin use was discouraged after the PCI procedure if the coronary lesion appeared angiographically stable. Early sheath removal was encouraged in both the IMPACT II and the PURSUIT studies while study drug was being infused. Prior to removing the sheath, it was recommended that heparin be discontinued for 3–4 hours and that an aPTT of <45 seconds be documented. In any case, both heparin and eptifibatide should be discontinued and sheath hemostasis should be achieved by standard compressive techniques at least 4 hours before hospital discharge.

Use of Thrombolytics, Anticoagulants, and Other Antiplatelet Agents. In the IMPACT II and PURSUIT studies, eptifibatide was used concomitantly with heparin and aspirin (see CLINICAL STUDIES). Because eptifibatide inhibits platelet aggregation, caution should be employed when it is used with other drugs that affect hemostasis, including **thrombolytics, oral anticoagulants, non-steroidal anti-inflammatory drugs, dipyridamole, ticlopidine,** and **clopidogrel.** To avoid potentially additive pharmacologic effects, concomitant treatment with **other inhibitors of platelet receptor GP IIb/IIIa** should be avoided.

There is only a small experience with concomitant use of eptifibatide and **thrombolytics.** In a study of 180 patients with acute myocardial infarction (AMI), eptifibatide (in regimens up to a bolus of 180 µg/kg followed by a continuous infusion of 0.75 µg/kg/min for 24 hours) was administered concomitantly with the approved "accelerated" regimen of alteplase, a thrombolytic agent. The studied regimens of eptifibatide did not increase the incidence of major bleeding or transfusion compared to the incidence seen when alteplase was given alone.

In the IMPACT II study, 15 patients received a thrombolytic agent in conjunction with the 135/0.5 dosing regimen, 2 of whom experienced a major bleed. In the PURSUIT study, 40 patients who received eptifibatide at the 180/2.0 dosing regimen received a thrombolytic agent, 10 of whom experienced a major bleed.

In another AMI study involving 181 patients, eptifibatide (in regimens up to a bolus of 180 µg/kg followed by a continuous infusion of up to 2.0 µg/kg/min for up to 72 hours) was administered concomitantly with streptokinase (1.5 million units over 60 minutes), another thrombolytic agent. At the highest studied infusion rates (1.3 µg/kg/min and 2.0 µg/kg/min), eptifibatide was associated with an increase in the incidence of bleeding and transfusions compared to the incidence seen when streptokinase was given alone.

These limited data on the use of eptifibatide in patients receiving thrombolytic agents do not allow an estimate of the bleeding risk associated with concomitant use of thrombolytics. Systemic thrombolytic therapy should be used with caution in patients who have received eptifibatide.

Minimization of Vascular and Other Trauma. Arterial and venous punctures, intramuscular injections, and the use of urinary catheters, nasotracheal intubation, and nasogastric tubes should be minimized. When obtaining intravenous access, noncompressible sites (e.g., subclavian or jugular veins) should be avoided.

Laboratory Tests. Before infusion of eptifibatide, the following laboratory tests should be performed to identify preexisting hemostatic abnormalities: hematocrit or hemoglobin, platelet count, serum creatinine, and PT/aPTT. In patients undergoing PCI, the activated clotting time (ACT) should also be measured.

Maintaining Target aPTT and ACT. The aPTT should be maintained between 50 and 70 seconds unless PCI is to be performed. In patients treated with heparin, bleeding can be minimized by close monitoring of the aPTT. Table 6 displays the risk of major bleeding according to the maximum aPTT attained within 72 hours in the PURSUIT study.

[See table 6 above]

During PCI, the PURSUIT study stipulated a target ACT of between 300 and 350 seconds. Patients receiving an eptifibatide 180 µg/kg bolus followed by a 2 µg/kg/min infusion experienced an increased incidence of bleeding relative to placebo, primarily at the femoral artery access site.

The aPTT or ACT should be checked prior to arterial sheath removal. The sheath should not be removed unless the aPTT is <45 seconds or the ACT is <150 seconds.

Thrombocytopenia. If the patient experiences a confirmed platelet decrease to <100,000/mm^3, INTEGRILIN and heparin should be discontinued and the condition appropriately monitored and treated.

Renal Insufficiency. Based on results of clinical studies with eptifibatide (which did not adjust dose for renal function) and the fact that the drug is cleared equally by renal and nonrenal mechanisms, dose adjustment is unnecessary for patients with mild to moderate renal impairment (serum creatinine <2.0 mg/dL for the 180 µg/kg bolus and the 2.0 µg/kg/min infusion and <4.0 mg/dL for the 135 µg/kg bolus and the 0.5 µg/kg/min infusion). For patients with serum creatinine >2.0 mg/dL and <4.0 mg/dL, eptifibatide should be administered as a 135 µg/kg bolus followed by a 0.5 µg/kg/min infusion. Plasma eptifibatide levels are expected to be higher in patients with more severe renal impairment, but no data are available for such patients or for patients on renal dialysis. *In vitro* studies have indicated that eptifibatide may be cleared from plasma by dialysis.

Table 6

Major Bleeding by Maximal aPTT Within 72 Hours in the PURSUIT Study

	Placebo n (%)	Eptifibatide 180/1.3* n (%)	Eptifibatide 180/2.0 n (%)
Maximum aPTT (seconds)			
<50	44/721(6.1%)	21/244(8.6%)	44/743(5.9%)
50-70 (recommended)	92/908(10.1%)	28/259(10.8%)	99/883(11.2%)
>70	281/2786(10.1%)	99/891(11.1%)	345/2811(12.3%)

*Administered only until the first interim analysis

Table 7

Bleeding Events and Transfusions in the PURSUIT and IMPACT II Studies

PURSUIT	Placebo n (%)	Eptifibatide 180/1.3* n (%)	Eptifibatide 180/2.0 n (%)
Patients	4696	1472	4679
Major bleeding[a]	425 (9.3%)	152 (10.5%)	498 (10.8%)
Minor bleeding[a]	347 (7.6%)	152 (10.5%)	604 (13.1%)
Requiring Transfusions[b]	490 (10.4%)	188 (12.8%)	601 (12.8%)
IMPACT II	**Placebo n (%)**	**Eptifibatide 135/0.5 n (%)**	**Eptifibatide 135/0.75 n (%)**
Patients	1285	1300	1286
Major bleeding[a]	55 (4.5%)	55 (4.4%)	58 (4.7%)
Minor bleeding[a]	115 (9.3%)	146 (11.7%)	177 (14.2%)
Requiring Transfusions[b]	66 (5.1%)	71 (5.5%)	74 (5.8%)

Note: denominator is based on patients for whom data are available

*Administered only until the first interim analysis

[a] For major and minor bleeding, patients are counted only once according to the most severe classification.

[b] Includes transfusions of whole blood, packed red blood cells, fresh frozen plasma, cryoprecipitate, platelets, and autotransfusion during the initial hospitalization.

Table 8

Major Bleeding by Procedures in the PURSUIT Study

	Placebo n (%)	Eptifibatide 180/1.3* n (%)	Eptifibatide 180/2.0 n (%)
Patients	4577	1451	4604
Overall Incidence of Major Bleeding	425 (9.3%)	152 (10.5%)	498 (10.8%)
Breakdown by Procedure:			
CABG	375 (8.2%)	123 (8.5%)	377 (8.2%)
Angioplasty without CABG	27 (0.6%)	16 (1.1%)	64 (1.4%)
Angiography without angioplasty or CABG	11 (0.2%)	7 (0.5%)	29 (0.6%)
Medical Therapy Only	12 (0.3%)	6 (0.4%)	28 (0.6%)

Denominators are based on the total number of patients whose TIMI classification was resolved.

*Administered only until the first interim analysis

Geriatric Use. The PURSUIT and IMPACT II clinical studies enrolled patients up to the age of 94 years (45% were age 65 and over; 12% were age 75 and older). There was no apparent difference in efficacy between older and younger patients treated with eptifibatide. The incidence of bleeding complications was higher in the elderly in both placebo and eptifibatide groups, and the incremental risk of eptifibatide-associated bleeding was greater in the older patients. No dose adjustment was made for elderly patients, but patients over 75 years of age had to weigh at least 50 kg to be enrolled in the PURSUIT study because of concern about an increased risk of bleeding in this subgroup (see also ADVERSE REACTIONS).

Carcinogenesis, Mutagenesis, Impairment of Fertility. No long-term studies in animals have been performed to evaluate the carcinogenic potential of eptifibatide. Eptifibatide was not genotoxic in the Ames test, the mouse lymphoma cell (L 5178Y, TK$^{+/-}$) forward mutation test, the human lymphocyte chromosome aberration test, or the mouse micronucleus test. Administered by continuous intravenous infusion at total daily doses up to 72 mg/kg/day (about 4 times the recommended maximum daily human dose on a body surface area basis), eptifibatide had no effect on fertility and reproductive performance of male and female rats.

Pregnancy. Pregnancy Category B. Teratology studies have been performed by continuous intravenous infusion of eptifibatide in pregnant rats at total daily doses of up to 72 mg/kg/day (about 4 times the recommended maximum daily human dose on a body surface area basis) and in pregnant rabbits at total daily doses of up to 36 mg/kg/day (also about 4 times the recommended maximum daily human dose on a body surface area basis). These studies revealed no evidence of harm to the fetus due to eptifibatide. There are, however, no adequate and well-controlled studies in pregnant women with eptifibatide. Because animal reproduction studies are not always predictive of human response, eptifibatide should be used during pregnancy only if clearly needed.

Pediatric Use. Safety and effectiveness of eptifibatide in pediatric patients have not been studied.

Nursing Mothers. It is not known whether eptifibatide is excreted in human milk. Because many drugs are excreted in human milk, caution should be exercised when eptifibatide is administered to a nursing mother.

ADVERSE REACTIONS

A total of 14,718 patients were treated in the two Phase III clinical trials (PURSUIT and IMPACT II). Of these, 8737 received eptifibatide: 1300 at 135/0.5 for up to 24 hours, 1286 at 135/0.75 for up to 24 hours, 1472 at 180/1.3 for up to 72 hours, and 4679 at 180/2.0 for up to 72 hours. The other 5981 patients received placebo. These 14,718 patients had a mean age of 62 years (range 20 to 94 years). Eighty-nine percent of the patients were Caucasian, with the remainder being predominantly Black (5%) and Hispanic (5%). Sixty-seven percent were men.

Because of the different regimens used in PURSUIT and IMPACT II, data from the two studies were not pooled.

Bleeding. The incidences of bleeding events and transfusions in the PURSUIT and IMPACT II studies are shown in Table 7. Bleeding was classified as major or minor by the criteria of the TIMI study group. Major bleeding events consisted of intracranial hemorrhage and other bleeding that led to decreases in hemoglobin greater than 5 g/dL. Minor bleeding events included spontaneous gross hematuria, spontaneous hematemesis, other observed blood loss with a hemoglobin decrease of more than 3 g/dL, and other hemoglobin decreases that were greater than 4 g/dL but less than 5 g/dL. In patients who received transfusions, the corresponding loss in hemoglobin was estimated through an adaptation period of the method of Landefeld *et al.*

[See table 7 above]

As shown in Tables 8 and 9, the overall incidence of major bleeding in these studies was strongly related to the inci-

Continued on next page

Integrilin—Cont.

dence of coronary artery bypass graft (CABG) surgery; the excess bleeding seen with eptifibatide, however, was seen only among the patients who did not undergo CABG.
In the PURSUIT study, the greatest increase in major bleeding in eptifibatide-treated patients compared to placebo was associated with bleeding at the femoral artery access site (2.8% versus 1.3%). Oropharyngeal (primarily gingival), genito-urinary, gastrointestinal, and retroperitoneal bleeding were also seen more commonly in eptifibatide-treated patients compared to placebo. Among patients experiencing a major bleed in the IMPACT II study, an increase in bleeding on eptifibatide versus placebo was observed only for the femoral artery access site (3.2% versus 2.8%).
Tables 8 and 9 display the incidence of TIMI major bleeding according to the cardiac procedures carried out in the PURSUIT and IMPACT II studies, respectively. The most common bleeding complications were related to cardiac revascularization (CABG-related or femoral artery access site bleeding).
[See table 8 on previous page]
[See table 9 at right]
In the PURSUIT study, the risk of major bleeding with eptifibatide increased inversely with patient weight. This relationship was most apparent for patients weighing less than 70 kg. These trends were not apparent in the IMPACT II study.
Bleeding adverse events resulting in discontinuation of study drug were more frequent among patients receiving eptifibatide than placebo (8% versus 1% in PURSUIT, 3.5% versus 1.9% in IMPACT II).
Intracranial Hemorrhage and Stroke. Intracranial hemorrhage was rare in the PURSUIT clinical study, with only 3 patients in the placebo group, 1 patient in the group treated with eptifibatide 180/1.3 and 5 patients in the group treated with eptifibatide 180/2.0 experiencing a hemorrhagic stroke within 30 days of randomization. The overall incidence of stroke was 0.5% in patients receiving eptifibatide 180/1.3, 0.7% in patients receiving eptifibatide 180/2.0, and 0.8% in placebo patients within 30 days of randomization.
In the IMPACT II study, intracranial hemorrhage was experienced by 1 patient treated with eptifibatide 135/0.5, 2 patients treated with eptifibatide 135/0.75 and 2 patients in the placebo group. The overall incidence of stroke was 0.5% in patients receiving 135/0.5 eptifibatide, 0.7% in patients receiving eptifibatide 135/0.75 and 0.7% in the placebo group.
Thrombocytopenia. In the PURSUIT and IMPACT II studies, the incidence of thrombocytopenia (<100,000/mm^3 or ≥50% reduction from baseline) and the incidence of platelet transfusions were similar between patients treated with eptifibatide and placebo.
Allergic Reactions. In the IMPACT II study, anaphylaxis was reported in 1 patient (0.08%) on placebo and in no patients on eptifibatide. In the PURSUIT study, anaphylaxis was reported in 7 patients receiving placebo (0.15%) and 7 patients receiving eptifibatide 180/2.0 (0.16%). In the IMPACT II study, 2 patients (1 patient (0.04%) receiving eptifibatide and 1 patient (0.08%) receiving placebo) discontinued study drug because of allergic reactions. In the PURSUIT study, anaphylaxis was given as a reason for drug discontinuation in 3 patients (0.05%) who received eptifibatide and in none of the patients who received placebo.
The potential for development of antibodies to eptifibatide has been studied in 433 subjects. Eptifibatide was non-antigenic in 412 patients receiving a single administration of eptifibatide (135 μg/kg bolus followed by a continuous infusion of either 0.5 μg/kg/min or 0.75 μg/kg/min), and in 21 subjects to whom eptifibatide (135 μg/kg bolus followed by a continuous infusion of 0.75 μg/kg/min) was administered twice, 28 days apart. In both cases, plasma for antibody detection was collected approximately 30 days after each dose. The development of antibodies to eptifibatide at higher doses has not been evaluated.
Other Adverse Reactions. Serious non-bleeding events occurred in 19% of the eptifibatide and 19% of the placebo patients in the PURSUIT study. The only serious non-bleeding adverse event that occurred at a rate of at least 1% and was more common with eptifibatide than placebo (7% versus 6%) was hypotension. Most of the serious non-bleeding events consisted of cardiovascular events typical of an unstable angina population. In the IMPACT II study, serious non-bleeding events that occurred in greater than 1% of patients were uncommon and similar in incidence between placebo- and eptifibatide-treated patients.
Discontinuation of study drug due to adverse events other than bleeding was uncommon in both the PURSUIT and IMPACT II studies, with no single event occurring in >0.5% of the study population. In the PURSUIT study, non-bleeding adverse events leading to discontinuation occurred in the eptifibatide and placebo groups in the following body systems with an incidence of ≥0.1%: cardiovascular system (0.3% and 0.3%), digestive system (0.1% and 0.1%), hemic/lymphatic system (0.1% and 0.1%), nervous system (0.3% and 0.4%), urogenital system (0.1% and 0.1%), and whole body system (0.2% and 0.2%). In the IMPACT II study, non-bleeding adverse events leading to discontinuation occurred in the 135/0.5 eptifibatide and placebo groups in the following body systems with an incidence of ≥0.1%: whole body (0.3% and 0.1%), cardiovascular system (1.4% and 1.4%), digestive system (0.2% and 0%), hemic/lymphatic system (0.2% and 0%), nervous system (0.3% and 0.2%), and respiratory system (0.1% and 0.1%).

Table 9
Major Bleeding by Procedures in the IMPACT II Study

	Placebo n (%)	Eptifibatide 135/0.5 n (%)	Eptifibatide 135/0.75 n (%)
Patients	1230	1249	1245
Overall Incidence of Major Bleeding	55 (4.5%)	55 (4.4%)	58 (4.7%)
Breakdown of Bleeding by Procedure:			
CABG	35 (2.8%)	23 (1.8%)	26 (2.1%)
Angioplasty without CABG	20 (1.6%)	32 (2.6%)	32 (2.7%)

Denominators are based on the total number of patients whose TIMI classification was resolved.

1. INTEGRILIN Dosing Chart by Weight for Patients With Acute Coronary Syndrome (180 μg/kg Bolus and 2μg/kg/min Infusion)

Patient Weight		180μg/kg Bolus Volume	2.0 μg/kg/min Infusion Volume	
(kg)	(lb)	(from 2 mg/mL vial)	(from 2 mg/mL 100-mL vial)	(from 0.75 mg/mL 100-mL vial)
37–41	81–91	3.4 mL	2.0 mL/h	6.0 mL/h
42–46	92–102	4.0 mL	2.5 mL/h	7.0 mL/h
47–53	103–117	4.5 mL	3.0 mL/h	8.0 mL/h
54–59	118–130	5.0 mL	3.5 mL/h	9.0 mL/h
60–65	131–143	5.6 mL	3.8 mL/h	10.0 mL/h
66–71	144–157	6.2 mL	4.0 mL/h	11.0 mL/h
72–78	158–172	6.8 mL	4.5 mL/h	12.0 mL/h
79–84	173–185	7.3 mL	5.0 mL/h	13.0 mL/h
85–90	186–198	7.9 mL	5.3 mL/h	14.0 mL/h
91–96	199–212	8.5 mL	5.6 mL/h	15.0 mL/h
97–103	213–227	9.0 mL	6.0 mL/h	16.0 mL/h
104–109	228–240	9.5 mL	6.4 mL/h	17.0 mL/h
110–115	241–253	10.2 mL	6.8 mL/h	18.0 mL/h
116–121	254–267	10.7 mL	7.0 mL/h	19.0 mL/h
>121	>267	11.3 mL	7.5 mL/h	20.0 mL/h

2. INTEGRILIN Dosing Chart by Weight for Patients Without Acute Coronary Syndromes Undergoing PCI (135 μg/kg Bolus and 0.5 μg/kg/min Infusion)

Patient Weight		135 μg/kg Bolus Volume	0.5 μg/kg/min Infusion Volume	
(kg)	(lb)	(from 2 mg/mL vial)	(from 2 mg/mL 100-mL vial)	(from 0.75 mg/mL 100-mL vial)
40–55	88–121	3.4 mL	0.7 mL/h	2.0 mL/h
56–68	122–150	4.2 mL	0.9 mL/h	2.5 mL/h
69–80	151–176	5.1 mL	1.1 mL/h	3.0 mL/h
81–93	177–205	5.9 mL	1.3 mL/h	3.5 mL/h
94–105	206–231	6.8 mL	1.5 mL/h	4.0 mL/h
106–118	232–260	7.6 mL	1.7 mL/h	4.5 mL/h
119–131	261–288	8.4 mL	1.9 mL/h	5.0 mL/h
132–143	289–315	9.2 mL	2.1 mL/h	5.5 mL/h

OVERDOSAGE

There has been only limited experience with overdosage of eptifibatide. There were 8 patients in the IMPACT II study and 9 patients in the PURSUIT study who received bolus doses and/or infusion doses more than double those called for in the protocols, or who were identified by the investigator as having received an overdose. None of these patients experienced an intracranial bleed or other major bleeding.

Eptifibatide was not lethal to rats, rabbits, or monkeys when administered by continuous intravenous infusion for 90 minutes at a total dose of 45 mg/kg (about 2 to 5 times the recommended maximum daily human dose on a body surface area basis). Symptoms of acute toxicity were loss of righting reflex, dyspnea, ptosis, and decreased muscle tone in rabbits and petechial hemorrhages in the femoral and abdominal areas of monkeys.

DOSAGE AND ADMINISTRATION

The safety and efficacy of eptifibatide has been established in clinical studies that employed concomitant use of heparin and aspirin. Different dose regimens of eptifibatide were used in the major clinical studies. (See CLINICAL STUDIES.)
Acute Coronary Syndrome. The recommended adult dosage of eptifibatide in patients with acute coronary syndrome is an intravenous bolus of 180 μg/kg as soon as possible following diagnosis, followed by a continuous infusion of 2.0 μg/kg/min until hospital discharge or initiation of CABG surgery, up to 72 hours. If a patient is to undergo a percutaneous coronary intervention (PCI) while receiving eptifibatide, consideration can be given to decreasing the infusion rate to 0.5 μg/kg/min (the infusion rate in IMPACT II) at the time of the procedure. Infusion should be continued for an additional 20–24 hours after the procedure, allowing for up to 96 hours of therapy. In the PURSUIT study, patients weighing more than 121 kg received a maximum bolus of 22.6 mg (11.3 mL of the 2 mg/mL injection) followed by a maximum infusion of 15 mg (20 mL of the 0.75 mg/mL injection) per hour.
Percutaneous Coronary Intervention (PCI) in patients not presenting with an acute coronary syndrome. The recommended adult dosage of eptifibatide in patients undergoing PCI and not presenting with an acute coronary syndrome is an intravenous bolus of 135 μg/kg administered immediately before the initiation of PCI followed by a continuous infusion of 0.5 μg/kg/min for 20–24 hours. In the IMPACT II study, there was little experience in patients weighing more than 143 kg.
In patients who undergo coronary artery bypass graft surgery, eptifibatide infusion should be discontinued prior to surgery.
In the clinical trials that showed eptifibatide to be effective, most patients received concomitant aspirin and heparin. The aspirin doses used in the clinical studies were as follows:

Acute Coronary Syndrome (PURSUIT Study)	Angioplasty (IMPACT II Study)
160 mg initially, then 75–325 mg daily	75–325 mg 1–24 hours prior to intervention

The initial target aPTT in the PURSUIT study was 50–70 seconds, and the recommended heparin dosing was:
- if weight ≥70 kg, 5000 U bolus followed by infusion of 1000 U/hr
- if weight <70 kg, 60 U/kg bolus followed by infusion of 12 U/kg/hr

When these patients were to undergo PCI, the target ACT was 300–350 seconds, and the recommended heparin doses were:

Initial Heparin Bolus

ACT (seconds)	Heparin Bolus
<150	100 U/kg (10,000 U maximum)
151–225	75 U/kg
226–299	50 U/kg
≥300	none

Repeat Heparin Bolus*

ACT (seconds)	Heparin Bolus
<275	50 U/kg
275–299	25 U/kg
≥300	none

*based on hourly ACT determinations

In the IMPACT II study, the target ACT was 300–350 seconds before the procedure and ≤ 350 seconds thereafter. The recommended heparin doses were:
• prior to intervention: 100 U/kg bolus
• during intervention: up to 2000 U bolus q15min
• after intervention: infusion at physician's discretion
Patients requiring thrombolytic therapy had eptifibatide infusions stopped and were discontinued from the studies.

Instructions for Administration

1. Like other parenteral drug products, INTEGRILIN solutions should be inspected visually for particulate matter and discoloration prior to administration, whenever solution and container permit.
2. INTEGRILIN may be administered in the same intravenous line as alteplase, atropine, dobutamine, heparin, lidocaine, meperidine, metoprolol, midazolam, morphine, nitroglycerin, or verapamil. INTEGRILIN should not be administered through the same intravenous line as furosemide.
3. INTEGRILIN may be administered in the same IV line with 0.9% NaCl or 0.9% NaCl/5% dextrose. With either vehicle, the infusion may also contain up to 60 mEq/L of potassium chloride. No incompatibilities have been observed with intravenous administration sets. No compatibility studies have been performed with PVC bags.
4. The bolus dose of INTEGRILIN should be withdrawn from the 10-mL vial into a syringe. The bolus dose should be administered by IV push over 1–2 minutes.
5. Immediately following the bolus dose administration, a continuous infusion of INTEGRILIN should be initiated. When using an intravenous infusion pump, INTEGRILIN should be administered undiluted directly from the 100-mL vial. The 100-mL vial should be spiked with a vented infusion set. Care should be taken to center the spike within the circle on the stopper top.

INTEGRILIN is to be administered by volume according to patient weight. Patients should receive study drug according to the following table:
[See table 1 on previous page]
[See table 2 on previous page]

HOW SUPPLIED

INTEGRILIN (eptifibatide) Injection is supplied as a sterile solution in 10-mL vials containing 20 mg of eptifibatide (NDC 0085-1177-01) and 100-mL vials containing either 75 mg of eptifibatide (NDC 0085-1136-01) or 200 mg of eptifibatide (NDC 0085-1177-02).
Vials should be stored refrigerated at 2–8°C (36–46°F). Vials may be transferred to room temperature storage* for a period not to exceed 2 months. Upon transfer, vial cartons must be marked by the dispensing pharmacist with a "DISCARD BY" date (2 months from the transfer date or the labeled expiration date, whichever comes first).
Do not use beyond the labeled expiration date. Protect from light until administration. Discard any unused portion left in the vial.

* USP controlled Room Temperature: 25°C (77°F) with excursions permitted between 15–30°C (59–86°F).

Rx only
Marketed By:
COR Therapeutics, Inc.
South San Francisco, CA 94080
and
Key Pharmaceuticals, Inc.
Kenilworth, NJ 07033
Distributed By:
Key Pharmaceuticals, Inc.
Kenilworth, NJ 07033

Issued December 1999
Rev 6

Shown in Product Identification Guide, page 311

K–DUR® ℞
Microburst Release System®
(Potassium Chloride) USP
Extended Release Tablets

DESCRIPTION

K-DUR® 20 is an immediately dispersing extended release oral dosage form of potassium chloride containing 1500 mg of microencapsulated potassium chloride USP equivalent to 20 mEq of potassium in a tablet.
K-DUR® 10 is an immediately dispersing extended release oral dosage form of potassium chloride containing 750 mg of microencapsulated potassium chloride USP equivalent to 10 mEq of potassium in a tablet.
These formulations are intended to slow the release of potassium so that the likelihood of a high localized concentration of potassium chloride within the gastrointestinal tract is reduced.
K-DUR is an electrolyte replenisher. The chemical name of the active ingredient is potassium chloride, and the structural formula is KCl. Potassium chloride USP occurs as a white, granular powder or as colorless crystals. It is odorless and has a saline taste. Its solutions are neutral to litmus. It is freely soluble in water and insoluble in alcohol.
K-DUR is a tablet formulation (not enteric coated or wax matrix) containing individually microencapsulated potassium chloride crystals which disperse upon tablet disintegration. In simulated gastric fluid at 37°C and in the absence of outside agitation, K-DUR begins disintegrating into microencapsulated crystals within seconds and completely disintegrates within one minute. The microencapsulated crystals are formulated to provide an extended release of potassium chloride.
Inactive Ingredients: Crospovidone, Ethylcellulose, Hydroxypropyl Cellulose, Magnesium Stearate, and Microcrystalline Cellulose.

CLINICAL PHARMACOLOGY

The potassium ion is the principal intracellular cation of most body tissues. Potassium ions participate in a number of essential physiological processes including the maintenance of intracellular tonicity, the transmission of nerve impulses, the contraction of cardiac, skeletal and smooth muscle and the maintenance of normal renal function.
The intracellular concentration of potassium is approximately 150 to 160 mEq per liter. The normal adult plasma concentration is 3.5 to 5 mEq per liter. An active ion transport system maintains this gradient across the plasma membrane.
Potassium is a normal dietary constituent and under steady state conditions the amount of potassium absorbed from the gastrointestinal tract is equal to the amount excreted in the urine. The usual dietary intake of potassium is 50 to 100 mEq per day.
Potassium depletion will occur whenever the rate of potassium loss through renal excretion and/or loss from the gastrointestinal tract exceeds the rate of potassium intake. Such depletion usually develops as a consequence of therapy with diuretics, primary or secondary hyperaldosteronism, diabetic ketoacidosis, or inadequate replacement of potassium in patients on prolonged parenteral nutrition. Depletion can develop rapidly with severe diarrhea, especially if associated with vomiting. Potassium depletion due to these causes is usually accompanied by a concomitant loss of chloride and is manifested by hypokalemia and metabolic alkalosis. Potassium depletion may produce weakness, fatigue, disturbances of cardiac rhythm (primarily ectopic beats), prominent U-waves in the electrocardiogram, and in advanced cases, flaccid paralysis and/or impaired ability to concentrate urine.
If potassium depletion associated with metabolic alkalosis cannot be managed by correcting the fundamental cause of the deficiency, e.g., where the patient requires long term diuretic therapy, supplemental potassium in the form of high potassium food or potassium chloride may be able to restore normal potassium levels.
In rare circumstances (e.g., patients with renal tubular acidosis) potassium depletion may be associated with metabolic acidosis and hyperchloremia. In such patients potassium replacement should be accomplished with potassium salts other than the chloride, such as potassium bicarbonate, potassium citrate, potassium acetate, or potassium gluconate.

INDICATIONS AND USAGE

BECAUSE OF REPORTS OF INTESTINAL AND GASTRIC ULCERATION AND BLEEDING WITH CONTROLLED RELEASE POTASSIUM CHLORIDE PREPARATIONS, THESE DRUGS SHOULD BE RESERVED FOR THOSE PATIENTS WHO CANNOT TOLERATE OR REFUSE TO TAKE LIQUID OR EFFERVESCENT POTASSIUM PREPARATIONS OR FOR PATIENTS IN WHOM THERE IS A PROBLEM OF COMPLIANCE WITH THESE PREPARATIONS.

1. For the treatment of patients with hypokalemia with or without metabolic alkalosis, in digitalis intoxication and in patients with hypokalemic familial periodic paralysis. If hypokalemia is the result of diuretic therapy, consideration should be given to the use of a lower dose of diuretic, which may be sufficient without leading to hypokalemia.
2. For the prevention of hypokalemia in patients who would be at particular risk if hypokalemia were to develop, e.g., digitalized patients or patients with significant cardiac arrhythmias.

The use of potassium salts in patients receiving diuretics for uncomplicated essential hypertension is often unnecessary when such patients have a normal dietary pattern and when low doses of the diuretic are used. Serum potassium should be checked periodically, however, and if hypokalemia occurs, dietary supplementation with potassium-containing foods may be adequate to control milder cases. In more severe cases, and if dose adjustment of the diuretic is ineffective or unwarranted, supplementation with potassium salts may be indicated.

CONTRAINDICATIONS

Potassium supplements are contraindicated in patients with hyperkalemia since a further increase in serum potassium concentration in such patients can produce cardiac arrest. Hyperkalemia may complicate any of the following conditions: chronic renal failure, systemic acidosis such as diabetic acidosis, acute dehydration, extensive tissue breakdown as in severe burns, adrenal insufficiency, or the administration of a potassium-sparing diuretic (e.g., spironolactone, triamterene, amiloride) (see **OVERDOSAGE).**
Controlled release formulations of potassium chloride have produced esophageal ulceration in certain cardiac patients with esophageal compression due to enlarged left atrium. Potassium supplementation, when indicated in such patients, should be given as a liquid preparation or as an aqueous (water) suspension of K-DUR (see **PRECAUTIONS; Information for Patients,** and **DOSAGE AND ADMINISTRATION** sections).
All solid oral dosage forms of potassium chloride are contraindicated in any patient in whom there is structural, pathological (e.g., diabetic gastroparesis) or pharmacologic (use of anticholinergic agents or other agents with anticholinergic properties at sufficient doses to exert anticholinergic effects) cause for arrest or delay in tablet passage through the gastrointestinal tract.

WARNINGS

Hyperkalemia (see **OVERDOSAGE**)—In patients with impaired mechanisms for excreting potassium, the administration of potassium salts can produce hyperkalemia and cardiac arrest. This occurs most commonly in patients given potassium by the intravenous route but may also occur in patients given potassium orally. Potentially fatal hyperkalemia can develop rapidly and be asymptomatic. The use of potassium salts in patients with chronic renal disease, or any other condition which impairs potassium excretion, requires particularly careful monitoring of the serum potassium concentration and appropriate dosage adjustment.
Interaction with Potassium Sparing Diuretics—Hypokalemia should not be treated by the concomitant administration of potassium salts and a potassium-sparing diuretic (e.g., spironolactone, triamterene or amiloride) since the simultaneous administration of these agents can produce severe hyperkalemia.
Interaction with Angiotensin Converting Enzyme Inhibitors—Angiotensin converting enzyme (ACE) inhibitors (e.g., captopril, enalapril) will produce some potassium retention by inhibiting aldosterone production. Potassium supplements should be given to patients receiving ACE inhibitors only with close monitoring.
Gastrointestinal Lesions—Solid oral dosage forms of potassium chloride can produce ulcerative and/or stenotic lesions of the gastrointestinal tract. Based on spontaneous adverse reaction reports, enteric coated preparations of potassium chloride are associated with an increased frequency of small bowel lesions (40–50 per 100,000 patient years) compared to sustained release wax matrix formulations (less than one per 100,000 patient years). Because of the lack of extensive marketing experience with microencapsulated products, a comparison between such products and wax matrix or enteric coated products is not available. K-DUR is a tablet formulated to provide a controlled rate of release of microencapsulated potassium chloride and thus to minimize the possibility of a high local concentration of potassium near the gastrointestinal wall.
Prospective trials have been conducted in normal human volunteers in which the upper gastrointestinal tract was evaluated by endoscopic inspection before and after one week of solid oral potassium chloride therapy. The ability of this model to predict events occurring in usual clinical practice is unknown. Trials which approximated usual clinical practice did not reveal any clear differences between the wax matrix and microencapsulated dosage forms. In contrast, there was a higher incidence of gastric and duodenal lesions in subjects receiving a high dose of a wax matrix controlled release formulation under conditions which did not resemble usual or recommended clinical practice (i.e., 96 mEq per day in divided doses of potassium chloride administered to fasted patients, in the presence of an anticholinergic drug to delay gastric emptying). The upper gastrointestinal lesions observed by endoscopy were asymptomatic and were not accompanied by evidence of bleeding (Hemoccult testing). The relevance of these findings to the usual conditions (i.e., non-fasting, no anticholinergic agent, smaller doses) under which controlled release potassium chloride products are used is uncertain; epidemiologic studies have not identified an elevated risk, compared to microencapsulated products, for upper gastrointestinal lesions in patients receiving wax matrix formulations. K-DUR should be discontinued immediately and the possibility of ulceration, obstruction or perforation considered if severe vomiting, abdominal pain, distention, or gastrointestinal bleeding occurs.
Metabolic Acidosis—Hypokalemia in patients with metabolic acidosis should be treated with an alkalinizing potassium salt such as potassium bicarbonate, potassium citrate, potassium acetate, or potassium gluconate.

PRECAUTIONS

General: The diagnosis of potassium depletion is ordinarily made by demonstrating hypokalemia in a patient with a clinical history suggesting some cause for potassium depletion. In interpreting the serum potassium level, the physician should bear in mind that acute alkalosis per se can produce hypokalemia in the absence of a deficit in total body potassium while acute acidosis per se can increase the serum potassium concentration into the normal range even in the presence of a reduced total body potassium. The treatment of potassium depletion, particularly in the presence of cardiac disease, renal disease, or acidosis requires careful attention to acid-base balance and appropriate monitoring of serum electrolytes, the electrocardiogram, and the clinical status of the patient.
Information for Patients: Physicians should consider reminding the patient of the following:
To take each dose with meals and with a full glass of water or other liquid.
To take each dose without crushing, chewing, or sucking the tablets. If those patients are having difficulty swallowing whole tablets, they may try one of the following alternate methods of administration:

Continued on next page

K-Dur—Cont.

a. Break the tablet in half, and take each half separately with a glass of water.
b. Prepare an aqueous (water) suspension as follows:
   1. Place the whole tablet(s) in approximately one-half glass of water (4 fluid ounces).
   2. Allow approximately 2 minutes for the tablet(s) to disintegrate.
   3. Stir for about half a minute after the tablet(s) has disintegrated.
   4. Swirl the suspension and consume the entire contents of the glass immediately by drinking or by the use of a straw.
   5. Add another one fluid ounce of water, swirl, and consume immediately.
   6. Then, add an additional one fluid ounce of water, swirl, and consume immediately.

Aqueous suspension of K-DUR tablets that is not taken immediately should be discarded. The use of other liquids for suspending K-DUR tablets is not recommended.
To take this medicine following the frequency and amount prescribed by the physician. This is especially important if the patient is also taking diuretics and/or digitalis preparations.
To check with the physician at once if tarry stools or other evidence of gastrointestinal bleeding is noticed.
Laboratory Tests: When blood is drawn for analysis of plasma potassium it is important to recognize that artifactual elevations can occur after improper venipuncture technique or as a result of in-vitro hemolysis of the sample.
Drug Interactions: Potassium-sparing diuretics, angiotensin converting enzyme inhibitors (see **WARNINGS**).
Carcinogenesis, Mutagenesis, Impairment of Fertility: Carcinogenicity, mutagenicity and fertility studies in animals have not been performed. Potassium is a normal dietary constituent.
Pregnancy Category C: Animal reproduction studies have not been conducted with K-DUR. It is unlikely that potassium supplementation that does not lead to hyperkalemia would have an adverse effect on the fetus or would affect reproductive capacity.
Nursing Mothers: The normal potassium ion content of human milk is about 13 mEq per liter. Since oral potassium becomes part of the body potassium pool, so long as body potassium is not excessive, the contribution of potassium chloride supplementation should have little or no effect on the level in human milk.
Pediatric Use: Safety and effectiveness in children have not been established.

ADVERSE REACTIONS

One of the most severe adverse effects is hyperkalemia (see **CONTRAINDICATIONS**, **WARNINGS**, and **OVERDOSAGE**). There have also been reports of upper and lower gastrointestinal conditions including obstruction, bleeding, ulceration, and perforation (see **CONTRAINDICATIONS** and **WARNINGS**).
The most common adverse reactions to oral potassium salts are nausea, vomiting, flatulence, abdominal pain/discomfort, and diarrhea. These symptoms are due to irritation of the gastrointestinal tract and are best managed by diluting the preparation further, taking the dose with meals or reducing the amount taken at one time.

OVERDOSAGE

The administration of oral potassium salts to persons with normal excretory mechanisms for potassium rarely causes serious hyperkalemia. However, if excretory mechanisms are impaired or if potassium is administered too rapidly intravenously, potentially fatal hyperkalemia can result (see **CONTRAINDICATIONS** and **WARNINGS**). It is important to recognize that hyperkalemia is usually asymptomatic and may be manifested only by an increased serum potassium concentration (6.5–8.0 mEq/L) and characteristic electrocardiographic changes (peaking of T-waves, loss of P-waves, depression of S-T segment, and prolongation of the QT-interval). Late manifestations include muscle-paralysis and cardiovascular collapse from cardiac arrest. (9–12 mEq/L).
Treatment measures for hyperkalemia include the following:

1. Elimination of foods and medications containing potassium and of any agents with potassium-sparing properties.
2. Intravenous administration of 300 to 500 mL/hr of 10% dextrose solution containing 10–20 units of crystalline insulin per 1,000 mL.
3. Correction of acidosis, if present, with intravenous sodium bicarbonate.
4. Use of exchange resins, hemodialysis, or peritoneal dialysis.

In treating hyperkalemia, it should be recalled that in patients who have been stabilized on digitalis, too rapid a lowering of the serum potassium concentration can produce digitalis toxicity.

DOSAGE AND ADMINISTRATION

The usual dietary intake of potassium by the average adult is 50 to 100 mEq per day. Potassium depletion sufficient to cause hypokalemia usually requires the loss of 200 or more mEq of potassium from the total body store.
Dosage must be adjusted to the individual needs of each patient. The dose for the prevention of hypokalemia is typically in the range of 20 mEq per day. Doses of 40–100 mEq per day or more are used for the treatment of potassium depletion. Dosage should be divided if more than 20 mEq per day is given such that no more than 20 mEq is given in a single dose.
Each K-DUR 20 tablet provides 20 mEq of potassium chloride.
Each K-DUR 10 tablet provides 10 mEq of potassium chloride.
K-DUR tablets should be taken with meals and with a glass of water or other liquid. This product should not be taken on an empty stomach because of its potential for gastric irritation (see **WARNINGS**).
Patients having difficulty swallowing whole tablets may try one of the following alternate methods of administration:
a. Break the tablet in half, and take each half separately with a glass of water.
b. Prepare an aqueous (water) suspension as follows:
   1. Place the whole tablet(s) in approximately one-half glass of water (4 fluid ounces).
   2. Allow approximately 2 minutes for the tablet(s) to disintegrate.
   3. Stir for about half a minute after the tablet(s) has disintegrated.
   4. Swirl the suspension and consume the entire contents of the glass immediately by drinking or by the use of a straw.
   5. Add another one fluid ounce of water, swirl, and consume immediately.
   6. Then, add an additional one fluid ounce of water, swirl, and consume immediately.

Aqueous suspension of K-DUR tablets that is not taken immediately should be discarded. The use of other liquids for suspending K-DUR tablets is not recommended.

HOW SUPPLIED

K-DUR 20 mEq Extended Release Tablets are available in bottles of 100 (NDC 0085-0787-01); bottles of 500 (NDC 0085-0787-06); bottles of 1000 (NDC 0085-0787-10) and boxes of 100 for unit dose dispensing (NDC 0085-0787-81). K-DUR 20 mEq tablets are white, oblong, imprinted K-DUR 20 and scored for flexibility of dosing.
K-DUR 10 mEq Extended Release Tablets are available in bottles of 100 (NDC 0085-0263-01) and boxes of 100 for unit dose dispensing (NDC 0085-0263-81). K-DUR 10 mEq tablets are white, oblong, imprinted K-DUR 10.

STORAGE CONDITIONS

Keep tightly closed. Store at controlled room temperature 15–30°C (59–86°F).

CAUTION

Federal law prohibits dispensing without prescription.
Rev. 4/90 14274766

Shown in Product Identification Guide, page 319

NITRO-DUR® ℞
(nitroglycerin)
Transdermal Infusion System

DESCRIPTION

Nitroglycerin is 1,2,3-propanetriol trinitrate, an organic nitrate whose structural formula is:

$$\begin{array}{c} H_2CONO_2 \\ | \\ HCONO_2 \\ | \\ H_2CONO_2 \end{array}$$

and whose molecular weight is 227.09. The organic nitrates are vasodilators, active on both arteries and veins.
The NITRO-DUR (nitroglycerin) Transdermal Infusion System is a flat unit designed to provide continuous controlled release of nitroglycerin through intact skin. The rate of release of nitroglycerin is linearly dependent upon the area of the applied system; each cm^2 of applied system delivers approximately 0.02 mg of nitroglycerin per hour. Thus, the 5-, 10-, 15-, 20-, 30-, and 40-cm^2 systems deliver approximately 0.1, 0.2, 0.3, 0.4, 0.6, and 0.8 mg of nitroglycerin per hour, respectively.
The remainder of the nitroglycerin in each system serves as a reservoir and is not delivered in normal use. After 12 hours, for example, each system has delivered approximately 6% of its original content of nitroglycerin.
The NITRO-DUR transdermal system contains nitroglycerin in acrylic-based polymer adhesives with a resinous cross-linking agent to provide a continuous source of active ingredient. Each unit is sealed in a paper polyethylene-foil pouch.

Cross section of the system.

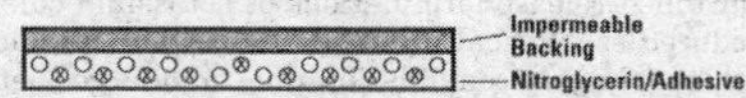

CLINICAL PHARMACOLOGY

The principal pharmacological action of nitroglycerin is relaxation of vascular smooth muscle and consequent dilatation of peripheral arteries and veins, especially the latter. Dilatation of the veins promotes peripheral pooling of blood and decreases venous return to the heart, thereby reducing left ventricular end-diastolic pressure and pulmonary capillary wedge pressure (preload). Arteriolar relaxation reduces systemic vascular resistance, systolic arterial pressure, and mean arterial pressure (afterload). Dilatation of the coronary arteries also occurs. The relative importance of preload reduction, afterload reduction, and coronary dilatation remains undefined.
Dosing regimens for most chronically used drugs are designed to provide plasma concentrations that are continuously greater than a minimally effective concentration. This strategy is inappropriate for organic nitrates. Several well-controlled clinical trials have used exercise testing to assess the antianginal efficacy of continuously delivered nitrates. In the large majority of these trials, active agents were indistinguishable from placebo after 24 hours (or less) of continuous therapy. Attempts to overcome nitrate tolerance by dose escalation, even to doses far in excess of those used acutely, have consistently failed. Only after nitrates have been absent from the body for several hours has their antianginal efficacy been restored.
Pharmacokinetics:
The volume of distribution of nitroglycerin is about 3 L/kg, and nitroglycerin is cleared from this volume at extremely rapid rates, with a resulting serum half-life of about 3 minutes. The observed clearance rates (close to 1 L/kg/min) greatly exceed hepatic blood flow; known sites of extrahepatic metabolism include red blood cells and vascular walls. The first products in the metabolism of nitroglycerin are inorganic nitrate and the 1,2- and 1,3-dinitroglycerols. The dinitrates are less effective vasodilators than nitroglycerin, but they are longer-lived in the serum, and their net contribution to the overall effect of chronic nitroglycerin regimens is not known. The dinitrates are further metabolized to (nonvasoactive) mononitrates and, ultimately, to glycerol and carbon dioxide.
To avoid development of tolerance to nitroglycerin, drug-free intervals of 10 to 12 hours are known to be sufficient; shorter intervals have not been well studied. In one well-controlled clinical trial, subjects receiving nitroglycerin appeared to exhibit a rebound or withdrawal effect, so that their exercise tolerance at the end of the daily drug-free interval was *less* than that exhibited by the parallel group receiving placebo.
In healthy volunteers, steady-state plasma concentrations of nitroglycerin are reached by about 2 hours after application of a patch and are maintained for the duration of wearing the system (observations have been limited to 24 hours). Upon removal of the patch, the plasma concentration declines with a half-life of about an hour.
Clinical Trials:
Regimens in which nitroglycerin patches were worn for 12 hours daily have been studied in well-controlled trials up to 4 weeks in duration. Starting about 2 hours after application and continuing until 10 to 12 hours after application, patches that deliver at least 0.4 mg of nitroglycerin per hour have consistently demonstrated greater antianginal activity than placebo. Lower-dose patches have not been as well studied, but in one large, well-controlled trial in which higher-dose patches were also studied, patches delivering 0.2 mg/hr had significantly *less* antianginal activity than placebo.
It is reasonable to believe that the rate of nitroglycerin absorption from patches may vary with the site of application, but this relationship has not been adequately studied.

INDICATIONS AND USAGE

Transdermal nitroglycerin is indicated for the prevention of angina pectoris due to coronary artery disease. The onset of action of transdermal nitroglycerin is not sufficiently rapid for this product to be useful in aborting an acute attack.

CONTRAINDICATIONS

Allergic reactions to organic nitrates are extremely rare, but they do occur. Nitroglycerin is contraindicated in patients who are allergic to it. Allergy to the adhesives used in nitroglycerin patches has also been reported, and it similarly constitutes a contraindication to the use of this product.

WARNINGS

Amplification of the vasodilatory effects of the NITRO-DUR patch by sildenafil can result in severe hypotension. The time course and dose dependence of this interaction have not been studied. Appropriate supportive care has not been studied, but it seems reasonable to treat this as a nitrate overdose, with elevation of the extremities and with central volume expansion.
The benefits of transdermal nitroglycerin in patients with acute myocardial infarction or congestive heart failure have not been established. If one elects to use nitroglycerin in these conditions, careful clinical or hemodynamic monitoring must be used to avoid the hazards of hypotension and tachycardia.
A cardioverter/defibrillator should not be discharged through a paddle electrode that overlies a NITRO-DUR patch. The arcing that may be seen in this situation is harmless in itself, but it may be associated with local current concentration that can cause damage to the paddles and burns to the patient.

PRECAUTIONS

General:
Severe hypotension, particularly with upright posture, may occur with even small doses of nitroglycerin. This drug should therefore be used with caution in patients who may

be volume depleted or who, for whatever reason, are already hypotensive. Hypotension induced by nitroglycerin may be accompanied by paradoxical bradycardia and increased angina pectoris.
Nitrate therapy may aggravate the angina caused by hypertrophic cardiomyopathy.
As tolerance to other forms of nitroglycerin develops, the effects of sublingual nitroglycerin on exercise tolerance, although still observable, is somewhat blunted.
In industrial workers who have had long-term exposure to unknown (presumably high) doses of organic nitrates, tolerance clearly occurs. Chest pain, acute myocardial infarction, and even sudden death have occurred during temporary withdrawal of nitrates from these workers, demonstrating the existence of true physical dependence.
Several clinical trials in patients with angina pectoris have evaluated nitroglycerin regimens which incorporated a 10- to 12-hour, nitrate-free interval. In some of these trials, an increase in the frequency of anginal attacks during the nitrate-free interval was observed in a small number of patients. In one trial, patients had decreased exercise tolerance at the end of the nitrate-free interval. Hemodynamic rebound has been observed only rarely; on the other hand, few studies were so designed that rebound, if it had occurred, would have been detected. The importance of these observations to the routine, clinical use of transdermal nitroglycerin is unknown.

Information for Patients:
Daily headaches sometimes accompany treatment with nitroglycerin. In patients who get these headaches, the headaches may be a marker of the activity of the drug. Patients should resist the temptation to avoid headaches by altering the schedule of their treatment with nitroglycerin, since loss of headache may be associated with simultaneous loss of antianginal efficacy.
Treatment with nitroglycerin may be associated with lightheadedness on standing, especially just after rising from a recumbent or seated position. This effect may be more frequent in patients who have also consumed alcohol.
After normal use, there is enough residual nitroglycerin in discarded patches that they are a potential hazard to children and pets.
A patient leaflet is supplied with the systems.

Drug Interactions:
The vasodilating effects of nitroglycerin may be additive with those of other vasodilators. Alcohol, in particular, has been found to exhibit additive effects of this variety.

Carcinogenesis, Mutagenesis, Impairment of Fertility:
Animal carcinogenesis studies with topically applied nitroglycerin have not been performed.
Rats receiving up to 434 mg/kg/day of dietary nitroglycerin for 2 years developed dose-related fibrotic and neoplastic changes in liver, including carcinomas, and interstitial cell tumors in testes. At high dose, the incidences of hepatocellular carcinomas in both sexes were 52% vs 0% in controls, and incidences of testicular tumors were 52% vs 8% in controls. Lifetime dietary administration of up to 1058 mg/kg/day of nitroglycerin was not tumorigenic in mice.
Nitroglycerin was weakly mutagenic in Ames tests performed in two different laboratories. Nevertheless, there was no evidence of mutagenicity in an *in vivo* dominant lethal assay with male rats treated with doses up to about 363 mg/kg/day, po, or in *in vitro* cytogenetic tests in rat and dog tissues.
In a three-generation reproduction study, rats received dietary nitroglycerin at doses up to about 434 mg/kg/day for 6 months prior to mating of the F_0 generation with treatment continuing through successive F_1 and F_2 generations. The high dose was associated with decreased feed intake and body weight gain in both sexes at all matings. No specific effect on the fertility of the F_0 generation was seen. Infertility noted in subsequent generations, however, was attributed to increased interstitial cell tissue and aspermatogenesis in the high-dose males. In this three-generation study there was no clear evidence of teratogenicity.

Pregnancy: Pregnancy Category C:
Animal teratology studies have not been conducted with nitroglycerin transdermal systems. Teratology studies in rats and rabbits, however, were conducted with topically applied nitroglycerin ointment at doses up to 80 mg/kg/day and 240 mg/kg/day, respectively. No toxic effects on dams or fetuses were seen at any dose tested. There are no adequate and well-controlled studies in pregnant women. Nitroglycerin should be given to a pregnant woman only if clearly needed.

Nursing Mothers:
It is not known whether nitroglycerin is excreted in human milk. Because many drugs are excreted in human milk, caution should be exercised when nitroglycerin is administered to a nursing woman.

Pediatric Use:
Safety and effectiveness in pediatric patients have not been established.

ADVERSE REACTIONS

Adverse reactions to nitroglycerin are generally dose related, and almost all of these reactions are the result of nitroglycerin's activity as a vasodilator. Headache, which may be severe, is the most commonly reported side effect. Headache may be recurrent with each daily dose, especially at higher doses. Transient episodes of lightheadedness, occasionally related to blood pressure changes, may also occur. Hypotension occurs infrequently, but in some patients it may be severe enough to warrant discontinuation of therapy. Syncope, crescendo angina, and rebound hypertension have been reported but are uncommon.
Allergic reactions to nitroglycerin are also uncommon, and the great majority of those reported have been cases of contact dermatitis or fixed drug eruptions in patients receiving nitroglycerin in ointments or patches. There have been a few reports of genuine anaphylactoid reactions, and these reactions can probably occur in patients receiving nitroglycerin by any route.
Extremely rarely, ordinary doses of organic nitrates have caused methemoglobinemia in normal-seeming patients. Methemoglobinemia is so infrequent at these doses that further discussion of its diagnosis and treatment is deferred (see **OVERDOSAGE**).
Application-site irritation may occur but is rarely severe.
In two placebo-controlled trials of intermittent therapy with nitroglycerin patches at 0.2 to 0.8 mg/hr, the most frequent adverse reactions among 307 subjects were as follows:

	Placebo	Patch
Headache	18%	63%
Lightheadedness	4%	6%
Hypotension, and/or Syncope	0%	4%
Increased Angina	2%	2%

OVERDOSAGE

Hemodynamic Effects:
The ill effects of nitroglycerin overdose are generally the results of nitroglycerin's capacity to induce vasodilatation, venous pooling, reduced cardiac output, and hypotension. These hemodynamic changes may have protean manifestations, including increased intracranial pressure, with any or all of persistent throbbing headache, confusion, and moderate fever; vertigo; palpitations; visual disturbances; nausea and vomiting (possibly with colic and even bloody diarrhea); syncope (especially in the upright posture); air hunger and dyspnea, later followed by reduced ventilatory effort; diaphoresis, with the skin either flushed or cold and clammy; heart block and bradycardia; paralysis; coma; seizures; and death.
Laboratory determinations of serum levels of nitroglycerin and its metabolites are not widely available, and such determinations have, in any event, no established role in the management of nitroglycerin overdose.
No data are available to suggest physiological maneuvers (eg, maneuvers to change the pH of the urine) that might accelerate elimination of nitroglycerin and its active metabolites. Similarly, it is not known which – if any – of these substances can usefully be removed from the body by hemodialysis.
No specific antagonist to the vasodilator effects of nitroglycerin is known, and no intervention has been subject to controlled study as a therapy of nitroglycerin overdose. Because the hypotension associated with nitroglycerin overdose is the result of venodilatation and arterial hypovolemia, prudent therapy in this situation should be directed toward increase in central fluid volume. Passive elevation of the patient's legs may be sufficient, but intravenous infusion of normal saline or similar fluid may also be necessary.
The use of epinephrine or other arterial vasoconstrictors in this setting is likely to do more harm than good.
In patients with renal disease or congestive heart failure, therapy resulting in central volume expansion is not without hazard. Treatment of nitroglycerin overdose in these patients may be subtle and difficult, and invasive monitoring may be required.

Methemoglobinemia:
Nitrate ions liberated during metabolism of nitroglycerin can oxidize hemoglobin into methemoglobin. Even in patients totally without cytochrome b_5 reductase activity, however, and even assuming that the nitrate moieties of nitroglycerin are quantitatively applied to oxidation of hemoglobin, about 1 mg/kg of nitroglycerin should be required before any of these patients manifests clinically significant (≥10%) methemoglobinemia. In patients with normal reductase function, significant production of methemoglobin should require even larger doses of nitroglycerin. In one study in which 36 patients received 2 to 4 weeks of continuous nitroglycerin therapy at 3.1 to 4.4 mg/hr, the average methemoglobin level measured was 0.2%; this was comparable to that observed in parallel patients who received placebo.
Notwithstanding these observations, there are case reports of significant methemoglobinemia in association with moderate overdoses of organic nitrates. None of the affected patients had been thought to be unusually susceptible.
Methemoglobin levels are available from most clinical laboratories. The diagnosis should be suspected in patients who exhibit signs of impaired oxygen delivery despite adequate cardiac output and adequate arterial PO_2. Classically, methemoglobinemic blood is described as chocolate brown, without color change on exposure to air.
When methemoglobinemia is diagnosed, the treatment of choice is methylene blue, 1–2 mg/kg intravenously.

DOSAGE AND ADMINISTRATION

The suggested starting dose is between 0.2 mg/hr* and 0.4 mg/hr*. Doses between 0.4 mg/hr* and 0.8 mg/hr* have shown continued effectiveness for 10 to 12 hours daily for at least 1 month (the longest period studied) of intermittent administration. Although the minimum nitrate-free interval has not been defined, data show that a nitrate-free interval of 10 to 12 hours is sufficient (see **CLINICAL PHARMACOLOGY**). Thus, an appropriate dosing schedule for nitroglycerin patches would include a daily patch-on period of 12 to 14 hours and a daily patch-off period of 10 to 12 hours.

*Release rates were formerly described in terms of drug delivered per 24 hours. In these terms, the supplied NITRO-DUR systems would be rated at 2.5 mg/24 hours (0.1 mg/hour), 5 mg/24 hours (0.2 mg/hour), 7.5 mg/24 hours (0.3 mg/hour), 10 mg/24 hours (0.4 mg/hour), and 15 mg/24 hours (0.6 mg/hour).

Although some well-controlled clinical trials using exercise tolerance testing have shown maintenance of effectiveness when patches are worn continuously, the large majority of such controlled trials have shown the development of tolerance (ie, complete loss of effect) within the first 24 hours after therapy was initiated. Dose adjustment, even to levels much higher than generally used, did not restore efficacy.

HOW SUPPLIED

NITRO-DUR System Rated Release *In Vivo**	Total Nitroglycerin Content	System Size	Package Size
0.1 mg/hr	20 mg	5 cm²	Unit Dose 30 (NDC 0085-3305-30) Hospital Unit Dose 100 (NDC 0085-3305-01) Institutional Package 30 (NDC 0085-3305-35)
0.2 mg/hr	40 mg	10 cm²	Unit Dose 30 (NDC 0085-3310-30) Hospital Unit Dose 100 (NDC 0085-3310-01) Institutional Package 30 (NDC 0085-3310-35)
0.3 mg/hr	60 mg	15 cm²	Unit Dose 30 (NDC 0085-3315-30) Hospital Unit Dose 100 (NDC 0085-3315-01) Institutional Package 30 (NDC 0085-3315-35)
0.4 mg/hr	80 mg	20 cm²	Unit Dose 30 (NDC 0085-3320-30) Hospital Unit Dose 100 (NDC 0085-3320-01) Institutional Package 30 (NDC 0085-3320-35)
0.6 mg/hr	120 mg	30 cm²	Unit Dose 30 (NDC 0085-3330-30) Hospital Unit Dose 100 (NDC 0085-3330-01) Institutional Package 30 (NDC 0085-3330-35)
0.8 mg/hr	160 mg	40 cm²	Unit Dose 30 (NDC 0085-0819-30) Hospital Unit Dose 100 (NDC 0085-0819-01) Institutional Package 30 (NDC 0085-0819-35)

*Release rates were formerly described in terms of drug delivered per 24 hours. In these terms, the supplied NITRO-DUR systems would be rated at 2.5 mg/ 24 hours (0.1 mg/hour), 5 mg/24 hours (0.2 mg/hour), 7.5 mg/24 hours (0.3 mg/hour), 10 mg/24 hours (0.4 mg/hour), and 15 mg/24 hours (0.6 mg/hour).

Store between 15° and 30°C (59° and 86°F). Do not refrigerate.
CAUTION: Federal law prohibits dispensing without prescription.
KEY®
Key Pharmaceuticals, Inc.
Kenilworth, NJ 07033 USA
Rev. 10/99 18143631
U.S. Patent No. 5,186,938

Shown in Product Identification Guide, page 319

THEO-DUR® ℞
(theophylline)
Extended-Release Tablets

Some of the information contained in this insert (eg, information regarding pediatric patients under the age of 12) was derived from FDA's Class Labeling Guidance for Immediate-Release Theophylline Products and is intended for informational purposes only.

DESCRIPTION

THEO-DUR® Extended-Release Tablets contain anhydrous theophylline in an extended-release formulation for oral administration which allows a 12-hour dosing interval for a majority of patients and a 24-hour dosing interval for selected patients (see **DOSAGE AND ADMINISTRATION** for a description of appropriate patient populations).

Continued on next page

Theo-Dur—Cont.

Theophylline:
Theophylline is a bronchodilator, structurally classified as a methylxanthine. It occurs as a white, odorless, crystalline powder with a bitter taste. Anhydrous theophylline has the chemical name 1*H*-Purine-2,6-dione,3,7-dihydro-1,3-dimethyl-, and is represented by the following structural formula:

The molecular formula of anhydrous theophylline is $C_7H_8N_4O_2$ with a molecular weight of 180.17.
THEO-DUR Extended-Release Tablets contain no color additives and are available in four strengths: 100 mg, 200 mg, 300 mg, and 450 mg.
The inactive ingredients for THEO-DUR 100 mg Extended-Release Tablets include: acacia, NF; acetone; alcohol, NF; cellulose acetate phthalate, NF; cetyl alcohol, NF; chloroform; confectioner's sugar 6X, NF; corn starch, NF; diethyl phthalate, NF; ethyl acetate, NF; glyceryl monostearate; isopropyl alcohol, USP; hydrous spray dried lactose, NF; magnesium stearate, NF; myristyl alcohol, NF; nonpareil seeds 18–20 mesh, NF; purified water, USP; sodium lauryl sulfate, NF; talc, USP; and white wax, NF.
The inactive ingredients for THEO-DUR 200 mg, 300 mg, and 450 mg Extended-Release Tablets include: acetone; cellulose acetate phthalate, NF; cetyl alcohol, NF; diethyl phthalate; glyceryl monostearate; hydroxypropyl methylcellulose 2910, USP; isopropyl alcohol, NF; anhydrous lactose, NF; magnesium stearate, NF; myristyl alcohol; nonpareil seeds 18–20 mesh, NF; purified water, USP; and white wax, NF.

CLINICAL PHARMACOLOGY

Mechanism of Action:
Theophylline has two distinct actions in the airways of patients with reversible obstruction; smooth muscle relaxation (ie, bronchodilation) and suppression of the response of the airways to stimuli (ie, nonbronchodilator prophylactic effects). While the mechanisms of action of theophylline are not known with certainty, studies in animals suggest that bronchodilation is mediated by the inhibition of two isozymes of phosphodiesterase (PDE III and, to a lesser extent, PDE IV) while nonbronchodilator prophylactic actions are probably mediated through one or more different molecular mechanisms that do not involve inhibition of PDE III or antagonism of adenosine receptors. Some of the adverse effects associated with theophylline appear to be mediated by inhibition of PDE III (eg, hypotension, tachycardia, headache, and emesis) and adenosine receptor antagonism (eg, alterations in cerebral blood flow).
Theophylline increases the force of contraction of diaphragmatic muscles. This action appears to be due to enhancement of calcium uptake through an adenosine-mediated channel.

Serum Concentration-Effect Relationship:
Bronchodilation occurs over the serum theophylline concentration range of 5–20 mcg/mL. Clinically important improvement in symptom control has been found in most studies to require peak serum theophylline concentrations >10 mcg/mL, but patients with mild disease may benefit from lower concentrations. At serum theophylline concentrations >20 mcg/mL, both the frequency and severity of adverse reactions increase. In general, maintaining peak serum theophylline concentrations between 10 and 15 mcg/mL will achieve most of the drug's potential therapeutic benefit while minimizing the risk of serious adverse events.

Pharmacokinetics:
Overview Theophylline is rapidly and completely absorbed after oral administration in solution or immediate-release solid oral dosage form. Theophylline does not undergo any appreciable presystemic elimination, distributes freely into fat-free tissues, and is extensively metabolized in the liver.
The pharmacokinetics of theophylline vary widely among similar patients and cannot be predicted by age, sex, body weight, or other demographic characteristics. In addition, certain concurrent illnesses and alterations in normal physiology (See **Table I**) and coadministration of other drugs (see **Table II**) can significantly alter the pharmacokinetic characteristics of theophylline. Within-subject variability in metabolism has also been reported in some studies, especially in acutely ill patients. It is, therefore, recommended that serum theophylline concentrations be measured frequently in acutely ill patients (eg, at 24-hour intervals) and periodically in patients receiving long-term therapy (eg, at 6- to 12-month intervals). More frequent measurements should be made in the presence of any condition that may significantly alter theophylline clearance (see **PRECAUTIONS, Monitoring Serum Theophylline Concentrations**, and **DOSAGE AND ADMINISTRATION**).
[See table I below]
Note: In addition to the factors listed above, theophylline clearance is increased and half-life decreased by low-carbohydrate/ high-protein diets, parenteral nutrition, and daily consumption of charcoal-broiled beef. A high-carbohydrate/ low-protein diet can decrease the clearance and prolong the half-life of theophylline.
Absorption Theophylline is rapidly and completely absorbed after oral administration in solution or immediate-release solid oral dosage form. After a single immediate-release theophylline dose of 5 mg/kg in adults, a mean peak serum concentration of about 10 mcg/mL (range 5–15 mcg/ mL) can be expected 1–2 hours after the dose. Coadministration of theophylline with food or antacids does not cause clinically significant changes in the absorption of theophylline from immediate-release dosage forms.

THEO-DUR Product Pharmacokinetics

THEO-DUR (100, 200, 300, and 450 mg) Extended-Release Tablets:
In single-dose studies with 18 normal fasting subjects, the THEO-DUR product at 8 mg/kg body weight (300–700 mg/ dose) produced mean peak theophylline plasma levels of 7.5 ± 1.9 mcg/mL at 9.2 ± 1.9 hours following administration. In multiple-dose, steady-state 3- and 5-day studies with 12 normal subjects, THEO-DUR administered at 8 mg/kg (300–600 mg/dose) twice daily, achieved an average peak-trough difference of 4 mcg/mL. The C_{max} and C_{min} were 13.9 ± 6.9 and 9.9 ± 6.0, respectively. The mean % fluctuation ± S.D. of the plasma concentration at steady state [% fluctuation = 100 $(C_{max}–C_{min})/C_{min}$] was 54.2 ± 45.7%. These pharmacokinetic parameters were measured under fasting conditions.

THEO-DUR (200, 300, and 450 mg) Extended-Release Tablets:
In a multiple-dose (300–500 mg BID) steady-state, 5-day study involving 14 normal, nonfasting subjects with theophylline half-lives between 5.8 and 12.3 hours (mean 8.0 ± 1.8 hours), THEO-DUR dosed twice daily, produced mean C_{max} and C_{min} levels of 12.2 ± 2.0 and 10.2 ± 1.6 mcg/mL, respectively, over the AM dosing interval and C_{max} and C_{min} of 11.6 ± 1.6 and 8.7 ± 1.8 mcg/mL, respectively, over the PM dosing interval. The mean % fluctuation ± S.D. over the AM dosing interval was 30.4 ± 12.9% and 33.7 ± 13.1% over the PM dosing interval. In the same subjects, the THEO-DUR product given once daily, in the morning, in doses ranging from 600–1000 mg (same daily dose as for BID above) produced a mean C_{max} and C_{min} of 14.4 ± 2.2 and 5.5 ± 2.0, respectively, and a mean % fluctuation ± S.D. of 195.8 ± 106.0%. Average peak-trough differences over 24 hours were 8.9 ± 1.3 and 3.7 ± 1.2 mcg/mL when THEO-DUR was given once or twice daily, respectively. In both the twice-daily and once-daily dosing regimens, THEO-DUR exhibited complete bioavailability when compared to an immediate-release product.

THEO-DUR (200, 300, and 450 mg) Extended-Release Tablets:
In a single-dose bioavailability study in eleven subjects, 1000 mg of the THEO-DUR product was administered under fasting conditions and immediately following a high-fat content (62 g) breakfast of approximately 1100 kcal. The rate and extent of absorption of theophylline from THEO-DUR administered in fasting and fed conditions were similar.
Distribution Once theophylline enters the systemic circulation, about 40% is bound to plasma protein, primarily albumin. Unbound theophylline distributes throughout body water, but distributes poorly into body fat. The apparent volume of distribution of theophylline is approximately 0.45 L/kg (range 0.3–0.7 L/kg) based on ideal body weight. Theophylline passes freely across the placenta, into breast milk, and into the cerebrospinal fluid (CSF). Saliva theophylline concentrations approximate unbound serum concentrations, but are not reliable for routine or therapeutic monitoring unless special techniques are used. An increase in the volume of distribution of theophylline, primarily due to reduction in plasma protein binding, occurs in premature neonates, patients with hepatic cirrhosis, uncorrected acidemia, the elderly, and in women during the third trimester of pregnancy. In such cases, the patient may show signs of toxicity at total (bound + unbound) serum concentrations of theophylline in the therapeutic range (10–20 mcg/mL) due to elevated concentrations of the pharmacologically active unbound drug. Similarly, a patient with decreased theophylline binding may have a subtherapeutic total drug concentration while the pharmacologically active unbound concentration is in the therapeutic range. If only total serum theophylline concentration is measured, this may lead to an unnecessary and potentially dangerous dose increase. In patients with reduced protein binding, measurement of unbound serum theophylline concentration provides a more reliable means of dosage adjustment than measurement of total serum theophylline concentration. Generally, concentrations of unbound theophylline should be maintained in the range of 6–12 mcg/mL.
Metabolism Following oral dosing, theophylline does not undergo any measurable first-pass elimination. In adults and children beyond 1 year of age, approximately 90% of the dose is metabolized in the liver. Biotransformation takes place through demethylation to 1-methylxanthine and 3-methylxanthine and hydroxylation to 1,3-dimethyluric acid. 1-methylxanthine is further hydroxylated, by xanthine oxidase, to 1-methyluric acid. About 6% of a theophylline dose is N-methylated to caffeine. Theophylline demethylation to 3-methylxanthine is catalyzed by cytochrome P450 1A2, while cytochromes P450 2E1 and P450 3A3 catalyze the hydroxylation to 1,3-dimethyluric acid. Demethylation to 1-methylxanthine appears to be catalyzed either by cyto-

Table I. Mean and range of total body clearance and half-life of theophylline related to age and altered physiological states.¶

Population characteristics	Total body clearance* mean (range)†† (mL/kg/min)	Half-life mean (range)†† (hr)
Age		
Premature neonates		
postnatal age 3–15 days	0.29 (0.09–0.49)	30 (17–43)
postnatal age 25–57 days	0.64 (0.04–1.2)	20 (9.4–30.6)
Term infants		
postnatal age 1–2 days	NR†	25.7 (25–26.5)
postnatal age 3–30 weeks	NR†	11 (6–29)
Children		
1–4 years	1.7 (0.5–2.9)	3.4 (1.2–5.6)
4–12 years	1.6 (0.8–2.4)	NR†
13–15 years	0.9 (0.48–1.3)	NR†
6–17 years	1.4 (0.2–2.6)	3.7 (1.5–5.9)
Adults (16–60 years)		
otherwise healthy nonsmoking asthmatics	0.65 (0.27–1.03)	8.7 (6.1–12.8)
Elderly (>60 years)		
nonsmokers with normal cardiac, liver, and renal function	0.41 (0.21–0.61)	9.8 (1.6–18)
Concurrent illness or altered physiological state		
Acute pulmonary edema	0.33** (0.07–2.45)	19** (3.1–82)
COPD >60 years, stable nonsmoker >1 year	0.54 (0.44–0.64)	11 (9.4–12.6)
COPD with cor pulmonale	0.48 (0.08–0.88)	NR†
Cystic fibrosis (14–28 years)	1.25 (0.31–2.2)	6.0 (1.8–10.2)
Fever associated with acute viral respiratory illness (children 9–15 years)	NR†	7.0 (1.0–13)
Liver disease - cirrhosis	0.31 **(0.1–0.7)	32**(10–56)
acute hepatitis	0.35 (0.25–0.45)	19.2 (16.6–21.8)
cholestasis	0.65 (0.25–1.45)	14.4 (5.7–31.8)
Pregnancy - 1st trimester	NR†	8.5 (3.1–13.9)
2nd trimester	NR†	8.8 (3.8–13.8)
3rd trimester	NR†	13.0 (8.4–17.6)
Sepsis with multi-organ failure	0.47 (0.19–1.9)	18.8 (6.3–24.1)
Thyroid disease - hypothyroid	0.38 (0.13–0.57)	11.6 (8.2–25)
hyperthyroid	0.8 (0.68–0.97)	4.5 (3.7–5.6)

¶ For various North American patient populations from literature reports. Different rates of elimination and consequent dosage requirements have been observed among other peoples.
* Clearance represents the volume of blood completely cleared of theophylline by the liver in 1 minute. Values listed were generally determined at serum theophylline concentrations <20 mcg/mL; clearance may decrease and half-life may increase at higher serum concentrations due to nonlinear pharmacokinetics.
†† Reported range or estimated range (mean ± 2 S.D.) where actual range not reported.
† NR = not reported or not reported in a comparable format.
** Median

chrome P450 1A2 or a closely related cytochrome. In neonates, the N-demethylation pathway is absent while the function of the hydroxylation pathway is markedly deficient. The activity of these pathways slowly increases to maximal levels by 1 year of age.
Caffeine and 3-methylxanthine are the only theophylline metabolites with pharmacologic activity. 3-methylxanthine has approximately one tenth the pharmacologic activity of theophylline and serum concentrations in adults with normal renal function are <1 mcg/mL. In patients with end-stage renal disease, 3-methylxanthine may accumulate to concentrations that approximate the unmetabolized theophylline concentration. Caffeine concentrations are usually undetectable in adults regardless of renal function. In neonates, caffeine may accumulate to concentrations that approximate the unmetabolized theophylline concentration and thus, exert a pharmacologic effect.
Both the N-demethylation and hydroxylation pathways of theophylline biotransformation are capacity-limited. Due to the wide intersubject variability of the rate of theophylline metabolism, nonlinearity of elimination may begin in some patients at serum theophylline concentrations <10 mcg/mL. Since this nonlinearity results in more than proportional changes in serum theophylline concentrations with changes in dose, it is advisable to make increases or decreases in dose in small increments in order to achieve desired changes in serum theophylline concentrations (see **DOSAGE AND ADMINISTRATION, Table V**). Accurate prediction of dose dependency of theophylline metabolism in patients *a priori* is not possible, but patients with very high initial clearance rates (ie, low steady-state serum theophylline concentrations at above average doses) have the greatest likelihood of experiencing large changes in serum theophylline concentration in response to dosage changes.
Excretion In neonates, approximately 50% of the theophylline dose is excreted unchanged in the urine. Beyond the first 3 months of life, approximately 10% of the theophylline dose is excreted unchanged in the urine. The remainder is excreted in the urine mainly as 1,3-dimethyluric acid (35%–40%), 1-methyluric acid (20%–25%), and 3-methylxanthine (15%–20%). Since little theophylline is excreted unchanged in the urine and since active metabolites of theophylline (ie, caffeine, 3-methylxanthine) do not accumulate to clinically significant levels even in the face of end-stage renal disease, no dosage adjustment for renal insufficiency is necessary in adults and children >3 months of age. In contrast, the large fraction of the theophylline dose excreted in the urine as unchanged theophylline and caffeine in neonates requires careful attention to dose reduction and frequent monitoring of serum theophylline concentrations in neonates with reduced renal function (see **WARNINGS**).
Serum Concentrations at Steady State After multiple doses of immediate-release theophylline, steady state is reached in 30–65 hours (average 40 hours) in adults. At steady state, on a dosage regimen with 6-hour intervals, the expected mean trough concentration is approximately 60% of the mean peak concentration, assuming a mean theophylline half-life of 8 hours. The difference between peak and trough concentrations is larger in patients with more rapid theophylline clearance. In patients with high theophylline clearance and half-lives of about 4–5 hours, such as children age 1 to 9 years, the trough serum theophylline concentration may be only 30% of peak with a 6-hour dosing interval. In these patients a slow-release formulation would allow a longer dosing interval (8–12 hours) with a smaller peak/trough difference.
Special Populations (see Table I for mean clearance and half-life values)
Geriatric: The clearance of theophylline is decreased by an average of 30% in healthy elderly adults (>60 yrs) compared to healthy young adults. Careful attention to dose reduction and frequent monitoring of serum theophylline concentrations are required in elderly patients (see **WARNINGS**).
Pediatrics: The clearance of theophylline is very low in neonates (see **WARNINGS**). Theophylline clearance reaches maximal values by 1 year of age, remains relatively constant until about 9 years of age and then slowly decreases by approximately 50% to adult values at about age 16. Renal excretion of unchanged theophylline in neonates amounts to about 50% of the dose, compared to about 10% in children older than 3 months and in adults. Careful attention to dosage selection and monitoring of serum theophylline concentrations are required in pediatric patients (see **WARNINGS** and **DOSAGE AND ADMINISTRATION**).
Gender: Gender differences in theophylline clearance are relatively small and unlikely to be of clinical significance. Significant reduction in theophylline clearance, however, has been reported in women on the 20th day of the menstrual cycle and during the third trimester of pregnancy.
Race: Pharmacokinetic differences in theophylline clearance due to race have not been studied.
Renal Insufficiency: Only a small fraction, eg, about 10%, of the administered theophylline dose is excreted unchanged in the urine of children greater than 3 months of age and adults. Since little theophylline is excreted unchanged in the urine and since active metabolites of theophylline (ie, caffeine, 3-methylxanthine) do not accumulate to clinically significant levels even in the face of end-stage renal disease, no dosage adjustment for renal insufficiency is necessary in adults and children >3 months of age. In contrast, approximately 50% of the administered theophylline dose is excreted unchanged in the urine in neonates. Careful attention to dose reduction and frequent monitoring of serum theophylline concentrations are required in neonates with decreased renal function (see **WARNINGS**).
Hepatic Insufficiency: Theophylline clearance is decreased by 50% or more in patients with hepatic insufficiency (eg, cirrhosis, acute hepatitis, cholestasis). Careful attention to dose reduction and frequent monitoring of serum theophylline concentrations are required in patients with reduced hepatic function (see **WARNINGS**).
Congestive Heart Failure (CHF): Theophylline clearance is decreased by 50% or more in patients with CHF. The extent of reduction in theophylline clearance in patients with CHF appears to be directly correlated to the severity of the cardiac disease. Since theophylline clearance is independent of liver blood flow, the reduction in clearance appears to be due to impaired hepatocyte function rather than reduced perfusion. Careful attention to dose reduction and frequent monitoring of serum theophylline concentrations are required in patients with CHF (see **WARNINGS**).
Smokers: Tobacco and marijuana smoking appear to increase the clearance of theophylline by induction of metabolic pathways. Theophylline clearance has been shown to increase by approximately 50% in young adult tobacco smokers and by approximately 80% in elderly tobacco smokers compared to nonsmoking subjects. Passive smoke exposure has also been shown to increase theophylline clearance by up to 50%. Abstinence from tobacco smoking for 1 week causes a reduction of approximately 40% in theophylline clearance. Careful attention to dose reduction and frequent monitoring of serum theophylline concentrations are required in patients who stop smoking (see **WARNINGS**). Use of nicotine gum has been shown to have no effect on theophylline clearance.
Fever: Fever, regardless of its underlying cause, can decrease the clearance of theophylline. The magnitude and duration of the fever appear to be directly correlated to the degree of decrease of theophylline clearance. Precise data are lacking, but a temperature of 39°C (102°F) for at least 24 hours or lesser temperature elevations for longer periods, are probably required to produce a clinically significant increase in serum theophylline concentrations. Children with rapid rates of theophylline clearance (ie, those who require a dose that is substantially larger than average [eg, >22 mg/kg/day] to achieve a therapeutic peak serum theophylline concentration when afebrile) may be at greater risk of toxic effects from decreased clearance during sustained fever. Careful attention to dose reduction and frequent monitoring of serum theophylline concentrations are required in patients with sustained fever (see **WARNINGS**).
Miscellaneous: Other factors associated with decreased theophylline clearance include the third trimester of pregnancy, sepsis with multiple organ failure, and hypothyroidism. Careful attention to dose reduction and frequent monitoring of serum theophylline concentrations are required in patients with any of these conditions (see **WARNINGS**). Other factors associated with increased theophylline clearance include hyperthyroidism and cystic fibrosis.
Clinical Studies:
In patients with chronic asthma, including patients with severe asthma requiring inhaled corticosteroids or alternate-day oral corticosteroids, many clinical studies have shown that theophylline decreases the frequency and severity of symptoms, including nocturnal exacerbations, and decreases the "as needed" use of inhaled $beta_2$-agonists. Theophylline has also been shown to reduce the need for short courses of daily oral prednisone to relieve exacerbations of airway obstruction that are unresponsive to bronchodilators in asthmatics.
In patients with chronic obstructive pulmonary disease (COPD), clinical studies have shown that theophylline decreases dyspnea, air trapping, the work of breathing, and improves contractility of diaphragmatic muscles with little or no improvement in pulmonary function measurements.

INDICATIONS AND USAGE

THEO-DUR Extended-Release Tablets are indicated for the treatment of the symptoms and reversible airflow obstruction associated with chronic asthma and other chronic lung diseases, eg, emphysema and chronic bronchitis.

CONTRAINDICATIONS

THEO-DUR Extended-Release Tablets are contraindicated in patients with a history of hypersensitivity to theophylline or other components in the product.

WARNINGS

Serious side effects such as ventricular arrhythmias, convulsions, or even death may appear as the first sign of toxicity without any recognized prior warning. Less serious signs of theophylline toxicity (eg, nausea and restlessness) may occur frequently when initiating therapy but are usually transient. When such signs are persistent during maintenance therapy, they are often associated with serum concentrations above 20 mcg/mL. Stated differently, serious toxicity is not reliably preceded by less severe side effects.
Concurrent Illness:
Theophylline should be used with extreme caution in patients with the following clinical conditions due to the increased risk of exacerbation of the concurrent condition:
Active peptic ulcer disease (peptic ulcer disease should be controlled with appropriate therapy since theophylline is known to increase peptic acid secretion)
Seizure disorders
Cardiac arrhythmias (not including bradyarrhythmias)
Conditions That Reduce Theophylline Clearance:
There are several readily identifiable causes of reduced theophylline clearance. ***If the total daily dose is not appropriately reduced so as to lower serum theophylline levels to within the therapeutic range in the presence of these risk factors, severe and potentially fatal theophylline toxicity can occur.*** Careful consideration must be given to the benefits and risks of theophylline use and the need for more intensive monitoring of serum theophylline concentrations in patients with the following risk factors:
Age:
Neonates (term and premature)
Children <1 year
Elderly (>60 years)
Concurrent Diseases:
Acute pulmonary edema
Congestive heart failure
Cor pulmonale
Fever; ≥102°F for 24 hours or more; or lesser temperature elevations for longer periods
Hypothyroidism
Liver disease; cirrhosis, acute hepatitis
Reduced renal function in infants <3 months of age
Sepsis with multi-organ failure
Shock
Cessation of Smoking
Drug Interactions:
Adding a drug that inhibits theophylline metabolism (eg, cimetidine, erythromycin, tacrine) or stopping a concurrently administered drug that enhances theophylline metabolism (eg, carbamazepine, rifampin). (See **PRECAUTIONS, Drug Interactions, Table II.**)
When Signs or Symptoms of Theophylline Toxicity Are Present:
Whenever a patient receiving theophylline develops nausea or vomiting, particularly repetitive vomiting, or other signs or symptoms consistent with theophylline toxicity (even if another cause may be suspected), additional doses of theophylline should be withheld and a serum theophylline concentration should be measured immediately. Patients should be instructed not to continue any dosage that causes adverse effects and to withhold subsequent doses until the symptoms have resolved, at which time the clinician may instruct the patient to resume the drug at a lower dosage (see **DOSAGE AND ADMINISTRATION, Dosage Guidelines, Table V**).
Dosage Increases:
Increases in the dose of theophylline should not be made in response to an acute exacerbation of symptoms of chronic lung disease since theophylline provides little added benefit to inhaled $beta_2$-selective agonists and systematically administered corticosteroids in this circumstance and increases the risk of adverse effects. A *peak* steady-state serum theophylline concentration should be measured before increasing the dose in response to persistent chronic symptoms to ascertain whether an increase in dose is safe. Before increasing the theophylline dose on the basis of a low serum concentration, the clinician should consider whether the blood sample was obtained at an appropriate time in relationship to the dose and whether the patient has adhered to the prescribed regimen (see **PRECAUTIONS, Monitoring Serum Theophylline Concentrations**).
As the rate of theophylline clearance may be dose dependent (ie, steady-state serum concentrations may increase disproportionately to the increase in dose), an increase in dose based upon a subtherapeutic serum concentration measurement should be conservative. In general, limiting dose increases to about 25% of the previous total daily dose will reduce the risk of unintended excessive increases in serum theophylline concentration (see **DOSAGE AND ADMINISTRATION, Table V**).

PRECAUTIONS

THEO-DUR TABLETS SHOULD *NOT* BE CHEWED OR CRUSHED AND SHOULD *BE BROKEN ONLY AT THE SCORE.*
General:
Careful consideration of the various interacting drugs (including recently discontinued medications), physiologic conditions, and other factors such as smoking that can alter theophylline clearance and require dosage adjustment should occur prior to initiation of theophylline therapy, prior to increases in theophylline dose, and during follow up (see **WARNINGS**). The dose of theophylline selected for initiation of therapy should be low and, ***if tolerated***, increased slowly over a period of a week or longer with the final dose guided by monitoring serum theophylline concentrations and the patient's clinical response (see **DOSAGE AND ADMINISTRATION, Table IV**).
Monitoring Serum Theophylline Concentrations:
Serum theophylline concentration measurements are readily available and should be used to determine whether the dosage is appropriate. Specifically, the serum theophylline concentration should be measured as follows:

1. When initiating therapy to guide final dosage adjustment after titration.
2. Before making a dose increase to determine whether the serum concentration is subtherapeutic in a patient who continues to be symptomatic.
3. Whenever signs or symptoms of theophylline toxicity are present.

Continued on next page

Theo-Dur—Cont.

4. Whenever there is a new illness, worsening of a chronic illness, or a change in the patient's treatment regimen that may alter theophylline clearance [eg, fever (see **CLINICAL PHARMACOLOGY**, *Fever*), hepatitis, or drugs listed in **Table II** are added or discontinued].

To guide a dose increase, the blood sample should be obtained at the time of the expected peak serum theophylline concentration; 4 to 8 hours when medication is taken every 12 hours or 8 hours when taken once daily. It is important that the patient has not missed or taken additional doses during the previous 48 hours and that the dosing intervals were reasonably equally spaced. A trough concentration (ie, at the end of the dosing interval) provides no additional useful information and may lead to an inappropriate dose increase since the peak serum theophylline concentration can be two or more times greater than the trough concentration with an immediate-release formulation. If the serum sample is drawn more than 8 hours after the dose, the results must be interpreted with caution since the concentration may not be reflective of the peak concentration. In contrast, when signs or symptoms of theophylline toxicity are present, the serum sample should be obtained as soon as possible, analyzed immediately, and the result reported to the clinician without delay. In patients in whom decreased serum protein binding is suspected (eg, cirrhosis, women during the third trimester of pregnancy), the concentration of unbound theophylline should be measured and the dosage adjusted to achieve an unbound concentration of 6–12 mcg/mL.

Saliva concentrations of theophylline cannot be used reliably to adjust dosage without special techniques.

Effects on Laboratory Tests:

As a result of its pharmacological effects, theophylline at serum concentrations within the 10–20 mcg/mL range modestly increases plasma glucose (from a mean of 88 mg% to 98 mg%), uric acid (from a mean of 4 mg/dL to 6 mg/dL), free fatty acids (from a mean of 451 μeq/L to 800 μeq/L), total cholesterol (from a mean of 140 vs 160 mg/dL), HDL (from a mean of 36 to 50 mg/dL), HDL/LDL ratio (from a mean of 0.5 to 0.7), and urinary free cortisol excretion (from a mean of 44 to 63 mcg/24 hr). Theophylline at serum concentrations within the 10–20 mcg/mL range may also transiently decrease serum concentrations of triiodothyronine (144 before, 131 after 1 week and 142 ng/dL after 4 weeks of theophylline). The clinical importance of these changes should be weighed against the potential therapeutic benefit of theophylline in individual patients.

Information for Patients:

This information is intended to aid in the safe and effective use of this medication. It is not a disclosure of all adverse or intended effects.

The patient (or parent/caregiver) should be instructed to seek medical advice whenever nausea, vomiting, persistent headache, insomnia, restlessness, or rapid heartbeat occurs during treatment with theophylline, even if another cause is suspected. The patient should be instructed to contact their clinician if they develop a new illness, especially if accompanied by a persistent fever, if they experience worsening of a chronic illness, if they start or stop smoking cigarettes or marijuana, or if another clinician adds a new medication or discontinues a previously prescribed medication. Patients should be informed that theophylline interacts with a wide variety of drugs (see **Table II**). They should be instructed to inform all clinicians involved in their care that they are taking theophylline, especially when a medication is being added or deleted from their treatment. Patients should be instructed to not alter the dose, timing of the dose, or frequency of administration without first consulting their clinician. If a dose is missed, the patient should be instructed to take the next dose at the usually scheduled time and to not attempt to make up for the missed dose.

THEO-DUR Tablets *should not be chewed or crushed*. When dosing THEO-DUR Extended-Release Tablets on a once-daily (q24h) basis, tablets should be taken whole and not split.

Drug Interactions

Drug/Drug Interactions:

Theophylline interacts with a wide variety of drugs. The interaction may be pharmacodynamic, ie, alterations in the therapeutic response to theophylline or another drug or occurrence of adverse effects without a change in serum theophylline concentration. More frequently, however, the interaction is pharmacokinetic, ie, the rate of theophylline clearance is altered by another drug resulting in increased or decreased serum theophylline concentrations. Theophylline only rarely alters the pharmacokinetics of other drugs. The drugs listed in **Table II** have the potential to produce clinically significant pharmacodynamic or pharmacokinetic interactions with theophylline. The information in the **"Effect"** column of **Table II** assumes that the interacting drug is being added to a steady-state theophylline regimen. If theophylline is being initiated in a patient who is already taking a drug that inhibits theophylline clearance (eg, cimetidine, erythromycin), the dose of theophylline required to achieve a therapeutic serum theophylline concentration will be smaller. Conversely, if theophylline is being initiated in a patient who is already taking a drug that enhances theophylline clearance (eg, rifampin), the dose of theophylline required to achieve a therapeutic serum theophylline concentration will be larger. Discontinuation of a concomitant drug that increases theophylline clearance will result in accumulation of theophylline to potentially toxic levels, unless the theophylline dose is appropriately reduced. Discontinuation of a concomitant drug that inhibits theophylline clearance will result in decreased serum theophylline concentrations, unless the theophylline dose is appropriately increased.

The listing of drugs in **Table II** is current as of February 9, 1995. New interactions are continuously being reported for theophylline, especially with new chemical entities. **The clinician should not assume that a drug does not interact with theophylline if it is not listed in Table II.** Before addition of a newly available drug in a patient receiving theophylline, the package insert of the new drug and/or the medical literature should be consulted to determine if an interaction between the new drug and theophylline has been reported.

[See table II on next page]

Drug/Food Interactions:

THEO-DUR 100 mg Extended-Release Tablets have not been adequately studied to determine whether their bioavailability is altered when given with food. Available data suggest that drug administration at the time of food ingestion may influence the absorption characteristics of theophylline controlled-release products resulting in serum values different from those found after administration in the fasting state.

A drug-food effect, if any, would likely have its greatest clinical significance when high theophylline serum levels are being maintained and/or when large single doses (> 13 mg/kg or 900 mg) of a controlled-release theophylline product are given.

THEO-DUR (200, 300, and 450 mg) Extended-Release Tablets: The rate and extent of absorption of theophylline from THEO-DUR 200 mg, 300 mg, and 450 mg tablets are similar when administered fasting or immediately after a high-fat content breakfast such as 8 oz. whole milk, egg/cheese/bacon on muffin, 1 blueberry muffin with margarine, and 1 serving of hash brown potatoes (about 1100 kcal, including approximately 62 g of fat) (see **CLINICAL PHARMACOLOGY, Pharmacokinetics**).

The Effect of Other Drugs on Theophylline Serum Concentration Measurements:

Most serum theophylline assays in clinical use are immunoassays which are specific for theophylline. Other xanthines such as caffeine, dyphylline, and pentoxifylline are not detected by these assays. Some drugs (eg, cefazolin, cephalothin), however, may interfere with certain HPLC techniques. Caffeine and xanthine metabolites in neonates or patients with renal dysfunction may cause the reading from some dry reagent office methods to be higher than the actual serum theophylline concentration.

Carcinogenesis, Mutagenesis, and Impairment of Fertility:

Long-term carcinogenicity studies have been carried out in mice (oral doses 30–150 mg/kg) and rats (oral doses 5–75 mg/kg). Results are pending.

Theophylline has been studied in Ames salmonella, *in vivo* and *in vitro* cytogenetics, micronucleus, and Chinese hamster ovary test systems and has not been shown to be genotoxic.

In a 14-week continuous breeding study, theophylline, administered to mating pairs of $B6C3F_1$ mice at oral doses of 120, 270, and 500 mg/kg (approximately 1.0–3.0 times the human dose on a mg/m^2 basis) impaired fertility, as evidenced by decreases in the number of live pups per litter, decreases in the mean number of litters per fertile pair, and increases in the gestation period at the high dose as well as decreases in the proportion of pups born alive at the mid and high dose. In 13-week toxicity studies, theophylline was administered to F344 rats and $B6C3F_1$ mice at oral doses of 40–300 mg/kg (approximately 2.0 times the human dose on a mg/m^2 basis). At the high dose, systemic toxicity was observed in both species including decreases in testicular weight.

Pregnancy:

Category C There are no adequate and well-controlled studies in pregnant women. Additionally, there are no teratogenicity studies in nonrodents (eg, rabbits). Theophylline was not shown to be teratogenic in CD-1 mice at oral doses up to 400 mg/kg, approximately 2.0 times the recommended human dose on a mg/m^2 basis or CD-1 rats at oral doses up to 260 mg/kg, approximately 3.0 times the recommended human dose on a mg/m^2 basis. At a dose of 220 mg/kg, embryotoxicity was observed in rats in the absence of maternal toxicity.

Nursing Mothers:

Theophylline is excreted into breast milk and may cause irritability or other signs of mild toxicity in nursing human infants. The concentration of theophylline in breast milk is about equivalent to the maternal serum concentration. An infant ingesting a liter of breast milk containing 10–20 mcg/mL of theophylline a day is likely to receive 10–20 mg of theophylline per day. Serious adverse effects in the infant are unlikely unless the mother has toxic serum theophylline concentrations.

Pediatric Use:

Safety and effectiveness of THEO-DUR Extended-Release Tablets administered:

1. Every 24 hours in pediatric patients under 12 years of age have not been established.
2. Every 12 hours in pediatric patients under 6 years of age have not been established.

Other theophylline formulations, however, are safe and effective for the approved indications in pediatric patients under the ages listed above. The maintenance dose of theophylline must be selected with caution in pediatric patients since the rate of theophylline clearance is highly variable across the age range of neonates to adolescents (see **CLINICAL PHARMACOLOGY, Table I, WARNINGS**, and **DOSAGE AND ADMINISTRATION, Table IV**).

Geriatric Use:

Elderly patients are at significantly greater risk of experiencing serious toxicity from theophylline than younger patients due to pharmacokinetic and pharmacodynamic changes associated with aging. Theophylline clearance is reduced in patients greater than 60 years of age, resulting in increased serum theophylline concentrations in response to a given theophylline dose. Protein binding may be decreased in the elderly resulting in a large proportion of the total serum theophylline concentration in the pharmacologically active unbound form. Elderly patients also appear to be more sensitive to the toxic effects of theophylline after chronic overdosage than younger patients. For these reasons, the maximum daily dose of theophylline in patients greater than 60 years of age ordinarily should not exceed 400 mg/day unless the patient continues to be symptomatic and the peak steady-state serum theophylline concentration is <10 mcg/mL (see **DOSAGE AND ADMINISTRATION**). Theophylline doses greater than 400 mg/day should be prescribed with caution in elderly patients.

ADVERSE REACTIONS

Adverse reactions associated with theophylline are generally mild when peak serum theophylline concentrations are <20 mcg/mL and mainly consist of transient caffeine-like adverse effects such as nausea, vomiting, headache, and insomnia. When peak serum theophylline concentrations exceed 20 mcg/mL, however, theophylline produces a wide range of adverse reactions including persistent vomiting, cardiac arrhythmias, and intractable seizures which can be lethal (see **OVERDOSAGE**). The transient caffeine-like adverse reactions occur in about 50% of patients when theophylline therapy is initiated at doses higher than recommended initial doses (eg, >300 mg/day in adults and >12 mg/kg/day in children beyond >1 year of age). During the initiation of theophylline therapy, caffeine-like adverse effects may transiently alter patient behavior, especially in school-age children, but this response rarely persists. Initiation of theophylline therapy at a low dose with subsequent slow titration to a predetermined age-related maximum dose will significantly reduce the frequency of these transient adverse effects (see **DOSAGE AND ADMINISTRATION, Table IV**). In a small percentage of patients (<3% of children and <10% of adults), the caffeine-like adverse effects persist during maintenance therapy, even at peak serum theophylline concentrations within the therapeutic range (ie, 10–20 mcg/mL). Dosage reduction may alleviate the caffeine-like adverse effects in these patients, however, persistent adverse effects should result in a reevaluation of the need for continued theophylline therapy and the potential therapeutic benefit of alternative treatment.

Other adverse reactions that have been reported to occur at serum theophylline concentrations less than 20 mcg/mL include diarrhea, irritability, restlessness, fine skeletal muscle tremors, alopecia, muscle twitching/spasms, palpitations, rash, reflex hyperexcitability, transient diuresis, and ventricular arrhythmia. Whether or not theophylline caused these reported events is not known. In patients with hypoxia secondary to COPD, multifocal atrial tachycardia and flutter have been reported at serum theophylline concentrations ≥ 15 mcg/mL. There have been a few isolated reports of seizures at serum theophylline concentrations <20 mcg/mL in patients with an underlying neurological disease or in elderly patients. The occurrence of seizures in elderly patients with serum theophylline concentrations <20 mcg/mL may be secondary to decreased protein binding resulting in a larger proportion of the total serum theophylline concentration in the pharmacologically active unbound form. The clinical characteristics of the seizures reported in patients with serum theophylline concentration <20 mcg/mL have generally been milder than seizures associated with excessive serum theophylline concentrations resulting from an overdose (ie, they have generally been transient, often stopped without anticonvulsant therapy, and did not result in neurological residua).

[See table III on page 1610]

OVERDOSAGE

General:

The chronicity and pattern of theophylline overdosage significantly influences clinical manifestations of toxicity, management, and outcome. There are two common presentations: (1) *acute overdose*, ie, ingestion of a single large excessive dose (>10 mg/kg) as occurs in the context of an attempted suicide or isolated medication error, and (2) *chronic overdosage*, ie, ingestion of repeated doses that are excessive for the patient's rate of theophylline clearance. The most common causes of chronic theophylline overdosage include patient or caregiver error in dosing, clinician prescribing of an excessive dose or a normal dose in the presence of factors known to decrease the rate of theophylline clearance, and increasing the dose in response to an exacerbation of symptoms without first measuring the serum theophylline concentration to determine whether a dose increase is safe.

Severe toxicity from theophylline overdose is a relatively rare event. In one health maintenance organization, the frequency of hospital admissions for chronic overdosage of theophylline was about 1 per 1000 person-years exposure. In another study, among 6000 blood samples obtained for measurement of serum theophylline concentration, for any reason, from patients treated in an emergency department, 7% were in the 20–30 mcg/mL range and 3% were >30 mcg/mL. Approximately two thirds of the patients with serum theophylline concentrations in the 20–30 mcg/mL range had one or more manifestations of toxicity while >90% of patients with serum theophylline concentrations >30 mcg/mL were clinically intoxicated. Similarly, in other reports, serious toxicity from theophylline is seen principally at serum concentrations >30 mcg/mL.

Table II. Clinically significant drug interactions with theophylline.*

Drug	Type of Interaction	Effect**
Adenosine	Theophylline blocks adenosine receptors.	Higher doses of adenosine may be required to achieve desired effect.
Alcohol	A single large dose of alcohol (eg, 3 mL/kg of whiskey) decreases theophylline clearance for up to 24 hours.	30% increase
Allopurinol	Decreases theophylline clearance at allopurinol doses ≥600 mg/day.	25% increase
Aminoglutethimide	Increases theophylline clearance by induction of microsomal enzyme activity.	25% decrease
Carbamazepine	Similar to aminoglutethimide.	30% decrease
Cimetidine	Decreases theophylline clearance by inhibiting cytochrome P45 1A2.	70% increase
Ciprofloxacin	Similar to cimetidine.	40% increase
Clarithromycin	Similar to erythromycin.	25% increase
Diazepam	Benzodiazepines increase CNS concentrations of adenosine, a potent CNS depressant, while theophylline blocks adnosine receptors.	Larger diazepam doses may be required to produce desired level of sedation. Discontinuation of theophylline without reduction of diazepam dose may result in respiratory depression.
Disulfiram	Decreases theophylline clearance by inhibiting hydroxylation and demethylation.	50% increase
Enoxacin	Similar to cimetidine.	300% increase
Ephedrine	Synergistic CNS effects.	Increased frequency of nausea, nervousness, and insomnia.
Erythromycin	Erythromycin metabolite decreases theophylline clearance by inhibiting cytochrome P450 3A3.	35% increase. Erythromycin steady-state serum concentrations decrease by a similar amount.
Estrogen	Estrogen-containing oral contraceptives decrease theophylline clearance in a dose-dependent fashion. The effect of progesterone on theophylline clearance is unknown.	30% increase
Flurazepam	Similar to diazepam.	Similar to diazepam.
Fluvoxamine	Similar to cimetidine.	Similar to cimetidine.
Halothane	Halothane sensitizes the myocardium to catecholamines; theophylline increases release of endogenous catecholamines.	Increased risk of ventricular arrhythmias.
Interferon, human recombinant alpha-A	Decreases theophylline clearance.	100% increase
Isoproterenol (IV)	Increases theophylline clearance.	20% decrease
Ketamine	Pharmacologic.	May lower theophylline seizure threshold.
Lithium	Theophylline increases renal lithium clearance.	Lithium dose required to achieve a therapeutic serum concentration increased an average of 60%.
Lorazepam	Similar to diazepam.	Similar to diazepam.
Methotrexate (MTX)	Decreases theophylline clearance.	20% increase after low dose MTX; higher dose MTX may have a greater effect.
Mexiletine	Similar to disulfiram.	80% increase
Midazolam	Similar to diazepam.	Similar to diazepam.
Moricizine	Increases theophylline clearance.	25% decrease
Norfloxacin	Increases serum theophylline levels.	
Ofloxacin	Increases serum theophylline levels.	
Pancuronium	Theophylline may antagonize nondepolarizing neuromuscular blocking effects; possibly due to phosphodiesterase inhibition.	Larger dose of pancuronium may be required to achieve neuromuscular blockade.
Pentoxifylline	Decreases theophylline clearance.	30% increase
Phenobarbital (PB)	Similar to aminoglutethimide.	25% decrease after 2 weeks of concurrent PB.
Phenytoin	Phenytoin increases theophylline clearance by increasing microsomal enzyme activity. Theophylline decreases phenytoin absorption.	Serum theophylline *and* phenytoin concentrations decrease about 40%.
Propafenone	Decreases theophylline clearance and pharmacologic interaction.	40% increase. $Beta_2$-blocking effect may decrease efficacy of theophylline.
Propranolol	Similar to cimetidine and pharmacologic interaction.	100% increase. $Beta_2$-blocking effect may decrease efficacy of theophylline.
Rifampin	Increases theophylline clearance by increasing cytochrome P450 1A2 and 3A3 activity.	20%–40% decrease
Ritonavir	Increases theophylline clearance (mechanism unknown).	43% decrease in AUC.
Sucralfate	Reduced absorption of theophylline.	
Sulfinpyrazone	Increases theophylline clearance by increasing demethylation and hydroxylation. Decreases renal clearance of theophylline.	20% decrease
Tacrine	Similar to cimetidine, also increases renal clearance of theophylline.	90% increase
Thiabendazole	Decreases theophylline clearance.	190% increase
Ticlopidine	Decreases theophylline clearance.	60% increase
Troleandomycin	Similar to erythromycin.	33%–100% increase depending on troleandomycin dose.
Verapamil	Similar to disulfiram.	20% increase

* Refer to **PRECAUTIONS, Drug Interactions** for further information regarding table.

** Average effect on steady-state theophylline concentration or other clinical effect for pharmacologic interactions. Individual patients may experience larger changes in serum theophylline concentration than the value listed.

Several studies have described the clinical manifestations of theophylline overdose and attempted to determine the factors that predict life-threatening toxicity. In general, patients who experience an acute overdose are less likely to experience seizures than patients who have experienced a chronic overdosage, unless the peak serum theophylline concentration is >100 mcg/mL. After a chronic overdosage, generalized seizures, life-threatening cardiac arrhythmias, and death may occur at serum theophylline concentrations >30 mcg/mL. The severity of toxicity after chronic overdosage is more strongly correlated with the patient's age than the peak serum theophylline concentration; patients >60 years are at the greatest risk for severe toxicity and mortality after a chronic overdosage. Pre-existing or concurrent disease may also significantly increase the susceptibility of a patient to a particular toxic manifestation, eg, patients with neurologic disorders have an increased risk of seizures and patients with cardiac disease have an increased risk of cardiac arrhythmias for a given serum theophylline concentration compared to patients without the underlying disease.

The frequency of various reported manifestations of theophylline overdose according to the mode of overdose are listed in **Table III.**

Other manifestations of theophylline toxicity include increases in serum calcium, creatine kinase, myoglobin, and leukocyte count; decreases in serum phosphate and magnesium, acute myocardial infarction, and urinary retention in men with obstructive uropathy.

Seizures associated with serum theophylline concentrations >30 mcg/mL are often resistant to anticonvulsant therapy and may result in irreversible brain injury if not rapidly controlled. Death from theophylline toxicity is most often secondary to cardiorespiratory arrest and/or hypoxic encephalopathy following prolonged generalized seizures or intractable cardiac arrhythmias causing hemodynamic compromise.

Overdose Management:

General Recommendations for Patients with Symptoms of Theophylline Overdose or Serum Theophylline Concentrations >30 mcg/mL. (Note: Serum theophylline concentrations may continue to increase after presentation of the patient for medical care.)

1. While simultaneously instituting treatment, contact a regional poison center to obtain updated information and advice on individualizing the recommendations that follow.
2. Institute supportive care, including establishment of intravenous access, maintenance of the airway, and electrocardiographic monitoring.
3. *Treatment of seizures:* Because of the high morbidity and mortality associated with theophylline-induced seizures, treatment should be rapid and aggressive. Anticonvulsant therapy should be initiated with an intravenous benzodiazepine, eg, diazepam, in increments of 0.1–0.2 mg/kg every 1–3 minutes until seizures are terminated. Repetitive seizures should be treated with a loading dose of phenobarbital (20 mg/kg infused over 30–60 minutes). Animal studies and case reports of theophylline overdose in humans suggest that phenytoin is ineffective in terminating theophylline-induced seizures. The doses of benzodiazepines and phenobarbital required to terminate theophylline-induced seizures are close to the doses that may cause severe respiratory depression or respiratory arrest; the clinician should therefore be prepared to provide assisted ventilation. Elderly patients and patients with COPD may be more susceptible to the respiratory depressant effects of anticonvulsants. Barbiturate-induced coma or administration of general anesthesia may be required to terminate repetitive seizures or status epilepticus. General anesthesia should be used with caution in patients with theophylline overdose because fluorinated volatile anesthetics may sensitize the myocardium to endogenous catecholamines released by theophylline. Enflurane appears less likely to be associated with this effect than halothane and may, therefore, be safer. Neuromuscular blocking agents alone should not be used to terminate seizures since they abolish the musculoskeletal manifestations without terminating seizure activity in the brain.
4. *Anticipate need for anticonvulsants:* In patients with theophylline overdose who are at high risk for theophylline-induced seizures, eg, patients with acute overdoses and serum theophylline concentrations >100 mcg/mL or chronic overdosage in patients >60 years of age with serum theophylline concentrations >30 mcg/mL, the need for anticonvulsant therapy should be anticipated. A benzodiazepine such as diazepam should be drawn into a syringe and kept at the patient's bedside and medical personnel qualified to treat seizures should be immediately available. In selected patients at high risk for theophylline-induced seizures, consideration should be given to the administration of prophylactic anticonvulsant therapy. Situations where prophylactic anticonvulsant therapy should be considered in high-risk patients include anticipated delays in instituting methods for extracorporeal removal of theophylline (eg, transfer of a high-risk patient from one healthcare facility to another for extra-

Continued on next page

Theo-Dur—Cont.

corporeal removal) and clinical circumstances that significantly interfere with efforts to enhance theophylline clearance (eg, a neonate where dialysis may not be technically feasible or a patient with vomiting unresponsive to antiemetics who is unable to tolerate multiple-dose oral activated charcoal). In animal studies, prophylactic administration of phenobarbital, *but not phenytoin,* has been shown to delay the onset of theophylline-induced generalized seizures and to increase the dose of theophylline required to induce seizures (ie, markedly increases the LD_{50}). Although there are no controlled studies in humans, a loading dose of intravenous phenobarbital (20 mg/kg infused over 60 minutes) may delay or prevent life-threatening seizures in high-risk patients while efforts to enhance theophylline clearance are continued. Phenobarbital may cause respiratory depression, particularly in elderly patients and patients with COPD.

5. *Treatment of cardiac arrhythmias:* Sinus tachycardia and simple ventricular premature beats are not harbingers of life-threatening arrhythmias, they do not require treatment in the absence of hemodynamic compromise, and they resolve with declining serum theophylline concentrations. Other arrhythmias, especially those associated with hemodynamic compromise, should be treated with antiarrhythmic therapy appropriate for the type of arrhythmia.
6. *Gastrointestinal decontamination:* Oral activated charcoal (0.5 g/kg up to 20 g and repeat at least once 1–2 hours after the first dose) is extremely effective in blocking the absorption of theophylline throughout the gastrointestinal tract, even when administered several hours after ingestion. If the patient is vomiting, the charcoal should be administered through a nasogastric tube or after administration of an antiemetic. Phenothiazine antiemetics such as prochlorperazine or perphenazine should be avoided since they can lower the seizure threshold and frequently cause dystonic reactions. A single dose of sorbitol may be used to promote stooling to facilitate removal of theophylline bound to charcoal from the gastrointestinal tract. Sorbitol, however, should be dosed with caution since it is a potent purgative which can cause profound fluid and electrolyte abnormalities, particularly after multiple doses. Commercially available fixed combinations of liquid charcoal and sorbitol should be avoided in young children and after the first dose in adolescents and adults since they do not allow for individualization of charcoal and sorbitol dosing. Ipecac syrup should be avoided in theophylline overdoses. Although ipecac induces emesis, it does not reduce the absorption of theophylline unless administered within 5 minutes of ingestion and even then is less effective than oral activated charcoal. Moreover, ipecac-induced emesis may persist for several hours after a single dose and significantly decrease the retention and the effectiveness of oral activated charcoal.
7. *Serum theophylline concentration monitoring:* The serum theophylline concentration should be measured immediately upon presentation, 2–4 hours later, and then at sufficient intervals, eg, every 4 hours, to guide treatment decisions and to assess the effectiveness of therapy. Serum theophylline concentrations may continue to increase after presentation of the patient for medical care as a result of continued absorption of theophylline from the gastrointestinal tract. Serial monitoring of serum theophylline serum concentrations should be continued until it is clear that the concentration is no longer rising and has returned to nontoxic levels.
8. *General monitoring procedures:* Electrocardiographic monitoring should be initiated on presentation and continued until the serum theophylline level has returned to a nontoxic level. Serum electrolytes and glucose should be measured on presentation and at appropriate intervals indicated by clinical circumstances. Fluid and electrolyte abnormalities should be promptly corrected. **Monitoring and treatment should be continued until the serum concentration decreases below 20 mcg/mL.**
9. *Enhance clearance of theophylline:* Multiple-dose oral activated charcoal (eg, 0.5 mg/kg up to 20 g, every 2 hours) increases the clearance of theophylline at least twofold by absorption of theophylline secreted into gastrointestinal fluids. Charcoal must be retained in, and pass through, the gastrointestinal tract to be effective; emesis should therefore be controlled by administration of appropriate antiemetics. Alternatively, the charcoal can be administered continuously through a nasogastric tube in conjunction with appropriate antiemetics. A single dose of sorbitol may be administered with the activated charcoal to promote stooling to facilitate clearance of the adsorbed theophylline from the gastrointestinal tract. Sorbitol alone does not enhance clearance of theophylline and should be dosed with caution to prevent excessive stooling which can result in severe fluid and electrolyte imbalances. Commercially available fixed combinations of liquid charcoal and sorbitol should be avoided in young children and after the first dose in adolescents and adults since they do not allow for individualization of charcoal and sorbitol dosing. In patients with intractable vomiting, extracorporeal methods of theophylline removal should be instituted (see **OVERDOSAGE, Extracorporeal Removal**).

Table III. Manifestations of theophylline toxicity.*

Sign/Symptom	Percentage of patients reported with sign or symptom: Acute Overdose (Large Single Ingestion) Study 1 (n=157)	Acute Overdose (Large Single Ingestion) Study 2 (n=14)	Chronic Overdosage (Multiple Excessive Doses) Study 1 (n=92)	Chronic Overdosage (Multiple Excessive Doses) Study 2 (n=102)
Asymptomatic	NR**	0	NR**	6
Gastrointestinal				
Vomiting	73	93	30	61
Abdominal pain	NR**	21	NR**	12
Diarrhea	NR**	0	NR**	14
Hematemesis	NR**	0	NR**	2
Metabolic/Other				
Hypokalemia	85	79	44	43
Hyperglycemia	98	NR**	18	NR**
Acid/base disturbance	34	21	9	5
Rhabdomyolysis	NR**	7	NR**	0
Cardiovascular				
Sinus tachycardia	100	86	100	62
Other supraventricular tachycardias	2	21	12	14
Ventricular premature beats	3	21	10	19
Atrial fibrillation or flutter	1	NR**	12	NR**
Multifocal atrial tachycardia	0	NR**	2	NR**
Ventricular arrhythmias with hemodynamic instability	7	14	40	0
Hypotension/shock	NR**	21	NR**	8
Neurologic				
Nervousness	NR**	64	NR**	21
Tremors	38	29	16	14
Disorientation	NR**	7	NR**	11
Seizures	5	14	14	5
Death	3	21	10	4

* These data are derived from two studies in patients with serum theophylline concentrations >30 mcg/mL. In the first study (Study #1-Shanon, *Ann Intern Med.* 1993;119:1161-67), data were prospectively collected from 249 consecutive cases of theophylline toxicity referred to a regional poison center for consultation. In the second study (Study #2-Sessler, *Am J Med.* 1990;88:567-76), data were retrospectively collected from 116 cases with serum theophylline concentrations >30 mcg/mL among 6000 blood samples obtained for measurement of serum theophylline concentrations in three emergency departments. Differences in the incidence of manifestations of theophylline toxicity between the two studies may reflect sample selection as a result of study design (eg, in Study #1, 48% of the patients had acute intoxications versus only 10% in Study #2) and different methods of reporting results.

**NR = Not reported in a comparable manner.

Specific Recommendations:

Acute Overdose

A. Serum Concentration >20 <30 mcg/mL
1. Administer a single dose of oral activated charcoal.
2. Monitor the patient and obtain a serum theophylline concentration in 2–4 hours to ensure that the concentration is not increasing.

B. Serum Concentration >30 <100 mcg/mL
1. Administer multiple-dose oral activated charcoal and measures to control emesis.
2. Monitor the patient and obtain serial theophylline concentrations every 2–4 hours to gauge the effectiveness of therapy and to guide further treatment decisions.
3. Institute extracorporeal removal if emesis, seizures, or cardiac arrhythmias cannot be adequately controlled (see **OVERDOSAGE, Extracorporeal Removal**).

C. Serum Concentration >100 mcg/mL
1. Consider prophylactic anticonvulsant therapy.
2. Administer multiple-dose oral activated charcoal and measures to control emesis.
3. Consider extracorporeal removal, even if the patient has not experienced a seizure (see **OVERDOSAGE, Extracorporeal Removal**).
4. Monitor the patient and obtain serial theophylline concentrations every 2–4 hours to gauge the effectiveness of therapy and to guide further treatment decisions.

Chronic Overdosage

A. Serum Concentration >20 <30 mcg/mL (with manifestations of theophylline toxicity)
1. Administer a single dose of oral activated charcoal.
2. Monitor the patient and obtain a serum theophylline concentration in 2–4 hours to ensure that the concentration is not increasing.

B. Serum Concentration >30 mcg/mL in patients <60 years of age
1. Administer multiple-dose oral activated charcoal and measures to control emesis.
2. Monitor the patient and obtain serial theophylline concentrations every 2–4 hours to gauge the effectiveness of therapy and to guide further treatment decisions.
3. Institute extracorporeal removal if emesis, seizures, or cardiac arrhythmias cannot be adequately controlled (see **OVERDOSAGE, Extracorporeal Removal**).

C. Serum Concentration >30 mcg/mL in patients ≥60 years of age
1. Consider prophylactic anticonvulsant therapy.
2. Administer multiple-dose oral activated charcoal and measures to control emesis.
3. Consider extracorporeal removal even if the patient has not experienced a seizure (see **OVERDOSAGE, Extracorporeal Removal**).
4. Monitor the patient and obtain serial theophylline concentrations every 2–4 hours to gauge the effectiveness of therapy and to guide further treatment decisions.

Extracorporeal Removal:

Increasing the rate of theophylline clearance by extracorporeal methods may rapidly decrease serum concentrations, but the risks of the procedure must be weighed against the potential benefit. Charcoal hemoperfusion is the most effective method of extracorporeal removal, increasing theophylline clearance up to sixfold, but serious complications, including hypotension, hypocalcemia, platelet consumption, and bleeding diatheses may occur. Hemodialysis is about as efficient as multiple-dose oral activated charcoal and has a lower risk of serious complications than charcoal hemoperfusion. Hemodialysis should be considered as an alternative when charcoal hemoperfusion is not feasible and multiple-dose oral charcoal is ineffective because of intractable emesis. Serum theophylline concentrations may rebound 5–10 mcg/mL after discontinuation of charcoal hemoperfusion or hemodialysis due to redistribution of theophylline from the tissue compartment. Peritoneal dialysis is ineffective for theophylline removal; exchange transfusions in neonates have been minimally effective.

DOSAGE AND ADMINISTRATION

THEO-DUR Extended-Release Tablets should not be chewed or crushed. When dosing THEO-DUR Extended-Release Tablets on a once-daily (q24h) basis, tablets should be taken whole and not split.

THEO-DUR (200, 300, and 450 mg) Extended-Release Tablets: The rate and extent of absorption of theophylline from THEO-DUR 200, 300, and 450 mg tablets when administered fasting or immediately after a high-fat content breakfast are similar (see **CLINICAL PHARMACOLOGY, Pharmacokinetics**).

THEO-DUR 100 mg Extended-Release Tablets have not been adequately studied for their bioavailability when administered with food (see **PRECAUTIONS, Drug/Food Interactions**).

General Considerations:

The steady-state peak serum theophylline concentration is a function of the dose, the dosing interval, and the rate of theophylline absorption and clearance in the individual patient. Because of marked individual differences in the rate of theophylline clearance, the dose required to achieve a peak serum theophylline concentration in the 10–20 mcg/mL range varies fourfold among otherwise similar patients in the absence of factors known to alter theophylline clearance (eg, 400–1600 mg/day in adults <60 years old and 10–36 mg/kg/day in children 1–9 years old). For a given population there is no single theophylline dose that will provide both safe and effective serum concentrations for all patients. Administration of the median theophylline dose required to achieve a therapeutic serum theophylline concentration in a given population may result in either subtherapeutic or potentially toxic serum theophylline concentrations in individual patients. For example, at a dose of 900 mg/day in adults <60 years or 22 mg/kg/day in children 1–9 years, the steady-state peak serum theophylline concentration will be <10 mcg/mL in about 30% of patients, 10–20 mcg/mL in about 50%, and 20–30 mcg/mL in about 20% of patients. **The**

Table IV. **Dosing initiation and titration (as anhydrous theophylline).***

A. Children (6–15 years) and adults (16–60 years) without risk factors for impaired clearance.

Titration Step	*Children <45 kg*	*Children >45 kg and adults*
1. Starting dosage:	12–14 mg/kg/day up to a maximum of 300 mg/day divided Q12 hrs*	300 mg/day divided Q12 hrs*
2. After 3 days, *if tolerated*, increase dose to:	16 mg/kg/day up to a maximum of 400 mg/day divided Q12 hrs*	400 mg/day divided Q12 hrs*
3. After 3 more days, *if tolerated*, increase dose to:	20 mg/kg/day up to a maximum of 600 mg/day divided Q12 hrs*	600 mg/day divided Q12 hrs*

B. **Patients With Risk Factors For Impaired Clearance, The Elderly (>60 Years), And Those In Whom It Is Not Feasible To Monitor Serum Theophylline Concentrations:**

In children 6–15 years of age, the final theophylline dose should not exceed 16 mg/kg/day up to a maximum of 400 mg/day in the presence of risk factors for reduced theophylline clearance (see **WARNINGS**) or if it is not feasible to monitor serum theophylline concentrations.

In adolescents ≥16 years and adults, including the elderly, the final theophylline dose should not exceed 400 mg/day in the presence of risk factors for reduced theophylline clearance (see **WARNINGS**) or if it is not feasible to monitor serum theophylline concentrations.

* Patients with more rapid metabolism, clinically identified by higher than average dose requirements, should receive a smaller dose more frequently (every 8 hours) to prevent breakthrough symptoms resulting from low trough concentrations before the next dose.

Table V. **Dosage adjustment guided by serum theophylline concentration.**

Peak Serum Concentration	**Dosage Adjustment**
<9.9 mcg/mL	If symptoms are not controlled and current dosage is tolerated, increase dose about 25%. Recheck serum concentration after 3 days for further dosage adjustment.
10 to 14.9 mcg/mL	If symptoms are controlled and current dosage is tolerated, maintain dose and recheck serum concentration at 6- to 12-month intervals.¶ If symptoms are not controlled and current dosage is tolerated, consider adding additional medication(s) to treatment regimen.
15–19.9 mcg/mL	Consider 10% decrease in dose to provide greater margin of safety even if current dosage is tolerated.¶
20–24.9 mcg/mL	Decrease dose by 25% even if no adverse effects are present. Recheck serum concentration after 3 days to guide further dosage adjustment.
25–30 mcg/mL	Skip next dose and decrease subsequent doses at least 25% even if no adverse effects are present. Recheck serum concentration after 3 days to guide further dosage adjustment. If symptomatic, consider whether overdose treatment is indicated (see recommendations for chronic overdosage).
>30 mcg/mL	Treat overdose as indicated (see recommendations for chronic overdosage). If theophylline is subsequently resumed, decrease dose by at least 50% and recheck serum concentration after 3 days to guide further dosage adjustment.

¶ Dose reduction and/or serum theophylline concentration measurement is indicated whenever adverse effects are present, physiologic abnormalities that can reduce theophylline clearance occur (eg, sustained fever), or a drug that interacts with theophylline is added or discontinued (see **WARNINGS**).

dose of theophylline must be individualized on the basis of peak serum theophylline concentration measurements in order to achieve a dose that will provide maximum potential benefit with minimal risk of adverse effects.

Transient caffeine-like adverse effects and excessive serum concentrations in slow metabolizers can be avoided in most patients by starting with a sufficiently low dose and slowly increasing the dose, *if judged to be clinically indicated*, in small increments (see **Table IV**). Dose increases should only be made if the previous dosage is well tolerated and at intervals of not less than 3 days to allow serum theophylline concentrations to reach the new steady state. Dosage adjustment should be guided by serum theophylline concentration measurement (see **PRECAUTIONS**, **Monitoring Serum Theophylline Concentrations**, and **DOSAGE AND ADMINISTRATION**, **Table V**). Healthcare providers should instruct patients and caregivers to discontinue any dosage that causes adverse effects, to withhold the medication until these symptoms are gone, and to then resume therapy at a lower, previously tolerated dosage (see **WARNINGS**).

If the patient's symptoms are well controlled, there are no apparent adverse effects, and no intervening factors that might alter dosage requirements (see **WARNINGS** and **PRECAUTIONS**), serum theophylline concentrations should be monitored at 6-month intervals for rapidly growing children and at yearly intervals for all others. In acutely ill patients, serum theophylline concentrations should be monitored at frequent intervals, eg, every 24 hours.

Theophylline distributes poorly into body fat, therefore, mg/kg dose should be calculated on the basis of ideal body weight.

Table IV contains theophylline dosing titration schema recommended for patients in various age groups and clinical circumstances.

Table V contains recommendations for theophylline dosage adjustment based upon serum theophylline concentrations.

Application of these general dosing recommendations to individual patients must take into account the unique clinical characteristics of each patient. In general, these recommendations should serve as the upper limit for dosage adjustments in order to decrease the risk of potentially serious adverse events associated with unexpected large increases in serum theophylline concentration.

[See table IV above]

[See table V above]

Once-Daily Dose:

The slow absorption rate of this preparation may allow once-daily administration in adult nonsmokers with appropriately total body clearance and other patients with low dosage requirements. Once-daily dosing should be considered only after the patient has been gradually and satisfactorily titrated to therapeutic levels with q12h dosing. Once-daily dosing (twice the q12h dose) should be based on the dosing guidelines in **Table IV** and **Table V** and should be initiated at the end of the last q12h dosing interval. The trough concentration (C_{min}) obtained following conversion to once-daily dosing may be lower (especially in high-clearance patients) and the peak concentration (C_{max}) may be higher (especially in low-clearance patients) than that obtained with q12h dosing. If symptoms recur, or signs of toxicity appear during the once-daily dosing interval, dosing on the q12h basis should be reinstituted.

It is essential that serum theophylline concentrations be monitored before and after transfer to once-daily dosing.

Food and posture, along with changes associated with circadian rhythm, may influence the rate of absorption and/or clearance rates of theophylline from controlled-release dosage forms administered at night. The exact relationship of these and other factors to nighttime serum concentrations and the clinical significance of such findings require additional study. Therefore, it is not recommended that THEO-DUR, when used as a once-a-day product, be administered at night. THEO-DUR, when used as a once-a-day product, must be taken whole and not broken.

HOW SUPPLIED

THEO-DUR 100 mg, 200 mg, and 300 mg Extended-Release Tablets are available in bottles of 100, 500, 1000, and 5000, and in unit-dose packages of 100. THEO-DUR 450 mg Extended-Release Tablets are available in bottles of 100, and unit-dose packages of 100.

100 mg tablet; NDC 0085-0487; round, white to off-white, debossed THEO-DUR 100 on one side and scored on the other side.

200 mg tablet; NDC 0085-0933; oval, white to off-white, debossed THEO-DUR 200 on one side and scored on the other side.

300 mg tablet; NDC 0085-0584; capsule shaped, white to off-white, debossed THEO-DUR 300 on one side and scored on the other side.

450 mg tablet; NDC 0085-0806; capsule shaped, white to off-white, scored debossed THEO-DUR 450 on one side.

STORAGE CONDITIONS

Keep tightly closed. Store at controlled room temperature 15°–30°C (59°–86°F).

CAUTION: Federal law prohibits dispensing without prescription.

Key Pharmaceuticals Inc,
Kenilworth, NJ 07033 USA

Rev. 3/97 19767710

Shown in Product Identification Guide, page 319

UNI-DUR® ℞

(theophylline)
Extended-release Tablets

Some of the information contained in this insert (eg, information regarding pediatric patients under the age of 12) was derived from FDA's Class Labeling Guidance for Immediate-Release Theophylline Products and is intended for informational purposes only.

DESCRIPTION

UNI-DUR® Extended-release Tablets for oral administration contain 400 or 600 mg anhydrous theophylline in an extended-release system which allows a 24-hour dosing interval for appropriate patients.

Theophylline is a bronchodilator, structurally classified as a methylxanthine. It occurs as a white, odorless, crystalline powder with a bitter taste. Anhydrous theophylline has the chemical name *1H*-Purine-2,6-dione,3,7-dihydro-1,3-dimethyl-, and is represented by the following structural formula:

The molecular formula of anhydrous theophylline is $C_7H_8N_4O_2$ with a molecular weight of 180.17.

The inactive ingredients for UNI-DUR 400 and 600 mg Extended-release Tablets include: acacia, NF; acetone; cellulose acetate phthalate, NF; cetyl alcohol, NF; confectioner's sugar, NF; corn starch, NF; diethyl phthalate, NF; glyceryl monostearate; lactose monohydrate, NF; magnesium stearate, NF; myristyl alcohol, NF; nonpareil seeds (sugar spheres), NF; and white wax, NF.

CLINICAL PHARMACOLOGY

Mechanism of Action:

Theophylline has two distinct actions in the airways of patients with reversible obstruction; smooth muscle relaxation (ie, bronchodilation) and suppression of the response of the airways to stimuli (ie, non-bronchodilator prophylactic effects). While the mechanisms of action of theophylline are not known with certainty, studies in animals suggest that bronchodilation is mediated by the inhibition of two isozymes of phosphodiesterase (PDE III and, to a lesser extent, PDE IV) while non-bronchodilator prophylactic actions are probably mediated through one or more different molecular mechanisms that do not involve inhibition of PDE III or antagonism of adenosine receptors. Some of the adverse effects associated with theophylline appear to be mediated by inhibition of PDE III (eg, hypotension, tachycardia, headache, and emesis) and adenosine receptor antagonism (eg, alterations in cerebral blood flow).

Theophylline increases the force of contraction of diaphragmatic muscles. This action appears to be due to enhancement of calcium uptake through an adenosine-mediated channel.

Serum Concentration-Effect Relationship:

Bronchodilation occurs over the serum theophylline concentration range of 5–20 mcg/mL. Clinically important improvement in symptom control has been found in most studies to require peak serum theophylline concentration >10 mcg/mL, but patients with mild disease may benefit from lower concentrations. At serum theophylline concentrations >20 mcg/mL, both the frequency and severity of adverse reactions increase. In general, maintaining peak serum theophylline concentrations between 10 and 15 mcg/mL will achieve most of the drug's potential therapeutic benefit while minimizing the risk of serious adverse events.

Pharmacokinetics:

Overview Theophylline is rapidly and completely absorbed after oral administration in solution or immediate-release solid oral dosage form. Theophylline does not undergo any appreciable pre-systemic elimination, distributes freely into fat-free tissues, and is extensively metabolized in the liver.

The pharmacokinetics of theophylline vary widely among similar patients and cannot be predicted by age, sex, body weight, or other demographic characteristics. In addition, certain concurrent illnesses and alterations in normal physiology (see **Table I**) and coadministration of other drugs (see **Table II**) can significantly alter the pharmacokinetic characteristics of theophylline. Within-subject variability in metabolism has also been reported in some studies, especially in acutely ill patients. It is, therefore, recommended that serum theophylline concentrations be measured frequently in acutely ill patients (eg, at 24-hour intervals) and periodically in patients receiving long-term therapy (eg, at 6- to 12-month intervals). More frequent measurements should be made in the presence of any condition that may significantly alter theophylline clearance (see **PRECAUTIONS, Monitoring Serum Theophylline Concentrations** and **DOSAGE AND ADMINISTRATION**).

Continued on next page

Uni-Dur—Cont.

[See table I at right]

Note: In addition to the factors listed above, theophylline clearance is increased and half-life decreased by low-carbohydrate/high-protein diets, parenteral nutrition, and daily consumption of charcoal-broiled beef. A high-carbohydrate/low-protein diet can decrease the clearance and prolong the half-life of theophylline.

Absorption Theophylline is rapidly and completely absorbed after oral administration in solution or immediate-release solid oral dosage form. After a single immediate-release theophylline dose of 5 mg/kg in adults, a mean peak serum concentration of about 10 mcg/mL (range 5–15 mcg/mL) can be expected 1–2 hours after the dose. Coadministration of theophylline with food or antacids does not cause clinically significant changes in the absorption of theophylline from immediate-release dosage forms.

UNI-DUR Pharmacokinetics

Following the single-dose crossover administration of a 600 mg UNI-DUR Tablet to 20 healthy male subjects after an overnight fast, a peak serum theophylline concentration of 5.3 ± 1.3 mcg/mL was obtained at 13.6 ± 3.7 hours and the mean area under the curve extrapolated to infinity (AUC_{inf}) was 132.7 ± 45.1 mcg hr/mL. When taken immediately after a high-fat breakfast, the mean AUC_{inf} was 136.0 ± 36.7 mcg hr/mL with a mean peak theophylline serum level of 5.2 ± 1.5 mcg/mL at 17.1 ± 6.3 hours. While food did not affect the extent of absorption as evidenced by the similar AUC_{inf} values, food did prolong the time to peak concentration. The absorption from half tablets of the 600 mg product was also evaluated and found to be bioequivalent to that of the whole tablets. The relative extent of absorption of theophylline from the 600 mg UNI-DUR Tablet, fasting, when compared to an immediate-release theophylline tablet, was 84.3%; and the nonfasting treatment was 88.7%.

In a separate multiple-dose study, two 400 mg UNI-DUR Tablets were compared to one 600 mg UNI-DUR Tablet. This study was a two-way, randomized, crossover multiple-dose study in 17 nonsmoking healthy males. Both products were dosed once a day in the morning after an overnight fast and 1 hour prior to a meal for 5 days. There was no significant difference in any of the pharmacokinetic parameters when corrected for dose.

The mean dose AUC_{ss} (corrected to the 600 mg dose) for the two 400 mg UNI-DUR Tablets was 179.7 ± 62.9 mcg hr/mL and for the 600 mg UNI-DUR Tablet was 170.9 ± 75.2 mcg hr/mL. The two 400 mg UNI-DUR Tablets reached dose corrected maximum serum concentration of 9.8 ± 2.6 mcg/mL and the 600 mg UNI-DUR Tablet reached a maximum of 9.7 ± 3.5 mcg/mL. The minimum concentrations were 4.9 ± 2.6 mcg/mL and 4.4 ± 2.6 mcg/mL for the two 400 mg and 600 mg UNI-DUR Tablets, respectively.

Steady-state pharmacokinetics were determined in a multiple-dose, crossover study with 24 healthy nonsmoking male subjects having an average theophylline clearance of 5.70 ± 2.36 (S.D.) liters per hour. Following an overnight fast, a UNI-DUR 600 mg Extended-release Tablet was administered once daily in the morning for 5 consecutive days. The UNI-DUR Tablet exhibited better extended-release characteristics compared with a reference extended-release q12h product (2 × 300 mg) administered once daily in the morning following an overnight fast for 5 consecutive days. The results are noted as follows (mean values ± S.D.):

[See second table above]

The mean percent fluctuation [$(C_{max}$-$C_{min}/C_{min}) \times 100$] was 130% for the once-daily UNI-DUR regimen and 389% for the reference q12h product administered once daily. The extent of theophylline absorption from UNI-DUR Tablets relative to the reference q12h product was 74.9% (95% C.I. = 67–84).

In a randomized, multiple-dose crossover study with 18 healthy male subjects, a 600 mg UNI-DUR Extended-release Tablet was administered once daily either in the morning or evening for 5 consecutive days. The theophylline AUC_{ss} for the 24-hour period following the dose given on day 5 was equivalent for morning (177 ± 89 mcg hr/mL) and evening (175 ± 76 mcg hr/mL) administration. The peak theophylline concentrations (C_{max}) at steady state were also equivalent for morning (10.6 ± 4.9 mcg/mL) and evening (10.3 ± 4.0 mcg/mL) administration.

Steady-state pharmacokinetics comparing UNI-DUR Tablets once-daily administration with twice-daily administration were determined in a multiple-dose, crossover study with 24 healthy, nonsmoking male subjects having an average theophylline clearance of 4.53 ± 1.21 (S.D.) liters per hour. Using UNI-DUR 400 mg Extended-release Tablets, a total daily theophylline dose of 800 mg was administered for 5 consecutive days either once daily as two tablets in the morning (8 AM) with a standardized breakfast or twice daily as one tablet in the morning (8 AM) with a standardized breakfast or twice daily as one tablet in the morning (8 AM) with a standardized breakfast and one tablet in the evening (8 PM). The once-daily UNI-DUR regimen was bioequivalent to the twice-daily UNI-DUR regimen. The results are noted as follows (mean values ± S.D.):

[See third table above]

The mean percent fluctuation [$(C_{max}$-$C_{min}/C_{min}) \times 100$] was 78% for the once-daily UNI-DUR regimen and 17% for the twice-daily UNI-DUR regimen. The extent of theophylline absorption from the once-daily UNI-DUR regimen relative to the twice-daily UNI-DUR regimen was 100% (95% C.I. = 95–105).

Table I. Mean and range of total body clearance and half-life of theophylline related to age and altered physiological states.¶

Population characteristics	Total body clearance* mean (range)††(mL/kg/min)		Half-life mean (range)†† (hr)	
Age				
Premature neonates				
postnatal age 3–15 days	0.29	(0.09–0.49)	30	(17–43)
postnatal age 25–57 days	0.64	(0.04–1.2)	20	(9.4–30.6)
Term infants				
postnatal age 1–2 days	NR†		25.7	(25–26.5)
postnatal age 3–30 weeks	NR†		11	(6–29)
Children				
1–4 years	1.7	(0.5–2.9)	3.4	(1.2–5.6)
4–12 years	1.6	(0.8–2.4)	NR†	
13–15 years	0.9	(0.48–1.3)	NR†	
6–17 years	1.4	(0.2–2.6)	3.7	(1.5–5.9)
Adults (16–60 years)				
otherwise healthy nonsmoking asthmatics	0.65	(0.27–1.03)	8.7	(6.1–12.8)
Elderly (>60 years) nonsmokers with normal cardiac, liver, and renal function	0.41	(0.21–0.61)	9.8	(1.6–18)
Concurrent illness or altered physiological state				
Acute pulmonary edema	0.33**	(0.07–2.45)	19**	(3.1–82)
COPD->60 years, stable nonsmoker >1 year	0.54	(0.44–0.64)	11	(9.4–12.6)
COPD with cor pulmonale	0.48	(0.08–0.88)	NR†	
Cystic fibrosis (14–28 years)	1.25	(0.31–2.2)	6.0	(1.8–10.2)
Fever associated with acute viral respiratory illness (children 9–15 years)	NR†		7.0	(1.0–13)
Liver disease- cirrhosis	0.31**	(0.1–0.7)	32**	(10–56)
acute hepatitis	0.35	(0.25–0.45)	19.2	(16.6–21.8)
cholestasis	0.65	(0.25–1.45)	14.4	(5.7–31.8)
Pregnancy- 1st trimester	NR†		8.5	(3.1–13.9)
2nd trimester	NR†		8.8	(3.8–13.8)
3rd trimester	NR†		13.0	(8.4–17.6)
Sepsis with multi-organ failure	0.47	(0.19–1.9)	18.8	(6.3–24.1)
Thyroid disease-hypothyroid	0.38	(0.13–0.57)	11.6	(8.2–25)
hyperthyroid	0.8	(0.68–0.97)	4.5	(3.7–5.6)

¶ For various North American patient populations from literature reports. Different rates of elimination and consequent dosage requirements have been observed among other peoples.

* Clearance represents the volume of blood completely cleared of theophylline by the liver in 1 minute. Values listed were generally determined at serum theophyllne concentrations <20 mcg/mL; clearance may decrease and half-life may increase at higher serum concentrations due to nonlinear pharmacokinetics.

†† Reported range or estimated range (mean ± 2 S.D.) where actual range not reported.

† NR = not reported or not reported in a comparable format.

** Median

	AUC_{ss} (mcg hr/mL)	C_{max} (mcg/mL)	C_{min} (mcg/mL)	T_{max} (hr)
UNI-DUR	119 ± 36	6.9 ± 2.4	3.7 ± 1.3	11.5 ± 5.7
Reference	154 ± 37	10.5 ±2.3	2.5 ± 1.1	7.6 ± 1.7

	AUC_{ss} (mcg hr/mL)	C_{max} (mcg/mL)	C_{min} (mcg/mL)	T_{max} (hr)
QD Regimen	187 ± 45	10.4 ± 2.9	6.0 ± 1.3	12.0 ± 3.7
q12h Regimen	187 ± 43	9.4 ± 2.2	8.4 ± 2.6	14.5 ± 6.6

Distribution Once theophylline enters the systemic circulation, about 40% is bound to plasma protein, primarily albumin. Unbound theophylline distributes throughout body water, but distributes poorly into body fat. The apparent volume of distribution of theophylline is approximately 0.45 L/kg (range 0.3–0.7 L/kg) based on ideal body weight. Theophylline passes freely across the placenta, into breast milk, and into the cerebrospinal fluid (CSF). Saliva theophylline concentrations approximate unbound serum concentrations, but are not reliable for routine or therapeutic monitoring unless special techniques are used. An increase in the volume of distribution of theophylline, primarily due to reduction in plasma protein binding, occurs in premature neonates, patients with hepatic cirrhosis, uncorrected acidemia, the elderly, and in women during the third trimester of pregnancy. In such cases, the patient may show signs of toxicity at total (bound + unbound) serum concentration of theophylline in the therapeutic range (10–20 mcg/mL) due to elevated concentrations of the pharmacologically active unbound drug. Similarly, a patient with decreased theophylline binding may have a subtherapeutic total drug concentration while the pharmacologically active unbound concentration is in the therapeutic range. If only total serum theophylline concentration is measured, this may lead to an unnecessary and potentially dangerous dose increase. In patients with reduced protein binding, measurement of unbound serum theophylline concentration provides a more reliable means of dosage adjustment than measurement of total serum theophylline concentration. Generally, concentrations of unbound theophylline should be maintained in the range of 6–12 mcg/mL.

Metabolism Following oral dosing, theophylline does not undergo any measurable first-pass elimination. In adults and children beyond 1 year of age, approximately 90% of the dose is metabolized in the liver. Biotransformation takes place through demethylation to 1-methylxanthine and 3-methylxanthine and hydroxylation to 1,3-dimethyluric acid. 1-methylxanthine is further hydroxylated by xanthine oxidase, to 1-methyluric acid. About 6% of a theophylline dose is N-methylated to caffeine. Theophylline demethylation to 3-methylxanthine is catalyzed by cytochrome P450 1A2, while cytochromes P450 2E1 and P450 3A3 catalyze the hydroxylation to 1,3-dimethyluric acid. Demethylation to 1-methylxanthine appears to be catalyzed either by cytochrome P450 1A2 or a closely related cytochrome. In neonates, the N-demethylation pathway is absent while the function of the hydroxylation pathway is markedly deficient. The activity of these pathways slowly increases to maximal levels by 1 year of age.

Caffeine and 3 methylxanthine are the only theophylline metabolites with pharmacologic activity. 3-methylxanthine has approximately one tenth the pharmacologic activity of theophylline and serum concentration in adults with normal renal function are <1 mcg/mL. In patients with end-stage renal disease, 3-methylxanthine may accumulate to concentrations that approximate the unmetabolized theophylline concentration. Caffeine concentrations are usually undetectable in adults regardless of renal function. In neonates, caffeine may accumulate to concentrations that approximate the unmetabolized theophylline concentration and thus, exert a pharmacologic effect.

Both the N-demethylation and hydroxylation pathways of theophylline biotransformation are capacity-limited. Due to the wide intersubject variability of the rate of theophylline metabolism, nonlinearity of elimination may begin in some patients at serum theophylline concentrations <10 mcg/mL. Since this nonlinearity results in more than proportional changes in serum theophylline concentrations with changes in dose, it is advisable to make increases or decreases in dose in small increments in order to achieve desired changes in serum theophylline concentrations (see **DOSAGE AND ADMINISTRATION**, **Table V**). Accurate prediction of dose-dependency of theophylline metabolism in patients *a priori* is not possible, but patients with very high initial clearance rates (ie, low steady-state serum theophylline concentrations at above average doses) have the greatest likelihood of experiencing large changes in serum theophylline concentration in response to dosage changes.

Excretion In neonates, approximately 50% of the theophylline dose is excreted unchanged in the urine. Beyond the first 3 months of life, approximately 10% of the theophylline dose is excreted unchanged in the urine. The remainder is excreted in the urine mainly as 1,3-dimethyluric acid (35%–40%), 1-methyluric acid (20%–25%), and 3-methylxanthine (15%–20%). Since little theophylline is excreted unchanged in the urine and since active metabolites of theophylline (ie, caffeine, 3-methylxanthine) do not accumulate to clinically significant levels even in the face of end-stage renal disease, no dosage adjustment for renal insufficiency is necessary in adults and children >3 months of age. In contrast, the large fraction of the theophylline dose excreted in the urine as unchanged theophylline and caffeine in neonates requires careful attention to dose reduction and frequent monitoring of serum theophylline concentrations in neonates with reduced renal function (see **WARNINGS**).

Serum Concentration at Steady State After multiple doses of immediate-release theophylline, steady state is reached in 30–65 hours (average 40 hours) in adults. At steady state, on a dosage regimen with 6-hour intervals, the expected mean trough concentration is approximately 60% of the mean peak concentration, assuming a mean theophylline half-life of 8 hours. The difference between peak and trough concentrations is larger in patients with more rapid theophylline clearance. In patients with high theophylline clearance and half-lives of about 4–5 hours, such as children aged 1 to 9 years, the trough serum theophylline concentration may be only 30% of peak with a 6-hour dosing interval. In these patients a slow-release formulation would allow a longer dosing interval (8–12 hours) with a smaller peak/trough difference.

Special Populations (See Table I for mean clearance and half-life values.)

Geriatric: The clearance of theophylline is decreased by an average of 30% in healthy elderly adults (>60 yrs) compared to healthy young adults. Careful attention to dose reduction and frequent monitoring of serum theophylline concentrations are required in elderly patients (see **WARNINGS**).

Pediatrics: The clearance of theophylline is very low in neonates (see **WARNINGS**). Theophylline clearance reaches maximal values by 1 year of age, remains relatively constant until about 9 years of age, and then slowly decreases by approximately 50% to adult values at about age 16. Renal excretion of unchanged theophylline in neonates amounts to about 50% of the dose, compared to about 10% in children older than 3 months and in adults. Careful attention to dosage selection and monitoring of serum theophylline concentrations are required in pediatric patients (see **WARNINGS** and **DOSAGE AND ADMINISTRATION**).

Gender: Gender differences in theophylline clearance are relatively small and unlikely to be of clinical significance. Significant reduction in theophylline clearance, however, has been reported in women on the 20th day of the menstrual cycle and during the third trimester of pregnancy.

Race: Pharmacokinetic differences in theophylline clearance due to race have not been studied.

Renal Insufficiency: Only a small fraction, eg, about 10%, of the administered theophylline dose is excreted unchanged in the urine of children greater than 3 months of age and adults. Since little theophylline is excreted unchanged in the urine and since active metabolites of theophylline (ie, caffeine, 3-methylxanthine) do not accumulate to clinically significant levels even in the face of end-stage renal disease, no dosage adjustment for renal insufficiency is necessary in adults and children >3 months of age. In contrast, approximately 50% of the administered theophylline dose is excreted unchanged in the urine in neonates. Careful attention to dose reduction and frequent monitoring of serum theophylline concentrations are required in neonates with decreased renal function (see **WARNINGS**).

Hepatic Insufficiency: Theophylline clearance is decreased by 50% or more in patients with hepatic insufficiency (eg, cirrhosis, acute hepatitis, cholestasis). Careful attention to dose reduction and frequent monitoring of serum theophylline concentrations are required in patients with reduced hepatic function (see **WARNINGS**).

Congestive Heart Failure (CHF): Theophylline clearance is decreased by 50% or more in patients with CHF. The extent of reduction in theophylline clearance in patients with CHF appears to be directly correlated to the severity of the cardiac disease. Since theophylline clearance is independent of liver blood flow, the reduction in clearance appears to be due to impaired hepatocyte function rather than reduced perfusion. Careful attention to dose reduction and frequent monitoring of serum theophylline concentrations are required in patients with CHF (see **WARNINGS**).

Smokers: Tobacco and marijuana smoking appear to increase the clearance of theophylline by induction of metabolic pathways. Theophylline clearance has been shown to increase by approximately 50% in young adult tobacco smokers and by approximately 80% in elderly tobacco smokers compared to nonsmoking subjects. Passive smoke exposure has also been shown to increase theophylline clearance by up to 50%. Abstinence from tobacco smoking for 1 week causes a reduction of approximately 40% in theophylline clearance. Careful attention to dose reduction and frequent monitoring of serum theophylline concentrations are required in patients who stop smoking (see **WARNINGS**). Use of nicotine gum has been shown to have no effect on theophylline clearance.

Fever: Fever, regardless of its underlying cause, can decrease the clearance of theophylline. The magnitude and duration of the fever appear to be directly correlated to the degree of decrease of theophylline clearance. Precise data are lacking, but a temperature of 39°C (102°F) for at least 24 hours or lesser temperature elevations for longer periods, are probably required to produce a clinically significant increase in serum theophylline concentrations. Children with rapid rates of theophylline clearance (ie, those who require a dose that is substantially larger than average [eg, >22 mg/kg/day] to achieve a therapeutic peak serum theophylline concentration when afebrile) may be at greater risk of toxic effects from decreased clearance during sustained fever. Careful attention to dose reduction and frequent monitoring of serum theophylline concentrations are required in patients with sustained fever (see **WARNINGS**).

Miscellaneous: Other factors associated with decreased theophylline clearance include the third trimester of pregnancy, sepsis with multiple organ failure, and hypothyroidism. Careful attention to dose reduction and frequent monitoring of serum theophylline concentrations are required in patients with any of these conditions (see **WARNINGS**). Other factors associated with increased theophylline clearance include hyperthyroidism and cystic fibrosis.

Clinical Studies:

In patients with chronic asthma, including patients with severe asthma requiring inhaled corticosteroids or alternate-day oral corticosteroids, many clinical studies have shown that theophylline decreases the frequency and severity of symptoms, including nocturnal exacerbations, and decreases the "as needed" use of inhaled beta$_2$-agonists. Theophylline has also been shown to reduce the need for short courses of daily oral prednisone to relieve exacerbations of airway obstruction that are unresponsive to bronchodilators in asthmatics.

In patients with chronic obstructive pulmonary disease (COPD), clinical studies have shown that theophylline decreases dyspnea, air trapping, the work of breathing, and improves contractility of diaphragmatic muscles with little or no improvement in pulmonary function measurements.

INDICATIONS AND USAGE

UNI-DUR Extended-release Tablets are indicated for the treatment of the symptoms and reversible airflow obstruction associated with chronic asthma and other chronic lung diseases, eg, emphysema and chronic bronchitis.

CONTRAINDICATIONS

UNI-DUR Extended-release Tablets are contraindicated in patients with a history of hypersensitivity to theophylline or other components in the product.

WARNINGS

Serious side effects such as ventricular arrhythmias, convulsions, or even death may appear as the first sign of toxicity without any recognized prior warnings. Less serious signs of theophylline toxicity (eg, nausea and restlessness) may occur frequently when initiating therapy but are usually transient. When such signs are persistent during maintenance therapy, they are often associated with serum concentrations above 20 mcg/mL. Stated differently, serious toxicity is not reliably preceded by less severe side effects.

Concurrent Illness:

Theophylline should be used with extreme caution in patients with the following clinical conditions due to the increased risk of exacerbation of the concurrent condition:

Active peptic ulcer disease (peptic ulcer disease should be controlled with appropriate therapy since theophylline is known to increase peptic acid secretion)
Seizure disorders
Cardiac arrhythmias (not including bradyarrhythmias)

Conditions That Reduce Theophylline Clearance:

There are several readily identifiable causes of reduced theophylline clearance. ***If the total daily dose is not appropriately reduced so as to lower serum theophylline levels to within the therapeutic range in the presence of these risk factors, severe and potentially fatal theophylline toxicity can occur.*** Careful consideration must be given to the benefits and risks of theophylline use and the need for more intensive monitoring of serum theophylline concentrations in patients with the following risk factors:

Age:
Neonates (term and premature)
Children <1 year
Elderly (>60 years)

Concurrent Diseases:
Acute pulmonary edema
Congestive heart failure
Cor pulmonale
Fever; ≥102°F for 24 hours or more; or lesser temperature elevations for longer periods
Hypothyroidism
Liver disease; cirrhosis, acute hepatitis
Reduced renal function in infants <3 months of age
Sepsis with multi-organ failure
Shock

Cessation of Smoking

Drug Interactions:
Adding a drug that inhibits theophylline metabolism (eg, cimetidine, erythromycin, tacrine) or stopping a concurrently administered drug that enhances theophylline metabolism (eg, carbamazepine, rifampin). (See **PRECAUTIONS, Drug Interactions, Table II.**)

When Signs or Symptoms of Theophylline Toxicity Are Present:

Whenever a patient receiving theophylline develops nausea or vomiting, particularly repetitive vomiting, or other signs or symptoms consistent with theophylline toxicity (even if another cause may be suspected), additional doses of theophylline should be withheld and a serum theophylline concentration should be measured immediately. Patients should be instructed not to continue any dosage that causes adverse effects and to withhold subsequent doses until the symptoms have resolved, at which time the clinician may instruct the patient to resume the drug at a lower dosage (see **DOSAGE AND ADMINISTRATION, Dosage Guidelines, Table V**).

Dosage Increases:

Increases in the dose of theophylline should not be made in response to an acute exacerbation of symptoms of chronic lung disease since theophylline provides little added benefit to inhaled beta$_2$-selective agonists and systemically administered corticosteroids in this circumstance and increases the risk of adverse effects. A *peak* steady-state serum theophylline concentration should be measured before increasing the dose in response to persistent chronic symptoms to ascertain whether an increase in dose is safe. Before increasing the theophylline dose on the basis of a low serum concentration, the clinician should consider whether the blood sample was obtained at an appropriate time in relationship to the dose and whether the patient has adhered to the prescribed regimen (see **PRECAUTIONS, Monitoring Serum Theophylline Concentrations**).

As the rate of theophylline clearance may be dose-dependent (ie, steady-state serum concentrations may increase disproportionately to the increase in dose), an increase in dose based upon a subtherapeutic serum concentration measurement should be conservative. In general, limiting dose increases to about 25% of the previous total daily dose will reduce the risk of unintended excessive increases in serum theophylline concentration (see **DOSAGE AND ADMINISTRATION, Table V**).

PRECAUTIONS

UNI-DUR TABLETS SHOULD *NOT* BE CHEWED OR CRUSHED AND SHOULD *BE BROKEN ONLY AT THE SCORE.*

General:

Careful consideration of the various interacting drugs (including recently discontinued medications), physiologic conditions, and other factors such as smoking that can alter theophylline clearance and require dosage adjustment should occur prior to initiation of theophylline therapy, prior to increases in theophylline dose, and during follow up (see **WARNINGS**). The dose of theophylline selected for initiation of therapy should be low and, ***if tolerated***, increased slowly over a period of a week or longer with the final dose guided by monitoring serum theophylline concentrations and the patient's clinical response (see **DOSAGE AND ADMINISTRATION, Table IV**).

Monitoring Serum Theophylline Concentrations:

Serum theophylline concentration measurements are readily available and should be used to determine whether the dosage is appropriate. Specifically, the serum theophylline concentration should be measured as follows:

1. When initiating therapy to guide final dosage adjustment after titration.
2. Before making a dose increase to determine whether the serum concentration is subtherapeutic in a patient who continues to be symptomatic.
3. Whenever signs or symptoms of theophylline toxicity are present.
4. Whenever there is a new illness, worsening of a chronic illness, or a change in the patient's treatment regimen that may alter theophylline clearance [eg, fever (see **CLINICAL PHARMACOLOGY,** *Fever*), hepatitis, or drugs listed in **Table II** are added or discontinued].

To guide a dose increase, the blood sample should be obtained at the time of the expected peak serum theophylline concentration; 8 to 12 hours after a UNI-DUR dose at steady state. For most patients, steady state will be reached after 4 days of dosing with UNI-DUR Tablets when no doses have been missed, no extra doses have been added, and none of the doses have been taken at unequal intervals. A trough concentration (ie, at the end of the dosing interval) provides no additional useful information and may lead to an inappropriate dose increase since the peak serum theophylline concentration can be two or more times greater than the trough concentration with an immediate-release formulation. If the serum sample is drawn more than 12 hours after the dose, the results must be interpreted with caution since the concentration may not be reflective of the peak concentration. In contrast, when signs or symptoms of theophylline toxicity are present, the serum sample should be obtained as soon as possible, analyzed immediately, and the result reported to the clinician without delay. In patients in whom decreased serum protein binding is suspected (eg, cirrhosis, women during the third trimester of pregnancy), the concentration of unbound theophylline should be measured and the dosage adjusted to achieve an unbound concentration of 6–12 mcg/mL.

Saliva concentrations of theophylline cannot be used reliably to adjust dosage without special techniques.

Effects on Laboratory Tests:

As a result of its pharmacological effects, theophylline at serum concentrations within the 10–20 mcg/mL range modestly increases plasma glucose (from a mean of 88 mg% to 98 mg%), uric acid (from a mean of 4 mg/dL to 6 mg/dL), free fatty acids (from a mean of 451 µEq/L to 800 µEq/L), total cholesterol (from a mean of 140 vs 160 mg/dL), HDL (from a mean of 36 to 50 mg/dL). HDL/LDL ratio (from a mean of 0.5 to 0.7), and urinary free cortisol excretion (from a mean of 44 to 63 mcg/24 hr). Theophylline at serum concentrations within the 10–20 mcg/mL range may also transiently decrease serum concentrations of triiodothyronine (144 before, 131 after 1 week and 142 ng/dL after 4 weeks of theophylline). The clinical importance of these changes should be weighed against the potential therapeutic benefit of theophylline in individual patients.

Information for Patients:

This information is intended to aid in the safe and effective use of this medication. It is not a disclosure of all adverse or intended effects.

Continued on next page

Uni-Dur—Cont.

The patient (or parent/caregiver) should be instructed to seek medical advice whenever nausea, vomiting, persistent headache, insomnia, restlessness, or rapid heartbeat occurs during treatment with theophylline, even if another cause is suspected. The patient should be instructed to contact their clinician if they develop a new illness, especially if accompanied by a persistent fever, if they experience worsening of a chronic illness, if they start or stop smoking cigarettes or marijuana, or if another clinician adds a new medication or discontinues a previously prescribed medication. Patients should be informed that theophylline interacts with a wide variety of drugs (see **Table II**). They should be instructed to inform all clinicians involved in their care that they are taking theophylline, especially when a medication is being added or deleted from their treatment. Patients should be instructed to not alter the dose, timing of the dose, or frequency of administration without first consulting their clinician. If a dose is missed, the patient should be instructed to take the next dose at the usually scheduled time and to not attempt to make up for the missed dose.

UNI-DUR Tablets *should not be chewed or crushed*. Information relating to taking UNI-DUR Tablets in relation to meals or fasting should be provided.

Drug Interactions

Drug/Drug Interactions:

Theophylline interacts with a wide variety of drugs. The interaction may be pharmacodynamic, ie, alterations in the therapeutic response to theophylline or another drug or occurrence of adverse effects without a change in serum theophylline concentration. More frequently, however, the interaction is pharmacokinetic, ie, the rate of theophylline clearance is altered by another drug resulting in increased or decreased serum theophylline concentrations. Theophylline only rarely alters the pharmacokinetics of other drugs. The drugs listed in **Table II** have the potential to produce clinically significant pharmacodynamic or pharmacokinetic interactions with theophylline. The information in the **"Effect"** column of **Table II** assumes that the interacting drug is being added to a steady-state theophylline regimen. If theophylline is being initiated in a patient who is already taking a drug that inhibits theophylline clearance (eg, cimetidine, erythromycin), the dose of theophylline required to achieve a therapeutic serum theophylline concentration will be smaller. Conversely, if theophylline is being initiated in a patient who is already taking a drug that enhances theophylline clearance (eg, rifampin), the dose of theophylline required to achieve a therapeutic serum theophylline concentration will be larger. Discontinuation of a concomitant drug that increases theophylline clearance will result in accumulation of theophylline to potentially toxic levels, unless the theophylline dose is appropriately reduced. Discontinuation of a concomitant drug that inhibits theophylline clearance will result in decreased serum theophylline concentrations, unless the theophylline dose is appropriately increased.

The listing of drugs in **Table II** is current as of February 9, 1995. New interactions are continuously being reported for theophylline, especially with new chemical entities. **The clinician should not assume that a drug does not interact with theophylline if it is not listed in Table II.** Before addition of a newly available drug in a patient receiving theophylline, the package insert of the new drug and/or the medical literature should be consulted to determine if an interaction between the new drug and theophylline has been reported.

[See table II at right]

Drug/Food Interactions:

The extent of theophylline absorption from UNI-DUR® Extended-release Tablets is similar when administered fasting or immediately after a high-fat content breakfast. However, the time to peak concentration was delayed following the high-fat content breakfast (see **CLINICAL PHARMACOLOGY, Pharmacokinetics**). This breakfast contained 729 total kilocalories of which 55% were derived from 45 g of fat; and it consisted of two scrambled eggs, two strips of bacon, one slice of toast with 1 pat of butter, 3 oz. of hash brown potatoes, and 180 mL of whole milk. The influence of the type and amount of other foods, as well as the time interval between drug and food has not been studied.

The Effect of Other Drugs on Theophylline Serum Concentration Measurements:

Most serum theophylline assays in clinical use are immunoassays which are specific for theophylline. Other xanthines such as caffeine, dyphylline, and pentoxifylline are not detected by these assays. Some drugs (eg, cefazolin, cephalothin), however, may interfere with certain HPLC techniques. Caffeine and xanthine metabolites in patients with renal dysfunction may cause the reading from some dry reagent office methods to be higher than the actual serum theophylline concentration.

Carcinogenesis, Mutagenesis, and Impairment of Fertility:

Long-term carcinogenicity studies have been carried out in mice (oral doses 30–150 mg/kg) and rats (oral doses 5–75 mg/kg). Results are pending.

Theophylline has been studied in Ames salmonella, *in vivo* and *in vitro* cytogenetics, micronucleus, and Chinese hamster ovary test systems and has not been shown to be genotoxic.

In a 14-week continuous breeding study, theophylline, administered to mating pairs of B6C3F$_1$ mice at oral doses of 120, 270, and 500 mg/kg (approximately 1.0–3.0 times the human dose on a mg/m^2 basis) impaired fertility, as evidenced by decreases in the number of live pups per litter, decreases in the mean number of litters per fertile pair, and increases in the gestation period at the high dose as well as decreases in the proportion of pups born alive at the mid and high dose. In 13-week toxicity studies, theophylline was administered to F344 rats and B6C3F$_1$ mice at oral doses of 40–300 mg/kg (approximately 2.0 times the human dose on a mg/m^2 basis). At the high dose, systemic toxicity was observed in both species including decreases in testicular weight.

Pregnancy:

Category C There are no adequate and well-controlled studies in pregnant women. Additionally, there are no teratoge-

Table II. Clinically significant drug interactions with theophylline.*

Drug	Type of Interaction	Effect**
Adenosine	Theophylline blocks adenosine receptors.	Higher doses of adenosine may be required to achieve desired effect.
Alcohol	A single large dose of alcohol (eg, 3 mL/kg of whiskey) decreases theophylline clearance for up to 24 hours.	30% increase
Allopurinol	Decreases theophylline clearance at allopurinol doses ≥600 mg/day.	25% increase
Aminoglutethimide	Increases theophylline clearance by induction of microsomal enzyme activity.	25% decrease
Carbamazepine	Similar to aminoglutethimide.	30% decrease
Cimetidine	Decreases theophylline clearance by inhibiting cytochrome P450 1A2.	70% increase
Ciprofloxacin	Similar to cimetidine.	40% increase
Clarithromycin	Similar to erythromycin.	25% increase
Diazepam	Benzodiazepines increase CNS concentrations of adenosine, a potent CNS depressant, while theophylline blocks adenosine receptors.	Larger diazepam doses may be required to produce desired level of sedation. Discontinuation of theophylline without reduction of diazepam dose may result in respiratory depression.
Disulfiram	Decreases theophylline clearance by inhibiting hydroxylation and demethylation.	50% increase
Enoxacin	Similar to cimetidine.	300% increase
Ephedrine	Synergistic CNS effects.	Increased frequency of nausea, nervousness, and insomnia.
Erythromycin	Erythromycin metabolite decreases theophylline clearance by inhibiting cytochrome P450 3A3.	35% increase. Erythromycin steady-state serum concentrations decrease by a similar amount.
Estrogen	Estrogen-containing oral contraceptives decrease theophylline clearance in a dose-dependent fashion. The effect of progesterone on theophylline clearance is unknown.	30% increase
Flurazepam	Similar to diazepam.	Similar to diazepam.
Fluvoxamine	Similar to cimetidine.	Similar to cimetidine.
Halothane	Halothane sensitizes the myocardium to catecholamines; theophylline increases release of endogenous catecholamines.	Increased risk of ventricular arrhythmias.
Interferon, human recombinant alpha-A	Decreases theophylline clearance.	100% increase
Isoproterenol (IV)	Increases theophylline clearance.	20% decrease
Ketamine	Pharmacologic.	May lower theophylline seizure threshold.
Lithium	Theophylline increases renal lithium clearance.	Lithium dose required to achieve a therapeutic serum concentration increased an average of 60%.
Lorazepam	Similar to diazepam.	Similar to diazepam.
Methotrexate (MTX)	Decreases theophylline clearance.	20% increase after low dose MTX; higher dose MTX may have a greater effect.
Mexiletine	Similar to disulfiram.	80% increase
Midazolam	Similar to diazepam.	Similar to diazepam.
Moricizine	Increases theophylline clearance.	25% decrease
Norfloxacin	Increases serum theophylline levels.	
Ofloxacin	Increases serum theophylline levels.	
Pancuronium	Theophylline may antagonize non-depolarizing neuromuscular blocking effects; possibly due to phosphodiesterase inhibition.	Larger dose of pancuronium may be required to achieve neuromuscular blockade.
Pentoxifylline	Decreases theophylline clearance.	30% increase
Phenobarbital (PB)	Similar to aminoglutethimide.	25% decrease after 2 weeks of concurrent PB.
Phenytoin	Phenytoin increases theophylline clearance by increasing microsomal enzyme activity. Theophylline decreases phenytoin absorption.	Serum theophylline *and* phenytoin concentrations decrease about 40%.
Propafenone	Decreases theophylline clearance and pharmacologic interaction.	40% increase. Beta$_2$-blocking effect may decrease efficacy of theophylline.
Propranolol	Similar to cimetidine and pharmacologic interaction.	100% increase. Beta$_2$-blocking effect may decrease efficacy of theophylline.
Rifampin	Increases theophylline clearance by increasing cytochrome P450 1A2 and 3A3 activity.	20%–40% decrease
Ritonavir	Increases theophylline clearance (mechanism unknown)	43% decrease in AUC
Sucralfate	Reduced absorption of theophylline.	
Sulfinpyrazone	Increases theophylline clearance by increasing demethylation and hydroxylation. Decreases renal clearance of theophylline.	20% decrease
Tacrine	Similar to cimetidine, also increases renal clearance of theophylline.	90% increase
Thiabendazole	Decreases theophylline clearance.	190% increase
Ticlopidine	Decreases theophylline clearance.	60% increase
Troleandomycin	Similar to erythromycin.	33%–100% increase depending on troleandomycin dose.
Verapamil	Similar to disulfiram.	20% increase

* Refer to **PRECAUTIONS,Drug Interactions** for further information regarding table.

** Average effect on steady-state theophylline concentration or other clinical effect for pharmacologic interactions. Individual patients may experience larger changes in serum theophylline concentration than the value listed.

nicity studies in nonrodents (eg, rabbits). Theophylline was not shown to be teratogenic in CD-1 mice at oral doses up to 400 mg/kg, approximately 2.0 times the recommended human dose on a mg/m^2 basis or CD-1 rats at oral doses up to 260 mg/kg, approximately 3.0 times the recommended human dose on a mg/m^2 basis. At a dose of 220 mg/kg, embryotoxicity was observed in rats in the absence of maternal toxicity.

Nursing Mothers:
Theophylline is excreted into breast milk and may cause irritability or other signs of mild toxicity in nursing human infants. The concentration of theophylline in breast milk is about equivalent to the maternal serum concentration. An infant ingesting a liter of breast milk containing 10–20 mcg/mL of theophylline a day is likely to receive 10–20 mg of theophylline per day. Serious adverse effects in the infant are unlikely unless the mother has toxic serum theophylline concentrations.

Pediatric Use:
Safety and effectiveness of UNI-DUR Extended-release Tablets in pediatric patients under 12 years of age have not been established. Other theophylline formulations, however, are safe and effective for the approved indications in pediatric patients under the age of 12. The maintenance dose of theophylline must be selected with caution in pediatric patients. The maintenance dose of theophylline must be selected with caution in pediatric patients since the rate of theophylline clearance is highly variable across the age range of neonates to adolescents (see **CLINICAL PHARMACOLOGY, Table I, WARNINGS,** and **DOSAGE AND ADMINISTRATION, Table IV**).

Geriatric Use:
Elderly patients are at significantly greater risk of experiencing serious toxicity from theophylline than younger patients due to pharmacokinetic and pharmacodynamic changes associated with aging. Theophylline clearance is reduced in patients greater than 60 years of age, resulting in increased serum theophylline concentrations in response to a given theophylline dose. Protein binding may be decreased in the elderly resulting in a larger proportion of the total serum theophylline concentration in the pharmacologically active unbound form. Elderly patients also appear to be more sensitive to the toxic effects of theophylline after chronic overdosage than younger patients. For these reasons, the maximum daily dose of theophylline in patients greater than 60 years of age ordinarily should not exceed 400 mg/day unless the patient continues to be symptomatic and the peak steady-state serum theophylline concentration is <10 mcg/mL (see **DOSAGE AND ADMINISTRATION**). Theophylline doses greater than 400 mg/day should be prescribed with caution in elderly patients.

ADVERSE REACTIONS

Adverse reactions associated with theophylline are generally mild when peak serum theophylline concentrations are <20 mcg/mL and mainly consist of transient caffeine-like adverse effects such as nausea, vomiting, headache, and insomnia. When peak serum theophylline concentrations exceed 20 mcg/mL, however, theophylline produces a wide range of adverse reactions including persistent vomiting, cardiac arrhythmias, and intractable seizures which can be lethal (see **OVERDOSAGE**). The transient caffeine-like adverse reactions occur in about 50% of patients when theophylline therapy is initiated at doses higher than recommended initial doses (eg, >300 mg/day in adults and >12 mg/kg/day in children beyond >1 year of age). During the initiation of theophylline therapy, caffeine-like adverse effects may transiently alter patient behavior, especially in school-age children, but this response rarely persists. Initiation of theophylline therapy at a low dose with subsequent slow titration to a predetermined age-related maximum dose will significantly reduce the frequency of these transient adverse effects (see **DOSAGE AND ADMINISTRATION, Table IV**). In a small percentage of patients (<3% of children and <10% of adults), the caffeine-like adverse effects persist during maintenance therapy, even at peak serum theophylline concentrations within the therapeutic range (ie, 10–20 mcg/mL). Dosage reduction may alleviate the caffeine-like adverse effects in these patients; however, persistent adverse effects should result in a re-evaluation of the need for continued theophylline therapy and the potential therapeutic benefit of alternative treatment.

Other adverse reactions that have been reported to occur at serum theophylline concentrations less than 20 mcg/mL include diarrhea, irritability, restlessness, fine skeletal muscle tremors, alopecia, muscle twitching/spasms, palpitations, rash, reflex hyperexcitability, transient diuresis, and ventricular arrhythmias. Whether or not theophylline caused these reported events is not known. In patients with hypoxia secondary to COPD, multifocal atrial tachycardia and flutter have been reported at serum theophylline concentrations ≥15mcg/mL. There have been a few isolated reports of seizures at serum theophylline concentrations <20 mcg/mL in patients with an underlying neurological disease or in elderly patients. The occurrence of seizures in elderly patients with serum theophylline concentrations <20 mcg/mL may be secondary to decreased protein binding resulting in a larger proportion of the total serum theophylline concentration in the pharmacologically active unbound form. The clinical characteristics of the seizures reported in patients with serum theophylline concentrations <20 mcg/mL have generally been milder than seizures associated with excessive serum theophylline concentrations resulting from an overdose (ie, they have generally been transient, often stopped without anticonvulsant therapy, and did not result in neurological residua).

Table III. Manifestations of theophylline toxicity.*

	Percentage of patients reported with sign or symptom			
	Acute Overdose (Large Single Ingestion)		Chronic Overdosage (Multiple Excessive Doses)	
Sign/Symptom	Study 1 (n=157)	Study 2 (n=14)	Study 1 (n=92)	Study 2 (n=102)
Asymptomatic	NR**	0	NR**	6
Gastrointestinal				
Vomiting	73	93	30	61
Abdominal pain	NR**	21	NR**	12
Diarrhea	NR**	0	NR**	14
Hematemesis	NR**	0	NR**	2
Metabolic/Other				
Hypokalemia	85	79	44	43
Hyperglycemia	98	NR**	18	NR**
Acid/base disturbance	34	21	9	5
Rhabdomyolysis	NR**	7	NR**	0
Cardiovascular				
Sinus tachycardia	100	86	100	62
Other supraventricular tachycardias	2	21	12	14
Ventricular premature beats	3	21	10	19
Atrial fibrillation or flutter	1	NR**	12	NR**
Multifocal atrial tachycardia	0	NR**	2	NR**
Ventricular arrhythmias with hemodynamic instability	7	14	40	0
Hypotension/shock	NR**	21	NR**	8
Neurologic				
Nervousness	NR**	64	NR**	21
Tremors	38	29	16	14
Disorientation	NR**	7	NR**	11
Seizures	5	14	14	5
Death	3	21	10	4

* These data are derived from two studies in patients with serum theophylline concentrations >30 mcg/mL. In the first study (Study #1-Shanon, *Ann Intern Med.* 1993;119:1161-67), data were prospectively collected from 249 consecutive cases of theophylline toxicity referred to a regional poison center for consultation. In the second study (Study #2-Sessler, *Am J Med.* 1990;88:567-76), data were retrospectively collected from 116 cases with serum theophylline concentrations >30 mcg/mL among 6000 blood samples obtained for measurement of serum theophylline concentrations in three emergency departments. Differences in the incidence of manifestations of theophylline toxicity between the two studies may reflect sample selection as a result of study design (eg, in Study #1, 48% of the patients had acute intoxications versus only 10% in Study #2) and different methods of reporting results.

**NR = Not reported in a comparable manner.

[See table III above]

OVERDOSAGE

General:
The chronicity and pattern of theophylline overdosage significantly influences clinical manifestations of toxicity, management, and outcome. There are two common presentations: (1) *acute overdose*, ie, ingestion of a single large excessive dose (>10 mg/kg) as occurs in the context of an attempted suicide or isolated medication error, and (2) *chronic overdosage*, ie, ingestion of repeated doses that are excessive for the patient's rate of theophylline clearance. The most common causes of chronic theophylline overdosage include patient or caregiver error in dosing, clinician prescribing of an excessive dose or a normal dose in the presence of factors known to decrease the rate of theophylline clearance, and increasing the dose in response to an exacerbation of symptoms without first measuring the serum theophylline concentration to determine whether a dose increase is safe.

Severe toxicity from theophylline overdose is a relatively rare event. In one health maintenance organization, the frequency of hospital admissions for chronic overdosage of theophylline was about 1 per 1000 person-years exposure. In another study, among 6000 blood samples obtained for measurement of serum theophylline concentration, for any reason, from patients treated in an emergency department, 7% were in the 20–30 mcg/mL range and 3% were >30 mcg/mL. Approximately two thirds of the patients with serum theophylline concentrations in the 20–30 mcg/mL range had one or more manifestations of toxicity while >90% of patients with serum theophylline concentrations >30 mcg/mL were clinically intoxicated. Similarly, in other reports, serious toxicity from theophylline is seen principally at serum concentrations >30 mcg/mL.

Several studies have described the clinical manifestations of theophylline overdose and attempted to determine the factors that predict life-threatening toxicity. In general, patients who experience an acute overdose are less likely to experience seizures than patients who have experienced a chronic overdosage, unless the peak serum theophylline concentration is >100 mcg/mL. After a chronic overdosage, generalized seizures, life-threatening cardiac arrhythmias, and death may occur at serum theophylline concentrations >30 mcg/mL. The severity of toxicity after chronic overdosage is more strongly correlated with the patient's age than the peak serum theophylline concentration; patients >60 years are at the greatest risk for severe toxicity and mortality after a chronic overdosage. Pre-existing or concurrent disease may also significantly increase the susceptibility of a patient to a particular toxic manifestation, eg, patients with neurologic disorders have an increased risk of seizures and patients with cardiac disease have an increased risk of cardiac arrhythmias for a given serum theophylline concentration compared to patients without the underlying disease.

The frequency of various reported manifestations of theophylline overdose according to the mode of overdose are listed in **Table III**.

Other manifestations of theophylline toxicity include increases in serum calcium, creatine kinase, myoglobin, and leukocyte count, decreases in serum phosphate and magnesium, acute myocardial infarction, and urinary retention in men with obstructive uropathy.

Seizures associated with serum theophylline concentrations >30 mcg/mL are often resistant to anticonvulsant therapy and may result in irreversible brain injury if not rapidly controlled. Death from theophylline toxicity is most often secondary to cardiorespiratory arrest and/or hypoxic encephalopathy following prolonged generalized seizures or intractable cardiac arrhythmias causing hemodynamic compromise.

Overdose Management:

General Recommendations for Patients With Symptoms of Theophylline Overdose or Serum Theophylline Concentrations >30 mcg/mL. (Note: Serum theophylline concentrations may continue to increase after presentation of the patient for medical care.)

1. While simultaneously instituting treatment, contact a regional poison center to obtain updated information and advice on individualizing the recommendations that follow.
2. Institute supportive care, including establishment of intravenous access, maintenance of the airway, and electrocardiographic monitoring.
3. *Treatment of seizures:* Because of the high morbidity and mortality associated with theophylline-induced seizures, treatment should be rapid and aggressive. Anticonvulsant therapy should be initiated with an intravenous benzodiazepine, eg, diazepam, in increments of 0.1–0.2 mg/kg every 1–3 minutes until seizures are terminated. Repetitive seizures should be treated with a loading dose of phenobarbital (20 mg/kg infused over 30–60 minutes). Animal studies and case reports of theophylline overdose in humans suggest that phenytoin is ineffective in terminating theophylline-induced seizures. The doses of benzodiazepines and phenobarbital required to terminate theophylline-induced seizures are close to the doses that may cause severe respiratory depression or respiratory arrest; the clinician should therefore be prepared to provide assisted ventilation. Elderly patients and patients with COPD may be more susceptible to the respiratory depressant effects of anticonvulsants. Barbiturate-induced coma or administration of general anesthesia may be required to terminate repetitive seizures or status epilepticus. General anesthesia should be used with caution in patients with theophylline overdose because fluorinated volatile anesthetics may sensitize the myocardium to endogenous catecholamines released by theophylline. Enflurane appears less likely to be associated with this effect than halothane and may, therefore, be safer. Neuromuscular blocking agents alone should not be used to terminate seizures since they abolish the musculoskeletal manifestations without terminating seizure activity in the brain.

Continued on next page

Uni-Dur—Cont.

4. *Anticipate need for anticonvulsants:* In patients with theophylline overdose who are at high risk for theophylline-induced seizures, eg, patients with acute overdoses and serum theophylline concentrations >100 mcg/mL or chronic overdosage in patients >60 years of age with serum theophylline concentrations >30 mcg/mL, the need for anticonvulsant therapy should be anticipated. A benzodiazepine such as diazepam should be drawn into a syringe and kept at the patient's bedside and medical personnel qualified to treat seizures should be immediately available. In selected patients at high risk for theophylline-induced seizures, consideration should be given to the administration of prophylactic anticonvulsant therapy. Situations where prophylactic anticonvulsant therapy should be considered in high-risk patient include anticipated delays in instituting methods for extracorporeal removal of theophylline (eg, transfer of a high-risk patient from one healthcare facility to another for extracorporeal removal) and clinical circumstances that significantly interfere with efforts to enhance theophylline clearance (eg, a neonate where dialysis may not be technically feasible or a patient with vomiting unresponsive to antiemetics who is unable to tolerate multiple-dose oral activated charcoal). In animal studies, prophylactic administration of phenobarbital, *but not phenytoin*, has been shown to delay the onset of theophylline-induced generalized seizures and to increase the dose of theophylline required to induce seizures (ie, markedly increases the LD_{50}). Although there are no controlled studies in humans, a loading dose of intravenous phenobarbital (20 mg/kg infused over 60 minutes) may delay or prevent life-threatening seizures in high-risk patients while efforts to enhance theophylline clearance are continued. Phenobarbital may cause respiratory depression, particularly in elderly patients and patients with COPD.
5. *Treatment of cardiac arrhythmias:* Sinus tachycardia and simple ventricular premature beats are not harbingers of life-threatening arrhythmias, they do not require treatment in the absence of hemodynamic compromise, and they resolve with declining serum theophylline concentrations. Other arrhythmias, especially those associated with hemodynamic compromise, should be treated with antiarrhythmic therapy appropriate for the type of arrhythmia.
6. *Gastrointestinal decontamination:* Oral activated charcoal (0.5 g/kg up to 20 g and repeat at least once 1–2 hours after the first dose) is extremely effective in blocking the absorption of theophylline throughout the gastrointestinal tract, even when administered several hours after ingestion. If the patient is vomiting, the charcoal should be administered through a nasogastric tube or after administration of an antiemetic. Phenothiazine antiemetics such as prochlorperazine or perphenazine should be avoided since they can lower the seizure threshold and frequently cause dystonic reactions. A single dose of sorbitol may be used to promote stooling to facilitate removal of theophylline bound to charcoal from the gastrointestinal tract. Sorbitol, however, should be dosed with caution since it is a potent purgative which can cause profound fluid and electrolyte abnormalities, particularly after multiple doses. Commercially available fixed combinations of liquid charcoal and sorbitol should be avoided in young children and after the first dose in adolescents and adults since they do not allow for individualization of charcoal and sorbitol dosing. Ipecac syrup should be avoided in theophylline overdoses. Although ipecac induces emesis, it does not reduce the absorption of theophylline unless administered within 5 minutes of ingestion and even then is less effective than oral activated charcoal. Moreover, ipecac-induced emesis may persist for several hours after a single dose and significantly decrease the retention and the effectiveness of oral activated charcoal.
7. *Serum theophylline concentration monitoring:* The serum theophylline concentration should be measured immediately upon presentation, 2–4 hours later, and then at sufficient intervals, eg, every 4 hours, to guide treatment decisions and to assess the effectiveness of therapy. Serum theophylline concentrations may continue to increase after presentation of the patient for medical care as a result of continued absorption of theophylline from the gastrointestinal tract. Serial monitoring of serum theophylline serum concentrations should be continued until it is clear that the concentration is no longer rising and has returned to nontoxic levels.
8. *General monitoring procedures:* Electrocardiographic monitoring should be initiated on presentation and continued until the serum theophylline level has returned to a nontoxic level. Serum electrolytes and glucose should be measured on presentation and at appropriate intervals indicated by clinical circumstances. Fluid and electrolyte abnormalities should be promptly corrected. **Monitoring and treatment should be continued until the serum concentration decreases below 20 mcg/mL.**
9. *Enhance clearance of theophylline:* Multiple-dose oral activated charcoal (eg, 0.5 mg/kg up to 20 g, every 2 hours) increases the clearance of theophylline at least twofold by absorption of theophylline secreted into gastrointestinal fluids. Charcoal must be retained in, and pass through, the gastrointestinal tract to be effective; emesis should therefore be controlled by administration of appropriate antiemetics. Alternatively, the charcoal can be administered continuously through a nasogastric tube in conjunction with appropriate antiemetics. A single dose of sorbitol may be administered with the activated charcoal to promote stooling to facilitate clearance of the adsorbed theophylline from the gastrointestinal tract. Sorbitol alone does not enhance clearance of theophylline and should be dosed with caution to prevent excessive stooling which can result in severe fluid and electrolyte imbalances. Commercially available fixed combinations of liquid charcoal and sorbitol should be avoided in young children and after the first dose in adolescents and adults since they do not allow for individualization of charcoal and sorbitol dosing. In patients with intractable vomiting, extracorporeal methods of theophylline removal should be instituted (see **OVERDOSAGE, Extracorporeal Removal**).

Table IV. **Dosing initiation and titration (as anhydrous theophylline).***

A. Children (12–15 years) and adults (16–60 years) without risk factors for impaired clearance.

Titration Step	*Children <45 kg*	*Children >45 kg and adults*
1. Starting dosage:	12–14 mg/kg/day up to a maximum of 300 mg/day administered QD*	300–400 mg/day[1] administered QD*
2. After 3 days, *if tolerated,* increase dose to:	16 mg/kg/day up to a maximum of 400 mg/day administered QD*	400–600 mg/day[1] administered QD*
3. After 3 more days, *if tolerated,* increase dose to:	20 mg/kg/day up to a maximum of 600 mg/day administered QD*	As with all theophylline products, doses greater than 600 mg should be titrated according to blood level (see **Table V**).

B. **Patients With Risk Factors For Impaired Clearance, The Elderly (>60 Years), And Those In Whom It Is Not Feasible To Monitor Serum Theophylline Concentrations:**

In children 12–15 years of age, the final theophylline dose should not exceed 16 mg/kg/day up to a maximum of 400 mg/day in the presence of risk factors for reduced theophylline clearance (see **WARNINGS**) or if it is not feasible to monitor serum theophylline concentrations.

In adolescents ≥16 years and adults, including the elderly, the final theophylline dose should not exceed 400 mg/day in the presence of risk factors for reduced theophylline clearance (see **WARNINGS**) or if it is not feasible to monitor serum theophylline concentrations.

*Patients with more rapid metabolism, clinically identified by higher than average dose requirements, should receive a smaller dose more frequently (every 12 hours) to prevent breakthrough symptoms resulting from low trough concentrations before the next dose.

[1]If caffeine-like adverse effects occur, then consideration should be given to a lower dose and titrating the dose more slowly (see **ADVERSE REACTIONS**).

Table V. **Dosage adjustment guided by serum theophylline concentration.**

Peak Serum Concentration	**Dosage Adjustment**
<9.9 mcg/mL	If symptoms are not controlled and current dosage is tolerated, increase dose about 25%. Recheck serum concentration after 3 days for further dosage adjustment.
10 to 14.9 mcg/mL	If symptoms are controlled and current dosage is tolerated, maintain dose and recheck serum concentration at 6- to 12-month intervals.¶ If symptoms are not controlled and current dosage is tolerated, consider adding additional medication(s) to treatment regimen.
15–19.9 mcg/mL	Consider 10% decrease in dose to provide greater margin of safety even if current dosage is tolerated.¶
20–24.9 mcg/mL	Decrease dose by 25% even if no adverse effects are present. Recheck serum concentration after 3 days to guide further dosage adjustment.
25–30 mcg/mL	Skip next dose and decrease subsequent doses at least 25% even if no adverse effects are present. Recheck serum concentration after 3 days to guide further dosage adjustment. If symptomatic, consider whether overdose treatment is indicated (see recommendations for chronic overdosage).
>30 mcg/mL	Treat overdose as indicated (see recommendations for chronic overdosage). If theophylline is subsequently resumed, decrease dose by at least 50% and recheck serum concentration after 3 days to guide further dosage adjustment.

¶ Dose reduction and/or serum theophylline concentration measurement is indicated whenever adverse effects are present, physiologic abnormalities that can reduce theophylline clearance occur (eg, sustained fever), or a drug that interacts with theophylline is added or discontinued (see **WARNINGS**).

Specific Recommendations:

Acute Overdose

A. Serum Concentration >20 <30 mcg/mL
   1. Administer a single dose of oral activated charcoal.
   2. Monitor the patient and obtain a serum theophylline concentration in 2–4 hours to ensure that the concentration is not increasing.

B. Serum Concentration >30 <100 mcg/mL
   1. Administer multiple-dose oral activated charcoal and measures to control emesis.
   2. Monitor the patient and obtain serial theophylline concentrations every 2–4 hours to gauge the effectiveness of therapy and to guide further treatment decisions.
   3. Institute extracorporeal removal if emesis, seizures, or cardiac arrhythmias cannot be adequately controlled (see **OVERDOSAGE, Extracorporeal Removal**).

C. Serum Concentration >100 mcg/mL
   1. Consider prophylactic anticonvulsant therapy.
   2. Administer multiple-dose oral activated charcoal and measures to control emesis.
   3. Consider extracorporeal removal, even if the patient has not experienced a seizure (see **OVERDOSAGE, Extracorporeal Removal**).
   4. Monitor the patient and obtain serial theophylline concentrations every 2–4 hours to gauge the effectiveness of therapy and to guide further treatment decisions.

Chronic Overdosage

A. Serum Concentration >20 <30 mcg/mL (with manifestations of theophylline toxicity)
   1. Administer a single dose of oral activated charcoal.
   2. Monitor the patient and obtain a serum theophylline concentration in 2–4 hours to ensure that the concentration is not increasing.

B. Serum Concentration >30 mcg/mL in patients <60 years of age
   1. Administer multiple-dose oral activated charcoal and measures to control emesis.
   2. Monitor the patient and obtain serial theophylline concentrations every 2–4 hours to gauge the effectiveness of therapy and to guide further treatment decisions.
   3. Institute extracorporeal removal if emesis, seizures, or cardiac arrhythmias cannot be adequately controlled (see **OVERDOSAGE, Extracorporeal Removal**).

C. Serum Concentration >30 mcg/mL in patients ≥60 years of age
   1. Consider prophylactic anticonvulsant therapy.
   2. Administer multiple-dose oral activated charcoal and measures to control emesis.
   3. Consider extracorporeal removal even if the patient has not experienced a seizure (see **OVERDOSAGE, Extracorporeal Removal**).
   4. Monitor the patient and obtain serial theophylline concentrations every 2–4 hours to gauge the effectiveness of therapy and to guide further treatment decisions.

Extracorporeal Removal:

Increasing the rate of theophylline by extracorporeal methods may rapidly decrease serum concentrations, but the risks of the procedure must be weighed against the potential benefit. Charcoal hemoperfusion is the most effective method of extracorporeal removal, increasing theophylline clearance up to sixfold, but serious complications, including hypotension, hypocalcemia, platelet consumption, and bleeding diatheses may occur. Hemodialysis is about as efficient as multiple-dose oral activated charcoal and has a lower risk of serious complications than charcoal hemoperfusion. Hemodialysis should be considered as an alternative when charcoal hemoperfusion is not feasible and multiple-dose oral charcoal is ineffective because of intractable emesis. Serum theophylline concentrations may rebound 5–10 mcg/mL after discontinuation of charcoal hemoperfusion or hemodialysis due to redistribution of theophylline from the tissue compartment. Peritoneal dialysis is ineffective for theophylline removal; exchange transfusions in neonates have been minimally effective.

DOSAGE AND ADMINISTRATION

The extent of absorption of theophylline from UNI-DUR Tablets when administered fasting or immediately after a high-fat content breakfast is similar. However, the time to peak concentration is delayed (see **PRECAUTIONS, Drug/Food Interactions**).

Effective use of theophylline (ie, the concentration of drug in the serum associated with optimal benefit and minimal risk of toxicity) is considered to occur when the theophylline concentration is maintained from 10 to 15 mcg/mL.

Patients who clear theophylline normally or relatively slowly, eg, nonsmokers, may be reasonable candidates for taking UNI-DUR Tablets once daily. However, certain patients, such as the young, smokers, and some nonsmoking adults are likely to metabolize theophylline more rapidly and may require dosing at 12-hour intervals. Such patients may experience symptoms of bronchospasm toward the end of a once-daily dosing interval and/or require a higher daily dose (higher than those recommended in labeling) and are more likely to experience relatively wide peak to trough differences in serum theophylline concentrations.

UNI-DUR Tablets may be administered either in the morning or in the evening.

UNI-DUR Tablets *should not be chewed or crushed.*

General Considerations:

The steady-state peak serum theophylline concentration is a function of the dose, the dosing interval, and the rate of theophylline absorption and clearance in the individual patient. Because of marked individual differences in the rate of theophylline clearance, the dose required to achieve a peak serum theophylline concentration in the 10–20 mcg/mL range varies fourfold among otherwise similar patients in the absence of factors known to alter theophylline clearance (eg, 400–1600 mg/day in adults <60 years old and 10–36 mg/kg/day in children 1–9 years old). For a given population there is no single theophylline dose that will provide both safe and effective serum concentrations for all patients. Administration of the median theophylline dose required to achieve a therapeutic serum theophylline concentration in a given population may result in either subtherapeutic or potentially toxic serum theophylline concentrations in individual patients. For example, at a dose of 900 mg/day in adults <60 years or 22 mg/kg/day in children 1–9 years, the steady-state peak serum theophylline concentration will be <10 mcg/mL in about 30% of patients, 10–20 mcg/mL in about 50%, and 20–30 mcg/mL in about 20% of patients. **The dose of theophylline must be individualized on the basis of peak serum theophylline concentration measurements in order to achieve a dose that will provide maximum potential benefit with minimal risk of adverse effects.**

Transient caffeine-like adverse effects and excessive serum concentrations in slow metabolizers can be avoided in most patients by starting with a sufficiently low dose and slowly increasing the dose, *if judged to be clinically indicated*, in small increments (see **Table IV**). Dose increases should only be made if the previous dosage is well tolerated and at intervals of no less than 3 days to allow serum theophylline concentrations to reach the new steady state. Dosage adjustment should be guided by serum theophylline concentration measurement (see **PRECAUTIONS, Monitoring Serum Theophylline Concentrations,** and **DOSAGE AND ADMINISTRATION, Table V**). Healthcare providers should instruct patients and caregivers to discontinue any dosage that causes adverse effects, to withhold the medication until these symptoms are gone, and to then resume therapy at lower, previously tolerated dosage (see **WARNINGS**).

If the patient's symptoms are well controlled, there are no apparent adverse effects, and no intervening factors that might alter dosage requirements (see **WARNINGS** and **PRECAUTIONS**), serum theophylline concentrations should be monitored at 6-month intervals for rapidly growing children and at yearly intervals for all others. In acutely ill patients, serum theophylline concentrations should be monitored at frequent intervals, eg, every 24 hours.

Theophylline distributes poorly into body fat, therefore, mg/kg dose should be calculated on the basis of ideal body weight.

Table IV contains theophylline dosing titration schema recommended for patients in various age groups and clinical circumstances. **Table V** contains recommendations for theophylline dosage adjustment based upon serum theophylline concentrations. **Application of these general dosing recommendations to individual patients must take into account the unique clinical characteristics of each patient. In general, these recommendations should serve as the upper limit for dose adjustments in order to decrease the risk of potentially serious adverse events associated with unexpected large increases in serum theophylline concentration.**

[See table IV on previous page]
[See table V on previous page]

HOW SUPPLIED

UNI-DUR Extended-release Tablets are supplied as controlled-release tablets containing either 400 mg or 600 mg of theophylline anhydrous. They are mottled white, capsule-shaped tablets; scored on one side and debossed with the product name and strength on the other.

UNI-DUR Extended-release Tablets 400 mg are available in bottles of 100's (NDC 0085-0694-01).

UNI-DUR Extended-release Tablets 600 mg are available in bottles of 100's (NDC 0085-0814-01).

STORAGE CONDITIONS

Keep bottles tightly closed. Store between 15° and 25°C (59° and 77°F).

CAUTION: Federal law prohibits dispensing without prescription.

Key Pharmaceuticals, Inc.
Kenilworth, NJ 07033 USA

Rev. 3/97 19767914

Shown in Product Identification Guide, page 319

Knoll Laboratories

**A Division of
Knoll Pharmaceutical Company
3000 CONTINENTAL DRIVE NORTH
MOUNT OLIVE, NJ 07828-1234**

Direct Inquiries to:
BASF Group
Customer Information Center:
General Information (800) 240-3820

Customer Operations: Orders, Credits/Returns, Wholesaler and Hospital Inquiries, Deductions, New Accounts (800) 526-0710

For Medical Information Contact:
(800) 526-0221

AKINETON® TABLETS AND AMPULES ℞

[*ā-kĭn 'ĕ-ton*]

biperiden hydrochloride and biperiden lactate

DESCRIPTION

Each AKINETON Tablet for oral administration contains 2 mg biperiden hydrochloride. Other ingredients may include corn syrup, lactose, magnesium stearate, potato starch and talc. Each 1 mL AKINETON Ampule for intramuscular or intravenous administration contains 5 mg biperiden lactate in an aqueous 1.4 percent sodium lactate solution. No added preservative. AKINETON is an anticholinergic agent. Biperiden is α-5-Norbornen-2-yl-α-phenyl-1-piperidine propanol. It is a white, crystalline, odorless powder, slightly soluble in water and alcohol. It is stable in air at normal temperatures. Biperiden may be represented by the following structural formula:

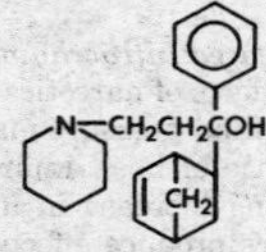

CLINICAL PHARMACOLOGY

AKINETON is a weak peripheral anticholinergic agent. It has, therefore, some antisecretory, antispasmodic and mydriatic effects. In addition, AKINETON possesses nicotinolytic activity. Parkinsonism is thought to result from an imbalance between the excitatory (cholinergic) and inhibitory (dopaminergic) systems in the corpus striatum. The mechanism of action of centrally active anticholinergic drugs such as AKINETON is considered to relate to competitive antagonism of acetylcholine at cholinergic receptors in the corpus striatum, which then restores the balance.

The parenteral form of AKINETON is an effective and reliable agent for the treatment of acute episodes of extrapyramidal disturbances sometimes seen during treatment with neuroleptic agents. Akathisia, akinesia, dyskinetic tremors, rigor, oculogyric crisis, spasmodic torticollis, and profuse sweating are markedly reduced or eliminated. With parenteral AKINETON, these drug-induced disturbances are rapidly brought under control. Subsequently, this can usually be maintained with oral doses which may be given with tranquilizer therapy in psychotic and other conditions requiring an uninterrupted therapeutic program.

Pharmacokinetics and Metabolism: Only limited pharmacokinetic studies of biperiden in humans are available The serum concentration at 1 to 1.5 hours following a single, 4 mg oral dose was 4–5 ng/mL. Plasma levels (0.1–0.2 ng/mL) could be determined up to 48 hours after dosing. Six hours after an oral dose of 250 mg/kg in rats, 87% of the drug had been absorbed. The metabolism of AKINETON is also incompletely understood, but does involve hydroxylation. In normal volunteers a single 10 mg intravenous dose of biperiden seemed to cause a transient rise in plasma cortisol and prolactin. No change in GH, LH, FSH, or TSH levels were seen. Biperiden lactate (10 mg/mL) was not irritating to the tissue of rabbits when injected intramuscularly (1.0 mL) into the sacrospinalis muscles and intradermally (0.25 mL) and subcutaneously (0.5 mL) into the shaved abdominal skin.

INDICATIONS AND USAGE

- As an adjunct in the therapy of all forms of parkinsonism (idiopathic, postencephalitic, arteriosclerotic)
- Control of extrapyramidal disorders secondary to neuroleptic drug therapy (e.g., phenothiazines)

CONTRAINDICATIONS

1) Hypersensitivity to biperiden 2) Narrow angle glaucoma 3) Bowel obstruction 4) Megacolon

WARNINGS

Isolated instances of mental confusion, euphoria, agitation and disturbed behavior have been reported in susceptible patients. Also, the central anticholinergic syndrome can occur as an adverse reaction to properly prescribed anticholinergic medication, although it is more frequently due to overdosage. It may also result from concomitant administration of an anticholinergic agent and a drug that has secondary anticholinergic actions (see Drug Interactions and Overdosage sections). Caution should be observed in patients with manifest glaucoma, though no prohibitive rise in intraocular pressure has been noted following either oral or parenteral administration. Patients with prostatism, epilepsy or cardiac arrhythmia should be given this drug with caution.

Occasionally, drowsiness may occur, and patients who drive a car or operate any other potentially dangerous machinery should be warned of this possibility. As with other drugs acting on the central nervous system, the consumption of alcohol should be avoided during AKINETON therapy.

PRECAUTIONS

Drug Interactions: The central anticholinergic syndrome can occur when anticholinergic agents such as AKINETON are administered concomitantly with drugs that have secondary anticholinergic actions, e.g., certain narcotic analgesics such as meperidine, the phenothiazines and other antipsychotics, tricyclic antidepressants, certain antiarrhythmics such as the quinidine salts, and antihistamines. See Overdosage section for signs and symptoms of the central anticholinergic syndrome, and for treatment.

Pregnancy: Pregnancy Category C. Animal reproduction studies have not been conducted with AKINETON. It is also not known whether AKINETON can cause fetal harm when administered to a pregnant woman or can affect reproduction capacity. AKINETON should be given to a pregnant woman only if clearly needed.

Nursing Mothers: It is not known whether this drug is excreted in human milk. Because many drugs are excreted in human milk, caution should be exercised when AKINETON is administered to a nursing woman.

Pediatric Use: Safety and effectiveness in children have not been established.

ADVERSE REACTIONS

Atropine-like side effects such as dry mouth; blurred vision; drowsiness; euphoria or disorientation; urinary retention; postural hypotension; constipation; agitation; disturbed behavior may be seen. There usually are no significant changes in blood pressure or heart rate in patients who have been given the parenteral form of AKINETON. Mild transient postural hypotension and bradycardia may occur. These side effects can be minimized or avoided by slow intravenous administration. No local tissue reactions have been reported following intramuscular injection. If gastric irritation occurs following oral administration, it can be avoided by administering the drug during or after meals. The central anticholinergic syndrome can occur as an adverse reaction to properly prescribed anticholinergic medication. See Overdosage section for signs and symptoms of the central anticholinergic syndrome, and for treatment.

OVERDOSAGE

Signs and Symptoms: Overdosage with AKINETON produces typical central symptoms of atropine intoxication (the central anticholinergic syndrome). Correct diagnosis depends upon recognition of the peripheral signs of parasympathetic blockade including dilated and sluggish pupils; warm, dry skin; facial flushing; decreased secretions of the mouth, pharynx, nose, and bronchi; foul-smelling breath; elevated temperature, tachycardia, cardiac arrhythmias, decreased bowel sounds, and urinary retention. Neuropsychiatric signs such as delirium, disorientation, anxiety, hallucinations, illusions, confusion, incoherence, agitation, hyperactivity, ataxia, loss of memory, paranoia, combativeness, and seizures may be present. The condition can progress to stupor, coma, paralysis, and cardiac and respiratory arrest and death.

Treatment: Treatment of acute overdose revolves around symptomatic and supportive therapy. If AKINETON was administered orally, gastric lavage or other measures to limit absorption should be instituted. A small dose of diazepam or a short acting barbiturate may be administered if CNS excitation is observed. Phenothiazines are contraindicated because the toxicity may be intensified due to their antimuscarinic action, causing coma. Respiratory support, artificial respiration or vasopressor agents may be necessary. Hyperpyrexia must be reversed, fluid volume replaced and acid-base balance maintained. Urinary catheterization may be necessary.

Routine use of physostigmine for overdose is controversial. Delirium, hallucinations, coma, and supraventricular tachycardia (not ventricular tachycardias or conduction defects) seem to respond. If indicated, 1 mg (half this amount for children or elderly) may be given intramuscularly or by slow intravenous infusion. If there is no response within 20 minutes, an additional 1 mg dose may be given; this may be repeated until a total of 4 mg has been administered, a reversal of the toxic effects occur or excessive cholinergic signs

Continued on next page

Akineton—Cont.

are seen. Frequent monitoring of clinical signs should be done. Since physostigmine is rapidly destroyed, additional injections may be required every one or two hours to maintain control. The relapse intervals tend to lengthen as the toxic anticholinergic agent is metabolized, so the patient should be carefully observed for 8 to 12 hours following the last relapse.

Toxicity in Animals: The LD_{50} of biperiden in the white mouse is 545 mg/kg orally, 195 mg/kg subcutaneously, and 56 mg/kg intravenously. The acute oral toxicity (LD_{50}) in rats is 750 mg/kg. The intraperitoneal toxicity (LD_{50}) of biperiden lactate in rats was 270 mg/kg and the intravenous toxicity (LD_{50}) in dogs is 222 mg/kg. In dogs under general anesthesia, respiratory arrest occurred at 33 mg/kg (intravenous) and circulatory standstill at 45 mg/kg (intravenous). The oral LD_{50} in dogs was 340 mg/kg. Chronic toxicity studies in both rat and dog have been reported.

DOSAGE AND ADMINISTRATION

Drug-Induced Extrapyramidal Symptoms:

Parenteral: The average adult dose is 2 mg intramuscularly or intravenously. May be repeated every half-hour until there is resolution of symptoms, but not more than four consecutive doses should be given in a 24-hour period.

Note: Parenteral drug products should be inspected visually for particulate matter and discoloration prior to administration, whenever solution and container permit.

Oral: One tablet one to three times daily.

Parkinson's Disease: Oral: The usual beginning dose is one tablet three or four times daily. The dosage should be individualized with the dose titrated upward to a maximum of 8 tablets (16 mg) per 24 hours.

HOW SUPPLIED

AKINETON Tablets, 2 mg each, white, embossed on one face with a triangle, bisected on the reverse and imprinted with the number "11."

Bottles of 100—NDC #0044-0120-02.

Bottles of 1000—NDC #0044-0120-04.

Storage: All dosage forms of AKINETON should be stored at 15°–30°C (59°–86°F). Dispense in tight, light-resistant container as defined in USP.

AKINETON is a registered trademark of Knoll AG

Revised: July 1996

Knoll Laboratories

A Division of

Knoll Pharmaceutical Company

Mount Olive, New Jersey 07828

BASF Pharma 0900002-2

Shown in Product Identification Guide, page 319

DILAUDID® Ⓒ℞

[*dī "law 'dĭd*]

hydromorphone hydrochloride

Rx only

DESCRIPTION

DILAUDID (hydromorphone hydrochloride), a hydrogenated ketone of morphine, is a narcotic analgesic. It is available in:

Ampules (for parenteral administration) containing:

1 mg, 2 mg, and 4 mg hydromorphone hydrochloride per mL with 0.2% sodium citrate, 0.2% citric acid solution. DILAUDID ampules are sterile.

Multiple Dose Vials (for parenteral administration) containing:

20 mL of solution. Each mL contains 2 mg hydromorphone hydrochloride and 0.5 mg edetate disodium with 1.8 mg methylparaben and 0.2 mg propylparaben as preservatives. Sodium hydroxide or hydrochloric acid is used for pH adjustment. DILAUDID multiple dose vials are sterile.

Color Coded Tablets (for oral administration) containing:

2 mg hydromorphone hydrochloride (orange tablet) and D&C red #30 Lake dye, D&C yellow #10 Lake dye, lactose, and magnesium stearate.

4 mg hydromorphone hydrochloride (yellow tablet) and D&C yellow #10 Lake dye, lactose, and magnesium stearate.

Suppositories (for rectal administration) containing:

3 mg hydromorphone hydrochloride in a cocoa butter base with silicon dioxide.

Non-Sterile Powder (for prescription compounding) containing hydromorphone hydrochloride. The structural formula of DILAUDID (hydromorphone hydrochloride) is:

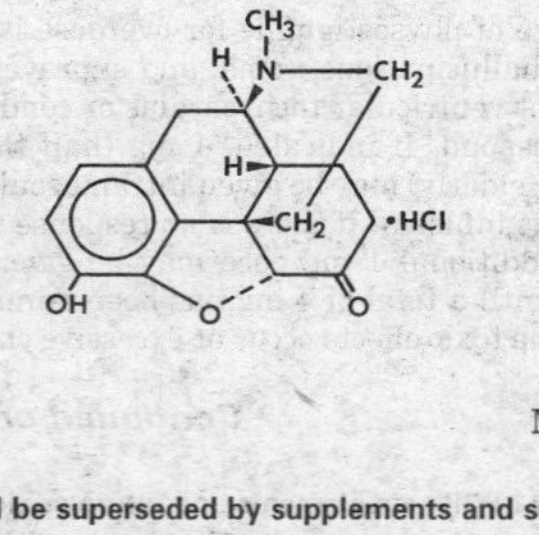

M.W. 321.8

CLINICAL PHARMACOLOGY

DILAUDID is a narcotic analgesic; its principal therapeutic effect is relief of pain. The precise mechanism of action of DILAUDID and other opiates is not known, although it is believed to relate to the existence of opiate receptors in the central nervous system. There is no intrinsic limit to the analgesic effect of DILAUDID; like morphine, adequate doses will relieve even the most severe pain. Clinically, however, dosage limitations are imposed by the adverse effects, primarily respiratory depression, nausea, and vomiting, which can result from high doses.

DILAUDID has diverse additional actions. It may produce drowsiness, changes in mood and mental clouding, depress the respiratory center and the cough center, stimulate the vomiting center, produce pinpoint constriction of the pupil, enhance parasympathetic activity, elevate cerebrospinal fluid pressure, increase biliary pressure, produce transient hyperglycemia.

Generally, the analgesic action of parenterally administered DILAUDID is apparent within 15 minutes and usually remains in effect for more than five hours. The onset of action of oral DILAUDID is somewhat slower, with measurable analgesia occurring within 30 minutes.

In human plasma the half-life of a DILAUDID 4 mg tablet is 2.6 hours. In a random crossover study in six subjects, 4 mg of oral DILAUDID produced a mean concentration/time curve similar to that of 2 mg DILAUDID I.V., after the first hour.

INDICATIONS AND USAGE

DILAUDID is indicatd for the relief of moderate to severe pain such as that due to:

Surgery
Cancer
Trauma (soft tissue & bone)
Biliary Colic
Myocardial Infarction
Burns
Renal Colic

CONTRAINDICATIONS

DILAUDID is contraindicated in patients with a known hypersensitivity to hydromorphone; in the presence of an intracranial lesion associated with increased intracranial pressure; and whenever ventilatory function is depressed (chronic obstructive pulmonary disease, cor pulmonale, emphysema, kyphoscoliosis, status asthmaticus).

WARNINGS

Respiratory Depression: DILAUDID produces dose-related respiratory depression by acting directly on brain stem respiratory centers. DILAUDID also affects centers that control respiratory rhythm, and may produce irregular and periodic breathing.

Head Injury and Increased Intracranial Pressure: The respiratory depressant effects of narcotics and their capacity to elevate cerebrospinal fluid pressure may be markedly exaggerated in the presence of head injury, other intracranial lesions or a preexisting increase in intracranial pressure. Furthermore, narcotics produce effects which may obscure the clinical course of patients with head injuries.

Acute Abdominal Conditions: The administration of narcotics may obscure the diagnosis or clinical course of patients with acute abdominal conditions.

PRECAUTIONS

Special Risk Patients: DILAUDID should be used with caution in elderly or debilitated patients and those with impaired renal or hepatic function, hypothyroidism, Addison's disease, prostatic hypertrophy or urethral stricture. As with any narcotic analgesic agent, the usual precautions should be observed and the possibility of respiratory depression should be kept in mind.

Cough Reflex: DILAUDID suppresses the cough reflex; as with all narcotics, caution should be exercised when DILAUDID is used postoperatively and in patients with pulmonary disease.

Usage in Ambulatory Patients: Narcotics may impair the mental and/or physical abilities required for the performance of potentially hazardous tasks such as driving a car or operating machinery; patients should be cautioned accordingly

Drug Interactions: Patients receiving other narcotic analgesics, general anesthetics, phenothiazines, tranquilizers, sedative hypnotics, tricyclic antidepressants or other CNS depressants (including alcohol) concomitantly with DILAUDID may exhibit an additive CNS depression. When such combined therapy is contemplated, the dose of one or both agents should be reduced.

Parenteral Administration: The parenteral form of DILAUDID may be given intravenously, but the injection should be given very slowly. Rapid intravenous injection of narcotic analgesics increases the possibility of side effects such as hypotension and respiratory depression.

Pregnancy: Pregnancy Category C. DILAUDID has been shown to be teratogenic in hamsters when given in doses 600 times the human dose. There are no adequate and well-controlled studies in pregnant women. DILAUDID should be used during pregnancy only if the potential benefit justifies the potential risk to the fetus.

Nonteratogenic effects: Babies born to mothers who have been taking opioids regularly prior to delivery will be physically dependent. The withdrawal signs include irritability and excessive crying, tremors, hyperactive reflexes, increased respiratory rate, increased stools, sneezing, yawning, vomiting, and fever. The intensity of the syndrome does not always correlate with the duration of maternal opioid use or dose. There is no consensus on the best method of managing withdrawal. Chlorpromazine 0.7 to 1.0 mg/kg q6h, phenobarbital 2 mg/kg q6h, and paregoric 2 to 4 drops/kg q4h, have been used to treat withdrawal symptoms in infants. The duration of therapy is 4 to 28 days, with the dosages decreased as tolerated.

Labor and Delivery: As with all narcotics, administration of DILAUDID to the mother shortly before delivery may result in some degree of respiratory depression in the newborn, especially if higher doses are used.

Nursing Mothers: It is not known whether this drug is excreted in human milk. Because many drugs are excreted in human milk and because of the potential for serious adverse reactions in nursing infants from DILAUDID, a decision should be made whether to discontinue nursing or to discontinue the drug, taking into account the importance of the drug to the mother.

Pediatric Use: Safety and effectiveness in children have not been established.

Geriatric Use: Clinical studies of DILAUDID did not include sufficient numbers of subjects aged 65 and over to determine whether they respond differently from younger subjects. Other reported clinical experience has not identified differences in responses between the elderly and younger patients. In general, dose selection for an elderly patient should be cautious, usually starting at the low end of the dosing range, reflecting the greater frequency of decreased hepatic, renal, or cardiac function, and of concomitant disease or other drug therapy.

ADVERSE REACTIONS

Central Nervous System: Sedation, drowsiness, mental clouding, lethargy, impairment of mental and physical performance, anxiety, fear, dysphoria, dizziness, psychic dependence, mood changes.

Gastrointestinal System: Nausea and vomiting occur infrequently; they are more frequent in ambulatory than in recumbent patients. The antiemetic phenothiazines are useful in suppressing these effects; however, some phenothiazine derivatives seem to be antianalgesic and to increase the amount of narcotic required to produce pain relief, while other phenothiazines reduce the amount of narcotic required to produce a given level of analgesia. Prolonged administration of DILAUDID may produce constipation. Opiate agonist-induced increase in intraluminal pressure may endanger surgical anastomosis.

Cardiovascular System: Circulatory depression, peripheral circulatory collapse and cardiac arrest have occurred after rapid intravenous injection Orthostatic hypotension and fainting may occur if a patient stands up suddenly after receiving an injection of DILAUDID.

Genitourinary System: Ureteral spasm, spasm of vesical sphincters and urinary retention have been reported.

Respiratory Depression: DILAUDID (hydromorphone hydrochloride) produces dose-related respiratory depression by acting directly on brain stem respiratory centers. DILAUDID also affects centers that control respiratory rhythm, and may produce irregular and periodic breathing. If significant respiratory depression occurs, it may be antagonized by the use of naloxone hydrochloride. The usual adult dose of 0.4 to 0.8 mg given *intramuscularly or intravenously*, promptly reverses the effects of morphine-like opioid agonists such as DILAUDID. In patients who are physically dependent, small doses of naloxone may be sufficient not only to antagonize respiratory depression, but also to precipitate withdrawal phenomena. The dose of naloxone should therefore be adjusted accordingly in such patients. Since the duration of action of DILAUDID may exceed that of the antagonist, the patient should be kept under continued surveillance, repeated doses of the antagonist may be required to maintain adequate respiration. Apply other supportive measures when indicated.

DRUG ABUSE AND DEPENDENCE

DILAUDID is a Schedule II narcotic. Psychic dependence, physical dependence, and tolerance may develop upon repeated administration of narcotics; therefore DILAUDID should be prescribed and administered with caution. However, psychic dependence is unlikely to develop when DILAUDID is used for a short time for the treatment of pain. Physical dependence, the condition in which continued administration of the drug is required to prevent the appearance of a withdrawal syndrome, usually assumes clinically significant proportions only after several weeks of continued narcotic use, although some mild degree of physical dependence may develop after a few days of narcotic therapy. Tolerance, in which increasingly large doses are required in order to produce the same degree of analgesia, is manifested initially by a shortened duration of analgesic effect, and subsequently by decreases in the intensity of analgesia. The rate of development of tolerance varies among patients.

OVERDOSAGE

Signs and Symptoms: Serious overdosage with DILAUDID is characterized by respiratory depression (a decrease in respiratory rate and/or tidal volume. Cheyne-Stokes respiration, cyanosis), extreme somnolence progressing to stupor or coma, skeletal muscle flaccidity, cold and clammy skin, and sometimes bradycardia and hypotension. In severe overdosage, particularly by the intravenous route, apnea, circulatory collapse, cardiac arrest, and death may occur.

Treatment: Primary attention should be given to the reestablishment of adequate respiratory exchange through provision of a patient airway and institution of assisted or controlled ventilation. The narcotic antagonist naloxone hydrochloride is a specific antidote against respiratory depression which may result from overdosage or unusual sensitivity to narcotics, including DILAUDID. Therefore, naloxone hydrochloride should be administered as described under *Adverse Reactions* (see *Respiratory Depression)* in conjunction with ventilatory assistance.

Since the duration of action of DILAUDID may exceed that of the antagonist, the patient should be kept under continued surveillance; repeated doses of the antagonist may be required to maintain adequate respiration. An antagonist should not be administered in the absence of clinically significant respiratory or cardiovascular depression. Oxygen, intravenous fluids vasopressors, and other supportive measures should be employed as indicated.

In cases of overdosage with oral DILAUDID, gastric lavage or induced emesis may be useful in removing unabsorbed drug from conscious patients.

DOSAGE AND ADMINISTRATION

Parenteral: The usual starting dose is 1–2 mg *subcutaneously* or *intramuscularly* every 4 to 6 hours as necessary for pain control. The dose should be adjusted according to the severity of pain, as well as the patient's underlying disease, age, and size. Patients with terminal cancer may be tolerant to narcotic analgesics and may, therefore, require higher doses for adequate pain relief. Intravenous or subcutaneous administration is usually not painful. Should intravenous administration be necessary, the injection should be given ***slowly***, over at least 2 to 3 minutes, depending on the dose. A gradual increase in dose may be required if analgesia is inadequate, tolerance occurs, or if pain severity increases. The first sign of tolerance is usually a reduced duration of effect.

NOTE: Parenteral drug products should be inspected visually for particulate matter and discoloration prior to administration, whenever solution and container permit. A slight yellowish discoloration may develop in DILAUDID ampules and multiple dose vials. No loss of potency has been demonstrated.

Oral: The usual oral dose is 2 mg every 4 to 6 hours as necessary. The dose must be individually adjusted according to severity of pain, patient response and patient size. More severe pain may require 4 mg or more every 4 to 6 hours. If the pain increases in severity, analgesia is not adequate or tolerance occurs, a gradual increase in dosage may be required. If pain is exceedingly severe, or if prompt response is desired, parenteral DILAUDID should be used initially in adequate amounts to control the pain.

Rectal: DILAUDID suppositories (3 mg) may provide longer duration of relief which could obviate additional medication during the sleeping hours. The usual adult dose is one (1) suppository inserted rectally every 6 to 8 hours or as directed by physician.

HOW SUPPLIED

Ampules: (One mL sterile solution for parenteral administration)

1 mg/mL ampules–Boxes of 10–
NDC #0044-1011-01.
2 mg/mL ampules–Boxes of 10–
NDC #0044-1012-01.
Boxes of 25-NDC #0044-1012-09.
4 mg/mL ampules–Boxes of 10–
NDC #0044-1014-01.

Multiple Dose Vials: (20 mL sterile solution for parenteral administration)

2 mg/mL–20 mL multiple dose vials-
NDC #0044-1062-05.

Caution: The packaging (vial stopper) of this product contains rubber latex which may cause allergic reactions.

Color Coded Tablets:

2 mg tablet (orange)–Bottles of 100–
NDC #0044-1022-02.
Unit Dose of 100 (4×25)-
NDC #0044-1022-45.
Bottles of 500–NDC #0044-1022-03.
4 mg tablet (yellow)–Bottles of 100–
NDC #0044-1024-02.
Unit Dose of 100 (4×25)-
NDC #0044-1024-45.
Bottles of 500–NDC #0044-1024-03.

Rectal Suppositories: 3 mg suppositories-Boxes of 6–NDC #0044-1053-01.

Non-Sterile Powder: For prescription compounding.
15 grain vial-NDC #0044-1040-01.

Storage: Parenteral and oral dosage forms of DILAUDID should be stored at 25°C (77°F); excursions permitted to 15°C–30°C (59°–86°F). [See USP Controlled Room Temperature]. Protect from light. DILAUDID suppositories should be stored in a refrigerator.

A Schedule CII Narcotic. DEA order form required.

Revised: December 1999

Parenteral Products Manufactured for
Knoll Laboratories
A Division of Knoll Pharmaceutical Company
By Abbott Laboratories
North Chicago, IL 60064, USA

Knoll Laboratories
A Division of
Knoll Pharmaceutical Company
Mount Olive, New Jersey 07828-1234
BASF Pharma

0900105-3

Shown in Product Identification Guide, page 319

DILAUDID–HP® INJECTION CII

[*dī "law 'dĭd*]
10mg/mL
hydromorphone hydrochloride

WARNING: DILAUDID-HP® (HIGH POTENCY) IS A HIGHLY CONCENTRATED SOLUTION OF HYDROMORPHONE INTENDED FOR USE IN NARCOTIC-TOLERANT PATIENTS. DO NOT CONFUSE DILAUDID-HP WITH STANDARD PARENTERAL FORMULATIONS OF DILAUDID OR OTHER NARCOTICS. OVERDOSE AND DEATH COULD RESULT.

DESCRIPTION

DILAUDID (hydromorphone hydrochloride), a hydrogenated ketone of morphine, is a narcotic analgesic. HIGH POTENCY DILAUDID is available in AMBER ampules or single dose vials for intravenous (IV), subcutaneous (SC), or intramuscular (IM) administration. Each 1 mL of sterile solution contains 10 mg hydromorphone hydrochloride with 0.2% sodium citrate, and 0.2% citric acid solution.

It is also available as lyophilized Dilaudid for intravenous (IV), subcutaneous (SC), or intramuscular (IM) administration. Each single dose vial contains 250mg sterile, lyophilized hydromorphone HCl to be reconstituted with 25mL of Sterile Water for Injection USP to provide a solution containing 10mg/mL.

The structural formula of DILAUDID (hydromorphone hydrochloride) is:

CH_3, H, N, CH_2, H, CH_2, •HCl, OH, O

MW 321.8

CLINICAL PHARMACOLOGY

Many of the effects described below are common to the class of narcotic analgesics. In some instances, data may not exist to demonstrate that DILAUDID-HP possesses similar or different effects than those observed with other narcotic analgesics. However, in the absence of data to the contrary, it is assumed that DILAUDID-HP would possess these effects.

Central Nervous System: Narcotic analgesics have multiple actions but exert their primary effects on the central nervous system and organs containing smooth muscle. The principal actions of therapeutic value are analgesia and sedation. A significant feature of the analgesia is that it occurs without loss of consciousness. Narcotic analgesics also suppress the cough reflex and cause respiratory depression, mood changes, mental clouding, euphoria, dysphoria, nausea, vomiting and electroencephalographic changes. The precise mode of analgesic action of narcotic analgesics is unknown. However, specific CNS opiate receptors have been identified. Narcotics are believed to express their pharmacological effects by combining with these receptors.

Narcotics depress the cough reflex by direct effect on the cough center in the medulla.

Narcotics produce respiratory depression by direct effect on brain stem respiratory centers. The mechanism of respiratory depression also involves a reduction in the responsiveness of the brain stem respiratory centers to increases in carbon dioxide tension.

Narcotics cause miosis. Pinpoint pupils are a common sign of narcotic overdose but are not pathognomonic (e.g., pontine lesions of hemorrhagic or ischemic origin may produce similar findings) and marked mydriasis occurs when asphyxia intervenes.

Gastrointestinal Tract and Other Smooth Muscle: Gastric, biliary and pancreatic secretions are decreased by narcotics. Narcotics cause a reduction in motility associated with an increase in tone in the antrum portion of the stomach and duodenum. Digestion of food in the small intestine is delayed and propulsive contractions are decreased. Propulsive peristaltic waves in the colon are decreased, and tone may be increased to the point of spasm. The end result is constipation. Narcotics can cause a marked increase in biliary tract pressure as a result of spasm of the sphincter of Oddi.

Cardiovascular System: Certain narcotics produce peripheral vasodilation which may result in orthostatic hypotension. Release of histamine may occur with narcotics and may contribute to narcotic-induced hypotension. Other manifestations of histamine release and/or peripheral vasodilation may include pruritis, flushing, and red eyes.

Effects on the myocardium after i.v. administration of narcotics are not significant in normal persons, vary with different narcotic analgesic agents and vary with the hemodynamic state of the patient, state of hydration and sympathetic drive.

Pharmacokinetics: In normal human volunteers hydromorphone is metabolized primarily in the liver. It is excreted primarily as the glucuronidated conjugate, with small amounts of parent drug and minor amounts of 6-hydroxy reduction metabolites.

Following intravenous administration of DILAUDID to normal volunteers, the mean half-life of elimination was 2.64 ± 0.88 hours. The mean volume of distribution was 91.5 liters, suggesting extensive tissue uptake. DILAUDID is rapidly removed from the blood stream and distributed to skeletal muscle, kidneys, liver, intestinal tract, lungs, spleen and brain. DILAUDID also crosses the placental membranes.

In terms of area under the analgesic time-effect curve, hydromorphone is approximately 8 times more potent than morphine (i.e., 1.3 mg of hydromorphone produces analgesia equal to that produced by 10 mg of morphine). After intramuscular administration, hydromorphone has a slightly more rapid onset and slightly shorter duration of action than morphine. The duration of DILAUDID analgesia in the non-tolerant patient with usual doses may be up to 4–5 hours. However, in tolerant subjects, duration will vary substantially depending on tolerance and dose. Dose should be adjusted so that 3–4 hours of pain relief may be achieved.

INDICATIONS AND USAGE

DILAUDID-HP is indicated for the relief of moderate-to-severe pain in narcotic-tolerant patients who require larger than usual doses of narcotics to provide adequate pain relief. Because DILAUDID-HP contains 10 mg of hydromorphone per mL, a smaller injection volume can be used than with other parenteral narcotic formulations. Discomfort associated with the intramuscular or subcutaneous injection of an unusually large volume of solution can therefore be avoided.

CONTRAINDICATIONS

DILAUDID-HP is contraindicated in: patients who are not already receiving large amounts of parenteral narcotics, patients with known hypersensitivity to the drug, patients with respiratory depression in the absence of resuscitative equipment, and in patients with status asthmaticus. DILAUDID-HP is also contraindicated for use in obstetrical analgesia.

WARNINGS—DRUG DEPENDENCE

DILAUDID-HP can produce drug dependence of the morphine type and therefore has the potential for being abused. Psychic dependence, physical dependence and tolerance may develop upon repeated administration of DILAUDID-HP, and it should be prescribed and administered with the same degree of caution appropriate for the use of morphine. Since DILAUDID-HP is indicated for use in patients who are already tolerant to and hence physically dependent on narcotics, abrupt discontinuance in the administration of DILAUDID-HP is likely to result in a withdrawal syndrome. (See **Drug Abuse and Dependence**).

Infants born to mothers physically dependent on DILAUDID-HP will also be physically dependent and may exhibit respiratory difficulties and withdrawal symptoms (See **Drug Abuse and Dependence**).

Impaired Respiration: Respiratory depression is the chief hazard of DILAUDID-HP. Respiratory depression occurs most frequently in the elderly, in the debilitated, and in those suffering from conditions accompanied by hypoxia or hypercapnia when even moderate therapeutic doses may dangerously decrease pulmonary ventilation.

DILAUDID-HP should be used with extreme caution in patients with chronic obstructive pulmonary disease or cor pulmonale, patients having a substantially decreased respiratory reserve, hypoxia, hypercapnia, or preexisting respiratory depression. In such patients even usual therapeutic doses of narcotic analgesics may decrease respiratory drive while simultaneously increasing airway resistance to the point of apnea.

Head Injury and Increased Intracranial Pressure: The respiratory depressant effects of DILAUDID-HP with carbon dioxide retention and secondary elevation of cerebrospinal fluid pressure may be markedly exaggerated in the presence of head injury, other intracranial lesions, or preexisting increase in intracranial pressure. Narcotic analgesics including DILAUDID-HP may produce effects which can obscure the clinical course and neurologic signs of further increase in pressure in patients with head injuries.

Hypotensive Effect: Narcotic analgesics, including DILAUDID-HP, may cause severe hypotension in an individual whose ability to maintain his blood pressure has already been compromised by a depleted blood volume, or a concurrent administration of drugs such as phenothiazines or general anesthetics (see also **Precautions —Drug Interactions**). DILAUDID-HP may produce orthostatic hypotension in ambulatory patients.

DILAUDID-HP should be administered with caution to patients in circulatory shock, since vasodilation produced by the drug may further reduce cardiac output and blood pressure.

PRECAUTIONS

General: Because of its high concentration, the delivery of precise doses of DILAUDID-HP may be difficult if low doses of hydromorphone are required. Therefore, DILAUDID-HP should be used only if the amount of hydromorphone required can be delivered accurately with this formulation.

Continued on next page

Dilaudid-HP—Cont.

In general, narcotics should be given with caution and the initial dose should be reduced in the elderly or debilitated and those with severe impairment of hepatic, pulmonary or renal function; myxedema or hypothyroidism; adrenocortical insufficiency (e.g., Addison's Disease); CNS depression or coma; toxic psychoses; prostatic hypertrophy or urethral stricture; gall bladder disease; acute alcoholism; delirium tremens; or kyphoscoliosis.

In the case of DILAUDID-HP, however, the patient is presumed to be receiving a narcotic to which he or she exhibits tolerance and the initial dose of DILAUDID-HP selected should be estimated based on the relative potency of hydromorphone and the narcotic previously used by the patient. See **(Dosage and Administration)** section.

The administration of narcotic analgesics including DILAUDID-HP may obscure the diagnosis or clinical course in patients with acute abdominal conditions and may aggravate preexisting convulsions in patients with convulsive disorders.

Reports of mild to severe seizures and myoclonus have been reported in severely compromised patients, administered high doses of parenteral hydromorphone, for cancer and severe pain. Opioid administration is associated with seizures and myoclonus in a variety of diseases where pain control is the primary focus.

Narcotic analgesics including DILAUDID-HP should also be used with caution in patients about to undergo surgery of the biliary tract since it may cause spasm of the sphincter of Oddi.

Drug Interactions: The concomitant use of other central nervous system depressants including sedatives or hypnotics, general anesthetics, phenothiazines, tranquilizers and alcohol may produce additive depressant effects. Respiratory depression, hypotension and profound sedation or coma may occur. When such combined therapy is contemplated, the dose of one or both agents should be reduced. Narcotic analgesics, including DILAUDID-HP may enhance the action of neuromuscular blocking agents and produce an increased degree of respiratory depression.

PREGNANCY—CATEGORY C:

Human: Adequate animal studies on reproduction have not been performed to determine whether hydromorphone affects fertility in males or females. There are no well-controlled studies in women. Reports based on marketing experience do not identify any specific teratogenic risks following routine (short-term) clinical use. Although there is no clearly defined risk, such reports do not exclude the possibility of infrequent or subtle damage to the human fetus. DILAUDID-HP should be used in pregnant women only when clearly needed (see ***Labor and Delivery*** and ***Drug Abuse and Dependence***).

Animal: Literature reports of hydromorphone hydrochloride administration to pregnant Syrian hamsters show that DILAUDID is teratogenic at a dose of 20 mg/kg which is 600 times the human dose. A maximal teratogenic effect (50% of fetuses affected) in the Syrian hamster was observed at a dose of 125 mg/kg.

Labor and Delivery: DILAUDID-HP is contraindicated in Labor and Delivery (see **Contraindications** section).

Nursing Mothers: Low levels of narcotic analgesics have been detected in human milk. As a general rule, nursing should not be undertaken while a patient is receiving DILAUDID-HP since it, and other drugs in this class, may be excreted in the milk.

Pediatric Use: Safety and effectiveness in children have not been established.

Geriatric Use: Clinical studies of Dilaudid-HP did not include sufficient numbers of subjects aged 65 and over to determine whether they respond differently from younger subjects. Other reported clinical experience has not identified differences in responses between the elderly and younger patients. In general, dose selection for an elderly patient should be cautious, usually starting at the low end of the dosing range, reflecting the greater frequency of decreased hepatic, renal, or cardiac function, and of concomitant disease or other drug therapy.

ADVERSE REACTIONS

The adverse effects of DILAUDID-HP are similar to those of other narcotic analgesics, and represent established pharmacological effects of the drug class. The major hazards include respiratory depression and apnea. To a lesser degree, circulatory depression, respiratory arrest, shock and cardiac arrest have occurred.

The most frequently observed adverse effects are lightheadedness, dizziness, sedation, nausea, vomiting, and sweating. These effects seem to be more prominent in ambulatory patients and in those not experiencing severe pain. Some adverse reactions in ambulatory patients may be alleviated if the patient lies down.

Less Frequently Observed with Narcotic Analgesics:

General and CNS: Dysphoria, euphoria, weakness, headache, agitation, tremor, uncoordinated muscle movements, alterations of mood (nervousness, apprehension, depression, floating feelings, dreams), muscle rigidity, paresthesia, muscle tremor, blurred vision, nystagmus, diplopia and miosis, transient hallucinations* and disorientation, visual disturbances, insomnia and increased intracranial pressure may occur.

STRONG ANALGESICS AND STRUCTURALLY RELATED DRUGS USED IN THE TREATMENT OF CANCER PAIN*

Nonproprietary (Trade) Names	IM OR SC ADMINISTRATION Dose, mg Equianalgesic to 10 mg of IM Morphine†	Duration Compared With Morphine
Morphine sulfate	10	Same
Papaveretum (Pantopon)	20	Same
Hydromorphone (DILAUDID) hydrochloride	1.3	Slightly Shorter
Oxymorphone (Numorphan) hydrochloride	1.1	Slightly Shorter
Nalbuphine (Nubain) hydrochloride	12	Same
Heroin, diamorphine hydrochloride (NA in U.S.)	4–5	Slightly Shorter
Levorphanol (Levo-Dromoran) tartrate	2.3	Same
Butorphanol (Stadol) tartrate	1.5–2.5	Same
Pentazocine (Talwin) lactate or hydrochloride	60	Shorter
Meperidine, pethidine (Demerol) hydrochloride	80	Shorter
Methadone (Dolophine) hydrochloride	10	Same

* From Beaver WT.
Management of cancer pain with parenteral medication. J. Am. Med. Assoc. 244:2653–2657 (1980).
† (In terms of the area under the analgesic time-effect curve.)

*Hallucinations, although unusual with pure agonist narcotics, have been observed in one patient following both a 6 mg and a 4 mg DILAUDID-HP dose. However, the patient was receiving several concomitant medications during the second episode and a causal relationship cannot be established.

Cardiovascular: Flushing of the face, chills, tachycardia, bradycardia, palpitation, faintness, syncope, hypotension and hypertension have been reported.

Respiratory: Bronchospasm and laryngospasm have been known to occur.

Gastrointestinal: Dry mouth, constipation, biliary tract spasm, anorexia, diarrhea, cramps and taste alterations have been reported.

Genitourinary: Urinary retention or hesitancy, and antidiuretic effects have been reported.

Dermatologic: Pruritis, urticaria, other skin rashes, wheal and flare over the vein with intravenous injection, and diaphoresis have been reported with narcotic analgesics.

Other: In clinical trials, neither local tissue irritation nor induration was observed at the site of subcutaneous injection of DILAUDID-HP; pain at the injection site was rarely observed. However, local irritation and induration have been seen following parenteral injection of other narcotic drug products.

DRUG ABUSE AND DEPENDENCE

Narcotic analgesics may cause psychological and physical dependence (see ***Warnings***). Physical dependence results in withdrawal symptoms in patients who abruptly discontinue the drug. Withdrawal symptoms also may be precipitated in the patient with physical dependence by the administration of a drug with narcotic antagonist activity, e.g., naloxone (see also ***Overdosage***). Physical dependence usually does not occur to a clinically significant degree until after several weeks of continued narcotic usage. Tolerance, in which increasingly large doses are required in order to produce the same degree of analgesia, is initially manifested by a shortened duration of analgesic effect, and subsequently, by decreases in the intensity of analgesia. In chronic pain patients, and in narcotic-tolerant cancer patients, the dose of DILAUDID-HP should be guided by the degree of tolerance manifested.

In chronic pain patients in whom narcotic analgesics including DILAUDID-HP are abruptly discontinued, a severe abstinence syndrome should be anticipated. This may be similar to the abstinence syndrome noted in patients who withdraw from heroin. The latter abstinence syndrome may be characterized by restlessness, lacrimation, rhinorrhea, yawning, perspiration, gooseflesh, restless sleep or "yen" and mydriasis during the first 24 hours. These symptoms may increase in severity and over the next 72 hours may be accompanied by increasing irritability, anxiety, weakness, twitching and spasms of muscles, kicking movements, severe backache, abdominal and leg pains, abdominal and muscle cramps, hot and cold flashes, insomnia, nausea, anorexia, vomiting, intestinal spasm, diarrhea, coryza and repetitive sneezing, increase in body temperature, blood pressure, respiratory rate and heart rate.

Because of excessive loss of fluids through sweating, or vomiting and diarrhea, there is usually marked weight loss, dehydration, ketosis, and disturbances in acid-base balance. Cardiovascular collapse can occur. Without treatment most observable symptoms disappear in 5–14 days; however, there appears to be a phase of secondary or chronic abstinence which may last for 2–6 months characterized by insomnia, irritability, muscular aches, and autonomic instability.

In the treatment of physical dependence on DILAUDID-HP, the patient may be detoxified by gradual reduction of the dosage, although this is unlikely to be necessary in the terminal cancer patient. If abstinence symptoms become severe, the patient may be given methadone. Temporary administration of tranquilizers and sedatives may aid in reducing patient anxiety. Gastrointestinal disturbances or dehydration should be treated accordingly.

OVERDOSAGE

Serious overdosage with DILAUDID-HP is characterized by respiratory depression, somnolence progressing to stupor or coma, skeletal muscle flaccidity, cold and clammy skin, constricted pupils, and sometimes bradycardia and hypotension. In serious overdosage, particularly following intravenous injection, apnea, circulatory collapse, cardiac arrest and death may occur.

In the treatment of overdosage primary attention should be given to the reestablishment of adequate respiratory exchange through provision of a patent airway and institution of assisted or controlled ventilation.

NARCOTIC-TOLERANT PATIENT: Since tolerance to the respiratory and CNS depressant effects of narcotics develops concomitantly with tolerance to their analgesic effects, serious respiratory depression due to an acute overdose is unlikely to be seen in narcotic-tolerant patients receiving DILAUDID-HP for chronic pain.

NOTE: In such an individual who is physically dependent on narcotics, administration of the usual dose of the antagonist will precipitate an acute withdrawal syndrome. The severity will depend on the degree of physical dependence and the dose of the antagonist administered. Use of a narcotic antagonist in such a person should be avoided. If necessary to treat serious respiratory depression in the physically dependent patient, the antagonist should be administered with extreme care and by titration with smaller than usual doses of the antagonist.

NON-TOLERANT PATIENT: The narcotic antagonist, naloxone, is a specific antidote against respiratory depression which may result from overdosage, or unusual sensitivity to DILAUDID-HP. A dose of naloxone (usually 0.4 to 2.0 mg) should be administered intravenously, if possible, simultaneously with respiratory resuscitation. The dose can be repeated in 3 minutes. Naloxone should not be administered in the absence of clinically significant respiratory or circulatory depression. Naloxone should be administered cautiously to persons who are known, or suspected to be physically dependent on DILAUDID-HP. In such cases, an abrupt or complete reversal of narcotic effects may precipitate an acute abstinence syndrome.

Since the duration of action of DILAUDID-HP may exceed that of the antagonist, the patient should be kept under continued surveillance; repeated doses of the antagonist may be required to maintain adequate respiration. Apply other supportive measures when indicated.

Supportive measures (including oxygen, vasopressors) should be employed in the management of circulatory shock and pulmonary edema accompanying overdose as indicated. Cardiac arrest or arrhythmias may require cardiac massage or defibrillation.

DOSAGE AND ADMINISTRATION

Parenteral: DILAUDID-HP SHOULD BE GIVEN ONLY TO PATIENTS WHO ARE ALREADY RECEIVING LARGE DOSES OF NARCOTICS. DILAUDID-HP is indicated for relief of moderate-to-severe pain in narcotic-tolerant patients. Thus, these patients will already have been treated with other narcotic analgesics. If the patient is being changed from regular DILAUDID to DILAUDID-HP, similar doses should be used, depending on the patient's clinical response to the drug. If DILAUDID-HP is substituted for a different narcotic analgesic, the following equivalency table should be used as a guide to determine the appropriate dose of DILAUDID-HP (hydromorphone hydrochloride).

[See table at top of previous page]

In open clinical trials with DILAUDID-HP in patients with terminal cancer, doses ranged from 1–14 mg subcutaneously or intramuscularly; one patient received 30 mg subcutaneously on two occasions. In these trials, both subcutaneous and intramuscular injections of DILAUDID-HP were well-tolerated, with minimal pain and/or burning at the injection site. Mild erythema was rarely noted after intramuscular injection. There was no induration after either intramuscular or subcutaneous administration of DILAUDID-HP. Subcutaneous injections of DILAUDID-HP were particularly well accepted when administered with a short, 30 gauge needle.

Experience with administration of DILAUDID-HP by the intravenous route is limited. Should intravenous administration be necessary, the injection should be given slowly, over at least 2 to 3 minutes. The intravenous route is usually painless.

A gradual increase in dose may be required if analgesia is inadequate, tolerance occurs, or if pain severity increases. The first sign of tolerance is usually a reduced duration of effect.

NOTE: Parenteral drug products should be inspected visually for particulate matter and discoloration prior to administration, whenever solution and container permit. A slight yellowish discoloration may develop in DILAUDID-HP ampules. No loss of potency has been demonstrated. Dilaudid injection is physically compatible and chemically stable for at least 24 hours at 25°C protected from light in most common large volume parenteral solutions.

500mg/50mL Vial: To use this single dose presentation, do not penetrate the stopper with a syringe. Instead, remove both the aluminum flipseal and rubber stopper in a suitable work area such as under a laminar flow hood (or equivalent clean air compounding area). The contents may then be withdrawn for preparation of a single, large volume parenteral solution. Any unused portion should be discarded in an appropriate manner.

CAUTION: The packaging (vial stopper) of this product contains rubber latex which may cause allergic reactions.

Reconstitution of sterile lyophilized Dilaudid HP 250mg: Reconstitution immediately prior to use with 25mL of Sterile Water for Injection USP to provide a sterile solution containing 10mg/mL.

HOW SUPPLIED

DILAUDID-HP *amber* ampules and single dose vials contain 10 mg hydromorphone hydrochloride per mL with 0.2% sodium citrate and 0.2% citric acid solution. No added preservative.

NOTE: DILAUDID-HP ampules are amber in color.

The lyophilized Dilaudid HP Single Dose Vial contains 250mg of sterile, lyophilized hydromorphone HCl.

HIGH POTENCY:

10 mg/1 mL
Box of 10 ampules
NDC 0044-1017-10
*50 mg/5mL
Box of 10 ampules
NDC 0044-1017-25
*500 mg/50 mL
Single dose vial
NDC 0044-1017-06
*lyophilized 250mg
Single Dose Vial
NDC 0044-1911-01

*FOR USE IN THE PREPARATION OF LARGE VOLUME PARENTERAL SOLUTIONS

STORAGE: Store at 25°C (77°F); excursions permitted to 15°–30°C (59°–86°F). [See USP Controlled Room Temperature].

A Schedule Ⓒ II Narcotic DEA Order Form Required.

Rx only

DILAUDID HP is a registered trademark of Knoll Pharmaceutical Company.

Revised: October 1999

Parenteral Products

Manufactured for
Knoll Laboratories
A Division of Knoll Pharmaceutical Company
Mount Olive, New Jersey 07828
By Abbott Laboratories
North Chicago, IL 60064, USA
BASF Pharma 0900012A-4

Shown in Product Identification Guide, page 319

DILAUDID® ORAL LIQUID and DILAUDID® 8 mg Tablets (hydromorphone hydrochloride)

Ⓒ II ℞

DESCRIPTION

DILAUDID (hydromorphone hydrochloride), a hydrogenated ketone of morphine, is a narcotic analgesic.

OPIOID ANALGESIC EQUIVALENTS WITH APPROXIMATELY EQUIANALGESIC POTENCY*

Nonproprietary (Trade) Name	IM or SC Dose	ORAL dose
Morphine Sulfate	10 mg	40–60 mg
Hydromorphone HCl (DILAUDID)	1.3–2 mg	6.5–7.5 mg
Oxymorphone HCl (Numorphan)	1–1.1 mg	6.6 mg
Levorphanol tartrate (Levo-Dromoran)	2–2.3 mg	4 mg
Meperidine HCl (Demerol)	75–100 mg	300–400 mg
Methadone HCl (Dolophine)	10 mg	10–20 mg

The structural formula of hydromorphone hydrochloride is:

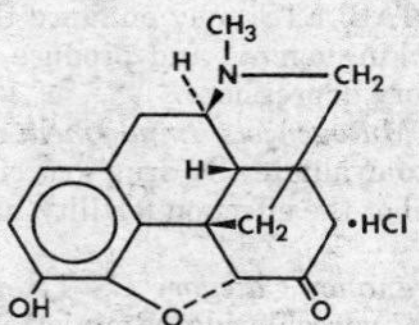

M.W. 321.8

Each 5 mL (1 teaspoon) of DILAUDID ORAL LIQUID contains 5 mg of hydromorphone hydrochloride. In addition, other ingredients include purified water, methylparaben, propylparaben, sucrose, and glycerin. DILAUDID ORAL LIQUID may contain traces of sodium bisulfite.

Each DILAUDID 8 mg TABLET contains 8 mg hydromorphone hydrochloride. In addition, the tablets include lactose anhydrous, and magnesium stearate. DILAUDID 8 mg TABLET may contain traces of sodium bisulfite.

CLINICAL PHARMACOLOGY

Many of the effects described below are common to this class of mu-opioid agonist analgesics. In some instances, data may not exist to distinguish the effects of DILAUDID ORAL LIQUID and DILAUDID 8 mg TABLETS from those observed with other opioid analgesics. However, in the absence of data to the contrary, it is assumed that DILAUDID ORAL LIQUID and DILAUDID 8 mg TABLETS would possess all the actions of mu-agonist opioids.

Opioid analgesics exert their primary effects on the central nervous system and organs containing smooth muscle. The principal actions of therapeutic value are analgesia and sedation. A significant feature of the analgesia is that it can occur without loss of consciousness. Opioid analgesics also suppress the cough reflex and may cause respiratory depression, mood changes, mental clouding, euphoria, dysphoria, nausea, vomiting and electroencephalographic changes. The precise mode of analgesic action of opioid analgesics is unknown. However, specific CNS opiate receptors have been identified. Opioids are believed to express their pharmacological effects by combining with these receptors.

Opioids depress the cough reflex by direct effect on the cough center in the medulla.

Opioids depress the respiratory reflex by a direct effect on brain stem respiratory centers. The mechanism of respiratory depression also involves a reduction in the responsiveness of the brain stem respiratory centers to increases in carbon dioxide tension.

Opioids cause miosis. Pinpoint pupils are a common sign of opioid overdose but are not pathognomonic (e.g., pontine lesions of hemorrhagic or ischemic origin may produce similar findings) and marked mydriasis occurs with asphyxia.

Gastric, biliary and pancreatic secretions are decreased by opioids. Opioids cause a reduction in motility associated with an increase in tone in the gastric antrum and duodenum. Digestion of food in the small intestine is delayed and propulsive contractions are decreased. Propulsive peristaltic waves in the colon are decreased, and tone may be increased to the point of spasm. The end result is constipation. Opioids can cause a marked increase in biliary tract pressure as a result of spasm of the sphincter of Oddi.

Certain opioids produce peripheral vasodilation which may result in orthostatic hypotension. Release of histamine may occur with opioids and may contribute to drug-induced hypotension. Other manifestations of histamine release may include pruritus, flushing, and red eyes.

The dosage of opioid analgesics like hydromorphone should be individualized for any given patient, since adverse events can occur at doses that may not provide complete freedom from pain (see INDIVIDUALIZATION OF DOSAGE).

PHARMACOKINETICS

In a single-dose crossover study in 27 normal subjects the pharmacokinetics of DILAUDID 8 mg TABLETS was compared to that of 8 mL of DILAUDID ORAL LIQUID (1 mg/mL). Plasma hydromorphone concentration was determined using a sensitive and specific assay. The pharmacokinetic parameters from this study are outlined below.

Parameter Mean & (CV)	8 mg Tablet	8 mg Oral Liquid (1 mg/mL)
C_{max} (ng/mL)	5.5 (33%)	5.7 (31%)
T_{max} (hr)	0.74 (34%)	0.73 (71%)
$AUC_{0-\infty}$ (ng*hr/mL)	23.7 (28%)	24.6 (29%)
$T_{1/2}$ (hr)	2.6 (18%)	2.8 (20%)

Dose proportionality between the DILAUDID 8 mg TABLETS and other strengths of Dilaudid tablets has not been established.

In normal human volunteers hydromorphone is metabolized primarily in the liver. It is excreted in the urine primarily as the glucuronidated conjugate, with small amounts of parent drug and minor amounts of 6-hydroxy reduction metabolites. The effects of renal disease on the clearance of hydromorphone are unknown, but caution should be taken to guard against unanticipated accumulation if renal and/or hepatic functions are seriously impaired. Hydromorphone has been shown to cross placental membranes.

CLINICAL TRIALS

Analgesic effects of single doses of DILAUDID ORAL LIQUID administered to patients with post-surgical pain have been studied in double-blind controlled trials. In one study with 61 patients, both 5 mg and 10 mg of DILAUDID ORAL LIQUID provided significantly more analgesia than placebo. In another trial with 80 patients, 5 mg and 10 mg of DILAUDID ORAL LIQUID were compared to 30 mg and 60 mg of morphine sulfate oral liquid. The pain relief provided by 5 mg and 10 mg DILAUDID ORAL LIQUID was comparable to 30 mg and 60 mg oral morphine sulfate, respectively.

INDIVIDUALIZATION OF DOSAGE

Safe and effective administration of opioid analgesics to patients with acute or chronic pain depends upon a comprehensive assessment of the patient. The nature of the pain (severity, frequency, etiology, and pathophysiology) as well as the concurrent medical status of the patient will affect selection of the starting dosage.

In non-opioid-tolerant patients, therapy with hydromorphone is typically initiated at an oral dose of 2–4 mg every four hours, but elderly patients may require lower doses (see **PRECAUTIONS**—Geriatric Use).

In patients receiving opioids, both the dose and duration of analgesia will vary substantially depending on the patient's opioid tolerance. The dose should be selected and adjusted so that at least 3–4 hours of pain relief may be achieved. In patients taking opioid analgesics, the starting dose of DILAUDID should be based on the prior opioid usage. This should be done by converting the total daily usage of the previous opioid to an equivalent total daily dosage of oral DILAUDID using an equianalgesic table (see below). For opioids not in the table, first estimate the equivalent total daily usage of oral morphine, then use the table to find the equivalent total daily dosage of Dilaudid.

Once the total daily dosage of DILAUDID has been estimated, it should be divided into the desired number of doses. Since there is individual variation in response to different opioid drugs, only $^1/_2$ to $^2/_3$ of the estimated dose of DILAUDID calculated from equivalence tables should be given for the first few doses, then increased as needed according to the patient's response.

In chronic pain, doses should be administered around-the-clock. A supplemental dose of 5–15% of the total daily usage may be administered every two hours on an "as-needed" basis.

Periodic reassessment after the initial dosing is always required. If pain management is not satisfactory and in the absence of significant opioid-induced adverse events, the hydromorphone dose may be increased gradually. If excessive opioid side effects are observed early in the dosing interval, the hydromorphone dose should be reduced. If this results in breakthrough pain at the end of the dosing interval, the dosing interval may need to be shortened. Dose titration should be guided more by the need for analgesia than the absolute dose of opioid employed.

[See table at top of page]

* Dosages, and ranges of dosages represented, are a compilation of estimated equipotent dosages from published references comparing opioid analgesics in cancer and severe pain.

INDICATIONS AND USAGE

DILAUDID ORAL LIQUID and DILAUDID 8 mg TABLETS are indicated for the management of pain in patients where an opioid analgesic is appropriate.

Continued on next page

Dilaudid—Cont.

CONTRAINDICATIONS

DILAUDID ORAL LIQUID and DILAUDID 8 mg TABLETS are contraindicated in: patients with known hypersensitivity to hydromorphone, patients with respiratory depression in the absence of resuscitative equipment, and in patients with status asthmaticus. DILAUDID ORAL LIQUID and DILAUDID 8 mg TABLETS are also contraindicated for use in obstetrical analgesia.

WARNINGS

Impaired Respiration: Respiratory depression is the chief hazard of DILAUDID ORAL LIQUID and DILAUDID 8 mg TABLETS. Respiratory depression occurs most frequently in overdose situations, in the elderly, in the debilitated, and in those suffering from conditions accompanied by hypoxia or hypercapnia when even moderate therapeutic doses may dangerously decrease pulmonary ventilation.

DILAUDID ORAL LIQUID and DILAUDID 8 mg TABLETS should be used with extreme caution in patients with chronic obstructive pulmonary disease or cor pulmonale, patients having a substantially decreased respiratory depression, hypoxia, hypercapnia, or in patients with preexisting respiratory depression. In such patients even usual therapeutic doses of opioid analgesics may decrease respiratory drive while simultaneously increasing airway resistance to the point of apnea.

Drug Dependence: DILAUDID is a Schedule II narcotic. DILAUDID ORAL LIQUID and DILAUDID 8 mg TABLETS can produce drug dependence of the morphine type and therefore have the potential for being abused. Psychic dependence, physical dependence and tolerance may develop upon repeated administration of DILAUDID, which should be prescribed and administered with the degree of caution appropriate to the use of morphine. Abrupt discontinuance in the administration of DILAUDID ORAL LIQUID and DILAUDID 8 mg TABLETS in patients who are physically dependent on opioids is likely to result in a withdrawal syndrome (see DRUG ABUSE AND DEPENDENCE).

Sulfites: Contains sodium bisulfite, a sulfite that may cause allergic-type reactions including anaphylactic symptoms and life-threatening or less severe asthmatic episodes in certain susceptible people. The overall prevalence of sulfite sensitivity in the general population is unknown and probably low. Sulfite sensitivity is seen more frequently in asthmatic than in nonasthmatic people.

PRECAUTIONS

Special Risk Patients: In general, opioids should be given with caution and the initial dose should be reduced in the elderly or debilitated and those with severe impairment of hepatic, pulmonary or renal functions; myxedema or hypothyroidism; adrenocortical insufficiency (e.g., Addison's Disease); CNS depression or coma; toxic psychoses; prostatic hypertrophy or urethral stricture; gall bladder disease; acute alcoholism; delirium tremens; kyphoscoliosis or following gastrointestinal surgery.

The administration of opioid analgesics including DILAUDID ORAL LIQUID and DILAUDID 8 mg TABLETS may obscure the diagnoses or clinical course in patients with acute abdominal conditions and may aggravate preexisting convulsions in patients with convulsive disorders.

Reports of mild to severe seizures and myoclonus have been reported in severely compromised patients, administered high doses of parenteral hydromorphone, for cancer and severe pain. Opioid administration is associated with seizures and myoclonus in a variety of diseases where pain control is the primary focus.

Head Injury and Increased Intracranial Pressure: The respiratory depressant effects of DILAUDID ORAL LIQUID and DILAUDID 8 mg TABLETS with carbon dioxide retention and secondary elevation of cerebrospinal fluid pressure may be markedly exaggerated in the presence of head injury, other intracranial lesions, or preexisting increase in intracranial pressure. Opioid analgesics including DILAUDID ORAL LIQUID and DILAUDID 8 mg TABLETS may produce effects which can obscure the clinical course and neurologic signs of further increase in intracranial pressure in patients with head injuries.

Hypotensive Effect: Opioid analgesics, including DILAUDID ORAL LIQUID and DILAUDID 8 mg TABLETS, may cause severe hypotension in an individual whose ability to maintain blood pressure has already been compromised by a depleted blood volume, or a concurrent administration of drugs such as phenothiazines or general anesthetics (see also PRECAUTIONS—Drug Interactions). Therefore, DILAUDID ORAL LIQUID and DILAUDID 8 mg TABLETS should be administered with caution to patients in circulatory shock, since vasodilation produced by the drug may further reduce cardiac output and blood pressure.

Use in Ambulatory Patients: DILAUDID ORAL LIQUID and DILAUDID 8 mg TABLETS may impair mental and/or physical ability required for the performance of potentially hazardous tasks (e.g. driving, operating machinery). Patients should be cautioned accordingly. DILAUDID may produce orthostatic hypotension in ambulatory patients. The addition of other CNS depressants to DILAUDID therapy may produce additive depressant effects, and DILAUDID should not be taken with alcohol.

Use in Biliary Surgery: Opioid analgesics including DILAUDID ORAL LIQUID and DILAUDID 8 mg TABLETS should also be used with caution in patients about to undergo surgery of the biliary tract since it may cause spasm of the sphincter of Oddi.

Use in Drug and Alcohol Dependent Patients: DILAUDID should be used with caution in patients with alcoholism and other drug dependencies due to the increased frequency of narcotic tolerance, dependence, and the risk of addiction observed in these patient populations. Abuse of DILAUDID in combination with other CNS depressant drugs can result in serious risk to the patient.

Drug Interactions: The concomitant use of other central nervous system depressants including sedatives or hypnotics, general anesthetics, phenothiazines, tranquilizers and alcohol may produce additive depressant effects. Respiratory depression, hypotension and profound sedation or coma may occur. When such combined therapy is contemplated, the dose of one or both agents should be reduced. Opioid analgesics, including DILAUDID ORAL LIQUID and DILAUDID 8 mg TABLETS, may enhance the action of neuromuscular blocking agents and produce an excessive degree of respiratory depression.

Carcinogenesis, Mutagenesis, Impairment of Fertility: Studies in animals to evaluate the drug's carcinogenic and mutagenic potential or the effect on fertility, have not been conducted.

Pregnancy—Pregnancy Category C: Literature reports of hydromorphone hydrochloride administration to pregnant Syrian hamsters show that DILAUDID is teratogenic at a dose of 20 mg/kg which is 600 times the human dose. A maximal teratogenic effect (50% of fetuses affected) in the Syrian hamster was observed at a dose of 125 mg/kg (738 mg/m^2). There are no well-controlled studies in women. Hydromorphone is known to cross placental membranes. DILAUDID ORAL LIQUID and DILAUDID 8 mg TABLETS should be used in pregnant women only if the potential benefit justifies the potential risk to the fetus (see *Labor and Delivery* and DRUG ABUSE AND DEPENDENCE).

Labor and Delivery: DILAUDID ORAL LIQUID and DILAUDID 8 mg TABLETS are contraindicated in Labor and Delivery (see CONTRAINDICATIONS).

Nursing Mothers: Low levels of opioid analgesics have been detected in human milk. As a general rule, nursing should not be undertaken while a patient is receiving DILAUDID ORAL LIQUID and DILAUDID 8 mg TABLETS since it, and other drugs in this class, may be excreted in the milk.

Pediatric Use: Safety and effectiveness in children have not been established.

Geriatric Use: Clinical studies of DILAUDID did not include sufficient numbers of subjects aged 65 and over to determine whether they respond differently from younger subjects. Other reported clinical experience has not identified differences in responses between the elderly and younger patients. Elderly subjects have been shown to have at least twice the sensitivity (as measured by EEG changes) of young adults for some opioids. In general, dose selection for an elderly patient should be cautious, usually starting at the low end of the dosing range, reflecting the greater frequency of decreased hepatic, renal, or cardiac function, and of concomitant disease or other drug therapy (see INDIVIDUALIZATION OF DOSAGES AND PRECAUTION).

ADVERSE REACTIONS

The adverse effects of DILAUDID ORAL LIQUID and DILAUDID 8 mg TABLETS are similar to those of other agonist analgesics, and represent established pharmacological effects of the drug class. The major hazards include respiratory depression and apnea. To a lesser degree, circulatory depression, respiratory arrest, shock and cardiac arrest have occurred.

The most frequently observed adverse effects are lightheadedness, dizziness, sedation, nausea, vomiting, sweating, dysphoria, euphoria, dry mouth, and pruritus. These effects seem to be more prominent in ambulatory patients and in those not experiencing severe pain. Syncopal reactions and related symptoms in ambulatory patients may be alleviated if the patient lies down.

Less Frequently Observed with Opioid Analgesics:

General and CNS: Weakness, headache, agitation, tremor, uncoordinated muscle movements, alterations of mood (nervousness, apprehension, depression, floating feelings, dreams), muscle rigidity, paresthesia, muscle tremor, blurred vision, nystagmus, diplopia and miosis, transient hallucinations and disorientation, visual disturbances, insomnia and increased intracranial pressure may occur.

Cardiovascular: Chills, tachycardia, bradycardia, palpitation, faintness, syncope, hypotension and hypertension have been reported.

Respiratory: Bronchospasm and laryngospasm have been known to occur.

Gastrointestinal: Constipation biliary tract spasm, ileus, anorexia, diarrhea, cramps and taste alteration have been reported.

Genitourinary: Urinary retention or hesitancy, and antidiuretic effects have been reported.

Dermatologic: Urticaria, other skin rashes, and diaphoresis.

DRUG ABUSE AND DEPENDENCE

DILAUDID is a Schedule II narcotic, similar to morphine. Opioid analgesics may cause psychological and physical dependence (see WARNINGS). Physical dependence results in withdrawal symptoms in patients who abruptly discontinue the drug. Withdrawal symptoms also may be precipitated in the patient with physical dependence by the administration of a drug with opioid antagonist activity, e.g., naloxone (see also OVERDOSAGE).

Physical dependence usually does not occur to a clinically significant degree until after several weeks of continued opioid usage, but it may become clinically detectable after as little as a week. Tolerance, in which increasingly large doses are required in order to produce the same degree of analgesia, is initially manifested by a shortened duration of analgesic effect, and subsequently, by decreases in the intensity of analgesia. In chronic pain patients, and in opioid-tolerant cancer patients, the dose of DILAUDID ORAL LIQUID and DILAUDID 8 mg TABLETS should be guided by the degree of tolerance manifested.

In chronic pain patients in whom opioid analgesics including DILAUDID ORAL LIQUID and DILAUDID 8 mg TABLETS are abruptly discontinued, a severe abstinence syndrome should be anticipated. This may be similar to the abstinence syndrome noted in patients who withdraw from heroin. Because of excessive loss of fluids through sweating, or vomiting and diarrhea, patients experiencing the syndrome usually exhibit marked weight loss, dehydration, ketosis, and disturbances in acid-base balance. Cardiovascular collapse can occur. Without treatment most observable symptoms disappear in 5–14 days; however, there appears to be a phase of secondary or chornic abstinence which may last for 2–6 months characterized by insomnia, irritability, muscular aches, and autonomic instability.

In the treatment of physical dependence on DILAUDID ORAL LIQUID and DILAUDID 8 mg TABLETS, the patient may be detoxified by gradual reduction of the dosage, although this is unlikely to be necessary in the terminal cancer patient. If abstinence symptoms become severe, the patient may be detoxified with methadone. Temporary administration of tranquilizers and sedatives may aid in reducing patient anxiety. Gastrointestinal disturbances or dehydration should be treated accordingly.

OVERDOSAGE

Serious overdosage with DILAUDID ORAL LIQUID and DILAUDID 8 mg TABLETS is characterized by respiratory depression, somnolence progressing to stupor or coma, skeletal muscle flaccidity, cold and clammy skin, constricted pupils, and sometimes bradycardia and hypotension. In serious overdosage, particularly following intravenous injection, apnea, circulatory collapse, cardiac arrest and death may occur.

In the treatment of overdosage, primary attention should be given to the reestablishment of adequate respiratory exchange through provision of a patent airway and institution of assisted or controlled ventilation. A potentially serious oral ingestion, if recent, should be managed with gut decontamination. In unconscious patients with a secure airway, instill activated charcoal (30–100 g in adults, 1–2 g/kg in infants) via a nasogastric tube. A saline cathartic or sorbitol may be added to the first dose of activated charcoal.

Opioid-tolerant patient: Since tolerance to the respiratory and CNS depressant effects of opioids develops concomitantly with tolerance to their analgesic effects, serious respiratory depression due to an acute overdose is unlikely to be seen in opioid-tolerant patients receiving the usual therapeutic dosage of DILAUDID ORAL LIQUID and DILAUDID 8 mg TABLETS for chronic pain.

Note: In an individual who is physically dependent on opioids, administration of the usual dose of an opioid antagonist will precipitate an acute withdrawal syndrome. The severity will depend on the degree of physical dependence and the dose of the antagonist administered. If necessary to treat serious respiratory depression in the physically-dependent patient, the opioid antagonist should be administered with care and by titration, using fractional (one fifth to one tenth) doses of the antagonist.

Non-tolerant patient: The opioid antagonist, naloxone, is a specific antidote against respiratory depression which may result from overdosage, or unusual sensitivity to DILAUDID ORAL LIQUID and DILAUDID 8 mg TABLETS. A dose of naloxone (usually given as a test dose of 0.4 mg, followed by up to 2.0 mg if needed) should be administered intravenously, if possible, simultaneously with respiratory resuscitation. The dose can be repeated in 3 minutes. Naloxone should not be administered in the absence of clinically significant respiratory or circulatory depression. Naloxone should be administered cautiously to persons who are known, or suspected to be physically dependent on DILAUDID ORAL LIQUID and DILAUDID 8 mg TABLETS (see Opioid tolerant patient).

Since the duration of action of DILAUDID ORAL LIQUID and DILAUDID 8 mg TABLETS may exceed that of the antagonist, the patient should be kept under continued surveillance; repeated doses of the antagonist may be required to maintain adequate respiration. Apply other supportive measures when indicated.

Supportive measures (including oxygen, vasopressors) should be employed in the management of circulatory shock and pulmonary edema accompanying overdose as indicated. Cardiac arrest or arrhythmias may require cardiac massage or defibrillation.

DOSAGE AND ADMINISTRATION

DILAUDID ORAL LIQUID: The usual adult oral dosage of DILAUDID ORAL LIQUID is one-half (2.5 mL) to two teaspoonfuls (10 mL) (2.5 mg–10 mg) every 3 to 6 hours as directed by the clinical situation. Oral dosages higher than the usual dosages may be required in some patients.

DILAUDID 8 mg TABLET: The usual starting dose for DILAUDID tablets is 2 mg to 4 mg, orally, every 4 to 6 hours. Appropriate use of the DILAUDID 8 mg TABLET must be decided by careful evaluation of each clinical situation.
A gradual increase in dose may be required if analgesia is inadequate, as tolerance develops, or if pain severity increases. The first sign of tolerance is usually a reduced duration of effect.

SAFETY AND HANDLING INSTRUCTIONS

DILAUDID ORAL LIQUID and DILAUDID 8 mg TABLETS pose little risk of direct exposure to health care personnel and should be handled and disposed of prudently in accordance with hospital or institutional policy. Significant absorption from dermal exposure is unlikely; accidental dermal exposure to DILAUDID ORAL LIQUID should be treated by removal of any contaminated clothing and rinsing the affected area with water. Patients and their families should be instructed to flush any DILAUDID ORAL LIQUID and DILAUDID 8 mg TABLETS that are no longer needed.
Access to abuseable drugs such as DILAUDID ORAL LIQUID and DILAUDID 8 mg TABLETS presents an occupational hazard for addiction in the health care industry. Routine procedures for handling controlled substances developed to protect the public may not be adequate to protect health care workers. Implementation of more effective accounting procedures and measures to restrict access to drugs of this class (appropriate to the practice setting) may minimize the risk of self-administration by health care providers.

HOW SUPPLIED

DILAUDID ORAL LIQUID is a clear, sweet, slightly viscous liquid. It is available in:
Bottles of 1 pint (473 mL)—NDC# 0044-1085-01
DILAUDID 8 mg TABLETS are white and triangular shaped, embossed with the number 8 on one side and bisected and embossed with a double "Knoll" triangle on the other side. They are available in:
Bottles of 100—NDC# 0044-1028-02
STORAGE: Store at 25°C (77°F); excursions permitted to 15°C–30°C (59°–86°F). [See USP Controlled Room Temperature]. Protect from light.
Rx only
A schedule II Narcotic DEA Order Form is Required.

Revised: October 1999
Knoll Laboratories
A Division of
Knoll Pharmaceutical Company
Mount Olive, New Jersey 07828
BASF Pharma 0900016-3
Shown in Product Identification Guide, page 319

ISOPTIN® SR ℞

(verapamil HCl)
Sustained Release Oral Tablets

DESCRIPTION

ISOPTIN SR® (verapamil hydrochloride) is a calcium ion influx inhibitor (slow channel blocker or calcium ion antagonist). ISOPTIN SR is available for oral administration as light green, capsule shaped, scored, film-coated tablets containing 240 mg verapamil hydrochloride, as light pink, oval shaped, scored, film-coated tablets containing 180 mg verapamil hydrochloride, and as light violet, oval shaped, film-coated tablets containing 120 mg verapamil hydrochloride. The tablets are designed for sustained release of the drug in the gastrointestinal tract, sustained release characteristics are not altered when the tablet is divided in half.
The structural formula of verapamil HCl is given below:

$C_{27}H_{38}N_2O_4 \cdot HCl$ M.W. = 491.08

Benzeneacetronitrile,
α-[[3-[[2-(3,4-dimethoxyphenyl) ethyl]
methylamino]
propyl]-3,4-dimethoxy-α-(1-methylethyl) hydrochloride

Verapamil HCl is an almost white, crystalline powder, practically free of odor, with a bitter taste. It is soluble in water, chloroform and methanol. Verapamil HCl is not chemically related to other cardioactive drugs.
In addition to verapamil HCl, the ISOPTIN SR tablet contains the following ingredients: alginate, hydroxypropyl methylcellulose, magnesium stearate, microcrystalline cellulose, polyethylene glycol, polyvinyl pyrroidone, talc, and titanium dioxide. The following are the color additives per tablet strength:

Strength (mg)	Color Additive(s)
120	Iron Oxide
180	Iron Oxide
240	D&C yellow #10 Lake dye, and FD&C blue #2 Lake dye

CLINICAL PHARMACOLOGY

ISOPTIN (verapamil HCl) is a calcium ion influx inhibitor (slow channel blocker or calcium ion antagonist) which exerts its pharmacologic effects by modulating the influx of ionic calcium across the cell membrane of the arterial smooth muscle as well as in conductile and contractile myocardial cells.
Mechanism of Action
Essential Hypertension
ISOPTIN exerts antihypertensive effects by decreasing systemic vascular resistance, usually without orthostatic decreases in blood pressure or reflex tachycardia; bradycardia (rate less than 50 beats/min) is uncommon (1.4%). During isometric or dynamic exercise ISOPTIN does not alter systolic cardiac function in patients with normal ventricular function. ISOPTIN does not alter total serum calcium levels. However, one report suggested that calcium levels above the normal range may alter the therapeutic effect of ISOPTIN.
Other Pharmacologic Actions of ISOPTIN Include the Following
ISOPTIN (verapamil HCl) dilates the main coronary arteries and coronary arterioles, both in normal and ischemic regions, and is a potent inhibitor of coronary artery spasm, whether spontaneous or ergonovine-induced. This property increases myocardial oxygen delivery in patients with coronary artery spasm, and is responsible for the effectiveness of ISOPTIN in vasospastic (Prinzmetal's or variant) as well as unstable angina at rest. Whether this effect plays any role in classical effort angina is not clear, but studies of exercise tolerance have not shown an increase in the maximum exercise rate-pressure product, a widely accepted measure of oxygen utilization. This suggests that, in general, relief of spasm or dilation of coronary arteries is not an important factor in classical angina.
ISOPTIN regularly reduces the total systemic resistance (afterload) against which the heart works both at rest and at a given level of exercise by dilating peripheral arterioles.
Electrical activity through the AV node depends, to a significant degree, upon calcium influx through the slow channel. By decreasing the influx of calcium, ISOPTIN prolongs the effective refractory period within the AV node and slows AV conduction in a rate-related manner.
Normal sinus rhythm is usually not affected, but in patients with sick sinus syndrome, ISOPTIN may interfere with sinus node impulse generation and may induce sinus arrest or sinoatrial block. Atrioventricular block can occur in patients without preexisting conduction defects (see WARNINGS).
ISOPTIN does not alter the normal atrial action potential or intraventricular conduction time, but depresses amplitude, velocity of depolarization and conduction in depressed atrial fibers. ISOPTIN may shorten the antegrade effective refractory period of accessory bypass tracts. Acceleration of ventricular rate and/or ventricular fibrillation has been reported in patients with atrial flutter or atrial fibrillation and a coexisting accessory AV pathway following administration of verapamil (see WARNINGS).
ISOPTIN has a local anesthetic action that is 1.6 times that of procaine on an equimolar basis. It is not known whether this action is important at the doses used in man.
Pharmacokinetics and Metabolism: With the immediate release formulation, more than 90% of the orally administered dose of ISOPTIN is absorbed. Because of rapid biotransformation of verapamil during its first pass through the portal circulation, bioavailability ranges from 20% to 35%. Peak plasma concentrations are reached between 1 and 2 hours after oral administration. Chronic oral administration of 120 mg of ISOPTIN every 6 hours resulted in plasma levels of verapamil ranging from 125 to 400 ng/mL with higher values reported occasionally. A nonlinear correlation between the verapamil dose administered and verapamil plasma levels does exist.
In early dose titration with verapamil a relationship exists between verapamil plasma concentrations and the prolongation of the PR interval. However, during chronic administration this relationship may disappear. The mean elimination half-life in single dose studies ranged from 2.8 to 7.4 hours. In these same studies, after repetitive dosing, the half-life increased to a range from 4.5 to 12.0 hours (after less than 10 consecutive doses given 6 hours apart). Half-life of verapamil may increase during titration. No relationship has been established between the plasma concentration of verapamil and a reduction in blood pressure.
Aging may affect the pharmacokinetics of verapamil. Elimination half-life may be prolonged in the elderly.
In multiple dose studies under fasting conditions the bioavailability measured by AUC of ISOPTIN SR was similar to ISOPTIN immediate release; rates of absorption were, of course, different. In a randomized, single-dose, crossover study using healthy volunteers, administration of 240 mg ISOPTIN SR with food produced peak plasma verapamil concentrations of 79 ng/mL, time to peak plasma verapamil concentrations of 7.71 hours, and AUC (0–24 hr) of 841 ng-hr/mL. When ISOPTIN SR was administered to fasting subjects, peak plasma verapamil concentration was 164 ng/mL; time to peak plasma verapamil concentration was 5.21 hours; and AUC (0–24 hr) was 1,478 ng-hr/mL. Similar results were demonstrated for plasma norverapamil. Food thus produces decreased bioavailability (AUC) but a narrower peak to trough ratio. Good correlation of dose and response is not available, but controlled studies of ISOPTIN SR have shown effectiveness of doses similar to the effective doses of ISOPTIN (immediate release).
In healthy man, orally administered ISOPTIN undergoes extensive metabolism in the liver. Twelve metabolites have been identified in plasma; all except norverapamil are present in trace amounts only. Norverapamil can reach steady-state plasma concentrations approximately equal to those of verapamil itself. The cardiovascular activity of norverapamil appears to be approximately 20% that of verapamil. Approximately 70% of an administered dose is excreted as metabolites in the urine and 16% or more in the feces within 5 days. About 3% to 4% is excreted in the urine as unchanged drug. Approximately 90% is bound to plasma proteins. In patients with hepatic insufficiency, metabolism of immediate release verapamil is delayed and elimination half-life prolonged up to 14 to 16 hours (see PRECAUTIONS); the volume of distribution is increased and plasma clearance reduced to about 30% of normal. Verapamil clearance values suggest that patients with liver dysfunction may attain therapeutic verapamil plasma concentrations with one-third of the oral daily dose required for patients with normal liver function.
After four weeks of oral dosing (120 mg q.i.d.), verapamil and norverapamil levels were noted in the cerebrospinal fluid with estimated partition coefficient of 0.06 for verapamil and 0.04 for norverapamil.
Hemodynamics and Myocardial Metabolism:
In ten healthy males, administration of oral verapamil (80 mg every 8 hours for 6 days) and a single oral dose of ethanol (0.8 g/kg) resulted in a 17% increase in mean peak ethanol concentrations (106.45 ± 21.40 to 124.23 ± 24.74 mg•hr/dL) compared to placebo. The area under the blood ethanol concentration versus time curve (AUC over 12 hours) increased by 30% (365.67 ± 93.52 to 475.07 ± 97.24 mg•hr/dL). Verapamil AUCs were positively correlated (r=0.71) to increased ethanol blood AUC values. (See PRECAUTIONS: Drug Interactions.)
ISOPTIN reduces afterload and myocardial contractility. Improved left ventricular diastolic function in patients with IHSS and those with coronary heart disease has also been observed with ISOPTIN therapy. In most patients, including those with organic cardiac disease, the negative inotropic action of ISOPTIN is countered by reduction of afterload and cardiac index is usually not reduced. However, in patients with severe left ventricular dysfunction (e.g., pulmonary wedge pressure above 20 mmHg or ejection fraction lower than 30%), or in patients taking beta-adrenergic blocking agents or other cardiodepressant drugs, deterioration of ventricular function may occur (see DRUG INTERACTIONS).
Pulmonary Function: ISOPTIN does not induce bronchoconstriction and hence, does not impair ventilatory function.

INDICATIONS AND USAGE

ISOPTIN SR (verapamil HCl) is indicated for the management of essential hypertension.

CONTRAINDICATIONS

Verapamil HCl is contraindicated in:
1. Severe left ventricular dysfunction (see WARNINGS)
2. Hypotension (systolic pressure less than 90 mm Hg) or cardiogenic shock
3. Sick sinus syndrome (except in patients with a functioning artificial ventricular pacemaker)
4. Second- or third-degree AV block (except in patients with a functioning artificial ventricular pacemaker).
5. Patients with atrial flutter or atrial fibrillation and an accessory bypass tract (e.g., Wolff-Parkinson-White, Lown-Ganong-Levine syndromes). (see WARNINGS).
6. Patients with known hypersensitivity to verapamil hydrochloride.

WARNINGS

Heart Failure: Verapamil has a negative inotropic effect which, in most patients, is compensated by its afterload reduction (decreased systemic vascular resistance) properties without a net impairment of ventricular performance. In clinical experience with 4,954 patients, 87 (1.8%) developed congestive heart failure or pulmonary edema. Verapamil should be avoided in patients with severe left ventricular dysfunction (e.g., ejection fraction less than 30%, or moderate to severe symptoms of cardiac failure) and in patients with any degree of ventricular dysfunction if they are receiving a beta adrenergic blocker (see DRUG INTERACTIONS). Patients with milder ventricular dysfunction should, if possible, be controlled with optimum doses of digitalis and/or diuretics before verapamil treatment (Note interactions with digoxin under: PRECAUTIONS).
Hypotension: Occasionally, the pharmacologic action of verapamil may produce a decrease in blood pressure below normal levels which may result in dizziness or symptomatic hypotension. The incidence of hypotension observed in 4,954 patients enrolled in clinical trials was 2.5%. In hypertensive patients, decreases in blood pressure below normal are unusual. Tilt table testing (60 degrees) was not able to induce orthostatic hypotension.
Elevated Liver Enzymes: Elevations of transaminases with and without concomitant elevations in alkaline phosphatase and bilirubin have been reported. Such elevations have sometimes been transient and may disappear even in the face of continued verapamil treatment. Several cases of

Continued on next page

Isoptin SR—Cont.

hepatocellular injury related to verapamil have been proven by rechallenge; half of these had clinical symptoms (malaise, fever, and/or right upper quadrant pain) in addition to elevations of SGOT, SGPT and alkaline phosphatase. Periodic monitoring of liver function in patients receiving verapamil is therefore prudent.

Accessory Bypass Tract (Wolff-Parkinson-White or Lown-Ganong-Levine): Some patients with paroxysmal and/or chronic atrial fibrillation or atrial flutter and a coexisting accessory AV pathway have developed increased antegrade conduction across the accessory pathway bypassing the AV node, producing a very rapid ventricular response or ventricular fibrillation after receiving intravenous verapamil (or digitalis). Although a risk of this occurring with oral verapamil has not been established, such patients receiving oral verapamil may be at risk and its use in these patients is contraindicated (see CONTRAINDICATIONS).

Treatment is usually DC-cardioversion. Cardioversion has been used safely and effectively after oral ISOPTIN.

Atrioventricular Block: The effect of verapamil on AV conduction and the SA node may lead to asymptomatic first-degree AV block and transient bradycardia, sometimes accompanied by nodal escape rhythms. PR interval prolongation is correlated with verapamil plasma concentrations, especially during the early titration phases of therapy. Higher degrees of AV block, however, were infrequently (0.8%) observed. Marked first-degree block or progressive development to second- or third-degree AV block requires a reduction in dosage or, in rare instances, discontinuation of verapamil HCl and institution of appropriate therapy depending upon the clinical situation.

Patients with Hypertrophic Cardiomyopathy (IHSS): In 120 patients with hypertrophic cardiomyopathy (most of them refractory or intolerant to propranolol) who received therapy with verapamil at doses up to 720 mg/day, a variety of serious adverse effects were seen. Three patients died in pulmonary edema; all had severe left ventricular outflow obstruction and a past history of left ventricular dysfunction. Eight other patients had pulmonary edema and/or severe hypotension; abnormally high (greater than 20 mmHg) pulmonary wedge pressure and a marked left ventricular outflow obstruction were present in most of these patients. Concomitant administration of quinidine (see DRUG INTERACTIONS) preceded the severe hypotension in 3 of the 8 patients (2 of whom developed pulmonary edema). Sinus bradycardia occurred in 11% of the patients, second-degree AV block in 4% and sinus arrest in 2%. It must be appreciated that this group of patients had a serious disease with a high mortality rate. Most adverse effects responded well to dose reduction and only rarely did verapamil have to be discontinued.

PRECAUTIONS

General

Use in Patients with Impaired Hepatic Functions: Since verapamil is highly metabolized by the liver, it should be administered cautiously to patients with impaired hepatic function. Severe liver dysfunction prolongs the elimination half-life of immediate release verapamil to about 14 to 16 hours; hence, approximately 30% of the dose given to patients with normal liver function should be administered to these patients. Careful monitoring for abnormal prolongation of the PR interval or other signs of excessive pharmacologic effects (see OVERDOSAGE) should be carried out.

Use in Patients with Attenuated (Decreased) Neuromuscular Transmission: It has been reported that verapamil decreases neuromuscular transmission in patients with Duchenne's muscular dystrophy, and that verapamil prolongs recovery from the neuromuscular blocking agent vecuronium. It may be necessary to decrease the dosage of verapamil when it is administered to patients with attenuated neuromuscular transmission.

Use in Patients with Impaired Renal Function: About 70% of an administered dose of verapamil is excreted as metabolites in the urine. Verapamil is not removed by hemodialysis. Until further data are available, verapamil should be administered cautiously to patients with impaired renal function. These patients should be carefully monitored for abnormal prolongation of the PR interval or other signs of overdosage (see OVERDOSAGE).

Drug Interactions

Beta Blockers: Concomitant therapy with beta-adrenergic blockers and verapamil may result in additive negative effects on heart rate, atrioventricular conduction, and/or cardiac contractility. The combination of sustained-release verapamil and beta-adrenergic blocking agents has not been studied. However, there have been reports of excessive bradycardia and AV block, including complete heart block, when the combination has been used for the treatment of hypertension. For hypertensive patients, the risks of combined therapy may outweigh the potential benefits. The combination should be used only with caution and close monitoring.

Asymptomatic bradycardia (36 beats/min) with a wandering atrial pacemaker has been observed in a patient receiving concomitant timolol (a beta-adrenergic blocker) eyedrops and oral verapamil.

A decrease in metoprolol and propranolol clearance has been observed when either drug is administered concomitantly with verapamil. A variable effect has been seen when verapamil and atenolol were given together.

Digitalis: Clinical use of verapamil in digitalized patients has shown the combination to be well tolerated if digoxin doses are properly adjusted. Chronic verapamil treatment can increase serum digoxin levels by 50 to 75% during the first week of therapy, and this can result in digitalis toxicity. In patients with hepatic cirrhosis the influence of verapamil on digoxin kinetics is magnified. Verapamil may reduce total body clearance and extrarenal clearance of digitoxin by 27% and 29%, respectively. Maintenance digitalis doses should be reduced when verapamil is administered, and the patient should be carefully monitored to avoid over- or underdigitalization. Whenever overdigitalization is suspected, the daily dose of digitalis should be reduced or temporarily discontinued. Upon discontinuation of ISOPTIN (verapamil HCl), the patient should be reassessed to avoid underdigitalization.

Antihypertensive Agents: Verapamil administered concomitantly with oral antihypertensive agents (e.g., vasodilators, angiotensin-converting enzyme inhibitors, diuretics, beta blockers) will usually have an additive effect on lowering blood pressure. Patients receiving these combinations should be appropriately monitored. Concomitant use of agents that attenuate alpha-adrenergic function with verapamil may result in a reduction in blood pressure that is excessive in some patients. Such an effect was observed in one study following the concomitant administration of verapamil and prazosin.

Antiarrhythmic Agents

Disopyramide: Until data on possible interactions between verapamil and disopyramide phosphate are obtained, disopyramide should not be administered within 48 hours before or 24 hours after verapamil administration.

Flecainide: A study of healthy volunteers showed that the concomitant administration of flecainide and verapamil may have additive effects on myocardial contractility, AV conduction, and repolarization. Concomitant therapy with flecainide and verapamil may result in additive negative inotropic effect and prolongation of atrioventricular conduction.

Quinidine: In a small number of patients with hypertrophic cardiomyopathy (IHSS), concomitant use of verapamil and quinidine resulted in significant hypotension. Until further data are obtained, combined therapy of verapamil and quinidine in patients with hypertrophic cardiomyopathy should probably be avoided.

The electrophysiological effects of quinidine and verapamil on AV conduction were studied in 8 patients. Verapamil significantly counteracted the effects of quinidine on AV conduction. There has been a report of increased quinidine levels during verapamil therapy.

Nitrates: Verapamil has been given concomitantly with short- and long-acting nitrates without any undesirable drug interactions. The pharmacologic profile of both drugs and the clinical experience suggest beneficial interactions.

Other

Alcohol: Verapamil has been found to significantly inhibit ethanol elimination resulting in elevated blood ethanol concentrations that may prolong the intoxicating effects of alcohol. (See CLINICAL PHARMACOLOGY, Pharmacokinetics and Metabolism).

Cimetidine: The interaction between cimetidine and chronically administered verapamil has not been studied. Variable results on clearance have been obtained in acute studies of healthy volunteers; clearance of verapamil was either reduced or unchanged.

Lithium: Increased sensitivity to the effects of lithium (neurotoxicity) has been reported during concomitant verapamil-lithium therapy; lithuim levels have been observed sometimes to increase, sometimes to decrease, and sometimes to be unchanged. Patients receiving both drugs must be monitored carefully.

Carbamazepine: Verapamil may increase carbamazepine concentrations during combined therapy. This may produce carbamazepine side effects such as diplopia, headache, ataxia, or dizziness.

Rifampin: Therapy with rifampin may markedly reduce oral verapamil bioavailability.

Phenobarbital: Phenobarbital therapy may increase verapamil clearance.

Cyclosporine: Verapamil therapy may increase serum levels of cyclosporine.

Theophylline: Verapamil therapy may inhibit the clearance and increase the plasma levels of theophylline.

Inhalation Anesthetics: Animal experiments have shown that inhalation anesthetics depress cardiovascular activity by decreasing the inward movement of calcium ions. When used concomitantly, inhalation anesthetics and calcium antagonists, such as verapamil, should be titrated carefully to avoid excessive cardiovascular depression.

Neuromuscular Blocking Agents: Clinical data and animal studies suggest that verapamil may potentiate the activity of neuromuscular blocking agents (curare-like and depolarizing). It may be necessary to decrease the dose of verapamil and/or the dose of the neuromuscular blocking agent when the drugs are used concomitantly.

Carcinogenesis, Mutagenesis, Impairment of Fertility: An 18–month toxicity study in rats, at a low multiple (6 fold) of the maximum recommended human dose, and not the maximum tolerated dose, did not suggest a tumorigenic potential. There was no evidence of a carcinogenic potential of verapamil administered in the diet of rats for two years at doses of 10, 35, and 120 mg/kg per day or approximately 1×, 3.5×, and 12×, respectively, the maximum recommended human daily dose (480 mg per day or 9.6 mg/kg/day).

Verapamil was not mutagenic in the Ames test in 5 test strains at 3 mg per plate, with or without metabolic activation.

Studies in female rats at daily dietary doses up to 5.5 times (55 mg/kg/day) the maximum recommended human dose did not show impaired fertility. Effects on male fertility have not been determined.

Pregnancy: Pregnancy Category C. Reproduction studies have been performed in rabbits and rats at oral doses up to 1.5 (15 mg/kg/day) and 6 (60 mg/kg/day) times the human oral daily dose, respectively, and have revealed no evidence of teratogenicity. In the rat, however, this multiple of the human dose was embryocidal and retarded fetal growth and development, probably because of adverse maternal effects reflected in the reduced weight gains of the dams. This oral dose has also been shown to cause hypotension in rats. There are no adequate and well-controlled studies in pregnant women. Because animal reproduction studies are not always predictive of human response, this drug should be used during pregnancy only if clearly needed. Verapamil crosses the placental barrier and can be detected in umbilical vein blood at delivery.

Labor and Delivery: It is not known whether the use of verapamil during labor or delivery has immediate or delayed adverse effects on the fetus, or whether it prolongs the duration of labor or increases the need for forceps delivery or other obstetric intervention. Such adverse experiences have not been reported in the literature, despite a long history of use of Verapamil in Europe in the treatment of cardiac side effects of beta-adrenergic agonist agents used to treat premature labor.

Nursing Mothers: Verapamil is excreted in human milk. Because of the potential for adverse reactions in nursing infants for verapamil, nursing should be discontinued while verapamil is administered.

Pediatric Use: Safety and efficacy of ISOPTIN tablets in pediatric patients below the age of 18 years have not been established.

Animal Pharmacology and/or Animal Toxicology: In chronic animal toxicology studies verapamil caused lenticular and/or suture line changes at 30 mg/kg/day or greater and frank cataracts at 62.5 mg/kg/day or greater in the beagle dog but not the rat. Development of cataracts due to verapamil has not been reported in man.

ADVERSE REACTIONS

Serious adverse reactions are uncommon when verapamil therapy is initiated with upward dose titration within the recommended single and total daily dose. See WARNINGS for discussion of heart failure, hypotension, elevated liver enzymes, AV block, and rapid ventricular response. Reversible (upon discontinuation of verapamil) non-obstructive, paralytic ileus has been infrequently reported in association with he use of verapamil. The following reactions to orally administered verapamil occurred at rates greater than 1.0% or occurred at lower rates but appeared clearly drug-related in clinical trials in 4,954 patients.

Constipation	7.3%	Fatigue	1.7%
Dizziness	3.3%	Dyspnea	1.4%
Nausea	2.7%	Bradycardia(HR <50/min)	1.4%
Hypotension	2.5%	AV Block-total (1°, 2°, 3°)	1.2%
Headache	2.2%	2° and 3°	0.8%
Edema	1.9%	Rash	1.2%
CHF/ Pulmonary Edema	1.8%	Flushing	0.6%

Elevated Liver Enzymes (see WARNING)

In clinical trials related to the control of ventricular response in digitalized patients who had atrial fibrillation or atrial flutter, ventricular rates below 50/min at rest occurred in 15% of patients and asymptomatic hypotension occurred in 5% of patients.

The following reactions, reported in 1.0% or less of patients, occurred under conditions (open trials, marketing experience) where a causal relationship is uncertain; they are listed to alert the physician to a possible relationship.

Cardiovascular: angina pectoris, atrioventricular dissociation, chest pain, claudication, myocardial infarction, palpitations, purpura (vasculitis), syncope.

Digestive System: diarrhea, dry mouth, gastrointestinal distress, gingival hyperplasia.

Hemic and Lymphatic: ecchymosis or bruising.

Nervous System: cerebrovascular accident, confusion, equilibrium disorders, insomnia, muscle cramps, paresthesia, psychotic symptoms, shakiness, somnolence.

Skin: arthralgia and rash, exanthema, hair loss, hyperkeratosis, maculae, sweating, urticaria, Stevens-Johnson syndrome, erythema multiforme.

Special Senses: blurred vision, tinnitus.

Urogenital: gynecomastia, impotence, galactorrheal hyperprolactinemia, increased urination, spotty menstruation.

Treatment of Acute Cardiovascular Adverse Reactions: The frequency of cardiovascular adverse reactions which require therapy is rare, hence, experience with their treatment is limited. Whenever severe hypotension or complete AV block occurs following oral administration of verapamil, the appropriate emergency measures should be applied immediately, e.g., intravenously administered isoproterenol HCl, norepinephrine bitartrate, atropine sulfate (all in the usual doses), or calcium gluconate (10% solution). In patients with hypertrophic cardiomyopathy (IHSS), alpha-adrenergic agents (phenylephrine HCl, metaraminol bitartrate or methoxamine HCl) should be used to maintain blood pressure, and isoproterenol and norepinephrine should be avoided. If further support is necessary, (dopamine HCl or dobutamine HCl) may be administered. Actual treatment and dosage should depend on the severity of the clinical situation and the judgment and experience of the treating physician.

OVERDOSAGE

Overdose with verapamil may lead to pronounced hypotension, bradycardia, and conduction system abnormalities (e.g., junctional rhythm with AV dissociation and high degree AV block, including asystole). Other symptoms secondary to hypoperfusion (e.g., metabolic acidosis, hyperglycemia, hyperkalemia, renal dysfunction, and convulsions) may be evident.

Treat all verapamil overdoses as serious and maintain observation for at least 48 hours (especially Isoptin SR), preferably under continuous hospital care. Delayed pharmacodynamic consequences may occur with the sustained released formulation. Verapamil is known to decrease gastrointestinal transit time.

In overdose, tablets of ISOPTIN SR have occasionally been reported to form concretions within the stomach or intestines. These concretions have not been visible on plain radiographs of the abdomen, and no medical means of gastrointestinal emptying is of proven efficacy in removing them. Endoscopy might reasonably be considered in cases of massive overdose when symptoms are unusually prolonged.

Treatment of overdosage should be supportive. Beta adrenergic stimulation or parenteral administration of calcium solutions may increase calcium ion flux across the slow channel, and have been used effectively in treatment of deliberate overdosage with verapamil. Continued treatment with large doses of calcium may produce a response. In a few reported cases, overdose with calcium channel blockers that was initially refractory to atropine became more responsive to this treatment when the patients received large doses (close to 1 gram/hour for more than 24 hours) of calcium chloride. Verapamil cannot be removed by hemodialysis. Clinically significant hypotensive reactions or high degree AV block should be treated with vasopressor agents or cardiac pacing, respectively. Asystole should be handled by the usual measures including cardiopulmonary resuscitation.

DOSAGE AND ADMINISTRATION

Essential Hypertension

The dose of ISOPTIN SR should be individualized by titration and the drug should be administered with food. Initiate therapy with 180 mg of sustained-release verapamil HCl, ISOPTIN SR, given in the morning. Lower, initial doses of 120 mg a day may be warranted in patients who may have an increased response to verapamil (e.g., the elderly or small people etc.). Upward titration should be based on therapeutic efficacy and safety evaluated weekly and approximately 24 hours after the previous dose. The antihypertensive effects of ISOPTIN SR are evident within the first week of therapy.

If adequate response is not obtained with 180 mg of ISOPTIN SR, the dose may be titrated upward in the following manner:

a) 240 mg each morning,
b) 180 mg each morning plus 180 mg each evening, or 240 mg each morning plus 120 mg each evening
c) 240 mg every twelve hours.

When switching from immediate release ISOPTIN to ISOPTIN SR, the total daily dose in milligrams may remain the same.

HOW SUPPLIED

ISOPTIN® SR 240 mg tablets are supplied as light green, capsule shaped, scored, film-coated tablets containing 240 mg of verapamil hydrochloride. The tablet is embossed with a double Knoll triangle on one side and "ISOPTIN SR" on the other side. ISOPTIN® SR 180 mg tablets are supplied as light pink, oval shaped, scored, film-coated tablets containing 180 mg of verapamil hydrochloride. The tablet is embossed with "ISOPTIN SR" on one side, and "180 mg" on the other side. The ISOPTIN® SR 120 mg tablets are supplied as light violet, oval shaped, film-coated tablets containing 120 mg of verapamil hydrochloride. The tablet is embossed with "KNOLL" on one side and "120 SR" on the other side.

240 mg (light green)- Bottle of 30-
NDC #0044-1826-93
Bottle of 100-
NDC #0044-1826-02
Bottle of 500-
NDC #0044-1826-03
Hospital Unit Dose (100 Tablets-
10 Strips of 10)-NDC #0044-1826-10

180 mg (light pink)- Bottle of 100-
NDC #0044-1825-02
Bottle of 500-
NDC #0044-1825-03
Hospital Unit Dose (100 Tablets-
10 Strips of 10)-NDC #0044-1825-12

120 mg (light violet)- Bottle of 100-
NDC #0044-1827-02
Bottle of 500-
NDC #0044-1827-03
Hospital Unit Dose (100 Tablets-
10 Strips of 10) - NDC #0044-1827-12

Storage: 15° to 25°C (59° to 77°F)

Protect from light and moisture.

Dispense in a light, light-resistant container as defined in the USP.

Revised: September 1997

Knoll Laboratories
A Division of
Knoll Pharmaceutical Company
Mount Olive, New Jersey 07828 **BASF** Pharma
0900023-6

Shown in Product Identification Guide, page 319

RYTHMOL® TABLETS ℞
(propafenone hydrochloride)

DESCRIPTION

RYTHMOL (propafenone hydrochloride) is an antiarrhythmic drug supplied in scored, film-coated tablets of 150, 225 and 300 mg for oral administration. Propafenone has some structural similarities to beta-blocking agents.

The structural formula of propafenone hydrochloride is given below:

O
‖
C–CH₂–CH₂–(phenyl)
O–CH₂–CH–CH₂–NH–CH₂–CH₂–CH₃ • HCL
OH

$C_{21}H_{27}NO_3{\cdot}HCl$ M. W. = 377.92

$C_{21}H_{27}NO_3{\cdot}HCl$ M.W. = 377.92

2′-[2–Hydroxy-3–(propylamino)
-propoxy]-3-phenylpropiophenone
hydrochloride

Propafenone hydrochloride occurs as colorless crystals or white crystalline powder with a very bitter taste. It is slightly soluble in water (20°C), chloroform and ethanol. The following inactive ingredients are contained in the tablet: corn starch, hydroxypropyl methylcellulose, magnesium stearate, polyethylene glycol, polysorbate, povidone, propylene glycol, sodium starch glycolate and titanium dioxide.

CLINICAL PHARMACOLOGY

Mechanism of Action: RYTHMOL (propafenone HCl) is a Class 1C antiarrhythmic drug with local anesthetic effects, and a direct stablizing action on myocardial membranes. The electrophysiological effect of RYTHMOL manifests itself in a reduction of upstroke velocity (Phase 0) of the monophasic action potential. In Purkinje fibers, and to a lesser extent myocardial fibers, RYTHMOL reduces the fast inward current carried by sodium ions. Diastolic excitability threshold is increased and effective refractory period prolonged. Propafenone reduces spontaneous automaticity and depresses triggered activity.

Studies in anesthetized dogs and isolated organ preparations show that RYTHMOL has beta-sympatholytic activity at about 1/50 the potency of propranolol. Clinical studies employing isoproternol challenge and exercise testing after single doses of propafenone indicate a beta-adrenergic blocking potency (per mg) about 1/40 that of propranolol in man. In clinical trials, resting heart rate decreases of about 8% were noted at the higher end of the therapeutic plasma concentration range. At very high concentrations in vitro, propafenone can inhibit the slow inward current carried by calcium but this calcium antagonist effect probably does not contribute to antiarrhythmic efficacy. Propafenone has local anesthetic activity approximately equal to procaine.

Electrophysiology: Electrophysiology studies in patients with ventricular tachycardia have shown that RYTHMOL prolongs atrioventricular conduction which having little or no effect on sinus node function. Both AV nodal conduction time (AH interval) and His-Purkinje conduction time (HV interval) are prolonged. Propafenone has little or no effect on the atrial functional refractory period, but AV nodal functional and effective refractory periods are prolonged. In patients with WPW, RYTHMOL reduces conduction and increses the effective refractory period of the accessory pathway in both directions. Propafenone slows conduction and consequently produces dose related changes in the PR interval and QRS duration. QTc interval does not change.

Mean Changes in ECG Intervals*
Total Daily Dose (mg)

	337.5 mg		450 mg		675 mg		900 mg	
Interval	msec	%	msec	%	msec	%	msec	%
RR	−14.5	−1.8	30.6	3.8	31.5	3.9	41.7	5.1
PR	3.6	2.1	19.1	11.6	28.9	17.8	35.6	21.9
QRS	5.6	6.4	5.5	6.1	7.7	8.4	15.6	17.3
QTc	2.7	0.7	−7.5	−1.8	5.0	1.2	14.7	3.7

* Change and percent change based on mean baseline values for each treatment group.

In any individual patient, the above ECG changes cannot be readily used to predict either efficacy or plasma concentration.

RYTHMOL causes a dose-related and concentration-related decrease in the rate of single and multiple PVCs and can suppress recurrence of ventricular tachycardia. Based on the percent of patients attaining substantial (80–90%) suppression of ventricular ectopic activity, it appears that trough plasma levels of 0.2 to 1.5 µg/mL can provide good suppression, with higher concentrations giving a greater rate of good response.

When 600 mg/day propafenone was administered to patients with paroxysmal atrial tachyarrhythmias, mean heart rate during arrhythmia decreased 14 beats/min and 37 beats/min for PAF patients and PSVT patients, respectively.

Hemodynamics: Sympathetic stimulation may be a vital component supporting circulatory function in patients with congestive heart failure, and its inhibition by the beta blockade produced by RYTHMOL may in itself aggravate congestive heart failure.

Additionally, like other Class 1C antiarrhythmic drugs, studies in humans have shown that RYTHMOL exerts a negative inotropic effect on the myocardium. Cardiac catheterization studies in patients with moderately impaired ventricular function (mean C.I.=2.61 L/min/m^2) utilizing intravenous propafenone infusions (2 mg/kg over 10 min+2 mg/min for 30 min) that gave mean plasma concentrations of 3.0 µg/mL (well above the therapeutic range of 0.2–1.5 µg/mL) showed significant increases in pulmonary capillary wedge pressure, systemic and pulmonary vascular resistances and depression of cardiac output and cardiac index.

Pharmacokinetics and Metabolism: RYTHMOL is nearly completely absorbed after oral administration with peak plasma levels occurring approximately 3.5 hours after administration in most individuals. Propafenone exhibits extensive saturable presystemic biotransformation (first pass effect) resulting in a dose dependent and dosage form dependent absolute bioavailability; e.g., a 150 mg tablet had absolute bioavailability of 3.4%, while a 300 mg tablet had absolute bioavailability of 10.6%. A 300 mg solution which was rapidly absorbed, had absolute bioavailability of 21.4%. At still larger doses, above those recommended, bioavailability increases still further. Decreased liver function also increases bioavailability, bioavailability inversely related to indocyanine green clearance reaching 60–70% at clearances of 7 mL/min and below. The clearance of propafenone is reduced and the elimination half-life increased in patients with significant heptic dysunction (see PRECAUTIONS).

RYTHMOL follows a nonlinear pharmacokinetic disposition presumably due to saturation of first pass hepatic metabolism as the liver is exposed to higher concentrations of propafenone and shows a very high degree of interindividual variability. For example, for a three-fold increase in daily dose from 300 to 900 mg/day there is a tenfold increase in steady-slate plasma concentration.The top 25% of patients given 375 mg/day, however, had a mean concentration of propafenone larger than the bottom 25%, and about equal to the second 25%, of patients given a dose of 900 mg. Although food increased peak blood level and bioavailability in a single dose study, during multiple dose administration of propafenone to healthy volunteers food did not change bioavailability significantly.

There are two genetically determined patterns of propafenone metabolism. In over 90% of patients, the drug is rapidly and extensively metabolized with an elimination half life from 2–10 hours. These patients metabolize propafenone into two active metabolites: 5-hydroxypropafenone and N-depropylpropafenone. In vitro preparations have shown these two metabolites to have antiarrhythmic activity comparable to propafenone but in man they both are usually present in concentrations less than 20% of propafenone. Nine additional metabolites have been identified, most in only trace amounts. It is the saturable hydroxylation pathway that is responsible for the nonlinear pharmacokinetic disposition.

In less than 10% of patients (and in any patient also receiving quindine, see PRECAUTIONS), metabolism of propafenone is slower because the 5-hydroxy metabolite is not formed or is minimally formed. The estimated propafenone elimination half-life ranges from 10–32 hours. Decreased ability to form the 5-hydroxy metabolite of propafernone is associated with a diminished ability to metabolize debrisoquine and a variety of other drugs (encainide, metoprolol, dextromethorphan). In these patients, the N-deproplpropafenone occurs in quantities comparable to the levels occurring in extensive metabolizers. In slow metabolizers propafenone pharmacokinetics are linear.

There are significant differences in plasma concentrations of propafenone in slow and extensive metabolizers, the former achieving concentrations 1.5 to 2.0 times those of the extensive metabolizers at daily doses of 675–900 mg/day. At low doses the differences are greater, with slow metabolizers attaining concentrations more than five times that of extensive metabolizers. Because the difference decreases at high doses and is mitigated by the lack of the active 5-hydroxy metabolite in the slow metabolizers, and because steady-state conditions are achieved after 4–5 days of dosing in all patients, the recommended dosing regimen is the same for all patients. The greater variability in blood levels require that the drug be titrated carefully in patients with close attention paid to clinical and ECG evidence of toxicity (See DOSAGE AND ADMINISTRATION).

Clinical Trials: In two randomized, crossover, placebo-controlled, double-blind trials of 60–90 days duration in patients with paroxysmal supraventricular arrhythmias [paroxysmal atrial fibrillation/flutter (PAF), or paroxysmal supraventricular tachycardia (PSVT)], propafenone reduced

Continued on next page

Rythmol—Cont.

the rate of both arrhythmias, as shown in the following table:

	Study 1		Study 2	
	Propafenone	Placebo	Propafenone	Placebo
PAF	n=30	n=30	n=9	n=9
Percent attack free	53%	13%	67%	22%
Median time to first recurrence	>98 days	8 days	62 days	5 days
PSVT	n=45	n=45	n=15	n=15
Percent attack free	47%	16%	38%	7%
Median time to first recurrence	>98 days	12 days	31 days	8 days

The patient population in the above trials was 50% male with a mean age of 57.3 years. Fifty percent of the patients had a diagnosis of PAF and 50% had PSVT. Eighty percent of the patients received 600 mg/day propafenone. No patient died in the above 2 studies.

In the U.S. long-term safety trials, 474 patients (mean age: 57.4 ± 14.5 years) with supraventricular arrhythmias [195 with PAF, 274 with PSVT and 5 with both PAF and PSVT] were treated up to 5 years (mean: 14.4 months) with propafenone. Fourteen of the patients died. When this mortality rate was compared to the rate in a similar patient population (n=194 patients; mean age: 43.0 ± 16.8 years) studied in an arrhythmia clinic, there was no age-adjusted difference in mortality. This comparison was not, however, a randomized trial and the 95% confidence interval around the comparison was large, such that neither a significant adverse or favorable effect could be ruled out.

INDICATIONS AND USAGE

In patients without structural heart disease, RYTHMOL (propafenone HCl) is indicated to prolong the time to recurrence of

— paroxysmal atrial fibrillation/flutter (PAF) associated with disabling symptoms.

— paroxysmal supraventricular tachycardia (PSVT) associated with disabling symptoms.

As with other agents, some patients with atrial flutter treated with propafenone have developed 1:1 conduction, producing an increase in ventricular rate. Concomitant treatment with drugs that increase the functional AV refractory period is recommended.

The use of RYTHMOL in patients with chronic atrial fibrillation has not been evaluated. RYTHMOL should not be used to control ventricular rate during atrial fibrillation.

RYTHMOL is also indicated for the treatment of

— documented ventricular arrhythmias, such as sustained ventricular tachycardia, that, in the judgement of the physician, are life-threatening. Because the proarrhythmic effects of RYTHMOL, its use with lesser ventricular arrhythmias is not recommended, even if patients are symptomatic, and any use of the drug should be reserved for patients in whom, in the opinion of the physician, the potential benefits outweigh the risks.

Initiation of RYTHMOL treatment, as with other anti-arrthythmics used to treat life-threatening ventricular arrhythmias, should be carried out in the hospital.

RYTHMOL, like other antiarrhythmic drugs, has not been shown to enhance survival in patients with ventricular or atrial arrhythmias.

CONTRAINDICATIONS

RYTHMOL (propafenone HCl) is contraindicated in the presence of uncontrolled congestive heart failure, cardiogenic shock, sinoatrial, atrioventricular and intraventricular disorders of impulse generation and/or conduction (e.g., sick sinus node syndrome, atrioventricular block) in the absence of an artificial pacemaker, bradycardia, marked hypotension, bronchospastic disorders, manifest electrolyte imbalance, and known hypersensitivity to the drug.

WARNINGS

Mortality: In the National Heart, Lung and Blood Institute's Cardiac Arrhythmia Suppression Trial (CAST), a long-term, multi-center, randomized, double-blind study in patients with asymptomatic non-life-threatening ventricular arrhythmias who had a myocardial infarction more than six days but less than two years previously, an increased rate of death or reversed cardiac arrest (7.7%; 56/730) was seen in patients treated with encainide or flecainide (class 1C antiarrhythmics) compared with that seen in patients assigned to placebo (3.0%; 22/725). The average duration of treatment with encainide or flecainide in this study was ten months. The applicability of the CAST results to other populations (e.g., those without recent myocardial infarction) or other antiarrhythmic drugs is uncertain, but at present it is prudent to consider any 1C antiarrhythmic to have a significant risk in patients with structural heart disease. Given the lack of any evidence that these drugs improve survival, antiarrhythmic agents should generally be avoided in patients with non-life-threatening ventricular arrhythmias, even if the patients are experiencing unpleasant, but not life-threatening, symptoms or signs.

Proarrhythmic Effects: RYTHMOL (propafenone HCl), like other antiarrhythmic agents, may cause new or worsened arrhythmias. Such proarrhythmic effects range from an increase in frequency of PVCs to the development of more severe ventricular tachycardia, ventricular fibrillation or torsade de pointes; i.e., tachycardia that is more sustained or more rapid which may lead to fatal consequences. It is therefore essential that each patient given RYTHMOL be evaluated electrocardiographically and clinically prior to, and during therapy to determine whether the response to RYTHMOL supports continued treatment.

Overall in clinical trials with propafenone. 4.7% of all patients had new or worsened ventricular arrhythmia possibly representing a proarrthythmic event (0.7% was an increase in PVCs; 4.0% a worsening, or new appearance, of VT or VF). Of the patients who had worsening of VT (4%), 92% had a history of VT and/or VT/VF, 71% had coronary artery disease, and 68% had a prior myocardial infarction. The incidence of proarrhythmia in patients with less serious or benign arrhythmias, which include patients with an increase in frequency of PVCs, was 1.6%. Although most proarrhythmic events occurred during the first week of therapy, late events also were seen and the CAST study (see above) suggests that an increased risk is present throughout treatment.

In the 474 patient U.S. multicenter trial in patients with symptomatic SVT, 1.9% (9/474) of these patients experienced ventricular tachycardia (VT) or ventricular fibrillation (VF) during the study. However, in 4 of the 9 patients, the ventricular tachycardia was of atrial origin. Six of the nine patients that developed ventricular arrhythmias did so within 14 days of onset of therapy. About 2.3% (11/474) of all patients had a recurrence of SVT during the study which could have been a change in the patients' arrhythmia behavior or could represent a proarrhythmic event. Case reports in patients treated with RYTHMOL for atrial fibrillation/flutter have included increased PVCs, VT, VF, and death.

Nonallergic Bronchospasm (e.g., chronic bronchitis, emphysema): PATIENTS WITH BRONCHOPASTIC DISEASE SHOULD, IN GENERAL, NOT RECEIVE PROPAFENONE or other agents with beta-adrenergic-blocking activity.

Congestive Heart Failure: During treatment with oral propafenone in patients with depressed baseline function (mean EF=33.5%), no significant decreases in ejection fraction were seen. In clinical trial experience, new or worsened CHF has been reported in 3.7% of patients with ventricular arrhythmia, of those 0.9% were considered probably or definitely related to RYTHMOL. Of the patients with congestive heart failure probably related to propafenone, 80% had preexisting heart failure and 85% had coronary artery disease. CHF attributable to RYTHMOL developed rarely (<0.2%) in ventricular arrhythmia patients who had no previous history of CHF. CHF occurred in 1.9% of patients studied with PAF or PSVT.

As RYTHMOL exerts both beta blockade and a (dose-related) negative inotropic effect on cardiac muscle, patients with congestive heart failure should be fully compensated before receiving RYTHMOL. If congestive heart failure worsens, RYTHMOL should be discontinued (unless congestive heart failure is due to the cardiac arrhythmia) and, if indicated, restarted at a lower dosage only after adequate cardiac compensation has been established.

Conduction Disturbances: RYTHMOL slows atrioventricular conduction and also causes first degree AV block. Average PR interval prolongation and increases in QRS duration are closely correlated with dosage increases and concomitant increases in propafenone plasma concentrations. The incidence of first degree, second degree, and third degree AV block observed in 2,127 patients was 2.5%, 0.6%, and 0.2%, respectively. Development of second or third degree AV block requires a reduction in dosage or discontinuation of RYTHMOL. Bundle branch block (1.2%) and intraventricular conduction delay (1.1%) have been reported in patients receiving propafenone. Bradycardia has also been reported (1.5%). Experience in patients with sick sinus node syndrome is limited and these patients should not be treated with propafenone.

Effects on Pacemaker Threshold: RYTHMOL may alter both pacing and sensing thresholds of artificial pacemakers. Pacemakers should be monitored and programmed accordingly during therapy.

Hematologic Disturbances: Agranulocytosis (fever, chills, weakness, and neutropenia) has been reported in patients receiving propafenone. Generally, the agranulocytosis occurred within the first two months of propafenone therapy and upon discontinuation of therapy, the white count usually normalized by 14 days. Unexplained fever and/or decrease in white cell count, particularly during the initial three months of therapy, warrant consideration of possible agranulocytosis/granulocytopenia. Patients should be instructed to promptly report the development of any signs of infection such as fever, sore throat, or chills.

PRECAUTIONS

Hepatic Dysfunction: Propafenone is highly metabolized by the liver and should, therefore, be administered cautiously to patients with impaired hepatic function. Severe liver dysfunction increases the bioavailability of propafenone to approximately 70% compared to 3–40% for patients with normal liver function. In eight patients with moderate to severe liver disease, the mean half-life was approximately 9 hours. As a result, the dose of propafenone given to patients with impaired hepatic function should be approximately 20–30% of the dose given to patients with normal hepatic function (see DOSAGE AND ADMINISTRATION). Careful monitoring for excessive pharmacological effects (see OVERDOSE) should be carried out.

Renal Dysfunction: A considerable percentage of propafenone metabolites (18.5%-38% of the dose/48 hours) are excreted in the urine.

Until further data are available, RYTHMOL (propafenone HCl) should be administered cautiously to patients with impaired renal function. These patients should be carefully monitored for signs of overdosage (see OVERDOSAGE).

Elevated ANA Titers: Positive ANA titers have been reported in patients receiving propafenone. They have been reversible upon cessation of treatment and may disappear even in the face of continued propafenone therapy. These laboratory findings were usually not associated with clinical symptoms, but there is one published case of drug-induced lupus erythematosis (positive rechallenge); if resolved completely upon discontinuation of therapy. Patients who develop an abnormal ANA test should be carefully evaluated and, if persistent or worsening elevation of ANA titers is detected, consideration should be given to discontinuing therapy.

Impaired Spermatogenesis: Reversible disorders of spermatogenesis have been demonstrated in monkeys, dogs and rabbits after high dose intravenous administration. Evaluation of the effects of short-term propafenone administration on spermatogenesis in 11 normal subjects suggests that propafenone produced a reversible, short-term drop (within normal range) in sperm count. Subsequent evaluations in 11 patients receiving propafenone chronically have suggested no effect of propafenone on sperm count.

Neuromuscular Dysfunction: Exacerbation of myasthenia gravis has been reported during propafenone therapy.

Drug interactions:

Quinidine: Small doses of quinidine completely inhibit the hydroxylation metabolic pathway, making all patients, in effect, slow metabolizers (see CLINCAL PHARMACOLOGY). There is, as yet, too little information to recommend concomitant use of propafenone and quinidine.

Local Anesthetics: Concomitant use of local anesthetics (i.e., during pacemaker implantations, surgery, or dental use) may increase the risks of central nervous system side effects.

Digitalis: RYTHMOL (propafenone hydrochloride) produces dose-related increases in serum digoxin levels ranging from about 35% at 450 mg/day to 85% at 900 mg/day of propafenone without affecting digoxin renal clearance. These elevations of digoxin levels were maintained for up to 16 months during concomitant administration. Plasma digoxin levels were maintained for up to 16 months during concomitant administration. Plasma digoxin levels of patients on concomitant therapy should be measured, and digoxin dosage should ordinarily be reduced when propafenone is started, especially if a relatively large digoxin dose is used or if plasma concentrations are relatively high.

Beta-Antagonists: In a study involving healthy subjects, concomitant administration of propafenone and propranolol has resulted in substantial increases in propranolol plasma concentration and elimination half-life with no change in propafenone plasma levels from control values. Similar observations have been reported with metoprolol. Propafenone appears to inhibit the hydroxylation pathway for the two beta-antagonists (just as quinidine inhibits propafenone metabolism). Increased plasma concentrations of metoprolol could overcome its relative cardioselectivity. In propafenone clinical trials, patients who were receiving beta-blockers concurrently did not experience an increased incidence of side effects. While the therapeutic range for beta-blockers is wide, a reduction in dosage may be necessary during concomitant administration with propafenone.

Warfarin: In a study of eight healthy subjects receiving propafenone and warfarin concomitantly, mean steady-state warfarin plasma concentrations increased 39% with a corresponding increase in prothrombin times of approximately 25%. It is therefore recommended that prothrombin times be routinely monitored and the dose of warfarin be adjusted if necessary.

Cimetidine: Concomitant administration of propafenone and cimetidine in 12 healthy subjects resulted in a 20% increase in steady-state plasma concentrations of propafenone with no detectable changes in electrocardiographic parameters beyond that measured on propafenone alone.

Desipramine: Concomitant administration of propafenone and desipramine may result in elevated serum desipramine levels. Both desipramine, a tricyclic antidepressant, and propafenone are cleared by oxidative pathways of demethylation and hydroxylation carried out by the hepatic P-450 cytochrome.

Cyclosporin: Propafenone therapy may increase levels of cyclosporin.

Theophylline: Propafenone may increase theophylline concentration during concomitant therapy with the development of theophylline toxicity.

Rifampin: Rifampin may accelerate the metabolism and decrease the plasma levels and antiarrhythmic efficacy of propafenone.

Adverse Reactions Reported for ≥1% of Ventricular Arrhythmia Patients N=2127

	Incidence by Total Daily Dose			Total Incidence	% of Pts. Who Discont.
	450 mg	600 mg	≥900 mg		
	(N = 1430)	(N = 1337)	(N = 1333)	(N = 2127)	
Dizziness	4%	7%	11%	13%	2.4%
Nausea and/or Vomiting	2%	6%	9%	11%	3.4%
Unusual Taste	3%	5%	6%	9%	0.7%
Constipation	2%	4%	5%	7%	0.5%
Fatigue	2%	3%	4%	6%	1.0%
Dyspnea	2%	2%	4%	5%	1.6%
Proarrhythmia	2%	2%	3%	5%	4.7%
Angina	2%	2%	3%	5%	0.5%
Headache(s)	2%	3%	3%	5%	1.0%
Blurred Vision	1%	2%	3%	4%	0.8%
CHF	1%	2%	3%	4%	1.4%
Ventricular Tachycardia	1%	2%	3%	3%	1.2%
Dyspepsia	1%	2%	3%	3%	0.9%
Palpitations	1%	2%	3%	3%	0.5%
Rash	1%	1%	2%	3%	0.8%
AV Block, First Degree	1%	1%	2%	3%	0.3%
Diarrhea	1%	2%	2%	3%	0.6%
Weakness	1%	2%	2%	2%	0.7%
Dry Mouth	1%	1%	1%	2%	0.2%
Syncope/Near Syncope	1%	1%	1%	2%	0.7%
QRS Duration, Increased	1%	1%	2%	2%	0.5%
Chest Pain	1%	1%	1%	2%	0.2%
Anorexia	1%	1%	2%	2%	0.4%
Abdominal Pain, Cramps	1%	1%	1%	2%	0.4%
Ataxia	0%	1%	2%	2%	0.2%
Insomnia	0%	1%	1%	2%	0.3%
Premature Ventricular Contraction(s)	1%	1%	1%	2%	0.1%
Bradycardia	1%	1%	1%	2%	0.5%
Anxiety	1%	1%	1%	2%	0.6%
Edema	1%	0%	1%	1%	0.2%
Tremor(s)	0%	1%	1%	1%	0.3%
Diaphoresis	1%	0%	1%	1%	0.3%
Bundle Branch Block	0%	1%	1%	1%	0.5%
Drowsiness	1%	1%	1%	1%	0.2%
Atrial Fibrillation	1%	1%	1%	1%	0.4%
Flatulence	0%	1%	1%	1%	0.1%
Hypotension	0%	1%	1%	1%	0.4%
Intraventricular Conduction Delay	0%	1%	1%	1%	0.1%
Pain, Joints	0%	0%	1%	1%	0.1%

Other: Limited experience with propafenone combined with calcium antagonists and diuretics has been reported without evidence of clinically significant adverse reactions.

Carcinogenesis, Mutagenesis, Impairment of Fertility: Lifetime maximally tolerated oral dose studies in mice (up to 360 mg/kg/day) and rats (up to 270 mg/kg/day) provided no evidence of a carcinogenic potential for propafenone. RYTHMOL was not mutagenic when assayed for genotoxicity in 1) mouse Dominant Lethal test, 2) rat bone marrow Chromosome Analysis, 3) Chinese hamster bone marrow and spermatogonia chromosome analysis, 4) Chinese hamster micronucleus test, and 5) Ames bacterial test.

Propafenone administered intravenously to rabbits, dogs, and monkeys has been shown to decrease spermatogenesis. These effects were reversible, were not found following oral dosing of propafenone, were seen only at lethal or sublethal dose levels and were not seen in rats treated either orally or intravenously (see PRECAUTIONS, Impaired Spermatogenesis). Propafenone did not affect fertility rates when administered orally to male and female rats at doses up to 270 mg/kg/day or when administered orally or intravenously to male rabbits at doses of 120 mg/kg/day or 3.5 mg/kg/day, respectively. On a body weight basis, the above noted oral doses in rat and rabbit are 18 times and 8 times, respectively, the maximum recommended daily human dose of 900 mg (based on 60 kg human body weight).

Pregnancy-Teratogenic Effects:
Pregnancy Category C:
Propafenone has been shown to be embryotoxic in rabbits and rats when given in doses 10 and 40 times, respectively, the maximum recommended human dose. No teratogenic potential was apparent in either species. There are no adequate and well-controlled studies in pregnant women. Propafenone should be used during pregnancy only if the potential benefit justifies the potential risk to the fetus.

Pregnancy-Nonteratogenic Effects: In a perinatal and postnatal study in rats, propafenone, at dose levels of 6 or more times the maximum recommended human dose, produced dose dependent increses in maternal and neonatal mortality, decreased maternal and pup body weight gain and reduced neonatal physiological development.

Labor and Delivery: It is not known whether the use of propafenone during labor or delivery has immediate or delayed adverse effects on the fetus, or whether it prolongs the duration of labor or increases the need for forceps delivery or other obstetrical intervention.

Nursing Mothers: It is not known whether this drug is excreted in human milk. Because many drugs are excreted in human milk and because of the potential for serious adverse reactions in nursing infants from RYTHMOL, a decision should be made whether to discontinue nursing or to discontinue the drug, taking into account the importance of the drug to the mother.

Pediatric Use: The safety and effectiveness of RYTHMOL in pediatric patients have not been established.

Geriatric Use: There does not appear to be any age-related differences in adverse reaction rates in the most commonly reported adverse reactions. Because of the possible increased risk of impaired hepatic or renal function in this age group, RYTHMOL should be used with caution. The effective dose may be lower in these patients.

Animal Toxicology: Renal changes have been observed in the rat following 6 months of oral administration of propafenone at doses of 180 and 360 mg/kg/day (12–24 times the maximum recommended human dose) but not 90 mg/kg/day. Both inflammatory and non-inflammatory changes in the renal tubules with accompanying interstitial nephritis were observed. These lesions were reversible in that they were not found in rats treated at these dosage levels and allowed to recover for 6 weeks. Fatty degenerative changes of the liver were found in rats following chronic administration of propafenone at dose levels 19 times the maximum recommended human dose.

ADVERSE REACTIONS

Adverse reactions associated with RYTHMOL occur most frequently in the gastrointestinal, cardiovascular, and central nervous systems. About 20% of patients treated with RYTHMOL have discontinued treatment because of adverse reactions.

Adverse reactions reported for > 1.5% of 474 SVT patients who received propafenone in U.S. clinical trials are presented in the following table by incidence and percent discontinuation, reported to the nearest percent.

Adverse Reactions Reported for > 1.5% of SVT Patients

	Incidence (N=480)	% of Pts. who Discontinued
Unusual taste	14%	1.3%
Nausea and/or Vomiting	11%	2.9%
Dizziness	9%	1.7%
Constipation	8%	0.2%
Headache	6%	0.8%
Fatigue	6%	1.5%
Blurred Vision	3%	0.6%
Weakness	3%	1.3%
Dyspnea	2%	1.0%
Wide Complex Tachycardia	2%	1.9%
CHF	2%	0.6%
Bradycardia	2%	0.2%
Palpitations	2%	0.2%
Tremor	2%	0.4%
Anorexia	2%	0.2%
Diarrhea	2%	0.4%
Ataxia	2%	0.0%

Results of controlled trials in ventricular arrhythmia patients comparing adverse reaction rates on propafenone and placebo, and on propafenone and quinidine are shown in the following table. Adverse reactions reported in ≥ 1% of the patients receiving propafenone are shown, unless they were more frequent on placebo than propafenone. The most common events were unusual taste, dizziness, first degree AV block, intraventricular conduction delay, nausea and/or vomiting, and constipation. Headache was relatively common also, but was not increased compared to placebo.

Continued on next page

Rythmol—Cont.

Adverse Reactions Reported for ≥1% of Ventricular Arrhythmia Patients

	Prop./Placebo Trials		Prop./Quinidine Trials	
	Prop.	Placebo	Prop.	Quinidine
	(N=247)	(N=111)	(N=53)	(N=52)
Unusual Taste	7%	1%	23%	0%
Dizziness	7%	5%	15%	10%
First Degree AV Block	5%	1%	2%	0%
Headache(s)	5%	5%	2%	8%
Constipation	4%	0%	6%	2%
Intraventricular Conduction Delay	4%	0%	-	-
Nausea and/or Vomiting	3%	1%	6%	15%
Fatigue	-	-	4%	2%
Palpitations	2%	1%	-	-
Blurred Vision	2%	1%	6%	2%
Dry Mouth	2%	1%	6%	6%
Dyspnea	2%	3%	4%	0%
Abdominal Pain/Cramps	-	-	2%	8%
Dyspepsia	-	-	2%	8%
CHF	-	-	2%	0%
Fever	-	-	2%	10%
Tinnitus	-	-	2%	2%
Vision, Abnormal	-	-	2%	2%
Esophagitis	-	-	2%	0%
Gastroenteritis	-	-	2%	0%
Anxiety	2%	2%	-	-
Anorexia	2%	1%	-	2%
Proarrhythmia	1%	0%	2%	0%
Flatulence	1%	0%	2%	0%
Angina	1%	0%	2%	4%
Second Degree AV Block	1%	0%	-	-
Bundle Branch Block	1%	0%	2%	2%
Loss of Balance	1%	0%	-	-
Diarrhea	1%	1%	6%	39%

Adverse reactions reported for ≥ 1% of 2,127 ventricular arrhythmia patients who received propafenone in U.S. clinical trials are presented in the following table by propafenone daily dose. The most common adverse reactions in controlled clinical trials appeared dose related (but note that most patients spent more time at the larger doses), especially dizziness, nausea and/or vomiting, unusual taste, constipation, and blurred vision. Some less common reactions may also have been dose related such as first degree AV block, congestive heart failure, dyspepsia, and weakness. The principal causes of discontinuation were the most common events and are shown in the table.

[See table at top of previous page]

In addition, the following adverse reactions were reported less frequently than 1% either in clinical trials or in marketing experience (*adverse events for marketing experience are given in italics*). Causality and relationship to propafenone therapy cannot necessarily be judged from these events.

Cardiovascular System: Atrial flutter, AV dissociation, cardiac arrest, flushing, hot flashes, sick sinus syndrome, sinus pause or arrest, supraventricular tachycardia.

Nervous System: Abnormal dreams, abnormal speech, abnormal vision, *apnea*, *coma*, confusion, depression, memory loss, numbness paresthesias, psychosis/mania, seizures (0.3%), tinnitus, unusual smell sensation, vertigo.

Gastrointestinal: A number of patients with liver abnormalities associated with propafenone therapy have been reported in foreign post-marketing experience. Some appeared due to hepatocellular injury, some were cholestatic and some showed a mixed picture. Some of these reports were simply discovered through clinical chemistries, others because of clinical symptoms including fulminant hepatitis and death. One case was rechallenged with a positive outcome. Cholestasis (0.1%), elevated liver enzymes (alkaline phophatase, serum transaminases) (0.2%), gastroenteritis, hepatitis (0.03%).

Hematologic: Agranulocytosis, anemia, bruising, granulocytopenia, *increased bleeding time*, leukopenia, purpura, thrombocytopenia.

Other: Alopecia, eye irritation, *hyponatremia/inappropriate ADH secretion*, impotence, increased glucose, kidney failure, positive ANA (0.7%), *lupus erythematosis*, muscle cramps, muscle weakness, nephrotic syndrome, pain, pruritus.

OVERDOSAGE

The symptoms of overdosage, which are usually most severe within 3 hours of ingestion, may include hypotension, somnolence, bradycardia, intra-atrial and intraventricular conduction disturbances, and rarely convulsions and high grade ventricular arrhythmias. Defibrillation as well as infusion of dopamine and isoproterenol have been effective in controlling rhythm and blood pressure. Convulsions have been alleviated with intravenous diazepam. General supportive measures such as mechanical respiratory assistance and external cardiac massage may be necessary.

DOSAGE AND ADMINISTRATION

The dose of RYTHMOL (propafenone HCl) must be individually titrated on the basis of response and tolerance. It is recommended that therapy be initiated with 150 mg propafenone given every eight hours (450 mg/day). Dosage may be increased at a minimum of 3 to 4 day intervals to 225 mg every 8 hours (675 mg/day) and, if necessary, to 300 mg every 8 hours (900 mg/day). The usefulness and safety of dosages exceeding 900 mg per day have not been established. In those patients in whom significant widening of the QRS complex or second or third degree AV block occurs, dose reduction should be considered.

As with other antiarrhythmic agents, in the elderly or in patients with marked previous myocardial damage, the dose of RYTHMOL should be increased more gradually during the initial phase of treatment.

HOW SUPPLIED

RYTHMOL (propafenone HCl) tablets are supplied as scored, round, film-coated tablets containing either 150 mg, 225 mg or 300 mg of propafenone hydrochloride and embossed with 150, 225 or 300 and an arched triangle on the same side.

150 mg (white)– Bottle of 100-NDC#0044-5022-02
Hospital Unit Dose (100 tablets-strips of 10)-NDC#0044-5022-10

225 mg (white)– Bottle of 100-NDC#0044-5024-02
Hospital Unit Dose (100 tablets-strips of 10)-NDC#0044-5024-10

300 mg (white)– Bottle of 100-NDC#0044-5023-02
Hospital Unit Dose (100 tablets-strips of 10)-NDC#0044-5023-10

Storage: Store at controlled room temperature 15°–30°C (59°–86°F). Dispense in a tight, light-resistant container as defined in the U.S.P.

Revised: January 1998

Knoll Laboratories
A Division of
Knoll Pharmaceutical Company
3000 Continental Drive- North
Mount Olive, NJ 07828-1234
BASF Pharma 0909001-5

Shown in Product Identification Guide, page 319

VICODIN HP® Ⓒ℞

[*vīkō-dīn*]

(hydrocodone bitartrate and acetaminophen tablets, USP)
10 mg/660 mg
Rx only

DESCRIPTION

Hydrocodone bitartrate and acetaminophen is supplied in tablet form for oral administration.

Hydrocodone bitartrate is an opioid analgesic and antitussive and occurs as fine, white crystals or as a crystalline powder. It is affected by light. The chemical name is 4,5α-epoxy-3-methoxy-17-methylmorphinan-6-one tartrate (1:1) hydrate (2:5). It has the following structural formula:

[See chemical structure at top of next column]

$C_{18}H_{21}NO_3 \cdot C_4H_6O_6 \cdot 2^1/_2H_2O)$ M.W.=494.50

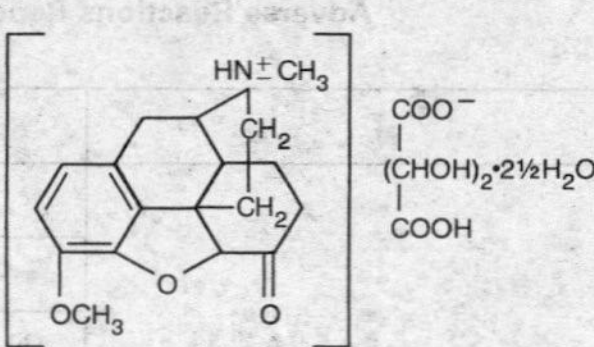

Acetaminophen, 4'-hydroxyacetanilide, a slightly bitter, white, odorless, crystalline powder, is a non-opiate, non-salicylate analgesic and antipyretic. It has the following structural formula:

$C_8H_9NO_2$ M.W.=151.17

Each VICODIN HP tablet contains:

Hydrocodone Bitartrate	10 mg
Acetaminophen	660 mg

In addition each tablet contains the following inactive ingredients: colloidal silicon dioxide, croscarmellose sodium, magnesium stearate, microcrystalline cellulose, povidone, pregelatinized starch, and stearic acid.

CLINICAL PHARMACOLOGY

Hydrocodone is a semisynthetic narcotic analgesic and antitussive with multiple actions qualitatively similar to those of codeine. Most of these involve the central nervous system and smooth muscle. The precise mechanism of action of hydrocodone and other opiates is not known, although it is believed to relate to the existance of opiate receptors in the central nervous system. In addition to analgesia, narcotics may produce drowsiness, changes in mood and mental clouding.

The analgesic action of acetaminophen involves peripheral influences, but the specific mechanism is as yet undetermined. Antipyretic activity is mediated through hypothalamic heat regulating centers. Acetaminophen inhibits prostaglandin synthetase. Therapeutic doses of acetaminophen have negligible effects on the cardiovascular or respiratory systems; however, toxic doses may cause circulatory failure and rapid, shallow breathing.

Pharmacokinetics: The behavior of the individual components is described below.

Hydrocodone: Following a 10mg oral dose of hydrocodone administered to five adult male subjects, the mean peak concentration was 23.6 ± 5.2ng/mL. Maximum serum levels were achieved at 1.3 ± 0.3 hours and the half-life was determined to be 3.8 ± 0.3 hours. Hydrocodone exhibits a complex pattern of metabolism including O-demethylation, N-demethylation and 6-keto reduction to the corresponding 6-α- and 6-β- hydroxy-metabolites. See OVERDOSAGE for toxicity information.

Acetaminophen: Acetaminophen is rapidly absorbed from the gastrointestinal tract and is distributed throughout most body tissues. The plasma half-life is 1.25 to 3 hours, but may be increased by liver damage and following overdosage. Elimination of acetaminophen is principally by liver metabolism (conjugation) and subsequent renal excretion of metabolites. Approximately 85% of an oral dose appears in the urine within 24 hours of adminstration, most as the glucuronide conjugate, with small amounts of other conjugates and unchanged drug. See OVERDOSAGE for toxicity information.

INDICATIONS AND USAGE

VICODIN HP® tablets are indicated for the relief of moderate to moderately severe pain.

CONTRAINDICATIONS

This product should not be administered to patients who have previously exhibited hypersensitivity to hydrocodone or acetaminophen.

Patients known to be hypersensitive to other opioids may exhibit cross-sensitivity to hydrocodone.

WARNINGS

Respiratory Depression: At high doses or in sensitive patients, hydrocodone may produce dose-related respiratory depression by acting directly on the brain stem respiratory center. Hydrocodone also affects the center that controls respiratory rhythm, and may produce irregular and periodic breathing.

Head Injury and Increased Intracranial Pressure: The respiratory depressant effects of narcotics and their capacity to elevate cerebrospinal fluid pressure may be markedly exaggerated in the presence of head injury, other intracranial lesions or a preexisting increase in intracranial pressure. Furthermore, narcotics produce adverse reactions which may obscure the clinical course of patients with head injuries.

Acute Abdominal Conditions: The administration of narcotics may obscure the diagnosis or clinical course of patients with acute abdominal conditions.

PRECAUTIONS

General:

Special Risk Patients: As with any narcotic analgesic agent, VICODIN HP Tablets should be used with caution in elderly or debilitated patients, and those with severe impairment of hepatic or renal function, hypothyroidism, Addison's disease, prostatic hypertrophy or urethral stricture. The usual precautions should be observed and the possibility of respiratory depression should be kept in mind.

Cough Reflex: Hydrocodone suppresses the cough reflex; as with all narcotics, caution should be exercised when VICODIN HP Tablets are used postoperatively and in patients with pulmonary disease.

Information for Patients: Hydrocodone, like all narcotics, may impair the mental and/or physical abilities required for the performance of potentially hazardous tasks such as driving a car or operating machinery; patients should be cautioned accordingly.

Alcohol and other CNS depressants may produce an additive CNS depression, when taken with this combination product, and should be avoided.

Hydrocodone may be habit forming. Patients should take the drug only for as long as it is prescribed, in the amounts prescribed, and no more frequently than prescribed.

Laboratory Tests: In patients with severe hepatic or renal disease, effects of therapy should be monitored with serial liver and/or renal function tests.

Drug Interactions: Patients receiving narcotics, antihistamines, antipsychotics, antianxiety agents, or other CNS depressants (including alcohol) concomitantly with VICODIN HP™ Tablets may exhibit an additive CNS depression. When combined therapy is contemplated, the dose of one or both agents should be reduced.

The use of MAO inhibitors or tricyclic antidepressants with hydrocodone preparations may increase the effect of either the antidepressant or hydrocodone.

Drug/Laboratory Test Interactions: Acetaminophen may produce false-positive test results for urinary 5-hydroxyindoleacetic acid.

Carcinogenesis, Mutagenesis, Impairment of Fertility: No adequate studies have been conducted in animals to determine whether hydrocodone or acetaminophen have a potential for carcinogenesis, mutagenesis, or impairment of fertility.

Pregnancy:

Teratogenic Effects: Pregnancy Category C. There are no adequate and well-controlled studies in pregnant women. VICODIN HP Tablets should be used during pregnancy only if the potential benefit justifies the potential risk to the fetus.

Nonteratogenic Effects: Babies born to mothers who have been taking opioids regularly prior to delivery will be physically dependent. The withdrawal signs include irritability and excessive crying, tremors, hyperactive reflexes, increased respiratory rate, increased stools, sneezing, yawning, vomiting, and fever. The intensity of the syndrome does not always correlate with the duration of maternal opioid use or dose. There is no consensus on the best method of managing withdrawal.

Labor and Delivery: As with all narcotics, administration of VICODIN HP® Tablets to the mother shortly before delivery may result in some degree of respiratory depression in the newborn, especially if higher doses are used.

Nursing Mothers: Acetaminophen is excreted in breast milk in small amounts, but the significance of its effects on nursing infants is not known. It is not known whether hydrocodone is excreted in human milk. Because many drugs are excreted in human milk and because of the potential for serious adverse reactions in nursing infants from hydrocodone and acetaminophen, a decision should be made whether to discontinue nursing or to discontinue the drug, taking into account the importance of the drug to the mother.

Pediatric Use: Safety and effectiveness in the pediatric population have not been established.

Geriatric Use: Clinical studies of Vicodin HP did not include sufficient numbers of subjects aged 65 and over to determine whether they respond differently from younger subjects. Other reported clinical experience has not identified differences in responses between the elderly and younger patients. In general, dose selection for an elderly patient should be cautious, usually starting at the low end of the dosing range, reflecting the greater frequency of decreased hepatic, renal, or cardiac function, and of concomitant disease or other drug therapy.

ADVERSE REACTIONS

The most frequently reported adverse reactions are lightheadedness, dizziness, sedation, nausea and vomiting. These effects seem to be more prominent in ambulatory than in nonambulatory patients, and some of these adverse reactions may be alleviated if the patient lies down.

Other adverse reactions include:

Central Nervous System: Drowsiness, mental clouding, lethargy, impairment of mental and physical performance, anxiety, fear, dysphoria, psychic dependence, mood changes.

Gastrointestinal System: Prolonged administration of VICODIN HP Tablets may produce constipation.

Genitourinary System: Ureteral spasm, spasm of vesical sphincters and urinary retention have been reported with opiates.

Respiratory Depression: Hydrocodone bitartrate may produce dose-related respiratory depression by acting directly on the brain stem respiratory centers (see OVERDOSAGE).

Special Senses: Very rare cases of hearing impairment or loss have been reported in patients predominantly receiving very high doses of hydrocodone/acetaminophen for long periods of time.

Dermatological: Skin rash, pruritus.

The following adverse drug events may be borne in mind as potential effects of acetaminophen: allergic reactions, rash, thrombocytopenia, agranulocytosis.

Potential effects of high dosage are listed in the OVERDOSAGE section.

DRUG ABUSE AND DEPENDENCE

Controlled Substance: VICODIN HP Tablets are classified as a Schedule Ⓒ III controlled substance.

Abuse and Dependence: Psychic dependence, physical dependence, and tolerance may develop upon repeated administration of narcotics; therefore, VICODIN HP Tablets should be prescribed and administered with caution. However, psychic dependence is unlikely to develop when VICODIN HP Tablets are used for a short time for the treatment of pain.

Physical dependence, the condition in which continued administration of the drug is required to prevent the appearance of a withdrawal syndrome, assumes clinically significant proportions only after several weeks of continued narcotic use, although some mild degree of physical dependence may develop after a few days of narcotic therapy. Tolerance, in which increasingly large doses are required in order to produce the same degree of analgesia, is manifested initially by a shortened duration of analgesic effect, and subsequently by decreases in the intensity of analgesia. The rate of development of tolerance varies among patients.

OVERDOSAGE

Following an acute overdosage, toxicity may result from hydrocodone or acetaminophen.

Signs and Symptoms:

Hydrocodone: Serious overdose with hydrocodone is characterized by respiratory depression (a decrease in respiratory rate and/or tidal volume, Cheyne-Stokes respiration, cyanosis), extreme somnolence progressing to stupor or coma, skeletal muscle flaccidity, cold and clammy skin, and sometimes bradycardia and hypotension. In severe overdosage, apnea, circulatory collapse, cardiac arrest and death may occur.

Acetaminophen: In acetaminophen overdosage: dose-dependent, potentially fatal hepatic necrosis is the most serious adverse effect. Renal tubular necrosis, hypoglycemic coma, and thrombocytopenia may also occur.

Early symptoms following a potentially hepatotoxic overdose may include: nausea, vomiting, diaphoresis and general malaise. Clinical and laboratory evidence of hepatic toxicity may not be apparent until 48 to 72 hours post-ingestion.

In adults, hepatic toxicity has rarely been reported with acute overdoses of less than 10 grams, or fatalities with less than 15 grams.

Treatment: A single or multiple overdose with hydrocodone and acetaminophen is a potentially lethal polydrug overdose, and consultation with a regional poison control center is recommended.

Immediate treatment includes support of cardiorespiratory function and measures to reduce drug absorption. Vomiting should be induced mechanically, or with syrup of ipecac, if the patient is alert (adequate pharyngeal and laryngeal reflexes). Oral activated charcoal (1 g/kg) should follow gastric emptying. The first dose should be accompanied by an appropriate cathartic. If repeated doses are used, the cathartic might be included with alternate doses as required. Hypotension is usually hypovolemic and should respond to fluids. Vasopressors and other supportive measures should be employed as indicated. A cuffed endo-tracheal tube should be inserted before gastric lavage of the unconscious patient and, when necessary, to provide assisted respiration.

Meticulous attention should be given to maintaining adequate pulmonary ventilation. In severe cases of intoxication, peritoneal dialysis, or preferably hemodialysis may be considered. If hypoprothrombinemia occurs due to acetaminophen overdose, vitamin K should be administered intravenously.

Naloxone, a narcotic antagonist, can reverse respiratory depression and coma associated with opioid overdose. Naloxone hydrochloride 0.4 mg to 2 mg is given parenterally. Since the duration of action of hydrocodone may exceed that of the naloxone, the patient should be kept under continuous surveillance and repeated doses of the antagonist should be administered as needed to maintain adequate respiration. A narcotic antagonist should not be administered in the absence of clinically significant respiratory or cardiovascular depression.

If the dose of acetaminophen may have exceeded 140 mg/kg, acetylcysteine should be administered as early as possible. Serum acetaminophen levels should be obtained, since levels four or more hours following ingestion help predict acetaminophen toxicity. Do not await acetaminophen assay results before initiating treatment. Hepatic enzymes should be obtained initially, and repeated at 24-hour intervals.

Methemoglobinemia over 30% should be treated with methylene blue by slow intravenous administration.

The toxic dose for adults for acetaminophen is 10 g.

DOSAGE AND ADMINISTRATION

Dosage should be adjusted according to severity of pain and the response of the patient. However, it should be kept in mind that tolerance to hydrocodone can develop with continued use and that the incidence of untoward effects is dose related.

The usual adult dosage is one tablet every four to six hours as needed for pain. The total daily dosage should not exceed 6 tablets.

HOW SUPPLIED

VICODIN HP® (hydrocodone bitartrate and acetaminophen, 10 mg/660 mg) is supplied as a white, oval-shaped, tablet bisected on one side and debossed with "VICODIN HP" on the other side.

Bottles of 100-NDC #0044-0725-02

Bottles of 500-NDC #0044-0725-03

Storage: Store at 25°C (77°F); excursions permitted to 15°–30°C (59°–86°F). [See USP Controlled Room Temperature].

Dispense in a tight, light-resistant container as defined in the USP.

A Schedule Ⓒ III Narcotic.

VICODIN HP is a registered trademark of Knoll Pharmaceutical Company

Revised: May 2000

Knoll Laboratories
A Division of **BASF** Pharma
Knoll Pharmaceutical Company
Mount Olive, New Jersey 07828 0900005-4

Shown in Product Identification Guide, page 319

VICODIN® Ⓒ III ℞

(hydrocodone bitartrate and acetaminophen tablets, USP)
5 mg/500 mg
Rx only

DESCRIPTION

Hydrocodone bitartrate and acetaminophen is supplied in tablet form for oral administration.

Hydrocodone bitartrate is an opioid analgesic and antitussive and occurs as fine, white crystals or as a crystalline powder. It is affected by light. The chemical name is: 4,5α-epoxy-3-methoxy-17-methylmorphinan-6-one tartrate (1:1) hydrate (2:5). It has the following structural formula:

$C_{18}H_{21}NO_3 C_4H_6O_6 \cdot 2^1/_2 H_2O$ M.W. 494.50

Acetaminophen, 4'-hydroxyacetanilide, a slightly bitter, white, odorless, crystalline powder, is a non-opiate, non-salicylate analgesic and antipyretic. It has the following structural formula:

$C_8H_9NO_2$ M.W. 151.16

Each VICODIN® tablet contains:

Hydrocodone Bitartrate 5 mg
Acetaminophen 500 mg

In addition each tablet contains the following inactive ingredients: colloidal silicon dioxide, starch, croscarmellose sodium, dibasic calcium phosphate, magnesium stearate, microcrystalline cellulose, povidone, and stearic acid.

CLINICAL PHARMACOLOGY

Hydrocodone is a semisynthetic narcotic analgesic and antitussive with multiple actions qualitatively similar to those of codeine. Most of these involve the central nervous system and smooth muscle. The precise mechanism of action of hydrocodone and other opiates is not known, although it is believed to relate to the existence of opiate receptors in the central nervous system. In addition to analgesia, narcotics may produce drowsiness, changes in mood and mental clouding.

The analgesic action of acetaminophen involves peripheral influences, but the specific mechanism is as yet undetermined. Antipyretic activity is mediated through hypothalmic heat regulating centers. Acetaminophen inhibits prostaglandin synthetase. Therapeutic doses of acetaminophen have negligible effects on the cardiovascular or respiratory systems; however, toxic doses may cause circulatory failure and rapid, shallow breathing.

Pharmacokinetics: The behavior of the individual components is described below.

Hydrocodone: Following a 10mg oral dose of hydrocodone administered to five adult male subjects, the mean peak concentration was 23.6 ± 5.2ng/mL. Maximum serum levels were achieved at 1.3 ± 0.3 hours and the half-life was determined to be 3.8 ± 0.3 hours. Hydrocodone exhibits a complex pattern of metabolism including O-demethylation, N-

Continued on next page

Vicodin—Cont.

demethylation and 6-keto reduction to the corresponding 6-α- and 6-β-hydroxymetabolites. See OVERDOSAGE for toxicity information.

Acetaminophen: Acetaminophen is rapidly absorbed from the gastrointestinal tract and is distributed throughout most body tissues. The plasma half-life is 1.25 to 3 hours, but may be increased by liver damage and following overdosage. Elimination of acetaminophen is principally by liver metabolism (conjugation) and subsequent renal excretion of metabolites. Approximately 85% of an oral dose appears in the urine within 24 hours of administration, most as the glucuronide conjugate, with small amounts of other conjugates and unchanged drug. See OVERDOSAGE for toxicity information.

INDICATIONS AND USAGE

VICODIN Tablets are indicated for the relief of moderate to moderately severe pain.

CONTRAINDICATIONS

This product should not be administered to patients who have previously exhibited hypersensitivity to hydrocodone or acetaminophen.

Patients known to be hypersensitive to other opioids may exhibit cross-sensitivity to hydrocodone.

WARNINGS

Respiratory Depression: At high doses or in sensitive patients, hydrocodone may produce dose-related respiratory depression by acting directly on the brain stem respiratory center. Hydrocodone also affects the center that controls respiratory rhythm, and may produce irregular and periodic breathing.

Head Injury and Increased Intracranial Pressure: The respiratory depressant effects of narcotics and their capacity to elevate cerebrospinal fluid pressure may be markedly exaggerated in the presence of head injury, other intracranial lesions or a preexisting increase in intracranial pressure. Furthermore, narcotics produce adverse reactions which may obscure the clinical course of patients with head injuries.

Acute Abdominal Conditions: The administration of narcotics may obscure the diagnosis or clinical course of patients with acute abdominal conditions.

PRECAUTIONS

General:

Special Risk Patients: As with any narcotic analgesic agent, VICODIN Tablets should be used with caution in elderly or debilitated patients and those with severe impairment of hepatic or renal function, hypothyroidism, Addison's disease, prostatic hypertrophy or urethral stricture. The usual precautions should be observed and the possibility of respiratory depression should be kept in mind.

Cough Reflex: Hydrocodone suppresses the cough reflex; as with all narcotics, caution should be exercised when VICODIN Tablets are used postoperatively and in patients with pulmonary disease.

Information for Patients: Hydrocodone, like all narcotics, may impair the mental and/or physical abilities required for the performance of potentially hazardous tasks such as driving a car or operating machinery; patients should be cautioned accordingly.

Alcohol and other CNS depressants may produce an additive CNS depression, when taken with this combination product, and should be avoided.

Hydrocodone may be habit forming. Patients should take the drug only for as long as it is prescribed, in the amounts prescribed, and no more frequently than prescribed.

Laboratory Tests: In patients with severe hepatic or renal disease, effects of therapy should be monitored with serial liver and/or renal function tests.

Drug Interactions: Patients receiving other narcotic analgesics, antihistamines, antipsychotics, antianxiety agents, or other CNS depressants (including alcohol) concomitantly with VICODIN Tablets may exhibit an additive CNS depression. When combined therapy is contemplated, the dose of one or both agents should be reduced.

The use of MAO inhibitors or tricyclic antidepressants with hydrocodone preparations may increase the effect of either the antidepressant or hydrocodone.

Drug/Laboratory Test Interactions: Acetaminophen may produce false-positive test results for urinary 5-hydroxyindoleacetic acid.

Carcinogenesis, Mutagenesis, Impairment of Fertility: No adequate studies have been conducted in animals to determine whether hydrocodone or acetaminophen have a potential for carcinogenesis, mutagenesis, or impairment of fertility.

Pregnancy:

Teratogenic Effects: Pregnancy Category C. There are no adequate and well-controlled studies in pregnant women. VICODIN Tablets should be used during pregnancy only if the potential benefit justifies the potential risk to the fetus.

Nonteratogenic Effects: Babies born to mothers who have been taking opioids regularly prior to delivery will be physically dependent. The withdrawal signs include irritability and excessive crying, tremors, hyperactive reflexes, increased respiratory rate, increased stools, sneezing, yawning, vomiting, and fever. The intensity of the syndrome does not always correlate with the duration of maternal opioid use or dose. There is not consensus on the best method of managing withdrawal.

Labor and Delivery: As with all narcotics, administration of VICODIN Tablets to the mother shortly before delivery may result in some degree of respiratory depression in the newborn, especially if higher doses are used.

Nursing Mothers: Acetaminophen is excreted in breast milk in small amounts, but the significance of its effects on nursing infants is not known. It is not known whether hydrocodone is excreted in human milk. Because many drugs are excreted in human milk and because of the potential for serious adverse reactions in nursing infants from hydrocodone and acetaminophen, a decision should be made whether to discontinue nursing or to discontinue the drug, taking into account the importance of the drug to the mother.

Pediatric Use: Safety and effectiveness in the pediatric population have not been established.

Geriatric Use: Clinical studies of VICODIN Tablets did not include sufficient numbers of subjects aged 65 and over to determine whether they respond differently from younger subjects. Other reported clinical experience has not identified differences in responses between the elderly and younger patients. In general, dose selection for an elderly patient should be cautious, usually starting at the low end of the dosing range, reflecting the greater frequency of decreased hepatic, renal, or cardia function, and of concomitant disease or other drug therapy.

ADVERSE REACTIONS

The most frequently reported adverse reactions include lightheadedness, dizziness, sedation, nausea and vomiting. These effects seem to be more prominent in ambulatory than in nonambulatory patients and some of these adverse reactions may be alleviated if the patient lies down.

Other adverse reactions include:

Central Nervous System: Drowsiness, mental clouding, lethargy, impairment of mental and physical performance, anxiety, fear, dysphoria, psychic dependence, mood changes.

Gastrointestinal System: Prolonged administration of VICODIN Tablets may produce constipation.

Genitourinary System: Ureteral spasm, spasm of vesical sphincters and urinary retention have been reported with opiates.

Respiratory Depression: Hydrocodone bitartrate may produce dose-related respiratory depression by acting directly on the brain stem respiratory center. (see OVERDOSAGE).

Special Senses: Very rare cases of hearing impairment or loss have been reported in patients predominantly receiving very high doses of hydrocodone/acetaminophen for long periods of time.

Dermatological: Skin rash, pruritus.

The following adverse drug events may be borne in mind as potential effects of acetaminophen: allergic reactions, rash, thrombocytopenia, agranulocytosis

Potential effects of high dosage are listed in the OVERDOSAGE section.

DRUG ABUSE AND DEPENDENCE

Controlled Substance: VICODIN Tablets are classified as a Schedule CIII **controlled substance.**

Abuse Dependence: Psychic dependence, physical dependence, and tolerance may develop upon repeated administration of narcotics; therefore, VICODIN Tablets should be prescribed and administered with caution. However, psychic dependence is unlikely to develop when VICODIN Tablets are used for a short time for the treatment of pain.

Physical dependence, the condition in which continued administration of the drug is required to prevent the appearance of a withdrawal syndrome, assumes clinically significant proportions only after several weeks of continued narcotic use, although some mild degree of physical dependence may develop after a few days of narcotic therapy. Tolerance, in which increasingly large doses are required in order to produce the same degree of analgesia, is manifested initially by a shortened duration of analgesic effect, and subsequently by decreases in the intensity of analgesia. The rate of development of tolerance varies among patients.

OVERDOSAGE

Following an acute overdosage, toxicity may result from hydrocodone or acetaminophen.

Signs and Symptoms:

Hydrocodone: Serious overdose with hydrocodone is characterized by respiratory depression (a decrease in respiratory rate and/or tidal volume, Cheyne-Stokes respiration, cyanosis), extreme somnolence progressing to stupor or coma, skeletal muscle flaccidity, cold and clammy skin, and sometimes bradycardia and hypotension. In severe overdosage, apnea, circulatory collapse, cardiac arrest and death may occur.

Acetaminophen: In acetaminophen overdosage, dose-dependent, potentially fatal hepatic necrosis is the most serious adverse effect. Renal tubular necrosis, hypoglycemic coma, and thrombocytopenia may also occur.

Early symptoms following a potentially hepatotoxic overdose may include: nausea, vomiting, diaphoresis and general malaise. Clinical and laboratory evidence of hepatic toxicity may not be apparent until 48 to 72 hours post-ingestion.

In adults, hepatic toxicity has rarely been reported with acute overdoses of less than 15 grams.

Treatment:

A single or multiple overdose with hydrocodone and acetaminophen is a potentially lethal polydrug overdose, and consultation with a regional poison control center is recommended.

Immediate treatment includes support of cardiorespiratory function and measures to reduce drug absorption. Vomiting should be induced mechanically, or with syrup of ipecac, if the patient is alert (adequate pharyngeal and laryngeal reflexes). Oral activated charcoal (1 g/kg) should follow gastric emptying. The first dose should be accompanied by an appropriate cathartic. If repeated doses are used, the cathartic might be included with alternate doses as required. Hypotension is usually hypovolemic and should respond to fluids. Vasopressors and other supportive measures should be employed as indicated. A cuffed endo-tracheal tube should be inserted before gastric lavage of the unconscious patient and, when necessary to provide assisted respiration.

Meticulous attention should be given to maintaining adequate pulmonary ventilation. In severe cases of intoxication, peritoneal dialysis, or preferably hemodialysis may be considered. If hypoprothrombinemia occurs due to acetaminophen overdose, vitamin K should be administered intravenously.

Naloxone, a narcotic antagonist, can reverse respiratory depression and coma associated with opioid overdose. Naloxone hydrochloride 0.4 mg to 2 mg is given parenterally. Since the duration of action of hydrocodone may exceed that of the naloxone, the patient should be kept under continuous surveillance and repeated doses of the antagonist should be administered as needed to maintain adequate respiration. A narcotic antagonist should not be administered in the absence of clinically significant respiratory or cardiovascular depression.

If the dose of acetaminophen may have exceeded 140 mg/kg, acetylcysteine should be administered as early as possible. Serum acetaminophen levels should be obtained, since levels four or more hours following ingestion help predict acetaminophen toxicity. Do not await acetaminophen assay results before initiating treatment. Hepatic enzymes should be obtained initially, and repeated at 24-hour intervals.

Methemoglobinemia over 30% should be treated with methylene blue by slow intravenous administration.

The toxic dose for adults for acetaminophen is 10 g.

DOSAGE AND ADMINISTRATION

Dosage should be adjusted according to the severity of the pain and the response of the patient. However, it should be kept in mind that tolerance to hydrocodone can develop with continued use and that the incidence of untoward effects is dose related.

The usual adult dosage is one or two tablets every four to six hours as needed for pain. The total daily dosage should not exceed 8 tablets.

HOW SUPPLIED

VICODIN is supplied as white, capsule-shaped tablets containing 5 mg hydrocodone bitartrate and 500 mg acetaminophen, bisected on one side and debossed with "VICODIN" on the other.

Bottles of 100—NDC #0044-0727-02.

Bottles of 500—NDC #0044-0727-03.

Hospital Unit Dose Package–100 tablets (4×25 tablets)—NDC#0044-0727-41.

Storage: Store at 25°C (77°F); excursions permitted to 15°–30°C (59°–86°F). [See USP Controlled Room Temperature].

Dispense in a tight, light-resistant container as defined in the USP.

A Schedule CIII Narcotic.

VICODIN is a registered trademark of Knoll Pharmaceutical Company

Revised: May 2000

Knoll Laboratories
A Division of Knoll Pharmaceutical Company **BASF** Pharma
Mount Olive, New Jersey 07828

0900010-3

Shown in Product Identification Guide, page 319

VICODIN ES® TABLETS CIII ℞

(hydrocodone bitartrate and acetaminophen tablets, USP)
7.5 mg/750 mg
Rx only

DESCRIPTION

Hydrocodone bitartrate and acetaminophen is supplied in tablet form for oral administration.

Hydrocodone bitartrate is an opioid analgesic and antitussive and occurs as fine, white crystals or as a crystalline powder. It is affected by light. The chemical name is: 4,5α-epoxy-3-methoxyl-17-methylmorphinan-6-one tartrate (1:1) hydrate (2:5). It has the following structural formula:

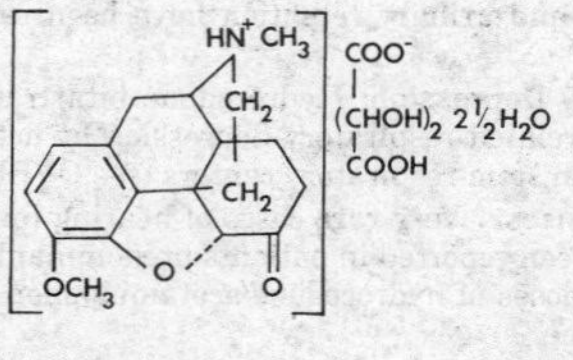

$C_{18}H_{21}NO_3 \cdot C_4H_6O_6 \cdot 2\frac{1}{2}\ H_2O$ M.W. 494.50

Acetaminophen, 4'-hydroxyacetanilide, is a slightly bitter, white, odorless, crystalline powder, is a non-opiate, non-salicylate analgesic and antipyretic. It has the following structural formula:

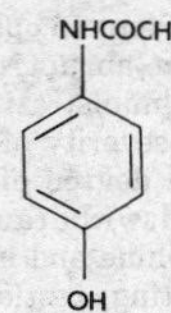

$C_8H_9NO_2$ M.W.151.16

Each VICODIN ES® tablet contains:
Hydrocodone Bitartrate 7.5 mg
Acetaminophen 750 mg

In addition each tablet contains the following inactive ingredients: colloidal silicon dioxide, pregelatinized starch, magnesium stearate, microcrystalline cellulose, povidone, and stearic acid.

CLINICAL PHARMACOLOGY

Hydrocodone is a semisynthetic narcotic analgesic and antitussive with multiple actions qualitatively similar to those of codeine. Most of these involve the central nervous system and smooth muscle. The precise mechanism of action of hydrocodone and other opiates is not known, although it is believed to relate to the existence of opiate receptors in the central nervous system. In addition to analgesia, narcotics may produce drowsiness, changes in mood and mental clouding.

The analgesic action of acetaminophen involves peripheral influences, but the specific mechanism is as yet undetermined. Antipyretic activity is mediated through hypothalmic heat regulating centers. Acetaminophen inhibits prostaglandin synthetase. Therapeutic doses of acetaminophen have negligible effects on the cardiovascular or respiratory systems; however, toxic doses may cause circulatory failure and rapid, shallow breathing.

Pharmacokinetics: The behavior of the individual components is described below.

Hydrocodone: Following a 10mg oral dose of hydrocodone administered to five adult male subjects, the mean peak concentration was 23.6 ± 5.2 ng/mL. Maximum serum levels were achieved at 1.3 ± 0.3 hours and the half-life was determined to be 3.8 ± 0.3 hours. Hydrocodone exhibits a complex pattern of metabolism including O-demethylation. N-demethylation and 6-keto reduction to the corresponding 6-α- and 6-β- hydroxymetabolites. See OVERDOSAGE for toxicity information.

Acetaminophen: Acetaminophen is rapidly absorbed from the gastrointestinal tract and is distributed throughout most body tissues. The plasma half-life is 1.25 to 3 hours, but may be increased by liver damage and following overdosage. Elimination of acetaminophen is principally by liver metabolism (conjugation) and subsequent renal excretion of metabolites. Approximately 85% of an oral dose appears in the urine within 24 hours of administration, most as the glucuronide conjugate, with small amounts of other conjugates and unchanged drug. See OVERDOSAGE for toxicity information.

INDICATIONS AND USAGE

VICODIN ES tablets are indicated for the relief of moderate to moderately severe pain.

CONTRAINDICATIONS

This product should not be administered to patients who have previously exhibited hypersensitivity to hydrocodone or acetaminophen.

Patients known to be hypersensitive to other opioids may exhibit cross-sensitivity to hydrocodone.

WARNINGS

Respiratory Depression: At high doses or in sensitive patients, hydrocodone may produce dose-related respiratory depression by acting directly on the brain stem respiratory center. Hydrocodone also affects the center that controls respiratory rhythm, and may produce irregular and periodic breathing.

Head Injury and Increased Intracranial Pressure: The respiratory depressant effects of narcotics and their capacity to elevate cerebrospinal fluid pressure may be markedly exaggerated in the presence of head injury, other intracranial lesions or a preexisting increase in intracranial pressure. Furthermore, narcotics produce adverse reactions which may obscure the clinical course of patients with head injuries.

Acute Abdominal Conditions: The administration of narcotics may obscure the diagnosis or clinical course of patients with acute abdominal conditions.

PRECAUTIONS

General:

Special Risk Patients: As with any narcotic analgesic agent, VICODIN ES tablets should be used with caution in elderly or debilitated patients and those with severe impairment of hepatic or renal function, hypothyroidism, Addison's disease, prostatic hypertrophy or urethral stricture. The usual precautions should be observed and the possibility of respiratory depression should be kept in mind.

Cough Reflex: Hydrocodone suppresses the cough reflex; as with all narcotics, caution should be exercised when VICODIN ES Tablets are used postoperatively and in patients with pulmonary disease.

Information for Patients: Hydrocodone, like all narcotics, may impair the mental and/or physical abilities required for the performance of potentially hazardous tasks such as driving a car or operating machinery; patients should be cautioned accordingly.

Alcohol and other CNS depressants may produce an additive CNS depression, when taken with this combination product, and should be avoided.

Hydrocodone may be habit forming. Patients should take the drug only for as long as it is prescribed. In the amounts prescribed, and no more frequently than prescribed.

Laboratory Tests: In patients with severe hepatic or renal disease, effects of therapy should be monitored with serial liver and/or renal function tests.

Drug Interactions: Patients receiving other narcotic analgesics, antihistamines, antipsychotics, antianxiety agents, or other CNS depressants (including alcohol) concomitantly with VICODIN ES tablets may exhibit an additive CNS depression. When combined therapy is contemplated, the dose of one or both agents should be reduced.

The use of MAO inhibitors or tricyclic antidepressants with hydrocodone preparations may increase the effect of either the antidepressant or hydrocodone.

Drug/Laboratory Test Interaction: Acetaminophen may produce false-positive test results for urinary 5-hydroxyindoleacetic acid.

Carcinogenesis, Mutagenesis, Impairment of Fertility: No adequate studies have been conducted in animals to determine whether hydrocodone or acetaminophen have a potential for carcinogenesis, mutagenesis, or impairment of fertility.

Pregnancy:

Teratogenic Effects: Pregnancy Category C. There are no adequate and well-controlled studies in pregnant women. VICODIN ES tablets should be used during pregnancy only if the potential benefit justifies the potential risk to the fetus.

Nonteratogenic Effects: Babies born to mothers who have been taking opioids regularly prior to delivery will be physically dependent. The withdrawal signs include irritability and excessive crying, tremors, hyperactive reflexes, increased respiratory rate, increased stools, sneezing, yawning, vomiting, and fever. The intensity of the syndrome does not always correlate with the duration of maternal opioid use or dose. There is no consensus on the best method of managing withdrawal.

Labor and Delivery: As with all narcotics, administration of VICODIN ES tablets to the mother shortly before delivery may result in some degree of respiratory depression in the newborn, especially if higher doses are used.

Nursing Mothers: Acetaminophen is excreted in breast milk in small amounts, but the significance of its effects on nursing infants is not known. It is not known whether hydrocodone is excreted in human milk. Because many drugs are excreted in human milk and because of the potential for serious adverse reactions in nursing infants from hydrocodone and acetaminophen, a decision should be made whether to discontinue nursing or to discontinue the drug, taking into account the importance of the drug to the mother.

Pediatric Use: Safety and effectiveness in the pediatric population have not been established.

Geriatric Use: Clinical studies of VICODIN ES® (hydrocodone bitartrate 7.5 mg and acetaminophen 750 mg) did not include sufficient numbers of subjects aged 65 and over to determine whether they respond differently from younger subjects. Other reported clinical experience has not identified differences in responses between the elderly and younger patients. In general, dose selection for an elderly patient should be cautious, usually starting at the low end of the dosing range, reflecting the greater frequency of decreased hepatic, renal, or cardiac function, and of concomitant disease or other drug therapy.

ADVERSE REACTIONS

The most frequently reported adverse reactions include: lightheadedness, dizziness, sedation, nausea and vomiting. These effects seem to be more prominent in ambulatory than in nonambulatory patients and some of these adverse reactions may be alleviated if the patient lies down.

Other adverse reactions include:

Central Nervous System: Drowsiness, mental clouding, lethargy, impairment of mental and physical performance, anxiety, fear, dysphoria, psychic dependence, mood changes.

Gastrointestinal System: Prolonged administration of VICODIN ES tablets may produce constipation.

Genitourinary System: Ureteral spasm, spasm of vesical sphincters and urinary retention have been reported with opiates.

Respiratory Depression: Hydrocodone bitartrate may produce dose-related respiratory depression by acting directly on the brain stem respiratory center. (see OVERDOSAGE).

Special Senses: Very rare cases of hearing impairment or loss have been reported in patients predominantly receiving very high doses of hydrocodone/acetaminophen for long periods of time.

Dermatological: Skin rash, pruritus.

The following adverse drug events may be borne in mind as potential effects of acetaminophen: allergic reactions, rash, thrombocytopenia, agranulocytosis.

Potential effects of high dosage are listed in the OVERDOSAGE section.

DRUG ABUSE AND DEPENDENCE

Controlled Substance: VICODIN ES tablets are classified as a Schedule Ⓒ III controlled substance.

Abuse and Dependence: Psychic dependence, physical dependence, and tolerance may develop upon repeated administration of narcotics; therefore, VICODIN ES tablets should be prescribed and administered with caution. However, psychic dependence is unlikely to develop when VICODIN ES tablets are used for a short time for the treatment of pain.

Physical dependence, the condition in which continued administration of the drug is required to prevent the appearance of a withdrawal syndrome, assumes clinically significant proportions only after several weeks of continued narcotic use, although some mild degree of physical dependence may develop after a few days of narcotic therapy. Tolerance, in which increasingly large doses are required in order to produce the same degree of analgesia, is manifested initially by a shortened duration of analgesic effect, and subsequently by decreases in the intensity f analgesia. The rate of development of tolerance varies among patients.

OVERDOSAGE

Following an acute overdosage, toxicity may result from hydrocodone or acetaminophen.

Signs and Symptoms:

Hydrocodone: Serious overdose with hydrocodone is characterized by respiratory depression (a decrease in respiratory rate and/or tidal volume. Cheyne-Stokes respiration, cyanosis), extreme somnolence progressing to stupor or coma, skeletal muscle flaccidity, cold and clammy skin, and sometimes bradycardia and hypotension. In severe overdosage, apnea, circulatory collapse, cardiac arrest and death may occur.

Acetaminophen: In acetaminophen overdosage: dose-dependent, potentially fatal hepatic necrosis is the most serious adverse effect. Renal tubular necrosis, hypoglycemic coma, and thrombocytopenia may also occur.

Early symptoms following a potentially hepatotoxic overdose may include: nausea, vomiting, diaphoresis and general malaise. Clinical and laboratory evidence of hepatic toxicity may not be apparent until 48 to 72 hours post-ingestion.

In adults, hepatic toxicity has rarely been reported with acute overdoses of less than 10 grams and fatalities with less than 15 grams.

Treatment:

A single or multiple overdose with hydrocodone and acetaminophen is a potentially lethal polydrug overdose, and consultation with a regional poison control center is recommended.

Immediate treatment includes support of cardiorespiratory function and measures to reduce drug absorption. Vomiting should be induced mechanically, or with syrup of ipecac, if the patient is alert (adequate pharyngeal and laryngeal reflexes). Oral activated charcoal (1 g/kg) should follow gastric emptying. The first dose should be accompanied by an appropriate cathartic. If repeated doses are used, the cathartic might be included with alternate doses as required. Hypotension is usually hypovolemic and should respond to fluids. Vasopressors and other supportive measures should be employed as indicated. A cuffed endo-tracheal tube should be inserted before gastric lavage of the unconscious patient and, when necessary, to provide assisted respiration.

Meticulous attention should be given to maintaining adequate pulmonary ventilation. In severe cases of intoxication, peritoneal dialysis, or preferably hemodialysis may be considered. If hypoprothrombinemia occurs due to acetaminophen overdose, vitamin K should be administered intravenously.

Naloxone, a narcotic antagonist, can reverse respiratory depression and coma associated with opioid overdose. Naloxone hydrochloride 0.4 mg to 2 mg is given parenterally. Since the duration of action of hydrocodone may exceed that of the naloxone, the patient should be kept under continuous surveillance and repeated doses of the antagonist should be administered as needed to maintain adequate respiration. A narcotic antagonist should not be administered in the absence of clinically significant respiratory or cardiovascular depression.

If the dose of acetaminophen may have exceeded 140 mg/kg, acetylcysteine should be administered as early as possible. Serum acetaminophen levels should be obtained, since levels four or more hours following ingestion help predict acetaminophen toxicity. Do not await acetaminophen assay results before initiating treatment. Hepatic enzymes should be obtained initially, and repeated at 24-hour intervals.

Methemoglobinemia over 30% should be treated with methylene blue by slow intravenous administration.

The toxic dose for adults for acetaminophen is 10 g.

DOSAGE AND ADMINISTRATION

Dosage should be adjusted according to the severity of the pain and the response of the patient. However, it should be kept in mind that tolerance to hydrocodone can develop with continued use and that the incidence of untoward effects is dose related.

The usual adult dosage is one tablet every four to six hours as needed for pain. The total daily dosage should not exceed 5 tablets.

Continued on next page

Vicodin ES—Cont.

HOW SUPPLIED

White, oval-shaped, faceted edged tablet bisected on one side and imprinted with "VICODIN ES" on the other side.
Bottles of 100-NDC #0044-0728-02
Bottles of 500-NDC #0044-0728-03
Hospital Unit Dosage Package—100 tablets (4×25 tablets)—NDC #0044-0728-41.
Storage: Store at 25°C (77°F); excursions permitted to 15°–30°C (59°–86°F). [See USP Controlled Room Temperature]. Dispense in a tight, light-resistant container as defined in the USP.
A Schedule Ⓒ Narcotic.
VICODIN ES is a registered trademark of Knoll Pharmaceutical Company.

Revised: May 2000

Knoll Laboratories
A Division of
Knoll Pharmaceutical Company
Mount Olive, New Jersey 07828

0900011-5

Shown in Product Identification Guide, page 319

VICODIN TUSS® Ⓒ

Expectorant
(hydrocodone bitartrate and guaifenesin)
Rx only

DESCRIPTION

VICODIN TUSS® Expectorant Syrup contains hydrocodone bitartrate, semi-synthetic centrally-acting narcotic antitussive and guaifenesin, an expectorant for oral administration.
Each teaspoonful (5 mL) contains:
Hydrocodone bitartrate USP .... 5 mg
Guaifenesin USP .... 100 mg
VICODIN TUSS Expectorant Syrup also contains: glycerin, L-menthol, methylparaben, propylparaben, propylene glycol, sodium saccharin, sorbitol solution, artificial flavoring, and purified water.

CLINICAL PHARMACOLOGY

Clinical trials have proven hydrocodone bitartrate to be an effective antitussive agent which is pharmacologically 2 to 8 times as potent as codeine. At equi-effective doses, its sedative action is greater than codeine. The precise mechanism of action of hydrocodone and other opiates is not known, however, hydrocodone is believed to act by directly depressing the cough center. In excessive doses hydrocodone, like other opium derivatives, can depress respiration. The effects of hydrocodone in therapeutic doses on the cardiovascular system is insignificant. The constipation effects of hydrocodone are much weaker than that of morphine and no stronger than that of codeine. Hydrocodone can produce miosis, euphoria, physical and psychological dependence. At therapeutic antitussive doses, it does exert analgesic effects. Following a 10 mg oral dose of hydrocodone administered to five male human subjects the mean peak concentration was 23.6 ± 5.2 ng/mL. Maximum serum levels were achieved at 1.3 ± 0.3 hours and half-life was determined to be 3.8 ± 0.3 hours. Hydrocodone exhibits a complex pattern of metabolism including O-demethylation, N-demethylation and 6-ketoreduction to the corresponding 6-α- and 6-β-hydroxymetabolites.
The exact mechanism of action is not established but guaifenesin is believed to act by stimulating receptors in the gastric mucosa that initates a reflex secretion of respiratory tract fluid, thereby increasing the volume and decreasing the viscosity of bronchial secretions. Studies with guaifenesin indicate that it is rapidly absorbed from the gastrointestinal tract and has a half-life of one hour.

INDICATIONS AND USAGE

VICODIN TUSS Expectorant is indicated for the symptomatic relief of irritating non-productive cough associated with upper and lower respiratory tract congestion.

CONTRAINDICATIONS

VICODIN TUSS Expectorant is contraindicated in patients hypersensitive to hydrocodone or guaifenesin. Patients known to be hypersensitive to other opioids may exhibit cross sensitivity to hydrocodone.

WARNINGS

Hydrocodone can produce drug dependence of the morphine type and therefore has the potential for being abused. Psychic dependence, physical dependence and tolerance may develop upon repeated administration of VICODIN TUSS Expectorant and it should be prescribed and administered with the same degree of caution appropriate to the use of other narcotic drugs (see DRUG ABUSE AND DEPENDENCE).
Respiratory Depression: VICODIN TUSS Expectorant produces dose-related respiratory depression by directly acting on the brain stem respiratory centers. If respiratory depression occurs, it may be antagonized by the use of naloxone hydrochloride and other supportive measures when indicated.
Head Injury and Increased Intracranial Pressure: The respiratory depressant properties of narcotics and their capacity to elevate cerebrospinal fluid pressure may be markedly exaggerated in the presence of head injury, other intracranial lesions or a pre-existing increase in intracranial pressure. Furthermore, narcotics produce adverse reactions which may obscure the clinical course of patients with head injuries.
Acute Abdominal Conditions: The administration of VICODIN TUSS Expectorant or other opioids may obscure the diagnosis or clinical course of patients with acute abdominal conditions.

PRECAUTIONS

Before prescribing medication to suppress or modify cough, it is important to ascertain that the underlying cause of cough is identified, that modification of cough does not increase the risk of clinical or physiologic complications, and that appropriate therapy for the primary disease is provided.
Usage in Ambulatory Patients: Hydrocodone, like all narcotics, may impair the mental and/or physical abilities required for the performance of potentially hazardous tasks such as driving a car or operating machinery, and patients should be warned accordingly.
Drug Interactions: Patients receiving other narcotic analgesics, general anesthetics, phenothiazines, other tranquilizers, sedative hypnotics or other CNS depressants (including alcohol) concomitantly with hydrocodone may exhibit an additive CNS depression. When such combined therapy is contemplated, the dose of one or both agents should be reduced (see WARNINGS).
Laboratory Interactions: The metabolite of guaifenesin has been found to produce an apparent increase in urinary 5-hydroxyindoleacetic acid, and guaifenesin therefore may interfere with the interpretation of this test for the diagnosis of carcinoid syndrome. Guaifenesin administration should be discontinued 24 hours prior to the collection of urine specimens for the determination of 5-hydroxyindoleacetic acid.
Carcinogenesis, mutagenesis, impairment of fertility: Carcinogenicity, mutagenicity and reproduction studies have not been conducted with VICODIN TUSS® Expectorant.
Usage in Pregnancy: Pregnancy Category C. Animal reproduction studies have not been conducted with VICODIN TUSS Expectorant. It is also not known whether VICODIN TUSS Expectorant can cause fetal harm when administered to a pregnant woman or can affect reproductive capacity. VICODIN TUSS Expectorant should be given to a pregnant woman only if clearly needed.
Nonteratogenic effects: Babies born to mothers who have been taking opioids regularly prior to delivery will be physically dependent. The withdrawal signs include irritability and excessive crying, tremors, hyperactive reflexes, increased respiratory rate, increased stools, sneezing, yawning, vomiting and fever. The intensity of the syndrome does not always correlate with the duration of maternal opioid use or dose. There is no consensus on the best method of managing withdrawal. Chlorpromazine 0.7–1.0 mg/kg q 6 h, phenobarbital 2 mg/kg q 6 h, and paregoric 2–4 drops/kg q 4 h, have been used to treat withdrawal symptoms in infants. The duration of therapy is 4 to 28 days, with the dosages decreased as tolerated.
Nursing mothers: It is not known whether this drug is excreted in human milk. Because many drugs are excreted in human milk and because of the potential for serious adverse reactions in nursing infants from VICODIN TUSS Expectorant, a decision should be made whether to discontinue nursing or discontinue the drug, taking into account the importance of the drug to the mother.
Geriatric Use: Clinical studies of VICODIN TUSS did not include sufficient numbers of subjects aged 65 and over to determine whether they respond differently from younger subjects. Other reported clinical experience has not identified differences in responses between the elderly and younger patients. In general, dose selection for an elderly patient should be cautious, usually starting at the low end of the dosing range, reflecting the greater frequency of decreased hepatic, renal, or cardiac function, and of concomitant disease or other drug therapy.

ADVERSE REACTIONS

Respiratory System: Hydrocodone produces dose-related respiratory depression by acting directly on brain stem respiratory centers.
Cardiovascular System: Hypertension, postural hypotension and palpitations.
Genitourinary System: Ureteral spasm, spasm of vesical sphincters and urinary retention have been reported with opiates.
Central Nervous System: Sedation, drowsiness, mental clouding, lethargy, impairment of mental and physical performance, anxiety, fear, dysphoria, dizziness, psychic dependence, mood changes and blurred vision.
Gastrointestinal System: Nausea and vomiting occur more frequently in ambulatory than in recumbent patients.

DRUG ABUSE DEPENDENCE

Special care should be exercised in prescribing hydrocodone for emotionally unstable patients and for those with a history of drug misuse. Such patients should be closely supervised when long-term therapy is contemplated.
VICODIN TUSS® Expectorant is a Schedule III narcotic. Psychic dependence, physical dependence and tolerance may develop upon repeated administration of narcotics; therefore, VICODIN TUSS Expectorant should always be prescribed and administered with caution. Physical dependence is the condition in which continued administration of the drug is required to prevent the appearance of a withdrawal syndrome.
Patients physically dependent on opioids will develop an abstinence syndrome upon abrupt discontinuation of the opioid or following the administration of a narcotic antagonist. The character and severity of the withdrawal symptoms are related to the degree of physical dependence. Manifestations of opioid withdrawal are similar to but milder than that of morphine and include lacrimation, rhinorrhea, yawning, sweating, restlessness, dilated pupils, anorexia, goose-flesh, irritability and tremor. In more severe forms, nausea, vomiting, intestinal spasm and diarrhea, increased heart rate and blood pressure, chills, and pains in bones and muscles of the back and extremities may occur. Peak effects will usually be apparent at 48 to 72 hours.
Treatment of withdrawal is usually managed by providing sufficient quantities of an opioid to suppress **severe** withdrawal symptoms and then gradually reducing the dose of opioid over a period of several days.

OVERDOSAGE

Signs and Symptoms: Serious overdosage with VICODIN TUSS Expectorant is characterized by respiratory depression (a decrease in respiratory rate and/or tidal volume, Cheyne-Stokes respiration, cyanosis), extreme somnolence progressing to stupor or coma, skeletal muscle flaccidity, cold and clammy skin, and sometimes bradycardia and hypotension. In severe overdosage apnea, circulatory collapse, cardiac arrest, and death may occur.
Treatment: Primary attention should be given to the reestablishment of adequate respiratory exchange through provision of a patent airway and the institution of assisted or controlled ventilation. The narcotic antagonist naloxone hydrochloride is a specific antidote for respiratory depression which may result from overdosage or unusual sensitivity to narcotics including hydrocodone. Therefore, an appropriate dose of naloxone hydrochloride should be administered, preferably by the intravenous route, simultaneously with efforts at respiratory resuscitation. For further information, see full prescribing information for naloxone hydrochloride. An antagonist should not be administered in the absence of clinically significant respiratory depression. Oxygen, intravenous fluids, vasopressors and other supportive measures should be employed as indicated. Gastric emptying may be useful in removing unabsorbed drug. Activated charcoal may be of benefit.

DOSAGE AND ADMINISTRATION

Usual Adult Dose: One teaspoonful (5 mL) after meals and at bedtime, not less than 4 hours apart (not to exceed 6 teaspoonsful in a 24 hour period). Treatment should be initiated with one teaspoonful and subsequent doses, up to a maximum single dose of 3 teaspoonsful, adjusted if required.
Usual Children's Dose:
Over 12 years: Initial dose 1 teaspoonful; maximum single dose, 2 teaspoonsful.
6 to 12 years: Initial dose $^1/_2$ teaspoonful; maximum single dose, 1 teaspoonful.

HOW SUPPLIED

VICODIN TUSS® Expectorant is available in bottles as a colorless, cherry-flavored syrup which contains no sugar, alcohol or dye.
One pint: NDC 0044-0730-16.
Store in a tight, light resistant container as defined in the USP. Keep tightly closed.
Storage: Store at 25°C (77°F); excursions permitted to 15°–30°C (59°–86°F). [See USP Controlled Room Temperature].

VICODIN TUSS is a registered trademark of Knoll Pharmaceutical Company

A Schedule Ⓒ Narcotic. Oral prescription where permitted by State Law.
Revised: May 2000
Knoll Laboratories
A Division of
Knoll Pharmaceutical Company
Mt. Olive, NJ 07828
BASF Pharma

0900007-3

Shown in Product Identification Guide, page 319

VICOPROFEN® Ⓒ ℞

[*vī-cō-prōfen*]
(hydrocodone bitartrate and ibuprofen tablets)
7.5 mg/200 mg
Rx only

DESCRIPTION

Each VICOPROFEN® tablet contains:
Hydrocodone Bitartrate, USP 7.5 mg
Ibuprofen, USP 200 mg
VICOPROFEN is supplied in a fixed combination tablet form for oral administration. VICOPROFEN combines the opioid analgesic agent, hydrocodone bitartrate, with the nonsteroidal anti-inflammatory (NSAID) agent, ibuprofen. Hydrocodone bitartrate is a semisynthetic and centrally acting opioid analgesic. Its chemical name is: 4,5 α-epoxy-3-

methoxy-17-methylmorphinan-6-one tartrate (1:1) hydrate (2:5). Its chemical formula is: $C_{18}H_{21}NO_3 \bullet C_4H_6O_6 \bullet 2^1/_2H_2O$, and the molecular weight is 494.50. Its structural formula is:

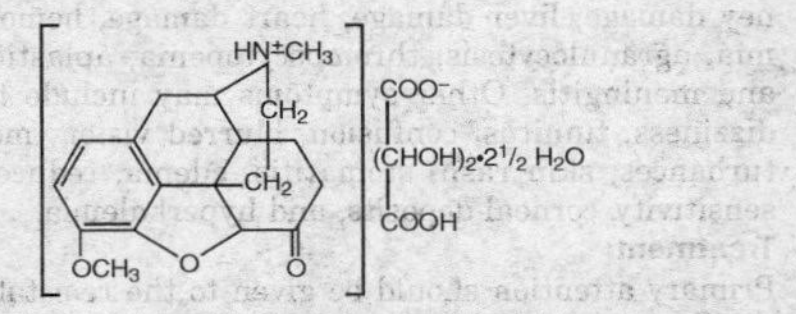

Ibuprofen is a nonsteroidal anti-inflammatory drug with analgesic and antipyretic properties. Its chemical name is: (±)-2-(*p*-isobutylphenyl) propionic acid. Its chemical formula is: $C_{13}H_{18}O_2$, and the molecular weight is: 206.29. Its structural formula is:

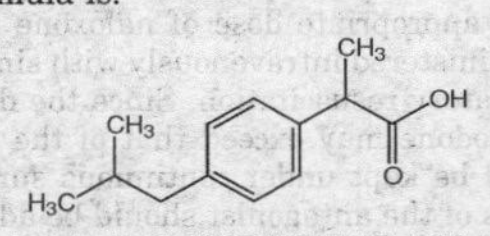

Inactive ingredients in VICOPROFEN tablets include: colloidal silicon dioxide, corn starch, croscarmellose sodium, hydroxypropyl methylcellulose, magnesium stearate, microcrystalline cellulose, polyethylene glycol, polysorbate 80, and titanium dioxide.

CLINICAL PHARMACOLOGY

Hydrocodone component: Hydrocodone is a semisynthetic opioid analgesic and antitussive with multiple actions qualitatively similar to those of codeine. Most of these involve the central nervous system and smooth muscle. The precise mechanism of action of hydrocodone and other opioids is not known, although it is believed to relate to the existence of opiate receptors in the central nervous system. In addition to analgesia, opioids may produce drowsiness, changes in mood, and mental clouding.

Ibuprofen component: Ibuprofen is a nonsteroidal anti-inflammatory agent that possesses analgesic and antipyretic activities. Its mode action, like that of other NSAIDs, is not completely understood, but may be related to inhibition of cyclooxygenase activity and prostaglandin synthesis. Ibuprofen is a peripherally acting analgesic. Ibuprofen does not have any known effects on opiate receptors.

Pharmacokinetics:

Absorption: After oral dosing with the VICOPROFEN tablet, a peak hydrocodone plasma level of 27 ng/mL is achieved at 1.7 hours, and a peak ibuprofen plasma level of 30 mcg/mL is achieved at 1.8 hours. The effect of food on the absorption of either component from the VICOPROFEN tablet has not been established.

Distribution: Ibuprofen is highly protein-bound (99%) like most other non-steroidal anti-inflammatory agents. Although the extent of protein binding of hydrocodone in human plasma has not been definitely determined, structural similarities to related opioid analgesics suggest that hydrocodone is not extensively protein bound. As most agents in the 5-ring morphinan group of semi-synthetic opioids bind plasma protein to a similar degree (range 19% [hydromorphone] to 45% [oxycodone]), hydrocodone is expected to fall within this range.

Metabolism: Hydrocodone exhibits a complex pattern of metabolism, including *O*-demethylation, *N*-demethylation, and 6-keto reduction to the corresponding 6-α-and 6-β-hydroxy metabolites. Hydromorphone, a potent opioid, is formed from the *O*-demethylation of hydrocodone and contributes to the total analgesic effect of hydrocodone. The *O*- and *N*-demethylation processes are mediated by separate P-450 isoenzymes: CYP2D6 and CYP3A4, respectively.

Ibuprofen is present in this product as a racemate, and following absorption it undergoes interconversion in the plasma from the R-isomer to the S-isomer. Both the R- and S- isomers are metabolized to two primary metabolites: (+)-2-4′-(2hydroxy-2-methyl-propyl) phenyl propionic acid and (+)-2-4′-(2carboxypropyl) phenyl propionic acid, both of which circulate in the plasma at low levels relative to the parent.

Elimination: Hydrocodone and its metabolites are eliminated primarily in the kidneys, with a mean plasma half-life of 4.5 hours. Ibuprofen is excreted in the urine, 50% to 60% as metabolites and approximately 15% as unchanged drug and conjugate. The plasma half-life is 2.2 hours.

Special Populations: No significant pharmacokinetic differences based on age or gender have been demonstrated. The pharmacokinetics of hydrocodone and ibuprofen from VICOPROFEN has not been evaluated in children.

Renal Impairment: The effect of renal insufficiency on the pharmacokinetics of the VICOPROFEN dosage form has not been determined.

CLINICAL STUDIES

In single-dose studies of post surgical pain (abdominal, gynecological, orthopedic), 940 patients were studied at doses of one or two tablets. VICOPROFEN produced greater efficacy than placebo and each of its individual components given at the same dose. No advantage was demonstrated for the two-tablet dose.

INDICATIONS AND USAGE

VICOPROFEN tablets are indicated for the short-term (generally less than 10 days) management of acute pain. VICOPROFEN is not indicated for the treatment of such conditions as osteoarthritis or rheumatoid arthritis.

CONTRAINDICATIONS

VICOPROFEN should not be administered to patients who previously have exhibited hypersensitivity to hydrocodone or ibuprofen. VICOPROFEN should not be given to patients who have experienced asthma, urticaria, or allergic-type reactions after taking aspirin or other NSAIDs. Severe, rarely fatal, anaphylactic-like reactions to NSAIDs have been reported in such patients (see WARNINGS - Anaphylactoid Reactions, and PRECAUTIONS - Pre-existing Asthma).

Patients known to be hypersensitive to other opioids may exhibit cross-sensitivity to hydrocodone.

WARNINGS

Abuse and Dependence: Hydrocodone can produce drug dependence of the morphine type and therefore has the potential for being abused. Psychic and physical dependence as well as tolerance may develop upon repeated administration of this drug and it should be prescribed and administered with the same degree of caution as other narcotic drugs (see DRUG ABUSE AND DEPENDENCE).

Respiratory Depression: At high doses or in opioid-sensitive patients, hydrocodone may produce dose-related respiratory depression by acting directly on the brain stem respiratory centers. Hydrocodone also affects the center that controls respiratory rhythm, and may produce irregular and periodic breathing.

Head Injury and Increased Intracranial Pressure: The respiratory depressant effects of opioids and their capacity to elevate cerebrospinal fluid pressure may be markedly exaggerated in the presence of head injury, intracranial lesions or a pre-existing increase in intracranial pressure. Furthermore, opioids produce adverse reactions which may obscure the clinical course of patients with head injuries.

Acute Abdominal Conditions: The administration of opioids may obscure the diagnosis or clinical course of patients with acute abdominal conditions.

Gastrointestinal (GI) Effects - Risk of GI Ulceration, Bleeding and Perforation: Serious gastrointestinal toxicity, such as inflammation, bleeding, ulceration, and perforation of the stomach, small intestine or large intestine, can occur at any time, with or without warning symptoms, in patients treated with nonsteroidal anti-inflammatory drugs (NSAIDs). Minor upper GI problems, such as dyspepsia, are common and may also occur at any time during NSAID therapy. Therefore, physicians and patients should remain alert for ulceration and bleeding even in the absence of previous GI tract symptoms. Patients should be informed about the signs and/or symptoms of serious GI toxicity and what steps to take if they occur. The utility of periodic laboratory monitoring has not been demonstrated, nor has it been adequately assessed. Only one in five patients, who develop a serious upper GI adverse event of NSAID therapy, is symptomatic. Even short term therapy is not without risk.

NSAIDs should be prescribed with extreme caution in those with a prior history of ulcer disease or gastrointestinal bleeding. Most spontaneous reports of fatal GI events are in elderly or debilitated patients and therefore special care should be taken in treating this population. To minimize the potential risk for an adverse GI event, the lowest effective dose should be used for the shortest possible duration. For high risk patients, alternate therapies that do not involve NSAIDs should be considered.

Studies have shown that patients with a prior history of peptic ulcer disease and/or gastrointestinal bleeding and who use NSAIDs, have a greater than 10-fold risk for developing a GI bleed than patients with neither of these risk factors. In addition to a past history of ulcer disease, pharmaco-epidemiological studies have identified several other co-therapies or co-morbid conditions that may increase the risk for GI bleeding such as: treatment with oral corticosteroids, treatment with anticoagulants, longer duration of NSAID therapy, smoking, alcoholism, older age, and poor general health status.

Anaphylactoid Reactions: Anaphylactoid reactions may occur in patients without known prior exposure to VICOPROFEN. VICOPROFEN should not be given to patients with the aspirin triad. The triad typically occurs in asthmatic patients who experience rhinitis with or without nasal polyps, or who exhibit severe, potentially fatal bronchospasm after taking aspirin or other NSAIDs. Fatal reactions to NSAIDs have been reported in such patients (see CONTRAINDICATIONS and PRECAUTIONS - Pre-existing Asthma). Emergency help should be sought when anaphylactoid reaction occurs.

Advanced Renal Disease: In cases with advanced kidney disease, treatment with VICOPROFEN is not recommended. If NSAID therapy, however, must be initiated, close monitoring of the patient's kidney function is advisable (see PRECAUTIONS - Renal Effects).

Pregnancy: As with other NSAID-containing products, VICOPROFEN should be avoided in late pregnancy because it may cause premature closure of the ductus arteriosus.

PRECAUTIONS

General Precautions

Special Risk Patients: As with any opioid analgesic agent, VICOPROFEN tablets should be used with caution in elderly or debilitated patients, and those with severe impairment of hepatic or renal function, hypothyroidism, Addison's disease, prostatic hypertrophy or urethral stricture. The usual precautions should be observed and the possibility of respiratory depression should be kept in mind.

Cough Reflex: Hydrocodone suppresses the cough reflex; as with opioids, caution should be exercised when VICOPROFEN is used postoperatively and in patients with pulmonary disease.

Effect on Diagnostic Signs: The antipyretic and anti-inflammatory activity of ibuprofen may reduce fever and inflammation, thus diminishing their utility as diagnostic signs in detecting complications of presumed noninfectious, noninflammatory painful conditions.

Hepatic Effects: As with other NSAIDs, ibuprofen has been reported to cause borderline elevations of one or more liver enzymes; this may occur in up to 15% of patients. These abnormalities may progress, may remain essentially unchanged, or may be transient with continued therapy. Notable (3 times the upper limit of normal) elevations of SGPT (ALT) or SGOT (AST) occurred in controlled clinical trials in less than 1% of patients. A patient with symptoms and/or signs suggesting liver dysfunction, or in whom an abnormal liver test has occurred, should be evaluated for evidence of the development of more severe hepatic reactions while on therapy with VICOPROFEN. Severe hepatic reactions, including jaundice and cases of fatal hepatitis, have been reported with ibuprofen as with other NSAIDs. Although such reactions are rare, if abnormal liver tests persist or worsen, if clinical signs and symptoms consistent with liver disease develop, or if systemic manifestations occur (e.g. eosinophilia, rash, etc.), VICOPROFEN should be discontinued.

Renal Effects: Caution should be used when initiating treatment with VICOPROFEN in patients with considerable dehydration. It is advisable to rehydrate patients first and then start therapy with VICOPROFEN. Caution is also recommended in patients with pre-existing kidney disease (see WARNINGS - Advanced Renal Disease).

As with other NSAIDs, long-term administration of ibuprofen has resulted in renal papillary necrosis and other renal pathologic changes. Renal toxicity has also been seen in patients in which renal prostaglandins have a compensatory role in the maintenance of renal perfusion. In these patients, administration of a nonsteroidal anti-inflammatory drug may cause a dose-dependent reduction in prostaglandin formation and, secondarily, in renal blood flow, which may precipitate overt renal decompensation. Patients at greatest risk of this reaction are those with impaired renal function, heart failure, liver dysfunction, those taking diuretics and ACE inhibitors, and the elderly. Discontinuation of nonsteroidal anti-inflammatory drug therapy is usually followed by recovery to the pretreatment state.

Ibuprofen metabolites are eliminated primarily by the kidneys. The extent to which the metabolites may accumulate in patients with renal failure has not been studied. Patients with significantly impaired renal function should be more closely monitored.

Hematological Effects: Ibuprofen, like other NSAIDs, can inhibit platelet aggregation but the effect is quantitatively less and of shorter duration than that seen with aspirin. Ibuprofen has been shown to prolong bleeding time in normal subjects. Because this prolonged bleeding effect may be exaggerated in patients with underlying hemostatic defects, VICOPROFEN should be used with caution in persons with intrinsic coagulation defects and those on anticoagulant therapy.

Anemia is sometimes seen in patients receiving NSAIDs, including ibuprofen. This may be due to fluid retention, GI loss, or an incompletely described effect upon erythropoiesis.

Fluid Retention and Edema: Fluid retention and edema have been reported in association with ibuprofen, therefore, the drug should be used with caution in patients with a history of cardiac decompensation, hypertension or heart failure.

Pre-existing Asthma: Patients with asthma may have aspirin-sensitive asthma. The use of aspirin in patients with aspirin-sensitive asthma has been associated with severe bronchospasm, which may be fatal. Since cross-reactivity between aspirin and other NSAIDs has been reported in such aspirin-sensitive patients, VICOPROFEN should not be administered to patients with this form of aspirin sensitivity and should be used with caution in patients with pre-existing asthma.

Aseptic Meningitis: Aseptic meningitis with fever and coma has been observed on rare occasions in patients on ibuprofen therapy. Although it is probably more likely to occur in patients with systemic lupus erythematosus and related connective tissue diseases, it has been reported in patients who do not have an underlying chronic disease. If signs or symptoms of meningitis develop in a patient on VICOPROFEN, the possibility of its being related to ibuprofen should be considered.

Information for Patients

VICOPROFEN, like other opioid-containing analgesics, may impair mental and/or physical abilities required for the performance of potentially hazardous tasks such as driving a car or operating machinery; patients should be cautioned accordingly.

Alcohol and other CNS depressants may produce an additive CNS depression, when taken with this combination product, and should be avoided.

VICOPROFEN may be habit-forming. Patients should take the drug only for as long as it is prescribed, in the amounts prescribed, and no more frequently than prescribed.

VICOPROFEN, like other drugs containing ibuprofen, is not free of side effects. The side effects of these drugs can cause discomfort and, rarely, there are more serious side ef-

Continued on next page

Vicoprofen—Cont.

fects, such as gastrointestinal bleeding, which may result in hospitalization and even fatal outcomes. Patients should be instructed to report any signs and symptoms of gastrointestinal bleeding, blurred vision or other eye symptoms, skin rash, weight gain, or edema.

Laboratory Tests

A decrease in hemoglobin may occur during VICOPROFEN® (hydrocodone bitartrate 7.5 mg and ibuprofen 200 mg) therapy, and elevations of liver enzymes may be seen in a small percentage of patients during VICOPROFEN therapy (see PRECAUTIONS - Hematological Effects and PRECAUTIONS - Hepatic Effects).

In patients with severe hepatic or renal disease, effects of therapy should be monitored with liver and/or renal function tests.

Drug Interactions

ACE-Inhibitors: Reports suggest that NSAIDs may diminish the antihypertensive effect of ACE-inhibitors. This interaction should be given consideration in patients taking VICOPROFEN concomitantly with ACE-inhibitors.

Anticholinergics: The concurrent use of anticholinergics with hydrocodone preparations may produce paralytic ileus.

Antidepressants: The use of MAO inhibitors or tricyclic antidepressants with VICOPROFEN may increase the effect of either the antidepressant or hydrocodone.

Aspirin: As with other products containing NSAIDs, concomitant administration of VICOPROFEN and aspirin is not generally recommended because of the potential of increased adverse effects.

CNS Depressants: Patients receiving other opioids, antihistamines, antipsychotics, antianxiety agents, or other CNS depressants (including alcohol) concomitantly with VICOPROFEN may exhibit an additive CNS depression. When combined therapy is contemplated, the dose of one or both agents should be reduced.

Furosemide: Ibuprofen has been shown to reduce the natriuretic effect of furosemide and thiazides in some patients. This response has been attributed to inhibition of renal prostaglandin synthesis. During concomitant therapy with VICOPROFEN the patient should be observed closely for signs of renal failure (see PRECAUTIONS- Renal Effects), as well as diuretic efficacy.

Lithium: Ibuprofen has been shown to elevate plasma lithium concentration and reduce renal lithium clearance. This effect has been attributed to inhibition of renal prostaglandin synthesis by ibuprofen. Thus, when VICOPROFEN and lithium are administered concurrently, patients should be observed for signs of lithium toxicity.

Methotrexate: Ibuprofen, as well as other NSAIDs, has been reported to competitively inhibit methotrexate accumulation in rabbit kidney slices. This may indicate that ibuprofen could enhance the toxicity of methotrexate. Caution should be used when VICOPROFEN is administered concomitantly with methotrexate.

Warfarin: The effects of warfarin and NSAIDs on GI bleeding are synergistic, such that users of both drugs together have a risk of serious GI bleeding higher than users of either drug alone.

Carcinogenicity, Mutagenicity, and Impairment of Fertility

The carcinogenic and mutagenic potential of VICOPROFEN has not been investigated. The ability of VICOPROFEN to impair fertility has not been assessed.

Pregnancy: Pregnancy Category C.

Teratogenic Effects: VICOPROFEN, administered to rabbits of 95 mg/kg (5.72 and 1.9 times the maximum clinical dose based on body weight and surface area, respectively), a maternally toxic dose, resulted in an increase in the percentage of litters and fetuses with any major abnormality and an increase in the number of litters and fetuses with one or more nonossified metacarpals (a minor abnormality). VICOPROFEN, administered to rats at 166 mg/kg (10.0 and 1.66 times the maximum clinical dose based on body weight and surface area, respectively), a maternally toxic dose, did not result in any reproductive toxicity. There are no adequate and well-controlled studies in pregnant women. VICOPROFEN should be used during pregnancy only if the potential benefit justifies the potential risk to the fetus.

Nonteratogenic Effects: Because of the known effects of nonsteroidal anti-inflammatory drugs on the fetal cardiovascular system (closure of the ductus arteriosus), use during pregnancy (particularly late pregnancy) should be avoided. Babies born to mothers who have been taking opioids regularly prior to delivery will be physically dependent. The withdrawal signs include irritability and excessive crying, tremors, hyperactive reflexes, increased respiratory rate, increased stools, sneezing, yawning, vomiting, and fever. The intensity of the syndrome does not always correlate with the duration of maternal opioid use or dose. There is no consensus on the best method of managing withdrawal.

Labor and Delivery

As with other drugs known to inhibit prostaglandin synthesis, an increased incidence of dystocia and delayed parturition occurred in rats. Administration of VICOPROFEN is not recommended during labor and delivery.

Nursing Mothers

It is not known whether hydrocodone is excreted in human milk. In limited studies, an assay capable of detecting 1 mcg/mL did not demonstrate ibuprofen in the milk of lactating mothers. However, because of the limited nature of the studies, and the possible adverse effects of protaglandin-inhibiting drugs on neonates, VICOPROFEN is not recommended for use in nursing mothers.

Pediatric Use

The safety and effectiveness of VICOPROFEN in pediatric patients below the age of 16 have not been established.

Geriatric Use

In controlled clinical trials there was no difference in tolerability between patients <65 years of age and those ≥65, apart from an increased tendency of the elderly to develop constipation. However, because the elderly may be more sensitive to the renal and gastrointestinal effects of nonsteroidal anti-inflammatory agents as well as possible increased risk of respiratory depression with opioids, extra caution and reduced dosages should be used when treating the elderly with VICOPROFEN.

ADVERSE REACTIONS

VICOPROFEN was administered to approximately 300 pain patients in a safety study that employed dosages and a duration of treatment sufficient to encompass the recommended usage (see DOSAGE AND ADMINISTRATION). Adverse event rates generally increased with increasing daily dose. The event rates reported below are from approximately 150 patients who were in a group that received one tablet of VICOPROFEN an average of three to four times daily. The overall incidence rates of adverse experiences in the trials were fairly similar for this patient group and those who received the comparison treatment, acetaminophen 600 mg with codeine 60 mg.

The following lists adverse events that occurred with an incidence of 1% or greater in clinical trials of VICOPROFEN, without regard to the causal relationship of the events to the drug. To distinguish different rates of occurrence in clinical studies, the adverse events are listed as follows:

name of adverse event = less than 3%

adverse events marked with an asterisk * = 3% to 9%

adverse event rates over 9% are in parentheses.

Body as a Whole: Abdominal pain*; Asthenia*; Fever; Flu syndrome; Headache (27%); Infection*; Pain.

Cardiovascular: Palpitations; Vasodilation.

Central Nervous System: Anxiety*; Confusion; Dizziness (14%); Hypertonia; Insomnia*; Nervousness*; Paresthesia; Somnolence (22%); Thinking abnormalities.

Digestive: Anorexia; Constipation (22%); Diarrhea*; Dry mouth*; Dyspepsia (12%); Flatulence*; Gastritis; Melena; Mouth ulcers; Nausea (21%); Thirst; Vomiting*.

Metabolic and Nutritional Disorders: Edema*.

Respiratory: Dyspnea; Hiccups; Pharyngitis; Rhinitis.

Skin and Appendages: Pruritus*; Sweating*.

Special Senses: Tinnitus.

Urogenital: Urinary frequency.

Incidence less than 1%

Body as a Whole: Allergic reaction.

Cardiovascular: Arrhythmia; Hypotension; Tachycardia.

Central Nervous System: Agitation; Abnormal dreams; Decreased libido; Depression; Euphoria; Mood changes; Neuralgia; Slurred speech; Tremor, Vertigo.

Digestive: Chalky stool; "Clenching teeth"; Dysphagia; Esophageal spasm; Esophagitis; Gastroenteritis; Glossitis; Liver enzyme elevation.

Metabolic and Nutritional: Weight decrease.

Musculoskeletal: Arthralgia; Myalgia.

Respiratory: Asthma; Bronchitis; Hoarseness; Increased cough; Pulmonary congestion; Pneumonia; Shallow breathing; Sinusitis.

Skin and Appendages: Rash; Urticaria.

Special Senses: Altered vision; Bad taste; Dry eyes.

Urogenital: Cystitis; Glycosuria; Impotence; Urinary incontinence; Urinary retention.

DRUG ABUSE AND DEPENDENCE

Controlled Substance: VICOPROFEN Tablets are a Schedule III controlled substance.

Abuse: Psychic dependence, physical dependence, and tolerance may develop upon repeated administration of opioids; therefore, VICOPROFEN Tablets should be prescribed and administered with the same degree of caution appropriate to use of other oral narcotic medications.

Dependence: Physical dependence, the condition in which continued administration of the drug is required to prevent the appearance of a withdrawal syndrome, assumes clinically significant proportions only after several weeks of continued opioid use, although a mild degree of physical dependence may develop after a few days of opioid therapy. Tolerance, in which increasingly large doses are required in order to produce the same degree of analgesia, is manifested initially by a shortened duration of analgesic effect, and subsequently by decreases in the intensity of analgesia. The rate of development of tolerance varies among patients. However, psychic dependence is unlikely to develop when VICOPROFEN Tablets are used for a short time for the treatment of acute pain.

OVERDOSAGE

Following an acute overdosage, toxicity may result from hydrocodone and/or ibuprofen.

Signs and Symptoms:

Hydrocodone component: Serious overdose with hydrocodone is characterized by respiratory depression (a decrease in respiratory rate and/or tidal volume, Cheyne-Stokes respiration, cyanosis) extreme somnolence progressing to stupor or coma, skeletal muscle flaccidity, cold and clammy skin, and sometimes bradycardia and hypotension. In severe overdosage, apnea, circulatory collapse, cardiac arrest and death may occur.

Ibuprofen component: Symptoms include gastrointestinal irritation with erosion and hemorrhage or perforation, kidney damage, liver damage, heart damage, hemolytic anemia, agranulocytosis, thrombocytopenia, aplastic anemia, and meningitis. Other symptoms may include headache, dizziness, tinnitus, confusion, blurred vision, mental disturbances, skin rash, stomatitis, edema, reduced retinal sensitivity, corneal deposits, and hyperkalemia.

Treatment:

Primary attention should be given to the re-establishment of adequate respiratory exchange through provision of a patent airway and the institution of assisted or controlled ventilation. Naloxone, a narcotic antagonist, can reverse respiratory depression and coma associated with opioid overdose or unusual sensitivity to opioids, including hydrocodone. Therefore, an appropriate dose of naloxone hydrochloride should be administered intravenously with simultaneous efforts at respiratory resuscitation. Since the duration of action of hydrocodone may exceed that of the naloxone, the patient should be kept under continuous surveillance and repeated doses of the antagonist should be administered as needed to maintain adequate respiration. Supportive measures should be employed as indicated. Gastric emptying may be useful in removing unabsorbed drug. In cases where consciousness is impaired it may be inadvisable to perform gastric lavage. If gastric lavage is performed, little drug will likely be recovered if more than an hour has elapsed since ingestion. Ibuprofen is acidic and is excreted in the urine; therefore, it may be beneficial to administer alkali and induce diuresis. In addition to supportive measures the use of oral activated charcoal may help to reduce the absorption and reabsorption of ibuprofen. Dialysis is not likely to be effective for removal of ibuprofen because it is very highly bound to plasma proteins.

DOSAGE AND ADMINISTRATION

For the short-term (generally less than 10 days) management of acute pain, the recommended dose of VICOPROFEN is one tablet every 4 to 6 hours, as necessary. Dosage should not exceed 5 tablets in a 24-hour period. It should be kept in mind that tolerance to hydrocodone can develop with continued use and that the incidence of untoward effects is dose related.

The lowest effective dose or the longest dosing interval should be sought for each patient, especially in the elderly. After observing the initial response to therapy with VICOPROFEN, the dose and frequency of dosing should be adjusted to suit the individual patient's need, without exceeding the total daily dose recommended.

HOW SUPPLIED

VICOPROFEN tablets are available as:

White film-coated round convex tablets, engraved with "VP" over the Knoll triangle on one side and plain on the other side.

Bottles of 100-NDC #0044-0723-02

Bottles of 500-NDC #0044-0723-03

Hospital Unit Dosage Package-100 tablets (4×25 tablets)-NDC #0044-0723-41

Storage: Store at 25° C (77° F); excursions permitted to 15° to 30° C (59°–86° F). [See USP Controlled Room Temperature].

Dispense in a tight, light-resistant container.

A Schedule ㉍ Narcotic.

VICOPROFEN is a registered trademark of Knoll Pharmaceutical Company

Revised: May 2000

Knoll Laboratories
A Division of
Knoll Pharmaceutical Company
3000 Continental Drive - North
Mount Olive, New Jersey 07828-1234 **BASF** Pharma
0900001-3

Shown in Product Identification Guide, page 319

IDENTIFICATION PROBLEM?
Turn to the **Product Identification Guide,** where you'll find more than 1600 products pictured in actual size and full color.

Knoll Pharmaceutical Company

**3000 CONTINENTAL DRIVE NORTH
MOUNT OLIVE, NJ 07828**

BASF Group

Direct Inquiries to:
BASF Group
Customer Information Center:
General Information (800) 240-3820

Customer Operations: Orders, Credits/Returns,
Wholesaler and Hospital Inquiries,
Deductions, New Accounts (800) 526-0710

For Medical Information Contact:
(800) 526-0221

MAVIK® ℞

[*mă 'vick*]
(Trandolapril) Tablets
PRESCRIBING INFORMATION

> **USE IN PREGNANCY**
> **When used in pregnancy during the second and third trimesters, ACE inhibitors can cause injury and even death to the developing fetus. When pregnancy is detected, MAVIK® should be discontinued as soon as possible. See WARNINGS, Fetal/Neonatal Morbidity and Mortality.**

DESCRIPTION

Trandolapril is the ethyl ester prodrug of a non-sulfhydryl angiotensin converting enzyme (ACE) inhibitor, trandolaprilat. Trandolapril is chemically described as (2S, 3aR, 7aS)-1-[(S)-N-[(S)-1-Carboxy-3-phenylpropyl]alanyl] hexahydro-2-indolinecarboxylic acid, 1-ethyl ester. Its empirical formula is $C_{24}H_{34}N_2O_5$ and its structural formula is

R:- C_2H_5: Trandolapril
-H: Trandolaprilat (diacid)

M.W.=430.54
Melting Point=125°C

Trandolapril is a colorless, crystalline substance that is soluble (>100 mg/mL) in chloroform, dichloromethane, and methanol. MAVIK® tablets contain 1 mg, 2 mg, or 4 mg of trandolapril for oral administration. Each tablet also contains corn starch, croscarmellose sodium, hydroxypropyl methyl-cellulose, iron oxide, lactose, povidone, sodium stearyl fumarate.

CLINICAL PHARMACOLOGY

Mechanism of Action:
Trandolapril is deesterified to the diacid metabolite, trandolaprilat, which is approximately eight times more active as an inhibitor of ACE activity. ACE is a peptidyl dipeptidase that catalyzes the conversion of angiotensin 1 to the vasoconstrictor, angiotensin II. Angiotensin II is a potent peripheral vasoconstrictor that also stimulates secretion of aldosterone by the adrenal cortex and provides negative feedback for renin secretion. The effect of tradolapril in hypertension appears to result primarily from the inhibition of circulating and tissue ACE activity thereby reducing angiotensin II formation, decreasing vasoconstriction, decreasing aldosterone secretion, and increasing plasma renin. Decreased aldosterone secretion leads to diuresis, natriuresis, and a small increase of serum potassium. In controlled clinical trials, treatment with MAVIK® alone resulted in mean increases in potassium of 0.1 mEq/L. (See **PRECAUTIONS**).
ACE is identical to kininase II, an enzyme that degrades bradykinin, a potent peptide vasodilator; whether increased levels of bradykinin play a role in the therapeutic effect of trandolapril remains to be elucidated.
While the principal mechanism of antihypertensive effect is thought to be through the renin-angiontensin-aldosterone system, trandolapril exerts antihypertensive actions even in patients with low-renin hypertension. MAVIK® was an effective antihypertensive in all races studied. Both black patients (usually a predominantly low-renin group) and non-black patients responded to 2 to 4 mg of MAVIK®.
Pharmacokinetics and Metabolism:
Pharmacokinetics Trandolapril's ACE-inhibiting activity is primarily due to its diacid metabolite, trandolaprilat. Cleavage of the ester group of trandolapril, primarily in the liver, is responsible for conversion. Absolute bioavailability after oral administration of trandolapril is about 10% as trandolapril and 70% as trandolaprilat. After oral trandolapril under fasting conditions, peak trandolapril levels occur at about one hour and peak trandolaprilat levels occur between 4 and 10 hours. The elimination half lives of trandolapril and transolaprilat are about 6 and 10 hours, respectively, but, like all ACE inhibitors, trandolaprilat also has a prolonged terminal elimination phase, involving a small fraction of administered drug, probably representing binding to plasma and tissue ACE. During multiple dosing of trandolapril, there is no significant accumulation of trandolaprilat. Food slows absorption of trandolapril, but does not affect AUC or Cmax of trandolaprilat or Cmax of trandolapril.
Metabolism and Excretion After oral administration of trandolapril, about 33% of parent drug and metabolites are recovered in urine, mostly as trandolaprilat, with about 66% in feces. The extent of the absorbed dose which is biliary excreted has not been determined. Plasma concentrations (Cmax and AUC of trandolapril and Cmax of trandolaprilat) are dose proportional over the 1–4 mg range, but the AUC of trandolaprilat is somewhat less than dose proportional. In addition to trandolaprilat, at least 7 other metabolites have been found, principally glucoronides or deesterification products.
Serum protein binding of trandolapril is about 80%, and is independent of concentration. Binding of trandolaprilat is concentration-dependent, varying from 65% at 1000 ng/mL to 94% at 0.1 ng/mL, indicating saturation of binding with increasing concentration.
The volume of distribution of trandolapril is about 18 liters. Total plasma clearances of trandolapril and trandolaprilat after approximately 2 mg IV doses are about 52 liters/hour and 7 liters/hour respectively. Renal clearance of trandolaprilat varies from 1–4 liters/hour, depending on dose.
Special populations:
Pediatric Trandolapril pharmacokinetics have not been evaluated in patients <18 years of age.
Geriatric and Gender Trandolapril pharmacokinetics have been investigated in the elderly (>65 years) and in both genders. The plasma concentration of trandolapril is increased in elderly hypertensive patients, but the plasma concentration of trandolaprilat and inhibition of ACE activity are similar in elderly and young hypertensive patients. The pharmacokinetics of trandolapril and trandolaprilat and inhibition of ACE activity are similar in male and female elderly hypertensive patients.
Race Pharmacokinetic differences have not been evaluated in different races.
Renal Insufficiency Compared to normal subjects, the plasma concentrations of trandolapril and trandolaprilat are approximately 2-fold greater and renal clearance is reduced by about 85% in patients with creatinine clearance below 30 ml/min and in patients on hemodialysis. Dosage adjustment is recommended in renally impaired patients. (See **DOSAGE** and **ADMINISTRATION**.)
Hepatic Insufficiency Following oral administration in patients with mild to moderate alcoholic cirrhosis, plasma concentrations of trandolapril and prandolaprilat were, respectively, 9-fold and 2-fold greater than in normal subjects, but inhibition of ACE activity was not affected. Lower doses should be considered in patients with hepatic insufficiency. (See **DOSAGE** and **ADMINISTRATION**.)
Drug Interactions Trandolapril did not affect the plasma concentration (pre-dose and 2 hours post-dose) of oral digoxin (0.25 mg). Coadministration of trandolapril and cimetidine led to an increase of about 44% in Cmax for trandolapril, but no difference in the pharmacokinetics of trandolaprilat or in ACE inhibition. Coadministration of trandolapril and furosemide led to an increase of about 25% in the renal clearance of trandolaprilat, but no effect was seen on the pharmacokinetics of furosemide or trandolaprilat or on ACE inhibition.
Pharmacodynamics and Clinical Effects:
A single 2–mg dose of MAVIK® produces 70 to 85% inhibition of plasma ACE activity at 4 hours with about 10% decline at 24 hours and about half the effect manifest at 8 days. Maximum ACE inhibition is achieved with a plasma trandolaprilat concentration of 2 ng/mL. ACE inhibition is a function of trandolaprilat concentration, not trandolapril concentration. The effect of trandolapril on exogenous angiotensin I was not measured.
Hypertension
Four placebo-controlled dose response studies were conducted using once-daily oral dosing of MAVIK® in doses from 0.25 to 16 mg per day in 827 black and non-black patients with mild to moderate hypertension. The minimal effective once-daily dose was 1 mg in non-black patients and 2 mg in black patients. Further decreases in trough supine diastolic blood pressure were obtained in non-black patients with higher doses, and no further response was seen with doses above 4 mg (up to 16 mg). The antihypertensive effect diminished somewhat at the end of the dosing interval, but trough/peak ratios are well above 50% for all effective doses. There was a slightly greater effect on the diastolic pressure, but no difference on systolic pressure with b.i.d. dosing. During chronic therapy, the maximum reduction in blood pressure with any dose is achieved within one week. Following 6 weeks of monotherapy in placebo-controlled trials in patients with mild to moderate hypertension, once-daily doses of 2 to 4 mg lowered supine or standing systolic/diastolic blood pressure 24 hours after dosing by an average of 7–10/4–5 mmHg below placebo responses in non-black patients. Once-daily doses of 2 to 4 mg lowered blood pressure 4–6/3–4 mmHg in black patients. Trough to peak ratios for effective doses ranged from 0.5 to 0.9. There were no differences in response between men and women, but responses were somewhat greater in patients under 60 than in patients over 60 years old. Abrupt withdrawal of MAVIK® has not been associated with a rapid increase in blood pressure.
Administration of MAVIK® to patients with mild to moderate hypertension results in a reduction of supine, sitting and standing blood pressure to about the same extent without compensatory tachycardia.
Symptomatic hypotension is infrequent, although it can occur in patients who are salt- and/or volume-depleted. (See **WARNINGS.**) Use of MAVIK® in combination with thiazide diuretics gives a blood pressure lowering effect greater than that seen with either agent alone, and the additional effect of trandolapril is similar to the effect of monotherapy.
Heart Failure Post Myocardial Infarction or Left Ventricular Dysfunction Post Myocardial Infarction:
The Trandolapril Cardiac Evaluation (TRACE) Trial was a Danish, 27-center, double-blind, placebo controlled, parallel-group study of the effect of trandolapril on all-cause mortality in stable patients with echocardiographic evidence of left ventricular dysfunction 3 to 7 days after a myocardial infarction. Subjects with residual ischemia or overt heart failure were included. Patients tolerant of a test dose of 1 mg trandolapril were randomized to placebo (n=873) or trandolapril (n=876) and followed for 24 months. Among patients randomized to trandolapril, who began treatment on 1 mg, 62% were successfully titrated to a target dose of 4 mg once daily over a period of weeks. The use of trandolapril was associated with a 16% reduction in the risk of all-cause mortality (p=0.042), largely cardiovascular mortality. Trandolapril was also associated with a 20% reduction in the risk of progression of heart failure (p=0.047), defined by a time-to-first-event analysis of death attributed to heart failure, hospitalization for heart failure, or requirement for open-label ACE inhibitor for the treatment of heart failure. There was no significant effect of treatment on other endpoints: subsequent hospitalization, incidence of recurrent myocardial infarction, exercise tolerance, ventricular function, ventricular dimensions, or NYHA class.
The population in TRACE was entirely Caucasian and had less usage than would be typical in a U.S. population of other post-infarction interventions: 42% thrombolysis, 16% beta-adrenergic blockade, and 6.7% PTCA or CABG during the entire period of follow-up. Blood pressure control, especially in the placebo group, was poor: 47 to 53% of patients randomized to placebo and 32 to 40% of patients randomized to trandolapril had blood pressures >140/95 at 90-day follow-up visits.

INDICATIONS AND USAGE

Hypertension
MAVIK® is indicated for the treatment of hypertension. It may be used alone or in combination with other antihypertensive medication such as hydrochlorothiazide.
In considering the use of MAVIK®, it should be noted that in controlled trials ACE inhibitors (for which adequate data are available) cause a higher rate of angioedema in black than in non-black patients. (See **Warnings**: **Angioedema**.)
When using MAVIK®, consideration should be given to the fact that another angiotensin converting enzyme inhibitor, captopril, has caused agranulocytosis, particularly in patients with renal impairment or collagen-vascular disease. Available data are insufficient to show that MAVIK® does not have a similar risk. (See **WARNINGS**.)
Heart Failure Post Myocardial Infarction or Left-Ventricular Dysfunction Post Myocardial Infarction:
MAVIK® is indicated in stable patients who have evidence of left-ventricular systolic dysfunction (identified by wall motion abnormalities) or who are symptomatic from congestive heart failure within the first few days after sustaining acute myocardial infarction. Administration of trandolapril to Caucasian patients has been shown to decrease the risk of death (principally cardiovascular death) and to decrease the risk of heart failure-related hospitalization (See **CLINICAL PHARMACOLOGY, Heart Failure or Left-Ventricular Dysfunction Post Myocardial Infarction** for details of the survival trial.)

CONTRAINDICATIONS

MAVIK® is contraindicated in patients who are hypersensitive to this product and in patients with a history of angioedema related to previous treatment with an ACE inhibitor.

WARNINGS

Anaphylactoid and Possibly Related Reactions:
Presumably because angiotensin converting enzyme inhibitors affect the metabolism of eicosanoids and polypeptides, including endogenous bradykinin, patients receiving ACE inhibitors, including MAVIK®, may be subject to a variety of adverse reactions, some of them serious.
Angioedema:
Angioedema of the face, extremities, lips, tongue, glottis, and larynx has been reported in patients treated with ACE inhibitors including MAVIK®. Symptoms suggestive of angioedema or facial edema occurred in 0.13% of MAVIK®-treated patients. Two of the four cases were life-threatening and resolved without treatment or with medication (corticosteroids). Angioedema associated with laryngeal edema can be fatal. If laryngeal stridor or angioedema of the face, tongue or glottis occurs, treatment with MAVIK® should be discontinued immediately, the patient treated in accordance with accepted medical care and carefully observed until the

Continued on next page

Mavik—Cont.

swelling disappears. In instances where swelling is confined to the face and lips, the condition generally resolves without treatment; antihistamines may be useful in relieving symptoms. **Where there is involvement of the tongue, glottis, or larynx, likely to cause airway obstruction, emergency therapy, including but not limited to subcutaneous epinephrine solution 1:1,000 (0.3 to 0.5 mL) should be promptly administered.** (See **PRECAUTIONS**: Information for Patients and **ADVERSE REACTIONS**.)

Anaphylactoid Reactions During Desensitization Two patients undergoing desentizing treatment with hymenoptera venom while receiving ACE inhibitors sustained life-threatening anaphylactoid reactions. In the same patients, these reactions did not occur when ACE inhibitors were temporarily withheld, but they reappeared when the ACE inhibitors were inadvertently readministered.

Anaphylactoid Reactions During Membrane Exposure- Anaphylactoid reactions have been reported in patients dialyzed with high-flux membranes and treated concomitantly with an ACE inhibitor. Anaphylactoid reactions have also been reported in patients undergoing low-density lipoprotein apheresis with dextran sulfate absorption.

Hypotension:

MAVIK® can cause symptomatic hypotension. Like other ACE inhibitors, MAVIK® has only rarely been associated with symptomatic hypotension in uncomplicated hypertensive patients. Symptomatic hypotension is most likely to occur in patients who have been sale- or volume-depleted as a result of prolonged treatment with diuretics, dietary sale restriction, dialysis, diarrhea, or vomiting. Volume and/or sale depletion should be corrected before initiating treatment with MAVIK®. (See **PRECAUTIONS**, Drug Interactions, and **ADVERSE REACTIONS**.) In controlled and uncontrolled studies, hypotension was reported as an adverse event in 0.6 percent of patients and led to discontinuations in 0.1% of patients.

In patients with concomitant congestive heart failure, with or without associated renal insufficiency, ACE inhibitor therapy may cause excessive hypotension, which may be associated with oliguria or azotemia, and rarely, with acute renal failure and death. In such patients, MAVIK® therapy should be started at the recommended dose under close medical supervision. These patients should be followed closely during the first 2 weeks of treatment and, thereafter, whenever the dosage of MAVIK® or diuretic is increased. (See **DOSAGE** and **ADMINISTRATION**.) Care in avoiding hypotension should also be taken in patients with ischemic heart disease, aortic stenosis, or cerebrovascular disease.

If symptomatic hypotension occurs, the patient should be placed in the supine position and, if necessary, normal saline may be administered intravenously. A transient hypotensive response is not a contraindication to further doses; however, lower doses of MAVIK® or reduced concomitant diuretic therapy should be considered.

Neutropenia/Agranulocytosis:

Another ACE inhibitor, captopril, has been shown to cause agranulocytosis and bone marrow depression rarely in patients with uncomplicated hypertension, but more frequently in patients with renal impairment, especially if they also have a collagen-vascular disease such as systemic lupus erythematosus or scleroderma. Available data from clinical trials of trandolapril are insufficient to show that trandolapril does not cause agranulocytosis at similar rates. As with other ACE inhibitors, periodic monitoring of white blood cell counts in patients with collagen-vascular disease and/or renal disease should be considered.

Hepatic Failure:

ACE inhibitors rarely have been associated with a syndrome of cholestatic jaundice, fulminant hepatic necrosis, and death. The mechanism of this syndrome is not understood. Patients receiving ACE inhibitors who develop jaundice should discontinue the ACE inhibitor and receive appropriate medical follow-up.

Fetal/Neonatal Morbidity and Mortality:

ACE inhibitors can cause fetal and neonatal morbidity and death when administered to pregnant women. Several dozen cases have been reported in the world literature. When pregnancy is detected, ACE inhibitors should be discontinued as soon as possible.

The use of ACE inhibitors during the second and third trimesters of pregnancy has been associated with fetal and neonatal injury, including hypotension, neonatal skull hypoplasia anuria, reversible or irreversible renal failure, and death. Oligohydramnios has also been reported, presumably resulting from decreased fetal renal function; oligohydramnios in this setting has been associated with fetal limb contractures, craniofacial deformation, and hypoplastic lung development. Prematurity, intrauterine growth retardation, and patent ductus arteriosus have also been reported, although it is not clear whether these occurrences were due to the ACE inhibitor exposure.

These adverse effects do not appear to have resulted from intrauterine ACE-inhibitor exposure that has been limited to the first trimester. Mothers whose embryos and fetuses are exposed to ACE inhibitors only during the first trimester should be so informed. Nonetheless, when patients become pregnant, physicians should make every effort to discontinue the use of trandolapril as soon as possible.

Rarely (probably less often than once in every thousand pregnancies), no alternative to ACE inhibitors will be found. In these rare cases, the mothers should be apprised of the potential hazards to their fetuses, and serial ultrasound examinations should be performed to assess the intra-amniotic environment.

If oligohydramnios is observed, trandolapril should be discontinued unless it is considered life-saving for the mother. Contraction stress testing (CST), a non-stress test (NST), or biophysical profiling (BPP) may be appropriate, depending upon the week of pregnancy.

Patients and physicians should be aware, however, that oligohydramnios may not appear until after the fetus has sustained irreversible injury.

Infants with histories of *in utero* exposure to ACE inhibitors should be closely observed for hypotension, oliguria, and hyperkalemia. If oliguria occurs, attention should be directed toward support of blood pressure and renal perfusion. Exchange transfusions or dialysis may be required as a means of reversing hypotension and/or substituting for disordered renal function.

Doses of 0.8 mg/kg/day (9.4 mg/m^2/day) in rabbits, 1000 mg/kg/day (7000 mg/m^2/day) in rats, and 25 mg/kg/day (295 mg/m^2/day) in cynomoglus monkeys did not produce teratogenic effects. These doses represent 10 and 3 times (rabbits), 1250 and 2564 times (rats), and 312 and 108 times (monkeys) the maximum projected human dose of 4 mg based on body-weight and body-surface-area, respectively assuming a 50 kg woman.

PRECAUTIONS

General

Impaired Renal Function:

As a consequence of inhibiting the renin-angiotensin-aldosterone system, changes in renal function may be anticipated in susceptible individuals. In patients with severe heart failure whose renal function may depend on the activity of the renin-angiotensin-aldosterone system, treatment with ACE inhibitors, including MAVIK®, may be associated with oliguria and/or progressive azotemia and rarely with acute renal failure and/or death.

In hypertensive patients with unilateral or bilateral renal artery stenosis, increases in blood urea nitrogen and serum creatinine have been observed in some patients following ACE inhibitor therapy. These increases were almost always reversible upon discontinuation of the ACE inhibitor and/or diuretic therapy. In such patients, renal function should be monitored during the first few weeks of therapy.

Some hypertensive patients with no apparent preexisting renal vascular disease have developed increases in blood urea and serum creatinine, usually minor and transient, especially when ACE inhibitors have been given concomitantly with a diuretic. This is more likely to occur in patients with preexisting renal impairment. Dosage reduction and/or discontinuation of any diuretic and/or the ACE inhibitor may be required.

Evaluation of hypertensive patients should always include assessment of renal function. (See **DOSAGE** and **ADMINISTRATION**.)

Hyperkalemia and potassium-sparing diuretics:

In clinical trials, hyperkalemia (serum potassium > 6.00 mEq/L) occurred in approximately 0.4 percent of hypertensive patients receiving MAVIK®. In most cases, elevated serum potassium levels were isolated values, which resolved despite continued therapy. None of these patients were discontinued from the trials because of hyperkalemia. Risk factors for the development of hyperkalemia include renal insufficiency, diabetes mellitus, and the concomitant use of potassium-sparing diuretics, potassium supplements, and/or potassium-containing salt substitutes, which should be used cautiously, if at all, with MAVIK®. (See **PRECAUTIONS:** Drug Interactions.)

Cough:

Presumably due to the inhibition of the degradation of endogenous bradykinin, persistent nonproductive cough has been reported with all ACE inhibitors, always resolving after discontinuation of therapy. ACE inhibitor-induced cough should be considered in the differential diagnosis of cough. In controlled trials of trandolapril, cough was present in 2% of trandolapril patients and 0% of patients given placebo. There was no evidence of a relationship to dose.

Surgery/anesthesia:

In patients undergoing major surgery or during anesthesia with agnets that produce hypotension, MAVIK® will block angiotensin II formation secondary to compensatory renin release. If hypotension occurs and is considered to be due to this mechanism, it can be corrected by volume expansion.

Information for Patients

Angioedema:

Angioedema, including laryngeal edema, may occur at any time during treatment with ACE inhibitors, including MAVIK®. Patients should be so advised and told to report immediately any signs or symptoms suggesting angioedema (swelling of face, extremities, eyes, lips, tongue, difficulty in swallowing or breathing) and to stop taking the drug until they have consulted with their physician. (See **WARNINGS** and **ADVERSE REACTIONS**.)

Symptomatic Hypotension:

Patients should be cautioned that light-headedness can occur, especially during the first days of MAVIK® therapy, and should be reported to a physician. If actual syncope occurs, patients should be told to stop taking the drug until they have consulted with their physician (See **WARNINGS**.)

All patients should be cautioned that inadequate fluid intake, excessive perspiration, diarrhea, or vomiting, resulting in reduced fluid volume, may precipitate an excessive fall in blood pressure with the same consequences of light-headedness and possible syncope.

Patients planning to undergo any surgery and/or anesthesia should be told to inform their physician that they are taking an ACE inhibitor that has a long duration of action.

Hyperkalemia:

Patients should be told not to use potassium supplements or salt substitutes containing potassium without consulting their physician. (See **PRECAUTIONS**.)

Neutropenia:

Patients should be told to report promptly any indication of infection (e.g., sore throat, fever) which could be a sign of neutropenia.

Pregnancy:

Female patients of childbearing age should be told about the consequences of second- and third-trimester exposure to ACE inhibitors, and they should also be told that these consequences do not appear to have resulted from intrauterine ACE-inhibitor exposure that has been limited to the first trimester. These patients should be asked to report pregnancies to their physicians as soon as possible.

NOTE: As with many other drugs, certain advice to patients being treated with MAVIK® is warranted. This information is intended to aid in the safe and effective use of this medication. It is not a disclosure of all possible adverse or intended effects.

Drug Interactions

Concomitant diuretic therapy:

As with other ACE inhibitors, patients on diuretics, especially those on recently instituted diuretic therapy, may experience an excessive reduction of blood pressure after initiation of therapy with MAVIK®. The possibility of exacerbation of hypotensive effects with MAVIK® may be minimized by either discontinuing the diuretic or cautiously increasing salt intake prior to initiation of treatment with MAVIK®. If it is not possible to discontinue the diuretic, the starting dose of trandolapril should be reduced (See **DOSAGE** and **ADMINISTRATION**.)

Agents increasing serum potassium:

Trandolapril can attenuate potassium loss caused by thiazide diuretics and increase serum potassium when used alone. Use of potassium-sparing diuretics (spironolactone, triamterene, or amiloride), potassium supplements, or potassium-containing salt substitutes concomitantly with ACE inhibitors can increase the risk of hyperkalemia. If concomitant use of such agents is indicated, they should be used with caution and with appropriate monitoring of serum potassium. (See **PRECAUTIONS**.)

Lithium:

Increased serum lithium levels and symptoms of lithium toxicity have been reported in patients receiving concomitant lithium and ACE inhibitor therapy. These drugs should be coadministered with caution, and frequent monitoring of serum lithium levels is recommended. If a diuretic is also used, the risk of lithium toxicity may be increased.

Other:

No clinically significant interaction has been found between trandolaprilat and food, cimetidine, digoxin, or furosemide. The anticoagulant effect of warfarin was not significantly changed by trandolapril.

Carcinogenesis, Mutagenesis, Impariment of Fertility

Long-term studies were conducted with oral trandolapril administered by gavage to mice (78 weeks) and rats (104 and 106 weeks). No evidence of carcinogenic potential was seen in mice dosed up to 25 mg/kg/day (85 mg/m^2/day) or rats dosed up to 8 mg/kg/day (60 mg/m^2/day). These doses are 313 and 32 times (mice), and 100 and 23 times (rats) the maximum recommended human daily dose (MRHDD) of 4 mg based on body-weight and body-surface-area, respectively assuming a 50 kg individual. The genotoxic potential of trandolapril was evaluated in the microbial mutagenicity (Ames) test, the point mutation and chromosome aberration assays in Chinese hamster V79 cells, and the micronucleus test in mice. There was no evidence of mutgenic or clastogenic potential in these in vitro and in vivo assays.

Reproduction studies in rats did not show any impairment of fertility at doses up to 100 mg/kg/day (710 mg/m^2/day) of trandolapril, or 1250 and 260 times the MRHDD on the basis of body-weight and body-surface-area, respectively

Pregnancy

Pregnancy Categories C (first trimester) and D (second and third trimesters): See WARNINGS, Fetal/Neonatal Morbidity and mortality.

Nursing Mothers

Radiolabeled trandolapril or its metabolites are secreted in rat milk. MAVIK® (trandolapril) should not be administered to nursing mothers.

Geriatric Use

In placebo-controlled studies of MAVIK®, 31.1% of patients were 60 years and older, 20.1% were 65 years and older, and 2.3% were 75 years and older. No overall differences in effectiveness or safety were observed between these patients and younger patients. (Greater sensitivity of some older individual patients cannot be ruled out).

Pediatric use

The safety and effectiveness of MAVIK® in pediatric patients have not been established.

ADVERSE REACTIONS

The safety experience in U.S. placebo-controlled trials included 1067 hypertensive patients, of whom 831 received MAVIK®. Nearly 200 hypertensive patients received MAVIK® for over one year in open-label trials. In controlled trials, withdrawals for adverse events were 2.1% on placebo and 1.4% on MAVIK®. Adverse events considered at least possibly related to treatment occurring in 1% of MAVIK®-treated patients and more common on MAVIK® than placeob, pooled for all doses, are shown below, together with the frequency of discontinuation of treatment because of these events.

ADVERSE EVENTS IN PLACEBO-CONTROLLED HYPERTENSION TRIALS
Occurring at 1% or greater

	MAVIK (N=832) % Incidence (% Discontinuance)	PLACEBO (N=237) % Incidence (% Discontinuance)
Cough	1.9 (0.1)	0.4 (0.4)
Dizziness	1.3 (0.2)	0.4 (0.4)
Diarrhea	1.0 (0.0)	0.4 (0.0)

Headache and fatigue were all seen in more than 1% of MAVIK®-treated patients but were more frequently seen on placebo. Adverse events were not usually persistent or difficult to manage.

Left Ventricular Dysfunction Post Myocardial Infarction: Adverse reactions related to Mavik®, occurring at a rate greater than that observed in placebo-treated patients with left ventricular dysfunction, are shown below. The incidences represent the experiences from the TRACE study. The follow-up time was between 24 and 50 months for this study.

Percentage of Patients with Adverse Events Greater Than Placebo

Adverse Event	Placebo-Controlled (TRACE) Mortality Study Trandolapril N=876	Placebo N=873
Cough	35	22
Dizziness	23	17
Hypotension	11	6.8
Elevated Serum uric acid	15	13
Elevated BUN	9.0	7.6
PICA or CABG	7.3	6.1
Dyspepsia	6.4	6.0
Syncope	5.9	3.3
Hyperkalemia	5.3	2.8
Bradycardia	4.7	4.4
Hypocalcemia	4.7	3.9
Myalgia	4.7	3.1
Elevated Creatinine	4.7	2.4
Gastritis	4.2	3.6
Cardiogenic shock	3.8	<2
Intermittent claudication	3.8	<2
Stroke	3.3	3.2
Asthenia	3.3	2.6

Clinical adverse experiences possibly or probably related or of uncertain relationship to therapy occurring in 0.3% to 1.0% (except as noted) of the patients treated with MAVIK® (with or without concomitant calcium ion antagonist or diuretic) in controlled or uncontrolled trials (N=1134) and less frequent, clinically significant events seen in clinical trials or post-marketing experience (the rarer events are in italics) include (listed by body system):

General Body Function: chest pain.

Cardiovascular: AV first degree block, bradycardia, edema, flushing, hypotension, palpitations.

Central Nervous System: drowsiness, insomnia, paresthesia, vertigo.

Dermatologic: pruritus, rash, pemphigus.

Eye, Ear, Nose, Throat: epistaxis, throat inflammation, upper respiratory tract infection.

Emotional, Mental, Sexual States: anxiety, impotence, decreased libido.

Gastrointestinal: abdominal distention, abdominal pain/cramps, constipation, dyspepsia, diarrhea, vomiting, *pancreatitis.*

Hemopoietic: *decreased leukocytes, decreased neutrophils.*

Metabolism and Endocrine: *increased creatinine, increased potassium,* increased SGPT (ALT).

Musculoskeletal System: extremity pain, muscle cramps, gout.

Pulmonary: dyspnea.

Angioedema: Angioedema has been reported in 4 (0.13%) patients receiving MAVIK® in U.S. and foreign studies. Angioedema associated with laryngeal edema may be fatal. If angioedema of the face, extremities, lips, tongue, glottis, and/or larynx occurs, treatment with MAVIK® should be discontinued and appropriate therapy instituted immediately. (See **WARNINGS.**)

Hypotension: In hypertensive patients, symptomatic hypotension occurred in 0.6 percent and near syncope occurred in 0.2 percent. Hypotension or syncope was a cause for discontinuation of therapy in 0.1 percent of hypertensive patients.

Fetal/Neonatal Morbidity and Mortality: See **WARNINGS,** Fetal Neonatal Morbidity and Mortality.

Cough: See **PRECAUTIONS,** Cough.

Clinical Laboratory Test Findings

Hematology: (See **WARNINGS.**) Low white blood cells, low neutrophils, low lymphocytes, thrombocytopenia.

Serum Electrolytes: Hyperkalemia (See **PRECAUTIONS,**) hyponatremia.

Creatinine and Blood Urea Nitrogen: Increases in creatinine levels occurred in 1.1 percent of patients receiving MAVIK® alone and 7.3 percent of patients treated with MAVIK®, a calcium ion antagonist and a diuretic. Increases in blood urea nitrogen levels occurred in 0.6 percent of patients receiving MAVIK® alone and 1.4 percent of patients receiving MAVIK®, a calcium ion antagonist, and a diuretic. None of these increases required discontinuation of treatment. Increases in these laboratory values are more likely to occur in patients with renal insufficiency or those pretreated with a diuretic and, based on experience with other ACE inhibitors, would be expected to be especially likely in patients with renal artery stenosis. (See **PRECAUTIONS** and **WARNINGS.**)

Liver function tests: Occasional elevation of transaminases at the rate of 3X upper normals occurred in 0.8% of patients and persistent increase in bilirubin occurred in 0.2% of patients. Discontinuation for elevated liver enzymes occurred in 0.2 percent of patients.

OVERDOSAGE

No data are available with respect to overdosage in humans. The oral LD_{50} of trandolapril in mice was 4875 mg/Kg in males and 3990 mg/Kg in females. In rats, an oral dose of 5000 mg/Kg caused low mortality (1 male out of 5; 0 females). In dogs, an oral dose of 1000 mg/Kg did not cause mortality and abnormal clinical signs were not observed. In humans the most likely clinical manifestation would be symptoms attributable to severe hypotension.

Laboratory determinations of serum levels of trandolapril and its metabolites are not widely available, and such determinations have, in any event, no established role in the management of trandolapril overdose. No data are available to suggest that physiological maneuvers (e.g., maneuvers to change the pH of the urine) might accelerate elimination of trandolapril and its metabolites. Trandolaprilat is removed by hemodialysis. Angiotension II could presumably serve as a specific antagonist antidote in the settling of trandolapril overdose, but angiotension II is essentially unavailable outside of scattered research facilities. Because the hypotensive effect of trandolapril is achieved through vasodilation and effective hypovolemia, it is reasonable to treat trandolapril overdose by infusion of normal saline solution.

DOSAGE AND ADMINISTRATION

The recommended initial dosage of MAVIK® for patients not receiving a diuretic is 1 mg once daily in non-black patients and 2 mg in black patients. Dosage should be adjusted according to the blood pressure response. Generally, dosage adjustments should be made at intervals of at least 1 week. Most patients have required dosages of 2 to 4 mg once daily. There is little clinical experience with doses above 8 mg.

Patients inadequately treated with once-daily dosing at 4 mg may be treated with twice-daily dosing. If blood pressure is not adequately controlled with MAVIK® monotherapy, a diuretic may be added.

In patients who are currently being treated with a diuretic, symptomatic hypotension occasionally can occur following the initial dose of MAVIK®. To reduce the likelihood of hypotension, the diuretic should, if possible, be discontinued two to three days prior to beginning therapy with MAVIK®. (See **WARNINGS.**) Then, if blood pressure is not controlled with MAVIK® alone, diuretic therapy should be resumed. If the diuretic cannot be discontinued, an initial dose of 0.5 mg MAVIK® should be used with careful medical supervision for several hours until blood pressure has stabilized. The dosage should subsequently be titrated (as described above) to the optimal response. (See **WARNINGS, PRECAUTIONS,** and **Drug Interactions.**)

Concomitant administration of MAVIK® with potassium supplements, potassium salt substitutes, or potassium-sparing diuretics can lead to increases of serum potassium. (See **PRECAUTIONS.**)

Dosage Adjustment in Renal Impairment or Hepatic Cirrhosis:

For patients with a creatinine clearance <30 mL/min. or with hepatic cirrhosis, the recommended starting dose, based on clinical and pharmacokinetic data, is 0.5 mg daily. Patients should subsequently have their dosage titrated (as described above) to the optimal response.

HOW SUPPLIED

MAVIK® tablets are supplied as follows:

1 mg tablet— salmon colored, round shaped, scored, compressed tablets, with code KNOLL 1 on one side.
NDC (0048-5805-01-bottles of 100)
NDC (0048-5805-41-unit dose packs of 100)

2 mg tablet— yellow colored, round shaped, compressed tablets with code KNOLL 2 on one side.
NDC (0048-5806-01-bottles of 100)
NDC (0048-5806-41-unit dose packs of 100)

4 mg tablet— rose colored, round shaped, compressed tablets, with code KNOLL 4 on one side.
NDC (0048-5807-01-bottles of 100)
NDC (0048-5807-41-unit dose packs of 100)

Dispense in well-closed container with safety closure.

Storage: Store at controlled room temperature 20–25°C (68–77°F) see USP.

Caution: Federal law prohibits dispensing without prescription.

Revised: June 1997

Knoll Pharmaceutical Company
3000 Continental Drive-North
Mount Olive, New Jersey 07828-1234
BASF Pharma

0983000-3

Shown in Product Identification Guide, page 319

MERIDIA® ℂ ℞

[mĕr-ĭdĭa]

(sibutramine hydrochloride monohydrate) Capsules
Rx only

DESCRIPTION

MERIDIA® (sibutramine hydrochloride monohydrate) is an orally administered agent for the treatment of obesity. Chemically, the active ingredient is a racemic mixture of the (+) and (−) enantiomers of cyclobutanemethanamine, 1-(4-chlorophenyl)-*N*, *N*-dimethyl-α-(2-methylpropyl)-, hydrochloride, monohydrate, and has an empirical formula of $C_{17}H_{29}Cl_2NO$. Its molecular weight is 334.33.

The structural formula is shown below:

Sibutramine hydrochloride monohydrate is a white to cream crystalline powder with a solubility of 2.9 mg/mL in pH 5.2 water. Its octanol:water partition coefficient is 30.9 at pH 5.0.

Each MERIDIA capsule contains 5 mg, 10 mg, 15 mg of sibutramine hydrochloride monohydrate. It also contains as inactive ingredients: lactose monohydrate, NF; microcrystalline cellulose, NF; colloidal silicon dioxide, NF; and magnesium stearate, NF in a hard-gelatin capsule [which contains titanium dioxide, USP; gelatin; FD&C Blue No. 2 (5- and 10-mg capsules only); D&C Yellow No. 10 (5- and 15-mg capsules only), and other inactive ingredients].

CLINICAL PHARMACOLOGY

Mode of Action

Sibutramine produces its therapeutic effects by norepinephrine, serotonin and dopamine reuptake inhibition. Sibutramine and its major pharmacologically active metabolites (M_1 and M_2) do not act via release of monoamines.

Pharmacodynamics

Sibutramine exerts its pharmacological actions predominantly via its secondary (M_1) and primary (M_2) amine metabolites. The parent compound, sibutramine, is a potent inhibitor of serotonin (5-hydroxytryptamine, 5-HT) and norepinephrine reuptake *in vivo*, but not *in vitro*. However, metabolites M_1 and M_2 inhibit the reuptake of these neurotransmitters both *in vitro* and *in vivo*.

In human brain tissue, M_1 and M_2 also inhibit dopamine reuptake *in vitro*, but with ~3-fold lower potency than for the reuptake inhibition of serotonin or norepinephrine.

Potencies of Sibutramine, M_1 and M_2 as *In Vitro* Inhibitors of Monoamine Reuptake in Human Brain

Potency to Inhibit Monoamine Reuptake (K_i; nM)

	Serotonin	Norepinephrine	Dopamine
Sibutramine	298	5451	943
M_1	15	20	49
M_2	20	15	45

A study using plasma samples taken from sibutramine-treated volunteers showed monoamine reuptake inhibition of norepinephrine > serotonin > dopamine; maximum inhibitions were norepinephrine = 73%, serotonin = 54% and dopamine = 16%.

Sibutramine and its metabolites (M_1 and M_2) are not serotonin, norepinephrine or dopamine releasing agents. Following chronic administration of sibutramine to rats, no depletion of brain monoamines has been observed.

Sibutramine, M_1 and M_2 exhibit no evidence of anticholinergic or antihistaminergic actions. In addition, receptor binding profiles show that sibutramine, M_1 and M_2 have low affinity for serotonin (5-HT_1, 5-HT_{1A}, 5-HT_{1B}, 5-HT_{2A}, 5-HT_{2C}), norepinephrine (β, $β_1$, $β_3$, $α_1$ and $α_2$), dopamine (D_1 and D_2), benzodiazepine, and glutamate (NMDA) receptors. These compounds also lack monoamine oxidase inhibitory activity *in vitro* and *in vivo*.

Pharmacokinetics

Absorption

Sibutramine is rapidly absorbed from the GI tract (T_{max} of 1.2 hours) following oral administration and undergoes extensive first-pass metabolism in the liver (oral clearance of 1750 L/h and half-life of 1.1 h) to form the pharmacologically active mono- and di- desmethyl metabolites M_1 and M_2. Peak plasma concentrations of M_1 and M_2 are reached within 3 to 4 hours. On the basis of mass balance studies, on average, at least 77% of a single oral dose of sibutramine is absorbed. The absolute bioavailability of sibutramine has not been determined.

Distribution

Radiolabeled studies in animals indicated rapid and extensive distribution into tissues: highest concentrations of radiolabeled material were found in the eliminating organs, liver and kidney. Tissue distribution was unaffected by pregnancy, with relatively low transfer to the fetus. *In vitro*,

Continued on next page

Meridia—Cont.

sibutramine, M_1 and M_2 are extensively bound (97%, 94% and 94%, respectively) to human plasma proteins at plasma concentrations seen following therapeutic doses.

Metabolism

Sibutramine is metabolized in the liver principally by the cytochrome P450(3A_4) isoenzyme, to desmethyl metabolites, M_1 and M_2. These active metabolites are further metabolized by hydroxylation and conjugation to pharmacologically inactive metabolites, M_5 and M_6. Following oral administration of radiolabeled sibutramine, essentially all of the peak radiolabeled material in plasma was accounted for by unchanged sibutramine (3%), M_1 (6%), M_2 (12%), M_5 (52%), and M_6 (27%).

M_1 and M_2 plasma concentrations reached steady-state within four days of dosing and were approximately two-fold higher than following a single dose. The elimination half-lives of M_1 and M_2, 14 and 16 hours, respectively, were unchanged following repeated dosing.

Excretion

Approximately 85% (range 68-95%) of a single orally administered radiolabeled dose was excreted in urine and feces over a 15-day collection period with the majority of the dose (77%) excreted in the urine. Major metabolites in urine were $M_5$and M_6; unchanged sibutramine, M_1, and M_2 were not detected. The primary route of excretion for M_1 and M_2 is hepatic metabolism and for M_5 and M_6 is renal excretion.

[See first table above]

Effect of Food

Administration of a single 20 mg dose of sibutramine with a standard breakfast resulted in reduced peak M_1 and M_2 concentrations (by 27% and 32%, respectively) and delayed the time to peak by approximately three hours. However, the AUCs of M_1 and M_2 were not significantly altered.

Special Populations

Geriatric: Plasma concentrations of M_1 and M_2 were similar between elderly (ages 61 to 77 yr) and young (ages 19 to 30 yr) subjects following a single 15-mg oral sibutramine dose. Plasma concentrations of the inactive metabolites M_5 and M_6 were higher in the elderly; these differences are not likely to be of clinical significance. In general, dose selection for an elderly patient should be cautious, reflecting the greater frequency of decreased hepatic, renal, or cardiac function, and of concomitant disease or other drug therapy.

Pediatric: The safety and effectiveness of MERIDIA in pediatric patients under 16 years old have not been established.

Gender: Pooled pharmacokinetic parameters from 54 young, healthy volunteers (37 males and 17 females) receiving a 15-mg oral dose of sibutramine showed the mean C_{max} and AUC of M_1 and M_2 to be slightly (≤19% and ≤36%, respectively) higher in females than males. Somewhat higher steady-state trough plasma levels were observed in female obese patients from a large clinical efficacy trial. However, these differences are not likely to be of clinical significance. Dosage adjustment based upon the gender of a patient is not necessary (see **"DOSAGE AND ADMINISTRATION"**).

Race: The relationship between race and steady-state trough M_1 and M_2 plasma concentrations was examined in a clinical trial in obese patients. A trend towards higher concentrations in Black patients over Caucasian was noted for $M_1$and M_2. However, these differences are not considered to be of clinical significance.

Renal Insufficiency: The effect of renal disease has not been studied. However, since sibutramine and its active metabolites M_1 and M_2 are eliminated by hepatic metabolism, renal disease is unlikely to have a significant effect on their disposition. Elimination of the inactive metabolites M_5 and M_6, which are renally excreted, may be affected in this population. MERIDIA, should not be used in patients with severe renal impairment.

Hepatic Insufficiency: In 12 patients with moderate hepatic impairment receiving a single 15-mg oral dose of sibutramine, the combined AUCs of M_1 and M_2 were increased by 24% compared to healthy subjects while M_5 and M_6 plasma concentrations were unchanged. The observed differences in M_1 and M_2 concentrations do not warrant dosage adjustment in patients with mild to moderate hepatic impairment. MERIDIA should not be used in patients with severe hepatic dysfunction.

CLINICAL STUDIES

Observational epidemiologic studies have established a relationship between obesity and the risks for cardiovascular disease, non-insulin dependent diabetes mellitus (NIDDM), certain forms of cancer, gallstones, certain respiratory disorders, and an increase in overall mortality. These studies suggest that weight loss, if maintained, may produce health benefits for some patients with chronic obesity who may also be at risk for other diseases.

The long-term effects of MERIDIA on the morbidity and mortality associated with obesity have not been established. Weight loss was examined in 11 double-blind, placebo-controlled obesity trials with study durations of 12 to 52 weeks and doses ranging from 1 to 30 mg once daily. Weight was significantly reduced in a dose-related manner in sibutramine-treated patients compared to placebo over the dose range of 5 to 20 mg once daily. In two 12-month studies, maximal weight loss was achieved by 6 months and statistically significant weight loss was maintained over 12 months. The amount of placebo-subtracted weight loss achieved on MERIDIA was consistent across studies.

Summary of Pharmacokinetic Parameters

Mean (% CV) and 95% Confidence Intervals of Pharmacokinetic Parameters (Dose = 15 mg)

Study Population	C_{max} (ng/mL)	T_{max} (h)	AUC† (ng*h/mL)	T½ (h)
Metabolite M_1				
Target Population:				
Obese Subjects	4.0 (42)	3.6 (28)	25.5 (63)	- -
(n=18)	3.2 – 4.8	3.1 – 4.1	18.1 – 32.9	
Special Population:				
Moderate Hepatic	2.2 (36)	3.3 (33)	18.7 (65)	- -
Impairment (n=12)	1.8 – 2.7	2.7 – 3.9	11.9 – 25.5	
Metabolite M_2				
Target Population:				
Obese Subjects	6.4 (28)	3.5 (17)	92.1 (26)	17.2 (58)
(n=18)	5.6 – 7.2	3.2 – 3.8	81.2 – 103	12.5 – 21.8
Special Population:				
Moderate Hepatic	4.3 (37)	3.8 (34)	90.5 (27)	22.7 (30)
Impairment (n=12)	3.4 – 5.2	3.1 – 4.5	76.9 – 104	18.9 – 26.5

† Calculated only up to 24 hr for M_1

Mean Weight Loss (lbs) in the Six-Month and One-Year Trials

		MERIDIA (mg)			
Study/Patient Group	Placebo (n)	5 (n)	10 (n)	15 (n)	20 (n)
Study 1					
All patients*	2.0	6.6	9.7	12.1	13.6
	(142)	(148)	(148)	(150)	(145)
Completers**	2.9	8.1	12.1	15.4	18.0
	(84)	(103)	(95)	(94)	(89)
Early responders***	8.5	13.0	16.0	18.2	20.1
	(17)	(60)	(64)	(73)	(76)
Study 2					
All patients*	3.5		9.8	14.0	
	(157)		(154)	(152)	
Completers**	4.8		13.6	15.2	
	(76)		(80)	(93)	
Early responders***	10.7		18.2	18.8	
	(24)		(57)	(76)	
Study 3****					
All patients*	15.2		28.4		
	(78)		(81)		
Completers**	16.7		29.7		
	(48)		(60)		
Early responders***	21.5		33.0		
	(22)		(46)		

* Data for all patients who received study drug and who had any post-baseline measurement (last observation carried forward analysis).

** Data for all patients who completed the entire 6-month (Study 1) or one-year period of dosing and have data recorded for the month 6 (Study 1) or month 12 visit.

*** Data for patients who lost at least 4 lbs in the first 4 weeks of treatment and completed the study.

**** Weight loss data shown describe changes in weight from the pre-VLCD; mean weight loss during the 4-week VLCD was 16.9 lbs for sibutramine and 16.3 lbs for placebo.

Analysis of the data in three long-term (≥6 months) obesity trials indicates that patients who lose at least 4 pounds in the first 4 weeks of therapy with a given dose of MERIDIA are most likely to achieve significant long-term weight loss on that dose of MERIDIA. Approximately 60% of such patients went on to achieve a placebo-subtracted weight loss of ≥5% of their initial body weight by month 6. Conversely, of those patients on a given dose of MERIDIA who did not lose at least 4 pounds in the first 4 weeks of therapy, approximately 80% did not go on to achieve a placebo-subtracted weight loss of ≥5% of their initial body weight on that dose by month 6.

Significant dose-related reductions in waist circumference, an indicator of intra-abdominal fat, have also been observed over 6 and 12 months in placebo-controlled clinical trials. In a 12-week placebo-controlled study of non-insulin dependent diabetes mellitus patients randomized to placebo or 15 mg per day of MERIDIA, Dual Energy X-Ray Absorptiometry (DEXA) assessment of changes in body composition showed that total body fat mass decreased by 1.8 kg in the MERIDIA group versus 0.2 kg in the placebo group ($p<0.001$). Similarly, truncal (android) fat mass decreased by 0.6 kg in the MERIDIA group versus 0.1 kg in the placebo group ($p<0.01$). The changes in lean mass, fasting blood sugar, and HbA_1 were not statistically different between the two groups.

Eleven double-blind, placebo-controlled obesity trials with study durations of 12 to 52 weeks have provided evidence that MERIDIA does not adversely affect glycemia, serum lipid profiles, or serum uric acid in obese patients. Treatment with MERIDIA (5 to 20 mg once daily) is associated with mean increases in blood pressure of 1 to 3 mm Hg and with mean increases in pulse rate of 4 to 5 beats per minute relative to placebo. These findings are similar in normotensives and in patients with hypertension controlled with medication. Those patients who lose significant (≥ 5% weight loss) amounts of weight on MERIDIA tend to have smaller increases in blood pressure and pulse rate (see **"WARNINGS"**).

In Study 1, a 6-month, double-blind, placebo-controlled study in obese patients, Study 2, a 1-year, double-blind, placebo-controlled study in obese patients, and Study 3, a 1-year, double-blind, placebo-controlled study in obese patients who lost at least 6 kg on a 4-week very low calorie diet (VLCD), MERIDIA produced significant reductions in weight, as shown above. In two 1-year studies, maximal weight loss was achieved by 6 months and statistically significant weight loss was maintained over 12 months.

[See second table above]

MERIDIA induced weight loss has been accompanied by beneficial changes in serum lipids that are similar to those seen with nonpharmacologically-mediated weight loss. A combined, weighted analysis of the changes in serum lipids in 11 placebo-controlled obesity studies ranging in length from 12 to 52 weeks is shown at the bottom of the next page for the last observation carried forward (LOCF) analysis.

[See table at top of next page]

MERIDIA induced weight loss has been accompanied by reductions in serum uric acid. In one study, serum uric acid has been identified as an independent risk factor for death from coronary artery disease.

Certain centrally-acting weight loss agents that cause release of serotonin from nerve terminals have been associated with cardiac valve dysfunction. The possible occurrence of cardiac valve disease was specifically investigated in two studies. In one study 2-D and color Doppler echocardiography were performed on 210 patients (mean age, 54 years) receiving MERIDIA 15 mg or placebo daily for periods of 2 weeks to 16 months (mean duration of treatment, 7.6 months). In patients without a prior history of valvular heart disease, the incidence of valvular heart disease was 3/132 (2.3%) in the sibutramine treatment group (all three cases were mild aortic insufficiency) and 2/77 (2.6%) in the placebo treatment group (one case of mild aortic insufficiency and one case of severe aortic insufficiency). In another study, 25 patients underwent 2-D and color Doppler echocardiography before treatment with MERIDIA and again after treatment with MERIDIA 5 to 30 mg daily for three months; there were no cases of valvular heart disease.

INDICATIONS AND USAGE

MERIDIA is indicated for the management of obesity, including weight loss and maintenance of weight loss, and should be used in conjunction with a reduced calorie diet. MERIDIA is recommended for obese patients with an initial body mass index ≥ 30 kg/m^2, or ≥ 27 kg/m^2 in the presence of other risk factors (e.g., hypertension, diabetes, dyslipidemia).

Below is a chart of Body Mass Index (BMI) based on various heights and weights.

BMI is calculated by taking the patient's weight, in kg, and dividing by the patient's height, in meters, squared. Metric conversions are as follows: pounds ÷ 2.2 = kg; inches × 0.0254 = meters.

BMI		25	26	27	28	29	30	31	32	33	34	35	40
		WEIGHT (lbs)											
	4'10"	119	124	129	134	138	143	149	153	158	163	167	191
	4'11"	124	128	133	138	143	148	154	158	164	169	173	198
	5'	128	133	138	143	148	153	159	164	169	175	179	204
	5'1"	132	137	143	148	153	158	165	169	175	180	185	211
	5'2"	136	142	147	153	158	164	170	175	181	186	191	218
H	5'3"	141	146	152	158	163	169	175	181	187	192	197	225
	5'4"	145	151	157	163	169	174	181	187	193	199	204	232
E	5'5"	150	156	162	168	174	180	187	193	199	205	210	240
	5'6"	155	161	167	173	179	186	192	199	205	211	216	247
I	5'7"	159	166	172	178	185	191	198	205	211	218	223	255
	5'8"	164	171	177	184	190	197	204	211	218	224	230	262
G	5'9"	169	176	182	189	196	203	210	217	224	231	236	270
	5'10"	174	181	188	195	202	207	216	223	230	237	243	278
H	5'11"	179	186	193	200	208	215	222	230	237	244	250	286
	6'	184	191	199	206	213	221	228	236	244	251	258	294
T	6'1"	189	197	204	212	219	227	236	243	251	258	265	302
	6'2"	194	202	210	218	225	233	241	250	258	265	272	311
	6'3"	200	208	216	224	232	240	248	256	264	272	279	319

CONTRAINDICATIONS

MERIDIA is contraindicated in patients receiving monoamine oxidase inhibitors (MAOIs) (see "**WARNINGS**").

MERIDIA is contraindicated in patients with hypersensitivity to sibutramine or any of the inactive ingredients of MERIDIA.

MERIDIA is contraindicated in patients who have anorexia nervosa.

MERIDIA is contraindicated in patients taking other centrally acting appetite suppressant drugs.

WARNINGS

Blood Pressure and Pulse

MERIDIA SUBSTANTIALLY INCREASES BLOOD PRESSURE IN SOME PATIENTS. REGULAR MONITORING OF BLOOD PRESSURE IS REQUIRED WHEN PRESCRIBING MERIDIA.

In placebo-controlled obesity studies, MERIDIA 5 to 20 mg once daily was associated with mean increases in systolic and diastolic blood pressure of approximately 1 to 3 mm Hg relative to placebo, and with mean increases in pulse rate relative to placebo of approximately 4 to 5 beats per minute. Larger increases were seen in some patients, particularly when therapy with MERIDIA was initiated at the higher doses (see table below). In pre-marketing placebo-controlled obesity studies, 0.4% of patients treated with MERIDIA were discontinued for hypertension (SBP ≥ 160 mm Hg or DBP ≥ 95 mm Hg), compared with 0.4% in the placebo group, and 0.4% of patients with MERIDIA were discontinued for tachycardia (pulse rate ≥ 100 bpm), compared with 0.1% in the placebo group. Blood pressure and pulse should be measured prior to starting therapy with MERIDIA and should be monitored at regular intervals thereafter. For patients who experience a sustained increase in blood pressure or pulse rate while receiving MERIDIA, either dose reduction or discontinuation should be considered. MERIDIA should be given with caution to those patients with a history of hypertension (see "**DOSAGE AND ADMINISTRATION**"), and should not be given to patients with uncontrolled or poorly controlled hypertension.

Percent Outliers in Studies 1 and 2

Dose (mg)	%Outliers* SBP	DBP	Pulse
Placebo	9	7	12
5	6	20	16
10	12	15	28
15	13	17	24
20	14	22	37

*Outlier defined as increase from baseline of ≥ 15 mm Hg for three consecutive visits (SBP), ≥ 10 mm Hg for three consecutive visits (DBP), or pulse ≥ 10 bpm for three consecutive visits.

Potential Interaction With Monoamine Oxidase Inhibitors

MERIDIA is a norepinephrine, serotonin and dopamine reuptake inhibitor and should not be used concomitantly with MAOIs (see "**PRECAUTIONS**", Drug Interactions subsection). There should be at least a 2-week interval after stopping MAOIs before commencing treatment with MERIDIA. Similarly, there should be at least a 2-week interval after stopping MERIDIA before starting treatment with MAOIs.

Concomitant Cardiovascular Disease

Treatment with MERIDIA has been associated with increases in heart rate and/or blood pressure. Therefore, MERIDIA should not be used in patients with a history of coronary artery disease, congestive heart failure, arrhythmias, or stroke.

Glaucoma

Because MERIDIA can cause mydriasis, it should be used with caution in patients with narrow angle glaucoma.

Combined Analysis (11 Studies) of Percentage Change in Serum Lipids (N) - LOCF

Category	TG	CHOL	LDL-C	HDL-C
All Placebo	0.53 (475)	-1.53 (475)	-0.09 (233)	-0.56 (248)
<5% Weight Loss	4.52 (382)	-0.42 (382)	-070 (205)	-0.71 (217)
≥5% Weight Loss	-15.30 (92)	-6.23 (92)	-6.19 (27)	0.94 (30)
All Sibutramine	-8.75 (1164)	-2.21 (1165)	-1.85 (642)	4.13 (664)
<5% Weight Loss	-0.54 (547)	0.17 (548)	-0.37 (320)	3.19 (331)
≥5% Weight Loss	-16.59 (612)	-4.87 (612)	-4.56 (317)	4.68 (328)

Baseline mean values:
Placebo: TG 187 mg/dL; CHOL 221 mg/dL; LDL-C 140 mg/dL; HDL-C 47 mg/dL
Sibutramine: TG 172 mg/dL; CHOL 215 mg/dL; LDL-C 140 mg/dL; HDL-C 47 mg/dL

Miscellaneous

Organic causes of obesity (e.g., untreated hypothyroidism) should be excluded before prescribing MERIDIA.

PRECAUTIONS

Pulmonary Hypertension

Certain centrally-acting weight loss agents that cause release of serotonin from nerve terminals have been associated with pulmonary hypertension (PPH), a rare but lethal disease. In pre-marketing clinical studies, no cases of PPH have been reported with MERIDIA. Because of the low incidence of this disease in the underlying population, however, it is not known whether or not MERIDIA may cause this disease.

Seizures

During premarketing testing, seizures were reported in < 0.1% of MERIDIA treated patients. MERIDIA should be used cautiously in patients with a history of seizures. It should be discontinued in any patient who develops seizures.

Gallstones

Weight loss can precipitate or exacerbate gallstone formation.

Renal/Hepatic Dysfunction

Patients with severe renal impairment or severe hepatic dysfunction have not been systematically studied; MERIDIA should therefore not be used in such patients.

Interference With Cognitive and Motor Performance

Although sibutramine did not affect psychomotor or cognitive performance in healthy volunteers, any CNS active drug has the potential to impair judgment, thinking or motor skills.

Information For Patients

Physicians should instruct their patients to read the patient package insert before starting therapy with MERIDIA and to reread it each time the prescription is renewed.

Physicians should also discuss with their patients any part of the package insert that is relevant to them. In particular, the importance of keeping appointments for follow-up visits should be emphasized.

Patients should be advised to notify their physician if they develop a rash, hives, or other allergic reactions.

Patients should be advised to inform their physicians if they are taking, or plan to take, any prescription or over-the-counter drugs, especially weight-reducing agents, decongestants, antidepressants, cough suppressants, lithium, dihydroergotamine, sumatriptan (Imitrex®), or tryptophan, since there is a potential for interactions.

Patients should be reminded of the importance of having their blood pressure and pulse monitored at regular intervals.

Drug Interactions

CNS Active Drugs: The use of MERIDIA in combination with other CNS-active drugs, particularly serotonergic agents, has not been systematically evaluated. Consequently, caution is advised if the concomitant administration of MERIDIA with other centrally-acting drugs is indicated (see "**CONTRAINDICATIONS**" and "**WARNINGS**").

In patients receiving monoamine oxidase inhibitors (MAOIs) (e.g. phenelzine, selegiline) in combination with serotonergic agents (e.g. fluoxetine, fluvoxamine, paroxetine, sertraline, venlafaxine), there have been reports of serious, sometimes fatal, reactions ("serotonin syndrome;" see below). Because MERIDIA inhibits serotonin reuptake, MERIDIA should not be used concomitantly with MAOI (see "**CONTRAINDICATIONS**"). At least 2 weeks should elapse between discontinuation of a MAOI and initiation of treatment with MERIDIA. Similarly, at least 2 weeks should elapse between discontinuation of MERIDIA and initiation of treatment with MAOI.

The rare, but serious, constellation of symptoms termed "serotonin syndrome" has also been reported with the concomitant use of selective serotonin reuptake inhibitors and agents for migraine therapy, such as Imitrex® (sumatriptan succinate) and dihydroergotamine, certain opioids, such as dextramethorphan, meperidine, pentazocine and fentanyl, lithium, or tryptophan. Serotonin syndrome has also been reported with the concomitant use of two serotonin reuptake inhibitors. The syndrome requires immediate medical attention and may include one or more of the following symptoms: excitement, hypomania, restlessness, loss of consciousness, confusion, disorientation, anxiety, agitation, motor weakness, myoclonus, tremor, hemiballismus, hyperreflexia, ataxia, dysarthria, incoordination, hyperthermia, shivering, pupillary dilation, diaphoresis, emesis, and tachycardia.

Because MERIDIA inhibits serotonin reuptake, it should not be administered with other serotonergic agents such as those listed above.

Drugs That May Raise Blood Pressure and/or Heart Rate: Concomitant use of MERIDIA and other agents that may raise blood pressure or heart rate have not been evaluated. These include certain decongestants, cough, cold, and allergy medications that contain agents such as phenylpropanolamine, ephedrine, or pseudoephedrine. Caution should be used when prescribing MERIDIA to patients who use these medications.

Drugs That Inhibit Cytochrome P450(3A$_4$) Metabolism: *In vitro* studies indicated that the cytochrome P450(3A$_4$)-mediated metabolism of sibutramine was inhibited by ketoconazole and to a lesser extent by erythromycin. Clinical interaction trials were conducted on these substrates. The data indicate that there is a potential for such interactions, but the magnitude appears to be small.

Ketoconazole: Concomitant administration of 200 mg doses of ketoconazole twice daily and 20 mg sibutramine once daily for 7 days in 12 uncomplicated obese subjects resulted in moderate increases in AUC and $C_{max}$of 58% and 36% for M_1 and of 20% and 19% for M_2, respectively.

Erythromycin: The steady-state pharmacokinetics of sibutramine and metabolites M_1 and M_2 were evaluated in 12 uncomplicated obese subjects following concomitant administration of 500 mg of erythromycin three times daily and 20 mg of sibutramine once daily for 7 days. Concomitant erythromycin resulted in small increases in the AUC (less than 14%) for M_1 and M_2. A small reduction in C_{max} for M_1 (11%) and a slight increase in C_{max} for M_2 (10%) were observed.

Cimetidine: Concomitant administration of cimetidine 400 mg twice daily and sibutramine 15 mg once daily for 7 days in 12 volunteers resulted in small increases in combined (M_1 and M_2) plasma C_{max} (3.4%) and AUC (7.3%); these differences are unlikely to be of clinical significance.

Alcohol: In a double-blind, placebo controlled, crossover study in 19 volunteers, administration of a single dose of ethanol (0.5 mL/kg) together with 20 mg of sibutramine resulted in no psychomotor interactions of clinical significance between alcohol and sibutramine. However, the concomitant use of MERIDIA and excess alcohol is not recommended.

Oral Contraceptives: The suppression of ovulation by oral contraceptives was not inhibited by MERIDIA. In a crossover study, 12 healthy female volunteers on oral steroid contraceptives received placebo in one period and 15 mg sibutramine in another period over the course of 8 weeks. No clinically significant systemic interaction was observed; therefore, no requirement for alternative contraceptive precautions are needed when patients taking oral contraceptives are concurrently prescribed sibutramine.

Drugs Highly Bound to Plasma Proteins: Although sibutramine and its active metabolites M_1 and M_2 are extensively bound to plasma proteins (≥94%), the low therapeutic concentrations and basic characteristics of these compounds make them unlikely to result in clinically significant protein binding interactions with other highly protein bound drugs such as warfarin and phenytoin. *In vitro* protein binding interaction studies have not been conducted.

Carcinogenesis, Mutagenesis, Impairment of Fertility

Carcinogenicity

Sibutramine was administered in the diet to mice (1.25, 5 or 20 mg/kg/day) and rats (1, 3, or 9 mg/kg/day) for two years generating combined maximum plasma AUC's of the two major active metabolites equivalent to 0.5 and 21 times, respectively, those following the maximum daily human dose (20 mg). There was no evidence of carcinogenicity in mice or in female rats. In male rats there was a higher incidence of benign tumors of the testicular interstitial cells; such tumors are commonly seen in rats and are hormonally mediated. The relevance of these tumors to humans is not known.

Mutagenicity

Sibutramine was not mutagenic in the Ames test, *in vitro* Chinese hamster V79 cell mutation assay, *in vitro* clastogenicity assay in human lymphocytes or micronucleus assay in mice. Its two major active metabolites were found to have equivocal bacterial mutagenic activity in the Ames test. However, both metabolites gave consistently negative results in the *in vitro* Chinese hamster V79 cell mutation assay, *in vitro* clastogenicity assay in human lymphocytes, *in vitro* DNA-repair assay in HeLa cells, micronucleus assay in mice and *in vivo* unscheduled DNA-synthesis assay in rat hepatocytes.

Impairment of Fertility

In rats, there were no effects on fertility at doses generating combined plasma AUC's of the two major active metabolites

Continued on next page

Meridia—Cont.

up to 43 times those following the maximum human dose (20 mg). At 13 times the human combined AUC, there was maternal toxicity, and the dam's nest-building behavior was impaired, leading to a higher incidence of perinatal mortality; there was no effect at approximately 4 times the human combined AUC.

Pregnancy

Teratogenic Effects-Pregnancy Category C

In rats, there was no evidence of teratogenicity at doses of 1, 3, or 10 mg/kg/day generating combined plasma AUC's of the two major active metabolites up to approximately 43 times those following the maximum human dose (20 mg). In rabbits dosed at 3, 15, or 75 mg/kg/day, plasma AUC's greater than approximately 5 times those following the maximum human dose caused maternal toxicity. At markedly toxic doses, Dutch Belted rabbits had a slightly higher than control incidence of pups with a broad short snout, short rounded pinnae, short tail and, in some, shorter thickened long bones in the limbs; at comparably high doses in New Zealand White rabbits, one study showed a slightly higher than control incidence of pups with cardiovascular anomalies while a second study showed a lower incidence than in the control group.

No adequate and well controlled studies with MERIDIA have been conducted in pregnant women. The use of MERIDIA during pregnancy is not recommended. Women of child-bearing potential should employ adequate contraception while taking MERIDIA. Patients should be advised to notify their physician if they become pregnant or intend to become pregnant during therapy.

Nursing Mothers

It is not known whether sibutramine or its metabolites are excreted in human milk. MERIDIA is not recommended for use in nursing mothers. Patients should be advised to notify their physician if they are breast-feeding.

Pediatric Use

The safety and effectiveness of MERIDIA in pediatric patients under 16 years of age have not been established.

Geriatric Use

Clinical studies of MERIDIA did not include sufficient numbers of patients aged 65 and over to determine whether they respond differently from younger patients. In general, dose selection for an elderly patient should be cautious, reflecting the greater frequency of decreased hepatic, renal, or cardiac function, and of concomitant disease or other drug therapy. Pharmacokinetics in elderly patients are discussed in "**CLINICAL PHARMACOLOGY**."

ADVERSE REACTIONS

In placebo-controlled studies, 9% of patients treated with MERIDIA (n=2068) and 7% of patients treated with placebo (n=884) withdrew for adverse events.

In placebo-controlled obesity studies, the most common events were dry mouth, anorexia, insomnia, constipation and headache. Adverse events in these studies occurring in ≥ 1% of MERIDIA treated patients and more frequently than in the placebo group are shown in the following table.

	Obese Patients in Placebo-Controlled Studies	
BODY SYSTEM	MERIDIA® (n = 2068)	Placebo (n = 884)
Adverse Event	% incidence	% incidence
BODY AS A WHOLE		
Headache	30.3	18.6
Back pain	8.2	5.5
Flu syndrome	8.2	5.8
Injury accident	5.9	4.1
Asthenia	5.9	5.3
Abdominal pain	4.5	3.6
Chest pain	1.8	1.2
Neck pain	1.6	1.1
Allergic reaction	1.5	0.8
CARDIOVASCULAR SYSTEM		
Tachycardia	2.6	0.6
Vasodilation	2.4	0.9
Migraine	2.4	2.0
Hypertension/increased blood pressure	2.1	0.9
Palpitation	2.0	0.8
DIGESTIVE SYSTEM		
Anorexia	13.0	3.5
Constipation	11.5	6.0
Increased appetite	8.7	2.7
Nausea	5.9	2.8
Dyspepsia	5.0	2.6
Gastritis	1.7	1.2
Vomiting	1.5	1.4
Rectal disorder	1.2	0.5
METABOLIC & NUTRITIONAL		
Thirst	1.7	0.9
Generalized edema	1.2	0.8
MUSCULOSKELETAL SYSTEM		
Arthralgia	5.9	5.0
Myalgia	1.9	1.1
Tenosynovitis	1.2	0.5
Joint disorder	1.1	0.6
NERVOUS SYSTEM		
Dry mouth	17.2	4.2
Insomnia	10.7	4.5
Dizziness	7.0	3.4
Nervousness	5.2	2.9
Anxiety	4.5	3.4
Depression	4.3	2.5
Paresthesia	2.0	0.5
Somnolence	1.7	0.9
CNS stimulation	1.5	0.5
Emotional lability	1.3	0.6
RESPIRATORY SYSTEM		
Rhinitis	10.2	7.1
Pharyngitis	10.0	8.4
Sinusitis	5.0	2.6
Cough increase	3.8	3.3
Laryngitis	1.3	0.9
SKIN & APPENDAGES		
Rash	3.8	2.5
Sweating	2.5	0.9
Herpes simplex	1.3	1.0
Acne	1.0	0.8
SPECIAL SENSES		
Taste perversion	2.2	0.8
Ear disorder	1.7	0.9
Ear pain	1.1	0.7
UROGENITAL SYSTEM		
Dysmenorrhea	3.5	1.4
Urinary tract infection	2.3	2.0
Vaginal monilia	1.2	0.5
Metrorrhagia	1.0	0.8

[See table below]

The following additional adverse events were reported in ≥ 1% of all patients who received MERIDIA in controlled and uncontrolled pre-marketing studies.

Body as a Whole: fever.

Digestive System: diarrhea, flatulence, gastroenteritis, tooth disorder.

Metabolic and Nutritional: peripheral edema.

Musculoskeletal System: arthritis.

Nervous System: agitation, leg cramps, hypertonia, thinking abnormal.

Respiratory System: bronchitis, dyspnea.

Skin and Appendages: pruritus.

Special Senses: amblyopia.

Urogenital System: menstrual disorders.

Postmarketing Reports

Voluntary reports of adverse events temporally associated with the use of MERIDIA are listed below. It is important to emphasize that although these events occurred during treatment with MERIDIA, they may have no causal relationship with the drug. Obesity itself, concurrent disease states/risk factors, or weight reduction may be associated with an increased risk for some of these events.

abnormal dreams, abnormal ejaculation, abnormal gait, abnormal vision, alopecia, amnesia, anaphylactic shock, anaphylactoid reaction, anemia, anger, angina pectoris, arthrosis, atrial fibrillation, blurred vision, bursitis, cerebrovascular accident, chest pressure, chest tightness, cholecystitis, cholelithiasis, concentration impaired, confusion, congestive heart failure, depression aggravated, dermatitis, dry eye, duodenal ulcer, epistaxis, eructation, eye pain, facial edema, gastrointestinal hemorrhage, Gilles de la Tourette's syndrome, goiter, heart arrest, heart rate decreased, hematuria, hyperglycemia, hyperthyroidism, hypesthesia, hypoglycemia, hypothyroidism, impotence, increased intraocular pressure, increased salivation, increased urinary frequency, intestinal obstruction, leukopenia, libido decreased, libido increased, limb pain, lymphadenopathy, manic reaction, micturition difficulty, mood changes, mouth ulcer, myocardial infarction, nasal congestion, nightmares, otitis externa, otitis media, petechiae, photosensitivity (eyes), photosensitivity (skin), respiratory disorder, serotonin syndrome, short term memory loss, speech disorder, stomach ulcer, sudden unexplained death, supraventricular tachycardia, syncope, thrombocytopenia, tinnitus, tongue edema, torsades de pointes, transient ischemic attack, tremor, twitch, urticaria, vascular headache, ventricular tachycardia, ventricular extrasystoles, ventricular fibrillation, vertigo, yawn.

Other Notable Adverse Events

Seizures: Convulsions were reported as an adverse event in three of 2068 (0.1%) MERIDIA treated patients and in none of 884 placebo-treated patients in placebo-controlled premarketing obesity studies. Two of the three patients with seizures had potentially predisposing factors (one had a prior history of epilepsy; one had a subsequent diagnosis of brain tumor). The incidence in all subjects who received MERIDIA (three of 4,588 subjects) was less than 0.1%.

Ecchymosis/Bleeding Disorders: Ecchymosis (bruising) was observed in 0.7% of MERIDIA treated patients and in 0.2% of placebo-treated patients in pre-marketing placebo-controlled obesity studies. One patient had prolonged bleeding of a small amount which occurred during minor facial surgery. MERIDIA may have an effect on platelet function due to its effect on serotonin uptake.

Interstitial Nephritis: Acute interstitial nephritis (confirmed by biopsy) was reported in one obese patient receiving MERIDIA during pre-marketing studies. After discontinuation of the medication, dialysis and oral corticosteroids were administered; renal function normalized. The patient made a full recovery.

Altered Laboratory Findings: Abnormal liver function tests, including increases in AST, ALT, GGT, LDH, alkaline phosphate and bilirubin, were reported as adverse events in 1.6% of MERIDIA-treated obese patients in placebo-controlled trials compared with 0.8% of placebo patients. In these studies, potentially clinically significant values (total bilirubin ≥ 2mg/dL; ALT, AST, GGT, LDH, or alkaline phosphatase ≥ 3× upper limit of normal) occurred in 0% (alkaline phosphatase) to 0.6% (ALT) of the MERIDIA treated patients and in none of the placebo-treated patients. Abnormal values tended to be sporadic, often diminished with continued treatment, and did not show a clear dose-response relationship.

DRUG ABUSE AND DEPENDENCE

Controlled Substance

MERIDIA is a controlled substance in Schedule IV of the Controlled Substances Act (CSA).

Abuse and Physical and Psychological Dependence

Physicians should carefully evaluate patients for history of drug abuse and follow such patients closely, observing them for signs of misuse or abuse (e.g., drug development of tolerance, incrementation of doses, drug seeking behavior).

OVERDOSAGE

Human Experience

There is very limited experience of overdose with MERIDIA. Three cases of overdose have been reported with MERIDIA. The first was in a 2-year-old child of one patient who ingested up to eight 10 mg capsules. No complications were observed during the overnight hospitalization, and the child was discharged the following day with no sequela. The second report was in a 30-year-old male in a depression study who ingested approximately 100 mg of sibutramine in an attempt to commit suicide. The patient suffered no adverse effects or ECG abnormalities post-ingestion. The third report was in the 45-year-old husband of a patient in an obese dyslipidemic study. He ingested 400 mg of his wife's drug supply and was hospitalized for observation; a heart rate of 120 bpm was noted. He was discharged the next day with no apparent sequela.

Overdose Management

There is no specific antidote to MERIDIA. Treatment should consist of general measures employed in the management of overdosage: an airway should be established; cardiac and vital sign monitoring is recommended; general symptomatic and supportive measures should be instituted. Cautious use of β-blockers may be indicated to control elevated blood pressure or tachycardia. The benefits of forced diuresis and hemodialysis are unknown.

DOSAGE AND ADMINISTRATION

The recommended starting dose of MERIDIA is 10 mg administered once daily with or without food. If there is inadequate weight loss, the dose may be titrated after four weeks to a total of 15 mg once daily. The 5 mg dose should be reserved for patients who do not tolerate the 10 mg dose. Blood pressure and heart rate changes should be taken into account when making decisions regarding dose titration (see "**PRECAUTIONS**").

Doses above 15 mg daily are not recommended. In most clinical trials, MERIDIA was given in the morning.

Analysis of numerous variables has indicated that approximately 60% of patients who lose at least 4 pounds in the first 4 weeks of treatment with a given dose of MERIDIA in combination with a reduced-calorie diet lose at least 5% (placebo-subtracted) of their initial body weight by the end of 6 months to 1 year of treatment on that dose of MERIDIA. Conversely, approximately, 80% of patients who do not lose at least 4 pounds in the first 4 weeks of treatment with a given dose of MERIDIA do not lose at least 5% (placebo-subtracted) of their initial body weight by the end of 6 months to 1 year of treatment on that dose. If a patient has not lost at least 4 pounds in the first 4 weeks of treatment, the physician should consider reevaluation of therapy which may include increasing the dose or discontinuation of MERIDIA.

The safety and effectiveness of MERIDIA, as demonstrated in double-blind, placebo-controlled trials, have not been determined beyond 1 year at this time.

HOW SUPPLIED

MERIDIA® (sibutramine hydrochloride monohydrate) Capsules contain 5 mg, 10 mg, or 15 mg sibutramine hydrochloride monohydrate and are supplied as follows:

5 mg, NDC 0048-0605-01, blue/yellow capsules imprinted with "MERIDIA" on the cap and "-5-" on the body, in bottles of 100 capsules.

10 mg, NDC 0048-0610-01, blue/white capsules imprinted with "MERIDIA" on the cap and "-10-" on the body, in bottles of 100 capsules.

15 mg, NDC 0048-0615-01, yellow/white capsules imprinted with "MERIDIA" on the cap and "-15-" on the body, in bottles of 100 capsules.

Storage: Store at 25°C (77°F); excursions permitted to 15-30°C (59-86°F) [see USP controlled room temperature]. Protect from heat and moisture. Dispense in a tight, light-resistant container as defined in USP.

MERIDIA is a registered trademark of Knoll Pharmaceutical Company.

IMITREX is a registered trademark of Glaxo Group Limited.

Sibutramine is covered by US Patent Nos. 4,746,680; 4,929,629; and 5,436,272.

Revised: November 1999
0995010-3
Knoll Pharmaceutical Company
3000 Continental Drive - North
Mount Olive, New Jersey 07828-1234
BASF Pharma

Shown in Product Identification Guide, page 319

SYNTHROID® ℞

[*sĭn 'throid*]

(levothyroxine sodium, USP)

SYNTHROID Tablets—for oral administration

SYNTHROID Injection—for parenteral administration

DESCRIPTION

SYNTHROID (levothyroxine sodium, USP) Tablets and Injection contain synthetic crystalline L-3,3′,5,5′,-tetraiodothyronine sodium salt [levothyroxine (T_4) sodium]. Synthetic T_4 is identical to that produced in the human thyroid gland.

Levothyroxine (T_4) Sodium has an empirical formula of $C_{15}H_{10}L_4NNaO_4xH_2O$, molecular weight of 798.86 (anhydrous), and structural formula as shown:

[See chemical structure at top of next column]

Inactive Ingredients (SYNTHROID Tablets): acacia, confectioner's sugar (contains corn starch), lactose, magnesium stearate, providone, talc. The following are the color additives by tablet strength:

HO—(I,I)—O—(I,I)—CH_2—C(NH_2)(H)—COONa·XH_2O

LEVOTHYROXINE SODIUM

Strength (mcg)	Color Additive(s)
25	FD&C Yellow No. 6
50	None
75	FD&C Red No. 40, FD&C Blue No. 2
88	FD&C Blue No. 1, FD&C Yellow No. 6, D&C Yellow No. 10
100	D&C Yellow No. 10, FD&C Yellow No. 6
112	D&C Red No. 27 & 30
125	FD&C Yellow No. 6, FD&C Red No. 40, FD&C Blue No. 1
150	FD&C Blue No. 2
175	FD&C Blue No. 1, D&C Red No. 27 & 30
200	FD&C Red No. 40
300	D&C Yellow No. 10, FD&C Yellow No. 6, FD&C Blue No. 1

Inactive Ingredients (SYNTHROID Injection): 10 mg mannitol USP, 0.7 mg tribasic sodium phosphate, anhydrous (200 mcg/vial), 1.75 mg tribasic sodium phosphate, anhydrous (500 mcg/vial), sodium hydroxide, Q.S. for pH adjustment. Levothyroxine sodium powder for reconstitution for injection is a sterile preparation.

CLINICAL PHARMACOLOGY

The synthesis and secretion of the major thyroid hormones, L-thyroxine (T_4) and L-triiodothyronine (T_3), from the normally functioning thyroid gland are regulated by complex feedback mechanisms of the hypothalamic-pituitary-thyroid axis. The thyroid gland is stimulated to secrete thyroid hormones by the action of thyrotropin (thyroid stimulating hormone, TSH), which is produced in the anterior pituitary gland. TSH secretion is in turn controlled by thyrotropin-releasing hormone (TRH) produced in the hypothalamus, circulating thyroid hormones, and possibly other mechanisms. Thyroid hormones circulating in the blood act as feedback inhibitors of both TSH and TRH secretion. Thus, when serum concentrations of T_3 and T_4 are increased, secretion of TSH and TRH decreases. Conversely, when serum thyroid hormone concentrations are decreased, secretion of TSH and TRH is increased. Administration of exogenous thyroid hormones to euthyroid individuals results in suppression of endogenous thyroid hormone secretion.

The mechanisms by which thyroid hormones exert their physiologic actions have not been completely elucidated. T_4 and T_3 are transported into cells by passive and active mechanisms. T_3 in cell cytoplasm and T_3 generated from T_4 within the cell diffuse into the nucleus and bind to thyroid receptor proteins, which appear to be primarily attached to DNA. Receptor binding leads to activation or repression of DNA transcription, thereby altering the amounts of mRNA and resultant proteins. Changes in protein concentrations are responsible for the metabolic changes observed in organs and tissues.

Thyroid hormones enhance oxygen consumption of most body tissues and increase the basal metabolic rate and metabolism of carbohydrates, lipids, and proteins. Thus, they exert a profound influence on every organ system and are of particular importance in the development of the central nervous system. Thyroid hormones also appear to have direct effects on tissues, such as increased myocardial contractility and decreased systemic resistance.

The physiologic effects of thyroid hormones are produced primarily by T_3, a large portion of which is derived from the deiodination of T_4 in peripheral tissues. About 70 to 90 percent of peripheral T_3 is produced by monodeiodination of T_4 at the 5 position (inner ring) results in the formation of reverse triiodothyronine (rT_3), which is calorigenically inactive.

PHARMACOKINETICS: Few clinical studies have evaluated the kinetics of orally administered thyroid hormone. In animals, the most active sites of absorption appear to be the proximal and mid-jejunum. T_4 is not absorbed from the stomach and little, if any, drug is absorbed from the duodenum. There seems to be no absorption of T_4 from the distal colon in animals. A number of human studies have confirmed the importance of an intact jejunum and ileum for T_4 absorption and have shown some absorption from the duodenum. Studies involving radioiodinated T_4 fecal excretion methods, equilibration, and AUC methods have shown that absorption varies from 48 to 80 percent of the administered dose. The extent of absorption is increased in the fasting state and decreased in malabsorption syndromes, such as sprue. Absorption may also decrease with age. The degree of T_4 absorption is dependent on the product formulation as well as on the character of the intestinal contents, including plasma protein and soluble dietary factors, which bind thyroid hormone making if unavailable for diffusion. Decreased absorption may result from administration of infant soybean formula, ferrous sulfate, sodium polystyrene sulfonate, aluminum hydroxide, sucralfate or bile acid sequestrants. T_4 absorption following intramuscular administration is variable.

Distribution of thyroid hormones in human body tissues and fluids has not been fully elucidated. More than 99 percent of circulating hormones is bound to serum proteins, including thyroxine-binding globulin (TBG), thyroxine-binding prealbumin (TBPA), and albumin (TBA). T_4 is more extensively and firmly bound to serum proteins than is T_3. Only unbound thyroid hormone is metabolically active. The higher affinity of TBG and TBPA for T_4 partly explains the higher serum levels, slower metabolic clearance, and longer serum elimination half-life of this hormone.

Certain drugs and physiologic conditions can alter the binding of thyroid hormones to serum proteins and/or the concentrations of the serum proteins available for thyroid hormone binding. These effects must be considered when interpreting the results of thyroid function tests. (See **Drug Interactions** and **Laboratory Test Interactions.)**

T_4 is eliminated slowly from the body, with a half-life of 6 to 7 day. T_3 has a half-life of 1 to 2 days. The liver is the major site of degradation for both hormones. T_4 and T_3 are conjugated with glucuronic and sulfuric acids and excreted in the bile. There is an enterohepatic circulation of thyroid hormones, as they are liberated by hydrolysis in the intestine and reabsorbed. A portion of the conjugated material reaches the colon unchanged, is hydrolyzed there, and is eliminated as free compounds in the feces. In man, approximately 20 to 40 percent of T_4 is eliminated in the stool. About 70 percent of the T_4 secreted daily is deiodinated to yield equal amounts of T_3 and rT_3. Subsequent deiodination of T_3 and rT_4 yields multiple forms of diiodothyronine. A number of the minor T_4 metabolites have also been identified. Although some of these metabolites have biologic activity, their overall contribution to the therapeutic effect of T_4 is minimal.

INDICATIONS AND USAGE

SYNTHROID is indicated:

1. As replacement or supplemental therapy in patients of any age or state (including pregnancy) with hypothyroidism of any etiology except transient hypothyroidism during the recovery phase of subacute thyroiditis: primary hypothyroidism resulting from thyroid dysfunction, primary atrophy, or partial or total absence of the thyroid gland, or from the effects of surgery, radiation or drugs, with or without the presence of goiter, including subclinical hypothyroidism; secondary (pituitary hypothyroidism; and tertiary (hypothalamic) hypothyroidism (see **CONTRAINDICATIONS** and **PRECAUTIONS**). SYNTHROID Injection can be used intravenously when rapid repletion is required, and either intravenously or intramuscularly when the oral route is precluded.
2. As a pituitary TSH suppressant in the treatment or prevention of various types of euthyroid goiters, including thyroid modules, subacute or chronic lymphocytic thyroiditis (Hashimoto's), multinodular goiter, and in conjunction with surgery and radioactive iodine therapy in the management of thyrotropin-dependent well-differentiated papillary or follicular carcinoma of the thyroid.

CONTRAINDICATIONS

SYNTHROID is contraindicated in patients with untreated thyrotoxicosis of any etiology or an apparent hypersensitivity to thyroid hormones or any of the inactive product constituents. (The 50 mcg tablet is formulated without color additives for patients who are sensitive to dyes.) There is no well-documented evidence of true allergic or idiosyncratic reactions to thyroid hormone. SYNTHROID is also contraindicated in the patients with uncorrected adrenal insufficiency, as thyroid hormones increase tissue demands for adrenocortical hormones and may thereby precipitate acute adrenal crisis (**see PRECAUTIONS**).

WARNINGS: Thyroid hormones, either alone or together with other therapeutic agents, should not be used for the treatment of obesity. In euthyroid patients, doses within the range of daily hormonal requirements are ineffective for weight reduction. Larger doses may produce serious or even life threatening manifestations of toxicity, particularly when given in association with sympathomimetic amines such as those used for their anorectic effects.

The use of SYNTHROID in the treatment of obesity, either alone or in combination with other drugs, is unjustified. The use of SYNTHROID is also unjustified in the treatment of male or female infertility unless this condition is associated with hypothyroidism.

PRECAUTIONS

General: SYNTHROID should be used with caution in patients with cardiovascular disorders, including angina, coronary artery disease, and hypertension, and in the elderly who have a greater likelihood of occult cardiac disease. Concomitant administration of thyroid hormone and sympathomimetic agents to patients with coronary artery disease may increase the risk of coronary insufficiency.

Use of SYNTHROID in patients with concomitant diabetes mellitus, diabetes insipidus or adrenal cortical insufficiency may aggravate the intensity of their symptoms. Appropriate adjustments of the various therapeutic measures directed at these concomitant endocrine diseases may therefore be required. Treatment of myxedema coma may require simultaneous administration of glucocorticoids (see **DOSAGE AND ADMINISTRATION**).

Continued on next page

Synthroid—Cont.

T_4 enhances the response to anticoagulant therapy. Prothrombin time should be closely monitored in patients taking both SYNTHROID and oral anticoagulants, and the dosage of anticoagulant adjusted accordingly.
Seizures have been reported rarely in association with the initiation of levothyroxine sodium therapy, and may be related to the effect of thyroid hormone on seizure threshold.
Lithium blocks the TSH-mediated release of T_4 and T_3. Thyroid function should therefore be carefully monitored during lithium initiation, stabilization, and maintenance. If hypothyroidism occurs during lithium treatment, a higher than usual SYNTHROID dose may be required.

Information for the Patient:
1. SYNTHROID is intended to replace a hormone that is normally produced by your thyroid gland. It is generally taken for life, except in cases of temporary hypothyroidism associated with an inflammation of the thyroid gland.
2. Before or at any time while using SYNTHROID you should tell your doctor if you are allergic to any foods or medicines, are pregnant or intend to become pregnant, are breastfeeding, are taking or start taking any other prescription or nonprescription (OTC) medications, or have any other medical problems (especially hardening of the arteries, heart disease, high blood pressure, or history of thyroid, adrenal or pituitary gland problems).
3. Use SYNTHROID only as prescribed by your doctor. Do not discontinue SYNTHROID or change the amount you take or how often you take it, except as directed by your doctor.
4. SYNTHROID, like all medicines obtained from your doctor, must be used only by you and for the condition determined appropriate by your doctor.
5. It may take a few weeks for SYNTHROID to begin working. Until it begins working, you may not notice any change in your symptoms.
6. You should notify your doctor if you experience any of the following symptoms, or if you experience any other unusual medical event: chest pain, shortness of breath, hives or skin rash, rapid or irregular heartbeat, headache, irritability, nervousness, sleeplessness, diarrhea, excessive sweating, heat intolerance, changes in appetite, vomiting, weight gain or loss, changes in menstrual periods, fever, hand tremors, leg cramps.
7. You should inform your doctor or dentist that you are taking SYNTHROID before having any kind of surgery.
8. You should notify your doctor if you become pregnant while taking SYNTHROID. Your dose of this medicine will likely have to be increased while you are pregnant.
9. If you have diabetes, your dose insulin or oral antidiabetic agent may need to be changed after starting SYNTHROID. You should monitor your blood or urinary glucose levels as directed by your doctor and report any changes to your doctor immediately.
10. If you are taking an oral anticoagulant drug such as warfarin, your dose may need to be changed after starting SYNTHROID. Your coagulation status should be checked often to determine if a change in dose is required.
11. Partial hair loss may occur rarely during the first few months of SYNTHROID therapy, but it is usually temporary.
12. SYNTHROID is the trade name for tablets, containing the thyroid hormone levothyroxine, manufactured by Knoll Pharmaceutical Company. Other manufacturers also makes tablets containing levothyroxine. You should not change to another manufacturer's product without discussing that change with your doctor first. Repeat blood tests and a change in the amount of levothyroxine you take may be required.
13. Keep SYNTHROID out of the reach of children. Store SYNTHROID away from heat and moisture.

Laboratory Tests: Treatment of patients with SYNTHROID requires periodic assessment of adequacy of titration by appropriate laboratory tests and clinical evaluation. Selection of appropriate tests for the diagnosis and management of thyroid disorders depends on patient variables such as presenting signs and symptoms, pregnancy, and concomitant medications. A combination of sensitive TSH assay and free T_4 estimate (free T_4, free T_4 index) are recommended to confirm a diagnosis of thyroid disease. Normal ranges for theses parameters are age-specific in newborns and younger children.
TSH alone or initially may be useful for thyroid disease screening and for monitoring therapy for primary hypothyroidism as a linear inverse correlation exists between serum TSH and free T_4. Measurement of total serum T_4 and T_3, resin T_3 uptake, and free T_3 concentrations may also be useful. Antithyroid microsomal antibodies are an indicator of autoimmune thyroid disease. The presence of positive microsomal antibodies in an euthyroid patient is a major risk factor for the future development of hypothyroidism. As elevated serum TSH in the presence of normal T_4 may indicate subclinical hypothyroidism. Intracellular resistance to thyroid hormone is quite rare, and is suggested by clinical signs and symptoms of hypothyroidism in the presence of high serum T_4 levels. Adequacy of SYNTHROID therapy for hypothyroidism of pituitary or hypothalamic origin should be assessed by measuring free T_4, which should be maintained in the upper half of the normal range. Measurement of TSH is not a reliable indicator of response to therapy for this condition. Adequacy of SYNTHROID therapy for congenital and acquired pediatric hypothyroidism should be assessed by measuring serum total T_4 or free T_4, which should be maintained in the upper half of the normal range. In congenital hypothyroidism, normalization of serum TSH levels may lag behind normalization of serum T_4 levels by 2 or 3 months or longer. In rare patients serum TSH remains relatively elevated despite clinical euthyroidism and age-specific normal levels of T_4 or free T_4.

Drug Interactions: The magnitude and relative clinical importance of the effects noted below are likely to be patient-specific and may vary by such factors as age, gender, race, intercurrent illnesses, dose of either agent, additional concomitant medications, and timing of drug administration. Any agent that alters thyroid hormone synthesis, secretion, distribution, effect on target tissues, metabolism, or elimination may alter the optimal therapeutic dose of SYNTHROID.
Levothyroxine sodium absorption—The following agents may bind and decrease absorption of levothyroxine sodium from the gastrointestinal tract: aluminum hydroxide, cholestyramine resin, colestipol hydrochloride, ferrous sulfate, sodium polystyrene sulfonate, soybean flour (e.g., infant formula), sucralfate.
Binding to serum proteins—The following agents may either inhibit levothyroxine sodium binding to serum proteins or alter the concentrations of serum binding proteins: androgens and related anabolic hormones, asparaginase, clofibrate, estrogens and estrogen-containing compounds, 5-fluorouracil, furosemide, glucocorticoids, meclofenamic acid, mefenamic acid, methadone, perphenazine, phenylbutazone, phenytoin, salicylates, tamoxifen.
Thyroid physiology—The following agents may alter thyroid hormone or TSH levels, generally by effects on thyroid hormone synthesis, secretion, distribution, metabolism, hormone action, or elimination, or altered TSH secretion: aminoglutethimide, p-aminosalicyclic acid, amiodarone, androgens and related anabolic hormones, complex anions (thiocyanate, perchlorate, pertechnetate), antithyroid drugs, β-adrenergic blocking agents, carbamazepine, chloral hydrate, diazepam, dopamine and dopamine agonists, ethionamide, glucocorticoids, heparin, hepatic enzyme inducers, insulin, iodinated cholestographic agents, iodine-containing compounds, levodopa, lovastatin, lithium, 6-mercaptopurine, metoclopramide, mitotane, nitroprusside, phenobarbital, phenytoin, resorcinol, rifampin, somatostatin analogs, sulfonamides, sulfonylureas, thiazide diuretics.
Adrenocorticoids—Metabolic clearance of adrenocorticoids is decreased in hypothyroid patients and increased in hyperthyroid patients, and may therefore change with changing thyroid status.
Amiodarone—Amiodarone therapy alone can cause hypothyroidism or hyperthyroidism.
Anticoagulants (oral)—The hypoprothrombinemic effect of anticoagulants may be potentiated, apparently by increased catabolism of vitamin K-dependent clotting factors.
Antidiabetic agents (insulin, sulfonylureas)—Requirements for insulin or oral antidiabetic agents may be reduced in hypothyroid patients with diabetes mellitus, and may subsequently increase with the initiation of thyroid hormone replacement therapy.
β-adrenergic blocking agents—Actions of some beta-blocking agents may be impaired when hypothyroid patients become euthyroid.
Cytokines (interferon, interleukin)—Cytokines have been reported to induce both hyperthyroidism and hypothyroidism.
Digitalis glycosides—Therapeutic effects of digitalis glycosides may be reduced. Serum digitalis levels may be decreased in hyperthyroidism or when a hypothyroid patient becomes euthyroid.
Ketamine—Marked hypertension and tachycardia have been reported in association with concomitant administration of levothyroxine sodium and ketamine.
Maprotiline—Risk of cardiac arrhythmias may increase.
Sodium iodide (^{123}I and ^{131}I), sodium pertechnetate Tc99m—Uptake of radiolabeled ions may be decreased.
Somatrem/somatropin—Excessive concurrent use of thyroid hormone may accelerate epiphyseal closure. Untreated hypothyroidism may interfere with the growth response to somatrem or somatropin.
Theophylline—Theophylline clearance may decrease in hypothyroid patients and return toward normal when a euthyroid state is achieved.
Tricyclic antidepressants—Concurrent use may increase the therapeutic and toxic effects of both drugs, possibly due to increased catecholamine sensitivity. Onset of action of tricyclics may be accelerated.
Sympathomimetic agents—Possible increased risk of coronary insufficiency in patients with coronary artery disease.

Laboratory Test Interactions: A number of drugs or moieties are known to alter serum levels of TSH, T_4 and T_3 and may thereby influence the interpretation of laboratory tests of thyroid function (see **Drug Interactions**).
1. Changes in TBG concentration should be taken into consideration when interpreting T_4 and T_3 values. Drugs such as estrogens and estrogen-containing oral contraceptives increase TBG concentrations. TBG concentrations may also be increased during pregnancy and in infectious hepatitis. Decreases in TBG concentrations are observed in nephrosis, acromegaly, and after androgen or corticosteroid therapy. Familial hyper- or hypo-thyroxine-binding-globulinemias have been described. The incidence of TBG deficiency is approximately 1 in 9000. Certain drugs such as salicylates inhibit the protein-binding of T_4. In such cases, the unbound (free) hormone should be measured. Alternatively, an indirect measure of free thyroxine, such as the FT_4I may be used.
2. Medicinal or dietary iodine interferes with *in vivo* tests of radioiodine uptake, producing low uptakes which may not indicate a true decrease in hormone synthesis.
3. Persistent clinical and laboratory evidence of hypothyroidism despite an adequate replacement dose suggests either poor patient compliance, impaired absorption, drug interactions, or decreased potency of the preparation due to improper storage.

Carcinogenesis, Mutagenesis, and Impairment of Fertility: Although animal studies to determine the mutagenic or carcinogenic potential of thyroid hormones have not been performed, synthetic T_4 is identical to that produced by the human thyroid gland. A reported association between prolonged thyroid hormone therapy and breast cancer has not been confirmed and patients receiving levothyroxine sodium for established indications should not discontinue therapy.

Pregnancy: Pregnancy Category A. Studies in pregnant women have not shown that levothyroxine sodium increases the risk of fetal abnormalities if administered during pregnancy. If levothyroxine sodium is used during pregnancy, the possibility of fetal harm appears remote. Because studies cannot rule out the possibility of harm, levothyroxine sodium should be used during pregnancy only if clearly needed.
Thyroid hormones cross the placental barrier to some extent. T_4 levels in the cord blood of athyroid fetuses have been shown to be about one-third of maternal levels. Nevertheless, maternal-fetal transfer of T_4 may not prevent *in utero* hypothyroidism.
Hypothyroidism during pregnancy is associated with a higher rate of complications, including spontaneous abortion and preeclampsia, and has been reported to have an adverse effect on fetal and childhood development. On the basis of current knowledge, SYNTHROID® (levothyroxine sodium, USP) should therefore not be discontinued during pregnancy, and hypothyroidism diagnosed during pregnancy should be treated. Studies have shown that during pregnancy T_4 concentrations may decrease and TSH concentrations may increase to values outside normal ranges. Postpartum values are similar to preconception values. Elevations in TSH may occur as early as 4 weeks gestation.
Pregnant women who are maintained on SYNTHROID should have their TSH measured periodically. An elevated TSH should be corrected by an increase in SYNTHROID dose. After pregnancy, the dose can be decreased to the optimal preconception dose.

Nursing Mothers: Minimal amounts of thyroid hormones are excreted in human milk. Thyroid hormones are not associated with serious adverse reactions and do not have known tumorigenic potential. While caution should be exercised when SYNTHROID is administered to a nursing woman, adequate replacement doses of levothyroxine sodium are generally needed to maintain normal lactation.

Pediatric Use: Congenital hypothyroidism: Rapid restoration of normal serum T_4 concentrations is essential for preventing the deleterious effects of neonatal thyroid hormone deficiency on intelligence, as well as on overall growth and development. SYNTHROID should be initiated immediately upon diagnosis, and is generally continued for life. The goal of therapy is to maintain the serum total T_4 or FT_4 in the upper half of the normal range and serum TSH in the normal range.
An initial starting dose of 10 to 15 mcg/kg/day (ages 0–3 months) will generally increase serum T_4 concentrations to the upper half of the normal range in less than 3 weeks. Clinical assessment of growth and development and thyroid status should be monitored frequently. In most cases, the dose of SYNTHROID per body weight will decrease gradually as the patient grows through infancy and childhood (see Table). Prolonged use of large doses in infants may be associated with later behavior problems.
Thyroid function tests (serum total T_4 or FT_4, and TSH) should be monitored closely and used to determine the adequacy of SYNTHROID therapy. Normalization of serum T_4 levels is usually followed by a rapid decline of TSH levels. Nevertheless, normalization of TSH may lag behind normalization of T_4 levels by 2 to 3 months or longer. The relative elevation of serum TSH is more marked during the early months of therapy, but can persist to some degree throughout life. In rare patients TSH remains relatively elevated despite clinical euthyroidism and age-specific normal levels of total T_4 or FT_4. Increasing the SYNTHROID dosage to suppress TSH into the normal range may result in overtreatment, with an elevated serum T_4 level and clinical features of hyperthyroidism, including irritability, increased appetite with diarrhea, and sleeplessness. Another risk of prolonged overtreatment in infants is premature cranial synostosis.
Assessment of permanence of hypothyroidism may be done when transient hypothyroidism is suspected. Levothyroxine therapy may be interrupted for 30 days after 3 years of age and serum measurement of T_4 and TSH levels obtained. If T_4 is low and the TSH level is elevated, permanent hypothyroidism is confirmed and therapy should be re-instituted. If T_4 and TSH remain in the normal range, a presumptive diagnosis of transient hypothyroidism can be

made. In this instance, continued clinical monitoring and periodic reevaluation of thyroid function may be warranted.

Acquired hypothyroidism. The initial dose of SYNTHROID varies with age and body weight, and should be adjusted to maintain serum total T_4 or free T_4 levels in the upper half of the normal range. In general, in the absence of overriding clinical concerns, children should be started on a full replacement dose. Children with underlying heart disease should be started at lower doses, with careful upward titration. Children with severe, long-standing hypothyroidism may also be started on a lower initial dose with upward titration in an attempt to avoid premature closure of epiphyses. The recommended dose per body weight decreases with age (see Table).

Treated children may resume growth at a rate greater than normal (period of transient catch-up growth). In some cases catch-up growth may be adequate to normalize growth; however, in children with severe and prolonged hypothyroidism, adult height may be reduced. Excessive thyroxine replacement may initiate accelerated bone maturation resulting in disproportionate advancement in skeletal age and shortened adult stature.

Assessment of permanence of hypothyroidism may be done when transient hypothyroidism is suspected. Levothyroxine therapy may be interrupted for 30 days and serum measurement of T_4 and TSH levels obtained. If T_4 is low and the TSH level is elevated, permanent hypothyroidism is confirmed and therapy should be re-instituted. If T_4 and TSH remain in the normal range, a presumptive diagnosis of transient hypothyroidism can be made. In this instance, continued clinical monitoring and periodic reevaluation of thyroid function may be warranted.

ADVERSE REACTIONS

Adverse reactions other than those indicative of thyrotoxicosis as a result of therapeutic overdosage, either initially or during the maintenance periods, are rare (see **OVERDOSAGE**). Craniosynostosis has been associated with iatrogenic hyperthyroidism in infants receiving thyroid hormone replacement therapy. Inadequate doses of SYNTHROID may produce or fail to resolve symptoms of hypothyroidism. Hypersensitivity reactions to the product excipients, such as rash and urticaria, may occur. Partial hair loss may occur during the initial months of therapy, but is generally transient. The incidence of continued hair loss is unknown. Pseudotumor cerebri has been reported in pediatric patients receiving thyroid hormone replacement therapy.

OVERDOSAGE

Signs and Symptoms: Excessive doses of SYNTHROID result in a hypermetabolic state indistinguishable from thyrotoxicosis of endogenous origin. Signs and symptoms of thyrotoxicosis include weight loss, increased appetite, palpitations, nervousness, diarrhea, abdominal cramps, sweating, tachycardia, increased pulse and blood pressure, cardiac arrhythmias, tremors, insomnia, heat intolerance, fever, and menstrual irregularities. Symptoms are not always evident or may not appear until several days after ingestion.

Treatment of Overdosage: SYNTHROID should be reduced in dose or temporarily discontinued if signs and symptoms of overdosage appear.

In the treatment of acute massive SYNTHROID overdosage, symptomatic and supportive therapy should be instituted immediately. Treatment is aimed at reducing gastrointestinal absorption and counteracting central and peripheral effects, mainly those of increased sympathetic activity. The stomach should be emptied immediately by emesis or gastric lavage if not otherwise contraindicated (e.g., by coma, convulsions or loss of gag reflex). Cholestyramine and activated charcoal have also been used to decrease levothyroxine sodium absorption. Oxygen should be administered and ventilation maintained as necessary, β-receptor antagonists, particularly propranolol, are useful in counteracting many of the effects of increased sympathetic activity. Propranolol may be administered intravenously at a dosage of 1 to 3 mg over a 10 minute period or orally, 80 to 160 mg/day, especially when no contraindications exist for its use. Cardiac glycosides may be administered if congestive heart failure develops. Measures to control fever, hypoglycemia, or fluid loss should be initiated as necessary. Glucocorticoids may be administered to inhibit the conversion of T_4 to T_3. Since T_4 is extensively protein bound, very little drug will be removed by dialysis.

DOSAGE AND ADMINISTRATION

The dosage and rate of administration of SYNTHROID is determined by the indication, and must in every case be individualized according to patient response and laboratory findings.

Hypothyroidism: The goal of therapy for primary hypothyroidism is to achieve and maintain a clinical and biochemical euthyroid state with consequent resolution of hypothyroid signs and symptoms. The starting dose of SYNTHROID, the frequency of dose titration, and the optimal full replacement dose must be individualized for every patient, and will be influenced by such factors as age, weight, cardiovascular status, presence of other illness, and the severity and duration of hypothyroid symptoms.

The usual full replacement dose of SYNTHROID for younger, healthy adults is approximately 1.6 mcg/kg/day administered once daily. In the elderly, the full replacement dose may be altered by decreases in T_4 metabolism and levothyroxine sodium absorption. Older patients may require less than 1 mcg/kg/day. Children generally require higher doses (see **Pediatric Dosage**). Women who are maintained on SYNTHROID during pregnancy may require increased doses (see **Pregnancy**).

Therapy is usually initiated in younger, healthy adults at the anticipated full replacement dose. Clinical and laboratory evaluations should be performed at 6 to 8 week intervals (2 to 3 weeks in severely hypothyroid patients), and the dosage adjusted by 12.5 to 25 mcg increments until the serum TSH concentration is normalized and signs and symptoms resolve. In older patients or in younger patients with a history of cardiovascular disease, the starting dose should be 12.5 to 50 mcg once daily with adjustments of 12.5 to 25 mcg every 3 to 6 weeks until TSH is normalized. If cardiac symptoms develop or worsen, the cardiac disease should be evaluated and the dose of SYNTHROID reduced. Rarely, worsening angina or other signs of cardiac ischemia may prevent achieving a TSH in the normal range.

Treatment of subclinical hypothyroidism, when indicated, may require lower than usual replacement doses, e.g. 1.0 mcg/kg/day. Patients for whom treatment is not initiated should be monitored yearly for changes in clinical status, TSH, and thyroid antibodies.

In patients with hypothyroidism resulting from pituitary or hypothalamic disease, the possibility of secondary adrenal insufficiency should be considered, and if present, treated with glucocorticoids prior to initiation of SYNTHROID. The adequacy of SYNTHROID therapy should be assessed in these patients by measuring FT_4I, which should be maintained in the upper half of the normal range, in addition to clinical assessment. Measurement of TSH is not a reliable indicator of response to therapy for this condition.

Few patients require doses greater than 200 mcg/day. An inadequate response to daily doses of 300 to 400 mcg/day is rare, and may suggest malabsorption, poor patient compliance, and/or drug interactions.

Once optimal replacement is achieved, clinical and laboratory evaluations should be conducted at least annually or whenever warranted by a change in patient status. Levothyroxine sodium products from different manufacturers should not be used interchangeably unless retesting of the patient and retitration of the dosage, as necessary, accompanies the product switch.

SYNTHROID Injection by the intravenous of intramuscular route can be substituted for the oral dosage form when the oral administration is precluded. The initial parenteral dosage should be approximately one-half the previously established oral dosage of SYNTHROID Tablets. Close observation of the patient is recommended, with adjustment of the dosage as needed. Administration of SYNTHROID Injection by the subcutaneous route is not recommended as studies have shown that the influx of T_4 from the subcutaneous site is very slow, and depends on many factors such as volume of injectate, the anatomic site of injection, ambient temperature, and presence of venospasm.

Myxedema Coma: Myxedema coma represents the extreme expression of severe hypothyroidism and is considered a medical emergency. It is characterized by hypothermia, hypotension, hypoventilation, hyponatremia, and bradycardia. In addition to restoration of normal thyroid hormone levels, therapy should be directed at the correction of electrolyte disturbances and possible infection. Because the mortality rate of patients with untreated myxedema coma is high, treatment must be started immediately, and should include appropriate supportive therapy and corticosteroids to prevent adrenal insufficiency. Possible precipitating factors should also be identified and treated. SYNTHROID may be given via nasogastric tube, but the preferred route of administration is intravenous. A bolus dose of SYNTHROID is given immediately to replete the peripheral pool of T_4, usually 300 to 500 mcg. Although such a dose is usually well-tolerated even in the elderly, the rapid intravenous administration of large doses of levothyroxine sodium to patients with cardiovascular disease is clearly not without risks. Under such circumstances, intravenous therapy should not be undertaken without weighing the alternate risks of myxedema coma and the cardiovascular disease. Clinical judgement in this situation may dictate smaller intravenous doses of SYNTHROID. The initial dose is followed by daily intravenous doses of 75 to 100 mcg until the patient is stable and oral administration is feasible. Normal T_4 levels are usually achieved in 24 hours, followed by progressive increases in T_3. Improvement in cardiac output, blood pressure, temperature, and mental status generally occur within 24 hours, with improvement in many manifestations of hypothyroidism in 4 to 7 days.

TSH Suppression in Thyroid Cancer and Thyroid Nodules: The rationale for TSH suppression therapy is that a reduction in TSH secretion may decrease the growth and function of abnormal thyroid tissue. Exogenous thyroid hormone may inhibit recurrence of tumor growth and may produce regression of metastases from well-differentiated (follicular and papillary) carcinoma of the thyroid. It is used as ancillary therapy of these conditions following surgery or radioactive iodine therapy. Medullary and anaplastic carcinoma of the thyroid is unresponsive to TSH suppression therapy. TSH suppression is also used in treating nontoxic solitary nodules and multinodular goiters.

No controlled studies have compared the various degrees of TSH suppression in the treatment of either benign or malignant thyroid nodular disease. Further, the effectiveness of TSH suppression for benign nodular disease is controversial. The dose of SYNTHROID used for TSH suppression should therefore be individualized by the nature of the disease, the patient being treated, and the desired clinical response, weighing the potential benefits of therapy against the risks of iatrogenic thyrotoxicosis. In general, SYNTHROID should be given in the smallest dose that will achieve the desired clinical response.

For well-differentiated thyroid cancer, TSH is generally suppressed to less than 0.1 mU/L. Doses of SYNTHROID greater than 2 mcg/kg/day are usually required. The efficacy of TSH suppression in reducing the size of benign thyroid nodules and in preventing nodule regrowth after surgery are controversial. Nevertheless, when treatment with levothyroxine sodium is considered warranted, TSH is generally suppressed to a higher target range (e.g., 0.1 to 0.3 mU/L) than that employed for the treatment of thyroid cancer.

SYNTHROID therapy may also be considered for patients with nontoxic multinodular goiter who have a TSH in the normal range, to moderately suppress TSH (e.g., 0.1 to 0.3 mU/L).

SYNTHROID should be administered with caution to patients in whom there is a suspicion of thyroid gland autonomy, in view of the fact that the effects of exogenous hormone administration will be additive to endogenous thyroid hormone production.

Pediatric Dosage: Congenital or acquired hypothyroidism: The dosage of SYNTHROID for pediatric hypothyroidism varies with age and body weight. SYNTHROID should be given at a dose that maintains the serum total T_4 or free T_4 concentrations in the upper half of the normal range and serum TSH in the normal range (see **Pediatric Use**).

SYNTHROID therapy is usually initiated at the full replacement dose (see Table). Infants and neonates with very low or undetectable serum T_4 levels (<5 mcg/dL) should start at the higher end of the dosage range (e.g., 50 mcg daily). A lower starting dosage (e.g., 25 mcg daily) should be considered for neonates at risk of cardiac failure, increasing every few days until a full maintenance dose is reached. In children with severe, long-standing hypothyroidism, SYNTHROID should be initiated gradually, with an initial dose of 25 mcg for two weeks, and then increasing the dose by 25 mcg every 2 to 4 weeks until the desired dose based on serum T_4 and TSH levels is achieved. (see **Pediatric Use**).

Serum T_4 and TSH measurements should be evaluated at the following intervals, with subsequent dosage adjustments to normalize serum total T_4 or FT_4, and TSH:

- 2 and 4 weeks after the initiation of SYNTHROID treatment;
- every 1 to 2 months during the first year of life;
- every 2 to 3 months between 1 and 3 years of age;
- every 3 to 12 months thereafter until growth is completed.

Evaluation at more frequent intervals is advisable when compliance is questioned or abnormal values are obtained. Patient evaluation is also advisable approximately 6 to 8 weeks after any change in SYNTHROID dose.

SYNTHROID tablets may be given to infants and children who cannot swallow intact tablets by crushing the tablet and suspending the freshly crushed tablet in a small amount of water (5 to 10 mL), breast milk or non-soybean formula. The suspension can be given by spoon or dropper. **DO NOT STORE THE SUSPENSION FOR ANY PERIOD OF TIME.** The crushed tablet may also be sprinkled over a small amount of food, such as apple sauce. Foods or formula containing large amounts of soybean, fiber, or iron should not be used for administering SYNTHROID.

Dosing Guidelines for Pediatric Hypothyroidism

Age	Daily dose per kg body weight*
0-3 mos	10-15 mcg
3-6 mos	8-10 mcg
6-12 mos	6-8 mcg
1-5 yrs	5-6 mcg
6-12 yrs	4-5 mcg
>12 years	2-3 mcg
Growth & puberty complete	1.6 mcg

* To be adjusted on the basis of clinical response and laboratory tests (see Laboratory Tests).

HOW SUPPLIED

SYNTHROID® (levothyroxine sodium, USP) **Tablets:** round, color coded, scored tablet debossed with "FLINT" and potency.

25 mcg, orange

Bottles of 100, Code 3P1023	NDC 0048-1020-03
Bottles of 1000, Code 3P1025	NDC 0048-1020-05

50 mcg, white

Bottles of 100, Code 3P1043	NDC 0048-1040-03
Bottles of 1000, Code 3P1045	NDC 0048-1040-05
Unit Dose Cartons of 100, Code 3P1033	NDC 0048-1040-13

75 mcg, violet

Bottles of 100, Code 3P1053	NDC 0048-1050-03
Bottles of 1000, Code 3P1055	NDC 0048-1050-05
Unit Dose Cartons of 100, Code 3P1003	NDC 0048-1050-13

88 mcg, olive

Bottles of 100, Code 3P0883	NDC 0048-1060-03

Continued on next page

Synthroid—Cont.

100 mcg, yellow
Bottles of 100, Code 3P1073 NDC 0048-1070-03
Bottles of 1000, Code 3P1075 NDC 0048-1070-05
Unit Dose Cartons of 100, Code 3P1063 NDC 0048-1070-13

112 mcg, rose
Bottles of 100, Code 3P1183 NDC 0048-1080-03
Bottles of 1000, Code 3P1185 NDC 0048-1080-05

125 mcg, brown
Bottles of 100, Code 3P1103 NDC 0048-1130-03
Bottles of 1000, Code 3P1105 NDC 0048-1130-05
Unit Dose Cartons of 100, Code 3P1113 NDC 0048-1130-13

150 mcg, blue
Bottles of 100, Code 3P1093 NDC 0048-1090-03
Bottles of 1000, Code 3P1095 NDC 0048-1090-05
Unit Dose Cartons of 100, Code 3P1083 NDC 0048-1090-13

175 mcg, lilac
Bottles of 100, Code 3P1153 NDC 0048-1100-03

200 mcg, pink
Bottles of 100, Code 3P1143 NDC 0048-1140-03
Bottles of 1000, Code 3P1145 NDC 0048-1140-05
Unit Dose Cartons of 100, Code 3P1133 NDC 0048-1140-13

300 mcg, green
Bottles of 100, Code 3P1173 NDC 0048-1170-03
Bottles of 1000, Code 3P1175 NDC 0048-1170-05

Store at controlled room temperature 15°-30°C (59°-86°F). SYNTHROID Tablets should be protected from light and moisture.

SYNTHROID® (levothyroxine sodium, USP) **Injection** is a lyophilized powder. It is supplied in color coded vials as follows:

200 mcg, gray
10 mL Single Dose Vial, Code 3P1312 NDC 0048-1014-99

500 mcg, yellow
10 mL Single Dose Vial, Code 3P1302 NDC 0048-1012-99

Store at controlled room temperature 15°- 30C (59 - 86°F).

DIRECTIONS FOR RECONSTITUTION: Reconstitute the lyophilized levothyroxine sodium by aseptically adding 5 mL of 0.9% Sodium Chloride Injection, USP (final volume approximately 5mL). Shake vial to insure complete mixing. Do not add to other intravenous fluids. Use immediately after reconstitution. Discard any unused portion.

CAUTION: Federal (USA) law prohibits dispensing without a prescription.

Tablets Manufactured by
BASF Pharmaceuticals
A Unit of BASF
Jayuya, Puerto Rico 00664
Injection Manufactured by
Ben Venue Laboratories, Inc.
Bedford, Ohio 44146 USA
For
Knoll Pharmaceutical Company
3000 Continental Drive-North
Mount Olive, NJ 07828–1234
BASF Pharma

Revised: April 1998 7920–10

Shown in Product Identification Guide, pages 319 and 320

TARKA® ℞
(Trandolapril/Verapamil Hydrochloride ER Tablets)

USE IN PREGNANCY

When used in pregnancy during the second and third trimesters, ACE inhibitors can cause injury and even death to the developing fetus. When pregnancy is detected, TARKA® should be discontinued as soon as possible. **See WARNINGS, Fetal/Neonatal Morbidity and Mortality.**

DESCRIPTION

TARKA® (trandolapril/verapamil hydrochloride ER) combines a slow release formulation of a calcium channel blocker, verapamil hydrochloride, and an immediate release formulation of an angiotensin converting enzyme inhibitor, trandolapril.

Verapamil Component—Verapamil hydrochloride is chemically described as benzeneacetonitrile, α[3-[[2-(3,4-dimethoxyphenyl) ethyl] methylamino] propyl]-3,4-dimethoxy-α-(1-methylethyl) hydrochloride. Its empirical formula is $C_{27}H_{38}N_2O_4$ HCl and its structural formula is:

Verapamil hydrochloride is an almost white crystalline powder, with a molecular weight of 491.08. It is soluble in water, chloroform, and methanol. It is practically free of odor, with a bitter taste.

Trandolapril Component—Trandolapril is the ethyl ester prodrug of a nonsulfhydryl angiotensin converting enzyme (ACE) inhibitor, trandolaprilat. It is chemically described as (2S,3aR,7aS)-1-[(S)-N-[(S)-Carboxy-3-phenylpropyl]alanyl] hexahydro-2-indolinecarboxylic acid, 1-ethyl ester. Its empirical formula is $C_{24}H_{34}N_2O_5$ and its structural formula is:

Trandolapril is a colorless, crystalline substance with a molecular weight of 430.54. It is soluble (>100 mg/mL) in chloroform, dichloromethane, and methanol.

TARKA tablets are formulated for oral administration, containing verapamil hydrochloride as a controlled release formulation and trandolapril as an immediate release formulation. The tablet strengths are trandolapril 2 mg/verapamil hydrochloride ER 180 mg, trandolapril 1 mg/verapamil hydrochloride ER 240 mg, trandolapril 2 mg/verapamil hydrochloride ER 240 mg, and trandolapril 4 mg/verapamil hydrochloride ER 240 mg. The tablets also contain the following ingredients: corn starch, dioctyl sodium sulfosuccinate, ethanol, hydroxypropyl cellulose, hydroxypropyl methylcellulose, lactose, magnesium stearate, microcrystalline cellulose, polyethylene glycol, povidone, purified water, silicon dioxide, sodium alginate, sodium stearyl fumarate, synthetic iron oxides, talc, and titanium dioxide.

CLINICAL PHARMACOLOGY

Verapamil hydrochloride and trandolapril have been used individually and in combination for the treatment of hypertension. For the four dosing strengths, the antihypertensive effect of the combination is approximately additive to the individual components.

Verapamil Component—Verapamil is a calcium channel blocker that exerts its pharmacologic effects by modulating the influx of ionic calcium across the cell membrane of the arterial smooth muscle as well as in conductile and contractile myocardial cells. Verapamil exerts antihypertensive effects by decreasing systemic vascular resistance, usually without orthostatic decreases in blood pressure or reflex tachycardia. During isometric or dynamic exercise, verapamil does not alter systolic cardiac function in patients with normal ventricular function. Verapamil does not alter total serum calcium levels.

Trandolapril Component—Trandolapril is de-esterified to its diacid metabolite, trandolaprilat. Both inhibit angiotensin-converting enzyme (ACE) in human subjects and in animals. Trandolaprilat is about 8 times more potent than trandolapril. ACE is a peptidyl dipeptidase that catalyzes the conversion of angiotensin I to the vasoconstrictor, angiotensin II. Angiotensin II also stimulates aldosterone secretion by the adrenal cortex.

Inhibition of ACE results in decreased plasma angiotensin II, which leads to decreased vasopressor activity and to decreased aldosterone secretion. The latter decrease may result in a small increase of serum potassium. In controlled clinical trials, treatment with TARKA resulted in mean increases in potassium of 0.1 mEq/L (see **PRECAUTIONS**). Removal of angiotensin II negative feedback on renin secretion leads to increased plasma renin activity (PRA).

ACE is identical to kininase II, an enzyme that degrades bradykinin. Whether increased levels of bradykinin, a potent vasodepressor peptide, play a role in the therapeutic effect of TARKA remains to be elucidated.

While the mechanism through which trandolapril lowers blood pressure is believed to be primarily suppression of the renin-angiotensin-aldosterone system, trandolapril has an antihypertensive effect even in patients with low renin hypertension. Trandolapril is an effective antihypertensive in all races studied. Both black patients (usually a predominantly low renin group) and non-black patients respond to 2 to 4 mg of trandolapril.

Pharmacokinetics and Metabolism: *TARKA*—Following a single oral dose of TARKA in healthy subjects, peak plasma concentrations are reached within 0.5–2 hours for trandolapril and within 4–15 hours for verapamil. Peak plasma concentrations of the active desmethyl metabolite of verapamil, norverapamil, are reached within 5–15 hours. Cleavage of the ester group converts trandolapril to its active diacid metabolite, trandolaprilat, which reaches peak plasma concentrations within 2–12 hours. The pharmacokinetics of trandolapril and trandolaprilat are not altered when trandolapril is administered in combination with verapamil, compared to monotherapy. The AUC and Cmax for both verapamil and norverapamil are increased when 240 mg of controlled release verapamil is administered concomitantly with 4 mg trandolapril. The increase in Cmax is 54 and 30% and the AUC is increased by 65 and 32% for verapamil and norverapamil, respectively. Administration of TARKA 4/240 (4 mg trandolapril and 240 mg verapamil hydrochloride ER) with a high-fat meal does not alter the bioavailability of trandolapril whereas verapamil peak concentrations and area under the curve (AUC) decrease 37% and 28%, respectively. Food thus decreases verapamil bioavailability and the time to peak plasma concentration for both verapamil and norverapamil are delayed by approximately 7 hours. Both optical isomers of verapamil are similarly affected.

Trandolaprilat has an effective elimination half-life of approximately 10 hours but like all ACE inhibitors, it has a prolonged terminal elimination half-life. The terminal half-life of verapamil is 6–11 hours. Steady-state plasma concentrations of the two components are achieved after about a week of once-daily dosing of TARKA. At steady-state, plasma concentrations of verapamil and trandolaprilat are up to two-fold higher than those observed after a single oral TARKA dose.

The pharmacokinetics of verapamil and trandolaprilat are significantly different in the elderly (≥65 years) than in younger subjects. The bioavailability of verapamil and norverapamil are increased by 87% and 77%, respectively, and that of trandolapril by approximately 35% in the elderly. AUCs are approximately 80% and 35% higher, respectively.

Verapamil Component—With the immediate release formulation, more than 90% of the orally administered dose is absorbed with peak plasma concentrations of verapamil observed 1 to 2 hours after dosing. A delayed rate but similar extent of absorption is observed for the sustained release formulation when compared to the immediate release formulation. Because of the rapid biotransformation of verapamil during its first pass through the portal circulation, absolute bioavailability ranges from 20% to 35%. A nonlinear correlation exists between verapamil dose and plasma concentrations.

In early dose titration with verapamil, a relationship exists between plasma concentrations of verapamil and prolongation of the PR interval. However, during chronic administration, this relationship may disappear. No relationship has been established between the plasma concentration of verapamil and reduction in blood pressure.

In healthy subjects, orally administered verapamil undergoes extensive metabolism in the liver. Twelve metabolites have been identified in plasma; all except norverapamil are present in trace amounts only. Approximately 70% of an administered dose is excreted as metabolites in the urine and 16% or more in the feces within 5 days. Urinary excretion of unchanged drug is about 3% to 4% of the dose. Verapamil is approximately 90% bound to plasma proteins.

In patients with hepatic insufficiency, verapamil clearance is decreased about 30% and the elimination half-life is prolonged up to 14 to 16 hours (see **PRECAUTIONS**). In patients with liver dysfunction, a dosage adjustment may be required. In the elderly (≥65 years), verapamil clearance is reduced resulting in increases in elimination half-life.

Trandolapril Component—Following oral administration of trandolapril, the absolute bioavailability of trandolapril is approximately 10% as trandolapril and 10% as trandolaprilat. Plasma concentrations of trandolaprilat but not trandolapril increase in proportion with dose. Plasma concentrations of trandolaprilat decline in a triphasic manner. The more prolonged terminal elimination phase probably represents a small fraction of dose saturably bound to ACE.

After an oral radiolabeled dose of trandolapril, excretion of trandolapril and metabolites account for 33% of the dose in the urine and about 66% in the feces. Less than 1% of the dose is excreted in the urine as unchanged drug. Serum protein binding of trandolapril is about 80%, and is independent of concentration. Binding of trandolaprilat is concentration-dependent, varying from 65% at 1000 ng/ml to 94% at 0.1 ng/ml, indicating saturation of binding with increasing concentration.

Compared to normal subjects, the plasma concentrations of trandolapril and trandolaprilat are approximately 2-fold greater and renal clearance is reduced by about 85% in patients with creatinine clearance below 30 ml/min and in patients on hemodialysis. Dosage adjustment is recommended in renally impaired patients. (See **DOSAGE AND ADMINISTRATION**).

Following oral administration in patients with mild to moderate alcoholic cirrhosis, plasma concentrations of trandolapril and trandolaprilat were, respectively, 9-fold and 2-fold greater than in normal subjects, but inhibition of ACE activity was not affected. Lower dosages should be considered in patients with hepatic insufficiency, (see **DOSAGE AND ADMINISTRATION**).

Pharmacodynamics: *TARKA*—Verapamil does not interfere with ACE inhibition by trandolapril. Trandolapril does not alter the effect of verapamil on intra-cardiac conduction.

Verapamil Component—Verapamil dilates the main coronary arteries, both in normal and ischemic regions, and is a potent inhibitor of coronary artery spasm. This property increases myocardial oxygen delivery in patients with coronary artery spasm, and is responsible for the effectiveness of verapamil in vasospastic (Prinzmetal's or variant) as well as unstable angina at rest.

Verapamil regularly reduces the total systemic resistance (afterload) by dilating peripheral arterioles. By decreasing the influx of calcium, verapamil prolongs the effective refractory period within the AV node and slows AV conduction in a rate-related manner.

Normal sinus rhythm is usually not affected, but in patients with sick sinus syndrome, verapamil may interfere with sinus node impluse generation and may induce sinus arrest or sinoatrial block. Atrioventricular block can occur in patients without preexisting conduction defects (see **WARNINGS**).

Verapamil does not alter the normal atrial action potential or intraventricular conduction time, but depresses amplitude, velocity of depolarization and conduction in depressed atrial fibers. Verapamil may shorten the antegrade effective refractory period of accessory bypass tracts. Acceleration of ventricular rate and/or ventricular fibrillation has been reported in patients with atrial flutter or atrial fibrillation and a coexisting accessory AV pathway following administration of verapamil (see **WARNINGS**).

Hemodynamics and Myocardial Metabolism: Verapamil reduces afterload and myocardial contractility. Improved left ventricular diastolic function in patients with idiopathic hypertrophic subaortic stenosis (IHSS) and those with coronary heart disease has also been observed with verapamil therapy. In most patients, including those with organic cardiac disease, the negative inotropic action of verapamil is countered by a reduction of afterload and cardiac index is usually not reduced. However, in patients with severe left ventricular dysfunction (e.g., pulmonary wedge pressure about 20 mmHg or ejection fraction less than 30%), or in patients taking beta-adrenergic blocking agents or other cardio-depressant drugs, deterioration of ventricular function may occur (see **DRUG INTERACTIONS**).

Pulmonary Function: Verapamil does not induce bronchoconstriction and hence, does not impair ventilatory function.

Trandolapril Component—After a single 2 mg dose of trandolapril, inhibition of ACE activity reaches a maximum (70–85%) at 4 hours with about 1% decline at 24 hours. Eight days after dosing, ACE inhibition is still 40%.

Four placebo-controlled dose response studies were conducted using once daily oral dosing of trandolapril in doses from 0.25 to 16 mg per day in 827 black and non-black patients with mild to moderate hypertension. The minimal effective once daily dose was 1.0 mg in non-black patients and 2.0 mg in black patients. Further decreases in trough supine diastolic blood pressure were obtained in non-black patients with higher doses, and no further response was seen in doses above 4 mg (up to 16 mg). The antihypertensive effect diminished somewhat at the end of the dosing interval.

During chronic therapy, the maximum reduction in blood pressure with any dose is achieved within one week. Following 6 weeks of monotherapy in placebo-controlled trials in patients with mild to moderate hypertension, once daily doses of 2 to 4 mg lowered supine or standing systolic/diastolic blood pressure 24 hours after dosing by an average 7–10/4–5 mmHg below placebo responses in non-black patients. Once daily doses of 2 to 4 mg lowered blood pressures 4–6/3–4 mmHg below placebo responses in black patients.

CLINICAL STUDIES

In controlled clinical trials, once daily doses of TARKA, trandolapril 4 mg/verapamil HCl ER 240 mg or trandolapril 2 mg/verapamil HCl ER 180 mg, decreased placebo-corrected seated pressure (systolic/diastolic) 24 hours after dosing by about 7–12/6–8 mmHg. Each of the components of TARKA added to the antihypertensive effect. Treatment effects were consistent across age groups (<65, ≥65 years), and gender (male, female).

Blood pressure reductions were significantly greater for the TARKA 4/240 combination than for either of the components used alone.

The antihypertensive effects of TARKA have continued during therapy for at least 1 year.

INDICATIONS AND USAGE

TARKA is indicated for treatment of hypertension.

This fixed combination drug is not indicated for the initial therapy of hypertension (see DOSAGE and ADMINISTRATION).

In using TARKA, consideration should be given to the fact that an angiotension converting enzyme inhibitor, captopril, has caused agranulocytosis, particularly in patients with renal impairment or collagen vascular disease, and that available data are insufficient to show that trandolapril does not have similar risk (see **WARNINGS: Neutropenia/Agranulocytosis**).

CONTRAINDICATIONS

TARKA is contraindicated in patients who are hypersensitive to any ACE inhibitor or verapamil.

Because of the verapamil component, TARKA is contraindicated in:

1. Severe left ventricular dysfunction (see **WARNINGS**).
2. Hypotension (systolic pressure less than 90 mmHg) or cardiogenic shock.
3. Sick sinus syndrome (except in patients with a functioning artificial ventricular pacemaker).
4. Second- or third-degree AV block (except in patients with a functioning artificial ventricular pacemaker).
5. Patients with atrial flutter or atrial fibrillation and an accessory bypass tract (e.g. Wolff-Parkinson-White, Lown-Ganong-Levine syndromes) (see **WARNINGS**).

Because of the trandolapril component, TARKA is contraindicated in patients with a history of angioedema related to previous treatment with angiotensin converting enzyme (ACE) inhibitor.

WARNINGS

Heart Failure: *Verapamil Component*—Verapamil has a negative inotropic effect which, in most patients, is compensated by its afterload reduction (decreased systemic vascular resistance) properties without a net impairment of ventricular performance. In clinical experience with 4,954 patients, 87 (1.8%) developed congestive heart failure of pulmonary edema. Verapamil should be avoided in patients with severe left ventricular dysfunction (e.g., ejection fraction less than 30%, pulmonary wedge pressure above 20 mmHg, or severe symptoms of cardiac failure) and in patients with any degree of ventricular dysfunction if they are receiving a beta adrenergic blocker (see **DRUG INTERACTIONS**). Patients with milder ventricular dysfunction should, if possible, be controlled with optimum doses of digitalis and/or diuretics before verapamil treatment (Note interactions with digoxin under: **PRECAUTIONS**).

Trandolapril Component—Trandolapril, as an ACE inhibitor, may cause excessive hypotension in patients with congestive heart failure (see **WARNINGS, Hypotension**).

Hypotension: *Verapamil Component*—Occasionally, the pharmacologic action of verapamil may produce a decrease in blood pressure below normal levels which may result in dizziness or symptomatic hypotension.

Trandolapril Component—Trandolapril can cause symptomatic hypotension. Like other ACE inhibitors, trandolapril has only rarely been associated with symptomatic hypotension in uncomplicated hypertensive patients. Symptomatic hypotension is most likely to occur in patients who are salt- or volume-depleted as a result of prolonged treatment with diuretics, dietary salt restriction, dialysis, diarrhea, or vomiting. Volume and/or salt depletion should be corrected before initiating treatment with trandolapril (see **PRECAUTIONS, Drug Interactions**, and **ADVERSE REACTIONS**).

In controlled studies, hypotension was observed in 0.6% of patients receiving any combination of trandolapril and verapamil HCl ER.

In patients with concomitant congestive heart failure, with or without associated renal insufficiency, ACE inhibitor therapy may cause excessive hypotension, which may be associated with oliguria or azotemia, and, rarely, with acute renal failure and death (see **DOSAGE AND ADMINISTRATION**).

If symptomatic hypotension occurs, the patients should be placed in the supine position and, if necessary, normal saline may be administered intravenously. A transient hypotensive response is not a contraindication to further doses; however, lower doses of verapamil HCl ER and/or trandolapril or reduced concomitant diuretic therapy should be considered.

Elevated Liver Enzymes/Hepatic Failure:

Verapamil Component—Elevations of transaminases with and without concomitant elevations in alkaline phosphatase and bilirubin have been reported. Such elevations have sometimes been transient and may disappear even in the face of continued verapamil treatment. Several cases of hepatocellular injury related to verapamil have been proven by rechallenge; half of these had clinical symptoms (malaise, fever, and/or right upper quadrant pain) in addition to elevations of SGOT, SGPT, and alkaline phosphatase.

Trandolapril Component—ACE inhibitors rarely have been associated with a syndrome of cholestatic jaundice, fulminant hepatic necrosis, and death. The mechanism of this syndrome is not understood. Patients receiving ACE inhibitors who develop jaundice should discontinue the ACE inhibitor and receive appropriate medical follow-up.

Liver abnormalities were noted in 3.2% of patients taking any of several combinations of trandolapril/verapamil doses. Periodic monitoring of liver function in patients taking TARKA is therefore prudent.

Accessory Bypass Tract (Wolff-Parkinson-White or Lown-Ganong-Levine Syndromes):

Verapamil Component—Some patients with paroxysmal and/or chronic atrial fibrillation or atrial flutter and a coexisting accessory AV pathway have developed increased antegrade conduction across the accessory pathway bypassing the AV node, producing a very rapid ventricular response or ventricular fibrillation after receiving intravenous verapamil (or digitalis). Although a risk of this occurring with oral verapamil has not been established, such patients receiving oral verapamil may be at risk and its use in these patients is contraindicated (see **CONTRAINDICATIONS**). Treatment is usually DC-cardioversion. Cardioversion has been used safely and effectively after oral verapamil.

Atrioventricular Block:

Verapamil Component—The effect of verapamil on AV conduction and the SA node may lead to asymptomatic first-degree AV block and transient bradycardia, sometimes accompanied by nodal escape rhythms. PR interval prolongation is correlated with verapamil plasma concentrations, especially during the early titration phases of therapy. Higher degrees of AV block, however, were infrequently (0.8%) observed. Marked first-degree block or progressive development to second- or third-degree AV block requires a reduction in dosage or, in rare instances, discontinuation of verapamil HCl and institution of appropriate therapy depending upon the clinical situation.

Patients with Hypertrophic Cardiomyopathy (IHSS):

Verapamil Component—In 120 patients with hypertrophic cardiomyopathy (most of them refractory or intolerant to propranolol) who received therapy with verapamil at doses up to 720 mg/day, a variety of serious adverse effects were seen. Three patients died in pulmonary edema; all had severe left ventricular outflow obstruction and a past history of left ventricular dysfunction. Eight other patients had pulmonary edema and/or severe hypotension; abnormally high (over 20 mmHg) capillary wedge pressure and a marked left ventricular outflow obstruction were present in most of these patients. Sinus bradycardia occurred in 11% of the patients, second-degree AV block in 4% and sinus arrest in 2%. It must be appreciated that this group of patients had a serious disease with a high mortality rate. Most adverse effects responded well to dose reduction and only rarely did verapamil have to be discontinued.

Anaphylactoid and Possibly Related Reactions:

Presumably because angiotensin-converting enzyme inhibitors affect the metabolism of eicosanoids and polypeptides, including endogenous bradykinin, patients receiving ACE inhibitors, including trandolapril may be subject to a variety of adverse reactions, some of them serious.

Angioedema:

Angioedema of the face, extremities, lips, tongue, glottis, and larynx has been reported in patients treated with ACE inhibitors including trandolapril. Symptoms suggestive of angioedema or facial edema occurred in 0.13% of trandolapril-treated patients. Two of the four cases were life-threatening and resolved without treatment or with medication (corticosteroids). Angioedema associated with laryngeal edema can be fatal. If laryngeal stridor or angioedema of the face, tongue or glottis occurs, treatment with TARKA should be discontinued immediately, the patient treated in accordance with accepted medical care and carefully observed until the swelling disappears. In instances where swelling is confined to the face and lips, the condition generally resolves without treatment; antihistamines may be useful in relieving symptoms **Where there is involvement of the tongue, glottis, or larynx, likely to cause airway obstruction, emergency therapy, including but not limited to subcutaneous epinephrine solution 1:1,000 (0.3 to 0.5 mL) should be promptly administered.** (see **PRECAUTIONS: Information for Patients** and **ADVERSE REACTIONS**).

Anaphylactoid Reactions During Desensitization: Two patients undergoing desensitizing treatment with hymenoptera venom while receiving ACE inhibitors sustained life-threatening anaphylactoid reactions. In the same patients, these reactions did not occur when ACE inhibitors were temporarily withheld, but they reappeared when the ACE inhibitors were inadvertently readministered.

Anaphylactoid Reactions During Membrane Exposure: Anaphylactoid reactions have been reported in patients dialyzed with high-flux membranes and treated concomitantly with an ACE inhibitor. Anaphylactoid reactions have also been reported in patients undergoing low-density lipoprotein apheresis with dextran sulfate absorption.

Neutropenia/Agranulocytosis:

Trandolapril Component—Another ACE inhibitor, captopril, has been shown to cause agranulocytosis and bone marrow depression rarely in patients with uncomplicated hypertension, but more frequently in patients with renal impairment, especially if they also have a collagen-vascular disease such as systemic lupus erythematosus or scleroderma. Available data from clinical trials of trandolapril or TARKA are insufficient to show that trandolapril does not cause agranulocytosis at similar rates. As with other ACE inhibitors, periodic monitoring of white blood cell counts in patients with collagen-vascular disease and/or renal disease should be considered.

Fetal/Neonatal Morbidity and Mortality:

Trandolapril Component—ACE inhibitors can cause fetal and neonatal morbidity and death when administered to pregnant women. Several dozen cases have been reported in the world literature. When pregnancy is detected, ACE inhibitors should be discontinued as soon as possible.

The use of ACE inhibitors during the second and third trimesters of pregnancy has been associated with fetal and neonatal injury, including hypotension, neonatal skull hypoplasia, anuria, reversible or irreversible renal failure, and death. Oligohydramnios has also been reported, presumably resulting from decreased fetal renal function; oligohydramnios in this setting has been associated with fetal limb contractures, craniofacial deformation, and hypoplastic lung development. Prematurity, intrauterine growth retardation, and patent ductus arteriosus have also been reported, although it is not clear whether these occurrences were due to the ACE-inhibitor exposure.

These adverse effects do not appear to have resulted from intrauterine ACE-inhibitor exposure that has been limited to the first trimester. Mothers whose embryos and fetuses are exposed to ACE inhibitors only during the first trimester should be so informed. Nonetheless, when patients become pregnant, physicians should make every effort to discontinue the use of TARKA as soon as possible.

Rarely (probably less often than once in every thousand pregnancies), no alternative to ACE inhibitors will be found. In these rare cases, the mothers should be apprised of the potential hazards to their fetuses, and serial ultrasound examinations should be performed to assess the intra-amniotic environment.

Continued on next page

Tarka—Cont.

If oligohydramnios is observed, TARKA should be discontinued unless it is considered life-saving for the mother. Contraction stress testing (CST), a non-stress test (NST), or biophysical profiling (BPP) may be appropriate, depending upon the week of pregnancy. Patients and physicians should be aware, however, that oligohydramnios may not appear until after the fetus has sustained irreversible injury.

Infants with histories of in utero exposure to ACE inhibitors should be closely observed for hypotension, oliguria, and hyperkalemia. If oliguria occurs, attention should be directed toward support of blood pressure and renal perfusion. Exchange transfusion or dialysis may be required as a means of reversing hypotension and/or substituting for disordered renal function.

Trandolapril in doses of 0.8 mg/kg/day in rabbits, 100.0 mg/kg/day in rats, and 25 mg/kg/day in cynomolgus monkeys (10, 1,250, and 312 times the maximum projected human dose, respectively, assuming a 50 kg woman) did not produce teratogenic effects.

PRECAUTIONS

Use in Patients with Impaired Hepatic Function:
TARKA has not been evaluated in subjects with impaired hepatic function.

Verapamil Component—Since verapamil is highly metabolized by the liver, it should be administered cautiously to patients with impaired hepatic function. Severe liver dysfunction prolongs the elimination half-life of immediate release verapamil to about 14 to 16 hours; hence, approximately 30% of the dose given to patients with normal liver function should be administered to these patients.

Careful monitoring for abnormal polongation of the PR interval or other signs of excessive pharmacologic effects (see **OVERDOSAGE**) should be carried out.

Trandolapril Component—Trandolapril and trandolaprilat concentrations increase in patients with impaired liver function.

Use in Patients with Impaired Renal Function:
TARKA has not been evaluated in patients with impaired renal function.

Verapamil Component—About 70% of an administered dose of verapamil is excreted as metabolites in the urine. Verapamil is not removed by hemodialysis. Until further data are available, verapamil should be administered cautiously to patients with impaired renal function. These patients should be carefully monitored for abnormal prolongation of the PR interval or other signs of overdosage (see **OVERDOSAGE**).

Trandolapril Component—As a consequence of inhibiting the renin-angiotensin-aldosterone system, changes in renal function may be anticipated in susceptible individuals. In patients with severe heart failure whose renal function may depend on the activity of the renin-angiotensin-aldosterone system, treatment with ACE inhibitors, including trandolapril, may be associated with oliguria and/or progressive azotemia and rarely with acute renal failure and/or death.

In hypertensive patients with unilateral or bilateral renal artery stenosis, increases in blood urea nitrogen and serum creatinine have been observed in some patients following ACE inhibitor therapy. These increases were almost always reversible upon discontinuation of the ACE inhibitor and/or diuretic therapy. In such patients, renal function should be monitored during the first few weeks of therapy.

Some hypertensive patients with no apparent preexisting renal vascular disease have developed increases in blood urea and serum creatinine, usually minor and transient, especially when ACE inhibitors have been given concomitantly with a diuretic. This is more likely to occur in patients with preexisting renal impairment. Dosage reduction and/or discontinuation of any diuretic and/or the ACE inhibitor may be required.

Evaluation of hypertensive patients should always include assessment of renal function (see DOSAGE AND ADMINISTRATION).

Use in Patients with Attenuated (Decreased) Neuromuscular Transmission:
Verapamil Component—It has been reported that verapamil decreases neuromuscular transmission in patients with Duchenne's muscular dystrophy, and that verapamil prolongs recovery from the neuromuscular blocking agent vecuronium. It may be necessary to decrease the dosage of verapamil when it is administered to patients with attenuated neuromuscular transmission. (See **PRECAUTIONS—Surgery/Anesthesia**)

Hyperkalemia and potassium-sparing diuretics:
Trandolapril Component—In clinical trials, hyperkalemia (serum potassium > 6.00 mEq/L) occurred in approximately 0.4 percent of hypertensive patients receiving trandolapril and in 0.8% of patients receiving a dose of trandolapril (0.5–8 mg) in combination with a dose of verapamil SR (120–240 mg). In most cases, elevated serum potassium levels were isolated values, which resolved despite continued therapy. None of these patients were discontinued from the trials because of hyperkalemia. Risk factors for the development of hyperkalemia include renal insufficiency, diabetes mellitus, and the concomitant use of potassium-sparing diuretics, potassium supplements, and/or potassium-containing salt substitutes, which should be used cautiously, if at all, with trandolapril (see **PRECAUTIONS, Drug Interactions**).

Cough:
Presumably due to the inhibition of the degradation of endogenous bradykinin, persistent nonproductive cough has been reported with all ACE inhibitors, always resolving after discontinuation of therapy. ACE inhibitor-induced cough should be considered in the differential diagnosis of cough. In controlled trials of trandolapril, cough was present in 2% of trandolapril patients and 0% of patients given placebo. There was no evidence of a relationship to dose.

Surgery/anesthesia:
Trandolapril Component—In patients undergoing major surgery or during anesthesia with agents that produce hypotension, trandolapril will block angiotensin II formation secondary to compensatory renin release. If hypotension occurs and is considered to be due to this mechanism, it can be corrected by volume expansion. (See **PRECAUTIONS—Use in Patients with Attenuated (Decreased) Neuromuscular Transmission**)

Drug Interactions:
Digitalis: Clinical use of verapamil in digitalized patients has shown the combination to be well tolerated if digoxin doses are properly adjusted. Chronic verapamil treatment can increase serum digoxin levels by 50 to 75% during the first week of therapy, and this can result in digoxin toxicity. In patients with hepatic cirrhosis, the influence of verapamil on digoxin kinetics is magnified. Verapamil may reduce total body clearance and extrarenal clearance of digitoxin by 27% and 29%, respectively. Maintenance digoxin doses should be reduced when verapamil is administered, and the patient should be carefully monitored to avoid over- or under-digitalization. Whenever overdigitalization is suspected, the daily dose of digoxin should be reduced or temporarily discontinued. Upon discontinuation of any verapamil-containing regime including TARKA, the patient should be reassessed to avoid underdigitalization. Neither trandolapril nor its metabolites have been found to interact with digoxin.

Lithium: Increased sensitivity to the effects of lithium (neurotoxicity) has been reported during concomitant verapamil-lithium therapy with either no change or an increase in serum lithium levels. Increased serum lithium levels and symptoms of lithium toxicity have been reported in patients receiving concomitant lithium and ACE inhibitor therapy. TARKA and lithium should be coadministered with caution, and frequent monitoring of serum lithium levels is recommended. If a diuretic is also used, the risk of lithium toxicity may be increased.

Cimetidine: The interaction between cimetidine and chronically administered verapamil has not been studied. Variable results on clearance have been obtained in acute studies of healthy volunteers; clearance of verapamil was either reduced or unchanged. Neither trandolapril nor its metabolites have been found to interact with cimetidine.

Beta Blockers: *Verapamil Component*—Concomitant therapy with beta-adrenergic blockers and verapamil may result in additive negative effects on heart rate, atrioventricular conduction, and/or cardiac contractility. The use of verapamil in combination with a beta-blocker should be used only with caution, and close monitoring.

Asymptomatic bradycardia (36 beats/min) with a wandering atrial pacemaker has been observed in a patient receiving concomitant timolol (a beta-adrenergic blocker) eyedrops and oral verapamil.

Antiarrhythmic Agents:
Verapamil Component—Disopyramide—Data on possible interactions between verapamil and disopyramide phosphate are not available. Therefore, disopyramide should not be administered within 48 hours before or 24 hours after verapamil administration.

Flecainide—A study of healthy volunteers showed that the concomitant administration of flecainide and verapamil may have additive effects on myocardial contractility, AV conduction, and repolarization. Concomitant therapy with flecainide and verapamil may result in additive negative inotropic effect and prolongation of atrioventricular conduction.

Quinidine—In a small number of patients with hypertrophic cardiomyopathy (IHSS), concomitant use of verapamil and quinidine resulted in significant hypotension. Until further data are obtained, combined therapy of verapamil and quinidine in patients with hypertrophic cardiomyopathy should probably be avoided.

The electrophysiological effects of quinidine and verapamil on AV conduction were studied in 8 patients. Verapamil significantly counteracted the effects of quinidine on AV conduction. There has been a report of increased quinidine levels during verapamil therapy.

Nitrates — Verapamil has been given concomitantly with short- and long-acting nitrates without any undesirable drug interactions. The pharmacologic profile of both drugs and the clinical experience suggest beneficial interactions.

Other: *Verapamil Component* — Carbamazepine — Verapamil may increase carbamazepine concentrations during combined therapy. This may produce carbamazepine side effects such as diplopia, headache, ataxia, or dizziness.

Rifampin — Therapy with rifampin may markedly reduce oral verapamil bioavailability.

Phenobarbital — Phenobarbital therapy may increase verapamil clearance.

Cyclosporin — Verapamil therapy may increase serum levels of cyclosporin.

Theophylline — Verapamil therapy may inhibit the clearance and increase the plasma levels of theophylline.

Inhalation Anesthetics — Animal experiments have shown that inhalation anesthetics depress cardiovascular activity by decreasing the inward movement of calcium ions. When used concomitantly, inhalation anesthetics and calcium antagonists, such as verapamil, should be titrated carefully to avoid excessive cardiovascular depression.

Neuromuscular Blocking Agents — Clinical data and animal studies suggest that verapamil may potentiate the activity of neuromuscular blocking agents (curare-like and depolarizing). It may be necessary to decrease the dose of verapamil and/or the dose of the neuromuscular blocking agent when the drugs are used concomitantly.

Concomitant diuretic therapy:
Trandolapril Component — As with other ACE inhibitors, patients on diuretics, especially those on recently instituted diuretic therapy, may occasionally experience an excessive reduction of blood pressure after initiation of therapy with TARKA. The possibility of exacerbation of hypotensive effects with TARKA may be minimized by either discontinuing the diuretic or cautiously increasing salt intake prior to initiation of treatment with TARKA. If it is not possible to discontinue the diuretic, the starting dose of TARKA should be reduced (see **DOSAGE AND ADMINISTRATION**).

Agents increasing serum potassium:
Trandolapril can attenuate potassium loss caused by thiazide diuretics and increase serum potassium when used alone. Use of potassium-sparing diuretics (spironolactone, triamterene, or amiloride), potassium supplements, or potassium-containing salt substitutes concomitantly with ACE inhibitors can increase the risk of hyperkalemia. If concomitant use of such agents is indicated, they should be used with caution and with appropriate monitoring of serum potassium. (See **PRECAUTIONS.**)

Other: *Trandolapril Component* — Neither trandolapril nor its metabolites have been found to interact with furosemide or nifledipine. The anticoagulant effect of warfarin was not significantly changed by trandolapril.

Carcinogenesis, Mutagenesis, Impairment of Fertility:
Verapamil Component — An 18–month toxicity study in rats, at a low multiple (6 fold) of the maximum recommended human dose, and not the maximum tolerated dose, did not suggest a tumorigenic potential. There was no evidence of a carcinogenic potential of verapamil administered in the diet of rats for two years at doses of 10, 35, and 120 mg/kg per day or approximately 1x, 3.5x and 12x, respectively, the maximum recommended human daily dose (480 mg per day or 9.6 mg/kg/day).

Verapamil was not mutagenic in the Ames test in 5 test strains at 3 mg per plate, with or without metabolic activation.

Studies in female rats at daily doses up to 5.5 times (55 mg/kg/day) the maximum recommended human dose did not show impaired fertility. Effects on male fertility have not been determined.

Long-term studies were conducted with oral trandolapril administered by gavage to mice (78 weeks) and rats (104 and 106 weeks). No evidence of carcinogenic potential was seen in mice dosed up to 25 mg/kg/day (85 mg/m^2/day) or rats dosed up to 8 mg/kg/day (60 mg/m^2/day). These doses are 313 and 32 times (mice), and 100 and 23 times (rats) the maximum recommended human daily dose (MRHDD) of 4 mg based on body-weight and body-surface-area, respectively assuming a 50 kg individual. The genotoxic potential of trandolapril was evaluated in the microbial mutagenicity (Ames) test, the point mutation and chromosome aberration assays in Chinese hamster V79 cells, and the micronucleus test in mice. There was no evidence of mutagenic or clastogenic potential in these in vitro and in vivo assays.

Reproduction studies in rats did not show any impairment of fertility at doses up to 100 mg/kg/day (710 mg/m^2/day) of trandolapril, or 1250 and 260 times the MRHDD on the basis of body-weight and body-surface-area, respectively.

Pregnancy; Pregnancy Categories C (first trimester) and D (second and third trimesters). See WARNINGS, Fetal/Neonatal Morbidity and Mortality.

Nursing Mothers: Verapamil is excreted in human milk. Radiolabeled trandolapril or its metabolites are secreted in rat milk. TARKA should not be administered to nursing mothers.

Geriatric Use: In placebo-controlled studies, where 23% of patients receiving TARKA were 65 years and older, and 2.4% were 75 years and older, no overall differences in effectiveness or safety were observed between these patients and younger patients. However, greater sensitivity of some older individual patients cannot be ruled out.

Pediatric Use: The safety and effectiveness of TARKA in children below the age of 18 have not been established.

Animal Pharmacology and/or Animal Toxicology: In chronic animal toxicology studies, verapamil caused lenticular and/or suture line changes at 30 mg/kg/day or greater and frank cataracts at 62.5 mg/kg/day or greater in the beagle dog but not the rat. Development of cataracts due to verapamil has not been reported in man.

ADVERSE REACTIONS

TARKA has been evaluated in over 1,957 subjects and patients. Of these, 541 patients, including 23% elderly patients, participated in U.S. controlled clinical trials, and 251 were studied in foreign controlled clinical trials. In clinical trials with TARKA, no adverse experiences peculiar to this combination drug have been observed. Adverse experiences that have occurred have been limited to those that have been previously reported with verapamil or trandolapril.

TARKA has been evaluated for long-term safety in 272 patients treated for 1 year or more. Adverse experiences were usually mild and transient.

Discontinuation of therapy because of adverse events in U.S. placebo-controlled hypertension studies was required in 2.6% and 1.9% of patients treated with TARKA and placebo, respectively.

Adverse experiences occurring in 1% or more of the 541 patients in placebo-controlled hypertension trials who were treated with a range of trandolapril (0.5–8 mg) and verapamil (120–240 mg) combinations are shown below.

[See table at right]

ADVERSE EVENTS OCCURRING IN ≥ 1% OF TARKA® PATIENTS IN U.S. PLACEBO-CONTROLLED TRIALS

	TARKA (N=541) % Incidence (% Discontinuance)	PLACEBO (N=206) % Incidence (% Discontinuance)
AV Block First Degree	3.9 (0.2)	0.5 (0.0)
Bradycardia	1.8 (0.0)	0.0 (0.0)
Bronchitis	1.5 (0.0)	0.5 (0.0)
Chest Pain	2.2 (0.0)	1.0 (0.0)
Constipation	3.3 (0.0)	1.0 (0.0)
Cough	4.6 (0.0)	2.4 (0.0)
Diarrhea	1.5 (0.2)	1.0 (0.0)
Dizziness	3.1 (0.0)	1.9 (0.5)
Dyspnea	1.3 (0.4)	0.0 (0.0)
Edema	1.3 (0.0)	2.4 (0.0)
Fatigue	2.8 (0.4)	2.4 (0.0)
Headache(s)+	8.9 (0.0)	9.7 (0.5)
Increased Liver Enzymes*	2.8 (0.2)	1.0 (0.0)
Nausea	1.5 (0.2)	0.5 (0.0)
Pain Extremity(ies)	1.1 (0.2)	0.5 (0.0)
Pain Back+	2.2 (0.0)	2.4 (0.0)
Pain Joint(s)	1.7 (0.0)	1.0 (0.0)
Upper Respiratory Tract infection(s)+	5.4 (0.0)	7.8 (0.0)
Upper Respiratory Tract Congestion+	2.4 (0.0)	3.4 (0.0)

* Also includes increase in SGPT, SGOT, Alkaline Phosphatase
\+ Incidence of adverse events is higher in Placebo group than TARKA patients

Other clinical adverse experiences possibly, probably, or definitely related to drug treatment occurring in 0.3% or more of patients treated with trandolapril/verapamil combinations with or without concomitant diuretic in controlled or uncontrolled trials (N=990) and less frequent, clinically significant events (in italics) include the following.

Cardiovascular: angina, *AV block second degree, bundle branch block*, edema, flushing, hypotension, *myocardial infarction*, palpitations, premature ventricular contractions, nonspecific ST-T changes, near syncope, tachycardia.

Central Nervous System: drowsiness, *hypesthesia, insomnia, loss of balance, paresthesia, vertigo.*

Dermatologic: pruritus, rash.

Emotional, Mental, Sexual States: anxiety, impotence, *abnormal mentation.*

Eye, Ear, Nose, Throat: epistaxis, tinnitus, upper respiratory tract infection, *blurred vision.*

Gastrointestinal: diarrhea, dyspepsia, dry mouth, nausea.

General Body Function: chest pain, malaise, weakness.

Genitourinary: endometriosis, hematuria, nocturia, polyuria, proteinuria.

Hemopoietic: decreased leukocytes, *decreased neutrophils.*

Musculoskeletal System: arthralgias/myalgias, *gout (increased uric acid).*

Pulmonary: dyspnea.

Angioedema: Angioedema has been reported in 3 (0.15%) patients receiving TARKA in the U.S. and foreign studies (N=1,957). Angioedema associated with laryngeal edema may be fatal. If angioedema of the face, extremities, lips, tongue, glottis, and/or larynx occurs, treatment with TARKA should be discontinued and appropriate therapy instituted immediately (see **WARNINGS**).

Hypotension: (See **WARNINGS**). In hypertensive patients, hypotension occurred in 0.6% and near syncope occurred in 0.1%. Hypotension or syncope was a cause for discontinuation of therapy in 0.4% of hypertensive patients.

Treatment of Acute Cardiovascular Adverse Reactions: The frequency of cardiovascular adverse reactions which require therapy is rare, hence, experience with their treatment is limited. Whenever severe hypotension or complete AV block occur following oral administration of TARKA (verapamil component), the appropriate emergency measures should be applied immediately, e.g., intravenously administered isoproterenol HCl, levarterenol bitartrate, atropine (all in the usual doses), or calcium gluconate (10% solution). In patients with hypertrophic cardiomyopathy (IHSS), alpha-adrenergic agents (phenylephrine, metaraminol bitartrate or methoxamine) should be used to maintain blood pressure, and isoproterenol and levarterenol should be avoided. If further support is necessary, inotropic agents (dopamine or dobutamine) may be administered. Actual treatment and dosage should depend on the severity and the clinical situation and the judgment and experience of the treating physician.

Fetal/Neonatal Morbidity and Mortality: See **WARNINGS, Fetal Neonatal Morbidity and Mortality.**

Other adverse experiences (in addition to those in table and listed above) that have been reported with the individual components are listed below.

Verapamil Component:

Cardiovascular: (See **WARNINGS.**) CHF/pulmonary edema, AV block 3°, atrioventricular dissociation, claudication, purpura (vasculitis), syncope.

Digestive System: gingival hyperplasia. Reversible, (upon discontinuation of verapamil) nonobstructive, paralytic ileus has been infrequently reported in association with the use of verapamil.

Hemic and Lymphatic: ecchymosis or bruising.

Nervous System: cerebrovascular accident, confusion, psychotic symptoms, shakiness, somnolence.

Skin: exanthema, hair loss, hyperkeratosis, maculae, sweating, urticaria, Stevens-Johnson syndrome, erythema multiform.

Urogenital: gynecomastia, galactorrhea/hyperprolactinemia, increased urination, spotty menstruation.

Trandolapril Component:

Emotional, Mental, Sexual States: decreased libido.

Gastrointestinal: pancreatitis.

Clinical Laboratory Test Findings

Hematology: (See **WARNINGS.**) Low white blood cells, low neutrophils, low lymphocytes, low platelets.

Serum Electrolytes: Hyperkalemia (See **PRECAUTIONS**), hyponatremia

Renal Function Tests: Increases in creatinine and blood urea nitrogen levels occurred in 1.1 percent and 0.3 percent, respectively, of patients receiving TARKA with or without hydrochlorothiazide therapy. None of these increases required discontinuation of treatment. Increases in these laboratory values are more likely to occur in patients with renal insufficiency or those pretreated with a diuretic and, based on experience with other ACE inhibitors, would be expected to be especially likely in patients with renal artery stenosis. (See **PRECAUTIONS** and **WARNINGS.**)

Liver function tests: Elevations of liver enzymes (SGOT, SGPT, LDH, and alkaline phosphatase) and/or serum bilirubin occurred. Discontinuation for elevated liver enzymes occurred in 0.9 percent of patients. (see **WARNINGS.**)

OVERDOSAGE

No specific information is available on the treatment of overdosage with TARKA.

Verapamil Component—Overdose with verapamil may lead to pronounced hypotension, bradycardia, and conduction system abnormalities (e.g., junctional rhythm with AV dissociation and high degree AV block, including asystole). Other symptoms secondary to hypoperfusion (e.g., metabolic acidosis, hyperglycemia, hyperkalemia, renal dysfunction, and convulsions) may be evident.

Treat all verapamil overdoses as serious and maintain observation for at least 48 hours, preferably under continuous hospital care. Delayed pharmacodynamic consequences may occur with the sustained release formulation. Verapamil is known to decrease gastrointestinal transit time. In cases of overdose, tablets of ISOPTIN SR have occasionally been reported to form concretions within the stomach or intestines. These concretions have not been visible on plain radiographs of the abdomen, and no medical means of gastrointestinal emptying is of proven efficacy in removing them. Endoscopy might reasonably be considered in cases of overdose when symptoms are unusually prolonged. Verapamil cannot be removed by hemodialysis.

Treatment of overdosage should be supportive. Beta adrenergic stimulation or parenteral administration of calcium solutions may increase calcium ion flux across the slow channel, and have been used effectively in treatment of deliberate overdosage with verapamil. The following measures may be considered:

Bradycardia and conduction system abnormalities: Atropine, isoproterenol, and cardiac pacing.

Hypotension: Intravenous fluids, vasopressors (e.g., dopamine, dobutamine), calcium solutions (e.g., 10% calcium chloride solution)

Cardiac failures: Inotropic agents (e.g., isoproterenol, dopamine, dobutamine), diuretics. Asystole should be handled by the usual measures including cardiopulmonary resuscitation.

Trandolapril Component—The oral LD_{50} of trandolapril in mice was 4875 mg/kg in males and 3990 mg/kg in females. In rats, an oral dose of 5000 mg/kg caused low mortality (1 male out of 5; 0 females). In dogs, an oral dose of 1000 mg/kg did not cause mortality and abnormal clinical signs were not observed.

In humans, the most likely clinical manifestation would be symptoms attributable to severe hypotension. Laboratory determinations of serum levels of trandolapril and its metabolites are not widely available, and such determinations have, in any event, no established role in the management of trandolapril overdose. No data are available to suggest that physiological maneuvers (e.g., maneuvers to change pH of the urine) might accelerate elimination of trandolapril and its metabolites. It is not known if trandolapril or trandolaprilat can be usefully removed from the body by hemodialysis.

Angiotensin II could presumably serve as a specific antagonist antidote in the setting of trandolapril overdose, but angiotensin II is essentially unavailable outside of scattered research facilities. Because the hypotensive effect of trandolapril is achieved through vasodilation and effective hypovolemia, it is reasonable to treat trandolapril overdose by infusion of normal saline solution.

DOSAGE AND ADMINISTRATION

The recommended usual dosage range of trandolapril for hypertension is 1 to 4 mg per day administered in a single dose or two divided doses. The recommended usual dosage range of Isoptin-SR for hypertension is 120 to 480 mg per day administered in a single dose or two divided doses.

The hazards (see **WARNINGS**) of trandolapril are generally independent of dose; those of verapamil are a mixture of dose-dependent phenomena (primarily dizziness, AV block, constipation) and dose-independent phenomena, the former much more common than the latter. Therapy with any combination of trandolapril and verapamil will thus be associated with both sets of dose-independent hazards. The dose-dependent side effects of verapamil have not been shown to be decreased by the addition of trandolapril nor visa versa.

Rarely, the dose-independent hazards of trandolapril are serious. To minimize dose-independent hazards, it is usually appropriate to begin therapy with TARKA only after a patient has either (a) failed to achieve the desired antihypertensive effect with one or the other monotherapy at its respective maximally recommended dose and shortest dosing interval, or (b) the dose of one or the other monotherapy cannot be increased further because of the dose-limiting side effects.

Clinical trials with TARKA have explored only once-a-day doses. The antihypertensive effect and or adverse effects of adding 4 mg of trandolapril once-a-day to a dose of 240 mg Isoptin-SR administered twice-a-day has not been studied, nor have the effects of adding as little of 180 mg of Isoptin-SR to 2 mg trandolapril administered twice-a-day been evaluated. Over the dose range of Isoptin-SR 120 to 240 mg once-a-day and trandolapril 0.5 to 8 mg once-a-day, the effects of the combination increase with increasing doses of either component.

Replacement therapy: For convenience, patients receiving trandolapril (up to 8 mg) and verapamil (up to 240 mg) in separate tablets, administered once-a-day, may instead wish to receive tablets of TARKA containing the same component doses. TARKA should be administered with food.

HOW SUPPLIED

TARKA 2/180 mg tablets are supplied as pink, oval, film-coated tablets containing 2 mg trandolapril in an immediate release form and 180 mg verapamil hydrochloride in a sustained release form. The tablet is embossed with the Knoll triangle and 182 on one side and TARKA on the other side.

NDC 0048-5921-80—bottles of 100

TARKA 1/240 mg tablets are supplied as white, oval, film-coated tablets containing 1 mg trandolapril in an immediate release form and 240 mg verapamil hydrochloride in a sustained release form. The tablet is embossed with the Knoll triangle and 241 on one side and TARKA on the other side.

NDC 0048-5912-40—bottles of 100

TARKA 2/240 mg tablets are supplied as gold, oval, film-coated tablets containing 2 mg trandolapril in an immediate release form and 240 mg verapamil hydrochloride in a sustained release form. The tablet is embossed with Knoll triangle and 242 on one side and TARKA on the other side.

NDC 0048-5922-40—bottles of 100

TARKA 4/240 mg tablets are supplied as reddish-brown, oval, film-coated tablets containing 4 mg trandolapril in an immediate release form and 240 mg verapamil hydrochloride in a sustained release form. The tablet is embossed with the Knoll triangle and 244 on one side and TARKA on the other side.

NDC 0048-5942-40—bottles of 100

Dispense in well-closed container with safety closure.

Continued on next page

Tarka—Cont.

Storage: Store at 15°–25°C (59°–77°F) see USP.
Caution: Federal law prohibits dispensing without prescription.

Revised: February 1997
Knoll Pharmaceutical Company
3000 Continental Drive – North
Mount Olive, New Jersey 07828-1234
BASF Pharma 0900055-3
Shown in Product Identification Guide, page 320

Kos Pharmaceuticals, Inc.
1001 BRICKELL BAY DRIVE
25TH FLOOR
MIAMI, FL 33131

For medical information contact:
Drug Information Services
1-888-4-LIPIDS
1-888-454-7437

NIASPAN® ℞ Only
[*niă-span*]
niacin extended-release tablets

DESCRIPTION
NIASPAN® (niacin extended-release tablets), contain niacin, a B-complex vitamin and antihyperlipidemic agent. Niacin (nicotinic acid, or 3-pyridinecarboxylic acid) is a white, crystalline powder, very soluble in water, with the following structural formula:

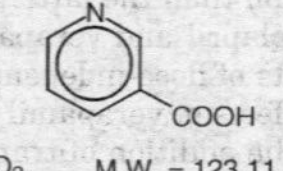

$C_6H_5NO_2$ M.W. = 123.11

NIASPAN® is an unscored, off-white tablet for oral administration that contains no color additives and is available in three tablet strengths containing 500, 750, and 1000mg niacin. NIASPAN tablets also contain the inactive ingredients methylcellulose, povidone, and stearic acid.

CLINICAL PHARMACOLOGY
Niacin functions in the body after conversion to nicotinamide adenine dinucleotide (NAD) in the NAD coenzyme system. Niacin (but not nicotinamide) in gram doses reduces total cholesterol (TC), low-density lipoprotein cholesterol (LDL-C) and triglycerides (TG), and increases high-density lipoprotein cholesterol (HDL-C). The magnitude of the individual lipid and lipoprotein responses may be influenced by the severity and type of underlying lipid abnormality. The increase in total HDL-C is associated with an increase in apolipoprotein A-I (Apo A-I) and a shift in the distribution of HDL subfractions. These shifts include an increase in the HDL_2:HDL_3 ratio, and an elevation in lipoprotein A-I (Lp A-I, an HDL particle containing only Apo A-I). Niacin treatment also decreases serum levels of apolipoprotein B-100 (Apo B), the major protein component of the very low-density lipoprotein (VLDL) and LDL fractions, and of Lp(a), a variant form of LDL independently associated with coronary risk.[1] In addition, preliminary reports suggest that niacin causes favorable LDL particle size transformations, although the clinical relevance of this effect requires further investigation. The effect of niacin-induced changes in lipids/lipoproteins on cardiovascular morbidity or mortality in individuals without pre-existing coronary disease has not been established.
A variety of clinical studies have demonstrated that elevated levels of TC, LDL-C, and Apo B promote human atherosclerosis. Similarly, decreased levels of HDL-C are associated with the development of atherosclerosis. Epidemiological investigations have established that cardiovascular morbidity and mortality vary directly with the level of TC and LDL-C, and inversely with the level of HDL-C.
Like LDL, cholesterol-enriched triglyceride-rich lipoproteins, including VLDL, intermediate density lipoprotein (IDL), and remnants, can also promote atherosclerosis. Elevated plasma TG are frequently found in a triad with low HDL-C levels and small LDL particles, as well as in association with non-lipid metabolic risk factors for coronary heart disease (CHD). As such total plasma TG has not consistently been shown to be an independent risk factor for CHD. Furthermore, the independent effect of raising HDL-C or lowering TG on the risk of coronary and cardiovascular morbidity and mortality has not been determined.

Mechanism of Action
The mechanism by which niacin alters lipid profiles has not been well defined. It may involve several actions including partial inhibition of release of free fatty acids from adipose tissue, and increased lipoprotein lipase activity, which may increase the rate of chylomicron triglyceride removal from plasma. Niacin decreases the rate of hepatic synthesis of VLDL and LDL, and does not appear to affect fecal excretion of fats, sterols, or bile acids.

Pharmacokinetics/Metabolism
Absorption
Niacin is rapidly and extensively absorbed (at least 60 to 76% of dose) when administered orally. To maximize bioavailability and reduce the risk of gastrointestinal (GI) upset, administration of NIASPAN with a low-fat meal or snack is recommended.
Single-dose bioavailability studies have demonstrated that NIASPAN tablet strengths are not interchangeable.
Distribution
Studies using radiolabeled niacin in mice show that niacin and its metabolites concentrate in the liver, kidney and adipose tissue.
Metabolism
The pharmacokinetic profile of niacin is complicated due to rapid and extensive first-pass metabolism, which is species and dose-rate specific. In humans, one pathway is through a simple conjugation step with glycine to form nicotinuric acid (NUA). NUA is then excreted in the urine, although there may be a small amount of reversible metabolism back to niacin. The other pathway results in the formation of nicotinamide adenine dinucleotide (NAD). It is unclear whether nicotinamide is formed as a precursor to, or following the synthesis of, NAD. Nicotinamide is further metabolized to at least N-methylnicotinamide (MNA) and nicotinamide-N-oxide (NNO). MNA is further metabolized to two other compounds, N-methyl-2-pyridone-5-carboxamide (2PY) and N-methyl-4-pyridone-5-carboxamide (4PY). The formation of 2PY appears to predominate over 4PY in humans. At the doses used to treat hyperlipidemia, these metabolic pathways are saturable, which explains the nonlinear relationship between niacin dose and plasma concentrations following multiple-dose NIASPAN administration (Table 1).
Nicotinamide does not have hypolipidemic activity; the activity of the other metabolites is unknown.

Table 1. Mean Steady-State Pharmacokinetic Parameters for Plasma Niacin

NIASPAN dose/day	given as	Niacin Peak Concentration (μg/mL)	Time to Peak (hrs)
1000mg	2×500mg	0.6	5
1500mg	2×750mg	4.9	4
2000mg	2×1000mg	15.5	5

Elimination
Niacin and its metabolites are rapidly eliminated in the urine. Following single and multiple doses, approximately 60 to 76% of the niacin dose administered as NIASPAN was recovered in urine as niacin and metabolites; up to 12% was recovered as unchanged niacin after multiple dosing. The ratio of metabolites recovered in the urine was dependent on the dose administered.

Special Populations
Hepatic
No studies have been performed. NIASPAN should be used with caution in patients with a past history of liver disease, who consume substantial quantities of alcohol, or have unexplained transaminase elevations. NIASPAN is contraindicated in patients with active liver disease (see WARNINGS).
Renal
There are no data in this population. NIASPAN should be used with caution in patients with renal disease (see PRECAUTIONS).
Gender
Steady-state plasma concentrations of niacin and metabolites after administration of NIASPAN are generally higher in women than in men, with the magnitude of the difference varying with dose and metabolite. Recovery of niacin and metabolites in urine, however, is generally similar for men and women, indicating that absorption is similar for both genders. The gender differences observed in plasma levels of niacin and its metabolites may be due to gender-specific differences in metabolic rate or volume of distribution. Data from the clinical trials suggest that women have a greater hypolipidemic response than men at equivalent doses of NIASPAN.

Niacin Clinical Studies
The role of LDL-C in atherogenesis is supported by pathological observations, clinical studies, and many animal experiments. Observational epidemiological studies have clearly established that high TC or LDL-C and low HDL-C are risk factors for CHD. Additionally, elevated levels of Lp(a) have been shown to be independently associated with CHD risk.[1] The efficacy of niacin in improving lipoprotein lipid profiles, either alone or in combination with other lipid-altering drugs, as an adjunct to diet therapy in the treatment of hyperlipoproteinemia has been well documented.
Niacin's ability to reduce mortality and the risk of definite, nonfatal myocardial infarction (MI) has also been assessed in long-term studies. The Coronary Drug Project,[2] completed in 1975, was designed to assess the safety and efficacy of niacin and other lipid-altering drugs in men 30 to 64 years old with a history of MI. Over an observation period of 5 years, niacin treatment was associated with a statistically significant reduction in nonfatal, recurrent MI. The incidence of definite, nonfatal MI was 8.9% for the 1,119 patients randomized to nicotinic acid versus 12.2% for the 2,789 patients who received placebo (p<0.004). Total mortality was similar in the two groups at 5 years (24.4% with nicotinic acid versus 25.4% with placebo; p=N.S.). At the time of a 15 year follow-up, there were 11% (69) fewer deaths in the niacin group compared to the placebo cohort (52.0% versus 58.2%; p=0.0004).[3] However, mortality at 15 years was not an original endpoint of the Coronary Drug Project. In addition, patients had not received niacin for approximately 9 years, and confounding variables such as concomitant medication use and medical or surgical treatments were not controlled.
The Cholesterol-Lowering Atherosclerosis Study (CLAS) was a randomized, placebo-controlled, angiographic trial testing combined colestipol and niacin therapy in 162 non-smoking males with previous coronary bypass surgery.[4] The primary, per-subject cardiac endpoint was global coronary artery change score. After 2 years, 61% of patients in the placebo cohort showed disease progression by global change score (n=82), compared with only 38.8% of drug-treated subjects (n=80), when both native arteries and grafts were considered (p<0.005); disease regression also occurred more frequently in the drug-treated group (16.2% versus 2.4%; p=0.002). In a follow-up to this trial in a subgroup of 103 patients treated for 4 years, again, significantly fewer patients in the drug-treated group demonstrated progression than in the placebo cohort (48% versus 85%, respectively; p<0.0001).[5]
The Familial Atherosclerosis Treatment Study (FATS) in 146 men ages 62 and younger with Apo B levels ≥125 mg/dL, established coronary artery disease, and family histories of vascular disease, assessed change in severity of disease in the proximal coronary arteries by quantitative arteriography.[6] Patients were given dietary counseling and randomized to treatment with either conventional therapy with double placebo (or placebo plus colestipol if the LDL-C was elevated); lovastatin plus colestipol; or niacin plus colestipol. In the conventional therapy group, 46% of patients had disease progression (and no regression) in at least one of nine proximal coronary segments; regression was the only change in 11%. In contrast, progression (as the only change) was seen in only 25% in the niacin plus colestipol group, while regression was observed in 39%. Though not an original endpoint of the trial, clinical events (death, MI, or revascularization for worsening angina) occurred in 10 of 52 patients who received conventional therapy, compared with 2 of 48 who received niacin plus colestipol.
The Harvard Atherosclerosis Reversibility Project (HARP) was a randomized placebo-controlled, 2.5-year study of the effect of a stepped-care antihyperlipidemic drug regimen on 91 patients (80 men and 11 women) with CHD and average baseline TC levels less than 250mg/dL and ratios of TC to HDL-C greater than 4.0.[7] Drug treatment consisted of an HMG-CoA reductase inhibitor administered alone as initial therapy followed by addition of varying dosages of either a slow-release nicotinic acid, cholestyramine, or gemfibrozil. Addition of nicotinic acid to the HMG-CoA reductase inhibitor resulted in further statistically significant mean reductions in TC, LDL-C, and TG, as well as a further increase in HDL-C in a majority of patients (40 of 44 patients). The ratios of TC to HDL-C and LDL-C to HDL-C were also significantly reduced by this combination drug regimen (see WARNINGS, *Skeletal Muscle*).

NIASPAN Clinical Studies
Placebo-controlled Clinical Studies in Patients with Primary Hypercholesterolemia and Mixed Dyslipidemia: In

Table 2. Lipid Response to NIASPAN Therapy

Treatment	n	Mean Percent Change from Baseline to Week 16* TC	LDL-C	HDL-C	TC/HDL-C	TG	Lp(a)	Apo B	Apo A-1
NIASPAN 1000mg qhs	41	−3	−5	+18	−17	−21	−13	−6	+9
NIASPAN 2000mg qhs	41	−10	−14	+22	−25	−28	−27	−16	+8
Placebo	40	0	−1	+4	−3	0	0	+1	+3
NIASPAN 1500mg qhs	76	−8	−12	+20	−20	−13	−15	−12	+8
Placebo	73	+2	+1	+2	+1	+12	+2	+1	+2

n = number of patients at baseline;
* Mean percent change from baseline for all NIASPAN doses was significantly different (p<0.05) from placebo for all lipid parameters shown except Apo A-1 at 2000mg.

two randomized, double-blind, parallel, multi-center, placebo-controlled trials, NIASPAN dosed at 1000, 1500 or 2000mg daily at bedtime with a low-fat snack for 16 weeks (including 4 weeks of dose escalation) favorably altered lipid profiles compared to placebo (Table 2). Women appeared to have a greater response than men at each NIASPAN dose level (see *Gender Effect*, below).

[See table 2 at bottom of previous page]

In a double-blind, multi-center, forced dose-escalation study, monthly 500mg increases in NIASPAN dose resulted in incremental reductions of approximately 5% in LDL-C and Apo B levels in the daily dose range of 500mg through 2000mg (Table 3). Women again tended to have a greater response to NIASPAN than men (see *Gender Effect*, below).

[See table 3 at right]

Pooled results for major lipids from these three placebo-controlled studies are shown below (Table 4).

[See table 4 at right]

Gender Effect: Combined data from the three placebo-controlled NIASPAN studies in patients with primary hypercholesterolemia and mixed dyslipidemia suggest that, at each NIASPAN dose level studied, changes in lipid concentrations are greater for women than for men (Table 5).

[See table 5 at right]

Long-term Study: In a recently completed long-term open-label study, patients with primary hypercholesterolemia and mixed dyslipidemia received NIASPAN in doses titrated to individual response and tolerance. An HMG-CoA reductase inhibitor or a bile acid sequestrant (BAS) was added to NIASPAN therapy for patients whose response to NIASPAN alone (usually at 2000mg qhs) was insufficient, or who would not tolerate higher niacin doses. Interim data from 48 and 96 weeks of treatment (Table 6) suggest combination therapy enhanced TC and LDL-C response (see WARNINGS, *Skeletal Muscle*).

[See table 6 at right]

Other Patient Populations: In a double-blind, multi-center, 19-week study the lipid-altering effects of NIASPAN (forced titration to 2000mg qhs) were compared to baseline in patients whose primary lipid abnormality was a low level of HDL-C (HDL-C≤40 mg/dL, TG ≤400 mg/dL, and LDL-C≤160, or <130 mg/dL in the presence of CHD). Results are shown below (Table 7).

[See table 7 at right]

At NIASPAN 2000 mg/day, median changes from baseline (25th, 75th percentiles) for LDL-C, HDL-C, and TG were −3% (−14, + 12%), +27% (+13, +38%), and −33% (−50, −19%), respectively.

INDICATIONS AND USAGE

Therapy with lipid-altering agents should be only one component of multiple risk factor intervention in individuals at significantly increased risk for atherosclerotic vascular disease due to hypercholesterolemia. Niacin therapy is indicated as an adjunct to diet when the response to a diet restricted in saturated fat and cholesterol and other nonpharmacologic measures alone has been inadequate (see also the NCEP treatment guidelines[8]). Prior to initiating therapy with niacin, secondary causes for hypercholesterolemia (e.g., poorly controlled diabetes mellitus, hypothyroidism, nephrotic syndrome, dysproteinemias, obstructive liver disease, other drug therapy, alcoholism) should be excluded, and a lipid profile obtained to measure TC, HDL-C, and TG.

1. NIASPAN is indicated as an adjunct to diet for reduction of elevated TC, LDL-C, Apo B and TG levels, and to increase HDL-C in patients with primary hypercholesterolemia (heterozygous familial and nonfamilial) and mixed dyslipidemia (Frederickson Types IIa and IIb; Table 8), when the response to an appropriate diet has been inadequate.
2. In patients with a history of myocardial infarction and hypercholesterolemia, niacin is indicated to reduce the risk of recurrent nonfatal myocardial infarction.
3. In patients with a history of coronary artery disease (CAD) and hypercholesterolemia, niacin, in combination with a bile acid binding resin, is indicated to slow progression or promote regression of atherosclerotic disease.
4. NIASPAN in combination with a bile acid binding resin is indicated as an adjunct to diet for reduction of elevated TC and LDL-C levels in adult patients with primary hypercholesterolemia (Type IIa; Table 8), when the response to an appropriate diet, or diet plus monotherapy, has been inadequate.
5. Niacin is also indicated as adjunctive therapy for treatment of adult patients with very high serum triglyceride levels (Types IV and V hyperlipidemia; Table 8) who present a risk of pancreatitis and who do not respond adequately to a determined dietary effort to control them. Such patients typically have serum TG levels over 2000 mg/dL and have elevations of VLDL-C as well as fasting chylomicrons (Type V hyperlipidemia; Table 8). Patients who consistently have total serum or plasma TG below 1000 mg/dL are unlikely to develop pancreatitis. Therapy with niacin may be considered for those patients with TG elevations between 1000 and 2000 mg/dL who have a history of pancreatitis or of recurrent abdominal pain typical of pancreatitis. Some Type IV patients with TG under 1000 mg/dL may, through dietary or alcohol indiscretion, convert to a Type V pattern with massive TG elevations accompanying fasting chylomicronemia, but the influence of niacin therapy on risk of pancreatitis in such situations has not been adequately studied. Drug therapy is not indicated for patients with Type I hyperlipoproteinemia, who have elevations of chylomicrons and plasma TG, but who have normal levels of VLDL-C. Inspection of plasma refrigerated for 14 hours is helpful in distinguishing Types I, IV, and V hyperlipoproteinemia.[9]

Table 3. Lipid Response in Dose-Escalation Study

Treatment	n	TC	LDL-C	HDL-C	TC/HDL-C	TG	Lp(a)	Apo B	Apo A-1
		Mean Percent Change from Baseline*							
Placebo‡	44	−2	−1	+5	−7	−6	−5	−2	+4
NIASPAN	87								
500mg qhs		−2	−3	+10	−10	−5	−3	−2	+5
1000mg qhs		−5	−9	+15	−17	−11	−12	−7	+8
1500mg qhs		−11	−14	+22	−26	−28	−20	−15	+10
2000mg qhs		−12	−17	+26	−29	−35	−24	−16	+12

n = number of patients enrolled;
‡ Placebo data shown are after 24 weeks of placebo treatment.
* For all NIASPAN doses except 500mg, mean percent change from baseline was significantly different ($p<0.05$) from placebo for all lipid parameters shown except Lp(a) and Apo A-1 which were significantly different from placebo starting with 1500mg and 2000mg, respectively.

Table 4. Selected Lipid Response to NIASPAN in Placebo-controlled Clinical Studies*

NIASPAN Dose	n	LDL-C	HDL-C	TG
		Mean Baseline and Median Percent Change from Baseline (25th, 75th Percentiles)		
1000mg qhs	104			
Baseline (mg/dL)		218	45	172
Percent Change		−7 (−15, 0)	+14 (+7,+23)	−16 (−34,+3)
1500mg qhs	120			
Baseline (mg/dL)		212	46	171
Percent Change		−13 (−21,−4)	+19 (+9,+31)	−25 (−45,−2)
2000mg qhs	85			
Baseline (mg/dL)		220	44	160
Percent Change		−16 (−26,−7)	+22 (+15,+34)	−38 (−52,−14)

* Represents pooled analyses of results; minimum duration on therapy at each dose was 4 weeks.

Table 5. Effect of Gender on NIASPAN Dose Response

NIASPAN Dose	n (M/F)	LDL-C M	LDL-C F	HDL-C M	HDL-C F	TG M	TG F	Apo B M	Apo B F
		Mean Percent Change from Baseline							
500mg qhs	50/37	−2	−5	+11	+8	−3	−9	−1	−5
1000mg qhs	76/52	−6*	−11*	+14	+20	−10	−20	−5*	−10*
1500mg qhs	104/59	−12	−16	+19	+24	−17	−28	−13	−15
2000mg qhs	75/53	−15	−18	+23	+26	−30	−36	−16	−16

n = Number of male/female patients enrolled.
* Percent change significantly different between genders ($p<0.05$).

Table 6. NIASPAN Efficacy with Combination Therapy

Treatment	Duration	n	TC	LDL-C	HDL-C	TC/HDL-C	TG	Lp(a)*	Apo B*
			Mean Percent Change from Baseline						
	Baseline	185	–	–	–	–	–	–	–
NIASPAN Alone	48 weeks	101	−11	−18	+29	−29	−24	−36	−15
	96 weeks	74	−10	−18	+32	−30	−27	na	na
	Baseline	53	–	–	–	–	–	–	–
NIASPAN & HMG-CoA	48 weeks	45	−23	−32	+26	−38	−30	−19	−26
	96 weeks	37	−24	−32	+25	−38	−32	na	na
	Baseline	16	–	–	–	–	–	–	–
NIASPAN & BAS	48 weeks	15	−11	−20	+36	−33	−13	−24	−19
	96 weeks	7	−15	−28	+31	−34	+5	na	na

Note: Median NIASPAN dose was 2000mg qhs in each dose group. Mean duration of HMG-CoA combination therapy was approximately 47 weeks. Mean duration of BAS combination therapy was approximately 40 weeks.
* number of patients (n) are up to 33% lower at baseline and at 48 weeks; na = data are not available.

Table 7. Lipid Response to NIASPAN in Patients with Low HDL-C

	n	TC	LDL-C	HDL-C	TC/HDL-C	TG	Lp(a)†	Apo B†	Apo A-I†	Lp A-I‡
		Mean Baseline and Mean Percent Change from Baseline								
Baseline (mg/dL)	88	190	120	31	6	194	8	106	105	32
Week 19 (% Change)	71	−3	0	+26	−22	−30	−20	−9	+11	+20

n = number of patients enrolled
* Mean percent change from baseline was significantly different ($p<0.05$) for all lipid parameters shown except LDL-C.
†n=72 at baseline and 69 at week 19.
‡n=30 at baseline and week 19.

Table 8. Classification of Hyperlipoproteinemias

Type	Lipoproteins Elevated	Lipid Elevations Major	Lipid Elevations Minor
I (rare)	chylomicrons	TG	↑→TC
IIa	LDL	TC	-
IIb	LDL, VLDL	TC	TG
III (rare)	IDL	TC/TG	-
IV	VLDL	TG	↑→TC
V (rare)	chylomicrons, VLDL	TG	↑→TC

TC = total cholesterol; TG = triglycerides; LDL = low-density lipoprotein; VLDL = very low-density lipoprotein; IDL = intermediate-density lipoprotein
↑→ = increased or no change

CONTRAINDICATIONS

NIASPAN is contraindicated in patients with a known hypersensitivity to niacin or any component of this medica-

Continued on next page

Niaspan—Cont.

tion, significant or unexplained hepatic dysfunction, active peptic ulcer disease, or arterial bleeding.

WARNINGS

NIASPAN preparations should not be substituted for equivalent doses of immediate-release (crystalline) niacin. For patients switching from immediate-release niacin to NIASPAN, therapy with NIASPAN should be initiated with low doses (i.e., 500 mg qhs) and the NIASPAN dose should then be titrated to the desired therapeutic response (see DOSAGE AND ADMINISTRATION).

Liver Dysfunction

Cases of severe hepatic toxicity, including fulminant hepatic necrosis, have occurred in patients who have substituted sustained-release (modified-release, timed-release) niacin products for immediate-release (crystalline) niacin at equivalent doses.

NIASPAN should be used with caution in patients who consume substantial quantities of alcohol and/or have a past history of liver disease. Active liver diseases or unexplained transaminase elevations are contraindications to the use of NIASPAN.

Niacin preparations, like some other lipid-lowering therapies, have been associated with abnormal liver tests. In three placebo-controlled clinical trials involving titration to final daily NIASPAN doses ranging from 500 to 3000mg, 245 patients received NIASPAN for a mean duration of 17 weeks. No patient with normal serum transaminase levels (AST, ALT) at baseline experienced elevations to more than 3 times the upper limit of normal (ULN) during treatment with NIASPAN. In these studies, fewer than 1% (2/245) of NIASPAN patients discontinued due to transaminase elevations greater than 2 times the ULN.

Interim results from a recently completed, long-term extension study involving more than 700 patients (617 who were treated for a mean duration of 50 weeks) showed that less than 1% (4/717) of NIASPAN-treated patients with normal serum transaminase levels at baseline experienced elevations greater than 3 times ULN (one of the four was receiving concomitant HMG-CoA reductase inhibitor therapy).

In the placebo-controlled clinical trials and the long-term extension study, elevations in transaminases did not appear to be related to treatment duration; elevations in AST levels did appear to be dose related. Transaminase elevations were reversible upon discontinuation of NIASPAN.

Liver tests should be performed on all patients during therapy with NIASPAN. Serum transaminase levels, including AST and ALT (SGOT and SGPT), should be monitored before treatment begins, every 6 weeks to 12 weeks for the first year, and periodically thereafter (e.g., at approximately 6-month intervals). Special attention should be paid to patients who develop elevated serum transaminase levels, and in these patients, measurements should be repeated promptly and then performed more frequently. If the transaminase levels show evidence of progression, particularly if they rise to 3 times the ULN and are persistent, or if they are associated with symptoms of nausea, fever, and/or malaise, the drug should be discontinued.

Skeletal Muscle

Rare cases of rhabdomyolysis have been associated with concomitant administration of lipid-altering doses (≥1 g/day) of niacin and HMG-CoA reductase inhibitors. However, no cases of rhabdomyolysis have been reported in 124 patients who were treated with NIASPAN in combination with various HMG-CoA reductase inhibitors. Physicians contemplating combined therapy with HMG-CoA reductase inhibitors and NIASPAN should carefully weigh the potential benefits and risks and should carefully monitor patients for any signs and symptoms of muscle pain, tenderness, or weakness, particularly during the initial months of therapy and during any periods of upward dosage titration of either drug. Periodic serum creatine phosphokinase (CPK) and potassium determinations should be considered in such situations, but there is no assurance that such monitoring will prevent the occurrence of severe myopathy.

PRECAUTIONS

General

Before instituting therapy with NIASPAN, an attempt should be made to control hyperlipidemia with appropriate diet, exercise, and weight reduction in obese patients, and to treat other underlying medical problems (see INDICATIONS AND USAGE).

Patients with a past history of jaundice, hepatobiliary disease, or peptic ulcer should be observed closely during NIASPAN therapy. Frequent monitoring of liver function tests and blood glucose should be performed to ascertain that the drug is producing no adverse effects on these organ systems. Diabetic patients may experience a dose-related rise in glucose tolerance, the clinical significance of which is unclear. Diabetic or potentially diabetic patients should be observed closely. Adjustment of diet and/or hypoglycemic therapy may be necessary.

Caution should also be used when NIASPAN is used in patients with unstable angina or in the acute phase of MI, particularly when such patients are also receiving vasoactive drugs such as nitrates, calcium channel blockers, or adrenergic blocking agents.

Elevated uric acid levels have occurred with niacin therapy, therefore use with caution in patients predisposed to gout.

NIASPAN has been associated with small but statistically significant dose-related reductions in platelet count (mean of -11% with 2000mg). In addition, NIASPAN has been associated with small but statistically significant increases in prothrombin time (mean of approximately +4%); accordingly, patients undergoing surgery should be carefully evaluated. Caution should be observed when NIASPAN is administered concomitantly with anticoagulants; prothrombin time and platelet counts should be monitored closely in such patients.

In placebo-controlled trials, NIASPAN has been associated with small but statistically significant, dose-related reductions in phosphorus levels (mean of −13% with 2000mg). Although these reductions were transient, phosphorus levels should be monitored periodically in patients at risk for hypophosphatemia.

Niacin is rapidly metabolized by the liver, and excreted through the kidneys. NIASPAN is contraindicated in patients with significant or unexplained hepatic dysfunction (see CONTRAINDICATIONS and WARNINGS) and should be used with caution in patients with renal dysfunction.

Information for Patients

Patients should be advised:

— to take NIASPAN at bedtime, after a low-fat snack. Administration on an empty stomach is not recommended;
— to carefully follow the prescribed dosing regimen, including the recommended titration schedule, in order to minimize side effects (see DOSAGE AND ADMINISTRATION);
— that flushing is a common side effect of niacin therapy that usually subsides after several weeks of consistent niacin use. Flushing may vary in severity, may last for several hours after dosing, and will, by taking NIASPAN® at bedtime, most likely occur during sleep; however, if awakened by flushing at night, to get up slowly, especially if feeling dizzy, feeling faint, or taking blood pressure medications;
— that taking aspirin (approximately 30 minutes before taking NIASPAN) or a non-steroidal anti-inflammatory drug (e.g., ibuprofen) may minimize flushing;
— to avoid ingestion of alcohol or hot drinks around the time of NIASPAN administration, to minimize flushing;
— that if NIASPAN therapy is discontinued for an extended length of time, their physician should be contacted prior to re-starting therapy; re-titration is recommended (see DOSAGE AND ADMINISTRATION; Table 10);
— to notify their physician if they are taking vitamins or other nutritional supplements containing niacin or related compounds such as nicotinamide (see Drug Interactions);
— to notify their physician if symptoms of dizziness occur;
— if diabetic, to notify their physician of changes in blood glucose;
— that NIASPAN tablets should not be broken, crushed or chewed, but should be swallowed whole.

Drug Interactions

HMG-CoA Reductase Inhibitors: See WARNINGS, *Skeletal Muscle.*

Antihypertensive Therapy: Niacin may potentiate the effects of ganglionic blocking agents and vasoactive drugs resulting in postural hypotension.

Aspirin: Concomitant aspirin may decrease the metabolic clearance of nicotinic acid. The clinical relevance of this finding is unclear.

Bile Acid Sequestrants: An *in vitro* study was carried out investigating the niacin-binding capacity of colestipol and cholestyramine. About 98% of available niacin was bound to colestipol, with 10 to 30% binding to cholestyramine. These results suggest that 4 to 6 hours, or as great an interval as possible, should elapse between the ingestion of bile acid-binding resins and the administration of NIASPAN.

Other: Concomitant alcohol or hot drinks may increase the side effects of flushing and pruritus and should be avoided around the time of NIASPAN ingestion. Vitamins or other nutritional supplements containing large doses of niacin or related compounds such as nicotinamide may potentiate the adverse effects of NIASPAN.

Drug/Laboratory Test Interactions

Niacin may produce false elevations in some fluorometric determinations of plasma or urinary catecholamines. Niacin may also give false-positive reactions with cupric sulfate solution (Benedict's reagent) in urine glucose tests.

Carcinogenesis, Mutagenesis, Impairment of Fertility

Niacin administered to mice for a lifetime as a 1% solution in drinking water was not carcinogenic. The mice in this study received approximately 6 to 8 times a human dose of 3000 mg/day as determined on a mg/m^2 basis. Niacin was negative for mutagenicity in the Ames test. No studies on impairment of fertility have been performed. No studies have been conducted with NIASPAN regarding carcinogenesis, mutagenesis, or impairment of fertility.

Pregnancy

Pregnancy Category C.

Animal reproduction studies have not been conducted with niacin or with NIASPAN. It is also not known whether niacin at doses typically used for lipid disorders can cause fetal harm when administered to pregnant women or whether it can affect reproductive capacity. If a woman receiving niacin for primary hypercholesterolemia (Types IIa or IIb) becomes pregnant, the drug should be discontinued. If a woman being treated with niacin for hypertriglyceridemia (Types IV or V) conceives, the benefits and risks of continued therapy should be assessed on an individual basis.

Nursing Mothers

Niacin has been reported to be excreted in human milk. Because of the potential for serious adverse reactions in nursing infants from lipid-altering doses of nicotinic acid, a decision should be made whether to discontinue nursing or to discontinue the drug, taking into account the importance of the drug to the mother. No studies have been conducted with NIASPAN in nursing mothers.

Pediatric Use

Safety and effectiveness of niacin therapy in pediatric patients (≤16 years) have not been established. No studies in patients under 21 years of age have been conducted with NIASPAN.

ADVERSE REACTIONS

NIASPAN is generally well tolerated; adverse reactions have been mild and transient. In the placebo-controlled clinical trials, flushing episodes (i.e., warmth, redness, itching and/or tingling) were the most common treatment-emergent adverse events (reported by as many as 88% of patients) for NIASPAN. Spontaneous reports suggest that flushing may also be accompanied by symptoms of dizziness, tachycardia, palpitations, shortness of breath, sweating, chills, and/or edema, which in rare cases may lead to syncope. In pivotal studies, fewer that 6% (14/245) of NIASPAN patients discontinued due to flushing. In comparisons of immediate-release (IR) niacin and NIASPAN, although the proportion of patients who flushed was similar, fewer flushing episodes were reported by patients who received NIASPAN. Following 4 weeks of maintenance therapy at daily doses of 1500mg, the incidence of flushing over the 4-week period averaged 8.56 events per patient for IR niacin versus 1.88 following NIASPAN.

Other adverse events occurring in 5% or greater of patients treated with NIASPAN, at least remotely related to NIASPAN, are shown in Table 9 below.

[See table 9 at left]

Table 9 Treatment-Emergent Adverse Events by Dose Level in ≥5% of Patients; Events Considered At Least Remotely Related to Study Medication

		Placebo-Controlled Studies NIASPAN Treatment[†]					
			Recommended Daily Maintenance Doses			Greater Than Recommended Daily Doses	
	Placebo (n=157) %	500mg‡ (n=87) %	1000mg (n=110) %	1500mg (n=136) %	2000mg (n=95) %	2500mg‡ (n=49) %	3000mg‡ (n=46) %
Headache	15	5*	9	11	8	4*	4
Pain	3	1	2	5	3	0	2
Pain, Abdominal	3	3	2	3	5	0	0
Diarrhea	8	6	7	6	8	10	11
Dyspepsia	8	2	4	5	5	6	0
Nausea	4	2	5	3	8	10	4
Vomiting	2	0	2	3	8*	8	2
Rhinitis	7	2	5	4	3	0	0
Pruritus	1	6	<1	3	1	0	0
Rash	<1	5	5	4	0	0	0

Note: Percentages are calculated from the total number of patients in each column. AEs are reported at the lowest dose where they occurred.

†Pooled results from placebo-controlled studies; for NIASPAN, n=245 and mean treatment duration = 17 weeks. Number of NIASPAN patients (n) are not additive across doses.

‡The 500mg, 2500mg and 3000mg/day doses are outside the recommended daily maintenance dosing range; see DOSAGE AND ADMINISTRATION.

* Significantly different from placebo at $p \leq 0.05$; Chi-square test (cell size>5), Fisher's Exact test (cell sizes≤5).

In general, the incidence of adverse events was higher in women compared to men.

Table 10. Recommended Dosing

	Week(s)	Daily dose	NIASPAN Dosage
INITIAL TITRATION SCHEDULE	1 to 4	500mg	1 NIASPAN 500mg tablet at bedtime
INITIAL TITRATION SCHEDULE	5 to 8	1000mg	2 NIASPAN 500mg tablets at bedtime
	*	1500mg	2 NIASPAN 750mg tablets or 3 NIASPAN 500mg tablets at bedtime
	*	2000mg	2 NIASPAN 1000mg tablets or 4 NIASPAN 500mg tablets at bedtime

* After Week 8, titrate to patient response and tolerance. If response to 1000mg daily is inadequate, increase dose to 1500mg daily; may subsequently increase dose to 2000mg daily. Daily dose should not be increased more than 500mg in a 4-week period, and doses above 2000mg daily are not recommended. Women may respond at lower doses than men.

The following adverse events have also been reported with niacin products, either during clinical trials or in routine patient management.

Body as a Whole: edema, asthenia, chills

Cardiovascular: atrial fibrillation, and other cardiac arrhythmias; tachycardia, palpitations; orthostasis; syncope; hypotension

Eye: toxic amblyopia, crystoid macular edema

Gastrointestinal: activation of peptic ulcers and peptic ulceration; jaundice

Metabolic: decreased glucose tolerance; gout

Musculoskeletal: myalgia

Nervous: dizziness, insomnia

Skin: hyper-pigmentation; maculopapular rash; acanthosis nigricans; urticaria; dry skin; sweating

Other: migraine

Clinical Laboratory Abnormalities

Chemistry: Elevations in serum transaminases (see WARNINGS - *Liver Dysfunction*), LDH, fasting glucose, uric acid, total bilirubin, and amylase; reductions in phosphorus

Hematology: Slight reductions in platelet counts and prolongation in prothrombin time (see WARNINGS)

DRUG ABUSE AND DEPENDENCE

Niacin is a non-narcotic drug. It has no known addiction potential in humans.

OVERDOSE

Supportive measures should be undertaken in the event of an overdosage.

DOSAGE AND ADMINISTRATION

NIASPAN should be taken at bedtime, after a low-fat snack, and doses should be individualized according to patient response. Therapy with NIASPAN must be initiated at 500 mg qhs in order to reduce the incidence and severity of side effects which may occur during early therapy. The recommended dose escalation is shown in Table 10 below.

[See table 10 above]

Maintenance Dose:

The daily dosage of NIASPAN should not be increased by more than 500mg in any 4-week period. The recommended maintenance dose is 1000mg (two 500mg tablets) to 2000mg (two 1000mg tablets or four 500mg tablets) once daily at bedtime. Doses greater than 2000mg daily are not recommended. Women may respond at lower NIASPAN doses than men (see CLINICAL PHARMACOLOGY, *Gender Effect*).

If lipid response to NIASPAN alone is insufficient, or if higher doses of NIASPAN are not well tolerated, some patients may benefit from combination therapy with a bile-acid binding resin or an HMG-CoA reductase inhibitor. (see WARNINGS, PRECAUTIONS, Drug Interactions, Concomitant Therapy below, and CLINICAL PHARMACOLOGY, NIASPAN Clinical Studies)

Flushing of the skin (see ADVERSE REACTIONS) may be reduced in frequency or severity by pretreatment with aspirin (taken 30 minutes prior to NIASPAN dose) or non-steroidal anti-inflammatory drugs. Tolerance to this flushing develops rapidly over the course of several weeks. Flushing, pruritus, and gastrointestinal distress are also greatly reduced by slowly increasing the dose of niacin and avoiding administration on an empty stomach.

Equivalent doses of NIASPAN should **not** be substituted for sustained-release (modified-release, timed-release) niacin preparations or immediate-release (crystalline) niacin (see WARNINGS). Patients previously receiving other niacin products should be started with the recommended NIASPAN titration schedule (see Table 10), and the dose should subsequently be individualized based on patient response. Single-dose bioavailability studies have demonstrated that NIASPAN tablet strengths are not interchangeable.

If NIASPAN therapy is discontinued for an extended period, reinstitution of therapy should include a titration phase (see Table 10).

NIASPAN tablets should be taken whole and should not be broken, crushed or chewed before swallowing.

Concomitant Therapy

Preliminary evidence suggests that the lipid-lowering effects of NIASPAN on TC and LDL-C are enhanced with an HMG-CoA reductase inhibitor, e.g., lovastatin, pravastatin, simvastatin, and fluvastatin. Additive effects on LDL-C are also seen when niacin is combined with bile acid binding resins. (see WARNINGS and PRECAUTIONS, Drug Interactions)

Dosage in Patients with Renal or Hepatic Insufficiency

Use of NIASPAN in patients with renal or hepatic insufficiency has not be studied. NIASPAN is contraindicated in patients with significant or unexplained hepatic dysfunction. NIASPAN should be used with caution in patients with renal insufficiency (see WARNINGS, PRECAUTIONS).

HOW SUPPLIED

NIASPAN is supplied as unscored, off-white capsule-shaped tablets containing 500, 750 or 1000mg of niacin in an extended-release formulation. Tablets are debossed KOS on one side and the tablet strength (500, 750 or 1000) on the other side. Tablets are supplied in bottles of 100 as shown below.

500mg tablets: bottles of 100 - NDC# 60598-001-01
750mg tablets: bottles of 100 - NDC# 60598-002-01
1000mg tablets: bottles of 100 - NDC# 60598-003-01

Store at room temperature, (20 to 25°C or 68 to 77°F).

REFERENCES

1. Bostom AG et al. *JAMA*. 1996; 276:544–548.
2. The Coronary Drug Project Research Group. *JAMA*. 1975; 231:360–381.
3. Canner PL et al. *J Am Coll Cardiol*. 1986; 8(6):1245–1255.
4. Blankenhorn DH et al. *JAMA*. 1987; 257(23):3233–3240.
5. Cashin-Hemphill L et al. *JAMA*. 1990; 264(23):3013–3017.
6. Brown G et al. *NEJM*. 1990; 323:1289–1298.
7. Pasternak RC et al. *Annals Int Med*. 1996; 125:529–540.
8. Summary of the Second Report of the National Cholesterol Education Program (NCEP) Expert Panel on Detection, Evaluation, and Treatment of High Blood Cholesterol in Adults (Adult Treatment Panel II), *JAMA*. 1993;269:3015–3023.
9. Nikkila EA, In: *The Metabolic Basis of Inherited Disease*. 5th ed. 1983. Chap. 30: 622–642.

Manufactured by:
Kos Pharmaceuticals, Inc.
Miami, FL 33131
400025/1199 ©1999 Kos Pharmaceuticals, Inc., Miami, FL 33131, USA

Shown in Product Identification Guide, page 320

Kramer Laboratories, Inc.

**8778 S.W. 8TH STREET
MIAMI, FL 33174**

Direct Inquiries to:
8778 S.W. 8th Street
Miami, FL 33174
(800) 824-4894
www.kramerlabs.com

For Medical Information Contact:
In Emergencies:
Professional Director
(800) 824-4894

HALFPRIN® OTC

162 mg. Enteric Coated Aspirin
Aspirin For Suspected Acute MI

DESCRIPTION

Halfprin® is the only 162 mg. enteric coated aspirin available for the indicated use to reduce the risk of vascular mortality in people with a suspected acute myocardial infarction (MI). The Halfprin® 162 mg. aspirin has been determined to be the indicated dose to reduce the risk of fatal and nonfatal cardiovascular and cerebrovascular events in subjects with a suspected acute MI.

INDICATIONS

Suspected Acute MI

The use of aspirin in patients with a suspected acute MI is supported by the results of a large, multicenter 2×2 factorial study of 17,187 subjects with suspected acute MI.(1). Subjects were randomized within 24 hours of the onset of symptoms so that 8,587 subjects received oral aspirin (162.5 milligrams, enteric-coated) daily for 1 month (the first dose crushed, sucked, or chewed) and 8,600 received oral placebo. Of the subjects 8,592 were also randomized to receive a single dose of streptokinase (1.5 million units) infused intravenously for about 1 hour, and 8,595 received a placebo infusion. Thus, 4,295 subject received aspirin plus placebo, 4,300 received streptokinase plus placebo, 4,292 received aspirin plus streptokinase, and 4,300 received double placebo.

Vascular mortality (attributed to cardiac, cerebral, hemorrhagic, other vascular, or unknown causes) occurred in 9.4 percent of subjects in the aspirin group and in 11.8 percent of subjects in the oral placebo group in the 35-day follow up. This represents an absolute reduction of 2.4 percent in the mean 35-day vascular mortality attributable to aspirin and a 23 percent reduction in odds of vascular death.

Significant absolute reductions in mortality and corresponding reductions in specific clinical events favoring aspirin were found for reinfarction (1.5 percent absolute reduction, 45 percent odds reduction, $2p<0.00001$), cardiac arrest (1.2 percent absolute reduction, 14.2 percent odds reduction, $2p<0.01$), and total stroke (0.4 percent absolute reduction, 41.5 percent odds reduction, $2p<0.01$). The effect of aspirin over and above its effect on mortality was evidenced by small, but significant, reductions in vascular morbidity in those subjects who were discharged.

The beneficial effects of aspirin on mortality were present with or without streptokinase infusion. Aspirin reduced vascular mortality from 10.4 to 8.0 percent for days 0 to 35 in subjects given streptokinase and reduced vascular mortality from 13.2 to 10.7 percent in the effects of aspirin and thrombolytic therapy with streptokinase in this study were approximately additive. Subjects who received the combination of streptokinase infusion and daily aspirin had significantly lower vascular mortality at 35 days than those who received either active treatment alone (combination 8.0 percent, aspirin 10.7 percent, streptokinase 10.4 percent, and no treatment 13.2 percent. While this study demonstrated that aspirin has an additive benefit in patients given streptokinase, there is no reason to restrict its use to that specific thrombolytic.

ADVERSE REACTIONS

Gastrointestinal Reactions

Doses of 1,000 milligrams per day of aspirin caused gastrointestinal symptoms and bleeding that in some cases were clinically significant. In the Aspirin Myocardial Infarction Study (AMIS) (4) with 4,500 post infarction subjects, the percentage incidences of gastrointestinal symptoms for the aspirin (1,000 milligrams of a standard, solid—tablet formulation) and placebo-treated subjects, respectively, were: Stomach pain (14.5 percent, 4.4 percent); heartburn (11.9 percent, 4.8 percent); nausea and/or vomiting (7.6 percent; 2.1 percent); hospitalization for gastrointestinal disorder (4.8 percent, 3.5 percent). Symptoms and signs of gastrointestinal irritation were not significantly increased in subjects treated for instable angina with 325 milligrams buffered aspirin in solution.

Bleeding

In the AMIS and other trails, aspirin treated subjects had increased rates of gross gastrointestinal bleeding. In the ISIS—2 study (1), there was no significant difference in the incidence of major bleeding (bleeds requiring transfusion) between 8,587 subjects taking 162.5 milligrams aspirin daily and 8,600 subjects taking placebo (31 versus 33 subjects). There were five confirmed cerebral hemorrhage in the aspirin group compared with two in the placebo group, but the incidence of stroke of all causes was significantly reduced from 81 to 47 for the placebo versus aspirin group (0.4 percent absolute change). There was a small and statistically significant excess (0.6 percent) of minor bleeding in people taking aspirin (2.5 percent for aspirin, 1.9 percent for placebo). No other significant adverse effects were reported.

Cardiovascular and Biochemical

In the AMIS trail(4), the dosage of 1,000 milligrams per day of aspirin was associated with small increases in systolic blood pressure (BP) (average 1.5 to 2.1 millimeters Hg) and diastolic BP (0.5 to 0.6 millimeters Hg), depending upon whether maximal or last available readings were used. Blood urea nitrogen and uric acid levels were also increased, but by less than 1.0 milligram percent.

Subjects with marked hypertension or renal insufficiency had been excluded from the trail so that clinical importance of these observations for such subjects or for any subjects treated over more prolonged periods is not known. It is recommended that patients placed on long-term aspirin treatment, even at doses of 160 milligrams per day, be seen at regular intervals to assess changes in these measurements.

DOSAGE AND ADMINISTRATION

The recommended dose of aspirin to treat suspected acute MI is 160 to 162.5 milligrams taken as soon as the first in-

Continued on next page

Halfprin—Cont.

farct is suspected and then daily for at least 30 days. (One-half of a conventional 325-milligram aspirin tablet or two 80–81 milligram aspirin tablets may be taken.) This use of aspirin applies to both solid, oral dosage forms (buffered, plain, and enteric-coated aspirin) and buffered aspirin in solution. If using a solid dosage form, the first dose should be crushed, sucked, or chewed. After the 30-day treatment, physicians should consider further therapy based on the labeling for dosage and administration of aspirin for prevention of recurrent MI (reinfarction).

REFERENCES

(1) ISIS-2 (Second International Study of Infarct Survival) Collaborative Group. "Randomized Trial of Intravenous Streptokinase, Oral Aspirin, Both, or Neither Among 17,187 Cases of Suspected Acute Myocardial Infarction: ISIS-2," lancet, 2:349–360, August 13, 1988.

HOW SUPPLIED

Halfprin Tablets
162 mg. in bottle of 60* and 200
81 mg. in bottle of 90
*Easy to open bottle/ Not child-resistant caps.

Comments questions or sample request call toll free 1-800-824-4894

Laser, Inc.

2200 W. 97TH PLACE, P.O. BOX 905
CROWN POINT, IN 46308

Direct Inquiries to:
Joseph N. Allegretti, R.Ph., President & C.O.O.
(219) 663-1165

DALLERGY® CAPLETS, SYRUP, TABLETS ℞

Each Extended-Release Caplet* (Capsule-shaped tablet) contains: Chlorpheniramine Maleate 8 mg, Phenylephrine Hydrochloride 20 mg, Methscopolamine Nitrate 2.5 mg. Each 5 mL of grape-flavored Syrup contains: Chlorpheniramine Maleate 2 mg, Phenylephrine Hydrochloride 10 mg, Methscopolamine Nitrate 0.625 mg. Each Tablet contains: Chlorpheniramine Maleate 4 mg, Phenylephrine Hydrochloride 10 mg, Methscopolamine Nitrate 1.25 mg.

*In a specially prepared base to provide a prolonged therapeutic effect.

DALLERGY® –JR. CAPSULES ℞

Each Extended-Release Capsule* contains: Brompheniramine Maleate 6 mg, Pseudoephedrine Hydrochloride 60 mg.

*In a specially prepared base to provide prolonged action.

DONATUSSIN DC SYRUP Ⓒ ℞

Each 5 mL contains: Hydrocodone* Bitartrate 2.5 mg
*(WARNING: May be habit forming), Phenylephrine Hydrochloride 7.5 mg, Guaifenesin 50 mg. Red Syrup.

DONATUSSIN DROPS ℞

Each mL contains: Chlorpheniramine Maleate 1 mg, Phenylephrine Hydrochloride 2 mg, Guaifenesin 20 mg. Peach-flavored, orange color.

DONATUSSIN SYRUP ℞

Each 5 mL contains: Dextromethorphan HBr 7.5 mg, Chlorpheniramine Maleate 2 mg, Phenylephrine HCl 10 mg, Guaifenesin 100 mg. Red Syrup.

FUMATINIC® CAPSULES ℞

Each Extended-Release FUMATINIC Capsule contains: Ferrous Fumarate* 200 mg (equivalent to 66 mg of elemental iron), Vitamin C* (Ascorbic Acid) 60 mg, Vitamin B-12 (Cyanocobalamin) 5 mcg with Intrinsic Factor.
*In a specially prepared base to provide prolonged action.

KIE® SYRUP ℞

Each 5 mL contains: Potassium Iodide 150 mg, Ephedrine Hydrochloride 8 mg. Green Syrup.

LACTOCAL–F TABLETS ℞

Multivitamin, Multimineral supplement for pregnant or lactating women. White coated dye free tablet.

RESPAIRE®–SR CAPSULES 60 & 120 ℞

Each Extended-Release RESPAIRE-60 SR Capsule contains: Pseudoephedrine Hydrochloride* 60 mg and Guaifenesin† 200 mg. Each Extended-Release RESPAIRE-120 SR Capsule contains: Pseudoephedrine Hydrochloride* 120 mg and Guaifenesin† 250 mg.

*In a specially prepared base to provide prolonged action.
†Designed for immediate release to provide rapid action.

Layton Bioscience, Inc.

709 EAST EVELYN AVENUE
SUNNYVALE, CA 94086

Direct Inquiries to:
ROBERT ALONSO, Vice President, Marketing
phone: (610) 975-9290

INVERSINE® TABLETS ℞
(MECAMYLAMINE HCl)

DESCRIPTION

INVERSINE® (Mecamylamine HCl) is a potent, oral antihypertension agent and ganglion blocker, and is a secondary amine. It is N.2.3.3–tetramethyl-bicyclo [2.2.1] heptan-2-amine hydrochloride. Its empirical formula is $C_{11}H_{21}N \bullet HCl$ and its structural formula is:

[structural formula: N–CH₃ (H), CH₃, CH₃, CH₃ •HCl]

It is a white, odorless, or practically odorless, crystalline powder, is highly stable, soluble in water and has a molecular weight of 203.75.
INVERSINE is supplied as tablets for oral use, each containing 2.5 mg mecamylamine HCl. Inactive ingredients are acacia, calcium phosphate, D&C Yellow 10, FD&C Yellow 6, lactose, magnesium stearate, starch, and talc.

CLINICAL PHARMACOLOGY

Mecamylamine reduces blood pressure in both normotensive and hypertensive individuals. It has a gradual onset of action (1/2 to 2 hours) and a longlasting effect (usually 6 to 12 hours or more). A small oral dosage often produces a smooth and predictable reduction of blood pressure. Although this antihypertensive effect is predominantly orthostatic, the supine pressure is also significantly reduced.
Pharmacokinetics and Metabolism
Mecamylamine is almost completely absorbed from the gastrointestinal tract, resulting in consistent lowering of blood pressure in most patients with hypertensive cardiovascular disease. Mecamylamine is excreted slowly in the urine in the unchanged form. The rate of its renal elimination is influenced markedly by urinary pH. Alkalinization of the urine reduces, and acidification promotes, renal excretion of mecamylamine.
Mecamylamine crosses the blood-brain and placental barriers.

INDICATIONS AND USAGE

For the management of moderately severe to severe essential hypertension and in uncomplicated cases of malignant hypertension.

CONTRAINDICATIONS

INVERSINE should not be used in mild, moderate, labile hypertension and may prove unsuitable in uncooperative patients. It is contraindicated in coronary insufficiency or recent myocardial infarction.
INVERSINE should be given with great discretion, if at all, when renal insufficiency is manifested by a rising or elevated BUN. The drug is contraindicated in uremia. Patients receiving antibiotics and sulfonamides should generally not be treated with ganglion blockers. Other contraindications are glaucoma, organic pyloric stenosis or hypersensitivity to the product.

WARNINGS

Mecamylamine, a secondary amine, readily penetrates into the brain and thus may produce central nervous system effects. Tremor, choreiform movements, mental aberrations, and convulsions may occur rarely. These have occurred most often when large doses of INVERSINE were used, especially in patients with cerebral or renal insufficiency.
When ganglion blockers or other potent antihypertensive drugs are discontinued suddenly, hypertensive levels return. In patients with malignant hypertension and others, this may occur abruptly and may cause fatal cerebral vascular accidents or acute congestive heart failure. When INVERSINE is withdrawn, this should be done gradually and other antihypertensive therapy usually must be substituted. On the other hand, the effects of INVERSINE sometimes may last from hours to days after therapy is discontinued.

PRECAUTIONS

General
The patient's condition should be evaluated carefully, particularly as to renal and cardiovascular function. When renal, cerebral, or coronary blood flow is deficient, any additional impairment, which might result from added hypotension, must be avoided. The use of INVERSINE in patients with marked cerebral and coronary arteriosclerosis or after a recent cerebral accident requires caution.
The action of INVERSINE may be potentiated by excessive heat, fever, infection, hemorrhage, pregnancy, anesthesia, surgery, vigorous exercise, other antihypertensive drugs, alcohol, and salt depletion as a result of diminished intake or increased excretion due to diarrhea, vomiting, excessive sweating, or diuretics.
During therapy with INVERSINE, sodium intake should not be restricted but, if necessary, the dosage of the ganglion blocker must be adjusted.
Since urinary retention may occur in patients on ganglion blockers, caution is required in patients with prostatic hypertrophy, bladder neck obstruction, and urethral stricture.
Frequent loose bowel movements with abdominal distention and decreased borborygmi may be the first signs of parlytic ileus. If these are present, INVERSINE should be discontinued immediately and remedial steps taken.
Information for patients
INVERSINE may cause dizziness, lightheadedness, or fainting, especially when rising from a lying or sitting position. This effect may be increased by alcoholic beverages, exercise or during hot weather. Getting up slowly may help alleviate such a reaction.
Drug Interactions
Patients receiving antibiotics and sulfonamides generally should not be treated with ganglion blockers.
The action of INVERSINE may be potentiated by anesthesia, other antihypertensive drugs and alcohol.
Carcinogenesis, Mutagenesis, Impairment of Fertility
Long-term studies in animals have not been performed to evaluate the effects upon fertility, mutagenic or carcinogenic potential of INVERSINE.
Pregnancy
Pregnancy Category C. Animal reproduction studies have not been conducted with INVERSINE. It is not known whether INVERSINE can cause fetal harm when given to a pregnant woman or can affect reproductive capacity. INVERSINE should be given to a pregnant woman only if clearly needed.
Nursing Mothers
Because of the potential for serious adverse reactions in nursing infants from INVERSINE, a decision should be made whether to discontinue nursing or to discontinue the drug, taking into account the importance of the drug to the mother.
Pediatric Use
Safety and effectiveness in pediatric patients have not been established.

ADVERSE REACTIONS

The following adverse reactions have been reported and within each category are listed in order of decreasing severity.
Gastrointestinal: Ileus, constipation (sometimes preceded by small, frequent liquid stools), vomiting, nausea, anorexia, glossitis and dryness of mouth.
Cardiovascular: Orthostatic dizziness and syncope, postural hypotension.
Nervous System/Psychiatric: Convulsions, choreiform movements, mental aberrations, tremor, and paresthesias (see WARNINGS).
Respiratory: Interstitial pulmonary edema and fibrosis.
Urogenital: Urinary retention, impotence, decreased libido.
Special Senses: Blurred vision, dilated pupils.
Miscellaneous: Weakness, fatigue, sedation.

OVERDOSAGE

Signs of overdosage include: hypotension (which may progress to peripheral vascular collapse), postural hypotension, nausea, vomiting, diarrhea, constipation, paralytic ileus, urinary retention, dizziness, anxiety, dry mouth, mydriasis, blurred vision, or palpitations. A rise in intraocular pressure may occur.
Pressor amines may be used to counteract excessive hypotension. Since patients being treated with ganglion blockers are more than normally reactive to pressor amines, small doses of the later are recommended to avoid excessive response.
The oral LD_{50} of mecamylamine in the mouse is 92 mg/kg.

DOSAGE AND ADMINISTRATION

Therapy is usually started with one 2.5 mg tablet of INVERSINE twice a day. This initial dosage should be modified by increments of one 2.5 mg tablet at intervals of not less than 2 days until the desired blood pressure response occurs (the criterion being a dosage just under that which causes signs of mild postural hypotension).
The average total daily dosage of INVERSINE is 25 mg, usually in three divided doses. However, as little as 2.5 mg daily may be sufficient to control hypertension in some patients. A range of two to four or even more doses may be required in severe cases when smooth control is difficult to obtain. In severe or urgent cases, larger increments at smaller intervals may be needed. Partial tolerance may develop in certain patients, requiring an increase in the daily dosage of INVERSINE.

Administration of INVERSINE after meals may cause a more gradual absorption and smoother control of excessively high blood pressure. The timing of doses in relation to meals should be consistent. Since the blood pressure response to antihypertensive drugs is increased in the early morning, the larger dose should be given at noontime and perhaps in the evening. The morning dose, as a rule, should be relatively small and in some instances may even be omitted.

The *initial regulation of dosage* should be determined by blood pressure readings in the erect position at the time of maximal effect of the drug, as well as by other signs and symptoms of orthostatic hypotension.

The *effective maintenance dosage* should be regulated by blood pressure readings in the erect position and by limitation of dosage to that which causes slight faintness or dizziness in this position. If the patient or a relative can use a sphygmomanometer, instructions may be given to reduce or omit a dose if readings fall below a designated level or if faintness or lightheadedness occurs. *However, no change should be instituted without the knowledge of the physician.*

Close supervision and education of the patient, as well as critical adjustment of dosage, are essential to successful therapy.

Other Antihypertensive Agents

When INVERSINE is given with other antihypertensive drugs, the dosage of these other agents, as well as that of INVERSINE, should be reduced to avoid excessive hypotension. However, thiazides should be continued in their usual dosage, while that of INVERSINE is decreased by at least 50 percent.

HOW SUPPLIED

8001—Tablets INVERSINE, 2.5 mg, are slightly yellow, round, compressed tablets, coded LBS01. They are supplied as follows:

NDC 17205-0626-1 in bottles of 100.

Manufactured by: Siegfried CMS Ltd., Zofingen, Switzerland for Layton BioScience, Inc.
Sunnyvale, CA 94086

2047

Inversine ® is a registered trademark of Layton BioScience, INC.

Lederle Piperacillin, Inc.
CAROLINA, PUERTO RICO 00630

Lederle Parenterals, Inc.
CAROLINA, PUERTO RICO 00630

LEDERLE PHARMACEUTICAL
Division American Cyanamid Company
Pearl River, NY 10965
US Gov't. License No. 17

For Medical Information Contact:

MARKETED ONCOLOGY PRODUCTS:
Immunex Corporation
Professional Services Department
51 University Street
Seattle, WA 98101
(800) IMMUNEX

OTHER MARKETED DRUG PRODUCTS:
Lederle Pharmaceutical/Wyeth-Ayerst Pharmaceuticals
Medical Affairs Department
P.O. Box 8299
Philadelphia, PA 19101
Day: (800) 934-5556
8:30 AM to 4:30 PM
(Eastern Standard Time),
Weekdays only
Night: (610) 688-4400 (Emergencies only; non-emergencies should wait until the next day)

MARKETED VACCINES AND TINE TESTS:
Lederle Pharmaceutical/Wyeth-Ayerst Pharmaceuticals
Medical Affairs Department
P.O. Box 8299
Philadelphia, PA 19101
Day: (800) 934-5556
8:30 AM to 4:30 PM
(Eastern Standard Time),
Weekdays only
Night: (610) 688-4400 (Emergencies only; non-emergencies should wait until the next day)

LEDERLE PRODUCTS

The following list of Lederle products includes the alphanumeric LEDERMARK® codes which provide quick and positive identification of Lederle capsules and tablets:

Product Identity Code No.	Product
	ACEL-IMUNE® Diphtheria and Tetanus Toxoids and Acellular Pertussis Vaccine Adsorbed
A11	ARTANE® Tabs., 2mg
A12	ARTANE® Tabs., 5mg
—	ARTANE® Elixir, 2mg/5mL
B1	ZEBETA® Tablets, 5mg
B3	ZEBETA® Tablets, 10mg
B12	ZIAC® Tablets, 2.5/6.25mg
B13	ZIAC® Tablets, 5/6.25mg
B14	ZIAC® Tablets, 10/6.25mg
D1	DIAMOX® Tablets, 125mg
D2	DIAMOX® Tablets, 250mg
D3	DIAMOX® SEQUELS® Capsules, 500mg
D11	DECLOMYCIN® Tabs., 150mg
D12	DECLOMYCIN® Tabs., 300mg
—	Diphtheria & Tetanus Toxoids Adsorbed, Alumium Phosphate-Adsorbed, for Pediatric Use
—	HibTITER® Haemophilus b Conjugate Vaccine
M1	RHEUMATREX® Tabs., 2.5mg
M45	MINOCIN® Pellet-Filled Caps., 50mg
M46	MINOCIN® Pellet-Filled Caps., 100mg
—	MINOCIN® IV, 100mg/vial
—	MINOCIN® Oral Suspension, 50mg/5mL
M55	MATERNA® Tabs.
—	PIPRACIL® 2g
—	PIPRACIL® 3g
—	PIPRACIL® 4g
—	PIPRACIL® 40g
—	PNU-IMUNE® 23 Pneumococcal Vaccine Polyvalent
S200	SUPRAX® Tablets, 200mg
S400	SUPRAX® Tablets, 400mg
—	SUPRAX® Powder for Oral Suspension
—	Tetanus Toxoid Adsorbed PUROGENATED®
—	Tetanus and Diphtheria Toxoids Adsorbed PUROGENATED® for Adult Use
—	Tuberculin, Old, TINE TEST®
—	Tuberculin, Purified Protein Derivative PPD TINE TEST®
T1	TriHEMIC® 600 Tabs.
—	ZOSYN® 2.25g vial
—	ZOSYN® 3.375g vial
—	ZOSYN® 4.5g vial
—	ZOSYN® 40.5g pharmacy bulk vial
—	ZOSYN® in Galaxy Containers

DIPHTHERIA and TETANUS TOXOIDS and ACELLULAR PERTUSSIS VACCINE ADSORBED ACEL-IMUNE® FOR ALL FIVE DOSES ℞

℞ only

DESCRIPTION

Diphtheria and Tetanus Toxoids and Acellular Pertussis Vaccine Adsorbed (DTaP), ACEL-IMUNE®, is a sterile combination of PUROGENATED® Diphtheria Toxoid, PUROGENATED® Tetanus Toxoid, and Acellular Pertussis Vaccine which is adsorbed to an aluminum adjuvant. The acellular pertussis vaccine component is produced by Takeda Chemical Industries, Ltd., Osaka, Japan and is combined with diphtheria and tetanus toxoids manufactured by Lederle Laboratories. The bulk vaccine is prepared by Lederle Laboratories. ACEL-IMUNE is filled, labeled, packaged, and released by Lederle Laboratories. ACEL-IMUNE is for intramuscular use only. After shaking, the vaccine is a homogeneous white suspension.

The diphtheria and tetanus toxoids are derived from *Corynebacterium diphtheriae* and *Clostridium tetani*, respectively, which are grown in media according to the method of Mueller and Miller.[1,2] *C. diphtheriae* is grown in a defined medium containing casamino acids and *C. tetani* in a medium containing beef heart infusion. They are detoxified by use of formaldehyde. The toxoids are refined by the Pillemer alcohol fractionation method[3] and are diluted with a solution containing sodium phosphate monobasic, sodium phosphate dibasic, glycine, and thimerosal (mercury derivative) as a preservative. The acellular pertussis vaccine component is prepared by growing Phase I *Bordetella pertussis* in Stainer-Scholte defined medium and harvesting the culture fluid. Purification of the acellular pertussis vaccine component is accomplished by ammonium sulfate fractionation steps and a final sucrose density gradient centrifugation. The acellular pertussis vaccine component is detoxified with formaldehyde and thimerosal (mercury derivative) is added as a preservative.

The diphtheria toxoid, tetanus toxoid, and acellular pertussis vaccine are combined, diluted in phosphate buffered saline (PBS), and adsorbed to aluminum adjuvant. The aluminum adjuvant is formulated to contain 0.23 mg aluminum per 0.5 mL dose as aluminum hydroxide and aluminum phosphate. The residual free formaldehyde content by assay is ≤0.02%. Thimerosal (mercury derivative) is present in a final concentration of 1:10,000. The final product may also contain gelatin and polysorbate 80 which are used in early stages of the manufacture of the pertussis component.

Each single dose of 0.5 mL of ACEL-IMUNE is formulated to contain 9 Lf of diphtheria toxoid and 5 Lf of tetanus toxoid (both toxoids induce not less than 2 units of antitoxin per mL in the guinea pig potency test) and 300 hemagglutinating (HA) units of acellular pertussis vaccine. A hemagglutination unit is that amount of material which completely agglutinates chicken red blood cells as measured by the HA assay.[4] The acellular pertussis vaccine component contains approximately 40 μg (but not more than 60 μg) of pertussis antigen protein per 0.5 mL dose with approximately 86% filamentous hemagglutinin (FHA), approximately 8% inactivated pertussis toxin (PT, also known as lymphocytosis promoting factor), approximately 4% per dose of 69-kilodalton outer membrane protein (pertactin), and approximately 2% type 2 fimbriae (pertussis-specific agglutinogen).

The potency of the pertussis component is evaluated by measurement of antibodies to FHA, PT, pertactin, and fimbriae in immunized mice by ELISA.

CLINICAL PHARMACOLOGY

Simultaneous immunization against diphtheria, tetanus, and pertussis (whooping cough) during infancy and childhood has been a routine practice in the United States since the late 1940s. It has played a major role in markedly reducing the incidence of cases and deaths from each of these diseases.

Diphtheria is primarily a localized and generalized intoxication caused by diphtheria toxin, an extracellular protein metabolite of toxinogenic strains of *C. diphtheriae.* While the incidence of diphtheria in the US has decreased from over 200,000 cases reported in 1921, before the general use of diphtheria toxoid, to only 15 cases reported from 1990 to 1994,[5] the case fatality rate has remained constant at about 5% to 10%. The highest case fatality rates are in the very young and in the elderly. Diphtheria remains a serious disease in some areas of the world as demonstrated by the recent epidemic in the former Soviet Union.[6]

Following adequate immunization with diphtheria toxoid it is thought that protection lasts for at least 10 years.[7] Antitoxin levels of at least 0.01 antitoxin units/mL are generally regarded as protective.[8] This significantly reduces both the risk of developing diphtheria and the severity of clinical illness. It does not, however, eliminate carriage of *C. diphtheriae* in the pharynx or on the skin.[7]

Tetanus is an intoxication manifested primarily by neuromuscular dysfunction caused by a potent exotoxin elaborated by *C. tetani.* The incidence of tetanus in the US has dropped dramatically with the routine use of tetanus toxoid, with an average of 57 cases reported annually from 1985–1994.[5] Spores of *C. tetani* are ubiquitous and there is essentially no natural immunity to tetanus toxin.

Thus, universal primary immunization with tetanus toxoid with subsequent maintenance of adequate antitoxin levels, by means of timed boosters, is recommended to protect all age groups.[7] Tetanus toxoid is a highly effective antigen and a completed primary series generally induces serum antitoxin levels of at least 0.01 antitoxin units, a level which has been reported to be protective.[9] It is thought that protection persists for at least 10 years.[7]

The toxoids of tetanus and diphtheria induce neutralizing antibodies to the toxins produced by the infecting organisms. In two clinical studies with ACEL-IMUNE®, serum antitoxin levels to diphtheria and tetanus toxins were shown to be greater than 0.01 antitoxin units/mL in 100% of 140 infants following three doses.[10] These levels are generally regarded to be protective.[9,11]

Pertussis (whooping cough) is a highly communicable disease of the respiratory tract. Attack rates of over 90% have been reported in unimmunized household contacts.[9,12] Since immunization against pertussis (whooping cough) became widespread, the number of reported cases and associated mortality in the US has declined from about 120,000 cases and 1100 deaths in 1950,[13] to a historical low of 1010 cases in 1976. However, since the early 1980s, reported pertussis incidence has increased with peaks occurring in 1983, 1986, 1990, and 1993. Following the peak in reported cases in 1993, the numbers declined during 1994 and the first 2 quarters of 1995 — a pattern consistent with the previously observed 3–4 year periodicity in pertussis incidence.[14] An average of 4515 cases were reported annually from 1990–1994.[5] Precise data do not exist, since bacteriological confirmation of pertussis can be obtained in less than half of the suspected cases. In the US, most reported illness from *B. pertussis* occurs in infants and young children; approximately 80% of reported deaths occur in children less than 1 year old.[7] Older children and adults, in whom classic signs are often absent, may go undiagnosed and serve as reservoirs of disease.[7,15]

Pertussis disease (whopping cough) is caused by a gram-negative coccobacillus, *B. pertussis.* Several antigens that are thought to play a role in protective immunity have been isolated from cultures of *B. pertussis.* These include FHA, PT, pertactin, and fimbriae.[16–18] Another biologically active component, endotoxin, may contribute to reactogenicity of pertussis vaccines.[19] The Takeda acellular pertussis vaccine

Continued on next page

Acel-Imune—Cont.

component used in ACEL-IMUNE contains inactivated FHA, PT, pertactin, and type 2 fimbriae, with minimal endotoxin compared to that in whole-cell pertussis vaccine. The pertussis component induces immunity against pertussis disease in humans.

Efficacy of ACEL-IMUNE was assessed in infants in a prospective study conducted in Germany at 227 investigator sites. A total of 8532 infants were randomized to receive ACEL-IMUNE (n=4273) or Lederle whole-cell DTP (n=4259) at mean ages of 3, 5 and 7 months followed by a fourth dose of ACEL-IMUNE (n=3991) or DTP (n=3925) at a mean age of 17 months. By parental choice, 1739 additional infants received German-manufactured Diphtheria and Tetanus Toxoids (DT) at mean ages of 3 and 5 months followed by a third dose at a mean age of 17 months. In order to adjust for potential confounding, several variables were examined to determine which ones differed between the randomized and non-randomized groups and affected the risk of developing pertussis. Telephone calls were performed every 14 days by investigator personnel to ensure close surveillance of pertussis disease among study subjects and household members. Evaluation of a 7-day cough which was not improving included a nasopharyngeal specimen for culture and blood sample for acute serology. Subjects with greater than 14 days of cough were evaluated by central investigators and convalescent serology was scheduled for 6–8 weeks after cough onset. Completeness of surveillance to ascertain the presence and duration of cough illness was not directly assessed; however, study sites were monitored for compliance with the protocol.

A total of 154 cases were identified using a case definition of 21 days or more of cough with paroxysms, whoop or post-tussive vomiting plus confirmation by positive culture for *B. pertussis*, or household contact with a person with positive culture for *B. pertussis*, or by serologic confirmation (significant rise in PT IgG between acute and convalescent samples or PT IgA value significantly elevated above the normal limits). Case rates per 100 person-years of follow-up for each vaccine were: DTaP, 0.48; DTP, 0.22; and DT, 2.98. Adjusting for single adult households and households in which all siblings were unimmunized, the vaccine efficacy after 3 doses and before receipt of the fourth dose of ACEL-IMUNE or until 19 months of age was 73% (95% Cl 51 to 86) and after 4 doses 85% (95% Cl 76 to 90). DTP efficacy after 3 doses was 83% (95% Cl 65 to 92) and after 4 doses was 94% (95% Cl 89 to 97). For ACEL-IMUNE, there is no significant difference in efficacy between 3 and 4 doses (p=0.16). Considering all observation time, i.e., including from after the third dose until the fourth dose (approximately 40% of follow-up time) and from after the fourth dose until the end of the study (approximately 60% of follow-up time), the adjusted efficacy estimated for ACEL-IMUNE was 81% (95% Cl 73 to 87) compared to 91% for DTP (95% Cl 85 to 95). The relative risk for pertussis in the ACEL-IMUNE group compared to the DTP group was 1.5 (95% Cl 0.7 to 3.4) after 3 doses and 2.8 (95% Cl 1.3 to 5.9) after 4 doses.

Some subjects with 21 days or more of cough with paroxysms, whoop or post-tussive vomiting did not have complete laboratory tests. Of those subjects whose available tests were negative (DT, 113 subjects; DTaP, 241 subjects; and DTP, 239 subjects), 68% in the DT group, 69% in the ACEL-IMUNE group, and 68% in the Lederle whole-cell DTP group had at least one missing laboratory test. In the efficacy analysis these subjects were classified as non-cases. The effect of this classification was evaluated by applying missing value imputation procedures in which it was assumed that the probability of being a pertussis case was the same among subjects with and without all laboratory results; missing values were found to have minimal effect on vaccine efficacy.[10] It is possible, however, that the misclassification of such subjects due to missing laboratory values may have resulted in overestimates of ACEL-IMUNE and whole-cell DTP efficacy.

Vaccine efficacy was also estimated in a household contact analysis within the prospective German study. A primary case of pertussis was defined as cough for 21 or more days with paroxysms, whoop, or post-tussive vomiting plus laboratory confirmation. A total of 167 households had a member other than a study infant who met this definition. A secondary case of pertussis was defined as cough for 21 or more days with paroxysms, whoop, or post-tussive vomiting plus laboratory confirmation, with an onset within 7–28 days after onset of pertussis in a primary case in the household. Thirteen secondary cases were identified among study infants, resulting in secondary attack rates of 9.5% (ACEL-IMUNE), 2.0% (DTP), and 32% (DT). Based on this analysis, the vaccine efficacy for ACEL-IMUNE was 70% (95% Cl 11 to 90). Analysis of potentially confounding variables revealed none that were associated with both vaccine group and pertussis case status.[10]

Following primary immunization, US children (n=126) had antibody titers to pertussis antigens which were similar to those achieved in German children who participated in a pilot study (n=52) and a subset of children in the efficacy trial (n=52) where vaccine efficacy was demonstrated.[10]

In a clinical study conducted in the US, 77 infants received ACEL-IMUNE, HibTITER and Hepatitis B vaccine simultaneously at 2, 4 and 6 months of age. Ninety-four percent of the children demonstrated anti-PRP antibodies ≥1 μg/mL. All of the 74 infants evaluated for HBs responses had anti-HBs titers of >10 mIU/mL.[10]

Sera from 30 infants who received OPV simultaneously with ACEL-IMUNE at 2 and 4 months showed that at 6 months, 90 to 100% had protective neutralizing antibody to all three poliovirus types (comparable to results seen with simultaneous DTP administration with OPV).[10]

Ninety-two to 100% of 15–18 month old children (n=48) who received MMR simultaneously with ACEL-IMUNE had protective titers to measles, mumps, and rubella; similar results were seen for children who received DTP and MMR simultaneously.[20]

INDICATIONS AND USAGE

Diphtheria and Tetanus Toxoids and Acellular Pertussis Vaccine Adsorbed, ACEL-IMUNE®, is indicated for active immunization of children from 6 weeks of age up to age 7 years (prior to seventh birthday) for protection against diphtheria, tetanus, and pertussis.

This product is not recommended for immunizing persons on or after their seventh birthday (see **DOSAGE AND ADMINISTRATION**).

Children who have recovered from culture-confirmed pertussis need not receive further doses of a pertussis-containing vaccine[7], but should complete the recommended series with Dipththeria and Tetanus Toxoids, Adsorbed for pediatric use (DT).

ACEL-IMUNE is intended for active immunization against diphtheria, tetanus, and pertussis, and is not to be used for treatment of actual infection.

If a contraindicating event to the pertussis vaccine component occurs, Diphtheria and Tetanus Toxoids Adsorbed for pediatric use (DT) should be substituted for each of the remaining doses. The Advisory Committee on Immunization Practices (ACIP) recommends that if an immediate anaphylactic reaction occurs, no further vaccination with any of the three antigens in DTP should be carried out.[7]

As with any vaccine, ACEL-IMUNE may not protect 100% of individuals receiving the vaccine.

If passive immunization is required, Tetanus Immune Globulin (TIG) or Diphtheria Antitoxin are recommended.

CONTRAINDICATIONS

HYPERSENSITIVITY TO ANY COMPONENT OF THE VACCINE, INCLUDING THIMEROSAL, A MERCURY DERIVATIVE, IS A CONTRAINDICATION.

THE DECISION TO ADMINISTER OR DELAY DTP VACCINATION BECAUSE OF A CURRENT OR RECENT FEBRILE ILLNESS DEPENDS LARGELY ON THE SEVERITY OF THE SYMPTOMS AND THEIR ETIOLOGY. ALTHOUGH A MODERATE OR SEVERE FEBRILE ILLNESS IS SUFFICIENT REASON TO POSTPONE VACCINATION, MINOR ILLNESSES SUCH AS A MILD UPPER RESPIRATORY INFECTION WITH OR WITHOUT LOW GRADE FEVER ARE NOT CONTRAINDICATIONS.[7,21,22]

ROUTINE IMMUNIZATION SHOULD BE DEFERRED DURING AN OUTBREAK OF POLIOMYELITIS PROVIDING THE PATIENT HAS NOT SUSTAINED AN INJURY THAT INCREASES THE RISK OF TETANUS AND PROVIDING AN OUTBREAK OF DIPHTHERIA OR PERTUSSIS DOES NOT OCCUR SIMULTANEOUSLY.[23]

DATA ON THE USE OF ACEL-IMUNE® IN CHILDREN FOR WHOM WHOLE-CELL PERTUSSIS VACCINE IS CONTRAINDICATED ARE NOT AVAILABLE. UNTIL SUCH DATA ARE AVAILABLE, IT WOULD BE PRUDENT TO CONSIDER THE ACIP AND AMERICAN ACADEMY OF PEDIATRICS (AAP) CONTRAINDICATIONS TO WHOLE-CELL PERTUSSIS VACCINE AS CONTRAINDICATIONS TO ACEL-IMUNE.

IMMUNIZATION WITH ACEL-IMUNE IS CONTRAINDICATED IF THE CHILD HAS EXPERIENCED ANY EVENT FOLLOWING PREVIOUS IMMUNIZATION WITH ANY VACCINE CONTAINING A PERTUSSIS COMPONENT, WHICH IS CONSIDERED BY THE AAP OR ACIP TO BE A CONTRAINDICATION TO FURTHER DOSES OF PERTUSSIS VACCINE. THESE EVENTS ARE:

AN IMMEDIATE ANAPHYLACTIC REACTION. BECAUSE OF THE UNCERTAINTY AS TO WHICH COMPONENT OF THE VACCINE MIGHT BE RESPONSIBLE, NO FURTHER VACCINATION WITH ANY OF THE ANTIGENS IN DTP SHOULD BE CARRIED OUT. ALTERNATIVELY, BECAUSE OF THE IMPORTANCE OF TETANUS VACCINATION, SUCH INDIVIDUALS MAY BE REFERRED FOR EVALUATION BY AN ALLERGIST.[7,21,22]

ENCEPHALOPATHY (NOT DUE TO ANOTHER IDENTIFIABLE CAUSE) OCCURRING WITHIN 7 DAYS FOLLOWING VACCINATION. THIS IS DEFINED AS AN ACUTE, SEVERE CENTRAL NERVOUS SYSTEM DISORDER OCCURRING WITHIN 7 DAYS FOLLOWING VACCINATION, AND GENERALLY CONSISTING OF MAJOR ALTERATIONS IN CONSCIOUSNESS, UNRESPONSIVENESS, GENERALIZED OR FOCAL SEIZURES THAT PERSIST MORE THAN A FEW HOURS, WITH FAILURE TO RECOVER WITHIN 24 HOURS. EVEN THOUGH CAUSATION BY DTP CANNOT BE ESTABLISHED, NO SUBSEQUENT DOSES OF PERTUSSIS VACCINE SHOULD BE GIVEN.[7,21,22]

THE CLINICAL JUDGMENT OF THE ATTENDING PHYSICIAN SHOULD PREVAIL AT ALL TIMES.

WARNINGS

THE ACIP AND THE AAP STATE THAT IF ANY OF THE FOLLOWING EVENTS OCCUR IN TEMPORAL RELATION TO RECEIPT OF DTP OR DTaP, THE DECISION TO GIVE SUBSEQUENT DOSES OF VACCINE CONTAINING THE PERTUSSIS COMPONENT SHOULD BE CAREFULLY CONSIDERED. ALTHOUGH THESE EVENTS WERE ONCE CONSIDERED CONTRAINDICATIONS TO WHOLE-CELL DTP, THERE MAY BE CIRCUMSTANCES, SUCH AS A HIGH INCIDENCE OF PERTUSSIS, IN WHICH THE POTENTIAL BENEFITS OUTWEIGH THE POSSIBLE RISKS, PARTICULARLY BECAUSE THESE EVENTS HAVE NOT BEEN SHOWN TO CAUSE PERMANENT SEQUELAE.[7,21,22]

1. TEMPERATURE OF ≥40.5°C (105°F) WITHIN 48 HOURS NOT DUE TO IDENTIFIABLE CAUSE.
2. COLLAPSE OR SHOCK-LIKE STATE (HYPOTONIC-HYPORESPONSIVE EPISODE) WITHIN 48 HOURS.
3. PERSISTENT, INCONSOLABLE CRYING LASTING ≥3 HOURS, OCCURRING WITHIN 48 HOURS.
4. CONVULSIONS WITH OR WITHOUT FEVER OCCURRING WITHIN 3 DAYS.[7,21,22,24]

Data on the use of ACEL-IMUNE® in children with a personal history of convulsion or an evolving or changing disorder of the central nervous system are not available. In the opinion of the manufacturer, the presence of a personal history of convulsion or an evolving disorder affecting the central nervous system is considered a warning against further immunization with this vaccine.

The ACIP and the AAP recommend considering deferral of immunization against pertussis in children with progressive neurologic disorders, personal history of convulsion, and known or suspected neurologic conditions which predispose to seizures or neurologic deterioration until the child's status has been fully assessed, a treatment regimen established, and the condition stabilized.[7,21,22,25]

Children with a personal or family history of convulsion may have an increased risk for seizures following DTP vaccination compared with children without such histories.[26,27] However, the ACIP states that children with stable central nervous system disorders, including well-controlled seizures or satisfactorily explained single seizures may receive pertussis vaccination. The ACIP and AAP do not consider a family history of seizures to be a contraindication to pertussis vaccination.[7,21,22] Data on the use of ACEL-IMUNE in such persons are not available.

Although there are no data on whether the prophylactic use of antipyretics can decrease the risk of febrile convulsions, data suggest that acetaminophen will reduce the incidence of postvaccination fever.[28] The ACIP and AAP recommend administering acetaminophen at age-appropriate doses at the time of vaccination and every 4 hours for 24 hours to children at higher risk for seizures than the general population.[7,22,29] The decision to administer a pertussis-containing vaccine to such children must be made by the physician on an individual basis, with consideration of all relevant factors, and assessment of potential risks and benefits for that individual. The physician should review the full text of ACIP and AAP guidelines prior to considering vaccination for such children.[7,22,29] The parent or guardian should be advised of the potential increased risk.

A detailed follow-up of the National Childhood Encephalopathy Study (NCES) indicated that children who had had a serious acute neurologic illness were significantly more likely than children in a control group without acute neurologic illness to have chronic nervous system dysfunction 10 years later.[30] These children with chronic nervous system dysfunction were more likely than children in the control group to have received DTP within 7 days of onset of the original serious acute neurologic illness (i.e., 12 [3.3%] of 367 children vs. six [0.8%] of 723 children).[21,30] After reviewing the follow-up data, a committee of the Institute of Medicine (IOM) concluded that the NCES provided evidence of an association between DTP and chronic nervous system dysfunction in children who had had a serious acute neurologic illness after vaccination with DTP.[31] However, IOM also concluded that the results were insufficient to determine whether DTP increases the overall risk for chronic nervous system dysfunction in children.[31] The ACIP indicated that the results of the NCES were insufficient to determine whether DTP administration before the acute neurological event influenced the potential for neurologic dysfunction 10 years later.[21] Acute encephalopathy or permanent neurological injury have not been reported in clinical trials after administration of ACEL-IMUNE, but the experience with this vaccine is insufficient to rule this out (see **ADVERSE REACTIONS**).

ACEL-IMUNE should not be given to infants or children with thrombocytopenia or any coagulation disorder that would contraindicate intramuscular injection unless the potential benefit clearly outweighs the risk of administration. If the decision is made to administer ACEL-IMUNE to children with coagulation disorders, it should be given with caution (see **DRUG INTERACTIONS**).

PRECAUTIONS

General

CARE IS TO BE TAKEN BY THE HEALTH PROVIDER FOR SAFE AND EFFECTIVE USE OF THIS PRODUCT.

1. PRIOR TO ADMINISTRATION OF ANY DOSE OF ACEL-IMUNE®, THE PARENT OR GUARDIAN SHOULD BE ASKED ABOUT THE PERSONAL HISTORY, FAMILY HISTORY, AND RECENT HEALTH STATUS OF THE VACCINE RECIPIENT. THE PHYSICIAN SHOULD ASCERTAIN PREVIOUS IMMUNIZATION HISTORY, CURRENT HEALTH STATUS, AND OCCURRENCE OF ANY SYMPTOMS AND/OR SIGNS OF AN ADVERSE EVENT AFTER PREVIOUS IMMUNIZATIONS IN THE CHILD TO BE IMMUNIZED, IN ORDER TO DETERMINE THE EX-

ISTENCE OF ANY CONTRAINDICATION TO IMMUNIZATION WITH ACEL-IMUNE AND TO ALLOW AN ASSESSMENT OF BENEFITS AND RISKS.

2. BEFORE THE INJECTION OF ANY BIOLOGICAL, THE PHYSICIAN SHOULD TAKE ALL PRECAUTIONS KNOWN FOR THE PREVENTION OF ALLERGIC OR ANY OTHER SIDE REACTIONS. This should include a review of the patient's history regarding possible sensitivity; the ready availability of epinephrine 1:1000 and other appropriate agents used for control of immediate allergic reactions; and a knowledge of the recent literature pertaining to use of the biological concerned, including the nature of side effects and adverse reactions that may follow its use.

3. Children with impaired immune responsiveness, whether due to the use of immunosuppressive therapy (including irradiation, corticosteroids, antimetabolites, alkylating agents, and cytotoxic agents), a genetic defect, human immunodeficiency virus (HIV) infection, or other causes, may have reduced antibody response to active immunization procedures.[7,22,32,33] Deferral of administration of vaccine may be considered in individuals receiving immunosuppressive therapy.[7] Other groups should receive this vaccine according to the usual recommended schedule[7,22,33,34] (see **DRUG INTERACTIONS**).

4. This product is not contraindicated for use in individuals with human immunodeficiency virus (HIV) infection.[35]

5. *Since this product is a suspension containing an adjuvant, shake vigorously to obtain a uniform suspension prior to withdrawing each dose from the multiple dose vial.*

6. A separate sterile syringe and needle or a sterile disposable unit should be used for each individual patient to prevent transmission of hepatitis or other infectious agents from one person to another. Needles should be disposed of properly and should not be recapped.

7. Special care should be taken to prevent injection into a blood vessel.

Information for Patient

PRIOR TO ADMINISTRATION OF ACEL-IMUNE®, HEALTH CARE PERSONNEL SHOULD INFORM THE PARENT, GUARDIAN, OR OTHER RESPONSIBLE ADULT OF THE RECOMMENDED IMMUNIZATION SCHEDULE FOR PROTECTION AGAINST DIPHTHERIA, TETANUS, AND PERTUSSIS AND THE BENEFITS AND RISKS TO THE CHILD RECEIVING THIS VACCINE CONTAINING AN ACELLULAR PERTUSSIS COMPONENT. GUIDANCE SHOULD BE PROVIDED ON MEASURES TO BE TAKEN SHOULD ADVERSE EVENTS OCCUR, SUCH AS ANTIPYRETIC MEASURES FOR ELEVATED TEMPERATURES AND THE NEED TO REPORT ADVERSE EVENTS TO THE HEALTH CARE PROVIDER. PARENTS SHOULD BE PROVIDED WITH VACCINE INFORMATION MATERIALS AT THE TIME OF EACH VACCINATION, AS STATED IN THE NATIONAL CHILDHOOD VACCINE INJURY ACT.[36]

THE HEALTH CARE PROVIDER SHOULD INFORM THE PATIENT, PARENT, OR GUARDIAN OF THE IMPORTANCE OF COMPLETING THE IMMUNIZATION SERIES UNLESS CONTRAINDICATED.

PATIENTS, PARENTS, OR GUARDIANS SHOULD BE INSTRUCTED TO REPORT ANY SERIOUS ADVERSE REACTIONS TO THEIR HEALTH CARE PROVIDER

Drug Interactions

Children receiving immunosuppressive therapy may have a reduced response to active immunization procedures.[7,22,32,33] Although no specific studies with pertussis vaccine are available, if immunosuppressive therapy will be discontinued shortly, it would be reasonable to defer immunization until the patient has been off therapy for one month; otherwise, the patient should be vaccinated while still on therapy.[32]

As with other intramuscular injections, ACEL-IMUNE® should be given with caution to children on anticoagulant therapy.

Tetanus Immune Globulin or Diphtheria Antitoxin, if used, should be given in a separate site with a separate needle and syringe if used at the same time as ACEL-IMUNE.

Please see **DOSAGE AND ADMINISTRATION** for information regarding simultaneous administration with other vaccines.

Carcinogenesis, Mutagenesis, Impairment of Fertility

ACEL-IMUNE has not been evaluated for its carcinogenic, mutagenic potential or impairment of fertility.

Pregnancy

Pregnancy Category C

Animal reproduction studies have not been conducted with ACEL-IMUNE®. It is not known whether ACEL-IMUNE vaccine can cause fetal harm when administered to a pregnant woman or can affect reproductive capacity. ACEL-IMUNE vaccine is NOT recommended for use in a pregnant woman.

THIS PRODUCT IS NOT RECOMMENDED FOR USE IN INDIVIDUALS 7 YEARS OF AGE OR OLDER.

Pediatric Use

The safety and effectiveness of ACEL-IMUNE® in children below the age of 6 weeks have not been established (see **DOSAGE AND ADMINISTRATION**).

For immunization of children 7 years of age and older, Tetanus and Diphtheria Toxoids Adsorbed for Adults Use (Td) is recommended.[7,22]

Protection against the indicated diseases (tetanus, diphtheria, pertussis) is based on a full course of immunization.

Table 1
Adverse Events Occurring Within 72 Hours Following DTaP and DTP

	% OF CHILDREN							
	ACEL-IMUNE®				Lederle-Whole Cell DTP			
EVENT	**Dose 1**	**Dose 2**	**Dose 3**	**Dose 4**	**Dose 1**	**Dose 2**	**Dose 3**	**Dose 4**
Number of Children[a]	**4273**	**4223**	**4155**	**3991**	**4259**	**4149**	**4087**	**3925**
Local								
Erythema >23 mm[b]	2	3	5	10	15	11	11	13
Induration >23 mm[b]	2	4	6	9	17	13	11	13
Systemic								
Fever[c] ≥38.0°C[b]	7	12	16	26	44	35	40	50
Fever[c]>39.0°C[b]	0.3	1	1	2	1	2	3	4
Fretfulness[b]	18	18	16	15	47	33	28	31
Drowsiness[b]	23	16	12	11	40	25	19	21
Decreased Appetite[b]	10	9	7	9	21	14	12	17

[a] For each adverse event, information was not available for a small number of subjects; 2/3 of all subjects received vaccinations in the thigh, 1/3 in the buttocks
[b] p <0.001—when compared to whole-cell DTP for all doses
[c] Rectal temperature

ADVERSE REACTIONS

Adverse reactions associated with ACEL-IMUNE® have been evaluated in a total of 6941 US and German infants administered a total of 20,390 doses for the first three doses in the series. A total of 5152 of these infants received ACEL-IMUNE for the fourth dose in a 4-dose DTaP series as toddlers and a total of 357 of these toddlers also received ACEL-IMUNE for the fifth dose in a 5-dose DTaP series at 4 to 6 years of age. Adverse event data were actively collected using parent diary cards, phone call follow-up, and/or by questioning the parents at clinic visits.

[See table above]

In the German efficacy study where 8532 infants were randomized to receive DTaP or DTP, a total of 16,642 doses of ACEL-IMUNE were given. When compared to Lederle whole-cell pertussis DTP vaccine, ACEL-IMUNE produced significantly fewer local reactions and systemic events (see Table 1).

In other clinical studies of ACEL-IMUNE conducted in the US, 2593 children received 8601 doses for doses 1 through 4. In general, rates of local reactions and systemic events were comparable to those reported in the German efficacy study and lower than for whole-cell DTP. Rates of local reactions increased over the first 4 doses of ACEL-IMUNE: erythema >20 mm from 1% (dose 1) to 8% (dose 4), induration >20 mm from 1% (dose 1) to 6% (dose 4), and tenderness from 4% (dose 2) to 16% (dose 4). Rates of temperature ≥38.0°C increased over the 4-dose series from 2% (dose 1) to 18% (dose 4). With the exception of drowsiness which decreased over the 4-dose series from 20% (dose 1) to 5% (dose 4), similar rates for doses 1 through 4 were reported for other systemic events: fretfulness from 18% (dose 4) to 23% (doses 1 and 2), and loss of appetite from 9% (dose 1) to 12% (dose 4).[10]

In four clinical studies conducted in Germany and the US, a total of 357 children received a fifth dose of ACEL-IMUNE in a 5-dose DTaP series at 4 to 6 years of age. Two hundred seventy-eight subjects received vaccine formulated to contain 0.15 mg aluminum per dose and 79 subjects received vaccine formulated to contain 0.23 mg aluminum per dose. While there were no comparative DTP groups in these study segments, the reactogenicity of ACEL-IMUNE was no greater than that described for historical controls who received a fifth dose of whole-cell DTP after 4 previous doses of whole-cell DTP.[10,37,38]

Table 2
Percent of Adverse Events Occurring within 72 Hours Following the Fifth Dose of ACEL-IMUNE® in Children Who Received Four Previous Consecutive Doses of ACEL-IMUNE®

Symptom	DTaP[1] N = 357
Erythema	
Any	35
Significant[2]	20
Induration	
Any	30
Significant[2]	14
Tenderness	38
Fever ≥38.0°C	9
>39.0°C	3
Fretfulness	9
Drowsiness	10
Decreased appetite	8
Vomiting	3

[1] For some adverse events, information was not available for a small number of subjects
[2] Significant varied by protocol from >20 mm–>24 mm

In the large German efficacy trial, 4273 subjects received 16,642 doses of ACEL-IMUNE and 4259 subjects received 16,420 doses of DTP. Adverse events (rates per 1000 doses) meeting AAP and ACIP criteria as absolute contraindications or precautions to further pertussis immunization and occurring within 72 hours following the immunizations were: persistent or unusual cry (1.14 for DTaP, 4.75 for DTP), fever ≥40.5°C (0.06 for DTaP, 0.18 for DTP), seizures, all of which were febrile (0.06 for DTaP, 0.18 for DTP) and hypotonic-hyporesponsive episode (0 for DTaP and 0.06 for DTP). When the total clinical trial experience with ACEL-IMUNE is considered (25,899 immunizations), rates per 1000 doses of ACEL-IMUNE were: persistent or unusual cry (1.27), fever ≥40.5°C (0.08), seizure (0.04), possible seizure (0.04), and hypotonic-hyporesponsive episode (0.04).[10]

Adverse reactions associated with ACEL-IMUNE have been evaluated in clinical trials in 911 children receiving this vaccine as the fourth or fifth dose in the DTP series when they had previously received 3 or 4 doses of whole-cell DTP. The percent of children experiencing common symptoms at any time within 72 hours following immunization is summarized in Table 3.

Table 3
Percent of Children with Symptoms Following a Fourth or Fifth Dose of ACEL-IMUNE® After 3 or 4 Doses of Whole-Cell DTP

Symptom	% of Children[1] Reporting Symptoms within 72 Hours of Immunization n = 911
Tenderness	26
Erythema (>2 cm)	10
Induration (>2 cm)	7
Increased injection site temperature	17
Fever[2] ≥38°C (100.4°F)	19
>39°C (102.2°F)	1.5
Drowsiness	6
Fretfulness	17
Vomiting	2

[1] Children 17 to 24 months of age (fourth dose) and 4 to 6 years of age (fifth dose)
[2] Rectal temperature for 17–24 month olds
Oral temperature for 4–6 year olds

In a large, post-marketing surveillance study, 28,095 doses of ACEL-IMUNE were administered to children as a fourth or fifth dose following previous doses with whole-cell DTP. The rates of local and systemic events reported in a subset of approximately 4400 subjects who were evaluated by telephone interview within 48 to 72 hours postimmunization were: tenderness, 31%; erythema ≥ 1 inch, 4%; induration ≥ 1 inch, 3.5%; perceived fever, 15%; irritability, 25%; and vomiting, 2%.[10]

As with other aluminum-containing vaccines, a nodule may occasionally be palpable at the injection site for several weeks. Sterile abscess formation or subcutaneous atrophy at the injection site may occur rarely.[39]

Urticaria, erythema multiforme or other rash, arthralgias,[40] and, more rarely, a severe anaphylactic reaction[7] (e.g., urticaria with swelling of the mouth, difficulty breathing, hypotension, or shock) have been reported following administration of preparations containing diphtheria, tetanus, and/or pertussis antigens.

Arthus-type hypersensitivity reactions, characterized by severe local reactions (generally starting 2 to 8 hours after an injection) may follow receipt of tetanus toxoid.

Whole-cell pertussis DTP has been associated with acute encephalopathy.[31] A detailed follow-up of the National Childhood Encephalopathy Study (NCES) indicated that children who had had a serious acute neurologic illness were significantly more likely than children in a control group without acute neurologic illness to have chronic nervous system dysfunction 10 years later.[30] These children with chronic nervous system dysfunction were more likely than children in the control group to have received DTP within 7 days of onset of the original serious acute neurologic illness (i.e., 12 [3.3%] of 367 children vs. six [0.8%] of 723 children).[21,30] After reviewing the follow-up data, a committee of the Institute of Medicine (IOM) concluded that the

Continued on next page

Acel-Imune—Cont.

NCES provided evidence of an association between DTP and chronic nervous system dysfunction in children who had a serious acute neurologic illness after vaccination with DTP.[31] However, IOM also concluded that the results were insufficient to determine whether DTP increases the overall risk for chronic nervous system dysfunction in children.[31] The ACIP indicated that the results of the NCES were insufficient to determine whether DTP administration before the acute neurological event influenced the potential for neurologic dysfunction 10 years later.[21]

Onset of infantile spasms has occurred in infants who have recently received DTP and DT. Analysis of data from the NCES on children with infantile spasms showed that receipt of DT or DTP was not causally related to infantile spasms.[31,41] The incidence of onset of infantile spasms increases at 3 to 9 months of age, the time period in which the second and third doses of DTP are generally given. Therefore, some cases of infantile spasms can be expected to be related by chance alone to recent receipt of DTP.[7,31]

A bulging fontanelle associated with increased intracranial pressure which occurred within 24 hours following DTP immunization has been reported, although a causal relationship has not been established.[31,42–44]

The above findings regarding possible association of unusual neurologic events related only to DTP vaccine containing whole-cell pertussis. At this time there are insufficient data to determine their relevance to ACEL-IMUNE.

Sudden Infant Death Syndrome (SIDS) has occurred in infants following administration of whole-cell pertussis DTP and DTaP. Large case-control studies of SIDS in the US have shown that receipt of whole-cell DTP was not causally related to SIDS.[45–47] A review by a committee of the IOM concluded that available evidence did not indicate a causal relation between DTP vaccine and SIDS.[31] The rate of SIDS in the German efficacy trial was 0.2 per thousand infants and in US safety studies was 0.8 per thousand infants vaccinated with ACEL-IMUNE.[10] The reported rate of SIDS in the US from 1985 through 1991 was 1.5 per thousand live births.[48] Since SIDS occurs most commonly at the age when DTP primary immunizations are recommended, by chance alone, some cases of SIDS can be expected to follow receipt of whole-cell pertussis DTP and DTaP.

Neurological complications,[49] such as convulsions,[40] encephalopathy[40,50] and various mono- and polyneuropathies,[50–56] including Guillain-Barré syndrome,[57,58] have been reported following administration of preparations containing diphtheria, tetanus, and/or pertussis antigens. A review by the IOM found a causal relation between tetanus toxoid and brachial neuritis and Guillain-Barré syndrome.[59] Permanent neurological disability and death have been reported rarely in temporal relation to immunization with vaccines containing pertussis antigens; however, a causal relationship has not been established.

As with any vaccine, there is the possibility that broad use of ACEL-IMUNE could reveal adverse reactions not observed in clinical trials.

In clinical trials involving 25,899 immunizations with ACEL-IMUNE, there were no occurrences of anaphylaxis or encephalopathy. Six deaths were reported to study investigators. Causes of death included three SIDS and three accidental deaths. None of these events was determined to be vaccine-related and all occurred more than 4 weeks postimmunization. No deaths from invasive bacterial infections were reported in studies with ACEL-IMUNE.

Adverse Event Reporting

Any adverse reactions following immunization should be reported by the health care provider to the US Department of Health and Human Services (DHHS). The **National Childhood Vaccine Injury Act** requires that the manufacturer and lot number of the vaccine administered be recorded by the health care provider in the vaccine recipient's permanent medical record (or in a permanent office log or file), along with the date of administration of the vaccine and the name, address, and title of the person administering the vaccine. The Act further requires the health care provider to report to the Secretary of the Department of Health and Human Services, the occurrence following immunization of any event set forth in the Vaccine Injury Table, including anaphylaxis or anaphylactic shock within 4 hours; encephalopathy or encephalitis within 72 hours; or any sequela (including death) of an illness, disability, injury or condition referred to above which illness, disability, injury, or condition arose within the time period prescribed or any event that would contraindicate further doses of vaccine, according to this ACEL-IMUNE package insert.[36,60]

The US Department of Health and Human Services has established Vaccine Adverse Event Reporting System (VAERS) to accept all reports of suspected adverse events after the administration of any vaccine including, but not limited to, the reporting of events required by the National Childhood Vaccine Injury Act of 1986.[36] The VAERS toll-free number for VAERS forms and information is 800-822-7967.

DOSAGE AND ADMINISTRATION

For intramuscular use only

The dose is 0.5 mL to be given intramuscularly.

Primary Immunization

For infants, the primary immunization series of ACEL-IMUNE® consists of three doses of 0.5 mL each. The customary age for the first dose is 2 months of age but can be given as young as 6 weeks of age. The recommended dosing interval is 4 to 8 weeks. It is also recommended that ACEL-IMUNE be given for all three doses since no interchangeability data on DTaP vaccines exist for the primary series.

ACEL-IMUNE may be used to complete the primary series in infants who have received one or two doses of whole-cell pertussis DTP. However, the safety and efficacy of ACEL-IMUNE in such infants has not been evaluated.

Booster Immunization

When ACEL-IMUNE® or DTP is given for the primary series, a fourth dose of ACEL-IMUNE is recommended at 15 to 20 months of age. The interval between the third and fourth dose should be at least 6 months. A fifth dose of 0.5 mL is recommended at 4 to 6 years of age, preferably prior to entrance into kindergarten or elementary school. If the fourth dose was administered on or after the fourth birthday, a fifth dose prior to school entry is not considered necessary.[7]

Preterm infants should be vaccinated according to their chronological age, calculated from date of birth.[7]

Interruption of the recommended schedules with a delay between doses does not interfere with the final immunity achieved: nor does it necessitate starting the series over again, regardless of the length of time elapsed between doses.[7]

In the case of anaphylaxis, no further vaccination with any of the three antigens in DTaP should be carried out. Alternatively, because of the importance of tetanus vaccination, such individuals may be referred for evaluation by an allergist.[7] If a contraindication to the pertussis vaccine component occurs, Diphtheria and Tetanus Toxoids, Adsorbed, for pediatric use (DT), should be substituted for each of the remaining doses.

The use of reduced volume (fractional doses) is not recommended. The effect of such practices on the frequency of serious adverse events and on protection against disease has not been determined.

Shake vigorously to obtain a uniform suspension prior to withdrawing each dose from the multiple dose vial. The vaccine should not be used if it cannot be resuspended.

Parenteral drug products should be inspected visually for particulate matter and discoloration prior to administration (see **DESCRIPTION**).

The vaccine should be injected intramuscularly. The preferred sites are the anterolateral aspect of the thigh or the deltoid muscle of the upper arm. The vaccine should not be injected in the gluteal area or areas where there may be a major nerve trunk. Before injection, the skin at the injection site should be cleansed and prepared with a suitable germicide.

After insertion of the needle, aspirate to help avoid inadvertent injection into a blood vessel.

For booster immunization against tetanus and diphtheria of individuals 7 years of age or older, the use of Tetanus and Diphtheria Toxoids Adsorbed for Adult Use (Td) is recommended.

Routine simultaneous administration of DTaP, OPV (or IPV), Hib vaccine, MMR, and Hepatitis B vaccine may be given to children who are the recommended age to receive these vaccines and for whom no specific contraindications exist at the time of the visit.[24]

HOW SUPPLIED

NDC 0005-1800-31 5.0 mL Vial

STORAGE

DO NOT FREEZE. STORE REFRIGERATED, AWAY FROM FREEZER COMPARTMENT, AT 2°C TO 8°C (36°F TO 46°F).

REFERENCES

1. Mueller JH, Miller PA. Production of diphtheria toxin of high potency (100 Lf) on a reproducible medium. *J Immunol.* 1941;40:21-32.
2. Mueller JH, Miller PA. Factors influencing the production of tetanus toxin. *J Immunol.* 1947;56:143-147.
3. Pillemer L, Grossberg DB, Wittler RG. The immunochemistry of toxins and toxoids. II. The preparation of immunologic evaluation of purified tetanal toxoid. *J Immunol.* 1946;54:213-224.
4. Arai H, Sato Y. Separation and characterization of two distinct hemagglutinins contained in purified leukocytosis promoter factor from *Bordetella pertussis. Biochimica et Biophysica Acta.* 1976;444:765-782.
5. CDC. Summary of Notifiable Diseases, United States, 1994. *MMWR.* 1995; 43(53):70-71.
6. Diphtheria Epidemic-New Independent States of the Former Soviet Union. 1990-1994. *MMWR.* 1995;44(10):177-181.
7. Diphtheria, tetanus and pertussis: Recommendations for vaccine use and other preventive measures—recommendations of the Immunization Practices Advisory Committee (ACIP). *MMWR.* 1991;40 (RR-10).
8. Ipsen J. Immunization of adults against diphtheria and tetanus. *NEJM.* 1954;251:459-466.
9. *Federal Register Notice,* Friday, December 13, 1985, Vol. 50, No. 240.
10. Unpublished data available from Lederle Laboratories.
11. Pappenheimer AM Jr. Diphtheria. In: Germanier R, ed. *Bacterial Vaccines.* New York, NY: Academic Press Inc; 1984:1-36.
12. Kendrick PL. Secondary familial attack rates from pertussis in vaccinated and unvaccinated children. *Am J. Hygiene.* 1940;32:89-91.
13. Reported incidence of notifiable diseases in the United States. *MMWR.* 1970;19(53):44.
14. Pertussis surveillance-United States, January 1992-June 1995. *MMWR.* 1995;44(28):525-529.
15. Mortimer JD Jr. Pertussis and its prevention: a family affair. *J Infect Dis.* 1990;161:473-479.
16. Cowell JL, Oda M, Burstyn DG, et al. Prospective protective antigens and animal models for pertussis. In: Leive L, Schlessinger D, eds, *Microbiology* - 1984. Washington, DC: American Society for Microbiology; 1984:172-175.
17. Shahin RD, Brennan MJ, Li ZM, et al. Characterization of the protective capacity and immunogenicity of the 69-kd outer membrane protein of *Bordetella pertussis. J Exper Med.* 1990;171(1):63-73.
18. Novotny P, Kobisch M, Cownley K, et al. Evaluation of *Bordetella bronchiseptica* vaccines in specific-pathogen-free piglets with bacterial cell surface antigens in enzyme linked immunosorbent assay. *Infect Immun.* 1985;50:190-198.
19. Manclark CR, Cowell JL. Pertussis vaccine. In: Germanier R, ed. *Bacterial Vaccines.* New York, NY: Academic Press, Inc; 1984;69-106.
20. Rothstein EP, Bernstein HH, Glode MP, et al. Simultaneous administration of a diphtheria and tetanus toxoids and acellular pertussis vaccine with measles-mumps-rubella and oral poliovirus vaccines. *AJDC.* 1993;(147):854-857.
21. Update: Vaccine side effects, adverse reactions, contraindications, and precautions. *MMWR.* 1996;45 (RR-12):22-31.
22. American Academy of Pediatrics. *Report of the Committee on Infectious Diseases.* 23rd ed. Elk Grove Village, IL: American Academy of Pediatrics; 1994.
23. Sutter RW, Patriarca PA, Suleiman, AJM, et al. Attributable risk of DTP (Diphtheria and Tetanus Toxoids and Pertussis Vaccines) injection in provoking paralytic poliomyelitis during a large outbreak in Oman. *J Infect Dis.* 1992;165:444-449.
24. Pertussis vaccination: acellular pertussis vaccine for reinforcing and booster use-supplementary ACIP statement. *MMWR* 1992;41(RR-1):1-10.
25. Livingstone S. Comprehensive management of epilepsy in infancy. Springfield, IL: Charles C. Thomas; 1972;159-66.
26. Livengood JR, Mullen JR, White JW, et al. Family history of convulsions and use of pertussis vaccine. *J Pediatr.* 1989;115:527-531.
27. Stetler HC, Orenstein WA, Bart KJ, et al. History of convulsion and use of pertussis vaccine. *J Pediatr.* 1985;107;175-179.
28. Ipp MM, Gold R, Greenberg S, et al. Acetaminophen prophylaxis of adverse reactions following vaccination of infants with diphtheria-pertussis-tetanus toxoids-polio vaccine. *Pediatr Infect Dis J.* 1987;6:721-725.
29. Pertussis immunization: family history of convulsions and use of antipyretics - supplementary ACIP statement. *MMWR.* 1987;36(18);281-282.
30. Miller D, Madge N, Diamond J, et al. Pertussis immunization and serious acute neurological illnesses in children. *BMJ.* 1993;307:1171-1176.
31. Howson CP, Howe CJ, Fineberg HV. Adverse effects of pertussis and rubella vaccines, pertussis vaccines and CNS disorders. Institute of Medicine (IOM). Washington, DC: National Academy Press; 1991.
32. Recommendations of the Advisory Committee on Immunization Practices (ACIP): Use of Vaccines and Immune Globulins in Persons with Altered Immunocompetence. *MMWR.* 1993;42(RR-4).
33. Immunization of children infected with human immunodeficiency virus - supplementary ACIP statement. *MMWR.* 1988;37(12):181-183.
34. Recommendation of the ACIP: immunization of children infected with human T-lymphotropic virus type III/lymphadenopathy-associated virus. *MMWR.* 1986;35(38):595-606.
35. General Recommendations on Immunization—Recommendations of the Immunization Practices Advisory Committee (ACIP). *MMWR.* 1989;38(13):221.
36. CDC. Vaccine Adverse Event Reporting System—United States. *MMWR.* 1990;39:730-733.
37. Morgan CM, Blumberg DA, Cherry JD, et al. Comparison of acellular and whole-cell pertussis-component DTP vaccines. *AJDC.* 1990;144:41-45.
38. Cody CL, Baraff LJ, Cherry JP, et al. Nature and rates of adverse reactions associated with DTP and DT immunizations in infants and children. *Pediatrics.* 1981;68:(5):650-660.
39. Fawcett HA, Smith NP. Injection-site granuloma due to aluminum. *Arch Dermatol.* 1984;120:1318-1322.
40. Adverse events following immunization. *MMWR.* 1985;34(3):43-47.
41. Bellman MH, Ross EM, Miller DL. Infantile spasms and pertussis immunization. *Lancet,* 1983; 1:1031-1034.
42. Jacob J, Mannino F. Increased intracranial pressure after diphtheria, tetanus and pertussis immunization. *AJDC.* 1979;(133):217-218.
43. Mathur R, Kumari S. Bulging fontanel following triple vaccine. *Indian Pediatr.* 1981;18(6):417-418.
44. Shendurnikar N, Gandhi DJ, Patel J, et al. Bulging fontanel following DTP vaccine. *Indian Pediatr.* 1986;23(11):960.
45. Griffin MR, Ray Wa, Livengood JR, et al. Risk of sudden infant death syndrome after immunization with the diphtheria-tetanus-pertussis vaccine. *NEJM* 1988;319(10):618-623.
46. Hoffman HJ, Hunter JC, Damus K, et al. Diphtheria-tetanus-pertussis immunization and sudden infant death: results of the National Institute of Child Health and Hu-

man Development Cooperative Epidemiological study of sudden infant death syndrome risk factors. *Pediatrics.* 1987:79:598-611.
47. Walker AM, Jick H, Perera DR, et al. Diphtheria-tetanus-pertussis immunization and sudden infant death syndrome. *Am J Pub Health.* 1987;77:945-951.
48. Willinger M, Hoffman HJ, Hartford RB. Infant sleep position and risk for sudden infant death syndrome: report of meeting held January 13 and 14, 1994, National Institutes of Health, Bethesda, MD. *Pediatrics.* 1994; 93(5):814-819.
49. Rutledge SL, Snead OC. Neurological complications of immunizations. *J Pediatr.* 1986;109:917-924.
50. Schlenska GK. Unusual neurological complications following tetanus toxoid administration. *J Neurol.* 1977;215: 299-302.
51. Blumstein GI, Kreithen H. Peripheral neuropathy following tetanus toxoid administration. *JAMA.* 1966;198: 1030-1031.
52. Reinstein L, Pargament JM, Goodman JS. Peripheral neuropathy after multiple tetanus toxoid injections. *Arch Phys Med Rehabil.* 1982;63:332-334.
53. Tsairis P, Dyck PJ, Mulder DW. Natural history of brachial plexus neuropathy. *Arch Neurol.* 1972;27:109-117.
54. Quast U, Hennessen W, Widmark RM. Mono- and polyneuritis after tetanus vaccination. *Dev Biol Stand.* 1979;43: 25-32.
55. Holliday PL, Bauer RB. Polyradiculoneuritis secondary to immunization with tetanus and diphtheria toxoids. *Arch Neurol.* 1983;40:56-57.
56. Fenichel GM. Neurological complications of tetanus toxoid. *Arch Neurol.* 1983;40:390.
57. Pollard JD, Selby G. Relapsing neuropathy due to tetanus toxoid. *J Neurol Sci.* 1978;37:113-125.
58. Newton N, Janati A. Guillain-Barré syndrome after vaccination with purified tetanus toxoid. *S Med J.* 1987;80: 1053-1054.
59. Stratton KR, Howe CJ, Johnston RB. Adverse events associated with childhood vaccines. Evidence bearing on causality. Institute of Medicine. Washington, DC: National Academy Press; 1994.
60. *Federal Register Final Rule,* Wednesday, February 8, 1995, Vo. 60, No. 26:7694.

Manufactured by:
LEDERLE LABORATORIES
Division American Cyanamid Company
Pearl River, NY 10965
US Gov't. License No. 17

Marketed by:
WYETH-LEDERLE VACCINES AND PEDIATRICS
Wyeth-Ayerst Laboratories
Philadelphia, PA 19101
CI 5200-1 Issued December 15, 1998

Shown in Product Identification Guide, page 320

ACHROMYCIN® V ℞

[*a-krō-mī-cin*]
tetracycline HCl
for ORAL USE

DESCRIPTION

ACHROMYCIN V tetracycline hydrochloride is an antibiotic isolated from *Streptomyces aureofaciens.* Chemically it is the monohydrochloride of [4S -(4α,4aα,5aα,6β,12aα,)] -4-(Dimethylamino)-1,4,4a,5,5a,6,11,12a-octahydro-3, 6, 10, 12, 12a-pentahydroxy-6-methyl-1, 11-dioxo-2-naphthacenecarboxamide.
ACHROMYCIN V oral dosage forms contain the following inactive ingredients:
Capsules: Blue 1, FD&C Yellow No. 6, Gelatin, Lactose, Magnesium Stearate, Red 28, Titanium Dioxide, Yellow 10 and other ingredients.

CLINICAL PHARMACOLOGY

The tetracyclines are primarily bacteriostatic and are thought to exert their antimicrobial effect by the inhibition of protein synthesis. Tetracyclines are active against a wide range of gram-negative and gram-positive organisms.
The drugs in the tetracycline class have closely similar antimicrobial spectra, and cross-resistance among them is common.
Microorganisms may be considered susceptible if the MIC (minimum inhibitory concentration) is not more than 4 mcg/mL and intermediate if the MIC is 4 to 12.5 mcg/mL.
Susceptibility plate testing: A tetracycline disc may be used to determine microbial susceptibility to drugs in the tetracycline class. If the Kirby-Bauer method of disc susceptibility testing is used, a 30 mcg tetracycline HCl disc should give a zone of at least 19 mm when tested against a tetracycline-susceptible bacterial strain.
Tetracyclines are readily absorbed and are bound to plasma proteins in varying degrees. They are concentrated by the liver in the bile and excreted in the urine and feces at high concentrations and in a biologically active form.

INDICATIONS

ACHROMYCIN V is indicated in infections caused by the following microorganisms.
Rickettsiae: (Rocky Mountain spotted fever, typhus fever and the typhus group, Q fever, rickettsialpox, tick fevers).
Mycoplasma pneumoniae (PPLO, Eaton agent).
Agents of psittacosis and ornithosis.
Agents of lymphogranuloma venereum and granuloma inguinale.
The spirochetal agent of relapsing fever (*Borrelia recurrentis*).
The following gram-negative microorganisms:
Haemophilus ducreyi (chancroid),
Yersinia pestis and *Francisella tularensis,* formerly *Pasteurella pestis* and *Pasteurella tularensis,*
Bartonella bacilliformis,
Bacteroides species,
Vibrio comma and *Vibrio fetus,*
Brucella species (in conjunction with streptomycin).
Because many strains of the following groups of microorganisms have been shown to be resistant to tetracyclines, culture and susceptibility testing are recommended.
ACHROMYCIN is indicated for treatment of infections caused by the following gram-negative microorganisms, when bacteriologic testing indicates appropriate susceptibility to the drug:
Escherichia coli,
Enterobacter aerogenes (formerly *Aerobacter aerogenes*),
Shigella species,
Mima species and *Herellea* species,
Haemophilus influenzae (respiratory infections),
Klebsiella species (respiratory and urinary infections).
ACHROMYCIN is indicated for treatment of infections caused by the following gram-positive microorganisms, when bacteriologic testing indicates appropriate susceptibility to the drug:
Streptococcus species:
Up to 44% of strains of *Streptococcus pyogenes* and 74% of *Streptococcus faecalis* have been found to be resistant to tetracycline drugs. Therefore, tetracyclines should not be used for streptococcal disease unless the organism has been demonstrated to be sensitive.
For upper respiratory infections due to Group A beta-hemolytic streptococci, penicillin is the usual drug of choice, including prophylaxis of rheumatic fever.
Streptococcus pneumoniae,
Staphylococcus aureus, skin and soft tissue infections.
Tetracyclines are not the drug of choice in the treatment of any type of staphylococcal infection.
When penicillin is contraindicated, tetracyclines are alternative drugs in the treatment of infections due to:

- *Neisseria gonorrhoeae,*
- *Treponema pallidum* and *Treponema pertenue* (syphilis and yaws),
- *Listeria monocytogenes,*
- *Clostridium* species,
- *Bacillus anthracis,*
- *Fusobacterium fusiforme* (Vincent's infection),
- *Actinomyces* species.

In acute intestinal amebiasis, the tetracyclines may be a useful adjunct to amebicides.
In severe acne, the tetracyclines may be useful adjunctive therapy.
ACHROMYCIN V is indicated in the treatment of trachoma, although the infectious agent is not always eliminated, as judged by immunofluorescence.
Inclusion conjunctivitis may be treated with oral tetracyclines or with a combination of oral and topical agents.
ACHROMYCIN is indicated for the treatment of uncomplicated urethral, endocervical or rectal infections in adults caused by *Chlamydia trachomatis.*[1]

CONTRAINDICATIONS

This drug is contraindicated in persons who have shown hypersensitivity to any of the tetracyclines.

WARNINGS

THE USE OF DRUGS OF THE TETRACYCLINE CLASS DURING TOOTH DEVELOPMENT (LAST HALF OF PREGNANCY, INFANCY AND CHILDHOOD TO THE AGE OF 8 YEARS) MAY CAUSE PERMANENT DISCOLORATION OF THE TEETH (YELLOW-GRAY-BROWN). This adverse reaction is more common during long-term use of the drugs but has been observed following repeated short-term courses. Enamel hypoplasia has also been reported. TETRACYCLINE DRUGS, THEREFORE, SHOULD NOT BE USED IN THIS AGE GROUP UNLESS OTHER DRUGS ARE NOT LIKELY TO BE EFFECTIVE OR ARE CONTRAINDICATED.
If renal impairment exists, even usual oral or parenteral doses may lead to excessive systemic accumulation of the drug and possible liver toxicity. Under such conditions, lower than usual total doses are indicated and, if therapy is prolonged, serum level determinations of the drug may be advisable.
Photosensitivity manifested by an exaggerated sunburn reaction has been observed in some individuals taking tetracyclines. Patients apt to be exposed to direct sunlight or ultraviolet light should be advised that this reaction can occur with tetracycline drugs, and treatment should be discontinued at the first evidence of skin erythema.
The anti-anabolic action of the tetracyclines may cause an increase in BUN. While this is not a problem in those with normal renal function, in patients with significantly impaired function, higher serum levels of tetracycline may lead to azotemia, hyperphosphatemia, and acidosis.
Usage in Pregnancy (See above **WARNINGS** about use during tooth development.) Results of animal studies indicate that tetracyclines cross the placenta, are found in fetal tissues and can have toxic effects on the developing fetus (often related to retardation of skeletal development). Evidence of embryotoxicity has also been noted in animals treated early in pregnancy.
Usage in Newborns, Infants, and Children (See above **WARNINGS** about use during tooth development.)
All tetracyclines form a stable calcium complex in any bone forming tissue. A decrease in the fibula growth rate has been observed in prematures given oral tetracycline in doses of 25 mg/kg every six hours. This reaction was shown to be reversible when the drug was discontinued.
Tetracyclines are present in the milk of lactating women who are taking a drug in this class.

PRECAUTIONS

General
Pseudotumor cerebri (benign intracranial hypertension) in adults has been associated with the use of tetracyclines. The usual clinical manifestations are headache and blurred vision. Bulging fontanels have been associated with the use of tetracyclines in infants. While both of these conditions and related symptoms usually resolve soon after discontinuation of the tetracycline, the possibility for permanent sequelae exists.
As with other antibiotics preparations, use of this drug may result in overgrowth of nonsusceptible organisms, including fungi. If superinfection occurs, the antibiotic should be discontinued and appropriate therapy should be instituted.
In venereal diseases when coexistent syphilis is suspected, darkfield examination should be done before treatment is started and the blood serology repeated monthly for at least 4 months.
In long-term therapy, periodic laboratory evaluation of organ systems, including hematopoietic, renal and hepatic studies should be performed.
All infections due to Group A beta-hemolytic streptococci should be treated for at least ten days.
Drug Interactions
Because tetracyclines have been shown to depress plasma prothrombin activity, patients who are on anticoagulant therapy may require downward adjustment of their anticoagulant dosage.
Since bacteriostatic drugs, such as the tetracycline class of antibiotics, may interfere with the bactericidal action of penicillins, it is not advisable to administer these drugs concomitantly.
Concurrent use of tetracyclines with oral contraceptives may render oral contraceptives less effective. Breakthrough bleeding has been reported.

ADVERSE REACTIONS

Gastrointestinal: Anorexia, nausea, vomiting, diarrhea, glossitis, dysphagia, enterocolitis, pancreatitis, and inflammatory lesions (with monilial overgrowth) in the anogenital region, increases in liver enzymes, and hepatic toxicity have been reported rarely. Rare instances of esophagitis and esophageal ulcerations have been reported in patients taking the tetracycline-class antibiotics in capsule and tablet form. Most of these patients took the medication immediately before going to bed (see **DOSAGE AND ADMINISTRATION**).
Skin: Maculopapular and erythematous rashes. Exfoliative dermatitis has been reported but is uncommon. Fixed drug eruptions, including balanitis, have been rarely reported. Photosensitivity is discussed above. (See **WARNINGS.**)
Renal toxicity: Rise in BUN has been reported and is apparently dose related. (See **WARNINGS.**)
Hypersensitivity reactions: Urticaria, angioneurotic edema, anaphylaxis, anaphylactoid purpura, pericarditis and exacerbation of systemic lupus erythematosus.
Blood: Hemolytic anemia, thrombocytopenia, neutropenia and eosinophilia have been reported.
CNS: Pseudotumor cerebri (benign intracranial hypertension) in adults and bulging fontanels in infants. (See **PRECAUTIONS—General.**) Dizziness, tinnitus, and visual disturbances have been reported. Myasthenic syndrome has been reported rarely.
Other: When given over prolonged periods, tetracyclines have been reported to produce brown-black microscopic discoloration of thyroid glands. No abnormalities of thyroid function studies are known to occur.

DOSAGE AND ADMINISTRATION

Therapy should be continued for at least 24 to 48 hours after symptoms and fever have subsided.
Concomitant therapy: Antacids containing aluminum, calcium, or magnesium impair absorption and should not be given to patients taking oral tetracycline.
Foods and some dairy products also interfere with absorption. Oral forms of tetracycline should be given 1 hour before or 2 hours after meals.
In patients with renal impairment: (See **WARNINGS**). Total dosage should be decreased by reduction of recommended individual doses and/or by extending time intervals between doses.
In the treatment of streptococcal infections, a therapeutic dose of tetracycline should be administered for at least ten days.
Adults: Usual daily dose, 1–2 grams divided in two or four equal doses, depending on the severity of the infection.
For children above eight years of age: Usual daily dose, 10–20 mg (25–50 mg/kg) per pound of body weight divided in two or four equal doses.

Continued on next page

Achromycin V—Cont.

For treatment of brucellosis, 500 mg tetracycline four times daily for 3 weeks should be accompanied by streptomycin, 1 gram intramuscularly twice daily the first week and once daily the second week.
For treatment of syphilis, a total of 30–40 grams in equally divided doses over a period of 10–15 days should be given. Close follow up, including laboratory tests, is recommended.
Gonorrhea patients sensitive to pencillin may be treated with tetracycline, administered as an initial oral dose of 1.5 grams followed by 0.5 gram every 6 hours for four days to a total dosage of 9 grams.
Uncomplicated urethral, endocervical, or rectal infection in adults caused by *Chlamydia trachomatis:* 500 mg, by mouth, 4 times a day for at least 7 days.[1]

HOW SUPPLIED

ACHROMYCIN® V tetracycline HCl oral dosage forms are available as follows:

CAPSULES

500 mg - Two-piece, hard shell, elongated, opaque capsules with a blue cap and a yellow body, printed with Lederle over A5 on one half and Lederle over 500 mg on the other in gray ink, supplied as follows:
NDC 0005-4875-23—Bottle of 100
NDC 0005-4875-34—Bottle of 1,000
250 mg - Two-piece, hard shell, opaque capsules with a blue cap and a yellow body, printed with Lederle over A3 on one half and Lederle over 250 mg on the other in gray ink, supplied as follows:
NDC 0005-4880-23—Bottle of 100
NDC 0005-4880-34—Bottle of 1,000

Store at Controlled Room Temperature 15°–30°C (59°–86°F).

Reference: 1. CDC Sexually Transmitted Diseases Treatment Guidelines 1982.

Manufactured by:
LEDERLE PHARMACEUTICAL DIVISION
American Cyanamid Company
Pearl River, NY 10965
CI 4945-1 Issued September 12, 1997

ARTANE® ℞

[*ar-tāne*]
(trihexyphenidyl HCl)
For Oral Use

DESCRIPTION

ARTANE trihexyphenidyl HCl is a synthetic antispasmodic drug available in the following forms:

Tablets:

Containing 2 mg and 5 mg ARTANE trihexyphenidyl HCl, each strength also containing as inactive ingredients: Corn Starch, Dibasic Calcium Phosphate, Magnesium Stearate and Pregelatinized Starch.

Elixir:

Containing 2 mg/5 mL ARTANE trihexyphenidyl HCl in a clear, colorless, lime-mint preparation, also containing as inactive ingredients: Alcohol 5%, Citric Acid, Flavorings, Methylparaben, Propylparaben, Sodium Chloride and Sorbitol Solution.

ACTIONS

ARTANE trihexyphenidyl HCl is the substituted piperidine salt, 3-(1-piperidyl)-1-phenyl-cyclohexyl-1-propanol hydrochloride, which exerts a direct inhibitory effect upon the parasympathetic nervous system. It also has a relaxing effect on smooth musculature; exerted both directly upon the muscle tissue itself and indirectly through an inhibitory effect upon the parasympathetic nervous system. Its therapeutic properties are similar to those of atropine although undesirable side effects are ordinarily less frequent and severe than with the latter.

INDICATIONS

This drug is indicated as an adjunct in the treatment of all forms of parkinsonism (postencephalitic, arteriosclerotic, and idiopathic). It is often useful as adjuvant therapy when treating these forms of parkinsonism with levodopa.
Additionally, it is indicated for the control of extrapyramidal disorders caused by central nervous system drugs such as the dibenzoxazepines, phenothiazines, thioxanthenes, and butyrophenones.

WARNING

Patients to be treated with ARTANE should have a gonioscope evaluation and close monitoring of intraocular pressures at regular periodic intervals.

PRECAUTIONS

Although trihexyphenidyl HCl is not contraindicated for patients with cardiac, liver, or kidney disorders, or with hypertension, such patients should be maintained under close observation.
Since the use of trihexyphenidyl HCl may in some cases continue indefinitely and since it has atropine-like properties, patients should be subjected to constant and careful long-term observation to avoid allergic and other untoward reactions. Inasmuch as trihexyphenidyl HCl possesses some parasympatholytic activity, it should be used with caution in patients with glaucoma, obstructive disease of the gastrointestinal or genitourinary tracts, and in elderly males with possible prostatic hypertrophy. Geriatric patients, particularly over the age of 60, frequently develop increased sensitivity to the actions of drugs of this type, and hence, require strict dosage regulation. Incipient glaucoma may be precipitated by parasympatholytic drugs such as trihexyphenidyl HCl.
Tardive dyskinesia may appear in some patients on long-term therapy with antipsychotic drugs or may occur after therapy with these drugs has been discontinued. Antiparkinsonism agents do not alleviate the symptoms of tardive dyskinesia, and in some instances may aggravate them. However, parkinsonism and tardive dyskinesia often coexist in patients receiving chronic neuroleptic treatment, and anticholinergic therapy with ARTANE may relieve some of these parkinsonism symptoms.

ADVERSE REACTIONS

Minor side effects, such as dryness of the mouth, blurring of vision, dizziness; mild nausea or nervousness, will be experienced by 30 to 50 percent of all patients. These sensations, however, are much less troublesome with ARTANE trihexyphenidyl HCl than with belladonna alkaloids and are usually less disturbing than unalleviated parkinsonism. Such reactions tend to become less pronounced, and even to disappear, as treatment continues. Even before these reactions have remitted spontaneously, they may often be controlled by careful adjustment of dosage form, amount of drug, or interval between doses.
Isolated instances of suppurative parotitis secondary to excessive dryness of the mouth, skin rashes, dilatation of the colon, paralytic ileus, and certain psychiatric manifestations such as delusions and hallucinations, plus one doubtful case of paranoia all of which may occur with any of the atropine-like drugs, have been reported rarely with ARTANE.
Patients with arteriosclerosis or with a history of idiosyncrasy to other drugs may exhibit reactions of mental confusion, agitation, disturbed behavior, or nausea and vomiting. Such patients should be allowed to develop a tolerance through the initial administration of a small dose and gradual increase in dose until an effective level is reached. If a severe reaction should occur, administration of the drug should be discontinued for a few days and then resumed at a lower dosage. Psychiatric disturbances can result from indiscriminate use (leading to overdosage) to sustain continued euphoria.
Potential side effects associated with the use of any atropine-like drugs include constipation, drowsiness, urinary hesitancy or retention, tachycardia, dilation of the pupil, increased intraocular tension, weakness, vomiting, and headache.
The occurrence of angle-closure glaucoma due to long-term treatment with trihexyphenidyl hydrochloride has been reported.

DOSAGE AND ADMINISTRATION

Dosage should be individualized. The initial dose should be low and then increased gradually, especially in patients over 60 years of age. Whether ARTANE® trihexyphenidyl HCl may best be given before or after meals should be determined by the way the patient reacts. Postencephalitic patients, who are usually more prone to excessive salivation, may prefer to take it after meals and may, in addition, require small amounts of atropine which, under such circumstances, is sometimes an effective adjuvant. If ARTANE tends to dry the mouth excessively, it may be better to take it before meals, unless it causes nausea. If taken after meals, the thirst sometimes induced can be allayed by mint candies, chewing gum or water.

ARTANE Trihexyphenidyl HCl in Idiopathic Parkinsonism

As initial therapy for parkinsonism, 1 mg of ARTANE in tablet or elixir form may be administered the first day. The dose may then be increased by 2 mg increments at intervals of three to five days, until a total of 6 to 10 mg is given daily. The total daily dose will depend upon what is found to be the optimal level. Many patients derive maximum benefit from this daily total of 6 to 10 mg, but some patients, chiefly those in the postencephalitic group, may require a total daily dose of 12 to 15 mg.

ARTANE Trihexyphenidyl HCl in Drug-Induced Parkinsonism

The size and frequency of dose of ARTANE needed to control extrapyramidal reactions to commonly employed tranquilizers, notably the phenothiazines, thioxanthenes, and butyrophenones, must be determined empirically. The total daily dosage usually ranges between 5 and 15 mg although, in some cases, these reactions have been satisfactorily controlled on as little as 1 mg daily. It may be advisable to commence therapy with a single 1 mg dose. If the extrapyramidal manifestations are not controlled in a few hours, the subsequent doses may be progressively increased until satisfactory control is achieved. Satisfactory control may sometimes be more rapidly achieved by temporarily reducing the dosage of the tranquilizer on instituting ARTANE trihexyphenidyl HCl therapy and then adjusting dosage of both drugs until the desired ataractic effect is retained without onset of extrapyramidal reactions.
It is sometimes possible to maintain the patient on a reduced ARTANE dosage after the reactions have remained under control for several days. Instances have been reported in which these reactions have remained in remission for long periods after ARTANE therapy was discontinued.

Concomitant Use of ARTANE Trihexyphenidyl HCl with Levodopa

When ARTANE is used concomitantly with levodopa, the usual dose of each may need to be reduced. Careful adjustment is necessary, depending on side effects and degree of symptom control. ARTANE dosage of 3 to 6 mg daily, in divided doses, is usually adequate.

Concomitant Use of ARTANE Trihexyphenidyl HCl with Other Parasympathetic Inhibitors

ARTANE trihexyphenidyl HCl may be substituted, in whole or in part, for other parasympathetic inhibitors. The usual technique is partial substitution initially, with progressive reduction in the other medication as the dose of trihexyphenidyl HCl is increased.
ARTANE TABLETS and ELIXIR—The total daily intake of ARTANE tablets or elixir is tolerated best if divided into 3 doses and taken at mealtimes. High doses (>10 mg daily) may be divided into 4 parts, with 3 doses administered at mealtimes and the fourth at bedtime.

HOW SUPPLIED

ARTANE trihexyphenidyl HCl is available as follows:

TABLETS

2 mg—round, flat, scored, white tablets; engraved ARTANE above 2 on one side and LL above A11 below the score on the other side, supplied as follows:
NDC 0005-4434-23—Bottle of 100
NDC 0005-4434-34—Bottle of 1000
5 mg—round, flat, scored, white tablets; engraved ARTANE above 5 on one side and LL above A12 below the score on the other side, supplied as follows:
NDC 0005-4436-23—Bottle of 100
NDC 0005-4436-34—Bottle of 1000

Store at controlled room temperature 20°–25°C (68°–77°F).
Dispense in tight containers as defined in the USP.

ELIXIR

2 mg/5 mL - NDC 0005-4440-65 - Bottle of 16 fl oz

Store at controlled room temperature 20°–25°C (68°–77°F).
DO NOT FREEZE.
Dispense in tight containers as defined in the USP.

Manufactured by:
LEDERLE PHARMACEUTICAL DIVISION
American Cyanamid Company
Pearl River, NY 10965
CI 4945-1 Issued August 21, 1997
Shown in Product Identification Guide, page 320

DECLOMYCIN® ℞

[*dĕk-lō-mī-sĭn*]
Demeclocycline Hydrochloride
For Oral Use

DESCRIPTION

DECLOMYCIN demeclocycline hydrochloride is an antibiotic isolated from a mutant strain of *Streptomyces aureofaciens.* Chemically it is 7-Chloro-4-(dimethylamino)-1,4, 4a,5,5a,6,11,12a-octahydro-3,6,10,12, 12a-pentahydroxy-1,11-dioxo-2-naphthacenecarboxamide monohydrochloride.
DECLOMYCIN contains the following inactive ingredients: Tablets: Alginic Acid, Corn Starch, Ethylcellulose, Hydroxypropyl Methylcellulose, Magnesium Stearate, Red 7, Sorbitol, Titanium Dioxide, Yellow 10 and other ingredients. May also contain Sodium Lauryl Sulfate.

CLINICAL PHARMACOLOGY

The tetracyclines are primarily bacteriostatic and are thought to exert their antimicrobial effect by the inhibition of protein synthesis. Tetracyclines are active against a wide range of gram-negative and gram-positive organisms.
The drugs in the tetracycline class have closely similar antimicrobial spectra, and cross-resistance among them is common. Microorganisms may be considered susceptible if the MIC (minimum inhibitory concentration) is not more than 4 mcg/mL and intermediate if the MIC is 4 to 12.5 mcg/mL.
Susceptibility plate testing: A tetracycline disc may be used to determine microbial susceptibility to drugs in the tetracycline class. If the Kirby-Bauer method of disc susceptibility testing is used, a 30 mcg tetracycline disc should give a zone of at least 19 mm when tested against a tetracycline-susceptible bacterial strain.
Tetracyclines are readily absorbed and are bound to plasma proteins in varying degrees. They are concentrated by the liver in the bile and excreted in the urine and feces at high concentrations and in a biologically active form.

INDICATIONS AND USAGE

DECLOMYCIN demeclocycline hydrochloride is indicated in infections caused by the following microorganisms:
Rickettsiae: (Rocky Mountain spotted fever, typhus fever and the typhus group, Q fever, rickettsialpox, tick fevers).
Mycoplasma pneumoniae (PPLO, Eaton agent).
Agents of psittacosis and ornithosis.
Agents of lymphogranuloma venereum and granuloma inguinale.
The spirochetal agent of relapsing fever (*Borrelia recurrentis*).
The following gram-negative microorganisms:
Haemophilus ducreyi (chancroid),
Yersinia pestis and *Francisella tularensis,* formerly *Pasteurella pestis* and *Pasteurella tularensis,*

Bartonella bacilliformis,
Bacteroides species,
Vibrio comma and *Vibrio fetus,*
Brucella species (in conjunction with streptomycin).
Because many strains of the following groups of microorganisms have been shown to be resistant to tetracyclines, culture and susceptibility testing are recommended.
Demeclocycline is indicated for treatment of infections caused by the following gram-negative microorganisms, when bacteriologic testing indicates appropriate susceptibility to the drug:
Escherichia coli,
Enterobacter aerogenes (formerly *Aerobacter aerogenes*),
Shigella species,
Mima species and *Herellea* species,
Haemophilus influenzae (respiratory infections),
Klebsiella species (respiratory and urinary infections).
DECLOMYCIN is indicated for treatment of infections caused by the following gram-positive microorganisms when bacteriologic testing indicates appropriate susceptibility to the drug:
Streptococcus species:
Up to 44% of strains of *Streptococcus pyogenes* and 74% of *Streptococcus faecalis* have been found to be resistant to tetracycline drugs. Therefore, tetracyclines should not be used for streptococcal disease unless the organism has been demonstrated to be sensitive.
For upper respiratory infections due to Group A beta-hemolytic streptococci, penicillin is the usual drug of choice, including prophylaxis of rheumatic fever.
Streptococcus pneumoniae,
Staphylococcus aureus, skin and soft tissue infections.
Tetracyclines are not the drugs of choice in the treatment of any type of staphylococcal infection.
When penicillin is contraindicated, tetracyclines are alternative drugs in the treatment of infections due to:
Neisseria gonorrhoeae,
Treponema pallidum and *Treponema pertenue* (syphilis and yaws),
Listeria monocytogenes,
Clostridium species,
Bacillus anthracis,
Fusobacterium fusiforme (Vincent's infection),
Actinomyces species.
In acute intestinal amebiasis, the tetracyclines may be a useful adjunct to amebicides.
DECLOMYCIN demeclocycline hydrochloride is indicated in the treatment of trachoma, although the infectious agent is not always eliminated, as judged by immunofluorescence.
Inclusion conjunctivitis may be treated with oral tetracyclines or with a combination of oral and topical agents.

CONTRAINDICATIONS

This drug is contraindicated in persons who have shown hypersensitivity to any of the tetracyclines.

WARNINGS

THE USE OF DRUGS OF THE TETRACYCLINE CLASS DURING TOOTH DEVELOPMENT (LAST HALF OF PREGNANCY, INFANCY, AND CHILDHOOD TO THE AGE OF 8 YEARS) MAY CAUSE PERMANENT DISCOLORATION OF THE TEETH (YELLOW-GRAY-BROWN).
This adverse reaction is more common during long-term use of the drugs but has been observed following repeated short-term courses. Enamel hypoplasia has also been reported.
TETRACYCLINE DRUGS, THEREFORE, SHOULD NOT BE USED IN THIS AGE GROUP UNLESS OTHER DRUGS ARE NOT LIKELY TO BE EFFECTIVE OR ARE CONTRAINDICATED.
If renal impairment exists, even usual oral or parenteral doses may lead to excessive systemic accumulation of the drug and possible liver toxicity. Under such conditions, lower than usual total doses are indicated and, if therapy is prolonged, serum level determinations of the drug may be advisable.
Phototoxic reactions can occur in individuals taking demeclocycline, and are characterized by severe burns of exposed surfaces resulting from direct exposure of patients to sunlight during therapy with moderate or large doses of demeclocycline. Patients apt to be exposed to direct sunlight or ultraviolet light should be advised that this reaction can occur, and treatment should be discontinued at the first evidence of skin erythema.
The anti-anabolic action of the tetracyclines may cause an increase in BUN. While this is not a problem in those with normal renal function, in patients with significantly impaired function, higher serum levels of tetracycline may lead to azotemia, hyperphosphatemia, and acidosis.
Administration of DECLOMYCIN has resulted in appearance of the diabetes insipidus syndrome (polyuria, polydipsia and weakness) in some patients on long-term therapy. The syndrome has been shown to be nephrogenic, dose-dependent and reversible on discontinuance of therapy.
Usage in pregnancy: (See above **WARNINGS** about use during tooth development.) Results of animal studies indicate that tetracyclines cross the placenta, are found in fetal tissues and can have toxic effects on the developing fetus (often related to retardation of skeletal development). Evidence of embryotoxicity has also been noted in animals treated early in pregnancy.
Usage in newborns, infants, and children: (See above **WARNINGS** about use during tooth development.)
All tetracyclines form a stable calcium complex in any bone forming tissue. A decrease in the fibula growth rate has been observed in prematures given oral tetracycline in doses of 25 mg/kg every six hours. This reaction was shown to be reversible when the drug was discontinued. Tetracyclines are present in the milk of lactating women who are taking a drug in this class.

PRECAUTIONS

General

Pseudotumor cerebri (benign intracranial hypertension) in adults has been associated with the use of tetracyclines. The usual clinical manifestations are headache and blurred vision. Bulging fontanels have been associated with the use of tetracyclines in infants. While both of these conditions and related symptoms usually resolve soon after discontinuation of the tetracycline, the possibility for permanent sequelae exists.
As with other antibiotic preparations, use of this drug may result in overgrowth of nonsusceptible organisms, including fungi. If superinfection occurs, the antibiotic should be discontinued and appropriate therapy should be instituted.
In venereal diseases when coexistent syphilis is suspected, darkfield examination should be done before treatment is started and the blood serology repeated monthly for at least 4 months.
In long-term therapy, periodic laboratory evaluation of organ systems, including hematopoietic, renal and hepatic studies should be performed.
All infections due to Group A beta-hemolytic streptococci should be treated for at least ten days.
Interpretation of Bacteriologic Studies: Following a course of therapy, persistence for several days in both urine and blood of bacterio-suppressive levels of demeclocycline may interfere with culture studies. These levels should not be considered therapeutic.

Drug Interactions

Because the tetracyclines have been shown to depress plasma prothrombin activity, patients who are on anticoagulant therapy may require downward adjustment of their anticoagulant dosage.
Since bacteriostatic drugs, such as the tetracycline class of antibiotics, may interfere with the bactericidal action of penicillins, it is not advisable to administer these drugs concomitantly.
Concurrent use of tetracyclines with oral contraceptives may render oral contraceptives less effective. Breakthrough bleeding has been reported.

ADVERSE REACTIONS

Gastrointestinal: Anorexia, nausea, vomiting, diarrhea, glossitis, dysphagia, enterocolitis, pancreatitis, and inflammatory lesions (with monilial overgrowth) in the anogenital region, increases in liver enzymes, and hepatic toxicity has been reported rarely. Rare instances of esophagitis and esophageal ulcerations have been reported in patients taking the tetracycline-class antibiotics in capsule and tablet form. Most of these patients took the medication immediately before going to bed (see **DOSAGE AND ADMINISTRATION**).
Skin: Maculopapular and erythematous rashes. Exfoliative dermatitis has been reported but is uncommon. Fixed drug eruptions, including balanitis, have been rarely reported. Photosensitivity is discussed above. (See **WARNINGS.**)
Renal toxicity: Rise in BUN has been reported and is apparently dose related. Nephrogenic diabetes insipidus. (See **WARNINGS.**)
Hypersensitivity reactions: Urticaria, angioneurotic edema, anaphylaxis, anaphylactoid purpura, pericarditis and exacerbation of systemic lupus erythematosus.
Blood: Hemolytic anemia, thrombocytopenia, neutropenia and eosinophilia have been reported.
CNS: Pseudotumor cerebri (benign intracranial hypertension) in adults and bulging fontanels in infants (see **PRECAUTIONS—General**). Dizziness, tinnitus, and visual disturbances have been reported. Myasthenic syndrome has been reported rarely.
Other: When given over prolonged periods, tetracyclines have been reported to produce brown-black microscopic discoloration of thyroid glands. No abnormalities of thyroid function studies are known to occur.

DOSAGE AND ADMINISTRATION

Therapy should be continued for at least 24 to 48 hours after symptoms and fever have subsided.
Concomitant therapy: Antacids containing aluminum, calcium, or magnesium impair absorption and should not be given to patients taking oral tetracycline.
Foods and some dairy products also interfere with absorption. Oral forms of tetracycline should be given one hour before or two hours after meals.
In patients with renal impairment: (See **WARNINGS.**) Total dosage should be decreased by reduction of recommended individual doses and/or by extending time intervals between doses.
In the treatment of streptococcal infections, a therapeutic dose of demeclocycline should be administered for at least ten days.
Adults: Usual daily dose—Four divided doses of 150 mg each or two divided doses of 300 mg each.
For children above eight years of age: Usual daily dose, 3–6 mg per pound body weight per day, depending upon the severity of the disease, divided into two to four doses.
Gonorrhea patients sensitive to penicillin may be treated with demeclocycline administered as an initial oral dose of 600 mg followed by 300 mg every 12 hours for four days to a total of 3 grams.

HOW SUPPLIED

DECLOMYCIN® demeclocycline hydrochloride Tablets, 150 mg are round, convex, red, film coated tablets, engraved with LL on one side and D11 on the other, supplied as follows:
NDC 0005-9218-23—Bottle of 100
DECLOMYCIN® demeclocycline hydrochloride Tablets, 300 mg are round, convex, red, film coated tablets, engraved with LL on one side and D12 on the other, supplied as follows:
NDC 0005-9270-29—Bottle of 48
Store at controlled room temperature 20°–25°C (68–77°F).

Manufactured by:
LEDERLE PHARMACEUTICAL DIVISION
American Cyanamid Company
Pearl River, NY 10965
CI 5189 Issued February 9, 1999

Shown in Product Identification Guide, page 320

DIAMOX® ℞
Acetazolamide Tablets USP
and
DIAMOX®
Sterile Acetazolamide Sodium USP
Intravenous

(For full prescribing information, please refer to the 2001 PDR for Ophthalmology.)

DIAMOX® ℞
Acetazolamide
SEQUELS®
Sustained Release Capsules

(For full prescribing information, please refer to the 2001 PDR for Ophthalmology.)

DIPHTHERIA AND TETANUS TOXOIDS ADSORBED ℞
Aluminum Phosphate-Adsorbed
For Pediatric Use
Rx only
For Intramuscular Injection Only

DESCRIPTION

Diphtheria and Tetanus Toxoids Adsorbed, Aluminum Phosphate Adsorbed, for pediatric use (DT), is a sterile combination of diphtheria toxoid and PUROGENATED® tetanus toxoid for intramuscular use only. After shaking, the vaccine is a homogeneous white suspension.
The diphtheria toxoid component is derived from *Corynebacterium diphtheriae*, which is grown in a growth medium containing an enzymatic digest of casein. The toxin is purified by ammonium sulfate precipitation and ion exchange chromatography. It is then detoxified with formaldehyde in the presence of L-lysine. The toxoid is maintained in sodium bicarbonate with L-lysine, formalin, and thimerosal (mercury derivative) as a preservative.
The tetanus toxoid component is derived from *Clostridium tetani*, which is grown in a growth medium containing beef heart infusion according to the method of Mueller and Miller.[1] It is detoxified with formaldehyde. The toxoid is refined by the Pillemer alcohol fractionation method[2] and diluted with a solution containing sodium containing sodium phosphate monobasic, sodium phosphate dibasic, glycine, and thimerosal (mercury derivative) as a preservative.
The diphtheria and tetanus toxoids are each adsorbed to aluminum phosphate and brought to final volume with physiological saline. Thimerosal (mercury derivative) is added as a preservative to a final concentration of 1:10,000. The final product is formulated to contain 0.23 mg per 0.5 mL dose of aluminum from the aluminum phosphate adjuvant. The residual free formaldehyde content by assay is less than 0.02%.
Each 0.5 mL dose is formulated to contain 12.5 Lf units of diphtheria toxoid and 5 Lf units of tetanus toxoid. The diphtheria and tetanus components induce at least 2 neutralizing units/mL of serum in the guinea pig potency test.

CLINICAL PHARMACOLOGY

Diphtheria is a disease resulting from infection of the respiratory tract with *Corynebacterium diphtheriae*. This disease can be localized to the site of infection or can be associated with systemic toxicity, which may include myocarditis and neuritis and is caused by diphtheria toxin, an extracellular protein metabolite of toxigenic strains of *C. diphtheriae*. The incidence of diphtheria in the United States has decreased from over 200,000 cases reported in 1921, before the general use of diphtheria toxoid, to only four cases of diphtheria reported in 1997. Of these four cases, two persons, both with localized mild illness, had culture-confirmed diphtheria.[3] The case fatality rate has re-

Continued on next page

Diphtheria & Tetanus Toxoids—Cont.

mained constant at about 5% to 10%. The highest case fatality rates are in the very young and the elderly. Diphtheria remains a serious disease in some areas of the world as demonstrated by the recent epidemic, during which over 7,000 cases of diphtheria were reported, in the former Soviet Union.[3,4]

Following adequate immunization with diphtheria toxoid, which induces antitoxin, it is thought that protection lasts for at least 10 years.[5] Serum antibody levels of at least 0.01 antitoxin units/mL are generally regarded as protective.[6] This significantly reduces both the risk of developing diphtheria and the severity of clinical illness. It does not, however, eliminate carriage of *C. diphtheriae* in the pharynx or on the skin.[5]

Tetanus manifests systemic toxicity primarily by neuromuscular dysfunction caused by a potent exotoxin elaborated by *C. tetani*. The incidence of tetanus in the U.S. has dropped dramatically with the routine use of tetanus toxoid, with an average of 57 cases reported annually from 1985–1994.[3] During the period from 1995 through 1997, 124 cases of tetanus were reported from 33 states and the District of Columbia, resulting in an average annual incidence of 0.15 cases per 1,000,000 population. The case-fatality ratio varied from 2.3% for persons aged 20–39 years to 16% for persons aged 40–59 years and to 18% for persons aged ≥60 years. Previous immunization status was directly related to the severity of the disease, with the case-fatality ratio ranging from 6% for persons who had received 1 to 2 doses of tetanus toxoid to 15% for persons who were unvaccinated. Tetanus remains a severe disease, with adults ≥60 years at the highest risk of severe disease.[7]

Spores of *C. tetani* are ubiquitous, and there is essentially no natural immunity to tetanus toxin. Thus, universal primary immunization with tetanus toxoid with subsequent maintenance of adequate antibody levels, by means of timed boosters, is recommended to protect all age groups.[5] Tetanus toxoid is a highly effective antigen and a completed primary series generally induces serum antibody levels of at least 0.01 antitoxin units/mL, a level that has been reported to be protective.[8] It is thought that protection persists for at least 10 years.[5]

The toxoids of tetanus and diphtheria induce neutralizing antibodies to the toxins produced by the infecting organisms. Serum antibody levels greater than 0.01 antitoxin units/mL are generally regarded as protective.[6,8] In one clinical study in Jamaica, West Indies, children ranging in age from three months to six years received two doses administered 28 days apart of DT in a primary series. Subjects 6 months of age or less were included if they had not received a previous dose of diphtheria or tetanus toxoids as determined through the immunization history provided by the mother and clinic records, and subjects over 6 months of age were included if they had a pre-immunization titer of less than 0.01 IU/mL. Protective levels of greater than 0.01 IU/mL were achieved in 22/23 (96%) of the children for diphtheria as measured by the rabbit skin method, and 26/26 (100%) of the children for tetanus as titrated in the mouse lethal method. The mean age of immunization was 21 months of age in the diphtheria subjects and 26 months in the tetanus subjects.[9]

INDICATIONS AND USAGE

Diphtheria and Tetanus Toxoids Adsorbed, Aluminum Phosphate Adsorbed, for pediatric use is indicated for active immunization against diphtheria and tetanus diseases in infants and children from 2 months of age up to 7 years of age (prior to their seventh birthday) for whom the use of a combined vaccine containing pertussis antigen is contraindicated.[5,10] (See **DOSAGE AND ADMINISTRATION** for "Tetanus Prophylaxis in Wound Management" and "Diphtheria Prophylaxis for Case Contacts.")

Protection against diphtheria and tetanus is based on a full course of immunization.

DT is intended only for active immunization against diphtheria and tetanus and is not to be used for treatment of actual infection or in people 7 years of age or older.

Persons recovering from tetanus or diphtheria. Diphtheria or tetanus infection may not confer immunity; therefore, initiation or completion of active immunization is indicated at the time of recovery from these infections.[5]

If a contraindication to using tetanus toxoid-containing preparations exists in a person who has not completed a primary immunizing course of tetanus toxoid, and other than a clean minor wound is sustained, only passive immunization should be given using human tetanus immune globulin (TIG). If passive immunization for diphtheria is needed, equine diphtheria antitoxin is recommended.[5] (see **DOSAGE AND ADMINISTRATION**)

As with any vaccine, DT may not protect 100% of individuals receiving the vaccine.

CONTRAINDICATIONS

HYPERSENSITIVITY TO ANY COMPONENT OF THE VACCINE, INCLUDING THIMEROSAL, A MERCURY DERIVATIVE, IS A CONTRAINDICATION.

THE OCCURRENCE OF ANY NEUROLOGICAL SYMPTOMS OR SIGNS, OR AN ALLERGIC OR ANAPHYLACTIC REACTION WHICH HAS FOLLOWED THE ADMINISTRATION OF THIS PRODUCT IS A CONTRAINDICATION TO FURTHER USE.

THE DECISION TO ADMINISTER OR DELAY VACCINATION BECAUSE OF A CURRENT OR RECENT FEBRILE ILLNESS DEPENDS LARGELY ON THE SEVERITY OF SYMPTOMS AND THEIR ETIOLOGY. ALTHOUGH A MODERATE OR SEVERE FEBRILE ILLNESS IS SUFFICIENT REASON TO POSTPONE VACCINATION, MINOR ILLNESSES SUCH AS A MILD UPPER RESPIRATORY INFECTION WITH OR WITHOUT LOW GRADE FEVER ARE NOT CONTRAINDICATIONS.[5,10,11]

ROUTINE IMMUNIZATION SHOULD BE DEFERRED DURING AN OUTBREAK OF POLIOMYELITIS, PROVIDED THE PATIENT HAS NOT SUSTAINED AN INJURY THAT INCREASES THE RISK OF TETANUS AND PROVIDED AN OUTBREAK OF DIPHTHERIA DISEASE DOES NOT OCCUR SIMULTANEOUSLY.[12]

THE CLINICAL JUDGMENT OF THE ATTENDING HEALTH CARE PROFESSIONAL SHOULD PREVAIL AT ALL TIMES.

WARNINGS

THIS PRODUCT IS NOT RECOMMENDED FOR IMMUNIZING PERSONS ON OR AFTER THEIR SEVENTH BIRTHDAY.

For individuals 7 years of age or older, Tetanus and Diphtheria Toxoids Adsorbed, for adult use (Td), should be used instead of DT. The concentration of diphtheria toxoid in preparations intended for use in persons 7 years of age or older is approximately 80% lower than that of the pediatric formulation. The lower dosage of diphtheria toxoid is recommended for persons 7 years of age or older because adverse reactions to the diphtheria component are thought to be related to both dose and age.[5]

Persons who experience Arthus-type hypersensitivity reactions or temperatures greater than 39.4°C (103°F) after a previous dose of tetanus toxoid usually have very high serum tetanus antibody levels and should not be given even emergency doses of a tetanus toxoid-containing preparation more frequently than every 10 years, even if they have a wound that is neither clean nor minor.[11]

If a contraindication to using tetanus toxoid-containing preparations exists in a person who has not completed a primary immunizing course of tetanus toxoid, and other than a clean, minor wound is sustained, only passive immunization should be given using human TIG[5] (see **INDICATIONS AND USAGE**).

DT should not be given to infants or children with thrombocytopenia or any coagulation disorder that would contraindicate intramuscular injection unless the potential benefits clearly outweigh the risk of administration. If the decision is made to administer DT to children with coagulation disorders, it should be given with caution (see **DRUG INTERACTIONS**).

Deaths have been reported in temporal association with the administration of preparations containing diphtheria and/or tetanus antigens (see **ADVERSE REACTIONS**).

Health care professionals should prescribe and/or administer this product with caution to patients with a possible history of latex sensitivity since this packaging contains dry natural rubber.

PRECAUTIONS

General

CARE IS TO BE TAKEN BY THE HEALTH CARE PROFESSIONAL FOR THE SAFE AND EFFECTIVE USE OF THIS PRODUCT.

1. PRIOR TO ADMINISTRATION OF ANY DOSE OF DT, THE PARENT OR GUARDIAN SHOULD BE ASKED ABOUT THE PERSONAL HISTORY, FAMILY HISTORY, AND RECENT HEALTH STATUS OF THE VACCINE RECIPIENT. THE HEALTH CARE PROFESSIONAL SHOULD ASCERTAIN PREVIOUS IMMUNIZATION HISTORY, CURRENT HEALTH STATUS, AND OCCURRENCE OF ANY SYMPTOMS AND/OR SIGNS OF AN ADVERSE EVENT AFTER PREVIOUS IMMUNIZATIONS IN THE CHILD TO BE IMMUNIZED, IN ORDER TO DETERMINE THE EXISTENCE OF ANY CONTRAINDICATION TO IMMUNIZATION WITH DT AND TO ALLOW AN ASSESSMENT OF BENEFITS AND RISKS.
2. HEALTH CARE PROFESSIONALS SHOULD ADMINISTER THIS PRODUCT WITH CAUTION TO PATIENTS WITH A PRIOR HISTORY OF GUILLAIN-BARRÉ SYNDROME (see **ADVERSE REACTIONS**).
3. BEFORE THE INJECTION OF ANY BIOLOGICAL, THE HEALTH CARE PROFESSIONAL SHOULD TAKE ALL PRECAUTIONS KNOWN FOR PREVENTION OF ALLERGIC OR ANY OTHER SIDE REACTIONS. This should include: a review of the patient's history regarding possible sensitivity; the ready availability of epinephrine 1:1000 and other appropriate agents used for control of immediate allergic reactions; and a knowledge of the recent literature pertaining to use of the biological concerned, including the nature of side effects and adverse reactions that may follow its use.
4. Children with impaired immune responsiveness, whether due to the use of immunosuppressive therapy (including irradiation, systemic corticosteroids, antimetabolites, alkylating agents, and cytotoxic agents), a genetic defect, human immunodeficiency virus (HIV) infection, leukemia, lymphoma, generalized malignancy, or other causes, may have a reduced antibody response to active immunization procedures.[5,10,13,14] Deferral of administration of DT may be considered in individuals receiving immunosuppressive therapy if it will be discontinued shortly.[5] Other groups should generally receive this vaccine according to the usual recommended schedule[5,10,14,15] (see **DRUG INTERACTIONS**).
5. This product is not contraindicated for use in individuals with HIV virus infection.[13,15]
6. *Since this product is a suspension containing an adjuvant, shake vigorously immediately prior to use to obtain a uniform suspension in the vaccine container.*
7. A separate sterile syringe and needle or a sterile disposable unit should be used for each individual patient to prevent transmission of hepatitis or other infectious agents from one person to another. Needles should be disposed of properly and should not be replaced.
8. Special care should be taken to prevent injection into or near a blood vessel or nerve.
9. Health care professionals should prescribe and/or administer this product with caution to patients with a possible history of latex sensitivity since this packaging contains dry natural rubber.

Information for Parents or Guardians

PRIOR TO THE ADMINISTRATION OF THIS VACCINE, HEALTH CARE PROFESSIONALS SHOULD INFORM THE PARENT OR GUARDIAN OF THE RECOMMENDED IMMUNIZATION SCHEDULE FOR PROTECTION AGAINST TETANUS AND DIPHTHERIA DISEASES AND THE BENEFITS AND RISKS OF VACCINATION AGAINST TETANUS AND DIPHTHERIA DISEASES. GUIDANCE SHOULD BE PROVIDED ON MEASURES TO BE TAKEN BY THE PARENT OR GUARDIAN SHOULD SUSPECTED ADVERSE EVENTS OCCUR, SUCH AS ANTIPYRETIC MEASURES FOR ELEVATED TEMPERATURES AND THE NEED TO REPORT ANY SUSPECTED ADVERSE OCCURRENCES TO THE HEALTH CARE PROFESSIONAL. PARENTS OR GUARDIANS SHOULD BE PROVIDED WITH VACCINE INFORMATION STATEMENTS PRIOR TO THE TIME OF VACCINATION, AS REQUIRED BY THE NATIONAL CHILDHOOD VACCINE INJURY ACT[17] (see **Adverse Event Reporting**).

THE HEALTH CARE PROFESSIONAL SHOULD INFORM THE PARENT OR GUARDIAN OF THE IMPORTANCE OF COMPLETING THE IMMUNIZATION SERIES UNLESS CONTRAINDICATED.

Drug Interactions

Infants or children receiving immunosuppressive therapy (including irradiation, systemic corticosteroids, antimetabolites, alkylating agents, and cytotoxic agents) may have a reduced response to active immunization procedures.[5,10,13,14] Although no specific studies are available, if immunosuppressive therapy will be discontinued shortly, it would be reasonable to defer immunization until the patient has been off therapy for one month; otherwise the patient should be vaccinated while still on therapy.[13] Short-term (less than 2 weeks) corticosteroid therapy or intra-articular, bursal, or tendon injections with corticosteroids is thought not to be immunosuppressive[13] (see **PRECAUTIONS, General**).

As with other intramuscular injections, diphtheria and tetanus toxoids should be given with caution to children on anticoagulant therapy (see **WARNINGS**).

Human TIG or equine diphtheria antitoxin, if used, should be given in a separate site with a separate needle and syringe.

See **DOSAGE AND ADMINISTRATION** for information regarding simultaneous administration with other vaccines.

Carcinogenesis, Mutagenesis, Impairment of Fertility

DT for pediatric use, has not been evaluated for its carcinogenic or mutagenic potential or for impairment of fertility.

Pregnancy

Pregnancy Category C.

Animal reproduction studies have not been conducted with DT vaccine. It is not known whether DT vaccine can cause fetal harm when administered to a pregnant woman or can affect reproductive capacity. DT is not recommended for use in a pregnant woman. THIS PRODUCT IS NOT RECOMMENDED FOR USE IN INDIVIDUALS 7 YEARS OF AGE OR OLDER.

Nursing Mothers

THIS PRODUCT IS NOT RECOMMENDED FOR USE IN INDIVIDUALS 7 YEARS OF AGE OR OLDER.

Pediatric Use

The safety and effectiveness of DT for pediatric use, in children below the age of 6 weeks have not been established (see **DOSAGE AND ADMINISTRATION**).

For either primary or booster immunization against tetanus and diphtheria diseases of individuals 7 years of age and older, the use of Tetanus and Diphtheria Toxoids Adsorbed, for adult use (Td) is recommended.[5,10]

This combined preparation for protection against both diphtheria and tetanus diseases is designed particularly to meet the needs of children less than 7 years of age for whom the use of a combined vaccine containing pertussis antigen is contraindicated. A combined antigen containing pertussis vaccine is the preferred vaccine for primary immunization.

Geriatric Use

This vaccine is NOT recommended for use in adult populations.

ADVERSE REACTIONS

In a prospective study that compared the reaction rates of a similar diphtheria and tetanus toxoid-containing vaccine to diphtheria and tetanus toxoids and pertussis vaccine (DTP), 784 children 0 to 6 years of age who were scheduled to receive routine DTP immunization instead received a dose of diphtheria and tetanus toxoid vaccine. Of these children, 684 and 110 were enrolled in the open-label and double-blind portions of the study, respectively. Most (98.8%) of the of the children received diphtheria and tetanus toxoid vaccine as a first, second, or third dose of the primary immunization series; the remainder of the immunizations were administered as a booster (4th or 5th) dose. Local and systemic reactions that occurred within 48 hours of immunization were reported by parents through home visit, telephone call or mail-in questionnaire. Local reactions occurring within 48 hours following immunization for both the blinded and unblinded groups included redness (7.6%), swelling (7.6%), and pain (9.9%). Systemic symptoms included drowsiness (14.9%), fretfulness (22.6%), vomiting (2.6%), anorexia (7.0%), and persistent crying (0.7%). The incidence rates of fever ≥38°C (100.4°F) and ≥39°C (102.2°F), reported in a subset of children (n=292) three to six hours post-immunization, were 9.3% and 0.7% respectively.[18,19]

Local reactions, manifested by varying degree of erythema, induration, and tenderness, may occur after administration of DT.[18,19] With vaccines in general, it is not uncommon for patients to note within 48 to 72 hours at or around the injection site the following minor reactions: edema; pain or tenderness; redness, inflammation or skin discoloration; mass or induration; or local hypersensitivity. Such local reactions are usually self-limited and require no therapy. As with other aluminum-containing vaccines,[20] a nodule may occasionally be palpable at the injection site for several weeks. Sterile abscess formation or subcutaneous atrophy at the injection site may also occur.

Arthus-type hypersensitivity reactions, characterized by severe local reactions (generally starting 2 to 8 hours after an injection) may follow receipt of tetanus toxoid in persons who have very high serum antitoxin antibodies due to overly frequent injections of tetanus toxoid[20] (see **WARNINGS**).

Pallor, coldness, and hyporesponsiveness have been reported in a child receiving a DT vaccine.[19]

Other adverse events which have been reported in temporal association with various tetanus toxoid-containing products include: warmth, swelling, cellulitis, malaise, weakness or fatigue, dizziness, irritability, aches and pains, arthralgia, flushing, tachycardia, syncope, nausea, vomiting, lymphadenopathy, phlebitis, pruritis/itching, hives, sweating, acute midbrain syndrome, EEG disturbances, accommodation pareses, paresthesia, radiculopathy, brachial plexus neuropathy, cranial nerve pareses, myelopathy, myelitis, and cochlear lesions.

NEUROLOGICAL COMPLICATIONS,[21] SUCH AS CONVULSIONS,[22] ENCEPHALOPATHY,[22,23] AND VARIOUS MONO- AND POLYNEUROPATHIES,[23–29] INCLUDING GUILLAIN-BARRÉ SYNDROME (GBS),[30–31] HAVE BEEN REPORTED FOLLOWING ADMINISTRATION OF PREPARATIONS CONTAINING DIPHTHERIA AND/OR TETANUS ANTIGENS. A REVIEW BY THE INSTITUTE OF MEDICINE (I.O.M.) FOUND EVIDENCE OF A CAUSAL RELATION BETWEEN TETANUS TOXOID AND BRACHIAL NEURITIS AND GBS, BUT DID NOT FIND EVIDENCE OF A CAUSAL RELATION BETWEEN DT AND SUDDEN INFANT DEATH SYNDROME (SIDS).[32]

ALLERGIC AND HYPERSENSITIVITY REACTIONS, URTICARIA, ERYTHEMA MULTIFORME OR OTHER RASH, ARTHRALGIAS[22] AND, MORE RARELY, A SEVERE ANAPHYLACTIC REACTION[32] (I.E., URTICARIA WITH SWELLING OF THE MOUTH, DIFFICULTY BREATHING, HYPOTENSION, SHOCK, OR DEATH) HAVE BEEN REPORTED FOLLOWING ADMINISTRATION OF PREPARATIONS CONTAINING DIPHTHERIA AND/OR TETANUS ANTIGENS.

DEATHS HAVE BEEN REPORTED IN TEMPORAL ASSOCIATION TO RECEIPT OF PREPARATIONS CONTAINING TETANUS AND DIPHTHERIA TOXOIDS. THE I.O.M. FOUND INADEQUATE EVIDENCE TO ACCEPT OR REJECT A CAUSAL RELATIONSHIP BETWEEN TETANUS TOXOID-CONTAINING PRODUCTS AND DEATH FROM CAUSES OTHER THAN ANAPHYLAXIS OR GBS.[32]

A review of two large, active surveillance studies of adults and children who received approximately 0.7 to 1.2 million and 8.1 million doses of tetanus toxoid-containing vaccines, respectively, found that the number of cases of GBS after the administration of such vaccines was less than that expected by chance alone.[33]

Adverse Event Reporting

Any suspected adverse events following immunization should be reported by the health care professioinal to the US Department of Health and Human Services (DHHS). The National Childhood Vaccine Injury Act requires that the manufacturer and lot number of the vaccine administered be recorded by the health care professional in the vaccine recipient's permanent medical record (or in a permanent office log or file), along with the date of the administration of the vaccine and the name, address, and title of the person administering the vaccine.

The statute further requires the health care professional to report to the Secretary of the US DHHS the occurrence following immunization of any events set forth in the statute's Vaccine Injury Table, including anaphylaxis or anaphylactic shock within 7 days, brachial neuritis within 28 days or any acute complication or sequela (including death) of the above events or any events that would contraindicate further doses of vaccine, according to this Diphtheria and Tetanus Toxoids, Aluminum Phosphate Adsorbed, for pediatric use, package insert.[17]

TABLE 1. ROUTINE DIPHTHERIA, TETANUS, AND PERTUSSIS VACCINATION SCHEDULE SUMMARY FOR CHILDREN UNDER 7 YEARS OF AGE—UNITED STATES§*

DOSE	CUSTOMARY AGE	AGE/INTERVAL+	PRODUCT
Primary 1	2 months	6 weeks old or older	DTaP/DTP§
Primary 2	4 months	4–8 weeks after first dose*	DTaP/DTP§
Primary 3	6 months	4–8 weeks after second dose*	DTaP/DTP§
Primary 4	15 months	6–12 months after third dose*	DTaP/DTP§
Booster	4–6 years old, before entering kindergarten or elementary school (not necessary if fourth primary vaccinating dose administered after fourth birthday)		DTa/P/DTP§

* Prolonging the interval dose not require restarting series.
\+ Use DT if pertussis vaccine is contraindicated. If the child is 1 year of age or older at the time that primary dose three is due, a third dose 6 to 12 months after the second completes primary vaccination with DT.
§ DTaP denotes diphtheria, tetanus, and accellular pertussis vaccine, which is the preferred pertussis-containing vaccine.[10,36] DTP denotes diphtheria, tetanus, and whole-cell pertussis vaccine.

SUMMARY GUIDE TO TETANUS PROPHYLAXIS IN ROUTINE WOUND MANAGEMENT§*

History of Tetanus Toxoid (doses)	Clean, Minor Wounds		All Other Wounds†	
	Td§	TIG	Td§	TIG
Unknown or <3	Yes	No	Yes	Yes
≥3¶	No**	No	No‡	No

* Important details are in the text.
† Such as, but not limited to, wounds contaminated with dirt, feces, soil, and saliva; puncture wounds; avulsions; and wounds resulting from missiles, crushing, burns and frostbite.
§ For children under 7 years old, DTP/DTaP (DT, if pertussis vaccine is contraindicated) is preferred to tetanus toxoid alone. For persons 7 years of age and older, Td is preferred to tetanus toxoid alone.
¶ If only three doses of fluid toxoid have been received, then a fourth dose of toxoid, preferably an adsorbed toxoid, should be given.
** Yes, if more than 10 years since last dose.
‡ Yes, if more than 5 years since last dose. (More frequent boosters are not needed and can accentuate side effects.)

The US DHHS has established the Vaccine Adverse Event Reporting System (VAERS) to accept all reports of suspected adverse events after the administration of any vaccine including, but not limited to, the reporting of events required by the National Childhood Vaccine Injury Act of 1986.[17] The VAERS toll-free number for VAERS forms and information is 800-822-7967.

DOSAGE AND ADMINISTRATION

For Intramuscular Use Only

The dose is 0.5 mL to be given intramuscularly.

Since this product is a suspension containing an adjuvant, shake vigorously immediately prior to use to obtain a uniform suspension in the vaccine container. The vaccine should not be used if it cannot be resuspended.

Parenteral drug products should be inspected visually for particulate matter and discoloration prior to administration (see **DESCRIPTION**). This product should not be used if particulate matter or discoloration is found.

The vaccine should be injected intramuscularly. The preferred sites are the anterolateral aspect of the thigh or the deltoid muscle of the upper arm. The vaccine should not be injected in the gluteal area or areas where there may be a major nerve trunk and/or blood vessel. Before injection, the skin at the injection site should be cleansed and prepared with a suitable germicide.

After insertion of the needle, aspirate and wait to see if any blood appears in the syringe, which will help avoid inadvertent injection into a blood vessel. If blood appears, withdraw the needle and prepare for a new injection at another site.

This combined preparation for protection against both diphtheria and tetanus diseases is designed particularly to meet the need of children between 2 months and less than 7 years of age for whom the use of a combined vaccine containing pertussis antigen is contraindicated.

It is recommended that active immunization against diphtheria and tetanus be started at 2 months of age.

No data are available for DT given simultaneously with OPV (or IPV), MMR, Hepatitis B, Hib, and rotavirus vaccines. Nonetheless, the ACIP encourages simultaneous administratioan of routine childhood vaccines for children who are at the recommended age for these vaccines and for whom no specific contraindications exist at the time of immunization.[16,34]

Unimmunized infants and children less than 1 year of age for whom vaccine containing pertussis antigen is contraindicated should receive three doses of 0.5 mL each of DT at 4- to preferably 8-week intervals, followed by a fourth (reinforcing) dose of 0.5 mL, 6 to 12 months after the third dose, for the primary series.[5,10]

Unimmunized children from 1 up to 7 years of age (prior to the 7th birthday) for whom vaccine containing pertussis antigen is contraindicated should receive two doses of 0.5 mL each of DT, at 4- to preferably 8-weeks intervals, followed by a third (reinforcing) dose 6 to 12 months later, for the primary series.[5,10]

If after beginning a DTP series, further doses of vaccine containing pertussis antigen become contraindicated, DT should be substituted for each of the remaining doses.[5,10]

The reinforcing dose is an integral part of the primary immunizing series.

Interruption of the recommended schedule with a delay between doses does not interfere with the final immunity achieved, nor does it necessitate starting the series over again, regardless of the length of time elapsed between doses.[5,10]

A booster dose of 0.5 mL is indicated at age 4 to 6 years (prior to the 7th birthday), preferably prior to entrance into kindergarten or elementary school. However, if the last dose of the primary immunizing series was administered after the fourth birthday, a booster prior to school entry is not considered necessary.[5,10]

For either primary or booster immunization against tetanus and diphtheria of individuals 7 years of age and older, the use of Tetanus and Diphtheria Toxoids Adsorbed, for adult use, is recommended.[5,10]

[See table 1 above]

Diphtheria Prophylaxis for Case Contacts

All case contacts, household and others, who have previously received fewer than three doses of diphtheria toxoid should receive an immediate dose of an appropriate diphtheria toxoid-containing preparation and should complete the series according to schedule. Case contacts who previously received three or more doses, but who have not received a dose of a preparation containing diphtheria toxoid within the previous five years, should receive a dose of a diphtheria toxoid-containing preparation appropriate for their age.[5] This combined preparation against both diphtheria and tetanus is designed particularly to meet the need of children less than 7 years of age for whom the use of a combined vaccine containing pertussis antigen is contraindicated.

Tetanus Prophylaxis in Wound Management

The need for diphtheria and tetanus toxoids (active immunization), with or without human TIG (passive immunization) depends upon the condition of the wound and the patient's immunization history. Tetanus has rarely occurred among persons with a documented primary series of tetanus toxoid injections.[5]

For routine wound management of children under 7 years of age who are not completely immunized, DT should be used instead of single-antigen tetanus toxoid (if pertussis antigen is contraindicated or individual circumstances are such that potential febrile reactions following DTP might confound the management of the patient).[5] Completion of primary vaccination thereafter should be ensured.

If emergency tetanus prophylaxis is indicated during the period between the last primary dose and the reinforcing dose, a 0.5 mL dose of DT should be given. If given before six months have elapsed, it should be counted as a primary dose; if given after six months, it should be regarded as the reinforcing dose.

For tetanus-prone wounds in children who have had fewer than three, or an unknown number of immunizations with a

Continued on next page

Diphtheria & Tetanus Toxoids—Cont.

tetanus toxoid-containing product, passive immunization with human TIG is also recommended.[5] A separate syringe and site of injection should be used.

If a contraindication to using tetanus toxoid-containing preparations exists in a person who has not completed a primary immunizing course of tetanus toxoid and other than a clean, minor wound is sustained, only passive immunization should be given using human TIG.[5]

[See second table at top of previous page]

HOW SUPPLIED

NDC 0005-1858-31 5.0 mL vial

STORAGE

DO NOT FREEZE. STORE REFRIGERATED, AWAY FROM FREEZER COMPARTMENT, AT 2°C to 8°C (36°F to 46°F).

REFERENCES

1. Mueller JH, Miller PA. Factors influencing the production of tetanal toxin. *J Immunol* 1947;56:143–147.
2. Pillemer L, Grossberg DB, Wittler RG: The immunochemistry of toxins and toxoids. II. The preparation and immunological evaluation of purified tetanal toxoid. *J Immunol* 1946;54:213–224.
3. CDC. Summary of Notifiable Diseases, United States, 1997. *MMWR*. 1998; 46(54): viii.
4. Diphtheria, Epidemic—New Independent States of the Former Soviet Union, 1990–1999 *MMWR*. 1995:44(10): 177–181.
5. CDC. Diphtheria, tetanus, and pertussis: Recommendations for vaccine use and other preventive measures—recommendations of the immunization Practices Advisory Committee (ACIP). *MMWR*. 1991:40(10).
6. Ipsen J. Immunization of adults against diphtheria and tetanus. *NEJM*. 1954;251:459–466.
7. Bardenheir, B et al: Tetanus surveillance—United States, 1995–1997. *MMWR*. 1998 47(ss-2):1.
8. Wassilak, SG et al: Tetanus Toxoid. Chpt. 18 (in) Plotkin, SA and Orenstein, WA. Vaccines, 3rd ed. Philadelphia, PA: WB Saunders Co. 1999.
9. Unpublished data on file; Lederle Laboratories.
10. American Academy of Pediatrics: Report of the Committee on Infectious Diseases. 24th ed. Elk Grove Village, Ill: American Academy of Pediatrics; 1997.
11. Update: Vaccine side effects, adverse reactions, contraindications, and precautions. *MMWR*. 1996;45 (RR-12): 22–31.
12. Sutter RW, Patriarca PA, Suleiman AJM, et al. Attributable risk of DTP (Diphtheria and Tetanus Toxoids and Pertussis Vaccine) injection in provoking paralytic poliomyelitis during a large outbreak on Oman. *J Infect Dis*. 1992;165:444–449.
13. CDC. Recommendations of the Advisory Committee on Immunization Practices (ACIP): Use of vaccines and immune globulins in persons with altered immunocompetence. *MMWR*. 1993;42(RR-4).
14. CDC. Immunization of children infected with human immunodeficiency virus—supplementary ACIP statement. *MMWR*. 1988;37(12):181–183.
15. CDC. Recommendation of the ACIP: immunization of children infected with human T-lymphotropic virus type III/lymphadenopathy-associated virus. *MMWR*. 1986;35(38):595–606.
16. CDC. General recommendations on immunization—Recommendations of the Immunization Practices Advisory Committee (ACIP). *MMWR*. 1994; 43(RR-1).
17. 42 U.S.C. §§ 300 aa -25,-26. See also: CDC. Vaccine Adverse Event Reporting System—United States. *MMWR*. 1190;39:730–733.
18. Cody C, Baroff LJ, Cherry JD, et al. Nature and rates of adverse reactions associated with DTP and DT immunizations in infants and children. *Pediatrics*. 1981;68:650–660.
19. Feery BJ. Incidence and type of reactions to triple antigen (DTP) and DT (CDT) vaccines. *Med J of Australia*. 1982;2:511–515.
20. Fawcett HA, Smith NP. Injection-site granuloma due to aluminum. *Arch Dermatol* 1984;120:1318–1322.
21. Rutledge SL, Snead OC. Neurologic complications of immunizations. *J Pediatr* 1986;109:917–924.
22. CDC. Adverse Events Following Immunization. *MMWR*. 1985;34(3):43–47.
23. Schlenska GK. Unusual neurological complications following tetanus toxoid administration. *J Neurol*. 1977;215:299–302.
24. Blumstein GI, Kreithen H. Peripheral neuropathy following tetanus toxoid administration. *JAMA*. 1966;198: 1030–1031.
25. Reinstein L, Pargament JM, Goodman JS. Peripheral neuropathy after multiple tetanus toxoid injections. *Arch Phys Med Rehabil*. 1982;63:332–334.
26. Tsairis P, Duck PJ, Mulder DW. Natural history of brachial plexus neuropathy. *Arch Neurol*. 1972;27:109–117.
27. Quast U, Hennessen W, Widmark RM. Mono- and polyneuritis after tetanus vaccination. *Devel Bio Stand*. 1979;43:25–32.
28. Holliday PL, Bauer RB. Polyradiculoneuritis secondary to immunization with tetanus and diphtheria toxoids. *Arch Neurol*. 1983;40:56–67.
29. Fenichel GM. Neurological complications of tetanus toxoid. *Arch Neurol* 1983;40:390.
30. Pollard JD, Selby G. Relapsing neuropathy due to tetanus toxoid. *J Neurol Sci*. 1978;37:113–125.
31. Newton N, Janati A. Guillain-Barré syndrome after vaccination with purified tetanus toxoid. *S Med J*. 1987;80: 1053–1054.
32. Stratton KR, Howe CJ, Johnston RB. Adverse effects associated with childhood vaccines. Institute of Medicine (IOM), Washington, DC: National Academy Press 1994.
33. Tuttle J, Chen RT, Rantala H, et al: The risk of Guillain-Barré syndrome after tetanus-toxoid-containing vaccines in adults and children in the United States. *Am J Pub Health*. 1997;87:2045–48.
34. CDC. Rotavirus vaccine for the prevention of rotavirus gastroenteritis among children. Recommendations of the Advisory Committee on Immunization Practices (ACIP). *MMWR*. 1999; 48(RR-2).
35. CDC. Pertussis vaccination: acellular pertussis vaccine for reinforcing and booster use-supplementary ACIP statement. *MMWR*. 1992; 41(RR-1):1–10.

Manufactured by:
LEDERLE LABORATORIES
Division American Cyanamid Company
Pearl River, NY 10965 USA
U.S. Gov't. License No. 17
Marketed by:
WYETH-LEDERLE VACCINES AND PEDIATRICS
Wyeth-Ayerst Laboratories
Philadelphia, PA 19101 USA
C1 6105-1 Issued February 10, 2000

HAEMOPHILUS b CONJUGATE VACCINE ℞
(Diphtheria CRM_{197} Protein Conjugate)
HibTITER®

℞ only

DESCRIPTION

Haemophilus b Conjugate Vaccine (Diphtheria CRM_{197} Protein Conjugate) HibTITER® is a sterile solution of a conjugate of oligosaccharides of the capsular antigen of *Haemophilus influenzae* type b (Haemophilus b) and diphtheria CRM_{197} protein (CRM_{197}) dissolved in 0.9% sodium chloride. The oligosaccharides are derived from highly purified capsular polysaccharide, polyribosylribitol phosphate, isolated from Haemophilus b strain Eagan grown in a chemically defined medium (a mixture of mineral salts, amino acids, and cofactors). The oligosaccharides are purified and sized by diafiltrations through a series of ultrafiltration membranes, and coupled by reductive amination directly to highly purified CRM_{197}.[1,2] CRM_{197} is a nontoxic variant of diphtheria toxin isolated from cultures of *Corynebacterium diphtheriae* C7 (β_{197}) grown in a casamino acids and yeast extract-based medium that is ultrafiltered before use. CRM_{197} is purified through ultrafiltration, ammonium sulfate precipitation, and ion-exchange chromatography to high purity. The conjugate is purified to remove unreacted protein, oligosaccharides, and reagents; sterilized by filtration; and filled into vials. HibTITER is intended for intramuscular use.

The vaccine is a clear, colorless solution. Each single dose of 0.5 mL is formulated to contain 10 µg of purified Haemophilus b saccharide and approximately 25 µg of CRM_{197} protein. Multidose vials contain thimerosal (mercurial derivative) 1:10,000 as a preservative. The potency of HibTITER is determined by chemical assay for polyribosylribitol.

CLINICAL PHARMACOLOGY

For several decades *Haemophilus influenzae* type b (Haemophilus b) was the most common cause of invasive bacterial disease, including meningitis, in young children in the United States. Although nonencapsulated *H. influenzae* are common and six capsular polysaccharide types are known, strains with the type b capsule caused most of the invasive Haemophilus diseases.[3]

Haemophilus b diseases occurred primarily in children under 5 years of age prior to immunization with *Haemophilus influenzae* type b vaccines. In the US, the cumulative risk of developing invasive Haemophilus b disease during the first 5 years of life was estimated to be about 1 in 200. Approximately 60% of cases were meningitis. Cellulitis, epiglottitis, pericarditis, pneumonia, sepsis, or septic arthritis made up the remaining 40%. An estimated 12,000 cases of Haemophilus b meningitis occurred annually prior to the routine use of conjugate vaccines in toddlers.[3,4] The mortality rate can be 5%, and neurologic sequelae have been observed in up to 38% of survivors.[5]

The incidence of invasive Haemophilus b disease peaks between 6 months and 1 year of age, and approximately 55% of disease occurs between 6 and 18 months of age.[3] Interpersonal transmission of Haemophilus b occurs and risk of invasive disease is increased in children younger than 4 years of age who are exposed in the household to a primary case of disease. Clusters of cases in children in day care have been reported and recent studies suggest that the rate of secondary cases may also be increased among children exposed to a primary case in the day-care setting.[3,6]

The incidence of invasive Haemophilus b disease is increased in certain children, such as those who are native Americans, black, or from lower socioeconomic status, and those with medical conditions such as asplenia, sickle cell disease, malignancies associated with immunosuppression, and antibody deficiency syndromes.[3,4,6]

The protective activity of antibody to Haemophilus b polysaccharide was demonstrated by passive antibody studies in animals and in children with agammaglobulinemia or with Haemophilus b disease[7] and confirmed with the efficacy study of Haemophilus b polysaccharide (HbPs) vaccine.[8] Data from passive antibody studies indicate that a preexisting titer of antibody to HbPs of 0.15 µg/mL correlates with protection.[9] Data from a Finnish field trial in children 18 to 71 months of age indicate that a titer of >1.0 µg/mL 3 weeks after vaccination is associated with long-term protection.[10,11]

Linkage of Haemophilus b saccharides to a protein such as CRM_{197} converts the saccharide (HbO) to a T-dependent (HbOC) antigen, and results in an enhanced antibody response to the saccharide in young infants that primes for an anamnestic response and is predominantly of the IgG class.[12] Laboratory evidence indicates that the native state of the CRM_{197} protein and the use of oligosaccharides in the formulation of HibTITER® enhances its immunogenicity.[13–15] Haemophilus b conjugate vaccines with other carrier proteins will be recognized differently by the immune system.

Prior to licensure, the immunogenicity of HibTITER was evaluated in US infants and children.[15] Infants 1 to 6 months of age at first immunization received three doses at approximately 2-month intervals.[16] Children 7 to 11 and 12 to 14 months of age received 2 doses at the same interval.[15] Children 15 to 23 months of age received a single dose.[17] HibTITER was highly immunogenic in all age groups studied, with 97% to 100% of 1,232 infants attaining titers of ≥1 µg/mL and 92% to 100% for bactericidal activity.[15–17]

Long-term persistence of the antibody response was observed. More than 80% of the 235 infants who received three doses of vaccine had an anti-HbPs antibody level ≥1 µg/mL at 2 years of age.[18]

The vaccine generated an immune response characteristic of a protein antigen. IgG anti-HbPs antibodies of IgG_1 subclass predominated and the immune system was primed for a booster response to HibTITER. There is some evidence suggesting natural increases in antibody levels over time after vaccination, most probably the result of contact with Haemophilus type b organisms or cross-reactive antigens.[18] These studies were carried out at a time when significant levels of Haemophilus b disease were still present in the community.

Antibody generated by HibTITER has been found to have high avidity, a measure of the functional affinity of antibody to bind to antigen. High-avidity antibody is more potent than low-avidity antibody in serum bactericidal assays.[19] The contribution to clinical protection is unknown.

Immunogenicity of HibTITER was evaluated in 26 children 22 months to 5 years of age who had not responded to earlier vaccination with Haemophilus b polysaccharide vaccine. One dose of HibTITER was immunogenic in all 26 children and generated titers of ≥1 µg/mL in 25 of the 26 infants.[20] HibTITER has been found to be immunogenic in children with sickle cell disease, a condition that may cause increased susceptibility to Haemophilus b disease.[21] HibTITER has also been shown to be immunogenic in native American infants, such as the group of 50 studied in Alaska who received three doses at 2, 4, and 6 months of age.[20] Antibody levels achieved were comparable to those seen in healthy US infants who received their first dose at 1 to 2 months of age and subsequent doses at 4 to 6 months of age.[15,16,20]

Postlicensure surveillance of immunogenicity was conducted during the distribution of the first 30 million doses of HibTITER and during the time period over which Haemophilus b disease in children has been decreasing significantly in areas of extensive vaccine usage.[20,22–29] After three doses, titers ranged from 2.37 to 8.45 µg/mL with 67% to 94% attaining ≥1 µg/mL.[20,24,25]

Persistence of antibody was examined in several cohorts of subjects that received either a selected commercial lot or that were part of the initial efficacy trial in northern California. Geometric mean titers for these cohorts were between 0.51 and 1.96 just prior to boosting at 15 to 18 months. These lots not only induced persistent antibody but also provided effective priming for a booster dose with commercial lots, with postboosting titers greater than 1.0 µg/mL in 80% to 97% of subjects.[20]

HibTITER (HbOC) was shown to be effective in a large-scale controlled clinical trial in a multiethnic population in northern California carried out between February 1988 and June 1990.[30,31] There were no (0) vaccine failures in infants who received three doses of HibTITER and 12 cases of Haemophilus b disease (6 cases of meningitis) in the control group. The estimate of efficacy is 100% (P = .0002) with 95% confidence intervals of 68% to 100%. Through the end of 1991, with an additional 49,000 person-years of follow-up, there were still no cases of Haemophilus b disease in fully vaccinated infants less than 2 years of age.[22,23] One case of disease has been reported in a 3½-year-old child who did not receive a booster dose as recommended.

A comparative clinical trial was performed in Finland where approximately 53,000 infants received HibTITER at 4 and 6 months of age and a booster dose at 14 months in a trial conducted from January 1988 through December 1990. Only two children developed Haemophilus b disease after receiving the two-dose primary immunization schedule. One child became ill at 15 months of age and the other at 18 months of age; neither child received the scheduled booster at 14 months of age. No vaccine failure has been reported in children who received the two-dose primary series and the booster dose at 14 months of age. Based on more than 32,000 person-years of follow-up time, the estimate of efficacy is about 95% when compared to historical control groups followed between 1985 and 1988.[20] Historical controls were used since all infants received one of two Haemophilus b conjugate vaccines during the period of the trial. Evidence of efficacy postlicensure includes significant reductions in Haemophilus b disease that are closely associated with increases in the net doses of Haemophilus b Conjugate Vaccine distributed in the US.[20,22–29] In the northern California Kaiser Permanente there has been a 94% decrease in Haemophilus disease incidence in 1991 for children younger than 18 months of age, compared to 1984–1988, when HibTITER was not available for this age group.[22,23] Furthermore, active surveillance by the Centers for Disease Control and Prevention (CDC) has shown a 71% decrease in Haemophilus b disease in children less than 15 months old, between 1989 and 1991, which corresponds temporally and geographically with increases in net doses of Haemophilus b conjugate vaccine distributed in the US.[26] As with all vaccines, this conjugate vaccine cannot be expected to be 100% effective. There have been rare reports to the Vaccine Adverse Event Reporting System (VAERS) of Haemophilus b disease following full primary immunization.

INDICATIONS AND USAGE

Haemophilus b Conjugate Vaccine (Diphtheria CRM_{197} Protein Conjugate) HibTITER® is indicated for the immunization of children 2 months to 71 months of age against invasive diseases caused by *H. influenzae* type b.

As with any vaccine, HibTITER may not protect 100% of individuals receiving the vaccine.

HibTITER may be administered simultaneously but at different sites from other routine pediatric vaccines, eg, Diphtheria and Tetanus Toxoids and Pertussis Vaccine Adsorbed (DTP), Oral Poliovirus Vaccine (OPV), and Measles-Mumps-Rubella Vaccine (MMR).[32,33]

CONTRAINDICATIONS

Hypersensitivity to any component of the vaccine, including diphtheria toxoid, or thimerosal in the multidose presentation, is a contraindication to use of HibTITER®.

WARNINGS

HibTITER® WILL NOT PROTECT AGAINST *H. INFLUENZAE* OTHER THAN TYPE b STRAINS, NOR WILL HibTITER PROTECT AGAINST OTHER MICROORGANISMS THAT CAUSE MENINGITIS OR SEPTIC DISEASE.

AS WITH ANY INTRAMUSCULAR INJECTION, HibTITER SHOULD BE GIVEN WITH CAUTION TO INFANTS OR CHILDREN WITH THROMBOCYTOPENIA OR ANY COAGULATION DISORDER THAT WOULD CONTRAINDICATE INTRAMUSCULAR INJECTION (SEE **DRUG INTERACTIONS**).

ANTIGENURIA HAS BEEN DETECTED FOLLOWING RECEIPT OF HAEMOPHILUS b CONJUGATE VACCINE[34] AND THEREFORE ANTIGEN DETECTION IN URINE MAY NOT HAVE DIAGNOSTIC VALUE IN SUSPECTED HAEMOPHILUS b DISEASE WITHIN 2 WEEKS OF IMMUNIZATION.

Health care professionals should administer HibTITER with caution to patients with a possible history of latex sensitivity, since its packaging contains dry natural rubber.

PRECAUTIONS

GENERAL

1. CARE IS TO BE TAKEN BY THE HEALTH CARE PROVIDER FOR SAFE AND EFFECTIVE USE OF THIS PRODUCT.
2. PRIOR TO ADMINISTRATION OF ANY DOSE OF HibTITER, THE PARENT OR GUARDIAN SHOULD BE ASKED ABOUT THE PERSONAL HISTORY, FAMILY HISTORY, AND RECENT HEALTH STATUS OF THE VACCINE RECIPIENT. THE HEALTH CARE PROVIDER SHOULD ASCERTAIN PREVIOUS IMMUNIZATION HISTORY, CURRENT HEALTH STATUS, AND OCCURRENCE OF ANY SYMPTOMS AND/OR SIGNS OF AN ADVERSE EVENT AFTER PREVIOUS IMMUNIZATION IN THE CHILD TO BE IMMUNIZED, IN ORDER TO DETERMINE THE EXISTENCE OF ANY CONTRAINDICATION TO IMMUNIZATION WITH HibTITER AND TO ALLOW AN ASSESSMENT OF BENEFITS AND RISKS.
3. BEFORE THE INJECTION OF ANY BIOLOGICAL, THE HEALTH CARE PROVIDER SHOULD TAKE ALL PRECAUTIONS KNOWN FOR THE PREVENTION OF ALLERGIC OR ANY OTHER SIDE REACTIONS. This should include: a review of the patient's history regarding possible sensitivity; the ready availability of epinephrine 1:1,000 and other appropriate agents used for control of immediate allergic reactions; and a knowledge of the recent literature pertaining to use of the biological concerned, including the nature of side effects and adverse reactions that may follow its use.
4. Children with impaired immune responsiveness, whether due to the use of immunosuppressive therapy (including irradiation, corticosteroids, antimetabolites, alkylating agents, and cytotoxic agents), a genetic defect, human immunodeficiency virus (HIV) infection, or other causes, may have reduced antibody response to active immunization procedures.[35,36] Deferral of administration of vaccine may be considered in individuals receiving immunosuppressive therapy.[35] Other groups should receive this vaccine according to the usual recommended schedule.[35–37] (See **DRUG INTERACTIONS.**)
5. This product is not contraindicated based on the presence of human immunodeficiency virus infection.[38]

TABLE 1
Number of Subjects (Percent) Manifesting Side Effects Associated with HibTITER® Administered Independently from DTP*
(Infants Vaccinated Initially at 1–6 Months of Age)

	Dose 1 n=401			Dose 2 n=383			Dose 3 n=334		
Symptoms	Same Day As Vacc.	+1 Day	+2 Days	Same Day As Vacc.	+1 Day	+2 Days	Same Day As Vacc.	+1 Day	+2 Days
Temp > 38.3°C	0	2	2	2	3	2	2	6	5
	—	<1%	<1%	<1%	<1%	<1%	<1%	1.8%	1.5%
Redness ≥ 2 cm	1	0	0	1	6	0	5	4	0
	<1%	—	—	<1%	1.6%	—	1.5%	1.2%	—
Warmth ≥ 2 cm	1	1	0	2	1	0	1	6	0
	<1%	<1%	—	<1%	<1%	—	<1%	1.8%	—
Swelling ≥ 2 cm	5	1	0	2	2	0	1	0	0
	1.2%	<1%	—	<1%	<1%	—	<1%	—	—

*DTP and HibTITER® given 2 weeks apart with DTP having been given first.

6. Any acute infection or febrile illness is reason for delaying use of HibTITER® except when in the opinion of the physician, withholding the vaccine entails a greater risk. A minor afebrile illness, such as a mild upper respiratory infection, is not usually reason to defer immunization.
7. As reported with Haemophilus b polysaccharide vaccine, cases of Haemophilus b disease may occur prior to the onset of the protective effects of the vaccine.[3,39]
8. The vaccine should not be injected intradermally since the safety and immunogenicity of this route have not been evaluated. The vaccine should be given intramuscularly.
9. A separate sterile syringe and needle or a sterile disposable unit should be used for each individual patient to prevent transmission of infectious agents from one person to another. Needles should be disposed of properly and should not be recapped.
10. Special care should be taken to prevent injection into a blood vessel.

The US Department of Health and Human Services has established a new Vaccine Adverse Event Reporting System (VAERS) to accept all reports of suspected adverse events after the administration of any vaccine, including but not limited to the reporting of events required by the National Childhood Vaccine Injury Act of 1986.[40] The VAERS toll-free number for VAERS forms and information is 800-822-7967.

ALTHOUGH SOME ANTIBODY RESPONSE TO DIPHTHERIA TOXIN OCCURS, IMMUNIZATION WITH HibTITER DOES NOT SUBSTITUTE FOR ROUTINE DIPHTHERIA IMMUNIZATION.

Packaging for HibTITER contains dry natural rubber. Health care professionals should administer HibTITER with caution to patients with a possible history of latex sensitivity

INFORMATION FOR PATIENT

PRIOR TO ADMINISTRATION OF HibTITER®, HEALTH CARE PERSONNEL SHOULD INFORM THE PARENT, GUARDIAN OR OTHER RESPONSIBLE ADULT, OF THE RECOMMENDED IMMUNIZATION SCHEDULE FOR PROTECTION AGAINST HAEMOPHILUS b DISEASE AND THE BENEFITS AND RISKS TO THE CHILD RECEIVING THIS VACCINE. GUIDANCE SHOULD BE PROVIDED ON MEASURES TO BE TAKEN SHOULD ADVERSE EVENTS OCCUR, SUCH AS, ANTIPYRETIC MEASURES FOR ELEVATED TEMPERATURES AND THE NEED TO REPORT ADVERSE EVENTS TO THE HEALTH CARE PROVIDER. Parents should be provided with vaccine information pamphlets at the time of each vaccination, as stated in the National Childhood Vaccine Injury Act.[40]

PATIENTS, PARENTS, OR GUARDIANS SHOULD BE INSTRUCTED TO REPORT ANY SERIOUS ADVERSE REACTIONS TO THEIR HEALTH CARE PROVIDER.

DRUG INTERACTIONS

No impairment of the antibody response to the individual antigens was demonstrated when HibTITER® was given at the same time but at separate sites as DTP plus OPV to children 2 to 20 months of age or MMR to children 15 ± 1 month of age.[20,41]

As with other intramuscular injections, HibTITER should be given with caution to children on anticoagulant therapy.

CARCINOGENESIS, MUTAGENESIS, IMPAIRMENT OF FERTILITY

HibTITER® has not been evaluated for its carcinogenic, mutagenic potential, or impairment of fertility.

PREGNANCY

REPRODUCTIVE STUDIES—PREGNANCY CATEGORY C

Animal reproduction studies have not been conducted with HibTITER®. It is also not known whether HibTITER can cause fetal harm when administered to a pregnant woman or can affect reproduction capability. HibTITER is NOT recommended for use in a pregnant woman.

GERIATRIC USE

This vaccine is NOT recommended for use in adult populations.

PEDIATRIC USE

The safety and effectiveness of HibTITER® in children below the age of 6 weeks have not been established.

ADVERSE REACTIONS

Adverse reactions associated with HibTITER® have been evaluated in 401 infants who were vaccinated initially at 1 to 6 months of age and were given 1,118 doses independent of DTP vaccine. Observations were made during the day of vaccination and days 1 and 2 postvaccination. A temperature >38.3°C was recorded at least once during the observation period following 2% of the vaccinations. Local erythema, warmth, or swelling (≥ 2 cm) was observed following 3.3% of vaccinations. The incidence of temperature > 38.3°C was greater during the first postvaccination day than during the day of vaccination or the second postvaccination day. The incidence of local erythema, warmth, or swelling was similar during the day of vaccination and the first postvaccination day; it was lower during the second postvaccination day. All side effects have been infrequent, mild, and transient with no serious sequelae (Table 1). No difference in the rates of these complaints was reported after dose 1, 2, or 3. [See table above]

The following complaints were also observed after 1,118 vaccinations with HibTITER: irritability (133), sleepiness (91), prolonged crying [≥ 4 hours] (38), appetite loss (23), vomiting (9), diarrhea (2), and rash (1).

Additional safety data with HibTITER are available from the efficacy studies conducted in young infants.[30] There were 79,483 doses given to 30,844 infants at approximately 2, 4, and 6 months of age in California, usually at the same time as DTP (but at a separate injection site) and OPV; approximately 100,000 doses have been given to 53,000 infants at 4 and 6 months in Finland at the same time as a combined DTP and inactivated polio (IPV) vaccine (but at a separate injection site). The rate and type of reactions associated with the vaccinations were no different from those seen when DTP or DTP-IPV was administered alone. These included fever, local reactions, rash, and one hyporesponsive episode with a single seizure. The safety of HibTITER was also evaluated in the California study by direct phone questioning of the parents or guardians of 6,887 vaccine recipients. The incidence and type of side effects reported within 24 hours of vaccination were similar to those cited in Table 1. In addition, analysis of emergency room (ER) visits within 30 days and hospitalization within 60 days after receipt of 23,800 doses of HibTITER showed no increase in the rates of any type of ER visit or hospitalization.

Table 2 details the side effects associated with a single vaccination of HibTITER given (without DTP) to infants of 15 to 23 months of age.

Similar results have been observed in the analysis of 2,285 subjects of 18 to 60 months of age, vaccinated as part of a postmarketing safety study of HibTITER.[20] These data were collected by telephone survey 24 to 48 hours postvaccination. Additional observations included irritability, restless sleep, and GI symptoms (diarrhea, vomiting, and loss of appetite) in the group that received HibTITER alone. A cause and effect relationship between these observations and the vaccinations has not been established.

TABLE 2
Selected Adverse Reactions* in Children of 15–23 Months of Age Following Vaccination with HibTITER®

Adverse Reaction	No. of Subjects	Reaction Within 24 h	% Postvaccination At 48 h
Fever			
>38.3°C	354	1.4	0.6
Erythema	354	2.0	—
Swelling	354	1.7	—
Tenderness	354	3.7	0.3

* The following complaints were reported after vaccination of these 354 children in the indicated number of children: diarrhea (9), vomiting (5), prolonged crying [>4 hours] (4), and rashes (2).

Rash, hives (urticaria), erythema multiforme, convulsions,[42] vomiting/diarrhea,[42] and Guillain-Barré syndrome[43] have

Continued on next page

HibTITER—Cont.

been observed following the administration of Haemophilus b polysaccharide and Haemophilus b conjugate vaccines. However, a cause and effect relationship among any of these events and the vaccination has not been established.

DOSAGE AND ADMINISTRATION

HibTITER® is for intramuscular use only.

Any parenteral drug product should be inspected visually for extraneous particulate matter and/or discoloration prior to administration whenever solution and container permit. If these conditions exist, HibTITER should not be administered.

Before injection, the skin over the site to be injected should be cleansed with a suitable germicide. After insertion of the needle, aspirate to help avoid inadvertent injection into a blood vessel.

The vaccine should be injected intramuscularly, preferably into the midlateral muscles of the thigh or deltoid, with care to avoid major peripheral nerve trunks.

HibTITER is indicated for children 2 months to 71 months of age for the prevention of invasive Haemophilus b disease. For infants 2 to 6 months of age, the immunizing dose is three separate injections of 0.5 mL given at approximately 2-month intervals. Previously unvaccinated infants from 7 through 11 months of age should receive two separate injections approximately 2 months apart. Children from 12 through 14 months of age who have not been vaccinated previously receive one injection. All vaccinated children receive a single booster dose at 15 months of age or older, but not less than 2 months after the previous dose. Previously unvaccinated children 15 to 71 months of age receive a single injection of HibTITER.[32,33] Preterm infants should be vaccinated with HibTITER according to their chronological age, from birth.[32]

Recommended Immunization Schedule

Age at First Immunization (Mo)	No. of Doses	Booster
2–6	3	Yes
7–11	2	Yes
12 –14	1	Yes
15 and over	1	No

Interruption of the recommended schedules with a delay between doses does not interfere with the final immunity achieved nor does it necessitate starting the series over again, regardless of the length of time elapsed between doses.[32,33]

NO DATA ARE AVAILABLE TO SUPPORT THE INTERCHANGEABILITY OF HibTITER OR OTHER HAEMOPHILUS b CONJUGATE VACCINES WITH ONE ANOTHER FOR THE PRIMARY IMMUNIZATION SERIES. THEREFORE, IT IS RECOMMENDED THAT THE SAME CONJUGATE VACCINE BE USED THROUGHOUT EACH IMMUNIZATION SCHEDULE, CONSISTENT WITH THE DATA SUPPORTING APPROVAL AND LICENSURE OF THE VACCINE.

Each dose of 0.5 mL is formulated to contain 10 µg of purified Haemophilus b saccharide and approximately 25 µg of CRM_{197} protein.

STORAGE

Stability studies indicate that HibTITER® can be shipped at ambient temperatures and stored at 2°–8°C (36°–46°F). DO NOT FREEZE.

HOW SUPPLIED

Vial, 1 Dose (4 per package) —Product No. 0005-0104-41
Vial, 10 Dose —Product No. 0005-0201-10

REFERENCES

1. United States Patent Number 4,902,506 by Anderson PW, Eby RJ filed May 5, 1986 issued February 20, 1990.
2. Seid RC Jr, Boykins RA, Liu DF, et al. Chemical evidence for covalent linkage of a semi-synthetic glycoconjugate vaccine for *Haemophilus influenzae* type b disease. *Glycoconjugate J.* 1989;6:489–498.
3. Wenger JD, Ward JL, Broome CV. Prevention of *Haemophilus influenzae* type b disease: vaccines and passive prophylaxis. In: Remington JS, Swartz MS, eds. *Current Clinical Topics in Infectious Diseases.* New York, NY: McGraw-Hill Inc; 1989;10:306–339.
4. Recommendation of the Immunization Practices Advisory Committee (ACIP)–polysaccharide vaccine for prevention of *Haemophilus influenzae* type b disease. *MMWR.* 1985;34:201–205.
5. Sell SH. Long term sequelae of bacterial meningitis in children. *Pediatr Infect Dis J.* 1983;2:90–93.
6. Broome CV. Epidemiology of *Haemophilus influenzae* type b infections in the United States. *Pediatr Infect Dis J.* 1987;6:779–782.
7. Alexander HE. The productive or curative element in type b *Haemophilus influenzae* rabbit serum. *Yale J Biol Med.* 1944;16:425–434.
8. Peltola H, Kayhty H, Sivonen A. *Haemophilus influenzae* type b capsular polysaccharide vaccine in children: a double-blind field study of 100,000 vaccinees 3 months to 5 years of age in Finland. *Pediatrics.* 1977;60:730–737.
9. Robbins JB, Parke JC Jr, Schneerson R. Quantitative measurement of "natural" and immunization-induced *Haemophilus influenzae* type b capsular polysaccharide antibodies. *Pediatr Res.* 1973;7:103-110.
10. Kayhty H, Peltola H, Karanko V, et al. The protective level of serum antibodies to the capsular polysaccharide of *Haemophilus influenzae* type b. *J Infect Dis.* 1983;147:1100.
11. Kayhty H, Karanko, V, Peltola H, et al. Serum antibodies after vaccination with *Haemophilus influenzae* type b capsular polysaccharide and responses to reimmunization: no evidence of immunologic tolerance or memory. *Pediatrics.* 1984;74:857–865.
12. Weinberg GA, Granoff DM. Polysaccharide-protein conjugate vaccines for the prevention of *Haemophilus influenzae* type b disease. *J Pediatr.* 1988;113:621–631.
13. Makela O, Péterfy F, Outshoorn IG, et al. Immunogenic properties of α (1–6) dextran, its protein conjugates, and conjugates of its breakdown products in mice. *Scand J Immunol.* 1984;19:541–550.
14. Anderson P, Pichichero ME, Insel RA. Immunogens consisting of oligosaccharides from *Haemophilus influenzae* type b coupled to diphtheria toxoid or the toxin protein CRM_{197}. *J Clin Invest.* 1985;76:52–59.
15. Madore DV, Phipps DC, Eby R, et al. Immune response of young children vaccinated with *Haemophilus influenzae* type b conjugate vaccines. In: Cruse JM, Lewis RE, eds. *Contributions to Microbiology and Immunology: Conjugate Vaccines.* New York, NY: Karger Medical and Scientific Publishers: 1989;10:125–150.
16. Madore DV, Phipps DC, Eby R, et al. Safety and immunologic response to *Haemophilus influenzae* type b oligosaccharide CRM_{197} conjugate vaccine in 1- to 6-month-old infants. *Pediatrics.* 1990;85:331–337.
17. Madore DV, Johnson CL, Phipps DC, et al. Safety and immunogenicity of *Haemophilus influenzae* type b oligosaccharide CRM_{197} conjugate vaccine in infants aged 15–23 months. *Pediatrics.* 1990;86:527–534.
18. Rothstein EP, Madore DV, Long S. Antibody persistence four years after primary immunization of infants and toddlers with *Haemophilus influenzae* type b CRM_{197} conjugate vaccine. *J Pediatr.* 1991;119:655–657.
19. Schlesinger Y, Granoff DM. Avidity and bactericidal activity of antibodies elicited by different *Haemophilus influenzae* type b conjugate vaccines. *JAMA.* 1992; 267: 1489–1494.
20. Unpublished data available from Lederle Laboratories.
21. Gigliotti F, Feldman S, Wang WC, et al. Immunization of young infants with sickle cell disease with a *Haemophilus influenzae* type b saccharide-diphtheria CRM_{197} protein conjugate vaccine. *J Pediatr.* 1989;114:1006-1010.
22. Black SB, Shinefield HR, The Kaiser Permanente Pediatric Vaccine Study Group. Immunization with oligosaccharide conjugate *Haemophilus influenzae* type b (HbOC) vaccine on a large health maintenance organization population: extended follow-up and impact on *Haemophilus influenzae* disease epidemiology. *Pediatr Infect Dis J.* 1992;11:610–613.
23. Black SB, Shinefield HR, Fireman B, et al. Safety, immunogenicity, and efficacy in infancy of oligosaccharide conjugate *Haemophilus influenzae* type b vaccine in a United States Population: possible implications for optimal use. *J Infect Dis.* 1992;165 (suppl 1):S139–S143.
24. Granoff DM, Anderson EL, Osterholm MT, et al. Differences in the immunogenicity of three *Haemophilus influenzae* type b conjugate vaccines in infants. *J Pediatr.* 1992;121:187–194.
25. Decker MD, Edwards KM, Bradley R, et al. Comparative trial in infants of four conjugate *Haemophilus influenzae* type b vaccines. *J Pediatr.* 1992;120:184–189.
26. Adams WG, Deaver KA, Cochi SL, et al. Decline of childhood *Haemophilus influenzae* type b (Hib) disease in the Hib vaccine era. *JAMA.* 1993;269:221–226.
27. Murphy TV, White KE, Pastor P, et al. Declining incidence of *Haemophilus influenzae* type b disease since introduction of vaccination. *JAMA.* 1993;269:246–248.
28. Broadhurst LE, Erickson RL, Kelley PW. Decreases in invasive *Haemophilus influenzae* diseases in US Army children, 1984 through 1991. *JAMA.* 1993;269:227–231.
29. Shapiro ED. Infections caused by *Haemophilus influenzae* type b: the beginning of the end? *JAMA.* 1993;269: 264–266.
30. Black SB, Shinefield HR, Lampert D, et al. Safety and immunogenicity of oligosaccharide conjugate *Haemophilus influenzae* type b (HbOC) vaccine in infancy. *Pediatr Infect Dis J.* 1991;10:92–96.
31. Black SB, Shinefield HR, Fireman B, et al. Efficacy in infancy of oligosaccharide conjugate *Haemophilus influenzae* type b (HbOC) vaccine in a United States Population of 61,080 children. *Pediatr Infect Dis J.* 1991;10:97–104.
32. Recommendations of the AAP: *Haemophilus influenzae* type b conjugate vaccines: recommendations for immunization of infants and children 2 months of age and older: update. *Pediatrics.* 1991;88:169–172.
33. Recommendation of the ACIP: Haemophilus b conjugate vaccines for prevention of *Haemophilus influenzae* type b disease among infants and children two months of age and older. *MMWR.* 1991;40:1–7.
34. Jones RG, Bass JW, Weisse ME, et al. Antigenuria after immunization with *Haemophilus influenzae* oligosaccharide CRM_{197} conjugate (HbOC) vaccine. *Pediatr Infect Dis J.* 1991;10:557–559.
35. American Academy of Pediatrics: Report of the Committee on Infectious Diseases. 22nd ed. Elk Grove Village, Ill: American Academy of Pediatrics; 1991.
36. Recommendation of the ACIP—immunization of children infected with human T-lymphotrophic virus type III/lymphadenopathy-associated virus. *MMWR.* 1986;35(38):595–606.
37. Immunization of children infected with human immunodeficiency virus—supplementary ACIP statement. *MMWR.* 1988;37(12):181–183.
38. General Recommendations on Immunization—recommendations of the Immunization Practices Advisory Committee (ACIP). *MMWR.* 1989;38(13):221.
39. Spinola SM, Sheaffer CI, Philbrick KB, et al. Antigenuria after *Haemophilus influenzae* type b polysaccharide immunization: a prospective study. *J Pediatr.* 1986;109:835–837.
40. CDC. Vaccine Adverse Event Reporting System—United States. *MMWR.* 1990;39:730–733.
41. Paradiso PR. Combined childhood immunizations. *JAMA.* 1992;268:1685.
42. Milstein JB, Gross TP, Kuritsky JN. Adverse reactions reported following receipt of *Haemophilus influenzae* type b vaccine: an analysis after one year of marketing. *Pediatrics.* 1987;80:270–274.
43. D'Cruz DF, Shapiro ED, Spiegelman KN, et al. Acute inflammatory demyelinating polyradiculoneuropathy (Guillain-Barré syndrome) after immunization with *Haemophilus influenzae* type b conjugate vaccine. *J Pediatr.* 1989;115:743–746.

Manufactured by:
LEDERLE LABORATORIES
Division American Cyanamid Company
Pearl River, NY 10965 USA
US Gov't. License No. 17
Marketed by:
WYETH-LEDERLE VACCINES AND PEDIATRICS
Wyeth-Ayerst Laboratories
Philadelphia, PA 19101
CI 6100-1 Issued September 29, 1999

Shown in Product Identification Guide, page 320

MATERNA® ℞

[mă-tĕr-nă]

Prenatal Vitamin and Mineral Tablets
For Use Before, During & After Pregnancy

DESCRIPTION

One tablet daily provides:

VITAMINS	
A*	5,000 IU
(50% as Beta Carotene)	
D	400 IU
E (*dl*-alpha tocopheryl acetate)	30 IU
C (ascorbic acid)	120 mg
Folic Acid	1 mg
B_1 (thiamine mononitrate)	3 mg
B_2 (riboflavin)	3.4 mg
B_6 (pyridoxine hydrochloride)	10 mg
Niacinamide	20 mg
B_{12} (cyanocobalamin)	12 mcg
Biotin	30 mcg
Pantothenic Acid (calcium pantothenate)	10 mg
MINERALS	
Calcium (calcium carbonate)	200 mg
Iodine (potassium iodide)	150 mcg
Iron (ferrous fumarate)	27 mg
Magnesium (magnesium oxide)	25 mg
Copper (cupric oxide)	2 mg
Zinc (zinc oxide)	25 mg
Chromium (chromium chloride)	25 mcg
Molybdenum (sodium molybdate)	25 mcg
Manganese (manganese sulfate)	5 mg
Selenium (sodium selenate)	20 mcg

*Input as vitamin A acetate and beta carotene

MATERNA contains no artificial dyes, flavors or added sweeteners.

INDICATIONS

To provide vitamin and mineral supplementation prior to conception, throughout pregnancy and during the postnatal period for both the lactating and nonlactating mother.

DOSAGE

Before, during and after pregnancy, one tablet daily, or as directed by a physician.

WARNING: Accidental overdose of iron-containing products is a leading cause of fatal poisoning in children under six. Keep this product out of the reach of children. In case of accidental overdose, call a doctor or poison control center immediately.

CAUTION

Federal law prohibits dispensing without prescription.

PRECAUTIONS

Folic acid may partially correct the hematological damage due to vitamin B_{12} deficiency of pernicious anemia, while the associated neurological damage progresses. In rare instances, allergic hypersensitivity has been reported following administration of folic acid.

NOTICE: Contact with moisture may produce surface discoloration or erosion of the tablet.

HOW SUPPLIED

MATERNA is available as oblong-shaped, scored, sand-colored, film-coated tablets, engraved with "M" to the left of the score and "55" to the right of the score on one side of each tablet and "MATERNA" on the other side, in bottles of 100, NDC 0005-5586-11.

Store at room temperature, approximately 25°C; avoid excess heat. Dispense in well-closed, light-resistant container.

A child-resistant safety cap is provided as a safeguard against accidental ingestion by children.

Questions or Comments: 1-800-999-9384

Manufactured by:
LEDERLE PHARMACEUTICAL DIVISION
American Cyanamid Company
Pearl River, NY 10965

Shown in Product Identification Guide, page 320

MINOCIN® ℞

[mĭ-nō-sĭn]

Sterile
Minocycline Hydrochloride
Intravenous
100 mg/Vial

DESCRIPTION

MINOCIN minocycline hydrochloride, a semisynthetic derivative of tetracycline, is named [4*S* -(4α,4aα,5aα,12aα)]-4,7-bis(dimethylamino)-1,4,4a,5,5a,6,11,12a-octahydro-3,10,-12,12a-tetrahydroxy-1, 11-dioxo-2-naphthacenecarboxamide monohydrochloride.

Each vial, dried by cryodesiccation, contains sterile minocycline HCl equivalent to 100 mg minocycline. When reconstituted with 5 mL of Sterile Water for Injection USP, the pH ranges from 2.0 to 2.8.

ACTIONS

Microbiology

The tetracyclines are primarily bacteriostatic and are thought to exert their antimicrobial effect by the inhibition of protein synthesis. Minocycline HCl is a tetracycline with antibacterial activity comparable to other tetracyclines with activity against a wide range of gram-negative and gram-positive organisms.

Tube dilution testing: Microorganisms may be considered susceptible (likely to respond to minocycline therapy) if the minimum inhibitory concentration (MIC) is not more than 4 mcg/mL. Microorganisms may be considered intermediate (harboring partial resistance) if the MIC is 4 to 12.5 mcg/mL and resistant (not likely to respond to minocycline therapy) if the MIC is greater than 12.5 mcg/mL.

Susceptibility plate testing: If the Kirby-Bauer method of susceptibility testing (using a 30 mcg tetracycline disc) gives a zone of 18 mm or greater, the bacterial strain is considered to be susceptible to any tetracycline. Minocycline shows moderate *in vitro* activity against certain strains of staphylococci which have been found resistant to other tetracyclines. For such strains, minocycline susceptibility powder may be used for additional susceptibility testing.

Human Pharmacology

Following a single dose of 200 mg administered intravenously to 10 healthy male volunteers, serum levels ranged from 2.52 to 6.63 mcg/mL (average 4.18), after 12 hours they ranged from 0.82 to 2.64 mcg/mL (average 1.38). In a group of five healthy male volunteers, serum levels of 1.4 to 1.8 mcg/mL were maintained at 12 and 24 hours with doses of 100 mg every 12 hours for three days. When given 200 mg once daily for three days, the serum levels had fallen to approximately 1 mcg/mL at 24 hours. The serum half-life following I.V. doses of 100 mg every 12 hours or 200 mg once daily did not differ significantly and ranged from 15 to 23 hours. The serum half-life following a single 200 mg oral dose in 12 essentially normal volunteers ranged from 11 to 17 hours, in 7 patients with hepatic dysfunction ranged from 11 to 16 hours, and in 5 patients with renal dysfunction from 18 to 69 hours.

Intravenously administered minocycline appears similar to oral doses in excretion. The urinary and fecal recovery of oral minocycline when administered to 12 normal volunteers is one-half to one-third that of other tetracyclines.

INDICATIONS

MINOCIN is indicated in infections caused by the following microorganisms:

- Rickettsiae: (Rocky Mountain spotted fever, typhus fever and the typhus group, Q fever, rickettsialpox, tick fevers).
- *Mycoplasma pneumoniae* (PPLO, Eaton agent).
- Agents of psittacosis and ornithosis.
- Agents of lymphogranuloma venereum and granuloma inguinale.
- The spirochetal agent of relapsing fever (*Borrelia recurrentis*).

The following gram-negative microorganisms:

- *Haemophilus ducreyi* (chancroid),
- *Yersinia pestis* and *Francisella tularensis,* formerly *Pasteurella pestis* and *Pasteurella tularensis,*
- *Bartonella bacilliformis,*
- *Bacteroides* species,
- *Vibrio comma* and *Vibrio fetus,*
- *Brucella* species (in conjunction with streptomycin).

Because many strains of the following groups of microorganisms have been shown to be resistant to tetracyclines, culture and susceptibility testing are recommended.

MINOCIN is indicated for treatment of infections caused by the following gram-negative microorganisms when bacteriologic testing indicates appropriate susceptibility to the drug:

- *Escherichia coli,*
- *Enterobacter aerogenes* (formerly *Aerobacter aerogenes*),
- *Shigella* species,
- *Mima species* and *Herellea* species,
- *Haemophilus influenzae* (respiratory infections),
- *Klebsiella* species (respiratory and urinary infections).

MINOCIN is indicated for treatment of infections caused by the following gram-positive microorganisms when bacteriologic testing indicates appropriate susceptibility to the drug:

Streptococcus species:

Up to 44% of strains of *Streptococcus pyogenes* and 74% of *Streptococcus faecalis* have been found to be resistant to tetracycline drugs. Therefore, tetracyclines should not be used for streptococcal disease unless the organism has been demonstrated to be sensitive.

For upper respiratory infections due to Group A beta-hemolytic streptococci, penicillin is the usual drug of choice, including prophylaxis of rheumatic fever.

- *Streptococcus pneumoniae,*
- *Staphylococcus aureus,* skin and soft tissue infections.

Tetracyclines are not the drugs of choice in the treatment of any type of staphylococcal infection.

When penicillin is contraindicated, tetracyclines are alternative drugs in the treatment of infections due to:

- *Neisseria gonorrhoeae,* and *Neisseria meningitidis,*
- *Treponema pallidum* and *Treponema pertenue* (syphilis and yaws),
- *Listeria monocytogenes,*
- *Clostridium* species,
- *Bacillus anthracis,*
- *Fusobacterium fusiforme* (Vincent's infection),
- *Actinomyces* species.

In acute intestinal amebiasis, the tetracyclines may be a useful adjunct to amebicides.

MINOCIN minocycline HCl is indicated in the treatment of trachoma, although the infectious agent is not always eliminated, as judged by immunofluorescence.

Inclusion conjunctivitis may be treated with oral tetracyclines or with a combination of oral and topical agents.

CONTRAINDICATIONS

This drug is contraindicated in persons who have shown hypersensitivity to any of the tetracyclines.

WARNINGS

In the presence of renal dysfunction, particularly in pregnancy, intravenous tetracycline therapy in daily doses exceeding 2 g has been associated with deaths through liver failure.

When the need for intensive treatment outweighs its potential dangers (mostly during pregnancy or in individuals with known or suspected renal or liver impairment), it is advisable to perform renal and liver function tests before and during therapy. Also, tetracycline serum concentrations should be followed.

If renal impairment exists, even usual oral or parenteral doses may lead to excessive systemic accumulation of the drug and possible liver toxicity. Under such conditions, lower than usual total doses are indicated, and if therapy is prolonged, serum level determinations of the drug may be advisable. This hazard is of particular importance in the parenteral administration of tetracyclines to pregnant or postpartum patients with pyelonephritis. When used under these circumstances, the blood level should not exceed 15 mcg/mL and liver function tests should be made at frequent intervals. Other potentially hepatotoxic drugs should not be prescribed concomitantly.

THE USE OF TETRACYCLINES DURING TOOTH DEVELOPMENT (LAST HALF OF PREGNANCY, INFANCY, AND CHILDHOOD TO THE AGE OF 8 YEARS) MAY CAUSE PERMANENT DISCOLORATION OF THE TEETH (YELLOW-GRAY-BROWN). This adverse reaction is more common during long-term use of the drugs but has been observed following repeated short-term courses. Enamel hypoplasia has also been reported. TETRACYCLINES, THEREFORE, SHOULD NOT BE USED IN THIS AGE GROUP UNLESS OTHER DRUGS ARE NOT LIKELY TO BE EFFECTIVE OR ARE CONTRAINDICATED.

Photosensitivity manifested by an exaggerated sunburn reaction has been observed in some individuals taking tetracyclines. Patients apt to be exposed to direct sunlight or ultraviolet light should be advised that this reaction can occur with tetracycline drugs, and treatment should be discontinued at the first evidence of skin erythema. Studies to date indicate that photosensitivity is rarely reported with MINOCIN minocycline HCl.

The anti-anabolic action of the tetracyclines may cause an increase in BUN. While this is not a problem in those with normal renal function, in patients with significantly impaired function, higher serum levels of tetracycline may lead to azotemia, hyperphosphatemia, and acidosis.

CNS side effects including light-headedness, dizziness or vertigo have been reported. Patients who experience these symptoms should be cautioned about driving vehicles or using hazardous machinery while on minocycline therapy. These symptoms may disappear during therapy and usually disappear rapidly when the drug is discontinued.

Usage in Pregnancy

(See above **WARNINGS** about use during tooth development.)

Results of animal studies indicate that tetracyclines cross the placenta, are found in fetal tissues and can have toxic effects on the developing fetus (often related to retardation of skeletal development). Evidence of embryotoxicity has also been noted in animals treated early in pregnancy.

The safety of MINOCIN for use during pregnancy has not been established.

Usage in Newborns, Infants, and Children

(See above **WARNINGS** about use during tooth development.)

All tetracyclines form a stable calcium complex in any bone-forming tissue. A decrease in the fibula growth rate has been observed in prematures given oral tetracycline in doses of 25 mg/kg every 6 hours. This reaction was shown to be reversible when the drug was discontinued.

Tetracyclines are present in the milk of lactating women who are taking a drug in this class.

PRECAUTIONS

General

Pseudotumor cerebri (benign intracranial hypertension) in adults has been associated with the use of tetracyclines. The usual clinical manifestations are headache and blurred vision. Bulging fontanels have been associated with the use of tetracyclines in infants. While both of these conditions and related symptoms usually resolve soon after discontinuation of the tetracycline, the possibility for permanent sequelae exists.

As with other antibiotic preparations, use of this drug may result in overgrowth of nonsusceptible organisms, including fungi. If superinfection occurs, the antibiotic should be discontinued and appropriate therapy should be instituted.

In venereal diseases when coexistent syphilis is suspected, darkfield examination should be done before treatment is started and the blood serology repeated monthly for at least 4 months.

In long-term therapy, periodic laboratory evaluation of organ systems, including hematopoietic, renal, and hepatic studies should be performed.

All infections due to Group A beta-hemolytic streptococci should be treated for at least ten days.

Drug Interactions

Because tetracyclines have been shown to depress plasma prothrombin activity, patients who are on anticoagulant therapy may require downward adjustment of their anticoagulant dosage.

Since bacteriostatic drugs may interfere with the bactericidal action of penicillin, it is advisable to avoid giving tetracycline in conjunction with penicillin.

Concurrent use of tetracyclines with oral contraceptives may render oral contraceptives less effective.

ADVERSE REACTIONS

Gastrointestinal: Anorexia, nausea, vomiting, diarrhea, glossitis, dysphagia, enterocolitis, pancreatitis, inflammatory lesions (with monilial overgrowth) in the anogenital region, and increases in liver enzymes. Rarely, hepatitis and liver failure have been reported.

These reactions have been caused by both the oral and parenteral administration of tetracyclines.

Skin: Maculopapular and erythematous rashes. Exfoliative dermatitis has been reported but is uncommon. Fixed drug eruptions, including balanitis, have been rarely reported. Erythema multiforme and rarely Stevens-Johnson syndrome have been reported. Photosensitivity is discussed above. (See **WARNINGS.**)

Pigmentation of the skin and mucous membranes has been reported.

Tooth discoloration has been reported, rarely, in adults.

Renal Toxicity: Rise in BUN has been reported and is apparently dose related. (See **WARNINGS.**) Reversible acute renal failure has been rarely reported.

Hypersensitivity Reactions: Urticaria, angioneurotic edema, polyarthralgia, anaphylaxis, anaphylactoid purpura, pericarditis, exacerbation of systemic lupus erythematosus, and rarely, pulmonary infiltrates with eosinophilia have been reported. A transient lupus-like syndrome has also been reported.

Blood: Hemolytic anemia, thrombocytopenia, neutropenia, and eosinophilia have been reported.

CNS: (See **WARNINGS.**) Pseudotumor cerebri (benign intracranial hypertension) in adults and bulging fontanels in infants. (See **PRECAUTIONS—General.**) Headache has also been reported.

Other: When given over prolonged periods, tetracyclines have been reported to produce brown-black microscopic discoloration of the thyroid glands. Very rare cases of abnormal thyroid function have been reported.

Decreased hearing has been rarely reported in patients on MINOCIN.

Continued on next page

Minocin Intravenous—Cont.

DOSAGE AND ADMINISTRATION

Note: Rapid administration is to be avoided. Parenteral therapy is indicated only when oral therapy is not adequate or tolerated. Oral therapy should be instituted as soon as possible. If intravenous therapy is given over prolonged periods of time, thrombophlebitis may result.

ADULTS: Usual adult dose: 200 mg followed by 100 mg every 12 hours and should not exceed 400 mg in 24 hours. The cryodesiccated powder should be reconstituted with 5 mL Sterile Water for Injection USP and immediately further diluted to 500 mL to 1,000 mL with Sodium Chloride Injection USP, Dextrose Injection USP, Dextrose and Sodium Chloride Injection USP, Ringer's Injection USP, or Lactated Ringer's Injection USP, but not other solutions containing calcium because a precipitate may form. When further diluted in 500 mL to 1,000 mL compatible solutions (except Lactated Ringers), the pH usually ranges from 2.5 to 4.0. The pH of MINOCIN IV 100 mg in Lactated Ringers 500 mL to 1,000 mL usually ranges from 4.5 to 6.0.

Final dilutions (500 mL to 1,000 mL) should be administered immediately but product and diluents are compatible at room temperature for 24 hours without a significant loss of potency. Any unused portions must be discarded after that period.

For children above eight years of age: Usual pediatric dose: 4 mg/kg followed by 2 mg/kg every 12 hours.

In patients with renal impairment: (See **WARNINGS.**)

Total dosage should be decreased by reduction of recommended individual doses and/or by extending time intervals between doses.

Parenteral drug products should be inspected visually for particulate matter and discoloration prior to administration, whenever solution and container permit.

HOW SUPPLIED

MINOCIN® minocycline HCl Intravenous is supplied as 100 mg vials of sterile cryodesiccated powder.

Product No. NDC 0205-5305-94

Store at Controlled Room Temperature 15–30°C (59–86°F).

Manufactured by:
LEDERLE PARENTERALS, INC.
Carolina, Puerto Rico 00987
50422-95 Revised January 1995

Shown in Product Identification Guide, page 320

MINOCIN® ℞
Minocycline Hydrochloride
Pellet-Filled Capsules

DESCRIPTION

MINOCIN minocycline hydrochloride, a semisynthetic derivative of tetracycline, is [4*S* -(4α,4aα,5aα,12aα)] -4,7-bis(dimethylamino)-1,4,4a,5,5a,6,11,12a-octahydro-3,10,12,12a-tetrahydroxy-1,11-dioxo-2-naphthacenecarboxamide monohydrochloride.

MINOCIN minocycline hydrochloride pellet-filled capsules for oral administration contain pellets of minocycline HCl equivalent to 50 mg or 100 mg of minocycline in microcrystalline cellulose.

The capsule shells contain the following inactive ingredients: Blue 1, Gelatin, Titanium Dioxide and Yellow 10. The 50 mg capsule shells also contain Black and Yellow Iron Oxides.

CLINICAL PHARMACOLOGY

MINOCIN minocycline hydrochloride pellet-filled capsules are rapidly absorbed from the gastrointestinal tract following oral administration. Following a single dose of two 100 mg pellet-filled capsules of MINOCIN minocycline HCl administered to 18 normal fasting adult volunteers, maximum serum concentrations were attained in 1 to 4 hours (average 2.1 hours) and ranged from 2.1 to 5.1 mcg/mL (average 3.5 mcg/mL). The serum half-life in the normal volunteers ranged from 11.1 to 22.1 hours (average 15.5 hours).

When MINOCIN minocycline hydrochloride pellet-filled capsules were given concomitantly with a meal which included dairy products, the extent of absorption of MINOCIN minocycline hydrochloride pellet-filled capsules was not noticeably influenced. The peak plasma concentrations were slightly decreased (11.2%) and delayed by one hour when administered with food, compared to dosing under fasting conditions.

In previous studies with other minocycline dosage forms, the minocycline serum half-life ranged from 11 to 16 hours in 7 patients with hepatic dysfunction, and from 18 to 69 hours in 5 patients with renal dysfunction. The urinary and fecal recovery of minocycline when administered to 12 normal volunteers is one-half to one-third that of other tetracyclines.

Microbiology

The tetracyclines are primarily bacteriostatic and are thought to exert their antimicrobial effect by the inhibition of protein synthesis. The tetracyclines, including minocycline, have similar antimicrobial spectra of activity against a wide range of gram-positive and gram-negative organisms. Cross-resistance of these organisms to tetracyclines is common.

While *in vitro* studies have demonstrated the susceptibility of most strains of the following microorganisms, clinical efficacy for infections other than those included in the **INDICATIONS AND USAGE** section has not been documented.

GRAM-NEGATIVE BACTERIA:
Bartonella bacilliformis
Brucella species
Calymmatobacterium granulomatis
Campylobacter fetus
Francisella tularensis
Haemophilus ducreyi
Haemophilus influenzae
Listeria monocytogenes
Neisseria gonorrhoeae
Vibrio cholerae
Yersinia pestis

Because many strains of the following groups of gram-negative microorganisms have been shown to be resistant to tetracyclines, culture and susceptibility tests are especially recommended:
Acinetobacter species
Bacteroides species
Enterobacter aerogenes
Escherichia coli
Klebsiella species
Shigella species

GRAM-POSITIVE BACTERIA:
Because many strains of the following groups of gram-positive microorganisms have been shown to be resistant to tetracyclines, culture and susceptibility testing are especially recommended. Up to 44 percent of *Streptococcus pyogenes* strains have been found to be resistant to tetracycline drugs. Therefore, tetracyclines should not be used for streptococcal disease unless the organism has been demonstrated to be susceptible.
Enterococcus group [*Enterococcus faecalis* (formerly *Streptococcus faecalis*) and *Enterococcus faecium* (formerly *Streptococcus faecium*)]
Streptococcus pneumoniae
Streptococcus pyogenes
Viridans group streptococci

OTHER MICROORGANISMS:
Actinomyces species
Bacillus anthracis
Balantidium coli
Borrelia recurrentis
Chlamydia psittaci
Chlamydia trachomatis
Clostridium species
Entamoeba species
Fusobacterium fusiforme
Mycoplasma pneumoniae
Propionibacterium acnes
Rickettsiae
Treponema pallidum
Treponema pertenue
Ureaplasma urealyticum

Susceptibility Tests

Diffusion Techniques

The use of antibiotic disk susceptibility test methods which measure zone diameter gives an accurate estimation of susceptibility of microorganisms to MINOCIN. One such standard procedure[1] has been recommended for use with disks for testing antimicrobials. Either the 30 mcg tetracycline-class disk or the 30 mcg minocycline disk should be used for the determination of the susceptibility of microorganisms to minocycline.

With this type of procedure a report of "susceptible" from the laboratory indicates that the infecting organism is likely to respond to therapy. A report of "intermediate susceptibility" suggests that the organism would be susceptible if a high dosage is used or if the infection is confined to tissues and fluids (e.g., urine) in which high antibiotic levels are attained. A report of "resistant" indicates that the infecting organism is not likely to respond to therapy. With either the tetracycline-class disk or the minocycline disk, zone sizes of 19 mm or greater indicate susceptibility, zone sizes of 14 mm or less indicate resistance, and zone sizes of 15 to 18 mm indicate intermediate susceptibility.

Standardized procedures require the use of laboratory control organisms. The 30 mcg tetracycline disk should give zone diameters between 19 and 28 mm for *Staphylococcus aureus* ATCC 25923 and between 18 and 25 mm for *Escherichia coli* ATCC 25922. The 30 mcg minocycline disk should give zone diameters between 25 and 30 mm for *S. aureus* ATCC 25923 and between 19 and 25 mm for *E. coli* ATCC 25922.

Dilution Techniques

When using the NCCLS agar dilution or broth dilution (including microdilution) method[2] or equivalent, a bacterial isolate may be considered susceptible if the MIC (minimal inhibitory concentration) of minocycline is 4 mcg/mL or less. Organisms are considered resistant if the MIC is 16 mcg/mL or greater. Organisms with an MIC value of less than 16 mcg/mL but greater than 4 mcg/mL are expected to be susceptible if a high dosage is used or if the infection is confined to tissues and fluids (e.g., urine) in which high antibiotic levels are attained.

As with standard diffusion methods, dilution procedures require the use of laboratory control organisms. Standard tetracycline or minocycline powder should give MIC values of 0.25 mcg/mL to 1.0 mcg/mL for *S. aureus* ATCC 25923, and 1.0 mcg/mL to 4.0 mcg/mL for *E. coli* ATCC 25922.

INDICATIONS AND USAGE

MINOCIN minocycline hydrochloride pellet-filled capsules are indicated in the treatment of the following infections due to susceptible strains of the designated microorganisms:

Rocky Mountain spotted fever, typhus fever and the typhus group, Q fever, rickettsialpox and tick fevers caused by *Rickettsiae.*
Respiratory tract infections caused by *Mycoplasma pneumoniae.*
Lymphogranuloma venereum caused by *Chlamydia trachomatis.*
Psittacosis (Ornithosis) due to *Chlamydia psittaci.*
Trachoma caused by *Chlamydia trachomatis,* although the infectious agent is not always eliminated, as judged by immunofluorescence.
Inclusion conjunctivitis caused by *Chlamydia trachomatis.*
Nongonococcal urethritis in adults caused by *Ureaplasma urealyticum* or *Chlamydia trachomatis.*
Relapsing fever due to *Borrelia recurrentis.*
Chancroid caused by *Haemophilus ducreyi.*
Plague due to *Yersinia pestis.*
Tularemia due to *Francisella tularensis.*
Cholera caused by *Vibrio cholerae.*
Campylobacter fetus infections caused by *Campylobacter fetus.*
Brucellosis due to *Brucella* species (in conjunction with streptomycin).
Bartonellosis due to *Bartonella bacilliformis.*
Granuloma inguinale caused by *Calymmatobacterium granulomatis.*

Minocycline is indicated for treatment of infections caused by the following gram-negative microorganisms, when bacteriologic testing indicates appropriate susceptibility to the drug:
Escherichia coli.
Enterobacter aerogenes.
Shigella species.
Acinetobacter species.
Respiratory tract infections caused by *Haemophilus influenzae.*
Respiratory tract and urinary tract infections caused by *Klebsiella* species.

MINOCIN minocycline hydrochloride pellet-filled capsules are indicated for the treatment of infections caused by the following gram-positive microorganisms when bacteriologic testing indicates appropriate susceptibility to the drug:
Upper respiratory tract infections caused by *Streptococcus pneumoniae.*
Skin and skin structure infections caused by *Staphylococcus aureus.* (Note: Minocycline is not the drug of choice in the treatment of any type of staphylococcal infection.)
Uncomplicated urethritis in men due to *Neisseria gonorrhoeae* and for the treatment of other gonococcal infections when penicillin is contraindicated.

When penicillin is contraindicated, minocycline is an alternative drug in the treatment of the following infections:
Infections in women caused by *Neisseria gonorrhoeae.*
Syphilis caused by *Treponema pallidum.*
Yaws caused by *Treponema pertenue.*
Listeriosis due to *Listeria monocytogenes.*
Anthrax due to *Bacillus anthracis.*
Vincent's infection caused by *Fusobacterium fusiforme.*
Actinomycosis caused by *Actinomyces israelii.*
Infections caused by *Clostridium* species.

In *acute intestinal amebiasis,* minocycline may be a useful adjunct to amebicides.

In severe *acne,* minocycline may be useful adjunctive therapy.

Oral minocycline is indicated in the treatment of asymptomatic carriers of *Neisseria meningitidis* to eliminate meningococci from the nasopharynx. In order to preserve the usefulness of minocycline in the treatment of asymptomatic meningococcal carrier, diagnostic laboratory procedures, including serotyping and susceptibility testing, should be performed to establish the carrier state and the correct treatment. It is recommended that the prophylactic use of minocycline be reserved for situations in which the risk of meningococcal meningitis is high.

Oral minocycline is not indicated for the treatment of meningococcal infection.

Although no controlled clinical efficacy studies have been conducted, limited clinical data show that oral minocycline hydrochloride has been used successfully in the treatment of infections caused by *Mycobacterium marinum.*

CONTRAINDICATIONS

This drug is contraindicated in persons who have shown hypersensitivity to any of the tetracyclines.

WARNINGS

MINOCIN PELLET-FILLED CAPSULES, LIKE OTHER TETRACYCLINE-CLASS ANTIBIOTICS, CAN CAUSE FETAL HARM WHEN ADMINISTERED TO A PREGNANT WOMAN. IF ANY TETRACYCLINE IS USED DURING PREGNANCY OR IF THE PATIENT BECOMES PREGNANT WHILE TAKING THESE DRUGS, THE PATIENT SHOULD BE APPRISED OF THE POTENTIAL HAZARD TO THE FETUS. THE USE OF DRUGS OF THE TETRACYCLINE CLASS DURING TOOTH DEVELOPMENT (LAST HALF OF PREGNANCY, INFANCY, AND

CHILDHOOD TO THE AGE OF 8 YEARS) MAY CAUSE PERMANENT DISCOLORATION OF THE TEETH (YELLOW-GRAY-BROWN).
This adverse reaction is more common during long-term use of the drug but has been observed following repeated short-term courses. Enamel hypoplasia has also been reported. TETRACYCLINE DRUGS, THEREFORE, SHOULD NOT BE USED DURING TOOTH DEVELOPMENT UNLESS OTHER DRUGS ARE NOT LIKELY TO BE EFFECTIVE OR ARE CONTRAINDICATED.
All tetracyclines form a stable calcium complex in any bone-forming tissue. A decrease in fibula growth rate has been observed in premature human infants given oral tetracycline in doses of 25 mg/kg every six hours. This reaction was shown to be reversible when the drug was discontinued.
Results of animal studies indicate that tetracyclines cross the placenta, are found in fetal tissues, and can have toxic effects on the developing fetus (often related to retardation of skeletal development). Evidence of embryotoxicity has been noted in animals treated early in pregnancy.
The anti-anabolic action of the tetracyclines may cause an increase in BUN. While this is not a problem in those with normal renal function, in patients with significantly impaired function, higher serum levels of tetracycline may lead to azotemia, hyperphosphatemia, and acidosis. If renal impairment exists, even usual oral or parenteral doses may lead to excessive systemic accumulations of the drug and possible liver toxicity. Under such conditions, lower than usual total doses are indicated, and if therapy is prolonged, serum level determinations of the drug may be advisable.
Photosensitivity manifested by an exaggerated sunburn reaction has been observed in some individuals taking tetracyclines. This has been reported rarely with minocycline.
Central nervous system side effects including light-headedness, dizziness, or vertigo have been reported with minocycline therapy. Patients who experience these symptoms should be cautioned about driving vehicles or using hazardous machinery while on minocycline therapy. These symptoms may disappear during therapy and usually disappear rapidly when the drug is discontinued.

PRECAUTIONS

General

As with other antibiotic preparations, use of this drug may result in overgrowth of non-susceptible organisms, including fungi. If superinfection occurs, the antibiotic should be discontinued and appropriate therapy instituted.
Pseudotumor cerebri (benign intracranial hypertension) in adults has been associated with the use of tetracyclines. The usual clinical manifestations are headache and blurred vision. Bulging fontanels have been associated with the use of tetracyclines in infants. While both of these conditions and related symptoms usually resolve after discontinuation of the tetracycline, the possibility for permanent sequelae exists.
Incision and drainage or other surgical procedures should be performed in conjunction with antibiotic therapy when indicated.

Information For Patients

Photosensitivity manifested by an exaggerated sunburn reaction has been observed in some individuals taking tetracyclines. Patients apt to be exposed to direct sunlight or ultraviolet light should be advised that this reaction can occur with tetracycline drugs, and treatment should be discontinued at the first evidence of skin erythema. This reaction has been reported rarely with use of minocycline.
Patients who experience central nervous system symptoms (see **WARNINGS**) should be cautioned about driving vehicles or using hazardous machinery while on minocycline therapy.
Concurrent use of tetracycline may render oral contraceptives less effective (see **Drug Interactions**).

Laboratory Tests

In venereal disease when coexistent syphilis is suspected, a dark-field examination should be done before treatment is started and the blood serology repeated monthly for at least four months.
In long-term therapy, periodic laboratory evaluations of organ systems, including hematopoietic, renal, and hepatic studies, should be performed.

Drug Interactions

Because tetracyclines have been shown to depress plasma prothrombin activity, patients who are on anticoagulant therapy may require downward adjustment of their anticoagulant dosage.
Since bacteriostatic drugs may interfere with the bactericidal action of penicillin, it is advisable to avoid giving tetracycline-class drugs in conjunction with penicillin.
Absorption of tetracyclines is impaired by antacids containing aluminum, calcium or magnesium, and iron-containing preparations.
The concurrent use of tetracycline and methoxyflurane has been reported to result in fatal renal toxicity.
Concurrent use of tetracyclines with oral contraceptives may render oral contraceptives less effective.

Drug/Laboratory Test Interactions

False elevations of urinary catecholamine levels may occur due to interference with the fluorescence test.

Carcinogenesis, Mutagenesis, Impairment of Fertility

Dietary administration of minocycline in long term tumorigenicity studies in rats resulted in evidence of thyroid tumor production. Minocycline has also been found to produce thyroid hyperplasia in rats and dogs. In addition, there has been evidence of oncogenic activity in rats in studies with a related antibiotic, oxytetracycline (i.e., adrenal and pituitary tumors). Likewise, although mutagenicity studies of minocycline have not been conducted, positive results in *in vitro* mammalian cell assays (i.e., mouse lymphoma and Chinese hamster lung cells) have been reported for related antibiotics (tetracycline hydrochloride and oxytetracycline). Segment I (fertility and general reproduction) studies have provided evidence that minocycline impairs fertility in male rats.

Teratogenic Effects: Pregnancy: *Pregnancy Category D:* (See **WARNINGS**.) *Nonteratogenic Effects:* (See **WARNINGS**.)

Labor and Delivery

The effect of tetracyclines on labor and delivery is unknown.

Nursing Mothers

Tetracyclines are excreted in human milk. Because of the potential for serious adverse reactions in nursing infants from the tetracyclines, a decision should be made whether to discontinue nursing or discontinue the drug, taking into account the importance of the drug to the mother (see **WARNINGS**).

Pediatric Use

See **WARNINGS.**

ADVERSE REACTIONS

Due to oral minocycline's virtually complete absorption, side effects to the lower bowel, particularly diarrhea, have been infrequent. The following adverse reactions have been observed in patients receiving tetracyclines.
Gastrointestinal: Anorexia, nausea, vomiting, diarrhea, glossitis, dysphagia, enterocolitis, pancreatitis, inflammatory lesions (with monilial overgrowth) in the anogenital region, and increases in liver enzymes. Rarely, hepatitis and liver failure have been reported. Rare instances of esophagitis and esophageal ulcerations have been reported in patients taking the tetracycline-class antibiotics in capsule and tablet form. Most of these patients took the medication immediately before going to bed (see **DOSAGE AND ADMINISTRATION**).
Skin: Maculopapular and erythematous rashes. Exfoliative dermatitis has been reported but is uncommon. Fixed drug eruptions have been rarely reported. Lesions occurring on the glans penis have caused balanitis. Erythema multiforme and rarely Stevens-Johnson syndrome have been reported. Photosensitivity is discussed above (see **WARNINGS**). Pigmentation of the skin and mucous membranes has been reported.
Renal toxicity: Elevations in BUN have been reported and are apparently dose related (see **WARNINGS**). Reversible acute renal failure has been rarely reported.
Hypersensitivity reactions: Urticaria, angioneurotic edema, polyarthralgia, anaphylaxis, anaphylactoid purpura, pericarditis, exacerbation of systemic lupus erythematosus and rarely pulmonary infiltrates with eosinophilia have been reported. A transient lupus-like syndrome has also been reported.
Blood: Hemolytic anemia, thrombocytopenia, neutropenia, and eosinophilia have been reported.
Central nervous system: Bulging fontanels in infants and benign intracranial hypertension (Pseudotumor cerebri) in adults (see **PRECAUTIONS—General**) have been reported. Headache has also been reported.
Other: When given over prolonged periods, tetracyclines have been reported to produce brown-black microscopic discoloration of the thyroid glands. Very rare cases of abnormal thyroid function have been reported.
Decreased hearing has been rarely reported in patients on MINOCIN®.
Tooth discoloration in children less than 8 years of age (see **WARNINGS**) and also, rarely, in adults has been reported.

OVERDOSAGE

Minocycline is not removed in significant quantities by hemodialysis or peritoneal dialysis. In one study, four patients received 200 mg oral doses 3 hours prior to hemodialysis, following flow rates of 100 to 200 mL/min there was no consistent difference between venous and arterial minocycline concentrations and no detectable minocycline was found in the dialysate. In another study, four patients were administered IP minocycline over 72 to 96 hours and achieved blood concentrations of 1.5 to 2 mcg/mL, over the following 12 hours drug free dialysate was used. No detectable minocycline was found to transfer from the blood to the dialysate.
In case of overdosage, discontinue medication, treat symptomatically, and institute supportive measures.

DOSAGE AND ADMINISTRATION

THE USUAL DOSAGE AND FREQUENCY OF ADMINISTRATION OF MINOCYCLINE DIFFERS FROM THAT OF THE OTHER TETRACYCLINES. EXCEEDING THE RECOMMENDED DOSAGE MAY RESULT IN AN INCREASED INCIDENCE OF SIDE EFFECTS.

MINOCIN minocycline hydrochloride pellet-filled capsules may be taken with or without food (see **CLINICAL PHARMACOLOGY**).

Adults

The usual dosage of MINOCIN minocycline hydrochloride pellet-filled capsules is 200 mg initially followed by 100 mg every 12 hours. Alternatively, if more frequent doses are preferred, two or four 50 mg pellet-filled capsules may be given initially followed by one 50 mg capsule four times daily.

For children above 8 years of age

The usual dosage of MINOCIN minocycline hydrochloride pellet-filled capsules is 4 mg/kg initially followed by 2 mg/kg every 12 hours.
Uncomplicated gonococcal infections other than urethritis and anorectal infections in men: 200 mg initially, followed by 100 mg every 12 hours for a minimum of four days, with post-therapy cultures within 2 to 3 days.
In the treatment of uncomplicated gonococcal urethritis in men, 100 mg every 12 hours for five days is recommended.
For the treatment of syphilis, the usual dosage of MINOCIN minocycline hydrochloride pellet-filled capsules should be administered over a period of 10 to 15 days. Close follow-up, including laboratory tests, is recommended.
In the treatment of meningococcal carrier state, the recommended dosage is 100 mg every 12 hours for five days.
Mycobacterium marinum infections: Although optimal doses have not been established, 100 mg every 12 hours for 6 to 8 weeks have been used successfully in a limited number of cases.
Uncomplicated nongonococcal urethral infection in adults caused by *Chlamydia trachomatis* or *Ureaplasma urealyticum:* 100 mg orally, every 12 hours for at least seven days.
Ingestion of adequate amounts of fluids along with capsule and tablet forms of drugs in the tetracycline-class is recommended to reduce the risk of esophageal irritation and ulceration.
In patients with renal impairment (see **WARNINGS**), the total dosage should be decreased by either reducing the recommended individual doses and/or by extending the time intervals between doses.

HOW SUPPLIED

MINOCIN® minocycline hydrochloride pellet-filled capsules are supplied as capsules containing minocycline hydrochloride equivalent to 100 mg and 50 mg minocycline.
100 mg, two-piece, hard-shell capsule with an opaque light green cap and a transparent green body, printed in white ink with Lederle over M46 on one half and Lederle over 100 mg on the other half. Each capsule contains pellets of minocycline HCl equivalent to 100 mg of minocycline, supplied as follows:
NDC 0005-5344-18—Bottle of 50
50 mg, two-piece, hard-shell capsule with an opaque yellow cap and a transparent green body, printed in black ink with Lederle over M45 on one half and Lederle over 50 mg on the other half. Each capsule contains pellets of minocycline HCl equivalent to 50 mg of minocycline, supplied as follows:
NDC 0005-5343-23—Bottle of 100
NDC 0005-5343-27—Bottle of 250

Store at Controlled Room Temperature 20°–25°C (68°–77°F).

Protect from light, moisture and excessive heat.

ANIMAL PHARMACOLOGY AND TOXICOLOGY

MINOCIN minocycline HCl has been observed to cause a dark discoloration of the thyroid in experimental animals (rats, minipigs, dogs, and monkeys). In the rat, chronic treatment with MINOCIN has resulted in goiter accompanied by elevated radioactive iodine uptake and evidence of thyroid tumor production. MINOCIN has also been found to produce thyroid hyperplasia in rats and dogs.

REFERENCES

1. National Committee for Clinical Laboratory Standards, Approved Standard: *Performance Standards for Antimicrobial Disk Susceptibility Tests,* 3rd Edition, Vol. 4(16): M2-A3, Villanova, PA, December 1984.
2. National Committee for Clinical Laboratory Standards, Approved Standard: *Methods for Dilution Antimicrobial Susceptibility Tests for Bacteria that Grow Aerobically,* 2nd Edition, Vol. 5(22):M7-A, Villanova, PA, December 1985.

Manufactured by:
LEDERLE PHARMACEUTICAL DIVISION
American Cyanamid Company
Pearl River, NY 10965
CI 4957-2 Revised August 18, 1998

Shown in Product Identification Guide, page 320

MINOCIN® ℞

[*mī′nō-sĭn*]

Minocycline Hydrochloride
Oral Suspension

DESCRIPTION

MINOCIN minocycline hydrochloride, a semisynthetic derivative of tetracycline, is named [4*S*-(4α, 4aα, 5aα, 12aα)]-4,7 - bis (dimethylamino) - 1,4,4a,5,5a,6,11,12a - octahydro-3,10,12,12a - tetrahydroxy - 1,11 - dioxo - 2 - naphthacenecarboxamide monohydrochloride.
Its structural formula is:

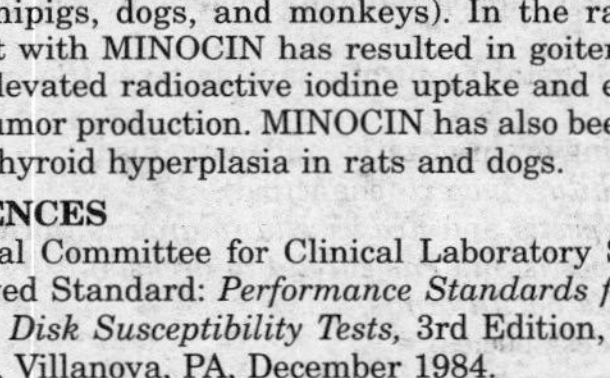

$C_{23}H_{27}N_3O_7 \cdot HCl$ M.W. 493.94

MINOCIN Oral Suspension contains minocycline HCl equivalent to 50 mg of minocycline per 5 mL (10 mg/mL)

Continued on next page

Minocin Oral—Cont.

and the following inactive ingredients: Alcohol, Butylparaben, Calcium Hydroxide, Cellulose, Decaglyceryl Tetraoleate, Edetate Calcium Disodium, Glycol, Guar Gum, Polysorbate 80, Propylparaben, Propylene Glycol, Sodium Saccharin, Sodium Sulfite (see **WARNINGS**) and Sorbitol.

ACTIONS

Microbiology

The tetracyclines are primarily bacteriostatic and are thought to exert their antimicrobial effect by the inhibition of protein synthesis. Minocycline HCl is a tetracycline with antibacterial activity comparable to other tetracyclines with activity against a wide range of gram-negative and gram-positive organisms.

Tube dilution testing: Microorganisms may be considered susceptible (likely to respond to minocycline therapy) if the minimum inhibitory concentration (MIC) is not more than 4 mcg/mL. Microorganisms may be considered intermediate (harboring partial resistance) if the MIC is 4 to 12.5 mcg/mL and resistant (not likely to respond to minocycline therapy) if the MIC is greater than 12.5 mcg/mL.

Susceptibility plate testing: If the Kirby-Bauer method of susceptibility testing (using a 30 mcg tetracycline disc) gives a zone of 18 mm or greater, the bacterial strain is considered to be susceptible to any tetracycline. Minocycline shows moderate *in vitro* activity against certain strains of staphylococci which have been found resistant to other tetracyclines. For such strains minocycline susceptibility powder may be used for additional susceptibility testing.

Human Pharmacology

Following a single dose of two 100 mg minocycline HCl capsules administered to ten normal adult volunteers, serum levels ranged from 0.74 to 4.45 mcg/mL in one hour (average 2.24), after 12 hours, they ranged from 0.34 to 2.36 mcg/mL (average 1.25). The serum half-life following a single 200 mg dose in 12 essentially normal volunteers ranged from 11 to 17 hours. In seven patients with hepatic dysfunction it ranged from 11 to 16 hours, and in 5 patients with renal dysfunction from 18 to 69 hours. The urinary and fecal recovery of minocycline when administered to 12 normal volunteers is one half to one third that of other tetracyclines.

INDICATIONS

MINOCIN is indicated in infections caused by the following microorganisms:

Rickettsiae: (Rocky Mountain spotted fever, typhus fever and the typhus group, Q fever, rickettsialpox, tick fevers).

Mycoplasma pneumoniae (PPLO, Eaton agent).

Agents of psittacosis and ornithosis.

Agents of lymphogranuloma venereum and granuloma inguinale.

The spirochetal agent of relapsing fever (*Borrelia recurrentis*).

The following gram-negative microorganisms:

Haemophilus ducreyi (chancroid),
Yersinia pestis and *Francisella tularensis* (formerly *Pasteurella pestis* and *Pasteurella tularensis*),
Bartonella bacilliformis,
Bacteroides species,
Vibrio comma and *Vibrio fetus,*
Brucella species (in conjunction with streptomycin).

Because many strains of the following groups of microorganisms have been shown to be resistant to tetracyclines, culture and susceptibility testing are recommended.

MINOCIN is indicated for treatment of infections caused by the following gram-negative microorganisms when bacteriologic testing indicates appropriate susceptibility to the drug:

Escherichia coli,
Enterobacter aerogenes (formerly *Aerobacter aerogenes*),
Shigella species,
Acinetobacter calcoaceticus (formerly Herellea, Mima),
Haemophilus influenzae (respiratory infections),
Klebsiella species (respiratory and urinary infections).

MINOCIN is indicated for treatment of infections caused by the following gram-positive microorganisms when bacteriologic testing indicates appropriate susceptibility to the drug:

Streptococcus species:

Up to 44% of strains of *Streptococcus pyogenes* and 74% of *Streptococcus faecalis* have been found to be resistant to tetracycline drugs. Therefore, tetracyclines should not be used for streptococcal disease unless the organism has been demonstrated to be sensitive.

For upper respiratory infections due to Group A beta-hemolytic streptococci, penicillin is the usual drug of choice, including prophylaxis of rheumatic fever.

Streptococcus pneumoniae (formerly Diplococcus pneumoniae),

Staphylococcus aureus, skin and soft tissue infections.

Tetracyclines are not the drugs of choice in the treatment of any type of staphylococcal infection.

MINOCIN is indicated for the treatment of uncomplicated gonococcal urethritis in men due to *Neisseria gonorrhoeae.*

When penicillin is contraindicated, tetracyclines are alternative drugs in the treatment of infections due to:

Neisseria gonorrhoeae (in women),
Treponema pallidum and *Treponema pertenue* (syphilis and yaws),
Listeria monocytogenes,
Clostridium species,
Bacillus anthracis,
Fusobacterium fusiforme (Vincent's infection),
Actinomyces species.

In acute intestinal amebiasis, the tetracyclines may be a useful adjunct to amebicides.

In severe acne, the tetracyclines may be useful adjunctive therapy.

MINOCIN minocycline HCl is indicated in the treatment of trachoma, although the infectious agent is not always eliminated, as judged by immunofluorescence.

MINOCIN is indicated for the treatment of uncomplicated urethral, endocervical or rectal infections in adults caused by *Chlamydia trachomatis* or *Ureaplasma urealyticum.*[1]

Inclusion conjunctivitis may be treated with oral tetracyclines or with a combination of oral and topical agents.

MINOCIN is indicated in the treatment of asymptomatic carriers of *Neisseria meningitidis* to eliminate meningococci from the nasopharynx.

In order to preserve the usefulness of MINOCIN in the treatment of asymptomatic meningococcal carriers, diagnostic laboratory procedures, including serotyping and susceptibility testing, should be performed to establish the carrier state and the correct treatment. It is recommended that the drug be reserved for situations in which the risk of meningococcal meningitis is high.

MINOCIN by oral administration is not indicated for the treatment of meningococcal infection.

Although no controlled clinical efficacy studies have been conducted, limited clinical data show that oral MINOCIN has been used successfully in the treatment of infections caused by Mycobacterium marinum.

CONTRAINDICATIONS

This drug is contraindicated in persons who have shown hypersensitivity to any of the tetracyclines.

WARNINGS

THE USE OF DRUGS OF THE TETRACYCLINE CLASS DURING TOOTH DEVELOPMENT (LAST HALF OF PREGNANCY, INFANCY, AND CHILDHOOD TO THE AGE OF 8 YEARS) MAY CAUSE PERMANENT DISCOLORATION OF THE TEETH (YELLOW-GRAY-BROWN). This adverse reaction is more common during long-term use of the drugs but has been observed following repeated short-term courses. Enamel hypoplasia has also been reported. TETRACYCLINE DRUGS, THEREFORE, SHOULD NOT BE USED IN THIS AGE GROUP UNLESS OTHER DRUGS ARE NOT LIKELY TO BE EFFECTIVE OR ARE CONTRAINDICATED.

If renal impairment exists, even usual oral or parenteral doses may lead to excessive systemic accumulations of the drug and possible liver toxicity. Under such conditions, lower than usual total doses are indicated, and if therapy is prolonged, serum level determinations of the drug may be advisable.

Photosensitivity manifested by an exaggerated sunburn reaction has been observed in some individuals taking tetracyclines. Patients apt to be exposed to direct sunlight or ultraviolet light should be advised that this reaction can occur with tetracycline drugs, and treatment should be discontinued at the first evidence of skin erythema. Studies to date indicate that photosensitivity is rarely reported with MINOCIN minocycline HCl.

The anti-anabolic action of the tetracyclines may cause an increase in BUN. While this is not a problem in those with normal renal function, in patients with significantly impaired function, higher serum levels of tetracycline may lead to azotemia, hyperphosphatemia, and acidosis.

CNS side effects including light-headedness, dizziness, or vertigo have been reported. Patients who experience these symptoms should be cautioned about driving vehicles or using hazardous machinery while on minocycline therapy. These symptoms may disappear during therapy and usually disappear rapidly when the drug is discontinued.

MINOCIN Oral Suspension contains sodium sulfite, a sulfite that may cause allergic-type reactions including anaphylactic symptoms and life-threatening or less severe asthmatic episodes in certain susceptible people. The overall prevalence of sulfite sensitivity in the general population is unknown and probably low. Sulfite sensitivity is seen more frequently in asthmatic than in nonasthmatic people.

Usage in Pregnancy (See above **WARNINGS** about use during tooth development.)

Results of animal studies indicate that tetracyclines cross the placenta, are found in fetal tissues and can have toxic effects on the developing fetus (often related to retardation of skeletal development). Evidence of embryotoxicity has also been noted in animals treated early in pregnancy.

The safety of MINOCIN for use during pregnancy has not been established.

Usage in Newborns, Infants, and Children (See above **WARNINGS** about use during tooth development.)

All tetracyclines form a stable calcium complex in any bone forming tissue. A decrease in the fibula growth rate has been observed in prematures given oral tetracycline in doses of 25 mg/kg every six hours. This reaction was shown to be reversible when the drug was discontinued.

Tetracyclines are present in the milk of lactating women who are taking a drug in this class.

PRECAUTIONS

General

Pseudotumor cerebri (benign intracranial hypertension) in adults has been associated with the use of tetracyclines. The usual clinical manifestations are headache and blurred vision. Bulging fontanels have been associated with the use of tetracyclines in infants. While both of these conditions and related symptoms usually resolve soon after discontinuation of the tetracycline, the possibility for permanent sequelae exists.

As with other antibiotic preparations, use of this drug may result in overgrowth of nonsusceptible organisms, including fungi. If superinfection occurs, the antibiotic should be discontinued and appropriate therapy should be instituted.

In venereal diseases when coexistent syphilis is suspected, darkfield examination should be done before treatment is started and the blood serology repeated monthly for at least 4 months.

In long-term therapy, periodic laboratory evaluation of organ systems, including hematopoietic, renal and hepatic studies should be performed.

All infections due to Group A beta-hemolytic streptococci should be treated for at least ten days.

Drug Interactions

Because tetracyclines have been shown to depress plasma prothrombin activity, patients who are on anticoagulant therapy may require downward adjustment of their anticoagulant dosage.

Since bacteriostatic drugs may interfere with the bactericidal action of penicillin, it is advisable to avoid giving tetracycline in conjunction with penicillin.

Concurrent use of tetracyclines with oral contraceptives may render oral contraceptives less effective.

ADVERSE REACTIONS

Gastrointestinal: Anorexia, nausea, vomiting, diarrhea, glossitis, dysphagia, enterocolitis, pancreatitis, inflammatory lesions (with monilial overgrowth) in the anogenital region and increases in liver enzymes. Rarely, hepatitis and liver failure have been reported.

These reactions have been caused by both the oral and parenteral administration of tetracyclines.

Skin: Maculopapular and erythematous rashes. Exfoliative dermatitis has been reported but is uncommon. Fixed drug eruptions, including balanitis, have been rarely reported. Erythema multiforme and rarely Stevens-Johnson syndrome have been reported. Photosensitivity is discussed above. (See **WARNINGS.**)

Pigmentation of the skin and mucous membranes has been reported.

Tooth discoloration has been reported rarely in adults.

Renal toxicity: Rise in BUN has been reported and is apparently dose related. (See **WARNINGS.**) Reversible acute renal failure has been rarely reported.

Hypersensitivity reactions: Urticaria, angioneurotic edema, polyarthralgia, anaphylaxis, anaphylactoid purpura, pericarditis, exacerbation of systemic lupus erythematosus and rarely pulmonary infiltrates with eosinophilia have been reported. A transient lupus-like syndrome has also been reported.

Blood: Hemolytic anemia, thrombocytopenia, neutropenia and eosinophilia have been reported.

CNS: (See **WARNINGS.**) Pseudotumor cerebri (benign intracranial hypertension) in adults and bulging fontanels in infants. (See **PRECAUTIONS—General.**) Headache has also been reported.

Other: When given over prolonged periods, tetracyclines have been reported to produce brown-black microscopic discoloration of the thyroid glands. Very rare cases of abnormal thyroid function have been reported.

Decreased hearing has been rarely reported in patients on MINOCIN.

DOSAGE AND ADMINISTRATION

Therapy should be continued for at least 24 to 48 hours after symptoms and fever have subsided.

Concomitant therapy: Antacids containing aluminum, calcium, or magnesium impair absorption and should not be given to patients taking oral tetracycline.

Studies to date have indicated that the absorption of MINOCIN is not notably influenced by foods and dairy products.

In patients with renal impairment: (See **WARNINGS.**) Total dosage should be decreased by reduction of recommended individual doses and/or extending time intervals between doses.

In the treatment of streptococcal infections, a therapeutic dose of tetracycline should be administered for at least ten days.

ADULTS: The usual dosage of MINOCIN is 200 mg initially followed by 100 mg every 12 hours.

For children above eight years of age: The usual dosage of MINOCIN minocycline HCl is 4 mg/kg initially followed by 2 mg/kg every 12 hours.

For treatment of syphilis, the usual dosage of MINOCIN should be administered over a period of 10 to 15 days. Close follow up, including laboratory tests, is recommended.

Gonorrhea patients sensitive to penicillin may be treated with MINOCIN, administered as 200 mg initially followed by 100 mg every twelve hours for a minimum of four days, with post-therapy cultures within 2 to 3 days.

In the treatment of meningococcal carrier state, recommended dosage is 100 mg every 12 hours for five days.

Mycobacterium marinum infections: Although optimal doses have not been established, 100 mg twice a day for 6 to 8 weeks have been used successfully in a limited number of cases.

Uncomplicated urethral, endocervical, or rectal infection in adults caused by *Chlamydia trachomatis* or *Ureaplasma urealyticum:* 100 mg, by mouth, 2 times a day for at least seven days.[1]

In the treatment of uncomplicated gonococcal urethritis in men, 100 mg twice a day orally for five days is recommended.

HOW SUPPLIED

MINOCIN® minocycline hydrochloride Oral Suspension contains minocycline hydrochloride equivalent to 50 mg minocycline per teaspoonful (5 mL). Preserved with propylparaben 0.10% and butylparaben 0.06% with Alcohol USP 5% v/v, Custard-flavored.

NDC 0005-5313-56 Bottle 2 fl. oz. (60 mL)

Store at controlled room temperature, between 20°C and 25°C (68°F and 77°F).

DO NOT FREEZE.

Animal Pharmacology and Toxicology

MINOCIN has been found to produce high blood concentrations following oral dosage to various animal species and to be extensively distributed to all tissues examined in ^{14}C-labeled drug studies in dogs. MINOCIN has been found experimentally to produce discoloration of the thyroid glands. This finding has been observed in rats and dogs. Changes in thyroid function have also been found in these animal species. However, no change in thyroid function has been observed in humans.

Reference: 1. CDC Sexually Transmitted Diseases Treatment Guidelines 1982.

Manufactured by:
LEDERLE PHARMACEUTICAL DIVISION
American Cyanamid Company
Pearl River, NY 10965
CI 6016-1 Issued February 23, 1999

Shown in Product Identification Guide, page 320

NEPTAZANE® ℞

[*něp-ta-zāne*]
methazolamide
Tablets, USP

(For full prescribing information, please refer to the 2001 PDR for Ophthalmology.)

PIPRACIL® ℞

[*pĭp' ră-sĭl*]
piperacillin sodium
For Intravenous and Intramuscular Use

DESCRIPTION

PIPRACIL piperacillin sodium is a semisynthetic broad-spectrum penicillin for parenteral use derived from D(-)α-aminobenzylpenicillin. The chemical name of piperacillin sodium is 4-Thia-1-azabicyclo[3.2.0]heptane-2-carboxylic acid, 6-[[[[(4-ethyl-2,3-dioxo-1-piperazinyl)carbonyl]amino]phenylacetyl]amino]-3,3-dimethyl-7-oxo-, monosodium salt, [2*S*-[2α, 5α, 6β(*S**)]].

PIPRACIL is a white to off-white solid having the characteristic appearance of products prepared by freeze-drying. Freely soluble in water and in alcohol. The pH of the aqueous solution is 5.5 to 7.5. One g contains 1.85 mEq (42.5 mg) of sodium (Na^+).

CLINICAL PHARMACOLOGY

Intravenous Administration. In healthy adult volunteers, mean serum levels immediately after a two to three minute intravenous injection of 2, 4, or 6 g were 305, 412, and 775 mcg/mL. Serum levels lack dose proportionality.

[See table at bottom of next page]

Intramuscular Administration. PIPRACIL is rapidly absorbed after intramuscular injection. In healthy volunteers, the mean peak serum concentration occurs approximately 30 minutes after a single dose of 2 g and is about 36 mcg/mL. The oral administration of 1 g probenecid before injection produces an increase in piperacillin peak serum level of about 30%. The area under the curve (AUC) is increased by approximately 60%.

General

PIPRACIL is not absorbed when given orally. Peak serum concentrations are attained approximately 30 minutes after intramuscular injections and immediately after completion of intravenous injection or infusion. The serum half-life in healthy volunteers ranges from 36 minutes to one hour and 12 minutes. The mean elimination half-life of PIPRACIL in healthy adult volunteers is 54 minutes following administration of 2 g and 63 minutes following 6 g. As with other penicillins, PIPRACIL is eliminated primarily by glomerular filtration and tubular secretion; it is excreted rapidly as unchanged drug in high concentrations in the urine. Approximately 60% to 80% of the administered dose is excreted in the urine in the first 24 hours. Piperacillin urine concentrations, determined by microbioassay, were as high as 14,100 mcg/mL following a 6 g intravenous dose and 8,500 mcg/mL following a 4 g intravenous dose. These urine drug concentrations remained well above 1,000 mcg/mL throughout the dosing interval. The elimination half-life is increased twofold in mild to moderate renal impairment and fivefold to sixfold in severe impairment.

PIPRACIL binding to human serum proteins is 16%. The drug is widely distributed in human tissues and body fluids, including bone, prostate, and heart and reaches high concentrations in bile. After a 4 g bolus, maximum biliary concentrations averaged 3,205 mcg/mL. It penetrates into the cerebrospinal fluid in the presence of inflamed meninges. Because PIPRACIL is excreted by the biliary route as well as by the renal route, it can be used safely in appropriate dosage (see **DOSAGE AND ADMINISTRATION**) in patients with severely restricted kidney function, and can be used effectively in treatment of hepatobiliary infections.

Microbiology

PIPRACIL is an antibiotic which exerts its bactericidal activity by inhibiting both septum and cell wall synthesis. It is active against a variety of gram-positive and gram-negative aerobic and anaerobic bacteria. *In vitro,* piperacillin is active against most strains of clinical isolates of the following microorganisms:

Aerobic and facultatively anaerobic organisms
- *Gram-negative bacteria*
  - *Escherichia coli*
  - *Proteus mirabilis*
  - *Proteus vulgaris*
  - *Morganella morganii* (formerly *Proteus morganii)*
  - *Providencia rettgeri* (formerly *Proteus rettgeri)*
  - *Serratia* species including *S marcescens* and *S liquefaciens*
  - *Klebsiella pneumoniae*
  - *Klebsiella* species
  - *Enterobacter* species including *E aerogenes* and *E cloacae*
  - *Citrobacter* species including *C freundii* and *C diversus*
  - *Salmonella species**
  - *Shigella species**
  - *Pseudomonas aeruginosa*
  - *Pseudomonas* species including *P cepacia,* P maltophilia,** and *P fluorescens*
  - *Acinetobacter* species (formerly *Mima-Herellea)*
  - *Haemophilus influenzae* (non-β-lactamase-producing strains)
  - *Neisseria gonorrhoeae*
  - *Neisseria meningitidis**
  - *Moraxella* species*
  - *Yersinia* species* (formerly *Pasteurella)*
- *Gram-positive bacteria*
  - Group D streptococci including
    - Enterococci *(Streptococcus faecalis, S faecium)*
    - Non-enterococci*
  - β-hemolytic streptococci including
    - Group A *Streptococcus (S pyogenes)*
    - Group B *Streptococcus (S agalactiae)*
  - *Streptococcus pneumoniae*
  - *Streptococcus viridans*
  - *Staphylococcus aureus* (non-penicillinase-producing)*
  - *Staphylococcus epidermidis* (non-penicillinase-producing)*

Anaerobic bacteria
- *Actinomyces* species*
- *Bacteroides* species including
  - *B fragilis group (B fragilis, B vulgatus)*
  - Non-*B fragilis* group *(B melaninogenicus)*
  - *B asaccharolyticus**
- *Clostridium* species including
  - *C perfringens* and *C difficile**
- *Eubacterium* species
- *Fusobacterium* species including *F nucleatum* and *F necrophorum*
- *Peptococcus* species
- *Peptostreptococcus* species
- *Veillonella* species

*Piperacillin has been shown to be active *in vitro* against these organisms; however, clinical efficacy has not yet been established.

In vitro, PIPRACIL is inactivated by staphylococcal β-lactamases and β-lactamases produced by gram-negative bacteria. However, it is active against β-lactamase-producing gonococci.

Many strains of gram-negative organisms resistant to certain antibiotics have been found to be susceptible to PIPRACIL.

PIPRACIL has excellent activity against gram-positive organisms, including enterococci *(S faecalis).* It is active against obligate anaerobes such as *Bacteroides* species and also against *C difficile* (which has been associated with pseudomembranous colitis).

Piperacillin is active against many gram-negative bacteria including *Enterobacteriaceae, Klebsiella, Serratia, Pseudomonas, E coli, Proteus,* and *Citrobacter,* and, in addition, it is active against anaerobes and enterococci.

In vitro tests show piperacillin to act synergistically with aminoglycoside antibiotics against most isolates of *P aeruginosa.*

Susceptibility Testing

The use of a 100 mcg piperacillin antibiotic disk with susceptibility test methods which measure zone diameter gives an accurate estimation of susceptibility of organisms to PIPRACIL. The following standard procedure† has been recommended for use with disks for testing antimicrobials.

† NCCLS Approved Standard; M2-A2 (Formerly ASM-2) Performance Standards for Antimicrobic Disk Susceptibility Tests, Second Edition, available from the National Committee of Clinical Laboratory Standards.

With this type of procedure, a report of "susceptible" from the laboratory indicates that the infecting organism is likely to respond to therapy. A report of "intermediate susceptibility" suggests that the organism would be susceptible if high dosage is used or if the infection is confined to tissue and fluids (eg, urine) in which high antibiotic levels are obtained. A report of "resistant" indicates that the infecting organism is not likely to respond to therapy. With the piperacillin disk, a zone of 18 mm or greater indicates susceptibility, zone sizes of 14 mm or less indicate resistance, and zone sizes of 15 to 17 mm indicate intermediate susceptibility.

Haemophilus and *Neisseria* species which give zones of ≥29 mm are susceptible; resistant strains give zones of ≤28 mm. The above interpretive criteria are based on the use of the standardized procedure. Antibiotic susceptibility testing requires carefully prescribed procedures. Susceptibility tests are biased to a considerable degree when different methods are used.

The standardized procedure requires the use of control organisms. The 100 mcg piperacillin disk should give zone diameters between 24 and 30 mm for *E coli* ATCC No. 25922 and between 25 and 33 mm for *Pseudomonas aeruginosa* ATCC No. 27853.

Dilution methods such as those described in the International Collaborative Study‡ have been used to determine susceptibility of organisms to PIPRACIL.

‡*Acta Pathol Microbiol Scand* [B] 1971; suppl 217.

Enterobacteriaceae, Pseudomonas species and *Acinetobacter* sp are considered susceptible if the minimal inhibitory concentration (MIC) of piperacillin is no greater than 64 mcg/mL and are considered resistant if the MIC is greater than 128 mcg/mL.

Haemophilus and *Neisseria* species are considered susceptible if the MIC of piperacillin is ≤ to 1 mcg/mL.

When anaerobic organisms are isolated from infection sites, it is recommended that other tests such as the modified Broth-Disk Method§ be used to determine the antibiotic susceptibility of these slowly growing organisms.

§ Wilkins TD and Thiel T. *Antimicrob Agents Chemother* 1973;3:350–356.

INDICATIONS AND USAGE

Therapeutic. PIPRACIL is indicated for the treatment of serious infections caused by susceptible strains of the designated organisms in the conditions as listed below.

Intra-Abdominal Infections including hepatobiliary and surgical infections caused by *E coli, P aeruginosa,* enterococci, *Clostridium* sp, anaerobic cocci, and *Bacteroides* sp, including *B fragilis.*

Urinary Tract Infections caused by *E coli, Klebsiella* sp, *P aeruginosa, Proteus* sp, including *P mirabilis,* and enterococci.

Gynecologic Infections including endometritis, pelvic inflammatory disease, pelvic cellulitis caused by *Bacteroides* sp including *B fragilis,* anaerobic cocci, *Neisseria gonorrhoeae,* and enterococci *(S faecalis).*

Septicemia including bacteremia caused by *E coli, Klebsiella* sp, *Enterobacter* sp, *Serratia* sp, *P mirabilis, S pneumoniae,* enterococci, *P aeruginosa, Bacteroides* sp, and anaerobic cocci.

Lower Respiratory Tract Infections caused by *E coli, Klebsiella* sp, *Enterobacter* sp, *Pseudomonas aeruginosa, Serratia* sp, *H influenzae, Bacteroides* sp, and anaerobic cocci. Although improvement has been noted in patients with cystic fibrosis, lasting bacterial eradication may not necessarily be achieved.

Skin and Skin Structure Infections caused by *E coli, Klebsiella* sp, *Serratia* sp, *Acinetobacter* sp, *Enterobacter* sp, *Pseudomonas aeruginosa,* indole-positive *Proteus* sp, *Proteus mirabilis, Bacteroides* sp, including *B fragilis,* anaerobic cocci, and enterococci.

Bone and Joint Infections caused by *P aeruginosa,* enterococci, *Bacteroides* sp, and anaerobic cocci.

Gonococcal Infections. PIPRACIL has been effective in the treatment of uncomplicated gonococcal urethritis.

PIPRACIL has also been shown to be clinically effective for the treatment of infections at various sites caused by *Streptococcus* species including Group A β-hemolytic *Streptococcus* and *S pneumoniae;* however, infections caused by these organisms are ordinarily treated with more narrow spectrum penicillins. Because of its broad spectrum of bactericidal activity against gram-positive and gram-negative aerobic and anaerobic bacteria, PIPRACIL is particularly useful for the treatment of mixed infections and presumptive therapy prior to the identification of the causative organisms.

Also, PIPRACIL may be administered as single drug therapy in some situations where normally two antibiotics might be employed.

Piperacillin has been successfully used with aminoglycosides, especially in patients with impaired host defenses. Both drugs should be used in full therapeutic doses.

Appropriate cultures should be made for susceptibility testing before initiating therapy and therapy adjusted, if appropriate, once the results are known.

Prophylaxis: PIPRACIL is indicated for prophylactic use in surgery including intra-abdominal (gastrointestinal and biliary) procedures, vaginal hysterectomy, abdominal hysterectomy, and cesarean section. Effective prophylactic use depends on the time of administration and PIPRACIL should be given one-half to one hour before the operation so that

Continued on next page

Pipracil—Cont.

effective levels can be achieved in the site prior to the procedure.
The prophylactic use of piperacillin should be stopped within 24 hours, since continuing administration of any antibiotic increases the possibility of adverse reactions, but in the majority of surgical procedures, does not reduce the incidence of subsequent infections. If there are signs of infection, specimens for culture should be obtained for identification of the causative organism so that appropriate therapy can be instituted.

CONTRAINDICATIONS

A history of allergic reactions to any of the penicillins and/or cephalosporins.

WARNINGS

Serious and occasionally fatal hypersensitivity (anaphylactic) reactions have been reported in patients receiving therapy with penicillins. These reactions are more apt to occur in persons with a history of sensitivity to multiple allergens.
There have been reports of patients with a history of penicillin hypersensitivity who have experienced severe hypersensitivity reactions when treated with a cephalosporin. Before initiating therapy with PIPRACIL, careful inquiry should be made concerning previous hypersensitivity reactions to penicillins, cephalosporins, and other allergens. If an allergic reaction occurs during therapy with PIPRACIL, the antibiotic should be discontinued. The usual agents (antihistamines, pressor amines, and corticosteroids) should be readily available. SERIOUS ANAPHYLACTOID REACTIONS REQUIRE IMMEDIATE EMERGENCY TREATMENT WITH EPINEPHRINE. OXYGEN AND INTRAVENOUS CORTICOSTEROIDS AND AIRWAY MANAGEMENT INCLUDING INTUBATION SHOULD ALSO BE ADMINISTERED AS NECESSARY.

PRECAUTIONS

General
While piperacillin possesses the characteristic low toxicity of the penicillin group of antibiotics, periodic assessment of organ system functions, including renal, hepatic, and hematopoietic, during prolonged therapy is advisable.
Bleeding manifestations have occurred in some patients receiving β-lactam antibiotics, including piperacillin. These reactions have sometimes been associated with abnormalities of coagulation tests such as clotting time, platelet aggregation and prothrombin time and are more likely to occur in patients with renal failure.
If bleeding manifestations occur, the antibiotic should be discontinued and appropriate therapy instituted.
The possibility of the emergence of resistant organisms which might cause superinfections should be kept in mind, particularly during prolonged treatment. If this occurs, appropriate measures should be taken.
As with other penicillins, patients may experience neuromuscular excitability or convulsions if higher than recommended doses are given intravenously.
PIPRACIL® is a monosodium salt containing 1.85 mEq of Na^+ per g. This should be considered when treating patients requiring restricted salt intake. Periodic electrolyte determinations should be made in patients with low potassium reserves, and the possibility of hypokalemia should be kept in mind with patients who have potentially low potassium reserves and who are receiving cytotoxic therapy or diuretics.
Antimicrobials used in high doses for short periods to treat gonorrhea may mask or delay the symptoms of incubating syphilis. Therefore, prior to treatment, patients with gonorrhea should also be evaluated for syphilis. Specimens for darkfield examination should be obtained from patients with any suspected primary lesion, and serologic tests should be performed. In all cases where concomitant syphilis is suspected, monthly serological tests should be made for a minimum of 4 months.
As with other semisynthetic penicillins, PIPRACIL therapy has been associated with an increased incidence of fever and rash in cystic fibrosis patients.

Drug Interactions
The mixing of piperacillin with an aminoglycoside *in vitro* can result in substantial inactivation of the aminoglycosides.
Piperacillin when used concomitantly with vecuronium has been implicated in the prolongation of the neuromuscular blockage of vecuronium. Due to their similar mechanism of action, it is expected that the neuromuscular blockade produced by any of the non-depolarizing muscle relaxants could be prolonged in the presence of piperacillin. (See package insert for vecuronium bromide.)

Pregnancy–Pregnancy Category B
Although reproduction studies in mice and rats performed at doses up to 4 times the human dose have shown no evidence of impaired fertility or harm to the fetus, safety of PIPRACIL use in pregnant women has not been determined by adequate and well-controlled studies. Because animal reproduction studies are not always predictive of human response, this drug should be used during pregnancy only if clearly needed. It has been found to cross the placenta in rats.

Nursing Mothers
Caution should be exercised when PIPRACIL is administered to nursing mothers. It is excreted in low concentrations in milk.

Pediatric Use
Dosages for children under the age of 12 have not been established. The safety of PIPRACIL in neonates is not known. In dog neonates, dilated renal tubules and peritubular hyalinization occurred following administration of PIPRACIL.

ADVERSE EFFECTS

PIPRACIL is generally well tolerated. The most common adverse reactions have been local in nature, following intravenous or intramuscular injection. The following adverse reactions may occur.
Local Reactions. In clinical trials thrombophlebitis was noted in 4% of patients. Pain, erythema, and/or induration at the injection site occurred in 2% of patients. Less frequent reactions including ecchymosis, deep vein thrombosis and hematomas have also occurred.
Gastrointestinal. Diarrhea and loose stools were noted in 2% of patients. Other less frequent reactions included vomiting, nausea, increases in liver enzymes (LDH, SGOT, SGPT), hyperbilirubinemia, cholestatic hepatitis, bloody diarrhea and, rarely, pseudomembranous colitis.
Hypersensitivity Reactions: Anaphylactoid Reactions, see **WARNINGS.**
Rash was noted in 1% of patients. Other less frequent findings included pruritus, vesicular eruptions, positive Coombs tests.
Other dermatologic manifestations such as erythema multiforme and Stevens-Johnson syndrome have been reported rarely.
Renal. Elevations of creatinine or BUN, and, rarely, interstitial nephritis.
Central Nervous System. Headache, dizziness, fatigue.
Hemic and Lymphatic. Reversible leukopenia, neutropenia, thrombocytopenia and/or eosinophilia have been reported. As with other β-lactam antibiotics, reversible leukopenia (neutropenia) is more apt to occur in patients receiving prolonged therapy at high dosages or in association with drugs known to cause this reaction.
Serum Electrolytes. Individuals with liver disease or individuals receiving cytotoxic therapy or diuretics were reported rarely to demonstrate a decrease in serum potassium concentrations with high doses of piperacillin.
Skeletal. Rarely, prolonged muscle relaxation.
Other. Superinfection, including candidiasis. Hemorrhagic manifestations.

DOSAGE AND ADMINISTRATION

PIPRACIL may be administered by the intramuscular route (see NOTE) or intravenously or given in a three- to five-minute intravenous injection. The usual dosage of PIPRACIL for serious infections is 3- to 4-g given every four to six hours as a 20- to 30-minute infusion. For serious infections, the intravenous route should be used.
PIPRACIL should not be mixed with an aminoglycoside in a syringe or infusion bottle since this can result in inactivation of the aminoglycoside.
The maximum daily dose for adults is usually 24 g/day, although higher doses have been used.
Intramuscular injections (See NOTE) should be limited to 2 g per injection site. This route of administration has been used primarily in the treatment of patients with uncomplicated gonorrhea and urinary tract infections.
NOTE: THE ADD-VANTAGE VIAL IS *NOT* FOR IM USE.

DOSAGE RECOMMENDATIONS

Type of Infection	Usual Total Daily Dose
Serious infections such as septicemia, nosocomial pneumonia, intra-abdominal infections, aerobic and anaerobic gynecologic infections, and skin and soft tissue infections	12–18 g/d IV (200 to 300 mg/kg/d) in divided doses every 4 to 6 h
Complicated urinary tract infections	8–16 g/d IV (125–200 mg/kg/d) in divided doses every 6 to 8 h
Uncomplicated urinary tract infections and most community-acquired pneumonia	6–8 g/d IM or IV (100 to 125 mg/kg/d) in divided doses every 6 to 12 h
Uncomplicated gonorrhea infections	2 g IM* as a one-time dose

* One g of probenecid given orally one-half hour prior to injection.

The average duration of PIPRACIL treatment is from seven to ten days, except in the treatment of gynecologic infections, in which it is from three to ten days; the duration should be guided by the patient's clinical and bacteriological progress. For most acute infections, treatment should be continued for at least 48 to 72 hours after the patient becomes asymptomatic. Antibiotic therapy for Group A β-hemolytic streptococcal infections should be maintained for at least ten days to reduce the risk of rheumatic fever or glomerulonephritis.
When PIPRACIL is given concurrently with aminoglycosides, both drugs should be used in full therapeutic doses.

Renal Impairment

Dosage in Renal Impairment

Creatinine Clearance mL/min	Urinary Tract Infection (uncomplicated)	Urinary Tract Infection (complicated)	Serious Systemic Infection
>40	No dosage adjustment necessary		
20–40	No dosage adjustment necessary	9 g/day 3 g every 8 h	12 g/day 4 g every 8 h
<20	6 g/day 3 g every 12 h	6 g/day 3 g every 12 h	8 g/day 4 g every 12 h

For patients on hemodialysis the maximum daily dose is 6 g/day (2 g every 8 hours). In addition, because hemodialysis removes 30%–50% of piperacillin in 4 hours, 1 g additional dose should be administered following each dialysis period.
For patients with renal failure and hepatic insufficiency, measurement of serum levels of PIPRACIL will provide additional guidance for adjusting dosage.

Prophylaxis
When possible, PIPRACIL should be administered as a 20- to 30-minute infusion just prior to anesthesia. Administration while the patient is awake will facilitate identification of possible adverse reactions during drug infusion.

PIPERACILLIN SERUM LEVELS IN ADULTS (mcg/mL) AFTER A TWO- TO THREE-MINUTE IV INJECTION

DOSE	0	10 min	20 min	30 min	1 h	1.5 h	2 h	3 h	4 h	6 h	8 h
2	305 (159–615)	202 (164–225)	156 (52–165)	67 (41–88)	40 (25–57)	24 (18–31)	20 (14–24)	8 (3–11)	3 (2–4)	2 (<0.6–3)	—
4	412 (389–484)	344 (315–379)	295 (269–330)	117 (98–138)	93 (78–110)	60 (50–67)	36 (26–51)	20 (17–24)	8 (7–11)	4 (3.7–4.1)	0.9 (0.7–1)
6	775 (695–849)	609 (530–670)	563 (492–630)	325 (292–363)	208 (180–239)	138 (115–175)	90 (71–113)	38 (29–53)	33 (25–44)	8 (3–19)	3.2 (<2–6)

PIPERACILLIN SERUM LEVELS IN ADULTS (mcg/mL) AFTER A 30-MINUTE IV INFUSION

DOSE	0	5 min	10 min	15 min	30 min	45 min	1 h	1.5 h	2 h	4 h	6 h	7.5 h
4	244 (155–298)	215 (169–247)	186 (140–209)	177 (142–213)	141 (122–156)	146 (110–265)	105 (85–133)	72 (53–105)	53 (36–69)	15 (6–24)	4 (1–9)	2 (0.5–3)
6	353 (324–371)	298 (242–339)	298 (232–331)	272 (219–314)	229 (185–249)	180 (144–209)	149 (117–171)	104 (89–113)	73 (66–94)	22 (12–39)	16 (5–49)	— —

A 30-minute infusion of 6 g every 6 h gave, on the fourth day, a mean peak serum concentration of 420 mcg/mL.

INDICATION	1st Dose	2nd Dose	3rd Dose
Intra-abdominal Surgery	2 g IV just prior to surgery	2 g during surgery	2 g every 6 h Post-Op for no more than 24 h
Vaginal Hysterectomy	2 g IV just prior to surgery	2 g 6 h after 1st dose	2 g 12 h after 1st dose
Cesarean Section	2 g IV after cord is clamped	2 g 4 h after 1st dose	2 g 8 h after 1st dose
Abdominal Hysterectomy	2 g IV just prior to surgery	2 g on return to recovery room	2 g after 6 h

Infants and Children: Dosages in infants and children under 12 years of age have not been established.

PRODUCT RECONSTITUTION/DOSAGE PREPARATION

Conventional Vials:

Diluents for Reconstitution

Sterile Water for Injection
Bacteriostatic¶ Water for Injection
Sodium Chloride Injection
Bacteriostatic¶ Sodium Chloride Injection
Dextrose 5% in Water
Dextrose 5% and 0.9% Sodium Chloride
#Lidocaine HCl 0.5% to 1% (without epinephrine)

¶ Either Parabens or Benzyl Alcohol
# For Intramuscular Use Only. Lidocaine is contraindicated in patients with a known history of hypersensitivity to local anesthetics of the amide type.

Conventional Vials:
Intravenous Solutions

Dextrose 5% in Water
0.9% Sodium Chloride
Dextrose 5% and 0.9% Sodium Chloride
Lactated Ringer's Injection††
Dextran 6% in 0.9% Sodium Chloride

†† When PIPRACIL® is further diluted with Lactated Ringer's Injection, the diluted solution must be administered within 2 hours.

Intravenous Admixtures

Normal Saline [+ KCl 40 mEq]
5% Dextrose in Water [+ KCl 40 mEq]
5% Dextrose/Normal Saline [+ KCl 40 mEq]
Ringer's Injection [+ KCl 40 mEq]
Lactated Ringer's Injection [+ KCl 40 mEq]††

†† When PIPRACIL® is further diluted with Lactated Ringer's Injection, the diluted solution must be administered within 2 hours.

ADD-Vantage Vials:**
ADD-Vantage System Admixtures

Dextrose 5% in Water (50 or 100 mL)
0.9% Sodium Chloride (50 or 100 mL)

** (ADD-Vantage is the registered trademark of Abbott Laboratories.)

INTRAVENOUS ADMINISTRATION

Reconstitution Directions for Conventional Vials: Reconstitute each gram of PIPRACIL with at least 5 mL of a suitable diluent (except Lidocaine HCl 0.5%–1% without epinephrine) listed above. Shake well until dissolved. Reconstituted solution may be further diluted to the desired volume (eg, 50 or 100 mL) in the above listed intravenous solutions and admixtures.

Reconstitution Directions for ADD-Vantage Vials: See Instruction Sheet provided in box.

Reconstitution Directions for PHARMACY BULK VIAL: Reconstitute the 40 g vial with 172 mL of a suitable diluent (except Lidocaine HCl 0.5%–1% without epinephrine) listed above to achieve a concentration of 1 g per 5 mL.

Directions for Administration:

Intermittent IV Infusion

Infuse diluted solution over a period of about 30 minutes. During infusion it is desirable to discontinue the primary intravenous solution.

Intravenous Injection (Bolus)

Reconstituted solution should be injected slowly over a 3- to 5-minute period to help avoid vein irritation.

INTRAMUSCULAR ADMINISTRATION (CONVENTIONAL VIALS ONLY)

Reconstitution Directions: Reconstitute each gram of PIPRACIL with 2 mL of a suitable diluent listed above to achieve a concentration of 1 g per 2.5 mL. Shake well until dissolved.

Directions for Administration

When indicated by clinical and bacteriological findings, intramuscular administration of 6 to 8 g daily of PIPRACIL, in divided doses, may be utilized for initiation of therapy. In addition, intramuscular administration of the drug may be considered for maintenance therapy after clinical and bacteriologic improvement has been obtained with intravenous piperacillin sodium treatment. Intramuscular administration should not exceed 2 g per injection at any one site.

The preferred site is the upper outer quadrant of the buttock (ie, *gluteus maximus*).

The deltoid area should be used only if well-developed, and then only with caution to avoid radial nerve injury. Intramuscular injections should not be made into the lower or mid-third of the upper arm.

Stability of PIPRACIL Following Reconstitution

PIPRACIL is stable in both glass and plastic containers when reconstituted with recommended diluents and when diluted with the intravenous solutions and intravenous admixtures indicated above.

Extensive stability studies have demonstrated chemical stability (potency, pH, and clarity) through 24 hours at room temperature, up to one week refrigerated, and up to one month frozen (−10° to −20°C). (Note: The 40 g Pharmacy Bulk Vial should not be frozen after reconstitution.) Appropriate consideration of aseptic technique and individual hospital policy, however, may recommend discarding unused portions after storage for 48 hours under refrigeration and discarding after 24 hours storage at room temperature.

ADD-Vantage System

Stability studies with the ad-mixed ADD-Vantage system have demonstrated chemical stability (potency, pH, and clarity) through 24 hours at room temperature. (Note: The ad-mixed ADD-Vantage should not be refrigerated or frozen after reconstitution.)

Additional stability data available upon request.

HOW SUPPLIED

PIPRACIL® (piperacillin sodium) is available in vials containing sterile freeze-dried piperacillin sodium powder equivalent to two, three, four and 40 g of piperacillin. One g of piperacillin (as a monosodium salt) contains 1.85 mEq (42.5 mg) of sodium.

Product Numbers

2 gram/Vial—10 per box—NDC 0206-3879-16
3 gram/Vial—10 per box—NDC 0206-3882-55
4 gram/Vial—10 per box—NDC 0206-3880-25
3 gram infusion Bottle—10 per box—NDC 0206-3882-65
4 gram infusion Bottle—10 per box—NDC 0206-3880-66
2 gram ADD-Vantage Vial—10 per box—NDC 0206-3879-27
3 gram ADD-Vantage Vial—10 per box—NDC 0206-3882-28
4 gram ADD-Vantage Vial—10 per box—NDC 0206-3880-29
40 gram Pharmacy Bulk Vial—NDC 0206-3877-60

Store at controlled room temperature 15°–30°C (59°–86°F).

Caution: Federal law prohibits dispensing without prescription.

Manufactured by:
LEDERLE PIPERACILLIN, INC.
Carolina, Puerto Rico 00987
CI 4579-2 Revised January 18, 1999

Shown in Product Identification Guide, page 320

PNEUMOCOCCAL VACCINE POLYVALENT PNU–IMUNE® 23 ℞

[*new-ĭ-mūne*]

DESCRIPTION

Pneumococcal Vaccine Polyvalent PNU-IMUNE® 23 is a sterile preparation intended for intramuscular or subcutaneous use. PNU-IMUNE 23 is indicated for immunization against infections caused by the 23 most prevalent types of *Streptococcus pneumoniae* (pneumococci) which are responsible for approximately 90% of serious pneumococcal disease in the United States and worldwide.[1–5] PNU-IMUNE 23 consists of a mixture of purified capsular polysaccharides from 23 types of *S pneumoniae*.

[See table at top of next page]

Each of the pneumococcal polysaccharide types is produced separately to assure a high degree of purity. After an individual pneumococcal type is grown, the polysaccharide is separated from the cell and purified by a series of steps including ethanol fractionation. The vaccine is formulated to contain 25 µg of each of the 23 purified polysaccharide types per 0.5 mL dose of vaccine. Thimerosal (a mercury derivative) at a final concentration of 0.01% is added as a preservative.

The vaccine is a clear, colorless liquid.

CLINICAL PHARMACOLOGY

Disease caused by *S pneumoniae* remains an important cause of morbidity and mortality in the US, particularly in the very young, the elderly, and persons with certain high-risk conditions. Pneumococcal pneumonia accounts for 10% to 25% of all pneumonias and an estimated 40,000 deaths annually.[2]

Studies suggest annual rates of bacteremia of 15–19/100,000 for the total population, and 50/100,000 for persons 65 and older. Certain population groups, eg, Native Americans may have considerably higher disease rates.[2]

Mortality from pneumococcal disease is highest in patients with bacteremia or meningitis, patients with underlying medical conditions, and older persons. In some high-risk patients, mortality has been reported to be over 40% for bacteremic disease and 55% for meningitis, despite appropriate antimicrobial therapy.[2]

In addition to the very young and persons 65 years of age or older, patients with certain chronic conditions are at increased risk of developing pneumococcal infection and severe pneumococcal illness. Patients with chronic cardiovascular or pulmonary disease, diabetes mellitus, alcoholism, and cirrhosis are generally immunocompetent but have increased risk. Other patients at greater risk because of decreased responsiveness to polysaccharide antigens or more rapid decline in serum antibody include those with functional or anatomic asplenia (eg, sickle cell disease or splenectomy), Hodgkin's disease, lymphoma, multiple myeloma, chronic renal failure, nephrotic syndrome, and organ transplantation. Studies indicate that patients with acquired immunodeficiency syndrome (AIDS) are also at increased risk of pneumococcal disease.[6,7] Recurrent pneumococcal meningitis may occur in patients with cerebrospinal fluid leakage that complicates skull fractures or neurologic procedures.

The polysaccharide capsules of pneumococci give these organisms resistance to the phagocytic action of polymorphonuclear leukocytes and monocytes. However, type-specific antibody facilitates their destruction in the body by the mechanism of complement-mediated lysis.

Most healthy adults, including the elderly, demonstrate at least a two-fold rise in type-specific antibodies within two to three weeks of immunization. Similar antibody responses have been reported in patients with alcoholic cirrhosis and diabetes mellitus. In contrast, elderly individuals with chronic pulmonary disease failed to mount a comparable immune response.[8] In immunocompromised patients, the response to immunization may also be lower. Children under two years of age respond poorly to most capsular polysaccharide types. Further, response to some pneumococcal types (eg, 6A and 14) important in pediatric infection is decreased in children less than 5 years of age.[9]

In clinical studies with PNU-IMUNE® 23, more than 90% of all adults showed two-fold or greater increase in geometric mean antibody titer for each capsular type contained in the vaccine.[10]

Patients over the age of 2 years, with anatomical or functional asplenia and otherwise intact lymphoid function, generally respond to pneumococcal vaccines with a serological conversion comparable to that observed in healthy individuals of the same age.[11]

Patients with acquired immunodeficiency syndrome (AIDS) may have an impaired antibody response to pneumococcal vaccine.[7,12] However, asymptomatic human immunodeficiency virus (HIV)-infected patients, or those with generalized lymphadenopathy, respond to the 23-valent pneumococcal vaccine.[13]

Following immunization of healthy adults, antibody levels remain elevated for at least 5 years, but in some individuals these may fall to preimmunization levels within 10 years.[14,15] A more rapid decline in antibodies may occur in children, particularly those who have undergone a splenectomy and those with sickle cell disease, in whom antibodies for some types can fall to preimmunization levels 3 to 5 years after immunization.[16,17] Similar rates of decline can occur in children with nephrotic syndrome.[18]

Controlled clinical trials in South Africa involving 12,000 gold miners have shown a 6-valent and a 13-valent pneumococcal vaccine to be 78.5% effective in preventing type-specific pneumococcal pneumonia and 82.3% effective in preventing pneumococcal bacteremia with the types contained in the vaccine.[19] In a preliminary study of an 8-valent polysaccharide vaccine in a group consisting of 77 patients with sickle cell disease and 19 asplenic persons, there were no pneumococcal infections in the immunized patients within two years of immunization. There were eight cases of pneumococcal infection in 106 unimmunized, age-matched patients with sickle cell disease. Antibody response of the asplenic patients was comparable to that of normal controls.[20]

In a study carried out by Austrian and colleagues with 13-valent pneumococcal vaccines prepared for the National Institute of Allergy and Infectious Disease, the reduction in pneumonias caused by the capsular types present in the vaccines was 79%. Reduction in type-specific pneumococcal bacteremia was 82%.[19]

In a double-blind study of a 14-valent pneumococcal vaccine carried out in Papua, New Guinea, pneumococcal infection was 84% lower in the immunized group and mortality from pneumonia 44% lower.[21]

Five case-control studies in the US have evaluated the efficacy of pneumococcal vaccine in the prevention of serious pneumococcal disease. Four of these studies showed the vaccine to be efficacious, with point estimates of efficacy ranging from 61% to 70%.[22–25] One study failed to show efficacy in preventing pneumococcal bacteremia.[26] This study was judged inadequate in determination of vaccination status, and the selection of controls was considered potentially biased.[2]

A prospective study failed to demonstrate efficacy against pneumococcal pneumonia and bronchitis;[8] this study has been criticized for methodological flaws.[2] In contrast, a prospective French study found pneumococcal vaccine to be 77% effective in reducing the incidence of pneumonia among nursing home residents.[27]

Despite conflicting findings, the data continue to support the use of pneumococcal vaccine for certain well-defined groups at risk.[2]

INDICATIONS AND USAGE

PNU-IMUNE® 23 is indicated for immunization against pneumococcal disease caused by those pneumococcal types included in the vaccine.

Adults

1. All adults 65 or older,[2] with emphasis on immunization of the older adult while in good health.

Continued on next page

Pnu-Imune 23—Cont.

2. Immunocompetent adults who are at increased risk of pneumococcal disease or its complications because of chronic illnesses (eg, cardiovascular or pulmonary disease, diabetes mellitus, alcoholism, cirrhosis, or cerebrospinal fluid leaks).[2]
3. Immunocompromised adults at increased risk of pneumococcal disease or its complications (eg, splenic dysfunction or anatomic asplenia, Hodgkin's disease, lymphoma, multiple myeloma, chronic renal failure, nephrotic syndrome, or conditions such as organ transplantation associated with immunosuppression).[2]

Children

1. Children 2 years of age or older with chronic illnesses specifically associated with increased risk of pneumococcal disease or its complications (eg, anatomic or functional asplenia [including sickle-cell disease], nephrotic syndrome, cerebrospinal fluid leaks, and conditions associated with immunosuppression).[2]

Special Groups

1. Persons living in special environments or social settings with an identified increased risk of pneumococcal disease or its complications.[2]
2. Patients with acquired immunodeficiency syndrome (AIDS) have been shown to have an impaired antibody response to pneumococcal vaccine. However, asymptomatic or symptomatic human immunodeficiency virus (HIV)-infected patients or those with persistent generalized lymphadenopathy respond to the 23-valent vaccine.[2]

Timing of Immunization

When elective splenectomy is being considered, pneumococcal vaccine should be given at least two weeks before surgery, if possible.[2]

For planning cancer chemotherapy or other immunosuppressive therapy, the interval between immunization and initiation of chemotherapy or immunosuppression should be at least two weeks.[2]

CONTRAINDICATIONS

HYPERSENSITIVITY TO ANY COMPONENT OF THE VACCINE, INCLUDING THIMEROSAL, A MERCURY DERIVATIVE, IS A CONTRAINDICATION TO THE USE OF THE PRODUCT.

THE OCCURRENCE OF ANY TYPE OF NEUROLOGICAL SYMPTOMS OR SIGNS FOLLOWING ADMINISTRATION OF THIS PRODUCT IS A CONTRAINDICATION TO FURTHER USE.

THE VACCINE SHOULD NOT BE ADMINISTERED TO PERSONS WITH ACUTE FEBRILE ILLNESSES UNTIL THEIR TEMPORARY SYMPTOMS AND/OR SIGNS HAVE ABATED.

The clinical judgment of the attending physician should prevail at all times.

WARNINGS

PNU-IMUNE® 23 is not an effective agent for prophylaxis against pneumococcal disease caused by types not present in the vaccine.

PNU-IMUNE 23 is not indicated for children under two years of age, since antibody response to most capsular polysaccharide types is poor in this age group.[2]

Patients with impaired immune responsiveness whether due to the use of immunosuppressive therapy, a genetic defect, human immunodeficiency virus (HIV) infection, or other causes may have a reduced antibody response to active immunization procedures.[2]

Patients who have received extensive chemotherapy and/or splenectomy for the treatment of Hodgkin's disease have been shown to have an impaired serum antibody response to pneumococcal vaccine.[28,29]

In one study, administration of the vaccine to patients on immunosuppressive drugs and/or irradiation for Hodgkin's disease resulted in reduction of preexisting antibody levels in several patients.[28] It is unclear whether this effect was due to the vaccine or to the effects of irradiation and/or chemotherapy.

At least two weeks should elapse between immunization and the initiation of chemotherapy or immunosuppressive therapy.[2]

Routine reimmunization with this vaccine is not recommended. For reimmunization recommendations (including recommendations regarding reimmunization of individuals at highest risk of fatal pneumococcal infection) see **DOSAGE AND ADMINISTRATION.**

In one study, local reactions after reimmunization were more severe than after initial immunization when the interval between immunizations was 13 months.[30]

Patients who have had episodes of pneumococcal pneumonia or other pneumococcal infection may have high levels of preexisting pneumococcal antibodies that may result in increased reactions to PNU-IMUNE® 23, mostly local, but occasionally systemic.[31] Caution should be exercised if such patients are considered for immunization with PNU-IMUNE 23.

Do not administer the vaccine intradermally since severe reactions may occur.

PRECAUTIONS

General

1. This product should not be used in children under 2 years of age.
2. PRIOR TO ADMINISTRATION OF ANY DOSE OF PNU-IMUNE® 23, THE PARENT, GUARDIAN, OR ADULT PATIENT SHOULD BE ASKED ABOUT THE RECENT HEALTH STATUS, MEDICAL AND IMMUNIZATION HISTORY OF THE PATIENT TO BE IMMUNIZED TO DETERMINE THE EXISTENCE OF ANY CONTRAINDICATION TO IMMUNIZATION WITH PNEUMOCOCCAL VACCINE (SEE **CONTRAINDICATIONS, WARNINGS**).
3. BEFORE ADMINISTRATION OF ANY BIOLOGICAL, THE PHYSICIAN SHOULD TAKE ALL KNOWN PRECAUTIONS FOR PREVENTION OF ALLERGIC OR ANY OTHER REACTIONS. This includes: a review of the patient's history regarding possible sensitivity, the ready availability of epinephrine 1:1,000 and other appropriate agents used for control of immediate allergic reactions, and a knowledge of the recent literature pertaining to use of the biological concerned, including the nature of side effects and adverse reactions that may follow its use.
4. A separate sterile syringe and needle or a sterile disposable unit should be used for each individual patient to prevent transmission of infectious agents from one person to another.

PRIOR TO ADMINISTRATION OF THIS VACCINE, HEALTH CARE PERSONNEL SHOULD INFORM THE PARENT, GUARDIAN, OR ADULT PATIENT OF THE BENEFITS AND RISKS OF IMMUNIZATION WITH PNEUMOCOCCAL VACCINE.

Pregnancy Category C: Animal reproduction studies have not been conducted with PNU-IMUNE® 23. It is also not known whether PNU-IMUNE 23 can cause fetal harm when administered to a pregnant woman or affect reproduction capacity. PNU-IMUNE 23 is not recommended for use in pregnant women.

It is not known whether the drug is excreted in human milk. Because many drugs are excreted in human milk, caution should be exercised when PNU-IMUNE 23 is administered to a nursing woman.

Nomenclature	*Pneumococcal Types*																						
Danish	1	2	3	4	5	6B	7F	8	9N	9V	10A	11A	12F	14	15B	17A	18C	19F	19A	20	22F	23F	33F
US	1	2	3	4	5	26	51	8	9	68	34	43	12	14	54	17	56	19	57	20	22	23	70

ADVERSE REACTIONS

Pneumococcal Vaccine Polyvalent PNU-IMUNE® 23 is associated with a relatively low incidence of adverse reactions. The adverse reactivity observed in clinical studies was of short duration and not serious.

In a study of 32 individuals who received PNU-IMUNE 23, 23 (72%) experienced local reaction characterized by soreness at the injection site within 3 days after immunization.[10]

Low grade fever (less than 37.8°C [100°F]) and mild myalgia occur occasionally and are usually confined to the 24-hour period following immunization. Rash and arthralgia have been reported infrequently.

Although rare, fever over 38.9°C (102°F) and marked local swelling have been reported with pneumococcal polysaccharide vaccine. Rash, urticaria, arthritis, arthralgia, and adenitis have been reported rarely.

Patients with otherwise stabilized idiopathic thrombocytopenic purpura have, on rare occasions, experienced a relapse in their thrombocytopenia, occurring 2 to 14 days after immunization, and lasting up to 2 weeks.[32]

Reactions of greater severity, or extent are unusual. Rarely, anaphylactoid reactions have been reported.

Temporal association of neurological disorders such as paresthesia and acute radiculoneuropathy, including Guillain-Barré syndrome, have been reported following parenteral injections of biological products including pneumococcal vaccine.

DOSAGE AND ADMINISTRATION

The immunization schedule consists of a single 0.5 mL dose given intramuscularly or subcutaneously. Intradermal administration should be avoided. *Do not inject intravenously.* Parenteral drug products should be inspected visually for particulate matter and discoloration prior to administration (see **DESCRIPTION**).

Before injection, the skin at the injection site should be cleansed with a suitable germicide. After insertion of the needle, aspirate to help avoid inadvertent injection into a blood vessel.

Simultaneous Administration with Other Vaccines

Many patients who receive pneumococcal vaccine should also be immunized with influenza vaccine which may be given simultaneously at a different site. In contrast to pneumococcal vaccine, influenza vaccine is recommended annually.[2]

Reimmunization

The incidence of local reactions after reimmunization were found to be more severe than after initial immunization when the interval between immunizations was 13 months.[29]

Reports of reimmunization after longer intervals in children and adults, including a large group of elderly persons reimmunized at least 4 years after primary immunization, suggest a similar incidence of such reactions.[2] The Immunization Practices Advisory Committee (ACIP) recommendations regarding reimmunization are as follows: Persons who receive the 14-valent vaccine should not *routinely* be reimmunized with the 23-valent vaccine. However, reimmunization with 23-valent vaccine should be strongly considered for persons who received the 14-valent vaccine *if they are at highest risk* of fatal pneumococcal infection (eg, asplenic patients). Reimmunization should also be carefully considered for adults at highest risk who received the 23-valent vaccine more than 6 years before and for those shown to have a rapid decline in antibody levels (eg, patients with nephrotic syndrome, renal failure, or transplant patients). Reimmunization should be carefully considered after 3 to 5 years for children with nephrotic syndrome, asplenia, or sickle cell anemia who would be 10 years old or younger at the time of reimmunization.[2]

HOW SUPPLIED

PNU-IMUNE® 23 is supplied as follows:

NDC 0005-2309-31 2.5 mL Vial, for use with syringe only.

NDC 0005-2309-33 5 × One Dose (0.5 mL) LEDERJECT® Disposable Syringes.

STORAGE

DO NOT FREEZE. STORE REFRIGERATED, AWAY FROM FREEZER COMPARTMENT AT 2°C TO 8°C (36°F TO 46°F).

Directions for Use of the LEDERJECT Disposable Syringe:

1. Twist the plunger rod clockwise to be sure the rod is secure to rubber plunger base.

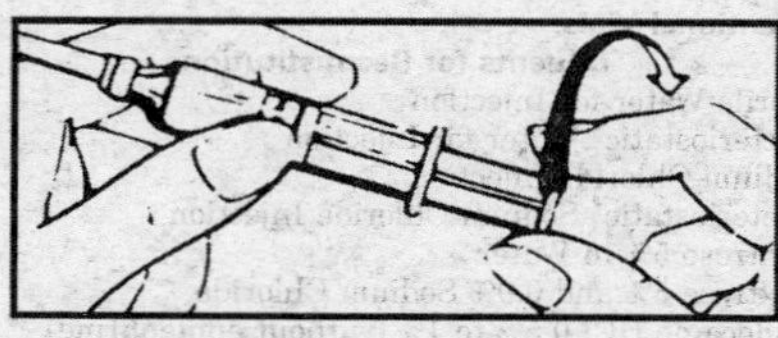

2. Hold needle shield in place with index finger and thumb of one hand while, with the other thumb, exert light pressure on plunger rod until the plunger base has been freed and demonstrates slight movement when pressure is applied.

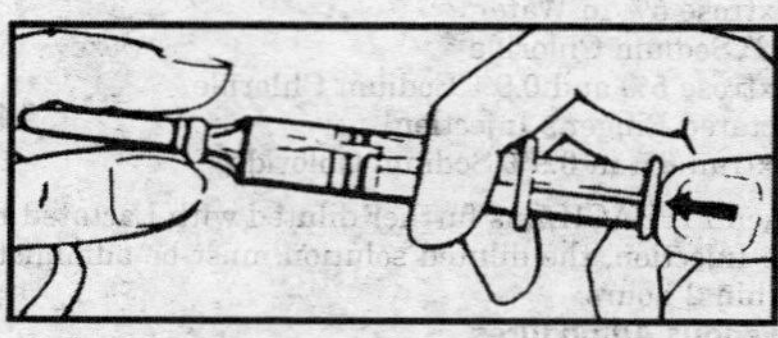

3. Grasp the rubber needle shield at its base; twist and pull to remove.

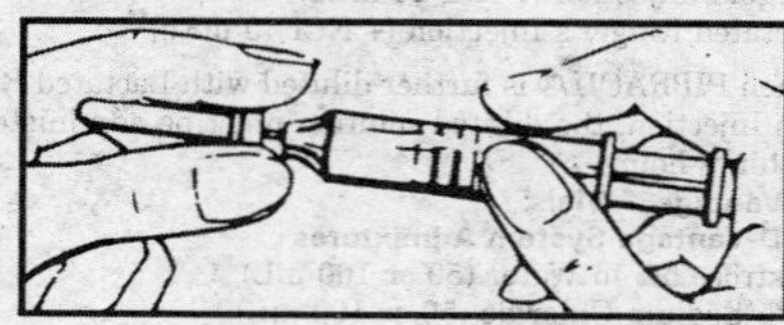

4. To prevent needle-stick injuries, needles should not be recapped, purposely bent, or broken by hand.

REFERENCES

1. Austrian R. Surveillance of pneumococcal infection for field trials of polyvalent vaccines. *Annual Contract Prog Report to the Nat Inst of Allerg and Inf Dis* 1975; Update to Dec. 1977, personal communication.
2. Immunization Practices Advisory Committee. Pneumococcal polysaccharide vaccine—recommendations of the ACIP. *MMWR.* 1989;38(5):64–76. Recommendations also published in: *JAMA.* 1989;261(9):1265–1267.
3. Lund E. Distribution of pneumococcal types at different times and different areas. In: Finland M, Marget W, Bartman K eds. *Bayer-Symposium III Bacterial Infections.* New York, NY:Springer-Verlag, 1971:49.
4. Mufson MA, Kruss DM, Wasil RE, et al. Capsular types and outcome of bacteremic pneumococcal disease in the antibiotic era. *Arch Int Med.* 1974;134:505–510.
5. Robbins JB, Austrian R, Lee CJ, et al. Consideration for formulating the second generation pneumococcal capsular polysaccharide vaccine with emphasis on the cross-reactive types within groups. *J Infec Dis.* 1983; 148(6): 1136–1159.
6. Lane CH, Masur H, Edgar LC, et al. Abnormalities of B-cell activation and immunoregulation in patients with the acquired immunodeficiency syndrome. *N Engl J Med.* 1983;309:453–458.
7. Ammann AJ, Schiffman G, Abrams D, et al. B-cell immunodeficiency in acquired immune deficiency syndrome. *JAMA.* 1984;251:1447–1449.
8. Simberkoff MS, Cross AP, Al-Ibrahim M, et al. Efficacy of pneumococcal vaccine in high-risk patients: results of a Veterans Administration cooperative study. *N Eng J Med.* 1986;315:1318–1327.
9. Douglas RM, Paton JC, Duncan SJ, et al. Antibody response to pneumococcal vaccination in children younger than five years of age. *J Infect Dis.* 1983;148:131–137.
10. Data on file, Lederle Laboratories.
11. Sullivan JL, Ochs HD, Schiffman G, et al. Immune response after splenectomy. *Lancet.* 1978;1:178–181.

12. Ballet J-J, Sulcebe G, Couderc L-J, et al. Impaired antipneumococcal antibody response in patients with AIDS-related persistent generalized lymphadenopathy. *Clin Exp Immunol.* 1987;68:479–487.
13. Huang K-L, Ruben FL, Rinaldo CR Jr, et al. Antibody responses after influenza and pneumococcal immunization in HIV-infected homosexual men. *JAMA.* 1987; 257: 2047–2050.
14. Mufson MA, Krause HE, Schiffman G. Long term persistence of antibodies following immunization with pneumococcal polysaccharide vaccine. *Proc Soc Exp Bio Med.* 1983;173:270–275.
15. Mufson MA, Krause HE, Schiffman G, et al. Pneumococcal antibody levels one decade after immunization of healthy adults. *Am J Med Sci.* 1987;293:279–284.
16. Giebiuk GS, Le CT, Schiffman G. Decline of serum antibody in splenectomized children after vaccination with pneumococcal capsular polysaccharides. *J Pediatr.* 1984;105:576–582.
17. Weintrub PS, Schiffman G, Addiego JE Jr, et al. Long-term follow-up and booster immunization with polyvalent pneumococcal polysaccharide in patient with sickle cell anemia. *J Pediatr.* 1984;105:261–263.
18. Spika JS, Halsey NA, Le CT, et al. Decline of vaccine-induced antipneumococcal antibody in children with nephrotic syndrome. *Am J Kidney Dis.* 1986;7:466–470.
19. Austrian R, Douglas RM, Schiffman G, et al. Prevention of pneumococcal pneumonia by vaccination. *Trans Assoc Am Phys.* 1976;89:184–194.
20. Ammann AJ, Addiego K, Wara DW, et al. Polyvalent pneumococcal-polysaccharide immunization of patients with sickle-cell anemia and patients with splenectomy. *N Engl J Med.* 1977;297:897–900.
21. Riley ID, Tarr PI, Andrews M, et al. Immunisation with a polyvalent pneumococcal vaccine: reduction of adult respiratory mortality in a New Guinea Highlands community. *Lancet.* 1977;1:1338–1341.
22. Shapiro ED, Clemens JD. A controlled evaluation of the protective efficacy of pneumococcal vaccine for patients at high risk of serious pneumococcal infections. *Ann Intern Med.* 1984;101:325–330.
23. Shapiro ED, Austrian R, Adair RK, et al. The protective efficacy of pneumococcal vaccine (Abstract). *Clin Res.* 1988;36:470A.
24. Sims RV, Steinmann WC, McConville JH, et al. The clinical effectiveness of pneumococcal vaccine in the elderly. *Ann Intern Med.* 1988;108:653–657.
25. Bolan G, Broome CV, Facklam RR, et al. Pneumococcal vaccine efficacy in selected populations in the United States. *Ann Intern Med.* 1986;104:1–6.
26. Forrester HL, Jahnigen DW, LaForce FM. Inefficacy of pneumococcal vaccine in a high-risk population. *Am J Med.* 1987;83:425–430.
27. Gaillat J, Zmirou D, Mallaret MR, et al. Essai clinique du vaccin antipneumococcique chez des personnes agées vivant en institution. *Rev Epidémiol* Santé Publique. 1985;33:437–444.
28. Siber GR, Weitzman SA, Aisenberg AC, et al. Impaired antibody response to pneumococcal vaccine after treatment for Hodgkin's disease. *N Eng J Med.* 1978;299: 442–448.
29. Siber GR, Gorham C, Martin P, et al. Antibody response to pretreatment immunization and post-treatment boosting with bacterial polysaccharide vaccines in patients with Hodgkin's disease. *Ann Intern Med.* 1986;104:467–475.
30. Borgono JM, McLean AA, Vella PP, et al. Vaccination and revaccination with polyvalent pneumococcal polysaccharide vaccines in adults and infants. *Proc Soc Exper Biol Med.* 1978;157:148–154.
31. Ponka A, Leinonen M: Adverse reactions to polyvalent pneumococcal vaccine. *Scand J Infect Dis.* 1982;14:67–71.
32. Kelton JG. Vaccination-associated relapse of immune thrombocytopenia. *JAMA.* 1981;245(4):369–371.

Manufactured by:
LEDERLE LABORATORIES
Division American Cyanamid Company
Pearl River, NY 10965
US Gov't. License No. 17
Marketed by:
WYETH-LEDERLE VACCINES AND PEDIATRICS
Wyeth-Ayerst Laboratories
Philadelphia, PA 19101
CI 4415-2 Revised October 5, 1998

Shown in Product Identification Guide, page 320

Pneumococcal 7-valent Conjugate Vaccine (Diphtheria CRM_{197} Protein)
PREVNAR™ ℞
[*prĕv' năr*]

℞ only
For Intramuscular Injection Only

DESCRIPTION

Prevnar™, Pneumococcal 7-valent Conjugate Vaccine (Diphtheria CRM_{197} Protein), is a sterile solution of saccharides of the capsular antigens of *Streptococcus pneumoniae* serotypes 4, 6B, 9V, 14, 18C, 19F, and 23F individually conjugated to diphtheria CRM_{197} protein. Each serotype is grown in soy peptone broth. The individual polysaccharides are purified through centrifugation, precipitation, ultrafiltration, and column chromatography. The polysaccharides are chemically activated to make saccharides which are directly conjugated to the protein carrier CRM_{197} to form the glycoconjugate. This is effected by reductive amination. CRM_{197} is a nontoxic variant of diphtheria toxin isolated from cultures of *Corynebacterium diphtheriae* strain C7 (β197) grown in a casamino acids and yeast extract-based medium. CRM_{197} is purified through ultrafiltration, ammonium sulfate precipitation, and ion-exchange chromatography. The individual glycoconjugates are purified by ultrafiltration and column chromatography and are analyzed for saccharide to protein ratios, molecular size, free saccharide, and free protein.

The individual glycoconjugates are compounded to formulate the vaccine, Prevnar™. Potency of the formulated vaccine is determined by quantification of each of the saccharide antigens, and by the saccharide to protein ratios in the individual glycoconjugates.

Prevnar™ is manufactured as a liquid preparation. Each 0.5 mL dose is formulated to contain: 2 µg of each saccharide for serotypes 4, 9V, 14, 18C, 19F, and 23F, and 4 µg of serotype 6B per dose (16 µg total saccharide); approximately 20 µg of CRM_{197} carrier protein; and 0.125 mg of aluminum per 0.5 mL dose as aluminum phosphate adjuvant. After shaking, the vaccine is a homogeneous, white suspension.

CLINICAL PHARMACOLOGY

S. pneumoniae is an important cause of morbidity and mortality in persons of all ages worldwide. The organism causes invasive infections, such as bacteremia and meningitis, as well as pneumonia and upper respiratory tract infections including otitis media and sinusitis. In children older than 1 month, *S. pneumoniae* is the most common cause of invasive disease.[1] Data from community-based studies performed between 1986 and 1995, indicate that the overall annual incidence of invasive pneumococcal disease in the United States is an estimated 10 to 30 cases per 100,000 persons, with the highest risk in children aged less than or equal to 2 years of age (140 to 160 cases per 100,000 persons).[2,3,4,5,6] Children in group child care can have an increased risk for invasive pneumococcal disease.[7,8] Immunocompromised individuals with neutropenia, asplenia, sickle cell disease, disorders of complement and humoral immunity, human immunodeficiency virus (HIV) infections or chronic underlying disease are also at risk for invasive pneumococcal disease.[8] *S. pneumoniae* is the most common cause of bacterial meningitis in the United States.[1] The annual incidence of pneumococcal meningitis in children between 1 to 23 months of age is approximately 7 cases per 100,000 persons.[1] Pneumococcal meningitis in childhood has been associated with 8% mortality and may result in neurological sequelae (25%) and hearing loss (32%) in survivors.[9]

S. pneumoniae is an important cause of acute otitis media, identified in 20 to 40% of middle ear fluid cultures.[10,11] The seven serotypes account for approximately 60% of acute otitis media due to *S. pneumoniae* (12–24% of all acute otitis media).[12] The exact contribution of *S. pneumoniae* to childhood pneumonia is unknown, as it is often not possible to identify the causative organisms. In studies of children less than 5 years of age with community-acquired pneumonia, where diagnosis was attempted using serological methods, antigen testing, or culture data, 30% of cases were classified as bacterial pneumonia, and 70% of these (21% of total community-acquired pneumonia) were found to be due to *S. pneumoniae*.[13,14]

In the past decade the proportion of *S. pneumoniae* isolates resistant to antibiotics has been on the rise in the United States worldwide. In a multi-center US surveillance study, the prevalence of penicillin and cephalosporin-nonsusceptible (intermediate or high level resistance) invasive disease isolates from children was 21% (range < 5% to 38% among centers), and 9.3% (range 0–18%), respectively. Over the 3-year surveillance period (1993–1996), there was a 50% increase in penicillin-nonsusceptible *S. pneumoniae* (PNSP) strains and a three-fold rise in cephalosporin-nonsusceptible strains.[8] Although generally less common than PNSP, pneumococci resistant to macrolides and trimethoprin-sulfazoxole have also been observed.[4] Day care attendance, a history of ear infection, and a recent history of antibiotic exposure, have also been associated with invasive infections with PNSP in children 2 months to 59 months of age.[7,8]

TABLE 1
Efficacy of Prevnar™ Against Invasive Disease Due to *S. pneumoniae* in Cases Accrued From October 15, 1995 Through August 20, 1998[18,19]

	Prevnar™	Control*		
	Number of Cases	Number of Cases	Efficacy	95% CI
Vaccine serotypes				
Per protocol	**0**	**17**	**100%**	**75.4, 100**
Intent-to-treat	**0**	**22**	**100%**	**81.7, 100**
All pneumococcal serotypes				
Per protocol	2	20	90.0%	58.3, 98.9
Intent-to-treat	3	27†	88.9%	63.8. 97.9

* Investigational meningococcal group C conjugate vaccine (MnCC).
† Includes one case in an immunocompromised subject.

TABLE 2
Geometric Mean Concentrations (µg/mL) of Pneumococcal Antibodies Following the Third and Fourth Doses of Prevnar™ or Control* When Administered Concurrently With DTP-HbOC in the Efficacy Study[19]

Serotype	Post dose 3 GMC† (95% CI for Prevnar™)		Post dose 4 GMC‡ (95% CI for Prevnar™)	
	Prevnar™§	Control*	Prevnar™§	Control*
	N=88	N=92	N=68	N=61
4	1.46 (1.19, 1.78)	0.03	2.38 (1.88, 3.03)	0.04
6B	4.70 (3.59, 6.14)	0.08	14.45 (11.17, 18.69)	0.17
9V	1.99 (1.64, 2.42)	0.05	3.51 (2.75, 4.48)	0.06
14	4.60 (3.70, 5.74)	0.05	6.52 (5.18, 8.21)	0.06
18C	2.16 (1.73, 2.69)	0.04	3.43 (2.70, 4.37)	0.07
19F	1.39 (1.16, 1.68)	0.09	2.07 (1.66, 2.57)	0.18
23F	1.85 (1.46, 2.34)	0.05	3.82 (2.85, 5.11)	0.09

* Control was investigational meningococcal group C conjugate vaccine (MnCC).
† Mean age of Prevnar™ group was 7.8 months and of control group was 7.7 months. N is slightly less for some serotypes in each group.
‡ Mean age of Prevnar™ group was 14.2 months and of control group was 14.4 months. N is slightly less for some serotypes in each group.
§ $p<0.001$ when Prevnar™ compared to control for each serotype using a Wilcoxon's test.

Continued on next page

Prevnar—Cont.

There has been no difference in mortality associated with PNSP strains.[8,9] However, the American Academy of Pediatrics (AAP) revised the antibiotic treatment guidelines in 1997 in response to the increased prevalence of antibiotic-resistant pneumococci.[15]
Approximately 90 serotypes of *S. pneumoniae* have been identified based on antigenic differences in their capsular polysaccharides. The distribution of serotypes responsible for disease differ with age and geographic location.[16]
Serotypes 4, 6B, 9V, 14, 18C, 19F, and 23F have been responsible for approximately 80% of invasive pneumococcal disease in children < 6 years of age in the United States.[12] These 7 serotypes also accounted for 74% of PNSP and 100% of pneumococci with high level penicillin resistance isolated from children < 6 years with invasive disease during a 1993–1994 surveillance by the Centers for Disease Control.

Results of Clinical Evaluations

Efficacy

Efficacy was assessed in a randomized, double-blind clinical trial in a multiethnic population at Northern California Kaiser Permanente (NCKP), beginning in October 1995, in which 37,816 infants were randomized to receive either Prevnar™ or a control vaccine (an investigational meningococcal group C conjugate vaccine [MnCC]) at 2, 4, 6, and 12–15 months of age. Prevnar™ was administered to 18,906 children and the control vaccine to 18,910 children. Routinely recommended vaccines were also administered which changed during the trial to reflect changing AAP and Advisory Committee on Immunization Practices (ACIP) recommendations. A planned interim analysis was performed upon accrual of 17 cases of invasive disease due to vaccine-type *S. pneumoniae* (August 1998). Ancillary endpoints for evaluation of efficacy against pneumococcal disease were also assessed in this trial.

Efficacy against invasive disease: Invasive disease was defined as isolation and identification of *S. pneumoniae* from normally sterile body sites in children presenting with an acute illness consistent with pneumococcal disease. Weekly surveillance of listings of cultures from the NCKP Regional Microbiology database was conducted to assure ascertainment of all cases. The primary endpoint was efficacy against invasive pneumococcal disease due to vaccine serotypes. The per protocol analysis of the primary endpoint included cases which occurred ≥ 14 days after the third dose. The intent-to-treat (ITT) analysis included all cases of invasive pneumococcal disease due to vaccine serotypes in children who received at least one dose of vaccine. Secondary analyses of efficacy against all invasive pneumococcal disease, regardless of serotype, were also performed according to these same per protocol and ITT definitions. Results of these analyses are presented in Table 1.

[See table 1 at top of previous page]

All 22 cases of invasive disease due to vaccine serotype strains in the ITT population were bacteremic. In addition, the following diagnoses were also reported: meningitis (2), pneumonia (2), and cellulitis (1).
Preliminary efficacy data through an extended follow-up period to April 20, 1999, resulted in a similar efficacy estimate (Per protocol: 1 case in Prevnar™ group, 39 cases in control group; ITT: 3 cases in Prevnar™ group, 49 cases in the control group).

Immunogenicity

Routine Schedule

Subjects from a subset of selected study sites in the NCKP efficacy study were approached for participation in the immunogenicity portion of the study on a volunteer basis. Immune responses following three or four doses of Prevnar™ or the control vaccine were evaluated in children who received either concurrent Diphtheria and Tetanus Toxoids and Pertussis Vaccine Adsorbed and Haemophilus b Conjugate Vaccine (Diphtheria CRM_{197} Protein Conjugate), (DTP-HbOC), or Diphtheria and Tetanus Toxoids and Acellular Pertussis Vaccine Adsorbed (DTaP), and Haemophilus b Conjugate Vaccine (Diphtheria CRM_{197} Protein Conjugate), (HbOC) vaccines at 2, 4, and 6 months of age. The use of Hepatitis B (Hep B), Oral Polio Vaccine (OPV), Inactivated Polio Vaccine (IPV), Measles-Mumps-Rubella (MMR), and Varicella vaccines were permitted according to the AAP and ACIP recommendations.
Table 2 presents the geometric mean concentrations (GMC) of pneumococcal antibodies following the third and fourth doses of Prevnar™ or the control vaccine when administered concurrently with DTP-HbOC vaccine in the efficacy study.

[See table 2 at top of previous page]

In another randomized study (Manufacturing Bridging Study, 118-16), immune responses were evaluated following three doses of Prevnar™ administered concomitantly with DTaP and HbOC vaccines at 2, 4, and 6 months of age, IPV at 2 and 4 months of age, and Hep B at 2 and 6 months of age. The control group received concomitant vaccines only. Table 3 presents the immune responses to pneumococcal polysaccharides observed in both this study and in the subset of subjects from the efficacy study that received concomitant DTaP and HbOC vaccines.

[See table 3 above]

In all studies in which the immune responses to Prevnar™ were contrasted to control, a significant antibody response was seen to all vaccine serotypes following three or four doses, although geometric mean concentrations of antibody

TABLE 3
Geometric Mean Concentrations (µg/mL) of Pneumococcal Antibodies Following the Third Dose of Prevnar™ or Control* When Administered Concurrently With DTaP and HbOC in the Efficacy Study† and Manufacturing Bridging Study[19,20]

Serotype	Efficacy Study Post dose 3 GMC† (95% CI for Prevnar™)		Manufacturing Bridging Study Post dose 3 GMC‡ (95% CI for Prevnar™)	
	Prevnar™‖	Control*	Prevnar™‖	Control*
	N=32	N=32	N=159	N=83
4	1.47 (1.08, 2.02)	0.02	2.03 (1.75, 2.37)	0.02
6B	2.18 (1.20, 3.96)	0.06	2.97 (2.43, 3.65)	0.07
9V	1.52 (1.04, 2.22)	0.04	1.18 (1.01, 1.39)	0.04
14	5.05 (3.32, 7.70)	0.04	4.64 (3.80, 5.66)	0.04
18C	2.24 (1.65, 3.02)	0.04	1.96 (1.66, 2.30)	0.04
19F	1.54 (1.09, 2.17)	0.10	1.91 (1.63, 2.25)	0.08
23F	1.48 (0.97, 2.25)	0.05	1.71 (1.44, 2.05)	0.05

* Control in efficacy was investigational meningococcal group C conjugate vaccine (MnCC) and in Manufacturing Bridging Study was concomitant vaccines only.
† Sufficient data are not available to reliably assess GMCs following 4 doses of Prevnar™ when administered with DTaP in the NCKP efficacy study.
‡ Mean age of Prevnar™ group was 7.4 months and of the control group was 7.6 months. N is slightly less for some serotypes in each group.
§ Mean age of the Prevnar™ group and the control group was 7.2 months.
‖ $p<0.001$ when Prevnar™ compared to control for each serotype using a Wilcoxon's test in the efficacy study and two-sample t-test in the Manufacturing Bridging Study.

TABLE 4
Geometric Mean Concentrations (µg/mL) of Pneumococcal Antibodies Following Immunization of Children From 7 Months Through 9 Years of Age With Prevnar™[26]

Age Group, Vaccinations	Study	Sample Size(s)	4	6B	9V	14	18C	19F	23F
7–11 mo. 3 doses	118-12	22	**2.34**	**3.66**	**2.11**	**9.33**	**2.31**	**1.60**	**2.50**
	118-16	39	**3.60**	**4.63**	**2.04**	**5.48**	**1.98**	**2.15**	**1.93**
12–17 mo. 2 doses	118-15*	82–84†	**3.91**	**4.67**	**1.94**	**6.92**	**2.25**	**3.78**	**3.29**
	118-18	33	**7.02**	**4.25**	**3.26**	**6.31**	**3.60**	**3.29**	**2.92**
18–23 mo. 2 doses	118-15*	52–54†	**3.36**	**4.92**	**1.80**	**6.69**	**2.65**	**3.17**	**2.71**
	118-18	45	**6.85**	**3.71**	**3.86**	**6.48**	**3.42**	**3.86**	**2.75**
24–35 mo. 1 dose	118-18	53	**5.34**	**2.90**	**3.43**	1.88	**3.03**	**4.07**	**1.56**
36–59 mo. 1 dose	118-18	52	**6.27**	**6.40**	**4.62**	**5.95**	**4.08**	**6.37**	**2.95**
5–9 yrs. 1 dose	118-18	101	**6.92**	**20.84**	**7.49**	**19.32**	**6.72**	**12.51**	**11.57**
118-8, DTaP	Post dose 3	31–32†	1.47	2.18	1.52	5.05	2.24	1.54	1.48

Bold = GMC not inferior to 118-8, DTaP post dose 3 (one-sided lower limit of the 95% CI of GMC ratio ≥ 0.50).
* Study in Navajo and Apache populations.
† Numbers vary with serotype.

varied among serotypes.[18,19,20,21,22,23,24,25] The minimum serum antibody concentration necessary for protection against invasive pneumococcal disease has not been determined for any serotype.
Prevnar™ induces functional antibodies to all vaccine serotypes, as measured by opsonophagocytosis following three doses.[25]

Previously Unvaccinated Older Infants and Children

To determine an appropriate schedule for children 7 months of age or older at the time of the first immunization with Prevnar™, 483 children in 4 ancillary studies received Prevnar™ at various schedules. GMCs attained using the various schedules among older infants and children were comparable to immune responses of children, who received concomitant DTaP, in the NCKP efficacy study (118-8) after 3 doses for most serotypes, as shown in Table 4. These data support the schedule for previously unvaccinated older infants and children who are beyond the age of the infant schedule. For usage in older infants and children see DOSAGE AND ADMINISTRATION.

[See table 4 above]

INDICATIONS AND USAGE

Prevnar™ is indicated for active immunization of infants and toddlers against invasive disease caused by *S. pneumoniae* due to capsular serotypes included in the vaccine (4, 6B, 9V, 14, 18C, 19F, and 23F). The routine schedule is 2, 4, 6, and 12–15 months of age. For additional information on usage, see DOSAGE AND ADMINISTRATION.
This vaccine is not intended to be used for treatment of active infection.
As with any vaccine, Prevnar™ may not protect 100% of individuals receiving the vaccine.

CONTRAINDICATIONS

Hypersensitivity to any component of the vaccine, including diphtheria toxoid, is a contraindication to use of this vaccine.
The decision to administer or delay vaccination because of a current or recent febrile illess depends largely on the severity of the symptoms and their etiology. Although a severe or even a moderate febrile illness is sufficient reason to postpone vaccinations, minor illnesses, such as a mild upper respiratory infection with or without low-grade fever, are not generally contraindications.[27,28]

WARNINGS

THIS VACCINE WILL NOT PROTECT AGAINST *S. PNEUMONIAE* DISEASE OTHER THAN THAT CAUSED BY THE SEVEN SEROTYPES INCLUDED IN THE VACCINE, NOR WILL IT PROTECT AGAINST OTHER MICROORGANISMS THAT CAUSE INVASIVE INFECTION SUCH AS BACTEREMIA AND MENINGITIS.
This vaccine should not be given to infants or children with thrombocytopenia or any coagulation disorder that would contraindicate intramuscular injection unless the potential benefit clearly outweighs the risk of administration. If the

decision is made to administer this vaccine to children with coagulation disorders, it should be given with caution. (See DRUG INTERACTIONS).

Immunization with Prevnar™ does not substitute for routine diphtheria immunization.

Healthcare professionals should prescribe and/or administer this product with caution to patients with a possible history of latex sensitivity since the packaging contains dry natural rubber.

PRECAUTIONS

Prevnar™ is for intramuscular use only. Prevnar™ SHOULD UNDER NO CIRCUMSTANCES BE ADMINISTERED INTRAVENOUSLY. The safety and immunogenicity for other routes of administration (e.g. subcutaneous) have not been evaluated.

General

CARE IS TO BE TAKEN BY THE HEALTHCARE PROFESSIONAL FOR THE SAFE AND EFFECTIVE USE OF THIS PRODUCT.

1. PRIOR TO ADMINISTRATION OF ANY DOSE OF THIS VACCINE, THE PARENT OR GUARDIAN SHOULD BE ASKED ABOUT THE PERSONAL HISTORY, FAMILY HISTORY, AND RECENT HEALTH STATUS OF THE VACCINE RECIPIENT. THE HEALTHCARE PROFESSIONAL SHOULD ASCERTAIN PREVIOUS IMMUNIZATION HISTORY, CURRENT HEALTH STATUS, AND OCCURRENCE OF ANY SYMPTOMS AND/OR SIGNS OF AN ADVERSE EVENT AFTER PREVIOUS IMMUNIZATIONS IN THE CHILD TO BE IMMUNIZED, IN ORDER TO DETERMINE THE EXISTENCE OF ANY CONTRAINDICATION TO IMMUNIZATION WITH THIS VACCINE AND TO ALLOW AN ASSESSMENT OF RISKS AND BENEFITS.
2. BEFORE THE ADMINISTRATION OF ANY BIOLOGICAL, THE HEALTHCARE PROFESSIONAL SHOULD TAKE ALL PRECAUTIONS KNOWN FOR THE PREVENTION OF ALLERGIC OR ANY OTHER ADVERSE REACTIONS. This should include a review of the patient's history regarding possible sensitivity; the ready availability of epinephrine 1:1000 and other appropriate agents used for control of immediate allergic reactions; and a knowledge of the recent literature pertaining to use of the biological concerned, including the nature of side effects and adverse reactions that may follow its use.
3. Children with impaired immune responsiveness, whether due to the use of immunosuppressive therapy (including irradiation, corticosteroids, antimetabolites, alkylating agents, and cytotoxic agents), a genetic defect, HIV infection, or other causes, may have reduced antibody response to active immunization.[27,28,29] (See DRUG INTERACTIONS).
4. The use of pneumococcal conjugate vaccine does not replace the use of 23-valent pneumococcal polysaccharide vaccine in children ≥ 24 months of age with sickle cell disease, asplenia, HIV infection, chronic illness or who are immunocompromised. Data on sequential vaccination with Prevnar™ followed by 23-valent pneumococcal polysaccharide vaccine are limited. In a randomized study, 23 children ≥ 2 years of age with sickle cell disease were administered either 2 doses of Prevnar™ followed by a dose of polysaccharide vaccine or a single dose of polysaccharide vaccine alone. In this small study, safety and immune responses with the combined schedule were similar to polysaccharide vaccine alone.[30]
5. Since this product is a suspension containing an aluminum adjuvant, shake vigorously immediately prior to use to obtain a uniform suspension prior to withdrawing the dose.
6. A separate sterile syringe and needle or a sterile disposable unit should be used for each individual to prevent transmission of hepatitis or other infectious agents from one person to another. Needles should be disposed of properly and should not be recapped.
7. Special care should be taken to prevent injection into or near a blood vessel or nerve.
8. Healthcare professionals should prescribe and/or administer this product with caution to patients with a possible history of latex sensitivity since the packaging contains dry natural rubber.

Information for Parents or Guardians

Prior to administration of this vaccine, the healthcare professional should inform the parent, guardian, or other responsible adult of the potential benefits and risks to the patient (see ADVERSE REACTIONS and WARNINGS sections), and the importance of completing the immunization series unless contraindicated. Parents or guardians should be instructed to report any suspected adverse reactions to their healthcare professional. The healthcare professional should provide vaccine information statements prior to each vaccination.

DRUG INTERACTIONS

Children receiving therapy with immunosuppressive agents (large amounts of corticosteroids, antimetabolites, alkylating agents, cytotoxic agents) may not respond optimally to active immunization.[28,29,31,32] (See PRECAUTIONS, General).

As with other intramuscular injections, Prevnar™ should be given with caution to children on anticoagulant therapy.

Simultaneous Administration with Other Vaccines

During clinical studies, Prevnar™ was administered simultaneously with DTP-HbOC or DTaP and HbOC, OPV or IPV, Hep B vaccines, MMR, and Varicella vaccine. Thus, the safety experience with Prevnar™ reflects the use of this product as part of the routine immunization schedule.[19,20,22,23,25]

The immune response to routine vaccines when administered with Prevnar™ (at separate sites) was assessed in 3 clinical studies in which there was a control group for comparison. Results for the concurrent immunizations in infants are shown in Table 5 and for toddlers in Table 6. Enhancement of antibody response to HbOC in the infant series was observed. Some suppression of *Haemophilus influenzae* type b (Hib) response was seen at the 4th dose, but over 97% of children achieved titers ≥ 1 μg/mL. Although some inconsistent differences in response to pertussis antigens were observed, the clinical relevance is unknown. The response to 2 doses of IPV given concomitantly with Prevnar™, assessed 3 months after the second dose,

Continued on next page

TABLE 5
Concurrent Administration of Prevnar™ With Other Vaccines to Infants in Non-Efficacy Studies[20,23]

Antigen*	GMC*		% Responders†		Study	Vaccine Schedule‡	N	
	Prevnar™	Control§	Prevnar™	Control§		(mo.)	Prevnar™	Control§
Hib	6.2	4.4	99.5, 88.3	97.0, 88.1	118-12	2,4,6	214	67
Diphtheria	0.9	0.8	100	97.0				
Tetanus	3.5	4.1‖	100	100				
PT	19.1	17.8	74.0	69.7				
FHA	43.8	46.7	66.4	69.7				
Pertactin	40.1	50.9	65.6	77.3				
Fimbriae 2	3.3	4.2	44.7	62.5¶				
Hib	11.9	7.8‖	100, 96.9	98.8, 92.8	118-16	2,4,6	159	83
Hep B	—	—	99.4	96.2	118-16	0,2,6	156	80
IPV Type 1	—	—	89.0	93.6¶	118-16	2,4	156	80
Type 2	—	—	94.2	93.6				
Type 3	—	—	83.8	80.8				

* Hib vaccine was HibTITER®, DTaP vaccine was Acel-Imune®. Hib (μg/mL) Dip, Tet (IU/mL); Pertussis Antigens (PT, FHA, Ptn, Fim) (units/mL).
† Responders = Hib (≥0.15 μg/mL, ≥1.0 μg/mL); Dip, Tet (≥0.1 IU/mL); Pertussis Antigens (PT, FHA, Ptn, Fim) [4-fold rise]; IPV (≥1:10); Hep B (≥10 mIU/mL).
‡ Schedule for concurrently administered vaccines; Prevnar™ administered at 2, 4, 6 mos.; blood for antibody assessment attained 1 month after third dose, except for IPV (3 months post-immunization).
§ Concurrent vaccines only.
‖ $p<0.05$ when Prevnar™ compared to control group using the following tests: ANCOVA for GMCs in 118-12; ANOVA for GMCs in 118-16; and Fisher's Exact test for % Responders in 118-12.
¶ Lower bound of 90% CI of difference >10%.

TABLE 6
Concurrent Administration of Prevnar™ With Other Vaccines to Toddlers in a Non-Efficacy Study[22]

Antigen*	GMC*		% Responders†		Study‡	Vaccine Schedule§	N	
	Prevnar™	Control‖	Prevnar™	Control‖		(mo.)	Prevnar™	Control‖
Hib	22.7	47.9¶	100, 97.9	100, 100	118-7	12–15	47	26
Diphtheria	2.0	3.2¶	100	100				
Tetanus	14.4	18.8	100	100				
PT	68.6	121.2¶	68.1	73.1				
FHA	29.0	48.2¶	68.1	84.6				
Pertactin	84.4	83.0	83.0	96.2				
Fimbriae 2	5.2	3.8	63.8	50.0				

* Hib vaccine was HibTITER®, DTaP vaccine was Acel-Imune®. Hib (μg/mL; Dip, Tet (IU/mL); Pertussis Antigens (PT, FHA, Ptn, Fim) (units/mL).
† Responders = Hib (≥0.15 μg/mL), ≥1.0 μg/mL); Dip, Tet (≥0.1 IU/mL); Pertussis Antigens (PT, FHA, Ptn, Fim) [4-fold rise].
‡ Children received a primary series of DTP-HbOC (Tetramune®).
§ Blood for antibody assessment obtained 1 month after dose.
‖ Concurrent vaccines only.
¶ $p<0.05$ when Prevnar™ compared to control group using a two-sample t-test.

TABLE 7
Percentage of Subjects Reporting Local Reactions Within 2 Days Following Immunization With Prevnar™ and DTP-HbOC* vaccines at 2, 4, 6, and 12–15 Months of Age[19]

Reaction	Dose 1		Dose 2		Dose 3		Dose 4	
	Prevnar™ Site	DTP-HbOC Site†	Prevnar™ Site	DTP-HbOC Site†	Prevnar™ Site	DTP-HbOC Site†	Prevnar™ Site	DTP-HbOC Site†
	N=2890	N=2890	N=2725	N=2725	N=2538	N=2538	N=599	N=599
Erythema								
Any	12.4	21.9	14.3	25.1	15.2	26.5	12.7	23.4
> 2.4 cm	1.2	4.6	1.0	2.9	2.0	4.4	1.7	6.4
Induration								
Any	10.9	22.4	12.3	23.0	12.8	23.3	11.4	20.5
> 2.4 cm	2.6	7.2	2.4	5.6	2.9	6.7	2.8	7.2
Tenderness								
Any	28.0	36.4	25.2	30.5	25.6	32.8	36.5	45.1
Interfered with limb movement	7.9	10.7	7.4	8.4	7.8	10.0	18.5	22.2

* If Hep B vaccine was administered simultaneously, it was administered into the same limb as the DTP-HbOC vaccine. If reactions occurred at either or both sites on that limb, the more severe reaction was recorded.
† $p<0.05$ when Prevnar™ site compared to the DTP-HbOC site using the sign test.

Prevnar—Cont.

was equivalent to controls for poliovirus Types 2 and 3, but lower for Type 1. MMR and Varicella immunogenicity data from controlled clinical trials with concurrent administration of Prevnar™ are not available.

[See table 5 at top of previous page]
[See table 6 at top of previous page]

CARCINOGENESIS, MUTAGENESIS, IMPAIRMENT OF FERTILITY

Prevnar™ has not been evaluated for any carcinogenic or mutagenic potential, or impairment of fertility.

PREGNANCY

Pregnancy Category C

Animal reproductive studies have not been conducted with this product. It is not known whether Prevnar™ can cause fetal harm when administered to a pregnant woman or whether it can affect reproductive capacity. This vaccine is not recommended for use in pregnant women.

Nursing Mothers

It is not known whether vaccine antigens or antibodies are excreted in human milk. This vaccine is not recommended for use in a nursing mother.

PEDIATRIC USE

Prevnar™ has been shown to be usually well-tolerated and immunogenic in infants. The safety and effectiveness of Prevnar™ in children below the age of 6 weeks have not been established. Immune responses elicited by Prevnar™ among infants born prematurely have not been studied. See DOSAGE AND ADMINISTRATION for the rcommended pediatric dosage.

GERIATRIC USE

This vaccine is NOT recommended for use in adult populations. It is not to be used as a substitute for the pneumococcal polysaccharide vaccine, in geriatric populations.

ADVERSE REACTIONS

The majority of the safety experience with Prevnar™ comes from the NCKP Efficacy Trial in which 17,066 infants received 55,352 doses of Prevnar™, along with other routine childhood vaccines through April 1998 (see CLINICAL PHARMACOLOGY section). The number of Prevnar™ recipients in the safety analysis differs from the number included in the efficacy analysis due to the different lengths of follow-up for these study endpoints. Safety was monitored in this study using several modalities. Local reactions and systemic events occurring within 48 hours of each dose of vaccine were ascertained by scripted telephone interview on a randomly selected subset of approximately 3,000 children in each vaccine group. The rate of relatively rare events requiring medical attention was evaluated across all doses in all study participants using automated databases. Specifically, rates of hospitalizations within 3, 14, 30, and 60 days of immunization, and of emergency room visits within 3, 14, and 30 days of immunization were assessed and compared between vaccine groups for each diagnosis. Seizures within 3 and 30 days of immunization were ascertained across multiple settings (hospitalizations, emergency room or clinic visits, telephone interviews). Deaths and SIDS were ascertained through April 1999. Hospitalizations due to diabetes, autoimmune disorders, and blood disorders were ascertained through August 1999.

In Tables 7 and 8, the rate of local reactions at the Prevnar™ injection site is compared at each dose to the DTP or DTaP injection site in the same children.

[See table 7 at top of previous page]
[See table 8 above]

Table 9 presents the rates of local reactions in previously unvaccinated older infants and children.

[See table 9 above]

Tables 10 and 11 present the rates of systemic events observed in the efficacy study when Prevnar™ was administered concomitantly with DTP or DTaP.

[See table 10 at top of next page]
[See table 11 at top of next page]

Table 12 presents results from a second study (Manufacturing Bridging Study) conducted at Northern California and Denver Kaiser sites, in which children were randomized to receive one of three lots of Prevnar™ with concomitant vaccines including DTaP, or the same concomitant vaccines alone. Information was ascertained by scripted telephone interview, as described below.

[See table 12 at top of next page]

Fever (≥ 38.0°C) within 48 hours of a vaccine dose was reported by a greater proportion of subjects who received Prevnar™, compared to control (investigational meningococcal group C conjugate vaccine [MnCC]), after each dose when administered concurrently with DTP-HbOC or DTaP in the efficacy study. In the Manufacturing Bridging Study, fever within 48–72 hours was also reported more commonly after each dose compared to infants in the control group who received only recommended vaccines. When administered concurrently with DTaP in either study, fever rates among Prevnar™ recipients ranged from 15% to 34%, and were greatest after the 2nd dose.

Table 13 presents the frequencies of systemic reactions in previously unvaccinated older infants and children.

[See table 13 at top of page 1678]

Of the 17,066 subjects who received at least one dose of Prevnar™ in the efficacy trial, there were 24 hospitalizations (for 29 diagnoses) within 3 days of a dose from October 1995 through April 1998. Diagnoses were as follows: bronchiolitis (5); congenital anomaly (4); elective procedure, UTI (3 each); acute gastroenteritis, asthma, pneumonia (2 each); aspiration, breath holding, influenza, inguinal hernia repair, otitis media, febrile seizure, viral syndrome, well child/reassurance (1 each). There were 162 visits to the emergency room (for 182 diagnoses) within 3 days of a dose from October 1995 through April 1998. Diagnoses were as follows: febrile illness (20); acute gastroenteritis (19); trauma, URI (16 each); otitis media (15); well child (13); irritable child, viral syndrome (10 each); rash (8); croup, pneumonia (6 each); poisoning/ingestion (5); asthma, bronchiolitis (4 each); febrile seizure, UTI (3 each); thrush, wheezing, breath holding, choking, conjunctivitis, inguinal hernia repair, pharyngitis (2 each); colic, colitis, congestive heart failure, elective procedure; hives, influenza, ingrown toenail, local swelling, roseola, sepsis (1 each).[19]

One case of hypotonic-hyporesponsive episode (HHE) was reported in the efficacy study following Prevnar™ and concurrent DTP vaccines in the study period from October 1995 through April 1998. Two additional cases of HHE were reported in four other studies and these also occurred in children who received Prevnar™ concurrently with DTP vaccine.[22,25]

In the Kaiser efficacy study in which 17,066 children received a total of 55,352 doses of Prevnar™ and 17,080 children received a total of 55,387 doses of the control vaccine (investigational meningococcal group C conjugate vaccine [MnCC]), seizures were reported in 8 Prevnar™ recipients and 4 control vaccine recipients within 3 days of immunization from October 1995 through April 1998. Of the 8 Prevnar™ recipients, 7 received concomitant DTP-containing vaccines and one received DTaP. Of the 4 control vaccine recipients, 3 received concomitant DTP-containing vaccines and one received DTaP.[19] In the other 4 studies combined, in which 1,102 children were immunized with 3,347 doses of Prevnar™ and 408 children were immunized with 1,310 doses of control vaccine (either investigational meningococcal group C conjugate vaccine [MnCC] or concurrent vaccines), there was one seizure event reported within 3 days of immunization.[23] This subject received Prevnar™ concurrent with DTaP vaccine.

Twelve deaths (5 SIDS and 7 with clear alternative cause) occurred among subjects receiving Prevnar™, of which 11 (4 SIDS and 7 with clear alternative cause) occurred in the Kaiser efficacy study from October 1995 until April 20, 1999. In comparison, 21 deaths (8 SIDS, 12 with clear alternative cause and one SIDS-like death in an older child), occurred in the control vaccine group during the same time period in the efficacy study.[19,20] The number of SIDS deaths in the efficacy study from October 1995 until April 20, 1999

TABLE 8
Percentage of Subjects Reporting Local Reactions Within 2 Days Following Immunization With Prevnar™* and DTaP Vaccines† at 2, 4, 6, and 12–15 Months of Age[19]

Reaction	Dose 1		Dose 2		Dose 3		Dose 4	
	Prevnar™ Site	DTaP Site	Prevnar™ Site	DTaP Site	Prevnar™ Site	DTaP Site	Prevnar™ Site	DTPaP Site‡
	N=693	N=693	N=526	N=526	N=422	N=422	N=165	N=165
Erythema								
Any	10.0	6.7§	11.6	10.5	13.8	11.4	10.9	3.6§
> 2.4 cm	1.3	0.4§	0.6	0.6	1.4	1.0	3.6	0.6
Induration								
Any	9.8	6.6§	12.0	10.5	10.4	10.4	12.1	5.5§
> 2.4 cm	1.6	0.9	1.3	1.7	2.4	1.9	5.5	1.8
Tenderness								
Any	17.9	16.0	19.4	17.3	14.7	13.1	23.3	18.4
Interfered with limb movement	3.1	1.8§	4.1	3.3	2.9	1.9	9.2	8.0

* HbOC was administered in the same limb as Prevnar™. If reactions occurred at either or both sites on that limb, the more severe reaction was recorded.
† If Hep B vaccine was administered simultaneously, it was administered into the same limb as the DTaP. If reactions occurred at either or both sites on that limb, the more severe reaction was recorded.
‡ Subjects may have received DTP or a mixed DTP/DTaP regimen for the primary series. Thus, this is the 4th dose of a pertussis vaccine, but not a 4th dose of DTaP.
§ $p<0.05$ when Prevnar™ site compared to the DTaP using the sign test.

TABLE 9
Percentage of Subjects Reporting Local Reactions Within 3 Days of Immunization in Infants and Children from 7 Months Through 9 Years of Age[26]

Age at 1st Vaccination	7 – 11 Mos.						12 – 23 Mos.			24 – 35 Mos.	35 – 59 Mos.	5 – 9 Yrs.
Study No.	118-12			118-16			118-9*	118-18		118-18	118-18	118-18
Dose Number	1	2	3†	1	2	3†	1	1	2	1	1	1
Number of Subjects	54	51	24	81	76	50	60	114	117	46	48	49
Reaction												
Erythema												
Any	16.7	11.8	20.8	7.4	7.9	14.0	48.3	10.5	9.4	6.5	29.2	24.2
>2.4 cm‡	1.9	0.0	0.0	0.0	0.0	0.0	6.7	1.8	1.7	0.0	8.3	7.1
Induration												
Any	16.7	11.8	8.3	7.4	3.9	10.0	48.3	8.8	6.0	10.9	22.9	25.5
>2.4 cm‡	3.7	0.0	0.0	0.0	0.0	0.0	3.3	0.9	0.9	2.2	6.3	9.3
Tenderness												
Any	13.0	11.8	12.5	8.6	10.5	12.0	46.7	25.7	26.5	41.3	58.3	82.8
Interfered with limb movements§	1.9	2.0	4.2	1.2	1.3	0.0	3.3	6.2	8.5	13.0	20.8	39.4

* For 118-9, 2 of 60 subjects were ≥24 months of age.
† For 118-12, dose 3 was administered at 15 – 18 mos. of age. For 118-16, dose 3 was administered at 12 – 15 mos. of age.
‡ For 118-16 and 118-18, ≥2 cm.
§ Tenderness interfering with limb movement.

TABLE 10
Percentage of Subjects* Reporting Systemic Events Within 2 Days Following Immunization With Prevnar™ or Control† Vaccine Concurrently With DTP-HbOC Vaccine at 2, 4, 6, and 12–15 Months of Age[18]

Reaction	Dose 1		Dose 2		Dose 3		Dose 4	
	Prevnar™	Control†	Prevnar™	Control†	Prevnar™	Control†	Prevnar™	Control†
	N=2998	N=2982	N=2788	N=2761	N=2596	N=2591	N=709	N=733
Fever								
≥ 38.0°C	33.4	28.7‡	34.7	27.4‡	40.6	32.4‡	41.9	36.9
> 39.0°C	1.3	1.3	3.0	1.6‡	5.3	3.4‡	4.5	4.5
Irritability	71.3	67.9‡	69.4	63.8‡	68.9	61.6‡	72.8	65.8‡
Drowsiness	49.2	50.6	32.5	33.6	25.9	23.4‡	21.3	22.7
Restless Sleep	18.1	17.9	27.3	24.3‡	33.3	30.1‡	29.9	28.0
Decreased Appetite	24.7	23.6	22.8	20.3‡	27.7	25.6	33.0	27.4‡
Vomiting	17.9	14.9‡	16.2	14.4	15.5	12.7‡	9.6	6.8
Diarrhea	12.0	10.7	10.9	9.9	11.5	10.4	12.1	11.2
Rash or Hives	0.7	0.6	0.8	0.8	1.4	1.1	1.4	0.8

* Approximately 90% of subjects received prophylactic or therapeutic antipyretics within 48 hours of each dose.
† Investigational meningococcal group C conjugate vaccine (MnCC).
‡ $p<0.05$ when Prevnar™ compared to control group using a Chi-Square test.

TABLE 11
Percentage of Subjects* Reporting Systemic Events Within 2 Days Following Immunization With Prevnar™ or Control† Vaccine Concurrently With DTaP Vaccine at 2, 4, 6, and 12–15 Months of Age[18]

Reaction	Dose 1		Dose 2		Dose 3		Dose 4‡	
	Prevnar™	Control†	Prevnar™	Control†	Prevnar™	Control†	Prevnar™	Control†
	N=710	N=711	N=559	N=508	N=461	N=414	N=224	N=230
Fever								
≥ 38.0°C	15.1	9.4§	23.9	10.8§	19.1	11.8§	21.0	17.0
> 39.0°C	0.9	0.3	2.5	0.8§	1.7	0.7	1.3	1.7
Irritability	48.0	48.2	58.7	45.3§	51.2	44.8	44.2	42.6
Drowsiness	40.7	42.0	25.6	22.8	19.5	21.9	17.0	16.5
Restless Sleep	15.3	15.1	20.2	19.3	25.2	19.0§	20.2	19.1
Decreased Appetite	17.0	13.5	17.4	13.4	20.7	13.8§	20.5	23.1
Vomiting	14.6	14.5	16.8	14.4	10.4	11.6	4.9	4.8
Diarrhea	11.9	8.4§	10.2	9.3	8.3	9.4	11.6	9.2
Rash or Hives	1.4	0.3§	1.3	1.4	0.4	0.5	0.5	1.7

* Approximately 75% of subjects received prophylactic or therapeutic antipyretics within 48 hours of each dose.
† Investigational meningococcal group C conjugate vaccine (MnCC).
‡ Most of these children had received DTP for the primary series. Thus, this is the 4th dose of a pertussis vaccine, but not of DTaP.
§ $p<0.05$ when Prevnar™ compared to control group using a Chi-Square test.

TABLE 12
Percentage of Subjects* Reporting Systemic Reactions Within 3 Days Following Immunization With Prevnar™, DTaP, HbOC, Hep B, and IPV vs. Control† in Manufacturing Bridging Study[20]

Reaction	Dose 1		Dose 2		Dose 3	
	Prevnar™	Control†	Prevnar™	Control†	Prevnar™	Control†
	N=498	N=108	N=452	N=99	N=445	N=89
Fever						
≥ 38.0°C	21.9	10.2‡	33.6	17.2‡	28.1	23.6
> 39.0°C	0.8	0.9	3.8	0.0	2.2	0.0
Irritability	59.7	60.2	65.3	52.5‡	54.2	50.6
Drowsiness	50.8	38.9‡	30.3	31.3	21.2	20.2
Decreased Appetite	19.1	15.7	20.6	11.1‡	20.4	9.0‡

* Approximately 72% of subjects received prophylactic or therapeutic antipyretics within 48 hours of each dose.
† Control group received concomitant vaccines only in the same schedule as the Prevnar™ group (DTaP, HbOC at dose 1, 2, 3; IPV at doses 1 and 2; Hep B at doses 1 and 3).
‡ $p<0.05$ when Prevnar™ compared to control group using Fisher's Exact test.

was similar to or lower than the age and season-adjusted expected rate from the California State data from 1995–1997 and are presented in Table 14.
[See table 14 at top of next page]

In a review of all hospitalizations that occurred between October 1995 and August 1999 in the efficacy study for the specific diagnoses of aplastic anemia, autoimmune disease, autoimmune hemolytic anemia, diabetes mellitus, neutropenia, and thrombocytopenia, the numbers of such cases were either equal to or less than the expected numbers based on the 1995 Kaiser Vaccine Safety Data Link (VSD) data set. Overall, the safety of Prevnar™ was evaluated in a total of five clinical studies in which 18,168 infants and children received a total of 58,699 doses of vaccine at 2, 4, 6, and 12–15 months of age. In addition, the safety of Prevnar™ was evaluated in 560 children from 4 ancillary studies who started immunization at 7 months to 9 years of age. Tables 15 and 16 summarize systemic reactogenicity data within 2 or 3 days across 4,748 subjects (13,039 infant doses and 1,706 toddler doses) for whom these data were collected and according to the pertussis vaccine administered concurrently.
[See table 15 at top of next page]
[See table 16 at top of page 1679]
With vaccines in general, including Prevnar™, it is not uncommon for patients to note within 48 to 72 hours at or around the injection site the following minor reactions: edema; pain or tenderness; redness, inflammation or skin discoloration; mass; or local hypersensitivity reaction. Such local reactions are usually self-limited and require no therapy.
As with other aluminum-containing vaccines, a nodule may occasionally be palpable at the injection site for several weeks.[33]

ADVERSE EVENT REPORTING

Any suspected adverse events following immunization should be reported by the healthcare professional to the US Department of Health and Human Services (DHHS). The National Vaccine Injury Compensation Program requires that the manufacturer and lot number of the vaccine administered by recorded by the healthcare professional in the vaccine recipient's permanent medical record (or in a permanent office log or file), along with the date of administration of the vaccine and the name, address, and title of the person administering the vaccine.
The US DHHS has established the Vaccine Adverse Event Reporting System (VAERS) to accept all reports of suspected adverse events after the administration of any vaccine including, but not limited to, the reporting of events required by the National Childhood Vaccine Injury Act of 1986. The FDA web site is:
http://www.fda.gov/cber/vaers/vaers.htm.
The VAERS toll-free number for VAERS forms and information is 800-822-7967.[34]

DOSAGE AND ADMINISTRATION

For intramuscular injection only. *Do not inject intravenously.*
The dose is 0.5 mL to be given intramuscularly.
Since this product is a suspension containing an adjuvant, shake vigorously immediately prior to use to obtain a uniform suspension in the vaccine container. The vaccine should not be used if it cannot be resuspended.
After shaking, the vaccine is a homogeneous, white suspension.
Parenteral drug products should be inspected visually for particulate matter and discoloration prior to administration (see DESCRIPTION). This product should not be used if particulate matter of discoloration is found.
The vaccine should be injected intramuscularly. The preferred sites are the anterolateral aspect of the thigh in infants or the deltoid muscle of the upper arm in toddlers and young children. The vaccine should not be injected in the gluteal area or areas where there may be a major nerve trunk and/or blood vessel. Before injection, the skin at the injection site should be cleansed and prepared with a suitable germicide. After insertion of the needle, aspirate and wait to see if any blood appears in the syringe, which will help avoid inadvertent injection into a blood vessel. If blood appears, withdraw the needle and prepare for a new injection at another site.

Vaccine Schedule

For infants, the immunization series of Prevnar™ consists of three doses of 0.5 mL each, at approximately 2-month intervals, followed by a fourth dose of 0.5 mL at 12–15 months of age. The customary age for the first dose is 2 months of age, but it can be given as young as 6 weeks of age. The recommended dosing interval is 4 to 8 weeks. The fourth dose should be administered at least 2 months after the third dose.

Previously Unvaccinated Older Infants and Children

For previously unvaccinated older infants and children, who are beyond the age of the routine infant schedule, the following schedule applies:[26]
[See page 17 at top of page 1679]
(See CLINICAL PHARMACOLOGY section for the limited available immunogenicity data and ADVERSE EVENTS section for limited safety data corresponding to the previously noted vaccination schedule for older children).
Safety and immunogenicity data are either limited or not available for children in specific high risk groups for inva-

Continued on next page

Prevnar—Cont.

sive pneumococcal disease (e.g. persons with sickle cell disease, asplenia, HIV-infected).

HOW SUPPLIED

Vial, 1 Dose (5 per package)—NDC 0005-1970-67

CPT Code 90669

STORAGE

DO NOT FREEZE. STORE REFRIGERATED, AWAY FROM FREEZER COMPARTMENT, AT 2°C TO 8°C (36°F TO 46°F).

TABLE 13
Percentage of Subjects Reporting Systemic Reactions Within 3 Days of Immunization in Infants and Children from 7 Months Through 9 Years of Age[26]

Age at 1st Vaccination	7 – 11 Mos.						12 – 23 Mos.			24 – 35 Mos.	35 – 59 Mos.	5 – 9 Yrs.
Study No.	118-12			118-16			118-9*	118-18		118-18	118-18	118-18
Dose Number	1	2	3†	1	2	3†	1	1	2	1	1	1
Number of Subjects	54	51	24	85	80	50	60	120	117	47	52	100
Reaction												
Fever												
≥ 38.0°C	20.8	21.6	25.0	17.6	18.8	22.0	36.7	11.7	6.8	14.9	11.5	7.0
> 39.0°C	1.9	5.9	0.0	1.6	3.9	2.6	0.0	4.4	0.0	4.2	2.3	1.2
Fussiness	29.6	39.2	16.7	54.1	41.3	38.0	40.0	37.5	36.8	46.8	34.6	29.3
Drowsiness	11.1	17.6	16.7	24.7	16.3	14.0	13.3	18.3	11.1	12.8	17.3	11.0
Decreased Appetite	9.3	15.7	0.0	15.3	15.0	30.0	25.0	20.8	16.2	23.4	11.5	9.0

* For 118-9, 2 of 60 subjects were ≥24 months of age.
† For 118-12, dose 3 was administered at 15 – 18 mos. of age. For 118-16, dose 3 was administered at 12 – 15 mos. of age.

TABLE 14
Age and Season-Adjusted Comparison of SIDS Rates in the NCKP Efficacy Trial With the Expected Rate from the California State Data for 1995–1997[19]

Vaccine	< One Week After Immunization		≤ Two Weeks After Immunization		≤ One Month After Immunization		≤ One Year After Immunization	
	Exp	Obs	Exp	Obs	Exp	Obs	Exp	Obs
Prevnar™	1.06	1	2.09	2	4.28	2	8.08	4
Control*	1.06	2	2.09	3†	4.28	3†	8.08	8†

* Investigational meningococcal group C conjugate vaccine (MnCC).
† Does not include one additional case of SIDS-like death in a child older than the usual SIDS age (448 days).

TABLE 15
Overall Percentage of Doses Associated With Systemic Events Within 2 or 3 Days For Efficacy Study and All Ancillary Studies When Prevnar™ Administered To Infants As a Primary Series at 2, 4, and 6 Months of Age[19,20,22,23,25]

Systemic Event	Prevnar™ Concurrently With DTP-HbOC (9,191 Doses)*	Prevnar™ Concurrently With DTaP-HbOC (3,848 Doses)†	DTaP and HbOC Control (538 Doses)‡
Fever			
≥ 38.0°C	35.6	21.1	**14.2**
> 39.0°C	3.1	1.8	**0.4**
Irritability	69.1	52.5	**45.2**
Drowsiness	36.9	32.9	**27.7**
Restless Sleep	25.8	20.6	**22.3**
Decreased Appetite	24.7	18.1	**13.6**
Vomiting	16.2	13.4	**9.8**
Diarrhea	11.4	9.8	**4.4**
Rash or Hives	0.9	0.6	**0.3**

* Total from which reaction data are available varies between reactions from 8,874–9,191 doses. Data from studies 118-3, 118-7, 118-8.
† Total from which reaction data are available varies between reactions from 3,121–3,848 doses. Data from studies 118-8, 118-12, 118-16.
‡ Total from which reaction data are available varies between reactions from 295–538 doses. Data from studies 118-12 and 118-16.

REFERENCES

1. Schuchat A, Robinson K, Wenger JD, et al. Bacterial meningitis in the United States in 1995. N Engl J Med. 1997; 337:970–6.
2. Zangwill KM, Vadheim CM, Vannier AM, et al. Epidemiology of invasive pneumococcal disease in Southern California: implications for the design and conduct of a pneumococcal conjugate vaccine efficacy trial. J Infect Dis. 1996; 174:752–9.
3. Pastor P, Medley F, Murphy T. Invasive pneumococcal disease in Dallas County, Texas: results from population-based surveillance in 1995. Clin Infect Dis. 1998; 26:590–5.
4. Hofmann J, Cetron MS, Farley MM, et al. The prevalence of drug-resistant *Streptococcus pneumoniae* in Atlanta. N Engl J Med. 1995; 333:481–515.
5. Breiman R, Spika J, Navarro V, et al. Pneumococcal bacteremia in Charleston County, South Carolina. Arch Intern Med. 1990; 150:1401–5.
6. Plouffe J, Breiman R, Facklam R. Franklin County Study Group. Bacteremia with *Streptococcus pneumoniae* in adults—implications for therapy and prevention. JAMA. 1996; 275:194–8.
7. Levine O, Farley M, Harrison LH, et al. Risk factors for invasive pneumococcal disease in children: a population-based case-control study in North America. Pediatrics. 1999; 103:1–5.
8. Kaplan SL, Mason EO, Barson WJ, et al. Three-year multicenter surveillance of systemic pneumococcal infections in children. Pediatrics. 1998; 102:538–44.
9. Arditi M, Edward M, Bradley J, et al. Three-year multicenter surveillance of pneumococcal meningitis in children: clinical characteristics and outcome related to penicillin susceptibility and dexamethasone use. Pediatrics. 1998; 102:1087–97.
10. Bluestone CD, Stephenson BS, Martin LM. Ten-year review of otitis media pathogens. Pediatr Infect Dis J. 1992; 11:S7–S11.
11. Giebink GS. The microbiology of otitis media. Pediatr Infect Dis J. 1989; 8:S18–S20.
12. Butler JC, Breiman RF, Lipman HB, et al. Serotype distribution of *Streptococcus pneumoniae* infections among preschool children in the United States, 1978–1994: implications for development of a conjugate vaccine. J Infect Dis. 1995; 171:885–9.
13. Paisley JW, Lauer BA, McIntosh K, et al. Pathogens associated with acute lower respiratory tract infection in young children. Pediatr Infect Dis J, 1984; 3:14–9.
14. Heiskanen-Kosma T, Korppi M, Jokinen C, et al. Etiology of childhood pneumonia: serologic results of a prospective, population-based study. Pediatr Infect Dis J. 1998; 17:986–91.
15. American Academy of Pediatrics Commitee on Infectious Diseases. Therapy for children with invasive pneumococcal infections. Pediatrics. 1997; 99:289–300.
16. Sniadack DH, Schwart B, Lipman H, et al. Potential interventions for the prevention of childhood pneumonia: geographic and temporal differences in serotype and serogroup distribution of sterile site pneumococcal isolates from children-implicatoins for vaccine strategies. Pediatr Infect Dis J. 1995; 14:503–10.
17. Butler JC, Hoffman J, Cetron MS, et al. The continued emergence of drug-resistant *Streptococcus pneumoniae* in the United States. An Update from the Centers for Disease Control and Prevention's Pneumococcal Sentinel Surveillance System. J Infect Dis. 1996; 174:986–93.
18. Black S, Shinefield H, Ray P, et al. Efficacy of Heptavalent Conjugate Pneumococcal Vaccine (Lederle Laboratories) in 37,000 Infants and Children. Results of the Northern California Kaiser Permanente Efficacy Trial. 38th ICAAC, San Diego, California, September 24–27, 1998.
19. Lederle Laboratories, Data on File: D118-P8.
20. Lederle Laboratories, Data on File: D118-P16.
21. Lederle Laboratories, Data on File: D118-P8 Addendum DTaP Immunogenicity.
22. Shinefield HR, Black S, Ray P. Safety and immunogenicity of heptavalent pneumococcal CRM_{197} conjugate vaccine in infants and toddlers. Pediatr Infect Dis J. 1999; 18:757–63.
23. Lederle Laboratories, Data on File: D118-P12.
24. Rennels MD, Edwards KM, Keyserling HL, et al. Safety and immunogenicity of heptavalent pneumococcal vaccine conjugated to CRM_{197} in United States infants. Pediatrics 1998; 101(4):604–11.
25. Lederle Laboratories, Data on File: D118-P3.
26. Lederle Laboratories, Data on File: Integrated Summary on Catch-Up.
27. Report of the Committee on Infectious Diseases 24th Edition. Elk Grove Village, IL: American Academy of Pediatrics, 1997; 31–3.
28. Update: Vaccine Side Effects, Adverse Reactions, Contraindications, and Precautions. MMWR. 1996; 45(RR-12):1–35.
29. Recommendations of the Advisory Committee on Immunization Practices (ACIP): use of vaccines and immunoglobulins in persons with altered immunocompetence. MMWR. 1993; 43(RR-4):1–18.
30. Vernacchio L, Neufeld EJ, MacDonald K, et al. Combined schedule of 7-valent pneumococcal conjugate vaccine followed by 23-valent pneumococcal vaccine in children and young adults with sickle cell disease. J Pediatr. 1998; 103:275–8.
31. Immunization of children infected with human immunodeficiency virus-supplementary ACIP statement. MMWR, 1988; 37(12):181–83.
32. Center for Disease Control. General recommendations on immunization. Recommendations of the Advisory Committee on Immunization Practices (ACIP). MMWR. 1994; 43(RR01):1–38.
33. Fawcett HA, Smith, NP. Injection-site granuloma due to aluminum. Archives Dermatology. 1984; 120:1318–22.
34. Vaccines Adverse Event Reporting System—United States. MMWR. 1190; 39:730–3.

Manufactured by:
LEDERLE LABORATORIES
Division American Cyanamid Company
Pearl River, NY 10965 USA
US GOVT. LICENSE NO. 17

Marketed by:
WYETH LEDERLE
VACCINES

TABLE 16
Overall Percentage of Doses Associated With Systemic Events Within 2 or 3 Days For Efficacy Study and All Ancillary Studies When Prevnar™ Administered To Toddlers as a Fourth Dose At 12 to 15 Months of Age[19,22]

Systemic Event	Prevnar™ Concurrently With DTP-HbOC (709 Doses)*	Prevnar™ Concurrently With DTaP and HbOC (270 Doses)†	Prevnar™ Only No Concurrent Vaccines (727 Doses)‡
Fever			
≥ 38.0°C	41.9	19.6	13.4
> 39.0°C	4.5	1.5	1.2
Irritability	72.8	45.9	45.8
Drowsiness	21.3	17.5	15.9
Restless Sleep	29.9	21.2	21.2
Decreased Appetite	33.0	21.1	18.3
Vomiting	9.6	5.6	6.3
Diarrhea	12.1	13.7	12.8
Rash or Hives	1.4	0.7	1.2

* Total from which reaction data are available varies between reactions from 706–709 doses. Data from studies 118-8.
† Total from which reaction data are available varies between reactions from 269–270 doses. Data from studies 118-7 and 118-8.
‡ Total from which reaction data are available varies between reactions from 725–727 doses. Data from studies 118-7 and 118-8.

Age at First Dose	Total Number of 0.5 mL Doses
7–11 months of age	3*
12–12 months of age	2†
≥ 24 months through 9 years of age	1

* 2 doses at least 4 weeks apart; third dose after the one-year birthday, separated from the second dose by at least 2 months.
† 2 doses at least 2 months apart.

Wyeth-Ayerst Pharmaceuticals
Philadelphia, PA 19101
CI 6044-1 Issued February 16, 2000
Shown in Product Identification Guide, page 320

PYRAZINAMIDE TABLETS, USP ℞
500 mg

DESCRIPTION

Pyrazinamide, the pyrazine analogue of nicotinamide, is an antituberculous agent. It is a white crystalline powder, stable at room temperature, and sparingly soluble in water. Pyrazinamide has the following chemical formula: $C_5H_5N_3O$, and the following molecular weight: 123.11.
Each Pyrazinamide tablet for oral administration contains 500 mg of pyrazinamide and the following inactive ingredients: Corn Starch, Magnesium Stearate, Modified Food Starch and Stearic Acid.

CLINICAL PHARMACOLOGY

Pyrazinamide is well absorbed from the GI tract and attains peak plasma concentrations within 2 hours. Plasma concentrations generally range from 30 to 50 mcg/mL with doses of 20 to 25 mg/kg. It is widely distributed in body tissues and fluids including the liver, lungs and cerebrospinal fluid (CSF). The CSF concentration is approximately equal to concurrent steady-state plasma concentrations in patients with inflamed meninges.[1] Pyrazinamide is approximately 10% bound to plasma proteins.[2]
The half-life (t1/2) of pyrazinamide is 9 to 10 hours in patients with normal renal and hepatic function. The plasma half-life may be prolonged in patients with impaired renal or hepatic function. Pyrazinamide is hydrolyzed in the liver to its major active metabolite, pyrazinoic acid. Pyrazinoic acid is hydroxylated to the main excretory product, 5-hydroxypyrazinoic acid.[3]
Approximately 70% of an oral dose is excreted in urine, mainly by glomerular filtration within 24 hours.[3]
Pyrazinamide may be bacteriostatic or bactericidal against *Mycobacterium tuberculosis* depending on the concentration of the drug attained at the site of infection. The mechanism of action is unknown. *In vitro* and *in vivo* the drug is active only at a slightly acidic pH.

INDICATIONS AND USAGE

Pyrazinamide is indicated for the initial treatment of active tuberculosis in adults and children when combined with other antituberculous agents. (The current recommendation of the CDC for drug-susceptible disease is to use a six-month regimen for initial treatment of active tuberculosis, consisting of isoniazid, rifampin and pyrazinamide given for 2 months, followed by isoniazid and rifampin for 4 months.*[4])
(Patients with drug-resistant disease should be treated with regimens individualized to their situation. Pyrazinamide frequently will be an important component of such therapy.)
(In patients with concomitant HIV infection, the physician should be aware of current recommendations of CDC. It is possible these patients may require a longer course of treatment.)
It is also indicated after treatment failure with other primary drugs in any form of active tuberculosis.
Pyrazinamide should only be used in conjunction with other effective antituberculous agents.

*See recommendations of Center for Disease Control (CDC) and American Thoracic Society for complete regimen and dosage recommendations.[4]

CONTRAINDICATIONS

Pyrazinamide is contraindicated in persons:
- with severe hepatic damage.
- who have shown hypersensitivity to it.
- with acute gout.

WARNINGS

Patients started on pyrazinamide should have baseline serum uric acid and liver function determinations. Those patients with preexisting liver disease or those at increased risk for drug related hepatitis (e.g., alcohol abusers) should be followed closely.
Pyrazinamide should be discontinued and not be resumed if signs of hepatocellular damage or hyperuricemia accompanied by an acute gouty arthritis appear.

PRECAUTIONS

General
Pyrazinamide inhibits renal excretion of urates, frequently resulting in hyperuricemia which is usually asymptomatic. If hyperuricemia is accompanied by acute gouty arthritis, pyrazinamide should be discontinued.
Pyrazinamide should be used with caution in patients with a history of diabetes mellitus, as management may be more difficult.
Primary resistance of *M. tuberculosis* to pyrazinamide is uncommon. In cases with known or suspected drug resistance, *in vitro* susceptibility tests with recent cultures of *M. tuberculosis* against pyrazinamide and the usual primary drugs should be performed. There are few reliable *in vitro* tests for pyrazinamide resistance. A reference laboratory capable of performing these studies must be employed.

Information for Patients
Patients should be instructed to notify their physicians promptly if they experience any of the following: fever, loss of appetite, malaise, nausea and vomiting, darkened urine, yellowish discoloration of the skin and eyes, pain or swelling of the joints.
Compliance with the full course of therapy must be emphasized, and the importance of not missing any doses must be stressed.

Laboratory Tests
Baseline liver function studies [especially ALT (SGPT), AST (SGOT) determinations] and uric acid levels should be determined prior to therapy. Appropriate laboratory testing should be performed at periodic intervals and if any clinical signs or symptoms occur during therapy.

Drug/Laboratory Test Interactions
Pyrazinamide has been reported to interfere with ACETEST® and KETOSTIX® urine tests to produce a pink-brown color.[5]

Carcinogenicity, Mutagenicity, Impairment of Fertility[6,7,8]
In lifetime bioassays in rats and mice, pyrazinamide was administered in the diet at concentrations of up to 10,000 ppm. This resulted in estimated daily doses for the mouse of 2 g/kg, or 40 times the maximum human dose, and for the rat of 0.5 g/kg, or 10 times the maximum human dose. Pyrazinamide was not carcinogenic in rats or male mice and no conclusion was possible for female mice due to insufficient numbers of surviving control mice.
Pyrazinamide was not mutagenic in the Ames bacterial test, but induced chromosomal aberrations in human lymphocyte cell cultures.

Pregnancy: Teratogenic Effects—Pregnancy Category C
Animal reproduction studies have not been conducted with pyrazinamide. It is also not known whether pyrazinamide can cause fetal harm when administered to a pregnant woman or can affect reproduction capacity. Pyrazinamide should be given to a pregnant woman only if clearly needed.

Nursing Mothers
Pyrazinamide has been found in small amounts in breast milk. Therefore, it is advised the pyrazinamide be used with caution in nursing mothers taking into account the risk-benefit of this therapy.[9]

Usage in Children
Pyrazinamide regimens employed in adults are probably equally effective in children.[4,10,11] Pyrazinamide appears to be well tolerated in children.

Geriatric Use[12]
Clinical studies of pyrazinamide did not include sufficient numbers of patients aged 65 and over to determine whether they respond differently from younger patients. Other reported clinical experience has not identified differences in responses between the elderly and younger patients. In general, dose selection for an elderly patient should be cautious, usually starting at the low end of the dosing range, reflecting the greater frequency of decreased hepatic or renal function, and of concomitant disease or other drug therapy.
It does not appear that patients with impaired renal function require a reduction in dose. It may be prudent to select doses at the low end of the dosing range, however.[13]

ADVERSE REACTIONS

General
Fever, porphyria and dysuria have rarely been reported. Gout (see PRECAUTIONS).

Gastrointestinal
The principal adverse effect is a hepatic reaction (see WARNINGS). Hepatotoxicity appears to be dose related, and may appear at any time during therapy. GI disturbances including nausea, vomiting and anorexia have also been reported.

Hematologic and Lymphatic
Thrombocytopenia and sideroblastic anemia with erythroid hyperplasia, vacuolation of erythrocytes and increased serum iron concentration have occurred rarely with this drug. Adverse effects on blood clotting mechanisms have also been rarely reported.

Other
Mild arthralgia and myalgia have been reported frequently. Hypersensitivity reactions including rashes, urticaria, and pruritus have been reported. Fever, acne, photosensitivity, porphyria, dysuria and interstitial nephritis have been reported rarely.

OVERDOSAGE

Overdosage experience is limited. In one case report of overdose, abnormal liver function tests developed. These spontaneously reverted to normal when the drug was stopped. Clinical monitoring and supportive therapy should be employed. Pyrazinamide is dialyzable.[13]

DOSAGE AND ADMINISTRATION

Pyrazinamide should always be administered with other effective antituberculous drugs. It is administered for the initial 2 months of a 6-month or longer treatment regimen for drug-susceptible patients. Patients who are known or suspected to have drug-resistant disease should be treated with regimens individualized to their situation. Pyrazinamide frequently will be an important component of such therapy. Patients with concomitant HIV infection may require longer courses of therapy. Physicians treating such patients should be alert to any revised recommendations from CDC for this group of patients.
Usual dose: Pyrazinamide is administered orally, 15 to 30 mg/kg once daily. Older regimens employed 3 to 4 divided doses daily, but most current recommendations are for once a day. Three grams per day should not be exceeded. The CDC recommendations do not exceed 2 g per day when given as a daily regimen (see table).
Alternatively, a twice weekly dosing regimen (50 to 70 mg/kg twice weekly based on lean body weight) has been developed to promote patient compliance with a regimen on an outpatient basis. In studies evaluating the twice weekly

Continued on next page

Pyrazinamide—Cont.

regimen, doses of pyrazinamide in excess of 3 g twice weekly have been administered. This exceeds the recommended maximum 3 g/daily dose. However, an increased incidence of adverse reactions has not been reported.
The table is taken from the CDC-American Thoracic Society joint recommendations:[4]
[See table at bottom of page 1594]

HOW SUPPLIED

Pyrazinamide Tablets, USP 500 mg are round, white, scored tablets, engraved P36 on the scored side, and LL on the other side, supplied as:
NDC 0005-5093-23 - Bottle of 100
NDC 0005-5093-31 - Bottle of 500
Store in a well-closed container at controlled room temperature 15°–30°C (59°–86°F).
Caution: Federal law prohibits dispensing without prescription.
Manufactured by:
LEDERLE PHARMACEUTICAL DIVISION
American Cyanamid Company
Pearl River, NY 10965

REFERENCES

1. *Drug Information, American Hospital Formulary Service.* American Society of Hospital Pharmacists. Bethesda, Md. 1991.
2. *USPDI, Drug Information for the Health Care Professional.* United States Pharmacopeial Convention, Inc. Rockville, Md. 1991:1B:2226–2227.
3. Goodman-Gilman A, Rall TW, Nies AS, Taylor P. *The Pharmacological Basis of Therapeutics,* ed 8. New York, Pergamon Press. 1990;1154.
4. Treatment of tuberculosis and tuberculosis infection in adults and children. *Am Rev Respir Dis.* 1986;134:363–368.
5. Reynolds JEF, Parfitt K, Parsons AV, Sweetman SC. *Martindale The Extra Pharmacopoeia,* ed 29. London, The Pharmaceutical Press. 1989;569-570.
6. Bioassay of pyrazinamide for possible carcinogenicity. National Cancer Institute Carcinogenesis Technical Report Series No. 48, 1978.
7. Zerger E, Anderson B, Haworth S, Lawlor T, Mortelmans K, Speck W. Salmonella mutagenicity tests: III. Results from the testing of 255 chemicals. *Environ Mutagen.* 1987;9(Suppl 9):1–109.
8. Roman IC, Georgian L. Cytogenetic effects of some antituberculosis drugs in vitro. *Mutation Research.* 1977;48:215–224.
9. Holdiness M. Antituberculosis drugs and breast-feeding. *Arch Intern Med.* 1984;144:1888.
10. Turcios N, Evans H. Preventing and managing tuberculosis in children. *J Resp Dis.* 1989;10(6)(Jun):23.
11. Starke JR. Multidrug therapy for tuberculosis in children. *Pediatr Infec Dis J.* 1990;9:785–793.
12. Specific requirements on content and format of labeling for human prescription drugs; proposed addition of "geriatric use" subsection in the labeling. *Federal Register.* 1990;55(212) (Nov 1):46134–46137.
13. Stamathakis G, Montes C, Trouvin JH, et al. Pyrazinamide and pyrazinoic acid pharmacokinetics in patients with chronic renal failure. *Clinical Nephrology.* 1988;30:230–234.

C1 4977-1 Issued September 29, 1998

SUPRAX® ℞

[sū 'prăcks]
Cefixime
Oral

DESCRIPTION

SUPRAX (cefixime) is a semisynthetic, cephalosporin antibiotic for oral administration. Chemically, it is (6*R*,7*R*)-7-[2-(2-Amino-4-thiazolyl)glyoxylamido]-8-oxo-3-vinyl-5-thia-1-azabicyclo[4.2.0]oct-2-ene-2-carboxylic acid, 7^2-(*Z*)-[*O*-(carboxymethyl)oxime]trihydrate. Molecular weight = 507.50 as the trihydrate.
SUPRAX is available in scored 200 mg and 400 mg film coated tablets and in a powder for oral suspension which when reconstituted provides 100 mg/5 mL.
Inactive ingredients contained in the 200 mg and 400 mg tablets are: dibasic calcium phosphate, hydroxypropyl methylcellulose 2910, light mineral oil, magnesium stearate, microcrystalline cellulose, pregelatinized starch, sodium lauryl sulfate, and titanium dioxide. The powder for oral suspension is strawberry flavored and contains sodium benzoate, sucrose, and xanthan gum.

CLINICAL PHARMACOLOGY

SUPRAX, given orally, is about 40% to 50% absorbed whether administered with or without food; however, time to maximal absorption is increased approximately 0.8 hours when administered with food. A single 200 mg tablet of SUPRAX produces an average peak serum concentration of approximately 2 mcg/mL (range 1 to 4 mcg/mL); a single 400 mg tablet produces an average peak concentration of approximately 3.7 mcg/mL (range 1.3 to 7.7 mcg/mL). The oral suspension produces average peak concentrations approximately 25%–50% higher than the tablets, when tested in normal *adult* volunteers. Two hundred and 400 mg doses of oral suspension produce average peak concentrations of 3 mcg/mL (range 1 to 4.5 mcg/mL) and 4.6 mcg/mL (range 1.9 to 7.7 mcg/mL), respectively, when tested in normal *adult* volunteers. The area under the time versus concentration curve is greater by approximately 10%–25% with the oral suspension than with the tablet after doses of 100 to 400 mg, when tested in normal *adult* volunteers. This increased absorption should be taken into consideration if the oral suspension is to be substituted for the tablet. Because of the lack of bioequivalence, tablets should not be substituted for oral suspension in the treatment of otitis media. (See **DOSAGE AND ADMINISTRATION**.) Cross-over studies of tablet versus suspension have not been performed in children.
Peak serum concentrations occur between 2 and 6 hours following oral administration of a single 200 mg tablet, a single 400 mg tablet, or 400 mg of suspension of SUPRAX. Peak serum concentrations occur between 2 and 5 hours following a single administration of 200 mg of suspension.

TABLE

Serum Levels of Cefixime after Administration of Tablets (mcg/mL)

DOSE	1h	2h	4h	6h	8h	12h	24h
100 mg	0.3	0.8	1.0	0.7	0.4	0.2	0.02
200 mg	0.7	1.4	2.0	1.5	1.0	0.4	0.03
400 mg	1.2	2.5	3.5	2.7	1.7	0.6	0.04

Serum Levels of Cefixime after Administration of Oral Suspension (mcg/mL)

DOSE	1h	2h	4h	6h	8h	12h	24h
100 mg	0.7	1.1	1.3	0.9	0.6	0.2	0.02
200 mg	1.2	2.1	2.8	2.0	1.3	0.5	0.07
400 mg	1.8	3.3	4.4	3.3	2.2	0.8	0.07

Approximately 50% of the absorbed dose is excreted unchanged in the urine in 24 hours. In animal studies, it was noted that cefixime is also excreted in the bile in excess of 10% of the administered dose. Serum protein binding is concentration independent with a bound fraction of approximately 65%. In a multiple dose study conducted with a research formulation which is less bioavailable than the tablet or suspension, there was little accumulation of drug in serum or urine after dosing for 14 days.

Recommended Drugs for the Initial Treatment of Tuberculosis in Children and Adults

Drug	Daily Dose* Children	Daily Dose* Adults	Maximal Daily Dose in Children and Adults	Twice Weekly Dose Children	Twice Weekly Dose Adults
Isoniazid	10 to 20 mg/kg PO or IM	5 mg/kg PO or IM	300 mg	20 to 40 mg/kg Max. 900 mg	15 mg/kg Max. 900 mg
Rifampin	10 to 20 mg/kg PO	10 mg/kg PO	600 mg	10 to 20 mg/kg Max. 600 mg	10 mg/kg Max. 600 mg
Pyrazinamide	15 to 30 mg/kg PO	15 to 30 mg/kg PO	2 g	50 to 70 mg/kg	50 to 70 mg/kg
Streptomycin	20 to 40 mg/kg IM	15 mg/kg** IM	1 g**	25 to 30 mg/kg IM	25 to 30 mg/kg IM
Ethambutol	15 to 25 mg/kg PO	15 to 25 mg/kg PO	2.5 g	50 mg/kg	50 mg/kg

Definition of abbreviations: PO = perorally; IM = intramuscularly.
* Doses based on weight should be adjusted as weight changes.
** In persons older than 60 yrs of age the daily dose of streptomycin should be limited to 10 mg/kg with a maximal dose of 750 mg.

The serum half-life of cefixime in healthy subjects is independent of dosage form and averages 3.0–4.0 hours but may range up to 9 hours in some normal volunteers. Average AUCs at steady state in elderly patients are approximately 40% higher than average AUCs in other healthy adults.
In subjects with moderate impairment of renal function (20 to 40mL/min creatinine clearance), the average serum half-life of cefixime is prolonged to 6.4 hours. In severe renal impairment (5 to 20 mL/min creatinine clearance), the half-life increased to an average of 11.5 hours. The drug is not cleared significantly from the blood by hemodialysis or peritoneal dialysis. However, a study indicated that with doses of 400 mg, patients undergoing hemodialysis have similar blood profiles as subjects with creatinine clearances of 21–60 mL/min. There is no evidence of metabolism of cefixime *in vivo*.
Adequate data on CSF levels of cefixime are not available.

Microbiology

As with other cephalosporins, bactericidal action of SUPRAX results from inhibition of cell-wall synthesis. SUPRAX is highly stable in the presence of beta-lactamase enzymes. As a result, many organisms resistant to penicillins and some cephalosporins due to the presence of beta-lactamases, may be susceptible to cefixime. SUPRAX has been shown to be active against most strains of the following organisms both *in vitro* and in clinical infections (see **INDICATIONS AND USAGE**):
Gram-positive Organisms.
Streptococcus pneumoniae,
Streptococcus pyogenes.
Gram-negative Organisms.
Haemophilus influenzae (beta-lactamase positive and negative strains),
Moraxella (Branhamella) catarrhalis (most of which are beta-lactamase positive),
Escherichia coli.
Proteus mirabilis.
Neisseria gonorrhoeae (including penicillinase- and non-penicillinase-producing strains).
SUPRAX has been shown to be active *in vitro* against most strains of the following organisms; however, clinical efficacy has not been established.
Gram-positive Organisms.
Streptococcus agalactiae.
Gram-negative Organisms.
Haemophilus parainfluenzae (beta-lactamase positive and negative strains),
Proteus vulgaris,
Klebsiella pneumoniae,
Klebsiella oxytoca,
Pasteurella multocida,
Providencia species,
Salmonella species,
Shigella species,
Citrobacter amalonaticus,
Citrobacter diversus,
Serratia marcescens.
Note: *Pseudomonas* species, strains of group D streptococci (including enterococci), *Listeria monocytogenes,* most strains of staphylococci (including methicillin-resistant strains) and most strains of *Enterobacter* are resistant to SUPRAX. In addition, most strains of *Bacteroides fragilis* and *Clostridia* are resistant to SUPRAX.

SUSCEPTIBILITY TESTING

Susceptibility Tests: Diffusion Techniques

Quantitative methods that require measurement of zone diameters give an estimate of antibiotic susceptibility. One such procedure[1–3] has been recommended for use with disks to test susceptibility to cefixime. Interpretation involves correlation of the diameters obtained in the disk test with minimum inhibitory concentration (MIC) for cefixime.
Reports from the laboratory giving results of the standard single-disk susceptibility test with a 5-mcg cefixime disk should be interpreted according to the following criteria:
[See first table at top of next page]
A report of "Susceptible" indicates that the pathogen is likely to be inhibited by generally achievable blood levels. A report of "Moderately Susceptible" indicates that inhibitory concentrations of the antibiotic may well be achieved if high dosage is used or if the infection is confined to tissues and fluids (eg, urine) in which high antibiotic levels are attained. A report of "Resistant" indicates that achievable concentrations of the antibiotic are unlikely to be inhibitory and other therapy should be selected.
Standardized procedures require the use of laboratory control organisms. The 5-mcg disk should give the following zone diameter:

Organism	Zone diameter (mm)
E. coli ATCC 25922	23–27
N. gonorrhoeae ATCC 49226[a]	37–45

[a] Using GC Agar Base with a defined 1% supplement with cysteine.

The class disk for cephalosporin susceptibility testing (the cephalothin disk) is not appropriate because of spectrum differences with cefixime. The 5-mcg cefixime disk should be used for all *in vitro* testing of isolates.

Dilution Techniques Broth or agar dilution methods can be used to determine the minimum inhibitory concentration (MIC) value for susceptibility of bacterial isolates to cefixime. The recommended susceptibility breakpoints are as follows:
[See second table in next column]
As with standard diffusion methods, dilution procedures require the use of laboratory control organisms. Standard cefixime powder should give the following MIC ranges in daily testing of quality control organisms:

Organism	MIC Range (µg/mL)
E. coli ATCC 25922	0.25 –1
S. aureus ATCC 29213	8–32
N. gonorrhoeae ATCC 49226[a]	0.008-0.03

[a] Using GC Agar Base with a defined 1% supplement without cysteine.

INDICATIONS AND USAGE

SUPRAX (cefixime) is indicated in the treatment of the following infections when caused by susceptible strains of the designated microorganisms:
Uncomplicated Urinary Tract Infections caused by *Escherichia coli* and *Proteus mirabilis.*
Otitis Media caused by *Haemophilus influenzae* (beta-lactamase positive and negative strains), *Moraxella (Branhamella) catarrhalis,* (most of which are beta-lactamase positive) and *S. pyogenes**.
Note: For information on otitis media caused by *Streptococcus pneumoniae,* see **CLINICAL STUDIES** section.
Pharyngitis and Tonsillitis, caused by *S. pyogenes.*
Note: Penicillin is the usual drug of choice in the treatment of *S. pyogenes* infections, including the prophylaxis of rheumatic fever. SUPRAX is generally effective in the eradication of *S. pyogenes* from the nasopharynx; however, data establishing the efficacy of SUPRAX in the subsequent prevention of rheumatic fever are not available.
Acute Bronchitis and Acute Exacerbations of Chronic Bronchitis, caused by *Streptococcus pneumoniae* and *Haemophilus influenzae* (beta-lactamase positive and negative strains).
Uncomplicated Gonorrhea (cervical/urethral), caused by *Neisseria gonorrhoeae* (penicillinase- and nonpenicillinase-producing strains).
Appropriate cultures and susceptibility studies should be performed to determine the causative organism and its susceptibility to SUPRAX; however, therapy may be started while awaiting the results of these studies. Therapy should be adjusted, if necessary, once these results are known.
*Efficacy for this organism in this organ system was studied in fewer than 10 infections.

CLINICAL STUDIES

In clinical trials of otitis media in nearly 400 children between the ages of 6 months to 10 years, *Streptococcus pneumoniae* was isolated from 47% of the patients, *Haemophilus influenzae* from 34%, *Moraxella (Branhamella) catarrhalis* from 15%, and *S. pyogenes* from 4%.
The overall response rate of *Streptococcus pneumoniae* to cefixime was approximately 10% lower and that of *Haemophilus influenzae* or *Moraxella (Branhamella) catarrhalis* approximately 7% higher (12% when beta-lactamase positive strains of *H. influenzae* are included) than the response rates of these organisms to the active control drugs.
In these studies, patients were randomized and treated with either cefixime at dose regimens of 4 mg/kg BID or 8 mg/kg QD, or with a standard antibiotic regimen. Sixty-nine to 70% of the patients in each group had resolution of signs and symptoms of otitis media when evaluated 2 to 4 weeks posttreatment, but persistent effusion was found in 15% of the patients. When evaluated at the completion of therapy, 17% of patients receiving cefixime and 14% of patients receiving effective comparative drugs (18% including those patients who had *Haemophilus influenzae* resistant to the control drug and who received the control antibiotic) were considered to be treatment failures. By the 2 to 4 week follow-up, a total of 30%–31% of patients had evidence of either treatment failure or recurrent disease.
[See third table above]

CONTRAINDICATIONS

SUPRAX is contraindicated in patients with known allergy to the cephalosporin group of antibiotics.

WARNINGS

BEFORE THERAPY WITH SUPRAX IS INSTITUTED, CAREFUL INQUIRY SHOULD BE MADE TO DETERMINE WHETHER THE PATIENT HAS HAD PREVIOUS HYPERSENSITIVITY REACTIONS TO CEPHALOSPORINS, PENICILLINS, OR OTHER DRUGS. IF THIS PRODUCT IS TO BE GIVEN TO PENICILLIN-SENSITIVE PATIENTS, CAUTION SHOULD BE EXERCISED BECAUSE CROSS-HYPERSENSITIVITY AMONG BETA-LACTAM ANTIBIOTICS HAS BEEN CLEARLY DOCUMENTED AND MAY OCCUR IN UP TO 10% OF PATIENTS WITH A HISTORY OF PENICILLIN ALLERGY. IF AN ALLERGIC REACTION TO SUPRAX OCCURS, DISCONTINUE THE DRUG. SERIOUS ACUTE HYPERSENSITIVITY REACTIONS MAY REQUIRE TREATMENT WITH EPINEPHRINE AND OTHER EMERGENCY MEASURES, INCLUDING OXYGEN, INTRAVENOUS FLUIDS, INTRAVENOUS ANTIHISTAMINES, CORTICOSTEROIDS, PRESSOR AMINES AND AIRWAY MANAGEMENT, AS CLINICALLY INDICATED.
Antibiotics, including SUPRAX, should be administered cautiously to any patient who has demonstrated some form of allergy, particularly to drugs.

SUPRAX® Recommended Susceptibility Ranges: Agar Disk Diffusion

Organisms	Resistant	Moderately Susceptible	Susceptible
Neisseria gonorrhoeae[a]	—	—	≥31 mm
All other organisms	≤ 15 mm	16–18 mm	≥19 mm

[a] Using GC Agar Base with a defined 1% supplement without cysteine.

MIC Interpretive Standards (µg/mL)

Organisms	Resistant	Moderately Susceptible	Susceptible
Neisseria gonorrhoeae[a]	—	—	≤ 0.25
All other organisms	≥ 4	2	≤ 1

Bacteriological Outcome of Otitis Media at Two to Four Weeks Post-Therapy Based on Repeat Middle Ear Fluid Culture or Extrapolation from Clinical Outcome

Organism	Cefixime[(a)] 4 mg/kg BID		Cefixime[(a)] 8 mg/kg QD		Control[(a)] drugs	
Streptococcus pneumoniae	48/70	(69%)	18/22	(82%)	82/100	(82%)
Haemophilus influenzae beta-lactamase negative	24/34	(71%)	13/17	(76%)	23/34	(68%)
Haemophilus influenzae beta-lactamase positive	17/22	(77%)	9/12	(75%)	1/1[(b)]	
Moraxella (Branhamella) catarrhalis	26/31	(84%)	5/5		18/24	(75%)
S. pyogenes	5/5		3/3		6/7	
All Isolates	120/162	(74%)	48/59	(81%)	130/166	(78%)

[(a)] Number eradicated/number isolated.
[(b)] An additional 20 beta-lactamase positive strains of *Haemophilus influenzae* were isolated, but were excluded from this analysis because they were resistant to the control antibiotic. In nineteen of these, the clinical course could be assessed, and a favorable outcome occurred in 10. When these cases are included in the overall bacteriological evaluation of therapy with the control drugs, 140/185 (76%) of pathogens were considered to be eradicated.

Treatment with broad-spectrum antibiotics, including SUPRAX, alters the normal flora of the colon and may permit overgrowth of clostridia. Studies indicate that a toxin produced by *Clostridium difficile* is a primary cause of severe antibiotic-associated diarrhea, including pseudomembranous colitis.
Pseudomembranous colitis has been reported with the use of SUPRAX and other broad-spectrum antibiotics (including macrolides, semisynthetic penicillins, and cephalosporins); therefore, it is important to consider this diagnosis in patients who develop diarrhea in association with the use of antibiotics. Symptoms of pseudomembranous colitis may occur during or after antibiotic treatment and may range in severity from mild to life- threatening. Mild cases of pseudomembranous colitis usually respond to drug discontinuation alone. In moderate to severe cases, management should include fluids, electrolytes, and protein supplementation. If the colitis does not improve after the drug has been discontinued, or if the symptoms are severe, oral vancomycin is the drug of choice for antibiotic-associated pseudomembranous colitis produced by *C difficile.* Other causes of colitis should be excluded.

PRECAUTIONS

General

The possibility of the emergence of resistant organisms, which might result in overgrowth should be kept in mind, particularly during prolonged treatment. In such use, careful observation of the patient is essential. If superinfection occurs during therapy, appropriate measures should be taken.
The dose of SUPRAX should be adjusted in patients with renal impairment as well as those undergoing continuous ambulatory peritoneal dialysis (CAPD) and hemodialysis (HD). Patients on dialysis should be monitored carefully. (See **DOSAGE AND ADMINISTRATION.**)
SUPRAX should be prescribed with caution in individuals with a history of gastrointestinal disease, particularly colitis.

Drug Interactions

Carbamazepine: Elevated carbamazepine levels have been reported in postmarketing experience when SUPRAX is administered concomitantly. Drug monitoring may be of assistance in detecting alterations in carbamazepine plasma concentrations.

Drug/Laboratory Test Interactions

A false-positive reaction for ketones in the urine may occur with tests using nitroprusside but not with those using nitroferricyanide.
The administration of SUPRAX may result in a false-positive reaction for glucose in the urine using Clinitest®,** Benedict's solution, or Fehling's solution. It is recommended that glucose tests based on enzymatic glucose oxidase reactions (such as Clinistix®** or Tes-Tape®**) be used.
A false-positive direct Coombs test has been reported during treatment with other cephalosporin antibiotics; therefore, it should be recognized that a positive Coombs test may be due to the drug.

Carcinogenesis, Mutagenesis, Impairment of Fertility

Lifetime studies in animals to evaluate carcinogenic potential have not been conducted. SUPRAX did not cause point mutations in bacteria or mammalian cells, DNA damage, or chromosome damage *in vitro* and did not exhibit clastogenic potential *in vivo* in the mouse micronucleus test. In rats, fertility and reproductive performance were not affected by cefixime at doses up to 125 times the adult therapeutic dose.

Usage in Pregnancy

Pregnancy Category B. Reproduction studies have been performed in mice and rats at doses up to 400 times the human dose and have revealed no evidence of harm to the fetus due to SUPRAX. There are no adequate and well-controlled studies in pregnant women. Because animal reproduction studies are not always predictive of human response, this drug should be used during pregnancy only if clearly needed.

Labor and Delivery

SUPRAX has not been studied for use during labor and delivery. Treatment should only be given if clearly needed.

Nursing Mothers

It is not known whether SUPRAX is excreted in human milk. Consideration should be given to discontinuing nursing temporarily during treatment with this drug.

Pediatric Use

Safety and effectiveness of SUPRAX in children aged less than 6 months old have not been established.
The incidence of gastrointestinal adverse reactions, including diarrhea and loose stools, in the pediatric patients receiving the suspension, was comparable to the incidence seen in adult patients receiving tablets.

ADVERSE REACTIONS

Most of the adverse reactions observed in clinical trials were of a mild and transient nature. Five percent (5%) of patients in the US trials discontinued therapy because of drug-related adverse reactions. The most commonly seen adverse reactions in US trials of the tablet formulation were gastrointestinal events, which were reported in 30% of adult patients on either the BID or the QD regimen. Clinically mild gastrointestinal side effects occurred in 20% of all patients, moderate events occurred in 9% of all patients, and severe adverse reactions occurred in 2% of all patients. Individual event rates included diarrhea 16%, loose or frequent stools 6%, abdominal pain 3%, nausea 7%, dyspepsia 3%, and flatulence 4%. The incidence of gastrointestinal adverse reactions, including diarrhea and loose stools, in pediatric patients receiving the suspension was comparable to the incidence seen in adult patients receiving tablets.
These symptoms usually responded to symptomatic therapy or ceased when SUPRAX was discontinued.
Several patients developed severe diarrhea and/or documented pseudomembranous colitis, and a few required hospitalization.
The following adverse reactions have been reported following the use of SUPRAX. Incidence rates were less than 1 in 50 (less than 2%), except as noted above for gastrointestinal events.
Gastrointestinal (See Above): Diarrhea, loose stools, abdominal pain, dyspepsia, nausea, and vomiting. Several cases of

Continued on next page

Suprax—Cont.

documented pseudomembranous colitis were identified during the studies. The onset of pseudomembranous colitis symptoms may occur during or after therapy.
Hypersensitivity Reactions: Skin rashes, urticaria, drug fever, and pruritus. Erythema multiforme, Stevens-Johnson syndrome, and serum sickness-like reactions have been reported.
Hepatic: Transient elevations in SGPT, SGOT, and alkaline phosphatase.
Renal: Transient elevations in BUN or creatinine.
Central Nervous System: Headaches or dizziness.
Hemic and Lymphatic Systems: Transient thrombocytopenia, leukopenia, and eosinophilia. Prolongation in prothrombin time was seen rarely.
Other: Genital pruritus, vaginitis, candidiasis.
In addition to the adverse reactions listed above, which have been observed in patients treated with SUPRAX, the following adverse reactions and altered laboratory tests have been reported for cephalosporin-class antibiotics:
Adverse reactions: Allergic reactions including anaphylaxis, toxic epidermal necrolysis, superinfection, renal dysfunction, toxic nephropathy, hepatic dysfunction including cholestasis, aplastic anemia, hemolytic anemia, hemorrhage, and colitis.
Several cephalosporins have been implicated in triggering seizures, particularly in patients with renal impairment when the dosage was not reduced. (See **DOSAGE AND ADMINISTRATION** and **OVERDOSAGE**.) If seizures associated with drug therapy occur, the drug should be discontinued. Anticonvulsant therapy can be given if clinically indicated.
Abnormal Laboratory Tests: Positive direct Coombs test, elevated bilirubin, elevated LDH, pancytopenia, neutropenia, agranulocytosis.

OVERDOSAGE

Gastric lavage may be indicated; otherwise, no specific antidote exists. Cefixime is not removed in significant quantities from the circulation by hemodialysis or peritoneal dialysis. Adverse reactions in small numbers of healthy adult volunteers receiving single doses up to 2 g of SUPRAX did not differ from the profile seen in patients treated at the recommended doses.

DOSAGE AND ADMINISTRATION

Adults: The recommended dose of SUPRAX is 400 mg daily. This may be given as a 400 mg tablet daily or as 200 mg tablet every 12 hours.
For the treatment of uncomplicated cervical/urethral gonococcal infections, a single oral dose of 400 mg is recommended.
Children: The recommended dose is 8 mg/kg/day of the suspension. This may be administered as a single daily dose or may be given in two divided doses, as 4 mg/kg every 12 hours.

PEDIATRIC DOSAGE CHART

Patient Weight (kg)	Dose/Day mg	Dose/Day mL	Dose/Day tsp of suspension
6.25	50	2.5	1/2
12.5	100	5.0	1
18.75	150	7.5	1 1/2
25.0	200	10.0	2
31.25	250	12.5	2 1/2
37.5	300	15.0	3

Children weighing more than 50 kg or older than 12 years should be treated with the recommended adult dose.
Otitis media should be treated with the suspension. Clinical studies of otitis media were conducted with the suspension, and the suspension results in higher peak blood levels than the tablet when administered at the same dose. Therefore, the tablet should not be substituted for the suspension in the treatment of otitis media. (See **CLINICAL PHARMACOLOGY**.)
Efficacy and safety in infants aged less than six months have not been established.
In the treatment of infections due to *S. pyogenes*, a therapeutic dosage of SUPRAX should be administered for at least 10 days.

Renal Impairment

SUPRAX may be administered in the presence of impaired renal function. Normal dose and schedule may be employed in patients with creatinine clearances of 60 mL/min or greater. Patients whose clearance is between 21 and 60 mL/min or patients who are on renal hemodialysis may be given 75% of the standard dosing interval (ie, 300 mg daily). Patients whose clearance is < 20 mL/min, or patients who are on continuous ambulatory peritoneal dialysis may be given half the standard dosage at the standard dosing interval (ie, 200 mg daily). Neither hemodialysis nor peritoneal dialysis removes significant amounts of drug from the body.

RECONSTITUTION DIRECTIONS FOR ORAL SUSPENSION

Bottle Size	Reconstitution Directions
100 mL	To reconstitute, suspend with **69 mL water**. Method: Tap the bottle several times to loosen powder contents prior to reconstitution. Add approximately half the total amount of water for reconstitution and shake well. Add the remainder of water and shake well.
75 mL	To reconstitute, suspend with **52 mL water**. Method: Tap the bottle several times to loosen powder contents prior to reconstitution. Add approximately half the total amount of water for reconstitution and shake well. Add the remainder of water and shake well.
50 mL	To reconstitute, suspend with **36 mL water**. Method: Tap the bottle several times to loosen powder contents prior to reconstitution. Add approximately half the total amount of water for reconstitution and shake well. Add the remainder of water and shake well.

After reconstitution, the suspension may be kept for 14 days either at room temperature, or under refrigeration, without significant loss of potency. Keep tightly closed. Shake well before using. Discard unused portion after 14 days.

HOW SUPPLIED

SUPRAX® (cefixime) Tablets, 200 mg, are convex, rectangular, white, film-coated tablets with rounded corners and beveled edges and a divided break line on each side, engraved with SUPRAX across one side and LL to the left and 200 to the right on the other side, supplied as follows:
NDC 0005-3899-23—Bottle of 100
Store at controlled room temperature 15°–30°C (59°–86°F).
SUPRAX® (cefixime) Tablets, 400 mg, are convex, rectangular, white, film-coated tablets with rounded corners and beveled edges and a divided break line on each side, engraved with SUPRAX across one side and LL to the left and 400 to the right on the other side, supplied as follows:
NDC 0005-3897-94—Unit-of-Issue 10s with CRC
NDC 0005-3897-18—Bottle of 50
NDC 0005-3897-23—Bottle of 100
NDC 0005-3897-60—10 (2 × 5) Strips
Store at controlled room temperature 15°–30°C (59°–86°F).
SUPRAX® (cefixime) for Oral Suspension is an off-white to cream-colored powder which when reconstituted as directed contains cefixime 100 mg/5 mL, supplied as follows:
NDC 0005-3898-40—50 mL Bottle
NDC 0005-3898-42—75 mL Bottle
NDC 0005-3898-46—100 mL Bottle
Prior to Reconstitution: Store at Controlled Room Temperature 15°–30°C (59°–86°F).
After reconstitution store at room temperature or under refrigeration.

REFERENCES

1. Bauer AW, Kirby WMM, Sherris JC, et al.: Antibiotic susceptibility testing by a standard single disk method. *Am J Clin Pathol* 1966;45:493.
2. National Committee for Clinical Laboratory Standards, Approved Standard: Performance Standards for Antimicrobial Disk Susceptibility Tests (M2-A3), December 1984.
3. Standardized disk susceptibility test. *Federal Register.* 1974;39(May 30): 19182–19184.

**Clinitest® and Clinistix® are registered trademarks of Ames Division, Miles Laboratories, Inc. Tes-Tape® is a registered trademark of Eli Lilly and Company.
Marketed by:
Wyeth Lederle Vaccines
Wyeth-Ayerst Laboratories
Philadelphia, PA 19101
Under License of
Fujisawa Pharmaceutical Co., Ltd.
Osaka, Japan
CI 4468-3 Revised October 22, 1998
Shown in Product Identification Guide, page 320

TETANUS AND DIPHTHERIA TOXOIDS ADSORBED ℞

FOR ADULT USE
Aluminum Phosphate-Adsorbed

℞ only
For Intramuscular Injection Only

DESCRIPTION

Tetanus and Diphtheria Toxoids Adsorbed For Adult Use, Aluminum Phosphate Adsorbed (Td), is a sterile combination of tetanus toxoid (PUROGENATED®) and diphtheria toxoid for intramuscular use only. After shaking, the vaccine is a homogeneous white suspension.
The tetanus toxoid component is derived from *Clostridium tetani*, which is grown in a growth medium containing beef heart infusion according to the method of Mueller and Miller.[1] It is detoxified with formaldehyde. The toxoid is refined by the Pillemer alcohol fractionation method[2] and diluted with a solution containing sodium phosphate monobasic, sodium phosphate dibasic, glycine, and thimerosal (mercury derivative) as a preservative.
The diphtheria toxoid component is derived from *Corynebacterium diphtheriae*, which is grown in a growth medium containing an enzymatic digest of casein. The toxin is purified by ammonium sulfate precipitation and ion exchange chromatography. It is then detoxified with formaldehyde in the presence of L-lysine. The toxoid is maintained in sodium bicarbonate with L-lysine, formaldehyde, and thimerosal (mercury derivative) as a preservative.
The tetanus and diphtheria toxoids are each adsorbed to aluminum phosphate and brought to final volume with physiological saline. Thimerosal (mercury derivative) is added as a preservative to a final concentration of 1:10,000. The final product is formulated to contain 0.3 mg of aluminum per 0.5 mL dose from the aluminum phosphate adjuvant. The residual free formaldehyde content by assay is less than 0.02%.
Each 0.5 mL dose is formulated to contain 5 Lf units of tetanus toxoid and not more than 2 Lf units of diphtheria toxoid. The tetanus component induces at least 2 neutralizing units/mL of serum and the diphtheria toxoid component induces at least 0.5 neutralizing units/mL of serum in the guinea pig potency test.

CLINICAL PHARMACOLOGY

Tetanus is an intoxication manifested primarily by neuromuscular dysfunction caused by a potent exotoxin elaborated by *C. tetani*. The incidence of tetanus in the United States has dropped dramatically with the routine use of tetanus toxoid with an average of 57 cases reported annually from 1985–1994.[3] During the period from 1995 through 1997, 124 cases of tetanus were reported from 33 states and the District of Columbia, resulting in an average annual incidence of 0.15 cases per 1,000,000 population. The case-fatality ratio varied from 2.3% for persons aged 20–39 years to 16% for persons ages 40–59 years and to 18% for persons aged ≥60 years. Previous immunization status was directly related to the severity of the disease, with the case-fatality ratio ranging from 6% for persons who had received 1 to 2 doses of tetanus toxoid to 15% for persons who were unvaccinated. Tetanus remains a severe disease, with adults ≥60 years at the highest risk of severe disease.[4]
Spores of *C. tetani* are ubiquitous, and there is essentially no natural immunity to tetanus toxin. Thus, universal primary immunization with tetanus toxoid with subsequent maintenance of adequate antitoxin levels, by means of timed boosters, is recommended to protect all age groups.[5]
Tetanus toxoid is a highly effective antigen and a completed primary series generally induces serum antitoxin levels of at least 0.01 antitoxin units/mL, a level that has been reported to be protective.[6] It is thought that protection persists for at least 10 years.[5]
Diphtheria is a disease resulting from infection of the respiratory tract with *Corynebacterium diphtheriae*. This disease can be localized to the site of infection or can be associated with systemic toxicity, which may include myocarditis and neuritis and is caused by diphtheria toxin, an extracellular protein metabolite of toxigenic strains of *C. diphtheriae*. While the incidence of diphtheria in the US has decreased from over 200,000 cases reported in 1921, before the general use of diphtheria toxoid, to only 15 cases reported from 1990 to 1994,[3] the case fatality rate has remained constant at about 5% to 10%. The highest case-fatality rates are in the very young and in the elderly. Diphtheria remains a serious disease in some areas of the world as demonstrated by the recent epidemic in the former Soviet Union.[7]
Following adequate immunization with diphtheria toxoid, which induces antitoxin, it is thought that protection lasts for at least 10 years.[5] Antitoxin levels of at least 0.01 antitoxin units/mL are generally regarded as protective.[8] This significantly reduces both the risk of developing diphtheria and the severity of clinical illness. It does not, however, eliminate carriage of *C. diphtheriae* in the pharynx or on the skin.[5]
The toxoids of tetanus and diphtheria induce neutralizing antibodies to the toxins produced by the infecting organism. Serum antitoxin levels greater than 0.01 antitoxin units/mL are generally regarded as protective.[6,8] In a study of adults, aged 18 to 55 years, whose previous immunization status for diphtheria and tetanus was not known, such levels were achieved in 33/35 (94%) and 34/34 (100%) of subjects for diphtheria and tetanus, respectively, following a booster dose of Lederle-produced Tetanus and Diphtheria Toxoid Adsorbed For Adults Use.[9] In another clinical study, such levels were achieved in 29/30 (97%) and 29/29 (100%) of subjects for diphtheria and tetanus, respectively, in adults previously primed for diphtheria and tetanus after a single booster dose of Lederle-produced Tetanus and Diphtheria Toxoids Adsorbed For Adult Use.[10]

INDICATIONS AND USAGE

Tetanus and Diphtheria Toxoids For Adult Use, Aluminum Phosphate Adsorbed, is indicated for active immunization against tetanus and diphtheria in adults and children 7 years of age and older.[5,11] (See **DOSAGE AND ADMINISTRATION** for "Tetanus Prophylaxis in Wound Management" and "Diphtheria Prophylaxis for Case Contacts.")
Tetanus and Diphtheria Toxoids Adsorbed For Adults Use is intended only for active immunization against tetanus and diphtheria, and is not to be used for treatment of actual infection.

The Advisory Committee on Immunization Practices (ACIP) recommends the use of the combined toxoids vaccine rather than single component vaccines for both primary and booster injections, including active tetanus immunization in wound management.[5]

Persons recovering from tetanus or diphtheria. Tetanus or diphtheria infection may not confer immunity; therefore, initiation or completion of active immunization is indicated at the time of recovery from these infections.[5]

Neonatal tetanus prevention. The risk to the fetus from tetanus/diphtheria toxoids in unknown.[12] The ACIP recommends that a previously unimmunized pregnant woman, who may deliver her child under nonhygienic circumstances and/or surroundings, should receive two properly spaced doses of Td before delivery, preferably during the last two trimesters.[5] Incompletely immunized pregnant women should complete the three-dose series. Those immunized more than 10 years previously should have a booster dose[5] (see **PRECAUTIONS—Pregnancy**).

If a contraindication to using tetanus toxoid-containing preparations exists in a person who has not completed a primary immunizing course of tetanus toxoid, and other than a clean minor wound is sustained, only passive immunization should be given using Tetanus Immune Globulin (TIG). If passive immunization for diphtheria is needed, Diphtheria Antitoxin is recommended[5] (see **DOSAGE AND ADMINISTRATION**).

As with any vaccine, Tetanus and Diphtheria Toxoids Adsorbed For Adult Use may not protect 100% of individuals receiving the vaccine.

CONTRAINDICATIONS

HYPERSENSITIVITY TO ANY COMPONENT OF THE VACCINE, INCLUDING THIMEROSAL, A MERCURY DERIVATIVE, IS A CONTRAINDICATION.

THE OCCURRENCE OF ANY NEUROLOGICAL SYMPTOMS OR SIGNS OR AN ANAPHYLACTIC REACTION FOLLOWING ADMINISTRATION OF THIS PRODUCT IS A CONTRAINDICATION TO FURTHER USE.

THE DECISION TO ADMINISTER OR DELAY VACCINATION BECAUSE OF A CURRENT OR RECENT FEBRILE ILLNESS DEPENDS LARGELY ON THE SEVERITY OF THE SYMPTOMS AND THEIR ETIOLOGY. ALTHOUGH A MODERATE OR SEVERE FEBRILE ILLNESS IS SUFFICIENT REASON TO POSTPONE VACCINATION, MINOR ILLNESSES SUCH AS A MILD UPPER RESPIRATORY INFECTION WITH OR WITHOUT LOW GRADE FEVER ARE NOT CONTRAINDICATIONS.[5,13,14]

ROUTINE IMMUNIZATION SHOULD BE DEFERRED DURING AN OUTBREAK OF POLIOMYELITIS, PROVIDING THE PATIENT HAS NOT SUSTAINED AN INJURY THAT INCREASES THE RISK OF TETANUS AND PROVIDING AN OUTBREAK OF DIPHTHERIA DOES NOT OCCUR SIMULTANEOUSLY.[15]

THE CLINICAL JUDGMENT OF THE ATTENDING PHYSICIAN SHOULD PREVAIL AT ALL TIMES.

WARNINGS

THIS PRODUCT IS NOT RECOMMENDED FOR IMMUNIZING PERSONS LESS THAN 7 YEARS OF AGE.

The concentration of diphtheria toxoid in preparations intended for use in persons 7 years of age or older is approximately 80% lower than that of the pediatric formulation (Diphtheria and Tetanus Toxoids Adsorbed, [DT]). The lower dosage of diphtheria toxoid is recommended for persons 7 years of age or older because adverse reactions to the diphtheria component are thought to be related to both dose and age.[5]

IT IS RECOMMENDED THAT BOOSTER DOSES BE ADMINISTERED EVERY 10 YEARS, EXCEPT UNDER CIRCUMSTANCES OF WOUND MANAGEMENT (see **DOSAGE AND ADMINISTRATION**). MORE FREQUENT ADMINISTRATION MAY BE ASSOCIATED WITH INCREASED INCIDENCE AND SEVERITY OF REACTIONS.[5]

Persons who experience Arthus-type hypersensitivity reactions or temperatures greater than 39.4°C (103°F), after a previous dose of tetanus toxoid usually have very high serum tetanus antitoxin levels and should not be given even emergency doses of Td more frequently than every 10 years, even if they have a wound that is neither clean nor minor.[13]

If a contraindication to using tetanus toxoid-containing preparations exists in a person who has not completed a primary immunizing course of tetanus toxoid, and other than a clean, minor wound is sustained, only passive immunization should be given using TIG.[5] (See **INDICATIONS AND USAGE.**)

Td should not be given to individuals with thrombocytopenia or any coagulation disorder that would contraindicate intramuscular injection unless the potential benefits clearly outweigh the risk of administration. If the decision is made to administer Td to individuals with coagulation disorders, it should be given with caution (see **DRUG INTERACTIONS**).

Deaths have been reported in temporal association with the administration of preparations containing diphtheria and/or tetanus antigens (see **ADVERSE REACTIONS**).

Health care professionals should administer this product with caution to patients with a possible history of latex sensitivity since this packaging contains dry natural rubber.

PRECAUTIONS

General

CARE IS TO BE TAKEN BY THE HEALTH CARE PROFESSIONAL FOR THE SAFE AND EFFECTIVE USE OF THIS PRODUCT.

1. PRIOR TO ADMINISTRATION OF ANY DOSE OF Td, THE PARENT OR GUARDIAN OR ADULT PATIENT SHOULD BE ASKED ABOUT THE PERSONAL HISTORY, FAMILY HISTORY, AND RECENT HEALTH STATUS OF THE VACCINE RECIPIENT. THE PHYSICIAN SHOULD ASCERTAIN PREVIOUS IMMUNIZATION HISTORY, CURRENT HEALTH STATUS, AND OCCURRENCE OF ANY SYMPTOMS AND/OR SIGNS OF AN ADVERSE EVENT AFTER PREVIOUS IMMUNIZATIONS IN THE INDIVIDUAL TO BE IMMUNIZED, IN ORDER TO DETERMINE THE EXISTENCE OF ANY CONTRAINDICATION TO IMMUNIZATION WITH Td AND TO ALLOW AN ASSESSMENT OF BENEFITS AND RISKS.
2. HEALTH CARE PROFESSIONALS SHOULD ADMINISTER THIS PRODUCT WITH CAUTION TO PATIENTS WITH A PRIOR HISTORY OF GUILLAIN-BARRÉ SYNDROME (see **ADVERSE REACTIONS**).
3. BEFORE THE INJECTION OF ANY BIOLOGICAL, THE PHYSICIAN SHOULD TAKE ALL PRECAUTIONS KNOWN FOR PREVENTION OF ALLERGIC OR ANY OTHER SIDE REACTIONS. This should include: a review of the patient's history regarding possible sensitivity; the ready availability of epinephrine 1:1000 and other appropriate agents used for control of immediate allergic reactions; and a knowledge of the recent literature pertaining to use of the biological concerned, including the nature of side effects and adverse reactions that may follow its use.
4. Patients with impaired immune responsiveness, whether due to the use of immunosuppressive therapy (including irradiation, corticosteroids, antimetabolites, alkylating agents, and cytotoxic agents), a genetic defect, or other causes, may have a reduced antibody response to active immunization procedures.[5,14,16,17] Deferral of administration of Td may be considered in individuals receiving immunosuppressive therapy.[5] Other groups should generally receive this vaccine according to the usual recommended schedule.[5,14,17,18] (see **DRUG INTERACTIONS.**)
5. This product is not contraindicated for use in individuals with human immunodeficiency (HIV) virus infection.[16,19]
6. *Since this product is a suspension containing an adjuvant, shake vigorously to obtain a uniform suspension in the vaccine container.*
7. A separate sterile syringe and needle or a sterile disposable unit should be used for each individual patient to prevent transmission of hepatitis or other infectious agents from one person to another. Needles should be disposed of properly and should not be recapped.
8. Special care should be taken to prevent injection into or near a blood vessel or nerve.
9. Health care professionals should administer this product with caution to patients with a possible history of latex sensitivity since this packaging contains dry natural rubber.

INFORMATION FOR PATIENTS

PRIOR TO THE ADMINISTRATION OF THIS VACCINE, HEALTH CARE PROFESSIONALS SHOULD INFORM THE PARENT, GUARDIAN, OR ADULT PATIENT OF THE RECOMMENDED IMMUNIZATION SCHEDULE FOR PROTECTION AGAINST TETANUS AND DIPHTHERIA AND THE BENEFITS AND RISKS OF VACCINATION AGAINST TETANUS AND DIPHTHERIA. GUIDANCE SHOULD BE PROVIDED ON MEASURES TO BE TAKEN SHOULD ADVERSE EVENTS OCCUR, SUCH AS ANTIPYRETIC MEASURES FOR ELEVATED TEMPERATURES AND THE NEED TO REPORT ADVERSE EVENTS TO THE HEALTH CARE PROFESSIONAL. PATIENTS, PARENTS, OR GUARDIANS SHOULD BE PROVIDED WITH VACCINE INFORMATION MATERIALS PRIOR TO THE TIME OF VACCINATION, AS MANDATED BY THE NATIONAL VACCINE INJURY COMPENSATION PROGRAM.[20]

THE HEALTH CARE PROFESSIONAL SHOULD INFORM THE PARENT, GUARDIAN, OR ADULT PATIENT OF THE IMPORTANCE OF COMPLETING THE IMMUNIZATION SERIES UNLESS CONTRAINDICATED.

PATIENTS, PARENTS, OR GUARDIANS SHOULD BE INSTRUCTED TO REPORT ANY ADVERSE REACTIONS OR SUSPECTED ADVERSE EVENTS TO THEIR HEALTH CARE PROFESSIONAL (see **ADVERSE REACTIONS, Adverse Event Reporting**).

Drug Interactions

Patients receiving immunosuppressive therapy (including irradiation, systemic corticosteroids, antimetabolites, alkylating agents, and cytotoxic agents) may have a reduced response to active immunization procedures.[5,14,16,17] Although no specific studies are available, if immunosuppressive therapy will be discontinued shortly, it would be reasonable to defer immunization until the patient has been off therapy for one month; otherwise the patient should be vaccinated while still on therapy.[16]

As with other intramuscular injections, tetanus and diphtheria toxoids should be given with caution to patients on anticoagulant therapy.

Tetanus Immune Globulin or Diphtheria Antitoxin, if used, should be given in a separate site with a separate needle and syringe.

Carcinogenesis, Mutagenesis, Impairment Of Fertility

Tetanus and Diphtheria Toxoids Adsorbed For Adult Use has not been evaluated for its carcinogenic or mutagenic potential or for impairment of fertility.

Pregnancy

Pregnancy Category C.

Animal reproductive studies have not been conducted with this product. The risk to the fetus from tetanus/diphtheria toxoids is unknown.[12] The ACIP recommends that Td should be given to inadequately immunized pregnant women because it affords protection against neonatal tetanus.[19] Waiting until the second trimester is a reasonable precaution to minimize any theoretical teratogenic concern.[13] Maintenance of adequate immunization by routine boosters in non-pregnant women of childbearing age (see **DOSAGE AND ADMINISTRATION**) can obviate the need to vaccinate women during pregnancy.

Nursing Mothers

Tetanus and diphtheria toxoids have not been isolated from breast milk. There is no evidence that breast milk from women receiving this product is harmful to infants.[19]

Pediatric Use

The safety and effectiveness of Tetanus and Diphtheria Toxoids Adsorbed For Adult Use in children less than 7 years of age have not been established and this product is not recommended for this population.

For either primary or booster immunization against tetanus and diphtheria in children less than 7 years of age, the use of Diphtheria and Tetanus Toxoids and Acellular Pertussis Vaccine (DTaP) is recommended.[5]

Geriatric Use

The response to immunization with tetanus toxoid has been demonstrated to be slower, of lower magnitude, and decreased duration in geriatric patients. A group of 17 geriatric subjects (mean age 70.6 ± 4.0 years) exhibited significantly lower antibody titers for up to 12 months after an injection of tetanus toxoid as compared to a group of 20 young subjects (mean age 31.3 ± 6.5 years).[21,23] In another study, subjects ages 65 to 84 years who received 5 Lf of adsorbed tetanus toxoid showed a decreased IgG antibody production as compared to adults ages 25 to 34 years.[22] In these studies, adequate protection was achieved in geriatric patients.[23–25] In a study of 161 nursing home residents, mean age 77 years, minor pain and/or tenderness at the injection site was reported by 9% of the patients and no systemic reactions were reported. Because patients were not examined for reactions and 23 vaccinated patients had decreased awareness and poor communication skills, the actual incidence of reactions may be higher.[26] The ACIP recommends that persons age 50 and over receive a Td booster every 10 years as part of routine health maintenance.[27]

ADVERSE REACTIONS

In an open-label study of Td in 35 adult subjects, aged 18–55 years, local reactions occurred in 28 (80%) of subjects. Injection site tenderness (80%) was the most common local reactions, followed by erythema and induration, each reported in 14% of subjects within 72 hours of injection of Td. There were reports of systemic reactions, including muscle pain (26%), headache (14%), and anorexia (6%) within 72 hours after immunization.[9]

Local reactions, manifested by varying degrees of erythema, induration, and tenderness, are common after the administration of Td.[11,28–32] With vaccines in general, it is not uncommon for patients to note within 48 to 72 hours at or around the injection site the following minor reactions: edema, pain, or tenderness; redness; inflammation or skin discoloration; mass; or hypersensitivity reaction. Such local reactions are usually self-limited and require no therapy. As with other aluminum-containing vaccines,[28] a nodule may occasionally be palpable at the injection site for several weeks. Sterile abscess formation or subcutaneous atrophy at the injection site may also occur.

Systemic reactions such as fever, chills, myalgia, and headache also may occur.[10,29–32] Other adverse events which have been reported in temporal association with various tetanus toxoid-containing products include: warmth, swelling, cellulitis, malaise, weakness or fatigue, dizziness, irritability, aches and pains, arthralgia, flushing, tachycardia, syncope, nausea, vomiting, lymphadenopathy, phlebitis, pruritis/itching, hives, sweating, acute midbrain syndrome, EEG disturbances, accommodation pareses, paresthesia, radiculopathy, brachial plexus neuropathy, cranial nerve pareses, myelopathy, myelitis, and cochlear lesions.

Arthus-type hypersensitivity reactions, characterized by severe local reactions (generally starting 2 to 8 hours after an injection), may follow receipt of tetanus toxoid in persons who have very high serum antitoxin antibodies due to overly frequent injections of tetanus toxoid (see **WARNINGS**).[13]

NEUROLOGICAL COMPLICATIONS,[33] SUCH AS CONVULSIONS,[34] ENCEPHALOPATHY,[34,35] AND VARIOUS MONO- AND POLYNEUROPATHIES,[35–41] INCLUDING GUILLAIN-BARRÉ SYNDROME (GBS),[42,43] HAVE BEEN REPORTED FOLLOWING ADMINISTRATION OF PREPARATIONS CONTAINING TETANUS AND/OR DIPHTHERIA ANTIGENS. A REVIEW BY THE INSTITUTE OF MEDICINE (I.O.M.) FOUND A CAUSAL RELATION BETWEEN TETANUS TOXOID AND BRACHIAL NEURITIS AND GBS.[44]

ALLERGIC AND HYPERSENSITIVITY REACTIONS, URTICARIA, ERYTHEMA MULTIFORME OR OTHER RASH[34], AND, MORE RARELY, A SEVERE ANAPHYLACTIC REACTION[44] (IE, URTICARIA WITH SWELLING OF THE MOUTH, DIFFICULTY BREATHING, HYPOTENSION, SHOCK, OR DEATH) HAVE BEEN REPORTED FOLLOWING ADMINISTRATION OF PREPARATIONS CONTAINING TETANUS AND/OR DIPHTHERIA ANTIGENS.

Continued on next page

Tetanus & Diphtheria Toxoids—Cont.

DEATHS HAVE BEEN REPORTED IN TEMPORAL ASSOCIATION TO RECEIPT OF PREPARATIONS CONTAINING TETANUS AND DIPHTHERIA TOXOIDS. THE I.O.M. FOUND INADEQUATE EVIDENCE TO ACCEPT OR REJECT A CAUSAL RELATIONSHIP BETWEEN TETANUS TOXOID-CONTAINING PRODUCTS AND DEATH FROM CAUSES OTHER THAN ANAPHYLAXIS OR GBS.[44]

A review of two large, active surveillance studies of adults and children who received approximately 0.7 to 1.2 million and 8.1 million doses of tetanus toxoid-containing vaccines, respectively, found that the number of cases of GBS after the administration of such vaccines was less than that expected by chance alone.[45]

Adverse Event Reporting

Any adverse reactions following immunization should be reported by the health care professional to the US Department of Health and Human Services (DHHS). The National Vaccine Injury Compensation Program requires that the manufacturer and lot number of the vaccine administered be recorded by the health care professional in the vaccine recipient's permanent medical record (or in a permanent office log or file), along with the date of administration of the vaccine and the name, address, and title of the person administering the vaccine. The statute further requires the health care professional to report to the Secretary of the Department of Health and Human Services the occurrence following immunization of any event set forth in the Vaccine Injury Table, including anaphylaxis or anaphylactic shock within 4 hours, brachial neuritis within 2 to 28 days or any acute complication or sequelae (including death) of an illness, disability, injury, or condition referred to above which illness, disability, injury, or condition arose within the time prescribed, or any event that would contraindicate further doses of vaccine, according to this Tetanus and Diphtheria Toxoids package insert.[20,46]

The US Department of Health and Human Services has established the Vaccine Adverse Event Reporting System (VAERS) to accept all reports of suspected adverse events after the administration of any vaccine including, but not limited to, the reporting of events required by the National Childhood Vaccine Injury Act of 1986.[20] The VAERS toll-free number for VAERS forms and information is 800-822-7967.

DOSAGE AND ADMINISTRATION

For Intramuscular Use Only

The dose is 0.5 mL to be given intramuscularly.

Since this product is a suspension containing an adjuvant, shake vigorously to obtain a uniform suspension in the vaccine container. The vaccine should not be used if it cannot be resuspended.

Parenteral drug products should be inspected visually for particulate matter and discoloration prior to administration whenever solution and container permit (see **DESCRIPTION**). This product should not be used if particulate matter or discoloration are found.

The vaccine should be injected intramuscularly. The preferred site is the deltoid muscle of the upper arm. The vaccine should not be injected in the gluteal area or areas where there may be a major nerve trunk and/or a blood vessel. Before injection, the skin at the injection site should be cleansed and prepared with a suitable germicide. After insertion of the needle, aspirate and wait to see if any blood appears in the syringe, which will help avoid inadvertent injection into a blood vessel. The needle length for adult vaccine administration should be of sufficient length to delivery the vaccine intramuscularly, in particular for intramuscular inejction into obese patients, a 1 inch or 1–1/2 inch needle may be necessary. Td is supplied in a multi-dose vial for use with syringe and needle; length of needle may be determined by the health care professional as needed for individual patients (see **HOW SUPPLIED**).[11,19]

PRIMARY IMMUNIZATION

The primary immunizing course for unimmunized individuals 7 years of age or older consists of two doses of 0.5 mL each, 4 to 8 weeks apart, followed by a third (reinforcing) dose of 0.5 mL 6 to 12 months after the second dose. The reinforcing dose is an integral part of the primary immunizing course.[5] Interruption of the recommended schedule with a delay between doses does not interfere with the final immunity achieved, nor does it necessitate starting the series over again, regardless of the length of time elapsed between doses.[5] In contrast, giving doses at less than recommended intervals may lessen the antibody response and therefore should be avoided.

Children who remain incompletely immunized at age 7 years and greater should be counted as having prior exposure to tetanus and diphtheria toxoids. For example, to complete the primary immunization series for tetanus and diphtheria, a child who previously received 2 doses of DTP or DTaP needs only 1 dose of Tetanus and Diphtheria Toxoids Adsorbed.

Any variation from the recommended volume or number of doses is discouraged. The serological response, clinical efficacy and/or frequency and severity of adverse reactions of schedules other than those described above have not been adequately studied.[19]

Booster Doses

A booster dose of 0.5 mL of Td is given 10 years after completion of primary immunization and every 10 years thereafter. If a dose is given sooner than 10 years, as part of wound management or on exposure to diphtheria, the next booster is not needed for 10 years thereafter. MORE FREQUENT BOOSTER DOSES ARE NOT INDICATED AND MAY BE ASSOCIATED WITH INCREASED INCIDENCE AND SEVERITY OF REACTIONS[5] (see **WARNINGS**).

Diphtheria Prophylaxis for Case Contacts

All case contacts, household and others, who have previously received fewer than three doses of diphtheria toxoid, should receive an immediate dose of an appropriate diphtheria toxoid-containing preparation and should complete the series according to schedule. Case contacts who have previously received three or more doses, but who have not received a dose of a preparation containing diphtheria toxoid within the previous five years, should receive a booster dose of a diphtheria toxoid-containing preparation appropriate for their age.[5] Td is an appropriate preparation in these circumstances for persons 7 years of age or older.

Tetanus Prophylaxis in Wound Management

The need for active immunization with a tetanus toxoid-containing preparation, with or without passive immunization with Tetanus Immune Globulin (TIG) depends on both the condition of the wound and the patient's immunization history. Tetanus has rarely occurred among persons with a documented primary series of tetanus toxoid injections. A thorough attempt must be made to determine whether a patient has completed primary immunization.

Individuals who have completed primary immunization against tetanus, and who sustain wounds which are minor and uncontaminated, should receive a booster dose of a tetanus-toxoid preparation only if they have not received tetanus toxoid within the preceding 10 years. For other wounds, a booster is appropriate if the patient has not received tetanus toxoid within the preceding 5 years. Antitoxin antibodies develop rapidly in persons who have previously received at least two doses of tetanus toxoid.[5] If a booster dose is given sooner than 10 years as part of wound management, the next booster should not be given for 10 years thereafter.

Individuals who have not completed primary immunization against tetanus, or whose immunization history is unknown or uncertain, should be immunized with a tetanus toxoid-containing product. Completion of primary immunization thereafter should be ensured. In addition, if these individuals have sustained a tetanus-prone wound, the use of TIG is recommended. A separate syringe and site of administration should be used.[5]

If a contraindication to using tetanus toxoid-containing preparations exists in a person who has not completed a primary immunizing course of tetanus toxoid and other than a clean, minor wound is sustained, only *passive* immunization should be given using TIG.[5]

SUMMARY GUIDE TO TETANUS PROPHYLAXIS IN ROUTINE WOUND MANAGEMENT[5]*

History of Tetanus Toxoid (doses)	Clean, Minor Wounds		All Other Wounds†	
	Td	TIG	Td	TIG
Unknown or <3	Yes	No	Yes	Yes
>3‡	No§	No	No°	No

* Important details are in the text.

† Such as, but not limited to, wounds contaminated with dirt, feces, soil, saliva; puncture wounds; avulsions; and wounds resulting from missiles, crushing, burns, and frostbite.

‡ If only three doses of *fluid* toxoid have been received, a fourth dose of toxoid, preferably an adsorbed toxoid, should be given.

§ Yes, if more than 10 years since last dose.

° Yes, if more than 5 years since last dose. (More frequent boosters are not needed and can accentuate side effects.)

Td is the preferred preparation for active tetanus immunization in wound management of patients 7 years of age or older. This is to enhance diphtheria protection, since a large proportion of adults are susceptible. Thus, by taking advantage of acute health care visits for wound management, some patients can be protected who otherwise would remain susceptible.[5]

HOW SUPPLIED

NDC 0005-1875-31 5.0 mL vial

NDC 0005-1875-47 Single-Dose LEDERJECT® Disposable Syringes.

STORAGE

DO NOT FREEZE. STORE REFRIGERATED, AWAY FROM FREEZER COMPARTMENT, AT 2°C to 8°C (36°F to 46°F).

REFERENCES

1. Mueller JH, Miller PA: Factors influencing the production of tetanal toxin. *J Immunol* 1947;56:143–147.
2. Pillemer L, Grossberg DB, Wittler RG: The immunochemistry of toxins and toxoids. II. The preparation and immunological evaluation of purified tetanal toxoid. *J Immunol* 1946;54:213–224.
3. CDC. Summary of notifiable diseases, United States, 1994. *MMWR.* 1995;43(53):70–71.
4. Bardenheier, B et al: Tetanus surveillance—United States, 1995–1997. *MMWR.* 1998; 47(SS-2):1.
5. Diphtheria, tetanus and pertussis: Recommendations for vaccine use and other preventive measures—recommendations of the Immunization Practices Advisory Committee (ACIP). *MMWR.* 1991;40(RR-10).
6. *Federal Register Notice.* Friday, December 13, 1985, Vol. 50, No. 240.
7. Diphtheria Epidemic-New Independent States of the Former Soviet Union. 1990–1994. *MMWR.* 1995;44(10):177–181.
8. Ipsen J. Immunization of adults against diphtheria and tetanus. *NEJM.* 1954;251:459–466.
9. Unpublished data on file; Lederle Laboratories.
10. Edwards KM, Decker MD, Graham BS, et al. Adult immunization with acellular pertussis vaccine. *JAMA.* 1993;269(1):53–56.
11. ACP Task Force on Adult Immunization and Infectious Diseases Society of America: *Guide for Adult Immunization*, 3rd ed. Philadelphia, PA: American College of Physicians; 1994.
12. Briggs GG, Freeman RK, Yaffee SJ. *Drugs in Pregnancy and Lactation*, 5th ed. Baltimore, MD: Williams and Wilkins; 1998.
13. Update: Vaccine side effects, adverse reactions, contraindications, and precautions. *MMWR.* 1996;45 (RR-12):22–31.
14. American Academy of Pediatrics. *Report of the Committee of Infectious Diseases*, 24th ed. Elk Grove Village, Ill; American Academy of Pediatric; 1997.
15. Sutter RW, Patriarca PA, Suleiman AJM, et al. Attributable risk of DTP (Diphtheria and Tetanus Toxoids and Pertussis Vaccine) injection in provoking paralytic poliomyelitis during a large outbreak in Oman. *J Infect Dis.* 1992;165:444–449.
16. Recommendations of the Advisory Committee on Immunization Practices (ACIP): Use of vaccines and immune globulins in persons with altered immunocompetence. *MMWR.* 1993;42(RR-4).
17. Immunization of children infected with human immunodeficiency virus—supplementary ACIP statement. *MMWR.* 1988;37(12):181–183.
18. Recommendation of the ACIP: Immunization of children infected with human T-lymphotropic virus type III/lymphadenopathy-associated virus. *MMWR.* 1986;35(38):595–606.
19. General Recommendations on Immunization—Recommendations of the Immunization Practices Advisory Committee (ACIP). *MMWR.* 1994;43(RR-1).
20. 42 U.S.C. §§ 300 aa -25, -26. See also: CDC. Vaccine Adverse Event Reporting System—United States. *MMWR.* 1990:39:730–733.
21. Burns, EA et al: Specific humoral immunity in the elderly: in vivo and in vitro response to vaccination. *J Gerontology.* 1993;48(6):B231–B236.
22. Kishimoto, S et al: Age-related decline in the in vitro and in vivo syntheses of anti-tetanus toxoid antibody in humans. *J Immunol.* 1980;125(5):2347–2352.
23. Murphy, SM et al: Tetanus immunity in elderly people. *Age and Aging.* 1995:24(2):99–102.
24. Simonsen, O et al: Revaccination of adults against diphtheria I: Responses and reactions to different doses of diphtheria toxoid in 30–70-year-old persons with low serum antitoxin levels. *Acta Pathologica Microbiologica, et Immunol Scand.* 1986;94(5):213–218.
25. Solomonova, K and Vizev, S: Secondary response to boostering by purified aluminum-hydroxide-adsorbed tetanus anatoxin in aging and in aged adults. *Immunobiol.* 1981;158(4):312–319.
26. Hagen-Coenen, J et al: Tetanus-diphtheria vaccinations in a veterans nursing home. *J Amer Geriatric Soc.* 1992;40(5):513–524.
27. ACIP: Assessing adult vaccination status at age 50 years. *MMWR.* 1995;44(29):561–563.
28. Fawcett HA, Smith NP: Injection-site granuloma due to aluminum. *Arch Dermatol* 1984;120:1318–1322.
29. Deacon SP, Langford DT, Shepherd WM, et al: A comparative clinical study of adsorbed tetanus vaccine and adult-type tetanus-diphtheria vaccine. *J Hyg (Cambridge)* 1982;89:513–519.
30. Macko MB, Powell CE: Comparison of the morbidity of tetanus toxoid boosters with tetanus-diphtheria toxoid boosters. *Ann Emerg Med* 1985;14(1):33–35.
31. Myers MG, Beckman CW, Vosdingh RA, et al: Primary immunization with tetanus and diphtheria toxoids. *JAMA.* 1982;248(19):2478–2480.
32. Sisk CW, Lewis CE: Reactions to tetanus-diphtheria toxoid (adult). *Arch Environ Health.* 1965;11:34–36.
33. Rutledge SL, Snead OC: Neurologic complications of immunizations. *J Pediatr.* 1986;109:917–924.
34. CDC. Adverse events following immunization. *MMWR.* 1985;34(3):43–47.
35. Schlenska GK: Unusual neurological complications following tetanus toxoid administration. *J Neurol.* 1977;215:299–302.
36. Blumstein GI, Kreithen H: Peripheral neuropathy following tetanus toxoid administration. *JAMA.* 1966;198:1030–1031.
37. Reinstein L, Pargament JM, Goodman JS: Peripheral neuropathy after multiple tetanus toxoid injections. *Arch Phys Med Rehabil.* 1982;63:332–334.
38. Tsairis P, Duck PJ, Mulder DW: Natural history of brachial plexus neuropathy. *Arch Neurol.* 1972;27:109–117.
39. Quast U, Hennessen W, Widmark RM: Mono- and polyneuritis after tetanus vaccination. *Devel Bio Stand* 1979;43:25–32.
40. Holliday PL, Bauer RB: Polyradiculoneuritis secondary to immunization with tetanus and diphtheria toxoids. *Arch Neurol.* 1983;40:56–67.

41. Fenichel GM: Neurological complications of tetanus toxoid. *Arch Neurol* 1983;40:390.
42. Pollard JD, Selby G: Relapsing neuropathy due to tetanus toxoid. *J Neurol Sci* 1978;37:113–125.
43. Newton N, Janati A: Guillain-Barré syndrome after vaccination with purified tetanus toxoid. *S Med J.* 1987;80: 1053–1054.
44. Stratton KR, Howe CJ, Johnston RB. Adverse effects associated with childhood vaccines. Institute of Medicine (IOM), Washington, DC: National Academy Press 1994.
45. Tuttle J, Chen RT, Rantala H, et al: The risk of Guillain-Barré Syndrome after tetanus-toxoid-containing vaccines in adults and children in the United States. *Am J Pub Health.* 1997;87:2045–48.
46. Department of Health and Human Services (1997). Federal Register: Feb. 20, 1997, p.7685 (Vol.62, No.34), [Online]. Available: http://frwebgate4.access.gpo.gov/cgi-bin.

Manufactured by:
LEDERLE LABORATORIES
Division American Cyanamid Company
Pearl River, NY 10965
US Gov't. License No. 17
Marketed by:
WYETH-LEDERLE VACCINES AND PEDIATRICS
Wyeth-Ayerst Laboratories
Philadelphia, PA 19101
CI 5202-2 Revised April 26, 1999

TETANUS TOXOID ADSORBED ℞
Tetanus Toxoid Aluminum Phosphate-Adsorbed
PUROGENATED®

DESCRIPTION
Tetanus Toxoid Adsorbed, aluminum phosphate-adsorbed, PUROGENATED® is a sterile preparation of refined tetanus toxoid for intramuscular use only. After shaking, the product is a homogenous white suspension.
The tetanus toxin is produced according to the method of Mueller and Miller[1] and is detoxified by use of formaldehyde. The toxoid is refined by the Pillemer alcohol fractionation method[2] and is diluted with a solution containing sodium phosphate dibasic, sodium phosphate monobasic, glycine, sodium chloride and thimerosal (mercury derivative) in a final concentration of 1:10,000 as a preservative and aluminum phosphate as adjuvant. The aluminum content does not exceed 0.80 mg per 0.5 mL dose.
Each 0.5 mL dose is formulated to contain 5 Lf units of tetanus toxoid.

CLINICAL PHARMACOLOGY
Tetanus is an intoxication manifested primarily by neuromuscular dysfunction caused by a potent exotoxin elaborated by *Clostridium tetani.* The incidence of tetanus in the U.S. has dropped dramatically with the routine use of tetanus toxoid, remaining relatively constant over the last decade at about 90 cases reported annually.[3] Spores of *C tetani* are ubiquitous and there is essentially no natural immunity to tetanus toxin. Thus, universal primary immunization with tetanus toxoid, and subsequent maintenance of adequate antitoxin levels by means of timed boosters, is necessary to protect all age groups.[3] Tetanus toxoid is a highly effective antigen, and a completed primary series generally induces protective levels of serum antitoxin that persist for at least 10 years.[3]

INDICATIONS AND USAGE
Tetanus Toxoid Adsorbed is indicated for active immunization against tetanus in adults and children 2 months of age or older.
Immunization of persons 7 years of age or older may be accomplished by the use of Tetanus and Diphtheria Toxoids Adsorbed, for Adult Use (Td), Tetanus Toxoid Adsorbed, or Tetanus Toxoid Fluid. The Immunization Practices Advisory Committee (ACIP) of the U.S. Public Health Service recommends the use of the combined toxoids vaccine rather than single component vaccines for both primary and booster injections, including active tetanus immunization in wound management.[3] Individuals for whom the use of a vaccine containing diphtheria toxoid is contraindicated should receive a single-component tetanus toxoid-containing vaccine.
Immunization of infants and children 2 months of age up to the seventh birthday is usually accomplished by the use of Diphtheria and Tetanus Toxoids and Pertussis Vaccine Adsorbed (DTP) or Diphtheria and Tetanus Toxoids Adsorbed, for pediatric use (DT). Tetanus Toxoid Adsorbed may be used for immunizing infants and children for whom the use of a vaccine containing diphtheria toxoid and pertussis antigen is contraindicated.
Comparative tests have shown that the adsorbed toxoids are superior to the fluid toxoids in antibody titers produced and in the durability of protection achieved. The promptness of antibody response to booster doses of either fluid or adsorbed toxoid is not sufficiently different to be of clinical importance. When Tetanus Immune Globulin (TIG) is to be administered at the same visit as tetanus toxoid, the adsorbed toxoid should be used.[3,4]
Persons recovering from tetanus. Tetanus infection may not confer immunity; therefore, initiation or completion of active immunization is indicated at the time of recovery from this infection.[3]
Neonatal tetanus prevention. There is no evidence that tetanus toxoid is teratogenic. A previously unimmunized pregnant woman who may deliver her child under nonhygienic circumstances and/or surroundings should receive two properly spaced doses of a tetanus toxoid-containing preparation before delivery, preferably during the last two trimesters. Incompletely immunized pregnant women should complete the three-dose series. Those immunized more than 10 years previously should have a booster dose.[3] (See also pregnancy information under **PRECAUTIONS**.)

CONTRAINDICATIONS
HYPERSENSITIVITY TO ANY COMPONENT OF THE VACCINE, INCLUDING THIMEROSAL, A MERCURY DERIVATIVE, IS A CONTRAINDICATION.
THE OCCURRENCE OF ANY TYPE OF NEUROLOGICAL SYMPTOMS OR SIGNS FOLLOWING ADMINISTRATION OF THIS PRODUCT IS A CONTRAINDICATION TO FURTHER USE.
IMMUNIZATION SHOULD BE DEFERRED DURING THE COURSE OF ANY FEBRILE ILLNESS OR ACUTE INFECTION. A MINOR AFEBRILE ILLNESS SUCH AS A MILD UPPER RESPIRATORY INFECTION IS NOT USUALLY REASON TO DEFER IMMUNIZATION.[3]
The clinical judgment of the attending physician should prevail at all times.
Routine immunization should be deferred during an outbreak of poliomyelitis providing the patient has not sustained an injury that increases the risk of tetanus.

WARNINGS
THE OCCURRENCE OF A NEUROLOGIC OR SEVERE HYPERSENSITIVITY REACTION FOLLOWING A PREVIOUS DOSE IS A CONTRAINDICATION TO FURTHER USE OF THIS PRODUCT.[3]
THE ADMINISTRATION OF BOOSTER DOSES MORE FREQUENTLY THAN RECOMMENDED (See **DOSAGE AND ADMINISTRATION**) MAY BE ASSOCIATED WITH INCREASED INCIDENCE AND SEVERITY OF REACTIONS.[3]
Persons who experience Arthus-type hypersensitivity reactions or temperature greater than 39.4°C (103°F) after a previous dose of tetanus toxoid usually have very high serum tetanus antitoxin levels and should not be given even emergency doses of tetanus toxoid more frequently than every 10 years, even if they have a wound that is neither clean nor minor.[3]
If a contraindication to using tetanus toxoid exists in a person who has not completed a primary immunizing course of tetanus toxoid, and other than a clean, minor wound is sustained, only passive immunization should be given using human Tetanus Immune Globulin (TIG).[3]
Tetanus Toxoid Adsorbed should not be given to individuals with thrombocytopenia or any coagulation disorder that would contraindicate intramuscular injection, unless the potential benefit clearly outweighs the risk of administration.
Patients with impaired immune responsiveness, whether due to the use of immunosuppressive therapy (including irradiation, corticosteroids, antimetabolites, alkylating agents, and cytotoxic agents), a genetic defect, human immunodeficiency virus (HIV) infection, or other causes, may have a reduced antibody response to active immunization procedures.[3–5] Deferral of administration of vaccine may be considered in individuals receiving immunosuppressive therapy.[3,4]
Special care should be taken to prevent injection into a blood vessel.

PRECAUTIONS
General
1. PRIOR TO ADMINISTRATION OF ANY DOSE OF VACCINE THE PARENT, GUARDIAN, OR ADULT PATIENT SHOULD BE ASKED ABOUT THE RECENT HEALTH STATUS AND IMMUNIZATION HISTORY OF THE PATIENT TO BE IMMUNIZED IN ORDER TO DETERMINE THE EXISTENCE OF ANY CONTRAINDICATIONS TO IMMUNIZATION (SEE **CONTRAINDICATIONS, WARNINGS**).
2. WHEN THE PATIENT RETURNS FOR THE NEXT DOSE IN A SERIES, THE PARENT, GUARDIAN, OR ADULT PATIENT SHOULD BE QUESTIONED CONCERNING OCCURRENCE OF ANY SYMPTOM AND/OR SIGN OF AN ADVERSE REACTION AFTER THE PREVIOUS DOSE (SEE **CONTRAINDICATIONS, ADVERSE REACTIONS**).
3. BEFORE THE INJECTION OF ANY BIOLOGICAL, THE PHYSICIAN SHOULD TAKE ALL PRECAUTIONS KNOWN FOR PREVENTION OF ALLERGIC OR ANY OTHER SIDE REACTIONS. This should include: a review of the patient's history regarding possible sensitivity; the ready availability of epinephrine 1:1,000 and other appropriate agents used for control of immediate allergic reactions; and a knowledge of the recent literature pertaining to use of the biological concerned, including the nature of side effects and adverse reactions that may follow its use.
4. A separate sterile syringe and needle or a sterile disposable unit should be used for each individual patient to prevent transmission of hepatitis or other infectious agents from one person to another.
5. *Shake vigorously before withdrawing each dose to resuspend the contents of the vial.*
6. NATIONAL CHILDHOOD VACCINE INJURY ACT OF 1986 (AS AMENDED IN 1987)
This Act requires that the manufacturer and lot number of the vaccine administered be recorded by the health care provider in the vaccine recipient's permanent record, along with the date of administration of the vaccine and the name, address and title of the person administering the vaccine.
The Act further requires the health care provider to report to a health department or to the FDA the occurrence following immunization of any event set forth in the Vaccine Injury Table including: anaphylaxis or anaphylactic shock within 24 hours, encephalopathy or encephalitis within 7 days, residual seizure disorder, any acute complication or sequelae (including death) of above events, or any event that would contraindicate further doses of vaccine, according to this package insert.[6]

Information for the Patient
PRIOR TO ADMINISTRATION OF THIS VACCINE, HEALTH CARE PERSONNEL SHOULD INFORM THE PARENT, GUARDIAN, OR ADULT PATIENT OF THE BENEFITS AND RISKS OF VACCINATION AGAINST TETANUS.

Use in Pregnancy
Pregnancy Category C.
Animal reproductive studies have not been conducted with this product. There is no evidence that tetanus toxoid is teratogenic. An appropriate tetanus toxoid-containing preparation (usually Td) should be given to inadequately immunized women because it affords protection against neonatal tetanus.[7] Waiting until the second trimester is a reasonable precaution to minimize any theoretical concern.[4] Maintenance of adequate immunization by routine boosters in nonpregnant women of child-bearing age (see **DOSAGE AND ADMINISTRATION**) can obviate the need to vaccinate women during pregnancy.

ADVERSE REACTIONS
Local reactions, such as erythema, induration and tenderness, are common after the administration of tetanus toxoid.[8,9,10] Such local reactions are usually self-limiting and require no therapy. Nodule,[11] sterile abscess formation, or subcutaneous atrophy may occur at the site of injection. Systemic reactions such as fever, chills, myalgia, and headaches also may occur.[8,9,10]
Arthus-type hypersensitivity reactions, or high fever, may occur in persons who have very high serum antitoxin antibodies due to overly frequent injections of toxoid.[3] (See **WARNINGS**.)
NEUROLOGICAL COMPLICATIONS[12] SUCH AS CONVULSIONS,[13] ENCEPHALOPATHY,[13,14] AND VARIOUS MONO- AND POLYNEUROPATHIES,[14–20] INCLUDING GUILLAIN-BARRÉ SYNDROME,[21,22] HAVE BEEN REPORTED FOLLOWING ADMINISTRATION OF PREPARATIONS CONTAINING TETANUS ANTIGEN.
URTICARIA, ERYTHEMA MULTIFORME OR OTHER RASH, ARTHRALGIAS[13] AND, MORE RARELY, A SEVERE ANAPHYLACTIC REACTION (I.E., URTICARIA WITH SWELLING OF THE MOUTH, DIFFICULTY BREATHING, HYPOTENSION OR SHOCK) HAVE BEEN REPORTED FOLLOWING ADMINISTRATION OF PREPARATIONS CONTAINING TETANUS ANTIGEN.

DOSAGE AND ADMINISTRATION
For Intramuscular Use Only
Shake vigorously before withdrawing each dose to resuspend the contents of the vial or syringe.
Parenteral drug products should be inspected visually for particulate matter and discoloration prior to administration. (See **DESCRIPTION.**)
Preferred injection sites for intramuscular injection include the anterolateral aspect of the upper thigh and the deltoid area of the upper arm. Care should be taken to avoid major peripheral nerve trunks.
Before injection, the skin at the injection site should be cleansed and prepared with a suitable germicide.
After insertion of the needle, aspirate to help avoid inadvertent injection into a blood vessel.
The primary immunizing course for unimmunized individuals one year of age or older consists of *two* doses of 0.5 mL each, 4 to 8 weeks apart, followed by a *third* (reinforcing) dose of 0.5 mL, 6 to 12 months after the second dose. The reinforcing dose is an integral part of the primary immunizing course.
If, after beginning combined immunization against diphtheria, tetanus, and pertussis, further doses of vaccine containing pertussis and diphtheria antigens become contraindicated, Tetanus Toxoid Adsorbed may be substituted for each of the remaining doses.
When immunization with Tetanus Toxoid Adsorbed is begun in the first year of life, the primary series consists of *three* doses of 0.5 mL each, 4 to 8 weeks apart, followed by a *fourth* (reinforcing) dose of 0.5 mL, 6 to 12 months after the third dose.
Interruption of the recommended schedule with a delay between doses does not interfere with the final immunity achieved with Tetanus Toxoid Adsorbed. There is no need to start the series over again, regardless of the length of time elapsed between doses.[3]

Booster Doses
A single injection of 0.5 mL of Tetanus Toxoid Adsorbed is given 10 years after completion of primary immunization and every 10 years thereafter. If a dose is given sooner as part of wound management, the next booster is not needed for 10 years thereafter. MORE FREQUENT BOOSTER

Continued on next page

Tetanus Toxoid Adsorbed—Cont.

DOSES ARE NOT INDICATED AND MAY BE ASSOCIATED WITH INCREASED INCIDENCE AND SEVERITY OF REACTIONS.[3]

Tetanus Prophylaxis in Wound Management

The need for active immunization with a tetanus toxoid-containing preparation, with or without passive immunization with human Tetanus Immune Globulin (TIG) depends on both the condition of the wound and the patient's immunization history. Tetanus has rarely occurred among persons with a documented primary series of toxoid injections. A thorough attempt must be made to determine whether a patient has completed primary immunization.[3]

Individuals who have completed primary immunization against tetanus, and who sustain wounds which are minor and uncontaminated, should receive a booster dose of the appropriate tetanus toxoid-containing preparation (see **INDICATIONS AND USAGE**) only if they have not received tetanus toxoid within the preceding 10 years. For other wounds, a booster is appropriate if the patient has not received tetanus toxoid within the preceding 5 years. Antitoxin antibodies develop rapidly in persons who have previously received at least two doses of tetanus toxoid.[3]

Individuals who have not completed primary immunization against tetanus, or whose immunization history is unknown or uncertain, should be immunized with the appropriate tetanus toxoid-containing product (see **INDICATIONS AND USAGE**). Completion of primary immunization thereafter should be ensured. In addition, if these individuals have sustained a tetanus-prone wound, the use of human Tetanus Immune Globulin (TIG) is recommended. A separate syringe and site of administration should be used. When TIG is to be administered at the same visit as tetanus toxoid, an adsorbed tetanus toxoid-containing preparation should be used.[3]

SUMMARY GUIDE TO TETANUS PROPHYLAXIS IN ROUTINE WOUND MANAGEMENT[3]*

History of tetanus toxoid (doses)	Clean, minor wounds		All other wounds†	
	Td§	TIG	Td§	TIG
Unknown or <three	Yes	No	Yes	Yes
≥three¶	No**	No	No††	No

* Important details are in the text.

† Such as, but not limited to, wounds contaminated with dirt, feces, soil, saliva, etc.; puncture wounds; avulsions; and wounds resulting from missiles, crushing, burns and frostbite.

§ For children under 7 years old DTP (DT, if pertussis vaccine is contraindicated) is preferred to tetanus toxoid alone. For persons 7 years and older, Td is preferred to tetanus toxoid alone.

¶ If only three doses of *fluid* toxoid have been received, a fourth dose of toxoid, preferably an adsorbed toxoid, should be given.

** Yes, if more than 10 years since last dose.

†† Yes, if more than 5 years since last dose. (More frequent boosters are not needed and can accentuate side effects.)

In order to enhance diphtheria protection in the population, the ACIP recommends Tetanus and Diphtheria Toxoids For Adult Use as the preferred preparation for active tetanus immunization in wound management of patients 7 years of age or older.[3]

HOW SUPPLIED

NDC 0005-1938-31 5.0 mL vial

NDC 0005-1938-47 10×0.5 mL LEDERJECT® disposable syringe. For directions on use of LEDERJECT® disposable syringe, please see package insert accompanying product.

STORAGE

DO NOT FREEZE. STORE REFRIGERATED, AWAY FROM FREEZER COMPARTMENT, AT 2°C to 8°C (36°F to 46°F).

REFERENCES

1. Mueller JH, Miller PA: Factors influencing the production of tetanal toxin. *J Immunol* 1947;56:143–147.
2. Pillemer L, Grossberg DB, Wittler RG: The immunochemistry of toxins and toxoids. II. The preparation and immunological evaluation of purified tetanal toxoid. *J Immunol* 1946;54:213–224.
3. Recommendation of the Immunization Practices Advisory Committee (ACIP): Diphtheria, tetanus and pertussis: Guidelines for vaccine prophylaxis and other preventive measures. *MMWR* 1985;34:405–426.
4. Committee on Immunization, Council of Medical Societies, American College of Physicians: Guide for Adult Immunization, 1st Edition 1985; Philadelphia, PA.
5. Recommendation of the ACIP: Immunization of children infected with Human T-Lymphotrophic Virus Type III/ Lymphadenopathy associated virus. *MMWR* 1986;35(38):595–606.
6. National Childhood Vaccine Injury Act: Requirements for permanent vaccination records and for reporting of selected events after vaccination. *MMWR* 1988;37(13):197–200.
7. Recommendations of the ACIP: General recommendations on immunization. *MMWR* 1983;32(1):1–17.
8. Macko MB, Powell CE: Comparison of the morbidity of tetanus toxoid boosters with tetanus-diphtheria toxoid boosters. *Ann Emerg Med* 1985;14:(1)33–35.
9. Deacon SP, et al: A comparative clinical study of adsorbed tetanus vaccine and adult-type tetanus-diphtheria vaccine. *J Hyg (Cambridge)* 1982;89:513–519.
10. Jacobs RL, et al: Adverse reactions to tetanus toxoid. *JAMA* 1982:247(1):40–42.
11. Fawcett HA, Smith N: Injection-site granuloma due to aluminum. *Arch Dermatol* 1984;120:1318–1322.
12. Rutledge SL, Snead OC: Neurologic complications of immunizations. *J Pediatr* 1986;109:917–924.
13. Adverse Events Following Immunization. *MMWR* 1985;34(3):43–47.
14. Schlenska GK: Unusual neurological complications following tetanus toxoid administration. *J Neurol* 1977;215:299–302.
15. Blumstein GI, Kreithen H: Peripheral neuropathy following tetanus toxoid administration. *JAMA* 1966;198:1030–1031.
16. Reinstein L, Pargament JM, Goodman JS: Peripheral neuropathy after multiple tetanus toxoid injections. *Arch Phys Med Rehabil* 1982;63:332–334.
17. Tsairis P, Duck PJ, Mulder DW: Natural history of brachial plexus neuropathy. *Arch Neurol* 1972;27:109–117.
18. Quast U, Hennessen W, Widmark RM: Mono- and polyneuritis after tetanus vaccination. *Devel Bio Stand* 1979;43:25–32.
19. Holliday PL, Bauer RB: Polyradiculoneuritis secondary to immunization with tetanus and diphtheria toxoids. *Arch Neurol* 1983;40:56–57.
20. Fenichel GM: Neurological complications of tetanus toxoid. *Arch Neurol* 1983;40:390.
21. Pollard JD, Selby G: Relapsing neuropathy due to tetanus toxoid. *J Neurol Sci* 1978;37:113–125.
22. Newton N, Janati A: Guillain-Barré syndrome after vaccination with purified tetanus toxoid. *S Med J* 1987;80:1053–1054.

Manufactured by:
LEDERLE LABORATORIES
Division American Cyanamid Company
Pearl River, NY 10965
US Gov't. License No. 17
Marketed by:
WYETH-LEDERLE VACCINES AND PEDIATRICS
Wyeth-Ayerst Laboratories
Philadelphia, PA 19101
CI 4417-1 Issued October 23, 1995

ZEBETA® ℞

[*zē-bā-tə*]
(Bisoprolol Fumarate)
Tablets

DESCRIPTION

ZEBETA (bisoprolol fumarate) is a synthetic $beta_1$-selective (cardioselective) adrenoceptor blocking agent. The chemical name for bisoprolol fumarate is (±)-1-[4-[[2-(1-Methylethoxy) ethoxy]methyl]phenoxy]-3-[(1-methylethyl)amino]-2-propanol (*E*) -2-butenedioate (2:1) (salt). It possesses an asymmetric carbon atom in its structure and is provided as a racemic mixture. The S(-) enantiomer is responsible for most of the beta-blocking activity. Its empirical formula is $(C_{18}H_{31}NO_4)_2 \cdot C_4H_4O_4$.

Bisoprolol fumarate has a molecular weight of 766.97. It is a white crystalline powder which is approximately equally hydrophilic and lipophilic, and is readily soluble in water, methanol, ethanol, and chloroform.

ZEBETA is available as 5 and 10 mg tablets for oral administration.

Inactive ingredients include Colloidal Silicon Dioxide, Corn Starch, Crospovidone, Diabasic Calcium Phosphate, Hydroxypropyl Methylcellulose, Magnesium Stearate, Microcrystalline Cellulose, Polyethylene Glycol, Polysorbate 80, and Titanium Dioxide. The 5 mg tablets also contain Red and Yellow Iron Oxide.

CLINICAL PHARMACOLOGY

ZEBETA is a $beta_1$-selective (cardioselective) adrenoceptor blocking agent without significant membrane stabilizing activity or intrinsic sympathomimetic activity in its therapeutic dosage range. Cardioselectivity is not absolute, however, and at higher doses (≥20 mg) bisoprolol fumarate also inhibits $beta_2$-adrenoceptors, chiefly located in the bronchial and vascular musculature; to retain selectivity, it is therefore important to use the lowest effective dose.

Pharmacokinetics and Metabolism

The absolute bioavailability after a 10 mg oral dose of bisoprolol fumarate is about 80%. Absorption is not affected by the presence of food. The first pass metabolism of bisoprolol fumarate is about 20%.

Binding to serum proteins is approximately 30%. Peak plasma concentrations occur within 2–4 hours of dosing with 5 to 20 mg, and mean peak values range from 16 ng/mL at 5 mg to 70 ng/mL at 20 mg. Once daily dosing with bisoprolol fumarate results in less than twofold intersubject variation in peak plasma levels. The plasma elimination half-life is 9–12 hours and is slightly longer in elderly patients, in part because of decreased renal function in that population. Steady state is attained within 5 days of once daily dosing. In both young and elderly populations, plasma accumulation is low; the accumulation factor ranges from 1.1 to 1.3, and is what would be expected from the first order kinetics and once daily dosing. Plasma concentrations are proportional to the administered dose in the range of 5 to 20 mg. Pharmacokinetic characteristics of the two enantiomers are similar.

Bisoprolol fumarate is eliminated equally by renal and non-renal pathways with about 50% of the dose appearing unchanged in the urine and the remainder appearing in the form of inactive metabolites. In humans, the known metabolites are labile or have no known pharmacologic activity. Less than 2% of the dose is excreted in the feces. Bisoprolol fumarate is not metabolized by cytochrome P450 II D6 (debrisoquin hydroxylase).

In subjects with creatinine clearance less than 40 mL/min, the plasma half-life is increased approximately threefold compared to healthy subjects.

In patients with cirrhosis of the liver, the elimination of ZEBETA (bisoprolol fumarate) is more variable in rate and significantly slower than that in healthy subjects, with plasma half-life ranging from 8.3 to 21.7 hours.

Pharmacodynamics

The most prominent effect of ZEBETA is the negative chronotropic effect, resulting in a reduction in resting and exercise heart rate. There is a fall in resting and exercise cardiac output with little observed change in stroke volume, and only a small increase in right atrial pressure or pulmonary capillary wedge pressure at rest or during exercise.

Findings in short-term clinical hemodynamics studies with ZEBETA are similar to those observed with other beta-blocking agents.

The mechanism of action of its antihypertensive effects has not been completely established. Factors which may be involved include:

1) Decreased cardiac output,
2) Inhibition of renin release by the kidneys,
3) Diminution of tonic sympathetic outflow from the vasomotor centers in the brain.

In normal volunteers, ZEBETA therapy resulted in a reduction of exercise- and isoproterenol-induced tachycardia. The maximal effect occurred within 1–4 hours post-dosing. Effects persisted for 24 hours at doses equal to or greater than 5 mg.

Electrophysiology studies in man have demonstrated that ZEBETA significantly decreases heart rate, increases sinus node recovery time, prolongs AV node refractory periods, and, with rapid atrial stimulation, prolongs AV nodal conduction.

$Beta_1$-selectivity of ZEBETA has been demonstrated in both animal and human studies. No effects at therapeutic doses on $beta_2$-adrenoceptor density have been observed. Pulmonary function studies have been conducted in healthy volunteers, asthmatics, and patients with chronic obstructive pulmonary disease (COPD). Doses of ZEBETA ranged from 5 to 60 mg, atenolol from 50 to 200 mg, metoprolol from 100 to 200 mg, and propranolol from 40 to 80 mg. In some studies, slight, asymptomatic increases in airways resistance (AWR) and decreases in forced expiratory volume (FEV_1) were observed with doses of bisoprolol fumarate 20 mg and higher, similar to the small increases in AWR also noted with the other cardioselective beta-blockers. The changes induced by beta-blockade with all agents were reversed by bronchodilator therapy.

ZEBETA had minimal effect on serum lipids during antihypertensive studies. In U.S. placebo-controlled trials, changes in total cholesterol averaged +0.8% for bisoprolol fumarate-treated patients, and +0.7% for placebo. Changes in triglycerides averaged +19% for bisoprolol fumarate-treated patients, and +17% for placebo.

ZEBETA has also been given concomitantly with thiazide diuretics. Even very low doses of hydrochlorothiazide (6.25 mg) were found to be additive with bisoprolol fumarate in lowering blood pressure in patients with mild-to-moderate hypertension.

CLINICAL STUDIES

In two randomized double-blind placebo-controlled trials conducted in the U.S., reductions in systolic and diastolic blood pressure and heart rate 24 hours after dosing in patients with mild-to-moderate hypertension are shown below. In both studies, mean systolic/diastolic blood pressures at baseline were approximately 150/100 mm Hg, and mean heart rate was 76 bpm. Drug effect is calculated by subtracting the placebo effect from the overall change in blood pressure and heart rate.

[See first table at top of next page]

Blood pressure responses were seen within one week of treatment and changed little thereafter. They were sustained for 12 weeks and for over a year in studies of longer duration. Blood pressure returned to baseline when bisoprolol fumarate was tapered over two weeks in a long-term study.

Overall, significantly greater blood pressure reductions were observed on bisoprolol fumarate than on placebo, regardless of race, age, or gender. There were no significant differences in response between black and nonblack patients.

INDICATIONS AND USAGE

ZEBETA is indicated in the management of hypertension. It may be used alone or in combination with other antihypertensive agents.

CONTRAINDICATIONS

ZEBETA is contraindicated in patients with cardiogenic shock, overt cardiac failure, second or third degree AV block, and marked sinus bradycardia.

WARNINGS

Cardiac Failure

Sympathetic stimulation is a vital component supporting circulatory function in the setting of congestive heart failure, and beta-blockade may result in further depression of myocardial contractility and precipitate more severe failure. In general, beta-blocking agents should be avoided in patients with overt congestive failure. However, in some patients with compensated cardiac failure it may be necessary to utilize them. In such a situation, they must be used cautiously.

In Patients Without a History of Cardiac Failure

Continued depression of the myocardium with beta-blockers can, in some patients, precipitate cardiac failure. At the first signs or symptoms of heart failure, discontinuation of ZEBETA should be considered. In some cases, beta-blocker therapy can be continued while heart failure is treated with other drugs.

Abrupt Cessation of Therapy

Exacerbation of angina pectoris, and, in some instances, myocardial infarction or ventricular arrhythmia, have been observed in patients with coronary artery disease following abrupt cessation of therapy with beta-blockers. Such patients should, therefore, be cautioned against interruption or discontinuation of therapy without the physician's advice. Even in patients without overt coronary artery disease, it may be advisable to taper therapy with ZEBETA over approximately one week with the patient under careful observation. If withdrawal symptoms occur, ZEBETA therapy should be reinstituted, at least temporarily.

Peripheral Vascular Disease

Beta-blockers can precipitate or aggravate symptoms of arterial insufficiency in patients with peripheral vascular disease. Caution should be exercised in such individuals.

Bronchospastic Disease

PATIENTS WITH BRONCHOSPASTIC DISEASE SHOULD, IN GENERAL, NOT RECEIVE BETA-BLOCKERS. Because of its relative beta$_1$-selectivity, however, ZEBETA may be used with caution in patients with bronchospastic disease who do not respond to, or who cannot tolerate other antihypertensive treatment. Since beta$_1$-selectivity is not absolute, the lowest possible dose of ZEBETA should be used, with therapy starting at 2.5 mg. A beta$_2$ agonist (bronchodilator) should be made available.

Anesthesia and Major Surgery

If ZEBETA treatment is to be continued perioperatively, particular care should be taken when anesthetic agents which depress myocardial function, such as ether, cyclopropane, and trichloroethylene, are used. See **OVERDOSAGE** for information on treatment of bradycardia and hypertension.

Diabetes and Hypoglycemia

Beta-blockers may mask some of the manifestations of hypoglycemia, particularly tachycardia. Nonselective beta-blockers may potentiate insulin-induced hypoglycemia and delay recovery of serum glucose levels. Because of its beta$_1$-selectivity, this is less likely with ZEBETA. However, patients subject to spontaneous hypoglycemia, or diabetic patients receiving insulin or oral hypoglycemic agents, should be cautioned about these possibilities and bisoprolol fumarate should be used with caution.

Thyrotoxicosis

Beta-adrenergic blockade may mask clinical signs of hyperthyroidism, such as tachycardia. Abrupt withdrawal of beta-blockade may be followed by an exacerbation of the symptoms of hyperthyroidism or may precipitate thyroid storm.

PRECAUTIONS

Impaired Renal or Hepatic Function

Use caution in adjusting the dose of ZEBETA in patients with renal or hepatic impairment (see **CLINICAL PHARMACOLOGY** and **DOSAGE AND ADMINISTRATION**).

Drug Interactions

ZEBETA should not be combined with other beta-blocking agents. Patients receiving catecholamine-depleting drugs, such as reserpine or guanethidine, should be closely monitored, because the added beta-adrenergic blocking action of ZEBETA may produce excessive reduction of sympathetic activity. In patients receiving concurrent therapy with clonidine, if therapy is to be discontinued, it is suggested that ZEBETA be discontinued for several days before the withdrawal of clonidine.

ZEBETA should be used with care when myocardial depressants or inhibitors of AV conduction, such as certain calcium antagonists [particularly of the phenylalkylamine (verapamil) and benzothiazepine (diltiazem) classes], or antiarrhythmic agents, such as disopyramide, are used concurrently.

Concurrent use of rifampin increases the metabolic clearance of ZEBETA, resulting in a shortened elimination half-life of ZEBETA. However, initial dose modification is generally not necessary. Pharmacokinetic studies document no clinically relevant interactions with other agents given concomitantly, including thiazide diuretics, digoxin and cimetidine. There was no effect of ZEBETA on prothrombin time in patients on stable doses of warfarin.

Risk of Anaphylactic Reaction: While taking beta-blockers, patients with a history of severe anaphylactic reaction to a variety of allergens may be more reactive to repeated challenge, either accidental, diagnostic, or therapeutic. Such patients may be unresponsive to the usual doses of epinephrine used to treat allergic reactions.

Sitting Systolic/Diastolic Pressure (BP) and Heart Rate (HR)
Mean Decrease (Δ) After 3 to 4 Weeks

Study A

	Placebo	Bisoprolol Fumarate 5 mg	10 mg	20 mg
n=	61	61	61	61
Total ΔBP (mm Hg)	5.4/3.2	10.4/8.0	11.2/10.9	12.8/11.9
Drug Effect[a]	—	5.0/4.8	5.8/7.7	7.4/8.7
Total ΔHR (bpm)	0.5	7.2	8.7	11.3
Drug Effect[a]	—	6.7	8.2	10.8

Study B

	Placebo	Bisoprolol Fumarate 2.5 mg	10 mg
n=	56	59	62
Total ΔBP (mm Hg)	3.0/3.7	7.6/8.1	13.5/11.2
Drug Effect[a]	—	4.6/4.4	10.5/7.5
Total ΔHR (bpm)	1.6	3.8	10.7
Drug Effect[a]	—	2.2	9.1

[a] Observed total change from baseline minus placebo.

Body System/Adverse Experience	All Adverse Experiences (% [a]) Placebo (n = 132) %	Bisoprolol Fumarate 5–20 mg (n = 273) %	2.5–40 mg (n = 404) %
Skin			
increased sweating	1.5	0.7	1.0
Musculo-skeletal			
arthralgia	2.3	2.2	2.7
Central Nervous System			
dizziness	3.8	2.9	3.5
headache	11.4	8.8	10.9
hypoaesthesia	0.8	1.1	1.5
Autonomic Nervous System			
dry mouth	1.5	0.7	1.3
Heart Rate/Rhythm			
bradycardia	0	0.4	0.5
Psychiatric			
vivid dreams	0	0	0
insomnia	2.3	1.5	2.5
depression	0.8	0	0.2
Gastrointestinal			
diarrhea	1.5	2.6	3.5
nausea	1.5	1.5	2.2
vomiting	0	1.1	1.5
Respiratory			
bronchospasm	0	0	0
cough	4.5	2.6	2.5
dyspnea	0.8	1.1	1.5
pharyngitis	2.3	2.2	2.2
rhinitis	3.0	2.9	4.0
sinusitis	1.5	2.2	2.2
URI	3.8	4.8	5.0
Body as a Whole			
asthenia	0	0.4	1.5
chest pain	0.8	1.1	1.5
fatigue	1.5	6.6	8.2
edema (peripheral)	3.8	3.7	3.0

[a] percentage of patients with event.

Information for Patients

Patients, especially those with coronary artery disease, should be warned about discontinuing use of ZEBETA without a physician's supervision. Patients should also be advised to consult a physician if any difficulty in breathing occurs, or if they develop signs or symptoms of congestive heart failure or excessive bradycardia.

Patients subject to spontaneous hypoglycemia, or diabetic patients receiving insulin or oral hypoglycemic agents, should be cautioned that beta-blockers may mask some of the manifestations of hypoglycemia, particularly tachycardia, and bisoprolol fumarate should be used with caution.

Patients should know how they react to this medicine before they operate automobiles and machinery or engage in other tasks requiring alertness.

Carcinogenesis, Mutagenesis, Impairment of Fertility

Long-term studies were conducted with oral bisoprolol fumarate administered in the feed of mice (20 and 24 months) and rats (26 months). No evidence of carcinogenic potential was seen in mice dosed up to 250 mg/kg/day or rats dosed up to 125 mg/kg/day. On a body-weight basis, these doses are 625 and 312 times, respectively, the maximum recommended human dose (MRHD) of 20 mg, (or 0.4 mg/kg/day based on a 50 kg individual); on a body-surface-area-basis, these doses are 59 times (mice) and 64 times (rats) the MRHD. The mutagenic potential of bisoprolol fumarate was evaluated in the microbial mutagenicity (Ames) test, the point mutation and chromosome aberration assays in Chinese hamster V79 cells, the unscheduled DNA synthesis test, the micronucleus test in mice, and the cytogenetics assay in rats. There was no evidence of mutagenic potential in these *in vitro* and *in vivo* assays.

Reproduction studies in rats did not show any impairment of fertility at doses up to 150 mg/kg/day of bisoprolol fumarate, or 375 and 77 times the MRHD on the basis of body-weight and body-surface-area, respectively.

Pregnancy Category C

In rats, bisoprolol fumarate was not teratogenic at doses up to 150 mg/kg/day which is 375 and 77 times the MRHD on the basis of body-weight and body-surface-area, respectively. Bisoprolol fumarate was fetotoxic (increased late resorptions) at 50 mg/kg/day and maternotoxic (decreased food intake and body-weight gain) at 150 mg/kg/day. The fetotoxicity in rats occurred at 125 times the MRHD on a body-weight-basis and 26 times the MRHD on the basis of body-surface-area. The maternotoxicity occurred at 375 times the MRHD on a body-weight basis and 77 times the MRHD on the basis of body-surface-area. In rabbits, bisoprolol fumarate was not teratogenic at doses up to 12.5 mg/kg/day, which is 31 and 12 times the MRHD based on body-weight and body-surface-area, respectively, but was embryolethal (increased early resorptions) at 12.5 mg/kg/day. There are no adequate and well-controlled studies in pregnant women. ZEBETA should be used during pregnancy only if the potential benefit justifies the potential risk to the fetus.

Nursing Mothers

Small amounts of bisoprolol fumarate (<2% of the dose) have been detected in the milk of lactating rats. It is not known whether this drug is excreted in human milk. Because many drugs are excreted in human milk caution should be exercised when bisoprolol fumarate is administered to nursing women.

Use in Elderly Patients

ZEBETA has been used in elderly patients with hypertension. Response rates and mean decreases in systolic and diastolic blood pressure were similar to the decreases in younger patients in the U.S. clinical studies. Although no dose response study was conducted in elderly patients, there was a tendency for older patients to be maintained on higher doses of bisoprolol fumarate.

Observed reductions in heart rate were slightly greater in the elderly than in the young and tended to increase with increasing dose. In general, no disparity in adverse experience reports or dropouts for safety reasons was observed between older and younger patients. Dose adjustment based on age is not necessary.

Continued on next page

Zebeta—Cont.

Pediatric Use
Safety and effectiveness in pediatric patients have not been established.

ADVERSE REACTIONS

Safety data are available in more than 30,000 patients or volunteers. Frequency estimates and rates of withdrawal of therapy for adverse events were derived from two U.S. placebo-controlled studies.
In Study A, doses of 5, 10 and 20 mg bisoprolol fumarate were administered for 4 weeks. In Study B, doses of 2.5, 10 and 40 mg of bisoprolol fumarate were administered for 12 weeks. A total of 273 patients were treated with 5–20 mg of bisoprolol fumarate; 132 received placebo.
Withdrawal of therapy for adverse events was 3.3% for patients receiving bisoprolol fumarate and 6.8% for patients on placebo. Withdrawals were less than 1% for either bradycardia or fatigue/lack of energy.
The following table presents adverse experiences, whether or not considered drug related, reported in at least 1% of patients in these studies, for all patients studied in placebo controlled clinical trials (2.5–40 mg), as well as for a subgroup that was treated with doses within the recommended dosage range (5–20 mg). Of the adverse events listed in the table, bradycardia, diarrhea, asthenia, fatigue and sinusitis appear to be dose related.
[See second table at top of previous page]
The following is a comprehensive list of adverse experiences reported with bisoprolol fumarate in worldwide studies, or in post marketing experience (in italics):
Central Nervous System: Dizziness, vertigo, headache, paresthesia, hypoaesthesia, somnolence, anxiety/restlessness, decreased concentration/memory.
Autonomic Nervous System: Dry mouth.
Cardiovascular: Bradycardia, palpitations and other rhythm disturbances, cold extremities, claudication, hypotension, orthostatic hypotension, chest pain, congestive heart failure, dyspnea on exertion.
Psychiatric: Vivid dreams, insomnia, depression.
Gastrointestinal: Gastric/epigastric/abdominal pain, gastritis, dyspepsia, nausea, vomiting, diarrhea, constipation.
Musculoskeletal: Muscle/joint pain, back/neck pain, muscle cramps, twitching/tremor.
Skin: Rash, acne, eczema, skin irritation, pruritus, flushing, sweating, alopecia, *angioedema, exfoliative dermatitis,* cutaneous vasculitis.
Special Senses: Visual disturbances, ocular pain/pressure, abnormal lacrimation, tinnitus, earache, taste abnormalities.
Metabolic: Gout.
Respiratory: Asthma/bronchospasm, bronchitis, coughing, dyspnea, pharyngitis, rhinitis, sinusitis, URI.
Genito-urinary: Decreased libido/impotence, *Peyronie's disease,* cystitis, renal colic.
Hematologic: Purpura.
General: Fatigue, asthenia, chest pain, malaise, edema, weight gain.
In addition, a variety of adverse effects have been reported with other beta-adrenergic blocking agents and should be considered potential adverse effects of ZEBETA:
Central Nervous System: Reversible mental depression progressing to catatonia, an acute reversible syndrome characterized by disorientation to time and place, emotional lability, slightly clouded sensorium.
Allergic: Fever, combined with aching and sore throat, laryngospasm, respiratory distress.
Hematologic: Agranulocytosis, thrombocytopenia, thrombocytopenic purpura.
Gastrointestinal: Mesenteric arterial thrombosis, ischemic colitis.
Miscellaneous: The oculomucocutaneous syndrome associated with the beta-blocker practolol has not been reported with ZEBETA during investigational use or extensive foreign marketing experience.
LABORATORY ABNORMALITIES: In clinical trials, the most frequently reported laboratory change was an increase in serum triglycerides, but this was not a consistent finding.
Sporadic liver test abnormalities have been reported. In the U.S. controlled trials experience with bisoprolol fumarate treatment for 4–12 weeks, the incidence of concomitant elevations in SGOT and SGPT of between 1–2 times normal was 3.9%, compared to 2.5% for placebo. No patient had concomitant elevations greater than twice normal.
In the long-term, uncontrolled experience with bisoprolol fumarate treatment for 6–18 months, the incidence of one or more concomitant elevations in SGOT and SGPT of between 1–2 times normal was 6.2%. The incidence of multiple occurrences was 1.9%. For concomitant elevations in SGOT and SGPT of greater than twice normal, the incidence was 1.5%. The incidence of multiple occurrences was 0.3%. In many cases these elevations were attributed to underlying disorders, or resolved during continued treatment with bisoprolol fumarate.
Other laboratory changes included small increases in uric acid, creatinine, BUN, serum potassium, glucose, and phosphorus and decreases in WBC and platelets. These were generally not of clinical importance and rarely resulted in discontinuation of bisoprolol fumarate.
As with other beta-blockers, ANA conversions have also been reported on bisoprolol fumarate. About 15% of patients in long-term studies converted to a positive titer, although about one-third of these patients subsequently reconverted to a negative titer while on continued therapy.

OVERDOSAGE

The most common signs expected with overdosage of a beta-blocker are bradycardia, hypotension, congestive heart failure, bronchospasm, and hypoglycemia. To date, a few cases of overdose (maximum: 2000 mg) with bisoprolol fumarate have been reported. Bradycardia and/or hypotension were noted. Sympathomimetic agents were given in some cases, and all patients recovered.
In general, if overdose occurs, ZEBETA therapy should be stopped and supportive and symptomatic treatment should be provided. Limited data suggest that bisoprolol fumarate is not dialyzable. Based on the expected pharmacologic actions and recommendations for other beta-blockers, the following general measures should be considered when clinically warranted:
Bradycardia
Administer IV atropine. If the response is inadequate, isoproterenol or another agent with positive chronotropic properties may be given cautiously. Under some circumstances, transvenous pacemaker insertion may be necessary.
Hypotension
IV fluids and vasopressors should be administered. Intravenous glucagon may be useful.
Heart Block (Second or Third Degree)
Patients should be carefully monitored and treated with isoproterenol infusion or transvenous cardiac pacemaker insertion, as appropriate.
Congestive Heart Failure
Initiate conventional therapy (ie, digitalis, diuretics, inotropic agents, vasodilating agents).
Bronchospasm
Administer bronchodilator therapy such as isoproterenol and/or aminophylline.
Hypoglycemia
Administer IV glucose.

DOSAGE AND ADMINISTRATION

The dose of ZEBETA must be individualized to the needs of the patient. The usual starting dose is 5 mg once daily. In some patients, 2.5 mg may be an appropriate starting dose (see **Bronchospastic Disease** in **WARNINGS**). If the antihypertensive effect of 5 mg is inadequate, the dose may be increased to 10 mg and then, if necessary, to 20 mg once daily.
Patients with Renal or Hepatic Impairment
In patients with hepatic impairment (hepatitis or cirrhosis) or renal dysfunction (creatinine clearance less than 40 mL/min), the initial daily dose should be 2.5 mg and caution should be used in dose-titration. Since limited data suggest that bisoprolol fumarate is not dialyzable, drug replacement is not necessary in patients undergoing dialysis.
Elderly Patients
It is not necessary to adjust the dose in the elderly, unless there is also significant renal or hepatic dysfunction (see above and **Use in Elderly Patients** in **PRECAUTIONS**).
Children
There is no pediatric experience with ZEBETA.

HOW SUPPLIED

ZEBETA® (bisoprolol fumarate) is supplied as 5 mg and 10 mg tablets.
The 5 mg tablet is pink, heart-shaped, biconvex, film-coated, and vertically scored in half on both sides, with an engraved B1 on one side and LL on the reverse side, supplied as follows:
NDC 0005-3816-38—Bottle of 30 with CRC
The 10 mg tablet is white, heart-shaped, biconvex, film-coated, with an engraved B3 on one side and LL on the reverse side, supplied as follows:
NDC 0005-3817-38—Bottle of 30 with CRC
Store at controlled room temperature 20°–25°C (68°– 77°F), protected from moisture.
Dispense in tight containers as defined in the USP.
Manufactured by:
LEDERLE PHARMACEUTICAL DIVISION
American Cyanamid Company
Pearl River, NY 10965
Under License of E. MERCK
Darmstadt, Germany
CI 5108-1 Issued July 7, 1998
Shown in Product Identification Guide, page 320

ZIAC® ℞

[zī 'ăk]
(Bisoprolol Fumarate and Hydrochlorothiazide) Tablets

DESCRIPTION

ZIAC (bisoprolol fumarate and hydrochlorothiazide) is indicated for the treatment of hypertension. It combines two antihypertensive agents in a once-daily dosage: a synthetic beta$_1$-selective (cardioselective) adrenoceptor blocking agent (bisoprolol fumarate) and a benzothiadiazine diuretic (hydrochlorothiazide).
Bisoprolol fumarate is chemically described as (±)-1-[4-[[2-(1-methylethoxy)ethoxy]methyl]phenoxy]-3-[(1-methyl) ethyl)amino]-2-propanol(*E*)-2-butenedioate (2:1) (salt). It possesses an asymmetric carbon atom in its structure and is provided as a racemic mixture. The S(-) enantiomer is responsible for most of the beta-blocking activity. Its empirical formula is $(C_{18}H_{31}NO_4)_2 \cdot C_4H_4O_4$ and it has a molecular weight of 766.97.
Bisoprolol fumarate is a white crystalline powder, approximately equally hydrophilic and lipophilic, and readily soluble in water, methanol, ethanol, and chloroform.
Hydrochlorothiazide (HCTZ) is 6-Chloro-3,4-dihydro-2*H*-1,2,4-benzothiadiazine-7-sulfonamide 1,1-dioxide. It is a white, or practically white, practically odorless crystalline powder. It is slightly soluble in water, sparingly soluble in dilute sodium hydroxide solution, freely soluble in n-butylamine and dimethylformamide, soluble in methanol, and insoluble in ether, chloroform, and dilute mineral acids. Its empirical formula is $C_7H_8ClN_3O_4S_2$ and it has a molecular weight of 297.73.

Each ZIAC®-2.5 mg/6.25 mg tablet for oral administration contains:
Bisoprolol fumarate .... 2.5 mg
Hydrochlorothiazide .... 6.25 mg
Each ZIAC®-5 mg/6.25 mg tablet for oral administration contains:
Bisoprolol fumarate .... 5 mg
Hydrochlorothiazide .... 6.25 mg
Each ZIAC®-10 mg/6.25 mg tablet for oral administration contains:
Bisoprolol fumarate .... 10 mg
Hydrochlorothiazide .... 6.25 mg

Inactive ingredients include Colloidal Silicon Dioxide, Corn Starch, Dibasic Calcium Phosphate, Hydroxypropyl Methylcellulose, Magnesium Stearate, Microcrystalline Cellulose, Polyethylene Glycol, Polysorbate 80, and Titanium Dioxide. The 5 mg/6.25 mg tablet also contains Red and Yellow Iron Oxide. The 2.5 mg/6.25 mg tablet also contains Crospovidone, Pregelatinized Starch and Yellow Iron Oxide.

CLINICAL PHARMACOLOGY

Bisoprolol fumarate and HCTZ have been used individually and in combination for the treatment of hypertension. The antihypertensive effects of these agents are additive; HCTZ 6.25 mg significantly increases the antihypertensive effect of bisoprolol fumarate. The incidence of hypokalemia with the bisoprolol fumarate and HCTZ 6.25 mg combination (B/H) is significantly lower than with HCTZ 25 mg. In clinical trials of ZIAC, mean changes in serum potassium for patients treated with ZIAC 2.5/6.25 mg, 5/6.25 mg or 10/6.25 mg or placebo were less than ± 0.1 mEq/L. Mean changes in serum potassium for patients treated with any dose of bisoprolol in combination with HCTZ 25 mg ranged from –0.1 to –0.3 mEq/L.
Bisoprolol fumarate is a beta$_1$-selective (cardioselective) adrenoceptor blocking agent without significant membrane stabilizing or intrinsic sympathomimetic activities in its therapeutic dose range. At higher doses (≥ 20 mg) bisoprolol fumarate also inhibits beta$_2$-adrenoreceptors located in bronchial and vascular musculature. To retain relative selectivity, it is important to use the lowest effective dose.
Hydrochlorothiazide is a benzothiadiazine diuretic. Thiazides affect renal tubular mechanisms of electrolyte reabsorption and increase excretion of sodium and chloride in approximately equivalent amounts. Natriuresis causes a secondary loss of potassium.
Pharmacokinetics and Metabolism
ZIAC
In healthy volunteers, both bisoprolol fumarate and hydrochlorothiazide are well absorbed following oral administration of ZIAC. No change is observed in the bioavailability of either agent when given together in a single tablet. Absorption is not affected whether ZIAC is taken with or without food. Mean peak bisoprolol fumarate plasma concentrations of about 9.0 ng/mL, 19 ng/mL and 36 ng/mL occur approximately 3 hours after the administration of the 2.5 mg/6.25 mg, 5 mg/6.25 mg and 10 mg/6.25 mg combination tablets, respectively. Mean peak plasma hydrochlorothiazide concentrations of 30 ng/mL occur approximately 2.5 hours following the administration of the combination. Dose proportional increases in plasma bisoprolol concentrations are observed between the 2.5 and 5, as well as between the 5 and 10 mg doses. The elimination $T_{1/2}$ of bisoprolol ranges from 7 to 15 hours and of hydrochlorothiazide ranges from 4 to 10 hours. The percent of dose excreted unchanged in urine is about 55% for bisoprolol and about 60% for o-hydrochlorothiazide.
Bisoprolol Fumarate
The absolute bioavailability after a 10 mg oral dose of bisoprolol fumarate is about 80%. The first pass metabolism of bisoprolol fumarate is about 20%.
The pharmacokinetic profile of bisoprolol fumarate has been examined following single doses and at steady state. Binding to serum proteins is approximately 30%. Peak plasma concentrations occur within 2–4 hours of dosing with 2.5 to 20 mg, and mean peak values range from 9.0 ng/mL at 2.5 mg to 70 ng/mL at 20 mg. Once-daily dosing with bisoprolol fumarate results in less than twofold intersubject variation in peak plasma concentrations. Plasma concentrations are proportional to the administered dose in the range of 2.5 to 20 mg. The plasma elimination half-life is 9–12 hours and is slightly longer in elderly patients, in part because of decreased renal function. Steady state is attained within 5 days with once-daily dosing. In both young and elderly populations, plasma accumulation is low; the accumulation factor ranges from 1.1 to 1.3, and is what would be expected from the half-life and once-daily dosing. Bisoprolol is eliminated equally by renal and nonrenal pathways with about

50% of the dose appearing unchanged in the urine and the remainder in the form of inactive metabolites. In humans, the known metabolites are labile or have no known pharmacologic activity. Less than 2% of the dose is excreted in the feces. The pharmacokinetic characteristics of the two enantiomers are similar. Bisoprolol is not metabolized by cytochrome P450 II D6 (debrisoquin hydroxylase).

In subjects with creatinine clearance less than 40 mL/min, the plasma half-life is increased approximately threefold compared to healthy subjects.

In patients with liver cirrhosis, the rate of elimination of bisoprolol is more variable and significantly slower than that in healthy subjects, with a plasma half-life ranging from 8 to 22 hours.

In elderly subjects, mean plasma concentrations at steady state are increased, in part attributed to lower creatinine clearance. However, no significant differences in the degree of bisoprolol accumulation is found between young and elderly populations.

Hydrochlorothiazide

Hydrochlorothiazide is well absorbed (65%–75%) following oral administration. Absorption of hydrochlorothiazide is reduced in patients with congestive heart failure.

Peak plasma concentrations are observed within 1–5 hours of dosing, and range from 70–490 ng/mL following oral doses of 12.5–100 mg. Plasma concentrations are linearly related to the administered dose. Concentrations of hydrochlorothiazide are 1.6–1.8 times higher in whole blood than in plasma. Binding to serum proteins has been reported to be approximately 40% to 68%. The plasma elimination half-life has been reported to be 6–15 hours. Hydrochlorothiazide is eliminated primarily by renal pathways. Following oral doses of 12.5–100 mg, 55%–77% of the administered dose appears in urine and greater than 95% of the absorbed dose is excreted in urine as unchanged drug. Plasma concentrations of hydrochlorothiazide are increased and the elimination half-life is prolonged in patients with renal disease.

Pharmacodynamics

Bisoprolol Fumarate

Findings in clinical hemodynamics studies with bisoprolol fumarate are similar to those observed with other beta-blockers. The most prominent effect is the negative chronotropic effect, giving a reduction in resting and exercise heart rate. There is a fall in resting and exercise cardiac output with little observed change in stroke volume, and only a small increase in right atrial pressure, or pulmonary capillary wedge pressure at rest or during exercise.

In normal volunteers, bisoprolol fumarate therapy resulted in a reduction of exercise- and isoproterenol-induced tachycardia. The maximal effect occurred within 1–4 hours post-dosing. Effects generally persisted for 24 hours at doses of 5 mg or greater.

In controlled clinical trials, bisoprolol fumarate given as a single daily dose has been shown to be an effective antihypertensive agent when used alone or concomitantly with thiazide diuretics (see **CLINICAL STUDIES**).

The mechanism of bisoprolol fumarate's antihypertensive effect has not been completely established. Factors that may be involved include:

1) Decreased cardiac output,
2) Inhibition of renin release by the kidneys,
3) Diminution of tonic sympathetic outflow from vasomotor centers in the brain.

$Beta_1$-selectivity of bisoprolol fumarate has been demonstrated in both animal and human studies. No effects at therapeutic doses on $beta_2$-adrenoreceptor density have been observed. Pulmonary function studies have been conducted in healthy volunteers, asthmatics, and patients with chronic obstructive pulmonary disease (COPD). Doses of bisoprolol fumarate ranged from 5 to 60 mg, atenolol from 50 to 200 mg, metoprolol from 100 to 200 mg, and propranolol from 40 to 80 mg. In some studies, slight, asymptomatic increases in airway resistance (AWR) and decreases in forced expiratory volume (FEV_1) were observed with doses of bisoprolol fumarate 20 mg and higher, similar to the small increases in AWR noted with other cardioselective beta-blocking agents. The changes induced by beta-blockade with all agents were reversed by bronchodilator therapy.

Electrophysiology studies in man have demonstrated that bisoprolol fumarate significantly decreases heart rate, increases sinus node recovery time, prolongs AV node refractory periods, and, with rapid atrial stimulation, prolongs AV nodal conduction.

Hydrochlorothiazide

Acute effects of thiazides are thought to result from a reduction in blood volume and cardiac output, secondary to a natriuretic effect, although a direct vasodilatory mechanism has also been proposed. With chronic administration, plasma volume returns toward normal, but peripheral vascular resistance is decreased.

Thiazides do not affect normal blood pressure. Onset of action occurs within 2 hours of dosing, peak effect is observed at about 4 hours, and activity persists for up to 24 hours.

CLINICAL STUDIES

In controlled clinical trials, bisoprolol fumarate/hydrochlorothiazide 6.25 mg has been shown to reduce systolic and diastolic blood pressure throughout a 24-hour period when administered once daily. The effects on systolic and diastolic blood pressure reduction of the combination of bisoprolol fumarate and hydrochlorothiazide were additive. Further, treatment effects were consistent across age groups (<60, ≥60 years), racial groups (black, nonblack), and gender (male, female).

In two randomized, double-blind, placebo-controlled trials conducted in the U.S., reductions in systolic and diastolic blood pressure and heart rate 24 hours after dosing in patients with mild-to-moderate hypertension are shown below. In both studies mean systolic/diastolic blood pressure and heart rate at baseline were approximately 151/101 mm Hg and 77 bpm.

[See table above]

Sitting Systolic/Diastolic Pressure (BP) and Heart Rate (HR)
Mean Decrease (Δ) After 3–4 Weeks

	Study 1		Study 2			
	Placebo	B5/H6.25 mg	Placebo	H6.25 mg	B2.5/H6.25 mg	B10/H6.25 mg
n=	75	150	56	23	28	25
Total ΔBP (mm Hg)	–2.9/–3.9	–15.8/–12.6	–3.0/–3.7	–6.6/–5.8	–14.1/–10.5	–15.3/–14.3
Drug Effect[a]	—/—	–12.9/–8.7	—/—	–3.6/–2.1	–11.1/–6.8	–12.3/–10.6
Total ΔHR (bpm)	–0.3	–6.9	–1.6	–0.8	–3.7	–9.8
Drug Effect[a]	—	–6.6	—	+0.8	–2.1	–8.2

[a] Observed mean change from baseline minus placebo.

Blood pressure responses were seen within 1 week of treatment but the maximum effect was apparent after 2 to 3 weeks of treatment. Overall, significantly greater blood pressure reductions were observed on ZIAC than on placebo. Further, blood pressure reductions were significantly greater for each of the bisoprolol fumarate plus hydrochlorothiazide combinations than for either of the components used alone regardless of race, age, or gender. There were no significant differences in response between black and nonblack patients.

INDICATIONS AND USAGE

ZIAC is indicated in the management of hypertension.

CONTRAINDICATIONS

ZIAC is contraindicated in patients in cardiogenic shock, overt cardiac failure (see **WARNINGS**), second or third degree AV block, marked sinus bradycardia, anuria, and hypersensitivity to either component of this product or to other sulfonamide-derived drugs.

WARNINGS

Cardiac Failure: In general, beta-blocking agents should be avoided in patients with overt congestive failure. However, in some patients with compensated cardiac failure, it may be necessary to utilize these agents. In such situations, they must be used cautiously.

Patients Without a History of Cardiac Failure: Continued depression of the myocardium with beta-blockers can, in some patients, precipitate cardiac failure. At the first signs or symptoms of heart failure, discontinuation of ZIAC should be considered. In some cases ZIAC therapy can be continued while heart failure is treated with other drugs.

Abrupt Cessation of Therapy: Exacerbations of angina pectoris and, in some instances, myocardial infarction or ventricular arrhythmia, have been observed in patients with coronary artery disease following abrupt cessation of therapy with beta-blockers. Such patients should, therefore, be cautioned against interruption or discontinuation of therapy without the physician's advice. Even in patients without overt coronary artery disease, it may be advisable to taper therapy with ZIAC over approximately 1 week with the patient under careful observation. If withdrawal symptoms occur, beta-blocking agent therapy should be reinstituted, at least temporarily.

Peripheral Vascular Disease: Beta-blockers can precipitate or aggravate symptoms of arterial insufficiency in patients with peripheral vascular disease. Caution should be exercised in such individuals.

Bronchospastic Disease: PATIENTS WITH BRONCHOSPASTIC PULMONARY DISEASE SHOULD, IN GENERAL, NOT RECEIVE BETA-BLOCKERS. Because of the relative $beta_1$-selectivity of bisoprolol fumarate, ZIAC may be used with caution in patients with bronchospastic disease who do not respond to, or who cannot tolerate other antihypertensive treatment. Since $beta_1$-selectivity is not absolute, the lowest possible dose of ZIAC should be used. A $beta_2$ agonist (bronchodilator) should be made available.

Anesthesia and Major Surgery: If ZIAC treatment is to be continued perioperatively, particular care should be taken when anesthetic agents that depress myocardial function, such as ether, cyclopropane, and trichloroethylene, are used. See **OVERDOSAGE** for information on treatment of bradycardia and hypotension.

Diabetes and Hypoglycemia: Beta-blockers may mask some of the manifestations of hypoglycemia, particularly tachycardia. Nonselective beta-blockers may potentiate insulin-induced hypoglycemia and delay recovery of serum glucose levels. Because of its $beta_1$-selectivity, this is less likely with bisoprolol fumarate. However, patients subject to spontaneous hypoglycemia, or diabetic patients receiving insulin or oral hypoglycemic agents, should be cautioned about these possibilities. Also, latent diabetes mellitus may become manifest and diabetic patients given thiazides may require adjustment of their insulin dose. Because of the very low dose of HCTZ employed, this may be less likely with ZIAC.

Thyrotoxicosis: Beta-adrenergic blockade may mask clinical signs of hyperthyroidism, such as tachycardia. Abrupt withdrawal of beta-blockade may be followed by an exacerbation of the symptoms of hyperthyroidism or may precipitate thyroid storm.

Renal Disease: Cumulative effects of the thiazides may develop in patients with impaired renal function. In such patients, thiazides may precipitate azotemia. In subjects with creatinine clearance less than 40 mL/min, the plasma half-life of bisoprolol fumarate is increased up to threefold, as compared to healthy subjects. If progressive renal impairment becomes apparent, ZIAC should be discontinued. (See **Pharmacokinetics and Metabolism.**)

Hepatic Disease: ZIAC should be used with caution in patients with impaired hepatic function or progressive liver disease. Thiazides may alter fluid and electrolyte balance, which may precipitate hepatic coma. Also, elimination of bisoprolol fumarate is significantly slower in patients with cirrhosis than in healthy subjects. (See **Pharmacokinetics and Metabolism.**)

PRECAUTIONS

General

Electrolyte and Fluid Balance Status: Although the probability of developing hypokalemia is reduced with ZIAC because of the very low dose of HCTZ employed, periodic determination of serum electrolytes should be performed, and patients should be observed for signs of fluid or electrolyte disturbances, ie, hyponatremia, hypochloremic alkalosis, and hypokalemia and hypomagnesemia. Thiazides have been shown to increase the urinary excretion of magnesium; this may result in hypomagnesemia.

Warning signs or symptoms of fluid and electrolyte imbalance include dryness of mouth, thirst, weakness, lethargy, drowsiness, restlessness, muscle pains or cramps, muscular fatigue, hypotension, oliguria, tachycardia, and gastrointestinal disturbances such as nausea and vomiting.

Hypokalemia may develop, especially with brisk diuresis when severe cirrhosis is present, during concomitant use of corticosteroids or adrenocorticotropic hormone (ACTH) or after prolonged therapy. Interference with adequate oral electrolyte intake will also contribute to hypokalemia. Hypokalemia and hypomagnesemia can provoke ventricular arrhythmias or sensitize or exaggerate the response of the heart to the toxic effects of digitalis. Hypokalemia may be avoided or treated by potassium supplementation or increased intake of potassium-rich foods.

Dilutional hyponatremia may occur in edematous patients in hot weather; appropriate therapy is water restriction rather than salt administration, except in rare instances when the hyponatremia is life-threatening. In actual salt depletion, appropriate replacement is the therapy of choice.

Parathyroid Disease: Calcium excretion is decreased by thiazides, and pathologic changes in the parathyroid glands, with hypercalcemia and hypophosphatemia, have been observed in a few patients on prolonged thiazide therapy.

Hyperuricemia: Hyperuricemia or acute gout may be precipitated in certain patients receiving thiazide diuretics. Bisoprolol fumarate, alone or in combination with HCTZ, has been associated with increases in uric acid. However, in U.S. clinical trials, the incidence of treatment-related increases in uric acid was higher during therapy with HCTZ 25 mg (25%) than with B/H 6.25 mg (10%). Because of the very low dose of HCTZ employed, hyperuricemia may be less likely with ZIAC.

Drug Interactions: ZIAC may potentiate the action of other antihypertensive agents used concomitantly. ZIAC should not be combined with other beta-blocking agents. Patients receiving catecholamine-depleting drugs, such as reserpine or guanethidine, should be closely monitored because the added beta-adrenergic blocking action of bisoprolol fumarate may produce excessive reduction of sympathetic activity. In patients receiving concurrent therapy with clonidine, if therapy is to be discontinued, it is suggested that ZIAC be discontinued for several days before the withdrawal of clonidine.

ZIAC should be used with caution when myocardial depressants or inhibitors of AV conduction, such as certain calcium antagonists [particularly of the phenylalkylamine (verapamil) and benzothiazepine (diltiazem) classes], or antiarrhythmic agents, such as disopyramide, are used concurrently.

Bisoprolol Fumarate

Concurrent use of rifampin increases the metabolic clearance of bisoprolol fumarate, shortening its elimination half-

Continued on next page

Ziac—Cont.

life. However, initial dose modification is generally not necessary. Pharmacokinetic studies document no clinically relevant interactions with other agents given concomitantly, including thiazide diuretics, digoxin and cimetidine. There was no effect of bisoprolol fumarate on prothrombin times in patients on stable doses of warfarin.

Risk of Anaphylactic Reaction: While taking beta-blockers, patients with a history of severe anaphylactic reaction to a variety of allergens may be more reactive to repeated challenge, either accidental, diagnostic, or therapeutic. Such patients may be unresponsive to the usual doses of epinephrine used to treat allergic reactions.

Hydrochlorothiazide

When given concurrently the following drugs may interact with thiazide diuretics.

Alcohol, barbiturates, or narcotics—potentiation of orthostatic hypotension may occur.

Antidiabetic drugs (oral agents and insulin)—dosage adjustment of the antidiabetic drug may be required.

Other antihypertensive drugs—additive effect or potentiation.

Cholestyramine and colestipol resins—Absorption of hydrochlorothiazide is impaired in the presence of anionic exchange resins. Single doses of cholestyramine and colestipol resins bind the hydrochlorothiazide and reduce its absorption in the gastrointestinal tract by up to 85 percent and 43 percent, respectively.

Corticosteroids, ACTH—intensified electrolyte depletion, particularly hypokalemia.

Pressor amines (eg, norepinephrine)—possible decreased response to pressor amines but not sufficient to preclude their use.

Skeletal muscle relaxants, nondepolarizing (eg, tubocurarine)—possible increased responsiveness to the muscle relaxant.

Lithium—generally should not be given with diuretics. Diuretic agents reduce the renal clearance of lithium and add a high risk of lithium toxicity. Refer to the package insert for lithium preparations before use of such preparations with ZIAC.

Nonsteroidal anti-inflammatory drugs—In some patients, the administration of a nonsteroidal anti-inflammatory agent can reduce the diuretic, natriuretic, and antihypertensive effects of loop, potassium-sparing and thiazide diuretics. Therefore, when ZIAC and nonsteroidal anti-inflammatory agents are used concomitantly, the patient should be observed closely to determine if the desired effect of the diuretic is obtained.

In patients receiving thiazides, sensitivity reactions may occur with or without a history of allergy or bronchial asthma. Photosensitivity reactions and possible exacerbation or activation of systemic lupus erythematosus have been reported in patients receiving thiazides. The antihypertensive effects of thiazides may be enhanced in the post-sympathectomy patient.

Laboratory Test Interactions: Based on reports involving thiazides, ZIAC may decrease serum levels of protein-bound iodine without signs of thyroid disturbance.

Because it includes a thiazide, ZIAC should be discontinued before carrying out tests for parathyroid function (see **PRECAUTIONS—Parathyroid Disease**).

INFORMATION FOR PATIENTS

Patients, especially those with coronary artery disease, should be warned against discontinuing use of ZIAC without a physician's supervision. Patients should also be advised to consult a physician if any difficulty in breathing occurs, or if they develop other signs or symptoms of congestive heart failure or excessive bradycardia.

Patients subject to spontaneous hypoglycemia, or diabetic patients receiving insulin or oral hypoglycemic agents, should be cautioned that beta-blockers may mask some of the manifestations of hypoglycemia, particularly tachycardia, and bisoprolol fumarate should be used with caution.

Patients should know how they react to this medicine before they operate automobiles and machinery or engage in other tasks requiring alertness. Patients should be advised that photosensitivity reactions have been reported with thiazides.

Carcinogenesis, Mutagenesis, Impairment of Fertility

Carcinogenesis

ZIAC: Long-term studies have not been conducted with the bisoprolol fumarate/hydrochlorothiazide combination.

Bisoprolol Fumarate: Long-term studies were conducted with oral bisoprolol fumarate administered in the feed of mice (20 and 24 months) and rats (26 months). No evidence of carcinogenic potential was seen in mice dosed up to 250 mg/kg/day or rats dosed up to 125 mg/kg/day. On a body-weight basis, these doses are 625 and 312 times, respectively, the maximum recommended human dose (MRHD) of 20 mg, or 0.4 mg/kg/day, based on 50 kg individuals; on a body-surface-area basis, these doses are 59 times (mice) and 64 times (rats) the MRHD.

Hydrochlorothiazide: Two-year feeding studies in mice and rats, conducted under the auspices of the National Toxicology Program (NTP), treated mice and rats with doses of hydrochlorothiazide up to 600 and 100 mg/kg/day, respectively. On a body-weight basis, these doses are 2400 times (in mice) and 400 times (in rats) the MRHD of hydrochlorothiazide (12.5 mg/day) in ZIAC®. On a body-surface-area basis, these doses are 226 times (in mice) and 82 times (in rats) the MRHD. These studies uncovered no evidence of carcinogenic potential of hydrochlorothiazide in rats or female mice, but there was equivocal evidence of hepatocarcinogenicity in male mice.

Body System/ Adverse Experience	% of Patients with Adverse Experiences* All Adverse Experiences Placebo† (n=144) %	B2.5–40/H6.25† (n=252) %	Drug Related Adverse Experiences Placebo† (n=144) %	B2.5–10/H6.25† (n=221) %
Cardiovascular				
bradycardia	0.7	1.1	0.7	0.9
arrhythmia	1.4	0.4	0.0	0.0
peripheral ischemia	0.9	0.7	0.9	0.4
chest pain	0.7	1.8	0.7	0.9
Respiratory				
bronchospasm	0.0	0.0	0.0	0.0
cough	1.0	2.2	0.7	1.5
rhinitis	2.0	0.7	0.7	0.9
URI	2.3	2.1	0.0	0.0
Body as a Whole				
asthenia	0.0	0.0	0.0	0.0
fatigue	2.7	4.6	1.7	3.0
peripheral edema	0.7	1.1	0.7	0.9
Central Nervous System				
dizziness	1.8	5.1	1.8	3.2
headache	4.7	4.5	2.7	0.4
Musculoskeletal				
muscle cramps	0.7	1.2	0.7	1.1
myalgia	1.4	2.4	0.0	0.0
Psychiatric				
insomnia	2.4	1.1	2.0	1.2
somnolence	0.7	1.1	0.7	0.9
loss of libido	1.2	0.4	1.2	0.4
impotence	0.7	1.1	0.7	1.1
Gastrointestinal				
diarrhea	1.4	4.3	1.2	1.1
nausea	0.9	1.1	0.9	0.9
dyspepsia	0.7	1.2	0.7	0.9

* Averages adjusted to combine across studies.
† Combined across studies.

Mutagenesis

ZIAC: The mutagenic potential of the bisoprolol fumarate/hydrochlorothiazide combination was evaluated in the microbial mutagenicity (Ames) test, the point mutation and chromosomal aberration assays in Chinese hamster V79 cells, and the micronucleus test in mice. There was no evidence of mutagenic potential in these *in vitro* and *in vivo* assays.

Bisoprolol Fumarate: The mutagenic potential of bisoprolol fumarate was evaluated in the microbial mutagenicity (Ames) test, the point mutation and chromosome aberration assays in Chinese hamster V79 cells, the unscheduled DNA synthesis test, the micronucleus test in mice, and the cytogenetics assay in rats. There was no evidence of mutagenic potential in these *in vitro* and *in vivo* assays.

Hydrochlorothiazide: Hydrochlorothiazide was not genotoxic in *in vitro* assays using strains TA 98, TA 100, TA 1535, TA 1537 and TA 1538 of *Salmonella typhimurium* (the Ames test); in the Chinese Hamster Ovary (CHO) test for chromosomal aberrations; or in *in vivo* assays using mouse germinal cell chromosomes, Chinese hamster bone marrow chromosomes, and the *Drosophila* sex-linked recessive lethal trait gene. Positive test results were obtained in the *in vitro* CHO Sister Chromatid Exchange (clastogenicity) test and in the mouse Lymphoma Cell (mutagenicity) assays, using concentrations of hydrochlorothiazide of 43–1300 µg/mL. Positive test results were also obtained in the *Aspergillus nidulans* nondisjunction assay, using an unspecified concentration of hydrochlorothiazide.

Impairment of Fertility

ZIAC: Reproduction studies in rats did not show any impairment of fertility with the bisoprolol fumarate/hydrochlorothiazide combination doses containing up to 30 mg/kg/day of bisoprolol fumarate in combination with 75 mg/kg/day of hydrochlorothiazide. On a body-weight basis, these doses are 75 and 300 times, respectively, the MRHD of bisoprolol fumarate and hydrochlorothiazide. On a body-surface-area basis, these study doses are 15 and 62 times, respectively, the MRHD.

Bisoprolol Fumarate: Reproduction studies in rats did not show any impairment of fertility at doses up to 150 mg/kg/day of bisoprolol fumarate, or 375 and 77 times the MRHD on the basis of body-weight and body-surface-area, respectively.

Hydrochlorothiazide: Hydrochlorothiazide had no adverse effects on the fertility of mice and rats of either sex in studies wherein these species were exposed, via their diet, to doses of up to 100 and 4 mg/kg/day, respectively, prior to mating and throughout gestation. Corresponding multiples of maximum recommended human doses are 400 (mice) and 16 (rats) on the basis of body-weight and 38 (mice) and 3.3 (rats) on the basis of body-surface-area.

Pregnancy: Teratogenic Effects-Pregnancy Category C

ZIAC: In rats, the bisoprolol fumarate/hydrochlorothiazide (B/H) combination was not teratogenic at doses up to 51.4 mg/kg/day of bisoprolol fumarate in combination with 128.6 mg/kg/day of hydrochlorothiazide. Bisoprolol fumarate and hydrochlorothiazide doses used in the rat study are, as multiples of the MRHD in the combination, 129 and 514 times greater, respectively, on a body-weight basis, and 26 and 106 times greater, respectively, on the basis of body-surface-area. The drug combination was maternotoxic (decreased body weight and food consumption) at B5.7/H14.3 (mg/kg/day) and higher, and fetotoxic (increased late resorptions) at B17.1/H42.9 (mg/kg/day) and higher. Maternotoxicity was present at 14/57 times the MRHD of B/H, respectively, on a body-weight basis, and 3/12 times the MRHD of B/H doses, respectively, on the basis of body-surface-area. Fetotoxicity was present at 43/172 times the MRHD of B/H, respectively, on a body-weight basis, and 9/35 times the MRHD of B/H doses, respectively, on the basis of body-surface-area. In rabbits, the B/H combination was not teratogenic at doses of B10/H25 (mg/kg/day). Bisoprolol fumarate and hydrochlorothiazide used in the rabbit study were not teratogenic at 25/100 times the B/H MRHD, respectively, on a body-weight basis, and 10/40 times the B/H MRHD, respectively, on the basis of body-surface-area. The drug combination was maternotoxic (decreased body weight) at B1/H2.5 (mg/kg/day) and higher, and fetotoxic (increased resorptions) at B10/H25 (mg/kg/day). The multiples of the MRHD for the B/H combination that were maternotoxic are, respectively, 2.5/10 (on the basis of body-weight) and 1/4 (on the basis of body-surface-area), and for fetotoxicity were, respectively, 25/100 (on the basis of body-weight) and 10/40 (on the basis of body-surface-area).

There are no adequate and well-controlled studies with ZIAC in pregnant women. ZIAC should be used during pregnancy only if the potential benefit justifies the risk to the fetus.

Bisoprolol Fumarate: In rats, bisoprolol fumarate was not teratogenic at doses up to 150 mg/kg/day, which were 375 and 77 times the MRHD on the basis of body-weight and body-surface-area, respectively. Bisoprolol fumarate was fetotoxic (increased late resorptions) at 50 mg/kg/day and maternotoxic (decreased food intake and body-weight gain) at 150 mg/kg/day. The fetotoxicity in rats occurred at 125 times the MRHD on a body-weight basis and 26 times the MRHD on the basis of body-surface-area. The maternotoxicity occurred at 375 times the MRHD on a body-weight basis and 77 times the MRHD on the basis of body-surface-area. In rabbits, bisoprolol fumarate was not teratogenic at doses up to 12.5 mg/kg/day, which is 31 and 12 times the MRHD based on body-weight and body-surface-area, respectively, but was embryolethal (increased early resorptions) at 12.5 mg/kg/day.

Hydrochlorothiazide: Hydrochlorothiazide was orally administered to pregnant mice and rats during respective periods of major organogenesis at doses up to 3000 and 1000 mg/kg/day, respectively. At these doses, which are multiples of the MRHD equal to 12,000 for mice and 4000 for rats, based on body-weight, and equal to 1129 for mice and 824 for rats, based on body-surface-area, there was no evidence of harm to the fetus. There are, however, no adequate and well-controlled studies in pregnant women. Because animal reproduction studies are not always predictive of human response, this drug should be used during pregnancy only if clearly needed.

Nonteratogenic Effects: Thiazides cross the placental barrier and appear in the cord blood. The use of thiazides in pregnant women requires that the anticipated benefit be weighed against possible hazards to the fetus. These hazards include fetal or neonatal jaundice, pancreatitis, thrombocytopenia, and possibly other adverse reactions which have occurred in the adult.

Nursing Mothers: Bisoprolol fumarate alone or in combination with HCTZ has not been studied in nursing mothers. Thiazides are excreted in human breast milk. Small amounts of bisoprolol fumarate (<2% of the dose) have been detected in the milk of lactating rats. Because of the potential for serious adverse reactions in nursing infants, a decision should be made whether to discontinue nursing or to discontinue the drug, taking into account the importance of the drug to the mother.

Use in Elderly Patients: In clinical trials, at least 270 patients treated with bisoprolol fumarate plus HCTZ were 60 years of age or older. HCTZ added significantly to the antihypertensive effect of bisoprolol in elderly hypertensive patients. No overall differences in effectiveness or safety were observed between these patients and younger patients. Other reported clinical experience has not identified differences in responses between the elderly and younger patients, but greater sensitivity of some older individuals cannot be ruled out.

Pediatric Use: Safety and effectiveness of ZIAC in children have not been established.

ADVERSE REACTIONS

ZIAC:

Bisoprolol fumarate/H6.25 mg is well tolerated in most patients. Most adverse effects (AEs) have been mild and transient. In more than 65,000 patients treated worldwide with bisoprolol fumarate, occurrences of bronchospasm have been rare. Discontinuation rates for AEs were similar for B/H6.25 mg and placebo-treated patients.

In the United States, 252 patients received bisoprolol fumarate (2.5, 5, 10, or 40 mg)/H6.25 mg and 144 patients received placebo in two controlled trials. In Study 1, bisoprolol fumarate 5/H6.25 mg was administered for 4 weeks. In Study 2, bisoprolol fumarate 2.5, 10 or 40/H6.25 mg was administered for 12 weeks. All adverse experiences, whether drug related or not, and drug related adverse experiences in patients treated with B2.5–10/H6.25 mg, reported during comparable, 4 week treatment periods by at least 2% of bisoprolol fumarate/H6.25 mg-treated patients (plus additional selected adverse experiences) are presented in the following table:

[See table at top of previous page]

Other adverse experiences that have been reported with the individual components are listed below.

Bisoprolol Fumarate:

In clinical trials worldwide, a variety of other AEs, in addition to those listed above, have been reported. While in many cases it is not known whether a causal relationship exists between bisoprolol and these AEs, they are listed to alert the physician to a possible relationship.

Central Nervous System: Unsteadiness, vertigo, syncope, paresthesia, hyperesthesia, sleep disturbance/vivid dreams, depression, anxiety/restlessness, decreased concentration/memory.

Cardiovascular: Palpitations and other rhythm disturbances, cold extremities, claudication, hypotension, orthostatic hypotension, chest pain, congestive heart failure.

Gastrointestinal: Gastric/epigastric/abdominal pain, peptic ulcer, gastritis, vomiting, constipation, dry mouth.

Musculoskeletal: Arthralgia, muscle/joint pain, back/neck pain, twitching/tremor.

Skin: Rash, acne, eczema, psoriasis, skin irritation, pruritus, purpura, flushing, sweating, alopecia, dermatitis, exfoliative dermatitis (very rarely), cutaneous vasculitis.

Special Senses: Visual disturbances, ocular pain/pressure, abnormal lacrimation, tinnitus, decreased hearing, earache, taste abnormalities.

Metabolic: Gout.

Respiratory: Asthma, bronchitis, dyspnea, pharyngitis, sinusitis.

Genito-urinary: Peyronie's disease (very rarely), cystitis, renal colic, polyuria.

General: Malaise, edema, weight gain, angioedema.

In addition, a variety of adverse effects have been reported with other beta-adrenergic blocking agents and should be considered potential adverse effects:

Central Nervous System: Reversible mental depression progressing to catatonia, hallucinations, an acute reversible syndrome characterized by disorientation to time and place, emotional lability, slightly clouded sensorium.

Allergic: Fever, combined with aching and sore throat, laryngospasm, and respiratory distress.

Hematologic: Agranulocytosis, thrombocytopenia.

Gastrointestinal: Mesenteric arterial thrombosis and ischemic colitis.

Miscellaneous: The oculomucocutaneous syndrome associated with the beta-blocker practolol has not been reported with bisoprolol fumarate during investigational use or extensive foreign marketing experience.

Hydrochlorothiazide

The following adverse experiences, in addition to those listed in the above table, have been reported with hydrochlorothiazide (generally with doses of 25 mg or greater).

General: Weakness.

Central Nervous System: Vertigo, paresthesia, restlessness.

Cardiovascular: Orthostatic hypotension (may be potentiated by alcohol, barbiturates, or narcotics).

Gastrointestinal: Anorexia, gastric irritation, cramping, constipation, jaundice (intrahepatic cholestatic jaundice), pancreatitis, cholecystitis, sialadenitis, dry mouth.

Musculoskeletal: Muscle spasm.

Serum Potassium Data from U.S. Placebo Controlled Studies

	Placebo† (n = 130*)	B2.5/H6.25 mg (n = 28*)	B5/H6.25 mg (n = 149*)	B10/H6.25 mg (n = 28*)	HCTZ25 mg† (n = 142*)
Potassium					
Mean Change[a] (mEq/L)	+0.04	+0.11	–0.08	0.00	–0.30
% Hypokalemia[b]	0.0%	0.0%	0.7%	0.0%	5.5%

* Patients with normal serum potassium at baseline.
[a] Mean change from baseline at Week 4.
[b] Percentage of patients with abnormality at Week 4.
† Combined across studies.

Hypersensitive Reactions: Purpura, photosensitivity, rash, urticaria, necrotizing angiitis (vasculitis and cutaneous vasculitis), fever, respiratory distress including pneumonitis and pulmonary edema, anaphylactic reactions.

Special Senses: Transient blurred vision, xanthopsia.

Metabolic: Gout.

Genito-urinary: Sexual dysfunction, renal failure, renal dysfunction, interstitial nephritis.

LABORATORY ABNORMALITIES:

ZIAC:

Because of the low dose of hydrochlorothiazide in ZIAC, adverse metabolic effects with B/H6.25 mg are less frequent and of smaller magnitude than with HCTZ 25 mg. Laboratory data on serum potassium from the U.S. placebo-controlled trials are shown in the following table:

[See table above]

Treatment with both beta blockers and thiazide diuretics is associated with increases in uric acid. However, the magnitude of the change in patients treated with B/H6.25 mg was smaller than in patients treated with HCTZ 25 mg. Mean increases in serum triglycerides were observed in patients treated with bisoprolol fumarate and hydrochlorothiazide 6.25 mg. Total cholesterol was generally unaffected, but small decreases in HDL cholesterol were noted.

Other laboratory abnormalities that have been reported with the individual components are listed below.

Bisoprolol Fumarate: In clinical trials, the most frequently reported laboratory change was an increase in serum triglycerides, but this was not a consistent finding.

Sporadic liver test abnormalities have been reported. In the U.S. controlled trials experience with bisoprolol fumarate treatment for 4–12 weeks, the incidence of concomitant elevations in SGOT and SGPT of between 1–2 times normal was 3.9%, compared to 2.5% for placebo. No patient had concomitant elevations greater than twice normal.

In the long-term, uncontrolled experience with bisoprolol fumarate treatment for 6–18 months, the incidence of one or more concomitant elevations in SGOT and SGPT of between 1–2 times normal was 6.2%. The incidence of multiple occurrence was 1.9%. For concomitant elevations in SGOT and SGPT of greater than twice normal, the incidence was 1.5%. The incidence of multiple occurrences was 0.3%. In many cases these elevations were attributed to underlying disorders, or resolved during continued treatment with bisoprolol fumarate.

Other laboratory changes included small increases in uric acid, creatinine, BUN, serum potassium, glucose, and phosphorus and decreases in WBC and platelets. There have been occasional reports of eosinophilia. These were generally not of clinical importance and rarely resulted in discontinuation of bisoprolol fumarate.

As with other beta-blockers, ANA conversions have also been reported on bisoprolol fumarate. About 15% of patients in long-term studies converted to a positive titer, although about one-third of these patients subsequently reconverted to a negative titer while on continued therapy.

Hydrochlorothiazide: Hyperglycemia, glycosuria, hyperuricemia, hypokalemia and other electrolyte imbalances (see **PRECAUTIONS**), hyperlipidemia, hypercalcemia, leukopenia, agranulocytosis, thrombocytopenia, aplastic anemia, and hemolytic anemia have been associated with HCTZ therapy.

OVERDOSAGE

There are limited data on overdose with ZIAC. However, several cases of overdose with bisoprolol fumarate have been reported (maximum: 2000 mg). Bradycardia and/or hypotension were noted. Sympathomimetic agents were given in some cases, and all patients recovered.

The most frequently observed signs expected with overdosage of a beta-blocker are bradycardia and hypotension. Lethargy is also common, and with severe overdoses, delirium, coma, convulsions, and respiratory arrest have been reported to occur. Congestive heart failure, bronchospasm, and hypoglycemia may occur, particularly in patients with underlying conditions. With thiazide diuretics, acute intoxication is rare. The most prominent feature of overdose is acute loss of fluid and electrolytes. Signs and symptoms include cardiovascular (tachycardia, hypotension, shock), neuromuscular (weakness, confusion, dizziness, cramps of the calf muscles, paresthesia, fatigue, impairment of consciousness), gastrointestinal (nausea, vomiting, thirst), renal (polyuria, oliguria, or anuria [due to hemoconcentration]), and laboratory findings (hypokalemia, hyponatremia, hypochloremia, alkalosis, increased BUN [especially in patients with renal insufficiency]).

If overdosage of ZIAC is suspected, therapy with ZIAC should be discontinued and the patient observed closely. Treatment is symptomatic and supportive; there is no specific antidote. Limited data suggest bisoprolol fumarate is not dialyzable; similarly, there is no indication that hydrochlorothiazide is dialyzable. Suggested general measures include induction of emesis and/or gastric lavage, administration of activated charcoal, respiratory support, correction of fluid and electrolyte imbalance, and treatment of convulsions. Based on the expected pharmacologic actions and recommendations for other beta-blockers and hydrochlorothiazide, the following measures should be considered when clinically warranted:

Bradycardia: Administer IV atropine. If the response is inadequate, isoproterenol or another agent with positive chronotropic properties may be given cautiously. Under some circumstances, transvenous pacemaker insertion may be necessary.

Hypotension, Shock: The patient's legs should be elevated. IV fluids should be administered and lost electrolytes (potassium, sodium) replaced. Intravenous glucagon may be useful. Vasopressors should be considered.

Heart Block (second or third degree): Patients should be carefully monitored and treated with isoproterenol infusion or transvenous cardiac pacemaker insertion, as appropriate.

Congestive Heart Failure: Initiate conventional therapy (ie, digitalis, diuretics, vasodilating agents, inotropic agents).

Bronchospasm: Administer a bronchodilator such as isoproterenol and/or aminophylline.

Hypoglycemia: Administer IV glucose.

Surveillance: Fluid and electrolyte balance (especially serum potassium) and renal function should be monitored until normalized.

DOSAGE AND ADMINISTRATION

Bisoprolol is an effective treatment of hypertension in once-daily doses of 2.5 to 40 mg, while hydrochlorothiazide is effective in doses of 12.5 to 50 mg. In clinical trials of bisoprolol/hydrochlorothiazide combination therapy using bisoprolol doses of 2.5 to 20 mg and hydrochlorothiazide doses of 6.25 to 25 mg, the antihypertensive effects increased with increasing doses of either component.

The adverse effects (see **WARNINGS**) of bisoprolol are a mixture of dose dependent phenomena (primarily bradycardia, diarrhea, asthenia and fatigue) and dose-independent phenomena (eg, occasional rash); those of hydrochlorothiazide are a mixture of dose dependent phenomena (primarily hypokalemia) and dose-independent phenomena (eg, possibly pancreatitis); the dose-dependent phenomena for each being much more common than the dose-independent phenomena. The latter consist of those few that are truly idiosyncratic in nature or those that occur with such low frequency that a dose relationship may be difficult to discern. Therapy with a combination of bisoprolol and hydrochlorothiazide will be associated with both sets of dose-independent adverse effects, and to minimize these, it may be appropriate to begin combination therapy only after a patient has failed to achieve the desired effect with monotherapy. On the other hand, regimens that combine low doses of bisoprolol and hydrochlorothiazide should produce minimal dose dependent adverse effects, eg, bradycardia, diarrhea, asthenia and fatigue, and minimal dose-dependent adverse metabolic effects, ie, decreases in serum potassium (see **CLINICAL PHARMACOLOGY**).

Therapy Guided by Clinical Effect: A patient whose blood pressure is not adequately controlled with 2.5–20 mg bisoprolol daily may instead be given ZIAC. Patients whose blood pressures are adequately controlled with 50 mg of hydrochlorothiazide daily, but who experience significant potassium loss with this regimen, may achieve similar blood pressure control without electrolyte disturbance if they are switched to ZIAC.

Initial Therapy: Antihypertensive therapy may be initiated with the lowest dose of ZIAC, one 2.5/6.25 mg tablet once daily. Subsequent titration (14 day intervals) may be carried out with ZIAC tablets up to the maximum recommended dose 20/12.5 mg (two 10/6.25 mg tablets) once daily, as appropriate.

Replacement Therapy: The combination may be substituted for the titrated individual components.

Cessation of Therapy: If withdrawal of ZIAC therapy is planned, it should be achieved gradually over a period of about 2 weeks. Patients should be carefully observed.

Patients with Renal or Hepatic Impairment: As noted in the **WARNINGS** section, caution must be used in dosing/titrating patients with hepatic impairment or renal dysfunction. Since there is no indication that hydrochlorothiazide is dialyzable, and limited data suggest that bisoprolol is not dialyzable, drug replacement is not necessary in patients undergoing dialysis.

Continued on next page

Ziac—Cont.

Elderly Patients: Dosage adjustment on the basis of age is not usually necessary, unless there is also significant renal or hepatic dysfunction (see above and **WARNINGS** section).
Children: There is no pediatric experience with ZIAC.

HOW SUPPLIED

ZIAC®-2.5 mg/6.25 mg Tablets (bisoprolol fumarate 2.5 mg and hydrochlorothiazide 6.25 mg) are yellow, round, convex, film coated tablets, engraved with a script "LL" within an engraved heart shape on one side and "B" above "12" on the other; approximately 1/4" in diameter, supplied as follows:
NDC 0005-3238-38—Bottle of 30 with child resistant closure
NDC 0005-3238-23—Bottle of 100
ZIAC®-5 mg/6.25 mg Tablets (bisoprolol fumarate 5 mg and hydrochlorothiazide 6.25 mg) are pink, round, convex, film coated tablets, engraved with a script "LL" within an engraved heart shape on one side and "B" above "13" on the other; approximately 9/32" in diameter, supplied as follows:
NDC 0005-3234-38—Bottle of 30 with child resistant closure
NDC 0005-3234-23—Bottle of 100
ZIAC®-10 mg/6.25 mg Tablets (bisoprolol fumarate 10 mg and hydrochlorothiazide 6.25 mg) are white, round, convex, film coated tablets, engraved with a script "LL" within an engraved heart shape on one side and "B" above "14" on the other; approximately 9/32" in diameter, supplied as follows:
NDC 0005-3235-38—Bottle of 30 with child resistant closure

Store at controlled room temperature 20°–25°C (68°–77°F). Dispense in tight containers as defined in the USP.

Manufactured by:
LEDERLE PHARMACEUTICAL DIVISION
American Cyanamid Company
Pearl River, NY 10965
Under License of Merck KGaA
Darmstadt, Germany
CI 6017-1 Issued April 6, 1999

Shown in Product Identification Guide, page 320

ZOSYN® ℞

[*zō 'sĭn*]
(Sterile Piperacillin Sodium and Tazobactam Sodium)

DESCRIPTION

Zosyn in an injectable antibacterial combination product consisting of the semisynthetic antibiotic piperacillin sodium and the β-lactamase inhibitor tazobactam sodium for intravenous administration.
Piperacillin sodium is derived from D(-)-α-aminobenzylpenicillin. The chemical name of piperacillin sodium is sodium (2*S*,5*R*,6*R*) -6- [(*R*) -2- (4-ethyl-2,3-dioxo-1-piperazine-carboxamido)-2-phenylacetamido]-3,3-dimethyl-7-oxo-4-thia-1-azabicyclo[3.2.0]heptane-2-carboxylate. The chemical formula is $C_{23}H_{26}N_5NaO_7S$ and the molecular weight is 539.6. Tazobactam sodium, a derivative of the penicillin nucleus, is a penicillanic acid sulfone. Its chemical name is sodium (2*S*,3*S*,5*R*)-3-methyl-7-oxo-3-(1*H*-1,2,3-triazol-1-ylmethyl)-4-thia-1-azabicyclo[3.2.0]heptane-2-carboxylate-4,4-dioxide. The chemical formula is $C_{10}H_{11}N_4NaO_5S$ and the molecular weight is 322.3.
Zosyn, piperacillin/tazobactam parenteral combination, is a white to off-white sterile, cryodesiccated powder consisting of piperacillin and tazobactam as their sodium salts packaged in glass vials. The product does not contain excipients or preservatives.
Each Zosyn 2.25 g single dose vial or ADD-Vantage® vial contains an amount of drug sufficient for withdrawal of piperacillin sodium equivalent to 2 grams of piperacillin and tazobactam sodium equivalent to 0.25 g of tazobactam.
Each Zosyn 3.375 g single dose vial or ADD-Vantage® vial contains an amount of drug sufficient for withdrawal of piperacillin sodium equivalent to 3 grams of piperacillin and tazobactam sodium equivalent to 0.375 g of tazobactam.
Each Zosyn 4.5 g single dose vial or ADD-Vantage® vial contains an amount of drug sufficient for withdrawal of piperacillin sodium equivalent to 4 grams of piperacillin and tazobactam sodium equivalent to 0.5 g of tazobactam.
Zosyn is a monosodium salt of piperacillin and a monosodium salt of tazobactam containing a total of 2.35 mEq (54 mg) of Na+ per gram of piperacillin in the combination product.

CLINICAL PHARMACOLOGY

Peak plasma concentrations of piperacillin and tazobactam are attained immediately after completion of an intravenous infusion of Zosyn. Piperacillin plasma concentrations, following a 30-minute infusion of Zosyn, were similar to those attained when equivalent doses of piperacillin were administered alone, with mean peak plasma concentrations of approximately 134, 242 and 298 µg/mL for the 2.25 g, 3.375 g and 4.5 g Zosyn (piperacillin/tazobactam) doses, respectively. The corresponding mean peak plasma concentrations of tazobactam were 15, 24, and 34 µg/mL, respectively.
Following a 30-minute I.V. infusion of 3.375 g Zosyn every 6 hours, steady-state plasma concentrations of piperacillin and tazobactam were similar to those attained after the first dose. In like manner, steady-state plasma concentrations were not different from those attained after the first dose when 2.25 g or 4.5 g doses of Zosyn were administered via 30-minute infusions every 6 hours. Steady-state plasma concentrations after 30-minute infusions every 6 hours are provided in Table 1.
Following single or multiple Zosyn doses to healthy subjects, the plasma half-life of piperacillin and of tazobactam ranged from 0.7 to 1.2 hours and was unaffected by dose or duration of infusion.
Piperacillin is metabolized to a minor microbiologically active desethyl metabolite. Tazobactam is metabolized to a single metabolite that lacks pharmacological and antibacterial activities. Both piperacillin and tazobactam are eliminated via the kidney by glomerular filtration and tubular secretion. Piperacillin is excreted rapidly as unchanged drug with 68% of the administered dose excreted in the urine. Tazobactam and its metabolite are eliminated primarily by renal excretion with 80% of the administered dose excreted as unchanged drug and the remainder as the single metabolite. Piperacillin, tazobactam, and desethyl piperacillin are also secreted into the bile.
Both piperacillin and tazobactam are approximately 30% bound to plasma proteins. The protein binding of either piperacillin or tazobactam is unaffected by the presence of the other compound. Protein binding of the tazobactam metabolite is negligible.
Piperacillin and tazobactam are widely distributed into tissues and body fluids including intestinal mucosa, gallbladder, lung, female reproductive tissues (uterus, ovary, and fallopian tube), interstitial fluid, and bile. Mean tissue concentrations are generally 50 to 100% of those in plasma. Distribution of piperacillin and tazobactam into cerebrospinal fluid is low in subjects with non-inflamed meninges, as with other penicillins.

TABLE 1
STEADY STATE MEAN PLASMA CONCENTRATIONS IN ADULTS AFTER 30-MINUTE INTRAVENOUS INFUSION OF PIPERACILLIN/TAZOBACTAM EVERY 6 HOURS

PIPERACILLIN

		Plasma Concentrations** (µg/mL)						AUC[a] (µg·hr/mL)
Piperacillin/ Tazobactam Dose[a]	No. of Evaluable Subjects	30 min	1 hr	2 hr	3 hr	4 hr	6 hr	AUC_{0-6}
2.25 g	8	134 (14)	57 (14)	17.1 (23)	5.2 (32)	2.5 (35)	0.9 (14)[b]	131 (14)
3.375 g	6	242 (12)	106 (8)	34.6 (20)	11.5 (19)	5.1 (22)	1.0 (10)	242 (10)
4.5 g	8	298 (14)	141 (19)	46.6 (28)	16.4 (29)	6.9 (29)	1.4 (30)	322 (16)

TAZOBACTAM

		Plasma Concentrations** (µg/mL)						AUC** (µg·hr/mL)
Piperacillin/ Tazobactam Dose[a]	No. of Evaluable Subjects	30 min	1 hr	2 hr	3 hr	4 hr	6 hr	AUC_{0-6}
2.25 g	8	14.8 (14)	7.2 (22)	2.6 (30)	1.1 (35)	0.7 (6)[c]	<0.5	16.0 (21)
3.375 g	6	24.2 (14)	10.7 (7)	4.0 (18)	1.4 (21)	0.7 (16)[b]	<0.5	25.0 (8)
4.5 g	8	33.8 (15)	17.3 (16)	6.8 (24)	2.8 (25)	1.3 (30)	<0.5	39.8 (15)

** Numbers in parentheses are coefficients of variation (CV%).
a: Piperacillin and tazobactam were given in combination.
b: N = 4
c: N = 3

After the administration of single doses of piperacillin/tazobactam to subjects with renal impairment, the half-life of piperacillin and of tazobactam increases with decreasing creatinine clearance. At creatinine clearance below 20 mL/min, the increase in half-life is twofold for piperacillin and fourfold for tazobactam compared to subjects with normal renal function. Dosage adjustments for Zosyn are recommended when creatinine clearance is below 40 mL/min in patients receiving the usual recommended daily dose of Zosyn. (See **DOSAGE AND ADMINISTRATION** section for specific recommendations for the treatment of patients with renal insufficiency.)
Hemodialysis removes 30 to 40% of a piperacillin/tazobactam dose with an additional 5% of the tazobactam dose removed as the tazobactam metabolite. Peritoneal dialysis removes approximately 6% and 21% of the piperacillin and tazobactam doses, respectively, with up to 16% of the tazobactam dose removed as the tazobactam metabolite. For dosage recommendations for patients undergoing hemodialysis, see **DOSAGE AND ADMINISTRATION** section.
The half-life of piperacillin and of tazobactam increases by approximately 25% and 18%, respectively, in patients with hepatic cirrhosis compared to healthy subjects. However, this difference does not warrant dosage adjustment of Zosyn due to hepatic cirrhosis.
[See table 1 below]

Microbiology

Piperacillin sodium exerts bactericidal activity by inhibiting septum formation and cell wall synthesis. *In vitro*, piperacillin is active against a variety of gram-positive and gram-negative aerobic and anaerobic bacteria. Tazobactam sodium has very little intrinsic microbiologic activity due to its very low level binding to penicillin-binding proteins; however, it is a β-lactamase inhibitor of the Richmond-Sykes class III (Bush class 2b & 2b′) penicillinases and cephalosporinases. It varies in its ability to inhibit class II and IV (2a & 4) penicillinases. Tazobactam does not induce chromosomally-mediated β-lactamases at tazobactam levels achieved with the recommended dosage regimen. Piperacillin/tazobactam has been shown to be active against most strains of the following piperacillin-resistant, β-lactamase producing microorganisms both *in vitro* and in clinical infections as described in the **INDICATIONS AND USAGE** section.

Gram-positive aerobes:
Staphylococcus aureus (NOT methicillin/oxacillin-resistant strains)
Gram-negative aerobes:
Escherichia coli
Haemophilus influenzae (NOT β-lactamase negative, ampicillin-resistant strains)
Gram-negative anaerobes:
Bacteroides fragilis group (*B. fragilis, B. ovatus, B. thetaiotaomicron*, or *B. vulgatus*)

The following *in vitro* data are available; **but their clinical significance is unknown.**
Piperacillin/tazobactam exhibits *in vitro* minimum inhibitory concentrations (MICs) of 16.0 µg/mL or less against most (≥90%) strains of *Enterobacteriaceae*, MICs of 1.0 µg/mL or less against most (≥90%) strains of *Haemophilus* species, MICs of 8.0 µg/mL or less against most (≥90%) strains of *Staphylococcus* species, and MICs of 16.0 µg/mL or less against most (≥90%) strains of *Bacteroides* species. Beta-lactamase negative strains should be tested against piperacillin alone; piperacillin break points should be used in evaluation of these results. However, the safey and efficacy of piperacillin/tazobactam in treating clinical infections due to these microorganisms have not been established in adequate and well-controlled clinical trials.

Gram-positive aerobes:
Enterococcus faecalis (piperacillin susceptible)
Staphylococcus epidermidis (NOT methicillin/oxacillin-resistant strains)
Streptococcus agalactiae†
Streptococcus pneumoniae†
Streptococcus pyogenes†
Viridans group streptococci†
Gram-negative aerobes:
Klebsiella oxytoca
Klebsiella pneumoniae
Moraxella catarrhalis
Morganella morganii
Neisseria gonorrhoeae
Neisseria meningitidis†
Proteus mirabilis
Proteus vulgaris
Pseudomonas aeruginosa (piperacillin susceptible)
Serratia marcescens
Gram-positive anaerobes:
Clostridium perfringens
Gram-negative anaerobes:
Bacteroides distasonis
Fusobacterium nucleatum
Prevotella melaninogenica (formerly *Bacteroides melaninogenicus)*

†These are not β-lactamase producing strains and, therefore, are susceptible to piperacillin alone.

Susceptibility Tests

Dilution Techniques
Quantitative methods are used to determine minimum inhibitory concentrations (MICs). These MICs provide estimates of the susceptibility of bacteria to antimicrobial compounds. The MICs should be determined using a standard-

ized procedure. Standardized procedures are based on a dilution method (broth or agar) or equivalent with standardized inoculum concentrations and standardized concentrations of piperacillin and tazobactam powders.[1] MIC values should be determined using serial dilutions of piperacillin combined with a fixed concentration of 4 μg/mL tazobactam. The MIC values obtained should be interpreted according to the following criteria:

For *Enterobacteriaceae:*

MIC (μg/mL)	Interpretation
≤16	Susceptible (S)
32–64	Intermediate (I)
≥128	Resistant (R)

For *Haemophilus* species:

MIC (μg/mL)	Interpretation
≤1	Susceptible (S)
≥2	Resistant (R)

For *Staphylococcus* species:

MIC (μg/mL)	Interpretation
≤8	Susceptible (S)
≥16	Resistant (R)

A report of "Susceptible" indicates that the pathogen is likely to be inhibited if the antimicrobial compound in the blood reaches the concentrations usually achievable. A report of "Intermediate" indicates that the result should be considered equivocal, and, if the microorganism is not fully susceptible to alternative, clinically feasible drugs, the test should be repeated. This category implies possible clinical applicability in body sites where the drug is physiologically concentrated or in situations where high dosage of drug can be used. This category also provides a buffer zone which prevents small uncontrolled technical factors from causing major discrepancies in interpretation. A report of "Resistant" indicates that the pathogen is not likely to be inhibited if the antimicrobial compound in the blood reaches the concentrations usually achievable; other therapy should be selected.

Standardized susceptibility test procedures require the use of laboratory control microorganisms to control the technical aspects of the laboratory procedures.

Laboratory control microorganisms are specific strains of microbiological assay organisms with intrinsic biological properties relating to resistance mechanisms and their genetic expression within bacteria; the specific strains are not clinically significant in their current microbiological status. Standard piperacillin and tazobactam powders should provide the following MIC values when tested against the designated quality control strains:

Microorganism	MIC (μg/mL)
Escherichia coli ATCC 25922	1–4
Escherichia coli ATCC 35218	0.5–2
Haemophilus influenzae ATCC 49247	0.06–0.5
Staphylococcus aureus ATCC 29213	0.25–2

Anaerobic Techniques

For anaerobic bacteria, the susceptibility to piperacillin/tazobactam can be determined by the reference agar dilution method or by alternate standardized test methods.[2]

For *Bacteroides* species, the dilution values should be interpreted as follows:

MIC (μg/mL)	Interpretation
≤16	Susceptible (S)
≥32	Resistant (R)

Serial dilutions of piperacillin combined with a fixed concentration of 4 μg/mL tazobactam should provide the following MIC values:

Microorganism	MIC (μg/mL)
Bacteroides fragilis ATCC 25285	0.12–0.5
Bacteroides thetaiotaomicron ATCC 29741	4–16

Diffusion Techniques

Quantitative methods that require measurement of zone diameters also provide reproducible estimates of the susceptibility of bacteria to antimicrobial compounds. One such standardized procedure requires the use of standardized inoculum concentrations.[3] This procedure uses paper disks impregnated with 100 μg of piperacillin and 10 μg of tazobactam to test the susceptibility of microorganisms to piperacillin/tazobactam. Interpretation is identical to that stated above for results using dilution techniques.

Reports from the laboratory providing results of the standard single-disk-susceptibility test with a 100/10-μg piperacillin/tazobactam disk should be interpreted according to the following criteria:

For *Enterobacteriaceae:*

Zone Diameter (mm)	Interpretation
≥21	Susceptible (S)
18–20	Intermediate (I)
≤17	Resistant (R)

For *Staphylococcus* species:

Zone Diameter (mm)	Interpretation
≥20	Susceptible (S)
≤19	Resistant (R)

As with standardized dilution techniques, diffusion methods require the use of laboratory control microorganisms to control the technical aspects of the laboratory procedures. Laboratory control microorganisms are specific strains of microbiological assay organisms with intrinsic biological properties relating to resistance mechanisms and their genetic expression within bacteria; the specific strains are not clinically significant in their current microbiological status. For the diffusion technique, the 100/10-μg piperacillin/tazobactam disk should provide the following zone diameters in these laboratory test quality control strains:

Microorganism	Zone Diameter (mm)
Escherichia coli ATCC 25922	24–30
Escherichia coli ATCC 35218	24–30
Staphylococcus aureus ATCC 25923	27–36

INDICATIONS AND USAGE

Zosyn is indicated for the treatment of patients with moderate to severe infections caused by piperacillin-resistant, piperacillin/tazobactam-susceptible, β-lactamase producing strains of the designated microorganisms in the specified conditions listed below:

Appendicitis (complicated by rupture or abscess) and peritonitis caused by piperacillin-resistant, β-lactamase producing strains of *Escherichia coli* or the following members of the *Bacteroides fragilis* group: *B. fragilis*, *B. ovatus*, *B. thetaiotamicron*, or *B. vulgatus*. The individual members of this group were studied in less than 10 cases.

Uncomplicated and complicated skin and skin structure infections, including cellulitis, cutaneous abscesses and ischemic/diabetic foot infections caused by piperacillin-resistant, β-lactamase producing strains of *Staphylococcus aureus.*

Postpartum endometritis or pelvic inflammatory disease caused by piperacillin-resistant, β-lactamase producing strains of *Escherichia coli.*

Community-acquired pneumonia (moderate severity only) caused by piperacillin-resistant, β-lactamase producing strains of *Haemophilius influenzae.*

Nosocomial pneumonia (moderate to severe) caused by piperacillin-resistant, β-lactamase producing strains of *Staphylococcus aureus.* (See **DOSAGE AND ADMINISTRATION.**)

As a combination product, Zosyn is indicated only for the specified conditions listed above. Infections caused by piperacillin-susceptible organisms, for which piperacillin has been shown to be effective, are also amenable to Zosyn treatment due to its piperacillin content. The tazobactam component of this combination product does not decrease the activity of the piperacillin component against piperacillin-susceptible organisms. Therefore, the treatment of mixed infections caused by piperacillin-susceptible organisms and piperacillin-resistant, β-lactamase producing organisms susceptible to Zosyn should not require the addition of another antibiotic. (See **DOSAGE AND ADMINISTRATION.**)

Zosyn is useful as presumptive therapy in the indicated conditions prior to the identification of causative organisms because of its broad spectrum of bactericidal activity against gram-positive and gram-negative aerobic and anaerobic organisms.

Appropriate cultures should usually be performed before initiating antimicrobial treatment in order to isolate and identify the organisms causing infection and to determine their susceptibility to Zosyn. Antimicrobial therapy should be adjusted, if appropriate, once the results of culture(s) and antimicrobial testing are known.

CONTRAINDICATIONS

Zosyn is contraindicated in patients with a history of allergic reactions to any of the penicillins, cephalosporins, or β-lactamase inhibitors.

WARNINGS

SERIOUS AND OCCASIONALLY FATAL HYPERSENSITIVITY (ANAPHYLACTIC) REACTIONS HAVE BEEN REPORTED IN PATIENTS ON PENICILLIN THERAPY. THESE REACTIONS ARE MORE LIKELY TO OCCUR IN INDIVIDUALS WITH A HISTORY OF PENICILLIN HYPERSENSITIVITY OR A HISTORY OF SENSITIVITY TO MULTIPLE ALLERGENS. THERE HAVE BEEN REPORTS OF INDIVIDUALS WITH A HISTORY OF PENICILLIN HYPERSENSITIVITY WHO HAVE EXPERIENCED SEVERE REACTIONS WHEN TREATED WITH CEPHALOSPORINS. BEFORE INITIATING THERAPY WITH ZOSYN, CAREFUL INQUIRY SHOULD BE MADE CONCERNING PREVIOUS HYPERSENSITIVITY REACTIONS TO PENICILLINS, CEPHALOSPORINS, OR OTHER ALLERGENS. IF AN ALLERGIC REACTION OCCURS, ZOSYN SHOULD BE DISCONTINUED AND APPROPRIATE THERAPY INSTITUTED. **SERIOUS ANAPHYLACTIC REACTIONS REQUIRE IMMEDIATE EMERGENCY TREATMENT WITH EPINEPHRINE. OXYGEN, INTRAVENOUS STEROIDS AND AIRWAY MANAGEMENT, INCLUDING INTUBATION, SHOULD ALSO BE ADMINISTERED AS INDICATED.**

Pseudomembranous colitis has been reported with nearly all antibacterial agents, including piperacillin/tazobactam, and may range in severity from mild to life-threatening. Therefore, it is important to consider this diagnosis in patients who present with diarrhea subsequent to the administration of antibacterial agents.

Treatment with antibacterial agents alters the normal flora of the colon and may permit overgrowth of clostridia. Studies indicate that a toxin produced by *Clostridium difficile* is one primary cause of "antibiotic-associated colitis."

After the diagnosis of pseudomembranous colitis has been established, therapeutic measures should be initiated. Mild cases of pseudomembranous colitis usually respond to drug discontinuation alone. In moderate to severe cases, consideration should be given to management with fluids and electrolytes, protein supplementation, and treatment with an antibacterial drug clinically effective against *Clostridium difficile* colitis.

PRECAUTIONS

General

Bleeding manifestations have occurred in some patients receiving β-lactam antibiotics, including piperacillin. These reactions have sometimes been associated with abnormalities of coagulation tests such as clotting time, platelet aggregation, and prothrombin time, and are more likely to occur in patients with renal failure. If bleeding manifestations occur, Zosyn should be discontinued and appropriate therapy instituted.

The possibility of the emergence of resistant organisms that might cause superinfections should be kept in mind. If this occurs, appropriate measures should be taken.

As with other penicillins, patients may experience neuromuscular excitability or convulsions if higher than recommended doses are given intravenously (particularly in the presence of renal failure).

Zosyn is a monosodium salt of piperacillin and a monosodium salt of tazobactam and contains a total of 2.35 mEq (54 mg) of Na^+ per gram of piperacillin in the combination product. This should be considered when treating patients requiring restricted salt intake. Periodic electrolyte determinations should be performed in patients with low potassium reserves, and the possibility of hypokalemia should be kept in mind with patients who have potentially low potassium reserves and who are receiving cytotoxic therapy or diuretics.

As with other semisynthetic penicillins, piperacillin therapy has been associated with an increased incidence of fever and rash in cystic fibrosis patients.

Laboratory Tests

Periodic assessment of hematopoietic function should be performed, especially with prolonged therapy, i.e., ≥21 days. (See **ADVERSE REACTIONS, Adverse Laboratory Events.**)

Drug Interactions

Aminoglycosides

The mixing of Zosyn with an aminoglycoside *in vitro* can result in substantial inactivation of the aminoglycoside. (See **DOSAGE AND ADMINISTRATION—Compatible Intravenous Diluent Solutions.**)

When Zosyn was co-administered with tobramycin, the area under the curve, renal clearance and urinary recovery of tobramycin were decreased by 11%, 32% and 38%, respectively. The alterations in the pharmacokinetics of tobramycin when administered in combination with piperacillin/tazobactam may be due to *in vivo* and *in vitro* inactivation of tobramycin in the presence of piperacillin/tazobactam. The inactivation of aminoglycosides in the presence of penicillin-class drugs has been recognized. It has been postulated that penicillin-aminoglycoside complexes form; these complexes are microbiologically inactive and of unknown toxicity. In patients with severe renal dysfunction (i.e., chronic hemodialysis patients), the pharmacokinetics of tobramycin are significantly altered when tobramycin is administered in combination with piperacillin.[4] The alteration of tobramycin pharmacokinetics and the potential toxicity of the penicillin-aminoglycoside complexes in patients with mild to moderate renal dysfunction who are administered an aminoglycoside in combination with piperacillin/tazobactam are unknown.

Probenecid

Probenecid administered concomitantly with Zosyn prolongs the half-life of piperacillin by 21% and that of tazobactam by 71%.

Vancomycin

No pharmacokinetic interactions have been noted between Zosyn and vancomycin.

Heparin

Coagulation parameters should be tested more frequently and monitored regularly during simultaneous administration of high doses of heparin, oral anticoagulants, or other drugs that may affect the blood coagulation system or the thrombocyte function.

Vecuronium

Piperacillin when used concomitantly with vecuronium has been implicated in the prolongation of the neuromuscular blockade of vecuronium. Zosyn (piperacillin/tazobactam) could produce the same phenomenon if given along with vecuronium. Due to their similar mechanism of action, it is expected that the neuromuscular blockade produced by any of the non-depolarizing muscle relaxants could be prolonged in the presence of piperacillin. (See package insert for vecuronium bromide.)

Drug/Laboratory Test Interactions

As with other penicillins, the administration of Zosyn may result in a false-positive reaction for glucose in the urine using a copper-reduction method (CLINITEST®). It is rec-

Continued on next page

Zosyn—Cont.

ommended that glucose tests based on enzymatic glucose oxidase reactions (such as DIASTIX® or TES-TAPE®) be used.

Carcinogenesis, Mutagenesis, Impairment of Fertility

Long term carcinogenicity studies in animals have not been conducted with piperacillin/tazobactam, piperacillin, or tazobactam.

Piperacillin/tazobactam was negative in microbial mutagenicity assays at concentrations up to 14.84/1.86 µg/plate. Piperacillin/tazobactam was negative in the unscheduled DNA synthesis (UDS) test at concentrations up to 5689/711 µg/mL. Piperacillin/tazobactam was negative in a mammalian point mutation (Chinese hamster ovary cell HPRT) assay at concentrations up to 8000/1000 µg/mL. Piperacillin/tazobactam was negative in a mammalian cell (BALB/c-3T3) transformation assay at concentrations up to 8/1 µg/mL. *In vivo,* piperacillin/tazobactam did not induce chromosomal aberrations in rats dosed I.V. with 1500/187.5 mg/kg; this dose is similar to the maximum recommended human daily dose on a body-surface-area basis (mg/m^2).

Piperacillin was negative in microbial mutagenicity assays at concentrations up to 50 µg/plate. There was no DNA damage in bacteria (Rec assay) exposed to piperacillin at concentrations up to 200 µg/disk. Piperacillin was negative in the UDS test at concentrations up to 10,000 µg/mL.

In a mammalian point mutation (mouse lymphoma cells) assay, piperacillin was positive at concentrations ≥2500 µg/mL. Piperacillin was negative in a cell (BALB/c-3T3) transformation assay at concentrations up to 3000 µg/mL. *In vivo,* piperacillin did not induce chromosomal aberrations in mice at I.V. doses up to 2000 mg/kg/day or rats at I.V. doses up to 1500 mg/kg/day. These doses are half (mice) or similar (rats) to the maximum recommended human daily dose based on body-surface area (mg/m^2). In another *in vivo* test, there was no dominant lethal effect when piperacillin was administered to rats at I.V. doses up to 2000 mg/kg/day, which is similar to the maximum recommended human daily dose based on body-surface area (mg/m^2). When mice were administered piperacillin at I.V. doses up to 2000 mg/kg/day, which is half the maximum recommended human daily dose based on body-surface area (mg/m^2), urine from these animals was not mutagenic when tested in a microbial mutagenicity assay. Bacteria injected into the peritoneal cavity of mice administered piperacillin at I.V. doses up to 2000 mg/kg/day did not show increased mutation frequencies.

Tazobactam was negative in microbial mutagenicity assays at concentrations up to 333 µg/plate. Tazobactam was negative in the UDS test at concentrations up to 2000 µg/mL. Tazobactam was negative in a mammalian point mutation (Chinese hamster ovary cell HPRT) assay at concentrations up to 5000 µg/mL. In another mammalian point mutation (mouse lymphoma cells) assay, tazobactam was positive at concentrations ≥3000 µg/mL. Tazobactam was negative in a cell (BALB/c-3T3) transformation assay at concentrations up to 900 µg/mL. In an *in vitro* cytogenetics (Chinese hamster lung cells) assay, tazobactam was negative at concentrations up to 3000 µg/mL. *In vivo,* tazobactam did not induce chromosomal aberrations in rats at I.V. doses up to 5000 mg/kg, which is 23 times the maximum recommended human daily dose based on body-surface area (mg/m^2).

Pregnancy

Teratogenic effects—Pregnancy Category B

Piperacillin/tazobactam

Reproduction studies have been performed in rats and have revealed no evidence of impaired fertility due to piperacillin/tazobactam administered up to a dose which is similar to the maximum recommended human daily dose based on body-surface area (mg/m^2).

Teratology studies have been performed in mice and rats and have revealed no evidence of harm to the fetus due to piperacillin/tazobactam administered up to a dose which is 1 to 2 times and 2 to 3 times the human dose of piperacillin and tazobactam, respectively, based on body-surface area (mg/m^2).

Piperacillin

Reproduction and teratology studies have been performed in mice and rats and have revealed no evidence of impaired fertility or harm to the fetus due to piperacillin administered up to a dose which is half (mice) or similar (rats) to the maximum recommended human daily dose based on body-surface area (mg/m^2).

Tazobactam

Reproduction studies have been performed in rats and have revealed no evidence of impaired fertility due to tazobactam administered at doses up to 3 times the maximum recommended human daily dose based on body-surface area (mg/m^2).

Teratology studies have been performed in mice and rats and have revealed no evidence of harm to the fetus due to tazobactam administered at doses up to 6 and 14 times, respectively, the human dose based on body-surface area (mg/m^2). In rats, tazobactam crosses the placenta. Concentrations in the fetus are less than or equal to 10% of those found in maternal plasma.

There are, however, no adequate and well-controlled studies with the piperacillin/tazobactam combination or with piperacillin or tazobactam alone in pregnant women. Because animal reproduction studies are not always predictive of the human response, this drug should be used during pregnancy only if clearly needed.

Nursing Mothers

Piperacillin is excreted in low concentrations in human milk; tazobactam concentrations in human milk have not been studied. Caution should be exercised when Zosyn is administered to a nursing woman.

Pediatric Use

Safety and efficacy in pediatric patients have not been established.

Geriatric Use

Patients over 65 years are **not** at an increased risk of developing adverse effects solely because of age. However, dosage should be adjusted in the presence of renal insufficiency. (See **DOSAGE AND ADMINISTRATION**.)

ADVERSE REACTIONS

During the initial clinical investigations, 2621 patients worldwide were treated with Zosyn in phase 3 trials. In the key North American clinical trials (n=830 patients), 90% of the adverse events reported were mild to moderate in severity and transient in nature. However, in 3.2% of the patients treated worldwide, Zosyn was discontinued because of adverse events primarily involving the skin (1.3%), including rash and pruritis; the gastrointestinal system (0.9%), including diarrhea, nausea, and vomiting; and allergic reactions (0.5%).

Adverse local reactions that were reported, irrespective of relationship to therapy with Zosyn, were phlebitis (1.3%), injection site reaction (0.5%), pain (0.2%), inflammation (0.2%), thrombophlebitis (0.2%), and edema (0.1%).

In the completed study of nosocomial lower respiratory tract infections, 155 patients were treated with Zosyn in a dosing regimen of 3.375 g every 4 hours in combination with an aminoglycoside. In this trial, 88.5% of the adverse experiences reported were mild to moderate in severity and transient in nature. However, in this trial, therapy with Zosyn was discontinued in four patients (2.6%) due to adverse experiences.

Irrespective of drug relationship or degree of severity, the adverse experiences which led to the discontinuation of Zosyn in these four patients were: thrombocytopenia and pancreatitis in one patient; fever in one patient; fever and eosinophilia in another patient; and diarrhea and elevated liver enzymes in the fourth patient.

Adverse Clinical Events

Based on patients from the North American trials (n=1063), the events with the highest incidence in patients, irrespective of relationship to Zosyn therapy, were diarrhea (11.3%); headache (7.7%); constipation (7.7%); nausea (6.9%); insomnia (6.6%); rash (4.2%), including maculopapular, bullous, urticarial, and eczematoid; vomiting (3.3%); dyspepsia (3.3%); pruritis (3.1%); stool changes (2.4%); fever (2.4%); agitation (2.1%); pain (1.7%); moniliasis (1.6%); hypertension (1.6%); dizziness (1.4%); abdominal pain (1.3%); chest pain (1.3%); edema (1.2%); anxiety (1.2%); rhinitis (1.2%); and dyspnea (1.1%).

Based on patients in the completed study of nosocomial lower respiratory tract infections (n=155), using every 4 hour dosing and aminoglycoside therapy, the events with the highest incidence in patients, irrespective of relationship to Zosyn and aminoglycoside therapy were: diarrhea (20%); constipation (8.4%); agitation (7.1%); nausea (5.8%); headache (4.5%); insomnia (4.5%); oral thrush (3.9%); erythematous rash (3.9%); anxiety (3.2%); fever (3.2%); pain (3.2%); pruritis (3.2%); hiccough (2.6%); vomiting (2.6%); dyspepsia (1.9%); edema (1.9%); fluid overload (1.9%); stool changes (1.9%); anorexia (1.3%); cardiac arrest (1.3%); confusion (1.3%); diaphoresis (1.3%); duodenal ulcer (1.3%); flatulence (1.3%); hypertension (1.3%); hypotension (1.3%); inflammation at injection site (1.3%); pleural effusion (1.3%); pneumothorax (1.3%); rash, not otherwise specified (1.3%); supraventricular tachycardia (1.3%); thrombophlebitis (1.3%); and urinary incontinence (1.3%).

Additional adverse systemic clinical events reported in 1.0% or less of the patients in the initial North American trials and/or in the patients administered Zosyn 3.375 g every 4 hours plus an aminoglycoside in the study of nosocomial lower respiratory tract are listed below within each body system (bracketed events occurred only in the nosocomial pneumonia trial);

Autonomic nervous system—hypotension, ileus, syncope

Body as a whole—rigors, back pain, malaise, [asthenia, chest pain]

Cardiovascular—tachycardia, including supraventricular and ventricular; bradycardia; arrhythmia, including atrial fibrillation, ventricular fibrillation, cardiac arrest, cardiac failure, circulatory failure, myocardial infarction, [angina]

Central nervous system—tremor, convulsions, vertigo, [aggressive reaction (combative)]

Gastrointestinal—melena, flatulence, hemorrhage, gastritis, hiccough, ulcerative stomatitis, [fecal incontinence, gastric ulcer, pancreatitis]

Pseudomembranous colitis was reported in one patient during the clinical trials. The onset of pseudomembranous colitis symptoms may occur during or after antibacterial treatment. (See **WARNINGS**.)

Hearing and Vestibular System—tinnitus, [deafness, earache]

Hypersensitivity—anaphylaxis

Metabolic and Nutritional—symptomatic hypoglycemia, thirst, [gout, vitamin B_{12} deficiency anemia]

Musculoskeletal—myalgia, arthralgia

Platelet, Bleeding, Clotting—mesenteric embolism, purpura, epistaxis, pulmonary embolism, [ecchymosis, hemoptysis] (See **PRECAUTIONS, General**.)

Psychiatric—confusion, hallucination, depression

Reproductive, Female—leukorrhea, vaginitis, [perineal irritation/pain]

Reproductive, Male—[balanoposthitis]

Respiratory—pharyngitis, pulmonary edema, bronchospasm, coughing, [atelectasis, dyspnea, hypoxia]

Skin and Appendages—genital pruritus, diaphoresis, [conjunctivitis, xerosis]

Special senses—taste perversion

Urinary—retention, dysuria, oliguria, hematuria, incontinence, [urinary tract infection with trichomonas, yeast in urine]

Vision—photophobia

Vascular (extracardiac)—flushing, [cerebrovascular accident]

Additional adverse events reported from worldwide marketing experience with Zosyn, occurring under circumstances where causal relationship to Zosyn is uncertain:

Gastrointestinal—hepatitis, cholestatic jaundice

Hematologic—hemolytic anemia

Renal—rarely, interstitial nephritis

Skin and Appendages—erythema multiforme and Stevens-Johnson syndrome, rarely reported

Adverse Laboratory Events (Seen During Clinical Trials)

Of the studies reported, including that of nosocomial lower respiratory tract infections in which a higher dose of Zosyn was used in combination with an aminoglycoside, changes in laboratory parameters, without regard to drug relationship include:

Hematologic—decreases in hemoglobin and hematocrit, thrombocytopenia, increases in platelet count, eosinophilia, leukopenia, neutropenia. The leukopenia/neutropenia associated with Zosyn administration appears to be reversible and most frequently associated with prolonged administration, i.e., ≥21 days of therapy. These patients were withdrawn from therapy; some had accompanying systemic symptoms (e.g., fever, rigors, chills).

Coagulation—positive direct Coombs' test, prolonged prothrombin time, prolonged partial thromboplastin time

Hepatic—transient elevations of AST (SGOT), ALT (SGPT), alkaline phosphatase, bilirubin

Renal—increases in serum creatinine, blood urea nitrogen

Urinalysis—proteinuria, hematuria, pyuria

Additional laboratory events include abnormalities in electrolytes (i.e., increases and decreases in sodium, potassium, and calcium), hyperglycemia, decreases in total protein or albumin.

The following adverse reaction has also been reported for PIPRACIL® (sterile piperacillin sodium):

Skeletal—prolonged muscle relaxation (See **PRECAUTIONS, Drug Interactions.**)

OVERDOSAGE

Information on overdosage of Zosyn in humans is not available.

Excessive serum levels of either piperacillin or tazobactam may be reduced by hemodialysis. (See **CLINICAL PHARMACOLOGY.**) No specific antidote is known. As with other penicillins, neuromuscular excitability or convulsions have occurred following large intravenous doses, primarily in patients with impaired renal function.

In the case of motor excitability or convulsions, general supportive measures, including administration of anticonvulsive agents (e.g., diazepam or barbiturates), may be considered.

DOSAGE AND ADMINISTRATION

Zosyn should be administered by intravenous infusion over 30 minutes

Normal Renal Function (Creatinine Clearance ≥90 mL/min)

The usual total dose of Zosyn for adults is 3.375 g every six hours totalling 13.5 g (12 g piperacillin sodium/1.5 g tazobactam sodium).

Initial presumptive treatment of patients with nosocomial pneumonia should start with Zosyn at a dosage of 3.375 g every four hours plus an aminoglycoside. Treatment with the aminoglycoside should be continued in patients from whom *Pseudomonas aeruginosa* is isolated. If *Pseudomonas aeruginosa* is not isolated, the aminoglycoside may be discontinued at the discretion of the treating physician. (See **DOSAGE AND ADMINISTRATION**.)

Renal Insufficiency

In patients with renal insufficiency (Creatinine Clearance <90 mL/min), the intravenous dose of Zosyn should be adjusted to the degree of actual renal function impairment. In patients with nosocomial pneumonia receiving concomitant aminoglycoside therapy, the aminoglycoside dosage should be adjusted according to the recommendations of the manufacturer. The recommended daily doses of Zosyn® for patients with renal insufficiency are as follows:

Zosyn Dosage Recommendations For All Indications Including Nosocomial Pneumonia

Creatinine Clearance (mL/min)	Recommended Dosage Regimen
>40–90	12 g/1.5 g/day in divided doses of 3.375 g q 6 h
20–40	8 g/1.0 g/day in divided doses of 2.25 g q 6 h
<20	6 g/0.75 g/day in divided doses of 2.25 g q 8 h

For patients on hemodialysis, irrespective of the condition under treatment, the maximum dose is 2.25 g Zosyn every eight hours. In addition, because hemodialysis removes 30% to 40% of a Zosyn dose in four hours, one additional dose of 0.75 g Zosyn should be administered following each dialysis period. For patients with renal failure, measurement of serum levels of piperacillin and tazobactam will provide additional guidance for adjusting dosage.

Duration of Therapy

The usual duration of Zosyn treatment is from seven to ten days. However, the recommended duration of Zosyn treatment of nosocomial pneumonia is seven to fourteen days. In all conditions, the duration of therapy should be guided by the severity of the infection and the patient's clinical and bacteriological progress.

Intravenous Administration

For conventional vials, reconstitute Zosyn per gram of piperacillin with 5 mL of a compatible reconstitution diluent from the list provided below. Shake well until dissolved. Single dose vials should be used immediately after reconstitution. Discard any unused portion after 24 hours if stored at room temperature (20° to 25° C [68° to 77° F]), or after 48 hours if stored at refrigerated temperature (2° to 8° C [36° to 46° F]).

Compatible Reconstitution Diluents

0.9% Sodium Chloride for Injection
Sterile Water for Injection
Dextrose 5%
Bacteriostatic Saline/Parabens
Bacteriostatic Water/Parabens
Bacteriostatic Saline/Benzyl Alcohol
Bacteriostatic Water/Benzyl Alcohol

Reconstituted Zosyn solution should be further diluted (recommended volume per dose of 50 mL to 150 mL) in a compatible intravenous diluent solution listed below.

Administer by infusion over a period of at least 30 minutes. During the infusion it is desirable to discontinue the primary infusion solution.

Compatible Intravenous Diluent Solutions

0.9% Sodium Chloride for Injection
Sterile Water for Injection‡
Dextrose 5%
Dextran 6% in Saline

‡ Maximum recommended volume per dose of Sterile Water for Injection is 50 mL.

Add-Vantage® System Admixtures

Dextrose 5% in Water (50 or 100 mL)
0.9% Sodium Chloride (50 or 100 mL)

For ADD-VANTAGE® vials reconstitution directions, see *INSTRUCTIONS FOR USE* sheet provided in the box.

LACTATED RINGERS SOLUTION IS NOT COMPATIBLE WITH ZOSYN.

When concomitant therapy with aminoglycosides is indicated, Zosyn and the aminoglycoside should be reconstituted and administered separately, due to the *in vitro* inactivation of the aminoglycoside by the penicillin. (See PRECAUTIONS, Drug Interactions.)

Zosyn can be used in ambulatory intravenous infusion pumps.

Stability of Zosyn Following Reconstitution

Zosyn is stable in glass and plastic containers (plastic syringes, I.V. bags and tubing) when used with compatible diluents.

Stability studies in the I.V. bags have demonstrated chemical stability (potency, pH of reconstituted solution and clarity of solution) for up to 24 hours at room temperature and up to one week at refrigerated temperature. Zosyn contains no preservatives. Appropriate consideration of aseptic technique should be used.

Stability of Zosyn in an ambulatory intravenous infusion pump has been demonstrated for a period of 12 hours at room temperature. Each dose was reconstituted and diluted to a volume of 37.5 mL or 25 mL. One-day supplies of dosing solution were aseptically transferred into the medication reservoir (I.V. bags or cartridge). The reservoir was fitted to a preprogrammed ambulatory intravenous infusion pump per the manufacturer's instructions. Stability of Zosyn is not affected when administered using an ambulatory intravenous infusion pump.

Stability studies with the admixed ADD-Vantage® system have demonstrated chemical stability (potency, pH and clarity) through 24 hours at room temperature. (Note: The admixed ADD-Vantage® should not be refrigerated or frozen after reconstitution.)

Parenteral drug products should be inspected visually for particulate matter and discoloration prior to administration, whenever solution and container permit.

HOW SUPPLIED

Zosyn® (sterile piperacillin sodium and tazobactam sodium) is supplied in the following sizes:

Each Zosyn 2.25 g vial provides piperacillin sodium equivalent to 2 grams of piperacillin and tazobactam sodium equivalent to 0.25 gram of tazobactam. Each vial contains 4.69 mEq (108 mg) of sodium.

Supplied 10 per box–NDC 0206-8452-16

Each Zosyn 3.375 g vial provides piperacillin sodium equivalent to 3 grams of piperacillin and tazobactam sodium equivalent to 0.375 gram of tazobactam. Each vial contains 7.04 mEq (162 mg) of sodium.

Supplied 10 per box–NDC 0206-8454-55

Each Zosyn 4.5 g vial provides piperacillin sodium equivalent to 4 grams of piperacillin and tazobactam sodium equivalent to 0.5 gram of tazobactam. Each vial contains 9.39 mEq (216 mg) of sodium.

Supplied 10 per box–NDC 0206-8455-25

Each Zosyn 2.25 g ADD-Vantage® vial provides piperacillin sodium equivalent to 2 grams of piperacillin and tazobactam sodium equivalent to 0.25 grams of tazobactam. Each ADD-Vantage® vial contains 4.69 mEq (108 mg) of sodium.

Supplied 10 per box—NDC 0206-8452-17.

Each Zosyn 3.375 g ADD-Vantage® vial provides piperacillin sodium equivalent to 3 grams of piperacillin and tazobactam sodium equivalent to 0.375 grams of tazobactam. Each ADD-Vantage® vial contains 7.04 mEq (162 mg) of sodium.

Supplied 10 per box—NDC 0206-8454-17.

Each Zosyn 4.5 g ADD-Vantage® vial provides piperacillin sodium equivalent to 4 grams of piperacillin and tazobactam sodium equivalent to 0.5 grams of tazobactam. Each ADD-Vantage® vial contains 9.39 mEq (216 mg) of sodium.

Supplied 10 per box—NDC 0206-8455-17.

Zosyn conventional and ADD-Vantage® vials should be stored at controlled room temperature (20° to 25°C [68° to 77°F]) prior to reconstitution.

Also Available

Zosyn is also supplied as follows:

Zosyn® (piperacillin sodium and tazobactam sodium injection) in Galaxy® Container (PL 2040 Plastic) is supplied as a frozen, iso-osmotic, sterile, nonpyrogenic solution in single-dose plastic containers as follows:

2.25 g (2 g piperacillin/0.25 g tazobactam) in 50 mL. Each container has 5.7 mEq (131 mg) of sodium.

Supplied 24/box—NDC 0206-8820-02

3.375 g (3 g piperacillin/0.375 g tazobactam) in 50 mL. Each container has 8.6 mEq (197 mg) of sodium.

Supplied 24/box—NDC 0206-8821-02

4.5 g (4 g piperacillin/0.5 g tazobactam) in 100 mL. Each container has 11.4 mEq (263 mg) of sodium.

Supplied 12/box—NDC 0206-8822-02

ALSO AVAILABLE

Zosyn is also supplied as follows:

40.5 g pharmacy bulk vial containing 36 grams of piperacillin and 4.5 grams of tazobactam. Each pharmacy bulk vial contains 84.5 mEq (1,944 mg) of sodium.

NDC 0206-8620-11

REFERENCES

1. National Committee for Clinical Laboratory Standards, Methods for Dilution Antimicrobial Susceptibility Tests for Bacteria that Grow Aerobically–Fourth Edition. Approved Standard NCCLS Document M7-A4, Vol. 17, No. 2, NCCLS, Wayne, PA, January, 1997.

2. National Committee for Clinical Laboratory Standards, Methods for Antimicrobial Susceptibility Testing for Anaerobic Bacteria–Third Edition. Approved Standard NCCLS Document M11-A3, Vol. 13, No. 26, NCCLS, Villanova, PA, December, 1993.

3. National Committee for Clinical Laboratory Standards. Performance Standard for Antimicrobial Disk Susceptibility Tests–Sixth Edition. Approved Standard NCCLS Document M2-A6, Vol. 17, No. 1, NCCLS, Wayne, PA, January, 1997.

4. Halstenson CE, Hirata CAI, Heim-Duthoy KL, Abraham PA, and Matzke GR. Effect of concomitant administraton of piperacillin on the dispositions of netilmicin and tobramycin in patients with end-stage renal disease. Antimicrob Agents Chemother 34(1):128-133, 1990.

CLINITEST® and DIASTIX® are registered trademarks of Ames Division, Miles Laboratories, Inc.

TES-TAPE® is a registered trademark of Eli Lilly and Company.

Galaxy® is a registered trademark of Baxter International, Inc.

ADD-VANTAGE is a registered trademark of Abbott Laboratories

Manufactured by:
LEDERLE PIPERACILLIN, INC.
Carolina, Puerto Rico 00987
CI 4630-2 Revised March 25, 1999

Shown in Product Identification Guide, page 321

ZOSYN® ℞

[*zō 'sĭn*]

(Piperacillin Sodium and Tazobactam Sodium Injection) in Galaxy® Containers (PL 2040 Plastic)

DESCRIPTION

Zosyn (piperacillin sodium and tazobactam sodium injection) in Galaxy® Containers (PL 2040 Plastic) is a sterile injectable antibacterial combination product consisting of the semisynthetic antibiotic piperacillin sodium and the β-lactamase inhibitor tazobactam sodium for intravenous administration.

Piperacillin sodium is derived from D(-)-α-aminobenzylpenicillin. The chemical name of piperacillin sodium is sodium (2*S*,5*R*,6*R*)-6-[(*R*)-2-(4-ethyl-2,3-dioxo-1-piperazine-carboxamido) -2-phenylacetamido]-3,3-dimethyl-7-oxo-4-thia-1-azabicyclo[3.2.0]heptane-2-carboxylate. The chemical formula is $C_{23}H_{26}N_5NaO_7S$ and the molecular weight is 539.6.

Tazobactam sodium, a derivative of the penicillin nucleus, is a penicillanic acid sulfone. Its chemical name is sodium (2*S*,3*S*,5*R*)-3-methyl-7-oxo-3-(1*H*-1,2,3-triazol-1-ylmethyl)-4-thia-1-azabicyclo [3.2.0]heptane-2-carboxylate-4,4-dioxide. The chemical formula is $C_{10}H_{11}N_4NaO_5S$ and the molecular weight is 322.3.

Zosyn in the Galaxy® Container (PL 2040 Plastic) is a frozen iso-osmotic sterile non-pyrogenic premixed solution. The components and dosage formulations are given in the table below:

[See table 1 at top of next page]

The pH has been adjusted between 4.5 to 6.8 with sodium bicarbonate and hydrochloric acid.

The solution is intended for intravenous use only.

The plastic container is fabricated from a specially designed multilayer plastic, PL 2040. Solutions are in contact with the polyethylene layer of this container and can leach out certain chemical components of the plastic in very small amounts within the expiration period. The suitability of the plastic has been confirmed in tests in animals according to the USP biological tests for plastic containers, as well as by tissue culture toxicity studies.

The approximate total sodium content for Zosyn (piperacillin sodium and tazobactam sodium injection) is 5.7 mEq (131 mg) per 50 mL in the 2.25 g dose, 8.6 mEq (197 mg) per 50 mL in the 3.375 g dose, and 11.4 mEq (263 mg) per 100 mL in the 4.5 g dose.

CLINICAL PHARMACOLOGY

Peak plasma concentrations of piperacillin and tazobactam are attained immediately after completion of an intravenous infusion of Zosyn. Piperacillin plasma concentrations, following a 30-minute infusion of Zosyn, were similar to those attained when equivalent doses of piperacillin were administered alone, with mean peak plasma concentrations of approximately 134 µg/mL, 242 µg/mL, and 298 µg/mL for the 2.25 g, 3.375 g, and 4.5 g Zosyn (piperacillin/tazobactam) doses, respectively. The corresponding mean peak plasma concentrations of tazobactam were 15 µg/mL, 24 µg/mL, and 34 µg/mL, respectively. Following a 30-minute I.V. infusion of 3.375 g Zosyn every 6 hours, steady-state plasma concentrations of piperacillin and tazobactam were similar to those attained after the first dose. In like manner, steady-state plasma concentrations were not different from those attained after the first dose when 2.25 g or 4.5 g doses of Zosyn were administered via 30-minute infusions every 6 hours. Steady-state plasma concentrations after 30-minute infusions every 6 hours are provided in Table 2.

Following single or multiple Zosyn doses to healthy subjects, the plasma half-life of piperacillin and of tazobactam ranged from 0.7 to 1.2 hours and was unaffected by dose or duration of infusion.

Piperacillin is metabolized to a minor microbiologically active desethyl metabolite. Tazobactam is metabolized to a single metabolite that lacks pharmacological and antibacterial activities. Both piperacillin and tazobactam are eliminated via the kidney by glomerular filtration and tubular secretion. Piperacillin is excreted rapidly as unchanged drug with 68% of the administered dose excreted in the urine. Tazobactam and its metabolite are eliminated primarily by renal excretion with 80% of the administered dose excreted as unchanged drug and the remainder as the single metabolite. Piperacillin, tazobactam, and desethyl piperacillin are also secreted into the bile.

Both piperacillin and tazobactam are approximately 30% bound to plasma proteins. The protein binding of either piperacillin or tazobactam is unaffected by the presence of the other compound. Protein binding of the tazobactam metabolite is negligible.

Piperacillin and tazobactam are widely distributed into tissues and body fluids including intestinal mucosa, gallbladder, lung, female reproductive tissues (uterus, ovary and fallopian tube), interstitial fluid, and bile. Mean tissue concentrations are generally 50 to 100% of those in plasma. Distribution of piperacillin and tazobactam into cerebrospinal fluid is low in subjects with non-inflamed meninges, as with other penicillins.

After the administration of single doses of piperacillin/tazobactam to subjects with renal impairment, the half-life of piperacillin and of tazobactam increases with decreasing creatinine clearance. At creatinine clearance below 20 mL/min, the increase in half-life is twofold for piperacillin and fourfold for tazobactam compared to subjects with normal renal function. Dosage adjustments for Zosyn are recommended when creatinine clearance is below 40 mL/min in patients receiving the usual recommended daily dose of Zosyn. (See **DOSAGE AND ADMINISTRATION** section for specific recommendations for the treatment of patients with renal insufficiency.)

Hemodialysis removes 30 to 40% of a piperacillin/tazobactam dose with an additional 5% of the tazobactam dose removed as the tazobactam metabolite. Peritoneal dialysis removes approximately 6% and 21% of the piperacillin and tazobactam doses, respectively, with up to 16% of the tazobactam dose removed as the tazobactam metabolite. For dosage recommendations for patients undergoing hemodialysis, see **DOSAGE AND ADMINISTRATION** section.

The half-life of piperacillin and of tazobactam increases by approximately 25% and 18%, respectively, in patients with hepatic cirrhosis compared to healthy subjects. However, this difference does not warrant dosage adjustment of Zosyn due to hepatic cirrhosis.

[See table 2 at top of next page]

Microbiology

Piperacillin sodium exerts bactericidal activity by inhibiting septum formation and cell wall synthesis. *In vitro*, piper-

Continued on next page

Zosyn—Cont.

acillin is active against a variety of gram-positive and gram-negative aerobic and anaerobic bacteria. Tazobactam sodium has very little intrinsic microbiologic activity due to its very low level of binding to penicillin-binding proteins; however, it is a β-lactamase inhibitor of the Richmond-Sykes class III (Bush class 2b & 2b') penicillinases and cephalosporinases. It varies in its ability to inhibit class II and IV (2a & 4) penicillinases. Tazobactam does not induce chromosomally-mediated β-lactamases at tazobactam levels achieved with the recommended dosage regimen. Piperacillin/tazobactam has been shown to be active against most strains of the following piperacillin resistant, β-lactamase producing microorganisms both *in vitro* and in clinical infections as described in the **INDICATIONS AND USAGE** section.

Gram-positive aerobes:
Staphylococcus aureus (NOT methicillin/oxacillin-resistant strains)
Gram-negative aerobes:
Escherichia coli
Haemophilus influenzae (NOT β-lactamase negative ampicillin-resistant strains)
Gram-negative anaerobes:
Bacteroides fragilis group (*B. fragilis, B. ovatus, B. thetaiotaomicron*, or *B. vulgatus*)

The following *in vitro* data are available; **but their clinical significance is unknown.**

Piperacillin/tazobactam exhibits *in vitro* minimal inhibitory concentrations (MICs) of 16.0 μg/mL or less against most (≥90%) strains of *Enterobacteriaceae*, (MICs of 1.0 μg/mL or less against most (≥90%) strains of *Haemophilus* species, MICs of 8.0 μg/mL or less against most (≥90%) strains *Staphylococcus* species, and MICs of 16.0 μg/mL or less against most (≥90%) strains of *Bacteroides* species. Beta-lactamase negative strains should be tested against piperacillin alone; piperacillin break points should be used in evaluation of these results. However, the safety and efficacy of piperacillin/tazobactam in treating clinical infection due to these microorganisms have not been established in adequate and well-controlled clinical trials.

Gram-positive aerobes:
Enterococcus faecalis (piperacillin susceptible)
Staphylococcus epidermidis (NOT methicillin/oxacillin-resistant strains)
Streptococcus agalactiae†
Streptococcus pneumoniae†
Streptococcus pyogenes†
Viridans group streptococci†
Gram-negative aerobes:
Klebsiella oxytoca
Klebsiella pneumoniae
Moraxella catarrhalis
Morganella morganii
Neisseria gonorrhoeae
Neisseria meningitidis†
Proteus mirabilis
Proteus vulgaris
Pseudomonas aeruginosa (piperacillin susceptible)
Serratia marcescens
Gram-positive anaerobes:
Clostridium perfringens
Gram-negative anaerobes:
Bacteroides distasonis
Fusobacterium nucleatum
Prevotella melaninogenica (formerly *Bacteroides melaninogenicus*)

†These are not β-lactamase producing strains and, therefore, are susceptible to piperacillin alone.

Susceptibility Tests

Dilution Techniques

Quantitative methods are used to determine minimum inhibitory concentrations (MICs). These MICs provide estimates of the susceptibility of bacteria to antimicrobial compounds. The MICs should be determined using a standardized procedure. Standardized procedures are based on a dilution method (broth or agar) or equivalent with standardized inoculum concentrations and standardized concentrations of piperacillin and tazobactam powders.[1] MIC values should be determined using serial dilutions of piperacillin combined with a fixed concentration of 4 μg/mL tazobactam. The MIC values obtained should be interpreted according to the following criteria:

For *Enterobacteriaceae:*

MIC (μg/mL)	Interpretation
≤16	Susceptible (S)
32–64	Intermediate (I)
≥128	Resistant (R)

For *Haemophilus* species:

MIC (μg/mL)	Interpretation
≤1	Susceptible (S)
≥2	Resistant (R)

For *Staphylococcus* species:

MIC (μg/mL)	Interpretation
≤8	Susceptible (S)
≥16	Resistant (R)

A report of "Susceptible" indicates that the pathogen is likely to be inhibited if the antimicrobial compound in the blood reaches the concentrations usually achievable. A report of "Intermediate" indicates that the result should be

Table 1: Zosyn® in Galaxy® Containers (PL 2040 Plastic) premixed frozen solution

Component*	Function	Dosage Formulations		
		2.25 g/50 mL	3.375 g/50 mL	4.5 g/100 mL
Piperacillin	active ingredient	2 g	3 g	4 g
Tazobactam	β-lactamase inhibitor	250 mg	375 mg	500 mg
Dextrose Hydrous USP	osmolality adjusting agent	1 g	350 mg	2 g
Sodium Citrate Dihydrate, USP	buffering agent	100 mg	150 mg	200 mg

*Piperacillin and tazobactam are present in the formulation as sodium salts. Dextrose Hydrous, USP and Sodium Citrate Dihydrate, USP amounts are approximate.

TABLE 2
STEADY STATE MEAN PLASMA CONCENTRATIONS IN ADULTS AFTER 30-MINUTE INTRAVENOUS INFUSION OF PIPERACILLIN/TAZOBACTAM EVERY 6 HOURS

PIPERACILLIN

		Plasma Concentrations** (μg/mL)						AUC** (μg•hr/mL)
Piperacillin/[c] Tazobactam Dose	No. of Evaluable Subjects	30 min	1 hr	2 hr	3 hr	4 hr	6 hr	AUC_{0-6}
2.25 g	8	134 (14)	57 (14)	17.1 (23)	5.2 (32)	2.5 (35)	0.9 (14)[a]	131 (14)
3.375 g	6	242 (12)	106 (8)	34.6 (20)	11.5 (19)	5.1 (22)	1.0 (10)	242 (10)
4.5 g	8	298 (14)	141 (19)	46.6 (28)	16.4 (29)	6.9 (29)	1.4 (30)	322 (16)

a: N = 4

TAZOBACTAM

		Plasma Concentrations** (μg/mL)						AUC** (μg•hr/mL)
Piperacillin/[c] Tazobactam Dose	No. of Evaluable Subjects	30 min	1 hr	2 hr	3 hr	4 hr	6 hr	AUC_{0-6}
2.25 g	8	14.8 (14)	7.2 (22)	2.6 (30)	1.1 (35)	0.7 (6)[c]	<0.5	16.0 (21)
3.375 g	6	24.2 (14)	10.7 (7)	4.0 (18)	1.4 (21)	0.7 (16)[a]	<0.5	25.0 (8)
4.5 g	8	33.8 (15)	17.3 (16)	6.8 (24)	2.8 (25)	1.3 (30)	<0.5	39.8 (15)

** Numbers in parentheses are coefficients of variation (CV%).
a: N = 4
b: N = 3
c: Piperacillin and tazobactam were given in combination.

considered equivocal, and, if the microorganism is not fully susceptible to alternative, clinically feasible drugs, the test should be repeated. This category implies possible clinical applicability in body sites where the drug is physiologically concentrated or in situations where high dosage of drug can be used. This category also provides a buffer zone which prevents small uncontrolled technical factors from causing major discrepancies in interpretation. A report of "Resistant" indicates that the pathogen is not likely to be inhibited if the antimicrobial compound in the blood reaches the concentrations usually achievable; other therapy should be selected.

Standardized susceptibility test procedures require the use of laboratory control microorganisms to control the technical aspects of the laboratory procedures. Laboratory control microorganisms are specific strains of microbiological assay organisms with intrinsic biological properties relating to resistance mechanisms and their genetic expression within bacteria; the specific strains are not clinically significant in their current microbiological status. Standard piperacillin and tazobactam powders should provide the following MIC values when tested against the designated quality control strains:

Microorganism	MIC (μg/mL)
Escherichia coli ATCC 25922	1 – 4
Escherichia coli ATCC 35218	0.5 – 2
Haemophilus influenzae ATCC 49247	0.06 – 0.5
Staphylococcus aureus ATCC 29213	0.25 – 2

Anaerobic Techniques

For anaerobic bacteria, the susceptibility to piperacillin/tazobactam can be determined by the reference agar dilution method or by alternate standardized test methods.[2] For *Bacteroides* species, the dilution values should be interpreted as follows:

MIC (μg/mL)	Interpretation
≤16	Susceptible (S)
≥32	Resistant (R)

Serial dilutions of piperacillin combined with a fixed concentration of 4 μg/mL tazobactam should provide the following MIC values:

Microorganism	MIC (μg/mL)
Bacteroides fragilis ATCC 25285	0.12 – 0.5
Bacteroides thetaiotaomicron ATCC 29741	4 – 16

Diffusion Techniques

Quantitative methods that require measurement of zone diameters also provide reproducible estimates of the susceptibility of bacteria to antimicrobial compounds. One such standardized procedure requires the use of standardized inoculum concentrations.[3] This procedure uses paper disks impregnated with 100 μg of piperacillin and 10 μg of tazobactam to test the susceptibility of microorganisms to piperacillin/tazobactam. Interpretation is identical to that stated above for results using dilution techniques.

Reports from the laboratory providing results of the standard single-disk susceptibility test with a 100/10-μg piperacillin/tazobactam disk should be interpreted according to the following criteria:

For *Enterobacteriaceae:*

Zone Diameter (mm)	Interpretation
≥21	Susceptible (S)
18 – 20	Intermediate (I)
≤17	Resistant (R)

For *Staphylococcus* species:

Zone Diameter (mm)	Interpretation
≥20	Susceptible (S)
≤19	Resistant (R)

As with standardized dilution techniques, diffusion methods require the use of laboratory control microorganisms to control the technical aspects of the laboratory procedures. Laboratory control microorganisms are specific strains of microbiological assay organisms with intrinsic biological properties relating to resistance mechanisms and their genetic expression within bacteria; the specific strains are not clinically significant in their current microbiological status. For the diffusion technique, the 100/10-μg piperacillin/tazobactam disk should provide the following zone diameters in these laboratory test quality control strains:

Microorganism	Zone Diameter (mm)
Escherichia coli ATCC 25922	24 – 30
Escherichia coli ATCC 35218	24 – 30
Staphylococcus aureus ATCC 25923	27 – 36

INDICATIONS AND USAGE

Zosyn is indicated for the treatment of patients with moderate to severe infections caused by piperacillin-resistant, piperacillin/tazobactam susceptible, β-lactamase producing strains of the designated microorganisms in the specified conditions listed below:

Appendicitis (complicated by rupture or abscess) and peritonitis caused by piperacillin-resistant, β-lactamase producing strains of *Escherichia coli* or the following members of the *Bacteroides fragilis* group: *B. fragilis, B. ovatus, B. thetaiotamicron, or B. vulgatus.* The individual members of this group were studied in less than 10 cases.

Uncomplicated and complicated skin and skin structure infections, including cellulitis, cutaneous abscesses and ischemic/diabetic foot infections caused by piperacillin-resistant, β-lactamase producing strains of *Staphylococcus aureus*.

Postpartum endometritis or pelvic inflammatory disease caused by piperacillin-resistant, β-lactamase producing strains of *Escherichia coli*.

Community-acquired pneumonia (moderate severity only) caused by piperacillin-resistant, β-lactamase producing strains of *Haemophilus influenzae*.

Nosocomial pneumonia (moderate to severe) caused by piperacillin-resistant, β-lactamase producing strains of *Staphylococcus aureus*. (See **DOSAGE AND ADMINISTRATION**).

As a combination product, Zosyn is indicated only for the specified conditions listed above. Infections caused by piperacillin-susceptible organisms, for which piperacillin has been shown to be effective, are also amenable to Zosyn treatment due to its piperacillin content. The tazobactam component of this combination product does not decrease the activity of the piperacillin component against piperacillin-susceptible organisms. Therefore, the treatment of mixed infections caused by piperacillin-susceptible organisms and piperacillin-resistant, β-lactamase producing organisms susceptible to Zosyn should not require the addition of another antibiotic. (See **DOSAGE AND ADMINISTRATION**.)

Zosyn is useful as presumptive therapy in the indicated conditions prior to the identification of causative organisms because of its broad spectrum of bactericidal activity against gram-positive and gram-negative aerobic and anaerobic organisms.

Appropriate cultures should usually be performed before initiating antimicrobial treatment in order to isolate and identify the organisms causing infection and to determine their susceptibility to Zosyn. Antimicrobial therapy should be adjusted, if appropriate, once the results of culture(s) and antimicrobial susceptibility testing are known.

CONTRAINDICATIONS

Zosyn is contraindicated in patients with a history of allergic reactions to any of the penicillins, cephalosporins, or β-lactamase inhibitors.

WARNINGS

SERIOUS AND OCCASIONALLY FATAL HYPERSENSITIVITY (ANAPHYLACTIC) REACTIONS HAVE BEEN REPORTED IN PATIENTS ON PENICILLIN THERAPY. THESE REACTIONS ARE MORE LIKELY TO OCCUR IN INDIVIDUALS WITH A HISTORY OF PENICILLIN HYPERSENSITIVITY OR A HISTORY OF SENSITIVITY TO MULTIPLE ALLERGENS. THERE HAVE BEEN REPORTS OF INDIVIDUALS WITH A HISTORY OF PENICILLIN HYPERSENSITIVITY WHO HAVE EXPERIENCED SEVERE REACTIONS WHEN TREATED WITH CEPHALOSPORINS. BEFORE INITIATING THERAPY WITH ZOSYN, CAREFUL INQUIRY SHOULD BE MADE CONCERNING PREVIOUS HYPERSENSITIVITY REACTIONS TO PENICILLINS, CEPHALOSPORINS, OR OTHER ALLERGENS. IF AN ALLERGIC REACTION OCCURS, ZOSYN SHOULD BE DISCONTINUED AND APPROPRIATE THERAPY INSTITUTED. **SERIOUS ANAPHYLACTIC REACTIONS REQUIRE IMMEDIATE EMERGENCY TREATMENT WITH EPINEPHRINE. OXYGEN, INTRAVENOUS STEROIDS AND AIRWAY MANAGEMENT, INCLUDING INTUBATION, SHOULD ALSO BE ADMINISTERED AS INDICATED.**

Pseudomembranous colitis has been reported with nearly all antibacterial agents, including piperacillin/tazobactam, and may range in severity from mild to life-threatening. Therefore, it is important to consider this diagnosis in patients who present with diarrhea subsequent to the administration of antibacterial agents.

Treatment with antibacterial agents alters the normal flora of the colon and may permit overgrowth of clostridia. Studies indicate that a toxin produced by *Clostridium difficile* is one primary cause of "antibiotic-associated colitis."

After the diagnosis of pseudomembranous colitis has been established, therapeutic measures should be initiated. Mild cases of pseudomembranous colitis usually respond to drug discontinuation alone. In moderate to severe cases, consideration should be given to management with fluids and electrolytes, protein supplementation, and treatment with an antibacterial drug clinically effective against *Clostridium difficile* colitis.

PRECAUTIONS

General

Bleeding manifestations have occurred in some patients receiving β-lactam antibiotics, including piperacillin. These reactions have sometimes been associated with abnormalities of coagulation tests such as clotting time, platelet aggregation, and prothrombin time, and are more likely to occur in patients with renal failure. If bleeding manifestations occur, Zosyn should be discontinued and appropriate therapy instituted.

The possibility of the emergence of resistant organisms that might cause superinfections should be kept in mind. If this occurs, appropriate measures should be taken.

As with other penicillins, patients may experience neuromuscular excitability or convulsions if higher than recommended doses are given intravenously (particularly in the presence of renal failure). Zosyn (piperacillin sodium and tazobactam sodium injection) in the Galaxy® container contains an approximate total sodium content of 5.7 mEq (131 mg) per 50 mL in the 2.25 g dose, 8.6 mEq (197 mg) per 50 mL in the 3.375 g dose, and 11.4 mEq (263 mg) per 100 mL in the 4.5 g dose. This should be considered when treating patients requiring restricted salt intake. Periodic electrolyte determinations should be performed in patients with low potassium reserves, and the possibility of hypokalemia should be kept in mind in patients who have potentially low potassium reserves and who are receiving cytotoxic therapy or diuretics.

As with other semisynthetic penicillins, piperacillin therapy has been associated with an increased incidence of fever and rash in cystic fibrosis patients.

Laboratory Tests

Periodic assessment of hematopoietic function should be performed, especially with prolonged therapy, i.e., ≥21 days. (See **ADVERSE REACTIONS**, **Adverse Laboratory Events**.)

Drug Interactions

Aminoglycosides

The mixing of Zosyn with an aminoglycoside *in vitro* can result in substantial inactivation of the aminoglycoside.

When Zosyn was co-administered with tobramycin, the area under the curve, renal clearance and urinary recovery of tobramycin were decreased by 11%, 32%, and 38%, respectively. The alterations in the pharmacokinetics of tobramycin when administered in combination with piperacillin/tazobactam may be due to *in vivo* and *in vitro* inactivation of tobramycin in the presence of piperacillin/tazobactam. The inactivation of aminoglycosides in the presence of penicillin-class drugs has been recognized. It has been postulated that penicillin-aminoglycoside complexes form; these complexes are microbiologically inactive and of unknown toxicity. In patients with severe renal dysfunction (i.e., chronic hemodialysis patients), the pharmacokinetics of tobramycin are significantly altered when tobramycin is administered in combination with piperacillin.[4] The alteration of tobramycin pharmacokinetics and the potential toxicity of the penicillin-aminoglycoside complexes in patients with mild to moderate renal dysfunction who are administered an aminoglycoside in combination with piperacillin/tazobactam are unknown.

Probenecid

Probenecid administered concomitantly with Zosyn prolongs the half-life of piperacillin by 21% and of tazobactam by 71%.

Vancomycin

No pharmacokinetic interactions have been noted between Zosyn and vancomycin.

Heparin

Coagulation parameters should be tested more frequently and monitored regularly during simultaneous administration of high doses of heparin, oral anticoagulants, or other drugs that may affect the blood coagulation system or the thrombocyte function.

Vecuronium

Piperacillin when used concomitantly with vecuronium has been implicated in the prolongation of the neuromuscular blockade of vecuronium. Zosyn (piperacillin/tazobactam) could produce the same phenomenon if given along with vecuronium. Due to their similar mechanism of action, it is expected that the neuromuscular blockade produced by any of the non-depolarizing muscle relaxants could be prolonged in the presence of piperacillin. (See package insert for vecuronium bromide.)

Drug/Laboratory Test Interactions

As with other penicillins, the administration of Zosyn may result in a false-positive reaction for glucose in the urine using a copper-reduction method (CLINITEST®). It is recommended that glucose tests based on enzymatic glucose oxidase reactions (such as DIASTIX® or TES-TAPE®) be used.

Carcinogenesis, Mutagenesis, Impairment of Fertility

Long term carcinogenicity studies in animals have not been conducted with piperacillin/tazobactam, piperacillin, or tazobactam. *Piperacillin/tazobactam* was negative in microbial mutagenicity assays at concentrations up to 14.84/1.86 μg/plate.

Piperacillin/tazobactam was negative in the unscheduled DNA synthesis (UDS) test at concentrations up to 5689/711 μg/mL. Piperacillin/tazobactam was negative in a mammalian point mutation (Chinese hamster ovary cell HPRT) assay at concentrations up to 8000/1000 μg/mL. Piperacillin/tazobactam was negative in a mammalian cell (BALB/c-3T3) transformation assay at concentrations up to 8/1 μg/mL. *In vivo*, piperacillin/tazobactam did not induce chromosomal aberrations in rats dosed I.V. with 1500/187.5 mg/kg; this dose is similar to the maximum recommended human daily dose on a body-surface-area basis (mg/m^2).

Piperacillin was negative in microbial mutagenicity assays at concentrations up to 50 μg/plate. There was no DNA damage in bacteria (Rec assay) exposed to piperacillin at concentrations up to 200 μg/disk. Piperacillin was negative in the UDS test at concentrations up to 10,000 μg/mL. In a mammalian point mutation (mouse lymphoma cells) assay, piperacillin was positive at concentrations ≥2500 μg/mL. Piperacillin was negative in a cell (BALB/c-3T3) transformation assay at concentrations up to 3000 μg/mL. *In vivo*, piperacillin did not induce chromosomal aberrations in mice at I.V. doses up to 2000 mg/kg/day or rats at I.V. doses up to 1500 mg/kg/day. These doses are half (mice) or similar (rats) to the maximum recommended human daily dose based on body-surface area (mg/m^2). In another *in vivo* test, there was no dominant lethal effect when piperacillin was administered to rats at I.V. doses up to 2000 mg/kg/day, which is similar to the maximum recommended human daily dose based on body-surface area (mg/m^2). When mice were administered piperacillin at I.V. doses up to 2000 mg/kg/day, which is half the maximum recommended human daily dose based on body-surface area (mg/m^2), urine from these animals was not mutagenic when tested in a microbial mutagenicity assay. Bacteria injected into the peritoneal cavity of mice administered piperacillin at I.V. doses up to 2000 mg/kg/day did not show increased mutation frequencies.

Tazobactam was negative in microbial mutagenicity assays at concentrations up to 333 μg/plate. Tazobactam was negative in the UDS test at concentrations up to 2000 μg/mL. Tazobactam was negative in a mammalian point mutation (Chinese hamster ovary cell HPRT) assay at concentrations up to 5000 μg/mL. In another mammalian point mutation (mouse lymphoma cells) assay, tazobactam was positive at concentrations ≥3000 μg/mL. Tazobactam was negative in a cell (BALB/c-3T3) transformation assay at concentrations up to 900 μg/mL. In an *in vitro* cytogenetics (Chinese hamster lung cells) assay, tazobactam was negative at concentrations up to 3000 μg/mL. *In vivo*, tazobactam did not induce chromosomal aberrations in rats at I.V. doses up to 5000 mg/kg, which is 23 times the maximum recommended human daily dose based on body-surface area (mg/m^2).

Pregnancy

Teratogenic effects—Pregnancy Category B

Piperacillin/tazobactam

Reproduction studies have been performed in rats and have revealed no evidence of impaired fertility due to piperacillin/tazobactam administered up to a dose which is similar to the maximum recommended human daily dose based on body-surface area (mg/m^2).

Teratology studies have been performed in mice and rats and have revealed no evidence of harm to the fetus due to piperacillin/tazobactam administered up to a dose which is 1 to 2 times and 2 to 3 times the human dose of piperacillin and tazobactam, respectively, based on body-surface area (mg/m^2).

Piperacillin

Reproduction and teratology studies have been performed in mice and rats and have revealed no evidence of impaired fertility or harm to the fetus due to piperacillin administered up to a dose which is half (mice) or similar (rats) to the maximum recommended human daily dose based on body-surface area (mg/m^2).

Tazobactam

Reproduction studies have been performed in rats and have revealed no evidence of impaired fertility due to tazobactam administered at doses up to 3 times the maximum recommended daily dose based on body-surface area (mg/m^2).

Teratology studies have been performed in mice and rats and have revealed no evidence of harm to the fetus due to tazobactam administered at doses up to 6 and 14 times, respectively, the human dose based on body-surface area (mg/m^2). In rats, tazobactam crosses the placenta. Concentrations in the fetus are less than or equal to 10% of those found in maternal plasma.

There are, however, no adequate and well-controlled studies with the piperacillin/tazobactam combination or with piperacillin or tazobactam alone in pregnant women. Because animal reproduction studies are not always predictive of the human response, this drug should be used during pregnancy only if clearly needed.

Nursing Mothers

Piperacillin is excreted in low concentrations in human milk; tazobactam concentrations in human milk have not been studied. Caution should be exercised when Zosyn is administered to a nursing woman.

Pediatric Use

Safety and efficacy in pediatric patients have not been established.

Geriatric Use

Patients over 65 years are not at an increased risk of developing adverse effects solely because of age. However, dosage should be adjusted in the presence of renal insufficiency. (See **DOSAGE AND ADMINISTRATION**).

ADVERSE REACTIONS

During the initial clinical investigations, 2621 patients worldwide were treated with Zosyn in phase 3 trials. In the key North American clinical trials (n=830 patients), 90% of the adverse events reported were mild to moderate in severity and transient in nature. However, in 3.2% of the patients treated worldwide, Zosyn was discontinued because of adverse events primarily involving the skin (1.3%), including rash and pruritus; the gastrointestinal system (0.9%), including diarrhea, nausea and vomiting; and allergic reactions (0.5%).

Adverse local reactions that were reported, irrespective of relationship to therapy with Zosyn, were phlebitis (1.3%), injection site reaction (0.5%), pain (0.2%), inflammation (0.2%), thrombophlebitis (0.2%), and edema (0.1%).

In the completed study of nosocomial lower respiratory tract infections, 155 patients were treated with Zosyn in a dosing regimen of 3.375 g every 4 hours in combination with an aminoglycoside. In this trial, 88.5% of the adverse experiences reported were mild to moderate in severity and transient in nature. However, in this trial, therapy with Zosyn was discontinued in four patients (2.6%) due to adverse experiences.

Continued on next page

Zosyn—Cont.

Irrespective of drug relationship or degree of severity, the adverse experiences which led to the discontinuation of Zosyn in these four patients were: thrombocytopenia and pancreatitis in one patient; fever in one patient; fever and eosinophilia in another patient; and diarrhea and elevated liver enzymes in the fourth patient.

Adverse Clinical Events

Based on patients from the North American trials (n=1063), the events with the highest incidence in patients, irrespective of relationship to Zosyn therapy, were diarrhea (11.3%); headache (7.7%); constipation (7.7%); nausea (6.9%); insomnia (6.6%); rash (4.2%), including maculopapular, bullous, urticarial, and eczematoid; vomiting (3.3%); dyspepsia (3.3%); pruritus (3.1%); stool changes (2.4%); fever (2.4%); agitation (2.1%); pain (1.7%); moniliasis (1.6%); hypertension (1.6%); dizziness (1.4%); abdominal pain (1.3%); chest pain (1.3%); edema (1.2%); anxiety (1.2%); rhinitis (1.2%); and dyspnea (1.1%).

Based on patients in the completed study of nosocomial lower respiratory tract infections (n=155), using every 4-hour dosing and aminoglycoside therapy, the events with the highest incidence in patients, irrespective of relationship to Zosyn and aminoglycoside therapy, were: diarrhea (20%); constipation (8.4%); agitation (7.1%); nausea (5.8%); headache (4.5%); insomnia (4.5%); oral thrush (3.9%); erythematous rash (3.9%); anxiety (3.2%); fever (3.2%); pain (3.2%); pruritus (3.2%); hiccough (2.6%); vomiting (2.6%); dyspepsia (1.9%); edema (1.9%); fluid overload (1.9%); stool changes (1.9%); anorexia (1.3%); cardiac arrest (1.3%); confusion (1.3%); diaphoresis (1.3%); duodenal ulcer (1.3%); flatulence (1.3%); hypertension (1.3%); hypotension (1.3%); inflammation at injection site (1.3%); pleural effusion (1.3%); pneumothorax (1.3%); rash, not otherwise specified (1.3%); supraventricular tachycardia (1.3%); thrombophlebitis (1.3%); and urinary incontinence (1.3%).

Additional adverse systemic clinical events reported in 1.0% or less of the patients in the initial North American trials and/or in the patients administered Zosyn 3.375 g every 4 hours plus an aminoglycoside in the study of nosocomial lower respiratory tract infections are listed below within each body system. (Bracketed events occurred only in the nosocomial pneumonia trial.)

Autonomic nervous system—hypotension, ileus, syncope
Body as a whole—rigors, back pain, malaise, [asthenia, chest pain]
Cardiovascular—tachycardia, including supraventricular and ventricular; bradycardia; arrhythmia, including atrial fibrillation, ventricular fibrillation, cardiac arrest, cardiac failure, circulatory failure, myocardial infarction, [angina]
Central nervous system—tremor, convulsions, vertigo, [aggressive reaction (combative)]
Gastrointestinal—melena, flatulence, hemorrhage, gastritis, hiccough, ulcerative stomatitis, [fecal incontinence, gastric ulcer, pancreatitis]

Pseudomembranous colitis was reported in one patient during the clinical trials. The onset of pseudomembranous colitis symptoms may occur during or after antibacterial treatment. (See **WARNINGS**.)

Hearing and Vestibular System—tinnitus, [deafness, earache]
Hypersensitivity—anaphylaxis
Metabolic and Nutritional—symptomatic hypoglycemia, thirst, [gout, vitamin B_{12} deficiency anemia]
Musculoskeletal—myalgia, arthralgia
Platelet, Bleeding, Clotting—mesenteric embolism, purpura, epistaxis, pulmonary embolism, [ecchymosis, hemoptysis] (See **PRECAUTIONS, General**.)
Psychiatric—confusion, hallucination, depression
Reproductive, Female—leukorrhea, vaginitis, [perineal irritation/pain]
Reproductive, Male—[balanoposthitis]
Respiratory—pharyngitis, pulmonary edema, bronchospasm, coughing, [atelectasis, dyspnea, hypoxia]
Skin and Appendages—genital pruritus, diaphoresis, [conjunctivitis, xerosis]
Special senses—taste perversion
Urinary—retention, dysuria, oliguria, hematuria, incontinence, [urinary tract infection with trichomonas, yeast in urine]
Vision—photophobia
Vascular (extracardiac)—flushing, [cerebrovascular accident]

Additional adverse events reported from worldwide marketing experience with Zosyn, occurring under circumstances where causal relationship to Zosyn is uncertain:

Gastrointestinal—hepatitis, cholestatic jaundice
Hematologic—hemolytic anemia
Renal—rarely, interstitial nephritis
Skin and Appendages—erythema multiforme and Stevens-Johnson syndrome, rarely reported

Adverse Laboratory Events (Seen During Clinical Trials)

Of the studies reported, including that of nosocomial lower respiratory tract infections in which a higher dose of Zosyn was used in combination with an aminoglycoside, changes in laboratory parameters, without regard to drug relationship, include:

Hematologic—decreases in hemoglobin and hematocrit, thrombocytopenia, increases in platelet count, eosinophilia, leukopenia, neutropenia

The leukopenia/neutropenia associated with Zosyn administration appears to be reversible and most frequently associated with prolonged administration, i.e., ≥21 days of therapy. These patients were withdrawn from therapy; some had accompanying systemic symptoms (e.g., fever, rigors, chills).

Coagulation—positive direct Coombs' test, prolonged prothrombin time, prolonged partial thromboplastin time
Hepatic—transient elevations of AST (SGOT), ALT (SGPT), alkaline phosphatase, bilirubin
Renal—increases in serum creatinine, blood urea nitrogen
Urinalysis—proteinuria, hematuria, pyuria

Additional laboratory events include abnormalities in electrolytes (i.e., increases and decreases in sodium, potassium and calcium), hyperglycemia, decreases in total protein or albumin.

The following adverse reaction has also been reported for PIPRACIL® (sterile piperacillin sodium):

Skeletal—prolonged muscle relaxation (See **PRECAUTIONS, Drug Interactions.**)

OVERDOSAGE

Information on overdosage of Zosyn in humans is not available.

Excessive serum levels of either piperacillin or tazobactam may be reduced by hemodialysis. (See **CLINICAL PHARMACOLOGY**.) No specific antidote is known. As with other penicillins, neuromuscular excitability or convulsions have occurred following large intravenous doses, primarily in patients with impaired renal function.

In the case of motor excitability or convulsions, general supportive measures, including administration of anticonvulsive agents (e.g., diazepam or barbiturates), may be considered.

DOSAGE AND ADMINISTRATION

Zosyn should be administered by intravenous infusion over 30 minutes.

Normal Renal Function (Creatinine Clearance ≥90 mL/min)

The usual daily dose of Zosyn for adults is 3.375 g every six hours totalling 13.5 g (12 g piperacillin sodium/1.5 g tazobactam sodium).

Initial presumptive treatment of patients with nosocomial pneumonia should start with Zosyn at a dosage of 3.375 g every 4 hours plus an aminoglycoside. Treatment with the aminoglycoside should be continued in patients from whom *Pseudomonas aeruginosa* is isolated. If *Pseudomonas aeruginosa* is not isolated, the aminoglycoside may be discontinued at the discretion of the treating physician. (See **DOSAGE AND ADMINISTRATION**.)

Zosyn should not be mixed with an aminoglycoside in a syringe or infusion bottle, since this can result in inactivation of the aminoglycoside. (See **PRECAUTIONS, Drug Interactions**.)

Renal Insufficiency

In patients with renal insufficiency (Creatinine Clearance <90 mL/min), the intravenous dose of Zosyn should be adjusted to the degree of actual renal function impairment. In patients with nosocomial pneumonia receiving concomitant aminoglycoside therapy, the aminoglycoside dosage should be adjusted according to the recommendations of the manufacturer. The recommended daily doses of Zosyn® for patients with renal insufficiency are as follows:

Zosyn Dosage Recommendations For All Indications Including Nosocomial Pneumonia

Creatinine Clearance (mL/min)	Recommended Dosage Regimen
>40–90	12 g/1.5 g/day in divided doses of 3.375 g q 6h
20–40	8 g/1.0 g/day in divided doses of 2.25 g q 6h
<20	6 g/0.75 g/day in divided doses of 2.25 g q 8h

For patients on hemodialysis, irrespective of the condition under treatment, the maximum dose is 2.25 g Zosyn every eight hours. In addition, because hemodialysis removes 30% to 40% of a piperacillin/tazobactam dose in four hours, one additional dose of 0.75 g Zosyn should be administered following each dialysis period. For patients with renal failure, measurement of serum levels of piperacillin and tazobactam will provide additional guidance for adjusting dosage.

Duration of Therapy

The usual duration of Zosyn treatment is from seven to ten days. However, the recommended duration of Zosyn treatment of nosocomial pneumonia is seven to fourteen days. In all conditions, the duration of therapy should be guided by the severity of the infection and the patient's clinical and bacteriological progress.

DIRECTIONS FOR USE OF ZOSYN (PIPERACILLIN SODIUM AND TAZOBACTAM SODIUM INJECTION) IN GALAXY® CONTAINERS (PL 2040 PLASTIC)

Zosyn Injection in Galaxy® Container (PL 2040 Plastic) is to be administered after thawing to room temperature using sterile equipment.

Administer by infusion over a period of at least 30 minutes. During the infusion it is desirable to discontinue the primary infusion solution.

STORAGE

Store in a freezer capable of maintaining a temperature of -20°C (-4°F).

THAWING OF PLASTIC CONTAINER

Thaw frozen container at room temperature 20°–25°C [68°–77°F] or under refrigeration (5°C or 41°F). **DO NOT FORCE THAW BY IMMERSION IN WATER BATHS OR BY MICROWAVE IRRADIATION.**

Check for minute leaks by squeezing container firmly. If leaks are detected, discard solution as sterility may be impaired.

The container should be visually inspected. Components of the solution may precipitate in the frozen state and will dissolve upon reaching room temperature with little or no agitation. Potency is not affected. Agitate after solution has reached room temperature. If after visual inspection the solution remains cloudy or if an insoluble precipitate is noted or if any seals or outlet ports are not intact, the container should be discarded.

The thawed solution is stable for 14 days under refrigeration (5°C or 41°F) or 24 hours at room temperature 20°–25°C [68°–77°F]. **DO NOT REFREEZE THAWED ANTIBIOTICS.**

DO NOT ADD SUPPLEMENTARY MEDICATION.

UNUSED PORTIONS OF ZOSYN SHOULD BE DISCARDED.

CAUTION: Do not use plastic containers in series connections. Such use could result in air embolism due to residual air being drawn from the primary container before administration of the fluid from the secondary container is complete.

Preparation for administration:

1. Suspend container from eyelet support.
2. Remove protector from outlet port at bottom of container.
3. Attach administration set. Refer to complete directions accompanying set.

Parenteral drug products should be inspected visually for particulate matter and discoloration prior to administration, whenever solution and container permit.

HOW SUPPLIED

Zosyn® (piperacillin sodium and tazobactam sodium injection) in Galaxy® Container (PL 2040 Plastic) is supplied as a frozen, iso-osmotic, sterile, nonpyrogenic solution in single-dose plastic container as follows:

2.25 g (2 g piperacillin/0.25 g tazobactam) in 50 mL. Each container has 5.7 mEq (131 mg) of sodium. Supplied 24/box—NDC 0206-8820-02

3.375 g (3 g piperacillin/0.375 g tazobactam) in 50 mL. Each container has 8.6 mEq (197 mg) of sodium. Supplied 24/box—0206-8821-02

4.5 g (4 g piperacillin/0.5 g tazobactam) in 100 mL. Each container has 11.4 mEq (263 mg) of sodium. Supplied 12/box—0206-8822-02

Store at or below -20°C (-4°F). [See **DOSAGE AND ADMINISTRATION, Direction for Use of Zosyn (piperacillin sodium and tazobactam sodium injection) in Galaxy® Container (PL 2040 Plastic).**]

Also Available

Zosyn (sterile piperacillin sodium and tazobactam sodium) is also supplied as follows:

2.25 g single-dose vial containing 2 g of piperacillin and 0.25 g of tazobactam. Each vial contains 4.69 mEq (108 mg) of sodium. Supplied 10/box—NDC 0206-8452-16

3.375 g single-dose vial containing 3 g of piperacillin and 0.375 g of tazobactam. Each vial contains 7.04 mEq (162 mg) of sodium. Supplied 10/box—NDC 0206-8454-55

4.5 g single-dose vial containing 4 g of piperacillin and 0.5 g of tazobactam. Each vial contains 9.39 mEq (216 mg) of sodium. Supplied 10/box—NDC 0206-8455-25

Zosyn is also supplied in the ADD-Vantage® Vial as follows:

2.25 g ADD-Vantage® vial (2 g piperacillin and 0.25 g of tazobactam). Each ADD-Vantage® vial contains 4.69 mEq (108 mg) of sodium. Supplied 10/box—NDC 0206-8452-17

3.375 g ADD-Vantage® vial (3 g piperacillin and 0.375 g of tazobactam). Each ADD-Vantage® vial contains 7.04 mEq (162 mg) of sodium. Supplied 10/box—NDC 0206-8454-17

4.5 g ADD-Vantage® vial (4 g piperacillin and 0.5 g of tazobactam). Each ADD-Vantage® vial contains 9.39 mEq (216 mg) of sodium. Supplied 10/box—NDC 0206-8455-17

Also Available

Zosyn is also supplied as follows:

40.5 g pharmacy-bulk vial containing 36 grams of piperacillin and 4.5 grams of tazobactam. Each pharmacy-bulk vial contains 84.5 mEq (1,944 mg) of sodium. NDC 0206-8620-11

Zosyn vials should be stored at controlled room temperature 15° to 30°C (59° to 86°F) prior to reconstitution.

REFERENCES

1. National Committee for Clinical Laboratory Standards. Methods for Dilution Antimicrobial Susceptibility Tests for Bacteria that Grow Aerobically—Fourth Edition. Approved Standard NCCLS Document M7-A4, Vol. 17, No. 2, NCCLS, Wayne, PA, January, 1997.
2. National Committee for Clinical Laboratory Standards. Methods for Antimicrobial Susceptibility Testing for Anaerobic Bacteria—Third Edition. Approved Standard NCCLS Document M11-A3, Vol. 13, No. 26, NCCLS, Villanova, PA, December, 1993.
3. National Committee for Clinical Laboratory Standards. Performance Standard for Antimicrobial Disk Susceptibility Tests—Sixth Edition. Approved Standard NCCLS Document M2-A6, Vol. 17, No. 1, NCCLS, Wayne, PA, January, 1997.
4. Halstenson, CE, Hirata CAI, Heim-Duthoy KL, Abraham PA, and Matzke GR. Effect of concomitant administration of piperacillin on the dispositions of netilmicin

and tobramycin in patients with end-stage renal disease. Antimicrob. Agents Chemother. 34(1):128–133, 1990.

CLINITEST® and DIASTIX® are registered trademarks of Ames Division, Miles Laboratories, Inc.
TES-TAPE® is a registered trademark of Eli Lilly and Company.
Galaxy® is a registered trademark of Baxter International, Inc.
ADD-Vantage® is a registered trademark of Abbott Laboratories.
Manufactured for Lederle Piperacillin Inc.
by Baxter Healthcare Corporation, Deerfield, IL 60015
CI 5029-4 Revised April 5, 1999

Shown in Product Identification Guide, page 321

ZOSYN® ℞
(Sterile Piperacillin Sodium and Tazobactam Sodium)

Pharmacy Bulk Package
Not for Direct Infusion

RECONSTITUTED STOCK SOLUTION MUST BE TRANSFERRED AND FURTHER DILUTED FOR I.V. INFUSION

DESCRIPTION

Package
The PHARMACY BULK VIAL is a container of sterile preparation which contains many single doses for parenteral use. The contents are intended for use in a pharmacy admixture program and are restricted to the preparation of admixtures for intravenous infusion.

Product Description
ZOSYN is an injectable antibacterial combination product consisting of the semisynthetic antibiotic piperacillin sodium and the β-lactamase inhibitor tazobactam sodium for intravenous administration.
Piperacillin sodium is derived from D(-)-α-aminobenzyl-penicillin. The chemical name of piperacillin sodium is sodium (2*S*, 5*R*, 6*R*)-6-[(*R*)-2-(4-ethyl-2,3-dioxo -1- piperazine-carboxamido)-2-phenylacetamido]-3,3-dimethyl-7-oxo-4-thia-1-azabicyclo[3.2.0]heptane-2-carboxylate. The chemical formula is $C_{23}H_{26}N_5NaO_7S$ and the molecular weight is 539.5.
Tazobactam sodium, a derivative of the penicillin nucleus, is a penicillanic acid sulfone. Its chemical name is sodium (2*S*, 3*S*, 5*R*)-3-methyl-7-oxo-3-(1*H*-1, 2, 3-triazol-1-ylmethyl)-4-thia-1-azabicyclo[3.2.0]heptane-2-carboxylate-4, 4-dioxide. The chemical formula is $C_{10}H_{11}N_4NaO_5S$ and the molecular weight is 322.3.
ZOSYN, piperacillin/tazobactam parenteral combination, is a white to off-white sterile, cryodesiccated powder consisting of piperacillin and tazobactam as their sodium salts packaged in glass vials. The product does not contain excipients or preservatives.
Each ZOSYN 40.5 g pharmacy bulk vial contains piperacillin sodium equivalent to 36 grams of piperacillin and tazobactam sodium equivalent to 4.5 g of tazobactam sufficient for delivery of multiple doses.
ZOSYN is a monosodium salt of piperacillin and a monosodium salt of tazobactam containing a total of 2.35 mEq (54 mg) of Na^+ per gram of piperacillin in the combination product.

HOW SUPPLIED

ZOSYN® (sterile piperacillin sodium and tazobactam sodium) is supplied as a powder in the pharmacy bulk vial as follows:
Each ZOSYN 40.5 g pharmacy bulk vial contains piperacillin sodium equivalent to 36 grams of piperacillin and tazobactam sodium equivalent to 4.5 grams tazobactam. Each pharmacy bulk vial contains 84.5 mEq (1,944 mg) of sodium.
NDC 0206-8620-11
ZOSYN pharmacy bulk vials should be stored at controlled room temperature 20° to 25°C (68° to 77°F) prior to reconstitution.

Also Available
Zosyn (sterile piperacillin sodium and tazobactam sodium) is also supplied as follows:
2.25 g single-dose vial containing 2 g of piperacillin and 0.25 g of tazobactam. Each vial contains 4.69 mEq (108 mg) of sodium. Supplied 10/box—NDC 0206-8452-16
3.375 g single-dose vial containing 3 g of piperacillin and 0.375 g of tazobactam. Each vial contains 7.04 mEq (162 mg) of sodium. Supplied 10/box—NDC 0206-8454-55
4.5 g single-dose vial containing 4 g of piperacillin and 0.5 g of tazobactam. Each vial contains 9.39 mEq (216 mg) of sodium. Supplied 10/box—NDC 0206-8455-25
Zosyn is also supplied in the ADD-Vantage® Vial as follows:
2.25 g ADD-Vantage® vial (2 g piperacillin and 0.25 g of tazobactam). Each ADD-Vantage® vial contains 4.69 mEq (108 mg) of sodium. Supplied 10/box—NDC 0206-8452-17
3.375 g ADD-Vantage® vial (3 g piperacillin and 0.375 g of tazobactam). Each ADD-Vantage® vial contains 7.04 mEq (162 mg) of sodium. Supplied 10/box—NDC 0206-8454-17
4.5 g ADD-Vantage® vial (4 g piperacillin and 0.5 g of tazobactam). Each ADD-Vantage® vial contains 9.39 mEq (216 mg) of sodium. Supplied 10/box—NDC 0206-8455-17

Also Available
Zosyn (piperacillin sodium and tazobactam sodium injection) is Galaxy® Container (PL 2040 Plastic) is supplied as a frozen, iso-osmotic, sterile, nonpyrogenic solution in single-dose plastic containers as follows:
2.25 g (2 g piperacillin/0.25 g tazobactam) in 50 mL. Each container has 5.7 mEq (131 mg) of sodium. Supplied 24/box—NDC 0206-8820-02
3.375 g (3 g piperacillin/0.375 g tazobactam) in 50 mL. Each container has 8.6 mEq (197 mg) of sodium. Supplied 24/box—NDC 0206-8821-02
4.5 g (4g piperacillin/0.5 g tazobactam) in 100 mL. Each container has 11.4 mEq (263 mg) of sodium. Supplied 12/box—NDC 0206-8822-02
For prescribing information write to Professional Service, Wyeth-Ayerst Pharmaceuticals, P.O. Box 8299, Philadelphia, PA 19101.

Shown in Product Identification Guide, page 321

Lederle Standard Products

Pearl River, NY 10965

The following list of Lederle Standard Products includes the alphanumeric LEDERMARK® codes which provide quick and positive identification of Lederle Standard Products capsules and tablets:

Product Identity Code No.	Product
A3	Tetracycline HCl Capsules, 250mg
A5	Tetracycline HCl Capsules, 500mg
A7	Atenolol Tablets, 25mg
A45	Albuterol Sulfate Tablets, 2mg
A46	Albuterol Sulfate Tablets, 4mg
A49	Atenolol Tablets, 50mg
A51	Alprazolam Tablets, USP, 0.25mg
A52	Alprazolam Tablets, USP, 0.5mg
A53	Alprazolam Tablets, USP, 1mg
A71	Atenolol Tablets, 100mg
C42	Clonidine HCl Tablets, USP, 0.1mg
C43	Clonidine HCl Tablets, USP, 0.2mg
C44	Clonidine HCl Tablets, USP, 0.3mg
CB300	Cimetidine Tablets, USP, 300mg
D44	Dipyridamole Tablets, 25mg
D45	Dipyridamole Tablets, 50mg
D46	Dipyridamole Tablets, 75mg
D51	Diazepam Tablets, USP, 2mg
D52	Diazepam Tablets, USP, 5mg
D53	Diazepam Tablets, USP, 10mg
D71	Diltiazem HCl Tablets, 30mg
D72	Diltiazem HCl Tablets, 60mg
D75	Diltiazem HCl Tablets, 90mg
D77	Diltiazem HCl Tablets, 120mg
—	Erythromycin Ethylsuccinate/Sulfisoxazole Acetyl for Oral Suspension, 200mg/600mg/5mL
—	Sterile Erythromycin Lactobionate for Injection, USP, 500mg/5 x 10mL vials
—	Sterile Erythromycin Lactobionate for Injection, USP, 1g/5 x 20mL vials
—	Folic Acid Injection, USP, 5mg/mL
F22	Fenoprofen Calcium Tablets, USP, 600mg
H11	Hydralazine HCl Tablets, USP, 25mg
H12	Hydralazine HCl Tablets, USP, 50mg
H14	Hydrochlorothiazide Tablets, USP, 25mg
H15	Hydrochlorothiazide Tablets, USP, 50mg
J1	Methazolamide Tablets, USP, 25mg
J2	Methazolamide Tablets, USP, 50mg
K1	Ketoprofen Capsules, 25mg
K2	Ketoprofen Capsules, 50mg
K3	Ketoprofen Capsules, 75mg
M20	Methocarbamol Tablets, USP, 750mg
M22	Methyldopa Tablets, USP, 250mg
M23	Methyldopa Tablets, USP, 500mg
N11	Naproxen Tablets, USP, 250mg
N17	Naproxen Tablets, USP, 375mg
N77	Naproxen Tablets, USP, 500mg
—	Nystatin Oral Suspension, 100,000 units/mL
P33	Propylthiouracil Tablets, USP, 50mg
P36	Pyrazinamide Tablets, 500mg
P69	Prazosin HCl Capsules, USP, 1mg
P70	Prazosin HCl Capsules, USP, 2mg
P71	Prazosin HCl Capsules, USP, 5mg
Q11	Quinidine Sulfate Tablets, USP, 200mg
S16	Sulindac Tablets, USP, 150mg
S17	Sulindac Tablets, USP, 200mg
T13	Sulfamethoxazole and Trimethoprim Tablets, USP, 400mg/80mg
—	Tobramycin Sulfate Injection, USP, 40mg/mL
—	Vancomycin HCl, USP, 500mg vial
—	Vancomycin HCl, USP, 1g vial
—	Vancomycin HCl, USP, 5g vial

Shown in Product Identification Guide, page 321

Ligand Pharmaceuticals Incorporated

10275 SCIENCE CENTER DRIVE
SAN DIEGO, CA 92121

Direct Inquiries to:
(858) 550-7500
Customer Service
(877) 454-4263
Medical Information
(800) 964-5836
Reimbursement Support
(877) 654-4263

ONTAK™ ℞
[*ŏn-tăck*]
(denileukin diftitox)

WARNING: Only physicians experienced in the use of antineoplastic therapy and management of patients with cancer should use ONTAK (denileukin diftitox). Patients treated with denileukin diftitox must be managed in a facility equipped and staffed for cardiopulmonary resuscitation and where the patient can be closely monitored for an appropriate period based on his or her health status.

DESCRIPTION

ONTAK™ (denileukin diftitox), a recombinant DNA-derived cytotoxic protein composed of the amino acid sequences for diphtheria toxin fragments A and B (Met_1-Thr_{387})-His followed by the sequences for interleukin-2 (IL-2; Ala_1-Thr_{133}), is produced in an *E. coli* expression system. ONTAK has a molecular weight of 58 kD. Neomycin is used in the fermentation process but is undetectable in the final product. The product is purified using reverse phase chromatography followed by a multistep diafiltration process.
ONTAK is supplied in single use vials as a sterile, frozen solution intended for intravenous (IV) administration. Each 2 mL vial of ONTAK contains 300 mcg of recombinant denileukin diftitox in a sterile solution of citric acid (20 mM), EDTA (0.05 mM) and polysorbate 20 (<1%) in Water for Injection, USP. The solution has a pH of 6.9 to 7.2.

CLINICAL PHARMACOLOGY

General: Denileukin diftitox is a fusion protein designed to direct the cytocidal action of diphtheria toxin to cells which express the IL-2 receptor. The human IL-2 receptor exists in three forms, low (CD25), intermediate (CD122/CD132) and high (CD25/CD122/CD132) affinity. The high affinity form of this receptor is usually found only on activated T lymphocytes, activated B lymphocytes and activated macrophages. Malignant cells expressing one or more of the subunits of the IL-2 receptor are found in certain leukemias and lymphomas including cutaneous T-cell lymphoma (CTCL)[1]. *Ex vivo* studies suggest that denileukin diftitox interacts with the high affinity IL-2 receptor on the cell surface and inhibits cellular protein synthesis, resulting in cell death within hours.
The biodistribution and excretion of radiolabeled denileukin diftitox were evaluated over 48 hours in rats. The liver and kidneys were the primary sites of distribution and accumulation of radiolabeled material outside of the vasculature. Denileukin diftitox was metabolized by proteolytic degradation. Excreted material was less than 25% of the total injected dose and consisted of low molecular weight breakdown products.
Pharmacokinetics: Pharmacokinetic parameters associated with denileukin diftitox were determined over a range of doses (3 to 31 mcg/kg/day) in patients with lymphoma. Denileukin diftitox was administered as an IV infusion following the schedule used in the clinical trials. Following the first dose, denileukin diftitox displayed 2-compartment behavior with a distribution phase (half-life approximately 2 to 5 minutes) and a terminal phase (half-life approximately 70 to 80 minutes). Systemic exposure was variable but proportional to dose. Clearance was approximately 1.5 to 2.0 mL/min/kg and the volume of distribution was similar to that of circulating blood (0.06 to 0.08 L/kg). No accumulation was evident between the first and fifth doses. Development of antibodies to denileukin diftitox has been shown to significantly impact clearance rates (see **CLINICAL STUDIES,** Immunogenicity). Gender, age, and race were introduced into a multivariate analysis with various pharmacokinetic parameters. The limited available data revealed no statistical relationships between these variables.

CLINICAL STUDIES

A randomized, double-blind study was conducted to evaluate doses of 9 or 18 mcg/kg/day in 71 patients with recurrent or persistent, Stage Ib to IVa CTCL. Entry to this study required demonstration of CD25 expression on at least 20% of the cells in any relevant tumor tissue sample (skin biopsy) or circulating cells. Tumor biopsies were not evaluated for expression of other IL-2 receptor subunit components (CD122/CD132). ONTAK was administered as an IV infu-

Continued on next page

Ontak—Cont.

sion daily for 5 days every 3 weeks. Patients received a median of 6 courses of ONTAK therapy (range 1 to 11). The study population had received a median of 5 prior therapies (range 1 to 12) with 63% of patients entering the trial with Stage IIb or more advanced stage disease. Overall, 30% (95% CI: 18–41%) of patients treated with ONTAK experienced an objective tumor response (50% reduction in tumor burden which was sustained for ≥ 6 weeks; Table 1). Seven patients (10%) achieved a complete response and 14 patients (20%) achieved a partial response. The overall median duration of response, measured from first day of response, was 4 months with a median duration for complete response of 9 months and for partial response of 4 months. In a Phase I/II dose-escalation study, 35 patients with Stage Ia to IVb CTCL were treated. ONTAK was administered as an IV infusion at doses ranging from 3 to 31 mcg/kg/day, daily for 5 days every 3 weeks. The overall response rate in patients with CTCL who expressed CD25 was 38% (12 of 32 patients); the complete response rate was 16% and the partial response rate was 22%. There were no responses in 21 patients with Hodgkin's Disease.

Table 1
Response in the Phase III Double-Blind Study
Patients with CTCL

Clinical Response	9 mcg/kg/day N = 35	18 mcg/kg/day N = 36
Complete Response	3 (9%)	4 (11%)
95% Confidence Interval	2 – 23%	3 – 26%
Partial Response	5 (14%)	9 (25%)
95% Confidence Interval	5 – 30%	12 – 42%
Overall Response	8 (23%)	13 (36%)
95% Confidence Interval	10 – 40%	21 – 54%

Immunogenicity: Prior to therapy, 39% (51/131) of lymphoma patients had low titers (<1:5) of antibody which cross-reacted with the diphtheria toxin domains of denileukin diftitox, presumably due to prior diphtheria immunization. Development of anti-denileukin diftitox antibodies was observed in 41/49 patients after a single course and in 33/34 patients after 3 cycles. Following anti-denileukin diftitox antibody formation, there was a significant increase (two to threefold) in clearance, which resulted in a decrease in mean systemic exposure of approximately 75%. Changes in clearance were related to the development of antibodies.

The antibody response in all such patients was directed against the diphtheria toxin domain. A low titer of antibodies to the IL-2 portion of the denileukin diftitox molecule also developed in approximately 50% of patients. The presence or absence of antibodies did not correlate with the risk of immediate hypersensitivity-type infusional adverse events.

INDICATIONS

ONTAK is indicated for the treatment of patients with persistent or recurrent cutaneous T-cell lymphoma whose malignant cells express the CD25 component of the IL-2 receptor (See **PRECAUTIONS**, Laboratory Tests, for CD25 expression testing). The safety and efficacy of denileukin diftitox in patients with CTCL whose malignant cells do not express the CD25 component of the IL-2 receptor have not been examined.

CONTRAINDICATIONS

ONTAK is contraindicated for use in patients with a known hypersensitivity to denileukin diftitox or any of its components: diphtheria toxin, interleukin-2, or excipients.

WARNINGS

Acute Hypersensitivity-type Reactions: Acute hypersensitivity reactions were reported in 98 of 143 patients (69%) during or within 24 hours of ONTAK infusion; approximately half of the events occurred on the first day of dosing regardless of the treatment cycle. The constellation of symptoms included one or more of the following, defined as the incidence (%) in these 98 patients: hypotension (50%), back pain (30%), dyspnea (28%) vasodilation (28%), rash (25%), chest pain or tightness (24%), tachycardia (12%), dysphagia or laryngismus (5%), syncope (3%), allergic reaction (1%) or anaphylaxis (1%). These events were severe in 2% of patients. Management consists of interruption or a decrease in the rate of infusion (depending on the severity of the reaction); 3% of infusions were terminated prematurely and reduction in rate occurred in 4% of the infusions during the clinical trials. The administration of IV antihistamines, corticosteroids, and epinephrine may also be required; two subjects received epinephrine and 18 (13%) received systemic corticosteroids in the clinical studies. These drugs and resuscitative equipment should be readily available during ONTAK administration.

Vascular Leak Syndrome: This syndrome, characterized by 2 or more of the following 3 symptoms (hypotension, edema, hypoalbuminemia) was reported in 27% (38/143) of patients in the clinical studies. Six percent (8/143) of patients were hospitalized for the management of these symptoms. The onset of symptoms in patients with vascular leak syndrome was delayed, usually occurring within the first two weeks of infusion and may persist or worsen after the cessation of denileukin diftitox. Special caution should be taken in patients with preexisting cardiovascular disease. (See **ADVERSE REACTIONS**, Cardiovascular System). Weight, edema, blood pressure and serum albumin levels should be carefully monitored on an outpatient basis. This syndrome is usually self-limited and treatment should be used only if clinically indicated. The type of treatment will depend on whether edema or hypotension is the primary clinical problem. Pre-existing low serum albumin levels appear to predict and may predispose patients to the syndrome (See **PRECAUTIONS**, Laboratory Tests).

PRECAUTIONS

General: Patients should be monitored carefully for infection since patients with CTCL have a predisposition to cutaneous infection. Also, the binding of denileukin diftitox to activated lymphocytes and macrophages can lead to cell death and may impair immune function in patients.

Laboratory Tests: Prior to administration of this product, the patient's malignant cells should be tested for CD25 expression. A testing service for the assay of CD25 on skin biopsy samples is available. For information on this service call 800-964-5836.

A complete blood count and a blood chemistry panel, including liver and renal function and serum albumin levels, should be performed prior to initiation of ONTAK treatment and weekly during therapy.

Eighty-three percent (118/143) of patients with lymphoma experienced hypoalbuminemia, which was considered moderate or severe in 17% (20/118) of the affected patients. For most patients, the nadir for hypoalbuminemia occurs one to two weeks after ONTAK administration. Serum albumin levels should be monitored prior to the initiation of each treatment course. Administration of ONTAK should be delayed until serum albumin levels are at least 3.0 g/dL (see **WARNINGS**).

Drug Interactions: No clinical drug interaction studies have been conducted. However, in a single *in vivo* rodent study denileukin diftitox had no effect on P450 levels.

Carcinogenesis, Mutagenesis, Impairment of Fertility: There have been no studies to assess the carcinogenic potential of denileukin diftitox. Denileukin diftitox showed no evidence of mutagenicity in the Ames test and the chromosomal aberration assay. There have been no studies to assess the effect of denileukin diftitox on fertility.

Pregnancy Category C: Animal reproduction studies have not been conducted with ONTAK. It is also not known whether ONTAK can cause fetal harm when administered to a pregnant woman or affect reproductive capacity. ONTAK should be given to a pregnant woman only if clearly needed.

Nursing Mothers: It is not known whether this drug is excreted in human milk. Because many drugs are excreted in human milk, and because of the potential for serious adverse reactions in nursing infants, patients receiving ONTAK should discontinue nursing.

Pediatric Use: Safety and effectiveness in pediatric patients have not been established.

Geriatric Use: Forty-nine percent (35/71) of the patients enrolled in the randomized two dose study were 65 years of age or older, and those patients had response rates similar to those seen in younger patients. The following adverse events (regardless of causality) tended to be more frequent and/or more severe in lymphoma patients who were 65 years of age or older: anorexia, hypotension, anemia, confusion, rash, nausea and/or vomiting.

ADVERSE REACTIONS

Adverse reactions are presented in Table 2. These data are based on adverse reactions observed in two clinical studies of 143 patients with lymphoma, including 105 patients with CTCL, treated at doses ranging from 3 to 31 mcg/kg/day.

All patients experienced one or more adverse events. Twenty-one percent of patients required hospitalization for drug-related adverse events; the most common reasons were evaluation of fever, management of vascular leak syndrome or dehydration secondary to gastrointestinal toxicity. Five percent of clinical adverse reactions were severe or life-threatening. The occurrence of adverse events tended to diminish in frequency after the first two courses, possibly related to antibody development.

Table 2
Adverse Reactions Occurring in
Lymphoma Patients
(Frequency ≥ 5% of Patients)
N = 143 patients

Body System	Combined Term	All Grades n (%)	Grades 3 and 4 n (%)
Body as a Whole			
	Chills/fever	116 (81)	31 (22)
	Asthenia	95 (66)	31 (22)
	Infection	69 (48)	34 (24)
	Pain	69 (48)	19 (13)
	Headache	37 (26)	5 (3)
	Chest pain	34 (24)	8 (6)
	Flu-like syndrome	11 (8)	0
	Injection site reaction	11 (8)	1 (1)
Cardiovascular			
	Hypotension	52 (36)	11 (8)
	Vasodilation	31 (22)	1 (1)
	Tachycardia	17 (12)	2 (1)
	Thrombotic events	10 (7)	6 (4)
	Hypertension	9 (6)	0
	Arrhythmia	8 (6)	5 (3)
Digestive			
	Nausea/vomiting	91 (64)	20 (14)
	Anorexia	51 (36)	12 (8)
	Diarrhea	42 (29)	5 (3)
	Constipation	13 (9)	2 (1)
	Dyspepsia	10 (7)	0
	Dysphagia	9 (6)	2 (1)
Hematologic and Lymphatic			
	Anemia	26 (18)	9 (6)
	Thrombocytopenia	12 (8)	3 (2)
	Leukopenia	9 (6)	4 (3)
Metabolic and Nutritional			
	Hypoalbuminemia	118 (83)	20 (14)
	Transaminase increase	87 (61)	22 (15)
	Edema	67 (47)	22 (15)
	Hypocalcemia	24 (17)	4 (3)
	Weight decrease	20 (14)	6 (4)
	Dehydration	13 (9)	10 (7)
	Hypokalemia	9 (6)	0
Musculoskeletal			
	Myalgia	25 (17)	3 (2)
	Arthralgia	11 (8)	2 (1)
Nervous			
	Dizziness	31 (22)	1 (1)
	Paresthesia	19 (13)	2 (1)
	Nervousness	16 (11)	2 (1)
	Confusion	11 (8)	8 (6)
	Insomnia	13 (9)	4 (3)
Respiratory			
	Dyspnea	42 (29)	20 (14)
	Cough increase	37 (26)	3 (2)
	Pharyngitis	25 (17)	0
	Rhinitis	19 (13)	2 (1)
	Lung disorder	11 (8)	0
Skin and Appendages			
	Rash	48 (34)	18 (13)
	Pruritus	29 (20)	5 (3)
	Sweating	15 (10)	1 (1)
Urogenital			
	Hematuria	15 (10)	5 (3)
	Albuminuria	14 (10)	1 (1)
	Pyuria	14 (10)	1 (1)
	Creatinine increase	10 (7)	1 (1)

Hypersensitivity: (see **WARNINGS**)

Vascular Leak Syndrome: (see **WARNINGS**)

Hypoalbuminemia: (see **PRECAUTIONS**, Laboratory tests)

Infectious Complications: Infections of various types were reported by 48% (69/143) of the study population, of which 23% (16/69) were considered severe. Six of the 143 patients (4%) discontinued ONTAK therapy because of infections.

Decreased lymphocyte counts (<900 cells/µL) occurred in 34% of lymphoma patients. In general, lymphocyte counts dropped during the dosing period (Days 1 to 5) and then returned to normal by Day 15. Smaller changes and more rapid recoveries were observed with subsequent courses.

Infusion-associated Reactions: (see **WARNINGS**) There are two distinct clinical syndromes associated with ONTAK infusion, an acute hypersensitivity-type symptom complex and a flu-like symptom complex. Overall, 69% of patients had infusion-related, hypersensitivity-type symptoms; for additional information, see **WARNINGS**. A flu-like syndrome was experienced by 91% of patients within several hours to days after ONTAK infusion. The symptom complex consists of one or more of the following: fever and/or chills (81%), asthenia (66%), digestive (64%), myalgias (18%) and arthralgias (8%). In the majority of patients, these symptoms were mild to moderate and responded to treatment with antipyretics and/or anti-emetics. Antipyretics and/or anti-emetics were used to relieve flu-like symptoms; however, the usefulness of these agents in ameliorating these toxicities or as prophylactic agents to decrease the incidence of the acute, flu-like toxicities has not b[illegible] prospectively studied.

Gastrointestinal: The onset of diarrhea may be delayed and the duration can be prolonged. Dehydration, usually concurrent with vomiting or anorexia, occurred in 9% of the patients. The majority of transient hepatic transaminase elevations occurred during the first course of ONTAK, were self-limited and resolved within two weeks.

Rash: A variety of rashes were reported, including generalized maculopapular, petechial, vesicular bullous, urticarial and/or eczematous with both acute and delayed onset. Antihistamines may be effective in relieving the symptoms, but more severe rashes may require the use of topical and/or oral corticosteroids.

Cardiovascular System: Two patients, both of whom had known or suspected pre-existing coronary artery disease, sustained acute myocardial infarctions while on study. Ten additional patients (7%) experienced thrombotic events. Two patients with progressive disease and multiple medical problems experienced deep vein thrombosis. Another patient sustained a deep vein thrombosis and pulmonary embolus during hospitalization for management of congestive heart failure and vascular leak syndrome. One patient with a history of severe peripheral vascular disease sustained an arterial thrombosis. Six patients experienced less severe superficial thrombophlebitis. Thrombotic events were also observed in preclinical animal studies.

Infrequent Serious Adverse Events: The following serious adverse events occurred at an incidence of less than 5%: pancreatitis, acute renal insufficiency, microscopic hematuria, hyperthyroidism and hypothyroidism.

OVERDOSAGE

There is no clinical experience with accidental ONTAK overdosage and no known antidote. At a dose of 31 mcg/kg/day, the dose-limiting toxicities were moderate-to-severe nausea, vomiting, fever, chills and/or persistent asthenia. Doses greater than 31 mcg/kg/day have not been evaluated in humans. If overdose occurs, hepatic and renal function and overall fluid balance should be closely monitored.

DOSAGE AND ADMINISTRATION

ONTAK is for intravenous (IV) use only. The recommended treatment regimen (one treatment cycle) is 9 or 18 mcg/kg/day administered intravenously for five consecutive days every 21 days. ONTAK should be infused over at least 15 minutes. If infusional adverse reactions occur (see **ADVERSE REACTIONS**), the infusion should be discontinued or the rate should be reduced depending on the severity of the reaction. There is no clinical experience with prolonged infusion times (> 80 minutes).

The optimal duration of therapy has not been determined; however, only 2% (1/51) of patients who did not demonstrate at least a 25% decrease in tumor burden prior to the fourth course of treatment subsequently responded.

Special Handling:

- ONTAK must be brought to room temperature, up to 25° C (77°F), before preparing the dose. The vials may be thawed in the refrigerator at 2 to 8°C (36 to 46°F) for not more than 24 hours or at room temperature for 1 to 2 hours. **ONTAK MUST NOT BE HEATED.**
- The solution in the vial may be mixed by gentle swirling; DO NOT VIGOROUSLY SHAKE **ONTAK** SOLUTION.
- After thawing, a haze may be visible. This haze should clear when the solution is at room temperature.
- ONTAK solution must not be used unless the solution is clear, colorless and without visible particulate matter.
- **ONTAK MUST NOT BE REFROZEN.**

Preparation and Administration:

- USE APPROPRIATE ASEPTIC TECHNIQUE IN DILUTION AND ADMINISTRATION OF **ONTAK**.
- Prepare and hold diluted ONTAK in plastic syringes or soft plastic IV bags. DO NOT USE A GLASS CONTAINER because adsorption to glass may occur in the dilute state.
- The concentration of ONTAK must be at least 15 mcg/mL during all steps in the preparation of the solution for IV infusion. This is best accomplished by withdrawing the calculated dose from the vial(s) and injecting it into an empty IV infusion bag. FOR EACH **1** ML OF **ONTAK** FROM THE VIAL(S), NO MORE THAN **9** ML OF STERILE SALINE WITHOUT PRESERVATIVE SHOULD THEN BE ADDED TO THE **IV** BAG.
- The ONTAK dose should be infused over at least 15 minutes.
- **ONTAK** SHOULD NOT BE ADMINISTERED AS A BOLUS INJECTION.
- Do not physically mix ONTAK with other drugs.
- DO NOT ADMINISTER **ONTAK** THROUGH AN IN-LINE FILTER.
- Prepared solutions of ONTAK should be administered within 6 hours, using a syringe pump or IV infusion bag.
- Unused portions of ONTAK should be discarded immediately.

HOW SUPPLIED

ONTAK is supplied as:
150 mcg/mL sterile, frozen solution (300 mcg in 2 mL) in a sterile, single-use vial
NDC 64365-503-01, 6 vials in a package.
Store frozen at or below -10°C.

REFERENCES

1. Nakase K, Kita K, Nasu K, Ueda T, Tanaka I, Shirakawa S and Tsudo M. Differential expression of interleukin-2 receptor (α and β chain) in mature lymphoid neoplasms. Amer. J. Hematol. 1994; 46: 179–183.

Issued February 05, 1999
Manufactured by:
Seragen, Incorporated
Hopkinton, MA 01748
US License No. 1258
Distributed by:
Ligand Pharmaceuticals Incorporated
San Diego, CA 92121
PV 3271 UCP

PANRETIN® ℞

[*păn-rĕtĭn*]
(alitretinoin) gel 0.1%
(For topical use only)

DESCRIPTION

Panretin® gel 0.1% contains alitretinoin and is intended for topical application only. The chemical name is 9-*cis*-retinoic acid and the structural formula is as follows:

[See chemical structure at top of next column]

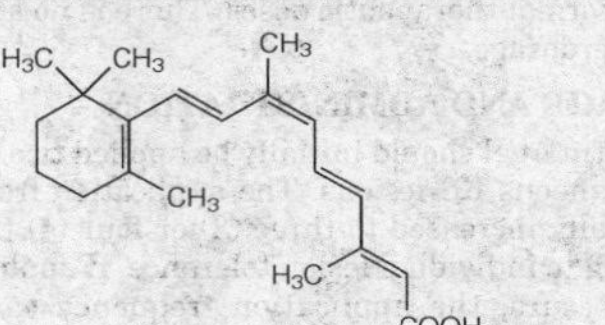

Chemically, alitretinoin is related to vitamin A. It is a yellow powder with a molecular weight of 300.44 and a molecular formula of $C_{20}H_{28}O_2$. It is slightly soluble in ethanol (7.01 mg/g at 25°C) and insoluble in water. Panretin® gel is a clear, yellow gel containing 0.1% (w/w) alitretinoin in a base of dehydrated alcohol USP, polyethylene glycol 400 NF, hydroxypropyl cellulose NF, and butylated hydroxytoluene NF.

CLINICAL PHARMACOLOGY

Mechanism of Action

Alitretinoin (9-*cis*-retinoic acid) is a naturally-occurring endogenous retinoid that binds to and activates all known intracellular retinoid receptor subtypes (RARα, RARβ, RARγ, RXRα, RXRβ and RXRγ). Once activated these receptors function as transcription factors that regulate the expression of genes that control the process of cellular differentiation and proliferation in both normal and neoplastic cells. Alitretinoin inhibits the growth of Kaposi's sarcoma (KS) cells in vitro.

Pharmacokinetics

No studies have examined plasma 9-*cis*-retinoic acid concentrations before and after treatment with Panretin® gel. There is, however, indirect evidence that absorption is not extensive. Plasma concentrations of 9-*cis*-retinoic acid were evaluated during clinical studies in patients with cutaneous lesions of AIDS-related KS after repeated multiple-daily dose application of Panretin® gel for up to 60 weeks. The range of 9-*cis*-retinoic acid plasma concentrations in these patients was similar to the range of circulating, naturally-occurring 9-*cis*-retinoic acid plasma concentrations in untreated healthy volunteers.

Although there are no detectable plasma concentrations of 9-*cis*-retinoic acid metabolites after topical application of Panretin® gel, in vitro studies indicate that the drug is metabolized to 4-hydroxy-9-*cis*-retinoic acid and 4-oxo-9-*cis*-retinoic acid by CYP 2C9, 3A4, 1A1, and 1A2 enzymes. In vivo, 4-oxo-9-*cis*-retinoic acid is the major circulating metabolite following oral administration of 9-*cis*-retinoic acid.

No formal pharmacokinetic drug interaction studies between Panretin® gel and antiretroviral agents have been conducted.

Clinical Studies

Panretin® gel is not a systemic therapy; it therefore cannot treat visceral Kaposi's sarcoma (KS) nor prevent the development of new KS lesions where it has not been applied. Visceral KS disease was not monitored in these trials, and the appearance of new KS lesions was not considered part of the response assessment in clinical trials.

Panretin® gel was evaluated in two multicenter, prospective, randomized, double-blind, vehicle-controlled studies in patients with cutaneous lesions of AIDS-related KS. In both studies the primary efficacy endpoint was the patients' cutaneous KS tumor response rate through 12 weeks of study drug treatment which was assessed by evaluating from 3 to 8 KS index lesions according to the modified AIDS Clinical Trials Group (ACTG) response criteria as applied to topical therapy (i.e., evaluation of height and area reductions of the index lesions only; progressive disease in non-index lesions and new lesions were not considered progressive disease; progressive disease was scored only in the treated index lesions). A global evaluation by physicians was also carried out. It considered all of the patient's treated lesions (index and other) compared to baseline. In this evaluation, patients with at least a 50% improvement in the KS lesions were considered responders. In addition, photographs of lesions in patients considered responders by the modified ACTG criteria were examined by the FDA for a cosmetically beneficial response, defined as at least a 50% improvement in appearance compared to baseline, considering both the KS lesions and dermal toxicity at the lesion site, in at least 50% of the index lesions and maintained for at least 3 weeks. Patients were also asked about their satisfaction with the treatment.

In Study 1, a total of 268 patients were entered from centers in the U.S. and Canada. Patients were treated topically three to four times a day with either Panretin® gel or a matching vehicle gel for a minimum of 12 weeks, followed by an open-label phase in patients who had not yet progressed on Panretin® gel. Responses during the double-blind phase are shown in Table 1. Responses to Panretin® gel were seen in both previously untreated patients and in patients with prior systemic and/or topical KS treatment. A total of 72 patients responded to Panretin® gel during the randomized or crossover portions of the study. At a median duration of monitoring of 16 weeks, only 15% of the 72 patients had relapsed. Panretin® gel would not be expected to affect development of new lesions in untreated areas and

TABLE 1: Summary of Tumor Responses

	STUDY 1		STUDY 2	
	Panretin® Gel N=134	Vehicle Gel N=134	Panretin® Gel N=36	Vehicle Gel N=46
Modified ACTG Response (index lesions)	34% PR 1% CR	16% PR p=0.0012	36% PR	7% PR
Physician's Global/ Subjective Assessment (all treated lesions)	19% PR	4% PR p=0.00014	47% PR	11% PR
Beneficial Response Photographs (index lesions only)	15%	4% p=0.0026	19%	2%

TABLE 2: Adverse Events with an Incidence of at Least 5% at the Application Site in Either Controlled Study in Patients Receiving Panretin® Gel or Vehicle Control

Adverse Event Term	Study 1		Study 2	
	Panretin® Gel N=134 Pts. %	Vehicle Gel N=134 Pts. %	Panretin® Gel N=36 Pts. %	Vehicle Gel N=46 Pts. %
Rash[1]	77	11	25	4
Pain[2]	34	7	0	4
Pruritus[3]	11	4	8	4
Exfoliative dermatitis[4]	9	2	3	0
Skin disorder[5]	8	1	0	0
Paresthesia[6]	3	0	22	7
Edema[7]	8	3	3	0

Includes Investigator terms:

1 Erythema, scaling, irritation, redness, rash, dermatitis
2 Burning, pain
3 Itching, pruritus
4 Flaking, peeling, desquamation, exfoliation
5 Excoriation, cracking, scab, crusting, drainage, eschar, fissure or oozing
6 Stinging, tingling
7 Edema, swelling, inflammation

Continued on next page

Panretin—Cont.

these were seen in about 50% of patients, at similar rates in treated and untreated patients, responders and non-responders. The patients' assessment of their overall satisfaction with the drug effect on all treated lesions significantly favored Panretin® gel.

Study 2 was an international study with a planned enrollment of 270 patients. Patients were treated topically twice a day with Panretin® gel or a matching vehicle for 12 weeks. The study was stopped early because of positive interim results in the initial 82 patient data set. Results of the study are shown in Table 1. Responses to Panretin® gel were seen both in previously untreated patients and in patients with prior systemic and/or topical KS treatment.

[See table 1 at top of previous page]

In the clinical trials, responses were seen as early as two (2) weeks; most patients, however, required four (4) to eight (8) weeks of treatment, and some patients did not experience significant improvement until 14 or more weeks of treatment. The cumulative percentage of patients who achieved a response was less than 1% at 2 weeks, 10% at 4 weeks, and 28% at 8 weeks.

In both studies, responses occurred in patients with a wide range of baseline CD4+ lymphocyte counts, including patients with CD4+ lymphocyte counts less than 50 cells/mm^3. Nearly all patients received concomitant combination antiretroviral therapy.

Photographs of patients revealed a substantial erythematous and edematous response in some cases, leading to a cosmetically mixed outcome even in apparent responders. Nonetheless, in Study 1 it appeared that a cosmetically satisfactory result occurred at about the same rate as the Physician's Global response rate and in both studies such a response was more frequent than in the vehicle control.

INDICATIONS AND USAGE

Panretin® gel is indicated for topical treatment of cutaneous lesions in patients with AIDS-related Kaposi's sarcoma. Panretin® gel is not indicated when systemic anti-KS therapy is required (e.g., more than 10 new KS lesions in the prior month, symptomatic lymphedema, symptomatic pulmonary KS, or symptomatic visceral involvement). There is no experience to date using Panretin® gel with systemic anti-KS treatment.

CONTRAINDICATIONS

Panretin® gel is contraindicated in patients with a known hypersensitivity to retinoids or to any of the ingredients of the product.

WARNINGS

Pregnancy: Panretin® gel could cause fetal harm if significant absorption were to occur in a pregnant woman. 9-*cis*-Retinoic acid has been shown to be teratogenic in rabbits and mice. An increased incidence of fused sternebrae and limb and craniofacial defects occurred in rabbits given oral doses of 0.5 mg/kg/day (about five times the estimated daily human topical dose on a mg/m^2 basis, assuming complete systemic absorption of 9-*cis*-retinoic acid, when Panretin® gel is administered as a 60 g tube over 1 month in a 60 kg human) during the period of organogenesis. Limb and craniofacial defects also occurred in mice given a single oral dose of 50 mg/kg on day eleven of gestation (about 127 times the estimated daily human topical dose on a mg/m^2 basis). Oral 9-*cis*-retinoic acid was also embryocidal, as indicated by early resorptions and post-implantation loss when it was given during the period of organogenesis to rabbits at doses of 1.5 mg/kg/day (about 15 times the estimated daily human topical dose on a mg/m^2 basis) and to rats at doses of 5 mg/kg/day (about 25 times the estimated daily human topical dose on a mg/m^2 basis). Animal reproduction studies with topical 9-*cis*-retinoic acid have not been conducted. It is not known whether topical Panretin® gel can modulate endogenous 9-*cis*-retinoic acid levels in a pregnant woman nor whether systemic exposure is increased by application to ulcerated lesions or by duration of treatment. There are no adequate and well-controlled studies in pregnant women. If Panretin® gel is used during pregnancy, or if the patient becomes pregnant while taking it, the patient should be apprised of the potential hazard to the fetus. Women of childbearing potential should be advised to avoid becoming pregnant.

PRECAUTIONS

Panretin® gel is indicated for topical treatment of Kaposi's sarcoma. Patients with cutaneous T-cell lymphoma were less tolerant of topical Panretin® gel; five of seven patients had 6 episodes of treatment-limiting toxicities—grade 3 dermal irritation—with Panretin® gel (0.01% or 0.05%).

Photosensitivity

Retinoids as a class have been associated with photosensitivity. There were no reports of photosensitivity associated with the use of Panretin® gel in the clinical studies. Nonetheless, because in vitro data indicate that 9-*cis*-retinoic acid may have a weak photosensitizing effect, patients should be advised to minimize exposure of treated areas to sunlight and sunlamps during the use of Panretin® gel.

Drug Interactions

Patients who are applying Panretin® gel should not concurrently use products that contain DEET (N,N-diethyl-m-toluamide), a common component of insect repellent products. Animal toxicology studies showed increased DEET toxicity when DEET was included as part of the formulation.

Although there was no clinical evidence in the vehicle-controlled studies of drug interactions with systemic antiretroviral agents, including protease inhibitors, macrolide antibiotics, and azole antifungals, the effect of Panretin® gel on the steady-state concentrations of these drugs is not known. No drug interaction data are available on concomitant administration of Panretin® gel and systemic anti-KS agents.

Drug/Laboratory Test Interactions

No interference with laboratory tests has been observed.

Carcinogenesis, Mutagenesis, Impairment of Fertility

Long-term studies in animals to assess the carcinogenic potential of 9-*cis*-retinoic acid have not been conducted. 9-*cis*-Retinoic acid was not mutagenic in vitro (bacterial assays, Chinese hamster ovary cell HGPRT mutation assay) and was not clastogenic in vitro (chromosome aberration test in human lymphocytes) nor in vivo (mouse micronucleus test).

Pregnancy Category D (see "Warnings" section)

Nursing Mothers

It is not known whether alitretinoin or its metabolites are excreted in human milk. Because many drugs are excreted in human milk and because of the potential for adverse reactions from Panretin® gel in nursing infants, mothers should discontinue nursing prior to using the drug.

Pediatric Use

Safety and effectiveness in pediatric patients have not been established.

Geriatric Use

Inadequate information is available to assess safety and efficacy in patients age 65 years or older.

ADVERSE REACTIONS

The safety of Panretin® gel has been assessed in clinical studies of 385 patients with AIDS-related KS. Adverse events associated with the use of Panretin® gel in patients with AIDS-related KS occurred almost exclusively at the site of application. The dermal toxicity begins as erythema; with continued application of Panretin® gel, erythema may increase and edema may develop. Dermal toxicity may become treatment-limiting, with intense erythema, edema, and vesiculation. Usually, however, adverse events are mild to moderate in severity; they led to withdrawal from the study in only 7% of the patients. Severe local (application site) skin adverse events occurred in about 10% of patients in the U.S. study (versus 0% in the vehicle control). Table 2 lists the adverse events that occurred at the application site with an incidence of at least 5% during the double-blind phase in the Panretin® gel-treated group and in the vehicle control group in either of the two controlled studies. Adverse events were reported at other sites but generally were similar in the two groups.

[See table 2 at top of previous page]

OVERDOSAGE

There has been no experience with acute overdose of Panretin® gel in humans. Systemic toxicity following acute overdosage with topical application of Panretin® gel is unlikely because of limited systemic plasma levels observed with normal therapeutic doses. There is no specific antidote for overdosage.

DOSAGE AND ADMINISTRATION

Panretin® gel should initially be applied two (2) times a day to cutaneous KS lesions. The application frequency can be gradually increased to three (3) or four (4) times a day according to individual lesion tolerance. If application site toxicity occurs, the application frequency can be reduced. Should severe irritation occur, application of drug can be temporarily discontinued for a few days until the symptoms subside.

Sufficient gel should be applied to cover the lesion with a generous coating. The gel should be allowed to dry for three to five minutes before covering with clothing. Because unaffected skin may become irritated, application of the gel to normal skin surrounding the lesions should be avoided. In addition, do not apply the gel on or near mucosal surfaces of the body.

A response of KS lesions may be seen as soon as two weeks after initiation of therapy but most patients require longer application. With continued application, further benefit may be attained. Some patients have required over 14 weeks to respond. In clinical trials, Panretin® gel was applied for up to 96 weeks. Panretin® gel should be continued as long as the patient is deriving benefit.

Occlusive dressings should not be used with Panretin® gel.

HOW SUPPLIED

Panretin® gel is available in tubes containing 60 grams. Store at 25° C (77° F); excursions permitted to 15–30° C (59–86° F) [see USP Controlled Room Temperature].

Manufactured for: **Ligand Pharmaceuticals Incorporated**
San Diego, CA 92121
by: Stiefel Laboratories Inc.
Coral Gables, FL 33134

NDC 64365-501-01
Ligand Part #3000101 (Rev. 0199)
Stiefel Part #80068 (Rev. 0298)

TARGRETIN® ℞

[*tahr-greh' tən*]
(bexarotene)
Capsules, 75 mg
Rx only.

(Please consult the Manufacturer's Index or the Brand and Generic Name Index for product page number)

TARGRETIN® ℞

[*tahr-greh' tən*]
(bexarotene) gel 1%
Rx only.

DESCRIPTION

Targretin® (bexarotene) gel 1% contains bexarotene and is intended for topical application only. Bexarotene is a member of a subclass of retinoids that selectively activate retinoid X receptors (RXRs). These retinoid receptors have biologic activity distinct from that of retinoic acid receptors (RARs).

The chemical name is 4-[1-(5,6,7,8-tetrahydro-3,5,5,8,8-pentamethyl-2-naphthalenyl)ethenyl] benzoic acid, and the structural formula is as follows:

Bexarotene is an off-white to white powder with a molecular weight of 348.48 and a molecular formula of $C_{24}H_{28}O_2$. It is insoluble in water and slightly soluble in vegetable oils and ethanol, USP.

Targretin® gel is a clear gelled solution containing 1.0% (w/w) bexarotene in a base of dehydrated alcohol, USP, polyethylene glycol 400, NF, hydroxypropyl cellulose, NF, and butylated hydroxytoluene, NF.

CLINICAL PHARMACOLOGY

Mechanism of Action

Bexarotene selectively binds and activates retinoid X receptor subtypes (RXRα, RXRβ, RXRγ). RXRs can form heterodimers with various receptor partners such as retinoic acid receptors (RARs), vitamin D receptor, thyroid receptor, and peroxisome proliferator activator receptors (PPARs). Once activated, these receptors function as transcription factors that regulate the expression of genes that control cellular differentiation and proliferation. Bexarotene inhibits the growth *in vitro* of some tumor cell lines of hematopoietic and squamous cell origin. It also induces tumor regression *in vivo* in some animal models. The exact mechanism of action of bexarotene in the treatment of cutaneous T-cell lymphoma (CTCL) is unknown.

Pharmacokinetics

General

Plasma concentrations of bexarotene were determined during clinical studies in patients with CTCL or following repeated single or multiple-daily dose applications of Targretin® gel 1% for up to 132 weeks. Plasma bexarotene concentrations were generally less than 5 ng/mL and did not exceed 55 ng/mL. However, only two patients with very intense dosing regimens (> 40% BSA lesions and QID dosing) were sampled. Plasma bexarotene concentrations and the frequency of detecting quantifiable plasma bexarotene concentrations increased with increasing percent body surface area treated and increasing quantity of Targretin® gel applied. The sporadically-observed and generally low plasma bexarotene concentrations indicated that, in patients receiving doses of low to moderate intensity, there is a low potential for significant plasma concentrations following repeated application of Targretin® gel. Bexarotene is highly bound (>99%) to plasma proteins. The plasma proteins to which bexarotene binds have not been elucidated, and the ability of bexarotene to displace drugs bound to plasma proteins and the ability of drugs to displace bexarotene binding have not been studied (see **PRECAUTIONS:** ***Protein Binding***). The uptake of bexarotene by organs or tissues has not been evaluated.

Metabolism

Four bexarotene metabolites have been identified in plasma following oral administration of bexarotene: 6- and 7-hydroxy-bexarotene and 6- and 7-oxo-bexarotene. *In vitro* studies suggest that cytochrome P450 3A4 is the major cytochrome P450 responsible for formation of the oxidative metabolites and that the oxidative metabolites may be glucuronidated. The oxidative metabolites are active in *in vitro* assays of retinoid receptor activation, but the relative contribution of the parent and any metabolites to the efficacy and safety of Targretin® gel is unknown.

Elimination

The renal elimination of bexarotene and its metabolites was examined in patients with Type 2 diabetes mellitus following oral administration of bexarotene. Neither bexarotene nor its metabolites were excreted in urine in appreciable amounts.

Special Populations

Elderly, Gender, Race: Because of a large number of immeasurable plasma concentrations (< 1ng/mL), any potential pharmacokinetic differences between Special Populations could not be assessed.

Pediatric: Studies to evaluate bexarotene pharmacokinetics in the pediatric population have not been conducted (see **PRECAUTIONS:** ***Pediatric Use***).

Renal Insufficiency: No formal studies have been conducted with Targretin® gel in patients with renal insufficiency. Urinary elimination of bexarotene and its known metabolites is a minor excretory pathway (<1% of an orally administered dose), but because renal insufficiency can result in significant protein binding changes, pharmacokinetics may be altered in patients with renal insufficiency (see **PRECAUTIONS:** ***Renal Insufficiency***).

Hepatic Insufficiency: No specific studies have been conducted with Targretin® gel in patients with hepatic insufficiency. Because less than 1% of the dose of oral bexarotene is excreted in the urine unchanged and there is *in vitro* evidence of extensive hepatic contribution to bexarotene elimination, hepatic impairment would be expected to lead to greatly decreased clearance (see **PRECAUTIONS: *Hepatic Insufficiency***).

Drug-Drug Interactions

No formal studies to evaluate drug interactions with bexarotene or Targretin® gel have been conducted. Bexarotene oxidative metabolites appear to be formed through cytochrome P450 3A4. Drugs that affect levels or activity of cytochrome P450 3A4 may potentially affect the disposition of bexarotene. Concomitant gemfibrozil was associated with increased bexarotene concentrations following oral administration of bexarotene.

Clinical Studies

Targretin® gel was evaluated for the treatment of patients with early stage (Stage IA-IIA) CTCL in one multicenter, open-label, clinical trial as well as in a Phase I-II program (dose-seeking trials with different response criteria than the multicenter trial). These clinical studies enrolled a total of 117 patients.

In the multicenter, open-label clinical trial, Targretin® gel was evaluated for the treatment of patients with early stage CTCL who were refractory to, intolerant to, or reached a response plateau for at least six months on at least two prior therapies. The study was conducted in the U.S., Canada, Europe, and Australia and enrolled a total of 50 patients; 46% of these patients were male, 80% were Caucasian, and the median age was 64 years (range 13 to 85).

Targretin® gel was also evaluated for the treatment of patients with CTCL in a U.S. Phase I-II program involving patients with early stage CTCL. This program enrolled a total of 67 patients; 55% of these patients were male, 85% were Caucasian, and the median age was 61 years (range 30 to 87).

In the multicenter, open-label clinical trial, considering prior systemic, irradiation, and topical treatments, patients had been exposed to a median of 3 prior therapies (range 2–7). All patients failed at least two treatments; the majority (68%) of patients were either refractory to two or more therapies, or were refractory to one therapy and intolerant to at least one therapy.

Patients were treated with Targretin® gel 1% for a planned 16-week period with an option to continue provided that no unacceptable toxicity was occurring.

Tumor response was assessed in the multicenter study by observation of up to five baseline-defined index lesions using a Composite Assessment of Index Lesion Disease Severity (CA). This endpoint was based on a summation of the grades, for all index lesions, of erythema, scaling, plaque elevation, hypopigmentation or hyperpigmentation, and area of involvement. New cutaneous lesions or tumors and extracutaneous disease manifestations were not considered in response or disease progression assessments.

All tumor responses required confirmation over at least two assessments separated by at least four weeks. A partial response was defined as an improvement of at least 50% in the index lesions. A complete clinical response required complete disappearance of the index lesions, but did not require confirmation by biopsy.

Targretin® gel produced an overall response rate of 26% (13/50) with a corresponding exact 95% confidence interval from 14.6% to 40.3% by the Composite Assessment of Index Lesion Severity. For the Stage IA and IB patients, the response rate was 28% (13/47) with a corresponding exact 95% confidence interval from 15.6% to 42.6%. For the Stage II patients the response rate was 0% (0/3). Two percent of patients (1/50) had a clinical complete response. The median time to best response on the Composite Assessment of Index Lesion Severity (n=13) was 85 days (range: 36–154). The rate of relapse in responding patients by the Composite Assessment of Index Lesion Severity was 23% (3/13) over a median observation period of 149 days (range 56–342). Fourteen patients developed new lesions in untreated areas (14/50; 28%). Four patients developed clinically abnormal lymph nodes (≥ 1cm diam) (4/50; 8%). One patient developed a cutaneous tumor (1/50; 2%).

The Phase I-II program (dose-seeking trials with different response criteria than the multicenter trial) was supportive of the multicenter study results.

INDICATIONS AND USAGE

Targretin® (bexarotene) gel 1% is indicated for the topical treatment of cutaneous lesions in patients with CTCL (Stage IA and IB) who have refractory or persistent disease after other therapies or who have not tolerated other therapies.

CONTRAINDICATIONS

Targretin® gel 1% is contraindicated in patients with a known hypersensitivity to bexarotene or other components of the product.

Pregnancy: Category X

Targretin® gel 1% may cause fetal harm when administered to a pregnant woman.

Targretin® gel must not be given to a pregnant woman or a woman who intends to become pregnant. If a woman becomes pregnant while taking Targretin® gel, Targretin® gel must be stopped immediately and the woman given appropriate counseling.

Bexarotene caused malformations when administered orally to pregnant rats during days 7–17 of gestation. Developmental abnormalities included incomplete ossification at 4 mg/kg/day and cleft palate, depressed eye bulge/microphthalmia, and small ears at 16 mg/kg/day. At doses greater than 10 mg/kg/day, bexarotene caused developmental mortality. The no-effect oral dose in rats was 1 mg/kg/day. Plasma bexarotene concentrations in patients with

Table 1. Incidence of All Adverse Events* and Application Site Adverse Events with Incidence ≥5% for All Application Frequencies of Targretin® Gel in the Multicenter CTCL Study

COSTART 5 Body System/Preferred Term	All Adverse Events N = 50 n (%)	Application Site Adverse Events N = 50 n (%)
Skin and Appendages		
Contact Dermatitis[1]	7 (14)	4 (8)
Exfoliative Dermatitis	3 (6)	0
Pruritus[2]	18 (36)	9 (18)
Rash[3]	36 (72)	28 (56)
Maculopapular Rash	3 (6)	0
Skin Disorder (NOS)[4]	13 (26)	9 (18)
Sweating	3 (6)	0
Body as a Whole		
Asthenia	3 (6)	0
Headache	7 (14)	0
Infection	9 (18)	0
Pain	15 (30)	9 (18)
Cardiovascular		
Edema	5 (10)	0
Peripheral Edema	3 (6)	0
Hemic and Lymphatic		
Leukopenia	3 (6)	0
Lymphadenopathy	3 (6)	0
WBC Abnormal	3 (6)	0
Metabolic and Nutritional		
Hyperlipemia	5 (10)	0
Nervous		
Paresthesia	3 (6)	3 (6)
Respiratory		
Cough Increased	3 (6)	0
Pharyngitis	3 (6)	0

* Regardless of association with treatment

Includes Investigator terms such as:

[1] Contact dermatitis, irritant contact dermatitis, irritant dermatitis

[2] Pruritus, itching, itching of lesion

[3] Erythema, scaling, irritation, redness, rash, dermatitis

[4] Skin inflammation, excoriation, sticky or tacky sensation of skin; NOS = Not Otherwise Specified

CTCL applying Targretin® gel 1% were generally less than one hundredth the Cmax associated with dysmorphogenesis in rats, although some patients had Cmax levels that were approximately one eighth the concentration associated with dysmorphogenesis in rats.

Women of child-bearing potential should be advised to avoid becoming pregnant when Targretin® gel is used. The possibility that a woman of child-bearing potential is pregnant at the time therapy is instituted should be considered. A negative pregnancy test (e.g., serum beta-human chorionic gonadotropin, beta-HCG) with a sensitivity of at least 50 mIU/L should be obtained within one week prior to Targretin® gel therapy, and the pregnancy test must be repeated at monthly intervals while the patient remains on Targretin® gel. Effective contraception must be used for one month prior to the initiation of therapy, during therapy and for at least one month following discontinuation of therapy; it is recommended that two reliable forms of contraception be used simultaneously unless abstinence is the chosen method. Male patients with sexual partners who are pregnant, possibly pregnant, or who could become pregnant must use condoms during sexual intercourse while applying Targretin® gel and for at least one month after the last dose of drug. Targretin® gel therapy should be initiated on the second or third day of a normal menstrual period. No more than a one month supply of Targretin® gel should be given to the patient so that the results of pregnancy testing can be assessed and counseling regarding avoidance of pregnancy and birth defects can be reinforced.

PRECAUTIONS

Pregnancy: **Category X.** See **CONTRAINDICATIONS**

General: Targretin® gel should be used with caution in patients with a known hypersensitivity to other retinoids. No clinical instances of cross-reactivity have been noted.

Vitamin A Supplementation: In clinical studies, patients were advised to limit vitamin A intake to ≤15,000 IU/day. Because of the relationship of bexarotene to vitamin A, patients should be advised to limit vitamin A supplements to avoid potential additive toxic effects.

Photosensitivity: Retinoids as a class have been associated with photosensitivity. *In vitro* assays indicate that bexarotene is a potential photosensitizing agent. There were no reports of photosensitivity in patients in the clinical studies. Patients should be advised to minimize exposure to sunlight and artificial ultraviolet light during the use of Targretin® gel.

Drug-Drug Interactions

Patients who are applying Targretin® gel should not concurrently use products that contain DEET (*N,N*-diethyl-*m*-toluamide), a common component of insect repellent products. An animal toxicology study showed increased DEET toxicity when DEET was included as part of the formulation.

No formal studies to evaluate drug interactions with bexarotene have been conducted. Bexarotene oxidative metabolites appear to be formed through cytochrome P450 3A4.

On the basis of the metabolism of bexarotene by cytochrome P450 3A4, concomitant ketoconazole, itraconazole, erythromycin and grapefruit juice could increase bexarotene plasma concentrations. Similarly, based on data that gemfibrozil increases bexarotene concentrations following oral bexarotene administration, concomitant gemfibrozil could increase bexarotene plasma concentrations. However, due to the low systemic exposure to bexarotene after low to moderately intense gel regimens (see Clinical Pharmacology), increases that occur are unlikely to be of sufficient magnitude to result in adverse effects.

No drug interaction data are available on concomitant administration of Targretin® gel and other CTCL therapies.

Targretin—Cont.

Renal Insufficiency
No formal studies have been conducted with Targretin® gel in patients with renal insufficiency. Urinary elimination of bexarotene and its known metabolites is a minor excretory pathway for bexarotene (<1% of an orally administered dose), but because renal insufficiency can result in significant protein binding changes, and bexarotene is >99% protein bound, pharmacokinetics may be altered in patients with renal insufficiency.
Hepatic Insufficiency
No specific studies have been conducted with Targretin® gel in patients with hepatic insufficiency. Because less than 1% of the dose of oral bexarotene is excreted in the urine unchanged and there is *in vitro* evidence of extensive hepatic contribution to bexarotene elimination, hepatic impairment would be expected to lead to greatly decreased clearance.
Protein Binding
Bexarotene is highly bound (>99%) to plasma proteins. The plasma proteins to which bexarotene binds have not been elucidated, and the ability of bexarotene to displace drugs bound to plasma proteins and the ability of drugs to displace bexarotene binding have not been studied.
Carcinogenesis, Mutagenesis, Impairment of Fertility
Long-term studies in animals to assess the carcinogenic potential of bexarotene have not been conducted. Bexarotene was not mutagenic to bacteria (Ames assay) or mammalian cells (mouse lymphoma assay). Bexarotene was not clastogenic *in vivo* (micronucleus test in mice). No formal fertility studies were conducted with bexarotene. Bexarotene caused testicular degeneration when oral doses of 1.5 mg/kg/day were given to dogs for 91 days.
Use in Nursing Mothers
It is not known whether bexarotene is excreted in human milk. Because many drugs are excreted in human milk and because of the potential for serious adverse reactions in nursing infants from bexarotene, a decision should be made whether to discontinue nursing or to discontinue the drug, taking into account the importance of the drug to the mother.
Pediatric Use
Safety and effectiveness in pediatric patients have not been established.
Geriatric Use
Of the total patients with CTCL in clinical studies of Targretin® gel, 62% were under 65 years and 38% were 65 years or older. No overall differences in safety were observed between patients 65 years of age or older and younger patients, but greater sensitivity of some older individuals to Targretin® gel cannot be ruled out. Responses to Targretin® gel were observed across all age groups decades, without preference for any individual age group decade.

ADVERSE REACTIONS
The safety of Targretin® gel has been assessed in clinical studies of 117 patients with CTCL who received Targretin® gel for up to 172 weeks. In the multicenter open label study, 50 patients with CTCL received Targretin® gel for up to 98 weeks. The mean duration of therapy for these 50 patients was 199 days. The most common adverse events reported with an incidence at the application site of at least 10% in patients with CTCL were rash, pruritus, skin disorder, and pain.
Adverse events leading to dose reduction or study drug discontinuation in at least two patients were rash, contact dermatitis, and pruritus.
Of the 49 patients (98%) who experienced any adverse event, most experienced events categorized as mild (9 patients, 18%) or moderate (27 patients, 54%). There were 12 patients (24%) who experienced at least one moderately severe adverse event. The most common moderately severe events were rash (7 patients, 14%) and pruritus (3 patients, 6%). Only one patient (2%) experienced a severe adverse event (rash).
In the patients with CTCL receiving Targretin® gel, adverse events reported regardless of relationship to study drug at an incidence of ≥5% are presented in Table 1.
A similar safety profile for Targretin® gel was demonstrated in the Phase I-II program. For the 67 patients enrolled in the Phase I-II program, the mean duration of treatment was 436 days (range 12–1203 days). As in the multicenter study, the most common adverse events regardless of relationship to study drug in the Phase I-II program were rash (78%), pain (40%), and pruritus (40%).
[See table 1 at top of previous page]

OVERDOSAGE
Systemic toxicity following acute overdosage with topical application of Targretin® gel is unlikely because of low systemic plasma levels observed with normal therapeutic doses. There is no specific antidote for overdosage.
There has been no experience with acute overdose of Targretin® gel in humans. Any overdose with Targretin® gel should be treated with supportive care for the signs and symptoms exhibited by the patient.

DOSAGE AND ADMINISTRATION
Targretin® gel should be initially applied once every other day for the first week. The application frequency should be increased at weekly intervals to once daily, then twice daily, then three times daily and finally four times daily according to individual lesion tolerance. Generally, patients were able to maintain a dosing frequency of two to four times per day. Most responses were seen at dosing frequencies of two times per day and higher. If application site toxicity occurs, the application frequency can be reduced. Should severe irritation occur, application of drug can be temporarily discontinued for a few days until the symptoms subside. See **CONTRAINDICATIONS: *Pregnancy: Category X*.**
Sufficient gel should be applied to cover the lesion with a generous coating. The gel should be allowed to dry before covering with clothing. Because unaffected skin may become irritated, application of the gel to normal skin surrounding the lesions should be avoided. In addition, do not apply the gel near mucosal surfaces of the body.
A response may be seen as soon as 4 weeks after initiation of therapy but most patients require longer application. With continued application, further benefit may be attained. The longest onset time for the first response among the responders was 392 days based on the Composite Assessment of Index Lesion Severity in the multicenter study. In clinical trials, Targretin® gel was applied for up to 172 weeks.
Targretin® gel should be continued as long as the patient is deriving benefit.
Occlusive dressings should not be used with Targretin® gel.
Targretin® gel is a topical therapy and is not intended for systemic use. Targretin® gel has not been studied in combination with other CTCL therapies.

HOW SUPPLIED
Targretin® gel is supplied in tubes containing 60 g (600 mg active bexarotene).
60 g tube .... NDC 64365-504-01
Store at 25°C (77°F); with excursions permitted to 15°-30°C (59°–86°F) [see USP]. Avoid exposing to high temperatures and humidity after the tube is opened. Protect from light.
Manufactured for: Ligand Pharmaceuticals Incorporated
San Diego, CA 92121
by: Stiefel Laboratories, Inc.
Coral Gables, Florida 33134
Ligand Part #3000204 (Rev. 0700)

Eli Lilly and Company
LILLY CORPORATE CENTER
INDIANAPOLIS, IN 46285

Direct Inquiries to:
Lilly Corporate Center
Indianapolis, IN 46285
(317) 276-2000
www.lilly.com
For Medical Information Contact:
Lilly Research Laboratories
Lilly Corporate Center
Indianapolis, IN 46285
(800) 545-5979

LEGEND
ADD-Vantage®—*Vials and Diluent Containers, Abbott*
Gelseal®—*Filled Elastic Capsule, Lilly*
Identi-Code®—*Formula Identification Code, Lilly*
Identi-Dose®—*Unit Dose Medication, Lilly*
Pulvule®—*Filled Gelatin Capsule, Lilly*
℞Pak—*Prescription Package, Lilly*
Solvet®—*Soluble Tablet, Lilly*
Traypak®—*Multivial Carton, Lilly*

IDENTI-CODE® Index
(formula identification code, Lilly)
Provides Positive Product Identification
A letter-number symbol, a 4-digit number, the name of the product, the strength of the product, or a combination of these appears on each Lilly capsule and most tablets and on each label of pediatric liquids, and powders for oral suspension. The letter/number or 4-digit number identifies the product.

Identi-Code® **Product Name**

Coated Tablets
1890 **Darvocet-N® 50**
Composition (Each Coated Tablet): Propoxyphene napsylate, 50 mg; acetaminophen, 325 mg (USP)
1883 **Darvon-N®**
Composition (Each Coated Tablet): Propoxyphene Napsylate, USP, 100 mg
1893 **Darvocet-N® 100**
Composition (Each Coated Tablet): Propoxyphene napsylate, 100 mg; acetaminophen, 650 mg (USP)

Pulvules®
365 **Darvon®**
Composition (Each Pulvule®): Propoxyphene Hydrochloride, USP, 65 mg
387 **Aventyl® HCl**
Composition (Each Pulvule®): Nortriptyline Hydrochloride, USP, 10 mg (equiv. to base)
389 **Aventyl® HCl**
Composition (Each Pulvule®): Nortriptyline Hydrochloride, USP, 25 mg (equiv. to base)
3061 **Ceclor®**
Composition (Each Pulvule®): Cefaclor, USP, 250 mg
3062 **Ceclor®**
Composition (Each Pulvule®): Cefaclor, USP, 500 mg
369 **Darvon® Compound-65**
Composition (Each Pulvule®): Propoxyphene hydrochloride, 65 mg; aspirin, 389 mg; caffeine, 32.4 mg
3125 **Vancocin® HCl**
Composition (Each Pulvule®): Vancomycin hydrochloride, 125 mg
3126 **Vancocin® HCl**
Composition (Each Pulvule®): Vancomycin hydrochloride, 250 mg
3144 **Axid®**
Composition (Each Pulvule®): Nizatidine, 150 mg
3145 **Axid®**
Composition (Each Pulvule®): Nizatidine, 300 mg

Compressed Tablets
967 **Sodium Chloride**
Composition (Each Compressed Tablet): Sodium Chloride, USP, 1 g
1265 **Sodium Bicarbonate**
Composition (Each Compressed Tablet): Sodium Bicarbonate, USP, 10 grs (648 mg)
1513 **Calcium Carbonate**
Composition (Each Compressed Tablet): Calcium Carbonate, USP, Aromatic, 10 grs (648 mg)
4006 **Prozac®**
Composition (Each Compressed Scored Tablet): Fluoxetine Hydrochloride, 10 mg
4165 **Evista®**
Composition (Each Compressed Tablet): Raloxifene Hydrochloride, 60 mg
4112 **Zyprexa®**
Composition (Each Compressed Tablet): Olanzapine, USP, 2.5 mg
4115 **Zyprexa®**
Composition (Each Compressed Tablet): Olanzapine, USP, 5 mg
4116 **Zyprexa®**
Composition (Each Compressed Tablet): Olanzapine, USP, 7.5 mg
4117 **Zyprexa®**
Composition (Each Compressed Tablet): Olanzapine, USP, 10 mg
4415 **Zyprexa®**
Composition (Each Compressed Tablet): Olanzapine, USP, 15 mg.

UNIT-DOSE PACKAGING
Identi-Dose® (unit dose medication, Lilly)
Reverse-Numbered Package
Closed-circuit control of medication from pharmacy to nurse to patient and return. Simplifies counting and dispensing whether in single-unit or prescription-size quantities. Fits into any dispensing system for ready identification and legibility, better inventory control, protection from contamination, easier handling and recording under Medicare, prevention of drug loss through pilferage or spilling, better control of Federal Controlled Substances, and less chance of medication errors.
The following products are available through normal channels of supply:
Identi-Dose® (ID100)
Pulvules®
No.
ⒸⅣ365 Darvon®, 65 mg
ⒸⅣ369 Darvon® Compound-65
3061 Ceclor®, 250 mg
Tablets
No.
ⒸⅣ1883 Darvon-N®, 100 mg
ⒸⅣ1893 Darvocet-N® 100
Reverse-Numbered Package (RN500)
Pulvules®
No.
Tablets
No.
ⒸⅣ**1893** Darvocet-N® 100
Single-Cut Identi-Dose® (ID500)
Tablets
No.
ⒸⅣ**1893** Darvocet-N® 100

ⒸⅡ, ⒸⅢ, ⒸⅣ Federal Controlled Substances.

AXID® ℞
[*ak 'sid*]
(nizatidine capsules, USP)

DESCRIPTION
Axid® (Nizatidine, USP) is a histamine H_2-receptor antagonist. Chemically, it is N-[2-[[[2-[(dimethylamino)methyl]-4-thiazolyl] methyl]thio]ethyl]-N′-methyl-2-nitro-1,1-ethenediamine.

The structural formula is as follows:

Nizatidine

Nizatidine has the empirical formula $C_{12}H_{21}N_5O_2S_2$ representing a molecular weight of 331.47. It is an off-white to buff crystalline solid that is soluble in water. Nizatidine has a bitter taste and mild sulfur-like odor. Each Pulvule® (capsule) contains for oral administration gelatin, pregelatinized starch, dimethicone, starch, titanium dioxide, yellow iron oxide, 150 mg (0.45 mmol) or 300 mg (0.91 mmol) of nizatidine, and other inactive ingredients. The 150-mg Pulvule also contains magnesium stearate, and the 300-mg Pulvule also contains croscarmellose sodium, povidone, red iron oxide, and talc.

CLINICAL PHARMACOLOGY

Axid is a competitive, reversible inhibitor of histamine at the histamine H_2-receptors, particularly those in the gastric parietal cells.

Antisecretory Activity —1. Effects on Acid Secretion: Axid significantly inhibited nocturnal gastric acid secretion for up to 12 hours. Axid also significantly inhibited gastric acid secretion stimulated by food, caffeine, betazole, and pentagastrin (Table 1).

Table 1
Effect of Oral Axid on Gastric Acid Secretion

	Time After Dose (h)	% Inhibition of Gastric Acid Output by Dose (mg) 20-50	75	100	150	300
Nocturnal	Up to 10	57		73		90
Betazole	Up to 3		93		100	99
Pentagastrin	Up to 6		25		64	67
Meal	Up to 4	41	64		98	97
Caffeine	Up to 3		73		85	96

2. Effects on Other Gastrointestinal Secretions—Pepsin: Oral administration of 75 to 300 mg of Axid did not affect pepsin activity in gastric secretions. Total pepsin output was reduced in proportion to the reduced volume of gastric secretions.

Intrinsic Factor: Oral administration of 75 to 300 mg of Axid increased betazole-stimulated secretion of intrinsic factor.

Serum Gastrin: Axid had no effect on basal serum gastrin. No rebound of gastrin secretion was observed when food was ingested 12 hours after administration of Axid.

3. Other Pharmacologic Actions—

a. Hormones: Axid was not shown to affect the serum concentrations of gonadotropins, prolactin, growth hormone, antidiuretic hormone, cortisol, triiodothyronine, thyroxin, testosterone, 5α-dihydrotestosterone, androstenedione, or estradiol.

b. Axid had no demonstrable antiandrogenic action.

4. Pharmacokinetics—The absolute oral bioavailability of nizatidine exceeds 70%. Peak plasma concentrations (700 to 1,800 μg/L for a 150-mg dose and 1,400 to 3,600 μg/L for a 300-mg dose) occur from 0.5 to 3 hours following the dose. A concentration of 1,000 μg/L is equivalent to 3 μmol/L; a dose of 300 mg is equivalent to 905 μmoles. Plasma concentrations 12 hours after administration are less than 10 μg/L. The elimination half-life is 1 to 2 hours, plasma clearance is 40 to 60 L/h, and the volume of distribution is 0.8 to 1.5 L/kg. Because of the short half-life and rapid clearance of nizatidine, accumulation of the drug would not be expected in individuals with normal renal function who take either 300 mg once daily at bedtime or 150 mg twice daily. Axid exhibits dose proportionality over the recommended dose range.

The oral bioavailability of nizatidine is unaffected by concomitant ingestion of propantheline. Antacids consisting of aluminum and magnesium hydroxides with simethicone decrease the absorption of nizatidine by about 10%. With food, the AUC and C_{max} increase by approximately 10%.

In humans, less than 7% of an oral dose is metabolized as N2-monodes-methylnizatidine, an H_2-receptor antagonist, which is the principal metabolite excreted in the urine. Other likely metabolites are the N2-oxide (less than 5% of the dose) and the S-oxide (less than 6% of the dose).

More than 90% of an oral dose of nizatidine is excreted in the urine within 12 hours. About 60% of an oral dose is excreted as unchanged drug. Renal clearance is about 500 mL/min, which indicates excretion by active tubular secretion. Less than 6% of an administered dose is eliminated in the feces.

Moderate to severe renal impairment significantly prolongs the half-life and decreases the clearance of nizatidine. In individuals who are functionally anephric, the half-life is 3.5 to 11 hours, and the plasma clearance is 7 to 14 L/h. To avoid accumulation of the drug in individuals with clinically significant renal impairment, the amount and/or frequency of doses of Axid should be reduced in proportion to the severity of dysfunction (*see* Dosage and Administration).

Approximately 35% of nizatidine is bound to plasma protein, mainly to α_1-acid glycoprotein. Warfarin, diazepam, acetaminophen, propantheline, phenobarbital, and propranolol did not affect plasma protein binding of nizatidine in vitro.

Clinical Trials —1. Active Duodenal Ulcer: In multicenter, double-blind, placebo-controlled studies in the United States, endoscopically diagnosed duodenal ulcers healed more rapidly following administration of Axid, 300 mg h.s. or 150 mg b.i.d., than with placebo (Table 2). Lower doses, such as 100 mg h.s., had slightly lower effectiveness.

Table 2
Healing Response of Ulcers to Axid
AXID

	300 mg h.s. Number Entered	300 mg h.s. Healed/Evaluable	150 mg b.i.d. Number Entered	150 mg b.i.d. Healed/Evaluable	Placebo Number Entered	Placebo Healed/Evaluable
STUDY 1						
Week 2			276	93/265 (35%)*	279	55/260 (21%)
Week 4				198/259 (76%)*		95/243 (39%)
STUDY 2						
Week 2	108	24/103 (23%)*	106	27/101 (27%)*	101	9/93 (10%)
Week 4		65/97 (67%)*		66/97 (68%)*		24/84 (29%)
STUDY 3						
Week 2	92	22/90 (24%)†			98	13/92 (14%)
Week 4		52/85 (61%)*				29/88 (33%)
Week 8		68/83 (82%)*				39/79 (49%)

* $P < 0.01$ as compared with placebo.
† $P < 0.05$ as compared with placebo.

[See table 2 above]

2. Maintenance of Healed Duodenal Ulcer:
Treatment with a reduced dose of Axid has been shown to be effective as maintenance therapy following healing of active duodenal ulcers. In multicenter, double-blind, placebo-controlled studies conducted in the United States, 150 mg of Axid taken at bedtime resulted in a significantly lower incidence of duodenal ulcer recurrence in patients treated for up to 1 year (Table 3).

Table 3
Percentage of Ulcers Recurring by 3, 6, and 12 Months in Double-Blind Studies Conducted in the United States

Month	Axid, 150 mg h.s.	Placebo
3	13% (28/208)*	40% (82/204)
6	24% (45/188)*	57% (106/187)
12	34% (57/166)*	64% (112/175)

* $P < 0.001$ as compared with placebo.

3. Gastroesophageal Reflux Disease (GERD):
In 2 multicenter, double-blind, placebo-controlled clinical trials performed in the United States and Canada, Axid was more effective than placebo in improving endoscopically diagnosed esophagitis and in healing erosive and ulcerative esophagitis.

In patients with erosive or ulcerative esophagitis, 150 mg b.i.d. of Axid given to 88 patients compared with placebo in 98 patients in Study 1 yielded a higher healing rate at 3 weeks (16% vs 7%) and at 6 weeks (32% vs 16%, $P<0.05$). Of 99 patients on Axid and 94 patients on placebo, Study 2 at the same dosage yielded similar results at 6 weeks (21% vs 11%, $P<0.05$) and at 12 weeks (29% vs 13%, $P<0.01$).

In addition, relief of associated heartburn was greater in patients treated with Axid. Patients treated with Axid consumed fewer antacids than did patients treated with placebo.

4. Active Benign Gastric Ulcer:
In a multicenter, double-blind, placebo-controlled study conducted in the United States and Canada, endoscopically diagnosed benign gastric ulcers healed significantly more rapidly following administration of nizatidine than of placebo (Table 4).

Table 4

Week	Treatment	Healing Rate	vs. Placebo p-value*
4	Niz 300 mg h.s.	52/153 (34%)	0.342
	Niz 150 mg b.i.d.	65/151 (43%)	0.022
	Placebo	48/151 (32%)	
8	Niz 300 mg h.s.	99/153 (65%)	0.011
	Niz 150 mg b.i.d.	105/151 (70%)	<0.001
	Placebo	78/151 (52%)	

*P-values are one-sided, obtained by Chi-square test, and not adjusted for multiple comparisons.

In a multicenter, double-blind, comparator-controlled study in Europe, healing rates for patients receiving nizatidine (300 mg h.s. or 150 mg b.i.d.) were equivalent to rates for patients receiving a comparator drug, and statistically superior to historical placebo control rates.

INDICATIONS AND USAGE

Axid is indicated for up to 8 weeks for the treatment of active duodenal ulcer. In most patients, the ulcer will heal within 4 weeks.

Axid is indicated for maintenance therapy for duodenal ulcer patients, at a reduced dosage of 150 mg h.s. after healing of an active duodenal ulcer. The consequences of continuous therapy with Axid for longer than 1 year are not known.

Axid is indicated for up to 12 weeks for the treatment of endoscopically diagnosed esophagitis, including erosive and ulcerative esophagitis, and associated heartburn due to GERD.

Axid is indicated for up to 8 weeks for the treatment of active benign gastric ulcer. Before initiating therapy, care should be taken to exclude the possibility of malignant gastric ulceration.

CONTRAINDICATION

Axid is contraindicated in patients with known hypersensitivity to the drug. Because cross sensitivity in this class of compounds has been observed, H_2-receptor antagonists, including Axid, should not be administered to patients with a history of hypersensitivity to other H_2-receptor antagonists.

PRECAUTIONS

General —1. Symptomatic response to nizatidine therapy does not preclude the presence of gastric malignancy.

2. Because nizatidine is excreted primarily by the kidney, dosage should be reduced in patients with moderate to severe renal insufficiency (*see* Dosage and Administration).

3. Pharmacokinetic studies in patients with hepatorenal syndrome have not been done. Part of the dose of nizatidine is metabolized in the liver. In patients with normal renal function and uncomplicated hepatic dysfunction, the disposition of nizatidine is similar to that in normal subjects.

Laboratory Tests —False-positive tests for urobilinogen with Multistix® may occur during therapy with nizatidine.

Drug Interactions —No interactions have been observed between Axid and theophylline, chlordiazepoxide, lorazepam, lidocaine, phenytoin, and warfarin. Axid does not inhibit the cytochrome P-450-linked drug-metabolizing enzyme system; therefore, drug interactions mediated by inhibition of hepatic metabolism are not expected to occur. In patients given very high doses (3,900 mg) of aspirin daily, increases in serum salicylate levels were seen when nizatidine, 150 mg b.i.d., was administered concurrently.

Carcinogenesis, Mutagenesis, Impairment of Fertility —A 2-year oral carcinogenicity study in rats with doses as high as 500 mg/kg/day (about 80 times the recommended daily therapeutic dose) showed no evidence of a carcinogenic effect. There was a dose-related increase in the density of enterochromaffin-like (ECL) cells in the gastric oxyntic mucosa. In a 2-year study in mice, there was no evidence of a carcinogenic effect in male mice; although hyperplastic nodules of the liver were increased in the high-dose males as compared with placebo. Female mice given the high dose of Axid (2,000 mg/kg/day, about 330 times the human dose) showed marginally statistically significant increases in hepatic carcinoma and hepatic nodular hyperplasia with no numerical increase seen in any of the other dose groups. The rate of hepatic carcinoma in the high-dose animals was within the historical control limits seen for the strain of mice used. The female mice were given a dose larger than the maximum tolerated dose, as indicated by excessive (30%) weight decrement as compared with concurrent controls and evidence of mild liver injury (transaminase elevations). The occurrence of a marginal finding at high dose only in animals given an excessive and somewhat hepatotoxic dose, with no evidence of a carcinogenic effect in rats, male mice, and female mice (given up to 360 mg/kg/day, about 60 times the human dose), and a negative mutagenicity battery are not considered evidence of a carcinogenic potential for Axid.

Axid was not mutagenic in a battery of tests performed to evaluate its potential genetic toxicity, including bacterial mutation tests, unscheduled DNA synthesis, sister chromatid exchange, the mouse lymphoma assay, chromosome aberration tests, and a micronucleus test.

In a 2-generation, perinatal and postnatal fertility study in rats, doses of nizatidine up to 650 mg/kg/day produced no adverse effects on the reproductive performance of parental animals or their progeny.

Continued on next page

*** Identi-Code® symbol. This product information was prepared in June 2000. Current information on these and other products of Eli Lilly and Company may be obtained by direct inquiry to Lilly Research Laboratories, Lilly Corporate Center, Indianapolis, Indiana 46285, (800) 545-5979.**

Axid—Cont.

Pregnancy—Teratogenic Effects—Pregnancy Category B—Oral reproduction studies in pregnant rats at doses up to 1500 mg/kg/day (9000 mg/m^2/day, 40.5 times the recommended human dose based on body surface area) and in pregnant rabbits at doses up to 275 mg/kg/day (3245 mg/m^2/day, 14.6 times the recommended human dose based on body surface area) have revealed no evidence of impaired fertility or harm to the fetus due to nizatidine. There are, however, no adequate and well-controlled studies in pregnant women. Because animal reproduction studies are not always predictive of human response, this drug should be used during pregnancy only if clearly needed.

Nursing Mothers —Studies conducted in lactating women have shown that 0.1% of the administered oral dose of nizatidine is secreted in human milk in proportion to plasma concentrations. Because of the growth depression in pups reared by lactating rats treated with nizatidine, a decision should be made whether to discontinue nursing or discontinue the drug, taking into account the importance of the drug to the mother.

Use in Pediatric Patients —Safety and effectiveness in pediatric patients have not been established.

Use in Elderly Patients —Ulcer healing rates in elderly patients are similar to those in younger age groups. The incidence rates of adverse events and laboratory test abnormalities are also similar to those seen in other age groups. Age alone may not be an important factor in the disposition of nizatidine. Elderly patients may have reduced renal function (*see* Dosage and Administration).

ADVERSE REACTIONS

Worldwide, controlled clinical trials of nizatidine included over 6,000 patients given nizatidine in studies of varying durations. Placebo-controlled trials in the United States and Canada included over 2,600 patients given nizatidine and over 1,700 given placebo. Among the adverse events in these placebo-controlled trials, anemia (0.2% vs 0%) and urticaria (0.5% vs 0.1%) were significantly more common in the nizatidine group.

Incidence in Placebo-Controlled Clinical Trials in the United States and Canada—Table 5 lists adverse events that occurred at a frequency of 1% or more among nizatidine-treated patients who participated in placebo-controlled trials. The cited figures provide some basis for estimating the relative contribution of drug and nondrug factors to the side effect incidence rate in the population studied.

Table 5
Incidence of Treatment-Emergent Adverse Events in Placebo-Controlled Clinical Trials
In The United States and Canada

Body System/Adverse Event*	Percentage of Patients Reporting Event	
	Nizatidine (N=2,694)	Placebo (N=1,729)
Body as a Whole		
Headache	16.6	15.6
Abdominal pain	7.5	12.5
Pain	4.2	3.8
Asthenia	3.1	2.9
Back pain	2.4	2.6
Chest pain	2.3	2.1
Infection	1.7	1.1
Fever	1.6	2.3
Surgical procedure	1.4	1.5
Injury, accident	1.2	0.9
Digestive		
Diarrhea	7.2	6.9
Nausea	5.4	7.4
Flatulence	4.9	5.4
Vomiting	3.6	5.6
Dyspepsia	3.6	4.4
Constipation	2.5	3.8
Dry mouth	1.4	1.3
Nausea and vomiting	1.2	1.9
Anorexia	1.2	1.6
Gastrointestinal disorder	1.1	1.2
Tooth disorder	1.0	0.8
Musculoskeletal		
Myalgia	1.7	1.5
Nervous		
Dizziness	4.6	3.8
Insomnia	2.7	3.4
Abnormal dreams	1.9	1.9
Somnolence	1.9	1.6
Anxiety	1.6	1.4
Nervousness	1.1	0.8
Respiratory		
Rhinitis	9.8	9.6
Pharyngitis	3.3	3.1
Sinusitis	2.4	2.1
Cough, increased	2.0	2.0
Skin and Appendages		
Rash	1.9	2.1
Pruritus	1.7	1.3
Special Senses		
Amblyopia	1.0	0.9

*Events reported by at least 1% of nizatidine-treated patients are included.

A variety of less common events were also reported; it was not possible to determine whether these were caused by nizatidine.

Hepatic —Hepatocellular injury, evidenced by elevated liver enzyme tests (SGOT [AST], SGPT [ALT], or alkaline phosphatase), occurred in some patients and was possibly or probably related to nizatidine. In some cases there was marked elevation of SGOT, SGPT enzymes (greater than 500 IU/L) and, in a single instance, SGPT was greater than 2,000 IU/L. The overall rate of occurrences of elevated liver enzymes and elevations to 3 times the upper limit of normal, however, did not significantly differ from the rate of liver enzyme abnormalities in placebo-treated patients. All abnormalities were reversible after discontinuation of Axid. Since market introduction, hepatitis and jaundice have been reported. Rare cases of cholestatic or mixed hepatocellular and cholestatic injury with jaundice have been reported with reversal of the abnormalities after discontinuation of Axid.

Cardiovascular —In clinical pharmacology studies, short episodes of asymptomatic ventricular tachycardia occurred in 2 individuals administered Axid and in 3 untreated subjects.

CNS —Rare cases of reversible mental confusion have been reported.

Endocrine —Clinical pharmacology studies and controlled clinical trials showed no evidence of antiandrogenic activity due to Axid. Impotence and decreased libido were reported with similar frequency by patients who received Axid and by those given placebo. Rare reports of gynecomastia occurred.

Hematologic —Anemia was reported significantly more frequently in nizatidine- than in placebo-treated patients. Fatal thrombocytopenia was reported in a patient who was treated with Axid and another H_2-receptor antagonist. On previous occasions, this patient had experienced thrombocytopenia while taking other drugs. Rare cases of thrombocytopenic purpura have been reported.

Integumental —Sweating and urticaria were reported significantly more frequently in nizatidine- than in placebo-treated patients. Rash and exfoliative dermatitis were also reported. Vasculitis has been reported rarely.

Hypersensitivity —As with other H_2-receptor antagonists, rare cases of anaphylaxis following administration of nizatidine have been reported. Rare episodes of hypersensitivity reactions (eg, bronchospasm, laryngeal edema, rash, and eosinophilia) have been reported.

Body as a Whole —Serum sickness-like reactions have occurred rarely in conjunction with nizatidine use.

Genitourinary —Reports of impotence have occurred.

Other —Hyperuricemia unassociated with gout or nephrolithiasis was reported. Eosinophilia, fever, and nausea related to nizatidine administration have been reported.

OVERDOSAGE

Overdoses of Axid have been reported rarely. The following is provided to serve as a guide should such an overdose be encountered.

Signs and Symptoms —There is little clinical experience with overdosage of Axid in humans. Test animals that received large doses of nizatidine have exhibited cholinergic-type effects, including lacrimation, salivation, emesis, miosis, and diarrhea. Single oral doses of 800 mg/kg in dogs and of 1,200 mg/kg in monkeys were not lethal. Intravenous median lethal doses in the rat and mouse were 301 mg/kg and 232 mg/kg respectively.

Treatment —To obtain up-to-date information about the treatment of overdose, a good resource is your certified Regional Poison Control Center. Telephone numbers of certified poison control centers are listed in the *Physicians' Desk Reference (PDR)*. In managing overdosage, consider the possibility of multiple drug overdoses, interaction among drugs, and unusual drug kinetics in your patient.

If overdosage occurs, use of activated charcoal, emesis, or lavage should be considered along with clinical monitoring and supportive therapy. The ability of hemodialysis to remove nizatidine from the body has not been conclusively demonstrated; however, due to its large volume of distribution, nizatidine is not expected to be efficiently removed from the body by this method.

DOSAGE AND ADMINISTRATION

Active Duodenal Ulcer —The recommended oral dosage for adults is 300 mg once daily at bedtime. An alternative dosage regimen is 150 mg twice daily.

Maintenance of Healed Duodenal Ulcer —The recommended oral dosage for adults is 150 mg once daily at bedtime.

Gastroesophageal Reflux Disease —The recommended oral dosage in adults for the treatment of erosions, ulcerations, and associated heartburn is 150 mg twice daily.

Active Benign Gastric Ulcer —The recommended oral dosage is 300 mg given either as 150 mg twice daily or 300 mg once daily at bedtime. Prior to treatment, care should be taken to exclude the possibility of malignant gastric ulceration.

Dosage Adjustment for Patients With Moderate to Severe Renal Insufficiency —The dose for patients with renal dysfunction should be reduced as follows:

Active Duodenal Ulcer, GERD and Benign Gastric Ulcer

C_{cr}	Dose
20–50 mL/min	150 mg daily
<20 mL/min	150 mg every other day

Maintenance Therapy

C_{cr}	Dose
20–50 mL/min	150 mg every other day
<20 mL/min	150 mg every 3 days

Some elderly patients may have creatinine clearances of less than 50 mL/min, and, based on pharmacokinetic data in patients with renal impairment, the dose for such patients should be reduced accordingly. The clinical effects of this dosage reduction in patients with renal failure have not been evaluated.

HOW SUPPLIED

Axid® Pulvules®* are available in:

The 150-mg Pulvules are imprinted with script "Lilly" and "3144" on the opaque dark yellow cap and "AXID 150 mg" on the opaque pale yellow body, using black ink. They are available as follows:

Bottles of 60†	NDC 0002-3144-60 (PU3144)
Bottles of 500	NDC 0002-3144-03 (PU3144)
ID‡100	NDC 0002-3144-33 (PU3144) (10 strips of 10 Pulvules)
ID‡620§	NDC 0002-3144-82 (PU3144) (20 cards of 31 Pulvules)

The 300-mg Pulvules are imprinted with script "Lilly" and "3145" on the opaque brown cap and "AXID 300 mg" on the opaque pale yellow body, using black ink. They are available as follows:

Bottles of 30†	NDC 0002-3145-30 (PU3145)

* Pulvules® (filled gelatin capsules, Lilly)
† RxPak (prescription package, Lilly)
‡ Identi-Dose® (unit dose medication, Lilly)
§FlexPak (flexible blister card, Lilly)

Store at controlled room temperature 20° to 25°C (68° to 77°F) in a tightly closed container [see USP].

The USP defines controlled room temperature as: A temperature maintained thermostatically that encompasses the usual and customary working environment of 20° to 25°C (68° to 77°F); that results in a mean kinetic temperature calculated to be not more than 25°C; and that allows for excursions between 15° and 30°C (59° and 86°F) that are experienced in pharmacies, hospitals, and warehouses.

CAUTION-Federal (USA) law prohibits dispensing without prescription.

Literature revised August 22, 1996 [082296]
PV 2099 AMP

Shown in Product Identification Guide, page 321

CECLOR® ℞
CEFACLOR, USP
[sē ´klôr]

DESCRIPTION

Ceclor® (Cefaclor, USP) is a semisynthetic cephalosporin antibiotic for oral administration. It is chemically designated as 3-chloro-7-D- (2-phenylglycinamido)-3-cephem-4-carboxylic acid monohydrate. The chemical formula for cefaclor is $C_{15}H_{14}ClN_3O_4S \cdot H_2O$ and the molecular weight is 385.82.

Each Pulvule® contains cefaclor monohydrate equivalent to 250 mg (0.68 mmol) or 500 mg (1.36 mmol) anhydrous cefaclor. The Pulvules also contain cornstarch, F D & C Blue No. 1, F D & C Red No. 40, gelatin, magnesium stearate, silicone, titanium dioxide, and other inactive ingredients. The 500-mg Pulvule also contains iron oxide.

After mixing, each 5 mL of Ceclor for Oral Suspension will contain cefaclor monohydrate equivalent to 125 mg (0.34 mmol), 187 mg (0.51 mmol), 250 mg (0.68 mmol), or 375 mg (1.0 mmol) anhydrous cefaclor. The suspensions also contain cellulose, cornstarch, F D & C Red No. 40, flavors, silicone, sodium lauryl sulfate, sucrose, and xanthan gum.

CLINICAL PHARMACOLOGY

Cefaclor is well absorbed after oral administration to fasting subjects. Total absorption is the same whether the drug is given with or without food; however, when it is taken with food, the peak concentration achieved is 50% to 75% of that observed when the drug is administered to fasting subjects and generally appears from three fourths to 1 hour later. Following administration of 250-mg, 500-mg, and 1-g doses to fasting subjects, average peak serum levels of approximately 7, 13, and 23 µg/mL respectively were obtained within 30 to 60 minutes. Approximately 60% to 85% of the drug is excreted unchanged in the urine within 8 hours, the greater portion being excreted within the first 2 hours. During this 8-hour period, peak urine concentrations following the 250-mg, 500-mg, and 1-g doses were approximately 600, 900, and 1,900 µg/mL respectively. The serum half-life in normal subjects is 0.6 to 0.9 hours. In patients with reduced renal function, the serum half-life of cefaclor is slightly prolonged. In those with complete absence of renal function, the plasma half-life of the intact molecule is 2.3 to 2.8 hours. Excretion pathways in patients with markedly impaired renal function have not been determined. Hemodialysis shortens the half-life by 25% to 30%.

Microbiology—In vitro tests demonstrate that the bactericidal action of the cephalosporins results from inhibition of cell-wall synthesis. Cefaclor has been shown to be active against most strains of the following microorganisms, both *in vitro* and in clinical infections as described in the INDICATIONS AND USAGE section.

Aerobes, Gram-positive

Staphylococci, including coagulase-positive, coagulase-negative, and penicillinase-producing strains
Streptococcus pneumoniae
Streptococcus pyogenes (group A β-hemolytic streptococci)

Aerobes, Gram-negative

Escherichia coli
Haemophilus influenzae, excluding β-lactamase-negative ampicillin-resistant strains
Klebsiella spp
Proteus mirabilis

The following *in vitro* data are available, **but their clinical significance is unknown.**

Cefaclor exhibits *in vitro* minimal inhibitory concentrations (MICs) of ≤8 μg/mL against most (≥90%) strains of the following microorganisms; however, the safety and effectiveness of cefaclor in treating clinical infections due to these microorganisms have not been established in adequate and well-controlled clinical trials.

Aerobes, Gram-negative

Citrobacter diversus
Moraxella (Branhamella) catarrhalis
Neisseria gonorrhoeae

Anaerobes, Gram-positive

Bacteroides spp. (excluding *Bacteroides fragilis*)
Peptococcus
Peptostreptococcus
Propionibacterium acnes

Note: Pseudomonas spp., *Acinetobacter calcoaceticus* and most strains of enterococci (*Enterococcus faecalis*, group D streptococci), *Enterobacter* spp., indole-positive *Proteus*, and *Serratia* spp. are resistant to cefaclor. When tested by *in vitro* methods, staphylococci exhibit cross-resistance between cefaclor and methicillin-type antibiotics.

Susceptibility Testing—

Dilution Techniques—Quantitative methods that are used to determine minimum inhibitory concentrations (MIC) provide reproducible estimates of the susceptibility of bacteria to antimicrobial compounds. One such standardized procedure that has been recommended for use with cefaclor powder uses a standardized dilution method[1] (broth, agar, or microdilution). The MIC values obtained should be interpreted according to the following criteria:

MIC (μg/mL)	Interpretation*
≤8	Susceptible (S)
16	Intermediate (I)
≥32	Resistant (R)

* When testing *H. influenzae* spp. these interpretive standards are applicable only to broth microdilution method using Haemophilus Test Medium (HTM)[1]

Note: β-lactamase-negative, ampicillin-resistant strains of *H. influenzae* should be considered resistant to cefaclor despite apparent *in vitro* susceptibility to this agent.

A report of "Susceptible" indicates that the pathogen is likely to be inhibited by usually achievable concentrations of the antimicrobial compound in blood. A report of "Intermediate" indicates that the result should be considered equivocal, and, if the microorganism is not fully susceptible to alternative, clinically feasible drugs, the test should be repeated. This category implies possible clinical applicability in body sites where the drug is physiologically concentrated or in situations where high dosage of drug can be used. This category also provides a buffer zone that prevents small uncontrolled technical factors from causing major discrepancies in interpretation. A report of "Resistant" indicates that usually achievable concentrations of the antimicrobial compound in the blood are unlikely to be inhibitory and that other therapy should be selected.

Standardized susceptibility test procedures require the use of laboratory control microorganisms. Standard cefaclor powder should provide the following MIC values:

Microorganism	MIC (μg/mL)
E. coli ATCC 25922	1–4
E. faecalis ATCC 29212	>32
S. aureus ATCC 29213	1–4
When testing *H. influenzae**	
Microorganism	MIC (μg/mL)
H. influenzae ATCC 49766	1–4

* Broth microdilution test performed using Haemophilus Test Medium (HTM)[1]

Diffusion Techniques—Quantitative methods that require measurement of zone diameters provide reproducible estimates of the susceptibility of bacteria to antimicrobial compounds. One such standardized procedure[2] that has been recommended for use with disks to test the susceptibility of microorganisms to cefaclor uses the 30-μg cefaclor disk. Interpretation involves correlation of the diameter obtained in the disk test with the MIC for cefaclor. Reports from the laboratory providing results of the standard single-disk susceptibility test with a 30-μg cefaclor disk should be interpreted according to the following criteria:

When Testing Organisms Other Than *Haemophilus* spp. and Streptococci

Zone Diameter (mm)	Interpretation
≥18	Susceptible (S)
15–17	Intermediate (I)
≤14	Resistant (R)
When testing *H. influenzae**	
Zone Diameter (mm)	Interpretation
≥20	Susceptible (S)
17–19	Intermediate (I)
≤16	Resistant (R)

* Disk susceptibility test performed using Haemophilus Test Medium (HTM)[2]

Note: β-lactamase-negative, ampicillin-resistant strains of *H. influenzae* should be considered resistant to cefaclor despite apparent *in vitro* susceptibility to this agent.

Interpretation should be as stated above for results using diffusion techniques.

As with standard dilution techniques, diffusion methods require the use of laboratory control microorganisms. The 30-μg cefaclor disk should provide the following zone diameters in these laboratory test quality control strains:

Microorganisms	Zone Diameter (mm)
E. coli ATCC 25922	23–27
S. aureus ATCC 25923	27–31
When testing *H. influenzae**	
Microorganisms	Zone Diameter (mm)
H. influenzae ATCC 49766	25–31

* Disk susceptibility test performed using Haemophilus Test Medium (HTM)[1]

INDICATIONS AND USAGE

Ceclor is indicated in the treatment of the following infections when caused by susceptible strains of the designated microorganisms.

Otitis media caused by *Streptococcus pneumoniae, Haemophilus influenzae*, staphylococci, and *Streptococcus pyogenes*

Note: β-lactamase-negative, ampicillin-resistant (BLNAR) strains of *Haemophilus influenzae* should be considered resistant to cefaclor despite apparent *in vitro* susceptibility of some BLNAR strains.

Lower respiratory tract infections, including pneumonia, caused by *Streptococcus pneumoniae, Haemophilus influenzae*, and *Streptococcus pyogenes*

Note: β-lactamase-negative, ampicillin-resistant (BLNAR) strains of *Haemophilus influenzae* should be considered resistant to cefaclor despite apparent *in vitro* susceptibility of some BLNAR strains.

Pharyngitis and Tonsillitis, caused by *Streptococcus pyogenes*

Note: Penicillin is the usual drug of choice in the treatment and prevention of streptococcal infections, including the prophylaxis of rheumatic fever. Ceclor is generally effective in the eradication of streptococci from the nasopharynx; however, substantial data establishing the efficacy of Ceclor in the subsequent prevention of rheumatic fever are not available at present.

Urinary tract infections, including pyelonephritis and cystitis, caused by *Escherichia coli, Proteus mirabilis, Klebsiella* spp., and coagulase-negative staphylococci

Skin and skin structure infections caused by *Staphylococcus aureus* and *Streptococcus pyogenes*

Appropriate culture and susceptibility studies should be performed to determine susceptibility of the causative organism to cefaclor.

CONTRAINDICATION

Ceclor is contraindicated in patients with known allergy to the cephalosporin group of antibiotics.

WARNINGS

BEFORE THERAPY WITH CECLOR IS INSTITUTED, CAREFUL INQUIRY SHOULD BE MADE TO DETERMINE WHETHER THE PATIENT HAS HAD PREVIOUS HYPERSENSITIVITY REACTIONS TO CEFACLOR, CEPHALOSPORINS, PENICILLINS, OR OTHER DRUGS. IF THIS PRODUCT IS TO BE GIVEN TO PENICILLIN-SENSITIVE PATIENTS, CAUTION SHOULD BE EXERCISED BECAUSE CROSS-HYPERSENSITIVITY AMONG β-LACTAM ANTIBIOTICS HAS BEEN CLEARLY DOCUMENTED AND MAY OCCUR IN UP TO 10% OF PATIENTS WITH A HISTORY OF PENICILLIN ALLERGY.

IF AN ALLERGIC REACTION TO CECLOR OCCURS, DISCONTINUE THE DRUG. SERIOUS ACUTE HYPERSENSITIVITY REACTIONS MAY REQUIRE TREATMENT WITH EPINEPHRINE AND OTHER EMERGENCY MEASURES, INCLUDING OXYGEN, INTRAVENOUS FLUIDS, INTRAVENOUS ANTIHISTAMINES, CORTICOSTEROIDS, PRESSOR AMINES, AND AIRWAY MANAGEMENT, AS CLINICALLY INDICATED.

Antibiotics, including Ceclor, should be administered cautiously to any patient who has demonstrated some form of allergy, particularly to drugs.

Pseudomembranous colitis has been reported with nearly all antibacterial agents, including cefaclor, and has ranged in severity from mild to life-threatening. Therefore, it is important to consider this diagnosis in patients who present with diarrhea subsequent to the administration of antibacterial agents.

Treatment with antibacterial agents alters the normal flora of the colon and may permit overgrowth of clostridia. Studies indicate that a toxin produced by *Clostridium difficile* is one primary cause of antibiotic-associated colitis.

After the diagnosis of pseudomembranous colitis has been established, therapeutic measures should be initiated. Mild cases of pseudomembranous colitis usually respond to drug discontinuation alone. In moderate to severe cases, consideration should be given to management with fluids and electrolytes, protein supplementation and treatment with an antibacterial drug effective against *C. difficile*.

PRECAUTIONS

General—Prolonged use of Ceclor may result in the overgrowth of nonsusceptible organisms. Careful observation of the patient is essential. If superinfection occurs during therapy, appropriate measures should be taken.

Positive direct Coombs' tests have been reported during treatment with the cephalosporin antibiotics. It should be recognized that a positive Coombs' test may be due to the drug, eg, in hematologic studies or in transfusion cross-matching procedures when antiglobulin tests are performed on the minor side or in Coombs' testing of newborns whose mothers have received cephalosporin antibiotics before parturition.

Ceclor should be administered with caution in the presence of markedly impaired renal function. Since the half-life of cefaclor in anuria is 2.3 to 2.8 hours, dosage adjustments for patients with moderate or severe renal impairment are usually not required. Clinical experience with cefaclor under such conditions is limited; therefore, careful clinical observation and laboratory studies should be made.

As with other β-lactam antibiotics, the renal excretion of cefaclor is inhibited by probenecid.

Antibiotics, including cephalosporins, should be prescribed with caution in individuals with a history of gastrointestinal disease, particularly colitis.

Drug/Laboratory Test Interactions—Patients receiving Ceclor may show a false-positive reaction for glucose in the urine with tests that use Benedict's and Fehling's solutions and also with Clinitest® tablets.

There have been reports of increased anticoagulant effect when Ceclor and oral anticoagulants were administered concomitantly.

Carcinogenesis, Mutagenesis, Impairment of Fertility—Studies have not been performed to determine potential for carcinogenicity, mutagenicity, or impairment of fertility.

Pregnancy—Teratogenic Effects—Pregnancy Category B—Reproduction studies have been performed in mice and rats at doses up to 12 times the human dose and in ferrets given 3 times the maximum human dose and have revealed no harm to the fetus due to Ceclor. There are, however, no adequate and well-controlled studies in pregnant women. Because animal reproduction studies are not always predictive of human response, this drug should be used during pregnancy only if clearly needed.

Labor and Delivery—The effect of Ceclor on labor and delivery is unknown.

Nursing Mothers—Small amounts of Ceclor have been detected in mother's milk following administration of single 500-mg doses. Average levels were 0.18, 0.20, 0.21, and 0.16 μg/mL at 2, 3, 4, and 5 hours respectively. Trace amounts were detected at 1 hour. The effect on nursing infants is not known. Caution should be exercised when Ceclor is administered to a nursing woman.

Pediatric Use—Safety and effectiveness of this product for use in infants less than 1 month of age have not been established.

ADVERSE REACTIONS

Adverse effects considered to be related to therapy with Ceclor are listed below:

Hypersensitivity reactions have been reported in about 1.5% of patients and include morbilliform eruptions (1 in 100). Pruritus, urticaria, and positive Coombs' tests each occur in less than 1 in 200 patients.

Cases of **serum-sickness-like** reactions have been reported with the use of Ceclor. These are characterized by findings of erythema multiforme, rashes, and other skin manifestations accompanied by arthritis/arthralgia, with or without fever, and differ from classic serum sickness in that there is infrequently associated lymphadenopathy and proteinuria, no circulating immune complexes, and no evidence to date of sequelae of the reaction. Occasionally, solitary symptoms may occur, but do not represent a **serum-sickness-like** reaction. While further investigation is ongoing, **serum-sickness-like** reactions appear to be due to hypersensitivity and more often occur during or following a second (or subsequent) course of therapy with Ceclor. Such reactions have been reported more frequently in pediatric patients than in adults with an overall occurrence ranging from 1 in 200 (0.5%) in one focused trial to 2 in 8,346 (0.024%) in overall clinical trials (with an incidence in pediatric patients in clinical trials of 0.055%) to 1 in 38,000 (0.003%) in spontaneous event reports. Signs and symptoms usually occur a

Continued on next page

*** Identi-Code® symbol. This product information was prepared in June 2000. Current information on these and other products of Eli Lilly and Company may be obtained by direct inquiry to Lilly Research Laboratories, Lilly Corporate Center, Indianapolis, Indiana 46285, (800) 545-5979.**

Ceclor—Cont.

few days after initiation of therapy and subside within a few days after cessation of therapy; occasionally these reactions have resulted in hospitalization, usually of short duration (median hospitalization = 2 to 3 days, based on postmarketing surveillance studies). In those requiring hospitalization, the symptoms have ranged from mild to severe at the time of admission with more of the severe reactions occurring in pediatric patients. Antihistamines and glucocorticoids appear to enhance resolution of the signs and symptoms. No serious sequelae have been reported.

More severe hypersensitivity reactions, including Stevens-Johnson syndrome, toxic epidermal necrolysis, and anaphylaxis have been reported rarely. Anaphylactoid events may be manifested by solitary symptoms, including angioedema, asthenia, edema (including face and limbs), dyspnea, paresthesias, syncope, hypotension, or vasodilatation. Anaphylaxis may be more common in patients with a history of penicillin allergy.

Rarely, hypersensitivity symptoms may persist for several months.

Gastrointestinal symptoms occur in about 2.5% of patients and include diarrhea (1 in 70).

Onset of pseudomembranous colitis symptoms may occur during or after antibiotic treatment. (*see* **WARNINGS**). Nausea and vomiting have been reported rarely. As with some penicillins and some other cephalosporins, transient hepatitis and cholestatic jaundice have been reported rarely.

Other effects considered related to therapy included eosinophilia (1 in 50 patients), genital pruritus or vaginitis (less than 1 in 100 patients), and, rarely, thrombocytopenia or reversible interstitial nephritis.

Causal Relationship Uncertain—

CNS—Rarely, reversible hyperactivity, agitation, nervousness, insomnia, confusion, hypertonia, dizziness, hallucinations, and somnolence have been reported.

Transitory abnormalities in clinical laboratory test results have been reported. Although they were of uncertain etiology, they are listed below to serve as alerting information for the physician.

Hepatic—Slight elevations of AST, ALT, or alkaline phosphatase values (1 in 40).

Hematopoietic–As has also been reported with other β-lactam antibiotics, transient lymphocytosis, leukopenia, and, rarely, hemolytic anemia, aplastic anemia, agranulocytosis, and reversible neutropenia of possible clinical significance.

There have been rare reports of increased prothrombin time with or without clinical bleeding in patients receiving Ceclor and Coumadin® concomitantly.

Renal—Slight elevations in BUN or serum creatinine (less than 1 in 500) or abnormal urinalysis (less than 1 in 200).

Cephalosporin-class Adverse Reactions

In addition to the adverse reactions listed above that have been observed in patients treated with cefaclor, the following adverse reactions and altered laboratory tests have been reported for cephalosporin-class antibiotics: fever, abdominal pain, superinfection, renal dysfunction, toxic nephropathy, hemorrhage, false positive test for urinary glucose, elevated bilirubin, elevated LDH, and pancytopenia.

Several cephalosporins have been implicated in triggering seizures, particularly in patients with renal impairment when the dosage was not reduced. If seizures associated with drug therapy occur, the drug should be discontinued. Anticonvulsant therapy can be given if clinically indicated (*see* **DOSAGE AND ADMINISTRATION** and **OVERDOSAGE** sections).

OVERDOSAGE

Signs and Symptoms—The toxic symptoms following an overdose of cefaclor may include nausea, vomiting, epigastric distress, and diarrhea. The severity of the epigastric distress and the diarrhea are dose related. If other symptoms are present, it is probable that they are secondary to an underlying disease state, an allergic reaction, or the effects of other intoxication.

Treatment—To obtain up-to-date information about the treatment of overdose, a good resource is your certified Regional Poison Control Center. Telephone numbers of certified poison control centers are listed in the *Physicians' Desk Reference* (*PDR*). In managing overdosage, consider the possibility of multiple drug overdoses, interaction among drugs, and unusual drug kinetics in your patient.

Unless 5 times the normal dose of cefaclor has been ingested, gastrointestinal decontamination will not be necessary.

Protect the patient's airway and support ventilation and perfusion. Meticulously monitor and maintain, within acceptable limits, the patient's vital signs, blood gases, serum electrolytes, etc. Absorption of drugs from the gastrointestinal tract may be decreased by giving activated charcoal, which, in many cases, is more effective than emesis or lavage; consider charcoal instead of or in addition to gastric emptying. Repeated doses of charcoal over time may hasten elimination of some drugs that have been absorbed. Safeguard the patient's airway when employing gastric emptying or charcoal.

Forced diuresis, peritoneal dialysis, hemodialysis, or charcoal hemoperfusion have not been established as beneficial for an overdose of cefaclor.

DOSAGE AND ADMINISTRATION

Ceclor is administered orally.

Adults—The usual adult dosage is 250 mg every 8 hours. For more severe infections (such as pneumonia) or those caused by less susceptible organisms, doses may be doubled.

Pediatric Patients—The usual recommended daily dosage for pediatric patients is 20 mg/kg/day in divided doses every 8 hours. In more serious infections, otitis media, and infections caused by less susceptible organisms, 40 mg/kg/day are recommended, with a maximum dosage of 1 g/day.

Ceclor Suspension

Weight	125 mg/5 mL	250 mg/5 mL
	20 mg/kg/day	
9 kg	1/2 tsp t.i.d.	
18 kg	1 tsp t.i.d.	1/2 tsp t.i.d.
	40 mg/kg/day	
9 kg	1 tsp t.i.d.	1/2 tsp t.i.d.
18 kg		1 tsp t.i.d.

B.I.D. Treatment Option—For the treatment of otitis media and pharyngitis, the total daily dosage may be divided and administered every 12 hours.

Ceclor Suspension

Weight	187 mg/5 mL	375 mg/5 mL
	20 mg/kg/day (Pharyngitis)	
9 kg	1/2 tsp b.i.d.	
18 kg	1 tsp b.i.d	1/2 tsp b.i.d.
	40 mg/kg/day (Otitis Media)	
9 kg	1 tsp b.i.d.	1/2 tsp b.i.d.
18 kg		1 tsp b.i.d.

Ceclor may be administered in the presence of impaired renal function. Under such a condition, the dosage usually is unchanged (*see* **PRECAUTIONS**).

In the treatment of β-hemolytic streptococcal infections, a therapeutic dosage of Ceclor should be administered for at least 10 days.

HOW SUPPLIED

Pulvules:

250 mg, purple and white (No. 3061)—(RxPak * of 15) NDC 0002-3061-15; (100s) NDC 0002-3061-02; (ID†100) NDC 0002-3061-33

500 mg, purple and gray (No. 3062)—(RxPak of 15) NDC 0002-3062-15

For Oral Suspension:

125 mg/5 mL, strawberry flavor (M-5057‡)—(150-mL size) NDC 0002-5057-68

187 mg/5 mL, strawberry flavor (M-5130‡)—(100-mL size) NDC 0002-5130-48

250 mg/5 mL, strawberry flavor (M-5058‡)—(75-mL size) NDC 0002-5058-18; (150-mL size) NDC 0002-5058-68

375 mg/5 mL, strawberry flavor (M-5132‡)—(100-mL size) NDC 0002-5132-48

*All RxPaks (prescription packages, Lilly) have safety closures.

†Identi-Dose® (unit dose medication, Lilly).

‡After mixing, store in a refrigerator. Shake well before using. Keep tightly closed. The mixture may be kept for 14 days without significant loss of potency. Discard unused portion after 14 days.

Store at 25°C (77°F); excursions permitted to 15-30°C (59–86°F) [See USP Controlled Room Temperature]

REFERENCES

1. National Committee for Clinical Laboratory Standards. Methods for Dilution Antimicrobial Susceptibility Tests for Bacteria that Grow Aerobically—Fourth Edition. Approved Standard NCCLS Document M7–A4, Vol. 17, No. 2, NCCLS, Wayne, PA, January, 1997.
2. National Committee for Clinical Laboratory Standards. Performance Standards for Antimicrobial Disk Susceptibility Tests—Sixth Edition Approved Standard NCCLS Document M2-A6, Vol. 17, No. 1, NCCLS, Wayne, PA, January, 1997.

Literature issued May 12, 2000

IT 0080 ITAMP [051200]

CEFACLOR, *see* Ceclor® (Cefaclor, USP). ℞

CEFAMANDOLE NAFATE, *see* Mandol® (Cefamandole Nafate, USP). ℞

CEFAZOLIN SODIUM, *see* Kefzol® (Cefazolin Sodium, USP). ℞

CEFTAZIDIME, *see* Tazidime® (Ceftazidime, USP). ℞

CEFUROXIME SODIUM, *see* Kefurox® (Cefuroxime Sodium, USP). ℞

DARVOCET-N® 50 Ⓒ
[där 'vō-sĕt ĕn]
and
DARVOCET-N® 100
(propoxyphene napsylate and acetaminophen tablets, USP)

DESCRIPTION

Darvon-N® Propoxyphene Napsylate, USP is an odorless, white crystalline powder with a bitter taste. It is very slightly soluble in water and soluble in methanol, ethanol, chloroform, and acetone. Chemically, it is (αS,1R)-α-[2-(Dimethylamino) -1 -methylethyl]- α -phenylphenethyl propionate compound with 2-naphthalenesulfonic acid (1:1) monohydrate, which can be represented by the accompanying structural formula. Its molecular weight is 565.74.

$$(CH_3)_2NCH_2-\underset{H}{\overset{CH_3}{C}}-\underset{C_6H_5}{\overset{OCOC_2H_5}{C}}-CH_2-C_6H_5 \cdot C_{10}H_7SO_3H \cdot H_2O$$

Propoxyphene napsylate differs from propoxyphene hydrochloride in that it allows more stable liquid dosage forms and tablet formulations. Because of differences in molecular weight, a dose of 100 mg (176.8 µmol) of propoxyphene napsylate is required to supply an amount of propoxyphene equivalent to that present in 65 mg (172.9 µmol) of propoxyphene hydrochloride.

Each tablet of Darvocet-N 50 contains 50 mg (88.4 µmol) propoxyphene napsylate and 325 mg (2,150 µmol) acetaminophen.

Each tablet of Darvocet-N 100 contains 100 mg (176.8 µmol) propopoxyphene napsylate and 650 mg (4,300 µmol) acetaminophen.

Each tablet also contains amberlite, cellulose, F D & C Yellow No. 6, magnesium stearate, stearic acid, titanium dioxide, and other inactive ingredients.

CLINICAL PHARMACOLOGY

Propoxyphene is a centrally acting narcotic analgesic agent. Equimolar doses of propoxyphene hydrochloride or napsylate provide similar plasma concentrations. Following administration of 65, 130, or 195 mg of propoxyphene hydrochloride, the bioavailability of propoxyphene is equivalent to that of 100, 200, or 300 mg respectively of propoxyphene napsylate. Peak plasma concentrations of propoxyphene are reached in 2 to 2 1/2 hours. After a 100-mg oral dose of propoxyphene napsylate, peak plasma levels of 0.05 to 0.1 µg/mL are achieved. As shown in Figure 1, the napsylate salt tends to be absorbed more slowly than the hydrochloride. At or near therapeutic doses, this absorption difference is small when compared with that among subjects and among doses.

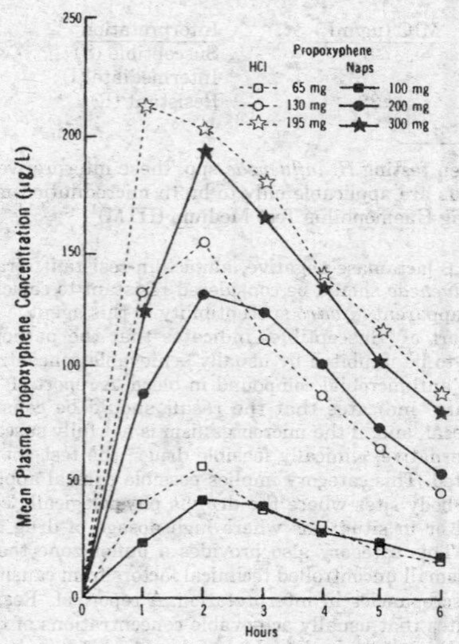

Figure 1. Mean plasma concentrations of propoxyphene in 8 human subjects following oral administration of 65 and 130 mg of the hydrochloride salt and 100 and 200 mg of the napsylate salt and in 7 given 195 mg of the hydrochloride and 300 mg of the napsylate salt.

Because of this several hundredfold difference in solubility, the absorption rate of very large doses of the napsylate salt is significantly lower than that of equimolar doses of the hydrochloride.

Repeated doses of propoxyphene at 6-hour intervals lead to increasing plasma concentrations, with a plateau after the ninth dose at 48 hours.

Propoxyphene is metabolized in the liver to yield norpropoxyphene. Propoxyphene has a half-life of 6 to 12 hours, whereas that of norpropoxyphene is 30 to 36 hours.

Norpropoxyphene has substantially less central-nervous-system-depressant effect than propoxyphene but a greater local anesthetic effect, which is similar to that of amitriptyline and antiarrhythmic agents, such as lidocaine and quinidine.

In animal studies in which propoxyphene and norpropoxyphene were continuously infused in large amounts, intracardiac conduction time (PR and QRS intervals) was prolonged. Any intracardiac conduction delay attributable to high concentrations of norpropoxyphene may be of relatively long duration.

ACTIONS

Propoxyphene is a mild narcotic analgesic structurally related to methadone. The potency of propoxyphene napsylate is from two-thirds to equal that of codeine.

Darvocet-N 50 and Darvocet-N 100 provide the analgesic activity of propoxyphene napsylate and the antipyretic-analgesic activity of acetaminophen.

The combination of propoxyphene and acetaminophen produces greater analgesia than that produced by either propoxyphene or acetaminophen administered alone.

INDICATION

These products are indicated for the relief of mild to moderate pain, either when pain is present alone or when it is accompanied by fever.

CONTRAINDICATIONS

Hypersensitivity to propoxyphene or acetaminophen

WARNINGS

- **Do not prescribe propoxyphene for patients who are suicidal or addiction-prone.**
- **Prescribe propoxyphene with caution for patients taking tranquilizers or antidepressant drugs and patients who use alcohol in excess.**
- **Tell your patients not to exceed the recommended dose and to limit their intake of alcohol.**

Propoxyphene products in excessive doses, either alone or in combination with other CNS depressants, including alcohol, are a major cause of drug-related deaths. Fatalities within the first hour of overdosage are not uncommon. In a survey of deaths due to overdosage conducted in 1975, in approximately 20% of the fatal cases, death occurred within the first hour (5% occurred within 15 minutes). Propoxyphene should not be taken in doses higher than those recommended by the physician. The judicious prescribing of propoxyphene is essential to the safe use of this drug. With patients who are depressed or suicidal, consideration should be given to the use of nonnarcotic analgesics. Patients should be cautioned about the concomitant use of propoxyphene products and alcohol because of potentially serious CNS-additive effects of these agents. Because of its added depressant effects, propoxyphene should be prescribed with caution for those patients whose medical condition requires the concomitant administration of sedatives, tranquilizers, muscle relaxants, antidepressants, or other CNS-depressant drugs. Patients should be advised of the additive depressant effects of these combinations.

Many of the propoxyphene-related deaths have occurred in patients with previous histories of emotional disturbances or suicidal ideation or attempts as well as histories of misuse of tranquilizers, alcohol, and other CNS-active drugs. Some deaths have occurred as a consequence of the accidental ingestion of excessive quantities of propoxyphene alone or in combination with other drugs. Patients taking propoxyphene should be warned not to exceed the dosage recommended by the physician.

Drug Dependence —Propoxyphene, when taken in higher-than-recommended doses over long periods of time, can produce drug dependence characterized by psychic dependence and, less frequently, physical dependence and tolerance. Propoxyphene will only partially suppress the withdrawal syndrome in individuals physically dependent on morphine or other narcotics. The abuse liability of propoxyphene is qualitatively similar to that of codeine although quantitatively less, and propoxyphene should be prescribed with the same degree of caution appropriate to the use of codeine.

Usage in Ambulatory Patients —Propoxyphene may impair the mental and/or physical abilities required for the performance of potentially hazardous tasks, such as driving a car or operating machinery. The patient should be cautioned accordingly.

PRECAUTIONS

General —Propoxyphene should be administered with caution to patients with hepatic or renal impairment since higher serum concentrations or delayed elimination may occur.

Drug Interactions —The CNS-depressant effect of propoxyphene is additive with that of other CNS depressants, including alcohol.

As is the case with many medicinal agents, propoxyphene may slow the metabolism of a concomitantly administered drug. Should this occur, the higher serum concentrations of that drug may result in increased pharmacologic or adverse effects of that drug. Such occurrences have been reported when propoxyphene was administered to patients on antidepressants, anticonvulsants, or warfarin-like drugs. Severe neurologic signs, including coma, have occurred with concurrent use of carbamazepine.

Usage in Pregnancy —Safe use in pregnancy has not been established relative to possible adverse effects on fetal development. Instances of withdrawal symptoms in the neonate have been reported following usage during pregnancy. Therefore, propoxyphene should not be used in pregnant women unless, in the judgment of the physician, the potential benefits outweigh the possible hazards.

Usage in Nursing Mothers —Low levels of propoxyphene have been detected in human milk. In postpartum studies involving nursing mothers who were given propoxyphene, no adverse effects were noted in infants receiving mother's milk.

Usage in Pediatric Patients —Safety and effectiveness in pediatric patients have not been established.

Usage in the Elderly —The rate of propoxyphene metabolism may be reduced in some patients. Increased dosing interval should be considered.

A Patient Information Sheet is available for this product. See text following "How Supplied" section below.

ADVERSE REACTIONS

In a survey conducted in hospitalized patients, less than 1% of patients taking propoxyphene hydrochloride at recommended doses experienced side effects. The most frequently reported were dizziness, sedation, nausea, and vomiting. Some of these adverse reactions may be alleviated if the patient lies down.

Other adverse reactions include constipation, abdominal pain, skin rashes, lightheadedness, headache, weakness, euphoria, dysphoria, hallucinations, and minor visual disturbances.

Liver dysfunction has been reported in association with both active components of Darvocet-N 50 and Darvocet-N 100. Propoxyphene therapy has been associated with abnormal liver function tests and, more rarely, with instances of reversible jaundice (including cholestatic jaundice). Hepatic necrosis may result from acute overdose of acetaminophen (*see* Management of Overdosage). In chronic ethanol abusers, this has been reported rarely with short-term use of acetaminophen dosages of 2.5 to 10 g/day. Fatalities have occurred.

Renal papillary necrosis may result from chronic acetaminophen use, particularly when the dosage is greater than recommended and when combined with aspirin.

Subacute painful myopathy has occurred following chronic propoxyphene overdosage.

DOSAGE AND ADMINISTRATION

These products are given orally. The usual dosage is 100 mg propoxyphene napsylate and 650 mg acetaminophen every 4 hours as needed for pain. The maximum recommended dose of propoxyphene napsylate is 600 mg per day.

Consideration should be given to a reduced total daily dosage in patients with hepatic or renal impairment.

MANAGEMENT OF OVERDOSAGE

In all cases of suspected overdosage, call your regional Poison Control Center to obtain the most up-to-date information about the treatment of overdose. This recommendation is made because, in general, information regarding the treatment of overdosage may change more rapidly than do package inserts.

Initial consideration should be given to the management of the CNS effects of propoxyphene overdosage. Resuscitative measures should be initiated promptly.

Symptoms of Propoxyphene Overdosage —The manifestations of acute overdosage with propoxyphene are those of narcotic overdosage. The patient is usually somnolent but may be stuporous or comatose and convulsing. Respiratory depression is characteristic. The ventilatory rate and/or tidal volume is decreased, which results in cyanosis and hypoxia. Pupils, initially pinpoint, may become dilated as hypoxia increases. Cheyne-Stokes respiration and apnea may occur. Blood pressure and heart rate are usually normal initially, but blood pressure falls and cardiac performance deteriorates, which ultimately results in pulmonary edema and circulatory collapse, unless the respiratory depression is corrected and adequate ventilation is restored promptly. Cardiac arrhythmias and conduction delay may be present. A combined respiratory-metabolic acidosis occurs owing to retained CO_2 (hypercapnia) and to lactic acid formed during anaerobic glycolysis. Acidosis may be severe if large amounts of salicylates have also been ingested. Death may occur.

Treatment of Propoxyphene Overdosage — Attention should be directed first to establishing a patent airway and to restoring ventilation. Mechanically assisted ventilation, with or without oxygen, may be required, and positive pressure respiration may be desirable if pulmonary edema is present. The narcotic antagonist naloxone will markedly reduce the degree of respiratory depression, and 0.4 to 2 mg should be administered promptly, preferably intravenously. If the desired degree of counteraction with improvement in respiratory functions is not obtained, naloxone should be repeated at 2- to 3-minute intervals. The duration of action of the antagonist may be brief. If no response is observed after 10 mg of naloxone have been administered, the diagnosis of propoxyphene toxicity should be questioned. Naloxone may also be administered by continuous intravenous infusion.

Treatment of Propoxyphene Overdosage in Pediatric Patients —The usual initial dose of naloxone in pediatric patients is 0.01 mg/kg body weight given intravenously. If this dose does not result in the desired degree of clinical improvement, a subsequent increased dose of 0.1 mg/kg body weight may be administered. If an IV route of administration is not available, naloxone may be administered IM or subcutaneously in divided doses. If necessary, naloxone can be diluted with Sterile Water for Injection.

Blood gases, pH, and electrolytes should be monitored in order that acidosis and any electrolyte disturbance present may be corrected promptly. Acidosis, hypoxia, and generalized CNS depression predispose to the development of cardiac arrhythmias. Ventricular fibrillation or cardiac arrest may occur and necessitate the full complement of cardiopulmonary resuscitation (CPR) measures. Respiratory acidosis rapidly subsides as ventilation is restored and hypercapnia eliminated, but lactic acidosis may require intravenous bicarbonate for prompt correction.

Electrocardiographic monitoring is essential. Prompt correction of hypoxia, acidosis, and electrolyte disturbance (when present) will help prevent these cardiac complications and will increase the effectiveness of agents administered to restore normal cardiac function.

In addition to the use of a narcotic antagonist, the patient may require careful titration with an anticonvulsant to control convulsions. Analeptic drugs (for example, caffeine or amphetamine) should not be used because of their tendency to precipitate convulsions.

General supportive measures, in addition to oxygen, include, when necessary, intravenous fluids, vasopressor-inotropic compounds, and, when infection is likely, anti-infective agents. Gastric lavage may be useful, and activated charcoal can adsorb a significant amount of ingested propoxyphene. Dialysis is of little value in poisoning due to propoxyphene. Efforts should be made to determine whether other agents, such as alcohol, barbiturates, tranquilizers, or other CNS depressants, were also ingested, since these increase CNS depression as well as cause specific toxic effects.

Symptoms of Acetaminophen Overdosage — Shortly after oral ingestion of an overdose of acetaminophen and for the next 24 hours, anorexia, nausea, vomiting, diaphoresis, general malaise, and abdominal pain have been noted. The patient may then present no symptoms, but evidence of liver dysfunction may become apparent up to 72 hours after ingestion, with elevated serum transaminase and lactic dehydrogenase levels, an increase in serum bilirubin concentrations, and a prolonged prothrombin time. Death from hepatic failure may result 3 to 7 days after overdosage.

Acute renal failure may accompany the hepatic dysfunction and has been noted in patients who do not exhibit signs of fulminant hepatic failure. Typically, renal impairment is more apparent 6 to 9 days after ingestion of the overdose.

Treatment of Acetaminophen Overdosage —Acetaminophen in massive overdosage may cause hepatic toxicity in some patients. *In all cases of suspected overdose, immediately call your regional poison center or the Rocky Mountain Poison Center's toll-free number* (800-525-6115) for assistance in diagnosis and for directions in the use of N-acetylcysteine as an antidote.

In adults, hepatic toxicity has rarely been reported with acute overdoses of less than 10 g and fatalities with less than 15 g. Importantly, young children seem to be more resistant than adults to the hepatotoxic effect of an acetaminophen overdose. Despite this, the measures outlined below should be initiated in any adult or pediatric patient suspected of having ingested an acetaminophen overdose.

Because clinical and laboratory evidence of hepatic toxicity may not be apparent until 48 to 72 hours postingestion, liver function studies should be obtained initially and repeated at 24-hour intervals.

Consider emptying the stomach promptly by lavage or by induction of emesis with syrup of ipecac. Patients' estimates of the quantity of a drug ingested are notoriously unreliable. Therefore, if an acetaminophen overdose is suspected, a serum acetaminophen assay should be obtained as early as possible, but no sooner than 4 hours following ingestion. The antidote, N-acetylcysteine, should be administered as early as possible, and within 16 hours of the overdose ingestion for optimal results. Following recovery, there are no residual, structural, or functional hepatic abnormalities.

ANIMAL TOXICOLOGY

The acute lethal doses of the hydrochloride and napsylate salts of propoxyphene were determined in 4 species. The results shown in Figure 2 indicate that, on a molar basis, the napsylate salt is less toxic than the hydrochloride. This may be due to the relative insolubility and retarded absorption of propoxyphene napsylate.

Figure 2. Acute oral toxicity of propoxyphene

	LD_{50} (mg/kg± SE) / LD_{50} (mmol/kg)	
Species	Propoxyphene Hydrochloride	Propoxyphene Napsylate
Mouse	282 ± 39 / 0.75	915 ± 163 / 1.62
Rat	230 ± 44 / 0.61	647 ± 95 / 1.14
Rabbit	*ca*82 / 0.22	>183 / >0.32
Dog	*ca*100 / 0.27	>183 / >0.32

Some indication of the relative insolubility and retarded absorption of propoxyphene napsylate was obtained by measuring plasma propoxyphene levels in 2 groups of 4 dogs fol-

Continued on next page

*** Identi-Code® symbol. This product information was prepared in June 2000. Current information on these and other products of Eli Lilly and Company may be obtained by direct inquiry to Lilly Research Laboratories, Lilly Corporate Center, Indianapolis, Indiana 46285, (800) 545-5979.**

Darvocet N—Cont.

lowing oral administration of equimolar doses of the 2 salts. As shown in Figure 3, the peak plasma concentration observed with propoxyphene hydrochloride was much higher than that obtained after administration of the napsylate salt.

Although none of the animals in this experiment died, 3 of the 4 dogs given propoxyphene hydrochloride exhibited convulsive seizures during the time interval corresponding to the peak plasma levels. The 4 animals receiving the napsylate salt were mildly ataxic but not acutely ill.

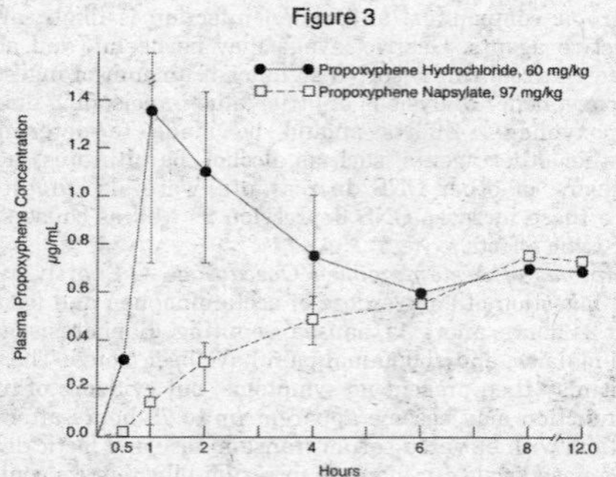

Figure 3. Plasma propoxyphene concentrations in dogs following large doses of the hydrochloride and napsylate salts.

HOW SUPPLIED

Darvocet-N® Tablets (No. 1890) are available in:
The 50 mg tablets are dark orange, capsule shaped, film coated, and imprinted with the script "Lilly" and "Darvocet-N 50" on one side of the tablet, using edible black ink. They are available as follows:

Bottles of 100 (RxPak*)	NDC 0002-0351-02 (TA1890)

Darvocet-N® Tablets (No. 1893) are available in:
The 100 mg tablets are dark orange, capsule shaped, film coated, and imprinted with the script "Lilly" on one side and "Darvocet-N 100" on the other side of the tablet, using edible black ink. They are available as follows:

Bottles of 100 (RxPak*)	NDC 0002-0363-02 (TA1893)
Bottles of 500	NDC 0002-0363-03 (TA1893)
ID† 100	NDC 0002-0363-33 (TA1893)
RN‡ 500	NDC 0002-0363-46 (TA1893)

* All RxPaks (prescription packages, Lilly) have safety closures.
† Identi-Dose® (unit dose medication, Lilly).
‡ Reverse-numbered package.

Store at controlled room temperature, 59° to 86°F (15° to 30°C).

The following information, including description of dosage forms and the maximum daily dosage of each, is available to patients receiving Darvon products.

Patient Information Sheet

YOUR PRESCRIPTION FOR A DARVON® (PROPOXYPHENE) PRODUCT CIV

Summary

Products containing Darvon are used to relieve pain.

LIMIT YOUR INTAKE OF ALCOHOL WHILE TAKING THIS DRUG. Make sure your doctor knows if you are taking tranquilizers, sleep aids, antidepressants, antihistamines, or any other drugs that make you sleepy. Combining propoxyphene with alcohol or these drugs in excessive doses is dangerous.

Use care while driving a car or using machines until you see how the drug affects you because propoxyphene can make you sleepy. Do not take more of the drug than your doctor prescribed. Dependence has occurred when patients have taken propoxyphene for a long period of time at doses greater than recommended.

The rest of this leaflet gives you more information about propoxyphene. Please read it and keep it for future use.

Uses of Darvon

Products containing Darvon are used for the relief of mild to moderate pain. Products that contain Darvon plus aspirin or acetaminophen are prescribed for the relief of pain or pain associated with fever.

Before Taking Darvon

Make sure your doctor knows if you have ever had an allergic reaction to propoxyphene, aspirin, or acetaminophen. Some forms of propoxyphene products contain aspirin to help relieve the pain. Your doctor should be advised if you have a history of ulcers or if you are taking an anticoagulant ("blood thinner"). The aspirin may irritate the stomach lining and may cause bleeding, particularly if an ulcer is present. Also, bleeding may occur if you are taking an anticoagulant. In a small group of people, aspirin may cause an asthma attack. If you are one of these people, be sure your drug does not contain aspirin.

The effect of propoxyphene in pediatric patients under 12 has not been studied. Therefore, use of the drug in this age group is not recommended.

Also, due to the possible association between aspirin and Reye Syndrome, those propoxyphene products containing aspirin should not be given to children, including teenagers, with chicken pox or flu unless prescribed by a physician.

The following propoxyphene product contains aspirin:
Darvon® Compound-65 (Propoxyphene Hydrochloride, Aspirin, and Caffeine, USP)

How to Take Darvon

Follow your doctor's directions exactly. Do not increase the amount you take without your doctor's approval. If you miss a dose of the drug, do not take twice as much the next time.

Pregnancy

Do not take propoxyphene during pregnancy unless your doctor knows you are pregnant and specifically recommends its use. Cases of temporary dependence in the newborn have occurred when the mother has taken propoxyphene consistently in the weeks before delivery. As a general principle, no drug should be taken during pregnancy unless it is clearly necessary.

General Cautions

Heavy use of alcohol with propoxyphene is hazardous and may lead to overdosage symptoms (*see* "Overdose" below). THEREFORE, LIMIT YOUR INTAKE OF ALCOHOL WHILE TAKING PROPOXYPHENE.

Combinations of excessive doses of propoxyphene, alcohol, and tranquilizers are dangerous. Make sure your doctor knows if you are taking tranquilizers, sleep aids, antidepressant drugs, antihistamines, or any other drugs that make you sleepy. The use of these drugs with propoxyphene increases their sedative effects and may lead to overdosage symptoms, including death (*see* "Overdose" below).

Propoxyphene may cause drowsiness or impair your mental and/or physical abilities; therefore, use caution when driving a vehicle or operating dangerous machinery. DO NOT perform any hazardous task until you have seen your response to this drug.

Propoxyphene may increase the concentration in the body of medications, such as anticoagulants ("blood thinners"), antidepressants, or drugs used for epilepsy. The result may be excessive or adverse effects of these medications. Make sure your doctor knows if you are taking any of these medications.

Dependence

You can become dependent on propoxyphene if you take it in higher than recommended doses over a long period of time. Dependence is a feeling of need for the drug and a feeling that you cannot perform normally without it.

Overdose

An overdose of Darvon, alone or in combination with other drugs, including alcohol, may cause weakness, difficulty in breathing, confusion, anxiety, and more severe drowsiness and dizziness. Extreme overdosage may lead to unconsciousness and death.

If the propoxyphene product contains acetaminophen, the overdosage symptoms include nausea, vomiting, lack of appetite, and abdominal pain. Liver damage may occur even after symptoms disappear. Death can occur days later.

When the propoxyphene product contains aspirin, symptoms of taking too much of the drug are headache, dizziness, ringing in the ears, difficulty in hearing, dim vision, confusion, drowsiness, sweating, thirst, rapid breathing, nausea, vomiting, and, occasionally, diarrhea.

In any suspected overdosage situation, contact your doctor or nearest hospital emergency room. GET EMERGENCY HELP IMMEDIATELY.

KEEP THIS DRUG AND ALL DRUGS OUT OF THE REACH OF THE PEDIATRIC POPULATION.

Possible Side Effects

When propoxyphene is taken as directed, side effects are infrequent. Among those reported are drowsiness, dizziness, nausea, and vomiting. If these effects occur, it may help if you lie down and rest.

Less frequently reported side effects are constipation, abdominal pain, skin rashes, lightheadedness, headache, weakness, hallucinations, minor visual disturbances, and feelings of elation or discomfort.

If side effects occur and concern you, contact your doctor.

Other Information

The safe and effective use of propoxyphene depends on your taking it exactly as directed. This drug has been prescribed specifically for you and your present condition. Do not give this drug to others who may have similar symptoms. Do not use it for any other reason.

If you would like more information about propoxyphene, ask your doctor or pharmacist. They have a more technical leaflet (professional labeling) you may read.

Selected Darvon Products

Maximum Daily Dosage		
6	Dark Orange, Capsule Shaped, Film Coated Tablets Imprinted with Script "Lilly" on the one side and "Darvocet-N 100" on the other, using edible black ink	DARVOCET-N® 100 CIV Propoxyphene Napsylate and Acetaminophen Tablets
6	Parobolic-Shaped Capsules Imprinted with Script "Lilly" and "3111" on the opaque gray cap and "Darvon Comp 65" on the opaque red body, using edible black ink	DARVON® COMPOUND-65 CIV Propoxyphene Hydrochloride, Aspirin, and Caffeine Pulvules®
6	Parobolic-Shaped Capsules Imprinted with Script "Lilly" and "H03" on the opaque pink cap and "Darvon" on the opaque pink body, using edible black ink	DARVON® CIV Propoxyphene Hydrochloride Pulvules, 65 mg

Literature revised May 3, 1999

PV 1518 AMP [050399]

Shown in Product Identification Guide, page 321

DARVON® CIV

[*där 'von*]
(propoxyphene hydrochloride)
Capsules, USP
PULVULES®

DESCRIPTION

Darvon® (Propoxyphene Hydrochloride, USP) is an odorless, white crystalline powder with a bitter taste. It is freely soluble in water. Chemically, it is (2*S*, 3*R*)-(+)-4-(Dimethylamino)-3-methyl-1,2-diphenyl-2-butanol propionate (ester) hydrochloride, which can be represented by the accompanying structural formula. Its molecular weight is 375.94.

$(CH_3)_2NCH_2$—CH(CH_3)—C($OCOC_2H_5$)(C_6H_5)—CH_2—C_6H_5 • HCl

Each Pulvule contains 65 mg (172.9 µmol) (No. 365) propoxyphene hydrochloride. It also contains D & C Red No. 33, F D & C Yellow No. 6, gelatin, magnesium stearate, silicone, starch, titanium dioxide, and other inactive ingredients.

CLINICAL PHARMACOLOGY

Propoxyphene is a centrally acting narcotic analgesic agent. Equimolar doses of propoxyphene hydrochloride or napsylate provide similar plasma concentrations. Following administration of 65, 130, or 195 mg of propoxyphene hydrochloride, the bioavailability of propoxyphene is equivalent to that of 100, 200, or 300 mg respectively of propoxyphene napsylate. Peak plasma concentrations of propoxyphene are reached in 2 to 2 $^1/_2$ hours. After a 65-mg oral dose of propoxyphene hydrochloride, peak plasma levels of 0.05 to 0.1 µg/mL are achieved.

Repeated doses of propoxyphene at 6-hour intervals lead to increasing plasma concentrations, with a plateau after the ninth dose at 48 hours.

Propoxyphene is metabolized in the liver to yield norpropoxyphene. Propoxyphene has a half-life of 6 to 12 hours, whereas that of norpropoxyphene is 30 to 36 hours.

Norpropoxyphene has substantially less central-nervous-system-depressant effect than propoxyphene but a greater local anesthetic effect, which is similar to that of amitriptyline and antiarrhythmic agents, such as lidocaine and quinidine.

In animal studies in which propoxyphene and norpropoxyphene were continuously infused in large amounts, intracardiac conduction time (PR and QRS intervals) was prolonged. Any intracardiac conduction delay attributable to high concentrations of norpropoxyphene may be of relatively long duration.

ACTIONS

Propoxyphene is a mild narcotic analgesic structurally related to methadone. The potency of propoxyphene hydrochloride is from two-thirds to equal that of codeine.

INDICATION

For the relief of mild to moderate pain.

CONTRAINDICATION

Hypersensitivity to propoxyphene.

WARNINGS

- **Do not prescribe propoxyphene for patients who are suicidal or addiction-prone.**
- **Prescribe propoxyphene with caution for patients taking tranquilizers or antidepressant drugs and patients who use alcohol in excess.**
- **Tell your patients not to exceed the recommended dose and to limit their intake of alcohol.**

Propoxyphene products in excessive doses, either alone or in combination with other CNS depressants, including alcohol, are a major cause of drug-related deaths. Fatalities within the first hour of overdosage are not uncommon. In a survey of deaths due to overdosage conducted in 1975, in approximately 20% of the fatal cases, death occurred within the first hour (5% occurred within 15 minutes). Propoxyphene should not be taken in doses higher than those recommended by the physician. The judicious prescribing of propoxyphene is essential to the safe use of this drug. With patients who are depressed or suicidal, consideration should be given to the use of nonnarcotic analgesics. Patients should be cautioned about the concomitant use of propoxyphene products and alcohol because of potentially serious CNS-additive effects of these agents. Because of its added depressant effects, propoxyphene should be prescribed with caution for those patients whose medical condition requires the concomitant administration of sedatives, tranquilizers, muscle relaxants, antidepressants, or other CNS-depressant drugs. Patients should be advised of the additive depressant effects of these combinations.

Many of the propoxyphene-related deaths have occurred in patients with previous histories of emotional disturbances or suicidal ideation or attempts as well as histories of misuse of tranquilizers, alcohol, and other CNS-active drugs. Some deaths have occurred as a consequence of the accidental ingestion of excessive quantities of propoxyphene alone or in combination with other drugs. Patients taking propoxyphene should be warned not to exceed the dosage recommended by the physician.

Drug Dependence —Propoxyphene, when taken in higher-than-recommended doses over long periods of time, can produce drug dependence characterized by psychic dependence and, less frequently, physical dependence and tolerance. Propoxyphene will only partially suppress the withdrawal syndrome in individuals physically dependent on morphine or other narcotics. The abuse liability of propoxyphene is qualitatively similar to that of codeine although quantitatively less, and propoxyphene should be prescribed with the same degree of caution appropriate to the use of codeine.

Usage in Ambulatory Patients —Propoxyphene may impair the mental and/or physical abilities required for the performance of potentially hazardous tasks, such as driving a car or operating machinery. The patient should be cautioned accordingly.

PRECAUTIONS

General —Propoxyphene should be administered with caution to patients with hepatic or renal impairment since higher serum concentrations or delayed elimination may occur.

Drug Interactions —The CNS-depressant effect of propoxyphene is additive with that of other CNS depressants, including alcohol.

As is the case with medicinal agents, propoxyphene may slow the metabolism of a concomitantly administered drug. Should this occur, the higher serum concentrations of that drug may result in increased pharmacologic or adverse effects of that drug. Such occurrences have been reported when propoxyphene was administered to patients on antidepressants, anticonvulsants, or warfarin-like drugs. Severe neurologic signs, including coma, have occurred with concurrent use of carbamazepine.

Usage in Pregnancy —Safe use in pregnancy has not been established relative to possible adverse effects on fetal development. Instances of withdrawal symptoms in the neonate have been reported following usage during pregnancy. Therefore, propoxyphene should not be used in pregnant women unless, in the judgment of the physician, the potential benefits outweigh the possible hazards.

Usage in Nursing Mothers —Low levels of propoxyphene have been detected in human milk. In postpartum studies involving nursing mothers who were given propoxyphene, no adverse effects were noted in infants receiving mother's milk.

Usage in Pediatric Patients —Safety and effectiveness in pediatric patients have not been established.

Usage in the Elderly —The rate of propoxyphene metabolism may be reduced in some patients. Increased dosing interval should be considered.

A Patient Information Sheet is available for this product. See text following "How Supplied" section below.

ADVERSE REACTIONS

In a survey conducted in hospitalized patients, less than 1% of patients taking propoxyphene hydrochloride at recommended doses experienced side effects. The most frequently reported were dizziness, sedation, nausea, and vomiting. Some of these adverse reactions may be alleviated if the patient lies down.

Other adverse reactions include constipation, abdominal pain, skin rashes, lightheadedness, headache, weakness, euphoria, dysphoria, hallucinations, and minor visual disturbances.

Propoxyphene therapy has been associated with abnormal liver function tests and, more rarely, with instances of reversible jaundice (including cholestatic jaundice).

Subacute painful myopathy has occurred following chronic propoxyphene overdosage.

DOSAGE AND ADMINISTRATION

Darvon is given orally. The usual dosage is 65 mg propoxyphene hydrochloride every 4 hours as needed for pain. The maximum recommended dose of propoxyphene hydrochloride is 390 mg/day.

Consideration should be given to a reduced total daily dosage in patients with hepatic or renal impairment.

MANAGEMENT OF OVERDOSAGE

In all cases of suspected overdosage, call your regional Poison Control Center to obtain the most up-to-date information about the treatment of overdose. This recommendation is made because, in general, information regarding the treatment of overdosage may change more rapidly than do package inserts.

Initial consideration should be given to the management of the CNS effects of propoxyphene overdosage. Resuscitative measures should be initiated promptly.

Symptoms of Propoxyphene Overdosage —The manifestations of acute overdosage with propoxyphene are those of narcotic overdosage. The patient is usually somnolent but may be stuporous or comatose and convulsing. Respiratory depression is characteristic. The ventilatory rate and/or tidal volume is decreased, which results in cyanosis and hypoxia. Pupils, initially pinpoint, may become dilated as hypoxia increases. Cheyne-Stokes respiration and apnea may occur. Blood pressure and heart rate are usually normal initially, but blood pressure falls and cardiac performance deteriorates, which ultimately results in pulmonary edema and circulatory collapse, unless the respiratory depression is corrected and adequate ventilation is restored promptly. Cardiac arrhythmias and conduction delay may be present. A combined respiratory-metabolic acidosis occurs owing to retained CO_2 (hypercapnia) and to lactic acid formed during anaerobic glycolysis. Acidosis may be severe if large amounts of salicylates have also been ingested. Death may occur.

Treatment of Propoxyphene Overdosage —Attention should be directed first to establishing a patent airway and to restoring ventilation. Mechanically assisted ventilation, with or without oxygen, may be required, and positive pressure respiration may be desirable if pulmonary edema is present. The narcotic antagonist naloxone will markedly reduce the degree of respiratory depression, and 0.4 to 2 mg should be administered promptly, preferably intravenously. If the desired degree of counteraction with improvement in respiratory functions is not obtained, naloxone should be repeated at 2- to 3-minute intervals. The duration of action of the antagonist may be brief. If no response is observed after 10 mg of naloxone have been administered, the diagnosis of propoxyphene toxicity should be questioned. Naloxone may also be administered by continuous intravenous infusion.

Treatment of Propoxyphene Overdosage in Pediatric Patients —The usual initial dose of naloxone in pediatric patients is 0.01 mg/kg body weight given intravenously. If this dose does not result in the desired degree of clinical improvement, a subsequent increased dose of 0.1 mg/kg body weight may be administered. If an IV route of administration is not available, naloxone may be administered IM or subcutaneously in divided doses. If necessary, naloxone can be diluted with Sterile Water for Injection.

Blood gases, pH, and electrolytes should be monitored in order that acidosis and any electrolyte disturbance present may be corrected promptly. Acidosis, hypoxia, and generalized CNS depression predispose to the development of cardiac arrhythmias. Ventricular fibrillation or cardiac arrest may occur and necessitate the full complement of cardiopulmonary resuscitation (CPR) measures. Respiratory acidosis rapidly subsides as ventilation is restored and hypercapnia eliminated, but lactic acidosis may require intravenous bicarbonate for prompt correction.

Electrocardiographic monitoring is essential. Prompt correction of hypoxia, acidosis, and electrolyte disturbance (when present) will help prevent these cardiac complications and will increase the effectiveness of agents administered to restore normal cardiac function.

In addition to the use of a narcotic antagonist, the patient may require careful titration with an anticonvulsant to control convulsions. Analeptic drugs (for example, caffeine or amphetamine) should not be used because of their tendency to precipitate convulsions.

General supportive measures, in addition to oxygen, include, when necessary, intravenous fluids, vasopressor-inotropic compounds, and, when infection is likely, anti-infective agents. Gastric lavage may be useful and activated charcoal can adsorb a significant amount of ingested propoxyphene. Dialysis is of little value in poisoning due to propoxyphene. Efforts should be made to determine whether other agents, such as alcohol, barbiturates, tranquilizers, or other CNS depressants, were also ingested, since these increase CNS depression as well as cause specific toxic effects.

HOW SUPPLIED

Darvon® Pulvules® (No. 365) are available in:

The 65 mg parabolic-shaped capsules are imprinted with the script "Lilly" and "H03" on the opaque pink cap and "Darvon" on the opaque pink body, using edible black ink. They are available as follows:

Bottles of 100 (RxPak*)	NDC 0002-0803-02 (PU0365)
Bottles of 500	NDC 0002-0803-03 (PU0365)
ID†100	NDC 0002-0803-33 (PU0365)

* All RxPaks (prescription packages, Lilly) have safety closures.

† Identi-Dose® (unit dose medication, Lilly)

Store at controlled room temperature, 59° to 86°F (15° to 30°C).

CAUTION—Federal (USA) law prohibits dispensing without prescription.

The following information, including description of dosage forms and the maximum daily dosage of each, is available to patients receiving Darvon products.

Patient Information Sheet

YOUR PRESCRIPTION FOR A DARVON® (PROPOXYPHENE) PRODUCT

Summary

Products containing Darvon are used to relieve pain.

LIMIT YOUR INTAKE OF ALCOHOL WHILE TAKING THIS DRUG. Make sure your doctor knows if you are taking tranquilizers, sleep aids, antidepressants, antihistamines, or any other drugs that make you sleepy. Combining propoxyphene with alcohol or these drugs in excessive doses is dangerous.

Use care while driving a car or using machines until you see how the drug affects you because propoxyphene can make you sleepy. Do not take more of the drug than your doctor prescribed. Dependence has occurred when patients have taken propoxyphene for a long period of time at doses greater than recommended.

The rest of this leaflet gives you more information about propoxyphene. Please read it and keep it for future use.

Uses of Darvon

Products containing Darvon are used for the relief of mild to moderate pain. Products that contain Darvon plus aspirin or acetaminophen are prescribed for the relief of pain or pain associated with fever.

Before Taking Darvon

Make sure your doctor knows if you have ever had an allergic reaction to propoxyphene, aspirin, or acetaminophen. Some forms of propoxyphene products contain aspirin to help relieve the pain. Your doctor should be advised if you have a history of ulcers or if you are taking an anticoagulant ("blood thinner"). The aspirin may irritate the stomach lining and may cause bleeding, particularly if an ulcer is present. Also, bleeding may occur if you are taking an anticoagulant. In a small group of people, aspirin may cause an asthma attack. If you are one of these people, be sure your drug does not contain aspirin.

The effect of propoxyphene in pediatric patients under 12 has not been studied. Therefore, use of the drug in this age group is not recommended.

Also, due to the possible association between aspirin and Reye Syndrome, those propoxyphene products containing aspirin should not be given to children, including teenagers, with chicken pox or flu unless prescribed by a physician.

The following propoxyphene product contains aspirin:

Darvon® Compound-65 (Propoxyphene Hydrochloride, Aspirin, and Caffeine, USP)

How to Take Darvon

Follow your doctor's directions exactly. Do not increase the amount you take without your doctor's approval. If you miss a dose of the drug, do not take twice as much the next time.

Pregnancy

Do not take propoxyphene during pregnancy unless your doctor knows you are pregnant and specifically recommends its use. Cases of temporary dependence in the newborn have occurred when the mother has taken propoxyphene consistently in the weeks before delivery. As a general principle, no drug should be taken during pregnancy unless it is clearly necessary.

General Cautions

Heavy use of alcohol with propoxyphene is hazardous and may lead to overdosage symptoms (*see* "Overdose" below). THEREFORE, LIMIT YOUR INTAKE OF ALCOHOL WHILE TAKING PROPOXYPHENE.

Combinations of excessive doses of propoxyphene, alcohol, and tranquilizers are dangerous. Make sure your doctor knows if you are taking tranquilizers, sleep aids, antidepressant drugs, antihistamines, or any other drugs that make you sleepy. The use of these drugs with propoxyphene increases their sedative effects and may lead to overdosage symptoms, including death (*see* "Overdose" below).

Propoxyphene may cause drowsiness or impair your mental and/or physical abilities; therefore, use caution when driving a vehicle or operating dangerous machinery. DO NOT perform any hazardous task until you have seen your response to this drug.

Propoxyphene may increase the concentration in the body of medications such as anticoagulants ("blood thinners"), antidepressants, or drugs used for epilepsy. The result may be excessive or adverse effects of these medications. Make sure your doctor knows if you are taking any of these medications.

Dependence

You can become dependent on propoxyphene if you take it in higher than recommended doses over a long period of time. Dependence is a feeling of need for the drug and a feeling that you cannot perform normally without it.

Overdose

An overdose of Darvon, alone or in combination with other drugs, including alcohol, may cause weakness, difficulty in

Continued on next page

*** Identi-Code® symbol. This product information was prepared in June 2000. Current information on these and other products of Eli Lilly and Company may be obtained by direct inquiry to Lilly Research Laboratories, Lilly Corporate Center, Indianapolis, Indiana 46285, (800) 545-5979.**

Darvon—Cont.

breathing, confusion, anxiety, and more severe drowsiness and dizziness. Extreme overdosage may lead to unconsciousness and death.

If the propoxyphene product contains acetaminophen, the overdosage symptoms include nausea, vomiting, lack of appetite, and abdominal pain. Liver damage may occur.

When the propoxyphene product contains aspirin, symptoms of taking too much of the drug are headache, dizziness, ringing in the ears, difficulty in hearing, dim vision, confusion, drowsiness, sweating, thirst, rapid breathing, nausea, vomiting, and, occasionally, diarrhea.

In any suspected overdosage situation, contact your doctor or nearest hospital emergency room. GET EMERGENCY HELP IMMEDIATELY.

KEEP THIS DRUG AND ALL DRUGS OUT OF THE REACH OF THE PEDIATRIC POPULATION.

Possible Side Effects

When propoxyphene is taken as directed, side effects are infrequent. Among those reported are drowsiness, dizziness, nausea, and vomiting. If these effects occur, it may help if you lie down and rest.

Less frequently reported side effects are constipation, abdominal pain, skin rashes, lightheadedness, headache, weakness, hallucinations, minor visual disturbances, and feelings of elation or discomfort.

If side effects occur and concern you, contact your doctor.

Other Information

The safe and effective use of propoxyphene depends on your taking it exactly as directed. This drug has been prescribed specifically for you and your present condition. Do not give this drug to others who may have similar symptoms. Do not use it for any other reason.

If you would like more information about propoxyphene, ask your doctor or pharmacist. They have a more technical leaflet (professional labeling) you may read.

Selected Darvon Products

Maximum Daily Dosage		
6	Dark Orange, Capsule Shaped, Film Coated Tablets Imprinted with Script "Lilly" on the one side and "Darvocet-N 100" on the other, using edible black ink	DARVOCET-N® 100 Ⓒ-IV Propoxyphene Napsylate and Acetaminophen Tablets
6	Parabolic-Shaped Capsules Imprinted with Script "Lilly" and "3111"on the opaque gray cap and"Darvon Comp 65" on the opaque red body, using edible black ink	DARVON® COMPOUND-65 Ⓒ-IV Propoxyphene Hydrochloride, Aspirin, and Caffeine Pulvules®
6	Parabolic-Shaped Capsules Imprinted with Script"Lilly" and "H03" on the opaque pink cap and "Darvon" on the opaque pink body, using edible black ink	DARVON® Ⓒ-IV Propoxyphene Hydrochloride Pulvules, 65 mg

Literature issued January 27, 1997

PV 3000 AMP [012797]

DARVON® COMPOUND-65 Ⓒ-IV

[där 'vŏn kŏm 'pound]

(propoxyphene hydrochloride, aspirin and caffeine capsules, USP)

DESCRIPTION

Darvon® (Propoxyphene Hydrochloride, USP) is an odorless, white crystalline powder with a bitter taste. It is freely soluble in water. Chemically, it is (2*S*,3*R*)-(+)-4-(Dimethylamino)-3-methyl-1,2-diphenyl-2-butanol propionate (ester) hydrochloride, which can be represented by the accompanying structural formula. Its molecular weight is 375.94.

$(CH_3)_2NCH_2-CH(CH_3)-C(OCOC_2H_5)(C_6H_5)-CH_2-C_6H_5 \cdot HCl$

Each Pulvule® contains 65 mg (172.9 µmol) propoxyphene hydrochloride, 389 mg (2,159 µmol) aspirin, and 32.4 mg (166.8 µmol) caffeine.

It also contains F D & C Red No. 3, F D & C Yellow No. 6, gelatin, glutamic acid hydrochloride, iron oxide, kaolin, silicone, titanium dioxide, and other inactive ingredients.

CLINICAL PHARMACOLOGY

Propoxyphene is a centrally acting narcotic analgesic agent. Equimolar doses of propoxyphene hydrochloride or napsylate provide similar plasma concentrations. Following administration of 65, 130, or 195 mg of propoxyphene hydrochloride, the bioavailability of propoxyphene is equivalent to that of 100, 200, or 300 mg respectively of propoxyphene napsylate. Peak plasma concentrations of propoxyphene are reached in 2 to 2 1/2 hours. After a 65-mg oral dose of propoxyphene hydrochloride, peak plasma levels of 0.05 to 0.1 µg/mL are achieved.

Repeated doses of propoxyphene at 6-hour intervals lead to increasing plasma concentrations, with a plateau after the ninth dose at 48 hours.

Propoxyphene is metabolized in the liver to yield norpropoxyphene. Propoxyphene has a half-life of 6 to 12 hours, whereas that of norpropoxyphene is 30 to 36 hours. Norpropoxyphene has substantially less central-nervous-system-depressant effect than propoxyphene but a greater local anesthetic effect, which is similar to that of amitriptyline and antiarrhythmic agents, such as lidocaine and quinidine.

In animal studies in which propoxyphene and norpropoxyphene were continuously infused in large amounts, intracardiac conduction time (PR and QRS intervals) was prolonged. Any intracardiac conduction delay attributable to high concentrations of norpropoxyphene may be of relatively long duration.

ACTIONS

Propoxyphene is a mild narcotic analgesic structurally related to methadone. The potency of propoxyphene hydrochloride is from two thirds to equal that of codeine.

The combination of propoxyphene with a mixture of aspirin and caffeine produces greater analgesia than that produced by either propoxyphene or aspirin and caffeine administered alone.

INDICATION

This product is indicated for the relief of mild to moderate pain, either when pain is present alone or when it is accompanied by fever.

CONTRAINDICATION

Hypersensitivity to propoxyphene, aspirin, or caffeine.

WARNINGS

- **Do not prescribe propoxyphene for patients who are suicidal or addiction-prone.**
- **Prescribe propoxyphene with caution for patients taking tranquilizers or antidepressant drugs and patients who use alcohol in excess.**
- **Tell your patients not to exceed the recommended dose and to limit their intake of alcohol.**

Propoxyphene products in excessive doses, either alone or in combination with other CNS depressants, including alcohol, are a major cause of drug-related deaths. Fatalities within the first hour of overdosage are not uncommon. In a survey of deaths due to overdosage conducted in 1975, in approximately 20% of the fatal cases, death occurred within the first hour (5% occurred within 15 minutes). Propoxyphene should not be taken in doses higher than those recommended by the physician. The judicious prescribing of propoxyphene is essential to the safe use of this drug. With patients who are depressed or suicidal, consideration should be given to the use of nonnarcotic analgesics. Patients should be cautioned about the concomitant use of propoxyphene products and alcohol because of potentially serious CNS-additive effects of these agents. Because of its added depressant effects, propoxyphene should be prescribed with caution for those patients whose medical condition requires the concomitant administration of sedatives, tranquilizers, muscle relaxants, antidepressants, or other CNS-depressant drugs. Patients should be advised of the additive depressant effects of these combinations.

Many of the propoxyphene-related deaths have occurred in patients with previous histories of emotional disturbances or suicidal ideation or attempts as well as histories of misuse of tranquilizers, alcohol, and other CNS-active drugs. Some deaths have occurred as a consequence of the accidental ingestion of excessive quantities of propoxyphene alone or in combination with other drugs. Patients taking propoxyphene should be warned not to exceed the dosage recommended by the physician.

Drug Dependence—Propoxyphene, when taken in higher-than-recommended doses over long periods of time, can produce drug dependence characterized by psychic dependence and, less frequently, physical dependence and tolerance. Propoxyphene will only partially suppress the withdrawal syndrome in individuals physically dependent on morphine or other narcotics. The abuse liability of propoxyphene is qualitatively similar to that of codeine although quantitatively less, and propoxyphene should be prescribed with the same degree of caution appropriate to the use of codeine.

Usage in Ambulatory Patients—Propoxyphene may impair the mental and/or physical abilities required for the performance of potentially hazardous tasks, such as driving a car or operating machinery. The patient should be cautioned accordingly.

Warning: Reye Syndrome is a rare but serious disease which can follow flu or chicken pox in children and teenagers. While the cause of Reye Syndrome is unknown, some reports claim aspirin (or salicylates) may increase the risk of developing this disease.

PRECAUTIONS

General—Salicylates should be used with extreme caution in the presence of peptic ulcer or coagulation abnormalities. Propoxyphene should be administered with caution to patients with hepatic or renal impairment since higher serum concentrations or delayed elimination may occur.

Drug Interactions—The CNS-depressant effect of propoxyphene is additive with that of other CNS depressants, including alcohol.

Salicylates may enhance the effect of anticoagulants and inhibit the uricosuric effect of uricosuric agents.

As is the case with medicinal agents, propoxyphene may slow the metabolism of a concomitantly administered drug. Should this occur, the higher serum concentrations of that drug may result in increased pharmacologic or adverse effects of that drug. Such occurrences have been reported when propoxyphene was administered to patients on antidepressants, anticonvulsants, or warfarin-like drugs. Severe neurologic signs, including coma, have occurred with concurrent use of carbamazepine.

Usage in Pregnancy—Safe use in pregnancy has not been established relative to possible adverse effects on fetal development. Instances of withdrawal symptoms in the neonate have been reported following usage during pregnancy. Therefore, propoxyphene should not be used in pregnant women unless, in the judgment of the physician, the potential benefits outweigh the possible hazards. Aspirin does not appear to have teratogenic effects. However, prolonged pregnancy and labor with increased bleeding before and after delivery, decreased birth weight, and increased rate of stillbirth were reported with high blood salicylate levels. Because of possible adverse effects on the neonate and the potential for increased maternal blood loss, aspirin should be avoided during the last 3 months of pregnancy.

Usage in Nursing Mothers—Low levels of propoxyphene have been detected in human milk. In postpartum studies involving nursing mothers who were given propoxyphene, no adverse effects were noted in infants receiving mother's milk.

Usage in Pediatric Patients—Safety and effectiveness in pediatric patients have not been established.

Usage in the Elderly—The rate of propoxyphene metabolism may be reduced in some patients. Increased dosing interval should be considered.

A Patient Information Sheet is available for this product. See text following "How Supplied" section below.

ADVERSE REACTIONS

In a survey conducted in hospitalized patients, less than 1% of patients taking propoxyphene hydrochloride at recommended doses experienced side effects. The most frequently reported were dizziness, sedation, nausea, and vomiting. Some of these adverse reactions may be alleviated if the patient lies down.

Other adverse reactions include constipation, abdominal pain, skin rashes, lightheadedness, headache, weakness, euphoria, dysphoria, hallucinations, and minor visual disturbances.

Propoxyphene therapy has been associated with abnormal liver function tests and, more rarely, with instances of reversible jaundice (including cholestatic jaundice).

Renal papillary necrosis may result from chronic aspirin use, particularly when the dosage is greater than recommended and when combined with acetaminophen.

Subacute painful myopathy has occurred following chronic propoxyphene overdosage.

DOSAGE AND ADMINISTRATION

This product is given orally. The usual dosage is 65 mg propoxyphene hydrochloride, 389 mg aspirin, and 32.4 mg caffeine every 4 hours as needed for pain.

The maximum recommended dose of propoxyphene hydrochloride is 390 mg/day.

Consideration should be given to a reduced total daily dosage in patients with hepatic or renal impairment.

MANAGEMENT OF OVERDOSAGE

In all cases of suspected overdosage, call your regional Poison Control Center to obtain the most up-to-date information about the treatment of overdose. This recommendation is made because, in general, information regarding the treatment of overdosage may change more rapidly than do package inserts.

Initial consideration should be given to the management of the CNS effects of propoxyphene overdosage. Resuscitative measures should be initiated promptly.

Symptoms of Propoxyphene Overdosage—The manifestations of acute overdosage with propoxyphene are those of narcotic overdosage. The patient is usually somnolent but may be stuporous or comatose and convulsing. Respiratory depression is characteristic. The ventilatory rate and/or tidal volume is decreased, which results in cyanosis and hypoxia. Pupils, initially pinpoint, may become dilated as hypoxia increases. Cheyne-Stokes respiration and apnea may occur. Blood pressure and heart rate are usually normal initially, but blood pressure falls and cardiac performance deteriorates, which ultimately results in pulmonary edema and circulatory collapse, unless the respiratory depression is corrected and adequate ventilation is restored promptly. Cardiac arrhythmias and conduction delay may be present. A combined respiratory-metabolic acidosis occurs owing to retained CO_2 (hypercapnia) and to lactic acid formed during anaerobic glycolysis. Acidosis may be severe if large amounts of salicylates have also been ingested. Death may occur.

Treatment of Propoxyphene Overdosage—Attention should be directed first to establishing a patent airway and to restoring ventilation. Mechanically assisted ventilation, with or without oxygen, may be required, and positive pressure respiration may be desirable if pulmonary edema is present. The narcotic antagonist naloxone will markedly reduce the degree of respiratory depression, and 0.4 to 2 mg should be administered promptly, preferably intravenously. If the desired degree of counteraction with improvement in respiratory functions is not obtained, naloxone should be repeated at 2- to 3-minute intervals. The duration of action of the antagonist may be brief. If no response is observed after 10 mg of naloxone have been administered, the diagnosis of propoxyphene toxicity should be questioned. Naloxone may also be administered by continuous intravenous infusion.

Treatment of Propoxyphene Overdosage in Pediatric Patients—The usual initial dose of naloxone in pediatric patients is 0.01 mg/kg body weight given intravenously. If this dose does not result in the desired degree of clinical improvement, a subsequent increased dose of 0.1 mg/kg body weight may be administered. If an IV route of administration is not available, naloxone may be administered IM or subcutaneously in divided doses. If necessary, naloxone can be diluted with Sterile Water for Injection.

Blood gases, pH, and electrolytes should be monitored in order that acidosis and any electrolyte disturbance present may be corrected promptly. Acidosis, hypoxia, and generalized CNS depression predispose to the development of cardiac arrhythmias. Ventricular fibrillation or cardiac arrest may occur and necessitate the full complement of cardiopulmonary resuscitation (CPR) measures. Respiratory acidosis rapidly subsides as ventilation is restored and hypercapnia eliminated, but lactic acidosis may require intravenous bicarbonate for prompt correction.

Electrocardiographic monitoring is essential. Prompt correction of hypoxia, acidosis, and electrolyte disturbance (when present) will help prevent these cardiac complications and will increase the effectiveness of agents administered to restore normal cardiac function.

In addition to the use of a narcotic antagonist, the patient may require careful titration with an anticonvulsant to control convulsions. Analeptic drugs (for example, caffeine or amphetamine) should not be used because of their tendency to precipitate convulsions.

General supportive measures, in addition to oxygen, include, when necessary, intravenous fluids, vasopressor-inotropic compounds, and, when infection is likely, anti-infective agents. Gastric lavage may be useful and activated charcoal can adsorb a significant amount of ingested propoxyphene. Dialysis is of little value in poisoning due to propoxyphene. Efforts should be made to determine whether other agents, such as alcohol, barbiturates, tranquilizers, or other CNS depressants, were also ingested, since these increase CNS depression as well as cause specific toxic effects.

Symptoms of Salicylate Overdosage—Such symptoms include central nausea and vomiting, tinnitus and deafness, vertigo and headaches, mental dullness and confusion, diaphoresis, rapid pulse, and increased respiration and respiratory alkalosis.

Treatment of Salicylate Overdosage—When Darvon Compound-65 has been ingested, the clinical picture may be complicated by salicylism.

The treatment of acute salicylate intoxication includes minimizing drug absorption, promoting elimination through the kidneys, and correcting metabolic derangements affecting body temperature, hydration, acid-base balance, and electrolyte balance. The technique to be employed for eliminating salicylate from the bloodstream depends on the degree of drug intoxication.

If the patient is seen within 4 hours of ingestion, the stomach should be emptied by inducing vomiting or by gastric lavage as soon as possible.

The nomogram of Done is a useful prognostic guide in which the expected severity of salicylate intoxication is based on serum salicylate levels and the time interval between ingestion and taking the blood sample.

Exchange transfusion is most feasible for a small infant. Intermittent peritoneal dialysis is useful for cases of moderate severity in adults. Intravenous fluids alkalinized by the addition of sodium bicarbonate or potassium citrate are helpful. Hemodialysis with the artificial kidney is the most effective means of removing salicylate and is indicated for the very severe cases of salicylate intoxication.

HOW SUPPLIED

Darvon® Compound-65 Pulvules® (No. 369) are available in:

The 65 mg parabolic-shaped capsules are imprinted with the script "Lilly" and "3111" on the opaque gray cap and "Darvon Comp 65" on the opaque red body, using edible black ink. They are available as follows:

Bottles of 100 (RxPak*)	NDC 0002-3111-02 (PU0369)
Bottles of 500	NDC 0002-3111-03 (PU0369)

*All RxPaks (prescription packages, Lilly) have safety closures.

Store at controlled room temperature, 59° to 86°F (15° to 30°C).

CAUTION—Federal (USA) law prohibits dispensing without prescription.

The following information, including description of dosage forms and the maximum daily dosage of each, is available to patients receiving Darvon products.

Patient Information Sheet ℂ

YOUR PRESCRIPTION FOR A DARVON® (PROPOXYPHENE) PRODUCT

Summary

Products containing Darvon are used to relieve pain.

LIMIT YOUR INTAKE OF ALCOHOL WHILE TAKING THIS DRUG. Make sure your doctor knows if you are taking tranquilizers, sleep aids, antidepressants, antihistamines, or any other drugs that make you sleepy. Combining propoxyphene with alcohol or these drugs in excessive doses is dangerous.

Use care while driving a car or using machines until you see how the drug affects you because propoxyphene can make you sleepy. Do not take more of the drug than your doctor prescribed. Dependence has occurred when patients have taken propoxyphene for a long period of time at doses greater than recommended.

The rest of this leaflet gives you more information about propoxyphene. Please read it and keep it for future use.

Uses of Darvon

Products containing Darvon are used for the relief of mild to moderate pain. Products that contain Darvon plus aspirin or acetaminophen are prescribed for the relief of pain or pain associated with fever.

Before Taking Darvon

Make sure your doctor knows if you have ever had an allergic reaction to propoxyphene, aspirin, or acetaminophen. Some forms of propoxyphene products contain aspirin to help relieve the pain. Your doctor should be advised if you have a history of ulcers or if you are taking an anticoagulant ("blood thinner"). The aspirin may irritate the stomach lining and may cause bleeding, particularly if an ulcer is present. Also, bleeding may occur if you are taking an anticoagulant. In a small group of people, aspirin may cause an asthma attack. If you are one of these people, be sure your drug does not contain aspirin.

The effect of propoxyphene in pediatric patients under 12 has not been studied. Therefore, use of the drug in this age group is not recommended.

Also, due to the possible association between aspirin and Reye Syndrome, those propoxyphene products containing aspirin should not be given to children, including teenagers, with chicken pox or flu unless prescribed by a physician.

The following propoxyphene product contains aspirin:

Darvon® Compound-65 (Propoxyphene Hydrochloride, Aspirin, and Caffeine, USP)

How to Take Darvon

Follow your doctor's directions exactly. Do not increase the amount you take without your doctor's approval. If you miss a dose of the drug, do not take twice as much the next time.

Pregnancy

Do not take propoxyphene during pregnancy unless your doctor knows you are pregnant and specifically recommends its use. Cases of temporary dependence in the newborn have occurred when the mother has taken propoxyphene consistently in the weeks before delivery. **IT IS ESPECIALLY IMPORTANT NOT TO USE DARVON COMPOUND-65 DURING THE LAST 3 MONTHS OF PREGNANCY UNLESS SPECIFICALLY DIRECTED TO DO SO BY A DOCTOR BECAUSE ASPIRIN MAY CAUSE PROBLEMS IN THE UNBORN CHILD OR COMPLICATIONS DURING DELIVERY.** As a general principle, no drug should be taken during pregnancy unless it is clearly necessary.

General Cautions

Heavy use of alcohol with propoxyphene is hazardous and may lead to overdosage symptoms (*see* "Overdose" below). THEREFORE, LIMIT YOUR INTAKE OF ALCOHOL WHILE TAKING PROPOXYPHENE.

Combinations of excessive doses of propoxyphene, alcohol, and tranquilizers are dangerous. Make sure your doctor knows if you are taking tranquilizers, sleep aids, antidepressant drugs, antihistamines, or any other drugs that make you sleepy. The use of these drugs with propoxyphene increases their sedative effects and may lead to overdosage symptoms, including death (*see* "Overdose" below).

Propoxyphene may cause drowsiness or impair your mental and/or physical abilities; therefore, use caution when driving a vehicle or operating dangerous machinery. DO NOT perform any hazardous task until you have seen your response to this drug.

Propoxyphene may increase the concentration in the body of medications such as anticoagulants ("blood thinners"), antidepressants, or drugs used for epilepsy. The result may be excessive or adverse effects of these medications. Make sure your doctor knows if you are taking any of these medications.

Dependence

You can become dependent on propoxyphene if you take it in higher than recommended doses over a long period of time. Dependence is a feeling of need for the drug and a feeling that you cannot perform normally without it.

Overdose

An overdose of Darvon, alone or in combination with other drugs, including alcohol, may cause weakness, difficulty in breathing, confusion, anxiety, and more severe drowsiness and dizziness. Extreme overdosage may lead to unconsciousness and death.

If the propoxyphene product contains acetaminophen, the overdose symptoms include nausea, vomiting, lack of appetite, and abdominal pain. Liver damage may occur.

When the propoxyphene product contains aspirin, symptoms of taking too much of the drug are headache, dizziness, ringing in the ears, difficulty in hearing, dim vision, confusion, drowsiness, sweating, thirst, rapid breathing, nausea, vomiting, and, occasionally, diarrhea.

In any suspected overdosage situation, contact your doctor or nearest hospital emergency room. GET EMERGENCY HELP IMMEDIATELY.

KEEP THIS DRUG AND ALL DRUGS OUT OF THE REACH OF THE PEDIATRIC POPULATION.

Possible Side Effects

When propoxyphene is taken as directed, side effects are infrequent. Among those reported are drowsiness, dizziness, nausea, and vomiting. If these effects occur, it may help if you lie down and rest.

Less frequently reported side effects are constipation, abdominal pain, skin rashes, lightheadedness, headache, weakness, hallucinations, minor visual disturbances, and feelings of elation or discomfort.

If side effects occur and concern you, contact your doctor.

Other Information

The safe and effective use of propoxyphene depends on your taking it exactly as directed. This drug has been prescribed specifically for you and your present condition. Do not give this drug to others who may have similar symptoms. Do not use it for any other reason.

If you would like more information about propoxyphene, ask your doctor or pharmacist. They have a more technical leaflet (professional labeling) you may read.

Selected Darvon Products

Maximum Daily Dosage		
6	Dark Orange, Capsule Shaped, Film Coated Tablets Imprinted with Script "Lilly" on one side and "Darvocet-N 100" on the other, using edible black ink	DARVOCET-N® 100 ℂ Propoxyphene Napsylate and Acetaminophen Tablets
6	Parabolic-Shaped Capsules Imprinted with Script "Lilly" and "3111" on the opaque gray cap and "Darvon Comp 65" on the opaque red body, using edible black ink	DARVON® COMPOUND-65 ℂ Propoxyphene Hydrochloride, Aspirin, and Caffeine Pulvules®
6	Parabolic-Shaped Capsules Imprinted with Script "Lilly" and "H03" on the opaque pink cap and "Darvon" on the opaque pink body, using edible black ink	DARVON® ℂ Propoxyphene Hydrochloride Pulvules, 65 mg

Literature revised July 18, 1996

PA 2116 AMP [071896]

DARVON-N® TABLETS ℂ

[*där ′vŏn*]

(propoxyphene napsylate tablets, USP)

DESCRIPTION

Darvon-N® (Propoxyphene Napsylate, USP) is an odorless, white crystalline powder with a bitter taste. It is very slightly soluble in water and soluble in methanol, ethanol, chloroform, and acetone. Chemically, it is (αS,1R)-α-[2-(Dimethylamino)-1-methylethyl]-α-phenylphenethyl propionate compound with 2-naphthalenesulfonic acid (1:1) monohydrate, which can be represented by the accompanying structural formula. Its molecular weight is 565.72.

$$(CH_3)_2NCH_2 - \overset{CH_3}{\underset{H}{C}} - \overset{OCC_2H_5}{\underset{C_6H_5}{C}} - CH_2 - C_6H_5 \cdot C_{10}H_7SO_3H \cdot H_2O$$

Propoxyphene napsylate differs from propoxyphene hydrochloride in that it allows more stable liquid dosage forms and tablet formulations. Because of differences in molecular weight, a dose of 100 mg (176.8 µmol) of propoxyphene napsylate is required to supply an amount of propoxyphene equivalent to that present in 65 mg (172.9 µmol) of propoxyphene hydrochloride.

Each tablet of Darvon-N contains 100 mg (176.8 µmol) propoxyphene napsylate. The tablet also contains cellulose, cornstarch, iron oxides, lactose, magnesium stearate, silicon dioxide, stearic acid, and titanium dioxide.

CLINICAL PHARMACOLOGY

Propoxyphene is a centrally acting narcotic analgesic agent. Equimolar doses of propoxyphene hydrochloride or napsy-

Continued on next page

ℂ Identi-Code® symbol. This product information was prepared in June 2000. Current information on these and other products of Eli Lilly and Company may be obtained by direct inquiry to Lilly Research Laboratories, Lilly Corporate Center, Indianapolis, Indiana 46285, (800) 545-5979.

Darvon-N—Cont.

late provide similar plasma concentrations. Following administration of 65, 130, or 195 mg of propoxyphene hydrochloride, the bioavailability of propoxyphene is equivalent to that of 100, 200, or 300 mg respectively of propoxyphene napsylate. Peak plasma concentrations of propoxyphene are reached in 2 to 2 1/2 hours. After a 100-mg oral dose of propoxyphene napsylate, peak plasma levels of 0.05 to 0.1 µg/mL are achieved. As shown in Figure 1, the napsylate salt tends to be absorbed more slowly than the hydrochloride. At or near therapeutic doses, this difference is small when compared with that among subjects and among doses.

Figure 1

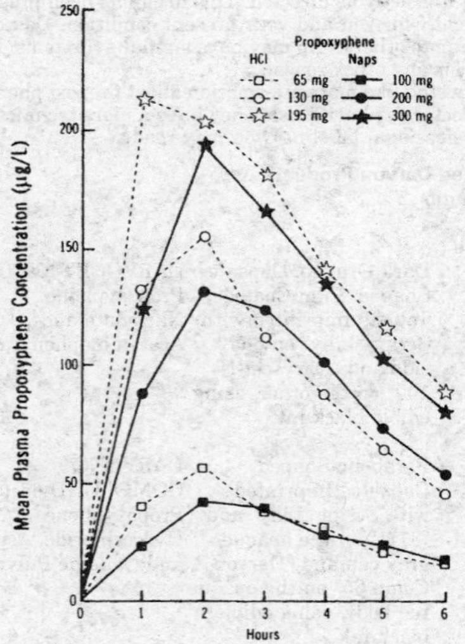

Figure 1. Mean plasma concentrations of propoxyphene in 8 human subjects following oral administration of 65 and 130 mg of the hydrochloride salt and 100 and 200 mg of the napsylate salt and in 7 given 195 mg of the hydrochloride and 300 mg of the napsylate salt.

Because of this several hundredfold difference in solubility, the absorption rate of very large doses of the napsylate salt is significantly lower than that of equimolar doses of the hydrochloride.

Repeated doses of propoxyphene at 6-hour intervals lead to increasing plasma concentrations, with a plateau after the ninth dose at 48 hours.

Propoxyphene is metabolized in the liver to yield norpropoxyphene. Propoxyphene has a half-life of 6 to 12 hours, whereas that of norpropoxyphene is 30 to 36 hours.

Norpropoxyphene has substantially less central-nervous-system-depressant effect than propoxyphene but a greater local anesthetic effect, which is similar to that of amitriptyline and antiarrhythmic agents, such as lidocaine and quinidine.

In animal studies in which propoxyphene and norpropoxyphene were continuously infused in large amounts, intracardiac conduction time (PR and QRS intervals) was prolonged. Any intracardiac conduction delay attributable to high concentrations of norpropoxyphene may be of relatively long duration.

ACTIONS

Propoxyphene is a mild narcotic analgesic structurally related to methadone. The potency of propoxyphene napsylate is from two thirds to equal that of codeine.

INDICATION

For the relief of mild to moderate pain.

CONTRAINDICATION

Hypersensitivity to propoxyphene.

WARNINGS

- **Do not prescribe propoxyphene for patients who are suicidal or addiction-prone.**
- **Prescribe propoxyphene with caution for patients taking tranquilizers or antidepressant drugs and patients who use alcohol in excess.**
- **Tell your patients not to exceed the recommended dose and to limit their intake of alcohol.**

Propoxyphene products in excessive doses, either alone or in combination with other CNS depressants, including alcohol, are a major cause of drug-related deaths. Fatalities within the first hour of overdosage are not uncommon. In a survey of deaths due to overdosage conducted in 1975, in approximately 20% of the fatal cases, death occurred within the first hour (5% occurred within 15 minutes). Propoxyphene should not be taken in doses higher than those recommended by the physician. The judicious prescribing of propoxyphene is essential to the safe use of this drug. With patients who are depressed or suicidal, consideration should be given to the use of non-narcotic analgesics. Patients should be cautioned about the concomitant use of propoxyphene products and alcohol because of potentially serious CNS-additive effects of these agents. Because of its added depressant effects, propoxyphene should be prescribed with caution for those patients whose medical condition requires the concomitant administration of sedatives, tranquilizers, muscle relaxants, antidepressants, or other CNS-depressant drugs. Patients should be advised of the additive depressant effects of these combinations.

Many of the propoxyphene-related deaths have occurred in patients with previous histories of emotional disturbances or suicidal ideation or attempts as well as histories of misuse of tranquilizers, alcohol, and other CNS-active drugs. Some deaths have occurred as a consequence of the accidental ingestion of excessive quantities of propoxyphene alone or in combination with other drugs. Patients taking propoxyphene should be warned not to exceed the dosage recommended by the physician.

Drug Dependence—Propoxyphene, when taken in higher-than-recommended doses over long periods of time, can produce drug dependence characterized by psychic dependence and, less frequently, physical dependence and tolerance. Propoxyphene will only partially suppress the withdrawal syndrome in individuals physically dependent on morphine or other narcotics. The abuse liability of propoxyphene is qualitatively similar to that of codeine although quantitatively less, and propoxyphene should be prescribed with the same degree of caution appropriate to the use of codeine.

Usage in Ambulatory Patients—Propoxyphene may impair the mental and/or physical abilities required for the performance of potentially hazardous tasks, such as driving a car or operating machinery. The patient should be cautioned accordingly.

PRECAUTIONS

General—Propoxyphene should be administered with caution to patients with hepatic or renal impairment since higher serum concentrations or delayed elimination may occur.

Drug Interactions—The CNS-depressant effect of propoxyphene is additive with that of other CNS depressants, including alcohol.

As is the case with many medicinal agents, propoxyphene may slow the metabolism of a concomitantly administered drug. Should this occur, the higher serum concentrations of that drug may result in increased pharmacologic or adverse effects of that drug. Such occurrences have been reported when propoxyphene was administered to patients on antidepressants, anticonvulsants, or warfarin-like drugs. Severe neurologic signs, including coma, have occurred with concurrent use of carbamazepine.

Usage in Pregnancy—Safe use in pregnancy has not been established relative to possible adverse effects on fetal development. Instances of withdrawal symptoms in the neonate have been reported following usage during pregnancy. Therefore, propoxyphene should not be used in pregnant women unless, in the judgment of the physician, the potential benefits outweigh the possible hazards.

Usage in Nursing Mothers—Low levels of propoxyphene have been detected in human milk. In postpartum studies involving nursing mothers who were given propoxyphene, no adverse effects were noted in infants receiving mother's milk.

Usage in Pediatric Patients— Safety and effectiveness in pediatric patients have not been established.

Usage in the Elderly—The rate of propoxyphene metabolism may be reduced in some patients. Increased dosing interval should be considered.

A Patient Information Sheet is available for this product. See text following "How Supplied" section below.

ADVERSE REACTIONS

In a survey conducted in hospitalized patients, less than 1% of patients taking propoxyphene hydrochloride at recommended doses experienced side effects. The most frequently reported were dizziness, sedation, nausea, and vomiting. Some of these adverse reactions may be alleviated if the patient lies down.

Other adverse reactions include constipation, abdominal pain, skin rashes, lightheadedness, headache, weakness, euphoria, dysphoria, hallucinations, and minor visual disturbances.

Propoxyphene therapy has been associated with abnormal liver function tests and, more rarely, with instances of reversible jaundice (including cholestatic jaundice).

Subacute painful myopathy has occurred following chronic propoxyphene overdosage.

DOSAGE AND ADMINISTRATION

Darvon-N is given orally. The usual dosage is 100 mg propoxyphene napsylate every 4 hours as needed for pain. The maximum recommended dose of propoxyphene napsylate is 600 mg per day.

Consideration should be given to a reduced total daily dosage in patients with hepatic or renal impairment.

MANAGEMENT OF OVERDOSAGE

In all cases of suspected overdosage, call your regional Poison Control Center to obtain the most up-to-date information about the treatment of overdose. This recommendation is made because, in general, information regarding the treatment of overdosage may change more rapidly than do package inserts.

Initial consideration should be given to the management of the CNS effects of propoxyphene overdosage. Resuscitative measures should be initiated promptly.

Symptoms of Propoxyphene Overdosage—The manifestations of acute overdosage with propoxyphene are those of narcotic overdosage. The patient is usually somnolent but may be stuporous or comatose and convulsing. Respiratory depression is characteristic. The ventilatory rate and/or tidal volume is decreased, which results in cyanosis and hypoxia. Pupils, initially pinpoint, may become dilated as hypoxia increases. Cheyne-Stokes respiration and apnea may occur. Blood pressure and heart rate are usually normal initially, but blood pressure falls and cardiac performance deteriorates, which ultimately results in pulmonary edema and circulatory collapse, unless the respiratory depression is corrected and adequate ventilation is restored promptly. Cardiac arrhythmias and conduction delay may be present. A combined respiratory-metabolic acidosis occurs owing to retained CO_2 (hypercapnia) and to lactic acid formed during anaerobic glycolysis. Acidosis may be severe if large amounts of salicylates have also been ingested. Death may occur.

Treatment of Propoxyphene Overdosage—Attention should be directed first to establishing a patent airway and to restoring ventilation. Mechanically assisted ventilation, with or without oxygen, may be required, and positive pressure respiration may be desirable if pulmonary edema is present. The narcotic antagonist naloxone will markedly reduce the degree of respiratory depression, and 0.4 to 2 mg should be administered promptly, preferably intravenously. If the desired degree of counteraction with improvement in respiratory functions is not obtained, naloxone should be repeated at 2- to 3-minute intervals. The duration of action of the antagonist may be brief. If no response is observed after 10 mg of naloxone have been administered, the diagnosis of propoxyphene toxicity should be questioned. Naloxone may also be administered by continuous intravenous infusion.

Treatment of Propoxyphene Overdosage in Pediatric Patients—The usual initial dose of naloxone in pediatric patients is 0.01 mg/kg body weight given intravenously. If this dose does not result in the desired degree of clinical improvement, a subsequent increased dose of 0.1 mg/kg body weight may be administered. If an IV route of administration is not available, naloxone may be administered IM or subcutaneously in divided doses. If necessary, naloxone can be diluted with Sterile Water for Injection.

Blood gases, pH, and electrolytes should be monitored in order that acidosis and any electrolyte disturbance present may be corrected promptly. Acidosis, hypoxia, and generalized CNS depression predispose to the development of cardiac arrhythmias. Ventricular fibrillation or cardiac arrest may occur and necessitate the full complement of cardiopulmonary resuscitation (CPR) measures. Respiratory acidosis rapidly subsides as ventilation is restored and hypercapnia eliminated, but lactic acidosis may require intravenous bicarbonate for prompt correction.

Electrocardiographic monitoring is essential. Prompt correction of hypoxia, acidosis, and electrolyte disturbance (when present) will help prevent these cardiac complications and will increase the effectiveness of agents administered to restore normal cardiac function.

In addition to the use of a narcotic antagonist, the patient may require careful titration with an anticonvulsant to control convulsions. Analeptic drugs (for example, caffeine or amphetamine) should not be used because of their tendency to precipitate convulsions.

General supportive measures, in addition to oxygen, include, when necessary, intravenous fluids, vasopressor-inotropic compounds, and, when infection is likely, anti-infective agents. Gastric lavage may be useful, and activated charcoal can adsorb a significant amount of ingested propoxyphene. Dialysis is of little value in poisoning due to propoxyphene. Efforts should be made to determine whether other agents, such as alcohol, barbiturates, tranquilizers, or other CNS depressants, were also ingested, since these increase CNS depression as well as cause specific toxic effects.

ANIMAL TOXICOLOGY

The acute lethal doses of the hydrochloride and napsylate salts of propoxyphene were determined in 4 species. The results shown in Figure 2 indicate that, on a molar basis, the napsylate salt is less toxic than the hydrochloride. This may be due to the relative insolubility and retarded absorption of propoxyphene napsylate.

Figure 2. Acute oral toxicity of propoxyphene

	LD_{50} (mg/kg) ± SE / LD_{50}(mmol/kg)	
Species	Propoxyphene Hydrochloride	Propoxyphene Napsylate
Mouse	282±39 / 0.75	915±163 / 1.62
Rat	230±44 / 0.61	647±95 / 1.14
Rabbit	*ca*82 / 0.22	>183 / >0.32
Dog	*ca* 100 / 0.27	>183 / >0.32

Some indication of the relative insolubility and retarded absorption of propoxyphene napsylate was obtained by measuring plasma propoxyphene levels in 2 groups of 4 dogs following oral administration of equimolar doses of the 2 salts. As shown in Figure 3, the peak plasma concentration observed with propoxyphene hydrochloride was much higher than that obtained after administration of the napsylate salt.

Although none of the animals in this experiment died, 3 of the 4 dogs given propoxyphene hydrochloride exhibited convulsive seizures during the time interval corresponding to the peak plasma levels. The 4 animals receiving the napsylate salt were mildly ataxic but not acutely ill.

Figure 3

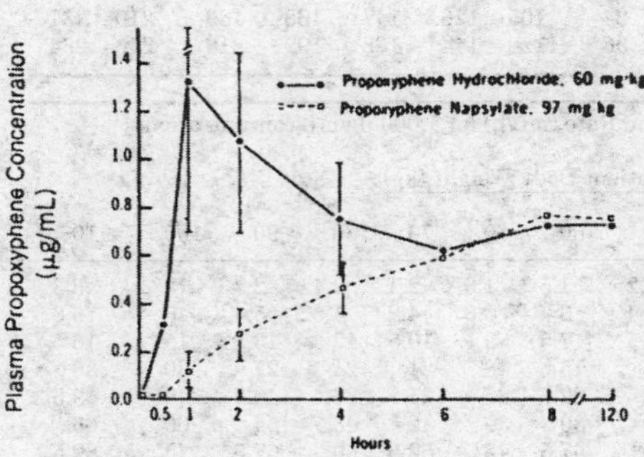

Figure 3. Plasma propoxyphene concentrations in dogs following large doses of the hydrochloride and napsylate salts

HOW SUPPLIED

Darvon-N® Tablets (No. 1883) are available in:

The 100 mg tablets are buff colored, elliptical shaped, film coated, and imprinted with the script "Lilly" and "Darvon-N 100" on one side of the tablet, using edible black ink. They are available as follows:

Bottles of 100 (RxPak*)	NDC 0002-0353-02 (TA1883)
Bottles of 500	NDC 0002-0353-03 (TA1883)
ID†100	NDC 0002-0353-33 (TA1883)

*All RxPaks (prescription packages, Lilly) have safety closures.

†Identi-Dose® (unit dose medication, Lilly).

Store at controlled room temperature, 59° to 86°F (15° to 30°C).

CAUTION—Federal (USA) law prohibits dispensing without prescription.

The following information, including description of dosage forms and the maximum daily dosage of each, is available to patients receiving Darvon products.

Patient Information Sheet ℂ-IV

YOUR PRESCRIPTION FOR A DARVON® (PROPOXYPHENE) PRODUCT

Summary

Products containing Darvon are used to relieve pain.

LIMIT YOUR INTAKE OF ALCOHOL WHILE TAKING THIS DRUG. Make sure your doctor knows if you are taking tranquilizers, sleep aids, antidepressants, antihistamines, or any other drugs that make you sleepy. Combining propoxyphene with alcohol or these drugs in excessive doses is dangerous.

Use care while driving a car or using machines until you see how the drug affects you because propoxyphene can make you sleepy. Do not take more of the drug than your doctor prescribed. Dependence has occurred when patients have taken propoxyphene for a long period of time at doses greater than recommended.

The rest of this leaflet gives you more information about propoxyphene. Please read it and keep it for future use.

Uses of Darvon

Products containing Darvon are used for the relief of mild to moderate pain. Products that contain Darvon plus aspirin or acetaminophen are prescribed for the relief of pain or pain associated with fever.

Before Taking Darvon

Make sure your doctor knows if you have ever had an allergic reaction to propoxyphene, aspirin, or acetaminophen. Some forms of propoxyphene products contain aspirin to help relieve the pain. Your doctor should be advised if you have a history of ulcers or if you are taking an anticoagulant ("blood thinner"). The aspirin may irritate the stomach lining and may cause bleeding, particularly if an ulcer is present. Also, bleeding may occur if you are taking an anticoagulant. In a small group of people, aspirin may cause an asthma attack. If you are one of these people, be sure your drug does not contain aspirin.

The effect of propoxyphene in pediatric patients under 12 has not been studied. Therefore, use of the drug in this age group is not recommended.

Also, due to the possible association between aspirin and Reye Syndrome, those propoxyphene products containing aspirin should not be given to children, including teenagers, with chicken pox or flu unless prescribed by a physician.

The following propoxyphene product contains aspirin: Darvon® Compound-65 (Propoxyphene Hydrochloride, Aspirin, and Caffeine, USP)

How to Take Darvon

Follow your doctor's directions exactly. Do not increase the amount you take without your doctor's approval. If you miss a dose of the drug, do not take twice as much the next time.

Pregnancy

Do not take propoxyphene during pregnancy unless your doctor knows you are pregnant and specifically recommends its use. Cases of temporary dependence in the newborn have occurred when the mother has taken propoxyphene consistently in the weeks before delivery. As a general principle, no drug should be taken during pregnancy unless it is clearly necessary.

General Cautions

Heavy use of alcohol with propoxyphene is hazardous and may lead to overdosage symptoms (*see* "Overdose" below). THEREFORE, LIMIT YOUR INTAKE OF ALCOHOL WHILE TAKING PROPOXYPHENE.

Combinations of excessive doses of propoxyphene, alcohol, and tranquilizers are dangerous. Make sure your doctor knows if you are taking tranquilizers, sleep aids, antidepressant drugs, antihistamines, or any other drugs that make you sleepy. The use of these drugs with propoxyphene increases their sedative effects and may lead to overdosage symptoms, including death (*see* "Overdose" below).

Propoxyphene may cause drowsiness or impair your mental and/or physical abilities; therefore, use caution when driving a vehicle or operating dangerous machinery. DO NOT perform any hazardous task until you have seen your response to this drug.

Propoxyphene may increase the concentration in the body of medications, such as anticoagulants ("blood thinners"), antidepressants, or drugs used for epilepsy. The result may be excessive or adverse effects of these medications. Make sure your doctor knows if you are taking any of these medications.

Dependence

You can become dependent on propoxyphene if you take it in higher than recommended doses over a long period of time. Dependence is a feeling of need for the drug and a feeling that you cannot perform normally without it.

Overdose

An overdose of Darvon, alone or in combination with other drugs, including alcohol, may cause weakness, difficulty in breathing, confusion, anxiety, and more severe drowsiness and dizziness. Extreme overdosage may lead to unconsciousness and death.

If the propoxyphene product contains acetaminophen, the overdosage symptoms include nausea, vomiting, lack of appetite, and abdominal pain. Liver damage may occur.

When the propoxyphene product contains aspirin, symptoms of taking too much of the drug are headache, dizziness, ringing in the ears, difficulty in hearing, dim vision, confusion, drowsiness, sweating, thirst, rapid breathing, nausea, vomiting, and, occasionally, diarrhea.

In any suspected overdosage situation, contact your doctor or nearest hospital emergency room. GET EMERGENCY HELP IMMEDIATELY.

KEEP THIS DRUG AND ALL DRUGS OUT OF THE REACH OF THE PEDIATRIC POPULATION.

Possible Side Effects

When propoxyphene is taken as directed, side effects are infrequent. Among those reported are drowsiness, dizziness, nausea, and vomiting. If these effects occur, it may help if you lie down and rest.

Less frequently reported side effects are constipation, abdominal pain, skin rashes, lightheadedness, headache, weakness, hallucinations, minor visual disturbances, and feelings of elation or discomfort.

If side effects occur and concern you, contact your doctor.

Other Information

The safe and effective use of propoxyphene depends on your taking it exactly as directed. This drug has been prescribed specifically for you and your present condition. Do not give this drug to others who may have similar symptoms. Do not use it for any other reason.

If you would like more information about propoxyphene, ask your doctor or pharmacist. They have a more technical leaflet (professional labeling) you may read.

Selected Darvon Products

Maximum Daily Dosage		
6	Dark Orange, Capsule Shaped, Film Coated Tablets Imprinted with Script "Lilly" on the one side and "Darvocet-N 100"on the other, using edible black ink	DARVOCET-N® 100 ℂ-IV Propoxyphene Napsylate and Acetaminophen Tablets
6	Parabolic-Shaped Capsules Imprinted with Script "Lilly" and "3111" on the opaque gray cap and "Darvon Comp 65" on the opaque red body, using edible black ink	DARVON® COMPOUND-65 ℂ-IV Propoxyphene Hydrochloride, Aspirin, and Caffeine Pulvules®
6	Parabolic-Shaped Capsules Imprinted with Script "Lilly" and "H03" on the opaque pink cap and "Darvon" on the opaque pink body, using edible black ink	DARVON® ℂ-IV Propoxyphene Hydrochloride Pulvules, 65 mg

Literature revised July 18, 1996
PV 1973 AMP [071896]

DOBUTREX® SOLUTION ℞

[*dō 'bū-trĕks*]

(dobutamine injection, USP)

DESCRIPTION

Dobutrex® Solution (Dobutamine Injection, USP) is the hydrochloride salt of 1, 2-benzenediol, 4-[2-[[3-(4-hydroxyphenyl)-1-methylpropyl]amino]ethyl]-, (±)-. It is a synthetic catecholamine.

HO / HO—⟨ring⟩—$(CH_2)_2NHCH(CH_2)_2$—⟨ring⟩—OH, with CH_3 on the CH

Molecular Formula: $C_{18}H_{23}NO_3$

Molecular Weight: 301.39

The clinical formulation is supplied in a sterile form for intravenous use only. Each mL contains 12.5 mg (41.5 µmol) dobutamine, 0.24 mg sodium bisulfite (added during manufacture), and water for injection, q.s. Hydrochloric acid and/or sodium hydroxide may have been added during manufacture to adjust the pH.

CLINICAL PHARMACOLOGY

Dobutrex Solution is a direct-acting inotropic agent whose primary activity results from stimulation of the β-receptors of the heart while producing comparatively mild chronotropic, hypertensive, arrhythmogenic, and vasodilative effects. It does not cause the release of endogenous norepinephrine, as does dopamine. In animal studies, dobutamine produces less increase in heart rate and less decrease in peripheral vascular resistance for a given inotropic effect than does isoproterenol.

In patients with depressed cardiac function, both dobutamine and isoproterenol increase the cardiac output to a similar degree. In the case of dobutamine, this increase is usually not accompanied by marked increases in heart rate (although tachycardia is occasionally observed), and the cardiac stroke volume is usually increased. In contrast, isoproterenol increases the cardiac index primarily by increasing the heart rate while stroke volume changes little or declines.

Facilitation of atrioventricular conduction has been observed in human electrophysiologic studies and in patients with atrial fibrillation.

Systemic vascular resistance is usually decreased with administration of dobutamine.

Occasionally, minimum vasoconstriction has been observed.

Most clinical experience with dobutamine is short-term—not more than several hours in duration. In the limited number of patients who were studied for 24, 48, and 72 hours, a persistent increase in cardiac output occurred in some, whereas output returned toward baseline values in others.

The onset of action of Dobutrex Solution is within 1 to 2 minutes; however, as much as 10 minutes may be required to obtain the peak effect of a particular infusion rate.

The plasma half-life of dobutamine in humans is 2 minutes. The principal routes of metabolism are methylation of the catechol and conjugation. In human urine, the major excretion products are the conjugates of dobutamine and 3-O-methyl dobutamine. The 3-O-methyl derivative of dobutamine is inactive.

Alteration of synaptic concentrations of catecholamines with either reserpine or tricyclic antidepressants does not alter the actions of dobutamine in animals, which indicates that the actions of dobutamine are not dependent on presynaptic mechanisms.

The effective infusion rate of dobutamine varies widely from patient to patient, and titration is always necessary (*see* Dosage and Administration). At least in pediatric patients, dobutamine-induced increases in cardiac output and systemic pressure are generally seen, in any given patient, at lower infusion rates than those that cause substantial tachycardia (*see* Pediatric Use under Precautions).

INDICATIONS AND USAGE

Dobutrex Solution is indicated when parenteral therapy is necessary for inotropic support in the short-term treatment of patients with cardiac decompensation due to depressed

Continued on next page

*** Identi-Code® symbol. This product information was prepared in June 2000. Current information on these and other products of Eli Lilly and Company may be obtained by direct inquiry to Lilly Research Laboratories, Lilly Corporate Center, Indianapolis, Indiana 46285, (800) 545-5979.**

Dobutrex—Cont.

contractility resulting either from organic heart disease or from cardiac surgical procedures. Experience with intravenous dobutamine in controlled trials does not extend beyond 48 hours of repeated boluses and/or continuous infusions. Whether given orally, continuously intravenously, or intermittently intravenously, neither dobutamine nor any other cyclic-AMP-dependent inotrope has been shown in controlled trials to be safe or effective in the long-term treatment of congestive heart failure. In controlled trials of chronic oral therapy with various such agents, symptoms were not consistently alleviated, and the cyclic-AMP-dependent inotropes were consistently associated with increased risk of hospitalization and death. Patients with NYHA Class IV symptoms appeared to be at particular risk.

CONTRAINDICATIONS

Dobutrex Solution is contraindicated in patients with idiopathic hypertrophic subaortic stenosis and in patients who have shown previous manifestations of hypersensitivity to Dobutrex Solution.

WARNINGS

1. Increase in Heart Rate or Blood Pressure
Dobutrex Solution may cause a marked increase in heart rate or blood pressure, especially systolic pressure. Approximately 10% of adult patients in clinical studies have had rate increases of 30 beats/minute or more, and about 7.5% have had a 50 mm Hg or greater increase in systolic pressure. Usually, reduction of dosage promptly reverses these effects. Because dobutamine facilitates atrioventricular conduction, patients with atrial fibrillation are at risk of developing rapid ventricular response. In patients who have atrial fibrillation with rapid ventricular response, a digitalis preparation should be used prior to institution of therapy with Dobutrex Solution. Patients with preexisting hypertension appear to face an increased risk of developing an exaggerated pressor response.
2. Ectopic Activity
Dobutrex Solution may precipitate or exacerbate ventricular ectopic activity, but it rarely has caused ventricular tachycardia.
3. Hypersensitivity
Reactions suggestive of hypersensitivity associated with administration of Dobutrex Solution, including skin rash, fever, eosinophilia, and bronchospasm, have been reported occasionally.
4. Dobutrex Solution contains sodium bisulfite, a sulfite that may cause allergic-type reactions, including anaphylactic symptoms and life-threatening or less severe asthmatic episodes, in certain susceptible people. The overall prevalence of sulfite sensitivity in the general population is unknown and probably low. Sulfite sensitivity is seen more frequently in asthmatic than in nonasthmatic people.

PRECAUTIONS

General—1. **During the administration of Dobutrex Solution, as with any adrenergic agent, ECG and blood pressure should be continuously monitored. In addition, pulmonary wedge pressure and cardiac output should be monitored whenever possible to aid in the safe and effective infusion of Dobutrex Solution.**
2. Hypovolemia should be corrected with suitable volume expanders before treatment with Dobutrex Solution is instituted.
3. No improvement may be observed in the presence of marked mechanical obstruction, such as severe valvular aortic stenosis.
Usage Following Acute Myocardial Infarction—Clinical experience with Dobutrex Solution following myocardial infarction has been insufficient to establish the safety of the drug for this use. There is concern that any agent that increases contractile force and heart rate may increase the size of an infarction by intensifying ischemia, but it is not known whether dobutamine does so.
Laboratory Tests—Dobutamine, like other β_2-agonists, can produce a mild reduction in serum potassium concentration, rarely to hypokalemic levels. Accordingly, consideration should be given to monitoring serum potassium.
Drug Interactions—Animal studies indicate that dobutamine may be ineffective if the patient has recently received a β-blocking drug. In such a case, the peripheral vascular resistance may increase.
Preliminary studies indicate that the concomitant use of dobutamine and nitroprusside results in a higher cardiac output and, usually, a lower pulmonary wedge pressure than when either drug is used alone.
There was no evidence of drug interactions in clinical studies in which Dobutrex Solution was administered concurrently with other drugs, including digitalis preparations, furosemide, spironolactone, lidocaine, glyceryl trinitrate, isosorbide dinitrate, morphine, atropine, heparin, protamine, potassium chloride, folic acid, and acetaminophen.
Carcinogenesis, Mutagenesis, Impairment of Fertility—Studies to evaluate the carcinogenic or mutagenic potential of dobutamine, or its potential to affect fertility, have not been conducted.
Pregnancy—Teratogenic Effects—Pregnancy Category B—Reproduction studies performed in rats at doses up to the normal human dose (10 μg/kg/min for 24 h, total daily dose of 14.4 mg/kg), and in rabbits at doses up to twice the normal human dose, have revealed no evidence of harm to the fetus due to dobutamine. There are, however, no adequate and well-controlled studies in pregnant women. Because animal reproduction studies are not always predictive of human response, this drug should be used during pregnancy only if clearly needed.
Labor and Delivery—The effect of Dobutrex Solution on labor and delivery is unknown.
Nursing Mothers—It is not known whether this drug is excreted in human milk. Because many drugs are excreted in human milk, caution should be exercised when Dobutrex Solution is administered to a nursing woman. If a mother requires Dobutrex Solution treatment, breast-feeding should be discontinued for the duration of the treatment.
Pediatric Use—Dobutamine has been shown to increase cardiac output and systemic pressure in pediatric patients of every age group. In premature neonates, however, dobutamine is less effective than dopamine in raising systemic blood pressure without causing undue tachycardia, and dobutamine has not been shown to provide any added benefit when given to such infants already receiving optimal infusions of dopamine.

ADVERSE REACTIONS

Increased Heart Rate, Blood Pressure, and Ventricular Ectopic Activity—A 10- to 20-mm increase in systolic blood pressure and an increase in heart rate of 5 to 15 beats/minute have been noted in most patients (*see* Warnings regarding exaggerated chronotropic and pressor effects). Approximately 5% of adult patients have had increased premature ventricular beats during infusions. These effects are dose related.
Hypotension—Precipitous decreases in blood pressure have occasionally been described in association with Dobutrex Solution therapy. Decreasing the dose or discontinuing the infusion typically results in rapid return of blood pressure to baseline values. In rare cases, however, intervention may be required and reversibility may not be immediate.
Reactions at Sites of Intravenous Infusion—Phlebitis has occasionally been reported. Local inflammatory changes have been described following inadvertent infiltration. Isolated cases of cutaneous necrosis (destruction of skin tissue) have been reported.
Miscellaneous Uncommon Effects—The following adverse effects have been reported in 1% to 3% of adult patients: nausea, headache, anginal pain, nonspecific chest pain, palpitations, and shortness of breath.
Isolated cases of thrombocytopenia have been reported.
Administration of Dobutrex Solution, like other catecholamines, can produce a mild reduction in serum potassium concentration, rarely to hypokalemic levels (*see* Precautions).

OVERDOSAGE

Overdoses of Dobutrex Solution have been reported rarely. The following is provided to serve as a guide if such an overdose is encountered.
Signs and Symptoms—Toxicity from Dobutrex Solution is usually due to excessive cardiac β-receptor stimulation. The duration of action of Dobutrex Solution is generally short ($T_{1/2}$ = 2 minutes) because it is rapidly metabolized by catechol-0-methyltransferase. The symptoms of toxicity may include anorexia, nausea, vomiting, tremor, anxiety, palpitations, headache, shortness of breath, and anginal and nonspecific chest pain. The positive inotropic and chronotropic effects of Dobutrex Solution on the myocardium may cause hypertension, tachyarrhythmias, myocardial ischemia, and ventricular fibrillation. Hypotension may result from vasodilation.
Treatment—To obtain up-to-date information about the treatment of overdose, a good resource is your certified Regional Poison Control Center. Telephone numbers of certified poison control centers are listed in the *Physicians' Desk Reference* (*PDR*). In managing overdosage, consider the possibility of multiple drug overdoses, interaction among drugs, and unusual drug kinetics in your patient.
The initial actions to be taken in a Dobutrex Solution overdose are discontinuing administration, establishing an airway, and ensuring oxygenation and ventilation. Resuscitative measures should be initiated promptly. Severe ventricular tachyarrhythmias may be successfully treated with propranolol or lidocaine. Hypertension usually responds to a reduction in dose or discontinuation of therapy.
Protect the patient's airway and support ventilation and perfusion. If needed, meticulously monitor and maintain, within acceptable limits, the patient's vital signs, blood gases, serum electrolytes, etc.
If the product is ingested, unpredictable absorption may occur from the mouth and the gastrointestinal tract. Absorption of drugs from the gastrointestinal tract may be decreased by giving activated charcoal, which, in many cases, is more effective than emesis or lavage; consider charcoal instead of or in addition to gastric emptying. Repeated doses of charcoal over time may hasten elimination of some drugs that have been absorbed. Safeguard the patient's airway when employing gastric emptying or charcoal.
Forced diuresis, peritoneal dialysis, hemodialysis, or charcoal hemoperfusion have not been established as beneficial for an overdose of Dobutrex Solution.

DOSAGE AND ADMINISTRATION

Note—Do not add Dobutrex Solution to 5% Sodium Bicarbonate Injection or to any other strongly alkaline solution.

Table 1
Dobutrex Solution Infusion Rate (mL/h) for 500 μg/mL concentration

Drug Delivery Rate (μg/kg/min)	Patient Body Weight (kg)											
	5	10	20	30	40	50	60	70	80	90	100	110
0.5	0.3	0.6	1.2	1.8	2.4	3	3.6	4.2	4.8	5.4	6	6.6
1	0.6	1.2	2.4	3.6	4.8	6	7.2	8.4	9.6	10.8	12	13.2
2.5	1.5	3	6	9	12	15	18	21	24	27	30	33
5	3	6	12	18	24	30	36	42	48	54	60	66
7.5	4.5	9	18	27	36	45	54	63	72	81	90	99
10	6	12	24	36	48	60	72	84	96	108	120	132
12.5	7.5	15	30	45	60	75	90	105	120	135	150	165
15	9	18	36	54	72	90	108	126	144	162	180	198
17.5	10.5	21	42	63	84	105	126	147	168	189	210	231
20	12	24	48	72	96	120	144	168	192	216	240	264

Dobutrex Solution Infusion Rate (mL/h) for 1,000 μg/mL concentration

Drug Delivery Rate (μg/kg/min)	Patient Body Weight (kg)											
	5	10	20	30	40	50	60	70	80	90	100	110
0.5	0.1	0.3	0.6	0.9	1.2	1.5	1.8	2.1	2.4	2.7	3	3.3
1	0.3	0.6	1.2	1.8	2.4	3	3.6	4.2	4.8	5.4	6	6.6
2.5	0.7	1.5	3	4.5	6	7.5	9	10.5	12	13.5	15	16.5
5	1.5	3	6	9	12	15	18	21	24	27	30	33
7.5	2.2	4.5	9	13.5	18	22.5	27	31.5	36	40.5	45	49.5
10	3	6	12	18	24	30	36	42	48	54	60	66
12.5	3.7	7.5	15	22.5	30	37.5	45	52.5	60	67.5	75	82.5
15	4.5	9	18	27	36	45	54	63	72	81	90	99
17.5	5.2	10.5	21	31.5	42	52.5	63	73.5	84	94.5	105	115.5
20	6	12	24	36	48	60	72	84	96	108	120	132

Dobutrex Solution Infusion Rate (mL/h) for 2,000 μg/mL concentration

Drug Delivery Rate (μg/kg/min)	Patient Body Weight (kg)											
	5	10	20	30	40	50	60	70	80	90	100	110
0.5	0.07	0.1	0.3	0.4	0.6	0.7	0.9	1	1.2	1.3	1.5	1.6
1	0.1	0.3	0.6	0.9	1.2	1.5	1.8	2.1	2.4	2.7	3	3.3
2.5	0.4	0.7	1.5	2	3	4	4.5	5	6	7	7.5	8
5	0.7	1.5	3	4.5	6	7.5	9	10.5	12	13.5	15	16.5
7.5	1.1	2.2	4.5	7	9	11	13.5	16	18	20	22.5	25
10	1.5	3	6	9	12	15	18	21	24	27	30	33
12.5	1.9	3.7	7	11	15	19	22.5	26	30	34	37.5	41
15	2.2	4.5	9	13.5	18	22.5	27	31.5	36	40.5	45	49.5
17.5	2.6	5.2	10.5	15.7	21	26.2	31.5	36.7	42	47.2	52.5	57.7
20	3	6	12	18	24	30	36	42	48	54	60	66

Because of potential physical incompatibilities, it is recommended that Dobutrex Solution not be mixed with other drugs in the same solution. Dobutrex Solution should not be used in conjunction with other agents or diluents containing both sodium bisulfate and ethanol.

Preparation and Stability—At the time of administration, Dobutrex Solution must be further diluted in an IV container to at least a 50-mL solution using one of the following intravenous solutions as a diluent: 5% Dextrose Injection, 5% Dextrose and 0.45% Sodium Chloride Injection, 5% Dextrose and 0.9% Sodium Chloride Injection, 10% Dextrose Injection, Isolyte® M with 5% Dextrose Injection, Lactated Ringer's Injection, 5% Dextrose in Lactated Ringer's Injection, Normosol®-M in D5-W, 20% Osmitrol® in Water for Injection, 0.9% Sodium Chloride Injection, or Sodium Lactate Injection. Intravenous solutions should be used within 24 hours.

Recommended Dosage—Infusion of dobutamine should be started at a low rate (0.5–1.0 μg/kg/min) and titrated at intervals of a few minutes, guided by the patient's response, including systemic blood pressure, urine flow, frequency of ectopic activity, heart rate, and (whenever possible) measurements of cardiac output, central venous pressure, and/or pulmonary capillary wedge pressure. In reported trials, the optimal infusion rates have varied from patient to patient, usually 2–20 μg/kg/min but sometimes slightly outside of this range. On rare occasions, infusion rates up to 40 μg/kg/min have been required to obtain the desired effect.

Rates of infusion (mL/h) for Dobutrex Solution concentrations of 500 μg/mL, 1,000 μg/mL, and 2,000 μg/mL necessary to attain various delivery rates of dobutamine (μg/kg/min) for patients of different weights are given in Table 1.

[See table 1 at top of previous page]
[See second table at top of previous page]
[See third table at top of previous page]

Concentrations of up to 5,000 μg/mL have been administered to humans (250 mg/50 mL). The final volume administered should be determined by the fluid requirements of the patient.

Intravenous drug products should be inspected visually and should not be used if particulate matter or discoloration is present.

HOW SUPPLIED

Vials: Each 20 mL vial contains 250 mg dobutamine.
NDC 0002-7175-01 (No. 7175)—1s
NDC 0002-7175-10 (No. 7175)—Traypak† of 10

†Traypak™ (multivial carton, Lilly).

Store at controlled room temperature, 59° to 86°F (15° to 30°C).

Literature revised February 18, 1999
PA 7368 AMP [021899]

EVISTA®
Raloxifene Hydrochloride
60 mg Tablets ℞

DESCRIPTION

EVISTA® (raloxifene hydrochloride) is a selective estrogen receptor modulator (SERM) that belongs to the benzothiophene class of compounds. The chemical structure is:

The chemical designation is methanone, [6-hydroxy-2-(4-hydroxyphenyl)benzo[*b*]thien-3-yl] - [4-[2-(1-piperidinyl) ethoxy]phenyl]-, hydrochloride. Raloxifene hydrochloride (HCl) has the empirical formula $C_{28}H_{27}NO_4S \bullet HCl$, which corresponds to a molecular weight of 510.05. Raloxifene HCl is an off-white to pale-yellow solid that is very slightly soluble in water.

EVISTA is supplied in a tablet dosage form for oral administration. Each EVISTA tablet contains 60 mg of raloxifene HCl, which is the molar equivalent of 55.71 mg of free base. Inactive ingredients include anhydrous lactose, carnauba wax, crospovidone, F D & C Blue No. 2 aluminum lake, hydroxypropyl methylcellulose, lactose monohydrate, magnesium stearate, modified pharmaceutical glaze, polyethylene glycol, polysorbate 80, povidone, propylene glycol, and titanium dioxide.

CLINICAL PHARMACOLOGY

Mechanism of Action

Decreases in estrogen levels after oophorectomy or menopause lead to increases in bone resorption and accelerated bone loss. Bone is initially lost rapidly because the compensatory increase in bone formation is inadequate to offset resorptive losses. In addition to loss of estrogen, this imbalance between resorption and formation may be due to age-related impairment of osteoblasts or their precursors. In some women, these changes will eventually lead to decreased bone mass, osteoporosis, and increased risk for fractures, particularly of the spine, hip, and wrist. Vertebral fractures are the most common type of osteoporotic fracture in postmenopausal women.

Raloxifene's biological actions are largely mediated through binding to estrogen receptors. This binding results in activation of certain estrogenic pathways and blockade of others. Thus, raloxifene is a selective estrogen receptor modulator (SERM).

Raloxifene decreases resorption of bone and reduces biochemical markers of bone turnover to the premenopausal range. These effects on bone are manifested as reductions in the serum and urine levels of bone turnover markers, decreases in bone resorption based on radiocalcium kinetics studies, increases in bone mineral density (BMD) and decreases in incidence of fractures. Raloxifene also has effects on lipid metabolism. Raloxifene decreases total and LDL cholesterol levels but does not increase triglyceride levels. It does not change total HDL cholesterol levels. Preclinical data demonstrate that raloxifene is an estrogen antagonist in uterine and breast tissues. Clinical trial data (through a median of 42 months) suggest that EVISTA lacks estrogen-like effects on the uterus and breast tissue.

Pharmacokinetics

The disposition of raloxifene has been evaluated in more than 3000 postmenopausal women in selected raloxifene osteoporosis treatment and prevention clinical trials using a population approach. Pharmacokinetic data were also obtained in conventional pharmacology studies in 292 postmenopausal women. Raloxifene exhibits high within-subject variability (approximately 30% coefficient of variation) of most pharmacokinetic parameters. Table 1 summarizes the pharmacokinetic parameters of raloxifene.

Absorption

Raloxifene is absorbed rapidly after oral administration. Approximately 60% of an oral dose is absorbed, but presystemic glucuronide conjugation is extensive. Absolute bioavailability of raloxifene is 2.0%. The time to reach average maximum plasma concentration and bioavailability are functions of systemic interconversion and enterohepatic cycling of raloxifene and its glucuronide metabolites.

Administration of raloxifene HCl with a standardized, high-fat meal increases the absorption of raloxifene (C_{max} 28% and AUC 16%), but does not lead to clinically meaningful changes in systemic exposure. EVISTA can be administered without regard to meals.

Distribution

Following oral administration of single doses ranging from 30 to 150 mg of raloxifene HCl, the apparent volume of distribution is 2348 L/kg and is not dose dependent.

Raloxifene and the monoglucuronide conjugates are highly (95%) bound to plasma proteins. Raloxifene binds to both albumin and α1-acid glycoprotein, but not to sex steroid binding globulin.

Metabolism

Biotransformation and disposition of raloxifene in humans have been determined following oral administration of ^{14}C-labeled raloxifene. Raloxifene undergoes extensive first-pass metabolism to the glucuronide conjugates: raloxifene-4′-glucuronide, raloxifene-6-glucuronide, and raloxifene-6, 4′-diglucuronide. No other metabolites have been detected, providing strong evidence that raloxifene is not metabolized by cytochrome P450 pathways. Unconjugated raloxifene comprises less than 1% of the total radiolabeled material in plasma. The terminal log-linear portions of the plasma concentration curves for raloxifene and the glucuronides are generally parallel. This is consistent with interconversion of raloxifene and the glucuronide metabolites.

Following intravenous administration, raloxifene is cleared at a rate approximating hepatic blood flow. Apparent oral clearance is 44.1 L/kg•hr. Raloxifene and its glucuronide conjugates are interconverted by reversible systemic metabolism and enterohepatic cycling, thereby prolonging its plasma elimination half-life to 27.7 hours after oral dosing.

Results from single oral doses of raloxifene predict multiple-dose pharmacokinetics. Following chronic dosing, clearance ranges from 40 to 60 L/kg • hr. Increasing doses of raloxifene HCl (ranging from 30 to 150 mg) result in slightly less than a proportional increase in the area under the plasma time concentration curve (AUC).

Excretion

Raloxifene is primarily excreted in feces, and less than 0.2% is excreted unchanged in urine. Less than 6% of the raloxifene dose is eliminated in urine as glucuronide conjugates.

[See table 1 at top of next page]

Special Populations

Geriatric—No differences in raloxifene pharmacokinetics were detected with regard to age (range 42 to 84 years).

Pediatric—The pharmacokinetics of raloxifene have not been evaluated in a pediatric population.

Gender—Total extent of exposure and oral clearance, normalized for lean body weight, are not significantly different between age-matched female and male volunteers.

Race—Pharmacokinetic differences due to race have been studied in 1712 women including 97.5% Caucasian, 1.0% Asian, 0.7% Hispanic, and 0.5% Black in the osteoporosis treatment trial and in 1053 women including 93.5% Caucasian, 4.3% Hispanic, 1.2% Asian, and 0.5% Black in the osteoporosis prevention trials. There were no discernible differences in raloxifene plasma concentrations among these groups; however, the influence of race cannot be conclusively determined.

Renal Insufficiency—Since negligible amounts of raloxifene and eliminated in urine, a study in patients with renal insufficiency was not conducted. In the osteoporosis treatment and prevention trials, raloxifene and metabolite concentrations in women with estimated creatinine clearance as low as 21 mL/min are similar to women with normal creatinine clearance.

Hepatic Dysfunction—Raloxifene was studied, as a single dose, in Child-Pugh Class A patients with cirrhosis and total serum bilirubin ranging from 0.6 to 2.0 mg/dL. Plasma raloxifene concentrations were approximately 2.5 times higher than in controls and correlated with bilirubin concentrations. Safety and efficacy have not been evaluated further in patients with hepatic insufficiency (see WARNINGS).

Drug-Drug Interactions

Clinically significant drug-drug interactions are discussed in PRECAUTIONS.

Ampicillin and Amoxicillin—Peak concentrations of raloxifene and the overall extent of absorption are reduced 28% and 14%, respectively, with coadministration of ampicillin. These reductions are consistent with decreased enterohepatic cycling associated with antibiotic reduction of enteric bacteria. However, the systemic exposure and the elimination rate of raloxifene were not affected. Therefore, EVISTA can be concurrently administered with ampicillin. In the osteoporosis treatment trial, co-administration of amoxicillin had no discernable differences in plasma raloxifene concentrations.

Antacids—Concurrent administration of calcium carbonate or aluminum and magnesium hydroxide-containing antacids does not affect the systemic exposure of raloxifene.

Corticosteroids—The chronic administration of raloxifene in postmenopausal women has no effect on the pharmacokinetics of methylprednisolone given as a single oral dose.

Cholestyramine—See PRECAUTIONS.

Cyclosporine—The coadministration of EVISTA with cyclosporine has not been evaluated.

Digoxin—Raloxifene has no effect on the pharmacokinetics of digoxin.

Warfarin—See PRECAUTIONS.

Animal Pharmacology

The skeletal effects of raloxifene treatment were assessed in ovariectomized rats and monkeys. In rats, raloxifene prevented increased bone resorption and bone loss after ovariectomy. There were positive effects of raloxifene on bone strength, but the effects varied with time. Cynomolgus monkeys were treated with raloxifene or conjugated estrogens for 2 years. In terms of bone cycles, this is equivalent to approximately 6 years in humans. Raloxifene and estrogen suppressed bone turnover, and increased BMD in the lumbar spine and in the central cancellous bone of the proximal tibia. In this animal model, there was a positive correlation between vertebral compressive breaking force and BMD of the lumbar spine.

Histologic examination of bone from rats and monkeys treated with raloxifene showed no evidence of woven bone, marrow fibrosis, or mineralization defects.

These results are consistent with data from human studies of radiocalcium kinetics and markers of bone metabolism, and are consistent with EVISTA's action as a skeletal antiresorptive agent.

Clinical Studies

In postmenopausal women with osteoporosis, EVISTA reduced the risk of vertebral fractures. EVISTA also increased BMD of the spine, hip and total body. Similarly, in early postmenopausal women without osteoporosis (women with normal or low BMD without fracture), EVISTA increased spine, hip and total body BMD relative to calcium alone at 24 months. The effect on hip bone mass was similar to that for the spine.

Treatment of Osteoporosis

The effects of EVISTA on fracture incidence and BMD in postmenopausal women with osteoporosis were examined at 3 years in a large randomized placebo-controlled, double-blind multinational osteoporosis treatment trial. All vertebral fractures were diagnosed radiographically; some of these fractures also were associated with symptoms (i.e., clinical fractures). The study population consisted of 7705 postmenopausal women with osteoporosis as defined by: a) low BMD (vertebral or hip bone mineral density at least 2.5 standard deviations below the mean value for healthy young women) without baseline vertebral fractures, or b) one or more baseline vertebral fractures. Women enrolled in this study had a median age of 67 years (range 31 to 80) and a median time since menopause of 19 years.

EVISTA, 60 mg administered once daily, increased spine and hip BMD by 2–3%. EVISTA decreased the incidence of the first vertebral fracture from 4.3% for placebo to 1.9% for EVISTA (relative risk reduction = 55%) and subsequent vertebral fractures from 20.2% for placebo to 14.1% for EVISTA (relative risk reduction = 30%) (Table 2). All women in the study received calcium (500 mg/day) and vitamin D (400–600 IU/day). EVISTA reduced the incidence of vertebral fractures whether or not patients had a vertebral fracture upon study entry. The decrease in incidence of vertebral fracture was greater than could be accounted for by increase in BMD alone.

[See table 2 at top of next page]

Continued on next page

*** Identi-Code® symbol. This product information was prepared in June 2000. Current information on these and other products of Eli Lilly and Company may be obtained by direct inquiry to Lilly Research Laboratories, Lilly Corporate Center, Indianapolis, Indiana 46285, (800) 545-5979.**

Evista—Cont.

The mean percentage change in BMD from baseline for EVISTA was statistically significantly greater than for placebo at each skeletal site (Table 3).

Table 3. EVISTA (60 mg once daily) related increases in BMD for the osteoporosis treatment study expressed as mean percentage increase versus placebo[ab]

	Time		
Site	12 Months %	24 Months %	36 Months %
Lumbar Spine	2.0	2.6	2.6
Femoral Neck	1.3	1.9	2.1
Ultradistal Radius	ND	2.2	ND
Distal Radius	ND	0.9	ND
Total Body	ND	1.1	ND

Note: all BMD increases were significant ($p<0.001$)
[a] Intent-to-treat analysis; last observation carried forward.
[b] All patients received calcium and vitamin D.
ND= not done (total body and radius BMD were measured only at 24 months)

Discontinuation from the study was required when excessive bone loss or multiple incident vertebral fractures occurred. Such discontinuation was statistically significantly more frequent in the placebo group (3.7%) than in the EVISTA group (1.1%).

Prevention of Osteoporosis

The effects of EVISTA on BMD in postmenopausal women were examined in three randomized, placebo-controlled, double-blind osteoporosis prevention trials: (1) a North American trial enrolled 544 women; (2) a European trial, 601 women; and (3) an international trial, 619 women who had undergone hysterectomy. In these trials, all women received calcium supplementation (400 to 600 mg/day). Women enrolled in these studies had a median age of 54 years and a median time since menopause of 5 years (less than 1 year up to 15 years postmenopause). The majority of the women were Caucasian (93.5%). Women were included if they had spine bone mineral density between 2.5 standard deviations below and 2 standard deviations above the mean value for healthy young women. The mean T scores (number of standard deviations above or below the mean in healthy young women) for the 3 studies ranged from −1.01 to −0.74 for spine BMD and included women both with normal and low BMD. EVISTA, 60 mg administered once daily, produced increases in bone mass versus calcium supplementation alone, as reflected by dual-energy x-ray absorptiometric (DXA) measurements of hip, spine and total body BMD. Compared with placebo, the increases in BMD for each of the 3 studies were statistically significant at 12 months and were maintained at 24 months (Table 4). The placebo groups lost approximately 1% of BMD over 24 months.

Table 4. EVISTA (60 mg once daily) related increases in BMD for the three osteoporosis prevention studies expressed as mean percentage increase versus placebo[a] at 24 months[b]

	Study		
Site	NA %	EU %	INT[c] %
Total Hip	2.0	2.4	1.3
Femoral Neck	2.1	2.5	1.6
Trochanter	2.2	2.7	1.3
Intertrochanter	2.3	2.4	1.3
Lumbar Spine	2.0	2.4	1.8

Abbreviations: NA = North American, EU = European, INT = International.
Note: all BMD increases were significant ($p\leq0.001$)
[a] All patients received calcium.
[b] Intent-to-treat analysis; last observation carried forward.
[c] All women in the study had previously undergone hysterectomy.

EVISTA also increased BMD compared with placebo in the total body by 1.3% to 2.0% and in Ward's Triangle (hip) by 3.1% to 4.0%. The effects of EVISTA on forearm BMD were inconsistent between studies. In Study EU, EVISTA prevented bone loss at the ultradistal radius, whereas in Study NA, it did not.

[See figures at top of next column]

Assessments of Bone Turnover

In a 31-week open-label radiocalcium kinetics study, 33 early postmenopausal women were randomized to treatment with once-daily EVISTA 60 mg, cyclic estrogen/progestin (0.625 mg conjugated estrogens daily with 5 mg medroxyprogesterone acetate daily for the first two weeks of each month [HRT]), or no treatment. Treatment with either EVISTA or HRT was associated with reduced bone resorption and a positive shift in calcium balance (−82 mg Ca/day and +60 mg Ca/day, respectively for EVISTA and −162 mg Ca/day and +91 mg Ca/day, respectively for HRT).

Table 1. Summary of raloxifene pharmacokinetic parameters in the healthy postmenopausal woman

	C_{max}[a] (ng/mL)/(mg/kg)	$t_{1/2}$ (hr)	$AUC_{0-\infty}$[a] (ng•hr/mL)/(mg/kg)	CL/F (L/kg•hr)	V/F (L/kg)
Single Dose					
Mean	0.50	27.7	27.2	44.1	2348
CV (%)	52	10.7 to 273[b]	44	46	52
Multiple Dose					
Mean	1.36	32.5	24.2	47.4	2853
CV (%)	37	15.8 to 86.6[b]	36	41	56

Abbreviations: C_{max} = maximum plasma concentration, $t_{1/2}$ = half-life, AUC = area under the curve, CL = clearance, V = volume of distribution, F = bioavailability, CV = coefficient of variation.
[a] Data normalized for dose in mg and body weight in kg.
[b] Range of observed half-life.

Table 2. Effect of EVISTA on Risk of Vertebral Fractures

	Number of Patients EVISTA	Number of Patients Placebo	Absolute Risk Reduction	Relative Risk Reduction (95% CI)
Fractures diagnosed radiographically				
Patients with no baseline fracture[a]	n=1401	n=1457		
Number (%) of patients with ≥1 new vertebral fracture	27 (1.9%)	62 (4.3%)	2.4%	55% (29%, 71%)
Patients with ≥1 baseline fracture[a]	n=858	n=835		
Number (%) of patients with ≥1 new vertebral fracture	121 (14.1%)	169 (20.2%)	6.1%	30% (14%, 44%)
Symptomatic vertebral fractures				
All randomized patients	n=2557	n=2576		
Number (%) of patients with ≥1 new clinical (painful) vertebral fracture	47 (1.8%)	81 (3.1%)	1.3%	41% (17%, 59%)

[a] Includes all patients with baseline and at least one follow-up radiograph.

Total hip mean percentage change from baseline All placebo and EVISTA subjects 24-month data from Studies NA and EU[a]

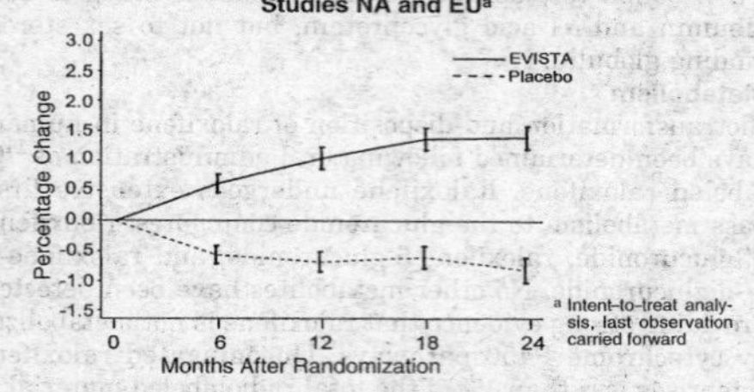

Total hip mean percentage change from baseline All placebo, EVISTA, and CE subjects 24-month data from Study INT (hysterectomized women)[a]

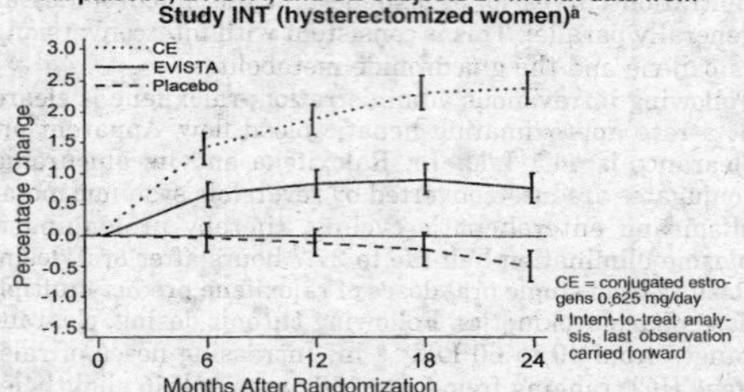

In both the osteoporosis treatment and prevention trials, EVISTA therapy resulted in consistent, statistically significant suppression of bone resorption and bone formation, as reflected by changes in serum and urine markers of bone turnover (e.g., bone-specific alkaline phosphatase, osteocalcin, and collagen breakdown products). The suppression of bone turnover markers was evident by 3 months and persisted throughout the 36-month and 24-month observation periods.

Bone Histomorphometry

In the treatment study, bone biopsies for qualitative and quantitative histomorphometry were obtained at baseline and after 2 years of treatment. There were 56 paired biopsies evaluable for all indices. In EVISTA-treated patients, there were statistically significant decreases in bone formation rate per tissue volume, consistent with a reduction in bone turnover. Normal bone quality was maintained; specifically, there was no evidence of osteomalacia, marrow fibrosis, cellular toxicity or woven bone after 2 years of treatment.

The tissue- and cellular-level effects of raloxifene were assessed by histomorphometric evaluation of human iliac crest bone biopsies taken after administration of a fluorochrome substance to label areas of mineralizing bone. The effects of EVISTA on bone histomorphometry were determined by pre- and post-treatment biopsies in a 6-month study of Caucasian postmenopausal women who received once-daily doses of EVISTA 60 mg or 0.625 mg conjugated estrogens. Ten raloxifene-treated and 8 estrogen-treated women had evaluable bone biopsies at baseline and after 6 months of therapy. Bone formation rate/bone volume and activation frequency, the primary efficacy parameters, decreased to a greater extent with conjugated estrogen treatment versus EVISTA treatment, although the differences were not statistically significant. Bone in EVISTA-and estrogen-treated women showed no evidence of mineralization defects, woven bone, or marrow fibrosis.

Effects on Lipid Metabolism

The effects of EVISTA on selected lipid fractions and clotting factors were evaluated in a 6-month study of 390 postmenopausal women. EVISTA was compared with oral continuous combined estrogen/progestin (0.625 mg conjugated estrogens plus 2.5 mg medroxyprogesterone acetate, [HRT]) and placebo (Table 5). EVISTA decreased serum total and LDL cholesterol without effects on serum total HDL cholesterol or triglycerides. In addition, EVISTA statistically significantly decreased serum fibrinogen and lipoprotein (a).

Table 5. EVISTA (60 mg once daily) and oral HRT effects on selected lipid fractions and clotting factors in a 6-month study—Median percentage change from baseline

	Treatment Group		
Endpoint	EVISTA (N=95) %	HRT (N=96) %	PLACEBO (N=98) %
Total Cholesterol	−6.6[a]	−4.4[a]	0.9
LDL Cholesterol	−10.9[a]	−12.7[a]	1.0
HDL Cholesterol	0.7[b]	10.6[a]	0.9
HDL-2 Cholesterol	15.4[b]	33.3[a]	0.0
HDL-3 Cholesterol	−2.5[ab]	2.7	0.0
Fibrinogen	−12.2[ab]	−2.8	−2.1
Lipoprotein (a)	−4.1[ab]	−16.3[a]	3.3
Triglycerides	−4.1[b]	20.0[a]	−0.3
Plasminogen Activator Inhibitor-1	−2.1[b]	−29.0[a]	−9.4

Abbreviations: HRT = continuous combined estrogen/progestin (0.625 mg conjugated estrogens plus 2.5 mg medroxyprogesterone acetate).
[a] Significantly different from placebo ($p<0.05$).
[b] Significantly different from HRT ($p<0.05$).

Consistent with results from the 6-month study, in the osteoporosis treatment (36 months) and prevention (24 months) studies, EVISTA statistically significantly decreased serum total and LDL cholesterol by 5% to 6% and 8% to 10% respectively, compared to placebo. EVISTA did not affect HDL cholesterol or triglyceride levels. The effect of EVISTA-induced reductions in total and LDL cholesterol on risk for cardiovascular disease is currently under study.

Effects on the Uterus

In the osteoporosis treatment trial, endometrial thickness was evaluated annually in a subset of the study population (1781 patients) for 3 years. Placebo-treated women had a

0.27 mm mean decrease from baseline in endometrial thickness over 3 years, whereas the EVISTA-treated women had a 0.06 mm mean increase. Patients in the osteoporosis treatment study were not screened at baseline or excluded for pre-existing endometrial or uterine disease. This study was not specifically designed to detect endometrial polyps. Over the 36 months of the study, clinically or histologically benign endometrial polyps were reported in 17 of 1999 placebo-treated women, 37 of 1948 EVISTA-treated women and in 31 of 2010 women treated with raloxifene HCl 120 mg/day.

There was no difference between EVISTA- and placebo-treated women in the incidences of endometrial carcinoma, vaginal bleeding or vaginal discharge.

In placebo-controlled osteoporosis prevention trials, endometrial thickness was evaluated every 6 months (for 24 months) by transvaginal ultrasonography (TVU). A total of 2978 TVU measurements were collected from 831 women in all dose groups. Placebo-treated women had a 0.04 mm mean increase from baseline in endometrial thickness over 2 years, whereas the EVISTA-treated women had a 0.09 mm mean increase. Endometrial thickness measurements in raloxifene-treated women were indistinguishable from placebo. There were no differences between the raloxifene and placebo groups with respect to the incidence of reported vaginal bleeding.

In a 6-month study of 18 postmenopausal women that compared EVISTA to conjugated estrogens (0.625 mg/day [ERT]), endpoint endometrial biopsies demonstrated stimulatory effects of ERT, which were not observed for EVISTA. All samples from EVISTA-treated women showed nonproliferative endometria.

A 12-month study of uterine effects compared a higher dose of raloxifene HCl (150 mg/day) with HRT. At baseline, 43 raloxifene-treated postmenopausal women and 37 HRT-treated women had a nonproliferative endometrium. At study completion, endometria in all of the raloxifene-treated women remained nonproliferative whereas 13 HRT-treated women had developed proliferative changes. Also, HRT significantly increased uterine volume; raloxifene did not increase uterine volume. Thus, no stimulatory effect of raloxifene on the endometrium was detected at more than twice the recommended dose.

Compared to placebo, EVISTA did not increase the risk of ovarian carcinoma.

Effects on the Breast

Across all placebo-controlled trials, EVISTA was indistinguishable from placebo with regard to frequency and severity of breast pain and tenderness. EVISTA was associated with significantly less breast pain and tenderness than reported by women receiving estrogens with or without added progestin (see ADVERSE REACTIONS and Table 6).

Mammograms were routinely performed on an annual or biennial basis in all placebo-controlled clinical trials lasting at least 12 months. Independent review has determined that 25 cases (raloxifene and placebo combined) represented newly-diagnosed invasive breast cancer. Among 7108 women randomized to raloxifene, there were 10 cases of invasive breast cancer per 19,381 person-years of follow-up (0.52 per 1000). Among 3467 women randomized to placebo, there were 15 cases of invasive breast cancer per 9250 person-years of follow-up (1.62 per 1000). The effectiveness of raloxifene in reducing the risk of breast cancer has not been established.

INDICATIONS AND USAGE

EVISTA is indicated for the treatment and prevention of osteoporosis in postmenopausal women.

For either osteoporosis treatment or prevention, supplemental calcium and/or vitamin D should be added to the diet if daily intake is inadequate.

Postmenopausal osteoporosis may be diagnosed by history or radiographic documentaton of osteoporotic fracture, bone mineral densitometry, or physical signs of vertebral crush fractures (e.g., height loss, dorsal kyphosis).

No single clinical finding or test result can quantify risk of postmenopausal osteoporosis with certainty. However, clinical assessment can help to identify women at increased risk. Widely accepted risk factors include Caucasian or Asian descent, slender body build, early estrogen deficiency, smoking, alcohol consumption, low calcium diet, sedentary lifestyle, and family history of osteoporosis. Evidence of increased bone turnover from serum and urine markers and low bone mass (e.g., at least 1 standard deviation below the mean for healthy, young adult women) as determined by densitometric techniques are also predictive. The greater the number of clinical risk factors, the greater the probability of developing postmenopausal osteoporosis.

CONTRAINDICATIONS

EVISTA is contraindicated in lactating women or women who are or may become pregnant. EVISTA may cause fetal harm when administered to a pregnant woman. In rabbit studies, abortion and a low rate of fetal heart anomalies (ventricular septal defects) occurred in rabbits at doses ≥0.1 mg/kg (≥0.04 times the human dose based on surface area, mg/m^2), and hydrocephaly was observed in fetuses at doses ≥10 mg/kg (≥4 times the human dose based on surface area, mg/m^2). In rat studies, retardation of fetal development and developmental abnormalities (wavy ribs, kidney cavitation) occurred at doses ≥1 mg/kg (≥0.2 times the human dose based on surface area, mg/m^2). Treatment of rats at doses of 0.1 to 10 mg/kg (0.02 to 1.6 times the human dose based on surface area, mg/m^2) during gestation and lactation produced effects that included delayed and disrupted parturition; decreased neonatal survival and altered physical development; sex- and age-specific reductions in growth and changes in pituitary hormone content; and decreased lymphoid compartment size in offspring. At 10 mg/kg, raloxifene disrupted parturition which resulted in maternal and progeny death and morbidity. Effects in adult offspring (4 months of age) included uterine hypoplasia and reduced fertility; however, no ovarian or vaginal pathology was observed. The patient should be apprised of the potential hazard to the fetus if this drug is used during pregnancy, or if the patient becomes pregnant while taking this drug.

Table 6. Adverse events occurring in placebo-controlled osteoporosis clinical trials at a frequency ≥2.0% and in more EVISTA-treated (60 mg once daily) women than placebo-treated women

Body System	Treament		Prevention	
	EVISTA N=2557 %	Placebo N=2576 %	EVISTA N=581 %	Placebo N=584 %
Body as a Whole				
Infection	A	A	15.1	14.6
Flu Syndrome	13.5	11.4	14.6	13.5
Headache	9.2	8.5	A	A
Leg Cramps	7.0	3.7	5.9	1.9
Chest Pain	A	A	4.0	3.6
Fever	3.9	3.8	3.1	2.6
Cardiovascular System				
Hot Flashes	9.7	6.4	24.6	18.3
Migraine	A	A	2.4	2.1
Syncope	2.3	2.1	B	B
Varicose Vein	2.2	1.5	A	A
Digestive System				
Nausea	8.3	7.8	8.8	8.6
Diarrhea	7.2	6.9	A	A
Dyspepsia	A	A	5.9	5.8
Vomiting	4.8	4.3	3.4	3.3
Flatulence	A	A	3.1	2.4
Gastrointestinal Disorder	A	A	3.3	2.1
Gastroenteritis	B	B	2.6	2.1
Metabolic and Nutritional				
Weight Gain	A	A	8.8	6.8
Peripheral Edema	5.2	4.4	3.3	1.9
Musculoskeletal System				
Arthralgia	15.5	14.0	10.7	10.1
Myalgia	A	A	7.7	6.2
Arthritis	A	A	4.0	3.6
Tendon Disorder	3.6	3.1	A	A
Nervous System				
Depression	A	A	6.4	6.0
Insomnia	A	A	5.5	4.3
Vertigo	4.1	3.7	A	A
Neuralgia	2.4	1.9	B	B
Hypesthesia	2.1	2.0	B	B
Respiratory System				
Sinusitis	7.9	7.5	10.3	6.5
Rhinitis	10.2	10.1	A	A
Bronchitis	9.5	8.6	A	A
Pharyngitis	5.3	5.1	7.6	7.2
Cough Increased	9.3	9.2	6.0	5.7
Pneumonia	A	A	2.6	1.5
Laryngitis	B	B	2.2	1.4
Skin and Appendages				
Rash	A	A	5.5	3.8
Sweating	2.5	2.0	3.1	1.7
Special Senses				
Conjunctivitis	2.2	1.7	A	A
Urogenital System				
Vaginitis	A	A	4.3	3.6
Urinary Tract Infection	A	A	4.0	3.9
Cystitis	4.6	4.5	3.3	3.1
Leukorrhea	A	A	3.3	1.7
Uterine Disorder[a,b]	3.3	2.3	A	A
Endometrial Disorder[a]	B	B	3.1	1.9
Vaginal Hemorrhage	2.5	2.4	A	A
Urinary Tract Disorder	2.5	2.1	A	A

A Placebo incidence greater than or equal to EVISTA incidence.
B Less than 2% incidence and more frequent with EVISTA.
[a] Treatment-emergent uterine-related adverse event, including only patients with an intact uterus: Prevention Trials: EVISTA, n=354, Placebo, n=364; Treatment Trial: EVISTA, n=1948, Placebo, n=1999.
[b] Actual terms most frequently referred to endometrial fluid.

EVISTA is contraindicated in women with active or past history of venous thromboembolic events, including deep vein thrombosis, pulmonary embolism, and retinal vein thrombosis.

EVISTA is contraindicated in women known to be hypersensitive to raloxifene or other constituents of the tablets.

WARNINGS

Venous Thromboembolism—In clinical trials, EVISTA-treated women had an increased risk of venous thromboembolism (deep vein thrombosis and pulmonary embolism). Other venous thromboembolic events could also occur. A less serious event, superficial thrombophlebitis, also has been reported more frequently with EVISTA. The greatest risk for deep vein thrombosis and pulmonary embolism occurs during the first 4 months of treatment, and the magnitude of risk appears to be similar to the reported risk associated with use of hormone replacement therapy. Because immobilization increases the risk for venous thromboembolic events independent of therapy, EVISTA should be discontinued at least 72 hours prior to and during prolonged immobilization (e.g., post-surgical recovery, prolonged bed rest), and EVISTA therapy should be resumed only after the patient is fully ambulatory. In addition, women taking EVISTA should be advised to move about periodically during prolonged travel. The risk-benefit balance should be considered in women at risk of thromboembolic disease for other reasons, such as congestive heart failure, superficial thrombophlebitis and active malignancy.

Premenopausal Use—There is no indication for premenopausal use of EVISTA. Safety of EVISTA in premenopausal women has not been established and its use is not recommended (see CONTRAINDICATIONS).

Hepatic Dysfunction—Raloxifene was studied, as a single dose, in Child-Pugh Class A patients with cirrhosis and serum total bilirubin ranging from 0.6 to 2.0 mg/dL. Plasma raloxifene concentrations were approximately 2.5 times higher than in controls and correlated with total bilirubin concentrations. Safety and efficacy have not been evaluated further in patients with severe hepatic insufficiency.

PRECAUTIONS

General

Concurrent Estrogen Therapy—The concurrent use of EVISTA and systemic estrogen or hormone replacement

Continued on next page

*** Identi-Code® symbol. This product information was prepared in June 2000. Current information on these and other products of Eli Lilly and Company may be obtained by direct inquiry to Lilly Research Laboratories, Lilly Corporate Center, Indianapolis, Indiana 46285, (800) 545-5979.**

Evista—Cont.

therapy (ERT or HRT) has not been studied in prospective clinical trials and therefore concomitant use of EVISTA with systemic estrogens is not recommended.

Lipid Metabolism—EVISTA lowers serum total and LDL cholesterol by 6% to 11%, but does not affect serum concentrations of total HDL cholesterol or triglycerides.

These effects should be taken into account in therapeutic decisions for patients who may require therapy for hyperlipidemia.

Concurrent use of EVISTA and lipid-lowering agents has not been studied.

Endometrium—EVISTA has not been associated with endometrial proliferation (see **Clinical Studies** and ADVERSE REACTIONS). Unexplained uterine bleeding should be investigated as clinically indicated.

Breast—EVISTA has not been associated with breast enlargement, breast pain, or an increased risk of breast cancer (see **Clinical Studies** and ADVERSE REACTIONS). Any unexplained breast abnormality occurring during EVISTA therapy should be investigated.

History of Breast Cancer—EVISTA has not been adequately studied in women with a prior history of breast cancer.

Use in Men—Safety and efficacy have not been evaluated in men.

Information for Patients

For safe and effective use of EVISTA, the physician should inform patients about the following:

Patient Immobilization—EVISTA should be discontinued at least 72 hours prior to and during prolonged immobilization (e.g., post-surgical recovery, prolonged bed rest), and patients should be advised to avoid prolonged restrictions of movement during travel because of the increased risk of venous thromboembolic events.

Hot Flashes or Flushes—EVISTA may increase the incidence of hot flashes and is not effective in reducing hot flashes or flushes associated with estrogen deficiency. In some asymptomatic patients, hot flashes may occur upon beginning EVISTA therapy.

Other Osteoporosis Treatment and Prevention Measures—Patients should be instructed to take supplemental calcium and/or vitamin D, if daily dietary intake is inadequate. Weight-bearing exercise should be considered along with the modification of certain behavioral factors, such as cigarette smoking, and and/or alcohol consumption, if these factors exist.

Physicians should instruct their patients to read the patient package insert before starting therapy with EVISTA and to re-read it each time the prescription is renewed.

Drug Interactions

Cholestyramine—Cholestyramine, an anion exchange resin, causes a 60% reduction in the absorption and enterohepatic cycling of raloxifene after a single dose. Co-administration of cholestyramine with EVISTA is not recommended. Although not specifically studied, it is anticipated that other anion exchange resins would have a similar effect.

Warfarin—In vitro, raloxifene did not interact with the binding of warfarin. The co-administration of EVISTA and warfarin, a coumarin derivative, has been assessed in a single dose study. In this study, raloxifene had no effect on the pharmacokinetics of warfarin. However, a 10% decrease in prothrombin time was observed in the single-dose study. If EVISTA is given concurrently with warfarin or other coumarin derivatives, prothrombin time should be monitored more closely when starting or stopping therapy with EVISTA. In the osteoporosis treatment trial, there were no clinically relevant effects of warfarin co-administration on plasma concentrations of raloxifene.

Other Highly Protein-Bound Drugs—Raloxifene is more than 95% bound to plasma proteins. Other highly protein-bound drugs should not cause clinically relevant changes in EVISTA plasma concentrations. Furthermore, in the osteoporosis treatment trial, there were no clinically relevant effects of co-administration of other highly protein-bound drugs (e.g., gemfibrozil) on plasma concentrations of raloxifene. In vitro, raloxifene did not interact with the binding of phenytoin, tamoxifen, or warfarin (see above). Although not examined, EVISTA might affect the protein binding of other drugs and should be used with caution with certain other highly protein-bound drugs such as diazepam, diazoxide and lidocaine.

Carcinogenesis, Mutagenesis, and Impairment of Fertility

Carcinogenesis:

In a 21-month carcinogenicity study in mice, there was an increased incidence of ovarian tumors in female animals given 9 to 242 mg/kg, which included benign and malignant tumors of granulosa/theca cell origin and benign tumors of epithelial cell origin. Systemic exposure (AUC) of raloxifene in this group was 0.3 to 34 times that in postmenopausal women administered a 60-mg dose. There was also an increased incidence of testicular interstitial cell tumors and prostatic adenomas and adenocarcinomas in male mice given 41 or 210 mg/kg (4.7 or 24 times the AUC in humans), and prostatic leiomyoblastoma in male mice given 210 mg/kg.

In a 2-year carcinogenicity study in rats, an increased incidence in ovarian tumors of granulosa/theca cell origin was observed in female rats given 279 mg/kg (approximately 400 times the AUC in humans). The female rodents in these studies were treated during their reproductive lives when their ovaries were functional and responsive to hormonal stimulation.

Table 7. Adverse events reported in the clinical trials for osteoporosis prevention with EVISTA (60 mg once daily) and continuous combined or cyclic estrogen plus progestin (HRT) at an incidence ≥2.0% in any treatment group[a]

Adverse Event	EVISTA (N=317) %	HRT-Continuous Combined (N=96) %	HRT-Cyclic (N=219) %
Urogenital			
Breast Pain	4.4	37.5	29.7
Vaginal Bleeding[b]	6.2	64.2	88.5
Digestive			
Flatulence	1.6	12.5	6.4
Cardiovascular			
Hot Flashes	28.7	3.1	5.9
Body as a Whole			
Infection	11.0	0	6.8
Abdominal Pain	6.6	10.4	18.7
Chest Pain	2.8	0	0.5

[a] These data are from both blinded and open-label studies.

[b] Treatment-emergent uterine-related adverse event, including only patients with an intact uterus: EVISTA, n=290, HRT-Continuous Combined, n=67, HRT-Cyclic, n=217.

Continuous Combined HRT = 0.625 mg conjugated estrogens plus 2.5 mg medroxyprogesterone acetate.

Cyclic HRT = 0.625 mg conjugated estrogens for 28 days with concomitant 5 mg medroxyprogesterone acetate or 0.15 mg norgestrel on days 1 through 14 or 17 through 28.

Mutagenesis:

Raloxifene HCl was not genotoxic in any of the following test systems: the Ames test for bacterial mutagenesis with and without metabolic activation, the unscheduled DNA synthesis assay in rat hepatocytes, the mouse lymphoma assay for mammalian cell mutation, the chromosomal aberration assay in Chinese hamster ovary cells, the in vivo sister chromatid exchange assay in Chinese hamsters, and the in vivo micronucleus test in mice.

Impairment of Fertility:

When male and female rats were given daily doses ≥5 mg/kg (≥0.8 times the human dose based on surface area, mg/m^2) prior to and during mating, no pregnancies occurred. In male rats, daily doses up to 100 mg/kg (16 times the human dose based on surface area, mg/m^2) for at least 2 weeks did not affect sperm production or quality, or reproductive performance. In female rats, at doses of 0.1 to 10 mg/kgday (0.02 to 1.6 times the human dose based on surface area, mg/m^2), raloxifene disrupted estrous cycles and inhibited ovulation. These effects of raloxifene were reversible. In another study in rats in which raloxifene was given during the preimplantation period at doses ≥0.1 mg/kg (≥0.02 times the human dose based on surface area, mg/m^2), raloxifene delayed and disrupted embryo implantation resulting in prolonged gestation and reduced litter size. The reproductive and developmental effects observed in animals are consistent with the estrogen receptor activity of raloxifene.

Pregnancy

Pregnancy Category X—EVISTA should not be used in women who are or may become pregnant (see CONTRAINDICATIONS).

Nursing Mothers—EVISTA should not be used by lactating women (see CONTRAINDICATIONS). It is not known whether raloxifene is excreted in human milk.

Pediatric Use—EVISTA should not be used in pediatric patients.

Geriatric Use—In the osteoporosis treatment trial of 7705 postmenopausal women, 4621 women were considered geriatric (greater than 65 years old). Of these, 845 women were greater than 75 years old. Safety and efficacy in older and younger postmenopausal women in the osteoporosis treatment trial appeared to be comparable.

ADVERSE REACTIONS

Adverse Events in the Osteoporosis Treatment Clinical Trial

The safety of raloxifene in the treatment of osteoporosis was assessed in a large (7705 patients) multinational placebo-controlled trial. Duration of treatment was 36 months and 5129 postmenopausal women were exposed to raloxifene (2557 received 60 mg/day and 2572 received 120 mg/day).

The majority of adverse events occurring during the study were mild and generally did not require discontinuation of therapy.

Therapy was discontinued due to an adverse event in 10.9% of EVISTA-treated women and 8.8% of placebo-treated women. Common adverse events considered to be related to EVISTA therapy were hot flashes and leg cramps. Hot flashes were most commonly reported during the first 6 months of treatment and were not different from placebo thereafter.

Adverse Events in Placebo-Controlled Clinical Trials to Support the Osteoporosis Prevention Indication

The safety of raloxifene has been assessed primarily in 12 Phase 2 and Phase 3 studies with placebo, estrogen, and estrogen-progestin replacement therapy (HRT) control groups. The duration of treatment ranged from 2 to 30 months and 2036 women were exposed to raloxifene (371 patients received 10 to 50 mg/day, 828 received 60 mg/day, and 837 received from 120 to 600 mg/day).

The majority of adverse events occurring during clinical trials were mild and generally did not require discontinuation of therapy.

Therapy was discontinued due to an adverse event in 11.4% of 581 EVISTA-treated women and 12.2% of 584 placebo-treated women. Common adverse events considered to be drug-related were hot flashes and leg cramps (see Table 6).

The first occurrence of hot flashes was most commonly reported during the first 6 months of treatment. Discontinuation rates due to hot flashes did not differ significantly between EVISTA and placebo groups (1.7% and 2.2%, respectively).

Table 6 lists adverse events occurring in either the osteoporosis treatment or the prevention placebo-controlled clinical trial databases at a frequency ≥2.0% in either group and in more EVISTA-treated women than in placebo-treated women. Adverse events are shown without attribution of causality.

[See table 6 at top of previous page]

Comparison of EVISTA and Hormone Replacement Therapy Adverse Events

EVISTA was compared with estrogen-progestin replacement therapy (HRT) in 3 clinical trials for prevention of osteoporosis. Table 7 shows adverse events occurring more frequently in one treatment group and at an incidence ≥2.0% in any group. Adverse events are shown without attribution of causality.

[See table 7 above]

Laboratory Changes

The following changes in analyte concentrations are commonly observed during EVISTA therapy: increased apolipoprotein A1; and reduced serum total cholesterol, LDL cholesterol, fibrinogen, apolipoprotein B, and lipoprotein (a). EVISTA modestly increases hormone-binding globulin concentrations, including sex steroid-binding globulin, thyroxine-binding globulin, and corticosteroid-binding globulin with corresponding increases in measured total hormone concentrations. There is no evidence that these changes in hormone-binding globulin concentrations affect concentrations of the corresponding free hormones.

There were small decreases in serum total calcium, inorganic phosphate, total protein, and albumin which were generally of lesser magnitude than decreases observed during ERT/HRT. Platelet count was also decreased slightly and was not different from ERT.

Additional Safety Information

In the osteoporosis treatment trial of 36 months duration, EVISTA was not associated with deterioration of cognitive function or a change in affect, based on prospective, objective testing.

Incidences of estrogen-dependent carcinoma of the endometrium and breast are being evaluated across all completed and ongoing clinical trials involving 17,151 patients, of which at least 10,850 women have received at least one dose of raloxifene. These trials provided over 21,000 person-years of raloxifene exposure with a maximum exposure of 58 months.

Endometrium—Compared to placebo, raloxifene did not increase the risk of endometrial cancer.

Breast—Compared to placebo, raloxifene did not increase the risk of breast cancer (see CLINICAL PHARMACOLOGY, **Effects on the Breast**).

OVERDOSAGE

Incidents of overdose in humans have not been reported. In an 8-week study of 63 postmenopausal women, a dose of raloxifene HCl 600 mg/day was safely tolerated. No mortality was seen after a single oral dose in rats or mice at 5000 mg/kg (810 times the human dose for rats and 405 times the human dose for mice based on surface area, mg/m^2) or in monkeys at 1000 mg/kg (80 times the AUC in humans). There is no specific antidote for raloxifene.

DOSAGE AND ADMINISTRATION

The recommended dosage is one 60-mg EVISTA tablet daily which may be administered any time of day without regard to meals.

HOW SUPPLIED

EVISTA 60-mg tablets are white, elliptical, and film coated. They are imprinted on one side with LILLY and the tablet code 4165 in edible blue ink. They are available as follows:

Bottle (count)	NDC Number
30 (unit of use)	NDC - 0002-4165-30
100 (unit of use)	NDC - 0002-4165-02
2000	NDC - 0002-4165-07

Store at controlled room temperature, 20° to 25° C (68° to 77° F) [see USP]. The USP defines controlled room temperature as a temperature maintained thermostatically that encompasses the usual and customary working environment of 20° to 25° C (68° to 77° F); that results in a mean kinetic temperature calculated to be not more than 25° C; and that allows for excursions between 15° and 30° C (59° and 86° F) that are experienced in pharmacies, hospitals, and warehouses.

Literature revised September 30, 1999

Eli Lilly and Company, Indianapolis, IN 46285, USA

PV 3082 AMP

Shown in Product Identification Guide, page 321

FLUOXETINE HYDROCHLORIDE, ℞
see Prozac® (Fluoxetine Hydrochloride).

GEMZAR® ℞
(GEMCITABINE HCl)
FOR INJECTION

DESCRIPTION

Gemzar® (gemcitabine HCl) is a nucleoside analogue that exhibits antitumor activity. Gemcitabine HCl is 2′-deoxy-2′,2′-difluorocytidine monohydrochloride (β-isomer).

The structural formula is as follows:

NH2 • HCl

The empirical formula for gemcitabine HCl is $C_9H_{11}F_2N_3O_4$ • HCl. It has a molecular weight of 299.66.

Gemcitabine HCl is a white to off-white solid. It is soluble in water, slightly soluble in methanol, and practically insoluble in ethanol and polar organic solvents.

The clinical formulation is supplied in a sterile form for intravenous use only. Vials of Gemzar contain either 200 mg or 1 g of gemcitabine HCl (expressed as free base) formulated with mannitol (200 mg or 1 g, respectively) and sodium acetate (12.5 mg or 62.5 mg, respectively) as a sterile lyophilized powder. Hydrochloric acid and/or sodium hydroxide may have been added for pH adjustment.

CLINICAL PHARMACOLOGY

Gemcitabine exhibits cell phase specificity, primarily killing cells undergoing DNA synthesis (S-phase) and also blocking the progression of cells through the G1/S-phase boundary. Gemcitabine is metabolized intracellularly by nucleoside kinases to the active diphosphate (dFdCDP) and triphosphate (dFdCTP) nucleosides. The cytotoxic effect of gemcitabine is attributed to a combination of two actions of the diphosphate and the triphosphate nucleosides, which leads to inhibition of DNA synthesis. First, gemcitabine diphosphate inhibits ribonucleotide reductase, which is responsible for catalyzing the reactions that generate the deoxynucleoside triphosphates for DNA synthesis. Inhibition of this enzyme by the diphosphate nucleoside causes a reduction in the concentrations of deoxynucleotides, including dCTP. Second, gemcitabine triphosphate competes with dCTP for incorporation into DNA. The reduction in the intracellular concentration of dCTP (by the action of the diphosphate) enhances the incorporation of gemcitabine triphosphate into DNA (self-potentiation). After the gemcitabine nucleotide is incorporated into DNA, only one additional nucleotide is added to the growing DNA strands. After this addition, there is inhibition of further DNA synthesis. DNA polymerase epsilon is unable to remove the gemcitabine nucleotide and repair the growing DNA strands (masked chain termination). In CEM T lymphoblastoid cells, gemcitabine induces internucleosomal DNA fragmentation, one of the characeristics of programmed cell death.

Gemcitabine demonstrated dose-dependent synergistic activity with cisplatin *in vitro*. No effect of cisplatin on gemcitabine triphosphate accumulation or DNA double-strand breaks was observed. *In vivo*, gemcitabine showed activity in combination with cisplatin against the LX-1 and CALU-6 human lung xenografts, but minimal activity was seen with the NCI-H460 or NCI-H520 xenografts. Gemcitabine was synergistic with cisplatin in the Lewis lung murine xenograft. Sequential exposure to gemcitabine 4 hours before cisplatin produced the greatest interaction.

Human Pharmacokinetics—Gemcitabine disposition was studied in five patients who received a single 1000 mg/m²/30 minute infusion of radiolabeled drug. Within one (1) week, 92% to 98% of the dose was recovered, almost entirely in the urine. Gemcitabine (<10%) and the inactive uracil metabolite, 2′-deoxy-2′,2′-difluorouridine (dFdU), accounted for 99% of the excreted dose. The metabolite dFdU is also found in plasma. Gemcitabine plasma protein binding is negligible.

The pharmacokinetics of gemcitabine were examined in 353 patients, about 2/3 men, with various solid tumors. Pharmacokinetic parameters were derived using data from patients treated for varying durations of therapy given weekly with periodic rest weeks and using both short infusions (<70 minutes) and long infusions (70 to 285 minutes). The total Gemzar dose varied from 500 to 3600 mg/m².

Gemcitabine pharmacokinetics are linear and are described by a 2-compartment model. Population pharmacokinetic analyses of combined single and multiple dose studies showed that the volume of distribution of gemcitabine was significantly influenced by duration of infusion and gender. Clearance was affected by age and gender. Differences in either clearance or volume of distribution based on patient characteristics or the duration of infusion result in changes in half-life and plasma concentrations. Table 1 shows plasma clearance and half-life of gemcitabine following short infusions for typical patients by age and gender.

Table 1
Gemcitabine Clearance and Half-Life for the "Typical" Patient

Age	Clearance Men (L/hr/m²)	Clearance Women (L/hr/m²)	Half-Life[a] Men (min)	Half-Life[a] Women (min)
29	92.2	69.4	42	49
45	75.7	57.0	48	57
65	55.1	41.5	61	73
79	40.7	30.7	79	94

[a]Half-life for patients receiving a short infusion (<70 min)

Gemcitabine half-life for short infusions ranged from 32 to 94 minutes, and the value for long infusions varied from 245 to 638 minutes, depending on age and gender, reflecting a greatly increased volume of distribution with longer infusions. The lower clearance in women and the elderly results in higher concentrations of gemcitabine for any given dose.

The volume of distribution was increased with infusion length. Volume of distribution of gemcitabine was 50 L/m² following infusions lasting <70 minutes, indicating that gemcitabine, after short infusions, is not extensively distributed into tissues. For long infusions, the volume of distribution rose to 370 L/m², reflecting slow equilibration of gemcitabine within the tissue compartment.

The maximum plasma concentrations of dFdU (inactive metabolite) were achieved up to 30 minutes after discontinuation of the infusions and the metabolite is excreted in urine without undergoing further biotransformation. The metabolite did not accumulate with weekly dosing, but its elimination is dependent on renal excretion, and could accumulate with decreased renal function.

The effects of significant renal or hepatic insufficiency on the disposition of gemcitabine have not been assessed.

The active metabolite, gemcitabine triphosphate, can be extracted from peripheral blood mononuclear cells. The half-life of the terminal phase for gemcitabine triphosphate from mononuclear cells ranges from 1.7 to 19.4 hours.

Table 2
Randomized Trials of Combination Therapy with Gemzar plus Cisplatin in NSCLC

Trial	28-day Schedule[a]			21-day Schedule[b]		
Treatment Arm	Gemzar/ Cisplatin	Cisplatin		Gemzar/ Cisplatin	Cisplatin/ Etoposide	
Number of patients	260	262		69	66	
Male	182	186		64	61	
Female	78	76		5	5	
Median age, years	62	63		58	60	
Range	36 to 88	35 to 79		33 to 76	35 to 75	
Stage IIIA	7%	7%		N/A	N/A	
Stage IIIB	26%	23%		48%	52%	
Stage IV	67%	70%		52%	49%	
Baseline KPS[c] 70 to 80	41%	44%		45%	52%	
Baseline KPS[c] 90 to 100	57%	55%		55%	49%	
Survival			p=0.008			p=0.18
Median, months	9.0	7.6		8.7	7.0	
(95% C.I.) months	8.2, 11.0	6.6, 8.8		7.8, 10.1	6.0, 9.7	
Time to Disease Progression			p=0.009			p=0.015
Median, months	5.2	3.7		5.0	4.1	
(95% C.I.) months	4.2, 5.7	3.0, 4.3		4.2, 6.4	2.4, 4.5	
Tumor Response	26%	10%	p<0.0001[d]	33%	14%	p=0.01[d]

[a]28-day schedule—Gemzar plus cisplatin: Gemzar 100 mg/m² on Days 1, 8, and 15 and cisplatin 100 mg/m² on Day 1 every 28 days; Single-agent cisplatin: cisplatin 100 mg/m² Day 1 every 28 days

[b]21-day schedule—Gemzar plus cisplatin: Gemzar 1250 mg/m² on Days 1 and 8 and cisplatin 100 mg/m² on Day 1 every 21 days; Etoposide plus Cisplatin: cisplatin 100 mg/m² on Day 1 and I.V. etoposide 100 mg/m² on Days 1, 2, and 3 every 21 days

[c]Karnofsky Performance Status

[d]p-value for tumor response was calculated using the 2-sided Fisher's exact test for difference in binomial proportions. All other p-values were calculated using the Logrank test for difference in overall time to an event.

N/A Not applicable

CLINICAL STUDIES

Non-Small Cell Lung Cancer (NSCLC)—Data from two randomized clinical studies (657 patients) support the use of Gemzar in combination with cisplatin for the first-line treatment of patients with locally advanced or metastatic NSCLC.

Gemzar plus cisplatin versus cisplatin: This study was conducted in Europe, the U.S., and Canada in 522 patients with inoperable Stage IIIA, IIIB, or IV NSCLC who had not received prior chemotherapy. Gemzar 1000 mg/m² was administered on days 1, 8, and 15 of a twenty-eight day cycle with cisplatin 100 mg/m² administered on day 1 of each cycle. Single-agent cisplatin 100 mg/m² was administered on day 1 of each 28-day cycle. The primary end point was survival. Patient demographics are shown in Table 2. An imbalance with regard to histology was observed with 48% of patients on the cisplatin arm and 37% of patients on the Gemzar plus cisplatin arm having adenocarcinoma.

The Kaplan-Meier survival curve is shown in Figure 1. Median survival time on the Gemzar plus cisplatin arm was 9.0 months compared to 7.6 months on the single-agent cisplatin arm (Logrank p=0.008, two-sided). Median time to disease progression was 5.2 months on the Gemzar plus cisplatin arm compared to 3.7 months on the cisplatin arm (Logrank p=0.009, two-sided). The objective response rate on the Gemzar plus cisplatin arm was 26% compared to 10% with cisplatin (Fisher's Exact p<0.0001, two-sided). No difference between treatment arms with regard to duration of response was observed.

Gemzar plus cisplatin versus etoposide plus cisplatin: A second, multicenter, study in Stage IIIB or IV NSCLC randomized 135 patients to Gemzar 1250 mg/m² on days 1 and 8, and cisplatin 100 mg/m² on day 1 of a 21-day cycle or to etoposide 100 mg/m² I.V. on days 1, 2, and 3 and cisplatin 100 mg/m² on day 1 on a 21-day cycle (Table 2).

There was no significant difference in survival between the two treatment arms (Logrank p=0.18, two-sided). The median survival was 8.7 months for the Gemzar plus cisplatin arm versus 7.0 months for the etoposide plus cisplatin arm. Median time to disease progression for the Gemzar plus cisplatin arm was 5.0 months compared to 4.1 months on the etoposide plus cisplatin arm (Logrank p=0.015, two-sided). The objective response rate for the Gemzar plus cisplatin arm was 33% compared to 14% on the etoposide plus cisplatin arm (Fisher's Exact p=0.01, two-sided).

Quality of Life (QOL): QOL was a secondary endpoint in both randomized studies. In the Gemzar plus cisplatin versus cisplatin study, QOL was measured using the FACT-L, which assessed physical, social, emotional and functional well-being, and lung cancer symptoms. In the study of Gemzar plus cisplatin versus etoposide plus cisplatin, QOL was measured using the EORTC QLQ-C30 and LC13, which assessed physical and psychological functioning and symptoms related to both lung cancer and its treatment. In both studies no significant differences were observed in QOL be-

Continued on next page

*** Identi-Code® symbol. This product information was prepared in June 2000. Current information on these and other products of Eli Lilly and Company may be obtained by direct inquiry to Lilly Research Laboratories, Lilly Corporate Center, Indianapolis, Indiana 46285, (800) 545-5979.**

Gemzar—Cont.

tween the Gemzar plus cisplatin arm and the comparator arm.

Figure 1

Kaplan-Meier Survival Curve in Gemzar plus Cisplatin versus Cisplatin NSCLC Study (N=522)

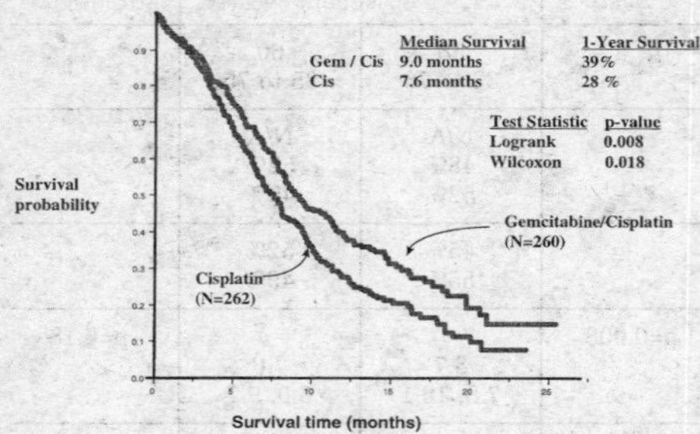

Pancreatic Cancer—Data from two clinical trials evaluated the use of Gemzar in patients with locally advanced or metastatic pancreatic cancer. The first trial compared Gemzar to 5-Fluorouracil (5-FU) in patients who had received no prior chemotherapy. A second trial studied the use of Gemzar in pancreatic cancer patients previously treated with 5-FU or a 5-FU-containing regimen. In both studies, the first cycle of Gemzar was administered intravenously at a dose of 1000 mg/m^2 over 30 minutes once weekly for up to 7 weeks (or until toxicity necessitated holding a dose) followed by a week of rest from treatment with Gemzar. Subsequent cycles consisted of injections once weekly for 3 consecutive weeks out of every 4 weeks.

[See table 2 at top of previous page]

The primary efficacy parameter in these studies was "clinical benefit response", which is a measure of clinical improvement based on analgesic consumption, pain intensity, performance status and weight change. Definitions for improvement in these variables were formulated prospectively during the design of the two trials. A patient was considered a clinical benefit responder if either:

i) the patient showed a ≥50% reduction in pain intensity (Memorial Pain Assessment Card) or analgesic consumption, or a twenty point or greater improvement in performance status (Karnofsky Performance Scale) for a period of at least four consecutive weeks, without showing any sustained worsening in any of the other parameters. Sustained worsening was defined as four consecutive weeks with either any increase in pain intensity or analgesic consumption or a 20 point decrease in performance status occurring during the first 12 weeks of therapy.

OR:

ii) the patient was stable on all of the aforementioned parameters, and showed a marked, sustained weight gain (≥7% increase maintained for ≥4 weeks) not due to fluid accumulation.

The first study was a multi-center (17 sites in US and Canada), prospective, single-blinded, two-arm, randomized, comparison of Gemzar and 5-FU in patients with locally advanced or metastatic pancreatic cancer who had received no prior treatment with chemotherapy. 5-FU was administered intravenously at a weekly dose of 600 mg/m^2 for 30 minutes. The results from this randomized trial are shown in Table 3. Patients treated with Gemzar had statistically significant increases in clinical benefit response, survival, and time to disease progression compared to 5-FU. The Kaplan-Meier curve for survival is shown in Figure 2. No confirmed objective tumor responses were observed with either treatment.

[See table 3 above]

Clinical benefit response was achieved by 14 patients treated with Gemzar and 3 patients treated with 5-FU. One patient of the Gemzar arm showed improvement in all three primary parameters (pain intensity, analgesic consumption, and performance status). Eleven patients on the Gemzar arm and two patients on the 5-FU arm showed improvement in analgesic consumption and/or pain intensity with stable performance status. Two patients on the Gemzar arm showed improvement in analgesic consumption or pain intensity with improvement in performance status. One patient on the 5-FU arm was stable with regard to pain intensity and analgesic consumption with improvement in performance status. No patient on either arm achieved a clinical benefit response based on weight gain.

[See figure 2 at top of next column]

The second trial was a multi-center (17 U.S. and Canadian centers), open-label study of Gemzar in 63 patients with advanced pancreatic cancer previously treated with 5-FU or a 5-FU-containing regimen. The study showed a clinical benefit response rate of 27% and median survival of 3.9 months.

Other Clinical Studies—When Gemzar was administered more frequently than once weekly or with infusions longer than 60 minutes, increased toxicity was observed. Results of a Phase 1 study of Gemzar to assess the maximum tolerated dose (MTD) on a daily x 5 schedule showed that patients developed significant hypotension and severe flu-like symptoms that were intolerable at doses above 10 mg/m^2. The incidence and severity of these events were dose-related.

Table 3
Gemzar Versus 5-FU in Pancreatic Cancer

	Gemzar	5-FU	
Number of patients	63	63	
Male	34	34	
Female	29	29	
Median age	62 years	61 years	
Range	37 to 79	36 to 77	
Stage IV disease	71.4%	76.2%	
Baseline KPS[a] ≤70	69.8%	68.3%	
Clinical benefit response	22.2% (N[c] = 14)	4.8% (N = 3)	p = 0.004
Survival			p = 0.0009
Median	5.7 months	4.2 months	
6-month probability[b]	(N = 30) 46%	(N = 19) 29%	
9-month probability[b]	(N = 14) 24%	(N = 4) 5%	
1-year probability[b]	(N = 9) 18%	(N = 2) 2%	
Range	0.2 to 18.6 months	0.4 to 15.1+ months	
95% C.I. of the median	4.7 to 6.9 months	3.1 to 5.1 months	
Time to Disease Progression			p = 0.0013
Median	2.1 months	0.9 months	
Range	0.1+to 9.4 months	0.1 to 12.0+months	
95% C.I. of the median	1.9 to 3.4 months	0.9 to 1.1 months	

[a]Karnofsky Performance Status
[b]Kaplan-Meier estimates
[c]N = number of patients
+ No progression at last visit; remains alive.
The p-value for clinical benefit response was calculated using the 2-sided test for difference in binomial proportions. All other p-values were calculated using the Logrank test for difference in overall time to an event.

Figure 2
Kaplan-Meier Survival Curve

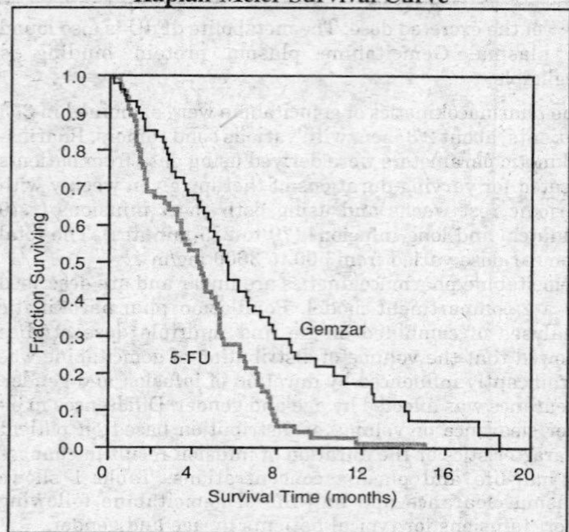

Other Phase 1 studies using a twice-weekly schedule reached MTDs of only 65 mg/m^2 (30-minute infusion) and 150 mg/m^2 (5-minute bolus). The dose-limiting toxicities were thrombocytopenia and flu-like symptoms, particularly asthenia. In a Phase 1 study to assess the maximum tolerated infusion time, clinically significant toxicity, defined as myelosuppression, was seen with weekly doses of 300 mg/m^2 at or above a 270-minute infusion time. The half-life of gemcitabine is influenced by the length of the infusion (*see* Clinical Pharmacology) and the toxicity appears to be increased if Gemzar is administered more frequently than once weekly or with infusions longer than 60 minutes (*see* Warnings). In a single trial, where Gemzar at a dose of 1000 mg/m^2 was administered for up to six (6) consecutive weeks concurrently with therapeutic thoracic radiation to patients with NSCLC, significant toxicity in the form of severe, and potentially life-threatening, esophagitis and pneumonitis was observed, particularly in patients receiving large volumes of radiotherapy. The optimum regimen for safe administration of Gemzar with therapeutic doses of radiation has not yet been determined (*see* Precautions).

INDICATIONS AND USAGE

Therapeutic Indications

Non-Small Cell Lung Cancer—Gemzar is indicated in combination with cisplatin for the first-line treatment of patients with inoperable, locally advanced (Stage IIIA or IIIB) or metastatic (Stage IV) non-small cell lung cancer.

Pancreatic Cancer—Gemzar is indicated as first-line treatment for patients with locally advanced (nonresectable Stage II or Stage III) or metastatic (Stage IV) adenocarcinoma of the pancreas. Gemzar is indicated for patients previously treated with 5-FU.

CONTRAINDICATION

Gemzar is contraindicated in those patients with a known hypersensitivity to the drug (*see* Adverse Reactions—Allergic).

WARNINGS

Caution—Prolongation of the infusion time beyond 60 minutes and more frequent than weekly dosing have been shown to increase toxicity (*see* Clinical Studies).

Gemzar can suppress bone marrow function as manifested by leukopenia, thrombocytopenia, and anemia (*see* Adverse Reactions), and myelosuppression is usually the dose-limiting toxicity. Patients should be monitored for myelosuppression during therapy. *See* Dosage and Administration for recommended dose adjustments.

Hemolytic-Uremic Syndrome (HUS) has been reported rarely with the use of Gemzar. (*see* Adverse Reactions—Renal)

Pregnancy—Pregnancy Category D. Gemzar can cause fetal harm when administered to a pregnant woman. Gemcitabine is embryotoxic causing fetal malformations (cleft palate, incomplete ossification) at doses of 1.5 mg/kg/day in mice (about 1/200 the recommended human dose on a mg/m^2 basis). Gemcitabine is fetotoxic causing fetal malformations (fused pulmonary artery, absence of gall bladder) at doses of 0.1 mg/kg/day in rabbits (about 1/600 the recommended human dose on a mg/m^2 basis). Embryotoxicity was characterized by decreased fetal viability, reduced live litter sizes, and developmental delays. There are no studies of Gemzar in pregnant women. If Gemzar is used during pregnancy, or if the patient becomes pregnant while taking Gemzar, the patient should be apprised of the potential hazard to the fetus.

PRECAUTIONS

General—Patients receiving therapy with Gemzar should be monitored closely by a physician experienced in the use of cancer chemotherapeutic agents. Most adverse events are reversible and do not need to result in discontinuation, although doses may need to be withheld or reduced. There was a greater tendency in women, especially older women, not to proceed to the next cycle.

Laboratory Tests—Patients receiving Gemzar should be monitored prior to each dose with a complete blood count (CBC), including differential and platelet count. Suspension or modification of therapy should be considered when marrow suppression is detected (*see* Dosage and Administration).

Laboratory evaluation of renal and hepatic function should be performed prior to initiation of therapy and periodically thereafter.

Carcinogenesis, Mutagenesis, Impairment of Fertility—Long-term animal studies to evaluate the carcinogenic potential of Gemzar have not been conducted. Gemcitabine induced forward mutations *in vitro* in a mouse lymphoma (L5178Y) assay and was clastogenic in an *in vivo* mouse micronucleus assay. Gemcitabine was negative when tested using the Ames, *in vivo* sister chromatid exchange, and *in vitro* chromosomal aberration assays, and did not cause unscheduled DNA synthesis *in vitro*. Gemcitabine I.P. doses of 0.5 mg/kg/day (about 1/700 the human dose on a mg/m^2 basis) in male mice had an effect on fertility with moderate to severe hypospermatogenesis, decreased fertility, and decreased implantations. In female mice fertility was not affected but maternal toxicities were observed at 1.5 mg/kg/day I.V. (about 1/200 the human dose on a mg/m^2 basis) and fetotoxicity or embryolethality was observed at 0.25 mg/kg/day I.V. (about 1/1300 the human dose on a mg/m^2 basis).

Pregnancy—Category D. *See* Warnings.

Nursing Mothers—It is not known whether Gemzar or its metabolites are excreted in human milk. Because many drugs are excreted in human milk and because of the potential for serious adverse reactions from Gemzar in nursing infants, the mother should be warned and a decision should be made whether to discontinue nursing or to discontinue the drug, taking into account the importance of the drug to the mother and the potential risk to the infant.

Table 4
Selected WHO-Graded Adverse Events in Patients Receiving Single Agent Gemzar
WHO Grades (% incidence)

	All Patients[a]			Pancreatic Cancer Patients[b]			Discontinuations (%)[c]
	All Grades	Grade 3	Grade 4	All Grades	Grade 3	Grade 4	All Patients
Laboratory[d]							
Hematologic							
Anemia	68	7	1	73	8	2	<1
Leukopenia	62	9	<1	64	8	1	<1
Neutropenia	63	19	6	61	17	7	—
Thrombocytopenia	24	4	1	36	7	<1	<1
Hepatic							<1
ALT	68	8	2	72	10	1	
AST	67	6	2	78	12	5	
Alkaline Phosphatase	55	7	2	77	16	4	
Bilirubin	13	2	<1	26	6	2	
Renal							<1
Proteinuria	45	<1	0	32	<1	0	
Hematuria	35	<1	0	23	0	0	
BUN	16	0	0	15	0	0	
Creatinine	8	<1	0	6	0	0	
Non-laboratory[e]							
Nausea and Vomiting	69	13	1	71	10	2	<1
Pain	48	9	<1	42	6	<1	<1
Fever	41	2	0	38	2	0	<1
Rash	30	<1	0	28	<1	0	<1
Dyspnea	23	3	<1	10	0	<1	<1
Constipation	23	1	<1	31	3	<1	0
Diarrhea	19	1	0	30	3	0	0
Hemorrhage	17	<1	<1	4	2	<1	<1
Infection	16	1	<1	10	2	<1	<1
Alopecia	15	<1	0	16	0	0	0
Stomatitis	11	<1	0	10	<1	0	<1
Somnolence	11	<1	<1	11	2	<1	<1
Paresthesias	10	<1	0	10	<1	0	0

Grade based on criteria from the World Health Organization (WHO)
[a]N = 699–974; all patients with laboratory or non-laboratory data
[b]N = 161–241; all pancreatic cancer patients with laboratory or non-laboratory data
[c]N = 979
[d]Regardless of causality
[e] Table includes non-laboratory data with incidence for all patients ≥10%. For approximately 60% of the patients, non-laboratory events were graded only if assessed to be possibly drug-related.

Table 5
Selected WHO-Graded Adverse Events from Comparative Trial of Gemzar and 5-FU in Pancreatic Cancer
WHO Grades (% incidence)

	Gemzar[a]			5-FU[b]		
	All Grades	Grade 3	Grade 4	All Grades	Grade 3	Grade 4
Laboratory[c]						
Hematologic						
Anemia	65	7	3	45	0	0
Leukopenia	71	10	0	15	2	0
Neutropenia	62	19	7	18	2	3
Thrombocytopenia	47	10	0	15	2	0
Hepatic						
ALT	72	8	2	38	0	0
AST	72	10	2	52	2	0
Alkaline Phosphatase	71	16	0	64	10	3
Bilirubin	16	2	2	25	6	3
Renal						
Proteinuria	10	0	0	2	0	0
Hematuria	13	0	0	0	0	0
BUN	8	0	0	10	0	0
Creatinine	2	0	0	0	0	0
Non-laboratory[d]						
Nausea and Vomiting	64	10	3	58	5	0
Pain	10	2	0	7	0	0
Fever	30	0	0	16	0	0
Rash	24	0	0	13	0	0
Dyspnea	6	0	0	3	0	0
Constipation	10	3	0	11	2	0
Diarrhea	24	2	0	31	5	0
Hemorrhage	0	0	0	2	0	0
Infection	8	0	0	3	2	0
Alopecia	18	0	0	16	0	0
Stomatitis	14	0	0	15	0	0
Somnolence	5	2	0	7	2	0
Paresthesias	2	0	0	2	0	0

Grade based on criteria from the World Health Organization (WHO)
[a]N = 58–63; all Gemzar patients with laboratory or non-laboratory data
[b]N = 61–63; all 5-FU patients with laboratory or non-laboratory data
[c]Regardless of causality
[d]Non-laboratory events were graded only if assessed to be possibly drug-related.

Elderly Patients—Gemzar clearance is affected by age (*see* Clinical Pharmacology). There is no evidence, however, that unusual dose adjustments, (i.e., other than those already recommended in the Dosage and Administration section) are necessary in patients over 65, and, in general adverse reaction rates in the single-agent safety database of 979 patients were similar in patients above and below 65. Grade 3/4 thrombocytopenia was more common in the elderly.

Gender—Gemzar clearance is affected by gender (*see* Clinical Pharmacology). In the single agent safety database (N=979 patients), however, there is no evidence that unusual dose adjustments (i.e., other than those already recommended in the Dosage and Administration section) are necessary in women. In general, in single agent studies of gemcitabine adverse reaction rates were similar in men and women, but women, especially older women, were more likely not to proceed to a subsequent cycle and to experience grade 3/4 neutropenia and thrombocytopenia.

Pediatric Patients—Gemzar has not been studied in pediatric patients. Safety and effectiveness in pediatric patients have not been established.

Patients with Renal or Hepatic Impairment—Gemzar should be used with caution in patients with preexisting renal impairment or hepatic insufficiency. Gemzar has not been studied in patients with significant renal or hepatic impairment.

Drug Interactions—No confirmed interactions have been reported with the use of Gemzar. No specific drug interaction studies have been conducted.

Radiation Therapy—Safe and effective regimens for the administration of Gemzar with therapeutic doses of radiation have not yet been determined (*See* Clinical Studies).

ADVERSE REACTIONS

Gemzar has been used in a wide variety of malignancies, both as a single agent and in combination with other cytotoxic drugs. The following discussion focuses on single agent use where the effects of Gemzar can be most readily determined and on the specific combination use that is the basis for its use in NSCLC.

Single-Agent Use: Myelosuppression is the principal dose-limiting toxicity with Gemzar therapy. Dosage adjustments for hematologic toxicity are frequently needed and are described in the Dosage and Administration section.

The data in Table 4 are based on 979 patients receiving Gemzar as a single-agent administered weekly as a 30-minute infusion for treatment of a wide variety of malignancies. The Gemzar starting doses ranged from 800 to 1250 mg/m^2. Data are also shown for the subset of patients with pancreatic cancer treated in 5 clinical studies. The frequency of all grades and severe (WHO grade 3 or 4) adverse events were generally similar in the single-agent safety database of 979 patients and the subset of patients with pancreatic cancer. Adverse reactions reported in the single-agent safety database resulted in discontinuation of Gemzar therapy in about 10% of patients. In the comparative trial in pancreatic cancer, the discontinuation rate for adverse reactions was 14.3% for the gemcitabine arm and 4.8% for the 5-FU arm.

All WHO-graded laboratory events are listed in Table 4, regardless of causality. Non-laboratory adverse events listed in Table 4 or discussed below were those reported, regardless of causality, for at least 10% of all patients, except the categories of Extravasation, Allergic, and Cardiovascular and certain specific events under the Renal, Pulmonary, and Infection categories. Table 5 presents the data from the comparative trial of Gemzar and 5-FU in pancreatic cancer for the same adverse events as those in Table 4, regardless of incidence.

Hematologic—In studies in pancreatic cancer myelosuppression is the dose-limiting toxicity with Gemzar, but <1% of patients discontinued therapy for either anemia, leukopenia, or thrombocytopenia. Red blood cell transfusions were required by 19% of patients. The incidence of sepsis was less than 1%. Petechiae or mild blood loss (hemorrhage), from any cause, was reported in 16% of patients; less than 1% of patients required platelet transfusions. Patients should be monitored for myelosuppression during Gemzar therapy and dosage modified or suspended according to the degree of hematologic toxicity (*see* Dosage and Administration).

Gastrointestinal—Nausea and vomiting were commonly reported (69%) but were usually of mild to moderate severity. Severe nausea and vomiting (WHO grade 3/4) occurred in <15% of patients. Diarrhea was reported by 19% of patients, and stomatitis by 11% of patients.

Hepatic—Gemzar was associated with transient elevations of one or both serum transaminases in approximately 70% of patients, but there was no evidence of increasing hepatic toxicity with either longer duration of exposure to Gemzar or with greater total cumulative dose.

Renal—Mild proteinuria and hematuria were commonly reported. Clinical findings consistent with the hemolytic uremic syndrome (HUS) were reported in 6 of 2429 patients (0.25%) receiving Gemzar in clinical trials. Four patients developed HUS on Gemzar therapy, two immediately post-therapy. The diagnosis of HUS should be considered if the patient develops anemia with evidence of microangiopathic hemolysis as indicated by elevation of bilirubin or LDH, reticulocytosis, severe thrombocytopenia, and/or evidence of renal failure (elevation of serum creatinine or BUN).

Continued on next page

*** Identi-Code® symbol. This product information was prepared in June 2000. Current information on these and other products of Eli Lilly and Company may be obtained by direct inquiry to Lilly Research Laboratories, Lilly Corporate Center, Indianapolis, Indiana 46285, (800) 545-5979.**

Gemzar—Cont.

Gemzar therapy should be discontinued immediately. Renal failure may not be reversible even with discontinuation of therapy and dialysis may be required.

Fever—The overall incidence of fever was 41%. This is in contrast to the incidence of infection (16%) and indicates that Gemzar may cause fever in the absence of clinical infection. Fever was frequently associated with other flu-like symptoms and was usually mild and clinically manageable.

Rash—Rash was reported in 30% of patients. The rash was typically a macular or finely granular maculopapular pruritic eruption of mild to moderate serverity involving the trunk and extremities. Pruritus was reported for 13% of patients.

Pulmonary—Dyspnea was reported in 23% of patients, severe dyspnea in 3%. Dyspnea may be due to underlying disease such as lung cancer (40% of study population) or pulmonary manifestations of other malignancies. Dyspnea was occasionally accompanied by bronchospasm (<2% of patients). Rare reports of parenchymal lung toxicity consistent with drug induced pneumonitis have been associated with the use of Gemzar. Rarely pulmonary edema of unknown etiology, sometimes severe, has occurred in association with Gemzar therapy. Gemzar therapy should be discontinued immediately and appropriate supportive care measures instituted.

Edema—Edema (13%), peripheral edema (20%) and generalized edema (<1%) were reported. Less than 1% of patients discontinued due to edema.

Flu-like Symptoms—"Flu syndrome" was reported for 19% of patients. Individual symptoms of fever, asthenia, anorexia, headache, cough, chills, and myalgia were commonly reported. Fever and asthenia were also reported frequently as isolated symptoms. Insomnia, rhinitis, sweating, and malaise were reported infrequently. Less than 1% of patients discontinued due to flu-like symptoms.

Infection—Infections were reported for 16% of patients. Sepsis was rarely reported (<1%).

Alopecia—Hair loss, usually minimal, was reported by 15% of patients.

Neurotoxicity—There was a 10% incidence of mild paresthesias and a <1% rate of severe paresthesias.

Extravasation—Injection-site related events were reported for 4% of patients. There were no reports of injection site necrosis. Gemzar is not a vesicant.

Allergic—Bronchospasm was reported for less than 2% of patients. Anaphylactoid reaction has been reported rarely. Gemzar should not be administered to patients with a known hypersensitivity to this drug (*see* Contraindication).

Cardiovascular—Two percent of patients discontinued therapy with Gemzar due to cardiovascular events such as myocardial infarction, cerebrovascular accident, arrhythmia, and hypertension. Many of these patients had a prior history of cardiovascular disease.

[See tables 4 & 5 at top of previous page]

Combination Use in Non-Small Cell Lung Cancer: In the Gemzar plus cisplatin vs. cisplatin study, dose adjustments occurred with 35% of Gemzar injections and 17% of cisplatin injections on the combination arm, versus 6% on the cisplatin only arm. Dose adjustments were required in greater than 90% of patients on the combination, versus 16% on cisplatin. Study discontinuations for possibly drug-related adverse events occurred in 15% of patients on the combination arm and 8% of patients on the cisplatin arm. In the Gemzar plus cisplatin vs. etoposide plus cisplatin study, dose adjustments occurred with 20% of Gemzar injections and 16% of cisplatin injections in the Gemzar plus cisplatin arm compared with 20% of etoposide injections and 15% of cisplatin injections in the etoposide plus cisplatin arm. In patients who completed more than one cycle, dose adjustments were reported in 81% of the Gemzar plus cisplatin patients, compared with 68% on the etoposide plus cisplatin arm. Study discontinuations for possibly drug-related adverse events occurred in 14% of patients on the gemcitabine plus cisplatin arm and in 8% of patients on the etoposide plus cisplatin arm. The incidence of myelosuppression was increased in frequency with Gemzar plus cisplatin treatment (~90%) compared to that with the Gemzar monotherapy (~60%). With combination therapy Gemzar dosage adjustments for hematologic toxicity were required more often while cisplatin dose adjustments were less frequently required.

Table 6 presents the safety data from the Gemzar plus cisplatin vs. cisplatin study in non-small cell lung cancer. The NCI Common Toxicity Criteria (CTC) were used. The two-drug combination was more myelosuppressive with four (1.5%) possibly treatment-related deaths, including three resulting from myelosuppression with infection and one case of renal failure associated with pancytopenia and infection. No deaths due to treatment were reported on the cisplatin arm. Nine cases of febrile neutropenia were reported on the combination therapy arm compared to two on the cisplatin arm. More patients required RBC and platelet transfusions on the Gemzar plus cisplatin arm.

Myelosuppression occurred more frequently on the combination arm, and in four possibly treatment-related deaths myelosuppression was observed. Sepsis was reported in 4% of patients on the Gemzar plus cisplatin arm compared to 1% on the cisplatin arm. Platelet transfusions were required in 21% of patients on the combination arm and <1% of patients on the cisplatin arm. Hemorrhagic events occurred in 14% of patients on the combination arm and 4% on the cisplatin arm. However, severe hemorrhagic events were rare. Red blood cell transfusions were required in 39% of the patients on the Gemzar plus cisplatin arm, versus 13% on the cisplatin arm. The data suggest cumulative anemia with continued Gemzar plus cisplatin use.

Nausea and vomiting despite the use of antiemetics occurred slightly more often with Gemzar plus cisplatin therapy (78%) than with cisplatin alone (71%). In studies with single-agent Gemzar, a lower incidence of nausea and vomiting (58%–69%) was reported. Renal function abnormalities, hypomagnesemia, neuromotor, neurocortical, and neurocerebellar toxicity occurred more often with Gemzar plus cisplatin than with cisplatin monotherapy. Neurohearing toxicity was similar on both arms.

Cardiac dysrrhythmias of grade 3 or greater were reported in seven (3%) patients treated with Gemzar plus cisplatin compared to one (<1%) grade 3 dysrrhythmia reported with cisplatin therapy. Hypomagnesemia and hypokalemia were associated with one grade 4 arrhythmia on the Gemzar plus cisplatin combination arm.

Table 7 presents data from the randomized study of Gemzar plus cisplatin versus etoposide plus cisplatin in 135 patients with NSCLC for the same WHO-graded adverse events as those in Table 5. One death (1.5%) was reported on the Gemzar plus cisplatin arm due to febrile neutropenia associated with renal failure which was possibly treatment-related. No deaths related to treatment occurred on the etoposide plus cisplatin arm. The overall incidence of grade 4 neutropenia on the Gemzar plus cisplatin arm was less than on the etoposide plus cisplatin arm (28% vs. 56%). Grade 3 anemia and grade 3/4 thrombocytopenia were more common on the Gemzar plus cisplatin arm. Grade 3/4 nausea and vomiting were also more common on the Gemzar plus cisplatin arm. On the Gemzar plus cisplatin arm, 7% of participants were hospitalized due to febrile neutropenia compared to 12% on the etoposide plus cisplatin arm. More than twice as many patients had dose reductions or omissions of a scheduled dose of Gemzar as compared to etoposide, which may explain the differences in the incidence of neutropenia and febrile neutropenia between treatment arms. Flu syndrome was reported by 3% of patients on the Gemzar plus cisplatin arm with none reported on the comparator arm. Eight patients (12%) on the Gemzar plus cisplatin arm reported edema compared to one patient (2%) on the etoposide plus cisplatin arm.

[See table 6 below]
[See table 7 at top of next page]

Table 6
Selected CTC-Graded Adverse Events from Comparative Trial of Gemzar plus Cisplatin versus Single-Agent Cisplatin in NSCLC
CTC Grades (% incidence)

	Gemzar plus Cisplatin[a]			Cisplatin[b]		
	All Grades	Grade 3	Grade 4	All Grades	Grade 3	Grade 4
Laboratory[c]						
Hematologic						
Anemia	89	22	3	67	6	1
Leukopenia	82	35	11	25	2	1
Neutropenia	79	22	35	20	3	1
Thrombocytopenia	85	25	25	13	3	1
Lymphocytes	75	25	18	51	12	5
Hepatic						
Transaminase	22	2	1	10	1	0
Alkaline Phosphatase	19	1	0	13	0	0
Renal						
Proteinuria	23	0	0	18	0	0
Hematuria	15	0	0	13	0	0
Creatinine	38	4	<1	31	2	<1
Other Laboratory						
Hyperglycemia	30	4	0	23	3	0
Hypomagnesemia	30	4	3	17	2	0
Hypocalcemia	18	2	0	7	0	<1
Non-laboratory[d]						
Hosp. For ADRs	48			30		
Sepsis	4			1		
RBC Transfusions	39			13		
Platelet Transfusions	21			<1		
Nausea	93	25	2	87	20	<1
Vomiting	78	11	12	71	10	9
Alopecia	53	1	0	33	0	0
Neuro Motor	35	12	0	15	3	0
Constipation	28	3	0	21	0	0
Neuro Hearing	25	6	0	21	6	0
Diarrhea	24	2	2	13	0	0
Neuro Sensory	23	1	0	18	1	0
Infection	18	3	2	12	1	0
Fever	16	0	0	5	0	0
Neuro Cortical	16	3	1	9	1	0
Neuro Mood	16	1	0	10	1	0
Local	15	0	0	6	0	0
Neuro Headache	14	0	0	7	0	0
Stomatitis	14	1	0	5	0	0
Hemorrhage	14	1	0	4	0	0
Dyspnea	12	4	3	11	3	2
Hypotension	12	1	0	7	1	0
Rash	11	0	0	3	0	0

Grade based on Common Toxicity Criteria (CTC). Table includes data for adverse events with incidence ≥10% in either arm.
[a]N = 217–253; all Gemzar plus cisplatin patients with laboratory or non-laboratory data. Gemzar at 1000 mg/m^2 on Days 1, 8, and 15 and cisplatin at 100 mg/m^2 on Day 1 every 28 days.
[b]N = 213–248; all cisplatin patients with laboratory or non-laboratory data. Cisplatin at 100 mg/m^2 on Day 1 every 28 days.
[c]Regardless of causality
[d]Non-laboratory events were graded only if assessed to be possibly drug-related.

OVERDOSAGE

There is no known antidote for overdoses of Gemzar. Myelosuppression, paresthesias and severe rash were the principal toxicities seen when a single dose as high as 5700 mg/m^2 was administered by I.V. infusion over 30 minutes every 2 weeks to several patients in a Phase 1 study. In the event of suspected overdose, the patient should be monitored with appropriate blood counts and should receive supportive therapy, as necessary.

DOSAGE AND ADMINISTRATION

Gemzar is for intravenous use only.

Adults

Single-Agent Use:

Pancreatic Cancer—Gemzar should be administered by intravenous infusion at a dose of 1000 mg/m^2 over 30 minutes once weekly for up to 7 weeks (or until toxicity necessitates reducing or holding a dose), followed by a week of rest from treatment. Subsequent cycles should consist of infusions once weekly for 3 consecutive weeks out of every 4 weeks.

Dose Modifications—Dosage adjustment is based upon the degree of hematologic toxicity experienced by the patient (*see* Warnings). Clearance in women and the elderly is reduced and women were somewhat less able to progress to subsequent cycles (*see* Human Pharmacokinetics and Precautions).

Patients receiving Gemzar should be monitored prior to each dose with a complete blood count (CBC), including differential and platelet count. If marrow suppression is detected, therapy should be modified or suspended according to the guidelines in Table 8.

Table 7
Selected WHO-Graded Adverse Events from Comparative Trial of Gemzar plus Cisplatin versus Etoposide plus Cisplatin in NSCLC
WHO Grades (% incidence)

	Gemzar plus Cisplatin[a]			Etoposide plus Cisplatin[b]		
	All Grades	Grade 3	Grade 4	All Grades	Grade 3	Grade 4
Laboratory[c]						
Hematologic						
Anemia	88	22	0	77	13	2
Leukopenia	86	26	3	87	36	7
Neutropenia	88	36	28	87	20	56
Thrombocytopenia	81	39	16	45	8	5
Hepatic						
ALT	6	0	0	12	0	0
AST	3	0	0	11	0	0
Alkaline Phosphatase	16	0	0	11	0	0
Bilirubin	0	0	0	0	0	0
Renal						
Proteinuria	12	0	0	5	0	0
Hematuria	22	0	0	10	0	0
BUN	6	0	0	4	0	0
Creatinine	2	0	0	2	0	0
Non-laboratory[d,e]						
Sepsis	2			2		
RBC Transfusions	29			21		
Platelet Transfusions	3			8		
Nausea and Vomiting	96	35	4	86	19	7
Fever	6	0	0	3	0	0
Rash	10	0	0	3	0	0
Dyspnea	1	0	1	3	0	0
Constipation	17	0	0	15	0	0
Diarrhea	14	1	1	13	0	2
Hemorrhage	9	0	3	3	0	3
Infection	28	3	1	21	8	0
Alopecia	77	13	0	92	51	0
Stomatitis	20	4	0	18	2	0
Somnolence	3	0	0	3	2	0
Paresthesias	38	0	0	16	2	0

Grade based on criteria from the World Health Organization (WHO)
[a]N = 67–69; all Gemzar plus cisplatin patients with laboratory or non-laboratory data. Gemzar at 1250 mg/m^2 on Days 1 and 8 and cisplatin at 100 mg/m^2 on Day 1 every 21 days.
[b]N = 57–63; all cisplatin plus etoposide patients with laboratory or non-laboratory data. Cisplatin at 100 mg/m^2 on Day 1 and I.V. etoposide at 100 mg/m^2 on Days 1, 2, and 3 every 21 days.
[c]Regardless of causality
[d]Non-laboratory events were graded only if assessed to be possibly drug-related.
[e]Pain data were not collected

Table 8
Dosage Reduction Guidelines

Absolute granulocyte count (× 10^6/L)		Platelet count (× 10 ^{6}/L)	% of full dose
≥1,000	and	≥100,000	100
500–999	or	50,000–99,000	75
<500	or	<50,000	Hold

Laboratory evaluation of renal and hepatic function, including transaminases and serum creatinine, should be performed prior to initiation of therapy and periodically thereafter. Gemzar should be administered with caution in patients with evidence of significant renal or hepatic impairment.
Patients treated with Gemzar who complete an entire cycle of therapy may have the dose for subsequent cycles increased by 25%, provided that the absolute granulocyte count (AGC) and platelet nadirs exceed 1500 x 10^6/L and 100,000 x 10^6/L, respectively, and if non-hematologic toxicity has not been greater than WHO grade 1. If patients tolerate the subsequent course of Gemzar at the increased dose, the dose for the next cycle can be further increased by 20%, provided again that the AGC and platelet nadirs exceed 1500 x 10^6/L and 100,000 x 10^6/L, respectively, and that non-hematologic toxicity has not been greater than WHO grade 1.

Combination Use:

Non-Small Cell Lung Cancer—Two schedules have been investigated and the optimum schedule has not been determined (*see* Clinical Studies). With the 4-week schedule, Gemzar should be administered intravenously at 1000 mg/m^2 over 30 minutes on days 1, 8, and 15 of each 28-day cycle. Cisplatin should be administered intravenously at 100 mg/m^2 on day 1 after the infusion of Gemzar. With the 3-week schedule, Gemzar should be administered intravenously at 1250 mg/m^2 over 30 minutes on days 1 and 8 of each 21-day cycle. Cisplatin at a dose of 100 mg/m^2 should be administered intravenously after the infusion of Gemzar on day 1. See prescribing information for cisplatin administration and hydration guidelines.
Dose Modifications—Dosage adjustments for hematologic toxicity may be required for Gemzar and for cisplatin. Gemzar dosage adjustment for hematological toxicity is based on the granulocyte and platelet counts taken on the day of therapy. Patients receiving Gemzar should be monitored prior to each dose with a complete blood count (CBC), including differential and platelet counts. If marrow suppression is detected, therapy should be modified or suspended according to the guidelines in Table 8. For cisplatin dosage adjustment, see manufacturer's prescribing information.
In general, for severe (grade 3 or 4) non-hematological toxicity, except alopecia and nausea/vomiting, therapy with Gemzar plus cisplatin should be held or decreased by 50% depending on the judgment of the treating physician. During combination therapy with cisplatin, serum creatinine, serum potassium, serum calcium, and serum magnesium should be carefully monitored (grade 3/4 serum creatinine toxicity for Gemzar plus cisplatin was 5% versus 2% for cisplatin alone).
Gemzar may be administered on an outpatient basis.
Instructions for Use/Handling—The recommended diluent for reconstitution of Gemzar is 0.9% Sodium Chloride Injection without preservatives. Due to solubility considerations, the maximum concentration for Gemzar upon reconstitution is 40 mg/mL. Reconstitution at concentrations greater than 40 mg/mL may result in incomplete dissolution, and should be avoided.
To reconstitute, add 5 mL of 0.9% Sodium Chloride Injection to the 200 mg vial or 25 mL of 0.9% Sodium Chloride Injection to the 1 g vial. Shake to dissolve. These dilutions each yield a gemcitabine concentration of 38 mg/mL which includes accounting for the displacement volume of the lyophilized powder (0.26 mL for the 200 mg vial or 1.3 mL for the 1 g vial). The total volume upon reconstitution will be 5.26 mL or 26.3 mL, respectively. Complete withdrawal of the vial contents will provide 200 mg or 1 g of gemcitabine, respectively. The appropriate amount of drug may be administered as prepared or further diluted with 0.9% Sodium Chloride Injection to concentrations as low as 0.1 mg/mL.
Reconstituted Gemzar is a clear, colorless to light straw-colored solution. After reconstitution with 0.9% Sodium Chloride Injection, the pH of the resulting solution lies in the range of 2.7 to 3.3. The solution should be inspected visually for particulate matter and discoloration, prior to administration, whenever solution or container permit. If particulate matter or discoloration is found, do not administer.
When prepared as directed, Gemzar solutions are stable for 24 hours at controlled room temperature 20° to 25°C (68° to 77°F) [*See* USP]. Discard unused portion. Solutions of reconstituted Gemzar should not be refrigerated, as crystallization may occur.
The compatibility of Gemzar with other drugs has not been studied. No incompatibilities have been observed with infusion bottles or polyvinyl chloride bags and administration sets.
Unopened vials of Gemzar are stable until the expiration date indicated on the package when stored at controlled room temperature 20° to 25°C (68° to 77°F) [*See* USP].
Caution should be exercised in handling and preparing Gemzar solutions. The use of gloves is recommended. If Gemzar solution contacts the skin or mucosa, immediately wash the skin thoroughly with soap and water or rinse the mucosa with copious amounts of water. Although acute dermal irritation has not been observed in animal studies, two of three rabbits exhibited drug-related systemic toxicities (death, hypoactivity, nasal discharge, shallow breathing) due to dermal absorption.
Procedures for proper handling and disposal of anti-cancer drugs should be considered. Several guidelines on this subject have been published.[1–7] There is no general agreement that all of the procedures recommended in the guidelines are necessary or appropriate.

HOW SUPPLIED

Vials:
200 mg white, lyophilized powder in a 10 mL size sterile single use vial (No. 7501)
NDC 0002-7501-01
1 g white, lyophilized powder in a 50-mL size sterile single use vial (No. 7502)
NDC 0002-7502-01
Store at controlled room temperature (20° to 25°C) (68° to 77°F). The USP has defined controlled room temperture as "A temperature maintained thermostatically that encompasses the usual and customary working environment of 20° to 25°C (68° to 77°F); that results in a mean kinetic temperature calculated to be not more than 25°C; and that allows for excursions between 15° and 30°C (59° and 86°F) that are experienced in pharmacies, hospitals, and warehouses."
Rx only

REFERENCES

1. Recommendations for the safe handling of parenteral antineoplastic drugs. NIH publication No. 83–2621. US Government Printing Office, Washington, DC 20402.
2. Council on Scientific Affairs: Guidelines for handling parenteral antineoplastics. *JAMA* 1985;253:1590.
3. National Study Commission on Cytotoxic Exposure—Recommendations for handling cytotoxic agents, 1987. Available from Louis P Jeffrey, ScD, Director of Pharmacy Services, Rhode Island Hospital, 593 Eddy Street, Providence, Rhode Island 02902.
4. Clinical Oncological Society of Australia: Guidelines and recommendations for safe handling of antineoplastic agents. *Med J Aust* 1983;1:426.
5. Jones RB, et al. Safe handling of chemotherapeutic agents: A report from the Mount Sinai Medical Center. *CA* 1983;33(Sept/Oct): 258.
6. American Society of Hospital Pharmacists: Technical assistance bulletin on handling cytotoxic drugs in hospitals. *Am J Hosp Pharm* 1990;47:1033.
7. Yodaiken RE, Bennet D, OSHA work-practice guidelines for personnel dealing with cytotoxic (antineoplastic) drugs. *Am J Hosp Pharm* 1988;43:1193-1204.

Literature revised August 26, 1998
PA 1635 AMP [082698]

GLUCAGON ℞
[*glōō 'ka-gŏn*]
FOR INJECTION
(rDNA ORIGIN)

DESCRIPTION

Glucagon for Injection (rDNA origin) is a polypeptide hormone identical to human glucagon that increases blood glucose and relaxes smooth muscle of the gastrointestinal tract. Glucagon is synthesized in a special non-pathogenic laboratory strain of *Escherichia coli* bacteria that has been genetically altered by the addition of the gene for glucagon. Glucagon is a single-chain polypeptide that contains 29 amino acid residues and has a molecular weight of 3,483. The empirical formula is $C_{153}H_{225}N_{43}O_{49}S$. The primary sequence of glucagon is shown below.

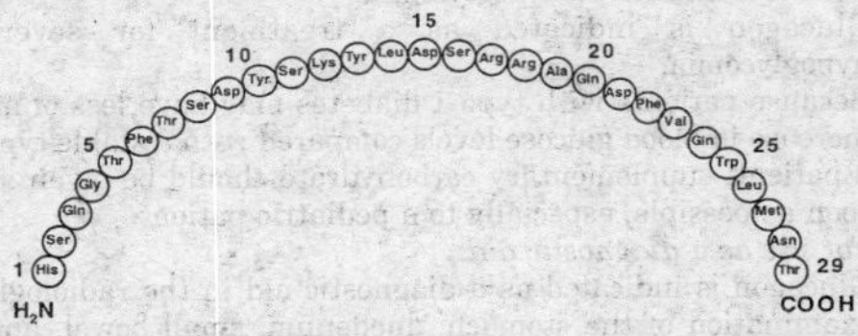

Crystalline glucagon is a white to off-white powder. It is relatively insoluble in water but is soluble at a pH of less than 3 or more than 9.5.
Glucagon is available for use intravenously, intramuscularly, or subcutaneously in a kit that contains a vial of ster-

Continued on next page

*** Identi-Code® symbol. This product information was prepared in June 2000. Current information on these and other products of Eli Lilly and Company may be obtained by direct inquiry to Lilly Research Laboratories, Lilly Corporate Center, Indianapolis, Indiana 46285, (800) 545-5979.**

Glucagon—Cont.

ile glucagon and a syringe of sterile diluent. The vial contains 1 mg (1 unit) of glucagon and 49 mg of lactose. Hydrochloric acid may have been added during manufacture to adjust the pH of the glucagon. One International Unit of glucagon is equivalent to 1 mg of glucagon.[1] The diluent syringe contains 12 mg/mL of glycerin, water for injection, and hydrochloric acid.

CLINICAL PHARMACOLOGY

Glucagon increases blood glucose concentration and is used in the treatment of hypoglycemia. Glucagon acts only on liver glycogen, converting it to glucose.

Glucagon administered through a parenteral route relaxes smooth muscle of the stomach, duodenum, small bowel, and colon.

Pharmacokinetics

Glucagon has been studied following intramuscular, subcutaneous, and intravenous administration in adult volunteers. Administration of the intravenous glucagon showed dose proportionality of the pharmacokinetics between 0.25 and 2.0 mg. Calculations from a 1 mg dose showed a small volume of distribution (mean, 0.25 L/kg) and a moderate clearance (mean, 13.5 mL/min/kg). The half-life was short, ranging from 8 to 18 minutes.

Maximum plasma concentrations of 7.9 ng/mL were achieved approximately 20 minutes after subcutaneous administration (*see* Figure 1A). With intramuscular dosing, maximum plasma concentrations of 6.9 ng/mL were attained approximately 13 minutes after dosing.

Glucagon is extensively degraded in liver, kidney, and plasma. Urinary excretion of intact glucagon has not been measured.

Pharmacodynamics

In a study of 25 volunteers, a subcutaneous dose of 1 mg glucagon resulted in a mean peak glucose concentration of 136 mg/dL 30 minutes after injection (*see* Figure 1B). Similarly, following intramuscular injection, the mean peak glucose level was 138 mg/dL, which occurred at 26 minutes after injection. No difference in maximum blood glucose concentration between animal-sourced and rDNA glucagon was observed after subcutaneous and intramuscular injection.

Figure 1
Mean (±SE) serum glucagon and blood glucose levels after subcutaneous injection of glucagon (1mg) in 25 normal volunteers

A

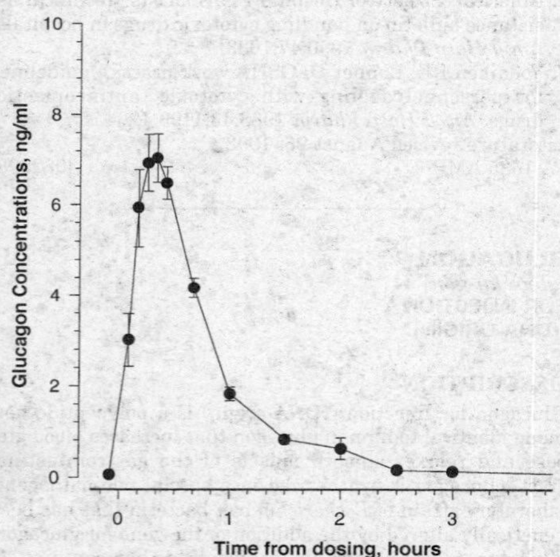

[See figure B at top of next column]

INDICATIONS AND USAGE

For the treatment of hypoglycemia:

Glucagon is indicated as a treatment for severe hypoglycemia.

Because patients with type 1 diabetes may have less of an increase in blood glucose levels compared with a stable type 2 patient, supplementary carbohydrate should be given as soon as possible, especially to a pediatric patient.

For use as a diagnostic aid:

Glucagon is indicated as a diagnostic aid in the radiologic examination of the stomach, duodenum, small bowel, and colon when diminished intestinal motility would be advantageous.

Glucagon is as effective for this examination as are the anticholinergic drugs. However, the addition of the anticholinergic agent may result in increased side effects.

CONTRAINDICATIONS

Glucagon is contraindicated in patients with known hypersensitivity to it or in patients with known pheochromocytoma.

WARNINGS

Glucagon should be administered cautiously to patients with a history suggestive of insulinoma, pheochromocytoma, or both. In patients with insulinoma, intravenous ad-

Dose	Route of Administration	Time of Onset of Action	Approximate Duration of Effect
0.25–0.5 mg (0.25–0.5 units)	IV	1 minute	9–17 minutes
1 mg (1 unit)	IM	8–10 minutes	12–27 minutes
2 mg* (2 units)	IV	1 minute	22–25 minutes
2 mg* (2 units)	IM	4–7 minutes	21–32 minutes

*Administration of 2 mg (2 units) doses produces a higher incidence of nausea and vomiting than do lower doses.

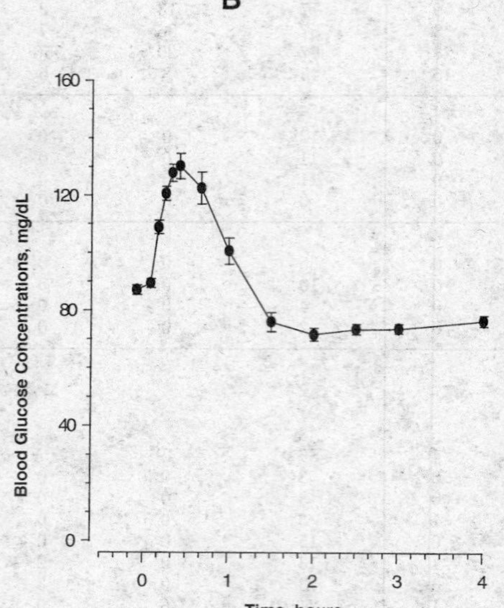

ministration of glucagon may produce an initial increase in blood glucose; however, because of glucagon's hyperglycemic effect the insulinoma may release insulin and cause subsequent hypoglycemia. A patient developing symptoms of hypoglycemia after a dose of glucagon should be given glucose orally, intravenously, or by gavage, whichever is most appropriate.

Exogenous glucagon also stimulates the release of catecholamines. In the presence of pheochromocytoma, glucagon can cause the tumor to release catecholamines, which may result in a sudden and marked increase in blood pressure. If a patient develops a sudden increase in blood pressure, 5 to 10 mg of phentolamine mesylate may be administered intravenously in an attempt to control the blood pressure.

Generalized allergic reactions, including urticaria, respiratory distress, and hypotension, have been reported in patients who received glucagon by injection.

PRECAUTIONS

General—Glucagon is effective in treating hypoglycemia only if sufficient liver glycogen is present. Because glucagon is of little or no help in states of starvation, adrenal insufficiency, or chronic hypoglycemia, hypoglycemia in these conditions should be treated with glucose.

Information for Patients—Refer patients and family members to the attached Information for the User for instructions describing the method of preparing and injecting glucagon. Advise the patient and family members to become familiar with the technique of preparing glucagon before an emergency arises. Instruct patients to use 1 mg (1 unit) for adults and 1/2 the adult dose (0.5 mg) [0.5 unit] for pediatric patients weighing less than 44 lb (20 kg).

Patients and family members should be informed of the following measures to prevent hypoglycemic reactions due to insulin:

1. Reasonable uniformity from day to day with regard to diet, insulin, and exercise.
2. Careful adjustment of the insulin program so that the type (or types) of insulin, dose, and time (or times) of administration are suited to the individual patient.
3. Frequent testing of the blood or urine for glucose so that a change in insulin requirements can be foreseen.
4. Routine carrying of sugar, candy, or other readily absorbable carbohydrate by the patient so that it may be taken at the first warning of an oncoming reaction.

To prevent severe hypoglycemia, patients and family members should be informed of the symptoms of mild hypoglycemia and how to treat it appropriately.

Family members should be informed to arouse the patient as quickly as possible because prolonged hypoglycemia may result in damage to the central nervous system. Glucagon or intravenous glucose should awaken the patient sufficiently so that oral carbohydrates may be taken.

Patients should be advised to inform their physician when hypoglycemic reactions occur so that the treatment regimen may be adjusted if necessary.

Laboratory Tests—Blood glucose determinations should be obtained to follow the patient with hypoglycemia until patient is asymptomatic.

Carcinogenesis, Mutagenesis, Impairment of Fertility—Because glucagon is usually given in a single dose and has a very short half-life, no studies have been done regarding carcinogenesis. In a series of studies examining effects on the bacterial mutagenesis (Ames) assay, it was determined that *an increase* in colony counts was related to technical difficulties in running this assay with peptides and was not due to mutagenic activities of the glucagon.

Reproduction studies have been performed in rats at doses up to 2 mg/kg glucagon administered two times a day (up to 40 times the human dose based on body surface area, mg/m^2) and have revealed no evidence of impaired fertility.

Pregnancy—Pregnancy Category B—Reproduction studies have not been performed with recombinant glucagon. However, studies with animal-sourced glucagon were performed in rats at doses up to 2 mg/kg glucagon administered two times a day (up to 40 times the human dose based on body surface area, mg/m^2), and have revealed no evidence of impaired fertility or harm to the fetus due to glucagon. There are, however, no adequate and well-controlled studies in pregnant women. Because animal reproduction studies are not always predictive of human response, this drug should be used during pregnancy only if clearly needed.

Nursing Mothers—It is not known whether this drug is excreted in human milk. Because many drugs are excreted in human milk, caution should be exercised when glucagon is administered to a nursing woman. If the drug is excreted in human milk during its short half-life, it will be hydrolyzed and absorbed like any other polypeptide. Glucagon is not active when taken orally because it is destroyed in the gastrointestinal tract before it can be absorbed.

Pediatric Use—For the treatment of hypoglycemia: The use of glucagon in pediatric patients has been reported to be safe and effective.[2-6]

For use as a diagnostic aid: Effectiveness has not been established in pediatric patients.

ADVERSE REACTIONS

Severe adverse reactions are very rare, although nausea and vomiting may occur occasionally. These reactions may also occur with hypoglycemia. Generalized allergic reactions have been reported (*see* WARNINGS). In a three month controlled study of 75 volunteers comparing animal-sourced glucagon with glucagon manufactured through rDNA technology, no glucagon-specific antibodies were detected in either treatment group.

OVERDOSAGE

Signs and Symptoms—If overdosage occurs, nausea, vomiting, gastric hypotonicity, and diarrhea would be expected without causing consequential toxicity.

Intravenous administration of glucagon has been shown to have positive inotropic and chronotropic effects. A transient increase in both blood pressure and pulse rate may occur following the administration of glucagon. Patients taking β-blockers might be expected to have a greater increase in both pulse and blood pressure, an increase of which will be transient because of glucagon's short half-life. The increase in blood pressure and pulse rate may require therapy in patients with pheochromocytoma or coronary artery disease.

When glucagon was given in large doses to patients with cardiac disease, investigators reported a positive inotropic effect. These investigators administered glucagon in doses of 0.5 to 16 mg/hour by continuous infusion for periods of 5 to 166 hours. Total doses ranged from 25 to 996 mg, and a 21-month-old infant received approximately 8.25 mg in 165 hours. Side effects included nausea, vomiting, and decreasing serum potassium concentration. Serum potassium concentration could be maintained within normal limits with supplemental potassium.

The intravenous median lethal dose for glucagon in mice and rats is approximately 300 mg/kg and 38.6 mg/kg, respectively.

Because glucagon is a polypeptide, it would be rapidly destroyed in the gastrointestinal tract if it were to be accidentally ingested.

Treatment—To obtain up-to-date information about the treatment of overdose, a good resource is your certified Regional Poison Control Center. Telephone numbers of certified poison control centers are listed in the *Physicians' Desk Reference (PDR)*. In managing overdosage, consider the possibility of multiple drug overdoses, interaction among drugs, and unusual drug kinetics in your patient.

In view of the extremely short half-life of glucagon and its prompt destruction and excretion, the treatment of overdosage is symptomatic, primarily for nausea, vomiting, and possible hypokalemia.

If the patient develops a dramatic increase in blood pressure, 5 to 10 mg of phentolamine mesylate has been shown to be effective in lowering blood pressure for the short time that control would be needed.

Forced diuresis, peritoneal dialysis, hemodialysis, or charcoal hemoperfusion have not been established as beneficial for an overdose of glucagon; it is extremely unlikely that one of these procedures would ever be indicated.

DOSAGE AND ADMINISTRATION

<u>General Instructions for Use:</u>

- The diluent is provided for use only in the preparation of glucagon for parenteral injection and for no other use.

- Glucagon should not be used at concentrations greater than 1 mg/mL (1 unit/mL).
- Reconstituted glucagon should be used immediately. **Discard any unused portion.**
- Reconstituted glucagon solutions should be used only if they are clear and of a water-like consistency.
- Parenteral drug products should be inspected visually for particulate matter and discoloration prior to administration.

Directions for Treatment of Severe Hypoglycemia:
Severe hypoglycemia should be treated initially with intravenous glucose, if possible.

1. If parenteral glucose can not be used, dissolve the lyophilized glucagon using the accompanying diluting solution and use immediately.
2. For adults and for pediatric patients weighing more than 44 lb (20 kg), give 1 mg (1 unit) by subcutaneous, intramuscular, or intravenous injection.
3. For pediatric patients weighing less than 44 lb (20 kg), give 0.5 mg (0.5 unit) or a dose equivalent to 20-30 µ/kg.[2-6]
4. **Discard any unused portion.**
5. An unconscious patient will usually awaken within 15 minutes following the glucagon injection. If the response is delayed, there is no contraindication to the administration of an additional dose of glucagon; however, in view of the deleterious effects of cerebral hypoglycemia emergency aid should be sought so that parenteral glucose can be given.
6. After the patient responds, supplemental carbohydrate should be given to restore liver glycogen and to prevent secondary hypoglycemia.

Directions for Use as a Diagnostic Aid:
Dissolve the lyophilized glucagon using the accompanying diluting solution and use immediately. **Discard any unused portion.**

The doses in the following table may be administered for relaxation of the stomach, duodenum, and small bowel, depending on the onset and duration of effect required for the examination. Since the stomach is less sensitive to the effect of glucagon, 0.5 mg (0.5 units) IV or 2 mg (2 units) IM are recommended.

[See table at top of previous page]

For examination of the colon, it is recommended that a 2 mg (2 units) dose be administered intramuscularly approximately 10 minutes prior to the procedure. Colon relaxation and reduction of patient discomfort may allow the radiologist to perform a more satisfactory examination.

HOW SUPPLIED

Glucagon Emergency Kit for Low Blood Sugar (Glucagon for Injection [rDNA origin]) (MS8031):
1 mg (1 unit)—(VL7529), with 1 mL of diluting solution (Hyporet®* HY7530) (1s) NDC 0002-8031-01
Glucagon Diagnostic Kit (Glucagon for Injection [rDNA origin]) (MS8085):
1 mg (1 unit)—(VL7529), with 1 mL of diluting solution (Hyporet®* HY7530) (1s)
NDC 0002-8085-01 (available in US market only).

*Hyporet® (disposable syringe, Lilly).

Stability and Storage:
Before Reconstitution—Vials of Glucagon, as well as the Diluting Solution for Glucagon, may be stored at controlled room temperature 20° to 25°C (68° to 77°F)[see USP].
The USP defines controlled room temperature by the following: A temperature maintained thermostatically that encompasses the usual and customary working environment of 20° to 25°C (68° to 77°F); that results in a mean kinetic temperature calculated to be not more than 25°C; and that allows for excursions between 15° and 30°C (59° and 86°F) that are experienced in pharmacies, hospitals, and warehouses.
After Reconstitution—Glucagon for Injection (rDNA origin) should be used immediately. **Discard any unused portion.**

REFERENCES

1. *Drug Information for the Health Care Professional.* 18th ed. Rockville, Maryland: The United States Pharmacopeial Convention, Inc; 1998; I:1512.
2. Gibbs et al: Use of glucagon to terminate insulin reactions in diabetic children. *Nebr Med J* 1958;43:56-57.
3. Cornblath M, et al: Studies of carbohydrate metabolism in the newborn: Effect of glucagon on concentration of sugar in capillary blood of newborn infant. *Pediatrics* 1958;21:885-892.
4. Carson MJ, Koch R: Clinical studies with glucagon in children. *J Pediatr* 1955;47:161-170
5. Shipp JC, et al: Treatment of insulin hypoglycemia in diabetic campers. *Diabetes* 1964;13:645-648.
6. Aman J, Wranne L: Hypoglycemia in childhood diabetes II: Effect of subcutaneous or intramuscular injection of different doses of glucagon. *Acta Pediatr Scand* 1988;77: 548-553.

Text issued September 11, 1998
Literature revised February 18, 1999
PA 2281 AMP [021899]

HEPARIN SODIUM ℞

[*hĕp 'ă-rŭn sō 'dē-ŭm*]
Injection, USP

WARNING—This is a potent drug, and serious consequences may result if used without constant medical supervision.

DESCRIPTION

Heparin is a heterogenous group of straight-chain anionic mucopolysaccharides, called glycosaminoglycans, having anticoagulant properties. Although others may be present, the main sugars in heparin are: (1) α-L-iduronic acid 2-sulfate, (2) 2-deoxy-2-sulfamino-α-glucose 6-sulfate, (3) β-D-glucuronic acid, (4) 2-acetamido-2-deoxy-α-D-glucose, and (5) α-L-iduronic acid. These sugars are present in decreasing amounts, usually in the order (2)>(1)>(4)>(3)>(5), and are joined by glycosidic linkages, forming polymers of varying sizes. Heparin is strongly acidic because of its covalently linked sulfate and carboxylic acid groups. In heparin sodium, the acidic protons of the sulfate units are partially replaced by sodium ions.

Structure of Heparin Sodium (representative subunits):

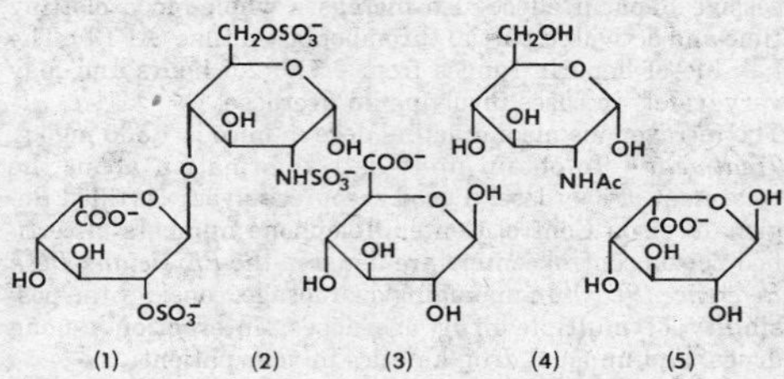

Heparin Sodium Injection, USP, is a sterile solution of heparin sodium derived from porcine intestinal mucosa, which is standardized for anticoagulant activity. It is to be administered by intravenous or deep subcutaneous routes. The potency is determined by a biological assay using a USP reference standard based on units of heparin activity per milligram.

Each mL of Vial No. 520 contains 10,000 USP heparin units (derived from porcine intestinal mucosa) and sodium chloride, 0.1%.

During manufacture, 1% benzyl alcohol is added as a preservative to each vial of heparin sodium. Sodium hydroxide and/or hydrochloric acid may be added during manufacture to adjust the pH.

CLINICAL PHARMACOLOGY

Heparin inhibits reactions that lead to the clotting of blood and the formation of fibrin clots both in vitro and in vivo. Heparin acts at multiple sites in the normal coagulation system. Small amounts of heparin in combination with antithrombin III (heparin cofactor) can inhibit thrombosis by inactivating activated Factor X and inhibiting the conversion of prothrombin to thrombin. Once active thrombosis has developed, larger amounts of heparin can inhibit further coagulation by inactivating thrombin and preventing the conversion of fibrinogen to fibrin. Heparin also prevents the formation of a stable fibrin clot by inhibiting the activation of the fibrin stabilizing factor.

Bleeding time is usually unaffected by heparin. Clotting time is prolonged by full therapeutic doses of heparin; in most cases, it is not measurably affected by low doses.

Peak plasma levels of heparin are achieved 2 to 4 hours following subcutaneous administration, although there are considerable individual variations. Log linear plots of heparin plasma concentrations with time for a wide range of dose levels are linear, which suggests the absence of zero order processes. The liver and the reticuloendothelial system are the sites of biotransformation. The biphasic elimination curve, a rapidly declining α phase ($t_{1/2}$ = 10′) and, after the age of 40, a slower β phase indicate uptake in organs. The absence of a relationship between anticoagulant half-life and concentration half-life may reflect factors such as protein binding of heparin.

Heparin does not have fibrinolytic activity; therefore, it will not lyse existing clots.

INDICATIONS AND USAGE

Heparin sodium is indicated for:
Anticoagulant therapy in prophylaxis and treatment of venous thrombosis and its extension
Prevention (in a low-dose regimen) of postoperative deep venous thrombosis and pulmonary embolism in patients undergoing major abdominothoracic surgery or who, for other reasons, are at risk of developing thromboembolic disease (*see* Dosage and Administration)
Prophylaxis and treatment of pulmonary embolism
Atrial fibrillation with embolization
Diagnosis and treatment of acute and chronic consumption coagulopathies (eg, disseminated intravascular coagulation)
Prevention of clotting in arterial and heart surgery
Prophylaxis and treatment of peripheral arterial embolism
As an anticoagulant in blood transfusions, extracorporeal circulation, and dialysis procedures and in blood samples for laboratory purposes

CONTRAINDICATIONS

Heparin sodium should not be used in patients with severe thrombocytopenia or patients for whom suitable blood coagulation tests (eg, tests for whole-blood clotting time and partial thromboplastin time) cannot be performed at appropriate intervals. (This restriction refers to full-dose administration of heparin; it is usually unnecessary to monitor coagulation parameters in patients receiving low-dose heparin). In addition, heparin sodium should not be administered to patients in an uncontrollable active bleeding state (*see* Warnings), except when this condition is the result of disseminated intravascular coagulation.

WARNINGS

Heparin is not intended for intramuscular use.

Hypersensitivity —Patients with documented hypersensitivity to heparin should be given the drug only in clearly life-threatening situations.

Hemorrhage —Hemorrhage can occur at virtually any site in patients receiving heparin. An unexplained fall in hematocrit, a fall in blood pressure, or any other unexplained symptom warrants consideration of a hemorrhagic event.

Heparin sodium should be used with extreme caution in disease states in which there is increased danger of hemorrhage. Some of the conditions in which this danger exists are as follows:

Cardiovascular —Subacute bacterial endocarditis. Severe hypertension.

Surgical —During and immediately following (a) a spinal tap or spinal anesthesia or (b) major surgery, especially involving the brain, spinal cord, or eye.

Hematologic —Conditions associated with increased bleeding tendencies, such as hemophilia, thrombocytopenia, and some vascular purpuras.

Gastrointestinal —Ulcerative lesions and continuous tube drainage of the stomach or small intestine.

Other —Menstruation and liver disease with impaired hemostasis.

Coagulation Testing —When heparin sodium is administered in therapeutic amounts, its dosage should be regulated by frequent blood coagulation tests. If the coagulation test result is unduly prolonged or if hemorrhage occurs, heparin sodium should be discontinued promptly (*see* Overdosage).

Thrombocytopenia —Thrombocytopenia occurs in patients receiving heparin with a reported incidence of 0% to 30%. Mild thrombocytopenia (count greater than 100,000/mm^3) may remain stable or reverse, even if heparin is continued. However, thrombocytopenia of any degree should be monitored closely. If the count falls below 100,000/mm^3 or if recurrent thrombosis develops (*see* Precautions, *White-Clot Syndrome*), the heparin product should be discontinued. If continued heparin therapy is essential, utilize heparin from a different organ source and reinstitute therapy with caution.

Miscellaneous —This product contains benzyl alcohol as a preservative. Benzyl alcohol has been reported to be associated with a fatal "gasping syndrome" in premature infants.

PRECAUTIONS

General —White-Clot Syndrome —It has been reported that patients taking heparin may develop new thrombus formation in association with thrombocytopenia. This development is the result of the irreversible aggregation of platelets induced by heparin, ie, the so-called "white-clot syndrome." The process may lead to severe thromboembolic complications such as skin necrosis, gangrene of the extremities that may lead to amputation, myocardial infarction, pulmonary embolism, stroke, and possibly death. Therefore, heparin administration should be promptly discontinued if a patient develops new thrombosis in association with thrombocytopenia.

Heparin Resistance —Increased resistance to heparin is frequently encountered in cases involving fever, thrombosis, thrombophlebitis, infections with thrombosing tendencies, myocardial infarction, and cancer. Increased resistance can also occur in postsurgical patients.

Increased Risk in Older Women —A higher incidence of bleeding has been reported in women over 60 years of age.

Laboratory Tests —Periodic platelet counts, hematocrit determinations, and tests for occult blood in the stool are recommended during the entire course of heparin therapy, regardless of the route of administration (*see* Dosage and Administration).

Drug Interactions —Oral anticoagulants: Heparin sodium may prolong the one-stage prothrombin time. Therefore, if a valid prothrombin time is to be obtained when heparin sodium is given with dicumarol or warfarin sodium, a period of at least 5 hours after the last intravenous dose or 24 hours after the last subcutaneous dose should elapse before blood is drawn.

Platelet inhibitors: Drugs such as acetylsalicylic acid, dextran, phenylbutazone, ibuprofen, indomethacin, dipyridamole, hydroxychloroquine, and others that interfere with platelet-aggregation reactions (the main hemostatic defense of heparinized patients) may induce bleeding and should be used with caution in patients receiving heparin sodium.

Other interactions: Digitalis, tetracyclines, nicotine, or antihistamines may partially counteract the anticoagulant action of heparin sodium.

Continued on next page

*** Identi-Code® symbol. This product information was prepared in June 2000. Current information on these and other products of Eli Lilly and Company may be obtained by direct inquiry to Lilly Research Laboratories, Lilly Corporate Center, Indianapolis, Indiana 46285, (800) 545-5979.**

Heparin Sodium—Cont.

Intravenous nitroglycerin administered to heparinized patients may result in a decrease of the partial thromboplastin time with subsequent rebound effect upon discontinuation of nitroglycerin. Careful monitoring of partial thromboplastin time and adjustment of heparin dosage are recommended during coadministration of heparin and intravenous nitroglycerin.
When clinical circumstances require reversal of heparinization, consult the labeling of Protamine Sulfate Injection, USP.
Drug/Laboratory Test Interactions —Hyperaminotransferasemia. Significant elevations of aminotransferase (SGOT and SGPT) levels have occurred in a high percentage of patients (and healthy subjects) who have received heparin. Since aminotransferase determinations are important in the differential diagnosis of myocardial infarction, liver disease, and pulmonary emboli, increases that might be caused by drugs (eg, heparin) should be interpreted with caution.
Carcinogenesis, Mutagenesis, Impairment of Fertility —No long-term studies in animals have been performed to evaluate the carcinogenic potential of heparin. Also, no reproduction studies in animals have been performed concerning mutagenesis or impairment of fertility.
Pregnancy —Teratogenic Effects: Pregnancy Category C —Animal reproduction studies have not been conducted with heparin sodium. It is also not known whether heparin sodium can cause fetal harm when administered to a pregnant woman or can affect reproduction capacity. Heparin sodium should be given to a pregnant woman only if clearly needed.
Nonteratogenic Effects: Heparin does not cross the placental barrier.
Nursing Mothers —Heparin is not excreted in human milk.
Pediatric Use —See Dosage and Administration.

ADVERSE REACTIONS

Hemorrhage —Hemorrhage is the chief complication that may result from heparin therapy (*see* Warnings). An overly prolonged clotting time or minor bleeding during therapy can usually be controlled by withdrawing the drug (*see* Overdosage). *Gastrointestinal or urinary tract bleeding during anticoagulant therapy may indicate the presence of an underlying occult lesion.* Bleeding can occur at any site, but certain specific hemorrhagic complications may be difficult to detect:

Adrenal hemorrhage, with resultant acute adrenal insufficiency, has occurred during anticoagulant therapy. Therefore, such treatment should be discontinued in patients who develop signs and symptoms of acute adrenal hemorrhage and insufficiency. Initiation of corrective therapy should not be delayed for laboratory confirmation of the diagnosis, since any delay in an acute situation may result in the patient's death.

Ovarian (corpus luteum) hemorrhage developed in a number of women of reproductive age receiving short- or long-term anticoagulant therapy. If unrecognized, this complication may be fatal.

Retroperitoneal hemorrhage has occurred.

Local Irritation —Local irritation, erythema, mild pain, hematoma, or ulceration may follow deep subcutaneous (intrafat) injection of heparin sodium. These complications are much more common after intramuscular use; therefore, such use is not recommended.
Hypersensitivity —Generalized hypersensitivity reactions have been reported, with chills, fever, and urticaria as the most common manifestations; asthma, rhinitis, lacrimation, headache, nausea and vomiting, and anaphylactoid reactions (including shock) have occurred more rarely. Itching and burning, especially on the plantar site of the feet, may occur.
The occurrence of thrombocytopenia has been reported in patients receiving heparin, with an incidence of 0% to 30%. Although often mild and of no obvious clinical significance, such thrombocytopenia can be accompanied by severe thromboembolic complications, such as skin necrosis, gangrene of the extremities that may lead to amputation, myocardial infarction, pulmonary embolism, stroke, and possibly death (*see* Warnings *and* Precautions).
Certain episodes of painful, ischemic, and cyanosed limbs have, in the past, been attributed to allergic vasospastic reactions. Whether these are, in fact, identical to the thrombocytopenia-associated complications remains to be determined.
Miscellaneous —Osteoporosis following long-term administration of high doses of heparin, cutaneous necrosis after systemic administration, suppression of aldosterone synthesis, delayed transient alopecia, priapism, and rebound hyperlipemia occurring after discontinuation of heparin sodium have also been reported.
Significant elevations of aminotransferase (SGOT and SGPT) levels have occurred in a high percentage of patients (and healthy subjects) who have received heparin.

OVERDOSAGE

Signs and Symptoms —Overdose of heparin may follow parenteral administration, but oral heparin has little systemic effect. Bleeding is the chief sign of heparin overdosage. Excessive heparin effect also increases whole-blood clotting time and activated partial thromboplastin time (APTT). The half-life of heparin ranges from 0.5 to 2.5 hours and may vary widely in cases involving an overdose.
The intravenous median lethal dose in mice is 1,500 mg/kg.
Treatment —To obtain up-to-date information about the treatment of overdose, a good resource is your certified Regional Poison Control Center. Telephone numbers of certified poison control centers are listed in the *Physicians' Desk Reference (PDR)*. In managing overdosage, consider the possibility of multiple drug overdoses, interaction among drugs, and unusual drug kinetics in your patient.
Minor bleeding occurring during therapy with heparin can often be treated by reducing the dose or increasing the dosing interval.
For major bleeding episodes, heparin may be neutralized by protamine; 1 mg of protamine will neutralize approximately 115 units of heparin of porcine intestinal mucosal origin. Protamine dosage may be guided by determining the amount of time by which clotting is shortened in vitro or by the results of other hematologic tests. Note that protamine may cause anaphylactoid reactions that may be life threatening. (See the protamine label for additional information.) The administration of whole blood or fresh frozen plasma should be considered for patients with significant blood losses. Vitamin K will not reverse the activity of heparin.

DOSAGE AND ADMINISTRATION

Parenteral drug products should be inspected visually for particulate matter and discoloration prior to administration if solution and container permit. Slight discoloration does not alter potency.
When heparin is added to an infusion solution for continuous intravenous administration, the container should be inverted at least 6 times to ensure adequate mixing and prevent pooling of the heparin in the solution.
Heparin sodium is not effective by oral administration and should be given by intermittent intravenous injection, intravenous infusion, or deep subcutaneous (intrafat, ie, above the iliac crest or abdominal fat layer) injection. *The intramuscular route of administration should be avoided because of the frequent occurrence of hematoma at the injection site.*
The dosage of heparin sodium should be adjusted according to the patient's coagulation test results. When heparin is given by continuous intravenous infusion, the coagulation time should be determined approximately every 4 hours in the early stages of treatment. When the drug is administered intermittently by intravenous injection, coagulation tests should be performed before each injection during the early stages of treatment and at appropriate intervals thereafter. Dosage is considered adequate when the APTT is 1.5 to 2 times normal or when the whole-blood clotting time is elevated approximately 2.5 to 3 times the control value.
After deep subcutaneous (intrafat) injections, tests for adequacy of dosage are best performed on samples drawn 4 to 6 hours after the injections.
Periodic platelet counts, hematocrit determinations, and tests for occult blood in the stool are recommended during the entire course of heparin therapy, regardless of the route of administration.
Converting to Oral Anticoagulant —When an oral anticoagulant of the coumarin (or similar) type is to be administered in patients already receiving heparin sodium, baseline and subsequent tests of prothrombin activity must be determined at times during which heparin activity is too low to affect the prothrombin time. Such a time usually occurs about 5 hours after the last IV bolus and 24 hours after the last subcutaneous dose. If heparin is continuously infused by IV, prothrombin time can usually be measured at any time.
In converting from heparin to an oral anticoagulant, the oral anticoagulant should be given in the usual initial amount; thereafter, prothrombin time should be determined at the usual intervals. To ensure continuous anticoagulation, it is advisable to continue full heparin therapy for several days after the prothrombin time has reached the limit of the therapeutic range. Heparin therapy may then be discontinued without tapering.
Therapeutic Anticoagulant Effect With Full-Dose Heparin—Although dosage must be adjusted for the individual patient according to the results of appropriate laboratory tests, the following dosage schedule may be used as a guideline:
[See table below]

Method of Administration	Frequency	Recommended Dose*
Deep Subcutaneous (Intrafat) Injection (A different site should be used for each injection to prevent the development of massive hematoma)	Initial dose	5,000 units by IV injection, followed by 10,000–20,000 units of a concentrated solution, subcutaneously
	Every 8 hours	8,000–10,000 units of a concentrated solution
	or Every 12 hours	15,000–20,000 units of a concentrated solution
Intermittent Intravenous Injection	Initial dose	10,000 units, either undiluted or in 50–100 mL of 0.9% Sodium Chloride Injection, USP
	Every 4 to 6 hours	5,000–10,000 units, either undiluted or in 50–100 mL of 0.9% Sodium Chloride Injection, USP
Continuous Intravenous Infusion	Initial dose	5,000 units by IV injection
	Continuous Infusion	20,000–40,000 units/24 hours in 1,000 mL of 0.9% Sodium-Chloride Injection, USP (or in any compatible solution) for infusion

* Based on 150-lb (68-kg) patient.

Pediatric Use —Follow recommendations of appropriate pediatric reference texts. In general, the following dosage schedule may be used as a guideline:

Initial Dose:	50 units/kg (IV, drip)
Maintenance Dose:	100 units/kg (IV, drip) every 4 hours, or 20,000 units/m^2/24 hours, infused continuously

Surgery of the Heart and Blood Vessels —Patients undergoing total body perfusion for open heart surgery should receive an initial dose of not less than 150 units of heparin sodium per kg of body weight. Frequently, a dose of 300 units/ kg is used for procedures estimated to last less than 60 minutes; a dose of 400 units/kg is often used for those procedures likely to last longer than 60 minutes.
Low-Dose Prophylaxis of Postoperative Thromboembolism—A number of well-controlled clinical trials have demonstrated that low-dose heparin prophylaxis, given prior to and after surgery, will reduce the incidences of postoperative deep-vein thrombosis in the legs (as measured by the I-125 fibrinogen technique and venography) and of clinical pulmonary embolism. The most widely used dosage is 5,000 units given 2 hours before surgery and 5,000 units given every 8 to 12 hours thereafter for 7 days or until the patient is fully ambulatory, whichever is longer. The heparin is given by deep subcutaneous (intrafat, ie, above the iliac crest or abdominal fat layer, arm, or thigh) injection with a fine (25- to 26-gauge) needle to minimize tissue trauma. A concentrated solution of heparin sodium is recommended. Such prophylaxis should be reserved for patients over the age of 40 who are undergoing major surgery. Patients with bleeding disorders and those having brain or spinal-cord surgery, spinal anesthesia, eye surgery, or potentially sanguineous operations should be excluded from this treatment, as should patients receiving oral anticoagulants or platelet-active drugs (*see* Warnings). The value of such prophylaxis in hip surgery has not been established. The possibility of increased bleeding during surgery or postoperatively should be borne in mind. If such bleeding occurs, discontinuance of heparin and neutralization with protamine sulfate are advisable. If clinical evidence of thromboembolism develops despite low-dose prophylaxis, full therapeutic doses of anticoagulants should be given unless contraindicated. Prior to initiating heparinization, the physician should rule out the probability of bleeding disorders by taking a thorough history and performing the appropriate laboratory tests. Appropriate coagulation tests should be repeated just prior to surgery. Coagulation test values should be normal or only slightly elevated at these times.
Extracorporeal Dialysis —Follow equipment manufacturers' operating directions carefully.
Blood Transfusion —The addition of 400 to 600 USP units to each 100 mL of whole blood for transfusion is usually employed to prevent coagulation. Usually, 7,500 USP units of heparin sodium are mixed with 100 mL of 0.9% Sodium Chloride Injection, USP (or 75,000 USP units/1,000 mL of 0.9% Sodium Chloride Injection, USP); 6 to 8 mL of this sterile solution is then added to each 100 mL of whole blood used.
Laboratory Samples —70 to 150 units of heparin sodium are usually added per 10- to 20-mL sample of whole blood to prevent coagulation of the sample. Leukocyte counts should be performed on heparinized blood within 2 hours after the addition of the heparin. Heparinized blood should not be used for isoagglutinin, complement, or erythrocyte fragility tests or for taking platelet counts.
Clearing Intermittent Infusion (Heparin Lock) Sets —To prevent clot formation in a heparin lock set following its proper insertion, dilute heparin solution (*see* USP monograph for Heparin Lock Flush Solution, USP) should be injected via the injection hub in a quantity sufficient to fill the entire set to the needle tip. This solution should be replaced each time the heparin lock is used. Aspirate before administering any solution via the lock in order to confirm the patency and location of the needle or catheter tip. If the drug to be administered is incompatible with heparin, the entire heparin lock set should be flushed with sterile water or normal saline before and after the medication is administered; following the second cleansing flush, the dilute heparin solution may be reinstilled in the set. The set manufacturer's instructions should be consulted for specifics concerning the heparin lock set being used at a given time.
NOTE: Since repeated injections of small doses of heparin can alter tests for activated partial thromboplastin time (APTT), a baseline value for APTT should be obtained prior to insertion of a heparin lock set.

HOW SUPPLIED
Multiple-Dose Vials:
10,000 USP heparin units/mL, 5 mL (No. 520)—(1s) NDC 0002-7217-01
Protect from light. Store at 25°C (77°F); excursions permitted to 15–30°C (59–86°F). [see USP Controlled Room Temperature].
Literature revised December 10, 1998
PA 0711 AMP [121098]

HUMALOG® ℞
[*hūm a lŏg*]
INSULIN LISPRO INJECTION
(rDNA ORIGIN)

DESCRIPTION
Humalog® (insulin lispro, rDNA origin) is a human insulin analog that is a rapid-acting, parenteral blood glucose-lowering agent. Chemically, it is Lys(B28), Pro(B29) human insulin analog, created when the amino acids at positions 28 and 29 on the insulin B-chain are reversed. Humalog is synthesized in a special non-pathogenic laboratory strain of *Escherichia coli* bacteria that has been genetically altered by the addition of the gene for insulin lispro.
Humalog has the following primary structure:

Figure 1

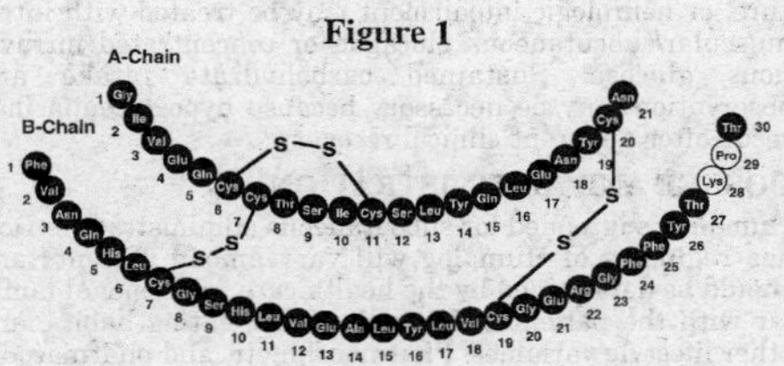

Insulin lispro has the empirical formula $C_{257}H_{383}N_{65}O_{77}S_6$ and a molecular weight of 5808, both identical to that of human insulin.
The vials and cartridges contain a sterile solution of Humalog for use as an injection. Humalog injection consists of zinc-insulin lispro crystals dissolved in a clear aqueous fluid.
Each milliliter of Humalog injection contains insulin lispro 100 Units, 16 mg glycerin, 1.88 mg dibasic sodium phosphate, 3.15 mg *m*-cresol, zinc oxide content adjusted to provide 0.0197 mg zinc ion, trace amounts of phenol, and water for injection. Insulin lispro has a pH of 7.0–7.8. Hydrochloric acid 10% and/or sodium hydroxide 10% may be added to adjust pH.

CLINICAL PHARMACOLOGY
Antidiabetic Activity—The primary activity of insulin, including Humalog, is the regulation of glucose metabolism. In addition, all insulins have several anabolic and anti-catabolic actions on many tissues in the body. In muscle and other tissues (except the brain), insulin causes rapid transport of glucose and amino acids intracellularly, promotes anabolism, and inhibits protein catabolism. In the liver, insulin promotes the uptake and storage of glucose in the form of glycogen, inhibits gluconeogenesis, and promotes the conversion of excess glucose into fat.
Humalog has been shown to be equipotent to human insulin on a molar basis. One unit of Humalog has the same glucose-lowering effect as one unit of human regular insulin, but its effect is more rapid and of shorter duration. The glucose-lowering activity of Humalog and human regular insulin is comparable when administered to normal volunteers by the intravenous route.
Pharmacokinetics-
Absorption and Bioavailability—Humalog is as bioavailable as human regular insulin, with absolute bioavailability ranging between 55%–77% with doses between 0.1–0.2 U/kg, inclusive. Studies in normal volunteers and patients with type I (insulin-dependent) diabetes demonstrated that Humalog is absorbed faster than human regular insulin (U100) (Figure 2). In normal volunteers given subcutaneous doses of Humalog ranging from 0.1–0.4 U/kg, peak serum levels were seen 30–90 minutes after dosing. When normal volunteers received equivalent doses of human regular insulin, peak insulin levels occurred between 50–120 minutes after dosing. Similar results were seen in patients with type I diabetes. The pharmacokinetic profiles of Humalog and human regular insulin are comparable to one another when administered to normal volunteers by the intravenous route. Humalog was absorbed at a consistently faster rate than human regular insulin in healthy male volunteers given 0.2 U/kg human regular insulin or Humalog at abdominal, deltoid, or femoral subcutaneous sites, the three sites often used by patients with diabetes. After abdominal administration of Humalog, serum drug levels are higher and the duration of action is slightly shorter than after deltoid or thigh administration (*see* DOSAGE AND ADMINISTRATION). Humalog has less intra- and inter-patient variability compared to human regular insulin.
[See figure 2 at top of next column]
Distribution—The volume of distribution for Humalog is identical to that of human regular insulin, with a range of 0.26–0.36 L/kg.

Figure 2
Serum Humalog and Insulin levels after subcutaneous injection of human regular insulin or Humalog (0.2 U/kg) immediately before a high carbohydrate meal in 10 patients with Type I diabetes.*

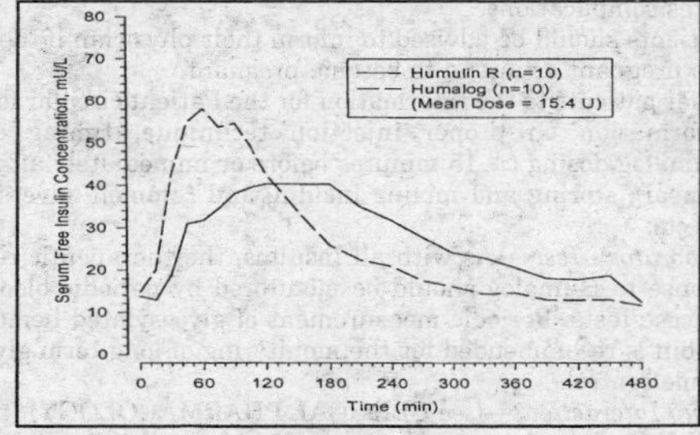

*Baseline insulin concentration was maintained by infusion of 0.2 mU/min/kg human insulin.

Metabolism—Human metabolism studies have not been conducted. However, animal studies indicate that the metabolism of Humalog is identical to that of human regular insulin.
Elimination—When Humalog is given subcutaneously, its $t_{1/2}$ is shorter than that of human regular insulin (1 vs 1.5 hours, respectively). When given intravenously, Humalog and human regular insulin show identical dose-dependent elimination, with a $t_{1/2}$ of 26 and 52 minutes at 0.1 U/kg and 0.2 U/kg, respectively.
Pharmacodynamics—Studies in normal volunteers and patients with diabetes demonstrated that Humalog has a more rapid onset of glucose-lowering activity, an earlier peak for glucose lowering, and a shorter duration of glucose-lowering activity than human regular insulin (Figure 3). The earlier onset of activity of Humalog is directly related to its more rapid rate of absorption. The time course of action of insulin and insulin analogs such as Humalog may vary considerably in different individuals or within the same individual. The parameters of Humalog activity (time of onset, peak time, and duration) as designated in Figure 3 should be considered only as general guidelines. The rate of insulin absorption and consequently the onset of activity is known to be affected by the site of injection, exercise, and other variables (*see* PRECAUTIONS, *General*).

Figure 3
Blood glucose levels after subcutaneous injection of human regular insulin or Humalog (0.2 U/kg) immediately before a high carbohydrate meal in 10 patients with Type I diabetes.*

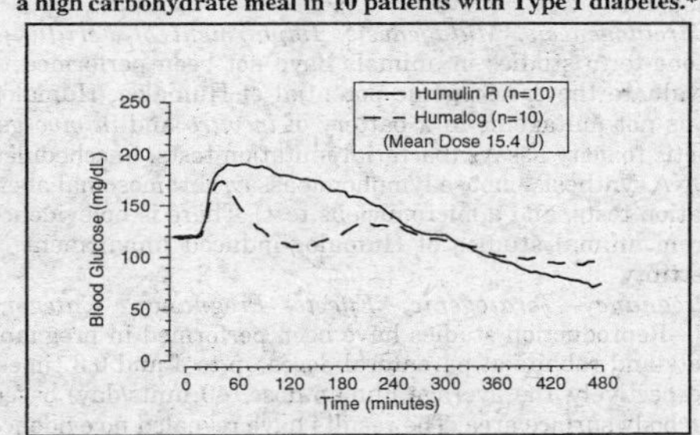

*Baseline insulin concentration was maintained by infusion of 0.2 mU/min/kg human insulin.

In open-label, crossover studies of 1008 patients with type I diabetes and 722 patients with type II (non-insulin-dependent) diabetes, Humalog reduced postprandial glucose compared with human regular insulin (*see* Table 1). The clinical significance of improvement in postprandial hyperglycemia has not been established.

Table 1

Comparison of Means of Glycemic Parameters at the End of Combined Treatment Periods. All Randomized Patients in Cross-over Studies (3 months for each treatment)

Type 1, N=1008 Glycemic Parameter, (mg/dL)	Humalog[a]	Humulin® R[a]*
Fasting Blood Glucose	209.5 ± 91.6	204.1 ± 89.3
1-Hour Postprandial	232.4 ± 97.7	250.0 ± 96.7
2-Hour Postprandial	200.9 ± 95.4	231.7 ± 103.9
HbA_{1c} (%)	8.2 ± 1.5	8.2 ± 1.5
Type 2, N=722 Glycemic Parameter, (mg/dL)	**Humalog[a]**	**Humulin R[a]**
Fasting Blood Glucose	192.1 ± 67.9	183.1 ± 66.1
1-Hour Postprandial	238.1 ± 79.7	250.0 ± 75.2
2-Hour Postprandial	217.4 ± 83.2	236.5 ± 80.6
HbA_{1c} (%)	8.2 ± 1.3	8.2 ± 1.4

[a]Mean ± Standard Deviation
*Humulin® (human injection [rDNA origin] injection)

In 12-month parallel studies in patients with Type 1 and type 2 diabetes, HbA_{1c} did not differ between patients treated with human regular insulin and those treated with Humalog.
Hypoglycemia—While the overall rate of hypoglycemia did not differ between patients with type 1 and type 2 diabetes treated with Humalog compared with human regular insulin, patients with type 1 diabetes treated with Humalog had fewer hypolgycemic episodes between midnight and 6 a.m. The lower rate of hypoglycemia in the Humalog-treated group may have been related to higher nocturnal blood glucose levels, as reflected by a small increase in mean fasting blood glucose levels.
Humalog in Combination with Sulfonylurea Agents—In a two month study in patients with fasting hyperglycemia despite maximal dosing with sulfonylureas (SU), patients were randomized to one of three treatment regimens; Humulin NPH at bedtime plus SU, Humalog three times a day before meals plus SU, or Humalog three times a day before meals and Humulin NPH at bedtime. The combination of Humalog and SU resulted in an improvement in HbA_{1c} accompanied by a weight gain. (*see* Table 2)

Table 2
Results of a Two-Month Study in Which Humalog Was Added to Sulfonylurea Therapy in Patients Not Adequately Controlled on Sulfonylurea Alone.

	Humulin® N h.s.+ SU	Humalog a.c. + SU	Humalog a.c. + Humulin® N h.s.
Randomized (n)	135	139	149
HbA_{1c} (%) at baseline	9.9	10.0	10.0
HbA_{1c} (%) at 2-months	8.7	8.4	8.5
HbA_{1c} (%) change from baseline	−1.2	−1.6	−1.4
Weight gain at 2-months (kg)	0.6	1.2	1.5
Hypoglycemia* (events/mo)	0.11	0.03	0.09
Number of injections	1	3	4
Total insulin dose (U)/kg at 2-months	0.23	0.33	0.52

a.c.-three times a day before meals, h.s.-at bedtime.
SU-oral sulfonylurea agent
*blood glucose ≤ 36 mg/dL or needing assistance from third party

Special Populations—
Age and Gender—Information on the effect of age and gender on the pharmacokinetics of Humalog is unavailable. However, in large clinical trials, subgroup analysis based on age and gender did not indicate any difference in postprandial glucose parameters between Humalog and human regular insulin.
Smoking—The effect of smoking on the pharmacokinetics and glucodynamics of Humalog has not been studied.
Pregnancy—The effect of pregnancy on the pharmacokinetics and glucodynamics of Humalog has not been studied.
Obesity—The effect of obesity and/or subcutaneous fat thickness on the pharmacokinetics and glucodynamics of Humalog has not been studied. In large clinical trials, which included patients with Body-Mass-Index up to and including 35 kg/m^2, no consistent differences were seen between Humalog and Humulin R with respect to postprandial glucose parameters.
Renal Impairment—Some studies with human insulin have shown increased circulating levels of insulin in patients with renal failure. In a study of 25 patients with type 2 diabetes and a wide range of renal function, the pharmacokinetic differences between Humalog and human regular insulin were generally maintained. However, the sensitivity of the patients to insulin did change, with an increased response to insulin as the renal function declined. Careful glucose monitoring and dose adjustments of insulin, including Humalog, may be necessary in patients with renal dysfunction.
Hepatic Impairment—Some studies with human insulin have shown increased circulating levels of insulin in patients with hepatic failure. In a study of 22 patients with type 2 diabetes, impaired hepatic function did not affect the subcutaneous absorption or general disposition of Humalog when compared to patients with no history of hepatic dys-

Continued on next page

*** Identi-Code® symbol. This product information was prepared in June 2000. Current information on these and other products of Eli Lilly and Company may be obtained by direct inquiry to Lilly Research Laboratories, Lilly Corporate Center, Indianapolis, Indiana 46285, (800) 545-5979.**

Humalog—Cont.

function. In that study, Humalog maintained its more rapid absorption and elimination when compared to human regular insulin. Careful glucose monitoring and dose adjustments of insulin, including Humalog, may be necessary in patients with hepatic dysfunction.

INDICATIONS AND USAGE

Humalog is an insulin analog that is indicated in the treatment of patients with diabetes mellitus for the control of hyperglycemia. Humalog has a more rapid onset and shorter duration of action than human regular insulin. Therefore, in patients with type 1 diabetes, Humalog should be used in regimens that include a longer-acting insulin. However, in patients with type 2 diabetes, Humalog may be used without a longer-acting insulin when used in combination therapy with sulfonylurea agents.

CONTRAINDICATIONS

Humalog is contraindicated during episodes of hypoglycemia and in patients sensitive to Humalog or one of its excipients.

WARNINGS

This human insulin analog differs from human regular insulin by its rapid onset of action as well as a shorter duration of activity. When used as a mealtime insulin, the dose of Humalog should be given within 15 minutes before or immediately after the meal. Because of the short duration of action of Humalog, patients with type I diabetes also require a longer-acting insulin to maintain glucose control.

Hypoglycemia is the most common adverse effect associated with insulins, including Humalog. As with all insulins, the timing of hypoglycemia may differ among various insulin formulations. Glucose monitoring is recommended for all patients with diabetes.

Any change of insulin should be made cautiously and only under medical supervision. Changes in insulin strength, manufacturer, type (e.g., regular, NPH, analog), species (animal, human), or method of manufacture (rDNA versus animal-source insulin) may result in the need for a change in dosage.

PRECAUTIONS

General—Hypoglycemia and hypokalemia are among the potential clinical adverse effects associated with the use of all insulins. Because of differences in the action of Humalog and other insulins, care should be taken in patients in whom such potential side effects might be clinically relevant (e.g., patients who are fasting, have autonomic neuropathy, or are using potassium-lowering drugs or patients taking drugs sensitive to serum potassium level). Lipodystrophy and hypersensitivity are among other potential clinical adverse effects associated with the use of all insulins.

As with all insulin preparations, the time course of Humalog action may vary in different individuals or at different times in the same individual and is dependent on site of injection, blood supply, temperature, and physical activity.

Adjustment of dosage of any insulin may be necessary if patients change their physical activity or their usual meal plan. Insulin requirements may be altered during illness, emotional disturbances, or other stress.

Hypoglycemia—As with all insulin preparations, hypoglycemic reactions may be associated with the administration of Humalog. Rapid changes in serum glucose levels may induce symptoms of hypoglycemia in persons with diabetes, regardless of the glucose value. Early warning symptoms of hypoglycemia may be different or less pronounced under certain conditions, such as long duration of diabetes, diabetic nerve disease, use of medications such as beta-blockers, or intensified diabetes control.

Renal Impairment—The requirements for insulin may be reduced in patients with renal impairment.

Hepatic Impairment—Although impaired hepatic function does not affect the absorption or disposition of Humalog, careful glucose monitoring and dose adjustments of insulin, including Humalog, may be necessary.

Allergy—Local Allergy—As with any insulin therapy, patients may experience redness, swelling, or itching at the site of injection. These minor reactions usually resolve in a few days to a few weeks. In some instances, these reactions may be related to factors other than insulin, such as irritants in a skin cleansing agent or poor injection technique.

Systemic Allergy—Less common, but potentially more serious, is generalized allergy to insulin, which may cause rash (including pruritus) over the whole body, shortness of breath, wheezing, reduction in blood pressure, rapid pulse, or sweating. Severe cases of generalized allergy, including anaphylactic reaction, may be life threatening. In controlled clinical trials, pruritus (with or without rash) was seen in 17 patients receiving Humulin R (N=2969) and 30 patients receiving Humalog (N=2944) (p=.053). Localized reactions and generalized myalgias have been reported with the use of cresol as an injectable excipient.

Antibody Production—In large clinical trials, antibodies that cross react with human insulin and insulin lispro were observed in both Humulin R- and Humalog-treatment groups. As expected, the largest increase in the antibody levels during the 12-month clinical trials was observed with patients new to insulin therapy.

Information for Patients—Patients should be informed of the potential risks and advantages of Humalog and alternative therapies. Patients should be informed about the importance of proper insulin storage, injection technique, timing of dosage, adherence to meal planning, regular physical activity, regular blood glucose monitoring, periodic glycosylated hemoglobin testing, recognition and management of hypo- and hyperglycemia, and periodic assessment for diabetes complications.

Patients should be advised to inform their physician if they are pregnant or intend to become pregnant.

Refer patients to the Information for the Patient circular for information on proper injection technique, timing of Humalog dosing (≤ 15 minutes before or immediately after a meal), storing and mixing insulin, and common adverse effects.

Laboratory Tests—As with all insulins, the therapeutic response to Humalog should be monitored by periodic blood glucose tests. Periodic measurement of glycosylated hemoglobin is recommended for the monitoring of long-term glycemic control.

Drug Interactions—(*see* CLINICAL PHARMACOLOGY) Insulin requirements may be increased by medications with hyperglycemic activity such as corticosteroids, isoniazid, certain lipid-lowering drugs (e.g., niacin), estrogens, oral contraceptives, phenothiazines, and thyroid replacement therapy.

Insulin requirements may be decreased in the presence of drugs with hypoglycemic activity, such as oral hypoglycemic agents, salicylates, sulfa antibiotics, and certain antidepressants (monoamine oxidase inhibitors), certain angiotensin-converting-enzyme inhibitors, beta-adrenergic blockers, inhibitors of pancreatic function (e.g., octreotide), and alcohol. Beta-adrenergic blockers may mask the symptoms of hypoglycemia in some patients.

Mixing of Insulins—Care should be taken when mixing all insulins as a change in peak action may occur. The American Diabetes Association warns in its Position Statement on Insulin Administration, "On mixing, physiochemical changes in the mixture may occur (either immediately or over time). As a result, the physiological response to the insulin mixture may differ from that of the injection of the insulins separately." Mixing Humalog with Humulin N or Humulin U does not decrease the absorption rate or the total bioavailability of Humalog. Given alone or mixed with Humulin N, Humalog results in a more rpaid absorption and glucose-lowering effect compared with human regular insulin.

The effects of mixing Humalog with insulins of animal source or insulin preparations produced by other manufacturers have not been studied (*see* WARNINGS).

If Humalog is mixed with a longer-acting insulin, such as Humulin N or Humulin U, Humalog should be drawn into the syringe first to prevent clouding of the Humalog by the longer-acting insulin. Injection should be made immediately after mixing. Mixtures should not be administered intravenously.

Carcinogenesis, Mutagenesis, Impairment of Fertility—Long-term studies in animals have not been performed to evaluate the carcinogenic potential of Humalog. Humalog was not mutagenic in a battery of *in vitro* and *in vivo* genetic toxicity assays (bacterial mutation tests, unscheduled DNA synthesis, mouse lymphoma assay, chromosomal aberration tests, and a micronucleus test). There is no evidence from animal studies of Humalog-induced impairment of fertility.

Pregnancy—Teratogenic Effects—Pregnancy Category B—Reproduction studies have been performed in pregnant rats and rabbits at parenteral doses up to 4 and 0.3 times, respectively, the average human dose (40 units/day) based on body surface area. The results have revealed no evidence of impaired fertility or harm to the fetus due to Humalog. There are, however, no adequate and well-controlled studies in pregnant women. Because animal reproduction studies are not always predictive of human response, this drug should be used during pregnancy only if clearly needed.

Although there are no clinical studies of the use of Humalog in pregnancy, published studies with human insulins suggest that optimizing overall glycemic control, including postprandial control, before conception and during pregnancy improves fetal outcome. Although the fetal complications of maternal hyperglycemia have been well documented, fetal toxicity also has been reported with maternal hypoglycemia. Insulin requirements usually fall during the first trimester and increase during the second and third trimesters. Careful monitoring of the patient is required throughout pregnancy. During the perinatal period, careful monitoring of infants born to mothers with diabetes is warranted.

Nursing Mothers—It is unknown whether Humalog is excreted in significant amounts in human milk. Many drugs, including human insulin, are excreted in human milk. For this reason, caution should be exercised when Humalog is administered to a nursing woman. Patients with diabetes who are lactating may require adjustments in Humalog dose, meal plan, or both.

Pediatric Use—In a 9-month, cross-over study of pre-pubescent children (n=60), aged 3 to 11 years, comparable glycemic control as measured by HbA_{1c} was achieved regardless of treatment group: human regular insulin 30 minutes before meals 8.4%, Humalog immediately before meals 8.4%, and Humalog immediately after meals 8.5%. In 8-month, cross-over study of adolescents (n=463), aged 9 to 19 years, comparable glycemic control as measured by HbA_{1c} was achieved regardless of treatment group; human regular insulin 30 to 45 minutes before meals 8.7% and Humalog immediately before meals 8.7%. The incidence of hypoglycemia was similar for all three treatment regimens. Adjustment of basal insulin may be required. To improve accuracy in dosing in pediatric patients, a diluent may be used. If the diluent is added directly to the Humalog vial, the shelf-life may be reduced. (see DOSAGE AND ADMINISTRATION).

Geriatric Use—Of the total number of subjects (n=2,834) in eight clinical studies of Humalog, twelve percent (n=338) were 65 years of age or over. The majority of these were type 2 patients. HbA_{1c} values and hypoglycemia rates did not differ by age. Pharmacokinetic/pharmacodynamic studies to assess the effect of age on the onset of Humalog action have not been performed.

ADVERSE REACTIONS

Clinical studies comparing Humalog with human regular insulin did not demonstrate a difference in frequency of adverse events between the two treatments.

Adverse events commonly associated with human insulin therapy include the following:

Body as a Whole—allergic reactions (*see* PRECAUTIONS)

Skin and Appendages—injection site reaction, lipodystrophy, pruritus, rash

Other—hypoglycemia (*see* WARNINGS *and* PRECAUTIONS)

OVERDOSAGE

Hypoglycemia may occur as a result of an excess of insulin relative to food intake, energy expenditure, or both. Mild episodes of hypoglycemia usually can be treated with oral glucose. Adjustments in drug dosage, meal patterns, or exercise, may be needed. More severe episodes with coma, seizure, or neurologic impairment may be treated with intramuscular/subcutaneous glucagon or concentrated intravenous glucose. Sustained carbohydrate intake and observation may be necessary because hypoglycemia may recur after apparent clinical recovery.

DOSAGE AND ADMINISTRATION

Humalog is intended for subcutaneous administration. Dosage regimens of Humalog will vary among patients and should be determined by the health care professional familiar with the patient's metabolic needs, eating habits, and other lifestyle variables. Pharmacokinetic and pharmacodynamic studies showed Humalog to be equipotent to human regular insulin (i.e., one unit of Humalog has the same glucose-lowering capability as one unit of human regular insulin), but with more rapid activity. The quicker glucose-lowering effect of Humalog is related to the more rapid absorption rate from subcutaneous tissue. An adjustment of dose or schedule of basal insulin may be needed when a patient changes from other insulins to Humalog, particularly to prevent pre-meal hyperglycemia.

When used as a meal-time insulin, Humalog should be given within 15 minutes before or immediately after a meal. Human regular insulin is best given 30–60 minutes before a meal. To achieve optimal glucose control, the amount of longer-acting insulin being given may need to be adjusted when using Humalog.

The rate of insulin absorption and consequently the onset of activity is known to be affected by the site of injection, exercise, and other variables. Humalog was absorbed at a consistently faster rate than human regular insulin in healthy male volunteers given 0.2 U/kg human regular insulin or Humalog at abdominal, deltoid, or femoral sites, the three sites often used by patients with diabetes. When not mixed in the same syringe with other insulins, Humalog maintains its rapid onset of action and has less variability in its onset of action among injection sites compared with human regular insulin (*see* PRECAUTIONS). After abdominal administration, Humalog concentrations are higher than those following deltoid or thigh injections. Also, the duration of action of Humalog is slightly shorter following abdominal injection, compared with deltoid and femoral injections. As with all insulin preparations, the time course of action of Humalog may vary considerably in different individuals or within the same individual. Patients must be educated to use proper injection techniques.

Humalog may be diluted with STERILE DILUENT for Humalog®, Humulin® N, Humulin® 50/50, Humulin® 70/30, and NPH Iletin® to concentration of 1:10 (equivalent to U-10) or 1:2 (equivalent to U-50). Diluted Humalog may remain in patient use for 28 days when stored at 5°C (41°F) and for 14 days when stored at 30°C (86°F).

Parenteral drug products should be inspected visually prior to administration whenever the solution and the container permit. If the solution is cloudy, contains particulate matter, is thickened, or is discolored, the contents must not be injected. Humalog should not be used after its expiration date.

HOW SUPPLIED

Humalog (insulin lispro injection, rDNA origin) vials are available in the following package size:

100 units per mL (U-100)

10 mL vials NDC 0002-7510-01 (VL-7510)

Humalog (insulin lispro injection, rDNA origin) cartridges are available in the following package size:

5 × 1.5 mL cartridges* NDC 0002-7515-59 (VL-7515)

Humalog (insulin lispro injection, rDNA origin) Pen, disposable insulin delivery device, is available in the following package size:

5 × 3.0 mL disposable insulin delivery devices NDC 0002-8725-59 (HP-8725)

*1.5 mL cartridges are for use in Becton Dickinson and Company's B-D®† Pen and Novo Nordisk A/S's NovoPen®, NovolinPen®‡, and NovoPen®‡ 1.5 insulin delivery devices.

† B-D® is a registered trademark of Becton Dickinson and Company.

‡ NovolinPen® and NovoPen® are registered trademarks of Novo Nordisk A/S.

Storage—Humalog should be stored in a refrigerator (2° to 8°C [36° to 46°F]), but not in the freezer. If refrigeration is impossible, the vial or cartridge of Humalog in use can be unrefrigerated for up to 28 days, as long as it is kept as cool as possible (not greater than 86°F [30°C]) and away from direct heat and light. Unrefrigerated vials and cartridges must be used within this time period or be discarded. Do not use Humalog if it has been frozen.

Rx only

Literature revised April 4, 2000

PA 9162 FSAMP [040400]

HUMALOG® Mix75/25™ ℞

[*hūm a lŏg*]

75% Insulin Lispro Protamine Suspension and 25% Insulin Lispro Injection (rDNA ORIGIN)

DESCRIPTION

Humalog® Mix75/25™ [75% insulin lispro protamine suspension and 25% insulin lispro injection, (rDNA origin)] is a mixture of insulin lispro solution, a rapid-acting blood glucose-lowering agent and insulin lispro protamine suspension, an intermediate-acting blood glucose-lowering agent. Chemically, insulin lispro is Lys(B28), Pro(B29) human insulin analog, created when the amino acids at positions 28 and 29 on the insulin B-chain are reversed. Insulin lispro is synthesized in a special non-pathogenic laboratory strain of *Escherichia coli* bacteria that has been genetically altered by the addition of the gene for insulin lispro. Insulin lispro protamine suspension (NPL component) is a suspension of crystals produced from combining insulin lispro and protamine sulfate under appropriate conditions for crystal formation.

Insulin lispro has the following primary structure:

Figure 1

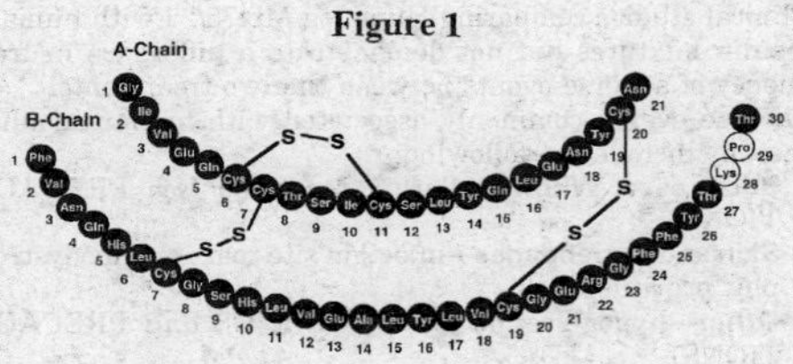

Insulin lispro has the empirical formula $C_{257}H_{383}N_{65}O_{77}S_6$ and a molecular weight of 5808, both identical to that of human insulin.

Humalog Mix75/25 disposable insulin delivery devices contain a sterile suspension of insulin lispro protamine suspension mixed with soluble insulin lispro for use as an injection.

Each milliliter of Humalog Mix75/25 injection contains insulin lispro 100 Units, 0.28 mg protamine sulfate, 16 mg glycerin, 3.78 mg dibasic sodium phosphate, 1.76 mg *m*-cresol, zinc oxide content adjusted to provide 0.025 mg zinc ion, 0.715 mg phenol, and water for injection. Humalog Mix75/25 has a pH of 7.0–7.8. Hydrochloric acid 10% and/or sodium hydroxide 10% may have been added to adjust pH.

CLINICAL PHARMACOLOGY

Antidiabetic Activity—The primary activity of insulin, including Humalog Mix75/25, is the regulation of glucose metabolism. In addition, all insulins have several anabolic and anti-catabolic actions on many tissues in the body. In muscle and other tissues (except the brain), insulin causes rapid transport of glucose and amino acids intracellularly, promotes anabolism, and inhibits protein catabolism In the liver, insulin promotes the uptake and storage of glucose in the form of glycogen, inhibits gluconeogenesis, and promotes the conversion of excess glucose into fat.

Insulin lispro, the rapid-acting component of Humalog Mix75/25, has been shown to be equipotent to regular human insulin on a molar basis. One unit of Humalog has the same glucose-lowering effect as one unit of regular human insulin, but its effect is more rapid and of shorter duration. Humalog Mix75/25 has a similar glucose-lowering effect as compared to Humulin 70/30 on a unit for unit basis.

Pharmacokinetics—

Absorption—Studies in nondiabetic subjects and patients with type 1 (insulin-dependent) diabetes demonstrated that Humalog®, the rapid-acting component of Humalog Mix75/25, is absorbed faster than regular human insulin (U100). In nondiabetic subjects given subcutaneous doses of Humalog ranging from 0.1–0.4 U/kg, peak serum concentrations were observed 30–90 minutes after dosing. When nondiabetic subjects received equivalent doses of regular human insulin, peak insulin concentrations occurred 50–120 minutes after dosing. Similar results were found in patients with type 1 diabetes.

Figure 4
Insulin activity after injection of Humalog Mix75/25 and Humulin 70/30 in nondiabetic subjects.

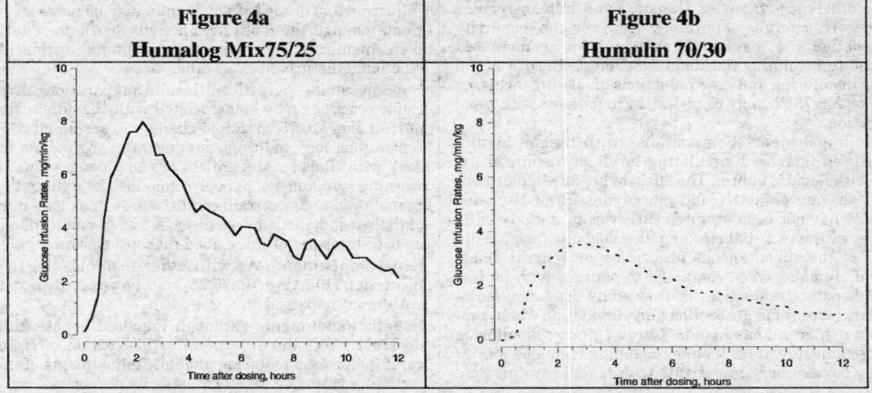

Figure 2
Serum immunoreactive insulin (IRI) concentrations, after subcutaneous injection of Humalog Mix75/25 or Humulin 70/30 in healthy nondiabetic subjects

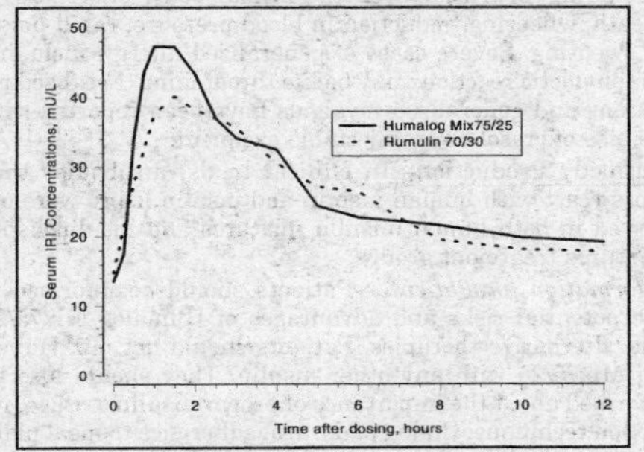

Humalog Mix75/25 has two phases of absorption. The early phase represents insulin lispro and its distinct characteristics of rapid onset. The late phase represents the prolonged action of insulin lispro protamine suspension. In 30 nondiabetic subjects given subcutaneous doses (0.3 U/kg) of Humalog Mix75/25, peak serum concentrations were observed 30 to 240 minutes (median, 60 minutes) after dosing (Figure 2). Identical results were found in patients with type 1 diabetes. The rapid absorption characteristics of Humalog are maintained with Humalog Mix75/25 (Figure 2).

Figure 2 represents serum insulin concentration versus time curves of Humalog Mix75/25 and Humulin 70/30. Humalog Mix75/25 has a more rapid absorption than Humulin 70/30, which has been confirmed in patients with type 1 diabetes.

Distribution—radiolabeled distribution studies of Humalog Mix75/25 have not been conducted. However, the volume of distribution following injection of Humalog is identical to that of regular human insulin, with a range of 0.26–0.36 L/kg.

Metabolism—Human metabolism studies of Humalog Mix75/25 have not been conducted. Studies in animals indicate that the metabolism of Humalog, the rapid-acting component of Humalog Mix75/25, is identical to that of regular human insulin.

Elimination—Humalog Mix75/25 has two absorption phases, a rapid and a prolonged phase, representative of the insulin lispro and insulin lispro protamine suspension components of the mixture. As with other intermediate-acting insulins, a meaningful terminal phase half-life cannot be calculated after administration of Humalog Mix75/25 because of the prolonged insulin lispro protamine suspension absorption.

Pharmacodynamics—Studies in nondiabetic subjects and patients with diabetes demonstrated that Humalog has a more rapid onset of glucose-lowering activity, an earlier peak for glucose lowering, and a shorter duration of glucose-lowering activity than regular human insulin. The early onset of activity of Humalog Mix75/25 is directly related to the rapid absorption of Humalog. The time course of action of insulin and insulin analogs such as Humalog (and hence Humalog Mix75/25) may vary considerably in different individuals or within the same individual. The parameters of Humalog Mix75/25 activity (time of onset, peak time, and duration) as presented in Figures 2, 3, and 4 should be considered only as general guidelines. The rate of insulin absorption and consequently the onset of activity is known to be affected by the site of injection, exercise, and other variables (*see* General *under* PRECAUTIONS).

In a glucose clamp study performed in 30 nondiabetic subjects, the onset of action and glucose-lowering activity of Humalog, Humalog Mix75/25, Humalog® Mix 50/50™ and insulin lispro protamine suspension were compared (Figure 3). Graphs of mean glucose infusion rate versus time showed a distinct insulin activity profile for each formulation. The rapid onset of glucose-lowering activity characteristic of Humalog was maintained in Humalog Mix75/25.

In separate glucose clamp studies performed in nondiabetic subjects, glucodynamics of Humalog Mix75/25 and Humulin 70/30 were assessed and are presented in Figure 4. Humalog Mix75/25 has a duration of activity similar to that of Humulin 70/30.

Figure 3
Insulin activity after injection of Humalog, Humalog Mix50/50, Humalog Mix75/25, or insulin lispro protamine suspension (NPL component) in 30 nondiabetic subjects.

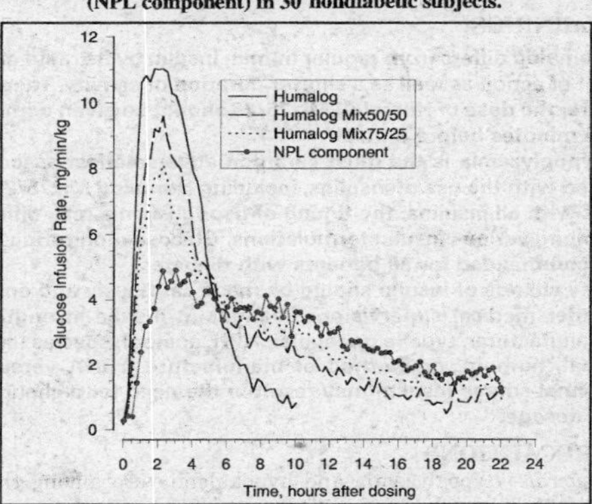

[See figure 4 above]

Figures 3 and 4 represent insulin activity profiles as measured by glucose clamp studies in healthy nondiabetic subjects.

Figure 3 shows the time activity profiles of Humalog, Humalog Mix75/25, Humalog Mix50/50, and insulin lispro protamine suspension (NPL component).

Figure 4 is a comparison of the time activity profiles of Humalog Mix75/25 (Figure 4a) and of Humulin 70/30 (Figure 4b) from two different studies.

Special Populations—

Age and Gender—Information on the effect of age on the pharmacokinetics of Humalog Mix75/25 is unavailable. Pharmacokinetic and pharmacodynamic comparisons between men and women administered Humalog Mix75/25 showed no gender differences. In large Humalog clinical trials, subgroup analyses based upon age and gender demonstrated that differences between Humalog and regular human insulin in postprandial glucose parameters are maintained across sub-groups.

Smoking—The effect of smoking on the pharmacokinetics and glucodynamics of Humalog Mix75/25 has not been studied.

Pregnancy—The effect of pregnancy on the pharmacokinetics and glucodynamics of Humalog Mix75/25 has not been studied.

Obesity—The effect of obesity and/or subcutaneous fat thickness on the pharmacokinetics and glucodynamics of Humalog Mix75/25 has not been studied. In large clinical trials, which included patients with Body-Mass-Index up to and including 35 kg/m², no consistent differences were observed between Humalog and Humulin R with respect to postprandial glucose parameters.

Renal Impairment—The effect of renal impairment on the pharmacokinetics and glucodynamics of Humalog Mix75/25

Continued on next page

*** Identi-Code® symbol. This product information was prepared in June 2000. Current information on these and other products of Eli Lilly and Company may be obtained by direct inquiry to Lilly Research Laboratories, Lilly Corporate Center, Indianapolis, Indiana 46285, (800) 545-5979.**

Humalog Mix—Cont.

has not been studied. In a study of 25 patients with type 2 diabetes and a wide range of renal function, the pharmacokinetic differences between Humalog and human regular insulin were generally maintained. However, the sensitivity of the patients to insulin did change, with an increased response to insulin as the renal function declined. Careful glucose monitoring and dose reductions of insulin, including Humalog Mix75/25, may be necessary in patients with renal dysfunction.

Hepatic Impairment—Some studies with human insulin have shown increased circulating levels of insulin in patients with hepatic failure. The effect of hepatic impairment on the pharmacokinetics and glucodynamics of Humalog Mix75/25 has not been studied. However, in a study of 22 patients with type 2 diabetes, impaired hepatic function did not affect the subcutaneous absorption or general disposition of Humalog when compared to patients with no history of hepatic dysfunction. In that study, Humalog maintained its more rapid absorption and elimination when compared to regular human insulin. Careful glucose monitoring and dose adjustments of insulin, including Humalog Mix75/25, may be necessary in patients with hepatic dysfunction.

INDICATIONS AND USAGE

Humalog Mix75/25, a mixture of 75% insulin lispro protamine suspension and 25% insulin lispro, is indicated in the treatment of patients with diabetes mellitus for the control of hyperglycemia. Humalog Mix75/25 has a more rapid onset of glucose-lowering activity compared to Humulin 70/30 while having a similar duration of action. This profile is achieved by combining the rapid onset of Humalog with the intermediate action of insulin lispro protamine suspension.

CONTRAINDICATIONS

Humalog Mix75/25 is contraindicated during episodes of hypoglycemia and in patients sensitive to insulin lispro or any of the excipients contained in the formulation.

WARNINGS

Humalog differs from regular human insulin by its rapid onset of action as well as a shorter duration of activity. Therefore, the dose of Humalog Mix75/25 should be given within 15 minutes before a meal.

Hypoglycemia is the most common adverse effect associated with the use of insulins, including Humalog Mix75/25. As with all insulins, the timing of hypoglycemia may differ among various insulin formulations. Glucose monitoring is recommended for all patients with diabetes.

Any change of insulin should be made cautiously and only under medical supervision. Changes in insulin strength, manufacturer, type (e.g., regular, NPH, analog), species (animal, human), or method of manufacture (rDNA versus animal-source insulin) may result in the need for a change in dosage.

PRECAUTIONS

General—Hypoglycemia and hypokalemia are among the potential clinical adverse effects associated with the use of all insulins. Because of differences in the action of Humalog Mix75/25 and other insulins, care should be taken in patients in whom such potential side effects might be clinically relevant (e.g., patients who are fasting, have autonomic neuropathy, or are using potassium-lowering drugs or patients taking drugs sensitive to serum potassium level). Lipodystrophy and hypersensitivity are among other potential clinical adverse effects associated with the use of all insulins.

As with all insulin preparations, the time course of action of Humalog Mix75/25 may vary in different individuals or at different times in the same individual and is dependent on site of injection, blood supply, temperature, and physical activity.

Adjustment of dosage of any insulin may be necessary if patients change their physical activity or their usual meal plan. Insulin requirements may be altered during illness, emotional disturbances, or other stress.

Hypoglycemia—As with all insulin preparations, hypoglycemic reactions may be associated with the administration of Humalog Mix75/25. Rapid changes in serum glucose concentrations may induce symptoms of hypoglycemia in persons with diabetes, regardless of the glucose value. Early warning symptoms of hypoglycemia may be different or less pronounced under certain conditions, such as long duration of diabetes, diabetic nerve disease, use of medications such as beta-blockers, or intensified diabetes control.

Renal Impairment—As with other insulins, the requirements for Humalog Mix75/25 may be reduced in patients with renal impairment.

Hepatic Impairment—Although impaired hepatic function does not affect the absorption or disposition of Humalog, careful glucose monitoring and dose adjustments of insulin, including Humalog Mix75/25, may be necessary.

Allergy—Local Allergy—As with any insulin therapy, patients may experience redness, swelling, or itching at the site of injection. These minor reactions usually resolve in a few days to a few weeks. In some instances, these reactions may be related to factors other than insulin, such as irritants in a skin cleansing agent or poor injection technique.

Systemic Allergy—Less common, but potentially more serious, is generalized allergy to insulin, which may cause rash (including pruritus) over the whole body, shortness of breath, wheezing, reduction in blood pressure, rapid pulse, or sweating. Severe cases of generalized allergy, including anaphylactic reaction, may be life threatening. Localized reactions and generalized myalgias have been reported with the use of cresol as an injectable excipient.

Antibody Production—In clinical trials, antibodies that cross react with human insulin and insulin lispro were observed in both human insulin mixtures and insulin lispro mixtures treatment groups.

Information for Patients—Patients should be informed of the potential risks and advantages of Humalog Mix75/25 and alternative therapies. Patients should not mix Humalog Mix75/25 with any other insulin. They should also be informed about the importance of proper insulin storage, injection technique, timing of dosage, adherence to meal planning, regular physical activity, regular blood glucose monitoring, periodic glycosylated hemoglobin testing, recognition and management of hypo- and hyperglycemia, and periodic assessment for diabetes complications.

Patients should be advised to inform their physician if they are pregnant or intend to become pregnant.

Refer patients to the Information for the Patient insert for information on normal appearance, proper resuspension and injection techniques, timing of dosing (within 15 minutes before a meal), storing, and common adverse effects.

Laboratory Tests—As with all insulins, the therapeutic response to Humalog Mix75/25 should be monitored by periodic blood glucose tests. Periodic measurement of glycosylated hemoglobin is recommended for the monitoring of long-term glycemic control.

Drug Interactions—Insulin requirements may be increased by medications with hyperglycemic activity such as corticosteroids, isoniazid, certain lipid-lowering drugs (e.g., niacin), estrogens, oral contraceptives, phenothiazines, and thyroid replacement therapy.

Insulin requirements may be decreased in the presence of drugs with hypoglycemic activity, such as oral antidiabetic agents, salicylates, sulfa antibiotics, certain antidepressants (monoamine oxidase inhibitors), certain angiotensin-converting-enzyme inhibitors, beta-adrenergic blockers, inhibitors of pancreatic function (e.g., octreotide), and alcohol. Beta-adrenergic blockers may mask the symptoms of hypoglycemia in some patients.

Carcinogenesis, Mutagenesis, Impairment of Fertility—Long-term studies in animals have not been performed to evaluate the carcinogenic potential of Humalog or Humalog Mix75/25. Insulin lispro was not mutagenic in a battery of *in vitro* and *in vivo* genetic toxicity assays (bacterial mutation tests, unscheduled DNA synthesis, mouse lymphoma assay, chromosomal aberration tests, and a micronucleus test). There is no evidence from animal studies of impairment of fertility induced by insulin lispro.

Pregnancy—Teratogenic Effects—Pregnancy Category B—Reproduction studies with insulin lispro have been performed in pregnant rats and rabbits at parenteral doses up to 4 and 0.3 times, respectively, the average human dose (40 units/day) based on body surface area. The results have revealed no evidence of impaired fertility or harm to the fetus due to insulin lispro. There are, however, no adequate and well-controlled studies with Humalog or Humalog Mix75/25 in pregnant women. Because animal reproduction studies are not always predictive of human response, this drug should be used during pregnancy only if clearly needed.

Nursing Mothers—It is unknown whether insulin lispro is excreted in significant amounts in human milk. Many drugs, including human insulin, are excreted in human milk. For this reason, caution should be exercised when Humalog Mix75/25 is administered to a nursing woman. Patients with diabetes who are lactating may require adjustments in Humalog Mix75/25 dose, meal plan, or both.

Pediatric Use—Safety and effectiveness of Humalog Mix75/25 in patients less than 18 years of age have not been established.

Geriatric Use—Clinical studies of Humalog Mix75/25 did not include sufficient numbers of patients aged 65 and over to determine whether they respond differently than younger patients. In general, dose selection for an elderly patient should take into consideration the greater frequency of decreased hepatic, renal, or cardiac function, and of concomitant disease or other drug therapy in this population.

ADVERSE REACTIONS

Clinical studies comparing Humalog Mix75/25 with human insulin mixtures did not demonstrate a difference in frequency of adverse events between the two treatments.

Adverse events commonly associated with human insulin therapy include the following:

Body as a Whole—allergic reactions (*see* PRECAUTIONS)

Skin and Appendages—injection site reaction, lipodystrophy, pruritus, rash

Other—hypoglycemia (*see* WARNINGS *and* PRECAUTIONS)

OVERDOSAGE

Hypoglycemia may occur as a result of an excess of insulin relative to food intake, energy expenditure, or both. Mild episodes of hypoglycemia usually can be treated with oral glucose. Adjustments in drug dosage, meal patterns, or exercise, may be needed. More severe episodes with coma, seizure, or neurologic impairment may be treated with intramuscular/subcutaneous glucagon or concentrated intravenous glucose. Sustained carbohydrate intake and observation may be necessary because hypoglycemia may recur after apparent clinical recovery.

DOSAGE AND ADMINISTRATION

[See table 1 below]

Humalog Mix75/25 is intended only for subcutaneous administration. Humalog Mix75/25 should not be administered intravenously. Dosage regimens of Humalog Mix75/25 will vary among patients and should be determined by the health care professional familiar with the patient's metabolic needs, eating habits, and other lifestyle variables. Humalog has been shown to be equipotent to regular human insulin on a molar basis. One unit of Humalog has the same glucose-lowering effect as one unit of regular human insulin, but its effect is more rapid and of shorter duration. Humalog Mix75/25 has a similar glucose-lowering effect as compared to Humulin 70/30 on a unit for unit basis. The quicker glucose-lowering effect of Humalog is related to the more rapid absorption rate of insulin lispro from subcutaneous tissue.

Humalog Mix75/25 starts lowering blood glucose more quickly than regular human insulin, allowing for convenient dosing immediately before a meal (within 15 minutes). In contrast, mixtures containing regular human insulin should be given 30–60 minutes before a meal.

The rate of insulin absorption and consequently the onset of activity are known to be affected by the site of injection, exercise, and other variables. As with all insulin preparations, the time course of action of Humalog Mix75/25 may vary considerably in different individuals or within the same individual. Patients must be educated to use proper injection techniques.

Humalog Mix75/25 should be inspected visually before use. Humalog Mix75/25 should be used only if it appears uniformly cloudy after mixing. Humalog Mix75/25 should not be used after its expiration date.

Table 1*
Summary of glucodynamic properties of insulin products (pooled cross-study comparison)

Insulin Products	Dose, U/kg	Time of peak activity, hours after dosing	Percent of total activity occurring in the first 4 hours
Humalog	0.3	2.4 (0.8–4.3)	70% (49–89%)
Humulin R	0.32 (0.26–0.37)	4.4 (4.0–5.5)	54% (38–65%)
Humalog Mix75/25	0.3	2.6 (1.0–6.5)	35% (21–56%)
Humulin 70/30	0.3	4.4 (1.5–16)	32% (14–60%)
Humalog Mix50/50	0.3	2.3 (0.8–4.8)	45% (27–69%)
Humulin 50/50	0.3	3.3 (2.0–5.5)	44% (21–60%)
NPH	0.32 (0.27–0.40)	5.5 (3.5–9.5)	14% (3.0–48%)
NPL component	0.3	5.8 (1.3–18.3)	22% (6.3–40%)

*The information supplied in Table 1 indicates when peak insulin activity can be expected and the percent of the total insulin activity occurring during the first 4 hours. The information was derived from 3 separate glucose clamp studies in nondiabetic subjects. Values represent means, with ranges provided in parentheses.

HOW SUPPLIED

Humalog Mix75/25 Pen, a disposable insulin delivery device, is available in the following package size:
5 × 3 mL disposable insulin delivery devices
NDC 0002-8794-59 (HP-8794)

Storage—Humalog Mix75/25 should be stored in a refrigerator (2° to 8°C [36° to 46°F]) before use, but not in the freezer. However, Humalog Mix75/25 Pens in use can be kept unrefrigerated at room temperature for up to 10 days, as long as they are kept as cool as possible and away from direct heat and light. Unrefrigerated Pens must be used within the specified time period or be discarded. Do not use Humalog Mix75/25 if it has been frozen.
Literature issued December, 1999

Manufactured by Lilly France S.A.
F-67640 Fegersheim, France
For Eli Lilly and Company
Indianapolis, IN 46285, USA

PA 9220 FSAMP

HUMATROPE® ℞

[*hū 'ma-trōp*]
somatropin (rDNA origin) for injection
VIALS
and
CARTRIDGES FOR USE WITH THE HumatroPen™ INJECTION DEVICE

DESCRIPTION

Humatrope® (Somatropin, rDNA Origin, for Injection) is a polypeptide hormone of recombinant DNA origin. Humatrope has 191 amino acid residues and a molecular weight of about 22,125 daltons. The amino acid sequence of the product is identical to that of human growth hormone of pituitary origin. Humatrope is synthesized in a strain of *Escherichia coli* that has been modified by the addition of the gene for human growth hormone.
Humatrope is a sterile, white, lyophilized powder intended for subcutaneous or intramuscular administration after reconstitution. Humatrope is a highly purified preparation. Phosphoric acid and/or sodium hydroxide may have been added to adjust the pH. Reconstituted solutions have a pH of approximately 7.5. This product is oxygen sensitive.
VIAL—Each vial of Humatrope contains 5 mg somatropin (15 IU or 225 nanomoles); 25 mg mannitol; 5 mg glycine; and 1.13 mg dibasic sodium phosphate. Each vial is supplied in a combination package with an accompanying 5-mL vial of diluting solution. The diluent contains water for injection with 0.3% Metacresol as a preservative and 1.7% glycerin.
CARTRIDGE—The cartridges of somatropin contain either 6 mg (18 IU), 12 mg (36 IU), or 24 mg (72 IU) of somatropin. The 6 mg, 12 mg and 24 mg cartridges contain respectively: mannitol 18 mg, 36 mg, and 72 mg; glycine 6 mg, 12 mg, and 24 mg; dibasic sodium phosphate 1.36 mg, 2.72 mg, and 5.43 mg. Each cartridge is supplied in a combination package with an accompanying syringe containing approximately 3 mL of diluting solution. The diluent contains Water for Injection; 0.3% Metacresol as a preservative; and 1.7%, 0.29%, and 0.29% gylcerin in the 6 mg, 12 mg, and 24 mg cartridges respectively.

CLINICAL PHARMACOLOGY

General: *Linear Growth*—Humatrope stimulates linear growth in pediatric patients who lack adequate normal endogenous growth hormone. In vitro, preclinical, and clinical testing have demonstrated that Humatrope is therapeutically equivalent to human growth hormone of pituitary origin and achieves equivalent pharmacokinetic profiles in normal adults. Treatment of growth hormone-deficient pediatric patients and patients with Turner syndrome with Humatrope produces increased growth rate and IGF-I (Insulin-like Growth Factor-I/Somatomedin-C) concentrations similar to those seen after therapy with human growth hormone of pituitary origin.
In addition, the following actions have been demonstrated for Humatrope and/or human growth hormone of pituitary origin.
A. *Tissue Growth*—1. Skeletal Growth: Humatrope stimulates skeletal growth in pediatric patients with growth hormone deficiency. The measurable increase in body length after administration of either Humatrope or human growth hormone of pituitary origin results from an effect on the growth plates of long bones. Concentrations of IGF-I, which may play a role in skeletal growth, are low in the serum of growth hormone-deficient pediatric patients but increase during treatment with Humatrope. Elevations in mean serum alkaline phosphatase concentrations are also seen. 2. Cell Growth: It has been shown that there are fewer skeletal muscle cells in short-statured pediatric patients who lack endogenous growth hormone as compared with normal pediatric populations. Treatment with human growth hormone of pituitary origin results in an increase in both the number and size of muscle cells.
B. *Protein Metabolism*—Linear growth is facilitated in part by increased cellular protein synthesis. Nitrogen retention, as demonstrated by decreased urinary nitrogen excretion and serum urea nitrogen, follows the initiation of therapy with human growth hormone of pituitary origin. Treatment with Humatrope results in a similar decrease in serum urea nitrogen.
C. *Carbohydrate Metabolism*—Pediatric patients with hypopituitarism sometimes experience fasting hypoglycemia that is improved by treatment with Humatrope. Large doses of human growth hormone may impair glucose tolerance. Untreated patients with Turner syndrome have an increased incidence of glucose intolerance. Administration of human growth hormone to normal adults or patients with Turner syndrome resulted in increases in mean serum fasting and postprandial insulin levels although mean values remained in the normal range. In addition, mean fasting and postprandial glucose and hemoglobin A_{1C} levels remained in the normal range.
D. *Lipid Metabolism*—In growth hormone-deficient patients, administration of human growth hormone of pituitary origin has resulted in lipid mobilization, reduction in body fat stores, and increased plasma fatty acids.
E. *Mineral Metabolism*—Retention of sodium, potassium, and phosphorus is induced by human growth hormone of pituitary origin. Serum concentrations of inorganic phosphate increased in patients with growth hormone deficiency after therapy with Humatrope or human growth hormone of pituitary origin. Serum calcium is not significantly altered in patients treated with either human growth hormone of pituitary origin or Humatrope.
PHARMACOKINETICS: Absorption—Humatrope has been studied following intramuscular, subcutaneous, and intravenous administration in adult volunteers. The absolute bioavailability of somatropin is 75% and 63% after subcutaneous and intramuscular administration, respectively.
Distribution—The volume of distribution of somatropin after intravenous injection is about 0.07 L/kg.
Metabolism—Extensive metabolism studies have not been conducted. The metabolic fate of somatropin involves classical protein catabolism in both the liver and kidneys. In renal cells, at least a portion of the breakdown products of growth hormone is returned to the systemic circulation. In normal volunteers, mean clearance is 0.14 L/hr/kg. The mean half-life of intravenous somatropin is 0.36 hours, whereas subcutaneously and intramuscularly administered somatropin have mean half-lives of 3.8 and 4.9 hours, respectively. The longer half-life observed after subcutaneous or intramuscular administration is due to slow absorption from the injection site.
Excretion—Urinary excretion of intact Humatrope has not been measured. Small amounts of somatropin have been detected in the urine of pediatric patients following replacement therapy.

Special Populations

Geriatric—The pharmacokinetics of Humatrope has not been studied in patients greater than 60 years of age.
Pediatric—The pharmacokinetics of Humatrope in pediatric patients is similar to adults.
Gender—No studies have been performed with Humatrope. The available literature indicates that the pharmacokinetics of growth hormone is similar in both men and women.
Race—No data are available.
Renal, Hepatic insufficiency—No studies have been performed with Humatrope.
[See table 1 above]

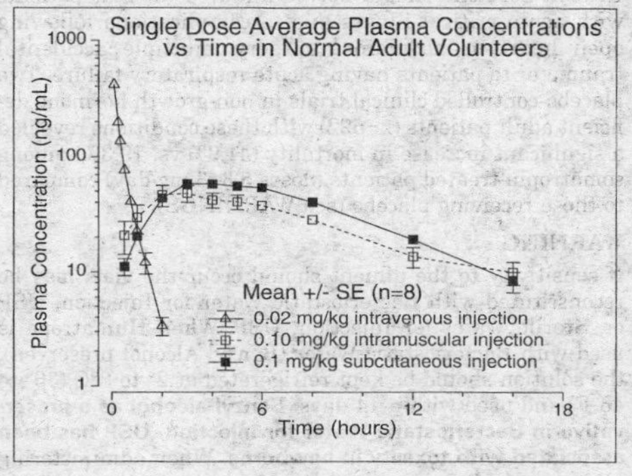

Table 1
Summary of Somatropin Parameters in the Normal Population

	C_{max} (ng/mL)	$t_{1/2}$ (hr)	$AUC_{0-\infty}$ (ng•hr/mL)	Cls (L/kg•hr)	Vβ (L/kg)
0.02 mg (0.05 IU*)/kg iv					
MEAN	415	0.363	156	0.135	0.0703
SD	75	0.053	33	0.029	0.0173
0.1 mg (0.27 IU*)/kg im					
MEAN	53.2	4.93	495	0.215	1.55
SD	25.9	2.66	106	0.047	0.91
0.1 mg (0.27 IU*)/kg sc					
MEAN	63.3	3.81	585	0.179	0.957
SD	18.2	1.40	90	0.028	0.301

Abbreviations: C_{max} = maximum concentration: $t_{1/2}$ = half-life; $AUC_{0-\infty}$= area under the curve; CIs = systemic clearance; Vβ = volume distribution; iv = intravenous; SD = standard deviation; im = intramuscular; sc = subcutaneous.
*Based on previous International Standard of 2.7 IU = 1 mg

Single Dose Average Plasma Concentrations vs Time in Normal Adult Volunteers

Plasma Concentration (ng/mL)
Time (hours)
Mean +/- SE (n=8)
0.02 mg/kg intravenous injection
0.10 mg/kg intramuscular injection
0.1 mg/kg subcutaneous injection

Effects of Humatrope treatment in adults with growth hormone deficiency

Two multicenter trials in adult onset growth hormone deficiency (n=98) and two studies in childhood onset growth hormone deficiency (n=67) were designed to assess the effects of replacement therapy with Humatrope. The primary efficacy measures were body composition (lean body mass and fat mass), lipid parameters, and the Nottingham Health Profile. The Nottingham Health Profile is a general health-related quality of life questionnaire. These four studies each included a 6-month randomized, blinded, placebo-controlled phase followed by 12 months of open-label therapy for all patients. The Humatrope dosages for all studies were identical: one month of therapy at 0.00625 mg/kg/day followed by the proposed maintenance dose of 0.0125 mg/kg/day. Adult onset patients and childhood onset patients differed by diagnosis (organic versus idiopathic pituitary disease), body size (normal versus small for mean height and weight), and age (mean = 44 versus 29 years). Lean body mass was determined by bioelectrical impedance analysis (BIA), validated with potassium 40. Body fat was assessed by BIA and sum of skinfold thickness. Lipid subfractions were analyzed by standard assay methods in a central laboratory.
Humatrope-treated adult onset patients, as compared to placebo, experienced an increase in lean body mass (2.59 versus -0.22 kg, $p<0.001$) and a decrease in body fat (-3.27 versus 0.56 kg, $p<0.001$). Similar changes were seen in childhood onset growth hormone deficient patients. These significant changes in lean body mass persisted throughout the 18 month period as compared to baseline for both groups, and for fat mass in the childhood onset group. Total cholesterol decreased short term (first 3 months) although the changes did not persist. However, the low HDL cholesterol levels observed at baseline (mean = 30.1 mg/mL and 33.9 mg/mL in adult onset and childhood onset patients) normalized by the end of 18 months of therapy (a change of 13.7 and 11.1 mg/dL for the adult onset and childhood onset groups, $p<0.001$). Adult onset patients reported significant improvements as compared to placebo in the following 2 of 6 possible health related domains: physical mobility and social isolation (Table 2). Patients with childhood onset disease failed to demonstrate improvements in Nottingham Health Profile outcomes.
Two additional studies on the effect of Humatrope on exercise capacity were also conducted. Improved physical function was documented by increased exercise capacity (VO_2 max, $p<0.005$) and work performance (Watts, $p<0.01$) (J Clin Endocrinol Metab 1995; 80:552-557).

Table 2
Changes[a] in Nottingham Health Profile Scores[b] in Adult Onset Growth Hormone Deficient Patients

Outcome Measure	Placebo (6 Months)	Humatrope Therapy (6 Months)	Significance
Energy Level	−11.4	−15.5	NS
Physical Mobility	−3.1	−10.5	p <0.01
Social Isolation	0.5	−4.7	p <0.01
Emotional Reactions	−4.5	−5.4	NS

Continued on next page

*** Identi-Code® symbol. This product information was prepared in June 2000. Current information on these and other products of Eli Lilly and Company may be obtained by direct inquiry to Lilly Research Laboratories, Lilly Corporate Center, Indianapolis, Indiana 46285, (800) 545-5979.**

Humatrope—Cont.

Sleep	−6.4	−3.7	NS
Pain	−2.8	−2.9	NS

[a]=An improvement in score is indicated by a more negative change in the score.
[b]=To account for multiple analyses, appropriate statistical methods were applied and the required level of significance is 0.01.
NS = not significant

Effects of growth hormone treatment in patients with Turner syndrome

One long-term, randomized, open-label multicenter concurrently controlled study, two long-term, open-label multicenter, historically controlled studies and one long-term, randomized, dose-response study were conducted to evaluate the efficacy of growth hormone for the treatment of patients with short stature due to Turner syndrome.

In the randomized study, GDCT, comparing growth hormone-treated patients to a concurrent control group who received no growth hormone, the growth hormone-treated patients who received a dose of 0.3 mg/kg/week given 6 times per week from a mean age of 11.7 years for a mean duration of 4.7 years attained a mean near final height of 146.0 ± 6.2 cm (n=27, mean ± SD) as compared to the control group who attained a near final height of 142.1 ± 4.8 cm (n=19). By analysis of covariance*, the effect of growth hormone therapy was a mean height increase of 5.4 cm (p = 0.001).

* Analysis of covariance includes adjustments for baseline height relative to age and for mid-parental height.

In two of the studies (85-023 and 85-044), the effect of long-term growth hormone treatment (0.375 mg/kg/week given either 3 times per week or daily) on adult height was determined by comparing adult heights in the treated patients with those of age-matched historical controls with Turner syndrome who never received any growth-promoting therapy. The greatest improvement in adult height was observed in patients who received early growth hormone treatment and estrogen after age 14 years. In Study 85-023, this resulted in a mean adult height gain of 7.4 cm (mean duration of GH therapy of 7.6 years) vs. matched historical controls by analysis of covariance.

In Study 85-044, patients treated with early growth hormone therapy were randomized to receive estrogen replacement therapy (conjugated estrogens, 0.3 mg escalating to 0.625 mg daily) at either age 12 or 15 years. Compared with matched historical controls, early GH therapy (mean duration of GH therapy 5.6 years) combined with estrogen replacement at age 12 years resulted in an adult height gain of 5.9 cm (n=26), whereas patients who initiated estrogen at age 15 years (mean duration of GH therapy 6.1 years) had a mean adult height gain of 8.3 cm (n=29). Patients who initiated GH therapy after age 11 (mean age 12.7 years; mean duration of GH therapy 3.8 years) had a mean adult height gain of 5.0 cm (n=51).

In a randomized blinded dose-response study, GDCI, patients were treated from a mean age of 11.1 years for a mean duration of 5.3 years with a weekly dose of either 0.27 mg/kg or 0.36 mg/kg administered 3 or 6 times weekly. The mean near final height of patients receiving growth hormone was 148.7 ±6.5 cm (n=31). When compared to historical control data, the mean gain in adult height was approximately 5 cm.

In some studies, Turner syndrome patients (n=181) treated to final adult height achieved statistically significant average height gains ranging from 5.0 - 8.3 cm.
[See table 3 above]

Table 3
Summary Table of Efficacy Results

Study/ Group	Study Design[a]	N at Adult Height	GH Age (yr)	Estrogen Age (yr)	GH Duration (yr)	Adult Height Gain (cm)[b]
GDCT	RCT	27	11.7	13	4.7	5.4
85-023	MHT	17	9.1	15.2	7.6	7.4
85-044: A*	MHT	29	9.4	15	6.1	8.3
B*		26	9.6	12.3	5.6	5.9
C*		51	12.7	13.7	3.8	5
GDCI	RDT	31	11.1	8–13.5	5.3	~5[c]

[a] RCT: randomized controlled trial; MHT: matched historical controlled trial; RDT: randomized dose-response trial.
[b] Analysis of covariance vs controls
[c] Compared with historical data
* A: GH age <11 yr, estrogen age 15 yr
B: GH age <11 yr, estrogen age 12 yr
C: GH age >11 yr, estrogen at month 12

Table 4
Treatment-Emergent Events of Special Interest by Treatment Group in Turner Syndrome

		Treatment Group		
Adverse Event	Overall	hGH[1]	Untreated[2]	Significance
Total Number of Patients	136	74	62	
Surgical Procedure	50 (36.8%)	33 (44.6%)	17 (27.4%)	p≤0.05
Otitis Media	48 (35.3%)	32 (43.2%)	16 (25.8%)	p≤0.05
Ear Disorders	16 (11.8%)	13 (17.6%)	3 (4.8%)	p≤0.05
Bone Disorder	13 (9.6%)	6 (8.1%)	7 (11.3%)	NS
Edema				
Conjunctival	1 (0.7%)	0	1 (1.6%)	NS
Non-specific	3 (2.2%)	2 (2.7%)	1 (1.6%)	NS
Facial	1 (0.7%)	1 (1.4%)	0	NS
Peripheral	6 (4.4%)	5 (6.8%)	1 (1.6%)	NS
Hyperglycemia	0	0	0	NS
Hypothyroidism	15 (11.0%)	10 (13.5%)	5 (8.1%)	NS
Increased Nevi[3]	10 (7.4%)	8 (10.8%)	2 (3.2%)	NS
Lymphedema	0	0	0	NS

[1] Dose = 0.3 mg/kg/week
[2] Open label study
[3] Includes any nevi coded to the following preferred terms: melanosis, skin hypertrophy, or skin benign neoplasm.
NS = not significant

Table 5
Treatment-Emergent Adverse Events with ≥5% Overall Incidence in Adult Onset Growth Hormone Deficient Patients Treated with Humatrope for 18 Months as Compared with 6 Month Placebo and 12 Month Humatrope Exposure

	18 Months Exposure [Placebo (6 Months)/hGH (12 Months)] (N=46)		18 Months hGH Exposure (N=52)	
Adverse Event	n	%	n	%
Edema[a]	7	15.2	11	21.2
Arthralgia	7	15.2	9	17.3
Paresthesia	6	13.0	9	17.3
Myalgia	6	13.0	7	13.5
Pain	6	13.0	7	13.5
Rhinitis	5	10.9	7	13.5
Peripheral Edema[b]	8	17.4	6	11.5
Back Pain	5	10.9	5	9.6
Headache	5	10.9	4	7.7
Hypertension	2	4.3	4	7.7
Acne	0	0	3	5.8
Joint Disorder	1	2.2	3	5.8
Surgical Procedure	1	2.2	3	5.8
Flu Syndrome	3	6.5	2	3.9

Abbreviations: hGH = Humatrope; N = number of patients receiving treatment in the period stated; n = number of patients reporting each treatment-emergent adverse event.
[a]p = 0.04 as compared to placebo (6 months)
[b]p = 0.02 as compared to placebo (6 months)

INDICATIONS AND USAGE

Pediatric Patients—Humatrope is indicated for the long-term treatment of pediatric patients who have growth failure due to an inadequate secretion of normal endogenous growth hormone.

Humatrope is indicated for the treatment of short stature associated with Turner syndrome in patients whose epiphyses are not closed.

Adult Patients—Humatrope is indicated for replacement of endogenous growth hormone in adults with growth hormone deficiency who meet both of the following two criteria:

1. Adult Onset: Patients who have growth hormone deficiency either alone or with multiple hormone deficiencies (hypopituitarism), as a result of pituitary disease, hypothalamic disease, surgery, radiation therapy, or trauma;

or

Childhood Onset: Patients who were growth hormone-deficient during childhood who have growth hormone deficiency confirmed as an adult before replacement therapy with Humatrope is started.

and

2. Biochemical diagnosis of growth hormone deficiency, by means of a negative response to a standard growth hormone stimulation test [maximum peak < 5 ng/mL when measured by RIA (polyclonal antibody) or < 2.5 ng/mL when measured by IRMA (monoclonal antibody)].

CONTRAINDICATIONS

Humatrope should not be used for growth promotion in pediatric patients with closed epiphyses.

Humatrope should not be used or should be discontinued when there is any evidence of active malignancy. Antimalignancy treatment must be complete with evidence of remission prior to the institution of therapy.

Humatrope should **not** be reconstituted with the supplied Diluent for Humatrope for use by patients with a known sensitivity to either Metacresol or glycerin.

Growth hormone should not be initiated to treat patients with acute critical illness due to complications following open heart or abdominal surgery, multiple accidental trauma or to patients having acute respiratory failure. Two placebo-controlled clinical trials in non-growth hormone deficient adult patients (n=522) with these conditions revealed a significant increase in mortality (41.9% vs. 19.3%) among somatropin treated patients (doses 5.3–8 mg/day) compared to those receiving placebo (see WARNINGS).

WARNING

If sensitivity to the diluent should occur the **vials** may be reconstituted with Bacteriostatic Water for Injection, USP or, Sterile Water for Injection, USP. When Humatrope is used with Bacteriostatic Water (Benzyl Alcohol preserved), the solution should be kept refrigerated at 2° to 8°C (36° to 46°F) and used within 14 days. **Benzyl alcohol as a preservative in Bacteriostatic Water for Injection, USP has been associated with toxicity in newborns.** When administering Humatrope to newborns, use the Humatrope diluent provided or if the patient is sensitive to the diluent, use Sterile Water for Injection, USP. When Humatrope is reconstituted with Sterile Water for Injection, USP in this manner, use only one dose per Humatrope vial and discard the unused portion. If the solution is not used immediately, it must be refrigerated (2° to 8°C [36° to 46°F]) and used within 24 hours.

Cartridges should be reconstituted only with the supplied diluent. Cartridges should not be reconstituted with the Diluent for Humatrope provided with Humatrope Vials, or with any other solution. Cartridges should not be used if the patient is allergic to Metacresol or glycerin.

See CONTRAINDICATIONS for information on increased mortality in patients with acute critical illnesses in intensive care units due to complications following open heart or abdominal surgery, multiple accidental trauma or with acute respiratory failure. The safety of continuing growth hormone treatment in patients receiving replacement doses for approved indications who concurrently develop these illnesses has not been established. Therefore, the potential benefit of treatment continuation with growth hormone in patients having acute critical illnesses should be weighed against the potential risk.

PRECAUTIONS

General—Therapy with Humatrope should be directed by physicians who are experienced in the diagnosis and man-

agement of patients with growth hormone deficiency, Turner syndrome or adult patients with either childhood-onset or adult-onset growth hormone deficiency.
Patients with preexisting tumors or with growth hormone deficiency secondary to an intracranial lesion should be examined routinely for progression or recurrence of the underlying disease process. In pediatric patients, clinical literature has demonstrated no relationship between somatropin replacement therapy and CNS tumor recurrence. In adults, it is unknown whether there is any relationship between somatropin replacement therapy and CNS tumor recurrence. Patients should be monitored carefully for any malignant transformation of skin lesions.
For patients with diabetes mellitus, the insulin dose may require adjustment when somatropin therapy is instituted. Because human growth hormone may induce a state of insulin resistance, patients should be observed for evidence of glucose intolerance. Patients with diabetes or glucose intolerance should be monitored closely during somatropin therapy.
In patients with hypopituitarism (multiple hormonal deficiencies) standard hormonal replacement therapy should be monitored closely when somatropin therapy is administered. Hypothyroidism may develop during treatment with somatropin, and inadequate treatment of hypothyroidism may prevent optimal response to somatropin.
Pediatric Patients (*see* General Precautions)—Pediatric patients with endocrine disorders, including growth hormone deficiency, may develop slipped capital epiphyses more frequently. Any pediatric patient with the onset of a limp during growth hormone therapy should be evaluated.
Growth hormone has not been shown to increase the incidence of scoliosis. Progression of scoliosis can occur in children who experience rapid growth. Because growth hormone increases growth rate, patients with a history of scoliosis who are treated with growth hormone should be monitored for progression of scoliosis. Skeletal abnormalities including scoliosis are commonly seen in untreated Turner syndrome patients.
Patients with Turner syndrome should be evaluated carefully for otitis media and other ear disorders since these patients have an increased risk of ear or hearing disorders (see Adverse Reactions). Patients with Turner syndrome are at risk for cardiovascular disorders (e.g. stroke, aortic aneurysm, hypertension) and these conditions should be monitored closely.
Patients with Turner syndrome have an inherently increased risk of developing autoimmune thyroid disease. Therefore, patients should have periodic thyroid function tests and be treated as indicated (*see* General Precautions).
Intracranial hypertension (IH) with papilledema, visual changes, headache, nausea and/or vomiting has been reported in a small number of pediatric patients treated with growth hormone products. Symptoms usually occurred within the first eight (8) weeks of the initiation of growth hormone therapy. In all reported cases, IH-associated signs and symptoms resolved after termination of therapy or a reduction of the growth hormone dose. Funduscopic examination of patients is recommended at the initiation and periodically during the course of growth hormone therapy. Patients with Turner syndrome may be at increased risk for development of IH.
Adult Patients (*see* General Precautions)—Patients with epiphyseal closure who were treated with growth hormone replacement therapy in childhood should be re-evaluated according to the criteria in *INDICATIONS AND USAGE* before continuation of somatropin therapy at the reduced dose level recommended for growth hormone-deficient adults.
Experience in patients above 60 years is lacking.
Experience with prolonged treatment in adults is limited.
Drug Interactions—Excessive glucocorticoid therapy may prevent optimal response to somatropin. If glucocorticoid replacement therapy is required, the glucocorticoid dosage and compliance should be monitored carefully to avoid either adrenal insufficiency or inhibition of growth promoting effects.
Limited published data indicate that growth hormone (GH) treatment increases cytochrome P450 (CP450) mediated antipyrine clearance in man. These data suggest that GH administration may alter the clearance of compounds known to be metabolized by CP450 liver enzymes (e.g., corticosteroids, sex steroids, anticonvulsants, cyclosporin). Careful monitoring is advisable when GH is administered in combination with other drugs known to be metabolized by CP450 liver enzymes.
Carcinogenesis, Mutagenesis, Impairment of Fertility—Long-term animal studies for carcinogenicity and impairment of fertility with this human growth hormone (Humatrope) have not been performed. There has been no evidence to date of Humatrope-induced mutagenicity.
Pregnancy—Pregnancy Category C—Animal reproduction studies have not been conducted with Humatrope. It is not known whether Humatrope can cause fetal harm when administered to a pregnant woman or can affect reproduction capacity. Humatrope should be given to a pregnant woman only if clearly needed.
Nursing Mothers—There have been no studies conducted with Humatrope in nursing mothers. It is not known whether this drug is excreted in human milk. Because many drugs are excreted in human milk, caution should be exercised when Humatrope is administered to a nursing woman.
Information for Patients—Patients being treated with growth hormone and/or their parents should be informed of the potential risks and benefits associated with treatment.

Table 6
Treatment-Emergent Adverse Events with ≥5% Overall Incidence in Childhood Onset Growth Hormone Deficient Patients Treated with Humatrope for 18 Months as Compared with 6 Month Placebo and 12 Month Humatrope Exposure

Adverse Event	18 Months Exposure [Placebo (6 Months)/hGH (12 Months)] (N=35)		18 Months hGH Exposure (N=32)	
	n	%	n	%
Flu Syndrome	8	22.9	5	15.6
AST Increased[a]	2	5.7	4	12.5
Headache	4	11.4	3	9.4
Asthenia	1	2.9	2	6.3
Cough Increased	0	0	2	6.3
Edema	3	8.6	2	6.3
Hypesthesia	0	0	2	6.3
Myalgia	2	5.7	2	6.3
Pain	3	8.6	2	6.3
Rhinitis	2	5.7	2	6.3
ALT Increased	2	5.7	2	6.3
Respiratory Disorder	2	5.7	1	3.1
Gastritis	2	5.7	0	0
Pharyngitis	5	14.3	1	3.1

Abbreviations: hGH = Humatrope; N = number of patients receiving treatment in the period stated; n = number of patients reporting each treatment-emergent adverse event; ALT = alanine amino transferase, formerly SGPT; AST = aspartate amino transferase, formerly SGOT.
[a]p = 0.03 as compared to placebo (6 months)

Table 7
Concentration of Reconstituted Humatrope Solutions, Incremental Dosage and Maximum Injectable Dose for Each Cartridge

Cartridge	Somatropin Concentration	Dose per click of dosage knob	Maximum Injectable Dose
6 mg	2.08 mg/mL	0.1 mg	1.2 mg
12 mg	4.17 mg/mL	0.2 mg	2.4 mg
24 mg	8.33 mg/mL	0.4 mg	4.8 mg

Instructions on appropriate use should be given, including a review of the contents of the patient information insert. This information is intended to aid in the safe and effective administration of the medication. It is not a disclosure of all possible adverse or intended effects.
Patients and/or parents should be thoroughly instructed in the importance of proper needle disposal. A puncture resistant container should be used for the disposal of used needles and/or syringes (consistent with applicable state requirements). Needles and syringes must not be reused (*see* Information for Patient insert).

ADVERSE REACTIONS
Growth-Hormone Deficient Pediatric Patients—As with all protein pharmaceuticals, a small percentage of patients may develop antibodies to the protein. During the first six months of Humatrope therapy in 314 naive patients, only 1.6% developed specific antibodies to Humatrope (binding capacity ≥ 0.02 mg/L). None had antibody concentrations which exceeded 2 mg/L. Throughout 8 years of this same study, 2 patients (0.6%) had binding capacity >2 mg/L. Neither patient demonstrated a decrease in growth velocity at or near the time of increased antibody production. It has been reported that growth attenuation from pituitary-derived growth hormone may occur when antibody concentrations are >1.5 mg/L.
In addition to an evaluation of compliance with the treatment program and of thyroid status, testing for antibodies to human growth hormone should be carried out in any patient who fails to respond to therapy.
In studies with growth hormone-deficient pediatric patients, injection site pain was reported infrequently. A mild and transient edema, which appeared in 2.5% of patients, was observed early during the course of treatment.
Leukemia has been reported in a small number of pediatric patients who have been treated with growth hormone, including growth hormone of pituitary origin as well as of recombinant DNA origin (somatrem and somatropin). The relationship, if any, between leukemia and growth hormone therapy is uncertain.
Turner Syndrome Patients—In a randomized, concurrent controlled trial, there was a statistically significant increase, in the occurence of otitis media (43% vs 26%), ear disorders (18% vs 5%) and surgical procedures (45% vs 27%) in patients receiving Humatrope compared with untreated control patients (Table 4). Other adverse events of special interest to Turner syndrome patients were not significantly different between treatment groups (Table 4). A similar increase in otitis media was observed in an 18 month placebo-controlled trial.
[See table 4 at top of previous page]
Adult Patients—In clinical studies in which high doses of Humatrope were administered to healthy adult volunteers, the following events occurred infrequently: headache, localized muscle pain, weakness, mild hyperglycemia, and glucosuria.
In the first 6 months of controlled blinded trial during which patients received either Humatrope or placebo, adult onset growth hormone-deficient adults who received Humotrope experienced a statistically significant increase in edema (Humatrope 17.3% vs. placebo 4.4%, p=0.043) and peripheral edema (11.5% vs. 0% respectively, p=0.017). In patients with adult onset growth hormone deficiency, edema, muscle pain, joint pain, and joint disorder were reported early in therapy and tended to be transient or responsive to dosage titration.
Two out of 113 adult onset patients developed carpal tunnel syndrome after beginning maintenance therapy without a low dose (0.00625 mg/kg/day) lead-in phase. Symptoms abated in these patients after dosage reduction.
All treatment-emergent adverse events with ≥5% overall incidence during 12 or 18 months of replacement therapy with Humatrope are shown in Table 5 (adult onset patients) and in Table 6 (childhood onset patients).
Adult patients treated with Humatrope who had been diagnosed with growth hormone deficiency in childhood reported side effects less frequently than those with adult onset growth hormone deficiency.
[See table 5 at top of previous page]
[See table 6 above]
Other adverse drug events that have been reported in growth hormone-treated patients include the following:
1) Metabolic: Infrequent, mild and transient peripheral or generalized edema. 2) Musculoskeletal: Rare carpal tunnel syndrome. 3) Skin: Rare increased growth of pre-existing nevi. Patients should be monitored carefully for malignant transformation. 4) Endrocrine: Rare gynecomastia. Rare pancreatitis.

OVERDOSAGE
Acute overdosage could lead initially to hypoglycemia and subsequently to hyperglycemia. Long-term overdosage could result in signs and symptoms of gigantism/acromegaly consistent with the known effects of excess human growth hormone. (See recommended and maximal dosage instructions given below.)

DOSAGE AND ADMINISTRATION
Pediatric Patients—The Humatrope dosage and administration schedule should be individualized for each patient. Therapy should not be continued if epiphyseal fusion has occurred. Response to growth hormone therapy tends to decrease with time. However, failure to increase growth rate, particularly during the first year of therapy, should prompt close assessment of compliance and evaluation of other causes of growth failure such as hypothyroidism, undernutrition and advanced bone age.
Growth hormone-deficient pediatric patients—The recommended weekly dosage is 0.18 mg/kg (0.54 IU/kg) of body weight. The maximal replacement weekly dosage is 0.3 mg/kg (0.90 IU/kg) of body weight. It should be divided into

Continued on next page

*** Identi-Code® symbol. This product information was prepared in June 2000. Current information on these and other products of Eli Lilly and Company may be obtained by direct inquiry to Lilly Research Laboratories, Lilly Corporate Center, Indianapolis, Indiana 46285, (800) 545-5979.**

Humatrope—Cont.

equal doses given either on 3 alternate days, 6 times per week or daily. The subcutaneous route of administration is preferable; intramuscular injection is also acceptable. The dosage and administration schedule for Humatrope should be individualized for each patient.
Turner Syndrome—A weekly dosage of up to 0.375 mg/kg (1.125 IU/kg) of body weight administered by subcutaneous injection is recommended. It should be divided into equal doses given either daily or on 3 alternate days.
Adult Patients—
Growth hormone-deficient adult patients—The recommended dosage at the start of therapy is not more than 0.006 mg/kg/day (0.018 IU/kg/day) given as a daily subcutaneous injection. The dose may be increased according to individual patient requirements to a maximum of 0.0125 mg/kg/day (0.0375 IU/kg/day).
During therapy, dosage should be titrated if required by the occurrence of side effects or to maintain the IGF-I response below the upper limit of normal IGF-I levels, matched for age and sex. To minimize the occurrence of adverse events in patients with increasing age or excessive body weight, dose reductions may be necessary.
Reconstitution—
Vial—Each 5-mg vial of Humatrope should be reconstituted with 1.5 to 5 mL of Diluent for Humatrope. The diluent should be injected into the vial of Humatrope by aiming the stream of liquid against the glass wall. Following reconstitution, the vial should be swirled with a GENTLE rotary motion until the contents are completely dissolved. DO NOT SHAKE. The resulting solution should be inspected for clarity. It should be clear. If the solution is cloudy or contains particulate matter, the contents MUST NOT be injected.
Before and after injection, the septum of the vial should be wiped with rubbing alcohol or an alcoholic antiseptic solution to prevent contamination of the contents by repeated needle insertions. Sterile disposable syringes and needles should be used for administration of Humatrope. The volume of the syringe should be small enough so that the prescribed dose can be withdrawn from the vial with reasonable accuracy.
Cartridge—Each cartridge of Humatrope should only be reconstituted using the diluent syringe and the diluent connector which accompany the cartridge **and should not be reconstituted with the Diluent for Humatrope provided with Humatrope Vials.** (See WARNING section). **See the HumatroPen™ User Guide for comprehensive directions on Humatrope cartridge reconstitution.**
The reconstituted solution should be inspected for clarity. It should be clear. If the solution is cloudy or contains particulate matter, the contents MUST NOT be injected.
The HumatroPen allows the sumatropin dosage volume to be dialed in increments of 0.048 mL per click of dosage knob, and the maximum dosage volume that can be injected is 0.576 mL (based on a 12 click maximum). (See Table 7 for additional information).
[See table 7 at top of previous page]
This cartridge has been designed for use only with the HumatroPen. A sterile disposable needle should be used for each administration of Humatrope.

STABILITY AND STORAGE

Vials—
Before Reconstitution—Vials of Humatrope and Diluent for Humatrope are stable when refrigerated (2° to 8°C [36° to 46°F]). Avoid freezing Diluent for Humatrope. Expiration dates are stated on the labels.
After Reconstitution —Vials of Humatrope are stable for up to 14 days when reconstituted with Diluent for Humatrope or Bacteriostatic Water for Injection, USP and stored in a refrigerator at 2° to 8°C (36° to 46°F). Avoid freezing the reconstituted vial of Humatrope.
After Reconstitution with Sterile Water, USP—Use only one dose per Humatrope vial and discard the unused portion. If the solution is not used immediately, it must be refrigerated (2° to 8°C [36° to 46°F]) and used within 24 hours.
Cartridges—
Before Reconstitution—Cartridges of Humatrope and Diluent for Humatrope are stable when refrigerated (2° to 8°C [36° to 46°F]). Avoid freezing Diluent for Humatrope. Expiration dates are stated on the labels.
After Reconstitution—Cartridges of Humatrope are stable for up to 28 days when reconstituted with Diluent for Humatrope and stored in a refrigerator at (2° to 8°C [36° to 46°F]). Store the HumatroPen without the needle attached. Avoid freezing the reconstituted cartridge of Humatrope.

HOW SUPPLIED

Vials:
5 mg (No. 7335)—(6s) NDC 0002-7335-16, and 5-mL vials of Diluent for Humatrope (No. 7336)
Cartridges:
Cartridge Kit (MS8089) NDC 0002-8089-01
6 mg cartridge (VL7554), and prefilled syringe of Diluent for Humatrope (VL7557)
Cartridge Kit (MS8090) NDC 0002-8090-01
12 mg cartridge (VL7555), and prefilled syringe of Diluent for Humatrope (VL7558)
Cartridge Kit (MS8091) NDC 0002-8091-01
24 mg cartridge (VL 7556), and prefilled syringe of Diluent for Humatrope (VL7558)

Text revised March, 1999
Literature issued May 10, 2000
PA 1649 AMP [051000]

HUMULIN® 50/50® OTC

[*hŭ 'mū-lĭn*]
(50% Human Insulin Isophane Suspension and 50% Human Insulin Injection [rDNA Origin])

INFORMATION FOR THE PATIENT

WARNINGS

THIS LILLY HUMAN INSULIN PRODUCT DIFFERS FROM ANIMAL-SOURCE INSULINS BECAUSE IT IS STRUCTURALLY IDENTICAL TO THE INSULIN PRODUCED BY YOUR BODY'S PANCREAS AND BECAUSE OF ITS UNIQUE MANUFACTURING PROCESS.
ANY CHANGE OF INSULIN SHOULD BE MADE CAUTIOUSLY AND ONLY UNDER MEDICAL SUPERVISION. CHANGES IN STRENGTH, MANUFACTURER, TYPE (E.G., REGULAR, NPH, LENTE®), SPECIES (BEEF, PORK, BEEF-PORK, HUMAN), OR METHOD OF MANUFACTURE (rDNA VERSUS ANIMAL-SOURCE INSULIN) MAY RESULT IN THE NEED FOR A CHANGE IN DOSAGE.
SOME PATIENTS TAKING HUMULIN® (HUMAN INSULIN, rDNA ORIGIN) MAY REQUIRE A CHANGE IN DOSAGE FROM THAT USED WITH ANIMAL-SOURCE INSULINS. IF AN ADJUSTMENT IS NEEDED, IT MAY OCCUR WITH THE FIRST DOSE OR DURING THE FIRST SEVERAL WEEKS OR MONTHS.

DIABETES

Insulin is a hormone produced by the pancreas, a large gland that lies near the stomach. This hormone is necessary for the body's correct use of food, especially sugar. Diabetes occurs when the pancreas does not make enough insulin to meet your body's needs.
To control your diabetes, your doctor has prescribed injections of insulin to keep your blood glucose at a nearly normal level. Proper control of your diabetes requires close and constant cooperation with your doctor. In spite of diabetes, you can lead an active, healthy, and useful life if you eat a balanced diet daily, exercise regularly, and take your insulin injections as prescribed.
You have been instructed to test your blood and/or your urine regularly for glucose. If your blood tests consistently show above- or below-normal glucose levels or your urine tests consistently show the presence of glucose, your diabetes is not properly controlled and you must let your doctor know.
Always keep an extra supply of insulin as well as a spare syringe and needle on hand. Always wear diabetic identification so that appropriate treatment can be given if complications occur away from home.

50/50 HUMAN INSULIN

Description
Humulin is synthesized in a non-disease-producing special laboratory strain of *Escherichia coli* bacteria that has been genetically altered by the addition of the gene for human insulin production. Humulin 50/50 is a mixture of 50% Human Insulin Isophane Suspension and 50% Human Insulin Injection. It is an intermediate-acting insulin combined with the more rapid onset of action of regular insulin. The duration of activity may last up to 24 hours following injection. The time course of action of any insulin may vary considerably in different individuals or at different times in the same individual. As with all insulin preparations, the duration of action of Humulin 50/50 is dependent on dose, site of injection, blood supply, temperature, and physical activity. Humulin 50/50 is a sterile suspension and is for subcutaneous injection only. It should not be used intravenously or intramuscularly. The concentration of Humulin 50/50 is 100 units/mL (U-100).
Identification
Human insulin manufactured by Eli Lilly and Company has the trademark Humulin and is available in 6 formulations—Regular (**R**), NPH (**N**), Lente (**L**), Ultralente® (**U**), 50% Human Insulin Isophane Suspension [NPH]/50% Human Insulin Injection [buffered regular] (**50/50**) and 70% Human Insulin Isophane Suspension [NPH]/30% Human Insulin Injection [buffered regular] (**70/30**). Your doctor has prescribed the type of insulin that he/she believes is best for you. **DO NOT USE ANY OTHER INSULIN EXCEPT ON HIS/HER ADVICE AND DIRECTION.**
Always check the carton and the bottle label for the name and letter designation of the insulin you receive from your pharmacy to make sure it is the same as that your doctor has prescribed. Humulin 50/50 can be identified as follows:
[See graphic at bottom of page]
Always examine the appearance of your bottle of insulin before withdrawing each dose. A bottle of Humulin 50/50 must be carefully shaken or rotated before each injection so that the contents are uniformly mixed. Humulin 50/50 should look uniformly cloudy or milky after mixing. Do not use it if the insulin substance (the white material) remains at the bottom of the bottle after mixing. Do not use a bottle of Humulin 50/50 if there are clumps in the insulin after mixing (Figure 1). Do not use a bottle of Humulin 50/50 if solid white particles stick to the bottom or wall of the bottle, giving it a frosted appearance (Figure 2). Always check the appearance of your bottle of insulin before using, and if you note anything unusual in the appearance of your insulin or notice your insulin requirements changing markedly, consult your doctor.

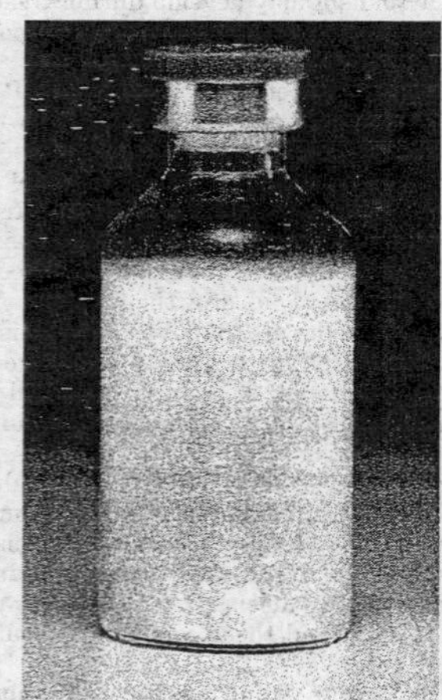

Fig. 1.—Do not use if there are clumps in the insulin after mixing.

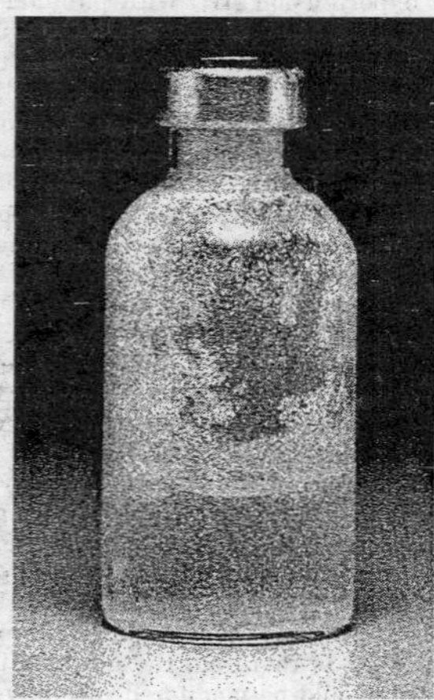

Fig. 2.—Do not use if particles on the bottom or wall give the bottle a frosted appearance

Storage
Insulin should be stored in a refrigerator but not in the freezer. If refrigeration is not possible, the bottle of insulin that you are currently using can be kept unrefrigerated as long as it is kept as cool as possible (below 86°F [30°C]) and away from heat and light. Do not use insulin if it has been frozen. Do not use a bottle of insulin after the expiration date stamped on the label.

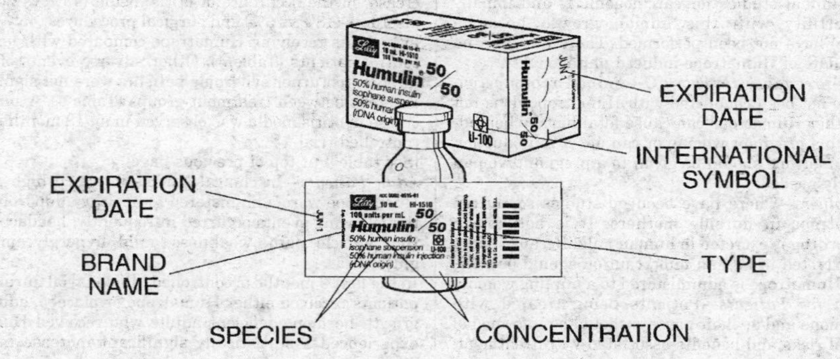

INJECTION PROCEDURES

Correct Syringe

Doses of insulin are measured in **units.** U-100 insulin contains 100 units/mL (1 mL = 1 cc). With Humulin 50/50, it is important to use a syringe that is marked for U-100 insulin preparations. Failure to use the proper syringe can lead to a mistake in dosage, causing serious problems for you, such as a blood glucose level that is too low or too high.

Syringe Use

To help avoid contamination and possible infection, follow these instructions exactly.

Disposable syringes and needles should be used only once and then discarded. **NEEDLES AND SYRINGES MUST NOT BE SHARED.**

Reusable syringes and needles must be sterilized before each injection. **Follow the package directions supplied with your syringe.** Described below are 2 methods of sterilizing.

Boiling

1. Put syringe, plunger, and needle in strainer, place in saucepan, and cover with water. Boil for 5 minutes.
2. Remove articles from water. When they have cooled, insert plunger into barrel, and fasten needle to syringe with a slight twist.
3. Push plunger in and out several times until water is completely removed.

Isopropyl Alcohol

If the syringe, plunger, and needle cannot be boiled, as when you are traveling, they may be sterilized by immersion for at least 5 minutes in Isopropyl Alcohol, 91%. Do not use bathing, rubbing, or medicated alcohol for this sterilization. If the syringe is sterilized with alcohol, it must be absolutely dry before use.

Preparing the Dose

1. Wash your hands.
2. Carefully shake or rotate the insulin bottle several times to completely mix the insulin.
3. Inspect the insulin. Humulin 50/50 should look uniformly cloudy or milky. Do not use it if you notice anything unusual in the appearance.
4. If using a new bottle, flip off the plastic protective cap, but **do not** remove the stopper. When using a new bottle, wipe the top of the bottle with an alcohol swab.
5. Draw air into the syringe equal to your insulin dose. Put the needle through rubber top of the insulin bottle and inject the air into the bottle.
6. Turn the bottle and syringe upside down. Hold the bottle and syringe firmly in 1 hand and shake gently.
7. Making sure the tip of the needle is in the insulin, withdraw the correct dose of insulin into the syringe.
8. Before removing the needle from the bottle, check your syringe for air bubbles which reduce the amount of insulin in it. If bubbles are present, hold the syringe straight up and tap its side until the bubbles float to the top. Push them out with the plunger and withdraw the correct dose.
9. Remove the needle from the bottle and lay the syringe down so that the needle does not touch anything.

Injection

Cleanse the skin with alcohol where the injection is to be made. Stabilize the skin by spreading it or pinching up a large area. Insert the needle as instructed by your doctor. Push the plunger in as far as it will go. Pull the needle out and apply gentle pressure over the injection site for several seconds. **Do not rub the area.** To avoid tissue damage, give the next injection at a site at least 1/2" from the previous site.

DOSAGE

Your doctor has told you which insulin to use, how much, and when and how often to inject it. Because each patient's case of diabetes is different, this schedule has been individualized for you.

Your usual insulin dose may be affected by changes in your food, activity, or work schedule. Carefully follow your doctor's instructions to allow for these changes. Other things that may affect your insulin dose are:

Illness

Illness, especially with nausea and vomiting, may cause your insulin requirements to change. Even if you are not eating, you will still require insulin. You and your doctor should establish a sick day plan for you to use in case of illness. When you are sick, test your blood/urine frequently and call your doctor as instructed.

Pregnancy

Good control of diabetes is especially important for you and your unborn baby. Pregnancy may make managing your diabetes more difficult. If you are planning to have a baby, are pregnant, or are nursing a baby, consult your doctor.

Medication

Insulin requirements may be increased if you are taking other drugs with hyperglycemic activity, such as oral contraceptives, corticosteroids, or thyroid replacement therapy. Insulin requirements may be reduced in the presence of drugs with hypoglycemic activity, such as oral hypoglycemics, salicylates (for example, aspirin), sulfa antibiotics, and certain antidepressants. Always discuss any medications you are taking with your doctor.

Exercise

Exercise may lower your body's need for insulin during and for some time after the activity. Exercise may also speed up the effect of an insulin dose, especially if the exercise involves the area of injection site (for example, the leg should not be used for injection just prior to running). Discuss with your doctor how you should adjust your regimen to accommodate exercise.

Travel

Persons traveling across more than 2 time zones should consult their doctor concerning adjustments in their insulin schedule.

COMMON PROBLEMS OF DIABETES

Hypoglycemia (Insulin Reaction)

Hypoglycemia (too little glucose in the blood) is one of the most frequent adverse events experienced by insulin users. It can be brought about by:

1. Taking too much insulin
2. Missing or delaying meals
3. Exercising or working more than usual
4. An infection or illness (especially with diarrhea or vomiting)
5. A change in the body's need for insulin
6. Diseases of the adrenal, pituitary, or thyroid gland, or progression of kidney or liver disease
7. Interactions with other drugs that lower blood glucose, such as oral hypoglycemics, salicylates (for example, aspirin), sulfa antibiotics, and certain antidepressants
8. Consumption of alcoholic beverages

Symptoms of mild to moderate hypoglycemia may occur suddenly and can include:

- sweating
- dizziness
- palpitation
- tremor
- hunger
- restlessness
- tingling in the hands, feet, lips, or tongue
- lightheadedness
- inability to concentrate
- headache
- drowsiness
- sleep disturbances
- anxiety
- blurred vision
- slurred speech
- depressed mood
- irritability
- abnormal behavior
- unsteady movement
- personality changes

Signs of severe hypoglycemia can include:

- disorientation
- unconsciousness
- seizures
- death

Therefore, it is important that assistance be obtained immediately.

Early warning symptoms of hypoglycemia may be different or less pronounced under certain conditions, such as long duration of diabetes, diabetic nerve disease, medications such as beta-blockers, change in insulin preparations, or intensified control (3 or more insulin injections per day) of diabetes.

A few patients who have experienced hypoglycemic reactions after transfer from animal-source insulin to human insulin have reported that the early warning symptoms of hypoglycemia were less pronounced or different from those experienced with their previous insulin.

Without recognition of early warning symptoms, you may not be able to take steps to avoid more serious hypoglycemia. Be alert for all of the various types of symptoms that may indicate hypoglycemia. Patients who experience hypoglycemia without early warning symptoms should monitor their blood glucose frequently, especially prior to activities such as driving. If the blood glucose is below your normal fasting glucose, you should consider eating or drinking sugar-containing foods to treat your hypoglycemia.

Mild to moderate hypoglycemia may be treated by eating foods or drinks that contain sugar. Patients should always carry a quick source of sugar, such as candy mints or glucose tablets. More severe hypoglycemia may require the assistance of another person. Patients who are unable to take sugar orally or who are unconscious require an injection of glucagon or should be treated with intravenous administration of glucose at a medical facility.

You should learn to recognize your own symptoms of hypoglycemia. If you are uncertain about these symptoms, you should monitor your blood glucose frequently to help you learn to recognize the symptoms that you experience with hypoglycemia.

If you have frequent episodes of hypoglycemia or experience difficulty in recognizing the symptoms, you should consult your doctor to discuss possible changes in therapy, meal plans, and/or exercise programs to help you avoid hypoglycemia.

Hyperglycemia and Diabetic Acidosis

Hyperglycemia (too much glucose in the blood) may develop if your body has too little insulin. Hyperglycemia can be brought about by:

1. Omitting your insulin or taking less than the doctor has prescribed
2. Eating significantly more than your meal plan suggests
3. Developing a fever, infection, or other significant stressful situation

In patients with insulin-dependent diabetes, prolonged hyperglycemia can result in diabetic acidosis. The first symptoms of diabetic acidosis usually come on gradually, over a period of hours or days, and include a drowsy feeling, flushed face, thirst, loss of appetite, and fruity odor on the breath. With acidosis, urine tests show large amounts of glucose and acetone. Heavy breathing and a rapid pulse are more severe symptoms. If uncorrected, prolonged hyperglycemia or diabetic acidosis can lead to nausea, vomiting, dehydration, loss of consciousness or death. Therefore, it is important that you obtain medical assistance immediately.

Lipodystrophy

Rarely, administration of insulin subcutaneously can result in lipoatrophy (depression in the skin) or lipohypertrophy (enlargement or thickening of tissue). If you notice either of these conditions, consult your doctor. A change in your injection technique may help alleviate the problem.

Allergy to Insulin

Local Allergy —Patients occasionally experience redness, swelling, and itching at the site of injection of insulin. This condition, called local allergy, usually clears up in a few days to a few weeks. In some instances, this condition may be related to factors other than insulin, such as irritants in the skin cleansing agent or poor injection technique. If you have local reactions, contact your doctor.

Systemic Allergy —Less common, but potentially more serious, is generalized allergy to insulin, which may cause rash over the whole body, shortness of breath, wheezing, reduction in blood pressure, fast pulse, or sweating. Severe cases of generalized allergy may be life threatening. If you think you are having a generalized allergic reaction to insulin, notify a doctor immediately.

ADDITIONAL INFORMATION

Additional information about diabetes may be obtained from your diabetes educator.

DIABETES FORECAST is a national magazine designed especially for patients with diabetes and their families and is available by subscription from the American Diabetes Association, National Service Center, 1660 Duke Street, Alexandria, Virginia 22314, 1-800-DIABETES (1-800-342-2383).

Another publication, **DIABETES COUNTDOWN**, is available from the Juvenile Diabetes Foundation International (JDF), 120 Wall Street, 19th Floor, New York, New York 10005-4001, 1-800-JDF-CURE (1-800-533-2873).

Additional information about Humulin can be obtained by calling 1-888-88-LILLY (1-888-885-4559).

Literature revised August 13, 1999

PA 6053 AMP [081399]

HUMULIN® 70/30 OTC

[*hū 'mŭ-lĭn*]

(70% Human Insulin Isophane Suspension and 30% Human Insulin Injection [rDNA origin])

INFORMATION FOR THE PATIENT

WARNINGS

THIS LILLY HUMAN INSULIN PRODUCT DIFFERS FROM ANIMAL-SOURCE INSULINS BECAUSE IT IS STRUCTURALLY IDENTICAL TO THE INSULIN PRODUCED BY YOUR BODY'S PANCREAS AND BECAUSE OF ITS UNIQUE MANUFACTURING PROCESS.

ANY CHANGE OF INSULIN SHOULD BE MADE CAUTIOUSLY AND ONLY UNDER MEDICAL SUPERVISION. CHANGES IN STRENGTH, MANUFACTURER, TYPE (E.G., REGULAR, NPH, LENTE®), SPECIES (BEEF, PORK, BEEF-PORK, HUMAN), OR METHOD OF MANUFACTURE (rDNA VERSUS ANIMAL-SOURCE INSULIN) MAY RESULT IN THE NEED FOR A CHANGE IN DOSAGE.

SOME PATIENTS TAKING HUMULIN® (HUMAN INSULIN, rDNA ORIGIN) MAY REQUIRE A CHANGE IN DOSAGE FROM THAT USED WITH ANIMAL-SOURCE INSULINS. IF AN ADJUSTMENT IS NEEDED, IT MAY OCCUR WITH THE FIRST DOSE OR DURING THE FIRST SEVERAL WEEKS OR MONTHS.

DIABETES

Insulin is a hormone produced by the pancreas, a large gland that lies near the stomach. This hormone is necessary for the body's correct use of food, especially sugar. Diabetes occurs when the pancreas does not make enough insulin to meet your body's needs.

To control your diabetes, your doctor has prescribed injections of insulin to keep your blood glucose at a nearly normal level. Proper control of your diabetes requires close and constant cooperation with your doctor. In spite of diabetes, you can lead an active, healthy, and useful life if you eat a balanced diet daily, exercise regularly, and take your insulin injections as prescribed.

You have been instructed to test your blood and/or your urine regularly for glucose. If your blood tests consistently show above- or below-normal glucose levels or your urine tests consistently show the presence of glucose, your diabetes is not properly controlled and you must let your doctor know.

Always keep an extra supply of insulin as well as a spare syringe and needle on hand. Always wear diabetic identification so that appropriate treatment can be given if complications occur away from home.

Continued on next page

*** Identi-Code® symbol. This product information was prepared in June 2000. Current information on these and other products of Eli Lilly and Company may be obtained by direct inquiry to Lilly Research Laboratories, Lilly Corporate Center, Indianapolis, Indiana 46285, (800) 545-5979.**

Humulin 70/30—Cont.

70/30 HUMAN INSULIN

Description

Humulin is synthesized in a non-disease-producing special laboratory strain of *Escherichia coli* bacteria that has been genetically altered by the addition of the gene for human insulin production. Humulin 70/30 is a mixture of 70% Human Insulin Isophane Suspension and 30% Human Insulin Injection. It is an intermediate-acting insulin combined with the more rapid onset of action of regular insulin. The duration of activity may last up to 24 hours following injection. The time course of action of any insulin may vary considerably in different individuals or at different times in the same individual. As with all insulin preparations, the duration of action of Humulin 70/30 is dependent on dose, site of injection, blood supply, temperature, and physical activity. Humulin 70/30 is a sterile suspension and is for subcutaneous injection only. It should not be used intravenously or intramuscularly. The concentration of Humulin 70/30 is 100 units/mL (U-100).

Identification

Human insulin manufactured by Eli Lilly and Company has the trademark Humulin and is available in 6 formulations—Regular (**R**), NPH (**N**), Lente (**L**), Ultralente® (**U**), 50% Human Insulin Isophane Suspension [NPH]/50% Human Insulin Injection [buffered regular] (**50/50**), and 70% Human Insulin Isophane Suspension [NPH]/30% Human Insulin Injection [buffered regular] (**70/30**). Your doctor has prescribed the type of insulin that he/she believes is best for you. **DO NOT USE ANY OTHER INSULIN EXCEPT ON HIS/HER ADVICE AND DIRECTION.**

Always check the carton and the bottle label for the name and letter designation of the insulin you receive from your pharmacy to make sure it is the same as that your doctor has prescribed. Humulin 70/30 can be identified as follows:

[See graphic at bottom of page]

Always examine the appearance of your bottle of insulin before withdrawing each dose. A bottle of Humulin 70/30 must be carefully shaken or rotated before each injection so that the contents are uniformly mixed. Humulin 70/30 should look uniformly cloudy or milky after mixing. Do not use it if the insulin substance (the white material) remains at the bottom of the bottle after mixing. Do not use a bottle of Humulin 70/30 if there are clumps in the insulin after mixing (Figure 1). Do not use a bottle of Humulin 70/30 if solid white particles stick to the bottom or wall of the bottle, giving it a frosted appearance (Figure 2). Always check the appearance of your bottle of insulin before using, and if you note anything unusual in the appearance of your insulin or notice your insulin requirements changing markedly, consult your doctor.

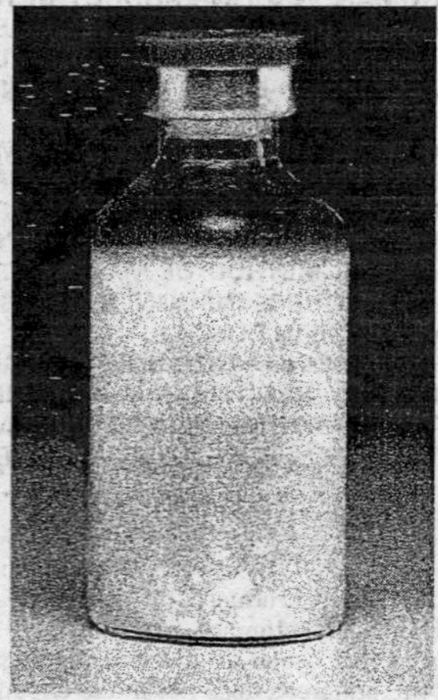

Fig. 1.—Do not use if there are clumps in the insulin after mixing.

Fig. 2.—Do not use if particles on the bottom or wall give the bottle a frosted appearance.

[See figure 2 at top of next column]

Storage

Insulin should be stored in a refrigerator but not in the freezer. If refrigeration is not possible, the bottle of insulin that you are currently using can be kept unrefrigerated as long as it is kept as cool as possible (below 86°F [30°C]) and away from heat and light. Do not use insulin if it has been frozen. Do not use a bottle of insulin after the expiration date stamped on the label.

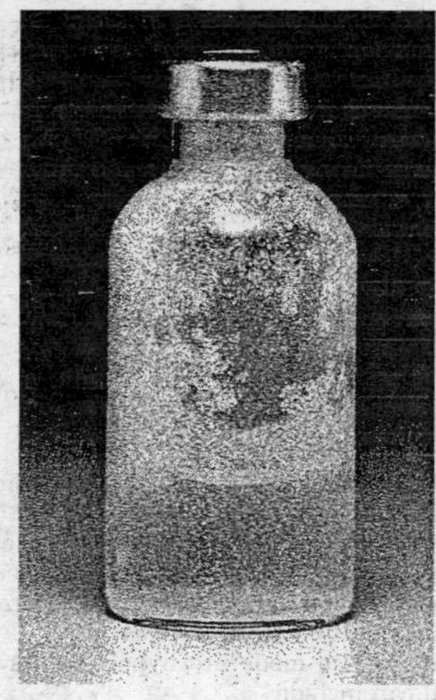

INJECTION PROCEDURES

Correct Syringe

Doses of insulin are measured in **units.** U-100 insulin contains 100 units/mL (1 mL=1 cc). With Humulin 70/30, it is important to use a syringe that is marked for U-100 insulin preparations. Failure to use the proper syringe can lead to a mistake in dosage, causing serious problems for you, such as a blood glucose level that is too low or too high.

Syringe Use

To help avoid contamination and possible infection, follow these instructions exactly.

Disposable syringes and needles should be used only once and then discarded. **NEEDLES AND SYRINGES MUST NOT BE SHARED.**

Reusable syringes and needles must be sterilized before each injection. **Follow the package directions supplied with your syringe.** Described below are 2 methods of sterilizing.

Boiling

1. Put syringe, plunger, and needle in strainer, place in saucepan, and cover with water. Boil for 5 minutes.
2. Remove articles from water. When they have cooled, insert plunger into barrel, and fasten needle to syringe with a slight twist.
3. Push plunger in and out several times until water is completely removed.

Isopropyl Alcohol

If the syringe, plunger, and needle cannot be boiled, as when you are traveling, they may be sterilized by immersion for at least 5 minutes in Isopropyl Alcohol, 91%. Do not use bathing, rubbing, or medicated alcohol for this sterilization. If the syringe is sterilized with alcohol, it must be absolutely dry before use.

Preparing the Dose

1. Wash your hands.
2. Carefully shake or rotate the insulin bottle several times to completely mix the insulin.
3. Inspect the insulin. Humulin 70/30 should look uniformly cloudy or milky. Do not use it if you notice anything unusual in the appearance.
4. If using a new bottle, flip off the plastic protective cap, but **do not** remove the stopper. When using a new bottle, wipe the top of the bottle with an alcohol swab.
5. Draw air into the syringe equal to your insulin dose. Put the needle through rubber top of the insulin bottle and inject the air into the bottle.
6. Turn the bottle and syringe upside down. Hold the bottle and syringe firmly in 1 hand and shake gently.
7. Making sure the tip of the needle is in the insulin, withdraw the correct dose of insulin into the syringe.
8. Before removing the needle from the bottle, check your syringe for air bubbles which reduce the amount of insulin in it. If bubbles are present, hold the syringe straight up and tap its side until the bubbles float to the top. Push them out with the plunger and withdraw the correct dose.
9. Remove the needle from the bottle and lay the syringe down so that the needle does not touch anything.

Injection

Cleanse the skin with alcohol where the injection is to be made. Stabilize the skin by spreading it or pinching up a large area. Insert the needle as instructed by your doctor. Push the plunger in as far as it will go. Pull the needle out and apply gentle pressure over the injection site for several seconds. **Do not rub the area.** To avoid tissue damage, give the next injection at a site at least $^{1}/_{2}$" from the previous site.

DOSAGE

Your doctor has told you which insulin to use, how much, and when and how often to inject it. Because each patient's case of diabetes is different, this schedule has been individualized for you.

Your usual insulin dose may be affected by changes in your food, activity, or work schedule. Carefully follow your doctor's instructions to allow for these changes. Other things that may affect your insulin dose are:

Illness

Illness, especially with nausea and vomiting, may cause your insulin requirements to change. Even if you are not eating, you will still require insulin. You and your doctor should establish a sick day plan for you to use in case of illness. When you are sick, test your blood/urine frequently and call your doctor as instructed.

Pregnancy

Good control of diabetes is especially important for you and your unborn baby. Pregnancy may make managing your diabetes more difficult. If you are planning to have a baby, are pregnant, or are nursing a baby, consult your doctor.

Medication

Insulin requirements may be increased if you are taking other drugs with hyperglycemic activity, such as oral contraceptives, corticosteroids, or thyroid replacement therapy. Insulin requirements may be reduced in the presence of drugs with hypoglycemic activity, such as oral hypoglycemics, salicylates (for example, aspirin), sulfa antibiotics, and certain antidepressants. Always discuss any medications you are taking with your doctor.

Exercise

Exercise may lower your body's need for insulin during and for some time after the activity. Exercise may also speed up the effect of an insulin dose, especially if the exercise involves the area of injection site (for example, the leg should not be used for injection just prior to running). Discuss with your doctor how you should adjust your regimen to accommodate exercise.

Travel

Persons traveling across more than 2 time zones should consult their doctor concerning adjustments in their insulin schedule.

COMMON PROBLEMS OF DIABETES

Hypoglycemia (Insulin Reaction)

Hypoglycemia (too little glucose in the blood) is one of the most frequent adverse events experienced by insulin users. It can be brought about by:

1. Taking too much insulin
2. Missing or delaying meals
3. Exercising or working more than usual
4. An infection or illness (especially with diarrhea or vomiting)
5. A change in the body's need for insulin
6. Diseases of the adrenal, pituitary, or thyroid gland, or progression of kidney or liver disease
7. Interactions with other drugs that lower blood glucose, such as oral hypoglycemics, salicylates (for example, aspirin), sulfa antibiotics, and certain antidepressants
8. Consumption of alcoholic beverages

Symptoms of mild to moderate hypoglycemia may occur suddenly and can include:

- sweating
- dizziness
- palpitation
- tremor
- hunger
- restlessness
- tingling in the hands, feet, lips, or tongue
- lightheadedness
- inability to concentrate
- headache
- drowsiness
- sleep disturbances
- anxiety
- blurred vision
- slurred speech
- depressed mood
- irritability
- abnormal behavior
- unsteady movement
- personality changes

Signs of severe hypoglycemia can include:

- disorientation
- unconsciousness
- seizures
- death

Therefore, it is important that assistance be obtained immediately.

Early warning symptoms of hypoglycemia may be different or less pronounced under certain conditions, such as long duration of diabetes, diabetic nerve disease, medications such as beta-blockers, change in insulin preparations, or intensified control (3 or more insulin injections per day) of diabetes.

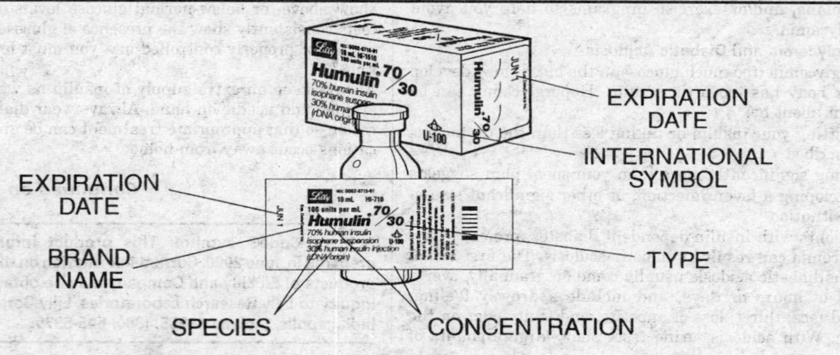

A few patients who have experienced hypoglycemic reactions after transfer from animal-source insulin to human insulin have reported that the early warning symptoms of hypoglycemia were less pronounced or different from those experienced with their previous insulin.

Without recognition of early warning symptoms, you may not be able to take steps to avoid more serious hypoglycemia. Be alert for all of the various types of symptoms that may indicate hypoglycemia. Patients who experience hypoglycemia without early warning symptoms should monitor their blood glucose frequently, especially prior to activities such as driving. If the blood glucose is below your normal fasting glucose, you should consider eating or drinking sugar-containing foods to treat your hypoglycemia.

Mild to moderate hypoglycemia may be treated by eating foods or drinks that contain sugar. Patients should always carry a quick source of sugar, such as candy mints or glucose tablets. More severe hypoglycemia may require the assistance of another person. Patients who are unable to take sugar orally or who are unconscious require an injection of glucagon or should be treated with intravenous administration of glucose at a medical facility.

You should learn to recognize your own symptoms of hypoglycemia. If you are uncertain about these symptoms, you should monitor your blood glucose frequently to help you learn to recognize the symptoms that you experience with hypoglycemia.

If you have frequent episodes of hypoglycemia or experience difficulty in recognizing the symptoms, you should consult your doctor to discuss possible changes in therapy, meal plans, and/or exercise programs to help you avoid hypoglycemia.

Hyperglycemia and Diabetic Acidosis

Hyperglycemia (too much glucose in the blood) may develop if your body has too little insulin. Hyperglycemia can be brought about by:

1. Omitting your insulin or taking less than the doctor has prescribed
2. Eating significantly more than your meal plan suggests
3. Developing a fever, infection, or other significant stressful situation.

In patients with insulin-dependent diabetes, prolonged hyperglycemia can result in diabetic acidosis. The first symptoms of diabetic acidosis usually come on gradually, over a period of hours or days, and include a drowsy feeling, flushed face, thirst, loss of appetite, and fruity odor on the breath. With acidosis, urine tests show large amounts of glucose and acetone. Heavy breathing and a rapid pulse are more severe symptoms. If uncorrected, prolonged hyperglycemia or diabetic acidosis can lead to nausea, vomiting, dehydration, loss of consciousness or death. Therefore, it is important that you obtain medical assistance immediately.

Lipodystrophy

Rarely, administration of insulin subcutaneously can result in lipoatrophy (depression in the skin) or lipohypertrophy (enlargement or thickening of tissue). If you notice either of these conditions, consult your doctor. A change in your injection technique may help alleviate the problem.

Allergy to Insulin

Local Allergy—Patients occasionally experience redness, swelling, and itching at the site of injection of insulin. This condition, called local allergy, usually clears up in a few days to a few weeks. In some instances, this condition may be related to factors other than insulin, such as irritants in the skin cleansing agent or poor injection technique. If you have local reactions, contact your doctor.

Systemic Allergy—Less common, but potentially more serious, is generalized allergy to insulin, which may cause rash over the whole body, shortness of breath, wheezing, reduction in blood pressure, fast pulse, or sweating. Severe cases of generalized allergy may be life threatening. If you think you are having a generalized allergic reaction to insulin, notify a doctor immediately.

ADDITIONAL INFORMATION

Additional information about diabetes may be obtained from your diabetes educator.

DIABETES FORECAST is a national magazine designed especially for patients with diabetes and their families and is available by subscription from the American Diabetes Association, National Service Center, 1660 Duke Street, Alexandria, Virginia 22314, 1-800-DIABETES (1-800-342-2383).

Another publication, **DIABETES COUNTDOWN**, is available from the Juvenile Diabetes Foundation International (JDF), 120 Wall Street, 19th Floor, New York, New York 10005-4001, 1-800-JDF-CURE (1-800-533-2873).

Additional information about Humulin can be obtained by calling 1-888-88-LILLY (1-888-885-4559).

Literature revised August 13, 1999

PA 6377 AMP [081399]

HUMULIN® 70/30 **OTC**

[*hū 'mū-lĭn*]

Cartridge

(70% Human Insulin Isophane Suspension and 30% Human Insulin Injection [rDNA origin])

1.5 mL Cartridge

For use in Becton Dickinson and Company's B-D®* Pen and Novo Nordisk A/S's NovoPen®†, NovolinPen®†, and NovoPen®† 1.5 insulin delivery devices.

INFORMATION FOR THE PATIENT

WARNINGS

THIS LILLY HUMAN INSULIN PRODUCT DIFFERS FROM ANIMAL-SOURCE INSULINS BECAUSE IT IS STRUCTURALLY IDENTICAL TO THE INSULIN PRODUCED BY YOUR BODY'S PANCREAS AND BECAUSE OF ITS UNIQUE MANUFACTURING PROCESS.

ANY CHANGE OF INSULIN SHOULD BE MADE CAUTIOUSLY AND ONLY UNDER MEDICAL SUPERVISION. CHANGES IN STRENGTH, MANUFACTURER, TYPE (E.G., REGULAR, NPH, LENTE, ETC), SPECIES (BEEF, PORK, BEEF-PORK, HUMAN), OR METHOD OF MANUFACTURE (rDNA VERSUS ANIMAL-SOURCE INSULIN) MAY RESULT IN THE NEED FOR A CHANGE IN DOSAGE.

SOME PATIENTS TAKING HUMULIN® (HUMAN INSULIN, rDNA ORIGIN) MAY REQUIRE A CHANGE IN DOSAGE FROM THAT USED WITH ANIMAL-SOURCE INSULINS. IF AN ADJUSTMENT IS NEEDED, IT MAY OCCUR WITH THE FIRST DOSE OR DURING THE FIRST SEVERAL WEEKS OR MONTHS.

TO OBTAIN AN ACCURATE DOSE, CAREFULLY READ AND FOLLOW THE INSULIN DELIVERY DEVICE ("INSULIN PEN") MANUFACTURER'S INSTRUCTIONS AND THIS INFORMATION FOR THE PATIENT INSERT BEFORE USING THIS PRODUCT IN AN INSULIN PEN. (*see* INSTRUCTIONS FOR USE section)

DIABETES

Insulin is a hormone produced by the pancreas, a large gland that lies near the stomach. This hormone is necessary for the body's correct use of food, especially sugar. Diabetes occurs when the pancreas does not make enough insulin to meet your body's needs.

To control your diabetes, your doctor has prescribed injections of insulin to keep your blood glucose at a nearly normal level. Proper control of your diabetes requires close and constant cooperation with your doctor. In spite of diabetes, you can lead an active, healthy, and useful life if you eat a balanced diet daily, exercise regularly, and take your insulin injections as prescribed.

You have been instructed to test your blood and/or your urine regularly for glucose. If your blood tests consistently show above- or below-normal glucose levels or your urine tests consistently show the presence of glucose, your diabetes is not properly controlled and you must let your doctor know.

Always keep an extra supply of insulin as well as a spare syringe and needle on hand. Always wear diabetic identification so that appropriate treatment can be given if complications occur away from home.

70/30 HUMAN INSULIN

Description

Humulin is synthesized in a non-disease-producing special laboratory strain of *Escherichia coli* bacteria that has been genetically altered by the addition of the human gene for insulin production. Humulin® 70/30 is a mixture of 70% Human Insulin Isophane Suspension and 30% Human Insulin Injection. It is an intermediate-acting insulin combined with the more rapid onset of action of regular insulin. The duration of activity may last up to 24 hours following injection. The time course of action of any insulin may vary considerably in different individuals or at different times in the same individual. As with all insulin preparations, the duration of action of Humulin 70/30 is dependent on dose, site of injection, blood supply, temperature, and physical activity. Humulin 70/30 is a sterile suspension and is for subcutaneous injection only. It should not be used intravenously or intramuscularly. The concentration of Humulin 70/30 in cartridges is 100 units/mL (U-100).

Identification

Cartridges of Humulin manufactured by Eli Lilly and Company are available in 3 formulations—Regular, NPH, and 70/30.

Your doctor has prescribed the type of insulin that he/she believes is best for you. **DO NOT USE ANY OTHER INSULIN EXCEPT ON HIS/HER ADVICE AND DIRECTION.**

Cartridges of Humulin 70/30, 1.5 mL, are available in boxes of 5. The cartridge containing Humulin 70/30 is not designed to allow any other insulin to be mixed in the cartridge or for the cartridge to be reused.

1.5 mL Cartridge

Humulin® 70/30 1.5 mL cartridges are for use in Becton Dickinson and Company's B-D® Pen and Novo Nordisk A/S's NovoPen®, NovolinPen®, and NovoPen® 1.5 insulin delivery devices.

Always examine the appearance of a cartridge of insulin before administering a dose. A cartridge of Humulin 70/30 contains a small glass bead to assist in mixing. A cartridge of Humulin 70/30 must be rolled between the palms 10 times and inverted 180° 10 times before each injection so that the contents are uniformly mixed (*see* Figures 1 and 2). Before inserting it in the insulin pen, inspect the cartridge for uniform mixing and repeat the above steps as necessary.

[See figure 1 at top of next column]

[See figure 2 at top of next column]

Humulin 70/30 should look uniformly cloudy or milky after mixing. Do not use if the insulin substance (the white material) remains visibly separated from the liquid after mixing. Do not use a cartridge of Humulin 70/30 if there are clumps in the insulin after mixing (*see* Figure 3). Do not use a cartridge of Humulin 70/30 if solid white particles stick to the walls of the cartridge, giving it a frosted appearance (*see* Figure 4).

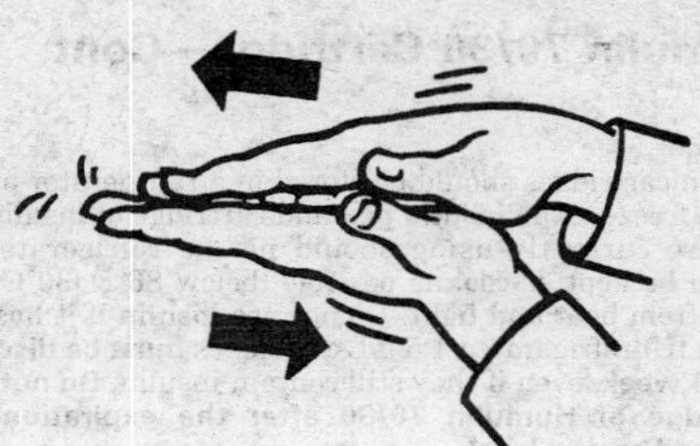

Figure 1.

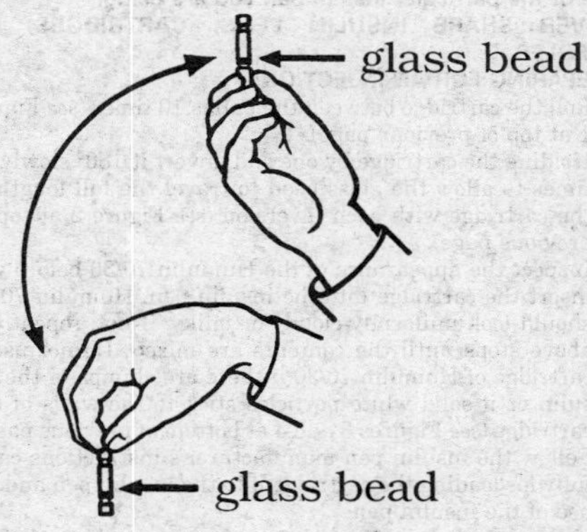

Figure 2.

Always check the appearance of the cartridge before using, and if you note anything unusual in the appearance of your insulin or notice your insulin requirements changing markedly, consult your doctor.

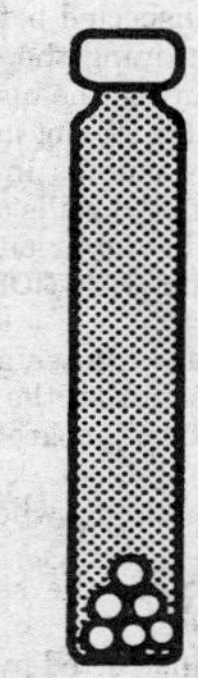

Figure 3.-- Do not use if there are clumps in the insulin after mixing.

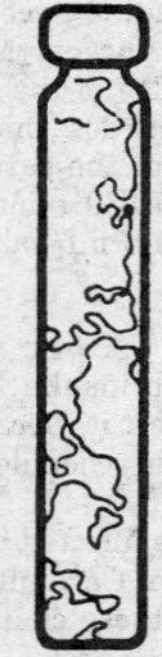

Figure 4.-- Do not use if particles on the bottom or wall give the cartridge a frosted appearance.

Continued on next page

* **Identi-Code® symbol. This product information was prepared in June 2000. Current information on these and other products of Eli Lilly and Company may be obtained by direct inquiry to Lilly Research Laboratories, Lilly Corporate Center, Indianapolis, Indiana 46285, (800) 545-5979.**

Humulin 70/30 Cartridge—Cont.

Storage
Insulin cartridges should be stored in a refrigerator but not in the freezer. The insulin pen and cartridge of insulin that you are currently using should not be refrigerated but should be kept as cool as possible (below 86°F [30°C]) and away from heat and light. Do not use insulin if it has been frozen. Unrefrigerated 1.5 mL cartridges **must be discarded after 1 week**, even if they still contain insulin. **Do not use a cartridge of Humulin 70/30 after the expiration date stamped on the label.**

INSTRUCTIONS FOR USE

Pens for insulin delivery differ in their operation. It is important to read, understand, and follow the instructions for use of the particular insulin pen you are using.

NEVER SHARE INSULIN PENS, CARTRIDGES, OR NEEDLES.

PREPARING FOR AN INJECTION:

1. Roll the cartridge between the palms 10 times (*see* Figure 1 at top of previous page).
2. Holding the cartridge by one end, invert it 180° slowly 10 times to allow the glass bead to travel the full length of the cartridge with each inversion (*see* Figure 2 at top of previous page).
3. Inspect the appearance of the Humulin 70/30 before you insert the cartridge into the insulin pen. Humulin 70/30 should look uniformly cloudy or milky. If not, repeat the above steps until the contents are mixed. Do not use a cartridge of Humulin 70/30 if there are clumps in the insulin or if solid white particles stick to the walls of the cartridge (*see* Figures 3 and 4 at bottom of previous page).
4. Follow the insulin pen manufacturer's instructions carefully for loading the cartridge into the insulin pen and for use of the insulin pen.
5. Use an alcohol swab to wipe the exposed rubber surface on the metal cap end of the cartridge.
6. Follow the insulin needle manufacturer's instructions for attaching and changing the needle.
7. Insulin cartridges may contain an air bubble(s) which must be removed from the cartridge and needle by proper priming prior to injection.
8. Once the cartridge is in use in an insulin pen, the insulin must be mixed and inspected before each injection. Roll the insulin pen, containing the cartridge, between the palms 10 times, and invert the insulin pen 180° slowly 10 times to mix the insulin. Do not use a cartridge of Humulin 70/30 if there are clumps in the insulin or if solid white particles stick to the walls of the cartridge (*see* Figures 3 and 4 at bottom of previous page).

GENERAL INJECTION INSTRUCTIONS:

1. Wash your hands.
2. To avoid tissue damage, choose a site for each injection that is at least 1/2 inch from the previous injection site. The usual sites of injection are abdomen, thighs, and arms.
3. Cleanse the skin with alcohol where the injection is to be made.
4. With one hand, stabilize the skin by spreading it or pinching up a large area.
5. Insert the needle as instructed by your doctor.
6. After dispensing a dose, pull the needle out and apply gentle pressure over the injection site for several seconds. **Do not rub the area.**
7. Immediately after an injection, remove the needle from the insulin pen. Doing so will guard against contamination, leakage, reentry of air, and needle clogs. **Do not reuse needles. Dispose of needles in a responsible manner.**
8. *1.5 mL cartridge* - Once the cartridge is in use, do not continue to use it if the leading edge of the plunger is beyond the black band on the cartridge. If a dose is started when the leading edge of the plunger is beyond the black band, an appropriate dose may not be delivered. Use the gauge on the side of the cartridge to help you judge how much Humulin 70/30 remains. The distance between each mark on the 1.5 mL cartridge is about 10 units.

DOSAGE

Your doctor has told you which insulin to use, how much, and when and how often to inject it. Because each patient's case of diabetes is different, this schedule has been individualized for you.

Your usual insulin dose may be affected by changes in your food, activity, or work schedule. Carefully follow your doctor's instructions to allow for these changes. Other things that may affect your insulin dose are:

Illness
Illness, especially with nausea and vomiting, may cause your insulin requirements to change. Even if you are not eating, you will still require insulin. You and your doctor should establish a sick day plan for you to use in case of illness. When you are sick, test your blood glucose/urine glucose and ketones frequently and call your doctor as instructed.

Pregnancy
Good control of diabetes is especially important for you and your unborn baby. Pregnancy may make managing your diabetes more difficult. If you are planning to have a baby, are pregnant, or are nursing a baby, consult your doctor.

Medication
Insulin requirements may be increased if you are taking other drugs with hyperglycemic activity, such as oral contraceptives, corticosteroids, or thyroid replacement therapy. Insulin requirements may be reduced in the presence of drugs with hypoglycemic activity, such as oral hypoglycemics, salicylates (for example, aspirin), sulfa antibiotics, and certain antidepressants. Always discuss any medications you are taking with your doctor.

Exercise
Exercise may lower your body's need for insulin during and for some time after the activity. Exercise may also speed up the effect of an insulin dose, especially if the exercise involves the area of injection site (for example, the leg should not be used for injection just prior to running). Discuss with your doctor how you should adjust your regimen to accommodate exercise.

Travel
Persons traveling across more than 2 time zones should consult their doctor concerning adjustments in their insulin schedule.

COMMON PROBLEMS OF DIABETES

Hypoglycemia (Insulin Reaction)
Hypoglycemia (too little glucose in the blood) is one of the most frequent adverse events experienced by insulin users. It can be brought about by:

1. Taking too much insulin
2. Missing or delaying meals
3. Exercising or working more than usual
4. An infection or illness (especially with diarrhea or vomiting)
5. A change in the body's need for insulin
6. Diseases of the adrenal, pituitary or thyroid gland, or progression of kidney or liver disease
7. Interactions with other drugs that lower blood glucose, such as oral hypoglycemics, salicylates (for example, aspirin), sulfa antibiotics, and certain antidepressants
8. Consumption of alcoholic beverages

Symptoms of mild to moderate hypoglycemia may occur suddenly and can include:

- sweating
- dizziness
- palpitation
- tremor
- hunger
- restlessness
- tingling in the hands, feet, lips, or tongue
- lightheadedness
- inability to concentrate
- headache
- drowsiness
- sleep disturbances
- anxiety
- blurred vision
- slurred speech
- depressed mood
- irritability
- abnormal behavior
- unsteady movement
- personality changes

Signs of severe hypoglycemia can include:

- disorientation
- unconsciousness
- seizures
- death

Therefore, it is important that assistance be obtained immediately.

Early warning symptoms of hypoglycemia may be different or less pronounced under certain conditions, such as long duration of diabetes, diabetic nerve disease, medications such as beta-blockers, change in insulin preparations, or intensified control (3 or more insulin injections per day) of diabetes.

A few patients who have experienced hypoglycemic reactions after transfer from animal-source insulin to human insulin have reported that the early warning symptoms of hypoglycemia were less pronounced or different from those experienced with their previous insulin.

Without recognition of early warning symptoms, you may not be able to take steps to avoid more serious hypoglycemia. Be alert for all of the various types of symptoms that may indicate hypoglycemia. Patients who experience hypoglycemia without early warning symptoms should monitor their blood glucose frequently, especially prior to activities such as driving. If the blood glucose is below your normal fasting glucose, you should consider eating or drinking sugar-containing foods to treat your hypoglycemia.

Mild to moderate hypoglycemia may be treated by eating foods or drinks that contain sugar. Patients should always carry a quick source of sugar, such as candy mints or glucose tablets. More severe hypoglycemia may require the assistance of another person. Patients who are unable to take sugar orally or who are unconscious require an injection of glucagon or should be treated with intravenous administration of glucose at a medical facility.

You should learn to recognize your own symptoms of hypoglycemia. If you are uncertain about these symptoms, you should monitor your blood glucose frequently to help you learn to recognize the symptoms that you experience with hypoglycemia.

If you have frequent episodes of hypoglycemia or experience difficulty in recognizing the symptoms, you should consult your doctor to discuss possible changes in therapy, meal plans, and/or exercise programs to help you avoid hypoglycemia.

Hyperglycemia and Diabetic Acidosis
Hyperglycemia (too much glucose in the blood) may develop if your body has too little insulin. Hyperglycemia can be brought about by:

1. Omitting your insulin or taking less than the doctor has prescribed
2. Eating significantly more than your meal plan suggests
3. Developing a fever, infection, or other significant stressful situation

In patients with insulin-dependent diabetes, prolonged hyperglycemia can result in diabetic acidosis. The first symptoms of diabetic acidosis usually come on gradually, over a period of hours or days, and include a drowsy feeling, flushed face, thirst, loss of appetite, and fruity odor on the breath. With acidosis, urine tests show large amounts of glucose and acetone. Heavy breathing and a rapid pulse are more severe symptoms. If uncorrected, prolonged hyperglycemia or diabetic acidosis can lead to nausea, vomiting, dehydration, loss of consciousness or death. Therefore, it is important that you obtain medical assistance immediately.

Lipodystrophy
Rarely, administration of insulin subcutaneously can result in lipoatrophy (depression in the skin) or lipohypertrophy (enlargement or thickening of tissue). If you notice either of these conditions, consult your doctor. A change in your injection technique may help alleviate the problem.

Allergy to Insulin
Local Allergy—Patients occasionally experience redness, swelling, and itching at the site of injection of insulin. This condition, called local allergy, usually clears up in a few days to a few weeks. In some instances, this condition may be related to factors other than insulin, such as irritants in the skin cleansing agent or poor injection technique. If you have local reactions, contact your doctor.

Systemic Allergy—Less common, but potentially more serious, is generalized allergy to insulin, which may cause rash over the whole body, shortness of breath, wheezing, reduction in blood pressure, fast pulse, or sweating. Severe cases of generalized allergy may be life threatening. If you think you are having a generalized allergic reaction to insulin, notify a doctor immediately.

ADDITIONAL INFORMATION

Additional information about diabetes may be obtained from your diabetes educator.

DIABETES FORECAST is a national magazine designed especially for patients with diabetes and their families and is available on subscription from the American Diabetes Association, National Service Center, 1660 Duke Street, Alexandria, Virginia 22314, 1-800-DIABETES (1-800-342-2383).

Another publication, **DIABETES COUNTDOWN**, is available from the Juvenile Diabetes Foundation International (JDF), 120 Wall Street, 19th Floor, New York, New York 10005-4001, 1-800-JDF-CURE (1-800-533-2873).

Additional information about Humulin can be obtained by calling 1-888-88-LILLY (1-888-885-4559).

Literature revised March 26, 1999
PA 9077 FSAMP [032699]

*B-D® is a registered trademark of Becton Dickinson and Company.
†NovolinPen® and NovoPen® are registered trademarks of Novo Nordisk A/S.

HUMULIN® 70/30 Pen ℞

[*hū'mŭ-lĭn*]

3.0 ML Disposable Insulin Delivery Device
70% Human Insulin Isophane Suspension and
30% Human Insulin Injection (rDNA origin)

INFORMATION FOR THE PATIENT

WARNINGS

THIS LILLY HUMAN INSULIN PRODUCT DIFFERS FROM ANIMAL-SOURCE INSULINS BECAUSE IT IS STRUCTURALLY IDENTICAL TO THE INSULIN PRODUCED BY YOUR BODY'S PANCREAS AND BECAUSE OF ITS UNIQUE MANUFACTURING PROCESS.

ANY CHANGE OF INSULIN SHOULD BE MADE CAUTIOUSLY AND ONLY UNDER MEDICAL SUPERVISION. CHANGES IN STRENGTH, MANUFACTURER, TYPE (E.G., REGULAR, NPH, LENTE, ETC), SPECIES (BEEF, PORK, BEEF-PORK, HUMAN), OR METHOD OF MANUFACTURE (rDNA VERSUS ANIMAL-SOURCE INSULIN) MAY RESULT IN THE NEED FOR A CHANGE IN DOSAGE.

SOME PATIENTS TAKING HUMULIN® (HUMAN INSULIN, rDNA ORIGIN) MAY REQUIRE A CHANGE IN DOSAGE FROM THAT USED WITH ANIMAL-SOURCE INSULINS. IF AN ADJUSTMENT IS NEEDED, IT MAY OCCUR WITH THE FIRST DOSE OR DURING THE FIRST SEVERAL WEEKS OR MONTHS.

TO OBTAIN AN ACCURATE DOSE, CAREFULLY READ AND FOLLOW THE "DISPOSABLE INSULIN DELIVERY DEVICE USER MANUAL" AND THIS INFORMATION FOR THE PATIENT INSERT BEFORE USING THIS PRODUCT. (*see also* INSTRUCTIONS FOR PEN USE section.)

DIABETES
Insulin is a hormone produced by the pancreas, a large gland that lies near the stomach. This hormone is necessary for the body's correct use of food, especially sugar. Diabetes occurs when the pancreas does not make enough insulin to meet your body's needs.

To control your diabetes, your doctor has prescribed injections of insulin to keep your blood glucose at a nearly normal level. Proper control of your diabetes requires close and constant cooperation with your doctor. In spite of diabetes, you can lead an active, healthy, and useful life if you eat a balanced diet daily, exercise regularly, and take your insulin injections as prescribed.

You have been instructed to test your blood and/or your urine regularly for glucose. If your blood tests consistently show above- or below-normal glucose levels or your urine tests consistently show the presence of glucose, your diabetes is not properly controlled and you must let your doctor know.

Always keep an extra supply of insulin as well as a spare syringe and needle on hand. Always wear diabetic identification so that appropriate treatment can be given if complications occur away from home.

70/30 HUMAN INSULIN

Description

Humulin is synthesized in a non-disease-producing special laboratory strain of *Escherichia coli* bacteria that has been genetically altered by the addition of the human gene for insulin production. Humulin® 70/30 is a mixture of 70% Human Insulin Isophane Suspension and 30% Human Insulin Injection. It is an intermediate-acting insulin combined with the more rapid onset of action of regular insulin. The duration of activity may last up to 24 hours following injection. The time course of action of any insulin may vary considerably in different individuals or at different times in the same individual. As with all insulin preparations, the duration of action of Humulin 70/30 is dependent on dose, site of injection, blood supply, temperature, and physical activity. Humulin 70/30 is a sterile suspension and is for subcutaneous injection only. It should not be used intravenously or intramuscularly. The concentration of Humulin 70/30 in the Humulin 70/30 Pen is 100 units/mL (U-100).

Identification

Humulin disposable insulin delivery devices, manufactured by Eli Lilly and Company, are available in 2 formulations—NPH, and 70/30.

Your doctor has prescribed the type of insulin that he/she believes is best for you. **DO NOT USE ANY OTHER INSULIN EXCEPT ON HIS/HER ADVICE AND DIRECTION.**

The Humulin 70/30 Pen is available in boxes of 5 disposable insulin delivery devices ("insulin pens"). The Humulin 70/30 Pen is not designed to allow any other insulin to be mixed in its cartridge, or for the cartridge to be removed.

Always examine the appearance of Humulin 70/30 suspension in the insulin pen before administering a dose. A cartridge of Humulin 70/30 contains a small glass bead to assist in mixing. Humulin 70/30 Pen must be rolled between the palms 10 times and inverted 180° 10 times before each injection so that the contents are uniformly mixed (*see* Figures 1 and 2). Inspect the Humulin 70/30 suspension for uniform mixing and repeat the above steps as necessary.

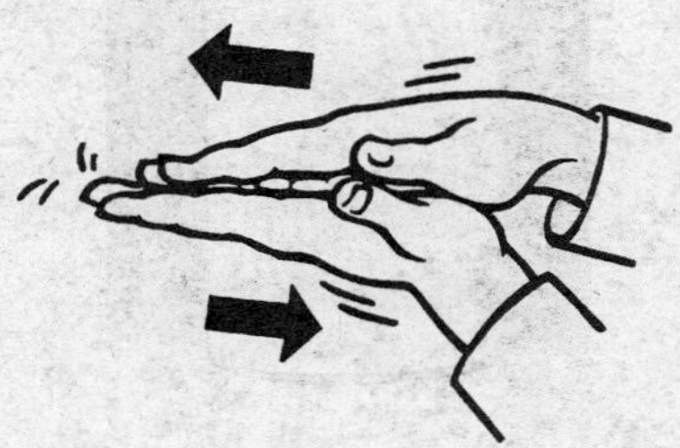

Figure 1.

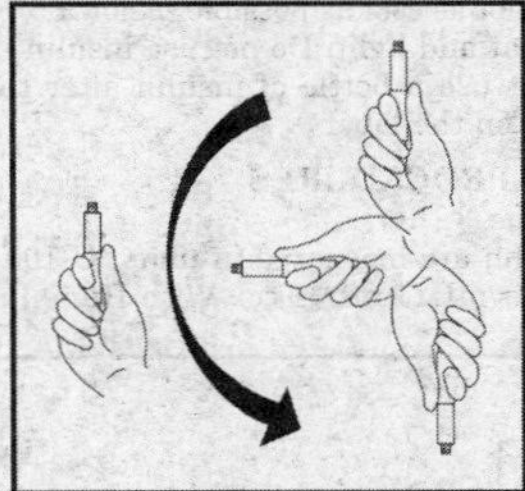

Figure 2.

Humulin 70/30 should look uniformly cloudy or milky after mixing. Do not use if the insulin substance (the white material) remains visibly separated from the liquid after mixing. Do not use Humulin 70/30 Pen if there are clumps in the insulin after mixing (*see* Figure 3). Do not use the Humulin 70/30 Pen if solid white particles stick to the walls of the cartridge, giving it a frosted appearance (*see* Figure 4).

Always check the appearance of the Humulin 70/30 suspension in the insulin pen before using, and if you note anything unusual in the appearance of Humulin 70/30 suspension or notice your insulin requirements changing markedly, consult your doctor.

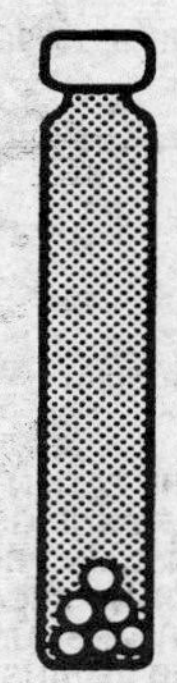

Figure 3.* – Do not use if there are clumps in the insulin after mixing.

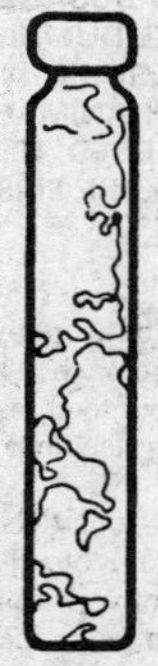

Figure 4.* – Do not use if particles on the bottom or wall give the cartridge a frosted appearance.

*Never attempt to remove the cartridge from the Humulin 70/30 Pen. Inspect the cartridge through the clear cartridge holder.

Storage

Humulin 70/30 Pens should be stored in a refrigerator but not in the freezer. The Humulin 70/30 Pen that you are currently using should not be refrigerated but should be kept as cool as possible (below 86°F [30°C]) and away from heat and light. Do not use an insulin pen if it has been frozen. Unrefrigerated Humulin 70/30 Pens **must be discarded after 10 days**, even if they still contain insulin. Do not use Humulin 70/30 Pens after the expiration date stamped on the label.

INSTRUCTIONS FOR PEN USE

It is important to read, understand, and follow the instructions in the "Disposable Insulin Delivery Device User Manual" before using. Failure to follow instructions may result in an inaccurate insulin dose.

NEVER SHARE INSULIN PENS, CARTRIDGES, OR NEEDLES.

PREPARING THE PEN FOR INJECTION:

1. Always check the appearance of the Humulin 70/30 suspension in the insulin pen before using.
2. Roll the Humulin 70/30 Pen between the palms 10 times (*see* Figure 1 above).
3. Holding the Humulin 70/30 Pen by one end, invert it 180° slowly 10 times to allow the glass bead to travel the full length of the cartridge with each inversion (*see* Figure 2 above). The cartridge is contained in the clear cartridge holder of the Humulin 70/30 Pen.
4. Inspect the appearance of the Humulin 70/30 suspension to make sure the contents look uniformly cloudy or milky. If not, repeat the above steps until the contents are mixed. Do not use a Humulin 70/30 Pen if there are clumps in the insulin or if solid white particles stick to the walls of the cartridge. (*see* Figures 3 and 4 above).
5. Follow the instruction in the "Disposable Insulin Delivery Device User Manual" for these steps:
   - Preparing the Pen
   - Attaching the Needle
   - Priming the Pen (Checking the Insulin Flow)
   - Setting (Dialing) a Dose
   - Injecting the Dose
   - Following an Injection

PREPARING FOR INJECTION:

1. Wash your hands.
2. To avoid tissue damage, choose a site for each injection that is at least 1/2 inch from the previous injection site. The usual sites of injection are abdomen, thighs, and arms.
3. Cleanse the skin with alcohol where the injection is to be made.
4. With one hand, stabilize the skin by spreading it or pinching up a large area.
5. Inject the dose as instructed by your doctor.
6. After dispensing a dose, pull the needle out and apply gentle pressure over the injection site for several seconds. Do not rub the area.
7. Immediately after an injection, remove the needle from the Humulin 70/30 Pen. Doing so will guard against contamination, leakage, reentry of air, and needle clogs. Do not reuse needles. Dispose of needles in a responsible manner.

DOSAGE

Your doctor has told you which insulin to use, how much, and when and how often to inject it. Because each patient's case of diabetes is different, this schedule has been individualized for you.

Your usual insulin dose may be affected by changes in your food, activity, or work schedule. Carefully follow your doctor's instructions to allow for these changes. Other things that may affect your insulin dose are:

Illness

Illness, especially with nausea and vomiting, may cause your insulin requirements to change. Even if you are not eating, you will still require insulin. You and your doctor should establish a sick day plan for you to use in case of illness. When you are sick, test your blood glucose/urine glucose and ketones frequently and call your doctor as instructed.

Pregnancy

Good control of diabetes is especially important for you and your unborn baby. Pregnancy may make managing your diabetes more difficult. If you are planning to have a baby, are pregnant, or are nursing a baby, consult your doctor.

Medication

Insulin requirements may be increased if you are taking other drugs with hyperglycemic activity, such as oral contraceptives, corticosteroids, or thyroid replacement therapy. Insulin requirements may be reduced in the presence of drugs with hypoglycemic activity, such as oral hypoglycemics, salicylates (for example, aspirin), sulfa antibiotics, and certain antidepressants. Always discuss any medications you are taking with your doctor.

Exercise

Exercise may lower your body's need for insulin during and for some time after the activity. Exercise may also speed up the effect of an insulin dose, especially if the exercise involves the area of injection site (for example, the leg should not be used for injection just prior to running). Discuss with your doctor how you should adjust your regimen to accommodate exercise.

Travel

Persons traveling across more than 2 time zones should consult their doctor concerning adjustments in their insulin schedule.

COMMON PROBLEMS OF DIABETES

Hypoglycemia (Insulin Reaction)

Hypoglycemia (too little glucose in the blood) is one of the most frequent adverse events experienced by insulin users. It can be brought about by:

1. Taking too much insulin
2. Missing or delaying meals
3. Exercising or working more than usual
4. An infection or illness (especially with diarrhea or vomiting)
5. A change in the body's need for insulin
6. Diseases of the adrenal, pituitary or thyroid gland, or progression of kidney or liver disease
7. Interactions with other drugs that lower blood glucose, such as oral hypoglycemics, salicylates (for example, aspirin), sulfa antibiotics, and certain antidepressants
8. Consumption of alcoholic beverages

Symptoms of mild to moderate hypoglycemia may occur suddenly and can include:

- sweating
- dizziness
- palpitation
- tremor
- hunger
- restlessness
- tingling in the hands, feet, lips, or tongue
- lightheadedness
- drowsiness
- sleep disturbances
- anxiety
- blurred vision
- slurred speech
- depressed mood
- irritability
- abnormal behavior
- inability to concentrate
- headache
- unsteady movement
- personality changes

Continued on next page

*** Identi-Code® symbol. This product information was prepared in June 2000. Current information on these and other products of Eli Lilly and Company may be obtained by direct inquiry to Lilly Research Laboratories, Lilly Corporate Center, Indianapolis, Indiana 46285, (800) 545-5979.**

Humulin 70/30 Pen—Cont.

Signs of severe hypoglycemia can include:

- disorientation
- unconsciousness
- seizures
- death

Therefore, it is important that assistance be obtained immediately.

Early warning symptoms of hypoglycemia may be different or less pronounced under certain conditions, such as long duration of diabetes, diabetic nerve disease, medications such as beta-blockers, change in insulin preparations, or intensified control (3 or more insulin injections per day) of diabetes.

A few patients who have experienced hypoglycemic reactions after transfer from animal-source insulin to human insulin have reported that the early warning symptoms of hypoglycemia were less pronounced or different from those experienced with their previous insulin.

Without recognition of early warning symptoms, you may not be able to take steps to avoid more serious hypoglycemia. Be alert for all of the various types of symptoms that may indicate hypoglycemia. Patients who experience hypoglycemia without early warning symptoms should monitor their blood glucose frequently, especially prior to activities such as driving. If the blood glucose is below your normal fasting glucose, you should consider eating or drinking sugar-containing foods to treat your hypoglycemia.

Mild to moderate hypoglycemia may be treated by eating foods or drinks that contain sugar. Patients should always carry a quick source of sugar, such as candy mints or glucose tablets. More severe hypoglycemia may require the assistance of another person. Patients who are unable to take sugar orally or who are unconscious require an injection of glucagon or should be treated with intravenous administration of glucose at a medical facility.

You should learn to recognize your own symptoms of hypoglycemia. If you are uncertain about these symptoms, you should monitor your blood glucose frequently to help you learn to recognize the symptoms that you experience with hypoglycemia.

If you have frequent episodes of hypoglycemia or experience difficulty in recognizing the symptoms, you should consult your doctor to discuss possible changes in therapy, meal plans, and/or exercise programs to help you avoid hypoglycemia.

Hyperglycemia and Diabetic Acidosis

Hyperglycemia (too much glucose in the blood) may develop if your body has too little insulin. Hyperglycemia can be brought about by:

1. Omitting your insulin or taking less than the doctor has prescribed
2. Eating significantly more than your meal plan suggests
3. Developing a fever, infection, or other significant stressful situation

In patients with insulin-dependent diabetes, prolonged hyperglycemia can result in diabetic acidosis. The first symptoms of diabetic acidosis usually come on gradually, over a period of hours or days, and include a drowsy feeling, flushed face, thirst, loss of appetite, and fruity odor on the breath. With acidosis, urine tests show large amounts of glucose and acetone. Heavy breathing and a rapid pulse are more severe symptoms. If uncorrected, prolonged hyperglycemia or diabetic acidosis can lead to nausea, vomiting, dehydration, loss of consciousness or death. Therefore, it is important that you obtain medical assistance immediately.

Lipodystrophy

Rarely, administration of insulin subcutaneously can result in lipoatrophy (depression in the skin) or lipohypertrophy (enlargement or thickening of tissue). If you notice either of these conditions, consult your doctor. A change in your injection technique may help alleviate the problem.

Allergy to Insulin

Local Allergy—Patients occasionally experience redness, swelling, and itching at the site of injection of insulin. This condition, called local allergy, usually clears up in a few days to a few weeks. In some instances, this condition may be related to factors other than insulin, such as irritants in the skin cleansing agent or poor injection technique. If you have local reactions, contact your doctor.

Systemic Allergy—Less common, but potentially more serious, is generalized allergy to insulin, which may cause rash over the whole body, shortness of breath, wheezing, reduction in blood pressure, fast pulse, or sweating. Severe cases of generalized allergy may be life threatening. If you think you are having a generalized allergic reaction to insulin, notify a doctor immediately.

ADDITIONAL INFORMATION

Additional information about diabetes may be obtained from your diabetes educator.

DIABETES FORECAST is a national magazine designed especially for patients with diabetes and their families and is available on subscription from the American Diabetes Association, National Service Center, 1660 Duke Street, Alexandria, Virginia 22314, 1-800-DIABETES (1-800-342-2383).

Another publication, **DIABETES COUNTDOWN**, is available from the Juvenile Diabetes Foundation International (JDF), 120 Wall Street, 19th Floor, New York, New York 10005-4001, 1-800-JDF-CURE (1-800-533-2873).

Additional information about Humulin and Humulin 70/30 Pen can be obtained by calling 1-888-88-LILLY (1-888-885-4559).

Literature issued March 26, 1999
PA 9141 FSAMP [032699]

HUMULIN® L OTC

[*hū 'mū-lĭn ĕl*]
Lente®
(human insulin [rDNA origin] zinc suspension)

INFORMATION FOR THE PATIENT

WARNINGS

THIS LILLY HUMAN INSULIN PRODUCT DIFFERS FROM ANIMAL-SOURCE INSULINS BECAUSE IT IS STRUCTURALLY IDENTICAL TO THE INSULIN PRODUCED BY YOUR BODY'S PANCREAS AND BECAUSE OF ITS UNIQUE MANUFACTURING PROCESS.

ANY CHANGE OF INSULIN SHOULD BE MADE CAUTIOUSLY AND ONLY UNDER MEDICAL SUPERVISION. CHANGES IN STRENGTH, MANUFACTURER, TYPE (E.G., REGULAR, NPH, LENTE®), SPECIES (BEEF, PORK, BEEF-PORK, HUMAN), OR METHOD OF MANUFACTURE (rDNA VERSUS ANIMAL-SOURCE INSULIN) MAY RESULT IN THE NEED FOR A CHANGE IN DOSAGE.

SOME PATIENTS TAKING HUMULIN® (HUMAN INSULIN, rDNA ORIGIN) MAY REQUIRE A CHANGE IN DOSAGE FROM THAT USED WITH ANIMAL-SOURCE INSULINS. IF AN ADJUSTMENT IS NEEDED, IT MAY OCCUR WITH THE FIRST DOSE OR DURING THE FIRST SEVERAL WEEKS OR MONTHS.

DIABETES

Insulin is a hormone produced by the pancreas, a large gland that lies near the stomach. This hormone is necessary for the body's correct use of food, especially sugar. Diabetes occurs when the pancreas does not make enough insulin to meet your body's needs.

To control your diabetes, your doctor has prescribed injections of insulin to keep your blood glucose at a nearly normal level. Proper control of your diabetes requires close and constant cooperation with your doctor. In spite of diabetes, you can lead an active, healthy, and useful life if you eat a balanced diet daily, exercise regularly, and take your insulin injections as prescribed.

You have been instructed to test your blood and/or your urine regularly for glucose. If your blood tests consistently show above- or below-normal glucose levels or your urine tests consistently show the presence of glucose, your diabetes is not properly controlled and you must let your doctor know.

Always keep an extra supply of insulin as well as a spare syringe and needle on hand. Always wear diabetic identification so that appropriate treatment can be given if complications occur away from home.

LENTE HUMAN INSULIN

Description

Humulin is synthesized in a special non-disease-producing laboratory strain of *Escherichia coli* bacteria that has been genetically altered by the addition of the gene for human insulin production. Humulin L is an amorphous and crystalline suspension of human insulin with zinc providing an intermediate-acting insulin with a slower onset and a longer duration of activity (up to 24 hours) than regular insulin. The time course of action of any insulin may vary considerably in different individuals or at different times in the same individual. As with all insulin preparations, the duration of action of Humulin L is dependent on dose, site of injection, blood supply, temperature, and physical activity. Humulin L is a sterile suspension and is for subcutaneous injection only. It should not be used intravenously or intramuscularly. The concentration of Humulin L is 100 units/mL (U-100).

Identification

Human insulin manufactured by Eli Lilly and Company has the trademark Humulin and is available in 6 formulations—Regular (**R**), NPH (**N**), Lente (**L**), Ultralente® (**U**), 50% Human Insulin Isophane Suspension [NPH]/50% Human Insulin Injection [buffered regular] (**50/50**), and 70% Human Insulin Isophane Suspension [NPH]/30% Human Insulin Injection [buffered regular] (**70/30**). Your doctor has prescribed the type of insulin that he/she believes is best for you. **DO NOT USE ANY OTHER INSULIN EXCEPT ON HIS/HER ADVICE AND DIRECTION.**

Always check the carton and the bottle label for the name and letter designation of the insulin you receive from your pharmacy to make sure it is the same as that your doctor has prescribed. Humulin L can be identified as follows:

[See graphic at bottom of page]

Always examine the appearance of your bottle of insulin before withdrawing each dose. A bottle of Humulin L must be carefully shaken or rotated before each injection so that the contents are uniformly mixed. Humulin L should look uniformly cloudy or milky after mixing. Do not use it if the insulin substance (the white material) remains at the bottom of the bottle after mixing (Figure 1). Do not use a bottle of Humulin L if there are clumps in the insulin after mixing (Figure 2). Always check the appearance of your bottle of insulin before using, and if you note anything unusual in the appearance of your insulin or notice your insulin requirements changing markedly, consult your doctor.

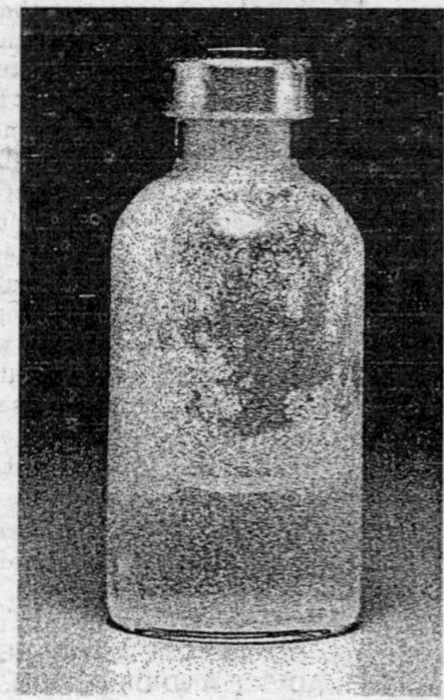

Fig. 1.—Do not use if the insulin material remains at the bottom of the bottle after mixing.

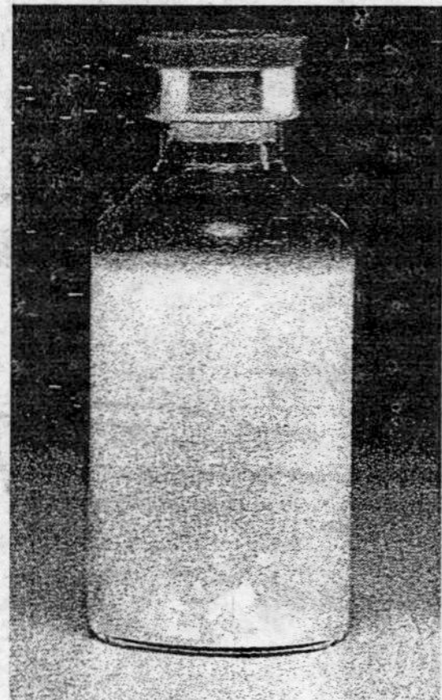

Fig. 2.—Do not use if there are clumps in the insulin after mixing.

Storage

Insulin should be stored in a refrigerator but not in the freezer. If refrigeration is not possible, the bottle of insulin that you are currently using can be kept unrefrigerated as long as it is kept as cool as possible (below 86°F [30°C]) and away from heat and light. Do not use insulin if it has been frozen. Do not use a bottle of insulin after the expiration date stamped on the label.

INJECTION PROCEDURES

Correct Syringe

Doses of insulin are measured in **units**. U-100 insulin contains 100 units/mL (1 mL=1 cc). With Humulin L, it is im-

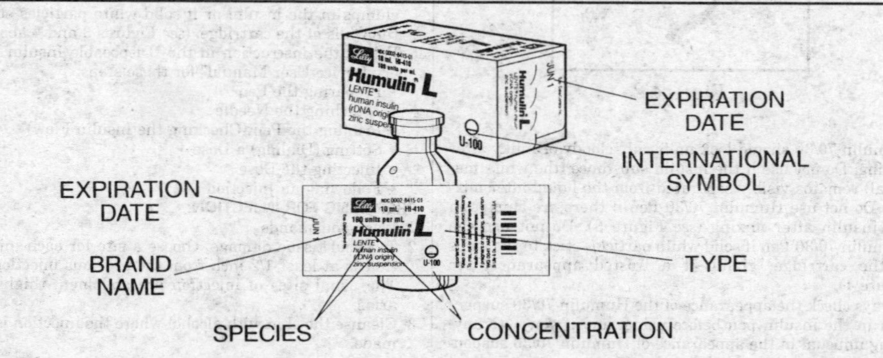

portant to use a syringe that is marked for U-100 insulin preparations. Failure to use the proper syringe can lead to a mistake in dosage, causing serious problems for you, such as a blood glucose level that is too low or too high.

Syringe Use

To help avoid contamination and possible infection, follow these instructions exactly.

Disposable syringes and needles should be used only once and then discarded. **NEEDLES AND SYRINGES MUST NOT BE SHARED.**

Reusable syringes and needles must be sterilized before each injection. **Follow the package directions supplied with your syringe.** Described below are 2 methods of sterilizing.

Boiling

1. Put syringe, plunger, and needle in strainer, place in saucepan, and cover with water. Boil for 5 minutes.
2. Remove articles from water. When they have cooled, insert plunger into barrel, and fasten needle to syringe with a slight twist.
3. Push plunger in and out several times until water is completely removed.

Isopropyl Alcohol

If the syringe, plunger, and needle cannot be boiled, as when you are traveling, they may be sterilized by immersion for at least 5 minutes in Isopropyl Alcohol, 91%. Do not use bathing, rubbing, or medicated alcohol for this sterilization. If the syringe is sterilized with alcohol, it must be absolutely dry before use.

Preparing the Dose

1. Wash your hands.
2. Carefully shake or rotate the insulin bottle several times to completely mix the insulin.
3. Inspect the insulin. Humulin L should look uniformly cloudy or milky. Do not use it if you notice anything unusual in the appearance.
4. If using a new bottle, flip off the plastic protective cap, but **do not** remove the stopper. When using a new bottle, wipe the top of the bottle with an alcohol swab.
5. If you are mixing insulins, refer to the instructions for mixing that follow.
6. Draw air into the syringe equal to your insulin dose. Put the needle through rubber top of the insulin bottle and inject the air into the bottle.
7. Turn the bottle and syringe upside down. Hold the bottle and syringe firmly in 1 hand and shake gently.
8. Making sure the tip of the needle is in the insulin, withdraw the correct dose of insulin into the syringe.
9. Before removing the needle from the bottle, check your syringe for air bubbles which reduce the amount of insulin in it. If bubbles are present, hold the syringe straight up and tap its side until the bubbles float to the top. Push them out with the plunger and withdraw the correct dose.
10. Remove the needle from the bottle and lay the syringe down so that the needle does not touch anything.

Mixing Humulin L with Regular or Ultralente Human Insulin

1. Lente human insulin should be mixed with regular or Ultralente human insulin only on the advice of your doctor.
2. Draw air into your syringe equal to the amount of Humulin L you are taking. Insert the needle into the Humulin L bottle and inject the air. Withdraw the needle.
3. Now inject air into your regular or Ultralente human insulin bottle in the same manner, but **do not** withdraw the needle.
4. Turn the bottle and syringe upside down.
5. Making sure the tip of the needle is in the insulin, withdraw the correct dose of regular or Ultralente insulin into the syringe.
6. Before removing the needle from the bottle, check your syringe for air bubbles which reduce the amount of insulin in it. If bubbles are present, hold the syringe straight up and tap its side until the bubbles float to the top. Push them out with the plunger and withdraw the correct dose.
7. Remove the needle from the bottle of regular or Ultralente insulin and insert it into the bottle of Humulin L. Turn the bottle and syringe upside down. Hold the bottle and syringe firmly in 1 hand and shake gently. Making sure the tip of the needle is in the insulin, withdraw your dose of Humulin L.
8. Remove the needle and lay the syringe down so that the needle does not touch anything.

Follow your doctor's instructions on whether to mix your insulins ahead of time or just before giving your injection. It is important to be consistent in your method.

Syringes from different manufacturers may vary in the amount of space between the bottom line and the needle. Because of this, do not change:

- the sequence of mixing, or
- the model and brand of syringe or needle that the doctor has prescribed.

Injection

Cleanse the skin with alcohol where the injection is to be made. Stabilize the skin by spreading it or pinching up a large area. Insert the needle as instructed by your doctor. Push the plunger in as far as it will go. Pull the needle out and apply gentle pressure over the injection site for several seconds. **Do not rub the area.** To avoid tissue damage, give the next injection at a site at least $^1/_2$" from the previous site.

DOSAGE

Your doctor has told you which insulin to use, how much, and when and how often to inject it. Because each patient's case of diabetes is different, this schedule has been individualized for you.

Your usual insulin dose may be affected by changes in your food, activity, or work schedule. Carefully follow your doctor's instructions to allow for these changes. Other things that may affect your insulin dose are:

Illness

Illness, especially with nausea and vomiting, may cause your insulin requirements to change. Even if you are not eating, you will still require insulin. You and your doctor should establish a sick day plan for you to use in case of illness. When you are sick, test your blood/urine frequently and call your doctor as instructed.

Pregnancy

Good control of diabetes is especially important for you and your unborn baby. Pregnancy may make managing your diabetes more difficult. If you are planning to have a baby, are pregnant, or are nursing a baby, consult your doctor.

Medication

Insulin requirements may be increased if you are taking other drugs with hyperglycemic activity, such as oral contraceptives, corticosteroids, or thyroid replacement therapy. Insulin requirements may be reduced in the presence of drugs with hypoglycemic activity, such as oral hypoglycemics, salicylates (for example, aspirin), sulfa antibiotics, and certain antidepressants. Always discuss any medications you are taking with your doctor.

Exercise

Exercise may lower your body's need for insulin during and for some time after the activity. Exercise may also speed up the effect of an insulin dose, especially if the exercise involves the area of injection site (for example, the leg should not be used for injection just prior to running). Discuss with your doctor how you should adjust your regimen to accommodate exercise.

Travel

Persons traveling across more than 2 time zones should consult their doctor concerning adjustments in their insulin schedule.

COMMON PROBLEMS OF DIABETES

Hypoglycemia (Insulin Reaction)

Hypoglycemia (too little glucose in the blood) is one of the most frequent adverse events experienced by insulin users. It can be brought about by:

1. Taking too much insulin
2. Missing or delaying meals
3. Exercising or working more than usual
4. An infection or illness (especially with diarrhea or vomiting)
5. A change in the body's need for insulin
6. Diseases of the adrenal, pituitary, or thyroid gland, or progression of kidney or liver disease
7. Interactions with other drugs that lower blood glucose, such as oral hypoglycemics, salicylates (for example, aspirin), sulfa antibiotics, and certain antidepressants
8. Consumption of alcoholic beverages

Symptoms of mild to moderate hypoglycemia may occur suddenly and can include:

- sweating
- dizziness
- palpitation
- tremor
- hunger
- restlessness
- tingling in the hands, feet, lips, or tongue
- lightheadedness
- inability to concentrate
- headache
- drowsiness
- sleep disturbances
- anxiety
- blurred vision
- slurred speech
- depressed mood
- irritability
- abnormal behavior
- unsteady movement
- personality changes

Signs of severe hypoglycemia can include:

- disorientation
- unconsciousness
- seizures
- death

Therefore, it is important that assistance be obtained immediately.

Early warning symptoms of hypoglycemia may be different or less pronounced under certain conditions, such as long duration of diabetes, diabetic nerve disease, medications such as beta-blockers, change in insulin preparations, or intensified control (3 or more insulin injections per day) of diabetes.

A few patients who have experienced hypoglycemic reactions after transfer from animal-source insulin to human insulin have reported that the early warning symptoms of hypoglycemia were less pronounced or different from those experienced with their previous insulin.

Without recognition of early warning symptoms, you may not be able to take steps to avoid more serious hypoglycemia. Be alert for all of the various types of symptoms that may indicate hypoglycemia. Patients who experience hypoglycemia without early warning symptoms should monitor their blood glucose frequently, especially prior to activities such as driving. If the blood glucose is below your normal fasting glucose, you should consider eating or drinking sugar-containing foods to treat your hypoglycemia.

Mild to moderate hypoglycemia may be treated by eating foods or drinks that contain sugar. Patients should always carry a quick source of sugar, such as candy mints or glucose tablets. More severe hypoglycemia may require the assistance of another person. Patients who are unable to take sugar orally or who are unconscious require an injection of glucagon or should be treated with intravenous administration of glucose at a medical facility.

You should learn to recognize your own symptoms of hypoglycemia. If you are uncertain about these symptoms, you should monitor your blood glucose frequently to help you learn to recognize the symptoms that you experience with hypoglycemia.

If you have frequent episodes of hypoglycemia or experience difficulty in recognizing the symptoms, you should consult your doctor to discuss possible changes in therapy, meal plans, and/or exercise programs to help you avoid hypoglycemia.

Hyperglycemia and Diabetic Acidosis

Hyperglycemia (too much glucose in the blood) may develop if your body has too little insulin. Hyperglycemia can be brought about by:

1. Omitting your insulin or taking less than the doctor has prescribed
2. Eating significantly more than your meal plan suggests
3. Developing a fever, infection, or other significant stressful situation

In patients with insulin-dependent diabetes, prolonged hyperglycemia can result in diabetic acidosis. The first symptoms of diabetic acidosis usually come on gradually, over a period of hours or days, and include a drowsy feeling, flushed face, thirst, loss of appetite, and fruity odor on the breath. With acidosis, urine tests show large amounts of glucose and acetone. Heavy breathing and a rapid pulse are more severe symptoms. If uncorrected, prolonged hyperglycemia or diabetic acidosis can lead to nausea, vomiting, dehydration, loss of consciousness or death. Therefore, it is important that you obtain medical assistance immediately.

Lipodystrophy

Rarely, administration of insulin subcutaneously can result in lipoatrophy (depression in the skin) or lipohypertrophy (enlargement or thickening of tissue). If you notice either of these conditions, consult your doctor. A change in your injection technique may help alleviate the problem.

Allergy to Insulin

Local Allergy —Patients occasionally experience redness, swelling, and itching at the site of injection of insulin. This condition, called local allergy, usually clears up in a few days to a few weeks. In some instances, this condition may be related to factors other than insulin, such as irritants in the skin cleansing agent or poor injection technique. If you have local reactions, contact your doctor.

Systemic Allergy —Less common, but potentially more serious, is generalized allergy to insulin, which may cause rash over the whole body, shortness of breath, wheezing, reduction in blood pressure, fast pulse, or sweating. Severe cases of generalized allergy may be life threatening. If you think you are having a generalized allergic reaction to insulin, notify a doctor immediately.

ADDITIONAL INFORMATION

Additional information about diabetes may be obtained from your diabetes educator.

DIABETES FORECAST is a national magazine designed especially for patients with diabetes and their families and is available by subscription from the American Diabetes Association, National Service Center, 1660 Duke Street, Alexandria, Virginia 22314, 1-800-DIABETES (1-800-342-2383).

Another publication, **DIABETES COUNTDOWN**, is available from the Juvenile Diabetes Foundation International (JDF), 120 Wall Street, 19th Floor, New York, New York 10005-4001, 1-800-JDF-CURE (1-800-533-2873).

Additional information about Humulin can be obtained by calling 1-888-88-LILLY (1-888-885-4559).

Literature revised August 13, 1999

PA 6355 AMP [081399]

HUMULIN® N OTC

[*hū 'mū-lĭn ĕn*]

NPH

(human insulin [rDNA origin] isophane suspension)

INFORMATION FOR THE PATIENT

WARNINGS

THIS LILLY HUMAN INSULIN PRODUCT DIFFERS FROM ANIMAL-SOURCE INSULINS BECAUSE IT IS STRUCTURALLY IDENTICAL TO THE INSULIN PRODUCED BY YOUR BODY'S PANCREAS AND BECAUSE OF ITS UNIQUE MANUFACTURING PROCESS.

ANY CHANGE OF INSULIN SHOULD BE MADE CAUTIOUSLY AND ONLY UNDER MEDICAL SUPERVISION. CHANGES IN STRENGTH, MANUFACTURER, TYPE (E.G., REGULAR, NPH, LENTE®), SPECIES (BEEF, PORK, BEEF-

Continued on next page

*** Identi-Code® symbol. This product information was prepared in June 2000. Current information on these and other products of Eli Lilly and Company may be obtained by direct inquiry to Lilly Research Laboratories, Lilly Corporate Center, Indianapolis, Indiana 46285, (800) 545-5979.**

Humulin N—Cont.

PORK, HUMAN), OR METHOD OF MANUFACTURE (rDNA VERSUS ANIMAL-SOURCE INSULIN) MAY RESULT IN THE NEED FOR A CHANGE IN DOSAGE.
SOME PATIENTS TAKING HUMULIN® (HUMAN INSULIN, rDNA ORIGIN) MAY REQUIRE A CHANGE IN DOSAGE FROM THAT USED WITH ANIMAL-SOURCE INSULINS. IF AN ADJUSTMENT IS NEEDED, IT MAY OCCUR WITH THE FIRST DOSE OR DURING THE FIRST SEVERAL WEEKS OR MONTHS.

DIABETES

Insulin is a hormone produced by the pancreas, a large gland that lies near the stomach. This hormone is necessary for the body's correct use of food, especially sugar. Diabetes occurs when the pancreas does not make enough insulin to meet your body's needs.
To control your diabetes, your doctor has prescribed injections of insulin to keep your blood glucose at a nearly normal level. Proper control of your diabetes requires close and constant cooperation with your doctor. In spite of diabetes, you can lead an active, healthy, and useful life if you eat a balanced diet daily, exercise regularly, and take your insulin injections as prescribed.
You have been instructed to test your blood and/or your urine regularly for glucose. If your blood tests consistently show above- or below-normal glucose levels or your urine tests consistently show the presence of glucose, your diabetes is not properly controlled and you must let your doctor know.
Always keep an extra supply of insulin as well as a spare syringe and needle on hand. Always wear diabetic identification so that appropriate treatment can be given if complications occur away from home.

NPH HUMAN INSULIN

Description
Humulin is synthesized in a special non-disease-producing laboratory strain of *Escherichia coli* bacteria that has been genetically altered by the addition of the gene for human insulin production. Humulin N is a crystalline suspension of human insulin with protamine and zinc providing an intermediate-acting insulin with a slower onset of action and a longer duration of activity (up to 24 hours) than that of regular insulin. The time course of action of any insulin may vary considerably in different individuals or at different times in the same individual. As with all insulin preparations, the duration of action of Humulin N is dependent on dose, site of injection, blood supply, temperature, and physical activity. Humulin N is a sterile suspension and is for subcutaneous injection only. It should not be used intravenously or intramuscularly. The concentration of Humulin N is 100 units/mL (U-100).

Identification
Human insulin manufactured by Eli Lilly and Company has the trademark Humulin and is available in 6 formulations—Regular (**R**), NPH (**N**), Lente (**L**), Ultralente® (**U**), 50% Human Insulin Isophane Suspension [NPH]/50% Human Insulin Injection [buffered regular] (**50/50**), and 70% Human Insulin Isophane Suspension [NPH]/30% Human Insulin Injection [buffered regular] (**70/30**). Your doctor has prescribed the type of insulin that he/she believes is best for you. **DO NOT USE ANY OTHER INSULIN EXCEPT ON HIS/HER ADVICE AND DIRECTION.**
Always check the carton and the bottle label for the name and letter designation of the insulin you receive from your pharmacy to make sure it is the same as that your doctor has prescribed. Humulin N can be identified as follows:
[See graphic below]
Always examine the appearance of your bottle of insulin before withdrawing each dose. A bottle of Humulin N must be carefully shaken or rotated before each injection so that the contents are uniformly mixed. Humulin N should look uniformly cloudy or milky after mixing. Do not use it if the insulin substance (the white material) remains at the bottom of the bottle after mixing. Do not use a bottle of Humulin N if there are clumps in the insulin after mixing (Figure 1). Do not use a bottle of Humulin N if solid white particles stick to the bottom or wall of the bottle, giving it a frosted appearance (Figure 2). Always check the appearance of your bottle of insulin before using, and if you note anything unusual in the appearance of your insulin or notice your insulin requirements changing markedly, consult your doctor.
[See figure at top of next column]

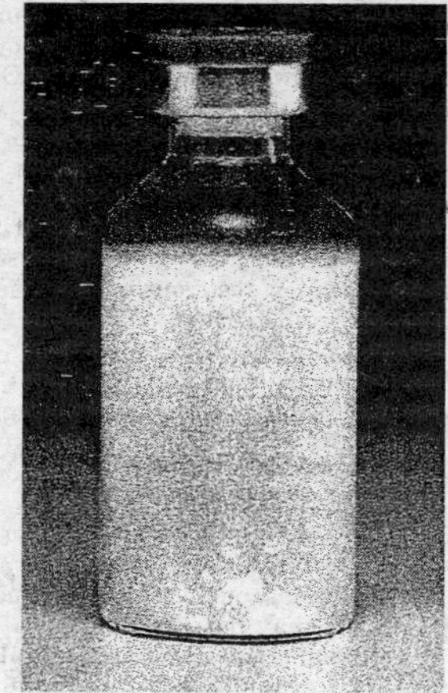

Fig. 1.—Do not use if there are clumps in the insulin after mixing.

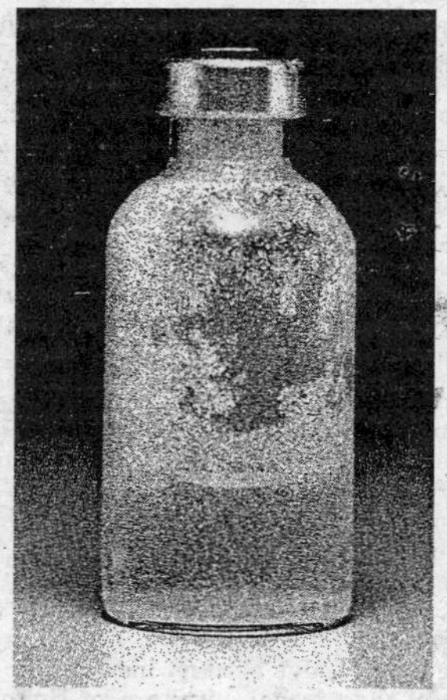
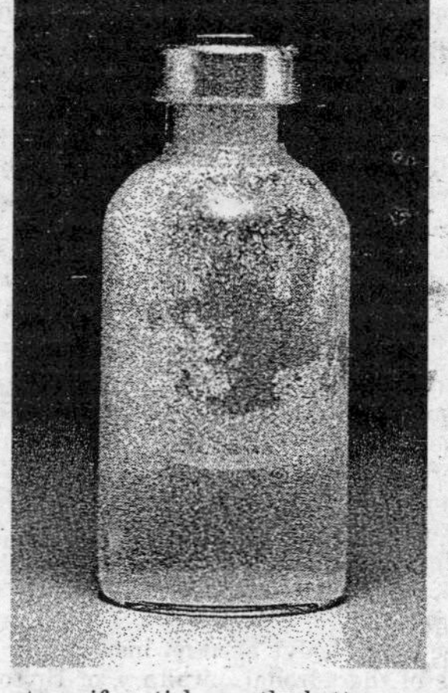

Fig. 2.—Do not use if particles on the bottom or wall give the bottle a frosted appearance.

Storage
Insulin should be stored in a refrigerator but not in the freezer. If refrigeration is not possible, the bottle of insulin that you are currently using can be kept unrefrigerated as long as it is kept as cool as possible (below 86°F [30°C]) and away from heat and light. Do not use insulin if it has been frozen. Do not use a bottle of insulin after the expiration date stamped on the label.

INJECTION PROCEDURES

Correct Syringe
Doses of insulin are measured in **units.** U-100 insulin contains 100 units/mL (1 mL = 1 cc). With Humulin N, it is important to use a syringe that is marked for U-100 insulin preparations. Failure to use the proper syringe can lead to a mistake in dosage, causing serious problems for you, such as a blood glucose level that is too low or too high.

Syringe Use
To help avoid contamination and possible infection, follow these instructions exactly.
Disposable syringes and needles should be used only once and then discarded. **NEEDLES AND SYRINGES MUST NOT BE SHARED.**
Reusable syringes and needles must be sterilized before each injection. **Follow the package directions supplied with your syringe.** Described below are 2 methods of sterilizing.

Boiling
1. Put syringe, plunger, and needle in strainer, place in saucepan, and cover with water. Boil for 5 minutes.
2. Remove articles from water. When they have cooled, insert plunger into barrel, and fasten needle to syringe with a slight twist.
3. Push plunger in and out several times until water is completely removed.

Isopropyl Alcohol
If the syringe, plunger, and needle cannot be boiled, as when you are traveling, they may be sterilized by immersion for at least 5 minutes in Isopropyl Alcohol, 91%. Do not use bathing, rubbing, or medicated alcohol for this sterilization. If the syringe is sterilized with alcohol, it must be absolutely dry before use.

Preparing the Dose
1. Wash your hands.
2. Carefully shake or rotate the insulin bottle several times to completely mix the insulin.
3. Inspect the insulin. Humulin N should look uniformly cloudy or milky. Do not use it if you notice anything unusual in the appearance.
4. If using a new bottle, flip off the plastic protective cap, but **do not** remove the stopper. When using a new bottle, wipe the top of the bottle with an alcohol swab.
5. If you are mixing insulins, refer to the instructions for mixing that follow.
6. Draw air into the syringe equal to your insulin dose. Put the needle through rubber top of the insulin bottle and inject the air into the bottle.
7. Turn the bottle and syringe upside down. Hold the bottle and syringe firmly in 1 hand and shake gently.
8. Making sure the tip of the needle is in the insulin, withdraw the correct dose of insulin into the syringe.
9. Before removing the needle from the bottle, check your syringe for air bubbles which reduce the amount of insulin in it. If bubbles are present, hold the syringe straight up and tap its side until the bubbles float to the top. Push them out with the plunger and withdraw the correct dose.
10. Remove the needle from the bottle and lay the syringe down so that the needle does not touch anything.

Mixing Humulin N and Regular Human Insulin
1. NPH human insulin should be mixed only with regular human insulin.
2. Draw air into your syringe equal to the amount of Humulin N you are taking. Insert the needle into the Humulin N bottle and inject the air. Withdraw the needle.
3. Now inject air into your regular human insulin bottle in the same manner, but **do not** withdraw the needle.
4. Turn the bottle and syringe upside down.
5. Making sure the tip of the needle is in the insulin, withdraw the correct dose of regular insulin into the syringe.
6. Before removing the needle from the bottle, check your syringe for air bubbles which reduce the amount of insulin in it. If bubbles are present, hold the syringe straight up and tap its side until the bubbles float to the top. Push them out with the plunger and withdraw the correct dose.
7. Remove the needle from the bottle of regular insulin and insert it into the bottle of Humulin N. Turn the bottle and syringe upside down. Hold the bottle and syringe firmly in 1 hand and shake gently. Making sure the tip of the needle is in the insulin, withdraw your dose of Humulin N.
8. Remove the needle and lay the syringe down so that the needle does not touch anything.

Follow your doctor's instructions on whether to mix your insulins ahead of time or just before giving your injection. It is important to be consistent in your method.
Syringes from different manufacturers may vary in the amount of space between the bottom line and the needle. Because of this, do not change:
- the sequence of mixing, or
- the model and brand of syringe or needle that the doctor has prescribed.

Injection
Cleanse the skin with alcohol where the injection is to be made. Stabilize the skin by spreading it or pinching up a large area. Insert the needle as instructed by your doctor. Push the plunger in as far as it will go. Pull the needle out and apply gentle pressure over the injection site for several seconds. **Do not rub the area.** To avoid tissue damage, give the next injection at a site at least 1/2" from the previous site.

DOSAGE

Your doctor has told you which insulin to use, how much, and when and how often to inject it. Because each patient's case of diabetes is different, this schedule has been individualized for you.
Your usual insulin dose may be affected by changes in your food, activity, or work schedule. Carefully follow your doctor's instructions to allow for these changes. Other things that may affect your insulin dose are:

Illness
Illness, especially with nausea and vomiting, may cause your insulin requirements to change. Even if you are not eating, you will still require insulin. You and your doctor should establish a sick day plan for you to use in case of illness. When you are sick, test your blood/urine frequently and call your doctor as instructed.

Pregnancy
Good control of diabetes is especially important for you and your unborn baby. Pregnancy may make managing your diabetes more difficult. If you are planning to have a baby, are pregnant, or are nursing a baby, consult your doctor.

Medication
Insulin requirements may be increased if you are taking other drugs with hyperglycemic activity, such as oral contraceptives, corticosteroids, or thyroid replacement therapy. Insulin requirements may be reduced in the presence of drugs with hypoglycemic activity, such as oral hypoglycemics, salicylates (for example, aspirin), sulfa antibiotics, and certain antidepressants. Always discuss any medications you are taking with your doctor.

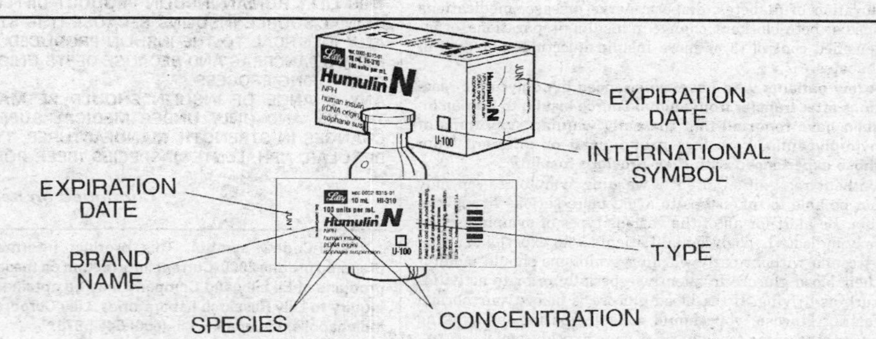

Exercise
Exercise may lower your body's need for insulin during and for some time after the activity. Exercise may also speed up the effect of an insulin dose, especially if the exercise involves the area of injection site (for example, the leg should not be used for injection just prior to running). Discuss with your doctor how you should adjust your regimen to accomodate exercise.
Travel
Persons traveling across more than 2 time zones should consult their doctor concerning adjustments in their insulin schedule.

COMMON PROBLEMS OF DIABETES
Hypoglycemia (Insulin Reaction)
Hypoglycemia (too little glucose in the blood) is one of the most frequent adverse events experienced by insulin users. It can be brought about by:
1. Taking too much insulin
2. Missing or delaying meals
3. Exercising or working more than usual
4. An infection or illness (especially with diarrhea or vomiting)
5. A change in the body's need for insulin
6. Diseases of the adrenal, pituitary, or thyroid gland, or progression of kidney or liver disease
7. Interactions with other drugs that lower blood glucose, such as oral hypoglycemics, salicylates (for example, aspirin), sulfa antibiotics, and certain antidepressants
8. Consumption of alcoholic beverages

Symptoms of mild to moderate hypoglycemia may occur suddenly and can include:
- sweating
- dizziness
- palpitation
- tremor
- hunger
- restlessness
- tingling in the hands, feet, lips, or tongue
- lightheadedness
- inability to concentrate
- headache
- drowsiness
- sleep disturbances
- anxiety
- blurred vision
- slurred speech
- depressed mood
- irritability
- abnormal behavior
- unsteady movement
- personality changes

Signs of severe hypoglycemia can include:
- disorientation
- unconsciousness
- seizures
- death

Therefore, it is important that assistance be obtained immediately.
Early warning symptoms of hypoglycemia may be different or less pronounced under certain conditions, such as long duration of diabetes, diabetic nerve disease, medications such as beta-blockers, change in insulin preparations, or intensified control (3 or more insulin injections per day) of diabetes.
A few patients who have experienced hypoglycemic reactions after transfer from animal-source insulin to human insulin have reported that the early warning symptoms of hypoglycemia were less pronounced or different from those experienced with their previous insulin.
Without recognition of early warning symptoms, you may not be able to take steps to avoid more serious hypoglycemia. Be alert for all of the various types of symptoms that may indicate hypoglycemia. Patients who experience hypoglycemia without early warning symptoms should monitor their blood glucose frequently, especially prior to activities such as driving. If the blood glucose is below your normal fasting glucose, you should consider eating or drinking sugar-containing foods to treat your hypoglycemia.
Mild to moderate hypoglycemia may be treated by eating foods or drinks that contain sugar. Patients should always carry a quick source of sugar, such as candy mints or glucose tablets. More severe hypoglycemia may require the assistance of another person. Patients who are unable to take sugar orally or who are unconscious require an injection of glucagon or should be treated with intravenous administration of glucose at a medical facility.
You should learn to recognize your own symptoms of hypoglycemia. If you are uncertain about these symptoms, you should monitor your blood glucose frequently to help you learn to recognize the symptoms that you experience with hypoglycemia.
If you have frequent episodes of hypoglycemia or experience difficulty in recognizing the symptoms, you should consult your doctor to discuss possible changes in therapy, meal plans, and/or exercise programs to help you avoid hypoglycemia.
Hyperglycemia and Diabetic Acidosis
Hyperglycemia (too much glucose in the blood) may develop if your body has too little insulin. Hyperglycemia can be brought about by:
1. Omitting your insulin or taking less than the doctor has prescribed
2. Eating significantly more than your meal plan suggests
3. Developing a fever, infection, or other significant stressful situation

In patients with insulin-dependent diabetes, prolonged hyperglycemia can result in diabetic acidosis. The first symptoms of diabetic acidosis usually come on gradually, over a period of hours or days, and include a drowsy feeling, flushed face, thirst, loss of appetite, and fruity odor on the breath. With acidosis, urine tests show large amounts of glucose and acetone. Heavy breathing and a rapid pulse are more severe symptoms. If uncorrected, prolonged hyperglycemia or diabetic acidosis can lead to nausea, vomiting, dehydration, loss of consciousness or death. Therefore, it is important that you obtain medical assistance immediately.
Lipodystrophy
Rarely, administration of insulin subcutaneously can result in lipoatrophy (depression in the skin) or lipohypertrophy (enlargement or thickening of tissue). If you notice either of these conditions, consult your doctor. A change in your injection technique may help alleviate the problem.
Allergy to Insulin
Local Allergy —Patients occasionally experience redness, swelling, and itching at the site of injection of insulin. This condition, called local allergy, usually clears up in a few days to a few weeks. In some instances, this condition may be related to factors other than insulin, such as irritants in the skin cleansing agent or poor injection technique. If you have local reactions, contact your doctor.
Systemic Allergy —Less common, but potentially more serious, is generalized allergy to insulin, which may cause rash over the whole body, shortness of breath, wheezing, reduction in blood pressure, fast pulse, or sweating. Severe cases of generalized allergy may be life threatening. If you think you are having a generalized allergic reaction to insulin, notify a doctor immediately.

ADDITIONAL INFORMATION
Additional information about diabetes may be obtained from your diabetes educator.
DIABETES FORECAST is a national magazine designed especially for patients with diabetes and their families and is available by subscription from the American Diabetes Association, National Service Center, 1660 Duke Street, Alexandria, Virginia 22314, 1-800-DIABETES (1-800-342-2383).
Another publication, **DIABETES COUNTDOWN**, is available from the Juvenile Diabetes Foundation International (JDF), 120 Wall Street, 19th Floor, New York, New York 10005-4001, 1-800-JDF-CURE (1-800-533-2873).
Additional information about Humulin can be obtained by calling 1-888-88-LILLY (1-888-885-4559).
Literature revised August 13, 1999
PA 6346 AMP [081399]

HUMULIN® N
NPH
[*hū ′mū-lĭn ĕn*]
Cartridge
(human insulin [rDNA origin]
isophane suspension)
1.5 mL CARTRIDGE

For use in Becton Dickinson and Company's B-D®* Pen and Novo Nordisk A/S's NovoPen®†, NovolinPen®†, and NovoPen®† 1.5 insulin delivery devices.

INFORMATION FOR THE PATIENT

WARNINGS
THIS LILLY HUMAN INSULIN PRODUCT DIFFERS FROM ANIMAL-SOURCE INSULINS BECAUSE IT IS STRUCTURALLY IDENTICAL TO THE INSULIN PRODUCED BY YOUR BODY'S PANCREAS AND BECAUSE OF ITS UNIQUE MANUFACTURING PROCESS.
ANY CHANGE OF INSULIN SHOULD BE MADE CAUTIOUSLY AND ONLY UNDER MEDICAL SUPERVISION. CHANGES IN STRENGTH, MANUFACTURER, TYPE (E.G., REGULAR, NPH, LENTE, ETC), SPECIES (BEEF, PORK, BEEF-PORK, HUMAN), OR METHOD OF MANUFACTURE (rDNA VERSUS ANIMAL-SOURCE INSULIN) MAY RESULT IN THE NEED FOR A CHANGE IN DOSAGE.
SOME PATIENTS TAKING HUMULIN® (HUMAN INSULIN, rDNA ORIGIN) MAY REQUIRE A CHANGE IN DOSAGE FROM THAT USED WITH ANIMAL-SOURCE INSULINS. IF AN ADJUSTMENT IS NEEDED, IT MAY OCCUR WITH THE FIRST DOSE OR DURING THE FIRST SEVERAL WEEKS OR MONTHS.
TO OBTAIN AN ACCURATE DOSE, CAREFULLY READ AND FOLLOW THE INSULIN DELIVERY DEVICE ("INSULIN PEN") MANUFACTURER'S INSTRUCTIONS AND THIS INFORMATION FOR THE PATIENT INSERT BEFORE USING THIS PRODUCT IN AN INSULIN PEN. (*see* INSTRUCTIONS FOR USE section)

DIABETES
Insulin is a hormone produced by the pancreas, a large gland that lies near the stomach. This hormone is necessary for the body's correct use of food, especially sugar. Diabetes occurs when the pancreas does not make enough insulin to meet your body's needs.
To control your diabetes, your doctor has prescribed injections of insulin to keep your blood glucose at a nearly normal level. Proper control of your diabetes requires close and constant cooperation with your doctor. In spite of diabetes, you can lead an active, healthy, and useful life if you eat a balanced diet daily, exercise regularly, and take your insulin injections as prescribed.
You have been instructed to test your blood and/or your urine regularly for glucose. If your blood tests consistently show above- or below-normal glucose levels or your urine tests consistently show the presence of glucose, your diabetes is not properly controlled and you must let your doctor know.
Always keep an extra supply of insulin as well as a spare syringe and needle on hand. Always wear diabetic identification so that appropriate treatment can be given if complications occur away from home.

NPH HUMAN INSULIN
Description
Humulin is synthesized in a non-disease-producing special laboratory strain of *Escherichia coli* bacteria that has been genetically altered by the addition of the human gene for insulin production. Humulin® N is a crystalline suspension of human insulin with protamine and zinc providing an intermediate-acting insulin with a slower onset of action and a longer duration of activity (up to 24 hours) than that of regular insulin. The time course of action of any insulin may vary considerably in different individuals or at different times in the same individual. As with all insulin preparations, the duration of action of Humulin N is dependent on dose, site of injection, blood supply, temperature, and physical activity. Humulin N is a sterile suspension and is for subcutaneous injection only. It should not be used intravenously or intramuscularly. The concentration of Humulin N in cartridges is 100 units/mL (U-100).
Identification
Cartridges of Humulin manufactured by Eli Lilly and Company are available in 3 formulations—Regular, NPH, and 70/30.
Your doctor has prescribed the type of insulin that he/she believes is best for you. **DO NOT USE ANY OTHER INSULIN EXCEPT ON HIS/HER ADVICE AND DIRECTION.**
Cartridges of Humulin N, 1.5 mL, are available in boxes of 5.
The cartridge containing Humulin N is not designed to allow any other insulin to be mixed in the cartridge or for the cartridge to be reused.
1.5 mL Cartridge
Humulin® N 1.5 mL cartridges are for use in Becton Dickinson and Company's B-D® Pen and Novo Nordisk A/S's NovoPen®, NovolinPen®, and NovoPen® 1.5 insulin delivery devices.
Always examine the appearance of a cartridge of insulin before administering a dose. A cartridge of Humulin N contains a small glass bead to assist in mixing. A cartridge of Humulin N must be rolled between the palms 10 times and inverted 180° 10 times before each injection so that the contents are uniformly mixed (*see* Figures 1 and 2). Before inserting it in the insulin pen, inspect the cartridge for uniform mixing and repeat the above steps as necessary.

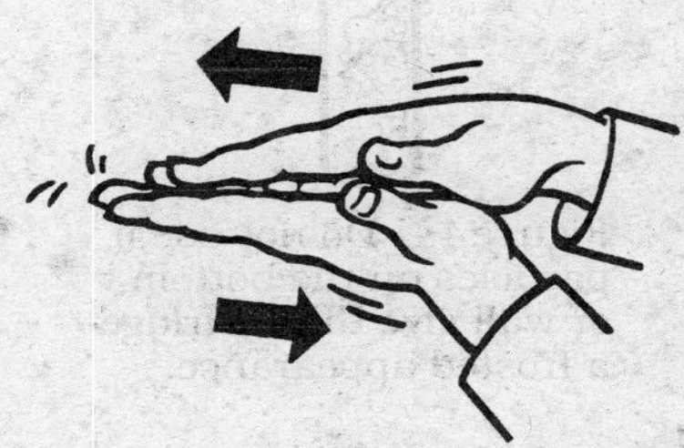

Figure 1.

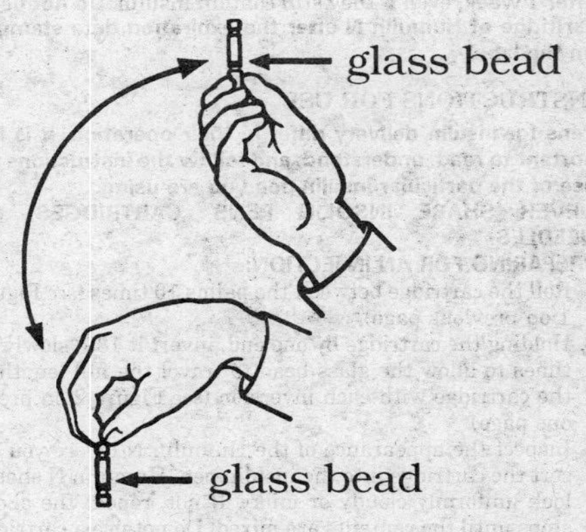

Figure 2.

Continued on next page

*** Identi-Code® symbol. This product information was prepared in June 2000. Current information on these and other products of Eli Lilly and Company may be obtained by direct inquiry to Lilly Research Laboratories, Lilly Corporate Center, Indianapolis, Indiana 46285, (800) 545-5979.**

Humulin N NPH Cartridge—Cont.

Humulin N should look uniformly cloudy or milky after mixing. Do not use if the insulin substance (the white material) remains visibly separated from the liquid after mixing. Do not use a cartridge of Humulin N if there are clumps in the insulin after mixing (*see* Figure 3). Do not use a cartridge of Humulin N if solid white particles stick to the walls of the cartridge, giving it a frosted appearance (*see* Figure 4). Always check the appearance of the cartridge before using, and if you note anything unusual in the appearance of your insulin or notice your insulin requirements changing markedly, consult your doctor.

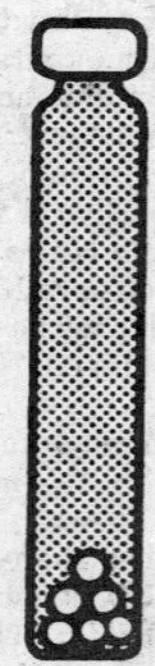

Figure 3.-- Do not use if there are clumps in the insulin after mixing.

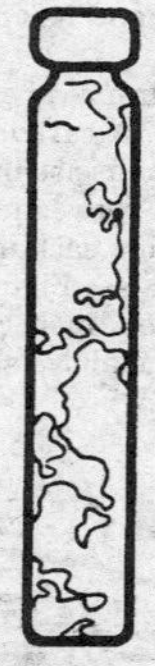

Figure 4.-- Do not use if particles on the bottom or wall give the cartridge a frosted appearance.

Storage

Insulin cartridges should be stored in a refrigerator but not in the freezer. The insulin pen and cartridge of insulin that you are currently using should not be refrigerated but should be kept as cool as possible (below 86°F [30°C]) and away from heat and light. Do not use insulin if it has been frozen. Unrefrigerated 1.5 mL cartridges **must be discarded after 1 week**, even if they still contain insulin. **Do not use a cartridge of Humulin N after the expiration date stamped on the label.**

INSTRUCTIONS FOR USE

Pens for insulin delivery differ in their operation. It is important to read, understand, and follow the instructions for use of the particular insulin pen you are using.

NEVER SHARE INSULIN PENS, CARTRIDGES, OR NEEDLES.

PREPARING FOR AN INJECTION:

1. Roll the cartridge between the palms 10 times (*see* Figure 1 on previous page).
2. Holding the cartridge by one end, invert it 180° slowly 10 times to allow the glass bead to travel the full length of the cartridge with each inversion (*see* Figure 2 on previous page).
3. Inspect the appearance of the Humulin N before you insert the cartridge into the insulin pen. Humulin N should look uniformly cloudy or milky. If not, repeat the above steps until the contents are mixed. Do not use a cartridge of Humulin N if there are clumps in the insulin or if solid white particles stick to the walls of the cartridge (*see* Figures 3 and 4 above).
4. Follow the insulin pen manufacturer's instructions carefully for loading the cartridge into the insulin pen and for use of the insulin pen.
5. Use an alcohol swab to wipe the exposed rubber surface on the metal cap end of the cartridge.
6. Follow the insulin needle manufacturer's instructions for attaching and changing the needle.
7. Insulin cartridges may contain an air bubble(s) which must be removed from the cartridge and needle by proper priming prior to injection.
8. Once the cartridge is in use in an insulin pen, the insulin must be mixed and inspected before each injection. Roll the insulin pen, containing the cartridge, between the palms 10 times, and invert the insulin pen 180° slowly 10 times to mix the insulin. Do not use a cartridge of Humulin N if there are clumps in the insulin or if solid white particles stick to the walls of the cartridge (*see* Figures 3 and 4 above).

GENERAL INJECTION INSTRUCTIONS:

1. Wash your hands.
2. To avoid tissue damage, choose a site for each injection that is at least 1/2 inch from the previous injection site. The usual sites of injection are abdomen, thighs, and arms.
3. Cleanse the skin with alcohol where the injection is to be made.
4. With one hand, stabilize the skin by spreading it or pinching up a large area.
5. Insert the needle as instructed by your doctor.
6. After dispensing a dose, pull the needle out and apply gentle pressure over the injection site for several seconds. **Do not rub the area.**
7. Immediately after an injection, remove the needle from the insulin pen. Doing so will guard against contamination, leakage, reentry of air, and needle clogs. **Do not reuse needles. Dispose of needles in a responsible manner.**
8. *1.5 mL cartridge* - Once the cartridge is in use, do not continue to use it if the leading edge of the plunger is beyond the black band on the cartridge. If a dose is started when the leading edge of the plunger is beyond the black band, an appropriate dose may not be delivered. Use the gauge on the side of the cartridge to help you judge how much Humulin N remains. The distance between each mark on the 1.5 mL cartridge is about 10 units.

DOSAGE

Your doctor has told you which insulin to use, how much, and when and how often to inject it. Because each patient's case of diabetes is different, this schedule has been individualized for you.

Your usual insulin dose may be affected by changes in your food, activity, or work schedule. Carefully follow your doctor's instructions to allow for these changes. Other things that may affect your insulin dose are:

Illness

Illness, especially with nausea and vomiting, may cause your insulin requirements to change. Even if you are not eating, you will still require insulin. You and your doctor should establish a sick day plan for you to use in case of illness. When you are sick, test your blood glucose/urine glucose and ketones frequently and call your doctor as instructed.

Pregnancy

Good control of diabetes is especially important for you and your unborn baby. Pregnancy may make managing your diabetes more difficult. If you are planning to have a baby, are pregnant, or are nursing a baby, consult your doctor.

Medication

Insulin requirements may be increased if you are taking other drugs with hyperglycemic activity, such as oral contraceptives, corticosteroids, or thyroid replacement therapy. Insulin requirements may be reduced in the presence of drugs with hypoglycemic activity, such as oral hypoglycemics, salicylates (for example, aspirin), sulfa antibiotics, and certain antidepressants. Always discuss any medications you are taking with your doctor.

Exercise

Exercise may lower your body's need for insulin during and for some time after the activity. Exercise may also speed up the effect of an insulin dose, especially if the exercise involves the area of injection site (for example, the leg should not be used for injection just prior to running). Discuss with your doctor how you should adjust your regimen to accommodate exercise.

Travel

Persons traveling across more than 2 time zones should consult their doctor concerning adjustments in their insulin schedule.

COMMON PROBLEMS OF DIABETES

Hypoglycemia (Insulin Reaction)

Hypoglycemia (too little glucose in the blood) is one of the most frequent adverse events experienced by insulin users. It can be brought about by:

1. Taking too much insulin
2. Missing or delaying meals
3. Exercising or working more than usual
4. An infection or illness (especially with diarrhea or vomiting)
5. A change in the body's need for insulin
6. Diseases of the adrenal, pituitary or thyroid gland, or progression of kidney or liver disease
7. Interactions with other drugs that lower blood glucose, such as oral hypoglycemics, salicylates (for example, aspirin), sulfa antibiotics, and certain antidepressants
8. Consumption of alcoholic beverages

Symptoms of mild to moderate hypoglycemia may occur suddenly and can include:

- sweating
- dizziness
- palpitation
- tremor
- hunger
- restlessness
- tingling in the hands, feet, lips, or tongue
- lightheadedness
- inability to concentrate
- headache
- drowsiness
- sleep disturbances
- anxiety
- blurred vision
- slurred speech
- depressed mood
- irritability
- abnormal behavior
- unsteady movement
- personality changes

Signs of severe hypoglycemia can include:

- disorientation
- unconsciousness
- seizures
- death

Therefore, it is important that assistance be obtained immediately.

Early warning symptoms of hypoglycemia may be different or less pronounced under certain conditions, such as long duration of diabetes, diabetic nerve disease, medications such as beta-blockers, change in insulin preparations, or intensified control (3 or more insulin injections per day) of diabetes.

A few patients who have experienced hypoglycemic reactions after transfer from animal-source insulin to human insulin have reported that the early warning symptoms of hypoglycemia were less pronounced or different from those experienced with their previous insulin.

Without recognition of early warning symptoms, you may not be able to take steps to avoid more serious hypoglycemia. Be alert for all of the various types of symptoms that may indicate hypoglycemia. Patients who experience hypoglycemia without early warning symptoms should monitor their blood glucose frequently, especially prior to activities such as driving. If the blood glucose is below your normal fasting glucose, you should consider eating or drinking sugar-containing foods to treat your hypoglycemia.

Mild to moderate hypoglycemia may be treated by eating foods or drinks that contain sugar. Patients should always carry a quick source of sugar, such as candy mints or glucose tablets. More severe hypoglycemia may require the assistance of another person. Patients who are unable to take sugar orally or who are unconscious require an injection of glucagon or should be treated with intravenous administration of glucose at a medical facility.

You should learn to recognize your own symptoms of hypoglycemia. If you are uncertain about these symptoms, you should monitor your blood glucose frequently to help you learn to recognize the symptoms that you experience with hypoglycemia.

If you have frequent episodes of hypoglycemia or experience difficulty in recognizing the symptoms, you should consult your doctor to discuss possible changes in therapy, meal plans, and/or exercise programs to help you avoid hypoglycemia.

Hyperglycemia and Diabetic Acidosis

Hyperglycemia (too much glucose in the blood) may develop if your body has too little insulin. Hyperglycemia can be brought about by:

1. Omitting your insulin or taking less than the doctor has prescribed
2. Eating significantly more than your meal plan suggests
3. Developing a fever, infection, or other significant stressful situation

In patients with insulin-dependent diabetes, prolonged hyperglycemia can result in diabetic acidosis. The first symptoms of diabetic acidosis usually come on gradually, over a period of hours or days, and include a drowsy feeling, flushed face, thirst, loss of appetite, and fruity odor on the breath. With acidosis, urine tests show large amounts of glucose and acetone. Heavy breathing and a rapid pulse are more severe symptoms. If uncorrected, prolonged hyperglycemia or diabetic acidosis can lead to nausea, vomiting, dehydration, loss of consciousness or death. Therefore, it is important that you obtain medical assistance immediately.

Lipodystrophy

Rarely, administration of insulin subcutaneously can result in lipoatrophy (depression in the skin) or lipohypertrophy (enlargement or thickening of tissue). If you notice either of these conditions, consult your doctor. A change in your injection technique may help alleviate the problem.

Allergy to Insulin

Local Allergy—Patients occasionally experience redness, swelling, and itching at the site of injection of insulin. This condition, called local allergy, usually clears up in a few days to a few weeks. In some instances, this condition may be related to factors other than insulin, such as irritants in the skin cleansing agent or poor injection technique. If you have local reactions, contact your doctor.

Systemic Allergy—Less common, but potentially more serious, is generalized allergy to insulin, which may cause rash over the whole body, shortness of breath, wheezing, reduction in blood pressure, fast pulse, or sweating. Severe cases of generalized allergy may be life threatening. If you think you are having a generalized allergic reaction to insulin, notify a doctor immediately.

ADDITIONAL INFORMATION

Additional information about diabetes may be obtained from your diabetes educator.

DIABETES FORECAST is a national magazine designed especially for patients with diabetes and their families and is available on subscription from the American Diabetes Association, National Service Center, 1660 Duke Street, Alexandria, Virginia 22314, 1-800-DIABETES (1-800-342-2383).

Another publication, **DIABETES COUNTDOWN**, is available from the Juvenile Diabetes Foundation International (JDF), 120 Wall Street, 19th Floor, New York, New York 10005-4001, 1-800-JDF-CURE (1-800-533-2873).

Additional information about Humulin can be obtained by calling 1-888-88-LILLY (1-888-885-4559).

Literature revised March 26, 1999

PA 9067 FSAMP [032699]

* B-D® is a registered trademark of Becton Dickinson and Company.

† NovolinPen® and NovoPen® are registered trademarks of Novo Nordisk A/S.

HUMULIN® N Pen ℞

[*hū 'mū-lĭn ĕn*]

3.0 ML Disposable Insulin Delivery Device

NPH

Human Insulin

(rDNA origin) Isophane Suspension

INFORMATION FOR THE PATIENT

WARNINGS

THIS LILLY HUMAN INSULIN PRODUCT DIFFERS FROM ANIMAL-SOURCE INSULINS BECAUSE IT IS STRUCTURALLY IDENTICAL TO THE INSULIN PRODUCED BY YOUR BODY'S PANCREAS AND BECAUSE OF ITS UNIQUE MANUFACTURING PROCESS.

ANY CHANGE OF INSULIN SHOULD BE MADE CAUTIOUSLY AND ONLY UNDER MEDICAL SUPERVISION. CHANGES IN STRENGTH, MANUFACTURER, TYPE (E.G., REGULAR, NPH, LENTE, ETC), SPECIES (BEEF, PORK, BEEF-PORK, HUMAN), OR METHOD OF MANUFACTURE (rDNA VERSUS ANIMAL-SOURCE INSULIN) MAY RESULT IN THE NEED FOR A CHANGE IN DOSAGE.

SOME PATIENTS TAKING HUMULIN® (HUMAN INSULIN, rDNA ORIGIN) MAY REQUIRE A CHANGE IN DOSAGE FROM THAT USED WITH ANIMAL-SOURCE INSULINS. IF AN ADJUSTMENT IS NEEDED, IT MAY OCCUR WITH THE FIRST DOSE OR DURING THE FIRST SEVERAL WEEKS OR MONTHS.

TO OBTAIN AN ACCURATE DOSE, CAREFULLY READ AND FOLLOW THE "DISPOSABLE INSULIN DELIVERY DEVICE USER MANUAL" AND THIS INFORMATION FOR THE PATIENT INSERT BEFORE USING THIS PRODUCT (*see also* INSTRUCTIONS FOR PEN USE section.)

DIABETES

Insulin is a hormone produced by the pancreas, a large gland that lies near the stomach. This hormone is necessary for the body's correct use of food, especially sugar. Diabetes occurs when the pancreas does not make enough insulin to meet your body's needs.

To control your diabetes, your doctor has prescribed injections of insulin to keep your blood glucose at a nearly normal level. Proper control of your diabetes requires close and constant cooperation with your doctor. In spite of diabetes, you can lead an active, healthy, and useful life if you eat a balanced diet daily, exercise regularly, and take your insulin injections as prescribed.

You have been instructed to test your blood and/or your urine regularly for glucose. If your blood tests consistently show above- or below-normal glucose levels or your urine tests consistently show the presence of glucose, your diabetes is not properly controlled and you must let your doctor know.

Always keep an extra supply of insulin as well as a spare syringe and needle on hand. Always wear diabetic identification so that appropriate treatment can be given if complications occur away from home.

NPH HUMAN INSULIN

Description

Humulin is synthesized in a non-disease-producing special laboratory strain of *Escherichia coli* bacterial that has been genetically altered by the addition of the human gene for insulin production. Humulin® N is a crystalline suspension of human insulin with protamine and zinc providing an intermediate-acting insulin with a slower onset of action and a longer duration of activity (up to 24 hours) than that of regular insulin. The time course of action of any insulin may vary considerably in different individuals or at different times in the same individual. As with all insulin preparations, the duration of action of Humulin N is dependent on dose, site of injection, blood supply, temperature, and physical activity. Humulin N is a sterile suspension and is for subcutaneous injection only. It should not be used intravenously or intramuscularly. The concentration of Humulin N in Humulin N Pen is 100 units/mL (U-100).

Identification

Humulin disposable insulin delivery devices, manufactured by Eli Lilly and Company, are available in 2 formulations—NPH and 70/30.

Your doctor has prescribed the type of insulin that he/she believes is best for you. **DO NOT USE ANY OTHER INSULIN EXCEPT ON HIS/HER ADVICE AND DIRECTION.**

The Humulin N Pen is available in boxes of 5 disposable insulin delivery devices ("insulin pens"). The Humulin N Pen is not designed to allow any other insulin to be mixed in its cartridge, or for the cartridge to be removed.

Always examine the appearance of Humulin N suspension in the insulin pen before administering a dose. A cartridge of Humulin N contains a small glass bead to assist in mixing. Humulin N Pen must be rolled between the palms 10 times and inverted 180° 10 times before each injection so that the contents are uniformly mixed (*see* Figures 1 and 2). Inspect the Humulin N suspension for uniform mixing and repeat the above steps as necessary.

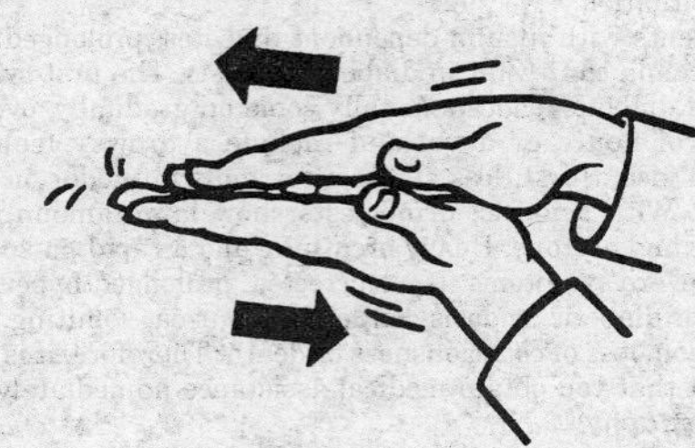

Figure 1.

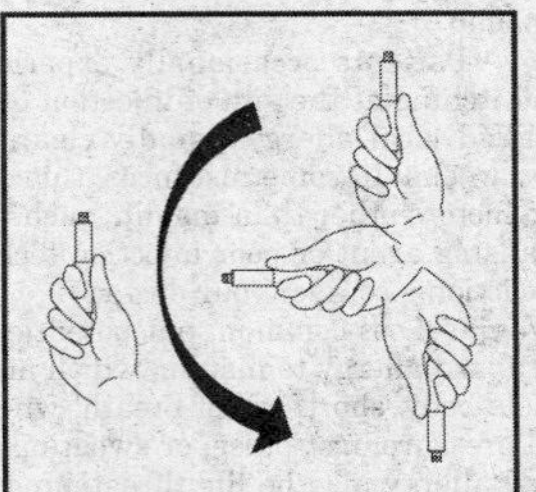

Figure 2.

Humulin N should look uniformly cloudy or milky after mixing. Do not use if the insulin substance (the white material) remains visibly separated from the liquid after mixing. Do not use the Humulin N Pen if there are clumps in the insulin after mixing (*see* Figure 3). Do not use the Humulin N Pen if solid white particles stick to the walls of the cartridge, giving it a frosted appearance (*see* Figure 4).

Always check the appearance of the Humulin N suspension in the insulin pen before using, and if you note anything unusual in the appearance of Humulin N suspension or notice your insulin requirements changing markedly, consult your doctor.

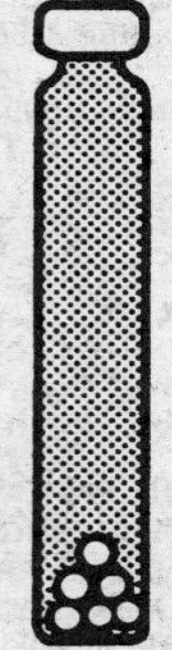

Figure 3.* – Do not use if there are clumps in the insulin after mixing.

[See figure 4 at top of next column]

*Never attempt to remove the cartridge from the Humulin N Pen. Inspect the cartridge through the clear cartridge holder.

Storage

Humulin N Pens should be stored in a refrigerator but not in the freezer. The Humulin N Pen that you are currently using should not be refrigerated but should be kept as cool as possible (below 86°F [30°C]) and away from heat and light. Do not use an insulin pen if it has been frozen. Unrefrigerated Humulin N Pens **must be discarded after 2 weeks,** even if they still contain insulin. Do not use Humulin N Pens after the expiration date stamped on the label.

INSTRUCTIONS FOR PEN USE

It is important to read, understand, and follow the instructions in the "Disposable Insulin Delivery Device User Manual" before using. Failure to follow instructions may result in an inaccurate insulin dose.

NEVER SHARE INSULIN PENS, CARTRIDGES, OR NEEDLES.

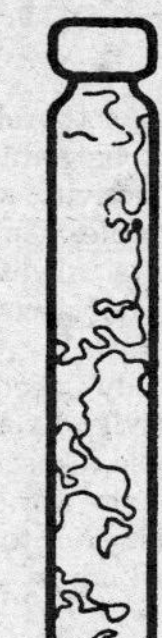

Figure 4.* – Do not use if particles on the bottom or wall give the cartridge a frosted appearance.

PREPARING THE PEN FOR INJECTION:

1. Always check the appearance of the Humulin N suspension in the insulin pen before using.
2. Roll the Humulin N Pen between the palms 10 times (*see* Figure 1 above).
3. Holding the Humulin N Pen by one end, invert it 180° slowly 10 times to allow the glass bead to travel the full length of the cartridge with each inversion (*see* Figure 2 above). This cartridge is contained in the clear cartridge holder of the Humulin N Pen.
4. Inspect the appearance of the Humulin N suspension to make sure the contents look uniformly cloudy or milky. If not, repeat the above steps until the contents are mixed. Do not use a Humulin N Pen if there are clumps in the insulin or if solid white particles stick to the walls of the cartridge (*see* Figures 3 and 4 above).
5. Follow the instructions in the "Disposable Insulin Delivery Device User Manual" for these steps:

- Preparing the Pen
- Attaching the Needle
- Priming the Pen (Checking the Insulin Flow)
- Setting (Dialing) a Dose
- Injecting the Dose
- Following an Injection

PREPARING FOR INJECTION:

1. Wash your hands.
2. To avoid tissue damage, choose a site for each injection that is at least 1/2 inch from the previous injection site. The usual sites of injection are abdomen, thighs, and arms.
3. Cleanse the skin with alcohol where the injection is to be made.
4. With one hand, stabilize the skin by spreading it or pinching up a large area.
5. Inject the dose as instructed by your doctor.
6. After dispensing a dose, pull the needle out and apply gentle pressure over the injection site for several seconds. Do not rub the area.
7. Immediately after an injection, remove the needle from the Humulin N Pen. Doing so will guard against contamination, leakage, reentry of air, and needle clogs. Do not reuse needles. Dispose of needles in a responsible manner.

DOSAGE

Your doctor has told you which insulin to use, how much, and when and how often to inject it. Because each patient's case of diabetes is different, this schedule has been individualized for you.

Your usual insulin dose may be affected by changes in your food, activity, or work schedule. Carefully follow your doctor's instructions to allow for these changes. Other things that may affect your insulin dose are:

Illness

Illness, especially with nausea and vomiting, may cause your insulin requirements to change. Even if you are not eating, you will still require insulin. You and your doctor should establish a sick day plan for you to use in case of illness. When you are sick, test your blood glucose/urine glucose and ketones frequently and call your doctor as instructed.

Pregnancy

Good control of diabetes is especially important for you and your unborn baby. Pregnancy may make managing your diabetes more difficult. If you are planning to have a baby, are pregnant, or are nursing a baby, consult your doctor.

Medication

Insulin requirements may be increased if you are taking other drugs with hyperglycemic activity, such as oral con-

Continued on next page

*** Identi-Code® symbol. This product information was prepared in June 2000. Current information on these and other products of Eli Lilly and Company may be obtained by direct inquiry to Lilly Research Laboratories, Lilly Corporate Center, Indianapolis, Indiana 46285, (800) 545-5979.**

Humulin N Pen—Cont.

traceptives, corticosteroids, or thyroid replacement therapy. Insulin requirements may be reduced in the presence of drugs with hypoglycemic activity, such as oral hypoglycemics, salicylates (for example, aspirin), sulfa antibiotics, and certain antidepressants. Always discuss any medications you are taking with your doctor.

Exercise

Exercise may lower your body's need for insulin during and for some time after the activity. Exercise may also speed up the effect of an insulin dose, especially if the exercise involves the area of injection site (for example, the leg should not be used for injection just prior to running). Discuss with your doctor how you should adjust your regimen to accommodate exercise.

Travel

Persons traveling across more than 2 time zones should consult their doctor concerning adjustments in their insulin schedule.

COMMON PROBLEMS OF DIABETES

Hypoglycemia (Insulin Reaction)

Hypoglycemia (too little glucose in the blood) is one of the most frequent adverse events experienced by insulin users. It can be brought about by:

1. Taking too much insulin
2. Missing or delaying meals
3. Exercising or working more than usual
4. An infection or illness (especially with diarrhea or vomiting)
5. A change in the body's need for insulin
6. Diseases of the adrenal, pituitary or thyroid gland, or progression of kidney or liver disease
7. Interactions with other drugs that lower blood glucose, such as oral hypoglycemics, salicylates (for example, aspirin), sulfa antibiotics, and certain antidepressants
8. Consumption of alcoholic beverages

Symptoms of mild to moderate hypoglycemia may occur suddenly and can include:

- sweating
- dizziness
- palpitation
- tremor
- hunger
- restlessness
- tingling in the hands, feet, lips, or tongue
- drowsiness
- sleep disturbances
- anxiety
- blurred vision
- slurred speech
- depressed mood
- irritability
- lightheadedness
- inability to concentrate
- headache
- abnormal behavior
- unsteady movement
- personality changes

Signs of severe hypoglycemia can include:

- disorientation
- unconsciousness
- seizures
- death

Therefore, it is important that assistance be obtained immediately.

Early warning symptoms of hypoglycemia may be different or less pronounced under certain conditions, such as long duration of diabetes, diabetic nerve disease, medications such as beta-blockers, change in insulin preparations, or intensified control (3 ore more insulin injections per day) of diabetes.

A few patients who have experienced hypoglycemic reactions after transfer from animal-source insulin to human insulin have reported that the early warning symptoms of hypoglycemia were less pronounced or different from those experienced with their previous insulin.

Without recognition of early warning symptoms, you may not be able to take steps to avoid more serious hypoglycemia. Be alert for all of the various types of symptoms that may indicate hypoglycemia. Patients who experience hypoglycemia without early warning symptoms should monitor their blood glucose frequently, especially prior to activities such as driving. If the blood glucose is below your normal fasting glucose, you should consider eating or drinking sugar-containing foods to treat your hypoglycemia.

Mild to moderate hypoglycemia may be treated by eating foods or drinks that contain sugar. Patients should always carry a quick source of sugar, such as candy mints or glucose tablets. More severe hypoglycemia may require the assistance of another person. Patients who are unable to take sugar orally or who are unconscious require an injection of glucagon or should be treated with intravenous administration of glucose at a medical facility.

You should learn to recognize your own symptoms of hypoglycemia. If you are uncertain about these symptoms, you should monitor your blood glucose frequently to help you learn to recognize the symptoms that you experience with hypoglycemia.

If you have frequent episodes of hypoglycemia or experience difficulty in recognizing the symptoms, you should consult your doctor to discuss possible changes in therapy, meal plans, and/or exercise programs to help you avoid hypoglycemia.

Hyperglycemia and Diabetic Acidosis

Hyperglycemia (too much glucose in the blood) may develop if your body has too little insulin. Hyperglycemia can be brought about by:

1. Omitting your insulin or taking less than the doctor has prescribed
2. Eating significantly more than your meal plan suggests
3. Developing a fever, infection, or other significant stressful situation

In patients with insulin-dependent diabetes, prolonged hyperglycemia can result in diabetic acidosis. The first symptoms of diabetic acidosis usually come on gradually, over a period of hours or days, and include a drowsy feeling, flushed face, thirst, loss of appetite, and fruity odor on the breath. With acidosis, urine tests show large amounts of glucose and acetone. Heavy breathing and a rapid pulse are more severe symptoms. If uncorrected, prolonged hyperglycemia or diabetic acidosis can lead to nausea, vomiting, dehydration, loss of consciousness or death. Therefore, it is important that you obtain medical assistance immediately.

Lipodystrophy

Rarely, administration of insulin subcutaneously can result in lipoatrophy (depression in the skin) or lipohypertrophy (enlargement or thickening of tissue). If you notice either of these conditions, consult your doctor. A change in your injection technique may help alleviate the problem.

Allergy to Insulin

Local Allergy—Patients occasionally experience redness, swelling, and itching at the site of injection of insulin. This condition, called local allergy, usually clears up in a few days to a few weeks. In some instances, this condition may be related to factors other than insulin, such as irritants in the skin cleansing agent or poor injection technique. If you have local reactions, contact your doctor.

Systemic Allergy—Less common, but potentially more serious, is generalized allergy to insulin, which may cause rash over the whole body, shortness of breath, wheezing, reduction in blood pressure, fast pulse, or sweating. Severe cases of generalized allergy may be life threatening. If you think you are having a generalized allergic reaction to insulin, notify a doctor immediately.

ADDITIONAL INFORMATION

Additional information about diabetes may be obtained from your diabetes educator.

DIABETES FORECAST is a national magazine designed especially for patients with diabetes and their families and is available on subscription from the American Diabetes Association, National Service Center, 1660 Duke Street, Alexandria, Virginia 22314, 1-800-DIABETES (1-800-342-2383).

Another publication, **DIABETES COUNTDOWN**, is available from the Juvenile Diabetes Foundation International (JDF), 120 Wall Street, 19th Floor, New York, New York 10005-4001, 1-800-JDF-CURE (1-800-533-2873).

Additional information about Humulin and Humulin N Pen can be obtained by calling 1-888-88-LILLY (1-888-885-4559).

Literature issued March 26, 1999

PA 9131 FSAMP [032699]

HUMULIN® R OTC

[*hū 'mū-lĭn är*]

Regular

(insulin human injection, USP [rDNA origin])

INFORMATION FOR THE PATIENT

WARNINGS

THIS LILLY HUMAN INSULIN PRODUCT DIFFERS FROM ANIMAL-SOURCE INSULINS BECAUSE IT IS STRUCTURALLY IDENTICAL TO THE INSULIN PRODUCED BY YOUR BODY'S PANCREAS AND BECAUSE OF ITS UNIQUE MANUFACTURING PROCESS.

ANY CHANGE OF INSULIN SHOULD BE MADE CAUTIOUSLY AND ONLY UNDER MEDICAL SUPERVISION. CHANGES IN STRENGTH, MANUFACTURER, TYPE (E.G., REGULAR, NPH, LENTE®), SPECIES (BEEF, PORK, BEEF-PORK, HUMAN), OR METHOD OF MANUFACTURE (rDNA VERSUS ANIMAL-SOURCE INSULIN) MAY RESULT IN THE NEED FOR A CHANGE IN DOSAGE.

SOME PATIENTS TAKING HUMULIN® (HUMAN INSULIN, rDNA ORIGIN) MAY REQUIRE A CHANGE IN DOSAGE FROM THAT USED WITH ANIMAL-SOURCE INSULINS. IF AN ADJUSTMENT IS NEEDED, IT MAY OCCUR WITH THE FIRST DOSE OR DURING THE FIRST SEVERAL WEEKS OR MONTHS.

DIABETES

Insulin is a hormone produced by the pancreas, a large gland that lies near the stomach. This hormone is necessary for the body's correct use of food, especially sugar. Diabetes occurs when the pancreas does not make enough insulin to meet your body's needs.

To control your diabetes, your doctor has prescribed injections of insulin to keep your blood glucose at a nearly normal level. Proper control of your diabetes requires close and constant cooperation with your doctor. In spite of diabetes, you can lead an active, healthy, and useful life if you eat a balanced diet daily, exercise regularly, and take your insulin injections as prescribed.

You have been instructed to test your blood and/or your urine regularly for glucose. If your blood tests consistently show above- or below-normal glucose levels or your urine tests consistently show the presence of glucose, your diabetes is not properly controlled and you must let your doctor know.

Always keep an extra supply of insulin as well as a spare syringe and needle on hand. Always wear diabetic identification so that appropriate treatment can be given if complications occur away from home.

REGULAR HUMAN INSULIN

Description

Humulin is synthesized in a special non-disease-producing laboratory strain of *Escherichia coli* bacteria that has been genetically altered by the addition of the gene for human insulin production. Humulin R consists of zinc-insulin crystals dissolved in a clear fluid. Humulin R has had nothing added to change the speed or length of its action. It takes effect rapidly and has a relatively short duration of activity (4 to 12 hours) as compared with other insulins. The time course of action of any insulin may vary considerably in different individuals or at different times in the same individual. As with all insulin preparations, the duration of action of Humulin R is dependent on dose, site of injection, blood supply, temperature, and physical activity. Humulin R is a sterile solution and is for subcutaneous injection. It should not be used intramuscularly. The concentration of Humulin R is 100 units/mL (U-100).

Identification

Human insulin manufactured by Eli Lilly and Company has the trademark Humulin and is available in 6 formulations—Regular (**R**), NPH (**N**), Lente (**L**), Ultralente® (**U**), 50% Human Insulin Isophane Suspension [NPH]/50% Human Insulin Injection [buffered regular] (**50/50**), and 70% Human Insulin Isophane Suspension [NPH]/30% Human Insulin Injection [buffered regular] (**70/30**). Your doctor has prescribed the type of insulin that he/she believes is best for you. **DO NOT USE ANY OTHER INSULIN EXCEPT ON HIS/HER ADVICE AND DIRECTION.**

Always check the carton and the bottle label for the name and letter designation of the insulin you receive from your pharmacy to make sure it is the same as that your doctor has prescribed. Humulin R can be identified as follows:

[See graphic at top of next page]

Always examine the appearance of your bottle of insulin before withdrawing each dose. Humulin R is a clear and colorless liquid with a water-like appearance and consistency. Do not use if it appears cloudy, thickened, or slightly colored or if solid particles are visible. Always check the appearance of your bottle of insulin before using, and if you note anything unusual in the appearance of your insulin or notice your insulin requirements changing markedly, consult your doctor.

Storage

Insulin should be stored in a refrigerator but not in the freezer. If refrigeration is not possible, the bottle of insulin that you are currently using can be kept unrefrigerated as long as it is kept as cool as possible (below 86°F [30°C]) and away from heat and light. Do not use insulin if it has been frozen. Do not use a bottle of insulin after the expiration date stamped on the label.

INJECTION PROCEDURES

Correct Syringe

Doses of insulin are measured in **units**. U-100 insulin contains 100 units/mL (1 mL = 1 cc). With Humulin R, it is important to use a syringe that is marked for U-100 insulin preparations. Failure to use the proper syringe can lead to a mistake in dosage, causing serious problems for you, such as a blood glucose level that is too low or too high.

Syringe Use

To help avoid contamination and possible infection, follow these instructions exactly.

Disposable syringes and needles should be used only once and then discarded. **NEEDLES AND SYRINGES MUST NOT BE SHARED.**

Reusable syringes and needles must be sterilized before each injection. **Follow the package directions supplied with your syringe.** Described below are 2 methods of sterilizing.

Boiling

1. Put syringe, plunger, and needle in strainer, place in saucepan, and cover with water. Boil for 5 minutes.
2. Remove articles from water. When they have cooled, insert plunger into barrel, and fasten needle to syringe with a slight twist.
3. Push plunger in and out several times until water is completely removed.

Isopropyl Alcohol

If the syringe, plunger, and needle cannot be boiled, as when you are traveling, they may be sterilized by immersion for at least 5 minutes in Isopropyl Alcohol, 91%. Do not use bathing, rubbing, or medicated alcohol for this sterilization. If the syringe is sterilized with alcohol, it must be absolutely dry before use.

Preparing the Dose

1. Wash your hands.
2. Inspect the insulin. Humulin R should look clear and colorless. Do not use Humulin R if it appears cloudy, thickened, or slightly colored or if solid particles are visible.
3. If using a new bottle, flip off the plastic protective cap, but **do not** remove the stopper. When using a new bottle, wipe the top of the bottle with an alcohol swab.
4. If you are mixing insulins, refer to instructions for mixing that follow.

5. Draw air into the syringe equal to your insulin dose. Put the needle through rubber top of the insulin bottle and inject the air into the bottle.
6. Turn the bottle and syringe upside down. Hold the bottle and syringe firmly in 1 hand.
7. Making sure the tip of the needle is in the insulin, withdraw the correct dose of insulin into the syringe.
8. Before removing the needle from the bottle, check your syringe for air bubbles which reduce the amount of insulin in it. If bubbles are present, hold the syringe straight up and tap its side until the bubbles float to the top. Push them out with the plunger and withdraw the correct dose.
9. Remove the needle from the bottle and lay the syringe down so that the needle dose not touch anything.

Mixing Humulin R with Longer-acting Human Insulins

1. Regular human insulin should be mixed with longer-acting human insulins only on the advice of your doctor.
2. Draw air into your syringe equal to the amount of longer-acting insulin you are taking. Insert the needle into the longer-acting insulin bottle and inject the air. Withdraw the needle.
3. Now inject air into your regular human insulin bottle in the same manner, but **do not** withdraw the needle.
4. Turn the bottle and syringe upside down.
5. Making sure the tip of the needle is in the insulin, withdraw the correct dose of regular insulin into the syringe.
6. Before removing the needle from the bottle, check your syringe for air bubbles which reduce the amount of insulin in it. If bubbles are present, hold the syringe straight up and tap its side until the bubbles float to the top. Push them out with the plunger and withdraw the correct dose.
7. Remove the needle from the bottle of regular insulin and insert it into the bottle of the longer-acting insulin. Turn the bottle and syringe upside down. Hold the bottle and syringe firmly in 1 hand and shake gently. Making sure the tip of the needle is in the insulin, withdraw your dose of longer-acting insulin.
8. Remove the needle and lay the syringe down so that the needle does not touch anything.

Follow your doctor's instructions on whether to mix your insulins ahead of time or just before giving your injection. It is important to be consistent in your method.

Syringes from different manufacturers may vary in the amount of space between the bottom line and the needle. Because of this, do not change:

- the sequence of mixing, or
- the model and brand of syringe or needle that the doctor has prescribed.

Injection

Cleanse the skin with alcohol where the injection is to be made. Stabilize the skin by spreading it or pinching up a large area. Insert the needle as instructed by your doctor. Push the plunger in as far as it will go. Pull the needle out and apply gentle pressure over the injection site for several seconds. **Do not rub the area.** To avoid tissue damage, give the next injection at a site at least 1/2" from the previous site.

DOSAGE

Your doctor has told you which insulin to use, how much, and when and how often to inject it. Because each patient's case of diabetes is different, this schedule has been individualized for you.

Your usual insulin dose may be affected by changes in your food, activity, or work schedule. Carefully follow your doctor's instructions to allow for these changes. Other things that may affect your insulin dose are:

Illness

Illness, especially with nausea and vomiting, may cause your insulin requirements to change. Even if you are not eating, you will still require insulin. You and your doctor should establish a sick day plan for you to use in case of illness. When you are sick, test your blood/urine frequently and call your doctor as instructed.

Pregnancy

Good control of diabetes is especially important for you and your unborn baby. Pregnancy may make managing your diabetes more difficult. If you are planning to have a baby, are pregnant, or are nursing a baby, consult your doctor.

Medication

Insulin requirements may be increased if you are taking other drugs with hyperglycemic activity, such as oral contraceptives, corticosteroids, or thyroid replacement therapy. Insulin requirements may be reduced in the presence of drugs with hypoglycemic activity, such as oral hypoglycemics, salicylates (for example, aspirin), sulfa antibiotics, and certain antidepressants. Always discuss any medications you are taking with your doctor.

Exercise

Exercise may lower your body's need for insulin during and for some time after the activity. Exercise may also speed up the effect of an insulin dose, especially if the exercise involves the area of injection site (for example, the leg should not be used for injection just prior to running). Discuss with your doctor how you should adjust your regimen to accommodate exercise.

Travel

Persons traveling across more than 2 time zones should consult their doctor concerning adjustments in their insulin schedule.

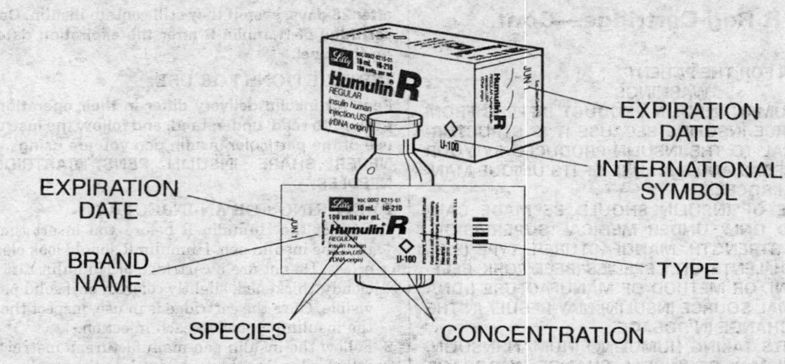

COMMON PROBLEMS OF DIABETES

Hypoglycemia (Insulin Reaction)

Hypoglycemia (too little glucose in the blood) is one of the most frequent adverse events experienced by insulin users. It can be brought about by:

1. Taking too much insulin
2. Missing or delaying meals
3. Exercising or working more than usual
4. An infection or illness (especially with diarrhea or vomiting)
5. A change in the body's need for insulin
6. Diseases of the adrenal, pituitary, or thyroid gland, or progression of kidney or liver disease
7. Interactions with other drugs that lower blood glucose, such as oral hypoglycemics, salicylates (for example, aspirin), sulfa antibiotics, and certain antidepressants
8. Consumption of alcoholic beverages

Symptoms of mild to moderate hypoglycemia may occur suddenly and can include:

- sweating
- dizziness
- palpitation
- tremor
- hunger
- restlessness
- tingling in the hands, feet, lips, or tongue
- lightheadedness
- inability to concentrate
- headache
- drowsiness
- sleep disturbances
- anxiety
- blurred vision
- slurred speech
- depressed mood
- irritability
- abnormal behavior
- unsteady movement
- personality changes

Signs of severe hypoglycemia can include:

- disorientation
- unconsciousness
- seizures
- death

Therefore, it is important that assistance be obtained immediately.

Early warning symptoms of hypoglycemia may be different or less pronounced under certain conditions, such as long duration of diabetes, diabetic nerve disease, medications such as beta-blockers, change in insulin preparations, or intensified control (3 or more insulin injections per day) of diabetes.

A few patients who have experienced hypoglycemic reactions after transfer from animal-source insulin to human insulin have reported that the early warning symptoms of hypoglycemia were less pronounced or different from those experienced with their previous insulin.

Without recognition of early warning symptoms, you may not be able to take steps to avoid more serious hypoglycemia. Be alert for all of the various types of symptoms that may indicate hypoglycemia. Patients who experience hypoglycemia without early warning symptoms should monitor their blood glucose frequently, especially prior to activities such as driving. If the blood glucose is below your normal fasting glucose, you should consider eating or drinking sugar-containing foods to treat your hypoglycemia.

Mild to moderate hypoglycemia may be treated by eating foods or drinks that contain sugar. Patients should always carry a quick source of sugar, such as candy mints or glucose tablets. More severe hypoglycemia may require the assistance of another person. Patients who are unable to take sugar orally or who are unconscious require an injection of glucagon or should be treated with intravenous administration of glucose at a medical facility.

You should learn to recognize your own symptoms of hypoglycemia. If you are uncertain about these symptoms, you should monitor your blood glucose frequently to help you learn to recognize the symptoms that you experience with hypoglycemia.

If you have frequent episodes of hypoglycemia or experience difficulty in recognizing the symptoms, you should consult your doctor to discuss possible changes in therapy, meal plans, and/or exercise programs to help you avoid hypoglycemia.

Hyperglycemia and Diabetic Acidosis

Hyperglycemia (too much glucose in the blood) may develop if your body has too little insulin. Hyperglycemia can be brought about by:

1. Omitting your insulin or taking less than the doctor has prescribed
2. Eating significantly more than your meal plan suggests
3. Developing a fever, infection, or other significant stressful situation

In patients with insulin-dependent diabetes, prolonged hyperglycemia can result in diabetic acidosis. The first symptoms of diabetic acidosis usually come on gradually, over a period of hours or days, and include a drowsy feeling, flushed face, thirst, loss of appetite, and fruity odor on the breath. With acidosis, urine tests show large amounts of glucose and acetone. Heavy breathing and a rapid pulse are more severe symptoms. If uncorrected, prolonged hyperglycemia or diabetic acidosis can lead to nausea, vomiting, dehydration, loss of consciousness or death. Therefore, it is important that you obtain medical assistance immediately.

Lipodystrophy

Rarely, administration of insulin subcutaneously can result in lipoatrophy (depression in the skin) or lipohypertrophy (enlargement or thickening of tissue). If you notice either of these conditions, consult your doctor. A change in your injection technique may help alleviate the problem.

Allergy to Insulin

Local Allergy—Patients occasionally experience redness, swelling, and itching at the site of injection of insulin. This condition, called local allergy, usually clears up in a few days to a few weeks. In some instances, this condition may be related to factors other than insulin, such as irritants in the skin cleansing agent or poor injection technique. If you have local reactions, contact your doctor.

Systemic Allergy—Less common, but potentially more serious, is generalized allergy to insulin, which may cause rash over the whole body, shortness of breath, wheezing, reduction in blood pressure, fast pulse, or sweating. Severe cases of generalized allergy may be life threatening. If you think you are having a generalized allergic reaction to insulin, notify a doctor immediately.

ADDITIONAL INFORMATION

Additional information about diabetes may be obtained from your diabetes educator.

DIABETES FORECAST is a national magazine designed especially for patients with diabetes and their families and is available by subscription from the American Diabetes Association, National Service Center, 1660 Duke Street, Alexandria, Virginia 22314, 1-800-DIABETES (1-800-342-2383).

Another publication, **DIABETES COUNTDOWN**, is available from the Juvenile Diabetes Foundation International (JDF), 120 Wall Street, 19th Floor, New York, New York 10005-4001, 1-800-JDF-CURE (1-800-533-2873).

Additional information about Humulin can be obtained by calling 1-888-88-LILLY (1-888-885-4559).

Literature revised August 13, 1999

PA 6326 AMP [081399]

HUMULIN® R **OTC**

[*hū 'mū-lĭn är*]

Regular
Cartridge
(insulin human injection, USP
[rDNA origin])
1.5 ML CARTRIDGE

For use in Becton Dickinson and Company's B-D®* Pen and Novo Nordisk A/S's NovoPen®†, NovolinPen®†, and NovoPen®† 1.5 insulin delivery devices.

Continued on next page

*** Identi-Code® symbol. This product information was prepared in June 2000. Current information on these and other products of Eli Lilly and Company may be obtained by direct inquiry to Lilly Research Laboratories, Lilly Corporate Center, Indianapolis, Indiana 46285, (800) 545-5979.**

Humulin R Reg Cartridge—Cont.

INFORMATION FOR THE PATIENT

WARNINGS

THIS LILLY HUMAN INSULIN PRODUCT DIFFERS FROM ANIMAL-SOURCE INSULINS BECAUSE IT IS STRUCTURALLY IDENTICAL TO THE INSULIN PRODUCED BY YOUR BODY'S PANCREAS AND BECAUSE OF ITS UNIQUE MANUFACTURING PROCESS.

ANY CHANGE OF INSULIN SHOULD BE MADE CAUTIOUSLY AND ONLY UNDER MEDICAL SUPERVISION. CHANGES IN STRENGTH, MANUFACTURER, TYPE (E.G., REGULAR, NPH, LENTE, ETC), SPECIES (BEEF, PORK, BEEF-PORK, HUMAN), OR METHOD OF MANUFACTURE (rDNA VERSUS ANIMAL-SOURCE INSULIN) MAY RESULT IN THE NEED FOR A CHANGE IN DOSAGE.

SOME PATIENTS TAKING HUMULIN® (HUMAN INSULIN, rDNA ORIGIN) MAY REQUIRE A CHANGE IN DOSAGE FROM THAT USED WITH ANIMAL-SOURCE INSULINS. IF AN ADJUSTMENT IS NEEDED, IT MAY OCCUR WITH THE FIRST DOSE OR DURING THE FIRST SEVERAL WEEKS OR MONTHS.

TO OBTAIN AN ACCURATE DOSE, CAREFULLY READ AND FOLLOW THE INSULIN DELIVERY DEVICE ("INSULIN PEN") MANUFACTURER'S INSTRUCTIONS AND THIS INFORMATION FOR THE PATIENT INSERT BEFORE USING THIS PRODUCT IN AN INSULIN PEN. (*see* INSTRUCTIONS FOR USE section)

DIABETES

Insulin is a hormone produced by the pancreas, a large gland that lies near the stomach. This hormone is necessary for the body's correct use of food, especially sugar. Diabetes occurs when the pancreas does not make enough insulin to meet your body's needs.

To control your diabetes, your doctor has prescribed injections of insulin to keep your blood glucose at a nearly normal level. Proper control of your diabetes requires close and constant cooperation with your doctor. In spite of diabetes, you can lead an active, healthy, and useful life if you eat a balanced diet daily, exercise regularly, and take your insulin injections as prescribed.

You have been instructed to test your blood and/or your urine regularly for glucose. If your blood tests consistently show above- or below-normal glucose levels or your urine tests consistently show the presence of glucose, your diabetes is not properly controlled and you must let your doctor know.

Always keep an extra supply of insulin as well as a spare syringe and needle on hand. Always wear diabetic identification so that appropriate treatment can be given if complications occur away from home.

REGULAR HUMAN INSULIN

Description

Humulin is synthesized in a non-disease-producing special laboratory strain of *Escherichia coli* bacteria that has been genetically altered by the addition of the human gene for insulin production. Humulin® R consists of zinc-insulin crystals dissolved in a clear fluid. Humulin R has had nothing added to change the speed or length of its action. It takes effect rapidly and has a relatively short duration of activity (4 to 12 hours) as compared with other insulins. The time course of action of any insulin may vary considerably in different individuals or at different times in the same individual. As with all insulin preparations, the duration of action of Humulin R is dependent on dose, site of injection, blood supply, temperature, and physical activity.

Humulin R is a sterile solution and is for subcutaneous injection. It should not be used intramuscularly. The concentration of Humulin R in cartridges is 100 units/mL (U-100).

Identification

Cartridges of Humulin manufactured by Eli Lilly and Company are available in 3 formulations—Regular, NPH, and 70/30.

Your doctor has prescribed the type of insulin that he/she believes is best for you. **DO NOT USE ANY OTHER INSULIN EXCEPT ON HIS/HER ADVICE AND DIRECTION.**

Cartridges of Humulin R, 1.5 mL, are available in boxes of 5.

The cartridge containing Humulin R is not designed to allow any other insulin to be mixed in the cartridge or for the cartridge to be reused.

1.5 mL Cartridge

Humulin® R 1.5 mL cartridges are for use in Becton Dickinson and Company's B-D® Pen and Novo Nordisk A/S's NovoPen®, NovolinPen®, and NovoPen® 1.5 insulin delivery devices.

Always examine the appearance of a cartridge of insulin before administering a dose. Humulin R is a clear and colorless liquid with a water-like appearance and consistency. Do not use if it appears cloudy, thickened, or slightly colored, or if solid particles are visible.

Always check the appearance of the cartridge before using, and if you note anything unusual in the appearance of your insulin or notice your insulin requirements changing markedly, consult your doctor.

Storage

Insulin cartridges should be stored in a refrigerator but not in the freezer. The insulin pen and cartridge of insulin that you are currently using should not be refrigerated but should be kept as cool as possible (below 86°F [30°C]) and away from heat and light. Do not use insulin if it has been frozen. Unrefrigerated 1.5 mL cartridges **must be discarded after 28 days**, even if they still contain insulin. **Do not use a cartridge of Humulin R after the expiration date stamped on the label.**

INSTRUCTIONS FOR USE

Pens for insulin delivery differ in their operation. It is important to read, understand, and follow the instructions for use of the particular insulin pen you are using.

NEVER SHARE INSULIN PENS, CARTRIDGES, OR NEEDLES.

PREPARING FOR AN INJECTION:

1. Inspect the Humulin R before you insert the cartridge into the insulin pen. Humulin R should look clear and colorless. Do not use a cartridge of Humulin R if it appears cloudy, thickened, slightly colored, or if solid particles are visible. Once the cartridge is in use, inspect the insulin in the insulin pen before each injection.
2. Follow the insulin pen manufacturer's instructions carefully for loading the cartridge into the insulin pen and for use of the insulin pen.
3. Use an alcohol swab to wipe the exposed rubber surface on the metal cap end of the cartridge.
4. Follow the insulin needle manufacturer's instructions for attaching and changing the needle.
5. Insulin cartridges may contain an air bubble(s) which must be removed from the cartridge and needle by proper priming prior to injection.

GENERAL INJECTION INSTRUCTIONS:

1. Wash your hands.
2. To avoid tissue damage, choose a site for each injection that is at least 1/2 inch from the previous injection site. The usual sites of injection are abdomen, thighs, and arms.
3. Cleanse the skin with alcohol where the injection is to be made.
4. With one hand, stabilize the skin by spreading it or pinching up a large area.
5. Insert the needle as instructed by your doctor.
6. After dispensing a dose, pull the needle out and apply gentle pressure over the injection site for several seconds. **Do not rub the area.**
7. Immediately after an injection, remove the needle from the insulin pen. Doing so will guard against contamination, leakage, reentry of air, and needle clogs. **Do not reuse needles. Dispose of needles in a responsible manner.**
8. *1.5 mL cartridge*—Once the cartridge is in use, do not continue to use it if the leading edge of the plunger is beyond the black band on the cartridge. If a dose is started when the leading edge of the plunger is beyond the black band, an appropriate dose may not be delivered. Use the gauge on the side of the cartridge to help you judge how much Humulin R remains. The distance between each mark on the 1.5 mL cartridge is about 10 units.

DOSAGE

Your doctor has told you which insulin to use, how much, and when and how often to inject it. Because each patient's case of diabetes is different, this schedule has been individualized for you.

Your usual insulin dose may be affected by changes in your food, activity, or work schedule. Carefully follow your doctor's instructions to allow for these changes. Other things that may affect your insulin dose are:

Illness

Illness, especially with nausea and vomiting, may cause your insulin requirements to change. Even if you are not eating, you will still require insulin. You and your doctor should establish a sick day plan for you to use in case of illness. When you are sick, test your blood glucose/urine glucose and ketones frequently and call your doctor as instructed.

Pregnancy

Good control of diabetes is especially important for you and your unborn baby. Pregnancy may make managing your diabetes more difficult. If you are planning to have a baby, are pregnant, or are nursing a baby, consult your doctor.

Medication

Insulin requirements may be increased if you are taking other drugs with hyperglycemic activity, such as oral contraceptives, corticosteroids, or thyroid replacement therapy. Insulin requirements may be reduced in the presence of drugs with hypoglycemic activity, such as oral hypoglycemics, salicylates (for example, aspirin), sulfa antibiotics, and certain antidepressants. Always discuss any medications you are taking with your doctor.

Exercise

Exercise may lower your body's need for insulin during and for some time after the activity. Exercise may also speed up the effect of an insulin dose, especially if the exercise involves the area of injection site (for example, the leg should not be used for injection just prior to running). Discuss with your doctor how you should adjust your regimen to accommodate exercise.

Travel

Persons traveling across more than 2 time zones should consult their doctor concerning adjustments in their insulin schedule.

COMMON PROBLEMS OF DIABETES

Hypoglycemia (Insulin Reaction)

Hypoglycemia (too little glucose in the blood) is one of the most frequent adverse events experienced by insulin users. It can be brought about by:

1. Taking too much insulin
2. Missing or delaying meals
3. Exercising or working more than usual
4. An infection or illness (especially with diarrhea or vomiting)
5. A change in the body's need for insulin
6. Diseases of the adrenal, pituitary or thyroid gland, or progression of kidney or liver disease
7. Interactions with other drugs that lower blood glucose, such as oral hypoglycemics, salicylates (for example, aspirin), sulfa antibiotics, and certain antidepressants
8. Consumption of alcoholic beverages

Symptoms of mild to moderate hypoglycemia may occur suddenly and can include:

- sweating
- dizziness
- palpitation
- tremor
- hunger
- restlessness
- tingling in the hands, feet, lips, or tongue
- lightheadedness
- inability to concentrate
- headache
- drowsiness
- sleep disturbances
- anxiety
- blurred vision
- slurred speech
- depressed mood
- irritability
- abnormal behavior
- unsteady movement
- personality changes

Signs of severe hypoglycemia can include:

- disorientation
- unconsciousness
- seizures
- death

Therefore, it is important that assistance be obtained immediately.

Early warning symptoms of hypoglycemia may be different or less pronounced under certain conditions, such as long duration of diabetes, diabetic nerve disease, medications such as beta-blockers, change in insulin preparations, or intensified control (3 or more insulin injections per day) of diabetes.

A few patients who have experienced hypoglycemic reactions after transfer from animal-source insulin to human insulin have reported that the early warning symptoms of hypoglycemia were less pronounced or different from those experienced with their previous insulin.

Without recognition of early warning symptoms, you may not be able to take steps to avoid more serious hypoglycemia. Be alert for all of the various types of symptoms that may indicate hypoglycemia. Patients who experience hypoglycemia without early warning symptoms should monitor their blood glucose frequently, especially prior to activities such as driving. If the blood glucose is below your normal fasting glucose, you should consider eating or drinking sugar-containing foods to treat your hypoglycemia.

Mild to moderate hypoglycemia may be treated by eating foods or drinks that contain sugar. Patients should always carry a quick source of sugar, such as candy mints or glucose tablets. More severe hypoglycemia may require the assistance of another person. Patients who are unable to take sugar orally or who are unconscious require an injection of glucagon or should be treated with intravenous administration of glucose at a medical facility.

You should learn to recognize your own symptoms of hypoglycemia. If you are uncertain about these symptoms, you should monitor your blood glucose frequently to help you learn to recognize the symptoms that you experience with hypoglycemia.

If you have frequent episodes of hypoglycemia or experience difficulty in recognizing the symptoms, you should consult your doctor to discuss possible changes in therapy, meal plans, and/or exercise programs to help you avoid hypoglycemia.

Hyperglycemia and Diabetic Acidosis

Hyperglycemia (too much glucose in the blood) may develop if your body has too little insulin. Hyperglycemia can be brought about by:

1. Omitting your insulin or taking less than the doctor has prescribed
2. Eating significantly more than your meal plan suggests
3. Developing a fever, infection, or other significant stressful situation

In patients with insulin-dependent diabetes, prolonged hyperglycemia can result in diabetic acidosis. The first symptoms of diabetic acidosis usually come on gradually, over a period of hours or days, and include a drowsy feeling, flushed face, thirst, loss of appetite, and fruity odor on the breath. With acidosis, urine tests show large amounts of glucose and acetone. Heavy breathing and a rapid pulse are more severe symptoms. If uncorrected, prolonged hyperglycemia or diabetic acidosis can lead to nausea, vomiting, dehydration, loss of consciousness or death. Therefore, it is important that you obtain medical assistance immediately.

Lipodystrophy

Rarely, administration of insulin subcutaneously can result in lipoatrophy (depression in the skin) or lipohypertrophy (enlargement or thickening of tissue). If you notice either of these conditions, consult your doctor. A change in your injection technique may help alleviate the problem.

Allergy to Insulin

Local Allergy—Patients occasionally experience redness, swelling, and itching at the site of injection of insulin. This condition, called local allergy, usually clears up in a few days to a few weeks. In some instances, this condition may be related to factors other than insulin, such as irritants in the skin cleansing agent or poor injection technique. If you have local reactions, contact your doctor.

Systemic Allergy—Less common, but potentially more serious, is generalized allergy to insulin, which may cause rash over the whole body, shortness of breath, wheezing, reduction in blood pressure, fast pulse, or sweating. Severe cases of generalized allergy may be life threatening. If you think you are having a generalized allergic reaction to insulin, notify a doctor immediately.

ADDITIONAL INFORMATION

Additional information about diabetes may be obtained from your diabetes educator.

DIABETES FORECAST is a national magazine designed especially for patients with diabetes and their families and is available on subscription from the American Diabetes Association, National Service Center, 1660 Duke Street, Alexandria, Virginia 22314, 1-800-DIABETES (1-800-342-2383).

Another publication, **DIABETES COUNTDOWN**, is available from the Juvenile Diabetes Foundation International (JDF), 120 Wall Street, 19th Floor, New York, New York 10005-4001, 1-800-JDF-CURE (1-800-533-2873).

Additional information about Humulin can be obtained by calling 1-888-88-LILLY (1-888-885-4559).

Literature revised March 26, 1999

PA 9057 FSAMP [032699]

* B-D® is a registered trademark of Becton Dickinson and Company.

† NovolinPen® and NovoPen® are registered trademarks of Novo Nordisk A/S.

HUMULIN® R ℞

[*hū 'mū-lĭn är*]

Regular U-500 (CONCENTRATED)
(insulin human injection, USP
[rDNA origin])

WARNINGS

THIS LILLY HUMAN INSULIN PRODUCT DIFFERS FROM ANIMAL-SOURCE INSULINS BECAUSE IT IS STRUCTURALLY IDENTICAL TO THE INSULIN PRODUCED BY YOUR BODY'S PANCREAS AND BECAUSE OF ITS UNIQUE MANUFACTURING PROCESS.

ANY CHANGE OF INSULIN SHOULD BE MADE CAUTIOUSLY AND ONLY UNDER MEDICAL SUPERVISION. CHANGES IN PURITY, STRENGTH, BRAND (MANUFACTURER), TYPE (REGULAR, NPH, LENTE®, ETC), SPECIES (BEEF, PORK, BEEF-PORK, HUMAN), AND/OR METHOD OF MANUFACTURE (rDNA VERSUS ANIMAL-SOURCE INSULIN) MAY RESULT IN THE NEED FOR A CHANGE IN DOSAGE.

SOME PATIENTS TAKING HUMULIN® (HUMAN INSULIN, rDNA ORIGIN, LILLY) MAY REQUIRE A CHANGE IN DOSAGE FROM THAT USED WITH ANIMAL-SOURCE INSULINS. IF AN ADJUSTMENT IS NEEDED, IT MAY OCCUR WITH THE FIRST DOSE OR DURING THE FIRST SEVERAL WEEKS OR MONTHS.

This insulin preparation contains 500 units of insulin in each milliliter. Extreme caution must be observed in the measurement of dosage because inadvertent overdose may result in irreversible insulin shock. Serious consequences may result if it is used other than under constant medical supervision.

DESCRIPTION

Humulin is synthesized in a special non-disease-producing laboratory strain of *Escherichia coli* bacteria that has been genetically altered by the addition of the gene for human insulin production. Humulin R (U-500) consists of zinc-insulin crystals dissolved in a clear fluid. Humulin R (U-500) is a sterile solution and is for subcutaneous injection. It should not be used intravenously or intramuscularly. The concentration of Humulin R (U-500) is 500 units/mL.

Each milliliter contains 500 units of biosynthetic human insulin, 16 mg glycerin, 2.5 mg *m*-cresol as a preservative, and zinc-oxide calculated to supplement endogenous zinc to obtain a total zinc content of 0.017 mg/100 units. Sodium hydroxide and/or hydrochloric acid may be added during manufacture to adjust the pH.

CLINICAL PHARMACOLOGY

Adequate insulin dosage permits the diabetic patient to utilize carbohydrates and fats in a comparatively satisfactory manner. Regardless of concentration, the action of insulin is basically the same: to enable carbohydrate metabolism to occur and thus to prevent the production of ketone bodies by the liver. Although, under usual circumstances, diabetes can be controlled with doses in the vicinity of 40 to 60 units or less, an occasional patient develops such resistance or becomes so unresponsive to the effect of insulin that daily doses of several hundred, or even several thousand, units are required. Patients who require doses in excess of 300 to 500 units daily usually have impaired insulin receptor function.

Occasionally, a cause of the insulin resistance can be found (such as hemochromatosis, cirrhosis of the liver, some complicating disease of the endocrine glands other than the pancreas, allergy, or infection), but in other cases, no cause of the high insulin requirement can be determined.

Humulin R (U-500) is unmodified by any agent that might prolong its action; however, clinical experience has shown that it frequently has a time action similar to a repository insulin preparation. It takes effect rapidly but has a relatively long duration of activity following a single dose (up to 24 hours) as compared with other Regular insulins. This effect has been credited to the high concentration of the preparation. The time course of action of any insulin may vary considerably in different individuals or at different times in the same individual. As with all insulin preparations, the duration of action of Humulin R (U-500) is dependent on dose, site of injection, blood supply, temperature, and physical activity.

INDICATIONS AND USAGE

Humulin R (U-500) is especially useful for the treatment of diabetic patients with marked insulin resistance (daily requirements more than 200 units), since a large dose may be administered subcutaneously in a reasonable volume.

CONTRAINDICATIONS

Humulin R (U-500) is contraindicated in hypoglycemia.

PRECAUTIONS

General—Every patient exhibiting insulin resistance who requires Humulin R (U-500) for control of diabetes should be under close observation until appropriate dosage is established. The response will vary among patients. Some patients can be controlled with a single dose daily; others may require 2 or 3 injections per day. Most patients will show a "tolerance" to insulin, so that minor variations in dosage can occur without the development of untoward symptoms of insulin shock.

Insulin resistance is frequently self-limited; after several weeks or months during which high dosage is required, responsiveness to the pharmacologic effect of insulin may be regained and dosage can be reduced.

Information for Patients—Patients should be instructed regarding their dosage and should be reminded that this formulation requires the administration of a smaller volume of solution than is the case with less concentrated formulations.

Laboratory Tests—Blood and urine glucose, glycohemoglobin, and urine ketones should be monitored frequently.

Drug Interactions—The concurrent use of oral hypoglycemic agents with Humulin R (U-500) is not recommended since there are no data to support such use.

Pregnancy-Teratogenic Effects—No reproduction studies have been conducted in animals, and there are no adequate and well-controlled studies in pregnant women. It would be anticipated that the benefits of this insulin preparation would outweigh any risk to the developing fetus.

Nonteratogenic Effects—Insulin does not cross the placenta as does glucose.

Labor and Delivery—Careful monitoring of the patient is required, since the insulin requirement may decrease following delivery.

Nursing Mothers—It is not known whether insulin is excreted in significant amounts in human milk. Because many drugs are excreted in human milk, caution should be exercised when Humulin R (U-500) insulin injection is administered to a nursing woman.

Pediatric Use—There are no special precautions relating to the use of this insulin formulation in the pediatric age group.

ADVERSE REACTIONS

As with other human insulin preparations, hypoglycemic reactions may be associated with the administration of Humulin R (U-500). However, deep secondary hypoglycemic reactions may develop 18 to 24 hours after the original injection of Humulin R (U-500). Consequently, patients should be carefully observed, and prompt treatment of such reactions should be initiated with glucagon injections and/or with glucose by intravenous injection or gavage.

Hypoglycemia

Hypoglycemia is one of the most frequent adverse events experienced by insulin users.

Symptoms of mild to moderate hypoglycemia may occur suddenly and can include:

- sweating
- dizziness
- palpitation
- tremor
- hunger
- restlessness
- tingling in the hands, feet, lips, or tongue
- lightheadedness
- inability to concentrate
- headache
- drowsiness
- sleep disturbances
- anxiety
- blurred vision
- slurred speech
- depressive mood
- irritability
- abnormal behavior
- unsteady movement
- personality changes

Signs of severe hypoglycemia can include:

- disorientation
- unconsciousness
- seizures
- death

Early warning symptoms of hypoglycemia may be different or less pronounced under certain conditions, such as long duration of diabetes, diabetic nerve disease, medications such as beta-blockers, change in insulin preparations, or intensified control (3 or more insulin injections per day) of diabetes.

A few patients who have experienced hypoglycemic reactions after transfer from animal-source insulin to human insulin have reported that the early warning symptoms of hypoglycemia were less pronounced or different from those experienced with their previous insulin.

Without recognition of early warning symptoms, the patient may not be able to take steps to avoid more serious hypoglycemia. Patients who experience hypoglycemia without early warning symptoms should monitor their blood glucose frequently, especially prior to activities such as driving. Mild to moderate hypoglycemia may be treated by eating foods or taking drinks that contain sugar. Patients should always carry a quick source of sugar, such as candy mints or glucose tablets.

Hypoglycemia when using Humulin R (U-500) can be prolonged and severe.

Lipodystrophy

Rarely, administration of insulin subcutaneously can result in lipoatrophy (depression in the skin) or lipohypertrophy (enlargement or thickening of tissue).

Allergy to Insulin

Local Allergy—Patients occasionally experience erythema, local edema, and pruritus at the site of injection of insulin. This condition usually is self-limiting. In some instances, this condition may be related to factors other than insulin, such as irritants in the skin cleansing agent or poor injection technique.

Systemic Allergy—Less common, but potentially more serious, is generalized allergy to insulin, which may cause rash over the whole body, shortness of breath, wheezing, reduction in blood pressure, fast pulse, or sweating. Severe cases of generalized allergy (anaphylaxis) may be life threatening.

DOSAGE AND ADMINISTRATION

Humulin R (U-500) should only be administered subcutaneously. It is inadvisable to inject Humulin R (U-500) intravenously because of possible inadvertent overdosage.

It is recommended that an insulin syringe or tuberculin-type syringe be used for the measurement of dosage. Variations in dosage are frequently possible in the insulin-resistant patient, since the individual is unresponsive to the pharmacologic effect of the insulin. Nevertheless, accuracy of measurement is to be encouraged because of the potential danger of the preparation.

STORAGE

Insulin should be kept in a cold place, preferably in a refrigerator, but must not be frozen.

Do not inject insulin that is not water-clear. Discoloration, turbidity, or unusual viscosity indicates deterioration or contamination.

Use of a package of insulin should not be started after the expiration date stamped on it.

HOW SUPPLIED

Vials, 500 units/mL, 20 mL (HI-500) (1s), NDC 0002-8501-01

Literature issued June 24, 1999

PA 2661 AMP [062499]

HUMULIN® U OTC

[*hū 'mū-lĭn ū*]

Ultralente®
(human insulin [rDNA origin]
extended zinc suspension)

INFORMATION FOR THE PATIENT

WARNINGS

THIS LILLY HUMAN INSULIN PRODUCT DIFFERS FROM ANIMAL-SOURCE INSULINS BECAUSE IT IS STRUCTURALLY IDENTICAL TO THE INSULIN PRODUCED BY YOUR BODY'S PANCREAS AND BECAUSE OF ITS UNIQUE MANUFACTURING PROCESS.

ANY CHANGE OF INSULIN SHOULD BE MADE CAUTIOUSLY AND ONLY UNDER MEDICAL SUPERVISION. CHANGES IN STRENGTH, MANUFACTURER, TYPE (E.G., REGULAR, NPH, LENTE®), SPECIES (BEEF, PORK, BEEF-PORK, HUMAN), OR METHOD OF MANUFACTURE (rDNA VERSUS ANIMAL-SOURCE INSULIN) MAY RESULT IN THE NEED FOR A CHANGE IN DOSAGE.

SOME PATIENTS TAKING HUMULIN® (HUMAN INSULIN, rDNA ORIGIN) MAY REQUIRE A CHANGE IN DOSAGE FROM THAT USED WITH ANIMAL-SOURCE INSULINS. IF AN ADJUSTMENT IS NEEDED, IT MAY OCCUR WITH THE FIRST DOSE OR DURING THE FIRST SEVERAL WEEKS OR MONTHS.

DIABETES

Insulin is a hormone produced by the pancreas, a large gland that lies near the stomach. This hormone is necessary

Continued on next page

*** Identi-Code® symbol. This product information was prepared in June 2000. Current information on these and other products of Eli Lilly and Company may be obtained by direct inquiry to Lilly Research Laboratories, Lilly Corporate Center, Indianapolis, Indiana 46285, (800) 545-5979.**

Humulin U—Cont.

for the body's correct use of food, especially sugar. Diabetes occurs when the pancreas does not make enough insulin to meet your body's needs.

To control your diabetes, your doctor has prescribed injections of insulin to keep your blood glucose at a nearly normal level. Proper control of your diabetes requires close and constant cooperation with your doctor. In spite of diabetes, you can lead an active, healthy, and useful life if you eat a balanced diet daily, exercise regularly, and take your insulin injections as prescribed.

You have been instructed to test your blood and/or your urine regularly for glucose. If your blood tests consistently show above- or below-normal glucose levels or your urine tests consistently show the presence of glucose, your diabetes is not properly controlled and you must let your doctor know.

Always keep an extra supply of insulin as well as a spare syringe and needle on hand. Always wear diabetic identification so that appropriate treatment can be given if complications occur away from home.

ULTRALENTE HUMAN INSULIN

Description

Humulin is synthesized in a special non-disease-producing laboratory strain of *Escherichia coli* bacteria that has been genetically altered by the addition of the gene for human insulin production. Humulin U is a crystalline suspension of human insulin with zinc providing a slower onset and a longer and less intense duration of activity (up to 28 hours) than regular insulin or the intermediate-acting insulins (NPH and Lente). The time course of action of any insulin may vary considerably in different individuals or at different times in the same individual. As with all insulin preparations, the duration of action of Humulin U is dependent on dose, site of injection, blood supply, temperature, and physical activity. Humulin U is a sterile suspension and is for subcutaneous injection only. It should not be used intravenously or intramuscularly. The concentration of Humulin U is 100 units/mL (U-100).

Identification

Human insulin manufactured by Eli Lilly and Company has the trademark Humulin and is available in 6 formulations—Regular (**R**), NPH (**N**), Lente (**L**), Ultralente (**U**), 50% Human Insulin Isophane Suspension [NPH]/50% Human Insulin Injection [buffered regular] (**50/50**), and 70% Human Insulin Isophane Suspension [NPH]/30% Human Insulin Injection [buffered regular] (**70/30**). Your doctor has prescribed the type of insulin that he/she believes is best for you. **DO NOT USE ANY OTHER INSULIN EXCEPT ON HIS/HER ADVICE AND DIRECTION.**

Always check the carton and the bottle label for the name and letter designation of the insulin you receive from your pharmacy to make sure it is the same as that your doctor has prescribed. Humulin U can be identified as follows:

[See graphic above]

Always examine the appearance of your bottle of insulin before withdrawing each dose. A bottle of Humulin U must be carefully shaken or rotated before each injection so that the contents are uniformly mixed. Humulin U should look uniformly cloudy or milky after mixing. Do not use it if the insulin substance (the white material) remains at the bottom of the bottle after mixing (Figure 1). Do not use a bottle of Humulin U if there are clumps in the insulin after mixing (Figure 2). Always check the appearance of your bottle of insulin before using, and if you note anything unusual in the appearance of your insulin or notice your insulin requirements changing markedly, consult your doctor.

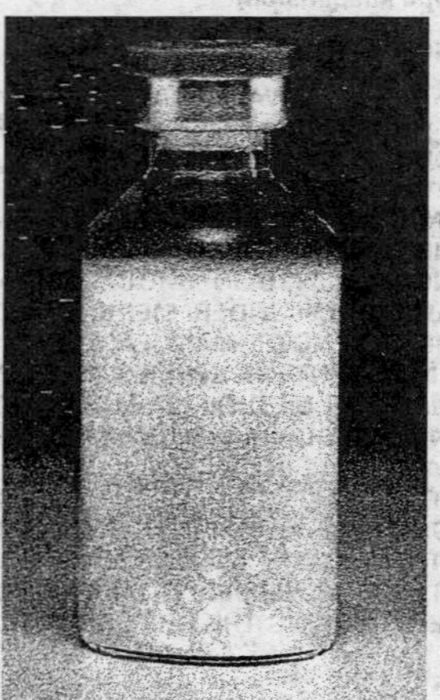

Fig 1.—Do not use if the insulin material remains at the bottom of the bottle after mixing.

Fig 2.—Do not use if there are clumps in the insulin after mixing.

[See figure 2 at top of next column]

Storage

Insulin should be stored in a refrigerator but not in the freezer. If refrigeration is not possible, the bottle of insulin that you are currently using can be kept unrefrigerated as long as it is kept as cool as possible (below 86°F [30°C]) and away from heat and light. Do not use insulin if it has been frozen. Do not use a bottle of insulin after the expiration date stamped on the label.

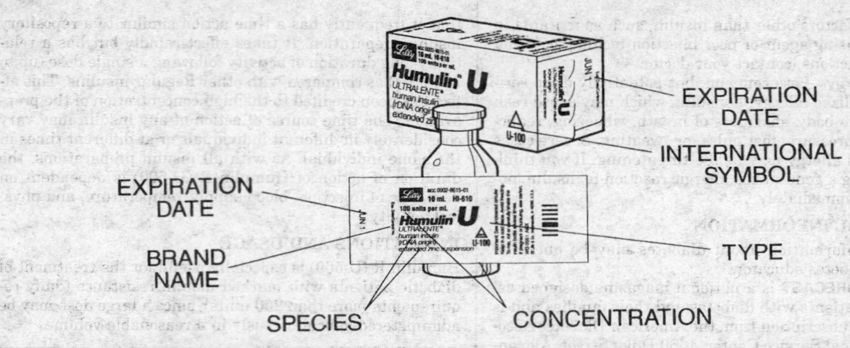

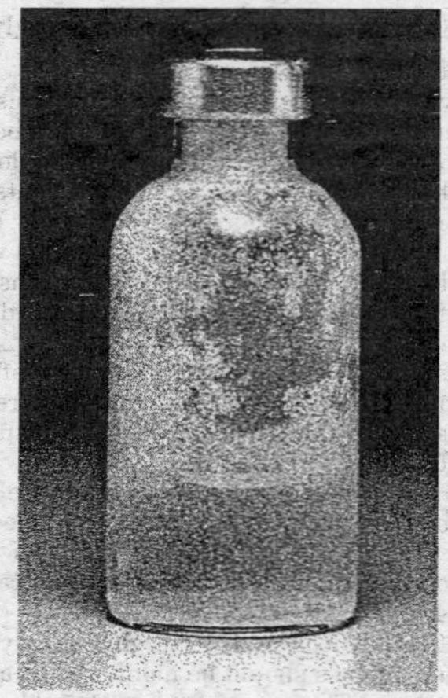

INJECTION PROCEDURES

Correct Syringe

Doses of insulin are measured in **units**. U-100 insulin contains 100 units/mL (1 mL = 1 cc). With Humulin U, it is important to use a syringe that is marked for U-100 insulin preparations. Failure to use the proper syringe can lead to a mistake in dosage, causing serious problems for you, such as a blood glucose level that is too low or too high.

Syringe Use

To help avoid contamination and possible infection, follow these instructions exactly.

Disposable syringes and needles should be used only once and then discarded. **NEEDLES AND SYRINGES MUST NOT BE SHARED.**

Reusable syringes and needles must be sterilized before each injection. **Follow the package directions supplied with your syringe.** Described below are 2 methods of sterilizing.

Boiling

1. Put syringe, plunger, and needle in strainer, place in saucepan, and cover with water. Boil for 5 minutes.
2. Remove articles from water. When they have cooled, insert plunger into barrel, and fasten needle to syringe with a slight twist.
3. Push plunger in and out several times until water is completely removed.

Isopropyl Alcohol

If the syringe, plunger, and needle cannot be boiled, as when you are traveling, they may be sterilized by immersion for at least 5 minutes in Isopropyl Alcohol, 91%. Do not use bathing, rubbing, or medicated alcohol for this sterilization. If the syringe is sterilized with alcohol, it must be absolutely dry before use.

Preparing the Dose

1. Wash your hands.
2. Carefully shake or rotate the insulin bottle several times to completely mix the insulin.
3. Inspect the insulin. Humulin U should look uniformly cloudy or milky. Do not use it if you notice anything unusual in the appearance.
4. If using a new bottle, flip off the plastic protective cap, but **do not** remove the stopper. When using a new bottle, wipe the top of the bottle with an alcohol swab.
5. If you are mixing insulins, refer to the instructions for mixing that follow.
6. Draw air into the syringe equal to your insulin dose. Put the needle through rubber top of the insulin bottle and inject the air into the bottle.
7. Turn the bottle and syringe upside down. Hold the bottle and syringe firmly in 1 hand and shake gently.
8. Making sure the tip of the needle is in the insulin, withdraw the correct dose of insulin into the syringe.
9. Before removing the needle from the bottle, check your syringe for air bubbles which reduce the amount of insulin in it. If bubbles are present, hold the syringe straight up and tap its side until the bubbles float to the top. Push them out with the plunger and withdraw the correct dose.
10. Remove the needle from the bottle and lay the syringe down so that the needle does not touch anything.

Mixing Humulin U with Regular or Lente Human Insulin

1. Ultralente human insulin should be mixed with regular or Lente human insulin only on the advice of your doctor.
2. Draw air into your syringe equal to the amount of Humulin U you are taking. Insert the needle into the Humulin U bottle and inject the air. Withdraw the needle.
3. Now inject air into your regular or Lente human insulin bottle in the same manner, but **do not** withdraw the needle.
4. Turn the bottle and syringe upside down.
5. Making sure the tip of the needle is in the insulin, withdraw the correct dose of regular or Lente insulin into the syringe.
6. Before removing the needle from the bottle, check your syringe for air bubbles which reduce the amount of insulin in it. If bubbles are present, hold the syringe straight up and tap its side until the bubbles float to the top. Push them out with the plunger and withdraw the correct dose.
7. Remove the needle from the bottle of regular or Lente insulin and insert it into the bottle of Humulin U. Turn the bottle and syringe upside down. Hold the bottle and syringe firmly in 1 hand and shake gently. Making sure the tip of the needle is in the insulin, withdraw your dose of Humulin U.
8. Remove the needle and lay the syringe down so that the needle does not touch anything.

Follow your doctor's instructions on whether to mix your insulins ahead of time or just before giving your injection. It is important to be consistent in your method.

Syringes from different manufacturers may vary in the amount of space between the bottom line and the needle. Because of this, do not change:

- the sequence of mixing, or
- the model and brand of syringe or needle that the doctor has prescribed.

Injection

Cleanse the skin with alcohol where the injection is to be made. Stabilize the skin by spreading it or pinching up a large area. Insert the needle as instructed by your doctor. Push the plunger in as far as it will go. Pull the needle out and apply gentle pressure over the injection site for several seconds. **Do not rub the area.** To avoid tissue damage, give the next injection at a site at least 1/2" from the previous site.

DOSAGE

Your doctor has told you which insulin to use, how much, and when and how often to inject it. Because each patient's case of diabetes is different, this schedule has been individualized for you.

Your usual insulin dose may be affected by changes in your food, activity, or work schedule. Carefully follow your doctor's instructions to allow for these changes. Other things that may affect your insulin dose are:

Illness

Illness, especially with nausea and vomiting, may cause your insulin requirements to change. Even if you are not eating, you will still require insulin. You and your doctor should establish a sick day plan for you to use in case of illness. When you are sick, test your blood/urine frequently and call your doctor as instructed.

Pregnancy

Good control of diabetes is especially important for you and your unborn baby. Pregnancy may make managing your diabetes more difficult. If you are planning to have a baby, are pregnant, or are nursing a baby, consult your doctor.

Medication

Insulin requirements may be increased if you are taking other drugs with hyperglycemic activity, such as oral contraceptives, corticosteroids, or thyroid replacement therapy. Insulin requirements may be reduced in the presence of drugs with hypoglycemic activity, such as oral hypoglycemics, salicylates (for example, aspirin), sulfa antibiotics, and certain antidepressants. Always discuss any medications you are taking with your doctor.

Exercise

Exercise may lower your body's need for insulin during and for some time after the activity. Exercise may also speed up the effect of an insulin dose, especially if the exercise involves the area of injection site (for example, the leg should not be used for injection just prior to running). Discuss with your doctor how you should adjust your regimen to accommodate exercise.

Travel
Persons traveling across more than 2 time zones should consult their doctor concerning adjustments in their insulin schedule.

COMMON PROBLEMS OF DIABETES

Hypoglycemia (Insulin Reaction)
Hypoglycemia (too little glucose in the blood) is one of the most frequent adverse events experienced by insulin users. It can be brought about by:

1. Taking too much insulin
2. Missing or delaying meals
3. Exercising or working more than usual
4. An infection or illness (especially with diarrhea or vomiting)
5. A change in the body's need for insulin
6. Diseases of the adrenal, pituitary, or thyroid gland, or progression of kidney or liver disease
7. Interactions with other drugs that lower blood glucose, such as oral hypoglycemics, salicylates (for example, aspirin) sulfa antibiotics, and certain antidepressants
8. Consumption of alcoholic beverages

Symptoms of mild to moderate hypoglycemia may occur suddenly and can include:

- sweating
- dizziness
- palpitation
- tremor
- hunger
- restlessness
- tingling in the hands, feet, lips, or tongue
- lightheadedness
- inability to concentrate
- headache
- drowsiness
- sleep disturbances
- anxiety
- blurred vision
- slurred speech
- depressed mood
- irritability
- abnormal behavior
- unsteady movement
- personality changes

Signs of severe hypoglycemia can include:

- disorientation
- unconsciousness
- seizures
- death

Therefore, it is important that assistance be obtained immediately.
Early warning symptoms of hypoglycemia may be different or less pronounced under certain conditions, such as long duration of diabetes, diabetic nerve disease, medications such as beta-blockers, change in insulin preparations, or intensified control (3 or more insulin injections per day) of diabetes.
A few patients who have experienced hypoglycemic reactions after transfer from animal-source insulin to human insulin have reported that the early warning symptoms of hypoglycemia were less pronounced or different from those experienced with their previous insulin.
Without recognition of early warning symptoms, you may not be able to take steps to avoid more serious hypoglycemia. Be alert for all of the various types of symptoms that may indicate hypoglycemia. Patients who experience hypoglycemia without early warning symptoms should monitor their blood glucose frequently, especially prior to activities such as driving. If the blood glucose is below your normal fasting glucose, you should consider eating or drinking sugar-containing foods to treat your hypoglycemia.
Mild to moderate hypoglycemia may be treated by eating foods or drinks that contain sugar. Patients should always carry a quick source of sugar, such as candy mints or glucose tablets. More severe hypoglycemia may require the assistance of another person. Patients who are unable to take sugar orally or who are unconscious require an injection of glucagon or should be treated with intravenous administration of glucose at a medical facility.
You should learn to recognize your own symptoms of hypoglycemia. If you are uncertain about these symptoms, you should monitor your blood glucose frequently to help you learn to recognize the symptoms that you experience with hypoglycemia.
If you have frequent episodes of hypoglycemia or experience difficulty in recognizing the symptoms, you should consult your doctor to discuss possible changes in therapy, meal plans, and/or exercise programs to help you avoid hypoglycemia.

Hyperglycemia and Diabetic Acidosis
Hyperglycemia (too much glucose in the blood) may develop if your body has too little insulin. Hyperglycemia can be brought about by:

1. Omitting your insulin or taking less than the doctor has prescribed
2. Eating significantly more than your meal plan suggests
3. Developing a fever, infection, or other significant stressful situation

In patients with insulin-dependent diabetes, prolonged hyperglycemia can result in diabetic acidosis. The first symptoms of diabetic acidosis usually come on gradually, over a period of hours or days, and include a drowsy feeling, flushed face, thirst, loss of appetite, and fruity odor on the breath. With acidosis, urine tests show large amounts of glucose and acetone. Heavy breathing and a rapid pulse are more severe symptoms. If uncorrected, prolonged hyperglycemia or diabetic acidosis can lead to nausea, vomiting, dehydration, loss of consciousness or death. Therefore, it is important that you obtain medical assistance immediately.

Lipodystrophy
Rarely, administration of insulin subcutaneously can result in lipoatrophy (depression in the skin) or lipohypertrophy (enlargement or thickening of tissue). If you notice either of these conditions, consult your doctor. A change in your injection technique may help alleviate the problem.

Allergy to Insulin
Local Allergy—Patients occasionally experience redness, swelling, and itching at the site of injection of insulin. This condition, called local allergy, usually clears up in a few days to a few weeks. In some instances, this condition may be related to factors other than insulin, such as irritants in the skin cleansing agent or poor injection technique. If you have local reactions, contact your doctor.
Systemic Allergy—Less common, but potentially more serious, is generalized allergy to insulin, which may cause rash over the whole body, shortness of breath, wheezing, reduction in blood pressure, fast pulse, or sweating. Severe cases of generalized allergy may be life threatening. If you think you are having a generalized allergic reaction to insulin, notify a doctor immediately.

ADDITIONAL INFORMATION

Additional information about diabetes may be obtained from your diabetes educator.
DIABETES FORECAST is a national magazine designed especially for patients with diabetes and their families and is available by subscription from the American Diabetes Association, National Service Center, 1660 Duke Street, Alexandria, Virginia 22314, 1-800-DIABETES (1-800-342-2383).
Another publication, **DIABETES COUNTDOWN**, is available from the Juvenile Diabetes Foundation International (JDF), 120 Wall Street, 19th Floor, New York, New York 10005-4001, 1-800-JDF-CURE (1-800-533-2873).
Additional information about Humulin can be obtained by calling 1-888-88-LILLY (1-888-885-4559).
Literature revised August 13, 1999
PA 6365 AMP [081399]

LENTE® ILETIN® II OTC

[*lĕn-tā ī 'lĕ-tĭn*]
(Insulin Zinc Suspension, USP, purified pork)

INFORMATION FOR THE PATIENT

WARNINGS

ANY CHANGE OF INSULIN SHOULD BE MADE CAUTIOUSLY AND ONLY UNDER MEDICAL SUPERVISION. CHANGES IN PURITY, STRENGTH, BRAND (MANUFACTURER), TYPE (REGULAR, NPH, LENTE®), SPECIES (BEEF, PORK, BEEF-PORK, HUMAN), AND/OR METHOD OF MANUFACTURE (RECOMBINANT DNA VERSUS ANIMAL-SOURCE INSULIN) MAY RESULT IN THE NEED FOR A CHANGE IN DOSAGE. IF AN ADJUSTMENT IS NEEDED, IT MAY OCCUR WITH THE FIRST DOSE OR DURING THE FIRST SEVERAL WEEKS OR MONTHS.

DIABETES
Insulin is a hormone produced by the pancreas, a large gland that lies near the stomach. This hormone is necessary for the body's correct use of food, especially sugar. Diabetes occurs when the pancreas does not make enough insulin to meet your body's needs.
To control your diabetes, your doctor has prescribed injections of insulin to keep your blood glucose at a nearly normal level. Proper control of your diabetes requires close and constant cooperation with your doctor. In spite of diabetes, you can lead an active, healthy, and useful life if you eat a balanced diet daily, exercise regularly, and take your insulin injections as prescribed.
You have been instructed to test your blood and/or your urine regularly for glucose. If your blood tests consistently show above- or below-normal glucose levels or your urine tests consistently show the presence of glucose, your diabetes is not properly controlled and you must let your doctor know.
Always keep an extra supply of insulin as well as a spare syringe and needle on hand. Always wear diabetic identification so that appropriate treatment can be given if complications occur away from home.

LENTE PORK INSULIN

Description
Lente pork insulin is obtained from pork pancreas.
Lente® Iletin® II (purified insulin, Lilly) is an amorphous and crystalline suspension of insulin with zinc providing an intermediate-acting insulin with a slower onset and a longer duration of activity (slightly more than 24 hours) than regular insulin. The time course of action of any insulin may vary considerably in different individuals or at different times in the same individual. As with all insulin preparations, the duration of action of Lente Iletin II is dependent on dose, site of injection, blood supply, temperature, and physical activity. Lente Iletin II is a sterile suspension and is for subcutaneous injection only. It should not be used intravenously or intramuscularly. The concentration of Lente Iletin II is 100 units/mL (U-100).

Identification
This insulin, manufactured by Eli Lilly and Company, has the trademark Iletin II and is available in various types—Regular, NPH, and Lente. Your doctor has prescribed the type of insulin that he/she believes is best for you. **DO NOT USE ANY OTHER INSULIN EXCEPT ON HIS/HER ADVICE AND DIRECTION.**
Always check the carton and the bottle label for the name and letter designation of the insulin you receive from your pharmacy to make sure it is the same as that your doctor has prescribed.
Always examine the appearance of your bottle of insulin before withdrawing each dose. A bottle of Lente Iletin II must be carefully shaken or rotated before each injection so that the contents are uniformly mixed. Lente Iletin II should look uniformly cloudy or milky after mixing. Do not use it if the insulin substance (the white material) remains at the bottom of the bottle after mixing. Do not use a bottle of Lente Iletin II if there are clumps in the insulin after mixing. Always check the appearance of your bottle of insulin before using, and if you note anything unusual in the appearance of your insulin or notice your insulin requirements changing markedly, consult your doctor.

Storage
Insulin should be stored in a refrigerator but not in the freezer. If refrigeration is not possible, the bottle of insulin that you are currently using can be kept unrefrigerated as long as it is kept as cool as possible (below 86°F [30°C]) and away from heat and light. Do not use insulin if it has been frozen. Do not use a bottle of insulin after the expiration date stamped on the label.

INJECTION PROCEDURES

Correct Syringe
Doses of insulin are measured in **units.** U-100 insulin contains 100 units/mL (1 mL = 1 cc). With Lente Iletin II, it is important to use a syringe that is marked for U-100 insulin preparations. Failure to use the proper syringe can lead to a mistake in dosage, causing serious problems for you, such as a blood glucose level that is too low or too high.

Syringe Use
To help avoid contamination and possible infection, follow these instructions exactly.
Disposable syringes and needles should be used only once and then discarded. **NEEDLES AND SYRINGES MUST NOT BE SHARED.**
Reusable syringes and needles must be sterilized before each injection. **Follow the package directions supplied with your syringe.** Described below are 2 methods of sterilizing.

Boiling

1. Put syringe, plunger, and needle in strainer, place in saucepan, and cover with water. Boil for 5 minutes.
2. Remove articles from water. When they have cooled, insert plunger into barrel, and fasten needle to syringe with a slight twist.
3. Push plunger in and out several times until water is completely removed.

Isopropyl Alcohol
If the syringe, plunger, and needle cannot be boiled, as when you are traveling, they may be sterilized by immersion for at least 5 minutes in Isopropyl Alcohol, 91%. Do not use bathing, rubbing, or medicated alcohol for this sterilization. If the syringe is sterilized with alcohol, it must be absolutely dry before use.

Preparing the Dose

1. Wash your hands.
2. Carefully shake or rotate the insulin bottle several times to completely mix the insulin.
3. Inspect the insulin. Lente Iletin II should look uniformly cloudy or milky. Do not use it if you notice anything unusual in the appearance.
4. If using a new bottle, flip off the plastic protective cap, but **do not** remove the stopper. When using a new bottle, wipe the top of the bottle with an alcohol swab.
5. If you are mixing insulins, refer to the Warnings below.
6. Draw air into the syringe equal to your insulin dose. Put the needle through rubber top of the insulin bottle and inject the air into the bottle.
7. Turn the bottle and syringe upside down. Hold the bottle and syringe firmly in 1 hand and shake gently.
8. Making sure the tip of the needle is in the insulin, withdraw the correct dose of insulin into the syringe.
9. Before removing the needle from the bottle, check your syringe for air bubbles which reduce the amount of insulin in it. If bubbles are present, hold the syringe straight up and tap its side until the bubbles float to the top. Push them out with the plunger and withdraw the correct dose.
10. Remove the needle from the bottle and lay the syringe down so that the needle does not touch anything.

WARNINGS—SEE ADDITIONAL WARNINGS ABOVE

Patients who have been directed by their doctors to mix 2 types of insulin should be aware that insulin hypodermic syringes of different manufacturers may vary in the amount of space between the bottom line and the needle.

Continued on next page

*** Identi-Code® symbol. This product information was prepared in June 2000. Current information on these and other products of Eli Lilly and Company may be obtained by direct inquiry to Lilly Research Laboratories, Lilly Corporate Center, Indianapolis, Indiana 46285, (800) 545-5979.**

Lente Iletin II (Pork)—Cont.

Because of this, do not change:
1. The order of mixing that the doctor has prescribed or
2. The model and brand of syringe or needle without first consulting your doctor.

The mixing should be done immediately prior to injection. Failure to heed this warning could result in a dosage error.

Injection

Cleanse the skin with alcohol where the injection is to be made. Stabilize the skin by spreading it or pinching up a large area. Insert the needle as instructed by your doctor. Push the plunger in as far as it will go. Pull the needle out and apply gentle pressure over the injection site for several seconds. **Do not rub the area.** To avoid tissue damage, give the next injection at a site at least $^1/_2$" from the previous site.

DOSAGE

Your doctor has told you which insulin to use, how much, and when and how often to inject it. Because each patient's case of diabetes is different, this schedule has been individualized for you.

Your usual insulin dose may be affected by changes in your food, activity, or work schedule. Carefully follow your doctor's instructions to allow for these changes. Other things that may affect your insulin dose are:

Illness

Illness, especially with nausea and vomiting, may cause your insulin requirements to change. Even if you are not eating, you will still require insulin. You and your doctor should establish a sick day plan for you to use in case of illness. When you are sick, test your blood/urine frequently and call your doctor as instructed.

Pregnancy

Good control of diabetes is especially important for you and your unborn baby. Pregnancy may make managing your diabetes more difficult. If you are planning to have a baby, are pregnant, or are nursing a baby, consult your doctor.

Medication

Insulin requirements may be increased if you are taking other drugs with hyperglycemic activity, such as oral contraceptives, corticosteroids, or thyroid replacement therapy. Insulin requirements may be reduced in the presence of drugs with hypoglycemic activity, such as oral hypoglycemics, salicylates (for example, aspirin), sulfa antibiotics, and certain antidepressants. Always discuss any medications you are taking with your doctor.

Exercise

Exercise may lower your body's need for insulin during and for some time after the activity. Exercise may also speed up the effect of an insulin dose, especially if the exercise involves the area of injection site (for example, the leg should not be used for injection just prior to running). Discuss with your doctor how you should adjust your regimen to accommodate exercise.

Travel

Persons traveling across more than 2 time zones should consult their doctor concerning adjustments in their insulin schedule.

COMMON PROBLEMS OF DIABETES

Hypoglycemia (Insulin Reaction)

Hypoglycemia (too little glucose in the blood) is one of the most frequent adverse events experienced by insulin users. It can be brought about by:
1. Taking too much insulin
2. Missing or delaying meals
3. Exercising or working more than usual
4. An infection or illness (especially with diarrhea or vomiting)
5. A change in the body's need for insulin
6. Diseases of the adrenal, pituitary, or thyroid gland, or progression of kidney or liver disease
7. Interactions with other drugs that lower blood glucose, such as oral hypoglycemics, salicylates (for example, aspirin), sulfa antibiotics, and certain antidepressants
8. Consumption of alcoholic beverages

Symptoms of mild to moderate hypoglycemia may occur suddenly and can include:
- sweating
- dizziness
- palpitation
- tremor
- hunger
- restlessness
- tingling in the hands, feet, lips, or tongue
- lightheadedness
- inability to concentrate
- headache
- drowsiness
- sleep disturbances
- anxiety
- blurred vision
- slurred speech
- depressive mood
- irritability
- abnormal behavior
- unsteady movement
- personality changes

Signs of severe hypoglycemia can include:
- disorientation
- unconsciousness
- seizures
- death

Therefore, it is important that assistance be obtained immediately.

Early warning symptoms of hypoglycemia may be different or less pronounced under certain conditions, such as long duration of diabetes, diabetic nerve disease, medications such as beta-blockers, change in insulin preparations, or intensified control (3 or more insulin injections per day) of diabetes.

Without recognition of early warning symptoms, you may not be able to take steps to avoid more serious hypoglycemia. Be alert for all of the various types of symptoms that may indicate hypoglycemia. Patients who experience hypoglycemia without early warning symptoms should monitor their blood glucose frequently, especially prior to activities such as driving. If the blood glucose is below your normal fasting glucose, you should consider eating or drinking sugar-containing foods to treat your hypoglycemia.

Mild to moderate hypoglycemia may be treated by eating foods or taking drinks that contain sugar. Patients should always carry a quick source of sugar, such as candy mints or glucose tablets. More severe hypoglycemia may require the assistance of another person. Patients who are unable to take sugar orally or who are unconscious require an injection of glucagon or should be treated with intravenous administration of glucose at a medical facility.

You should learn to recognize your own symptoms of hypoglycemia. If you are uncertain about these symptoms, you should monitor your blood glucose frequently to help you learn to recognize the symptoms that you experience with hypoglycemia.

If you have frequent episodes of hypoglycemia or experience difficulty in recognizing the symptoms, you should consult your doctor to discuss possible changes in therapy, meal plans, and/or exercise programs to help you avoid hypoglycemia.

Hyperglycemia and Diabetic Acidosis

Hyperglycemia (too little glucose in the blood) may develop if your body has too little insulin. Hyperglycemia can be brought about by:
1. Omitting your insulin or taking less than the doctor has prescribed
2. Eating significantly more than your meal plan suggests
3. Developing a fever or infection

In patients with insulin-dependent diabetes, prolonged hyperglycemia can result in diabetic acidosis. The first symptoms of diabetic acidosis usually come on gradually, over a period of hours or days, and include a drowsy feeling, flushed face, thirst, loss of appetite, and fruity odor on the breath. With acidosis, urine tests show large amounts of glucose and acetone. Heavy breathing and a rapid pulse are more severe symptoms. If uncorrected, prolonged hyperglycemia or diabetic acidosis can result in loss of consciousness or death. Therefore, it is important that you obtain medical assistance immediately.

Lipodystrophy

Rarely, administration of insulin subcutaneously can result in lipoatrophy (depression in the skin) or lipohypertrophy (enlargement or thickening of tissue). If you notice either of these conditions, consult your doctor. A change in your injection technique may help alleviate the problem.

Allergy to Insulin

Local Allergy—Patients occasionally experience redness, swelling, and itching at the site of injection of insulin. This condition, called local allergy, usually clears up in a few days to a few weeks. In some instances, this condition may be related to factors other than insulin, such as irritants in the skin cleansing agent or poor injection technique. If you have local reactions, contact your doctor.

Systemic Allergy—Less common, but potentially more serious, is generalized allergy to insulin, which may cause rash over the whole body, shortness of breath, wheezing, reduction in blood pressure, fast pulse, or sweating. Severe cases of generalized allergy may be life threatening. If you think you are having a generalized allergic reaction to insulin, notify a doctor immediately.

ADDITIONAL INFORMATION

Additional information about diabetes may be obtained from your diabetes educator.

DIABETES FORECAST is a national magazine designed especially for patients with diabetes and their families and is available by subscription from the American Diabetes Association, National Service Center, 1660 Duke Street, Alexandria, Virginia 22314.

Another publication, **DIABETES COUNTDOWN,** is available from the Juvenile Diabetes Foundation International (JDF), 120 Wall Street, 19th Floor, New York, New York 10005-40001, 1-800-JDF-CURE (1-800-533-2873).

Additional information about Iletin can be obtained by calling 1-888-88-LILLY (1-888-885-4559).

Literature revised August 13, 1999

PA 8549 AMP [081399]

NPH ILETIN® II OTC

[*ĕn ′pē-āch ī ′lĕ-tĭn*]

(Isophane Insulin Suspension, USP, purified pork)

INFORMATION FOR THE PATIENT

WARNINGS

ANY CHANGE OF INSULIN SHOULD BE MADE CAUTIOUSLY AND ONLY UNDER MEDICAL SUPERVISION. CHANGES IN PURITY, STRENGTH, BRAND (MANUFACTURER), TYPE (REGULAR, NPH, LENTE®), SPECIES (BEEF, PORK, BEEF-PORK, HUMAN), AND/OR METHOD OF MANUFACTURE (RECOMBINANT DNA VERSUS ANIMAL-SOURCE INSULIN) MAY RESULT IN THE NEED FOR A CHANGE IN DOSAGE. IF AN ADJUSTMENT IS NEEDED, IT MAY OCCUR WITH THE FIRST DOSE OR DURING THE FIRST SEVERAL WEEKS OR MONTHS.

DIABETES

Insulin is a hormone produced by the pancreas, a large gland that lies near the stomach. This hormone is necessary for the body's correct use of food, especially sugar. Diabetes occurs when the pancreas does not make enough insulin to meet your body's needs.

To control your diabetes, your doctor has prescribed injections of insulin to keep your blood glucose at a nearly normal level. Proper control of your diabetes requires close and constant cooperation with your doctor. In spite of diabetes, you can lead an active, healthy, and useful life if you eat a balanced diet daily, exercise regularly, and take your insulin injections as prescribed.

You have been instructed to test your blood and/or your urine regularly for glucose. If your blood tests consistently show above- or below-normal glucose levels or your urine tests consistently show the presence of glucose, your diabetes is not properly controlled and you must let your doctor know.

Always keep an extra supply of insulin as well as a spare syringe and needle on hand. Always wear diabetic identification so that appropriate treatment can be given if complications occur away from home.

NPH PORK INSULIN

Description

NPH pork insulin is obtained from pork pancreas.

NPH Iletin® II (purified insulin, Lilly) is a crystalline suspension of insulin with protamine and zinc providing an intermediate-acting insulin with a slower onset of action and a longer duration of activity (slightly more than 24 hours) than that of regular insulin. The time course of action of any insulin may vary considerably in different individuals or at different times in the same individual. As with all insulin preparations, the duration of action of NPH Iletin II is dependent on dose, site of injection, blood supply, temperature, and physical activity. NPH Iletin II is a sterile suspension and is for subcutaneous injection only. It should not be used intravenously or intramuscularly. The concentration of NPH Iletin II is 100 units/mL (U-100).

Identification

This insulin, manufactured by Eli Lilly and Company, has the trademark Iletin II and is available in various types—Regular, NPH, and Lente. Your doctor has prescribed the type of insulin that he/she believes is best for you. **DO NOT USE ANY OTHER INSULIN EXCEPT ON HIS/HER ADVICE AND DIRECTION.**

Always check the carton and the bottle label for the name and letter designation of the insulin you receive from your pharmacy to make sure it is the same as that your doctor has prescribed.

Always examine the appearance of your bottle of insulin before withdrawing each dose. A bottle of NPH Iletin II must be carefully shaken or rotated before each injection so that the contents are uniformly mixed. NPH Iletin II should look uniformly cloudy or milky after mixing. Do not use it if the insulin substance (the white material) remains at the bottom of the bottle after mixing. Do not use a bottle of NPH Iletin II if there are clumps in the insulin after mixing. Always check the appearance of your bottle of insulin before using, and if you note anything unusual in the appearance of your insulin or notice your insulin requirements changing markedly, consult your doctor.

Storage

Insulin should be stored in a refrigerator but not in the freezer. If refrigeration is not possible, the bottle of insulin that you are currently using can be kept unrefrigerated as long as it is kept as cool as possible (below 86°F [30°C]) and away from heat and light. Do not use insulin if it has been frozen. Do not use a bottle of insulin after the expiration date stamped on the label.

INJECTION PROCEDURES

Correct Syringe

Doses of insulin are measured in **units**. U-100 insulin contains 100 units/mL (1 mL = 1 cc). With NPH Iletin II, it is important to use a syringe that is marked for U-100 insulin preparations. Failure to use the proper syringe can lead to a mistake in dosage, causing serious problems for you, such as a blood glucose level that is too low or too high.

Syringe Use

To help avoid contamination and possible infection, follow these instructions exactly.

Disposable syringes and needles should be used only once and then discarded. **NEEDLES AND SYRINGES MUST NOT BE SHARED.**

Reusable syringes and needles must be sterilized before each injection. **Follow the package directions supplied with your syringe.** Described below are 2 methods of sterilizing.

Boiling

1. Put syringe, plunger, and needle in strainer, place in saucepan, and cover with water. Boil for 5 minutes.
2. Remove articles from water. When they have cooled, insert plunger into barrel, and fasten needle to syringe with a slight twist.
3. Push plunger in and out several times until water is completely removed.

Isopropyl Alcohol
If the syringe, plunger, and needle cannot be boiled, as when you are traveling, they may be sterilized by immersion for at least 5 minutes in Isopropyl Alcohol, 91%. Do not use bathing, rubbing, or medicated alcohol for this sterilization. If the syringe is sterilized with alcohol, it must be absolutely dry before use.

Preparing the Dose

1. Wash your hands.
2. Carefully shake or rotate the insulin bottle several times to completely mix the insulin.
3. Inspect the insulin. NPH Iletin II should look uniformly cloudy or milky. Do not use it if you notice anything unusual in the appearance.
4. If using a new bottle, flip off the plastic protective cap, but **do not** remove the stopper. When using a new bottle, wipe the top of the bottle with an alcohol swab.
5. If you are mixing insulins, refer to the Warnings below.
6. Draw air into the syringe equal to your insulin dose. Put the needle through rubber top of the insulin bottle and inject the air into the bottle.
7. Turn the bottle and syringe upside down. Hold the bottle and syringe firmly in 1 hand and shake gently.
8. Making sure the tip of the needle is in the insulin, withdraw the correct dose of insulin into the syringe.
9. Before removing the needle from the bottle, check your syringe for air bubbles which reduce the amount of insulin in it. If bubbles are present, hold the syringe straight up and tap its side until the bubbles float to the top. Push them out with the plunger and withdraw the correct dose.
10. Remove the needle from the bottle and lay the syringe down so that the needle does not touch anything.

WARNINGS—SEE ADDITIONAL WARNINGS ABOVE
Patients who have been directed by their doctors to mix 2 types of insulin should be aware that insulin hypodermic syringes of different manufacturers may vary in the amount of space between the bottom line and the needle.
Because of this, do not change:
1. The order of mixing that the doctor has prescribed or
2. The model and brand of syringe or needle without first consulting your doctor.

The mixing should be done immediately prior to injection. Failure to heed this warning could result in a dosage error.

Injection
Cleanse the skin with alcohol where the injection is to be made. Stabilize the skin by spreading it or pinching up a large area. Insert the needle as instructed by your doctor. Push the plunger in as far as it will go. Pull the needle out and apply gentle pressure over the injection site for several seconds. **Do not rub the area**. To avoid tissue damage, give the next tissue damage, give the next injection at a site at least $^1/_2$" from the previous site.

DOSAGE
Your doctor has told you which insulin to use, how much, and when and how often to inject it. Because each patient's case of diabetes is different, this schedule has been individualized for you.
Your usual insulin dose may be affected by changes in your food, activity, or work schedule. Carefully follow your doctor's instructions to allow for these changes. Other things that may affect your insulin dose are:

Illness
Illness, especially with nausea and vomiting, may cause your insulin requirements to change. Even if you are not eating, you will still require insulin. You and your doctor should establish a sick day plan for you to use in case of illness. When you are sick, test your blood/urine frequently and call your doctor as instructed.

Pregnancy
Good control of diabetes is especially important for you and your unborn baby. Pregnancy may make managing your diabetes more difficult. If you are planning to have a baby, are pregnant, or are nursing a baby, consult your doctor.

Medication
Insulin requirements may be increased if you are taking other drugs with hyperglycemic activity, such as oral contraceptives, corticosteroids, or thyroid replacement therapy. Insulin requirements may be reduced in the presence of drugs with hypoglycemic activity, such as oral hypoglycemics, salicylates (for example, aspirin), sulfa antibiotics, and certain antidepressants. Always discuss any medications you are taking with your doctor.

Exercise
Exercise may lower your body's need for insulin during and for some time after the activity. Exercise may also speed up the effect of an insulin dose, especially if the exercise involves the area of injection site (for example, the leg should not be used for injection prior to running). Discuss with your doctor how you should adjust your regimen to accommodate exercise.

Travel
Persons traveling across more than 2 time zones should consult their doctor concerning adjustments in their insulin schedule.

COMMON PROBLEMS OF DIABETES

Hypoglycemia (Insulin Reaction)
Hypoglycemia (too little glucose in the blood) is one of the most frequent adverse events experienced by insulin users. It can be brought about by:
1. Taking too much insulin
2. Missing or delaying meals
3. Exercising or working more than usual
4. An infection or illness (especially with diarrhea or vomiting)
5. A change in the body's need for insulin
6. Diseases of the adrenal, pituitary, or thyroid gland, or progression of kidney or liver disease
7. Interactions with other drugs that lower blood glucose, such as oral hypoglycemics, salicylates (for example, aspirin), sulfa antibiotics, and certain antidepressants
8. Consumption of alcoholic beverages

Symptoms of mild to moderate hypoglycemia may occur suddenly and can include:
- sweating
- dizziness
- palpitation
- tremor
- hunger
- restlessness
- tingling in the hands, feet, lips, or tongue
- lightheadedness
- inability to concentrate
- headache
- drowsiness
- sleep disturbances
- anxiety
- blurred vision
- slurred speech
- depressive mood
- irritability
- abnormal behavior
- unsteady movement
- personality changes

Signs of severe hypoglycemia can include:
- disorientation
- unconsciousness
- seizures
- death

Therefore, it is important that assistance be obtained immediately
Early warning symptoms of hypoglycemia may be different or less pronounced under certain conditions, such as long duration of diabetes, diabetic nerve disease, medications such as beta-blockers, change in insulin preparations, or intensified control (3 or more insulin injections per day) of diabetes.
Without recognition of early warning symptoms, you may not be able to take steps to avoid more serious hypoglycemia. Be alert for all of the various types of symptoms that may indicate hypoglycemia. Patients who experience hypoglycemia without early warning symptoms should monitor their blood glucose frequently, especially prior to activities such as driving. If the blood glucose is below your normal fasting glucose, you should consider eating or drinking sugar-containing foods to treat your hypoglycemia.
Mild to moderate hypoglycemia may be treated by eating foods or taking drinks that contain sugar. Patients should always carry a quick source of sugar, such as candy mints or glucose tablets. More severe hypoglycemia may require the assistance of another person. Patients who are unable to take sugar orally or who are unconscious require an injection of glucagon or should be treated with intravenous administration of glucose at a medical facility.
You should learn to recognize your own symptoms of hypoglycemia. If you are uncertain about these symptoms, you should monitor your blood glucose frequently to help you learn to recognize the symptoms that you experience with hypoglycemia.
If you have frequent episodes of hypoglycemia or experience difficulty in recognizing the symptoms, you should consult your doctor to discuss possible changes in therapy, meal plans, and/or exercise programs to help you avoid hypoglycemia.

Hyperglycemia and Diabetic Acidosis
Hyperglycemia (too much glucose in the blood) may develop if your body has too little insulin. Hyperglycemia can be brought about by:
1. Omitting your insulin or taking less than the doctor has prescribed
2. Eating significantly more than your meal plan suggests
3. Developing a fever or infection

In patients with insulin-dependent diabetes, prolonged hyperglycemia can result in diabetic acidosis. The first symptoms of diabetic acidosis usually come on gradually, over a period of hours or days, and include a drowsy feeling, flushed face, thirst, loss of appetite, and fruity odor on the breath. With acidosis, urine tests show large amounts of glucose and acetone. Heavy breathing and a rapid pulse are more severe symptoms. If uncorrected, prolonged hyperglycemia or diabetic acidosis can result in loss of consciousness or death. Therefore, it is important that you obtain medical assistance immediately.

Lipodystrophy
Rarely, administration of insulin subcutaneously can result in lipoatrophy (depression in the skin) or lipohypertrophy (enlargement or thickening of tissue). If you notice either of these conditions, consult your doctor. A change in your injection technique may help alleviate the problem.

Allergy to Insulin
Local Allergy—Patients occasionally experience redness, swelling, and itching at the site of injection of insulin. This condition, called local allergy, usually clears up in a few days to a few weeks. In some instances, this condition may be related to factors other than insulin, such as irritants in the skin cleansing agent or poor injection technique. If you have local reactions, contact your doctor.
Systemic Allergy—Less common, but potentially more serious, is generalized allergy to insulin, which may cause rash over the whole body, shortness of breath, wheezing, reduction in blood pressure, fast pulse, or sweating. Severe cases of generalized allergy may be life threatening. If you think you are having a generalized allergic reaction to insulin, notify a doctor immediately.

ADDITIONAL INFORMATION
Additional information about diabetes may be obtained from your diabetes educator.
DIABETES FORECAST is a national magazine designed especially for patients with diabetes and their families and is available by subscription from the American Diabetes Association, National Service Center, 1660 Duke Street, Alexandria, Virginia 22314.
Another publication, **DIABETES COUNTDOWN**, is available from the Juvenile Diabetes Foundation International (JDF), 120 Wall Street, 19th Floor, New York, New York 10005-4001, 1-800-JDF-CURE (1-800-533-2873).
Literature revised August 13, 1999
PA 8517 AMP [081399]

REGULAR ILETIN® II — OTC

[*rĕg-ū-lĕr ī 'lĕ-tĭn*]
(Insulin Injection, USP, purified pork)

INFORMATION FOR THE PATIENT
WARNINGS
ANY CHANGE OF INSULIN SHOULD BE MADE CAUTIOUSLY AND ONLY UNDER MEDICAL SUPERVISION. CHANGES IN PURITY, STRENGTH, BRAND (MANUFACTURER), TYPE (REGULAR, NPH, LENTE®), SPECIES (BEEF, PORK, BEEF-PORK, HUMAN), AND/OR METHOD OF MANUFACTURE (RECOMBINANT DNA VERSUS ANIMAL-SOURCE INSULIN) MAY RESULT IN THE NEED FOR A CHANGE IN DOSAGE. IF AN ADJUSTMENT IS NEEDED, IT MAY OCCUR WITH THE FIRST DOSE OR DURING THE FIRST SEVERAL WEEKS OR MONTHS.

DIABETES
Insulin is a hormone produced by the pancreas, a large gland that lies near the stomach. This hormone is necessary for the body's correct use of food, especially sugar. Diabetes occurs when the pancreas does not make enough insulin to meet your body's needs.
To control your diabetes, your doctor has prescribed injections of insulin to keep your blood glucose at a nearly normal level. Proper control of your diabetes requires close and constant cooperation with your doctor. In spite of diabetes, you can lead an active, healthy, and useful life if you eat a balanced diet daily, exercise regularly, and take your insulin injections as prescribed.
You have been instructed to test your blood and/or your urine regularly for glucose. If your blood tests consistently show above- or below-normal glucose levels or your urine tests consistently show the presence of glucose, your diabetes is not properly controlled and you must let your doctor know.
Always keep an extra supply of insulin as well as a spare syringe and needle on hand. Always wear diabetic identification so that appropriate treatment can be given if complications occur away from home.

REGULAR PORK INSULIN

Description
Regular pork insulin is obtained from pork pancreas.
Regular Iletin® II (purified insulin, Lilly) consists of zinc-insulin crystals dissolved in a clear fluid. Regular Iletin II has had nothing added to change the speed or length of its action. It takes effect rapidly and has a relatively short duration of activity (4 to 12 hours) as compared with other insulins. The time course of action of any insulin may vary considerably in different individuals or at different times in the same individual. As with all insulin preparations, the duration of action of Regular Iletin II is dependent on dose, site of injection, blood supply, temperature, and physical activity. Regular Iletin II is a sterile solution and is for subcutaneous injection. It should not be used intramuscularly. The concentration of Regular Iletin II is 100 units/mL (U-100).

Identification
This insulin, manufactured by Eli Lilly and Company, has the trademark Iletin II and is available in various types—Regular, NPH, and Lente. Your doctor has prescribed the type of insulin that he/she believes is best for you. **DO NOT USE ANY OTHER INSULIN EXCEPT ON HIS/HER ADVICE AND DIRECTION.**

Continued on next page

*** Identi-Code® symbol. This product information was prepared in June 2000. Current information on these and other products of Eli Lilly and Company may be obtained by direct inquiry to Lilly Research Laboratories, Lilly Corporate Center, Indianapolis, Indiana 46285, (800) 545-5979.**

Regular Iletin II (Pork)—Cont.

Always check the carton and the bottle label for the name and letter designation of the insulin you receive from your pharmacy to make sure it is the same as that your doctor has prescribed.
Always examine the appearance of your bottle of insulin before withdrawing each dose. Regular Iletin II is a clear and colorless liquid with a water-like appearance and consistency. Do not use if it appears cloudy, thickened, or slightly colored or if solid particles are visible. Always check the appearance of your bottle of insulin before using, and if you note anything unusual in the appearance of your insulin or notice your insulin requirements changing markedly, consult your doctor.

Storage

Insulin should be stored in a refrigerator but not in the freezer. If refrigeration is not possible, the bottle of insulin that you are currently using can be kept unrefrigerated as long as it is kept as cool as possible (below 86°F [30°C]) and away from heat and light. Do not use insulin if it has been frozen. Do not use a bottle of insulin after the expiration date stamped on the label.

INJECTION PROCEDURES

Correct Syringe

Doses of insulin are measured in **units.** U-100 insulin contains 100 units/mL (1 mL=1 cc). With Regular Iletin II, it is important to use a syringe that is marked for U-100 insulin preparations. Failure to use the proper syringe can lead to a mistake in dosage, causing serious problems for you, such as a blood glucose level that is too low or too high.

Syringe Use

To help avoid contamination and possible infection, follow these instructions exactly.
Disposable syringes and needles should be used only once and then discarded.
NEEDLES AND SYRINGES MUST NOT BE SHARED.
Reusable syringes and needles must be sterilized before each injection. **Follow the package directions supplied with your syringe.** Described below are 2 methods of sterilizing.

Boiling

1. Put syringe, plunger, and needle in strainer, place in saucepan, and cover with water. Boil for 5 minutes.
2. Remove articles from water. When they have cooled, insert plunger into barrel, and fasten needle to syringe with a slight twist.
3. Push plunger in and out several times until water is completely removed.

Isopropyl Alcohol

If the syringe, plunger, and needle cannot be boiled, as when you are traveling, they may be sterilized by immersion for at least 5 minutes in Isopropyl Alcohol, 91%. Do not use bathing, rubbing, or medicated alcohol for this sterilization. If the syringe is sterilized with alcohol, it must be absolutely dry before use.

Preparing the Dose

1. Wash your hands.
2. Inspect the insulin. Regular Iletin II should look clear and colorless. Do not use Regular Iletin II if it appears cloudy, thickened, or slightly colored or if solid particles are visible.
3. If using a new bottle, flip off the plastic protective cap, but **do not** remove the stopper. When using a new bottle, wipe the top of the bottle with an alcohol swab.
4. If you are mixing insulins, refer to the Warnings below.
5. Draw air into the syringe equal to your insulin dose. Put the needle through rubber top of the insulin bottle and inject the air into the bottle.
6. Turn the bottle and syringe upside down. Hold the bottle and syringe firmly in 1 hand.
7. Making sure the tip of the needle is in the insulin, withdraw the correct dose of insulin into the syringe.
8. Before removing the needle from the bottle, check your syringe for air bubbles which reduce the amount of insulin in it. If bubbles are present, hold the syringe straight up and tap its side until the bubbles float to the top. Push them out with the plunger and withdraw the correct dose.
9. Remove the needle from the bottle and lay the syringe down so that the needle does not touch anything.

WARNINGS—SEE ADDITIONAL WARNINGS ABOVE

Patients who have been directed by their doctors to mix 2 types of insulin should be aware that insulin hypodermic syringes of different manufacturers may vary in the amount of space between the bottom line and the needle.
Because of this, do not change:
1. The order of mixing that the doctor has prescribed or
2. The model and brand of syringe or needle without first consulting your doctor.

The mixing should be done immediately prior to injection. Failure to heed this warning could result in a dosage error.

Injection

Cleanse the skin with alcohol where the injection is to be made. Stabilize the skin by spreading it or pinching up a large area. Insert the needle as instructed by your doctor. Push the plunger in as far as it will go. Pull the needle out and apply gentle pressure over the injection site for several seconds. **Do not rub the area.** To avoid tissue damage, give the next injection at a site at least $^1/_2$" from the previous site.

DOSAGE

Your doctor has told you which insulin to use, how much, and when and how often to inject it. Because each patient's case of diabetes is different, this schedule has been individualized for you.
Your usual insulin dose may be affected by changes in your food, activity, or work schedule. Carefully follow your doctor's instructions to allow for these changes. Other things that may affect your insulin dose are:

Illness

Illness, especially with nausea and vomiting, may cause your insulin requirements to change. Even if you are not eating, you will still require insulin. You and your doctor should establish a sick day plan for you to use in case of illness. When you are sick, test your blood/urine frequently and call your doctor as instructed.

Pregnancy

Good control of diabetes is especially important for you and your unborn baby. Pregnancy may make managing your diabetes more difficult. If you are planning to have a baby, are pregnant, or are nursing a baby, consult your doctor.

Medication

Insulin requirements may be increased if you are taking other drugs with hyperglycemic activity, such as oral contraceptives, corticosteroids, or thyroid replacement therapy. Insulin requirements may be reduced in the presence of drugs with hypoglycemic activity, such as oral hypoglycemics, salicylates (for example, aspirin), sulfa antibiotics, and certain antidepressants. Always discuss any medications you are taking with your doctor.

Exercise

Exercise may lower your body's need for insulin during and for some time after the activity. Exercise may also speed up the effect of an insulin dose, especially if the exercise involves the area of injection site (for example, the leg should not be used for injection just prior to running). Discuss with your doctor how you should adjust your regimen to accommodate exercise.

Travel

Persons traveling across more than 2 time zones should consult their doctor concerning adjustments in their insulin schedule.

COMMON PROBLEMS OF DIABETES

Hypoglycemia (Insulin Reaction)

Hypoglycemia (too little glucose in the blood) is one of the most frequent adverse events experienced by insulin users. It can be brought about by:
1. Taking too much insulin
2. Missing or delaying meals
3. Exercising or working more than usual
4. An infection or illness (especially with diarrhea or vomiting)
5. A change in the body's need for insulin
6. Diseases of the adrenal, pituitary, or thyroid gland, or progression of kidney or liver disease
7. Interactions with other drugs that lower blood glucose, such as oral hypoglycemics, salicylates (for example, aspirin), sulfa antibiotics, and certain antidepressants
8. Consumption of alcoholic beverages

Symptoms of mild to moderate hypoglycemia may occur suddenly and can include:
- sweating
- dizziness
- palpitation
- tremor
- hunger
- restlessness
- tingling in the hands, feet, lips, or tongue
- lightheadedness
- inability to concentrate
- headache
- drowsiness
- sleep disturbances
- anxiety
- blurred vision
- slurred speech
- depressive mood
- irritability
- abnormal behavior
- unsteady movement
- personality changes

Signs of severe hypoglycemia can include:
- disorientation
- unconsciousness
- seizures
- death

Therefore, it is important that assistance be obtained immediately.
Early warning symptoms of hypoglycemia may be different or less pronounced under certain conditions, such as long duration of diabetes, diabetic nerve disease, medications such as beta-blockers, change in insulin preparations, or intensified control (3 or more insulin injections per day) of diabetes.
Without recognition of early warning symptoms, you may not be able to take steps to avoid more serious hypoglycemia. Be alert for all of the various types of symptoms that may indicate hypoglycemia. Patients who experience hypoglycemia without early warning symptoms should monitor their blood glucose frequently, especially prior to activities such as driving. If the blood glucose is below your normal fasting glucose, you should consider eating or drinking sugar-containing foods to treat your hypoglycemia.
Mild to moderate hypoglycemia may be treated by eating foods or taking drinks that contain sugar. Patients should always carry a quick source of sugar, such as candy mints or glucose tablets. More severe hypoglycemia may require the assistance of another person. Patients who are unable to take sugar orally or who are unconscious require an injection of glucagon or should be treated with intravenous administration of glucose at a medical facility.
You should learn to recognize your own symptoms of hypoglycemia. If you are uncertain about these symptoms, you should monitor your blood glucose frequently to help you learn to recognize the symptoms that you experience with hypoglycemia.
If you have frequent episodes of hypoglycemia or experience difficulty in recognizing the symptoms, you should consult your doctor to discuss possible changes in therapy, meal plans, and/or exercise programs to help you avoid hypoglycemia.

Hyperglycemia and Diabetic Acidosis

Hyperglycemia (too much glucose in the blood) may develop if your body has too little insulin. Hyperglycemia can be brought about by:
1. Omitting your insulin or taking less than the doctor has prescribed
2. Eating significantly more than your meal plan suggests
3. Developing a fever or infection

In patients with insulin-dependent diabetes, prolonged hyperglycemia can result in diabetic acidosis. The first symptoms of diabetic acidosis usually come on gradually, over a period of hours or days, and include a drowsy feeling, flushed face, thirst, loss of appetite, and fruity odor on the breath. With acidosis, urine tests show large amounts of glucose and acetone. Heavy breathing and a rapid pulse are more severe symptoms. If uncorrected, prolonged hyperglycemia or diabetic acidosis can result in loss of consciousness or death. Therefore, it is important that you obtain medical assistance immediately.

Lipodystrophy

Rarely, administration of insulin subcutaneously can result in lipoatrophy (depression in the skin) or lipohypertrophy (enlargement or thickening of tissue). If you notice either of these conditions, consult your doctor. A change in your injection technique may help alleviate the problem.

Allergy to Insulin

Local Allergy —Patients occasionally experience redness, swelling, and itching at the site of injection of insulin. This condition, called local allergy, usually clears up in a few days to a few weeks. In some instances, this condition may be related to factors other than insulin, such as irritants in the skin cleansing agent or poor injection technique. If you have local reactions, contact your doctor.
Systemic Allergy —Less common, but potentially more serious, is generalized allergy to insulin, which may cause rash over the whole body, shortness of breath, wheezing, reduction in blood pressure, fast pulse, or sweating. Severe cases of generalized allergy may be life threatening. If you think you are having a generalized allergic reaction to insulin, notify a doctor immediately.

ADDITIONAL INFORMATION

Additional information about diabetes may be obtained from your diabetes educator.
DIABETES FORECAST is a national magazine designed especially for patients with diabetes and their families and is available by subscription from the American Diabetes Association, National Service Center, 1660 Duke Street, Alexandria, Virginia 22314.
Another publication, **DIABETES COUNTDOWN,** is available from the Juvenile Diabetes Foundation International (JDF), 120 Wall Street, 19th Floor, New York, New York 10005–4001.
Literature revised October 28, 1992
PA 8486 AMP [102892]

KEFUROX® ℞

[*kĕf 'yū-rōeks*]
(cefuroxime for injection, USP)

DESCRIPTION

Cefuroxime is a semisynthetic, broad spectrum cephalosporin antibiotic for intravenous administration. It is the sodium salt of (6R,7R)3-carbamoyloxymethyl-7-[Z-2-methoxyimino-2-(fur-2-yl)acetamido]ceph-3-em-4-carboxylate, and it has the following structural formula:

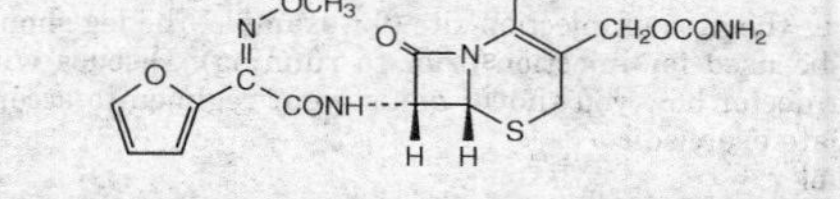

The chemical formula is $C_{16}H_{15}N_4NaO_8S$, and the molecular weight is 446.37.
Kefurox contains approximately 54.2 mg (2.4 mEq) of sodium per gram of cefuroxime activity.
Kefurox in sterile crystalline form is supplied in vials equivalent to 750 mg, 1.5 g, or 7.5 g of cefuroxime as cefuroxime sodium. Solutions of Kefurox range in color from light yellow to amber, depending on the concentration and diluent used. The pH of freshly constituted solutions usually ranges from 4.5–8.5.

CLINICAL PHARMACOLOGY

Following IV doses of 750 mg and 1.5 g, serum concentrations were approximately 50 and 100 mcg/mL, respectively, at 15 minutes. Therapeutic serum concentrations of approximately 2 mcg/mL or more were maintained for 5.3 hours and 8 hours or more, respectively. There was no evidence of accumulation of cefuroxime in the serum following IV administration of 1.5-g doses every 8 hours to normal volunteers. The serum half-life after IV injections is approximately 80 minutes.

Approximately 89% of a dose of cefuroxime is excreted by the kidneys over an 8-hour period, resulting in high urinary concentrations.

Intravenous doses of 750 mg and 1.5 g produced urinary levels averaging 1,150 and 2,500 mcg/mL, respectively, during the first 8-hour period.

The concomitant oral administration of probenecid with cefuroxime slows tubular secretion, decreases renal clearance by approximately 40%, increases the peak serum level by approximately 30%, and increases the serum half-life by approximately 30%. Cefuroxime is detectable in therapeutic concentrations in pleural fluid, joint fluid, bile, sputum, bone, cerebrospinal fluid (in patients with meningitis), and aqueous humor.

Cefuroxime is approximately 50% bound to serum protein.

Microbiology: Cefuroxime has *in vitro* activity against a wide range of gram-positive and gram-negative organisms, and it is highly stable in the presence of beta-lactamases of certain gram-negative bacteria. The bactericidal action of cefuroxime results from inhibition of cell-wall synthesis.

Cefuroxime is usually active against the following organisms *in vitro*.

Aerobes, Gram-positive: *Staphylococcus aureus; Staphylococcus epidermidis; Streptococcus pneumoniae;* and *Streptococcus pyogenes* (and other streptococci).

NOTE: Most strains of enterococci, e.g., *Enterococcus faecalis* (formerly *Streptococcus faecalis*), are resistant to cefuroxime. Methicillin-resistant staphylococci and *Listeria monocytogenes* are resistant to cefuroxime.

Aerobes, Gram-negative: *Citrobacter* spp; *Enterobacter* spp.; *Escherichia coli; Haemophilus influenzae* (including ampicillin-resistant strains); *Haemophilus parainfluenzae; Klebsiella* spp. (including *Klebsiella pneumoniae); Moraxella (Branhamella) catarrhalis* (including ampicillin- and cephalothin-resistant strains); *Morganella morganii* (formerly *Proteus morganii*); *Neisseria gonorrhoeae* (including penicillinase- and non-penicillinase-producing strains); *Neisseria meningitidis; Proteus mirabilis; Providencia rettgeri* (formerly *Proteus rettgeri*); *Salmonella* spp.; and *Shigella* spp.

NOTE: Some strains of *Morganella morganii, Enterobacter cloacae,* and *Citrobacter* spp. have been shown by *in vitro* tests to be resistant to cefuroxime and other cephalosporins. *Pseudomonas* and *Campylobacter* spp., *Acinetobacter calcoaceticus,* and most strains of *Serratia* spp. and *Proteus vulgaris* are resistant to most first- and second-generation cephalosporins.

Anaerobes: Gram-positive and gram-negative cocci (including *Peptococcus* and *Peptostreptococcus* spp); gram-positive bacilli (including *Clostridium* spp); gram-negative bacilli (including *Bacteroides* and *Fusobacterium* spp).

NOTE: *Clostridium difficile* and most strains of *Bacteroides fragilis* are resistant to cefuroxime.

Susceptibility Tests: ***Diffusion Techniques:*** Quantitative methods that require measurement of zone diameters give an estimate of antibiotic susceptibility. One such standard procedure[1] that has been recommended for use with disks to test susceptibility of organisms to cefuroxime uses the 30-mcg cefuroxime disk. Interpretation involves the correlation of the diameters obtained in the disk test with minimum inhibitory concentration (MIC) for cefuroxime.

A report of "Susceptible" indicates that the pathogen is likely to be inhibited by generally achievable blood levels. A report of "Moderately Susceptible" suggests that the organism would be susceptible if high dosage is used or if the infection is confined to tissues and fluids in which high antibiotic levels are attained. A report of "Intermediate" suggests an equivocable or indeterminate result. A report of "Resistant" indicates that achievable concentrations of the antibiotic are unlikely to be inhibitory and other therapy should be selected.

Reports from the laboratory giving results of the standard single-disk susceptibility test for organisms other than *Haemophilus* spp. and *Neisseria gonorrhoeae* with a 30-mcg cefuroxime disk should be interpreted according to the following criteria:

Zone Diameter (mm)	Interpretation
≥ 18	(S) Susceptible
15-17	(MS) Moderately Susceptible
≤ 14	(R) Resistant

Results for *Haemophilus* spp. should be interpreted according to the following criteria:

Zone Diameter (mm)	Interpretation
≥ 24	(S) Susceptible
21-23	(I) Intermediate
≤ 20	(R) Resistant

Results for *Neisseria gonorrhoeae* should be interpreted according to the following criteria:

Zone Diameter (mm)	Interpretation
≥ 31	(S) Susceptible
26-30	(MS) Moderately Susceptible
≤ 25	(R) Resistant

Organisms should be tested with the cefuroxime disk since cefuroxime has been shown by *in vitro* tests to be active against certain strains found resistant when other beta-lactam disks are used. The cefuroxime disk should not be used for testing susceptibility to other cephalosporins.

Standardized procedures require the use of laboratory control organisms. The 30-mcg cefuroxime disk should give the following zone diameters

1. Testing for organisms other than *Haemophilus* ssp. and *Neisseria gonorrhoeae:*

Organism	Zone Diameter (mm)
Staphylococcus aureus ATCC 25923	27-35
Escherichia coli ATCC 25922	20-26

2. Testing for *Haemophilus* spp.:

Organism	Zone Diameter (mm)
Haemophilus influenzae ATCC 49766	28-36

3. Testing for *Neisseria gonorrhoeae:*

Organism	Zone Diameter (mm)
Neisseria gonorrhoeae ATCC 49226	33-41
Staphylococcus aureus ATCC 25923	29-33

Dilution Techniques: Use a standardized dilution method[1] (broth, agar, microdilution) or equivalent with cefuroxime powder. The MIC values obtained for bacterial isolates other than *Haemophilus* spp. and *Neisseria gonorrhoeae* should be interpreted according to the following criteria:

MIC (mcg/mL)	Interpretation
≤ 8	(S) Susceptible
16	(MS) Moderately Susceptible
≥ 32	(R) Resistant

MIC values obtained for *Haemophilus* spp. should be interpreted according to the following criteria:

MIC (mcg/mL)	Interpretation
≤ 4	(S) Susceptible
8	(I) Intermediate
≥ 16	(R) Resistant

MIC values obtained for *Neisseria gonorrhoeae* should be interpreted according to the following criteria:

MIC (mcg/mL)	Interpretation
≤ 1	(S) Susceptible
2	(MS) Moderately Susceptible
≥ 4	(R) Resistant

As with standard diffusion techniques, dilution methods require the use of laboratory control organisms. Standard cefuroxime powder should provide the following MIC values.

1. For organisms other than *Haemophilus* spp. and *Neisseria gonorrhoeae:*

Organism	MIC (mcg/mL)
Staphylococcus aureus ATCC 29213	0.5-2.0
Escherichia coli ATCC 25922	2.0-8.0

2. For *Haemophilus* spp.:

Organism	MIC (mcg/mL)
Haemophilus influenzae ATCC 49766	0.25-1.0

3. For *Neisseria gonorrhoeae*:

Organism	MIC (mcg/mL)
Neisseria gonorrhoeae ATCC 49226	0.25-1.0
Staphylococcus aureus ATCC 29213	0.25-1.0

INDICATIONS AND USAGE

Kefurox is indicated for the treatment of patients with infections caused by susceptible strains of the designated organisms in the following diseases:

1. **Lower Respiratory Tract Infections**, including pneumonia, caused by *Streptococcus pneumoniae, Haemophilus influenzae* (including ampicillin-resistant strains), *Klebsiella* spp., *Staphylococcus aureus* (penicillinase- and non-penicillinase-producing strains), *Streptococcus pyogenes*, and *Escherichia coli.*
2. **Urinary Tract Infections** caused by *Escherichia coli* and *Klebsiella* spp.
3. **Skin and Skin Structure Infections** caused by *Staphylococcus aureus* (penicillinase- and non-penicillinase-producing strains), *Streptococcus pyogenes, Escherichia coli, Klebsiella* spp., and *Enterobacter* spp.
4. **Septicemia** caused by *Staphylococcus aureus* (penicillinase- and non-penicillinase-producing strains), *Streptococcus pneumoniae, Escherichia coli, Haemophilus influenzae* (including ampicillin-resistant strains), and *Klebsiella* spp.
5. **Meningitis** caused by *Streptococcus pneumoniae, Haemophilus influenzae* (including ampicillin-resistant strains), *Neisseria meningitidis*, and *Staphylococcus aureus* (penicillinase- and non-penicillinase-producing strains) (See PRECAUTIONS).
6. **Gonorrhea**—Uncomplicated and disseminated gonococcal infections due to *Neisseria gonorrhoeae* (penicillinase- and non-penicillinase-producing strains) in both males and females.
7. **Bone and Joint Infections** caused by *Staphylococcus aureus* (penicillinase- and non-penicillinase-producing strains).

Clinical microbiological studies in skin and skin structure infections frequently reveal the growth of susceptible strains of both aerobic and anaerobic organisms. Kefurox has been used successfully in these mixed infections in which several organisms have been isolated. Appropriate cultures and susceptibility studies should be performed to determine the susceptibility of the causative organisms to Kefurox (cefuroxime for injection).

Therapy may be started while awaiting the results of these studies; however, once these results become available, the antibiotic treatment should be adjusted accordingly. In certain cases of confirmed or suspected gram-positive or gram-negative sepsis or in patients with other serious infections in which the causative organism has not been identified, Kefurox may be used concomitantly with an aminoglycoside (*see* PRECAUTIONS). The recommended doses of both antibiotics may be given depending on the severity of the infection and the patient's condition.

Prevention: The preoperative prophylactic administration of Kefurox may prevent the growth of susceptible disease-causing bacteria and, thereby may reduce the incidence of certain postoperative infections in patients undergoing surgical procedures (e.g., vaginal hysterectomy) that are classified as clean-contaminated or potentially contaminated procedures. Effective prophylactic use of antibiotics in surgery depends on the time of administration. Kefurox should usually be given one-half to 1 hour before the operation to allow sufficient time to achieve effective antibiotic concentrations in the wound tissues during the procedure. The dose should be repeated intraoperatively if the surgical procedure is lengthy.

Prophylactic administration is usually not required after the surgical procedure ends and should be stopped within 24 hours. In the majority of surgical procedures, continuing prophylactic administration of any antibiotic does not reduce the incidence of subsequent infections but will increase the possibility of adverse reactions and the development of bacterial resistance.

The perioperative use of Kefurox has also been effective during open heart surgery for surgical patients in whom infections at the operative site would present a serious risk. For these patients, it is recommended that Kefurox therapy be continued for at least 48 hours after the surgical procedure ends. If an infection is present, specimens for culture should be obtained for the identification of the causative organism, and appropriate antimicrobial therapy should be instituted.

CONTRAINDICATIONS

Kefurox is contraindicated in patients with known allergy to the cephalosporin group of antibiotics.

WARNINGS

BEFORE THERAPY WITH KEFUROX IS INSTITUTED, CAREFUL INQUIRY SHOULD BE MADE TO DETERMINE WHETHER THE PATIENT HAS HAD PREVIOUS HYPERSENSITIVITY REACTIONS TO CEPHALOSPORINS, PENICILLINS, OR OTHER DRUGS. THIS PRODUCT SHOULD BE GIVEN CAUTIOUSLY TO PENICILLIN-SENSITIVE PATIENTS. ANTIBIOTICS SHOULD BE ADMINISTERED WITH CAUTION TO ANY PATIENT WHO HAS DEMONSTRATED SOME FORM OF ALLERGY, PARTICULARLY TO DRUGS. IF AN ALLERGIC REACTION TO KEFUROX (CEFUROXIME FOR INJECTION) OCCURS, DISCONTINUE THE DRUG. SERIOUS ACUTE HYPERSENSITIVITY REACTIONS MAY REQUIRE EPINEPHRINE AND OTHER EMERGENCY MEASURES.

Pseudomembranous colitis has been reported with the use of cephalosporins (and other broad-spectrum antibiotics); therefore, it is important to consider its diagnosis in patients who develop diarrhea in association with antibiotic use.

Treatment with broad-spectrum antibiotics alters the normal flora of the colon and may permit overgrowth of clostridia. Studies indicate a toxin produced by *Clostridium difficile* is one primary cause of antibiotic-associated colitis. Cholestyramine and colestipol resins have been shown to bind the toxin *in vitro*.

Mild cases of colitis may respond to drug discontinuation alone. Moderate to severe cases should be managed with fluid, electrolyte, and protein supplementation as indicated. When the colitis is not relieved by drug discontinuation or when it is severe, oral vancomycin is the treatment of choice for antibiotic-associated pseudomembranous colitis produced by *Clostridium difficile.* Other causes of colitis should also be considered.

PRECAUTIONS

General: Although Kefurox rarely produces alterations in kidney function, evaluation of renal status during therapy is recommended, especially in seriously ill patients receiv-

Continued on next page

*** Identi-Code® symbol. This product information was prepared in June 2000. Current information on these and other products of Eli Lilly and Company may be obtained by direct inquiry to Lilly Research Laboratories, Lilly Corporate Center, Indianapolis, Indiana 46285, (800) 545-5979.**

Kefurox—Cont.

ing the maximum doses. Cephalosporins should be given with caution to patients receiving concurrent treatment with potent diuretics as these regimens are suspected of adversely affecting renal function.
The total daily dose of Kefurox should be reduced in patients with transient or persistent renal insufficiency (*see* DOSAGE AND ADMINISTRATION), because high and prolonged serum antibiotic concentrations can occur in such individuals from usual doses.
As with other antibiotics, prolonged use of Kefurox may result in overgrowth of nonsusceptible organisms. Careful observation of the patient is essential. If superinfection occurs during therapy, appropriate measures should be taken.
Broad-spectrum antibiotics should be prescribed with caution in individuals with a history of gastrointestinal disease, particularly colitis.
Nephrotoxicity has been reported following concomitant administration of aminoglycoside antibiotics and cephalosporins.
As with other therapeutic regimens used in the treatment of meningitis, mild-to-moderate hearing loss has been reported in some pediatric patients treated with cefuroxime sodium. Persistence of positive CSF (cerebrospinal fluid) cultures at 18 to 36 hours, particularly in patients with *Haemophilus influenzae* isolates, has also been noted; however, the precise clinical impact of this is unknown.
Drug/Laboratory Test Interactions: A false-positive reaction for glucose in the urine may occur with copper reduction tests (Benedict's or Fehling's solution or with Clintest® tablets) but not with enzyme-based tests for glycosuria (e.g., Tes-Tape®, Glucose Enzymatic Test Strips, USP). As a false-negative result may occur in the ferricyanide test, it is recommended that either the glucose oxidase or hexokinase method be used to determine blood plasma glucose levels in patients receiving Kefurox.
Cefuroxime does not interfere with the assay of serum and urine creatinine by the the alkaline picrate method.
Carcinogenesis, Mutagenesis, and Impairment of Fertility: Although no long-term studies in animals have been performed to evaluate carcinogenic potential, no mutagenic potential of cefuroxime was found in standard laboratory tests.
Reproductive studies revealed no impairment of fertility in animals.
Pregnancy: Teratogenic Effects: Pregnancy Category B—Reproduction studies have been performed in mice and rabbits at doses up to 60 times the human dose and have revealed no evidence of impaired fertility or harm to the fetus due to cefuroxime. There are, however, no adequate well-controlled studies in pregnant women. Because animal reproduction studies are not always predictive of human response, this drug should be used during pregnancy only if clearly needed.
Nursing Mothers: Since Kefurox is excreted in human milk, caution should be exercised when Kefurox is administered to a nursing woman.
Pediatric Use: Safety and effectiveness in pediatric patients below the age of 3 months have not been established. Accumulation of other members of the cephalosporin class in newborn infants (with resulting prolongation of drug half-life) has been reported.

ADVERSE REACTIONS

Kefurox is generally well tolerated. The most common adverse effects have been local reactions following IV administration. Other adverse reactions have been encountered only rarely.
Local Reactions—Thrombophlebitis has occurred with IV administration in 1 in 60 patients.
Gastrointestinal—Gastrointestinal symptoms occurred in 1 in 150 patients and included diarrhea (1 in 220 patients) and nausea (1 in 440 patients). Onset of pseudomembranous colitis symptoms may occur during or after antibiotic treatment. (see WARNINGS).
Hypersensitivity Reactions—Hypersensitivity reactions have been reported in fewer than 1% of the patients treated with Kefurox and include rash (1 in 125). Pruritus, urticaria and positive Coombs' test each occurred in less than 1 in 250 patients, and, as with other cephalosporins, rare cases of anaphylaxis, drug fever, erythema multiforme, toxic epidermal necrolysis, and Stevens-Johnson syndrome have occurred.
Blood—A decrease in hemoglobin and hematocrit has been observed in 1 in 10 patients and transient eosinophilia in 1 in 14 patients. Less common reactions seen were transient neutropenia (fewer than 1 in 100 patients) and leukopenia (1 in 750 patients). A similar pattern and incidence were seen with other cephalosporins used in controlled studies. As with other cephalosporins, there have been rare reports of thrombocytopenia.
Hepatic—Transient rise in AST (SGOT) and ALT (SGPT) (1 in 25 patients), alkaline phosphatase (1 in 50 patients), LDH (1 in 75 patients), and bilirubin (1 in 500 patients) levels has been noted.
Kidney—Elevations in serum creatinine and/or blood urea nitrogen and a decreased creatinine clearance have been observed, but their relationship to cefuroxime is unknown.
In addition to the adverse reactions listed above that have been observed in patients treated with cefuroxime, the following adverse reactions and altered laboratory tests have been reported for cephalosporin-class antibiotics:
Adverse Reactions: Vomiting, abdominal pain, colitis, vaginitis including vaginal candidiasis, toxic nephropathy, hepatic dysfunction including cholestasis, aplastic anemia, hemolytic anemia, hemorrhage.
Several cephalosporins have been implicated in triggering seizures, particularly in patients with renal impairment when the dosage was not reduced (see DOSAGE AND ADMINISTRATION). If seizures associated with drug therapy should occur, the drug should be discontinued. Anticonvulsant therapy can be given if clinically indicated.
Altered Laboratory Tests: Prolonged prothrombin time, pancytopenia, agranulocytosis.

OVERDOSAGE

Overdosage of cephalosporins can cause cerebral irritation leading to convulsions. Serum levels of cefuroxime can be reduced by hemodialysis and peritoneal dialysis.

DOSAGE AND ADMINISTRATION

DOSAGE: Adults—The usual adult dosage range for Kefurox (cefuroxime for injection) is 750 mg to 1.5 grams every 8 hours, usually for 5 to 10 days. In uncomplicated urinary tract infections, skin and skin structure infections, disseminated gonococcal infections, and uncomplicated pneumonia, a 750-mg dose every 8 hours is recommended. In severe or complicated infections, a 1.5-gram dose every 8 hours is recommended.
In bone and joint infections, a 1.5 gram dose every 8 hours is recommended. In clinical trials, surgical intervention was performed when indicated as an adjunct to Kefurox therapy. A course of oral antibiotics was administered when appropriate following the completion of parenteral administration of Kefurox.
In life-threatening infections or infections due to less susceptible organisms, 1.5 grams every 6 hours may be required. In bacterial meningitis, the dose should not exceed 3 grams every 8 hours. For preventive use for clean-contaminated or potentially contaminated surgical procedures, a 1.5-gram dose administered intravenously just before surgery (approximately one-half to 1 hour before the initial incision) is recommended. Thereafter, give 750 mg intravenously every 8 hours when the procedure is prolonged. For preventive use during open heart surgery, a 1.5-gram dose administered intravenously at the induction of anesthesia and every 12 hours thereafter for a total of 6 grams is recommended.
Impaired Renal Function— A reduced dosage must be employed when renal function is impaired. Dosage should be determined by the degree of renal impairment and the susceptibility of the causative organism (see Table 1).

TABLE 1: Dosage of Kefurox in Adults With Reduced Renal Function

Creatinine Clearance (mL/min)	Dose	Frequency
>20	750 mg–1.5 g	q8h
10–20	750 mg	q12h
<10	750 mg	q24h*

* Since Kefurox is dialyzable, patients on hemodialysis should be given a further dose at the end of the dialysis.

When only serum creatinine is available, the following formula[2] (based on sex, weight, and age of the patient) may be used to convert this value into creatinine clearance. The serum creatinine should represent a steady state of renal function.

$$\text{Males: Creatinine Clearance (mL/min)} = \frac{\text{Weight (kg)} \times (140 - \text{age})}{72 \times \text{serum creatinine (mg/dL)}}$$

Females: 0.85 × male value

Note: As with antibiotic therapy in general, administration of Kefurox should be continued for a minimum of 48 to 72 hours after the patient becomes asymptomatic or after evidence of bacterial eradication has been obtained; a minimum of 10 days of treatment is recommended in infections caused by *Streptococcus pyogenes* in order to guard against the risk of rheumatic fever or glomerulonephritis; frequent bacteriologic and clinical appraisal is necessary during therapy of chronic urinary tract infection and may be required for several months after therapy has been completed; persistent infections may require treatment for several weeks; and doses smaller than those indicated above should not be used. In staphylococcal and other infections involving a collection of pus, surgical drainage should be carried out where indicated.
Infants and Children Above 3 Months of Age—Administration of 50 to 100 mg/kg/day in equally divided doses, every 6 to 8 hours, has been successful for most infections susceptible to cefuroxime. The higher dosage of 100 mg/kg/day (not to exceed the maximum adult dosage) should be used for the more severe or serious infections.
In bone and joint infections, 150 mg/kg per day (not to exceed the maximum adult dose) is recommended in equally divided doses every 8 hours. In clinical trials, a course of oral antibiotics was administered to children following the completion of parenteral administration of Kefurox.
In cases of bacterial meningitis, a larger dosage of Kefurox is recommended, 200 to 240 mg/kg per day intravenously in divided doses every 6 to 8 hours.
In children with renal insufficiency, the frequency of dosing should be modified to be consistent with the recommendations for adults.
Preparation of Solution: The directions for preparing Kefurox (cefuroxime for injection) for IV use is summarized in Table 2.
For Intravenous Use: Each 750-mg vial/10-mL should be constituted with 7 mL of sterile water for injection. Withdraw completely the resulting solution for injection.
Each 1.5-g vial should be constituted with 14 mL of sterile water for injection, and the solution should be completely withdrawn for injection.
[See table 2 below]
Administration: After constitution, Kefurox may be given intravenously.
Intravenous Administration—The IV route may be preferable for patients with bacterial septicemia or other severe or life-threatening infections or for patients who may be poor risks because of lowered resistance, particularly if shock is present or impending.
For Direct Intermittent IV Administration—Slowly inject the solution into a vein over a period of 3 to 5 minutes or give it through the tubing system by which the patient is also receiving IV solutions.
For Intermittent IV Infusion with a Y-Type Administration Set—Dosing can be accomplished through the tubing system by which the patient may be receiving other IV solutions.
However, during infusion of the solution containing Kefurox, it is advisable to temporarily discontinue administration of any other solutions at the same site.
ADD-Vantage® vials are to be constituted only with 50 or 100 mL of 5% dextrose injection, 0.9% sodium chloride injection, or 0.45% sodium chloride injection in Abbott ADD-Vantage flexible diluent containers (see Instructions for Constitution). ADD-Vantage vials that have been joined to Abbott ADD-Vantage diluent containers and activated to dissolve the drug are stable for 24 hours at room temperature or for 7 days under refrigeration. Joined vials that have not been activated may be used within a 14-day period; this period corresponds to that for use of Abbott ADD-Vantage containers following removal of the outer packaging (overwrap).
Freezing solutions of Kefurox in the ADD-Vantage system is not recommended.

DIRECTIONS FOR USE OF KEFUROX (cefuroxime for injection) IN ADD-VANTAGE® VIALS

To Open Diluent Container:
Peel overwrap at corner and remove solution container. Some opacity of the plastic due to moisture absorption during the sterilization process may be observed. This is normal and does not affect the solution quality or safety. The opacity will diminish gradually.

To Assemble Vial and Flexible Diluent Container: (Use Aseptic Technique)

1. Remove the protective covers from the top of the vial and the vial port on the diluent container as follows:
   a. To remove the breakaway vial cap, swing the pull ring over the top of the vial and pull down far enough to

TABLE 2: Preparation of Solution

Strength	Amount of Diluent to Be Added (mL)	Volume to Be Withdrawn (mL)	Approximate Concentration (mg/mL)
750 mg/10 mL vial	7 (IV)	Total	100
1.5 g/20 mL vial	14 (IV)	Total	100
750 mg/100 mL bottle	50 (IV)	—	15
750 mg/100 mL bottle	100 (IV)	—	7.5
1.5 g/100 mL bottle	50 (IV)	—	30
1.5 g/100 mL bottle	100 (IV)	—	15
750 mg/ADD-Vantage	50 (IV)	—	15
750 mg/ADD-Vantage	100 (IV)	—	7.5
1.5 g/ADD-Vantage	50 (IV)	—	30
1.5 g/ADD-Vantage	100 (IV)	—	15

start the opening (SEE FIGURE 1), then pull straight up to remove the cap. (SEE FIGURE 2.)

NOTE: Do not access vial with syringe.

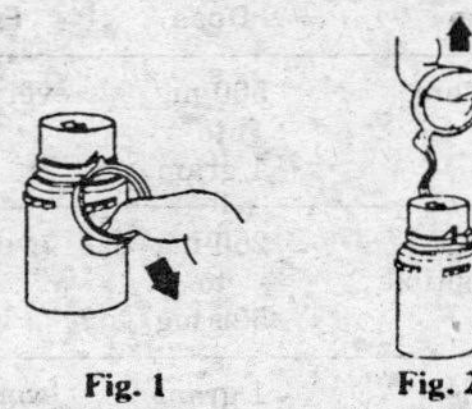

Fig. 1 Fig. 2

b. To remove the vial port cover, grasp the tab on the pull ring, pull up to break the 3 tie strings, then pull back to remove the cover. (SEE FIGURE 3.)

2. Screw the vial into the vial port until it will go no further. THE VIAL MUST BE SCREWED IN TIGHTLY TO ASSURE A SEAL. This occurs approximately ½ turn (180°) after the first audible click. (SEE FIGURE 4.) The clicking sound does not assure a seal; the vial must be turned as far as it will go.

   NOTE: Once vial is sealed, do not attempt to remove. (SEE FIGURE 4.)
3. Recheck the vial to assure that it is tight by trying to turn it further in the direction of assembly.
4. Label appropriately

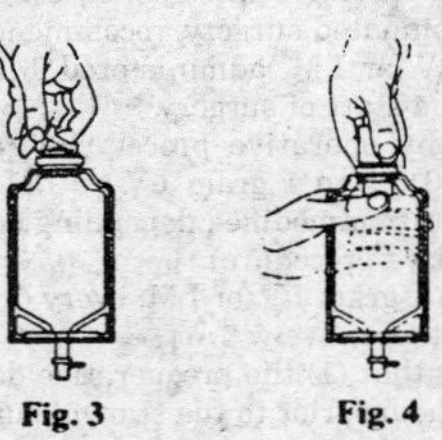

Fig. 3 Fig. 4

To Reconstitute the Drug:

1. Squeeze the bottom of the diluent container gently to inflate the portion of container surrounding the end of the drug vial.
2. With the other hand, push the drug vial down into the container telescoping the walls of the container. Grasp the inner cap of the vial through the walls of the container. (SEE FIGURE 5.)
3. Pull the inner cap from the drug vial. (SEE FIGURE 6.) Verify that the rubber stopper has been pulled out, allowing the drug and diluent to mix.
4. Mix container contents throroughly and use within the specified time.

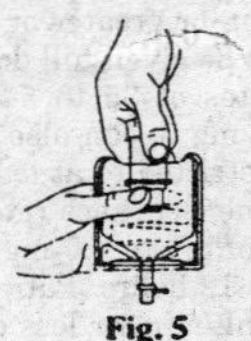

Fig. 5

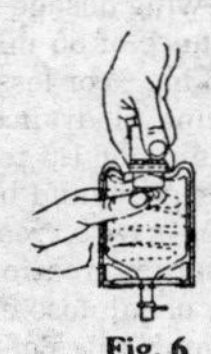

Fig. 6

For Continuous IV Infusion —A solution of Kefurox may be added to an IV bottle containing one of the following fluids: 0.9% sodium chloride injection, 5% dextrose injection, 10% dextrose injection, 5% dextrose and 0.9% sodium chloride injection, 5% dextrose and 0.45% sodium chloride injection, or 1/6 M sodium lactate injection

Solutions of Kefurox, like those of most beta-lactam antibiotics, should not be added to solutions of aminoglycoside antibiotics because of potential interaction.

However, if concurrent therapy with Kefurox (cefuroxime for injection) and an aminoglycoside is indicated, each of these antibiotics can be administered separately to the same patient.

Compatibility and Stability —Intravenous—When the 750-mg and 1.5-g vials are constituted as directed with sterile water for injection, the Kefurox solutions for IV administration maintain satisfactory potency for 24 hours at room temperature and for 48 hours (750-mg and 1.5-g vials under refrigeration (5°C). More dilute solutions, such as 750 mg or 1.5 g plus 100 mL of sterile water for injection, 5% dextrose injection, or 0.9% sodium chloride injection, also maintain satisfactory potency for 24 hours at room temperature and for 7 days under refrigeration.

These solutions may be further diluted to concentrations of between 1 and 30 mg/mL in the following solutions and will lose not more than 10% activity for 24 hours at room temperature or for at least 7 days under refrigeration: 0.9% sodium chloride injection; 1/6 M sodium lactate injection; ringer's injection, USP; lactated ringer's injection, USP; 5% dextrose and 0.9% sodium chloride injection; 5% dextrose injection; 5% dextrose and 0.45% sodium chloride injection; 5% dextrose and 0.225% sodium chloride injection; 10% dextrose injection; and 10% invert sugar in water for injection. Unused solutions should be discarded after the time periods mentioned above.

Kefurox has also been found to be compatible for 24 hours at room temperature when admixed in IV infusion with the following: heparin (10 and 50 units/mL) in 0.9% sodium chloride injection, or potassium chloride (10 and 40 mEq/L) in 0.9% sodium chloride injection. Sodium bicarbonate injection, USP, is not recommended for the dilution of Kefurox.

The 750-mg and 1.5-g Kefurox ADD-Vantage vials, when diluted in 50 or 100 mL of 5% dextrose injection, 0.9% sodium chloride injection, or 0.45% sodium chloride injection, may be stored for up to 24 hours at room temperature or for 7 days under refrigeration.

Frozen Stability: Constitute the 750-mg and 1.5-g vial as directed for IV administration in Table 2. Immediately withdraw the total contents of the 750-mg or 1.5-g vial and add to a Viaflex® Mini-bag™ containing 50 or 100 mL of 0.9% sodium chloride injection or 5% dextrose injection and freeze. Frozen solutions are stable for 6 months when stored at –20 C. Frozen solutions should be thawed at room temperature and not refrozen. Do not force thaw by immersion in water baths or by microwave irradiation. Thawed solutions may be stored for up to 24 hours at room temperature or for 7 days in a refrigerator.

Note: Parenteral drug products should be inspected visually for particulate matter and discoloration before administration whenever solution and container permit.

As with other cephalosporins, Kefurox powder as well as solutions and suspensions tend to darken, depending on storage conditions, without adversely affecting product potency.

HOW SUPPLIED

Kefurox (cefuroxime for injection) in the dry state should be stored between 15° and 30° C (59° and 86° F) and protected from light. Kefurox is a dry, white to off-white powder supplied in vials as follows:

Vials:

750 mg,* 10-mL size (No. 7271)—(Traypak§ of 25) NDC 0002-7271-25

1.5 g,* 20-mL size (No. 7272)—(Traypak of 10) NDC 0002-7272-10

750 mg,* 100-mL size (No. 7273)—(Traypak of 10) NDC 0002-7273-10

1.5 g,* 100-mL size (No. 7274)—(Traypak of 10) NDC 0002-7274-10

ADD-Vantage‖ Vials:

750 mg,* (No. 7278)—(Traypak of 25) NDC 0002-7278-25

1.5 g,* (No. 7279)—(Traypak of 10) NDC 0002-7279-10

The above ADD-Vantage Vials are to be used only with Abbott Laboratories' ADD-Vantage Antibiotic Diluent Container.

Also available:

Pharmacy Bulk Package:

7.5 g,* 100-mL size (No. 7275)—(Traypak of 6) NDC 0002-7275-16

* Equivalent to cefuroxime.

§ Traypak™ (multivial carton, Lilly).

‖ ADD-Vantage® (vials and diluent containers, Abbott).

REFERENCES:

1. National Committee for Clinical Laboratory Standards, *Performance Standards for Antimicrobial Susceptibility Testing.* Third Informational Supplement. NCCLS Document M100–S3, Vol. 11, No. 17 Villanova, Pa: NCCCLS; 1991.
2. Cockcroft DW, Gault MH. Prediction of creatinine clearance from serum creatinine. Nephron; 1976. 16:31–41.

Rx only

Literature issued May, 1998.

Manufactured for **ELI LILLY AND COMPANY,**
Indianapolis, IN 46285, USA.
by BMH Limited, Philadelphia, PA 19101
KX:L4

KEFZOL® ℞

[kĕf 'zōl]

(cefazolin for injection, USP)

DESCRIPTION

Kefzol (cefazolin for injection, USP) is a semi-synthetic cephalosporin for parenteral administration. It is the sodium salt of 3-{[(5-methyl-1,3,4-thiadiazol-2-yl)thio] methyl}-8-oxo-7-[2-(1H-tetrazol-1-yl)acetamido]-5-thia-1-azabicyclo[4.2.0]oct-2-ene-2-caboxylic acid.

Structural Formula:

The sodium content is 48 mg per gram of cefazolin.

Kefzol in lyophilized form is supplied in vials equivalent to 1 gram of cefazolin: in "Piggyback" Vials for intravenous admixture equivalent to 1 gram of cefazolin; and in Pharmacy Bulk Vials equivalent to 10 grams of cefazolin.

CLINICAL PHARMACOLOGY

Human Pharmacology: After intramuscular administration of *Kefzol* to normal volunteers, the mean serum concentrations were 37 mcg/mL at 1 hour and 3 mcg/mL at 8 hours following a 500 mg dose, and 64 mcg/mL at 1 hour and 7 mcg/mL at 8 hours following a 1 gram dose.

Studies have shown that the following intravenous administration of *Kefzol* to normal volunteers, mean serum concentrations peaked at approximately 185 mcg/mL and were approximately 4 mcg/mL at 8 hours for a 1 gram dose.

The serum half-life for *Kefzol* is approximately 1.8 hours following I.V. administration and approximately 2.0 hours following I.M. administration.

In a study (using normal volunteers) of constant intravenous infusion with dosages of 3.5 mg/kg for 1 hour (approximately 250 mg) and 1.5 mg/kg the next 2 hours (approximately 100 mg), *Kefzol* produced a steady serum level at the third hour of approximately 28 mcg/mL.

Studies in patients hospitalized with infections indicate that Kefzol (cefazolin for injection) produces mean peak serum levels approximately equivalent to those seen in normal volunteers.

Bile levels in patients without obstructive biliary disease can reach or exceed serum levels by up to five times; however, in patients with obstructive biliary disease, bile levels of *Kefzol* are considerably lower than serum levels (<1.0 mcg/mL).

In synovial fluid, the *Kefzol* level becomes comparable to that reached in serum at about 4 hours after drug administration.

Studies of cord blood show prompt transfer of *Kefzol* across the placenta. *Kefzol* is present in very low concentrations in the milk of nursing mothers.

Kefzol is excreted unchanged in the urine. In the first 6 hours approximately 60% of the drug is excreted in the urine and this increases to 70%–80% within 24 hours. *Kefzol* achieves peak urine concentrations of approximately 2400 mcg/mL and 4000 mcg/mL respectively following 500 mg and 1 gram intramuscular doses.

In patients undergoing peritoneal dialysis (2 L/hr.), *Kefzol* produced mean serum levels of approximately 10 and 30 mcg/mL after 24 hours' instillation of a dialyzing solution containing 50 mg/L and 150 mg/L, respectively. Mean peak levels were 29 mcg/mL (range 13–44 mcg/mL) with 50 mg/L (three patients), and 72 mcg/mL (range 26–142 mcg/mL) with 150 mg/L (six patients). Intraperitoneal administration of *Kefzol* is usually well tolerated.

Controlled studies on adult normal volunteers, receiving 1 gram 4 times a day for 10 days, monitoring CBC, SGOT, SGPT, bilirubin, alkaline, phosphatase, BUN, creatinine and urinalysis, indicated no clinically significant changes attributed to *Kefzol*.

Microbiology: *In vitro* tests demonstrate that the bactericidal action of cephalosporins results from inhibition of cell wall synthesis. Kefzol (cefazolin for injection) is active against the following organisms *in vitro* and in clinical infections:

Staphylococcus aureus (including penicillinase-producing strains)

Staphylococcus epidermidis

Methicillin-resistant staphylococci are uniformly resistant to cefazolin

Group A beta-hemolytic streptococci and other strains of streptococci (many strains of enterococci are resistant)

Streptococcus pneumoniae · *Klebsiella species*
Escherichia coli · *Enterobacter aerogenes*
Proteus mirabilis · *Haemophilus influenzae*

Most strains of indole positive *Proteus (Proteus vulgaris), Enterobacter cloacae, Morganella morganii* and *Providencia rettgeri* are resistant. *Serratia, Pseudomonas, Mima, Herellea* species are almost uniformly resistant to cefazolin.

Disk Susceptibility Tests

Disk diffusion technique—Quantitative methods that require measurement of zone diameters give the most precise estimates of antibiotic susceptibility. One such procedure[1] has been recommended for use with disks to test susceptibility to cefazolin.

Reports from a laboratory using the standardized single-disk susceptibility test[1] with a 30 mcg cefazolin disk should be interpreted according to the following criteria:

Susceptible organisms produce zones of 18 mm or greater, indicating that the tested organism is likely to respond to therapy.

Organisms of intermediate susceptibility produce zones 15 to 17 mm, indicating that the tested organism would be susceptible if high dosage is used or if the infection is confined to tissues and fluids (e.g., urine), in which high antibiotic levels are attained.

Resistant organisms produce zones of 14 mm or less, indicating that other therapy should be selected.

For gram-positive isolates, a zone of 18 mm is indicative of a cefazolin-susceptible organism when tested with either the cephalosporin-class disk (30 mcg cephalothin) or the cefazolin disk (30 mcg cefazolin).

Gram-negative organisms should be tested with the cefazolin disk (using the above criteria), since cefazolin has been shown by *in vitro* tests to have activity against certain strains of Enterobacteriaceae found resistant when tested

Continued on next page

*** Identi-Code® symbol. This product information was prepared in June 2000. Current information on these and other products of Eli Lilly and Company may be obtained by direct inquiry to Lilly Research Laboratories, Lilly Corporate Center, Indianapolis, Indiana 46285, (800) 545-5979.**

Kefzol—Cont.

with the cephalothin disk. Gram-negative organisms having zones of less than 18 mm around the cephalothin disk may be susceptible to cefazolin.

Standardized procedures require use of control organisms. The 30 mcg cefazolin disk should give zone diameter between 23 and 29 mm for *E. coli* ATCC 25922 and between 29 and 35 mm for *S. aureus* ATCC 25923.

The cefazolin disk should not be used for testing susceptibility to other cephalosporins

Dilution Techniques—A bacterial isolate may be considered susceptible if the minimal inhibitory concentration (MIC) for cefazolin is not more than 16 mcg per mL. Organisms are considered resistant if the MIC is equal to or greater than 64 mcg per mL.

The range of MIC's for the control strains are as follows:

S. aureus ATCC 25923, 0.25–1.0 mcg/mL
E. coli ATCC 25922, 1.0–4.0 mcg/mL

[1] Bauer, A.W.; Kirby, W.M.M.; Sherris, J.C., and Turck, M.: Antibiotic Testing by a Standardized Single Disc Method, Am J. Clin. Path. 45:493, 1966. Standardized Disc Susceptibility Test, Federal Register 39:19182-19184, 1974.

INDICATIONS AND USAGE

Kefzol (cefazolin for injection) is indicated in the treatment of the following serious infections due to susceptible organisms:

RESPIRATORY TRACT INFECTIONS due to *Streptococcus pneumoniae, Klebsiella* species *Haemophilus influenzae, Staphylococcus aureus* (penicillin-sensitive and penicillin-resistant) and group A beta-hemolytic streptococci.

Injectable benzathine penicillin is considered to be the drug of choice in treatment and prevention of streptococcal infections, including the prophylaxis of rheumatic fever.

Kefzol is effective in the eradication of streptococci from the nasopharynx; however, data establishing the efficacy of *Kefzol* in the subsequent prevention of rheumatic fever are not available at present.

URINARY TRACT INFECTIONS due to *Escherichia coli, Proteus mirabilis, Klebsiella* species and some strains of enterobacter and enterococci.

SKIN AND SKIN STRUCTURE INFECTIONS due to *Staphylococcus aureus* (penicillin-sensitive and penicillin-resistant), group A beta hemolytic streptococci and other strains of streptococci.

BILIARY TRACT INFECTIONS due to *Escherichia coli*, various strains of streptococci, *Proteus mirabilis, Klebsiella* species and *Staphylococcus aureus.*

BONE AND JOINT INFECTIONS due to *Staphylococcus aureus.*

GENITAL INFECTIONS (i.e., prostatitis epididymitis) due to *Escherichia coli, Proteus mirabilis, Klebsiella* species and some strains of enterococci.

SEPTICEMIA due to *Streptococcus pneumoniae, Staphylococcus aureus* (penicillin-sensitive and penicillin-resistant), *Proteus mirabilis, Escherichia coli* and *Klebsiella* species.

ENDOCARDITIS due to *Staphylococcus aureus* (penicillin-sensitive and penicillin-resistant and group A beta-hemolytic streptococci.

Appropriate culture and susceptible studies should be performed to determine susceptibility of the causative organism to *Kefzol*.

PERIOPERATIVE PROPHYLAXIS: The prophylactic administration of *Kefzol* preoperatively, intraoperatively and postoperatively may reduce the incidence of certain postoperative infections in patients undergoing surgical procedures which are classified as contaminated or potentially contaminated (e.g., vaginal hysterectomy, and cholecystectomy in high-risk patients such as those over 70 year of age, with acute cholecystitis, obstructive jaundice or common duct bile stones).

The perioperative use of *Kefzol* may also be effective in surgical patients in whom infection at the operative site would present a serious risk (e.g., during open-heart surgery and prosthetic arthroplasty).

The prophylactic administration of *Kefzol* should usually be discontinued within a 24-hour period after the surgical procedure. In surgery where the occurrence of infection may be particularly devastating (e.g., open-heart surgery and prosthetic arthroplasty), the prophylactic administration of *Kefzol* may be continued for 3 to 5 days following the completion of surgery.

If there are signs of infection, specimens for cultures should be obtained for the identification of the causative organism so that appropriate therapy may be instituted.

(See DOSAGE AND ADMINISTRATION.)

CONTRAINDICATIONS

KEFZOL (CEFAZOLIN FOR INJECTION) IS CONTRAINDICATED IN PATIENTS WITH KNOWN ALLERGY TO THE CEPHALOSPORIN GROUP OF ANTIBIOTICS.

WARNINGS

BEFORE THERAPY WITH *KEFZOL* IS INSTITUTED, CAREFUL INQUIRY SHOULD BE MADE TO DETERMINE WHETHER THE PATIENT HAS HAD PREVIOUS HYPERSENSITIVITY REACTIONS TO CEFAZOLIN, CEPHALOSPORINS, PENICILLINS, OR OTHER DRUGS, IF THIS PRODUCT IS GIVEN TO PENICILLIN-SENSITIVE PATIENTS. CAUTION SHOULD BE EXERCISED BECAUSE CROSS-HYPERSENSITIVITY AMONG BETA-LACTAM ANTIBIOTICS HAS BEEN CLEARLY DOCUMENTED AND MAY OCCUR IN UP TO 10% OF PATIENTS WITH A HISTORY OF PENICILLIN ALLERGY IF AN ALLERGIC REACTION TO *KEFZOL* OCCURS, DISCONTINUE TREATMENT WITH THE DRUG. SERIOUS ACUTE HYPERSENSITIVITY REACTIONS MAY REQUIRE TREATMENT WITH EPINEPHRINE AND OTHER EMERGENCY MEASURES, INCLUDING OXYGEN, IV FLUIDS, IV ANTIHISTAMINES, CORTICOSTEROIDS, PRESSOR AMINES AND AIRWAY MANAGEMENT, AS CLINICALLY INDICATED.

Pseudomembranous colitis has been reported with nearly all antibacterial agents, including cefazolin, and may range in severity from mild to life-threatening. Therefore, it is important to consider this diagnosis in patients who present with diarrhea subsequent to the administration of antibacterial agents.

Treatment with antibacterial agents alters the normal flora of the colon and may permit overgrowth of clostridia. Studies indicate that a toxin produced by *Clostridium difficile* is one primary cause of "antibiotic-associated colitis."

After the diagnosis of pseudomembranous colitis has been established, therapeutic measures should be initiated. Mild cases of pseudomembranous colitis usually respond to drug discontinuation alone. In moderate to severe cases, consideration should be given to management with fluids and electrolytes, protein supplementation and treatment with an antibacterial drug clinically effective against *C. difficile* colitis.

PRECAUTIONS

General—Prolonged use of Kefzol (cefazolin for injection) may result in the overgrowth of nonsusceptible organisms. Careful clinical observation of the patient is essential.

When *Kefzol* is administered to patients with low urinary output because of impaired renal function, lower daily dosage is required (see DOSAGE AND ADMINISTRATION).

As with other beta-lactam antibiotics, seizures may occur if inappropriately high doses are administered to patients with impaired renal function (see DOSAGE AND ADMINISTRATION).

Kefzol, as with all cephalosporins, should be prescribed with caution in individuals with a history of gastrointestinal disease, particularly colitis.

Drug Interactions—Probenecid may decrease renal tubular secretion of cephalosporins when used concurrently, resulting in increased and more prolonged cephalosporin blood levels.

Drug/Laboratory Test Interactions—A false positive reaction for glucose in the urine may occur with Benedict's solution, Fehling's solution, or with Clinitest® tablets, but not with enzyme-based tests such as Clinistix® and Tes-Tape®. Positive direct and indirect antiglobulin (Coombs) tests have occurred; these may also occur in neonates whose mothers received cephalosporins before delivery.

Carcinogenesis/Mutagenesis—Mutagenicity studies and long-term studies in animals to determine the carcinogenic potential of Kefzol (cefazolin for injection) have not been performed.

Pregnancy—Teratogenic Effects—Pregnancy Category B. Reproduction studies have been performed in rats, mice and rabbits at doses up to 25 times the human dose and have revealed no evidence of impaired fertility or harm to the fetus due to *Kefzol*. There are, however, no adequate and well-controlled studies in pregnant women. Because animal reproduction studies are not always predictive of human response, this drug should be used during pregnancy only if clearly needed.

Labor and Delivery—When cefazolin has been administered prior to caesarean section, drug levels in cord blood have been approximately one quarter to one third of maternal drug levels. The drug appears to have no adverse effect on the fetus.

Nursing Mothers—*Kefzol* (cefazolin for injection) is present in very low concentrations in the milk of nursing mothers. Caution should be exercised when *Kefzol* is administered to a nursing woman.

Pediatric Use—Safety and effectiveness for use in premature infants and neonates have not been established. See DOSAGE AND ADMINISTRATION for recommended dosage in pediatric patients over 1 month.

ADVERSE REACTIONS

The following reactions have been reported:

Gastrointestinal: Diarrhea, oral candidiasis (oral thrush), vomiting, nausea, stomach cramps, anorexia and pseudomembranous colitis. Onset of pseudomembranous colitis symptoms may occur during or after antibiotic treatment (see WARNINGS). Nausea and vomiting have been reported rarely.

Allergic: Anaphylaxis, eosinophilia, itching, drug fever, skin rash, Stevens-Johnson syndrome.

Hematologic: Neutropenia, leukopenia, thrombocytopenia, thrombocythemia.

Hepatic and Renal: Transient rise in SGOT, SGPT, BUN and alkaline phosphatase levels has been observed without clinical evidence of renal or hepatic impairment.

Local Reactions: Rare instances of phlebitis have been reported at site of injection. Pain at the site of injection after intramuscular administration has occurred infrequently. Some induration has occurred.

Other Reactions: Genital and anal pruritus (including vulvar pruritus, genital moniliasis and vaginitis).

DOSAGE AND ADMINISTRATION

Usual Adult Dosage

Type of Infection	Dose	Frequency
Moderate to severe infections	500 mg to 1 gram	every 6 to 8 hrs.
Mild infections caused by susceptible gram + cocci	250 mg to 500 mg	every 8 hours
Acute, uncomplicated urinary tract infections	1 gram	every 12 hours
Pneumococcal pneumonia	500 mg	every 12 hours
Severe, life-threatening infections (e.g., endocarditis, septicemia)*	1 gram to 1.5 grams	every 6 hours

*In rare instances, doses up to 12 grams of *Kefzol* per day have been used.

Perioperative Prophylactic Use

To prevent postoperative infection in contaminated or potentially contaminated surgery, recommended doses are:

a. 1 gram I.V. or I.M. administered 1/2 hour to 1 hour prior to the start of surgery.
b. For lengthy operative procedures (e.g., 2 hours or more), 500 mg to 1 gram I.V. or I.M. during surgery (administration modified depending on the duration of the operative procedure).
c. 500 mg to 1 gram I.V. or I.M. every 6 to 8 hours for 24 hours postoperatively.

It is important that (1) the preoperative dose be given just (1/2 hour to 1 hour) prior to the start of surgery so that adequate antibiotic levels are present in the serum and tissues at the time of the initial surgical incision; and (2) *Kefzol* be administered, if necessary, at appropriate intervals during surgery to provide sufficient levels of the antibiotic at the anticipated moments of greatest exposure to infective organisms.

In surgery where the occurrence of infection may be particularly devastating (e.g., open-heart surgery and prosthetic arthroplasty), the prophylactic administration of Kefzol (cefazolin for injection) may be continued for 3 to 5 days following the completion of surgery.

Dosage Adjustment for Patients With Reduced Renal Function

Kefzol may be used in patients with reduced renal function with the following dosage adjustments: Patients with a creatinine clearance of 55 mL/min, or greater or a serum creatinine of 1.5 mg % or less can be given full doses. Patients with creatinine clearance rates of 35 to 54 mL/min, or serum creatinine of 1.6 to 3.0 mg % can also be given full doses but dosage should be restricted to at least 8 hour intervals. Patients with creatinine clearance rates of 11 to 34 mL/min, or serum creatinine of 3.1 to 4.5 mg % should be given 1/2 the usual dose every 12 hours. Patients with creatinine clearance rates of 10 mL/min, or less or serum creatinine of 4.6 mg % or greater should be given 1/2 the usual dose every 18 to 24 hours. All reduced dosage recommendations apply after an initial loading dose appropriate to the severity of the infection. Patients undergoing peritoneal dialysis: see Human Pharmacology.

Pediatric Dosage

In pediatric patients, a total daily dosage of 25 to 50 mg per kg (approximately 10 to 20 mg per pound) of body weight, divided into three or four equal doses, is effective for most mild to moderately severe infections. Total daily dosage may be increased to 100 mg per kg (45 mg per pound) of body weight for severe infections. Since safety for use in premature infants and in neonates has not been established, the use of Kefzol (cefazolin for injection) in these patients is not recommended.

[See first table at top of next page]
[See second table at top of next page]

In pediatric patients, with mild to moderate renal impairment (creatinine clearance of 70 to 40 mL/min.), 60 percent of the normal daily dose given in equally divided doses every 12 hours should be sufficient. In patients with moderate impairment (creatinine clearance of 40 to 20 mL/min.), 25 percent of the normal daily dose given in equally divided doses every 12 hours should be adequate. Pediatric patients with severe renal impairment (creatinine clearance of 20 to 5 mL/min.) may be given 10 percent of the normal daily dose every 24 hours. All dosage recommendations apply after an initial loading dose.

RECONSTITUTION

Preparation of Parenteral Solution

Parenteral drug products should be SHAKEN WELL when reconstituted, and inspected visually for particulate matter prior to administration. If particulate matter is evident in reconstituted fluids, the drug solution should be discarded. When reconstituted or diluted according to the instructions below, Kefzol (cefazolin for injection) is stable for 24 hours at room temperature or for 10 days if stored under refrigeration (5°C or 41°F). Reconstituted solutions may range in color from pale yellow to yellow without a change in potency.

PEDIATRIC DOSAGE GUIDE

Weight		25 mg/kg/Day Divided Into 3 Doses		25 mg/kg/Day Divided Into 4 Doses	
Lbs	Kg	Approximate Single Dose mg/q8h	Vol. (mL) needed with dilution of 125 mg/mL	Approximate Single Dose mg/q6h	Vol. (mL) needed with dilution of 125 mg/mL
10	4.5	40 mg	0.35 mL	30 mg	0.25 mL
20	9.0	75 mg	0.60 mL	55 mg	0.45 mL
30	13.6	115 mg	0.90 mL	85 mg	0.70 mL
40	18.1	150 mg	1.20 mL	115 mg	0.90 mL
50	22.7	190 mg	1.50 mL	140 mg	1.10 mL

PEDIATRIC DOSAGE GUIDE

Weight		50 mg/kg/Day Divided Into 3 Doses		50 mg/kg/Day Divided Into 4 Doses	
Lbs	Kg	Approximate Single Dose mg/q8h	Vol. (mL) needed with dilution of 225 mg/mL	Approximate Single Dose mg/q6h	Vol. (mL) needed with dilution of 225 mg/mL
10	4.5	75 mg	0.35 mL	55 mg	0.25 mL
20	9.0	150 mg	0.70 mL	110 mg	0.50 mL
30	13.6	225 mg	1.00 mL	170 mg	0.75 mL
40	18.1	300 mg	1.35 mL	225 mg	1.00 mL
50	22.7	375 mg	1.70 mL	285 mg	1.25 mL

Single-Dose Vials

For I.M. injection, I.V. direct (bolus) injection or I.V. infusion, reconstitute with Sterile Water for Injection according to the following table. SHAKE WELL.

Vial Size	Amount of Diluent	Approximate Concentration	Approximate Available Volume
1 gram	2.5 mL	330 mg/mL	3.0 mL

Pharmacy Bulk Vials

Add Sterile Water for Injection, Bacteriostatic Water for Injection or Sodium Chloride Injection according to the table below. SHAKE WELL.

Vial Size	Amount of Diluent	Approximate Concentration	Approximate Available Volume
10 grams	45 mL	1 gram/5 mL	51 mL
	96 mL	1 gram/10 mL	102 mL

"Piggyback" Vials

Reconstitute with 50 to 100 mL of Sodium Chloride Injection or other I.V. solution listed under ADMINISTRATION. When adding diluent to vial, allow air to escape by using a small vent needle or by pumping the syringe. SHAKE WELL. Administer with primary I.V. fluids, as a single dose.

ADMINISTRATION

Intramuscular Administration—Reconstitute vials with Sterile Water for Injection according to the dilution table above. Shake well until dissolved. *Kefzol* should be injected into a large muscle mass. Pain on injection is infrequent in *Kefzol*.

Intravenous Administration—Direct (bolus) injection: Following reconstitution according to the above table, further dilute vials with approximately 5 mL Sterile Water for Injection. Inject the solution slowly over 3 to 5 minutes, directly or through tubing for patients receiving parenteral fluids (see list below).

Intermittent or continuous infusion: Dilute reconstituted *Kefzol* in 50 to 100 mL of one of the following solutions:

- Sodium Chloride Injection, USP
- 5% or 10% Dextrose Injection, USP
- 5% Dextrose in Lactated Ringer's Injection, USP
- 5% Dextrose and 0.9% Sodium Chloride Injection, USP
- 5% Dextrose and 0.45% Sodium Chloride Injection, USP
- 5% Dextrose and 0.2% Sodium Chloride Injection, USP
- Lactated Ringer's Injection, USP
- Invert Sugar 5% or 10% in Sterile Water for Injection
- Ringer's Injection, USP
- 5% Sodium Bicarbonate Injection, USP

HOW SUPPLIED

Kefzol (cefazolin for injection)—supplied in vials equivalent to 1 gram of cefazolin; in "Piggyback" Vials for intravenous admixture equivalent to 1 gram of cefazolin; and in Pharmacy Bulk Vials equivalent to 10 grams of cefazolin.

Vials:

1 gram, 10-mL size (No. 768)—(Traypak* of 25) NDC 0002-1498-25

1 gram, 100-mL size (No. 7011)†—(Traypak of 10) NDC 0002-7011-10

Pharmacy Bulk Vials:

10 gram, 100-mL size (No. 7014)—(Traypak of 6) NDC 0002-7014-16

Also Available:

Faspak‡:

1 gram (No. 7202)†—(Faspak of 96) NDC 0002-7202-74

ADD-Vantage§ Vial:

1 gram (No. 7266)—(Traypak of 25) NDC 0002-7266-25

The above ADD-Vantage Vials are to be used *only* with Abbott Laboratories' 50-mL or 100-mL Flexible Diluent Containers containing 0.9% Sodium Chloride Injection or 5% Dextrose Injection.

As with other cephalosporins, Kefzol (cefazolin for injection) tends to darken depending on storage conditions; within the stated recommendations, however, product potency is not adversely affected.

Before reconstitution protect from light and store at Controlled Room Temperature 20° to 25°C (68° and 77°F).

*Traypak™ (multivial carton. Lilly).
†For IV use
‡Faspak® (flexible plastic bag. Lilly)
§ADD-Vantage® (vials and diluent containers, Abbott).
Rx only
Date of issuance Sept. 1998
KL:L5 [0998]

Manufactured for
ELI LILLY AND COMPANY
Indianapolis, IN 46285, USA
by
BMH Limited
Philadelphia, PA 19101

LENTE® ILETIN® II OTC
(insulin zinc suspension, Lilly)
See under Iletin® (insulin)

MANDOL® ℞

[*măn 'dōl*]
(Cefamandole Nafate for Injection, USP)

DESCRIPTION

Mandol® (Cefamandole Nafate for Injection, USP) is a semisynthetic broad-spectrum cephalosporin antibiotic for parenteral administration. It is 5-thia-1-azabicyclo [4.2.0]oct-2-ene-2-carboxylic acid, 7-[[(formyloxy)phenylacetyl]amino]-3-[[(1-methyl-1*H*-tetrazol-5-yl)thio]methyl]-8-oxo-, monosodium salt, [6*R*-[6α,7β(*R**)]]. Cefamandole has the empirical formula $C_{19}H_{17}N_6NaO_6S_2$ representing a molecular weight of 512.49.

Mandol also contains 63 mg sodium carbonate/g of cefamandole activity. The total sodium content is approximately 77 mg (3.3 mEq sodium ion) per g of cefamandole activity. After addition of diluent, cefamandole nafate rapidly hydrolyzes to cefamandole, and both compounds have microbiologic activity in vivo. Solutions of Mandol range from light-yellow to amber, depending on concentration and diluent used. The pH of freshly reconstituted solutions usually ranges from 6.0 to 8.5.

CLINICAL PHARMACOLOGY

After intramuscular administration of a 500-mg dose of cefamandole to normal volunteers, the mean peak serum concentration was 13 µg/mL. After a 1-g dose, the mean peak concentration was 25 µg/mL. These peaks occurred at 30 to 120 minutes. Following intravenous doses of 1, 2, and 3 g, serum concentrations were 139, 240, and 533 mcg/mL respectively at 10 minutes. These concentrations declined to 0.8, 2.2, and 2.9 mcg/mL at 4 hours. Intravenous administration of 4-g doses every 6 hours produced no evidence of accumulation in the serum. The half-life after an intravenous dose is 32 minutes; after intramuscular administration, the half-life is 60 minutes.

Sixty-five percent to 85% of cefamandole is excreted by the kidneys over an 8-hour period, resulting in high urinary concentrations. Following intramuscular doses of 500 mg and 1 g, urinary concentrations averaged 254 and 1,357 mcg/mL respectively. Intravenous doses of 1 and 2 g produced urinary levels averaging 750 and 1,380 mcg/mL respectively. Probenecid slows tubular excretion and doubles the peak serum level and the duration of measurable serum concentrations.

The antibiotic reaches therapeutic levels in pleural and joint fluids and in bile and bone.

Microbiology—The bactericidal action of cefamandole results from inhibition of cell-wall synthesis. Cephalosporins have in vitro activity against a wide range of gram-positive and gram-negative organisms. Cefamandole is usually active against the following organisms in vitro and in clinical infections:

Gram-positive
- *Staphylococcus aureus*, including penicillinase- and non-penicillinase-producing strains
- *Staphylococcus epidermidis*
- β-hemolytic and other streptococci (Most strains of enterococci, eg, *Enterococcus faecalis* [formerly *Streptococcus faecalis*], are resistant.)
- *Streptococcus pneumoniae*

Gram-negative
- *Escherichia coli*
- *Klebsiella* spp.
- *Enterobacter* spp. (Initially susceptible organisms occasionally may become resistant during therapy.)
- *Haemophilus influenzae*
- *Proteus mirabilis*
- *Providencia rettgeri (formerly Proteus rettgeri)*
- *Morganella morganii (formerly Proteus morganii)*
- *Proteus vulgaris* (Some strains of *P. vulgaris* have been shown by in vitro tests to be resistant to cefamandole and certain other cephalosporins.)

Anaerobic organisms
- Gram-positive and gram-negative cocci (including *Peptococcus* and *Peptostreptococcus* spp.)
- Gram-positive bacilli (including *Clostridium* spp.)
- Gram-negative bacilli (including *Bacteroides* and *Fusobacterium* spp.). Most strains of *Bacteroides fragilis* are resistant.

Pseudomonas, Acinetobacter calcoaceticus (formerly *Mima* and *Herellea* spp.), and most *Serratia* strains are resistant to cefamandole and certain other cephalosporins. Cefamandole is resistant to degradation by β-lactamases from certain members of the *Enterobacteriaceae.*

Susceptibility Tests —Quantitative methods that require measurement of zone diameters give the most precise estimates of antibiotic susceptibility. One such procedure[1] has been recommended for use with disks to test susceptibility to cefamandole. Interpretation involves correlation of the diameters obtained in the disk test with minimal inhibitory concentration (MIC) values for cefamandole.

Reports from the laboratory giving results of the standardized single-disk susceptibility test[1] using a 30-mcg cefamandole disk should be interpreted according to the following criteria:

- Susceptible organisms produce zones of 18 mm or greater, indicating that the tested organism is likely to respond to therapy.
- Organisms of intermediate susceptibility produce zones of 15 to 17 mm, indicating that the tested organism would be susceptible if high dosage is used or if the infection is confined to tissues and fluids (eg, urine) in which high antibiotic levels are attained.
- Resistant organisms produce zones of 14 mm or less, indicating that other therapy should be selected.

For gram-positive isolates, the test may be performed with either the cephalosporin-class disk (30 mcg cephalothin) or the cefamandole disk (30 mcg cefamandole), and a zone of 18 mm is indicative of a cefamandole-susceptible organism.

Continued on next page

*** Identi-Code® symbol. This product information was prepared in June 2000. Current information on these and other products of Eli Lilly and Company may be obtained by direct inquiry to Lilly Research Laboratories, Lilly Corporate Center, Indianapolis, Indiana 46285, (800) 545-5979.**

Mandol—Cont.

Gram-negative organisms should be tested with the cefamandole disk (using the above criteria), since cefamandole has been shown by in vitro tests to have activity against certain strains of *Enterobacteriaceae* found resistant when tested with the cephalosporin-class disk. Gram-negative organisms having zones of less than 18 mm around the cephalothin disk are not necessarily of intermediate susceptibility or resistant to cefamandole.

The cefamandole disk should not be used for testing susceptibility to other cephalosporins.

A bacterial isolate may be considered susceptible if the MIC value for cefamandole[2] is not more than 16 mcg/mL. Organisms are considered resistant if the MIC is greater than 32 mcg/mL.

INDICATIONS AND USAGE

Mandol is indicated for the treatment of serious infections caused by susceptible strains of the designated microorganisms in the diseases listed below:

- Lower respiratory infections, including pneumonia, caused by *S. pneumoniae, H. influenzae, Klebsiella* spp., *S. aureus* (penicillinase- and non-penicillinase-producing), β-hemolytic streptococci, and *P. mirabilis*
- Urinary tract infections caused by *E. coli, Proteus* spp. (both indole-negative and indole-positive), *Enterobacter* spp., *Klebsiella* spp., group D streptococci (Note: Most enterococci, eg, *E. faecalis,* are resistant), and *S. epidermidis*
- Peritonitis caused by *E. coli* and *Enterobacter* spp.
- Septicemia caused by *E. coli, S. aureus* (penicillinase- and non-penicillinase-producing), *S. pneumoniae, S. pyogenes* (group A β-hemolytic streptococci), *H. influenzae,* and *Klebsiella* spp.
- Skin and skin structure infections caused by *S. aureus* (penicillinase- and non-penicillinase-producing), *S. pyogenes* (group A β-hemolytic streptococci), *H. influenzae, E. coli, Enterobacter* spp., and *P. mirabilis*
- Bone and joint infections caused by *S. aureus* (penicillinase- and non-penicillinase-producing)

Clinical microbiologic studies in nongonococcal pelvic inflammatory disease in females, lower respiratory infections, and skin infections frequently reveal the growth of susceptible strains of both aerobic and anaerobic organisms. Mandol has been used successfully in those infections in which several organisms have been isolated. Most strains of *B. fragilis* are resistant in vitro; however, infections caused by susceptible strains have been treated successfully.

Specimens for bacteriologic cultures should be obtained in order to isolate and identify causative organisms and to determine their susceptibilities to cefamandole. Therapy may be instituted before results of susceptibility studies are known; however, once these results become available, the antibiotic treatment should be adjusted accordingly.

In certain cases of confirmed or suspected gram-positive or gram-negative sepsis or in patients with other serious infections in which the causative organism has not been identified, Mandol may be used concomitantly with an aminoglycoside (*see* Precautions). The recommended doses of both antibiotics may be given, depending on the severity of the infection and the patient's condition. The renal function of the patient should be carefully monitored, especially if higher dosages of the antibiotics are to be administered.

Antibiotic therapy of β-hemolytic streptococcal infections should continue for at least 10 days.

Preventive Therapy—The administration of Mandol preoperatively, intraoperatively, and postoperatively may reduce the incidence of certain postoperative infections in patients undergoing surgical procedures that are classified as contaminated or potentially contaminated (eg, gastrointestinal surgery, cesarean section, vaginal hysterectomy, or cholecystectomy in high-risk patients such as those with acute cholecystitis, obstructive jaundice, or common-bile-duct stones).

In major surgery in which the risk of postoperative infection is low but serious (cardiovascular surgery, neurosurgery, or prosthetic arthroplasty), Mandol may be effective in preventing such infections.

If signs of infection occur, specimens for culture should be obtained for identification of the causative organism so that appropriate antibiotic therapy may be instituted.

CONTRAINDICATION

Mandol is contraindicated in patients with known allergy to the cephalosporin group of antibiotics.

WARNINGS

BEFORE THERAPY WITH MANDOL IS INSTITUTED, CAREFUL INQUIRY SHOULD BE MADE TO DETERMINE WHETHER THE PATIENT HAS HAD PREVIOUS HYPERSENSITIVITY REACTIONS TO CEPHALOSPORINS, PENICILLINS, OR OTHER DRUGS. THIS PRODUCT SHOULD BE GIVEN CAUTIOUSLY TO PENICILLIN-SENSITIVE PATIENTS. ANTIBIOTICS SHOULD BE ADMINISTERED WITH CAUTION TO ANY PATIENT WHO HAS DEMONSTRATED SOME FORM OF ALLERGY, PARTICULARLY TO DRUGS. SERIOUS ACUTE HYPERSENSITIVITY REACTIONS MAY REQUIRE EPINEPHRINE AND OTHER EMERGENCY MEASURES.

In neonates, accumulation of other cephalosporin-class antibiotics (with resulting prolongation of drug half-life) has been reported.

Pseudomembranous colitis has been reported with virtually all broad-spectrum antibiotics (including macrolides, semisynthetic penicillins, and cephalosporins); therefore, it is important to consider its diagnosis in patients who develop diarrhea in association with the use of antibiotics. Such colitis may range in severity from mild to life threatening.

Treatment with broad-spectrum antibiotics alters the normal flora of the colon and may permit overgrowth of clostridia. Studies indicate that a toxin produced by *Clostridium difficile* is a primary cause of antibiotic-associated colitis.

Mild cases of pseudomembranous colitis usually respond to drug discontinuance alone. In moderate to severe cases, management should include sigmoidoscopy, appropriate bacteriologic studies, and fluid, electrolyte, and protein supplementation. When the colitis does not improve after the drug has been discontinued, or when it is severe, oral vancomycin is the drug of choice for antibiotic-associated pseudomembranous colitis produced by *C. difficile.* Other causes of colitis should be ruled out.

PRECAUTIONS

General—Although Mandol rarely produces alteration in kidney function, evaluation of renal status is recommended, especially in seriously ill patients receiving maximum doses.

Prolonged use of Mandol may result in the overgrowth of nonsusceptible organisms. Careful observation of the patient is essential. If superinfection occurs during therapy, appropriate measures should be taken.

Nephrotoxicity has been reported following concomitant administration of aminoglycoside antibiotics and cephalosporins.

A false-positive reaction for glucose in the urine may occur with Benedict's or Fehling's solution or with Clinitest® tablets. There may be a false-positive test for proteinuria with acid and denaturization-precipitation tests.

As with other broad-spectrum antibiotics, hypoprothrombinemia, with or without bleeding, has been reported rarely, but it has been promptly reversed by administration of vitamin K. Such episodes usually have occurred in elderly, debilitated, or otherwise compromised patients with deficient stores of vitamin K. Treatment of such individuals with antibiotics possessing significant gram-negative and/or anaerobic activity is thought to alter the number and/or type of intestinal bacterial flora, with consequent reduction in synthesis of vitamin K. Prophylactic administration of vitamin K may be indicated in such patients, especially when intestinal sterilization and surgical procedures are performed.

In a few patients receiving Mandol, nausea, vomiting, and vasomotor instability with hypotension and peripheral vasodilatation occurred following the ingestion of ethanol.

Cefamandole inhibits the enzyme acetaldehyde dehydrogenase in laboratory animals. This causes accumulation of acetaldehyde when ethanol is administered concomitantly.

Broad-spectrum antibiotics should be prescribed with caution in individuals with a history of gastrointestinal disease, particularly colitis.

Carcinogenesis, Mutagenesis, Impairment of Fertility—Certain β-lactam antibiotics containing the N-methylthiotetrazole side chain have been reported to cause delayed maturity of the testicular germinal epithelium when given to neonatal rats during initial spermatogenic development (6 to 36 days of age). In animals that were treated from 6 to 36 days of age with 1,000 mg/kg/day of cefamandole (approximately 5 times the maximum clinical dose), the delayed maturity was pronounced and was associated with decreased testicular weights and a reduced number of germinal cells in the leading waves of spermatogenic development. The effect was slight in rats given 50 or 100 mg/kg/day. Some animals that were given 1,000 mg/kg/day during days 6 to 36 were infertile after becoming sexually mature. No adverse effects have been observed in rats exposed in utero, in neonatal rats (4 days of age or younger) treated prior to the initiation of spermatogenesis, or in older rats (more than 36 days of age) after exposure for up to 6 months. The significance to humans of these findings in rats is unknown because of differences in the time of initiation of spermatogenesis, rate of spermatogenic development, and duration of puberty.

Usage in Pregnancy—Pregnancy Category B—Reproduction studies have been performed in rats given doses of 500 or 1,000 mg/kg/day and have revealed no evidence of impaired fertility or harm to the fetus due to Mandol. There are, however, no adequate and well-controlled studies in pregnant women. Because animal reproduction studies are not always predictive of human response, this drug should be used during pregnancy only if clearly needed.

Nursing Mothers—Caution should be exercised when Mandol is administered to a nursing woman.

Usage in Infants—Mandol has been effectively used in this age group, but all laboratory parameters have not been extensively studied in infants between 1 and 6 months of age; safety of this product has not been established in premature infants and term neonates under 1 month of age. Therefore, if Mandol is administered to infants, the physician should determine whether the potential benefits outweigh the possible risks involved.

ADVERSE REACTIONS

Gastrointestinal—Symptoms of pseudomembranous colitis may appear either during or after antibiotic treatment. Nausea and vomiting have been reported rarely. As with some penicillins and some other cephalosporins, transient hepatitis and cholestatic jaundice have been reported rarely.

Hypersensitivity—Anaphylaxis, maculopapular rash, urticaria, eosinophilia, and drug fever have been reported. These reactions are more likely to occur in patients with a history of allergy, particularly to penicillin.

Blood—Thrombocytopenia has been reported rarely. Neutropenia has been reported, especially in long courses of treatment. Some individuals have developed positive direct Coombs' tests during treatment with the cephalosporin antibiotics.

Liver—Transient rise in SGOT, SGPT, and alkaline phosphatase levels has been noted.

Kidney—Decreased creatinine clearance has been reported in patients with prior renal impairment. As with some other cephalosporins, transitory elevations of BUN have occasionally been observed with Mandol; their frequency increases in patients over 50 years of age. In some of these cases, there was also a mild increase in serum creatinine.

Local Reactions—Pain on intramuscular injection is infrequent. Thrombophlebitis occurs rarely.

OVERDOSAGE

The administration of inappropriately large doses of parenteral cephalosporins may cause seizures, particularly in patients with renal impairment. Dosage reduction is necessary when renal function is impaired (*see* Dosage and Administration). If seizures occur, the drug should be promptly discontinued; anticonvulsant therapy may be administered if clinically indicated. Hemodialysis may be considered in cases of overwhelming overdosage.

DOSAGE AND ADMINISTRATION

Dosage—Adults: The usual dosage range for cefamandole is 500 mg to 1 g every 4 to 8 hours.

In infections of skin structures and in uncomplicated pneumonia, a dosage of 500 mg every 6 hours is adequate.

In uncomplicated urinary tract infections, a dosage of 500 mg every 8 hours is sufficient. In more serious urinary tract infections, a dosage of 1 g every 8 hours may be needed.

In severe infections, 1-g doses may be given at 4 to 6-hour intervals.

In life-threatening infections or infections due to less susceptible organisms, doses up to 2 g every 4 hours (ie, 12 g/day) may be needed.

Infants and Children: Administration of 50 to 100 mg/kg/day in equally divided doses every 4 to 8 hours has been effective for most infections susceptible to Mandol. This may be increased to a total daily dose of 150 mg/kg (not to exceed the maximum adult dose) for severe infections. (*See* recommendations regarding this age group in Warnings *and* Precautions.)

Note: As with antibiotic therapy in general, administration of Mandol should be continued for a minimum of 48 to 72 hours after the patient becomes asymptomatic or after evidence of bacterial eradication has been obtained; a minimum of 10 days of treatment is recommended in infections caused by group A β-hemolytic streptococci in order to guard against the risk of rheumatic fever or glomerulonephritis; frequent bacteriologic and clinical appraisal is necessary during therapy of chronic urinary tract infection and may be required for several months after therapy has been completed; persistent infections may require treatment for several weeks; and doses smaller than those indicated above should not be used.

For perioperative use of Mandol, the following dosages are recommended:

Adults—1 or 2 g intravenously or intramuscularly $^1/_2$ to 1 hour prior to the surgical incision followed by 1 or 2 g every 6 hours for 24 to 48 hours.

Pediatric Patients (3 months of age and older)—50 to 100 mg/kg/day in equally divided doses by the routes and schedule designated above.

Note: In patients undergoing prosthetic arthroplasty, administration is recommended for as long as 72 hours.

In patients undergoing cesarean section, the initial dose may be administered just prior to surgery or immediately after the cord has been clamped.

Impaired Renal Function—When renal function is impaired, a reduced dosage must be employed and the serum levels closely monitored. After an initial dose of 1 to 2 g (depending on the severity of infection), a maintenance dosage schedule should be followed (see chart). Continued dosage should be determined by degree of renal impairment, severity of infection, and susceptibility of the causative organism.

[See table at top of next page]

When only serum creatinine is available, the following formula (based on sex, weight, and age of the patient) may be used to convert this value into creatinine clearance. The serum creatinine should represent a steady state of renal function.

$$\text{Males: } \frac{\text{Weight (kg)} \times (140 - \text{age})}{72 \times \text{serum creatinine}}$$

Females: 0.9 × above value

Modes of Administration—Mandol may be given intravenously or by deep intramuscular injection into a large muscle mass (such as the gluteus or lateral part of the thigh) to minimize pain.

Intramuscular Administration—Each g of Mandol should be diluted with 3 mL of 1 of the following diluents: Sterile

MAINTENANCE DOSAGE GUIDE FOR PATIENTS WITH RENAL IMPAIRMENT

Creatinine Clearance (mL/min/1.73 m^2)	Renal Function	Life-Threatening Infections— Maximum Dosage	Less Severe Infections
>80	Normal	2 g q4h	1–2 g q6h
80–50	Mild Impairment	1.5 g q4h OR 2 g q6h	0.75–1.5 g q6h
50–25	Moderate Impairment	1.5 g q6h OR 2 g q8h	0.75–1.5 g q8h
25–10	Severe Impairment	1 g q6h OR 1.25 g q8h	0.5–1 g q8h
10–2	Marked Impairment	0.67 g q8h OR 1 g q12h	0.5–0.75 g q12h
<2	None	0.5 g q8h OR 0.75 g q12h	0.25–0.5 g q12h

Water for Injection, Bacteriostatic Water for Injection, 0.9% Sodium Chloride Injection, or Bacteriostatic Sodium Chloride Injection. Shake well until dissolved.

Intravenous Administration —The intravenous route may be preferable for patients with bacterial septicemia, localized parenchymal abscesses (such as intra-abdominal abscess), peritonitis, or other severe or life-threatening infections when they may be poor risks because of lowered resistance. In those with normal renal function, the intravenous dosage for such infections is 3 to 12 g of Mandol daily. In conditions such as bacterial septicemia, 6 to 12 g/day may be given initially by the intravenous route for several days, and dosage may then be gradually reduced according to clinical response and laboratory findings.

If combination therapy with Mandol and an aminoglycoside is indicated, each of these antibiotics should be administered in different sites. *Do not mix an aminoglycoside with Mandol in the same intravenous fluid container.*

A SOLUTION OF 1 G OF MANDOL IN 22 ML OF STERILE WATER FOR INJECTION IS ISOTONIC.

The choice of saline, dextrose, or electrolyte solution and the volume to be employed are dictated by fluid and electrolyte management.

For direct intermittent intravenous administration, each g of cefamandole should be reconstituted with 10 mL of Sterile Water for Injection, 5% Dextrose Injection, or 0.9% Sodium Chloride Injection. Slowly inject the solution into the vein over a period of 3 to 5 minutes, or give it through the tubing of an administration set while the patient is also receiving 1 of the following intravenous fluids: 0.9% Sodium Chloride Injection; 5% Dextrose Injection; 10% Dextrose Injection; 5% Dextrose and 0.9% Sodium Chloride Injection; 5% Dextrose and 0.45% Sodium Chloride Injection; 5% Dextrose and 0.2% Sodium Chloride Injection; or Sodium Lactate Injection (M/6).

Intermittent intravenous infusion with a Y-type administration set or volume control set can also be accomplished while any of the above-mentioned intravenous fluids are being infused. However, during infusion of the solution containing Mandol, it is desirable to discontinue the other solution. When this technique is employed, careful attention should be paid to the volume of the solution containing Mandol so that the calculated dose will be infused. If Sterile Water for Injection is used as the diluent, reconstitute with approximately 20 mL/g to avoid a hypotonic solution.

For continuous intravenous infusion, each g of cefamandole should be diluted with 10 mL of Sterile Water for Injection. An appropriate quantity of the resulting solution may be added to an IV bottle containing 1 of the following fluids: 0.9% Sodium Chloride Injection; 5% Dextrose Injection; 10% Dextrose Injection; 5% Dextrose and 0.9% Sodium Chloride Injection; 5% Dextrose and 0.45% Sodium Chloride Injection; 5% Dextrose and 0.2% Sodium Chloride Injection; or Sodium Lactate Injection (M/6).

STABILITY

Reconstituted Mandol is stable for 24 hours at room temperature (25°C) and for 96 hours if stored under refrigeration (5°C). *During storage at room temperature, carbon dioxide develops inside the vial after reconstitution. This pressure may be dissipated prior to withdrawal of the vial contents, or it may be used to aid withdrawal if the vial is inverted over the syringe needle and the contents are allowed to flow into the syringe.*

Solutions of Mandol in Sterile Water for Injection, 5% Dextrose Injection, or 0.9% Sodium Chloride Injection that are frozen immediately after reconstitution in the conventional vials in which the drugs are supplied are stable for 6 months when stored at −20°C. **If the product is warmed (to a maximum of 37°C), care should be taken to avoid heating it after the thawing is complete. Once thawed, the solution should not be refrozen.**

HOW SUPPLIED

Vials (Dry Powder):

1 g,* 10-mL size (No. 7061)—(Traypak† of 25) NDC 0002-7061-25

2 g,* 20-mL size (No. 7064)—(Traypak of 10) NDC 0002-7064-10

*Equivalent to cefamandole activity.

†Traypak™ (multivial carton, Lilly).

Literature revised August 13, 1999

IT 0480 ITAMP [081399]

1. Bauer AW, Kirby WMM, et al: Antibiotic susceptibility testing by a standardized single disk method. *Am J Clin Pathol* 1966;45:493. Standardized disk susceptibility test. *Federal Register* 1974;39:19182–19184. National Committee for Clinical Laboratory Standards. Approved Standard: M2-A3 Performance standards for antimicrobial disk susceptibility tests—Fourth Edition, December, 1988.

2. Determined by the ICS agar-dilution method (Ericsson HM, Sherris JC: *Acta Pathol Microbiol Scand* 1971;[suppl 217]:B), or any other method that has been shown to give equivalent results.

NEBCIN® ℞

[*nĕb 'sĭn*]

(Tobramycin Sulfate Injection, USP)

WARNINGS

Patients treated with Nebcin® (Tobramycin Sulfate Injection, USP) and other aminoglycosides should be under close clinical observation, because these drugs have an inherent potential for causing ototoxicity and nephrotoxicity.

Neurotoxicity, manifested as both auditory and vestibular ototoxicity, can occur. The auditory changes are irreversible, are usually bilateral, and may be partial or total. Eighth-nerve impairment and nephrotoxicity may develop, primarily in patients having preexisting renal damage and in those with normal renal function to whom aminoglycosides are administered for longer periods or in higher doses than those recommended. Other manifestations of neurotoxicity may include numbness, skin tingling, muscle twitching, and convulsions. The risk of aminoglycoside-induced hearing loss increases with the degree of exposure to either high peak or high trough serum concentrations. Patients who develop cochlear damage may not have symptoms during therapy to warn them of eighth-nerve toxicity, and partial or total irreversible bilateral deafness may continue to develop after the drug has been discontinued.

Rarely, nephrotoxicity may not become apparent until the first few days after cessation of therapy. Aminoglycoside-induced nephrotoxicity usually is reversible.

Renal and eighth-nerve function should be closely monitored in patients with known or suspected renal impairment and also in those whose renal function is initially normal but who develop signs of renal dysfunction during therapy. Peak and trough serum concentrations of aminoglycosides should be monitored periodically during therapy to assure adequate levels and to avoid potentially toxic levels. Prolonged serum concentrations above 12 µg/mL should be avoided. Rising trough levels (above 2 µg/mL) may indicate tissue accumulation. Such accumulation, excessive peak concentrations, advanced age, and cumulative dose may contribute to ototoxicity and nephrotoxicity (*see* **PRECAUTIONS**). Urine should be examined for decreased specific gravity and increased excretion of protein, cells, and casts. Blood urea nitrogen, serum creatinine, and creatinine clearance should be measured periodically. When feasible, it is recommended that serial audiograms be obtained in patients old enough to be tested, particularly high-risk patients. Evidence of impairment of renal, vestibular, or auditory function requires discontinuation of the drug or dosage adjustment.

Nebcin should be used with caution in premature and neonatal infants because of their renal immaturity and the resulting prolongation of serum half-life of the drug.

Concurrent and sequential use of other neurotoxic and/or nephrotoxic antibiotics, particularly other aminoglycosides (eg, amikacin, streptomycin, neomycin, kanamycin, gentamicin, and paromomycin), cephaloridine, viomycin, polymyxin B, colistin, cisplatin, and vancomycin, should be avoided. Other factors that may increase patient risk are advanced age and dehydration.

Aminoglycosides should not be given concurrently with potent diuretics, such as ethacrynic acid and furosemide. Some diuretics themselves cause ototoxicity, and intravenously administered diuretics enhance aminoglycoside toxicity by altering antibiotic concentrations in serum and tissue.

Aminoglycosides can cause fetal harm when administered to a pregnant woman (*see* **PRECAUTIONS**).

DESCRIPTION

Tobramycin sulfate, a water-soluble antibiotic of the aminoglycoside group, is derived from the actinomycete *Streptomyces tenebrarius.* Nebcin, Injection, is a clear and colorless sterile aqueous solution for parenteral administration. Tobramycin sulfate is *O*-3-amino-3-deoxy-α-D-glucopyranosyl-(1→4)-*O*-[2,6-diamino-2,3,6-trideoxy-α-D-*ribo*-hexopyranosyl-(1→6)]-2-deoxy-L-streptamine, sulfate (2:5)(salt) and has the chemical formula $(C_{18}H_{37}N_5O_9)_2 \bullet 5H_2SO_4$. The molecular weight is 1425.45. The structural formula for tobramycin is as follows:

Each mL also contains phenol as a preservative (5 mg, multiple-dose vials; 1.25 mg, ADD-Vantage® vials), sodium bisulfite (3.2 mg, multiple-dose vials; 1.6 mg, ADD-Vantage vials), 0.1 mg edetate disodium, and water for injection, qs. Sulfuric acid and/or sodium hydroxide may have been added to adjust the pH.

CLINICAL PHARMACOLOGY

Tobramycin is rapidly absorbed following intramuscular administration. Peak serum concentrations of tobramycin occur between 30 and 90 minutes after intramuscular administration. Following an intramuscular dose of 1 mg/kg of body weight, maximum serum concentrations reach about 4 mcg/mL, and measurable levels persist for as long as 8 hours. Therapeutic serum levels are generally considered to range from 4 to 6 mcg/mL. When Nebcin is administered by intravenous infusion over a 1-hour period, the serum concentrations are similar to those obtained by intramuscular administration. Nebcin is poorly absorbed from the gastrointestinal tract.

In patients with normal renal function, except neonates, Nebcin administered every 8 hours does not accumulate in the serum. However, in those patients with reduced renal function and in neonates, the serum concentration of the antibiotic is usually higher and can be measured for longer periods of time than in normal adults. Dosage for such patients must, therefore, be adjusted accordingly (*see* **DOSAGE AND ADMINISTRATION**).

Following parenteral administration, little, if any, metabolic transformation occurs, and tobramycin is eliminated almost exclusively by glomerular filtration. Renal clearance is similar to that of endogenous creatinine. Ultrafiltration studies demonstrate that practically no serum protein binding occurs. In patients with normal renal function, up to 84% of the dose is recoverable from the urine in 8 hours and up to 93% in 24 hours.

Peak urine concentrations ranging from 75 to 100 mcg/mL have been observed following the intramuscular injection of a single dose of 1 mg/kg. After several days of treatment, the amount of tobramycin excreted in the urine approaches the daily dose administered. When renal function is impaired, excretion of Nebcin is slowed, and accumulation of the drug may cause toxic blood levels.

The serum half-life in normal individuals is 2 hours. An inverse relationship exists between serum half-life and creat-

Continued on next page

*** Identi-Code® symbol. This product information was prepared in June 2000. Current information on these and other products of Eli Lilly and Company may be obtained by direct inquiry to Lilly Research Laboratories, Lilly Corporate Center, Indianapolis, Indiana 46285, (800) 545-5979.**

Nebcin—Cont.

inine clearance, and the dosage schedule should be adjusted according to the degree of renal impairment (*see* **DOSAGE AND ADMINISTRATION**). In patients undergoing dialysis, 25% to 70% of the administered dose may be removed, depending on the duration and type of dialysis.

Tobramycin can be detected in tissues and body fluids after parenteral administration. Concentrations in bile and stools ordinarily have been low, which suggests minimum biliary excretion. Tobramycin has appeared in low concentration in the cerebrospinal fluid following parenteral administration, and concentrations are dependent on dose, rate of penetration, and degree of meningeal inflammation. It has also been found in sputum, peritoneal fluid, synovial fluid, and abscess fluids, and it crosses the placental membranes. Concentrations in the renal cortex are several times higher than the usual serum levels.

Probenecid does not affect the renal tubular transport of tobramycin.

Microbiology – Tobramycin acts by inhibiting synthesis of protein in bacterial cells. *In vitro* tests demonstrate that tobramycin is bactericidal.

Tobramycin has been shown to be active against most strains of the following organisms both *in vitro* and in clinical infections as described in the Indications and Usage section:

Aerobic Gram-positive microorganisms

Staphylococcus aureus

Aerobic Gram-negative microorganisms

Citrobacter species
Enterobacter species
Escherichia coli
Klebsiella species
Morganella morganii
Pseudomonas aeruginosa
Proteus mirabilis
Proteus vulgaris
Providencia species
Serratia species

Aminoglycosides have a low order of activity against most gram-positive organisms, including *Streptococcus pyogenes, Streptococcus pneumoniae,* and enterococci.

Although most strains of enterococci demonstrate *in vitro* resistance, some strains in this group are susceptible. *In vitro* studies have shown that an aminoglycoside combined with an antibiotic that interferes with cell-wall synthesis affects some enterococcal strains synergistically. The combination of penicillin G and tobramycin results in a synergistic bactericidal effect *in vitro* against certain strains of *Enterococcus faecalis*. However, this combination is not synergistic against other closely related organisms, eg, *Enterococcus faecium*. Speciation of enterococci alone cannot be used to predict susceptibility. Susceptibility testing and tests for antibiotic synergism are emphasized.

Cross resistance between aminoglycosides may occur.

Susceptibility Tests —

Diffusion techniques: Quantitative methods that require measurement of zone diameters give the most precise estimates of susceptibility of bacteria to antimicrobial agents. One such procedure is the National Committee for Clinical Laboratory Standards (NCCLS)-approved procedure.[1] This method has been recommended for use with disks to test susceptibility to tobramycin. Interpretation involves correlation of the diameters obtained in the disk test with minimum inhibitory concentrations (MIC) for tobramycin.

Reports from the laboratory giving results of the standard single-disk susceptibility test with a 10-mcg tobramycin disk should be interpreted according to the following criteria:

Zone Diameter (mm)	Interpretation
≥15	(S) Susceptible
13–14	(I) Intermediate
≤12	(R) Resistant

A report of "Susceptible" indicates that the pathogen is likely to be inhibited by generally achievable blood levels. A report of "Intermediate" suggests that the organism would be susceptible if high dosage is used or if the infection is confined to tissues and fluids in which high antimicrobial levels are obtained. A report of "Resistant" indicates that achievable concentrations are unlikely to be inhibitory and other therapy should be selected.

Standardized procedures require the use of laboratory control organisms. The 10-mcg tobramycin disk should give the following zone diameters:

Organism	Zone Diameter (mm)
E. coli ATCC 25922	18–26
P. aeruginosa ATCC 27853	19–25
S. aureus ATCC 25923	19–29

Dilution techniques: Broth and agar dilution methods, such as those recommended by the NCCLS,[2] may be used to determine MICs of tobramycin. MIC test results should be interpreted according to the following criteria:

MIC (mcg/mL)	Interpretation
≤4	(S) Susceptible
8	(I) Intermediate
≥16	(R) Resistant

As with standard diffusion methods, dilution procedures require the use of laboratory control organisms. Tobramycin laboratory reagent should give the following MIC values:

Organism	MIC Range (mcg/mL)
E. faecalis ATCC 29212	8–32
E. coli ATCC 25922	0.25–1
P. aeruginosa ATCC 27853	0.25–1
S. aureus ATCC 29213	0.12–1

INDICATIONS AND USAGE

Nebcin is indicated for the treatment of serious bacterial infections caused by susceptible strains of the designated microorganisms in the diseases listed below:

Septicemia in the pediatric patient and adult caused by *P. aeruginosa, E. coli,* and *Klebsiella* spp

Lower respiratory tract infections caused by *P. aeruginosa, Klebsiella* spp, *Enterobacter* spp, *Serratia* spp, *E. coli,* and *S. aureus* (penicillinase- and non-penicillinase-producing strains)

Serious central-nervous-system infections (meningitis) caused by susceptible organisms

Intra-abdominal infections, including peritonitis, caused by *E. coli, Klebsiella* spp, and *Enterobacter* spp

Skin, bone, and skin structure infections caused by *P. aeruginosa, Proteus* spp, *E. coli, Klebsiella* spp, *Enterobacter* spp, and *S. aureus*

Complicated and recurrent urinary tract infections caused by *P. aeruginosa, Proteus* spp (indole-positive and indole-negative), *E. coli, Klebsiella* spp, *Enterobacter* spp, *Serratia* spp, *S. aureus, Providencia* spp, and *Citrobacter* spp

Aminoglycosides, including Nebcin, are not indicated in uncomplicated initial episodes of urinary tract infections unless the causative organisms are not susceptible to antibiotics having less potential toxicity. Nebcin may be considered in serious staphylococcal infections when penicillin or other potentially less toxic drugs are contraindicated and when bacterial susceptibility testing and clinical judgment indicate its use.

Bacterial cultures should be obtained prior to and during treatment to isolate and identify etiologic organisms and to test their susceptibility to tobramycin. If susceptibility tests show that the causative organisms are resistant to tobramycin, other appropriate therapy should be instituted. In patients in whom a serious life-threatening gram-negative infection is suspected, including those in whom concurrent therapy with a penicillin or cephalosporin and an aminoglycoside may be indicated, treatment with Nebcin may be initiated before the results of susceptibility studies are obtained. The decision to continue therapy with Nebcin should be based on the results of susceptibility studies, the severity of the infection, and the important additional concepts discussed in the Warnings box above.

CONTRAINDICATIONS

A hypersensitivity to any aminoglycoside is a contraindication to the use of tobramycin. A history of hypersensitivity or serious toxic reactions to aminoglycosides may also contraindicate the use of any other aminoglycoside because of the known cross-sensitivity of patients to drugs in this class.

WARNINGS

See **WARNINGS** box above.

Nebcin contains sodium bisulfite, a sulfite that may cause allergic-type reactions, including anaphylactic symptoms and life-threatening or less severe asthmatic episodes, in certain susceptible people. The overall prevalence of sulfite sensitivity in the general population is unknown and probably low. Sulfite sensitivity is seen more frequently in asthmatic than in nonasthmatic people.

Serious allergic reactions including anaphylaxis and dermatologic reactions including exfoliative dermatitis, toxic epidermal necrolysis, erythema multiforme, and Stevens-Johnson Syndrome have been reported rarely in patients on tobramycin therapy. Although rare, fatalities have been reported. (*See* **CONTRAINDICATIONS**.)

If an allergic reaction occurs, the drug should be discontinued and appropriate therapy instituted.

PRECAUTIONS

Serum and urine specimens for examination should be collected during therapy, as recommended in the WARNINGS box. Serum calcium, magnesium, and sodium should be monitored.

Peak and trough serum levels should be measured periodically during therapy. Prolonged concentrations above 12 mcg/mL should be avoided. Rising trough levels (above 2 mcg/mL) may indicate tissue accumulation. Such accumulation, advanced age, and cumulative dosage may contribute to ototoxicity and nephrotoxicity. It is particularly important to monitor serum levels closely in patients with known renal impairment.

A useful guideline would be to perform serum level assays after 2 or 3 doses, so that the dosage could be adjusted if necessary, and at 3- to 4-day intervals during therapy. In the event of changing renal function, more frequent serum levels should be obtained and the dosage or dosage interval adjusted according to the guidelines provided in the Dosage and Administration section.

In order to measure the peak level, a serum sample should be drawn about 30 minutes following intravenous infusion or 1 hour after an intramuscular injection. Trough levels are measured by obtaining serum samples at 8 hours or just prior to the next dose of Nebcin. These suggested time intervals are intended only as guidelines and may vary according to institutional practices. It is important, however, that there be consistency within the individual patient program unless computerized pharmacokinetic dosing programs are available in the institution. These serum-level assays may be especially useful for monitoring the treatment of severely ill patients with changing renal function or of those infected with less susceptible organisms or those receiving maximum dosage.

Neuromuscular blockade and respiratory paralysis have been reported in cats receiving very high doses of tobramycin (40 mg/kg). The possibility of prolonged or secondary apnea should be considered if tobramycin is administered to anesthetized patients who are also receiving neuromuscular blocking agents, such as succinylcholine, tubocurarine, or decamethonium, or to patients receiving massive transfusions of citrated blood. If neuromuscular blockade occurs, it may be reversed by the administration of calcium salts.

Cross-allergenicity among aminoglycosides has been demonstrated.

In patients with extensive burns, or cystic fibrosis, altered pharmacokinetics may result in reduced serum concentrations of aminoglycosides. In such patients treated with Nebcin, measurement of serum concentration is especially important as a basis for determination of appropriate dosage.

Elderly patients may have reduced renal function that may not be evident in the results of routine screening tests, such as BUN or serum creatinine. A creatinine clearance determination may be more useful. Monitoring of renal function during treatment with aminoglycosides is particularly important in such patients.

An increased incidence of nephrotoxicity has been reported following concomitant administration of aminoglycoside antibiotics and cephalosporins.

Aminoglycosides should be used with caution in patients with muscular disorders, such as myasthenia gravis or parkinsonism, since these drugs may aggravate muscle weakness because of their potential curare-like effect on neuromuscular function.

Aminoglycosides may be absorbed in significant quantities from body surfaces after local irrigation or application and may cause neurotoxicity and nephrotoxicity.

Aminoglycosides have not been approved for intraocular and/or subconjunctival use. Physicians are advised that macular necrosis has been reported following administration of aminoglycosides, including tobramycin, by these routes.

See **WARNINGS** box regarding concurrent use of potent diuretics and concurrent and sequential use of other neurotoxic or nephrotoxic drugs.

The inactivation of tobramycin and other aminoglycosides by β-lactam-type antibiotics (penicillins or cephalosporins) has been demonstrated *in vitro* and in patients with severe renal impairment. Such inactivation has not been found in patients with normal renal function who have been given the drugs by separate routes of administration.

Therapy with tobramycin may result in overgrowth of nonsusceptible organisms. If overgrowth of nonsusceptible organisms occurs, appropriate therapy should be initiated.

Pregnancy Category D —Aminoglycosides can cause fetal harm when administered to a pregnant woman. Aminoglycoside antibiotics cross the placenta, and there have been several reports of total irreversible bilateral congenital deafness in children whose mothers received streptomycin during pregnancy. Serious side effects to mother, fetus, or newborn have not been reported in the treatment of pregnant women with other aminoglycosides. If tobramycin is used during pregnancy or if the patient becomes pregnant while taking tobramycin, she should be apprised of the potential hazard to the fetus.

Pediatric Use —See **INDICATIONS AND USAGE** *and* **DOSAGE AND ADMINISTRATION**.

ADVERSE REACTIONS

Neurotoxicity —Adverse effects on both the vestibular and auditory branches of the eighth nerve have been noted, especially in patients receiving high doses or prolonged therapy, in those given previous courses of therapy with an ototoxin, and in cases of dehydration. Symptoms include dizziness, vertigo, tinnitus, roaring in the ears, and hearing loss. Hearing loss is usually irreversible and is manifested initially by diminution of high-tone acuity. Tobramycin and gentamicin sulfates closely parallel each other in regard to ototoxic potential.

Nephrotoxicity —Renal function changes, as shown by rising BUN, NPN, and serum creatinine and by oliguria, cylindruria, and increased proteinuria, have been reported, especially in patients with a history of renal impairment who are treated for longer periods or with higher doses than those recommended. Adverse renal effects can occur in patients with initially normal renal function.

Clinical studies and studies in experimental animals have been conducted to compare the nephrotoxic potential of tobramycin and gentamicin. In some of the clinical studies and in the animal studies, tobramycin caused nephrotoxicity significantly less frequently than gentamicin. In some other clinical studies, no significant difference in the incidence of nephrotoxicity between tobramycin and gentamicin was found.

Other reported adverse reactions possibly related to Nebcin include anemia, granulocytopenia, and thrombocytopenia; and fever, rash, exfoliative dermatitis, itching, urticaria, nausea, vomiting, diarrhea, headache, lethargy, pain at the injection site, mental confusion, and disorientation. Laboratory abnormalities possibly related to Nebcin include increased serum transaminases (AST, ALT); increased serum LDH and bilirubin; decreased serum calcium, magnesium, sodium, and potassium; and leukopenia, leukocytosis, and eosinophilia.

OVERDOSAGE

Signs and Symptoms —The severity of the signs and symptoms following a tobramycin overdose are dependent on the dose administered, the patient's renal function, state of hydration, and age and whether or not other medications with similar toxicities are being administered concurrently. Toxicity may occur in patients treated more than 10 days, in adults given more than 5 mg/kg/day, in pediatric patients given more than 7.5 mg/kg/day, or in patients with reduced renal function where dose has not been appropriately adjusted.

Nephrotoxicity following the parenteral administration of an aminoglycoside is most closely related to the area under the curve of the serum concentration versus time graph. Nephrotoxicity is more likely if trough blood concentrations fail to fall below 2 mcg/mL and is also proportional to the average blood concentration. Patients who are elderly, have abnormal renal function, are receiving other nephrotoxic drugs, or are volume depleted are at greater risk for developing acute tubular necrosis. Auditory and vestibular toxicities have been associated with aminoglycoside overdose. These toxicities occur in patients treated longer than 10 days, in patients with abnormal renal function, in dehydrated patients, or in patients receiving medications with additive auditory toxicities. These patients may not have signs or symptoms or may experience dizziness, tinnitus, vertigo, and a loss of high-tone acuity as ototoxicity progresses. Ototoxicity signs and symptoms may not begin to occur until long after the drug has been discontinued.

Neuromuscular blockade or respiratory paralysis may occur following administration of aminoglycosides. Neuromuscular blockade, respiratory failure, and prolonged respiratory paralysis may occur more commonly in patients with myasthenia gravis or Parkinson's disease. Prolonged respiratory paralysis may also occur in patients receiving decamethonium, tubocurarine, or succinylcholine. If neuromuscular blockade occurs, it may be reversed by the administration of calcium salts but mechanical assistance may be necessary.

If tobramycin were ingested, toxicity would be less likely because aminoglycosides are poorly absorbed from an intact gastrointestinal tract.

Treatment —In all cases of suspected overdosage, call your Regional Poison Control Center to obtain the most up-to-date information about the treatment of overdose. This recommendation is made because, in general, information regarding the treatment of overdose may change more rapidly than the package insert. In managing overdosage, consider the possibility of multiple drug overdoses, interaction among drugs, and unusual drug kinetics in your patient.

The initial intervention in a tobramycin overdose is to establish an airway and ensure oxygenation and ventilation. Resuscitative measures should be initiated promptly if respiratory paralysis occurs.

Patients who have received an overdose of tobramycin and who have normal renal function should be adequately hydrated to maintain a urine output of 3 to 5 mL/kg/hr. Fluid balance, creatinine clearance, and tobramycin plasma levels should be carefully monitored until the serum tobramycin level falls below 2 mcg/mL.

Patients in whom the elimination half-life is greater than 2 hours or whose renal function is abnormal may require more aggressive therapy. In such patients, hemodialysis may be beneficial.

DOSAGE AND ADMINISTRATION

Nebcin may be given intramuscularly or intravenously. ADD-Vantage vials are not for intramuscular administration. Recommended dosages are the same for both routes. The patient's pretreatment body weight should be obtained for calculation of correct dosage. It is desirable to measure both peak and trough serum concentrations (*see* **WARNINGS** box *and* **PRECAUTIONS**).

Administration for Patients With Normal Renal Function —Adults With Serious Infections: 3 mg/kg/day in 3 equal doses every 8 hours (*see* Table 1).

Adults With Life-Threatening Infections: Up to 5 mg/kg/day may be administered in 3 or 4 equal doses (*see* Table 1). The dosage should be reduced to 3 mg/kg/day as soon as clinically indicated. To prevent increased toxicity due to excessive blood levels, dosage should not exceed 5 mg/kg/day unless serum levels are monitored (*see* **WARNINGS** box *and* **PRECAUTIONS**).

[See table 1 above]

Pediatric patients (greater than 1 week of age): 6 to 7.5 mg/kg/day in 3 or 4 equally divided doses (2 to 2.5 mg/kg every 8 hours or 1.5 to 1.89 mg/kg every 6 hours).

Premature or Full-Term Neonates 1 Week of Age or Less: Up to 4 mg/kg/day may be administered in 2 equal doses every 12 hours.

It is desirable to limit treatment to a short term. The usual duration of treatment is 7 to 10 days. A longer course of therapy may be necessary in difficult and complicated infections. In such cases, monitoring of renal, auditory, and vestibular functions is advised, because neurotoxicity is more likely to occur when treatment is extended longer than 10 days.

TABLE 1. DOSAGE SCHEDULE GUIDE FOR ADULTS WITH NORMAL RENAL FUNCTION
(Dosage at 8-Hour Intervals)

For Patient Weighing kg	lb	Usual Dose for Serious Infections 1 mg/kg q8h (Total, 3 mg/kg/day) mg/dose	q8h mL/dose*	Maximum Dose for Life-Thr!eatening Infections (Reduce as soon as possible) 1.66 mg/kg q8h (Total, 5 mg/kg/day) mg/dose	q8h mL/dose*
120	264	120 mg	3 mL	200 mg	5 mL
115	253	115 mg	2.9 mL	191 mg	4.75 mL
110	242	110 mg	2.75 mL	183 mg	4.5 mL
105	231	105 mg	2.6 mL	175 mg	4.4 mL
100	220	100 mg	2.5 mL	166 mg	4.2 mL
95	209	95 mg	2.4 mL	158 mg	4 mL
90	198	90 mg	2.25 mL	150 mg	3.75 mL
85	187	85 mg	2.1 mL	141 mg	3.5 mL
80	176	80 mg	2 mL	133 mg	3.3 mL
75	165	75 mg	1.9 mL	125 mg	3.1 mL
70	154	70 mg	1.75 mL	116 mg	2.9 mL
65	143	65 mg	1.6 mL	108 mg	2.7 mL
60	132	60 mg	1.5 mL	100 mg	2.5 mL
55	121	55 mg	1.4 mL	91 mg	2.25 mL
50	110	50 mg	1.25 mL	83 mg	2.1 mL
45	99	45 mg	1.1 mL	75 mg	1.9 mL
40	88	40 mg	1 mL	66 mg	1.6 mL

*Applicable to all product forms except Nebcin, Pediatric, Injection (*see* How Supplied).

Dosage in Patients with Cystic Fibrosis—In patients with cystic fibrosis, altered pharmacokinetics may result in reduced serum concentrations of aminoglycosides. Measurement of tobramycin serum concentration during treatment is especially important as a basis for determining appropriate dose. In patients with severe cystic fibrosis, an initial dosing regimen of 10 mg/kg/day in 4 equally divided doses is recommended. This dosing regimen is suggested only as a guide. The serum levels of tobramycin should be measured directly during treatment due to wide interpatient variability.

Administration for Patients With Impaired Renal Function —Whenever possible, serum tobramycin concentrations should be monitored during therapy.

Following a loading dose of 1 mg/kg, subsequent dosage in these patients must be adjusted, either with reduced doses administered at 8-hour intervals or with normal doses given at prolonged intervals. Both of these methods are suggested as guides to be used when serum levels of tobramycin cannot be measured directly. They are based on either the creatinine clearance level or the serum creatinine level of the patient because these values correlate with the half-life of tobramycin. The dosage schedule derived from either method should be used in conjunction with careful clinical and laboratory observations of the patient and should be modified as necessary. Neither method should be used when dialysis is being performed.

Reduced dosage at 8-hour intervals: When the creatinine clearance rate is 70 mL or less per minute or when the serum creatinine value is known, the amount of the reduced dose can be determined by multiplying the normal dose from Table 1 by the percent of normal dose from the accompanying nomogram.

REDUCED DOSAGE NOMOGRAM*
Creatinine Clearance (mL/min/1.73 m²)

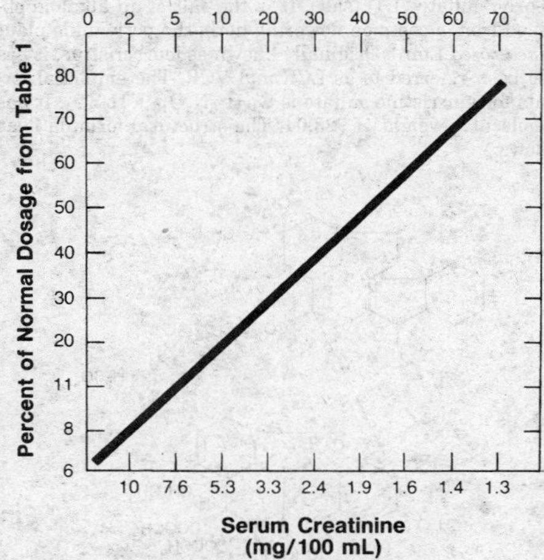

***Scales have been adjusted to facilitate dosage calculations.**

An alternate rough guide for determining reduced dosage at 8-hour intervals (for patients whose steady-state serum creatinine values are known) is to divide the normally recommended dose by the patient's serum creatinine.

Normal dosage at prolonged intervals: If the creatinine clearance rate is not available and the patient's condition is stable, a dosage frequency *in hours* for the dosage given in Table 1 can be determined by multiplying the patient's serum creatinine by 6.

Dosage in Obese Patients —The appropriate dose may be calculated by using the patient's estimated lean body weight plus 40% of the excess as the basic weight on which to figure mg/kg.

Intramuscular Administration —Nebcin may be administered by withdrawing the appropriate dose directly from a vial. ADD-Vantage vials are not for intramuscular administration.

Intravenous Administration—For intravenous administration, the usual volume of diluent (0.9% Sodium Chloride Injection or 5% Dextrose Injection) is 50 to 100 mL for adult doses. For pediatric patients, the volume of diluent should be proportionately less than that for adults. The diluted solution usually should be infused over a period of 20 to 60 minutes. Infusion periods of less than 20 minutes are not recommended, because peak serum levels may exceed 12 mcg/mL (*see* **WARNINGS** box).

Use of ADD-Vantage Nebcin Vials —ADD-Vantage Nebcin vials are not intended for multiple use and should not be used with a syringe in the conventional way. These products are intended for use only with Abbott ADD-Vantage diluent containers and in those instances in which the physician's order specified 60-mg or 80-mg doses. Use within 24 hours after activation.

Nebcin should not be physically premixed with other drugs but should be administered separately according to the recommended dose and route.

Prior to administration, parenteral drug products should be inspected visually for particulate matter and discoloration whenever solution and container permit.

INSTRUCTIONS FOR USE-*ADD-Vantage*® Vial

To Open:

Peel overwrap from the corner and remove container. Some opacity of the plastic due to moisture absorption during the sterilization process may be observed. This is normal and does not affect the solution quality or safety. The opacity will diminish gradually.

To Assemble Vial and Flexible Diluent Container: USE ASEPTIC TECHNIQUE

1. Remove the protective covers from the top of the vial and the vial port on the diluent container as follows:
a. To remove the breakaway vial cap, swing the pull ring over the top of the vial and pull down far enough to start the opening (SEE FIGURE 1.), then pull straight up to remove the cap. (SEE FIGURE 2.) NOTE: Do not access vial with syringe.

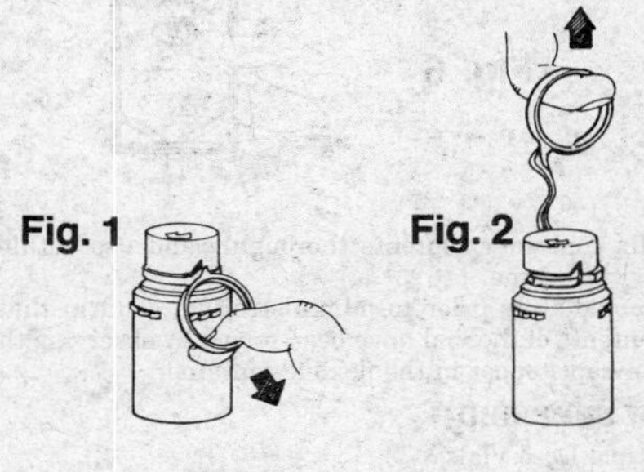

Continued on next page

*** Identi-Code® symbol. This product information was prepared in June 2000. Current information on these and other products of Eli Lilly and Company may be obtained by direct inquiry to Lilly Research Laboratories, Lilly Corporate Center, Indianapolis, Indiana 46285, (800) 545-5979.**

Nebcin—Cont.

b. To remove the vial port cover, grasp the tab on the pull ring, pull up to break the three tie strings, then pull back to remove the cover. (SEE FIGURE 3.)

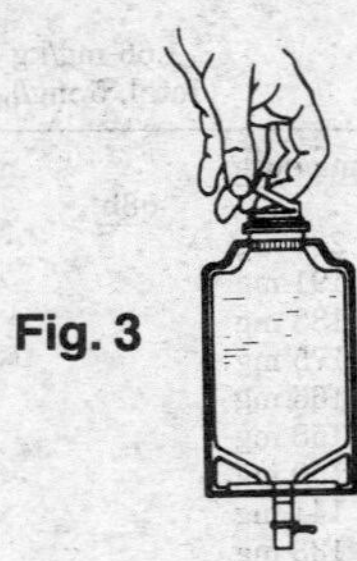

Fig. 3

2. Screw the vial into the vial port until it will go no further. THE VIAL MUST BE SCREWED IN TIGHTLY TO ASSURE A SEAL. This occurs approximately 1/2 turn (180°) after the first audible click. (SEE FIGURE 4.) The clicking sound does not assure a seal; the vial must be turned as far as it will go. NOTE: Once vial is seated, do not attempt to remove. (SEE FIGURE 4.)

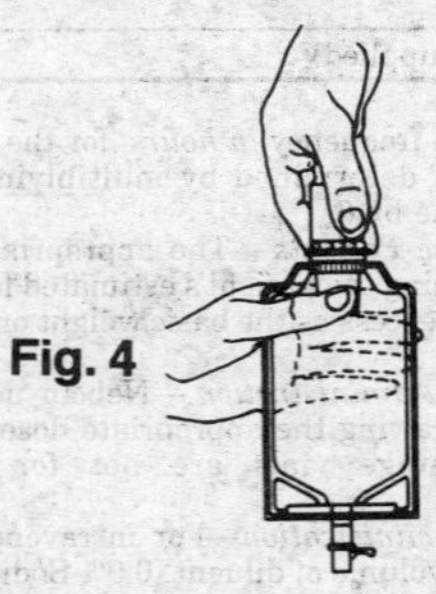

Fig. 4

3. Recheck the vial to assure that it is tight by trying to turn it further in the direction of assembly.
4. Label appropriately.

To Mix the Drug:

1. Squeeze the bottom of the diluent container gently to inflate the portion of the container surrounding the end of the drug vial.
2. With the other hand, push the drug vial down into the container telescoping the walls of the container. Grasp the inner cap of the vial through the walls of the container. (SEE FIGURE 5.)

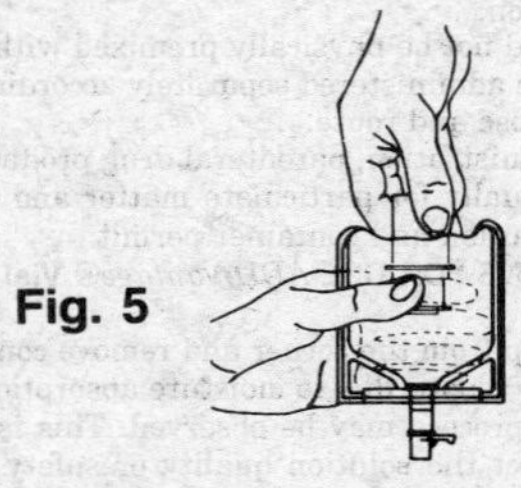

Fig. 5

3. Pull the inner cap from the drug vial (SEE FIGURE 6.) Verify that the rubber stopper has been pulled out, allowing the drug and diluent to mix.

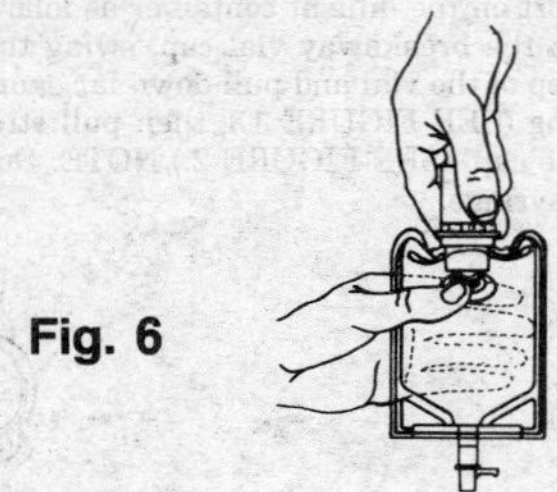

Fig. 6

4. Mix container contents thoroughly and use within the specified time.
5. Immediately prior to administration, confirm that the contents of the vial have been mixed by observing the inner cap/stopper in the flexible container.

HOW SUPPLIED

Multiple-Dose Vials:

80 mg*/2 mL, 2 mL (No. 781)—(Traypak† of 25) NDC 0002-1499-25

Pediatric, 20 mg*/2 mL, 2 mL (No. 782)—(1s) NDC 0002-0501-01

40 mg*/mL, 1.2 g/30 mL (No. 7090)—(Traypak of 6) NDC 0002-7090-16

ADD-Vantage Vials:

60 mg*/6 mL, 6 mL (No. 7293)—(Traypak of 25) NDC 0002-7293-25

80 mg*/8 mL, 8 mL (No. 7294)—(Traypak of 25) NDC 0002-7294-25

The above ADD-Vantage vials are to be used only with Abbott Laboratories' diluent containers.

Instructions for the use of ADD-Vantage vials are described above. (*See* **DOSAGE AND ADMINISTRATION**.)

Also Available:

Pharmacy Bulk Vial:

1.2 g* (Dry Powder) (40-mL size) (No. 7040)—(Traypak of 6) NDC 0002-7040-16

Store at controlled room temperature 59° to 86°F (15° to 30°C).

* Equivalent to tobramycin.

† Traypak™ (multivial carton, Lilly).

REFERENCES

1. National Committee for Clinical Laboratory Standards, Performance Standards for Antimicrobial Disk Susceptibility Tests—Sixth Edition. Approved Standard NCCLS Document M2-A6, Vol. 17, No 1, NCCLS, Wayne, PA, 1997.
2. National Committee for Clinical Laboratory Standards, Methods for Dilution Antimicrobial Susceptibility Tests for Bacteria that Grow Aerobically—Fourth Edition. Approved Standard NCCLS Document M7-A4, Vol. 17, No 2, NCCLS, Wayne, PA, 1997.

ADD-Vantage® (vials and diluent containers) is a registered trademark of Abbott Laboratories.

Literature revised March 25, 1999

PA 2012 AMP [032599]

NPH ILETIN® II OTC

(isophane insulin suspension, Lilly) See Under Iletin® (insulin)

ONCOVIN® ℞

[ŏn ′kō-vĭn]

(Vincristine Sulfate Injection, USP)

Solution

WARNINGS

Caution—This preparation should be administered by individuals experienced in the administration of Oncovin. It is extremely important that the intravenous needle or catheter be properly positioned before any Oncovin is injected. Leakage into surrounding tissue during intravenous administration of Oncovin may cause considerable irritation. If extravasation occurs, the injection should be discontinued immediately, and any remaining portion of the dose should then be introduced into another vein. Local injection of hyaluronidase and the application of moderate heat to the area of leakage help disperse the drug and are thought to minimize discomfort and the possibility of cellulitis. FATAL IF GIVEN INTRATHECALLY. FOR INTRAVENOUS USE ONLY. *See Warnings section for the treatment of patients given intrathecal Oncovin.*

DESCRIPTION

Oncovin® (Vincristine Sulfate, USP) is vincaleukoblastine, 22-oxo-, sulfate (1:1) (salt). It is the salt of an alkaloid obtained from a common flowering herb, the periwinkle plant (*Vinca rosea* Linn). Originally known as leurocristine, it has also been referred to as LCR and VCR. The empirical formula for vincristine sulfate is $C_{46}H_{56}N_4O_{10} \bullet H_2SO_4$. It has a molecular weight of 923.04. The structural formula is as follows:

[structural formula: OH, N, $-CH_2CH_3$, N H, $COOCH_3$, $\cdot H_2SO_4$, N, H, CH_2CH_3, CH_3O, N, CHO HO, $OCOCH_3$, $COOCH_3$]

Vincristine sulfate is a white to off-white powder. It is soluble in methanol, freely soluble in water, but only slightly soluble in 95% ethanol.

Each mL contains vincristine sulfate, 1 mg (1.08 µmol); mannitol, 100 mg; methylparaben, 1.3 mg; propylparaben, 0.2 mg; and water for injection, qs. Acetic acid and sodium acetate have been added for pH control. The pH of Oncovin Solution ranges from 3.5 to 5.5. This product is a sterile solution for cancer/oncolytic use.

CLINICAL PHARMACOLOGY

The mechanisms of action of Oncovin remain under investigation. The mechanism of action of Oncovin has been related to the inhibition of microtubule formation in the mitotic spindle, resulting in an arrest of dividing cells at the metaphase stage.

Central nervous system leukemia has been reported in patients undergoing otherwise successful therapy with Oncovin. This suggests that Oncovin does not penetrate well into the cerebrospinal fluid.

Pharmacokinetic studies in patients with cancer have shown a triphasic serum decay pattern following rapid intravenous injection. The initial, middle, and terminal half-lives are 5 minutes, 2.3 hours, and 85 hours respectively; however, the range of the terminal half-life in humans is from 19 to 155 hours. The liver is the major excretory organ in humans and animals. The metabolism of vinca alkaloids has been shown to be mediated by hepatic cytochrome P450 isoenzymes in the CYP 3A subfamily. This metabolic pathway may be impaired in patients with hepatic dysfunction or who are taking concomitant potent inhibitors of these isoenzymes (*see* Precautions). About 80% of an injected dose of Oncovin appears in the feces and 10% to 20% can be found in the urine. Within 15 to 30 minutes after injection, over 90% of the drug is distributed from the blood into tissue, where it remains tightly, but not irreversibly, bound.

Current principles of cancer chemotherapy involve the simultaneous use of several agents. Generally, each agent used has a unique toxicity and mechanism of action so that therapeutic enhancement occurs without additive toxicity. It is rarely possible to achieve equally good results with single-agent methods of treatment. Thus, Oncovin is often chosen as part of polychemotherapy because of lack of significant bone-marrow suppression (at recommended doses) and of unique clinical toxicity (neuropathy). *See* Dosage and Administration for possible increased toxicity when used in combination therapy.

INDICATIONS AND USAGE

Oncovin is indicated in acute leukemia.

Oncovin has also been shown to be useful in combination with other oncolytic agents in Hodgkin's disease, non-Hodgkin's malignant lymphomas (lymphocytic, mixed-cell, histiocytic, undifferentiated, nodular, and diffuse types), rhabdomyosarcoma, neuroblastoma, and Wilms' tumor.

CONTRAINDICATIONS

Patients with the demyelinating form of Charcot-Marie-Tooth syndrome should not be given Oncovin. Careful attention should be given to those conditions listed under Warnings *and* Precautions.

WARNINGS

This preparation is for intravenous use only. It should be administered by individuals experienced in the administration of Oncovin. The intrathecal administration of Oncovin usually results in death. Syringes containing this product should be labeled, using the auxiliary sticker provided, to state "FATAL IF GIVEN INTRATHECALLY. FOR INTRAVENOUS USE ONLY."

Extemporaneously prepared syringes containing this product must be packaged in an overwrap which is labeled "DO NOT REMOVE COVERING UNTIL MOMENT OF INJECTION. FATAL IF GIVEN INTRATHECALLY. FOR INTRAVENOUS USE ONLY."

After inadvertent intrathecal administration, immediate neurosurgical intervention is required in order to prevent ascending paralysis leading to death. In a very small number of patients, life-threatening paralysis and subsequent death was averted but resulted in devastating neurological sequelae, with limited recovery afterwards.

Based on the published management of these survival cases[1–3], if Oncovin is mistakenly given by the intrathecal route, the following treatment should be initiated **immediately after the injection:**

1. Removal of as much CSF as is safely possible through the lumbar access.
2. Insertion of an epidural catheter into the subarachnoid space via the intervertebral space above initial lumbar access and CSF irrigation with lactated Ringer's solution. Fresh frozen plasma should be requested and, when available, 25 mL should be added to every 1 liter of lactated Ringer's solution.
3. Insertion of an intraventricular drain or catheter by a neurosurgeon and continuation of CSF irrigation with fluid removal through the lumbar access connected to a closed drainage system. Lactated Ringer's solution should be given by continuous infusion at 150 mL/hour, or at a rate of 75 mL/hour when fresh frozen plasma has been added as above.

The rate of infusion should be adjusted to maintain a spinal fluid protein level of 150 mg/dL.

The following measures have also been used in addition but may not be essential:

Glutamic acid, 10 grams, has been given intravenously over 24 hours, followed by 500 mg three times daily by mouth for 1 month. Folinic acid has been administered intravenously as a 100 mg bolus and then infused at a rate of 25 mg/hour for 24 hours, then bolus doses of 25 mg every 6 hours for 1 week. Pyridoxine has been given at a dose of 50 mg every 8 hours by intravenous infusion over 30 minutes. Their roles in the reduction of neurotoxicity are unclear.

Pregnancy Category D—Oncovin can cause fetal harm when administered to a pregnant woman. When pregnant mice and hamsters were given doses of Oncovin that caused the resorption of 23% to 85% of fetuses, fetal malformations were produced in those that survived. Five monkeys were given single doses of Oncovin between days 27 and 34 of their pregnancies; 3 of the fetuses were normal at term, and 2 viable fetuses had grossly evident malformations at term. In several animal species, Oncovin can induce teratogenesis as well as embryo death at doses that are nontoxic to the pregnant animal. There are no adequate and well-controlled studies in pregnant women. If this drug is used during pregnancy or if the patient becomes pregnant while receiving this drug, she should be apprised of the potential hazard to the fetus. Women of childbearing potential should be advised to avoid becoming pregnant.

PRECAUTIONS

General—Acute uric acid nephropathy, which may occur after the administration of oncolytic agents, has also been reported with Oncovin. In the presence of leukopenia or a complicating infection, administration of the next dose of Oncovin warrants careful consideration.

If central nervous system leukemia is diagnosed, additional agents may be required because Oncovin does not appear to cross the blood-brain barrier in adequate amounts.

Particular attention should be given to dosage and neurologic side effects if Oncovin is administered to patients with preexisting neuromuscular disease and when other drugs with neurotoxic potential are also being used.

Acute shortness of breath and severe bronchospasm have been reported following the administration of vinca alkaloids. These reactions have been encountered most frequently when the vinca alkaloid was used in combination with mitomycin C and may require aggressive treatment, particularly when there is preexisting pulmonary dysfunction. The onset of these reactions may occur minutes to several hours after the vinca alkaloid is injected and may occur up to 2 weeks following the dose of mitomycin. Progressive dyspnea requiring chronic therapy may occur. Oncovin should not be readministered.

Care must be taken to avoid contamination of the eye with concentrations of Oncovin used clinically. If accidental contamination occurs, severe irritation (or, if the drug was delivered under pressure, even corneal ulceration) may result. The eye should be washed immediately and thoroughly.

Laboratory Tests—Because dose-limiting clinical toxicity is manifested as neurotoxicity, clinical evaluation (eg, history, physical examination) is necessary to detect the need for dosage modification. Following administration of Oncovin, some individuals may have a fall in the white-blood-cell count or platelet count, particularly when previous therapy or the disease itself has reduced bone-marrow function. Therefore, a complete blood count should be done before administration of each dose. Acute elevation of serum uric acid may also occur during induction of remission in acute leukemia; thus, such levels should be determined frequently during the first 3 to 4 weeks of treatment or appropriate measures taken to prevent uric acid nephropathy. The laboratory performing these tests should be consulted for its range of normal values.

Drug Interaction—The simultaneous oral or intravenous administration of phenytoin and antineoplastic chemotherapy combinations that included vincristine sulfate has been reported to reduce blood levels of the anticonvulsant and to increase seizure activity. Dosage adjustment should be based on serial blood level monitoring. The contribution of vincristine sulfate to this interaction is not certain. The interaction may result from reduced absorption of phenytoin and an increase in the rate of its metabolism and elimination.

Caution should be exercised in patients concurrently taking drugs known to inhibit drug metabolism by hepatic cytochrome P450 isoenzymes in the CYP 3A subfamily, or in patients with hepatic dysfunction. Concurrent administration of vincristine sulfate with itraconazole (a known inhibitor of the metabolic pathway) has been reported to cause an earlier onset and/or an increased severity of neuromuscular side effects (*see* Adverse Reactions). This interaction is presumed to be related to inhibition of the metabolism of vincristine.

Carcinogenesis, Mutagenesis, Impairment of Fertility—Neither in vivo nor in vitro laboratory tests have conclusively demonstrated the mutagenicity of this product. Fertility following treatment with Oncovin alone for malignant disease has not been studied in humans. Clinical reports of both male and female patients who received multiple-agent chemotherapy that included Oncovin indicate that azoospermia and amenorrhea can occur in postpubertal patients. Recovery occurred many months after completion of chemotherapy in some but not all patients. When the same treatment is administered to prepubertal patients, permanent azoospermia and amenorrhea are much less likely.

Patients who received chemotherapy with Oncovin in combination with anticancer drugs known to be carcinogenic have developed second malignancies. The contributing role of Oncovin in this development has not been determined. No evidence of carcinogenicity was found following intraperitoneal administration of Oncovin in rats and mice, although this study was limited.

Usage in Pregnancy—*Pregnancy Category D*—*See* Warnings.

Nursing Mothers—It is not known whether this drug is excreted in human milk. Because many drugs are excreted in human milk and because of the potential for serious adverse reactions due to Oncovin in nursing infants, a decision should be made either to discontinue nursing or the drug, taking into account the importance of the drug to the mother.

Pediatric Use—See Dosage and Administration section.

ADVERSE REACTIONS

Prior to the use of this drug, patients and/or their parents/guardian should be advised of the possibility of untoward symptoms.

In general, adverse reactions are reversible and are related to dosage. The most common adverse reaction is hair loss; the most troublesome adverse reactions are neuromuscular in origin.

When single, weekly doses of the drug are employed, the adverse reactions of leukopenia, neuritic pain, and constipation occur but are usually of short duration (ie, less than 7 days). When the dosage is reduced, these reactions may lessen or disappear. The severity of such reactions seems to increase when the calculated amount of drug is given in divided doses. Other adverse reactions, such as hair loss, sensory loss, paresthesia, difficulty in walking, slapping gait, loss of deep-tendon reflexes, and muscle wasting, may persist for at least as long as therapy is continued. Generalized sensorimotor dysfunction may become progressively more severe with continued treatment. Although most such symptoms usually disappear by about the sixth week after discontinuance of treatment, some neuromuscular difficulties may persist for prolonged periods in some patients. Regrowth of hair may occur while maintenance therapy continues.

The following adverse reactions have been reported:

Hypersensitivity—Rare cases of allergic-type reactions, such as anaphylaxis, rash, and edema, that are temporally related to vincristine therapy have been reported in patients receiving vincristine as a part of multidrug chemotherapy regimens.

Gastrointestinal—Constipation, abdominal cramps, weight loss, nausea, vomiting, oral ulceration, diarrhea, paralytic ileus, intestinal necrosis and/or perforation, and anorexia have occurred. Constipation may take the form of upper-colon impaction, and, on physical examination, the rectum may be empty. Colicky abdominal pain coupled with an empty rectum may mislead the physician. A flat film of the abdomen is useful in demonstrating this condition. All cases have responded to high enemas and laxatives. A routine prophylactic regimen against constipation is recommended for all patients receiving Oncovin.

Paralytic ileus (which mimics the "surgical abdomen") may occur, particularly in young pediatric patients. The ileus will reverse itself with temporary discontinuance of Oncovin and with symptomatic care.

Genitourinary—Polyuria, dysuria, and urinary retention due to bladder atony have occurred. Other drugs known to cause urinary retention (particularly in the elderly) should, if possible, be discontinued for the first few days following administration of Oncovin.

Cardiovascular—Hypertension and hypotension have occurred. Chemotherapy combinations that have included vincristine sulfate, when given to patients previously treated with mediastinal radiation, have been associated with coronary artery disease and myocardial infarction. Causality has not been established.

Neurologic—Frequently, there is a sequence to the development of neuromuscular side effects. Initially, only sensory impairment and paresthesia may be encountered. With continued treatment, neuritic pain and, later, motor difficulties may occur. There have been no reports of any agent that can reverse the neuromuscular manifestations that may accompany therapy with Oncovin.

Loss of deep-tendon reflexes, foot drop, ataxia, and paralysis have been reported with continued administration. Cranial nerve manifestations, such as isolated paresis and/or paralysis of muscles controlled by cranial motor nerves, including potentially life-threatening bilateral vocal cord paralysis, may occur in the absence of motor impairment elsewhere; extraocular and laryngeal muscles are those most commonly involved. Jaw pain, pharyngeal pain, parotid gland pain, bone pain, back pain, limb pain, and myalgias have been reported; pain in these areas may be severe. Convulsions, frequently with hypertension, have been reported in a few patients receiving Oncovin. Several instances of convulsions followed by coma have been reported in pediatric patients. Transient cortical blindness and optic atrophy with blindness have been reported. Treatment with vinca alkaloids has resulted rarely in both vestibular and auditory damage to the eighth cranial nerve. Manifestations include partial or total deafness which may be temporary or permanent, and difficulties with balance including dizziness, nystagmus, and vertigo. Particular caution is warranted when Oncovin is used in combination with other agents known to be ototoxic such as the platinum-containing oncolytics.

Pulmonary—*See* Precautions.

Endocrine—Rare occurrences of a syndrome attributable to inappropriate antidiuretic hormone secretion have been observed in patients treated with Oncovin. This syndrome is characterized by high urinary sodium excretion in the presence of hyponatremia; renal or adrenal disease, hypotension, dehydration, azotemia, and clinical edema are absent. With fluid deprivation, improvement occurs in the hyponatremia and in the renal loss of sodium.

Hematologic—Oncovin does not appear to have any constant or significant effect on platelets or red blood cells. Serious bone-marrow depression is usually not a major dose-limiting event. However, anemia, leukopenia, and thrombocytopenia have been reported. Thrombocytopenia, if present when therapy with Oncovin is begun, may actually improve before the appearance of marrow remission.

Skin—Alopecia and rash have been reported.

Other—Fever and headache have occurred.

OVERDOSAGE

Side effects following the use of Oncovin are dose related. In pediatric patients under 13 years of age, death has occurred following doses of Oncovin that were 10 times those recommended for therapy. Severe symptoms may occur in this patient group following dosages of 3 to 4 mg/m^2. Adults can be expected to experience severe symptoms after single doses of 3 mg/m^2 or more (*see* Adverse Reactions). Therefore, following administration of doses higher than those recommended, patients can be expected to experience exaggerated side effects. Supportive care should include the following: (1) prevention of side effects resulting from the syndrome of inappropriate antidiuretic hormone secretion (preventive treatment would include restriction of fluid intake and perhaps the administration of a diuretic affecting the function of Henle's loop and the distal tubule); (2) administration of anticonvulsants; (3) use of enemas or cathartics to prevent ileus (in some instances, decompression of the gastrointestinal tract may be necessary); (4) monitoring the cardiovascular system; and (5) determining daily blood counts for guidance in transfusion requirements.

Folinic acid has been observed to have a protective effect in normal mice that were administered lethal doses of Oncovin (*Cancer Res* 1963; 23:1390). Isolated case reports suggest that folinic acid may be helpful in treating humans who have received an overdose of Oncovin. It is suggested that 100 mg of folinic acid be administered intravenously every 3 hours for 24 hours and then every 6 hours for at least 48 hours. Theoretically (based on pharmacokinetic data), tissue levels of Oncovin can be expected to remain significantly elevated for at least 72 hours. Treatment with folinic acid does not eliminate the need for the above-mentioned supportive measures.

Most of an intravenous dose of Oncovin is excreted into the bile after rapid tissue binding (*see* Clinical Pharmacology). Because only very small amounts of the drug appear in dialysate, hemodialysis is not likely to be helpful in cases of overdosage. An increase in the severity of side effects may be experienced by patients with liver disease that is severe enough to decrease biliary excretion.

Enhanced fecal excretion of parenterally administered vincristine has been demonstrated in dogs pretreated with cholestyramine. There are no published clinical data on the use of cholestyramine as an antidote in humans.

There are no published clinical data on the consequences of oral ingestion of vincristine. Should oral ingestion occur, the stomach should be evacuated. Evacuation should be followed by oral administration of activated charcoal and a cathartic.

DOSAGE AND ADMINISTRATION

This preparation is for intravenous use only (see Warnings). *Neurotoxicity appears to be dose related. Extreme care must be used in calculating and administering the dose of Oncovin since overdosage may have a very serious or fatal outcome.*

Special Dispensing Information—WHEN DISPENSING ONCOVIN IN OTHER THAN THE ORIGINAL CONTAINER, IT IS IMPERATIVE THAT IT BE PACKAGED IN THE PROVIDED OVERWRAP WHICH BEARS THE FOLLOWING STATEMENT: "DO NOT REMOVE COVERING UNTIL MOMENT OF INJECTION. FATAL IF GIVEN INTRATHECALLY. FOR INTRAVENOUS USE ONLY". (*see* Warnings) A syringe containing a specific dose must be labeled, using the auxiliary sticker provided, to state: "FATAL IF GIVEN INTRATHECALLY. FOR INTRAVENOUS USE ONLY."

The concentration of vincristine contained in all vials of Oncovin is 1 mg/mL. Do not add extra fluid to the vial prior to removal of the dose. Withdraw the solution of Oncovin into an accurate dry syringe, measuring the dose carefully. Do not add extra fluid to the vial in an attempt to empty it completely.

Caution—It is extremely important that the intravenous needle or catheter be properly positioned before any Oncovin is injected. Leakage into surrounding tissue during intravenous administration of Oncovin may cause considerable irritation. If extravasation occurs, the injection should be discontinued immediately, and any remaining portion of the dose should then be introduced into another vein. Local injection of hyaluronidase and the application of moderate heat to the area of leakage will help disperse the drug and may minimize discomfort and the possibility of cellulitis.

Oncovin must be administered via an intact, free-flowing intravenous needle or catheter. Care should be taken that there is no leakage or swelling occurring during administration (*see* boxed Warnings).

The solution may be injected either directly into a vein or into the tubing of a running intravenous infusion (*see* Drug Interactions below). Injection of Oncovin should be accomplished within 1 minute.

The drug is administered intravenously *at weekly intervals.* The usual dose of Oncovin for pediatric patients is 1.5–2 mg/

Continued on next page

*** Identi-Code® symbol. This product information was prepared in June 2000. Current information on these and other products of Eli Lilly and Company may be obtained by direct inquiry to Lilly Research Laboratories, Lilly Corporate Center, Indianapolis, Indiana 46285, (800) 545-5979.**

Oncovin—Cont.

m^2. For pediatric patients weighing 10 kg or less, the starting dose should be 0.05 mg/kg, administered once a week. The usual dose of Oncovin for adults is 1.4 mg/m^2. A 50% reduction in the dose of Oncovin is recommended for patients having a direct serum bilirubin value above 3 mg/100 mL.

Oncovin should not be given to patients while they are receiving radiation therapy through ports that include the liver. When Oncovin is used in combination with L-asparaginase, Oncovin should be given 12 to 24 hours before administration of the enzyme in order to minimize toxicity; administering L-asparaginase before Oncovin may reduce hepatic clearance of Oncovin.

Drug Incompatibilities —Oncovin should not be diluted in solutions that raise or lower the pH outside the range of 3.5 to 5.5. It should not be mixed with anything other than normal saline or glucose in water.

Whenever solution and container permit, parenteral drug products should be inspected visually for particulate matter and discoloration prior to administration.

Procedures for proper handling and disposal of anticancer drugs should be considered. Several guidelines on this subject have been published.[4–10] There is no general agreement that all of the procedures recommended in the guidelines are necessary or appropriate.

HOW SUPPLIED

Multiple-Dose Vials:

1 mg/1 mL, 1 mL (No. 7194)—(1s) NDC 0002-7194-01
2 mg/2 mL, 2 mL (No. 7195)—(1s) NDC 0002-7195-01
5 mg/5 mL, 5 mL (No. 7196)—(1s) NDC 0002-7196-01

This product should be refrigerated.

REFERENCES

1. Dyke. Treatment of inadvertent intrathecal injection of vincristine. N Engl J Med, 1989, 321: 1270–71.
2. Michelagnoli MP, Bailey CC, Wilson L, Livingston J, Kinsey SB. Potential salvage therapy for inadvertent intrathecal administration of vincristine. Br. J. Haematology, 1997, 99: 364–367. (Mfr. Control No. GB97113451A)
3. Zaragoza MR, Ritchey ML, Walter A. Neurourologic consequences of accidental intrathecal vincristine: A case report. Med. Pediatr. Oncol., 1995, 24(1): 61–62.
4. Recommendations for the Safe Handling of Parenteral Antineoplastic Drugs, NIH Publication No. 83-2621. For sale by the Superintendent of Documents, U.S. Government Printing Office, Washington, DC 20402.
5. AMA Council Report, Guidelines for Handling Parenteral Antineoplastics. JAMA, 1985;253(11):1590–1592.
6. National Study Commission on Cytotoxic Exposure—Recommendations for Handling Cytotoxic Agents. Available from Louis P. Jeffrey, ScD., Chairman, National Study Commission on Cytotoxic Exposure, Massachusetts College of Pharmacy and Allied Health Sciences, 179 Longwood Avenue, Boston, Massachusetts 02115.
7. Clinical Oncological Society of Australia, Guidelines and Recommendations for Safe Handling of Antineoplastic Agents. Med J Australia, 1983;1:426–428.
8. Jones RB, et al: Safe Handling of Chemotherapeutic Agents: A Report from the Mount Sinai Medical Center. CA—A Cancer Journal for Clinicians, 1983; (Sept/Oct)258–263.
9. American Society of Hospital Pharmacists Technical Assistance Bulletin on Handling Cytotoxic and Hazardous Drugs. Am J Hosp Pharm, 1990;47:1033–1049.
10. OSHA Work-Practice Guidelines for Personnel Dealing with Cytotoxic (Antineoplastic) Drugs. Am J Hosp Pharm, 1986;43:1193–1204.

Literature revised May 19, 1999
PA 0103 AMP [051999]

PROTAMINE SULFATE ℞

[*prō 'ta-mēn sŭl 'fāt*]
Injection, USP

DESCRIPTION

Protamines are simple proteins of low molecular weight that are rich in arginine and strongly basic. They occur in the sperm of salmon and certain other species of fish.

Protamine sulfate occurs as fine white or off-white amorphous or crystalline powder. It is sparingly soluble in water. The pH is between 6 and 7. The cationic hydrogenated protamine at a pH of 6.8 to 7.1 reacts with anionic heparin at a pH of 5.0 to 7.5 to form an inactive complex.

Protamine Sulfate Injection, USP, is a sterile, isotonic solution of protamine sulfate. It acts as a heparin antagonist. It is also a weak anticoagulant.

Each 25-mL vial contains protamine sulfate equivalent to 250 mg of activity. This product also contains 0.9% Sodium Chloride Reagent in Water for Injection, USP. Sodium phosphate and/or sulfuric acid may have been added during manufacture to adjust the pH. Contains no preservative. Protamine sulfate is administered intravenously.

CLINICAL PHARMACOLOGY

When administered alone, protamine has an anticoagulant effect. However, when it is given in the presence of heparin (which is strongly acidic), a stable salt is formed and the anticoagulant activity of both drugs is lost.

Protamine sulfate has a rapid onset of action. Neutralization of heparin occurs within 5 minutes after intravenous administration of an appropriate dose of protamine sulfate. Although the metabolic fate of the heparin-protamine complex has not been elucidated, it has been postulated that protamine sulfate in the heparin-protamine complex may be partially metabolized or may be attacked by fibrinolysin, thus freeing heparin.

INDICATIONS AND USAGE

Protamine sulfate is indicated in the treatment of heparin overdosage.

CONTRAINDICATION

Protamine sulfate is contraindicated in patients who have shown previous intolerance to the drug.

WARNINGS

Hyperheparinemia or bleeding has been reported in experimental animals and in some patients 30 minutes to 18 hours after cardiac surgery (under cardiopulmonary bypass) in spite of complete neutralization of heparin by adequate doses of protamine sulfate at the end of the operation. It is important to keep the patient under close observation after cardiac surgery. Additional doses of protamine sulfate should be administered if indicated by coagulation studies, such as the heparin titration test with protamine and the determination of plasma thrombin time.

Too-rapid administration of protamine sulfate can cause severe hypotensive and anaphylactoid reactions (*see* Dosage and Administration). Facilities to treat shock should be available.

PRECAUTIONS

***General*—Because of the anticoagulant effect of protamine, it is unwise to give more than 50 mg over a short period unless a larger dose is clearly needed.**

Patients with a history of allergy to fish may develop hypersensitivity reactions to protamine, although to date no relationship has been established between allergic reactions to protamine and fish allergy.

Previous exposure to protamine can induce a humoral immune response and predispose susceptible individuals to the development of untoward reactions from the subsequent use of this drug. Patients exposed to protamine through the use of protamine-containing insulin or during heparin neutralization may experience life-threatening reactions and fatal anaphylaxis upon receiving large doses of protamine intravenously. Severe reactions to intravenous protamine can occur in the absence of local or systemic allergic reactions to subcutaneous injection of protamine-containing insulin. Reports of the presence of antiprotamine antibodies in the sera of infertile or vasectomized men suggest that some of these individuals may react to use of protamine sulfate.

Fatal anaphylaxis has been reported in one patient with no prior history of allergies.

Drug Interactions —Protamine sulfate has been shown to be incompatible with certain antibiotics, including several of the cephalosporins and penicillins (*see* Dosage and Administration).

Carcinogenesis, Mutagenesis, Impairment of Fertility —Studies have not been performed to determine potential for carcinogenicity, mutagenicity, or impairment of fertility.

Pregnancy —Pregnancy Category C —Animal reproduction studies have not been conducted with protamine sulfate. It is also not known whether protamine sulfate can cause fetal harm when administered to a pregnant woman or can affect reproduction capacity. Protamine sulfate should be given to a pregnant woman only if clearly needed.

Nursing Mothers —It is not known whether this drug is excreted in human milk. Because many drugs are excreted in human milk, caution should be exercised when protamine sulfate is administered to a nursing woman.

Pediatric Use —Safety and effectiveness in pediatric patients have not been established.

ADVERSE REACTIONS

The intravenous administration of protamine sulfate may cause a sudden fall in blood pressure and bradycardia. Other reactions include transitory flushing and feeling of warmth, dyspnea, nausea, vomiting, and lassitude. Back pain has been reported in conscious patients undergoing such procedures as cardiac catheterization.

Severe adverse reactions have been reported including: (1) Anaphylaxis that resulted in severe respiratory distress, circulatory collapse, and capillary leak (*see* Precautions). Fatal anaphylaxis has been reported in one patient with no prior history of allergies; (2) Anaphylactoid reactions with circulatory collapse, capillary leak, and noncardiogenic pulmonary edema; acute pulmonary hypertension.

Complement activation by the heparin-protamine complexes, release of lysosomal enzymes from neutrophils, and prostaglandin and thromboxane generation have been associated with the development of anaphylactoid reactions.

Severe and potentially irreversible circulatory collapse associated with myocardial failure and reduced cardiac output can also occur. The mechanism(s) of this reaction and the role played by concurrent factors are unclear.

High-protein, noncardiogenic pulmonary edema associated with the use of protamine has been reported in patients on cardiopulmonary bypass who are undergoing cardiovascular surgery. The etiologic role of protamine in the pathogenesis of this condition is uncertain, and multiple factors have been present in most cases. The condition has been reported in association with administration of certain blood products, other drugs, cardiopulmonary bypass alone, and other etiologic factors. It is difficult to treat, and it can be life threatening. Because fatal anaphylactic and anaphylactoid reactions have been reported after the administration of protamine sulfate, the drug should be given only when resuscitation techniques and treatment of anaphylactic and anaphylactoid shock are readily available.

OVERDOSAGE

Signs and Symptoms—Overdose of protamine sulfate may cause bleeding. Protamine has a weak anticoagulant effect due to an interaction with platelets and with many proteins including fibrinogen. This effect should be distinguished from the rebound anticoagulation that may occur 30 minutes to 18 hours following the reversal of heparin with protamine.

Rapid administration of protamine is more likely to result in bradycardia, dyspnea, a sensation of warmth, flushing, and severe hypotension. Hypertension has also occurred.

The median lethal intravenous dose of protamine sulfate is 50 mg/kg in mice. Serum concentrations of protamine sulfate are not clinically useful. Information is not available on the amount of drug in a single dose that is associated with overdosage or is likely to be life threatening.

Treatment—To obtain up-to-date information about the treatment of overdose, a good resource is your certified Regional Poison Control Center. Telephone numbers of certified poison control centers are listed in the *Physicians' Desk Reference (PDR)*. In managing overdosage, consider the possibility of multiple drug overdoses, interaction among drugs, and unusual drug kinetics in your patient.

Replace blood loss with blood transfusions or fresh frozen plasma.

If the patient is hypotensive, consider fluids, epinephrine, dobutamine, or dopamine.

DOSAGE AND ADMINISTRATION

Each mg of protamine sulfate neutralizes approximately 90 USP units of heparin activity derived from lung tissue or about 115 USP units of heparin activity derived from intestinal mucosa.

Protamine Sulfate Injection should be given by very slow intravenous injection over a 10-minute period in doses not to exceed 50 mg (*see* Warnings).

Protamine sulfate is intended for injection without further dilution; however, if further dilution is desired, D5-W or normal saline may be used. Diluted solutions should not be stored since they contain no preservative.

Protamine sulfate should not be mixed with other drugs without knowledge of their compatibility, because protamine sulfate has been shown to be incompatible with certain antibiotics, including several of the cephalosporins and penicillins.

Because heparin disappears rapidly from the circulation, the dose of protamine sulfate required also decreases rapidly with the time elapsed following intravenous injection of heparin. For example, if the protamine sulfate is administered 30 minutes after the heparin, one half the usual dose may be sufficient.

The dosage of protamine sulfate should be guided by blood coagulation studies (*see* Warnings).

Parenteral drug products should be inspected visually for particulate matter and discoloration prior to administration whenever solution and container permit.

HOW SUPPLIED

Vials:

25 mL (No. 735)—(1s) NDC 0002-1462-01

Vials should be stored in the refrigerator between 2° and 8°C (35.6° and 46.4°F).

CAUTION—The total dose of protamine sulfate contained in Vials No. 735 is 250 mg of activity in 25 mL.

The large-size vials (No. 735) are designed for antiheparin treatment only when large doses of heparin have been given during surgery and are to be neutralized by large doses of protamine sulfate after surgical procedures.

CAUTION—Federal (USA) law prohibits dispensing without prespcription.

Literature revised August 6, 1996
PA 8182 AMP [080696]

QUINIDINE GLUCONATE INJECTION, USP ℞

[*kwin-ə dēn glü-kə, nāt*]

This product is to be used by the physician or under his/her direction.

DESCRIPTION

Quinidine is an antimalarial schizonticide and an antiarrhythmic agent with class 1a activity; it is the d-isomer of quinine and its molecular weight is 324.43. Quinidine gluconate is the gluconate salt of quinidine; its chemical name is cinchonan-9-ol, 6′-methoxy-, (9*S*)-, mono-D-gluconate; its structural formula is:

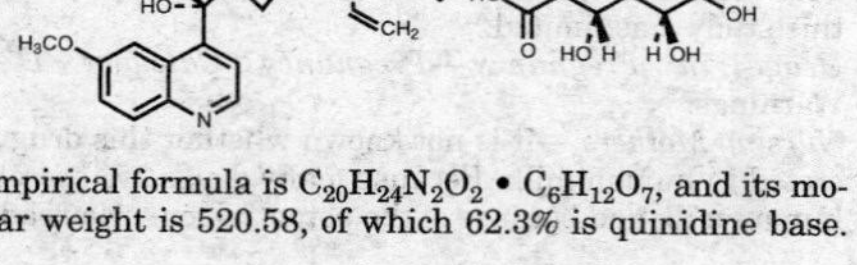

Its empirical formula is $C_{20}H_{24}N_2O_2 \cdot C_6H_{12}O_7$, and its molecular weight is 520.58, of which 62.3% is quinidine base.

Each vial of Quinidine Gluconate Injection contains 800 mg (1.5 mmol) of quinidine gluconate (500 mg of quinidine) in 10 mL of Sterile Water for Injection, 0.005% of edetate disodium, 0.25% phenol, and (as needed) D-gluconic acid δ-lactone to adjust the pH.

CLINICAL PHARMACOLOGY

Pharmacokinetics and Metabolism—After intramuscular injection of quinidine gluconate, peak serum levels of quinidine are achieved in a little less than two hours. This time to peak levels is identical to the time measured when quinidine salts are administered orally.

The volume of distribution of quinidine is typically 2–3 L/kg in healthy young adults, but this may be reduced to as little as 0.5 L/kg in patients with congestive heart failure, or increased to 3–5 L/kg in patients with cirrhosis of the liver. At concentrations of 2–5 mg/L (6.5–16.2 μmol/L), the fraction of quinidine bound to plasma proteins (mainly to α_1-acid glycoprotein and to albumin) is 80–88% in adults and older children, but it is lower in pregnant women, and in infants and neonates it may be as low as 50–70%. Because α_1-acid glycoprotein levels are increased in response to stress, serum levels of total quinidine may be greatly increased in settings such as acute myocardial infarction, even though the serum content of unbound (active) drug may remain normal. Protein binding is also increased in chronic renal failure, but binding abruptly descends toward or below normal when heparin is administered for hemodialysis.

Quinidine clearance typically proceeds at 3–5 mL/min/kg in adults, but clearance in pediatric patients may be twice or three times as rapid. The elimination half-life is about 6–8 hours in adults and 3–4 hours in pediatric patients. Quinidine clearance is unaffected by hepatic cirrhosis, so the increased volume of distribution seen in cirrhosis leads to a proportionate increase in the elimination half-life.

Most quinidine is eliminated hepatically via the action of cytochrome P450IIIA4; there are several different hydroxylated metabolites, and some of these have antiarrhythmic activity.

The most important of quinidine's metabolites is 3-hydroxyquinidine (3HQ), serum levels of which can approach those of quinidine in patients receiving conventional doses of quinidine gluconate. The volume of distribution of 3HQ appears to be larger than that of quinidine, and the elimination half-life of 3HQ is about 12 hours.

As measured by antiarrhythmic effects in animals, by QT_c prolongation in human volunteers, or by various *in vitro* techniques, 3HQ has at least half the antiarrhythmic activity of the parent compound, so it may be responsible for a substantial fraction of the effect of quinidine gluconate in chronic use.

When the urine pH is less than 7, about 20% of administered quinidine appears unchanged in the urine, but this fraction drops to as little as 5% when the urine is more alkaline. Renal clearance involves both glomerular filtration and active tubular secretion, moderated by (pH-dependent) tubular reabsorption. The net renal clearance is about 1 mL/min/kg in healthy adults.

When renal function is taken into account, quinidine clearance is apparently independent of patient age.

Assays of serum quinidine levels are widely available, but the results of modern assays may not be consistent with results cited in the older medical literature. The serum levels of quinidine cited in this package insert are those derived from specific assays, using either benzene extraction or (preferably) reverse-phase high-pressure liquid chromatography. In matched samples, older assays might unpredictably have given results that were as much as two or three times higher. A typical "therapeutic" concentration range is 2–6 mg/L (6.2–18.5 μmol/L).

Mechanisms of Action—In patients with malaria, quinidine acts primarily as an intraerythrocytic schizonticide, with little effect upon sporozoites or upon pre-erythrocytic parasites. Quinidine is gametocidal to *Plasmodium vivax* and *P. malariae,* but not to *P. falciparum*.

In cardiac muscle and in Purkinje fibers, quinidine depresses the rapid inward depolarizing sodium current, thereby slowing phase-0 depolarization and reducing the amplitude of the action potential without affecting the resting potential. In normal Purkinje fibers, it reduces the slope of phase-4 depolarization, shifting the threshold voltage upward toward zero. The result is slowed conduction and reduced automaticity in all parts of the heart, with increase of the effective refractory period relative to the duration of the action potential in the atria, ventricles, and Purkinje tissues. Quinidine also raises the fibrillation thresholds of the atria and ventricles, and it raises the ventricular *de*fibrillation threshold as well. Quinidine's actions fall into class Ia in the Vaughan-Williams classification.

By slowing conduction and prolonging the effective refractory period, quinidine can interrupt or prevent reentrant arrhythmias and arrythmias due to increased automaticity, including atrial flutter, atrial fibrillation, and paroxysmal supraventricular tachycardia.

In patients with the sick sinus syndrome, quinidine can cause marked sinus node depression and bradycardia. In most patients, however, use of quinidine is associated with an increase in sinus rate.

Quinidine prolongs the QT interval in dose-related fashion. This may lead to increased ventricular automaticity and polymorphic ventricular tachycardias, including *torsades de pointes* (*see* Warnings).

In addition, quinidine has anticholinergic activity, it has negative inotropic activity, and it acts peripherally as an α-adrenergic antagonist (that is, as a vasodilator).

Clinical Effects

Malaria: Intravenous quinidine has been associated with clearing of parasitemia and high rates of survival in patients with severe *P. falciparum* malaria and hyperparasitemia. Placebo-controlled trials have not been performed, but clearing of these levels of parasitemia is unprecedented in the absence of effective therapy. Use of quinidine in patients infected with chloroquine-sensitive malaria or in chloroquine-resistant non-falciparum malaria has not been reported.

Maintenance of sinus rhythm after conversion from atrial fibrillation: In six clinical trials (published between 1970 and 1984) with a total of 808 patients, quinidine (418 patients) was compared to nontreatment (258 patients) or placebo (132 patients) for the maintenance of sinus rhythm after cardioversion from chronic atrial fibrillation. Quinidine was consistently more efficacious in maintaining sinus rhythm, but a meta-analysis found that mortality in the quinidine-exposed patients (2.9%) was significantly greater than mortality in the patients who had not been treated with active drug (0.8%). Suppression of atrial fibrillation with quinidine has theoretical patient benefits (*eg,* improved exercise tolerance; reduction in hospitalization for cardioversion; lack of arrhythmia-related palpitations, dyspnea, and chest pain; reduced incidence of systemic embolism and/or stroke), but these benefits have never been demonstrated in clinical trials. Some of these benefits (*eg,* reduction in stroke incidence) may be achievable by other means (anticoagulation).

By slowing the rate of atrial flutter/fibrillation, quinidine can decrease the degree of atrioventricular block and cause an increase, sometimes marked, in the rate at which supraventricular impulses are successfully conducted by the atrioventricular node, with a resultant paradoxical increase in ventricular rate (*see* Warnings).

Non-life-threatening ventricular arrhythmias: In studies of patients with a variety of ventricular arrhythmias (mainly frequent ventricular premature beats and non-sustained ventricular tachycardia), quinidine (total N=502) has been compared to flecainide (N=141), mexiletine (N=246), propafenone (N=53), and tocainide (N=67). In each of these studies, the mortality in the quinidine group was numerically greater than the mortality in the comparator group. When the studies were combined in the meta-analysis, quinidine was associated with a statistically significant threefold relative risk of death.

At therapeutic doses, quinidine's only consistent effect upon the surface electrocardiogram is an increase in the QT interval. This prolongation can be monitored as a guide to safety, and it may provide better guidance than serum drug levels (*see* Warnings).

INDICATIONS AND USAGE

Treatment of malaria—Quinidine gluconate injection is indicated for the treatment of life-threatening *Plasmodium flaciparum* malaria.

Conversion of atrial fibrillation/flutter—Quinidine gluconate injection is also indicated (when rapid therapeutic effect is required, or when oral therapy is not feasible) as a means of restoring normal sinus rhythm in patients with symptomatic atrial fibrillation/flutter whose symptoms are not adequately controlled by measures that reduce the rate of ventricular response. If this use of quinidine gluconate does not restore sinus rhythm within a reasonable time, then its use should be discontinued.

Treatment of ventricular arrhythmias—Quinidine gluconate injection is also indicated for the treatment of documented ventricular arrhythmias, such as sustained ventricular tachycardia, that in the judgement of the physician are life-threatening. Because of the proarrhythmic effects of quinidine, its use with ventricular arrhythmias of lesser severity is generally not recommended, and treatment of patients with asymptomatic ventricular premature contractions should be avoided. Where possible, therapy should be guided by the results of programmed electrical stimulation and/or Holter monitoring with exercise.

Antiarrhythmic drugs (including quinidine) have not been shown to enhance survival in patients with ventricular arrhythmias.

CONTRAINDICATIONS

Quinidine is contraindicated in patients who are known to be allergic to it, or who have developed thrombocytopenic purpura during prior therapy with quinidine or quinine.

In the absence of a functioning artificial pacemaker, quinidine is also contraindicated in any patient whose cardiac rhythm is dependent upon a junctional or idioventricular pacemaker, including patients in complete atrioventricular block.

Quinidine is also contraindicated in patients who, like those with myasthenia gravis, might be adversely affected by an anticholinergic agent.

WARNINGS

Inappropriate infusion rate—Overly rapid infusion of quinidine (*see* Dosage and Administration) may cause peripheral vascular collapse and severe hypotension.

Proarrhythmic effects—Like many other drugs (including all other class 1a antiarrhythmics), quinidine prolongs the QT_c interval, and this can lead to *torsades de pointes,* a life-threatening ventricular arrhythmia (*see* Overdosage). The risk of *torsades* is increased by any of bradycardia, hypokalemia, hypomagnesemia, and high serum levels of quinidine, but it may appear in the absence of any of these risk factors. The best predictor of this arrhythmia appears to be the length of the QT_c interval, and quinidine should be used with extreme care in patients who have preexisting long-QT syndromes, who have histories of *torsades de pointes* of any cause, or who have previously responded to quinidine (or other drugs that prolong ventricular repolarization) with marked lengthening of the QT_c interval. Estimation of the incidence of *torsades* in patients with therapeutic levels of quinidine is not possible from the available data.

Other ventricular arrhythmias that have been reported with quinidine include frequent extrasystoles, ventricular tachycardia, ventricular flutter, and ventricular fibrillation.

Paradoxical increase in ventricular rate in atrial flutter/fibrillation—When quinidine is administered to patients with atrial flutter/fibrillation, the desired pharmacologic reversion to sinus rhythm may (rarely) be preceded by a slowing of the atrial rate with a consequent increase in the rate of beats conducted to the ventricles. The resulting ventricular rate may be very high (greater than 200 beats per minute) and poorly tolerated. This hazard may be decreased if partial atrioventricular block is achieved prior to initiation of quinidine therapy, using conduction-reducing drugs such as **digitalis, verapamil, diltiazem,** or a β-receptor blocking agent.

Exacerbated bradycardia in sick sinus syndrome—In patients with the sick sinus syndrome, quinidine has been associated with marked sinus node depression and bradycardia.

Pharmacokinetic considerations—Renal or hepatic dysfunction causes the elimination of quinidine to be slowed, while congestive heart failure causes a reduction in quinidine's apparent volume of distribution. Any of these conditions can lead to quinidine toxicity if dosage is not appropriately reduced. In addition, interactions with coadministered drugs can alter the serum concentration and activity of quinidine, leading either to toxicity or to lack of efficacy if the dose of quinidine is not appropriately modified (*see* Precautions/Drug Interactions).

Vagolysis—Because quinidine opposes the atrial and A-V nodal effects of vagal stimulation, physical or pharmacological vagal maneuvers undertaken to terminate paroxysmal supraventricular tachycardia may be ineffective in patients receiving quinidine.

PRECAUTIONS

Heart block—In patients without implanted pacemakers who are at high risk of complete atrioventricular block (*eg,* those with digitalis intoxication, second-degree atrioventricular block, or severe intraventricular conduction defects), quinidine should be used only with caution.

Drug Interactions—Altered pharmacokinetics of quinidine: Drugs that alkalinize the urine (**carbonic-anhydrase inhibitors, sodium bicarbonate, thiazide diuretics**) reduce renal elimination of quinidine.

By pharmacokinetic mechanisms that are not well understood, quinidine levels are increased by coadministration of **amiodarone** or **cimetidine**. Very rarely, and again by mechanisms not understood, quinidine levels are decreased by coadministration of **nifedipine**.

Hepatic elimination of quinidine may be accelerated by coadministration of drugs (**phenobarbital, phenytoin, rifampin**) that induce production of cytochrome P450IIIA4.

Perhaps because of competition of the P450IIIA4 metabolic pathway, quinidine levels rise when **ketaconazole** is coadministered.

Coadministration of **propranolol** usually does not affect quinidine pharmacokinetics, but in some studies, the β-blocker appeared to cause increases in peak serum levels of quinidine, decreases in quinidine's volume of distribution and decreases in total quinidine clearance. The effects (if any) of coadministration of **other β-blockers** on quinidine pharmacokinetics have not been adequately studied.

Hepatic clearance of quinidine is significantly reduced during coadministration of **verapamil**, with corresponding increases in serum levels and half-life.

Altered pharmacokinetics of other drugs: Quinidine slows the elimination of **digoxin** and simultaneously reduces digoxin's apparent volume of distribution. As a result, serum digoxin levels may be as much as doubled. When quinidine and digoxin are coadministered, digoxin doses usually need to be reduced. Serum levels of **digitoxin** are also raised when quinidine is coadministered, although the effect appears to be smaller.

By a mechanism that is not understood, quinidine potentiates the anticoagulatory action of warfarin, and the anticoagulant dosage may need to be reduced.

Cytochrome P450IID6 is an enzyme critical to the metabolism of many drugs, notably including **mexiletine**, some **phenothiazines**, and most **polycyclic antidepressants**. Constitutional deficiency of cytochrome P450IID6 is found in less than 1% of Orientals, in about 2% of American blacks, and in about 8% of American whites. Testing with debrisoquine is sometimes used to distinguish the P450IID6-deficient "poor metabolizers" from the majority-phenotype "extensive metabolizers."

Continued on next page

*** Identi-Code® symbol. This product information was prepared in June 2000. Current information on these and other products of Eli Lilly and Company may be obtained by direct inquiry to Lilly Research Laboratories, Lilly Corporate Center, Indianapolis, Indiana 46285, (800) 545-5979.**

Quinidine Gluconate—Cont.

When drugs whose metabolism is P450IID6-dependent are given to poor metabolizers, the serum levels achieved are higher, sometimes much higher, than the serum levels achieved when identical doses are given to extensive metabolizers. To obtain similar clinical benefit without toxicity, doses given to poor metabolizers may need to be greatly reduced. In the cases of prodrugs whose actions are actually mediated by P450IID6-produced metabolites (for example, **codeine** and **hydrocodone**, whose analgesic and antitussive effects appear to be mediated by morphine and hydromorphone, respectively), it may not be possible to achieve the desired clinical benefits in poor metabolizers.

Quinidine is not metabolized by cytochrome P450IID6, but therapeutic serum levels of quinidine inhibit the action of cytochrome P450IID6, effectively converting extensive metabolizers into poor metabolizers. Caution must be exercised whenever quinidine is prescribed together with drugs metabolized by cytochrome P450IID6.

Perhaps by competing for pathways of renal clearance, coadministration of quinidine causes an increase in serum levels of **procainamide**.

Serum levels of **haloperidol** are increased when quinidine is coadministered.

Presumably because both drugs are metabolized by cytochrome P450IIIA4, coadministration of quinidine causes variable slowing of the metabolism of **nifedipine**. Interactions with other dihydropyridine calcium-channel blockers have not been reported, but these agents (including **felodipine, nicardipine,** and **nimodipine**) are all dependent upon P450IIIA4 for metabolism, so similar interactions with quinidine should be anticipated.

Altered pharmacodynamics of other drugs: Quinidine's anticholinergic, vasodilating, and negative inotropic actions may be additive to those of other drugs with these effects, and antagonistic to those of drugs with cholinergic, vasoconstricting, and positive inotropic effects. For example, when quinidine and **verapamil** are coadministered in doses that are each well tolerated as monotherapy, hypotension attributable to additive peripheral α-blockade is sometimes reported.

Quinidine potentiates the actions of depolarizing (succinylcholine, decamethonium) and nondepolarizing (*d*-tubocurarine, pancuronium) neuromuscular blocking agents. These phenomena are not well understood, but they are observed in animal models as well as in humans. In addition, *in vitro* addition of quinidine to the serum of pregnant women reduces the activity of pseudocholinesterase, an enzyme that is essential to the metabolism of succinylcholine.

Diltiazem significantly decreases the clearance and increases the $t_{1/2}$ of quinidine, but quinidine does not alter the kinetics of diltiazem. Non-interactions of quinidine with other drugs: Quinidine has no clinically significant effect on the pharmacokinetics of **diltiazem, flecainide, mephenytoin, metoprolol, propafenone, propranolol, quinine, timolol,** or **tocainide**.

Conversely, the pharmacokinetics of quinidine are not significantly affected by **caffeine, ciprofloxacin, digoxin, felodipine, omeprazole, or quinine.** Quinidine's pharmacokinetics are also unaffected by cigarette smoking.

Carcinogenesis, mutagenesis, impairment of fertility—Animal studies to evaluate quinidine's carcinogenic or mutagenic potential have not been performed. Similarly, there are no animal data as to quinidine's potential to impair fertility.

Pregnancy—Pregnancy Category C—Animal reproductive studies have not been conducted with quinidine. There are no adequate and well-controlled studies in pregnant women. Quinidine should be given to a pregnant woman only if clearly needed.

In one neonate whose mother had received quinidine throughout her pregnancy, the serum level of quinidine was equal to that of the mother, with no apparent ill effect. The level of quinidine in amniotic fluid was about three times higher than that found in serum.

Labor and Delivery—Quinine is said to be oxytocic in humans, but there are no adequate data as to quinidine's effect (if any) on human labor and delivery.

Nursing mothers—Quinidine is present in human milk at levels slightly lower than those in maternal serum; a human infant ingesting such milk should (scaling directly by weight) be expected to develop serum quinidine levels at least an order of magnitude lower than those of the mother. On the other hand, the pharmacokinetics and pharmacodynamics of quinidine in human infants have not been adequately studied, and neonates' reduced protein binding of quinidine may increase their risk of toxicity at low total serum levels. Administration of quinidine should (if possible) be avoided in lactating women who continue to nurse.

Pediatric use—In antimalarial trials, quinidine was as safe and effective in pediatric patients as in adults. Notwithstanding the known pharmacokinetic differences between pediatric patients and adults (*see* Pharmacokinetics and Metabolism), pediatric patients in these trials received the same doses (on a mg/kg basis) as adults.

Safety and effectiveness of antiarrhythmic use in pediatric patients have not been established.

Geriatric use—Safety and efficacy of quinidine in elderly patients has not been systematically studied. Clinical studies of quinidine did not include sufficient numbers of subjects aged 65 and over to determine whether they respond differently from younger subjects. The reported clinical experience has not identified differences in responses between the elderly and younger patients. In general, dose selection for an elderly patient should be cautious, usually starting at the low end of the dosing range, reflecting the greater frequency of decreased hepatic, renal or cardiac function and of concomitant disease or other drug therapy.

ADVERSE REACTIONS

Quinidine preparations have been used for many years, but there are only sparse data from which to estimate the incidence of various adverse reactions. The adverse reactions most frequently reported have consistently been gastrointestinal, including diarrhea, nausea, vomiting, and heartburn/esophagitis. In one study of 245 adult outpatients who received quinidine to suppress premature ventricular contractions, the incidences of reported adverse experiences were as shown in the table below. The most serious quinidine-associated adverse reactions are described above under Warnings.

Adverse Experiences in a 245-Patient PVC Trial

	Incidence (%)
diarrhea	85 (35)
"upper gastrointestinal distress"	55 (22)
lightheadedness	37 (15)
headache	18 (7)
fatigue	17 (7)
palpitations	16 (7)
angina-like pain	14 (6)
weakness	13 (5)
rash	11 (5)
visual problems	8 (3)
change in sleep habits	7 (3)
tremor	6 (2)
nervousness	5 (2)
discoordination	3 (1)

Intramuscular injections of quinidine gluconate are typically followed by moderate to severe local pain. Some patients will develop tender nodules at the site of injection that persist for several weeks.

Vomiting and diarrhea can occur as isolated reactions to therapeutic levels of quinidine, but they may also be the first signs of **cinchonism**, a syndrome that may also include tinnitus, reversible high-frequency hearing loss, deafness, vertigo, blurred vision, diplopia, photophobia, headache, confusion, and delirium. Cinchonism is most often a sign of chronic quinidine toxicity, but it may appear in sensitive patients after a single moderate dose.

A few cases of **hepatotoxicity**, including granulomatous hepatitis, have been reported in patients receiving quinidine. All of these have appeared during the first few weeks of therapy, and most (not all) have remitted once quinidine was withdrawn.

Autoimmune and inflammatory syndromes associated with quinidine therapy have included fever, urticaria, flushing, exfoliative rash, bronchospasm, pneumonitis, psoriasiform rash, pruritus and lymphadenopathy, hemolytic anemia, vasculitis, thrombocytopenic purpura, uveitis, angioedema, agranulocytosis, the sicca syndrome, arthralgia, myalgia, elevation in serum levels of skeletal-muscle enzymes, and a disorder resembling systemic lupus erythematosus.

Convulsions, apprehension, and ataxia have been reported, but it was not clear that these were not simply the results of hypotension and consequent cerebral hypoperfusion. There are many reports of syncope. Acute psychotic reactions have been reported to follow the first dose of quinidine, but these reactions appear to be extremely rare.

Other adverse reactions occasionally reported include depression, mydriasis, disturbed color perception, night blindness, scotomata, optic neuritis, visual field loss, photosensitivity, and abnormalities of pigmentation.

OVERDOSAGE

There are only scattered reports of overdosage with intravenous quinidine, but overdoses with oral quinidine have been well described. Death has been described after a 5-gram ingestion by a toddler, while an adolescent was reported to survive after ingesting 8 grams of quinidine.

The most important ill effects of acute quinidine overdoses are ventricular arrhythmias and hypotension. Other signs and symptoms of overdose may include vomiting, diarrhea, tinnitus, high-frequency hearing loss, vertigo, blurred vision, diplopia, photophobia, headache, confusion, and delirium.

Arrhythmias—Serum quinidine levels can be conveniently assayed and monitored, but the electrocardiographic QT_c interval is a better predictor of quinidine-induced ventricular arrhythmias.

The necessary treatment of hemodynamically unstable polymorphic ventricular tachycardia (including *torsades de pointes*) is withdrawal of treatment with quinidine and either immediate cardioversion or, if a cardiac pacemaker is in place or immediately available, immediate overdrive pacing. After pacing or cardioversion, further management must be guided by the length of the QT_c interval.

Quinidine-associated ventricular tachyarrhythmias with normal underlying QT_c intervals have not been adequately studied. Because of the theoretical possibility of QT-prolonging effects that might be additive to those of quinidine, other antiarrhythmics with Class I (disopyramide, procainamide) or Class III activities should (if possible) be avoided. Similarly, although the use of bretylium in quinidine overdose has not been reported, it is reasonable to expect that the α-blocking properties of bretylium might be additive to those of quinidine, resulting in problematic hypotension.

If the post-cardioversion QT_c interval is prolonged, then the pre-cardioversion polymorphic ventricular tachyarrhythmia was (by definition) *torsades de pointes*. In this case, lidocaine and bretylium are unlikely to be of value, and other Class I antiarrhythmics (disopyramide, procainamide) are likely to exacerbate the situation. Factors contributing to QT_c prolongation (especially hypokalemia and hypomagnesemia) should be sought out and (if possible) aggressively corrected. Prevention of recurrent *torsades* may require sustained overdrive pacing or the cautious administration of isoproterenol (30–150 ng/kg/min).

Hypotension—Quinidine-induced hypotension that is not due to an arrhythmia is likely to be a consequence of quinidine-related α-blockade and vasorelaxation. Simple repletion of central volume (Trendelenburg positioning, saline infusion) may be sufficient therapy; other interventions reported to have been beneficial in this setting are those that increase peripheral vascular resistance, including α-agonist catecholamines (norepiniphrine, metaraminol) and the Military Anti-Shock Trousers.

Treatment—To obtain up-to-date information about the treatment of overdose, a good resource is your certified Regional Poison Control Center. Telephone numbers of certified poison control centers are listed in the *Physicians' Desk Reference (PDR)*. In managing overdose, consider the possibilities of multiple-drug overdoses, drug-drug interactions, and unusual drug kinetics in your patient.

Accelerated removal—Adequate studies of orally-administered activated charcoal in human overdoses of quinidine have not been reported, but there are animal data showing significant enhancement of systemic elimination following this intervention, and there is at least one human case report in which the elimination half-life of quinidine in the serum was apparently shortened by repeated gastric lavage. Activated charcoal should be avoided if an ileus is present; the conventional dose is 1 gram/kg, administered every 2–6 hours as a slurry with 8 mL/kg of tap water.

Although renal elimination of quinidine might theoretically be accelerated by maneuvers to acidify the urine, such maneuvers are potentially hazardous and of no demonstrated benefit.

Quinidine is not usefully removed from the circulation of dialysis.

Following quinidine overdose, **drugs that delay elimination of quinidine (cimetidine, carbonic-anhydrase inhibitors, diltiazem, thiazide diuretics) should be withdrawn** unless absolutely required.

DOSAGE AND ADMINISTRATION

Because the kinetics of absorption may vary with the patient's peripheral perfusion, intramuscular injection of quinidine gluconate is not recommended.

Treatment of P. falciparum malaria—Two regimens have each been shown to be effective, with or without concomitant exchange transfusion. There are no data indicating that either should be preferred to the other.

In **Regimen A**, each patient received a **loading dose** of 15 mg/kg of quinidine base (that is, 24 mg/kg of quinidine gluconate) in 250 mL of normal saline infused over 4 hours. Thereafter, each patient received a **maintenance regimen** of 7.5 mg/kg of base (12 mg/kg of quinidine gluconate) infused over 4 hours every 8 hours, starting 8 hours after the beginning of the loading dose. This regimen was continued for 7 days, except that in patients able to swallow, the maintenance infusions were discontinued, and approximately the same daily doses of quinidine were supplied orally, using 300-mg tablets of quinidine sulfate.

In **Regimen B**, each patient received a **loading dose** of 6.25 mg/kg of quinidine base (that is, 10 mg/kg of quinidine gluconate) in approximately 5 mL/kg of normal saline over 1–2 hours. Thereafter, each patient received a **maintenance infusion** of 12.5 μg/kg/min of base (that is, 20 μg/kg/min of quinidine gluconate). In patients able to swallow, the maintenance infusion was discontinued, and eight-hourly oral quinine sulfate was administered to provide approximately as much daily quinine base as the patient had been receiving quinidine base (for example, each adult patient received 650 mg of quinine sulfate every eight hours). Quinidine/quinine therapy was continued for 72 hours or until parasitemia had decreased to 1% or less, whichever came first. After completion of quinidine/quinine therapy, adults able to swallow received a single 1500-mg/75-mg dose of sulfadoxine/pyrimethamine (FANSIDAR®, Roche Laboratories) or a seven-day course of tetracycline (250 mg four times daily), while those unable to swallow received seven-day courses of intravenous doxycycline hyclate (VIBRAMYCIN®, Roerig), 100 mg twice daily. Most of the patients described as having been treated with this regimen also underwent exchange transfusion. Small children have received this regimen without dose adjustment and with apparent good results, notwithstanding the known differences in quinidine pharmacokinetics between pediatric patients and adults (*see* Clinical Pharmacology).

Even in patients without preexisting cardiac disease, antimalarial use of quinidine has occasionally been associated with hypotension, QT_c prolongation, and cinchonism; *see* Warnings.

Treatment of symptomatic atrial fibrillation/flutter—A patient receiving an intravenous infusion of quinidine must be carefully monitored, with frequent or continuous electrocardiography and blood-pressure measurement. The infusion should be discontinued as soon as sinus rhythm is restored:

the QRS complex widens to 130% of its pre-treatment duration; the QT_c interval widens to 130% of its pre-treatment duration, and is then longer than 500 ms; P waves disappear; or the patient develops significant tachycardia, symptomatic bradycardia, or hypotension.

To prepare quinidine for infusion, the contents of the supplied vial (80 mg/mL) should be diluted to 50 mL (16 mg/mL) with 5% dextrose. The resulting solution may be stored for up to 24 hours at room temperature or up to 48 hours at 4°C (40°F).

Because quinidine may be absorbed to PVC tubing, tubing length should be minimized. In one study (*Am J Health Syst Pharm.* 1996; 53:655–8), use of 112 inches of tubing resulted in 30% loss of quinidine, but drug loss was less than 3% when only 12 inches of tubing was used.

An infusion of quinidine must be delivered slowly, preferable under control of a volumetric pump, no faster than 0.25 mg/kg/min (that is, no faster than 1 mL/kg/hour). During the first few minutes of the infusion, the patient should be monitored especially closely for possible hypersensitive or idiosyncratic reactions.

Most arrhythmias that will respond to intravenous quinidine will respond to a total dose of less than 5 mg/kg, but some patients may require as much as 10 mg/kg. If conversion to sinus rhythm has not been achieved after infusion of 10 mg/kg, then the infusion should be discontinued, and other means of conversion (*eg*, direct-current cardioversion) should be considered.

Treatment of life-threatening ventricular arrhythmias—Dosing regimens for the use of intravenous quinidine gluconate in controlling life-threatening ventricular arrhythmias have not been adequately studied. Described regimens have generally been similar to the regimen described just above for the treatment of symptomatic atrial fibrillation/flutter.

HOW SUPPLIED

The 80 mg/mL, 10 mL Multiple-Dose Vial is available as:
1 NDC 0002-1407-01 (VL530)
Store at 25°C (77°F); excursions permitted to 15–30°C (59–86°F). [see USP Controlled Room Temperature].
Rx only
Literature revised June 9, 1999
PA 0576 AMP [060999]

REGULAR ILETIN® II OTC
(insulin injection, Lilly) See under Iletin® (insulin)

REOPRO® ℞
Abciximab
For intravenous administration

DESCRIPTION

Abciximab, ReoPro®, is the Fab fragment of the chimeric human-murine monoclonal antibody 7E3. Abciximab binds to the glycoprotein (GP) IIb/IIIa ($\alpha_{IIb}\beta_3$) receptor of human platelets and inhibits platelet aggregation. Abciximab also binds to the vitronectin ($\alpha_v\beta_3$) receptor found on platelets and vessel wall endothelial and smooth muscle cells.

The chimeric 7E3 antibody is produced by continuous perfusion in mammalian cell culture. The 47,615 dalton Fab fragment is purified from cell culture supernatant by a series of steps involving specific viral inactivation and removal procedures, digestion with papain and column chromatography.

ReoPro® is a clear, colorless, sterile, non-pyrogenic solution for intravenous (IV) use. Each single use vial contains 2 mg/mL of Abciximab in a buffered solution (pH 7.2) of 0.01 M sodium phosphate, 0.15 M sodium chloride and 0.001% polysorbate 80 in Water for Injection. No preservatives are added.

CLINICAL PHARMACOLOGY

General: Abciximab binds to the intact platelet GPIIb/IIIa receptor, which is a member of the integrin family of adhesion receptors and the major platelet surface receptor involved in platelet aggregation. Abciximab inhibits platelet aggregation by preventing the binding of fibrinogen, von Willebrand factor, and other adhesive molecules to GPIIb/IIIa receptor sites on activated platelets. The mechanism of action is thought to involve steric hindrance and/or conformational effects to block access of large molecules to the receptor rather than direct interaction with the RGD (arginine-glycine-aspartic acid) binding site of GPIIb/IIIa.

Abciximab binds with similar affinity to the vitronectin receptor, also known as the $\alpha_v\beta_3$ integrin. The vitronectin receptor mediates the procoagulant properties of platelets and the proliferative properties of vascular endothelial and smooth muscle cells. In *in vitro* studies using a model cell line derived from melanoma cells, Abciximab blocked $\alpha_v\beta_3$-mediated effects including cell adhesion (IC_{50}=0.34 µg/mL). At concentrations which, *in vitro*, provide >80% GPIIb/IIIa receptor blockade, but above the *in vivo* therapeutic range, Abciximab more effectively blocked the burst of thrombin generation that followed platelet activation than select comparator antibodies which inhibit GPIIb/IIIa alone(1). The relationship of these *in vitro* data to clinical efficacy is uncertain.

Pre-clinical experience: Maximal inhibition of platelet aggregation was observed when ≥ 80% of GPIIb/IIIa receptors were blocked by Abciximab. In non-human primates, Abciximab bolus doses of 0.25 mg/kg generally achieved a blockade of at least 80% of platelet receptors and fully inhibited platelet aggregation. Inhibition of platelet function was temporary following a bolus dose, but receptor blockade could be sustained at ≥ 80% by continuous intravenous infusion. The inhibitory effects of Abciximab were substantially reversed by the transfusion of platelets in monkeys. The antithrombotic efficacy of prototype antibodies [murine 7E3 Fab and $F(ab')_2$] and Abciximab was evaluated in dog, monkey and baboon models of coronary, carotid, and femoral artery thrombosis. Doses of the murine version of 7E3 or Abciximab sufficient to produce high-grade (≥ 80%) GPIIb/IIIa receptor blockade prevented acute thrombosis and yielded lower rates of thrombosis compared with aspirin and/or heparin.

Pharmacokinetics: Following intravenous bolus administration, free plasma concentrations of Abciximab decrease rapidly with an initial half-life of less than 10 minutes and a second phase half-life of about 30 minutes, probably related to rapid binding to the platelet GPIIb/IIIa receptors. Platelet function generally recovers over the course of 48 hours (2,3), although Abciximab remains in the circulation for 15 days or more in a platelet-bound state. Intravenous administration of a 0.25 mg/kg bolus dose of Abciximab followed by continuous infusion of 10 µg/min (or a weight-adjusted infusion of 0.125 µg/kg/min to a maximum of 10 µg/min) produces approximately constant free plasma concentrations throughout the infusion. At the termination of the infusion period, free plasma concentrations fall rapidly for approximately six hours then decline at a slower rate.

Pharmacodynamics: Intravenous administration in humans of single bolus doses of Abciximab from 0.15 mg/kg to 0.30 mg/kg produced rapid dose-dependent inhibition of platelet function as measured by *ex vivo* platelet aggregation in response to adenosine diphosphate (ADP) or by prolongation of bleeding time. At the two highest doses (0.25 and 0.30 mg/kg) at two hours post injection, over 80% of the GPIIb/IIIa receptors were blocked and platelet aggregation in response to 20 µM ADP was almost abolished. The median bleeding time increased to over 30 minutes at both doses compared with a baseline value of approximately five minutes.

Intravenous administration in humans of a single bolus dose of 0.25 mg/kg followed by a continuous infusion of 10 µg/min for periods of 12 to 96 hours produced sustained high-grade GPIIb/IIIa receptor blockade (≥ 80%) and inhibition of platelet function (*ex vivo* platelet aggregation in response to 5 µM or 20 µM ADP less than 20% of baseline and bleeding time greater than 30 minutes) for the duration of the infusion in most patients. Similar results were obtained when a weight-adjusted infusion dose (0.125 µg/kg/min to a maximum of 10 µg/min) was used in patients weighing up to 80 kg. Results in patients who received the 0.25 mg/kg bolus followed by a 5 µg/min infusion for 24 hours showed a similar initial receptor blockade and inhibition of platelet aggregation, but the response was not maintained throughout the infusion period.

Low levels of GPIIb/IIIa receptor blockade are present for more than 10 days following cessation of the infusion. After discontinuation of Abciximab infusion, platelet function returns gradually to normal. Bleeding time returned to ≤ 12 minutes within 12 hours following the end of infusion in 15 of 20 patients (75%), and within 24 hours in 18 of 20 patients (90%). *Ex vivo* platelet aggregation in response to 5 µM ADP returned to ≥ 50% of baseline within 24 hours following the end of infusion in 11 of 32 patients (34%) and within 48 hours in 23 of 32 patients (72%). In response to 20 µM ADP, *ex vivo* platelet aggregation returned to ≥ 50% of baseline within 24 hours in 20 of 32 patients (62%) and within 48 hours in 28 of 32 patients (88%).

CLINICAL STUDIES

Abciximab has been studied in three Phase 3 clinical trials, all of which evaluated the effect of Abciximab in patients undergoing percutaneous coronary intervention: in patients at high risk for abrupt closure of the treated coronary vessel (EPIC), in a broader group of patients (EPILOG), and in unstable angina patients not responding to conventional medical therapy (CAPTURE). Percutaneous intervention included balloon angioplasty, atherectomy, or stent placement. All trials involved the use of various, concomitant heparin dose regimens and, unless contraindicated, aspirin (325 mg) was administered orally two hours prior to the planned procedure and then once daily.

Table 1
PRIMARY ENDPOINT EVENT RATE AT 30 DAYS - EPIC TRIAL

	Placebo (n=696)	Abciximab Bolus (n=695)	Abciximab Bolus + Infusion (n=708)
	Number of Patients (%)		
Death, MI, or urgent intervention[a]	89 (12.8)	79 (11.5)	59 (8.3)
p-value vs. placebo		0.428	0.008
Components of Primary Endpoint[b]			
Death	12 (1.7)	9 (1.3)	12 (1.7)
Acute myocardial infarctions in surviving patients	55 (7.9)	40 (5.8)	31 (4.4)
Urgent interventions in surviving patients without an acute myocardial infarction	22 (3.2)	30 (4.4)	16 (2.2)

[a]Patients who experienced more than one event in the first 30 days are counted only once.
[b]Patients are counted only once under the most serious component (death > acute MI > urgent intervention).

EPIC was a multicenter, double-blind, placebo-controlled trial of Abciximab in patients undergoing percutaneous transluminal coronary angioplasty or atherectomy (4). In the EPIC trial, 2099 patients between 26 and 83 years of age who were at high risk for abrupt closure of the treated coronary vessel were randomly allocated to one of three treatments: 1) an Abciximab bolus (0.25 mg/kg) followed by an Abciximab infusion (10 µg/min) for 12 hours (bolus plus infusion group); 2) an Abciximab bolus (0.25 mg/kg) followed by a placebo infusion (bolus group), or; 3) a placebo bolus followed by a placebo infusion (placebo group). Patients at high risk during or following percutaneous coronary intervention were defined as those with unstable angina or non-Q wave myocardial infarction (n=489), those with an acute Q-wave myocardial infarction within 12 hours of symptom onset (n=66), and those who were at high risk because of coronary morphology and/or clinical characteristics (n=1544). Treatment with study agent in each of the three arms was initiated 10–60 minutes before the onset of percutaneous coronary intervention. All patients initially received an intravenous heparin bolus (10,000 to 12,000 units) and boluses of up to 3,000 units thereafter to a maximum of 20,000 units during percutaneous coronary intervention. Heparin infusion was continued for 12 hours to maintain a therapeutic elevation of activated partial thromboplastin time (APTT, 1.5–2.5 times normal).

The primary endpoint was the occurrence of any of the following events within 30 days of percutaneous coronary intervention: death, myocardial infarction (MI), or the need for urgent intervention for recurrent ischemia [i.e., urgent percutaneous transluminal coronary angioplasty, urgent coronary artery bypass graft (CABG) surgery, a coronary stent, or an intra-aortic balloon pump]. The 30-day (Kaplan-Meier) primary endpoint event rates for each treatment group by intention-to-treat analysis of all randomized patients are shown in Table 1. The 4.5% lower incidence of the primary endpoint rates in the bolus plus infusion treatment group, compared with the placebo group, was statistically significant, whereas the 1.3% lower incidence in the bolus treatment group was not. A lower incidence of the primary endpoint was observed in the bolus plus infusion treatment arm for all three high-risk subgroups: patients with unstable angina, patients presenting within 12 hours of the onset of symptoms of an acute myocardial infarction, and patients with other high-risk clinical and/or morphologic characteristics (4). The treatment effect was largest in the first two subgroups and smallest in the third subgroup.

[See table 1 above]

The primary endpoint event rates in the bolus plus infusion treatment group were reduced mostly in the first 48 hours and this benefit was sustained through blinded evaluations at 30 days(4), six months(5) and three years(6). At the six-month follow-up visit this event rate remained lower in the bolus infusion arm (12.3%) than in the placebo arm (17.6%) (p=0.006 vs. placebo). Median long-term follow up was 3.1 years (99% of patients had follow up between 2.5 and 3.5 years). Using Kaplan-Meier estimates, at 3 years the absolute reduction in events was maintained with an event rate of 19.6% in the bolus plus infusion arm and 24.4% in the placebo arm (p=0.027 vs. placebo).

EPILOG was a randomized, double-blind, multicenter, placebo-controlled trial which evaluated Abciximab in a broad population of patients undergoing percutaneous coronary intervention (excluding patients with myocardial infarction and unstable angina meeting the EPIC high risk criteria)(7). EPILOG tested the hypothesis that use of a low-dose, weight-adjusted heparin regimen, early femoral arterial sheath removal, improved access site management and weight-adjustment of the Abciximab infusion dose could significantly lower the bleeding rate yet maintain the efficacy seen in the EPIC trial. EPILOG was a three treatment-arm trial: Abciximab plus standard dose, weight-adjusted heparin[1]; Abciximab plus low dose, weight-adjusted heparin[2];

Continued on next page

*** Identi-Code® symbol. This product information was prepared in June 2000. Current information on these and other products of Eli Lilly and Company may be obtained by direct inquiry to Lilly Research Laboratories, Lilly Corporate Center, Indianapolis, Indiana 46285, (800) 545-5979.**

ReoPro—Cont.

and placebo plus standard dose, weight-adjusted heparin. The Abciximab bolus dose was the same as that used in the EPIC trial (0.25 mg/kg), but the continuous infusion dose was weight adjusted in patients up to 80 kg[3] (0.125 μg/kg/min). Specific patient and access site management procedures as well as a strong recommendation for early sheath removal were also incorporated into the trial as described in PRECAUTIONS. The EPILOG trial achieved the objective of lowering the bleeding rate while maintaining efficacy: in the Abciximab treatment arms major bleeding was not significantly different from that in the placebo arm (see ADVERSE REACTIONS: Bleeding).

[1] Bolus administration of 100 U/kg weight-adjusted heparin to achieve an activated clotting time (ACT) of 300 seconds (maximum initial bolus 10,000 units).
[2] Bolus administration of 70 U/kg weight-adjusted heparin to achieve an activated clotting time (ACT) of 200 seconds (maximum initial bolus 7,000 units).
[3] Bolus administration of 0.25 mg/kg Abciximab 10 to 60 minutes before percutaneous coronary intervention immediately followed by a 0.125 μg/kg/min infusion (maximum 10 μg/min) for 12 hours.

The primary endpoint of the EPILOG trial was the composite of death or MI occurring within 30 days of percutaneous coronary intervention. The composite of death, MI, or urgent intervention was an important secondary endpoint. As seen in the EPIC trial, the endpoint events in the Abciximab treatment group were reduced mostly in the first 48 hours and this benefit was sustained through blinded evaluations at 30 days and six months. The (Kaplan-Meier) endpoint event rates at 30 days are shown in Table 2 for each treatment group by intention-to-treat analysis of all 2792 randomized patients. At the six-month follow-up visit, the event rate for death, MI, or repeat (urgent or non-urgent) intervention remained lower in the Abciximab treatment arms (22.3% and 22.8%, respectively, for the standard- and low-dose heparin arms) than in the placebo arm (25.8%) and the event rate for death, MI, or urgent intervention was substantially lower in the Abciximab treatment arms (8.3% and 8.4%, respectively, for the standard- and low-dose heparin arms) than in the placebo arm (14.7%). The proportionate reductions in endpoint event rates were similar irrespective of the type of coronary intervention used (balloon angioplasty, atherectomy, or stent placement). Risk assessment using the American College of Cardiology/American Heart Association clinical/morphological criteria had large inter-observer variability. Consequently, a low risk subgroup could not be reproducibly identified in which to evaluate efficacy.

[See table 2 above]

CAPTURE was a randomized, double-blind, multicenter, placebo-controlled trial of the use of Abciximab in unstable angina patients not responding to conventional medical therapy for whom percutaneous coronary intervention was planned, but not immediately performed (8) In contrast to the EPIC and EPILOG trials, the CAPTURE trial involved the administration of placebo or Abciximab starting 18 to 24 hours prior to percutaneous coronary intervention and continuing until one hour after completion of the intervention. Patients were assessed as having unstable angina not responding to conventional medical therapy if they had at least one episode of myocardial ischemia despite bed rest and at least two hours of therapy with intravenous heparin and oral or intravenous nitrates. These patients were enrolled into the CAPTURE trial, if during a screening angiogram, they were determined to have a coronary lesion amenable to percutaneous coronary intervention. Patients received a bolus dose and intravenous infusion of placebo or Abciximab for 18 to 24 hours. At the end of the infusion period, the intervention was performed. The Abciximab or placebo infusion was discontinued one hour following the intervention. Patients were treated with intravenous heparin and oral or intravenous nitrates throughout the 18 to 24-hour Abciximab infusion period prior to the percutaneous coronary intervention.

The Abciximab dose was a 0.25 mg/kg bolus followed by a continuous infusion at a rate of 10 μg/min. The CAPTURE trial incorporated weight adjustment of the standard heparin dose only during the performance of the intervention, but did not investigate the effect of a lower heparin dose, and arterial sheaths were left in place for approximately 40 hours. The primary endpoint of the CAPTURE trial was the occurrence of any of the following events within 30 days of percutaneous coronary intervention: death, MI, or urgent intervention. The 30-day (Kaplan-Meier) primary endpoint event rates for each treatment group by intention-to-treat analysis of all 1265 randomized patients are shown in Table 3.

[See table 3 above]

The 30-day results are consistent with EPIC results, with the greatest effects on the myocardial infarction and urgent intervention components of the composite endpoint. As secondary endpoints, the components of the composite endpoint were analyzed separately for the period prior to the percutaneous coronary intervention and the period from the beginning of the intervention through Day 30. The greatest difference in MI occurred in the post-intervention period: the rates of MI were lower in the Abciximab group compared with placebo (Abciximab 3.6%, placebo 6.1%). There was also a reduction in MI occurring prior to the percutaneous coronary intervention (Abciximab 0.6%, placebo 2.0%). An Abciximab-associated reduction in the incidence of urgent intervention occurred in the post-intervention period. No effect on mortality was observed in either period. At six months of follow up, the composite endpoint of death, MI, or repeat intervention (urgent or non-urgent) was not different between the Abciximab and placebo groups (Abciximab 31.0%, placebo 30.8%, p=0.77).

Table 2
ENDPOINT EVENT RATES AT 30 DAYS - EPILOG TRIAL

	Placebo + Standard Dose Heparin (n=939)	Abciximab + Standard Dose Heparin (n=918)	Abciximab + Low Dose Heparin (n=935)
	Number of Patients (%)		
Death or MI[a]	85 (9.1)	38 (4.2)	35 (3.8)
p-value vs. placebo		<0.001	<0.001
Death, MI, or urgent intervention[a]	109 (11.7)	49 (5.4)	48 (5.2)
p-value vs. placebo		<0.001	<0.001
Components of Composite Endpoints[b]			
Death	7 (0.8)	4 (0.4)	3 (0.3)
Acute myocardial infarctions in surviving patients	78 (8.4)	34 (3.7)	32 (3.4)
Urgent interventions in surviving patients without an acute myocardial infarction	24 (2.6)	11 (1.2)	13 (1.4)

[a]Patients who experienced more than one event in the first 30 days are counted only once.
[b]Patients are counted only once under the most serious component (death > acute MI > urgent intervention).

Table 3
PRIMARY ENDPOINT EVENT RATE AT 30 DAYS - CAPTURE TRIAL

	Placebo (n=635)	Abciximab (n=630)
	Number of Patients (%)	
Death, MI, or urgent intervention[a]	101 (15.9)	71 (11.3)
p-value vs. placebo		0.012
Components of Primary Endpoint[b]		
Death	8 (1.3)	6 (1.0)
MI in surviving patients	49 (7.7)	24 (3.8)
Urgent intervention in surviving patients without acute MI	44 (6.9)	41 (6.6)

[a] Patients who experienced more than one event in the first 30 days are counted only once. Urgent interventions included any unplanned percutaneous coronary intervention after the planned intervention, as well as any stent placement for immediate patency and any unplanned CABG or use of an intra-aortic balloon pump.
[b] Patients are counted only once under the most serious component (death>acute MI>urgent intervention).

Mortality was uncommon in all three trials, EPIC, EPILOG and CAPTURE. Similar mortality rates were observed in all arms within each trial. In all three trials, the rates of acute MI were significantly lower in the groups treated with Abciximab. Urgent intervention rates were also lower in Abciximab-treated groups in these trials.

Anticoagulation: Due to the incidence of bleeding seen in the EPIC trial, the dosing regimens of concomitant heparin and the target levels for anticoagulation were successively varied in the CAPTURE and EPILOG trials. These modified dosing regimens combined with other measures for patient management were associated with reduced bleeding rates (see ADVERSE REACTIONS: Bleeding)

EPILOG trial: Heparin was weight adjusted in all treatment arms. A baseline ACT was determined prior to percutaneous coronary intervention. In the low-dose heparin arm of the trial, heparin was administered as follows:

The initial heparin bolus was based upon the results of the baseline ACT, according to the following regimen:

- ACT < 150 seconds: administer 70 U/kg heparin
- ACT 150 - 199 seconds: administer 50 U/kg heparin
- ACT ≥ 200 seconds: administer no heparin

Additional 20 U/kg heparin boluses were given to achieve and maintain an ACT of 200 seconds during the procedure.

Discontinuation of heparin immediately after the procedure and removal of the arterial sheath within six hours were strongly recommended in the trial. If prolonged heparin therapy or delayed sheath removal was clinically indicated, heparin was adjusted to keep the APTT at a target of 60 to 85 seconds.

CAPTURE trial: Anticoagulation was initiated prior to the administration of Abciximab. Anticoagulation was initiated with an intravenous heparin infusion to achieve a target APTT of 60 to 85 seconds. The heparin infusion was not uniformly weight adjusted in this trial. The heparin infusion was maintained during the Abciximab infusion and was adjusted to achieve an ACT of 300 seconds or an APTT of 70 seconds during the percutaneous coronary intervention. Following the intervention, heparin management was as outlined above for the EPILOG trial.

INDICATIONS AND USAGE

Abciximab is indicated as an adjunct to percutaneous coronary intervention for the prevention of cardiac ischemic complications.

- in patients undergoing percutaneous coronary intervention
- in patients with unstable angina not responding to conventional medical therapy when percutaneous coronary intervention is planned within 24 hours

Abciximab use in patients not undergoing percutaneous coronary intervention has not been studied.

Abciximab is intended for use with aspirin and heparin and has been studied only in that setting, as described in CLINICAL STUDIES.

CONTRAINDICATIONS

Because Abciximab may increase the risk of bleeding, Abciximab is contraindicated in the following clinical situations:

- Active internal bleeding
- Recent (within six weeks) gastrointestinal (GI) or genitourinary (GU) bleeding of clinical significance
- History of cerebrovascular accident (CVA) within two years, or CVA with a significant residual neurological deficit
- Bleeding diathesis
- Administration of oral anticoagulants within seven days unless prothrombin time is ≤ 1.2 times control
- Thrombocytopenia (< 100,000 cells/μL)
- Recent (within six weeks) major surgery or trauma
- Intracranial neoplasm, arteriovenous malformation, or aneurysm
- Severe uncontrolled hypertension
- Presumed or documented history of vasculitis
- Use of intravenous dextran before percutaneous coronary intervention, or intent to use it during an intervention

Abciximab is also contraindicated in patients with known hypersensitivity to any component of this product or to murine proteins.

WARNINGS

Abciximab has the potential to increase the risk of bleeding, particularly in the presence of anticoagulation, e.g., from heparin, other anticoagulants, or thrombolytics (see ADVERSE REACTIONS: Bleeding).

The risk of major bleeds due to Abciximab therapy may be increased in patients receiving thrombolytics and should be weighed against the anticipated benefits.

Should serious bleeding occur that is not controllable with pressure, the infusion of Abciximab and any concomitant heparin should be stopped.

PRECAUTIONS

Bleeding Precautions: Results of the EPILOG trial show that bleeding can be reduced by the use of low-dose, weight-adjusted heparin regimens, adherence to stricter anticoagulation guidelines, early femoral arterial sheath removal, careful patient and access site management and weight-adjustment of the Abciximab infusion dose.

Therapy with Abciximab requires careful attention to all potential bleeding sites (including catheter insertion sites, arterial and venous puncture sites, cutdown sites, needle puncture sites, and gastrointestinal, genitourinary, and retroperitoneal sites).

Arterial and venous punctures, intramuscular injections, and use of urinary catheters, nasotracheal intubation, nasogastric tubes and automatic blood pressure cuffs should be minimized. When obtaining intravenous access, non-compressible sites (e.g., subclavian or jugular veins) should be avoided. Saline or heparin locks should be considered for blood drawing. Vascular puncture sites should be documented and monitored. Gentle care should be provided when removing dressings.

Femoral artery access site:

Arterial access site care is important to prevent bleeding. Care should be taken when attempting vascular access that only the anterior wall of the femoral artery is punctured, avoiding a Seldinger (through and through) technique for obtaining sheath access. Femoral vein sheath placement should be avoided unless needed. While the vascular sheath is in place, patients should be maintained on complete bed rest with the head of the bed ≤30° and the affected limb restrained in a straight position. Patients may be medicated for back/groin pain as necessary.

Discontinuation of heparin immediately upon completion of the procedure and removal of the arterial sheath within six hours is strongly recommended if APTT ≤ 50 sec or ACT ≤ 175 sec (See PRECAUTIONS: Laboratory Tests). In all circumstances, heparin should be discontinued at least two hours prior to arterial sheath removal.

Following sheath removal, pressure should be applied to the femoral artery for at least 30 minutes using either manual compression or a mechanical device for hemostasis. A pressure dressing should be applied following hemostasis. The patient should be maintained on bed rest for six to eight hours following sheath removal or discontinuation of Abciximab, or four hours following discontinuation of heparin, whichever is later. The pressure dressing should be removed prior to ambulation. The sheath insertion site and distal pulses of affected leg(s) should be frequently checked while the femoral artery sheath is in place and for six hours after femoral artery sheath removal. Any hematoma should be measured and monitored for enlargement.

The following conditions have been associated with an increased risk of bleeding and may be additive with the effect of Abciximab in the angioplasty setting: percutaneous coronary intervention within 12 hours of the onset of symptoms for acute myocardial infarction, prolonged percutaneous coronary intervention (lasting more than 70 minutes) and failed percutaneous coronary intervention.

Use of Thrombolytics, Anticoagulants and Other Antiplatelet Agents: In the EPIC, EPILOG and CAPTURE trials, Abciximab was used concomitantly with heparin and aspirin. For details of the anticoagulation algorithms used in these clinical trials, see CLINICAL STUDIES: Anticoagulation. Because Abciximab inhibits platelet aggregation, caution should be employed when it is used with other drugs that affect hemostasis, including thrombolytics, oral anticoagulants, non-steroidal anti-inflammatory drugs, dipyridamole, and ticlopidine.

In the EPIC trial, there was limited experience with the administration of Abciximab with low molecular weight dextran. Low molecular weight dextran was usually given for the deployment of a coronary stent, for which oral anticoagulants were also given. In the 11 patients who received low molecular weight dextran with Abciximab, five had major bleeding events and four had minor bleeding events. None of the five placebo patients treated with low molecular weight dextran had a major or minor bleeding event (see CONTRAINDICATIONS).

There are limited data on the use of Abciximab in patients receiving thrombolytic agents. Because of concern about synergistic effects on bleeding, systemic thrombolytic therapy should be used judiciously.

Thrombocytopenia: Platelet counts should be monitored prior to treatment, two to four hours following the bolus dose of Abciximab and at 24 hours or prior to discharge, whichever is first. If a patient experiences an acute platelet decrease (e.g., a platelet decrease to less than 100,000 cells/µL and a decrease of at least 25% from pre-treatment value), additional platelet counts should be determined. These platelet counts should be drawn in three separate tubes containing ethylenediaminetetraacetic acid (EDTA), citrate and heparin, respectively, to exclude pseudothrombocytopenia due to *in vitro* anticoagulant interaction. If true thrombocytopenia is verified, Abciximab should be immediately discontinued and the condition appropriately monitored and treated. For patients with thrombocytopenia in the clinical trials, a daily platelet count was obtained until it returned to normal. If a patient's platelet count dropped to 60,000 cells/µL, heparin and aspirin were discontinued. If a patient's platelet count dropped below 50,000 cells/µL, platelets were transfused. Most cases of severe thrombocytopenia (<50,000 cells/µL) occurred within the first 24 hours of Abciximab administration.

Restoration of Platelet Function: In the event of serious uncontrolled bleeding or the need for emergency surgery, Abciximab should be discontinued. If platelet function does not return to normal, it may be restored, at least in part, with platelet transfusion.

Laboratory Tests: Before infusion of Abciximab, platelet count, prothrombin time, ACT and APTT should be measured to identify pre-existing hemostatic abnormalities.

Based on an integrated analysis of data from all studies, the following guidelines may be utilized to minimize the risk for bleeding:

When Abciximab is initiated 18 to 24 hours before percutaneous coronary intervention, the APTT should be maintained between 60 and 85 seconds during the Abciximab and heparin infusion period.

Table 4
NON-CABG BLEEDING IN THE EPIC, EPILOG AND CAPTURE TRIALS
Number of Patients with Bleeds (%)

EPIC:

	Placebo (n = 696)	Abciximab (Bolus + Infusion) (n = 708)
Major[a]	23 (3.3)	75 (10.6)
Minor	64 (9.2)	119 (16.8)
Requiring Transfusion[b]	14 (2.0)	55 (7.8)

CAPTURE:

	Placebo (n = 635)	Abciximab (n = 630)
Major[a]	12 (1.9)	24 (3.8)
Minor	13 (2.0)	30 (4.8)
Requiring Transfusion[b]	9 (1.4)	15 (2.4)

EPILOG:

	Placebo (n = 939)	Abciximab + Standard-dose Heparin (n = 918)	Abciximab + Low-dose Heparin (n = 935)
Major[a]	10 (1.1)	17 (1.9)	10 (1.1)
Minor	32 (3.4)	70 (7.6)	37 (4.0)
Requiring Transfusion[b]	10 (1.1)	7 (0.8)	6 (0.6)

[a] Patients who had bleeding in more than one classification are counted only once according to the most severe classification. Patients with multiple bleeding events of the same classification are also counted once within that classification.

[b] Packed red blood cells or whole blood

During percutaneous coronary intervention the ACT should be maintained between 200 and 300 seconds.

If anticoagulation is continued in these patients following percutaneous coronary intervention, the APTT should be maintained between 60 and 85 seconds.

The APTT or ACT should be checked prior to arterial sheath removal. The sheath should not be removed unless APTT ≤ 50 seconds or ACT ≤ 175 seconds.

Readministration: Administration of Abciximab may result in human anti-chimeric antibody (HACA) formation that could potentially cause allergic or hypersensitivity reactions (including anaphylaxis), thrombocytopenia or diminished benefit upon readministration of Abciximab. In the EPIC, EPILOG, and CAPTURE trials, positive HACA responses occurred in approximately 5.8% of the Abciximab-treated patients. There was no excess of hypersensitivity or allergic reactions related to Abciximab treatment.

Readministration of Abciximab to 29 healthy volunteers who had not developed a HACA response after first administration has not led to any change in Abciximab pharmacokinetics or to any reduction in antiplatelet potency. However, results in this small group of patients suggest that the incidence of HACA response may be increased after readministration. Readministration to patients who have developed a positive HACA response after initial administration has not been evaluated in clinical trials.

Allergic Reactions: Anaphylaxis has not been reported for Abciximab-treated patients in any of the Phase 3 clinical trials. However, anaphylaxis may occur. If it does, administration of Abciximab should be immediately stopped and standard appropriate resuscitative measures should be initiated.

Drug Interactions: Although drug interactions with Abciximab have not been studied systematically, Abciximab has been administered to patients with ischemic heart disease treated concomitantly with a broad range of medications used in the treatment of angina, myocardial infarction and hypertension. These medications have included heparin, warfarin, beta-adrenergic receptor blockers, calcium channel antagonists, angiotensin converting enzyme inhibitors, intravenous and oral nitrates, and aspirin. Heparin, other anticoagulants, thrombolytics, and antiplatelet agents may be associated with an increase in bleeding. Patients with HACA titers may have allergic or hypersensitivity reactions when treated with other diagnostic or therapeutic monoclonal antibodies.

Carcinogenesis, Mutagenesis and Impairment of Fertility: *In vitro* and *in vivo* mutagenicity studies have not demonstrated any mutagenic effect. Long-term studies in animals have not been performed to evaluate the carcinogenic potential or effects on fertility in male or female animals.

Pregnancy Category C: Animal reproduction studies have not been conducted with Abciximab. It is also not known whether Abciximab can cause fetal harm when administered to a pregnant woman or can affect reproduction capacity. Abciximab should be given to a pregnant woman only if clearly needed.

Nursing Mothers: It is not known whether this drug is excreted in human milk or absorbed systemically after ingestion. Because many drugs are excreted in human milk, caution should be exercised when Abciximab is administered to a nursing woman.

Pediatric Use: Safety and effectiveness in pediatric patients have not been studied.

ADVERSE REACTIONS

Bleeding: Abciximab has the potential to increase the risk of bleeding, particularly in the presence of anticoagulation, e.g. from heparin, other anticoagulants or thrombolytics. Bleeding in the Phase 3 trials was classified as major, minor or insignificant by the criteria of the Thrombolysis in Myocardial Infarction study group(9). Major bleeding events were defined as either an intracranial hemorrhage or a decrease in hemoglobin greater than 5 g/dL. Minor bleeding events included spontaneous gross hematuria, spontaneous hematemesis, observed blood loss with a hemoglobin decrease of more than 3 g/dL, or a decrease in hemoglobin of at least 4 g/dL without an identified bleeding site. Insignificant bleeding events were defined as a decrease in hemoglobin of less than 3 g/dL or a decrease in hemoglobin between 3–4 g/dL without observed bleeding. In patients who received transfusions, the number of units of blood lost was estimated through an adaptation of the method of Landefeld, et al.(10).

In the EPIC trial, in which a non-weight-adjusted, standard heparin dose regimen was used, the most common complication during Abciximab therapy was bleeding during the first 36 hours. The incidences of major bleeding, minor bleeding and transfusion of blood products were significantly increased. Approximately 70% of Abciximab-treated patients with major bleeding had bleeding at the arterial access site in the groin. Abciximab-treated patients also had a higher incidence of major bleeding events from gastrointestinal, genitourinary, retroperitoneal, and other sites.

Bleeding rates were reduced in the CAPTURE trial, and further reduced in the EPILOG trial by use of modified dosing regimens and specific patient management techniques. In EPILOG, using the heparin and Abciximab dosing, sheath removal and arterial access site guidelines described under PRECAUTIONS, the incidence of major bleeding in patients treated with Abciximab and low-dose, weight-adjusted heparin was not significantly different from that in patients receiving placebo.

Subgroup analyses in the EPIC and CAPTURE trials showed that non-CABG major bleeding was more common in Abciximab patients weighing ≤ 75 kg. In the EPILOG trial which used weight-adjusted heparin dosing, the non-CABG major bleeding rates for Abciximab-treated patients did not differ substantially by weight subgroup.

Although data are limited, Abciximab treatment was not associated with excess major bleeding in patients who underwent CABG surgery. (The range among all treatment arms was 3–5% in EPIC and 1–2% in the CAPTURE and EPILOG trials.) Some patients with prolonged bleeding times received platelet transfusions to correct the bleeding time prior to surgery. (See PRECAUTIONS: Restoration of Platelet Function.)

The rates of major bleeding, minor bleeding and bleeding events requiring transfusions in the EPIC, CAPTURE and EPILOG trials are shown in Table 4. The rates of insignificant bleeding events are not included in Table 4.

[See table 4 above]

Intracranial Hemorrhage and Stroke: The total incidence of intracranial hemorrhage and non-hemorrhagic stroke across all three trials was not significantly different, 7/2225 for placebo patients and 10/3112 for Abciximab treated patients. The incidence of intracranial hemorrhage was 3/2225 for placebo patients and 6/3112 for Abciximab patients.

Thrombocytopenia: In the clinical trials, patients treated with Abciximab were more likely than patients treated with placebo to experience decreases in platelet counts. The rates of thrombocytopenia and transfusions were lower in the subsequent CAPTURE and EPILOG trials (Table 5).

[See table 5 at top of next page]

Other Adverse Reactions: Table 6 shows adverse events other than bleeding and thrombocytopenia from the combined EPIC, EPILOG and CAPTURE trials which occurred

Continued on next page

*** Identi-Code® symbol. This product information was prepared in June 2000. Current information on these and other products of Eli Lilly and Company may be obtained by direct inquiry to Lilly Research Laboratories, Lilly Corporate Center, Indianapolis, Indiana 46285, (800) 545-5979.**

ReoPro—Cont.

in patients in the bolus plus infusion arm at an incidence of more than 0.5% higher than in those treated with placebo. [See table 6 above]

The following additional adverse events from the EPIC, EPILOG and CAPTURE trials were reported by investigators for patients treated with a bolus plus infusion of Abciximab at incidences which were less than 0.5% higher than for patients in the placebo arm.

Cardiovascular System—ventricular tachycardia (1.4%), pseudoaneurysm (0.8%), palpitation (0.5%), arteriovenous fistula (0.4%), incomplete AV block (0.3%), nodal arrhythmia (0.2%), complete AV block (0.1%), embolism (limb)(0.1%); thrombophlebitis (0.1%);

Gastrointestinal System—dyspepsia (2.1%), diarrhea (1.1%), ileus (0.1%), gastroesophageal reflux (0.1%);

Hemic and Lymphatic System—anemia (1.3%), leukocytosis (0.5%), petechiae (0.2%);

Nervous System—dizziness (2.9%), anxiety (1.7%), abnormal thinking (1.3%), agitation (0.7%), hypesthesia (0.6%), confusion (0.5%), muscle contractions (0.4%), coma (0.2%), hypertonia (0.2%), diplopia (0.1%);

Respiratory System—pneumonia (0.4%), rales (0.4%), pleural effusion (0.3%), bronchitis (0.3%) bronchospasm (0.3%), pleurisy (0.2%), pulmonary embolism (0.2%), rhonchi (0.1%);

Musculoskeletal System—myalgia (0.2%);

Urogenital System—urinary retention (0.7%), dysuria (0.4%), abnormal renal function (0.4%), frequent micturition (0.1%), cystalgia (0.1%), urinary incontinence (0.1%), prostatitis (0.1%);

Miscellaneous—pain (5.4%), sweating increased (1.0%), asthenia (0.7%), incisional pain (0.6%), pruritus (0.5%), abnormal vision (0.3%), edema (0.3%), wound (0.2%), abscess (0.2%), cellulitis (0.2%), peripheral coldness (0.2%), injection site pain (0.1%), dry mouth (0.1%), pallor (0.1%), diabetes mellitus (0.1%), hyperkalemia (0.1%), enlarged abdomen (0.1%), bullous eruption (0.1%), inflammation (0.1%), drug toxicity (0.1%).

OVERDOSAGE

There has been no experience of overdosage in human clinical trials.

DOSAGE AND ADMINISTRATION

The safety and efficacy of Abciximab have only been investigated with concomitant administration of heparin and aspirin as described in CLINICAL STUDIES.

In patients with failed percutaneous coronary interventions, the continuous infusion of Abciximab should be stopped because there is no evidence for Abciximab efficacy in that setting.

In the event of serious bleeding that cannot be controlled by compression, Abciximab and heparin should be discontinued immediately.

The recommended dosage of Abciximab in adults is a 0.25 mg/kg intravenous bolus administered 10–60 minutes before the start of percutaneous coronary intervention, followed by a continuous intravenous infusion of 0.125 μg/kg/min (to a maximum of 10 μg/min) for 12 hours.

Patients with unstable angina not responding to conventional medical therapy and who are planned to undergo percutaneous coronary intervention within 24 hours may be treated with an Abciximab 0.25 mg/kg intravenous bolus followed by an 18 to 24-hour intravenous infusion of 10 μg/min, concluding one hour after the percutaneous coronary intervention.

Instructions for Administration

1. Parenteral drug products should be inspected visually for particulate matter prior to administration. Preparations of Abciximab containing visibly opaque particles should NOT be used.

2. Hypersensitivity reactions should be anticipated whenever protein solutions such as Abciximab are administered. Epinephrine, dopamine, theophylline, antihistamines, and corticosteroids should be available for immediate use. If symptoms of an allergic reaction or anaphylaxis appear, the infusion should be stopped and appropriate treatment given.

3. As with all parenteral drug products, aseptic procedures should be used during the administration of Abciximab.

4. Withdraw the necessary amount of Abciximab for bolus injection into a syringe. Filter the bolus injection using a sterile, non-pyrogenic, low protein-binding 0.2 or 0.22 μm filter (Millipore SLGV025LS or equivalent).

5. Withdraw the necessary amount of Abciximab for the continuous infusion into a syringe. Inject into an appropriate container of sterile 0.9% saline or 5% dextrose and infuse at the calculated rate via a continuous infusion pump. The continuous infusion should be filtered either upon admixture using a sterile, non-pyrogenic, low protein-binding 0.2 or 0.22 μm syringe filter (Millipore SLGV025LS or equivalent) or upon administration using an in-line, sterile, non-pyrogenic, low protein-binding 0.2 or 0.22 μm filter (Abbott #4524 or equivalent). Discard the unused portion at the end of the infusion.

6. No incompatibilities have been shown with intravenous infusion fluids or commonly used cardiovascular drugs. Nevertheless, Abciximab should be administered in a separate intravenous line whenever possible and not mixed with other medications.

Table 5
THROMBOCYTOPENIA AND PLATELET TRANSFUSIONS[a]

	Placebo + Standard-dose Heparin	Abciximab + Standard-dose Heparin	Abciximab + Low-dose Heparin
	Total number of patients enrolled		
EPIC	n = 696	n = 708	—
CAPTURE	n = 635	n = 630	—
EPILOG	n = 939	n = 918	n = 935
	% of patients with events		
Patients with decrease of platelets to <50,000 cells/μL[a]			
EPIC	0.7	1.6	—
CAPTURE	0.3	1.7	—
EPILOG	0.4	0.9	0.4
Patients with decrease of platelets to <100,000 cells/μL[a]			
EPIC	3.4	5.2	—
CAPTURE	1.3	5.6	—
EPILOG	1.5	2.6	2.5
Patients who received platelet tranfusions[b]			
EPIC	2.6	5.5	—
CAPTURE	0.3	2.1	—
EPILOG	1.1	1.6	0.9

[a] Patients with a platelet count of <50,000 cells/μL are also included in the category of patients with a platelet count of <100,000 cells/μL.

[b] Includes patients receiving platelet transfusions for thrombocytopenia or any other reason.

Table 6
ADVERSE EVENTS AMONG TREATED PATIENTS IN THE EPIC, EPILOG AND CAPTURE TRIALS

Event	Placebo (n = 2226)	Bolus + Infusion (n = 3111)
	Number of Patients (%)	
Cardiovascular System		
Hypotension	230 (10.3)	447 (14.4)
Bradycardia	79 (3.5)	140 (4.5)
Gastrointestinal System		
Nausea	255 (11.5)	423 (13.6)
Vomiting	152 (6.8)	226 (7.3)
Abdominal Pain	49 (2.2)	97 (3.1)
Miscellaneous		
Back Pain	304 (13.7)	546 (17.6)
Chest Pain	208 (9.3)	356 (11.4)
Headache	122 (5.5)	200 (6.4)
Puncture Site Pain	58 (2.6)	113 (3.6)
Peripheral Edema	25 (1.1)	49 (1.6)

7. No incompatibilities have been observed with glass bottles or polyvinyl chloride bags and administration sets.

HOW SUPPLIED

Abciximab (ReoPro®) 2 mg/mL is supplied in 5 mL vials containing 10 mg (NDC 0002-7140-01).

Vials should be stored at 2 to 8°C (36 to 46°F). Do not freeze. Do not shake. Do not use beyond the expiration date. Discard any unused portion left in the vial.

REFERENCES

1. Reverter JC, Beguin S, Kessels H, Kumar R, Hemmer HC, Coller BS. Inhibition of platelet-mediated, tissue-factor-induced thrombin generation by the mouse/human chimeric 7E3 antibody; potential implications for the effect of c7E3 Fab treatment on acute thrombosis and "clinical restenosis". *J Clin Invest*; 1996;**98**:863–874.
2. Tcheng J, Ellis SG, George BS. Pharmacodynamics of chimeric glycoprotein IIb/IIIa integrin antiplatelet antibody Fab 7E3 in high risk coronary angioplasty. *Circulation*; 1994;**90**:1757–1764.
3. Simoons ML, de Boer MJ, van der Brand MJBM, et al. Randomized trial of a GPIIb/IIIa platelet receptor blocker in refractory unstable angina. *Circulation*; 1994;**89**:596–603.
4. EPIC Investigators. Use of a monoclonal antibody directed against the platelet glycoprotein IIb/IIIa receptor in high-risk coronary angioplasty. *N Engl J Med*; 1994;**330**:956–961.
5. Topol EJ, Califf RM, Weisman HF, et al. Randomised trial of coronary intervention with antibody against platelet IIb/IIIa integrin for reduction of clinical restenosis: results at six months. *Lancet* 1994;**343**:881–886.
6. Topol EJ, Ferguson JJ, Weisman HF, et al. for the EPIC Investigators. Long term protection from myocardial ischemic events in a randomized trial of brief integrin blockade with percutaneous coronary intervention. *JAMA*. 1997;**278**:479–484.
7. EPILOG Investigators. Platelet glycoprotein IIb/IIIa receptor blockade and low dose heparin during percutaneous coronary revascularization. *N Eng J Med*. 1997;**336**:1689–1696.
8. CAPTURE Investigators. Randomised placebo-controlled trial of abciximab before, during and after coronary intervention in refractory unstable angina: the CAPTURE study. *Lancet* 1997;**349**;1429–1435.
9. Rao, AK, Pratt C, Berke A, et al. Thrombolysis in Myocardial Infarction (TIMI) Trial – Phase I: Hemorrhagic manifestations and changes in plasma fibrinogen and the fibrinolytic system in patients treated with recombinant tissue plasminogen activator and streptokinase. *J Am Coll Cardiol*. 1988;**11**:1–11.
10. Landefeld, CS, Cook EF, Flatley M, et al. Identification and preliminary validation of predictors of major bleeding in hospitalized patients starting anticoagulant therapy. *Am J Med*. 1987;**82**:703–713.

Revision Date: February 12, 1998

Manufactured by:
Centocor B.V.
Leiden, The Netherlands
U.S. License Number: 1178

Distributed by:
Eli Lilly and Company
Indianapolis, IN 46285

Shown in Product Identification Guide, page 321

SARAFEM™ ℞

[sair-a-fem]
fluoxetine hydrochloride

DESCRIPTION

SARAFEM™ (Fluoxetine Hydrochloride) is a selective serotonin reuptake inhibitor (SSRI) for oral administration; fluoxetine was initially developed and marketed as an antidepressant (Prozac®, fluoxetine hydrochloride). It is designated (±)-N-methyl-3-phenyl-3-[(α,α,α-trifluoro-*p*-tolyl)oxy]propylamine hydrochloride and has the empirical formula of $C_{17}H_{18}F_3NO \bullet HCl$. Its molecular weight is 345.79. The structural formula is:

F_3C—(C₆H₄)—O—CHCH₂CH₂NHCH₃ • HCl (with phenyl ring on CH)

Fluoxetine hydrochloride is a white to off-white crystalline solid with a solubility of 14 mg/mL in water.

Each Pulvule® contains fluoxetine hydrochloride equivalent to 10 mg (32.3 μmol) or 20 mg (64.7 μmol) of fluoxetine. The Pulvules also contain dimethicone, F D & C Blue No. 1, F D & C Red No. 3, F D & C Yellow No. 6, gelatin, sodium lauryl sulfate, starch, and titanium dioxide.

CLINICAL PHARMACOLOGY

Pharmacodynamics:

The mechanism of action of fluoxetine in premenstrual dysphoric disorder (PMDD) is unknown, but is presumed to be linked to its inhibition of CNS neuronal uptake of serotonin. Studies at clinically relevant doses in humans have demonstrated that fluoxetine blocks the uptake of serotonin into human platelets. Studies in animals also suggest that fluoxetine is a much more potent uptake inhibitor of serotonin than of norepinephrine.

Antagonism of muscarinic, histaminergic, and α_1-adrenergic receptors has been hypothesized to be associated with various anticholinergic, sedative, and cardiovascular effects of certain psychoactive drugs. Fluoxetine has little affinity for these receptors.

Absorption, Distribution, Metabolism, and Excretion:

Systemic Bioavailability—In humans, following a single oral 40 mg dose, peak plasma concentrations of fluoxetine from 15 to 55 ng/mL are observed after 6 to 8 hours.

Food does not appear to affect the systemic bioavailability of fluoxetine, although it may delay its absorption inconsequentially. Thus, fluoxetine may be administered with or without food.

Protein Binding—Over the concentration range from 200 to 1,000 ng/mL, approximately 94.5% of fluoxetine is bound in vitro to human serum proteins, including albumin and α_1-glycoprotein. The interaction between fluoxetine and other highly protein-bound drugs has not been fully evaluated, but may be important (*see* Precautions).

Enantiomers—Fluoxetine is a racemic mixture (50/50) of *R*-fluoxetine and *S*-fluoxetine enantiomers. In animal models, both enantiomers are specific and potent serotonin uptake inhibitors with essentially equivalent pharmacologic activity. The *S*-fluoxetine enantiomer is eliminated more slowly and is the predominant enantiomer present in plasma at steady state.

Metabolism—Fluoxetine is extensively metabolized in the liver to norfluoxetine and a number of other, unidentified metabolites. The only identified active metabolite, norfluoxetine, is formed by demethylation of fluoxetine. In animal models, *S*-norfluoxetine is a potent and selective inhibitor of serotonin uptake and has activity essentially equivalent to *R*- or *S*-fluoxetine. *R*-norfluoxetine is significantly less potent than the parent drug in the inhibition of serotonin uptake. The primary route of elimination appears to be hepatic metabolism to inactive metabolites excreted by the kidney.

Clinical Issues Related to Metabolism/Elimination—The complexity of the metabolism of fluoxetine has several consequences that may potentially affect fluoxetine's clinical use.

Variability in Metabolism—A subset (about 7%) of the population has reduced activity of the drug metabolizing enzyme cytochrome P450IID6. Such individuals are referred to as "poor metabolizers" of drugs such as debrisoquin, dextromethorphan, and the tricyclic antidepressants. In a study involving labeled and unlabeled enantiomers administered as a racemate, these individuals metabolized *S*-fluoxetine at a slower rate and thus achieved higher concentrations of *S*-fluoxetine. Consequently, concentrations of *S*-norfluoxetine at steady state were lower. The metabolism of *R*-fluoxetine in these poor metabolizers appears normal. When compared with normal metabolizers, the total sum at steady state of the plasma concentrations of the 4 active enantiomers was not significantly greater among poor metabolizers. Thus, the net pharmacodynamic activities were essentially the same. Alternative, nonsaturable pathways (non-IID6) also contribute to the metabolism of fluoxetine. This explains how fluoxetine achieves a steady-state concentration rather than increasing without limit.

Because fluoxetine's metabolism, like that of a number of other compounds including tricyclic antidepressants and other selective serotonin reuptake inhibitors, involves the P450IID6 system, concomitant therapy with drugs also metabolized by this enzyme system (such as the tricyclic antidepressants) may lead to drug interactions (*see* Drug Interactions *under* Precautions).

Accumulation and Slow Elimination—The relatively slow elimination of fluoxetine (elimination half-life of 1 to 3 days after acute administration and 4 to 6 days after chronic administration) and its active metabolite, norfluoxetine (elimination half-life of 4 to 16 days after acute and chronic administration), leads to significant accumulation of these active species in chronic use and delayed attainment of steady state, even when a fixed dose is used. After 30 days of dosing at 40 mg/day, plasma concentrations of fluoxetine in the range of 91 to 302 ng/mL and norfluoxetine in the range of 72 to 258 ng/mL have been observed. Plasma concentrations of fluoxetine were higher than those predicted by single-dose studies, because fluoxetine's metabolism is not proportional to dose. Norfluoxetine, however, appears to have linear pharmacokinetics. Its mean terminal half-life after a single dose was 8.6 days and after multiple dosing was 9.3 days. Steady state levels after prolonged dosing are similar to levels seen at 4–5 weeks.

The long elimination half-lives of fluoxetine and norfluoxetine assure that, even when dosing is stopped, active drug substance will persist in the body for weeks (primarily depending on individual patient characteristics, previous dosing regimen, and length of previous therapy at discontinuation). This is of potential consequence when drug discontinuation is required or when drugs are prescribed that might interact with fluoxetine and norfluoxetine following the discontinuation of SARAFEM.

Liver Disease—As might be predicted from its primary site of metabolism, liver impairment can affect the elimination of fluoxetine. The elimination half-life of fluoxetine was prolonged in a study of cirrhotic patients, with a mean of 7.6 days compared to the range of 2 to 3 days seen in subjects without liver disease; norfluoxetine elimination was also delayed, with a mean duration of 12 days for cirrhotic patients compared to the range of 7 to 9 days in normal subjects. This suggests that the use of fluoxetine in patients with liver disease must be approached with caution. If fluoxetine is administered to patients with liver disease, a lower or less frequent dose should be used (*see* Use in Patients with Concomitant Illness *under* Precautions *and* Dosage and Administration).

Renal Disease—In depressed patients on dialysis (N=12), fluoxetine administered as 20 mg once daily for two months produced steady-state fluoxetine and norfluoxetine plasma concentrations comparable to those seen in patients with normal renal function. While the possibility exists that renally excreted metabolites of fluoxetine may accumulate to higher levels in patients with severe renal dysfunction, use of a lower or less frequent dose is not routinely necessary in renally impaired patients (*see* Use in Patients with Concomitant Illness *under* Precautions *and* Dosage and Administration).

Clinical Trials:

Premenstrual Dysphoric Disorder (PMDD)—The effectiveness of SARAFEM for the treatment of PMDD was established in two placebo-controlled trials. Patients in these trials met DSM-IIIR criteria for Late Luteal Phase Dysphoric Disorder (LLPDD), the clinical entity now referred to as Premenstrual Dysphoric Disorder (PMDD) in DSM-IV. Patients on oral contraceptives were excluded from these trials; therefore, the efficacy of fluoxetine in combination with oral contraceptives for the treatment of PMDD is unknown. In the first double-blind, parallel group study of 6 months duration involving n=320 patients, fixed doses of fluoxetine 20 mg and 60 mg/day given continuously throughout the menstrual cycle were shown to be significantly more effective than placebo as measured by a Visual Analogue Scale (VAS) total score (including mood and physical symptoms). The average total VAS score decreased 7% on placebo treatment, 36% on 20 mg and 39% on 60 mg fluoxetine. The difference between the 20 mg and 60 mg doses was not statistically significant. The following table shows the percentage of patients meeting criteria for either moderate or marked improvement on the VAS total score:

Percentage of Patients Moderately and Markedly Improved (>50% and 75% reduction, respectively, from baseline Luteal Phase VAS total score)

Improvement	N	Placebo	N	Fluox 20 mg	N	Fluox 60 mg
Moderate	94	11%	95	37%	85	38%
Marked	94	4%	95	6%	85	18%

In a second double-blind, cross-over study, patients (n=19) were treated with fluoxetine 20 mg to 60 mg/day (mean dose=27 mg/day) and placebo continuously throughout the menstrual cycle for a period of three months each. Fluoxetine was significantly more effective than placebo as measured by within cycle follicular to luteal phase changes in the VAS total score (mood, physical, and social impairment symptoms). The average VAS total score (follicular to luteal phase increase) was 3.8 times higher during placebo treatment than what was observed during fluoxetine treatment.

In a third double-blind, parallel group study, patients with LLPDD (n=42) were treated with fluoxetine 20 mg/day, bupropion 300 mg/day, or placebo for two months. Neither fluoxetine nor bupropion was shown to be superior to placebo on the primary endpoint, i.e., response rate [defined as a rating of 1 (very much improved) or 2 (much improved) on the CGI], possibly due to sample size.

INDICATIONS AND USAGE

SARAFEM is indicated for the treatment of premenstrual dysphoric disorder (PMDD).

The efficacy of fluoxetine in the treatment of PMDD was established in 2 placebo-controlled trials (*see* Clinical Trials *under* Clinical Pharmacology).

The essential features of PMDD, according to the Diagnostic and Statistical Manual-4th edition (DSM-IV) include markedly depressed mood, anxiety or tension, affective lability, and persistent anger or irritability. Other features include decreased interest in usual activities, difficulty concentrating, lack of energy, change in appetite or sleep, and feeling out of control. Physical symptoms associated with PMDD include breast tenderness, headache, joint and muscle pain, bloating, and weight gain. These symptoms occur regularly during the luteal phase and remit within a few days following onset of menses; the disturbance markedly interferes with work or school or with usual social activities and relationships with others. In making the diagnosis, care should be taken to rule out other cyclical mood disorders that may be exacerbated by treatment with an antidepressant.

The effectiveness of SARAFEM in long-term use, that is, for more than 6 months, has not been systematically evaluated in controlled trials. Therefore, the physician who elects to use SARAFEM for extended periods should periodically re-evaluate the long-term usefulness of the drug for the individual patient.

CONTRAINDICATIONS

SARAFEM is contraindicated in patients known to be hypersensitive to it.

Monoamine Oxidase Inhibitors—There have been reports of serious, sometimes fatal, reactions (including hyperthermia, rigidity, myoclonus, autonomic instability with possible rapid fluctuations of vital signs, and mental status changes that include extreme agitation progressing to delirium and coma) in patients receiving fluoxetine in combination with a monoamine oxidase inhibitor (MAOI), and in patients who have recently discontinued fluoxetine and are then started on an MAOI. Some cases presented with features resembling neuroleptic malignant syndrome. Therefore, fluoxetine should not be used in combination with an MAOI, or within a minimum of 14 days of discontinuing therapy with an MAOI. Since fluoxetine and its major metabolite have very long elimination half-lives, at least 5 weeks (perhaps longer, especially if fluoxetine has been prescribed chronically and/or at higher doses [*see* Accumulation and Slow Elimination *under* Clinical Pharmacology]) should be allowed after stopping fluoxetine before starting an MAOI.

Thioridazine—Thioridazine should not be administered with SARAFEM or within a minimum of 5 weeks after SARAFEM has been discontinued (*see* WARNINGS).

WARNINGS

Rash and Possibly Allergic Events—In three premarketing clinical trials for PMDD, 5% of 243 patients treated with SARAFEM reported rash and/or urticaria. None of these cases were classified as serious and 2 of 243 patients (both receiving 60 mg) were withdrawn from treatment because of rash and/or urticaria.

In US fluoxetine clinical trials for conditions other than PMDD, 7% of 10,782 patients developed various types of rashes and/or urticaria. Among the cases of rash and/or urticaria reported in premarketing clinical trials, almost a third were withdrawn from treatment because of the rash and/or systemic signs or symptoms associated with the rash. Clinical findings reported in association with rash include fever, leukocytosis, arthralgias, edema, carpal tunnel syndrome, respiratory distress, lymphadenopathy, proteinuria, and mild transaminase elevation. Most patients improved promptly with discontinuation of fluoxetine and/or adjunctive treatment with antihistamines or steroids, and all patients experiencing these events were reported to recover completely.

In premarketing clinical trials of fluoxetine for conditions other than PMDD, 2 patients are known to have developed a serious cutaneous systemic illness. In neither patient was there an unequivocal diagnosis, but 1 was considered to have a leukocytoclastic vasculitis, and the other, a severe desquamating syndrome that was considered variously to be a vasculitis or erythema multiforme. Other patients have had systemic syndromes suggestive of serum sickness.

Since the introduction of fluoxetine for other indications, systemic events, possibly related to vasculitis, have developed in patients with rash. Although these events are rare, they may be serious, involving the lung, kidney, or liver. Death has been reported to occur in association with these systemic events.

Anaphylactoid events, including bronchospasm, angioedema, and urticaria alone and in combination, have been reported.

Pulmonary events, including inflammatory processes of varying histopathology and/or fibrosis, have been reported rarely. These events have occurred with dyspnea as the only preceding symptom.

Whether these systemic events and rash have a common underlying cause or are due to different etiologies or pathogenic processes is not known. Furthermore, a specific underlying immunologic basis for these events has not been identified. Upon the appearance of rash or of other possibly allergic phenomena for which an alternative etiology cannot be identified, SARAFEM should be discontinued.

Potential Interaction with Thioridazine—In a study of 19 healthy male subjects, which included 6 slow and 13 rapid hydroxylators of debrisoquin, a single 25-mg oral dose of thioridazine produced a 2.4-fold higher C_{max} and a 4.5-fold higher AUC for thioridazine in the slow hydroxylators compared to the rapid hydroxylators. The rate of debrisoquin hydroxylation is felt to depend on the level of cytochrome P450IID6 isozyme activity. Thus, this study suggests that drugs which inhibit P450IID6, such as certain SSRIs, including fluoxetine, will produce elevated plasma levels of thioridazine (*see* PRECAUTIONS).

Thioridazine administration produces a dose-related prolongation of the QTc interval, which is associated with serious ventricular arrhythmias, such as torsades de pointes-type arrhythmias, and sudden death. This risk is expected to increase with fluoxetine-induced inhibition of thioridazine metabolism (*see* CONTRAINDICATIONS).

Continued on next page

*** Identi-Code® symbol. This product information was prepared in June 2000. Current information on these and other products of Eli Lilly and Company may be obtained by direct inquiry to Lilly Research Laboratories, Lilly Corporate Center, Indianapolis, Indiana 46285, (800) 545-5979.**

Sarafem—Cont.

PRECAUTIONS

General

Anxiety and Insomnia—In a placebo-controlled trial of fluoxetine in premenstrual dysphoric disorder (PMDD), treatment-emergent adverse events were assessed. Rates were as follows for SARAFEM 20 mg (the recommended dose), SARAFEM 60 mg and placebo, respectively: anxiety (5%, 9%, and 6%), nervousness (7%, 9%, and 4%), and insomnia (9%, 26%, and 7%). Events associated with discontinuation for SARAFEM 20 mg, 60 mg, and placebo, respectively were: anxiety (0%, 6%, and 2%), nervousness (2%, 0%, and 1%), and insomnia (1%, 4%, and 1%). In US placebo-controlled clinical trials of fluoxetine for other approved indications, anxiety, nervousness, and insomnia have been among the most commonly reported adverse events (*see* Table 2 *under* Adverse Reactions).

Altered Appetite and Weight—In a placebo-controlled trial of fluoxetine in PMDD, 4% of patients on SARAFEM 20 mg (the recommended dose), 13% on SARAFEM 60 mg, and 3% of placebo patients reported anorexia. In two placebo-controlled trials, potentially clinically significant weight gain (≥ 7%) occurred in 8% of patients on SARAFEM 20 mg, 6% of patients on SARAFEM 60 mg, and 1% of patients on placebo. Potentially clinically significant weight loss (≥ 7%) occurred in 7% of patients on SARAFEM 20 mg, 12% of patients on SARAFEM 60 mg, and 3% of patients on placebo. In US placebo-controlled clinical trials of fluoxetine for other approved indications, changes in appetite and weight have also been reported (*see* Table 2 and Other Events Observed in US Clinical Trials *under* Adverse Reactions).

Activation of Mania/Hypomania—No patients treated with SARAFEM in three PMDD clinical trials (N=243) reported mania/hypomania. In all US fluoxetine clinical trials for conditions other than PMDD, 0.7% of 10,782 patients reported mania/hypomania. Activation of mania/hypomania may occur with medications used to treat depression, especially in patients predisposed to Bipolar Affective Disorder.

Seizures—No patients treated with SARAFEM in three PMDD clinical trials (N=243) reported seizures. In all US fluoxetine clinical trials for conditions other than PMDD, 0.2% of 10,782 patients reported seizures. Antidepressant medication should be introduced with care in patients with a history of seizures.

Suicide—No patients treated with SARAFEM in three PMDD clinical trials (N=243) attempted suicide. The possibility of a suicide attempt is inherent in mood disorders and may persist until significant remission occurs. In PMDD patients with a significant mood disturbance, close supervision should accompany drug therapy. In high-risk patients, prescriptions for antidepressant medication should be written for the smallest quantity of medication consistent with good patient management, in order to reduce the risk of overdose.

The Long Elimination Half-Lives of Fluoxetine and Its Metabolites—Because of the long elimination half-lives of the parent drug and its major active metabolite, changes in dose will not be fully reflected in plasma for several weeks, affecting both strategies for titration to final dose and withdrawal from treatment (*see* Clinical Pharmacology *and* Dosage and Administration).

Use in Patients With Concomitant Illness—Clinical experience with fluoxetine in patients with concomitant systemic illness is limited. Caution is advisable in using fluoxetine in patients with diseases or conditions that could affect metabolism or hemodynamic responses.

Fluoxetine has not been evaluated or used to any appreciable extent in patients with a recent history of myocardial infarction or unstable heart disease. Patients with these diagnoses were systematically excluded from clinical studies during the product's premarket testing. However, the electrocardiograms of 312 patients who received fluoxetine in double-blind trials for a condition other than PMDD were retrospectively evaluated; no conduction abnormalities that resulted in heart block were observed. The mean heart rate was reduced by approximately 3 beats/min.

In subjects with cirrhosis of the liver, the clearances of fluoxetine and its active metabolite, norfluoxetine, were decreased, thus increasing the elimination half-lives of these substances (*see* Liver Disease *under* Clinical Pharmacology). A lower or less frequent dose should be used in patients with cirrhosis (*see* Dosage and Administration).

Studies in depressed patients on dialysis did not reveal excessive accumulation of fluoxetine or norfluoxetine in plasma (*see* Renal Disease *under* Clinical Pharmacology). Use of a lower or less frequent dose for renally impaired patients is not routinely necessary (*see* Dosage and Administration).

In patients with diabetes, fluoxetine may alter glycemic control. Hypoglycemia has occurred during therapy with fluoxetine, and hyperglycemia has developed following discontinuation of the drug. As is true with many other types of medication when taken concurrently by patients with diabetes, insulin and/or oral hypoglycemic dosage may need to be adjusted when therapy with fluoxetine is instituted or discontinued.

Interference With Cognitive and Motor Performance—Any psychoactive drug may impair judgment, thinking, or motor skills, and patients should be cautioned about operating hazardous machinery, including automobiles, until they are reasonably certain that the drug treatment does not affect them adversely.

Information for Patients—Patient information is printed at the end of this insert. To assure safe and effective use of SARAFEM, the information and instructions provided in the patient information section should be discussed with patients.

Laboratory Tests—There are no specific laboratory tests recommended.

Drug Interactions—As with all drugs, the potential for interaction by a variety of mechanisms (eg, pharmacodynamic, pharmacokinetic drug inhibition or enhancement, etc) is a possibility (*see* Accumulation and Slow Elimination *under* Clinical Pharmacology).

Drugs Metabolized by P450IID6—Approximately 7% of the normal population has a genetic defect that leads to reduced levels of activity of the cytochrome P450 isoenzyme P450IID6. Such individuals have been referred to as "poor metabolizers" of drugs such as debrisoquin, dextromethorphan, and tricyclic antidepressants. Many drugs, including fluoxetine and other selective uptake inhibitors of serotonin, are metabolized by this isoenzyme; thus, both the pharmacokinetic properties and relative proportion of metabolites are altered in poor metabolizers. However, for fluoxetine and its metabolite the sum of the plasma concentrations of the 4 active enantiomers is comparable between poor and extensive metabolizers (*see* Variability in Metabolism *under* Clinical Pharmacology).

Fluoxetine, like other agents that are metabolized by P450IID6, inhibits the activity of this isoenzyme, and thus may make normal metabolizers resemble "poor metabolizers." Therapy with medications that are predominantly metabolized by the P450IID6 system and that have a relatively narrow therapeutic index (*see* list below), should be initiated at the low end of the dose range if a patient is receiving fluoxetine concurrently or has taken it in the previous 5 weeks. Thus, her dosing requirements resemble those of "poor metabolizers." If fluoxetine is added to the treatment regimen of a patient already receiving a drug metabolized by P450IID6, the need for decreased dose of the original medication should be considered. Drugs with a narrow therapeutic index represent the greatest concern (eg, flecainide, vinblastine, and tricyclic antidepressants). Due to the risk of serious ventricular arrhythmias and sudden death potentially associated with elevated plasma levels of thioridazine, thioridazine should not be administered with fluoxetine or within a minimum of 5 weeks after fluoxetine has been discontinued (*see* Contraindications *and* Warnings).

Drugs Metabolized by Cytochrome P450IIIA4—In an in vivo interaction study involving co-administration of fluoxetine with single doses of terfenadine (a cytochrome P450IIIA4 substrate), no increase in plasma terfenadine concentrations occurred with concomitant fluoxetine. In addition, in vitro studies have shown ketoconazole, a potent inhibitor of P450IIIA4 activity, to be at least 100 times more potent than fluoxetine or norfluoxetine as an inhibitor of the metabolism of several substrates for this enzyme, including astemizole, cisapride, and midazolam. These data indicate that fluoxetine's extent of inhibition of cytochrome P450IIIA4 activity is not likely to be of clinical significance.

CNS Active Drugs—The risk of using fluoxetine in combination with other CNS active drugs has not been systematically evaluated. Nonetheless, caution is advised if the concomitant administration of fluoxetine and such drugs is required. In evaluating individual cases, consideration should be given to using lower initial doses of the concomitantly administered drugs, using conservative titration schedules, and monitoring of clinical status (*see* Accumulation and Slow Elimination *under* Clinical Pharmacology).

Anticonvulsants—Patients on stable doses of phenytoin and carbamazepine have developed elevated plasma anticonvulsant concentrations and clinical anticonvulsant toxicity following initiation of concomitant fluoxetine treatment.

Antipsychotics—Some clinical data suggests a possible pharmacodynamic and/or pharmacokinetic interaction between serotonin specific reuptake inhibitors (SSRIs) and antipsychotics. Elevation of blood levels of haloperidol and clozapine has been observed in patients receiving concomitant fluoxetine. A single case report has suggested possible additive effects of pimozide and fluoxetine leading to bradycardia. For thioridazine, see Contraindications and Warnings.

Benzodiazepines—The half-life of concurrently administered diazepam may be prolonged in some patients (*see* Accumulation and Slow Elimination *under* Clinical Pharmacology). Coadministration of alprazolam and fluoxetine has resulted in increased alprazolam plasma concentrations and in further psychomotor performance decrement due to increased alprazolam levels.

Lithium—There have been reports of both increased and decreased lithium levels when lithium was used concomitantly with fluoxetine. Cases of lithium toxicity and increased serotonergic effects have been reported. Lithium levels should be monitored when these drugs are administered concomitantly.

Tryptophan—Five patients receiving fluoxetine in combination with tryptophan experienced adverse reactions, including agitation, restlessness, and gastrointestinal distress.

Monoamine Oxidase Inhibitors—*See* Contraindications.

Antidepressants—In two studies, previously stable plasma levels of imipramine and desipramine have increased greater than 2 to 10-fold when fluoxetine has been administered in combination. This influence may persist for three weeks or longer after fluoxetine is discontinued. Thus, the dose of tricyclic antidepressant (TCA) may need to be reduced and plasma TCA concentrations may need to be monitored temporarily when fluoxetine is coadministered or has been recently discontinued (*see* Accumulation and Slow Elimination *under* Clinical Pharmacology, and Drugs Metabolized by P450IID6 *under* Drug Interactions).

Sumatriptan—There have been rare postmarketing reports describing patients with weakness, hyperreflexia, and incoordination following the use of a selective serotonin reuptake inhibitor (SSRI) and sumatriptan. If concomitant treatment with sumatriptan and an SSRI (e.g., fluoxetine, fluvoxamine, paroxetine, sertraline, or citalopram) is clinically warranted, appropriate observation of the patient is advised.

Potential Effects of Coadministration of Drugs Tightly Bound to Plasma Proteins—Because fluoxetine is tightly bound to plasma protein, the administration of fluoxetine to a patient taking another drug that is tightly bound to protein (eg, warfarin, digitoxin) may cause a shift in plasma concentrations potentially resulting in an adverse effect. Conversely, adverse effects may result from displacement of protein bound fluoxetine by other tightly bound drugs (*see* Accumulation and Slow Elimination *under* Clinical Pharmacology).

Warfarin—Altered anti-coagulant effects, including increased bleeding, have been reported when fluoxetine is coadministered with warfarin. Patients receiving warfarin therapy should receive careful coagulation monitoring when fluoxetine is initiated or stopped.

Electroconvulsive Therapy—There are no clinical studies establishing the benefit of the combined use of ECT and fluoxetine. There have been rare reports of prolonged seizures in patients on fluoxetine receiving ECT treatment.

Carcinogenesis, Mutagenesis, Impairment of Fertility—There is no evidence of carcinogenicity, mutagenicity, or impairment of fertility with fluoxetine.

Carcinogenicity—The dietary administration of fluoxetine to rats and mice for 2 years at doses of up to 10 and 12 mg/kg/day, respectively (approximately 1.2 and 0.7 times, respectively, the maximum recommended human dose [MRHD] of 80 mg on a mg/m^2 basis), produced no evidence of carcinogenicity.

Mutagenicity—Fluoxetine and norfluoxetine have been shown to have no genotoxic effects based on the following assays: bacterial mutation assay, DNA repair assay in cultured rat hepatocytes, mouse lymphoma assay, and in vivo sister chromatid exchange assay in Chinese hamster bone marrow cells.

Impairment of Fertility—Two fertility studies conducted in rats at doses of up to 7.5 and 12.5 mg/kg/day (approximately 0.9 and 1.5 times the MRHD on a mg/m^2 basis) indicated that fluoxetine had no adverse effects on fertility.

Pregnancy—Pregnancy Category C: In embryo-fetal development studies in rats and rabbits, there was no evidence of teratogenicity following administration of up to 12.5 and 15 mg/kg/day, respectively (1.5 and 3.6 times, respectively, the maximum recommended human dose [MRHD] of 80 mg on a mg/m^2 basis) throughout organogenesis. However, in rat reproduction studies, an increase in stillborn pups, a decrease in pup weight, and an increase in pup deaths during the first 7 days postpartum occurred following maternal exposure to 12 mg/kg/day (1.5 times the MRHD on a mg/m^2 basis) during gestation or 7.5 mg/kg/day (0.9 times the MRHD on a mg/m^2 basis) during gestation and lactation. There was no evidence of developmental neurotoxicity in the surviving offspring of rats treated with 12 mg/kg/day during gestation. The no-effect dose for rat pup mortality was 5 mg/kg/day (0.6 times the MRHD on a mg/m^2 basis). Fluoxetine should be used during pregnancy only if the potential benefit justifies the potential risk to the fetus.

Labor and Delivery—The effect of fluoxetine on labor and delivery in humans is unknown. However, because fluoxetine crosses the placenta and because of the possibility that fluoxetine may have adverse effects on the newborn, fluoxetine should be used during labor and delivery only if the potential benefit justifies the potential risk to the fetus.

Nursing Mothers—Because fluoxetine is excreted in human milk, nursing while on fluoxetine is not recommended. In 1 breast milk sample, the concentration of fluoxetine plus norfluoxetine was 70.4 ng/mL. The concentration in the mother's plasma was 295.0 ng/mL. No adverse effects on the infant were reported. In another case, an infant nursed by a mother on fluoxetine developed crying, sleep disturbance, vomiting, and watery stools. The infant's plasma drug levels were 340 ng/mL of fluoxetine and 208 ng/mL of norfluoxetine on the second day of feeding.

Pediatric Use—Safety and effectiveness in pediatric patients have not been established.

Geriatric Use—The diagnosis of PMDD is not applicable to postmenopausal women.

Hyponatremia—Several cases of hyponatremia (some with serum sodium lower than 110 mmol/L) have been reported. The hyponatremia appeared to be reversible when fluoxetine was discontinued. Although these cases were complex with varying possible etiologies, some were possibly due to the syndrome of inappropriate antidiuretic hormone secretion (SIADH). The majority of these occurrences have been in older patients and in patients taking diuretics or who were otherwise volume depleted. In a placebo-controlled, double-blind trial, 10 of 313 fluoxetine patients and 6 of 320 placebo recipients had a lowering of serum sodium below the reference range; this difference was not statistically significant. The lowest observed concentration was 129 mmol/L. The observed decreases were not clinically significant.

Platelet Function—There have been rare reports of altered platelet function and/or abnormal results from laboratory studies in patients taking fluoxetine. While there have been reports of abnormal bleeding in several patients taking fluoxetine, it is unclear whether fluoxetine had a causative role.

ADVERSE REACTIONS

In one of 3 placebo-controlled trials of fluoxetine in PMDD, treatment-emergent adverse events reporting rates were assessed. The information from Table 1 included under Adverse Reactions is based on data from this trial at the recommended dose of SARAFEM (SARAFEM 20 mg, N=104; placebo, N=108). In addition, a broader set of information on treatment-emergent adverse events in the population of female patients, 18–45 years of age, from the US placebo-controlled depression, OCD, and bulimia clinical trials is presented for comparison (Table 2).

Adverse events were recorded by clinical investigators using descriptive terminology of their own choosing. Consequently, it is not possible to provide a meaningful estimate of the proportion of individuals experiencing adverse events without first grouping similar types of events into a limited (i.e., reduced) number of standardized event categories.

In the tables and tabulations that follow, COSTART Dictionary terminology has been used to classify reported adverse events. The stated frequencies represent the proportion of individuals who experienced, at least once, a treatment-emergent adverse event of the type listed. An event was considered treatment-emergent if it occurred for the first time or worsened while receiving therapy following baseline evaluation. It is important to emphasize that events reported during therapy were not necessarily caused by it.

The prescriber should be aware that the figures in the tables and tabulations cannot be used to predict the incidence of side effects in the course of usual medical practice where patient characteristics and other factors differ from those that prevailed in the clinical trials. Similarly, the cited frequencies cannot be compared with figures obtained from other clinical investigations involving different treatments, uses, and investigators. The cited figures, however, do provide the prescribing physician with some basis for estimating the relative contribution of drug and nondrug factors to the side effect incidence rate in the population studied.

Incidence in a Placebo-Controlled PMDD Clinical Trial—Table 1 enumerates the most common treatment-emergent adverse events associated with the use of SARAFEM 20 mg (incidence of at least 5% for SARAFEM 20 mg and greater than placebo) for the treatment of PMDD.

Table 1
MOST COMMON TREATMENT-EMERGENT ADVERSE EVENTS: INCIDENCE IN A PMDD PLACEBO-CONTROLLED CLINICAL TRIAL

Body System/ Adverse Event*	Percentage of patients reporting event	
	Sarafem 20 mg (N=104)	Placebo (N=108)
Body as a Whole		
Headache	13	9
Asthenia	12	3
Pain	9	7
Accidental injury	8	4
Infection	7	4
Digestive System		
Nausea	13	7
Nervous System		
Insomnia	9	7
Dizziness	7	4
Nervousness	7	4
Thinking abnormal†	6	—
Respiratory System		
Rhinitis	23	17
Pharyngitis	10	6

*Included are events reported by at least 5% of patients taking SARAFEM 20 mg, except the following events, which had an incidence on placebo > SARAFEM 20 mg: diarrhea and flu syndrome.

† Thinking abnormal is the COSTART term that captures concentration difficulties.

—Incidence less than 0.5%.

Incidence in US Depression, OCD, and Bulimia Placebo-Controlled Clinical Trials (excluding data from extensions of trials)—Table 2 enumerates the most common treatment-emergent adverse events associated with the use of fluoxetine up to 80 mg (incidence of at least 2% for fluoxetine and greater than placebo) in female patients ages 18–45 years from US placebo-controlled clinical trials in the treatment of depression, OCD, and bulimia.

Table 2
TREATMENT-EMERGENT ADVERSE EVENTS: INCIDENCE IN FEMALE PATIENTS AGES 18–45 YEARS IN US DEPRESSION, OCD, AND BULIMIA PLACEBO-CONTROLLED CLINICAL TRIALS

Body System/ Adverse Event*	Percentage of patients reporting event	
	Fluoxetine (N=1145)	Placebo (N=553)
Body as a Whole		
Headache	24	21
Asthenia	14	6
Flu syndrome	7	3
Abdominal pain	6	5
Accidental injury	4	3
Fever	3	2
Cardiovascular System		
Palpitation	3	2
Vasodilatation	3	1
Digestive System		
Nausea	27	11
Anorexia	11	4
Dry mouth	11	8
Diarrhea	10	7
Dyspepsia	7	5
Constipation	5	3
Vomiting	3	2
Metabolic and Nutritional Disorders		
Weight loss	3	1
Nervous System		
Insomnia	24	11
Nervousness	14	10
Anxiety	13	9
Somnolence	13	6
Tremor	12	1
Dizziness	11	5
Libido decreased	4	1
Abnormal dreams	3	2
Thinking abnormal†	3	2
Respiratory System		
Pharyngitis	6	5
Yawn	5	—
Skin and Appendages		
Sweating	8	3
Rash	5	3
Special Senses		
Abnormal vision	3	1
Urogenital System		
Urinary frequency	2	1

*Included are events reported by at least 2% of patients taking fluoxetine, except the following events, which had an incidence on placebo > fluoxetine (depression, OCD, and bulimia combined): back pain, cough increased, depression (includes suicidal thoughts), dysmenorrhea, flatulence, infection, myalgia, pain, pruritus, rhinitis, sinusitis.

† Thinking abnormal is the COSTART term that captures concentration difficulties.

—Incidence less than 0.5%.

Associated with Discontinuation in a Placebo-Controlled PMDD Clinical Trial—The most common adverse event (incidence at least 2% for SARAFEM 20 mg and greater than placebo) associated with discontinuation in a PMDD placebo-controlled trial was nausea (3% for SARAFEM 20 mg, N=104 and 1% for placebo, N=108). In this clinical trial, more than one event may have been recorded as the cause of discontinuation.

Associated with Discontinuation in US Depression, OCD, and Bulimia Placebo-Controlled Clinical Trials (excluding data from extensions of trials)—In female patients age 18–45 years in US depression, OCD, and bulimia placebo-controlled clinical trials combined, which collected a single primary event associated with discontinuation (incidence at least 1% for fluoxetine and at least twice that for placebo), insomnia (1%, N=561) was the only event reported.

Female Sexual Dysfunction with SSRIs—Although changes in sexual desire, sexual performance and sexual satisfaction often occur as manifestations of a mood-related disorder, they may also be a consequence of pharmacologic treatment. In particular, some evidence suggests that selective serotonin reuptake inhibitors (SSRIs) can cause such untoward sexual experiences. Reliable estimates of the incidence and severity of untoward experiences involving sexual desire, performance, and satisfaction are difficult to obtain, however, in part because patients and physicians may be reluctant to discuss them. Accordingly, estimates of the incidence of untoward sexual experience and performance cited in product labeling, are likely to underestimate their actual incidence. For example, in women (age 18–45) receiving fluoxetine for indications other than PMDD, decreased libido for at least one indication, showed an incidence for fluoxetine of 4% and at least twice that of placebo. There have been spontaneous reports in women (age 18–45) taking fluoxetine for indications other than PMDD of orgasmic dysfunction, including anorgasmia.

There are no adequate, controlled studies examining sexual dysfunction with fluoxetine treatment.

While it is difficult to know the precise risk of sexual dysfunction associated with the use of SSRIs, physicians should routinely inquire about such possible side effects.

Other Events Observed In US Clinical Trials—Following is a list of all treatment-emergent adverse events reported at anytime by females and males taking fluoxetine in all US clinical trials for conditions other than PMDD as of May 8, 1995 (10,782 patients) except (1) those listed in the body or footnotes of Tables 1 or 2 above or elsewhere in labeling; (2) those for which the COSTART terms were uninformative or misleading; (3) those events for which a causal relationship to fluoxetine use was considered remote; (4) events occurring in only 1 patient treated with fluoxetine and which did not have a substantial probability of being acutely life-threatening; and (5) events that could only occur in males. Events are classified within body system categories using the following definitions: frequent adverse events are defined as those occurring on 1 or more occasions in at least 1/100 patients; infrequent adverse events are those occurring in 1/100 to 1/1,000 patients; rare events are those occurring in less than 1/1,000 patients.

Body as a Whole—*Frequent:* chest pain and chills; *Infrequent:* chills and fever, face edema, intentional overdose, malaise, pelvic pain, suicide attempt; *Rare:* abdominal syndrome acute, hypothermia, intentional injury, neuroleptic malignant syndrome, photosensitivity reaction.

Cardiovascular System—*Frequent:* hemorrhage, hypertension; *Infrequent:* angina pectoris, arrhythmia, congestive heart failure, hypotension, migraine, myocardial infarct, postural hypotension, syncope, tachycardia, vascular headache; *Rare:* atrial fibrillation, bradycardia, cerebral embolism, cerebral ischemia, cerebrovascular accident, extrasystoles, heart arrest, heart block, pallor, peripheral vascular disorder, phlebitis, shock, thrombophlebitis, thrombosis, vasospasm, ventricular arrhythmia, ventricular extrasystoles, ventricular fibrillation.

Digestive System—*Frequent:* increased appetite, nausea and vomiting; *Infrequent:* aphthous stomatitis, cholelithiasis, colitis, dysphagia, eructation, esophagitis, gastritis, gastroenteritis, glossitis, gum hemorrhage, hyperchlorhydria, increased salivation, liver function tests abnormal, melena, mouth ulceration, nausea/vomiting/diarrhea, stomach ulcer, stomatitis, thirst; *Rare:* biliary pain, bloody diarrhea, cholecystitis, duodenal ulcer, enteritis, esophageal ulcer, fecal incontinence, gastrointestinal hemorrhage, hematemesis, hemorrhage of colon, hepatitis, intestinal obstruction, liver fatty deposit, pancreatitis, peptic ulcer, rectal hemorrhage, salivary gland enlargement, stomach ulcer hemorrhage, tongue edema.

Endocrine System—*Infrequent:* hypothyroidism; *Rare:* diabetic acidosis, diabetes mellitus.

Hemic and Lymphatic System—*Infrequent:* anemia, ecchymosis; *Rare:* blood dyscrasia, hypochromic anemia, leukopenia, lymphedema, lymphocytosis, petechia, purpura, thrombocythemia, thrombocytopenia.

Metabolic and Nutritional—*Frequent:* weight gain; *Infrequent:* dehydration, generalized edema, gout, hypercholesteremia, hyperlipemia, hypokalemia, peripheral edema; *Rare:* alcohol intolerance, alkaline phosphatase increased, BUN increased, creatine phosphokinase increased, hyperkalemia, hyperuricemia, hypocalcemia, iron deficiency anemia, SGPT increased.

Musculoskeletal System—*Infrequent:* arthritis, bone pain, bursitis, leg cramps, tenosynovitis; *Rare:* arthrosis, chondrodystrophy, myasthenia, myopathy, myositis, osteomyelitis, osteoporosis, rheumatoid arthritis.

Nervous System—*Frequent:* agitation, amnesia, confusion, emotional lability, paresthesia, and sleep disorder; *Infrequent:* abnormal gait, acute brain syndrome, akathisia, apathy, ataxia, buccoglossal syndrome, CNS depression, CNS stimulation, depersonalization, euphoria, hallucinations, hostility, hyperkinesia, hypertonia, hypesthesia, incoordination, libido increased, myoclonus, neuralgia, neuropathy, neurosis, paranoid reaction, personality disorder,† psychosis, vertigo; *Rare:* abnormal electroencephalogram, antisocial reaction, circumoral paresthesia, coma, delusions, dysarthria, dystonia, extrapyramidal syndrome, foot drop, hyperesthesia, neuritis, paralysis, reflexes decreased, reflexes increased, stupor.

Respiratory System—*Infrequent:* asthma, epistaxis, hiccup, hyperventilation; *Rare:* apnea, atelectasis, cough decreased, emphysema, hemoptysis, hypoventilation, hypoxia, larynx edema, lung edema, pneumothorax, stridor.

Skin and Appendages—*Infrequent:* acne, alopecia, contact dermatitis, eczema, maculopapular rash, skin discoloration, skin ulcer, vesiculobullous rash; *Rare:* furunculosis, herpes zoster, hirsutism, petechial rash, psoriasis, purpuric rash, pustular rash, seborrhea.

Special Senses—*Frequent:* ear pain, taste perversion, tinnitus; *Infrequent:* conjunctivitis, dry eyes, mydriasis, photophobia; *Rare:* blepharitis, deafness, diplopia, exophthalmos, eye hemorrhage, glaucoma, hyperacusis, iritis, parosmia, scleritis, strabismus, taste loss, visual field defect.

Continued on next page

*** Identi-Code® symbol. This product information was prepared in June 2000. Current information on these and other products of Eli Lilly and Company may be obtained by direct inquiry to Lilly Research Laboratories, Lilly Corporate Center, Indianapolis, Indiana 46285, (800) 545-5979.**

Sarafem—Cont.

Urogenital System—*Infrequent:* abortion*, albuminuria, amenorrhea*, anorgasmia, breast enlargement, breast pain, cystitis, dysuria, female lactation*, fibrocystic breast*, hematuria, leukorrhea*, menorrhagia*, metrorrhagia*, nocturia, polyuria, urinary incontinence, urinary retention, urinary urgency, vaginal hemorrhage*; *Rare:* breast engorgement, glycosuria, hypomenorrhea*, kidney pain, oliguria, uterine hemorrhage*, uterine fibroids enlarged*.

† Personality disorder is the COSTART term for designating non-aggressive objectionable behavior.
* Adjusted for gender

Postintroduction Reports—Voluntary reports of adverse events temporally associated with fluoxetine that have been received since market introduction of fluoxetine and that may have no causal relationship with the drug include the following: aplastic anemia, atrial fibrillation, cerebral vascular accident, cholestatic jaundice, confusion, dyskinesia (including, for example, a case of buccal-lingual-masticatory syndrome with involuntary tongue protrusion reported to develop in a 77-year-old female after 5 weeks of fluoxetine therapy and which completely resolved over the next few months following drug discontinuation), eosinophilic pneumonia, epidermal necrolysis, erythema nodosum, exfoliative dermatitis, gynecomastia, heart arrest, hepatic failure/necrosis, hyperprolactinemia, immune-related hemolytic anemia, kidney failure, misuse/abuse, movement disorders developing in patients with risk factors including drugs associated with such events and worsening of preexisting movement disorders, neuroleptic malignant syndrome-like events, pancreatitis, pancytopenia, priapism, pulmonary embolism, pulmonary hypertension, QT prolongation, Stevens-Johnson syndrome, sudden unexpected death, suicidal ideation, thrombocytopenia, thrombocytopenic purpura, vaginal bleeding after drug withdrawal, ventricular tachycardia (including torsades de pointes-type arrhythmias), and violent behaviors.

DRUG ABUSE AND DEPENDENCE

Controlled Substance Class—Fluoxetine is not a controlled substance.

Physical and Psychological Dependence—Fluoxetine has not been systematically studied, in animals or humans, for its potential for abuse, tolerance, or physical dependence. While the premarketing clinical experience with fluoxetine did not reveal any tendency for a withdrawal syndrome or any drug seeking behavior, these observations were not systematic and it is not possible to predict on the basis of this limited experience the extent to which a CNS active drug will be misused, diverted, and/or abused once marketed. Consequently, physicians should carefully evaluate patients for history of drug abuse and follow such patients closely, observing them for signs of misuse or abuse of fluoxetine (eg, development of tolerance, incrementation of dose, drug-seeking behavior).

OVERDOSAGE

Human Experience—As of December 1987, there were 2 deaths among approximately 38 reports of acute overdose with fluoxetine, either alone or in combination with other drugs and/or alcohol. One death involved a combined overdose with approximately 1,800 mg of fluoxetine and an undetermined amount of maprotiline. Plasma concentrations of fluoxetine and maprotiline were 4.57 mg/L and 4.18 mg/L, respectively. A second death involved 3 drugs yielding plasma concentrations as follows: fluoxetine, 1.93 mg/L; norfluoxetine, 1.10 mg/L; codeine, 1.80 mg/L; temazepam, 3.80 mg/L.

One other patient who reportedly took 3,000 mg of fluoxetine experienced 2 grand mal seizures that remitted spontaneously without specific anticonvulsant treatment (*see* Management of Overdose). The actual amount of drug absorbed may have been less due to vomiting.

Nausea and vomiting were prominent in overdoses involving higher fluoxetine doses. Other prominent symptoms of overdose included agitation, restlessness, hypomania, and other signs of CNS excitation. Except for the 2 deaths noted above, all other overdose cases recovered without residua.

Since introduction, reports of death attributed to overdosage of fluoxetine alone have been extremely rare.

Animal Experience—Studies in animals do not provide precise or necessarily valid information about the treatment of human overdose. However, animal experiments can provide useful insights into possible treatment strategies.

The oral median lethal dose in rats and mice was found to be 452 and 248 mg/kg, respectively. Acute high oral doses produced hyperirritability and convulsions in several animal species.

Among 6 dogs purposely overdosed with oral fluoxetine, 5 experienced grand mal seizures. Seizures stopped immediately upon the bolus intravenous administration of a standard veterinary dose of diazepam. In this short term study, the lowest plasma concentration at which a seizure occurred was only twice the maximum plasma concentration seen in humans taking 80 mg/day, chronically.

In a separate single-dose study, the ECG of dogs given high doses did not reveal prolongation of the PR, QRS, or QT intervals. Tachycardia and an increase in blood pressure were observed. Consequently, the value of the ECG in predicting cardiac toxicity is unknown. Nonetheless, the ECG should ordinarily be monitored in cases of human overdose (*see* Management of Overdose).

Management of Overdose—Treatment should consist of those general measures employed in the management of overdosage with any SSRI.

Ensure an adequate airway, oxygenation, and ventilation. Monitor cardiac rhythm and vital signs. General supportive and symptomatic measures are also recommended. Induction of emesis is not recommended. Gastric lavage with a large-bore orogastric tube with appropriate airway protection, if needed, may be indicated if performed soon after ingestion, or in symptomatic patients.

Activated charcoal should be administered. Due to the large volume of distribution of this drug, forced diuresis, dialysis, hemoperfusion and exchange transfusion are unlikely to be of benefit. No specific antidotes for fluoxetine are known.

A specific caution involves patients who are taking or have recently taken fluoxetine and might ingest excessive quantities of a tricyclic antidepressant. In such a case, accumulation of the parent tricyclic and/or an active metabolite may increase the possibility of clinically significant sequelae and extend the time needed for close medical observation (*see* Precautions).

Based on experience in animals, which may not be relevant to humans, fluoxetine-induced seizures that fail to remit spontaneously may respond to diazepam.

In managing overdosage, consider the possibility of multiple drug involvement. The physician should consider contacting a poison control center for additional information on the treatment of any overdose. Telephone numbers for certified poison control centers are listed in the *Physicians' Desk Reference (PDR)*.

DOSAGE AND ADMINISTRATION

Premenstrual Dysphoric Disorder—

Initial Treatment—The recommended dose of SARAFEM for the treatment of PMDD is 20 mg/day. In a study comparing fluoxetine 20 and 60 mg/day to placebo, both doses were proven to be effective but there was no statistically significant added benefit for the 60 mg/day compared to the 20 mg/day dose. Fluoxetine doses above 60 mg/day have not been systematically studied in patients with PMDD. The maximum fluoxetine dose should not exceed 80 mg/day.

As with many other medications, a lower or less frequent dosage should be considered in patients with hepatic impairment. A lower or less frequent dosage should also be considered for patients with concurrent disease or on multiple concomitant medications. Dosage adjustments for renal impairment are not routinely necessary (*see* Liver Disease and Renal Disease *under* Clinical Pharmacology, *and* Use in Patients with Concomitant Illness *under* Precautions).

Maintenance/Continuation Treatment—Systematic evaluation of SARAFEM has shown that its efficacy in PMDD is maintained for periods of up to 6 months at a dose of 20 mg/day (*see* Clinical Trials *under* Clinical Pharmacology). Patients should be periodically reassessed to determine the need for continued treatment.

HOW SUPPLIED

SARAFEM™ (Fluoxetine Hydrochloride) Pulvules® are available in 10 mg* and 20 mg* capsule strengths.

The 10 mg Pulvule has an opaque lavender body and cap, and is imprinted with "10 mg" on the body and "LILLY 3210" on the cap:
NDC 0002-3210-07 (PU3210)—Bottles of 2000
NDC 0002-3210-45 (PU3210)—Blisters of 28

The 20 mg Pulvule has an opaque pink body with opaque lavender cap, and is imprinted with "20 mg" on the body and "LILLY 3220" on the cap:
NDC 0002-3220-45 (PU3220)—Blisters of 28

* equivalent to fluoxetine base
† Identi-Dose (unit dose medication, Lilly)

Store at controlled room temperature, 59° to 86°F (15° to 30°C).
Protect from light.
Rx only

ANIMAL TOXICOLOGY

Phospholipids are increased in some tissues of mice, rats, and dogs given fluoxetine chronically. This effect is reversible after cessation of fluoxetine treatment. Phospholipid accumulation in animals has been observed with many cationic amphiphilic drugs, including fenfluramine, imipramine, and ranitidine. The significance of this effect in humans is unknown.

INFORMATION FOR THE PATIENT
SARAFEM™
fluoxetine hydrochloride

READ THIS INFORMATION COMPLETELY BEFORE USING SARAFEM (SAIR-a-fem). This leaflet provides a summary about SARAFEM and does not contain complete information about your medicine. This information is not meant to take the place of discussions between you and your doctor. Talk with your doctor, pharmacist or other healthcare professional if there is something you do not understand or if you want to learn more about SARAFEM. Always follow your doctor's instructions on how to take SARAFEM.

What is SARAFEM?

SARAFEM is a prescription medicine used by women who have menstrual periods or cycles to treat the symptoms of premenstrual dysphoric disorder (PMDD).

What is PMDD?

PMDD is a medical condition that affects only women who have menstrual periods or cycles. Symptoms of PMDD are limited to the week or two before a woman's menstrual period and commonly include mood symptoms such as irritability, mood swings, and tension as well as physical symptoms of bloating and breast tenderness. When the symptoms of PMDD appear they cause interference in day to day activities and relationships.

What is the active ingredient in SARAFEM?

SARAFEM contains fluoxetine hydrochloride, the same active ingredient found in Prozac®.

How does SARAFEM work?

While it is unknown what causes PMDD, many doctors believe it may be related to an imbalance in a natural chemical in the body called serotonin. The actions of SARAFEM on serotonin may explain its effects in improving the symptoms of this condition.

Who should not take SARAFEM?

You should not take SARAFEM if you:
- are allergic to fluoxetine hydrochloride, the active ingredient in SARAFEM.
- are taking a type of antidepressant medicine known as a monoamine oxidase inhibitor (MAOI), such as Nardil (phenelzine) or Parnate (tranylcypromine). Using an MAOI together with many prescription medicines including SARAFEM can cause serious or even life-threatening reactions. You must wait at least 14 days after you have stopped taking an MAOI before you can take SARAFEM. Also, you need to wait at least 5 weeks after you stop taking SARAFEM before you take an MAOI.
- are taking a type of antipsychotic medicine known as Mellaril (thioridazine). You need to wait at least 5 weeks after you stop taking SARAFEM before you take Mellaril.

How should I take SARAFEM?

- Take SARAFEM exactly as directed by your doctor.
- SARAFEM comes as a 10 mg lavender capsule and a 20 mg pink and lavender capsule. The usual dose is 20 mg a day, but your doctor will prescribe the dose that is right for you.
- If you miss a dose, take it as soon as you remember. However, if it is time for your next dose, skip the missed dose and take only your regularly scheduled dose. Do not take more than the daily amount of SARAFEM that has been prescribed for you.
- SARAFEM can be taken with or without food.
- To help you remember to take SARAFEM, it may be best to take it at about the same time each day, such as every morning.
- Remember to get your refills before you run out of SARAFEM.
- Talk with your doctor about how long you should keep taking SARAFEM.
- Talk with your doctor before you stop taking SARAFEM.

What should I talk to my doctor about when taking SARAFEM?

- If you get a rash or hives while taking SARAFEM, call your doctor right away because this can be a sign of a serious medical condition.
- Be sure to tell your doctor if you are taking Prozac, since this contains fluoxetine, the same active ingredient found in SARAFEM.
- Be sure to tell your doctor if you are taking or plan to take any prescription or nonprescription medicines, vitamins, natural supplements, herbal remedies or alcohol. As with most other prescription medications, SARAFEM may interact with some of these products.
- You should tell your doctor if you are pregnant, plan to become pregnant or are breast feeding while taking SARAFEM.
- Tell your doctor if you have diabetes. The dose of diabetes medicine you need may change when you start or stop taking SARAFEM.
- Tell your doctor about any other medical conditions you may have, especially liver disease, or a history of seizures or mania.

What are possible side effects of SARAFEM?

All prescription medicines may cause side effects in some patients.
- In medical studies of women taking SARAFEM for PMDD, the most common side effects likely caused by SARAFEM were tiredness, upset stomach, nervousness, dizziness, and difficulty concentrating. Other side effects were reported less frequently in those same studies. Side effects were generally mild, often disappeared after a few weeks, and most did not cause women to stop taking SARAFEM.
- SARAFEM can cause changes in sexual desire or satisfaction.
- Do not drive a car or operate dangerous machinery until you know what effect SARAFEM may have on you.
- Contact your doctor or healthcare professional if you get a rash or hives, or if you get other side effects that concern you while taking SARAFEM.

What else can I do?

In addition to taking SARAFEM:
- eat a well-balanced diet (including fruits, vegetables and fiber) and get regular exercise.
- drink plenty of water daily and lower the amount of caffeine and salt in your diet, especially before your menstrual period.

Talk to your doctor before you begin any diet or exercise program.

How do I store SARAFEM?

- Store SARAFEM at room temperature.
- Keep all medicines, including SARAFEM, out of the reach of children.

General Information

This is a summary of information about SARAFEM. Medicines are sometimes prescribed for purposes other than those listed in a patient information summary. This medicine was prescribed for your use only. Do not let anyone else use your SARAFEM.

If you have any questions or concerns, want to report any problems with the use of SARAFEM or want more information about SARAFEM, contact your doctor, pharmacist or other healthcare professional.

This patient information summary has been approved by the US Food and Drug Administration.

www.sarafem.com

Literature issued July, 2000

Eli Lilly and Company
Indianapolis, IN 46285, USA

PV 3280 AMP

Shown in Product Identification Guide, page 321

TAZIDIME® ℞

[*tă 'zĭ-dēm*]

brand of

ceftazidime for injection, USP

for intravenous or intramuscular use

DESCRIPTION

Ceftazidime is a semisynthetic, broad-spectrum, beta-lactam antibiotic for parenteral administration. It is the pentahydrate of pyridinium, 1-[[7-[[(2-amino-4-thiazolyl)](1-carboxy-1-methylethoxy) imino]ace-tyl]amino]-2-carboxy-8-oxo-5-thia-1-azabicyclo (4.2.0)oct-2-en-3-yl] methyl]-, hydroxide, inner salt, [6R-[6α,7β(Z)]]. It has the following structural formula:

The empirical formula is $C_{22}H_{32}N_6O_{12}S_2$ representing a molecular weight of 636.6.

Tazidime (ceftazidime for injection is a sterile, dry powdered mixture of ceftazidime pentahydrate and sodium carbonate. The sodium carbonate at a concentration of 118 mg/gram of ceftazidime activity has been admixed to facilitate dissolution. The total sodium content of the mixture is approximately 54 mg (2.3 mEq)/gram of ceftazidime activity. *Tazidime* in sterile crystalline form is supplied in vials equivalent to 1 gram or 2 grams of anhydrous ceftazidime, in piggyback vials equivalent to 1 gram or 2 grams of anhydrous ceftazidime and ADD-Vantage® vials equivalent to 1 gram or 2 grams of anhydrous ceftazidime. Solutions of *Tazidime* range in color from light yellow to amber, depending on the diluent and volume used. The pH of freshly reconstituted solutions usually ranges from 5.0 to 8.0.

CLINICAL PHARMACOLOGY

After IV administration of 500 mg and 1 gram doses of ceftazidime over 5 minutes to normal adult male volunteers, mean peak serum concentrations of 45 mcg/mL and 90 mcg/mL, respectively, were achieved. After IV infusion of 500 mg, 1 gram and 2 gram doses of ceftazidime over 20 to 30 minutes to normal adult male volunteers, mean peak serum concentrations of 42 mcg/mL, 69 mcg/mL and 170 mcg/mL, respectively, were achieved. The average serum concentrations following IV infusion of 500 mg, 1 gram and 2 gram doses to these volunteers over an 8-hour interval are given in Table 1.

Table 1

Ceftazidime IV Dosage	Serum Concentrations (mcg/mL)				
	0.5 hr.	1 hr.	2 hr.	4 hr.	8 hr.
500 mg	42	25	12	6	2
1 gram	60	39	23	11	3
2 grams	129	75	42	13	5

The absorption and elimination of ceftazidime were directly proportional to the size of the dose. The half-life following IV administration was approximately 1.9 hours. Less than 10% of ceftazidime was protein bound. The degree of protein binding was independent of concentration. There was no evidence of accumulation of ceftazidime in the serum in individuals with normal renal function following multiple IV doses of 1 gram and 2 grams every 8 hours for 10 days.

Following IM administration of 500 mg and 1 gram doses of ceftazidime to normal adult volunteers, the mean peak serum concentrations were 17 mcg/mL and 39 mcg/mL, respectively, at approximately 1 hour. Serum concentrations remained above 4 mcg/mL for 6 and 8 hours after the IM administration of 500 mg and 1 gram doses, respectively. The half-life of ceftazidime in these volunteers was approximately 2 hours.

Table 2. Ceftazidime Concentrations in Body Tissues and Fluids

Tissue or Fluid	Dose/ Route	No. Patients	Time of Sample Post-Dose	Average Tissue of Fluid Level (mcg/mL or mcg/g)
Urine	500 mg IM.	6	0 to 2 hours	2,100.0
	2 grams IV	6	0 to 2 hours	12,000.0
Bile	2 grams IV	3	90 min.	36.4
Synovial fluid	2 grams IV	13	2 hours	25.6
Peritoneal fluid	2 grams IV	8	2 hours	48.6
Sputum	1 gram IV	8	1 hour	9.0
Cerebrospinal fluid	2 grams q8h IV	5	120 min.	9.8
(inflamed meninges)	2 grams q8h IV	6	180 min.	9.4
Aqueous humor	2 grams IV	13	1 to 3 hours	11.0
Blister fluid	1 gram IV	7	2 to 3 hours	19.7
Lymphatic fluid	1 gram IV	7	2 to 3 hours	23.4
Bone	2 grams IV	8	0.67 hour	31.1
Heart muscle	2 grams IV	35	30 to 280 min.	12.7
Skin	2 grams IV	22	30 to 180 min.	6.6
Skeletal muscle	2 grams IV	35	30 to 280 min.	9.4
Myometrium	2 grams IV	31	1 to 2 hours	18.7

The presence of hepatic dysfunction had no effect on the pharmacokinetics of ceftazidime in individuals administered 2 grams intravenously every 8 hours for 5 days. Therefore, a dosage adjustment from the normal recommended dosage is not required for patients with hepatic dysfunction, provided renal function is not impaired.

Approximately 80% to 90% of an IM or IV dose of ceftazidime is excreted unchanged by the kidneys over a 24-hour period. After the IV administration of single 500 mg or 1 gram doses, approximately 50% of the dose appeared in the urine in the first 2 hours. An additional 20% was excreted between 2 and 4 hours after dosing, and approximately another 12% of the dose appeared in the urine between 4 and 8 hours later. The elimination of ceftazidime by the kidneys resulted in high therapeutic concentrations in the urine.

The mean renal clearance of ceftazidime was approximately 100 mL/min. The calculated plasma clearance of approximately 115 mL/min, indicated nearly complete elimination of ceftazidime by the renal route. Administration of probenecid before dosing had no effect on the elimination kinetics of ceftazidime. This suggested that ceftazidime is eliminated by glomerular filtration and is not actively secreted by renal tubular mechanisms.

Since ceftazidime is eliminated almost solely by the kidneys, its serum half-life is significantly prolonged in patients with impaired renal function. Consequently, dosage adjustments to such patients as described in the DOSAGE AND ADMINISTRATION section are suggested.

Therapeutic concentrations of ceftazidime are achieved in the following body tissues and fluids.

[See table 2 above]

Microbiology: Ceftazidime is bactericidal in action, exerting its effect by inhibition of enzymes responsible for cell-wall synthesis. A wide range of gram-negative organisms is susceptible to ceftazidime *in vitro*, including strains resistant to gentamicin and other aminoglycosides. In addition, ceftazidime has been shown to be active against gram-positive organisms. It is highly stable to most clinically important beta-lactamases, plasmid or chromosomal, which are produced by both gram-negative and gram-positive organisms and, consequently, is active against many strains resistant to ampicillin and other cephalosporins.

Ceftazidime has been shown to be active against the following organisms both *in vitro* and in clinical infections (see INDICATIONS AND USAGE).

Aerobes, Gram-Negative: *Citrobacter* spp. (including *Citrobacter freundii* and *Citrobacter diversus*); *Enterobacter* spp. (including *Enterobacter cloacae* and *Enterobacter aerogenes*); *Escherichia coli; Haemophilus influenzae,* including ampicillin-resistant strains; *Klebsiella* spp. (including *Klebsiella pneumoniae*); *Neisseria meningitidis; Proteus mirabilis; Proteus vulgaris; Pseudomonas* spp. (including *Pseudomonas aeruginosa*); and *Serratia* spp.

Aerobes, Gram-Positive: *Staphylococcus aureus,* including penicillinase- and non-penicillinase-producing strains; *Streptococcus agalactiae* (group B streptococci); *Streptococcus pneumoniae;* and *Streptococcus pyogenes* (group A beta-hemolytic streptococci).

Anaerobes: *Bacteroides* spp. (NOTE: Many strains of *Bacteroides fragilis* are resistant).

Ceftazidime has been shown to be active *in vitro* against most strains of the following organisms; however, the clinical significance of these data is unknown. *Acinetobacter* spp.; *Clostridium* spp. (not including *Clostridium difficile*); *Haemophilus parainfluenzae; Morganella morganii* (formerly *Proteus morganii*); *Neisseria gonorrhoeae; Peptococcus* spp.; *Peptostreptococcus* spp.; *Providencia* spp. (including *Providencia rettgeri,* formerly *Proteus rettgeri*); *Salmonella* spp.; *Shigella* spp.; *Staphylococcus epidermidis;* and *Yersinia enterocolitica.*

Ceftazidime and the aminoglycosides have been shown to be synergistic *in vitro* against *Pseudomonas aeruginosa* and the enterobacteriaceae. Ceftazidime and carbenicillin have also been shown to be synergistic *in vitro* against *Pseudomonas aeruginosa.*

Ceftazidime is not active *in vitro* against: methicillin-resistant staphylococci, *Streptococcus faecalis* and many other enterococci, *Listeria monocytogenes, Campylobacter* spp., or *Clostridium difficile.*

Susceptibility Tests: ***Diffusion Techniques:*** Quantitative methods that require measurement of zone diameters give an estimate of antibiotic susceptibility. One such procedure[1–3] has been recommended for use with disks to test susceptibility to ceftazidime.

Reports from the laboratory giving results of the standard single-disk susceptibility test with a 30 mcg ceftazidime disk should be interpreted according to the following criteria:

Susceptible organisms produce zones of 18 mm or greater, indicating that the test organism is likely to respond to therapy.

Organisms that produce zones of 15 mm to 17 mm are expected to be susceptible if high dosage is used or if the infection is confined to tissues and fluids (e.g., urine) in which high antibiotic levels are attained.

Resistant organisms produce zones of 14 mm or less, indicating that other therapy should be selected.

Organisms should be tested with the ceftazidime disk, since ceftazidime has been shown by *in vitro* tests to be active against certain strains found resistant when other beta-lactam disks are used.

Standardized procedures require the use of laboratory control organisms. The 30 mcg ceftazidime disk should give zone diameters between 25 mm and 32 mm for *Escherichia coli* ATCC 25922. For *Pseudomonas aeruginosa* ATCC 27853, the zone diameters should be between 22 mm and 29 mm. For *Staphylococcus aureus* ATCC 25923, the zone diameters should be between 16 mm and 20 mm.

Dilution Techniques

In other susceptibility testing procedures, e.g., ICS agar dilution or the equivalent, bacterial isolate may be considered susceptible if the minimum inhibitory concentration (MIC) value for ceftazidime is not more than 16 mcg/mL. Organisms are considered resistant to ceftazidime if the MIC is ≥ 64 mcg/mL. Organisms having an MIC value of < 64 mcg/mL but > 16 mcg/mL are expected to be susceptible if high dosage is used or if the infection is confined to tissues and fluids (e.g., urine) in which high antibiotic levels are attained.

As with standard diffusion methods, dilution procedures require the use of laboratory control organisms. Standard ceftazidime powder should give MIC values in the range of 4 mcg/mL and 16 mcg/mL for *Staphylococcus aureus* ATCC 25923. For *Escherichia coli* ATCC 25922, the MIC range should be between 0.125 mcg/mL and 0.5 mcg/mL. For *Pseudomonas aeruginosa* ATCC 27853, the MIC range should be between 0.5 mcg/mL and 2 mcg/mL.

INDICATIONS AND USAGE

Tazidime (ceftazidime for injection) is indicated for the treatment of patients with infections caused by susceptible strains of the designated organisms in the following diseases:

1. Lower Respiratory Tract Infections, including pneumonia, caused by *Psuedomonas aeruginosa* and other *Pseudomonas* spp.; *Haemophilus influenzae,* including ampicillin-resistant strains; *Klebsiella* spp.; *Enterobacter* spp.; *Proteus mirabilis; Escherichia coli; Serratia* spp.; *Citrobacter* spp.; *Streptococcus pneumoniae;* and *Staphylococcus aureus* (methicillin-susceptible strains).

2. Skin and Skin-Structure Infections, caused by *Pseudomonas aeruginosa, Klebsiella* spp.; *Escherichia coli; Proteus* spp., including *Proteus mirabilis* and indole-positive *Proteus; Enterobacter* spp.; *Serratia* spp.; *Staphylococcus aureus* (methicillin-susceptible strains); and *Streptococcus pyogenes* (group A beta-hemolytic streptococci).

3. Urinary Tract Infections, both complicated and uncomplicated, caused by *Pseudomonas aeruginosa; Enterobacter* spp.; *Proteus* spp., including *Proteus mirabilis* and indole-positive *Proteus; Klebsiella* spp. and *Escherichia coli.*

Continued on next page

*** Identi-Code® symbol. This product information was prepared in June 2000. Current information on these and other products of Eli Lilly and Company may be obtained by direct inquiry to Lilly Research Laboratories, Lilly Corporate Center, Indianapolis, Indiana 46285, (800) 545-5979.**

Tazidime—Cont.

4. Bacterial Septicemia caused by *Pseudomonas aeruginosa, Klebsiella* spp.; *Haemophilus influenzae; Escherichia coli, Serratia* spp., *Streptococcus pneumoniae,* and *Staphylococus aureus* (methicillin-susceptible strains).
5. Bone and Joint Infections caused by *Pseudomonas aeruginosa; Klebsiella* spp.; *Enterobacter* spp.; and *Staphylococcus aureus* (methicillin-susceptible strains).
6. Gynecologic Infections, including endometritis, pelvic cellulitis, and other infections of the female genital tract caused by *Escherichia coli.*
7. Intra-abdominal Infections, including peritonitis caused by *Escherichia coli, Klebsiella* spp.; *Staphylococcus aureus* (methicillin-susceptible strains), and polymicrobial infections caused by aerobic and anaerobic organisms, and *Bacteroides* spp. (many strains of *Bacteroides fragilis* are resistant).
8. Central Nervous System Infections, including meningitis caused by *Haemophilus influenzae* and *Neisseria meningitidis.* Ceftazidime has also been used successfully in a limited number of cases of meningitis due to *Pseudomonas aeruginosa* and *Streptococcus pneumoniae.*
Specimens for bacterial cultures should be obtained before therapy in order to isolate and identify causative organisms and to determine their susceptibility to ceftazidime. Therapy may be instituted before results of susceptibility studies are known; however, once these results become available, the antibiotic treatment should be adjusted accordingly.
Tazidime (ceftazidime for injection) may be used alone in cases of confirmed or suspected sepsis. Ceftazidime has been used successfully in clinical trials as empiric therapy in cases where various concomitant therapies with other antibiotics have been used.
Tazidime may also be used concomitantly with other antibiotics, such as aminoglycosides, vancomycin and clindamycin, in severe and life-threatening infections and in the immunocompromised patient. When such concomitant treatment is appropriate, prescribing information in the labeling for the other antibiotics should be followed. The dose depends on the severity of the infection and the patient's condition.

CONTRAINDICATION

Tazidime is contraindicated in patients who have shown hypersensitivity to ceftazidime or the cephalosporin group of antibiotics.

WARNINGS

BEFORE THERAPY WITH *TAZIDIME* IS INSTITUTED, CAREFUL INQUIRY SHOULD BE MADE TO DETERMINE WHETHER THE PATIENT HAS HAD PREVIOUS HYPERSENSITIVITY REACTIONS TO CEFTAZIDIME, CEPHALOSPORINS, PENICILLINS, OR OTHER DRUGS. IF THIS PRODUCT IS GIVEN TO PENICILLIN-SENSITIVE PATIENTS, CAUTION SHOULD BE EXERCISED BECAUSE CROSS-HYPERSENSITIVITY AMONG BETA-LACTAM ANTIBIOTICS HAS BEEN CLEARLY DOCUMENTED AND MAY OCCUR IN UP TO 10% OF PATIENTS WITH A HISTORY OF PENICILLIN ALLERGY. IF AN ALLERGIC REACTION TO *TAZIDIME* OCCURS, DISCONTINUE TREATMENT WITH THE DRUG. SERIOUS ACUTE HYPERSENSITIVITY REACTIONS MAY REQUIRE TREATMENT WITH EPINEPHRINE AND OTHER EMERGENCY MEASURES, INCLUDING OXYGEN, IV FLUIDS, IV ANTIHISTAMINES, CORTICOSTEROIDS, PRESSOR AMINES AND AIRWAY MANAGEMENT, AS CLINICALLY INDICATED.
Pseudomembranous colitis has been reported with nearly all antibacterial agents, including ceftazidime, and may range in severity from mild to life-threatening. Therefore, it is important to consider this diagnosis in patients who present with diarrhea subsequent to the administration of antibacterial agents.
Treatment with antibacterial agents alters the normal flora of the colon and may permit overgrowth of clostridia. Studies indicate that a toxin produced by *Clostridium difficile* is a primary cause of "antibiotic-associated colitis."
After the diagnosis of pseudomembranous colitis has been established appropriate therapeutic measures should be initiated. Mild cases of pseudomembranous colitis usually respond to drug discontinuation alone. In moderate to severe cases, consideration should be given to management with fluids and electrolytes, protein supplementation and treatment with an oral antibacterial drug clinically effective against *Clostridium difficile* colitis.
Elevated levels of ceftazidime in patients with renal insufficiency can lead to seizures, encephalopathy, asterixis and neuromuscular excitability (see PRECAUTIONS).

PRECAUTIONS

General: Ceftazidime has not been shown to be nephrotoxic; however, high and prolonged serum antibiotic concentrations can occur from usual dosages in patients with transient or persistent reduction of urinary output because of renal insufficiency. The total daily dosage should be reduced when ceftazidime is administered to patients with renal insufficiency (see DOSAGE AND ADMINISTRATION). Elevated levels of ceftazidime in these patients can lead to seizures, encephalophathy, asterixis and neuromuscular excitability. Continued dosage should be determined by degree of renal impairment, severity of infection and susceptibility of the causative organisms.

Table 3. Recommended Dosage Schedule

	Dose	Frequency
Adults		
Usual recommended dose	1gram IV or IM	q8 or 12h
Uncomplicated urinary tract infections	250 mg IV or IM	q12h
Bone and joint infections	2 grams IV	q12h
Complicated urinary tract infections	500 mg IV or IM	q8 or 12h
Uncomplicated pneumonia; mild skin and skin structure infections	500 mg to 1 gram IV or IM	q8h
Serious gynecological and intra-abdominal infections	2 grams IV	q8h
Meningitis	2 grams IV	q8h
Very severe life-threatening infections especially in immuno-compromised patients	2 grams IV	q8h
Lung infections caused by Pseudomonas spp. in patients with cystic fibrosis with normal renal function*	30 to 50 mg/kg IV to a maximum of 6 grams per day	q8h
Neonates (0–4 weeks)	30 mg/kg IV	q12h
Infants and children (1 month to 12 years)	30 to 50 mg/kg IV to a maximum of 6 grams per day†	q8h

*Although clinical improvement has been shown, bacteriological cures cannot be expected in patients with chronic respiratory disease and cystic fibrosis.
†The higher dose should be reserved for immunocompromised pediatric patients or pediatric patients with cystic fibrosis or meningitis.

As with other antibiotics, prolonged use of Tazidime (ceftazidime for injection) may result in overgrowth of nonsusceptible organisms. Repeated evaluation of the patient's condition is essential. If superinfection occurs during therapy, appropriate measures should be taken.
Inducible type-1 beta-lactamase resistance has been noted with some organisms (e.g., *Enterobacter* spp., *Pseudomonas* spp., and *Serratia* spp.). As with other extended-spectrum beta-lactam antibiotics, resistance can develop during therapy, leading to clinical failure in some cases. When treating infections caused by these organisms, periodic susceptibility testing should be performed when clinically appropriate. If patients fail to respond to monotherapy, an aminoglycoside or similar agent should be considered.
Cephalosporins may be associated with a fall in prothrombin activity. Those at risk include patients with renal or hepatic impairment, or poor nutritional state, as well as patients receiving a protracted course of antimicrobial therapy. Prothrombin time should be monitored in patients at risk and exogenous vitamin K administered as indicated.
Tazidime should be prescribed with caution in individuals with a history of gastrointestinal disease, particularly colitis.
Distal necrosis can occur after inadvertent intra-arterial administration of ceftazidime.
Drug Interactions: Nephrotoxicity has been reported following concomitant administration of cephalosporins with aminoglycoside antibiotics or potent diuretics, such as furosemide. Renal function should be carefully monitored, especially if higher dosages of the aminoglycosides are to be administered or if therapy is prolonged, because of the potential nephrotoxicity and ototoxicity of aminoglycoside antibiotics. Nephrotoxicity and ototoxicity were not noted when ceftazidime was given alone in clinical trials.
Chloramphenicol has been shown to be antagonistic to beta-lactam antibiotics, including ceftazidime, based on *in vitro* studies and time kill curves with enteric gram-negative bacilli. Due to the possibility of antagonism *in vivo*, particularly when bactericidal activity is desired, this drug combination should be avoided.
Drug/Laboratory Test Interactions: The administration of ceftazidime may result in a false-positive reaction for glucose in the urine when using Clinitest® tablets, Benedict's solution or Fehling's solution. It is recommended that glucose tests based on enzymatic glucose oxidase reactions (such as Clinistix® or Tes-Tape®) be used.
Carcinogenesis, Mutagenesis, Impairment of Fertility: Long-term studies in animals have not been performed to evaluate carcinogenic potential. However, a mouse micronucleus test and an Ames test were both negative for mutagenic effects.
Pregnancy: ***Teratogenic Effects:*** Pregnancy Category B. Reproduction studies have been performed in mice and rats at doses up to 40 times the human dose and have revealed no evidence of impaired fertility or harm to the fetus due to Tazidime. There are, however, no adequate and well-controlled studies in pregnant women. Because animal reproduction studies are not always predictive of human response, this drug should be used during pregnancy only if clearly needed.
Nursing Mothers: Ceftazidime is excreted in human milk in low concentrations. Caution should be exercised when *Tazidime* is administered to a nursing woman.
Pediatric Use: See DOSAGE AND ADMINISTRATION.

ADVERSE REACTIONS

Ceftazidime is generally well tolerated. The incidence of adverse reactions associated with the administration of ceftazidime was low in clinical trials. The most common were local reactions following IV injection, and allergic and gastrointestinal reactions. Other adverse reactions were encountered infrequently. No disulfiram-like reactions were reported.
The following adverse effects from clinical trials were considered to be either related to ceftazidime therapy or were of uncertain etiology.
Local Effects, reported in fewer than 2% of patients, were phlebitis and inflammation at the site of injection (1 in 69 patients).
Hypersensitivity Reactions, reported in 2% of patients, were pruritus, rash and fever. Toxic epidermal necrolysis, Stevens-Johnson syndrome, and erythema multiforme have also been reported with cephalosporin antibiotics, including ceftazidime. Immediate reactions, generally manifested by rash and/or pruritus, occurred in 1 in 285 patients. Angioedema and anaphylaxis (bronchospasm and/or hypotension) have been reported very rarely.
Gastrointestinal Symptoms, reported in fewer than 2% of patients, were diarrhea (1 in 78), nausea (1 in 156), vomiting (1 in 500) and abdominal pain (1 in 416).
The onset of pseudomembranous colitis symptoms may occur during or after treatment (See WARNINGS).
Central Nervous System Reactions (fewer than 1%) include headache, dizziness and paresthesia. Seizures have been reported with several cephalosporins, including ceftazidime. In addition, encephalopathy, asterixis and neuromuscular excitability have been reported in renally impaired patients treated with unadjusted dosage regimens of ceftazidime (see PRECAUTIONS: General).
Less Frequent Adverse Events (fewer than 1%) were candidiasis (including oral thrush) and vaginitis.
Hematologic: Rare cases of hemolytic anemia have been reported.
Laboratory Test Changes noted during Tazidime (ceftazidime for injection) clinical trials were transient and included: eosinophilia (1 in 13), positive Coombs' test without hemolysis (1 in 23), thrombocytosis (1 in 45), and slight elevations in one or more of the hepatic enzymes, aspartate aminotransferase (AST, SGOT) (1 in 16), alanine aminotransferase (ALT, SGPT) (1 in 15), LDH (1 in 18). GGT (1 in 19) and alkaline phosphatase (1 in 23). As with some other cephalosporins, transient elevations of blood urea, blood urea nitrogen and/or serum creatinine were observed occa-

sionally. Transient leukopenia, neutropenia, agranulocytosis, thrombocytopenia and lymphocytosis were seen very rarely.

Observed During Clinical Practice In addition to the adverse events reported from clinical trials, the following events have been identified during post-approval use of ceftazidime. Because they are reported voluntarily from a population of unknown size, estimates of frequency cannot be made. These events have been chose for inclusion due to a combination of their seriousness, frequency of reporting, or potential causal connection to ceftazidime.

General: Anaphylactic or anaphylactoid reactions, which, in rare instances, were severe (e.g., cardiopulmonary arrest), including laryngeal edema, stridor, and urticaria; pain at injection site.

Hepatobiliary Tract and Pancreas: Hyperbilirubinemia.

Renal and Genitourinary: Renal Impairment.

Cephalosporin-Class Adverse Reactions: In addition to the adverse reactions listed above that have been observed in patients treated with ceftazidime, the following adverse reactions and altered laboratory tests have been reported for cephalosporin-class antibiotics:

Adverse Reactions: Urticaria, colitis, renal dysfunction, toxic nephropathy, hepatic dysfunction including cholestasis, aplastic anemia, hemorrhage.

Altered Laboratory Tests: Prolonged prothrombin time, false-positive test for urinary glucose, elevated bilirubin, pancytopenia.

OVERDOSAGE

Ceftazidime overdosage has occurred in patients with renal failure. Reactions have included seizure activity, encephalopathy, asterixis and neuromuscular excitability. Patients who receive an acute overdosage should be carefully observed and given supportive treatment. In the presence of renal insufficiency, hemodialysis or peritoneal dialysis may aid in the removal of ceftazidime from the body.

DOSAGE AND ADMINISTRATION

Dosage: The usual adult dosage is 1 gram administered intravenously or intramuscularly every 8 or 12 hours. The dosage and route should be determined by the susceptibility of the causative organisms, the severity of infection and the condition and renal function of the patient.

The guidelines for dosage of Tazidime (ceftazidime for injection) are listed in Table 3. The following dosage schedule is recommended.

[See table 3 at top of previous page]

Impaired Hepatic Function: No adjustment in dosage is required for patients with hepatic dysfunction.

Impaired Renal Function: Ceftazidime is excreted by the kidneys, almost exclusively by glomerular filtration. Therefore, in patients with impaired renal function (glomerular filtration rate [GFR] <50 mL/min.), it is recommended that the dosage of ceftazidime be reduced to compensate for its slower excretion. In patients with suspected renal insufficiency, an initial loading dose of 1 gram of ceftazidime may be given. An estimate of GFR should be made to determine the appropriate maintenance dose. The recommended dosage is presented in Table 4.

Table 4. Recommended Maintenance Doses of Tazidime (ceftazidime for injection) in Renal Insufficiency

NOTE: IF THE DOSE RECOMMENDED IN TABLE 3 ABOVE IS LOWER THAN THAT RECOMMENDED FOR PATIENTS WITH RENAL INSUFFICIENCY AS OUTLINED IN TABLE 4, THE LOWER DOSE SHOULD BE USED.

Creatinine Clearance (mL/min.)	Recommended Unit Dose of *Tazidime*	Frequency of Dosing
50 to 31	1 gram	q12h
30 to 16	1 gram	q24h
15 to 6	500 mg	q24h
<5	500 mg	q48h

When only serum creatinine is available, the following formula (Cockcroft's equation)[4] may be used to estimate creatinine clearance. The serum creatinine should represent a steady state of renal function:

$$\text{Males: Creatinine clearance (mL/min.)} = \frac{\text{Weight (kg)} \times (140 - \text{age})}{72 \times \text{serum creatinine (mg/dL)}}$$

$$\text{Females: } 0.85 \times \text{male value}$$

In patients with severe infections who would normally receive 6 grams of *Tazidime* daily were it not for renal insufficiency, the unit dose given in the table above may be increased by 50% or the dosing frequency increased appropriately. Further dosing should be determined by therapeutic monitoring, severity of the infection and susceptibility of the causative organism.

In pediatric patients as for adults, the creatinine clearance should be adjusted for body surface area or lean body mass and the dosing frequency reduced in cases of renal insufficiency.

In patients undergoing hemodialysis, a loading dose of 1 gram is recommended, followed by 1 gram after each hemodialysis period.

Tazidime (ceftazidime for injection) can also be used in patients undergoing intra-peritoneal dialysis (IPD) and continuous ambulatory peritoneal dialysis. In such patients, a loading dose of 1 gram of *Tazidime* may be given, followed by 500 mg every 24 hours. In addition to IV use, *Tazidime* can be incorporated in the dialysis fluid at a concentration of 250 mg for 2 liters of dialysis fluid.

NOTE: Generally, *Tazidime* should be continued for 2 days after the signs and symptoms of infection have disappeared, but in complicated infections longer therapy may be required.

Administration: *Tazidime* may be given intravenously or by deep IM injection into a large muscle mass such as the upper outer quadrant of the gluteus maximus or lateral part of the thigh.

NOTE: *Tazidime* in ADD-Vantage® vials is not intended for direct IV or IM injection.

Intramuscular Administration: For IM administration, *Tazidime* should be reconstituted with Sterile Water for Injection Refer to Table 5.

Intravenous Administration: The IV route is preferable for patients with bacterial septicemia, bacterial meningitis, peritonitis, or other severe or life-threatening infections, or for patients who may be poor risks because of lowered resistance resulting from such debilitating conditions as malnutrition, trauma, surgery, diabetes, heart failure or malignancy, particularly if shock is present or pending.

For direct intermittent IV administration, reconstitute *Tazidime* as directed in Table 5 with Sterile Water for Injection. Slowly inject directly into the vein over a period of 3 to 5 minutes or give through the tubing of an administration set while the patient is also receiving one of the compatible IV fluids (See COMPATIBILITY AND STABILITY).

For IV infusion, reconstitute the 1- or 2-gram piggyback vial with 100 mL of Sodium Chloride Injection or one of the compatible IV fluids listed under the COMPATIBILITY AND STABILITY section. Alternatively, reconstitute the 1 gram or 2 gram vial and add an appropriate quantity of the resulting solution to an IV container with one of the compatible IV fluids.

Intermittent intravenous infusion with a Y-type administration set can be accomplished with compatible solutions. However, during infusion of a solution containing ceftazidime it is desirable to discontinue the other solution.

All vials of Tazidime as supplied are under reduced pressure. When Tazidime is dissolved, carbon dioxide is released and a positive pressure develops. See RECONSTITUTION.

Solutions of *Tazidime*, like those of most beta-lactam antibiotics should not be added to solutions of aminoglycoside antibiotics because of potential interaction.

However, if concurrent therapy with *Tazidime* and an aminoglycoside is indicated, each of these antibiotics can be administered separately to the same patient.

***TAZIDIME* INJECTION IN ADD-VANTAGE® VIALS**

NOTE: Tazidime (ceftazidime for injection) in the ADD-Vantage® vial is intended to be administered as a single-dose intravenous infusion with the ADD-Vantage® flexible diluent container.

Tazidime in single-dose ADD-Vantage® vials should be prepared as directed (see RECONSTITUTION, for ADD-Vantage® Vials) with either 0.9% Sodium Chloride Injection in the 50 mL or 100 mL flexible diluent containers, 0.45% Sodium Chloride Injection in the 50 mL container or 5% Dextrose Injection in the 50 mL or 100 mL containers.

RECONSTITUTION

Single Dose Vials:

For IM Injection, IV direct (bolus) injection, or IV infusion, reconstitute with Sterile Water for Injection according to the following table. The vacuum may assist entry of the diluent. SHAKE WELL.

Table 5

Vial Size	Amount of Diluent to Be Added	Approx. Avail. Volume	Approximate Ceftazidime Concentration
Intramuscular or Intravenous Direct (bolus) Injection			
1 gram	3.0 mL	3.6 mL	280 mg/mL
Intravenous Infusion			
1 gram	10 mL	10.6 mL	95 mg/mL
2 gram	10 mL	11.2 mL	180 mg/mL

Withdraw the total volume of solution into the syringe (the pressure in the vial may aid withdrawal). The withdrawn solution may contain some bubbles of carbon dioxide.

NOTE: As with the administration of all parenteral products, accumulated gases should be expressed from the syringe immediately before injection of *Tazidime*.

These solutions of *Tazidime* are stable for 24 hours at room temperature or 7 days if refrigerated (5°C). Slight yellowing does not affect potency.

For IV infusion, dilute reconstituted solution in 50 to 100 mL of one of the parenteral fluids listed under COMPATIBILITY AND STABILITY.

"Piggyback" Vials:

For IV infusion, reconstitute with 10 mL of Sodium Chloride Injection according to the following table. The vacuum may assist entry of the diluent. SHAKE WELL.

Table 6

Vial Size	Diluent to Be Added	Approx. Avail. Volume	Approx. Avg. Concentration
1 gram	100 mL*	100 mL	10 mg/mL
2 gram	100 mL*	100 mL	20 mg/mL

*Addition should be in two stages.

Insert a gas relief needle through the vial closure to relieve the internal pressure. With the gas relief needle in position, add the remaining 90 mL of Sodium Chloride Injection. Remove the gas relief needle and syringe needle; shake the vial and set up for infusion in the normal way.

NOTE: To preserve product sterility, it is important that a gas relief needle is not inserted through the vial closure before the product has dissolved.

These solutions of Tazidime (ceftazidime for injection) are stable for 24 hours at room temperature or 7 days if refrigerated (5°C). Slight yellowing does not affect potency.

ADD-Vantage® Vials: ADD-Vantage® vials of Tazidime (ceftazidime for injection) are to be reconstituted only with 0.9% Sodium Chloride Injection or 5% Dextrose Injection in the 50 mL or 100 mL flexible diluent containers, or with 0.45% Sodium Chloride Injection in the 50 mL container.

DIRECTIONS FOR USE OF TAZIDIME® (CEFTAZIDIME FOR INJECTION) IN ADD-VANTAGE® VIALS

To Open Diluent Container:

Peel overwrap at corner and remove solution container. Some opacity of the plastic due to moisture absorption during the sterilization process may be observed. This is normal and does not affect the solution quality or safety. The opacity will diminish gradually.

To Assemble Vial and Flexible Diluent Container: (Use Aseptic Technique)

1. Remove the protective covers from the top of the vial and the vial port on the diluent container as follows:
   a. To remove the breakaway vial cap, swing the pull ring over the top of the vial and pull down far enough to start the opening (SEE FIGURE 1), then pull straight up to remove the cap. (SEE FIGURE 2.)
   NOTE: Do not access vial with syringe.

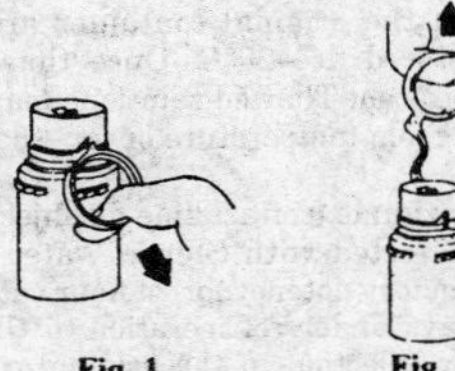

Fig. 1 Fig. 2

   b. To remove the vial port cover, grasp the tab on the pull ring, pull up to break the three tie strings, then pull back to remove the cover. (SEE FIGURE 3.)
2. Screw the vial into the vial port until it will go no further. THE VIAL MUST BE SCREWED IN TIGHTLY TO ASSURE A SEAL. This occurs approximately 1/2 turn (180°) after the first audible click. (SEE FIGURE 4.) The clicking sound does not assure a seal; the vial must be turned as far as it will go.
   NOTE: Once vial is sealed, do not attempt to remove. (SEE FIGURE 4.)
3. Recheck the vial to assure that it is tight by trying to turn it further in the direction of assembly.
4. Label appropriately.

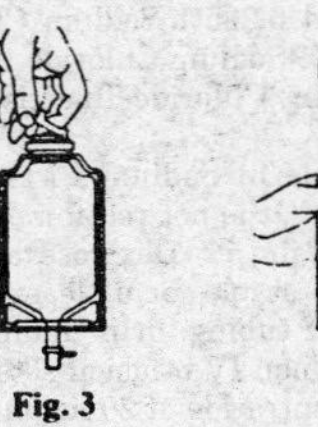

Fig. 3 Fig. 4

To Reconstitute the Drug:

1. Squeeze the bottom of the diluent container gently to inflate the portion of the container surrounding the end of the drug vial.
2. With the other hand, push the drug vial down into the container telescoping the walls of the container. Grasp the inner cap of the vial through the walls of the container. (SEE FIGURE 5.)
3. Pull the inner cap from the drug vial. (SEE FIGURE 6.) Verify that the rubber stopper has been pulled out, allowing the drug and diluent to mix.

Continued on next page

*** Identi-Code® symbol. This product information was prepared in June 2000. Current information on these and other products of Eli Lilly and Company may be obtained by direct inquiry to Lilly Research Laboratories, Lilly Corporate Center, Indianapolis, Indiana 46285, (800) 545-5979.**

Tazidime—Cont.

4. Mix container contents thoroughly and use within the specified time.

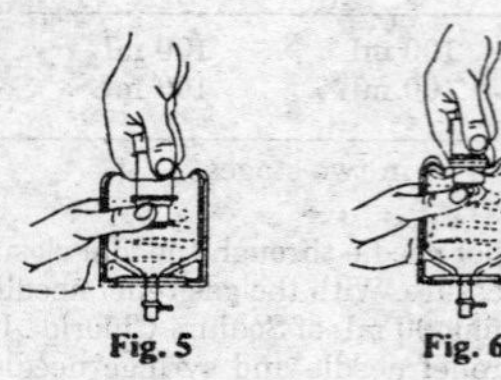
Fig. 5 Fig. 6

Preparation for Administration:
(Use Aseptic Technique)
1. Confirm the activation and admixture of vial contents.
2. Check for leaks by squeezing container firmly. If leaks are found discard unit as sterility may be impaired.
3. Close flow control clamp of administration set.
4. Remove cover from outlet port at bottom of container.
5. Insert piercing pin of administration set into port with a twisting motion until the pin is firmly seated. **NOTE:** See full directions on administration set carton.
6. Lift the free end of the hanger loop on the bottom of the vial, breaking the two tie strings. Bend the loop outward to lock it in the upright position, then suspend container from hanger.
7. Squeeze and release drip chamber to establish proper fluid level in chamber.
8. Open flow control clamp and clear air from set. Close clamp.
9. Attach set to venipuncture device. If device is not indwelling, prime and make venipuncture.
10. Regulate rate of administration with flow control clamp.

WARNING: Do not use flexible container in series connections.

COMPATIBILITY AND STABILITY

Intramuscular: Tazidime (ceftazidime for injection), when reconstituted as directed with Sterile Water for Injection, maintains satisfactory potency for 24 hours at room temperature or for 7 days under refrigeration (5°C). Solutions in Sterile Water for Injection that are frozen immediately after reconstitution in the original container are stable for 3 months when stored at –20°C. Once thawed, solutions should not be refrozen. Thawed solutions may be stored for up to 8 hours at room temperature or for 4 days in a refrigerator (5°C).

Intravenous: Tazidime (ceftazidime for injection) when reconstituted as directed with Sterile Water for Injection, maintains satisfactory potency for 24 hours at room temperature or for 7 days under refrigeration (5°C). Solutions in Sterile Water for Injection in the original container or in 0.9% Sodium Chloride Injection in Viaflex® small volume containers that are frozen immediately after reconstitution are stable for 3 months when stored at –20°C. For larger volumes where it may be necessary to warm the frozen product (to a maximum of 40°C), care should be taken to avoid heating after thawing is complete. Do not force thaw by immersion in water baths or by microwave irradiation. Once thawed, solutions should not be refrozen. Thawed solutions may be stored for up to 8 hours at room temperature or for 4 days in a refrigerator (5°C).

Tazidime is compatible with the more commonly used IV infusion fluids. Solutions at concentrations between 1 mg/mL and 40 mg/mL in the following infusion fluids may be stored for up to 24 hours at room temperature or 7 days if refrigerated: 0.9% Sodium Chloride Injection; Ringer's Injection USP; Lactated Ringer's Injection USP; 5% Dextrose Injection; 5% Dextrose and 0.225% Sodium Chloride Injection; 5% Dextrose and 0.45% Sodium Chloride Injection; 5% Dextrose and 0.9% Sodium Chloride Injection; 10% Dextrose Injection.

Tazidime is less stable in Sodium Bicarbonate Injection than in other IV fluids. It is not recommended as a diluent Solutions of *Tazidime* in 5% Dextrose and 0.9% Sodium Chloride Injection are stable for at least 6 hours at room temperature in plastic tubing, drip chambers and volume control devices of common IV infusion sets.

Ceftazidime at a concentration of 20 mg/mL has been found physically compatible for 24 hours at room temperature or 7 days under refrigeration in Sterile Water for Injection when admixed with: cefazolin sodium 330 mg/mL; heparin 1000 units/mL; and cimetidine HCl 150 mg/mL.

Ceftazidime at a concentration of 20 mg/mL has been found physically compatible for 24 hours at room temperature or 7 days under refrigeration in 5% Dextrose Injection when admixed with potassium chloride 40 mEq/l.

Vancomycin solution exhibits a physical incompatibility when mixed with a number of drugs, including ceftazidime. The likelihood of precipitation with ceftazidime is dependent on the concentrations of vancomycin and ceftazidime present. It is therefore recommended, when both drugs are to be administered by intermittent IV infusion, that they be given separately, flushing the IV lines (with one of the compatible IV fluids) between the administration of these two agents.

ADD-Vantage® Vials: Ordinarily. ADD-Vantage® vials should be reconstituted only when it is certain that the patient is ready to receive the drug. However, *Tazidime* in ADD-Vantage® vials is stable for 24 hours at room temperature when reconstituted as directed (see RECONSTITUTION, ADD-Vantage® Vials and DIRECTIONS FOR USE OF TAZIDIME® INJECTION IN ADD-VANTAGE® VIALS).

Note: Parenteral drug products should be inspected visually for particulate matter prior to administration wherever solution and container permit.

As with other cephalosporins, *Tazidime* powder, as well as solutions, tend to darken depending on storage conditions; within the stated recommendations, however, product potency is not adversely affected.

HOW SUPPLIED

Tazidime in the dry state should be stored at Controlled Room Temperature 20° to 25°C (68° to 77°F). Tazidime (ceftazidime for injection) is supplied in vials equivalent to 1 gram and 2 grams of ceftazidime; in "Piggyback" Vials for I.V. admixture equivalent to 1 gram and 2 grams of ceftazidime; and in ADD-Vantage,* Vials containing ceftazidime pentahydrate equivalent to 1 gram and 2 grams of ceftazidime.

1g† (No. 7290)—(Traypak of 25) NDC 0002-7290-25
2g† (No. 7291)—(Traypak of 10) NDC 0002-7291-10

The above ADD-Vantage,* Vials are to be used only with Abbott Laboratories' ADD-Vantage, Diluent Containers.

Vials (Dry Powder):
1g,† 20-mL size (No. 7231)—(Traypak of 25) NDC 0002-7231-25
1g,† 100-mL size (No. 7238)—(Traypak of 10) NDC 0002-7238-10
2g,† 60-mL size (No. 7234)—(Traypak of 10) NDC 0002-7234-10
2g,† 100-mL size (No. 7239)—(Traypak of 10) NDC 0002-7239-10

Also available:
Faspak§:
1 g† (No. 7245)—(Faspak of 24) NDC 0002-7245-24
2 g† (No. 7246)—(Faspak of 24) NDC 0002-7246-24
Pharmacy Bulk Package:
6g,† 100-mL size (No. 7241)—(Traypak of 6) NDC 0002-7241-16

*ADD-Vantage, (vials and diluent containers. Abbott). ADD-Vantage, is a trademark of Abbott Laboratories.
†Equivalent to ceftazidime activity.
‡Traypak™ (multivial carton, Lilly).
§Faspak, (flexible plastic bag, Lilly).

REFERENCES

1. Bauer, A.W.; Kirby, W.M.M., and Sherris, J.C., et al.: Antibiotic susceptibility testing by a standardized single disc method, Am. J. Clin. Pathol. 45:493, 1966.
2. National Committee for Clinical Laboratory Standards, Approved Standard: Performance Standards for Antimicrobial Disc Susceptibility Tests (M2–A3), December, 1984.
3. Standardized disc susceptibility test. Federal Register 39:19182–19184, 1974.
4. Cockcroft, D.W., and Gault, M.H.: Prediction of creatinine clearance from serum creatinine, Nephron 16:31–41, 1976.

Rx only
DATE OF ISSUANCE DEC. 1999

Manufactured for
ELI LILLY AND COMPANY
Indianapolis, IN 46285, USA
by
BMH Limited
Philadelphia, PA 19101

TD:L6

TOBRAMYCIN SULFATE ℞
See Nebcin® (Tobramycin Sulfate Injection, USP).

VANCOCIN® HCl ℞

[*văn 'kō-sĭn ăch 'sē-ĕl*]
(Sterile Vancomycin Hydrochloride, USP)
IntraVenous

VIALS

DESCRIPTION

Vancocin® HCl (Sterile Vancomycin Hydrochloride, USP), IntraVenous, is a chromatographically purified, tricyclic glycopeptide antibiotic derived from *Amycolatopsis orientalis* (formerly *Nocardia orientalis*) and has the chemical formula $C_{66}H_{75}Cl_2N_9O_{24}$ • HCl. The molecular weight is 1,485.73; 500 mg of the base is equivalent to 0.34 mmol.

Vancomycin hydrochloride has the following structural formula:

[See chemical structure at top of next column]

The vials contain sterile vancomycin hydrochloride equivalent to either 500 mg or 1 g vancomycin activity. Vancomycin hydrochloride is an off-white lyophilized plug. When reconstituted in water, it forms a clear solution with a pH range of 2.5 to 4.5. This product is oxygen sensitive.

CLINICAL PHARMACOLOGY

Vancomycin is poorly absorbed after oral administration; it is given intravenously for therapy of systemic infections. Intramuscular injection is painful.

[Chemical structure of vancomycin hydrochloride • HCl]

In subjects with normal kidney function, multiple intravenous dosing of 1 g of vancomycin (15 mg/kg) infused over 60 minutes produces mean plasma concentrations of approximately 63 µg/mL immediately after the completion of infusion, mean plasma concentrations of approximately 23 µg/mL 2 hours after infusion, and mean plasma concentrations of approximately 8 µg/mL 11 hours after the end of the infusion. Multiple dosing of 500 mg infused over 30 minutes produces mean plasma concentrations of about 49 µg/mL at the completion of infusion, mean plasma concentrations of about 19 µg/mL 2 hours after infusion, and mean plasma concentrations of about 10 µg/mL 6 hours after infusion. The plasma concentrations during multiple dosing are similar to those after a single dose.

The mean elimination half-life of vancomycin from plasma is 4 to 6 hours in subjects with normal renal function. In the first 24 hours, about 75% of an administered dose of vancomycin is excreted in urine by glomerular filtration. Mean plasma clearance is about 0.058 L/kg/h, and mean renal clearance is about 0.048 L/kg/h. Renal dysfunction slows excretion of vancomycin. In anephric patients, the average half-life of elimination is 7.5 days. The distribution coefficient is from 0.3 to 0.43 L/kg. There is no apparent metabolism of the drug. About 60% of an intraperitoneal dose of vancomycin administered during peritoneal dialysis is absorbed systemically in 6 hours. Serum concentrations of about 10 µg/mL are achieved by intraperitoneal injection of 30 mg/kg of vancomycin. Although vancomycin is not effectively removed by either hemodialysis or peritoneal dialysis, there have been reports of increased vancomycin clearance with hemoperfusion and hemofiltration.

Total systemic and renal clearance of vancomycin may be reduced in the elderly.

Vancomycin is approximately 55% serum protein bound as measured by ultrafiltration at vancomycin serum concentrations of 10 to 100 µg/mL. After IV administration of Vancocin HCl, inhibitory concentrations are present in pleural, pericardial, ascitic, and synovial fluids; in urine; in peritoneal dialysis fluid; and in atrial appendage tissue. Vancocin HCl does not readily diffuse across normal meninges into the spinal fluid; but, when the meninges are inflamed, penetration into the spinal fluid occurs.

Microbiology —The bactericidal action of vancomycin results primarily from inhibition of cell-wall biosynthesis. In addition, vancomycin alters bacterial-cell-membrane permeability and RNA synthesis. There is no cross-resistance between vancomycin and other antibiotics. Vancomycin is active against staphylococci, including *Staphylococcus aureus* and *Staphylococcus epidermidis* (including heterogeneous methicillin-resistant strains); streptococci, including *Streptococcus pyogenes, Streptococcus pneumoniae* (including penicillin-resistant strains), *Streptococcus agalactiae*, the viridans group, *Streptococcus bovis*, and enterococci (eg, *Enterococcus faecalis* [formerly *Streptococcus faecalis*]); *Clostridium difficile* (eg, toxigenic strains implicated in pseudomembranous enterocolitis); and diphtheroids. Other organisms that are susceptible to vancomycin in vitro include *Listeria monocytogenes, Lactobacillus* species, *Actinomyces* species, *Clostridium* species, and *Bacillus* species. Vancomycin is not active in vitro against gram-negative bacilli, mycobacteria, or fungi.

Synergy —The combination of vancomycin and an aminoglycoside acts synergistically in vitro against many strains of *S. aureus*, nonenterococcal group D streptococci, enterococci, and *Streptococcus* species (viridans group).

Disk Susceptibility Tests —The standardized disk method described by the National Committee for Clinical Laboratory Standards has been recommended to test susceptibility to vancomycin. Results of standard susceptibility tests with a 30-µg vancomycin hydrochloride disk should be interpreted according to the following criteria: Susceptible organisms produce zones greater than or equal to 12 mm, indicating that the test organism is likely to respond to therapy. Organisms that produce zones of 10 or 11 mm are considered to be of intermediate susceptibility. Organisms in this category are likely to respond if the infection is confined to tissues or fluids in which high antibiotic concentrations are attained. Resistant organisms produce zones of 9 mm or less, indicating that other therapy should be selected.

Using a standardized dilution method, a bacterial isolate may be considered susceptible if the MIC value for vancomycin is 4 µg/mL or less. Organisms are considered resistant to vancomycin if the MIC is greater than or equal to 16 µg/mL. Organisms having an MIC value of less than 16 µg/mL but greater than 4 µg/mL are considered to be of intermediate susceptibility.[1–2]

Standardized procedures require the use of laboratory control organisms. The 30-µg vancomycin disk should give zone diameters between 15 and 19 mm for *S. aureus* ATCC 25923. As with the standard diffusion methods, dilution procedures require the use of laboratory control organisms. Standard vancomycin powder should give MIC values in the range of 0.5 µg/mL to 2.0 µg/mL for *S. aureus* ATCC 29213. For *E. faecalis* ATCC 29212, the MIC range should be 1.0 to 4.0 µg/mL.

INDICATIONS AND USAGE

Vancocin HCl is indicated for the treatment of serious or severe infections caused by susceptible strains of methicillin-resistant (beta-lactam-resistant) staphylococci. It is indicated for penicillin-allergic patients, for patients who cannot receive or who have failed to respond to other drugs, including the penicillins or cephalosporins, and for infections caused by vancomycin-susceptible organisms that are resistant to other antimicrobial drugs. Vancocin HCl is indicated for initial therapy when methicillin-resistant staphylococci are suspected, but after susceptibility data are available, therapy should be adjusted accordingly.

Vancocin HCl is effective in the treatment of staphylococcal endocarditis. Its effectiveness has been documented in other infections due to staphylococci, including septicemia, bone infections, lower respiratory tract infections, and skin and skin structure infections. When staphylococcal infections are localized and purulent, antibiotics are used as adjuncts to appropriate surgical measures.

Vancocin HCl has been reported to be effective alone or in combination with an aminoglycoside for endocarditis caused by *Streptococcus viridans* or *S. bovis*. For endocarditis caused by enterococci (eg, *E. faecalis*), Vancocin HCl has been reported to be effective only in combination with an aminoglycoside.

Vancocin HCl has been reported to be effective for the treatment of diphtheroid endocarditis. Vancocin HCl has been used successfully in combination with either rifampin, an aminoglycoside, or both in early-onset prosthetic valve endocarditis caused by *S. epidermidis* or diphtheroids.

Specimens for bacteriologic cultures should be obtained in order to isolate and identify causative organisms and to determine their susceptibilities to Vancocin HCl.

The parenteral form of Vancocin HCl may be administered orally for treatment of antibiotic-associated pseudomembranous colitis caused by *C. difficile* and for staphylococcal enterocolitis. Parenteral administration of Vancocin HCl alone is of unproven benefit for these indications. **Vancocin HCl is not effective by the oral route for other types of infection.**

Although no controlled clinical efficacy studies have been conducted, intravenous vancomycin has been suggested by the American Heart Association and the American Dental Association as prophylaxis against bacterial endocarditis in penicillin-allergic patients who have congenital heart disease or rheumatic or other acquired valvular heart disease when these patients undergo dental procedures or surgical procedures of the upper respiratory tract.

Note: When selecting antibiotics for the prevention of bacterial endocarditis, the physician or dentist should read the full joint statement of the American Heart Association and the American Dental Association.[3]

CONTRAINDICATION

Vancocin HCl is contraindicated in patients with known hypersensitivity to this antibiotic.

WARNINGS

Rapid bolus administration (eg, over several minutes) may be associated with exaggerated hypotension, and, rarely, cardiac arrest.

Vancocin HCl should be administered in a dilute solution over a period of not less than 60 minutes to avoid rapid-infusion-related reactions. Stopping the infusion usually results in prompt cessation of these reactions.

Ototoxicity has occurred in patients receiving Vancocin HCl. It may be transient or permanent. It has been reported mostly in patients who have been given excessive doses, who have an underlying hearing loss, or who are receiving concomitant therapy with another ototoxic agent, such as an aminoglycoside. Vancomycin should be used with caution in patients with renal insufficiency because the risk of toxicity is appreciably increased by high, prolonged blood concentrations.

Dosage of Vancocin HCl must be adjusted for patients with renal dysfunction (*see* PRECAUTIONS *and* DOSAGE AND ADMINISTRATION).

Pseudomembranous colitis has been reported with nearly all antibacterial agents, including vancomycin, and may range in severity from mild to life-threatening. Therefore, it is important to consider this diagnosis in patients who present with diarrhea subsequent to the administration of antibacterial agents.

Treatment with antibacterial agents alters the normal flora of the colon and may permit overgrowth of clostridia. Studies indicate that a toxin produced by *Clostridium difficile* is a primary cause of "antibiotic-associated colitis." After the diagnosis of pseudomembranous colitis has been established, therapeutic measures should be initiated. Mild cases of pseudomembranous colitis usually respond to drug discontinuation alone. In moderate to severe cases, consideration should be given to management with fluids and electrolytes, protein supplementation, and treatment with an antibacterial drug clinically effective against *C. difficile* colitis.

PRECAUTIONS

General —Clinically significant serum concentrations have been reported in some patients who have taken multiple oral doses of vancomycin for active *C. difficile*-induced pseudomembranous colitis.

Prolonged use of Vancocin HCl may result in the overgrowth of nonsusceptible organisms. Careful observation of the patient is essential. If superinfection occurs during therapy, appropriate measures should be taken.

In order to minimize the risk of nephrotoxicity when treating patients with underlying renal dysfunction or patients receiving concomitant therapy with an aminoglycoside, serial monitoring of renal function should be performed and particular care should be taken in following appropriate dosing schedules (*see* DOSAGE AND ADMINISTRATION).

Serial tests of auditory function may be helpful in order to minimize the risk of ototoxicity.

Reversible neutropenia has been reported in patients receiving Vancocin HCl (*see* ADVERSE REACTIONS). Patients who will undergo prolonged therapy with Vancocin HCl or those who are receiving concomitant drugs that may cause neutropenia should have periodic monitoring of the leukocyte count.

Vancocin HCl is irritating to tissue and must be given by a secure intravenous route of administration. Pain, tenderness, and necrosis occur with intramuscular injection of Vancocin HCl or with inadvertent extravasation. Thrombophlebitis may occur, the frequency and severity of which can be minimized by administering the drug slowly as a dilute solution (2.5 to 5 g/L) and by rotating the sites of infusion.

There have been reports that the frequency of infusion-related events (including hypotension, flushing, erythema, urticaria, and pruritus) increases with the concomitant administration of anesthetic agents. Infusion-related events may be minimized by the administration of Vancocin HCl as a 60-minute infusion prior to anesthetic induction.

The safety and efficacy of vancomycin administration by the intrathecal (intralumbar or intraventricular) routes have not been assessed.

Reports have revealed that administration of sterile vancomycin HCl by the intraperitoneal route during continuous ambulatory peritoneal dialysis (CAPD) has resulted in a syndrome of chemical peritonitis. To date, this syndrome has ranged from a cloudy dialysate alone to a cloudy dialysate accompanied by variable degrees of abdominal pain and fever. This syndrome appears to be short-lived after discontinuation of intraperitoneal vancomycin.

Drug Interactions—Concomitant administration of vancomycin and anesthetic agents has been associated with erythema and histamine-like flushing (*see* USAGE IN PEDIATRICS *under* PRECAUTIONS) and anaphylactoid reactions (*see* ADVERSE REACTIONS).

Concurrent and/or sequential systemic or topical use of other potentially neurotoxic and/or nephrotoxic drugs, such as amphotericin B, aminoglycosides, bacitracin, polymyxin B, colistin, viomycin, or cisplatin, when indicated, requires careful monitoring.

Usage in Pregnancy—Pregnancy Category C—Animal reproduction studies have not been conducted with Vancocin HCl. It is not known whether Vancocin HCl can affect reproduction capacity. In a controlled clinical study, the potential ototoxic and nephrotoxic effects of Vancocin HCl on infants were evaluated when the drug was administered to pregnant women for serious staphylococcal infections complicating intravenous drug abuse. Vancocin HCl was found in cord blood. No sensorineural hearing loss or nephrotoxicity attributable to Vancocin HCl was noted. One infant whose mother received Vancocin HCl in the third trimester experienced conductive hearing loss that was not attributed to the administration of Vancocin HCl. Because the number of patients treated in this study was limited and Vancocin HCl was administered only in the second and third trimesters, it is not known whether Vancocin HCl causes fetal harm. Vancocin HCl should be given to a pregnant woman only if clearly needed.

Nursing Mothers—Vancocin HCl is excreted in human milk. Caution should be exercised when Vancocin HCl is administered to a nursing woman. Because of the potential for adverse events, a decision should be made whether to discontinue nursing or to discontinue the drug, taking into account the importance of the drug to the mother.

Usage in Pediatrics —In premature neonates and young infants, it may be appropriate to confirm desired vancomycin serum concentrations. Concomitant administration of vancomycin and anesthetic agents has been associated with erythema and histamine-like flushing in children (*see* ADVERSE REACTIONS).

Geriatrics —The natural decrement of glomerular filtration with increasing age may lead to elevated vancomycin serum concentrations if dosage is not adjusted. Vancomycin dosage schedules should be adjusted in elderly patients (*see* DOSAGE AND ADMINISTRATION).

ADVERSE REACTIONS

Infusion-Related Events —During or soon after rapid infusion of Vancocin HCl, patients may develop anaphylactoid reactions, including hypotension (*see* ANIMAL PHARMACOLOGY), wheezing, dyspnea, urticaria, or pruritus. Rapid infusion may also cause flushing of the upper body ("Red Man Syndrome") or pain and muscle spasm of the chest and back. These reactions usually resolve within 20 minutes but may persist for several hours. Such events are infrequent if Vancocin HCl is given by a slow infusion over 60 minutes. In studies of normal volunteers, infusion-related events did not occur when Vancocin HCl was administered at a rate of 10 mg/min or less.

Nephrotoxicity —Rarely, renal failure, principally manifested by increased serum creatinine or BUN concentrations, especially in patients given large doses of Vancocin HCl, has been reported. Rare cases of interstitial nephritis have been reported. Most of these have occurred in patients who were given aminoglycosides concomitantly or who had preexisting kidney dysfunction. When Vancocin HCl was discontinued, azotemia resolved in most patients.

Gastrointestinal —Onset of pseudomembranous colitis symptoms may occur during or after antibiotic treatment (*see* WARNINGS).

Ototoxicity —A few dozen cases of hearing loss associated with Vancocin HCl have been reported. Most of these patients had kidney dysfunction or a preexisting hearing loss or were receiving concomitant treatment with an ototoxic drug. Vertigo, dizziness, and tinnitus have been reported rarely.

Hematopoietic —Reversible neutropenia, usually starting 1 week or more after onset of therapy with Vancocin HCl or after a total dosage of more than 25 g, has been reported for several dozen patients. Neutropenia appears to be promptly reversible when Vancocin HCl is discontinued. Thrombocytopenia has rarely been reported.

Although a causal relationship has not been established, reversible agranulocytosis (granulocytes $<500/mm^3$) has been reported rarely.

Phlebitis —Inflammation at the injection site has been reported.

Miscellaneous —Infrequently, patients have been reported to have had anaphylaxis, drug fever, nausea, chills, eosinophilia, rashes (including exfoliative dermatitis), Stevens-Johnson syndrome, toxic epidermal necrolysis, and rare cases of vasculitis in association with administration of Vancocin HCl.

Chemical peritonitis has been reported following intraperitoneal administration of vancomycin (*see* PRECAUTIONS).

OVERDOSAGE

Supportive care is advised, with maintenance of glomerular filtration. Vancomycin is poorly removed by dialysis. Hemofiltration and hemoperfusion with polysulfone resin have been reported to result in increased vancomycin clearance. The median lethal intravenous dose is 319 mg/kg in rats and 400 mg/kg in mice.

To obtain up-to-date information about the treatment of overdose, a good resource is your certified Regional Poison Control Center. Telephone numbers of certified poison control centers are listed in the *Physicians' Desk Reference (PDR)*. In managing overdosage, consider the possibility of multiple drug overdoses, interaction among drugs, and unusual drug kinetics in your patient.

DOSAGE AND ADMINISTRATION

Infusion-related events are related to both concentration and rate of administration of vancomycin. Concentrations of no more than 5 mg/mL and rates of no more than 10 mg/min are recommended in adults (see also age-specific recommendations). In selected patients in need of fluid restriction, a concentration up to 10 mg/mL may be used; use of such higher concentrations may increase the risk of infusion-related events. Infusion-related events may occur, however, at any rate or concentration.

Patients With Normal Renal Function

Adults —The usual daily intravenous dose is 2 g divided either as 500 mg every 6 hours or 1 g every 12 hours. Each dose should be administered at no more than 10 mg/min or over a period of at least 60 minutes, whichever is longer. Other patient factors, such as age or obesity, may call for modification of the usual intravenous daily dose.

Children —The usual intravenous dosage of Vancocin HCl is 10 mg/kg per dose given every 6 hours. Each dose should be administered over a period of at least 60 minutes.

Infants and Neonates —In neonates and young infants, the total daily intravenous dosage may be lower. In both neonates and infants, an initial dose of 15 mg/kg is suggested, followed by 10 mg/kg every 12 hours for neonates in the 1st week of life and every 8 hours thereafter up to the age of 1 month. Each dose should be administered over 60 minutes. Close monitoring of serum concentrations of vancomycin may be warranted in these patients.

Patients With Impaired Renal Function and Elderly Patients

Dosage adjustment must be made in patients with impaired renal function. In premature infants and the elderly, greater dosage reductions than expected may be necessary because of decreased renal function. Measurement of vancomycin serum concentrations can be helpful in optimizing therapy, especially in seriously ill patients with changing renal function. Vancomycin serum concentrations can be de-

Continued on next page

*** Identi-Code® symbol. This product information was prepared in June 2000. Current information on these and other products of Eli Lilly and Company may be obtained by direct inquiry to Lilly Research Laboratories, Lilly Corporate Center, Indianapolis, Indiana 46285, (800) 545-5979.**

Vanocin HCl Intravenous—Cont.

termined by use of microbiologic assay, radioimmunoassay, fluorescence polarization immunoassay, fluorescence immunoassay, or high-pressure liquid chromatography.

If creatinine clearance can be measured or estimated accurately, the dosage for most patients with renal impairment can be calculated using the following table. The dosage of Vancocin HCl per day in mg is about 15 times the glomerular filtration rate in mL/min:

DOSAGE TABLE FOR VANCOMYCIN
IN PATIENTS WITH IMPAIRED RENAL FUNCTION
(Adapted from Moellering et al)[4]

Creatinine Clearance mL/min	Vancomycin Dose mg/24 h
100	1,545
90	1,390
80	1,235
70	1,080
60	925
50	770
40	620
30	465
20	310
10	155

The initial dose should be no less than 15 mg/kg, even in patients with mild to moderate renal insufficiency.

The table is not valid for functionally anephric patients. For such patients, an initial dose of 15 mg/kg of body weight should be given to achieve prompt therapeutic serum concentrations. The dose required to maintain stable concentrations is 1.9 mg/kg/24 h. In patients with marked renal impairment, it may be more convenient to give maintenance doses of 250 to 1,000 mg once every several days rather than administering the drug on a daily basis. In anuria, a dose of 1,000 mg every 7 to 10 days has been recommended.

When only the serum creatinine concentration is known, the following formula (based on sex, weight, and age of the patient) may be used to calculate creatinine clearance. Calculated creatinine clearances (mL/min) are only estimates. The creatinine clearance should be measured promptly.

Men: $\dfrac{\text{Weight (kg)} \times (140 - \text{age in years})}{72 \times \text{serum creatinine concentration (mg/dL)}}$

Women: $0.85 \times$ above value

The serum creatinine must represent a steady state of renal function. Otherwise, the estimated value for creatinine clearance is not valid. Such a calculated clearance is an overestimate of actual clearance in patients with conditions: (1) characterized by decreasing renal function, such as shock, severe heart failure, or oliguria; (2) in which a normal relationship between muscle mass and total body weight is not present, such as obese patients or those with liver disease, edema, or ascites; and (3) accompanied by debilitation, malnutrition, or inactivity.

The safety and efficacy of vancomycin administration by the intrathecal (intralumbar or intraventricular) routes have not been assessed.

Intermittent infusion is the recommended method of administration.

PREPARATION AND STABILITY

At the time of use, reconstitute by adding either 10 mL of Sterile Water for Injection to the 500-mg vial or 20 mL of Sterile Water for Injection to the 1-g vial of dry, sterile vancomycin powder. Vials reconstituted in this manner will give a solution of 50 mg/mL. FURTHER DILUTION IS REQUIRED.

After reconstitution with Sterile Water for Injection, 5% Dextrose Injection, or 0.9% Sodium Chloride for Injection, the vials may be stored in a refrigerator for 14 days without significant loss of potency. Reconstituted solutions containing 500 mg of vancomycin must be diluted with at least 100 mL of diluent. Reconstituted solutions containing 1 g of vancomycin must be diluted with at least 200 mL of diluent. The desired dose, diluted in this manner, should be administered by intermittent intravenous infusion over a period of at least 60 minutes.

Compatibility With Intravenous Fluids —Solutions that are diluted with 5% Dextrose Injection or 0.9% Sodium Chloride Injection may be stored in a refrigerator for 14 days without significant loss of potency. Solutions that are diluted with the following infusion fluids may be stored in a refrigerator for 96 hours:

- 5% Dextrose Injection and 0.9% Sodium Chloride Injection, USP
- Lactated Ringer's Injection, USP
- Lactated Ringer's and 5% Dextrose Injection, USP
- Normosol®-M* and 5% Dextrose
- Isolyte® E**
- Acetated Ringer's Injection

Vancomycin solution has a low pH and may cause chemical or physical instability when it is mixed with other compounds.

Prior to administration, parenteral drug products should be inspected visually for particulate matter and discoloration whenever solution or container permits.

For Oral Administration —Oral Vancocin HCl is used in treating antibiotic-associated pseudomembranous colitis caused by *C. difficile* and for staphylococcal enterocolitis. Vancocin HCl is not effective by the oral route for other types of infections. The usual adult total daily dosage is 500 mg to 2 g given in 3 or 4 divided doses for 7 to 10 days. The total daily dosage in children is 40 mg/kg of body weight in 3 or 4 divided doses for 7 to 10 days. The total daily dosage should not exceed 2 g. The appropriate dose may be diluted in 1 oz of water and given to the patient to drink. Common flavoring syrups may be added to the solution to improve the taste for oral administration. The diluted solution may be administered via a nasogastric tube.

*Normosol®-M, Abbott Hospital Products (Division of Abbott Laboratories)
**Isolyte® E, McGaw, Inc.

HOW SUPPLIED

Vancocin® HCl Vials (or Sterile Vancomycin Hydrochloride, USP) are available in:

The 500 mg,* 10-mL vials are available as follows:
10-mL vials NDC 0002-1444-01 (VL 657)
Traypak† of 25 NDC 0002-1444-25 (VL 657)

The 1 g,* 20-mL vials are available as follows:
Traypak of 25 NDC 0002-7321-25 (VL 7321)

Also available:

Vancocin-HCl ADD-Vantage‡ Vials (or Sterile Vancomycin Hydrochloride, USP) are available in:

The 500 mg,* 15-mL vials are available as follows:
Traypak of 10 NDC 0002-7297-10 (VL 7297)

The 1 g,* 15-mL vials are available as follows:
Traypak of 10 NDC 0002-7298-10 (VL 7298)

Vancocin HCl Pharmacy Bulk Package (or Vancomycin Hydrochloride for Injection, USP) are available in:

The 10 g,* 100-mL vials are available as follows:
100-mL vial NDC 0002-7355-01 (VL 7355)

Prior to reconstitution, the vials may be stored at room temperature, 59° to 86°F (15° to 30°C).

*Equivalent to vancomycin.
†Traypak™ (multivial carton, Lilly).
‡ADD-Vantage® (vials and diluent containers, Abbott).

CAUTION—Federal (USA) law prohibits dispensing without prescription.

ANIMAL PHARMACOLOGY

In animal studies, hypotension and bradycardia occurred in dogs receiving an intravenous infusion of vancomycin hydrochloride, 25 mg/kg, at a concentration of 25 mg/mL and an infusion rate of 13.3 mL/min.

REFERENCES

1. National Committee for Clinical Laboratory Standards. Performance Standards for Antimicrobial Disk Susceptibility Tests–Fifth Edition. Approved Standard NCCLS Document M2-A5, Vol. 13, No. 24, NCCLS, Villanova, PA, December, 1993.
2. National Committee for Clinical Laboratory Standards. Methods for Dilution Antimicrobial Susceptibility Tests for Bacteria that Grow Aerobically–Third Edition. Approved Standard NCCLS Document M7-A3, Vol. 13, No. 25, NCCLS, Villanova, PA, December, 1993.
3. Dajani, Adnan S, et al: Prevention of bacterial endocarditis. Recommendations by the American Heart Association. *JAMA* 264 (22):2919–2922, December 12, 1990.
4. Moellering RC, Krogstad DJ, Greenblatt DJ: Vancomycin therapy in patients with impaired renal function: A nomogram for dosage. *Ann Intern Med* 1981;94:343.

Literature revised June 17, 1997
PA 7897 AMP [061797]

VANCOCIN® HCl ℞

[*văn 'kō-sĭn ăch 'sē-ĕl*]
(vancomycin hydrochloride)
For Oral Solution, USP

This preparation for the treatment of colitis is for oral use only and is not systemically absorbed. Vancocin® HCl must be given orally for treatment of staphylococcal enterocolitis and antibiotic-associated pseudomembranous colitis caused by *Clostridium difficile.* Orally administered Vancocin HCl is *not* effective for other types of infection.

Parenteral administration of Vancocin HCl is not effective for treatment of staphylococcal enterocolitis and antibiotic-associated pseudomembranous colitis caused by *C. difficile.* If parenteral vancomycin therapy is desired, use Vancocin® HCl (Sterile Vancomycin Hydrochloride, USP), IntraVenous, and consult package insert accompanying that preparation.

DESCRIPTION

Vancocin® HCl for Oral Solution (Vancomycin Hydrochloride for Oral Solution, USP), contains chromatographically purified vancomycin hydrochloride, a tricyclic glycopeptide antibiotic derived from *Amycolatopsis orientalis* (formerly *Nocardia orientalis*), which has the chemical formula $C_{66}H_{75}Cl_2N_9O_{24} \cdot HCl$. The molecular weight of vancomycin hydrochloride is 1,485.73; 500 mg of the base is equivalent to 0.34 mmol.

Vancocin HCl for Oral Solution contains vancomycin hydrochloride equivalent to 10 g (6.7 mmol) or 1 g (0.67 mmol) vancomycin. Calcium disodium edetate, equivalent to 0.2 mg edetate per gram of vancomycin, is added at the time of manufacture. The 10-g bottle may contain up to 40 mg of ethanol per gram of vancomycin.

Vancomycin hydrochloride has the following structure:

CLINICAL PHARMACOLOGY

Vancomycin is poorly absorbed after oral administration. During multiple dosing of 250 mg every 8 hours for 7 doses, fecal concentrations of vancomycin in volunteers exceeded 100 mg/kg in the majority of samples. No blood concentrations were detected and urinary recovery did not exceed 0.76%. In anephric patients with no inflammatory bowel disease, blood concentrations of vancomycin were barely measurable (0.66 μg/mL) in 2 of 5 subjects who received 2 g of Vancocin HCl for Oral Solution daily for 16 days. No measurable blood concentrations were attained in the other 3 patients. With doses of 2 g daily, very high concentrations of drug can be found in the feces (>3,100 mg/kg) and very low concentrations (<1 μg/mL) can be found in the serum of patients with normal renal function who have pseudomembranous colitis. Orally administered vancomycin does not usually enter the systemic circulation even when inflammatory lesions are present. After multiple-dose oral administration of vancomycin, measurable serum concentrations may infrequently occur in patients with active *C. difficile*-induced pseudomembranous colitis, and, in the presence of renal impairment, the possibility of accumulation exists.

Microbiology —The bactericidal action of vancomycin results primarily from inhibition of cell-wall biosynthesis. In addition, vancomycin alters bacterial-cell-membrane permeability and RNA synthesis. There is no cross-resistance between vancomycin and other antibiotics. Vancomycin is active against *C. difficile* (eg, toxigenic strains implicated in pseudomembranous enterocolitis). It is also active against staphylococci, including *Staphylococcus aureus.*

For further information, see prescribing information for Vancocin HCl, IntraVenous.

Vancomycin is not active in vitro against gram-negative bacilli, mycobacteria, or fungi.

Disk Susceptibility Tests —The standardized disk and/or dilution methods described by the National Committee for Clinical Laboratory Standards have been recommended to test susceptibility to vancomycin.

INDICATIONS AND USAGE

Vancocin HCl for Oral Solution is administered orally for treatment of staphylococcal enterocolitis and antiobiotic-associated pseudomembranous colitis caused by *C. difficile.* Parenteral administration of Vancocin HCl is not effective for the above indications; therefore, Vancocin HCl must be given orally for these indications. **Orally administered Vancocin HCl is not effective for other types of infection.**

CONTRAINDICATION

Vancocin HCl is contraindicated in patients with known hypersensitivity to this antibiotic.

PRECAUTIONS

General —Clinically significant serum concentrations have been reported in some patients who have taken multiple oral doses of vancomycin for active *C. difficile*-induced pseudomembranous colitis; therefore, monitoring of serum concentrations may be appropriate.

Some patients with inflammatory disorders of the intestinal mucosa may have significant systemic absorption of vancomycin and, therefore, may be at risk for the development of adverse reactions associated with the parenteral administration of vancomycin (See package insert accompanying the intravenous preparation.) The risk is greater if renal impairment is present. It should be noted that the total systemic and renal clearances of vancomycin are reduced in the elderly.

Ototoxicity has occurred in patients receiving Vancocin HCl. It may be transient or permanent. It has been reported mostly in patients who have been given excessive intravenous doses, who have an underlying hearing loss, or who are receiving concomitant therapy with another ototoxic agent, such as an aminoglycoside. Serial tests of auditory function may be helpful in order to minimize the risk of ototoxicity.

When patients with underlying renal dysfunction or those receiving concomitant therapy with an aminoglycoside are being treated, serial monitoring of renal function should be performed.

Usage in Pregnancy —*Pregnancy Category C* —Animal reproduction studies have not been conducted with Vancocin HCl. It is not known whether Vancocin HCl can affect reproduction capacity. In a controlled clinical study, the potential ototoxic and nephrotoxic effects of Vancocin HCl on infants were evaluated when the drug was administered intravenously to pregnant women for serious staphylococcal infections complicating intravenous drug abuse. Vancocin HCl was found in cord blood. No sensorineural hearing loss or nephrotoxicity attributable to Vancocin HCl was noted. One infant whose mother received Vancocin HCl in the third trimester experienced conductive hearing loss that was not attributed to the administration of Vancocin HCl. Because the number of patients treated in this study was limited and Vancocin HCl was administered only in the second and third trimesters, it is not known whether Vancocin HCl causes fetal harm. Vancocin HCl should be given to a pregnant woman only if clearly needed.

Nursing Mothers —Vancocin HCl is excreted in human milk based on information obtained with the intravenous administration of Vancocin HCl. Blood concentrations achieved with oral administration are very low (*see* CLINICAL PHARMACOLOGY). Caution should be exercised when Vancocin HCl is administered to a nursing woman. Because of the potential for adverse events, a decision should be made whether to discontinue nursing or discontinue the drug, taking into account the importance of the drug to the mother.

ADVERSE REACTIONS

Nephrotoxicity —Rarely, renal failure, principally manifested by increased serum creatinine or BUN concentrations, especially in patients given large doses of intravenously administered Vancocin HCl, has been reported. Rare cases of interstitial nephritis have been reported. Most of these have occurred in patients who were given aminoglycosides concomitantly or who had preexisting kidney dysfunction. When Vancocin HCl was discontinued, azotemia resolved in most patients.

Ototoxicity —A few dozen cases of hearing loss associated with intravenously administered Vancocin HCl have been reported. Most of these patients had kidney dysfunction or a preexisting hearing loss or were receiving concomitant treatment with an ototoxic drug. Vertigo, dizziness, and tinnitus have been reported rarely.

Hematopoietic —Reversible neutropenia, usually starting 1 week or more after onset of intravenous therapy with Vancocin HCl or after a total dosage of more than 25 g, has been reported for several dozen patients. Neutropenia appears to be promptly reversible when Vancocin HCl is discontinued. Thrombocytopenia has rarely been reported.

Miscellaneous —Infrequently, patients have been reported to have had anaphylaxis, drug fever, chills, nausea, eosinophilia, rashes (including exfoliative dermatitis), Stevens-Johnson syndrome, toxic epidermal necrolysis, and rare cases of vasculitis in association with the administration of Vancocin HCl.

A condition has been reported that is similar to the IV-induced syndrome with symptoms consistent with anaphylactoid reactions, including hypotension, wheezing, dyspnea, urticaria, pruritus, flushing of the upper body ("Red Man Syndrome"), pain and muscle spasm of the chest and back. These reactions usually resolve within 20 minutes but may persist for several hours.

OVERDOSAGE

Supportive care is advised, with maintenance of glomerular filtration. Vancomycin is poorly removed by dialysis. Hemofiltration and hemoperfusion with polysulfone resin have been reported to result in increased vancomycin clearance.

Treatment —To obtain up-to-date information about the treatment of overdose, a good resource is your certified Regional Poison Control Center. Telephone numbers of certified poison control centers are listed in the *Physicians' Desk Reference (PDR)*. In managing overdosage, consider the possibility of multiple drug overdoses, interaction among drugs, and unusual drug kinetics in your patient.

DOSAGE AND ADMINISTRATION

Adults —Oral Vancocin HCl is used in treating antibiotic-associated pseudomembranous colitis caused by *C. difficile* and staphylococcal enterocolitis. Vancocin HCl is not effective by the oral route for other types of infections. The usual adult total daily dosage is 500 mg to 2 g administered orally in 3 or 4 divided doses for 7 to 10 days.

Pediatric Patients —The usual daily dosage is 40 mg/kg in 3 or 4 divided doses for 7 to 10 days. The total daily dosage should not exceed 2 g.

PREPARATION AND STABILITY

The contents of the 10-g bottle may be mixed with distilled or deionized water (115 mL) for oral administration. When mixed with 115 mL of water, each 6 mL provides approximately 500 mg of vancomycin. The contents of the 1-g bottle may be mixed with distilled or deionized water (20 mL). When reconstituted with 20 mL, each 5 mL contains approximately 250 mg of vancomycin. Mix thoroughly to dissolve. These mixtures may be kept for 2 weeks in a refrigerator without significant loss of potency.

The appropriate oral solution dose may be diluted in 1 oz of water and given to the patient to drink. Common flavoring syrups may be added to the solution to improve the taste for oral administration. The diluted material may be administered via nasogastric tube.

HOW SUPPLIED

Vancocin® HCl For Oral Solution (or Vancomycin Hydrochloride for Oral Solution, USP) is available in:

10-g* Bottle NDC 0002-2372-37 (M-206)
1 g* Bottle Traypak† of 6 NDC 0002-5105-16 (M-5105)

Prior to reconstitution, store at controlled room temperature, 59° to 86°F (15° to 30°C).

Also available:

Vancocin HCl Pulvules® (or Vancomycin Hydrochloride Capsules, USP) are available in:

The 125 mg* Pulvules have an opaque blue cap and opaque brown body imprinted with "3125" on the cap and "VANCOCIN HCL 125 MG" on the body in white ink. They are available in:

ID‡20 NDC 0002-3125-42 (PU3125)

The 250 mg* Pulvules have an opaque blue cap and opaque lavender body imprinted with "3126" on the cap and "VANCOCIN HCL 250 MG" on the body in white ink. They are available in:

ID20 NDC 0002-3126-42 (PU3126)

*Equivalent to vancomycin.
†Traypak™ (multivial carton, Lilly).
‡Identi-Dose® (unit dose medication, Lilly).
Literature revised December 21, 1998
PA 0550 AMP [122198]

VANCOCIN® HCl ℞

[văn 'kō-sĭn ăch 'sē-ĕl]
(vancomycin hydrochloride)
Capsules, USP
Pulvules®

This preparation for the treatment of colitis is for oral use only and is not systemically absorbed. Vancocin® HCl must be given orally for treatment of staphylococcal enterocolitis and antibiotic-associated pseudomembranous colitis caused by *Clostridium difficile*. Orally administered Vancocin HCl is *not* effective for other types of infection.

Parenteral administration of Vancocin HCl is not effective for treatment of staphylococcal enterocolitis and antibiotic-associated pseudomembranous colitis caused by *C. difficile*. If parenteral vancomycin therapy is desired, use Vancocin® HCl (Sterile Vancomycin Hydrochloride, USP), IntraVenous, and consult package insert accompanying that preparation.

DESCRIPTION

Pulvules® Vancocin® HCl (Vancomycin Hydrochloride Capsules, USP) contain chromatographically purified vancomycin hydrochloride, a tricyclic glycopeptide antibiotic derived from *Amycolatopsis orientalis* (formerly *Nocardia orientalis*), which has the chemical formula $C_{66}H_{75}Cl_2N_9O_{24}$ • HCl. The molecular weight of vancomycin hydrochloride is 1,485.73; 500 mg of the base is equivalent to 0.34 mmol.

The Pulvules contain vancomycin hydrochloride equivalent to 125 mg (0.08 mmol) or 250 mg (0.17 mmol) vancomycin. The Pulvules also contain F D & C Blue No. 2, gelatin, iron oxide, polyethylene glycol, titanium dioxide, and other inactive ingredients.

Vancomycin hydrochloride has the following structural formula:

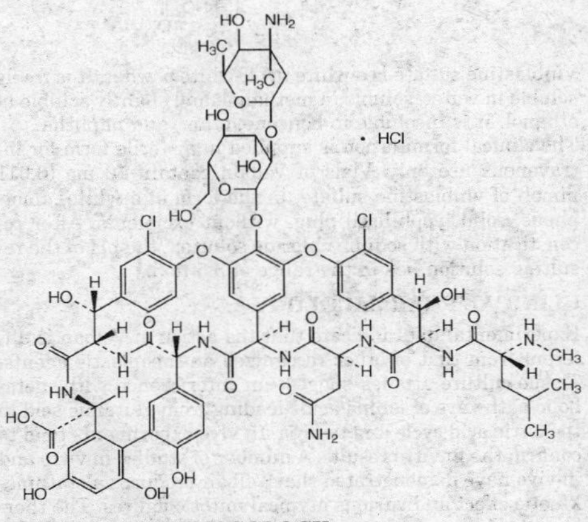

CLINICAL PHARMACOLOGY

Vancomycin is poorly absorbed after oral administration. During multiple dosing of 250 mg every 8 hours for 7 doses, fecal concentrations of vancomycin in volunteers exceeded 100 mg/kg in the majority of samples. No blood concentrations were detected and urinary recovery did not exceed 0.76%. Additional data using the oral solution dosage form follow. In anephric patients with no inflammatory bowel disease, blood concentrations of vancomycin were barely measurable (0.66 μg/mL) in 2 of 5 subjects who received 2 g of Vancocin HCl for Oral Solution daily for 16 days. No measurable blood concentrations were attained in the other 3 patients. With doses of 2 g daily, very high concentrations of drug can be found in the feces (>3,100 mg/kg) and very low concentrations (<1 μg/mL) can be found in the serum of patients with normal renal function who have pseudomembranous colitis. Orally administered vancomycin does not usually enter the systemic circulation even when inflammatory lesions are present. After multiple-dose oral administration of vancomycin, measurable serum concentrations may infrequently occur in patients with active *C. difficile*-induced pseudomembranous colitis, and, in the presence of renal impairment, the possibility of accumulation exists.

Microbiology—The bactericidal action of vancomycin results primarily from inhibition of cell-wall biosynthesis. In addition, vancomycin alters bacterial-cell-membrane permeability and RNA synthesis. There is no cross-resistance between vancomycin and other antibiotics. Vancomycin is active against *C. difficile* (eg, toxigenic strains implicated in pseudomembranous enterocolitis). It is also active against staphylococci, including *Staphylococcus aureus*.

For further information, see prescribing information for Vancocin HCl, IntraVenous.

Vancomycin is not active in vitro against gram-negative bacilli, mycobacteria, or fungi.

Disk Susceptibility Tests—The standardized disk and/or dilution methods described by the National Committee for Clinical Laboratory Standards have been recommended to test susceptibility to vancomycin.

INDICATIONS AND USAGE

Pulvules Vancocin HCl may be administered orally for treatment of staphylococcal enterocolitis and antibiotic-associated pseudomembranous colitis caused by *C. difficile*. Parenteral administration of Vancocin HCl is not effective for the above indications; therefore, Vancocin HCl must be given orally for these indications. **Orally administered Vancocin HCl is not effective for other types of infection.**

CONTRAINDICATION

Vancocin HCl is contraindicated in patients with known hypersensitivity to this antibiotic.

PRECAUTIONS

General—Clinically significant serum concentrations have been reported in some patients who have taken multiple oral doses of vancomycin for active *C. difficile*-induced pseudomembranous colitis; therefore, monitoring of serum concentrations may be appropriate in some instances, eg, in patients with renal insufficiency and/or colitis.

Some patients with inflammatory disorders of the intestinal mucosa may have significant systemic absorption of vancomycin and, therefore, may be at risk for the development of adverse reactions associated with the parenteral administration of vancomycin. (See package insert accompanying the intravenous preparation.) The risk is greater if renal impairment is present. It should be noted that the total systemic and renal clearances of vancomycin are reduced in the elderly.

Ototoxicity has occurred in patients receiving Vancocin HCl. It may be transient or permanent. It has been reported mostly in patients who have been given excessive intravenous doses, who have an underlying hearing loss, or who are receiving concomitant therapy with another ototoxic agent, such as an aminoglycoside. Serial tests of auditory function may be helpful in order to minimize the risk of ototoxicity.

When patients with underlying renal dysfunction or those receiving concomitant therapy with an aminoglycoside are being treated, serial monitoring of renal function should be performed.

Carcinogenesis, Mutagenesis, Impairment of Fertility—No long-term carcinogenesis studies in animals have been conducted.

At concentrations up to 1,000 μg/mL, vancomycin had no mutagenic effect *in vitro* in the mouse lymphoma forward mutation assay or the primary rat hepatocyte unscheduled DNA synthesis assay. The concentrations tested *in vitro* were above the peak plasma vancomycin concentrations of 20 to 40 μg/mL usually achieved in humans after slow infusion of the maximum recommended dose of 1 g. Vancomycin had no mutagenic effect *in vivo* in the Chinese hamster sister chromatid exchange assay (400 mg/kg IP) or the mouse micronucleus assay (800 mg/kg IP).

No definitive fertility studies have been conducted.

Pregnancy—Teratogenic Effects—Pregnancy Category B—The highest doses of vancomycin tested were not teratogenic in rats given up to 200 mg/kg/day IV (1,180 mg/m^2 or 1 times the recommended maximum human dose based on a mg/m^2 basis) or in rabbits given up to 120 mg/kg/day IV (1,320 mg/m^2 or 1.1 times the recommended maximum human dose based on a mg/m^2 basis). No effects on fetal weight or development were seen in rats at the highest dose tested or in rabbits given 80 mg/kg/day (880 mg/m^2 or 0.74 times the recommended maximum human dose based on mg/m^2).

In a controlled clinical study, the potential ototoxic and nephrotoxic effects of Vancocin HCl on infants were evaluated when the drug was administered intravenously to pregnant women for serious staphylococcal infections complicating intravenous drug abuse. Vancocin HCl was found in cord blood. No sensorineural hearing loss or nephrotoxicity attributable to Vancocin HCl was noted. One infant whose mother received Vancocin HCl in the third trimester experienced conductive hearing loss that was not attributed to the administration of Vancocin HCl. Because the number of patients treated in this study was limited and Vancocin HCl was administered only in the second and third trimesters, it is not known whether Vancocin HCl causes fetal

Continued on next page

*** Identi-Code® symbol. This product information was prepared in June 2000. Current information on these and other products of Eli Lilly and Company may be obtained by direct inquiry to Lilly Research Laboratories, Lilly Corporate Center, Indianapolis, Indiana 46285, (800) 545-5979.**

Vancocin HCl Caps/Pulvules—Cont.

harm. Because animal reproduction studies are not always predictive of human response, Vancocin HCl should be given to a pregnant woman only if clearly needed.
Nursing Mothers—Vancocin HCl is excreted in human milk based on information obtained with the intravenous administration of Vancocin HCl. Blood concentrations achieved with oral administration are very low (*see* CLINICAL PHARMACOLOGY). It is not known whether oral vancomycin is excreted in human milk, as no studies of vancomycin concentration in human milk after oral administration have been done. Caution should be exercised when Vancocin HCl is administered to a nursing woman. Because of the potential for adverse events, a decision should be made whether to discontinue nursing or discontinue the drug, taking into account the importance of the drug to the mother.
Pediatric Use—Safety and effectiveness in pediatric patients have not been established.

ADVERSE REACTIONS

Nephrotoxicity—Rarely, renal failure, principally manifested by increased serum creatinine or BUN concentrations, especially in patients given large doses of intravenously administered Vancocin HCl has been reported. Rare cases of interstitial nephritis have been reported. Most of these have occurred in patients who were given aminoglycosides concomitantly or who had preexisting kidney dysfunction. When Vancocin HCl was discontinued, azotemia resolved in most patients.
Ototoxicity—A few dozen cases of hearing loss associated with intravenously administered Vancocin HCl have been reported. Most of these patients had kidney dysfunction or a preexisting hearing loss or were receiving concomitant treatment with an ototoxic drug. Vertigo, dizziness, and tinnitus have been reported rarely.
Hematopoietic—Reversible neutropenia, usually starting 1 week or more after onset of intravenous therapy with Vancocin HCl or after a total dose of more than 25 g, has been reported for several dozen patients. Neutropenia appears to be promptly reversible when Vancocin HCl is discontinued. Thrombocytopenia has rarely been reported.
Miscellaneous—Infrequently, patients have been reported to have had anaphylaxis, drug fever, chills, nausea, eosinophilia, rashes (including exfoliative dermatitis), Stevens-Johnson syndrome, toxic epidermal necrolysis, and rare cases of vasculitis in association with the administration of Vancocin HCl.
A condition has been reported that is similar to the IV-induced syndrome with symptoms consistent with anaphylactoid reactions, including hypotension, wheezing, dyspnea, urticaria, pruritus, flushing of the upper body ("Red Man Syndrome"), pain and muscle spasm of the chest and back. These reactions usually resolve within 20 minutes but may persist for several hours.

OVERDOSAGE

Supportive care is advised, with maintenance of glomerular filtration. Vancomycin is poorly removed by dialysis. Hemofiltration and hemoperfusion with polysulfone resin have been reported to result in increased vancomycin clearance.
Treatment—To obtain up-to-date information about the treatment of overdose, a good resource is your certified Regional Poison Control Center. Telephone numbers of certified poison control centers are listed in the *Physicians' Desk Reference (PDR)*. In managing overdosage, consider the possibility of multiple drug overdoses, interaction among drugs, and unusual drug kinetics in your patient.

DOSAGE AND ADMINISTRATION

Adults—Oral Vancocin HCl is used in treating antibiotic-associated pseudomembranous colitis caused by *C. difficile* and staphylococcal enterocolitis. Vancocin HCl is not effective by the oral route for other types of infections. The usual adult total daily dosage is 500 mg to 2 g administered orally in 3 or 4 divided doses for 7 to 10 days.
Pediatric Patients—The usual daily dosage is 40 mg/kg in 3 or 4 divided doses for 7 to 10 days. The total daily dosage should not exceed 2 g.

HOW SUPPLIED

Vancocin® HCl Pulvules® (or Vancomycin Hydrochloride Capsules, USP) are available in:
The 125 mg* Pulvules have an opaque blue cap and opaque brown body imprinted with "3125" on the cap and "VANCOCIN HCL 125 MG" on the body in white ink. They are available in:
ID†20 NDC 0002-3125-42 (PU3125)
The 250 mg* Pulvules have an opaque blue cap and opaque lavender body imprinted with "3126" on the cap and "VANCOCIN HCL 250 MG" on the body in white ink. They are available in:
ID†20 NDC 0002-3126-42 (PU3126)
Also Available:
Vancocin HCl For Oral Solution (or Vancomycin Hydrochloride for Oral Solution, USP) is available in:
10-g* Bottle NDC 0002-2372-37 (M-206)
1-g* Bottle Traypak‡ of 6 NDC 0002-5105-16 (M-5105)
Store at controlled room temperature, 59° to 86°F (15° to 30°C).

*Equivalent to vancomycin.
†Identi-Dose® (unit dose medication, Lilly).
‡Traypak™ (multivial carton, Lilly).
Literature revised December 21, 1998
PV 1982 AMP [122198]

VANCOMYCIN HYDROCHLORIDE ℞

See Vancocin® HCl (Vancomycin Hydrochloride, USP).

VELBAN® ℞

[*vĕl 'băn*]
(vinblastine sulfate for injection, USP)

WARNINGS

Caution—This preparation should be administered by individuals experienced in the administration of Velban. It is extremely important that the intravenous needle or catheter be properly positioned before any Velban is injected. Leakage into surrounding tissue during intravenous administration of Velban may cause considerable irritation. If extravasation occurs, the injection should be discontinued immediately, and any remaining portion of the dose should then be introduced into another vein. Local injection of hyaluronidase and the application of moderate heat to the area of leakage help disperse the drug and are thought to minimize discomfort and the possibility of cellulitis.
FATAL IF GIVEN INTRATHECALLY. FOR INTRAVENOUS USE ONLY. *See Warnings section for the treatment of patients given intrathecal Velban.*

DESCRIPTION

Velban® (Vinblastine Sulfate for Injection, USP) is vincaleukoblastine, sulfate (1:1) (salt). It is the salt of an alkaloid extracted from *Vinca rosea* Linn, a common flowering herb known as the periwinkle (more properly known as *Catharanthus roseus* G. Don). Previously, the generic name was vincaleukoblastine, abbreviated VLB. It is a stathmokinetic oncolytic agent. When treated in vitro with this preparation, growing cells are arrested in metaphase.
Chemical and physical evidence indicate that Velban has the empirical formula $C_{46}H_{58}N_4O_9 \cdot H_2SO_4$ and that it is a dimeric alkaloid containing both indole and dihydroindole moieties. It has a molecular weight of 909.07. The structural formula is as follows:

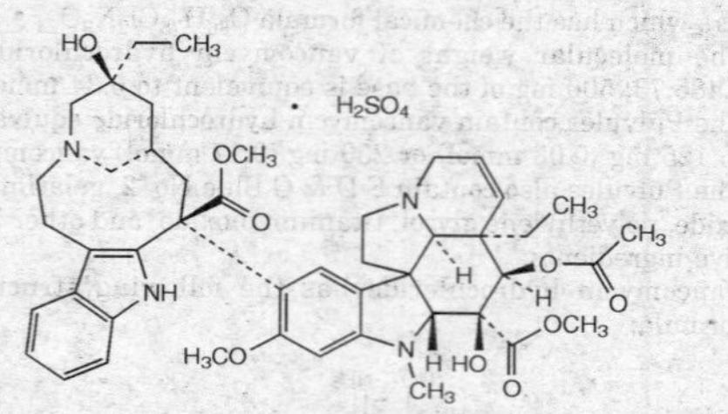

Vinblastine sulfate is a white to off-white powder. It is freely soluble in water, soluble in methanol, and slightly soluble in ethanol. It is insoluble in benzene, ether, and naphtha.
The clinical formulation is supplied in a sterile form for intravenous use only. Vials of Velban contain 10 mg (0.011 mmol) of vinblastine sulfate, in the form of a white, amorphous, solid lyophilized plug, without excipients. After reconstitution with sodium chloride solution, the pH of the resulting solution lies in the range of 3.5 to 5.

CLINICAL PHARMACOLOGY

Experimental data indicate that the action of Velban is different from that of other recognized antineoplastic agents. Tissue-culture studies suggest an interference with metabolic pathways of amino acids leading from glutamic acid to the citric acid cycle and to urea. In vivo experiments tend to confirm the in vitro results. A number of studies in vitro and in vivo have demonstrated that Velban produces a stathmokinetic effect and various atypical mitotic figures. The therapeutic responses, however, are not fully explained by the cytologic changes, since these changes are sometimes observed clinically and experimentally in the absence of any oncolytic effects.
Reversal of the antitumor effect of Velban by glutamic acid or tryptophan has been observed. In addition, glutamic acid and aspartic acid have protected mice from lethal doses of Velban. Aspartic acid was relatively ineffective in reversing the antitumor effect.
Other studies indicate that Velban has an effect on cell-energy production required for mitosis and interferes with nucleic acid synthesis. The mechanism of action of Velban has been related to the inhibition of microtubule formation in the mitotic spindle, resulting in an arrest of dividing cells at the metaphase stage.
Pharmacokinetic studies in patients with cancer have shown a triphasic serum decay pattern following rapid intravenous injection. The initial, middle, and terminal half-lives are 3.7 minutes, 1.6 hours, and 24.8 hours respectively. The volume of the central compartment is 70% of body weight, probably reflecting very rapid tissue binding to formed elements of the blood. Extensive reversible tissue binding occurs. Low body stores are present at 48 and 72 hours after injection. Since the major route of excretion may be through the biliary system, toxicity from this drug may be increased when there is hepatic excretory insufficiency. The metabolism of vinca alkaloids has been shown to be mediated by hepatic cytochrome P450 isoenzymes in the CYP 3A subfamily. This metabolic pathway may be impaired in patients with hepatic dysfunction or who are taking concomitant potent inhibitors of these isoenzymes such as erythromicin. Enhanced toxicity has been reported in patients receiving concomitant erythromycin (See PRECAUTIONS). Following injection of tritiated vinblastine in the human cancer patient, 10% of the radioactivity was found in the feces and 14% in the urine; the remaining activity was not accounted for. Similar studies in dogs demonstrated that, over 9 days, 30% to 36% of radioactivity was found in the bile and 12% to 17% in the urine. A similar study in the rat demonstrated that the highest concentrations of radioactivity were found in the lung, liver, spleen, and kidney 2 hours after injection.
Hematologic Effects—Clinically, leukopenia is an expected effect of Velban, and the level of the leukocyte count is an important guide to therapy with this drug. In general, the larger the dose employed, the more profound and longer lasting the leukopenia will be. The fact that the white-blood-cell count returns to normal levels after drug-induced leukopenia is an indication that the white-cell-producing mechanism is not permanently depressed. Usually, the white count has completely returned to normal after the virtual disappearance of white cells from the peripheral blood. Following therapy with Velban, the nadir in white-blood-cell count may be expected to occur 5 to 10 days after the last day of drug administration. Recovery of the white blood count is fairly rapid thereafter and is usually complete within another 7 to 14 days. With the smaller doses employed for maintenance therapy, leukopenia may not be a problem.
Although the thrombocyte count ordinarily is not significantly lowered by therapy with Velban, patients whose bone marrow has been recently impaired by prior therapy with radiation or with other oncolytic drugs may show thrombocytopenia (less than 200,000 platelets/mm^3). When other chemotherapy or radiation has not been employed previously, thrombocyte reduction below the level of 200,000/mm^3 is rarely encountered, even when Velban may be causing significant leukopenia. Rapid recovery from thrombocytopenia within a few days is the rule.
The effect of Velban upon the red-cell count and hemoglobin is usually insignificant when other therapy does not complicate the picture. It should be remembered, however, that patients with malignant disease may exhibit anemia even in the absence of any therapy.

INDICATIONS AND USAGE

Velban is indicated in the palliative treatment of the following:

I. Frequently Responsive Malignancies—
- Generalized Hodgkin's disease (Stages III and IV, Ann Arbor modification of Rye staging system)
- Lymphocytic lymphoma (nodular and diffuse, poorly and well differentiated)
- Histiocytic lymphoma
- Mycosis fungoides (advanced stages)
- Advanced carcinoma of the testis
- Kaposi's sarcoma
- Letterer-Siwe disease (histiocytosis X)

II. Less Frequently Responsive Malignancies—
- Choriocarcinoma resistant to other chemotherapeutic agents
- Carcinoma of the breast, unresponsive to appropriate endocrine surgery and hormonal therapy

Current principles of chemotherapy for many types of cancer include the concurrent administration of several antineoplastic agents. For enhanced therapeutic effect without additive toxicity, agents with different dose-limiting clinical toxicities and different mechanisms of action are generally selected. Therefore, although Velban is effective as a single agent in the aforementioned indications, it is usually administered in combination with other antineoplastic drugs. Such combination therapy produces a greater percentage of response than does a single-agent regimen. These principles have been applied, for example, in the chemotherapy of Hodgkin's disease.
Hodgkin's Disease—Velban has been shown to be one of the most effective single agents for the treatment of Hodgkin's disease. Advanced Hodgkin's disease has also been successfully treated with several multiple-drug regimens that included Velban. Patients who had relapses after treatment with the MOPP program—mechlorethamine hydrochloride (nitrogen mustard), vincristine sulfate (Oncovin [Vincristine Sulfate Injection]), prednisone, and procarbazine—have likewise responded to combination-drug therapy that included Velban. A protocol using cyclophosphamide in place of nitrogen mustard and Velban instead of Oncovin is an alternative therapy for previously untreated patients with advanced Hodgkin's disease.
Advanced testicular germinal-cell cancers (embryonal carcinoma, teratocarcinoma, and choriocarcinoma) are sensitive to Velban alone, but better clinical results are achieved when Velban is administered concomitantly with other antineoplastic agents. The effect of bleomycin is significantly enhanced if Velban is administered 6 to 8 hours prior to the administration of bleomycin; this schedule permits more cells to be arrested during metaphase, the stage of the cell cycle in which bleomycin is active.

CONTRAINDICATIONS

Velban is contraindicated in patients who have significant granulocytopenia unless this is a result of the disease being treated. It should not be used in the presence of bacterial infections. Such infections must be brought under control prior to the initiation of therapy with Velban.

WARNINGS

This preparation is for intravenous use only. It should be administered by individuals experienced in the administration of Velban. The intrathecal administration of Velban usually results in death. Syringes containing this product should be labeled using the auxiliary sticker provided, to state "FATAL IF GIVEN INTRATHECALLY. FOR INTRAVENOUS USE ONLY.

Extemporaneously prepared syringes containing this product must be packaged in an overwrap that is labeled "DO NOT REMOVE COVERING UNTIL MOMENT OF INJECTION. FATAL IF GIVEN INTRATHECALLY. FOR INTRAVENOUS USE ONLY."

After inadvertent intrathecal administration of vinca alkaloids, immediate neurosurgical intervention is required in order to prevent ascending paralysis leading to death. In a very small number of patients, life-threatening paralysis and subsequent death was averted but resulted in devastating neurological sequelae, with limited recovery afterwards.

There are no published cases of survival following intrathecal administration of Velban to base treatment on. However, based on the published management of survival cases involving the related vinca alkaloid vincristine sulfate[1-3], if Velban is mistakenly given by the intrathecal route, the following treatment should be initiated **immediately after the injection:**

1. Removal of as much CSF as is safely possible through the lumbar access.
2. Insertion of an epidural catheter into the subarachnoid space via the intervertebral space above initial lumbar access and CSF irrigation with lactated Ringer's solution. Fresh frozen plasma should be requested and, when available, 25 mL should be added to every 1 liter of lactated Ringer's solution.
3. Insertion of an intraventricular drain or catheter by a neurosurgeon and continuation of CSF irrigation with fluid removal through the lumbar access connected to a closed drainage system. Lactated Ringer's solution should be given by continuous infusion at 150 mL/hour, or at a rate of 75 mL/hour when fresh frozen plasma has been added as above.

The rate of infusion should be adjusted to maintain a spinal fluid protein level of 150 mg/dL.

The following measures have also been used in addition but may not be essential:

Glutamic acid, 10 grams, has been given intravenously over 24 hours, followed by 500 mg three times daily by mouth for 1 month. Folinic acid has been administered intravenously as a 100 mg bolus and then infused at a rate of 25 mg/hour for 24 hours, then bolus doses of 25 mg every 6 hours for 1 week. Pyridoxine has been given at a dose of 50 mg every 8 hours by intravenous infusion over 30 minutes. Their roles in the reduction of neurotoxicity are unclear.

Pregnancy Category D—Caution is necessary with the administration of all oncolytic drugs during pregnancy. Information on the use of Velban during human pregnancy is very limited. Animal studies with Velban suggest that teratogenic effects may occur. Vinblastine sulfate can cause fetal harm when administered to a pregnant woman. Laboratory animals given this drug early in pregnancy suffer resorption of the conceptus: surviving fetuses demonstrate gross deformities. There are no adequate and well-controlled studies in pregnant women. If this drug is used during pregnancy, or if the patient becomes pregnant while receiving this drug, she should be apprised of the potential hazard to the fetus. Women of childbearing potential should be advised to avoid becoming pregnant.

Aspermia has been reported in man. Animal studies show metaphase arrest and degenerative changes in germ cells.

Leukopenia (granulocytopenia) may reach dangerously low levels following administration of the higher recommended doses. It is therefore important to follow the dosage technique recommended under the Dosage and Administration section. Stomatitis and neurologic toxicity, although not common or permanent, can be disabling.

PRECAUTIONS

General—Toxicity may be enhanced in the presence of hepatic insufficiency.

If leukopenia with less than 2,000 white blood cells/mm^3 occurs following a dose of Velban, the patient should be watched carefully for evidence of infection until the white-blood-cell count has returned to a safe level.

When cachexia or ulcerated areas of the skin surface are present, there may be a more profound leukopenic response to the drug; therefore, its use should be avoided in older persons suffering from either of these conditions.

In patients with malignant-cell infiltration of the bone marrow, the leukocyte and platelet counts have sometimes fallen precipitously after moderate doses of Velban. Further use of the drug in such patients is inadvisable.

Acute shortness of breath and severe bronchospasm have been reported following the administration of vinca alkaloids. These reactions have been encountered most frequently when the vinca alkaloid was used in combination with mitomycin C and may require aggressive treatment, particularly when there is pre-existing pulmonary dysfunction. The onset may be within minutes or several hours after the vinca is injected and may occur up to 2 weeks following a dose of mitomycin. Progressive dyspnea requiring chronic therapy may occur. Velban should not be readministered.

The use of small amounts of Velban daily for long periods is not advised, even though the resulting total weekly dosage may be similar to that recommended. Little or no added therapeutic effect has been demonstrated when such regimens have been used. *Strict adherence to the recommended dosage schedule is very important.* When amounts equal to several times the recommended weekly dosage were given in 7 daily installments for long periods, convulsions, severe and permanent central-nervous-system damage, and even death occurred.

Care must be taken to avoid contamination of the eye with concentrations of Velban used clinically. If accidental contamination occurs, severe irritation (or, if the drug was delivered under pressure, even corneal ulceration) may result. The eye should be washed with water immediately and thoroughly.

It is not necessary to use preservative-containing solvents if unused portions of the remaining solutions are discarded immediately. Unused preservative-containing solutions should be refrigerated for future use.

Information for Patients—The patient should be warned to report immediately the appearance of sore throat, fever, chills, or sore mouth. Advice should be given to avoid constipation, and the patient should be made aware that alopecia may occur and that jaw pain and pain in the organs containing tumor tissue may occur. The latter is thought possibly to result from swelling of tumor tissue during its response to treatment. Scalp hair will regrow to its pretreatment extent even with continued treatment with Velban. Nausea and vomiting, although not common, may occur. Any other serious medical event should be reported to the physician.

Laboratory Tests—Since dose-limiting clinical toxicity is the result of depression of the white-blood-cell count, it is imperative that this count be obtained just before the planned dose of Velban. Following administration of Velban, a fall in the white-blood-cell count may occur. The nadir of this fall is observed from 5 to 10 days following a dose. Recovery to pretreatment levels is usually observed from 7 to 14 days after treatment. These effects will be exaggerated when preexisting bone marrow damage is present and also with the higher recommended doses (*see* Dosage and Administration). The presence of this drug or its metabolites in blood or body tissues is not known to interfere with clinical laboratory tests.

Drug Interactions—Solutions should be made with normal saline (with or without preservative) and should not be combined in the same container with any other chemical. Unused portions of the remaining solutions that do not contain preservatives should be discarded immediately.

The simultaneous oral or intravenous administration of phenytoin and antineoplastic chemotherapy combinations that included vinblastine sulfate has been reported to have reduced blood levels of the anticonvulsant and to have increased seizure activity. Dosage adjustment should be based on serial blood level monitoring. The contribution of vinblastine sulfate to this interaction is not certain. The interaction may result from either reduced absorption of phenytoin or an increase in the rate of its metabolism and elimination.

Caution should be exercised in patients concurrently taking drugs known to inhibit drug metabolism by hepatic cytochrome P450 isoenzymes in the CYP 3A subfamily, or in patients with hepatic dysfunction. Concurrent administration of vinblastine sulfate with an inhibitor of this metabolic pathway may cause an earlier onset and/or an increased severity of side effects. Enhanced toxicity has been reported in patients receiving concomitant erythromycin (*see* Adverse Reactions).

Carcinogenesis, Mutagenesis, Impairment of Fertility—Aspermia has been reported in man. Animal studies suggest that teratogenic effects may occur. *See* Warnings regarding impaired fertility. Animal studies have shown metaphase arrest and degenerative changes in germ cells. Amenorrhea has occurred in some patients treated with the combination consisting of an alkylating agent, procarbazine, prednisone, and Velban. Its occurrence was related to the total dose of these 4 agents used. Recovery of menses was frequent. The same combination of drugs given to male patients produced azoospermia; if spermatogenesis did return, it was not likely to do so with less than 2 years of unmaintained remission.

Mutagenicity—Tests in *Salmonella typhimurium* and with the dominant lethal assay in mice failed to demonstrate mutagenicity. Sperm abnormalities have been noted in mice. Velban has produced an increase in micronuclei formation in bone marrow cells of mice; however, since Velban inhibits mitotic spindle formation, it cannot be concluded that this is evidence of mutagenicity. Additional studies in mice demonstrated no reduction in fertility of males. Chromosomal translocations did occur in male mice. First-generation male offspring of these mice were not heterozygous translocation carriers.

In vitro tests using hamster lung cells in culture have produced chromosomal changes, including chromatid breaks and exchanges, whereas tests using another type of hamster cell failed to demonstrate mutation. Breaks and aberrations were not observed on chromosome analysis of marrow cells from patients being treated with this drug.

It is not clear from the literature how this drug affects synthesis of DNA and RNA. Some believe that there is no interference. Others believe that vinblastine interferes with nucleic acid metabolism but may not do so by direct effect but possibly as the result of biochemical disturbance in some other part of the molecular organization of the cell. No inhibition of RNA synthesis occurred in rat hepatoma cells exposed in culture to noncytotoxic levels of vinblastine. Conflicting results have been noted by others regarding interference with DNA synthesis.

Carcinogenesis—There is no currently available evidence to indicate that Velban itself has been carcinogenic in humans since the inception of its clinical use in the late 1950s. Patients treated for Hodgkin's disease have developed leukemia following radiation therapy and administration of Velban in combination with other chemotherapy including agents known to intercalate with DNA. It is not known to what extent Velban may have contributed to the appearance of leukemia. Available data in rats and mice have failed to demonstrate clearly evidence of carcinogenesis when the animals were treated with the maximum tolerated dose and with one half that dose for 6 months. This testing system demonstrated that other agents were clearly carcinogenic, whereas Velban was in the group of drugs causing slightly increased or the same tumor incidence as controls in one study and 1.5 to twofold increase in tumor incidence over controls in another study.

Usage in Pregnancy—*Pregnancy Category D* (*see* Warnings). Velban should be given to a pregnant woman only if clearly needed. Animal studies suggest that teratogenic effects may occur.

Pediatric Use—The dosage schedule for pediatric patients is indicated under Dosage and Administration.

Nursing Mothers—It is not known whether this drug is excreted in human milk. Because many drugs are excreted in human milk and because of the potential for serious adverse reactions from Velban in nursing infants, a decision should be made whether to discontinue nursing or the drug, taking into account the importance of the drug to the mother.

ADVERSE REACTIONS

Prior to the use of the drug, patients should be advised of the possibility of untoward symptoms.

In general, the incidence of adverse reactions attending the use of Velban appears to be related to the size of the dose employed. With the exception of epilation, leukopenia, and neurologic side effects, adverse reactions generally have not persisted for longer than 24 hours. Neurologic side effects are not common; but when they do occur, they often last for more than 24 hours. Leukopenia, the most common adverse reaction, is usually the dose-limiting factor.

The following are manifestations that have been reported as adverse reactions, in decreasing order of frequency. The most common adverse reactions are underlined:

Hematologic—<u>Leukopenia</u> (granulocytopenia), anemia, thrombocytopenia (myelosuppression).

Dermatologic—<u>Alopecia</u> is common. A single case of light sensitivity associated with this product has been reported.

Gastrointestinal—<u>Constipation</u>, anorexia, nausea, vomiting, abdominal pain, ileus, vesiculation of the mouth, pharyngitis, diarrhea, hemorrhagic enterocolitis, bleeding from an old peptic ulcer, rectal bleeding.

Neurologic—Numbness of digits (paresthesias), loss of deep tendon reflexes, peripheral neuritis, mental depression, headache, convulsions.

Treatment with vinca alkaloids has resulted rarely in both vestibular and auditory damage to the eighth cranial nerve. Manifestations include partial or total deafness which may be temporary or permanent, and difficulties with balance including dizziness, nystagmus, and vertigo. Particular caution is warranted when vinblastine sulfate is used in combination with other agents known to be ototoxic such as the platinum-containing oncolytics.

Cardiovascular—<u>Hypertension</u>. Cases of unexpected myocardial infarction and cerebrovascular accidents have occurred in patients undergoing combination chemotherapy with vinblastine, bleomycin, and cisplatin. Raynaud's phenomenon has also been reported with this combination.

Pulmonary—*See* Precautions.

Miscellaneous—<u>Malaise</u>, <u>bone pain</u>, weakness, <u>pain in tumor-containing tissue</u>, dizziness, <u>jaw pain</u>, skin vesiculation, hypertension, Raynaud's phenomenon when patients are being treated with Velban in combination with bleomycin and cis-platinum for testicular cancer. The syndrome of inappropriate secretion of antidiuretic hormone has occurred with higher than recommended doses.

Nausea and vomiting usually may be controlled with ease by antiemetic agents. When epilation develops, it frequently is not total; and, in some cases, hair regrows while maintenance therapy continues.

Continued on next page

*** Identi-Code® symbol. This product information was prepared in June 2000. Current information on these and other products of Eli Lilly and Company may be obtained by direct inquiry to Lilly Research Laboratories, Lilly Corporate Center, Indianapolis, Indiana 46285, (800) 545-5979.**

Velban—Cont.

Extravasation during intravenous injection may lead to cellulitis and phlebitis. If the amount of extravasation is great, sloughing may occur.

OVERDOSAGE

Signs and Symptoms—Side effects following the use of Velban are dose related. Therefore, following administration of more than the recommended dose, patients can be expected to experience these effects in an exaggerated fashion. (*See* Clinical Pharmacology, Contraindications, Warnings, Precautions, and Adverse Reactions.) There is no specific antidote. In addition, neurotoxicity similar to that with Oncovin may be observed. Since the major route of excretion may be through the biliary system, toxicity from this drug may be increased when there is hepatic insufficiency.

Treatment—To obtain up-to-date information about the treatment of overdose, a good resource is your certified Regional Poison Control Center. Telephone numbers of certified poison control centers are listed in the *Physicians' Desk Reference (PDR)*. In managing overdosage, consider the possibility of multiple drug overdoses, interaction among drugs, and unusual drug kinetics in your patient. Overdoses of Velban have been reported rarely. The following is provided to serve as a guide should such an overdose be encountered.

Supportive care should include the following: (1) prevention of side effects that result from the syndrome of inappropriate secretion of antidiuretic hormone (this would include restriction of the volume of daily fluid intake to that of the urine output plus insensible loss and perhaps the administration of a diuretic affecting the function of the loop of Henle and the distal tubule); (2) administration of an anticonvulsant; (3) prevention of ileus; (4) monitoring the cardiovascular system; and (5) determining daily blood counts for guidance in transfusion requirements and assessing the risk of infection. The major effect of excessive doses of Velban will be myelosuppression, which may be life threatening. There is no information regarding the effectiveness of dialysis nor of cholestyramine for the treatment of overdosage.

Velban in the dry state is irregularly and unpredictably absorbed from the gastrointestinal tract following oral administration. Absorption of the solution has not been studied. If Velban is swallowed, activated charcoal in a water slurry may be given by mouth along with a cathartic. The use of cholestyramine in this situation has not been reported.

Symptoms of overdose will appear when greater-than-recommended doses are given. Any dose of Velban that results in elimination of platelets and neutrophils from blood and marrow and their precursors from marrow should be considered life threatening. The exact dose that will do this in all patients is unknown. Overdoses occurring during prolonged, consecutive-day infusions may be more toxic than the same total dose given by rapid intravenous injection. The intravenous median lethal dose in mice is 10 mg/kg body weight; in rats, it is 2.9 mg/kg. The oral median lethal dose in rats is 7 mg/kg.

Protect the patient's airway and support ventilation and perfusion. Meticulously monitor and maintain, within acceptable limits, the patient's vital signs, blood gases, serum electrolytes, etc. Absorption of drugs from the gastrointestinal tract may be decreased by giving activated charcoal, which, in many cases, is more effective than emesis or lavage; consider charcoal instead of or in addition to gastric emptying if the drug has been swallowed. Repeated doses of charcoal over time may hasten elimination of some drugs that have been absorbed. Safeguard the patient's airway when employing gastric emptying or charcoal.

DOSAGE AND ADMINISTRATION

This preparation is for intravenous use only (see Warnings).

Special Dispensing Information—WHEN DISPENSING VELBAN IN OTHER THAN THE ORIGINAL CONTAINER, IT IS IMPERATIVE THAT IT BE PACKAGED IN THE PROVIDED OVERWRAP WHICH BEARS THE FOLLOWING STATEMENT: "DO NOT REMOVE COVERING UNTIL MOMENT OF INJECTION. FATAL IF GIVEN INTRATHECALLY. FOR INTRAVENOUS USE ONLY" (*see* Warnings). A syringe containing a specific dose must be labeled, using the auxiliary sticker provided, to state: "FATAL IF GIVEN INTRATHECALLY. FOR INTRAVENOUS USE ONLY".

Caution—It is extremely important that the intravenous needle or catheter be properly positioned before any Velban is injected. Leakage into surrounding tissue during intravenous administration of Velban may cause considerable irritation. If extravasation occurs, the injection should be discontinued immediately and any remaining portion of the dose should then be introduced into another vein. Local injection of hyaluronidase and the application of moderate heat to the area of leakage will help disperse the drug and may minimize discomfort and the possibility of cellulitis.

There are variations in the depth of the leukopenic response that follows therapy with Velban. For this reason, it is recommended that the drug be given no more frequently than *once every 7 days.*

Adult Patients —It is wise to initiate therapy for adults by administering a single intravenous dose of 3.7 mg/m^2 of body surface area (bsa). Thereafter, white-blood-cell counts should be made to determine the patient's sensitivity to Velban.

A simplified and conservative incremental approach to dosage *at weekly intervals* for adults may be outlined as follows:

First dose	3.7 mg/m^2 bsa
Second dose	5.5 mg/m^2 bsa
Third dose	7.4 mg/m^2 bsa
Fourth dose	9.25mg/m^2 bsa
Fifth dose	11.1 mg/m^2 bsa

The above mentioned increases may be used until a maximum dose not exceeding 18.5 mg/m^2 bsa for adults is reached. The dose should not be increased after that dose which reduces the white-cell count to approximately 3,000 cells/mm^3. In some adults, 3.7 mg/m^2 bsa may produce this leukopenia; other adults may require more than 11.1 mg/m^2 bsa; and, very rarely, as much as 18.5 mg/m^2 bsa may be necessary. For most adult patients, however, the weekly dosage will prove to be 5.5 to 7.4 mg/m^2 bsa.

When the dose of Velban which will produce the above degree of leukopenia has been established, a dose of *1 increment smaller* than this should be administered at weekly intervals for maintenance. Thus, the patient is receiving the maximum dose that does not cause leukopenia. *It should be emphasized that, even though 7 days have elapsed, the next dose of Velban should not be given until the white-cell count has returned to at least 4,000/mm^3.* In some cases, oncolytic activity may be encountered before leukopenic effect. When this occurs, there is no need to increase the size of subsequent doses (*see* Precautions).

Pediatric Patients—A review of published literature from 1993 to 1995 showed that initial doses of Velban in pediatric patients varied depending on the schedule used and whether Velban was administered as a single agent or incorporated within a particular chemotherapeutic regimen. As a single agent for Letterer-Siwe disease (histiocytosis X), the initial dose of Velban was reported as 6.5 mg/m^2. When Velban was used in combination with other chemotherapeutic agents for the treatment of Hodgkin's disease, the initial dose was reported as 6 mg/m^2. For testicular germ cell carcinomas, the initial dose of Velban was reported as 3 mg/m^2 in a combination regimen. Dose modifications should be guided by hematologic tolerance.

Patients with Renal or Hepatic Impairment—A reduction of 50% in the dose of Velban is recommended for patients having a direct serum bilirubin value above 3 mg/100 mL. Since metabolism and excretion are primarily hepatic, no modification is recommended for patients with impaired renal function.

The duration of maintenance therapy varies according to the disease being treated and the combination of antineoplastic agents being used. There are differences of opinion regarding the duration of maintenance therapy with the same protocol for a particular disease; for example, various durations have been used with the MOPP program in treating Hodgkin's disease. Prolonged chemotherapy for maintaining remissions involves several risks, among which are life-threatening infectious diseases, sterility, and possibly the appearance of other cancers through suppression of immune surveillance.

In some disorders, survival following complete remission may not be as prolonged as that achieved with shorter periods of maintenance therapy. On the other hand, failure to provide maintenance therapy in some patients may lead to unnecessary relapse; complete remissions in patients with testicular cancer, unless maintained for at least 2 years, often result in early relapse.

To prepare a solution containing 1 mg of Velban/mL, add 10 mL of Bacteriostatic Sodium Chloride Injection (preserved with benzyl alcohol) or 10 mL of Sodium Chloride Injection (unpreserved) to the 10 mg of Velban in the sterile vial. Do not use other solutions. The drug dissolves instantly to give a clear solution.

Parenteral drug products should be inspected visually for particulate matter and discoloration prior to administration, whenever solution and container permit.

Unused portions of the remaining solutions made with normal saline that do not contain preservatives should be discarded immediately. Unused preservative-containing solutions made with normal saline may be stored in a refrigerator for future use for a maximum of 28 days.

The dose of Velban (calculated to provide the desired amount) may be injected either into the tubing of a running intravenous infusion or directly into a vein. The latter procedure is readily adaptable to outpatient therapy. In either case, the injection may be completed in about 1 minute. If care is taken to insure that the needle is securely within the vein and that no solution containing Velban is spilled extravascularly, cellulitis and/or phlebitis will not occur. To minimize further the possibility of extravascular spillage, it is suggested that the syringe and needle be rinsed with venous blood before withdrawal of the needle. The dose should not be diluted in large volumes of diluent (ie, 100 to 250 mL) or given intravenously for prolonged periods (ranging from 30 to 60 minutes or more), since this frequently results in irritation of the vein and increases the chance of extravasation.

Because of the enhanced possibility of thrombosis, it is considered inadvisable to inject a solution of Velban into an extremity in which the circulation is impaired or potentially impaired by such conditions as compressing or invading neoplasm, phlebitis, or varicosity.

Procedures for proper handling and disposal of anticancer drugs should be considered. Several guidelines on this subject have been published.[4–10] There is no general agreement that all of the procedures recommended in the guidelines are necessary or appropriate.

HOW SUPPLIED

Vials, 10 mg, 10-mL size (No. 687)—(1s) NDC 0002-1452-01

The vials should be stored in a refrigerator (2° to 8°C, or 36° to 46°F) to assure extended stability.

REFERENCES

1. Dyke. Treatment of inadvertent intrathecal injection of vincristine. N Engl J Med, 1989, 321: 1270–71.
2. Michelagnoli MP, Bailey CC, Wilson L, Livingston J, Kinsey SB. Potential salvage therapy for inadvertent intrathecal administration of vincristine. Br. J. Haematology, 1997, 99: 364–367. (Mfr. Control No. GB97113451A)
3. Zaragoza MR, Ritchey ML, Walter A. Neurourologic consequences of accidental intrathecal vincristine: A case report. Med. Pediatr. Oncol., 1995, 24(1): 61–62.
4. Recommendations for the Safe Handling of Parenteral Antineoplastic Drugs, NIH Publication No. 83-2621. For sale by the Superintendent of Documents, U.S. Government Printing Office, Washington, DC 20402.
5. AMA Council Report, Guidelines for Handling Parenteral Antineoplastics. JAMA, 1985;253(11):1590–1592.
6. National Study Commission on Cytotoxic Exposure—Recommendations for Handling Cytotoxic Agents. Available from Louis P. Jeffrey, ScD., Chairman, National Study Commission on Cytotoxic Exposure, Massachusetts College of Pharmacy and Allied Health Sciences, 179 Longwood Avenue, Boston, Massachusetts 02115.
7. Clinical Oncological Society of Australia, Guidelines and Recommendations for Safe Handling of Antineoplastic Agents. Med J Australia, 1983;1:426–428.
8. Jones RB, et al: Safe Handling of Chemotherapeutic Agents: A Report from the Mount Sinai Medical Center. CA—A Cancer Journal for Clinicians, 1983; (Sept/Oct)258–263.
9. American Society of Hospital Pharmacists Technical Assistance Bulletin on Handling Cytotoxic and Hazardous Drugs. Am J Hosp Pharm, 1990;47:1033–1049.
10. OSHA Work-Practice Guidelines for Personnel Dealing with Cytotoxic (Antineoplastic) Drugs. Am J Hosp Pharm, 1986;43:1193–1204.

Text revised May 19, 1999

PA 2565 AMP [051999]

ZINC-INSULIN CRYSTALS OTC

See under Iletin® (insulin).

ZYPREXA® ℞

[*zī-prex-ah*]

(Olanzapine) Tablets

ZYPREXA® ZYDIS® ℞

(Olanzapine) Orally Disintegrating Tablets

DESCRIPTION

ZYPREXA (olanzapine) is a psychotropic agent that belongs to the thienobenzodiazepine class. The chemical designation is 2-methyl-4-(4-methyl-1-piperazinyl)-10*H*-thieno[2,3-*b*] [1,5]benzodiazepine. The molecular formula is $C_{17}H_{20}N_4S$, which corresponds to a molecular weight of 312.44. The chemical structure is:

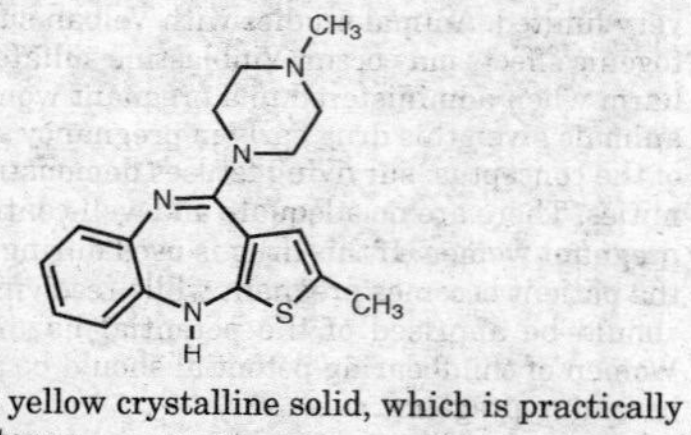

Olanzapine is a yellow crystalline solid, which is practically insoluble in water.

ZYPREXA tablets are intended for oral administration only. Each tablet contains olanzapine equivalent to 2.5 mg (8 µmol), 5 mg (16 µmol), 7.5 mg (24 µmol), 10 mg (32 µmol), or 15 mg (48 µmol). Inactive ingredients are carnauba wax, crospovidone, hydroxypropyl cellulose, hydroxypropyl methylcellulose, lactose, magnesium stearate, microcrystalline cellulose, and other inactive ingredients. The color coating contains Titanium Dioxide (all strengths) and F D & C Blue No. 2 Aluminum Lake (15 mg). The 2.5, 5.0, 7.5, and 10 mg tablets are imprinted with edible ink which contains F D & C Blue No. 2 Aluminum Lake.

ZYPREXA ZYDIS (olanzapine orally disintegrating tablets) is intended for oral administration only.

Each orally disintegrating tablet contains olanzapine equivalent to 5 mg (16 µmol) or 10 mg (32 µmol). It begins disintegrating in the mouth within seconds, allowing its contents to be subsequently swallowed with or without liquid.

ZYPREXA ZYDIS (olanzapine orally disintegrating tablets) also contains the following inactive ingredients: gelatin, mannitol, aspartame, sodium methyl paraben and sodium propyl paraben.

CLINICAL PHARMACOLOGY

Pharmacodynamics:

Olanzapine is a selective monoaminergic antagonist with high affinity binding to the following receptors: serotonin

$5HT_{2A/2C}$ (K_i=4 and 11 nM, respectively), dopamine D_{1-4} (K_i=11–31 nM), muscarinic M_{1-5} (K_i=1.9–25 nM), histamine H_1 (K_i=7 nM), and adrenergic α_1 receptors (K_i=19 nM). Olanzapine binds weakly to $GABA_A$, BZD, and β adrenergic receptors (K_i > 10 μM).

The mechanism of action of olanzapine, as with other drugs having efficacy in schizophrenia, is unknown. However, it has been proposed that this drug's efficacy in schizophrenia is mediated through a combination of dopamine and serotonin type 2 ($5HT_2$) antagonism. The mechanism of action of olanzapine in the treatment of acute manic episodes associated with Bipolar I Disorder is unknown.

Antagonism at receptors other than dopamine and $5HT_2$ with similar receptor affinities may explain some of the other therapeutic and side effects of olanzapine. Olanzapine's antagonism of muscarinic M_{1-5} receptors may explain its anticholinergic effects. Olanzapine's antagonism of histamine H_1 receptors may explain the somnolence observed with this drug. Olanzapine's antagonism of adrenergic α_1 receptors may explain the orthostatic hypotension observed with this drug.

Pharmacokinetics:

Olanzapine is well absorbed and reaches peak concentrations in approximately 6 hours following an oral dose. It is eliminated extensively by first pass metabolism, with approximately 40% of the dose metabolized before reaching the systemic circulation. Food does not affect the rate or extent of olanzapine absorption. Pharmacokinetic studies showed that ZYPREXA tablets and ZYPREXA ZYDIS (olanzapine orally disintegrating tablets) dosage forms of olanzapine are bioequivalent.

Olanzapine displays linear kinetics over the clinical dosing range. Its half-life ranges from 21 to 54 hours (5th to 95th percentile; mean of 30 hr), and apparent plasma clearance ranges from 12 to 47 L/hr (5th to 95th percentile; mean of 25 L/hr).

Administration of olanzapine once daily leads to steady-state concentrations in about one week that are approximately twice the concentrations after single doses. Plasma concentrations, half-life, and clearance of olanzapine may vary between individuals on the basis of smoking status, gender and age (*see* Special Populations).

Olanzapine is extensively distributed throughout the body, with a volume of distribution of approximately 1000 L. It is 93% bound to plasma proteins over the concentration range of 7 to 1100 ng/mL, binding primarily to albumin and α_1-acid glycoprotein.

Metabolism and Elimination—Following a single oral dose of ^{14}C labeled olanzapine, 7% of the dose of olanzapine was recovered in the urine as unchanged drug, indicating that olanzapine is highly metabolized. Approximately 57% and 30% of the dose was recovered in the urine and feces, respectively. In the plasma, olanzapine accounted for only 12% of the AUC for total radioactivity, indicating significant exposure to metabolites. After multiple dosing, the major circulating metabolites were the 10-N-glucuronide, present at steady state at 44% of the concentration of olanzapine, and 4′-N-desmethyl olanzapine, present at steady state at 31% of the concentration of olanzapine. Both metabolites lack pharmacological activity at the concentrations observed.

Direct glucuronidation and cytochrome P450 (CYP) mediated oxidation are the primary metabolic pathways for olanzapine. In vitro studies suggest that CYPs 1A2 and 2D6, and the flavin-containing monooxygenase system are involved in olanzapine oxidation. CYP2D6 mediated oxidation appears to be a minor metabolic pathway in vivo, because the clearance of olanzapine is not reduced in subjects who are deficient in this enzyme.

Special Populations—

Renal Impairment—Because olanzapine is highly metabolized before excretion and only 7% of the drug is excreted unchanged, renal dysfunction alone is unlikely to have a major impact on the pharmacokinetics of olanzapine. The pharmacokinetic characteristics of olanzapine were similar in patients with severe renal impairment and normal subjects, indicating that dosage adjustment based upon the degree of renal impairment is not required. In addition, olanzapine is not removed by dialysis. The effect of renal impairment on metabolite elimination has not been studied.

Hepatic Impairment—Although the presence of hepatic impairment may be expected to reduce the clearance of olanzapine, a study of the effect of impaired liver function in subjects (n=6) with clinically significant (Childs Pugh Classification A and B) cirrhosis revealed little effect on the pharmacokinetics of olanzapine.

Age—In a study involving 24 healthy subjects, the mean elimination half-life of olanzapine was about 1.5 times greater in elderly (>65 years) than in non-elderly subjects (≤65 years). Caution should be used in dosing the elderly, especially if there are other factors that might additively influence drug metabolism and/or pharmacodynamic sensitivity (*see* DOSAGE AND ADMINISTRATION).

Gender—Clearance of olanzapine is approximately 30% lower in women than in men. There were, however, no apparent differences between men and women in effectiveness or adverse effects. Dosage modifications based on gender should not be needed.

Smoking Status—Olanzapine clearance is about 40% higher in smokers than in nonsmokers, although dosage modifications are not routinely recommended.

Race—No specific pharmacokinetic study was conducted to investigate the effects of race. A cross-study comparison between data obtained in Japan and data obtained in the US suggests that exposure to olanzapine may be about 2-fold greater in the Japanese when equivalent doses are administered. Clinical trial safety and efficacy data, however, did not suggest clinically significant differences among Caucasian patients, patients of African descent, and a third pooled category including Asian and Hispanic patients. Dosage modifications for race are, therefore, not recommended.

Combined Effects—The combined effects of age, smoking, and gender could lead to substantial pharmacokinetic differences in populations. The clearance in young smoking males, for example, may be 3 times higher than that in elderly nonsmoking females. Dosing modification may be necessary in patients who exhibit a combination of factors that may result in slower metabolism of olanzapine (*see* DOSAGE AND ADMINISTRATION).

Clinical Efficacy Data:

Schizophrenia

The efficacy of olanzapine in the management of the manifestations of psychotic disorders was established in 2 short-term (6-week) controlled trials of inpatients who met DSM III-R criteria for schizophrenia. A single haloperidol arm was included as a comparative treatment in one of the two trials, but this trial did not compare these two drugs on the full range of clinically relevant doses for both.

Several instruments were used for assessing psychiatric signs and symptoms in these studies, among them the Brief Psychiatric Rating Scale (BPRS), a multi-item inventory of general psychopathology traditionally used to evaluate the effects of drug treatment in psychosis. The BPRS psychosis cluster (conceptual disorganization, hallucinatory behavior, suspiciousness, and unusual though content) is considered a particularly useful subset for assessing actively psychotic schizophrenic patients. A second traditional assessment, the Clinical Global Impression (CGI), reflects the impression of a skilled observer, fully familiar with the manifestations of schizophrenia, about the overall clinical state of the patient. In addition, two more recently developed but less well evaluated scales were employed; these included the 30-item Positive and Negative Symptoms Scale (PANSS), in which is embedded the 18 items of the BPRS, and the Scale for Assessing Negative Symptoms (SANS). The trial summaries below focus on the following outcomes: PANSS total and/or BPRS total; BPRS psychosis cluster; PANSS negative subscale or SANS; and CGI Severity. The results of the trials follow:

(1) In a 6-week, placebo-controlled trial (n=149) involving two fixed olanzapine doses of 1 and 10 mg/day (once daily schedule), olanzapine, at 10 mg/day (but not at 1 mg/day), was superior to placebo on the PANSS total score (also on the extracted BPRS total), on the BPRS psychosis cluster, on the PANSS Negative subscale, and on CGI Severity.

(2) In a 6-week, placebo-controlled trial (n=253) involving 3 fixed dose ranges of olanzapine (5.0±2.5 mg/day, 10.0±2.5 mg/day, and 15.0±2.5 mg/day) on a once daily schedule, the two highest olanzapine dose groups (actual mean doses of 12 and 16 mg/day, respectively) were superior to placebo on BPRS total score, BPRS psychosis cluster, and CGI severity score; the highest olanzapine dose group was superior to placebo on the SANS. There was no clear advantage for the high dose group over the medium dose group.

Examination of population subsets (race and gender) did not reveal any differential responsiveness on the basis of these subgroupings.

Bipolar Mania

The efficacy of olanzapine in the treatment of acute manic episodes was established in 2 short-term (one 3-week and one 4-week) placebo-controlled trials in patients who met the DSM-IV criteria for Bipolar I Disorder with manic or mixed episodes. These trials included patients with or without psychotic features and with or without a rapid-cycling course.

The primary rating instrument used for assessing manic symptoms in these trials was the Young Mania Rating Scale (Y-MRS), and 11-item clinician-rated scale traditionally used to assess the degree of manic symptomatology in a range from 0 (no manic features) to 60 (maximum score). The primary outcome in these trials was change from baseline in the Y-MRS total score. The results of the trials follow:

(1) In one 3-week placebo-controlled trial (n=67) which involved a dose range of olanzapine (5–20 mg/day, once daily, starting at 10 mg/day), olanzapine was superior to placebo in the reduction of Y-MRS total score. In an identically designed trial conducted simultaneously with the first trial, olanzapine demonstrated a similar treatment difference, but possibly due to sample size and site variability, was not shown to be superior to placebo on this outcome.

(2) In a 4-week placebo-controlled trial (n=115) which involved a dose range of olanzapine (5–20 mg/day, once daily, starting at 15 mg/day), olanzapine was superior to placebo in the reduction of Y-MRS total score.

INDICATIONS AND USAGE

Schizophrenia

ZYPREXA is indicated for the management of the manifestations of psychotic disorders.

The efficacy of ZYPREXA was established in short-term (6-week) controlled trials of schizophrenic inpatients (*see* CLINICAL PHARMACOLOGY).

The effectiveness of ZYPREXA in long-term use, that is, for more than 6 weeks, has not been systematically evaluated in controlled trials. Therefore, the physician who elects to use ZYPREXA for extended periods should periodically re-evaluate the long-term usefulness of the drug for the individual patient (*see* DOSAGE AND ADMINISTRATION).

Bipolar Mania

ZYPREXA is indicated for the short-term treatment of acute manic episodes associated with Bipolar I Disorder.

The efficacy of ZYPREXA was established in two placebo-controlled trials (one 3-week and one 4-week) with patients meeting DSM-IV criteria for Bipolar I Disorder who currently displayed an acute manic or mixed episode with or without psychotic features (*see* CLINCIAL PHARMACOLOGY).

The effectiveness of ZYPREXA for longer-term use, that is, for more than 4 weeks treatment of an acute episode, and for prophylactic use in mania, has not been systematically evaluated in controlled clinical trials. Therefore, physicians who elect to use ZYPREXA for extended periods should periodically re-evaluate the long-term risks and benefits of the drug for the individual patient (*see* DOSAGE AND ADMINISTRATION).

CONTRAINDICATIONS

ZYPREXA is contraindicated in patients with a known hypersensitivity to the product.

WARNINGS

Neuroleptic Malignant Syndrome (NMS)—A potentially fatal symptom complex sometimes referred to as Neuroleptic Malignant Syndrome (NMS) has been reported in association with administration of antipsychotic drugs, including olanzapine. Clinical manifestations of NMS are hyperpyrexia, muscle rigidity, altered mental status and evidence of autonomic instability (irregular pulse or blood pressure, tachycardia, diaphoresis and cardiac dysrhythmia). Additional signs may include elevated creatinine phosphokinase, myoglobinuria (rhabdomyolysis), and acute renal failure.

The diagnostic evaluation of patients with this syndrome is complicated. In arriving at a diagnosis, it is important to exclude cases where the clinical presentation includes both serious medical illness (e.g., pneumonia, systemic infection, etc.) and untreated or inadequately treated extrapyramidal signs and symptoms (EPS). Other important considerations in the differential diagnosis include central anticholinergic toxicity, heat stroke, drug fever, and primary central nervous system pathology.

The management of NMS should include: 1) immediate discontinuation of antipsychotic drugs and other drugs not essential to concurrent therapy; 2) intensive symptomatic treatment and medical monitoring; and 3) treatment of any concomitant serious medical problems for which specific treatments are available. There is no general agreement about specific pharmacological treatment regimens for NMS.

If a patient requires antipsychotic drug treatment after recovery from NMS, the potential reintroduction of drug therapy should be carefully considered. The patient should be carefully monitored, since recurrences of NMS have been reported.

Tardive Dyskinesia—A syndrome of potentially irreversible, involuntary, dyskinetic movements may develop in patients treated with antipsychotic drugs. Although the prevalence of the syndrome appears to be highest among the elderly, especially elderly women, it is impossible to rely upon prevalence estimates to predict, at the inception of antipsychotic treatment, which patients are likely to develop the syndrome. Whether antipsychotic drug products differ in their potential to cause tardive dyskinesia is unknown.

The risk of developing tardive dyskinesia and the likelihood that it will become irreversible are believed to increase as the duration of treatment and the total cumulative dose of antipsychotic drugs administered to the patient increase. However, the syndrome can develop, although much less commonly, after relatively brief treatment periods at low doses.

There is no known treatment for established cases of tardive dyskinesia, although the syndrome may remit, partially or completely, if antipsychotic treatment is withdrawn. Antipsychotic treatment, itself, however, may suppress (or partially suppress) the signs and symptoms of the syndrome and thereby may possibly mask the underlying process. The effect that symptomatic suppression has upon the long-term course of the syndrome is unknown.

Given these considerations, olanzapine should be prescribed in a manner that is most likely to minimize the occurrence of tardive dyskinesia. Chronic antipsychotic treatment should generally be reserved for patients (1) who suffer from a chronic illness that is known to respond to antipsychotic drugs, and (2) for whom alternative, equally effective, but potentially less harmful treatments are not available or appropriate. In patients who do require chronic treatment, the smallest dose and the shortest duration of treatment producing a satisfactory clinical response should be sought. The need for continued treatment should be reassessed periodically.

Continued on next page

*** Identi-Code® symbol. This product information was prepared in June 2000. Current information on these and other products of Eli Lilly and Company may be obtained by direct inquiry to Lilly Research Laboratories, Lilly Corporate Center, Indianapolis, Indiana 46285, (800) 545-5979.**

Zyprexa—Cont.

If signs and symptoms of tardive dyskinesia appear in a patient on olanzapine, drug discontinuation should be considered. However, some patients may require treatment with olanzapine despite the presence of the syndrome.

PRECAUTIONS

General

Orthostatic Hypotension—Olanzapine may induce orthostatic hypotension associated with dizziness, tachycardia, and in some patients, syncope, especially during the initial dose-titration period, probably reflecting its α_1-adrenergic antagonistic properties. Syncope was reported in 0.6% (15/2500) of olanzapine-treated patients in phase 2-3 studies. The risk of orthostatic hypotension and syncope may be minimized by initiating therapy with 5 mg QD (*see* DOSAGE AND ADMINISTRATION). A more gradual titration to the target dose should be considered if hypotension occurs. Olanzapine should be used with particular caution in patients with known cardiovascular disease (history of myocardial infarction or ischemia, heart failure, or conduction abnormalities), cerebrovascular disease, and conditions which would predispose patients to hypotension (dehydration, hypovolemia, and treatment with antihypertensive medications).

Seizures—During premarketing testing, seizures occurred in 0.9% (22/2500) of olanzapine-treated patients. There were confounding factors that may have contributed to the occurrence of seizures in many of these cases. Olanzapine should be used cautiously in patients with a history of seizures or with conditions that potentially lower the seizure threshold, e.g., Alzheimer's dementia. Conditions that lower the seizure threshold may be more prevalent in a population of 65 years or older.

Hyperprolactinemia—As with other drugs that antagonize dopamine D_2 receptors, olanzapine elevates prolactin levels, and a modest elevation persists during chronic administration. Tissue culture experiments indicate that approximately one-third of human breast cancers are prolactin dependent in vitro, a factor of potential importance if the prescription of these drugs is contemplated in a patient with previously detected breast cancer of this type. Although disturbances such as galactorrhea, amenorrhea, gynecomastia, and impotence have been reported with prolactin-elevating compounds, the clinical significance of elevated serum prolactin levels is unknown for most patients. As is common with compounds which increase prolactin release, an increase in mammary gland neoplasia was observed in the olanzapine carcinogenicity studies conducted in mice and rats (*see* Carcinogenesis). However, neither clinical studies nor epidemiologic studies have shown an association between chronic administration of this class of drugs and tumorigenesis in humans; the available evidence is considered too limited to be conclusive.

Transaminase Elevations—In placebo-controlled studies, clinically significant ALT (SGPT) elevations ($\geq$3 times the upper limit of the normal range) were observed in 2% (6/243) of patients exposed to olanzapine compared to none (0/115) of the placebo patients. None of these patients experienced jaundice. In two of these patients, liver enzymes decreased toward normal despite continued treatment and in two others, enzymes decreased upon discontinuation of olanzapine. In the remaining two patients, one, seropositive for hepatitis C, had persistent enzyme elevation for four months after discontinuation, and the other had insufficient follow-up to determine if enzymes normalized.

Within the larger premarketing database of about 2400 patients with baseline SGPT $\leq$90 IU/L, the incidence of SGPT elevation to >200 IU/L was 2% (50/2381). Again, none of these patients experienced jaundice or other symptoms attributable to liver impairment and most had transient changes that tended to normalize while olanzapine treatment was continued.

Among all 2500 patients in clinical trials, about 1% (23/2500) discontinued treatment due to transaminase increases.

Caution should be exercised in patients with signs and symptoms of hepatic impairment, in patients with preexisting conditions associated with limited hepatic functional reserve, and in patients who are being treated with potentially hepatotoxic drugs. Periodic assessment of transaminases is recommended in patients with significant hepatic disease (*see* Laboratory Tests).

Potential for Cognitive and Motor Impairment—Somnolence was a commonly reported adverse event associated with olanzapine treatment, occurring at an incidence of 26% in olanzapine patients compared to 15% in placebo patients. This adverse event was also dose related. Somnolence led to discontinuation in 0.4% (9/2500) of patients in the premarketing database.

Since olanzapine has the potential to impair judgment, thinking, or motor skills, patients should be cautioned about operating hazardous machinery, including automobiles, until they are reasonably certain that olanzapine therapy does not affect them adversely.

Body Temperature Regulation—Disruption of the body's ability to reduce core body temperature has been attributed to antipsychotic agents. Appropriate care is advised when prescribing olanzapine for patients who will be experiencing conditions which may contribute to an elevation in core body temperature, e.g., exercising strenuously, exposure to extreme heat, receiving concomitant medication with anticholinergic activity, or being subject to dehydration.

Dysphagia—Esophageal dysmotility and aspiration have been associated with antipsychotic drug use. Two olanzapine-treated patients (2/407) in two studies in patients with Alzheimer's disease died from aspiration pneumonia during or within 30 days of the termination of the double-blind portion of their respective studies; there were no deaths in the placebo-treated patients. One of these patients had experienced dysphagia prior to the development of aspiration pneumonia. Aspiration pneumonia is a common cause of morbidity and mortality in patients with advanced Alzheimer's disease. Olanzapine and other antipsychotic drugs should be used cautiously in patients at risk for aspiration pneumonia.

Suicide—The possibility of a suicide attempt is inherent in schizophrenia and in bipolar disorder, and close supervision of high-risk patients should accompany drug therapy. Prescriptions for olanzapine should be written for the smallest quantity of tablets consistent with good patient management, in order to reduce the risk of overdose.

Use in Patients with Concomitant Illness—Clinical experience with olanzapine in patients with certain concomitant systemic illnesses (*see* Renal Impairment and Hepatic Impairment *under* CLINICAL PHARMACOLOGY, Special Populations) is limited.

Olanzapine exhibits in vitro muscarinic receptor affinity. In premarketing clinical trials with olanzapine, olanzapine was associated with constipation, dry mouth, and tachycardia, all adverse events possibly related to cholinergic antagonism. Such adverse events were not often the basis for discontinuations from olanzapine, but olanzapine should be used with caution in patients with clinically significant prostatic hypertrophy, narrow angle glaucoma, or a history of paralytic ileus.

In a fixed-dose study of olanzapine (olanzapine at doses of 5, 10, and 15 mg/day) and placebo in nursing home patients (mean age: 83 years, range: 61–97; median Mini-Mental State Examination (MMSE): 5, range: 0–22) having various psychiatric symptoms in association with Alzheimer's disease, the following treatment-emergent adverse events were reported in all (each and every) olanzapine-treated groups at an incidence of either (1) two-fold or more in excess of the placebo-treated group, where at least 1 placebo-treated patient was reported to have experienced the event, or (2) at least 2 cases if no placebo-treated patient was reported to have experienced the event: somnolence, abnormal gait, fever, dehydration, and back pain. The rate of discontinuation in this study for olanzapine was 12% vs 4% with placebo. Discontinuations due to abnormal gait (1% for olanzapine vs 0% for placebo), accidental injury (1% for olanzapine vs 0% for placebo), and somnolence (3% for olanzapine vs 0% for placebo) were considered to be drug related. As with other CNS-active drugs, olanzapine should be used with caution in elderly patients with dementia (*see* PRECAUTIONS).

Olanzapine has not been evaluated or used to any appreciable extent in patients with a recent history of myocardial infarction or unstable heart disease. Patients with these diagnoses were excluded from premarketing clinical studies. Because of the risk of orthostatic hypotension with olanzapine, caution should be observed in cardiac patients (*see* Orthostatic Hypotension).

Information for Patients—Physicians are advised to discuss the following issues with patients for whom they prescribe olanzapine:

Orthostatic Hypotension—Patients should be advised of the risk of orthostatic hypotension, especially during the period of initial dose titration and in association with the use of concomitant drugs that may potentiate the orthostatic effect of olanzapine, e.g., diazepam or alcohol (*see* Drug Interactions).

Interference with Cognitive and Motor Performance—Because olanzapine has the potential to impair judgment, thinking, or motor skills, patients should be cautioned about operating hazardous machinery, including automobiles, until they are reasonably certain that olanzapine therapy does not affect them adversely.

Pregnancy—Patients should be advised to notify their physician if they become pregnant or intend to become pregnant during therapy with olanzapine.

Nursing—Patients should be advised not to breast-feed an infant if they are taking olanzapine.

Concomitant Medication—Patients should be advised to inform their physicians if they are taking, or plan to take, any prescription or over-the-counter drugs, since there is a potential for interactions.

Alcohol—Patients should be advised to avoid alcohol while taking olanzapine.

Heat Exposure and Dehydration—Patients should be advised regarding appropriate care in avoiding overheating and dehydration.

Phenylketonurics—ZYPREXA ZYDIS (olanzapine orally disintegrating tablets) contains phenylalanine (0.34 and 0.45 mg per 5 and 10 mg tablet, respectively).

Laboratory Tests—Periodic assessment of transaminases is recommended in patients with significant hepatic disease (*see* Transaminase Elevations).

Drug Interactions—The risks of using olanzapine in combination with other drugs have not been extensively evaluated in systematic studies. Given the primary CNS effects of olanzapine, caution should be used when olanzapine is taken in combination with other centrally acting drugs and alcohol.

Because of its potential for inducing hypotension, olanzapine may enhance the effects of certain antihypertensive agents.

Olanzapine may antagonize the effects of levodopa and dopamine agonists.

The Effect of Other Drugs on Olanzapine—Agents that induce CYP1A2 or glucuronyl transferase enzymes, such as omeprazole and rifampin, may cause an increase in olanzapine clearance. Inhibitors of CYP1A2 (e.g., fluvoxamine) could potentially inhibit olanzapine elimination. Because olanzapine is metabolized by multiple enzyme systems, inhibition of a single enzyme may not appreciably decrease olanzapine clearance.

Charcoal—The administration of activated charcoal (1 g) reduced the C_{max} and AUC of olanzapine by about 60%. As peak olanzapine levels are not typically obtained until about 6 hours after dosing, charcoal may be a useful treatment for olanzapine overdose.

Cimetidine and Antacids—Single doses of cimetidine (800 mg) or aluminum- and magnesium-containing antacids did not affect the oral bioavailability of olanzapine.

Carbamazepine—Carbamazepine therapy (200 mg bid) causes an approximately 50% increase in the clearance of olanzapine. This increase is likely due to the fact that carbamazepine is a potent inducer of CYP1A2 activity. Higher daily doses of carbamazepine may cause an even greater increase in olanzapine clearance.

Ethanol—Ethanol (45 mg/70 kg single dose) did not have an effect on olanzapine pharmacokinetics.

Fluoxetine—Fluoxetine (60 mg single dose or 60 mg daily for 8 days) causes a small (mean 16%) increase in the maximum concentration of olanzapine and a small (mean 16%) decrease in olanzapine clearance. The magnitude of the impact of this factor is small in comparison to the overall variability between individuals, and therefore dose modification is not routinely recommended.

Valproate—Studies in vitro using human liver microsomes determined that olanzapine has little potential to inhibit the major metabolic pathway, glucuronidation, of valproate. Further, valproate has little effect on the metabolism of olanzapine in vitro. Thus, a clinically signficant pharmacokinetic interaction between olanzapine and valproate is unlikely.

Warfarin—Warfarin (20 mg single dose) did not affect olanzapine pharmacokinetics.

Effect of Olanzapine on Other Drugs—In vitro studies utilizing human liver microsomes suggest that olanzapine has little potential to inhibit CYP1A2, CYP2C9, CYP2C19, CYP2D6, and CYP3A. Thus, olanzapine is unlikely to cause clinically important drug interactions mediated by these enzymes.

Single doses of olanzapine did not affect the pharmacokinetics of imipramine or its active metabolite desipramine, and warfarin. Multiple doses of olanzapine did not influence the kinetics of diazepam and its active metabolite N-desmethyldiazepam, lithium, ethanol, or biperiden. However, the coadministration of either diazepam or ethanol with olanzapine potentiated the orthostatic hypotension observed with olanzapine. Multiple doses of olanzapine did not affect the pharmacokinetics of theophylline or its metabolites.

Carcinogenesis, Mutagenesis, Impairment of Fertility—

Carcinogenesis—Oral carcinogenicity studies were conducted in mice and rats. Olanzapine was administered to mice in two 78-week studies at doses of 3, 10, 30/20 mg/kg/day (equivalent to 0.8-5 times the maximum recommended human daily dose on a mg/m^2 basis) and 0.25, 2, 8 mg/kg/day (equivalent to 0.06-2 times the maximum recommended human daily dose on a mg/m^2 basis). Rats were dosed for 2 years at doses of 0.25, 1, 2.5, 4 mg/kg/day (males) and 0.25, 1, 4, 8 mg/kg/day (females) (equivalent to 0.13-2 and 0.13-4 times the maximum recommended human daily dose on a mg/m^2 basis, respectively). The incidence of liver hemangiomas and hemangiosarcomas was significantly increased in one mouse study in female mice dosed at 8 mg/kg/day (2 times the maximum recommended human daily dose on a mg/m^2 basis). These tumors were not increased in another mouse study in females dosed at 10 or 30/20 mg/kg/day (2-5 times the maximum recommended human daily dose on a mg/m^2 basis); in this study, there was a high incidence of early mortalities in males of the 30/20 mg/kg/day group. The incidence of mammary gland adenomas and adenocarcinomas was significantly increased in female mice dosed at $\geq$2 mg/kg/day and in female rats dosed at $\geq$4 mg/kg/day (0.5 and 2 times the maximum recommended human daily dose on a mg/m^2 basis, respectively). Antipsychotic drugs have been shown to chronically elevate prolactin levels in rodents. Serum prolactin levels were not measured during the olanzapine carcinogenicity studies; however, measurements during subchronic toxicity studies showed that olanzapine elevated serum prolactin levels up to 4-fold in rats at the same doses used in the carcinogenicity study. An increase in mammary gland neoplasms has been found in rodents after chronic administration of other antipsychotic drugs and is considered to be prolactin mediated. The relevance for human risk of the finding of prolactin mediated endocrine tumors in rodents is unknown (*see* Hyperprolactinemia *under* PRECAUTIONS, General).

Mutagenesis—No evidence of mutagenic potential for olanzapine was found in the Ames reverse mutation test, in vivo micronucleus test in mice, the chromosomal aberration test in Chinese hamster ovary cells, unscheduled DNA synthesis test in rat hepatocytes, induction of forward mutation test in mouse lymphoma cells, or in vivo sister chromatid exchange test in bone marrow of Chinese hamsters.

Impairment of Fertility—In a fertility and reproductive performance study in rats, male mating performance, but not fertility, was impaired at a dose of 22.4 mg/kg/day and female fertility was decreased at a dose of 3 mg/kg/day (11 and 1.5 times the maximum recommended human daily dose on a mg/m^2 basis, respectively). Discontinuance of olanzapine treatment reversed the effects on male mating performance. In female rats, the precoital period was increased and the mating index reduced at 5 mg/kg/day (2.5 times the maximum recommended human daily dose on a mg/m^2 basis). Diestrous was prolonged and estrous delayed at 1.1 mg/kg/day (0.6 times the maximum recommended human daily dose on a mg/m^2 basis); therefore olanzapine may produce a delay in ovulation.

Pregnancy—

Pregnancy Category C—In reproduction studies in rats at doses up to 18 mg/kg/day and in rabbits at doses up to 30 mg/kg/day (9 and 30 times the maximum recommended human daily dose on a mg/m^2 basis, respectively) no evidence of teratogenicity was observed. In a rat teratology study, early resorptions and increased numbers of nonviable fetuses were observed at a dose of 18 mg/kg/day (9 times the maximum recommended human daily dose on a mg/m^2 basis). Gestation was prolonged at 10 mg/kg/day (5 times the maximum recommended human daily dose on a mg/m^2 basis). In a rabbit teratology study, fetal toxicity (manifested as increased resorptions and decreased fetal weight) occurred at a maternally toxic dose of 30 mg/kg/day (30 times the maximum recommended human daily dose on a mg/m^2 basis).

Placental transfer of olanzapine occurs in rat pups.

There are no adequate and well-controlled trials with olanzapine in pregnant females. Seven pregnancies were observed during clinical trials with olanzapine, including 2 resulting in normal births, 1 resulting in neonatal death due to a cardiovascular defect, 3 therapeutic abortions, and 1 spontaneous abortion. Because animal reproduction studies are not always predictive of human response, this drug should be used during pregnancy only if the potential benefit justifies the potential risk to the fetus.

Labor and Delivery—Parturition in rats was not affected by olanzapine. The effect of olanzapine on labor and delivery in humans is unknown.

Nursing Mothers—Olanzapine was excreted in milk of treated rats during lactation. It is not known if olanzapine is excreted in human milk. It is recommended that women receiving olanzapine should not breast-feed.

Pediatric Use—Safety and effectiveness in pediatric patients have not been established.

Geriatric Use—Of the 2500 patients in premarketing clinical studies with olanzapine, 11% (263) were 65 years of age or over. In patients with schizophrenia, there was no indication of any different tolerability of olanzapine in the elderly compared to younger patients. Studies in patients with various psychiatric symptoms in association with Alzheimer's disease have suggested that there may be a different tolerability profile in this population compared to younger patients with schizophrenia. As with other CNS-active drugs, olanzapine should be used with caution in elderly patients with dementia. Also, the presence of factors that might decrease pharmacokinetic clearance or increase the pharmacodynamic response to olanzapine should lead to consideration of a lower starting dose for any geriatric patient (*see* PRECAUTIONS and DOSAGE AND ADMINISTRATION).

ADVERSE REACTIONS

The information below is derived from a clinical trial database for olanzapine consisting of 4189 patients with approximately 2665 patient-years of exposure. This database includes: (1) 2500 patients who participated in multiple-dose premarketing trials in schizophrenia and Alzheimer's disease representing approximately 1122 patient-years of exposure as of February 14, 1995; (2) 182 patients who participated in premarketing bipolar mania trials representing approximately 66 patient-years of exposure; (3) 191 patients who participated in a trial of patients having various psychiatric symptoms in association with Alzheimer's disease representing approximately 29 patient-years of exposure; and (4) 1316 patients from 43 additional clinical trials as of May 1, 1997.

The conditions and duration of treatment with olanzapine varied greatly and included (in overlapping categories) open-label and double-blind phases of studies, inpatients and outpatients, fixed-dose and dose-titration studies, and short-term or longer-term exposure. Adverse reactions were assessed by collecting adverse events, results of physical examinations, vital signs, weights, laboratory analytes, ECGs, chest x-rays, and results of ophthalmologic examinations.

Certain portions of the discussion below relating to objective or numeric safety parameters, namely, dose-dependent adverse events, vital sign changes, weight gain, laboratory changes, and ECG changes are derived from studies in patients with schizophrenia and have not been duplicated for bipolar mania. However, this information is also generally applicable to bipolar mania.

Adverse events during exposure were obtained by spontaneous report and recorded by clinical investigators using terminology of their own choosing. Consequently, it is not possible to provide a meaningful estimate of the proportion of individuals experiencing adverse events without first grouping similar types of events into a smaller number of standardized event categories. In the tables and tabulations that follow, standard COSTART dictionary terminology has been used to classify reported adverse events.

The stated frequencies of adverse events represent the proportion of individuals who experienced, at least once, a treatment-emergent adverse event of the type listed. An event was considered treatment emergent if it occurred for the first time or worsened while receiving therapy following baseline evaluation. The reported events do not include those event terms which were so general as to be uninformative. Events listed elsewhere in labeling may not be repeated below. It is important to emphasize that, although the events occurred during treatment with olanzapine, they were not necessarily caused by it. The entire label should be read to gain a complete understanding of the safety profile of olanzapine.

The prescriber should be aware that the figures in the tables and tabulations cannot be used to predict the incidence of side effects in the course of usual medical practice where patient characteristics and other factors differ from those that prevailed in the clinical trials. Similarly, the cited frequencies cannot be compared with figures obtained from other clinical investigations involving different treatments, uses, and investigators. The cited figures, however, do provide the prescribing physician with some basis for estimating the relative contribution of drug and nondrug factors to the adverse event incidence in the population studied.

Incidence of Adverse Events in Short-Term, Placebo-Controlled Trials—The following findings are based on the short-term, placebo-controlled premarketing trials for schizophrenia and bipolar mania and a subsequent trial of patients having various psychiatric symptoms in association with Alzheimer's disease.

Adverse Events Associated with Discontinuation of Treatment in Short-Term, Placebo-Controlled Trials—Schizophrenia—Overall, there was no difference in the incidence of discontinuation due to adverse events (5% for olanzapine vs 6% for placebo). However, discontinuations due to increases in SGPT were considered to be drug related (2% for olanzapine vs 0% for placebo) (*see* PRECAUTIONS).

Bipolar Mania—Overall, there was no difference in the incidence of discontinuation due to adverse events (2% for olanzapine vs 2% for placebo).

Commonly Observed Adverse Events in Short-Term, Placebo-Controlled Trials—The most commonly observed adverse events associated with the use of olanzapine (incidence of 5% or greater) and not observed at an equivalent incidence among placebo-treated patients (olanzapine incidence at least twice that for placebo) were:

Common Treatment-Emergent Adverse Events Associated with the Use of Olanzapine in 6-Week Trials—SCHIZOPHRENIA

Adverse Event	Percentage of Patients Reporting Event	
	Olanzapine (N=248)	Placebo (N=118)
Postural hypotension	5	2
Constipation	9	3
Weight gain	6	1
Dizziness	11	4
Personality disorder[1]	8	4
Akathisia	5	1

[1] Personality disorder is the COSTART term for designating non-aggressive objectionable behavior.

Common Treatment-Emergent Adverse Events Associated with the Use of Olanzapine in 3-Week and 4-Week Trials—BIPOLAR MANIA

Adverse Event	Percentage of Patients Reporting Event	
	Olanzapine (N=125)	Placebo (N=129)
Asthenia	15	6
Dry Mouth	22	7
Constipation	11	5
Dyspepsia	11	5
Increased appetite	6	3
Somnolence	35	13
Dizziness	18	6
Tremor	6	3

Adverse Events Occurring at an Incidence of 2% or More Among Olanzapine-Treated Patients in Short-Term, Placebo-Controlled Trials—Table 1 enumerates the incidence, rounded to the nearest percent, of treatment-emergent adverse events that occurred in 2% or more of patients treated with olanzapine (doses ≥2.5 mg/day) and with incidence greater than placebo who participated in the acute phase of placebo-controlled trials.

Table 1
Treatment-Emergent Adverse Events: Incidence in Short-Term, Placebo-Controlled Clinical Trials[1]

Body System/Adverse Event	Percentage of Patients Reporting Event	
	Olanzapine (N=532)	Placebo (N=294)
Body as a Whole		
Accidental Injury	12	8
Asthenia	10	9
Fever	6	2
Back pain	5	2
Chest pain	3	1
Cardiovascular System		
Postural hypotension	3	1
Tachycardia	3	1
Hypertension	2	1
Digestive System		
Dry mouth	9	5
Constipation	9	4
Dyspepsia	7	5
Vomiting	4	3
Increased appetite	3	2
Hemic and Lymphatic System		
Ecchymosis	5	3
Metabolic and Nutritional Disorders		
Weight gain	5	3
Peripheral edema	3	1
Musculoskeletal System		
Extremity pain (other than joint)	5	3
Joint pain	5	3
Nervous System		
Somnolence	29	13
Insomnia	12	11
Dizziness	11	4
Abnormal gait	6	1
Tremor	4	3
Akathisia	3	2
Hypertonia	3	2
Articulation impairment	2	1
Respiratory System		
Rhinitis	7	6
Cough increased	6	3
Pharyngitis	4	3
Special Senses		
Amblyopia	3	2
Urogenital System		
Urinary incontinence	2	1
Urinary tract infection	2	1

[1] Events reported by at least 2% of patients treated with olanzapine, except the following events which had an incidence equal to or less than placebo: abdominal pain, agitation, anorexia, anxiety, apathy, confusion, depression, diarrhea, dysmenorrhea[2], hallucinations, headache, hostility, hyperkinesia, myalgia, nausea, nervousness, paranoid reaction, personality disorder[3], rash, thinking abnormal, weight loss.

[2] Denominator used was for females only (olanzapine, N=201; placebo, N=114).

[3] Personality disorder is the COSTART term for designating non-aggressive objectionable behavior.

Additional Findings Observed in Clinical Trials—The following findings are based on clinical trials.

Dose Dependency of Adverse Events in Short-Term, Placebo-Controlled Trials—

Extrapyramidal Symptoms: The following table enumerates the percentage of patients with treatment-emergent extrapyramidal symptoms as assessed by categorical analyses of formal rating scales during acute therapy in a controlled clinical trial comparing olanzapine at 3 fixed doses with placebo in the treatment of schizophrenia.

Continued on next page

*** Identi-Code® symbol. This product information was prepared in June 2000. Current information on these and other products of Eli Lilly and Company may be obtained by direct inquiry to Lilly Research Laboratories, Lilly Corporate Center, Indianapolis, Indiana 46285, (800) 545-5979.**

Zyprexa—Cont.

TREATMENT-EMERGENT EXTRAPYRAMIDAL SYMPTOMS ASSESSED BY RATING SCALES INCIDENCE IN A FIXED DOSAGE RANGE, PLACEBO-CONTROLLED CLINICAL TRIAL—ACUTE PHASE*

	Percentage of Patients			
	Placebo	Olanzapine 5± 2.5 mg/day	Olanzapine 10 ± 2.5 mg/day	Olanzapine 15 ± 2.5 mg/day
Parkinsonism[1]	15	14	12	14
Akathisia[2]	23	16	19	27

*No statistically significant differences.
[1] Percentage of patients with a Simpson-Angus Scale total score >3.
[2] Percentage of patients with a Barnes Akathisia Scale global score ≥2.

The following table enumerates the percentage of patients with treatment-emergent extrapyramidal symptoms as assessed by spontaneously reported adverse events during acute therapy in the same controlled clinical trial comparing olanzapine at 3 fixed doses with placebo in the treatment of schizophrenia.

TREATMENT-EMERGENT EXTRAPYRAMIDAL SYMPTOMS ASSESSED BY ADVERSE EVENTS INCIDENCE IN A FIXED DOSAGE RANGE, PLACEBO-CONTROLLED CLINICAL TRIAL—ACUTE PHASE

	Percentage of Patients Reporting Event			
	Placebo (N=68)	Olanzapine 5±2.5 mg/day (N=65)	Olanzapine 10±2.5 mg/day (N=64)	Olanzapine 15±2.5 mg/day (N=69)
Dystonic events[1]	1	3	2	3
Parkinsonism events[2]	10	8	14	20
Akathisia events[3]	1	5	11*	10*
Dyskinetic events[4]	4	0	2	1
Residual events[5]	1	2	5	1
Any extra-pyramidal event	16	15	25	32*

*Statistically significantly different from placebo.
[1] Patients with the following COSTART terms were counted in this category: dystonia, generalized spasm, neck rigidity, oculogyric crisis, opisthotonos, torticollis.
[2] Patients with the following COSTART terms were counted in this category: akinesia, cogwheel rigidity, extrapyramidal syndrome, hypertonia, hypokinesia, masked facies, tremor.
[3] Patients with the following COSTART terms were counted in this category: akathisia, hyperkinesia.
[4] Patients with the following COSTART terms were counted in this category: buccoglossal syndrome, choreoathetosis, dyskinesia, tardive dyskinesia.
[5] Patients with the following COSTART terms were counted in this category: movement disorder, myoclonus, twitching.

Other Adverse Events: The following table addresses dose relatedness for other adverse events using data from a schizophrenia trial involving fixed dosage ranges. It enumerates the percentage of patients with treatment-emergent adverse events for the three fixed-dose range groups and placebo. The data were analyzed using the Cochran-Armitage test, excluding the placebo group, and the table includes only those adverse events for which there was a statistically significant trend.

	Percentage of Patients Reporting Event			
Adverse Event	Placebo (N=68)	Olanzapine 5±2.5 mg/day (N=65)	Olanzapine 10±2.5 mg/day (N=64)	Olanzapine 15±2.5 mg/day (N=69)
Asthenia	15	8	9	20
Dry mouth	4	3	5	13
Nausea	9	0	2	9
Somnolence	16	20	30	39
Tremor	3	0	5	7

Vital Sign Changes—Olanzapine is associated with orthostatic hypotension and tachycardia (*see* PRECAUTIONS).

Weight Gain—In placebo-controlled, 6-week studies, weight gain was reported in 5.6% of olanzapine patients compared to 0.8% of placebo patients. Olanzapine patients gained an average of 2.8 kg, compared to an average 0.4 kg weight loss in placebo patients; 29% of olanzapine patients gained greater than 7% of their baseline weight, compared to 3% of placebo patients. A categorization of patients at baseline on the basis of body mass index (BMI) revealed a significantly greater effect in patients with low BMI compared to normal or overweight patients; nevertheless, weight gain was greater in all 3 olanzapine groups compared to the placebo group. During long-term continuation therapy with olanzapine (238 median days of exposure), 56% of olanzapine patients met the criterion for having gained greater than 7% of their baseline weight. Average weight gain during long-term therapy was 5.4 kg.

Laboratory Changes—An assessment of the premarketing experience for olanzapine revealed an association with asymptomatic increases in SGPT, SGOT, and GGT (*see* PRECAUTIONS). Olanzapine administration was also associated with increases in serum prolactin (*see* PRECAUTIONS), with an asymptomatic elevation of the eosinophil count in 0.3% of patients, and with an increase in CPK.

Given the concern about neutropenia associated with other psychotropic compounds and the finding of leukopenia associated with the administration of olanzapine in several animal models (*see* ANIMAL TOXICOLOGY), careful attention was given to examination of hematologic parameters in premarketing studies with olanzapine. There was no indication of a risk of clinically significant neutropenia associated with olanzapine treatment in the premarketing database for this drug.

In the olanzapine clinical trial database, as of September 30, 1999, 4577 olanzapine-treated patients (representing approximately 2255 patient-years of exposure) and 445 placebo-treated patients who had no history of diabetes mellitus and whose baseline random plasma glucose levels were 140 mg/dL or lower were identified. Persistent random glucose levels ≥ 200 mg/dL (suggestive of possible diabetes) were observed in 0.8% of olanzapine-treated patients (placebo 0.7%). Transient (i.e., resolved while the patients remained on treatment) random glucose levels ≥ 200 mg/dL were found in 0.3% of olanzapine-treated patients (placebo 0.2%). Persistent random glucose levels ≥ 160 mg/dL but < 200 mg/dL (possibly hyperglycemia, not necessarily diabetes) were observed in 1.0% of olanzapine-treated patients (placebo 1.1%). Transient random glucose levels ≥ 160 mg/dL but < 200 mg/dL were found in 1.0% of olanzapine-treated patients (placebo 0.4%).

ECG Changes—Between-group comparisons for pooled placebo-controlled trials revealed no statistically significant olanzapine/placebo differences in the proportions of patients experiencing potentially important changes in ECG parameters, including QT, QTc, and PR intervals. Olanzapine use was associated with a mean increase in heart rate of 2.4 beats per minute compared to no change among placebo patients. This slight tendency to tachycardia may be related to olanzapine's potential for inducing orthostatic changes (*see* PRECAUTIONS).

Other Adverse Events Observed During the Clinical Trial Evaluation of Olanzapine—Following is a list of terms that reflect treatment-emergent adverse events reported by patients treated with olanzapine (at multiple doses ≥ 1 mg/day) in clinical trials (4189 patients, 2665 patient-years of exposure). This listing does not include those events already listed in previous tables or elsewhere in labeling, those events for which a drug cause was remote, those event terms which were so general as to be uninformative, and those events reported only once which did not have a substantial probability of being acutely life-threatening.

Events are further categorized by body system and listed in order of decreasing frequency according to the following definitions: frequent adverse events are those occurring in at least 1/100 patients (only those not already listed in the tabulated results from placebo-controlled trials appear in this listing); infrequent adverse events are those occurring in 1/100 to 1/1000 patients; rare events are those occurring in fewer than 1/1000 patients.

Body as a Whole—*Frequent:* dental pain, flu syndrome, intentional injury, and suicide attempt; *Infrequent:* abdomen enlarged, chills, chills and fever, face edema, malaise, moniliasis, neck pain, neck rigidity, pelvic pain, and photosensitivity reaction; *Rare:* hangover effect and sudden death.

Cardiovascular System—*Frequent:* hypotension; *Infrequent:* bradycardia, cerebrovascular accident, congestive heart failure, heart arrest, hemorrhage, migraine, pallor, palpitation, vasodilatation, and ventricular extrasystoles; *Rare:* arteritis, atrial fibrillation, heart failure, and pulmonary embolus.

Digestive System—*Frequent:* increased salivation and thirst; *Infrequent:* dysphagia, eructation, fecal impaction, fecal incontinence, flatulence, gastritis, gastroenteritis, gingivitis, hepatitis, melena, mouth ulceration, nausea and vomiting, oral moniliasis, periodontal abscess, rectal hemorrhage, stomatitis, tongue edema, and tooth caries; *Rare:* aphthous stomatitis, enteritis, esophageal ulcer, esophagitis, glossitis, ileus, intestinal obstruction, liver fatty deposit, and tongue discoloration.

Endocrine System—*Infrequent:* diabetes mellitus; *Rare:* diabetic acidosis and goiter.

Hemic and Lymphatic System—*Frequent:* leukopenia; *Infrequent:* anemia, cyanosis, leukocytosis, lymphadenopathy, thrombocythemia, and thrombocytopenia; *Rare:* normocytic anemia.

Metabolic and Nutritional Disorders—*Infrequent:* acidosis, alkaline phosphatase increased, bilirubinemia, dehydration, hypercholesteremia, hyperglycemia, hyperlipemia, hyperuricemia, hypoglycemia, hypokalemia, hyponatremia, lower extremity edema, upper extremity edema, and water intoxication; *Rare:* gout, hyperkalemia, hypernatremia, hypoproteinemia, and ketosis.

Musculoskeletal System—*Frequent:* joint stiffness and twitching; *Infrequent:* arthritis, arthrosis, bursitis, leg cramps, and myasthenia; *Rare:* bone pain, myopathy, osteoporosis, and rheumatoid arthritis.

Nervous System—*Frequent:* abnormal dreams, emotional lability, euphoria, libido decreased, paresthesia, and schizophrenia reaction; *Infrequent:* alcohol misuse, amnesia, antisocial reaction, ataxia, CNS stimulation, cogwheel rigidity, coma, delerium, depersonalization, dysarthria, facial paralysis, hypesthesia, hypokinesia, hypotonia, incoordination, libido increased, obsessive compulsive symptoms, phobias, somatization, stimulant misuse, stupor, stuttering, tardive dyskinesia, tobacco misuse, vertigo, and withdrawal syndrome; *Rare:* akinesia, circumoral paresthesia, encephalopathy, neuralgia, neuropathy, nystagmus, paralysis, and subarachnoid hemorrhage.

Respiratory System—*Frequent:* dyspnea; *Infrequent:* apnea, aspiration pneumonia, asthma, atelectasis, epistaxis, hemoptysis, hyperventilation, laryngitis, pneumonia, and voice alteration; *Rare:* hiccup, hypoventilation, hypoxia, lung edema, and stridor.

Skin and Appendages—*Frequent:* sweating; *Infrequent:* alopecia, contact dermatitis, dry skin, eczema, maculopapular rash, pruritus, seborrhea, skin ulcer, and vesiculobullous rash; *Rare:* hirsutism, pustular rash, skin discoloration, and urticaria.

Special Senses—*Frequent:* conjunctivitis; *Infrequent:* abnormality of accommodation, blepharitis, cataract, corneal lesion, deafness, diplopia, dry eyes, ear pain, eye hemorrhage, eye inflammation, eye pain, ocular muscle abnormality, taste perversion, and tinnitus; *Rare:* glaucoma, keratoconjunctivitis, macular hypopigmentation, miosis, mydriasis, and pigment deposits lens.

Urogenital System—*Frequent:* amenorrhea*, hematuria, metrorrhagia*, and vaginitis*; *Infrequent:* abnormal ejaculation*, breast pain, cystitis, decreased menstruation*, dysuria, female lactation, glycosuria, impotence*, increased menstruation*, menorrhagia*, polyuria, premenstrual syndrome*, pyuria, urinary frequency, urinary retention, urination impaired, uterine fibroids enlarged*, and vaginal hemorrhage*; *Rare:* albuminuria, gynecomastia, mastitis, oliguria, and urinary urgency.

*Adjusted for gender.

Postintroduction Reports—Adverse events reported since market introduction which were temporally (but not necessarily causally) related to ZYPREXA therapy include the following: diabetic coma and priapism.

DRUG ABUSE AND DEPENDENCE

Controlled Substance Class—Olanzapine is not a controlled substance.

Physical and Psychological Dependence—In studies prospectively designed to assess abuse and dependence potential, olanzapine was shown to have acute depressive CNS effects but little or no potential of abuse or physical dependence in rats administered oral doses up to 15 times the maximum recommended human daily dose (20 mg) and rhesus monkeys administered oral doses up to 8 times the maximum recommended human daily dose on a mg/m^2 basis. Olanzapine has not been systematically studied in humans for its potential for abuse, tolerance, or physical dependence. While the clinical trials did not reveal any tendency for any drug-seeking behavior, these observations were not systematic, and it is not possible to predict on the basis of this limited experience the extent to which a CNS-active drug will be misused, diverted, and/or abused once marketed. Consequently, patients should be evaluated carefully for a history of drug abuse, and such patients should be observed closely for signs of misuse or abuse of olanzapine (e.g., development of tolerance, increases in dose, drug-seeking behavior).

OVERDOSAGE

Human Experience—In premarketing trials involving more than 3100 patients and/or normal subjects, accidental or intentional acute overdosage of olanzapine was identified in 67 patients. In the patient taking the largest identified amount, 300 mg, the only symptoms reported were drowsiness and slurred speech. In the limited number of patients who were evaluated in hospitals, including the patient taking 300 mg, there were no observations indicating an adverse change in laboratory analytes or ECG. Vital signs were usually within normal limits following overdoses.

Overdosage Management—The possibility of multiple drug involvement should be considered. In case of acute overdosage, establish and maintain an airway and ensure adequate oxygenation and ventilation. Gastric lavage (after intubation, if patient is unconscious) and administration of activated charcoal together with a laxative should be consid-

	TABLE STRENGTH				
	2.5 mg	5 mg	7.5 mg	10 mg	15 mg
Tablet No.	4112	4115	4116	4117	4415
Identification	LILLY 4112	LILLY 4115	LILLY 4116	LILLY 4117	LILLY 4415
NDC Codes:					
Bottles 30	—	—	—	—	NDC-0002-4415-30
Bottles 60	NDC-0002-4112-60	NDC-0002-4115-60	NDC-0002-4116-60	NDC-0002-4117-60	—
Blisters-ID*100	—	NDC-0002-4115-33	NDC-0002-4116-33	NDC-0002-4117-33	NDC-0002-4415-33

*Identi-Dose® (unit dose medication, Lilly)

ered. The possibility of obtundation, seizures, or dystonic reaction of the head and neck following overdose may create a risk of aspiration with induced emesis. Cardiovascular monitoring should commence immediately and should include continuous electrocardiographic monitoring to detect possible arrhythmias.

There is no specific antidote to olanzapine. Therefore, appropriate supportive measures should be initiated. Hypotension and circulatory collapse should be treated with appropriate measures such as intravenous fluids and/or sympathomimetic agents. (Do not use epinephrine, dopamine, or other sympathomimetics with beta-agonist activity, since beta stimulation may worsen hypotension in the setting of olanzapine-induced alpha blockade.) Close medical supervision and monitoring should continue until the patient recovers.

DOSAGE AND ADMINISTRATION

Schizophrenia

Usual Dose—Olanzapine should be administered on a once-a-day schedule without regard to meals, generally beginning with 5 to 10 mg initially, with a target dose of 10 mg/day within several days. Further dosage adjustments, if indicated, should generally occur at intervals of not less than 1 week, since steady state for olanzapine would not be achieved for approximately 1 week in the typical patient. When dosage adjustments are necessary, dose increments/decrements of 5 mg QD are recommended.

Antipsychotic efficacy was demonstrated in a dose range of 10 to 15 mg/day in clinical trials. However, doses above 10 mg/day were not demonstrated to be more efficacious than the 10 mg/day dose. An increase to a dose greater than the target dose of 10 mg/day (i.e., to a dose of 15 mg/day or greater) is recommended only after clinical assessment. The safety of doses above 20 mg/day has not been evaluated in clinical trials.

Dosing in Special Populations—The recommended starting dose is 5 mg in patients who are debilitated, who have a predisposition to hypotensive reactions, who otherwise exhibit a combination of factors that may result in slower metabolism of olanzapine (e.g., nonsmoking female patients ≥65 years of age), or who may be more pharmacodynamically sensitive to olanzapine (*see* CLINICAL PHARMACOLOGY; also *see* Use in Patients with Concomitant Illness and Drug Interactions *under* PRECAUTIONS). When indicated, dose escalation should be performed with caution in these patients.

Maintenance Treatment—While there is no body of evidence available to answer the question of how long the patient treated with olanzapine should remain on it, the effectiveness of maintenance treatment is well established for many other antipsychotic drugs. It is recommended that responding patients be continued on olanzapine, but at the lowest dose needed to maintain remission. Patients should be periodically reassessed to determine the need for maintenance treatment.

Bipolar Mania

Usual Dose—Olanzapine should be administered on a once-a-day schedule without regard to meals, generally beginning with 10 or 15 mg. Dosage adjustments, if indicated, should generally occur at intervals of not less than 24 hours, reflecting the procedures in the placebo-controlled trials. When dosage adjustments are necessary, dose increments/decrements of 5 mg QD are recommended.

Short-term (3–4 weeks) antimanic efficacy was demonstrated in a dose range of 5 mg to 20 mg/day in clinical trials. The safety of doses above 20 mg/day has not been evaluated in clinical trials.

Dosing in Special Populations—*See* Dosing in Special Populations *under* DOSAGE AND ADMINISTRATION, Schizophrenia.

Maintenance Treatment—There is no body of evidence available from controlled trials to guide a clinician in the longer-term management of a patient who improves during treatment of an acute manic episode with olanzapine. While it is generally agreed that pharmacological treatment beyond an acute response in mania is desirable, both for maintenance of the initial response and for prevention of new manic episodes, there are no systematically obtained data to support the use of olanzapine in such longer-term treatment (i.e., beyond 3–4 weeks).

Administration of ZYPREXA ZYDIS (olanzapine orally disintegrating tablets)—After opening sachet, peel back foil on blister. Do not push tablet through foil. Immediately upon opening the blister, using dry hands, remove tablet and place entire ZYPREXA ZYDIS in the mouth. Tablet disintegration occurs rapidly in saliva so it can be easily swallowed with or without liquid.

HOW SUPPLIED

The ZYPREXA 2.5 mg, 5 mg, 7.5 mg, and 10 mg tablets are white, round, and imprinted in blue ink with LILLY and tablet number. The 15 mg tablets are elliptical, blue, and debossed with LILLY and tablet number. The tablets are available as follows:

[See table above]

ZYPREXA ZYDIS (olanzapine orally disintegrating tablets) are yellow, round, and debossed with the tablet strength. The tablets are available as follows:

ZYPREXA ZYDIS Tablets*	TABLET STRENGTH 5 mg	10 mg
Tablet No.	4453	4454
Debossed	5	10
NDC Codes:		
Dose Pack 30 (Child-Resistant)	NDC-0002-4453-85	NDC-0002-4454-85

ZYPREXA is a registered trademark of Eli Lilly and Company.

ZYDIS is a registered trademark of R. P. Scherer Corporation.

*ZYPREX ZYDIS (olanzapine orally disintegrating tablets) is manufactured for Eli Lilly and Company by Scherer DDS Limited, United Kingdom, SN5 8RU.

Store at controlled room temperature, 20° to 25°C (68° to 77°F) [*see* USP]. The USP defines controlled room temperature as a temperature maintained thermostatically that encompasses the usual and customary working environment of 20° to 25°C (68° to 77°F); that results in a mean kinetic temperature calculated to be not more than 25°C; and that allows for excursions between 15° and 30°C (59° and 86°F) that are experienced in pharmacies, hospitals, and warehouses.

Protect from light and moisture.

ANIMAL TOXICOLOGY

In animal studies with olanzapine, the principal hematologic findings were reversible peripheral cytopenias in individual dogs dosed at 10 mg/kg (17 times the maximum recommended human daily dose on a mg/m^2 basis), dose-related decreases in lymphocytes and neutrophils in mice, and lymphopenia in rats. A few dogs treated with 10 mg/kg developed reversible neutropenia and/or reversible hemolytic anemia between 1 and 10 months of treatment. Dose-related decreases in lymphocytes and neutrophils were seen in mice given doses of 10 mg/kg (equal to 2 times the maximum recommended human daily dose on a mg/m^2 basis) in studies of 3 months' duration. Nonspecific lymphopenia, consistent with decreased body weight gain, occurred in rats receiving 22.5 mg/kg (11 times the maximum recommended human daily dose on a mg/m^2 basis) for 3 months or 16 mg/kg (8 times the maximum recommended human daily dose on a mg/m^2 basis) for 6 or 12 months. No evidence of bone marrow cytotoxicity was found in any of the species examined. Bone marrows were normocellular or hypercellular, indicating that the reductions in circulating blood cells were probably due to peripheral (non-marrow) factors.

Literature revised April 12, 2000

PV 3390 AMP [041200]

Shown in Product Identification Guide, page 321

EDUCATIONAL MATERIALS

Diabetes Patient Education Materials

Managing Your Diabetes^{SM} Patient Education System (available in English and Spanish)

◊ Comprehensive workbook on diabetes self-care and basic facts, along with three insulin product brochures
◊ 5- part video series
◊ Meal planning guides
◊ Self-care diaries

Professional Education Materials and Services

◊ CE programs
◊ Speaker programs
◊ Professional slide series

For information on these and other educational materials, see your Lilly sales representative.

Managing Your Diabetes^{SM} Patient Education System is a trademark of Eli Lilly and Company.

Humatrope®/Growth Hormone Patient Education Materials

Pediatric Patient Materials

- Preparation and injection booklet and video
- *HumatroPen™ User Guide* and video
- *Ready, Set, Grow!* booklet about growth in children
- *The Highs and Lows of Growing Up* booklet about the psychological effects of short stature in children
- *What, Why, and How: The Stimulation Test* booklet about what to anticipate before, during and after stimulation testing

Adult Patient Materials

- Preparation and injection booklet and video
- *HumatroPen™ User Guide*
- *Are You Being Treated for Hypopituitarism?* booklet about hypopituitarism and Humatrope® treatment

Professional Education Materials and Services

- CME program

For information about these and other educational materials, please see your Lilly sales representative.

The Liposome Company, Inc.

ONE RESEARCH WAY
PRINCETON, NJ 08540-6619

Direct Inquiries to:
Professional Services
(800) 335-5476
FAX: (609) 452-8512

For Medical Information Contact:
Professional Services
(800) 335-5476
(609) 520-6586
FAX: (609) 452–8512

ABELCET® ℞

['ā-bəl-"set]
(Amphotericin B Lipid Complex Injection)

DESCRIPTION

ABELCET® is a sterile, pyrogen-free suspension for intravenous infusion. ABELCET® consists of amphotericin B complexed with two phospholipids in a 1:1 drug-to-lipid molar ratio. The two phospholipids, L-α-dimyristoylphosphatidylcholine (DMPC) and L-α-dimyristoylphosphatidylglycerol (DMPG), are present in a 7:3 molar ratio. ABELCET® is yellow and opaque in appearance, with a pH of 5–7.

NOTE: Liposomal encapsulation or incorporation in a lipid complex can substantially affect a drug's functional properties relative to those of the unencapsulated or nonlipid-associated drug. In addition, different liposomal or lipid-complexed products with a common active ingredient may vary from one another in the chemical composition and physical form of the lipid component. Such differences may affect functional properties of these drug products.

Amphotericin B is a polyene, antifungal antibiotic produced from a strain of *Streptomyces nodosus*. Amphotericin B is designated chemically as [1R-(1R*, 3S*, 5R*, 6R*, 9R*, 11R*, 15S*, 16R*, 17R*, 18S*, 19E, 21E, 23E, 25E, 27E, 29E, 31E, 33R*, 35S*, 36R*, 37S*)]-33-[(3-Amino-3, 6-dideoxy-β-D-mannopyranosyl) oxy]-1,3,5,6,9,11,17,37-octahydroxy - 15,16,18 - trimethyl - 13 - oxo - 14,39 - dioxabicyclo[33.3.1] nonatriaconta-19,21,23,25,27,29,31-heptaene-36-carboxylic acid.

It has a molecular weight of 924.09 and a molecular formula of $C_{47}H_{73}NO_{17}$. The structural formula is:

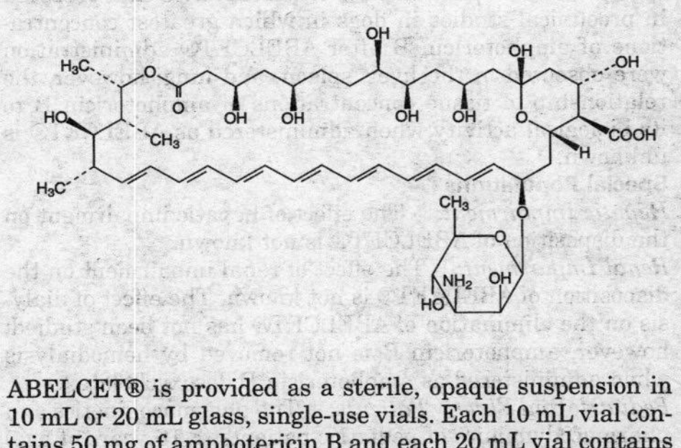

ABELCET® is provided as a sterile, opaque suspension in 10 mL or 20 mL glass, single-use vials. Each 10 mL vial contains 50 mg of amphotericin B and each 20 mL vial contains 100 mg of amphotericin B (see DOSAGE AND ADMINISTRATION), and each mL of ABELCET® contains:

Amphotericin B USP	5 mg
L-α-dimyristoylphosphatidylcholine (DMPC)	3.4 mg
L-α-dimyristoylphosphatidylglycerol (DMPG)	1.5 mg
Sodium Chloride USP	9 mg
Water for Injection USP, q.s. 1 mL	

Continued on next page

Abelcet—Cont.

MICROBIOLOGY

Mechanism of Action

The active component of ABELCET®, amphotericin B, acts by binding to sterols in the cell membrane of susceptible fungi, with a resultant change in the permeability of the membrane. Mammalian cell membranes also contain sterols, and damage to human cells is believed to occur through the same mechanism of action.

Activity *in vitro* and *in vivo*

ABELCET® shows *in vitro* activity against *Aspergillus* sp. (n=3) and *Candida* sp. (n=10), with MICs generally <1 μg/mL. Depending upon the species and strain of *Aspergillus* and *Candida* tested, significant *in vitro* differences in susceptibility to amphotericin B have been reported (MICs ranging from 0.1 to >10 μg/mL). However, standardized techniques for susceptibility testing for antifungal agents have not been established, and results of susceptibility studies do not necessarily correlate with clinical outcome.

ABELCET® is active in animal models against *Aspergillus fumigatus, Candida albicans, C. guillermondii, C. stellatoideae,* and *C. tropicalis, Cryptococcus sp., Coccidioidomyces sp., Histoplasma sp., and Blastomyces sp.* in which endpoints were clearance of microorganisms from target organ(s) and/or prolonged survival of infected animals.

Drug Resistance

Fungal species with decreased susceptibility to amphotericin B have been isolated after serial passage in culture media containing the drug, and from some patients receiving prolonged therapy. Although the relevance of drug resistance to clinical outcome has not been established, fungal species which are resistant to amphotericin B may also be resistant to ABELCET®.

CLINICAL PHARMACOLOGY

Pharmacokinetics

The assay used to measure amphotericin B in the blood after the administration of ABELCET® does not distinguish amphotericin B that is complexed with the phospholipids of ABELCET® from amphotericin B that is uncomplexed.

The pharmacokinetics of amphotericin B after the administration of ABELCET® are nonlinear. Volume of distribution and clearance from blood increase with increasing dose of ABELCET®, resulting in less than proportional increases in blood concentrations of amphotericin B over a dose range of 0.6–5 mg/kg/day. The pharmacokinetics of amphotericin B in whole blood after the administration of ABELCET® and amphotericin B desoxycholate are:

[See table above]

The large volume of distribution and high clearance from blood of amphotericin B after the administration of ABELCET® probably reflect uptake by tissues. The long terminal elimination half-life probably reflects a slow redistribution from tissues. Although amphotericin B is excreted slowly, there is little accumulation in the blood after repeated dosing. AUC of amphotericin B increased approximately 34% from day 1 after the administration of ABELCET® 5 mg/kg/day for 7 days. The effect of gender or ethnicity on the pharmacokinetics of ABELCET® has not been studied.

Tissue concentrations of amphotericin B have been obtained at autopsy from one heart transplant patient who received three doses of ABELCET® at 5.3 mg/kg/day:

Concentration in Human Tissues

Organ	Amphotericin B Tissue Concentration (μg/g)
Spleen	290
Lung	222
Liver	196
Lymph Node	7.6
Kidney	6.9
Heart	5
Brain	1.6

This pattern of distribution is consistent with that observed in preclinical studies in dogs in which greatest concentrations of amphotericin B after ABELCET® administration were observed in the liver, spleen, and lung; however, the relationship of tissue concentrations of amphotericin B to its biological activity when administered as ABELCET® is unknown.

Special Populations

Hepatic Impairment: The effect of hepatic impairment on the disposition of ABELCET® is not known.

Renal Impairment: The effect of renal impairment on the disposition of ABELCET® is not known. The effect of dialysis on the elimination of ABELCET® has not been studied; however, amphotericin B is not removed by hemodialysis when administered as amphotericin B desoxycholate.

Pediatric and Elderly Patients: The pharmacokinetics and pharmacodynamics of pediatric patients (≤16 years of age) and elderly patients (≥65 years of age) have not been studied.

INDICATIONS AND USAGE

ABELCET® is indicated for the treatment of invasive fungal infections in patients who are refractory to or intolerant of conventional amphotericin B therapy. This is based on open-label treatment of patients judged by their physicians to be intolerant to or failing conventional amphotericin B therapy (See DESCRIPTION OF CLINICAL STUDIES).

Pharmacokinetic Parameters of Amphotericin B in Whole Blood in Patients Administered Multiple Doses of ABELCET® or Amphotericin B Desoxycholate

Pharmacokinetic Parameter	ABELCET® 5 mg/kg/day for 5–7 days Mean ± SD	Amphotericin B 0.6 mg/kg/day for 42 days[a] Mean ± SD
Peak Concentration (μg/mL)	1.7 ± 0.8 (n=10)[b]	1.1 ± 0.2 (n=5)
Concentration at End of Dosing Interval (μg/mL)	0.6 ± 0.3 (n=10)[b]	0.4 ± 0.2 (n=5)
Area Under Blood Concentration-Time Curve (AUC_{0-24h}) (μg*h/mL)	14 ± 7 (n=14)[b,c]	17.1 ± 5 (n=5)
Clearance (mL/h*kg)	436 ± 188.5 (n=14)[b,c]	38 ± 15 (n=5)
Apparent Volume of Distribution (Vd_{area}) (L/kg)	131 ± 57.7 (n=8)[c]	5 ± 2.8 (n=5)
Terminal Elimination Half-Life (h)	173.4 ± 78 (n=8)[c]	91.1 ± 40.9 (n=5)
Amount Excreted in Urine Over 24 h After Last Dose (% of dose)[d]	0.9 ± 0.4 (n=8)[c]	9.6 ± 2.5 (n=8)

[a] Data from patients with mucocutaneous leishmaniasis. Infusion rate was 0.25 mg/kg/h.

[b] Data from studies in patients with cytologically proven cancer being treated with chemotherapy or neutropenic patients with presumed or proven fungal infection. Infusion rate was 2.5 mg/kg/h.

[c] Data from patients with mucocutaneous leishmaniasis. Infusion rate was 4 mg/kg/h.

[d] Percentage of dose excreted in 24 hours after last dose.

DESCRIPTION OF CLINICAL STUDIES

Fungal Infections

Data from 473 patients were pooled from three open-label studies in which ABELCET® was provided for the treatment of patients with invasive fungal infections who were judged by their physicians to be refractory to or intolerant of conventional amphotericin B, or who had preexisting nephrotoxicity. Results of these studies demonstrated effectiveness of ABELCET® in the treatment of invasive fungal infections as a second line therapy.

Patients were defined by their individual physician as being refractory to or failing conventional amphotericin B therapy based on overall clinical judgement after receiving a minimum total dose of 500 mg of amphotericin B. Nephrotoxicity was defined as a serum creatinine that had increased to >2.5 mg/dL in adults and >1.5 mg/dL in pediatric patients, or a creatinine clearance of <25 mL/min while receiving conventional amphotericin B therapy.

Of the 473 patients, four were enrolled more than once; each enrollment contributed separately to the denominator. The median age was 39 years (range of <1 to 93 years); 307 patients were male and 166 female. Patients were Caucasian (381, 81%), African-American (41, 9%), Hispanic (27, 6%), Asian (10, 2%), and various other races (14, 3%). The median baseline neutrophil count was 4,000 PMN/mm^3; of these, 101 (21%) had a baseline neutrophil count <500/mm^3.

Two-hundred eighty-two patients of the 473 patients were considered evaluable for response to therapy; the other 191 patients were excluded on the basis of unconfirmed diagnosis, confounding factors, concomitant systemic antifungal therapy, or receiving 4 doses or less of ABELCET®. For evaluable patients, the following fungal infections were treated (n=282): aspergillosis (n=111), candidiasis (n=87), zygomycosis (n=25), cryptococcosis (n=16), and fusariosis (n=11). There were fewer than 10 evaluable patients for each of several other fungal species treated.

For each type of fungal infection listed above there were some patients successfully treated. However, in the absence of controlled studies it is unknown how response would have compared to either continuing conventional amphotericin B therapy or the use of alternative antifungal agents.

Renal Function: Patients with aspergillosis who initiated treatment with ABELCET® when serum creatinine was above 2.5 mg/dL experienced a decline in serum creatinine during treatment (Figure 1). Serum creatinine levels were also lower during treatment with ABELCET® when compared to the serum creatinine levels of patients treated with conventional amphotericin B in a retrospective historical control study. Meaningful statistical testing of the differences between these two groups is precluded since these data were obtained from two separate studies.

Figure 1
Changes in Mean Serum Creatinine Over Time
Patients with Aspergillosis and Serum Creatinine >2.5 mg/dL at Baseline

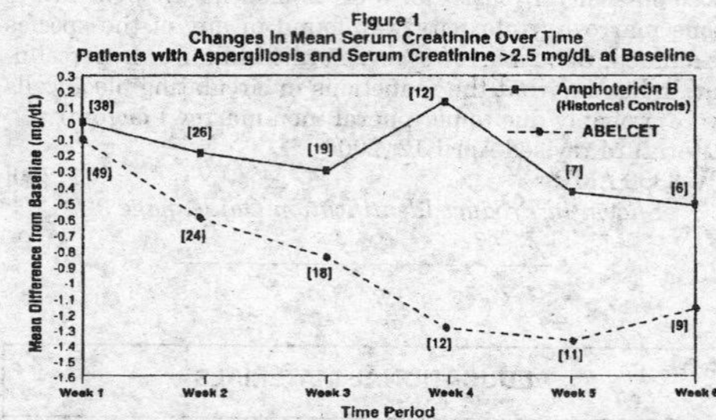

[ ]= Number of patients at each time point.
Note: These curves do not represent the clinical course of a given patient, but that of an open-label cohort of patients.

[See figure 2 at top of next column]

In a randomized study of ABELCET® for the treatment of invasive candidiasis in patients with normal baseline renal function, the incidence of nephrotoxicity was significantly less for ABELCET® at a dose of 5 mg/kg/day than for conventional amphotericin B at a dose of 0.7 mg/kg/day.

Despite generally less nephrotoxicity of ABELCET® observed at a dose of 5 mg/kg/day compared with conventional

Figure 2
Changes in Mean Serum Creatinine Over Time
Patients with Fungal Infections and Serum Creatinine >2.5 mg/dL at Baseline

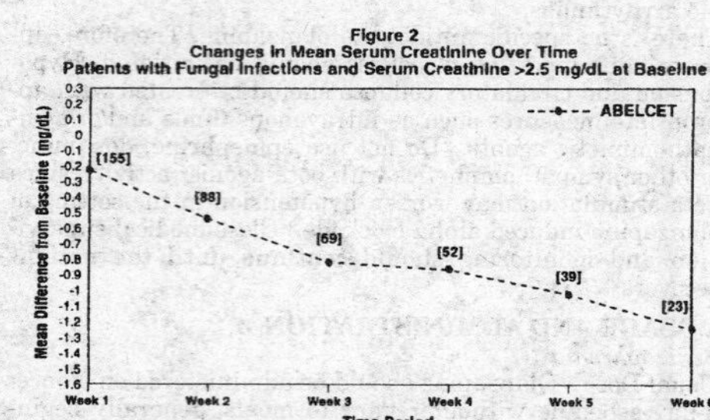

[ ]= Number of patients at each time point.
Note: These curves do not represent the clinical course of a given patient, but that of an open-label cohort of patients.

amphotericin B therapy at a dose range of 0.6–1 mg/kg/day, dose-limiting renal toxicity may still be observed with ABELCET®. Renal toxicity of doses greater than 5 mg/kg/day of ABELCET® has not been formally studied.

CONTRAINDICATIONS

ABELCET® is contraindicated in patients who have shown hypersensitivity to amphotericin B or any other component in the formulation.

WARNINGS

Anaphylaxis has been reported with amphotericin B desoxycholate and other amphotericin B-containing drugs. Anaphylaxis has been reported with ABELCET® with an incidence rate of <0.1%. If severe respiratory distress occurs, the infusion should be immediately discontinued. The patient should not receive further infusions of ABELCET®.

PRECAUTIONS

General: As with any amphotericin B-containing product, during the initial dosing of ABELCET®, the drug should be administered under close clinical observation by medically trained personnel.

Acute reactions including fever and chills may occur 1 to 2 hours after starting an intravenous infusion of ABELCET®. These reactions are usually more common with the first few doses of ABELCET® and generally diminish with subsequent doses. Infusion has been rarely associated with hypotension, bronchospasm, arrhythmias, and shock.

Laboratory Tests: Serum creatinine should be monitored frequently during ABELCET® therapy (see ADVERSE REACTIONS). It is also advisable to regularly monitor liver function, serum electrolytes (particularly magnesium and potassium), and complete blood counts.

Drug Interactions: No formal clinical studies of drug interactions have been conducted with ABELCET®. However, when administered concomitantly, the following drugs are known to interact with amphotericin B; therefore, the following drugs may interact with ABELCET®:

Antineoplastic agents: Concurrent use of antineoplastic agents and amphotericin B may enhance the potential for renal toxicity, bronchospasm, and hypotension. Antineoplastic agents should be given concomitantly with ABELCET® with great caution.

Corticosteroids and corticotropin (ACTH): Concurrent use of corticosteroids and corticotropin (ACTH) with amphotericin B may potentiate hypokalemia which could predispose the patient to cardiac dysfunction. If used concomitantly with ABELCET®, serum electrolytes and cardiac function should be closely monitored.

Cyclosporin A: Data from a prospective study of prophylactic ABELCET® in 22 patients undergoing bone marrow transplantation suggested that concurrent initiation of cyclosporin A and ABELCET® within several days of bone marrow ablation may be associated with increased nephrotoxicity.

Digitalis glycosides: Concurrent use of amphotericin B may induce hypokalemia and may potentiate digitalis toxicity. When administered concomitantly with ABELCET®, serum potassium levels should be closely monitored.

Flucytosine: Concurrent use of flucytosine with amphotericin B-containing preparations may increase the toxicity of

flucytosine by possibly increasing its cellular uptake and/or impairing its renal excretion. Flucytosine should be given concomitantly with ABELCET® with caution.
Imidazoles (e.g., ketoconazole, miconazole, clotrimazole, fluconazole, etc): Antagonism between amphotericin B and imidazole derivatives such as miconazole and ketoconazole, which inhibit ergosterol synthesis, has been reported in both *in vitro* and *in vivo* animal studies. The clinical significance of these findings has not been determined.
Leukocyte transfusions: Acute pulmonary toxicity has been reported in patients receiving intravenous amphotericin B and leukocyte transfusions. Leukocyte transfusions and ABELCET® should not be given concurrently.
Other nephrotoxic medications: Concurrent use of amphotericin B and agents such as aminoglycosides and pentamidine may enhance the potential for drug-induced renal toxicity. Aminoglycosides and pentamidine should be used concomitantly with ABELCET® only with great caution. Intensive monitoring of renal function is recommended in patients requiring any combination of nephrotoxic medications.
Skeletal muscle relaxants: Amphotericin B-induced hypokalemia may enhance the curariform effect of skeletal muscle relaxants (e.g., tubocurarine) due to hypokalemia. When administered concomitantly with ABELCET®, serum potassium levels should be closely monitored.
Zidovudine: Increased myelotoxicity and nephrotoxicity were observed in dogs when either ABELCET® (at doses of 0.16 or 0.5 times the recommended human dose) or amphotericin B desoxycholate (at 0.5 times the recommended human dose) were administered concomitantly with zidovudine for 30 days. If zidovudine is used concomitantly with ABELCET®, renal hematologic function should be closely monitored.

Carcinogenesis, Mutagenesis, and Impairment of Fertility: No long-term studies in animals have been performed to evaluate the carcinogenic potential of ABELCET®. The following *in vitro* (with and without metabolic activation) and *in vivo* studies to assess ABELCET® for mutagenic potential were conducted: bacterial reverse mutation assay, mouse lymphoma forward mutation assay, chromosomal aberration assay in CHO cells, and *in vivo* mouse micronucleus assay. ABELCET® was found to be without mutagenic effects in all assay systems. Studies demonstrated that ABELCET® had no impact on fertility in male and female rats at doses up to 0.32 times the recommended human dose (based on body surface area considerations).

Pregnancy: There are no reports of pregnant women having been treated with ABELCET®. Teratogenic Effects. Pregnancy Category B: Reproductive studies in rats and rabbits at doses of ABELCET® up to 0.64 times the human dose revealed no harm to the fetus. Because animal reproductive studies are not always predictive of human response, and adequate and well-controlled studies have not been conducted in pregnant women, ABELCET® should be used during pregnancy only after taking into account the importance of the drug to the mother.

Nursing Mothers: It is not known whether ABELCET® is excreted in human milk. Because many drugs are excreted in human milk, and because of the potential for serious adverse reactions in breast-fed infants from ABELCET®, a decision should be made whether to discontinue nursing or to discontinue the drug, taking into account the importance of the drug to the mother.

Pediatric Use: One hundred eleven children (2 were enrolled twice and counted as separate patients), age 16 years and under, of whom 11 were less than 1 year, have been treated with ABELCET® at 5 mg/kg/day in two open-label studies and one small, prospective, single-arm study. In one single-center study, 5 children with hepatosplenic candidiasis were effectively treated with 2.5 mg/kg/day of ABELCET®. No serious unexpected adverse events have been reported.

Geriatric Use: Forty-nine elderly patients, age 65 years or over, have been treated with ABELCET® at 5 mg/kg/day in two open-label studies and one small, prospective, single-arm study. No serious unexpected adverse events have been reported.

ADVERSE REACTIONS

The total safety data base is composed of 921 patients treated with ABELCET® (5 patients were enrolled twice and counted as separate patients), of whom 775 were treated with 5 mg/kg/day. Of these 775 patients, 194 patients were treated in four comparative studies; 25 were treated in open-label, non-comparative studies; and 556 patients were treated in an open-label, emergency-use program. Most had underlying hematologic neoplasms, and many were receiving multiple concomitant medications. Of the 556 patients treated with ABELCET®, 9% discontinued treatment due to adverse events regardless of presumed relationship to study drug.
In general, the adverse events most commonly reported with ABELCET® were transient chills and/or fever during infusion of the drug.

Adverse Events[a] with an Incidence of ≥3% (N=556)

Adverse Event	Percentage (%) of Patients
Chills	18
Fever	14
Increased Serum Creatinine	11
Multiple Organ Failure	11
Nausea	9
Hypotension	8
Respiratory Failure	8
Vomiting	8
Dyspnea	7
Sepsis	7
Diarrhea	6
Headache	6
Heart Arrest	6
Hypertension	5
Hypokalemia	5
Infection	5
Kidney Failure	5
Pain	5
Thrombocytopenia	5
Abdominal Pain	4
Anemia	4
Bilirubinemia	4
Gastrointestinal Hemorrhage	4
Leukopenia	4
Rash	4
Respiratory Disorder	4
Chest Pain	3
Nausea and Vomiting	3

[a] The causal association between these adverse events and ABELCET® is uncertain.

The following adverse events have also been reported in patients using ABELCET® in open-label, uncontrolled clinical studies. The causal association between these adverse events and ABELCET® is uncertain.
Body as a whole: malaise, weight loss, deafness, injection site reaction including inflammation
Allergic: bronchospasm, wheezing, asthma, anaphylactoid and other allergic reactions
Cardiopulmonary: cardiac failure, pulmonary edema, shock, myocardial infarction, hemoptysis, tachypnea, thrombophlebitis, pulmonary embolus, cardiomyopathy, pleural effusion, arrhythmias including ventricular fibrillation
Dermatological: maculopapular rash, pruritus, exfoliative dermatitis, erythema multiforme
Gastrointestinal: acute liver failure, hepatitis, jaundice, melena, anorexia, dyspepsia, cramping, epigastric pain, veno-occlusive liver disease, diarrhea, hepatomegaly, cholangitis, cholecystitis
Hematologic: coagulation defects, leukocytosis, blood dyscrasias including eosinophilia
Musculoskeletal: myasthenia, including bone, muscle, and joint pains
Neurologic: convulsions, tinnitus, visual impairment, hearing loss, peripheral neuropathy, transient vertigo, diplopia, encephalopathy, cerebral vascular accident, extrapyramidal syndrome and other neurologic symptoms
Urogenital: oliguria, decreased renal function, anuria, renal tubular acidosis, impotence, dysuria
Serum electrolyte abnormalities: hypomagnesemia, hyperkalemia, hypocalcemia, hypercalcemia
Liver function test abnormalities: increased AST, ALT, alkaline phosphatase, LDH
Renal function test abnormalities: increased BUN
Other test abnormalities: acidosis, hyperamylasemia, hypoglycemia, hyperglycemia, hyperuricemia, hypophosphatemia

OVERDOSAGE

Amphotericin B desoxycholate overdose has been reported to result in cardio-respiratory arrest. Fifteen patients have been reported to have received one or more doses of ABELCET® between 7–13 mg/kg. None of these patients had a serious acute reaction to ABELCET®. If an overdose is suspected, discontinue therapy, monitor the patient's clinical status, and administer supportive therapy as required. ABELCET® is not hemodialyzable.

DOSAGE AND ADMINISTRATION

The recommended daily dosage for adults and children is 5 mg/kg given as a single infusion. ABELCET® should be administered by intravenous infusion at a rate of 2.5 mg/kg/h. If the infusion time exceeds 2 hours, mix the contents by shaking the infusion bag every 2 hours.
Renal toxicity of ABELCET®, as measured by serum creatinine levels, has been shown to be dose dependent. Decisions about dose adjustments should be made only after taking into account the overall clinical condition of the patient.

Preparation of Admixture for Infusion: Shake the vial gently until there is no evidence of any yellow sediment at the bottom. Withdraw the appropriate dose of ABELCET® from the required number of vials into one or more sterile syringes using an 18-gauge needle. Remove the needle from each syringe filled with ABELCET® and replace with the 5-micron filter needle supplied with each vial. Each filter needle may be used to filter the contents of up to four 100 mg vials or eight 50 mg vials. Insert the filter needle of the syringe into an IV bag containing 5% Dextrose Injection USP, and empty the contents of the syringe into the bag. The final infusion concentration should be 1 mg/mL. For pediatric patients and patients with cardiovascular disease the drug may be diluted with 5% Dextrose Injection to a final infusion concentration of 2 mg/mL. Before infusion, shake the bag until the contents are thoroughly mixed. Do not use the admixture after dilution with 5% Dextrose Injection if there is any evidence of foreign matter. Vials are for single use. Unused material should be discarded. Aseptic technique must be strictly observed throughout handling of ABELCET®, since no bacteriostatic agent or preservative is present.
DO NOT DILUTE WITH SALINE SOLUTIONS OR MIX WITH OTHER DRUGS OR ELECTROLYTES as the compatibility of ABELCET® with these materials has not been established. An existing intravenous line should be flushed with 5% Dextrose Injection before infusion of ABELCET®, or a separate infusion line should be used. DO NOT USE AN IN-LINE FILTER.
The diluted ready-for-use admixture is stable for up to 48 hours at 2° to 8°C (36° to 46°F) and an additional 6 hours at room temperature.

HOW SUPPLIED

Single-use vials along with 5-micron filter needles are individually packaged.
100 mg of ABELCET® in 20 mL of suspension NDC 61799-101-41
50 mg of ABELCET® in 10 mL of suspension NDC 61799-101-31

STORAGE

Prior to admixture, ABELCET® should be stored at 2° to 8°C (36° to 46°F) and protected from exposure to light. Do not freeze. ABELCET® should be retained in the carton until time of use.
The admixed ABELCET® and 5% Dextrose Injection may be stored for up to 48 hours at 2° to 8° (36° to 46°F) and an additional 6 hours at room temperature. Do not freeze. Any unused material should be discarded.
U.S. Patent Nos. 4,973,465
5,616,334
The Liposome Company, Inc. 9/99
Princeton, NJ, USA I-101-41-US-H
Shown in Product Identification Guide, page 321

Lotus Biochemical Corporation

P.O. BOX 3586
RADFORD, VA 24143

Direct Inquiries to:
Jay Kirk
(800) 455-5525
FAX: (800) 962-2200

For Medical Information Contact:
In Emergencies:
Lawrence P. Olon
(423) 989-9190
FAX: (423) 989-3532

EASPRIN® ℞

[ē-ăsprin]
(Aspirin Delayed-release Tablets, USP)
Enteric Coated Tablets

DESCRIPTION

Easprin®, Aspirin Delayed-release Tablets, USP, enteric coated (E/C), contain 975 mg (15 grains) aspirin for oral administration. The enteric coating is designed to prevent the release of aspirin in the stomach and thereby reduce gastric irritation and total occult blood loss. The pharmacologic effects of aspirin include analgesia, antipyresis, antiinflammatory activity, and antirheumatic activity. The structural formula of aspirin (salicylic acid acetate) is:

$C_9H_8O_4$
MOL. WT. 180.16
COOH
$OCOCH_3$

INACTIVE INGREDIENTS

Microcrystalline cellulose, starch, croscarmellose sodium, silicon dioxide, talc, shellac, titanium dioxide, hydroxypropyl methylcellulose phthalate, polyvinyl acetate phthalate, cellulose acetate phthalate.

CLINICAL PHARMACOLOGY

Aspirin is a salicylate that has demonstrated antiinflammatory, analgesic, antipyretic, and antirheumatic activity.
Aspirin's mode of action as an antiinflammatory and antirheumatic agent may be due to inhibition of synthesis and release of prostaglandins.
Aspirin appears to produce analgesia by virtue of both a peripheral and CNS effect. Peripherally, aspirin acts by inhibiting the synthesis and release of prostaglandins. Acting centrally, it would appear to produce analgesia at a hypothalamic site in the brain, although the mode of action is not known.
Aspirin also acts on the hypothalamus to produce antipyresis; heat dissipation is increased as a result of vasodilation and increased peripheral blood flow. Aspirin's antipyretic activity may also be related to inhibition of synthesis and release of prostaglandins.
EASPRIN Tablets are enteric coated. This coating acts to prevent the release of aspirin in the stomach but permits

Continued on next page

Easprin—Cont.

the tablet to dissolve with resultant absorption in the upper portion of the small intestine. This reduces any gastric irritation that may occur with uncoated aspirin but does delay the onset of action. Aspirin is rapidly hydrolyzed primarily in the liver to salicylic acid, which is conjugated with glycine (forming salicyluric acid) and glucuronic acid and excreted largely in the urine. As a result of the rapid hydrolysis, plasma concentrations of aspirin are always low and rarely exceed 20 mcg/ml at ordinary therapeutic doses. The peak salicylate level for uncoated aspirin occurs in about 2 hours, however, with enteric coated aspirin tablets this is delayed. A direct correlation between salicylate plasma levels and clinical analgesic effectiveness has not been definitely established, but effective analgesia is usually achieved at plasma levels of 15 to 30 mg per 100 ml. Effective antiinflammatory activity is usually achieved at salicylate plasma levels of 20 to 30 mg per 100 ml. There is also poor correlation between toxic symptoms and plasma salicylate concentrations, but most patients exhibit symptoms of salicylism at plasma salicylate levels of 35 mg per 100 ml. The plasma half-life for aspirin is approximately 15 minutes; that for salicylate lengthens as the dose increases. Doses of 300 to 600 mg have a half-life of 3.1 to 3.2 hours, with doses of 1 gram, the half-life is increased to 5 hours and with 2 grams it is increased to about 9 hours.

Salicylates are excreted mainly by the kidney. Studies in man indicate that salicylate is excreted in the urine as free salicylic acid (10%), salicyluric acid (75%), salicylic phenolic (10%), and acyl (5%) glucuronides and gentisic acid.

INDICATIONS AND USAGE

EASPRIN Tablet indicated in patients who need the higher 975 mg dose of aspirin in the long-term palliative treatment of mild to moderate pain and inflammation of arthritic and other inflammatory conditions.

CONTRAINDICATIONS

EASPRIN Tablet should not be used in patients who have previously exhibited hypersensitivity to aspirin and/or nonsteroidal antiinflammatory agents.

EASPRIN Tablets should not be given to patients with a recent history of gastrointestinal bleeding or in patients with bleeding disorders (eg, hemophilia).

WARNINGS

EASPRIN Tablets should be used with caution when anticoagulants are prescribed concurrently, for aspirin may depress the concentration of prothrombin in plasma and thereby increase bleeding time. Large doses of salicylates have a hypoglycemic action and may enhance the effect of the oral hypoglycemics. Consequently, they should not be given concomitantly; if however, this is necessary, the dosage of the hypoglycemic agent must be reduced while the salicylate is given. This hypoglycemic action may also effect the insulin requirements of diabetics.

Although salicylates in large doses are uricosuric agents, smaller amounts may decrease the uricosuric effects of probenecid, sulfinpyrazone, and phenylbutazone.

PRECAUTIONS

General: EASPRIN Tablets should be administered with caution to patients with asthma, nasal polyps, or nasal allergies.

In patients receiving large doses of aspirin and/or prolonged therapy, mild salicylate intoxication (salicylism) may develop that may be reversed by reduction in dosage.

Although the fecal blood loss with EASPRIN Tablets is less than that with uncoated aspirin tablets, EASPRIN Tablets should be administered with caution to patients with a history of gastric distress, ulcer, or bleeding problems. Occult gastrointestinal bleeding occurs in many patients but is not correlated with gastric distress. The amount of blood lost is usually insignificant clinically, but with prolonged administration, it may result in iron deficiency anemia.

Sodium excretion produced by spironolactone may be decreased in the presence of salicylates.

Salicylates can produce changes in thyroid function tests.

Salicylates should be used with caution in patients with severe hepatic damage, pre-existing hypoprothrombinemia or K deficiency, and in those undergoing surgery.

DRUG INTERACTIONS:

Anticoagulants: See WARNINGS.

Hypoglycemic Agents: See WARNINGS.

Uricosuric Agents: Aspirin may decrease the effects of probenecid, sulfinpyrazone, and phenylbutazone.

Spironolactone: See General PRECAUTIONS above.

Alcohol: Has a synergistic effect with aspirin in causing gastrointestinal bleeding.

Corticosteroids: Concomitant administration with aspirin may increase the risk of gastrointestinal ulceration.

Pyrazolone Derivatives (phenylbutazone, oxyphenbutazone, and possibly dipyrone): Concomitant administration with aspirin may increase the risk of gastrointestinal ulceration.

Nonsteroidal Antiinflammatory Agents: Aspirin is contraindicated in patients who are hypersensitive to nonsteroidal antiinflammatory agents.

Urinary Alkalinizers: Decrease aspirin effectiveness by increasing the rate of salicylate renal excretion.

Phenobarbital: Decreases aspirin effectiveness by enzyme induction.

Propranolol: May decrease aspirin's antiinflammatory action by competing for the same receptors.

Antacid: EASPRIN Tablets should not be given concurrently with antacids, since an increase in the pH of the stomach may effect the enteric coating of the tablets.

Usage in Pregnancy: Aspirin does not appear to have any teratogenic effects. However, it has been reported that adverse effects were increased in the mother and fetus following chronic ingestion of aspirin. Prolonged pregnancy and labor with increased bleeding before and after delivery, as well as decreased birth weight and increased risk of stillbirth were correlated with high blood salicylate levels. Because of possible adverse effects on the neonate and the potential for increased maternal blood loss, aspirin should be avoided during the last three months of pregnancy.

ADVERSE REACTIONS

Gastrointestinal: Dyspepsia, nausea, vomiting, diarrhea, gastrointestinal bleeding, and/or ulceration.

Ear: Tinnitus, vertigo, reversible hearing loss.

Hematologic: Prolongation of bleeding time, leukopenia, thrombocytopenia, purpura, decreased plasma iron concentration and shortened erythrocyte survival time.

Dermatologic and Hypersensitivity: Urticaria, angioedema, pruritus, various skin eruptions, asthma, and anaphylaxis.

Miscellaneous: Acute reversible hepatotoxicity, mental confusion, drowsiness, sweating, dizziness, headache, fever, thirst, and dimness of vision.

OVERDOSAGE

Overdosage of 200 to 500 mg/kg is in the fatal range. Early symptoms are CNS stimulation with vomiting, hyperpnea, hyperactivity, and possibly convulsions. This progresses quickly to depression, coma, respiratory failure, and collapse. These symptoms are accompanied by severe electrolyte disturbances.

In the treatment of salicylate overdosage, intensive supportive therapy should be instituted immediately. Plasma salicylate levels should be measured in order to determine the severity of the poisoning and to provide a guide for therapy. Emptying of the stomach should be accomplished as soon as possible with ipecac syrup unless the patient is depressed. In depressed patients use airway protected gastric lavage. Delay absorption with activated charcoal and give a saline cathartic. Proceed according to Standard Reference Procedures for Salicylate intoxication.

DOSAGE AND ADMINISTRATION

Usual Adult Dosage: One tablet 3 to 4 times daily.

Patients who have displayed no significant adverse effects on a long term qid regimen and who receive a total daily dosage of aspirin no greater than 3.9 grams may be considered for a bid regimen (2 EASPRIN Tablets twice daily). Patients on the bid regimen should be closely monitored for serum salicylate levels, increased incidence of CNS-related adverse effects, increased fecal blood loss, or any other signs or symptoms suggestive of significant blood loss.

If necessary, dosage may be increased until relief is obtained, but dosage should be maintained slightly below that which produces tinnitus. Plasma salicylate levels may also be helpful in determining proper dosage (see Clinical Pharmacology section).

HOW SUPPLIED

EASPRIN Tablets, white, imprinted, each containing 975 mg (15 grains) aspirin are available in bottles of 100's (NDC 59417-975-71).

Storage: Store at controlled room temperature 15°–30°C (59°–86°F).

Rx only

Manufactured for:
LOTUS BIOCHEMICAL CORPORATION
Radford, VA 24143, USA
By:
Time-Cap Labs, Inc.
Farmingdale, NY 11735, USA

Rev. 07/98

ERGOMAR® Sublingual Tablets, 2 mg ℞

[*er 'go-mar"*]
(ergotamine tartrate tablets, USP)

DESCRIPTION

Each sublingual tablet of ERGOMAR contains 2 mg ergotamine tartrate, USP.

Inactive Ingredients: Corn starch, D & C Yellow No. 10, FD & C Blue No. 1, lactose monohydrate NF, magnesium stearate, peppermint oil, saccharin sodium.

Pharmacological Category: Vasoconstrictor, uterine stimulant, alpha adrenoreceptor antagonist.

Therapeutic Class: Anti-migraine.

Chemical Name: Ergotaman-3′,6′, 18-trione, 12′-hydroxy-2′-methyl-5′-(phenyl-methyl)-,(5′α)-,[R-(R*,R*)]-2, 3-dihydroxybutanedioate(2:1)(tartrate).

Structural Formula:

[See chemical structure at top of next column]

CLINICAL PHARMACOLOGY

The pharmacological properties of ergotamine are extremely complex; some of its actions are unrelated to each other, and even mutually antagonistic. The drug has partial agonist and/or antagonist activity against tryptaminergic, dopaminergic and alpha adrenergic receptors depending

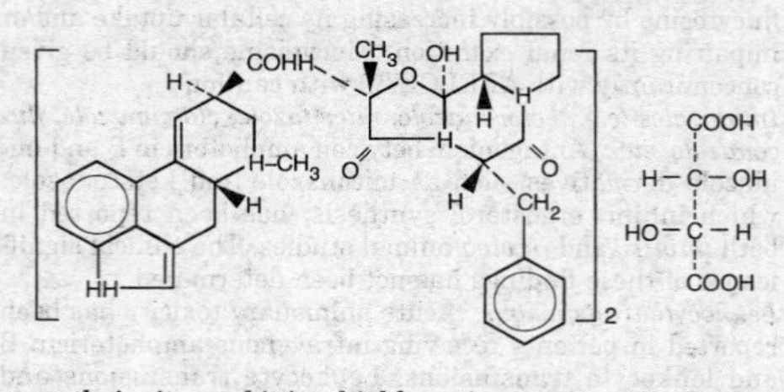

upon their site, and it is a highly active uterine stimulant. It causes constriction of peripheral and cranial blood vessels and produces depression of central vasomotor centers. The pain of a migraine attack is believed to be due to greatly increased amplitude of pulsations in the cranial arteries, especially the meningeal branches of the external carotid artery. Ergotamine reduces extracranial blood flow, causes a decline in the amplitude of pulsation in the cranial arteries, and decreases hyperperfusion of the territory of the basilar artery. It does not reduce cerebral hemispheric blood flow.

Long term usage has established the fact that ergotamine tartrate is effective in controlling up to 70% of acute migraine attacks, so that it is now considered specific for the treatment of this headache syndrome. Ergotamine produces constriction of both arteries and veins. In doses used in the treatment of vascular headaches, ergotamine usually produces only small increases in blood pressure but it does increase peripheral resistance and decrease blood flow in various organs. Small doses of the drug increase the force and frequency of uterine contraction; larger doses increase the resting tone of the uterus also. The gravid uterus is particularly sensitive to these effects of ergotamine. Although specific teratogenic effects attributable to ergotamine have not been found, the fetus suffers if ergotamine is given to the mother. Retarded fetal growth and an increase in intrauterine death and resorption have been seen in animals. These are thought to result from ergotamine induced increases in uterine motility and vasoconstriction in the placental vascular bed.

The bioavailability of sublingually administered ergotamine has not been determined.

Ergotamine is metabolized by the liver by largely undefined pathways, and 90% of the metabolites are excreted in the bile. The unmetabolized drug is erratically secreted in the saliva, and only traces of unmetabolized drug appear in the urine and feces. Ergotamine is secreted into breast milk. The elimination half-life of ergotamine from plasma is about 2 hours, but the drug may be stored in some tissues, which would account for its long lasting therapeutic and toxic actions.

INDICATIONS AND USAGE

ERGOMAR is indicated as therapy to abort or prevent vascular headache, e.g., migraine, migraine variants, or so called "histaminic cephalalgia."

CONTRAINDICATIONS

ERGOMAR is contraindicated in peripheral vascular disease (thromboangitis obliterans, luetic arteritis, severe arteriosclerosis, thrombophlebitis, Raynaud's disease), coronary heart disease, hypertension, impaired hepatic or renal function, severe pruritis, and sepsis. It is also contraindicated in patients who are hypersensitive to any of its components. ERGOMAR may cause fetal harm when administered to a pregnant woman by virtue of its powerful uterine stimulant actions. ERGOMAR is contraindicated in women who are, or may become, pregnant.

PRECAUTIONS

General: Although signs and symptoms of ergotism rarely develop even after long term intermittent use of ergotamine, care should be exercised to remain within the limits of recommended dosage.

Drug Interactions: The effects of ERGOMAR may be potentiated by triacetyloleandomycin which inhibits the metabolism of ergotamine. The pressor effects of ERGOMAR and other vasoconstrictor drugs can combine to cause dangerous hypertension.

Carcinogenesis: No studies have been performed to investigate ERGOMAR for carcinogenic effects.

Pregnancy: Pregnancy Category X—See CONTRAINDICATIONS section.

Nursing Mothers: Ergotamine is secreted into human milk. It can reach the breast-fed infant by this route and exert pharmacologic effects in it. Caution should be exercised when ERGOMAR is administered to a nursing woman. Excessive dosing or prolonged administration of ergotamine may inhibit lactation.

ADVERSE REACTIONS

Nausea and vomiting occur in up to 10% of patients after ingestion of therapeutic doses of ergotamine. Weakness of the legs and pain in limb muscles are also frequent complaints. Numbness and tingling of the fingers and toes, precordial pain, transient changes in heart rate and localized edema and itching may also occur, particularly in patients who are sensitive to the drug.

DRUG ABUSE AND DEPENDENCE

Patients who take ergotamine for extended periods of time may become dependent upon it and require progressively increasing doses for relief of vascular headaches, and for prevention of dysphoric effects which follow withdrawal of the drug.

OVERDOSAGE

Overdosage with ergotamine causes nausea, vomiting, weakness of the legs, pain in limb muscles, numbness and tingling of the fingers and toes, precordial pain, tachycardia or bradycardia, hypertension or hypotension and localized edema and itching together with signs and symptoms of ischemia due to vasoconstriction of peripheral arteries and arterioles. The feet and hands become cold, pale and numb. Muscle pain occurs while walking and later at rest also. Gangrene may ensue. Confusion, depression, drowsiness and convulsions are occasional signs of ergotamine toxicity. Overdosage is particularly likely to occur in patients with sepsis or impaired renal or hepatic function. Patients with peripheral vascular disease are specially at risk of developing peripheral ischemia following treatment with ergotamine. Some cases of ergotamine poisoning have been reported in patients who have taken less than 5 mg of the drug. Usually, however, toxicity is seen in doses of ergotamine tartrate in excess of about 15 mg in 24 hours or 40 mg in a few days.

Treatment of ergotamine overdosage consists of the withdrawal of the drug followed by symptomatic measures including attempts to maintain an adequate circulation in the affected parts. Anticoagulant drugs, low molecular weight dextran and potent vasodilator drugs may all be beneficial. Intravenous infusion of sodium nitroprusside has also been reported to be successful. Vasodilators must be used with special care in the presence of hypotension.

Nausea and vomiting may be relieved by atropine or antiemetic compounds of the phenothiazine group. Ergotamine is dialyzable.

DOSAGE AND ADMINISTRATION

All efforts should be made to initiate therapy as soon as possible after the first symptoms of the attack are noted, since success is proportional to rapidity of treatment, and lower dosages will be effective. At the first sign of an attack or to relieve symptoms after onset of an attack one 2 mg tablet is placed under the tongue. Another tablet should be taken at half-hour intervals thereafter, if necessary, but dosage must not exceed three tablets in any 24 hour period. Dosage should be limited to not more than five tablets (10mg) in any one week.

HOW SUPPLIED

20 tablets (green) each containing 2 mg ergotamine tartrate, supplied in foil strips in a plastic child resistant container. Each tablet is debossed with the following product identification code: LB 2. Protect from light and heat. Keep out of the reach of children.

NDC 59417-120-20 Containers of 20.

CAUTION:

Rx only

Manufactured for:

LOTUS BIOCHEMICAL CORPORATION

Radford, VA 24143, USA

By: Mikart, Inc.

Atlanta, GA 30318 USA

Rev. 7/00

3M Pharmaceuticals

3M CENTER 275-2E-13
P.O. BOX 33275
ST. PAUL, MN 55133-3275

Commercial Customers:
Orders, Returns, Accounting
(800) 447-4537

Trade and Government:
(800) 328-6523

For Medical Matters Contact:
Drug Surveillance & Information
3M Pharmaceuticals
3M Center, Bldg. 275-2E-13
PO Box 33275
St. Paul MN, 55133-3275
(800) 328-0255
For Aldara™:
(800) 814-1795

In Emergencies:
(651) 736-4930 (all hours)

Website:
www.3M.com/pharma

ALDARA™ ℞

[al dar' a]
(imiquimod)
Cream, 5%
For Dermatologic Use Only - Not for Ophthalmic Use

DESCRIPTION

Aldara™ is the brand name for imiquimod which is an immune response modifier. Each gram of the 5% cream contains 50 mg of imiquimod in an off-white oil-in-water vanishing cream base consisting of isostearic acid, cetyl alcohol, stearyl alcohol, white pretrolatum, polysorbate 60, sorbitan monostearate, glycerin, xanthan gum, purified water, benzyl alcohol, methylparaben, and propylparaben.

Chemically, imiquimod is 1-(2-methylpropyl)-1*H*-imidazo[4,5-*c*]quinolin-4-amine. Imiquimod has a molecular formula of $C_{14}H_{16}N_4$ and a molecular weight of 240.3. Its structural formula is:

[Structural formula: NH2, N, CH3, CH3]

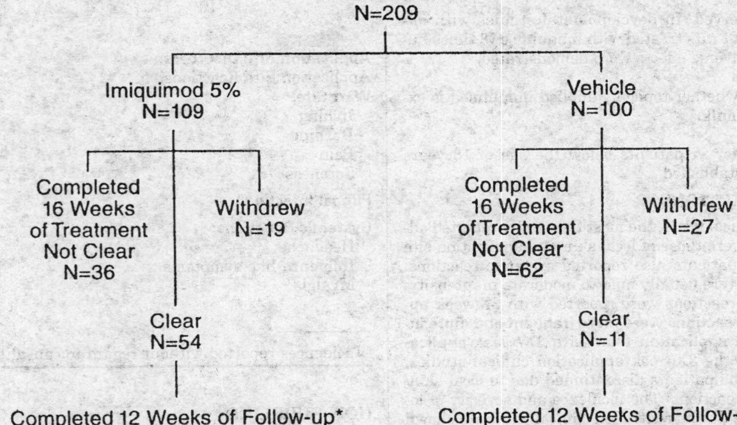

*The other patients were either lost to follow-up or experienced recurrences.

CLEARANCE—STUDY 1004

Treatment	Patients with Complete Clearance of Warts	Patients Without Follow-up	Patients with Warts Remaining at Week 16
Overall			
imiquimod 5% (N =109)	50%	17%	33%
vehicle (N =100)	11%	27%	62%
Females			
imiquimod 5% (N =46)	72%	11%	17%
vehicle (N =40)	20%	33%	48%
Males			
imiquimod 5% (N =63)	33%	22%	44%
vehicle (N =60)	5%	23%	72%

CLINICAL PHARMACOLOGY

Pharmacodynamics

The mechanism of action of imiquimod in treating genital/perianal warts is unknown. Imiquimod has no direct antiviral activity in cell culture. Mouse skin studies suggest that imiquimod induces cytokines including interferon-α. However, the clinical relevance of these findings is unknown.

Pharmacokinetics

Percutaneous absorption of [^{14}C] imiquimod was minimal in a study involving 6 healthy subjects treated with a single topical application (5 mg) of [^{14}C] imiquimod cream formulation. No radioactivity was detected in the serum (lower limit of quantitation: 1 ng/mL) and <0.9% of the radiolabelled dose was excreted in the urine and feces following topical application.

CLINICAL STUDIES

In a double-blind, placebo-controlled clinical trial, 209 otherwise healthy patients 18 years of age and older with genital/perianal warts were treated with Aldara 5% cream or vehicle control 3X/week for a maximum of 16 weeks. The median baseline wart area was 69 mm^2 (range 8 to 5525 mm^2). Patient accountability is shown in the figure below. [See graphic above]

Data on complete clearance are listed in the table below. The median time to complete wart clearance was 10 weeks. [See table above]

INDICATIONS AND USAGE

Aldara 5% cream is indicated for the treatment of external genital and perianal warts/condyloma acuminata in adults.

CONTRAINDICATIONS

None known

WARNINGS

Aldara cream has not been evaluated for the treatment of urethral, intra-vaginal, cervical, rectal, or intra-anal human papilloma viral disease and is not recommended for these conditions.

PRECAUTIONS

General

Local skin reactions such as erythema, erosion, excoriation/flaking, and edema are common. Should severe local skin reaction occur, the cream should be removed by washing the treatment area with mild soap and water. Treatment with Aldara cream can be resumed after the skin reaction has subsided. There is no clinical experience with Aldara cream therapy immediately following the treatment of genital/perianal warts with other cutaneously applied drugs; therefore, Aldara cream administration is not recommended until genital/perianal tissue is healed from any previous drug or surgical treatment. Aldara has the potential to exacerbate inflammatory conditions of the skin.

Information for Patients

Patients using Aldara 5% cream should receive the following information and instructions: The effect of Aldara 5% cream on the transmission of genital/perianal warts is unknown. Aldara 5% cream may weaken condoms and vaginal diaphragms. Therefore, concurrent use is not recommended.

1. This medication is to be used as directed by a physician. It is for external use only. Eye contact should be avoided.
2. The treatment area should not be bandaged or otherwise covered or wrapped as to be occlusive.
3. Sexual (genital, anal, oral) contact should be avoided while the cream is on the skin.
4. It is recommended that 6–10 hours following Aldara 5% cream application the treatment area be washed with mild soap and water.
5. It is common for patients to experience local skin reactions such as erythema, erosion, excoriation/flaking, and edema at the site of application or surrounding areas. Most skin reactions are mild to moderate. Severe skin reactions can occur and should be reported promptly to the prescribing physician.
6. Uncircumcised males treating warts under the foreskin should retract the foreskin and clean the area daily.
7. Patients should be aware that new warts may develop during therapy, as Aldara is not a cure.

Carcinogenicity, Mutagenesis, and Impairment of Fertility

Rodent carcinogenicity data are not available. Imiquimod was without effect in a series of eight different mutagenicity assays including Ames, mouse lymphoma, CHO chromosome aberration, human lymphocyte chromosome aberration, SHE cell transformation, rat and hamster bone marrow cytogenetics, and mouse dominant lethal test. Daily oral administration of imiquimod to rats, at doses up to 8 times the recommended human dose on a mg/m^2 basis throughout mating, gestation, parturition and lactation, demonstrated no impairment of reproduction.

Pregnancy

Pregnancy Category B: There are no adequate and well-controlled studies in pregnant women. Imiquimod was not found to be teratogenic in rat or rabbit teratology studies. In rats at a high maternally toxic dose (28 times human dose on a mg/m^2 basis), reduced pup weights and delayed ossifi-

Continued on next page

Aldara—Cont.

cation were observed. In developmental studies with off-spring of pregnant rats treated with imiquimod (8 times human dose), no adverse effects were demonstrated.

Nursing Mothers

It is not known whether topically applied imiquimod is excreted in breast milk.

Pediatric Use

Safety and efficacy in patients below the age of 18 years have not been established.

ADVERSE REACTIONS

In controlled clinical trials, the most frequently reported adverse reactions were those of local skin and application site reactions; some patients also reported systemic reactions. These reactions were usually mild to moderate in intensity; however, severe reactions were reported with 3X/week application. **These reactions were more frequent and more intense with daily application than with 3X/week application.** Overall, in the 3X/week application clinical studies, 1.2% (4/327) of the patients discontinued due to local skin/application site reactions. The incidence and severity of local skin reactions during controlled clinical trials are shown in the following table.

[See table below]

Remote site skin reactions were also reported in female and male patients treated 3X/week with imiquimod 5% cream. The severe remote site skin reactions reported for females were erythema (3%), ulceration (2%), and edema (1%); and for males, erosion (2%), and erythema, edema, induration, and excoriation/flaking (each 1%).

Adverse events judged to be probably or possibly related to Aldara reported by more than 5% of patients are listed below; also included are soreness, influenza-like symptoms and myalgia.

[See table above]

Adverse events judged to be possibly or probably related to Aldara and reported by more than 1% of patients include: **Application Site Disorders: Wart Site Reactions** (burning, hypopigmentation, irritation, itching, pain, rash, sensitivity, soreness, stinging, tenderness); **Remote Site Reactions** (bleeding, burning, itching, pain, tenderness, tinea cruris); **Body as a Whole:** fatigue, fever, influenza-like symptoms; **Central and Peripheral Nervous System Disorders:** headache; **Gastro-Intestinal System Disorders:** diarrhea; **Musculo-Skeletal System Disorders:** myalgia.

OVERDOSAGE

Overdosage of Aldara 5% cream in humans is unlikely due to minimal percutaneous absorption. Animal studies reveal a rabbit dermal lethal imiquimod dose of greater than 1600 mg/m^2. Persistent topical overdosing of Aldara 5% cream could result in severe local skin reactions. The most clinically serious adverse event reported following multiple oral imiquimod doses of >200 mg was hypotension which resolved following oral or intravenous fluid administration.

DOSAGE AND ADMINISTRATION

Aldara cream is to be applied 3 times per week, prior to normal sleeping hours, and left on the skin for 6–10 hours. Following the treatment period cream should be removed by washing the treated area with mild soap and water. Examples of 3 times per week application schedules are: Monday, Wednesday, Friday; or Tuesday, Thursday, Saturday application prior to sleeping hours. Aldara treatment should continue until there is total clearance of the genital/perianal warts or for a maximum of 16 weeks. Local skin reactions (erythema) at the treatment site are common. A rest period of several days may be taken if required by the patient's discomfort or severity of the local skin reaction. Treatment may resume once the reaction subsides. Non-occlusive dressings such as cotton gauze or cotton underwear may be used in the management of skin reactions. The technique for proper dose administration should be demonstrated by the prescriber to maximize the benefit of Aldara therapy. Handwashing before and after cream application is recommended. Aldara 5% cream is packaged in single-use packets which contain sufficient cream to cover a wart area of up to 20 cm^2; use of excessive amounts of cream should be avoided. Patients should be instructed to apply Aldara cream to external genital/perianal warts. A thin layer is applied to the wart area and rubbed in until the cream is no longer visible. The application site is not to be occluded.

3X/WEEK APPLICATION

	Females		Males	
	5% Imiquimod (N=117)	Vehicle (N=103)	5% Imiquimod (N=156)	Vehicle (N=158)
Application Site Disorders:				
Application Site Reactions				
Wart Site:				
Itching	32%	20%	22%	10%
Burning	26%	12%	9%	5%
Pain	8%	2%	2%	1%
Soreness	3%	0%	0%	1%
Fungal Infection[a]	11%	3%	2%	1%
Systemic Reactions:				
Headache	4%	3%	5%	2%
Influenza-like symptoms	3%	2%	1%	0%
Myalgia	1%	0%	1%	1%

[a] Incidences reported without regard to causality with Aldara.

HOW SUPPLIED

Aldara (imiquimod) cream, 5%, is supplied in single-use packets which contain 250 mg of the cream. Available as: box of 12 packets NDC 0089-0610-12. Store below 25°C (77°F). Avoid freezing.

Rx only

Distributed by
3M Pharmaceuticals
Northridge, CA 91324
3/98 614501

Shown in Product Identification Guide, page 321

ALU-TAB™ Tablets (aluminum hydroxide) and ALU-CAP™ Capsules (aluminum hydroxide) OTC

For indications, actions, warnings, dosage, and precautions see container label or call 800-328-0255 for a copy.

HOW SUPPLIED

Bottles of 250 green film-coated Alu-Tab tablets (NDC **0089-0107-25**). Bottles of 100 red and green Alu-Cap capsules (NDC **0089-0105-10**).

CALCIUM DISODIUM VERSENATE ℞
(edetate calcium disodium injection, USP)

> **WARNINGS:**
> Calcium Disodium Versenate is capable of producing toxic effects which can be fatal. Lead encephalopathy is reltively rare in adults, but occurs more often in pediatric patients in whom it may be incipient and thus overlooked. The mortality rate in pediatric patients has been high. Patients with lead encephalopathy and cerebral edema may experience a lethal increase in intracranial pressure following intravenous infusion: the intramuscular route is preferred for these patients. In cases where the intravenous route is necessary, avoid rapid infusion. The dosage schedule should be followed and at no time should the recommended daily dose be exceeded.

DESCRIPTION

Calcium Disodium Versenate (edetate calcium disodium injection, USP) is a sterile, injectable, chelating agent in concentrated solution for intravenous infusion or intramuscular injection. Each 5 ml ampul contains 1000 mg of edetate calcium disodium (equivalent to 200 mg/ml) in water for injection. Chemically, this product is called [[N,N′-1,2-ethanediyl-bis [N-(carboxymethyl)-glycinato] (4-)-N,N′,O,O′,O^N,O$^{N′}$]-,disodium,hydrate, (OC-6-21)-Calciate(2-).

Structural Formula:

NaOOCCH$_2$ CH$_2$COONa Ca • x H$_2$O

$C_{10}H_{12}CaN_2Na_2O_8 \bullet x\ H_2O$

Molecular weight 374.27 (anhydrous)

CLINICAL PHARMACOLOGY

The pharmacologic effects of edetate calcium disodium are due to the formation of chelates with divalent and trivalent metals. A stable chelate will form with any metal that has the ability to displace calcium from the molecule, a feature shared by lead, zinc, cadmium, manganese, iron and mercury. The amounts of manganese and iron metabolized are not significant. Copper[1] is not mobilized and mercury is unavailable for chelation because it is too tightly bound to body ligands or it is stored in inaccessible body compartments. The excretion of calcium by the body is not increased following intravenous administration of edetate calcium disodium, but the excretion of zinc is considerably increased.[1]

Edetate calcium disodium is poorly absorbed from the gastrointestinal tract. In blood, all the drug is found in the plasma. Edetate calcium disodium does not appear to penetrate cells; it is distributed primarily in the extracellular fluid with only about 5% of the plasma concentration found in the spinal fluid.

The half life of edetate calcium disodium is 20 to 60 minutes. It is excreted primarily by the kidney, with about 50% excreted in one hour and over 95% within 24 hours.[2] Almost none of the compound is metabolized.

The primary source of lead chelated by Calcium Disodium Versenate is from bone; subsequently, soft-tissue lead is redistributed to bone when chelation is stopped.[3,4] There is also some reduction in kidney lead levels following chelation therapy.

It has been shown in animals that following a single dose of Calcium Disodium Versenate urinary lead output increases, blood lead concentration decreases, but brain lead is significantly increased due to internal redistribution of lead.[5] (See **WARNINGS**.) These data are in agreement with the recent results of others in experimental animals showing that after a five day course of treatment there is no net reduction in brain lead.[6]

INDICATIONS AND USAGE

Edetate calcium disodium is indicated for the reduction of blood levels and depot stores of lead in lead poisoning (acute and chronic) and lead encephalopathy, in both pediatric populations and adults.

Chelation therapy should not replace effective measures to eliminate or reduce further exposure to lead.

CONTRAINDICATIONS

Edetate calcium disodium should not be given during periods of anuria, nor to patients with active renal disease or hepatitis.

WARNINGS

See boxed warning.

3X/WEEK APPLICATION
Wart Site Reaction As Assessed By Investigator

	Mild/Moderate				Severe			
	Females		Males		Females		Males	
	5% Imiquimod N=114	Vehicle N=99	5% Imiquimod N=156	Vehicle N=157	5% Imiquimod N=114	Vehicle N=99	5% Imiquimod N=156	Vehicle N=157
Erythema	61%	21%	54%	22%	4%	0%	4%	0%
Erosion	30%	8%	29%	6%	1%	0%	1%	0%
Excoriation/ Flaking	18%	8%	25%	8%	0%	0%	1%	0%
Edema	17%	5%	12%	1%	1%	0%	0%	0%
Induration	5%	2%	7%	2%	0%	0%	0%	0%
Ulceration	5%	1%	4%	1%	3%	0%	0%	0%
Scabbing	4%	0%	13%	3%	0%	0%	0%	0%
Vesicles	3%	0%	2%	0%	0%	0%	0%	0%

PRECAUTIONS

General Precautions: Edetate calcium disodium may produce the same renal damage as lead poisoning, such as proteinuria and microscopic hematuria. Treatment-induced nephrotoxicity is dose-dependent and may be reduced by assuring adequate diuresis before therapy begins. Urine flow must be monitored throughout therapy which must be stopped if anuria or severe oliguria develop. The proximal tubule hydropic degeneration usually recovers upon cessation of therapy. Edetate calcium disodium must be used in reduced doses in patients with pre-existing mild renal disease.

Patients should be monitored for cardiac rhythm irregularities and other ECG changes during intravenous therapy.

Information for patients: Patients should be instructed to immediately inform their physician if urine output stops for a period of 12 hours.

Laboratory tests: Urinalysis and urine sediment, renal and hepatic function and serum electrolyte levels should be checked before each course of therapy and then be monitored daily during therapy in severe cases, and in less serious cases after the second and fifth day of therapy. Therapy must be discontinued at the first sign of renal toxicity. The presence of large renal epithelial cells or increasing number of red blood cells in urinary sediment or greater proteinuria call for immediate stopping of edetate calcium disodium administration. Alkaline phosphatase values are frequently depressed (possibly due to decreased serum zinc levels), but return to normal within 48 hours after cessation of therapy. Elevated erythrocyte protoporphyrin levels (>35 mcg/dl of whole blood) indicate the need to perform a venous blood lead determination. If the whole blood lead concentration is between 25–55 mcg/dl a mobilization test can be considered.[7,8] (See **Diagnostic Test**.) An elevation of urinary coproporphyrin (adults: >250 mcg/day; pediatric patients under 80 lbs: >75 mcg/day) and elevation of urinary delta aminolevulinic acid (ALA) (adults: >4 mg/day; pediatric patients: >3 mg/m^2/day) are associated with blood lead levels >40 mcg/dl. Urinary coproporphyrin may be falsely negative in terminal patients and in severely iron-depleted pediatric patients who are not regenerating heme.[9] In growing pediatric patients long bone x-rays showing lead lines and abdominal x-rays showing radio-opaque material in the abdomen may be of help in estimating the level of exposure to lead.

Drug Interactions: There is no known drug interference with standard clinical laboratory tests. Steroids enhance the renal toxicity of edetate calcium disodium in animals.[7] Edetate calcium disodium interferes with the action of zinc insulin preparations by chelating the zinc.[7]

Carcinogenesis, Mutagenesis, Impairment of Fertility: Long term animal studies have not been conducted with edetate calcium disodium to evaluate its carcinogenic potential, mutagenic potential or its effect on fertility.

Pregnancy: Category B: One reproduction study was performed in rats at doses up to 13 times the human dose and revealed no evidence of impaired fertility or harm to the fetus due to Calcium Disodium Versenate.[10] Another reproduction study performed in rats at doses up to about 25 to 40 times the human dose revealed evidence of fetal malformations due to Calcium Disodium Versenate, which were prevented by simultaneous supplementation of dietary zinc.[11] There are, however, no adequate and well-controlled studies in pregnant women. Because animal reproduction studies are not always predictive of human response, this drug should be used during pregnancy only if clearly needed.

Labor and Delivery: Calcium Disodium Versenate has no recognized use during labor and delivery, and its effects during these processes are unknown.

Nursing Mothers: It is not known whether this durg is excreted in human milk. Because many drugs are excreted in human milk, caution should be exercised when Calcium Disodium Versenate is administered to a nursing woman.

Pediatric Use: Since lead poisoning occurs in pediatric populations and adults but is frequently more severe in pediatric patients, Calcium Disodium Versenate is used in patients of all ages. The intramuscular route is preferred by some for young pediatric patients. In cases where the intravenous route is necessary, avoid rapid infusion. (See **WARNINGS**.) Urine flow must be monitored throughout therapy; Calcium Disodium Versenate therapy must be stopped if anuria or severe oliguria develops. (See **General Precautions**.) At no time should the recommended daily dosage be exceeded. (See **DOSAGE AND ADMINISTRATION**.)

ADVERSE REACTIONS

The following adverse effects have been associated with the use of edetate calcium disodium:

Body as a Whole: pain at intramuscular injection site, fever, chills, malaise, fatigue, myalgia, arthralgia.

Cardiovascular: hypotension, cardiac rhythm irregularities.

Renal: acute necrosis of proximal tubules (which may result in fatal nephrosis), infrequent changes in distal tubules and glomeruli.

Urinary: glycosuria, proteinuria, microscopic hematuria and large epithelial cells in urinary sediment.

Nervous System: tremors, headache, numbness, tingling.

Gastrointestinal: cheilosis, nausea, vomiting, anorexia, excessive thirst.

Hepatic: mild increases in SGOT and SGPT are common, and return to normal within 48 hours after cessation of therapy.

Immunogenic: histamine-like reactions (sneezing, nasal congestion, lacrimation), rash.

Hematopoietic: transient bone marrow depression, anemia.

Metabolic: zinc deficiency, hypercalcemia.

OVERDOSAGE

Symptoms: inadvertent administration of 5 times the recommended dose, infused intravenously over a 24 hour period, to an asymptomatic 16 month old patient with a blood lead content of 56 mcg/dl did not cause any ill effects. Edetate calcium disodium can aggravate the symptoms of severe lead poisoning, therefore, most toxic effects (cerebral edema, renal tubular necrosis) appear to be associated with lead poisoning.

Because of cerebral edema, a therapeutic dose may be lethal to an adult or a pediatric patient with lead encephalopathy. Higher dosage of edetate calcium disodium may produce a more severe zinc deficiency.

Treatment: Cerebral edema should be treated with repeated doses of mannitol. Steroids enhance the renal toxicity of edetate calcium disodium in animals and, therefore, are no longer recommended.[7] Zinc levels must be monitored. Good urinary output must be maintained because diuresis will enhance drug elimination. It is not known if edetate calcium disodium is dialyzable.

DOSAGE AND ADMINISTRATION

When a source for the lead intoxication has been identified, the patient should be removed from the source, if possible. The recommended dose of Calcium Disodium Versenate for asymptomatic adults and pediatric patients whose blood lead level is <70 mcg/dl but >20 mcg/dl (World Health Organization recommended upper allowable level) is 1000 mg/m^2/day whether given intravenously or intramuscularly. (See Surface Area Nomogram.)

SURFACE AREA NOMOGRAM

HEIGHT IN CENTIMETERS — SURFACE AREA IN METER^2 — WEIGHT IN KILOGRAMS

Drawn from Gehan & George, Cancer Chemotherapy Reports 54:225, 1970.

For adults with lead nephropathy, the following dosing regimen has been suggested: 500 mg/m^2 every 24 hours for 5 days for patients with serum creatinine levels of 2–3 mg/dl, every 48 hours for 3 doses for patients with creatinine levels of 3–4 mg/dl, and once weekly for patients with creatinine levels above 4 mg/dl. These regimens may be repeated at one month intervals.[12]

Calcium Disodium Versenate, used alone, may aggravate symptoms in patients with very high blood lead levels. When the blood lead level is >70 mcg/dl or clinical symptoms consistent with lead poisoning are present, it is recommended that Calcium Disodium Versenate be used in conjunction with BAL (dimercaprol). Please consult published protocols and specialized references for dosage recommendations of combination therapy.[14–18]

Therapy of lead poisoning in adults and pediatric patients with Calcium Disodium Versenate is continued over a period of five days. Therapy is then interrupted for 2 to 4 days to allow redistribution of the lead and to prevent severe depletion of zinc and other essential metals. Two courses of treatment are usually employed; however, it depends on severity of the lead toxicity and the patient's tolerance of the drug.

Calcium Disodium Versenate is equally effective whether administered intravenously or intramuscularly. The intramuscular route is used for all patients with overt lead encephalopathy and this route is preferred by some for young pediatric patients.

Acutely ill individuals may be dehydrated from vomiting. Since edetate calcium disodium is excreted almost exclusively in the urine, it is very important to establish urine flow with intravenous fluid administration before the first dose of the chelating agent is given; however, excessive fluid must be avoided in patients with encephalopathy. Once urine flow is established, further intravenous fluid is restricted to basal water and electrolyte requirements. Administration of Calcium Disodium Versenate should be stopped whenever there is cessation of urine flow in order to avoid unduly high tissue levels of the drug. Edetate calcium disodium must be used in reduced doses in patients with pre-existing mild renal disease.

Intravenous Administration: Add the total daily dose of Calcium Disodium Versenate (1000 mg/m^2/day) to 250–500 ml of 5% dextrose or 0.9% sodium chloride injection. The total daily dose should be infused over a period of 8–12 hours. Calcium Disodium Versenate Injection is incompatible with 10% dextrose, 10% invert sugar in 0.9% sodium chloride, lactate Ringer's, Ringer's, one-sixth molar sodium lactate injections, and with injectable amphotericin B and hydralazine hydrochloride.

Intramuscular Administration: The total daily dosage (1000 mg/m^2/day) should be divided into equal doses spaced 8–12 hours apart. Lidocaine or procaine should be added to the Calcium Disodium Versenate Injection to minimize pain at the injection site. The final lidocaine or procaine concentration of 5 mg/ml (0.5%) can be obtained as follows: 0.25 ml of 10% lidocaine solution per 5 ml (entire content of ampul) concentrated Calcium Disodium Versenate; 1 ml of 1% lidocaine or procaine solution per ml of concentrated Calcium Disodium Versenate. When used alone, regardless of method of administration, Calcium Disodium Versenate should not be given at doses larger than those recommended.

Diagnostic Test: Several methods have been described for lead mobilization tests using edetate calcium disodium to assess body stores.[7,9,12,13,18]

These procedures have advantages and disadvantages that should be reviewed in current references. Edetate calcium disodium mobilization tests should not be performed in symptomatic patients and in patients with blood lead levels above 55 mcg/dl for whom appropriate therapy is indicated.

Parenteral drugs should be inspected visually for particulate matter and discoloration prior to administration, whenever solution and container permit.

HOW SUPPLIED

Calcium Disodium Versenate Injection, 5 ml ampul containing 200 mg of edetate calcium disodium per ml (1 g per ampul), in boxes containing 6 ampuls (NDC **0089-0510-06**).

Store at controlled room temperature 15°–30°C (59°–86°F).

Rx only

REFERENCES

1. Thomas DJ, Chisolm JJ. Lead, zinc and copper decorporation during calcium disodium ethylenediamine tetraacetate treatment of lead-poisoned children. J Pharmacol Exp Therapeu 1986; 239: 829–835.
2. The Pharmacological Basis of Therapeutics, 7th edition, Goodman and Gilman, editors. MacMillan Publishing Company, New York, 1985, pp. 1619–1622.
3. Hammond PB, Aronson AL, Olson WC. The mechanism of mobilization of lead by ethylenediaminetetraacetate. J Pharmacol Exp Therapeu 1967; 157: 196–206.
4. Van deVyver FL, D'Haese PC, Visser WJ, et al. Bone lead in dialysis patients. Kidney Intl 1988; 33:601–607.
5. Cory-Slecta DA, Weiss B, Cox C. Mobilization and redistribution of lead over the course of calcium disodium ethylenediamine tetraacetate chelation therapy. J Pharmacol Exp Therapeu 1987; 243:804–813.
6. Chisolm JJ, Mobilization of lead by calcium disodium edetate. Am J Dis Child 1987; 141:1256–1257.
7. Drug Evaluations, 6th Edition, American Medical Association, Saunders, Philadelphia, 1986, pp. 1637–1639.
8. Centers for Disease Control: Preventing lead poisoning in young children. Atlanta, GA, Department of Health and Human Services, 1985 Jan.
9. Finberg L, Rajagopal V. Diagnosis and treatment of lead poisoning in children. J Family Med 1985 April: 3–12.
10. Schardein JL, Sakowski R, Petrere J, et al. Teratogenesis studies with EDTA and its salts in rats. Toxicol Appl Pharmacol 1981; 61:423–428.
11. Swenerton H, Hurley LS. Teratogenic effects of a chelating agent and their prevention by zinc. Science 1971; 173:62–64.
12. American Hospital Formulary Service, Drug Information, 1988, pp. 1695–1698.
13. Markowitz ME, Rosen JF. Assessment of lead stores in chidren: Validation of an 8-hour $CaNa_2EDTA$ (Calcium Disodium Versenate) provocative test. J Pediatrics 1984; 104:337–341.
14. Piomelli S, Rosen JF, Chisolm JJ, et al. Management of childhood lead poisoning. J Pediatrics 1984; 105:523–532.
15. Sachs HK, Blanksma LA, Murray EF, et al. Ambulatory treatment of lead poisoning: Report of 1,155 cases. Pediatrics 1970; 46:389.
16. Chisolm JJ. The use of chelating agents in the treatment of acute and chronic lead intoxication in childhood. J Pediatrics 1968; 73:1.
17. Coffin R, Phillips JL, Staples WI, et al. Treatment of lead encephalopathy in children. J Pediatrics 1966;69: 198–206.

Continued on next page

Calcium Disodium Versenate—Cont.

18. Chisolm JJ. Increased lead absorption and acute lead poisoning. Current Pediatric Therapy 12, Gillis and Kagan, editors, WB Saunders, Philadelphia, 1986, pp. 667–671.

Manufactured for
3M Pharmaceuticals
Northridge, CA 91324
By Abbott Laboratories
North Chicago, IL 60064
994004 January 2000

DISALCID™ ℞
(salsalate)
Tablets and Capsules

DESCRIPTION

DISALCID (salsalate) is a nonsteroidal anti-inflammatory agent for oral administration. Chemically, salsalate (salicylsalicylic acid or 2-hydroxybenzoic acid, 2-carboxyphenyl ester) is a dimer of salicylic acid; its structural formula is shown below.

Chemical Structure:

salsalate

Each DISALCID capsule contains 500 mg salsalate and also contains colloidal silicon dioxide, gelatin, magnesium stearate, pregelatinized starch, corn starch, titanium dioxide, FD&C blue #1, and D&C yellow #10.

Each DISALCID tablet contains 500 or 750 mg salsalate and also contains croscarmellose sodium, hydroxypropyl methylcellulose, magnesium stearate, microcrystalline cellulose, polyethylene glycol, polysorbate 80, propylene glycol, talc, titanium dioxide, FD&C blue #1, and D&C yellow #10. (See HOW SUPPLIED.)

CLINICAL PHARMACOLOGY

DISALCID is insoluble in acid gastric fluids (<0.1 mg/ml at pH 1.0), but readily soluble in the small intestine where it is partially hydrolyzed to two molecules of salicylic acid. A significant portion of the parent compound is absorbed unchanged and undergoes rapid esterase hydrolysis in the body; its half-life is about one hour. About 13% is excreted through the kidneys as a glucuronide conjugate of the parent compound, the remainder as salicylic acid and its metabolites. Thus, the amount of salicylic acid available from DISALCID is about 15% less than from aspirin, when the two drugs are administered on a salicylic acid molar equivalent basis (3.6 g salsalate/5 g aspirin). Salicylic acid biotransformation is saturated at anti-inflammatory doses of DISALCID. Such capacity-limited biotransformation results in an increase in the half-life of salicylic acid from 3.5 to 16 or more hours. Thus, dosing with DISALCID twice a day will satisfactorily maintain blood levels within the desired therapeutic range (10 to 30 mg/100 ml) throughout the 12-hour intervals. Therapeutic blood levels continue for up to 16 hours after the last dose. The parent compound does not show capacity-limited biotransformation, nor does it accumulate in the plasma on multiple dosing. Food slows the absorption of all salicylates including DISALCID.

The mode of anti-inflammatory action of DISALCID and other nonsteroidal anti-inflammatory drugs is not fully defined. Although salicylic acid (the primary metabolite of DISALCID) is a weak inhibitor of prostaglandin synthesis **in vitro,** DISALCID appears to selectively inhibit prostaglandin synthesis **in vivo,**[1] providing anti-inflammatory activity equivalent to aspirin[2] and indomethacin.[3] Unlike aspirin, DISALCID does not inhibit platelet aggregation.[4]

The usefulness of salicylic acid, the active **in vivo** product of DISALCID, in the treatment of arthritic disorders has been established.[5,6] In contrast to aspirin, DISALCID causes no greater fecal gastrointestinal blood loss than placebo.[7]

INDICATIONS AND USAGE

DISALCID is indicated for relief of the signs and symptoms of rheumatoid arthritis, osteoarthritis and related rheumatic disorders.

CONTRAINDICATIONS

DISALCID is contraindicated in patients hypersensitive to salsalate.

WARNINGS

Reye's Syndrome may develop in individuals who have chicken pox, influenza, or flu symptoms. Some studies suggest a possible association between the development of Reye's Syndrome and the use of medicines containing salicylate or apirin. DISALCID contains a salicylate and therefore is not recommended for use in patients with chicken pox, influenza, or flu symptoms.

PRECAUTIONS

General Precautions: Patients on treatment with DISALCID should be warned not to take other salicylates so as to avoid potentially toxic concentrations. Great care should be exercised when DISALCID is prescribed in the presence of chronic renal insufficiency or peptic ulcer disease. Protein binding of salicylic acid can be influenced by nutritional status, competitive binding of other drugs, and fluctuations in serum proteins caused by disease (rheumatoid arthritis, etc.).

Although cross reactivity, including bronchospasm, has been reported occasionally with non-acetylated salicylates, including salsalate, in aspirin-sensitive patients,[8,9] salsalate is less likely than aspirin to induce asthma in such patients.[10]

Laboratory Tests: Plasma salicylic acid concentrations should be periodically monitored during long-term treatment with DISALCID to aid maintenance of therapeutically effective levels: 10 to 30 mg/100 ml. Toxic manifestations are not usually seen until plasma concentrations exceed 30 mg/100 ml (see OVERDOSAGE). Urinary pH should also be regularly monitored: sudden acidification, as from pH 6.5 to 5.5, can double the plasma level, resulting in toxicity.

Drug Interactions: Salicylates antagonize the uricosuric action of drugs used to treat gout. ASPIRIN AND OTHER SALICYLATE DRUGS WILL BE ADDITIVE TO DISALCID AND MAY INCREASE PLASMA CONCENTRATIONS OF SALICYLIC ACID TO TOXIC LEVELS. Drugs and foods that raise urine pH will increase renal clearance and urinary excretion of salicylic acid, thus lowering plasma levels; acidifying drugs or foods will decrease urinary excretion and increase plasma levels. Salicylates given concomitantly with anticoagulant drugs may predispose to systemic bleeding. Salicylates may enhance the hypoglycemic effect of oral anti-diabetic drugs of the sulfonylurea class. Salicylate competes with a number of drugs for protein binding sites, notably penicillin, thiopental, thyroxine, triiodothyronine, phenytoin, sulfinpyrazone, naproxen, warfarin, methotrexate, and possibly corticosteroids.

Drug/Laboratory Test Interactions: Salicylate competes with thyroid hormone for binding to plasma proteins, which may be reflected in a depressed plasma T_4 value in some patients; thyroid function and basal metabolism are unaffected.

Carcinogenesis: No long-term animal studies have been performed with DISALCID to evaluate its carcinogenic potential.

Use in Pregnancy: Pregnancy Category C: Salsalate and salicylic acid have been shown to be teratogenic and embryocidal in rats when given in doses 4 to 5 times the usual human dose. These effects were not observed at doses twice as great as the usual human dose. There are no adequate and well-controlled studies in pregnant women. DISALCID should be used during pregnancy only if the potential benefit justifies the potential risk to the fetus.

Labor and Delivery: There exist no adequate and well-controlled studies in pregnant women. Although adverse effects on mother or infant have not been reported with DISALCID use during labor, caution is advised when anti-inflammatory dosage is involved. However, other salicylates have been associated with prolonged gestation and labor, maternal and neonatal bleeding sequelae, potentiation of narcotic and barbiturate effects (respiratory or cardiac arrest in the mother), delivery problems and stillbirth.

Nursing Mothers: It is not known whether salsalate per se is excreted in human milk; salicylic acid, the primary metabolite of DISALCID, has been shown to appear in human milk in concentrations approximating the maternal blood level. Thus, the infant of a mother on DISALCID therapy might ingest in mother's milk 30 to 80% as much salicylate per kg body weight as the mother is taking. Accordingly, caution should be exercised when DISALCID is administered to a nursing woman.

Pediatric Use: Safety and effectiveness in pediatric patients have not been established. (See WARNINGS section.)

ADVERSE REACTIONS

In two well-controlled clinical trials (n=280 patients), the following reversible adverse experiences characteristic of salicylates were most commonly reported with DISALCID, listed in descending order of frequency: tinnitus, nausea, hearing impairment, rash, and vertigo. These common symptoms of salicylates, i.e., tinnitus or reversible hearing impairment, are often used as a guide to therapy.

Although cause-and-effect relationships have not been established, spontaneous reports over a ten-year period have included the following additional medically significant adverse experiences: abdominal pain, abnormal hepatic function, anaphylactic shock, angioedema, bronchospasm, decreased creatinine clearance, diarrhea, G.I. bleeding, hepatitis, hypotension, nephritis and urticaria.

DRUG ABUSE AND DEPENDENCE

Drug abuse and dependence have not been reported with DISALCID.

OVERDOSAGE

Death has followed ingestion of 10 to 30 g of salicylates in adults, but much larger amounts have been ingested without fatal outcome.

Symptoms: The usual symptoms of salicylism—tinnitus, vertigo, headache, confusion, drowsiness, sweating, hyperventilation, vomiting and diarrhea—will occur. More severe intoxication will lead to disruption of electrolyte balance and blood pH, and hyperthermia and dehydration.

Treatment: Further absorption of DISALCID from the G.I. tract should be prevented by emesis (syrup of ipecac) and, if necessary, by gastric lavage.

Fluid and electrolyte imbalance should be corrected by the administration of appropriate I.V. therapy. Adequate renal function should be maintained. Hemodialysis or peritoneal dialysis may be required in extreme cases.

DOSAGE AND ADMINISTRATION

Adults: The usual dosage is 3000 mg daily, given in divided doses as follows: 1) two doses of two 750 mg tablets; 2) two doses of three 500 mg tablets/capsules; or 3) three doses of two 500 mg tablets/capsules. Some patients, e.g., the elderly, may require a lower dosage to achieve therapeutic blood concentrations and to avoid the more common side effects such as auditory.

Alleviation of symptoms is gradual, and full benefit may not be evident for 3 to 4 days, when plasma salicylate levels have achieved steady state. There is no evidence for development of tissue tolerance (tachyphylaxis) but salicylate therapy may induce increased activity of metabolizing liver enzymes, causing a greater rate of salicyluric acid production and excretion, with a resultant increase in dosage requirement for maintenance of therapeutic serum salicylate levels.

Children: Dosage recommendations and indications for DISALCID use in children have not been established.

HOW SUPPLIED

Each DISALCID 500 mg aqua/white capsule printed with Disalcid/3M is available in:
Bottles of 100 (NDC #0089–0148–10)

Each DISALCID 500 mg aqua, film coated, round, bisected tablet embossed with DISALCID on one side and 3M on the other side is available in:
Bottles of 100 (NDC #0089–0149–10)
Bottles of 500 (NDC #0089–0149–50)

Each DISALCID 750 mg aqua, film coated, capsule shaped, bisected tablet embossed with DISALCID 750 on one side and 3M on the other side is available in:
Bottles of 100 (NDC #0089–0151–10)
Bottles of 500 (NDC #0089–0151–50)

Store at controlled room temperature 15°-30°C (59°-86°F).
Rx only

REFERENCES

1. Morris HG, et al. Effects of salsalate (non-acetylated salicylate) and aspirin on serum prostaglandins in humans. Thera Drug Mon 1985;7:435–438.
2. April PA, et al. Does the acetyl group of aspirin contribute to the anti-inflammatory efficacy of salicylic acid in the treatment of rheumatoid arthritis? Sem Arth & Rheum 1990;19:(4):2:20–28.
3. Deodhar SD, et al. A short term comparative trial of salsalate and indomethacin in rheumatoid arthritis. Curr Med Res Opin 1977;5:185–188.
4. Estes D, Kaplan K. Lack of platelet effect with the aspirin analog, salsalate. Arth & Rheum 1980;23:1303–1307.
5. Dick C, et al. Effect of anti-inflammatory drug therapy on clearance of ^{133}Xe from knee joints of patients with rheumatoid arthritis. Br Med J 1969;3:278–280.
6. Dick WC, et al. Indices of inflammatory activity. Ann of Rheum Dis 1970;29:643–648.
7. Cohen A, Fecal blood loss and plasma salicylate study of salicylsalicylic acid and aspirin. J Clin Pharmacol 1979;19:242–247.
8. Chudwin DS, et al. Sensitivity to non-acetylated salicylates in a patient with asthma, nasal polyps, and rheumatoid arthritis. Ann of Allergy 1986;57:133–134.
9. Spector SL, et al. Aspirin and concomitant idiosyncrasies in adult asthmatic patients. J Allergy Clin Immunol 1979;64:500–506.
10. Stevenson DD, et al. Salsalate cross sensitivity in aspirin-sensitive asthmatics. J Allergy Clin Immunol 1990;86:749–758.

00300 June 1998
3M Pharmaceuticals
Northridge, CA 91324

MAXAIR™ AUTOHALER™ ℞
(pirbuterol acetate inhalation aerosol)
For Oral Inhalation Only

DESCRIPTION

The active component of MAXAIR AUTOHALER (pirbuterol acetate) is (R,S)α^6-[[(1,1-dimethylethyl)amino]methyl]-3-hydroxy-2,6-pyridinedimethanol monoacetate salt, a beta-2-adrenergic bronchodilator, having the following chemical structure:

Pirbuterol acetate is a white, crystalline racemic mixture of two optically active isomers. It is a powder, freely soluble in water, with a molecular weight of 300.3 and empirical formula of $C_{12}H_{20}N_2O_3 \bullet C_2H_4O_2$.

MAXAIR AUTOHALER is a prescribed metered-dose aerosol unit for oral inhalation. It provides a fine-particle suspension of pirbuterol acetate in the propellant mixture of trichloromonofluoromethane and dichlorodifluoromethane, with sorbitan trioleate. Each actuation delivers 253 mcg of pirbuterol (as pirbuterol acetate) from the value and 200 mcg of pirbuterol (as pirbuterol acetate) from the mouthpiece. The unit is breath-actuated such that the medication is delivered automatically during inspiration without the need for the patient to coordinate actuation with inspiration. Each 14.0 g canister provides 400 inhalations and each 2.8 g canister provides 80 inhalations.

Change in device and instructions: a test fire slide has been added to the bottom of the Autohaler (actuator/mouthpiece) device to enable priming of the Autohaler.

As with all aerosol medications, it is recommended to prime (test) MAXAIR AUTOHALER before using for the first time. MAXAIR AUTOHALER should also be primed if it has not been used in 48 hours. As described in the priming procedure, use the test fire slide to release two priming sprays into the air away from yourself and other people. (See "Patient's Instructions For Use" portion of this package insert.)

CLINICAL PHARMACOLOGY

In vitro studies and *in vivo* pharmacologic studies have demonstrated that pirbuterol has a preferential effect on beta-2 adrenergic receptors compared with isoproterenol. While it is recognized that beta-2 adrenergic receptors are the predominant receptors in bronchial smooth muscle, data indicate that there is a population of beta-2 receptors in the human heart, existing in a concentration between 10–50%. The precise function of these receptors has not been established (see WARNINGS section).

The pharmacologic effects of beta adrenergic agonist drugs, including pirbuterol, are at least in part attributable to stimulation through beta adrenergic receptors of intracellular adenyl cyclase, the enzyme which catalyzes the conversion of adenosine triphosphate (ATP) to cyclic-3′,5′-adenosine monophosphate (c-AMP). Increased c-AMP levels are associated with relaxation of bronchial smooth muscle and inhibition of release of mediators of immediate hypersensitivity from cells, especially from mast cells.

Bronchodilator activity of pirbuterol was manifested clinically by an improvement in various pulmonary function parameters (FEV_1, MMF, FEFR, airway resistance [RAW] and conductance [GA/V_{tg}]).

Clinical Trials: In controlled double-blind single-dose clinical trials, the onset of improvement in pulmonary function occurred within 5 minutes in most patients as determined by forced expiratory volume in one second (FEV_1). FEV_1 and MMF measurements also showed that maximum improvement in pulmonary function generally occurred 30–60 minutes following one (1) or two (2) inhalations of pirbuterol (200–400 mcg). The duration of action of pirbuterol is maintained for 5 hours (the time at which the last observations were made) in a substantial number of patients, based on a 15% or greater increase in FEV_1. In controlled repetitive-dose studies of 12 weeks' duration, 74% of 156 patients on pirbuterol and 62% of 141 patients on metaproterenol showed a clinically significant improvement based on a 15% or greater increase in FEV_1 on at least half of the days. Onset and duration were equivalent to that seen in single-dose studies. Continued effectiveness was demonstrated over the 12-week period in the majority (94%) of responding patients; however, chronic dosing was associated with the development of tachyphylaxis (tolerance) to the bronchodilator effect in some patients in both treatment groups.

A placebo-controlled, double-blind, single-dose study (24 patients per treatment group), utilizing continuous Holter monitoring for 5 hours after drug administration, showed no significant difference in ectopic activity between the placebo control group and pirbuterol at the recommended dose (200-400 mcg), and twice the recommended dose (800 mcg). As with other inhaled beta adrenergic agonists, supraventricular and ventricular ectopic beats have been seen with pirbuterol (see WARNINGS).

Two randomized, double-blind, cross-over studies in a total of 97 patients, have compared the clinical effects of either one inhalation or two inhalations of the pirbuterol formulations in the AUTOHALER actuator and the conventional inhaler and demonstrated no significant difference between the formulations for the means of peak changes in FEV_1, time to peak FEV_1, onset, duration, or area under the FEV_1 curve.

Preclinical: Studies in laboratory animals (minipigs, rodents, and dogs) have demonstrated the occurrence of cardiac arrhythmias and sudden death (with histologic evidence of myocardial necrosis) when beta-agonists and methylxanthines were administered concurrently. The clinical significance of these findings when applied to humans is unknown.

Pharmacokinetics: As expected by extrapolation from oral data, systemic blood levels of pirbuterol are below the limit of assay sensitivity (2–5 ng/ml) following inhalation of doses up to 800 mcg (twice the maximum recommended dose).

A mean of 51% of the dose is recovered in urine as pirbuterol plus its sulfate conjugated following administration by aerosol. Pirbuterol is not metabolized by catechol-O-methyltransferase.

The percent of administered dose recovered as pirbuterol plus its sulfate conjugate does not change significantly over the dose range of 400 mcg to 800 mcg and is not significantly different from that after oral administration of pributerol. The plasma half-life measured after oral administration is about two hours.

INDICATIONS AND USAGE

MAXAIR AUTOHALER is indicated for the prevention and reversal of bronchospasm in patients 12 years of age and older with reversible bronchospasm including asthma. It may be used with or without concurrent theophylline and/or corticosteroid therapy.

CONTRAINDICATIONS

MAXAIR AUTOHALER is contraindicated in patients with a history of hypersensitivity to pirbuterol to any of its ingredients.

WARNINGS

Cardiovascular: MAXAIR AUTOHALER, like other inhaled beta adrenergic agonists, can produce a clinically significant cardiovascular effect in some patients, as measured by pulse rate, blood pressure and/or symptoms. Although such effects are uncommon after administration of MAXAIR AUTOHALER at recommended doses, if they occur, the drug may need to be discontinued. In addition, beta-agonists have been reported to produce ECG changes, such as flattening of the T wave, prolongation of the QTc interval, and ST segment depression. The clinical significance of these findings is unknown. Therefore, MAXAIR AUTOHALER, like all sympathomimetic amines, should be used with caution in patients with cardiovascular disorders, especially coronary insufficiency, cardiac arrhythmias, and hypertension.

Paradoxical Bronchospasm: MAXAIR AUTOHALER can produce paradoxical bronchospasm, which can be life threatening. If paradoxical bronchospasm occurs, MAXAIR AUTOHALER should be discontinued immediately and alternative therapy instituted. It should be recognized that paradoxical bronchospasm, when associated with inhaled formulations, frequently occurs with the first use of a new canister or vial.

Use of Anti-Inflammatory Agents: The use of beta adrenergic agonist bronchodilators alone may not be adequate to control asthma in many patients. Early consideration should be given to adding anti-inflammatory agents, e.g., corticosteroids.

Deterioration of Asthma: Asthma may deteriorate acutely over a period of hours or chronically over several days or longer. If the patient needs more doses of MAXAIR AUTOHALER than usual, this may be a marker of destabilization of asthma and requires reevaluation of the patient and the treatment regimen, giving special consideration to the possible need for anti-inflammatory treatment, e.g., corticosteroids.

PRECAUTIONS

General: Since pirbuterol is a sympathomimetic amine, it should be used with caution in patients with cardiovascular disorders, including ischemic heart disease, hypertension, or cardiac arrhythmias, in patients with hyperthyroidism or diabetes mellitus, and in patients who are unusually responsive to sympathomimetic amines or who have convulsive disorders. Significant changes in systolic and diastolic blood pressure could be expected to occur in some patients after use of any beta adrenergic aerosol bronchodilator.

Beta adrenergic agonist medications may produce significant hypokalemia in some patients, possibly through intracellular shunting, which has the potential to produce adverse cardiovascular effects. The decrease is usually transient, not requiring supplementation.

Information for Patients: The action of MAXAIR AUTOHALER should last up to five hours or longer. MAXAIR AUTOHALER should not be used more frequently than recommended. Do not increase the dose of frequency of MAXAIR AUTOHALER without consulting your physician. If you find that treatment with MAXAIR AUTOHALER becomes less effective for symptomatic relief, or your symptoms become worse, and/or you need to use the product more frequently than usual, you should seek medical attention immediately. While you are using MAXAIR AUTOHALER, other inhaled drugs and asthma medications should be taken only as directed by your physician. Common adverse effects include palpitations, chest pain, rapid heart rate, tremor or nervousness. If you are pregnant or nursing, contact your physician about use of MAXAIR AUTOHALER. Effective and safe use includes an understanding of the way the medication should be administered. **Change in device and instructions: a test fire slide has been added to the bottom of the Autohaler (actuator/mouthpiece) device to enable priming of the Autohaler.** As with all aerosol medications. It is recommended to prime (test) MAXAIR AUTOHALER before using for the first time. MAXAIR AUTOHALER should also be primed if it has not been used in 48 hours. As described in the priming procedure, use the test fire slide to release two priming sprays into the air away from yourself and other people (See "Patient's Instructions For Use" portion of this package insert.)

The MAXAIR AUTOHALER actuator should not be used with any other inhalation aerosol canister. In addition, canisters for use with MAXAIR AUTOHALER should not be utilized with any other actuator.

Drug Interactions: Other short-acting beta adrenergic aerosol bronchodilators should not be used concomitantly with MAXAIR AUTOHALER because they may have additive effects.

Monoamine Oxidase Inhibitors or Tricyclic Antidepressants: Pirbuterol should be administered with extreme caution to patients being treated with monoamine oxidase inhibitors or tricyclic antidepressants, or within 2 weeks of discontinuation of such agents, because the action of pirbuterol on the vascular system may be potentiated.

Beta Blockers: Beta adrenergic receptor blocking agents not only block the pulmonary effect of beta-agonists, such as MAXAIR AUTOHALER, but may produce severe bronchospasm in asthmatic patients. Therefore, patients with asthma should not normally be treated with beta blockers. However, under certain circumstances, e.g., as prophylaxis after myocardial infarction, there may be no acceptable alternatives to the use of beta adrenergic blocking agents in patients with asthma. In this setting, cardioselective beta blockers could be considered, although they should be administered with caution.

Diuretics: The ECG changes and/or hypokalemia that may result from the administration of non-potassium sparing diuretics (such as loop or thiazide diuretics) can be acutely worsened by beta-agonists, especially when the recommended dose of the beta-agonist is exceeded. Although the clinical significance of these effects is not known, caution is advised in the coadministration of beta-agonists with non-potassium sparing diuretics.

Carcinogenesis, Mutagenesis and Impairment of Fertility: In a 2-year study in Sprague-Dawley rats, pirbuterol hydrochloride administered at dietary doses of 1.0, 3.0, and 10 mg/kg (approximately 3, 10, and 35 times the maximum recommended daily inhalation dose for adults and children on a mg/m^2 basis) showed no evidence of carcinogenicity. In an 18-month study in mice at dietary doses of 1.0, 3.0, and 10 mg/kg (approximately 2, 5, and 15 times the maximum recommended daily inhalation dose for adults and children on a mg/m^2 basis) no evidence of tumorigenicity was seen. Reproduction studies in rats administered pirbuterol hydrochloride at oral doses of 1, 3, and 10 mg/kg (approximately 3, 10, and 35 times the maximum recommended daily inhalation dose for adults on a mg/m^2 basis) revealed no evidence of impaired fertility.

Pirbuterol dihydrochloride showed no evidence of mutagenicity in *in vitro* assays and host-mediated microbial (Ames) assays for point mutations and *in vivo* tests for somatic or germ cell effects following acute and subchronic treatment in mice (cytogenicity assays).

Teratogenic Effects—Pregnancy Category C: Pirbuterol was not teratogenic in rats administered oral doses of 30, 100, and 300 mg/kg (approximately 100, 340, and 1000 times the maximum recommended daily inhalation dose for adults on a mg/m^2 basis). Pirbuterol was not teratogenic in rabbits administered oral doses of 30 and 100 mg/kg (approximately 200 and 680 times the maximum recommended inhalation dose of adults on a mg/m^2 basis). However, pirbuterol at an oral dose of 300 mg/kg (approximately 2000 times the maximum recommended daily inhalation dose in adults on a mg/m^2 basis) caused abortions and fetal death. There are no adequate and well-controlled studies in pregnant women. Pirbuterol should be used during pregnancy only if the potential benefit justifies the potential risk to the fetus.

Labor and Delivery: Because of the potential for beta-agonist interference with uterine contractility, use of MAXAIR AUTOHALER for relief of bronchospasm during labor should be restricted to these patients in whom the benefits clearly outweigh the risk.

Nursing Mothers: It is known whether pirbuterol is excreted in human milk. Therefore, MAXAIR AUTOHALER should be used during nursing only if the potential benefit justifies the possible risk to the newborn.

Pediatric Use: MAXAIR AUTOHALER is not recommended for patients under the age of 12 years because of insufficient clinical data to establish safety and effectiveness.

ADVERSE REACTIONS

The following rates of adverse reactions to pirbuterol are based on single- and multiple-dose clinical trials involving 761 patients, 400 of whom received multiple doses (mean duration of treatment was 2.5 months and maximum was 19 months).

The following were the adverse reactions reported more frequently than 1 in 100 patients:

CNS: nervousness (6.9%), tremor (6.0%), headache (2.0%), dizziness (1.2%).

Cardiovascular: palpitations (1.7%), tachycardia (1.2%).

Respiratory: cough (1.2%).

Gastrointestinal: nausea (1.7%).

The following adverse reactions occurred less frequently than 1 in 100 patients and there may be a causal relationship with pirbuterol:

CNS: depression, anxiety, confusion, insomnia, weakness, hyperkinesia, syncope.

Cardiovascular: hypotension, skipped beats, chest pain.

Gastrointstinal: dry mouth, glossitis, abdominal pain/cramps, anorexia, diarrhea, stomatitis, nausea and vomiting.

Ear, Nose and Throat: smell/taste changes, sore throat.

Dermatological: rash, pruritus.

Other: numbness in extremities, alopecia, bruising, fatigue edema, weight gain, flushing.

Other adverse reactions were reported with a frequency of less than 1 in 100 patients but a causal relationship between pirbuterol and the reaction could not be determined: migraine, productive cough, wheezing, and dermatitis.

The following rates of adverse reactions during three-month controlled clinical trials involving 310 patients are noted. The table does not include mild reactions.

PERCENT OF PATIENTS WITH MODERATE TO SEVERE ADVERSE REACTIONS

Reaction	Pirbuterol N=157	Metaproterenol N=153
Central Nervous System		
tremors	1.3%	3.3%
nervousness	4.5%	2.6%
headache	1.3%	2.0%
weakness	.0%	1.3%
drowsiness	.0%	0.7%
dizziness	0.6%	.0%

Continued on next page

Maxair Autoinhaler—Cont.

Cardiovascular		
palpitations	1.3%	1.3%
tachycardia	1.3%	2.0%
Respiratory		
chest pain/tightness	1.3%	.0%
cough	.0%	0.7%
Gastrointestinal		
nausea	1.3%	2.0%
diarrhea	1.3%	0.7%
dry mouth	1.3%	1.3%
vomiting	.0%	0.7%
Dermatological		
skin reaction	.0%	0.7%
rash	.0%	1.3%
Other		
bruising	0.6%	.0%
smell/taste change	0.6%	.0%
backache	.0%	0.7%
fatigue	.0%	0.7%
hoarseness	.0%	0.7%
nasal congestion	.0%	0.7%

Electrocadiograms: Electrocardiograms, obtained during a randomized, double-blind, cross-over study in 57 patients, showed no observations or findings considered clinically significant, or related to drug administration. Most electrocardiographic observations, obtained during a randomized, double-blind, cross-over study in 40 patients, were judged not clinically significant or related to drug administration. One patient was noted to have some changes on the one hour postdose electrocardiograph consisting of ST and T wave abnormality suggesting possible inferior ischemia. This abnormality was not observed on the predose or the six hours postdose ECG. A treadmill was subsequently performed and all the findings were normal.

OVERDOSAGE

The expected symptoms with overdosage are those of excessive beta-stimulation and/or any of the symptoms listed under ADVERSE REACTIONS, e.g., seizures, angina, hypertension or hypotension, tachycardia with rates up to 200 beats per minute, arrhythmias, nervousness, headache, tremor, dry mouth. palpitation, nausea, dizziness, fatigue, malaise, and insomnia. Hypokalemia may also occur. As with all sympathomimetic aerosol medication, cardiac arrest and even death may be associated with abuse of MAXAIR AUTOHALER.

Treatment consists of discontinuation of pirbuterol together with appropriate symptomatic therapy. The judicious use of a cardioselective beta-receptor block may be considered, bearing in mind that such medication can produce bronchospasm. There is unsufficient evidence to determine if dialysis is beneficial for overdosage.

The oral median lethal dose of pirbuterol dihydrochloride in mice and rats is greater than 2000 mg/kg (approximately 3400 and 6800 times the maximum recommended daily inhalation dose for adults on a mg/m^2 basis).

DOSAGE AND ADMINISTRATION

The usual dose of adults and children 12 years and older is two inhalations (400 mcg) repeated every 4–6 hours. On inhalation (200 mcg) repeated every 4–6 hours may be sufficient for some patients.

A total daily dose of 12 inhalations should not be exceeded. It a previously effective dosage regimen fails to provide the usual relief, medical advice should be sought immediately as this is often a sign of seriously worsening asthma which would require reassessment of therapy.

HOW SUPPLIED

MAXAIR AUTOHALER, box of one, is supplied in a pressurized aluminum canister with a light blue plastic breath-activated actuator and a light blue mouthpiece cover. DO NOT USE WITH OTHER CANISTERS OR MOUTHPIECES. Each actuation delivers 253 mcg of pirbuterol (as pirbuterol acetate) from the value and 200 mcg of pirbuterol (as pirbuterol acetate) from the mouthpiece.

Canister net content weight 14.0 g, 400 inhalations (NDC **0089-0815-21**) and canister net content weight 2.8 g, 80 inhalations (Hospital Pack: NDC **0089-0817-10**, Sample Pack: NDC **0089-0815-08**).

The correct amount of medication in each canister cannot be assured after 80 actuations from the 2.8 g canister and 400 actuations from the 14.0 g canister, even though the canister is not completely empty. The canister should be discarded when the labeled numbers of actuations have been used.

Note: The indented statement below is required by the Federal government's Clean Air Act for all products containing or manufactured with chlorofluorocarbons (CFC's).

> **WARNING:** Contains trichloromonofluoromethane and dichlorodifluoromethane, substances which harm public health and environment by destroying ozone in the upper atmosphere.

A notice similar to the above WARNING has been placed in the "Patient's Instructions For Use" portion of this package insert under the Environmental Protection Agency's (EPA's) regulations. The patient's warning states that the patients should consult his or her physician if there are questions about alternatives.

Rx only

Store between 15° and 30°C (59° to 86°F). Failure to use this product within this temperature range may result in improper dosing. For optimal results, the canister should be at room temperature before use. Shake well before using.

The contents of MAXAIR AUTOHALER are under pressure. Do not puncture. Do not use or store near heat or open flame. Exposure to temperature above 120°F may cause bursting. Never throw container into fire or incinerator. Keep out of reach of children. Avoid spraying in eyes.

The light blue plastic actuator supplied with MAXAIR AUTOHALER should not be used with any other product canisters, and actuators from other product should not be used with MAXAIR AUTOHALER canister.

3M Pharmaceuticals
Northridge, CA 91324
654100 APRIL 2000

MAXAIR™ AUTOHALER™ (pirbuterol acetate inhalation aerosol)

Patient's Instructions For Use

Questions? Call our Patient Assistance Line at 1-(800)-841-3885 24 hours a day. To talk to an operator call between 8:30 AM and 5PM EST (Weekdays).

Change in device and instructions: a test fire slide has been added to the bottom of the Autohaler (actuator/mouthpiece) device to enable priming of the Autohaler.

Priming Procedure for MAXAIR™ AUTOHALER™

As with all aerosol medications, it is recommended to prime (test) MAXAIR AUTOHALER before using for the first time. MAXAIR AUTOHALER should also be primed if it has not been used in 48 hours. As described in the priming procedure, use the test fire slide to release two priming sprays into the air away from yourself and other people.

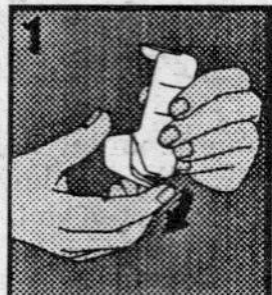

Remove mouthpiece cover by pulling down lip on **back** of cover.

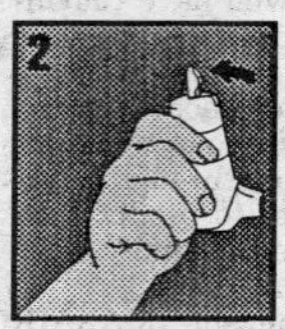

Point the mouthpiece away from yourself and other people so that the priming sprays will go into the air. Push the lever up so that it stays up.

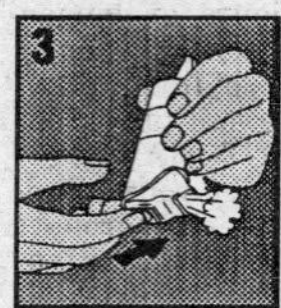

To release a priming spray, push the white test fire slide on the bottom of the mouthpiece in the direction indicated by the arrow on the test fire slide.

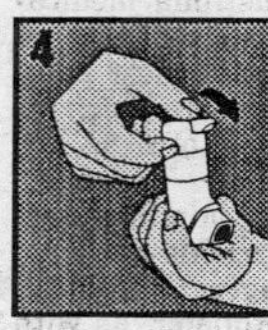

To release the second priming spray, return the lever to its down position and repeat steps 2 and 3. After releasing the second priming spray, return the lever to its down position.

Using Your MAXAIR™ AUTOHALER™

IMPORTANT NOTE: Use MAXAIR AUTOHALER according to the instructions given to you by your physician, who will advise you on the number of inhalations to take. If you have previously been using MAXAIR Inhaler, you should take the same number of inhalations through your MAXAIR AUTOHALER as you did through the MAXAIR Inhaler.

Before using your MAXAIR AUTOHALER, read complete instructions carefully.

The light blue plastic actuator supplied with MAXAIR AUTOHALER should not be used with any other product canisters, and actuators from other products should not be used with a MAXAIR AUTOHALER canister.

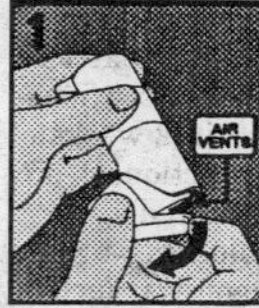

Remove mouthpiece cover by pulling down lip on **back** of cover.
Inspect mouthpiece for foreign objects.
Locate "Up" arrows on MAXAIR AUTOHALER.
Locate air vents at bottom of MAXAIR AUTOHALER.

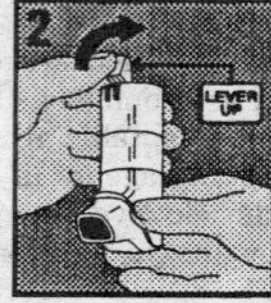

Hold MAXAIR AUTOHALER **upright** as shown in figure 2. The arrows should point up.
MAXAIR AUTOHALER must be held upright while raising lever.
Raise lever so that is stays up. It will "snap" into place.
Do not lower lever until step 6.

Hold MAXAIR AUTOHALER around the middle as shown in figure 3.
Shake MAXAIR AUTOHALER gently several times.

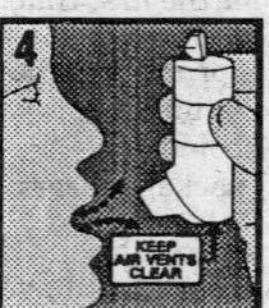

Continue to hold MAXAIR AUTOHALER upright as shown in figure 4.
Do not block air vents at bottom of MAXAIR AUTOHALER.
Exhale normally before use.

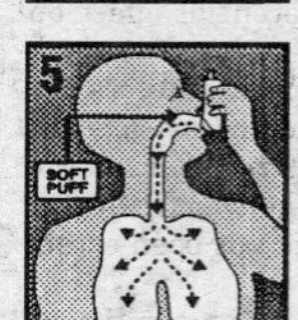

Seal your lips tightly around mouthpiece as shown in figure 5.
Inhale deeply through mouthpiece with **steady, moderate force.** You will hear a "click" and feel a **soft** puff when your inhaling triggers the release of medicine.
Do not stop when you hear and feel the puff. Continue to take a **full, deep breath.**
Take MAXAIR AUTOHALER away from your mouth when done inhaling. Hold your breath for 10 seconds, then exhale slowly.

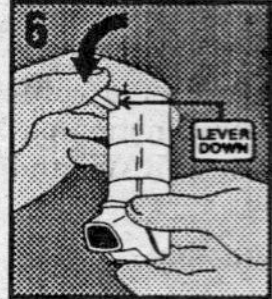

Continue to hold MAXAIR AUTOHALER upright while lowering the lever as shown in figure 6. Lower lever after each inhalation.
If your physician has prescribed additional inhalations, wait one minute then repeat steps 2 through 6. Following use, make sure lever is down and replace mouthpiece cover.

How to Clean and Care for MAXAIR™ AUTOHALER™

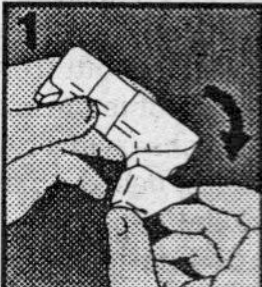

Remove mouthpiece cover by pulling down lip on **back** of cover.

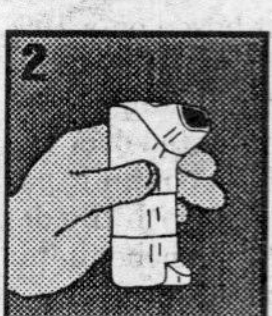

Turn MAXAIR AUTOHALER upside down. Wipe mouthpiece with a clean dry cloth.

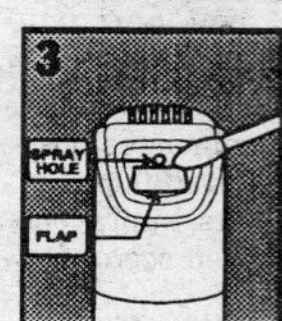

Gently tap back of MAXAIR AUTOHALER so flap comes down and spray hole can be seen. With white flap down as shown in the picture, clean the surface of the flap with a dry cotton swab.

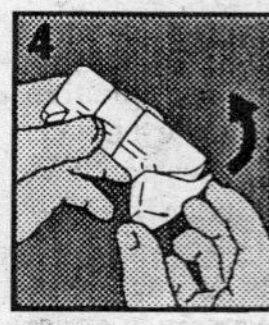

Replace mouthpiece cover. When you are not using MAXAIR AUTOHALER, make sure lever is down and mouthpiece cover is in place.
Repeat cleaning instructions weekly or as often as required.

Note: The indented statement below is required by the Federal Government's Clean Air Act for all products containing or manufactured with chlorofluorocarbons (CFC's).

> This product contains trichloromonofluromethane and dichlorodifluoromethane, substances which harm the environment by destroying ozone in the upper atmosphere.

Your physician has determined that this product is likely to help your personal health. USE THIS PRODUCT AS DIRECTED, UNLESS INSTRUCTED TO DO OTHERWISE BY YOUR PHYSICIAN. If you have any questions about alternatives, consult with your physician.

The correct amount of medication in each canister cannot be assured after 80 actuations from the 2.8 g canister and 400 actuations from the 14.0 g canister, even though the canister is not completely empty. You should keep track of the number of actuations used from each MAXAIR AUTOHALER and discard the MAXAIR AUTOHALER after 80 actuations from the 2.8 g canister and 400 actuations from the 14.0 g canister. MAXAIR AUTOHALER should be discarded when the labeled numbers of actuations have been used. Before you reach the specified number of actuations, you should consult your physician to determine whether a refill is needed. Just as you should not take extra doses without consulting your physician, you also should not stop using MAXAIR AUTOHALER without consulting your physician.

Dosage: Use only as directed by your physician.

WARNINGS: The effects of MAXAIR AUTOHALER may last up to five hours or longer. Therefore, it should not be used more frequently than recommended. Do not increase the number of frequency of doses without speaking with the prescribing physician. If the recommended dosage does not provide relief of symptoms, or your symptoms get worse, speak with your physician. While taking MAXAIR AUTOHALER, other inhaled medicines should not be used unless prescribed.

Important Information:

Store between 15° and 30° C (59° to 86° F). Failure to use this product within this temperature range may result in improper dosing. For optimal results, the canister should be at room temperature before use. Shake well before using.

Caution: Contents of canister under pressure. Do not puncture. Do not use near heat or open flame. Exposure to temperatures above 120°F may cause bursting. Never throw container into fire or incinerator. Avoid spraying in eyes. Keep out of reach of children.

Rx only

Use MAXAIR AUTOHALER only as prescribed by your physician.

Handle with care.

DO NOT USE WITH OTHER CANISTERS OR MOUTHPIECES.

For information on the drug, refer to your doctor or pharmacist.

General Information about MAXAIR™ AUTOHALER™ (pirbuterol acetate inhalation aerosol)

Your MAXAIR AUTOHALER is a new type of inhaler designed to be very easy to use. MAXAIR AUTOHALER automatically releases an inhalation of medicine when you inhale.

What will I feel when I use MAXAIR AUTOHALER?

MAXAIR AUTOHALER provides a soft spray of medicine. It is designed to automatically deliver a precisely measured dose of your medicine with each inhalation, so you can be assured of a consistent dose of medicine.

When medicine is delivered, you will hear a "click" a feel a **soft** inhalation.

How will I know when there's no more medicine in MAXAIR AUTOHALER?

The MAXAIR AUTOHALER you receive from the pharmacy contains 400 inhalations (the MAXAIR AUTOHALER sample contains 80 inhalations and says "SAMPLE" on the back; the MAXAIR AUTOHALER hospital unit also contains 80 inhalations and says "Hospital Pack" on the back). You can estimate how many days it will last by dividing 80 or 40 (total inhalations in a unit) by the number of inhalations you normally use in a day. The chart below can help you calculate about how long your 400 inhalation MAXAIR AUTOHALER will last. Actual usage may vary depending on how many inhalations you use each day. A total daily dose of 12 inhalations should not be exceeded.

Average Number of Inhalations Per Day	Approximate Days of Therapy Available
2 inhalations/day	200 days
4 inhalations/day	100 days
6 inhalations/day	65 days
8 inhalations/day	50 days

3M Pharmaceuticals
Northridge, CA 91324 APRIL 2000
Shown in Product Identification Guide, page 321

MAXAIR™ Inhaler ℞

(pirbuterol acetate inhalation aerosol)
Bronchodilator Aerosol
For Inhalation Only

DESCRIPTION

The active component of MAXAIR Inhaler is (R,S)α^6-{[(1,1-dimethylethyl) amino] methyl} - 3 - hydroxy - 2,6 - pyridinedimethanol monoacetate salt, a beta-2 adrenergic bronchodilator, having the following chemical structure:

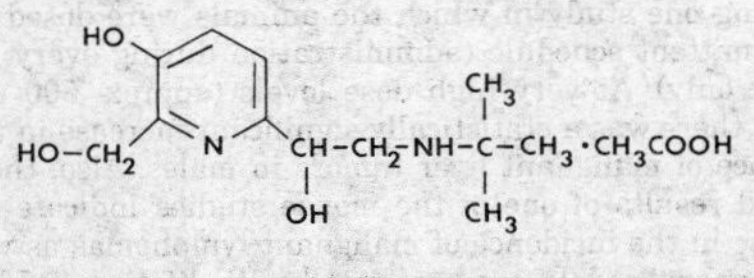

Pirbuterol acetate is a white, crystalline racemic mixture of two optically active isomers. It is a powder, freely soluble in water, with a molecular weight of 300.3 and empirical formula of $C_{12}H_{20}N_2O_3 \cdot C_2H_4O_2$.

MAXAIR Inhaler is a metered dose aerosol unit for oral inhalation. It provides a fine-particle suspension of pirbuterol acetate in the propellant mixture of trichloromonofluoromethane and dichlorodifluoromethane, with sorbitan trioleate. Each actuation delivers from the mouthpiece pirbuterol acetate equivalent to 0.2 mg of pirbuterol with the majority of particles less than 5 microns in diameter. Each canister provides at least 300 inhalations.

CLINICAL PHARMACOLOGY

In vitro studies and *in vivo* pharmacologic studies have demonstrated that MAXAIR has a preferential effect on beta-2 adrenergic receptors compared with isoproterenol. While it is recognized that beta-2 adrenergic receptors are the predominant receptors in bronchial smooth muscle, recent data indicate that there is a population of beta-2 receptors in the human heart, existing in a concentration between 10–50%. The precise function of these, however, is not yet established (see WARNINGS section).

The pharmacologic effects of beta adrenergic agonist drugs, including pirbuterol, are at least in part attributable to stimulation through beta adrenergic receptors of intracellular adenyl cyclase, the enzyme which catalyzes the conversion of adenosine triphosphate (ATP) to cyclic-3′,5′-adenosine monophosphate (c-AMP). Increased c-AMP levels are associated with relaxation of bronchial smooth muscle and inhibition of release of mediators of immediate hypersensitivity from cells, especially from mast cells.

Bronchodilator activity of MAXAIR was manifested clinically by an improvement in various pulmonary function parameters (FEV_1, MMF, PEFR, airway resistance [RAW] and conductance [GA/V_{tg}]).

In controlled double-blind single dose clinical trials, the onset of improvement in pulmonary function occurred within 5 minutes in most patients as determined by forced expiratory volume in one second (FEV_1). FEV_1 and MMF measurements also showed that maximum improvement in pulmonary function generally occurred 30–60 minutes following one (1) or two (2) inhalations of pirbuterol (0.2–0.4 mg). The duration of action of MAXAIR is maintained for 5 hours (the time at which the last observations were made) in a substantial number of patients, based on a 15% or greater increase in FEV_1. In controlled repetitive dose studies of 12 weeks' duration, 74% of 156 patients on pirbuterol and 62% of 141 patients on metaproterenol showed a clinically significant improvement based on a 15% or greater increase in FEV_1 on at least half of the days. Onset and duration were equivalent to that seen in single dose studies. Continued effectiveness was demonstrated over the 12-week period in the majority (94%) of responding patients; however, chronic dosing was associated with the development of tachyphylaxis (tolerance) to the bronchodilator effect in some patients in both treatment groups.

A placebo-controlled double-blind single dose study (24 patients per treatment group), utilizing continuous Holter monitoring for 5 hours after drug administration, showed no significant difference in ectopic activity between the placebo control group and MAXAIR at the recommended dose (0.2–0.4 mg), and twice the recommended dose (0.8 mg). As with other inhaled beta adrenergic agonists, supraventricular and ventricular ectopic beats have been seen with MAXAIR (see WARNINGS).

Recent studies in laboratory animals (minipigs, rodents, and dogs) recorded the occurrence of cardiac arrhythmias and sudden death (with histologic evidence of myocardial necrosis) when beta agonists and methylxanthines were administered concurrently. The significance of these findings when applied to humans is currently unknown.

Pharmacokinetics

As expected by extrapolation from oral data, systemic blood levels of pirbuterol are below the limit of assay sensitivity (2–5 ng/ml) following inhalation of doses up to 0.8 mg (twice the maximum recommended dose). A mean of 51% of the dose is recovered in urine as pirbuterol plus its sulfate conjugate following administration by aerosol. Pirbuterol is not metabolized by catechol-O-methyltransferase. The percent of administered dose recovered as pirbuterol plus its sulfate conjugate does not change significantly over the dose range of 0.4 mg to 0.8 mg and is not significantly different from that after oral administration of pirbuterol. The plasma half-life measured after oral administration is about two hours.

INDICATIONS AND USAGE

MAXAIR Inhaler is indicated for the prevention and reversal of bronchospasm in patients with reversible bronchospasm including asthma. It may be used with or without concurrent theophylline and/or steroid therapy.

CONTRAINDICATIONS

MAXAIR is contraindicated in patients with a history of hypersensitivity to any of its ingredients.

WARNINGS

As with other beta adrenergic aerosols, MAXAIR should not be used in excess. Controlled clinical studies and other clinical experience have shown that MAXAIR like other inhaled beta adrenergic agonists can produce a significant cardiovascular effect in some patients, as measured by pulse rate, blood pressure, symptoms, and/or ECG changes. As with other beta adrenergic aerosols, the potential for paradoxical bronchospasm (which can be life threatening) should be kept in mind. If it occurs, the preparation should be discontinued immediately and alternative therapy instituted.

Fatalities have been reported in association with excessive use of inhaled sympathomimetic drugs.

The contents of MAXAIR Inhaler are under pressure. Do not puncture. Do not use or store near heat or open flame. Exposure to temperature above 120°F may cause bursting. Never throw container into fire or incinerator. Keep out of reach of children.

PRECAUTIONS

General

Since pirbuterol is a sympathomimetic amine, it should be used with caution in patients with cardiovascular disorders, including ischemic heart disease, hypertension, or cardiac arrhythmias, in patients with hyperthyroidism or diabetes mellitus, and in patients who are unusually responsive to sympathomimetic amines or who have convulsive disorders. Significant changes in systolic and diastolic blood pressure could be expected to occur in some patients after use of any beta adrenergic aerosol bronchodilator.

Information for Patients

MAXAIR effects may last up to five hours or longer. It should not be used more often than recommended and the patient should not increase the number of inhalations or frequency of use without first asking the physician. If symptoms of asthma get worse, adverse reactions occur, or the patient does not respond to the usual dose, the patient should be instructed to contact the physician immediately. The patient should be advised to see the Illustrated Directions for Use.

Drug Interactions

Other beta adrenergic aerosol bronchodilators should not be used concomitantly with MAXAIR because they may have additive effects. Beta adrenergic agonists should be administered with caution to patients being treated with monoamine oxidase inhibitors or tricyclic antidepressants, since the action of beta adrenergic agonists on the vascular system may be potentiated.

Carcinogenesis, Mutagenesis and Impairment of Fertility

Pirbuterol hydrochloride administered in the diet to rats for 24 months and to mice for 18 months was free of carcinogenic activity at doses corresponding to 200 times the maximum human inhalation dose. In addition, the intragastric intubation of the drug at doses corresponding to 6250 times the maximum recommended human daily inhalation dose resulted in no increase in tumors in a 12-month rat study. Studies with pirbuterol revealed no evidence of mutagenesis. Reproduction studies in rats revealed no evidence of impaired fertility.

Teratogenic Effects—Pregnancy Category C

Reproduction studies have been performed in rats and rabbits by the inhalation route at doses up to 12 times (rat) and 16 times (rabbit) the maximum human inhalation dose and have revealed no significant findings. Animal reproduction studies in rats at *oral doses* up to 300 mg/kg and in rabbits at oral doses up to 100 mg/kg have shown no adverse effect on reproductive behavior, fertility, litter size, peri- and postnatal viability or fetal development. In rabbits at the highest dose level given, 300 mg/kg, abortions and fetal mortality were observed. There are no adequate and well controlled studies in pregnant women and MAXAIR should be used during pregnancy only if the potential benefit justifies the potential risk to the fetus.

Nursing Mothers

It is not known whether MAXAIR is excreted in human milk. Therefore, MAXAIR should be used during nursing only if the potential benefit justifies the possible risk to the newborn.

Pediatric Use

MAXAIR Inhaler is not recommended for patients under the age of 12 years because of insufficient clinical data to establish safety and effectiveness.

ADVERSE REACTIONS

The following rates of adverse reactions to pirbuterol are based on single and multiple dose clinical trials involving 761 patients, 400 of whom received multiple doses (mean duration of treatment was 2.5 months and maximum was 19 months).

The following were the adverse reactions reported more frequently than 1 in 100 patients:

CNS: nervousness (6.9%), tremor (6.0%), headache (2.0%), dizziness (1.2%).

Cardiovascular: palpitations (1.7%), tachycardia (1.2%).

Respiratory: cough (1.2%).

Gastrointestinal: nausea (1.7%).

The following adverse reactions occurred less frequently than 1 in 100 patients and there may be a causal relationship with pirbuterol:

CNS: depression, anxiety, confusion, insomnia, weakness, hyperkinesia, syncope.

Cardiovascular: hypotension, skipped beats, chest pain.

Gastrointestinal: dry mouth, glossitis, abdominal pain/cramps, anorexia, diarrhea, stomatitis, nausea and vomiting.

Ear, Nose and Throat: smell/taste changes, sore throat.

Dermatological: rash, pruritus.

Other: numbness in extremities, alopecia, bruising, fatigue, edema, weight gain, flushing.

Other adverse reactions were reported with a frequency of less than 1 in 100 patients but a causal relationship between pirbuterol and the reaction could not be determined: migraine, productive cough, wheezing, and dermatitis.

Continued on next page

Maxair Inhaler—Cont.

The following rates of adverse reactions during three-month controlled clinical trials involving 310 patients are noted. The table does not include mild reactions.

PERCENT OF PATIENTS WITH MODERATE TO SEVERE ADVERSE REACTIONS

Reaction	Pirbuterol N=157	Metaproterenol N=153
Central Nervous System		
tremors	1.3%	3.3%
nervousness	4.5%	2.6%
headache	1.3%	2.0%
weakness	.0%	1.3%
drowsiness	.0%	0.7%
dizziness	0.6%	.0%
Cardiovascular		
palpitations	1.3%	1.3%
tachycardia	1.3%	2.0%
Respiratory		
chest pain/tightness	1.3%	.0%
cough	.0%	0.7%
Gastrointestinal		
nausea	1.3%	2.0%
diarrhea	1.3%	0.7%
dry mouth	1.3%	1.3%
vomiting	.0%	0.7%
Dermatological		
skin reaction	.0%	0.7%
rash	.0%	1.3%
Other		
bruising	0.6%	.0%
smell/taste change	0.6%	.0%
backache	.0%	0.7%
fatigue	.0%	0.7%
hoarseness	.0%	0.7%
nasal congestion	.0%	0.7%

OVERDOSAGE

The expected symptoms with overdosage are those of excessive beta-stimulation and/or any of the symptoms listed under adverse reactions, e.g., angina, hypertension or hypotension, arrhythmias, nervousness, headache, tremor, dry mouth, palpitation, nausea, dizziness, fatigue, malaise, and insomnia.

Treatment consists of discontinuation of pirbuterol together with appropriate symptomatic therapy.

The oral acute lethal dose in male and female rats and mice was greater than 2000 mg base/kg. The aerosol acute lethal dose was not determined.

DOSAGE AND ADMINISTRATION

The usual dose for adults and children 12 years and older is two inhalations (0.4 mg) repeated every 4–6 hours. One inhalation (0.2 mg) repeated every 4–6 hours may be sufficient for some patients.

A total daily dose of 12 inhalations should not be exceeded. If a previously effective dosage regimen fails to provide the usual relief, medical advice should be sought immediately as this is often a sign of seriously worsening asthma which would require reassessment of therapy.

HOW SUPPLIED

MAXAIR Inhaler box of one, is supplied in a pressurized aluminum canister with a light-blue plastic actuator and attached white mouthpiece. Each actuation delivers pirbuterol acetate equivalent to 256 mcg of pirbuterol (as pirbuterol acetate) from the value and 200 mcg of pirbuterol (as pirbuterol acetate) from the mouthpiece.

Net content weight 25.6 g, 300 actuations (NDC **0089-0790-21**). The correct amount of medication in each canister cannot be assured after 300 actuations even though the canister is not completely empty. The canister should be discarded when the labeled number of actuations has been used.

Note: The indented statement below is required by the Federal government's Clean Air Act for all products containing or manufactured with chlorofluorocarbons (CFC's).

> **WARNING:** Contains trichloromonofluoromethane and dichlorodifluoromethane, substances which harm public health and environment by destroying ozone in the upper atmosphere.

A notice similar to the above WARNING has been placed in the "Patient's Instructions for Use" of this product pursuant to EPA regulations. The patient's warning states that the patient should consult his or her physician if there are questions about alternatives.

Rx only

Store between 15° and 30°C (59° to 86°F).

Failure to use this product within this temperature range may result in improper dosing. For optimal results, the canister should be at room temperature before use. Shake well before using.

The contents of MAXAIR Inhaler are under pressure. Do not puncture. Do not use or store near heat or open flame. Exposure to temperature above 120°F may cause bursting. Never throw container into fire or incinerator. Keep out of reach of children. Avoid spraying in eyes.

The light blue plastic actuator supplied with MAXAIR Inhaler should not be used with any other product canisters, and actuators from other products should not be used with the MAXAIR Inhaler canister.

3M Pharmaceuticals
Northridge, CA 91324
620901 May 1998

Shown in Product Identification Guide, page 321

METROGEL-VAGINAL® ℞

(metronidazole vaginal gel)
0.75% Vaginal Gel
FOR INTRAVAGINAL USE ONLY
NOT FOR OPHTHALMIC, DERMAL, OR ORAL USE

DESCRIPTION

METROGEL-VAGINAL is the intravaginal dosage form of the synthetic antibacterial agent, metronidazole, USP at a concentration of 0.75%. Metronidazole is a member of the imidazole class of antibacterial agents and is classified therapeutically as an anti-protozoal and anti-bacterial agent. Chemically, metronidazole is a 2-methyl-5-nitroimidazole-1-ethanol. It has a chemical formula of $C_6H_9N_3O_3$, a molecular weight of 171.16, and has the following structure:

METROGEL-VAGINAL is a gelled, purified water solution, containing metronidazole at a concentration of 7.5 mg/g (0.75%). The gel is formulated at pH 4.0. The gel also contains carbomer 934P, edetate disodium, methylparaben, propylparaben, propylene glycol, and sodium hydroxide. Each applicator full of 5 grams of vaginal gel contains approximately 37.5 mg of metronidazole.

CLINICAL PHARMACOLOGY

Normal Subjects:

Following a single, intravaginal 5 gram dose of metronidazole vaginal gel (equivalent to 37.5 mg of metronidazole) to 12 normal subjects, a mean maximum serum metronidazole concentration of 237 ng/mL was reported (range: 152 to 368 ng/mL). This is approximately 2% of the mean maximum serum metronidazole concentration reported in the same subjects administered a single, oral 500 mg dose of metronidazole (mean C_{max} = 12,785 ng/mL, range: 10,013 to 17,400 ng/mL). These peak concentrations were obtained in 6 to 12 hours after dosing with metronidazole vaginal gel and 1 to 3 hours after dosing with oral metronidazole.

The extent of exposure [area under the curve (AUC)] of metronidazole, when administered as a single intravaginal 5 gram dose of metronidazole vaginal gel (equivalent to 37.5 mg of metronidazole), was approximately 4% of the AUC of a single oral 500 mg dose of metronidazole (4977 ng-hr/mL and approximately 125,000 ng-hr/mL, respectively).

Dose-adjusted comparisons of AUCs demonstrated that, on a mg to mg comparison basis, the absorption of metronidazole, when administered vaginally, was approximately half that of an equivalent oral dosage.

Patients with Bacterial Vaginosis:

Following single and multiple 5 gram doses of metronidazole vaginal gel to 4 patients with bacterial vaginosis, a mean maximum serum metronidazole concentration of 214 ng/mL on day 1 and 294 ng/mL (range: 228 to 349 ng/mL) on day five were reported. Steady-state metronidazole serum concentrations following oral dosages of 400 to 500 mg BID have been reported to range from 6,000 to 20,000 ng/mL.

Microbiology:

The intracellular targets of action of metronidazole on anaerobes are largely unknown. The 5-nitro group of metronidazole is reduced by metabolically active anaerobes, and studies have demonstrated that the reduced form of the drug interacts with bacterial DNA. However, it is not clear whether interaction with DNA alone is an important component in the bactericidal action of metronidazole on anaerobic organisms.

Culture and sensitivity testing of bacteria are not routinely performed to establish the diagnosis of bacterial vaginosis. (See **INDICATIONS AND USAGE**.)

Standard methodology for the susceptibility testing of the potential bacterial vaginosis pathogens, *Gardnerella vaginalis, Mobiluncus* spp., and *Mycoplasma hominis*, has not been defined. Nonetheless, metronidazole is an antimicrobial agent active *in vitro* against most strains of the following organisms that have been reported to be associated with bacterial vaginosis:

Bacteroides spp.
Gardnerella vaginalis
Mobiluncus spp.
Peptostreptococcus spp.

INDICATIONS AND USAGE

METROGEL-VAGINAL is indicated in the treatment of bacterial vaginosis (formerly referred to as *Haemophilus* vaginitis, *Gardnerella* vaginitis, nonspecific vaginitis, *Corynebacterium* vaginitis, or anaerobic vaginosis).

NOTE: For purposes of this indication, a clinical diagnosis of bacterial vaginosis is usually defined by the presence of a homogeneous vaginal discharge that (a) has a pH of greater than 4.5, (b) emits a "fishy" amine odor when mixed with a 10% KOH solution, and (c) contains clue cells on microscopic examination. Gram's stain results consistent with a diagnosis of bacterial vaginosis include (a) markedly reduced or absent *Lactobacillus* morphology, (b) predominance of *Gardnerella* morphotype, and (c) absent or few white blood cells. Other pathogens commonly associated with vulvovaginitis, e.g., *Trichomonas vaginalis, Chlamydia trachomatis, N. gonorrhoeae, Candida albicans*, and *Herpes simplex* virus should be ruled out.

CONTRAINDICATIONS

METROGEL-VAGINAL is contraindicated in patients with a prior history of hypersensitivity to metronidazole, parabens, other ingredients of the formulation, or other nitroimidazole derivatives.

WARNINGS

Convulsive Seizures and Peripheral Neuropathy:

Convulsive seizures and peripheral neuropathy, the latter characterized mainly by numbness or paresthesia of an extremity, have been reported in patients treated with oral or intravenous metronidazole. The appearance of abnormal neurologic signs demands the prompt discontinuation of metronidazole vaginal gel therapy. Metronidazole vaginal gel should be administered with caution to patients with central nervous system diseases.

Psychotic Reactions:

Psychotic reactions have been reported in alcoholic patients who were using oral metronidazole and disulfiram concurrently. Metronidazole vaginal gel should not be administered to patients who have taken disulfiram within the last two weeks.

PRECAUTIONS

METROGEL-VAGINAL affords minimal peak serum levels and systemic exposure (AUCs) of metronidazole compared to 500 mg oral metronidazole dosing. Although these lower levels of exposure are less likely to produce the common reactions seen with oral metronidazole, the possibility of these and other reactions cannot be excluded presently. Data from well-controlled trials directly comparing metronidazole administered orally to metronidazole administered vaginally are not available.

General: Patients with severe hepatic disease metabolize metronidazole slowly. This results in the accumulation of metronidazole and its metabolites in the plasma. Accordingly, for such patients, metronidazole vaginal gel should be administered cautiously.

Known or previously unrecognized vaginal candidiasis may present more prominent symptoms during therapy with metronidazole vaginal gel. Approximately 6–10% of patients treated with METROGEL-VAGINAL developed symptomatic *Candida* vaginitis during or immediately after therapy.

Disulfiram-like reaction to alcohol has been reported with oral metronidazole, thus the possibility of such a reaction occurring while on metronidazole vaginal gel therapy cannot be excluded.

METROGEL-VAGINAL contains ingredients that may cause burning and irritation of the eye. In the event of accidental contact with the eye, rinse the eye with copious amounts of cool tap water.

Information for the Patient: The patient should be cautioned about drinking alcohol while being treated with metronidazole vaginal gel. While blood levels are significantly lower with METROGEL-VAGINAL than with usual doses of oral metronidazole, a possible interaction with alcohol cannot be excluded.

The patient should be instructed not to engage in vaginal intercourse during treatment with this product.

Drug Interactions: Oral metronidazole has been reported to potentiate the anticoagulant effect of warfarin and other coumarin anticoagulants, resulting in a prolongation of prothrombin time. This possible drug interaction should be considered when metronidazole vaginal gel is prescribed for patients on this type of anticoagulant therapy.

In patients stabilized on relatively high doses of lithium, short-term oral metronidazole therapy has been associated with elevation of serum lithium levels and, in a few cases, signs of lithium toxicity.

Use of cimetidine with oral metronidazole may prolong the half-life and decrease plasma clearance of metronidazole.

Drug/Laboratory Test Interactions: Metronidazole may interfere with certain types of determinations of serum chemistry values, such as aspartate aminotransferase (AST, SGOT), alanine aminotransferase (ALT, SGPT), lactate dehydrogenase (LDH), triglycerides, and glucose hexokinase. Values of zero may be observed. All of the assays in which interference has been reported involve enzymatic coupling of the assay to oxidation-reduction of nicotinamide-adenine dinucleotides (NAD+NADH). Interference is due to the similarity in absorbance peaks of NADH (340 nm) and metronidazole (322 nm) at pH 7.

Carcinogenesis, Mutagenesis, Impairment of Fertility: Metronidazole has shown evidence of carcinogenic activity in a number of studies involving chronic oral administration in mice and rats. Prominent among the effects in the mouse was the promotion of pulmonary tumorigenesis. This has been observed in all six reported studies in that species, including one study in which the animals were dosed on an intermittent schedule (administration during every fourth week only). At very high dose levels (approx. 500 mg/kg/day), there was a statistically significant increase in the incidence of malignant liver tumors in males. Also, the published results of one of the mouse studies indicate an increase in the incidence of malignant lymphomas as well as pulmonary neoplasms associated with lifetime feeding of the drug. All these effects are statistically significant. Several long-term oral dosing studies in the rat have been completed. There were statistically significant increases in the incidence of various neoplasms, particularly in mammary

and hepatic tumors, among female rats administered metronidazole over those noted in the concurrent female control groups. Two lifetime tumorigenicity studies in hamsters have been performed and reported to be negative.
These studies have not been conducted with 0.75% metronidazole vaginal gel, which would result in significantly lower systemic blood levels than those obtained with oral formulations.
Although metronidazole has shown mutagenic activity in a number of *in vitro* assay systems, studies in mammals (*in vivo*) have failed to demonstrate a potential for genetic damage.
Fertility studies have been performed in mice up to six times the recommended human oral dose (based on mg/m^2) and have revealed no evidence of impaired fertility.
Pregnancy: Teratogenic Effects Pregnancy Category B
There has been no experience to date with the use of METROGEL-VAGINAL in pregnant patients. Metronidazole crosses the placental barrier and enters the fetal circulation rapidly. No fetotoxicity or teratogenicity was observed when metronidazole was administered orally to pregnant mice at six times the recommended human dose (based on mg/m^2); however, in a single small study where the drug was administered intraperitoneally, some intrauterine deaths were observed. The relationship of these findings to the drug is unknown.
There are, however, no adequate and well-controlled studies in pregnant women. Because animal reproduction studies are not always predictive of human response, and because metronidazole is a carcinogen in rodents, this drug should be used during pregnancy only if clearly needed.
Nursing mothers: Specific studies of metronidazole levels in human milk following intravaginally administered metronidazole have not been performed. However, metronidazole is secreted in human milk in concentrations similar to those found in plasma following oral administration of metronidazole.
Because of the potential for tumorigenicity shown for metronidazole in mouse and rat studies, a decision should be made whether to discontinue nursing or to discontinue the drug, taking into account the importance of the drug to the mother.
Pediatric use: Safety and effectiveness in children have not been established.

ADVERSE EVENTS
Clinical Trials:
There were no deaths or serious adverse events related to drug therapy in clinical trials involving 800 non-pregnant women who received METROGEL-VAGINAL.
In a randomized, single-blind clinical trial of 505 non-pregnant women who received METROGEL-VAGINAL once or twice a day, 2 patients (1 from each regimen) discontinued therapy early due to drug-related adverse events. One patient discontinued drug because of moderate abdominal cramping and loose stools, while the other patient discontinued drug because of mild vaginal burning. These symptoms resolved after discontinuation of drug.
Medical events judged to be related, probably related, or possibly related to administration of METROGEL-VAGINAL once or twice a day were reported for 195/505 (39%) patients. The incidence of individual adverse reactions were not significantly different between the two regimens. Unless percentages are otherwise stipulated, the incidence of individual adverse reactions listed below was less than 1%:
Reproductive: Vaginal discharge (12%), symptomatic *Candida* cervicitis/vaginitis (10%), vulva/vaginal irritative symptoms (9%), pelvic discomfort (3%).
Gastrointestinal: Gastrointestinal discomfort (7%), nausea and/or vomiting (4%), unusual taste (2%), diarrhea/loose stools (1%), decreased appetite (1%), abdominal bloating/gas; thirsty, dry mouth. *Neurologic:* Headache (5%), dizziness (2%), depression. *Dermatologic:* Generalized itching or rash. *Other:* Unspecified cramping (1%), fatigue, darkened urine.
In previous clinical trials submitted for approved labeling of MetroGel-Vaginal the following was also reported: *Laboratory:* Increased/decreased white blood cell counts (1.7%).
Other Metronidazole Formulations: Other effects that have been reported in association with the use of **topical (dermal)** formulations of metronidazole include skin irritation, transient skin erythema, and mild skin dryness and burning. None of these adverse events exceeded an incidence of 2% of patients.
METROGEL-VAGINAL affords minimal peak serum levels and systemic exposure (AUC) of metronidazole compared to 500 mg oral metronidazole dosing. Although these lower levels of exposure are less likely to produce the common reactions seen with oral metronidazole, the possibility of these and other reactions cannot be excluded presently.
The following adverse reactions and altered laboratory tests have been reported with the **oral or parenteral** use of metronidazole:
Cardiovascular: Flattening of the T-wave may be seen in electrocardiographic tracings.
Central Nervous System: (See **WARNINGS**). Headache, dizziness, syncope, ataxia, confusion, convulsive seizures, peripheral neuropathy, vertigo, incoordination, irritability, depression, weakness, insomnia.
Gastrointestinal: Abdominal discomfort; nausea; vomiting; diarrhea; an unpleasant metallic taste; anorexia; epigastric distress; abdominal cramping; constipation; "furry" tongue; glossitis; stomatitis; pancreatitis; and modification of taste of alcoholic beverages.

MINITRAN System Rated Release In Vivo	System Size	Total Nitroglycerin in System	NDC Number (30 per carton)
0.1 mg/hr	3.3 cm^2	9 mg	NDC-0089-0301-02
0.2 mg/hr	6.7 cm^2	18 mg	NDC-0089-0302-02
0.4 mg/hr	13.3 cm^2	36 mg	NDC-0089-0303-02
0.6 mg/hr	20.0 cm^2	54 mg	NDC-0089-0304-02

Genitourinary: Overgrowth of *Candida* in the vagina, dyspareunia, decreased libido, proctitis.
Hematopoietic: Reversible neutropenia, reversible thrombocytopenia.
Hypersensitivity Reactions: Urticaria; erythematous rash; flushing; nasal congestion; dryness of the mouth, vagina, or vulva; fever; pruritus; fleeting joint pains.
Renal: Dysuria, cystitis, polyuria, incontinence, a sense of pelvic pressure, darkened urine.

OVERDOSAGE
There is no human experience with overdosage of metronidazole vaginal gel. Vaginally applied metronidazole gel, 0.75% could be absorbed in sufficient amounts to produce systemic effects.
(See **WARNINGS**.)

DOSAGE AND ADMINISTRATION
The recommended dose is one applicator full of METROGEL-VAGINAL (approximately 5 grams containing approximately 37.5 mg of metronidazole) intravaginally once or twice a day for 5 days. For once a day dosing, MetroGel-Vaginal should be administered at bedtime.

HOW SUPPLIED
METROGEL-VAGINAL (metronidazole vaginal gel, 0.75%) 0.75% Vaginal Gel is supplied in a 70 gram tube and packaged with 5 vaginal applicators. NDC number for the 70 gram tube is 0089-0200-25. Store at controlled room temperature 15° to 30°C (59° to 86°F). Protect from freezing.
Clinical Studies
In a randomized, single-blind, clinical trial of non-pregnant women with bacterial vaginosis who received MetroGel-Vaginal daily for 5 days, the clinical cure rates for evaluable patients, determined at 4 weeks after completion of therapy for the QD and BID regimens were 98/185 (53%) and 109/190 (57%), respectively.
Rx only
620700 March 1998

Manufactured for
3M Pharmaceuticals
Northridge, CA 91324
Manufactured by
DPT Laboratories, Inc.
San Antonio, TX, 78215
Shown in Product Identification Guide, page 321

MINITRAN™ ℞
(nitroglycerin)
Transdermal Delivery System

For full prescribing information see leaflet accompanying product or call 800-328-0255 for a copy.

HOW SUPPLIED
[See table above]

NORFLEX™ ℞
(orphenadrine citrate)
Extended-release
Tablets and Injection

DESCRIPTION
Orphenadrine citrate is the citrate salt of orphenadrine (2-dimethylaminoethyl 2-methylbenzhydryl ether citrate). It occurs as a white, crystalline powder having a bitter taste. It is practically odorless; sparingly soluble in water, slightly soluble in alcohol.
Each Norflex Extended-release tablet contains 100 mg orphenadrine citrate. Norflex Extended-release tablets also contain: calcium stearate, ethylcellulose, and lactose. Norflex Injection contains 60 mg of orphenadrine citrate in aqueous solution in each ampul. Norflex Injection also contains: sodium bisulfite NF, 2.0 mg; sodium chloride USP, 5.8 mg; sodium hydroxide, to adjust pH; and water for injection USP, q.s. to 2 mL.

ACTIONS
The mode of therapeutic action has not been clearly identified, but may be related to its analgesic properties. Orphenadrine citrate also possesses anticholinergic actions.

INDICATIONS
Orphenadrine citrate is indicated as an adjunct to rest, physical therapy, and other measures for the relief of discomfort associated with acute painful musculoskeletal conditions. The mode of action of the drug has not been clearly identified, but may be related to its analgesic properties. Orphenadrine citrate does not directly relax tense skeletal muscles in man.

CONTRAINDICATIONS
Contraindicated in patients with glaucoma, pyloric or duodenal obstruction, stenosing peptic ulcers, prostatic hypertrophy or obstruction of the bladder neck, cardio-spasm (megaesophagus) and myasthenia gravis. Contraindicated in patients who have demonstrated a previous hypersensitivity to the drug.

WARNINGS
Some patients may experience transient episodes of lightheadedness, dizziness or syncope. Norflex may impair the ability of the patient to engage in potentially hazardous activities such as operating machinery or driving a motor vehicle; ambulatory patients should therefore be cautioned accordingly.
Norflex Injection contains sodium bisulfite, a sulfite that may cause allergic-type reactions including anaphylactic symptoms and life-threatening or less severe asthmatic episodes in certain susceptible people. The overall prevalence of sulfite sensitivity in the general population is unknown and probably low. Sulfite sensitivity is seen more frequently in asthmatic than nonasthmatic people.

PREGNANCY
Pregnancy Category C. Animal reproduction studies have not been conducted with Norflex. It is also not known whether Norflex can cause fetal harm when administered to a pregnant woman or can affect reproduction capacity. Norflex should be given to a pregnant woman only if clearly needed.

PEDIATRIC USE
Safety and effectiveness in pediatric patients have not been established.

PRECAUTIONS
Confusion, anxiety and tremors have been reported in few patients receiving propoxyphene and orphenadrine concomitantly. As these symptoms may be simply due to an additive effect, reduction of dosage and/or discontinuation of one or both agents is recommended in such cases.
Orphenadrine citrate should be used with caution in patients with tachycardia, cardiac decompensation, coronary insufficiency, cardiac arrhythmias.
Safety of continuous long-term therapy with orphenadrine has not been established. Therefore, if orphenadrine is prescribed for prolonged use, periodic monitoring of blood, urine and liver function values is recommended.

ADVERSE REACTIONS
Adverse reactions of orphenadrine are mainly due to the mild anticholinergic action of orphenadrine, and are usually associated with higher dosage. Dryness of the mouth is usually the first adverse effect to appear. When the daily dose is increased, possible adverse effects include: tachycardia, palpitation, urinary hesitancy or retention, blurred vision, dilatation of pupils, increased ocular tension, weakness, nausea, vomiting, headache, dizziness, constipation, drowsiness, hypersensitivity reactions, pruritus, hallucinations, agitation, tremor, gastric irritation, and rarely urticaria and other dermatoses. Infrequently, an elderly patient may experience some degree of mental confusion. These adverse reactions can usually be eliminated by reduction in dosage. Very rare cases of aplastic anemia associated with the use of orphenadrine tablets have been reported. No causal relationship has been established.
Rare instances of anaphylactic reaction have been reported associated with the intramuscular injection of Norflex Injection.

DOSAGE AND ADMINISTRATION
TABLETS: Adults—Two tablets per day; one in the morning and one in the evening.
INJECTION: Adults—One 2 mL ampul (60 mg) intravenously or intramuscularly; may be repeated every 12 hours. Relief may be maintained by 1 Norflex Extended-release tablet twice daily.

HOW SUPPLIED
TABLETS: Each round, white tablet imprinted with "3M" on one side and "221" on the other. Bottles of 100 (NDC **0089-0221-10**) and 500 (NDC **0089-0221-50**). Each tablet contains 100 mg of orphenadrine citrate.
INJECTION: Boxes of 6 (NDC **0089-0540-06**) 2 mL ampuls, each ampul containing 60 mg of orphenadrine citrate in aqueous solution.
Store at controlled room temperature, 15°–30°C (59°–86°F).
Rx only
60050 March 1998
994102

Tablets Manufactured by
3M Pharmaceuticals
Northridge, CA 91324

Injection Manufactured for
3M Pharmaceuticals
Northridge, CA 91324
By Abbott Laboratories
North Chicago, IL 60064

Continued on next page

NORGESIC™ ℞
and
NORGESIC™ FORTE ℞
Tablets

ACTIONS
Orphenadrine citrate is a centrally acting (brain stem) compound which in animals selectively blocks facilitatory functions of the reticular formation. Orphenadrine does not produce myoneural block, nor does it affect crossed extensor reflexes. Orphenadrine prevents nicotine-induced convulsions but not those produced by strychnine.
Chronic administration of Norgesic to dogs and rats has revealed no drug-related toxicity. No blood or urine changes were observed, nor were there any macroscopic or microscopic pathological changes detected. Extensive experience with combinations containing aspirin and caffeine has established them as safe agents. The addition of orphenadrine citrate does not alter the toxicity of aspirin and caffeine.
The mode of therapeutic action of orphenadrine has not been clearly identified, but may be related to its analgesic properties. Orphenadrine citrate also possesses anticholinergic actions.

INDICATIONS
1. Symptomatic relief of mild to moderate pain of acute musculoskeletal disorders.
2. The orphenadrine component is indicated as an adjunct to rest, physical therapy, and other measures for the relief of discomfort associated with acute painful musculoskeletal conditions.
   The mode of action of orphenadrine has not been clearly identified, but may be related to its analgesic properties. Norgesic and Norgesic Forte do not directly relax tense skeletal muscles in man.

CONTRAINDICATIONS
Because of the mild anticholinergic effect of orphenadrine, Norgesic or Norgesic Forte should not be used in patients with glaucoma, pyloric or duodenal obstruction, achalasia, prostatic hypertrophy or obstructions at the bladder neck. Norgesic or Norgesic Forte is also contraindicated in patients with myasthenia gravis and in patients known to be sensitive to aspirin or caffeine.
The drug is contraindicated in patients who have demonstrated a previous hypersensitivity to the drug.

WARNINGS
Reye's Syndrome may develop in individuals who have chicken pox, influenza, or flu symptoms. Some studies suggest a possible association between the development of Reye's Syndrome and the use of medicines containing salicylate or aspirin. Norgesic and Norgesic Forte contain aspirin and therefore are not recommended for use in patients with chicken pox, influenza, or flu symptoms.
Norgesic and Norgesic Forte may impair the ability of the patient to engage in potentially hazardous activities such as operating machinery or driving a motor vehicle; ambulatory patients should therefore be cautioned accordingly.
Aspirin should be used with extreme caution in the presence of peptic ulcers and coagulation abnormalities.

USAGE IN PREGNANCY
Since safety of the use of this preparation in pregnancy, during lactation, or in the childbearing age has not been established, use of the drug in such patients requires that the potential benefits of the drug be weighed against its possible hazard to the mother and child.

PEDIATRIC USE
Safety and effectiveness in pediatric patients have not been established.

PRECAUTIONS
Confusion, anxiety and tremors have been reported in a few patients receiving propoxyphene and orphenadrine concomitantly. As these symptoms may be simply due to an additive effect, reduction of dosage and/or discontinuation of one or both agents is recommended in such cases.
Safety of continuous long term therapy with Norgesic or Norgesic Forte has not been established; therefore, if Norgesic or Norgesic Forte is prescribed for prolonged use, periodic monitoring of blood, urine and liver function values is recommended.

ADVERSE REACTIONS
Side effects of Norgesic or Norgesic Forte are those seen with aspirin and caffeine or those usually associated with mild anticholinergic agents. These may include tachycardia, palpitation, urinary hesitancy or retention, dry mouth, blurred vision, dilatation of the pupil, increased intraocular tension, weakness, nausea, vomiting, headache, dizziness, constipation, drowsiness, and rarely, urticaria and other dermatoses. Infrequently, an elderly patient may experience some degree of confusion. Mild central excitation and occasional hallucinations may be observed. These mild side effects can usually be eliminated by reduction in dosage. One case of aplastic anemia associated with the use of Norgesic has been reported. No causal relationship has been established. Rare G.I. hemorrhage due to aspirin content may be associated with the administration of Norgesic or Norgesic Forte. Some patients may experience transient episodes of light-headedness, dizziness or syncope.

DOSAGE AND ADMINISTRATION
Norgesic: Adults 1 to 2 tablets 3 to 4 times daily.
Norgesic Forte: Adults ½ to 1 tablet 3 to 4 times daily.

HOW SUPPLIED
Norgesic tablets can be identified by their two layers colored white and yellow. Each round tablet is embossed "NORGESIC" on one side and "3M" on the other and contains orphenadrine citrate (2-dimethylaminoethyl 2-methylbenzhydryl ether citrate) 25 mg, aspirin 385 mg, and caffeine 30 mg.
Norgesic Forte tablets are exactly twice the strength of Norgesic. They are identified by their scored capsule shape and by their two layers colored white and yellow. Each capsule shaped tablet is embossed "NORGESIC FORTE" on one side and "3M" on the other and contains orphenadrine citrate 50 mg, aspirin 770 mg, and caffeine 60 mg.
Norgesic and Norgesic Forte also contain: lactose, polyethylene glycol, povidone, starch, sucrose, zinc stearate, and D&C yellow #10.
Norgesic: Bottles of 100 tablets (NDC **0089-0231-10**) and 500 tablets (NDC **0089-0231-50**).
Norgesic Forte: Bottles of 100 tablets (NDC **0089-0233-10**) and 500 tablets (NDC **0089-0233-50**).
Store below 30°C (86°F).
Rx only
600600 May 1998
3M Pharmaceuticals
Northridge, CA 91324

TAMBOCOR™ ℞
[*tăm-ba-kōr*]
(flecainide acetate)
Tablets

DESCRIPTION
TAMBOCOR™ (flecainide acetate) is an antiarrhythmic drug available in tablets of 50, 100 or 150 mg for oral administration.
Flecainide acetate is benzamide, N-(2-piperidinylmethyl)-2,5-bis(2,2,2-trifluoroethoxy)-monoacetate. The structural formula is given below.

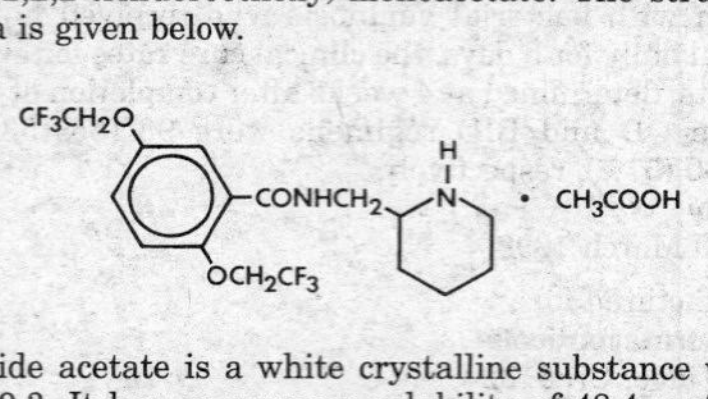

Flecainide acetate is a white crystalline substance with a pK_a of 9.3. It has an aqueous solubility of 48.4 mg/mL at 37°C.
TAMBOCOR tablets also contain: croscarmellose sodium, hydrogenated vegetable oil, magnesium stearate, microcrystalline cellulose and starch.

CLINICAL PHARMACOLOGY
TAMBOCOR has local anesthetic activity and belongs to the membrane stabilizing (Class 1) group of antiarrhythmic agents; it has electrophysiologic effects characteristic of the IC class of antiarrhythmics.
Electrophysiology. In man, TAMBOCOR produces a dose-related decrease in intracardiac conduction in all parts of the heart with the greatest effect on the His-Purkinje system (H-V conduction). Effects upon atrioventricular (AV) nodal conduction time and intra-atrial conduction times, although present, are less pronounced than those on ventricular conduction velocity. Significant effects on refractory periods were observed only in the ventricle. Sinus node recovery times (corrected) following pacing and spontaneous cycle lengths are somewhat increased. This latter effect may become significant in patients with sinus node dysfunction. (See Warnings.)
TAMBOCOR causes a dose-related and plasma-level related decrease in single and multiple PVCs and can suppress recurrence of ventricular tachycardia. In limited studies of patients with a history of ventricular tachycardia, TAMBOCOR has been successful 30–40% of the time in fully suppressing the inducibility of arrhythmias by programmed electrical stimulation. Based on PVC suppression, it appears that plasma levels of 0.2 to 1.0 µg/mL may be needed to obtain the maximal therapeutic effect. It is more difficult to assess the dose needed to suppress serious arrhythmias, but trough plasma levels in patients successfully treated for recurrent ventricular tachycardia were between 0.2 and 1.0 µg/mL. Plasma levels above 0.7–1.0 µg/mL are associated with a higher rate of cardiac adverse experiences such as conduction defects or bradycardia. The relation of plasma levels to proarrhythmic events is not established, but dose reduction in clinical trials of patients with ventricular tachycardia appears to have led to a reduced frequency and severity of such events.
Hemodynamics. TAMBOCOR does not usually alter heart rate, although bradycardia and tachycardia have been reported occasionally.
In animals and isolated myocardium, a negative inotropic effect of flecainide has been demonstrated. Decreases in ejection fraction, consistent with a negative inotropic effect, have been observed after single administration of 200 to 250 mg of the drug in man; both increases and decreases in ejection fraction have been encountered during multidose therapy in patients at usual therapeutic doses. (See Warnings.)
Metabolism in Humans. Following oral administration, the absorption of TAMBOCOR is nearly complete. Peak plasma levels are attained at about three hours in most individuals (range, 1 to 6 hours). Flecainide does not undergo any consequential presystemic biotransformation (first-pass effect). Food or antacid do not affect absorption. Milk, however, may inhibit absorption in infants. A reduction in TAMBOCOR dosage should be considered when milk is removed from the diet of infants.
The apparent plasma half-life averages about 20 hours and is quite variable (range, 12 to 27 hours) after multiple oral doses in patients with premature ventricular contractions (PVCs). With multiple dosing, plasma levels increase because of its long half-life with steady-state levels approached in 3 to 5 days; once at steady-state, no additional (or unexpected) accumulation of drug in plasma occurs during chronic therapy. Over the usual therapeutic range, data suggest that plasma levels in an individual are approximately proportional to dose, deviating upwards from linearity only slightly (about 10 to 15% per 100 mg on average).
In healthy subjects, about 30% of a single oral dose (range, 10 to 50%) is excreted in urine as unchanged drug. The two major urinary metabolites are meta-O-dealkylated flecainide (active, but about one-fifth as potent) and the meta-O-dealkylated lactam of flecainide (non-active metabolite). These two metabolites (primarily conjugated) account for most of the remaining portion of the dose. Several minor metabolites (3% of the dose or less) are also found in urine; only 5% of an oral dose is excreted in feces. In patients, free (unconjugated) plasma levels of the two major metabolites are very low (less than 0.05 µg/mL).
In vitro metabolic studies have confirmed that cytochrome P450IID6 is involved in the metabolism of flecainide.
When urinary pH is very alkaline (8 or higher), as may occur in rare conditions (e.g., renal tubular acidosis, strict vegetarian diet), flecainide elimination from plasma is much slower.
The elimination of flecainide from the body depends on renal function (i.e., 10 to 50% appears in urine as unchanged drug). With increasing renal impairment, the extent of unchanged drug excretion in urine is reduced and the plasma half-life of flecainide is prolonged. Since flecainide is also extensively metabolized, there is no simple relationship between creatinine clearance and the rate of flecainide elimination from plasma. (See Dosage and Administration.)
In patients with NYHA class III congestive heart failure (CHF), the rate of flecainide elimination from plasma (mean half-life, 19 hours) is moderately slower than for healthy subjects (mean half-life, 14 hours), but similar to the rate for patients with PVCs without CHF. The extent of excretion of unchanged drug in urine is also similar. (See Dosage and Administration.)
Under one year of age, currently available data are limited but suggest that the half-life at birth may be as long as 29 hours, decreasing to 11–12 hours by three months of age and 6 hours by one year of age. The pharmacokinetics in hydropic infants have not been studied, but case reports suggest prolonged elimination. In children aged 1 year to 12 years the half-life is approximately 8 hours. In adolescents (age 12 to 15) the plasma elimination half-life is approximately 11–12 hours. Since milk may inhibit absorption in infants, a reduction in TAMBOCOR dosage should be considered when milk is removed from the diet (e.g., gastroenteritis, weaning). Plasma trough flecainide levels should be monitored during major changes in dietary milk intake.
From age 20 to 80, plasma levels are only slightly higher with advancing age; flecainide elimination from plasma is somewhat slower in elderly subjects than in younger subjects. Patients up to age 80+ have been safely treated with usual dosages.
The extent of flecainide binding to human plasma proteins is about 40% and is independent of plasma drug level over the range of 0.015 to about 3.4 µg/mL. Thus, clinically significant drug interactions based on protein binding effects would not be expected.
Hemodialysis removes only about 1% of an oral dose as unchanged flecainide.
Small increases in plasma digoxin levels are seen during coadministration of TAMBOCOR with digoxin. Small increases in both flecainide and propranolol plasma levels are seen during coadministration of these two drugs. (See Precautions, Drug Interactions.)
Clinical Trials. In two randomized, crossover, placebo-controlled clinical trials of 16 weeks double-blind duration, 79% of patients with paroxysmal supraventricular tachycardia (PSVT) receiving flecainide were attack free, whereas 15% of patients receiving placebo remained attack free. The median time-before-recurrence of PSVT in patients receiving placebo was 11 to 12 days, whereas over 85% of patients receiving flecainide had no recurrence at 60 days.
In two randomized, crossover, placebo-controlled clinical trials of 16 weeks double-blind duration, 31% of patients with paroxysmal atrial fibrillation/flutter (PAF) receiving flecainide were attack free, whereas 8% receiving placebo remained attack free. The median time-before-recurrence of PAF in patients receiving placebo was about 2 to 3 days, whereas for those receiving flecainide the median time-before-recurrence was 15 days.

INDICATIONS AND USAGE
In patients without structural heart disease, TAMBOCOR is indicated for the prevention of
— paroxysmal supraventricular tachycardias (PSVT), including atrioventricular nodal reentrant tachycardia, atrioventricular reentrant tachycardia and other supraventricular tachycardias of unspecified mechanism associated with disabling symptoms

— paroxysmal atrial fibrillation/flutter (PAF) associated with disabling symptoms

TAMBOCOR is also indicated for the prevention of

— documented ventricular arrhythmias, such as sustained ventricular tachycardia (sustained VT), that in the judgment of the physician are life-threatening.

Use of TAMBOCOR for the treatment of sustained VT, like other antiarrhythmics, should be initiated in the hospital. The use of TAMBOCOR is not recommended in patients with less severe ventricular arrhythmias even if the patients are symptomatic.

Because of the proarrhythmic effects of TAMBOCOR, its use should be reserved for patients in whom, in the opinion of the physician, the benefits of treatment outweigh the risks.

TAMBOCOR should not be used in patients with recent myocardial infarction. (See Boxed Warnings.)

Use of TAMBOCOR in chronic atrial fibrillation has not been adequately studied and is not recommended. (See Boxed Warnings.)

As is the case for other antiarrhythmic agents, there is no evidence from controlled trials that the use of TAMBOCOR favorably affects survival or the incidence of sudden death.

CONTRAINDICATIONS

TAMBOCOR is contraindicated in patients with pre-existing second- or third-degree AV block, or with right bundle branch block when associated with a left hemiblock (bifascicular block), unless a pacemaker is present to sustain the cardiac rhythm should complete heart block occur. TAMBOCOR is also contraindicated in the presence of cardiogenic shock or known hypersensitivity to the drug.

WARNINGS

Mortality. TAMBOCOR was included in the National Heart Lung and Blood Institute's Cardiac Arrhythmia Suppression Trial (CAST), a long-term, multicenter, randomized, double-blind study in patients with asymptomatic non-life-threatening ventricular arrhythmias who had a myocardial infarction more than six days but less than two years previously. An excessive mortality or non-fatal cardiac arrest rate was seen in patients treated with TAMBOCOR compared with that seen in patients assigned to a carefully matched placebo-treated group. This rate was 16/315 (5.1%) for TAMBOCOR and 7/309 (2.3%) for the matched placebo. The average duration of treatment with TAMBOCOR in this study was ten months.

The applicability of the CAST results to other populations (e.g., those without recent myocardial infarction) is uncertain, but at present, it is prudent to consider the risks of Class IC agents (including TAMBOCOR), coupled with the lack of any evidence of improved survival, generally unacceptable in patients without life-threatening ventricular arrhythmias, even if the patients are experiencing unpleasant, but not life-threatening, symptoms or signs.

Ventricular Pro-arrhythmic Effects in Patients with Atrial Fibrillation/Flutter. A review of the world literature revealed reports of 568 patients treated with oral TAMBOCOR for paroxysmal atrial fibrillation/flutter (PAF). Ventricular tachycardia was experienced in 0.4% (2/568) of these patients. Of 19 patients in the literature with chronic atrial fibrillation (CAF), 10.5% (2) experienced VT or VF. FLECAINIDE IS NOT RECOMMENDED FOR USE IN PATIENTS WITH CHRONIC ATRIAL FIBRILLATION. Case reports of ventricular proarrhythmic effects in patients treated with TAMBOCOR for atrial fibrillation/flutter have included increased PVCs, VT, ventricular fibrillation (VF), and death.

As with other Class I agents, patients treated with TAMBOCOR for atrial flutter have been reported with 1:1 atrioventricular conduction due to slowing the atrial rate. A paradoxical increase in the ventricular rate also may occur in patients with atrial fibrillation who receive TAMBOCOR. Concomitant negative chronotropic therapy such as digoxin or beta-blockers may lower the risk of this complication.

PROARRHYTHMIC EFFECTS

TAMBOCOR, like other antiarrhythmic agents, can cause new or worsened supraventricular or ventricular arrhythmias. Ventricular proarrhythmic effects range from an increase in frequency of PVCs to the development of more severe ventricular tachycardia, e.g., tachycardia that is more sustained or more resistant to conversion to sinus rhythm, with potentially fatal consequences. In studies of ventricular arrhythmia patients treated with TAMBOCOR, three-fourths of proarrhythmic events were new or worsened ventricular tachyarrhythmias, the remainder being increased frequency of PVCs or new supraventricular arrhythmias. In patients treated with flecainide for sustained ventricular tachycardia, 80% (51/64) of proarrhythmic events occurred within 14 days of the onset of therapy. In studies of 225 patients with supraventricular arrhythmia (108 with paroxysmal supraventricular tachycardia and 117 with paroxysmal atrial fibrillation), there were 9 (4%) proarrhythmic events, 8 of them in patients with paroxysmal atrial fibrillation. Of the 9, 7 (including the one in a PSVT patient) were exacerbations of supraventricular arrhythmias (longer duration, more rapid rate, harder to reverse) while 2 were ventricular arrhythmias, including one fatal case of VT/VF and one wide complex VT (the patient showed inducible VT, however, after withdrawal of flecainide), both in patients with paroxysmal atrial fibrillation and known coronary artery disease.

It is uncertain if TAMBOCOR's risk of proarrhythmia is exaggerated in patients with chronic atrial fibrillation (CAF), high ventricular rate, and/or exercise. Wide complex tachycardia and ventricular fibrillation have been reported in two of 12 CAF patients undergoing maximal exercise tolerance testing.

In patients with complex ventricular arrhythmias, it is often difficult to distinguish a spontaneous variation in the patient's underlying rhythm disorder from drug-induced worsening, so that the following occurrence rates must be considered approximations. Their frequency appears to be related to dose and to the underlying cardiac disease.

Among patients treated for sustained VT (who frequently also had CHF, a low ejection fraction, a history of myocardial infarction and/or an episode of cardiac arrest), the incidence of proarrhythmic events was 13% when dosage was initiated at 200 mg/day with slow upward titration, and did not exceed 300 mg/day in most patients. In early studies in patients with sustained VT utilizing a higher initial dose (400 mg/day) the incidence of proarrhythmic events was 26%; moreover, in about 10% of the patients treated proarrhythmic events resulted in death, despite prompt medical attention. With lower initial doses, the incidence of proarrhythmic events resulting in death decreased to 0.5% of these patients. Accordingly, it is extremely important to follow the recommended dosage schedule. (See Dosage and Administration.)

The relatively high frequency of proarrhythmic events in patients with sustained VT and serious underlying heart disease, and the need for careful titration and monitoring, requires that therapy of patients with sustained VT be started in the hospital. (See Dosage and Administration.)

HEART FAILURE

TAMBOCOR has a negative inotropic effect and may cause or worsen CHF, particularly in patients with cardiomyopathy, preexisting severe heart failure (NYHA functional class III or IV) or low ejection fractions (less than 30%). In patients with supraventricular arrhythmias new or worsened CHF developed in 0.4% (1/225) of patients. In patients with sustained ventricular tachycardia during a mean duration of 7.9 months of TAMBOCOR therapy, 6.3% (20/317) developed new CHF. In patients with sustained ventricular tachycardia and a history of CHF, during a mean duration of 5.4 months of TAMBOCOR therapy, 25.7% (78/304) developed worsened CHF. Exacerbation of preexisting CHF occurred more commonly in studies which included patients with class III or IV failure than in studies which excluded such patients. TAMBOCOR should be used cautiously in patients who are known to have a history of CHF or myocardial dysfunction. The initial dosage in such patients should be no more than 100 mg bid (see Dosage and Administration) and patients should be monitored carefully. Close attention must be given to maintenance of cardiac function, including optimization of digitalis, diuretic, or other therapy. In cases where CHF has developed or worsened during treatment with TAMBOCOR, the time of onset has ranged from a few hours to several months after starting therapy. Some patients who develop evidence of reduced myocardial function while on TAMBOCOR can continue on TAMBOCOR with adjustment of digitalis or diuretics, others may require dosage reduction or discontinuation of TAMBOCOR. When feasible, it is recommended that plasma flecainide levels be monitored. Attempts should be made to keep trough plasma levels below 0.7 to 1.0 μg/mL.

Effects on Cardiac Conduction. TAMBOCOR slows cardiac conduction in most patients to produce dose-related increases in PR, QRS, and QT intervals.

PR interval increases on average about 25% (0.04 seconds) and as much as 118% in some patients. Approximately one-third of patients may develop new first-degree AV heart block (PR interval ≥ 0.20 seconds). The QRS complex increases on average about 25% (0.02 seconds) and as much as 150% in some patients. Many patients develop QRS complexes with a duration of 0.12 seconds or more. In one study, 4% of patients developed new bundle branch block while on TAMBOCOR. The degree of lengthening of PR and QRS intervals does not predict either efficacy or the development of cardiac adverse effects. In clinical trials, it was unusual for PR intervals to increase to 0.30 seconds or more, or for QRS intervals to increase to 0.18 seconds or more. Thus, caution should be used when such intervals occur, and dose reductions may be considered. The QT interval widens about 8%, but most of this widening (about 60% to 90%) is due to widening of the QRS duration. The JT interval (QT minus QRS) only widens about 4% on the average. Significant JT prolongation occurs in less than 2% of patients. There have been rare cases of Torsade de Pointes-type arrhythmia associated with TAMBOCOR therapy.

Clinically significant conduction changes have been observed at these rates: sinus node dysfunction such as sinus pause, sinus arrest and symptomatic bradycardia (1.2%), second-degree AV block (0.5%) and third-degree AV block (0.4%). An attempt should be made to manage the patient on the lowest effective dose in an effort to minimize these effects. (See Dosage and Administration.) If second- or third-degree AV block, or right bundle branch block associated with a left hemiblock occur, TAMBOCOR therapy should be discontinued unless a temporary or implanted ventricular pacemaker is in place to ensure an adequate ventricular rate.

Sick Sinus Syndrome (Bradycardia-Tachycardia Syndrome). TAMBOCOR should be used only with extreme caution in patients with sick sinus syndrome because it may cause sinus bradycardia, sinus pause, or sinus arrest.

Effects on Pacemaker Thresholds. TAMBOCOR is known to increase endocardial pacing thresholds and may suppress ventricular escape rhythms. These effects are reversible if flecainide is discontinued. It should be used with caution in patients with permanent pacemakers or temporary pacing electrodes and should not be administered to patients with existing poor thresholds or nonprogrammable pacemakers unless suitable pacing rescue is available.

The pacing threshold in patients with pacemakers should be determined prior to instituting therapy with TAMBOCOR, again after one week of administration and at regular intervals thereafter. Generally threshold changes are within the range of multiprogrammable pacemakers and, when these occur, a doubling of either voltage or pulse width is usually sufficient to regain capture.

Electrolyte Disturbances. Hypokalemia or hyperkalemia may alter the effects of Class I antiarrhythmic drugs. Preexisting hypokalemia or hyperkalemia should be corrected before administration of TAMBOCOR.

Pediatric Use. The safety and efficacy of TAMBOCOR in the fetus, infant, or child have not been established in double-blind, randomized, placebo-controlled trials. The proarrhythmic effects of TAMBOCOR, as described previously, apply also to children. In pediatric patients with structural heart disease, TAMBOCOR has been associated with cardiac arrest and sudden death. TAMBOCOR should be started in the hospital with rhythm monitoring. Any use of TAMBOCOR in children should be directly supervised by a cardiologist skilled in the treatment of arrhythmias in children.

PRECAUTIONS

Drug Interactions. TAMBOCOR has been administered to patients receiving **digitalis** preparations or **beta-adrenergic blocking agents** without adverse effects. During administration of multiple oral doses of TAMBOCOR to healthy subjects stabilized on a maintenance dose of **digoxin**, a 13%–19% increase in plasma **digoxin** levels occurred at six hours postdose.

In a study involving healthy subjects receiving TAMBOCOR and **propranolol** concurrently, plasma flecainide levels were increased about 20% and **propranolol** levels were increased about 30% compared to control values. In this formal interaction study, TAMBOCOR and **propranolol** were each found to have negative inotropic effects; when the drugs were administered together, the effects were additive. The effects of concomitant administration of TAMBOCOR and **propranolol** on the PR interval were less than additive. In TAMBOCOR clinical trials, patients who were receiving **beta blockers** concurrently did not experience an increased incidence of side effects. Nevertheless, the possibility of additive negative inotropic effects of **beta blockers** and flecainide should be recognized.

Flecainide is not extensively bound to plasma proteins. In vitro studies with several drugs which may be administered concomitantly showed that the extent of flecainide binding to human plasma proteins is either unchanged or only slightly less. Consequently, interactions with other drugs which are highly protein bound (e.g., **anticoagulants**) would not be expected. TAMBOCOR has been used in a large number of patients receiving **diuretics** without apparent interaction. Limited data in patients receiving known enzyme inducers (**phenytoin, phenobarbital, carbamazepine**) indicate only a 30% increase in the rate of flecainide elimination. In healthy subjects receiving **cimetidine** (1 gm daily) for one week, plasma flecainide levels increased by about 30% and half-life increased by about 10%.

When **amiodarone** is added to flecainide therapy, plasma flecainide levels may increase two-fold or more in some patients, if flecainide dosage is not reduced. (See Dosage and Administration.)

Drugs that inhibit cytochrome P450IID6, such as **quinidine**, might increase the plasma concentrations of flecainide in patients that are on chronic flecainide therapy; especially if these patients are extensive metabolizers.

There has been little experience with the coadministration of TAMBOCOR and either **disopyramide** or **verapamil.** Because both of these drugs have negative inotropic properties and the effects of coadministration with TAMBOCOR are unknown, neither **disopyramide** nor **verapamil** should be administered concurrently with TAMBOCOR unless, in the judgment of the physician, the benefits of this combination outweigh the risks. There has been too little experience with the coadministration of TAMBOCOR with **nifedipine** or **diltiazem** to recommend concomitant use.

Carcinogenesis, Mutagenesis, Impairment of Fertility. Long-term studies with flecainide in rats and mice at doses up to 60 mg/kg/day have not revealed any compound-related carcinogenic effects. Mutagenicity studies (Ames test, mouse lymphoma and in vivo cytogenetics) did not reveal any mutagenic effects. A rat reproduction study at doses up to 50 mg/kg/day (seven times the usual human dose) did not reveal any adverse effect on male or female fertility.

Pregnancy. Pregnancy Category C. Flecainide has been shown to have teratogenic effects (club paws, sternebrae and vertebrae abnormalities, pale hearts with contracted ventricular septum) and an embryotoxic effect (increased resorptions) in one breed of rabbit (New Zealand White) when

Continued on next page

Tambocor—Cont.

given doses of 30 and 35 mg/kg/day, but not in another breed of rabbit (Dutch Belted) when given doses up to 30 mg/kg/day. No teratogenic effects were observed in rats and mice given doses up to 50 and 80 mg/kg/day, respectively; however, delayed sternebral and vertebral ossification was observed at the high dose in rats. Because there are no adequate and well-controlled studies in pregnant women, TAMBOCOR should be used during pregnancy only if the potential benefit justifies the potential risk to the fetus.

Labor and Delivery. It is not known whether the use of TAMBOCOR during labor or delivery has immediate or delayed adverse effects on the mother or fetus, affects the duration of labor or delivery, or increases the possibility of forceps delivery or other obstetrical intervention.

Nursing Mothers. Results from a multiple dose study conducted in mothers soon after delivery indicates that flecainide is excreted in human breast milk in concentrations as high as 4 times (with average levels about 2.5 times) corresponsing plasma levels; assuming a maternal plasma level at the top of the therapeutic range (1 μg/mL), the calculated daily dose to a nursing infant (assuming about 700 mL breast milk over 24 hours) would be less than 3 mg.

Pediatric Use. The safety and efficacy of TAMBOCOR in the fetus, infant, or child have not been established in double-blind, randomized, placebo-controlled trials (see CLINICAL PHARMACOLOGY, WARNINGS, and DOSAGE AND ADMINISTRATION).

Hepatic Impairment. Since flecainide elimination from plasma can be markedly slower in patients with significant hepatic impairment, TAMBOCOR should not be used in such patients unless the potential benefits clearly outweigh the risks. If used, frequent and early plasma level monitoring is required to guide dosage (see Plasma Level Monitoring); dosage increases should be made very cautiously when plasma levels have plateaued (after more than four days).

ADVERSE REACTIONS

In post-myocardial infarction patients with asymptomatic PVCs and non-sustained ventricular tachycardia, TAMBOCOR therapy was found to be associated with a 5.1% rate of death and non-fatal cardiac arrest, compared with a 2.3% rate in a matched placebo group. (See Warnings.)

Adverse effects reported for TAMBOCOR, described in detail in the Warnings section, were new or worsened arrhythmias which occurred in 1% of 108 patients with PSVT and in 7% of 117 patients with PAF; and new or exacerbated ventricular arrhythmias which occurred in 7% of 1330 patients with PVCs, non-sustained or sustained VT. In patients treated with flecainide for sustained VT, 80% (51/64) of proarrhythmic events occurred within 14 days of the onset of therapy. 198 patients with sustained VT experienced a 13% incidence of new or exacerbated ventricular arrhythmias when dosage was initiated at 200 mg/day with slow upward titration, and did not exceed 300 mg/day in most patients. In some patients, TAMBOCOR treatment has been associated with episodes of unresuscitatable VT or ventricular fibrillation (cardiac arrest). (See Warnings.)

New or worsened CHF occurred in 6.3% of 1046 patients with PVCs, non-sustained or sustained VT. Of 297 patients with sustained VT, 9.1% experienced new or worsened CHF. New or worsened CHF was reported in 0.4% of 225 patients with supraventricular arrhythmias. There have also been instances of second- (0.5%) or third-degree (0.4%) AV block. Patients have developed sinus bradycardia, sinus pause, or sinus arrest, about 1.2% altogether (see Warnings). The frequency of most of these serious adverse events probably increases with higher trough plasma levels, especially when these trough levels exceed 1.0 μg/mL.

There have been rare reports of isolated elevations of serum alkaline phosphatase and isolated elevations of serum transaminase levels. These elevations have been asymptomatic and no cause and effect relationship with TAMBOCOR has been established. In foreign postmarketing surveillance studies, there have been rare reports of hepatic dysfunction including reports of cholestasis and hepatic failure, and extremely rare reports of blood dyscrasias. Although no cause and effect relationship has been established, it is advisable to discontinue TAMBOCOR in patients who develop unexplained jaundice or signs of hepatic dysfunction or blood dyscrasias in order to eliminate TAMBOCOR as the possible causative agent.

Incidence figures for other adverse effects in patients with ventricular arrhythmias are based on a multicenter efficacy study, utilizing starting doses of 200 mg/day with gradual upward titration to 400 mg/day. Patients were treated for an average of 4.7 months, with some receiving up to 22 months of therapy. In this trial, 5.4% of patients discontinued due to non-cardiac adverse effects.

[See table 1 below]

The following additional adverse experiences, possibly related to TAMBOCOR therapy and occurring in 1% to less than 3% of patients, have been reported in acute and chronic studies: *Body as a Whole* —malaise, fever; *Cardiovascular*—tachycardia, sinus pause or arrest; *Gastrointestinal* —vomiting, diarrhea, dyspepsia, anorexia; *Skin* —rash; *Visual*—diplopia; *Nervous System* —hypoesthesia, paresthesia, paresis, ataxia, flushing, increased sweating, vertigo, syncope, somnolence, tinnitus; *Psychiatric* —anxiety, insomnia, depression.

The following additional adverse experiences, possibly related to TAMBOCOR, have been reported in less than 1% of patients: *Body as a Whole* —swollen lips, tongue and mouth; arthralgia, bronchospasm, myalgia; *Cardiovascular* —angina pectoris, second-degree and third-degree AV block, bradycardia, hypertension, hypotension; *Gastrointestinal* —flatulence; *Urinary System* —polyuria, urinary retention; *Hematologic* —leukopenia, granulocytopenia, thrombocytopenia; *Skin* —urticaria, exfoliative dermatitis, pruritus, alopecia; *Visual* —eye pain or irritation, photophobia, nystagmus; *Nervous System* —twitching, weakness, change in taste, dry mouth, convulsions, impotence, speech disorder, stupor, neuropathy; *Respiratory* —pneumonitis/pulmonary infiltration possibly due to chronic flecainide treatment: *Psychiatric*—amnesia, confusion, decreased libido, depersonalization, euphoria, morbid dreams, apathy.

For patients with supraventricular arrhythmias, the most commonly reported noncardiac adverse experiences remain consistent with those known for patients treated with TAMBOCOR for ventricular arrhythmias. Dizziness is possibly more frequent in PAF patients.

OVERDOSAGE

No specific antidote has been identified for the treatment of TAMBOCOR overdosage. Overdoses ranging up to 8000 mg have been survived, with peak plasma flecainide concentrations as high as 5.3 μg/mL. Untoward effects in these cases included nausea and vomiting, convulsions, hypotension, bradycardia, syncope, extreme widening of the QRS complex, widening of the QT interval, widening of the PR interval, ventricular tachycardia, AV nodal block, asystole, bundle branch block, cardiac failure, and cardiac arrest. The spectrum of events observed in fatal cases was much the same as that seen in the non-fatal cases. Death has resulted following ingestion of as little as 1000 mg; concomitant overdose of other drugs and/or alcohol in many instances undoubtedly contributed to the fatal outcome. Treatment of overdosage should be supportive and may include the following: removal of unabsorbed drug from the gastrointestinal tract, administration of inotropic agents or cardiac stimulants such as dopamine, dobutamine or isoproterenol; mechanically assisted respiration; circulatory assists such as intra-aortic balloon pumping; and transvenous pacing in the event of conduction block. Because of the long plasma half-life of flecainide (12 to 27 hours in patients receiving usual doses), and the possibility of markedly non-linear elimination kinetics at very high doses, these supportive treatments may need to be continued for extended periods of time.

Hemodialysis is not an effective means of removing flecainide from the body. Since flecainide elimination is much slower when urine is very alkaline (pH 8 or higher), theoretically, acidification of urine to promote drug excretion may be beneficial in overdose cases with very alkaline urine. There is no evidence that acidification from normal urinary pH increases excretion.

DOSAGE AND ADMINISTRATION

For patients with sustained VT, no matter what their cardiac status, TAMBOCOR, like other antiarrhythmics, should be initiated in-hospital with rhythm monitoring.

Flecainide has a long half-life (12 to 27 hours in patients). Steady-state plasma levels, in patients with normal renal and hepatic function, may not be achieved until the patient has received 3 to 5 days of therapy at a given dose. Therefore, **increases in dosage should be made no more frequently than once every four days,** since during the first 2 to 3 days of therapy the optimal effect of a given dose may not be achieved.

For patients with PSVT and patients with PAF the recommended starting dose is 50 mg every 12 hours. TAMBOCOR doses may be increased in increments of 50 mg bid every four days until efficacy is achieved. For PAF patients, a substantial increase in efficacy without a substantial increase in discontinuations for adverse experiences may be achieved by increasing the TAMBOCOR dose from 50 mg to 100 mg bid. The maximum recommended dose for patients with paroxysmal supraventricular arrhythmias is 300 mg/day.

For sustained VT the recommended starting dose is 100 mg every 12 hours. This dose may be increased in increments of 50 mg bid every four days until efficacy is achieved. Most patients with sustained VT do not require more than 150 mg every 12 hours (300 mg/day), and the maximum dose recommended is 400 mg/day.

In patients with sustained VT, use of higher initial doses and more rapid dosage adjustments have resulted in an increased incidence of proarrhythmic events and CHF, particularly during the first few days of dosing (see Warnings). Therefore, a loading dose is not recommended.

Intravenous lidocaine has been used occasionally with TAMBOCOR while awaiting the therapeutic effect of TAMBOCOR. No adverse drug interactions were apparent. However, no formal studies have been performed to demonstrate the usefulness of this regimen.

An occasional patient not adequately controlled by (or intolerant to) a dose given at 12-hour intervals may be dosed at eight-hour intervals.

Once adequate control of the arrhythmia has been achieved, it may be possible in some patients to reduce the dose as necessary to minimize side effects or effects on conduction. In such patients, efficacy at the lower dose should be evaluated.

TAMBOCOR should be used cautiously in patients with a history of CHF or myocardial dysfunction (see Warnings).

Any use of TAMBOCOR in children should be directly supervised by a cardiologist skilled in the treatment of arrhythmias in children. Because of the evolving nature of information in this area, specialized literature should be consulted. Under six months of age, the initial starting dose of TAMBOCOR in children is approximately 50 mg/M^2 body surface area daily, divided into two or three equally spaced doses. Over six months of age, the initial starting dose may be increased to 100 mg/M^2 per day. The maximum recommended dose is 200 mg/M^2 per day. This dose should not be exceeded. In some children on higher doses, despite previously low plasma levels, the level has increased rapidly to far above therapeutic values while taking the same dose. Small changes in dose may also lead to disproportionate increases in plasma levels. Plasma trough (less than one hour pre-dose) flecainide levels and electrocardiograms should be obtained at presumed steady state (after at least five doses) either after initiation or change in TAMBOCOR dose, whether the dose was increased for lack of effectiveness, or increased growth of the patient. For the first year on therapy, whenever the patient is seen for reasons of clinical follow-up, it is suggested that a 12-lead electrocardiogram and plasma trough flecainide level are obtained. The usual therapeutic level of flecainide in children is 200–500 ng/mL. In some cases, levels as high as 800 ng/mL may be required for control.

In patients with severe renal impairment (creatinine clearance of 35 mL/min/1.73 square meters or less), the initial dosage should be 100 mg once daily (or 50 mg bid); when used in such patients, frequent plasma level monitoring is required to guide dosage adjustments (see Plasma Level Monitoring). In patients with less severe renal disease, the initial dosage should be 100 mg every 12 hours; plasma level monitoring may also be useful in these patients during dosage adjustment. In both groups of patients, dosage increases should be made very cautiously when plasma levels have plateaued (after more than four days), observing the patient closely for signs of adverse cardiac effects or other toxicity. It should be borne in mind that in these patients it may take longer than four days before a new steady-state plasma level is reached following a dosage change.

Based on theoretical considerations, rather than experimental data, the following suggestion is made: when transferring patients from another antiarrhythmic drug to TAMBOCOR allow at least two to four plasma half-lives to elapse for the drug being discontinued before starting TAMBOCOR at the usual dosage. In patients where withdrawal of a previous antiarrhythmic agent is likely to produce life-threatening arrhythmias, the physician should consider hospitalizing the patient.

When flecainide is given in the presence of amiodarone, reduce the usual flecainide dose by 50% and monitor the patient closely for adverse effects. Plasma level monitoring is strongly recommended to guide dosage with such combination therapy (see below).

Plasma Level Monitoring. The large majority of patients successfully treated with TAMBOCOR were found to have trough plasma levels between 0.2 and 1.0 μg/mL. The prob-

Table 1
Most Common Non-Cardiac Adverse Effects in Ventricular Arrhythmia Patients Treated with TAMBOCOR in the Multicenter Study

Adverse Effect	Incidence All 429 Patients at Any Dose	Incidence By Dose During Upward Titration: 200 mg/Day (N=426)	300 mg/Day (N=293)	400 mg/Day (N=100)
Dizziness*	18.9%	11.0%	10.6%	13.0%
Visual Disturbances†	15.9%	5.4%	12.3%	18.0%
Dyspnea	10.3%	5.2%	7.5%	4.0%
Headache	9.6%	4.5%	6.1%	9.0%
Nausea	8.9%	4.9%	4.8%	6.0%
Fatigue	7.7%	4.5%	4.4%	3.0%
Palpitation	6.1%	3.5%	2.4%	7.0%
Chest Pain	5.4%	3.1%	3.8%	1.0%
Asthenia	4.9%	2.6%	2.0%	4.0%
Tremor	4.7%	2.4%	3.4%	2.0%
Constipation	4.4%	2.8%	2.1%	1.0%
Edema	3.5%	1.9%	1.4%	2.0%
Abdominal pain	3.3%	1.9%	2.4%	1.0%

* Dizziness includes reports of dizziness, lightheadedness, faintness, unsteadiness, near syncope, etc.
† Visual disturbance includes reports of blurred vision, difficulty in focusing, spots before eyes, etc.

ability of adverse experiences, especially cardiac, may increase with higher trough plasma levels, especially when these exceed 1.0 µg/mL. Periodic monitoring of trough plasma levels may be useful in patient management. Plasma level monitoring is required in patients with severe renal failure or severe hepatic disease, since elimination of flecainide from plasma may be markedly slower. Monitoring of plasma levels is strongly recommended in patients on concurrent amiodarone therapy and may also be helpful in patients with CHF and in patients with moderate renal disease.

HOW SUPPLIED

All tablets are embossed with 3M on one side and TR 50, TR 100 or TR 150 on the other side.

Tambocor, 50 mg per white, round tablet, is available in
Bottles of 100—NDC #0089-0305-10.
Boxes of 100 in unit dose blister strips—NDC #0089-0305-16.

Tambocor, 100 mg per white, round, scored tablet, is available in
Bottles of 100—NDC #0089-0307-10.
Boxes of 100 in unit dose blister strips—NDC #0089-0307-16.

Tambocor, 150 mg per white, oval, scored tablet, is available in
Bottles of 100—NDC #0089-0314-10.

Store at controlled room temperature 15°–30°C (59°–86°F) in a tight, light-resistant container.

Rx only
600900 June 1998

Manufactured by
3M Pharmaceuticals
Northridge, CA 91324

Shown in Product Identification Guide, page 321

THEOLAIR™ ℞
(theophylline tablets USP)
TABLETS

For full prescribing information see leaflet accompanying product or call 800-328-0255 for a copy.

HOW SUPPLIED
THEOLAIR™ Tablets:

125 mg tablets—Each round, white, scored tablet imprinted with "3M" on one side and "342" on the other. Bottles of 100 (NDC 0089-0342-10).

250 mg tablets—Each capsule-shaped, white, scored tablet imprinted with "3M" on one side and "THEOLAIR 250" on the other. Bottles of 100 (NDC 0089-0344-10).

Mallinckrodt Inc.

675 McDONNELL BLVD
PO BOX 5840
ST. LOUIS, MO 63134
www.mallinckrodt-rx.com

Direct Inquiries to:
For additional information call:
Customer Service 1-800-325-8888
Professional Services 1-800-744-1414

BUTALBITAL, ACETAMINOPHEN AND CAFFEINE TABLETS USP ℞

DESCRIPTION

Butalbital, acetaminophen and caffeine is supplied in tablet form for oral administration.

Butalbital (5-allyl-5-isobutylbarbituric acid), a slightly bitter, white, odorless, crystalline powder, is a short to intermediate-acting barbiturate. It has the following structural formula:

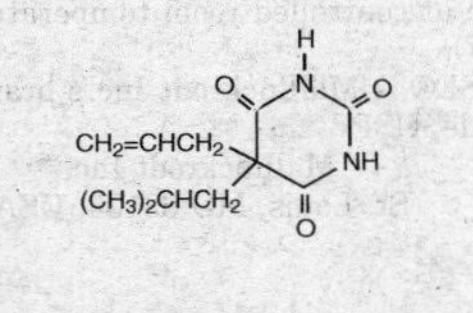

$C_{11}H_{16}N_2O_3$ MW=224.26

Acetaminophen (4′-hydroxyacetanalide), a slightly bitter, white, odorless, crystalline powder, is a non-opiate, non-salicylate analgesic and antipyretic. It has the following structural formula:

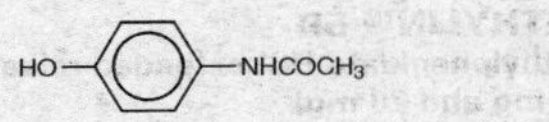

$C_8H_9NO_2$ MW=151.17

Caffeine (1,3,7-trimethylxanthine), a bitter, white powder or white-glistening needles, is a central nervous system stimulant. It has the following structural formula:

[See chemical structure at top of next column]

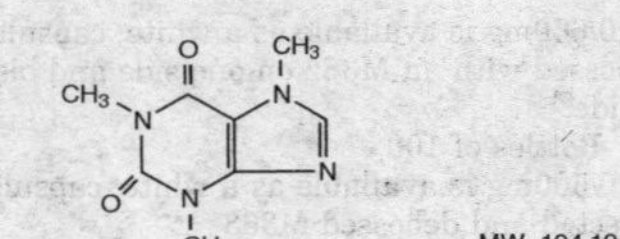

$C_8H_{10}N_4O_2$ MW=194.19

Each tablet contains:

Butalbital, USP	50 mg
Warning: May be habit forming	
Acetaminophen, USP	325 mg
Caffeine (Anhydrous), USP	40 mg

In addition each tablet contains the following inactive ingredients:
Microcrystalline cellulose, starch (corn), pregelatinized starch, gelatin, sodium starch glycolate, magnesium stearate.

HOW SUPPLIED

Butalbital, Acetaminophen and Caffeine Tablets USP are white, round, unscored, compressed tablets imprinted Ⓜ on one side and 970 on the opposite side.

Each tablet contains Butalbital 50 mg (WARNING: May be habit forming), Acetaminophen 325 mg and Caffeine 40 mg.

Bottles of 100	NDC 0406-0970-01
Bottles of 500	NDC 0406-0970-05

STORAGE: Store at controlled room temperature 15°–30°C (59°–86°F). Protect from moisture.

CAUTION: Federal law prohibits dispensing without prescription.

Manufactured by
Mallinckrodt Inc.
St. Louis, MO 63134, U.S.A.

2/98

DIPHENOXYLATE HYDROCHLORIDE AND ATROPINE SULFATE TABLETS, USP Ⓒ ℞

DESCRIPTION

Each tablet, for oral administration, contains:

Diphenoxylate Hydrochloride, USP	2.5 mg
WARNING: May be habit forming	
Atropine Sulfate, USP	0.025 mg

In addition, each tablet, contains the following inactive ingredients: confectioner's sugar, corn starch, lactose monohydrate, magnesium stearate and sodium starch glycolate.

Diphenoxylate hydrochloride, an antidiarrheal, is ethyl 1-(3-cyano-3,3-diphenylpropyl)-4-phenylisonipecotate monohydrochloride and has the following structural formula:

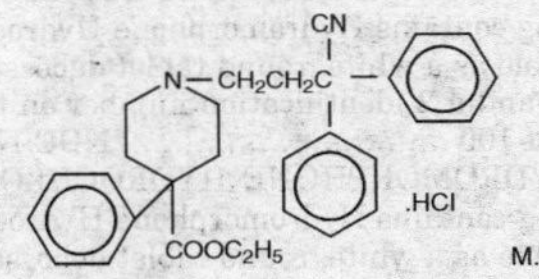

$C_{30}H_{32}N_2O_2$•HCl M.W. 489.06

Atropine sulfate, an anticholinergic, is Benzeneacetic acid,-(hydroxymethyl)-8-methyl-8-azabicyclol [3.2.1] oct-3-yl ester, endo-±, sulfate(2:1) (salt), monohydrate and has the following structural formula:

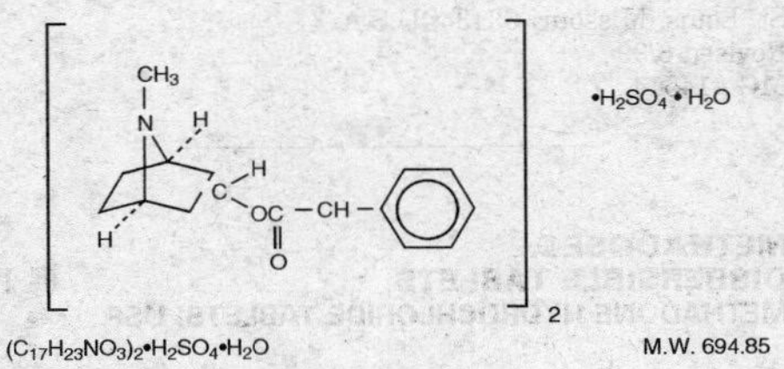

$(C_{17}H_{23}NO_3)_2$•H_2SO_4•H_2O M.W. 694.85

A subtherapeutic amount of atropine sulfate is present to discourage deliberate overdosage.

HOW SUPPLIED

Diphenoxylate Hydrochloride and Atropine Sulfate Tablets, USP are available as white, round tablets, debossed "3966" containing 2.5 mg diphenoxylate hydrochloride, USP (WARNING: May be habit forming), and 0.025 mg atropine sulfate, USP, packaged in bottles of 100 and 1000 tablets.

PHARMACIST: Dispense in a well-closed, light-resistant container as defined in the USP. Use child-resistant closure.

Store at controlled room temperature
15°–30°C (59°–86°F). 0172

Rx only 05/98

MANUFACTURED BY D6
ZENITH GOLDLINE PHARMACEUTICALS, INC.
MIAMI, FL 33137
DIPHENOXYLATE HYDROCHLORIDE and
ATROPINE SULFATE TABLETS, USP

HYDROCODONE* BITARTRATE AND ACETAMINOPHEN CAPSULES
5 mg/500 mg Ⓒℿ ℞
***Warning:** May be habit forming.

DESCRIPTION

Hydrocodone Bitartrate and Acetaminophen Capsules are supplied in capsule form for oral administration.

Hydrocodone bitartrate is an opioid analgesic and antitussive and occurs as fine, white crystals or as a crystalline powder. It is affected by light. The chemical name is 4, 5α-epoxy-3-methoxy-17-methylmorphinan-6-one tartrate (1:1) hydrate (2:5). It has the following structural formula:

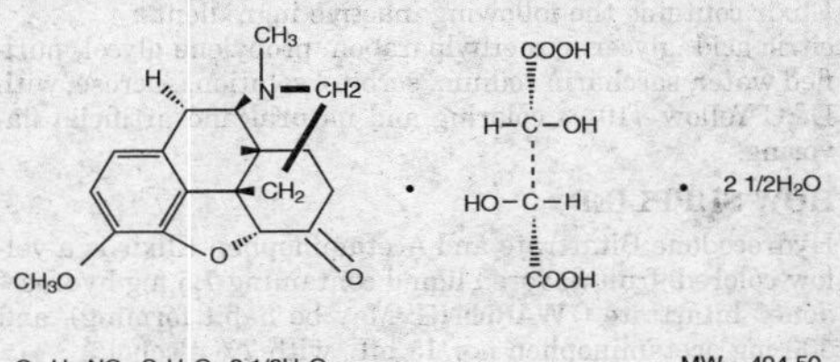

$C_{18}H_{21}NO_3$•$C_4H_6O_6$•2 1/2H_2O MW = 494.50

Acetaminophen, 4′-hydroxyacetanilide, a slightly bitter, white, odorless, crystalline powder, is a non-opiate, non-salicylate analgesic and antipyretic. It has the following structural formula:

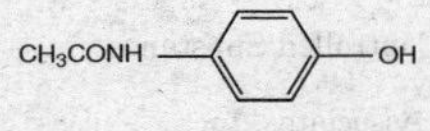

$C_8H_9NO_2$ MW = 151.17

Each HYDROCODONE* BITARTRATE AND ACETAMINOPHEN 5 mg/500 mg capsule contains:

Hydrocodone Bitartrate, USP	5 mg
(***Warning**: May be habit forming)	
Acetaminophen, USP	500 mg

In addition each capsule contains the following inactive ingredients: Benzyl Alcohol, Butylparaben, Edetate Calcium Disodium, FD&C Blue 1, FD&C Red 3, Gelatin, Methylparaben, Propylparaben, Sodium Lauryl Sulfate, Sodium Propionate, Titanium Dioxide.

HOW SUPPLIED

Each HYDROCODONE* BITARTRATE AND ACETAMINOPHEN 5mg/500 mg capsule contains Hydrocodone Bitartrate 5 mg (***Warning:** May be habit forming) and Acetaminophen 500 mg. It is available as an opaque maroon capsule imprinted in white Ⓜ 4357.

Bottles of 100 NDC No. 0406-4357-01

Dispense in a tight, light-resistant container as defined in the USP.

Storage: Store at controlled room temperature 15° to 30°C (59° to 86°F).

A Schedule III Narcotic.

Federal (U.S.A.) law prohibits dispensing without prescription.

Manufactured by
Mallinckrodt Inc.
St. Louis, MO 63134, U.S.A.

4/98

HYDROCODONE BITARTRATE AND ACETAMINOPHEN ELIXIR
7.5 mg/500 mg per 15 mL Ⓒℿ ℞

DESCRIPTION

Hydrocodone bitartrate and acetaminophen is supplied in liquid form for oral administration. Hydrocodone bitartrate is an opioid analgesic and antitussive which occurs as fine, white crystals or as a crystalline powder. It is affected by light. The chemical name is 4,5α-epoxy-3-methoxy-17-methylmorphinan-6-one tartrate (1:1) hydrate (2:5). It has the following structural formula:

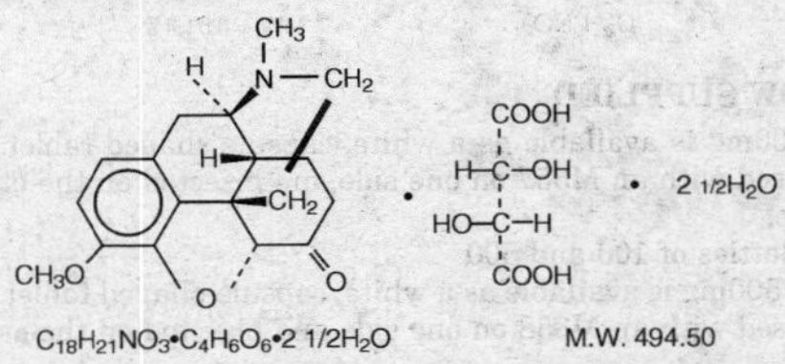

$C_{18}H_{21}NO_3$•$C_4H_6O_6$•2 1/2H_2O M.W. 494.50

Acetaminophen, 4′-hydroxyacetanalide, a slightly bitter, white, odorless, crystalline powder, is a non-opiate, non-salicylate analgesic and antipyretic. It has the following structural formula:

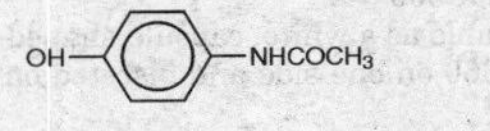

$C_8H_9NO_2$ M.W. 151.17

Continued on next page

Hydrocodone/APAP Elixir—Cont.

Hydrocodone Bitartrate and Acetaminophen Elixir contains:

	Per 5 mL	Per 15 mL
Hydrocodone* Bitartrate *(**WARNING**: May be habit forming)	2.5 mg	7.5 mg
Acetaminophen	167 mg	500 mg
Alcohol	7%	7%

In addition Hydrocodone Bitartrate and Acetaminophen Elixir contains the following inactive ingredients: citric acid, glycerin, methylparaben, propylene glycol, purified water, saccharin sodium, sorbitol solution, sucrose, with D&C Yellow #10 as coloring and natural and artificial flavoring.

HOW SUPPLIED

Hydrocodone Bitartrate and Acetaminophen Elixir is a yellow-colored, fruit flavored liquid containing 7.5 mg hydrocodone* bitartrate (***WARNING**: May be habit forming), and 500 mg acetaminophen per 15 mL, with 7% alcohol.

16 fl oz (473 mL) Bottle .... NDC No.0406-0375-16.

Storage: Store at controlled room temperature 15°–30°C (59°–86°F).

Dispense in a tight, light-resistant container with a child-resistant closure.

CAUTION: Federal law prohibits dispensing without prescription.

A Schedule III Controlled Substance.

Manufactured by
Pharmaceutical Associates, Inc.
Greenville, SC 29605
Manufactured for:
Mallinckrodt Inc.
St. Louis, MO 63134, U.S.A. 11/97

HYDROCODONE BITARTRATE AND ACETAMINOPHEN TABLETS, USP ℂ℟

5/500mg
7.5/500mg
7.5/650mg
7.5/750mg
10/650mg
10/660mg
10/500mg

DESCRIPTION

Hydrocodone Bitartrate and Acetaminophen Tablets are supplied in tablet form for oral administration.

Hydrocodone bitartrate is an opioid analgesic and antitussive and occurs as fine, white crystals or as a crystalline powder. It is affected by light. The chemical name is 4, 5α-epoxy-3-methoxy-17-methylmorphinan-6-one tartrate (1:1) hydrate (2:5). It has the following structural formula:

$C_{18}H_{21}NO_3 \cdot C_4H_6O_6 \cdot 2\ 1/2\ H_2O$ MW = 494.50

Acetaminophen, 4′-hydroxyacetanilide, a slightly bitter, white, odorless, crystalline powder, is a non-opiate, non-salicylate analgesic and antipyretic. It has the following structural formula:

$C_8H_9NO_2$ MW = 151.17

HOW SUPPLIED

5/500mg is available as a white, capsule-shaped tablet debossed with an M357 on one side and bisected on the other side.

Bottles of 100 and 500

7.5/500mg is available as a white, capsule-shaped tablet debossed with an M358 on one side and bisected on the other side.

Bottles of 100 and 500

7.5/650mg is available as a white, capsule-shaped tablet debossed with an M359 on one side and bisected on the other side.

Bottles of 100 and 500

7.5/750mg is available as a white, capsule-shaped tablet debossed with an M360 on one side and bisected on the other side.

Bottles of 100 and 500

10/650mg is available as a blue, capsule-shaped tablet debossed with an M361 on one side and bisected on the other side.

Bottles of 100 and 500

10/660mg is available as a white, capsule-shaped tablet debossed with an M362 on one side and bisected on the other side.

Bottles of 100

10/500mg is available as a white, capsule-shaped tablet bisected and debossed M363

Bottles of 100 and 500

Dispense in a tight, light-resistant container with a child-resistant closure.

Storage: Store at controlled room temperature 15° to 30°C (59° to 86°F). Protect from light.

A Schedule III Narcotic.
Rx only
Mallinckrodt, Inc.
St. Louis, Missouri 63134, U.S.A.

110899

HYDROMORPHONE HYDROCHLORIDE TABLETS, USP ℂ℟

Rx only

DESCRIPTION

Hydromorphone Hydrochloride Tablets, a hydrogenated ketone of morphine, is a narcotic analgesic. It has the following structural formula:

$C_{17}H_{19}NO_3 \cdot HCl$ MW = 321.81

Each HYDROMORPHONE HYDROCHLORIDE TABLET, USP 2 mg contains:

Hydromorphone Hydrochloride, USP. . . 2 mg

In addition, each HYDROMORPHONE HYDROCHLORIDE TABLET, USP 2 mg contains the following inactive ingredients: Lactose Monohydrate NF, Magnesium Stearate NF, Microcrystalline Cellulose NF and Stearic Acid NF.

Each HYDROMORPHONE HYDROCHLORIDE TABLET, USP 4 mg contains:

Hydromorphone Hydrochloride, USP. . . 4 mg

In addition, each HYDROMORPHONE HYDROCHLORIDE TABLET, USP 4 mg contains the following inactive ingredients: Lactose Monohydrate NF, Magnesium Stearate NF, Microcrystalline Cellulose NF and Stearic Acid NF.

HOW SUPPLIED

Each HYDROMORPHONE HYDROCHLORIDE TABLET, USP 2 mg contains Hydromorphone Hydrochloride 2 mg. It is available as a white, round tablet debossed with an M on one side and a 2 identification number on the reverse side.

Bottles of 100 .... NDC No. 0406-3243-01

Each HYDROMORPHONE HYDROCHLORIDE TABLET, USP 4 mg contains Hydromorphone Hydrochloride 4 mg. It is available as a white, round tablet debossed with an M on one side and a 4 identification number on the reverse side.

Bottles of 100 .... NDC No. 0406-3244-01

Dispense in a tight, light-resistant container as defined in USP.

Storage: Store at controlled room temperature 20° to 25° C (68° to 77° F).

A Schedule II Narcotic.
Mallinckrodt Inc.
St. Louis, Missouri 63134, U.S.A.
Revised 3/99
MG #14514

METHADOSE® DISPERSIBLE TABLETS ℂ℟

METHADONE HYDROCHLORIDE TABLETS, USP

DESCRIPTION

Methadone Hydrochloride, USP 6-(dimethylamino)-4, 4-diphenyl-3-heptanone hydrochloride, is a white, crystalline material that is water soluble. However, the METHADOSE® Dispersible Tablet preparation of Methadone Hydrochloride, USP has been specially formulated with insoluble excipients to deter the use of this drug by injection. Its molecular weight is 345.91.

Each METHADOSE® Dispersible Tablet contains: 40 mg (0.116 mmol) Methadone Hydrochloride, USP.

Each tablet also contains Dibasic Calcium Phosphate USP, Microcrystalline Cellulose NF, Magnesium Stearate NF, Colloidal Silicon Dioxide NF, Pregelatinized Starch NF, and Stearic Acid NF.

HOW SUPPLIED

METHADOSE® Dispersible Tablets:

40 mg (white, quadrisect) (Identified METHADOSE 40) NDC 0406–0540–34: Bottles of 100 tablets

Store at controlled room temperature, 15° to 30° C (59° to 86° F)

METHADOSE® is Mallinckrodt Inc.'s brand of Methadone Hydrochloride, USP.

Manufactured by
Mallinckrodt Inc.
St. Louis, MO 63134, USA

9/98
98017

METHADOSE® ORAL CONCENTRATE ℂ℟

(methadone hydrochloride oral concentrate, USP)
Rx only
FOR ORAL USE ONLY

DESCRIPTION

METHADOSE® is a cherry flavored liquid concentrate of methadone hydrochloride. The liquid concentrate contains 10 mg of methadone hydrochloride per mL. Methadone hydrochloride, 3-heptanone, 6-(dimethylamino)-4, 4-diphenyl-, hydrochloride is a white, crystalline, odorless powder. It is soluble in water; freely soluble in alcohol and in chloroform; practically insoluble in ether and in glycerin. It is present in Methadose® as the racemic mixture. Methadone hydrochloride has a melting point of 235° C, a pKa of 8.25 to 10.12, a solution (1 in 100) pH between 4.5 and 6.5, a partition coefficient of 117 at pH 7.4 in octanol/water and a molecular weight of 345.91. Its molecular formula is $C_{21}H_{27}NO \cdot HCl$ and its structural formulae is:

Other Ingredients: Artificial Cherry Flavor, Citric Acid Anhydrous USP, FD&C Red No. 40, D&C Red No. 33, Methylparaben NF, Poloxamer 407 NF, Propylene Glycol USP, Propylparaben NF, Purified Water USP, Sodium Citrate Dihydrate USP, Sucrose NF.

HOW SUPPLIED

METHADOSE® is supplied in one liter bottles (NDC 0406-0527-10).

Preserve in tight containers, protected from light. Store at Controlled Room Temperature 20° – 25° C (68°– 77° F); brief excursions permitted between 15 – 30° C (59° – 86° F).

Mallinckrodt Inc.
St. Louis, MO 63134, USA

032900

METHADOSE® ORAL TABLETS ℂ℟

METHADONE HYDROCHLORIDE TABLETS, USP

DESCRIPTION

Methadone Hydrochloride, USP 6-(dimethylamino)-4, 4-diphenyl-3-heptanone hydrochloride, is a white, crystalline material that is water soluble. Its molecular weight is 345.91.

Each METHADONE® Oral Tablet contains: 5 mg (0.0145 mmol) or 10 mg (0.029 mmol) Methadone Hydrochloride, USP.

Each tablet also contains Dibasic Calcium Phosphate USP, Microcrystalline Cellulose NF, Magnesium Stearate NF, Colloidal Silicon Dioxide NF, Pregelatinized Starch NF, and Stearic Acid NF.

HOW SUPPLIED

METHADOSE® Oral Tablets (Methadone Hydrochloride Tablets, USP):

5 mg white, scored tablets (identified METHADOSE 5) NDC 0406-6974-34; Bottles of 100 tablets

10 mg white, scored tablets (identified METHADOSE 10) NDC 0406-3454-34; Bottles of 100 tablets

Keep tightly closed. Dispense in a tight, light-resistant container. Store at controlled room temperature, 15° to 30° C (59° to 86° F).

METHADOSE® is Mallinckrodt Inc.'s brand of Methadone Hydrochloride, USP.

Mallinckrodt Inc.
St. Louis, MO 63134, USA

9/98
98018

METHYLIN™ ℂ℟

methylphenidate HCl tablets, USP
(5 mg, 10 mg, and 20 mg)

METHYLIN™ ER ℂ℟

methylphenidate HCl extended-release tablets, USP
(10 mg and 20 mg)
Rx Only

DESCRIPTION

Methylphenidate hydrochloride is a mild central nervous system (CNS) stimulant, available as tablets of 5 mg, 10 mg, and 20 mg and as extended release tablets of 10 mg and 20 mg. Methylphenidate hydrochloride is methyl α-phenyl-2-

piperidineacetate hydrochloride, and its structural formula is

Methylphenidate Hydrochloride

$C_{14}H_{19}NO_2 \cdot HCl$ MW = 269.77

Methylphenidate Hydrochloride USP is a white, odorless, fine crystalline powder. Its solutions are acid to litmus. It is freely soluble in water and in methanol, soluble in alcohol, and slightly soluble in chloroform and in acetone.

Each Methylin™ tablet, for oral administration, contains 5 mg, 10 mg, or 20 mg of methylphenidate hydrochloride. In addition, each tablet contains the following inactive ingredients: Lactose Monohydrate NF, Magnesium Stearate NF, Microcrystalline Cellulose NF, and Talc USP. Each Methylin™ ER tablet, for oral administration, contains 10 mg or 20 mg in an extended release formulation. In addition, each extended-release tablet contains the following inactive ingredients: Hydroxypropyl Methylcellulose 2208 USP, Magnesium Stearate NF, Microcrystalline Cellulose NF, and Talc USP.

CLINICAL PHARMACOLOGY

Methylin™ is a mild central nervous system stimulant.

The mode of action in man is not completely understood, but Methylin™ presumably activates the brain stem arousal system and cortex to produce its stimulant effect.

There is neither specific evidence which clearly establishes the mechanism whereby Methylin™ produces its mental and behavioral effects in children, nor conclusive evidence regarding how these effects relate to the condition of the central nervous system.

Methylphenidate hydrochloride in the ER tablets is more slowly but as extensively absorbed as in the regular tablets. Relative bioavailability of the extended release tablet compared to the immediate release tablet, measured by the urinary excretion of methylphenidate major metabolite (α-phenyl-2-piperidine acetic acid) was 105% (49% to 168%) in children and 101% (85% to 152%) in adults. The time to peak rate in children was 4.7 hours (1.3 to 8.2 hours) for the extended release tablets and 1.9 hours (0.3 to 4.4 hours) for the tablets. An average of 67% of extended release tablet dose was excreted in children as compared to 86% in adults.

In a clinical study involving adult subjects who received extended-release tablets, plasma concentrations of methylphenidate's major metabolite appeared to be greater in females than in males. No gender differences were observed for methylphenidate plasma concentration in the same subjects.

INDICATIONS AND USAGE

Attention Deficit Disorders, Narcolepsy

Attention Deficit Disorders (previously known as Minimal Brain Dysfunction in Children). Other terms being used to describe the behavioral syndrome below include: Hyperkinetic Child Syndrome, Minimal Brain Damage, Minimal Cerebral Dysfunction, Minor Cerebral Dysfunction.

Methylin™ is indicated as an integral part of a total treatment program which typically includes other remedial measures (psychological, educational, social) for a stabilizing effect in children with a behavioral syndrome characterized by the following group of developmentally inappropriate symptoms: moderate-to-severe distractibility, short attention span, hyperactivity, emotional lability, and impulsivity. The diagnosis of this syndrome should not be made with finality when these symptoms are only of comparatively recent origin. Nonlocalizing (soft) neurological signs, learning disability, and abnormal EEG may or may not be present, and a diagnosis of central nervous system dysfunction may or may not be warranted.

Special Diagnostic Considerations

Specific etiology of this syndrome is unknown, and there is no single diagnostic test. Adequate diagnosis requires the use not only of medical but of special psychological, educational, and social resources.

Characteristics commonly reported include: chronic history of short attention span, distractibility, emotional lability, impulsivity, and moderate-to-severe hyperactivity; minor neurological signs and abnormal EEG. Learning may or may not be impaired. The diagnosis must be based upon a complete history and evaluation of the child and not solely on the presence of one or more of these characteristics.

Drug treatment is not indicated for all children with this syndrome. Stimulants are not intended for use in the child who exhibits symptoms secondary to environmental factors and/or primary psychiatric disorders, including psychosis. Appropriate educational placement is essential and psychosocial intervention is generally necessary. When remedial measures alone are insufficient, the decision to prescribe stimulant medication will depend upon the physician's assessment of the chronicity and severity of the child's symptoms.

CONTRAINDICATIONS

Marked anxiety, tension, and agitation are contraindications to Methylin™, since the drug may aggravate these symptoms. Methylin™ is contraindicated also in patients known to be hypersensitive to the drug, in patients with glaucoma, and in patients with motor tics or with a family history or diagnosis of Tourette's syndrome.

WARNINGS

Methylin™ should not be used in children under six years, since safety and efficacy in this age group have not been established.

Sufficient data on safety and efficacy of long-term use of Methylin™ in children are not yet available. Although a causal relationship has not been established, suppression of growth (*i.e.*, weight gain, and/or height) has been reported with the long-term use of stimulants in children. Therefore, patients requiring long-term therapy should be carefully monitored.

Methylin™ should not be used for severe depression of either exogenous or endogenous origin. Clinical experience suggests that in psychotic children, administration of Methylin™ may exacerbate symptoms of behavior disturbance and thought disorder.

Methylin™ should not be used for the prevention or treatment of normal fatigue states.

There is some clinical evidence that Methylin™ may lower the convulsive threshold in patients with prior history of seizures, with prior EEG abnormalities in absence of seizures, and, very rarely, in absence of history of seizures and no prior EEG evidence of seizures. Safe concomitant use of anticonvulsants and Methylin™ has not been established. In the presence of seizures, the drug should be discontinued.

Use cautiously in patients with hypertension. Blood pressure should be monitored at appropriate intervals in all patients taking Methylin™, especially those with hypertension.

Symptoms of visual disturbances have been encountered in rare cases. Difficulties with accommodation and blurring of vision have been reported.

Drug Interactions

Methylin™ may decrease the hypotensive effect of guanethidine. Use cautiously with pressor agents and MAO inhibitors.

Human pharmacologic studies have shown that methylphenidate hydrochloride may inhibit the metabolism of coumarin anticoagulants, anticonvulsants (phenobarbital, diphenylhydantoin, primidone), phenylbutazone, and tricyclic drugs (imipramine, clomipramine, desipramine). Downward dosage adjustments of these drugs may be required when given concomitantly with Methylin™.

Usage in Pregnancy

Adequate animal reproduction studies to establish safe use of Methylin™ during pregnancy have not been conducted. Therefore, until more information is available, Methylin™ should not be prescribed for women of childbearing age unless, in the opinion of the physician, the potential benefits outweigh the possible risks.

Drug Dependence

Methylin™ should be given cautiously to emotionally unstable patients, such as those with a history of drug dependence or alcoholism, because such patients may increase dosage on their own initiative. Chronically abusive use can lead to marked tolerance and psychic dependence with varying degrees of abnormal behavior. Frank psychotic episodes can occur, especially with parenteral abuse. Careful supervision is required during drug withdrawal, since severe depression as well as the effects of chronic overactivity can be unmasked. Long-term follow-up may be required because of the patient's basic personality disturbances.

PRECAUTIONS

Patients with an element of agitation may react adversely; discontinue therapy if necessary.

Periodic CBC, differential, and platelet counts are advised during prolonged therapy.

Drug treatment is not indicated in all cases of this behavioral syndrome and should be considered only in light of the complete history and evaluation of the child. The decision to prescribe Methylin™ should depend on the physician's assessment of the chronicity and severity of the child's symptoms and their appropriateness for his/her age. Prescription should not depend solely on the presence of one or more of the behavioral characteristics.

When these symptoms are associated with acute stress reactions, treatment with Methylin™ is usually not indicated. Long-term effects of Methylin™ in children have not been well established.

Carcinogenesis, Mutagenesis, Impairment of Fertility

In a lifetime carcinogenicity study carried out in B6C3F1 mice, methylphenidate caused an increase in hepatocellular adenomas and, in males only, an increase in hepatoblastomas, at a daily dose of approximately 60 mg/kg/day. This dose is approximately 30 times and 2.5 times the maximum recommended human dose on a mg/kg and mg/m^2 basis, respectively. Hepatoblastoma is a relatively rare rodent malignant tumor type. There was no increase in total malignant hepatic tumors. The mouse strain used is sensitive to the development of hepatic tumors, and the significance of these results to humans is unknown.

Methylphenidate did not cause any increases in tumors in a lifetime carcinogenicity study carried out in F344 rats; the highest dose used was approximately 45 mg/kg/day, which is approximately 22 times and 4 times the maximum recommended human dose on a mg/kg and mg/m^2 basis, respectively.

Methylphenidate was not mutagenic in the *in vitro* Ames reverse mutation assay or in the *in vitro* mouse lymphoma cell forward mutation assay. Sister chromatid exchanges and chromosome aberrations were increased, indicative of a weak clastogenic response, in an *in vitro* assay in cultured Chinese Hamster Ovary (CHO) cells. The genotoxic potential of methylphenidate has not been evaluated in an *in vivo* assay.

ADVERSE REACTIONS

Nervousness and insomnia are the most common adverse reactions but are usually controlled by reducing dosage and omitting the drug in the afternoon or evening. Other reactions include hypersensitivity (including skin rash, urticaria, fever, arthralgia, exfoliative dermatitis, erythema multiforme with histopathological findings of necrotizing vasculitis, and thrombocytopenic purpura); anorexia; nausea; dizziness; palpitations; headache; dyskinesia; drowsiness; blood pressure and pulse changes, both up and down; tachycardia; angina; cardiac arrhythmia; abdominal pain; weight loss during prolonged therapy. There have been rare reports of Tourette's syndrome. Toxic psychosis has been reported. Although a definite causal relationship has not been established, the following have been reported in patients taking this drug: instances of abnormal liver function, ranging from transaminase elevation to hepatic coma; isolated cases of cerebral arteritis and/or occlusion; leukopenia and/or anemia; transient depressed mood; a few instances of scalp hair loss. Very rare reports of neuroleptic malignant syndrome (NMS) have been received, and, in most of these, patients were concurrently receiving therapies associated with NMS. In a single report, a ten year old boy who had been taking methylphenidate for approximately 18 months experienced an NMS-like event within 45 minutes of ingesting his first dose of venlafaxine. It is uncertain whether this case represented a drug-drug interaction, a response to either drug alone, or some other cause.

In children, loss of appetite, abdominal pain, weight loss during prolonged therapy, insomnia, and tachycardia may occur more frequently; however, any of the other adverse reactions listed above may also occur.

OVERDOSAGE

Signs and symptoms of acute overdosage, resulting principally from overstimulation of the central nervous system and from excessive sympathomimetic effects, may include the following: vomiting, agitation, tremors, hyperreflexia, muscle twitching, convulsions (may be followed by coma), euphoria, confusion, hallucinations, delirium, sweating, flushing, headache, hyperpyrexia, tachycardia, palpitations, cardiac arrhythmias, hypertension, mydriasis, and dryness of mucous membranes.

Consult with a Certified Poison Control Center regarding treatment for up-to-date guidance and advice.

Treatment consists of appropriate supportive measures. The patient must be protected against self-injury and against external stimuli that would aggravate overstimulation already present. Gastric contents may be evacuated by gastric lavage. In the presence of severe intoxication, use a carefully titrated dosage of a *short-acting* barbiturate before performing gastric lavage. Other measures to detoxify the gut include administration of activated charcoal and a cathartic.

Intensive care must be provided to maintain adequate circulation and respiratory exchange; external cooling procedures may be required for hyperpyrexia.

Efficacy of peritoneal dialysis or extracorporeal hemodialysis for Methylin™ overdosage has not been established.

DOSAGE AND ADMINISTRATION

Dosage should be individualized according to the needs and responses of the patient.

Adults

tablets: Administer in divided doses 2 or 3 times daily, preferably 30 to 45 minutes before meals. Average dosage is 20 to 30 mg daily. Some patients may require 40 to 60 mg daily. In others, 10 to 15 mg daily will be adequate. Patients who are unable to sleep if medication is taken late in the day should take the last dose before 6 p.m.

ER tablets: Methylin™ ER tablets have a duration of action of approximately 8 hours. Therefore, Methylin™ ER tablets may be used in place of Methylin™ tablets when the 8-hour dosage of Methylin™ ER corresponds to the titrated 8-hour dosage of Methylin™. Methylin™ ER tablets must be swallowed whole and never crushed or chewed.

Children (6 years and over)

Methylin™ should be initiated in small doses, with gradual weekly increments. Daily dosage above 60 mg is not recommended.

If improvement is not observed after appropriate dosage adjustment over a one-month period, the drug should be discontinued.

tablets: Start with 5 mg twice daily (before breakfast and lunch) with gradual increments of 5 to 10 mg weekly.

ER tablets: Methylin™ ER tablets have a duration of action of approximately 8 hours. Therefore, Methylin™ ER tablets may be used in place of Methylin™ tablets when the 8-hour dosage of Methylin™ ER corresponds to the titrated 8-hour dosage of Methylin™. Methylin™ ER tablets must be swallowed whole and never crushed or chewed.

If paradoxical aggravation of symptoms or other adverse effects occur, reduce dosage, or, if necessary, discontinue the drug.

Methylin™ should be periodically discontinued to assess the child's condition. Improvement may be sustained when the drug is either temporarily or permanently discontinued.

Continued on next page

Methylin—Cont.

Drug treatment should not and need not be indefinite and usually may be discontinued after puberty.

HOW SUPPLIED

Each Methylin™ (methylphenidate HCl tablet, USP) 5 mg is available as a round, white unscored tablet debossed with 5 on one side and a boxed "M" on the other side.

Bottles of 100 .... NDC 0406-1121-01
Bottles of 1000 .... NDC 0406-1121-10

Each Methylin™ (methylphenidate HCl tablet, USP) 10 mg is available as a round, white scored tablet debossed with 10 on one side of the tablet and a M on the other side.

Bottles of 100 .... NDC 0406-1122-01
Bottles of 1000 .... NDC 0406-1122-10

Each Methylin™ (methylphenidate HCl tablet, USP) 20 mg is available as a round, white scored tablet debossed with 20 on one side of the tablet and a boxed "M" on the other side.

Bottles of 100 .... NDC 0406-1124-01
Bottles of 1000 .... NDC 0406-1124-10

Protect from light. Dispense in tight, light-resistant container with child-resistant closure.

Storage: Store at controlled room temperature 15° to 30°C (59° to 86°F). (See USP).

Each Methylin™ ER (methylphenidate HCl extended-release tablet, USP) 10 mg is available as a round, white to off-white tablet, debossed with 1423 on one side and a boxed "M" on the other side.

Bottles of 100 .... NDC 0406-1423-01

Each Methylin™ ER (methylphenidate HCl extended-release tablet, USP) 20 mg is available as a round, white to off-white tablet, debossed with 1451 on one side and a boxed "M" on the other side.

Bottles of 100 .... NDC 0406-1451-01

Note: Methylin™ and Methylin™ ER tablets are color-additive free.

Dispense in tight, light-resistant container with child-resistant closure.

Storage: Store at controlled room temperature 15° to 30°C (59° to 86°F)(see USP).

Protect from moisture.

Mallinckrodt Inc.
St. Louis, MO 63134 U.S.A.

020100

Shown in Product Identification Guide, page 321

OXYCODONE AND ACETAMINOPHEN TABLETS, USP 5 mg*/325 mg

Ⓒ℞

Rx only

DESCRIPTION

The oxycodone component is 4,5α-epoxy-14-hydroxy-3-methoxy-17-methylmorphinan-6-one hydrochloride, a white, odorless, crystalline powder having a saline, bitter taste. It is derived from the opium alkaloid, thebaine, and may be represented by the structural formula shown below:

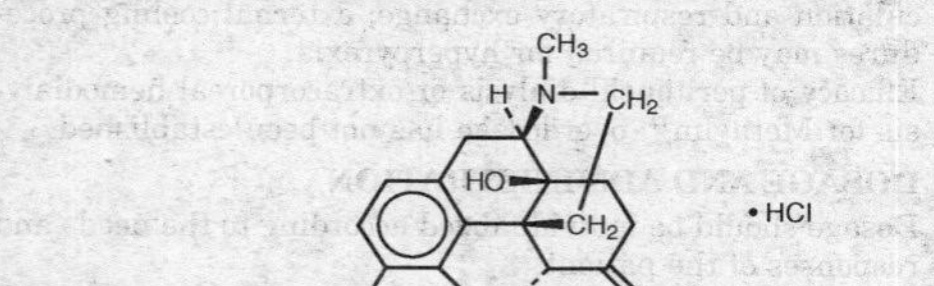

$C_{18}H_{21}NO_4 \cdot HCl$ MW = 351.83

Acetaminophen, 4′-hydroxyacetanilide, is a non-opiate, non-salicylate analgesic and antipyretic which occurs as a white, odorless, crystalline powder, possessing a slightly bitter taste. It has the following structural formula:

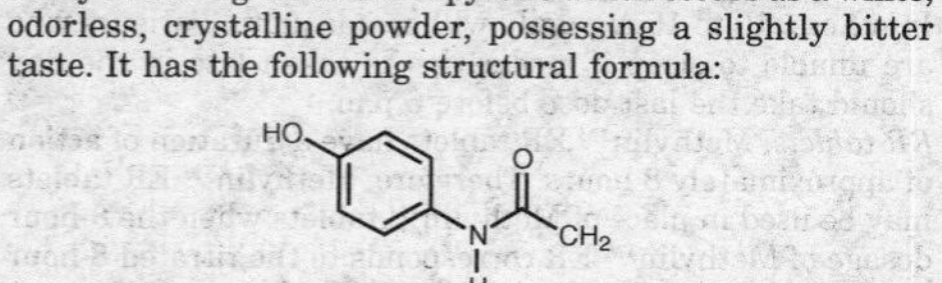

$C_8H_9NO_2$ MW = 151.17

Each oxycodone and acetaminophen tablet, USP 5 mg/325 mg for oral administration contains:

Oxycodone Hydrochloride, USP .... 5 mg*
Acetaminophen, USP .... 325 mg

*5 mg Oxycodone Hydrochloride, USP is equivalent to 4.4815 mg Oxycodone.

In addition, each tablet contains the following inactive ingredients: Microcrystalline Cellulose NF, Pregelatinized Starch NF, Silicon Dioxide NF, Stearic Acid NF, Crospovidone NF, and Povidone USP.

HOW SUPPLIED

Each OXYCODONE AND ACETAMINOPHEN, USP tablet contains Oxycodone Hydrochloride 5 mg (equivalent to 4.4815 mg Oxycodone) and Acetaminophen 325 mg. It is available as a round, white scored tablet debossed with a 512 identification number.

Bottles of 100 .... NDC No. 0406-0512-01
Bottles of 500 .... NDC No. 0406-0512-05

Dispense in a tight, light-resistant container with a child-resistant closure.

Protect from moisture. Store at controlled room temperature 15° to 30°C (59° to 86°F).

Mallinckrodt Inc.
St. Louis, Missouri 63134, U.S.A.
MG #13468

081899

OXYCODONE AND ACETAMINOPHEN CAPSULES, USP

Ⓒ℞

5 mg/500 mg
Rx only

DESCRIPTION

Each Oxycodone and Acetaminophen Capsule, USP 5 mg/500 mg contains:

Oxycodone Hydrochloride, USP .... 5 mg*
Acetaminophen, USP .... 500 mg

*5 mg Oxycodone Hydrochloride, USP is equivalent to 4.4815 mg oxycodone.

In addition, each capsule contains the following inactive ingredients: Gelatin NF, Magnesium Stearate NF, Silicon Dioxide NF, Sodium Lauryl Sulfate NF, Pregelatinized Starch NF, Stearic Acid NF, FD&C Blue No. 1, FD&C Red No. 40, FD&C Yellow No. 6, and Titanium Dioxide USP.

The oxycodone component is 14-hydroxydihydrocodeinone, a white, odorless, crystalline powder having a saline, bitter taste. It is derived from the opium alkaloid, thebaine, and may be represented by the structural formula shown below:

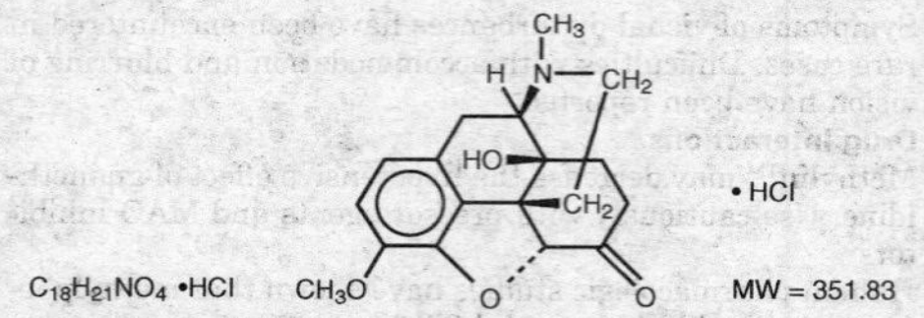

$C_{18}H_{21}NO_4 \cdot HCl$ MW = 351.83

Acetaminophen, 4′-hydroxyacetanilide, is a non-opiate, non-salicylate analgesic and antipyretic which occurs as a white, odorless, crystalline powder with a slightly bitter taste. It has the following structural formula:

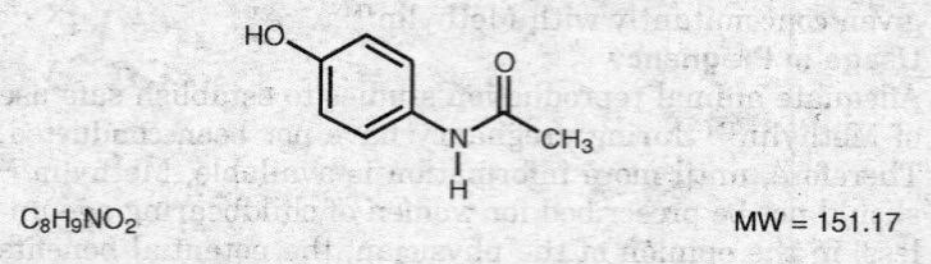

$C_8H_9NO_2$ MW = 151.17

HOW SUPPLIED

Each OXYCODONE AND ACETAMINOPHEN, USP capsule contains Oxycodone Hydrochloride 5 mg (equivalent to 4.4815 mg oxycodone) and Acetaminophen 500 mg. It is available as a Red/Beige hard gelatin capsule imprinted with Ⓜ 532 identification number.

Bottles of 100 .... NDC No. 0406-0532-01
Bottles of 500 .... NDC No. 0406-0532-05

Dispense in a tight, light-resistant container with a child-resistant closure.

Protect from moisture. Store at controlled room temperature 15° to 30°C (59° to 86°F).

DEA Order Form Required. Revised 8/99

Manufactured by
Mallinckrodt Inc.
St. Louis, Missouri 63134, U.S.A.
MG #13469

PENTAZOCINE AND NALOXONE HYDROCHLORIDES TABLETS USP

ⒸⅣ℞

Analgesic for Oral Use Only
Rx only

DESCRIPTION

Pentazocine and naloxone hydrochlorides tablets, USP contain pentazocine hydrochloride, USP, equivalent to 50 mg base and is a member of the benzazocine series (also known as the benzomorphan series), and naloxone hydrochloride, USP, equivalent to 0.5 mg base.

Pentazocine and naloxone hydrochlorides tablets are an analgesic for oral administration.

Chemically, pentazocine hydrochloride is (2*R**,6*R**,11*R**)- 1, 2, 3, 4, 5, 6-Hexahydro-6,11-dimethyl-3-(3-methyl-2-butenyl)-2,6-methano-3-benzazocin-8-ol hydrochloride, a white, crystalline substance soluble in acidic aqueous solutions, and has the following structural formula:

$C_{19}H_{27}NO \cdot HCl$ M.W. = 321.88

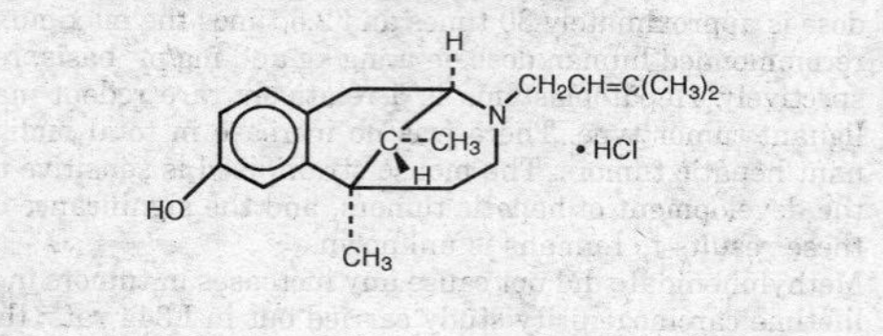

Chemically, naloxone hydrochloride is 17-Allyl-4,5α-epoxy-3,14-dihydroxy-morphinan-6-one hydrochloride. It is a slightly off-white powder, and is soluble in water and dilute acids, and has the following structural formula:

[See chemical structure at top of next column]

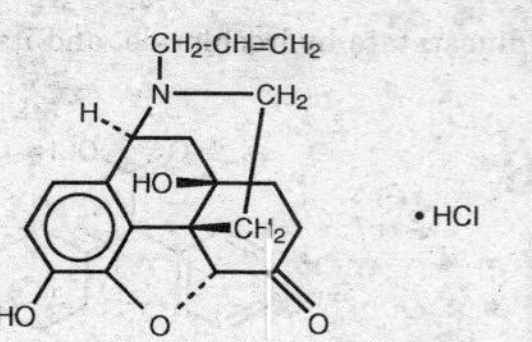

Each tablet, for oral administration, contains pentazocine hydrochloride, USP, equivalent to 50 mg of pentazocine, and naloxone hydrochloride, USP, equivalent to 0.5 mg of naloxone. In addition, each tablet contains the following inactive ingredients: Colloidal Silicon Dioxide, Corn Starch, Dibasic Calcium Phosphate, D&C Yellow #10, Aluminum lake, Magnesium Stearate, Microcrystalline Cellulose, Sodium Lauryl Sulfate.

HOW SUPPLIED

Pentazocine and Naloxone Hydrochlorides Tablets, USP are capsule-shaped, light yellow tablets, debossed with "M118" on one side and a score line on the other side, each containing pentazocine hydrochloride equivalent to 50 mg base and naloxone hydrochloride equivalent to 0.5 mg base.

Bottles of 100 (NDC 0406-3118-01).

Store at controlled room temperature 15° C to 30° C (59° F to 86° F).

Manufactured by:
OHM Laboratories, Inc.
North Brunswick, NJ 08902 USA
Manufactured for:
Mallinckrodt Inc.
St. Louis, MO 63134, U.S.A.
March 2000 P1007

PROPADE™

℞

Phenylpropanolamine Hydrochloride and Chlorpheniramine Maleate Extended-Release Capsules
Rx only

DESCRIPTION

Each extended-release capsule contains Phenylpropanolamine Hydrochloride 75 mg and Chlorpheniramine Maleate 12 mg.

Phenylpropanolamine Hydrochloride is (±)-Norephedrine Hydrochloride, an adrenergic agent. Chlorpheniramine Maleate is 2-(p-Chloro-a-(2-(dimethylamino)ethyl)benzyl) pyridine maleate (1:1), an antihistamine.

The structural formulas are as follows:

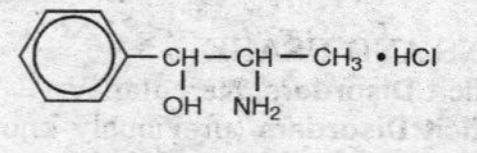

Phenylpropanolamine HCl
M.W. 187.67

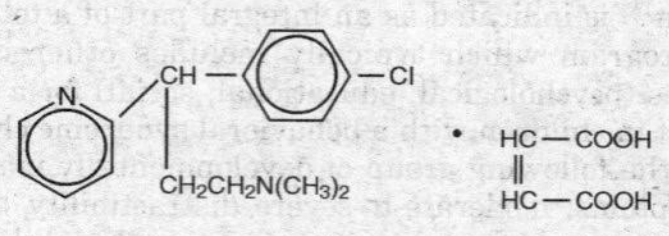

Chlorpheniramine Maleate
M.W. 390.87

HOW SUPPLIED

Each Phenylpropanolamine Hydrochloride 75 mg and Chlorpheniramine Maleate 12 mg Extended-release Capsule is a blue and clear capsule imprinted Ⓜ 0421.

Bottles of 100 .... NDC 0406-0421-01
Bottles of 1000 .... NDC 0406-0421-10

Dispense in a tight, light-resistant container as defined in the USP.

Store at controlled room temperature 15°–30°C (59°–86°F).

Mallinckrodt Inc.
St. Louis, MO 63134, U.S.A.
MG #12985 090899

IDENTIFICATION PROBLEM?
Turn to the **Product Identification Guide**, where you'll find more than 1600 products pictured in actual size and full color.

Marlyn Nutraceuticals

4404 E. ELWOOD
PHOENIX, AZ 85040

Direct Inquiries to:
Dr. Aftab Ahmed
4404 E. Elwood
Phoenix, AZ 85040
(800) 4-MARLYN
480 991-0200
EMAIL info@Marlyn.com

HEP–FORTE® OTC
[*hep-for 'tay*]

DESCRIPTION

Hep Forte is a comprehensive formulation of protein, B factors and other nutritional factors which can be important as a dietary supplement for maintenance and support of normal hepatic function.

COMPOSITION

Each capsule contains:

Vitamin A (Palmitate)	1,200I.U.
Vitamin E (d-Alpha Tocopherol)	10I.U.
Vitamin C (Ascorbic Acid)	10mg.
Folic Acid	0.06mg.
Vitamin B1 (Thiamine Mononitrate)	1mg.
Vitamin B2 (Riboflavin)	1mg.
Niacinamide	10mg.
Vitamin B6 (Pyridoxine HCl)	0.5mg.
Vitamin B12 (Cobalamin)	1mcg.
Biotin	3.3mcg.
Pantothenic Acid	2mg.
Choline Bitartrate	21mg.
Zinc (Zinc Sulfate)	2mg.
Desiccated Liver	194.4mg.
Liver Concentrate	64.8mg.
Liver Fraction Number 2	64.8mg.
Yeast (Dried)	64.8mg.
dl-Methionine	10mg.
Inositol	10mg.

INDICATIONS

Hep Forte is a balanced formulation of vitamins, minerals, lipotropic factors, and vitamin-protein supplements. It is of value as a nutritional supplement for persons who are receiving professional treatment for alcoholism, hepatic dysfunction due to hepatotoxic drugs and liver poisons, male and female infertility due to hormonal imbalance caused by hepatic dysfunction, and for nutritional supplementation after treatment.

CONTRAINDICATIONS

There are no known contraindications to Hep Forte.

DOSAGE

Three to six capsules daily.

HOW SUPPLIED

Bottles of 100, 300 or 500 capsules.
Literature Available.

MARLYN FORMULA 50® OTC

PRODUCT OVERVIEW

KEY FACTS

MARLYN FORMULA 50 is a dietary supplement providing a combination of amino acids and B6 in a gelatin capsule which provides protein "building blocks" important to growth and development of all protein containing tissue including nails, hair, and skin.

MAJOR USES

Dermatologists recommend Formula 50 for splitting, peeling nails. Since splitting and peeling nails are often associated with nail fungus, Formula 50 may be recommended in conjunction with drug therapy for nail fungus in order to provide protein necessary to growth and development of nails. OB-Gyn's recommend it for help in controlling excessive hair fall-out after child birth.

SAFETY INFORMATION

There are no known contraindications or adverse reactions.

PRESCRIBING INFORMATION

MARLYN FORMULA 50®

COMPOSITION

Each capsule contains:

Amino Acids	0.3 Gm*
Vitamin B6 (pyridoxine HCl)	1.0 mg.

*Approximate analysis of the amino acids: indispensable amino acids (lysine, tryptophan, phenylalanine, methionine, threonine, leucine, isoleucine, valine), 35.30%; semi-dispensable amino acids (arginine, histidine, tyrosine, cystine, glycine), 19.18%; dispensable amino acids (glutamic acid, alanine, aspartic acid, serine, proline), 45.56%.

Amino acids: Protein "building blocks" important to growth and development of all protein containing tissue including nails, hair, and skin.

DOSAGE AND ADMINISTRATION

The recommended daily dose is 6 capsules daily.

SUPPLY

Bottles of 100, 250 and 500 capsules.

McNeil Consumer Healthcare

Division of McNeil-PPC, Inc.
FORT WASHINGTON, PA 19034

Direct Inquiries to:
Consumer Affairs Department
Fort Washington, PA 19034
(215) 273-7000

AFLEXA™ OTC
[*ə-fleks' -ə*]
(Glucosamine)

DESCRIPTION

Aflexa is a dietary supplement containing glucosamine a natural building block of healthy cartilage. Each AFLEXA™ Tablet contains 340 mg of glucosamine (300 mg as glucosamine sulfate and 200 mg as glucosamine hydrochloride).

ACTIONS

Taken daily, AFLEXA™ offers a number of valuable benefits:

- Helps maintain lubricating fluid in joints*
- Promotes joint flexibility and range of motion*
- Provides a natural building block of healthy cartilage*
- Promotes comfortable joint function*

USES

AFLEXA™ is intended to help maintain healthy cartilage in people whose joints may be affected by the natural aging process.

DIRECTIONS

Take one tablet three times a day. Benefits may begin within 2–4 weeks of daily use.

PRECAUTIONS

Do not use if you are allergic to shellfish. If you are pregnant or breast-feeding, ask your doctor before use. Use only as directed. Keep out of reach of children.

INGREDIENTS

GLUCOSAMINE SULFATE, GLUCOSAMINE HYDROCHLORIDE, CELLULOSE, HYDROXYPROPYL METHYLCELLULOSE, POLYETHYLENE GLYCOL, SILICON DIOXIDE, PROPYLENE GLYCOL, CROSPOVIDONE, HYDROXYPROPYL CELLULOSE, TITANIUM DIOXIDE, MAGNESIUM STEARATE, POLYSORBATE 80, POVIDONE.

HOW SUPPLIED

AFLEXA glucosamine is available in bottles of 50, 110 and 250.
Store at room temperature.
DO NOT USE IF CARTON IS OPENED OR IF NECK WRAP OR FOIL INNER SEAL IS BROKEN OR MISSING.

* **These Statements Have Not Been Evaluated By The Food & Drug Administration. This Product Is Not Intended To Diagnose, Treat, Cure Or Prevent Any Disease.**

Shown in Product Identification Guide, page 321

Children's MOTRIN® OTC
Ibuprofen Oral Suspension and Chewable Tablets

DESCRIPTION

Children's MOTRIN® Ibuprofen Oral Suspension is an alcohol-free, berry, bubblegum or grape-flavored suspension. Each 5 mL (teaspoon) of ***Children's MOTRIN® Ibuprofen Oral Suspension*** contains ibuprofen 100 mg. Each ***Children's MOTRIN® Ibuprofen Chewable Tablet*** contains 50 mg of ibuprofen and are available as orange or grape-flavored chewable tablets.

USES

Children's MOTRIN® Ibuprofen Oral Suspension and Children's MOTRIN® Ibuprofen Chewable Tablets: Temporarily:

- **Reduces fever**
- **Relieves minor aches and pains** due to the common cold, flu, sore throat, headaches and toothaches

DIRECTIONS

Do not take/chew more than directed. If needed, repeat dose every **6–8 hours.** Do not use more than **4 times a day.** If possible, use weight to dose; otherwise use age. If stomach upset occurs while taking this product, give with food or milk. ***Children's MOTRIN® Ibuprofen Oral Suspension:*** Shake well before using. Only use enclosed measuring cup. Replace bottle cap tightly to maintain child resistance. 2–3 years (24–35 lbs): 1 tsp; 4–5 years (36–47 lbs): 1½ tsp; 6–8 years (48–59 lbs): 2 tsp; 9–10 years (60–71 lbs): 2½ tsp; 11 years (72–95 lbs): 3 tsp. Under 2 years (under 24 lbs), consult a physician. ***Children's MOTRIN® Ibuprofen Chewable Tablets:*** 2–3 years (24–35 lbs): 2 tablets; 4–5 years (36–47 lbs): 3 tablets; 6–8 years (48–59 lbs): 4 tablets; 9–10 years (60–71 lbs): 5 tablets; 11 years (72–95 lbs): 6 tablets. Under 2 years (under 24 lbs), call a doctor.

Children's MOTRIN® Ibuprofen Oral Suspension:

WARNINGS

Allergy Alert: ibuprofen may cause a severe allergic reaction which may include:

- hives • facial swelling
- asthma (wheezing) • shock

Do not use if you have ever had an allergic reaction to any other pain reliever/fever reducer.

Stop use and ask a doctor if an allergic reaction occurs. Seek medical help right away.

Call Your Doctor If:

- Your child is under a doctor's care for any serious condition or is taking any other drug.
- Your child has problems or serious side effects from taking fever reducers or pain relievers.
- Your child does not get any relief within first day (24 hours) of treatment, or pain or fever gets worse.
- Stomach upset gets worse or lasts.
- Redness or swelling is present in the painful area.
- Sore throat is severe, lasts for more than 2 days or occurs with fever, headache, rash, nausea or vomiting.
- Any new symptoms appear.

Do Not Use:

- With any other product that contains ibuprofen, or other pain reliever/fever reducer, unless directed by a doctor.
- For more than **3 days** for fever or pain unless directed by a doctor.
- For stomach pain unless directed by a doctor.
- If your child is dehydrated (significant fluid loss) due to continued vomiting, diarrhea or lack of fluid intake.
- **If plastic carton wrap or bottle wrap imprinted "Safety Seal®", is broken or missing.**

Keep this and all drugs out of the reach of children. In case of accidental overdose, seek professional assistance or contact a poison control center immediately

Children's MOTRIN® Ibuprofen Chewable Tablets:

Allergy alert: ibuprofen may cause a severe allergic reaction which may include:

- hives • facial swelling
- asthma (wheezing) • shock

Sore throat warning: severe or persistent sore throat or sore throat accompanied by high fever, headache, nausea, and vomiting may be serious. Consult doctor promptly. Do not use more than 2 days or administer to children under 3 years of age unless directed by doctor.

Do not use if the child has ever had an allergic reaction to any pain reliever/fever reducer

Ask a doctor before use if the child has

- not been drinking fluids
- lost a lot of fluid due to continued vomiting or diarrhea
- stomach pain
- problems or serious side effects from taking fever reducers or pain relievers

Ask a doctor or pharmacist before use if the child is

- under a doctor's care for any serious condition
- taking any other drug
- taking any other product that contains ibuprofen, or any other pain reliever/fever reducer

When using this product

- mouth or throat burning may occur; give with food or water
- if stomach upset occurs, give with food or milk

Stop use and ask a doctor if

- an allergic reaction occurs. Seek medical help right away
- fever or pain gets worse or lasts more than 3 days
- the child does not get any relief within first day (24 hours) of treatment
- stomach pain or upset gets worse or lasts
- redness or swelling is present in the painful area
- any new symptoms appear

Keep out of reach of children. In case of overdose, get medical help or contact a Poison Control Center right away.

OTHER INFORMATION

- phenylketonurics: contains phenylalanine 1.4 mg per tablet
- do not use if neck wrap or foil inner seal imprinted **"Safety Seal®"** is broken or missing
- store at 20–25°C (68–77°F)

PROFESSIONAL INFORMATION

OVERDOSAGE INFORMATION

The *toxicity of ibuprofen overdose* is dependent upon the amount of drug ingested and the time elapsed since ingestion, though individual response may vary, which makes it necessary to evaluate each case individually. Although uncommon, serious toxicity and death have been reported in the medical literature with ibuprofen overdosage. The most frequently reported symptoms of ibuprofen overdose include abdominal pain, nausea, vomiting, lethargy and drowsiness. Other central nervous system symptoms include headache, tinnitus, CNS depression and seizures. Metabolic acidosis, coma, acute renal failure and apnea (primarily in

Continued on next page

Children's Motrin—Cont.

very young children) may rarely occur. Cardiovascular toxicity, including hypotension, bradycardia, tachycardia and atrial fibrillation, also have been reported.

The *treatment of acute ibuprofen overdose* is primarily supportive. Management of hypotension, acidosis and gastrointestinal bleeding may be necessary. In cases of acute overdose, the stomach should be emptied through ipecac-induced emesis or lavage. Emesis is most effective if initiated within 30 minutes of ingestion. Orally administered activated charcoal may help in reducing the absorption and reabsorption of ibuprofen.

In children, the estimated amount of ibuprofen ingested per body weight may be helpful to predict the potential for development of toxicity although each case must be evaluated. Ingestion of less than 100 mg/kg is unlikely to produce toxicity. Children ingesting 100 to 200 mg/kg may be managed with induced emesis and a minimal observation time of four hours. Children ingesting 200 to 400 mg/kg of ibuprofen should have immediate gastric emptying and at least four hours observation in a health care facility. Children ingesting greater than 400 mg/kg require immediate medical referral, careful observation and appropriate supportive therapy. Ipecac-induced emesis is not recommended in overdoses greater than 400 mg/kg because of the risk of convulsions and the potential for aspiration of gastric contents.

In adult patients the history of the dose reportedly ingested does not appear to be predictive of toxicity. The need for referral and follow-up must be judged by the circumstances at the time of the overdose ingestion. Symptomatic adults should be admitted to a health care facility for observation.

INACTIVE INGREDIENTS

Children's MOTRIN® Berry-Flavored Ibuprofen Oral Suspension: Acesulfame potassium, citric acid, cornstarch, D&C Yellow #10, FD&C Red #40, glycerin, natural and artificial flavors polysorbate 80, purified water, sodium benzoate, sucrose, xanthan gum.

Children's MOTRIN® Bubble Gum-Flavored Ibuprofen Oral Suspension: Acesulfame potassium, citric acid, cornstarch, FD&C Red #40, natural and artificial flavors, glycerin, polysorbate 80, purified water, sodium benzoate, sucrose, xanthan gum.

Children's MOTRIN® Grape-Flavored Ibuprofen Oral Suspension: Acesulfame potassium, citric acid, cornstarch, D&C Red #33, FD&C Blue #1, FD&C Red #40, natural and artificial flavors, glycerin, polysorbate 80, purified water, sodium benzoate, sucrose, xanthan gum.

Children's MOTRIN® Ibuprofen Orange-Flavored Chewable Tablets: acesulfame K, aspartame, cellulose, citric acid, FD&C Yellow #6, flavor, fumaric acid, hydroxyethyl cellulose, hydroxypropyl methylcellulose, magnesium stearate, mannitol, povidone, sodium lauryl sulfate, sodium starch glycolate.

Children's MOTRIN® Grape-Flavored Chewable Tablets: acesulfame K, aspartame, cellulose, citric acid, D&C red #7, red #30, FD&C blue #1, flavor, fumaric acid, hydroxyethyl cellulose, hydroxypropyl methylcellulose, magnesium stearate, mannitol, povidone, sodium lauryl sulfate, sodium starch glycolate.

HOW SUPPLIED

Children's MOTRIN® Ibuprofen Oral Suspension: Berry-flavored, orange-colored; Bubble Gum flavored, pink-colored and Grape-flavored, purple-colored liquid in tamper evident bottles of 2 and 4 fl. oz. Store between 20–25°C (68°–77°F).

Children's MOTRIN® Ibuprofen Chewable Tablets: Orange-flavored, orange-colored, and Grape-flavored, purple-colored, chewable tablets in 24 count bottles.

Shown in Product Identification Guide, pages 321 & 322

Children's TYLENOL® ALLERGY-D Liquid and Chewable Tablets — OTC

DESCRIPTION

Children's TYLENOL® ALLERGY-D Liquid is Bubble Gum Blast-flavored and contains no alcohol or aspirin. Each teaspoonful (5 mL) contains acetaminophen 160 mg, diphenhydramine HCl 12.5 mg and pseudoephedrine HCl 15 mg. ***Children's TYLENOL® ALLERGY-D Chewable Tablets*** are Bubble Gum Blast-flavored and each tablet contains acetaminophen 80 mg, diphenhydramine HCl 6.25 mg and pseudoephedrine HCl 7.5 mg.

ACTIONS

Children's TYLENOL® ALLERGY-D Liquid and ***Chewable Tablets*** combine the analgesic-antipyretic acetaminophen with the antihistamine diphenhydramine hydrochloride and the decongestant pseudoephedrine hydrochloride to provide fast, effective, temporary relief of all your child's symptoms associated with hay fever and other respiratory allergies including sneezing, sore throat, itchy throat, itchy/watery eyes, runny nose, stuffy nose and nasal congestion. Acetaminophen is equal to aspirin in analgesic and antipyretic effectiveness and it is unlikely to produce the side effects often associated with aspirin or aspirin-containing products.

USES

For the reduction of fever. For the temporary relief of these hay fever and other upper respiratory allergy symptoms: stuffy nose, sneezing, sore throat, nasal congestion, itchy/watery eyes, runny nose, stuffy nose, nasal congestion.

DIRECTIONS

If possible, use weight to dose; otherwise use age. All doses may be repeated every 4-6 hours, if needed. Do not use more than 4 times in 24 hours. Under 6 years (under 48 lbs), consult a physician. ***Children's TYLENOL® ALLERGY-D Liquid:*** 6-11 years (48–95 lbs): 2 teaspoonfuls. An AccuDose™ measuring cup is provided for accurate dosing. ***Children's TYLENOL® ALLERGY-D Chewable Tablets:*** 6-11 years (48–95 lbs): 4 tablets.

Professional Dosage Schedule: ***Children's TYLENOL® ALLERGY-D Liquid:*** If possible, use weight to dose; otherwise use age. 4–11 months (12–17 lbs): 1/2 teaspoonful; 12–23 months (18–23 lbs): 3/4 teaspoonful; 2–3 years (24–35 lbs): 1 teaspoonful; 4–5 years (36–47 lbs): $1^1/_2$ teaspoonfuls; 6–8 years (48–59 lbs): 2 teaspoonfuls; 9–10 years (60–71 lbs): $2^1/_2$ teaspoonfuls; 11 years (72–95 lbs): 3 teaspoonfuls. ***Children's TYLENOL® ALLERGY-D Chewable Tablets:*** If possible, use weight to dose; otherwise use age. 2–3 years (24–35 lbs): 2 tablets; 4–5 years (36–47 lbs): 3 tablets; 6–8 years (48–59 lbs): 4 tablets; 9–10 years (60–71 lbs): 5 tablets; 11 years (72–95 lbs): 6 tablets.

PRECAUTIONS

If a rare sensitivity reaction occurs, the drug should be discontinued.

WARNINGS

Do not take for pain for more than 5 days or for fever for more than 3 days unless directed by a doctor. If pain or fever persists, or gets worse, if new symptoms occur, or if redness or swelling is present, consult a doctor because these could be signs of a serious condition. If sore throat is severe, persists for more than 2 days, is accompanied or followed by fever, headache, rash, nausea or vomiting, consult a doctor promptly. If nervousness, dizziness or sleeplessness occur, discontinue use and consult a doctor. May cause excitability especially in children. Do not give this product to children who have a breathing problem such as chronic bronchitis, or who have glaucoma, heart disease, high blood pressure, thyroid disease, or diabetes without first consulting the child's doctor. May cause marked drowsiness; sedatives and tranquilizers may increase the drowsiness effect. Do not give this product to children who are taking sedatives or tranquilizers without first consulting the child's doctor. **Do not exceed recommended dosage.** Taking more than the recommended dose (overdose) may not provide more relief and could cause serious health problems. Keep this and all drugs out of the reach of children. In case of accidental overdose, contact a doctor or poison control center immediately. Prompt medical attention is critical for adults as well as for children even if you do not notice any signs or symptoms. Do not use with other products containing acetaminophen.

NOTE: In addition to the above:

Children's TYLENOL® ALLERGY-D Liquid: **Do not use if plastic carton wrap, bottle wrap, or foil inner seal imprinted "Safety Seal®" is broken or missing.**

Children's TYLENOL® ALLERGY-D Chewable Tablets: **Do not use if carton is opened or if blister unit is broken.** Phenylketonurics: Contains Phenylalanine 5 mg per tablet.

DRUG INTERACTION PRECAUTIONS

Do not give this product to a child who is taking a prescription monoamine oxidase inhibitor (MAOI) (certain drugs for depression, psychiatric or emotional conditions), or for 2 weeks after stopping the MAOI drug. If you are uncertain whether your child's prescription drug contains an MAOI, consult a health professional before giving this product.

PROFESSIONAL INFORMATION

OVERDOSAGE INFORMATION

Acetaminophen in massive overdosage may cause hepatic toxicity in some patients. In adults and adolescents (≥12 years of age), hepatic toxicity may occur following ingestion of greater than 7.5 to 10 grams over a period of 8 hours or less. Fatalities are infrequent (less than 3–4% of untreated cases) and have rarely been reported with overdoses of less than 15 grams. In children (<12 years of age), an acute overdosage of less than 150 mg/kg has not been associated with hepatic toxicity. Early symptoms following a potentially hepatotoxic overdose may include: nausea, vomiting, diaphoresis and general malaise. Clinical and laboratory evidence of hepatic toxicity may not be apparent until 48 to 72 hours postingestion. In adults and adolescents, any individual presenting with an unknown amount of acetaminophen ingested or with a questionable or unreliable history about the time of ingestion should have a plasma acetaminophen level drawn and be treated with *N*-acetylcysteine. For full prescribing information, refer to the *N*-acetylcysteine package insert. Do not await the results of assays for acetaminophen levels before initiating treatment with *N*-acetylcysteine. The following additional procedures are recommended: Promptly initiate gastric decontamination of the stomach. A plasma acetaminophen assay should be obtained as early as possible, but no sooner than four hours following ingestion. If an acetaminophen *extended release* product is involved, it may be appropriate to obtain an additional plasma acetaminophen level 4–6 hours following the initial acetaminophen level. If either acetaminophen level plots above the treatment line on the acetaminophen overdose nomogram, *N*-acetylcysteine treatment should be continued for a full course of therapy. Liver function studies should be obtained initially and repeated at 24–hour intervals.

Serious toxicity or fatalities have been extremely infrequent following an acute acetaminophen overdose in young children, possibly because of differences in the way they metabolize acetaminophen. In children, the maximum potential amount ingested can be more easily estimated. If more than 150 mg/kg or an unknown amount was ingested, obtain a plasma acetaminophen level as soon as possible, but no sooner than 4 hours following ingestion. If an acetaminophen *extended release* product is involved, it may be appropriate to obtain an additional plasma acetaminophen level 4–6 hours following the initial acetaminophen level. If either acetaminophen level plots above the treatment line on the acetaminophen overdose nomogram, *N*-acetylcysteine treatment should be initiated and continued for a full course of therapy. If an assay cannot be obtained and the estimated acetaminophen ingestion exceeds 150 mg/kg, dosing with *N*-acetylcysteine should be initiated and continued for a full course of therapy.

For additional emergency information, call your regional poison center or call the Rocky Mountain Poison Center toll-free (1–800–525–6115).

Diphenhydramine toxicity should be treated as you would an antihistamine/anticholinergic overdose and is likely to be present within a few hours after acute ingestion.

Symptoms from pseudoephedrine overdose consist most often of mild anxiety, tachycardia and/or mild hypertension. Symptoms usually appear within 4 to 8 hours of ingestion and are transient usually requiring no treatment.

INACTIVE INGREDIENTS

Liquid: Benzoic Acid, Citric Acid, Corn Syrup, D&C Red #33, FD&C Red #40, Flavors, Polyethylene Glycol, Propylene Glycol, Purified Water, Sodium Benzoate, Sorbitol.

Chewable Tablets: Aspartame, Cellulose, Cellulose Acetate, D&C Red #7, Flavors, Magnesium Stearate, Mannitol, Polymethacrylate, Povidone.

HOW SUPPLIED

Liquid: Pink-colored–child-resistant bottles of 4 fl. oz. Store at room temperature. Avoid excessive heat, 104°F (40°C).

Chewable Tablets: Pink-colored, imprinted "CTA" on one side—blister packs of 24. Store at room temperature.

Shown in Product Identification Guide, page 322

Children's TYLENOL® — OTC

acetaminophen
Soft-Chews Chewable Tablets and Suspension Liquid

Infants' TYLENOL®

acetaminophen
Concentrated Drops

Product information for all dosage forms of CHILDREN'S TYLENOL acetaminophen have been combined under this heading

DESCRIPTION

Infants' TYLENOL® Grape Concentrated Drops are stable, alcohol-free, grape-flavored and purple in color. ***Infants' TYLENOL® Cherry Concentrated Drops*** are stable, alcohol-free, cherry-flavored and red in color. Each 1.6 mL (2 dropperfuls) contains 160 mg acetaminophen. ***Infants' TYLENOL® Concentrated Drops*** features the SAFE-TY-LOCK™ Bottle. The SAFE-TY-LOCK™ Bottle has a unique safety barrier inside the bottle which helps make administration easier. The integrated dropper promotes proper administration. The innovative design eliminates excess product on dropper. The star-shaped barrier inside the bottle minimizes spills and discourages pouring into a spoon. ***Children's TYLENOL® Suspension Liquid*** is stable, alcohol-free, cherry-flavored and red in color, or bubble gum-flavored and pink in color, or grape-flavored and purple in color. Each 5 mL (one teaspoonful) contains 160 mg acetaminophen. Each ***Children's TYLENOL® Soft-Chews Chewable Tablet*** contains 80 mg acetaminophen in a grape, bubble gum, or fruit flavor.

ACTIONS

Acetaminophen is a clinically proven analgesic/antipyretic. Acetaminophen produces analgesia by elevation of the pain threshold and antipyresis through action on the hypothalamic heat regulating center. Acetaminophen is equal to aspirin in analgesic and antipyretic effectiveness and it is unlikely to produce many of the side effects associated with aspirin and aspirin-containing products.

USES

Children's TYLENOL® Soft-Chews Chewable Tablets, Suspension Liquid and ***Infants' TYLENOL® Concentrated Drops:*** For the reduction of fever. For the temporary relief of minor aches and pains associated with a cold, flu, headache, sore throat, immunizations, toothache.

DIRECTIONS

If possible, use weight to dose; otherwise use age. All dosages may be repeated every 4 hours, if needed. Do not use more than 5 times a day. Under 2 years (under 24 lbs), consult a physician. ***Children's TYLENOL® Soft-Chews Chewable Tablets:*** Chew tablets before swallowing. ***Children's TYLENOL® Soft-Chews Chewable Tablets*** are not the same concentration as Junior Strength Tylenol® Chewable Tablets or Caplets. For accurate dosing follow dosing instructions on label. 2–3 years (24–35 lbs): 2 tablets; 4–5 years (36–47 lbs): 3 tablets; 6–8 years (48–59 lbs): 4 tablets; 9–10 years (60–71 lbs): 5 tablets; 11 years (72–95 lbs): 6 tablets. ***Children's TYLENOL® Suspension Liquid:*** Children's Tylenol® Liquids are **less** concentrated than Infants' Tylenol® Concentrated Drops. For accurate dosing follow dosing instructions on label. This product has been specifically designed for use with the enclosed measuring cup. Use only enclosed measuring cup to dose this product. Do not use any other dosing device. 2–3 years (24–35 lbs): 1 teaspoonful; 4–5 years (36–47 lbs): 1 $^{1}/_{2}$ teaspoonfuls; 6–8 years (48–59 lbs): 2 teaspoonfuls; 9–10 years (60–71 lbs): 2 $^{1}/_{2}$ teaspoonfuls; 11 years (72–95 lbs): 3 teaspoonfuls. ***Infants' TYLENOL® Concentrated Drops:*** Infants' Tylenol® Drops are **more** concentrated than Children's Tylenol® Liquids. For accurate dosing follow dosing instructions on label. This product has been specifically designed for use only with enclosed dropper. Do not use any other dosing device with this product. 2–3 years (24–35 lbs): 2 dropperfuls (2 × 0.8 mL).

Professional Dosage Schedule: ***Children's TYLENOL® Suspension Liquid:*** Children's Tylenol® Liquids are **less** concentrated than Infants' Tylenol® Concentrated Drops. For accurate dosing follow dosing instructions on label. This product has been specifically designed for use with the enclosed measuring cup. Use only enclosed measuring cup to dose this product. Do not use any other dosing device. If possible, use weight to dose; otherwise use age. 4–11 months (12–17 lbs): $^{1}/_{2}$ teaspoonful; 12–23 months (18–23 lbs): $^{3}/_{4}$ teaspoonful. ***Infants' TYLENOL® Concentrated Drops:*** Infants' Tylenol® Drops are **more** concentrated than Children's Tylenol® Liquids. For accurate dosing follow dosing instructions on label. This product has been specifically designed for use only with enclosed dropper. Do not use any other dosing device with this product. If possible, use weight to dose; otherwise use age. 0–3 months (6–11 lbs): 0.4 mL; 4–11 months (12–17 lbs): 0.8 mL; 12–23 months (18–23 lbs): 1.2 mL. All dosages may be repeated every 4 hours, if needed. Do not use more than 5 times a day.

PRECAUTIONS

If a rare sensitivity reaction occurs, the drug should be discontinued.

WARNINGS

Children's TYLENOL® Soft-Chew Chewable Tablets, Suspension Liquid and Infants' TYLENOL® Concentrated Drops:

Do Not Use:

- with any other products containing acetaminophen.
- for more than 3 days for fever unless directed by a doctor.
- for more than 5 days for pain unless directed by a doctor.

Stop Using This Product and Ask a Doctor If:

- symptoms do not improve.
- new symptoms occur.
- pain or fever persists or gets worse.
- redness or swelling is present.
- sore throat is severe, lasts for more than 2 days or occurs with fever, headache, rash, nausea or vomiting.

Do not exceed recommended dose. Taking more than the recommended dose (overdose) may not provide more relief and could cause serious health problems. Keep this and all drugs out of the reach of children. In case of accidental overdose, contact a physician or poison control center immediately. Prompt medical attention is critical even if you do not notice any signs or symptoms.

NOTE: In addition to the above:

Infants' TYLENOL® Concentrated Drops: **Do not use if plastic carton wrap or bottle wrap imprinted "Safety Seal®" is broken or missing.**

Children's TYLENOL® Suspension Liquid: **Do not use if plastic carton wrap, bottle wrap, or foil inner seal imprinted "Safety Seal®" is broken or missing.**

Children's TYLENOL® Soft-Chews Chewable Tablets: **Do not use if carton is opened or if neck wrap or foil inner seal imprinted "Safety Seal®" is broken or missing.** Phenylketonurics: grape contains phenylalanine 5 mg per tablet, bubble gum contains 6 mg per tablet, fruit contains 6 mg per tablet.

PROFESSIONAL INFORMATION

OVERDOSAGE INFORMATION

Acetaminophen in massive overdosage may cause hepatic toxicity in some patients. In adults and adolescents (≥ 12 years of age), hepatic toxicity may occur following ingestion of greater than 7.5 to 10 grams over a period of 8 hours or less. Fatalities are infrequent (less than 3–4% of untreated cases) and have rarely been reported with overdoses of less than 15 grams. In children (< 12 years of age), an acute overdosage of less than 150 mg/kg has not been associated with hepatic toxicity. Early symptoms following a potentially hepatotoxic overdose may include: nausea, vomiting, diaphoresis and general malaise. Clinical and laboratory evidence of hepatic toxicity may not be apparent until 48 to 72 hours postingestion. In adults and adolescents, any individual presenting with an unknown amount of acetaminophen ingested or with a questionable or unreliable history about the time of ingestion should have a plasma acetaminophen level drawn and be treated with *N*-acetylcysteine. For full prescribing information, refer to the *N*-acetylcysteine package insert. Do not await results of assays for acetaminophen levels before initiating treatment with *N*-acetylcysteine. The following additional procedures are recommended: Promptly initiate gastric decontamination of the stomach. A plasma acetaminophen assay should be obtained as early as possible, but no sooner than four hours following ingestion. If an acetaminophen *extended release* product is involved, it may be appropriate to obtain an additional plasma acetaminophen level 4–6 hours following the initial acetaminophen level. If either acetaminophen level plots above the treatment line on the acetaminophen overdose nomogram, *N*-acetylcysteine treatment should be continued for a full course of therapy. Liver function studies should be obtained initially and repeated at 24-hour intervals.

Serious toxicity or fatalities have been extremely infrequent following an acute acetaminophen overdose in young children, possibly because of differences in the way they metabolize acetaminophen. In children, the maximum potential amount ingested can be more easily estimated. If more than 150 mg/kg or an unknown amount was ingested, obtain a plasma acetaminophen level as soon as possible, but no sooner than 4 hours following ingestion. If an acetaminophen *extended release* product is involved, it may be appropriate to obtain an additional plasma acetaminophen level 4–6 hours following the initial acetaminophen level. If either acetaminophen level plots above the treatment line on the acetaminophen overdose nomogram, *N*-acetylcysteine treatment should be initiated and continued for a full course of therapy. If an assay cannot be obtained and the estimated acetaminophen ingestion exceeds 150 mg/kg, dosing with *N*-acetylcysteine should be initiated and continued for a full course of therapy.

For additional emergency information, call your regional poison center or call the Rocky Mountain Poison Center toll free, (1-800-525-6115).

Inactive Ingredients: ***Children's TYLENOL® Soft-Chews Fruit Flavored Chewable Tablets:*** Aspartame, Cellulose, Citric Acid, D&C Red #7, Flavors, D&C Red #7, Flavors, Magnesium Stearate, Mannitol. May contain Ethylcellulose or Cellulose Acetate and Povidone.

Children's TYLENOL® Soft-Chews Grape Flavored Chewable Tablets: Aspartame, Cellulose, Citric Acid, D&C Red #7, D&C Red #30, FD&C Blue #1, Flavors, Magnesium Stearate, Mannitol. May contain Ethylcellulose or Cellulose Acetate and Povidone.

Children's TYLENOL® Soft-Chews Bubble Gum Flavored Chewable Tablets: Aspartame, Cellulose, D&C Red #7, Flavors, Magnesium Stearate, Mannitol. May contain Ethylcellulose or Cellulose Acetate and Povidone.

Children's TYLENOL® Suspension Liquid: Butylparaben, Cellulose, Citric Acid, Corn Syrup, Flavors, Glycerin, Propylene Glycol, Purified Water, Sodium Benzoate, Sorbitol, Xanthan Gum. In addition to the above ingredients cherry-flavored suspension contains FD&C Red #40, bubble gum-flavored suspension contains D&C Red #33 and FD&C Red #40, and grape-flavored suspension contains D&C Red #33 and FD&C Blue #1.

Infants' TYLENOL® Cherry Concentrated Drops: Butylparaben, Cellulose, Citric Acid, Corn Syrup, FD&C Red #40, Flavors, Glycerin, Propylene Glycol, Purified Water, Sodium Benzoate, Sorbitol, Xanthan Gum.

Infants' TYLENOL® Grape Concentrated Drops: Butylparaben, Cellulose, Citric Acid, Corn Syrup, D&C Red #33, FD&C Blue #1, Flavors, Glycerin, Propylene Glycol, Purified Water, Sodium Benzoate, Sorbitol, Xanthan Gum.

HOW SUPPLIED

Soft-Chew Chewable Tablets (pink-colored fruit, purple-colored grape, pink-colored bubble gum, scored, imprinted "TY80"): Bottles of 30 and also blister packaged 60's and 96's. (fruit). Bubble gum and fruit: Store at room temperature; grape: store at room temperature and keep product away from direct light. **Suspension liquid** (red-colored cherry): bottles of 2 and 4 fl. oz. (pink-colored bubble gum and purple-colored grape): bottles of 4 fl. oz. Store at room temperature. **Concentrated drops** (purple-colored grape): bottles of $^{1}/_{2}$ oz (15 mL) and 1 oz (30 mL); (red-colored cherry): bottles of $^{1}/_{2}$ oz and 1 oz, each with calibrated plastic dropper. Store at room temperature.

All packages listed above have child-resistant safety caps or blisters.

Shown in Product Identification Guide, page 322

Children's TYLENOL® COLD Suspension Liquid and Chewable Tablets OTC

DESCRIPTION

Children's TYLENOL® COLD Suspension Liquid is Great Grape-flavored and contains no alcohol or aspirin. Each teaspoonful (5 mL) contains acetaminophen 160 mg, chlorpheniramine maleate 1 mg, and pseudoephedrine HCl 15 mg. ***Children's TYLENOL® COLD Chewable Tablets*** are Great Grape-flavored and each tablet contains acetaminophen 80 mg, chlorpheniramine maleate 0.5 mg and pseudoephedrine HCl 7.5 mg.

ACTIONS

Children's TYLENOL® COLD Multi Symptom Suspension Liquid and Chewable Tablets combine the analgesic-antipyretic acetaminophen with the decongestant pseudoephedrine hydrochloride and the antihistamine chlorpheniramine maleate to help relieve nasal congestion, dry runny noses and prevent sneezing as well as to relieve the fever, aches, pains and general discomfort associated with colds and upper respiratory infections. Acetaminophen is equal to aspirin in analgesic and antipyretic effectiveness and it is unlikely to produce the side effects often associated with aspirin or aspirin-containing products.

USES

For temporary relief of these cold symptoms: nasal congestion, runny nose, sore throat, sneezing, minor aches and pains, headaches and fever.

DIRECTIONS

If possible, use weight to dose; otherwise use age. All doses may be repeated every 4–6 hours, if needed. Do not use more than 4 times in 24 hours. Under 6 years (under 48 lbs), consult a physician. ***Children's TYLENOL® COLD Suspension Liquid Formula:*** 6–11 years (48–95 lbs): 2 teaspoonfuls. An AccuDose™ measuring cup is provided and marked for accurate dosing. ***Children's TYLENOL® COLD Chewable Tablets:*** 6–11 years (48–95 lbs): 4 tablets.

Professional Dosage Schedule: ***Children's TYLENOL® COLD Suspension Liquid:*** 4–11 months (12–17 lbs): $^{1}/_{2}$ teaspoonful; 12–23 months (18–23 lbs): $^{3}/_{4}$ teaspoonful; 2–3 years (24–35 lbs): 1 teaspoonful; 4–5 years (36–47 lbs): 1$^{1}/_{2}$ teaspoonfuls; 6–8 years (48–59 lbs): 2 teaspoonfuls; 9–10 years (60–71 lbs): 2$^{1}/_{2}$ teaspoonfuls; 11 years (72–95 lbs): 3 teaspoonfuls. All doses may be repeated every 4–6 hours, if needed. Do not use more than 4 times in 24 hours. ***Children's TYLENOL® COLD Chewable Tablets:*** If possible, use weight to dose; otherwise use age. 2–3 years (24–35 lbs): 2 tablets; 4–5 years (36–47 lbs): 3 tablets; 6–8 years (48–59 lbs): 4 tablets; 9–10 years (60–71 lbs): 5 tablets; 11 years (72–95 lbs): 6 tablets.

PRECAUTIONS

If a rare sensitivity reaction occurs, the drug should be discontinued.

WARNINGS

Do not take for pain for more than 5 days or for fever for more than 3 days unless directed by a doctor. If pain or fever persists, or gets worse, if new symptoms occur, or if redness or swelling is present, consult a doctor because these could be signs of a serious condition. If sore throat is severe, persists for more than 2 days, is accompanied or followed by fever, headache, rash, nausea, or vomiting, consult a doctor promptly. If nervousness, dizziness, or sleeplessness occur, discontinue use and consult a doctor. May cause excitability especially in children. Do not give this product to children who have a breathing problem such as chronic bronchitis, or who have glaucoma, heart disease, high blood pressure, thyroid disease, or diabetes without first consulting the child's doctor. May cause drowsiness. Sedatives and tranquilizers may increase the drowsiness effect. Do not give this product to children who are taking sedatives or tranquilizers, without first consulting the child's doctor. **Do not exceed recommended dosage.** Taking more than the recommended dose (overdose) may not provide more relief and could cause serious health problems. Keep this and all drugs out of the reach of children. In case of accidental overdose, contact a doctor or poison control center immediately. Prompt medical attention is critical even if you do not notice any signs or symptoms. Do not use with other products containing acetaminophen.

NOTE: In addition to the above:

Children's TYLENOL® COLD Suspension Liquid: **Do not use if plastic carton wrap, bottle wrap, or foil inner seal imprinted "Safety Seal®" is broken or missing.**

Children's TYLENOL® COLD Chewable Tablets: **Do not use if carton is opened or if blister unit is broken.** Phenylketonurics: contains phenylalanine 6 mg per tablet.

DRUG INTERACTION PRECAUTION

Do not give this product to a child who is taking a prescription monamine omidase inhibitor (MAOI) (certain drugs for depression, psychiatric or emotional conditions), or for 2 weeks after stopping the MAOI drug. If you are uncertain whether your child's prescription drug contains an MAOI, consult a health professional before giving this product.

PROFESSIONAL INFORMATION

OVERDOSAGE INFORMATION

Acetaminophen in massive overdosage may cause hepatic toxicity in some patients. In adults and adolescents (≥ 12 years of age), hepatic toxicity may occur following ingestion of greater than 7.5 to 10 grams over a period of 8 hours or less. Fatalities are infrequent (less than 3–4% of untreated cases) and have rarely been reported with overdoses of less than 15 grams. In children (<12 years of age), an acute overdosage of less than 150 mg/kg has not been associated with hepatic toxicity. Early symptoms following a potentially hepatotoxic overdose may include: nausea, vomiting, diaphoresis and general malaise. Clinical and laboratory evidence of hepatic toxicity may not be apparent until 48 to 72 hours postingestion. In adults and adolescents, any individual presenting with an unknown amount of acetaminophen ingested or with a questionable or unreliable history about the time of ingestion should have a plasma acetaminophen level drawn and be treated with *N*-acetylcysteine. For full prescribing information, refer to the *N*-acetylcysteine package insert. Do not await the results of assays for acetaminophen levels before initiating treatment with *N*-acetylcysteine. The following additional procedures are recommended: Promptly initiate gastric decontamination of the stomach. A plasma acetaminophen assay should be obtained as early as possible, but no sooner than four hours following ingestion. If an acetaminophen *extended release* product is

Continued on next page

Children's Tylenol Cold—Cont.

involved, it may be appropriate to obtain an additional plasma acetaminophen level 4–6 hours following the initial acetaminophen level. If either acetaminophen level plots above the treatment line on the acetaminophen overdose nomogram, *N*-acetylcysteine treatment should be continued for a full course of therapy. Liver function studies should be obtained initially and repeated at 24-hour intervals.

Serious toxicity or fatalities have been extremely infrequent following an acute acetaminophen overdose in young children, possibly because of differences in the way they metabolize acetaminophen. In children, the maximum potential amount ingested can be more easily estimated. If more than 150 mg/kg or an unknown amount was ingested, obtain a plasma acetaminophen level as soon as possible, but no sooner than 4 hours following ingestion. If an acetaminophen *extended release* product is involved, it may be appropriate to obtain an additional plasma acetaminophen level 4–6 hours following the initial acetaminophen level. If either acetaminophen level plots above the treatment line on the nomogram, *N*-acetylcysteine treatment should be initiated and continued for a full course of therapy. If an assay cannot be obtained and the estimated acetaminophen ingestion exceeds 150 mg/kg, dosing with *N*-acetylcysteine should be initiated and continued for a full course of therapy.

For additional emergency information, call your regional poison center or call the Rocky Mountain Poison Center toll-free, (1-800-525-6115).

Chlorpheniramine toxicity should be treated as you would an antihistamine/anticholinergic overdose and is likely to be present within a few hours after acute ingestion.

Symptoms from pseudoephedrine overdose consist most often of mild anxiety, tachycardia and/or mild hypertension. Symptoms usually appear within 4 to 8 hours of ingestion and are transient, usually requiring no treatment.

INACTIVE INGREDIENTS

Liquid: acesulfame potassium, butylparaben, cellulose, citric acid, corn syrup, D&C Red #33, FD&C Blue #1, FD&C Red #40, flavors, glycerin, propylene glycol, purified water, sodium benzoate, sodium carboxymethylcellulose, sorbitol, xanthan gum.

Chewable Tablets: Aspartame, Basic Polymethacrylate, Cellulose, Cellulose Acetate, Citric Acid, D&C Red #7, FD&C Blue #1, Flavors, Hydroxypropyl Methylcellulose, Magnesium Stearate, Mannitol.

HOW SUPPLIED

Liquid: Purple-colored—bottles of 4 fl. oz. Store at room temperature.

Chewable Tablets: Purple-colored, imprinted "TYLENOL COLD" on one side and "TC" on opposite side—blisters of 24. Store at room temperature.

Shown in Product Identification Guide, page 322

Children's TYLENOL® COLD Plus Cough Suspension Liquid and Chewable Tablets — OTC

DESCRIPTION

Children's TYLENOL® COLD Plus Cough Suspension Liquid is Wild Cherry-flavored and contains no alcohol or aspirin. Each teaspoonful (5 mL) contains acetaminophen 160 mg, chlorpheniramine maleate 1 mg, dextromethorphan HBr 5 mg and pseudoephedrine HCl 15 mg.

Children's TYLENOL® COLD Plus Cough Chewable Tablets are Wild Cherry-flavored and each tablet contains: acetaminophen 80 mg, chlorpheniramine maleate 0.5 mg, dextromethorphan HBr 2.5 mg, and pseudoephedrine HCl 7.5 mg.

ACTIONS

Children's TYLENOL® COLD Plus Cough Suspension Liquid and Chewable Tablets combines the analgesic-antipyretic acetaminophen with the decongestant pseudoephedrine hydrochloride, the cough suppressant dextromethorphan hydrobromide, and the antihistamine chlorpheniramine maleate to help relieve coughs, nasal congestion, and sore throat, dry runny noses, and prevent sneezing as well as to relieve the fever, aches, pains and general discomfort associated with colds and upper respiratory infections. Acetaminophen is equal to aspirin in analgesic and antipyretic effectiveness and it is unlikely to produce the side effects often associated with aspirin or aspirin-containing products.

USES

For the temporary relief of these cold symptoms: minor aches and pains, sore throat, coughs, nasal congestion, headaches, fever, sneezing, runny nose.

DIRECTIONS

If possible, use weight to dose; otherwise use age. All doses may be repeated every 4–6 hours, if needed. Do not use more than 4 times in 24 hours. Under 6 years (under 48 lbs), consult a doctor.

Children's TYLENOL® COLD Plus Cough Suspension Liquid: 6–11 years (48–95 lbs): 2 teaspoonfuls. An AccuDose™ measuring cup is provided and marked for accurate dosing. ***Children's TYLENOL® COLD Plus Cough Chewable Tablets:*** 6–11 years (48–95 lbs): 4 tablets.

Professional Dosage Schedule: ***Children's TYLENOL® COLD Plus Cough Suspension Liquid:*** If possible, use weight to dose; otherwise use age. 4–11 months (12–17 lbs): $^1/_2$ teaspoonful; 12–23 months (18–23 lbs): $^3/_4$ teaspoonful; 2–3 years (24–35 lbs): 1 teaspoonful; 4–5 years (36–47 lbs): $1^1/_2$ teaspoonfuls; 6–8 years (48–59 lbs): 2 teaspoonfuls; 9–10 years (60–71 lbs): $2^1/_2$ teaspoonfuls; 11 years (72–95 lbs): 3 teaspoonfuls. All doses may be repeated every 4–6 hours, if needed. Do not use more than 4 times in 24 hours. ***Children's TYLENOL® COLD Plus Cough Chewable Tablets:*** If possible, use weight to dose; otherwise use age. 2–3 years (24–35 lbs): 2 tablets; 4–5 years (36–47 lbs): 3 tablets; 6–8 years (48–59 lbs): 4 tablets; 9–10 years (60–71 lbs): 5 tablets; 11 years (72–95 lbs): 6 tablets.

PRECAUTIONS

If a rare sensitivity reaction occurs, the drug should be discontinued.

WARNINGS

Do not take for pain for more than 5 days or for fever for more than 3 days unless directed by a doctor. If pain or fever persists, or gets worse, if new symptoms occur, or if redness or swelling is present, consult a doctor because these could be signs of a serious condition. If sore throat is severe, persists for more than 2 days, is accompanied or followed by fever, headache, rash, nausea or vomiting, consult a doctor promptly. If nervousness, dizziness, or sleeplessness occur, discontinue use and consult a doctor. May cause excitability especially in children. Do not give this product to children who have a breathing problem such as chronic bronchitis, or who have glaucoma, heart disease, high blood pressure, thyroid disease, or diabetes, without first consulting the child's doctor. May cause drowsiness. Sedatives and tranquilizers may increase the drowsiness effect. Do not give this product to children who are taking sedatives or tranquilizers without first consulting the child's doctor. A persistent cough may be a sign of a serious condition. If cough persists for more than 1 week, tends to recur, or is accompanied by fever, rash or persistent headache, consult a doctor. Do not give this product for persistent or chronic cough such as occurs with asthma or if cough is accompanied by excessive phlegm (mucus) unless directed by a doctor. **Do not exceed recommended dosage.** Taking more than the recommended dose (overdose) may not provide more relief and could cause serious health problems. Keep this and all drugs out of the reach of children. In case of accidental overdose, contact a doctor or poison control center immediately. Prompt medical attention is critical even if you do not notice any signs or symptoms. Do not use with other products containing acetaminophen.

NOTE: In addition to the above:

Liquid: Do not use if plastic carton wrap, bottle wrap, or foil inner seal imprinted "Safety Seal®" is broken or missing.

Chewable Tablets: Do not use if carton is opened or if blister unit is broken. Phenylketonurics: contains phenylalanine 4 mg per tablet.

DRUG INTERACTION PRECAUTION

Do not give this product to a child who is taking a prescription monoamine oxidase inhibitor (MAOI) (certain drugs for depression, psychiatric or emotional conditions), or for 2 weeks after stopping the MAOI drug. If you are uncertain whether your child's prescription drug contains an MAOI, consult a health professional before giving this product.

PROFESSIONAL INFORMATION
OVERDOSAGE INFORMATION

Acetaminophen in massive overdosage may cause hepatic toxicity in some patients. In adults and adolescents ($\geq$ 12 years of age), hepatic toxicity may occur following ingestion of greater than 7.5 to 10 grams over a period of 8 hours or less. Fatalities are infrequent (less than 3–4% of untreated cases) and have rarely been reported with overdoses of less than 15 grams. In children (<12 years of age), an acute overdosage of less than 150 mg/kg has not been associated with hepatic toxicity. Early symptoms following a potentially hepatotoxic overdose may include: nausea, vomiting, diaphoresis and general malaise. Clinical and laboratory evidence of hepatic toxicity may not be apparent until 48 to 72 hours postingestion. In adults and adolescents, any individual presenting with an unknown amount of acetaminophen ingested or with a questionable or unreliable history about the time of ingestion should have a plasma acetaminophen level drawn and be treated with *N*-acetylcysteine. For full prescribing information, refer to the *N*-acetylcysteine package insert. Do not await the results of assays for plasma acetaminophen levels before initiating treatment with *N*-acetylcysteine. The following additional procedures are recommended: Promptly initiate gastric decontamination of the stomach. A plasma acetaminophen assay should be obtained as early as possible, but no sooner than four hours following ingestion. If an acetaminophen *extended release* product is involved, it may be appropriate to obtain an additional plasma acetaminophen level 4–6 hours following the initial acetaminophen level. If either acetaminophen level plots above the treatment line on the acetaminophen overdose nomogram, *N*-acetylcysteine treatment should be continued for a full course of therapy. Liver function studies should be obtained initially and repeated at 24-hour intervals.

Serious toxicity or fatalities have been extremely infrequent following an acute acetaminophen overdose in young children, possibly because of differences in the way they metabolize acetaminophen. In children, the maximum potential amount ingested can be more easily estimated. If more than 150 mg/kg or an unknown amount was ingested, obtain a plasma acetaminophen level as soon as possible, but no sooner than 4 hours following ingestion. If an acetaminophen *extended release* product is involved, it may be appropriate to obtain an additional plasma acetaminophen level 4–6 hours following the initial acetaminophen level. If either acetaminophen level plots above the treatment line on the acetaminophen overdose nomogram, *N*-acetylcysteine treatment should be initiated and continued for a full course of therapy. If an assay cannot be obtained and the estimated acetaminophen ingestion exceeds 150 mg/kg, dosing with *N*-acetylcysteine should be initiated and continued for a full course of therapy.

For additional emergency information, call your regional poison center or call the Rocky Mountain Poison Center toll-free, (1-800-525-6115).

Chlorpheniramine toxicity should be treated as you would an antihistamine/anticholinergic overdose and is likely to be present within a few hours after acute ingestion.

Symptoms from pseudoephedrine overdose consist most often of mild anxiety, tachycardia and/or mild hypertension. Symptoms usually appear within 4 to 8 hours of ingestion and are transient, usually requiring no treatment.

Acute dextromethorphan overdose usually does not result in serious signs and symptoms unless massive amounts have been ingested. Signs and symptoms of a substantial overdose may include nausea and vomiting, visual disturbances, CNS disturbances, and urinary retention.

INACTIVE INGREDIENTS

Liquid: Acesulfame K, Butylparaben, Cellulose, Citric Acid, Corn Syrup, D&C Red #33, FD&C Red #40, Flavors, Glycerin, Propylene Glycol, Purified Water, Sodium Benzoate, Sodium Carboxymethylcellulose, Sorbitol, Xanthan Gum.

Chewable Tablets: Aspartame, Basic Polymethacrylate, Cellulose, Cellulose Acetate, D&C Red #7, Flavors, Hydroxypropyl Methylcellulose, Magnesium Stearate, Mannitol.

HOW SUPPLIED

Liquid: Red-colored suspension—bottles of 4 fl. oz. Store at room temperature.

Chewable Tablets: Red-colored, imprinted "TYLENOL C/C" on one side and "TC/C" on the opposite side—blisters of 24. Store at room temperature.

Shown in Product Identification Guide, page 322

Children's TYLENOL® FLU Suspension Liquid — OTC

DESCRIPTION

Children's TYLENOL® FLU Suspension Liquid is Bubble Gum Blast-flavored and contains no alcohol or aspirin. Each teaspoonful (5 mL) contains acetaminophen 160 mg, chlorpheniramine maleate 1 mg, dextromethorphan HBr 7.5 mg and pseudoephedrine HCl 15 mg.

ACTIONS

Children's TYLENOL® FLU Suspension Liquid combines the analgesic-antipyretic acetaminophen with the decongestant pseudoephedrine hydrochloride, the cough suppressant dextromethorphan hydrobromide and the antihistamine chlorpheniramine maleate to provide fast, effective, temporary relief of all your child's symptoms associated with flu including fever, body aches, headache, stuffy nose, runny nose, sore throat and coughs. Acetaminophen is equal to aspirin in analgesic and antipyretic effectiveness and it is unlikely to produce the side effects often associated with aspirin or aspirin-containing products.

USES

For the temporary relief of these cold and flu symptoms: minor aches and pains, sore throat, coughs, nasal congestion, headaches, fever, and runny nose.

DIRECTIONS

If possible, use weight to dose; otherwise use age. All doses may be repeated every 6–8 hours, if needed. Do not use more than 4 times in 24 hours. Under 6 years (under 48 lbs), consult a physician. An AccuDose™ measuring cup is provided for accurate dosing. ***Children's TYLENOL® FLU Suspension Liquid:*** 6–11 years (48–95 lbs): 2 teaspoonfuls.

Professional Dosage Schedule: If possible, use weight to dose; otherwise use age. 4–11 months (12–17 lbs): ½ teaspoon; 12–23 months (18–23 lbs): ¾ teaspoonful; 2–3 years (24–35 lbs): 1 teaspoonful; 4–5 years (36–47 lbs): 1½ teaspoonfuls; 6–8 years (48–59 lbs): 2 teaspoonfuls; 9–10 years (60–71 lbs): 2½ teaspoonfuls; 11 years (72–95 lbs): 3 teaspoonfuls. All doses may be repeated every 6–8 hours, if needed. Do not use more than 4 times in 24 hours.

PRECAUTIONS

If a rare sensitivity reaction occurs, the drug should be discontinued.

WARNINGS

Do not use if plastic carton wrap, bottle wrap, or foil inner seal imprinted "Safety Seal"® is broken or missing. Do not take for pain for more than 5 days or for fever for more than 3 days unless directed by a doctor. If pain or fever persists, or gets worse, if new symptoms occur, or if redness or swelling is present, consult a doctor because these could be signs of a serious condition. If sore throat is severe, persists for more than 2 days, is accompanied or followed by fever, headache, rash, nausea or vomiting, consult a doctor promptly. If nervousness, dizziness or sleeplessness occur, discontinue use and consult a doctor. May cause excitability especially in children. Do not give this product to children who have a breathing problem such as chronic bronchitis, or who have glaucoma, heart disease, high blood pressure, thyroid disease or diabetes without first consulting the child's doctor. May cause drowsiness. Sedatives and tranquilizers may increase the drowsiness effect. Do not give this product to children who are taking sedatives or tranquilizers without first consulting the child's doctor. A persistent cough may be a sign of a serious condition. If cough persists for more than 1 week, tends to recur, or is accompanied by fever, rash, or persistent headache, consult a doctor. Do not give this product for persistent or chronic cough such as occurs with asthma or if cough is accompanied by excessive phlegm (mucus) unless directed by a doctor. **Do not exceed recommended dosage.** Taking more than the recommended dose (overdose) may not provide more relief and could cause serious health problems. Keep this and all drugs out of the reach of children. In case of accidental overdose, contact a doctor or poison control center immediately. Prompt medical attention is critical even if you do not notice any signs or symptoms. Do not use with other products containing acetaminophen.

DRUG INTERACTION PRECAUTION

Do not give this product to a child who is taking a prescription monoamine oxidase inhibitor (MAOI) (certain drugs for depression, psychiatric or emotional conditions) or for 2 weeks after stopping the MAOI drug. If you are uncertain whether your child's prescription drug contains an MAOI, consult a health professional before giving this product.

PROFESSIONAL INFORMATION

OVERDOSAGE INFORMATION

Acetaminophen in massive overdosage may cause hepatic toxicity in some patients. In adults and adolescents, (≥12 years of age), hepatic toxicity may occur following ingestion of greater than 7.5 to 10 grams over a period of 8 hours or less. Fatalities are infrequent (less than 3–4% of untreated cases) and have rarely been reported with overdoses of less than 15 grams. In children (<12 years of age), an acute overdosage of less than 150 mg/kg has not been associated with hepatic toxicity. Early symptoms following a potentially hepatotoxic overdose may include: nausea, vomiting, diaphoresis and general malaise. Clinical and laboratory evidence of hepatic toxicity may not be apparent until 48 to 72 hours postingestion. In adults and adolescents, any individual presenting with an unknown amount of acetaminophen ingested or with a questionable or unreliable history about the time of ingestion should have a plasma acetaminophen level drawn and be treated with *N*-acetylcysteine. For full prescribing information, refer to the *N*-acetylcysteine package insert. Do not await the results of assays for plasma acetaminophen levels before initiating treatment with *N*-acetylcysteine. The following additional procedures are recommended: Promptly initiate gastric decontamination of the stomach. A plasma acetaminophen assay should be obtained as early as possible, but no sooner than four hours following ingestion. If an acetaminophen *extended release* product is involved, it may be appropriate to obtain an additional plasma acetaminophen level 4–6 hours following the initial acetaminophen level. If either acetaminophen level plots above the treatment line on the acetaminophen overdose nomogram, *N*-acetylcysteine treatment should be continued for a full course of therapy. Liver function studies should be obtained initially and repeated at 24–hour intervals.

Serious toxicity or fatalities have been extremely infrequent following an acute acetaminophen overdose in young children, possibly because of differences in the way they metabolize acetaminophen. In children, the maximum potential amount ingested can be more easily estimated. If more than 150 mg/kg or an unknown amount was ingested, obtain a plasma acetaminophen level as soon as possible, but no sooner than 4 hours following ingestion. If an acetaminophen *extended release* product is involved, it may be appropriate to obtain an additional plasma acetaminophen level 4–6 hours following the initial acetaminophen level. If either acetaminophen level plots above the treatment line on the acetaminophen overdose nomogram, *N*-acetylcysteine treatment should be initiated and continued for a full course of therapy. If an assay cannot be obtained and the estimated acetaminophen ingestion exceeds 150 mg/kg, dosing with *N*-acetylcysteine should be initiated and continued for a full course of therapy.

For additional emergency information, call your regional poison center or call the Rocky Mountain Poison Center toll-free, (1-800-525-6115).

Chlorpheniramine toxicity should be treated as you would an antihistamine/anticholinergic overdose and is likely to be present within a few hours after acute ingestion.

Symptoms from pseudoephedrine overdose consist most often of mild anxiety, tachycardia, and/or mild hypertension. Symptoms usually appear within 4 to 8 hours of ingestion and are transient, usually requiring no treatment.

Acute dextromethorphan overdose usually does not result in serious signs and symptoms unless massive amounts have been ingested. Signs and symptoms of a substantial overdose may include nausea and vomiting, visual disturbances, CNS disturbances, and urinary retention.

INACTIVE INGREDIENTS

Acesulfame K, Butylparaben, Cellulose, Citric Acid, Corn Syrup, D&C Red #33, FD&C Red #40, Flavors, Glycerin, Propylene Glycol, Purified Water, Sodium Benzoate, Sodium Carboxymethylcellulose, Sorbitol, Xanthan Gum.

HOW SUPPLIED

Pinkish-red-colored suspension liquid in bottles of 4 fl. oz. Store at room temperature.

Shown in Product Identification Guide, page 322

Children's TYLENOL® OTC

SINUS Suspension Liquid and Chewable Tablets

DESCRIPTION

Children's TYLENOL® SINUS Liquid is Fruit Burst-flavored and contains no alcohol or aspirin. Each teaspoonful (5 mL) contains acetaminophen 160 mg and pseudoephedrine HCl 15 mg. ***Children's TYLENOL® SINUS Chewable Tablets*** are Fruit Burst-flavored and each tablet contains acetaminophen 80 mg and pseudoephedrine HCl 7.5 mg.

ACTIONS

Children's TYLENOL® SINUS Suspension Liquid and Chewable Tablets combine the analgesic-antipyretic acetaminophen with the decongestant pseudoephedrine hydrochloride to provide fast, effective, temporary relief of all your child's sinus symptoms including stuffy nose, sinus headache, sinus pressure, sinus pain, and nasal congestion. Acetaminophen is equal to aspirin in analgesic and antipyretic effectiveness and is unlikely to produce the side effects often associated with aspirin or aspirin-containing products.

USES

For the reduction of fever. For the temporary relief of minor aches, pains and headaches, sinus congestion, stuffy nose, sinus pressure.

DIRECTIONS

If possible, use weight to dose; otherwise use age. All doses may be repeated every 4–6 hours, if needed. Do not use more than 4 times in 24 hours. Under 2 years (under 24 lbs), consult a physician. ***Children's TYLENOL® SINUS Suspension Liquid:*** 2–5 years (24–47 lbs): 1 teaspoonful; 6–11 years (48–95 lbs): 2 teaspoonfuls. An AccuDose™ measuring cup is provided for accurate dosing. ***Children's TYLENOL® SINUS Chewable Tablets:*** 2–5 years (24–47 lbs): 2 tablets; 6–11 years (48–95 lbs): 4 tablets.

Professional Dosage Schedule: ***Children's TYLENOL® SINUS Suspension Liquid:*** If possible, use weight to dose; otherwise use age. 4–11 months (12–17 lbs): 1/2 teaspoonful; 12–23 months (18–23 lbs): 3/4 teaspoonful; 2–3 years (24–35 lbs): 1 teaspoonful; 4–5 years (36–47 lbs): 1 1/2 teaspoonfuls; 6–8 years (48–59 lbs): 2 teaspoonfuls; 9–10 years (60–71 lbs): 2 1/2 teaspoonfuls; 11 years (72–95 lbs): 3 teaspoonfuls. ***Children's TYLENOL® SINUS Chewable Tablets:*** If possible, use weight to dose; otherwise use age. 2–3 years (24–35 lbs): 2 tablets; 4–5 years (36–47 lbs): 3 tablets; 6–8 years (48–59 lbs): 4 tablets; 9–10 years (60–71 lbs): 5 tablets; 11 years (72–95 lbs): 6 tablets.

PRECAUTIONS

If a rare sensitivity reaction occurs, the drug should be discontinued.

WARNINGS

Do not take for pain for more than 5 days or for fever for more than 3 days unless directed by a doctor. If pain or fever persists, or gets worse, if new symptoms occur, or if redness or swelling is present, consult a doctor because these could be signs of a serious condition. If nervousness, dizziness or sleeplessness occur, discontinue use and consult a doctor. Do not give this product to children who have heart disease, high blood pressure, thyroid disease, or diabetes without first consulting the child's doctor. **Do not exceed recommended dosage.** Taking more than the recommended dose (overdose) may not provide more relief and could cause serious health problems. Keep this and all drugs out of the reach of children. In case of accidental overdose, contact a doctor or poison control center immediately. Prompt medical attention is critical even if you do not notice any signs or symptoms. Do not use with other products containing acetaminophen.

NOTE: In addition to the above:

Children's TYLENOL® SINUS Suspension Liquid: **Do not use if plastic carton wrap, bottle wrap, or foil inner seal imprinted "Safety Seal®" is broken or missing.**

Children's TYLENOL® SINUS Chewable Tablets: **Do not use if carton is opened or if blister unit is broken.** Phenylketonurics: contains phenylalanine 5 mg per tablet.

DRUG INTERACTION PRECAUTION

Do not give this product to a child who is taking a prescription monoamine oxidase inhibitor (MAOI) (certain drugs for depression, psychiatric or emotional conditions), or for 2 weeks after stopping the MAOI drug. If you are uncertain whether your child's prescription drug contains an MAOI, consult a health professional before giving this product.

PROFESSIONAL INFORMATION

OVERDOSAGE INFORMATION

Acetaminophen in massive overdosage may cause hepatic toxicity in some patients. In adults and adolescents (≥ 12 years of age), hepatic toxicity may occur following ingestion of greater than 7.5 to 10 grams over a period of 8 hours or less. Fatalities are infrequent (less than 3–4% of untreated cases) and have rarely been reported with overdoses of less than 15 grams. In children (< 12 years of age), an acute overdosage of less than 150 mg/kg has not been associated with hepatic toxicity. Early symptoms following a potentially hepatotoxic overdose may include: nausea, vomiting, diaphoresis and general malaise. Clinical and laboratory evidence of hepatic toxicity may not be apparent until 48 to 72 hours postingestion. In adults and adolescents, any individual presenting with an unknown amount of acetaminophen ingested or with a questionable or unreliable history about the time of ingestion should have a plasma acetaminophen level drawn and be treated with *N*-acetylcysteine. For full prescribing information, refer to the *N*-acetylcysteine package insert. Do not await the results of assays for acetaminophen levels before initiating treatment with *N*-acetylcysteine. The following additional procedures are recommended: Promptly initiate gastric decontamination of the stomach. A plasma acetaminophen assay should be obtained as early as possible, but no sooner than 4 hours following ingestion. If an acetaminophen *extended release* product is involved, it may be appropriate to obtain an additional plasma level 4–6 hours following the initial acetaminophen level. If either acetaminophen level plots above the treatment line on the acetaminophen overdose nomogram, *N*-acetylcysteine treatment should be continued for a full course of therapy. Liver function studies should be obtained initially and repeated at 24–hour intervals.

Serious toxicity or fatalities have been extremely infrequent following an acute acetaminophen overdose in young children, possibly because of differences in the way they metabolize acetaminophen. In children, the maximal potential amount ingested can be more easily estimated. If more than 150 mg/kg or an unknown amount was ingested, obtain a plasma acetaminophen level as soon as possible, but no sooner than 4 hours following ingestion. If an acetaminophen *extended release* product is involved, it may be appropriate to obtain an additional plasma acetaminophen level 4–6 hours following the initial acetaminophen level. If either acetaminophen level plots above the treatment line on the acetaminophen overdose nomogram, *N*-acetylcysteine treatment should be initiated and continued for a full course of therapy. If an assay cannot be obtained and the estimated acetaminophen ingestion exceeds 150 mg/kg, dosing with *N*-acetylcysteine should be initiated and continued for a full course of therapy.

For additional emergency information, call your regional poison center or call the Rocky Mountain Poison Center toll-free, (1–800–525–6115).

Symptoms from pseudoephedrine overdose consist most often of mild anxiety, tachycardia and/or mild hypertension. Symptoms usually appear within 4 to 8 hours of ingestion and are transient, usually requiring no treatment.

INACTIVE INGREDIENTS

Liquid: acesulfame potassium, butylparaben, cellulose, citric acid, corn syrup, D&C Red #33, FD&C Red #40, flavors, glycerin, propylene glycol, purified water, sodium benzoate, sodium carboxymethylcellulose, sorbitol, xanthan gum.

Chewable Tablets: Aspartame, Cellulose, Cellulose Acetate, Citric Acid, D&C Red #7, Flavors, Magnesium Stearate, Mannitol, Polymethacrylate, Povidone.

HOW SUPPLIED

Liquid: Red-colored–child resistant bottles of 4 fl. oz. Store at room temperature. Avoid excessive heat, 104°F (40°C).

Chewable Tablets: Pink-colored, imprinted with "CTS" on one side–blister packs of 24. Store at room temperature.

Shown in Product Identification Guide, page 322

IMODIUM® A–D OTC

(loperamide hydrochloride)

DESCRIPTION

Each 5 mL (teaspoon) of ***IMODIUM® A-D*** liquid contains loperamide hydrochloride 1 mg. ***IMODIUM® A-D*** liquid is stable, cherry-mint flavored, and clear in color.

Each caplet of ***IMODIUM® A-D*** contains 2 mg of loperamide and is scored and colored green.

ACTIONS

IMODIUM® A-D contains a clinically proven antidiarrheal medication. Loperamide HCl acts by slowing intestinal motility and by affecting water and electrolyte movement through the bowel.

INDICATION

IMODIUM® A-D controls the symptoms of diarrhea, including Traveler's Diarrhea.

DIRECTIONS

Use the enclosed cup to accurately measure Imodium® A-D Liquid. Drink plenty of clear fluids to help prevent dehydration, which may accompany diarrhea.

ADULTS AND CHILDREN 12 YEARS OF AGE AND OLDER: Take 4 teaspoonfuls (1 dosage cup) or 2 caplets after the first loose bowel movement and 2 teaspoonfuls or 1 caplet after each subsequent loose bowel movement but no more than 8 teaspoonfuls or 4 caplets a day for no more than 2 days.

CHILDREN 9–11 YEARS OLD (60–95 LBS): Take 2 teaspoonfuls (1/2 dosage cup) or 1 caplet after the first loose bowel

Continued on next page

Imodium A-D—Cont.

movement and 1 teaspoonful or 1/2 caplet after each subsequent loose bowel movement but no more than 6 teaspoonfuls or 3 caplets a day for no more than 2 days.

CHILDREN 6–8 YEARS OLD (48–59 LBS): Take 2 teaspoonfuls (1/2 dosage cup) or 1 caplet after the first loose bowel movement and 1 teaspoonful or 1/2 caplet after each subsequent loose bowel movement but no more than 4 teaspoonfuls or 2 caplets a day for no more than 2 days.

Professional Dosage Schedule for children 2–5 years old (24–47 lbs): 1 teaspoonful after first loose bowel movement, followed by 1 after each subsequent loose bowel movement. Do not exceed 3 teaspoonfuls a day.

WARNINGS

KEEP THIS AND ALL DRUGS OUT OF THE REACH OF CHILDREN. Do not use for more than two days unless directed by a physician. DO NOT USE IF DIARRHEA IS ACCOMPANIED BY HIGH FEVER (GREATER THAN 101°F), OR IF BLOOD OR MUCUS IS PRESENT IN THE STOOL, OR IF YOU HAVE HAD A RASH OR OTHER ALLERGIC REACTION TO LOPERAMIDE HCl. If you are taking antibiotics or have a history of liver disease, consult a physician before using this product. As with any drug, if you are pregnant or nursing a baby, seek the advice of a health professional before using this product. In case of accidental overdose, seek professional assistance or contact a poison control center immediately.

PROFESSIONAL INFORMATION

OVERDOSAGE INFORMATION

Overdosage of loperamide HCl in man may result in constipation, CNS depression and nausea. A slurry of activated charcoal administered promptly after ingestion of loperamide hydrochloride can reduce the amount of drug which is absorbed. If vomiting occurs spontaneously upon ingestion, a slurry of 100 grams of activated charcoal should be administered orally as soon as fluids can be retained. If vomiting has not occurred, and CNS depression is evident, gastric lavage should be performed followed by administration of 100 gms of the activated charcoal slurry through the gastric tube. In the event of overdosage, patients should be monitored for signs of CNS depression for at least 24 hours. Children may be more sensitive to central nervous system effects than adults. If CNS depression is observed, naloxone may be administered. If responsive to naloxone, vital signs must be monitored carefully for recurrence of symptoms of drug overdose for at least 24 hours after the last dose of naloxone.

INACTIVE INGREDIENTS

Liquid: Benzoic acid, citric acid, flavors, glycerin, propylene glycol, purified water, sodium benzoate, sorbitol, sucrose, contains 0.5% alcohol.

Caplets: Dibasic calcium phosphate, magnesium stearate, microcrystalline cellulose, colloidal silicon dioxide, FD&C Blue #1 and D&C Yellow #10.

HOW SUPPLIED

Liquid: Cherry-mint flavored liquid (clear) 2 fl. oz., and 4 fl. oz. tamper evident bottles with child resistant safety caps and special dosage cups. Store between 20–25 °C (69–77 °F). Avoid excessive heat.

Caplets: Green scored caplets in 6's and 12's, 18's and 24's blister packaging which is tamper evident and child resistant. Store at 15–30°C (59–86°F)

Shown in Product Identification Guide, page 321

IMODIUM® ADVANCED OTC

Chewable Tablets
(loperamide HCl/simethicone)

DESCRIPTION

Each mint-flavored chewable tablet of ***Imodium® Advanced*** contains loperamide HCl 2 mg/simethicone 125 mg.

ACTIONS

Imodium® Advanced combines original prescription strength Imodium® to control the symptoms of diarrhea plus simethicone to relieve bloating, pressure and cramps commonly referred to as gas. Loperamide HCl acts by slowing intestinal motility and by affecting water and electrolyte movement through the bowel. Simethicone acts in the stomach and intestines by altering the surface tension of gas bubbles enabling them to coalesce, thereby freeing and eliminating the gas more easily by belching or passing flatus.

USES

Controls the symptoms of diarrhea plus bloating, pressure, and cramps commonly referred to as gas.

Directions: Chew the first dose and take with water after the first loose stool. If needed, chew the next dose and take with water after the next loose stool. Drink plenty of clear liquids to prevent dehydration.

Adults aged 12 years and over: Chew 2 tablets and take with water after the first loose stool. If needed, chew 1 tablet and take with water after the next loose stool. Do not exceed 4 tablets a day.

Children 9-11 years (60-95 lbs): Chew 1 tablet and take with water after the first loose stool. If needed, chew 1/2 tablet and take with water after the next loose stool. Do not exceed 3 tablets a day.

Children 6-8 years (48-59 lbs): Chew 1 tablet and take with water after the first loose stool. If needed, chew 1/2 tablet and take with water after the next loose stool. Do not exceed 2 tablets a day.

Children under 6 years old (up to 47 lbs): Consult a physician. Not intended for use in children under 6 years old.

WARNINGS

Do Not Use If:
- You have a high fever (over 101° F)
- Blood or mucus is in your stool
- You have had a rash or other allergic reaction to Loperamide HCl

Do Not Use Without Asking A Doctor:
- For more than 2 days
- If you are taking antibiotics
- If you have a history of liver disease

As with any drug, If you are pregnant or nursing a baby, seek the advice of a health professional before using this product.
- **Keep this and all drugs out of the reach of children.**
- In case of accidental overdose, seek professional assistance or call a poison control center immediately.

PROFESSIONAL INFORMATION

OVERDOSAGE INFORMATION

Overdosage of loperamide HCl in man may result in constipation, CNS depression and nausea. A slurry of activated charcoal administered promptly after ingestion of loperamide hydrochloride can reduce the amount of drug which is absorbed. If vomiting occurs spontaneously upon ingestion, a slurry of 100 grams of activated charcoal should be administered orally as soon as fluids can be retained. If vomiting has not occurred, and CNS depression is evident, gastric lavage should be performed followed by administration of 100 gms of the activated charcoal slurry through the gastric tube. In the event of overdosage, patients should be monitored for signs of CNS depression for at least 24 hours. Children may be more sensitive to central nervous system effects than adults. If CNS depression is observed, naloxone may be administered. If responsive to naloxone, vital signs must be monitored carefully for recurrence of symptoms of drug overdose for at least 24 hours after the last dose of naloxone. No treatment is necessary for the simethicone ingestion in this circumstance.

INACTIVE INGREDIENTS

Cellulose acetate, corn starch, D&C Yellow No. 10, dextrates, FD&C Blue No. 1, flavors, microcrystalline cellulose, polymethacrylates, saccharin sodium, sorbitol, stearic acid, sucrose, tribasic calcium phosphate.

HOW SUPPLIED

Mint chewable tablets in 6's, 12's, 18's, 30's, and 42's blister packaging which is tamper evident and child resistant. Each Imodium® Advanced tablet is round, light green in color and has "IMODIUM" embossed on one side and "2/125" on the other side.
Store at 15–30°C (59–86°F).

Shown in Product Identification Guide, page 321

Infants' MOTRIN® CONCENTRATED DROPS OTC

DESCRIPTION

Infants' MOTRIN® Concentrated Drops is an alcohol-free, berry flavored suspension. Each 1.25 mL (dropperful) contains ibuprofen 50 mg.

USES

temporarily:
- reduces fever
- relieves minor aches and pains due to the common cold, flu, sore throat, headaches and toothaches

DIRECTIONS
- do not give more than directed
- shake well before using
- if possible, use weight to dose; otherwise use age
- use only with enclosed dropper. Fill to dose level. Do not use any other dosing device.
- dispense liquid slowly into the child's mouth, toward inner cheek
- replace original bottle cap to maintain child resistance
- if needed, repeat dose every **6–8 hours**
- do not use more than **4 times a day**

Dosing

under 6 mos: call a doctor; **6–11** mos (**12–17** lbs): **1** dropperful (1.25mL); **12–23** mos (**18–23** lbs): **1½** dropperfuls (1.875 mL)

Attention: Specifically designed for use with enclosed dropper. Use only enclosed dropper to dose this product. Do not use any other dosing device.

WARNINGS

Allergy alert: ibuprofen may cause a severe allergic reaction which may include:
- hives • facial swelling
- asthma (wheezing) • shock

Sore throat warning: severe or persistent sore throat or sore throat accompanied by high fever, headache, nausea, and vomiting may be serious. Consult doctor promptly. Do not use more than 2 days or administer to children under 3 years of age unless directed by doctor.

Do not use if the child has ever had an allergic reaction to any pain reliever/fever reducer

Ask a doctor before use if the child has
- not been drinking fluids
- lost a lot of fluid due to continued vomiting or diarrhea
- stomach pain
- problems or serious side effects from taking fever reducers or pain relievers

Ask a doctor or pharmacist before use if child is
- under a doctor's care for any serious condition
- taking any other drug
- taking any other product that contains ibuprofen, or any other pain reliever/fever reducer

When using this product give with food or milk if stomach upset occurs

Stop use and ask a doctor if
- an allergic reaction occurs. Seek medical help right away.
- fever or pain gets worse or lasts more than 3 days
- the child does not get any relief within first day (24 hours) of treatment
- stomach pain or upset gets worse or lasts
- redness or swelling is present in the painful area
- any new symptoms appear

Keep out of reach of children. In case of overdose, get medical help or contact a Poison Control Center right away.

OTHER INFORMATION
- **Do not use if plastic bottle wrap imprinted "Safety Seal®" and "Use With Enclosed Dropper Only" is broken or missing.**
- Store at 20°–25°C (68°–77°F)

INACTIVE INGREDIENTS

Artificial flavors, citric acid, corn starch, FD&C Red #40, glycerin, polysorbate 80, purified water, sodium benzoate, sorbitol, sucrose, xanthan gum

HOW SUPPLIED

Berry-flavored, pink-colored liquid in ½ fl. oz. bottles.

PROFESSIONAL INFORMATION

OVERDOSAGE INFORMATION

The toxicity of ibuprofen overdose is dependent upon the amount of drug ingested and the time elapsed since ingestion, though individual response may vary, which makes it necessary to evaluate each case individually. Although uncommon, serious toxicity and death have been reported in the medical literature with ibuprofen overdosage. The most frequently reported symptoms of ibuprofen overdose include abdominal pain, nausea, vomiting, lethargy and drowsiness. Other central nervous system symptoms include headache, tinnitus, CNS depression and seizures. Metabolic acidosis, coma, acute renal failure and apnea (primarily in very young children) may rarely occur. Cardiovascular toxicity, including hypotension, bradycardia, tachycardia and atrial fibrillation, also have been reported.

The treatment of acute ibuprofen overdose is primarily supportive. Management of hypotension, acidosis and gastrointestinal bleeding may be necessary. In cases of acute overdose, the stomach should be emptied through ipecac-induced emesis or lavage. Emesis is most effective if initiated within 30 minutes of ingestion. Orally administered activated charcoal may help in reducing the absorption and reabsorption of ibuprofen. In children, the estimated amount of ibuprofen ingested per body weight may be helpful to predict the potential for development of toxicity although each case must be evaluated. Ingestion of less than 100 mg/kg is unlikely to produce toxicity. Children ingesting 100 to 200 mg/kg may be managed with induced emesis and a minimal observation time of four hours. Children ingesting 200 to 400 mg/kg of ibuprofen should have immediate gastric emptying and at least four hours observation in a health care facility. Children ingesting greater than 400 mg/kg require immediate medical referral, careful observation and appropriate supportive therapy. Ipecac-induced emesis is not recommended in overdoses greater than 400 mg/kg because of the risk of convulsions and the potential for aspiration of gastric contents.

In adult patients the history of the dose reportedly ingested does not appear to be predictive of toxicity. The need for referral and follow-up must be judged by the circumstances at the time of the overdose ingestion. Symptomatic adults should be admitted to a health care facility for observation.

Shown in Product Identification Guide, page 321

Infants' TYLENOL® COLD OTC

Decongestant & Fever Reducer Concentrated Drops

DESCRIPTION

Infants' TYLENOL® COLD Decongestant & Fever Reducer Concentrated Drops are alcohol-free, aspirin-free, Bubble Gum Blast-flavored and red in color. Each 1.6 mL (2 dropperfuls) contains acetaminophen 160 mg and pseudoephedrine HCl 15 mg.

ACTIONS

Acetaminophen is a clinically proven analgesic/antipyretic. Acetaminophen produces analgesia by elevation of the pain threshold and antipyresis through action on the hypothalamic heat regulating center. Acetaminophen is equal to aspirin in analgesic and antipyretic effectiveness and it is unlikely to produce many of the side effects associated with aspirin and aspirin-containing products. Pseudoephedrine hydrochloride is a sympathomimetic amine which provides temporary relief of nasal congestion.

USES

For the reduction of fever. For the temporary relief of these cold symptoms: minor aches and pains, nasal congestion, headaches.

DIRECTIONS

Infants' Tylenol® Cold Decongestant and Fever Reducer Drops are more concentrated than Children's Tylenol® Cold Liquid Products. For accurate dosing, follow the dosing instructions on the label. If possible, use weight to dose; otherwise use age. All dosages may be repeated every 4–6 hours, if needed. Do not use more than 4 times in 24 hours. Under 2 years (under 24 lbs), consult a physician. A calibrated dropper is provided for accurate dosing. **Attention: This product has been specially designed for use only with the enclosed dropper. Do not use any other dosing device with this product.**

Infants' TYLENOL® COLD Decongestant & Fever Reducer Concentrated Drops: 2–3 years (24–35 lbs): 2 dropperfuls (2 ×0.8 mL).

Professional Dosage Schedule: If possible, use weight to dose; otherwise use age. 0–3 months (6-11 lbs): 1/2 dropperful (0.4 mL); 4–11 months (12–17 lbs): 1 dropperful (0.8 mL); 12–23 months (18–23 lbs): 1 1/2 dropperfuls (1.2 mL). All dosages may be repeated every 4–6 hours, if needed. Do not use more than 4 times in 24 hours.

PRECAUTIONS

If a rare sensitivity reaction occurs, the drug should be discontinued.

WARNINGS

Do not use if plastic carton wrap or bottle wrap imprinted "Safety Seal®" is broken or missing. Do not take for pain for more than 5 days or for fever for more than 3 days unless directed by a doctor. If pain or fever persists or gets worse, if new symptoms occur, or if redness or swelling is present, consult a doctor because these could be signs of a serious condition. If nervousness, dizziness or sleeplessness occur, discontinue use and consult a doctor. Do not give this product to children who have heart disease, high blood pressure, thyroid disease, or diabetes without first consulting the child's doctor. **Do not exceed recommended dosage.** Taking more than the recommended dose (overdose) may not provide more relief and could cause serious health problems. Keep this and all drugs out of the reach of children. In case of accidental overdose, contact a doctor or poison control center immediately. Prompt medical attention is critical even if you do not notice any signs or symptoms. Do not use with other products containing acetaminophen.

DRUG INTERACTION PRECAUTION

Do not give this product to a child who is taking a prescription monoamine oxidase inhibitor (MAOI) (certain drugs for depression, psychiatric or emotional conditions), or for 2 weeks after stopping the MAOI drug. If you are uncertain whether your child's prescription drug contains an MAOI, consult a health professional before giving this product.

PROFESSIONAL INFORMATION
OVERDOSAGE INFORMATION

Acetaminophen in massive overdosage may cause hepatic toxicity in some patients. In adults and adolescents (≥12 years of age), hepatic toxicity may occur following ingestion of greater than 7.5 to 10 grams over a period of 8 hours or less. Fatalities are infrequent (less than 3–4% of untreated cases) and have rarely been reported with overdoses of less than 15 grams. In children (<12 years of age), an acute overdosage of less than 150 mg/kg has not been associated with hepatic toxicity. Early symptoms following a potentially hepatotoxic overdose may include: nausea, vomiting, diaphoresis and general malaise. Clinical and laboratory evidence of hepatic toxicity may not be apparent until 48 to 72 hours postingestion. In adults and adolescents, any individual presenting with an unknown amount of acetaminophen ingested or with a questionable or unreliable history about the time of ingestion should have a plasma acetaminophen level drawn and be treated with *N*-acetylcysteine. For full prescribing information, refer to the *N*-acetylcysteine package insert. Do not await results of assays for plasma acetaminophen levels before initiating treatment with *N*-acetylcysteine. The following additional procedures are recommended: Promptly initiate gastric decontamination of the stomach. A plasma acetaminophen assay should be obtained as early as possible, but no sooner than four hours following ingestion. If an acetaminophen *extended release* product is involved, it may be appropriate to obtain an additional plasma acetaminophen level 4–6 hours following the initial acetaminophen level. If either acetaminophen level plots above the treatment line on the acetaminophen overdose nomogram, *N*-acetylcysteine treatment should be continued for a full course of therapy. Liver function studies should be obtained initially and repeated at 24-hour intervals.

Serious toxicity or fatalities have been extremely infrequent following an acute acetaminophen overdose in young children, possibly because of differences in the way they metabolize acetaminophen. In children, the maximum potential amount ingested can be more easily estimated. If more than 150 mg/kg or an unknown amount was ingested, obtain a plasma acetaminophen level as soon as possible, but no sooner than 4 hours following ingestion. If an acetaminophen *extended release* product is involved, it may be appropriate to obtain an additional plasma acetaminophen level 4–6 hours following the initial acetaminophen level. If either acetaminophen level plots above the treatment line on the acetaminophen overdose nomogram, *N*-acetylcysteine treatment should be initiated and continued for a full course of therapy. If an assay cannot be obtained and the estimated acetaminophen ingested exceeds 150 mg/kg, dosing with *N*-acetylcysteine should be initiated and continued for a full course of therapy.

For additional emergency information, call your regional poison center or call the Rocky Mountain Poison Center toll-free, (1-800-525-6115).

Symptoms from pseudoephedrine overdose consist most often of mild anxiety, tachycardia and/or mild hypertension. Symptoms usually appear within 4 to 8 hours of ingestion and are transient, usually requiring no treatment.

INACTIVE INGREDIENTS

Citric Acid, Corn Syrup, FD&C Red #40, Flavors, Polyethylene Glycol, Propylene Glycol, Saccharin, Sodium Benzoate.

HOW SUPPLIED

Red-colored drops in bottles of 1/2 fl. oz. Store at room temperature.

Shown in Product Identification Guide, page 322

INFANTS' TYLENOL® COLD — OTC
Decongestant and Fever Reducer Concentrated Drops *PLUS COUGH*

DESCRIPTION

Infants' TYLENOL® COLD Decongestant & Fever Reducer Concentrated Drops PLUS COUGH are alcohol-free, aspirin-free, Wild Cherry-flavored and red in color. Each 1.6 mL (2 dropperfuls) contains acetaminophen 160 mg, dextromethorphan HBr 5 mg, and pseudoephedrine HCl 15 mg.

ACTIONS

Acetaminophen is a clinically proven analgesic/antipyretic. Acetaminophen produces analgesia by elevation of the pain threshold and antipyresis through action on the hypothalamic heat regulating center. Acetaminophen is equal to aspirin in analgesic and antipyretic effectiveness and it is unlikely to produce many of the side effects associated with aspirin and aspirin-containing products. Pseudoephedrine hydrochloride is a sympathomimetic amine which provides temporary relief of nasal congestion. Dextromethorphan hydrobromide is a cough suppressant which helps relieve coughs.

USES

For the reduction of fever. For the temporary relief of these cold symptoms: coughs, nasal congestion, minor aches and pains, sore throat, headaches.

DIRECTIONS

Infants' Tylenol® Cold Decongestant and Fever Reducer Drops are more concentrated than Children's Tylenol® Cold Liquid Products. For accurate dosing, follow the dosing instructions on the label. If possible, use weight to dose; otherwise use age. All dosages may be repeated every 4–6 hours, if needed. Do not use more than 4 times in 24 hours. Under 2 years (under 24 lbs), consult a physician. A calibrated dropper is provided for accurate dosing. **Attention: This product has been specially designed for use only with the enclosed dropper. Do not use any other dosing device with this product.**

Infants' TYLENOL® COLD Decongestant & Fever Reducer Concentrated Drops PLUS COUGH: 2–3 years (24–35 lbs) 2 dropperfuls (2 x 0.8 mL).

Professional Dosage Schedule: If possible, use weight to dose; otherwise use age. 0–3 months (6–11 lbs): 1/2 dropperful (0.4 mL); 4–11 months (12–17 lbs): 1 dropperful (0.8 mL); 12–23 months (18–23 lbs): 1 1/2 dropperfuls (1.2 mL). All dosages may be repeated every 4–6 hours, if needed. Do not use more than 4 times in 24 hours.

PRECAUTIONS

If a rare sensitivity reaction occurs, the drug should be discontinued.

WARNINGS

Do not use if plastic carton wrap or bottle wrap imprinted "Safety Seal®" is broken or missing. Do not take for pain for more than 5 days or for fever for more than 3 days unless directed by a doctor. If pain or fever persists, or gets worse, if new symptoms occur, or if redness or swelling is present, consult a doctor because these could be signs of a serious condition. If sore throat is severe, persists for more than 2 days, is accompanied or followed by fever, headache, rash, nausea, or vomiting, consult a doctor promptly. If nervousness, dizziness or sleeplessness occur, discontinue use and consult a doctor. Do not give this product to children who have heart disease, high blood pressure, thyroid disease, or diabetes without first consulting the child's doctor. A persistent cough may be a sign of a serious condition. If cough persists for more than 1 week, tends to recur or is accompanied by fever, rash or persistent headache, consult a doctor. Do not give this product for persistent or chronic cough such as occurs with asthma or if cough is accompanied by excessive phlegm (mucus) unless directed by a doctor. **Do not exceed recommended dosage.** Taking more than the recommended dose (overdose) may not provide more relief and could cause serious health problems. Keep this and all drugs out of the reach of children. In case of accidental overdose, contact a doctor or poison control center immediately. Prompt medical attention is critical even if you do not notice any signs or symptoms. Do not use with other products containing acetaminophen.

DRUG INTERACTION PRECAUTION

Do not give this product to a child who is taking a prescription monoamine oxidase inhibitor (MAOI) (certain drugs for depression, psychiatric or emotional conditions), or for 2 weeks after stopping the MAOI drug. If you are uncertain whether your child's prescription drug contains an MAOI, consult a health professional before giving this product.

PROFESSIONAL INFORMATION
OVERDOSAGE INFORMATION

Acetaminophen in massive overdosage may cause hepatic toxicity in some patients. In adults and adolescents (≥ 12 years of age), hepatic toxicity may occur following ingestion of greater than 7.5 to 10 grams over a period of 8 hours or less. Fatalities are infrequent (less than 3–4% of untreated cases) and have rarely been reported with overdoses of less than 15 grams. In children (< 12 years of age), an acute overdosage of less than 150 mg/kg has not been associated with hepatic toxicity.

Early symptoms following a potentially hepatotoxic overdose may include: nausea, vomiting, diaphoresis and general malaise. Clinical and laboratory evidence of hepatic toxicity may not be apparent until 48 to 72 hours postingestion. In adults and adolescents, any individual presenting with an unknown amount of acetaminophen ingested or with a questionable or unreliable history about the time of ingestion should have a plasma acetaminophen level drawn and be treated with *N*-acetylcysteine. For full prescribing information, refer to the *N*-acetylcysteine package insert. Do not await results of assays for plasma acetaminophen levels before initiating treatment with *N*-acetylcysteine. The following additional procedures are recommended: Promptly initiate gastric decontamination of the stomach. A plasma acetaminophen assay should be obtained as early as possible, but no sooner than four hours following ingestion. If an acetaminophen *extended release* product is involved, it may be appropriate to obtain an additional plasma acetaminophen level 4–6 hours following the initial acetaminophen level. If either acetaminophen level plots above the treatment line on the acetaminophen overdose nomogram, *N*-acetylcycsteine treatment should be continued for a full course of therapy. Liver function studies should be obtained initially and repeated at 24-hour intervals.

Serious toxicity or fatalities have been extremely infrequent following an acute acetaminophen overdose in young children, possibly because of differences in the way they metabolize acetaminophen. In children, the maximum potential amount ingested can be more easily estimated. If more than 150 mg/kg or an unknown amount was ingested, obtain a plasma acetaminophen level as soon as possible, but no sooner than 4 hours following ingestion. If an acetaminophen *extended release* product is involved, it may be appropriate to obtain an additional plasma acetaminophen level 4–6 hours following the initial acetaminophen level. If either acetaminophen level plots above the treatment line on the acetaminpohen overdose nomogram, *N*-acetylcysteine treatment should be initiated and continued for a full course of therapy. If an assay cannot be obtained and the estimated acetaminophen ingestion exceeds 150 mg/kg, dosing with *N*-acetylcysteine should be initiated and continued for a full course of therapy.

For additional emergency information, call your regional poison center or call the Rocky Mountain Poison Center toll-free, (1-800-525-6115).

Symptoms from pseudoephedrine overdose consist most often of mild anxiety, tachycardia and/or mild hypertension. Symptoms usually appear within 4 to 8 hours of ingestion and are transient, usually requiring no treatment.

Acute dextromethorphan overdose usually does not result in serious signs and symptoms unless massive amounts have been ingested. Signs and symptoms of a substantial overdose may include nausea and vomiting, visual disturbances, CNS disturbances and urinary retention.

INACTIVE INGREDIENTS

Acesulfame Potassium, Citric Acid, Corn Syrup, FD&C Red #40, Flavors, Polyethylene Glycol, Propylene Glycol, Sodium Benzoate.

HOW SUPPLIED

Red-colored drops in bottles of ½ fl. oz. Store at room temperature.

Shown in Product Identification Guide, page 322

Junior Strength MOTRIN® CHEWABLE TABLETS and Junior Strength MOTRIN® CAPLETS — OTC

DESCRIPTION

Junior Strength MOTRIN® Chewable Tablets and Junior Strength MOTRIN® Caplets contain ibuprofen 100 mg. ***Junior Strength MOTRIN® Chewable Tablets*** are available in

Continued on next page

Junior Strength Motrin—Cont.

orange or grape flavors. ***Junior Strength MOTRIN® Caplets*** are available as easy-to-swallow caplets (capsule shaped tablet).

USES

temporarily:
• reduces fever
• relieves minor aches and pains due to the common cold, flu, sore throat, headaches and toothaches

DIRECTIONS

• do not chew/give more than directed.
• If possible, use weight to dose; otherwise use age
• if needed, repeat dose every **6–8 hours**
• do not use more than **4 times a day**

Dosing

Under 6 yrs (under 48 lbs): call a doctor; 6–8 yrs (48–59 lbs): 2 tablets; 9–10 yrs (60–71 lbs): $2^1/_2$ tablets; 11 yrs (72–95 lbs): 3 tablets

WARNINGS

Allergy alert: ibuprofen may cause a severe allergic reaction which may include:
• hives •facial swelling
• asthma (wheezing) •shock

Sore throat warning: severe or persistent sore throat or sore throat accompanied by high fever, headache, nausea, and vomiting may be serious. Consult doctor promptly. Do not use more than 2 days or administer to children under 3 years of age unless directed by doctor.

Do not use if the child has ever had an allergic reaction to any pain reliever/fever reducer

Ask a doctor before use if the child has
• not been drinking fluids
• lost a lot of fluid due to continued vomiting or diarrhea
• stomach pain
• problems or serious side effects from taking fever reducers or pain relievers

Ask a doctor or pharmacist before use if child is
• under a doctor's care for any serious condition
• taking any other drug
• taking any other product that contains ibuprofen, or any other pain reliever/fever reducer

Junior Strength MOTRIN® Chewable Tablets

When using this product mouth or throat burning may occur; give with food or water
• if stomach upset occurs, give with food or milk

Junior Strength MOTRIN® Caplets:

When using this product give with food or milk if stomach upset occurs

Stop use and ask a doctor if
• an allergic reaction occurs. Seek medical help right away.
• fever or pain gets worse or lasts more than 3 days
• the child does not get any relief within first day (24 hours) of treatment
• stomach pain or upset gets worse or lasts
• redness or swelling is present in the painful area
• any new symptoms appear

Keep out of reach of children. In case of overdose, get medical help or contact a Poison Control Center right away.
• **Do not use if neck wrap or foil inner seal imprinted "Safety Seal®" is broken or missing**

Junior Strength MOTRIN® Chewable Tablets
• phenylketonurics: contains phenylalanine 2.8 mg per tablet

INACTIVE INGREDIENTS

Orange-flavored tablets: acesulfame K, aspartame, cellulose, citric acid, FD&C yellow #6, flavor, fumaric acid, hydroxyethyl cellulose, hydroxypropyl methylcellulose, magnesium stearate, mannitol, povidone, sodium lauryl sulfate, sodium starch glycolate

Grape-flavored tablets: acesulfame K, aspartame, cellulose, citric acid, D&C red #7, D&C red #30, FD&C blue #1, flavor, fumaric acid, hydroxyethyl cellulose, hydroxypropyl methylcellulose, magnesium stearate, mannitol, povidone, sodium lauryl sulfate, sodium starch glycolate

Easy-To-Swallow Caplets: carnauba wax, corn starch, D&C Yellow #10, FD&C Yellow #6, hydroxypropyl methylcellulose, microcrystalline cellulose, polydextrose, polyethylene glycol, propylene glycol, silicon dioxide, sodium starch glycolate, titanium dioxide, triacetin

HOW SUPPLIED

Junior Strength MOTRIN® Chewable Tablets are available as orange-flavored, orange-colored chewable tablets or grape-flavored, purple-colored chewable tablets in 24-count bottles. Store at 20–25°C (68–77°F).

Junior Strength MOTRIN® Caplets are available as easy-to-swallow caplets (capsule shaped tablets) in 24-count bottles. Store at 20–25°C (68–77°F).

PROFESSIONAL INFORMATION

OVERDOSAGE INFORMATION

The *toxicity of ibuprofen overdose* is dependent upon the amount of drug ingested and the time elapsed since ingestion, though individual response may vary, which makes it necessary to evaluate each case individually. Although uncommon, serious toxicity and death have been reported in the medical literature with ibuprofen overdosage. The most frequently reported symptoms of ibuprofen overdose include abdominal pain, nausea, vomiting, lethargy and drowsiness. Other central nervous system symptoms include headache, tinnitus, CNS depression and seizures. Metabolic acidosis, coma, acute renal failure and apnea (primarily in very young children) may rarely occur. Cardiovascular toxicity, including hypotension, bradycardia, tachycardia and atrial fibrillation, also have been reported.

The *treatment of acute ibuprofen overdose* is primarily supportive. Management of hypotension, acidosis and gastrointestinal bleeding may be necessary. In cases of acute overdose, the stomach should be emptied through ipecac-induced emesis or lavage. Emesis is most effective if initiated within 30 minutes of ingestion. Orally administered activated charcoal may help in reducing the absorption and reabsorption of ibuprofen. In children, the estimated amount of ibuprofen ingested per body weight may be helpful to predict the potential for development of toxicity although each case must be evaluated. Ingestion of less than 100 mg/kg is unlikely to produce toxicity. Children ingesting 100 to 200 mg/kg may be managed with induced emesis and a minimal observation time of four hours. Children ingesting 200 to 400 mg/kg of ibuprofen should have immediate gastric emptying and at least four hours observation in a health care facility. Children ingesting greater than 400 mg/kg require immediate medical referral, careful observation and appropriate supportive therapy. Ipecac-induced emesis is not recommended in overdoses greater than 400 mg/kg because of the risk of convulsions and the potential for aspiration of gastric contents.

In adult patients the history of the dose reportedly ingested does not appear to be predictive of toxicity. The need for referral and follow-up must be judged by the circumstances at the time of the overdose ingestion. Symptomatic adults should be admitted to a health care facility for observation.

Shown in Product Identification Guide, page 322

Junior Strength TYLENOL® OTC
acetaminophen
Soft-Chews
Chewable Tablets

DESCRIPTION

Each ***Junior Strength TYLENOL® Soft-Chews Chewable Tablet*** contains 160 mg acetaminophen in a grape or fruit-flavored chewable tablet.

ACTIONS

Acetaminophen is a clinically proven analgesic/antipyretic. Acetaminophen produces analgesia by elevation of the pain threshold and antipyresis through action on the hypothalamic heat-regulating center. Acetaminophen is equal to aspirin in analgesic and antipyretic effectiveness and it is unlikely to produce many of the side effects associated with aspirin and aspirin-containing products.

USES

Junior Strength TYLENOL® Soft-Chews Chewable Tablets: For the temporary relief of minor aches and pains associated with: a cold, flu, headache, muscle aches, sprains, overexertion. For the reduction of fever.

DIRECTIONS

Junior Strength Tylenol® Soft-Chews Chewable Tablets contain more medicine than Children's Tylenol® Soft-Chews Chewable Tablets.

Chew tablets before swallowing. If possible, use weight to dose; otherwise use age. All dosages may be repeated every 4 hours, if needed. Do not use more than 5 times a day. Under 6 years (under 48 lbs), consult a physician. ***Junior Strength TYLENOL® Soft-Chews Chewable Tablets:*** 6–8 years (48–59 lbs): 2 tablets; 9–10 years (60–71 lbs): $2\ ^1/_2$ tablets; 11 years (72–95 lbs): 3 tablets; 12 years (96 lbs and over): 4 tablets.

PRECAUTIONS

If a rare sensitivity reaction occurs, the drug should be discontinued.

WARNINGS

Do Not Use:
• with any other products containing acetaminophen.
• for more than 3 days for fever unless directed by a doctor.
• for more than 5 days for pain unless directed by a doctor.

Stop Using This Product and Ask a Doctor If:
• symptoms do not improve.
• new symptoms occur.
• pain or fever persists or gets worse.
• redness or swelling is present.

Do not exceed recommended dose. Taking more than the recommended dose (overdose) may not provide more relief and could cause serious health problems. Keep this and all drugs out of the reach of children. In case of accidental overdose, contact a physician or poison control center immediately. Prompt medical attention is critical even if you do not notice any signs or symptoms.

NOTE: In addition to the above: Phenylketonurics: grape soft-chew contains phenylalanine 10 mg per tablet, fruit soft-chew contains phenylalanine 12 mg per tablet. **Do not use if carton is opened or if blister unit is broken.**

PROFESSIONAL INFORMATION

OVERDOSAGE INFORMATION

Acetaminophen in massive overdosage may cause hepatic toxicity in some patients. In adults and adolescents (≥ 12 years of age), hepatic toxicity may occur following ingestion of greater than 7.5 to 10 grams over a period of 8 hours or less. Fatalities are infrequent (less than 3–4% of untreated cases) and have rarely been reported with overdoses of less than 15 grams. In children (< 12 years of age), an acute overdosage of less than 150 mg/kg has not been associated with hepatic toxicity. Early symptoms following a potentially hepatotoxic overdose may include: nausea, vomiting, diaphoresis and general malaise. Clinical and laboratory evidence of hepatic toxicity may not be apparent until 48 to 72 hours postingestion. In adults and adolescents, any individual presenting with an unknown amount of acetaminophen ingested or with a questionable or unreliable history about the time of ingestion should have a plasma acetaminophen level drawn and be treated with *N*-acetylcysteine. For full prescribing information, refer to the *N*-acetylcysteine package insert. Do not await the results of assays for acetaminophen levels before initiating treatment with *N*-acetylcysteine. The following additional procedures are recommended: Promptly initiate gastric decontamination of the stomach. A plasma acetaminophen assay should be obtained as early as possible, but no sooner than four hours following ingestion. If an acetaminophen *extended release* product is involved, it may be appropriate to obtain an additional plasma acetaminophen level 4–6 hours following the initial acetaminophen level. If either acetaminophen level plots above the treatment line on the acetaminophen overdose nomogram, *N*-acetylcysteine treatment should be continued for a full course of therapy. Liver function studies should be obtained initially and repeated at 24-hour intervals.

Serious toxicity or fatalities have been extremely infrequent following an acute acetaminophen overdose in young children, possibly because of differences in the way they metabolize acetaminophen. In children, the maximum potential amount ingested can be more easily estimated. If more than 150 mg/kg or an unknown amount was ingested, obtain a plasma acetaminophen level as soon as possible, but no sooner than 4 hours following ingestion. If an acetaminophen *extended release* product is involved, it may be appropriate to obtain an additional plasma acetaminophen level 4–6 hours following the initial acetaminophen level. If either acetaminophen level plots above the treatment line on the acetaminophen overdose nomogram, *N*-acetylcysteine treatment should be initiated and continued for a full course of therapy. If an assay cannot be obtained and the estimated acetaminophen ingestion exceeds 150 mg/kg, dosing with *N*-acetylcysteine should be initiated and continued for a full course of therapy.

For additional emergency information, call your regional poison center or call the Rocky Mountain Poison Center toll-free, (1-800-525-6115).

INACTIVE INGREDIENTS

Junior Strength TYLENOL® Fruit-Flavored Soft-Chews Chewable Tablets: Aspartame, Cellulose, Citric Acid, D&C Red #7, Flavors, Magnesium Stearate, Mannitol. May contain Ethylcellulose or Cellulose Acetate and Povidone.

Junior Strength TYLENOL® Grape-Flavored Soft-Chews Chewable Tablets: Aspartame, Cellulose, Citric Acid, D&C Red #7, D&C Red #30, FD&C Blue #1, Flavors, Magnesium Stearate, Mannitol. May contain Ethylcellulose or Cellulose Acetate and Povidone.

HOW SUPPLIED

Soft-Chews Chewable Tablets (purple-colored grape or pink-colored fruit, imprinted "TYLENOL 160") Package of 24. All packages are safety sealed and use child resistant blister packaging. Fruit: Store at room temperature. Avoid excessive heat: 40°C (104°F); grape: Store at room temperature. Avoid excessive heat: 40°C (104°F). Keep product away from direct light.

Shown in Product Identification Guide, page 322

LACTAID® Drops OTC
(lactase enzyme)

DESCRIPTION

LACTAID® is the original dairy digestive supplement that makes milk more digestible. ***LACTAID® Drops*** may be added to milk for *in vitro* hydrolysis of lactose.

LACTAID® Drops contain sufficient lactase enzyme (derived from *Kluyveromyces lactis*) to hydrolyze lactose in milk.

ACTIONS

LACTAID® Drops are a liquid form of the natural lactase enzyme that makes milk more digestible. The lactase enzyme hydrolyzes the lactose sugar (a double sugar) into its simple sugar components, glucose and galactose.

USES

Lactaid contains a natural enzyme that helps break down lactose, the complex sugar found in dairy foods. If not properly digested, lactose can cause gas, bloating, cramps or diarrhea.*

*This statement has not been evaluated by the Food and Drug Administraiton. This product is not intended to diagnose, treat, cure, or prevent any disease.

DIRECTIONS

Add 5–7 drops of ***LACTAID® Drops*** to a quart of milk, shake gently and refrigerate for 24 hours. Because sensitivity to lactose can vary, you may have to adjust the number of drops you use. If you are still experiencing discomfort after consuming milk with 5–7 ***LACTAID® Drops*** per quart, you may want to add 10 or even 15 drops per quart. Lactaid may be used with any kind of milk: whole, 1%, 2%, non-fat, skim, powdered and chocolate milk.

WARNINGS

Consult your doctor: If you experience any symptoms which are unusual or seem unrelated to the condition for which you took this product. **Do not use if carton is opened, or if bottle wrap imprinted "Safety Seal®" is broken or missing.**

INGREDIENTS

Glycerin, Water, Lactase Enzyme

HOW SUPPLIED

LACTAID® Drops are available in .22 fl. oz. (7 mL), (30 quart supply). Store at or below room temperature (below 77°F). Refrigerate after opening.
Lactaid Drops are certified kosher from the Orthodox Union.
Also available: 70% lactose-reduced Lactaid Milk and 100% lactose-reduced Lactaid Milk.

Shown in Product Identification Guide, page 321

LACTAID® Original Strength Caplets OTC
(lactase enzyme)

LACTAID® Extra Strength Caplets
(lactase enzyme)

LACTAID® Ultra Caplets and Chewable Tablets
(lactase enzyme)

DESCRIPTION

Each ***LACTAID® Original Strength Caplet*** contains 3000 FCC (Food Chemical Codex) units of lactase enzyme (derived from *Aspergillus oryzae*).
Each ***LACTAID® Extra Strength Caplet*** contains 4500 FCC units of lactase enzyme (derived from *Aspergillus oryzae*).
Each ***LACTAID® Ultra Caplet*** contains 9000 FCC units of lactase enzyme (derived from *Aspergillus oryzae*).
Each ***LACTAID® Ultra Chewable Tablet*** contains 9000 FCC units of lactase enzyme (derived from *Aspergillus oryzae*).
LACTAID® is the original lactase dietary supplement that makes milk and dairy foods more digestible. ***LACTAID®*** lactase enzyme hydrolyzes lactose into two digestible simple sugars: glucose and galactose. ***LACTAID® Caplets*** are taken orally for *in vivo* hydrolysis of lactose.

ACTIONS

LACTAID® Caplets/Chewable Tablets work to naturally replenish lactase enzyme that aids in dairy food digestion. Lactase enzyme hydrolyzes lactose sugar (a double sugar) into its simple sugar components, glucose and galactose.

USES

Lactaid contains a natural enzyme that helps your body break down lactose, the complex sugar found in dairy foods. If not properly digested, lactose can cause gas, bloating, cramps or diarrhea.*

*This statement has not been evaluated by the Food and Drug Administration. This product is not intended to diagnose, treat, cure, or prevent and disease.

DIRECTIONS

Original Strength: Swallow or chew 3 caplets with the first bite of dairy food. For best results, you may have to adjust the number of caplets up or down. **Extra Strength:** Swallow or chew 2 caplets with first bite of dairy food. For best results, you may have to adjust the number of caplets up or down. **Ultra Caplets:** Swallow 1 caplet with the first bite of dairy food. If you suffer from severe digestive discomfort, you may have to take more than one caplet, but no more than two at a time. **Ultra Chewables:** Chew and swallow 1 chewable tablet with your first bite of dairy food. If you suffer from severe digestive discomfort, you may have to take more than one tablet but no more than two at a time. Don't be discouraged if at first Lactaid does not work to your satisfaction. Because the degree of enzyme deficiency naturally varies from person to person and from food to food, you may have to adjust the number of caplets/chewable tablets up or down to find your own level of comfort. Since Lactaid Caplets/Chewable Tablets work only on the food as you eat it, use them every time you enjoy dairy foods.

WARNINGS

Consult your doctor if you experience any symptoms which are unusual or seem unrelated to the condition for which you took this product. **Do not use if carton is open or if printed plastic neckwrap is broken or if single serve packet is open.**
LACTAID® Ultra Chewable Tablets: Contains Phenylalanine 0.49 mg/tablet

INGREDIENTS

LACTAID® Original Strength Caplets: Mannitol, Cellulose, Lactase Enzyme (3,000 FCC Lactase units/Caplet), Dextrose, Sodium Citrate, Magnesium Stearate.
LACTAID® Extra Strength Caplets: Lactase Enzyme (4,500 FCC Lactase units/Caplet), Mannitol, Cellulose, Dextrose, Sodium Citrate, Magnesium Stearate.
LACTAID® Ultra Caplets: Cellulose, Lactase Enzyme (9,000 FCC Lactase units/Caplet), Dextrose, Sodium Citrate, Magnesium Stearate, Colloidal Silicon Dioxide.
LACTAID® Ultra Chewable Tablets: Mannitol, Cellulose, Lactase Enzyme (9,000 FCC Lactase units/tablet), Sodium Citrate, Dextrose, Magnesium Stearate, Flavor, Citric Acid, Acesulfame K, Aspartame.

HOW SUPPLIED

LACTAID® Original Strength Caplets are available in bottles of 120 count. Store at or below room temperature (below 77°F) but do not refrigerate. Keep away from heat.
LACTAID® Extra Strength Caplets are available in bottles of 50 count. Store at or below room temerature (below 77°F) but do not refrigerate. ***LACTAID® ULTRA Caplets*** are available in single serve packets in 12, 32 and 60 count packages. Store at or below room temperature (below 77°F) but do not refrigerate. ***LACTAID® Ultra Chewable Tablets*** are available in bottles of 12 and 32 counts. Store at or below room temperature (below 77°F), but do not refrigerate. Keep away from heat and moisture.
LACTAID® Caplets and ***LACTAID® Ultra Chewable Tablets*** are certified kosher from the Orthodox Union.
Also available: 70% lactose-reduced Lactaid Milk and 100% lactose-reduced Lactaid Milk.

Shown in Product Identification Guide, page 321

MOTRIN® Cold & Flu Caplets OTC

DESCRIPTION

Each ***MOTRIN® Cold & Flu Caplet*** contains ibuprofen 200 mg and pseudoephedrine HCl 30 mg.

INDICATIONS

MOTRIN® Cold & Flu Caplets: For the temporary relief of symptoms associated with the common cold or flu, including nasal congestion, headache, body aches, pains and fever; and sinusitis.

DIRECTIONS

Adults and children 12 years of age and older: Take 1 caplet every 4 to 6 hours while symptoms persist. If symptoms do not respond to 1 caplet, 2 caplets may be used but do not exceed 6 caplets in 24 hours, unless directed by a doctor. The smallest effective dose should be used. Take with food or milk if occasional and mild heartburn, upset stomach, or stomach pain occurs with use. Consult a doctor if these symptoms are more than mild or if they persist. *Children:* Do not give this product to children under 12 years of age except under the advice and supervision of a doctor.

WARNINGS

Do not take for more than 7 days. If symptoms do not improve, or are accompanied by fever that persists for more than 3 days, or if new symptoms occur, consult a doctor. These could be signs of a serious illness. As with aspirin and acetaminophen, if you have any condition which requires you to take prescription drugs or if you have had any problems or serious side effects from taking any non-prescription pain reliever, do not take this product without first discussing it with your doctor. IF YOU EXPERIENCE ANY SYMPTOMS WHICH ARE UNUSUAL OR SEEM UNRELATED TO THE CONDITION FOR WHICH YOU TOOK THIS PRODUCT CONSULT A DOCTOR BEFORE TAKING ANY MORE OF IT. If you are under a doctor's care for any serious condition, consult a doctor before taking this product. **Do not exceed recommended dosage.** If nervousness, dizziness or sleeplessness occur, discontinue use and consult a doctor. Do not take this product if you have heart disease, high blood pressure, thyroid disease, diabetes, or difficulty in urination due to enlargement of the prostate gland, unless directed by a doctor. Do not combine this product with other non-prescription pain relievers. Do not combine this product with any other ibuprofen-containing product. Keep this and all drugs out of the reach of children. In case of accidental overdose, seek professional assistance or contact a poison control center immediately. As with any drug, if you are pregnant or nursing a baby, seek the advice of a health professional before using this product. IT IS ESPECIALLY IMPORTANT NOT TO USE THIS PRODUCT DURING THE LAST 3 MONTHS OF PREGNANCY UNLESS SPECIFICALLY DIRECTED TO DO SO BY A DOCTOR BECAUSE IT MAY CAUSE PROBLEMS IN THE UNBORN CHILD OR COMPLICATIONS DURING DELIVERY.
Allergy Alert: ibuprofen may cause a severe allergic reaction which may include: hives, facial swelling, asthma (wheezing), shock.
Do not use if you have ever had an allergic reaction to any other pain reliever/fever reducer.
Stop use and ask a doctor if an allergic reaction occurs. Seek medical help right away.

Alcohol Warning: If you consume 3 or more alcoholic drinks every day, ask your doctor whether you should take ibuprofen or other pain relievers/fever reducers. Ibuprofen may cause stomach bleeding.

DRUG INTERACTION PRECAUTION

Do not use this product if you are now taking a prescription monoamine oxidase inhibitor (MAOI) (certain drugs for depression, psychiatric or emotional conditions, or Parkinson's disease), or for 2 weeks after stopping the MAOI drug. If you are uncertain whether your drug contains an MAOI, consult a health professional before taking this product.

PROFESSIONAL INFORMATION
OVERDOSAGE INFORMATION

The *toxicity of ibuprofen overdose* is dependent upon the amount of drug ingested and the time elapsed since ingestion, though individual response may vary, which makes it necessary to evaluate each case individually. Although uncommon, serious toxicity and death have been reported in the medical literature with ibuprofen overdosage. The most frequently reported symptoms of ibuprofen overdose include abdominal pain, nausea, vomiting, lethargy and drowsiness. Other central nervous system symptoms include headache, tinnitus, CNS depression and seizures. Metabolic acidosis, coma, acute renal failure and apnea (primarily in very young children) may rarely occur. Cardiovascular toxicity, including hypotension, bradycardia, tachycardia and atrial fibrillation, also have been reported.
The *treatment of acute ibuprofen overdose* is primarily supportive. Management of hypotension, acidosis and gastrointestinal bleeding may be necessary. In cases of acute overdose, the stomach should be emptied through ipecac-induced emesis or lavage. Emesis is most effective if initiated within 30 minutes of ingestion. Orally administered activated charcoal may help in reducing the absorption and reabsorption of ibuprofen. In children, the estimated amount of ibuprofen ingested per body weight may be helpful to predict the potential for development of toxicity although each case must be evaluated. Ingestion of less than 100 mg/kg is unlikely to produce toxicity. Children ingesting 100 to 200 mg/kg may be managed with induced emesis and a minimal observation time of four hours. Children ingesting 200 to 400 mg/kg of ibuprofen should have immediate gastric emptying and at least four hours observation in a health care facility. Children ingesting greater than 400 mg/kg require immediate medical referral, careful observation and appropriate supportive therapy. Ipecac-induced emesis is not recommended in overdoses greater than 400 mg/kg because of the risk of convulsions and the potential for aspiration of gastric contents.
In adult patients the history of the dose reportedly ingested does not appear to be predictive of toxicity. The need for referral and follow-up must be judged by the circumstances at the time of the overdose ingestion. Symptomatic adults should be admitted to a health care facility for observation. Symptoms from pseudoephedrine overdose consist most often of mild anxiety, tachycardia and/or hypertension. Symptoms usually appear within 4 to 8 hours of ingestion and are transient, usually requiring no treatment.

INACTIVE INGREDIENTS

Caplets: Carnauba Wax, Cellulose, Corn Starch, D&C Yellow #10, FD&C Red #40, Hydroxypropyl Methylcellulose, Silicon Dioxide, Sodium Lauryl Sulfate, Sodium Starch Glycolate, Stearic Acid, Titanium Dioxide, Triacetin.

HOW SUPPLIED

Caplets: (yellow, printed "Motrin Cold & Flu" in red) in blister packs of 10 and 20.
Store between 20–25°C (68–77°F). Avoid excessive heat.

Shown in Product Identification Guide, page 322

MOTRIN® MIGRAINE PAIN CAPLETS OTC

DESCRIPTION

Each ***Motrin® Migraine Pain Caplet*** contains ibuprofen 200 mg.

USE

treats pain of migraine headache

DIRECTIONS

Adults:
- take 1 or 2 caplets with a glass of water
- the smallest effective dose should be used
- if symptoms persist or worsen, ask your doctor
- do not take more than 2 caplets in 24 hours for pain of migraine unless directed by a doctor

Under 18 years of age:
- ask a doctor

WARNINGS

Allergy alert: ibuprofen may cause a severe allergic reaction which may include:
- hives • facial swelling
- asthma (wheezing) • shock

Alcohol warning: If you consume 3 or more alcoholic drinks every day, ask your doctor whether you should take ibuprofen or other pain relievers/fever reducers. Ibuprofen may cause stomach bleeding.
Do not use if you have ever had an allergic reaction to any other pain relievers/fever reducers
Ask a doctor before use if you have
- never had migraines diagnosed by a health professional
- a headache that is different from your usual migraines
- the worst headache of your life
- fever and stiff neck
- headaches beginning after or caused by head injury, exertion, coughing or bending
- experienced your first headache after the age of 50
- daily headaches
- a migraine headaches so severe as to require bed rest
- problems or serious side effects from taking pain relievers or fever reducers

Continued on next page

Motrin Migraine—Cont.

- stomach pain
- vomiting with your migraine headache

Ask a doctor or pharmacist before use if you are
- under a doctor's care for any serious condition
- take any other drug
- taking any other product that contain ibuprofen, or any other pain reliever/fever reducer

Stop use and ask a doctor if
- an allergic reaction occurs. Seek medical help right away.
- migraine headache pain is not relieved or gets worse after first dose
- stomach pain or upset gets worse or lasts
- new or unexpected symptoms occur

If pregnant or breast-feeding, ask a health professional before use. It is especially important not to use ibuprofen during the last 3 months of pregnancy unless definitely directed to do so by a doctor because it may cause problems in the unborn child or complications during delivery.
Keep out of reach of children. In case of overdose, get medical help or contact a Poison Control Center right away.

OTHER INFORMATION
- do not use if neck wrap or foil inner seal imprinted **"Safety Seal"** is broken or missing
- store at 20–25°C (68–77°F)

INACTIVE INGREDIENTS
carnauba wax, corn starch, hydroxypropyl methylcellulose, iron oxide black, pregelatinized starch, propylene glycol, silicon dioxide, stearic acid, titanium dioxide

HOW SUPPLIED
Caplets (white printed "Motrin IB" in black) in tamper evident packaging of 24, 50, and 100

PROFESSIONAL INFORMATION
OVERDOSAGE INFORMATION
The toxicity of ibuprofen overdose is dependent upon the amount of drug ingested and the time elapsed since ingestion, though individual response may vary, which makes it necessary to evaluation each case individually. Although uncommon, serious toxicity and death have been reported in the medical literature which ibuprofen overdosage. The most frequently reported symptoms of ibuprofen overdose include abdominal pain, nausea, vomiting, lethargy and drowsiness. Other central nervous system symptoms include headache, tinnitus. CNS depression and seizures. Metabolic acidosis, coma, acute renal failure and apnea (primarily in very young children) may rarely occur. Cardiovascular toxicity, including hypotension, bradycardia, tachycardia and atrial fibrillation, also have been reported.
The *treatment of acute ibuprofen overdose* is primarily supportive. Management of hypotension, acidosis and gastrointestinal bleeding may be necessary. In cases of acute overdose, the stomach should be emptied through ipecac-induced emesis or lavage. Emesis is most effective if initiated without 30 minutes of ingestion. Orally administered activated charcoal may help in reducing the absorption and reabsorption of ibuprofen. In children, the estimated amount of ibuprofen ingested per body weight may be helpful to predict the potential for development of toxicity although each case must be evaluated. Ingestion of less than 100 mg/kg is unlikely to produce toxicity. Children ingesting 100 to 200 mg/kg may be managed with induced emesis and a minimal observation time of four hours. Children ingesting 200 to 400 mg/kg ibuprofen should have immediate gastric emptying and at least four hours observation in a health care facility. Children ingesting greater than 400 mg/kg require immediately medical referral, careful observation and appropriate supportive therapy. Ipecac-induced emesis is not recommended in overdoses greater than 400 mg/kg because of the risk of convulsions and the potential for aspiration of gastric contents.
In adult patients the history of the dose reportedly ingested does not appear to be predictive of toxicity. The need for referral and follow-up must be judged by the circumstances at the time of the overdose ingestion. Symptomatic adults should be admitted to a health care facility for observation.
Shown in Product Identification Guide, page 322

MOTRIN® Sinus Headache Caplets OTC

DESCRIPTION
Each ***MOTRIN® Sinus Headache Caplet*** contains ibuprofen 200 mg and pseudoephedrine HCl 30 mg.

INDICATIONS
MOTRIN® Sinus Headache Caplets are indicated for the temporary relief of symptoms associated with sinusitis, the common cold or flu including nasal congestion, headache, body aches, pains and fever.

DIRECTIONS
Do not take more than directed. *Adults and children 12 years of age and older:* Take 1 caplet every 4 to 6 hours while symptoms persist. If symptoms do not respond to 1 caplet, 2 caplets may be used but do not exceed 6 caplets in 24 hours, unless directed by a doctor. The smallest effective dose should be used. Take with food or milk if occasional and mild heartburn, upset stomach, or stomach pain occurs with use. Consult a doctor if these symptoms are more than mild or if they persist. *Children:* Do not give this product to children under 12 years of age except under the advice and supervision of a doctor.

WARNINGS
Do not take for more than 7 days. If symptoms do not improve, or are accompanied by fever that persists for more than 3 days, or if new symptoms occur, consult a doctor. These could be signs of a serious illness. As with aspirin and acetaminophen, if you have any condition which requires you to take prescription drugs or if you have had any problems or serious side effects from taking any non-prescription pain reliever, do not take this product without first discussing it with your doctor. IF YOU EXPERIENCE ANY SYMPTOMS WHICH ARE UNUSUAL OR SEEM UNRELATED TO THE CONDITION FOR WHICH YOU TOOK THIS PRODUCT CONSULT A DOCTOR BEFORE TAKING ANY MORE OF IT. If you are under a doctor's care for any serious condition, consult a doctor before taking this product.
Do not exceed recommended dosage. If nervousness, dizziness, or sleeplessness occur, discontinue use and consult a doctor. Do not take this product if you have heart disease, high blood pressure, thyroid disease, diabetes, or difficulty in urination due to enlargement of the prostate gland, unless directed by a doctor. Do not combine this product with other non-prescription pain relievers. Do not combine this product with any other ibuprofen-containing product. Keep this and all drugs out of the reach of children. In case of accidental overdose, seek professional assistance or contact a poison control center immediately. As with any drug, if you are pregnant or nursing a baby, seek the advice of a health professional before using this product. IT IS ESPECIALLY IMPORTANT NOT TO USE THIS PRODUCT DURING THE LAST 3 MONTHS OF PREGNANCY UNLESS SPECIFICALLY DIRECTED TO DO SO BY A DOCTOR BECAUSE IT MAY CAUSE PROBLEMS IN THE UNBORN CHILD OR COMPLICATIONS DURING DELIVERY.
Allergy Alert: ibuprofen may cause a severe allergic reaction which may include: hives, facial swelling, asthma (wheezing), shock.
Do not use if you have ever had an allergic reaction to any other pain reliever/fever reducer.
Stop use and ask a doctor if an allergic reaction occurs. Seek medical help right away.

Alcohol Warning: If you consume 3 or more alcoholic drinks every day, ask your doctor whether you should take ibuprofen or other pain relievers/fever reducers. Ibuprofen may cause stomach bleeding.

DRUG INTERACTION PRECAUTION
Do not use this product if you are now taking a prescription monoamine oxidase inhibitor (MAOI) (certain drugs for depression, psychiatric or emotional conditions, or Parkinson's disease), or for 2 weeks after stopping the MAOI drug. If you are uncertain whether your drug contains an MAOI, consult a health professional before taking this product.

PROFESSIONAL INFORMATION
OVERDOSAGE INFORMATION
The *toxicity of ibuprofen overdose* is dependent upon the amount of drug ingested and the time elapsed since ingestion, though individual response may vary, which makes it necessary to evaluate each case individually. Although uncommon, serious toxicity and death have been reported in the medical literature with ibuprofen overdosage. The most frequently reported symptoms of ibuprofen overdose include abdominal pain, nausea, vomiting, lethargy and drowsiness. Other central nervous system symptoms include headache, tinnitus, CNS depression and seizures. Metabolic acidosis, coma, acute renal failure and apnea (primarily in very young children) may rarely occur. Cardiovascular toxicity, including hypotension, bradycardia, tachycardia and atrial fibrillation, also have been reported.
The *treatment of acute ibuprofen overdose* is primarily supportive. Management of hypotension, acidosis and gastrointestinal bleeding may be necessary. In cases of acute overdose, the stomach should be emptied through ipecac-induced emesis or lavage. Emesis is most effective if initiated within 30 minutes of ingestion. Orally administered activated charcoal may help in reducing the absorption and reabsorption of ibuprofen. In children, the estimated amount of ibuprofen ingested per body weight may be helpful to predict the potential for development of toxicity although each case must be evaluated. Ingestion of less than 100 mg/kg is unlikely to produce toxicity. Children ingesting 100 to 200 mg/kg may be managed with induced emesis and a minimal observation time of four hours. Children ingesting 200 to 400 mg/kg of ibuprofen should have immediate gastric emptying and at least four hours observation in a health care facility. Children ingesting greater than 400 mg/kg require immediate medical referral, careful observation and appropriate supportive therapy. Ipecac-induced emesis is not recommended in overdoses greater than 400 mg/kg because of the risk of convulsions and the potential for aspiration of gastric contents.
In adult patients the history of the dose reportedly ingested does not appear to be predictive of toxicity. The need for referral and follow-up must be judged by the circumstances at the time of the overdose ingestion. Symptomatic adults should be admitted to a health care facility for observation. Symptoms from pseudoephedrine overdose consist most often of mild anxiety, tachycardia and/or hypertension. Symptoms usually appear within 4 to 8 hours of ingestion and are transient, usually requiring no treatment.

INACTIVE INGREDIENTS
Caplets: Carnauba Wax, Cellulose, Corn Starch, FD&C Red #40, Hydroxypropyl Methylcellulose, Silicon Dioxide, Sodium Lauryl Sulfate, Sodium Starch Glycolate, Stearic Acid, Titanium Dioxide, Triacetin.

HOW SUPPLIED
Caplets: (white, printed "Motrin Sinus Headache" in red) in blister packs of 20 and 40.
Store between 20–25°C (68–77°F). Avoid excessive heat.
Shown in Product Identification Guide, page 322

MOTRIN® IB Pain Reliever/Fever Reducer Tablets, Caplets and Gelcaps OTC

DESCRIPTION
Each ***Motrin® IB Pain Reliever/Fever Reducer Tablet, Caplet and Gelcap*** contains ibuprofen 200 mg.

INDICATIONS
Motrin® IB Pain Reliever/Fever Reducer Tablets, Caplets and Gelcaps: For the temporary relief of headache, muscular aches, the minor pain of arthritis, toothache, backache, minor aches and pains associated with the common cold, the pain of menstrual cramps, and for reduction of fever.

DIRECTIONS
Do not take more than directed. Adults: Take 1 tablet, caplet or gelcap every 4 to 6 hours while symptoms persist. If pain or fever does not respond to 1 tablet, caplet or gelcap, 2 tablets, caplets or gelcaps may be used, but do not exceed 6 tablets, caplets or gelcaps in 24 hours, unless directed by a doctor. The smallest effective dose should be used. Take with food or milk if occasional and mild heartburn, upset stomach or stomach pain occurs with use. Consult a doctor if these symptoms are more than mild or if they persist.
Children: Do not give this product to children under 12 except under the advice and supervision of a doctor.

WARNINGS
Do not take for pain for more than 10 days or for fever for more than 3 days unless directed by a doctor. If pain or fever persists or gets worse, if new symptoms occur, or if the painful area is red or swollen, consult a doctor. These could be signs of a serious illness. If you are under a doctor's care for any serious condition, consult a doctor before taking this product. As with aspirin and acetaminophen, if you have any condition which requires you to take prescription drugs, or if you have had any problems or serious side effects from taking any non-prescription pain reliever, do not take MOTRIN® IB without first discussing it with your doctor. If you experience any symptoms which are unusual or seem unrelated to the condition for which you took ibuprofen, consult a doctor before taking any more of it. Although ibuprofen is indicated for the same conditions as aspirin and acetaminophen, it should not be taken with them except under a doctor's direction. Do not combine this product with any other ibuprofen-containing product. Keep this and all drugs out of the reach of children. In case of accidental overdose, seek professional assistance or contact a poison control center immediately. As with any drug, if you are pregnant or nursing a baby, seek the advice of a health professional before using this product. IT IS ESPECIALLY IMPORTANT NOT TO USE IBUPROFEN DURING THE LAST 3 MONTHS OF PREGNANCY UNLESS SPECIFICALLY DIRECTED TO DO SO BY A DOCTOR BECAUSE IT MAY CAUSE PROBLEMS IN THE UNBORN CHILD OR COMPLICATIONS DURING DELIVERY.
Allergy Alert: ibuprofen may cause a severe allergic reaction which may include: hives, facial swelling, asthma (wheezing), shock.
Do not use if you have ever had an allergic reaction to any other pain reliever/fever reducer.
Stop use and ask a doctor if an allergic reaction occurs. Seek medical help right away.

ALCOHOL WARNING: If you consume 3 or more alcoholic drinks every day, ask your doctor whether you should take ibuprofen or other pain relievers/fever reducers. Ibuprofen may cause stomach bleeding.

PROFESSIONAL INFORMATION
OVERDOSAGE INFORMATION
The *toxicity of ibuprofen overdose* is dependent upon the amount of drug ingested and the time elapsed since ingestion, though individual response may vary, which makes it necessary to evaluate each case individually. Although uncommon, serious toxicity and death have been reported in the medical literature with ibuprofen overdosage. The most frequently reported symptoms of ibuprofen overdose include abdominal pain, nausea, vomiting, lethargy and drowsiness. Other central nervous system symptoms include headache, tinnitus, CNS depression and seizures. Metabolic acidosis, coma, acute renal failure and apnea (primarily in very young children) may rarely occur. Cardiovascular toxicity, including hypotension, bradycardia, tachycardia and atrial fibrillation, also have been reported.
The *treatment of acute ibuprofen overdose* is primarily supportive. Management of hypotension, acidosis and gastrointestinal bleeding may be necessary. In cases of acute overdose, the stomach should be emptied through ipecac-induced emesis or lavage. Emesis is most effective if initiated

within 30 minutes of ingestion. Orally administered activated charcoal may help in reducing the absorption and reabsorption of ibuprofen. In children, the estimated amount of ibuprofen ingested per body weight may be helpful to predict the potential for development of toxicity although each case must be evaluated. Ingestion of less than 100 mg/kg is unlikely to produce toxicity. Children ingesting 100 to 200 mg/kg may be managed with induced emesis and a minimal observation time of four hours. Children ingesting 200 to 400 mg/kg of ibuprofen should have immediate gastric emptying and at least four hours observation in a health care facility. Children ingesting greater than 400 mg/kg require immediate medical referral, careful observation and appropriate supportive therapy. Ipecac-induced emesis is not recommended in overdoses greater than 400 mg/kg because of the risk of convulsions and the potential for aspiration of gastric contents.

In adult patients the history of the dose reportedly ingested does not appear to be predictive of toxicity. The need for referral and follow-up must be judged by the circumstances at the time of the overdose ingestion. Symptomatic adults should be admitted to a health care facility for observation.

INACTIVE INGREDIENTS

Tablets and Caplets: Carnauba wax, corn starch, FD&C Yellow #6, hydroxypropyl methylcellulose, iron oxide, polydextrose, polyethylene glycol, silicon dioxide, stearic acid, titanium dioxide.

Gelcaps: Benzyl alcohol, butylparaben, butyl alcohol, castor oil, colloidal silicon dioxide, cornstarch, edetate calcium disodium, FDC Yellow No. 6, gelatin, hydroxypropyl methylcellulose, iron oxide black, magnesium stearate, methylparaben, microcrystalline cellulose, povidone, pregelatinized starch, propylene glycol, propylparaben, SDA 3A alcohol, sodium lauryl sulfate, sodium propionate, sodium starch glycolate, and titanium dioxide.

HOW SUPPLIED

Tablets: (orange, printed "Motrin IB" in black) in tamper evident packaging of 24, 50, 100, 130, 135, and 165. Store between 20°–25° C (68°–77° F)

Caplets: (orange, printed "Motrin IB" in black) in tamper evident packaging of 24, 50, 60, 100, 130, 135, 165, 250 and 500. Store between 20°–25° C (68°–77° F)

Gelcaps: (colored orange and white, printed "Motrin IB" in black) in tamper evident packaging of 24 and 50. Store between 20–25° C (68–77° F)

Shown in Product Identification Guide, page 322

MOTRIN® Ibuprofen Suspension ℞
100 mg/5 mL

MOTRIN® Ibuprofen Oral Drops ℞
40 mg/mL

MOTRIN® Ibuprofen Chewable Tablets ℞
50 mg and 100 mg

MOTRIN® Ibuprofen Caplets ℞
100 mg

DESCRIPTION

The active ingredient in MOTRIN is ibuprofen, which is a member of the propionic acid group of nonsteroidal anti-inflammatory drugs (NSAIDs). Ibuprofen is a racemic mixture of [+]S- and [−]R-enantiomers. It is a white to off-white crystalline powder, with a melting point of 74° to 77°C. It is practically insoluble in water (<0.1 mg/mL), but readily soluble in organic solvents such as ethanol and acetone. Ibuprofen has a pKa of 4.43±0.03 and an n-octanol/water partition coefficient of 11.7 at pH 7.4. The chemical name for ibuprofen is (±)-2-(p-isobutylphenyl) propionic acid. The molecular weight of ibuprofen is 206.28. Its molecular formula is $C_{13}H_{18}O_2$ and it has the following structural formula:

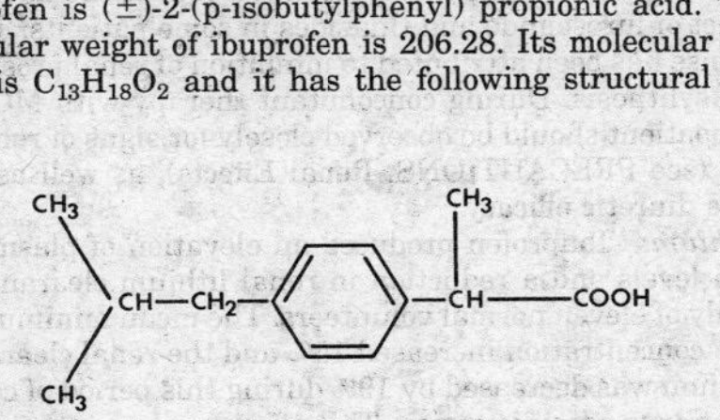

MOTRIN Suspension is a sucrose-sweetened, orange-colored, berry-flavored liquid suspension containing 100 mg of ibuprofen in 5 mL (20 mg/mL). Inactive ingredients include citric acid, glycerin, polysorbate 80, pregelatinized starch, purified water, sodium benzoate, sucrose, xanthan gum, D&C Yellow #10 and FD&C Red #40, and artificial flavors.

MOTRIN Oral Drops (intended for pediatric use only) is a sucrose-sweetened, pink-colored, berry-flavored liquid suspension containing 40 mg of ibuprofen per mL. Inactive ingredients include citric acid, glycerin, polysorbate 80, pregelatinized starch, purified water, sodium benzoate, sorbitol, sucrose, xanthan gum, FD&C Red #40, and artificial flavors.

MOTRIN Chewable Tablets are aspartame-sweetened, citrus-tasting, orange-colored tablets, that contain 50 mg or 100 mg of ibuprofen per tablet. Inactive ingredients include aspartame, citric acid, hydroxyethyl cellulose, hydroxypropyl methylcellulose, magnesium stearate, mannitol, microcrystalline cellulose, povidone, sodium lauryl sulfate, sodium starch glycolate, FD&C Yellow #6, and artificial flavors.

Table 1
Pharmacokinetic Parameters of Ibuprofen Formulations
[Mean Values (% coefficient of variation)]

Dose	200mg (≈2.8 mg/kg) in Adults				10 mg/kg in Febrile Children	
Formulation	**Suspension**	**Drops**	**Caplet**	**Chewable Tablet**	**Suspension**	**Chewable Tablet**
Number of Patients	24	24	25	24	18	18
AUCinf (µg·h/mL)	64 (27%)	74 (19%)	60 (19%)	66 (22%)	155 (24%)	176 (25%)
Cmax (µg/mL)	19 (22%)	24 (21%)	20 (18%)	15 (24%)	55 (23%)	43 (39%)
Tmax (h)	0.79 (69%)	1.0 (60%)	1.04 (50%)	2.0 (56%)	0.97 (57%)	1.43 (69%)
Cl/F (mL/h/kg)	45.6 (22%)	43.4 (18%)	45.0 (19%)	42.8 (18%)	68.6 (22%)	60.9 (27%)

Legend: AUCinf = Area-under-the-curve to infinity
Tmax = Time-to-peak plasma concentration
Cmax = Peak plasma concentration
Cl/F = Clearance divided by fraction at drug absorbed

MOTRIN Caplets are unsweetened, white-colored, unflavored, film-coated, capsule-shaped tablets, containing 100 mg of ibuprofen per tablet. Inactive ingredients include carnauba wax, colloidal silicone dioxide, cornstarch, hydroxypropyl methylcellulose, microcrystalline cellulose, polydextrose, polyethylene glycol, pregelatinized starch, propylene glycol, sodium starch glycolate, titanium dioxide, triacetin, D&C Yellow #10, and FD&C Yellow #6.

CLINICAL PHARMACOLOGY

Pharmacodynamics—Ibuprofen is a nonsteroidal anti-inflammatory drug (NSAID) that possesses anti-inflammatory, analgesic and antipyretic activity. Its mode of action, like that of other NSAIDs, is not completely understood, but may be related to prostaglandin synthetase inhibition. After absorption of the racemic ibuprofen, the [−]R-enantiomer undergoes interconversion to the [+]S-form. The biological activities of ibuprofen are associated with the [+]S-enantiomer.

In clinical studies in adult patients with rheumatoid arthritis and osteoarthritis, ibuprofen has been shown to be comparable to aspirin in controlling pain and inflammation, though causing fewer of the mild gastrointestinal side effects (see ADVERSE REACTIONS). MOTRIN may be well tolerated in some patients who have had gastrointestinal side effects with aspirin, but these patients, when treated with MOTRIN, should be carefully followed for signs and symptoms of gastrointestinal ulceration and bleeding. Although it is not definitely known whether ibuprofen causes less peptic ulceration than aspirin, in one study involving 885 adult patients with rheumatoid arthritis treated for up to one year (438 patients on ibuprofen and 447 patients on aspirin), there were no reports of gastric ulceration with ibuprofen whereas frank ulceration was reported in 13 patients in the aspirin group (statistically significant p<.001). Gastroscopic studies at varying doses of ibuprofen showed an increased tendency toward endoscopic lesions at higher doses. However, at clinically comparable doses (2,400 mg of ibuprofen vs. 3,600 mg of aspirin), endoscopic lesions were approximately half that seen with aspirin. Studies using ^{51}Cr-tagged red cells indicate that fecal blood loss associated with ibuprofen in doses up to 2400 mg daily did not exceed the range of normal, and was significantly less than that seen in aspirin-treated patients. The clinical significance of these findings is unknown.

Pharmacokinetics—As noted in the DESCRIPTION section, ibuprofen is a racemic mixture of [−]R-and [+]S-isomers. *In vivo* and *in vitro* studies indicate that the [+]S-isomer is responsible for clinial activity. The [−]R-form, while thought to be pharmacologically inactive, is slowly and incompletely (60%) interconverted into the active [+]S species in adults. The degree of interconversion in children is unknown, but is thought to be similar. The [−]R-isomer serves as a circulating reservoir to maintain levels of active drug. Ibuprofen is well absorbed orally, with less than 1% being excreted in the urine unchanged. It has a biphasic elimination time curve with a plasma half-life of approximately 2 hours. Studies in febrile children have established the dose-proportionality of 5 and 10 mg/kg doses of ibuprofen. Studies in adults have established the dose-proportionality of ibuprofen as a single oral dose from 50 to 600 mg for total drug and up to 1200 mg for free drug.

Absorption—*In vivo* studies indicate that ibuprofen is well absorbed orally from the suspension, drops, caplet and chewable tablet formulations, with peak plasma levels usually occurring within 1 to 2 hours. The pharmacokinetic differences between the products in adults (see Table 1) are due to differences in the rate of absorption of ibuprofen from the various dosage forms. The observed differences in the table between adults and children, in terms of AUC and C_{max}, are due to both differences in dose per body weight and age-or fever-related change in volume of distribution (Vd/F). All of the formulations are equally bioavailable in terms of peak plasma levels (C_{max}) and extent of absorption (AUC), however, the time-to-peak (T_{max}) is different between the products. Clinically, this has been shown to have no effect on either onset or peak fever reduction in children. [See table 1 above]

Antacid—A bioavailability study in adults has shown that there was no interference with the absorption of ibuprofen when given in conjunction with an antacid containing both aluminum hydroxide and magnesium hydroxide.

Food Effects—Absorption is most rapid when MOTRIN is given under fasting conditions. Administration of MOTRIN Suspension, MOTRIN Oral Drops, MOTRIN Chewable Tablets and MOTRIN Caplets with food affects the rate but not the extent of absorption. When taken with food, T_{max} is delayed by approximately 30 to 60 minutes, and peak levels are reduced by approximately 30 to 50%.

Distribution—Ibuprofen, like most other drugs of its class, is highly protein bound (>99% bound at 20 µg/mL). Protein binding is saturable and at concentrations >20 µg/mL binding is non-linear. Based on oral dosing data there is an age-or fever-related change in volume of distribution for ibuprofen. Febrile children <11 years old have a volume of approximately 0.2 L/kg while adults have a volume of approximately 0.12 L/kg. The clinical significance of these findings is unknown.

Metabolism—Following oral administration, the majority of the dose was recovered in the urine within 24 hours as the hydroxy-(25%) and carboxypropyl-(37%) phenylpropionic acid metabolites. The percentages of free and conjugated ibuprofen found in the urine were approximately 1% and 14%, respectively. The remainder of the drug was found in the stool as both metabolites and unabsorbed drug.

Elimination—Ibuprofen is rapidly metabolized and eliminated in the urine. The excretion of ibuprofen is virtually complete 24 hours after the last dose. It has a biphasic plasma elimination time curve with a half-life of approximately 2.0 hours. There is no difference in the observed terminal elimination rate or half-life between children and adults, however, there is an age-or fever-related change in total clearance. This suggests that the observed change in clearance is due to changes in the volume of distribution of ibuprofen (see Table 1 for Cl/F values).

Clinical Studies—Controlled clinical trials comparing doses of 5 and 10 mg/kg ibuprofen suspension and 10-15 mg/kg of acetaminophen elixir have been conducted in children 6 months to 12 years of age with fever primarily do to viral illnesses. In these studies there were no differences between treatment in fever reduction for the first hour and maximum fever reduction occurred between 2 and 4 hours. Response after 1 hour was dependent on both the level of temperature elevation as well as the treatment. In children with baseline temperatures at or below 102.5°F both ibuprofen doses and acetaminophen were equally effective in their maximum effect. In children with temperatures above 102.5°F, the ibuprofen 10 mg/kg dose was more effective. By 6 hours, children treated with ibuprofen 5mg/kg tended to have recurrence in fever, whereas children treated with ibuprofen 10 mg/kg still had significant fever reduction at 8 hours. In control groups treated with 10 mg/kg acetaminophen, fever reduction resembled that seen in children treated with 5 mg/kg of ibuprofen, with the exception that temperature elevation tended to return 1-2 hours earlier.

A comparison of MOTRIN Chewable Tablets and MOTRIN Suspension in febrile children showed similar antipyretic effects of the two formulations, lasting between 6 and 8 hours. No clinical studies of fever reduction in children have been performed with MOTRIN Caplets or MOTRIN Oral Drops.

Controlled single-dose clinical analgesia trials comparing doses of 5 and 10 mg/kg ibuprofen suspension with acetaminophen suspension 12.5 mg/kg and placebo, have been conducted in children 5 to 12 years of age, with sore throat pain due to an infectious agent, or ear pain due to acute otitis media. Onset of pain relief provided by ibuprofen was similar to that of acetaminophen, occurring within the first hour, usually around the half-hour mark. All active treatments showed significant pain relief verus placebo, and the

Continued on next page

Motrin—Cont.

10 mg/kg dose of ibuprofen had a duration of analgesic effect of 6 to 8 hours. Ibuprofen 10 mg/kg provided more overall pain relief than the 5 mg/kg dose.
Controlled studies have demonstrated that ibuprofen is a more effective analgesic than propoxyphene for the relief of episiotomy pain, pain following dental extraction procedures, and for the relief of the symptoms of primary dysmenorrhea.
In patients with primary dysmenorrhea, ibuprofen has been shown to reduce elevated levels of prostaglandin activity in the menstrual fluid and to reduce resting and active intrauterine pressure, as well as the frequency of uterine contractions. The probable mechanism of action is to inhibit prostaglandin synthesis rather than simply to provide analgesia.
In clinical studies in adult patients with rheumatoid arthritis, ibuprofen has been shown to be comparable to indomethacin in controlling the signs and symptoms of disease activity, with a lower incidence of milder gastrointestinal and CNS side effects than indomethacin.
MOTRIN may be used in combination with gold salts and/or corticosteroids.

INDICATIONS AND USAGE

In Children

MOTRIN is indicated:

- For the reduction of fever in patients aged 6 months and older.
- For relief of mild to moderate pain in patients aged 6 months and older.
- For relief of signs and symptoms of juvenille arthritis.

In Adults

MOTRIN is indicated:

- For relief of mild to moderate pain.
- For treatment of primary dysmenorrhea.
- For relief of the signs and symptoms of rheumatoid arthritis and osteoarthritis.

Since there have been no controlled trials to demonstrate whether there is any beneficial effect or harmful interaction with the use of ibuprofen in conjuction with aspirin, the combination cannot be recommended (see PRECAUTIONS—Drug Interactions).

CONTRAINDICATIONS

MOTRIN should not be used in patients with previously demonstrated hypersensitivity to ibuprofen, or in individuals with a history of allergic manifestations to aspirin or other NSAIDs. Severe anaphylactic-like reactions to ibuprofen have been reported in such patients, some with fatal outcome.

WARNINGS

Risk of GI Ulceration, Bleeding and Perforation with NSAID Therapy. Serious gastrointestinal toxicity such as bleeding, ulceration, and perforation, can occur at any time, with or without warning symptoms, in patients treated chronically with NSAID therapy. Although minor upper gastrointestinal problems, such as dyspepsia, are common, usually developing early in therapy, physicians should remain alert for ulceration and bleeding in patients treated chronically with NSAIDs even in the absence of previous GI tract symptoms. In patients observed in clinical trials of several months to two years duration, symptomatic upper GI ulcers, gross bleeding or perforation appear to occur in approximately 1% of patients treated for 3–6 months, and in about 2–4% of patients treated for one year. Physicians should inform patients about the signs and/or symptoms of serious GI toxicity and what steps to take if they occur.
Studies to date have not identified any subset of patients not at risk of developing peptic ulceration and bleeding. Except for a prior history of serious GI events and other risk factors known to be associated with peptic ulcer disease, such as alcoholism, smoking, etc., no risk factors (e.g., age, sex) have been associated with increased risk. Elderly or debilitated patients seem to tolerate ulceration or bleeding less well than other individuals and most spontaneous reports of fatal GI events are in this population. Studies to date are inconclusive concerning the relative risk of various NSAIDs in causing such reactions. High doses of any NSAID probably carry a greater risk of these reactions, although controlled clinical trials showing this do not exist in most cases. In considering the use of relatively large doses (within the recommended dosage range), sufficient benefit should be anticipated to offset the potential increased risk of GI toxicity.
Anaphylactoid Reactions: Anaphylactoid reactions may occur even in patients without prior exposure to ibuprofen. Extreme caution should be exercised when giving MOTRIN to patients with bronchospastic reactivity (e.g., asthma), nasal polyps, or those with a history of angiodema. Emergency help should be sought in case such anaphylactoid reaction occurs.
Advanced Renal Disease: In cases with advanced kidney disease, treatment with MOTRIN should not be initiated; if MOTRIN is used in such cases, close monitoring of the patient's kidney functions is advisable (see PRECAUTIONS—Renal Effects).

PRECAUTIONS

Renal Effects: Caution should be used when initiating treatment with MOTRIN in patients with considerable dehydration. It is advisable to rehydrate patients first and then start therapy with MOTRIN. Caution is also recommended in patients with pre-existing kidney disease (see WARNINGS—Advanced Renal Disease).
As with other NSAIDs, long-term administration of ibuprofen to animals has resulted in renal papillary necrosis and other abnormal renal pathology. In humans, there have been reports of acute interstitial nephritis with hematuria, proteinuria, and occasionally nephrotic syndrome.
A second form of renal toxicity has been seen in patients with prerenal conditions leading to a reduction in renal blood flow or blood volume, where the renal prostaglandins have a supportive role in the maintenance of renal perfusion. In these patients, administration of an NSAID may cause a dose-dependent reduction in prostaglandin formation and may precipitate overt renal decompensation. Patients at greatest risk of this reaction are those with impaired renal function, heart failure, liver dysfunction, those taking diuretics and the elderly. Discontinuation of NSAID therapy is typically followed by recovery to the pre-treatment state.
Those patients at high risk, who chronically take ibuprofen, should have renal function monitored if they have signs or symptoms which may be consistent with mild azotemia, such as malaise, fatigue, loss of appetite, etc. Occasional patients may develop some elevation of serum creatinine and BUN levels without signs or symptoms.
Since ibuprofen is eliminated primarily by the kidneys, patients with significantly impaired renal function should be closely monitored and a reduction in dosage should be anticipated to avoid drug accumulation. Prospective studies on the safety of ibuprofen in patients with chronic renal failure have not been conducted.
Fluid Retention: Fluid retention and edema have been reported in association with ibuprofen, therefore, the drug should be used with caution in patients with a history of cardiac decompensation or hypertension.
Hematologic Effects: MOTRIN can inhibit platelet aggregation but, unlike aspirin, its effect on platelet function is reversible, quantitatively less, and of shorter duration. Because this prolonged bleeding effect may be exaggerated in patients with underlying hemostatic defects, MOTRIN should be used with caution in persons with intrinsic coagulation defects and those on anticoagulant therapy.
Hepatic Effects: As with other nonsteroidal anti-inflammatory drugs, borderline elevations of one or more liver laboratory tests may occur in up to 15% of patients. These abnormalities may progress, may remain essentially unchanged, or may be transient with continued therapy. The ALT (SGPT) test is probably the most sensitive indicator of liver dysfunction. Meaningful (3 times the upper limit of normal) elevations of ALT and AST (SGOT) occurred in controlled clinical trials in less than 1% of patients. A patient with symptoms and/or signs suggesting liver dysfunction, or in whom an abnormal liver test has occurred, should be evaluated for evidence of the development of more severe hepatic reactions while on therapy with MOTRIN. Severe hepatic reactions, including jaundice and cases of fatal hepatitis, have been reported with ibuprofen as with other nonsteroidal anti-inflammatory drugs. Although such reactions are rare, if abnormal liver tests persist or worsen, if clinical signs and symptoms consistent with liver disease develop, or if systemic manifestations occur (e.g., eosinophilia, rash, etc.), treatment with MOTRIN should be discontinued.
Aseptic Meningitis: Aseptic meningitis, with fever and coma, has been observed on rare occasions in patients on ibuprofen therapy. Although it is probably more likely to occur in patients with systemic lupus erythematosus and related connective tissue diseases, it has been reported in patients who do not have an underlying chronic disease. If signs or symptoms of meningitis develop in a patient receiving MOTRIN, the possibility of its being related to ibuprofen should be considered.
Other Precautions—The pharmacological activity of MOTRIN may induce fever reduction and inflammation, thus diminishing their utility as diagnostic signs in detecting underlying conditions.
In order to avoid exacerbation of manifestations of adrenal insufficiency, patients who have been on prolonged corticosteroid therapy should have their therapy tapered slowly rather than discontinued abruptly when ibuprofen is added to the treatment program.
Blurred and/or diminished vision, scotomata, and/or changes in color vision have been reported. If a patient develops such complaints while receiving MOTRIN Chewable Tablets, the drug should be discontinued and the patient should have an ophthalmologic examination which includes central visual fields and color vision testing.
Phenylketonurics: MOTRIN Chewable Tablets 50 mg contain phenylalanine 3 mg per tablet, and the 100 mg tablets contain phenylalanine 6 mg per tablet.
Diabetics: MOTRIN Suspension and MOTRIN Oral Drops contain 0.3 g sucrose and 1.6 calories per mL, or 1.5 g sucrose and 8 calories per teaspoon, which should be taken into consideration when treating diabetic patients with this product.
Information for Patients—MOTRIN, like other drugs of its class, is not free of side effects. The side effects of these drugs can cause discomfort and, rarely, there are more serious side effects, such as gastrointestinal bleeding, which may result in hospitalization and even fatal outcomes.
NSAIDs are often essential agents in the management of arthritis, pain and fever, but they also may be commonly employed for conditions which are less serious. Physicians may wish to discuss with their patients the potential risks (see WARNINGS, PRECAUTIONS, and ADVERSE REACTIONS) and likely benefits of NSAID treatment, particularly when the drugs are used for less serious conditions where treatment without NSAIDs may represent an acceptable alternative to both the patient and physician.
Patients on MOTRIN should report to their physicians signs or symptoms of gastrointestinal ulceration or bleeding, blurred vision or other eye symptoms, skin rash, weight gain, or edema.
Because serious GI tract ulceration and bleeding can occur without warning symptoms, physicians should follow chronically treated patients for the signs and symptoms of ulceration and bleeding and should inform them of the importance of this follow-up (see WARNINGS).
Patients should also be instructed to seek medical emergency help in case of an occurrence of an anaphylactoid reaction (see WARNINGS).

LABORATORY TESTS

Hemoglobin Levels: In cross-study comparisons, in adults, with doses ranging from 1200 mg to 3200 mg daily for several weeks, a slight dose-response decrease in hemoglobin/hematocrit was noted. This has been observed with other nonsteroidal anit-inflammatory drugs; the mechanism is unknown. However, even with daily doses of 3200 mg, the total decrease in hemoglobin usually does not exceed 1 g/dL; if there are no signs of bleeding, it is probably not clinically important.
In two postmarketing clinical studies with ibuprofen, the incidence of a decreased hemoglobin level was greater than previously reported. Decrease in hemoglobin of 1 g/dL or more was observed in 17.1% of 193 patients on 1600 mg ibuprofen daily (osteoarthritis), and 22.8% of 189 patients taking 2400mg of ibuprofen daily (rheumatoid arthritis). Positive stool occult blood tests and elevated serum creatinine levels were also observed in these studies.

DRUG INTERACTIONS

Coumarin-type anticoagulants: Several short-term controlled studies failed to show that iburprofen significantly affected prothrombin times or a variety of other clotting factors administered to individuals on coumarin-type anticoagulants. Because bleeding has been reported when ibuprofen and other nonsteroidal anti-inflammatory agents have been administered to patients on coumarin-type anticoagulants, the physician should be cautious when administering MOTRIN to patients on anticoagulants.
Aspirin: Animal studies show that aspirin given with NSAIDs, including ibuprofen, yields a net decrease in anti-inflammatory activity with lowered blood levels of the non-aspirin drug. Single-dose bioavailability studies in normal volunteers have failed to show an effect of aspirin on ibuprofen blood levels. Correlative clinical studies have not been done.
Methotrexate: Ibuprofen, as well as other NSAIDs, has been reported to competitively inhibit methotrexate accumulation in rabbit kidney slices. This may indicate that ibuprofen could enhance the toxicity of methotrexate. Caution should be used, therefore, if MOTRIN is administered concomitantly with methotrexate.
H-2 Antagonists: In studies with human volunteers, coadministration of cimetidine or ranitidine with ibuprofen had no substantive effect on ibuprofen serum concentrations.
ACE-inhibitors: Reports suggest that NSAIDs, including ibuprofen, may diminish the antihypertensive effect of ACE-inhibitors. This interaction should be given consideration in patients taking MOTRIN concomitantly with ACE-inhibitors.
Furosemide: Clinical studies, as well as random observations, have shown that ibuprofen can reduce the natriuretic effect of furosemide and thiazides in some patients. This response has been attributed to inhibition of renal prostaglandin synthesis. During concomitant therapy with MOTRIN, the patient should be observed closely for signs of renal failure (see PRECAUTIONS, Renal Effects), as well as to assure diuretic efficacy.
Lithium: Ibuprofen produced an elevation of plasma lithium levels and a reduction in renal lithium clearance in a study of eleven normal volunteers. The mean minimum lithium concentration increased 15% and the renal clearance of lithium was decreased by 19% during this period of concomitant drug administration. This effect has been attributed to inhibition of renal prostaglandin synthesis by ibuprofen. Thus, when MOTRIN and lithium are administered concurrently, subjects should be observed carefully for signs of lithium toxicity. (Read circulars for lithium preparation before use of such concurrent therapy.)
Teratogenic Effects—Pregnancy Category B: Reproductive studies conducted in rats and rabbits at doses somewhat less than the maximal clinical dose did not demonstrate evidence of developmental abnormalities. However, animal reproduction studies are not always predictive of human response. As there are no adequate and well-controlled studies in pregnant women, this drug should be used during pregnancy only if clearly needed. Because of the known effects of nonsteroidal anti-inflammatory drugs on the fetal cardiovascular system (closure of ductus arteriosus), use during late pregnancy should be avoided. Administration of MOTRIN is not recommended during pregnancy.
Labor and Delivery: As with other drugs known to inhibit prostaglandin synthesis, an increased incidence of dystocia and delayed parturition occurred in rats. Administration of MOTRIN is not recommended during labor and delivery.

Nursing Mothers: In limited studies, an assay capable of detecting 1 μg/mL did not demonstrate ibuprofen in the milk of lactating mothers. Because of the limited nature of these studies, however, and the possible adverse effects of prostaglandin inhibiting drugs on neonates, MOTRIN is not recommended for use in nursing mothers.

Pediatric Use: Safety and efficacy of MOTRIN in children below the age of 6 months has not been established (see CLINICAL PHARMACOLOGY-Clinical Studies). There is no evidence of age-dependent kinetics in patients 2 to 11 years old (see CLINICAL PHARMACOLOGY-Pharmacokinetics). Dosing of MOTRIN in children 6 months or older should be guided by their body weight (see DOSAGE AND ADMINISTRATION).

ADVERSE REACTIONS

The most frequent type of adverse reaction occurring with ibuprofen is gastrointestinal. In controlled clinical trials, the percentage of adult patients reporting one or more gastrointestinal complaints ranged from 4% to 16%.

In controlled studies in adults, when ibuprofen was compared to aspirin and indomethacin in equally effective doses, the overall incidence of gastrointestinal complaints was about half that seen in either the aspirin- or indomethacin-treated patients.

Adverse reactions observed during controlled clinical trials in adults at an incidence greater than 1% are listed in the chart. Those reactions listed under the heading "Incidence Greater than 1% (but less than 3%) Probable Causal Relationship," encompass observations in approximately 3,000 patients. More than 500 of these patients were treated for periods of at least 54 weeks.

Still other reactions, occurring less frequently than 1 in 100, were reported in controlled clinical trials and from marketing experience. These reactions have been divided into two categories: "Incidence less than 1%—Probable Causal Relationships," lists reactions with Ibuprofen therapy for which the probability of a causal relationship exists; this category was completed over time with postmarketing serious adverse reactions. "Incidence less than 1% —Causal Relationship Unknown," lists reactions with ibuprofen therapy for which a causal relationship has not been established, but are presented as alerting information for physicians.

INCIDENCE OF 1% OR GREATER

Probable Causal Relationship

*Incidence between 3 and 9%=ADR marked with**
Incidence between 1 and <3%=unmarked ADR

Cardiovascular system: Edema, fluid retention (generally responds promptly to drug discontinuation) (See PRECAUTIONS).

Digestive system: Nausea*, epigastric pain*, heartburn*, diarrhea, abdominal distress, nausea and vomiting, indigestion, constipation, abdominal cramps or pain, fullness of GI tract (bloating and flatulence).

Nervous system: Dizziness*, headache, nervousness.

Skin and appendages: Rash* (including maculopapular type), pruritus

Specal senses: Tinnitus.

INCIDENCE LESS THAN 1%

Probable Causal Relationship: The following adverse reactions were reported in clincial trials at an incidence of less than 1%, or were reported from postmarketing or foreign experience. The probability exists between the drug and these adverse reactions.

Body as a whole: Anaphylaxis and anaphylactoid reactions (see WARNINGS).

Cardiovascular system: Cerebrovascular accident, hypotension, congestive heart failure in patients with marginal cardiac function, elevated blood pressure, palpitations.

Digestive system: Gastric or duodenal ulcer with bleeding and/or perforation, gastrointestinal hemorrhage, pancreatitis, melena, gastritis, duodenitis, esophagitis, hematemesis, hepatorenal syndrome, liver necrosis, liver failure, hepatitis, jaundice, abnormal liver tests.

Hematologic system: Neutropenia, agranulocytosis, aplastic anemia, hemolytic anemia (sometimes Coombs positive), thrombocytopenia with or without purpura, eosinophilia, decrease in hemoglobin and hematocrit (see PRECAUTIONS), pancytopenia.

Nervous system: Depression, insomia, confusion, emotional liability, somnolence, convulsions, aseptic meningitis with fever and coma (see PRECAUTIONS).

Respiratory: Bronchospasm, dyspnea, apnea.

Skin and appendages: Vesiculobullous eruptions, urticaria, erythema multiforme, Stevens-Johnson syndrome, alopecia, exfoliative dermatitis, Lyell's syndrome (toxic epidermal necrolysis), photosensitivity reactions.

Special senses: Hearing loss, amblyopia (blurred and/or diminished vision, scotomata and/or changes in color vision) (see PRECAUTIONS—Other Precautions).

Urogenital system: Acute renal failure in patients with pre-existing significantly impaired renal function (see PRECAUTIONS), renal papillary necrosis, tubular necrosis, glomerulitis, decreased creatinine clearance, polyuria, azotemia, cystitis, hematuria.

Miscellaneous: Dry eyes and mouth, gingival ulcer, rhinitis.

INCIDENCE LESS THAN 1%

Causal Relationship Unknown: The following adverse reactions occurred at an incidence of less than 1% in clinical trials, or were suggested by marketing experience under circumstances where a causal relationship could not be definitely established. They are listed as alerting information for the physician.

Allergic: Serum sickness, lupus erythematosus syndrome, Henoch-Schönlein vasculitis, angioedema.

Cardiovascular system: Arrhythmias (sinus tachycardia, sinus bradycardia).

Hematologic system: Bleeding episodes (e.g., epistaxis, menorrhagia).

Metabolic/endocrine: Gynecomastia, hypoglycemic reaction, acidosis.

Nervous system: Paresthesias, hallucinations, dream abnormalities, pseudo-tumor cerebri.

Special senses: Conjunctivitis, diplopia, optic neuritis, cataracts.

OVERDOSAGE

The *toxicity of ibuprofen overdose* is dependent upon the amount of drug ingested and the time elapsed since ingestion, though individual response may vary, which makes it necessary to evaluate each case individually. Although uncommon, serious toxicity and death have been reported in the medical literature with ibuprofen overdosage. The most frequently reported symptoms of ibuprofen overdose include abdominal pain, nausea, vomiting, lethargy and drowsiness. Other central nervous system symptoms include headache, tinnitus, CNS depression and seizures. Metabolic acidosis, coma, acute renal failure and apnea (primarily in very young children) may rarely occur. Cardiovascular toxicity, including hypotension, bradycardia, tachycardia and atrial fibrillation, also have been reported.

The *treatment of acute ibuprofen overdose* is primarily supportive. Management hypotension acidosis and gastrointestinal bleeding may be necessary. In cases of acute overdose, the stomach should be emptied through ipecac-induced emesis or lavage. Emesis is most effective if initiated within 30 minutes of ingestion. Orally administered activated charcoal may help in reducing the absorption and reabsorption of ibuprofen.

In children, the estimated amount of ibuprofen ingested per body weight may be helpful to predict the potential for development of toxicity although each case must be evaluated. Ingestion of less than 100 mg/kg is unlikely to produce toxicity. Children ingesting 100 to 200 mg/kg may be managed with induced emesis and a minimal observation time of four hours. Children ingesting 200 to 400 mg/kg of ibuprofen should have immediate gastric emptying and at least four hours observation in a health care facility. Children ingesting greater than 400 mg/kg require immediate medical referral, careful observation and appropriate supportive therapy. Ipecac-induced emesis is not recommended in overdoses greater than 400 mg/kg because of the risk for convulsions and the potential for aspiration of gastric contents.

In adult patients the history of the dose reportedly ingested does not appear to be predictive of toxicity. The need for referral and follow-up must be judged by the circumstances at the time of the overdose ingestion. Symptomatic adults should be admitted to a health care facility for observation.

DOSAGE AND ADMINISTRATION

CHILDREN

Fever reduction: For reduction of fever in children, 6 months to 12 years of age, the dosage should be adjusted on the basis of the initial temperature level (see CLINICAL PHARMACOLOGY). The recommended dose is 5 mg/kg if the baseline temperature is less than 102.5°F, or 10 mg/kg if the baseline temperature is 102.5°F or greater. The duration of fever reduction is generally 6 to 8 hours. The recommended maximum daily dose is 40 mg/kg.

Analgesia: For relief of mild to moderate pain in children, 6 months to 12 years of age, the recommended dosage is 10 mg/kg, every 6 to 8 hours. The recommended maximum daily dose is 40 mg/kg. Doses should be given so as not to disturb the child's sleep pattern. Taking fluids after chewing MOTRIN Chewable Tablets may help to promote absorption of the drug (see CLINICAL PHARMACOLOGY—Pharmacokinetics, and "Individualization of Dosage" in this section).

Juvenile Arthritis: The recommended dose is 30 to 40 mg/kg/day divided into three to four doses (see Individualization of Dosage). Patients with milder disease may be adequately treated with 20 mg/kg/day.

ADULTS

Analgesia: 400 mg every 4 to 6 hours as necessary for the relief of mild to moderate pain in adults. In controlled analgesic clincial trials, doses of MOTRIN greater than 400 mg were no more effective than the 400 mg dose.

Primary Dysmenorrhea: For the treatment of primary dysmenorrhea, beginning with the earliest onset of such pain, MOTRIN should be given in a dose of 400 mg every 4 hours, as necessary, for the relief of pain.

Rheumatoid arthritis and osteoarthritis, including flare-ups of chronic disease: Suggested dosage: 1200-3200 mg daily (300 mg q.i.d or 400 mg, 600 mg or 800 mg t.i.d. or q.i.d). Individual patients may show a better response to 3200 mg daily, as compared with 2400 mg, although in well-controlled clinical trials patients on 3200 mg did not show a better mean response in terms of efficacy. Therefore, when treating patients with 3200 mg/day, the physician should observe sufficient increased clinical benefits to offset potential increased risk.

Individualization of Dosage The dose of MOTRIN should be tailored to each patient, and may be lowered or raised from the suggested doses depending on the severity of symptoms either at time of initiating drug therapy or as the patient responds or fails to respond.

One fever study showed that, after the initial dose of MOTRIN, subsequent doses may be lowered and still provide adequate fever control.

In a situation when low fever would require the MOTRIN 5 mg/kg dose in a child with pain, the dose that will effectively treat the predominant symptom should be chosen.

In chronic conditions, a therapeutic response to MOTRIN therapy is sometimes seen in a few days to a week, but most often is observed by two weeks. After a satisfactory response has been achieved, the patient's dose should be reviewed and adjusted as required.

In patients with juvenile arthritis, doses above 50 mg/kg/day are not recommended because they have not been studied and doses exceeding the upper recommended dose of 40 mg/kg/day may increase the risk of causing serious adverse events. The therapeutic response may require from a few days to several weeks to be achieved. Once a clincial effect is obtained, the dosage should be lowered to the smallest dose of MOTRIN needed to maintain adequate control of symptoms.

In general, patients with rheumatoid arthritis seem to require higher doses than do patients with osteoarthritis. The smallest dose of MOTRIN that yields acceptable control should be employed.

HOW SUPPLIED

MOTRIN® (ibuprofen) Suspension 100 mg/5 mL
Orange-colored, berry-flavored suspension
–Bottles of 120 mL—NDC 0045-0448-04
–Bottles of 480 mL—NDC 0045-0448-16
Shake well before using. Store at controlled room temperature [15° to 30°C (59° to 86°F)]

MOTRIN® (ibuprofen) Oral Drops, 40mg/mL
(intended for pediatric use only)
Pink-colored, berry flavored suspension
–Bottles of 15 ml—NDC 0045-0446-15
Shake well before using. Store at controlled room temperature [15° to 30°C (59° to 86°F)].

MOTRIN® (ibuprofen) Chewable Tablets, 50 mg
Round, orange-colored, citrus-tasting, scored tablet, debossed "MOTRIN 50"
–Bottles of 100 Chewable Tablets—NDC 0045-0361-10
Store at controlled room temperature [15° to 30°C (59° to 86°F)]

MOTRIN® (ibuprofen) Chewable Tablets, 100 mg
Round, orange-colored, citrus-tasting, scored tablet, debossed "MOTRIN 100"
–Bottles of 100 Chewable Tablets—NDC 0045-0431-10
Store at controlled room temperature [15° to 30°C (59° to 86°F)]

MOTRIN® (ibuprofen) Caplets, 100 mg
White-colored, scored capsule-shaped tablet, imprinted "M 100"
–Bottles of 100 Caplets—NDC 0045-0445-10
Store at controlled room temperature [15° to 30°C (59° to 86°F)]

Caution: Federal Law prohibits dispensing without prescription.

McNEIL CONSUMER PRODUCTS CO.
DIVISION OF McNEIL-PPC, INC.
FORT WASHINGTON, PA 19034-USA
DECEMBER 1994

Shown in Product Identification Guide, page 322

NICOTROL® INHALER ℞

(nicotine inhalation system) 10 mg/cartridge
(4 mg delivered)

DESCRIPTION

NICOTROL® Inhaler (nicotine inhalation system) consists of a mouthpiece and a plastic cartridge delivering 4 mg of nicotine from a porous plug containing 10 mg nicotine. The cartridge is inserted into the mouthpiece prior to use.

Nicotine is a tertiary amine composed of a pyridine and a pyrrolidine ring. It is a colorless to pale yellow, freely water-soluble, strongly alkaline, oily, volatile, hygroscopic liquid obtained from the tobacco plant. Nicotine has a characteristic pungent odor and turns brown on exposure to air or light. Of its two stereoisomers, S(-)nicotine is the more active. It is the prevalent form in tobacco, and is the form in the NICOTROL Inhaler. The free alkaloid is absorbed rapidly through the skin, mucous membranes, and respiratory tract.

Structural formula:

N CH3 N

Chemical Name: S-3-(1-methyl-2-pyrrolidinyl) pyridine
Molecular Formula: $C_{10}H_{14}N_2$
Molecular Weight: 162.23
Ionization Constants: $pKa_1 = 7.84$, $pKa_2 = 3.04$ at 15°C
Octanol-Water Partition Coefficient: 15:1 at pH 7

Nicotine is the active ingredient; inactive components of the product are menthol and a porous plug which are pharmacologically inactive. Nicotine is released when air is inhaled through the Inhaler.

Continued on next page

Nicotrol Inhaler—Cont.

CLINICAL PHARMACOLOGY

Pharmacologic Action

Nicotine, the chief alkaloid in tobacco products, binds stereo-selectively to nicotinic-cholinergic receptors at the autonomic ganglia, in the adrenal medulla, at neuromuscular junctions, and in the brain. Two types of central nervous system effects are believed to be the basis of nicotine's positively reinforcing properties. A stimulating effect is exerted mainly in the cortex via the locus ceruleus and a reward effect is exerted in the limbic system. At low doses the stimulant effects predominate while at high doses the reward effects predominate. Intermittent intravenous administration of nicotine activates neurohormonal pathways, releasing acetylcholine, norepinephrine, dopamine, serotonin, vasopressin, beta-endorphin, growth hormone, and ACTH.

Pharmacodynamics

The cardiovascular effects of nicotine include peripheral vasoconstriction, tachycardia, and elevated blood pressure. Acute and chronic tolerance to nicotine develops from smoking tobacco or ingesting nicotine preparations. Acute tolerance (a reduction in response for a given dose) develops rapidly (less than 1 hour), but not at the same rate for different physiologic effects (skin temperature, heart rate, subjective effects). Withdrawal symptoms such as cigarette craving can be reduced in most individuals by plasma nicotine levels lower than those from smoking.

Withdrawal from nicotine in addicted individuals can be characterized by craving, nervousness, restlessness, irritability, mood lability, anxiety, drowsiness, sleep disturbances, impaired concentration, increased appetite, minor somatic complaints (headache, myalgia, constipation, fatigue), and weight gain. Nicotine toxicity is characterized by nausea, abdominal pain, vomiting, diarrhea, diaphoresis, flushing, dizziness, disturbed hearing and vision, confusion, weakness, palpitations, altered respiration and hypotension.

Both smoking and nicotine can increase circulating cortisol and catecholamines, and tolerance does not develop to the catecholamine-releasing effects of nicotine. Changes in the response to a concomitantly administered adrenergic agonist or antagonist should be watched for when nicotine intake is altered during NICOTROL Inhaler therapy and/or smoking cessation (See PRECAUTIONS, Drug Interactions).

PHARMACOKINETICS

Absorption

Most of the nicotine released from the NICOTROL Inhaler is deposited in the mouth. Only a fraction of the dose released, less than 5%, reaches the lower respiratory tract. An intensive inhalation regimen (80 deep inhalations over 20 minutes) releases on the average 4 mg of the nicotine content of each cartridge of which about 2 mg is systemically absorbed. Peak plasma concentrations are typically reached within 15 minutes of the end of inhalation.

Absorption of nicotine through the buccal mucosa is relatively slow and the high and rapid rise followed by the decline in nicotine arterial plasma concentrations seen with cigarette smoking are not achieved with the inhaler. After use of the single inhaler the arterial nicotine concentrations rise slowly to an average of 6 ng/mL in contrast to those of a cigarette, which increase rapidly and reach a mean C_{max} of approximately 49 ng/mL within 5 minutes.

The temperature dependency of nicotine release from the NICOTROL Inhaler was studied between 68°F and 104°F in eighteen patients. Average achievable steady state plasma levels after 20 minutes of an intensive inhalation regimen each hour at ambient room temperature are on the order of 23 ng/mL. The corresponding nicotine plasma levels achievable at 86°F and 104°F are on the order of 30 and 34 ng/mL. Nicotine peak plasma concentration (C_{max}) at steady-state, after 20 minutes of an intensive inhalation regimen per hour, for 10 hours.

	C_{max} (ng/mL)		
	20°C/68°F	30°C/86°F	40°C/104°F
	N = 18	N = 18	N = 18
Mean	22.5	29.7	34.0
S.D.	7.7	8.3	6.9
Min	11.1	17.6	24.1
Max	40.4	47.2	48.6

Ad libitum use of the NICOTROL Inhaler typically produces nicotine plasma levels of 6-8 ng/mL, corresponding to about 1/3 of those achieved with cigarette smoking.

Distribution

The volume of distribution following IV administration of nicotine is approximately 2 to 3 L/kg. Plasma protein binding of nicotine is <5%. Therefore, changes in nicotine binding from use of concomitant drugs or alterations of plasma proteins by disease states would not be expected to have significant effects on nicotine kinetics.

Metabolism

More than 20 metabolites of nicotine have been identified, all of which are less active than the parent compound. The primary urinary metabolites are cotinine (15% of the dose) and trans-3-hydroxycotinine (45% of the dose). Cotinine has a half-life of 15 to 20 hours and concentrations that exceed nicotine by 10-fold. The major site for the metabolism of nicotine is the liver. The kidney and lung are also sites of nicotine metabolism.

Elimination

About 10% of the nicotine absorbed is excreted unchanged in the urine. This may be increased to up to 30% with high urine flow rates and urinary acidification below pH 5. The average plasma clearance is about 1.2 L/min in a healthy adult smoker. The apparent elimination half-life of nicotine is 1 to 2 hours.

Gender Differences

Intersubject variability coefficients of variation (C.V.) for the pharmacokinetic parameters (AUC and C_{max}) were approximately 40% and 30%, respectively, for males and females. There were no medically significant differences between females and males in the kinetics of NICOTROL Inhaler.

CLINICAL TRIALS

The efficacy of NICOTROL Inhaler therapy as an aid to smoking cessation was demonstrated in two single-center, placebo-controlled, double-blind trials with a total of 445 healthy patients. The number of Nicotrol Inhaler cartridges used was a minimum dose of 4 cartridges/day and a maximum dose of 20 cartridges/day.

In both studies, the recommended duration of treatment was 3 months; however, the patients were permitted to continue to use the product for up to 6 months, if they wished. The quit rates are the percentage of all persons initially enrolled who continuously abstained after week 2. NICOTROL Inhaler was more effective than placebo at 6 weeks, 3 months and 6 months. The efficacy is shown in the following table.

Quit Rates by Treatment
(N = 445 Patients in 2 Studies)

Group	Number of Patients	At 6 Weeks	At 3 Months	At 6 Months	At 12 Months*
Nicotrol Inhaler	223	44-45%	31-32%	20-21%	11-13%
Placebo	222	14-23%	8-15%	6-11%	5-10%

* Follow-up, patients not on treatment.

Patients who used NICOTROL Inhaler had a significant reduction in the "urge to smoke", a major nicotine withdrawal symptom, compared with placebo-treated patients throughout the first week, (see Figure 1).

Figure 1

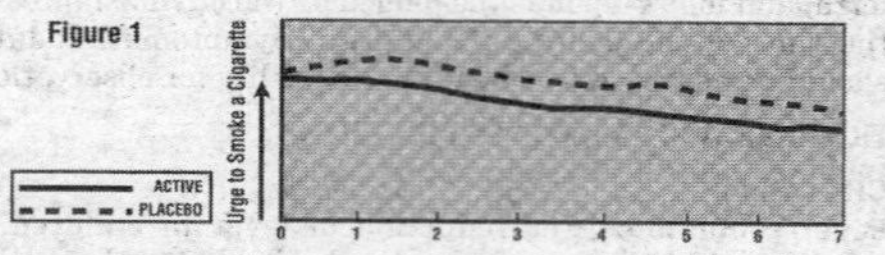

INDICATIONS AND USAGE

NICOTROL Inhaler is indicated as an aid to smoking cessation for the relief of nicotine withdrawal symptoms. NICOTROL Inhaler therapy is recommended for use as part of a comprehensive behavioral smoking cessation program.

CONTRAINDICATIONS

Use of NICOTROL Inhaler therapy is contraindicated in patients with known hypersensitivity or allergy to nicotine or to menthol.

WARNINGS

Nicotine from any source can be toxic and addictive. Smoking causes lung disease, cancer and heart disease, and may adversely affect pregnant women or the fetus. For any smoker, with or without concomitant disease or pregnancy, the risk of nicotine replacement in a smoking cessation program should be weighed against the hazard of continued smoking, and the likelihood of achieving cessation of smoking without nicotine replacement.

Pregnancy, Warning

Tobacco smoke, which has been shown to be harmful to the fetus, contains nicotine, hydrogen cyanide, and carbon monoxide. The Nicotrol Inhaler does not deliver hydrogen cyanide and carbon monoxide. However, nicotine has been shown in animal studies to cause fetal harm. It is therefore presumed that NICOTROL Inhaler can cause fetal harm when administered to a pregnant woman. The effect of nicotine delivery by NICOTROL Inhaler has not been examined in pregnancy (See **PRECAUTIONS**). **Therefore, pregnant smokers should be encouraged to attempt cessation using educational and behavioral interventions before using pharmacological approaches.** If NICOTROL Inhaler is used during pregnancy, or if the patient becomes pregnant while using it, the patient should be apprised of the potential hazard to the fetus.

Safety Note Concerning Children

This product contains nicotine and should be kept out of the reach of children and pets. The amounts of nicotine that are tolerated by adult smokers can produce symptoms of poisoning and could prove fatal if the nicotine from the Nicotrol Inhaler is inhaled, ingested or buccally absorbed by children or pets. A cartridge contains about 60% of its initial drug content when it is discarded, which is about 6 mg. Patients should be cautioned to keep both the used and unused cartridges of NICOTROL Inhaler out of the reach of children and pets.

All components of the NICOTROL Inhaler system should also be kept out of the reach of children and pets to avoid accidental swallowing and choking.

PRECAUTIONS

General

The patient should be urged to stop smoking completely when initiating NICOTROL Inhaler therapy (See **DOSAGE AND ADMINISTRATION**). Patients should be informed that if they continue to smoke while using the product, they may experience adverse effects due to peak nicotine levels higher than those experienced from smoking alone. If there is a clinically significant increase in cardiovascular or other effects attributable to nicotine, the treatment should be discontinued (See **WARNINGS**). Physicians should anticipate that concomitant medications may need dosage adjustment (See **Drug Interactions**). Sustained use (beyond 6 months) of NICOTROL Inhaler by patients who stop smoking has not been studied and is not recommended.(See **DRUG ABUSE AND DEPENDENCE**).

Bronchospastic Disease

Nicotrol Inhaler has not been specifically studied in asthma or chronic pulmonary disease. Nicotine is an airway irritant and might cause bronchospasm. Nicotrol Inhaler should be used with caution in patients with bronchospastic disease. Other forms of nicotine replacement might be preferable in patients with severe bronchospastic airway disease.

Cardiovascular or Peripheral Vascular Diseases

The risks of nicotine replacement in patients with cardiovascular and peripheral vascular diseases should be weighed against the benefits of including nicotine replacement in a smoking cessation program for them. Specifically, patients with coronary heart disease (history of myocardial infarction and/or angina pectoris), serious cardiac arrhythmias, or vasospastic diseases (Buerger's disease, Prinzmetal's variant angina and Raynaud's phenomena) should be evaluated carefully before nicotine replacement is prescribed.

Tachycardia and palpitations have been reported occasionally with the use of NICOTROL Inhaler as well as with other nicotine replacement therapies. No serious cardiovascular events were reported in clinical studies with NICOTROL Inhaler, but if such symptoms occur, its use should be discontinued.

NICOTROL Inhaler generally should not be used in patients during the immediate post-myocardial infarction period, nor in patients with serious arrhythmias, or with severe or worsening angina.

Renal or Hepatic Insufficiency

The pharmacokinetics of nicotine have not been studied in the elderly or in patients with renal or hepatic impairment. However, given that nicotine is extensively metabolized and that its total system clearance is dependent on liver blood flow, some influence of hepatic impairment on drug kinetics (reduced clearance) should be anticipated. Only severe renal impairment would be expected to affect the clearance of nicotine or its metabolites from the circulation (See **PHARMACOKINETICS**).

Endocrine Diseases

NICOTROL Inhaler therapy should be used with caution in patients with hyperthyroidism, pheochromocytoma or insulin-dependent diabetes, since nicotine causes the release of catecholamines by the adrenal medulla.

Peptic Ulcer Disease

Nicotine delays healing in peptic ulcer disease; therefore, NICOTROL Inhaler therapy should be used with caution in patients with active peptic ulcers and only when the benefits of including nicotine replacement in a smoking cessation program outweigh the risks.

Accelerated Hypertension

Nicotine therapy constitutes a risk factor for development of malignant hypertension in patients with accelerated hypertension; therefore, NICOTROL Inhaler therapy should be used with caution in these patients and only when the benefits of including nicotine replacement in a smoking cessation program outweigh the risks.

Information for Patient

A patient information sheet is included in the package of NICOTROL Inhaler cartridges dispensed to the patient. Patients should be encouraged to read the information sheet carefully and to ask their physician and pharmacist about the proper use of the product (See **DOSAGE AND ADMINISTRATION**). Patients must be advised to keep both used and unused cartridges out of the reach of children and pets.

Drug Interactions

Physiological changes resulting from smoking cessation, with or without nicotine replacement, may alter the pharmacokinetics of certain concomitant medications, such as tricyclic antidepressants and theophylline. Doses of these and perhaps other medications may need to be adjusted in patients who successfully quit smoking.

Carcinogenesis, Mutagenesis, Impairment of Fertility

Nicotine itself does not appear to be a carcinogen in laboratory animals. However, nicotine and its metabolites increased the incidences of tumors in the cheek pouches of hamsters and forestomach of F344 rats, respectively when given in combination with tumor initiators. One study, which could not be replicated, suggested that cotinine, the primary metabolite of nicotine, may cause lymphoreticular sarcoma in the large intestine of rats.

Neither nicotine nor cotinine was mutagenic in the Ames salmonella test. Nicotine induced reparable DNA damage in an *E. coli* test system. Nicotine was shown to be genotoxic in a test system using Chinese hamster ovary cells. In rats and rabbits, implantation can be delayed or inhibited by a reduction in DNA synthesis that appears to be caused by nicotine. Studies have shown a decrease in litter size in rats treated with nicotine during gestation.

PREGNANCY

Pregnancy Category D (See **WARNINGS** sections).

The harmful effects of cigarette smoking on maternal and fetal health are clearly established. These include low birth weight, an increased risk of spontaneous abortion, and increased perinatal mortality. The specific effects of NICOTROL Inhaler therapy on fetal development are unknown. Therefore pregnant smokers should be encouraged to attempt cessation using educational and behavioral interventions before using pharmacological approaches.

Spontaneous abortion during nicotine replacement therapy has been reported; as with smoking, nicotine as a contributing factor cannot be excluded.

NICOTROL Inhaler therapy should be used during pregnancy only if the likelihood of smoking cessation justifies the potential risk of using it by the pregnant patient, who might continue to smoke.

Teratogenicity

Animal Studies: Nicotine was shown to produce skeletal abnormalitites in the offspring of mice when toxic doses were given to the dams (25 mg/kg IP or SC).

Human Studies: Nicotine teratogenicity has not been studied in humans except as a component of cigarette smoke (each cigarette smoked delivers about 1 mg of nicotine). It has not been possible to conclude whether cigarette smoking is teratogenic to humans.

Other Effects

Animal Studies: A nicotine bolus (up to 2 mg/kg) to pregnant rhesus monkeys caused acidosis, hypercarbia, and hypotension (fetal and maternal concentrations were about 20 times those achieved after smoking one cigarette in 5 minutes). Fetal breathing movements were reduced in the fetal lamb after intravenous injection of 0.25 mg/kg nicotine to the ewe (equivalent to smoking 1 cigarette every 20 seconds for 5 minutes). Uterine blood flow was reduced about 30% after infusion of 0.1 μg/kg/min nicotine to pregnant rhesus monkeys (equivalent to smoking about six cigarettes every minute for 20 minutes).

Human Experience: Cigarette smoking during pregnancy is associated with an increased risk of spontaneous abortion, low birth weight infants and perinatal mortality. Nicotine and carbon monoxide are considered the most likely mediators of these outcomes. The effects of cigarette smoking on fetal cardiovascular parameters have been studied near term. Cigarettes increased fetal aortic blood flow and heart rate and decreased uterine blood flow and fetal breathing movements. NICOTROL Inhaler has not been studied in pregnant women.

Labor and Delivery

NICOTROL Inhaler is not recommended for use during labor and delivery. The effect of nicotine on a mother or the fetus during labor is unknown.

Use in Nursing Mothers

Caution should be exercised when the NICOTROL Inhaler is administered to nursing mothers. The safety of NICOTROL Inhaler therapy in nursing infants has not been examined. Nicotine passes freely into breast milk; the milk to plasma ratio averages 2.9. Nicotine is absorbed orally. An infant has the ability to clear nicotine by hepatic first-pass clearance; however, the efficiency of removal is probably lowest at birth. Nicotine concentrations in milk can be expected to be lower with NICOTROL Inhaler when used as recommended than with cigarette smoking, as maternal plasma nicotine concentrations are generally reduced with nicotine replacement. The risk of exposure of the infant to nicotine from NICOTROL Inhaler therapy should be weighed against the risks associated with the infant's exposure to nicotine from continued smoking by the mother (passive smoke exposure and contamination of breast milk with other components of tobacco smoke) and from NICOTROL Inhaler alone, or in combination with continued smoking.

Pediatric Use

Safety and effectiveness in pediatric and adolescent patients below the age of 18 years have not been established for any nicotine replacement product. However, no specific medical risk is known or expected in nicotine dependent adolescents. Nicotrol Inhaler should be used for the treatment of tobacco dependence in the older adolescent only if the potential benefit justifies the potential risk.

Geriatric Use

One hundred and thirty-two patients aged 60 or more participated in clinical trials of NICOTROL Inhaler. Nicotrol Inhaler appeared to be as effective in this age group as in younger smokers. Because medical conditions that are precautions to nicotine use are more common in the elderly, physicians should use care in prescribing this product to these patients.

ADVERSE REACTIONS

Assessment of adverse events in the 1,439 patients (730 on active drug) who participated in controlled clinical trials (including three dose finding studies) is complicated by the occurrence of signs and symptoms of nicotine withdrawal in some patients and nicotine excess in others. The incidence of adverse events is confounded by: (1) the many minor complaints that smokers commonly have, (2) continued smoking by many patients (3) the local irritation from both the active drug and the placebo.

RECOMMENDED DOSING

Duration	Recommended Cartridges/day	
INITIAL TREATMENT	Up to 12 weeks	6-16
Gradual Reduction (if needed)	6-12 weeks	No tapering strategy has been shown to be superior to any other in clinical studies.

Local Irritation

NICOTROL Inhaler and the placebo were both associated with local irritant side effects. Local irritation in mouth and throat was reported by 40% of patients on active drug as compared to 18% of patients on placebo. Irritant effects were higher in the two pivotal trials with higher doses, being 66% on active drug and 42% on placebo. Coughing (32% active versus 12% placebo) and rhinitis (23% active versus 16% placebo) were also higher on active drug. The majority of patients rated these symptoms as mild.

The frequency of cough and mouth and throat irritation declined with continued use of NICOTROL Inhaler. Other adverse events that occurred in over 3% of patients on active drug in placebo controlled pivotal trials considered possibly related to the local irritant effects of the NICOTROL Inhaler are taste comments, pain in jaw and neck, tooth disorders and sinusitis.

Withdrawal

Symptoms of withdrawal were common in both active and placebo groups. Common withdrawal symptoms seen in over 3% of patients on active drug included: dizziness, anxiety, sleep disorder, depression, withdrawal syndrome, drug dependence, fatigue and myalgia.

Nicotine Related Adverse Events

The most common nicotine-related adverse event was dyspepsia. This was present in 18% of patients in the active group compared to 9% of patients in the placebo group. Other nicotine related events present in greater than 3% of patients on active drug include nausea, diarrhea, and hiccup.

Smoking Related Adverse Events

Smoking related adverse events present in greater than 3% of patients on active drug include chest discomfort, bronchitis, and hypertension.

Other Adverse Events

Adverse events of unknown relationship to nicotine occurring in greater than 3% of patients on active drug include headache (26% of patients on active drug and 15% of patients on placebo), influenza-like symptoms, pain, backpain, allergy, paraesthesias, flatulence and fever.

DRUG ABUSE AND DEPENDENCE

The NICOTROL Inhaler is likely to have a low abuse potential based on differences between the product and cigarettes in three characteristics commonly considered important in contributing to abuse: slower absorption, smaller fluctuations in blood levels and lower blood levels of nicotine. NICOTROL Inhaler, like many other nicotine-based smoking cessation therapies, does not produce arterial concentrations similar to cigarettes. However, nicotine withdrawal symptoms were noted in clinical trials at the time of NICOTROL Inhaler tapering and after NICOTROL Inhaler discontinuation.

Dependence might occur from transference of tobacco-related nicotine dependence to the NICOTROL Inhaler. The use of the inhaler beyond 6 months has not been evaluated in clinical trials and is not recommended. To minimize the risk of dependence, patients should be encouraged to withdraw gradually from NICOTROL Inhaler therapy after 3 months of usage (See **DOSAGE AND ADMINISTRATION**). If necessary, dose reduction can be achieved by gradual reduction of the dose over a 6 to 12 week period.

OVERDOSAGE

Signs and Symptoms of Nicotine Toxicity

Signs and symptoms of an overdose of the NICOTROL Inhaler would be expected to be the same as those of acute nicotine poisoning including: pallor, cold sweat, nausea, salivation, vomiting, abdominal pain, diarrhea, headache, dizziness, disturbed hearing and vision, tremor, mental confusion, and weakness. Prostration, hypotension, and respiratory failure may ensue with large overdoses. Lethal doses produce convulsions quickly and death follows as a result of peripheral or central respiratory paralysis or, less frequently, cardiac failure.

Overdose from Inhalation

The oral LD_{50} for nicotine is >5 mg/kg in dogs and >24 mg/kg in rodents. Death is due to respiratory paralysis. The oral minimum acute lethal dose for nicotine in adult humans is reported to be 40 to 60 mg (<1 mg/kg). The effects of using several cartridges in rapid succession are unknown (See **WARNINGS, Safety Note Concerning Children**).

One cartridge of NICOTROL Inhaler contains 10 mg nicotine, of which, approximately 4 mg is delivered nicotine. It is unlikely that an excessive nicotine overdose will occur via inhalation. Should such an overdose occur, however, with signs of nicotine poisoning, the patient should be instructed to contact his/her physician immediately. For additional emergency information, call your regional poison center.

Overdose from Ingestion

Persons ingesting NICOTROL Inhaler cartridges should be referred to a health care facility for management. In unconscious patients with a secure airway, instill activated charcoal via a nasogastric tube. A saline cathartic or sorbitol may be added to the first dose of activated charcoal. Repeated doses of activated charcoal should be administered as long as the cartridge remains in the gastrointestinal tract since it will continue to release nicotine for many hours. The NICOTROL Inhaler cartridges can be identified with a radiogram.

Management of Nicotine Poisoning

Other supportive measures include diazepam or barbiturates for seizures, atropine for excessive bronchial secretions or dairrhea, respiratory support for respiratory failure, and vigorous fluid support for hypotension and cardiovascular collapse.

DOSAGE AND ADMINISTRATION

Patients must desire to stop smoking and should be instructed to ***stop smoking completely*** as they begin using NICOTROL Inhaler. It is important that patients understand the instructions, and have their questions answered. They should clearly understand the directions for using the NICOTROL Inhaler and safely disposing of the used cartridges.

The initial dosage of NICOTROL Inhaler is individualized. Patients may self-titrate to the level of nicotine they require. Most successful patients in the clinical trials used between 6 and 16 cartridges a day. Best effect was achieved by frequent continuous puffing (20 minutes). The recommended duration of treatment is 3 months, after which patients may be weaned from the NICOTROL Inhaler by gradual reduction of the daily dose over the following 6 to 12 weeks. The safety and efficacy of the continued use of NICOTROL Inhaler for periods longer than 6 months have not been studied and such use is not recommended.

Dosing recommendations are summarized in the table below.

[See table above]

Initial Treatment (Up to 12 Weeks)

For best results, patients should be encouraged to use at least 6 cartridges per day at least for the first 3 to 6 weeks of treatment. In clinical trials, the average daily dose was >6 (range 3 to 18) cartridges for patients who successfully quit smoking. Additional doses may be needed to control the urge to smoke with a maximum of 16 cartridges daily for up to 12 weeks. Regular use of NICOTROL Inhaler during the first week of treatment may help patients adapt to the irritant effects of the product. Some patients may exhibit signs or symptoms of nicotine withdrawal or excess which will require an adjustment of the dosage (see **Individualization of Dosage**).

Gradual Reduction of Dose (Up to 12 Weeks)

Most patients will need to gradually discontinue use of the NICOTROL Inhaler after the initial treatment period. Gradual reduction of dose may begin after twelve weeks of initial treatment and may last for up to twelve weeks. Recommended strategies for discontinuing use include suggesting to patients that they use the product less frequently, keep a tally of daily usage, try to meet a steadily reducing target or set a planned quit date for stopping use of the product.

Individualization of Dosage

The Nicotrol Inhaler provides the smoker with adequate amounts of nicotine to reduce the urge to smoke, and may provide some degree of comfort by providing a hand-to-mouth ritual similar to smoking, although the importance of such an effect in smoking cessation is, as yet, unknown. The success or failure of smoking cessation is influenced by the quality, intensity and frequency of supportive care. Patients are more likely to quit smoking if they are seen frequently and participate in formal smoking cessation programs.

The goal of NICOTROL Inhaler therapy is complete abstinence. If a patient is unable to stop smoking by the fourth week of therapy, treatment should probably be discontinued.

Patients who fail to quit on any attempt may benefit from interventions to improve their chances for success on subsequent attempts. Patients who were unsuccessful should be counseled and should then probably be given a therapeutic holiday before the next attempt. A new quit attempt should be encouraged when conditions are more favorable.

Based on the clinical trials, a reasonable approach to assisting patients in their attempt to quit smoking is to begin initial treatment, using the recommended dosage (See **DOSAGE AND ADMINISTRATION**). Dosage can then be adjusted in those patients with signs or symptoms of nicotine withdrawal or excess. Patients who are successfully abstinent on NICOTROL Inhaler should be treated at the se-

Continued on next page

Nicotrol Inhaler—Cont.

lected dosage for up to 12 weeks, after which use of the Inhaler should be gradually reduced over the next 6 to 12 weeks. Some patients may not require gradual reduction of dosage and may abruptly stop treatment successfully. The safe use of this product for longer than six months has not been established.

The symptoms of nicotine withdrawal overlap those of nicotine excess (See **Pharmacodynamics** and **ADVERSE REACTION** sections). Since patients using NICOTROL Inhaler may also smoke intermittently, it is sometimes difficult to determine if they are experiencing nicotine withdrawal or nicotine excess. Controlled clinical trials of nicotine products suggest that palpitations, nausea and sweating are more often symptoms of nicotine excess, whereas anxiety, nervousness and irritability are more often symptoms of nicotine withdrawal.

SAFETY AND HANDLING

Disposal

See patient information sheet for instructions on handling and disposal. After using the NICOTROL Inhaler, carefully separate the mouthpiece, remove the used cartridge and throw it away, out of the reach of children and pets. Store the mouthpiece in the plastic storage case for further use. The mouthpiece is reusable and should be cleaned regularly with soap and water. The NICOTROL Inhaler cartridges can be detected on a radiogram.

HOW SUPPLIED

NDC 0045–0901–01

NICOTROL INHALER (nicotine inhalation system) is supplied as 42 cartridges each containing 10 mg (4 mg is delivered) nicotine. Each unit consists of 1 mouthpiece, 7 storage trays each containing 6 cartridges and 1 plastic storage case. A patient information leaflet is enclosed with the package.

Store at room temperatue not to exceed 30°C (86°F). Protect cartridges from light.

CAUTION: Federal law prohibits dispensing without a prescription.

Manufactured by: Pharmacia & Upjohn AB, Sweden
Distributed by: McNEIL Consumer Healthcare
Division of McNEIL-PPC, Inc.
Fort Washington, PA 19034 USA

MADE IN SWEDEN
U.S. Patent No. 5,400,808

Shown in Product Identification Guide, page 322

NICOTROL® NS ℞

(nicotine nasal spray)
10 mg/mL

DESCRIPTION

Nicotrol® NS (nicotine nasal spray) is an aqueous solution of nicotine intended for administration as a metered spray to the nasal mucosa.

Nicotine is a tertiary amine composed of pyridine and a pyrroline ring. It is a colorless to pale yellow, freely water-soluble, strongly alkaline, oily, volatile, hygroscopic liquid obtained from the tobacco plant. Nicotine has a characteristic pungent odor and turns brown on exposure to air or light. Of its two stereoisomers, S(-)nicotine is the more active. It is the prevalent form in tobacco, and is the form in NICOTROL NS. The free alkaloid is absorbed rapidly through skin, mucous membranes, and the respiratory tract.

Chemical Name: S-3-(1-methyl-2-pyrrolidinyl) pyridine
Molecular Formula $C_{10}H_{14}N_2$
Molecular Weight: 162.23
Ionization Constants: pKa_1 =7.84, pKa_2 =3.04 at 15°C
Octanol-Water Partition Coefficient: 15:1 at pH 7

N CH3 N

Each 10 mL spray bottle contains 100 mg nicotine (10 mg/mL) in an inactive vehicle containing disodium phosphate, sodium dihydrogen phosphate, citric acid, methylparaben, propylparaben, edetate disodium, sodium chloride, polysorbate 80, aroma and water. The solution is isotonic with a pH of 7. It contains no chlorofluorocarbons.

After priming the delivery system for NICOTROL NS, each actuation of the unit delivers a metered dose spray containing approximately 0.5 mg of nicotine. The size of the droplets produced by the unit is in excess of 8 microns. One NICOTROL NS unit delivers approximately 200 applications.

CLINICAL PHARMACOLOGY

Pharmacologic Action

Nicotine, the chief alkaloid in tobacco products, binds stereo-selectively to nicotinic-cholinergic receptors at the autonomic ganglia, in the adrenal medulla, at neuromuscular junctions, and in the brain. Two types of central nervous system effects are believed to be the basis of nicotine's positively reinforcing properties. A stimulating effect is exerted mainly in the cortex via the locus ceruleus and a reward effect is exerted in the limbic system. At low doses, the stimulant effects predominate while at high doses the reward effects predominate. Intermittent intravenous administration of nicotine activates neurohormonal pathways, releasing acetylcholine, norepinephrine, dopamine, serotonin, vasopressin, beta-endorphin, growth hormone, and ACTH.

Pharmacodynamics

The cardiovascular effects of nicotine include peripheral vasoconstriction, tachycardia and elevated blood pressure. Acute and chronic tolerance to nicotine develops from smoking tobacco or ingesting nicotine preparations. Acute tolerance (a reduction in response for a given dose) develops rapidly (less than 1 hour), but not at the same rate for different physiologic effects (skin temperature, heart rate, subjective effects). Withdrawal symptoms such as cigarette craving can be reduced in most individuals by plasma nicotine levels lower than those from smoking.

Withdrawal from nicotine in addicted individuals can be characterized by craving, nervousness, restlessness, irritability, mood lability, anxiety, drowsiness, sleep disturbances, impaired concentration, increased appetite, minor somatic complaints (headache, myalgia, constipation, fatigue), and weight gain. Nicotine toxicity is characterized by nausea, abdominal pain, vomiting, diarrhea, diaphoresis, flushing, dizziness, disturbed hearing and vision, confusion, weakness, palpitations, altered respiration and hypotension.

Both smoking and nicotine can increase circulating cortisol and catecholamines, and tolerance does not develop to the catecholamine-releasing effects of nicotine. Changes in the response to a concomitantly administered adrenergic agonist or antagonist should be watched for when nicotine intake is altered during NICOTROL NS therapy and/or smoking cessation (See **PRECAUTIONS, Drug Interactions**).

PHARMACOKINETICS

Each actuation of NICOTROL NS delivers a metered 50 microliter spray containing approximately 0.5 mg of nicotine. One dose is considered 1 mg of nicotine (2 sprays, one in each nostril).

Absorption

Following administration of 2 sprays of NICOTROL NS approximately 53% ±16% (Mean ±SD) enters the systemic circulation. No significant difference in rate or extent of absorption could be seen due to the deposition of nicotine on different parts of the nasal mucosa. Plasma concentrations of nicotine obtained from 1 dose (1 mg nicotine) of NICOTROL NS rise rapidly, reaching maximum venous concentrations of 2–12 ng/mL in 4–15 minutes. The apparent absorption half-life of nicotine is approximately 3 minutes. There is wide variation among subjects in their plasma nicotine concentrations from the spray. As a result, after a 1 mg dose of spray approximately 20% of the subjects reached peak nicotine concentrations similar to those seen after smoking one cigarette (7–17 ng/mL) (See **DRUG ABUSE AND DEPENDENCE** Section). Figure 1 below plots the mean and 5th and 95th percentile nicotine concentrations after a 1 mg single dose of the nasal spray (n=30).

Figure 1: Mean and Range of the 95th and 5th Percentile Nicotine Concentrations After a 1 mg Dose of NICOTROL NS (n=30)

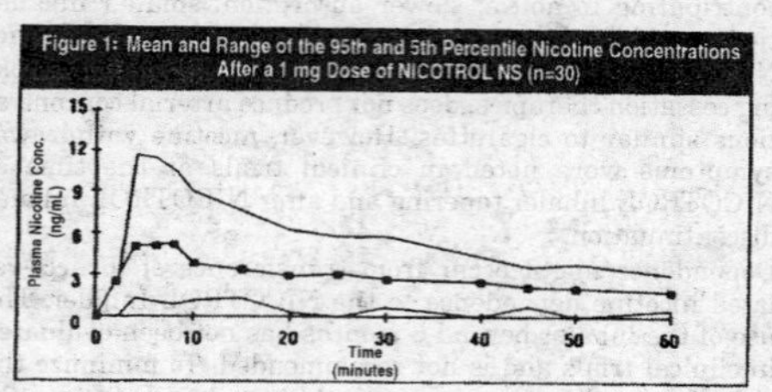

Table 1: Trough Plasma Nicotine Concentrations after 11 Hours of Dosing With 1 mg, 2 mg and 3 mg of NICOTROL NS per hour (n=16)

Dose	Mean (ng/mL) ±SD	(Range)
1 mg every 60 minutes (1 mg/hr)	6 ± 3	(1.7–12)
1 mg every 30 minutes (2 mg/hr)	14 ± 6	(1.5–24)
1 mg every 20 minutes (3 mg/hr)	18 ± 10	(1.2–35)

The data from Table 1 is derived from a three-way crossover study of repeated applications of NICOTROL NS in sixteen smokers (8 male, 8 female) ranging in age from 18 to 48 years. There is a slight deviation from dose-concentration proportionality from one dose to three doses of NICOTROL NS per hour as shown in Figure 2.

[See figure at top of next column]

Sixteen smokers (7 males and 9 females) ranging in age from 22 to 44 years were dosed with 1 mg of NICOTROL NS every hour for 10 hours. The pharmacokinetic parameters that were obtained are presented in Table 2.

Figure 2: Mean 95th and 5th Percentile Trough Nicotine Plasma Concentrations in Subjects Taking NICOTROL NS for 12 Hours (n=16)

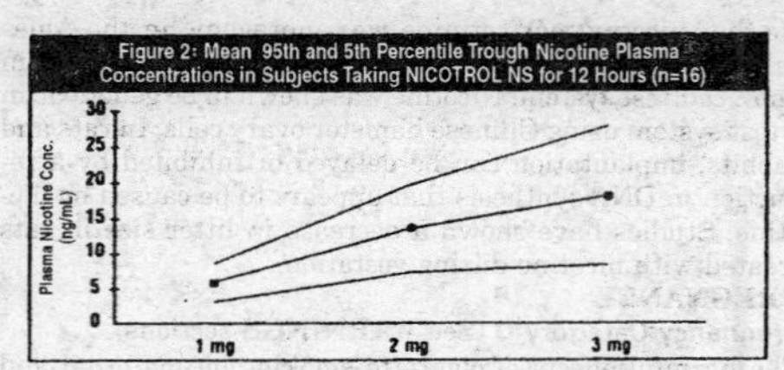

Table 2 Nicotine Pharmacokinetic Parameters at Steady-State for 1 mg hour of NICOTROL NS Administered Hourly for Ten Hours (Mean ± SD and Range) (n=16)

Parameter	1 mg (2 sprays)	(Range)
Cavg (ng/mL)	8 ± 3	(2.5–12)
Cmax (ng/mL)	9 ± 3	(3.1–14)
Tmax (minutes)	13 ± 5	(10–20)

Cavg: average plasma nicotine concentration for the dosing interval of 10–11 hours
Cmax: maximum measured plasma concentration after last dose administration
Tmax: time of maximum plasma concentration after last dose administration

Distribution

The volume of distribution following IV administration of nicotine is approximately 2 to 3 L/kg. Plasma protein binding of nicotine is <5%. Therefore, changes in nicotine binding from use of concomitant drugs or alterations of plasma proteins by disease states would not be expected to have significant effects on nicotine kinetics.

Metabolism

More than 20 metabolites of nicotine have been identified, all of which are less active than the parent compound. The primary urinary metabolites are cotinine (15% of the dose) and trans-3-hydroxycotinine (45% of the dose). Cotinine has a half-life of 15 to 20 hours and concentrations that exceed nicotine by 10-fold. The major site for the metabolism of nicotine is the liver. The kidney and lung are also sites of nicotine metabolism.

Elimination

About 10% of the nicotine absorbed is excreted unchanged in the urine. This may be increased to up to 30% with high urine flow rates and urinary acidification below pH 5. The average plasma clearance is about 1.2 L/min in a healthy adult smoker. The apparent elimination half-life of nicotine from NICOTROL NS is 1 to 2 hours.

Pharmacokinetic Model

The data were well described by a two-compartment model with first-order input.

Based on individual fits (N=18) the following parameters were derived after the administration of a 1 mg dose: Absorption rate constant Ka =14.4 ±7.3 hr^{-1} (Mean ±SD). Elimination rate constant (Ke) =0.60 ±0.53 hr^{-1}. Distribution rate constants K_{12}=4.84 ±2.57 hr^{-1}, (K_{21}) =4.35 ±2.30 hr^{-1}. Volume of distribution over fraction absorbed (V/F) =2.73 ±0.82 L/kg in 8 female and 10 male adults weighing 76 ±15 kg.

Gender Differences

Intersubject variability (50% coefficient of variation) among the pharmacokinetic parameters (AUC, C_{max} and Clearance/kg) were observed for both genders. There were no differences between females or males in the kinetics of NICOTROL NS.

Drug/Drug Interactions

The extent of absorption is slightly reduced (approximately 10%) in patients with the common cold/rhinitis. In patients with rhinitis the peak plasma concentration is reduced by approximately 20% (concentrations are lower by 1.5 ng/mL on average) and the time to peak concentration prolonged by approximately 30% (delayed by 7 minutes on average). The use of a nasal vasoconstrictor such as xylometazoline in patients with rhinitis will further prolong the time to peak by approximately 40% (delayed by 15 minutes on average), but the peak plasma concentration remains on average the same as those with rhinitis.

CLINICAL TRIALS

The efficacy of NICOTROL NS therapy as an aid to smoking cessation was demonstrated in three single-center, placebo-controlled, double-blind trials with a total of 730 patients. One of the trials used NICOTROL NS with individual counseling while the other two used group support. Patients with severe or symptomatic cardiovascular disease, hypertension, asthma, diabetes or severe allergy were not included in the studies. The amount of NICOTROL NS used was left to the discretion of each patient, with a minimum dose of 8 mg/day and a maximum dose of 40 mg/day.

In all three studies, the recommended duration of treatment was 3 months; however in two of these trials, 241 patients were permitted to continue to use the product for up to 1 year, if they wished. Among the 64 patients abstinent from cigarettes at the end of a year, 23 (36%) were still using the spray, and probable dependence on the spray was seen in several patients. (See **DRUG ABUSE AND DEPENDENCE**).

Quitting was defined as *total abstinence* from smoking for at least 4 weeks. The "quit rates" are the percentage of all persons initially enrolled who continuously abstained after week 2 or 4.
In all three studies, NICOTROL NS was more effective than placebo at 6 weeks, 3 months, 6 months, and 1 year. The two studies where NICOTROL NS could be used for more than 6 months did not have a better outcome at 1 year than the study in which NICOTROL NS was discontinued at 6 months.
[See table 3 above]

Table 3 Quit Rates by Treatment (N=730 smokers in 3 Studies)

Group	Size (n)	At 6 Weeks	At 3 Months	At 6 Months	At 1 Year
NICOTROL NS	369	49–58%	41–45%	31–35%	23–27%
Placebo	361	21–32%	17–20%	12–15%	10–15%

Patients treated with NICOTROL NS had more relief of the urge to smoke and withdrawal symptoms compared with placebo-treated patients.
NICOTROL NS allows the patient to vary the dose of nicotine on a short-term basis. As with other variable dose smoking cessation products, NICOTROL NS may be useful in the management of highly dependent smokers.

INDICATIONS AND USAGE

NICOTROL NS is indicated as an aid to smoking cessation for the relief of nicotine withdrawal symptoms. NICOTROL NS therapy should be used as a part of a comprehensive behavioral smoking cessation program.
The safety and efficacy of the continued use of NICOTROL NS for periods longer than 6 months have not been adequately studied and such use is not recommended.

CONTRAINDICATIONS

Use of NICOTROL NS therapy is contraindicated in patients with known hypersensitivity or allergy to nicotine or to any component of the product.

WARNINGS

Nicotine from any source can be toxic and addictive. Smoking causes lung disease, cancer, and heart disease and may adversely affect pregnant women or the fetus. For any smoker, with or without concomitant disease or pregnancy, the risk of nicotine replacement in a smoking cessation program should be weighed against the hazard of continued smoking, and the likelihood of achieving cessation of smoking without nicotine replacement.

Pregnancy, Warning

Tobacco smoke, which has been shown to be harmful to the fetus, contains nicotine, hydrogen cyanide, and carbon monoxide. Nicotine has been shown in animal studies to cause fetal harm. It is therefore presumed that NICOTROL NS can cause fetal harm when administered to a pregnant woman. The effect of nicotine delivery by NICOTROL NS has not been examined in pregnancy (See **PRECAUTIONS**). **Therefore, pregnant smokers should be encouraged to attempt cessation using educational and behavioral interventions before using pharmacological approaches.** If NICOTROL NS is used during pregnancy, or if the patient becomes pregnant while using it, the patient should be apprised of the potential hazard to the fetus.

Safety Note Concerning Children

The amounts of nicotine that are tolerated by adult smokers can produce symptoms of poisoning and could prove fatal if NICOTROL NS is used or ingested by children or pets. A full bottle of NICOTROL NS contains 100 mg of nicotine, some of which will still be in the bottle when it is discarded. Therefore, patients should be cautioned to keep both used and unused containers of NICOTROL NS out of the reach of children and pets.

PRECAUTIONS

General

The patient should be urged to stop smoking completely when initiating NICOTROL NS therapy (See **DOSAGE AND ADMINISTRATION**). Patients should be informed that if they continue to smoke while using the product, they may experience adverse effects due to peak nicotine levels higher than those experienced from smoking alone. If there is a clinically significant increase in cardiovascular or other effects attributable to nicotine, the treatment should be discontinued (See **WARNINGS**). Physicians should anticipate that concomitant medications may need dosage adjustment (See **Drug Interactions**).
Sustained use (beyond 6 months) of NICOTROL NS by patients who stop smoking is not recommended and should be discouraged (See **DRUG ABUSE AND DEPENDENCE**).
Use of NICOTROL NS is not recommended in patients with known chronic nasal disorders (e.g. allergy, rhinitis, nasal polyps and sinusitis) since such use has not been adequately studied.

Asthma, Bronchospasm and Reactive Airway Disease

Exacerbation of bronchospasm in patients with pre-existing asthma has been reported. Use of NICOTROL NS in patients with severe reactive airway disease is not recommended.

Effect of NICOTROL NS on the Nasal Mucosa

Topical application of either nicotine or tobacco products is irritating to the nasal mucosa and physicians should consider both the risks and benefits to the patient before initiating or continuing NICOTROL NS therapy.
The effect of NICOTROL NS on the nasal mucosa was studied in 39 cigarette smokers who used NICOTROL NS for 1 month. When compared to baseline, random biopsies taken after four weeks of treatment revealed 1 patient with persistence of pre-existing dysplasia and 1 patient with a newly found dysplasia. In both, dysplasia was not seen after a recovery period of eight weeks.
Forty-two patients who used NICOTROL NS for more than 6 months underwent follow-up ear, nose and throat examinations 1 to 3 months after discontinuing the use of the spray. Many reported local irritant effects of the spray during spray use, but none showed persistent mucosal injury that the examining physician could attribute to use of the product.
The clinical significance of these findings is not known, but extended use of the product beyond six months is not recommended.

Cardiovascular or Peripheral Vascular Diseases

The risks of nicotine replacement in patients with cardiovascular and peripheral vascular diseases should be weighed against the benefits of including nicotine replacement in a smoking cessation program for them. Specifically, patients with coronary heart disease (history of myocardial infarction and/or angina pectoris), serious cardiac arrhythmias, or vasospastic diseases (Buerger's disease, Prinzmetal's variant angina and Raynaud's phenomena) should be evaluated carefully before nicotine replacement is prescribed.
Tachycardia occurring in association with nicotine replacement therapy has been reported. No serious cardiovascular events were reported in clinical studies with NICOTROL NS, but if symptoms occur, its use should be discontinued.
NICOTROL NS generally should not be used in patients during the immediate post-myocardial infarction period, nor in patients with serious arrhythmias, or with severe or worsening angina.

Renal or Hepatic Insufficiency

The pharmacokinetics of nicotine have not been studied in the elderly or in patients with renal or hepatic impairment. However, given that nicotine is extensively metabolized and that its total system clearance is dependent on liver blood flow, some influence of hepatic impairment on drug kinetics (reduced clearance) should be anticipated. Only severe renal impairment would be expected to affect the clearance of nicotine or its metabolites from the circulation (See **PHARMACOKINETICS**).

Endocrine Diseases

NICOTROL NS therapy should be used with caution in patients with hyperthyroidism, pheochromocytoma or insulin-dependent diabetes, since nicotine causes the release of catecholamines by the adrenal medula.

Peptic Ulcer Disease

Nicotine delays healing in peptic ulcer disease, therefore, NICOTROL NS therapy should be used with caution in patients with active peptic ulcers and only when the benefits of including nicotine replacement in a smoking cessation program outweigh the risks.

Accelerated Hypertension

Nicotine therapy constitutes a risk factor for development of malignant hypertension in patients with accelerated hypertension; therefore, NICOTROL NS therapy should be used with caution in these patients and only when the benefits of including nicotine replacement in a smoking cessation program outweigh the risks.

Information to Patient

A patient instruction sheet is included in the package of NICOTROL NS dispensed to the patient. Patients should be encouraged to read the instruction sheet carefully and to ask their physician and pharmacist about the proper use of the product (See **DOSAGE AND ADMINISTRATION**).
It should be explained to patients that they are likely to experience nasal irritation, which may become less bothersome with continued use.
Patients must be advised to keep both used and unused containers out of the reach of children and pets.

Drug Interactions

The extent of absorption and peak plasma concentration is slightly reduced in patients with the common cold/rhinitis. In addition, the time to peak concentration is prolonged. The use of a nasal vasoconstrictor such as xylometazoline in patients with rhinitis will further prolong the time to peak (See **PHARMACOKINETICS**). Smoking cessation, with or without nicotine replacement, may alter the pharmacokinetics of certain concomitant medications.

May Require a Decrease in Dose at Cessation of Smoking	Possible Mechanism
Acetaminophen caffeine imipramine, oxazepam, pentazocine, propranolol, or other beta-blockers, theophylline	Deinduction of hepatic enzymes or smoking cessation
Insulin	Increase of subcutaneous insulin absorption with smoking cessation
Adrenergic antagonists (e.g. prazosin labetalol)	Decrease in circulating catecholamines with smoking cessation

May Require an Increase in Dose at Cessation of Smoking	Possible Mechanism
Adrenergic agonists (e.g. isoproterenol, phenylephrine)	Decrease in circulating catecholamines with smoking cessation

Carcinogenesis, Mutagenesis, Impairment of Fertility

Nicotine itself does not appear to be a carcinogen in laboratory animals. However, nicotine and its metabolites increased the incidence of tumors in the cheek pouches of hamsters and forestomach of F344 rats, respectively, when given in combination with tumor-initiators. One study, which could not be replicated, suggested that cotinine, the primary metabolite of nicotine, may cause lymphoreticular sarcoma in the large intestine of rats.
Neither nicotine nor cotinine were mutagenic in the Ames salmonella test. Nicotine induced repairable DNA damage in an E. coli test system. Nicotine was shown to be genotoxic in a test system using Chinese hamster ovary cells. In rats and rabbits, implantation can be delayed or inhibited by a reduction in DNA synthesis that appears to be caused by nicotine. Studies have shown a decrease in litter size in rats treated with nicotine during gestation.

PREGNANCY

Pregnancy Category D (See **WARNINGS** sections).
The harmful effects of cigarette smoking on maternal and fetal health are clearly established. These include low birth weight, an increased risk of spontaneous abortion, and increased perinatal mortality. The specific effects of NICOTROL NS on fetal development are unknown. Therefore pregnant smokers should be encouraged to attempt cessation using educational and behavioral interventions before using pharmacological approaches.
Spontaneous abortion during nicotine replacement therapy has been reported; as with smoking, nicotine as a contributing factor cannot be excluded.
NICOTROL NS should be used during pregnancy only if the likelihood of smoking cessation justifies the potential risk of using it by the pregnant patient, who might continue to smoke.

Teratogenicity

Animal Studies Nicotine was shown to produce skeletal abnormalities in the offspring of mice when toxic doses were given to the dams (25 mg/kg IP or SC).
Human Studies Nicotine teratogenicity has not been studied in humans except as a component of cigarette smoke (each cigarette smoked delivers about 1 mg of nicotine). It has not been possible to conclude whether cigarette smoking is teratogenic to humans.

Other Effects

Animal Studies A nicotine bolus (up to 2 mg/kg) to pregnant rhesus monkeys caused acidosis, hypercarbia, and hypotension (fetal and maternal concentrations were about 20 times those achieved after smoking one cigarette in 5 minutes). Fetal breathing movements were reduced in the fetal lamb after intravenous injection of 0.25 mg/kg nicotine to the ewe (equivalent to smoking 1 cigarette every 20 seconds for 5 minutes). Uterine blood flow was reduced about 30% after infusion of 0.1 µg/kg/min nicotine to pregnant rhesus monkeys (equivalent to smoking about six cigarettes every minute for 20 minutes)
Human Experience Cigarette smoking during pregnancy is associated with an increased risk of spontaneous abortion, low birth weight infants and perinatal mortality. Nicotine and carbon monoxide are considered the most likely mediators of these outcomes. The effects of cigarette smoking on fetal cardiovascular parameters have been studied near term. Cigarettes increased fetal aortic blood flow and heart rate and decreased uterine blood flow and fetal breathing movements. NICOTROL NS has not been studied in pregnant women.

Labor and Delivery

NICOTROL NS is not recommended for use during labor and delivery. The effect of nicotine on a mother or the fetus during labor is unknown.

Use in Nursing Mothers

Caution should be exercised when NICOTROL NS is administered to nursing mothers. The safety of NICOTROL NS therapy in nursing infants has not been examined. Nicotine passes freely into breast milk; the milk to plasma ratio averages 2.9. Nicotine is absorbed orally. An infant has the ability to clear nicotine by hepatic first-pass clearance; however, the efficiency of removal is probably lowest at birth. Nicotine concentrations in milk can be expected to be lower with NICOTROL NS when used as recommended than with cigarette smoking, as maternal plasma nicotine concentrations are generally reduced with nicotine replacement. The risk of exposure of the infant to nicotine from NICOTROL NS therapy should be weighed against the risks associated

Continued on next page

Nicotrol NS—Cont.

with the infant's exposure to nicotine from continued smoking by the mother (passive smoke exposure and contamination of breast milk with other components of tobacco smoke) and from NICOTROL NS alone, or in combination with continued smoking.

Pediatric Use

NICOTROL NS therapy is not recommended for use in the pediatric population because its safety and effectiveness in children and adolescents who smoke have not been evaluated.

Geriatric Use

Forty-one patients over the age of 60 participated in clinical trials of NICOTROL NS. The spray appeared to be as effective in this age group as in younger smokers. Because medical conditions that are precautions to nicotine use are more common in the elderly, physicians should use care in prescribing this product to these patients.

ADVERSE REACTIONS

Assessment of adverse events in the 730 patients who participated in controlled clinical trials is complicated by the occurrence of signs and symptoms of nicotine withdrawal in some patients and nicotine excess in others. The incidence of adverse events is confounded by the many minor complaints that smokers commonly have, by continued smoking by many patients and the local irritation from both active drug and the pepper placebo. No serious adverse events were reported during the trials.

Common Smoker's Complaints

Common complaints experienced by the smokers in the study (users of both active and placebo spray) include, chest tightness, dyspepsia, paraesthesia (tingling) in limbs, constipation, and stomatitis.

Tobacco Withdrawal Symptoms

Symptoms of tobacco withdrawal were frequent in users of both active and placebo sprays. Common withdrawal symptoms seen in over 5% of patients included: anxiety, irritability, restlessness, cravings, dizziness, impaired concentration, weight increase, emotional lability, somnolence and fatigue, increased sweating, and insomnia. Less frequently seen probable withdrawal symptoms (under 5%) included: confusion, depression, apathy, tremor, increased appetite, incoordination and increased dreaming.

Anxiety, irritability, restlessness and tobacco cravings occurred about equally in both groups, while other symptoms tended to be slightly more common on placebo spray.

Effects of the Spray

NICOTROL NS and the pepper-containing placebo were both associated with irritant side effects on the nasopharyngeal and ocular tissues. During the first 2 days of treatment, nasal irritation was reported by nearly all (94%) of the patients, the majority of whom rated it as either moderate or severe. Both the frequency and severity of nasal irritation declined with continued use of NICOTROL NS but was still experienced by most (81%) of the patients after 3 weeks of treatment, with most patients rating it as moderate or mild. Other common side-effects for both active and placebo groups were runny nose, throat irritation, watering eyes, sneezing, and cough.

The following local events were reported somewhat more commonly for active than for placebo spray: nasal congestion, subjective comments related to the taste or use of the dosage form, sinus irritation, transient epistaxis, eye irritation, transient changes in sense of smell, pharyngitis, paraethesias of the nose, mouth or head, numbness of the nose, or mouth, burning of the nose or eyes, earache, facial flushing, transient changes in sense of taste, hoarseness, nasal ulcer or blister.

Effects of Nicotine

Feelings of dependence on the spray were reported by more patients on active spray than placebo. Drug-like effects such as calming were also more frequent on active spray. (See **DRUG ABUSE AND DEPENDENCE**)

Other Adverse Effects

Adverse events which could not be classified and listed above and which were reported by >1% of patients on active spray are listed in the following table

Adverse Events Not Attributable to Intercurrent Illness

Adverse Event	Active	Placebo
HEADACHE	18%	15%
BACK PAIN	6%	4%
DYSPNEA	5%	6%
NAUSEA	5%	5%
ARTHRALGIA	5%	1%
MENSTRUAL DISORDER	4%	4%
PALPITATION	4%	4%
FLATULENCE	4%	3%
TOOTH DISORDER	4%	1%
GUM PROBLEMS	4%	1%
MYALGIA	3%	4%
ABDOMINAL PAIN	3%	3%
CONFUSION	3%	3%
ACNE	3%	1%
DYSMENORRHEA	3%	0%
PRURITUS	2%	3%

Adverse events reported with a frequency of <1% among active spray users are listed below:

Body as a Whole: edema peripheral, pain, numbness, allergy

Gastrointestinal: dry mouth, hiccup, diarrhea

Hematologic: purpura

Neurological: aphasia, amnesia, migraine, numbness

Respiratory: bronchitis, bronchospasm, sputum increased

Skin and appendages: rash, purpura

Special Senses: vision abnormal

DRUG ABUSE AND DEPENDENCE

NICOTROL NS has a dependence potential intermediate between other nicotine-based therapies and cigarettes. This is the result of differences between cigarettes, NICOTROL NS, nicotine gum and nicotine patches in pharmacokinetic and dosing characteristics commonly associated with abuse and dependence. NICOTROL NS is distinct from other nicotine-based smoking cessation therapies in its greater speed of onset, greater capacity for self-titration of dose, and frequent and rapid fluctuations in plasma nicotine concentration.

Dependence on nicotine nasal spray occurred in the clinical trials. Feelings of dependency on the spray were reported by 32% of active spray users and 13% of placebo spray users. Such dependence may represent transference of tobacco-related nicotine dependence to NICOTROL NS.

Fifteen to 20% of patients used the active spray for longer periods than recommended (6 months to 1 year) and 5% used the spray at a higher dose than recommended. Some of these patients experienced anxiety about stopping the spray and some reported craving for the spray rather than for cigarettes.

OVERDOSAGE

The oral LD_{50} for nicotine is >5 mg/kg in dogs and >24 mg/kg in rodents. Death is due to respiratory paralysis. The oral minimum acute lethal dose for nicotine in adult humans is reported to be 40 to 60 mg (<1 mg/kg). A full bottle of NICOTROL NS contains 100 mg of nicotine.

NICOTROL NS would be expected to be irritating if sprayed in the eyes, mouth or ears. Eye exposure should be treated with copious irrigation with water for 20 minutes. Large oral nicotine ingestions cause vomiting, and the consequences of an overdose will vary; should this occur, patients should contact their physician immediately. For additional emergency information, call your regional poison center.

Signs and Symptoms of Nicotine Toxicity

Signs and symptoms of an overdose of NICOTROL NS would be expected to be the same as those of acute nicotine poisoning including: pallor, cold sweat, nausea, salivation, vomiting, abdominal pain, diarrhea, headache, dizziness, disturbed hearing and vision, tremor, mental confusion, and weakness. Prostration, hypotension, and respiratory failure may ensue with large overdoses. Lethal doses produce convulsions quickly and death follows as a result of peripheral or central respiratory paralysis or, less frequently, cardiac failure.

Overdose from Ingestion

If emesis has not occurred, it should be induced in conscious patients with a suitable emetic followed by an appropriate dose of activated charcoal. In unconscious patients with a secure airway, instill activated charcoal via a nasogastric tube. A saline cathartic or sorbitol may be added to the first dose of activated charcoal.

Management of Nicotine Poisoning

Other supportive measures include diazepam or barbiturates for seizures, atropine for excessive bronchial secretions or diarrhea, respiratory support for respiratory failure, and vigorous fluid support for hypotension and cardiovascular collapse.

DOSAGE AND ADMINISTRATION

It is important that patients understand the instructions for use of NICOTROL NS, and have their questions answered. They should clearly understand the directions for using NICOTROL NS and safely disposing of the used container. They should be instructed to stop smoking completely when they begin using the product.

Patients should be instructed not to sniff, swallow or inhale through the nose as the spray is being administered. They should also be advised to administer the spray with the head tilted back slightly.

The dose of NICOTROL NS, should be **individualized** on the basis of each patient's nicotine dependence and the occurrence of symptoms of nicotine excess (See Individualization of Dosage).

Each actuation of NICOTROL NS delivers a metered 50 microliter spray containing 0.5 mg of nicotine. One dose is 1 mg of nicotine (2 sprays, one in each nostril).

Patients should be started with 1 or 2 doses per hour, which may be increased up to a maximum recommended dose of 40 mg (80 sprays, somewhat less than 1/2 bottle) per day. For best results, patients should be encouraged to use at least the recommended minimum of 8 doses per day, as less is unlikely to be effective. In clinicals trials, the patients who successfully quit smoking used the product heavily when nicotine withdrawal was at its peak, sometimes up to the recommended maximum of 40 doses per day (in heavier smokers). Dosing recommendations are summarized in Table 4.

[See table 4 below]

No tapering strategy has been shown to be optimal in clinical studies. Many patients simply stopped using the spray at their last clinic visit.

Recommended strategies for discontinuation of use include suggesting that patients: use only 1/2 a dose (1 spray) at a time, use the spray less frequently, keep a tally of daily usage, try to meet a steadily reducing usage target, skip a dose by not medicating every hour, or set a planned "quit date" for stopping use of the spray.

Individualization of Dosage

The success or failure of smoking cessation is influenced by the quality, intensity and frequency of supportive care. Patients are more likely to quit smoking if they are seen frequently and participate in formal smoking cessation programs.

The goal of NICOTROL NS therapy is complete abstinence. If a patient is unable to stop smoking by the fourth week of therapy, treatment should probably be discontinued.

Patients who fail to quit on any attempt may benefit from interventions to improve their chances for success on subsequent attempts. Patients who were unsuccessful should be counseled and should then probably be given a "therapy holiday" before the next attempt. A new quit attempt should be encouraged when conditions are more favorable.

Based on the clinical trials, a reasonable approach to assisting patients in their attempt to quit smoking is to begin initial treatment, using the recommended dosage (See **DOSAGE AND ADMINISTRATION**). Regular use of the spray during the first week of treatment may help patients adapt to the irritant effects of the spray. Dosage can then be adjusted in those subjects with signs or symptoms of nicotine withdrawal or excess. Patients who are successfully abstinent on NICOTROL NS should be treated at the selected dosage for up to 8 weeks, following which use of the spray should be discontinued over the next 4 to 6 weeks. Some patients may not require gradual reduction of dosage and may abruptly stop treatment successfully. Treatment with NICOTROL NS for longer periods has not been shown to improve outcome, and the safety of use for periods longer than 6 months has not been established.

The symptoms of nicotine withdrawal overlap those of nicotine excess (See **Pharmacodynamics and ADVERSE REACTIONS** sections). Since patients using NICOTROL NS may also smoke intermittently, it is sometimes difficult to determine if patients are experiencing nicotine withdrawal or nicotine excess. Controlled clinical trials of nicotine products suggest that palpitations, nausea and sweating are more often symptoms of nicotine excess, whereas anxiety, nervousness and irritability are more often symptoms of nicotine withdrawal

SAFETY AND HANDLING

As with all medicines, especially ones in liquid form, care should be taken in handling NICOTROL NS during periods of opening and closing the container (See **WARNINGS and Safety Note Concerning Children**). If it is dropped it may break. If this occurs, the spill should be cleaned up immediately with an absorbent cloth/paper towel. Care should be taken to avoid contact of the solution with the skin. Broken glass should be picked up carefully, using a broom. The area of the spill should be washed several times. Absorbent material may be disposed of as any other household waste. Should even a small amount of NICOTROL NS come in contact with the skin, lips, mouth, eyes or ears, the affected area(s) should be immediately rinsed with water only.

Disposal

Used bottles of NICOTROL NS should be disposed of with their child-resistant caps in place. Used bottles should be disposed of in such a way as to prevent access by children or pets. See patient information for further information on handling and disposal.

HOW SUPPLIED

NDC 0045-0899-01

Nicotrol® NS (nicotine nasal spray) 10 mg/mL, is supplied in individual 10 mL bottles.

Each unit consists of a glass container, mounted with a metered spray pump

A patient information leaflet is enclosed with the package

Store at room temperature not to exceed 30°C/86°F.

CAUTION: Federal law prohibits dispensing without prescription.

Manufactured by Pharmacia and Upjohn AB, Sweden

Distributed by: McNEIL Consumer Healthcare
Division of McNEIL-PPC, Inc.
Fort Washington, PA 19034 USA
©McN-PPC, Inc. '96
MADE IN SWEDEN
U.S. Patent No. 5,374,659

Shown in Product Identification Guide, page 322

Table 4

Maximum Recommended Duration of Treatment	Recommended Doses per Hour	Maximum Doses per Hour	Maximum Doses per Day
3 months	1–2*	5	40

* One dose = 2 sprays (one in each nostril). One dose delivers 1 mg of nicotine to the nasal mucosa.

NICOTROL® OTC
NICOTINE TRANSDERMAL SYSTEM

DESCRIPTION

NICOTROL® (nicotine transdermal system) is a multilayered, rectangular, thin film laminated unit containing nicotine as the active ingredient. ***NICOTROL®*** Patch provides systemic delivery of 15 mg of nicotine over 16 hours. ***NICOTROL®*** Patch is for people who smoke over 10 cigarettes a day.

ACTIONS

NICOTROL® (nicotine transdermal system) Patch helps smokers quit by reducing nicotine withdrawal symptoms. Many ***NICOTROL®*** Patch users will be able to stop smoking for a few days but often will start smoking again. Most smokers have to try to quit several times before they completely stop.
Your own chances of quitting smoking depend on how much you want to quit, how strongly you are addicted to nicotine and how closely you follow a quitting program like the PATHWAYS TO CHANGE® Program that comes with the ***NICOTROL®*** Patch.
If you find you cannot stop or if you start smoking again after using ***NICOTROL®*** Patch, please talk to a health care professional who can help you find a program that may work better for you. Remember that breaking this addiction doesn't happen overnight.
Because the ***NICOTROL®*** Patch provides some nicotine, the ***NICOTROL®*** Patch will help you stop smoking by reducing nicotine withdrawal symptoms such as nicotine cravings, nervousness and irritability.

USE

To reduce withdrawal symptoms, including nicotine craving, associated with quitting smoking.

DIRECTIONS

- Stop smoking completely when you begin using the ***NICOTROL®*** Patch.
- Refer to enclosed patient information leaflet before using this product.
- Use one ***NICOTROL®*** Patch every day for six weeks. Remove backing from the patch and immediately press onto clean dry hairless skin. Hold for ten seconds. Wash hands.
- The ***NICOTROL®*** Patch should be worn during awake hours and removed prior to sleep.

For Best Results In Quitting Smoking:
1. Firmly commit to quitting smoking.
2. Use enclosed support materials.
3. Use the ***NICOTROL®*** Patches for six weeks.
4. Stop using ***NICOTROL®*** Patches at the end of week six. If you still feel the need for ***NICOTROL®*** Patches talk to your doctor.

WARNINGS

- Keep this and all medication out of reach of children and pets. Even used patches have enough nicotine to poison children and pets. Be sure to fold sticky ends together and throw away out of reach of children and pets. In case of accidental overdose, seek professional assistance or contact a poison control center immediately.
- Nicotine can increase your baby's heart rate. First try to stop smoking without the nicotine patch. As with any drug, if you are pregnant or nursing a baby, seek the advice of a health professional before using this product.
- Do not smoke even when you are not wearing the patch. The nicotine in your skin will still be entering your bloodstream for several hours after you take the patch off.
- If you forget to remove the patch at bedtime you may have vivid dreams or other sleep disruptions.

Do Not Use if You:
- Continue to smoke, chew tobacco, use snuff, or use a nicotine gum or other nicotine containing products.

Ask Your Doctor Before Use if You:
- Are under 18 years of age.
- Have heart disease, recent heart attack or irregular heartbeat. Nicotine can increase your heart rate.
- Have high blood pressure not controlled with medication. Nicotine can increase blood pressure.
- Take prescription medicine for depression or asthma. Your prescription dose may need to be adjusted.
- Are allergic to adhesive tape or have skin problems, because you are more likely to get rashes.

Stop Use and See Your Doctor if You Have:
- Skin redness caused by the patch that does not go away after four days, or if your skin swells or you get a rash.
- Irregular heartbeat or palpitations.
- Symptoms of nicotine overdose such as nausea, vomiting, dizziness, weakness and rapid heartbeat.

INACTIVE INGREDIENTS

polyisobutylenes, polybutene non-woven polyester, pigmented aluminized and clear polyesters.

HOW SUPPLIED

Starter Kit-7, Refill Kit-7. DO NOT USE IF POUCH IS DAMAGED OR OPEN. Do not Store above 86°F (30°C)
- **Not for sale to those under 18 years of age.**
- **Proof of age required.**
- **Not for sale in vending machines or from any source where proof of age cannot be verified.**

Shown in Product Identification Guide, page 322

NIZORAL® A-D OTC
KETOCONAZOLE SHAMPOO 1%

DESCRIPTION

Nizoral® A-D (Ketoconazole Shampoo 1%) Anti-Dandruff Shampoo is a light-blue liquid for topical application, containing the broad spectrum synthetic antifungal agent Ketoconazole in a concentration of 1%.

Use: ***Nizoral® A-D*** controls the flaking, scaling, and itching associated with dandruff.

DIRECTIONS

Adults and children over 12 years of age:
- wet hair thoroughly
- apply shampoo, generously lather, rinse thoroughly. Repeat.
- use every 3–4 days for up to 8 weeks if needed, or as directed by a doctor. Then use only as needed to control dandruff.

Children under 12 years of age: Ask a doctor.

WARNINGS

Do Not Use:
- on scalp that is broken or inflamed
- if you are allergic to ingredients in this product

When Using This Product:
- do not get into eyes
- if product gets into eyes, rinse thoroughly with water

Stop Using This Product If:
- rash appears
- condition worsens or does not improve in 2–4 weeks

Ask a doctor. These may be signs of a serious condition.
For external use only.
As with any drug, if you are pregnant or nursing a baby, seek the advice of a health professional before using this product.
Keep this and all drugs out of the reach of children.
In case of accidental ingestion, seek professional assistance or contact a Poison Control Center immediately.
STORAGE: Store between 35° and 86°F (2° and 30°C). Protect from light. Protect from freezing.

PROFESSIONAL INFORMATION

OVERDOSAGE INFORMATION

Nizoral® A-D (Ketoconazole) 1% Shampoo is intended for external use only. In the event of accidental ingestion, supportive measures should be employed. Induced emesis and gastric lavage should usually be avoided.

INACTIVE INGREDIENTS

Water, Sodium Laureth Sulfate, Cocamide MEA, Sodium Cocoyl Sarcosinate, Glycol Distearate, Acrylic Acid Polymer (Carbomer 1342), Fragrance, Sodium Chloride, Tetrasodium EDTA, Butylated Hydroxytoluene, Quaternium-15, Polyquaternium-7, Sodium Hydroxide and/or Hydrochloric Acid, FD&C Blue No. 1.

HOW SUPPLIED

Available in 4 and 7 fl. oz. bottles.
Shown in Product Identification Guide, page 322

NIZORAL® ℞
[nī 'zōr-ăl]
(ketoconazole) 2% Cream

DESCRIPTION

NIZORAL® (ketoconazole) 2% Cream contains the broad-spectrum synthetic antifungal agent, ketoconazole 2%, formulated in an aqueous cream vehicle consisting of propylene glycol, stearyl and cetyl alcohols, sorbitan monostearate, polysorbate 60, isopropyl myristate, sodium sulfite anhydrous, polysorbate 80 and purified water.
Ketoconazole is *cis* -1-acetyl-4-[4-[[2-(2,4-dichlorophenyl)-2-(1*H* -imidazol -1- ylmethyl) -1, 3- dioxolan -4- yl] methoxy]phenyl]piperazine.

CLINICAL PHARMACOLOGY

When NIZORAL® (ketoconazole) 2% Cream was applied dermally to intact or abraded skin of Beagle dogs for 28 consecutive days at a dose of 80 mg, there were no detectable plasma levels using an assay method having a lower detection limit of 2 ng/ml.
After a single topical application to the chest, back and arms of normal volunteers, systemic absorption of ketoconazole was not detected at the 5 ng/ml level in blood over a 72-hour period.
Two dermal irritancy studies, a human sensitization test, a phototoxicity study and a photoallergy study conducted in 38 male and 62 female volunteers showed no contact sensitization of the delayed hypersensitivity type, no irritation, no phototoxicity and no photoallergenic potential due to NIZORAL® (ketoconazole) 2% Cream.
Microbiology: Ketoconazole is a broad spectrum synthetic antifungal agent which inhibits the *in vitro* growth of the following common dermatophytes and yeasts by altering the permeability of the cell membrane: dermatophytes: *Trichophyton rubrum, T. mentagrophytes, T. tonsurans, Microsporum canis, M. audouini, M. gypseum* and *Epidermophyton floccosum;* yeasts: *Candida albicans, Malassezia ovale* (*Pityrosporum ovale*) and *C. tropicalis;* and the organism responsible for tinea versicolor, *Malassezia furfur* (*Pityrosporum orbiculare*). Only those organisms listed in the INDICATIONS AND USAGE Section have been proven to be clinically affected. Development of resistance to ketoconazole has not been reported.
Mode of Action: *In vitro* studies suggest that ketoconazole impairs the synthesis of ergosterol, which is a vital component of fungal cell membranes. It is postulated that the therapeutic effect of ketoconazole in seborrheic dermatitis is due to the reduction of M. ovale, but this has not been proven.

INDICATIONS AND USAGE

NIZORAL® (ketoconazole) 2% Cream is indicated for the topical treatment of tinea corporis, tinea cruris and tinea pedis caused by *Trichophyton rubrum, T. mentagrophytes* and *Epidermophyton floccosum;* in the treatment of tinea (pityriasis) versicolor caused by *Malassezia furfur (Pityrosporum orbiculare);* in the treatment of cutaneous candidiasis caused by *Candida spp.* and in the treatment of seborrheic dermatitis.

CONTRAINDICATIONS

NIZORAL® (ketoconazole) 2% Cream is contraindicated in persons who have shown hypersensitivity to the active or excipient ingredients of this formulation.

WARNINGS

NIZORAL® (ketoconazole) 2% Cream is not for ophthalmic use.
NIZORAL® (ketoconazole) 2% Cream contains sodium sulfite anhydrous, a sulfite that may cause allergic-type reactions including anaphylactic symptoms and life-threatening or less severe asthmatic episodes in certain susceptible people. The overall prevalence of sulfite sensitivity in the general population is unknown and probably low. Sulfite sensitivity is seen more frequently in asthmatic than in nonasthmatic people.

PRECAUTIONS

General: If a reaction suggesting sensitivity or chemical irritation should occur, use of the medication should be discontinued. Hepatitis (1:10,000 reported incidence) and, at high doses, lowered testosterone and ACTH induced corticosteroid serum levels have been seen with orally administered ketoconazole; these effects have not been seen with topical ketoconazole.
Carcinogenesis, Mutagenesis, Impairment of Fertility: A long-term feeding study in Swiss Albino mice and in Wistar rats showed no evidence of oncogenic activity. The dominant lethal mutation test in male and female mice revealed that single oral doses of ketoconazole as high as 80 mg/kg produced no mutation in any stage of germ cell development. The Ames' *Salmonella* microsomal activator assay was also negative.
Pregnancy: Teratogenic effects: Pregnancy Category C: Ketoconazole has been shown to be teratogenic (syndactylia and oligodactylia) in the rat when given orally in the diet at 80 mg/kg/day, (10 times the maximum recommended human oral dose). However, these effects may be related to maternal toxicity, which was seen at this and higher dose levels.
There are no adequate and well-controlled studies in pregnant women. Ketoconazole should be used during pregnancy only if the potential benefit justifies the potential risk to the fetus.
Nursing Mothers: It is not known whether NIZORAL® (ketoconazole) 2% Cream administered topically could result in sufficient systemic absorption to produce detectable quantities in breast milk. Nevertheless, a decision should be made whether to discontinue nursing or discontinue the drug, taking into account the importance of the drug to the mother.
Pediatric Use: Safety and effectiveness in children have not been established.

ADVERSE REACTIONS

During clinical trials 45 (5.0%) of 905 patients treated with NIZORAL® (ketoconazole) 2% Cream and 5 (2.4%) of 208 patients treated with placebo reported side effects consisting mainly of severe irritation, pruritus and stinging. One of the patients treated with NIZORAL® Cream developed a painful allergic reaction.
In worldwide postmarketing experience, rare reports of contact dermatitis have been associated with NIZORAL Cream or one of its excipients, namely sodium sulfite or propylene glycol.

DOSAGE AND ADMINISTRATION

Cutaneous candidiasis, tinea corporis, tinea cruris, tinea pedis, and *tinea (pityriasis) versicolor:* It is recommended that NIZORAL® (ketoconazole) 2% Cream be applied once daily to cover the affected and immediate surrounding area. Clinical improvement may be seen fairly soon after treatment is begun; however, candidal infections and tinea cruris and corporis should be treated for two weeks in order to reduce the possibility of recurrence. Patients with tinea versicolor usually require two weeks of treatment. Patients with tinea pedis require six weeks of treatment.
Seborrheic dermatitis: NIZORAL® (ketoconazole) 2% Cream should be applied to the affected area twice daily for four weeks or until clinical clearing.
If a patient shows no clinical improvement after the treatment period, the diagnosis should be redetermined.

Continued on next page

Nizoral Cream—Cont.

HOW SUPPLIED

NIZORAL® (ketoconazole) 2% Cream is supplied in 15 (NDC 50580-374-15), 30 (NDC 50580-374-30) and 60 (NDC 50580-374-60) gm tubes.
Store below 77°F (25°C)
Revised July 1994, April 1995
U.S. Patent No. 4,335,125
McNeil Consumer Healthcare
Fort Washington, PA 19034
Shown in Product Identification Guide, page 322

NIZORAL® ℞
[*nī 'zōr-ăl*]
(ketoconazole) 2% Shampoo

DESCRIPTION

NIZORAL® (ketoconazole) 2% Shampoo is a red-orange liquid for topical application, containing the broad-spectrum synthetic antifungal agent ketoconazole in a concentration of 2% in an aqueous suspension. It also contains: coconut fatty acid diethanolamide, disodium monolauryl ether sulfosuccinate, F.D. & C. Red No. 40, hydrochloric acid, imidurea, laurdimonium hydrolyzed animal collagen, macrogol 120 methyl-glucose dioleate, perfume bouquet, sodium chloride, sodium hydroxide, sodium lauryl ether sulfate, and purified water.
Ketoconazole is cis-1-acetyl-4-[4-[[2-(2,4-di-chlorophenyl)-2-(1H-imidazol-1-ylmethyl)-1,3-dioxolan-4-yl]methoxy]phenyl]piperazine.

CLINICAL PHARMACOLOGY

Tinea (pityriasis) versicolor is a non-contagious infection of the skin caused by *Pityrosporum orbiculare (Malassezia furfur)*. This commensal organism is part of the normal skin flora. In susceptible individuals the condition is often recurrent and may give rise to hyperpigmented or hypopigmented patches on the trunk which may extend to the neck, arms and upper thighs. Treatment of the infection may not immediately result in restoration of pigment to the affected sites. Normalization of pigment following successful therapy is variable and may take months, depending on individual skin type and incidental skin exposure. The rate of recurrence of infection is variable.
When ketoconazole 2% shampoo was applied dermally to intact or abraded skin of rabbits for 28 days at doses up to 50 mg/kg and allowed to remain one hour before being washed away, there were no detectable plasma ketoconazole levels using an assay method having a lower detection limit of 5 ng/mL. NIZORAL® (ketoconazole) was not detected in plasma in 39 patients who shampooed 4–10 times per week for 6 months or in 33 patients who shampooed 2–3 times per week for 3–26 months (mean: 16 months).
An exaggerated use washing test on the sensitive antecubital skin of 10 subjects twice daily for five consecutive days showed that the irritancy potential of ketoconazole 2% shampoo was significantly less than that of 2.5% selenium sulfide shampoo.
A human sensitization test, a phototoxicity study, and a photoallergy study conducted in 38 male and 22 female volunteers showed no contact sensitization of the delayed hypersensitivity type, no phototoxicity and no photoallergenic potential due to NIZORAL® (ketoconazole) 2% Shampoo.
Mode of Action: Interpretations of *in vivo* studies suggest that ketoconazole impairs the synthesis of ergosterol, which is a vital component of fungal cell membranes. It is postulated, but not proven, that the therapeutic effect of ketoconazole in tinea (pityriasis) versicolor is due to the reduction of *Pityrosporum orbiculare (Malassezia furfur)* and that the therapeutic effect in dandruff is due to the reduction of *Pityrosporum ovale*. Support for the therapeutic effect in tinea versicolor comes from a three-arm, parallel, double-blind, placebo-controlled study in patients who had moderately severe tinea (pityriasis) versicolor. Successful response rates in the primary efficacy population for each of both three-day and single-day regimens of ketoconazole 2% shampoo were statistically significantly greater (73% and 69%, respectively) than a placebo regimen (5%). There had been mycological confirmation of fungal disease in all cases at baseline. Mycological clearing rates were 84% and 78%, respectively, for the three-day and one-day regimens of the 2% shampoo and 11% in the placebo regimen. While the differences in the rates of successful response between either of the two active treatments and placebo were statistically significant, the difference between the two active regimens was not.
Microbiology: NIZORAL® (ketoconazole) is a broad-spectrum synthetic antifungal agent which inhibits the growth of the following common dermatophytes and yeasts by altering the permeability of the cell membrane: dermatophytes: *Trichophyton rubrum, T. mentagrophytes, T. tonsurans, Microsporum canis, M. audouini, M. gypseum* and *Epidermophyton floccosum;* yeasts: *Candida albicans, C. tropicalis, Pityrosporum ovale (Malassezia ovale)* and *Pityrosporum orbiculare (M. furfur)*. Development of resistance by these microorganisms to ketoconazole has not been reported.

INDICATIONS AND USAGE

NIZORAL® (ketoconazole) 2% Shampoo is indicated for the treatment of tinea (pityriasis) versicolor caused by or presumed to be caused by *Pityrosporum orbiculare* (also known as *Malassezia furfur* or *M. orbiculare*).
Note: Tinea (pityriasis) versicolor may give rise to hyperpigmented or hypopigmented patches on the trunk which may extend to the neck, arms and upper thighs. Treatment of the infection may not immediately result in normalization of pigment to the affected sites. Normalization of pigment following successful therapy is variable and may take months, depending on individual skin type and incidental sun exposure. Although tinea versicolor is not contagious, it may recur because the organism that causes the disease is part of the normal skin flora.

CONTRAINDICATIONS

NIZORAL® (ketoconazole) 2% Shampoo is contraindicated in persons who have shown hypersensitivity to the active ingredient or excipients of this formulation.

PRECAUTIONS

General: If a reaction suggesting sensitivity or chemical irritation should occur, use of the medication should be discontinued.
Information for Patients: May be irritating to mucous membranes of the eyes and contact with this area should be avoided.
There have been reports that use of the shampoo resulted in removal of the curl from permanently waved hair.
Carcinogenesis, Mutagenesis, Impairment of Fertility: The dominant lethal mutation test in male and female mice revealed that single oral doses of ketoconazole as high as 80 mg/kg produced no mutation in any stage of germ cell development. The Ames Salmonella microsomal activator assay was also negative. A long-term feeding study of ketoconazole in Swiss Albino mice and in Wistar rats showed no evidence of oncogenic activity.
Pregnancy: Teratogenic effects: Pregnancy Category C: Ketoconazole is not detected in plasma after chronic shampooing. Ketoconazole has been shown to be teratogenic (syndactylia and oligodactylia) in the rat when given orally in the diet at 80 mg/kg/day (10 times the maximum recommended human oral dose). However, these effects may be related to maternal toxicity, which was seen at this and higher dose levels.
There are no adequate and well-controlled studies in pregnant women. Ketoconazole should be used during pregnancy only if the potential benefit justifies the potential risk to the fetus.
Nursing mothers: Ketoconazole is not detected in plasma after chronic shampooing. Nevertheless, caution should be exercised when NIZORAL® (ketoconazole) 2% Shampoo is administered to a nursing woman.
Pediatric Use: Safety and effectiveness in children have not been established.

ADVERSE REACTIONS

In 11 double-blind trials in 264 patients using ketoconazole 2% shampoo for the treatment of dandruff or seborrheic dermatitis, an increase in normal hair loss and irritation occurred in less than 1% of patients. In three open-label safety trials in which 41 patients shampooed 4–10 times weekly for six months, the following adverse experiences each occurred once: abnormal hair texture, scalp pustules, mild dryness of the skin, and itching. As with other shampoos, oiliness and dryness of hair and scalp have been reported.
In a double-blind, placebo-controlled trial in which patients with tinea versicolor were treated with either a single application of NIZORAL® (ketoconazole) 2% Shampoo (n=106), a daily application for three consecutive days (n=107), or placebo (n=105), drug-related adverse events occurred in 5 (5%), 7 (7%) and 4 (4%) of patients, respectively. The only events that occurred in more than one patient in any one of the three treatment groups were pruritus, application site reaction, and dry skin; none of these events occurred in more than 3% of the patients in any one of the three groups.

OVERDOSAGE

NIZORAL® (ketoconazole) 2% Shampoo is intended for external use only. In the event of accidental ingestion, supportive measures should be employed. Induced emesis and gastric lavage should usually be avoided.

DOSAGE AND ADMINISTRATION

Apply the shampoo to the damp skin of the affected area and a wide margin surrounding this area. Lather, leave in place for 5 minutes, and then rinse off with water.
One application of the shampoo should be sufficient.

HOW SUPPLIED

NIZORAL® (ketoconazole) 2% Shampoo is a red-orange liquid supplied in a 4-fluid ounce nonbreakable plastic bottle (NDC 50580-432-04).
Storage conditions: Store at a temperature not above 25°C (77°F). Protect from light.
Manufactured by:
Janssen Cilag SPA
Latina, Italy
Distributed by:
McNeil Consumer Healthcare
Fort Washington, PA 19034
Revised June 1996, August 1997
U.S. Patent No. 4,335,125
Shown in Product Identification Guide, page 322

SIMPLY SLEEP™ OTC
Nighttime Sleep Aid

DESCRIPTION

SIMPLY SLEEP™ is a non habit-forming nighttime sleep aid. Each ***SIMPLY SLEEP™*** Caplet contains diphenhydramine HCl 25 mg.

ACTIONS

SIMPLY SLEEP™ contains an antihistamine (diphenhydramine HCl) which has sedative properties.

USES

For relief of occasional sleeplessness.

DIRECTIONS

Adults and Children 12 years of age and older: Take 2 Caplets at bedtime if needed or as directed by a doctor.
Children under 12 years of age: Do not give this product to children under 12 years of age.

PRECAUTIONS

If a rare sensitivity reaction occurs, the drug should be discontinued.

WARNINGS

Do not give to children under 12 years of age. If sleeplessness persists continuously for more than 2 weeks, consult your doctor. Insomnia may be a symptom of serious underlying medical illness. Do not take this product, unless directed by a doctor, if you have a breathing problem such as emphysema or chronic bronchitis, or if you have glaucoma or difficulty in urination due to enlargement of the prostate gland. Avoid alcoholic beverages while taking this product. Do not take this product if you are taking sedatives or tranquilizers, without first consulting your doctor.
Keep this and all drugs out of the reach of children. In case of accidental overdose, contact a doctor or poison control center immediately. As with any drug, if you are pregnant or nursing a baby, seek the advice of a health care professional before using this product.
Do not use if carton is opened or blister unit is broken.

INACTIVE INGREDIENTS

Cellulose, Croscarmellose Sodium, Dibasic Calcium Phosphate, Dihydrate, FD&C Blue #1, Hydroxypropyl Methylcellulose, Magnesium Stearate, Polyethylene Glycol, Polysorbate 80, Titanium Dioxide.

HOW SUPPLIED

Light blue mini-caplets embossed with "SL" on one side in blister packs of 24 and 48. Store at room temperature.
Shown in Product Identification Guide, page 322

Extra Strength **OTC**
TYLENOL® acetaminophen
Gelcaps, Geltabs, Caplets, Tablets

Extra Strength
TYLENOL® acetaminophen
Adult Liquid Pain Reliever

Regular Strength
TYLENOL® acetaminophen
Caplets and Tablets

TYLENOL® Arthritis Pain Extended Relief Caplets
acetaminophen extended release
Caplets

Product information for all dosage forms of Adult TYLENOL acetaminophen have been combined under this heading.

DESCRIPTION

Each ***Extra Strength TYLENOL® Gelcap, Geltab, Caplet, or Tablet*** contains acetaminophen 500 mg.
Each 15 mL ($^1/_2$ fl oz or one tablespoonful) of ***Extra Strength TYLENOL® Adult Liquid Pain Reliever*** contains 500 mg acetaminophen (alcohol 7%).
Each ***Regular Strength TYLENOL® Caplet or Tablet*** contains acetaminophen 325 mg.
Each ***TYLENOL® Arthritis Pain Extended Relief Caplet*** contains acetaminophen 650 mg.

ACTIONS

Acetaminophen is a clinically proven analgesic and antipyretic. Acetaminophen produces analgesia by elevation of the pain threshold and antipyresis through action on the hypothalamic heat regulating center. Acetaminophen is equal to aspirin in analgesic and antipyretic effectiveness and it is unlikely to produce many of the side effects associated with aspirin and aspirin-containing products.
Tylenol Arthritis Extended Relief uses a unique, patented bilayer caplet. The first layer dissolves quickly to provide prompt relief while the second layer is time released to provide up to 8 hours of relief.

USES

For the temporary relief of minor aches and pains associated with headache, muscular aches, backache, minor arthritis pain, common cold, toothache, menstrual cramps and for the reduction of fever.

DIRECTIONS

Extra Strength TYLENOL® Gelcaps, Geltabs, Caplets, or Tablets: **Adults and children 12 years of age and older:** Take 2 gelcaps, geltabs, caplets, or tablets every 4 to 6 hours as needed. Do not take more than 8 gelcaps, geltabs, caplets or tablets in 24 hours, or as directed by a doctor. **Children under 12 years:** Do not use this adult Extra Strength product in children under 12 years of age. This will provide more than the recommended dose (overdose) of TYLENOL® and could cause serious health problems.
Extra Strength TYLENOL® Adult Liquid Pain Reliever: **Adults and children 12 years of age and older:** Take 2 Table-

spoons (tbsp.) in dose cup provided every 4 to 6 hours as needed. Do not take more than 8 Tablespoons in 24 hours, or as directed by a doctor. **Children under 12 years:** Do not use this adult Extra Strength product in children under 12 years of age. This will provide more than the recommended dose (overdose) of TYLENOL® and could cause serious health problems.

Regular Strength TYLENOL® Tablets: **Adults and Children 12 years of Age and Older:** Take 2 tablets every 4 to 6 hours as needed. Do not take more than 12 tablets in 24 hours, or as directed by a doctor. **Children 6–11 years of age.** Take 1 tablet every 4 to 6 hours as needed. Do not take more than 5 tablets in 24 hours. **Children under 6 years of age:** Do not use this adult Regular Strength product in children under 6 years of age. This will provide more than the recommended dose (overdose) of TYLENOL® and could cause serious health problems.

TYLENOL® Arthritis Pain Extended Relief Caplets: **Adults and Children 12 years of Age and Older:** Take 2 caplets every 8 hours, not to exceed 6 caplets in any 24-hour period. TAKE TWO CAPLETS WITH WATER, SWALLOW EACH CAPLET WHOLE. DO NOT CRUSH, CHEW, OR DISSOLVE THE CAPLET. Not for use in children under 12 years of age.

PRECAUTIONS

If a rare sensitivity reaction occurs, the drug should be discontinued.

WARNINGS

Extra Strength TYLENOL® Gelcaps, Geltabs, Caplets, or Tablets, Extra Strength TYLENOL® Adult Liquid Pain Reliever, Regular Strength TYLENOL® Tablets:

Alcohol Warning: If you consume 3 or more alcoholic drinks every day, ask your doctor whether you should take acetaminophen or other pain relievers/fever reducers. Acetaminophen may cause liver damage.

Do not use if carton is opened or red neck wrap or foil seal imprinted with "Safety Seal®" is broken.

Do not Use:

- with any other product containing acetaminophen
- for more than 10 days for pain unless directed by a doctor.
- for more than 3 days for fever unless directed by a doctor.

Stop Using and Ask a Doctor If:

- symptoms do not improve
- new symptoms occur
- pain or fever persists or gets worse
- redness or swelling is present

Do not exceed recommended dose. Keep this and all drugs out of the reach of children. In case of accidental overdose, contact a physician or poison control center immediately. Prompt medical attention is critical for adults as well as for children even if you do not notice any signs or symptoms. As with any drug, if you are pregnant or nursing a baby, seek the advice of a health professional before using this product.

TYLENOL® Arthritis Pain Extended Relief Caplets: **Alcohol Warning:** If you consume 3 or more alcoholic drinks every day, ask your doctor whether you should take acetaminophen or other pain relievers/fever reducers. Acetaminophen may cause liver damage.

Do not use if carton is opened or red neck wrap or foil inner seal imprinted with "Safety Seal®" is broken. Do not take for pain for more than 10 days or for fever for more than 3 days unless directed by a physician. If pain or fever persists, or gets worse, if new symptoms occur, or if redness or swelling is present, consult a physician because these could be signs of a serious condition. As with any drug, if you are pregnant or nursing a baby, seek the advice of a health professional before using this product. Keep this and all drugs out of the reach of children. In case of accidental overdose, contact a physician or poison control center immediately. Prompt medical attention is critical for adults as well as for children even if you do not notice any signs or symptoms. Do not use with other products containing acetaminophen.

PROFESSIONAL INFORMATION

OVERDOSAGE INFORMATION

Acetaminophen in massive overdosage may cause hepatic toxicity in some patients. In adults and adolescents (≥12 years of age), hepatic toxicity may occur following ingestion of greater than 7.5 to 10 grams over a period of 8 hours or less. Fatalities are infrequent (less than 3–4% of untreated cases) and have rarely been reported with overdoses of less than 15 grams. In children (<12 years of age), an acute overdosage of less than 150 mg/kg has not been associated with hepatic toxicity. Early symptoms following a potentially hepatotoxic overdose may include: nausea, vomiting, diaphoresis and general malaise. Clinical and laboratory evidence of hepatic toxicity may not be apparent until 48 to 72 hours postingestion. In adults and adolescents, any individual presenting with an unknown amount of acetaminophen ingested or with a questionable or unreliable history about the time of ingestion should have a plasma acetaminophen level drawn and be treated with *N*-acetylcysteine. For full prescribing information, refer to the *N*-acetylcysteine package insert. Do not await results of assays for plasma acetaminophen levels before initiating treatment with *N*-acetylcysteine. The following additional procedures are recommended: Promptly initiate gastric decontamination of the stomach. A plasma acetaminophen assay should be obtained as early as possible, but no sooner than four hours following ingestion. If an acetaminophen *extended release* product is involved, it may be appropriate to obtain an additional plasma acetaminophen level 4–6 hours following the initial acetaminophen level. If either acetaminophen level plots above the treatment line on the acetaminophen overdose nomogram, *N*-acetylcysteine treatment should be continued for a full course of therapy. Liver function studies should be obtained initially and repeated at 24-hour intervals.

Serious toxicity or fatalities have been extremely infrequent following an acute acetaminophen overdose in young children, possibly because of differences in the way they metabolize acetaminophen. In children, the maximum potential amount ingested can be more easily estimated. If more than 150 mg/kg or an unknown amount was ingested, obtain a plasma acetaminophen level as soon as possible, but no sooner than 4 hours following ingestion. If an acetaminophen *extended release* product is involved, it may be appropriate to obtain an additional plasma acetaminophen level 4–6 hours following the initial acetaminophen level. If either acetaminophen level plots above the treatment line on the acetaminophen overdose nomogram, *N*-acetylcysteine treatment should be initiated and continued for a full course of therapy. If an assay cannot be obtained and the estimated acetaminophen ingestion exceeds 150 mg/kg, dosing with *N*-acetylcysteine should be initiated and continued for a full course of therapy.

For additional emergency information, call your regional poison center or call the Rocky Mountain Poison Center toll-free, (1-800-525-6115).

Alcohol Information: Chronic heavy alcohol abusers may be at increased risk of liver toxicity from excessive acetaminophen use, although reports of this event are rare. Reports usually involve cases of severe chronic alcoholics and the dosages of acetaminophen most often exceed recommended doses and often involve substantial overdose. Healthcare professionals should alert their patients who regularly consume large amounts of alcohol not to exceed recommended doses of acetaminophen.

INACTIVE INGREDIENTS

Extra Strength TYLENOL®: **Tablets:** Cellulose, Corn Starch, Magnesium Stearate, Sodium Starch Glycolate. **Caplets:** Cellulose, Corn Starch, FD&C Red No. 40, Hydroxypropyl Methylcellulose, Magnesium Stearate, Polyethylene Glycol, Sodium Starch Glycolate. **Gelcaps:** Benzyl Alcohol, Blue #1 and #2, Butylparaben, Castor Oil, Cellulose, Corn Starch, Edetate Calcium Disodium, Gelatin, Hydroxypropyl Methylcellulose, Magnesium Stearate, Methylparaben, Propylparaben, Red #40, Sodium Lauryl Sulfate, Sodium Propionate, Sodium Starch Glycolate, Titanium Dioxide, and Yellow #10. **Geltabs:** Benzyl Alcohol, Blue #1 and 2, Butylparaben, Castor Oil, Cellulose, Corn Starch, Edetate Calcium Disodium, Gelatin, Hydroxypropyl Methylcellulose, Magnesium Stearate, Methylparaben, Propylparaben, Red #40, Sodium Lauryl Sulfate, Sodium Propionate, Sodium Starch Glycolate, Titanium Dioxide, and Yellow #10.

Extra Strength TYLENOL® Adult Liquid Pain Reliever: Alcohol (7%), Citric Acid, D&C Yellow #10, FD&C Blue #1, FD&C Yellow #6, Flavor, Glycerin, Polyethylene Glycol, Purified Water, Sodium Benzoate, Sorbitol, Sucrose.

Regular Strength TYLENOL®: **Tablets:** Cellulose, Corn Starch, Magnesium Stearate, Sodium Starch Glycolate.

TYLENOL® Arthritis Pain Extended Relief Caplets: Corn Starch, Hydroxyethyl Cellulose, Hydroxypropyl Methylcellulose, Magnesium Stearate, Microcrystalline Cellulose, Povidone, Powdered Cellulose, Pregelatinized Starch, Sodium Starch Glycolate, Titanium Dioxide, Triacetin.

HOW SUPPLIED

Extra Strength TYLENOL®: **Tablets** (colored white, imprinted "TYLENOL" and "500")—vials of 10, and tamper-evident bottles of 30, 60, 100, and 200. Store at room temperature. **Caplets** (colored white, imprinted "TYLENOL 500 mg")—vials of 10, 10 blister packs, and tamper-evident bottles of 24, 50, 100, 175, and 250. Store at room temperature. **Gelcaps** (colored yellow and red, imprinted "Tylenol 500") vials of 10 and tamper-evident bottles of 24, 50, 100, and 225. Store at room temperature; avoid high humidity and excessive heat 40°C (104°F). **Geltabs** (colored yellow and red, imprinted "Tylenol 500") tamper-evident bottles of 24, 50, and 100. Store at room temperature; avoid high humidity and excessive heat 40°C (104°F).

Extra Strength TYLENOL® Adult Liquid Pain Reliever: Mint-flavored liquid (colored green) 8 fl. oz. tamper-evident bottle with child resistant safety cap and special dosage cup. Store at room temperature.

Regular Strength TYLENOL®: **Tablets** (colored white, scored, imprinted "TYLENOL" and "325")—tamper-evident bottles of 24, 50, 100 and 200. Store at room temperature.

TYLENOL® Arthritis Pain Extended Relief Caplets: (colored white, engraved "TYLENOL ER") tamper-evident bottles of 24, 50, and 100's. Store at room temperature. Avoid excessive heat (40°C).

Shown in Product Identification Guide, page 322

TYLENOL® SEVERE ALLERGY OTC
Caplets

Maximum Strength
TYLENOL® ALLERGY SINUS
NightTime Caplets

Maximum Strength
TYLENOL® ALLERGY SINUS
Caplets, Gelcaps and Geltabs

Product information for all dosage forms of TYLENOL ALLERGY have been combined under this heading.

DESCRIPTION

Each ***TYLENOL® SEVERE ALLERGY Caplet*** contains acetaminophen 500 mg and diphenhydramine HCl 12.5 mg. Each ***Maximum Strength TYLENOL® ALLERGY SINUS NightTime Caplet*** contains acetaminophen 500 mg, diphenhydramine HCl 25 mg, and pseudoephedrine HCl 30 mg. Each ***Maximum Strength TYLENOL® ALLERGY SINUS Caplet Gelcap and Geltab*** contains acetaminophen 500 mg, chlorpheniramine maleate 2 mg, and pseudoephedrine HCl 30 mg.

ACTIONS

TYLENOL® SEVERE ALLERGY Caplets contain a clinically proven analgesic-antipyretic and antihistamine. Acetaminophen produces analgesia by elevation of the pain threshold and antipyresis through action on the hypothalamic heat regulating center. Acetaminophen is equal to aspirin in analgesic and antipyretic effectiveness, and it is unlikely to produce many of the side effects associated with aspirin and aspirin-containing products.

Diphenhydramine is an antihistamine which helps provide temporary relief of itchy, watery eyes, runny nose, sneezing, itching of the nose or throat due to hay fever or other respiratory allergies.

Maximum Strength TYLENOL® ALLERGY SINUS NightTime Caplets contain, in addition to the above ingredients, a decongestant, pseudoephedrine. Pseudoephedrine is a sympathomimetic amine which provides temporary relief of nasal and sinus congestion.

Maximum Strength TYLENOL® ALLERGY SINUS Caplets, Gelcaps and Geltabs contain acetaminophen, pseudoephedrine and the antihistamine, chlorpheniramine. Chlorpheniramine is an antihistamine which helps provide temporary relief of runny nose, sneezing and watery and itchy eyes.

USES

TYLENOL® SEVERE ALLERGY: For the temporary relief of itchy, watery eyes, runny nose, sneezing, sore or scratchy throat and itching of the nose or throat due to hay fever or other upper respiratory allergies.

Maximum Strength TYLENOL® ALLERGY SINUS NightTime and ***TYLENOL® ALLERGY SINUS:*** For the temporary relief of nasal congestion, sinus congestion and pressure, sinus pain, headache, runny nose, sneezing, itching of the nose or throat and itchy watery eyes due to hay fever or other respiratory allergies.

PRECAUTIONS

TYLENOL® SEVERE ALLERGY, Maximum Strength TYLENOL® ALLERGY SINUS NightTime and ***Maximum Strength TYLENOL® ALLERGY SINUS:*** If a rare sensitivity reaction occurs, the drug should be discontinued.

DIRECTIONS

TYLENOL® SEVERE ALLERGY: **Adults and children 12 years of age and older:** Take 2 caplets every 4–6 hours. Do not take more than 8 caplets in 24 hours, or as directed by a doctor. **Children under 12 years:** Do not use this adult product in children under 12 years of age. This will provide more than the recommended dose (overdose) and could cause serious health problems.

Maximum Strength TYLENOL® ALLERGY SINUS NightTime: **Adults and children 12 years of age and older:** Take 2 caplets at bedtime. May repeat every 4–6 hours. Do not take more than 8 caplets in 24 hours, or as directed by a doctor. **Children under 12 years:** Do not use this adult product in children under 12 years of age. This will provide more than the recommended dose (overdose) and could cause serious health problems.

Maximum Strength TYLENOL® ALLERGY SINUS: **Adults and children 12 years of age and older:** Take two every 4–6 hours. Do not take more than 8 in 24 hours, or as directed by a doctor. **Children under 12 years:** Do not use this adult product in children under 12 years of age. This will provide more than the recommended dose (overdose) and could cause serious health problems.

WARNINGS

Alcohol Warning: If you consume 3 or more alcoholic drinks every day, ask your doctor whether you should take acetaminophen or other pain relievers/fever reducers. Acetaminophen may cause liver damage.

TYLENOL® SEVERE ALLERGY: **Do not use if carton is opened or if blister unit is broken.** Do not take for pain for more than 7 days or for fever for more than 3 days unless directed by a doctor. If pain or fever persists, or gets worse, if new symptoms occur, or if redness or swelling is present, consult a doctor because these could be signs of a serious condition. If sore throat is severe, persists for more than 2 days, is accompanied or followed by fever, headache, rash, nausea or vomiting, consult a doctor promptly. May cause excitability especially in children. If nervousness, dizziness or sleeplessness occur, discontinue use and consult a doctor. May cause marked drowsiness; alcohol, sedatives and tranquilizers may increase the drowsiness effect. Avoid alcoholic beverages while taking this product. Do not take this product if you are taking sedatives or tranquilizers without first consulting your doctor. Use caution while driving a motor vehicle or operating machinery. Do not take this product, unless directed by a doctor, if you have a breathing problem such as emphysema or chronic bronchitis, or if you have glaucoma or difficulty in urination due to enlargement of the prostate gland.

Continued on next page

Tylenol Allergy—Cont.

Do not exceed recommended dosage. Keep this and all drugs out of the reach of children. In case of accidental overdose, contact a doctor or poison control center immediately. Prompt medical attention is critical for adults as well as for children even if you do not notice any signs or symptoms. As with any drug, if you are pregnant or nursing a baby, seek the advice of a health professional before using this product. Do not use with other products containing acetaminophen.

***Maximum Strength TYLENOL® ALLERGY SINUS NightTime:* Do not use if carton is open or if a blister unit is broken.** Do not take for pain for more than 7 days or for fever for more than 3 days unless directed by a doctor. If pain or fever persists, or gets worse, if new symptoms occur, or if redness or swelling is present, consult a doctor because these could be signs of a serious condition. May cause excitability especially in children. If nervousness, dizziness or sleeplessness occur, discontinue use and consult a doctor. May cause marked drowsiness; alcohol, sedatives and tranquilizers may increase the drowsiness effect. Avoid alcoholic beverages while taking this product. Do not take this product if you are taking sedatives or tranquilizers without first consulting your doctor. Use caution when driving a motor vhicle or operating machinery. Do not take this product, unless directed by a doctor, if you have a breathing problem such as emphysema or chronic bronchitis, or if you have glaucoma, or difficulty in urination due to enlargement of the prostate gland. Do not take this product if you have heart disease, high blood pressure, thyroid disease or diabetes unless directed by a doctor.

Do not exceed recommended dosage. Keep this and all drugs out of the reach of children. In case of accidental overdose, contact a doctor or poison control center immediately. Prompt medical attention is critical for adults as well as for children even if you do not notice any signs or symptoms. As with any drug, if you are pregnant or nursing a baby, seek the advice of a health professional before using this product. Do not use with other products containing acetaminophen.

***Maximum Strength TYLENOL® ALLERGY SINUS:* Do not use if carton is opened or if blister unit is broken.** Do not take for pain for more than 7 days or for fever for more than 3 days unless directed by a doctor. If pain or fever persists, or gets worse, if new symptoms occur, or if redness or swelling is present, consult a doctor because these could be signs of a serious condition. May cause excitability especially in children. If nervousness, dizziness or sleeplessness occur, discontinue use and consult a doctor. May cause drowsiness; alcohol, sedatives and tranquilizers may increase the drowsiness effect. Avoid alcoholic beverages while taking this product. Do not take this product if you are taking sedatives or tranquilizers, without first consulting your doctor. Use caution when driving a motor vehicle or operating machinery. Do not take this product, unless directed by a doctor, if you have a breathing problem such as emphysema or chronic bronchitis, or if you have glaucoma, or difficulty in urination due to enlargement of the prostate gland. Do not take this product if you have heart disease, high blood pressure, thyroid disease or diabetes unless directed by a doctor.

Do not exceed recommended dosage. Keep this and all drugs out of the reach of children. In case of accidental overdose, contact a doctor or poison control center immediately. Prompt medical attention is critical for adults as well as for children even if you do not notice any signs or symptoms. As with any drug, if you are pregnant or nursing a baby, seek the advice of a health professional before using this product. Do not use with other products containing acetaminophen.

DRUG INTERACTION PRECAUTION

Maximum Strength TYLENOL® ALLERGY SINUS NightTime* and *TYLENOL® ALLERGY SINUS: Do not use this product if you are now taking a prescription monamine oxidase inhibitor (MAOI) (certain drugs for depression, psychiatric or emotional condition, or Parkinson's disease), or for 2 weeks after stopping the MAOI drug. If you are uncertain whether your prescription drug contains an MAOI, consult a health professional before taking this product.

PROFESSIONAL INFORMATION

OVERDOSAGE INFORMATION

Acetaminophen in massive overdosage may cause hepatic toxicity in some patients. In adults and adolescents (≥12 years of age), hepatic toxicity may occur following ingestion of greater than 7.5 to 10 grams over a period of 8 hours or less. Fatalities are infrequent (less than 3–4% of untreated cases) and have rarely been reported with overdoses of less than 15 grams. In children (<12 years of age), an acute overdosage of less than 150 mg/kg has not been associated with hepatic toxicity. Early symptoms following a potentially hepatotoxic overdose may include: nausea, vomiting, diaphoresis and general malaise. Clinical and laboratory evidence of hepatic toxicity may not be apparent until 48 to 72 hours postingestion. In adults and adolescents, any individual presenting with an unknown amount of acetaminophen ingested or with a questionable or unreliable history about the time of ingestion should have a plasma acetaminophen level drawn and be treated with *N*-acetylcysteine. For full prescribing information, refer to the *N*-acetylcysteine package insert. Do not await results of assays for plasma acetaminophen levels before initiating treatment with *N*-acetylcysteine. The following additional procedures are recommended: Promptly initiate gastric decontamination of the stomach. A plasma acetaminophen assay should be obtained as early as possible, but no sooner than four hours following ingestion. If an acetaminophen *extended release* product is involved, it may be appropriate to obtain an additional plasma acetaminophen level 4–6 hours following the initial acetaminophen level. If either acetaminophen level plots above the treatment line on the acetaminophen overdose nomogram, *N*-acetylcysteine treatment should be continued for a full course of therapy. Liver function studies should be obtained initially and repeated at 24-hour intervals.

Serious toxicity or fatalities have been extremely infrequent following an acute acetaminophen overdose in young children, possibly because of differences in the way they metabolize acetaminophen. In children, the maximum potential amount ingested can be more easily estimated. If more than 150 mg/kg or an unknown amount was ingested, obtain a plasma acetaminophen level as soon as possible, but no sooner than 4 hours following ingestion. If an acetaminophen *extended release* product is involved, it may be appropriate to obtain an additional plasma acetaminophen level 4–6 hours following the initial acetaminophen level. If either acetaminophen level plots above the treatment line on the acetaminophen overdose nomogram, *N*-acetylcysteine treatment should be initiated and continued for a full course of therapy. If an assay cannot be obtained and the estimated acetaminophen ingestion exceeds 150 mg/kg, dosing with *N*-acetylcysteine should be initiated and continued for a full course of therapy.

For additional emergency information, call your regional poison center or call the Rocky Mountain Poison Center toll-free (1–800–525–6115).

Symptoms for pseudoephedrine overdose consist most often of mild anxiety, tachycardia and/or hypertension. Symptoms usually appear within 4 to 8 hours of ingestion and are transient, usually requiring no treatment.

Diphenhydramine and chlorpheniramine toxicity should be treated as you would an antihistamine/anticholinergic overdose and is likely to be present within a few hours after acute ingestion.

Alcohol Information: Chronic heavy alcohol abusers maybeatincreasedriskoflivertoxicityfromexcessiveacetaminophen use, although reports of this event are rare. Reports usually involve cases of severe chronic alcoholics and the dosages of acetaminophen most often exceed recommended doses and often involve substantial overdose. Healthcare professionals should alert their patients who regularly consume large amounts of alcohol not to exceed recommended doses of acetaminophen.

INACTIVE INGREDIENTS

***TYLENOL® SEVERE ALLERGY:* Caplets:** Carnauba Wax, Cellulose, Corn Starch, D&C Yellow #10, FD&C Yellow #6, Hydroxpropyl Cellulose, Hydroxypropyl Methylcellulose, Iron Oxide, Magnesium Stearate, Polyethylene Glycol, Sodium Citrate, Sodium Starch Glycolate, Titanium Dioxide.

***Maximum Strength TYLENOL® ALLERGY SINUS NightTime:* Caplets:** Carnauba Wax, Cellulose, Corn Starch, D&C Yellow #10, FD&C Blue #1, Hydroxypropyl Methylcellulose, Iron Oxide, Magnesium Stearate, Polyethylene Glycol, Polysorbate 80, Sodium Citrate, Sodium Starch Glycolate, Titanium Dioxide.

***Maximum Strength TYLENOL® ALLERGY SINUS:* Caplets:** Carnauba Wax, Cellulose, Corn Starch, D&C Yellow #10, FD&C Yellow #6, Hydroxypropyl Cellulose, Hydroxypropyl Methylcellulose, Magnesium Stearate, Polyethylene Glycol, Sodium Starch Glycolate, Titanium Dioxide. **Gelcaps and Geltabs:** Benzyl Alcohol, Butylparaben, Castor Oil, Cellulose, Corn Starch, D&C Yellow #10, Edetate Calcium Disodium, FD&C Blue #1, FD&C Blue #2, Gelatin, Hydroxypropyl Methylcellulose, Magnesium Stearate, Methylparaben, Propylparaben, Sodium Lauryl Sulfate, Sodium Propionate, Sodium Starch Glycolate, Titanium Dioxide.

HOW SUPPLIED

***TYLENOL® SEVERE ALLERGY:* Caplets:** Yellow film-coated, imprinted with "TYLENOL Severe Allergy" on one side—blister packs of 24. Store at room temperature.

***Maximum Strength TYLENOL® ALLERGY SINUS NightTime:* Caplets:** Light blue film-coated, imprinted with "TYLENOL A/S NightTime" on one side—blister packs of 24. Store at room temperature.

***Maximum Strength TYLENOL® ALLERGY SINUS:* Caplets:** Yellow film-coated, imprinted with "TYLENOL Allergy Sinus" on one side—blister packs of 24. Store at room temperature.

Gelcaps and Geltabs: Green and yellow-colored, imprinted with "TYLENOL A/S"—blister packs of 24 and 48. Store at room temperature; avoid high humidity and excessive heat 40°C (104°F).

Shown in Product Identification Guide, page 323

Multi-Symptom TYLENOL® COLD Non-Drowsy OTC
Caplets and Gelcaps

Multi-Symptom TYLENOL® COLD Complete Formula
Caplets

Product information for all dosage forms of TYLENOL COLD have been combined under this heading.

DESCRIPTION

Each ***Multi-Symptom TYLENOL® COLD Non-Drowsy Caplet and Gelcap*** contains acetaminophen 325 mg, dextromethorphan HBr 15 mg, and pseudoephedrine HCl 30 mg Each ***Multi-Symptom TYLENOL® COLD Complete Formula Caplet*** contains acetaminophen 325 mg, chlorpheniramine maleate 2 mg, dextromethorphan HBr 15 mg, and pseudoephedrine HCl 30 mg.

ACTIONS

Multi-Symptom TYLENOL® COLD Non-Drowsy contains a clinically proven analgesic-antipyretic, decongestant and cough suppressant. Acetaminophen produces analgesia by elevation of the pain threshold and antipyresis through action on the hypothalamic heat regulating center. Acetaminophen is equal to aspirin in analgesic and antipyretic effectiveness and it is unlikely to produce many of the side effects associated with aspirin and aspirin-containing products. Pseudoephedrine is a sympathomimetic amine which provides temporary relief of nasal congestion. Dextromethorphan is a cough suppressant which provides temporary relief of coughs due to minor throat irritations that may occur with the common cold.

Multi-Symptom TYLENOL® COLD Complete Formula Caplets contain, in addition to the above ingredients, an antihistamine. Chlorpheniramine is an antihistamine which helps provide temporary relief of runny nose, sneezing and watery and itchy eyes.

USES

Multi-Symptom TYLENOL® COLD Non-Drowsy: For the temporary relief of these cold symptoms: minor aches and pains, headaches, sore throat, nasal congestion, coughs. For the reduction of fever.

Multi-Symptom TYLENOL® COLD Complete Formula: For the temporary relief of these cold symptoms: minor aches and pains, headaches, sore throat, nasal congestion, runny nose, coughs, sneezing, watery and itchy eyes. For the reduction of fever.

DIRECTIONS

***Multi-Symptom TYLENOL® COLD Non Drowsy and Multi-Symptom TYLENOL® COLD Complete Formula:* Adults and children 12 years of age and older:** Take 2 every 6 hours. Do not take more than 8 in 24 hours, or as directed by a doctor. **Children 6–11 years of age:** Take 1 every 6 hours. Do not take more than 4 in 24 hours, or as directed by a doctor. **Children under 6 years of age:** Do not use this product in children under 6 years of age. This will provide more than the recommended dose (overdose) and could cause serious health problems.

PRECAUTIONS

If a rare sensitivity reaction occurs, the drug should be discontinued.

WARNINGS

Alcohol Warning: If you consume 3 or more alcoholic drinks every day, ask your doctor whether you should take acetaminophen or other pain relievers/fever reducers. Acetaminophen may cause liver damage.

***Multi-Symptom TYLENOL® COLD Non Drowsy:* Do not use if carton is opened or if blister unit is broken.** Do not take for pain for more than 7 days or for fever for more than 3 days unless directed by a doctor. If pain or fever persists, or gets worse, if new symptoms occur, or if redness or swelling is present, consult a doctor because these could be signs of a serious condition. If sore throat is severe, persists for more than 2 days, is accompanied or followed by fever, headache, rash, nausea or vomiting, consult a doctor promptly. A persistent cough may be a sign of a serious condition. If cough persists for more than 1 week, tends to recur or is accompanied by fever, rash or persistent headache, consult a doctor. Do not take this product for persistent or chronic cough such as occurs with smoking, asthma, emphysema or if cough is accompanied by excessive phlegm (mucus) unless directed by a doctor.

Do not exceed recommended dosage. If nervousness, dizziness or sleeplessness, occur, discontinue use and consult a doctor. Do not take this product if you have heart disease, high blood pressure, thyroid disease, diabetes or difficulty in urination due to enlargement of the prostate gland unless directed by a doctor.

Keep this and all drugs out of the reach of children. In case of accidental overdose, contact a doctor or poison control center immediately. Prompt medical attention is critical for adults as well as for children even if you do not notice any signs or symptoms. As with any drug, if you are pregnant or nursing a baby, seek the advice of a health professional before using this product. Do not use with other products containing acetaminophen.

***Multi-Symptom TYLENOL® COLD Complete Formula:* Do not use if carton is opened or if blister unit is broken.** Do not take for pain for more than 7 days or for fever for more than 3 days unless directed by a doctor. If pain or fever persists, or gets worse, if new symptoms occur, or if redness or swelling is present, consult a doctor because these could be signs of a serious condition. If sore throat is severe, persists for more than 2 days, is accompanied or followed by fever, headache, rash, nausea or vomiting, consult a doctor promptly. A persistent cough may be a sign of a serious condition. If cough persists for more than 1 week, tends to recur or is accompanied by fever, rash or persistent headache, consult a doctor. Do not take this product for persistent or chronic cough such as occurs with smoking, asthma, emphysema or if cough is accompanied by excessive phlegm (mucus) unless directed by a doctor.

Do not exceed recommended dosage. If nervousness, dizziness or sleeplessness occur, discontinue use and consult a doctor. May cause excitability especially in children. Do not take this product unless directed by a doctor, if you have a breathing problem such as emphysema or chronic bronchitis, or if you have glaucoma or difficulty in urination due to enlargement of the prostate gland. Do not take this product if you have heart disease, high blood pressure, thyroid disease or diabetes unless directed by a doctor. May cause drowsiness; alcohol, sedatives and tranquilizers may increase the drowsiness effect. Avoid alcoholic beverages while taking this product. Do not take this product if you are taking sedatives or tranquilizers without first consulting your doctor. Use caution when driving a motor vehicle or operating machinery.

Keep this and all drugs out of the reach of children. In case of accidental overdose, contact a doctor or poison control center immediately. Prompt medical attention is critical for adults as well as for children even if you do not notice any signs or symptoms. As with any drug, if you are pregnant or nursing a baby, seek the advice of a health professional before using this product. Do not use with other products containing acetaminophen.

DRUG INTERACTION PRECAUTION

Do not use this product if you are now taking a prescription monoamine oxidase inhibitor (MAOI) (certain drugs for depression, psychiatric or emotional conditions, or Parkinson's disease), or for 2 weeks after stopping the MAOI drug. If you are uncertain whether your prescription drug contains an MAOI, consult a health professional before taking this product.

PROFESSIONAL INFORMATION

OVERDOSAGE INFORMATION

Acetaminophen in massive overdosage may cause hepatic toxicity in some patients. In adults and adolescents (≥ 12 years of age), hepatic toxicity may occur following ingestion of greater than 7.5 to 10 grams over a period of 8 hours or less. Fatalities are infrequent (less than 3–4% of untreated cases) and have rarely been reported with overdoses of less than 15 grams. In children (<12 years of age), an acute overdosage of less than 150 mg/kg has not been associated with hepatic toxicity. Early symptoms following a potentially hepatotoxic overdose may include: nausea, vomiting, diaphoresis and general malaise. Clinical and laboratory evidence of hepatic toxicity may not be apparent until 48 to 72 hours postingestion. In adults and adolescents, any individual presenting with an unknown amount of acetaminophen ingested or with a questionable or unreliable history about the time of ingestion should have a plasma acetaminophen level drawn and be treated with *N*-acetylcysteine. For full prescribing information, refer to the *N*-acetylcysteine package insert. Do not await results of assays for plasma acetaminophen levels before initiating treatment with *N*-acetylcysteine. The following additional procedures are recommended: Promptly initiate gastric decontamination of the stomach. A plasma acetaminophen assay should be obtained as early as possible, but no sooner than four hours following ingestion. If an acetaminophen *extended release* product is involved, it may be appropriate to obtain an additional plasma acetaminophen level 4–6 hours following the initial acetaminophen level. If either acetaminophen level plots above the treatment line on the acetaminophen overdose nomogram, *N*-acetylcysteine treatment should be continued for a full course of therapy. Liver function studies should be obtained initially and repeated at 24-hour intervals.

Serious toxicity or fatalities have been extremely infrequent following an acute acetaminophen overdose in young children, possibly because of differences in the way they metabolize acetaminophen. In children, the maximum potential amount ingested can be more easily estimated. If more than 150 mg/kg or an unknown amount was ingested, obtain a plasma acetaminophen level as soon as possible, but no sooner than 4 hours following ingestion. If an acetaminophen *extended release* product is involved, it may be appropriate to obtain an additional plasma acetaminophen level 4–6 hours following the initial acetaminophen level. If either acetaminophen level plots above the treatment line on the acetaminophen overdose nomogram, *N*-acetylcysteine treatment should be initiated and continued for a full course of therapy. If an assay cannot be obtained and the estimated acetaminophen ingestion exceeds 150 mg/kg, dosing with *N*-acetylcysteine should be initiated and continued for a full course of therapy.

For additional emergency information, call your regional poison center or call the Rocky Mountain Poison Center toll-free, (1-800-525-6115).

Symptoms from pseudoephedrine overdose consist most often of mild anxiety, tachycardia and/or mild hypertension. Symptoms usually appear within 4 to 8 hours of ingestion and are transient, usually requiring no treatment.

Acute dextromethorphan overdose usually does not result in serious signs and symptoms unless massive amounts have been ingested. Signs and symptoms of a substantial overdose may include nausea and vomiting, visual disturbances, CNS disturbances, and urinary retention.

Chlorpheniramine toxicity should be treated as you would an antihistamine/anticholinergic overdose and is likely to be present within a few hours after acute ingestion.

Alcohol Information: Chronic heavy alcohol abusers may be at increased risk of liver toxicity from excessive acetaminophen use, although reports of this event are rare. Reports usually involve cases of severe chronic alcoholics and the dosages of acetaminophen most often exceed recommended doses and often involve substantial overdose. Healthcare professionals should alert their patients who regularly consume large amounts of alcohol not to exceed recommended doses of acetaminophen.

INACTIVE INGREDIENTS

Multi-Symptom TYLENOL® COLD Non Drowsy Formula:
Caplets: Carnauba Wax, Cellulose, Corn Starch, D&C Yellow #10, FD&C Blue #1, Hydroxypropyl Methylcellulose, Iron Oxide, Magnesium Stearate, Sodium Starch Glycolate, Titanium Dioxide, Triacetin.

Gelcaps: Benzyl Alcohol, Butylparaben, Castor Oil, Cellulose, Corn Starch, D&C Yellow #10, Edetate Calcium Disodium, FD&C Red #40, Gelatin, Hydroxypropyl Methylcellulose, Iron Oxide, Magnesium Stearate, Methylparaben, Propylparaben, Sodium Lauryl Sulfate, Sodium Propionate, Sodium Starch Glycolate, Titanium Dioxide.

Multi-Symptom TYLENOL® COLD Complete Formula:
Caplets: Carnauba Wax, Cellulose, Corn Starch, D&C Yellow #10, FD&C Blue #1, FD&C Yellow #6, Hydroxypropyl Methylcellulose, Iron Oxide, Magnesium Stearate, Sodium Starch Glycolate, Titanium Dioxide, Triacetin.

HOW SUPPLIED

Multi-Symptom TYLENOL® COLD Non Drowsy: **Caplets:** White-colored, imprinted with "TYLENOL Cold"—blister packs of 24. Store at room temperature. **Gelcaps:** Red- and tan-colored, imprinted with "TYLENOL COLD"—blister packs of 24. Store at room temperature. Avoid high humidity and excessive heat 40°C (104°F).

Multi-Symptom TYLENOL® COLD Complete Formula: **Caplets:** Yellow-colored, imprinted with "TYLENOL Cold"—blister packs of 24. Store at room temperature.

Shown in Product Identification Guide, page 322

Multi-Symptom TYLENOL® COLD — OTC
SEVERE CONGESTION NON-DROWSY

DESCRIPTION

Each **Multi-Symptom TYLENOL® COLD SEVERE CONGESTION Non-Drowsy Caplet** contains acetaminophen 325 mg, dextromethorphan HBr 15 mg, guaifenesin 200 mg and pseudoephedrine HCl 30 mg.

ACTIONS

Multi-Symptom TYLENOL® COLD SEVERE CONGESTION NON-DROWSY Caplets contains a clinically proven analgesic-antipyretic, decongestant, expectorant and cough suppressant. Acetaminophen produces analgesia by elevation of the pain threshold and antipyresis through action on the hypothalamic heat regulating center. Acetaminophen is equal to aspirin in analgesic and antipyretic effectiveness and is unlikely to produce many of the side effects associated with aspirin and aspirin-containing products. Pseudoephedrine is a sympathomimetic amine which provides temporary relief of nasal congestion. Guaifenesin is an expectorant which helps loosen phlegm (mucus) and thin bronchial secretions to make coughs more productive. Dextromethorphan is a cough suppressant which provides temporary relief of coughs due to minor throat irritations that may occur with the common cold.

USES

Multi-Symptom TYLENOL® COLD SEVERE CONGESTION NON-DROWSY Caplets: For the temporary relief of these cold symptoms: minor aches and pains, headaches, sore throat, nasal congestion, chest congestion, cough. For the reduction of fever.

DIRECTIONS

Adults and children 12 years of age and older: Take 2 caplets every 6–8 hours. Do not take more than 8 caplets in 24 hours, or as directed by a doctor. **Children 6–11 years of age:** Take 1 caplet every 6–8 hours. Do not take more than 4 caplets in 24 hours, or as directed by a doctor. **Children under 6 years of age:** Do not use this product in children under 6 years of age. This will provide more than the recommended dose (overdose) and could cause serious health problems.

PRECAUTIONS

If a rare sensitivity reaction occurs, the drug should be discontinued.

WARNINGS

Alcohol Warning: If you consume 3 or more alcoholic drinks every day, ask your doctor whether you should take acetaminophen or other pain relievers/fever reducers. Acetaminophen may cause liver damage.

Do not use if carton is opened or if blister unit is broken. Do not take for pain for more than 7 days or for fever for more than 3 days unless directed by a doctor. If pain or fever persists, or gets worse, if new symptoms occur, or if redness or swelling is present, consult a doctor because these could be signs of a serious condition. If sore throat is severe, persists for more than 2 days, is accompanied or followed by fever, headache, rash, nausea or vomiting, consult a doctor promptly. A persistent cough may be a sign of a serious condition. If cough persists for more than 1 week, tends to recur or is accompanied by fever, rash or persistent headache, consult a doctor. Do not take this product for persistent or chronic cough such as occurs with smoking, asthma, emphysema or if cough is accompanied by excessive phlegm (mucus) unless directed by a doctor.

Do not exceed recommended dosage. If nervousness, dizziness, or sleeplessness occur, discontinue use and consult a doctor. Do not take this product if you have heart disease, high blood pressure, thyroid disease, diabetes or difficulty in urination due to enlargement of the prostate gland unless directed by a doctor.

Keep this and all drugs out of the reach of children. In case of accidental overdose, contact a doctor or poison control center immediately. Prompt medical attention is critical for adults as well as for children even if you do not notice any signs or symptoms. As with any drug, if you are pregnant or nursing a baby, seek the advice of a health professional before using this product. Do not use with other products containing acetaminophen.

DRUG INTERACTION PRECAUTION

Do not use this product if you are now taking a prescription monoamine oxidase inhibitor (MAOI) (certain drugs for depression, psychiatric or emotional conditions, or Parkinson's disease), or for 2 weeks after stoppping the MAOI drug. If you are uncertain whether your prescription drug contains an MAOI, consult a health professional before taking this product.

PROFESSIONAL INFORMATION

OVERDOSAGE INFORMATION

Acetaminophen in massive overdosage may cause hepatic toxicity in some patients. In adults and adolescents (≥ 12 years of age), hepatic toxicity may occur following ingestion of greater than 7.5 to 10 grams over a period of 8 hours or less. Fatalities are infrequent (less than 3–4% of untreated cases) and have rarely been reported with overdoses of less than 15 grams. In children (< 12 years of age), an acute overdosage of less than 150 mg/kg has not been associated with hepatic toxicity. Early symptoms following a potentially hepatotoxic overdose may include: nausea, vomiting, diaphoresis and general malaise. Clinical and laboratory evidence of hepatic toxicity may not be apparent until 48 to 72 hours postingestion. In adults and adolescents, any individual presenting with an unknown amount of acetaminophen ingested or with a questionable or unreliable history about the time of ingestion should have a plasma acetaminophen level drawn and be treated with *N*-acetylcysteine. For full prescribing information, refer to the *N*-acetylcysteine package insert. Do not await results of assays for plasma acetaminophen levels before initiating treatment with *N*-acetylcysteine. The following additional procedures are recommended: Promptly initiate gastric decontamination of the stomach. A plasma acetaminophen assay should be obtained as early as possible, but no sooner than four hours following ingestion. If an acetaminophen *extended release* product is involved, it may be appropriate to obtain an additional plasma acetaminophen level 4–6 hours following the initial acetaminophen level. If either acetaminophen level plots above the treatment line on the acetaminophen overdose nomogram, *N*-acetylcysteine treatment should be continued for a full course of therapy. Liver function studies should be obtained initially and repeated at 24-hour intervals.

Serious toxicity or fatalities have been extremely infrequent following an acute acetaminophen overdose in young children, possibly because of differences in the way they metabolize acetaminophen. In children, the maximum potential amount ingested can be more easily estimated. If more than 150 mg/kg or an unknown amount was ingested, obtain a plasma acetaminophen level as soon as possible, but no sooner than 4 hours following ingestion. If an acetaminophen *extended release* product is involved, it may be appropriate to obtain an additional plasma acetaminophen level 4–6 hours following the initial acetaminophen level. If either acetaminophen level plots above the treatment line on the acetaminophen overdose nomogram, *N*-acetylcysteine treatment should be initiated and continued for a full course of therapy. If an assay cannot be obtained and the estimated acetaminophen ingestion exceeds 150 mg/kg, dosing with *N*-acetylcysteine should be initiated and continued for a full course of therapy.

For additional emergency information, call your regional poison center or call the Rocky Mountain Poison Center toll-free, (1-800-525-6115).

Symptoms from pseudoephedrine overdose consist most often of mild anxiety, tachycardia and/or mild hypertension. Symptoms usually appear within 4 to 8 hours of ingestion and are transient, usually requiring no treatment.

Acute dextromethorphan overdose usually does not result in serious signs and symptoms unless massive amounts have been ingested. Signs and symptoms of a substantial overdose may include nausea and vomiting, visual disturbance, CNS disturbances, and urinary retention.

Chlorpheniramine toxicity should be treated as you would an antihistamine/anticholinergic overdose and is likely to be present within a few hours after acute ingestion. Guaifenesin should be treated as a non-toxic ingestion.

Alcohol Information: Chronic heavy alcohol abusers may be at increased risk of liver toxicity from excessive acetaminophen use, although reports of this event are rare. Reports usually involve cases of severe chronic alcoholics and the dosages of acetaminophen most often exceed recom-

Continued on next page

Tylenol Cold Severe—Cont.

mended doses and often involve substantial overdose. Healthcare professionals should alert their patients who regularly consume large amounts of alcohol not to exceed recommended doses of acetaminophen.

INACTIVE INGREDIENTS

Carnauba Wax, Cellulose, Corn Starch, D&C Yellow #10, FD&C Blue #1, FD&C Yellow #6, Hydroxypropyl Methylcellulose, Iron Oxide, Povidone, Silicon Dioxide, Sodium Starch Glycolate, Stearic Acid, Titanium Dioxide, Triacetin.

HOW SUPPLIED

Caplets: Buttery-tan-colored, imprinted with "TYLENOL COLD SC" in green ink—blister packs of 24. Store at room temperature. Avoid high humidity and excessive heat (40°C).

Shown in Product Identification Guide, page 323

Maximum Strength TYLENOL® FLU NON-DROWSY Gelcaps OTC

Maximum Strength TYLENOL® FLU NightTime Gelcaps

Maximum Strength TYLENOL® FLU NightTime Liquid

Product information for all dosage forms of TYLENOL FLU have been combined under this heading.

DESCRIPTION

Each ***Maximum Strength TYLENOL® FLU NON-DROWSY Gelcap*** contains acetaminophen 500 mg, dextromethorphan HBr 15 mg and pseudoephedrine HCl 30 mg. Each ***Maximum Strength TYLENOL® FLU NightTime Gelcap*** contains acetaminophen 500 mg, diphenhydramine HCl 25 mg and pseudoephedrine HCl 30 mg. ***Maximum Strength TYLENOL® FLU NightTime Liquid:*** Each 30 mL (2 tablespoonsful) contains acetaminophen 1000 mg, dextromethorphan HBr 30 mg, doxylamine succinate 12.5 mg, and pseudoephedrine HCl 60 mg.

ACTIONS

Maximum Strength TYLENOL® FLU NON-DROWSY Gelcaps contain clinically proven analgesic-antipyretic, decongestant and cough suppressant. Acetaminophen produces analgesia by elevation of the pain threshold and antipyresis through action on the hypothalamic heat regulating center. Acetaminophen is equal to aspirin in analgesic and antipyretic effectiveness and it is unlikely to produce many of the side effects associated with aspirin and aspirin-containing products. Pseudoephedrine hydrochloride is a sympathomimetic amine which provides temporary relief of nasal congestion. Dextromethorphan is a cough suppressant which provides temporary relief of coughs due to minor throat irritations that may occur with the common cold.
Maximum Strength TYLENOL® FLU NightTime Gelcaps contains the same clinically proven analgesic-antipyretic and decongestant as ***Maximum Strength TYLENOL FLU NON-DROWSY Gelcaps*** along with an antihistamine. Diphenhydramine is an antihistamine which helps provide temporary relief of runny nose and sneezing. ***Maximum Strength TYLENOL® FLU NightTime Liquid*** contains the same clinically proven analgesic-antipyretic, decongestant and cough suppressant as ***Maximum Strength TYLENOL FLU NON-DROWSY Gelcaps*** along with an antihistamine. Doxylamine succinate is an antihistamine which helps provide temporary relief of runny nose and sneezing.

USES

Maximum Strength TYLENOL® FLU NON-DROWSY Gelcaps: For the temporary relief of these cold and flu symptoms: minor aches and pains, headaches, sore throat, nasal congestion, coughs. For the reduction of fever.
Maximum Strength TYLENOL® FLU NightTime Gelcaps: For the temporary relief of these cold and flu symptoms: minor aches and pains, headaches, sore throat, nasal congestion, runny nose, sneezing. For the reduction of fever.
Maximum Strength TYLENOL® FLU NightTime Liquid: For the temporary relief of: body aches and headache, coughing, nasal congestion, sore throat, runny nose/sneezing. For the reduction of fever.

DIRECTIONS

Maximum Strength TYLENOL® FLU NON-DROWSY Gelcaps: **Adults and children 12 years of age and older:** Take 2 gelcaps every 6 hours. Do not take more than 8 gelcaps in 24 hours, or as directed by a doctor. **Children under 12 years:** Do not use this adult product in children under 12 years of age. This will provide more than the recommended dose (overdose) and could cause serious health problems.
Maximum Strength TYLENOL® FLU NightTime Gelcaps: **Adults and children 12 years of age and older:** Take 2 gelcaps at bedtime. May repeat every 6 hours. Do not take more than 8 gelcaps in 24 hours, or as directed by a doctor. **Children under 12 years:** Do not use this adult product in children under 12 years of age. This will provide more than the recommended dose (overdose) and could cause serious health problems.
Maximum Strength TYLENOL® FLU NightTime Liquid: **Adults and children 12 years of age and older:** Take 2 Tablespoons (tbsp). May repeat every 6 hours. Do not use more than 4 times in 24 hours, or as directed by a doctor. **Children under 12 years:** Do not use this adult product in children under 12 years of age. This will provide more than the recommended dose (overdose) and could cause serious health problems.

PRECAUTIONS

If a rare sensitivity reaction occurs, the drug should be discontinued.

WARNINGS

Alcohol Warning: If you consume 3 or more alcoholic drinks every day, ask your doctor whether you should take acetaminophen or other pain relievers/fever reducers. Acetaminophen may cause liver damage.
Maximum Strength TYLENOL® FLU NON-DROWSY Gelcaps: **Do not use if carton is opened or if blister unit is broken.** Do not take for pain for more than 7 days or for fever for more than 3 days unless directed by a doctor. If pain or fever persists, or gets worse, if new symptoms occur, or if redness or swelling is present, consult a doctor because these could be signs of a serious condition. If sore throat is severe, persists for more than 2 days, is accompanied or followed by fever, headache, rash, nausea or vomiting, consult a doctor promptly. A persistent cough may be a sign of a serious condition. If cough persists for more than 1 week, tends to recur or is accompanied by fever, rash or persistent headache, consult a doctor. Do not take this product for persistent or chronic cough such as occurs with smoking, asthma, emphysema or if cough is accompanied by excessive phlegm (mucus) unless directed by a doctor.
Do not exceed recommended dosage. If nervousness, dizziness or sleeplessness occur, discontinue use and consult a doctor. Do not take this product if you have heart disease, high blood pressure, thyroid disease, diabetes, or difficulty in urination due to enlargement of the prostate gland unless directed by a doctor.
Keep this and all drugs out of the reach of children. In case of accidental overdose, contact a doctor or poison control center immediately. Prompt medical attention is critical for adults as well as for children even if you do not notice any signs or symptoms. As with any drug, if you are pregnant or nursing a baby, seek the advice of a health professional before using this product. Do not use with other products containing acetaminophen.
Maximum Strength TYLENOL® FLU NightTime Gelcaps: **Do not use if carton is opened or if blister unit is broken.** Do not take for pain for more than 7 days or for fever for more than 3 days unless directed by a doctor. If pain or fever persists, or gets worse, if new symptoms occur, or if redness or swelling is present, consult a doctor because these could be signs of a serious condition. If sore throat is severe, persists for more than 2 days, is accompanied by fever, headache, rash, nausea or vomiting, consult a doctor promptly.
Do not exceed recommended dosage. If nervousness, dizziness, or sleeplessness occur, discontinue use and consult a doctor. May cause excitability, especially in children. Do not take this product, unless directed by a doctor, if you have a breathing problem such as emphysema or chronic bronchitis, or if you have glaucoma or difficulty in urination due to enlargement of the prostate gland. Do not take this product if you have heart disease, high blood pressure, thyroid disease, or diabetes unless directed by a doctor. May cause marked drowsiness; alcohol, sedatives and tranquilizers may increase the drowsiness effect. Avoid alcoholic beverages while taking this product. Do not take this product if you are taking sedatives or tranquilizers without first consulting your doctor. Use caution when driving a motor vehicle or operating machinery.
Keep this and all drugs out of the reach of children. In case of accidental overdose, contact a doctor or poison control center immediately. Prompt medical attention is critical for adults as well as for children even if you do not notice any signs or symptoms. As with any drug, if you are pregnant or nursing a baby, seek the advice of a health professional before using this product. Do not use with other products containing acetaminophen.
Maximum Strength TYLENOL® FLU NightTime Liquid: **Do not use if carton is opened or if bottle wrap or foil inner seal imprinted "Safety Seal®" is broken or missing.** Do not take for pain for more than 7 days or for fever for more than 3 days unless directed by a doctor. If pain or fever persists, or gets worse, if new symptoms occur, or if redness or swelling is present, consult a doctor because these could be signs of a serious condition. If sore throat is severe, persists for more than 2 days, is accompanied or followed by fever, headache, rash, nausea, or vomiting, consult a doctor promptly. A persistent cough may be a sign of a serious condition. If cough persists for more than 1 week, tends to recur or is accompanied by fever, rash or persistent headache, consult a doctor. Do not take this product for persistent or chronic cough such as occurs with smoking, asthma, or emphysema or if cough is accompanied by excessive phlegm (mucus) unless directed by a doctor.
Do not exceed recommended dosage. If nervousness, dizziness or sleeplessness occur, discontinue use and consult a doctor. May cause excitability especially in children. Do not take this product, unless directed by a doctor, if you have a breathing problem such as emphysema or chronic bronchitis, or if you have glaucoma or difficulty in urination due to enlargement of the prostate gland. Do not take this product if you have heart disease, high blood pressure, thyroid disease or diabetes unless directed by a doctor.
May cause marked drowsiness; alcohol, sedatives and tranquilizers may increase the drowsiness effect. Avoid alcoholic beverages while taking this product. Do not take this product if you are taking sedatives or tranquilizers, without first consulting your doctor. Use caution when driving a motor vehicle or operating machinery.
Keep this and all drugs out of the reach of children. In case of accidental overdose, contact a doctor or poison control center immediately. Prompt medical attention is critical for adults as well as for children even if you do not notice any signs or symptoms. As with any drug, if you are pregnant or nursing a baby, seek the advice of a health professional before using this product. Do not use with other products containing acetaminophen.

DRUG INTERACTION PRECAUTION

Do not use this product if you are now taking a prescription monoamine oxidase inhibitor (MAOI) (certain drugs for depression, psychiatric or emotional conditions, or Parkinson's disease), or for 2 weeks after stopping the MAOI drug. If you are uncertain whether your prescription drug contains an MAOI, consult a health professional before taking this product.

PROFESSIONAL INFORMATION
OVERDOSAGE INFORMATION

Acetaminophen in massive overdosage may cause hepatic toxicity in some patients. In adults and adolescents (≥12 years of age), hepatic toxicity may occur following ingestion of greater than 7.5 to 10 grams over a period of 8 hours or less. Fatalities are infrequent (less than 3–4% of untreated cases) and have rarely been reported with overdosage of less than 15 grams. In children (<12 years of age), an acute overdosage of less than 150 mg/kg has not been associated with hepatic toxicity. Early symptoms following a potentially hepatotoxic overdose may include: nausea, vomiting, diaphoresis and general malaise. Clinical and laboratory evidence of hepatic toxicity may not be apparent until 48 to 72 hours postingestion. In adults and adolescents, any individual presenting with an unknown amount of acetaminophen ingested or with a questionable or unreliable history about the time of ingestion should have a plasma acetaminophen level drawn and be treated with *N*-acetylcysteine. For full prescribing information, refer to the *N*-acetylcysteine package insert. Do not await results of assays for plasma acetaminophen levels before initiating treatment with *N*-acetylcysteine. The following additional procedures are recommended: Promptly initiate gastric decontamination of the stomach. A plasma acetaminophen assay should be obtained as early as possible, but not sooner than four hours following ingestion. If an acetaminophen *extended release* product is involved, it may be appropriate to obtain an additional plasma acetaminophen level 4–6 hours following the initial acetaminophen level. If either acetaminophen level plots above the treatment line on the acetaminophen overdose nomogram, *N*-acetylcysteine treatment should be continued for a full use of therapy. Liver function studies should be obtained initially and repeated at 24-hour intervals.
Serious toxicity or fatalities have been extremely infrequent following an acute acetaminophen overdose in young children, possibly because of differences in the way they metabolize acetaminophen. In children, the maximum potential amount ingested can be more easily estimated. If more than 150 mg/kg or an unknown amount was ingested, obtain an plasma acetaminophen level as soon as possible, but no sooner than 4 hours following ingestion. If an acetaminophen *extended release* product is involved, it may be appropriate to obtain an additional plasma acetaminophen level 4–6 hours following the initial acetaminophen level. If either acetaminophen level plots above the treatment line on the acetaminophen overdose nomogram, the *N*-acetylcysteine treatment should be initiated and continued for a full course of therapy. If an assay cannot be obtained and the estimated acetaminophen ingestion exceeds 150 mg/kg, dosing with *N*-acetylcysteine should be initiated and continued for a full course of therapy.
For additional emergency information, call your regional poison center or call the Rocky Mountain Poison Center toll-free, (1-800-525-6115).
Symptoms from pseudoephedrine overdose consist most often of mild anxiety, tachycardia and/or mild hypertension. Symptoms usually appear within 4 to 8 hours of ingestion and are transient, usually requiring no treatment.
Acute dextromethorphan overdose usually does not result in serious signs and symptoms unless massive amounts have been ingested. Signs and symptoms of a substantial overdose may include nausea and vomiting, visual disturbances, CNS disturbances, and urinary retention.
Diphenhydramine and doxylamine toxicity should be treated as you would an antihistamine/anticholinergic overdose and is likely to be present within a few hours after acute ingestion.
Alcohol Information: Chronic heavy alcohol abusers may be at increased risk of liver toxicity from excessive acetaminophen use, although reports of this event are rare. Reports usually involve cases of severe chronic alcoholics and the dosages of acetaminophen most often exceed recommended doses and often involve substantial overdose. Healthcare professionals should alert their patients who regularly consume large amounts of alcohol not to exceed recommended doses of acetaminophen.

INACTIVE INGREDIENTS

Maximum Strength TYLENOL® FLU NON-DROWSY Gelcaps: Benzyl Alcohol, Butylparaben, Castor Oil, Cellulose,

Corn Starch, Edetate Calcium Disodium, FD&C Blue #1, FD&C Red #40, Gelatin, Hydroxypropyl Methylcellulose, Iron Oxide, Magnesium Stearate, Methylparaben, Propylparaben, Sodium Lauryl Sulfate, Sodium Propionate, Sodium Starch Glycolate, Titanium Dioxide.
Maximum Strength TYLENOL® FLU NightTime Gelcaps: Benzyl Alcohol, Butylparaben, Castor Oil, Cellulose, Corn Starch, D&C Red #28, Edetate Calcium Disodium, FD&C Blue #1, Gelatin, Hydroxypropyl Methylcellulose, Iron Oxide, Magnesium Stearate, Methylparaben, Propylparaben, Sodium Citrate, Sodium Lauryl Sulfate, Sodium Propionate, Sodium Starch Glycolate, Titanium Dioxide.
Maximum Strength TYLENOL® FLU NightTime Liquid: Citric Acid, Corn Syrup, D&C Red #33, FD&C Red #40, Flavors, Polyethylene Glycol, Propylene Glycol, Purified Water, Saccharin Sodium, Sodium Benzoate, Sorbitol.

HOW SUPPLIED

***Maximum Strength TYLENOL® FLU NON-DROWSY:* Gelcaps:** Burgundy- and white-colored gelcap, imprinted with "TYLENOL FLU" in gray ink—blister packs of 24. Store at room temperature. Avoid high humidity and excessive heat 40°C (104°F).
***Maximum Strength TYLENOL® FLU NightTime:* Gelcaps:** Blue and white-colored gelcap, imprinted with "TYLENOL FLU NT" gray ink—blister packs of 12 and 24. Store at room temperature. Avoid high humidity and excessive heat 40°C (104°F). **Liquid:** Red-colored—bottles of 8 fl. oz with child resistant safety cap and tamper evident packaging. Store at room temperature.

Shown in Product Identification Guide, page 323

Maximum Strength TYLENOL® SORE THROAT Adult Liquid — OTC

DESCRIPTION

Maximum Strength TYLENOL® SORE THROAT Liquid is available in Honey Lemon Flavor or Cherry Flavor and contains acetaminophen 1000 mg in each 30 mL (2 Tablespoonsful).

ACTIONS

Acetaminophen is a clinically proven analgesic/antipyretic. Acetaminophen produces analgesia by elevation of the pain threshold and antipyresis through action on the hypothalamic heat regulating center. Acetaminophen is equal to aspirin in analgesic and antipyretic effectiveness and it is unlikely to produce many of the side effects associated with aspirin and aspirin-containing products.

USES

For the temporary relief of minor aches and pains associated with sore throat, headache, muscular aches, common cold. For the reduction of fever.

DIRECTIONS

Adults and children 12 years of age and older: Take 2 Tablespoons (tbsp.) every 4 to 6 hours as needed. Do not use more than 4 times in 24 hours, or as directed by a doctor.
Children under 12 years: Do not use this adult product in children under 12 years of age. This will provide more than the recommended dose (overdose) of TYLENOL® and could cause serious health problems.

PRECAUTIONS

If a rare sensitivity reaction occurs, the drug should be discontinued.

WARNINGS

Alcohol Warning: If you consume 3 or more alcoholic drinks every day, ask your doctor whether you should take acetaminophen or other pain relievers/fever reducers. Acetaminophen may cause liver damage.
Do Not Use:
- with any other product containing acetaminophen
- for more than 10 days for pain unless directed by a doctor
- for more than 3 days for fever unless directed by a doctor

Stop Using and Ask a Doctor if:
- symptoms do not improve
- new symptoms occur
- pain or fever persists or gets worse
- redness or swelling is present
- sore throat is severe, persists for more than 2 days, is accompanied or followed by fever, headache, rash, nausea or vomiting

Do not exceed recommended dose. Keep this and all drugs out of the reach of children. In case of accidental overdose, contact a physician or poison control center immediately. Prompt medical attention is critical for adults as well as for children even if you do not notice any signs or symptoms. As with any drug, if you are pregnant or nursing a baby, seek the advice of a health professional before using this product.
Do not use if carton is opened or if bottle wrap or foil inner seal imprinted "Safety Seal®" is broken or missing.

PROFESSIONAL INFORMATION
OVERDOSAGE INFORMATION

Acetaminophen in massive overdosage may cause hepatic toxicity in some patients. In adults and adolescents (≥ 12 years of age), hepatic toxicity may occur following ingestion of greater than 7.5 to 10 grams over a period of 8 hours or less. Fatalities are infrequent (less than 3–4% of untreated cases) and have rarely been reported with overdoses of less than 15 grams. In children (< 12 years of age), an acute overdosage of less than 150 mg/kg has not been associated with hepatic toxicity. Early symptoms following a potentially hepatotoxic overdose may include: nausea, vomiting, diaphoresis and general malaise. Clinical and laboratory evidence of hepatic toxicity may not be apparent until 48 to 72 hours postingestion. In adults and adolescents, any individual presenting with an unknown amount of acetaminophen ingested or with a questionable or unreliable history about the time of ingestion should have a plasma acetaminophen level drawn and be treated with *N*-acetylcysteine. For full prescribing information, refer to the *N*-acetylcysteine package insert. Do not await results of assays for plasma acetaminophen levels before initiating treatment with *N*-acetylcysteine. The following additional procedures are recommended: Promptly initiate gastric decontamination of the stomach. A plasma acetaminophen assay should be obtained as early as possible, but no sooner than four hours following ingestion. If an acetaminophen *extended release* product is involved, it may be appropriate to obtain an additional plasma acetaminophen level 4–6 hours following the initial acetaminophen level. If either acetaminophen level plots above the treatment line on the acetaminophen overdose nomogram, *N*-acetylcysteine treatment should be continued for a full course of therapy. Liver function studies should be obtained initially and repeated at 24-hour intervals.
Serious toxicity or fatalities have been extremely infrequent following acute acetaminophen overdosage in young children, possibly because of differences in the way they metabolize acetaminophen. In children, the maximum potential amount ingested can be more easily estimated. If more than 150 mg/kg or an unknown amount was ingested, obtain a plasma acetaminophen level as soon as possible, but no sooner than 4 hours following ingestion. If an acetaminophen *extended release* product is involved, it may be appropriate to obtain an additional plasma acetaminophen level 4–6 hours following the initial acetaminophen level. If either acetaminophen level plots above the treatment line on the acetaminophen overdose nomogram, *N*-acetylcysteine treatment should be initiated and continued for a full course of therapy. If an assay cannot be obtained and the estimated acetaminophen ingestion exceeds 150 mg/kg, dosing with *N*-acetylcysteine should be initiated and continued for a full course of therapy.
For additional emergency information, call your regional poison center or call the Rocky Mountain Poison Center toll-free, (1-800-525-6115).
Alcohol Information: Chronic heavy alcohol abusers may be at increased risk of liver toxicity from excessive acetaminophen use, although reports of this event are rare. Reports usually involve cases of severe chronic alcoholics and the dosages of acetaminophen most often exceed recommended doses and often involve substantial overdose. Healthcare professionals should alert their patients who regularly consume large amounts of alcohol not to exceed recommended doses of acetaminophen.

INACTIVE INGREDIENTS

Maximum Strength TYLENOL® SORE THROAT Honey-Lemon-Flavored Adult Liquid: Carmel color, Citric Acid, Flavor, High Fructose Corn Syrup, Polyethylene Glycol, Propylene Glycol, Purified Water, Saccharin Sodium, Sodium Benzoate, Sorbitol
Maximum Strength TYLENOL® SORE THROAT Cherry-Flavored Adult Liquid: Citric Acid, D&C Red No. 33, FD&C Red No. 40, Flavor, High Fructose Corn Syrup, Polyethylene Glycol, Propylene Glycol, Purified Water, Saccharin Sodium, Sodium Benzoate, Sorbitol

HOW SUPPLIED

Honey lemon-flavored or cherry-flavored liquid in child-resistant tamper-evident bottles of 8 fl. oz. Store at room temperature.

Shown in Product Identification Guide, page 323

Extra Strength TYLENOL® PM
Pain Reliever/Sleep Aid Caplets, Geltabs and Gelcaps

DESCRIPTION

Each ***Extra Strength TYLENOL® PM Caplet, Geltab*** or ***Gelcap*** contains acetaminophen 500 mg and diphenhydramine HCl 25 mg.

ACTIONS

Extra Strength TYLENOL® PM Caplets, Geltabs and ***Gelcaps*** contain a clinically proven analgesic-antipyretic and an antihistamine. Maximum allowable non-prescription levels of acetaminophen and diphenhydramine provide temporary relief of occasional headaches and minor aches and pains accompanying sleeplessness. Acetaminophen is equal to aspirin in analgesic and antipyretic effectiveness and it is unlikely to produce many of the side effects associated with aspirin containing products. Acetaminophen produces analgesia by elevation of the pain threshold. Diphenhydramine HCl is an antihistamine with sedative properties.

USES

Extra Strength TYLENOL® PM Caplets, Geltabs and ***Gelcaps:*** For the temporary relief of occasional headaches and minor aches and pains with accompanying sleeplessness.

DIRECTIONS

Adults and children 12 years of age and older: Take 2 caplets, geltabs or gelcaps at bedtime or as directed by a doctor. **Children under 12 years of age:** Do not use this adult product in children under 12 years of age. This will provide more than the recommended dose (overdose) and could cause serious health problems.

PRECAUTIONS

If a rare sensitivity reaction occurs, the drug should be discontinued.

WARNINGS

Alcohol Warning: If you consume 3 or more alcoholic drinks every day, ask your doctor whether you should take acetaminophen or other pain relievers/fever reducers. Acetaminophen may cause liver damage.
Do not use if carton is opened or neck wrap or foil inner seal imprinted with "Safety Seal®" is broken. If sleeplessness persists continuously for more than 2 weeks, consult your doctor. Insomnia may be a symptom of serious underlying medical illness. Do not take for pain for more than 10 days or for fever for more than 3 days unless directed by a doctor. If pain or fever persists, or gets worse, if new symptoms occur, or if redness or swelling is present, consult a doctor because these could be signs of a serious condition. Do not take this product, unless directed by a doctor, if you have a breathing problem such as emphysema or chronic bronchitis, or if you have glaucoma or difficulty in urination due to enlargement of the prostate gland. Avoid alcoholic beverages while taking this product. Do not take this product if your are taking sedatives or tranquilizers without first consulting your doctor.
Do not exceed recommended dose. Keep this and all drugs out of the reach of children. In case of accidental overdose, contact a physician or poison control center immediately. Prompt medical attention is critical for adults as well as for children even if you do not notice any signs or symptoms. As with any drug, if you are pregnant or nursing a baby, seek the advice of a health professional before using this product. Do not use with other products containing acetaminophen.
CAUTION: This product will cause drowsiness. Do not drive a motor vehicle or operate machinery after use.

PROFESSIONAL INFORMATION
OVERDOSAGE INFORMATION

Acetaminophen in massive overdosage may cause hepatic toxicity in some patients. In adults and adolescents (≥ 12 years of age), hepatic toxicity may occur following ingestion of greater than 7.5 to 10 grams over a period of 8 hours or less. Fatalities are infrequent (less than 3–4% of untreated cases) and have rarely been reported with overdoses of less than 15 grams. In children (<12 years of age), an acute overdosage of less than 150 mg/kg has not been associated with hepatic toxicity.
Early symptoms following a potentially hepatotoxic overdose may include: nausea, vomiting, diaphoresis and general malaise. Clinical and laboratory evidence of hepatic toxicity may not be apparent until 48 to 72 hours postingestion. In adults and adolescents, any individual presenting with an unknown amount of acetaminophen ingested or with a questionable or unreliable history about the time of ingestion should have a plasma acetaminophen level drawn and be treated with *N*-acetylcysteine. For full prescribing information, refer to the *N*-acetylcysteine package insert. Do not await results of assays for plasma acetaminophen levels before initiating treatment with *N*-acetylcysteine. The following additional procedures are recommended: Promptly initiate gastric decontamination of the stomach. A plasma acetaminophen assay should be obtained as early as possible, but no sooner than four hours following ingestion. If an acetaminophen *extended release* product is involved, it may be appropriate to obtain an additional plasma acetaminophen level 4–6 hours following the initial acetaminophen level. If either acetaminophen level plots above the treatment line on the acetaminophen overdose nomogram, *N*-acetylcysteine treatment should be continued for a full course of therapy. Liver function studies should be obtained initially and repeated at 24-hour intervals.
Serious toxicity or fatalities have been extremely infrequent following an acute acetaminophen overdose in young children, possibly because of differences in the way they metabolize acetaminophen. In children, the maximum potential amount ingested can be more easily estimated. If more than 150 mg/kg or an unknown amount was ingested, obtain a plasma acetaminophen level as soon as possible, but no sooner than 4 hours following ingestion. If an acetaminophen *extended release* product is involved, it may be appropriate to obtain an additional plasma acetaminophen level 4–6 hours following the initial acetaminophen level. If either acetaminophen level plots above the treatment line on the acetaminophen overdose nomogram, *N*-acetylcysteine treatment should be initiated and continued for a full course of therapy. If an assay cannot be obtained and the estimated acetaminophen ingestion exceeds 150 mg/kg, dosing with *N*-acetylcysteine should be initiated and continued for a full course of therapy.
For additional emergency information, call your regional poison center or call the Rocky Mountain Poison Center toll-free, (1-800-525-6115).
Diphenhydramine toxicity should be treated as you would an antihistamine/anticholinergic overdose and is likely to be present within a few hours after acute ingestion.

Continued on next page

Tylenol PM—Cont.

Alcohol Information: Chronic heavy alcohol abusers may be at increased risk of liver toxicity from excessive acetaminophen use, although reports of this event are rare. Reports usually involve cases of severe chronic alcoholics and the dosages of acetaminophen most often exceed recommended doses and often involve substantial overdose. Healthcare professionals should alert their patients who regularly consume large amounts of alcohol not to exceed recommended doses of acetaminophen.

INACTIVE INGREDIENTS

Caplets: Cellulose, Cornstarch, FD&C Blue #1, FD&C Blue #2, Hydroxypropyl Methylcellulose, Magnesium Stearate, Polyethylene Glycol, Polysorbate 80, Sodium Citrate, Sodium Starch Glycolate, Titanium Dioxide.

Geltabs/Gelcaps: Benzyl Alcohol, Butylparaben, Castor Oil, Cellulose, Corn Starch, D&C Red #28, Edetate Calcium Disodium, FD&C Blue #1, Gelatin, Hydroxypropyl Methylcellulose, Magnesium Stearate, Methylparaben, Propylparaben, Sodium Citrate, Sodium Lauryl Sulfate, Sodium Propionate, Sodium Starch Glycolate, Titanium Dioxide.

HOW SUPPLIED

Caplets (colored light blue imprinted "Tylenol PM") vials of 10 and tamper-evident bottles of 24, 50, 100, and 150. Store at room temperature.

Gelcaps (colored blue and white imprinted "TYLENOL PM") tamper-evident bottles of 24 and 50. Store at room temperature; avoid high humidity and excessive heat 40°C (104°F).

Geltabs (colored blue and white imprinted "TYLENOL PM") tamper-evident bottles of 24, 50, and 100. Store at room temperature; avoid high humidity and excessive heat 40°C (104°F).

Shown in Product Identification Guide, page 323

Maximum Strength TYLENOL® SINUS NON-DROWSY OTC
Geltabs, Gelcaps, Caplets and Tablets

Maximum Strength TYLENOL® SINUS
NightTime Caplets

Product information for all dosage forms of TYLENOL SINUS have been combined under this heading.

DESCRIPTION

Each ***Maximum Strength TYLENOL® SINUS NON-DROWSY Geltab, Gelcap, Caplet or Tablet*** contains acetaminophen 500 mg and pseudoephedrine HCl 30 mg. Each ***Maximum Strength TYLENOL® SINUS NightTime Caplet*** contains acetaminophen 500 mg, doxylamine succinate 6.25 mg and pseudoephedrine HCl 30 mg.

ACTIONS

Maximum Strength TYLENOL® SINUS NON-DROWSY contains a clinically proven analgesic-antipyretic and a decongestant. Maximum allowable non-prescription levels of acetaminophen and pseudoephedrine provide temporary relief of sinus headache and congestion. Acetaminophen is equal to aspirin in analgesic and antipyretic effectiveness and it is unlikely to produce many of the side effects associated with aspirin and aspirin-containing products. Acetaminophen produces analgesia by elevation of the pain threshold and antipyresis through action on the hypothalamic heat regulating center. Pseudoephedrine hydrochloride is a sympathomimetic amine which promotes sinus cavity drainage by reducing nasopharyngeal mucosal congestion.

Maximum Strength TYLENOL® SINUS NightTime Caplets contain, in addition to the above ingredients, an antihistamine which provides temporary relief of runny nose and itching of the nose or throat.

USES

Maximum Strength TYLENOL® SINUS NON-DROWSY: For the temporary relief of sinus pain and headaches and nasal and sinus congestion.

Maximum Strength TYLENOL® SINUS NightTime: For the temporary relief of nasal congestion, sinus congestion and pressure, sinus pain, headache, runny nose, and itching of the nose or throat.

PRECAUTIONS

If a rare sensitivity reaction occurs, the drug should be discontinued.

DIRECTIONS

Maximum Strength TYLENOL® SINUS NON-DROWSY:

Adults and children 12 years of age and older: Take 2 every 4–6 hours. Do not take more than 8 in 24 hours, or as directed by a doctor.

Children under 12 years: Do not use this adult product in children under 12 years of age. This will provide more than the recommended dose (overdose) and could cause serious health problems.

***Maximum Strength TYLENOL® SINUS NightTime:* Adults and children 12 years of age and older:** Take 2 caplets at bedtime. May repeat every 4 to 6 hours. Do not take more than 8 caplets in 24 hours, or as directed by a doctor.

Children under 12 years: Do not use this adult product in children under 12 years of age. This will provide more than the recommended dose (overdose) and could cause serious health problems.

WARNINGS

Alcohol Warning: If you consume 3 or more alcoholic drinks every day, ask your doctor whether you should take acetaminophen or other pain relievers/fever reducers. Acetaminophen may cause liver damage.

***Maximum Strength TYLENOL® SINUS NON-DROWSY:* Do not use if carton is opened or if blister unit is broken.** Do not take for pain for more than 7 days or for fever for more than 3 days unless directed by a doctor. If pain or fever persists, or gets worse, if new symptoms occur, or if redness or swelling is present, consult a doctor because these could be signs of a serious condition. If nervousness, dizziness or sleeplessness occur, discontinue use and consult a doctor. Do not take this product if you have heart disease, high blood pressure, thyroid disease, diabetes, or difficulty in urination due to enlargement of the prostate gland unless directed by a doctor.

Do not exceed recommended dosage. Keep this and all drugs out of the reach of children. In case of accidental overdose, contact a doctor or poison control center immediately. Prompt medical attention is critical for adults as well as for children even if you do not notice any signs or symptoms. As with any drug, if you are pregnant or nursing a baby, seek the advice of a health professional before using this product. Do not use with other products containing acetaminophen.

***Maximum Strength TYLENOL® SINUS NightTime Caplets:* Do not use if carton is opened or if blister unit is broken.** Do not take for pain for more than 7 days or for fever for more than 3 days unless directed by a doctor. If pain or fever persists, or gets worse, if new symptoms occur, or if redness or swelling is present, consult a doctor because these could be signs of a serious condition. May cause excitability especially in children. If nervousness, dizziness or sleeplessness occur, discontinue use and consult a doctor. May cause marked drowsiness; alcohol, sedatives and tranquilizers may increase the drowsiness effect. Avoid alcoholic beverages while taking this product. Do not take this product if you are taking sedatives or tranquilizers, without first consulting your doctor. Use caution when driving a motor vehicle or operating machinery. Do not take this product, unless directed by a doctor, if you have a breathing problem such as emphysema or chronic bronchitis, or if you have glaucoma, or difficulty in urination due to enlargement of the prostate gland. Do not take this product if you have heart disease, high blood pressure, thyroid disease or diabetes unless directed by a doctor.

Do not exceed recommended dosage. Keep this and all drugs out of the reach of children. In case of accidental overdose, contact a doctor or poison control center immediately. Prompt medical attention is critical for adults as well as for children even if you do not notice any signs or symptoms. As with any drug. If you are pregnant or nursing a baby, seek the advice of a health professional before using this product. Do not use with other products containing acetaminophen.

DRUG INTERACTION PRECAUTION

Do not use this product if you are now taking a prescription monoamine oxidase inhibitor (MAOI) (certain drugs for depression, psychiatric or emotional conditions, or Parkinson's disease), or for 2 weeks after stopping the MAOI drug. If you are uncertain whether your prescription drug contains an MAOI, consult a health professional before taking this product.

PROFESSIONAL INFORMATION
OVERDOSAGE INFORMATION

Acetaminophen in massive overdosage may cause hepatic toxicity in some patients. In adults and adolescents ($\geq$ 12 years of age), hepatic toxicity may occur following ingestion of greater than 7.5 to 10 grams over a period of 8 hours or less. Fatalities are infrequent (less than 3–4% of untreated cases) and have rarely been reported with overdoses of less than 15 grams. In children (< 12 years of age), an acute overdosage of less than 150 mg/kg has not been associated with hepatic toxicity. Early symptoms following a potentially hepatotoxic overdose may include: nausea, vomiting, diaphoresis and general malaise. Clinical and laboratory evidence of hepatic toxicity may not be apparent until 48 to 72 hours postingestion. In adults and adolescents, any individual presenting with an unknown amount of acetaminophen ingested or with a questionable or unreliable history about the time of ingestion should have a plasma acetaminophen level drawn and be treated with *N*-acetylcysteine. For full prescribing information, refer to the *N*-acetylcysteine package insert. Do not await results of assays for plasma acetaminophen levels before initiating treatment with *N*-acetylcysteine. The following additional procedures are recommended: Promptly initiate gastric decontamination of the stomach. A plasma acetaminophen assay should be obtained as early as possible, but no sooner than four hours following ingestion. If an acetaminophen *extended release* product is involved, it may be appropriate to obtain an additional plasma acetaminophen level 4–6 hours following the initial acetaminophen level. If either acetaminophen level plots above the treatment line on the acetaminophen overdose nomogram, *N*-acetylcysteine treatment should be continued for a full course of therapy. Liver function studies should be obtained initially and repeated at 24-hour intervals.

Serious toxicity or fatalities have been extremely infrequent following an acute acetaminophen overdose in young children, possibly because of differences in the way they metabolize acetaminophen. In children, the maximum potential amount ingested can be more easily estimated. If more than 150 mg/kg or an unknown amount was ingested, obtain a plasma acetaminophen level as soon as possible, but no sooner than 4 hours following ingestion. If an acetaminophen *extended release* product is involved, it may be appropriate to obtain an additional plasma acetaminophen level 4–6 hours following the initial acetaminophen level. If either acetaminophen level plots above the treatment line on the acetaminophen overdose nomogram, *N*-acetylcysteine treatment should be initiated and continued for a full course of therapy. If an assay cannot be obtained and the estimated acetaminophen ingestion exceeds 150 mg/kg, dosing with *N*-acetylcysteine should be initiated and continued for a full course of therapy.

For additional emergency information, call your regional poison center or call the Rocky Mountain Poison Center toll-free (1-800-525-6115).

Symptoms from pseudoephedrine overdose consist most often of mild anxiety, tachycardia and/or mild hypertension. Symptoms usually appear within 4 to 8 hours after ingestion and are transient, usually requiring no treatment.

Doxylamine toxicity should be treated as you would an antihistamine/anticholinergic overdose and is likely to be present within a few hours after acute ingestion.

Alcohol Information: Chronic heavy alcohol abusers may be at increased risk of liver toxicity from excessive acetaminophen use, although reports of this event are rare. Reports usually involve cases of severe chronic alcoholics and the dosages of acetaminophen most often exceed recommended doses and often involve substantial overdose. Healthcare professionals should alert their patients who regularly consume large amounts of alcohol not to exceed recommended doses of acetaminophen.

INACTIVE INGREDIENTS

***Maximum Strength TYLENOL® SINUS NON-DROWSY Formula:* Caplets:** Carnauba Wax, Cellulose, Corn Starch, D&C Yellow #10, FD&C Blue #1, FD&C Red #40, Hydroxypropyl Methylcellulose, Iron Oxide, Magnesium Stearate, Polyethylene Glycol, Polysorbate 80, Sodium Starch Glycolate, Titanium Dioxide.

Tablets: Cellulose, Corn Starch, D&C Yellow #10, FD&C Blue #1, FD&C Yellow #6, Magnesium Stearate, Sodium Starch Glycolate.

Gelcaps and Geltabs: Benzyl Alcohol, Butylparaben, Castor Oil, Cellulose, Corn Starch, D&C Yellow #10, Edetate Calcium Disodium, FD&C Blue #1, Gelatin, Hydroxypropyl Methylcellulose, Iron Oxide, Magnesium Stearate, Methylparaben, Propylparaben, Sodium Lauryl Sulfate, Sodium Propionate, Sodium Starch Glycolate, Titanium Dioxide.

Maximum Strength TYLENOL® SINUS NightTime Caplets: Cellulose, Corn Starch, FD&C Blue #1, FD&C Blue #2, Hydroxypropyl Methylcellulose, Iron Oxide, Silicon Dioxide, Sodium Starch Glycolate, Stearic Acid, Titanium Dioxide, Triacetin.

HOW SUPPLIED

***Maximum Strength TYLENOL® SINUS NON-DROWSY Formula:* Tablets:** Light green-colored, imprinted with "MAXIMUM STRENGTH" on one side and "TYLENOL SINUS" on the opposite side—blister packs of 48. Store at room temperature.

Caplets: Light green-colored, imprinted with "TYLENOL SINUS" in green ink—blister packs of 24 and 48. Store at room temperature.

Gelcaps: Green- and white-colored, imprinted with "TYLENOL SINUS" in dark green ink—blister packs of 24 and 48. Store at room temperature; avoid high humidity and excessive heat 40°C (104°F).

Geltabs: Green-colored on one side and white-colored on opposite side, imprinted with "TYLENOL SINUS" in gray ink—blister packs of 24 and 48. Store at room temperature; avoid high humidity and excessive heat 40°C (104°F).

Maximum Strength TYLENOL® SINUS NightTime Caplets: Green-colored, imprinted with "Tylenol Sinus NT"—blister packs of 24. Store at room temperature.

Shown in Product Identification Guide, page 323

Women's TYLENOL® Multi-Symptom Menstrual Relief Pain Reliever/Diuretic OTC
Caplets

DESCRIPTION

Each ***Women's Tylenol® Multi-Symptom Menstrual Relief Caplet*** contains acetaminophen 500 mg and pamabrom 25 mg.

ACTIONS

Women's TYLENOL® Multi-Symptom Menstrual Relief Caplets contain a clinically proven analgesic-antipyretic and a diuretic. Maximum allowable non-prescription levels of acetaminophen and pamabrom provide temporary relief of minor aches and pains due to cramps, headache, and backache and water retention, weight gain, bloating, swelling and full feeling associated with the premenstrual and menstrual periods. Acetaminophen is equal to aspirin in analgesic and antipyretic effectiveness and it is unlikely to produce many of the side effects associated with aspirin containing products. Acetaminophen produces analgesia by elevation of the pain threshold. Pamabrom is a diuretic which relieves water retention.

USES

Women's TYLENOL® Multi-Symptom Menstrual Relief Caplets: For the temporary relief of minor aches and pains due to cramps, headache, backache. Temporarily relieves water weight gain, bloating, swelling and full feeling associated with the premenstrual and menstrual periods.

DIRECTIONS

Do not take more than directed. **Adults and children 12 years and over:** Take 2 caplets every 4 to 6 hours, do not take more than 8 caplets in 24 hours, or as directed by a doctor. **Children under 12 years:** Do not use this adult product in children under 12 years of age; this will provide more than the recommended dose (overdose) and could cause serious health problems.

WARNINGS

Alcohol Warning: If you consume 3 or more alcoholic drinks every day, ask your doctor whether you should take acetaminophen or other pain relievers/fever reducers. Acetaminophen may cause liver damage. **Do not use if carton is opened, or if neck wrap or foil inner seal imprinted "Safety Seal®" is broken or missing.**

Do not use

- with any other product containing acetaminophen

Stop use and ask a doctor if

- new symptoms occur
- redness or swelling is present
- pain gets worse or lasts for more than 10 days

If pregnant or breast-feeding, ask a health professional before use

Keep out of reach of children.

In case of overdose, immediately get medical help or contact a Poison Control Center right away. Prompt medical attention is critical for adults as well as for children even if you do not notice any signs or symptoms.

PROFESSIONAL INFORMATION

OVERDOSAGE INFORMATION

Acetaminophen in massive overdosage may cause hepatic toxicity in some patients. In adults and adolescents (≥12 years of age), hepatic toxicity may occur following ingestion of greater than 7.5 to 10 grams over a period of 8 hours or less. Fatalities are infrequent (less than 3–4% of untreated cases) and have rarely been reported with overdoses of less than 15 grams. In children (<12 years of age), an acute overdosage of less than 150 mg/kg has not been associated with hepatic toxicity. Early symptoms following a potentially hepatotoxic overdosage may include: nausea, vomiting, diaphoresis and general malaise. Clinical and laboratory evidence of hepatic toxicity may not be apparent until 48 to 72 hours postingestion. In adults and adolescents, any individual presenting with an unknown amount of acetaminophen ingested or with a questionable or unreliable history about the time of ingestion should have a plasma acetaminophen level drawn and be treated with *N*-acetylcysteine. For full prescribing information, refer to the *N*-acetylcysteine package insert. Do not await results of assays for plasma acetaminophen levels before initiating treatment with *N*-acetylcysteine. The following additional procedures are recommended: Promptly initiate gastric decontamination of the stomach. A plasma acetaminophen assay should be obtained as early as possible, but no sooner than four hours following ingestion. If an acetaminophen *extended release* product is involved, it may be appropriate to obtain an additional plasma acetaminophen level 4–6 hours following the initial acetaminophen level. If either acetaminophen level plots above the treatment line on the acetaminophen overdose nomogram, *N*-acetylcysteine treatment should be continued for a full course of therapy. Liver function studies should be obtained initially and repeated at 24-hour intervals.

Serious toxicity or fatalities have been extremely infrequent following a acute acetaminophen overdose in young children, possibly because of differences in the way they metabolize acetaminophen. In children, the maximum potential amount ingested can be more easily estimated. If more than 150 mg/kg or an unknown amount ingested, obtain a plasma acetaminophen level as soon as possible, but no sooner than 4 hours following ingestion. If an acetaminophen *extended release* product is involved, it may be appropriate to obtain an additional plasma acetaminophen level 4–6 hours following the initial acetaminophen level. If either acetaminophen level plots above the treatment line on the acetaminophen overdose nomogram, *N*-acetylcysteine treatment should be initiated and continued for a full course of therapy. If an assay cannot be obtained and the estimated acetaminophen ingestion exceeds 150 mg/kg, dosing with *N*-acetylcysteine should be initiated and continued for a full course of therapy.

For additional emergency information, call your regional poison center or call the Rocky Mountain Poison Center toll-free, (1-800-525-6115).

Acute overexposure of diuretics is primarily associated with fluid and electrolyte loss. Fluid loss should be corrected with the appropriate intravenous and/or oral fluids.

Alcohol Information: Chronic heavy alcohol abusers may be at increased risk of liver toxicity from excessive acetaminophen use, although reports of this event are rare. Reports usually involve cases of severe chronic alcoholics and the dosages of acetaminophen most often exceed recommended doses and often involve substantial overdose. Healthcare professionals should alert their patients who regularly consume large amounts of alcohol not to exceed recommended doses of acetaminophen.

INACTIVE INGREDIENTS

cellulose, corn starch, hydroxypropyl methylcellulose, magnesium stearate, polydextrose, polyethylene glycol, sodium starch glycolate, titanium dioxide, triacetin.

HOW SUPPLIED

Caplets—white capsule shaped caplets with TYME printed on one side in tamper-evident bottles of 24 and 40. Store at room temperature; avoid excessive heat 40 C (104 F).

Shown in Product Identification Guide, page 323

VERMOX® ℞

[*věr 'mŏx*]
(mebendazole)
Chewable Tablets

DESCRIPTION

VERMOX® (mebendazole) is a (synthetic) broad-spectrum anthelmintic available as chewable tablets, each containing 100 mg of mebendazole. Inactive ingredients are: colloidal silicon dioxide, corn starch, hydrogenated vegetable oil, magnesium stearate, microcrystalline cellulose, sodium lauryl sulfate, sodium saccharin, sodium starch glycolate, talc, tetrarome orange, and FD&C yellow No. 6.

Mebendazole is methyl 5-benzoylbenzimidazole-2-carbamate.

Mebendazole is a white to slightly yellow powder with a molecular weight of 295.29. It is less than 0.05% soluble in water, dilute mineral acid solutions, alcohol, ether and chloroform, but is soluble in formic acid.

CLINICAL PHARMACOLOGY

Following administration of 100 mg twice daily for three consecutive days, plasma levels of VERMOX® (mebendazole) and its primary metabolite, the 2-amine, do not exceed 0.03 μg/ml and 0.09 μg/ml, respectively. All metabolites are devoid of anthelmintic activity. In man, approximately 2% of administered VERMOX® is excreted in urine and the remainder in the feces as unchanged drug or a primary metabolite.

Mode of Action: VERMOX® inhibits the formation of the worms' microtubules and causes the worms' glucose depletion.

INDICATIONS AND USAGE

VERMOX® (mebendazole) is indicated for the treatment of *Enterobius vermicularis* (pinworm), *Trichuris trichiura* (whipworm), *Ascaris lumbricoides* (common roundworm), *Ancylostoma duodenale* (common hookworm), *Necator americanus* (American hookworm) in single or mixed infections.

Efficacy varies as a function of such factors as pre-existing diarrhea and gastrointestinal transit time, degree of infection, and helminth strains. Efficacy rates derived from various studies are shown in the table below:

[See first table below]

CONTRAINDICATIONS

VERMOX® (mebendazole) is contraindicated in persons who have shown hypersensitivity to the drug.

WARNINGS

There is no evidence that VERMOX® (mebendazole), even at high doses, is effective for hydatid disease. There have been rare reports of neutropenia and agranulocytosis, when VERMOX® was taken for prolonged periods and at dosages substantially above those recommended.

PRECAUTIONS

General: Periodic assessment of organ system functions, including hematopoietic and hepatic, is advisable during prolonged therapy.

Information for Patients: Patients should be informed of the potential risk to the fetus in women taking VERMOX® (mebendazole) during pregnancy, especially during the first trimester (see Pregnancy).

Patients should also be informed that cleanliness is important to prevent reinfection and transmission of the infection.

Drug Interactions: Preliminary evidence suggests that cimetidine inhibits mebendazole metabolism and may result in an increase in plasma concentrations of mebendazole.

Carcinogenesis, Mutagenesis, Impairment of Fertility: In carcinogenicity tests of mebendazole in mice and rats, no carcinogenic effects were seen at doses as high as 40 mg/kg (one to two times the human dose, based on mg/m^2) given daily over two years. Dominant lethal mutation tests in mice showed no mutagenicity at single doses as high as 640 mg/kg (18 times the human dose, based on mg/m^2). Neither the spermatocyte test, the F_1 translocation test, nor the Ames test indicated mutagenic properties. Doses up to 40 mg/kg in mice (equal to the human dose, based on mg/m^2), given to males for 60 days and to females for 14 days prior to gestation, had no effect upon fetuses and offspring, though there was slight maternal toxicity.

Pregnancy: Teratogenic effects. Pregnancy Category C. Mebendazole has shown embryotoxic and teratogenic activity in pregnant rats at single oral doses as low as 10 mg/kg (approximately equal to the human dose, based on mg/m^2). In view of these findings the use of VERMOX® is not recommended in pregnant women. Although there are no adequate and well-controlled studies in pregnant women, a post-marketing survey has been done of a limited number of women who inadvertently had consumed VERMOX® during the first trimester of pregnancy. The incidence of spontaneous abortion and malformation did not exceed that in the general population. In 170 deliveries on term, no teratogenic risk of VERMOX® was identified.

Nursing Mothers: It is not known whether VERMOX® is excreted in human milk. Because many drugs are excreted in human milk, caution should be exercised when VERMOX® is administered to a nursing woman.

Pediatric Use: The drug has not been extensively studied in children under two years; therefore, in the treatment of children under two years the relative benefit/risk should be considered.

ADVERSE REACTIONS

Gastrointestinal: Transient symptoms of abdominal pain and diarrhea in cases of massive infection and expulsion of worms.

Hypersensitivity: Rash, urticaria and angioedema have been observed on rare occasions.

Central Nervous System: Very rare cases of convulsions have been reported.

Liver: There have been liver function test elevations [AST (SGOT), ALT (SGPT), AND GGT] and rare reports of hepatitis when VERMOX® was taken for prolonged periods and at dosages substantially above those recommended.

Hematologic: Neutropenia and agranulocytosis. (See WARNINGS).

OVERDOSAGE

In the event of accidental overdosage gastrointestinal complaints lasting up to a few hours may occur. Vomiting and purging should be induced.

DOSAGE AND ADMINISTRATION

The same dosage schedule applies to children and adults. The tablet may be chewed, swallowed, or crushed and mixed with food.

[See second table below]

If the patient is not cured three weeks after treatment, a second course of treatment is advised. No special procedures, such as fasting or purging, are required.

HOW SUPPLIED

VERMOX® (mebendazole) is available as chewable tablets, each containing 100 mg of mebendazole, and is supplied in boxes of twelve tablets and boxes of sixty tablets.

Store at controlled room temperature 59°–77°F (15°–25°C).

McNeil Consumer Healthcare
Fort Washington, PA 19034
Rev. October 1999
NDC 50580-070-12 (blister package of 12)
NDC 50580-070-60 (blister package of 60)
U.S. Patent 3,657,267

Shown in Product Identification Guide, page 323

Vermox®	Pinworm (enterobiasis)	Whipworm (trichuriasis)	Common Roundworm (ascariasis)	Hookworm
Cure rates mean	95%	68%	98%	96%
Egg reduction mean	—	93%	99%	99%

Vermox®

	Pinworm (enterobiasis)	Whipworm (trichuriasis)	Common Roundworm (ascariasis)	Hookworm
Dose	1 tablet, once	1 tablet morning and evening for 3 consecutive days.	1 tablet morning and evening for 3 consecutive days.	1 tablet morning and evening for 3 consecutive days.

MDR Fitness Corp.

MEDICAL DOCTORS' RESEARCH
14101 NW 4th STREET
SUNRISE, FL 33325

Direct Inquiries to:
1-800-637-8227 ext 5111 or 5436
www.mdri.com

MDR FITNESS TABS FOR MEN OTC
MDR FITNESS TABS FOR WOMEN

DESCRIPTION

The original AM/PM Fitness Tabs® from Medical Doctors' Research are patented because of their ability to increase blood levels of nutrients that can increase immune defenses and reduce the risk of coronary heart disease within weeks of taking the formula. MDR Fitness Tabs. The A.M. and P.M. dosage allows more absorption of the water soluble vitamins (B-complex and C) which are not readily stored by the body. The AM tablet provides more micronutrients required for energy producing reactions when physical activity is greater. The MDR formulas are free of dyes, yeast, preservatives, fillers, soy, wheat gluten, lactose and other sugars.

INDICATIONS AND USAGE

MDR Fitness Tabs are designed for the maintenance of good health and nutrition for men and women, 11 years of age or older, whenever a multi-vitamin, mineral supplement is indicated to help provide nutrients missing from the diet or to replace nutrient loss from oral contraceptives, antacids, excessive alcohol, smoking, physical or emotional stress, exercise, weight loss diets, or illness. Daily use of MDR Fitness Tabs may also play a protective role for good health by assuring adequate intake of essential nutrients, including antioxidant nutrients shown in recent research to enhance the body's natural defenses.

Directions: After the first meal of the day, take one "AM" Fitness Tab. After lunch or dinner, take one "PM" Fitness Tab. Swallow Fitness Tab with a full glass of water.

PRECAUTIONS

Not recommended for persons with severe kidney disease or those undergoing renal dialysis, unless under a physician's supervision. Diabetics may need to adjust insulin dosage and should be monitored. Not recommended for those suffering from pernicious anemia, or Parkinson patients on levodopa therapy, due to the presence of vitamin B-6 which may decrease levodopa's efficacy. Pregnant and lactating women may need additional supplementation.

Note: MDR also provides a Stress Defense supplement to be taken with MDR Fitness Tabs when higher dosages are indicated. MDR has formulated Vital Factors, to supplement MDR Fitness Tabs in persons over 40 years of age. The formula contains secretagogues that help enhance the body's natural release of Human Growth Hormone, and other vital factors which decline with age. Patients report increased vitality, energy, better sleep, improved flexibility and mental function after using Vital Factors.

Also available: Nite-Cal Calcium, Children's Chewable, Chondro-Pro Arthritis Formula and CardioTone Cardiovascular Nutritional Support.

For Samples, Product or Order Information Call
1-800-MDR-TABS ext. 5111 or 5436 or fax (954) 845-9505
att: L. Giordano
www.mdri.com
or write: (MDR) Medical Doctors' Research
14101 NW 4th Street
SUNRISE, FL 33325

Medeva Pharmaceuticals, Inc.

P.O. Box 31710
ROCHESTER, NY 14603

Direct Inquiries to:
Customer Service Department
P.O. Box 31766
Rochester, NY 14603
(716) 274-5300
(888) 9-MEDEVA
In Emergencies:
(800) 932-1950 (24 hours)

AMERICAINE® ANESTHETIC LUBRICANT ℞

[*uh-mer 'ĭ-kān"*]
(benzocaine)
R238D
Rev. 5/99

DESCRIPTION

AMERICAINE Anesthetic Lubricant contains benzocaine 20% with benzethonium chloride 0.1% as a preservative in a water soluble base of polyethylene glycol 300 and 3350.

Benzocaine, a local anesthetic, is chemically ethyl *p*-aminobenzoate, $C_9H_{11}NO_2$, with a molecular weight of 165.19 and has the following structural formula:

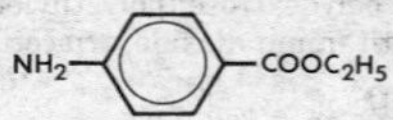

CLINICAL PHARMACOLOGY

Benzocaine reversibly stabilizes the neuronal membrane which decreases its permeability to sodium ions. Depolarization of the neuronal membrane is inhibited thereby blocking the initiation and conduction of nerve impulses.

INDICATIONS AND USAGE

AMERICAINE Anesthetic Lubricant is indicated for general use as a lubricant and topical anesthetic on intratracheal catheters and pharyngeal and nasal airways to obtund the pharyngeal and tracheal reflexes; on nasogastric and endoscopic tubes; urinary catheters; laryngoscopes; proctoscopes; sigmoidoscopes and vaginal specula.

CONTRAINDICATIONS

Known allergy or hypersensitivity to benzocaine.

PRECAUTIONS

General: Medication should be discontinued if sensitivity or irritation occurs.

Carcinogenesis, Mutagenesis, Impairment of Fertility: Long-term studies in animals or humans to evaluate the carcinogenic and mutagenic potential or the effect on fertility have not been conducted.

Pregnancy: Pregnancy Category C. Animal reproduction studies have not been conducted with AMERICAINE Anesthetic Lubricant. It is also not known whether AMERICAINE Anesthetic Lubricant can cause fetal harm when administered to a pregnant woman or can affect reproduction capacity. AMERICAINE Anesthetic Lubricant should be given to a pregnant woman only if clearly needed.

Nursing Mothers: It is not known whether this drug is excreted in human milk. Because many drugs are excreted in human milk, caution should be exercised when AMERICAINE Anesthetic Lubricant is administered to a nursing woman.

Pediatric Use: Do not use in infants under 1 year of age.

ADVERSE REACTIONS

Contact dermatitis and/or hypersensitivity to benzocaine can cause burning, stinging, pruritus, tenderness, erythema, rash, urticaria and edema. Rarely, benzocaine may induce methemoglobinemia causing respiratory distress and cyanosis. Intravenous methylene blue is the specific therapy for this condition.

DOSAGE AND ADMINISTRATION

Apply evenly to exterior of tube or instrument prior to use.

HOW SUPPLIED

AMERICAINE Anesthetic Lubricant (benzocaine) is available in:

NDC 53014-376-16	28 g tube
NDC 53014-376-62	2.5 g unit dose foil packs, 144 per carton

Store at 15°–25°C (59°–77°F).
Rx only
MEDEVA PHARMACEUTICALS
Medeva Pharmaceuticals, Inc.
Rochester, NY 14623 USA
®Ciba-Geigy Corporation
©1999, Medeva Pharmaceuticals, Inc.

Rev. 5/99
R238D

AMERICAINE® OTIC ℞

[*uh-mer ' ĭ-kān "*]
(benzocaine)
Topical Anesthetic Ear Drops
Rev. 8/99
R248

DESCRIPTION

AMERICAINE Otic, topical anesthetic ear drops, contain benzocaine 20% (w/w) in a water soluble base of glycerin 1% (w/w) and polyethylene glycol 300 with benzethonium chloride 0.1% as a preservative.

Benzocaine, a local anesthetic, is chemically ethyl *p*-aminobenzoate, $C_9H_{11}NO_2$, with a molecular weight of 165.19 and has the following structural formula:

CLINICAL PHARMACOLOGY

Benzocaine reversibly stabilizes the neuronal membrane which decreases its permeability to sodium ions. Depolarization of the neuronal membrane is inhibited thereby blocking the initiation and conduction of nerve impulses.

INDICATIONS AND USAGE

AMERICAINE Otic is indicated for relief of pain and pruritus in acute congestive and serous otitis media, acute swimmer's ear, and other forms of otitis externa.

CONTRAINDICATIONS

In the presence of a perforated tympanic membrane or ear discharge.
Known allergy or hypersensitivity to benzocaine.

WARNINGS

Indiscriminate use of anesthetic ear drops may mask symptoms of fulminating infection of the middle ear.

PRECAUTIONS

General: Medication should be discontinued if sensitivity or irritation occurs.

Carcinogenesis, Mutagenesis, Impairment of Fertility: Long-term studies in animals or humans to evaluate the carcinogenic and mutagenic potential or the effect on fertility have not been conducted.

Pregnancy: Pregnancy Category C. Animal reproduction studies have not been conducted with AMERICAINE Otic. It is also not known whether AMERICAINE Otic can cause fetal harm when administered to a pregnant woman or can affect reproduction capacity. AMERICAINE Otic should be given to a pregnant woman only if clearly needed.

Nursing Mothers: It is not known whether this drug is excreted in human milk. Because many drugs are excreted in human milk, caution should be exercised when AMERICAINE Otic is administered to a nursing woman.

Pediatric Use: Do not use in infants under 1 year of age.

ADVERSE REACTIONS

Contact dermatitis and/or hypersensitivity to benzocaine can cause burning, stinging, pruritus, tenderness, erythema, rash, urticaria and edema. Rarely, benzocaine may induce methemoglobinemia causing respiratory distress and cyanosis. Intravenous methylene blue is the specific therapy for this condition.

DOSAGE AND ADMINISTRATION

Instill 4–5 drops of AMERICAINE Otic in the external auditory canal, then insert a cotton pledget into the meatus. Application may be repeated every one to two hours if necessary.

HOW SUPPLIED

AMERICAINE Otic (benzocaine), topical anesthetic ear drops, is available in dropper-top bottles.

NDC 53014-377-51 — 15 mL bottle

Keep bottle tightly closed. Store at 15°–30°C (59°–86°F).
Keep out of the reach of children.
Rx only
Marketed by:
MEDEVA PHARMACEUTICALS
Medeva Pharmaceuticals, Inc.
Rochester, NY 14623 USA
Manufactured by:
Taylor Pharmaceuticals
Decatur, IL 62525 USA
® Ciba-Geigy Corporation
© 1999, Medeva Pharmaceuticals, Inc.

Rev. 8/99
R248

GASTROCROM® ℞

[*gas-tro-crōm*]
(cromolyn sodium, USP)
Oral Concentrate
Rx Only

Rev 4/99
R081C

For Oral Use Only – Not for Inhalation or Injection.

DESCRIPTION

Each 5 mL ampule of GASTROCROM contains 100 mg cromolyn sodium, USP, in purified water. Cromolyn sodium is a hygroscopic, white powder having little odor. It may leave a slightly bitter aftertaste. GASTROCROM (cromolyn sodium, USP) Oral Concentrate is clear, colorless, and sterile. It is intended for oral use.

Chemically, cromolyn sodium is disodium 5,5'-[(2- hydroxytrimethylene)dioxy]bis[4-oxo-4*H*-1-benzopyran-2- carboxylate]. The empirical formula is $C_{23}H_{14}Na_2O_{11}$; the molecular weight is 512.34. Its chemical structure is:

Pharmacologic Category: Mast cell stabilizer
Therapeutic Category: Antiallergic

CLINICAL PHARMACOLOGY

In vitro and *in vivo* animal studies have shown that cromolyn sodium inhibits the release of mediators from sensitized mast cells. Cromolyn sodium acts by inhibiting the release of histamine and leukotrienes (SRS-A) from the mast cell.

Cromolyn sodium has no intrinsic vasoconstrictor, antihistamine, or glucocorticoid activity.
Cromolyn sodium is poorly absorbed from the gastrointestinal tract. No more than 1% of an administered dose is absorbed by humans after oral administration, the remainder being excreted in the feces. Very little absorption of cromolyn sodium was seen after oral administration of 500 mg by mouth to each of 12 volunteers. From 0.28 to 0.50% of the administered dose was recovered in the first 24 hours of urinary excretion in 3 subjects. The mean urinary excretion of an administered dose over 24 hours in the remaining 9 subjects was 0.45%.

CLINICAL STUDIES

Four randomized, controlled clinical trials were conducted with GASTROCROM in patients with either cutaneous or systemic mastocytosis; two of which utilized a placebo-controlled crossover design, one utilized in active-controlled (chlorpheniramine plus cimetidine) crossover design, and one utilized a placebo-controlled parallel group design. Due to the rare nature of this disease, only 36 patients qualified for study entry, of whom 32 were considered evaluable. Consequently, formal statistical analyses were not performed. Clinically significant improvement in gastrointestinal symptoms (diarrhea, abdominal pain) were seen in the majority of patients with some improvement also seen for cutaneous manifestations (urticaria, pruritus, flushing) and cognitive function. The benefit seen with GASTROCROM 200 mg QID was similar to chlorpheniramine (4 mg QID) plus cimetidine (300 mg QID) for both cutaneous and systemic symptoms of mastocytosis.
Clinical improvement occurred within 2–6 weeks of treatment initiation and persisted for 2–3 weeks after treatment withdrawal. GASTROCROM did not affect urinary histamine levels or peripheral eosinophilia, although neither of these variables appeared to correlate with disease severity. Positive clinical benefits were also reported for 37 of 51 patients who received GASTROCROM in United States and foreign humanitarian programs.

INDICATIONS AND USAGE

GASTROCROM is indicated in the management of patients with mastocytosis. Use of this product has been associated with improvement in diarrhea, flushing, headaches, vomiting, urticaria, abdominal pain, nausea, and itching in some patients.

CONTRAINDICATIONS

GASTROCROM is contraindicated in those patients who have shown hypersensitivity to cromolyn sodium.

WARNINGS

The recommended dosage should be decreased in patients with decreased renal or hepatic function. Severe anaphylactic reactions may occur rarely in association with cromolyn sodium administration.

PRECAUTIONS

In view of the biliary and renal routes of excretion of GASTROCROM, consideration should be given to decreasing the dosage of the drug in patients with impaired renal or hepatic function.
Carcinogenesis, Mutagenesis, and Impairment of Fertility: In carcinogenicity studies in mice, hamsters, and rats, cromolyn sodium had no neoplastic effects at intraperitoneal doses up to 150 mg/kg three days per week for 12 months in mice, at intraperitoneal doses up to 53 mg/kg three days per week to 15 weeks followed by 17.5 mg/kg three days per week for 37 weeks in hamsters, and at subcutaneous doses up to 75 mg/kg six days per week for 18 months in rats. These doses in mice, hamsters, and rats are less than the maximum recommended daily oral dose in adults and children on a mg/m^2 basis.
Cromolyn sodium showed no mutagenic potential in Ames Salmonella/microsome plate assays, mitotic gene conversion in *Saccharomyces cerevisiae* and in an *in vitro* cytogenetic study in human peripheral lymphocytes.
In rats, cromolyn sodium showed no evidence of impaired fertility at subcutaneous doses up to 175 mg/kg in males (approximately equal to the maximum recommended daily oral dose in adults on a mg/m^2 basis) and 100 mg/kg in females (less than the maximum recommended daily oral dose in adults on a mg/m^2 basis).
Pregnancy: Pregnancy Category B. In reproductive studies in pregnant mice, rats, and rabbits, cromolyn sodium produced no evidence of fetal malformations at subcutaneous doses up to 540 mg/kg in mice (approximately equal to the maximum recommended daily oral dose in adults on a mg/m^2 basis) and 164 mg/kg in rats (less than the maximum recommended daily oral dose in adults on a mg/m^2 basis) or at intravenous doses up to 485 mg/kg in rabbits (approximately 4 times the maximum recommended daily oral dose in adults on a mg/m^2 basis). There are, however, no adequate and well controlled studies in pregnant women.
Because animal reproduction studies are not always predictive of human response, this drug should be used during pregnancy only if clearly needed.
Drug Interaction During Pregnancy: In pregnant mice, cromolyn sodium alone did not cause significant increases in resorptions or major malformations at subcutaneous doses up to 540 mg/kg (approximately equal to the maximum recommended daily oral dose in adults on a mg/m^2 basis). Isoproterenol alone increased both resorptions and major malformations (primarily cleft palate) at a subcutaneous dose of 2.7 mg/kg (approximately 7 times the maximum recommended daily inhalation dose in adults on a mg/m^2 basis). The incidence of major malformations increased further when cromolyn sodium at a subcutaneous dose of 540 mg/kg was added to isoproterenol at a subcutaneous dose of 2.7 mg/kg. No such interaction was observed in rats or rabbits.
Nursing Mothers: It is not known whether this drug is excreted in human milk. Because many drugs are excreted in human milk, caution should be exercised when GASTROCROM is administered to a nursing woman.
Pediatric Use: In adult rats no adverse effects of cromolyn sodium were observed at oral doses up to 6144 mg/kg (approximately 25 times the maximum recommended daily oral dose in adults on a mg/m^2 basis). In neonatal rats, cromolyn sodium increased mortality at oral doses of 1000 mg/kg or greater (approximately 9 times the maximum recommended daily oral dose in infants on a mg/m^2 basis) but not at doses of 300 mg/kg or less (approximately 3 times the maximum recommended daily oral dose in infants on a mg/m^2 basis). Plasma and kidney concentrations of cromolyn after oral administration to neonatal rats were up to 20 times greater than those in older rats. In term infants up to six months of age, available clinical data suggest that the dose should not exceed 20 mg/kg/day. The use of this product in pediatric patients less than two years of age should be reserved for patients with severe disease in which the potential benefits clearly outweigh the risks.

ADVERSE REACTIONS

Most of the adverse events reported in mastocytosis patients have been transient and could represent symptoms of the disease. The most frequently reported adverse events in mastocytosis patients who have received GASTROCROM during clinical studies were headache and diarrhea, each of which occurred in 4 of the 87 patients. Pruritus, nausea, and myalgia were each reported in 3 patients and abdominal pain, rash, and irritability in 2 patients each. One report of malaise was also recorded.
Other Adverse Events: Additional adverse events have been reported during studies in other clinical conditions and from worldwide postmarketing experience. In most cases the available information is incomplete and attribution to the drug cannot be determined. The majority of these reports involve the gastrointestinal system and include: diarrhea, nausea, abdominal pain, constipation, dyspepsia, flatulence, glossitis, stomatitis, vomiting, dysphagia, esophagospasm.
Other less commonly reported events (the majority representing only a single report) include the following:

Skin:	pruritus, rash, urticaria/angioedema, erythema/burning, photosensitivity
Musculoskeletal:	arthralgia, myalgia, stiffness/ weakness of legs
Neurologic:	headache, dizziness, hypoesthesia, paresthesia, migraine, convulsions, flushing
Psychiatric:	psychosis, anxiety, depression, hallucinations, behavior change, insomnia, nervousness
Heart Rate:	tachycardia, premature ventricular contractions (PVCs), palpitations
Respiratory:	pharyngitis, dyspnea
Miscellaneous:	fatigue, edema, unpleasant taste, chest pain, postprandial lightheadedness and lethargy, dysuria, urinary frequency, purpura, hepatic function test abnormal, polycythemia, neutropenia, pancytopenia, tinnitus, lupus erythematosus (LE) syndrome

DOSAGE AND ADMINISTRATION

NOT FOR INHALATION OR INJECTION. SEE DIRECTIONS FOR USE.
The usual starting dose is as follows:
Adults and Adolescents (13 Years and Older): Two ampules four times daily, taken one-half hour before meals and at bedtime.
Children 2–12 Years: One ampule four times daily, taken one-half hour before meals and at bedtime.
Pediatric Patients Under 2 Years: Not recommended.
If satisfactory control of symptoms is not achieved within two to three weeks, the dosage may be increased but should not exceed 40 mg/kg/day.
Patients should be advised that the effect of GASTROCROM therapy is dependent upon its administration at regular intervals, as directed.
Maintenance Dose: Once a therapeutic response has been achieved, the dose may be reduced to the minimum required to maintain the patient with a lower degree of symptomatology. To prevent relapses, the dosage should be maintained.
Administration: GASTROCROM should be administered as a solution at least $^1/_2$ hour before meals and at bedtime after preparation according to the following directions:
1. Break open ampule(s) and squeeze liquid contents of ampule(s) into a glass of water.
2. Stir solution.
3. Drink all of the liquid.

HOW SUPPLIED

GASTROCROM Oral Concentrate is an unpreserved, colorless solution supplied in a low density polyethylene plastic unit dose ampule with 8 ampules per foil pouch. Each 5 mL ampule contains 100 mg cromolyn sodium, USP, in purified water.

NDC 53014-678-70 96 ampules × 5 mL

GASTROCROM Oral Concentrate should be stored between 15°–30°C (59°–86°F) and protected from light. Do not use if it contains a precipitate or becomes discolored. Keep out of the reach of children.
Store ampules in foil pouch until ready for use.
Marketed by:
Medeva Pharmaceuticals, Inc.
Rochester, NY 14623 USA
Manufactured by:
Automatic Liquid Packaging, Inc.
Woodstock, IL 60098 USA
® Fisons Investments Inc. Rev. 4/99

R081C

Patient Instructions
GASTROCROM®
(cromolyn sodium, USP)
Oral Concentrate

For Oral Use Only – Not for Inhalation or Injection.
How to Use GASTROCROM:
As with all prescription drugs, follow the directions for dosage that your physician recommends.
The effect of GASTROCROM therapy is dependent upon its administration at REGULAR intervals, for as long as recommended by your physician.
Usual Starting Dose:
Adults and Adolescents (13 Years and Older):
Two ampules four times daily, taken one-half hour before meals and at bedtime.
Children 2–12 Years:
One ampule four times daily, taken one-half hour before meals and at bedtime.
Note:
Your physician may decide to increase OR decrease your dosage to achieve optimum results with GASTROCROM. However, do not change your dose or stop taking GASTROCROM without first consulting your physician.
Care & Storage:
GASTROCROM Oral Concentrate should be stored between 15°–30°C (59°–86°F) and protected from light. Do not use if it contains a precipitate (particles or cloudiness) or becomes discolored. Keep out of the reach of children.
Store ampules in foil pouch until ready for use.
Recycling Information: GASTROCROM Oral Concentrate ampules are made with a low density polyethylene plastic (recycling material code: 4 LDPE).
Directions for Use:

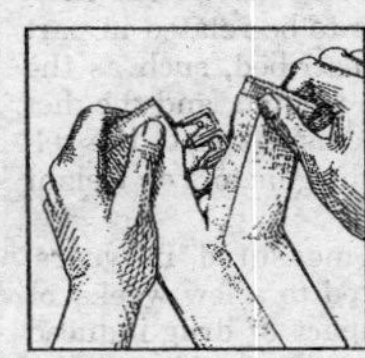
1. Open foil pouch by tearing at serrated edge as shown.

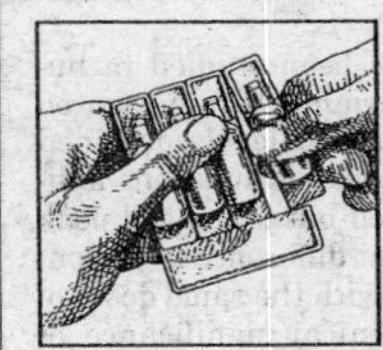
2. Remove ampule(s) from the strip.

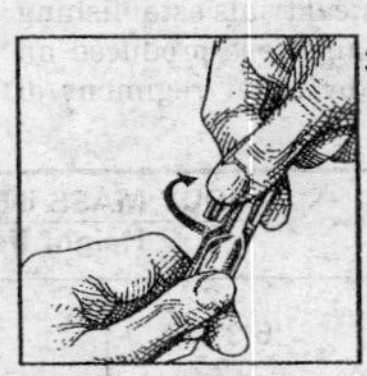
3. Open the ampule by twisting off the tabbed top section.

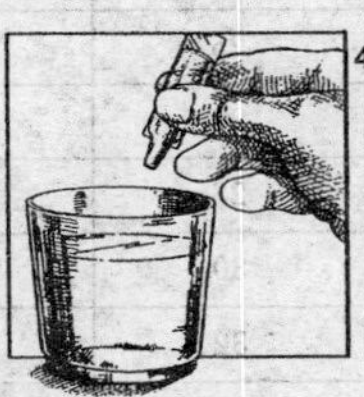
4. Squeeze liquid contents into a glass of water. Stir solution. Drink all of the liquid. Discard the empty ampule.

Marketed by:
Medeva Pharmaceuticals, Inc.
Rochester, NY 14623 USA

Continued on next page

Information on the Medeva Pharmaceuticals, Inc. products listed on these pages contains the full prescribing information from product circulars in use as of July 2000. For further information, please consult the package insert currently accompanying the product.

Gastrocrom—Cont.

Manufactured by:
Automatic Liquid Packaging, Inc., Woodstock, IL 60098 USA
® Fisons Investments Inc. Rev. 4/99
 R081C

IONAMIN® CAPSULES Ⓒ ℞
(phentermine resin)
Rx Only

R195G
Rev. 2/99

DESCRIPTION
IONAMIN '15' and IONAMIN '30' contain 15 mg and 30 mg respectively of phentermine as the cationic exchange resin complex. Phentermine is α, α-dimethyl phenethylamine (phenyl-tertiary-butylamine).
Inactive Ingredients: D&C Yellow No. 10, dibasic calcium phosphate, FD&C Yellow No. 6, gelatin, iron oxides (15 mg capsules only), lactose, magnesium stearate, titanium dioxide.

ACTIONS
IONAMIN is a sympathomimetic amine with pharmacologic activity similar to the prototype drug of this class used in obesity, amphetamine (d- and dl-amphetamine). Actions include central nervous system stimulation and elevation of blood pressure. Tachyphylaxis and tolerance have been demonstrated with all drugs of this class in which these phenomena have been looked for.
Drugs of this class used in obesity are commonly known as "anorectics" or "anorexigenics." It has not been established, however, that the action of such drugs in treating obesity is primarily one of appetite suppression. Other central nervous system actions, or metabolic effects may be involved.
Adult obese subjects instructed in dietary management and treated with "anorectic" drugs, lose more weight on the average than those treated with placebo and diet, as determined in relatively short-term clinical trials.
The magnitude of increased weight loss of drug-treated patients over placebo-treated patients is only a fraction of a pound a week. The rate of weight loss is greatest in the first weeks of therapy for both drug and placebo subjects and tends to decrease in succeeding weeks. The possible origins of the increased weight loss due to the various drug effects are not established. The amount of weight loss associated with the use of an "anorectic" drug varies from trial to trial, and the increased weight loss appears to be related in part to variables other than the drugs prescribed, such as the physician-investigator, the population treated, and the diet prescribed. Studies do not permit conclusions as to the relative importance of the drug and non-drug factors on weight loss.
The natural history of obesity is measured in years, whereas the studies cited are restricted to a few weeks' or months' duration; thus, the total impact of drug-induced weight loss over that of diet alone must be considered clinically limited.
The bioavailability of IONAMIN has been studied in humans in which blood levels of phentermine were measured by a gas chromatography method. Blood levels obtained with the 15 mg and 30 mg resin complex formulations indicated slower absorption with a reduced but prolonged peak concentration and without a significant difference in prolongation of blood levels when compared with the same doses of phentermine hydrochloride. The clinical significance of these differences is not known. In clinical trials establishing the efficacy of IONAMIN, a single daily dose produced an effect comparable to that produced by other regimens of "anorectic" drug therapy.

INDICATION
IONAMIN Capsules are indicated as a short-term (a few weeks) adjunct in a regimen of weight reduction based on exercise, behavioral modification, and caloric restriction in the management of exogenous obesity for patients with an initial body mass index ≥30 kg/m^2, or ≥27 kg/m^2 in the presence of other risk factors (e.g., hypertension, diabetes, hyperlipidemia).
Below is a chart of Body Mass Index (BMI) based on various heights and weights.
BMI is calculated by taking the patient's weight, in kilograms (kg), divided by the patient's height, in meters (m), squared. Metric conversions are as follows: pounds ÷ 2.2 = kg; inches × 0.0254 = meters.
[See table below]
The limited usefulness of agents of this class (see ACTIONS) should be measured against possible risk factors inherent in their use such as those described below.

CONTRAINDICATIONS
Advanced arteriosclerosis, cardiovascular disease, moderate to severe hypertension, hyperthyroidism, known hypersensitivity, or idiosyncrasy to the sympathomimetic amines, glaucoma.
Agitated states.
Patients with a history of drug abuse.
During or within 14 days following the administration of monoamine oxidase inhibitors (hypertensive crises may result).

WARNINGS
IONAMIN Capsules are indicated only as short-term monotherapy for the management of exogenous obesity. The safety and efficacy of combination therapy with phentermine and any other drug products for weight loss, including selective serotonin reuptake inhibitors (e.g., fluoxetine, sertraline, fluvoxamine, paroxetine), have not been established. Therefore, the coadministration of these drug products for weight loss is not recommended.
Primary Pulmonary Hypertension (PPH)—a rare, frequently fatal disease of the lungs—has been reported to occur in patients receiving a combination of phentermine with fenfluramine or dexfenfluramine. The possibility of an association between PPH and the use of phentermine alone cannot be ruled out. The initial symptom of PPH is usually dyspnea. Other initial symptoms include: angina pectoris, syncope, or lower extremity edema. Patients should be advised to report immediately any deterioration in exercise tolerance. Treatment should be discontinued in patients who develop new, unexplained symptoms of dyspnea, angina pectoris, syncope, or lower extremity edema.
Valvular Heart Disease: Serious regurgitant cardiac valvular disease, primarily affecting the mitral, aortic and/or tricuspid valves, has been reported in otherwise healthy persons who had taken a combination of phentermine with fenfluramine or dexfenfluramine for weight loss. The etiology of these valvulopathies has not been established and their course in individuals after the drugs are stopped is not known.
If tolerance to the "anorectic" effect develops, the recommended dose should not be exceeded in an attempt to increase the effect: rather, the drug should be discontinued.
IONAMIN may impair the ability of the patient to engage in potentially hazardous activities such as operating machinery or driving a motor vehicle; the patient should therefore be cautioned accordingly.
When using CNS active agents, consideration must always be given to the possibility of adverse interactions with alcohol.
Drug Dependence: IONAMIN is related chemically and pharmacologically to amphetamine (d- and dl-amphetamine) and other stimulant drugs that have been extensively abused. The possibility of abuse of IONAMIN should be kept in mind when evaluating the desirability of including a drug as part of a weight reduction program. Abuse of amphetamine (d- and dl-amphetamine) and related drugs may be associated with intense psychological dependence and severe social dysfunction. There are reports of patients who have increased the dosage of some of these drugs to many times that recommended. Abrupt cessation following prolonged high dosage administration results in extreme fatigue and mental depression; changes are also noted on the sleep EEG. Manifestations of chronic intoxication with anorectic drugs include severe dermatoses, marked insomnia, irritability, hyperactivity, and personality changes. The most severe manifestation of chronic intoxications is psychosis, often clinically indistinguishable from schizophrenia.
Usage in Pregnancy: Safe use in pregnancy has not been established. Use of IONAMIN by women who are or may become pregnant requires that the potential benefit be weighed against the possible hazard to mother and infant.
Pediatric Use: IONAMIN® Capsules (phentermine resin) are not recommended for use in pediatric patients under 16 years of age.

PRECAUTIONS
Caution is to be exercised in prescribing IONAMIN for patients with even mild hypertension. Insulin requirements in diabetes mellitus may be altered in association with the use of IONAMIN and the concomitant dietary regimen.
IONAMIN may decrease the hypotensive effect of adrenergic neuron blocking drugs.
The least amount feasible should be prescribed or dispensed at one time in order to minimize the possibility of overdosage.

ADVERSE REACTIONS
Cardiovascular: Primary pulmonary hypertension (see WARNINGS), palpitation, tachycardia, elevation of blood pressure.
Central Nervous System: Overstimulation, restlessness, dizziness, insomnia, euphoria, dysphoria, tremor, headache; rarely psychotic episodes at recommended doses with some drugs in this class.
Gastrointestinal: Dryness of the mouth, unpleasant taste, diarrhea, constipation, other gastrointestinal disturbances.
Allergic: Urticaria.
Endocrine: Impotence, changes in libido.

DOSAGE AND ADMINISTRATION
One capsule daily, before breakfast or 10–14 hours before retiring. For individuals exhibiting greater drug responsiveness, IONAMIN '15' will usually suffice. IONAMIN '30' is recommended for less responsive patients. IONAMIN is not recommended for use in pediatric patients under 16 years of age.
IONAMIN Capsules should be swallowed whole.

OVERDOSAGE
Manifestations of acute overdosage may include restlessness, tremor, hyperreflexia, rapid respiration, confusion, assaultiveness, hallucinations, panic states.
Fatigue and depression usually follow the central stimulation.
Cardiovascular effects include arrhythmias, hypertension, or hypotension and circulatory collapse. Gastrointestinal symptoms include nausea, vomiting, diarrhea, and abdominal cramps. Overdosage of pharmacologically similar compounds has resulted in fatal poisoning, usually terminating in convulsions and coma.
Management of acute IONAMIN intoxication is largely symptomatic and includes lavage and sedation with a barbiturate. Experience with hemodialysis or peritoneal dialysis is inadequate to permit recommendation in this regard. Intravenous phentolamine (Regitine) has been suggested on pharmacologic grounds for possible acute, severe hypertension, if this complicates overdosage.

HOW SUPPLIED
IONAMIN Capsules (phentermine resin) are available in two strengths:
15 mg, yellow/grey capsules, imprinted with "IONAMIN 15."
NDC 53014-903-71 Bottle of 100's
NDC 53014-903-84 Bottle of 400's
30 mg, yellow/yellow capsules, imprinted with "IONAMIN 30."
NDC 53014-904-71 Bottle of 100's
NDC 53014-904-84 Bottle of 400's
Dispense in a tight container. Store at room temperature.
Keep out of the reach of children.
Medeva Pharmaceuticals, Inc.
Rochester, NY 14623 USA

® Fisons Investments Inc.

Rev. 2/99
R195G

BODY MASS INDEX (BMI), kg/m^2
Height (feet, inches)

Weight (pounds)	5'0"	5'3"	5'6"	5'9"	6'0"	6'3"
140	27	25	23	21	19	18
150	29	27	24	22	20	19
160	31	28	26	24	22	20
170	33	30	28	25	23	21
180	35	32	29	27	25	23
190	37	34	31	28	26	24
200	39	36	32	30	27	25
210	41	37	34	31	29	26
220	43	39	36	33	30	28
230	45	41	37	34	31	29
240	47	43	39	36	33	30
250	49	44	40	37	34	31

METADATE™ ER TABLETS Ⓒ ℞
[*mĕt ə dāte*]
methylphenidate HCl extended-release tablets, USP
10 mg and 20 mg
Rx only

R425B
Rev. 8/99

DESCRIPTION
METADATE ER Tablets (methylphenidate hydrochloride extended-release tablets, USP) are a mild central nervous system (CNS) stimulant. METADATE ER is available as extended-release tablets of 10 and 20 mg for oral administration.

Methylphenidate hydrochloride is methyl α-phenyl-2-piperidineacetate hydrochloride, and its structural formula is:

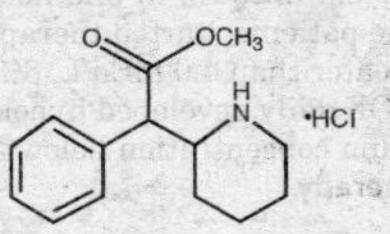

Methylphenidate hydrochloride is a white, odorless, fine crystalline powder. Its solutions are acid to litmus. It is freely soluble in water and in methanol, soluble in alcohol, and slightly soluble in chloroform and in acetone. Its chemical formula is $C_{14}H_{19}NO_2$•HCl, and its molecular weight is 269.77.

Inactive Ingredients: Cetyl alcohol, ethylcellulose, anhydrous lactose and magnesium stearate.

CLINICAL PHARMACOLOGY

METADATE ER is a mild central nervous system stimulant.

The mode of action in man is not completely understood, but methylphenidate presumably activates the brain stem arousal system and cortex to produce its stimulant effect.

There is neither specific evidence which clearly establishes the mechanism whereby methylphenidate produces its mental and behavioral effects in children, nor conclusive evidence regarding how these effects relate to the condition of the central nervous system.

METADATE ER in extended-release tablets is more slowly but as extensively absorbed as in the regular tablets. Bioavailability of METADATE 20 mg Extended-Release Tablets was compared to a sustained-release reference product and an immediate-release product. The extent of absorption for the three products was similar, and the rate of absorption of the two sustained-release products was not statistically different.

Based on rate of bioavailability ($AUC_{0\to\infty}$, T_{max}, and C_{max}), no significant statistical difference was found following single dose administration, in fasting and fed adults, of two METADATE 10 mg Extended-Release Tablets, or one methylphenidate hydrochloride, USP sustained-release 20 mg tablet. The administration of the extended-release methylphenidate HCl, USP, tablets with food, resulted in a greater C_{max} and $AUC_{0\to\infty}$, than when administered in a fasting condition.

Pharmacokinetic and statistical analyses for a multiple dose study demonstrated that 3 times daily administration of two METADATE 10 mg Extended-Release Tablets met the requirements for bioequivalence to one methylphenidate hydrochloride, USP sustained-release 20 mg tablet when administered every eight hours. Pharmacokinetic parameters (i.e., $AUC_{0\to\infty}$, T_{max}, C_{max}, C_{min}, and C_{av}) demonstrated achievement of steady state following 3 times daily administration of two METADATE 10 mg Extended-Release Tablets was confirmed.

In a clinical study involving adult subjects who received ER tablets, plasma concentrations of methylphenidate hydrochloride's major metabolite appeared to be greater in females than in males. No gender differences were observed for methylphenidate hydrochloride's plasma concentration in the same subjects.

INDICATIONS AND USAGE

Attention Deficit Disorders, Narcolepsy: *Attention Deficit Disorders* (previously known as Minimal Brain Dysfunction in Children). Other terms being used to describe the behavioral syndrome below include: Hyperkinetic Child Syndrome, Minimal Brain Damage, Minimal Cerebral Dysfunction, Minor Cerebral Dysfunction.

METADATE ER is indicated as an integral part of a total treatment program which typically includes other remedial measures (psychological, educational, social) for a stabilizing effect in children with a behavioral syndrome characterized by the following group of developmentally inappropriate symptoms: moderate-to-severe distractibility, short attention span, hyperactivity, emotional lability, and impulsivity. The diagnosis of this syndrome should not be made with finality when these symptoms are only of comparatively recent origin. Nonlocalizing (soft) neurological signs, learning disability, and abnormal EEG may or may not be present, and a diagnosis of central nervous system dysfunction may or may not be warranted.

Special Diagnostic Considerations: Specific etiology of this syndrome is unknown, and there is no single diagnostic test. Adequate diagnosis requires the use not only of medical but of special psychological, educational, and social resources.

Characteristics commonly reported include: chronic history of short attention span, distractibility, emotional lability, impulsivity, and moderate-to-severe hyperactivity; minor neurological signs and abnormal EEG. Learning may or may not be impaired. The diagnosis must be based upon a complete history and evaluation of the child and not solely on the presence of one or more of these characteristics.

Drug treatment is not indicated for all children with this syndrome. Stimulants are not intended for use in the child who exhibits symptoms secondary to environmental factors and/or primary psychiatric disorders, including psychosis. Appropriate educational placement is essential and psychosocial intervention is generally necessary. When remedial measures alone are insufficient, the decision to prescribe stimulant medication will depend upon the physician's assessment of the chronicity and severity of the child's symptoms.

CONTRAINDICATIONS

Marked anxiety, tension and agitation are contraindications to METADATE ER, since the drug may aggravate these symptoms. METADATE ER is contraindicated also in patients known to be hypersensitive to the drug, in patients with glaucoma, and in patients with motor tics or with a family history or diagnosis of Tourette's syndrome.

WARNINGS

METADATE ER should not be used in children under six years, since safety and efficacy in this age group have not been established.

Sufficient data on safety and efficacy of long-term use of methylphenidate in children are not yet available. Although a causal relationship has not been established, suppression of growth (i.e. weight gain, and/or height) has been reported with the long-term use of stimulants in children. Therefore, patients requiring long-term therapy should be carefully monitored.

METADATE ER should not be used for severe depression of either exogenous or endogenous origin. Clinical experience suggests that in psychotic children, administration of methylphenidate may exacerbate symptoms of behavior disturbance and thought disorder.

METADATE ER should not be used for the prevention or treatment of normal fatigue states.

There is some clinical evidence that methylphenidate may lower the convulsive threshold in patients with prior history of seizures, with prior EEG abnormalities in absence of seizures, and, very rarely, in absence of history of seizures and no prior EEG evidence of seizures. Safe concomitant use of anticonvulsants and METADATE ER has not been established. In the presence of seizures, the drug should be discontinued.

Use cautiously in patients with hypertension. Blood pressure should be monitored at appropriate intervals in all patients taking METADATE ER, especially those with hypertension.

Symptoms of visual disturbances have been encountered in rare cases. Difficulties with accommodation and blurring of vision have been reported.

Drug Interactions: METADATE ER may decrease the hypotensive effect of guanethidine. Use cautiously with pressor agents and MAO inhibitors.

Human pharmacologic studies have shown that methylphenidate may inhibit the metabolism of coumarin anticoagulants, anticonvulsants (phenobarbital, phenytoin, primidone), phenylbutazone, and tricyclic antidepressants (imipramine, clomipramine, desipramine). Downward dosage adjustments of these drugs may be required when given concomitantly with METADATE ER.

Usage in Pregnancy: Adequate animal reproduction studies to establish safe use of methylphenidate during pregnancy have not been conducted. Therefore, until more information is available, METADATE ER should not be prescribed for women of childbearing age unless, in the opinion of the physician, the potential benefits outweigh the possible risks.

Drug Dependence: METADATE ER should be given cautiously to emotionally unstable patients, such as those with a history of drug dependence or alcoholism, because such patients may increase dosage on their own initiative.

Chronically abusive use can lead to marked tolerance and psychic dependence with varying degrees of abnormal behavior. Frank psychotic episodes can occur, especially with parenteral abuse. Careful supervision is required during drug withdrawal, since severe depression as well as the effects of chronic overactivity can be unmasked. Long-term follow-up may be required because of the patient's basic personality disturbances.

PRECAUTIONS

Patients with an element of agitation may react adversely; discontinue therapy if necessary.

Periodic CBC, differential, and platelet counts are advised during prolonged therapy.

Drug treatment is not indicated in all cases of this behavioral syndrome and should be considered only in light of the complete history and evaluation of the child. The decision to prescribe METADATE™ ER Tablets (methylphenidate hydrochloride extended-release tablets, USP) should depend on the physician's assessment of the chronicity and severity of the child's symptoms and their appropriateness for his/her age. Prescription should not depend solely on the presence of one or more of the behavioral characteristics.

When these symptoms are associated with acute stress reactions, treatment with methylphenidate is usually not indicated.

Long-term effects of methylphenidate in children have not been well established.

Carcinogenesis, Mutagenesis, Impairment of Fertility: In a lifetime carcinogenicity study carried out in B6C3F1 mice, methylphenidate caused an increase in hepatocellular adenomas and, in males only, an increase in hepatoblastomas, at a daily dose of approximately 60 mg/kg/day. This dose is approximately 30 times and 2.5 times the maximum recommended human dose on a mg/kg and mg/m^2 basis respectively.

Hepatoblastoma is a relatively rare rodent malignant tumor type. There was no increase in total malignant hepatic tumors. The mouse strain used is sensitive to the development of hepatic tumors, and the significance of these results to humans is unknown.

Methylphenidate did not cause any increases in tumors in a lifetime carcinogenicity study carried out in F344 rats; the highest dose used was approximately 45 mg/kg/day, which is approximately 22 times and 4 times the maximum recommended human dose on a mg/kg and mg/m^2 basis, respectively.

Methylphenidate was not mutagenic in the *in vitro* Ames reverse mutation assay or in the *in vitro* mouse lymphoma cell forward mutation assay. Sister chromatid exchanges and chromosome aberrations were increased, indicative of a weak clastogenic response, in an *in vitro* assay in cultured Chinese Hamster Ovary (CHO) cells. The genotoxic potential of methylphenidate has not been evaluated in an *in vivo* assay.

ADVERSE REACTIONS

Nervousness and insomnia are the most common adverse reactions but are usually controlled by reducing dosage and omitting the drug in the afternoon or evening. Other reactions include hypersensitivity (including skin rash, urticaria, fever, arthralgia, exfoliative dermatitis, erythema multiforme with histopathological findings of necrotizing vasculitis, and thrombocytopenic purpura); anorexia; nausea; dizziness; palpitations; headache; dyskinesia; drowsiness; blood pressure and pulse changes, both up and down; tachycardia; angina; cardiac arrhythmia; abdominal pain; weight loss during prolonged therapy. There have been rare reports of Tourette's syndrome. Toxic psychosis has been reported. Although a definite causal relationship has not been established, the following have been reported in patients taking this drug: instances of abnormal liver function, ranging from transaminase elevation to hepatic coma; isolated cases of cerebral arteritis and/or occlusion; leukopenia and/or anemia; transient depressed mood; a few instances of scalp hair loss. Very rare reports of neuroleptic malignant syndrome (NMS) have been received, and, in most of these, patients were concurrently receiving therapies associated with NMS. In a single report, a ten year old boy who had been taking methylphenidate for approximately 18 months experienced an NMS-like event within 45 minutes of ingesting his first dose of venlafaxine. It is uncertain whether this case represented a drug-drug interaction, a response to either drug alone, or some other cause.

In children, loss of appetite, abdominal pain, weight loss during prolonged therapy, insomina, and tachycardia may occur more frequently; however, any of the other adverse reactions listed above may also occur.

OVERDOSAGE

Signs and symptoms of acute overdosage, resulting principally from overstimulation of the central nervous system and from excessive sympathomimetic effects, may include the following: vomiting, agitation, tremors, hyperreflexia, muscle twitching, convulsions (may be followed by coma), euphoria, confusion, hallucinations, delirium, sweating, flushing, headache, hyperpyrexia, tachycardia, palpitations, cardiac arrhythmias, hypertension, mydriasis, and dryness of mucous membranes.

Consult with a Certified Poison Control Center regarding treatment for up-to-date guidance and advice.

Treatment consists of appropriate supportive measures. The patient must be protected against self-injury and against external stimuli that would aggravate overstimulation already present. Gastric contents may be evacuated by gastric lavage. In the presence of severe intoxication, use a carefully titrated dosage of a *short-acting* barbiturate *before* performing gastric lavage.

Other measures to detoxify the gut include administration of activated charcoal and a cathartic.

Intensive care must be provided to maintain adequate circulation and respiratory exchange; external cooling procedures may be required for hyperpyrexia.

Efficacy of peritoneal dialysis or extracorporeal hemodialysis for methylphenidate overdosage has not been established.

DOSAGE AND ADMINISTRATION

Dosage should be individualized according to the needs and responses of the patient.

Adults: *Methylphenidate Hydrochloride, USP Immediate-Release Tablets:* Administer in divided doses 2 or 3 times daily, preferably 30 to 45 minutes before meals. Average dosage is 20 to 30 mg daily. Some patients may require 40 to 60 mg daily. In others, 10 to 15 mg daily will be adequate. Patients who are unable to sleep if medication is taken late in the day should take the last dose before 6 p.m.

Extended-Release Tablets: METADATE ER Tablets have a duration of action of approximately 8 hours. Therefore, the extended-release tablets may be used in place of the immediate-release tablets when the 8-hour dosage of METADATE ER Tablets corresponds to the titrated 8-hour

Continued on next page

Information on the Medeva Pharmaceuticals, Inc. products listed on these pages contains the full prescribing information from product circulars in use as of July 2000. For further information, please consult the package insert currently accompanying the product.

Metadate ER—Cont.

dosage of the immediate-release tablets. METADATE ER Tablets must be swallowed whole and never crushed or chewed.

Children (6 years and over): Methylphenidate hydrochloride tablets should be initiated in small doses, with gradual weekly increments. Daily dosage above 60 mg is not recommended.

If improvement is not observed after appropriate dosage adjustment over a one-month period, the drug should be discontinued.

Methylphenidate Hydrochloride, USP Immediate-Release Tablets: Start with 5 mg twice daily (before breakfast and lunch) with gradual increments of 5 to 10 mg weekly.

Extended-Release Tablets: METADATE ER Tablets have a duration of action of approximately 8 hours. Therefore, the extended-release tablets may be used in place of the immediate-release tablets when the 8-hour dosage of METADATE ER Tablets corresponds to the titrated 8-hour dosage of the immediate-release tablets. METADATE ER Tablets must be swallowed whole and never crushed or chewed.

If paradoxical aggravation of symptoms or other adverse effects occur, reduce dosage, or, if necessary, discontinue the drug.

METADATE ER should be periodically discontinued to assess the child's condition. Improvement may be sustained when the drug is either temporarily or permanently discontinued.

Drug treatment should not and need not be indefinite and usually may be discontinued after puberty.

HOW SUPPLIED

METADATE ER Tablets (methylphenidate hydrochloride extended-release tablets, USP) are available as follows:

10 mg: Oval, white, uncoated, unscored, debossed "561 MD".
NDC 53014-593-07 Bottle of 100's

20 mg: Round, white, uncoated, unscored, debossed "562 MD".
NDC 53014-594-07 Bottle of 100's

NOTE: METADATE ER Tablets are color-additive free.

PHARMACIST: Dispense in a tight, light-resistant container as defined in the USP with a child-resistant closure.

Store at controlled room temperature 15°–30°C (59°–86°F). Protect from moisture.

Medeva Pharmaceuticals, Inc.
Rochester, NY 14623 USA

METADATE is a Trademark of Medeva Pharma Limited.

Rev. 8/99
R425B

MYKROX® TABLETS ℞

[mī 'krahks]
(metolazone tablets, USP)
R156H
Rev. 7/99
Rx only

DO NOT INTERCHANGE

MYKROX TABLETS ARE A RAPIDLY AVAILABLE FORMULATION OF METOLAZONE FOR ORAL ADMINISTRATION. MYKROX TABLETS AND OTHER FORMULATIONS OF METOLAZONE THAT SHARE ITS MORE RAPID AND COMPLETE BIOAVAILABILITY ARE NOT THERAPEUTICALLY EQUIVALENT TO ZAROXOLYN® TABLETS AND OTHER FORMULATIONS OF METOLAZONE THAT SHARE ITS SLOW AND INCOMPLETE BIOAVAILABILITY. FORMULATIONS BIOEQUIVALENT TO MYKROX AND FORMULATIONS BIOEQUIVALENT TO ZAROXOLYN SHOULD NOT BE INTERCHANGED FOR ONE ANOTHER.

DESCRIPTION

MYKROX Tablets (metolazone tablets, USP) for oral administration contain $^1/_2$ mg of metolazone, USP, a diuretic/saluretic/antihypertensive drug of the quinazoline class.

Metolazone has the molecular formula $C_{16}H_{16}ClN_3O_3S$, the chemical name 7-chloro-1,2,3,4-tetrahydro-2-methyl-3-(2-methylphenyl)-4-oxo-6-quinazolinesulfonamide, and a molecular weight of 365.83. The structural formula is:

Metolazone is only sparingly soluble in water, but more soluble in plasma, blood, alkali and organic solvents.

Inactive Ingredients: Dibasic calcium phosphate, magnesium stearate, microcrystalline cellulose, pregelatinized starch, sodium starch glycolate.

CLINICAL PHARMACOLOGY

MYKROX (metolazone) is a quinazoline diuretic, with properties generally similar to the thiazide diuretics. The actions of MYKROX result from interference with the renal tubular mechanism of electrolyte reabsorption. MYKROX acts primarily to inhibit sodium reabsorption at the cortical diluting site and to a lesser extent in the proximal convoluted tubule. Sodium and chloride ions are excreted in approximately equivalent amounts. The increased delivery of sodium to the distal tubular exchange site results in increased potassium excretion. MYKROX does not inhibit carbonic anhydrase. A proximal action of metolazone has been shown in humans by increased excretion of phosphate and magnesium ions and by a markedly increased fractional excretion of sodium in patients with severely compromised glomerular filtration. This action has been demonstrated in animals by micropuncture studies.

The antihypertensive mechanism of action of metolazone is not fully understood but is presumed to be related to its saluretic and diuretic properties.

In two double-blind, controlled clinical trials of MYKROX Tablets, the maximum effect on mean blood pressure was achieved within 2 weeks of treatment and showed some evidence of an increased response at 1 mg compared to $^1/_2$ mg. There was no indication of an increased response with 2 mg. After six weeks of treatment, the mean fall in serum potassium was 0.42 mEq/L at $^1/_2$ mg, 0.66 mEq/L at 1 mg and 0.7 mEq/L at 2 mg. Serum uric acid increased by 1.1 to 1.4 mg/dL at increasing doses. There were small falls in serum sodium and chloride and a 1.3–2.1 mg/dL increase in BUN at increasing doses.

The rate and extent of absorption of metolazone from MYKROX Tablets were equivalent to those from an oral solution of metolazone. Peak blood levels are obtained within 2 to 4 hours of oral administration with an elimination half-life of approximately 14 hours. MYKROX Tablets have been shown to produce blood levels that are dose proportional between $^1/_2$–2 mg. Steady state blood levels are usually reached in 4–5 days.

In contrast, other formulations of metolazone produce peak blood concentrations approximately 8 hours following oral administration; absorption continues for an additional 12 hours.

INDICATIONS AND USAGE

MYKROX Tablets are indicated for the treatment of hypertension, alone or in combination with other antihypertensive drugs of a different class.

MYKROX TABLETS HAVE NOT BEEN EVALUATED FOR THE TREATMENT OF CONGESTIVE HEART FAILURE OR FLUID RETENTION DUE TO RENAL OR HEPATIC DISEASE AND THE CORRECT DOSAGE FOR THESE CONDITIONS AND OTHER EDEMA STATES HAS NOT BEEN ESTABLISHED. SINCE A SAFE AND EFFECTIVE DIURETIC DOSE HAS NOT BEEN ESTABLISHED, MYKROX TABLETS SHOULD NOT BE USED WHEN DIURESIS IS DESIRED.

Usage in Pregnancy

The routine use of diuretics in an otherwise healthy woman is inappropriate and exposes mother and fetus to unnecessary hazard. Diuretics do not prevent development of toxemia of pregnancy, and there is no evidence that they are useful in the treatment of developed toxemia (see PRECAUTIONS).

Edema during pregnancy may arise from pathologic causes or from the physiologic and mechanical consequences of pregnancy. MYKROX is not indicated for the treatment of edema in pregnancy. Dependent edema in pregnancy resulting from restriction of venous return by the expanded uterus is properly treated through elevation of the lower extremities and use of support hose; use of diuretics to lower intravascular volume in this case is illogical and unnecessary. There is hypervolemia during normal pregnancy which is harmful to neither the fetus nor the mother (in the absence of cardiovascular disease), but which is associated with edema, including generalized edema, in the majority of pregnant women. If this edema produces discomfort, increased recumbency will often provide relief. In rare instances, this edema may cause extreme discomfort which is not relieved by rest. In these cases, a short course of diuretics may be appropriate.

CONTRAINDICATIONS

Anuria, hepatic coma or precoma, known allergy or hypersensitivity to metolazone.

WARNINGS

Rapid Onset Hyponatremia

Rarely, the rapid onset of severe hyponatremia and/or hypokalemia has been reported following initial doses of thiazide and non-thiazide diuretics. When symptoms consistent with severe electrolyte imbalance appear rapidly, drug should be discontinued and supportive measures should be initiated immediately. Parenteral electrolytes may be required. Appropriateness of therapy with this class of drugs should be carefully reevaluated.

Hypokalemia

Hypokalemia may occur, with consequent weakness, cramps, and cardiac dysrhythmias. Serum potassium should be determined at regular intervals, and dose reduction, potassium supplementation or addition of a potassium sparing diuretic instituted whenever indicated. Hypokalemia is a particular hazard in patients who are digitalized or who have or have had a ventricular arrhythmia; dangerous or fatal arrhythmias may be precipitated. Hypokalemia is dose related.

In controlled clinical trials, 1.5% of patients taking $^1/_2$ mg and 3.1% of patients taking 1 mg of MYKROX daily developed clinical hypokalemia (defined as hypokalemia accompanied by signs or symptoms); 21% of the patients taking $^1/_2$ mg and 30% of the patients taking 1 mg of MYKROX daily developed hypokalemia (defined as a serum potassium concentration below 3.5 mEq/L); in another controlled clinical trial in which the patients started therapy with a serum potassium level greater than 4.0 mEq/L, 8% of patients taking $^1/_2$ mg of MYKROX daily developed hypokalemia (defined as a serum potassium concentration below 3.5 mEq/L).

Concomitant Therapy

Lithium

In general, diuretics should not be given concomitantly with lithium because they reduce its renal clearance and add a high risk of lithium toxicity. Read prescribing information for lithium preparations before use of such concomitant therapy.

Furosemide: Unusually large or prolonged losses of fluids and electrolytes may result when metolazone is administered concomitantly to patients receiving furosemide (see PRECAUTIONS, DRUG INTERACTIONS).

Other Antihypertensive Drugs: When MYKROX Tablets are used with other antihypertensive drugs, particular care must be taken to avoid excessive reduction of blood pressure, especially during initial therapy.

Cross-Allergy

Cross-allergy, while not reported to date, theoretically may occur when MYKROX Tablets are given to patients known to be allergic to sulfonamide-derived drugs, thiazides, or quinethazone.

Sensitivity Reactions

Sensitivity reactions (e.g., angioedema, bronchospasm) may occur with or without a history of allergy or bronchial asthma and may occur with the first dose of MYKROX.

PRECAUTIONS

DO NOT INTERCHANGE

MYKROX TABLETS ARE A RAPIDLY AVAILABLE FORMULATION OF METOLAZONE FOR ORAL ADMINISTRATION. MYKROX TABLETS AND OTHER FORMULATIONS OF METOLAZONE THAT SHARE ITS MORE RAPID AND COMPLETE BIOAVAILABILITY ARE NOT THERAPEUTICALLY EQUIVALENT TO ZAROXOLYN TABLETS AND OTHER FORMULATIONS OF METOLAZONE THAT SHARE ITS SLOW AND INCOMPLETE BIOAVAILABILITY. FORMULATIONS BIOEQUIVALENT TO MYKROX AND FORMULATIONS BIOEQUIVALENT TO ZAROXOLYN SHOULD NOT BE INTERCHANGED FOR ONE ANOTHER.

GENERAL:

Fluid and Electrolytes

All patients receiving therapy with MYKROX Tablets should have serum electrolyte measurements done at appropriate intervals and be observed for clinical signs of fluid and/or electrolyte imbalance: namely, hyponatremia, hypochloremic alkalosis, and hypokalemia. In patients with severe edema accompanying cardiac failure or renal disease, a low-salt syndrome may be produced, especially with hot weather and a low-salt diet. Serum and urine electrolyte determinations are particularly important when the patient has protracted vomiting, severe diarrhea, or is receiving parenteral fluids. Warning signs of imbalance are: dryness of mouth, thirst, weakness, lethargy, drowsiness, restlessness, muscle pains or cramps, muscle fatigue, hypotension, oliguria, tachycardia, and gastrointestinal disturbances such as nausea and vomiting. Hyponatremia may occur at any time during long term therapy and, on rare occasions, may be life threatening.

The risk of hypokalemia is increased when larger doses are used, when diuresis is rapid, when severe liver disease is present, when corticosteroids are given concomitantly, when oral intake is inadequate or when excess potassium is being lost extrarenally, such as with vomiting or diarrhea.

Thiazide-like diuretics have been shown to increase the urinary excretion of magnesium; this may result in hypomagnesemia.

Glucose Tolerance

Metolazone may raise blood glucose concentrations possibly causing hyperglycemia and glycosuria in patients with diabetes or latent diabetes.

Hyperuricemia

MYKROX regularly causes an increase in serum uric acid and can occasionally precipitate gouty attacks even in patients without a prior history of them.

Azotemia

Azotemia, presumably prerenal azotemia, may be precipitated during the administration of MYKROX Tablets. If azotemia and oliguria worsen during treatment of patients with severe renal disease, MYKROX Tablets should be discontinued.

Renal Impairment

Use caution when administering MYKROX Tablets to patients with severely impaired renal function. As most of the drug is excreted by the renal route, accumulation may occur.

Orthostatic Hypotension

Orthostatic hypotension may occur; this may be potentiated by alcohol, barbiturates, narcotics, or concurrent therapy with other antihypertensive drugs. In controlled clinical trials, 1.4% of patients treated with MYKROX Tablets ($^1/_2$ mg) had orthostatic hypotension; this effect was not reported in the placebo group.

Hypercalcemia

Hypercalcemia may infrequently occur with metolazone, especially in patients taking high doses of vitamin D or with high bone turnover states, and may signify hidden hyperparathyroidism. Metolazone should be discontinued before tests for parathyroid function are performed.

Systemic Lupus Erythematosus
Thiazide diuretics have exacerbated or activated systemic lupus erythematosus and this possibility should be considered with MYKROX Tablets.
INFORMATION FOR PATIENTS: Patients should be informed of possible adverse effects, advised to take the medication as directed and promptly report any possible adverse reactions to the treating physician.
DRUG INTERACTIONS:
Diuretics
Furosemide and probably other loop diuretics given concomitantly with metolazone can cause unusually large or prolonged losses of fluid and electrolytes (see WARNINGS).
Other Antihypertensives
When MYKROX Tablets are used with other antihypertensive drugs, care must be taken, especially during initial therapy. Dosage adjustments of other antihypertensives may be necessary.
Alcohol, Barbiturates, and Narcotics
The hypotensive effects of these drugs may be potentiated by the volume contraction that may be associated with metolazone therapy.
Digitalis Glycosides
Diuretic-induced hypokalemia can increase the sensitivity of the myocardium to digitalis. Serious arrhythmias can result.
Corticosteroids or ACTH
May increase the risk of hypokalemia and increase salt and water retention.
Lithium
Serum lithium levels may increase (see WARNINGS).
Curariform Drugs
Diuretic-induced hypokalemia may enhance neuromuscular blocking effects of curariform drugs (such as tubocurarine)—the most serious effect would be respiratory depression which could proceed to apnea. Accordingly, it may be advisable to discontinue MYKROX Tablets three days before elective surgery.
Salicylates and Other Non-Steroidal Anti-Inflammatory Drugs
May decrease the antihypertensive effects of MYKROX Tablets.
Sympathomimetics
Metolazone may decrease arterial responsiveness to norepinephrine, but this diminution is not sufficient to preclude effectiveness of the pressor agent for therapeutic use.
Insulin and Oral Antidiabetic Agents
See Glucose Tolerance under PRECAUTIONS, GENERAL.
Methenamine
Efficacy may be decreased due to urinary alkalizing effect of metolazone.
Anticoagulants
Metolazone, as well as other thiazide-like diuretics, may affect the hypoprothrombinemic response to anticoagulants; dosage adjustments may be necessary.
DRUG/LABORATORY TEST INTERACTIONS: None reported.
CARCINOGENESIS, MUTAGENESIS, IMPAIRMENT OF FERTILITY: Mice and rats administered metolazone 5 days/week for up to 18 and 24 months, respectively, at daily doses of 2, 10 and 50 mg/kg, exhibited no evidence of a tumorigenic effect of the drug. The small number of animals examined histologically and poor survival in the mice limit the conclusions that can be reached from these studies.
Metolazone was not mutagenic *in vitro* in the Ames Test using Salmonella typhimurium strains TA-97, TA-98, TA-100, TA-102 and TA-1535.
Reproductive performance has been evaluated in mice and rats. There is no evidence that metolazone possesses the potential for altering reproductive capacity in mice. In a rat study, in which males were treated orally with metolazone at doses of 2, 10 and 50 mg/kg for 127 days prior to mating with untreated females, an increased number of resorption sites was observed in dams mated with males from the 50 mg/kg group. In addition, the birth weight of offspring was decreased and the pregnancy rate was reduced in dams mated with males from the 10 and 50 mg/kg groups.
PREGNANCY
Teratogenic Effects—Pregnancy Category B.
Reproduction studies performed in mice, rabbits and rats treated during the appropriate periods of gestation at doses up to 50 mg/kg/day have revealed no evidence of harm to the fetus due to metolazone. There are, however, no adequate and well-controlled studies in pregnant women. Because animal reproduction studies are not always predictive of human response, MYKROX Tablets should be used during pregnancy only if clearly needed. Metolazone crosses the placental barrier and appears in cord blood.
Non-Teratogenic Effects
The use of MYKROX Tablets in pregnant women requires that the anticipated benefit be weighed against possible hazards to the fetus. These hazards include fetal or neonatal jaundice, thrombocytopenia, and possibly other adverse reactions which have occurred in the adult. It is not known what effect the use of the drug during pregnancy has on the later growth, development and functional maturation of the child. No such effects have been reported with metolazone.
LABOR AND DELIVERY: Based on clinical studies in which women received metolazone in late pregnancy until the time of delivery, there is no evidence that the drug has any adverse effects on the normal course of labor or delivery.
NURSING MOTHERS: Metolazone appears in breast milk. Because of the potential for serious adverse reactions in nursing infants from metolazone, a decision should be made whether to discontinue nursing or to discontinue the drug, taking into account the importance of the drug to the mother.
PEDIATRIC USE: Safety and effectiveness of MYKROX Tablets in pediatric patients have not been established, and such use is not recommended.

ADVERSE REACTIONS

Adverse experience information is available from more than 14 years of accumulated marketing experience with other formulations of metolazone for which reliable quantitative information is lacking and from controlled clinical trials with MYKROX from which incidences can be calculated.
In controlled clinical trials with MYKROX, adverse experiences resulted in discontinuation of therapy in 6.7–6.8% of patients given $^1/_2$ to 1 mg of MYKROX.
Adverse experiences occurring in controlled clinical trials with MYKROX with an incidence of > 2%, whether or not considered drug-related, are summarized in the following table.

Incidence of Adverse Experiences Volunteered or Elicited (by Patient in Percent)*

	MYKROX n=226†
Dizziness (lightheadedness)	10.2
Headaches	9.3
Muscle Cramps	5.8
Fatigue (malaise, lethargy, lassitude)	4.4
Joint Pain, swelling	3.1
Chest Pain (precordial discomfort)	2.7

* Percent of patients reporting an adverse experience one or more times.
† All doses combined ($^1/_2$, 1 and 2 mg).

Some of the adverse effects reported in association with MYKROX also occur frequently in untreated hypertensive patients, such as headache and dizziness, which occurred in 14.8 and 7.4% of patients in a smaller parallel placebo group.
The following adverse effects were reported in less than 2% of the MYKROX treated patients.
Cardiovascular: Cold extremities, edema, orthostatic hypotension, palpitations.
Central and Peripheral Nervous System: Anxiety, depression, dry mouth, impotence, nervousness, neuropathy, weakness, "weird" feeling.
Dermatological: Pruritus, rash, skin dryness.
Eyes, Ears, Nose, Throat: Cough, epistaxis, eye itching, sinus congestion, sore throat, tinnitus.
Gastrointestinal: Abdominal discomfort (pain, bloating), bitter taste, constipation, diarrhea, nausea, vomiting.
Genitourinary: Nocturia.
Musculoskeletal: Back pain.
Other Adverse Experiences:
Adverse experiences reported with other marketed metolazone formulations and most thiazide diuretics, for which quantitative data are not available, are listed in decreasing order of severity within body systems. Several are single or rare occurrences.
Cardiovascular: excessive volume depletion, hemoconcentration, venous thrombosis.
Central and Peripheral Nervous System: syncope, paresthesias, drowsiness, restlessness (sometimes resulting in insomnia).
Dermatologic/Hypersensitivity: necrotizing angiitis (cutaneous vasculitis), purpura, dermatitis, photosensitivity, urticaria.
Gastrointestinal: hepatitis, intrahepatic cholestatic jaundice, pancreatitis, anorexia.
Hematologic: aplastic (hypoplastic) anemia, agranulocytosis, leukopenia.
Metabolic: hypokalemia (see WARNINGS, Hypokalemia), hyponatremia, hyperuricemia, hypochloremia, hypochloremic alkalosis, hyperglycemia, glycosuria, increase in serum urea nitrogen (BUN) or creatinine, hypophosphatemia, hypomagnesemia, hypercalcemia.
Musculoskeletal: acute gouty attacks.
Other: transient blurred vision, chills.
In addition, rare adverse experiences reported in association with similar anti-hypertensive-diuretics but not reported to date for metolazone include: sialadenitis, xanthopsia, respiratory distress (including pneumonitis), thrombocytopenia, and anaphylactic reactions. These experiences could occur with clinical use of metolazone.

OVERDOSAGE

Intentional overdosage has been reported rarely with metolazone and similar diuretic drugs.
Signs and Symptoms
Orthostatic hypotension, dizziness, drowsiness, syncope, electrolyte abnormalities, hemoconcentration and hemodynamic changes due to plasma volume depletion may occur. In some instances depressed respiration may be observed. At high doses, lethargy of varying degree may progress to coma within a few hours. The mechanism of CNS depression with thiazide overdosage is unknown. Also, GI irritation and hypermotility may occur. Temporary elevation of BUN has been reported, especially in patients with impairment of renal function. Serum electrolyte changes and cardiovascular and renal function should be closely monitored.
Treatment
There is no specific antidote available but immediate evacuation of stomach contents is advised. Dialysis is not likely to be effective. Care should be taken when evacuating the gastric contents to prevent aspiration, especially in the stuporous or comatose patient. Supportive measures should be initiated as required to maintain hydration, electrolyte balance, respiration and cardiovascular and renal function.

DOSAGE AND ADMINISTRATION

Therapy should be individualized according to patient response.
For initial treatment of mild to moderate hypertension, the recommended dose is one MYKROX Tablet ($^1/_2$ mg) once daily, usually in the morning. If patients are inadequately controlled with one $^1/_2$ mg tablet, the dose can be increased to two MYKROX Tablets (1 mg) once a day. An increase in hypokalemia may occur. Doses larger than 1 mg do not give increased effectiveness.
The same dose titration is necessary if MYKROX Tablets are to be substituted for other dosage forms of metolazone in the treatment of hypertension.
If blood pressure is not adequately controlled with two MYKROX Tablets alone, the dose should not be increased; rather, another antihypertensive agent with a different mechanism of action should be added to therapy with MYKROX Tablets.

HOW SUPPLIED

MYKROX Tablets (metolazone tablets, USP), $^1/_2$ mg are white, flat-faced, round tablets, debossed "MYKROX" on one side, and "$^1/_2$" on reverse side.
NDC 53014-847-71 Bottle of 100's
Store at 25°C (77°F); excursions permitted to 15–30°C (59–86°F) [See USP Controlled Room Temperature]. Protect from light. Keep out of the reach of children.
MEDEVA PHARMACEUTICALS
Medeva Pharmaceuticals, Inc.
Rochester, NY 14623 USA
®Fisons Investments Inc.
Rev. 7/99
R156H

PEDIAPRED® ℞
(prednisolone sodium phosphate, USP)
Oral Solution
Rx Only
R024K
Rev. 3/99

DESCRIPTION

PEDIAPRED (prednisolone sodium phosphate, USP) Oral Solution is a dye free, colorless to light straw colored, raspberry flavored solution. Each 5 mL (teaspoonful) of PEDIAPRED contains 6.7 mg prednisolone sodium phosphate (5 mg prednisolone base) in a palatable, aqueous vehicle.
PEDIAPRED also contains dibasic sodium phosphate, edetate disodium, methylparaben, purified water, sodium biphosphate, sorbitol, natural and artificial raspberry flavor.
Prednisolone sodium phosphate occurs as white or slightly yellow, friable granules or powder. It is freely soluble in water; soluble in methanol; slightly soluble in alcohol and in chloroform; and very slightly soluble in acetone and in dioxane. The chemical name of prednisolone sodium phosphate is pregna -1,4- diene-3,20-dione, 11,17-dihydroxy -21-(phosphonooxy)-, disodium salt, (11b)-. The empirical formula is $C_{21}H_{27}Na_2O_8P$; the molecular weight is 484.39. Its chemical structure is:

Pharmacological Category: Glucocorticoid

CLINICAL PHARMACOLOGY

Naturally occurring glucocorticoids (hydrocortisone), which also have salt-retaining properties, are used as replacement therapy in adrenocortical deficiency states. Their synthetic analogs are primarily used for their potent anti-inflammatory effects in disorders of many organ systems.
Prednisolone is a synthetic adrenocortical steroid drug with predominantly glucocorticoid properties. Some of these properties reproduce the physiological actions of endogenous glucocorticosteroids, but others do not necessarily reflect any of the adrenal hormones' normal functions; they are seen only after administration of large therapeutic doses of the drug. The pharmacological effects of predniso-

Continued on next page

Information on the Medeva Pharmaceuticals, Inc. products listed on these pages contains the full prescribing information from product circulars in use as of July 2000. For further information, please consult the package insert currently accompanying the product.

Pediapred—Cont.

lone which are due to its glucocorticoid properties include: promotion of gluconeogenesis; increased deposition of glycogen in the liver; inhibition of the utilization of glucose; anti-insulin activity; increased catabolism of protein; increased lipolysis; stimulation of fat synthesis and storage; increased glomerular filtration rate and resulting increase in urinary excretion of urate (creatinine excretion remains unchanged); and increased calcium excretion.

Depressed production of eosinophils and lymphocytes occurs, but erythropoiesis and production of polymorphonuclear leukocytes are stimulated. Inflammatory processes (edema, fibrin deposition, capillary dilatation, migration of leukocytes and phagocytosis) and the later stages of wound healing (capillary proliferation, deposition of collagen, cicatrization) are inhibited.

Prednisolone can stimulate secretion of various components of gastric juice. Suppression of the production of corticotropin may lead to suppression of endogenous corticosteroids. Prednisolone has slight mineralocorticoid activity, whereby entry of sodium into cells and loss of intracellular potassium is stimulated. This is particularly evident in the kidney, where rapid ion exchange leads to sodium retention and hypertension.

Prednisolone is rapidly and well absorbed from the gastrointestinal tract following oral administration. PEDIAPRED Oral Solution produces a 14% higher peak plasma level of prednisolone which occurs 20% faster than that seen with tablets. Prednisolone is 70–90% protein-bound in the plasma and it is eliminated from the plasma with a half-life of 2 to 4 hours. It is metabolized mainly in the liver and excreted in the urine as sulfate and glucuronide conjugates.

INDICATIONS AND USAGE

PEDIAPRED Oral Solution is indicated in the following conditions:

1. ***Endocrine Disorders***
   Primary or secondary adrenocortical insufficiency (hydrocortisone or cortisone is the first choice; synthetic analogs may be used in conjunction with mineralocorticoids where applicable; in infancy mineralocorticoid supplementation is of particular importance); congenital adrenal hyperplasia; hypercalcemia associated with cancer; nonsuppurative thyroiditis.
2. ***Rheumatic Disorders***
   As adjunctive therapy for short term administration (to tide the patient over an acute episode or exacerbation) in: psoriatic arthritis; rheumatoid arthritis, including juvenile rheumatoid arthritis (selected cases may require low dose maintenance therapy); ankylosing spondylitis; acute and subacute bursitis; acute nonspecific tenosynovitis; acute gouty arthritis; epicondylitis. For the treatment of systemic lupus erythematosus, dermatomyositis (polymyositis), polymyalgia rheumatica, Sjogren's syndrome, relapsing polychondritis, and certain cases of vasculitis.
3. ***Dermatologic Diseases***
   Pemphigus; bullous dermatitis herpetiformis; severe erythema multiforme (Stevens-Johnson syndrome); exfoliative erythroderma; mycosis fungoides.
4. ***Allergic States***
   Control of severe or incapacitating allergic conditions intractable to adequate trials of conventional treatment in adult and pediatric populations with: seasonal or perennial allergic rhinitis; asthma; contact dermatitis; atopic dermatitis; serum sickness; drug hypersensitivity reactions.
5. ***Ophthalmic Diseases***
   Uveitis and ocular inflammatory conditions unresponsive to topical corticosteroids; temporal arteritis; sympathetic ophthalmia.
6. ***Respiratory Diseases***
   Symptomatic sarcoidosis; idiopathic eosinophilic pneumonias; fulminating or disseminated pulmonary tuberculosis when used concurrently with appropriate antituberculous chemotherapy; asthma (as distinct from allergic asthma listed above under "Allergic States"), hypersensitivity pneumonitis, idiopathic pulmonary fibrosis, acute exacerbations of chronic obstructive pulmonary disease (COPD), and Pneumocystis carinii pneumonia (PCP) associated with hypoxemia occurring in an HIV (+) individual who is also under treatment with appropriate anti-PCP antibiotics. Studies support the efficacy of systemic corticosteroids for the treatment of these conditions: allergic bronchopulmonary aspergillosis, idiopathic bronchiolitis obliterans with organizing pneumonia.
7. ***Hematologic Disorders***
   Idiopathic thrombocytopenic purpura in adults; selected cases of secondary thrombocytopenia; acquired (autoimmune) hemolytic anemia; pure red cell aplasia; Diamond-Blackfan anemia.
8. ***Neoplastic Diseases***
   For the treatment of acute leukemia and aggressive lymphomas in adults and children.
9. ***Edematous States***
   To induce diuresis or remission of proteinuria in nephrotic syndrome in adults with lupus erythematosus and in adults and pediatric populations, with idiopathic nephrotic syndrome, without uremia.
10. ***Gastrointestinal Diseases***
    To tide the patient over a critical period of the disease in: ulcerative colitis; regional enteritis.
11. ***Nervous System***
    Acute exacerbations of multiple sclerosis.
12. ***Miscellaneous***
    Tuberculous meningitis with subarachnoid block or impending block, tuberculosis with enlarged mediastinal lymph nodes causing respiratory difficulty, and tuberculosis with pleural or pericardial effusion (appropriate antituberculous chemotherapy must be used concurrently when treating any tuberculosis complications); Trichinosis with neurologic or myocardial involvement; acute or chronic solid organ rejection (with or without other agents).

CONTRAINDICATIONS

Systemic fungal infections.
Hypersensitivity to the drug or any of its components.

WARNINGS

General: In patients on corticosteroid therapy subjected to unusual stress, increased dosage of rapidly acting corticosteroids before, during and after the stressful situation is indicated.

Endocrine: Corticosteroids can produce reversible hypothalamic-pituitary adrenal (HPA) axis suppression with the potential for glucocorticosteroid insufficiency after withdrawal of treatment.

Metabolic clearance of corticosteroids is decreased in hypothyroid patients and increased in hyperthyroid patients. Changes in thyroid status of the patient may necessitate adjustment in dosage.

Infections (General): Persons who are on drugs which suppress the immune system are more susceptible to infections than healthy individuals. There may be decreased resistance and inability to localize infection when corticosteroids are used. Infection with any pathogen including viral, bacterial, fungal, protozoan or helminthic infection, in any location of the body, may be associated with the use of corticosteroids alone or in combination with other immunosuppressive agents that affect humoral or cellular immunity, or neutrophil function. These infections may be mild to severe, and, with increasing doses of corticosteroids, the rate of occurrence of infectious complications increases. Corticosteroids may also mask some signs of infection after it has already started.

Viral Infections: Chicken pox and measles, for example, can have a more serious or even fatal course in non-immune children or adults on corticosteroids. In such children or adults who have not had these diseases, particular care should be taken to avoid exposure. How the dose, route and duration of corticosteroid administration affect the risk of developing a disseminated infection is not known. The contribution of the underlying disease and/or prior corticosteroid treatment to the risk is also not known. If exposed to chicken pox, prophylaxis with varicella zoster immune globulin (VZIG) may be indicated. If exposed to measles, prophylaxis with immunoglobulin (IG) may be indicated. (See the respective package inserts for complete VZIG and IG prescribing information). If chicken pox develops, treatment with antiviral agents should be considered.

Special Pathogens: Latent disease may be activated or there may be an exacerbation of intercurrent infections due to pathogens, including those caused by Candida, Mycobacterium, Ameba, Toxoplasma, Pneumocystis, Cryptococus, Nocardia, etc.

Corticosteroids may activate latent amebiasis. Therefore, it is recommended that latent or active amebiasis be ruled out before initiating corticosteroid therapy in any patient who has spent time in the tropics or in any patient with unexplained diarrhea.

Similarly, corticosteroids should be used with great care in patients with known or suspected Strongyloides (threadworm) infestation. In such patients, corticosteroid-induced immunosuppression may lead to Strongyloides hyperinfection and dissemination with widespread larval migration, often accompanied by severe enterocolitis and potentially fatal gram-negative septicemia.

Corticosteroids should not be used in cerebral malaria.

Tuberculosis: The use of prednisolone in active tuberculosis should be restricted to those cases of fulminating or disseminated tuberculosis in which the corticosteroid is used for the management of the disease in conjunction with an appropriate antituberculous regimen.

If corticosteroids are indicated in patients with latent tuberculosis or tuberculin reactivity, close observation is necessary as reactivation of the disease may occur. During prolonged corticosteroid therapy these patients should receive chemoprophylaxis.

Vaccination: **Administration of live or live, attenuated vaccines is contraindicated in patients receiving immunosuppressive doses of corticosteroids. Killed or inactivated vaccines may be administered, however, the response to such vaccines can not be predicted.** Immunization procedures may be undertaken in patients who are receiving corticosteroids as replacement therapy, e.g., for Addison's disease.

Ophthalmic: Use of corticosteroids may produce posterior subcapsular cataracts, glaucoma with possible damage to the optic nerves, and may enhance the establishment of secondary ocular infections due to bacteria, fungi, or viruses. The use of oral corticosteroids is not recommended in the treatment of optic neuritis and may led to an increase in the risk of new episodes. Corticosteroids should not be used in active ocular herpes simplex.

Cardio-renal: Average and large doses of hydrocortisone or cortisone can cause elevation of blood pressure, salt and water retention, and increased excretion of potassium. These effects are less likely to occur with the synthetic derivatives except when used in large doses. Dietary salt restriction and potassium supplementation may be necessary. All corticosteroids increase calcium excretion.

PRECAUTIONS

General: The lowest possible dose of corticosteroid should be used to control the condition under treatment, and when reduction in dosage is possible, the reduction should be gradual.

Since complications of treatment with glucocorticoids are dependent on the size of the dose and the duration of treatment, a risk/benefit decision must be made in each individual case as to dose and duration of treatment and as to whether daily or intermittent therapy should be used.

There is an enhanced effect of corticosteroids in patients with hypothyroidism and in those with cirrhosis.

Kaposi's sarcoma has been reported to occur in patients receiving corticosteroid therapy, most often for chronic conditions. Discontinuation of corticosteroids may result in clinical improvement.

Endocrine: Drug-induced secondary adrenocortical insufficiency may be minimized by gradual reduction of dosage. This type of relative insufficiency may persist for months after discontinuation of therapy; therefore, in any situation of stress occurring during that period, hormone therapy should be reinstituted. Since mineralocorticoid secretion may be impaired, salt and/or a mineralocorticoid should be administered concurrently.

Ophthalmic: Intraocular pressure may become elevated in some individuals. If steroid therapy is continued for more than 6 weeks, intraocular pressure should be monitored.

Neuro-psychiatric: Although controlled clinical trials have shown corticosteroids to be effective in speeding the resolution of acute exacerbations of multiple sclerosis, they do not show that they affect the ultimate outcome or natural history of the disease. The studies do show that relatively high doses of corticosteroids are necessary to demonstrate a significant effect. (See DOSAGE AND ADMINSTRATION).

An acute myopathy has been observed with the use of high doses of corticosteroids, most often occurring in patients with disorders of neuromuscular transmission (e.g., myasthenia gravis), or in patients receiving concomitant therapy with neuromuscular blocking drugs (e.g., pancuronium). This acute myopathy is generalized, may involve ocular and respiratory muscles, and may result in quadriparesis. Elevation of creatinine kinase may occur. Clinical improvement or recovery after stopping corticosteroids may require weeks to years.

Psychic derangements may appear when corticosteroids are used, ranging from euphoria, insomnia, mood swings, personality changes, and severe depression, to frank psychotic manifestations. Also, existing emotional instability or psychotic tendencies may be aggravated by corticosteroids.

Gastrointestinal: Steroids should be used with caution in nonspecific ulcerative colitis, if there is a probability of impending perforation, abscess or other pyogenic infection; diverticulitis; fresh intestinal anastomoses; active or latent peptic ulcer.

Signs of peritoneal irritation following gastrointestinal perforation in patients receiving corticosteroids may be minimal or absent.

Cardio-renal: As sodium retention with resultant edema and potassium loss may occur in patients receiving corticosteroids, these agents should be used with caution in patients with hypertension, congestive heart failure, or renal insufficiency.

Musculoskeletal: Corticosteroids decrease bone formation and increase bone resorption both through their effect on calcium regulation (i.e. decreasing absorption and increasing excretion) and inhibition of osteoblast function. This, together with a decrease in the protein matrix of the bone secondary to an increase in protein catabolism, and reduced sex hormone production, may lead to inhibition of bone growth in children and adolescents and the development of osteoporosis at any age. Special consideration should be given to patients at increased risk of osteoporosis (i.e., postmenopausal women) before initiating corticosteroid therapy.

Information for Patients: Patients should be warned not to discontinue the use of PEDIAPRED® (prednisolone sodium phosphate, USP) Oral Solution abruptly or without medical supervision, to advise any medical attendants that they are taking PEDIAPRED and to seek medical advice at once should they develop fever or other signs of infection.

Persons who are on immunosuppressant doses of corticosteroids should be warned to avoid exposure to chicken pox or measles. Patients should also be advised that if they are exposed, medical advice should be sought without delay.

Drug Interactions: Drugs such as barbiturates, phenytoin, ephedrine, and rifampin, which induce hepatic microsomal drug metabolizing enzyme activity may enhance metabolism of prednisolone and require that the dosage of PEDIAPRED be increased.

Increased activity of both cyclosporin and corticosteroids may occur when the two are used concurrently. Convulsions have been reported with this concurrent use.

Estrogens may decrease the hepatic metabolism of certain corticosteroids thereby increasing their effect.

Ketoconazole have been reported to decrease the metabolism of certain corticosteroids by up to 60% leading to an increased risk of corticosteroid side effects.

Coadministration of corticosteroids and warfarin usually results in inhibition of response to warfarin, although there have been some conflicting reports. Therefore, coagulation indices should be monitored frequently to maintain the desired anticoagulant effect.
Concomitant use of aspirin (or other non-steroidal anti-inflammatory agents) and corticosteroids increases the risk of gastrointestinal side effects. Aspirin should be used cautiously in conjunction with corticosteroids in hypoprothrombinemia. The clearance of salicylates may be increased with concurrent use of corticosteroids.
When corticosteroids are administered concomitantly with potassium-depleting agents (i.e., diuretics, amphotericin-B), patients should be observed closely for development of hypokalemia. Patients on digitalis glycosides may be at increased risk of arrhythmias due to hypokalemia.
Concomitant use of anticholinesterase agents and corticosteroids may produce severe weakness in patients with myasthenia gravis. If possible, anticholinesterase agents should be withdrawn at least 24 hours before initiating corticosteroid therapy.
Due to inhibition of antibody response, patients on prolonged corticosteroid therapy may exhibit a diminished response to toxoids and live or inactivated vaccines. Corticosteroids may also potentiate the replication of some organisms contained in live attenuated vaccines. If possible, routine administration of vaccines or toxoids should be deferred until corticosteroid therapy is discontinued.
Because corticosteroids may increase blood glucose concentrations, dosage adjustments of antidiabetic agents may be required.
Corticosteroids may suppress reactions to skin tests.
***Pregnancy:* Teratogenic Effects: Pregnancy Category C.** Prednisolone has been shown to be teratogenic in many species when given in doses equivalent to the human dose. Animal studies in which prednisolone has been given to pregnant mice, rats, and rabbits have yielded an increased incidence of cleft palate in the offspring. There are no adequate and well controlled studies in pregnant women. PEDIAPRED should be used during pregnancy only if the potential benefit justifies the potential risk to the fetus. Infants born to mothers who have received corticosteroids during pregnancy should be carefully observed for signs of hypoadrenalism.
Nursing Mothers: Systematically administered corticosteroids appear in human milk and could suppress growth, interfere with endogenous corticosteroid production, or cause other untoward effects. Caution should be exercised when PEDIAPRED is administered to a nursing woman.
Pediatric Use: The efficacy and safety of prednisolone in the pediatric population are based on the well-established course of effect of corticosteroids which is similar in pediatric and adult populations. Published studies provide evidence of efficacy and safety in pediatric patients for the treatment of nephrotic syndrome (>2 years of age), and aggressive lymphomas and leukemias (> 1 month of age). However, some of these conclusions and other indications for pediatric use of corticosteroid, e.g., severe asthma and wheezing, are based on adequate and well-controlled trials conducted in adults, on the premises that the course of the diseases and their pathophysiology are considered to be substantially similar in both populations.
The adverse effects of prednisolone in pediatric patients are similar to those in adults (see ADVERSE REACTIONS). Like adults, pediatric patients should be carefully observed with frequent measurements of blood pressure, weight, height, intraocular pressure, and clinical evaluation for the presence of infection, psychosocial disturbances, thromboembolism, peptic ulcers, cataracts, and osteoporosis. Children who are treated with corticosteroids by any route, including systemically administered corticosteroids, may experience a decrease in their growth velocity. This negative impact of corticosteroids on growth has been observed at low systemic doses and in the absence of laboratory evidence of HPA axis suppression (i.e., cosyntropin stimulation and basal cortisol plasma levels). Growth velocity may therefore be a more sensitive indicator of systemic corticosteroid exposure in children than some commonly used tests of HPA axis function. The linear growth of children treated with corticosteroids by any route should be monitored, and the potential growth effects of prolonged treatment should be weighed against clinical benefits obtained and the availability of other treatment alternatives. In order to minimize the potential growth effects of corticosteroids, children should be titrated to the lowest effective dose.

ADVERSE REACTIONS

(listed alphabetically under each subsection): Fluid and Electrolyte Disturbances: Congestive heart failure in susceptible patients; fluid retention; hypertension; hypokalemic alkalosis; potassium loss; sodium retention.
Cardiovascular: Hypertrophic cardiomyopathy in premature infants.
Musculoskeletal: Aseptic necrosis of femoral and humeral heads; loss of muscle mass; muscle weakness; osteoporosis; pathologic fracture of long bones; steroid myopathy; tendon rupture; vertebral compression fractures.
Gastrointestinal: Abdominal distention; elevation in serum liver enzyme levels (usually reversible upon discontinuation); pancreatitis; peptic ulcer with possible perforation and hemorrhage; ulcerative esophagitis.
Dermatologic: Facial erythema; increased sweating; impaired wound healing; may suppress reactions to skin tests; petechiae and ecchymoses; thin fragile skin; urticaria; edema.
Metabolic: Negative nitrogen balance due to protein catabolism.
Neurological: Convulsions; headache; increased intracranial pressure with papilledema (pseudotumor cerebri) usually following discontinuation of treatment; psychic disorders; vertigo.
Endocrine: Decreased carbohydrate tolerance; development of cushingoid state; hirsutism; increased requirements for insulin or oral hypoglycemic agents in diabetes; manifestations of latent diabetes mellitus; menstrual irregularities; secondary adrenocortical and pituitary unresponsiveness, particularly in times of stress, as in trauma, surgery or illness; suppression of growth in children.
Ophthalmic: Exophthalmos; glaucoma; increased intraocular pressure; posterior subcapsular cataracts.
Other: Increased appetite; malaise; nausea; weight gain.

OVERDOSAGE

The effects of accidental ingestion of large quantities of prednisolone over a very short period of time have not been reported, but prolonged use of the drug can produce mental symptoms, moon face, abnormal fat deposits, fluid retention, excessive appetite, weight gain, hypertrichosis, acne, striae, ecchymosis, increased sweating, pigmentation, dry scaly skin, thinning scalp hair, increased blood pressure, tachycardia, thrombophlebitis, decreased resistance to infection, negative nitrogen balance with delayed bone and wound healing, headache, weakness, menstrual disorders, accentuated menopausal symptoms, neuropathy, fractures, osteoporosis, peptic ulcer, decreased glucose tolerance, hypokalemia, and adrenal insufficiency. Hepatomegaly and abdominal distention have been observed in children.
Treatment of acute overdosage is by immediate gastric lavage or emesis followed by supportive and symptomatic therapy. For chronic overdosage in the face of severe disease requiring continuous steroid therapy the dosage of prednisolone may be reduced only temporarily, or alternate day treatment may be introduced.

DOSAGE AND ADMINISTRATION

The initial dosage of PEDIAPRED may vary from 5 mL to 60 mL (5 to 60 mg prednisolone base) per day depending on the specific disease entity being treated. In situations of less severity, lower doses will generally suffice while in selected patients higher initial doses may be required. The initial dosage should be maintained or adjusted until a satisfactory response is noted. If after a reasonable period of time, there is a lack of satisfactory clinical response, PEDIAPRED should be discontinued and the patient placed on other appropriate therapy. **IT SHOULD BE EMPHASIZED THAT DOSAGE REQUIREMENTS ARE VARIABLE AND MUST BE INDIVIDUALIZED ON THE BASIS OF THE DISEASE UNDER TREATMENT AND THE RESPONSE OF THE PATIENT.** After a favorable response is noted, the proper maintenance dosage should be determined by decreasing the initial drug dosage in small decrements at appropriate time intervals until the lowest dosage which will maintain an adequate clinical response is reached. It should be kept in mind that constant monitoring is needed in regard to drug dosage. Included in the situations which may make dosage adjustments necessary are changes in clinical status secondary to remissions or exacerbations in the disease process, the patient's individual drug responsiveness, and the effect of patient exposure to stressful situations not directly related to the disease entity under treatment; in this latter situation it may be necessary to increase the dosage of PEDIAPRED for a period of time consistent with the patient's condition. If after long term therapy the drug is to be stopped, it is recommended that it be withdrawn gradually rather than abruptly.
In the treatment of acute exacerbations of multiple sclerosis, daily doses of 200 mg of prednisolone for a week followed by 80 mg every other day or 4 to 8 mg dexamethasone every other day for one month have been shown to be effective.
In pediatric patients, the initial dose of PEDIAPRED may vary depending on the specific disease entity being treated. The range of initial doses is 0.14 to 2 mg/kg/day in three or four divided doses (4 to 60 mg/m^{2}bsa/day).
The standard regimen used to treat nephrotic syndrome in pediatric patients is 60 mg/m^2/day given in three divided doses for 4 weeks, followed by 4 weeks of single doses alternate-day therapy at 40 mg/m^2/day.
The National Heart, Lung, and Blood Institute (NHLBI) recommended dosing for sytemic prednisone, prednisolone or methylprednisolone in children whose asthma is uncontrolled by inhaled corticosteroids and long-acting bronchodilators is 1–2 mg/kg/day in single or divided doses. It is further recommended that short course, or "burst" therapy, be continued until a child achieves a peak expiratory flow rate of 80% of his or her personal best or symptoms resolve. This usually requires 3 to 10 days of treatment, although it can take longer. There is no evidence that tapering the dose after improvement will prevent a relapse.
For the purpose of comparison, the following is the equivalent milligram dosage of the various glucocorticoids:

Cortisone, 25	Triamcinolone, 4
Hydrocortisone, 20	Paramethasone, 2
Prednisolone, 5	Betamethasone, 0.75
Prednisone, 5	Dexamethasone, 0.75
Methylprednisolone, 4	

These dose relationships apply only to oral or intravenous administration of these compounds. When these substances or their derivatives are injected intramuscularly or into joint spaces, their relative properties may be greatly altered.

HOW SUPPLIED

PEDIAPRED (prednisolone sodium phosphate, USP) Oral Solution is a colorless to light straw colored solution containing 6.7 mg prednisolone sodium phosphate (5 mg prednisolone base) per 5 mL (teaspoonful).
NDC 53014-250-01 120 mL bottle
Store at 4°–25°C (39°–77°F). May be refrigerated. Keep tightly closed and out of the reach of children.
Medeva Pharmaceuticals, Inc.
Rochester, NY 14623 USA

SEMPREX®-D CAPSULES ℞

[*sĕm-prĕx*]
(acrivastine and pseudoephedrine hydrochloride)

R314
Rev. 3/98
466051

DESCRIPTION

SEMPREX-D Capsules (acrivastine and pseudoephedrine hydrochloride) are a fixed combination product formulated for oral administration. Acrivastine is an antihistamine and pseudoephedrine is a decongestant. Each capsule contains 8 mg acrivastine and 60 mg pseudoephedrine hydrochloride and the inactive ingredients: lactose, magnesium stearate and sodium starch glycolate. The green and white capsule shell consists of gelatin, D&C Yellow No. 10, FD&C Green No. 3, and titanium dioxide. The yellow band around the capsule consists of gelatin and D&C Yellow No. 10. The capsules may contain one or more parabens and are printed with edible black and white inks.
The chemical name of acrivastine is (*E,E*)-3-[6-[1-(4-methylphenyl)-3-(1-pyrrolidinyl)-1-propenyl]-2-pyridinyl]-2-propenoic acid; the molecular formula is $C_{22}H_{24}N_2O_2$. As an analog of triprolidine hydrochloride, acrivastine is classified as an alkylamine antihistamine. Acrivastine is an odorless, white to pale cream crystalline powder that is soluble in chloroform and alcohol and slightly soluble in water.
The chemical name of pseudoephedrine hydrochloride is [*S*-(*R**,*R**)]-α-[1-(methylamino)ethyl]benzenemethanol hydrochloride; the molecular formula is $C_{10}H_{15}NO \cdot HCl$. Pseudoephedrine is one of the naturally occurring dextrorotatory diastereoisomers of ephedrine and is classified as an indirect sympathomimetic amine. Pseudoephedrine hydrochloride occurs as odorless, fine white to off-white crystals or powder; the drug is soluble in water, alcohol and chloroform.
Structural formulae for the active ingredients of SEMPREX-D Capsules are as follows:

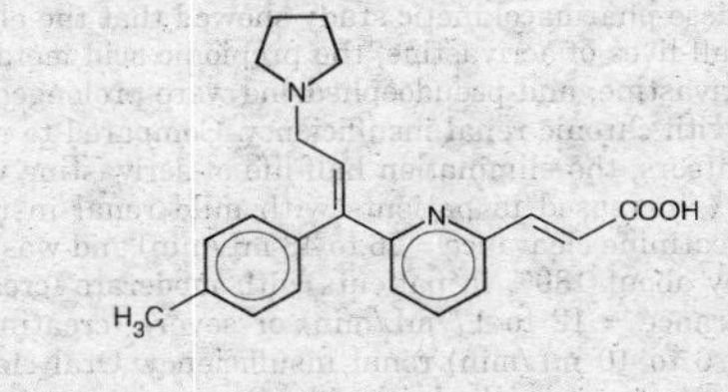

(a) Acrivastine
(Molecular Weight = 348.44)

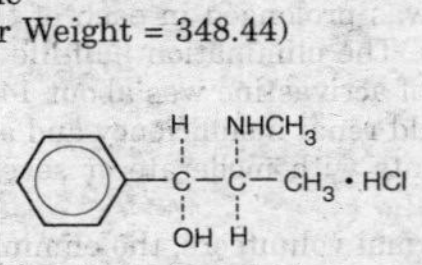

(b) Pseudoephedrine hydrochloride
(Molecular Weight = 201.70)

CLINICAL PHARMACOLOGY

Acrivastine, a structural analog of triprolidine hydrochloride, exhibits H_1-antihistaminic activity in isolated tissues, animals, and humans, and has sedative effects in humans (see PRECAUTIONS). The propionic acid derivative of acrivastine is a metabolite in several animal species (as well as in man) and also exhibits H_1-antihistaminic activity.
Pseudoephedrine hydrochloride is an indirect sympathomimetic agent; that is, it releases norepinephrine from adrenergic nerves.
In vitro tests and in vivo studies in animals of acrivastine and pseudoephedrine in combination failed to demonstrate evidence of any beneficial or deleterious pharmacologic interaction between the two agents.

Continued on next page

Information on the Medeva Pharmaceuticals, Inc. products listed on these pages contains the full prescribing information from product circulars in use as of July 2000. For further information, please consult the package insert currently accompanying the product.

Semprex-D—Cont.

Pharmacokinetics and Metabolism

Acrivastine was absorbed rapidly from the combination capsule following oral administration and was as bioavailable as a solution of acrivastine. After administration of SEMPREX-D Capsules, maximum plasma acrivastine concentrations were achieved at 1.14 ± 0.23 hours. A mass balance study in 7 healthy volunteers showed that acrivastine is primarily eliminated by the kidneys. Over a 72-hour collection period, about 84% of the administered total radioactivity was recovered in urine and about 13% in feces, for a combined recovery of about 97%. Further, 67% of the administered radioactive dose was recovered in urine as the unchanged drug, 11% as the propionic acid metabolite, and 6% as other unknown metabolites.

Acrivastine exhibits linear kinetics over dosages ranging from 2 to 32 mg t.i.d. The mean ± SD terminal half-life for acrivastine was 1.9 ± 0.3 hours following single oral doses and increased to 3.5 ± 1.9 hours at steady state. The terminal half-life for the propionic acid metabolite was 3.8 ± 1.4 hours. Because of the short half-lives of both acrivastine and its metabolites, accumulation in the plasma following multiple dosing is not expected.

The steady-state maximum acrivastine plasma concentration was 227 ± 47 ng/mL. The oral clearance and apparent volume of distribution were 2.9 ± 0.7 mL/min/kg and 0.46 ± 0.05 L/kg, respectively, following a single oral dose; oral clearance did not change at steady state (2.86 ± 0.75 mL/min/kg). The apparent volume of distribution increased to 0.82 ± 0.6 L/kg to parallel the increase in the elimination half-life of the drug.

Acrivastine binding to human plasma proteins was 50 ± 2.0% and was concentration-independent over the range of 5 to 1000 ng/mL. The main binding protein was serum albumin although the drug was slightly bound to α1-acid glycoprotein. No displacement interaction was observed between acrivastine and either phenytoin or theophylline. The binding of acrivastine was not affected by the presence of pseudoephedrine.

Pseudoephedrine hydrochloride was also rapidly absorbed from the combination capsule, and the capsule was as bioavailable as a solution of pseudoephedrine. Steady state maximum plasma concentration for pseudoephedrine was 498 ± 129 ng/mL. The terminal half-life, oral clearance and apparent volume of distribution were 6.2 ± 1.8 hours, 5.9 ± 1.7 mL/min/kg, and 3.0 ± 0.4 L/kg, respectively. Elimination of pseudoephedrine is primarily through the renal route as 55% to 75% of an administered dose appears unchanged in the urine. Pseudoephedrine elimination, however, is highly dependent upon urine pH; the plasma half-life decreased to about 4 hours at pH 5 and increased to 13 hours at pH 8.

Pseudoephedrine did not bind to human plasma proteins over the concentration range of 50 to 2000 ng/mL.

Acrivastine and pseudoephedrine do not influence the pharmacokinetics of the other drug when administered concomitantly.

Special Populations

A single dose pharmacokinetic study showed that the elimination half-lives of acrivastine, the propionic acid metabolite of acrivastine, and pseudoephedrine were prolonged in patients with chronic renal insufficiency. Compared to normal volunteers, the elimination half-life of acrivastine was about 50% increased in patients with mild renal insufficiency (creatinine clearance = 26 to 48 mL/min) and was increased by about 130% in patients with moderate (creatinine clearance = 12 to 17 mL/min) or severe (creatinine clearance 6 to 10 mL/min) renal insufficiency. Oral clearance of acrivastine was diminished by the same magnitude as the half-life was prolonged in each of the three renally impaired groups. The elimination half-life of the propionic acid metabolite of acrivastine was about 140% increased in patients with mild renal insufficiency and about 5 times increased in patients with moderate or severe renal insufficiency.

Compared to normal volunteers, the elimination half-life of pseudoephedrine was about 3 times increased in patients with mild renal insufficiency, about 7 times increased in patients with moderate renal insufficiency, and about 10 times increased in patients with severe renal insufficiency. Oral clearance of pseudoephedrine was diminished by about the same magnitude as the half-life was prolonged in each of the three renally impaired groups (see PRECAUTIONS: Use in Patients with Diminished Renal Function).

The total body load removed by dialysis is approximately 20%, 27%, and 38% for acrivastine, the propionic acid metabolite of acrivastine, and pseudoephedrine, respectively, and therefore, a supplemental dose after a dialysis session is not required.

Based on a multiple dose cross study comparison, the apparent volume of distribution for acrivastine was 44% lower in elderly (n = 36, 65–75 yr) than in young volunteers (n = 16, 19–33 yr). This difference could be attributed to the decrease in total body water that occurs with aging. Despite this difference, no appreciable differences in plasma acrivastine concentrations were seen in the elderly compared to the young, and no appreciable accumulation of acrivastine occurred in plasma at steady-state. The elimination half-life for pseudoephedrine was 18% longer in elderly (7.9 hours) than in younger subjects (6.7 hours), presumably due to the decline in average renal function that occurs with aging. Despite this difference, clearance of pseudoephedrine was not appreciably different in elderly and younger subjects. Elderly patients should therefore be given the same dosage as younger patients. SEMPREX-D Capsules are not recommended, however, in patients with renal impairment (see PRECAUTIONS: Use in Patients with Diminished Renal Function).

The effect of age and sex on the pharmacokinetic parameters of acrivastine and pseudoephedrine was determined in 93 healthy volunteers who participated in various studies. All of the 93 volunteers were Caucasian (81 males and 12 females); 57 were between the ages of 18 and 38 years and 36 were between the ages of 65 and 75 years. There were no age- or sex-related differences in the pharmacokinetic parameters of either acrivastine or pseudoephedrine.

The effect of race on acrivastine and pseudoephedrine pharmacokinetics was examined by screening data obtained from 1035 patients, age 12 to 71 years, who participated in the eight safety and efficacy studies. No race-related differences were observed in the pharmacokinetics of either acrivastine or pseudoephedrine.

Clinical Studies

In healthy volunteers, histamine-induced wheal and flare areas were significantly reduced relative to placebo at 30 minutes after administration of a single dose of acrivastine 8 mg. Maximum reductions of wheal and flare occurred by 1 to 2 hours and significant reductions relative to placebo persisted for up to 6 hours after a single oral dose of acrivastine 8 mg. No additional reductions of wheal and flare were observed following single doses of acrivastine up to 24 mg. The exact correlation between responses on skin testing and clinical efficacy is not established.

Five randomized, placebo- and/or active-controlled trials compared SEMPREX-D with its acrivastine and pseudoephedrine components for the symptomatic relief of seasonal allergic rhinitis. In these studies, 696 patients received four daily doses of acrivastine 8 mg plus pseudoephedrine hydrochloride 60 mg (i.e., SEMPREX-D Capsules or bioequivalent formulations administered concurrently) or the same doses of the components for 14 days. The combination reduced the intensity of sneezing, rhinorrhea, pruritus, and lacrimation more than pseudoephedrine and reduced the intensity of nasal congestion more than acrivastine, demonstrating a contribution of each of the components. The onset of antihistaminic and nasal decongestant actions occurred within one or two hours after the first dose of SEMPREX-D Capsules. Somnolence occurred in about 12% of patients given SEMPREX-D compared with about 6% on placebo.

INDICATIONS AND USAGE

SEMPREX-D Capsules are indicated for relief of symptoms associated with seasonal allergic rhinitis such as sneezing, rhinorrhea, pruritus, lacrimation, and nasal congestion. SEMPREX-D Capsules should be administered when both the antihistaminic activity of acrivastine and the nasal decongestant activity of pseudoephedrine are desired (see CLINICAL PHARMACOLOGY). The efficacy of SEMPREX-D Capsules beyond 14 days of continuous treatment in patients with seasonal allergic rhinitis has not been adequately investigated in clinical trials.

SEMPREX-D Capsules have not been adequately studied for effectiveness in relieving the symptoms of the common cold.

CONTRAINDICATIONS

SEMPREX-D Capsules are contraindicated in patients with a known sensitivity to acrivastine, other alkylamine antihistamines (e.g., triprolidine), pseudoephedrine, other sympathomimetic amines (e.g., phenylpropanolamine), or to any other components of the formulation. SEMPREX-D Capsules are contraindicated in patients with severe hypertension or severe coronary artery disease. SEMPREX-D Capsules are contraindicated in patients taking monoamine oxidase (MAO) inhibitors and for 14 days after stopping use of an MAO inhibitor (see Drug Interactions).

WARNINGS

SEMPREX-D Capsules should be used with caution in patients with hypertension, diabetes mellitus, ischemic heart disease, increased intraocular pressure, hyperthyroidism, prostatic hypertrophy, stenosing peptic ulcer, or pyloroduodenal obstruction. Overdose of sympathomimetic amines may produce CNS stimulation with convulsions or cardiovascular collapse with accompanying hypotension. The elderly are more likely to have adverse reactions to sympathomimetic amines.

PRECAUTIONS

General: Acrivastine is sedating in some patients. In controlled clinical trials, somnolence (i.e., drowsiness, sedation, sleepiness) was more common with SEMPREX-D Capsules (by an average of 6%) than with placebo (see ADVERSE EXPERIENCES).

Patients should be advised to assess their individual responses to SEMPREX-D Capsules before engaging in any activity requiring mental alertness, such as driving a motor vehicle or operating machinery. Concurrent use of SEMPREX-D Capsules with alcohol or other CNS depressants may cause additional reductions in alertness and impairment of CNS performance and should be avoided (see Drug Interactions).

Use in Patients with Diminished Renal Function: Acrivastine and pseudoephedrine are excreted primarily through the kidney. Both compounds therefore accumulate in patients with impaired renal function. Due to the differential effects of renal failure on the serum half-life and clearance of acrivastine and pseudoephedrine, use of SEMPREX-D Capsules, a fixed combination product, in patients with renal impairment (creatinine clearance ≤ 48 mL/min) is not recommended (see OVERDOSAGE and CLINICAL PHARMACOLOGY).

Information to Patients: Patients taking SEMPREX®-D Capsules (acrivastine and pseudoephedrine hydrochloride) should receive the following information. SEMPREX-D Capsules are prescribed to reduce symptoms associated with seasonal allergic rhinitis. Patients should be instructed to take SEMPREX-D Capsules only as prescribed and not to exceed the prescribed dose. Patients should be advised against the concurrent use of SEMPREX-D with over-the-counter antihistamines and decongestants. Patients who are or may become pregnant should be told that this product should be used in pregnancy or during lactation only if the potential benefit justifies the potential risks to the fetus or nursing infant. Due to the risk of hypertensive crisis, patients should be instructed not to take SEMPREX-D Capsules if they are presently taking a monoamine oxidase inhibitor or for 14 days after stopping use of an MAO inhibitor. Patients should be advised to assess their individual responses to SEMPREX-D Capsules before engaging in any activity requiring mental alertness, such as driving a car or operating machinery. Patients should be advised that the concurrent use of SEMPREX-D Capsules with alcohol and other CNS depressants may lead to additional reductions in alertness and impairment of CNS performance and should be avoided.

Use in the Elderly (Approximately 60 Years or Older): Elderly patients who participated in clinical trials did not differ in effectiveness or adverse effects from younger patients. Antihistamines, however, as a pharmaceutical class, are more likely to cause dizziness, sedation, bladder-neck obstruction, and hypotension in elderly patients. The elderly are also more likely to have adverse reactions to sympathomimetics such as pseudoephedrine (see CLINICAL PHARMACOLOGY and WARNINGS).

Drug Interactions: MAO inhibitors and beta-adrenergic agonists increase the effects of sympathomimetic amines. Concomitant use of sympathomimetic amines with MAO inhibitors can result in a hypertensive crisis (see CONTRAINDICATIONS). Because MAO inhibitors are long-acting, SEMPREX-D Capsules should not be taken with an MAO inhibitor or for 14 days after stopping use of an MAO inhibitor.

Because of their pseudoephedrine content, SEMPREX-D Capsules may reduce the antihypertensive effects of drugs that interfere with sympathetic activity. Care should be taken in the administration of SEMPREX-D Capsules concomitantly with other sympathomimetic amines because the combined effects on the cardiovascular system may be harmful to the patient.

Concomitant administration of SEMPREX-D Capsules with alcohol and other CNS depressants may result in additional reductions in alertness and impairment of CNS performance and should be avoided.

No formal drug interaction studies between SEMPREX-D Capsules and other possibly co-administered drugs have been performed.

Carcinogenesis, Mutagenesis, and Impairment of Fertility: Carcinogenicity studies with the combination of acrivastine and pseudoephedrine have not been performed. Oral doses of acrivastine alone at levels up to 40 mg/kg/day (236 mg/m^2/day or 10 times the recommended human daily dose) for 20 to 22 months in rats and up to 250 mg/kg/day (750 mg/m^2/day or 32 times the recommended human daily dose) for 20 to 24 months in mice revealed no evidence of carcinogenic potential. No evidence of mutagenicity (with or without metabolic activation) was observed in the Ames Salmonella mutagenicity assay or in the L5178Y/tk+/− mouse lymphoma assay. In an in vitro cytogenetic study performed in cultured human lymphocytes, acrivastine induced structural chromosomal abnormalities in the absence of metabolic activation, but not in its presence. In an in vivo cytogenetic study in rats given single oral doses of acrivastine up to 1000 mg/kg (5900 mg/m^2 or 249 times the recommended human daily dose) there were no structural chromosomal alterations.

Reproduction-fertility studies in rats given acrivastine alone at levels up to 200 mg/kg/day (1180 mg/m^2/day or 50 times the recommended human daily dose) had no effect on male or female fertility. Similarly no effect on fertility was seen in male rats given acrivastine 20 mg/kg/day and pseudoephedrine 100 mg/kg/day (118 and 590 mg/m^2/day or 5 and 3 times the recommended human daily doses, respectively) or in female rats given acrivastine 4 mg/kg/day and pseudoephedrine 20 mg/kg/day (23.6 and 118 mg/m^2/day or 1 and 0.7 times the recommended human daily doses, respectively).

Pregnancy: Pregnancy Category B:

Teratogenic Effects: No evidence of teratogenicity was seen in rats and rabbits given acrivastine 1000 and 400 mg/kg/day, respectively (5900 and 4720 mg/m^2/day or 249 and 200 times the recommended human daily dose). No evidence of teratogenicity was seen in rats given a combination of acrivastine 30 mg/kg/day and pseudoephedrine 150 mg/kg/day (177 and 885 mg/m^2/day or 8 and 5 times the recommended human daily dose, respectively). Similarly, no evidence of teratogenicity was observed in rabbits given acrivastine 20 mg/kg/day and pseudoephedrine 100 mg/kg/day (236 and 1180 mg/m^2/day or 10 and 7 times the recommended human daily doses, respectively). There are, however, no adequate and well-controlled studies in pregnant women. Because animal teratology studies are not always predictive of human

ADVERSE EVENTS REPORTED IN CLINICAL TRIALS* (PERCENT OF PATIENTS REPORTING)†

	Controlled Studies			
	Placebo (n = 1767)	Acrivastine (n = 1935)	Pseudoephedrine (n = 887)	Acrivastine plus Pseudoephedrine (n = 1650)
CNS				
Somnolence‡	6	12	8	12
Headache	18	19	19	19
Dizziness	2	3	3	3
Nervousness‡	1	2	4	3
Insomnia‡	1	1	6	4
MISCELLANEOUS				
Nausea	2	3	3	2
Dry Mouth‡	2	3	5	7
Asthenia	2	3	2	2
Dyspepsia	1	1	2	2
Pharyngitis	2	1	1	3
Cough Increase	1	2	1	2
Dysmenorrhea	1	2	3	2

* Includes all events regardless of causal relationship to treatment.
† Includes all adverse events with a reported frequency of >1% for the acrivastine plus pseudoephedrine treatment group.
‡ SEMPREX-D demonstrates a statistically higher frequency of events than placebo, P ≤0.05.

responses, SEMPREX-D Capsules should be used during pregnancy only if the potential benefit justifies the potential risks to the fetus.

Nonteratogenic Effects: In a perinatal-postnatal study in rats, acrivastine given alone at levels up to 500 mg/kg/day (2950 mg/m^2/day or 124 times the recommended human daily dose) was associated with maternal and neonatal mortality at the maximum dose level. Neonatal survival was decreased in rats given a combination of acrivastine 20 mg/kg/day and pseudoephedrine 100 mg/kg/day (118 and 590 mg/m^2/day or 5 and 3 times the human dose, respectively).

Nursing Mothers: It is not known whether acrivastine is excreted in human milk; pseudoephedrine is excreted in human milk. SEMPREX-D Capsules should only be used in nursing mothers when the potential benefit justifies the potential risks to the nursing infant.

Pediatric Use: Safety and effectiveness of SEMPREX-D Capsules in pediatric patients under the age of 12 years have not been established.

ADVERSE EXPERIENCES

Information on the incidence of adverse events in clinical investigations conducted in the U.S. was obtained from 33 controlled and 15 uncontrolled clinical studies in which 2499 patients received acrivastine and 2631 patients received acrivastine plus pseudoephedrine hydrochloride for treatment periods ranging from one day to one year. The majority of patients in clinical trials were exposed to acrivastine or acrivastine plus pseudoephedrine for less than 90 days. Acrivastine dosage ranged from 3 to 96 mg/day; 1336 patients received dosages equal to or greater than acrivastine 24 mg/day. Acrivastine plus pseudoephedrine hydrochloride dosages ranged from acrivastine 8 to 48 mg/day plus pseudoephedrine hydrochloride 60 to 240 mg/day. A total of 2335 patients received three or four daily doses of acrivastine 8 mg plus pseudoephedrine hydrochloride 60 mg. In controlled clinical trials, only 12 spontaneously elicited adverse events were reported with frequencies greater than 1% in the acrivastine plus pseudoephedrine hydrochloride treatment group (see table).

[See table above]

The nature and overall frequencies of adverse events from international clinical trials (35 studies involving approximately 1600 patients) were similar to the results obtained in the U.S. studies.

Post-marketing clinical experience reports with acrivastine and acrivastine plus pseudoephedrine have included rare serious hypersensitivity reactions manifested by anaphylaxis, angioedema, bronchospasm, and erythema multiforme. No deaths associated with use of acrivastine or acrivastine plus pseudoephedrine have been reported.

Pseudoephedrine may cause ephedrine-like reactions such as tachycardia, palpitations, headache, dizziness, or nausea (see WARNINGS and OVERDOSAGE).

OVERDOSAGE

There have been no reports of overdosage with SEMPREX-D Capsules. In the clinical trial program and in international post-marketing experience, there have been two reported overdoses with acrivastine. Doses were 72 mg and 322 mg. Both patients recovered without sequelae. Adverse events included trembling, stridor, loss of consciousness and possible convulsions in the first patient and somnolence in the second.

Since acrivastine and pseudoephedrine have pharmacologically different actions, it is difficult to predict how an individual will respond to overdosage with SEMPREX-D Capsules. However, acute overdosage with SEMPREX-D Capsules may produce clinical signs of either CNS stimulation or depression. Overdosage of sympathomimetics has been associated with the following events: fear, anxiety, tenseness, restlessness, tremor, weakness, pallor, respiratory difficulty, dysuria, insomnia, hallucinations, convulsions. CNS depression, arrhythmias, and cardiovascular collapse with hypotension. Treatment for overdosage with SEMPREX-D Capsules should follow general symptomatic and supportive principles.

In a placebo-controlled, double-blind clinical trial in 18 healthy male subjects, single doses of acrivastine up to 400 mg (50 times the recommended antihistaminic dose) produced only a weak vagolytic effect, manifested as an increase in heart rate, and did not cause cardiac repolarization delays (i.e., increased QTc). Daily doses of acrivastine up to 2400 mg (75 times the recommended antihistamine dose) in an uncontrolled study in 38 cancer patients produced a 15–beats-per-minute increase in mean heart rate and occasional episodes of nausea and vomiting. The effects of acrivastine plus pseudoephedrine at single or multiple doses higher than the recommended daily dose of SEMPREX-D Capsules (i.e., 32 mg acrivastine plus 240 mg pseudoephedrine) on heart rate and cardiac repolarization have not been investigated in clinical trials.

The mean LD_{50} (single, oral dose) of acrivastine is greater than 4000 mg/kg (23600 mg/m^2 or 1000 times the recommended human daily dose) in rats and greater than 1200 mg/kg (3600 mg/m^2 or 153 times the recommended human daily dose) in mice. The mean LD_{50} (single, oral dose) of pseudoephedrine hydrochloride is 2206 mg/kg (13015 mg/m^2 or 73 times the recommended human daily dose) in rats and 726 mg/kg (2178 mg/m^2 or 12 times the recommended human daily dose) in mice. The toxic and lethal concentrations of acrivastine and pseudoephedrine in human biologic fluids are not known. Based upon pharmacokinetic screening data from clinical trials, the maximum plasma acrivastine concentration after dosing with acrivastine 8 mg was 393 ng/mL and the maximum plasma pseudoephedrine concentration after dosing with pseudoephedrine hydrochloride 60 mg was 1308 ng/mL.

DOSAGE AND ADMINISTRATION

The recommended dosage for adults and adolescents 12 years and older is one capsule administered orally, every 4 to 6 hours four times a day.

HOW SUPPLIED

SEMPREX-D Capsules (dark green opaque cap and white opaque body with a yellow band) contain acrivastine 8 mg and pseudoephedrine hydrochloride 60 mg. The cap is printed with "MEDEVA" in white ink, and the body is printed with "SEMPREX-D" in black ink.

NDC 53014-404-10 Bottle of 100's.

Store at 15° to 25°C (59° to 77°F) in a dry place and protected from light. Keep out of the reach of children.

Rx Only

Marketed by:
Medeva Pharmaceuticals, Inc.
Rochester, NY 14623 USA
Manufactured by:
Catalytica Pharmaceuticals, Inc.
Greenville, NC 27834 USA
U.S. Patent Nos. 4501893 and 4650807.
® Medeva California, Inc.

 Rev. 3/98
R314
466051

TUSSIONEX® PENNKINETIC®

(hydrocodone polistirex and chlorpheniramine polistirex)
Extended-Release Suspension

Ⓒ℞

LR226B
Rev. 6/98

DESCRIPTION

Each teaspoonful (5 mL) of TUSSIONEX Pennkinetic Extended-Release Suspension contains hydrocodone polistirex equivalent to 10 mg of hydrocodone bitartrate and chlorpheniramine polistirex equivalent to 8 mg of chlorpheniramine maleate. TUSSIONEX Pennkinetic Extended-Release Suspension provides up to 12-hour relief per dose. Hydrocodone is a centrally-acting narcotic antitussive. Chlorpheniramine is an antihistamine. TUSSIONEX Pennkinetic Extended-Release Suspension is for oral use only.

Hydrocodone Polistirex: sulfonated styrene-divinylbenzene copolymer complex with 4,5α-epoxy-3-methoxy-17-methylmorphinan-6-one.

Chlorpheniramine Polistirex: sulfonated styrene-divinylbenzene copolymer complex with 2-[*p*-chloro-α-[2-(dimethylamino)ethyl]-benzyl]pyridine.

Inactive Ingredients: Ascorbic acid, D&C Yellow No. 10, ethylcellulose, FD&C Yellow No. 6, flavor, high fructose corn syrup, methylparaben, polyethylene glycol 3350, polysorbate 80, pregelatinized starch, propylene glycol, propylparaben, purified water, sucrose, vegetable oil, xanthan gum.

CLINICAL PHARMACOLOGY

Hydrocodone is a semisynthetic narcotic antitussive and analgesic with multiple actions qualitatively similar to those of codeine. The precise mechanism of action of hydrocodone and other opiates is not known; however, hydrocodone is believed to act directly on the cough center. In excessive doses, hydrocodone, like other opium derivatives, will depress respiration. The effects of hydrocodone in therapeutic doses on the cardiovascular system are insignificant. Hydrocodone can produce miosis, euphoria, physical and psychological dependence.

Chlorpheniramine is an antihistamine drug (H_1 receptor antagonist) that also possesses anticholinergic and sedative activity. It prevents released histamine from dilating capillaries and causing edema of the respiratory mucosa.

Hydrocodone release from TUSSIONEX Pennkinetic Extended-Release Suspension is controlled by the Pennkinetic System, an extended-release drug delivery system which combines an ion-exchange polymer matrix with a diffusion rate-limiting permeable coating. Chlorpheniramine release is prolonged by use of an ion-exchange polymer system.

Following multiple dosing with TUSSIONEX Pennkinetic Extended-Release Suspension, hydrocodone mean (S.D.) peak plasma concentrations of 22.8 (5.9) ng/mL occurred at 3.4 hours. Chlorpheniramine mean (S.D.) peak plasma concentrations of 58.4 (14.7) ng/mL occurred at 6.3 hours following multiple dosing. Peak plasma levels obtained with an immediate-release syrup occurred at approximately 1.5 hours for hydrocodone and 2.8 hours for chlorpheniramine. The plasma half-lives of hydrocodone and chlorpheniramine have been reported to be approximately 4 and 16 hours, respectively.

INDICATIONS AND USAGE

TUSSIONEX Pennkinetic Extended-Release Suspension is indicated for relief of cough and upper respiratory symptoms associated with allergy or a cold.

Continued on next page

Information on the Medeva Pharmaceuticals, Inc. products listed on these pages contains the full prescribing information from product circulars in use as of July 2000. For further information, please consult the package insert currently accompanying the product.

Tussionex—Cont.

CONTRAINDICATIONS

Known allergy or sensitivity to hydrocodone or chlorpheniramine.

WARNINGS

Respiratory Depression: As with all narcotics, TUSSIONEX Pennkinetic Extended-Release Suspension produces dose-related respiratory depression by directly acting on brain stem respiratory centers. Hydrocodone affects the center that controls respiratory rhythm, and may produce irregular and periodic breathing. Caution should be exercised when TUSSIONEX Pennkinetic Extended-Release Suspension is used postoperatively and in patients with pulmonary disease or whenever ventilatory function is depressed. If respiratory depression occurs, it may be antagonized by the use of naloxone hydrochloride and other supportive measures when indicated (see OVERDOSAGE).

Head Injury and Increased Intracranial Pressure: The respiratory depressant effects of narcotics and their capacity to elevate cerebrospinal fluid pressure may be markedly exaggerated in the presence of head injury, other intracranial lesions or a pre-existing increase in intracranial pressure. Furthermore, narcotics produce adverse reactions which may obscure the clinical course of patients with head injuries.

Acute Abdominal Conditions: The administration of narcotics may obscure the diagnosis or clinical course of patients with acute abdominal conditions.

Obstructive Bowel Disease: Chronic use of narcotics may result in obstructive bowel disease especially in patients with underlying intestinal motility disorder.

Pediatric Use: In pediatric patients, as well as adults, the respiratory center is sensitive to the depressant action of narcotic cough suppressants in a dose-dependent manner. Benefit to risk ratio should be carefully considered especially in pediatric patients with respiratory embarrassment (e.g., croup) (see PRECAUTIONS).

PRECAUTIONS

General: Caution is advised when prescribing this drug to patients with narrow-angle glaucoma, asthma or prostatic hypertrophy.

Special Risk Patients: As with any narcotic agent, TUSSIONEX Pennkinetic Extended-Release Suspension should be used with caution in elderly or debilitated patients and those with severe impairment of hepatic or renal function, hypothyroidism, Addison's disease, prostatic hypertrophy or urethral stricture. The usual precautions should be observed and the possibility of respiratory depression should be kept in mind.

Information for Patients: As with all narcotics, TUSSIONEX Pennkinetic Extended-Release Suspension may produce marked drowsiness and impair the mental and/or physical abilities required for the performance of potentially hazardous tasks such as driving a car or operating machinery; patients should be cautioned accordingly. TUSSIONEX Pennkinetic Extended-Release Suspension must not be diluted with fluids or mixed with other drugs as this may alter the resin-binding and change the absorption rate, possibly increasing the toxicity. Keep out of the reach of children.

Cough Reflex: Hydrocodone suppresses the cough reflex; as with all narcotics, caution should be exercised when TUSSIONEX Pennkinetic Extended-Release Suspension is used postoperatively, and in patients with pulmonary disease.

Drug Interactions: Patients receiving narcotics, antihistaminics, antipsychotics, antianxiety agents or other CNS depressants (including alcohol) concomitantly with TUSSIONEX Pennkinetic Extended-Release Suspension may exhibit an additive CNS depression. When combined therapy is contemplated, the dose of one or both agents should be reduced.
The use of MAO inhibitors or tricyclic antidepressants with hydrocodone preparations may increase the effect of either the antidepressant or hydrocodone.
The concurrent use of other anticholinergics with hydrocodone may produce paralytic ileus.

Carcinogenesis, Mutagenesis, Impairment of Fertility: Carcinogenicity, mutagenicity and reproductive studies have not been conducted with TUSSIONEX® Pennkinetic® (hydrocodone polistirex and chlorpheniramine polistirex) Extended-Release Suspension.

Pregnancy: Teratogenic Effects—Pregnancy Category C. Hydrocodone has been shown to be teratogenic in hamsters when given in doses 700 times the human dose. There are no adequate and well-controlled studies in pregnant women. TUSSIONEX Pennkinetic Extended-Release Suspension should be used during pregnancy only if the potential benefit justifies the potential risk to the fetus.

Nonteratogenic Effects: Babies born to mothers who have been taking opioids regularly prior to delivery will be physically dependent. The withdrawal signs include irritability and excessive crying, tremors, hyperactive reflexes, increased respiratory rate, increased stools, sneezing, yawning, vomiting and fever. The intensity of the syndrome does not always correlate with the duration of maternal opioid use or dose.

Labor and Delivery: As with all narcotics, administration of TUSSIONEX Pennkinetic Extended-Release Suspension to the mother shortly before delivery may result in some degree of respiratory depression in the newborn, especially if higher doses are used.

Nursing Mothers: It is not known whether this drug is excreted in human milk. Because many drugs are excreted in human milk and because of the potential for serious adverse reactions in nursing infants from TUSSIONEX Pennkinetic Extended-Release Suspension, a decision should be made whether to discontinue nursing or to discontinue the drug, taking into account the importance of the drug to the mother.

Pediatric Use: Safety and effectiveness of TUSSIONEX Pennkinetic Extended-Release Suspension in pediatric patients under six have not been established.

ADVERSE REACTIONS

Central Nervous System: Sedation, drowsiness, mental clouding, lethargy, impairment of mental and physical performance, anxiety, fear, dysphoria, euphoria, dizziness, psychic dependence, mood changes.

Dermatologic System: Rash, pruritus.

Gastrointestinal System: Nausea and vomiting may occur; they are more frequent in ambulatory than in recumbent patients. Prolonged administration of TUSSIONEX Pennkinetic Extended-Release Suspension may produce constipation.

Genitourinary System: Ureteral spasm, spasm of vesicle sphincters and urinary retention have been reported with opiates.

Respiratory Depression: TUSSIONEX Pennkinetic Extended-Release Suspension may produce dose-related respiratory depression by acting directly on brain stem respiratory centers (see OVERDOSAGE).

Respiratory System: Dryness of the pharynx, occasional tightness of the chest.

DRUG ABUSE AND DEPENDENCE

TUSSIONEX Pennkinetic Extended-Release Suspension is a Schedule III narcotic. Psychic dependence, physical dependence and tolerance may develop upon repeated administration of narcotics; therefore, TUSSIONEX Pennkinetic Extended-Release Suspension should be prescribed and administered with caution. However, psychic dependence is unlikely to develop when TUSSIONEX Pennkinetic Extended-Release Suspension is used for a short time for the treatment of cough. Physical dependence, the condition in which continued administration of the drug is required to prevent the appearance of a withdrawal syndrome, assumes clinically significant proportions only after several weeks of continued oral narcotic use, although some mild degree of physical dependence may develop after a few days of narcotic therapy.

OVERDOSAGE

Signs and Symptoms: Serious overdosage with hydrocodone is characterized by respiratory depression (a decrease in respiratory rate and/or tidal volume, Cheyne-Stokes respiration, cyanosis), extreme somnolence progressing to stupor or coma, skeletal muscle flaccidity, cold and clammy skin, and sometimes bradycardia and hypotension. Although miosis is characteristic of narcotic overdosage, mydriasis may occur in terminal narcosis or severe hypoxia. In severe overdosage apnea, circulatory collapse, cardiac arrest and death may occur. The manifestations of chlorpheniramine overdosage may vary from central nervous system depression to stimulation.

Treatment: Primary attention should be given to the reestablishment of adequate respiratory exchange through provision of a patent airway and the institution of assisted or controlled ventilation. The narcotic antagonist naloxone hydrochloride is a specific antidote for respiratory depression which may result from overdosage or unusual sensitivity to narcotics including hydrocodone. Therefore, an appropriate dose of naloxone hydrochloride should be administered, preferably by the intravenous route, simultaneously with efforts at respiratory resuscitation. Since the duration of action of hydrocodone in this formulation may exceed that of the antagonist, the patient should be kept under continued surveillance and repeated doses of the antagonist should be administered as needed to maintain adequate respiration. For further information, see full prescribing information for naloxone hydrochloride. An antagonist should not be administered in the absence of clinically significant respiratory depression. Oxygen, intravenous fluids, vasopressors and other supportive measures should be employed as indicated. Gastric emptying may be useful in removing unabsorbed drug.

DOSAGE AND ADMINISTRATION

Shake well before using.
Adults: 1 teaspoonful (5 mL) every 12 hours; do not exceed 2 teaspoonfuls in 24 hours.
Children 6–12: 1/2 teaspoonful every 12 hours; **do not exceed 1 teaspoonful in 24 hours.**
Not recommended for children under 6 years of age (see PRECAUTIONS).

HOW SUPPLIED

TUSSIONEX Pennkinetic (hydrocodone polistirex and chlorpheniramine polistirex) Extended-Release Suspension is a gold-colored suspension.
NDC 53014-548-67 473 mL bottle
Shake well. Dispense in a well-closed container. Store at 59°–86°F (15°–30°C).
Rx only
Medeva Pharmaceuticals, Inc.
Rochester, NY 14623 USA
© 1998, Medeva Pharmaceuticals, Inc. Rev. 6/98
® Fisons Investments Inc. LR226B

VALSTAR™ ℞

(valrubicin)
Sterile Solution for Intravesical Instillation
Rx Only
For Intravesical Use Only
Not for IV or IM Use

Rev. 5/99
R309A

DESCRIPTION

Valrubicin (N-trifluoroacetyladriamycin-14-valerate), a semisynthetic analog of the anthracycline doxorubicin, is a cytotoxic agent with the chemical name, (2*S-cis*)-2-[1,2,3,4,6,11-hexahydro-2,5,12-trihydroxy-7-methoxy-6,11-dioxo-4-[[2,3,6-trideoxy-3-[(trifluoroacetyl)amino]-α-L-*lyxo*-hexopyranosyl]oxyl]-2-naphthacenyl]-2-oxoethyl pentanoate. Valrubicin is an orange or orange-red powder that is highly lipophilic, soluble in methylene chloride, ethanol, methanol and acetone, and relatively insoluble in water. Its chemical formula is $C_{34}H_{36}F_3NO_{13}$ and its molecular weight is 723.65. The chemical structure is shown in FIGURE 1.

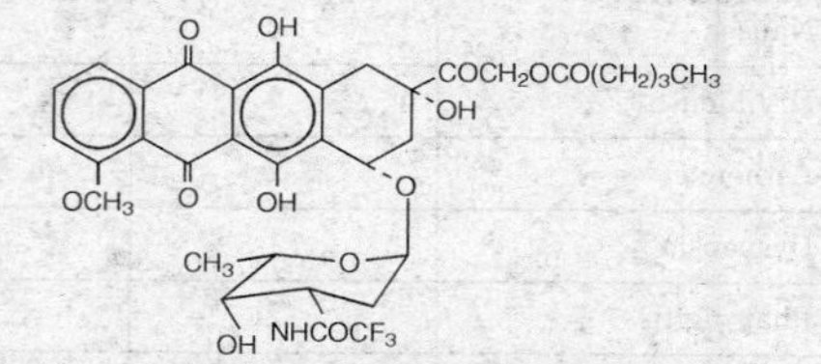

FIGURE 1. Chemical Structure of Valrubicin

VALSTAR (valrubicin) Sterile Solution for Intravesical Instillation is intended for intravesical administration in the urinary bladder. It is supplied as a nonaqueous solution that should be diluted before intravesical administration. Each vial of VALSTAR contains valrubicin at a concentration of 40 mg/mL in 50% Cremophor® EL (polyoxyethyleneglycol triricinoleate)/50% dehydrated alcohol, USP without preservatives or other additives. The solution is sterile and nonpyrogenic.

CLINICAL PHARMACOLOGY

Mechanism of Action: Valrubicin is an anthracycline that affects a variety of inter-related biological functions, most of which involve nucleic acid metabolism. It readily penetrates into cells, where it inhibits the incorporation of nucleosides into nucleic acids, causes extensive chromosomal damage, and arrests cell cycle in G_2. Although valrubicin does not bind strongly to DNA, a principal mechanism of its action, mediated by valrubicin metabolites, is interference with the normal DNA breaking-resealing action of DNA topoisomerase II.

Pharmacokinetics after Intravesical Administration of VALSTAR: When 800 mg VALSTAR was administered intravesically to patients with carcinoma *in situ*, VALSTAR penetrated into the bladder wall. The mean total anthracycline concentration measured in bladder tissue exceeded the levels causing 90% cytotoxicity to human bladder cells cultured *in vitro*. During the two-hour dose-retention period, the metabolism of VALSTAR to its major metabolites N-trifluoroacetyladriamycin and N-trifluoroacetyladriamycinol was negligible. After retention, the drug was almost completely excreted by voiding the instillate. Mean percent recovery of VALSTAR, N-trifluoroacetyladriamycin, and total anthracyclines in 14 urine samples from six patients was 98.6%, 0.4%, and 99.0% of the total administered drug, respectively. During the two-hour dose-retention period, only nanogram quantities of VALSTAR were absorbed into the plasma. VALSTAR metabolites N-trifluoroacetyladriamycin and N-trifluoroacetyladriamycinol were measured in blood. Total systemic exposure to anthracyclines during and after intravesical administration of VALSTAR is dependent upon the condition of the bladder wall. The mean $AUC_{0-6\ hours}$ (total anthracyclines exposure) for an intravesical dose of 900 mg of VALSTAR administered 2 weeks after transurethral resection of bladder tumors (n=6) was 78 nmol/L•hr. In patients receiving 800 mg of VALSTAR 5 to 51 minutes after typical (n=8) and extensive (n=5) transurethral resection of bladder tumors (TURBs), the mean $AUC_{0-6\ hours}$ values for total anthracyclines were 409 and 788 nmol/L•hr, respectively. The $AUC_{0-6\ hours}$ total exposure to anthracyclines was 18,382 nmol/L•hr in one patient who experienced a perforated bladder following a transurethral resection that occurred 5 minutes before administration of an intravesical dose of 800 mg of VALSTAR. Administration of a comparable intravenous dose of VALSTAR (600 mg/m^2; n=2) as a 24-hour infusion resulted in an $AUC_{0-6\ hours}$ for total anthracyclines of 11,975 nmol/L•hr. These results are shown in FIGURE 2.

[See figure at top of next page]

The patient with a perforated bladder who received 800 mg of VALSTAR intravesically developed severe leukopenia and neutropenia approximately two weeks after drug administration. Systemic hematologic toxcity from VALSTAR was not seen after an intravesical dose of 800 mg of VALSTAR unless perforation of the urinary bladder occurred.

CLINICAL TRIALS

VALSTAR has been administered intravesically to a total of 230 patients with transitional cell carcinoma of the bladder, including 205 patients who received multiple weekly doses ranging from 200 to 900 mg. One hundred seventy-nine of the 205 patients received the approved dose and schedule of 800 mg weekly for multiple weeks.

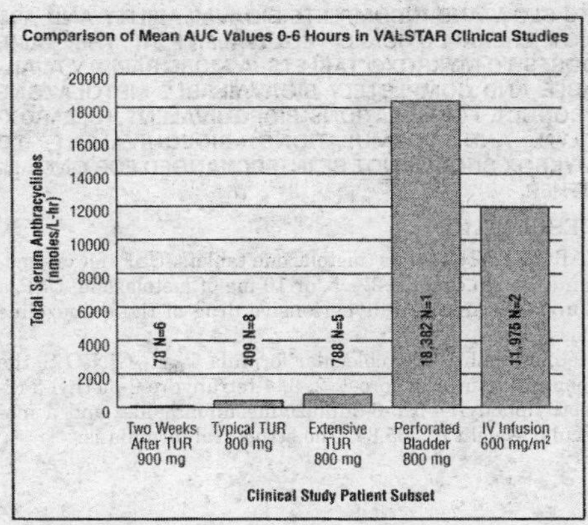

FIGURE 2. Comparison of Mean $AUC_{0\text{-}6\ hours}$ in VALSTAR Clinical Studies (N=number of patients)

In the 90 study patients with BCG-refractory carcinoma *in situ* (CIS), 70% had received at least 2 courses of BCG and 30% had received one course of BCG and at least one additional course of treatment with another agent(s) - e.g., mitomycin, thiotepa, or interferon. VALSTAR was administered beginning at least two weeks after transurethral resection and/or fulguration. After intravesical administration of VALSTAR, 16 patients (18%) had a complete response documented by bladder biopsies and cytology at 6 months following initiation of therapy. Median duration of response from start of treatment varied according to the method of analysis (13.5 months if measured to last bladder biopsy without tumor and 21 months if measured until time of documented recurrence). A retrospective analysis in the 16 patients with complete response to VALSTAR demonstrated that time to recurrence of their disease after treatment with VALSTAR was longer than time to recurrence after previous courses of intravesical therapy.

Of the 90 patients with BCG-refractory CIS, 11% (10 patients) developed metastatic or deeply-invasive bladder cancer during follow-up; four of these patients, none who underwent cystectomy, died with metastatic bladder cancer and six were found to have developed stage progression to deeply-invasive disease (T3), with lymph node involvement in one patient, at the time of cystectomy. It is difficult to ascertain to what extent the development of advanced bladder cancer in these patients was due to the delay in cystectomy required to receive treatment with VALSTAR (3 months was the time to follow-up to determine response), as cystectomy was often delayed or was never performed despite failure of treatment with VALSTAR. In the 10 patients documented to have invasive bladder cancer or metastatic disease, the delay between the time of treatment failure (when cystectomy should have been performed) and cystectomy or documentation of advanced bladder cancer was a median of 17.5 months.

INDICATIONS AND USAGE

VALSTAR is indicated for intravesical therapy of BCG-refractory carcinoma *in situ* (CIS) of the urinary bladder in patients for whom immediate cystectomy would be associated with unacceptable morbidity or mortality.

CONTRAINDICATIONS

VALSTAR is contraindicated in patients with known hypersensitivity to anthracyclines or Cremophor® EL (polyoxyethyleneglycol triricinoleate).

Patients with concurrent urinary tract infections should not receive VALSTAR.

VALSTAR should not be administered to patients with a small bladder capacity, i.e., unable to tolerate a 75 mL instillation.

WARNINGS

Patients should be informed that VALSTAR has been shown to induce complete response in only about 1 in 5 patients with BCG-refractory CIS, and that delaying cystectomy could lead to development of metastatic bladder cancer, which is lethal. The exact risk of developing metastatic bladder cancer from such a delay may be difficult to assess (See CLINICAL TRIALS) but increases the longer cystectomy is delayed in the presence of persisting CIS. **If there is not a complete response of CIS to treatment after 3 months or if CIS recurs, cystectomy must be reconsidered.**

VALSTAR should not be administered to patients with a perforated bladder or to those in whom the integrity of the bladder mucosa has been compromised (see PRECAUTIONS and CLINICAL PHARMACOLOGY, Pharmacokinetics Figure 2).

In order to avoid possible dangerous systemic exposure to VALSTAR for the patients undergoing transurethral resection of the bladder, the status of the bladder should be evaluated before the intravesical instillation of drug. In case of bladder perforation, the administration of VALSTAR should be delayed until bladder integrity has been restored.

VALSTAR should be administered under the supervision of a physician experienced in the use of intravesical cancer chemotherapeutic agents.

PRECAUTIONS

General: Aseptic techniques must be used during administration of intravesical VALSTAR to avoid introducing contaminants into the urinary tract or traumatizing unduly the urinary mucosa.

TABLE 1
Occurrence of Local Adverse Reactions Before and During Treatment with Intravesical VALSTAR (% of Patients)

Reaction	Patients Who Received Multiple-Cycle Treatment Regimen at 800 mg/dose (N = 170) Before Treatment	During 6-week Course of Treatment
ANY LOCAL BLADDER SYMPTOM	45%	88%
Urinary Frequency	30%	61%
Dysuria	11%	56%
Urinary Urgency	27%	57%
Bladder Spasm	3%	31%
Hematuria	11%	29%
Bladder Pain	6%	28%
Urinary Incontinence	7%	22%
Cystitis	4%	15%
Nocturia	2%	7%
Local Burning Symptoms—Procedure Related	0%	5%
Urethral Pain	0%	3%
Pelvic Pain	1%	1%
Hematuria (Gross)	0%	1%

TABLE 2
Most Commonly Reported Systemic Adverse Reactions Following Intravesical Administration of VALSTAR (% of Patients)

Body System / Preferred Term	All Patients Who Received VALSTAR (N = 230)
Body as a Whole	
Abdominal Pain	5%
Asthenia	4%
Back Pain	3%
Chest Pain	3%
Fever	2%
Headache	4%
Malaise	4%
Cardiovascular	
Vasodilation	2%
Digestive	
Diarrhea	3%
Flatulence	1%
Nausea	5%
Vomiting	2%
Hemic and Lymphatic	
Anemia	2%
Metabolic and Nutritional	
Hyperglycemia	1%
Peripheral Edema	1%
Musculoskeletal	
Myalgia	1%
Nervous	
Dizziness	3%
Respiratory	
Pneumonia	1%
Skin and Appendages	
Rash	3%
Urogenital	
Hematuria (microscopic)	3%
Urinary Retention	4%
Urinary Tract Infection	15%

Information for Patients: Patients should be informed that VALSTAR has been shown to induce complete responses in only about 1 in 5 patients, and that delaying cystectomy could lead to development of metastatic bladder cancer, which is lethal. They should discuss with their physician the relative risk of cystectomy versus the risk of metastatic bladder cancer (see CLINICAL TRIALS) and be aware that the risk increases the longer cystectomy is delayed in the presence of persisting CIS.

Patients should be informed that the major acute toxicities from VALSTAR are related to irritable bladder symptoms that may occur during instillation and retention of VALSTAR and for a limited period following voiding. For the first 24 hours following administration, red-tinged urine is typical. Patients should report prolonged irritable bladder symptoms or prolonged passage of red-colored urine immediately to their physician.

Women of childbearing potential should be advised not to become pregnant during treatment. Men should be advised to refrain from engaging in procreative activities while receiving therapy with VALSTAR. All patients of reproductive age should be advised to use an effective contraception method during the treatment period.

Irritable Bladder Symptoms: VALSTAR should be used with caution in patients with severe irritable bladder symptoms. Bladder spasm and spontaneous discharge of the intravesical instillate may occur; clamping of the urinary catheter is not advised and, if performed, should be executed under medical supervision and with caution.

Drug Interactions: Because systemic exposure to VALSTAR is negligible following intravesical administration, the potential for drug interactions is low. No drug interaction studies were conducted.

Carcinogenesis, Mutagenesis, Impairment of Fertility: The carcinogenic potential of VALSTAR has not been evaluated, but the drug does cause damage to DNA *in vitro*. VALSTAR was mutagenic in *in vitro* assays in *Salmonella typhimurium* and *Escherichia coli*. VALSTAR was clastogenic in the chromosomal aberration assay in CHO cells. Studies of the effects of VALSTAR on male or female fertility have not been done.

Pregnancy: Pregnancy Category C. Valrubicin can cause fetal harm if a pregnant woman is exposed to the drug systemically. Such exposure could occur after perforation of the urinary bladder during valrubicin therapy. Daily intravenous doses of 12 mg/kg (about one sixth of the recommended human intravesical dose on a mg/m^2 basis) given to rats during fetal development caused fetal malformations. A dose of 24 mg/kg (about one third the recommended human intravesical dose on a mg/m^2 basis) caused numerous, severe alterations in the skull and skeleton of the developing fetuses. This dose also caused an increase in fetal resorptions and a decrease in viable fetuses. Thus, valrubicin is embryotoxic and teratogenic. There are no preclinical studies of the effects of intravesical valrubicin on fetal develop-

Continued on next page

Information on the Medeva Pharmaceuticals, Inc. products listed on these pages contains the full prescribing information from product circulars in use as of July 2000. For further information, please consult the package insert currently accompanying the product.

Valstar—Cont.

ment and no adequate and well controlled studies of valrubicin in pregnant women. If valrubicin is used during pregnancy, or if the patient becomes pregnant while receiving this drug, the patient should be apprised of the potential hazard to the fetus. It should be used during pregnancy only if the potential benefit justifies the potential risk to the fetus. Women who might become pregnant should be advised to avoid doing so during therapy with VALSTAR.

Nursing Mothers: It is not known whether VALSTAR is excreted in human milk. Nevertheless, the drug is highly lipophilic and any exposure of infants to VALSTAR could pose serious health risks. Women should discontinue nursing before the initiation of VALSTAR therapy.

Pediatric Use: Safety and effectiveness in pediatric patients have not been established.

Geriatric Use: Because carcinoma *in situ* of the bladder generally occurs in older individuals, 85% of the patients enrolled in the clinical studies of VALSTAR were more than 60 years of age (49% of the patients were more than 70 years of age). In the primary efficacy studies, the mean age of the population was 69.5 years. There are no specific precautions regarding use of VALSTAR in geriatric patients who are otherwise in good health.

ADVERSE REACTIONS

Approximately 84% of patients who received intravesical VALSTAR in clinical studies experienced local adverse events, but approximately half of the patients reported irritable bladder symptoms prior to treatment. The local adverse reactions associated with VALSTAR usually occur during or shortly after instillate and resolve within 1 to 7 days after the instillation is removed from the bladder.

TABLE 1 displays the frequency of the local adverse experiences at baseline and during treatment among 170 patients who received 800 mg doses of VALSTAR™ (valrubicin) Sterile Solution for Intravesical Instillation in a multiple-cycle treatment regimen. Ony 7 of 143 patients who were scheduled to receive six doses failed to receive all of the planned doses because of the occurrence of local bladder symptoms.

[See table 1 at top of previous page]

Most systemic adverse events associated with use of VALSTAR have been mild in nature and self-limited, resolving within 24 hours after drug administration. TABLE 2 displays the adverse events other than local bladder symptoms that occurred in 1% or more of the 230 patients who received at least one dose of VALSTAR (200 to 900 mg) in a clinical trial. It cannot be determined whether these events are drug-related.

[See table 2 at top of previous page]

Adverse reactions other than local reactions that occurred in less than 1% of the patients who received VALSTAR intravesically in clinical trials are listed below. This list includes only adverse reactions that were suspected of being related to treatment.

Digestive System: Tenesmus.
Metabolic and Nutritional: Nonprotein nitrogen increased.
Skin and Appendages: Pruritus.
Special Senses: Taste loss.
Urogenital System: Local skin irritation, poor urine flow, and urethritis.

Inadvertent paravenous extravasation of VALSTAR was not associated with skin ulceration or necrosis.

OVERDOSAGE

There is no known antidote for overdoses of VALSTAR. The primary anticipated complications of overdosage associated with intravesical administration would be consistent with irritable bladder symptoms.

Myelosuppression is possible if VALSTAR is inadvertently administered systemically or if significant systemic exposure occurs following intravesical administration (e.g., in patients with bladder rupture/perforation). The maximum tolerated dose in humans by either intraperitoneal or intravenous administration is 600 mg/m^2. Dose limiting toxicities are leukopenia and neutropenia, beginning within 1 week of dose administration, with nadirs by the second week, and recovery generally by the third week. If VALSTAR is administered when bladder rupture or perforation is suspected, weekly monitoring of complete blood counts should be performed for 3 weeks.

DOSAGE AND ADMINISTRATION

VALSTAR is recommended at a dose of 800 mg administered intravesically once a week for six weeks. Administration should be delayed at least two weeks after transurethral resection and/or fulguration. For each instillation, four 5 mL vials (200 mg valrubicin/5 mL vial) should be allowed to warm slowly to room temperature, but should not be heated. Twenty milliliters of VALSTAR should then be withdrawn from the four vials and diluted with 55 mL 0.9% Sodium Chloride Injection, USP providing 75 mL of a diluted VALSTAR solution. A urethral catheter should then be inserted into the patient's bladder under aseptic conditions, the bladder drained, and the diluted 75 mL VALSTAR solution instilled slowly via gravity flow over a period of several minutes. The catheter should then be withdrawn. The patient should retain the drug for two hours before voiding. At the end of two hours, all patients should void. (Some patients will be unable to retain the drug for the full two hours.) Patients should be instructed to maintain adequate hydration following treatment.

Patients receiving VALSTAR for refractory carcinoma *in situ* must be monitored closely for disease recurrence or progression. Recommended evaluations include cystoscopy, biopsy, and urine cytology every 3 months.

Administration Precautions: As recommended with other cytotoxic agents, caution should be exercised in handling and preparing the solution of VALSTAR. Contact toxicity, common and severe with other anthracyclines, is not typical with VALSTAR and, when observed, has been mild. Skin reactions may occur with accidental exposure, and the use of gloves during dose preparation and administration is recommended. Irritation of the eye has also been reported with accidental exposure. If this happens, the eye should be flushed with water immediately and thoroughly.

VALSTAR sterile solution contains Cremophor® EL, which has been known to cause leaching of di(2-ethylhexyl)phthalate (DEHP) a hepatotoxic plasticizer, from polyvinyl chloride (PVC) bags and intravenous tubing. VALSTAR solutions should be prepared and stored in glass, polypropylene, or polyolefin containers and tubing. It is recommended that non-DEHP containing administration sets, such as those that are polyethylene-lined, be used.

Procedures for proper handling and disposal of anticancer drugs should be used.[1–7] Spills should be cleaned up with undiluted chlorine bleach.

Preparation for Administration: VALSTAR Sterile Solution for Intravesical Instillation is a clear red solution. It should be visually inspected for particulate matter and discoloration prior to administration. At temperatures below 4°C, Cremophor® EL may begin to form a waxy precipitate. If this happens, the vial should be warmed in the hand until the solution is clear. If particulate matter is still seen, VALSTAR should not be administered.

Stability: Unopened vials of VALSTAR are stable until the date indicated on the package when stored under refrigerated conditions at 2°–8°C (36°–46°F). Vials should not be heated. VALSTAR diluted in 0.9% Sodium Chloride Injection, USP for administration is stable for 12 hours at temperatures up to 25°C (77°F). Since compatability data are not available, VALSTAR should not be mixed with other drugs.

HOW SUPPLIED

VALSTAR Sterile Solution for Intravesical Instillation is a clear red solution in Cremophor® EL / dehydrated alcohol, USP, containing 40 mg valrubicin per mL. VALSTAR Sterile Solution for Intravesical Instillation is available in single-use, clear glass vials, individually packaged in the following sizes:

NDC 53014-216-04	Carton of 4, 5 mL Single-Use Vials (200 mg/5 mL)
NDC 53014-216-24	Carton of 24, 5 mL Single-Use Vials (200 mg/5 mL)

Store vials under refrigeration at 2°–8°C (36°–46°F) in the carton. DO NOT FREEZE.

Marketed by:
Medeva Pharmaceuticals, Inc.
Rochester, NY 14623 USA
Manufactured by:
Ben Venue Laboratories, Inc.
Bedford, OH 44146 USA
for: Anthra Pharmaceuticals, Inc.
Princeton, NJ 08540 USA

Rev. 5/99

 R309A

REFERENCES

1. *Recommendations for the Safe Handling of Parenteral Antineoplastic Drugs,* NIH Publication No. 83-2621. For sale by the Superintendent of Documents, U.S. Government Printing Office, Washington, DC 20402.
2. "AMA Council Report, Guidelines for Handing Parenteral Antineoplastics." *JAMA,* 1985; 2.53(11): 1590–1592.
3. *National Study Commission on Cytotoxic Exposure—Recommendations for Handling Cytotoxic Agents.* Available from Louis P. Jeffrey, ScD., Chairman, National Study Commission on Cytotoxic Exposure, Massachusetts College of Pharmacy and Allied Health Sciences, 179 Longwood Avenue, Boston, Massachusetts 02115.
4. "Clinical Oncological Society of Australia, Guidelines and Recommendations for Safe Handling of Antineoplastic Agents." *Med J Australia,* 1983; 1:426–428.
5. Jones R.B., et al. "Safe Handling of Chemotherapeutic Agents: A Report from the Mount Sinai Medical Center." *CA—A Cancer Journal for Clinicians,* 1983; (Sept/Oct): 258–263.
6. "American Society of Hospital Pharmacists Technical Assistance Bulletin on Handling Cytotoxic and Hazardous Drugs." *Am J. Hosp Pharm,* 1990; 47:1033–1049.
7. "Controlling Occupational Exposure to Hazardous Drugs." *(OSHA Work-Practice Guidelines), Am J Health-Syst Pharm,* 1996; 53:1669–1685.

ZAROXOLYN® TABLETS ℞

[zar "ox 'uh-lin]
(metolazone tablets, USP)
Rx Only
R241J
Rev. 2/00

DO NOT INTERCHANGE:

DO NOT INTERCHANGE ZAROXOLYN TABLETS AND OTHER FORMULATIONS OF METOLAZONE THAT SHARE ITS SLOW AND INCOMPLETE BIOAVAILABILITY AND ARE NOT THERAPEUTICALLY EQUIVALENT AT THE SAME DOSES TO MYKROX® TABLETS, A MORE RAPIDLY AVAILABLE AND COMPLETELY BIOAVAILABLE METOLAZONE PRODUCT. FORMULATIONS BIOEQUIVALENT TO ZAROXOLYN AND FORMULATIONS BIOEQUIVALENT TO MYKROX SHOULD NOT BE INTERCHANGED FOR ONE ANOTHER.

DESCRIPTION

ZAROXOLYN Tablets (metolazone tablets, USP) for oral administration contain 2½, 5, or 10 mg of metolazone, USP, a diuretic/saluretic/antihypertensive drug of the quinazoline class.

Metolazone has the molecular formula $C_{16}H_{16}ClN_3O_3S$, the chemical name 7-chloro-1, 2, 3, 4-tetrahydro-2-methyl-3-(2-methylphenyl)-4-oxo-6-quinazolinesulfonamide, and a molecular weight of 365.83. The structural formula is:

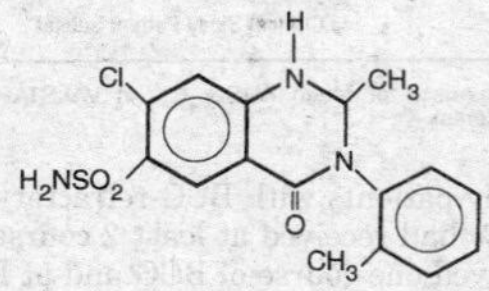

Metolazone is only sparingly soluble in water, but more soluble in plasma, blood, alkali, and organic solvents.

Inactive Ingredients: Magnesium stearate, microcrystalline cellulose and dye: 2½ mg-D&C Red No. 33; 5 mg-FD&C Blue No. 2; 10 mg-D&C Yellow No. 10 and FD&C Yellow No. 6.

CLINICAL PHARMACOLOGY

ZAROXOLYN (metolazone) is a quinazoline diuretic, with properties generally similar to the thiazide diuretics. The actions of ZAROXOLYN result from interference with the renal tubular mechanism of electrolyte reabsorption. ZAROXOLYN acts primarily to inhibit sodium reabsorption at the cortical diluting site and to a lesser extent in the proximal convoluted tubule. Sodium and chloride ions are excreted in approximately equivalent amounts. The increased delivery of sodium to the distal tubular exchange site results in increased potassium excretion. ZAROXOLYN does not inhibit carbonic anhydrase. A proximal action of metolazone has been shown in humans by increased excretion of phosphate and magnesium ions and by a markedly increased fractional excretion of sodium in patients with severely compromised glomerular filtration. This action has been demonstrated in animals by micropuncture studies.

When ZAROXOLYN Tablets are given, diuresis and saluresis usually begin within one hour and may persist for 24 hours or more. For most patients, the duration of effect can be varied by adjusting the daily dose. High doses may prolong the effect. A single daily dose is recommended. When a desired therapeutic effect has been obtained, It may be possible to reduce dosage to a lower maintenance level.

The diuretic potency of ZAROXOLYN at maximum therapeutic dosage is approximately equal to thiazide diuretics. However, unlike thiazides, ZAROXOLYN may produce diuresis in patients with glomerular filtration rates below 20 mL/min.

ZAROXOLYN and furosemide administered concurrently have produced marked diuresis in some patients where edema or ascites was refractory to treatment with maximum recommended doses of these or other diuretics administered alone. The mechanism of this interaction is unknown (see WARNINGS and PRECAUTIONS, Drug Interactions).

Maximum blood levels of metolazone are found approximately eight hours after dosing. A small fraction of metolazone is metabolized. Most of the drug is excreted in the unconverted form in the urine.

INDICATIONS AND USAGE

ZAROXOLYN is indicated for the treatment of salt and water retention including:

- edema accompanying congestive heart failure;
- edema accompanying renal diseases, including the nephrotic syndrome and states of diminished renal function.

ZAROXOLYN is also indicated for the treatment of hypertension, alone or in combination with other antihypertensive drugs of a different class. MYKROX Tablets, a more rapidly available form of metolazone, are intended for the treatment of new patients with mild to moderate hypertension. A dose titration is necessary if MYKROX Tablets are to be substituted for ZAROXOLYN in the treatment of hypertension. See package circular for MYKROX Tablets (Medeva).

Usage in Pregnancy: The routine use of diuretics in an otherwise healthy woman is inappropriate and exposes mother and fetus to unnecessary hazard. Diuretics do not prevent development of toxemia of pregnancy, and there is no evidence that they are useful in the treatment of developed toxemia.

Edema during pregnancy may arise from pathologic causes or from the physiologic and mechanical consequences of pregnancy. ZAROXOLYN is indicated in pregnancy when edema is due to pathologic causes, just as it is in the absence of pregnancy (see PRECAUTIONS). Dependent edema in pregnancy resulting from restriction of venous return by the expanded uterus is properly treated through elevation of the lower extremities and use of support hose; use of diuretics to lower intravascular volume in this case is illogical and unnecessary. There is hypervolemia during normal pregnancy which is harmful to neither the fetus nor the mother (in the absence of cardiovascular disease), but which is associated with edema, including generalized edema, in the majority of pregnancy women. If this edema produces discomfort, increased recumbency will often provide relief. In rare instances, this edema may cause extreme discomfort which is not relieved by rest. In these cases, a short course of diuretics may be appropriate.

CONTRAINDICATIONS

Anuria, hepatic coma or precoma, known allergy or hypersensitivity to metolazone.

WARNINGS

Rapid Onset Hyponatremia: Rarely, the rapid onset of severe hyponatremia and/or hypokalemia has been reported following initial doses of thiazide and non-thiazide diuretics. When symptoms consistent with severe electrolyte imbalance appear rapidly, drug should be discontinued and supportive measures should be initiated immediately. Parenteral electrolytes may be required. Appropriateness of therapy with this class of drugs should be carefully reevaluated.

Hypokalemia: Hypokalemia may occur with consequent weakness, cramps, and cardiac dysrhythmias. Serum potassium should be determined at regular intervals, and dose reduction, potassium supplementation or addition of a potassium-sparing diuretic instituted whenever indicated. Hypokalemia is a particular hazard in patients who are digitalized or who have or have had a ventricular arrhythmia; dangerous or fatal arrhythmias may be precipitated. Hypokalemia is dose related.

Concomitant Therapy: Lithium: In general, diuretics should not be given concomitantly with lithium because they reduce its renal clearance and add a high risk of lithium toxicity. Read prescribing information for lithium preparations before use of such concomitant therapy.

Furosemide: Unusually large or prolonged losses of fluids and electrolytes may result when ZAROXOLYN is administered concomitantly to patients receiving furosemide (see PRECAUTIONS, Drug Interactions).

Other Antihypertensive Drugs: When ZAROXOLYN is used with other antihypertensive drugs, particular care must be taken to avoid excessive reduction of blood pressure, especially during initial therapy.

Cross-Allergy: Cross-allergy, white not reported to date, theoretically may occur when ZAROXOLYN is given to patients known to be allergic to sulfonamide-derived drugs, thiazides, or quinethazone.

Sensitivity Reactions: Sensitivity reactions (e.g., angioedema, bronchospasm) may occur with or without a history of allergy or bronchial asthma and may occur with the first dose of ZAROXOLYN.

PRECAUTIONS

DO NOT INTERCHANGE

DO NOT INTERCHANGE ZAROXOLYN TABLETS AND OTHER FORMULATIONS OF METOLAZONE THAT SHARE ITS SLOW AND INCOMPLETE BIOAVAILABILITY AND ARE NOT THERAPEUTICALLY EQUIVALENT AT THE SAME DOSES TO MYKROX TABLETS, A MORE RAPIDLY AVAILABLE AND COMPLETELY BIOAVAILABLE METOLAZONE PRODUCT. FORMULATIONS BIOEQUIVALENT TO ZAROXOLYN AND FORMULATIONS BIOEQUIVALENT TO MYKROX SHOULD NOT BE INTERCHANGED FOR ONE ANOTHER.

General: *Fluid and Electrolytes:* All patients receiving therapy with ZAROXOLYN Tablets should have serum electrolyte measurements done at appropriate intervals and be observed for clinical signs of fluid and/or electrolyte imbalance: namely, hyponatremia, hypochloremic alkalosis, and hypokalemia. In patients with severe edema accompanying cardiac failure or renal disease, a low-salt syndrome may be produced, especially with hot weather and a low-salt diet. Serum and urine electrolyte determinations are particularly important when the patient has protracted vomiting, severe diarrhea, or is receiving parenteral fluids. Warning signs of imbalance are: dryness of mouth, thirst, weakness, lethargy, drowsiness, restlessness, muscle pains or cramps, muscle fatigue, hypotension, oliguria, tachycardia, and gastrointestinal disturbances such as nausea and vomiting. Hyponatremia may occur at any time during long term therapy and, on rare occasions, may be life threatening.

The risk of hypokalemia is increased when larger doses are used, when diuresis is rapid, when severe liver disease is present, when corticosteroids are given concomitantly, when oral intake is inadequate or when excess potassium is being lost extrarenally, such as with vomiting or diarrhea.

Thiazide-like diuretics have been shown to increase the urinary excretion of magnesium; this may result in hypomagnesemia

Glucose Tolerance: Metolazone may raise blood glucose concentrations possibly causing hyperglycemia and glycosuria in patients with diabetes or latent diabetes.

Hyperuricemia: ZAROXOLYN regularly causes an increase in serum uric acid and can occasionally precipitate gouty attacks even in patients without a prior history of them.

Azotemia: Azotemia, presumably prerenal azotemia, may be precipitated during the administration of ZAROXOLYN. If azotemia and oliguria worsen during treatment of patients with severe renal disease, ZAROXOLYN should be discontinued.

Renal Impairment: Use caution when administering ZAROXOLYN Tablets to patients with severely impaired renal function. As most of the drug is excreted by the renal route, accumulation may occur.

Orthostatic Hypotension: Orthostatic hypotension may occur; this may be potentiated by alcohol, barbiturates, narcotics, or concurrent therapy with other antihypertensive drugs.

Hypercalcemia: Hypercalcemia may infrequently occur with metolazone, especially in patients taking high doses of vitamin D or with high bone turnover states, and may signify hidden hyperparathyroidism. Metolazone should be discontinued before tests for parathyroid function are performed.

Systemic Lupus Erythematosus: Thiazide diuretics have exacerbated or activated systemic lupus erythematosus and this possibility should be considered with ZAROXOLYN Tablets.

Information for Patients: Patients should be informed of possible adverse effects, advised to take the medication as directed, and promptly report any possible adverse reactions to the treating physician.

Drug Interactions: *Diuretics:* Furosemide and probably other loop diuretics given concomitantly with metolazone can cause unusually large or prolonged losses of fluid and electrolytes (see WARNINGS).

Other Antihypertensives: When ZAROXOLYN Tablets are used with other antihypertensive drugs, care must be taken, especially during initial therapy. Dosage adjustments of other antihypertensives may be necessary.

Alcohol, Barbiturates, and Narcotics: The hypotensive effects of these drugs may be potentiated by the volume contraction that may be associated with metolazone therapy.

Digitalis Glycosides: Diuretic-induced hypokalemia can increase the sensitivity of the myocardium to digitalis. Serious arrhythmias can result.

Corticosteroids or ACTH: May increase the risk of hypokalemia and increase salt and water retention.

Lithium: Serum lithium levels may increase (see WARNINGS).

Curariform Drugs: Diuretic-induced hypokalemia may enhance neuromuscular blocking effects of curariform drugs (such as tubocurarine) – the most serious effect would be respiratory depression which could proceed to apnea. Accordingly, it may be advisable to discontinue ZAROXOLYN® Tablets (metolazone tablets, USP) three days before elective surgery.

Salicylates and Other Non-Steroidal Anti-Inflammatory Drugs: May decrease the antihypertensive effects of ZAROXOLYN Tablets.

Sympathomimetics: Metolazone may decrease arterial responsiveness to norepinephrine, but this diminution is not sufficient to preclude effectiveness of the pressor agent for therapeutic use.

Insulin and Oral Antidiabetic Agents: See Glucose Tolerance under PRECAUTIONS, General.

Methenamine: Efficacy may be decreased due to urinary alkalizing effect of metolazone.

Anticoagulants: Metolazone, as well as other thiazide-like diuretics, may affect the hypoprothrombinemic response to anticoagulants; dosage adjustments may be necessary.

Drug/Laboratory Test Interactions: None reported.

Carcinogenesis, Mutagenesis, Impairment of Fertility: Mice and rats administered metolazone 5 days/week for up to 18 and 24 months, respectively, at daily doses of 2, 10, and 50 mg/kg, exhibited no evidence of a tumorigenic effect of the drug. The small number of animals examined histologically and poor survival in the mice limit the conclusions that can be reached from these studies.

Metolazone was not mutagenic *in vitro* in the Ames Test using Salmonella typhimurium strains TA-97, TA-98, TA-100, TA-102, and TA-1535.

Reproductive performance has been evaluated in mice and rats. There is no evidence that metolazone possesses the potential for altering reproductive capacity in mice. In a rat study, in which males were treated orally with metolazone at doses of 2, 10, and 50 mg/kg for 127 days prior to mating with untreated females, an increased number of resorption sites was observed in dams mated with males from the 50 mg/kg group. In addition, the birth weight of offspring was decreased and the pregnancy rate was reduced in dams mated with males from the 10 and 50 mg/kg groups.

Pregnancy: Teratogenic Effects—Pregnancy Category B. Reproduction studies performed in mice, rabbits, and rats treated during the appropriate period of gestation at doses up to 50 mg/kg/day have revealed no evidence of harm to the fetus due to metolazone. There are, however, no adequate and well-controlled studies in pregnant women. Because animal reproduction studies are not always predictive of human response, ZAROXOLYN Tablets should be used during pregnancy only if clearly needed. Metolazone crosses the placental barrier and appears in cord blood.

Non-Teratogenic Effects: The use of ZAROXOLYN Tablets in pregnant women requires that the anticipated benefit be weighed against possible hazards to the fetus. These hazards include fetal or neonatal jaundice, thrombocytopenia, and possibly other adverse reactions which have occurred in the adult. It is not known what effect the use of the drug during pregnancy has on the later growth, development, and functional maturation of the child. No such effects have been reported with metolazone.

Labor and Delivery: Based on clinical studies in which women received matolazone in late pregnancy until the time of delivery, there is no evidence that the drug has any adverse effects on the normal course of labor or delivery.

Nursing Mothers: Metolazone appears in breast milk. Because of the potential for serious adverse reactions in nursing infants from metolazone, a decision should be made whether to discontinue nursing or to discontinue the drug, taking into account the importance of the drug to the mother.

Pediatric Use: Safety and effectiveness in pediatric patients have not been established in controlled clinical trials. There is limited experience with the use of ZAROXOLYN in pediatric patients with congestive heart failure, hypertension, bronchopulmonary dysplasia, nephrotic syndrome and nephrogenic diabetes insipidus. Doses used generally ranged from 0.05 to 0.1 mg/kg administered once daily and usually resulted in a 1 to 2.8 kg weight loss and 150 to 300 cc increase in urine output. Not all patients responded and some gained weight. Those patients who did respond did so in the first few days of treatment. Prolonged use (beyond a few days) was generally associated with no further beneficial effect or a return to baseline status and is not recommended.

There is limited experience with the combination of ZAROXOLYN and furosemide in pediatric patients with furosemide-resistant edema. Some benefited while others did not or had an exaggerated response with hypovolemia, tachycardia, and orthostatic hypotension requiring fluid replacement. Severe hypokalemia was reported and there was a tendency for diuresis to persist for up to 24 hours after ZAROXOLYN was discontinued. Hyperbilirubinemia has been reported in 1 neonate. Close clinical and laboratory monitoring of all children treated with diuretics is indicated. See CONTRAINDICATIONS, WARNINGS, PRECAUTIONS.

ADVERSE REACTIONS

ZAROXOLYN is usually well tolerated, and most reported adverse reactions have been mild and transient. Many ZAROXOLYN related adverse reactions represent extensions of its expected pharmacologic activity and can be attributed to either its antihypertensive action or its renal/metabolic actions. The following adverse reactions have been reported. Several are single or comparably rare occurrences. Adverse reactions are listed in decreasing order of severity within body systems.

Cardiovascular: Chest pain/discomfort, orthostatic hypotension, excessive volume depletion, hemoconcentration, venous thrombosis, palpitations.

Central and Peripheral Nervous System: Syncope, neuropathy, vertigo, paresthesias, psychotic depression, impotence, dizziness/lightheadedness, drowsiness, fatigue, weakness, restlessness (sometimes resulting in insomnia), headache.

Dermatologic/Hypersensitivity: Necrotizing angiitis (cutaneous vasculitis), purpura, dermatitis (photosensitivity), urticaria, and skin rashes.

Gastrointestinal: Hepatitis, intrahepatic cholestatic jaundice, pancreatitis, vomiting, nausea, epigastric distress, diarrhea, constipation, anorexia, abdominal bloating.

Hematologic: Aplastic/hypoplastic anemia, agranulocytosis, leukopenia.

Metabolic: Hypokalemia, hyponatremia, hyperuricemia, hypochloremia, hypochloremic alkalosis, hyperglycemia, glycosuria, increase in serum urea nitrogen (BUN) or creatinine, hypophosphatemia, hypomagnesemia, hypercalcemia.

Musculoskeletal: Joint pain, acute gouty attacks, muscle cramps or spasm.

Other: Transient blurred vision, chills.

In addition, adverse reactions reported with similar antihypertensive-diuretics, but which have not been reported to date for ZAROXOLYN include: bitter taste, dry mouth, sialadenitis, xanthopsia, respiratory distress (including pneumonitis), thrombocytopenia, and anaphylactic reactions. These reactions should be considered as possible occurrences with clinical usage of ZAROXOLYN.

Whenever adverse reactions are moderate or severe, ZAROXOLYN dosage should be reduced or therapy withdrawn.

OVERDOSAGE

Intentional overdosage has been reported rarely with metolazone and similar diuretic drugs.

Signs and Symptoms: Orthostatic hypotension, dizziness, drowsiness, syncope, electrolyte abnormalities, hemoconcentration and hemodynamic changes due to plasma volume depletion may occur. In some instances depressed respiration may be observed. At high doses, lethargy of varying degree may progress to coma within a few hours. The mechanism of CNS depression with thiazide overdosage is unknown. Also, GI irritation and hypermotility may occur. Temporary elevation of BUN has been reported, especially in patients with impairment of renal function. Serum electrolyte changes and cardiovascular and renal function should be closely monitored.

Treatment: There is no specific antidote available but immediate evacuation of stomach contents is advised. Dialysis is not likely to be effective. Care should be taken when evacuating the gastric contents to prevent aspiration, especially

Continued on next page

Information on the Medeva Pharmaceuticals, Inc. products listed on these pages contains the full prescribing information from product circulars in use as of July 2000. For further information, please consult the package insert currently accompanying the product.

Zaroxolyn—Cont.

in the stuporous or comatose patient. Supportive measures should be initiated as required to maintain hydration, electrolyte balance, respiration, and cardiovascular and renal function.

DOSAGE AND ADMINISTRATION

Effective dosage of ZAROXOLYN should be individualized according to indication and patient response. A single daily dose is recommended. Therapy with ZAROXOLYN should be titrated to gain an initial therapeutic response and to determine the minimal dose possible to maintain the desired therapeutic response.

Usual Single Daily Dosage Schedules: Suitable initial dosages will usually fall in the ranges given.

Edema of cardiac failure:
ZAROXOLYN 5 to 20 mg once daily.
Edema of renal disease:
ZAROXOLYN 5 to 20 mg once daily.
Mild to moderate essential hypertension;
ZAROXOLYN 2½ to 5 mg once daily.
New patients—MYKROX® Tablets (metolazone tablets, USP) (see MYKROX package circular). If considered desirable to switch patients currently on ZAROXOLYN to MYKROX, the dose should be determined by titration starting at one tablet (½ mg) once daily and increasing to two tablets (1 mg) once daily if needed.

Treatment of Edematous States: The time interval required for the initial dosage to produce an effect may vary. Diuresis and saluresis usually begin within one hour and persist for 24 hours or longer. When a desired therapeutic effect has been obtained, it may be advisable to reduce the dose if possible. The daily dose depends on the severity of the patient's condition, sodium intake, and responsiveness. A decision to change the daily dose should be based on the results of thorough clinical and laboratory evaluations. If antihypertensive drugs or diuretics are given concurrently with ZAROXOLYN, more careful dosage adjustment may be necessary. For patients who tend to experience paroxysmal nocturnal dyspnea, it may be advisable to employ a larger dose to ensure prolongation of diuresis and saluresis for a full 24-hour period.

Treatment of Hypertension: The time interval required for the initial dosage regimen to show effect may vary from three or four days to three to six weeks in the treatment of elevated blood pressure. Doses should be adjusted at appropriate intervals to achieve maximum therapeutic effect.

HOW SUPPLIED

ZAROXOLYN Tablets (metolazone tablets, USP) are shallow biconvex, round tablets, and are available in three strengths:

2½ mg, pink, debossed "ZAROXOLYN" on one side, and "2½" on reverse side.

NDC 53014-975-71	Bottle of 100's
NDC 53014-975-90	Bottle of 1000's
NDC 53014-975-72	Carton of 100's, unit dose

5 mg, blue, debossed "ZAROXOLYN" on one side, and "5" on reverse side.

NDC 53014-850-71	Bottle of 100's
NDC 53014-850-90	Bottle of 1000's
NDC 53014-850-72	Carton of 100's, unit dose

10 mg, yellow, debossed "ZAROXOLYN" on one side, and "10" on reverse side.

NDC 53014-835-71	Bottle of 100's
NDC 53014-835-90	Bottle of 1000's
NDC 53014-835-72	Carton of 100's, unit dose

Store at 25°C (77°F); excursions permitted to 15°–30°C (59°–86°F) [See USP Controlled Room Temperature]. Protect from light. Keep out of the reach of children.

Medeva Pharmaceuticals, Inc.
Rochester, NY 14623 USA
® Fisons Investments Inc. Rev. 2/00

EDUCATIONAL MATERIAL

For educational information, please write to Medeva Pharmaceuticals, Inc., PO Box 31766, Rochester, NY 14603.

NOTICE

Before prescribing or administering any product described in PHYSICIANS' DESK REFERENCE check the **PDR Supplements** for revised information.

MEDICIS, The Dermatology Company®

8125 NORTH HAYDEN ROAD
SCOTTSDALE, AZ 85258

For Medical Information Contact:
Generally:
Medical Affairs Department
(602) 808-8800
FAX: (602) 808-0822

In Emergencies:
(602) 808-8800

DYNACIN® ℞

[dī 'nă-cən]
(minocycline HCl capsules, USP)
Prescribing information as of July 1998

DESCRIPTION

Minocycline hydrochloride, a semisynthetic derivative of tetracycline, is [4S-(4α, 4aα, 5aα, 12aα)]-4,7-bis(dimethylamino) -1,4,4a,5,5a,6,11,12a -octahydro -3,10,12,12a -tetrahydroxy-1,11-dioxo-2-naphthacenecarboxamide monohydrochloride. The structural formula is represented below:

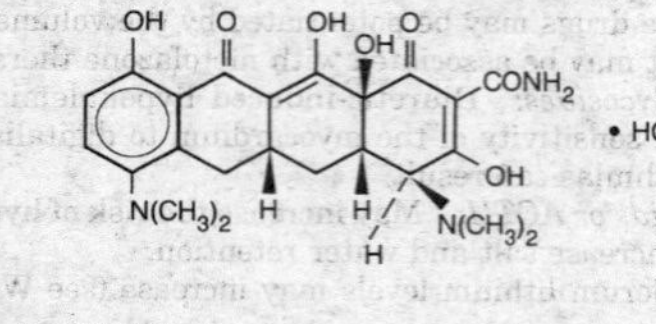

$C_{23}H_{27}N_3O_7 \cdot HCl$ M.W. 493.94

Each minocycline hydrochloride capsule, for oral administration, contains the equivalent of 50 mg, 75 mg or 100 mg of minocycline. In addition each capsule contains the following inactive ingredients: magnesium stearate and starch (corn).

The 50 mg, 75 mg and 100 mg capsule shells contain: gelatin, silicon dioxide, sodium lauryl sulfate and titanium dioxide.

The 75 mg and 100 mg capsule shell also contains: black iron oxide.

CLINICAL PHARMACOLOGY

Following oral administration of minocycline hydrochloride capsules, absorption from the gastrointestinal tract is rapid. Maximum serum concentrations following a single dose of minocycline hydrochloride to normal fasting adult volunteers were attained in 1 to 4 hours. The serum half-life in normal volunteers ranges from approximately 11 hours to 22 hours.

When minocycline hydrochloride capsules were given concomitantly with a meal which included dairy products, the extent of absorption of minocycline hydrochloride capsules was not noticeably influenced. The peak plasma concentrations were slightly decreased and delayed by one hour when administered with food, compared to dosing under fasting conditions.

In previous studies with other minocycline dosage forms, the minocycline serum half-life ranged from 11 to 16 hours in 7 patients with hepatic dysfunction, and from 18 to 69 hours in 5 patients with renal dysfunction. The urinary and fecal recovery of minocycline when administered to 12 normal volunteers is one-half to one-third that of other tetracyclines.

Microbiology: The tetracyclines are primarily bacteriostatic and are thought to exert their antimicrobial effect by the inhibition of protein synthesis. The tetracyclines, including minocycline, have similar antimicrobial spectra of activity against a wide range of gram-positive and gram-negative organisms. Cross-resistance of these organisms to tetracyclines is common.

While *in vitro* studies have demonstrated the susceptibility of most strains of the following microorganisms, clinical efficacy for infections other than those included in the **INDICATIONS AND USAGE** section has not been documented.

Gram-Negative Bacteria
Bartonella bacilliformis
Brucella species
Campylobacter fetus
Francisella tularensis
Haemophilus ducreyi
Haemophilus influenzae
Listeria monocytogenes
Neisseria gonorrhoeae
Vibrio cholerae
Yersinia pestis

Because many strains of the following groups of gram-negative microorganisms have been shown to be resistant to tetracyclines, culture and susceptibility tests are especially recommended:
Acinetobacter species
Bacteroides species
Enterobacter aerogenes
Escherichia coli
Klebsiella species
Shigella species

Gram-Positive Bacteria

Because many strains of the following groups of gram-positive microorganisms have been shown to be resistant to tetracyclines, culture and susceptibility testing are especially recommended. Up to 44 percent of *Streptococcus pyogenes* strains have been found to be resistant to tetracycline drugs. Therefore, tetracyclines should not be used for streptococcal disease unless the organism has been demonstrated to be susceptible.

Alpha-hemolytic streptococci (viridans group)
Streptococcus pneumoniae
Streptococcus pyogenes

Other Microorganisms
Actinomyces species
Bacillus anthracis
Balantidium coli
Borrelia recurrentis
Chlamydia psittaci
Chlamydia trachomatis
Clostridium species
Entamoeba species
Fusobacterium fusiforme
Propionibacterium acnes
Treponema pallidum
Treponema pertenue
Ureaplasma urealyticum

Susceptibility Tests:

Diffusion Techniques: The use of antibiotic disk susceptibility test methods which measure zone diameter gives an accurate estimation of susceptibility of microorganisms to minocycline. One such standard procedure[1] has been recommended for use with disks for testing antimicrobials. Either the 30 mcg tetracycline-class disk or the 30 mcg minocycline disk should be used for the determination of the susceptibility of microorganisms to minocycline.

With this type of procedure a report of "susceptible" from the laboratory indicates that the infecting organism is likely to respond to therapy. A report of "intermediate susceptibility" suggests that the organism would be susceptible if a high dosage is used or if the infection is confined to tissues and fluids (e.g., urine) in which high antibiotic levels are attained. A report of "resistant" indicates that the infecting organism is not likely to respond to therapy. With either the tetracycline-class disk or the minocycline disk, zone sizes of 19 mm or greater indicate susceptibility, zone sizes of 14 mm or less indicate resistance, and zone sizes of 15 to 18 mm indicate intermediate susceptibility.

Standardized procedures require the use of laboratory control organisms. The 30 mcg tetracycline disk should give zone diameters between 19 and 28 mm for *Staphylococcus aureus* ATCC 25923 and between 18 and 25 mm for *Escherichia coli* ATCC 25922. The 30 mcg minocycline disk should give zone diameters between 25 and 30 mm for *S. aureus* ATCC 25923 and between 19 and 25 mm for *E. coli* ATCC 25922.

Dilution Techniques: When using the NCCLS agar dilution or broth dilution (including microdilution) method[2] or equivalent, a bacterial isolate may be considered susceptible if the MIC (minimal inhibitory concentration) of minocycline is 4 mcg/mL or less. Organisms are considered resistant if the MIC is 16 mcg/mL or greater. Organisms with an MIC value of less than 16 mcg/mL but greater than 4 mcg/mL are expected to be susceptible if a high dosage is used or if the infection is confined to tissues and fluids (e.g., urine) in which high antibiotic levels are attained.

As with standard diffusion methods, dilution procedures require the use of laboratory control organisms. Standard tetracycline or minocycline powder should give MIC values of 0.25 mcg/mL to 1.0 mcg/mL for *S. aureus* ATCC 25923, and 1.0 mcg/mL to 4.0 mcg/mL for *E. coli* ATCC 25922.

INDICATIONS AND USAGE

Minocycline Hydrochloride Capsules are indicated in the treatment of the following infections due to susceptible strains of the designated microorganisms:

Rocky Mountain spotted fever, typhus fever and the typhus group, Q fever, rickettsialpox and tick fevers caused by *Rickettsiae*
Respiratory tract infections caused by *Mycoplasma pneumoniae*
Lymphogranuloma venereum caused by *Chlamydia trachomatis*
Psittacosis (Ornithosis) due to *Chlamydia psittaci*
Trachoma caused by *Chlamydia trachomatis*, although the infectious agent is not always eliminated, as judged by immunofluorescence
Inclusion conjunctivitis caused by *Chlamydia trachomatis*
Nongonococcal urethritis in adults caused by *Ureaplasma urealyticum* or *Chlamydia trachomatis*
Relapsing fever due to *Borrelia recurrentis*
Chancroid caused by *Haemophilus ducreyi*
Plague due to *Yersinia pestis*
Tularemia due to *Francisella tularensis*
Cholera caused by *Vibrio cholerae*
Campylobacter fetus infections caused by *Campylobacter fetus*
Brucellosis due to *Brucella* species (in conjunction with streptomycin)
Bartonellosis due to *Bartonella bacilliformis*
Granuloma inguinale caused by *Calymmatobacterium granulomatis*

Minocycline is indicated for treatment of infections caused by the following gram-negative microorganisms, when bacteriologic testing indicates appropriate susceptibility to the drug:
Escherichia coli
Enterobacter aerogenes
Shigella species
Acinetobacter species
Respiratory tract infections caused by *Haemophilus influenzae*
Respiratory tract and urinary tract infections caused by *Klebsiella* species
Minocycline hydrochloride capsules are indicated for the treatment of infections caused by the following gram-positive microorganisms when bacteriologic testing indicates appropriate susceptibility to the drug:
Upper respiratory tract infections caused by *Streptococcus pneumoniae*
Skin and skin structure infections caused by *Staphylococcus aureus*. (Note: Minocycline is not the drug of choice in the treatment of any type of staphylococcal infection.)
Uncomplicated urethritis in men due to *Neisseria gonorrhoeae* and for the treatment of other gonococcal infections when penicillin is contraindicated.
When penicillin is contraindicated, minocycline is an alternative drug in the treatment of the following infections:
Infections in women caused by *Neisseria gonorrhoeae*
Syphilis caused by *Treponema pallidum*
Yaws caused by *Treponema pertenue*
Listeriosis due to *Listeria monocytogenes*
Anthrax due to *Bacillus anthracis*
Vincent's infection caused by *Fusobacterium fusiforme*
Actinomycosis caused by *Actinomyces israelii*
Infections caused by *Clostridium* species
In *acute intestinal amebiasis*, minocycline may be a useful adjunct to amebicides.
In severe *acne*, minocycline may be useful adjunctive therapy.
Oral minocycline is indicated in the treatment of asymptomatic carriers of *Neisseria meningitidis* to eliminate meningococci from the nasopharynx. In order to preserve the usefulness of minocycline in the treatment of asymptomatic meningococcal carrier, diagnostic laboratory procedures, including serotyping and susceptibility testing, should be performed to establish the carrier state and the correct treatment. It is recommended that the prophylactic use of minocycline be reserved for situations in which the risk of meningococcal meningitis is high.
Oral minocycline is not indicated for the treatment of meningococcal infection.
Although no controlled clinical efficacy studies have been conducted, limited clinical data show that oral minocycline hydrochloride has been used successfully in the treatment of infections caused by *Mycobacterium marinum*.

CONTRAINDICATIONS

This drug is contraindicated in persons who have shown hypersensitivity to any of the tetracyclines.

WARNINGS

MINOCYCLINE, LIKE OTHER TETRACYCLINE-CLASS ANTIBIOTICS, CAN CAUSE FETAL HARM WHEN ADMINISTERED TO A PREGNANT WOMAN. IF ANY TETRACYCLINE IS USED DURING PREGNANCY OR IF THE PATIENT BECOMES PREGNANT WHILE TAKING THESE DRUGS, THE PATIENT SHOULD BE APPRISED OF THE POTENTIAL HAZARD TO THE FETUS. THE USE OF DRUGS OF THE TETRACYCLINE CLASS DURING TOOTH DEVELOPMENT (LAST HALF OF PREGNANCY, INFANCY, AND CHILDHOOD TO THE AGE OF 8 YEARS) MAY CAUSE PERMANENT DISCOLORATION OF THE TEETH (YELLOW-GRAY-BROWN).
This adverse reaction is more common during long-term use of the drug but has been observed following repeated short-term courses. Enamel hypoplasia has also been reported. TETRACYCLINE DRUGS, THEREFORE, SHOULD NOT BE USED DURING TOOTH DEVELOPMENT UNLESS OTHER DRUGS ARE NOT LIKELY TO BE EFFECTIVE OR ARE CONTRAINDICATED.
All tetracyclines form a stable calcium complex in any bone-forming tissue. A decrease in fibula growth rate has been observed in young animals (rats and rabbits) given oral tetracycline in doses of 25 mg/kg every six hours. This reaction was shown to be reversible when the drug was discontinued.
Results of animal studies indicate that tetracyclines cross the placenta, are found in fetal tissues, and can have toxic effects on the developing fetus (often related to retardation of skeletal development). Evidence of embryotoxicity has been noted in animals treated early in pregnancy.
The anti-anabolic action of the tetracyclines may cause an increase in BUN. While this is not a problem in those with normal renal function, in patients with significantly impaired function, higher serum levels of tetracycline may lead to azotemia, hyperphosphatemia, and acidosis. If renal impairment exists, even usual oral or parenteral doses may lead to excessive systemic accumulations of the drug and possible liver toxicity. Under such conditions, lower than usual total doses are indicated, and if therapy is prolonged, serum level determinations of the drug may be advisable.
Photosensitivity manifested by an exaggerated sunburn reaction has been observed in some individuals taking tetracyclines. This has been reported rarely with minocycline.
Central nervous system side effects including light-headedness, dizziness, or vertigo have been reported with minocycline therapy. Patients who experience these symptoms should be cautioned about driving vehicles or using hazardous machinery while on minocycline therapy. These symptoms may disappear during therapy and usually disappear rapidly when the drug is discontinued.

PRECAUTIONS

General: As with other antibiotic preparations, use of this drug may result in overgrowth of nonsusceptible organisms, including fungi. If superinfection occurs, the antibiotic should be discontinued and appropriate therapy instituted.
Pseudotumor cerebri (benign intracranial hypertension) in adults has been associated with the use of tetracyclines. The usual clinical manifestations are headache and blurred vision. Bulging fontanels have been associated with the use of tetracyclines in infants. While both of these conditions and related symptoms usually resolve after discontinuation of tetracycline, the possibility for permanent sequelae exists.
Incision and drainage or other surgical procedures should be performed in conjunction with antibiotic therapy when indicated.
Information for Patients: Photosensitivity manifested by an exaggerated sunburn reaction has been observed in some individuals taking tetracyclines. Patients apt to be exposed to direct sunlight or ultraviolet light should be advised that this reaction can occur with tetracycline drugs, and treatment should be discontinued at the first evidence of skin erythema. This reaction has been reported rarely with use of minocycline.
Patients who experience central nervous system symptoms (see **WARNINGS**) should be cautioned about driving vehicles or using hazardous machinery while on minocycline therapy.
Concurrent use of tetracycline may render oral contraceptives less effective (see **Drug Interactions**).
Laboratory Tests: In venereal disease when coexistent syphilis is suspected, a dark-field examination should be done before treatment is started and the blood serology repeated monthly for at least four months.
In long-term therapy, periodic laboratory evaluations of organ systems, including hematopoietic, renal, and hepatic studies should be performed.
Drug Interactions: Because tetracyclines have been shown to depress plasma prothrombin activity, patients who are on anticoagulant therapy may require downward adjustment of their anticoagulant dosage.
Since bacteriostatic drugs may interfere with the bactericidal action of penicillin, it is advisable to avoid giving tetracycline-class drugs in conjunction with penicillin.
Absorption of tetracyclines is impaired by antacids containing aluminum, calcium or magnesium, and iron-containing preparations.
The concurrent use of tetracycline and methoxyflurane has been reported to result in fatal renal toxicity.
Concurrent use of tetracyclines may render oral contraceptives less effective.
Drug/Laboratory Test Interactions: False elevations of urinary catecholamine levels may occur due to interference with the fluorescence test.
Carcinogenesis, Mutagenesis, Impairment of Fertility: Dietary administration of minocycline in long-term tumorigenicity studies in rats resulted in evidence of thyroid tumor production. Minocycline has also been found to produce thyroid hyperplasia in rats and dogs. In addition, there has been evidence of oncogenic activity in rats in studies with a related antibiotic, oxytetracycline (i.e., adrenal and pituitary tumors). Likewise, although mutagenicity studies of minocycline have not been conducted, positive results in *in vitro* mammalian cell assays (i.e., mouse lymphoma and Chinese hamster lung cells) have been reported for related antibiotics (tetracycline hydrochloride and oxytetracycline).
Segment I (fertility and general reproduction) studies have provided evidence that minocycline impairs fertility in male rats.
Teratogenic Effects: *Pregnancy:* Pregnancy Category D (see **WARNINGS**.)
Labor and Delivery: The effect of tetracyclines on labor and delivery is unknown.
Nursing Mothers: Tetracyclines are excreted in human milk. Because of the potential for serious adverse reactions in nursing infants from the tetracyclines, a decision should be made whether to discontinue nursing or discontinue the drug, taking into account the importance of the drug to the mother (see **WARNINGS**).
Pediatric Use: (see **WARNINGS**).

ADVERSE REACTIONS

Due to oral minocycline's virtually complete absorption, side effects to the lower bowel, particularly diarrhea, have been infrequent. The following adverse reactions have been observed in patients receiving tetracyclines.
Gastrointestinal: Anorexia, nausea, vomiting, diarrhea, glossitis, dysphagia, enterocolitis, pancreatitis, inflammatory lesions (with monilial overgrowth) in the anogenital region, and increases in liver enzymes. Rarely, hepatitis and liver failure have been reported. Rare instances of esophagitis and esophageal ulcerations have been reported in patients taking the tetracycline-class antibiotics in capsule and tablet form. Most of these patients took the medication immediately before going to bed (see **DOSAGE AND ADMINISTRATION**).
Skin: Maculopapular and erythematous rashes. Exfoliative dermatitis has been reported but is uncommon. Fixed drug eruptions, including balanitis, have been rarely reported. Erythema multiforme and rarely Stevens-Johnson syndrome have been reported. Photosensitivity is discussed above (see **WARNINGS**). Pigmentation of the skin and mucous membranes has been reported.
Renal toxicity: Elevations in BUN have been reported and are apparently dose related (see **WARNINGS**).
Hypersensitivity reactions: Urticaria, angioneurotic edema, polyarthralgia, anaphylaxis, anaphylactoid purpura, pericarditis, exacerbation of systemic lupus erythematosus and rarely pulmonary infiltrates with eosinophilia have been reported. A transient lupus-like syndrome has also been reported.
Blood: Hemolytic anemia, thrombocytopenia, neutropenia, and eosinophilia have been reported.
Central Nervous System: Bulging fontanels in infants and benign intracranial hypertension (Pseudotumor cerebri) in adults (see **PRECAUTIONS-General**) have been reported. Headache has also been reported.
Other: When given over prolonged periods, tetracyclines have been reported to produce brown-black microscopic discoloration of the thyroid glands. Very rare cases of abnormal thyroid function have been reported.
Decreased hearing has been rarely reported in patients on minocycline hydrochloride.
Tooth discoloration in children less than 8 years of age (see **WARNINGS**) and also, rarely, in adults has been reported.

OVERDOSAGE

In case of overdosage, discontinue medication, treat symptomatically and institute supportive measures.

DOSAGE AND ADMINISTRATION

THE USUAL DOSAGE AND FREQUENCY OF ADMINISTRATION OF MINOCYCLINE DIFFERS FROM THAT OF THE OTHER TETRACYCLINES. EXCEEDING THE RECOMMENDED DOSAGE MAY RESULT IN AN INCREASED INCIDENCE OF SIDE EFFECTS.
Minocycline hydrochloride capsules may be taken with or without food. (See **CLINICAL PHARMACOLOGY**.)
Adults: The usual dosage of minocycline hydrochloride is 200 mg initially followed by 100 mg every 12 hours. Alternatively, if more frequent doses are preferred, two or four 50 mg capsules may be given initially followed by one 50 mg capsule four times daily.
For children above 8 years of age: The usual dosage of minocycline hydrochloride is 4 mg/kg initially followed by 2 mg/kg every 12 hours.
Uncomplicated gonococcal infections other than urethritis and anorectal infections in men: 200 mg initially, followed by 100 mg every 12 hours for a minimum of four days, with post-therapy cultures within 2 to 3 days.
In the treatment of uncomplicated gonococcal urethritis in men, 100 mg every 12 hours for five days is recommended.
For the treatment of syphilis, the usual dosage of minocycline hydrochloride capsules should be administered over a period of 10 to 15 days. Close follow-up, including laboratory tests, is recommended.
In the treatment of meningococcal carrier state, the recommended dosage is 100 mg every 12 hours for five days.
Mycobacterium marinum infections: Although optimal doses have not been established, 100 mg every 12 hours for 6 to 8 weeks have been used successfully in a limited number of cases.
Uncomplicated nongonococcal urethral infection in adults caused by *Chlamydia trachomatis* or *Ureaplasma urealyticum:* 100 mg orally, every 12 hours for at least seven days.
Ingestion of adequate amounts of fluids along with capsule and tablet forms of drugs in the tetracycline-class is recommended to reduce the risk of esophageal irritation and ulceration.
In patients with renal impairment (see **WARNINGS**), the total dosage should be decreased by either reducing the recommended individual doses and/or by extending the time intervals between doses.

HOW SUPPLIED

DYNACIN® (Minocycline HCl Capsules, USP) equivalent to 50 mg minocycline are opaque white capsules imprinted "0497" and "DYNACIN® 50 mg" supplied in bottles of 100 and 500.
DYNACIN® (Minocycline HCl Capsules, USP) equivalent to 75 mg minocycline are light gray opaque capsules imprinted "0499" and "DYNACIN® 75 mg" supplied in bottles of 100 and 500.
DYNACIN® (Minocycline HCl Capsules, USP) equivalent to 100 mg minocycline are opaque dark gray and opaque white capsules imprinted "0498" and "DYNACIN® 100 mg" supplied in bottles of 50 and 500.
Dispense in tight, light-resistant container with child-resistant closure.
Store at controlled room temperature 15°–30°C (59°–86°F). Protect from light, moisture and excessive heat.
Rx Only

ANIMAL PHARMACOLOGY AND TOXICOLOGY

Minocycline hydrochloride has been observed to cause a dark discoloration of the thyroid in experimental animals (rats, minipigs, dogs and monkeys). In the rat, chronic treatment with minocycline hydrochloride has resulted in goiter accompanied by elevated radioactive iodine uptake, and evidence of thyroid tumor production. Minocycline hydrochloride has also been found to produce thyroid hyperplasia in rats and dogs.

Continued on next page

Dynacin—Cont.

REFERENCES

1. National Committee for Clinical Laboratory Standards, Approved Standard: *Performance Standards for Antimicrobial Disk Susceptibility Tests,* 3rd Edition, Vol. 4(16): M2-A3, Villanova, PA, December 1984.
2. National Committee for Clinical Laboratory Standards, Approved Standard: *Methods for Dilution Antimicrobial Susceptibility Tests for Bacteria that Grow Aerobically,* 2nd Edition, Vol. 5(22):M7-A, Villanova, PA, December 1985.

Manufactured for:
MEDICIS, The Dermatology Company®
Scottsdale, AZ 85258
by: DANBURY PHARMACAL, INC.
Danbury, CT 06810

LIDEX® ℞
[lī 'dex]
(fluocinonide)
Cream 0.05%
Gel 0.05%
Ointment 0.05%
Topical Solution 0.05%

LIDEX-E® ℞
(fluocinonide)
Cream 0.05%

SYNALAR® ℞
[sin 'ă-lahr]
(fluocinolone acetonide)
Cream 0.025%
Ointment 0.025%
Topical Solution 0.01%

SYNEMOL® ℞
[sin 'ĕ-mōl]
(fluocinolone acetonide)
Cream 0.025%
Prescribing information as of January 1999

Rx only

DESCRIPTION

These preparations are all intended for topical administration.

LIDEX preparations have as their active component the corticosteroid fluocinonide, which is the 21-acetate ester of fluocinolone acetonide and has the chemical name pregna-1,4-diene-3,20-dione, 21- (acetyloxy) -6,9-difluoro-11-hydroxy-16,17-[(1-methylethylidene)bis(oxy)]-, (6α,11β, 16α)-. It has the following chemical structure:

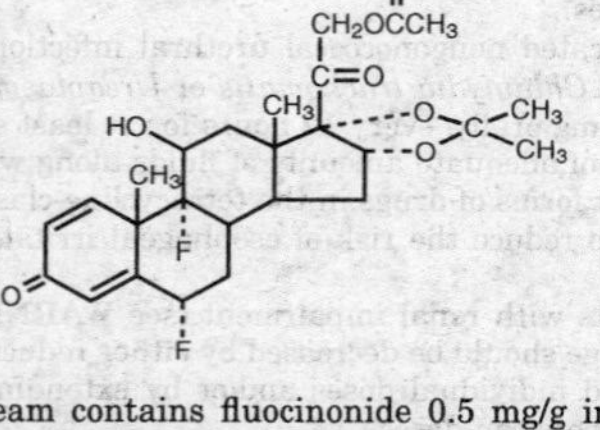

LIDEX Cream contains fluocinonide 0.5 mg/g in FAPG® cream, a specially formulated cream base consisting of citric acid, 1,2,6-hexanetriol, polyethylene glycol 8000, propylene glycol and stearyl alcohol. This white cream vehicle is greaseless, non-staining, anhydrous and completely water miscible. The base provides emollient and hydrophilic properties. In this formulation, the active ingredient is totally in solution.

LIDEX Gel contains fluocinonide 0.5 mg/g in a specially formulated gel base consisting of carbomer 940, edetate disodium, propyl gallate, propylene glycol, sodium hydroxide and/or hydrochloric acid (to adjust the pH), and water (purified). This clear, colorless, thixotropic vehicle is greaseless, non-staining and completely water miscible. In this formulation, the active ingredient is totally in solution.

LIDEX Ointment contains fluocinonide 0.5 mg/g in a specially formulated ointment base consisting of glyceryl monostearate, white petrolatum, propylene carbonate, propylene glycol and white wax. It provides the occlusive and emollient effects desirable in an ointment. In this formulation, the active ingredient is totally in solution.

LIDEX Topical Solution contains fluocinonide 0.5 mg/mL in a solution of alcohol (35%), citric acid, diisopropyl adipate, and propylene glycol. In this formulation, the active ingredient is totally in solution.

LIDEX-E Cream contains fluocinonide 0.5 mg/g in a water-washable aqueous emollient base of cetyl alcohol, citric acid, mineral oil, polysorbate 60, propylene glycol, sorbitan monostearate, stearyl alcohol and water (purified).

SYNALAR preparations have as their active component the corticosteroid fluocinolone acetonide, which has the chemical name pregna-1,4-diene-3,20-dione,6,9-difluoro-11,21-dihydroxy-16,17- [(1-methylethylidene)bis(oxy)] -, (6α,11β, 16α)-. It has the following chemical structure:

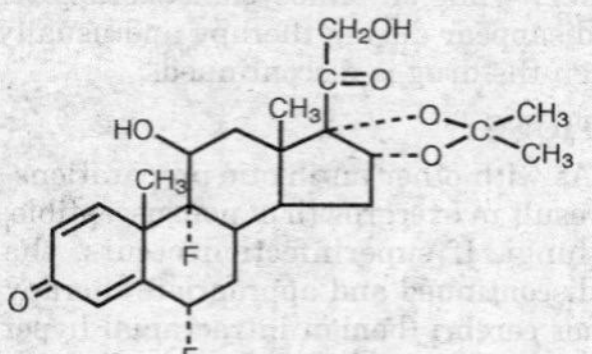

SYNALAR Cream contains fluocinolone acetonide 0.25 mg/g in a water-washable aqueous base of butylated hydroxytoluene, cetyl alcohol, citric acid, edetate disodium, methylparaben and propylparaben (preservatives), mineral oil, polyoxyl 20 cetostearyl ether, propylene glycol, simethicone, stearyl alcohol, water (purified) and white wax.

SYNALAR Ointment contains fluocinolone acetonide 0.25 mg/g in a white petroleum USP vehicle.

SYNALAR Topical Solution contains fluocinolone acetonide 0.1 mg/mL in a water-washable base of citric acid and propylene glycol.

SYNEMOL Cream contains fluocinolone acetonide 0.25 mg/g in a water-washable aqueous emollient base of cetyl alcohol, citric acid, mineral oil, polysorbate 60, propylene glycol, sorbitan monostearate, stearyl alcohol and water (purified).

CLINICAL PHARMACOLOGY

Topical corticosteroids share anti-inflammatory, anti- pruritic and vasoconstrictive actions.

The mechanism of anti-inflammatory activity of the topical corticosteroids is unclear. Various laboratory methods, including vasoconstrictor assays, are used to compare and predict potencies and/or clinical efficacies of the topical corticosteroids. There is some evidence to suggest that a recognizable correlation exists between vasoconstrictor potency and therapeutic efficacy in man.

Pharmacokinetics: The extent of percutaneous absorption of topical corticosteroids is determined by many factors including the vehicle, the integrity of the epidermal barrier, and the use of occlusive dressings. A significantly greater amount of fluocinonide is absorbed from the solution than from the cream or gel formulations.

Topical corticosteroids can be absorbed from normal intact skin. Inflammation and/or other disease processes in the skin increase percutaneous absorption. Occlusive dressings substantially increase the percutaneous absorption of topical corticosteroids. Thus, occlusive dressings may be a valuable therapeutic adjunct for treatment of resistant dermatoses. (See **DOSAGE AND ADMINISTRATION.**)

Once absorbed through the skin, topical corticosteroids are handled through pharmacokinetic pathways similar to systemically administered corticosteroids. Corticosteroids are bound to plasma proteins in varying degrees. Corticosteroids are metabolized primarily in the liver and are then excreted by the kidneys. Some of the topical corticosteroids and their metabolites are also excreted into the bile.

INDICATIONS AND USAGE

These products are indicated for the relief of the inflammatory and pruritic manifestations of corticosteroid-responsive dermatoses.

CONTRAINDICATIONS

Topical corticosteroids are contraindicated in those patients with a history of hypersensitivity to any of the components of the preparation.

PRECAUTIONS

General: Systemic absorption of topical corticosteroids has produced reversible hypothalamic-pituitary-adrenal (HPA) axis suppression, manifestations of Cushing's syndrome, hyperglycemia, and glucosuria in some patients.

Conditions which augment systemic absorption include the application of the more potent steroids, use over large surface areas, prolonged use, and the addition of occlusive dressings.

Therefore, patients receiving a large dose of a potent topical steroid applied to a large surface area or under an occlusive dressing should be evaluated periodically for evidence of HPA axis suppression by using the urinary free cortisol and ACTH stimulation tests. If HPA axis suppression is noted, an attempt should be made to withdraw the drug, to reduce the frequency of application, or to substitute a less potent steroid.

Recovery of HPA axis function is generally prompt and complete upon discontinuation of the drug. Infrequently, signs and symptoms of steroid withdrawal may occur, requiring supplemental systemic corticosteroids.

Children may absorb proportionally larger amounts of topical corticosteroids and thus be more susceptible to systemic toxicity. (See **PRECAUTIONS—Pediatric Use.**) These preparations are not for ophthalmic use. Severe irritation is possible if fluocinonide solution contacts the eye. If that should occur, immediate flushing of the eye with a large volume of water is recommended.

If irritation develops, topical corticosteroids should be discontinued and appropriate therapy instituted.

As with any topical corticosteroid product, prolonged use may produce atrophy of the skin and subcutaneous tissues. When used on intertriginous or flexor areas, or on the face, this may occur even with short-term use.

In the presence of dermatological infections, the use of an appropriate antifungal or antibacterial agent should be instituted. If a favorable response does not occur promptly, the corticosteroid should be discontinued until the infection has been adequately controlled.

Information for the Patient: Patients using topical corticosteroids should receive the following information and instructions:

1. This medication is to be used as directed by the physician. It is for external use only. Avoid contact with the eyes.
2. Patients should be advised not to use this medication for any disorder other than that for which it was prescribed.
3. The treated skin area should not be bandaged or otherwise covered or wrapped as to be occlusive unless directed by the physician.
4. Patients should report any signs of local adverse reactions especially under occlusive dressing.
5. Parents of pediatric patients should be advised not to use tight-fitting diapers or plastic pants on a child being treated in the diaper area as these garments may constitute occlusive dressings.

Laboratory Tests: The following tests may be helpful in evaluating HPA axis suppression: Urinary free cortisol test and ACTH stimulation test.

Carcinogenesis, Mutagenesis, and Impairment of Fertility: Long-term animal studies have not been performed to evaluate the carcinogenic potential or the effect on fertility of topical corticosteroids.

Studies to determine mutagenicity with prednisolone and hydrocortisone have revealed negative results.

Pregnancy Category C: Corticosteroids are generally teratogenic in laboratory animals when administered systemically at relatively low dosage levels. The more potent corticosteroids have been shown to be teratogenic after dermal application in laboratory animals. There are no adequate and well-controlled studies in pregnant women on teratogenic effects from topically applied corticosteroids. Therefore, topical corticosteroids should be used during pregnancy only if the potential benefit justifies the potential risk to the fetus. Drugs of this class should not be used extensively on pregnant patients, in large amounts, or for prolonged periods of time.

Nursing Mothers: It is not known whether topical administration of corticosteroids could result in sufficient systemic absorption to produce detectable quantities in breast milk. Systemically administered corticosteroids are secreted into breast milk in quantities *not* likely to have a deleterious effect on the infant. Nevertheless, caution should be exercised when topical corticosteroids are administered to a nursing woman.

Pediatric Use: Pediatric patients may demonstrate greater susceptibility to topical corticosteroid-induced hypothalamic-pituitary-adrenal (HPA) axis suppression and Cushing's syndrome than mature patients because of a larger skin surface area to body weight ratio. HPA axis suppression, Cushing's syndrome, and intracranial hypertension have been reported in children receiving topical corticosteroids. Manifestations of adrenal suppression in children include linear growth retardation, delayed weight gain, low plasma cortisol levels, and absence of response to ACTH stimulation. Manifestations of intracranial hypertension include bulging fontanelles, headaches, and bilateral papilledema.

Administration of topical corticosteroids to children should be limited to the least amount compatible with an effective therapeutic regimen. Chronic corticosteroid therapy may interfere with the growth and development of children.

ADVERSE REACTIONS

The following local adverse reactions are reported infrequently with topical corticosteroids, but may occur more frequently with the use of occlusive dressings. These reactions are listed in an approximate decreasing order of occurrence: burning, itching, irritation, dryness, folliculitis, hypertrichosis, acneiform eruptions, hypopigmentation, perioral dermatitis, allergic contact dermatitis, maceration of the skin, secondary infection, skin atrophy, striae, miliaria.

OVERDOSAGE

Topically applied corticosteroids can be absorbed in sufficient amounts to produce systemic effects. (See **PRECAUTIONS.**)

DOSAGE AND ADMINISTRATION

Topical corticosteroids are generally applied to the affected area as a thin film from two to four times daily depending on the severity of the condition. In hairy sites, the hair should be parted to allow direct contact with the lesion.

Occlusive dressings may be used for the management of psoriasis or recalcitrant conditions. Some plastic films may be flammable and due care should be exercised in their use. Similarly, caution should be employed when such films are used on children or left in their proximity, to avoid the possibility of accidental suffocation.

If an infection develops, the use of occlusive dressings should be discontinued and appropriate antimicrobial therapy instituted.

HOW SUPPLIED

LIDEX® (fluocinonide) Topical Solution 0.05%—Plastic squeeze bottles: 20cc (NDC 99207-517-44), 60cc (NDC 99207-517-46). Store at room temperature. Avoid excessive heat, above 40°C (104°F).

Manufactured by: West Pharmaceutical Services Lakewood, Inc.
Lakewood, NJ 08701

LIDEX® (fluocinonide) Cream 0.05%—15 g Tube (NDC 99207-511-13), 30 g Tube (NDC 99207-511-14), 60 g Tube (NDC 99207-511-17), 120 g Tube (NDC 99207-511-22). Store at room temperature. Avoid excessive heat, above 40°C (104°F).
LIDEX® (fluocinonide) Gel 0.05%—15 g Tube
(NDC 99207-507-13), 30 g Tube (NDC 99207-507-14), 60 g Tube (NDC 99207-507-17). Store at controlled room temperature:
15°–30°C (59°–86°F).
LIDEX® (fluocinonide) Ointment 0.05%—15 g Tube
(NDC 99207-514-13), 30 g Tube (NDC 99207-514-14), 60 g Tube (NDC 99207-514-17), 120 g Tube (NDC 99207-514-22). Store at room temperature. Avoid temperature over 30°C (86°F).
LIDEX-E® (fluocinonide) Cream 0.05%—15 g Tube
(NDC 99207-513-13), 30 g Tube (NDC 99207-513-14), 60 g Tube (NDC 99207-513-17). Store at room temperature. Avoid excessive heat, above 40°C (104°F).
SYNALAR® (fluocinolone acetonide) Cream 0.025%—15 g Tube (NDC 99207-501-13), 60 g Tube (NDC 99207-501-17). Store at room temperature; avoid freezing and excessive heat, above 40°C (104°F).
SYNALAR® (fluocinolone acetonide) Topical Solution 0.01%—20cc (NDC 99207-506-44), 60cc
(NDC 99207-506-46). Store at room temperature. Avoid freezing.
SYNALAR® (fluocinolone acetonide) Ointment 0.025%—15 g Tube (NDC 99207-504-13), 60 g Tube
(NDC 99207-504-17). Store at room temperature, avoid freezing and excessive heat, above 40°C (104°F).
SYNEMOL® (fluocinolone acetonide) Cream 0.025%—60 g Tube (NDC 99207-509-17). Store at room temperature. Avoid excessive heat, above 40°C (104°F).
Manufactured for:
MEDICIS, The Dermatology Company®
Scottsdale, AZ 85258
by: Patheon, Inc.
Mississauga, Ontario
CANADA L5N 7K9
U.S. Patent No. 4,017,615 for LIDEX Ointment.

LOPROX® ℞

[*lō 'prŏx*]
(ciclopirox)
Cream 0.77%
Lotion 0.77%
Prescribing information as of April 1999

FOR DERMATOLOGIC USE ONLY.
NOT FOR USE IN EYES.
Rx Only

DESCRIPTION

LOPROX® (ciclopirox) Cream 0.77% and LOPROX® (ciclopirox) Lotion 0.77% are for topical use.
Each gram of LOPROX Cream contains 7.70 mg of Ciclopirox (as Ciclopirox Olamine) in a water miscible vanishing cream base consisting of Purified Water USP, Octyldodecanol NF, Mineral Oil USP, Stearyl Alcohol NF, Cetyl Alcohol NF, Cocamide DEA, Polysorbate 60 NF, Myristyl Alcohol NF, Sorbitan Monostearate NF, Lactic Acid USP, and Benzyl Alcohol NF (1%) as preservative.
Each gram of LOPROX Lotion contains 7.70 mg of Ciclopirox (as Ciclopirox Olamine) in a water miscible lotion base consisting of Purified Water USP, Cocamide DEA, Octyldodecanol NF, Mineral Oil USP, Stearyl Alcohol NF, Cetyl Alcohol NF, Polysorbate 60 NF, Myristyl Alcohol NF, Sorbitan Monostearate NF, Lactic Acid USP, and Benzyl Alcohol NF (1%) as preservative.
LOPROX Cream and Lotion contain a synthetic, broad-spectrum, antifungal agent ciclopirox (as ciclopirox olamine). The chemical name is 6-cyclohexyl-1-hydroxy-4-methyl-2(1*H*)-pyridone, 2-aminoethanol salt.
The CAS Registry Number is 41621-49-2.
The chemical structure is:

LOPROX Cream and Lotion have a pH of 7.

CLINICAL PHARMACOLOGY

Ciclopirox is a broad-spectrum, antifungal agent that inhibits the growth of pathogenic dermatophytes, yeasts, and *Malassezia furfur*. Ciclopirox exhibits fungicidal activity *in vitro* against isolates of *Trichophyton rubrum, Trichophyton mentagrophytes, Epidermophyton floccosum, Microsporum canis,* and *Candida albicans*.
Pharmacokinetic studies in men with tagged ciclopirox solution in polyethylene glycol 400 showed an average of 1.3% absorption of the dose when it was applied topically to 750 cm^2 on the back followed by occlusion for 6 hours. The biological half-life was 1.7 hours and excretion occurred via the kidney. Two days after application only 0.01% of the dose applied could be found in the urine. Fecal excretion was negligible.
Penetration studies in human cadaverous skin from the back, with LOPROX Cream with tagged ciclopirox showed the presence of 0.8 to 1.6% of the dose in the stratum corneum 1.5 to 6 hours after application. The levels in the dermis were still 10 to 15 times above the minimum inhibitory concentrations.
Autoradiographic studies with human cadaverous skin showed that ciclopirox penetrates into the hair and through the epidermis and hair follicles into the sebaceous glands and dermis, while a portion of the drug remains in the stratum corneum.
Draize Human Sensitization Assay, 21-Day Cumulative Irritancy study, Phototoxicity study, and Photo-Draize study conducted in a total of 142 healthy male subjects showed no contact sensitization of the delayed hypersensitivity type, no irritation, no phototoxicity, and no photo-contact sensitization due to LOPROX Cream.
In vitro penetration studies in frozen or fresh excised human cadaver and pig skin indicated that the penetration of LOPROX Lotion is equivalent to that of LOPROX Cream. Therapeutic equivalence of cream and lotion formulations also was indicated by studies of experimentally induced guinea pig and human trichophytosis.

INDICATIONS AND USAGE

LOPROX Cream and Lotion are indicated for the topical treatment of the following dermal infections: tinea pedis, tinea cruris, and tinea corporis due to *Trichophyton rubrum, Trichophyton mentagrophytes, Epidermophyton floccosum,* and *Microsporum canis*; cutaneous candidiasis (moniliasis) due to *Candida albicans*; and tinea (pityriasis) versicolor due to *Malassezia furfur.*

CONTRAINDICATIONS

LOPROX Cream and Lotion are contraindicated in individuals who have shown hypersensitivity to any of its components.

WARNINGS

General: LOPROX Cream and Lotion are not for ophthalmic use. **Keep out of reach of children.**

PRECAUTIONS

If a reaction suggesting sensitivity or chemical irritation should occur with the use of LOPROX Cream or Lotion, treatment should be discontinued and appropriate therapy instituted.
Information for Patients:
The patient should be told to:
1. Use the medication for the full treatment time even though signs/symptoms may have improved and notify the physician if there is no improvement after four weeks.
2. Inform the physician if the area of application shows signs of increased irritation (redness, itching, burning, blistering, swelling, or oozing) indicative of possible sensitization.
3. Avoid the use of occlusive wrappings or dressings.

Carcinogenesis, Mutagenesis, Impairment of Fertility: A carcinogenicity study in female mice dosed cutaneously twice per week for 50 weeks followed by a 6-month drug-free observation period prior to necropsy revealed no evidence of tumors at the application site.
The following *in vitro* and *in vivo* genotoxicity tests have been conducted with ciclopirox olamine: studies to evaluate gene mutation in the Ames *Salmonella*/Mammalian Microsome Assay (negative) and Yeast Saccharomyces Cerevisiae Assay (negative) and studies to evaluate chromosome aberrations *in vivo* in the Mouse Dominant Lethal Assay and in the Mouse Micronucleus Assay at 500 mg/kg (negative).
The following battery of *in vitro* genotoxicity tests were conducted with ciclopirox: a chromosome aberration assay in V79 Chinese Hamster Cells, with and without metabolic activation (positive); a gene mutation assay in the HGPRT - test with V79 Chinese Hamster Cells (negative); and a primary DNA damage assay (i.e., unscheduled DNA Synthesis Assay in A549 Human Cells (negative)). An *in vitro* Cell Transformation Assay in BALB/C3T3 Cells was negative for cell transformation. In an *in vivo* Chinese Hamster Bone Marrow Cytogenetic Assay, ciclopirox was negative for chromosome aberrations at 5000 mg/kg.
Pregnancy Category B: Reproduction studies have been performed in the mouse, rat, rabbit, and monkey, (via various routes of administration) at doses 10 times or more the topical human dose and have revealed no significant evidence of impaired fertility or harm to the fetus due to ciclopirox. There are, however, no adequate or well-controlled studies in pregnant women. Because animal reproduction studies are not always predictive of human response, this drug should be used during pregnancy only if clearly needed.
Nursing Mothers: It is not known whether this drug is excreted in human milk. Because many drugs are excreted in human milk, caution should be exercised when LOPROX Cream or Lotion is administered to a nursing woman.
Pediatric Use: Safety and effectiveness in pediatric patients below the age of 10 years have not been established.

ADVERSE REACTIONS

In all controlled clinical studies with 514 patients using LOPROX Cream and in 296 patients using the vehicle cream, the incidence of adverse reactions was low. This included pruritus at the site of application in one patient and worsening of the clinical signs and symptoms in another patient using ciclopirox cream and burning in one patient and worsening of the clinical signs and symptoms in another patient using the vehicle cream.
In the controlled clinical trial with 89 patients using LOPROX Lotion and 89 patients using the vehicle, the incidence of adverse reactions was low. Those considered possibly related to treatment or occurring in more than one patient were pruritus, which occurred in two patients using ciclopirox lotion and one patient using the lotion vehicle, and burning, which occurred in one patient using ciclopirox lotion.

DOSAGE AND ADMINISTRATION

Gently massage LOPROX Cream or Lotion into the affected and surrounding skin areas twice daily, in the morning and evening. Clinical improvement with relief of pruritus and other symptoms usually occurs within the first week of treatment. If a patient shows no clinical improvement after four weeks of treatment with LOPROX Cream or Lotion, the diagnosis should be redetermined. Patients with tinea versicolor usually exhibit clinical and mycological clearing after two weeks of treatment.

HOW SUPPLIED

LOPROX® (ciclopirox) Cream 0.77% is supplied in 15 gram (NDC 99207-009-15), 30 gram (NDC 99207-009-30), and 90 gram (NDC 99207-009-90) tubes.
Store at controlled room temperature 15°– 30°C (59°– 86°F).
LOPROX® (ciclopirox) Lotion 0.77% is supplied in 30 mL bottles (NDC 99207-008-30), and 60 mL bottles (NDC 99207-008-60).
Bottle space provided to allow for vigorous shaking before each use.
Store between 5° and 25°C (41° and 77°F).
REG TM THE AVENTIS GROUP
Manufactured for:
MEDICIS, The Dermatology Company®
Scottsdale, AZ 85258
LOPROX Cream by:
Hoechst Marion Roussel
Deutschland GmbH
D-65926 Frankfurt am Main
LOPROX Lotion by:
West Pharmaceutical Services Lakewood, Inc.
Lakewood, NJ 08701

LOPROX® ℞

[*lō' prŏx*]
(ciclopirox)
Gel 0.77%
Prescribing information as of March 2000

FOR DERMATOLOGIC USE ONLY
NOT FOR USE IN EYES
Rx Only

DESCRIPTION

LOPROX® (ciclopirox) Gel 0.77% contains a synthetic antifungal agent, ciclopirox. It is intended for topical dermatologic use only.
Each gram of LOPROX Gel contains 7.70 mg of Ciclopirox in a gel consisting of Purified Water USP, Isopropyl Alcohol USP, Octyldodecanol NF, Dimethicone Copolyol 190, Carbomer 980, Sodium Hydroxide NF, and Docusate Sodium USP.
LOPROX Gel is a white, slightly fluid gel.
The chemical name for ciclopirox is 6-cyclohexyl-1-hydroxy-4-methyl-2(1*H*)-pyridinone, with the empirical formula $C_{12}H_{17}NO_2$ and a molecular weight of 207.27. The CAS Registry Number is [29342-05-0]. The chemical structure is:

CLINICAL PHARMACOLOGY

Mechanism of Action: Ciclopirox acts by chelation of polyvalent cations (Fe^{3+} or Al^{3+}) resulting in the inhibition of the metal-dependent enzymes that are responsible for the degradation of peroxides within the fungal cell.
In vitro studies showed that ciclopirox inhibited the formation of 5-lipoxygenase inflammatory mediators (5-HETE and LTB_4) and also inhibited PGE_2 release in a cell culture model. *In vivo*, ciclopirox inhibited inflammation in an arachidonic acid-induced murine ear edema model. The clinical significance of these findings is unknown.
Pharmacokinetics: A comparative study of the pharmacokinetics of LOPROX Gel and LOPROX® (ciclopirox) Cream 0.77% in 18 healthy males indicated that systemic absorption of ciclopirox from LOPROX Gel was higher than that of LOPROX Cream. A 5 gm dose of LOPROX Gel produced a mean (±SD) peak serum concentration of 25.02 (±20.6) ng/mL total ciclopirox and 5 gm of LOPROX Cream produced 18.62 (±13.56) ng/mL total ciclopirox. Approximately 3% of the applied ciclopirox was excreted in the urine within 48 hours after application, with a renal elimination half-life of about 5.5 hours.

Continued on next page

Loprox Lotion—Cont.

In a study of LOPROX Gel, 16 men with moderate to severe tinea cruris applied approximately 15 grams/day of the gel for 14.5 days. The mean (±SD) dose-normalized values of C_{max} for total ciclopirox in serum were 100 (±42) ng/mL on Day 1 and 238 (±144) ng/mL on Day 15. During the 10 hours after dosing on Day 1, approximately 10% of the administered dose was excreted in the urine.

Microbiology: Ciclopirox is a hydroxypyridinone antifungal agent that inhibits the growth of pathogenic dermatophytes. Ciclopirox has been shown to be active against most strains of the following microorganisms both *in vitro* and in clinical infections as described in the INDICATIONS AND USAGE section:

Trichophyton rubrum, Trichophyton mentagrophytes, and Epidermophyton floccosum.

INDICATIONS AND USAGE

Superficial Dermatophyte Infections

LOPROX® (ciclopirox) Gel 0.77% is indicated for the topical treatment of interdigital tinea pedis and tinea corporis due to *Trichophyton rubrum, Trichophyton mentagrophytes,* or *Epidermophyton floccosum.*

Seborrheic Dermatitis

LOPROX Gel is indicated for the topical treatment of seborrheic dermatitis of the scalp.

CONTRAINDICATIONS

LOPROX Gel is contraindicated in individuals who have shown hypersensitivity to any of its components.

WARNINGS

LOPROX Gel is not for ophthalmic, oral, or intravaginal use.

Keep out of reach of children.

PRECAUTIONS

If a reaction suggesting sensitivity or chemical irritation should occur with the use of LOPROX Gel, treatment should be discontinued and appropriate therapy instituted. A transient burning sensation may occur, especially after application to sensitive areas. Avoid contact with eyes. Efficacy of LOPROX Gel in immunosuppressed individuals has not been studied. Seborrheic dermatitis in association with acne, atopic dermatitis, Parkinsonism, psoriasis and rosacea has not been studied with LOPROX Gel. Efficacy in the treatment of plantar and vesicular types of tinea pedis has not been established.

Informaton for Patients:

The patient should be told the following:

1. Use LOPROX Gel as directed by the physician. Avoid contact with the eyes and mucous membranes. LOPROX Gel is for external use only.
2. Use the medication for fungal infections for the full treatment time even though symptoms may have improved, and notify the physician if there is no improvement after 4 weeks.
3. A transient burning/stinging sensation may be felt. This may occur in approximately 15% to 20% of cases, when LOPROX Gel is used to treat seborrheic dermatitis of the scalp.
4. Inform the physician if the area of application shows signs of increased irritation or possible sensitization (redness with itching, burning, blistering, swelling, and/or oozing).
5. Avoid the use of occlusive dressings.
6. Do not use this medication for any disorder other than that for which it is prescribed.

Carcinogenesis, Mutagenesis, Impairment of Fertility: A carcinogenicity study of ciclopirox (1% and 5% solutions in polyethylene glycol 400) in female mice dosed cutaneously twice per week for 50 weeks followed by a 6-month drug-free observation period prior to necropsy revealed no evidence of tumors at the application site.

The following battery of *in vitro* genotoxicity tests was conducted with ciclopirox: evaluation of gene mutation in the Ames *Salmonella* and *E. coli* assays (negative); chromosome aberration assays in V79 Chinese hamster cells, with and without metabolic activation (positive); gene mutation assays in the HGPRT-test with V79 Chinese hamster cells (negative); and a primary DNA damage assay (i.e., unscheduled DNA synthesis assay in A549 human cells) (negative). An *in vitro* cell transformation assay in BALB/c 3T3 cells was negative for cell transformation. In an *in vivo* Chinese hamster bone marrow cytogenetic assay, ciclopirox was negative for chromosome aberrations at 5000 mg/kg.

Pregnancy: Teratogenic effects: Pregnancy Category B

Reproduction studies of ciclopirox revealed no significant evidence of impaired fertility in rats exposed orally up to 5 mg/kg body weight (approximately 5 times the maximum recommended topical human dose based on surface area). No fetotoxicity was shown due to ciclopirox in the mouse, rat, rabbit, and monkey at oral doses up to 100, 30, 30, and 50 mg/kg body weight, respectively (approximately 37.5 30, 44, and 77 times the maximum recommended topical human dose based on surface area). By the dermal route of administration, no fetotoxicity was shown due to ciclopirox in the rat and rabbit at doses up to 120 and 100 mg/kg body weight, respectively (approximately 121 and 147 times, respectively, the maximum recommended topical human dose based on surface area).

There are no adequate or well-controlled studies of topically applied ciclopirox in pregnant women. LOPROX Gel should be used during pregnancy only if the potential benefit justifies the potential risk to the fetus.

Nursing Mothers: It is not known whether this drug is excreted in human milk. Since many drugs are excreted in human milk, caution should be exercised when LOPROX Gel is administered to a nursing woman.

Pediatric Use: The efficacy and safety of LOPROX Gel in pediatric patients below the age of 16 years have not been established.

ADVERSE REACTIONS

In clinical trials, 140 (39%) of 359 subjects treated with LOPROX Gel reported adverse experiences, irrespective of relationship to test materials, which resulted in 8 subjects discontinuing treatment. The most frequent experience reported was skin burning sensation upon application, which occurred in approximately 34% of seborrheic dermatitis patients and 7% of tinea pedis patients. Adverse experiences occurring between 1% to 5% were contact dermatitis and pruritus. Other reactions that occurred in less than 1% included dry skin, acne, rash, alopecia, pain upon application, eye pain, and facial edema.

DOSAGE AND ADMINISTRATION

Superficial Dermatophyte Infections

Gently massage LOPROX Gel into the affected areas and surrounding skin twice daily, in the morning and evening immediately after cleaning or washing the areas to be treated. Interdigital tinea pedis and tinea corporis should be treated for 4 weeks. If a patient shows no clinical improvement after 4 weeks of treatment, the diagnosis should be reviewed.

Seborrheic Dermatitis of the Scalp

Apply LOPROX Gel to affected scalp areas twice daily, in the morning and evening for 4 weeks. Clinical improvement usually occurs within the first week with continuing resolution of signs and symptoms through the fourth week of treatment. If a patient shows no clinical improvement after 4 weeks of treatment, the diagnosis should be reviewed.

HOW SUPPLIED

Loprox® (ciclopirox) Gel 0.77% is supplied in 30 g tubes (NDC 99207-013-30), and 45 g tubes (NDC 99207-013-45). Store between 15° and 30°C (59° and 86°F).

Manufactured for:
MEDICIS, The Dermatology Company®
Scottsdale, AZ 85258
by: Hoechst Marion Roussel Deutschland GmbH,
D-65926 Frankfurt am Main
Made in Germany
REG TM THE AVENTIS GROUP
01330-08A

LUSTRA® ℞

[lŭs' tră]
(hydroquinone USP 4%)
LUSTRA-AF™
(hydroquinone USP 4%)
Prescribing information as of April 2000

Rx Only
FOR EXTERNAL USE ONLY

DESCRIPTION

Hydroquinone is 1,4-benzenediol. Hydroquinone is structurally related to monobenzone. Hydroquinone occurs as fine, white needles. The drug is freely soluble in water and in alcohol and has a pK_a of 9.96. Chemically, hydroquinone is designated as p-dihydroxybenzene; the empirical formula is $C_6H_6O_2$; molecular weight 110.1. The structural formula is:

OH
OH
$C_6H_6O_2$

CONTENTS

ACTIVE INGREDIENT: Hydroquinone USP 4%.

OTHER INGREDIENTS (LUSTRA® (hydroquinone USP 4%)): Purified Water, Phenyl Trimethicone, Glycerin 99% USP, Glyceryl Stearate (and) PEG-100 Stearate, Alcohol, Cetyl Alcohol, Cyclopentasiloxane (and) Polysilicone-11, Linoleic Acid, Glycolic Acid, Polyacrylamide (and) C 13-14 Isoparaffin (and) Laureth-7, Cetearyl Alcohol (and) Ceteareth 20, Ascorbyl Palmitate, Triethanolamine 99%, Tocopheryl Acetate, Phenoxyethanol, Benzyl Alcohol, Hydrogenated Lecithin, Dimethiconol, Sodium Metabisulfite, Sodium Citrate, Disodium EDTA, Ascorbic Acid, Butylated Hydroxytoluene, Alpha Tocopherol, Carbomer, Fragrance.

OTHER INGREDIENTS (LUSTRA-AF™ (hydroquinone USP 4%)): Purified Water, Octyl Methoxycinnamate USP, Phenyl Trimethicone, Glycerin 99% USP, Glyceryl Stearate (and) PEG-100 Stearate, Cetyl Alcohol, Avobenzone USP, Alcohol, Cyclopentasiloxane (and) Polysilicone-11, Linoleic Acid, Glycolic Acid, Polyacrylamide (and) C 13-14 Isoparaffin (and) Laureth-7, Cetearyl Alcohol (and) Ceteareth 20, Ascorbyl Palmitate, Triethanolamine 99%, Tocopheryl Acetate, Phenoxyethanol, Benzyl Alcohol, Hydrogenated Lecithin, Dimethiconol, Sodium Metabisulfite, Sodium Citrate, Ascorbic Acid, Disodium EDTA, Alpha Tocopherol, Butylated Hydroxytoluene, Carbomer, Fragrance.

CLINICAL PHARMACOLOGY

Topical application of hydroquinone produces a reversible depigmentation of the skin by inhibition of the enzymatic oxidation of tyrosine to 3-(3,4-dihydroxyphenyl) alanine (dopa)[1] and suppression of other melanocyte metabolic processes.[2] Exposure to sunlight or ultraviolet light will cause repigmentation which may be prevented by the broad spectrum sunscreen agents contained in LUSTRA-AF.[3]

INDICATIONS AND USAGE

LUSTRA and LUSTRA-AF are indicated for the gradual treatment of ultraviolet induced dyschromia and discoloration resulting from the use of oral contraceptives, pregnancy, hormone replacement therapy, or skin trauma.

DOSAGE AND ADMINISTRATION

LUSTRA or LUSTRA-AF should be applied to the affected areas twice daily, morning and before bedtime, or as directed by a physician. During and after the use of LUSTRA sun exposure should be limited, and a sunscreen agent or sun-protective clothing should be used to cover the treated areas, to prevent repigmentation. There is no recommended dosage for pediatric patients under 12 years of age except under the advice and supervision of a physician.

CONTRAINDICATIONS

LUSTRA and LUSTRA-AF are contraindicated in any patient that has a prior history of hypersensitivity or allergic reaction to hydroquinone or any of the other ingredients. The safety of topical hydroquinone use during pregnancy or on children (12 years and under) has not been established.

WARNINGS

A. CAUTION: Hydroquinone is a depigmenting agent which may produce unwanted cosmetic effects if not used as directed. The physician should be familiar with the contents of this insert before prescribing or dispensing this medication.

B. Test for skin sensitivity before using LUSTRA or LUSTRA-AF by applying a small amount to an unbroken patch of skin and check within 24 hours. Minor redness is not a contraindication, but where there is itching, vesicle formation, or excessive inflammatory response further treatment is not advised. Close patient supervision is recommended. Contact with the eyes should be avoided. If no lightening effect is noted after two months of treatment, use of LUSTRA or LUSTRA-AF should be discontinued. LUSTRA-AF is formulated for use as a treatment for dyschromia and should not be used for the prevention of sunburn.

C. Sunscreen use is an essential aspect of hydroquinone therapy, because even minimal sunlight sustains melanocytic activity. During treatment and maintenance therapy, sun exposure should be avoided on treated skin by application of a broad spectrum sunscreen (SPF 15 or greater) or by use of protective clothing to prevent repigmentation. Although LUSTRA has an antioxidant system in its vehicle, there are no sunblocking or sunscreening agents in LUSTRA. The sunscreens in LUSTRA-AF provide the necessary sun protection during therapy. During and after the use of LUSTRA-AF, sun exposure should be limited or sun-protective clothing should be used to cover the treated areas to prevent repigmentation.

D. Keep this and all medications out of the reach of children. In case of accidental ingestion, contact a physician or a poison control center immediately.

E. WARNING: Contains sodium metabisulfite, a sulfite which may cause serious allergic reactions (e.g., hives, itching, wheezing, anaphylaxis, severe asthma attack) in certain susceptible persons.

F. On rare occasions, a gradual blue-black darkening of the skin may occur. In which case, use of LUSTRA or LUSTRA-AF should be discontinued and a physician contacted immediately.

PRECAUTIONS

SEE WARNINGS

A. Pregnancy Category C: Animal reproduction studies have not been conducted with topical hydroquinone. It is also not known whether hydroquinone can cause fetal harm when used topically on a pregnant woman or can affect reproductive capacity. It is not known to what degree, if any, topical hydroquinone is absorbed systemically. Topical hydroquinone should be used in pregnant women only where clearly indicated.

B. Nursing mothers: It is not known whether topical hydroquinone is absorbed or excreted in human milk. Caution is advised when hydroquinone is used by a nursing mother.

C. Pediatric usage: Safety and effectiveness in pediatric patients below the age of 12 years have not been established.

ADVERSE REACTIONS

No systemic reactions have been reported. Occasional cutaneous hypersensitivity (localized contact dermatitis) may occur, in which case the medication should be discontinued and the physician notified immediately.

OVERDOSAGE

There have been no systemic reactions reported from the use of topical hydroquinone. However, treatment should be limited to relatively small areas of the body at one time, since some patients experience a transient skin reddening and a mild burning sensation which does not preclude treatment.

HOW SUPPLIED

LUSTRA is available as follows:
1 ounce jar (28.4 g) NDC 99207-250-10
2 ounce jar (56.8 g) NDC 99207-250-20
LUSTRA-AF is available as follows:
1 ounce jar (28.4 g) NDC 99207-255-10
2 ounce jar (56.8 g) NDC 99207-255-20

REFERENCES

1. Denton, C., A.B. Lerner, and T.B. Fitzpatrick. "Inhibition of Melanin Formation by Chemical Agents." *Journal of Investigative Dermatology.* 1952;18:119–135.
2. Jimbow, K., H. Obata, M. Pathak, and T.B. Fitzpatrick. "Mechanism of Depigmentation by Hydroquinone." *Journal of Investigative Dermatology.* 1974;62:436–449.
3. Parrish, J.A., R.R. Anderson, F. Urbach, and D. Pitts. UVA, Biological Effects of Ultraviolet Radiation with Emphasis on Human Responses to Longwave Ultraviolet. Plenum Press, New York and London, 1978, p. 151.

LUSTRA and LUSTRA-AF should be stored at: 15°–25°C (59°–77°F).
Covered by US Patent 5,932,612.
Manufactured for:
MEDICIS, The Dermatology Company®
Scottsdale, AZ 85258
by: Contract Pharmaceuticals Limited
Mississauga, Ontario CANADA
25010–08D 4/00

OVIDE® ℞

[*ō 'vīd*]
(malathion)
Lotion, 0.5%
Prescribing information as of May 1999

Rx Only
For topical use only. Not for oral or ophthalmic use.

DESCRIPTION

OVIDE Lotion contains 0.005 g of malathion per mL in a vehicle of isopropyl alcohol (78%), terpineol, dipentene, and pine needle oil. The chemical name of malathion is (±) - [(dimethoxyphosphinothioyl) - thio] butanedioic acid diethyl ester. Malathion has a molecular weight of 330.36, represented by $C_{10}H_{19}O_6PS_2$, and has the following chemical structure:

[Chemical structure: $(H_3CO)_2P(=S)-S-CH(COOCH_2CH_3)CH_2COOCH_2CH_3$]

CLINICAL PHARMACOLOGY

Malathion is an organophosphate agent which acts as a pediculicide by inhibiting cholinesterase activity *in vivo*. Inadvertent transdermal absorption of malathion has occurred from its agricultural use. In such cases, acute toxicity was manifested by excessive cholinergic activity, i.e., increased sweating, salivary and gastric secretion, gastrointestinal and uterine motility, and bradycardia (see **OVERDOSAGE**). Because the potential for transdermal absorption of malathion from OVIDE Lotion is not known at this time, strict adherence to the dosing instructions regarding its use in children, method of application, duration of exposure, and frequency of application is required.

INDICATIONS AND USAGE

OVIDE Lotion is indicated for patients infected with *Pediculus humanus capitis* (head lice and their ova) of the scalp hair.

CONTRAINDICATIONS

OVIDE Lotion is contraindicated for neonates and infants because their scalps are more permeable and may have increased absorption of malathion. OVIDE Lotion should also not be used on individuals known to be sensitive to malathion or any of the ingredients in the vehicle.

WARNINGS

1. OVIDE Lotion is **flammable**. The lotion and wet hair should not be exposed to open flames or electric heat sources, including hair dryers and electric curlers. Do not smoke while applying lotion or while hair is wet. Allow hair to dry naturally and to remain uncovered after application of OVIDE Lotion.
2. OVIDE Lotion should only be used on children under the direct supervision of an adult.
3. If OVIDE Lotion comes into contact with the eyes, flush immediately with water. Consult a physician if eye irritation persists.
4. If skin irritation occurs, discontinue use of product until irritation clears. Reapply the OVIDE Lotion, and if irritation reoccurs, consult a physician.
5. Slight stinging sensations may occur with the use of OVIDE Lotion.

General: Keep out of reach of children. Close eyes tightly during product application. If accidentally placed in the eye, flush immediately with water. Use only on scalp hair.

Information to Patients:
1. OVIDE Lotion is **flammable.** The lotion and hair wet with lotion should not be exposed to open flames or electric heat sources, including hair dryers and electric curlers. Do not smoke while applying lotion or while hair is wet. The person applying OVIDE Lotion should wash hands after application. Allow hair to dry naturally and to remain uncovered after application of OVIDE Lotion.
2. OVIDE Lotion should only be used on children under the direct supervision of an adult. Children should be warned to stay away from lighted cigarettes, open flames, and electric heat sources while the hair is wet.
3. In case of accidental ingestion of OVIDE Lotion by mouth, seek medical attention immediately.
4. If you are pregnant or nursing, you should contact your physician before using OVIDE Lotion.
5. If OVIDE Lotion comes into contact with the eyes, flush immediately with water. Consult a physician if eye irritation persists or if visual changes occur.
6. If skin irritation occurs, wash scalp and hair immediately. If the irritation clears, OVIDE Lotion may be re-applied. If irritation reoccurs, consult a physician.
7. Slight stinging sensations may be produced when using OVIDE Lotion.
8. Apply OVIDE Lotion on the scalp hair in an amount just sufficient to thoroughly wet hair and scalp. Pay particular attention to the back of the head and neck when applying OVIDE Lotion. Anyone applying OVIDE Lotion should wash hands immediately after the application process is complete.
9. Allow hair to dry naturally and to remain uncovered. Shampoo hair after 8 to 12 hours, again paying attention to the back of the head and neck while shampooing.
10. Rinse hair and use a fine-toothed (nit) comb to remove dead lice and eggs.
11. If lice are still present after 7–9 days, repeat with a second application of OVIDE Lotion.
12. Further treatment is generally not necessary. Other family members should be evaluated by a physician to determine if infested, and if so, receive treatment.

Laboratory Tests: There are no special laboratory tests needed in order to use this medication.

Carcinogenesis, Mutagenesis, and Impairment of Fertility: Although carcinogenesis, mutagenesis, and impairment of fertility have not been studied with OVIDE Lotion, malathion has been shown to be genotoxic in a number of *in vitro* and *in vivo* mutation and clastogenicity assays. However, there was no evidence of a carcinogenic effect following long-term oral administration of malathion in F344 rats after 2 years feeding with up to 0.4% (~ 200 – 400 mg/kg/day) nor was it tumorigenic in Osborne-Mendel rats or B6C3F1 mice after similar feeding for 80 weeks with 0.8% (~ 400 – 600 mg/kg/day) or 1.6% (~ 1,000 – 2,000 mg/kg/day), respectively. Based on body surface area, doses tested are approximately 4 to 40 fold greater than those anticipated in humans (assuming 100% bioavailability).

Reproduction studies performed with malathion in rats at doses approximately 30 fold greater than those anticipated in humans (based on body surface area and assuming 100% bioavailability) revealed no evidence of impaired fertility.

Pregnancy: Pregnancy Category B. There was no evidence of teratogenicity in studies in rats and rabbits at doses up to 900 mg/kg/day and 100 mg/kg/day malathion, respectively. A study in rats failed to show any gross fetal abnormalities attributable to feeding malathion up to 2,500 ppm (~ 200 mg/kg/day) in the diet during a three-generation evaluation period. These doses were approximately 2 to 10 times higher than the anticipated human dose (based on body surface area and assuming 100% bioavailability). Because animal reproduction studies are not always predictive of human responses, this drug should be used (or handled) during pregnancy only if clearly needed.

Nursing Mothers: Malathion in an acetone vehicle has been reported to be absorbed through human skin to the extent of 8% of the applied dose. However, percutaneous absorption from the OVIDE Lotion, 0.5% formulation has not been studied, and it is not known whether malathion is excreted in human milk. Because many drugs are excreted in human milk, caution should be exercised when OVIDE Lotion is administered to (or handled by) a nursing mother.

Pediatric Use: The safety and effectiveness of OVIDE Lotion in children less than 6 years of age has not been established via well-controlled trials.

ADVERSE REACTIONS

Malathion has been shown to be irritating to the skin and scalp. Accidental contact with the eyes can result in mild conjunctivitis.

It is not known if OVIDE Lotion has the potential to cause contact allergic sensitization.

OVERDOSAGE

Consideration should be given, as part of the treatment program, to the high concentration of isopropyl alcohol in the vehicle.

Malathion, although a weaker cholinesterase inhibitor than some other organophosphates, may be expected to exhibit the same symptoms of cholinesterase depletion after accidental ingestion orally. If accidentally swallowed, vomiting should be induced promptly or the stomach lavaged with 5% sodium bicarbonate solution.

Severe respiratory distress is the major and most serious symptom of organophosphate poisoning requiring artificial respiration, and atropine may be needed to counteract the symptoms of cholinesterase depletion.

Repeat analyses of serum and RBC cholinesterase may assist in establishing the diagnosis and formulating a long-range prognosis.

DOSAGE AND ADMINISTRATION

1. Apply OVIDE Lotion on **DRY** hair in amount just sufficient to thoroughly wet the hair and scalp. Pay particular attention to the back of the head and neck while applying OVIDE Lotion. Wash hands after applying to scalp.
2. Allow hair to dry naturally—use no electric heat source, and allow hair to remain uncovered.
3. After 8 to 12 hours, the hair should be shampooed.
4. Rinse and use a fine-toothed (nit) comb to remove dead lice and eggs.
5. If lice are still present after 7–9 days, repeat with a second application of OVIDE Lotion.

Further treatment is generally not necessary. Other family members should be evaluated by a physician to determine if infested, and if so, receive treatment.

Clinical Studies: Two controlled clinical trials evaluated the pediculicidal activity of OVIDE Lotion. Patients applied the lotion to the hair and scalp in quantities, up to a maximum of 2 fl. oz., sufficient to thoroughly wet the hair and scalp. The lotion was allowed to air dry and was shampooed with Prell shampoo 8 to 12 hours after application. Patients in both the OVIDE Lotion group and in the vehicle group were examined immediately after shampooing, 24 hours after, and 7 days after for the presence of live lice. Results are shown in the following table:

[See table above]

Number of Patients Without Live Scalp Lice

Treatment	Immediately After	24 Hrs. After	7 Days After
OVIDE Lotion	129/129	122/129	114/126
OVIDE Vehicle	105/105	63/105	31/105

The presence or absence of ova at day 7 was not evaluated in these studies. The presence or absence of live lice or ova at 14 days following treatment was not evaluated in these studies. The residual amount of malathion on hair and scalp is unknown.

HOW SUPPLIED

OVIDE® (malathion) Lotion, 0.5%, is supplied in bottles of 2 fl. oz. (59 mL) NDC 99207-650-02.
Store at controlled room temperature 20°–25°C (68°–77°F).
Flammable. Keep away from heat and open flame.
Manufactured for:
MEDICIS, The Dermatology Company®
Scottsdale, AZ 85258
by: West Pharmaceutical Services Lakewood, Inc.
Lakewood, NJ 08701
65002-08A

PLEXION™ ℞

[*plĕx' ēōn*]
(sodium sulfacetamide 10% and sulfur 5%)
Cleanser
Lotion
Prescribing information as of September 2000

Rx Only

DESCRIPTION

Sodium sulfacetamide is a sulfonamide with antibacterial activity while sulfur acts as a keratolytic agent. Chemically sodium sulfacetamide is N-[(4-aminophenyl) sulfonyl]-acetamide, monosodium salt, monohydrate. The structural formula is:

[Chemical structure: $NH_2-C_6H_4-SO_2N(Na)COCH_3 \cdot H_2O$]

Each gram of Plexion™ (Sodium Sulfacetamide 10% and Sulfur 5%) Cleanser contains 100 mg. of Sodium Sulfacetamide and 50 mg. of Sulfur in a cleanser base containing Water, Sodium Methyl Oleyltaurate, Sodium Cocoyl Isethionate, Disodium Oleamido MEA Sulfosuccinate, Cetyl Alcohol NF, Glyceryl Stearate (and) PEG-100 Stearate, Stearyl Alcohol NF, PEG-55 Propylene Glycol Oleate, Magnesium Aluminum Silicate NF, Methylparaben NF, Disodium EDTA, Butylated Hydroxytoluene NF, Sodium Thiosulfate, Fragrance, Xanthan Gum NF, and Propylparaben NF.

Each gram of Plexion™ (Sodium Sulfacetamide 10% and Sulfur 5%) Lotion contains 100 mg. of Sodium Sulfacetamide and 50 mg. of Sulfur in a lotion containing Water, Propylene Glycol, Isopropyl Myristate, Light Mineral Oil, Polysorbate 60, Sorbitan Monostearate, Cetyl Alcohol, Hydrogenated Coco-Glycerides, Stearyl Alcohol, Fragrances, Benzyl Alcohol, Glyceryl Stearate (and) PEG-100 Stearate, Dimethicone, Zinc Ricinoleate, Xanthan Gum, Disodium EDTA, and Sodium Thiosulfate.

Continued on next page

Plexion—Cont.

CLINICAL PHARMACOLOGY

The most widely accepted mechanism of action of sulfonamides is the Woods-Fildes theory which is based on the fact that sulfonamides act as competitive antagonists to para-aminobenzoic acid (PABA), an essential component for bacterial growth. While absorption through intact skin has not been determined, sodium sulfacetamide is readily absorbed from the gastrointestinal tract when taken orally and excreted in the urine, largely unchanged. The biological half-life has variously been reported as 7 to 12.8 hours. The exact mode of action of sulfur in the treatment of acne is unknown, but it has been reported that it inhibits the growth of Propionibacterium acnes and the formation of free fatty acids.

INDICATIONS

PLEXION Cleanser and Lotion are indicated in the topical control of acne vulgaris, acne rosacea and seborrheic dermatitis.

CONTRAINDICATIONS

PLEXION Cleanser and Lotion are contraindicated for use by patients having known hypersensitivity to sulfonamides, sulfur or any other component of this preparation. PLEXION Cleanser and Lotion are not to be used by patients with kidney disease.

WARNINGS

Although rare, sensitivity to sodium sulfacetamide may occur. Therefore, caution and careful supervision should be observed when prescribing this drug for patients who may be prone to hypersensitivity to topical sulfonamides. Systemic toxic reactions such as agranulocytosis, acute hemolytic anemia, purpura hemorrhagica, drug fever, jaundice, and contact dermatitis indicate hypersensitivity to sulfonamides. Particular caution should be employed if areas of denuded or abraded skin are involved.

FOR EXTERNAL USE ONLY. Keep away from eyes. Keep out of reach of children. Keep tube tightly closed.

PRECAUTIONS

General: If irritation develops, use of the product should be discontinued and appropriate therapy instituted. Patients should be carefully observed for possible local irritation or sensitization during long-term therapy. The object of this therapy is to achieve desquamation without irritation, but sodium sulfacetamide and sulfur can cause reddening and scaling of the epidermis. These side effects are not unusual in the treatment of acne vulgaris, but patients should be cautioned about the possibility.

Carcinogenesis, Mutagenesis and Impairment of Fertility: Long-term studies in animals have not been performed to evaluate carcinogenic potential.

Pregnancy: Category C. Animal reproduction studies have not been conducted with PLEXION Cleanser or Lotion. It is also not known whether PLEXION Cleanser and Lotion can cause fetal harm when administered to a pregnant woman or can affect reproduction capacity. PLEXION Cleanser and Lotion should be given to a pregnant woman only if clearly needed.

Nursing Mothers: It is not known whether sodium sulfacetamide is excreted in the human milk following topical use of PLEXION Cleanser or Lotion. However, small amounts of orally administered sulfonamides have been reported to be eliminated in human milk. In view of this and because many drugs are excreted in human milk, caution should be exercised when PLEXION Cleanser or Lotion are administered to a nursing woman.

Pediatric Use: Safety and effectiveness in children under the age of 12 have not been established.

ADVERSE REACTIONS

Although rare, sodium sulfacetamide may cause local irritation.

DOSAGE AND ADMINISTRATION

PLEXION Cleanser: Wash affected areas once or twice daily, or as directed by your physician. Avoid contact with eyes or mucous membranes. Wet skin and liberally apply to areas to be cleansed, massage gently into skin for 10–20 seconds working into a full lather, rinse thoroughly and pat dry. If drying occurs, it may be controlled by rinsing cleanser off sooner or using less often.

PLEXION Lotion: Cleanse affected areas. Apply a thin film of PLEXION Lotion to affected areas 1 to 3 times daily, or as directed by a physician.

HOW SUPPLIED

Plexion™ (sodium sulfacetamide 10% and sulfur 5%) Cleanser is available in 6 oz. (170.3 g) tube, NDC 99207-741-06 and 12 oz. (340.2 g) bottle, NDC 99207-741-12.

Plexion™ (sodium sulfacetamide 10% and sulfur 5%) Lotion is available in 30 g tube (NDC 99207-742-30) and 60 g tube (NDC 99207-742-60).

Store at: 15°–25°C (59°–77°F).

Manufactured for:
MEDICIS, The Dermatology Company®
Scottsdale, AZ 85258
by: Contract Pharmaceuticals Limited
Mississauga, Ontario CANADA
74106-08M 9/00

SYNALAR® ℞
(fluocinolone acetonide)
Cream 0.025%
Ointment 0.025%
Topical Solution 0.01%

Refer to entry under LIDEX® (fluocinonide)

SYNEMOL® ℞
(fluocinolone acetonide)
Cream 0.025%

Refer to entry under LIDEX® (fluocinonide)

TOPICORT® ℞
[tŏp 'i-cŏrt]
(desoximetasone)
Emollient Cream 0.25%
Gel 0.05%
Ointment 0.25%

TOPICORT® LP ℞
(desoximetasone)
Emollient Cream 0.05%
Prescribing information as of April 1999

FOR DERMATOLOGIC USE ONLY
NOT FOR USE IN EYES
Rx Only

DESCRIPTION

Topicort® (desoximetasone) Emollient Cream 0.25%, Topicort® (desoximetasone) Gel 0.05%, Topicort® (desoximetasone) Ointment 0.25%, and Topicort® LP (desoximetasone) Emollient Cream 0.05% contain the active synthetic corticosteroid desoximetasone. The topical corticosteroids constitute a class of primarily synthetic steroids used as anti-inflammatory and anti-pruritic agents.

Each gram of TOPICORT Emollient Cream 0.25% contains 2.5 mg of Desoximetasone in an emollient cream consisting of White Petrolatum USP, Purified Water USP, Isopropyl Myristate NF, Lanolin Alcohols NF, Mineral Oil USP, Cetostearyl Alcohol NF, Aluminum Stearate, and Magnesium Stearate.

Each gram of TOPICORT Gel 0.05% contains 0.5 mg Desoximetasone in a gel consisting of Purified Water USP, SD Alcohol 40 (20% w/w), Isopropyl Myristate NF, Carbomer 940, Trolamine NF, Edetate Disodium USP, and Docusate Sodium USP.

Each gram of TOPICORT Ointment 0.25% contains 2.5 mg of Desoximetasone in a base consisting of White Petrolatum USP, Propylene Glycol USP, Sorbitan Sesquioleate, Beeswax, Fatty Alcohol Citrate, Fatty Acid Pentaerythritol Ester, Aluminum Stearate, Citric Acid, and Butylated Hydroxyanisole.

Each gram of TOPICORT LP Emollient Cream 0.05% contains 0.5 mg Desoximetasone in an emollient cream consisting of White Petrolatum USP, Purified Water USP, Isopropyl Myristate NF, Lanolin Alcohols NF, Mineral Oil USP, Cetostearyl Alcohol NF, Aluminum Stearate, Edetate Disodium USP, Lactic Acid USP, and Magnesium Stearate.

The chemical name of desoximetasone is Pregna-1, 4-diene-3, 20-dione, 9-fluoro-11, 21-dihydroxy-16-methyl-, (11β, 16α)-. Desoximetasone has the empirical formula $C_{22}H_{29}FO_4$ and a molecular weight of 376.47. The CAS Registry Number is 382-67-2. The chemical structure is:

[Chemical structure: CH_2OH, C=O, CH_3, HO, H, CH_3, CH_3, H, H, F, H, O]

CLINICAL PHARMACOLOGY

Topical corticosteroids share anti-inflammatory, anti-pruritic, and vasoconstrictive actions.

The mechanism of anti-inflammatory activity of the topical corticosteroids is unclear. Various laboratory methods, including vasoconstrictor assays, are used to compare and predict potencies and/or clinical efficacies of the topical corticosteroids. There is some evidence to suggest that a recognizable correlation exists between vasoconstrictor potency and therapeutic efficacy in man.

Pharmacokinetics: The extent of percutaneous absorption of topical corticosteroids is determined by many factors, including the vehicle, the integrity of the epidermal barrier, and the use of occlusive dressings.

Topical corticosteroids can be absorbed from normal intact skin. Inflammation and/or other disease processes in the skin increase percutaneous absorption. Occlusive dressings substantially increase the percutaneous absorption of topical corticosteroids. Thus, occlusive dressings may be a valuable therapeutic adjunct for treatment of resistant dermatoses.

Once absorbed through the skin, topical corticosteroids are handled through pharmacokinetic pathways similar to systemically administered corticosteroids. Corticosteroids are bound to plasma proteins in varying degrees. Corticosteroids are metabolized primarily in the liver and are then excreted by the kidneys. Some of the topical corticosteroids and their metabolites are also excreted into the bile.

Pharmacokinetic studies in men with TOPICORT (desoximetasone) Emollient Cream 0.25% with tagged desoximetasone showed a total of 5.2% ± 2.9% excretion in urine (4.1% ± 2.3%) and feces (1.1% ± 0.6%) and no detectable level (limit of sensitivity: 0.005 µg/mL) in the blood when it was applied topically on the back followed by occlusion for 24 hours. Seven days after application, no further radioactivity was detected in urine or feces. The half-life of the material was 15 ± 2 hours (for urine) and 17 ± 2 hours (for feces) between the third and fifth trial day.

Pharmacokinetic studies in men with TOPICORT (desoximetasone) Ointment 0.25% with tagged desoximetasone showed no detectable level (limit of sensitivity: 0.003 µg/mL) in 1 subject and 0.004 and 0.006 µg/mL in the remaining 2 subjects in the blood when it was applied topically on the back followed by occlusion for 24 hours. The extent of absorption for the ointment was 7% based on radioactivity recovered from urine and feces. Seven days after application, no further radioactivity was detected in urine or feces.

Studies with other similarly structured steroids have shown that predominant metabolite reaction occurs through conjugation to form the glucuronide and sulfate ester.

INDICATIONS AND USAGE

TOPICORT Emollient Cream 0.25%, TOPICORT Gel 0.05%, TOPICORT Ointment 0.25% and TOPICORT LP Emollient Cream 0.05% are indicated for the relief of the inflammatory and pruritic manifestations of corticosteroid-responsive dermatoses.

CONTRAINDICATIONS

Topical corticosteroids are contraindicated in those patients with a history of hypersensitivity to any of the components of the preparation.

WARNINGS

TOPICORT Emollient Cream 0.25%, TOPICORT Gel 0.05%, TOPICORT Ointment 0.25% and TOPICORT LP Emollient Cream 0.05% are not for ophthalmic use. **Keep out of reach of children.**

PRECAUTIONS

General: Systemic absorption of topical corticosteroids has produced reversible hypothalamic-pituitary-adrenal (HPA) axis suppression, manifestations of Cushing's syndrome, hyperglycemia, and glucosuria in some patients.

Conditions which augment systemic absorption include the application of the more potent steroids, use over large surface areas, prolonged use, and the addition of occlusive dressings.

Therefore, patients receiving a large dose of a potent topical steroid applied to a large surface area or under an occlusive dressing should be evaluated periodically for evidence of HPA axis suppression by using the urinary free cortisol and ACTH stimulation tests. If HPA axis suppression is noted, an attempt should be made to withdraw the drug, to reduce the frequency of application, or to substitute a less potent steroid. Recovery of HPA axis function is generally prompt and complete upon discontinuation of the drug. Infrequently, signs and symptoms of steroid withdrawal may occur, requiring supplemental systemic corticosteroids.

Pediatric patients may absorb proportionally larger amounts of topical corticosteroids and thus be more susceptible to systemic toxicity (See **PRECAUTIONS-Pediatric Use**). If irritation develops, topical corticosteroids should be discontinued and appropriate therapy instituted.

In the presence of dermatological infections, the use of an appropriate antifungal or antibacterial agent should be instituted. If a favorable response does not occur promptly, the corticosteroid should be discontinued until the infection has been adequately controlled.

Information for the Patient: Patients using topical corticosteroids should receive the following information and instructions:

1. This medication is to be used as directed by the physician. It is for external use only. Avoid contact with the eyes.
2. Patients should be advised not to use this medication for any disorder other than for which it was prescribed.
3. The treated skin area should not be bandaged or otherwise covered or wrapped as to be occlusive unless directed by the physician.
4. Patients should report any signs of local adverse reactions, especially under occlusive dressing.
5. Parents of pediatric patients should be advised not to use tight-fitting diapers or plastic pants on a child being treated in the diaper area, as these garments may constitute occlusive dressings.

Laboratory Tests: The following tests may be helpful in evaluating the HPA axis suppression: Urinary free cortisol test and ACTH stimulation test.

Carcinogenesis, Mutagenesis, and Impairment of Fertility: Long-term animal studies have not been performed to evaluate the carcinogenic potential or the effect on fertility of topical corticosteroids.

Studies to determine mutagenicity with prednisolone and hydrocortisone have revealed negative results. Desoximetasone did not show potential for mutagenic activity *in vitro* in the Ames microbial mutagen test with or without metabolic activation.

Pregnancy Category C: Corticosteroids are generally teratogenic in laboratory animals when administered systemically at relatively low dosage levels. The more potent corti-

costeroids have been shown to be teratogenic after dermal application in laboratory animals.
Desoximetasone has been shown to be teratogenic and embryotoxic in mice, rats, and rabbits when given by subcutaneous or dermal routes of administration in doses 3 to 30 times the human dose of TOPICORT Emollient Cream 0.25% or TOPICORT Ointment 0.25% or 15 to 150 times the human dose of TOPICORT LP Emollient Cream 0.05% or TOPICORT Gel 0.05%.
There are no adequate and well-controlled studies in pregnant women on teratogenic effects from topically applied corticosteroids. Therefore, TOPICORT Emollient Cream 0.25%, TOPICORT Ointment 0.25%, TOPICORT Gel 0.05%, and TOPICORT LP Emollient Cream 0.05% should be used during pregnancy only if the potential benefit justifies the potential risk to the fetus. Drugs of this class should not be used extensively on pregnant patients, in large amounts, or for prolonged periods of time.
Nursing Mothers: It is not known whether topical administration of corticosteroids could result in sufficient systemic absorption to produce detectable quantities in breast milk. Systemically administered corticosteroids are secreted into breast milk in quantities not likely to have a deleterious effect on the infant. Nevertheless, caution should be exercised when topical corticosteroids are administered to a nursing woman.
Pediatric Use: Pediatric patients may demonstrate greater susceptibility to topical corticosteroid-induced HPA axis suppression and Cushing's syndrome than mature patients because of a larger skin surface area to body weight ratio.
HPA axis suppression, Cushing's syndrome, and intracranial hypertension have been reported in pediatric patients receiving topical corticosteroids. Manifestations of adrenal suppression in pediatric patients include linear growth retardation, delayed weight gain, low plasma cortisol levels, and absence of response to ACTH stimulation. Manifestations of intracranial hypertension include bulging fontanelles, headaches, and bilateral papilledema.
Administration of topical corticosteroids to pediatric patients should be limited to the least amount compatible with an effective therapeutic regimen. Chronic corticosteroid therapy may interfere with the growth and development of pediatric patients. Safety and effectiveness of TOPICORT Ointment 0.25% in pediatric patients below the age of 10 have not been established.

ADVERSE REACTIONS

The following local adverse reactions are reported infrequently with topical corticosteroids, but may occur more frequently with the use of occlusive dressings. These reactions are listed in an approximate decreasing order of occurrence: burning, itching, irritation, dryness, folliculitis, hypertrichosis, acneiform eruptions, hypopigmentation, perioral dermatitis, allergic contact dermatitis, maceration of the skin, secondary infection, skin atrophy, striae, and miliaria.
In controlled clinical studies the incidence of adverse reactions was low (0.8%) for TOPICORT Emollient Cream 0.25% and included burning, folliculitis, and folliculopustular lesions. The incidence of adverse reactions was also 0.8% for TOPICORT LP Emollient Cream 0.05% and included pruritus, erythema, vesiculation, and burning sensation. The incidence of adverse reactions was low (0.3%) for TOPICORT Ointment 0.25% and consisted of development of comedones at the site of application.

OVERDOSAGE

Topically applied corticosteroids can be absorbed in sufficient amounts to produce systemic effects (See **PRECAUTIONS**).

DOSAGE AND ADMINISTRATION

Apply a thin film of TOPICORT Emollient Cream, TOPICORT Ointment, TOPICORT Gel, or TOPICORT LP Emollient Cream to the affected skin areas twice daily. Rub in gently.

HOW SUPPLIED

TOPICORT (desoximetasone) Emollient Cream 0.25% is supplied in 15 gram (NDC 99207-011-15) and 60 gram (NDC 99207-011-60) tubes.
TOPICORT (desoximetasone) Ointment 0.25% is supplied in 15 gram (NDC 99207-025-15) and 60 gram (NDC 99207-025-60) tubes.
TOPICORT (desoximetasone) Gel 0.05% is supplied in 15 gram (NDC 99207-014-15) and 60 gram (NDC 99207-014-60) tubes.
TOPICORT LP (desoximetasone) Emollient Cream 0.05% is supplied in 15 gram (NDC 99207-012-15) and 60 gram (NDC 99207-012-60) tubes.
Store at controlled room temperature 15°– 30° C (59°– 86° F).
Manufactured for:
MEDICIS, The Dermatology Company®
Scottsdale, AZ 85258
by: Hoechst Marion Roussel
Deutschland GmbH,
D-65926 Frankfurt am Main
Made in Germany
REG TM THE AVENTIS GROUP

TRIAZ® ℞

[trī 'ăz]
(benzoyl peroxide)
Gel 3%
Gel 6%
Gel 10%
Cleanser 3%
Cleanser 6%
Cleanser 10%
Prescribing information as of May 2000

Rx Only

DESCRIPTION

TRIAZ® (benzoyl peroxide) 3%, 6%, and 10% Gels and TRIAZ® (benzoyl peroxide) 3%, 6%, and 10% Cleansers are topical, gel-based, benzoyl peroxide containing preparations for use in the treatment of acne vulgaris. Benzoyl peroxide is an oxidizing agent that possesses antibacterial properties and is classified as a keratolytic. Benzoyl peroxide ($C_{14}H_{10}O_4$) is represented by the following chemical structure:

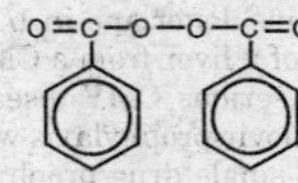

TRIAZ 3% Gel contains Benzoyl Peroxide 3% as the active ingredient in a gel-based formulation consisting of: Water, C12–15 Alkyl Benzoate, Glycerin, Cetearyl 50, Polyacrylamide (and) C12–14 Isoparaffin (and) Laureth-7, PEG-100 Stearate, Steareth S-2, Steareth S-20, Dimethicone 200, Glycolic Acid, Zinc Lactate, Lactic Acid, Disodium EDTA, Sodium Hydroxide.
TRIAZ 6% and 10% Gels contain, respectively, Benzoyl Peroxide 6% and 10% as the active ingredient in a gel-based formulation consisting of: Water, C12-15 Alkyl Benzoate, Glycerin, Cetyl Stearyl Alcohol, Glycolic Acid, Polyacrylamide (and) C13-14 Isoparaffin (and) Laureth-7, Glyceryl Stearate (and) PEG-100 Stearate, Steareth S-2, Sodium Hydroxide, Steareth S-20, Dimethicone, Zinc Lactate, Disodium EDTA.
TRIAZ 3% Cleanser contains Benzoyl Peroxide 3% as the active ingredient in a vehicle consisting of: Glycerin, Petrolatum, C12–15 Alkyl Benzoate, Tauranol I-78, Alfa Olefin Sulfonate, Special Petrolatum Fraction, Zinc Lactate, Carbomer, Potassium Polymetaphosphate, Titanium Dioxide, Triethanolamine, Glycolic Acid, Lavender Extract, Menthol.
TRIAZ 6% and 10% Cleansers contain, respectively, Benzoyl Peroxide 6% and 10% as the active ingredient in a vehicle consisting of: Glycerin, Petrolatum, C12-15 Alkyl Benzoate, Sodium Cocoyl Isethionate, Water, Special Petrolatum Fraction, Sodium C14-16 Olefin Sulfonate, Zinc Lactate, Carbomer, Potassium Polymetaphosphate, Titanium Dioxide, Triethanolamine, Glycolic Acid, Lavender Extract, Menthol.

CLINICAL PHARMACOLOGY

The mechanism of action of benzoyl peroxide is not totally understood but its antibacterial activity against *Propionibacterium acnes* is thought to be a major mode of action. In addition, patients treated with benzoyl peroxide show a reduction in lipids and free fatty acids, and mild desquamation (drying and peeling activity) with simultaneous reduction in comedones and acne lesions. Little is known about the percutaneous penetration, metabolism, and excretion of benzoyl peroxide, although it has been shown that benzoyl peroxide absorbed by the skin is metabolized to benzoic acid and then excreted as benzoate in the urine. There is no evidence of systemic toxicity caused by benzoyl peroxide in humans.

INDICATIONS AND USAGE

TRIAZ 3%, 6%, and 10% Gels and TRIAZ 3%, 6%, and 10% Cleansers are indicated for the topical treatment of acne vulgaris.

CONTRAINDICATIONS

These preparations are contraindicated in patients with a history of hypersensitivity to any of their components.

WARNINGS

When using this product, avoid unnecessary sun exposure and use a sunscreen.

PRECAUTIONS

General: For external use only. If severe irritation develops, discontinue use and institute appropriate therapy. After reaction clears, treatment may often be resumed with less frequent application. These preparations should not be used in or near the eyes or on mucous membranes.
Information for Patients: Avoid contact with eyes, eyelids, lips and mucous membranes. If accidental contact occurs, rinse with water. Contact with any colored material (including hair and fabric) may result in bleaching or discoloration. If excessive irritation develops, discontinue use and consult your physician.
Carcinogenesis, Mutagenesis, Impairment of Fertility: Data from several studies employing a strain of mice that are highly susceptible to developing cancer suggest that benzoyl peroxide acts as a tumor promoter. The clinical significance of these findings to humans is unknown. Benzoyl peroxide has not been found to be mutagenic (Ames Test) and there are no published data indicating it impairs fertility.
Pregnancy: Teratogenic Effects: *Pregnancy Category C:* Animal reproduction studies have not been conducted with benzoyl peroxide. It is not known whether benzoyl peroxide can cause fetal harm when administered to a pregnant woman or can effect reproduction capacity. Benzoyl peroxide should be used by a pregnant woman only if clearly needed. There are no available data on the effect of benzoyl peroxide on the later growth, development and functional maturation of the unborn child.
Nursing Mothers: It is not known whether this drug is excreted in human milk. Because many drugs are excreted in human milk, caution should be exercised when benzoyl peroxide is administered to a nursing woman.
Pediatric Use: Safety and effectiveness in children have not been established.

ADVERSE REACTIONS

Allergic contact dermatitis and dryness have been reported with topical benzoyl peroxide therapy.

OVERDOSAGE

If excessive scaling, erythema or edema occurs, the use of these preparations should be discontinued. To hasten resolution of the adverse effects, cool compresses may be used. After symptoms and signs subside, a reduced dosage schedule may be cautiously tried if the reaction is judged to be due to excessive use and not allergenicity.

DOSAGE AND ADMINISTRATION

TRIAZ Gels: Apply once or twice daily to cover affected areas, or as directed by your dermatologist. Use after washing with a mild cleanser, such as one of the TRIAZ Cleansers, and water.
TRIAZ Cleansers: Wash affected areas once or twice daily, or as directed by your dermatologist. Avoid contact with eyes or mucous membranes. Wet skin and liberally apply to areas to be cleansed, massage gently into skin for 10–20 seconds working into a full lather, rinse thoroughly and pat dry. If drying occurs, it may be controlled by rinsing cleanser off sooner or using less often.

HOW SUPPLIED

TRIAZ 3% Gel—1.5 oz. (42.5 g) tube, NDC 99207-209-01.
TRIAZ 6% Gel—1.5 oz. (42.5 g) tube, NDC 99207-051-01.
TRIAZ 10% Gel—1.5 oz. (42.5 g) tube, NDC 99207-210-01.
TRIAZ 3% Cleanser—6 oz. (170.3 g) tube, NDC 99207-206-12.
TRIAZ 3% Cleanser—12 oz. (340.2 g) bottle, NDC 99207-206-09.
TRIAZ 6% Cleanser—6 oz. (170.3 g) tube, NDC 99207-116-12.
TRIAZ 6% Cleanser—12 oz. (340.2 g) bottle, NDC 99207-116-09.
TRIAZ 10% Cleanser—3 oz. (85.1 g) tube, NDC 99207-106-02.
TRIAZ 10% Cleanser—6 oz. (170.3 g) tube, NDC 99207-106-12.
TRIAZ 10% Cleanser—12 oz. (340.2 g) bottle, NDC 99207-106-09.
Store at 15°–25°C (59°–77°F).
Covered by US Patents: 5,648,389; 5,254,334; 5,409,706; and 5,632,996.
Manufactured for:
MEDICIS, The Dermatology Company®
Scottsdale, AZ 85258
by: Contract Pharmaceuticals Limited,
Mississauga, Ontario CANADA
by: West Pharmaceutical Services Lakewood, Inc.
Lakewood, NJ 08701

MedImmune, Inc.

35 WEST WATKINS MILL ROAD
GAITHERSBURG, MD 20878

For Medical Information Contact:
(800) 949-3789
Adverse Drug Experience:
(800) 949-3789
In Emergencies:
24-hour emergency
(800) 949-3789
Sales and Ordering/Customer Service:
(800) 527-7130
Customer Support Network
(877) 633-4411

CYTOGAM® ℞

CYTOMEGALOVIRUS IMMUNE GLOBULIN INTRAVENOUS (HUMAN) (CMV-IGIV)
Liquid Formulation Solvent Detergent Treated

DESCRIPTION

CytoGam®, Cytomegalovirus Immune Globulin Intravenous (Human) (CMV-IGIV), is an immunoglobulin G (IgG) containing a standardized amount of antibody to Cytomegalovirus (CMV). CMV-IGIV is formulated in final vial as a sterile liquid. The globulin is stabilized with 5% sucrose and 1% Albumin (Human). CytoGam® contains no preservative. The purified immunoglobulin is derived from pooled adult human plasma selected for high titers of antibody for Cyto-

Continued on next page

CytoGam—Cont.

megalovirus (CMV) (1). Source material for fractionation may be obtained from another U.S. licensed manufacturer. Pooled plasma was fractionated by ethanol precipitation of the proteins according to Cohn Methods 6 and 9, modified to yield a product suitable for intravenous administration. A widely utilized solvent-detergent viral inactivation process is also used (2). Certain manufacturing operations may be performed by other firms. Each milliliter contains: 50 ± 10 mg of immunoglobulin, primarily IgG, and trace amount of IgA and IgM; 50 mg of sucrose; 10 mg of Albumin (Human). The sodium content is 20–30 mEq per liter, i.e., 0.4–0.6 mEq per 20 ml or 1.0–1.5 mEq per 50 ml. The solution should appear colorless and translucent.

CLINICAL PHARMACOLOGY

CytoGam® contains IgG antibodies representative of the large number of normal persons who contributed to the plasma pools from which the product was derived. The globulin contains a relatively high concentration of antibodies directed against Cytomegalovirus (CMV). In the case of persons who may be exposed to CMV, CytoGam® can raise the relevant antibodies to levels sufficient to attenuate or reduce the incidence of serious CMV disease.

INDICATIONS AND USAGE

Cytomegalovirus Immune Globulin Intravenous (Human) is indicated for the prophylaxis of cytomegalovirus disease associated with transplantation of kidney, lung, liver, pancreas and heart. In transplants of these organs other than kidney from CMV seropositive donors into seronegative recipients, prophylactic CMV-IGIV should be considered in combination with ganciclovir.

CLINICAL STUDIES

Clinical studies have shown a 50% reduction in primary CMV disease in renal transplant patients given CMV-IGIV (3) and a 56% reduction in serious CMV disease (4) in liver transplant patients given CMV-IGIV. CMV-IGIV prophylaxis was associated with increased survival in liver transplant recipients (5).

In two separate clinical trials, CytoGam® was shown to provide effective prophylaxis in renal-transplant recipients at risk for primary CMV disease. In the first randomized trial, (3) the incidence of virologically confirmed CMV-associated syndromes was reduced from 60% in controls (n=35) to 21% in recipients of CMV immune globulin (n=24) ($p<0.01$); marked leukopenia was reduced from 37% in controls to 4% in globulin recipients ($p<0.01$); and fungal or parasitic superinfections were not seen in globulin recipients but occurred in 20% of controls ($p=0.05$). Serious CMV disease was reduced from 46% to 13%. There was a concomitant but not statistically significant reduction in the incidence of CMV pneumonia (17% of controls as compared with 4% of globulin recipients). There was no effect on rates of viral isolation or seroconversion although the rate of viremia was less in CytoGam® recipients. In a subsequent non-randomized trial in renal transplant recipients (n=36), (6) the incidence of virologically confirmed CMV-associated syndrome was reduced to 36% in the globulin recipients in comparison to a 60% incidence in control patients (n=35) in the randomized trial. The rates of serious CMV disease, and concomitant fungal and parasitic superinfection were similar to patients receiving CMV-IGIV in the first trial.

In a randomized, double-blind, placebo-controlled trial, in liver transplant recipients (4), the incidence of serious CMV-associated disease was reduced from 26% in the 72 control patients to 12% in the 69 CMV-IGIV recipients ($p=0.02$); serious CMV-associated disease included CMV disease in 2 or more organs, CMV pneumonia, or CMV-associated invasive fungal infection, the incidence of which was 18% in controls and 7% in CMV-IGIV recipients ($p=0.04$). In follow-up (5) of the liver transplant patients studied in this randomized controlled trial and a subsequent open-label trial (7), the one year survival of the 72 control patients was 72% versus 86% in the 90 recipients of CMV-IGIV ($p=0.03$). In the randomized control trial, the reduction in serious CMV-associated disease in CMV seronegative recipients of livers from a CMV seropositive donor (7/19 in the CMV-IGIV group vs. 9/19 in control) was less than in transplants with other donor and recipient serologic status (1/50 in the CMV-IGIV group vs. 10/53 in the control group). This finding was similar to that of Merigan et al. (8) in a study of ganciclovir prophylaxis after heart transplantation. In this study, patients received ganciclovir IV at 5mg/kg bid for the initial 14 days post-transplant, then at 6 mg/kg each day for 5 days per week through day 28.

Recent studies of combined prophylaxis with CMV-IGIV and ganciclovir have shown reductions in the incidence of serious CMV associated disease in CMV seronegative recipients of CMV seropositive organs below that expected from one drug alone (9–12).

Ham et al. (9) used CMV-IGIV with a dosage schedule of 150 mg/kg CMV-IGIV within 72 hours of transplant; 100 mg/kg at two, four, six and eight weeks following liver transplant and then 50 mg/kg at 12 and 16 weeks post-transplant in combination with ganciclovir (10 mg/kg/day for 14 days). The incidence of CMV disease was reduced from an expected 60–80% rate to 7% in 15 seronegative recipients of a seropositive organ.

Snydman (10) using the CMV-IGIV dosage schedule listed under DOSAGE AND ADMINISTRATION Section in combination with ganciclovir (10 mg/kg/day for 14 days) reduced the incidence of serious CMV disease in D+R− liver transplant recipients receiving placebo or one drug from 16/47 (34%) to 3/41 (7%) in patients receiving both drugs for prophylaxis.

		Type of Transplant	
		Kidney	Liver, Pancreas Lung, Heart
Within:	72 hours of transplant:	150 mg/kg	150 mg/kg
	2 weeks post transplant:	100 mg/kg	150 mg/kg
	4 weeks post transplant	100 mg/kg	150 mg/kg
	6 weeks post transplant:	100 mg/kg	150 mg/kg
	8 weeks post transplant:	100 mg/kg	150 mg/kg
	12 weeks post transplant:	50 mg/kg	100 mg/kg
	16 weeks post transplant:	50 mg/kg	100 mg/kg

Martin (11) using CMV-IGIV 100 mg/kg every two weeks for six weeks followed by 50 mg/kg every two weeks with a final dose at week 16, in combination with ganciclovir 10 mg/kg/day for 14 days after transplantation, observed severe CMV disease in 1/74 (1%) of CMV seronegative recipients of a kidney from a CMV seropositive donor, in 0/14 (0%) of CMV seronegative recipients of a kidney-pancreas transplant from a CMV seropositive donor and in 1/12 (8%) of CMV seronegative recipients of a liver from a CMV seropositive donor. The incidence of serious CMV disease with combined CMV-IGIV and ganciclovir prophylaxis was lower than previous experience with single drug prophylaxis.

Valantine and Luikart (12) compared prophylaxis with CMV-IGIV (biweekly for three months) in combination with ganciclovir prophylaxis (IV at 5mg/kg bid for the initial 14 days post-transplant, then at 6 mg/kg through day 28) in 16 CMV seronegative recipients of hearts from CMV seropositive donors with 16 matched controls receiving ganciclovir alone. The actuarial incidence of CMV disease was reduced from 55% in the ganciclovir group to 46% in the combined group ($p\leq0.06$) and survival was increased from 61% to 94% ($p\leq0.001$). In heart-lung or lung transplant patients in whom either the donor or recipient was CMV seropositive, the actuarial incidence of CMV disease in patients receiving ganciclovir alone (n=25) was 85% as compared to 36% of the 33 patients receiving both CMV-IGIV and ganciclovir ($p\leq0.05$). Survival was 60% in the ganciclovir group and 80% in patients receiving CMV-IGIV and ganciclovir ($p\leq0.01$).

CONTRAINDICATIONS

CytoGam® should not be used in individuals with a history of a prior severe reaction associated with the administration of this or other human immunoglobulin preparations. Persons with selective immunoglobulin A deficiency have the potential for developing antibodies to immunoglobulin A and could have anaphylactic reactions to subsequent administration of blood products that contain immunoglobulin A, including CytoGam®.

WARNINGS

CMV-IGIV is made from human plasma and, like other plasma products, carries the possibility for transmission of blood-borne viral agents and theoretically, the Creutzfeldt-Jakob disease (CJD) agent. The risk of transmission of recognized blood-borne viruses is considered to be low because of the viral inactivation and removal properties in the Cohn-Oncley cold ethanol precipitation procedure used for purification of immune globulin products (13–15). Until 1993, cold ethanol manufactured immune globulins licensed in the United States had not been documented to transmit any viral agent. However, during a brief period in late 1993 to early 1994, intravenous immune globulin made by one U.S. manufacturer was associated with transmission of Hepatitis C virus (16). To further guard against possible transmission of blood-borne viruses, including Hepatitis C, CMV-IGIV is treated with a solvent detergent viral inactivation procedure (2) known to inactivate a wide spectrum of lipid enveloped viruses, including HIV-1, HIV-2, Hepatitis B, and Hepatitis C (17). However, because new blood-borne viruses may yet emerge, some of which may not be inactivated by the manufacturing process or by solvent detergent treatment, CMV-IGIV, like any other blood product, should be given only if a benefit is expected. All infections should be reported directly to your physician and to the Massachusetts Public Health Biologic Laboratories (617-983-6400). Please discuss the risk and benefits of this product with your physician.

Immune Globulin Intravenous (Human) products have been reported to be associated with renal dysfunction, acute renal failure, osmotic nephrosis and death (18–20). Patients predisposed to acute renal failure include patients with any degree of pre-existing renal insufficiency, diabetes mellitus, age greater than 65, volume depletion, sepsis, paraproteinemia or patients receiving known nephrotoxic drugs. Especially in such patients, IGIV products should be administered at the minimum concentrations available and the minimum rate of infusion practical. While these reports of renal dysfunction and acute renal failure have been associated with the use of many IGIV products, those containing sucrose as a stabilizer (and given at daily doses of 400 mg/kg or greater) account for a disproportionate share of the total number. CytoGam® contains sucrose as a stabilizer. See Precautions and Dosage and Administration sections for important information intended to reduce the risk of acute renal failure.

During administration, the patient's vital signs should be monitored continuously and careful observation made for any symptoms throughout the infusion. Epinephrine should be available for the treatment of an acute anaphylactic reaction (see PRECAUTIONS section).

PRECAUTIONS

Assure that patients are not volume depleted prior to the initiation of IGIV. Periodic monitoring of renal function tests and urine output is particularly important in patients judged to have a potential increased risk for developing acute renal failure. Renal function, including the measurement of blood urea nitrogen (BUN) or serum creatinine should be assessed prior to the initial infusion of CytoGam® and again at appropriate intervals thereafter. If renal function deteriorates, discontinuation of the product should be considered. For patients judged to be at risk for developing renal dysfunction, it may be prudent to reduce the amount of product infused per unit time by infusing CytoGam® at rate of 180mg Ig/kg/hour or less. The recommended rate of Cytogam® infusion for prophylaxis of CMV disease in solid organ transplant patients is 60 mg Ig/kg/hr (see DOSAGE AND ADMINISTRATION)

Although systemic allergic reactions are rare (see ADVERSE REACTIONS section), epinephrine and diphenhydramine should be available for treatment of acute allergic symptoms. If hypotension or anaphylaxis occur, the administration of the immunoglobulin should be discontinued immediately and an antidote should be given as noted above.

An aseptic meningitis syndrome (AMS) has been reported to occur infrequently in association with Immune Globulin Intravenous (Human) (IGIV) treatment (21–24). The syndrome usually begins within several hours to two days following IGIV treatment. It is characterized by symptoms and signs including severe headache, nuchal rigidity, drowsiness, fever, photophobia, painful eye movements, and nausea and vomiting. Cerebrospinal fluid (CSF) studies are frequently positive with pleocytosis up to several thousand cells per cu.mm., predominantly from the granulocytic series, and elevated protein levels up to several hundred mg/dl. Patients exhibiting such symptoms and signs should receive a thorough neurological examination, including CSF studies, to rule out other causes of meningitis. AMS may occur more frequently in association with high dose (2 g/kg) IGIV treatment. Discontinuation of IGIV treatment has resulted in remission of AMS within several days without sequelae.

CytoGam® does not contain a preservative. The vial should be entered only once for administration purposes and the infusion should begin within 6 hours. The infusion schedule should be adhered to closely (see INFUSION section). Do not use if the solution is turbid.

Drug Interactions: Antibodies present in immune globulin preparation may interfere with the immune response to live virus vaccines such as measles, mumps, and rubella; therefore, vaccination with live virus vaccines should be deferred until approximately three months after administration of CytoGam®. If such vaccinations were given shortly after CytoGam®, a revaccination may be necessary. Admixtures of CytoGam® with other drugs have not been evaluated. It is recommended that CytoGam® be administered separately from other drugs or medications which the patient may be receiving (see DOSING AND ADMINISTRATION section).

Pregnancy Category C: Animal reproduction studies have not been conducted with Cytomegalovirus Immune Globulin Intravenous (Human). It is also not known whether Cytomegalovirus Immune Globulin Intravenous (Human) can cause fetal harm when administered to a pregnant woman or can affect reproduction capacity. Cytomegalovirus Immune Globulin Intravenous (Human) should be given to a pregnant woman only if clearly needed.

ADVERSE REACTIONS

Minor reactions such as flushing, chills, muscle cramps, back pain, fever, nausea, vomiting, arthralgia, and wheezing were the most frequent adverse reactions observed during the clinical trials of CytoGam®. The incidence of these reactions during the clinical trials was less than 6.0% of all infusions and such reactions were most often related to infusion rates. A decrease in blood pressure was observed in 1 of 1039 infusions in clinical trials of CytoGam®. If a patient develops a minor side effect, *slow the rate* immediately or temporarily interrupt the infusion.

Increases in serum creatinine and blood urea nitrogen (BUN) have been observed as soon as one to two days following IGIV infusion. Progression to oliguria or anuria requiring dialysis has been observed. Types of severe renal adverse events that have been seen following IGIV therapy include acute renal failure, acute tubular necrosis, proximal tubular nephropathy and osmotic nephrosis (18–20).

Severe reactions such as angioneurotic edema and anaphylactic shock, although not observed during clinical trials, are a possibility. Clinical anaphylaxis may occur even when

NDC No.	Total Quantity of Immunoglobulin	Volume	Concentration
60574-3102-1	1000 mg ± 200 mg	20 ml	50 ± 10 mg/ml
60574-3101-1	2500 mg ± 500 mg	50 ml	50 ± 10 mg/ml

the patient is not known to be sensitized to immune globulin products. A reaction may be related to the rate of infusion; therefore, carefully adhere to the infusion rates as outlined under "DOSAGE AND ADMINISTRATION." If anaphylaxis or drop in blood pressure occurs, *discontinue infusion* and use antidote such as diphenhydramine and adrenalin.

OVERDOSAGE

Although few data are available, clinical experience with other immunoglobulin preparations suggests that the major manifestations would be those related to volume overload.

DOSAGE AND ADMINISTRATION

The maximum recommended total dosage per infusion is 150 mg Ig/kg, administered according to the following schedule.
[See table at top of previous page]

Preparation for Administration. Remove the tab portion of the vial cap and clean the rubber stopper with 70% alcohol or equivalent. DO NOT SHAKE VIAL; AVOID FOAMING. Parenteral drug products should be inspected visually for particulate matter and discoloration prior to administration whenever solution and container permit. Infuse the solution only if it is colorless, free of particulate matter and not turbid.

Infusion. Infusion should begin within 6 hours after entering the vial and should be complete within 12 hours of entering the vial. Vital signs should be taken preinfusion, midway and post-infusion as well as before any rate increase. CytoGam® should be administered through an intravenous line using an administration set that contains an in-line filter (pore size 15µ) and a constant infusion pump (i.e., IVAC pump or equivalent). A smaller in-line filter (0.2µ) is also acceptable. Pre-dilution of CytoGam® before infusion is not recommended.

CytoGam® should be administered through a separate intravenous line. If this is not possible, CytoGam® may be "piggybacked" into a pre-existing line if that line contains either Sodium Chloride, Injection, USP, or one of the following dextrose solutions (with or without NaCl added): 2.5% dextrose in water, 5% dextrose in water, 10% dextrose in water, 20% dextrose in water. If a pre-existing line must be used, the CytoGam® should not be diluted more than 1:2 with any of the above-named solutions. Admixtures of CytoGam® with any other solutions have not been evaluated.

Initial Dose. Administer intravenously at 15 mg Ig per kg body weight per hour. If no adverse reactions occur after 30 minutes, the rate may be increased to 30 mg Ig/kg/hr; if no adverse reactions occur after a subsequent 30 minutes, then the infusion may be increased to 60 mg Ig/kg/hr (volume not to exceed 75 ml/hour). DO NOT EXCEED THIS RATE OF ADMINISTRATION. The patient should be monitored closely during and after each rate change.

Subsequent Doses. Administer at 15 mg Ig/kg/hr for 15 minutes. If no adverse reactions occur, increase to 30 mg Ig/kg/hr for 15 minutes and then increase to a maximum rate of 60 mg Ig/kg/hr (volume not to exceed 75 ml/hour). DO NOT EXCEED THIS RATE OF ADMINISTRATION. The patient should be monitored closely during each rate change.

CytoGam® should be used with caution in patients with pre-existing renal insufficiency and in patients judged to be at increased risk of developing renal insufficiency (including, but not limited to those with diabetes mellitus, age greater than 65, volume depletion, paraproteinemia, sepsis and patients receiving known nephrotoxic drugs). In these cases especially, it is important to assure that patients are not volume depleted prior to CytoGam® infusion. While most cases of renal insufficiency have occurred in patients receiving total doses of 400 mg Ig/kg or greater, no prospective data are presently available to identify a maximum safe dose, concentration or rate of infusion in patients determined to be at increased risk of acute renal failure. In the absence of prospective data, recommended doses should not be exceeded and the concentration and infusion rate selected should be the minimum practicable. The product should be infused at a rate of 180 mg Ig/kg/hr or less.

Potential adverse reactions are: flushing, chills, muscle cramps, back pain, fever, nausea, vomiting, wheezing, drop in blood pressure. Minor adverse reactions have been infusion rate related—if the patient develops a minor side effects (i.e., nausea, back pain, flushing), slow the rate or temporarily interrupt the infusion. If anaphylaxis or drop in blood pressure occurs, discontinue infusion and use antidote such as diphenhydramine and adrenalin.

To prevent the transmission of hepatitis viruses or other infectious agents from one person to another, sterile disposable syringes and needles should be used. The syringes and needles should not be reused.

HOW SUPPLIED

CytoGam®, Cytomegalovirus Immune Globulin Intravenous (Human), is supplied in two single-dose vial forms:
[See table above]

STORAGE

CytoGam® should be stored between 2° C and 8° C (35.6° F and 46.4° F), and used within 6 hours after entering the vial.

REFERENCES

1. Snydman DR, Melver J, Leszczynski J, et al. A pilot trial of a novel cytomegalovirus immune globulin in renal transplant recipients. Transplantation 38:553–557, 1984. **2.** Horowitz B, Wiebe ME, Lippin A, et al. Inactivation of viruses in labile blood derivatives. Transfusion; 25:516–522, 1985. **3.** Snydman DR, Werner BG, and Heinze-Lacey BH, et al. Use of cytomegalovirus immune globulin to prevent cytomegalovirus disease in renal transplant recipients. NEJM 317:1049–1054, 1987. **4.** Snydman DR, Werner BG, Dougherty NN et al. Cytomegalovirus Immune Globulin prophylaxis in liver transplantation. A randomized, double-blind, placebo-controlled trial. Ann Int Med 119:984–991, 1993. **5.** Falagas ME, Snydman DR, Ruthazer R. et al. Cytomegalovirus Immune Globulin (CMVIG) prophylaxis is associated with increased survival after orthotopic liver transplantation. Clin Transplantation, 11:432–437, 1997. **6.** Snydman DR, Werner BG, Tilney NL, et al. A final analysis of primary cytomegalovirus disease prevention in renal transplant recipients with a cytomegalovirus immune globulin: Comparison of randomized and open-label trials. Transplant Proceed 23:1357–1360, 1991. **7.** Snydman DR, Werner BG, Dougherty NN, et al. A further analysis of the use of Cytomegalovirus Immune Globulin in orthotopic liver transplant patients at risk for primary infection. Transplant Proceed 26, suppl 1:23–27, 1994. **8.** Merigan TC, Renlund DG, Keay S et al. A controlled trial of ganciclovir to prevent cytomegalovirus disease after heart transplantation. NEJM 326:1182–1186, 1992. **9.** Ham JM, Shelden SR, Godkin RR, et al. Cytomegalovirus prophylaxis with ganciclovir, acyclovir and CMV hyperimmune globulin in liver transplant patients receiving OKT3 induction. Transplant Proc 1995; 27 (5 suppl 1):31–33. **10.** Snydman DR. Combined CMV-IGIV and ganciclovir prophylaxis in CMV seronegative transplant recipients from CMV seropositive donors. Report on file, MedImmune, Inc. **11.** Martin M. CMV prophylaxis with combination ganciclovir and CMV hyperimmune globulin followed by high-dose acyclovir in solid organ transplant recipients. Report on file, MedImmune, Inc. **12.** Valantine H and Luikart H. Impact of CMV hyperimmune globulin on outcome after cardiothoracic transplantation: A comparative study of combined prophylaxis with CMVIG plus ganciclovir vs. ganciclovir alone. Report on file, MedImmune, Inc. **13.** Bossell, et al. Safety of therapeutic immune globulin preparations with respect to transmission of human T-lymphotropic virus type III/lymphadenopathy-associated virus infection. MMWR vol. 35:231–233, April 11, 1996. **14.** Wells MA, Wittek AE, Epstein JS, et al. Inactivation and partition of human T-cell lymphotropic virus, type III, during ethanol fractionation of plasma. Transfusion 26:210–213, 1986. **15.** McIver J, Grady G. Immunoglobulin preparations. In: Churchill WH and Kurtz SR, (ed): Transfusion Medicine. Boston: Blackwell; 1988. **16.** Schneider L, Geha R. Outbreak of Hepatitis C associated with intravenous immunoglobulin administration—United States, October 1993–June 1994. MMWR vol. 43:505–509, July 22, 1994. **17.** Edwards CA, Piet MPJ, Chin S, et al. Tri(nButyl) phosphate detergent treatment of licensed therapeutic and experimental blood derivatives. Vox Sang 52:53–59, 1987.**18.** Cayco AV, Perazella MA, Hayslett JP. Renal insufficiency after intravenous immune globulin therapy: A report of two cases and an analysis of the literature. J Am Soc Nephrology; 8: 1788–1793, 1997. **19.** Cantu TG, Hoehn-Saric EW, Burgess KM et al. Acute renal failure associated with immunoglobulin therapy. Am J. Kidney Dis; 25: 228–234, 1995. **20.** Hansen-Schmidt S., Silomon J, Keller F. Osmotic nephrosis due to high-dose immunoglobulin therapy containing sucrose (but not with glycine) in a patient with immunoglobulin a nephritis. Am. J. Kidney Dis.; 28: 451–453, 1996. **21.** Sekul E, Culper E, Dalaks M. Aseptic meningitis associated with high-dose intravenous immunoglobulin therapy; Frequency and risk factors. Ann Int Med; 123:259–262, 1994. **22.** Kato E, Shindo S, Eto Y, et al. Administration of immune globulin associated with aseptic meningitis. JAMA; 259:3269–3270, 1988. **23.** Casteels Van Daele M, Wijndaele L, Hunnick K, et al. Intravenous immunoglobulin and acute aseptic meningitis. NEJM; 323:614–615, 1990. **24.** Scribner C, Kapit R, Philips E, et al. Aseptic meningitis and intravenous immunoglobulin therapy. Ann Intern Med; 121:305–306, 1994.

For additional information concerning Cytomegalovirus Immune Globulin Intravenous (Human) contact:
Professional Services
MedImmune, Inc.
35 West Watkins Mill Road
Gaithersburg, MD 20878, USA
1-800-949-3789
Manufactured by:
MASSACHUSETTS PUBLIC HEALTH BIOLOGIC LABORATORIES
Boston, Massachusetts 02130, USA
U.S. Govt. License No. 64
Marketed by:
MedImmune Inc.
35 W. Watkins Mill Road
Gaithersburg, MD 20878
Revised April 2000

Shown in Product Identification Guide, page 323

SYNAGIS® ℞
(palivizumab)
for Intramuscular Administration

DESCRIPTION

Synagis® (palivizumab) is a humanized monoclonal antibody (IgG1κ) produced by recombinant DNA technology, directed to an epitope in the A antigenic site of the F protein of respiratory syncytial virus (RSV). Palivizumab is a composite of human (95%) and murine (5%) antibody sequences. The human heavy chain sequence was derived from the constant domains of human IgG1 and the variable framework regions of the V_H genes Cor (1) and Cess (2). The human light chain sequence was derived from the constant domain of Cκ and the variable framework regions of the V_L gene K104 with Jκ -4 (3). The murine sequences were derived from a murine monoclonal antibody, Mab 1129 (4), in a process which involved the grafting of the murine complementarity determining regions into the human antibody frameworks. Synagis® is composed of two heavy chains and two light chains and has a molecular weight of approximately 148,000 Daltons.

Synagis® is supplied as a sterile lyophilized product for reconstitution with sterile water for injection. Reconstituted Synagis® is to be administered by intramuscular injection only. Upon reconstitution, Synagis® contains the following excipients: 47 mM histidine, 3.0 mM glycine and 5.6% mannitol and the active ingredient, palivizumab, at a concentration of 100 milligrams per vial. The reconstituted solution should appear clear or slightly opalescent.

CLINICAL PHARMACOLOGY

Mechanism of Action: Synagis® exhibits neutralizing and fusion-inhibitory activity against RSV. These activities inhibit RSV replication in laboratory experiments. Although resistant RSV strains may be isolated in laboratory studies, a panel of 57 clinical RSV isolates were all neutralized by Synagis® (5). Synagis® serum concentrations of ≥ 40 µg/ml have been shown to reduce pulmonary RSV replication in the cotton rat model of RSV infection by 100-fold (5). The *in vivo* neutralizing activity of the active ingredient in Synagis® was assessed in a randomized, placebo-controlled study of 35 pediatric patients tracheally intubated because of RSV disease. In these patients, palivizumab significantly reduced the quantity of RSV in the lower respiratory tract compared to control patients (6).

Pharmacokinetics: In studies in adult volunteers Synagis® had a pharmacokinetic profile similar to a human IgG1 antibody in regard to the volume of distribution and the half-life (mean 18 days). In pediatric patients less than 24 months of age, the mean half-life of Synagis® was 20 days and monthly intramuscular doses of 15 mg/kg achieved mean ±SD 30 day trough serum drug concentrations of 37 ±21 µg/mL after the first injection, 57 ±41 µg/mL after the second injection, 68 ±51 µg/mL after the third injection and 72 ±50 µg/mL after the fourth injection (7). In pediatric patients given Synagis® for a second season, the mean ±SD serum concentrations following the first and fourth injections were 61 ±17 µg/mL and 86 ±31 µg/mL, respectively.

CLINICAL STUDIES

The safety and efficacy of Synagis® were assessed in a randomized, double-blind, placebo-controlled trial (IMpact-RSV Trial) of RSV disease prophylaxis among high-risk pediatric patients (7). This trial, conducted at 139 centers in the United States, Canada and the United Kingdom, studied patients ≤ 24 months of age with bronchopulmonary dysplasia (BPD) and patients with premature birth (≤ 35 weeks gestation) who were ≤ 6 months of age at study entry. Patients with uncorrected congenital heart disease were excluded from enrollment. In this trial, 500 patients were randomized to receive five monthly placebo injections and 1,002 patients were randomized to receive five monthly injections of 15 mg/kg of Synagis®. Subjects were randomized into the study from November 15 to December 13, 1996, and were followed for safety and efficacy for 150 days. Ninety-nine percent of all subjects completed the study and 93% received all five injections. The primary endpoint was the incidence of RSV hospitalization.

RSV hospitalizations occurred among 53 of 500 (10.6%) patients in the placebo group and 48 of 1002 (4.8%) patients in the Synagis® group, a 55% reduction ($p<0.001$). The reduction of RSV hospitalization was observed both in patients enrolled with a diagnosis of BPD (34/266 [12.8%] placebo vs 39/496 [7.9%] Synagis®) and patients enrolled with a diagnosis of prematurity without BPD (19/234 [8.1%] placebo vs 9/506 [1.8%] Synagis®). The reduction of RSV hospitalization was observed throughout the course of the RSV season. Among secondary endpoints, the incidence of ICU admission during hospitalization for RSV infection was lower among subjects receiving Synagis® (1.3%) than among those receiving placebo (3.0%), but there was no difference in the mean duration of ICU care between the two groups for patients requiring ICU care. Overall, the data do not suggest that RSV illness was less severe among patients who received Synagis® and who required hospitalization due to RSV infection than among placebo patients who required hospitalization due to RSV infection. Synagis® did not alter the incidence and mean duration of hospitalization for non-RSV respiratory illness or the incidence of otitis media.

Continued on next page

Synagis—Cont.

INDICATIONS AND USAGE

Synagis® is indicated for the prevention of serious lower respiratory tract disease caused by respiratory syncytial virus (RSV) in pediatric patients at high risk of RSV disease. Safety and efficacy were established in infants with bronchopulmonary dysplasia (BPD) and infants with a history of prematurity (≤ 35 weeks gestational age). (See *Clinical Studies* section)

CONTRAINDICATIONS

Synagis® should not be used in pediatric patients with a history of a severe prior reaction to Synagis® or other components of this product.

WARNINGS

Anaphylactoid reactions following the administration of Synagis® have not been observed but can occur following the administration of proteins. **If anaphylaxis or severe allergic reaction occurs, administer epinephrine (1:1000) and provide supportive care as required.**

PRECAUTIONS

General: Synagis® is for intramuscular use only. As with any intramuscular injection, Synagis® should be given with caution to patients with thrombocytopenia or any coagulation disorder.

The safety and efficacy of Synagis® have not been demonstrated for treatment of established RSV disease.

The single-use vial of Synagis® does not contain a preservative. Injections should be given within 6 hours after reconstitution.

Immunogenicity: In the IMpact-RSV trial, the incidence of anti-humanized antibody following the fourth injection was 1.1% in the placebo group and 0.7% in the Synagis® group. In pediatric patients receiving Synagis® for a second season, one of fifty-six patients had transient, low titer reactivity. This reactivity was not associated with adverse events or alteration in Synagis® serum concentrations.

Drug Interactions: No formal drug-drug interaction studies were conducted. In the IMpact-RSV trial, the proportions of patients in the placebo and Synagis® groups who received routine childhood vaccines, influenza vaccine, bronchodilators or corticosteroids were similar and no incremental increase in adverse reactions was observed among patients receiving these agents.

Carcinogenesis, Mutagenesis, Impairment of Fertility: Carcinogenesis, mutagenesis and reproductive toxicity studies have not performed.

Pregnancy: Pregnancy Category C: Synagis® is not indicated for adult usage and animal reproduction studies have not been conducted. It is also not known whether Synagis® can cause fetal harm when administered to a pregnant woman or could affect reproductive capacity.

ADVERSE REACTIONS

In the combined pediatric prophylaxis studies of pediatric patients with BPD or prematurity involving 520 subjects receiving placebo and 1168 subjects receiving Synagis®, the proportions of subjects in the placebo and Synagis® groups who experienced any adverse event or any serious adverse event were similar.

Most of the safety information was derived from the IMpact-RSV trial. In this study, Synagis® (palivizumab) was discontinued in five patients: two because of vomiting and diarrhea, one because of erythema and moderate induration at the site of the fourth injection, and two because of preexisting medical conditions which required management (one with congenital anemia and one with pulmonary venous stenosis requiring cardiac surgery). Deaths in study patients occurred in five of 500 placebo recipients and four of 1002 Synagis® recipients. Sudden infant death syndrome was responsible for two of these deaths in the placebo group and one death in the Synagis® group. Adverse events which occurred in more than 1% of patients receiving Synagis® in the IMpact-RSV study for which the incidence in the Synagis® group was 1% greater than in the placebo group are shown in Table 1.

Table 1. Adverse Events Occurring in IMpact-RSV Study at Greater Frequency in the Synagis® Group

% of patients with:	Placebo n = 500	Synagis® n = 1002
upper respiratory infection	49.0%	52.6%
otitis media	40.0%	41.9%
rhinitis	23.4%	28.7%
rash	22.4%	25.6%
pain	6.8%	8.5%
hernia	5.0%	6.3%
SGOT increased	3.8%	4.9%
pharyngitis	1.4%	2.6%

Other adverse events reported in more than 1% of the Synagis® group included: fever, cough, wheeze, bronchiolitis, pneumonia, bronchitis, asthma, croup, dyspnea, sinusitis, apnea, failure to thrive, nervousness, diarrhea, vomiting, and gastroenteritis, SGPT increase, liver function abnormality, study drug injections site reaction, conjunctivitis, viral infection, oral monilia, fungal dermatitis, eczema, seborrhea, anemia and flu syndrome. The incidence of these adverse events was similar between the Synagis® and placebo groups.

OVERDOSAGE

No data from clinical studies are available on overdosage. No toxicity was observed in rabbits administered a single intramuscular or subcutaneous injection of Synagis® at a dose of 50 mg/kg. No data are available from human subjects who have received more than 5 monthly Synagis® doses during a single RSV season.

DOSAGE AND ADMINISTRATION

The recommended dose of Synagis® is 15 mg/kg of body weight. Patients, including those who develop an RSV infection, should receive monthly doses throughout the RSV season. The first dose should be administered prior to commencement of the RSV season. In the northern hemisphere, the RSV season typically commences in November and lasts through April, but it may begin earlier or persist later in certain communities.

Synagis® should be administered in a dose of 15 mg/kg intramuscularly using aseptic technique, preferably in the anterolateral aspect of the thigh. The gluteal muscle should not be used routinely as an injection site because of the risk of damage to the sciatic nerve. The dose per month = [patient weight (kg) × 15 mg/kg ÷ 100 mg/mL of Synagis®]. Injection volumes over 1 mL should be given as a divided dose.

Preparation for Administration

- To reconstitute, remove the tab portion of the vial cap and clean the rubber stopper with 70% ethanol or equivalent.
- Both the 50 mg and 100 mg vials contain an overfill to allow the withdrawal of 50 milligrams or 100 milligrams respectively when reconstituted following the directions described below.
- Slowly add 0.6 mL of sterile water for injection to the 50 mg vial or add 1.0 mL of sterile water for injection to the 100 mg vial. The vial should be gently swirled for 30 seconds to avoid foaming. DO NOT SHAKE VIAL.
- Reconstituted Synagis® should stand at room temperature for a minimum of 20 minutes until the solution clarifies.
- Reconstituted Synagis® does not contain a preservative and should be administered within 6 hours of reconstitution

To prevent the transmission of hepatitis viruses or other infectious agents from one person to another, sterile disposable syringes and needles should be used. Do not reuse syringes and needles.

HOW SUPPLIED

Synagis® is supplied in single use vials as lyophilized powder to deliver either 50 milligrams or 100 milligrams when reconstituted with sterile water for injection.

50 mg vial NDC 60574-4112-1

Upon reconstitution the 50 mg vial contains 50 milligrams Synagis® in 0.5 mL.

100 mg vial NDC 60574-4111-1

Upon reconstitution the 100 mg vial contains 100 milligrams Synagis® in 1.0 mL.

Upon receipt and until reconstitution for use, Synagis® should be stored between 2 and 8°C (35.6° and 46.4°F) in its original container. Do not freeze. Do not use beyond the expiration date.

REFERENCES

1. Press E, and Hogg N. The amino acid sequences of the Fd Fragments of Two Human gamma-1 heavy chains. Biochem. J. 1970;117:641–660.
2. Takahashi N, Noma T, and Honjo T. Rearranged immunoglobulin heavy chain variable region (V_H) pseudogene that deletes the second complementarity-determining region. Proc. Nat. Acad. Sci. USA 1984;81:5194–5198.
3. Bentley D, and Rabbitts T. Human immunoglobulin variable region genes – DNA sequences of two V_k genes and a pseudogene. Nature 1980;288:730–733.
4. Beeler JA and Van Wyke Coelingh K. Neutralization epitopes of the F Protein of Respiratory Syncytial Virus: Effect of mutation upon fusion function. J. Virology 1989;63:2941–2950
5. Johnson S, Oliver C, Prince GA, et al. Development of a humanized monoclonal antibody (MEDI-493) with potent in vitro and in vivo activity against respiratory syncytial virus. J. Infect. Dis. 1997; 176:1215–1224.
6. DeVincenzo, JP, Malley R, Ramilo O, et al. Viral Concentraction in Upper and Lower Respiratory Secretions from Respiratory Syncytial Virus (RSV) Infected Children Treated with RSV Monoclonal Antibody (MEDI-493). Pediatric Research 1998; 43: 144A [Abstract 830].
7. The IMpact RSV Study Group. Palivizumab, a Humanized Respiratory Syncytial Virus Monoclonal Antibody, Reduces Hospitalization From Respiratory Syncytial Virus Infection in High-risk Infants. *Pediatrics in press.*

® Synagis is a registered trademark of MedImmune Inc.

Manufactured by:
MedImmune, Inc.
Gaithersburg, MD 20878
(1-877-633-4411)

Co-Marketed by:
Ross Products Division
Abbott Laboratories, Inc.
Columbus, Ohio 43215-1724

Rev. date: December 2, 1999 3AG1103

Shown in Product Identification Guide, page 323

MedImmune Oncology, Inc.

ONE TOWER BRIDGE
100 FRONT STREET
WEST CONSHOHOCKEN, PA 19428

Direct Inquiries to:
MedImmune Oncology, Inc.
(877)-633-4411

For Medical Information, adverse drug experiences, product sales, and ordering, and other inquiries please contact:
(800)-949-3789.
internet—www.medimmune.com

For Emergencies, 24 hours.
(800)-949-3789

Ethyol® (amifostine), see Listing under ALZA Pharmaceuticals

HEXALEN® ℞

[hex 'a-len]
(ALTRETAMINE)
CAPSULES
50 mg

WARNINGS

1. HEXALEN® should only be given under the supervision of a physician experienced in the use of antineoplastic agents.
2. Peripheral blood counts should be monitored at least monthly, prior to the initiation of each course of HEXALEN, and as clinically indicated (see Adverse Reactions).
3. Because of the possibility of HEXALEN-related neurotoxicity, neurologic examination should be performed regularly during HEXALEN administration (see Adverse Reactions).

DESCRIPTION

HEXALEN (altretamine), is a synthetic cytotoxic antineoplastic s-triazine derivative. HEXALEN capsules contain 50 mg of altretamine for oral administration. Inert ingredients include lactose, anhydrous and calcium stearate. Altretamine, known chemically as N,N,N′,N′,N″,N″-hexamethyl-1,3,5-triazine-2,4,6-triamine, has the following structural formula:

$(CH_3)_2N$ — triazine ring — $N(CH_3)_2$, with $N(CH_3)_2$

Its empirical formula is $C_9H_{18}N_6$ with a molecular weight of 210.28. Altretamine is a white crystalline powder, melting at 172° ± 1°C. Altretamine is practically insoluble in water but is increasingly soluble at pH 3 and below.

CLINICAL PHARMACOLOGY

The precise mechanism by which HEXALEN exerts its cytotoxic effect is unknown, although a number of theoretical possibilities have been studied. Structurally, HEXALEN resembles the alkylating agent triethylenemelamine, yet *in vitro* tests for alkylating activity of HEXALEN and its metabolites have been negative. HEXALEN has been demonstrated to be efficacious for certain ovarian tumors resistant to classical alkylating agents. Metabolism of altretamine is a requirement for cytotoxicity. Synthetic monohydroxymethylmelamines, and products of altretamine metabolism, *in vitro* and *in vivo*, can form covalent adducts with tissue macromolecules including DNA, but the relevance of these reactions to antitumor activity is unknown.

HEXALEN is well-absorbed following oral administration in humans, but undergoes rapid and extensive demethylation in the liver, producing variation in altretamine plasma levels. The principal metabolites are pentamethylmelamine and tetramethylmelamine.

Pharmacokinetic studies were performed in a limited number of patients and should be considered preliminary. After oral administration of HEXALEN to 11 patients with advanced ovarian cancer in doses of 120–300 mg/m², peak plasma levels (as measured by gas-chromatographic assay) were reached between 0.5 and 3 hours, varying from 0.2 to 20.8 mg/l. Half-life of the β-phase of elimination ranged from 4.7 to 10.2 hours. Altretamine and metabolites show binding to plasma proteins. The free fractions of altretamine, pentamethylmelamine and tetramethylmelamine are 6%, 25% and 50%, respectively.

Following oral administration of ^{14}C-ring-labeled altretamine (4 mg/kg), urinary recovery of radioactivity was 61% at 24 hours and 90% at 72 hours. Human urinary metabolites were N-demethylated homologues of altretamine with <1% unmetabolized altretamine excreted at 24 hours.
After intraperitoneal administration of ^{14}C-ring-labeled altretamine to mice, tissue distribution was rapid in all organs, reaching a maximum at 30 minutes. The excretory organs (liver and kidney) and the small intestine showed high concentrations of radioactivity, whereas relatively low concentrations were found in other organs, including the brain.
There have been no formal pharmacokinetic studies in patients with compromised hepatic and/or renal function, though HEXALEN has been administered both concurrently and following nephrotoxic drugs such as cisplatin.
HEXALEN has been administered in 4 divided doses, with meals and at bedtime, though there is no pharmacokinetic data on this schedule nor information from formal interaction studies about the effect of food on its bioavailability or pharmacokinetics.
In two studies in patients with persistent or recurrent ovarian cancer following first-line treatment with cisplatin and/or alkylating agent-based combinations, HEXALEN was administered as a single agent for 14 or 21 days of a 28 day cycle. In the 51 patients with measurable or evaluable disease, there were 6 clinical complete responses, 1 pathologic complete response, and 2 partial responses for an overall response rate of 18%. The duration of these responses ranged from 2 months in a patient with a palpable pelvic mass to 36 months in a patient who achieved a pathologic complete response. In some patients, tumor regression was associated with improvement in symptoms and performance status.

INDICATIONS AND USAGE

HEXALEN (altretamine) is indicated for use as a single agent in the palliative treatment of patients with persistent or recurrent ovarian cancer following first-line therapy with a cisplatin and/or alkylating agent-based combination.

CONTRAINDICATIONS

HEXALEN is contraindicated in patients who have shown hypersensitivity to it. HEXALEN should not be employed in patients with preexisting severe bone marrow depression or severe neurologic toxicity. HEXALEN has been administered safely, however, to patients heavily pretreated with cisplatin and/or alkylating agents, including patients with preexisting cisplatin neuropathies. Careful monitoring of neurologic function in these patients is essential.

WARNINGS

See boxed Warnings.
Concurrent administration of HEXALEN and antidepressants of the monoamine oxidase (MAO) inhibitor class may cause severe orthostatic hypotension. Four patients, all over 60 years of age, were reported to have experienced symptomatic hypotension after 4 to 7 days of concomitant therapy with HEXALEN and MAO inhibitors.
HEXALEN causes mild to moderate myelosuppression and neurotoxicity. Blood counts and a neurologic examination should be performed prior to the initiation of each course of therapy and the dose of HEXALEN adjusted as clinically indicated (see Dosage and Administration).

Pregnancy: Category D

HEXALEN has been shown to be embryotoxic and teratogenic in rats and rabbits when given at doses 2 and 10 times the human dose. HEXALEN may cause fetal damage when administered to a pregnant woman. If HEXALEN is used during pregnancy, or if the patient becomes pregnant while taking the drug, the patient should be apprised of the potential hazard to the fetus. Women of childbearing potential should be advised to avoid becoming pregnant.

PRECAUTIONS

General

Neurologic examination should be performed regularly (see Adverse Reactions).

Laboratory Tests

Peripheral blood counts should be monitored at least monthly, prior to the initiation of each course of HEXALEN, and as clinically indicated (see Adverse Reactions).

Drug Interactions

Concurrent administration of HEXALEN and antidepressants of the MAO inhibitor class may cause severe orthostatic hypotension (see Warnings section). Cimetidine, an inhibitor of microsomal drug metabolism, increased altretamine's half-life and toxicity in a rat model.
Data from a randomized trial of HEXALEN and cisplatin plus or minus pyridoxine in ovarian cancer indicated that pyridoxine significantly reduced neurotoxicity; however, it adversely affected response duration suggesting that pyridoxine should not be administered with HEXALEN and/or cisplatin (1).

Carcinogenesis, Mutagenesis and Impairment of Fertility

The carcinogenic potential of HEXALEN has not been studied in animals, but drugs with similar mechanisms of action have been shown to be carcinogenic. HEXALEN was weakly mutagenic when tested in strain TA100 of *Salmonella typhimurium*. HEXALEN administered to female rats 14 days prior to breeding through the gestation period had no adverse effect on fertility, but decreased post-natal survival at 120 mg/m^2/day and was embryocidal at 240 mg/m^2/day. Administration of 120 mg/m^2/day HEXALEN to male rats for 60 days prior to mating resulted in testicular atrophy, reduced fertility and a possible dominant lethal mutagenic effect. Male rats treated with HEXALEN at 450 mg/m^2/day for 10 days had decreased spermatogenesis, atrophy of testes, seminal vesicles and ventral prostate.

Pregnancy

Pregnancy Category D: see Warnings section.

Nursing Mothers

It is not known whether altretamine is excreted in human milk. Because there is a possibility of toxicity in nursing infants secondary to HEXALEN treatment of the mother, it is recommended that breast feeding be discontinued if the mother is treated with HEXALEN.

Pediatric Use

The safety and effectiveness of HEXALEN in children have not been established.

ADVERSE REACTIONS

Gastrointestinal

With continuous high-dose daily HEXALEN, nausea and vomiting of gradual onset occur frequently. Although in most instances these symptoms are controllable with antiemetics, at times the severity requires HEXALEN dose reduction or, rarely, discontinuation of HEXALEN therapy. In some instances, a tolerance of these symptoms develops after several weeks of therapy. The incidence and severity of nausea and vomiting are reduced with moderate-dose administration of HEXALEN. In 2 clinical studies of single-agent HEXALEN utilizing a moderate, intermittent dose and schedule, only 1 patient (1%) discontinued HEXALEN due to severe nausea and vomiting.

Neurotoxicity

Peripheral neuropathy and central nervous system symptoms (mood disorders, disorders of consciousness, ataxia, dizziness, vertigo) have been reported. They are more likely to occur in patients receiving continuous high-dose daily HEXALEN than moderate-dose HEXALEN administered on an intermittent schedule. Neurologic toxicity has been reported to be reversible when therapy is discontinued. Data from a randomized trial of HEXALEN and cisplatin plus or minus pyridoxine in ovarian cancer indicated that pyridoxine significantly reduced neurotoxicity; however, it adversely affected response duration suggesting that pyridoxine should not be administered with HEXALEN and/or cisplatin (1).

Hematologic

HEXALEN causes mild to moderate dose-related myelosuppression. Leukopenia below 3000 WBC/mm^3 occurred in <15% of patients on a variety of intermittent or continuous dose regimens. Less than 1% had leukopenia below 1000 WBC/mm^3. Thrombocytopenia below 50,000 platelets/mm^3 was seen in <10% of patients. When given in doses of 8–12 mg/kg/day over a 21 day course, nadirs of leukocyte and platelet counts were reached by 3–4 weeks, and normal counts were regained by 6 weeks. With continuous administration at doses of 6–8 mg/kg/day, nadirs are reached in 6–8 weeks (median).
Data in the following table are based on the experience of 76 patients with ovarian cancer previously treated with a cisplatin-based combination regimen who received single-agent HEXALEN. In one study, HEXALEN, 260 mg/m^2/day, was administered for 14 days of a 28 day cycle. In another study, HEXALEN, 6–8 mg/kg/day, was administered for 21 days of a 28 day cycle.

ADVERSE EXPERIENCES IN 76 PREVIOUSLY TREATED OVARIAN CANCER PATIENTS RECEIVING SINGLE-AGENT HEXALEN

Adverse Experiences	% Patients
Gastrointestinal	
Nausea and Vomiting	33
Mild to Moderate	32
Severe	1
Increased Alkaline Phosphatase	9
Neurologic	
Peripheral Sensory Neuropathy	31
Mild	22
Moderate to Severe	9
Anorexia and Fatigue	1
Seizures	1
Hematologic	
Leukopenia	5
WBC 2000–2999/mm^3	4
WBC <2000/mm^3	1
Thrombocytopenia	9
Platelets 75,000–99,000/mm ^{3}	6
Platelets <75,000/mm ^{3}	3
Anemia	33
Mild	20
Moderate to Severe	13
Renal	
Serum Creatinine 1.6–3.75 mg/dl	7
BUN	9
25–40 mg%	5
41–60 mg%	3
>60 mg%	1

Additional adverse reaction information is available from 13 single-agent altretamine studies (total of 1014 patients) conducted under the auspices of the National Cancer Institute. The treated patients had a variety of tumors and many were heavily pretreated with other chemotherapies; most of these trials utilized high, continuous daily doses of altretamine (6–12 mg/kg/day). In general, adverse reaction experiences were similar in the two trials described above. Additional toxicities, not reported in the above table, included hepatic toxicity, skin rash, pruritus and alopecia, each occurring in <1% of patients.

OVERDOSAGE

No case of acute overdosage in humans has been described. The oral LD50 dose in rats was 1050 mg/kg and 437 mg/kg in mice.

DOSAGE AND ADMINISTRATION

HEXALEN is administered orally. Doses are calculated on the basis of body surface area.
HEXALEN may be administered either for 14 or 21 consecutive days in a 28 day cycle at a dose of 260 mg/m^2/day. The total daily dose should be given as 4 divided oral doses after meals and at bedtime. There is no pharmacokinetic information supporting this dosing regimen and the effect of food on HEXALEN bioavailability or pharmacokinetics has not been evaluated.
HEXALEN should be temporarily discontinued (for 14 days or longer) and subsequently restarted at 200 mg/m^2/day for any of the following situations:

1) Gastrointestinal intolerance unresponsive to symptomatic measures;
2) White blood count <2000/mm^3 or granulocyte count <1000/mm^3;
3) Platelet count <75,000/mm^3;
4) Progressive neurotoxicity.

If neurologic symptoms fail to stabilize on the reduced dose schedule, HEXALEN should be discontinued indefinitely.
Procedures for proper handling and disposal of anticancer drugs should be considered. Several guidelines on this subject have been published (2–8). There is no general agreement that all of the procedures recommended in the guidelines are necessary or appropriate.

HOW SUPPLIED

HEXALEN (altretamine) is available in 50 mg clear, hard gelatin capsules imprinted with the following inscription: USB001.
Bottles of 100 capsules (NDC 58178-001-70)
Store at controlled room temperature 15° to 30°C (59° to 86°F).

REFERENCES

1. Wiernik PH, et al. Hexamethylmelamine and Low or Moderate Dose Cisplatin With or Without Pyridoxine for Treatment of Advanced Ovarian Carcinoma: A Study of the Eastern Cooperative Oncology Group. *Cancer Investigation* 10(1): 1–9, 1992.
2. Recommendations for the Safe Handling of Parenteral Antineoplastic Drugs. NIH Publication No. 83-2621. For sale by the Superintendent of Documents, U.S. Government Printing Office, Washington, D.C. 20402.
3. AMA Council Report. Guidelines for Handling Parenteral Antineoplastics. *Journal of the American Medical Association* March 15, 1985.
4. National Study Commission on Cytotoxic Exposure—Recommendation for Handling Cytotoxic Agents. Available from Louis P. Jeffrey, Sc.D., Director of Pharmacy Services, Rhode Island Hospital, 593 Eddy Street, Providence, Rhode Island 02902.
5. Clinical Oncological Society of Australia: Guidelines and Recommendations for Safe Handling of Antineoplastic Agents. *Medical Journal of Australia* 1:426–428, 1983.
6. Jones, RB, et al. Safe Handling of Chemotherapeutic Agents: A Report from the Mount Sinai Medical Center. *CA —A Cancer Journal for Clinicians* Sept/Oct, 258–263, 1983.
7. American Society of Hospital Pharmacists Technical Assistance Bulletin on Handling Cytotoxic Drugs in Hospitals. *American Journal of Hospital Pharmacy* 42:131–137, 1985.
8. OSHA Work Practice Guidelines for Personnel Dealing with Cytotoxic (Antineoplastic) Drugs. *American Journal of Hospital Pharmacy* 43:1193–1204, 1986.

Distributed By: **MedImmune Oncology, Inc.**
West Conshohocken, PA 19428
1-877-633-4411

Revision Date 7/2000 PE

Shown in Product Identification Guide, page 323

NEUTREXIN® ℞

[n(y)ü-trex 'in]
(trimetrexate glucuronate for injection)

WARNINGS
NEUTREXIN (TRIMETREXATE GLUCURONATE FOR INJECTION) MUST BE USED WITH CONCURRENT LEUCOVORIN (LEUCOVORIN PROTECTION) TO AVOID POTENTIALLY SERIOUS OR LIFE-THREATENING TOXICITIES (SEE PRECAUTIONS AND DOSAGE AND ADMINISTRATION).

DESCRIPTION

Neutrexin is the brand name for trimetrexate glucuronate. Trimetrexate, a 2,4-diaminoquinazoline, non-classical folate

Continued on next page

Neutrexin—Cont.

antagonist, is a synthetic inhibitor of the enzyme dihydrofolate reductase (DHFR). Neutrexin is available as a sterile lyophilized powder in multi-dose vials, containing trimetrexate glucuronate equivalent to either 200 mg or 25 mg of trimetrexate without any preservatives or excipients. The powder is reconstituted prior to intravenous infusion (see **DOSAGE AND ADMINISTRATION, RECONSTITUTION AND DILUTION**).

Trimetrexate glucuronate is chemically known as 2,4-diamino-5-methyl-6-[(3,4,5-trimethoxyanilino)methyl] quinazoline mono-D-glucuronate, and has the following structure:

The empirical formula for trimetrexate glucuronate is $C_{19}H_{23}N_5O_3 \cdot C_6H_{10}O_7$ with a molecular weight of 563.56. The active ingredient, trimetrexate free base, has an empirical formula of $C_{19}H_{23}N_5O_3$ with a molecular weight of 369.42. Trimetrexate glucuronate for injection is a pale greenish-yellow powder or cake. Trimetrexate glucuronate is soluble in water (>50 mg/mL), whereas trimetrexate free base is practically insoluble in water (<0.1 mg/mL). The pKa of trimetrexate free base in 50% methanol/water is 8.0. The logarithm_{10} of the partition coefficient of trimetrexate free base between octanol and water is 1.63.

CLINICAL PHARMACOLOGY

Mechanism of Action

In vitro studies have shown that trimetrexate is a competitive inhibitor of dihydrofolate reductase (DHFR) from bacterial, protozoan, and mammalian sources. DHFR catalyzes the reduction of intracellular dihydrofolate to the active coenzyme tetrahydrofolate. Inhibition of DHFR results in the depletion of this coenzyme, leading directly to interference with thymidylate biosynthesis, as well as inhibition of folate-dependent formyltransferases, and indirectly to inhibition of purine biosynthesis. The end result is disruption of DNA, RNA, and protein synthesis, with consequent cell death.

Leucovorin (folinic acid) is readily transported into mammalian cells by an active, carrier-mediated process and can be assimilated into cellular folate pools following its metabolism. *In vitro* studies have shown that leucovorin provides a source of reduced folates necessary for normal cellular biosynthetic processes. Because the *Pneumocystis carinii* organism lacks the reduced folate carrier-mediated transport system, leucovorin is prevented from entering the organism. Therefore, at concentrations achieved with therapeutic doses of trimetrexate plus leucovorin, the selective transport of trimetrexate, but not leucovorin, into the *Pneumocystis carinii* organism allows the concurrent administration of leucovorin to protect normal host cells from the cytotoxicity of trimetrexate without inhibiting the antifolate's inhibition of *Pneumocystis carinii*. It is not known if considerably higher doses of leucovorin would affect trimetrexate's effect on *Pneumocystis carinii*.

Microbiology

Trimetrexate inhibits, in a dose-related manner, *in vitro* growth of the trophozoite stage of rat *Pneumocystis carinii* cultured on human embryonic lung fibroblast cells. Trimetrexate concentrations between 3 and 54.1 µM were shown to inhibit the growth of trophozoites. Leucovorin alone at a concentration of 10 µM did not alter either the growth of the trophozoites or the anti-pneumocystis activity of trimetrexate. Resistance to trimetrexate's antimicrobial activity against *Pneumocystis carinii* has not been studied.

Pharmacokinetics

Trimetrexate pharmacokinetics were assessed in six patients with acquired immunodeficiency syndrome (AIDS) who had *Pneumocystis carinii* pneumonia (4 patients) or toxoplasmosis (2 patients). Trimetrexate was administered intravenously as a bolus injection at a dose of 30 mg/m^2/day along with leucovorin 20 mg/m^2 every 6 hours for 21 days. Trimetrexate clearance (mean ± SD) was 38 ± 15 mL/min/m^2 and volume of distribution at steady state (Vd_{ss}) was 20 ± 8 L/m^2. The plasma concentration time profile declined in a biphasic manner over 24 hours with a terminal half-life of 11 ± 4 hours.

The pharmacokinetics of trimetrexate without the concomitant administration of leucovorin have been evaluated in cancer patients with advanced solid tumors using various dosage regimens. The decline in plasma concentrations over time has been described by either biexponential or triexponential equations. Following the single-dose administration of 10 to 130 mg/m^2 to 37 patients, plasma concentrations were obtained for 72 hours. Nine plasma concentration time profiles were described as biexponential. The alpha phase half-life was 57 ± 28 minutes, followed by a terminal phase with a half-life of 16 ± 3 hours. The plasma concentrations in the remaining patients exhibited a triphasic decline with half-lives of 8.6 ± 6.5 minutes, 2.4 ± 1.3 hours, and 17.8 ± 8.2 hours.

Trimetrexate clearance in cancer patients has been reported as 53 ± 41 mL/min (14 patients) and 32 ± 18 mL/min/m^2

TABLE 1
TREATMENT IND
Baseline Characteristics

	IST (n = 227)	RIST (n = 146)	RST (n = 204)	TOTAL (n = 577)
Ventilatory Support Required n (%)	39 (17)	50 (34)	129 (63)	218 (38)
Median Days on Standard Therapy	10	12	16	14
First Episode of PCP n (%)	104 (46)	103 (71)	190 (93)	397 (69)

TABLE 2
TREATMENT IND
Survival Rate One Month After Completion of Neutrexin Therapy

	IST	RIST	RST
All Patients	153/227 (67%)	73/146 (50%)	50/204 (25%)
Baseline Ventilatory Support	9/39 (23%)	15/50 (30%)	18/129 (14%)
No Baseline Ventilatory Support	144/188 (77%)	58/96 (60%)	32/75 (43%)

TABLE 3
NEUTREXIN COMPARATIVE TRIAL
Comparison of Adverse Events Reported for ≥1% of Patients

Adverse Events	Number and Percent (%) of Patients with Adverse Events			
	TMTX/LV (n = 109)		TMP/SMX (n = 111)	
Non-Laboratory Adverse Events:				
Fever	9	(8.3)	14	(12.6)
Rash/Pruritus	6	(5.5)	14	(12.6)
Nausea/Vomiting	5	(4.6)[a]	15	(13.5)[a]
Confusion	3	(2.8)	3	(2.7)
Fatigue	2	(1.8)	0	(0.0)
Hematologic Toxicity:				
Neutropenia (≤1000/mm^3)	33	(30.3)	37	(33.3)
Thrombocytopenia (≤75,000/mm^3)	11	(10.1)	17	(15.3)
Anemia (Hgb <8 g/dL)	8	(7.3)	10	(9.0)
Hepatotoxicity:				
Increased AST (>5 × ULN[b])	15	(13.8)	10	(9.0)
Increased ALT (>5 × ULN)	12	(11.0)	13	(11.7)
Increased Alkaline Phosphatase (>5 × ULN)	5	(4.6)	3	(2.7)
Increased Bilirubin (2.5 × ULN)	2	(1.8)	1	(0.9)
Renal:				
Increased Serum Creatinine (>3 × ULN)	1	(0.9)	2	(1.8)
Electrolyte Imbalance:				
Hyponatremia	5	(4.6)	10	(9.0)
Hypocalcemia	2	(1.8)	0	(0.0)
No. of Patients With at least one Adverse Event[c]	**58**	**(53.2)**	**60**	**(54.1)**

a Statistically significant difference between treatment groups (Chi-square: p = 0.022)
b ULN = Upper limit of normal range
c Patients could have reported more than one adverse event; therefore, the sum of adverse events exceeds the number of patients

(23 patients) following single-dose administration. After a five-day infusion of trimetrexate to 16 patients, plasma clearance was 30 ± 8 mL/min/m^2.

Renal clearance of trimetrexate in cancer patients has varied from about 4 ± 2 mL/min/m^2 to 10 ± 6 mL/min/m^2. Ten to 30% of the administered dose is excreted unchanged in the urine. Considering the free fraction of trimetrexate, active tubular secretion may possibly contribute to the renal clearance of trimetrexate. Renal clearance has been associated with urine flow, suggesting the possibility of tubular reabsorption as well.

The Vd_{ss} of trimetrexate in cancer patients after single-dose administration and for whom plasma concentrations were obtained for 72 hours was 36.9 ± 17.6 L/m^2 (n=23) and 0.62 ± 0.24 L/kg (n=14). Following a constant infusion of trimetrexate for five days, Vd_{ss} was 32.8 ± 16.6 L/m^2. The volume of the central compartment has been estimated as 0.17 ± 0.08 L/kg and 4.0 ± 2.9 L/m^2.

There have been inconsistencies in the reporting of trimetrexate protein binding. The *in vitro* plasma protein binding of trimetrexate using ultrafiltration is approximately 95% over the concentration range of 18.75 to 1000 ng/mL. There is a suggestion of capacity limited binding (saturable binding) at concentrations greater than about 1000 ng/mL, with free fraction progressively increasing to about 9.3% as concentration is increased to 15 µg/mL. Other reports have declared trimetrexate to be greater than 98% bound at concentrations of 0.1 to 10 µg/mL; however, specific free fractions were not stated. The free fraction of trimetrexate also has been reported to be about 15 to 16% at a concentration of 60 ng/mL, increasing to about 20% at a trimetrexate concentration of 6 µg/mL.

Trimetrexate metabolism in man has not been characterized. Preclinical data strongly suggest that the major metabolic pathway is oxidative O-demethylation, followed by conjugation to either glucuronide or the sulfate. N-demethylation and oxidation is a related minor pathway. Preliminary findings in humans indicate the presence of a glucuronide conjugate with DHFR inhibition and a demethylated metabolite in urine.

The presence of metabolite(s) in human plasma following the administration of trimetrexate is suggested by the differences seen in trimetrexate plasma concentrations when measured by HPLC and a nonspecific DHFR inhibition assay. The profiles are similar initially, but diverge with time; concentrations determined by DHFR being higher than those determined by HPLC. This suggests the presence of one or more metabolites with DHFR inhibition activity. After intravenous administration of trimetrexate to humans, urinary recovery averaged about 40%, using a DHFR assay, in comparison to 10% urinary recovery as determined by HPLC, suggesting the presence of one or more metabolites that retain inhibitory activity against DHFR. Fecal recovery of trimetrexate over 48 hours after intravenous administration ranged from 0.09 to 7.6% of the dose as determined by DHFR inhibition and 0.02 to 5.2% of the dose as determined by HPLC.

The pharmacokinetics of trimetrexate have not been determined in patients with renal insufficiency or hepatic dysfunction.

INDICATIONS AND USAGE

Neutrexin (trimetrexate glucuronate for injection) with concurrent leucovorin administration (leucovorin protection) is indicated as an alternative therapy for the treatment of moderate-to-severe *Pneumocystis carinii* pneumonia (PCP) in immunocompromised patients, including patients with the acquired immunodeficiency syndrome (AIDS), who are intolerant of, or are refractory to, trimethoprim-sulfamethoxazole therapy or for whom trimethoprim-sulfamethoxazole is contraindicated.

This indication is based on the results of a randomized, controlled double-blind trial comparing Neutrexin with concurrent leucovorin protection (TMTX/LV) to trimethoprim-sulfamethoxazole (TMP/SMX) in patients with moderate-to-severe *Pneumocystis carinii* pneumonia, as well as results of a Treatment IND. These studies are summarized below:

Neutrexin Comparative Study with TMP/SMX: This double-blind, randomized trial initiated by the AIDS Clinical Trials Group (ACTG) in 1988 was designed to compare the safety and efficacy of TMTX/LV to that of TMP/SMX for the treatment of histologically confirmed, moderate-to-severe PCP, defined as (A-a) baseline gradient >30 mmHg, in patients with AIDS.

Of the 220 patients with histologically confirmed PCP, 109 were randomized to receive TMTX/LV and 111 to TMP/SMX. Study patients randomized to TMTX/LV treatment were to receive 45 mg/m² of TMTX daily for 21 days plus 20 mg/m² of LV every 6 hours for 24 days. Those randomized to TMP/SMX were to receive 5 mg/kg TMP plus 25 mg/kg SMX four times daily for 21 days.

Response to therapy, defined as alive and off ventilatory support at completion of therapy, with no change in anti-pneumocystis therapy, or addition of supraphysiologic doses of steroids, occurred in fifty percent of patients in each treatment group.

The observed mortality in the TMTX/LV treatment group was approximately twice that in the TMP/SMX treatment group (95% CI: 0.99–4.11). Thirty of 109 (27%) patients treated with TMTX/LV and 18 of 111 (16%) patients receiving TMP/SMX died during the 21-day treatment course or 4-week follow-up period. Twenty-seven of 30 deaths in the TMTX/LV arm were attributed to PCP; all 18 deaths in the TMP/SMX arm were attributed to PCP.

A significantly smaller proportion of patients who received TMTX/LV compared to TMP/SMX failed therapy due to toxicity (10% vs. 25%), and a significantly greater proportion of patients failed due to lack of efficacy (40% vs. 24%). Six patients (12%) who responded to TMTX/LV relapsed during the one-month follow-up period; no patient responding to TMP/SMX relapsed during this period. Information is not available as to whether these patients received prophylaxis therapy for PCP.

Treatment IND: The FDA granted a Treatment IND for Neutrexin with leucovorin protection in February 1988 to make Neutrexin therapy available to HIV-infected patients with histologically confirmed PCP who had disease refractory to or who are intolerant of TMP/SMX and/or intravenous pentamidine.

Over 500 physicians in the United States participated in the Treatment IND. Of the first 753 patients enrolled, 577 were evaluable for efficacy. Of these, 227 patients were intolerant of both TMP/SMX and pentamidine (IST—patients intolerant of both standard therapies), 146 were intolerant of one therapy and refractory to the other (RIST-patients refractory to one therapy and intolerant of the other) and 204 were refractory to both therapies (RST-refractory to both standard therapies). This was a very ill patient population; 38% required ventilatory support at entry (Table 1). These studies did not have concurrent control groups.

[See table 1 at top of previous page]

The overall survival rate one month after completion of TMTX/LV as salvage therapy was 48%. Patients who had not responded to treatment with both TMP/SMX and pentamidine, of whom 63% required mechanical ventilation at entry, achieved a survival rate of 25% following treatment with TMTX/LV. Survival was 67% in patients who were intolerant to both TMP/SMX and pentamidine (Table 2).

[See table 2 at top of previous page]

In the Treatment IND, 12% of the patients discontinued Neutrexin therapy (with leucovorin protection) for toxicity.

TABLE 4
NEUTREXIN COMPARATIVE TRIAL
Adverse Events Resulting in Discontinuation of Therapy

Adverse Events	Number and Percent (%) of Patients Discontinued for Adverse Events[b] TMTX/LV (n = 109)	TMP/SMX (n = 111)
Non-Laboratory Adverse Events:		
Rash/Pruritus	3 (2.8)	5 (4.5)
Fever	2 (1.8)	4 (3.6)
Nausea/Vomiting	1 (0.9)	8 (7.2)
Neurologic Toxicity	1 (0.9)[c]	2 (1.8)
Hematologic Toxicity:		
Neutropenia (≤1000/mm³)	4 (3.7)	6 (5.4)
Thrombocytopenia (≤75,000/mm³)	0 (0.0)	4 (3.6)
Anemia (Hgb <8 g/dL)	0 (0.0)	4 (3.6)
Hepatotoxicity:		
Increased AST (>5 × ULN[a])	3 (2.8)	9 (8.1)
Increased ALT (>5 × ULN)	1 (0.9)	4 (3.6)
Increased Alkaline Phosphatase (>5 × ULN)	0 (0.0)	1 (0.9)
Electrolyte Imbalance:		
Hyponatremia	0 (0.0)	3 (2.7)
No. of Patients Discontinuing Therapy Due to an Adverse Event[b]	**11 (10.1)[d]**	**32 (28.8)[d]**

a ULN = Upper limit of normal range
b Patients could discontinue therapy due to more than one toxicity; therefore the sum exceeds number of patients who discontinued due to toxicity
c Patient discontinued TMTX/LV due to seizure, though causal relationship could not be established
d Statistically significant difference between treatment groups (Chi-square: $p < 0.001$)
Hematologic toxicity was the principal dose-limiting side effect.

TABLE 5
DOSE MODIFICATIONS FOR HEMATOLOGIC TOXICITY

Toxicity Grade	Neutrophils (Polys and Bands)	Platelets	Recommended Dosages of Neutrexin	Leucovorin
1	>1000/mm³	>75,000/mm³	45 mg/m² once daily	20 mg/m² every 6 hours
2	750–1000/mm³	50,000–75,000/mm³	45 mg/m² once daily	40 mg/m² every 6 hours
3	500–749/mm³	25,000–49,999/mm³	22 mg/m² once daily	40 mg/m² every 6 hours
4	<500/mm³	≤25,000/mm³	Day 1–9 Discontinue Day 10–21 Interrupt up to 96 hours[a]	40 mg/m²every 6 hours

a If Grade 4 hematologic toxicity occurs prior to Day 10, Neutrexin should be discontinued. Leucovorin (40 mg/m², q6h) should be administered for an additional 72 hours. If Grade 4 hematologic toxicity occurs at Day 10 or later, Neutrexin may be held up to 96 hours to allow counts to recover. If counts recover to Grade 3 within 96 hours, Neutrexin should be administered at a dose of 22 mg/m² and leucovorin maintained at 40 mg/m², q6h. When counts recover to Grade 2 toxicity, Neutrexin dose may be increased to 45 mg/m², but the leucovorin dose should be maintained at 40 mg/m² for the duration of treatment. If counts do not improve to ≤ Grade 3 toxicity within 96 hours, Neutrexin should be discontinued. Leucovorin at a dose of 40 mg/m², q6h should be administered for 72 hours following the last dose of Neutrexin.

CONTRAINDICATIONS

Neutrexin (trimetrexate glucuronate for injection) is contraindicated in patients with clinically significant sensitivity to trimetrexate, leucovorin, or methotrexate.

WARNINGS

Neutrexin (trimetrexate glucuronate for injection) must be used with concurrent leucovorin to avoid potentially serious or life-threatening complications including bone marrow suppression, oral and gastrointestinal mucosal ulceration, and renal and hepatic dysfunction. Leucovorin therapy must extend for 72 hours past the last dose of Neutrexin. Patients should be informed that failure to take the recommended dose and duration of leucovorin can lead to fatal toxicity. Patients should be closely monitored for the development of serious hematologic adverse reactions (see **PRECAUTIONS** and **DOSAGE AND ADMINISTRATION**).

Neutrexin can cause fetal harm when administered to a pregnant woman. Trimetrexate has been shown to be fetotoxic and teratogenic in rats and rabbits. Rats administered 1.5 and 2.5 mg/kg/day intravenously on gestational days 6–15 showed substantial postimplantation loss and severe inhibition of maternal weight gain. Trimetrexate administered intravenously to rats at 0.5 and 1.0 mg/kg/day on gestational days 6–15 retarded normal fetal development and was teratogenic. Rabbits administered trimetrexate intravenously at daily doses of 2.5 and 5.0 mg/kg/day on gestational days 6–18 resulted in significant maternal and fetal toxicity. In rabbits, trimetrexate at 0.1 mg/kg/day was teratogenic in the absence of significant maternal toxicity. These effects were observed using doses 1/20 to 1/2 the equivalent human therapeutic dose based on a mg/m² basis. Teratogenic effects included skeletal, visceral, ocular, and cardiovascular abnormalities. If Neutrexin is used during pregnancy, or if the patient becomes pregnant while taking this drug, the patient should be apprised of the potential hazard to the fetus. Women of childbearing potential should be advised to avoid becoming pregnant.

PRECAUTIONS

General

Patients receiving Neutrexin (trimetrexate glucuronate for injection) may experience severe hematologic, hepatic, renal, and gastrointestinal toxicities. Caution should be used in treating patients with impaired hematologic, renal, or hepatic function. Patients who require concomitant therapy with nephrotoxic, myelosuppressive, or hepatotoxic drugs should be treated with Neutrexin at the discretion of the physician and monitored carefully. To allow for full therapeutic doses of Neutrexin, treatment with zidovudine should be discontinued during Neutrexin therapy.

Neutrexin-associated myelosuppression, stomatitis, and gastrointestinal toxicities generally can be ameliorated by adjusting the dose of leucovorin. Mild elevations in transaminases and alkaline phosphatase have been observed with Neutrexin administration and are usually not cause for modification of Neutrexin therapy (see **DOSAGE AND ADMINISTRATION**). Seizures have been reported rarely (<1%) in AIDS patients receiving Neutrexin; however, a causal relationship has not been established. Trimetrexate is a known inhibitor of histamine metabolism. Hypersensitivity/allergic type reactions including but not limited to rash, chills/rigors, fever, diaphoresis and dyspnea, have occurred with trimetrexate primarily when it is administered as a bolus infusion or at doses higher than those recommended for PCP, and most frequently in combination with 5FU and leucovorin. In rare cases, anaphylactoid reactions, including acute hypotension and loss of consciousness have occurred.

Neutrexin has not been evaluated clinically for the treatment of concurrent pulmonary conditions such as bacterial, viral, or fungal pneumonia or mycobacterial diseases. *In vitro* activity has been observed against *Toxoplasma gondii, Mycobacterium avium* complex, gram positive cocci, and gram negative rods. If clinical deterioration is observed in patients, they should be carefully evaluated for other possible causes of pulmonary disease and treated with additional agents as appropriate.

Laboratory Tests

Patients receiving Neutrexin with leucovorin protection should be seen frequently by a physician. Blood tests to assess the following parameters should be performed at least twice a week during therapy: hematology (absolute neutrophil counts [ANC], platelets), renal function (serum creatinine, BUN), and hepatic function (AST, ALT, alkaline phosphatase).

Drug Interactions

Since trimetrexate is metabolized by a P450 enzyme system, drugs that induce or inhibit this drug metabolizing enzyme system may elicit important drug-drug interactions that may alter trimetrexate plasma concentrations. Agents that might be coadministered with trimetrexate in AIDS patients for other indications that could elicit this activity include erythromycin, rifampin, rifabutin, ketoconazole, and fluconazole. *In vitro* perfusion of isolated rat liver has shown that cimetidine caused a significant reduction in trimetrexate metabolism and that acetaminophen altered the relative concentration of trimetrexate metabolites possibly by competing for sulfate metabolites. Based on an *in vitro* rat liver model, nitrogen substituted imidazole drugs (clotrimazole, ketoconazole, miconazole) were potent, non-competitive inhibitors of trimetrexate metabolism. Patients medicated with these drugs and trimetrexate should be carefully monitored.

Carcinogenesis, Mutagenesis, Impairment of Fertility

Carcinogenesis: Long term studies in animals to evaluate the carcinogenic potential of trimetrexate have not been performed.

Mutagenesis: Trimetrexate was not mutagenic when tested using the standard Ames *Salmonella* mutagenicity assay with and without metabolic activation. Trimetrexate did not induce mutations in Chinese hamster lung cells or

Continued on next page

Neutrexin—Cont.

sister-chromatid exchange in Chinese hamster ovary cells. Trimetrexate did induce an increase in the chromosomal aberration frequency of cultured Chinese hamster lung cells; however, trimetrexate showed no clastogenic activity in a mouse micronucleus assay.
Impairment of fertility: No studies have been conducted to evaluate the potential of trimetrexate to impair fertility. However, during standard toxicity studies conducted in mice and rats, degeneration of the testes and spermatocytes including the arrest of spermatogenesis was observed.
Pregnancy, Teratogenic Effects- See **WARNINGS.**
Pregnancy Category D
Nursing Mothers
It is not known if trimetrexate is excreted in human milk. Because many drugs are excreted in human milk and because of the potential for serious adverse reactions in nursing infants from trimetrexate, it is recommended that breast feeding be discontinued if the mother is treated with Neutrexin.
Pediatric Use
The safety and effectiveness of Neutrexin for the treatment of histologically confirmed PCP has not been established for patients under 18 years of age. Two children, ages 15 months and 9 months, were treated with trimetrexate and leucovorin using a dose of 45 mg/m^2 of trimetrexate per day for 21 days and 20 mg/m^2 of leucovorin every 6 hours for 24 days. There were no serious or unexpected adverse effects.

ADVERSE REACTIONS

Because many patients who participated in clinical trials of Neutrexin (trimetrexate glucuronate for injection) had complications of advanced HIV disease, it is difficult to distinguish adverse events caused by Neutrexin from those resulting from underlying medical conditions.
Table 3 lists the adverse events that occurred in ≥1% of the patients who participated in the Comparative Study of Neutrexin plus leucovorin versus TMP/SMX.
[See table 3 at top of page 1866]
Laboratory toxicities were generally manageable with dose modification of trimetrexate/leucovorin (see **DOSAGE AND ADMINISTRATION**).
Table 4 lists the adverse events resulting in discontinuation of study therapy in the Neutrexin Comparative Study with TMP/SMX. Twenty-nine percent of the patients on the TMP/SMX arm discontinued therapy due to adverse events compared to 10% of the patients treated with TMTX/LV ($p < 0.001$).
[See table 4 at top of previous page]

OVERDOSAGE

Neutrexin (trimetrexate glucuronate for injection) administered without concurrent leucovorin can cause lethal complications. There has been no extensive experience in humans receiving single intravenous doses of trimetrexate greater than 90 mg/m^2/day with concurrent leucovorin. The toxicities seen at this dose were primarily hematologic. In the event of overdose, Neutrexin should be stopped and leucovorin should be administered at a dose of 40 mg/m^2 every 6 hours for 3 days. The LD_{50} of intravenous trimetrexate in mice is 62 mg/kg (186 mg/m^2).

DOSAGE AND ADMINISTRATION

Caution: Neutrexin (trimetrexate glucuronate for injection) must be administered with concurrent leucovorin (leucovorin protection) to avoid potentially serious or life-threatening toxicities. Leucovorin therapy must extend for 72 hours past the last dose of Neutrexin.
Neutrexin (trimetrexate glucuronate for injection) is administered at a dose of 45 mg/m^2 once daily by intravenous infusion over 60 minutes. Leucovorin must be administered daily during treatment with Neutrexin and for 72 hours past the last dose of Neutrexin. Leucovorin may be administered intravenously at a dose of 20 mg/m^2 over 5 to 10 minutes every 6 hours for a total daily dose of 80 mg/m^2, or orally as 4 doses of 20 mg/m^2 spaced equally throughout the day. The oral dose should be rounded up to the next higher 25 mg increment. The recommended course of therapy is 21 days of Neutrexin and 24 days of leucovorin.
Neutrexin and leucovorin may alternatively be dosed on a mg/kg basis, depending on the patients body weight, using the conversion factors shown in the table below:

Body Weight (kg)	Neutrexin Dose (mg/kg/day)	Leucovorin Dose (mg/kg/qid)
<50	1.5	0.6
50-80	1.2	0.5
>80	1.0	0.5

Dosage Modifications
Hematologic toxicity: Neutrexin (trimetrexate glucuronate for injection) and leucovorin doses should be modified based on the worst hematologic toxicity according to the following table. If leucovorin is given orally, doses should be rounded up to the next higher 25 mg increment.
[See table 5 at top of previous page]
Hepatic toxicity: Transient elevations of transaminases and alkaline phosphatase have been observed in patients treated with Neutrexin. Interruption of treatment is advisable if transaminase levels or alkaline phosphatase levels increase to >5 times the upper limit of normal range.
Renal toxicity: Interruption of Neutrexin is advisable if serum creatinine levels increase to >2.5 mg/dL and the elevation is considered to be secondary to Neutrexin.
Other toxicities: Interruption of treatment is advisable in patients who experience severe mucosal toxicity that interferes with oral intake. Treatment should be discontinued for fever (oral temperature ≥ 105°F/40.5°C) that cannot be controlled with antipyretics.
Leucovorin therapy must extend for 72 hours past the last dose of Neutrexin.
RECONSTITUTION AND DILUTION
Each vial of Neutrexin (trimetrexate glucuronate for injection) should be reconstituted in accordance with labeled instructions with either 5% Dextrose Injection, USP, or Sterile Water for Injection, USP, to yield a concentration of 12.5 mg of trimetrexate per mL (complete dissolution should occur within 30 seconds). The reconstituted product will appear as a pale greenish-yellow solution and must be inspected visually prior to dilution. **Do not use if cloudiness or precipitate is observed.** Neutrexin should not be reconstituted with solutions containing either chloride ion or leucovorin, since precipitation occurs instantly.
After reconstitution, the solution should be used immediately; however, the solution is stable for 6 hours at room temperature (20 to 25°C), or 24 hours under refrigeration (2–8°C).
Prior to administration, the reconstituted solution should be further diluted with 5% Dextrose Injection, USP, to yield a final concentration of 0.25 to 2 mg of trimetrexate per mL. The diluted solution should be administered by intravenous infusion over 60 minutes. Neutrexin should not be mixed with solutions containing either chloride ion or leucovorin, since precipitation occurs instantly. The diluted solution is stable under refrigeration or at room temperature for up to 24 hours. Do not freeze. Discard any unused portion after 24 hours. The intravenous line must be flushed thoroughly with at least 10 mL of 5% Dextrose Injection, USP, before and after administering Neutrexin.
Leucovorin protection may be administered prior to or following Neutrexin. In either case, the intravenous line must be flushed thoroughly with at least 10 mL of 5% Dextrose Injection, USP. Leucovorin calcium for injection should be diluted according to the instructions in the leucovorin package insert, and administered over 5 to 10 minutes every 6 hours.
Caution: Parenteral products should be inspected visually for particulate matter and discoloration prior to administration, whenever solution and container permit. Neutrexin forms a precipitate instantly upon contact with chloride ion or leucovorin, therefore it should not be added to solutions containing sodium chloride or other anions. Neutrexin and leucovorin solutions must be administered separately. Intravenous lines should be flushed with at least 10 mL of 5% Dextrose Injection, USP, between Neutrexin and leucovorin infusions.

HANDLING AND DISPOSAL

If Neutrexin (trimetrexate glucuronate for injection) contacts the skin or mucosa, immediately wash thoroughly with soap and water. Procedures for proper disposal of cytotoxic drugs should be considered. Several guidelines on this subject have been published (1–5).

HOW SUPPLIED

Neutrexin (trimetrexate glucuronate for injection) is supplied as a sterile lyophilized powder in either 5 mL or 30 mL vials. Each 5 mL vial contains trimetrexate glucuronate equivalent to 25 mg of trimetrexate. Each 30 mL vial contains trimetrexate glucuronate equivalent to 200 mg trimetrexate. The 5 mL vials are packaged and available in two market presentations as listed below:
10 Pack—10 vials in a white chip-board carton (NDC 58178-020-10)
50 Pack—2 trays of 25 vials per shrink-wrapped tray (NDC 58178-020-50)
The 30 mL vials are packaged and available as listed below:
Single Pack—1 vial (NDC 58178-021-01)
Store at controlled room temperature 20° to 25°C (68° to 77°F). **Protect from exposure to light.**
U.S. Patents 4,376,858; 4,694,007; 6,017,922

REFERENCES

1. AMA Council Report. Guidelines for Handling Parenteral Antineoplastics. *Journal of the American Medical Association* March 15, 1985.
2. Clinical Oncological Society of Australia: Guidelines and Recommendations for Safe Handling of Antineoplastic Agents. *Medical Journal of Australia* 1:426–428, 1983.
3. Jones RB, et al. Safe Handling of Chemotherapeutic Agents: A Report from the Mount Sinai Medical Center. *CA–A Cancer Journal for Clinicians* Sept/Oct, 258–263, 1983.
4. American Society of Hospital Pharmacists Technical Assistance Bulletin on Handling Cytotoxic Drugs in Hospitals. *American Journal of Hospital Pharmacy* 42: 131–137, 1985.
5. OSHA Work Practice Guidelines for Personnel Dealing with Cytotoxic (Antineoplastic) Drugs. *American Journal of Hospital Pharmacy* 43: 1193–1204, 1986.

Distributed by:
MedImmune Oncology, Inc.
West Conshohocken, PA 19428
1-877-633-4411

Revision Date 5/2000
Shown in Product Identification Guide, page 323

Merck & Co., Inc.
WEST POINT, PA 19486

For Medical Information Contact:
Generally:
Product and service information:
Call the Merck National Service Center, 8:00 AM to 7:00 PM (ET), Monday through Friday:
(800) NSC-MERCK
(800) 672-6372
FAX: (800) MERCK-68
FAX: (800) 637-2568
Adverse Drug Experiences:
Call the Merck National Service Center, 8:00 AM to 7:00 PM (ET), Monday through Friday:
(800) NSC-MERCK
(800) 672-6372
In Emergencies:
24-hour emergency information for healthcare professionals:
(800) NSC-MERCK
(800) 672-6372
Sales and Ordering:
For product orders and direct account inquiries only, call the Order Management Center,
8:00 AM to 7:00 PM (ET), Monday through Friday:
(800) MERCK RX
(800) 637-2579

AGGRASTAT® ℞
(tirofiban hydrochloride injection premixed)
AGGRASTAT®
(tirofiban hydrochloride injection)

DESCRIPTION

AGGRASTAT* (tirofiban hydrochloride), a non-peptide antagonist of the platelet glycoprotein (GP) llb/llla receptor, inhibits platelet aggregation.
Tiroban hydrochloride monohydrate, a non-peptide molecule, is chemically described as *N*-(butylsulfonyl)-*O*-[4-(4-piperidinyl)butyl]-L-tyrosine monohydrochloride monohydrate.
Its molecular formula is $C_{22}H_{36}N_2O_5S \cdot HCl \cdot H_2O$ and its structural formula is:

HN—CH₂CH₂CH₂CH₂O—(C₆H₄)—CH₂—C(H)(COOH)—NHSO₂CH₂CH₂CH₂CH₃ •HCl •H₂O

Tirofiban hydrochloride monohydrate is a white to off-white, non-hygroscopic, free-flowing powder, with a molecular weight of 495.08. It is very slightly soluble in water.
AGGRASTAT Injection Premixed is supplied as a sterile solution in water for injection, for intravenous use only, in plastic containers of 250 mL or 500 mL.
Each 250 mL of the premixed, iso-osmotic intravenous injection contains 14.045 mg tirofiban hydrochloride monohydrate equivalent to 12.5 mg tirofiban (50 mcg/mL) and the following inactive ingredients: 2.25 g sodium chloride, 135 mg sodium citrate dihydrate, and 8 mg citric acid anhydrous.
Each 500 mL of the premixed, iso-osmotic intravenous injection contains 28.09 mg tirofiban hydrochloride monohydrate equivalent to 25 mg tirofiban (50 mcg/mL) and the following inactive ingredients: 4.5 g sodium chloride, 270 mg sodium citrate dihydrate, and 16 mg citric acid anhydrous. The pH of the solution ranges from 5.5 to 6.5 and may have been adjusted with hydrochloric acid and/or sodium hydroxide.
The flexible container is manufactured from a specially designed multilayer plastic (PL2408). Solutions in contact with the plastic container leach out certain chemical components from the plastic in very small amounts; however, biological testing was supportive of the safety of the plastic container materials.
AGGRASTAT Injection is a sterile concentrated solution for intravenous infusion after dilution and is supplied in a 50 mL vial. Each mL of the solution contains 0.281 mg of tirofiban hydrochloride monohydrate equivalent to 0.25 mg of tirofiban and the following inactive ingredients: 0.16 mg citric acid anhydrous, 2.7 mg sodium citrate dihydrate, 8 mg sodium chloride, and water for injection. The pH ranges from 5.5 to 6.5 and may have been adjusted with hydrochloric acid and/or sodium hydroxide.

*Registered trademark of MERCK & CO., Inc.

CLINICAL PHARMACOLOGY

Mechanism of Action
AGGRASTAT is a reversible antagonist of fibrinogen binding to the GP llb/llla receptor, the major platelet surface re-

ceptor involved in platelet aggregation. When administered intravenously, AGGRASTAT inhibits *ex vivo* platelet aggregation in a dose- and concentration-dependent manner. When given according to the recommended regimen, >90% inhibition is attained by the end of the 30-minute infusion. Platelet aggregation inhibition is reversible following cessation of the infusion of AGGRASTAT.

Pharmacokinetics

Tirofiban has a half-life of approximately 2 hours. It is cleared from the plasma largely by renal excretion, with about 65% of an administered dose appearing in urine and about 25% in feces, both largely as unchanged tirofiban. Metabolism appears to be limited.

Tirofiban is not highly bound to plasma proteins and protein binding is concentration independent over the range of 0.01 to 25 mcg/mL. Unbound fraction in human plasma is 35%. The steady state volume of distribution of tirofiban ranges from 22 to 42 liters.

In healthy subjects, the plasma clearance of tirofiban ranges from 213 to 314 mL/min. Renal clearance accounts for 39 to 69% of plasma clearance. The recommended regimen of a loading infusion followed by a maintenance infusion produces a peak tirofiban plasma concentration that is similar to the steady state concentration during the infusion. In patients with coronary artery disease, the plasma clearance of tirofiban ranges from 152 to 267 mL/min; renal clearance accounts for 39% of plasma clearance.

Special Populations

Gender

Plasma clearance of tirofiban in patients with coronary artery disease is similar in males and females.

Elderly

Plasma clearance of tirofiban is about 19 to 26% lower in elderly (>65 years) patients with coronary artery disease than in younger (≤65 years) patients.

Race

No difference in plasma clearance was detected in patients of different races.

Hepatic Insufficiency

In patients with mild to moderate hepatic insufficiency, plasma clearance of tirofiban is not significantly different from clearance in healthy subjects.

Renal Insufficiency

Plasma clearance of tirofiban is significantly decreased (>50%) in patients with creatinine clearance <30 mL/min, including patients requiring hemodialysis (see DOSAGE AND ADMINISTRATION, *Recommended Dosage*). Tirofiban is removed by hemodialysis.

Pharmacodynamics

AGGRASTAT inhibits platelet function, as demonstrated by its ability to inhibit *ex vivo* adenosine phosphate (ADP)-induced platelet aggregation and prolong bleeding time in healthy subjects and patients with coronary artery disease. The time course of inhibition parallels the plasma concentration profile of the drug. Following discontinuation of an infusion of AGGRASTAT, 0.10 mcg/kg/min, *ex vivo* platelet aggregation returns to near baseline in approximately 90% of patients with coronary artery disease in 4 to 8 hours. The addition of heparin to this regimen does not significantly alter the percentage of subjects with >70% inhibition of platelet aggregation (IPA), but does increase the average bleeding time, as well as the number of patients with bleeding times prolonged to >30 minutes.

In patients with unstable angina, a two-staged intravenous infusion regimen of AGGRASTAT (loading infusion of 0.4 mcg/kg/min for 30 minutes followed by 0.1 mcg/kg/min for up to 48 hours in the presence of heparin and aspirin), produces approximately 90% inhibition of *ex vivo* ADP-induced platelet aggregation with a 2.9-fold prolongation of bleeding time during the loading infusion. Inhibition persists over the duration of the maintenance infusion.

Clinical Trials

Three large-scale clinical studies were conducted to study the efficacy and safety of AGGRASTAT in the management of patients with Acute Coronary Syndrome (unstable angina/non-Q-wave myocardial infarction). Acute Coronary Syndrome is characterized by prolonged (≥10 minutes) or repetitive symptoms of cardiac ischemia occurring at rest or with minimal exertion, associated with either ischemic ST-T wave changes on electrocardiogram (ECG) or elevated cardiac enzymes. The definition includes "unstable angina" and "non-Q-wave myocardial infarction" but excludes myocardial infarction that is associated with Q-waves or non-transient ST-segment elevation. The three studies examined AGGRASTAT alone and as an addition to heparin, prior to and after angioplasty (if indicated) (PRISM-PLUS), in comparison to heparin in a similar population (PRISM), and in addition to heparin in patients undergoing percutaneous transluminal coronary angioplasty (PTCA) or atherectomy (RESTORE). These trials are discussed in detail below.

PRISM-PLUS (Platelet Receptor Inhibition for Ischemic Syndrome Management–Patients Limited by Unstable Signs and Symptoms)

In the multi-center, randomized, parallel, double-blind PRISM-PLUS trial, the use of AGGRASTAT in combination with heparin (n=773) was compared to heparin alone (n=797) in patients with documented unstable angina/non-Q-wave myocardial infarction within 12 hours of entry into the study and initiation of treatment. All patients with unstable angina/non-Q-wave myocardial infarction had cardiac ischemia documented by ECG or had elevated cardiac enzymes. Patients who were medically managed or who subsequently underwent revascularization procedures were studied. The mean age of the population was 63 years; 32% of patients were female and approximately half of the population presented with non-Q-wave myocardial infarction. Exclusions included contraindications to anticoagulation (see CONTRAINDICATIONS), decompensated heart failure, platelet count <150,000/mm^3, and creatinine >2.5 mg/dL. In this study, patients were randomized to either AGGRASTAT (30 minute loading infusion of 0.4 mcg/kg/min followed by a maintenance infusion of 0.10 mcg/kg/min) and heparin (bolus of 5,000 units (U) followed by an infusion of 1,000 U/hr titrated to maintain an activated partial thromboplastin time (APTT) of approximately 2 times control), or heparin alone (bolus of 5,000 U followed by an infusion of 1,000 U/hr titrated to maintain an APTT of approximately 2 times control). All patients received concomitant aspirin unless contraindicated. Patients underwent 48 hours of medical stabilization on study drug therapy, and they were to undergo angiography before 96 hours (and, if indicated, angioplasty/atherectomy, while continuing on AGGRASTAT and heparin for 12–24 hours after the procedure). Some patients went on to coronary artery bypass grafting (CABG) after cessation of drug therapy. AGGRASTAT and heparin could be continued for up to 108 hours. On average, patients received AGGRASTAT for 71.3 hours. A third group of patients was initially randomized to AGGRASTAT alone (no heparin). This arm was stopped when the group was found, at an interim look, to have greater mortality than the other two groups. Note, however, that a direct comparison of heparin and tirofiban alone in the PRISM study (see below) did not show excess mortality

The primary endpoint of the study was a composite of refractory ischemia, new myocardial infarction and death at 7 days after initiation of AGGRASTAT and heparin. At the primary endpoint, there was a 32% risk reduction in the overall composite. The components of the composite were examined separately (they total more than the composite because a patient could have more than one, e.g., by dying after having a new infarction). There was a 47% risk reduction in myocardial infarction and a 30% risk reduction in refractory ischemia. The results are shown in Table 1.

[See table 1 above]

Table 1
Cardiac Ischemic Events (7 Days)

Endpoint	AGGRASTAT+ Heparin (n=773)	Heparin (n=797)	Risk Reduction	p-value
Composite Endpoint	12.9%	17.9%	32%	0.004
Components				
Myocardial Infarction and Death	4.9%	8.3%	43%	0.006
Myocardial Infarction	3.9%	7.0%	47%	0.006
Death	1.9%	1.9%	—	—
Refractory Ischemia	9.3%	12.7%	30%	0.023

The benefit seen at 7 days was maintained over time. At 30 days, the risk of the composite endpoint was reduced by 22% (p=0.029) and there was a 30% reduction in the composite of myocardial infarction and death (p=0.027). At 6 months, the risk of the composite endpoint was reduced by 19% (p=0.024). The risk reduction in the composite endpoint at 30 days and 6 months is shown in the Kaplan-Meier curve below.

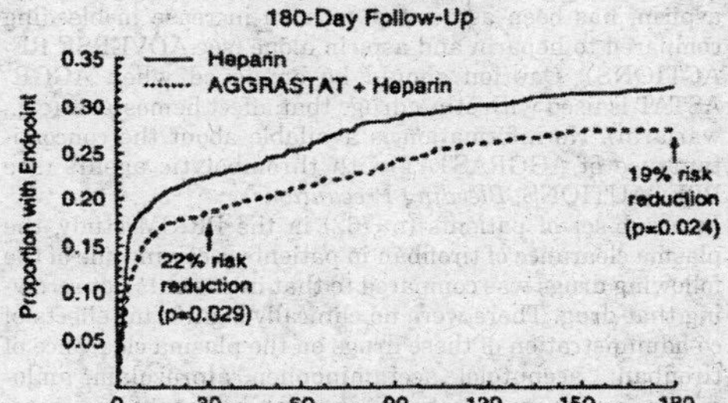

Composite Endpoint
180-Day Follow-Up

Heparin
AGGRASTAT + Heparin
Proportion with Endpoint
Study Day
22% risk reduction (p=0.029)
19% risk reduction (p=0.024)

PRISM-PLUS was not designed to provide definitive results in subsets of the overall population. Nonetheless, results were examined for demographic (age, gender, race) subsets and for people who did and did not receive PTCA, atherectomy, or CABG.

In PRISM-PLUS, there was a consistent treatment effect in patients either greater or less than 65 years old, and in men and women. Too few non-Caucasians were enrolled to make a definite statement about racial differences in treatment effect.

Approximately 90% of patients in the PRISM-PLUS study underwent coronary angiography and 30% underwent angioplasty/atherectomy during the first 30 days of the study. The majority of these patients continued on study drug throughout these procedures. AGGRASTAT was continued for 12-24 hours (average 15 hours) after angioplasty/atherectomy. The effects of AGGRASTAT at Day 30 did not appear to differ among the sub-populations that did or did not receive PTCA or CABG, both prior to and after the procedure.

A sub-study in PRISM-PLUS of angiograms after 48 to 96 hours found that there was a significant decrease in the extent of angiographically apparent thrombus in patients treated with AGGRASTAT in combination with heparin compared to heparin alone. In addition, flow in the affected coronary artery was significantly improved.

PRISM (Platelet Receptor Inhibition for Ischemic Syndrome Management)

In the PRISM study, a randomized, parallel, double-blind, active control study, AGGRASTAT alone (n=1616) was compared to heparin (n=1616) alone as medical management in patients with unstable angina/non-Q-wave myocardial infarction. In this study, the drug was started within 24 hours of the time the patient experienced chest pain. The mean age of the population was 62 years; 32% of the population was female and 25% had non-Q-wave myocardial infraction on presentation. Thirty percent had no ECG evidence of cardiac ischemia. Exclusion criteria were similar to PRISM-PLUS. The primary, prospectively identified endpoint was the composite endpoint of refractory ischemia, myocardial infarction or death after a 48-hour drug infusion with AGGRASTAT. The results are shown in Table 2.

[See table 2 above]

Table 2
Cardiac Ischemic Events

Composite Endpoint	AGGRASTAT (n=1616)	Heparin (n=1616)	Risk Reduction	p-value
2 Days	3.8%	5.6%	33%	0.015
7 Days	10.3%	11.3%	10%	0.33
30 Days	15.9%	17.1%	8%	0.34

In the PRISM study, no adverse effect of AGGRASTAT on mortality at either 7 or 30 days was detected. This result is in conflict with the PRISM-PLUS study, where the arm that included AGGRASTAT without heparin (n=345) was dropped at an interim analysis by the Data Safety Monitoring Committee due to increased mortality at 7 days. A pooled analysis of the data from these two trials (PRISM and PRISM-PLUS) demonstrated that the effect of AGGRASTAT alone on mortality (at 7 and 30 days) was comparable to that of heparin alone.

RESTORE (Randomized Efficacy Study of Tirofiban for Outcomes and Restenosis)

The RESTORE study (n=2141) was a randomized, controlled comparison of AGGRASTAT and placebo, each added to heparin, in patients undergoing PTCA or atherectomy within 72 hours of presentation with unstable angina or acute myocardial infarction. The mean age of the population was 59 years; 27% were female. Two-thirds of patients underwent angioplasty for unstable angina and the remainder in association with acute myocardial infarction. Exclusions included anatomy not amenable to angioplasty, contraindications to anticoagulation (see CONTRAINDICATIONS), platelet count <150,000/mm^3, and creatinine >2.0 mg/dL. AGGRASTAT (with heparin) was initiated immediately prior to the angioplasty/atherectomy at a dose of 10 mcg/kg bolus (over 3 minutes) followed by an infusion of 0.15 mcg/kg/min along with a heparin bolus (bolus of 10,000 U, or 150 U/kg for patients <70 kg). The infusion dose of AGGRASTAT is 50% higher than the dose used in the PRISM-PLUS trial. AGGRASTAT was administered for a total of 36 hours. In general, heparin was to be discontinued at the conclusion of the angioplasty/atherectomy. Reasons for continued heparin included: imperfect outcome (e.g., large tear, intraluminal filling defect, or residual stenosis >40%), large thrombus load, continuing rest angina through the procedure, abrupt closure or very active artery during the procedure, or side branch occlusion. The primary endpoint was the composite of all deaths, non-fatal myocardial infarctions, and all repeat revascularization procedures at 30

Continued on next page

Aggrastat—Cont.

days. For results see Table 3. A sub-study in RESTORE of angiograms after approximately 6 months found that AGGRASTAT had no significant effect on the extent of coronary artery restenosis following angioplasty.
[See table 3 above]
The risk reduction in the composite endpoint at 180 days is shown in the Kaplan-Meier curve below.

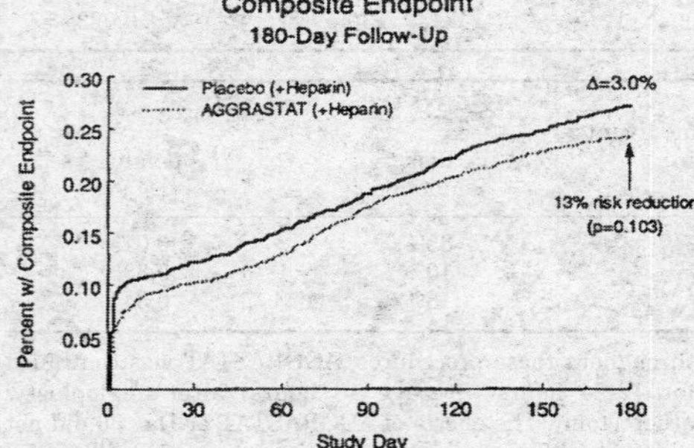

INDICATIONS AND USAGE

AGGRASTAT, in combination with heparin, is indicated for the treatment of acute coronary syndrome, including patients who are to be managed medically and those undergoing PTCA or atherectomy. In this setting, AGGRASTAT has been shown to decrease the rate of a combined endpoint of death, new myocardial infarction or refractory ischemia/repeat cardiac procedure (for discussion of trial results and for definition of acute coronary syndrome see CLINICAL PHARMACOLOGY, *Clinical Trials*).
AGGRASTAT has been studied in a setting, as described in *Clinical Trials*, that included aspirin and heparin.

CONTRAINDICATIONS

AGGRASTAT is contraindicated in patients with:
- known hypersensitivity to any component of the product
- active internal bleeding or a history of bleeding diathesis within the previous 30 days
- a history of intracranial hemorrhage, intracranial neoplasm, arteriovenous malformation, or aneurysm
- a history of thrombocytopenia following prior exposure to AGGRASTAT
- history of stroke within 30 days or any history of hemorrhagic stroke
- major surgical procedure or severe physical trauma within the previous month
- history, symptoms, or findings suggestive of aortic dissection
- severe hypertension (systolic blood pressure >180 mmHg and/or diastolic blood pressure >110 mmHg)
- concomitant use of another parenteral GP IIb/IIIa inhibitor
- acute pericarditis

WARNINGS

Bleeding is the most common complication encountered during therapy with AGGRASTAT. Administration of AGGRASTAT is associated with an increase in bleeding events classified as both major and minor bleeding events by criteria developed by the Thrombolysis in Myocardial Infarction Study group (TIMI).** Most major bleeding associated with AGGRASTAT occurs at the arterial access site for cardiac catheterization.
AGGRASTAT should be used with caution in patients with platelet count <150,000/mm³ and in patients with hemorrhagic retinopathy.
Because AGGRASTAT inhibits platelet aggregation, caution should be employed when it is used with other drugs that affect hemostasis. The safety of AGGRASTAT when used in combination with thrombolytic agents has not been established.
During therapy with AGGRASTAT, patients should be monitored for potential bleeding. When bleeding cannot be controlled with pressure, infusion of AGGRASTAT and heparin should be discontinued.

** Bovill, E.G.; et al.: Hemorrhagic Events during Therapy with Recombinant Tissue-Type Plasminogen Activator, Heparin, and Aspirin for Acute Myocardial Infarction, Results of the Thrombolysis in Myocardial Infarction (TIMI) Phase II Trial, Annals of Internal Medicine,*115*(4):256-265, 1991.

PRECAUTIONS

Bleeding Precautions
Percutaneous Coronary Intervention—Care of the femoral artery access site: Therapy with AGGRASTAT is associated with increases in bleeding rates particularly at the site of arterial access for femoral sheath placement. Care should be taken when attempting vascular access that only the anterior wall of the femoral artery is punctured. Prior to pulling the sheath, heparin should be discontinued for 3-4 hours

Table 3
Cardiac Ischemic Events

Composite Endpoint	AGGRASTAT (n=1071)	Placebo (n=1070)	Risk Reduction	p-value
2 Days	5.4%	8.7%	38%	0.004
7 Days	7.6%	10.4%	28%	0.023
30 Days	10.3%	12.2%	17%	0.17

Bleeding	PRISM-PLUS* (UAP/Non-Q-Wave MI Study)		RESTORE* (Angioplasty/Atherectomy Study)	
	AGGRASTAT** + Heparin*** (n=773) % (n)	Heparin*** (n=797) % (n)	AGGRASTAT† + Heparin†† (n=1071) % (n)	Heparin†† (n=1070) % (n)
Major Bleeding (TIMI Criteria)‡	1.4 (11)	0.8 (6)	2.2 (24)	1.6 (17)
Minor Bleeding (TIMI Criteria)§	10.5 (81)	8.0 (64)	12.0 (129)	6.3 (67)
Transfusions	4.0 (31)	2.8 (22)	4.3 (46)	2.5 (27)

* Patients received aspirin unless contraindicated.
** 0.4 mcg/kg/min loading infusion; 0.10 mcg/kg/min maintenance infusion.
*** 5,000 U bolus followed by 1,000 U/hr titrated to maintain an APTT of approximately 2 times control.
† 10 mcg/kg bolus followed by infusion of 0.15 mcg/kg/min.
†† Bolus of 10,000 U or 150 U/kg for patients <70 kg followed by administration as necessary to maintain ACT in approximate range of 300 to 400 seconds during procedure.
‡ Hemoglobin drop of >50 g/L with or without an identified site, intracranial hemorrhage, or cardiac tamponade.
§ Hemoglobin drop of >30 g/L with bleeding from a known site, spontaneous gross hematuria, hematemesis or hemoptysis.

and activated clotting time (ACT) <180 seconds or APTT <45 seconds should be documented. Care should be taken to obtain proper hemostasis after removal of the sheaths using standard compressive techniques followed by close observation. While the vascular sheath is in place, patients should be maintained on complete bed rest with the head of the bed elevated 30° and the affected limb restrained in a straight position. Sheath hemostasis should be achieved at least 4 hours before hospital discharge.
Minimize Vascular and Other Trauma: Other arterial and venous punctures, intramuscular injections, and the use of urinary catheters, nasotracheal intubation and nasogastric tubes should be minimized. When obtaining intravenous access, non-compressible sites (e.g., subclavian or jugular veins) should be avoided.
Laboratory Monitoring: Platelet counts, and hemoglobin and hematocrit should be monitored prior to treatment, within 6 hours following the loading infusion, and at least daily thereafter during therapy with AGGRASTAT (or more frequently if there is evidence of significant decline). If the patient experiences a platelet decrease to <90,000/mm³, additional platelet counts should be performed to exclude pseudothrombocytopenia. If thrombocytopenia is confirmed, AGGRASTAT and heparin should be discontinued and the condition appropriately monitored and treated.
To monitor unfractionated heparin, APTT should be monitored 6 hours after the start of the heparin infusion; heparin should be adjusted to maintain APTT at approximately 2 times control.
Severe Renal Insufficiency
In clinical studies, patients with severe renal insufficiency (creatinine clearance <30 mL/min) showed decreased plasma clearance of AGGRASTAT. The dosage of AGGRASTAT should be reduced in these patients (see DOSAGE AND ADMINISTRATION and CLINICAL PHARMACOLOGY, *Clinical Trials*).
Drug Interactions
AGGRASTAT has been studied on a background of aspirin and heparin.
The use of AGGRASTAT, in combination with heparin and aspirin, has been associated with an increase in bleeding compared to heparin and aspirin alone (see ADVERSE REACTIONS). Caution should be employed when AGGRASTAT is used with other drugs that affect hemostasis (e.g., warfarin). No information is available about the concomitant use of AGGRASTAT with thrombolytic agents (see PRECAUTIONS, *Bleeding Precautions*).
In a sub-set of patients (n=762) in the PRISM study, the plasma clearance of tirofiban in patients receiving one of the following drugs was compared to that in patients not receiving that drug. There were no clinically significant effects of co-administration of these drugs on the plasma clearance of tirofiban: acebutolol, acetaminophen, alprazolam, amlodipine, aspirin preparations, atenolol, bromazepam, captopril, diazepam, digoxin, diltiazem, docusate sodium, enalapril, furosemide, glyburide, heparin, insulin, isosorbide, lorazepam, lovastatin, metoclopramide, metoprolol, morphine, nifedipine, nitrate preparations, oxazepam, potassium chloride, propranolol, ranitidine, simvastatin, sucralfate and temazepam. Patients who received levothyroxine or omeprazole along with AGGRASTAT had a higher rate of clearance of AGGRASTAT. The clinical significance of this is unknown.
Carcinogenesis, Mutagenesis, Impairment of Fertility
The carcinogenic potential of AGGRASTAT has not been evaluated.
Tirofiban HCl was negative in the *in vitro* microbial mutagenesis and V-79 mammalian cell mutagenesis assays. In addition, there was no evidence of direct genotoxicity in the *in vitro* alkaline elution and *in vitro* chromosomal aberration assays. There was no induction of chromosomal aberrations in bone marrow cells of male mice after the administration of intravenous doses up to 5 mg tirofiban/kg (about 3 times the maximum recommended daily human dose when compared on a body surface area basis).
Fertility and reproductive performance were not affected in studies with male and female rats given intravenous doses of tirofiban hydrochloride up to 5 mg/kg/day (about 5 times the maximum recommended daily human dose when compared on a body surface area basis).
Pregnancy
Pregnancy Category B
Tirofiban has been shown to cross the placenta in pregnant rats and rabbits. Studies with tirofiban HCl at intravenous doses up to 5 mg/kg/day (about 5 and 13 times the maximum recommended daily human dose for rat and rabbit, respectively, when compared on a body surface area basis) have revealed no harm to the fetus. There are, however, no adequate and well-controlled studies in pregnant women. Because animal reproduction studies are not always predictive of human response, this drug should be used during pregnancy only if clearly needed.
Nursing Mothers
It is not known whether tirofiban is excreted in human milk. However, significant levels of tirofiban were shown to be present in rat milk. Because many drugs are excreted in human milk, and because of the potential for adverse effects on the nursing infant, a decision should be made whether to discontinue nursing or discontinue the drug, taking into account the importance of the drug to the mother.
Pediatric Use
Safety and effectiveness of AGGRASTAT in pediatric patients (<18 years old) have not been established.
Geriatric Use
Of the total number of patients in controlled clinical studies of AGGRASTAT, 42.8% were 65 years and over, while 11.7% were 75 and over. With respect to efficacy, the effect of AGGRASTAT in the elderly (≥65 years) appeared similar to that seen in younger patients (<65 years). Elderly patients receiving AGGRASTAT with heparin or heparin alone had a higher incidence of bleeding complications than younger patients, but the incremental risk of bleeding in patients treated with AGGRASTAT in combination with heparin compared to the risk in patients treated with heparin alone was similar regardless of age. The overall incidence of nonbleeding adverse events was higher in older patients (compared to younger patients) but this was true both for AGGRASTAT with heparin and heparin alone. No dose adjustment is recommended for the elderly population (see DOSAGE AND ADMINISTRATION, *Recommended Dosage*).

ADVERSE REACTIONS

In clinical trials, 1946 patients received AGGRASTAT in combination with heparin and 2002 patients received AGGRASTAT alone. Duration of exposure was up to 116 hours. 43% of the population was >65 years of age and approximately 30% of patients were female.
BLEEDING
The most common drug-related adverse event reported during therapy with AGGRASTAT when used concomitantly with heparin and aspirin, was bleeding (usually reported by the investigators as oozing or mild). The incidences of major and minor bleeding using the TIMI criteria in the PRISM-PLUS and RESTORE studies are shown below.
[See second table above]
There were no reports of intracranial bleeding in the PRISM-PLUS study for AGGRASTAT in combination with

heparin or in the heparin control group. The incidence of intracranial bleeding in the RESTORE study was 0.1% for AGGRASTAT in combination with heparin and 0.3% for the control group (which received heparin). In the PRISM-PLUS study, the incidences of retroperitoneal bleeding reported for AGGRASTAT in combination with heparin, and for the heparin control group were 0.0% and 0.1%, respectively. In the RESTORE study, the incidences of retroperitoneal bleeding reported for AGGRASTAT in combination with heparin, and the control group were 0.6% and 0.3%, respectively. The incidences of TIMI major gastrointestinal and genitourinary bleeding for AGGRASTAT in combination with heparin in the PRISM-PLUS study were 0.1% and 0.1%, respectively; the incidences in the RESTORE study for AGGRASTAT in combination with heparin were 0.2% and 0.0%, respectively.

The incidence rates of TIMI major bleeding in patients undergoing percutaneous procedures in PRISM-PLUS are shown below.

[See first table above]

The incidence rates of TIMI major bleeding (in some cases possibly reflecting hemodilution rather than actual bleeding) in patients undergoing CABG in the PRISM-PLUS and RESTORE studies within one day of discontinuation of AGGRASTAT are shown below.

[See second table above]

Female patients and elderly patients receiving AGGRASTAT with heparin or heparin alone had a higher incidence of bleeding complications than male patients or younger patients. The incremental risk of bleeding in patients treated with AGGRASTAT in combination with heparin over the risk in patients treated with heparin alone was comparable regardless of age or gender. No dose adjustment is recommended for these populations (see DOSAGE AND ADMINISTRATION, *Recommended Dosage*).

NON-BLEEDING

The incidences of non-bleeding adverse events that occurred at an incidence of >1% and numerically higher than control, regardless of drug relationship, are shown below:

	AGGRASTAT+ Heparin (n=1953) %	Heparin (n=1887) %
Body as a Whole		
Edema/swelling	2	1
Pain, pelvic	6	5
Reaction, vasovagal	2	1
Cardiovascular System		
Bradycardia	4	3
Dissection, coronary artery	5	4
Musculoskeletal System		
Pain, leg	3	2
Nervous System/Psychiatric		
Dizziness	3	2
Skin and Skin Appendage		
Sweating	2	1

Other non-bleeding side effects (considered at least possibly related to treatment) reported at a >1% rate with AGGRASTAT administered concomitantly with heparin were nausea, fever, and headache; these side effects were reported at a similar rate in the heparin group.

In clinical studies, the incidences of adverse events were generally similar among different races, patients with or without hypertension, patients with or without diabetes mellitus, and patients with or without hypercholesteremia. The overall incidence of non-bleeding adverse events was higher in female patients (compared to male patients) and older patients (compared to younger patients). However, the incidences of non-bleeding adverse events in these patients were comparable between the AGGRASTAT with heparin and the heparin alone groups. (See above for bleeding adverse events.)

Allergic Reactions/Readministration

No patients in the clinical database developed anaphylaxis and/or hives requiring discontinuation of the infusion of tirofiban (see also *Post-Marketing Experience, Hypersensitivity*). No information is available regarding the development of antibodies to tirofiban; very few patients received tirofiban twice.

Laboratory Findings

The most frequently observed laboratory adverse events in patients receiving AGGRASTAT concomitantly with heparin were related to bleeding. Decreases in hemoglobin (2.1%) and hematocrit (2.2%) were observed in the group receiving AGGRASTAT compared to 3.1% and 2.6%, respectively, in the heparin group. Increases in the presence of urine and fecal occult blood were also observed (10.7% and 18.3%, respectively) in the group receiving AGGRASTAT compared to 7.8% and 12.2%, respectively, in the heparin group.

Patients treated with AGGRASTAT, with heparin, were more likely to experience decreases in platelet counts than the control group. These decreases were reversible upon discontinuation of AGGRASTAT. The percentage of patients with a decrease of platelets to <90,000/mm^3 was 1.5%, compared with 0.6% in the patients who received heparin alone. The percentage of patients with a decrease of platelets to <50,000/mm^3 was 0.3%, compared with 0.1% of the patients who received heparin alone.

	AGGRASTAT + Heparin n	%	Heparin n	%
Prior to Procedures	2/773	0.3	1/797	0.1
Following Angiography	9/697	1.3	5/708	0.7
Following PTCA	6/239	2.5	5/236	2.2

	AGGRASTAT + Heparin n	%	Heparin n	%
PRISM-PLUS	5/29	17.2	11/31	35.4
RESTORE	3/12	25.0	6/16	37.5

	Most Patients		**Severe Renal Impairment**	
Patient Weight (kg)	30 Min Loading Infusion Rate (mL/hr)	Maintenance Infusion Rate (mL/hr)	30 Min Loading Infusion Rate (mL/hr)	Maintenance Infusion Rate (mL/hr)
30–37	16	4	8	2
38–45	20	5	10	3
46–54	24	6	12	3
55–62	28	7	14	4
63–70	32	8	16	4
71–79	36	9	18	5
80–87	40	10	20	5
88–95	44	11	22	6
96–104	48	12	24	6
105–112	52	13	26	7
113–120	56	14	28	7
121–128	60	15	30	8
129–137	64	16	32	8
138–145	68	17	34	9
146–153	72	18	36	9

Post-Marketing Experience

The following additional adverse reactions have been reported in post-marketing experience: *Bleeding:* intracranial bleeding, retroperitoneal bleeding, and hemopericardium; *Body as a Whole:* Acute decreases in platelet counts (see *Laboratory Findings* above) which may be associated with chills and low-grade fever; *Hypersensitivity:* Rash and/or hives.

OVERDOSAGE

In clinical trials, inadvertent overdosage with AGGRASTAT occurred in doses up to 5 times and 2 times the recommended dose for bolus administration and loading infusion, respectively. Inadvertent overdosage occurred in doses up to 9.8 times the 0.15 µg/kg/min maintenance infusion rate.

The most frequently reported manifestation of overdosage was bleeding, primarily minor mucocutaneous bleeding events and minor bleeding at the sites of cardiac catheterization (see PRECAUTIONS, *Bleeding Precautions*).

Overdosage of AGGRASTAT should be treated by assessment of the patient's clinical condition and cessation or adjustment of the drug infusion as appropriate.

AGGRASTAT can be removed by hemodialysis.

DOSAGE AND ADMINISTRATION

AGGRASTAT Injection must first be diluted to the same strength as AGGRASTAT Injection Premixed, as noted under *Directions for Use.*

Use with Aspirin and Heparin

In the clinical studies, patients received aspirin, unless it was contraindicated, and heparin. AGGRASTAT and heparin can be administered through the same intravenous catheter.

Precautions

AGGRASTAT is intended for intravenous delivery using sterile equipment and technique. Do not add other drugs or remove solution directly from the bag with a syringe. Do not use plastic containers in series connections; such use can result in air embolism by drawing air from the first container if it is empty of solution. Any unused solution should be discarded.

Directions for Use

AGGRASTAT Injection is first diluted to the same strength as AGGRASTAT Injection Premixed as follows: withdraw and discard 100 mL from a 500 mL bag of sterile 0.9% sodium chloride or 5% dextrose in water and replace this volume with 100 mL of AGGRASTAT Injection (from two 50 mL vials) or withdraw and discard 50 mL from a 250 mL bag of sterile 0.9% sodium chloride of 5% dextrose in water and replace this volume with 50 mL of AGGRASTAT Injection (from one 50 mL vial), to achieve a final concentration of 50 mcg/mL. Mix well prior to administration.

AGGRASTAT Injection Premixed is supplied as 250 mL or 500 mL of 0.9% sodium chloride containing 50 mcg/mL tirofiban. It is supplied in IntraVia *** containers (PL 2408 plastic). To open the IntraVia® container, first tear off its foil overpouch or dust cover. The plastic may be somewhat opaque because of moisture absorption during sterilization; the opacity will diminish gradually. Check for leaks by squeezing the inner bag firmly; if any leaks are found, the sterility is suspect and the solution should be discarded. Do not use unless the solution is clear and the seal is intact. Suspend the container from its eyelet support, remove the plastic protector from the outlet port, and attach a conventional administration set.

AGGRASTAT may be administered in the same intravenous line as dopamine, lidocaine, potassium chloride, and PEPCID* (famotidine) Injection. AGGRASTAT should not be administered in the same intravenous line as diazepam.

Recommended Dosage

In most patients, AGGRASTAT should be administered intravenously, at an initial rate of 0.4 mcg/kg/min for 30 minutes and then continued at 0.1 mcg/kg/min. Patients with severe renal insufficiency (creatinine clearance <30 mL/min) should receive half the usual rate of infusion (see PRECAUTIONS, *Severe Renal Insufficiency* and CLINICAL PHARMACOLOGY, *Pharmacokinetics, Special Populations, Renal Insufficiency*). The table below is provided as a guide to dosage adjustment by weight.

[See third table above]

No dosage adjustment is recommended for elderly or female patients (see PRECAUTIONS, *Geriatric Use*). In PRISM-PLUS, AGGRASTAT was administered in combination with heparin for 48 to 108 hours. The infusion should be continued through angiography and for 12 to 24 hours after angioplasty or atherectomy.

*** Registered trademark of Baxter International, Inc.
*Registered trademark of MERCK & CO., Inc.

Continued on next page

Information on the Merck & Co., Inc. products listed on these pages is the full prescribing information from product circulars in use September 30, 2000. For information, please call 1-800-NSC MERCK [1-800-672-6372].

Aggrastat—Cont.

HOW SUPPLIED

FOR INTRAVENOUS USE ONLY
No. 3713—AGGRASTAT Injection 12.5 mg per 50 mL (250 µg per mL) is a non-preserved, clear, colorless concentrated sterile solution for intravenous infusion after dilution and is supplied as follows:
NDC 0006-3713-50, 50 mL vials.
No. 3739—AGGRASTAT Injection Premixed 12.5 mg tirofiban per 250 mL (50 mcg per mL) and 25 mg tirofiban per 500 mL (50 mcg per mL) are clear, non-preserved, sterile solutions premixed in a vehicle made iso-osmotic with sodium chloride, and are supplied as follows:
NDC 0006-3739-96, 250 mL single-dose IntraVia® containers (PL 2408 Plastic).
NDC 0006-3739-43, 500 mL single-dose IntraVia® containers (PL 2408 Plastic).
Storage
AGGRASTAT Injection
Store at 25°C (77°F) with excursions permitted between 15–30°C (59–86°F) (see USP Controlled Room Temperature). Do not freeze. Protect from light during storage.
AGGRASTAT Injection Premixed
Store at 25°C (77°F) with excursions permitted between 15–30°C (59–86°F) (see USP Controlled Room Temperature). Do not freeze. Protect from light during storage.
AGGRASTAT (Tirofiban Hydrochloride Injection Premixed) is manufactured for:
MERCK & CO., INC., West Point, PA 19486, USA
by:
BAXTER HEALTHCARE CORPORATION
Deerfield, Illinois 60015 USA
AGGRASTAT (Tirofiban Hydrochloride Injection) is manufactured for:
MERCK & CO., INC., West Point, PA 19486, USA
by:
BEN VENUE LABORATORIES
Bedford, Ohio 44146 USA
9123305 Issued April 2000

ALDOCLOR® Tablets ℞
(Methyldopa-Chlorothiazide)

> **WARNING**
>
> This fixed combination drug is not indicated for initial therapy of hypertension. Hypertension requires therapy titrated to the individual patient. If the fixed combination represents the dosage so determined, its use may be more convenient in patient management. The treatment of hypertension is not static, but must be re-evaluated as conditions in each patient warrant.

DESCRIPTION

ALDOCLOR* (Methyldopa-Chlorothiazide) combines two antihypertensives: methyldopa and chlorothiazide.

Methyldopa
Methyldopa is an antihypertensive and is the *L* - isomer of alpha-methyldopa. It is levo-3-(3,4-dihydroxyphenyl)-2- methylalanine. Its empirical formula is $C_{10}H_{13}NO_4$, with a molecular weight of 211.22, and its structural formula is:

Methyldopa is a white to yellowish white, odorless fine powder, and is soluble in water.

Chlorothiazide
Chlorothiazide is a diuretic and antihypertensive. It is 6-chloro-2*H* -1, 2, 4-benzothiadiazine-7-sulfonamide 1, 1-dioxide. Its empirical formula is $C_7H_6ClN_3O_4S_2$ and its structural formula is:

It is a white, or practically white crystalline powder with a molecular weight of 295.73, which is very slightly soluble in water, but readily soluble in dilute aqueous sodium hydroxide. It is soluble in urine to the extent of about 150 mg per 100 mL at pH 7.

ALDOCLOR is supplied as tablets for oral use, each containing 250 mg of methyldopa and 250 mg of chlorothiazide. Each tablet contains the following inactive ingredients: calcium disodium edetate, cellulose, citric acid, D&C Yellow 10 aluminum lake, ethylcellulose, FD&C Yellow 6 aluminum lake, gelatin, glycerin, guar gum, hydroxypropyl methylcellulose, magnesium stearate, starch, talc, titanium dioxide, and FD&C Blue 2 aluminum lake.

---

*Registered trademark of MERCK & CO., Inc.

CLINICAL PHARMACOLOGY

Methyldopa
Methyldopa is an aromatic-amino-acid decarboxylase inhibitor in animals and in man. Although the mechanism of action has yet to be conclusively demonstrated, the antihypertensive effect of methyldopa probably is due to its metabolism to alpha-methylnorepinephrine, which then lowers arterial pressure by stimulation of central inhibitory alpha-adrenergic receptors, false neurotransmission, and/or reduction of plasma renin activity. Methyldopa has been shown to cause a net reduction in the tissue concentration of serotonin, dopamine, norepinephrine, and epinephrine.

Only methyldopa, the *L* -isomer of alpha-methyldopa, has the ability to inhibit dopa decarboxylase and to deplete animal tissues of norepinephrine. In man, the antihypertensive activity appears to be due solely to the *L* -isomer. About twice the dose of the racemate (*DL* -alpha-methyldopa) is required for equal antihypertensive effect.

Methyldopa has no direct effect on cardiac function and usually does not reduce glomerular filtration rate, renal blood flow, or filtration fraction. Cardiac output usually is maintained without cardiac acceleration. In some patients the heart rate is slowed.

Normal or elevated plasma renin activity may decrease in the course of methyldopa therapy.

Methyldopa reduces both supine and standing blood pressure. It usually produces highly effective lowering of the supine pressure with infrequent symptomatic postural hypotension. Exercise hypotension and diurnal blood pressure variations rarely occur.

Chlorothiazide
The mechanism of the antihypertensive effect of thiazides is unknown. Chlorothiazide does not usually affect normal blood pressure.

Chlorothiazide affects the distal renal tubular mechanism of electrolyte reabsorption. At maximal therapeutic dosage all thiazides are approximately equal in their diuretic efficacy.

Chlorothiazide increases excretion of sodium and chloride in approximately equivalent amounts. Natriuresis may be accompanied by some loss of potassium and bicarbonate.

After oral use diuresis begins within 2 hours, peaks in about 4 hours and lasts about 6 to 12 hours.

Pharmacokinetics and Metabolism
Methyldopa
The maximum decrease in blood pressure occurs four to six hours after oral dosage. After withdrawal, blood pressure usually returns to pretreatment levels within 24–48 hours.

Methyldopa is extensively metabolized. The known urinary metabolites are: α-methyldopa mono-0-sulfate; 3-0 methyl-α- methyldopa; 3,4,-dihydroxyphenylacetone; α-methyldopamine; 3-0-methyl-α-methyldopamine and their conjugates.

Approximately 70 percent of the drug which is absorbed is excreted in the urine as methyldopa and its mono-0-sulfate conjugate. The renal clearance is about 130 mL/min in normal subjects and is diminished in renal insufficiency. The plasma half-life of methyldopa is 105 minutes. After oral doses, excretion is essentially complete in 36 hours.

Methyldopa crosses the placental barrier, appears in cord blood, and appears in breast milk.

Chlorothiazide
Chlorothiazide is not metabolized but is eliminated rapidly by the kidney. The plasma half-life is 45–120 minutes. After oral doses, 20–24 percent of the dose is excreted unchanged in the urine. Chlorothiazide crosses the placental but not the blood-brain barrier and is excreted in breast milk.

INDICATION AND USAGE

Hypertension (see box warning).

CONTRAINDICATIONS

ALDOCLOR is contraindicated in patients:
— with active hepatic disease, such as acute hepatitis and active cirrhosis
— with liver disorders previously associated with methyldopa therapy (see WARNINGS)
— with anuria
— with hypersensitivity to methyldopa, or to chlorothiazide or other sulfonamide-derived drugs
— on therapy with monoamine oxidase (MAO) inhibitors.

WARNINGS

Methyldopa
It is important to recognize that a positive Coombs test, hemolytic anemia, and liver disorders may occur with methyldopa therapy. The rare occurrences of hemolytic anemia or liver disorders could lead to potentially fatal complications unless properly recognized and managed. Read this section carefully to understand these reactions.

With prolonged methyldopa therapy, 10 to 20 percent of patients develop a positive direct Coombs test which usually occurs between 6 and 12 months of methyldopa therapy. Lowest incidence is at daily dosage of 1 g or less. This on rare occasions may be associated with hemolytic anemia, which could lead to potentially fatal complications. One cannot predict which patients with a positive direct Coombs test may develop hemolytic anemia.

Prior existence or development of a positive direct Coombs test is not in itself a contraindication to use of methyldopa. If a positive Coombs test develops during methyldopa therapy, the physician should determine whether hemolytic anemia exists and whether the positive Coombs test may be a problem. For example, in addition to a positive direct Coombs test there is less often a positive indirect Coombs test which may interfere with cross matching of blood.

Before treatment is started, it is desirable to do a blood count (hematocrit, hemoglobin, or red cell count) for a baseline or to establish whether there is anemia. Periodic blood counts should be done during therapy to detect hemolytic anemia. It may be useful to do a direct Coombs test before therapy and at 6 and 12 months after the start of therapy.

If Coombs-positive hemolytic anemia occurs, the cause may be methyldopa and the drug should be discontinued. Usually the anemia remits promptly. If not, corticosteroids may be given and other causes of anemia should be considered. If the hemolytic anemia is related to methyldopa, the drug should not be reinstituted.

When methyldopa causes Coombs positivity alone or with hemolytic anemia, the red cell is usually coated with gamma globulin of the IgG (gamma G) class only. The positive Coombs test may not revert to normal until weeks to months after methyldopa is stopped.

Should the need for transfusion arise in a patient receiving methyldopa, both a direct and an indirect Coombs test should be performed. In the absence of hemolytic anemia, usually only the direct Coombs test will be positive. A positive direct Coombs test alone will not interfere with typing or cross matching. If the indirect Coombs test is also positive, problems may arise in the major cross match and the assistance of a hematologist or transfusion expert will be needed.

Occasionally, fever has occurred within the first three weeks of methyldopa therapy, associated in some cases with eosinophilia or abnormalities in one or more liver function tests, such as serum alkaline phosphatase, serum transaminases (SGOT, SGPT), bilirubin, and prothrombin time. Jaundice, with or without fever, may occur with onset usually within the first two to three months of therapy. In some patients the findings are consistent with those of cholestasis. In others the findings are consistent with hepatitis and hepatocellular injury.

Rarely, fatal hepatic necrosis has been reported after use of methyldopa. These hepatic changes may represent hypersensitivity reactions. Periodic determination of hepatic function should be done particularly during the first 6 to 12 weeks of therapy or whenever an unexplained fever occurs. If fever, abnormalities in liver function tests, or jaundice appear, stop therapy with methyldopa. If caused by methyldopa, the temperature and abnormalities in liver function characteristically have reverted to normal when the drug was discontinued. Methyldopa should not be reinstituted in such patients.

Rarely, a reversible reduction of the white blood cell count with a primary effect on the granulocytes has been seen. The granulocyte count returned promptly to normal on discontinuance of the drug. Rare cases of granulocytopenia have been reported. In each instance, upon stopping the drug, the white cell count returned to normal. Reversible thrombocytopenia has occurred rarely.

Chlorothiazide
Use with caution in severe renal disease. In patients with renal disease, thiazides may precipitate azotemia. Cumulative effects of the drug may develop in patients with impaired renal function.

Thiazides should be used with caution in patients with impaired hepatic function or progressive liver disease, since minor alterations of fluid and electrolyte balance may precipitate hepatic coma.

Thiazides may add to or potentiate the action of other antihypertensive drugs.

Sensitivity reactions may occur in patients with or without a history of allergy or bronchial asthma.

The possibility of exacerbation or activation of systemic lupus erythematosus has been reported.

Lithium generally should not be given with diuretics (see PRECAUTIONS, *Drug Interactions*).

PRECAUTIONS

General
Methyldopa
Methyldopa should be used with caution in patients with a history of previous liver disease or dysfunction (see WARNINGS).

Some patients taking methyldopa experience clinical edema or weight gain which may be controlled by use of a diuretic. Methyldopa should not be continued if edema progresses or signs of heart failure appear.

Hypertension has recurred occasionally after dialysis in patients given methyldopa because the drug is removed by this procedure.

Rarely, involuntary choreoathetotic movements have been observed during therapy with methyldopa in patients with severe bilateral cerebrovascular disease. Should these movements occur, stop therapy.

Chlorothiazide
All patients receiving diuretic therapy should be observed for evidence of fluid or electrolyte imbalance: namely, hyponatremia, hypochloremic alkalosis, and hypokalemia. Serum and urine electrolyte determinations are particularly important when the patient is vomiting excessively or receiving parenteral fluids. Warning signs or symptoms of fluid and electrolyte imbalance, irrespective of cause include dryness of mouth, thirst, weakness, lethargy, drowsiness, restlessness, confusion, seizures, muscle pains or cramps, muscular fatigue, hypotension, oliguria, tachycardia, and gastrointestinal disturbances such as nausea and vomiting. Hypokalemia may develop, especially after prolonged therapy or when severe cirrhosis is present (see CONTRAINDICATIONS and WARNINGS).
Interference with adequate oral electrolyte intake will also contribute to hypokalemia. Hypokalemia may cause cardiac arrhythmia and may also sensitize or exaggerate the response of the heart to the toxic effects of digitalis (e.g., increased ventricular irritability). Hypokalemia may be avoided or treated by use of potassium sparing diuretics or potassium supplements such as foods with a high potassium content.
Although any chloride deficit is generally mild and usually does not require specific treatment except under extraordinary circumstances (as in liver disease or renal disease), chloride replacement may be required in the treatment of metabolic alkalosis.
Dilutional hyponatremia may occur in edematous patients in hot weather; appropriate therapy is water restriction, rather than administration of salt, except in rare instances when the hyponatremia is life threatening. In actual salt depletion, appropriate replacement is the therapy of choice.
Hyperuricemia may occur or acute gout may be precipitated in certain patients receiving thiazides.
In diabetic patients dosage adjustments of insulin or oral hypoglycemic agents may be required. Hyperglycemia may occur with thiazide diuretics. Thus latent diabetes mellitus may become manifest during thiazide therapy.
The antihypertensive effects of the drug may be enhanced in the postsympathectomy patient.
If progressive renal impairment becomes evident, consider withholding or discontinuing diuretic therapy.
Thiazides have been shown to increase the urinary excretion of magnesium; this may result in hypomagnesemia.
Thiazides may decrease urinary calcium excretion. Thiazides may cause intermittent and slight elevation of serum calcium in the absence of known disorders of calcium metabolism. Marked hypercalcemia may be evidence of hidden hyperparathyroidism. Thiazides should be discontinued before carrying out tests for parathyroid function.
Increases in cholesterol and triglyceride levels may be associated with thiazide diuretic therapy.
Laboratory Tests
Methyldopa
Blood count, Coombs test and liver function tests are recommended before initiating therapy and at periodic intervals (see WARNINGS).
Chlorothiazide
Periodic determination of serum electrolytes to detect possible electrolyte imbalance should be done at appropriate intervals.
Drug Interactions
Methyldopa
When methyldopa is used with other antihypertensive drugs, potentiation of antihypertensive effect may occur. Patients should be followed carefully to detect side reactions or unusual manifestations of drug idiosyncrasy.
Patients may require reduced doses of anesthetics when on methyldopa. If hypotension does occur during anesthesia, it usually can be controlled by vasopressors. The adrenergic receptors remain sensitive during treatment with methyldopa.
When methyldopa and lithium are given concomitantly the patient should be carefully monitored for symptoms of lithium toxicity. Read the prescribing information for lithium preparations.
Several studies demonstrate a decrease in the bioavailability of methyldopa when it is ingested with ferrous sulfate or ferrous gluconate. This may adversely affect blood pressure control in patients treated with methyldopa. Coadministration of methyldopa with ferrous sulfate or ferrous gluconate is not recommended.
Monoamine oxidase (MAO) inhibitors: See CONTRAINDICATIONS.
Chlorothiazide
When given concurrently the following drugs may interact with thiazide diuretics.
Alcohol, barbiturates, or narcotics —potentiation of orthostatic hypotension may occur.
Antidiabetic drugs (oral agents and insulin)—dosage adjustment of the antidiabetic drug may be required.
Other antihypertensive drugs —additive effect or potentiation.
Cholestyramine and colestipol resins —Both cholestyramine and colestipol resins have the potential of binding thiazide diuretics and reducing diuretic absorption from the gastrointestinal tract.
Corticosteroids, ACTH —intensified electrolyte depletion, particularly hypokalemia.
Pressor amines (e.g., norepinephrine) —possible decreased response to pressor amines but not sufficient to preclude their use.
Skeletal muscle relaxants, nondepolarizing (e.g., tubocurarine) —possible increased responsiveness to the muscle relaxant.
Lithium —generally should not be given with diuretics. Diuretic agents reduce the renal clearance of lithium and add a high risk of lithium toxicity. Refer to the package insert for lithium preparations before use of such preparations with ALDOCLOR.
Non-steroidal Anti-inflammatory Drugs —In some patients, the administration of a non-steroidal anti-inflammatory agent can reduce the diuretic, natriuretic, and antihypertensive effects of loop, potassium-sparing and thiazide diuretics. Therefore, when ALDOCLOR and non-steroidal anti-inflammatory agents are used concomitantly, the patient should be observed closely to determine if the desired effect of the diuretic is obtained.
Drug/Laboratory Test Interactions
Methyldopa
Methyldopa may interfere with measurement of: urinary uric acid by the phosphotungstate method, serum creatinine by the alkaline picrate method, and SGOT by colorimetric methods. Interference with spectrophotometric methods for SGOT analysis has not been reported.
Since methyldopa causes fluorescence in urine samples at the same wave lengths as catecholamines, falsely high levels of urinary catecholamines may be reported. This will interfere with the diagnosis of pheochromocytoma. It is important to recognize this phenomenon before a patient with a possible pheochromocytoma is subjected to surgery. Methyldopa does not interfere with measurement of VMA (vanillylmandelic acid), a test for pheochromocytoma, by those methods which convert VMA to vanillin. Methyldopa is not recommended for the treatment of patients with pheochromocytoma. Rarely, when urine is exposed to air after voiding, it may darken because of breakdown of methyldopa or its metabolites.
Chlorothiazide
Thiazides should be discontinued before carrying out tests for parathyroid function (see PRECAUTIONS, *General*).
Carcinogenesis, Mutagenesis, Impairment of Fertility
Studies to evaluate the carcinogenic or mutagenic potential of the methyldopa-chlorothiazide combination, or the effects of this combination on fertility have not been performed.
Methyldopa
No evidence of a tumorigenic effect was seen when methyldopa was given for two years to mice at doses up to 1800 mg/kg/day or to rats at doses up to 240 mg/kg/day (30 and 4 times the maximum recommended human dose in mice and rats, respectively, when compared on the basis of body weight; 2.5 and 0.6 times the maximum recommended human dose in mice and rats, respectively, when compared on the basis of body surface area; calculations assume a patient weight of 50 kg).
Methyldopa was not mutagenic in the Ames Test and did not increase chromosomal aberration or sister chromatid exchanges in Chinese hamster ovary cells. These *in vitro* studies were carried out both with and without exogenous metabolic activation.
Fertility was unaffected when methyldopa was given to male and female rats at 100 mg/kg/day (1.7 times the maximum daily human dose when compared on the basis of body weight; 0.2 times the maximum daily human dose when compared on the basis of body surface area). Methyldopa decreased sperm count, sperm motility, the number of late spermatids and the male fertility index when given to male rats of 200 and 400 mg/kg/day (3.3 and 6 times the maximum daily human dose when compared on the basis of body weight; 0.5 and 1 times the maximum daily human dose when compared on the basis of body surface area).
Chlorothiazide
Carcinogenicity studies have not been done with chlorothiazide.
Chlorothiazide was not mutagenic *in vitro* in the Ames microbial mutagen test (using a maximum concentration of 5 mg/plate and *Salmonella typhimurium* strains TA 98 and TA 100) and was not mutagenic and did not induce miotic nondis junction to diploid-strains of *Aspergillus nidulans.*
Chlorothiazide had no adverse effects on fertility in female rats at doses up to 60/mg/kg/day and no adverse effects on fertility in male rats at doses up to 40 mg/kg/day. These doses are 1.5 and 1.0 times* the recommended maximum human dose, respectively, when compared on a body weight basis.

*Calculations based on a human body weight of 50 kg.

Pregnancy
Use of diuretics during normal pregnancy is inappropriate and exposes mother and fetus to unnecessary hazard. Diuretics do not prevent development of toxemia of pregnancy and there is no satisfactory evidence that they are useful in treatment of toxemia.
Teratogenic Effects —Pregnancy Category C: Reproduction studies in the rat, at doses up to 40 mg/kg/day (3–4 times the maximum recommended human dose), did not impair fertility or cause abnormalities of the fetus due to ALDOCLOR.
There are no adequate and well-controlled studies with ALDOCLOR in pregnant women. Because animal reproduction studies are not always predictive of human response, this drug should be used during pregnancy only if clearly needed.
Chlorothiazide: Thiazides cross the placental barrier and appear in cord blood.
Although reproduction studies performed with chlorothiazide doses of 50 mg/kg/day in rabbits, 60 mg/kg/day in rats and 500 mg/kg/day in mice revealed no external abnormalities or impairment of neonatal growth and survival due to chlorothiazide, such studies did not include complete visceral and skeletal examinations.
Methyldopa: Reproduction studies performed with methyldopa at oral doses up to 1000 mg/kg in mice, 200 mg/kg in rabbits, and 100 mg/kg in rats revealed no evidence of harm to the fetus. These doses are 16.6 times, 3.3 times and 1.7 times, respectively, the maximum daily human dose when compared on the basis of body weight: 1.4 times, 1.1 times and 0.2 times, respectively, when compared on the basis of body surface area: calculations assume a patient weight of 50 kg. There are, however, no adequate and well-controlled studies in pregnant women in the first trimester of pregnancy. Because animal reproduction studies are not always predictive of human response, methyldopa should be used during pregnancy only if clearly needed.
Published reports of the use of methyldopa during all trimesters indicate that if this drug is used during pregnancy the possibility of fetal harm appears remote. In five studies, three of which were controlled, involving 332 pregnant hypertensive women, treatment with methyldopa was associated with an improved fetal outcome. The majority of these women were in the third trimester when methyldopa therapy was begun.
In one study, women who had begun methyldopa treatment between weeks 16 and 20 of pregnancy gave birth to infants whose average head circumference was reduced by a small amount (34.2 ± 1.7 cm vs. 34.6 ± 1.3 cm [mean ± 1 S.D.]). Long-term follow up of 195 (97.5%) of the children born to methyldopa-treated pregnant women (including those who began treatment between weeks 16 and 20) failed to uncover any significant adverse effect on the children. At four years of age, the developmental delay commonly seen in children born to hypertensive mothers was less evident in those whose mothers were treated with methyldopa during pregnancy than those whose mothers were untreated. The children of the treated group scored consistently higher than the children of the untreated group on five major indices of intellectual and motor development. At age seven and one-half developmental scores and intelligence indices showed no significant differences in children of treated or untreated hypertensive women.
Nonteratogenic Effects: These may include fetal or neonatal jaundice, thrombocytopenia, and possibly other adverse reactions which have occurred in the adult.
Nursing Mothers
Methyldopa and thiazides appear in breast milk. Therefore, because of the potential for serious adverse reactions in nursing infants from chlorothiazide, a decision should be made whether to discontinue nursing or to discontinue the drug, taking into account the importance of the drug to the mother.
Pediatric Use
Safety and effectiveness of ALDOCLOR in pediatric patients have not been established.

ADVERSE REACTIONS

The following adverse reactions have been reported and, within each category, are listed in order of decreasing severity.
Methyldopa
Sedation, usually transient, may occur during the initial period of therapy or whenever the dose is increased. Headache, asthenia, or weakness may be noted as early and transient symptoms. However, significant adverse effects due to methyldopa have been infrequent and this agent usually is well tolerated.
Cardiovascular: Aggravation of angina pectoris, congestive heart failure, prolonged carotid sinus hypersensitivity, orthostatic hypotension (decrease daily dosage), edema or weight gain, bradycardia.
Digestive: Pancreatitis, colitis, vomiting, diarrhea, sialadenitis, sore or "black" tongue, nausea, constipation, distension, flatus, dryness of mouth.
Endocrine: Hyperprolactinemia.
Hematologic: Bone marrow depression, leukopenia, granulocytopenia, thrombocytopenia, hemolytic anemia; positive tests for antinuclear antibody, LE cells, and rheumatoid factor, positive Coombs test.
Hepatic: Liver disorders including hepatitis, jaundice, abnormal liver function tests (see WARNINGS).
Hypersensitivity: Myocarditis, pericarditis, vasculitis, lupus-like syndrome, drug-related fever, eosinophilia.
Nervous System/Psychiatric: Parkinsonism, Bell's palsy, decreased mental acuity, involuntary choreoathetotic movements, symptoms of cerebrovascular insufficiency, psychic disturbances including nightmares and reversible mild psychoses or depression, headache, sedation, asthenia or weakness, dizziness, lightheadedness, paresthesias.
Metabolic: Rise in BUN.
Musculoskeletal: Arthralgia, with or without joint swelling; myalgia.

Continued on next page

Information on the Merck & Co., Inc. products listed on these pages is the full prescribing information from product circulars in use September 30, 2000. For information, please call 1-800-NSC MERCK [1-800-672-6372].

Aldoclor—Cont.

Respiratory: Nasal stuffiness.
Skin: Toxic epidermal necrolysis, rash.
Urogenital: Amenorrhea, breast enlargement, gynecomastia, lactation, impotence, decreased libido.
Chlorothiazide
Body as a Whole: Weakness.
Cardiovascular: Hypotension including orthostatic hypotension (may be aggravated by alcohol, barbiturates, narcotics or antihypertensive drugs).
Digestive: Pancreatitis, jaundice (intrahepatic cholestatic jaundice), diarrhea, vomiting, sialadenitis, cramping, constipation, gastric irritation, nausea, anorexia.
Hematologic: Aplastic anemia, agranulocytosis, leukopenia, hemolytic anemia, thrombocytopenia.
Hypersensitivity: Anaphylactic reactions, necrotizing angiitis (vasculitis and cutaneous vasculitis), respiratory distress including pneumonitis and pulmonary edema, photosensitivity, fever, urticaria, rash, purpura.
Metabolic: Electrolyte imbalance (see PRECAUTIONS), hyperglycemia, glycosuria, hyperuricemia.
Musculoskeletal: Muscle spasm.
Nervous System/Psychiatric: Vertigo, paresthesias, dizziness, headache, restlessness.
Renal: Renal failure, renal dysfunction, interstitial nephritis. (See WARNINGS.)
Skin: Erythema multiforme including Stevens-Johnson syndrome, exfoliative dermatitis including toxic epidermal necrolysis, alopecia.
Special Senses: Transient blurred vision, xanthopsia.
Urogenital: Impotence.

OVERDOSAGE

Acute overdosage may produce acute hypotension with other responses attributable to brain and gastrointestinal malfunction (excessive sedation, weakness, bradycardia, dizziness, lightheadedness, constipation, distention, flatus, diarrhea, nausea, vomiting).
In the event of overdosage, symptomatic and supportive measures should be employed. When ingestion is recent, gastric lavage or emesis may reduce absorption. Otherwise, management includes special attention to cardiac rate and output, blood volume, electrolyte imbalance, paralytic ileus, urinary function and cerebral activity.
Sympathomimetic drugs [e.g., levarterenol, epinephrine, ARAMINE* (Metaraminol Bitartrate)] may be indicated. Methyldopa is dialyzable. The degree to which chlorothiazide is removed by hemodialysis has not been established.
The oral LD_{50} of methyldopa is greater than 1.5 g/kg in both the mouse and the rat. The oral LD_{50} of chlorothiazide is 8.5 g/kg, greater than 10 g/kg, and greater than 1 g/kg in the mouse, rat, and dog respectively.

*Registered trademark of MERCK & CO., INC.

DOSAGE AND ADMINISTRATION

DOSAGE MUST BE INDIVIDUALIZED, AS DETERMINED BY TITRATION OF THE INDIVIDUAL COMPONENTS (see box warning). Once the patient has been successfully titrated, ALDOCLOR may be substituted if the previously determined titrated doses are the same as in the combination. The usual starting dosage is one tablet of ALDOCLOR 250 two or three times a day.
When administered individually, the usual daily dosage of chlorothiazide is 0.5 g to 1.0 g in single or divided doses and that of methyldopa is 500 mg to 2 g. To minimize the sedation associated with methyldopa, start dosage increases in the evening.
Occasionally tolerance to methyldopa may occur, usually between the second and third month of therapy. Additional separate doses of methyldopa or replacement of ALDOCLOR with single entity agents is necessary until the new effective dose ratio is re-established by titration. The maximum recommended daily dose of methyldopa is 3 g. When ALDOCLOR 250 is used to provide 1 g of methyldopa, 1 g of chlorothiazide is delivered. It is prudent, if greater than 1 g of methyldopa per day is required, to provide the additional methyldopa as methyldopa alone.
If ALDOCLOR does not adequately control blood pressure, additional doses of other agents may be given. When ALDOCLOR is given with antihypertensives other than thiazides, the initial dosage of methyldopa should be limited to 500 mg daily in divided doses and the dose of these other agents may need to be adjusted to effect a smooth transition.
Since both components of ALDOCLOR have a relatively short duration of action, withdrawal is followed by return of hypertension usually within 48 hours. This is not complicated by an overshoot of blood pressure.
Since methyldopa is largely excreted by the kidney, patients with impaired renal function may respond to smaller doses. Syncope in older patients may be related to an increased sensitivity and advanced arteriosclerotic vascular disease. This may be avoided by lower doses.

HOW SUPPLIED

No. 3319—Tablets ALDOCLOR 250 are green, oval, film coated tablets coded MSD 634 on one side and ALDOCLOR on the other. Each tablet contains 250 mg of methyldopa and 250 mg of chlorothiazide. They are supplied as follows:
NDC 0006-0634-68 bottles of 100.
Shown in Product Identification Guide, page 323
Storage
Keep container tightly closed. Protect from moisture, light, and freezing, −20°C (−4°F) and store at room temperature, 15–30°C (59–86°F).
7899646 Issued February 1999

ALDOMET® Tablets ℞
(Methyldopa)

DESCRIPTION

ALDOMET* (Methyldopa) is an antihypertensive drug.
Methyldopa, the *L*-isomer of alpha-methyldopa is levo-3-(3,4 - dihydroxyphenyl) -2-methylalanine. Its empirical formula is $C_{10}H_{13}NO_4$, with a molecular weight of 211.22, and its structural formula is:

Methyldopa is a white to yellowish white, odorless fine powder, and is soluble in water.
ALDOMET is supplied as tablets, for oral use, in three strengths: 125 mg, 250 mg, or 500 mg of methyldopa per tablet. Inactive ingredients in the tablets are: calcium disodium edetate, cellulose, citric acid, colloidal silicon dioxide, D&C Yellow 10, ethylcellulose, guar gum, hydroxypropyl methylcellulose, iron oxide, magnesium stearate, propylene glycol, talc, and titanium dioxide.

*Registered trademark of MERCK & CO., INC.

CLINICAL PHARMACOLOGY

ALDOMET is an aromatic-amino-acid decarboxylase inhibitor in animals and in man. Although the mechanism of action has yet to be conclusively demonstrated, the antihypertensive effect of methyldopa probably is due to its metabolism to alpha-methylnorepinephrine, which then lowers arterial pressure by stimulation of central inhibitory alpha-adrenergic receptors, false neurotransmission, and/or reduction of plasma renin activity. Methyldopa has been shown to cause a net reduction in the tissue concentration of serotonin, dopamine, norepinephrine, and epinephrine.
Only methyldopa, the *L*-isomer of alpha-methyldopa, has the ability to inhibit dopa decarboxylase and to deplete animal tissues of norepinephrine. In man the antihypertensive activity appears to be due solely to the *L*-isomer. About twice the dose of the racemate (*DL*-alpha-methyldopa) is required for equal antihypertensive effect.
Methyldopa has no direct effect on cardiac function and usually does not reduce glomerular filtration rate, renal blood flow, or filtration fraction. Cardiac output usually is maintained without cardiac acceleration. In some patients the heart rate is slowed.
Normal or elevated plasma renin activity may decrease in the course of methyldopa therapy.
ALDOMET reduces both supine and standing blood pressure. Methyldopa usually produces highly effective lowering of the supine pressure with infrequent symptomatic postural hypotension. Exercise hypotension and diurnal blood pressure variations rarely occur.
Pharmacokinetics and Metabolism
The maximum decrease in blood pressure occurs four to six hours after oral dosage. Once an effective dosage level is attained, a smooth blood pressure response occurs in most patients in 12 to 24 hours. After withdrawal, blood pressure usually returns to pretreatment levels within 24–48 hours.
Methyldopa is extensively metabolized. The known urinary metabolites are: α-methyldopa mono-0-sulfate; 3-0-methyl-α-methyldopa; 3,4-dihydroxyphenylacetone; α-methyldopamine; 3-0-methyl-α-methyldopamine and their conjugates.
Approximately 70% of the drug which is absorbed is excreted in the urine as methyldopa and its mono-0-sulfate conjugate. The renal clearance is about 130 mL/min in normal subjects and is diminished in renal insufficiency. The plasma half-life of methyldopa is 105 minutes. After oral doses, excretion is essentially complete in 36 hours.
Methyldopa crosses the placental barrier, appears in cord blood, and appears in breast milk.

INDICATION AND USAGE

Hypertension.

CONTRAINDICATIONS

ALDOMET is contraindicated in patients:
— with active hepatic disease, such as acute hepatitis and active cirrhosis
— with liver disorders previously associated with methyldopa therapy (see WARNINGS)
— with hypersensitivity to any component of these products
— on therapy with monoamine oxidase (MAO) inhibitors.

WARNINGS

It is important to recognize that a positive Coombs test, hemolytic anemia, and liver disorders may occur with methyldopa therapy. The rare occurrences of hemolytic anemia or liver disorders could lead to potentially fatal complications unless properly recognized and managed. Read this section carefully to understand these reactions.
With prolonged methyldopa therapy, 10 to 20 percent of patients develop a positive direct Coombs test which usually occurs between 6 and 12 months of methyldopa therapy. Lowest incidence is at daily dosage of 1 g or less. This on rare occasions may be associated with hemolytic anemia, which could lead to potentially fatal complications. One cannot predict which patients with a positive direct Coombs test may develop hemolytic anemia.
Prior existence or development of a positive direct Coombs test is not in itself a contraindication to use of methyldopa. If a positive Coombs test develops during methyldopa therapy, the physician should determine whether hemolytic anemia exists and whether the positive Coombs test may be a problem. For example, in addition to a positive direct Coombs test there is less often a positive indirect Coombs test which may interfere with cross matching of blood.
Before treatment is started, it is desirable to do a blood count (hematocrit, hemoglobin, or red cell count) for a baseline or to establish whether there is anemia. Periodic blood counts should be done during therapy to detect hemolytic anemia. It may be useful to do a direct Coombs test before therapy and at 6 and 12 months after the start of therapy.
If Coombs-positive hemolytic anemia occurs, the cause may be methyldopa and the drug should be discontinued. Usually the anemia remits promptly. If not, corticosteroids may be given and other causes of anemia should be considered. If the hemolytic anemia is related to methyldopa, the drug should not be reinstituted.
When methyldopa causes Coombs positivity alone or with hemolytic anemia, the red cell is usually coated with gamma globulin of the IgG (gamma G) class only. The positive Coombs test may not revert to normal until weeks to months after methyldopa is stopped.
Should the need for transfusion arise in a patient receiving methyldopa, both a direct and an indirect Coombs test should be performed. In the absence of hemolytic anemia, usually only the direct Coombs test will be positive. A positive direct Coombs test alone will not interfere with typing or cross matching. If the indirect Coombs test is also positive, problems may arise in the major cross match and the assistance of a hematologist or transfusion expert will be needed.
Occasionally, fever has occurred within the first 3 weeks of methyldopa therapy, associated in some cases with eosinophilia or abnormalities in one or more liver function tests, such as serum alkaline phosphatase, serum transaminases (SGOT, SGPT), bilirubin, and prothrombin time. Jaundice, with or without fever, may occur with onset usually within the first 2 to 3 months of therapy. In some patients the findings are consistent with those of cholestasis. In others the findings are consistent with hepatitis and hepatocellular injury.
Rarely, fatal hepatic necrosis has been reported after use of methyldopa. These hepatic changes may represent hypersensitivity reactions. Periodic determinations of hepatic function should be done particularly during the first 6 to 12 weeks of therapy or whenever an unexplained fever occurs. If fever, abnormalities in liver function tests, or jaundice appear, stop therapy with methyldopa. If caused by methyldopa, the temperature and abnormalities in liver function characteristically have reverted to normal when the drug was discontinued. Methyldopa should not be reinstituted in such patients.
Rarely, a reversible reduction of the white blood cell count with a primary effect on the granulocytes has been seen. The granulocyte count returned promptly to normal on discontinuance of the drug. Rare cases of granulocytopenia have been reported. In each instance, upon stopping the drug, the white cell count returned to normal. Reversible thrombocytopenia has occurred rarely.

PRECAUTIONS

General
Methyldopa should be used with caution in patients with a history of previous liver disease or dysfunction (see WARNINGS).
Some patients taking methyldopa experience clinical edema or weight gain which may be controlled by use of a diuretic. Methyldopa should not be continued if edema progresses or signs of heart failure appear.
Hypertension has recurred occasionally after dialysis in patients given methyldopa because the drug is removed by this procedure.
Rarely involuntary choreoathetotic movements have been observed during therapy with methyldopa in patients with severe bilateral cerebrovascular disease. Should these movements occur, stop therapy.
Laboratory Tests
Blood count, Coombs test, and liver function tests are recommended before initiating therapy and at periodic intervals (see WARNINGS).

Drug Interactions
When methyldopa is used with other antihypertensive drugs, potentiation of antihypertensive effect may occur. Patients should be followed carefully to detect side reactions or unusual manifestations of drug idiosyncrasy.
Patients may require reduced doses of anesthetics when on methyldopa. If hypotension does occur during anesthesia, it usually can be controlled by vasopressors. The adrenergic receptors remain sensitive during treatment with methyldopa.
When methyldopa and lithium are given concomitantly the patient should be carefully monitored for symptoms of lithium toxicity. Read the circular for lithium preparations.
Several studies demonstrate a decrease in the bioavailability of methyldopa when it is ingested with ferrous sulfate or ferrous gluconate. This may adversely affect blood pressure control in patients treated with methyldopa. Coadministration of methyldopa with ferrous sulfate or ferrous gluconate is not recommended.
Monoamine oxidase (MAO) inhibitors: see CONTRAINDICATIONS.
Drug/Laboratory Test Interactions
Methyldopa may interfere with measurement of: urinary uric acid by the phosphotungstate method, serum creatinine by the alkaline picrate method, and SGOT by colorimetric methods. Interference with spectrophotometric methods for SGOT analysis has not been reported.
Since methyldopa causes fluorescence in urine samples at the same wave lengths as catecholamines, falsely high levels of urinary catecholamines may be reported. This will interfere with the diagnosis of pheochromocytoma. It is important to recognize this phenomenon before a patient with a possible pheochromocytoma is subjected to surgery. Methyldopa does not interfere with measurement of VMA (vanillylmandelic acid), a test for pheochromocytoma, by those methods which convert VMA to vanillin. Methyldopa is not recommended for the treatment of patients with pheochromocytoma. Rarely, when urine is exposed to air after voiding, it may darken because of breakdown of methyldopa or its metabolites.
Carcinogenesis, Mutagenesis, Impairment of Fertility
No evidence of a tumorigenic effect was seen when methyldopa was given for two years to mice at doses up to 1800 mg/kg/day or to rats at doses up to 240 mg/kg/day (30 and 4 times the maximum recommended human dose in mice and rats, respectively, when compared on the basis of body weight; 2.5 and 0.6 times the maximum recommended human dose in mice and rats, respectively, when compared on the basis of body surface area; calculations assume a patient weight of 50 kg).
Methyldopa was not mutagenic in the Ames Test and did not increase chromosomal aberration or sister chromatid exchanges in Chinese hamster ovary cells. These *in vitro* studies were carried out both with and without exogenous metabolic activation.
Fertility was unaffected when methyldopa was given to male and female rats at 100 mg/kg/day (1.7 times the maximum daily human dose when compared on the basis of body weight; 0.2 times the maximum daily human dose when compared on the basis of body surface area). Methyldopa decreased sperm count, sperm motility, the number of late spermatids and the male fertility index when given to male rats at 200 and 400 mg/kg/day (3.3 and 6.7 times the maximum daily human dose when compared on the basis of body weight; 0.5 and 1 times the maximum daily human dose when compared on the basis of body surface area).
Pregnancy
Pregnancy Category B. Reproduction studies performed with methyldopa at oral doses up to 1000 mg/kg in mice, 200 mg/kg in rabbits and 100 mg/kg in rats revealed no evidence of harm to the fetus. These doses are 16.6 times, 3.3 times and 1.7 times, respectively, the maximum daily human dose when compared on the basis of body weight; 1.4 times, 1.1 times and 0.2 times, respectively, when compared on the basis of body surface area; calculations assume a patient weight of 50 kg. There are, however, no adequate and well-controlled studies in pregnant women in the first trimester of pregnancy. Because animal reproduction studies are not always predictive of human response, ALDOMET should be used during pregnancy only if clearly needed.
Published reports of the use of methyldopa during all trimesters indicate that if this drug is used during pregnancy the possibility of fetal harm appears remote. In five studies, three of which were controlled, involving 332 pregnant hypertensive women, treatment with ALDOMET was associated with an improved fetal outcome. The majority of these women were in the third trimester when methyldopa therapy was begun.
In one study, women who had begun methyldopa treatment between weeks 16 and 20 of pregnancy gave birth to infants whose average head circumference was reduced by a small amount (34.2 ± 1.7 cm vs. 34.6 ± 1.3 cm [mean ± 1 S.D.]). Long-term follow up of 195 (97.5%) of the children born to methyldopa-treated pregnant women (including those who began treatment between weeks 16 and 20) failed to uncover any significant adverse effect on the children. At four years of age, the developmental delay commonly seen in children born to hypertensive mothers was less evident in those whose mothers were treated with methyldopa during pregnancy than those whose mothers were untreated. The children of the treated group scored consistently higher than the children of the untreated group on five major indices of intellectual and motor development. At age seven and one-half developmental scores and intelligence indices showed no significant differences in children of treated or untreated hypertensive women.
Nursing Mothers
Methyldopa appears in breast milk. Therefore, caution should be exercised when methyldopa is given to a nursing woman.
Pediatric Use
There are no well-controlled clinical trials in pediatric patients. Information on dosing in pediatric patients is supported by evidence from published literature regarding the treatment of hypertension in pediatric patients. (See DOSAGE AND ADMINISTRATION.)

ADVERSE REACTIONS

Sedation, usually transient, may occur during the initial period of therapy or whenever the dose is increased. Headache, asthenia, or weakness may be noted as early and transient symptoms. However, significant adverse effects due to ALDOMET have been infrequent and this agent usually is well tolerated.
The following adverse reactions have been reported and, within each category, are listed in order of decreasing severity.
Cardiovascular: Aggravation of angina pectoris, congestive heart failure, prolonged carotid sinus hypersensitivity, orthostatic hypotension (decrease daily dosage), edema or weight gain, bradycardia.
Digestive: Pancreatitis, colitis, vomiting, diarrhea, sialadenitis, sore or "black" tongue, nausea, constipation, distension, flatus, dryness of mouth.
Endocrine: Hyperprolactinemia.
Hematologic: Bone marrow depression, leukopenia, granulocytopenia, thrombocytopenia, hemolytic anemia; positive tests for antinuclear antibody, LE cells, and rheumatoid factor, positive Coombs test.
Hepatic: Liver disorders including hepatitis, jaundice, abnormal liver function tests (see WARNINGS).
Hypersensitivity: Myocarditis, pericarditis, vasculitis, lupus-like syndrome, drug-related fever, eosinophilia.
Nervous System/Psychiatric: Parkinsonism, Bell's palsy, decreased mental acuity, involuntary choreoathetotic movements, symptoms of cerebrovascular insufficiency, psychic disturbances including nightmares and reversible mild psychoses or depression, headache, sedation, asthenia or weakness, dizziness, lightheadedness, paresthesias.
Metabolic: Rise in BUN.
Musculoskeletal: Arthralgia, with or without joint swelling; myalgia.
Respiratory: Nasal stuffiness.
Skin: Toxic epidermal necrolysis, rash.
Urogenital: Amenorrhea, breast enlargement, gynecomastia, lactation, impotence, decreased libido.

OVERDOSAGE

Acute overdosage may produce acute hypotension with other responses attributable to brain and gastrointestinal malfunction (excessive sedation, weakness, bradycardia, dizziness, lightheadedness, constipation, distention, flatus, diarrhea, nausea, vomiting).
In the event of overdosage, symptomatic and supportive measures should be employed. When ingestion is recent, gastric lavage or emesis may reduce absorption. When ingestion has been earlier, infusions may be helpful to promote urinary excretion. Otherwise, management includes special attention to cardiac rate and output, blood volume, electrolyte balance, paralytic ileus, urinary function and cerebral activity.
Sympathomimetic drugs [e.g., levarterenol, epinephrine, ARAMINE* (Metaraminol Bitartrate)] may be indicated. Methyldopa is dialyzable.
The oral LD_{50} of methyldopa is greater than 1.5 g/kg in both the mouse and the rat.

*Registered trademark of MERCK & CO., INC.

DOSAGE AND ADMINISTRATION

ADULTS

Initiation of Therapy
The usual starting dosage of ALDOMET is 250 mg two or three times a day in the first 48 hours. The daily dosage then may be increased or decreased, preferably at intervals of not less than two days, until an adequate response is achieved. To minimize the sedation, start dosage increases in the evening. By adjustment of dosage, morning hypotension may be prevented without sacrificing control of afternoon blood pressure.
When methyldopa is given to patients on other antihypertensives, the dose of these agents may need to be adjusted to effect a smooth transition. When ALDOMET is given with antihypertensives other than thiazides, the initial dosage of ALDOMET should be limited to 500 mg daily in divided doses; when ALDOMET is added to a thiazide, the dosage of thiazide need not be changed.
Maintenance Therapy
The usual daily dosage of ALDOMET is 500 mg to 2 g in two to four doses. Although occasional patients have responded to higher doses, the maximum recommended daily dosage is 3 g. Once an effective dosage range is attained, a smooth blood pressure response occurs in most patients in 12 to 24 hours. Since methyldopa has a relatively short duration of action, withdrawal is followed by return of hypertension usually within 48 hours. This is not complicated by an overshoot of blood pressure.
Occasionally tolerance may occur, usually between the second and third month of therapy. Adding a diuretic or increasing the dosage of methyldopa frequently will restore effective control of blood pressure. A thiazide may be added at any time during methyldopa therapy and is recommended if therapy has not been started with a thiazide or if effective control of blood pressure cannot be maintained on 2 g of methyldopa daily.
Methyldopa is largely excreted by the kidney and patients with impaired renal function may respond to smaller doses. Syncope in older patients may be related to an increased sensitivity and advanced arteriosclerotic vascular disease. This may be avoided by lower doses.

PEDIATRIC PATIENTS

Initial dosage is based on 10 mg/kg of body weight daily in two to four doses. The daily dosage then is increased or decreased until an adequate response is achieved. The maximum dosage is 65 mg/kg or 3 g daily, whichever is less. (See **PRECAUTIONS**, *Pediatric Use.*)

HOW SUPPLIED

No. 3341—Tablets ALDOMET, 125 mg, are yellow, film coated, round tablets, coded MSD 135 on one side and ALDOMET on the other. They are supplied as follows:
NDC 0006-0135-68 bottles of 100.
Shown in Product Identification Guide, page 323
No. 3290—Tablets ALDOMET, 250 mg, are yellow, film coated, round tablets, coded MSD 401 on one side and ALDOMET on the other. They are supplied as follows:
NDC 0006-0401-68 bottles of 100
(6505-00-890-1856, 250 mg 100's)
NDC 0006-0401-82 bottles of 1000
(6505-00-931-6646, 250 mg 1000's).
Shown in Product Identification Guide, page 323
No. 3292—Tablets ALDOMET, 500 mg, are yellow, film coated, round tablets, coded MSD 516 on one side and ALDOMET on the other. They are supplied as follows:
NDC 0006-0516-68 bottles of 100
(6505-01-003-4119, 500 mg 100's)
NDC 0006-0516-74 bottles of 500
(6505-01-199-8339, 500 mg 500's).
Shown in Product Identification Guide, page 323
Storage
Store Tablets ALDOMET in a well-closed container at controlled room temperature [15–30°C (59–86°F)].
7843431 Issued July 1998

ALDOMET® Ester HCl Injection (Methyldopate HCl) ℞

DESCRIPTION

Injection ALDOMET* Ester Hydrochloride (Methyldopate HCl) is an antihypertensive agent for intravenous use.
Methyldopate hydrochloride [levo-3-(3,4-dihydroxyphenyl)-2-methylalanine, ethyl ester hydrochloride]is the ethyl ester of methyldopa, supplied as the hydrochloride salt with a molecular weight of 275.73. Methyldopate hydrochloride is more soluble and stable in solution than methyldopa and is the preferred form for intravenous use.
The empirical formula for methyldopate hydrochloride is $C_{12}H_{17}NO_4{\cdot}HCl$ and its structural formula is:

Injection ALDOMET Ester Hydrochloride is supplied as a sterile solution in 5 mL vials each of which contains:

Methyldopate hydrochloride	250.0 mg
Inactive ingredients:	
Citric acid anhydrous	25.0 mg
Disodium edetate	2.5 mg
Monothioglycerol	10.0 mg
Sodium hydroxide to adjust pH	
Water for Injection, q.s. to 5 mL	

Methylparaben 7.5 mg, propylparaben 1 mg, and sodium bisulfite 16 mg added as preservatives.

*Registered trademark of MERCK & CO., INC.

CLINICAL PHARMACOLOGY

ALDOMET (Methyldopa), an antihypertensive, is an aromatic-amino-acid decarboxylase inhibitor in animals and in

Continued on next page

Information on the Merck & Co., Inc. products listed on these pages is the full prescribing information from product circulars in use September 30, 2000. For information, please call 1-800-NSC MERCK [1-800-672-6372].

Aldomet Ester HCl—Cont.

man. Although the mechanism of action has yet to be conclusively demonstrated, the antihypertensive effect of methyldopa probably is due to its metabolism to alpha-methyl-norepinephrine, which then lowers arterial pressure by stimulation of central inhibitory alpha-adrenergic receptors, false neurotransmission, and/or reduction of plasma renin activity. Methyldopa has been shown to cause a net reduction in the tissue concentration of serotonin, dopamine, norepinephrine, and epinephrine.

Only methyldopa, the *L*-isomer of alpha-methyldopa, has the ability to inhibit dopa decarboxylase and to deplete animal tissues of norepinephrine. In man the antihypertensive activity appears to be due solely to the *L*-isomer. About twice the dose of the racemate (*DL*-alpha-methyldopa) is required for equal antihypertensive effect.

Methyldopa has no direct effect on cardiac function and usually does not reduce glomerular filtration rate, renal blood flow, or filtration fraction. Cardiac output usually is maintained without cardiac acceleration. In some patients the heart rate is slowed.

Normal or elevated plasma renin activity may decrease in the course of methyldopa therapy.

Methyldopa reduces both supine and standing blood pressure. It usually produces highly effective lowering of the supine pressure with infrequent symptomatic postural hypotension. Exercise hypotension and diurnal blood pressure variations rarely occur.

Pharmacokinetics and Metabolism

Methyldopate hydrochloride is the ethyl ester of methyldopa hydrochloride and possesses the same pharmacologic attributes.

Methyldopa is extensively metabolized. The known urinary metabolites are: α-methyldopa mono-0-sulfate; 3-0-methyl-α-methyldopa; 3,4-dihydroxyphenylacetone; α-methyldopamine; 3-0-methyl-α-methyldopamine and their conjugates.

Following intravenous administration of methyldopate hydrochloride a decrease in blood pressure may occur in four to six hours and last 10 to 16 hours.

Approximately 49 percent of the dose of methyldopate hydrochloride is excreted in the urine as methyldopa and its mono-0-sulfate. The renal clearance of methyldopa following methyldopate hydrochloride is about 156 mL/min in normal subjects and is diminished in renal insufficiency. Following methyldopate hydrochloride injection the plasma half-life of methyldopa is 90–127 mins. Approximately 17 percent of a dose of methyldopate hydrochloride given to normal subjects appears in plasma as free methyldopa.

Methyldopa crosses the placental barrier, appears in cord blood, and appears in breast milk.

INDICATION AND USAGE

Hypertension, when parenteral medication is indicated.

The treatment of hypertensive crises may be initiated with Injection ALDOMET Ester Hydrochloride.

CONTRAINDICATIONS

Injection ALDOMET Ester Hydrochloride is contraindicated in patients:

— with active hepatic disease, such as acute hepatitis and active cirrhosis

— with liver disorders previously associated with methyldopa therapy (see WARNINGS)

— with hypersensitivity to any component of this product, including sulfites (see WARNINGS)

— on therapy with monoamine oxidase (MAO) inhibitors.

WARNINGS

It is important to recognize that a positive Coombs test, hemolytic anemia, and liver disorders may occur with methyldopa therapy. The rare occurrences of hemolytic anemia or liver disorders could lead to potentially fatal complications unless properly recognized and managed. Read this section carefully to understand these reactions.

With prolonged methyldopa therapy, 10 to 20 percent of patients develop a positive direct Coombs test which usually occurs between 6 and 12 months of methyldopa therapy. Lowest incidence is at daily dosage of 1 g or less. This on rare occasions may be associated with hemolytic anemia, which could lead to potentially fatal complications. One cannot predict which patients with a positive direct Coombs test may develop hemolytic anemia.

Prior existence or development of a positive direct Coombs test is not in itself a contraindication to use of methyldopa.

If a positive Coombs test develops during methyldopa therapy, the physician should determine whether hemolytic anemia exists and whether the positive Coombs test may be a problem. For example, in addition to a positive direct Coombs test there is less often a positive indirect Coombs test which may interfere with cross matching of blood.

Before treatment is started, it is desirable to do a blood count (hematocrit, hemoglobin, or red cell count) for a baseline or to establish whether there is anemia. Periodic blood counts should be done during therapy to detect hemolytic anemia. It may be useful to do a direct Coombs test before therapy and at 6 and 12 months after the start of therapy.

If Coombs-positive hemolytic anemia occurs, the cause may be methyldopa and the drug should be discontinued. Usually the anemia remits promptly. If not, corticosteroids may be given and other causes of anemia should be considered. If the hemolytic anemia is related to methyldopa, the drug should not be reinstituted.

When methyldopa causes Coombs positivity alone or with hemolytic anemia, the red cell is usually coated with gamma globulin of the IgG (gamma G) class only. The positive Coombs test may not revert to normal until weeks to months after methyldopa is stopped.

Should the need for transfusion arise in a patient receiving methyldopa, both a direct and an indirect Coombs test should be performed. In the absence of hemolytic anemia, usually only the direct Coombs test will be positive. A positive direct Coombs test alone will not interfere with typing or cross matching. If the indirect Coombs test is also positive, problems may arise in the major cross match and the assistance of a hematologist or transfusion expert will be needed.

Occasionally, fever has occurred within the first three weeks of methyldopa therapy, associated in some cases with eosinophilia or abnormalities in one or more liver function tests, such as serum alkaline phosphatase, serum transaminases (SGOT, SGPT), bilirubin and prothrombin time. Jaundice, with or without fever, may occur with onset usually within the first two to three months of therapy. In some patients the findings are consistent with those of cholestasis. In others the findings are consistent with hepatitis and hepatocellular injury.

Rarely fatal hepatic necrosis has been reported after use of methyldopa. These hepatic changes may represent hypersensitivity reactions. Periodic determination of hepatic function should be done particularly during the first 6 to 12 weeks of therapy or whenever an unexplained fever occurs. If fever, abnormalities in liver function tests, or jaundice appear, stop therapy with methyldopa. If caused by methyldopa, the temperature and abnormalities in liver function characteristically have reverted to normal when the drug was discontinued. Methyldopa should not be reinstituted in such patients.

Rarely, a reversible reduction of the white blood cell count with a primary effect on the granulocytes has been seen. The granulocyte count returned promptly to normal on discontinuance of the drug. Rare cases of granulocytopenia have been reported. In each instance, upon stopping the drug, the white cell count returned to normal. Reversible thrombocytopenia has occurred rarely.

Injection ALDOMET Ester Hydrochloride contains sodium bisulfite, a sulfite that may cause allergic-type reactions including anaphylactic symptoms and life-threatening or less severe asthmatic episodes in certain susceptible people. The overall prevalence of sulfite sensitivity in the general population is unknown and probably low. Sulfite sensitivity is seen more frequently in asthmatic than in nonasthmatic people.

PRECAUTIONS

General

Methyldopa should be used with caution in patients with a history of previous liver disease or dysfunction (see WARNINGS).

Some patients taking methyldopa experience clinical edema or weight gain which may be controlled by use of a diuretic. Methyldopa should not be continued if edema progresses or signs of heart failure appear.

A paradoxical pressor response has been reported with intravenous administration of ALDOMET Ester Hydrochloride.

Hypertension has recurred occasionally after dialysis in patients given methyldopa because the drug is removed by this procedure.

Rarely involuntary choreoathetotic movements have been observed during therapy with methyldopa in patients with severe bilateral cerebrovascular disease. Should these movements occur, stop therapy.

Laboratory Tests

Blood count, Coombs test, and liver function tests are recommended before initiating therapy and at periodic intervals (see WARNINGS).

Drug Interactions

When methyldopa is used with other antihypertensive drugs, potentiation of antihypertensive effect may occur. Patients should be followed carefully to detect side reactions or unusual manifestations of drug idiosyncrasy.

Patients may require reduced doses of anesthetics when on methyldopa. If hypotension does occur during anesthesia, it usually can be controlled by vasopressors. The adrenergic receptors remain sensitive during treatment with methyldopa.

When methyldopa and lithium are given concomitantly the patient should be carefully monitored for symptoms of lithium toxicity. Read the circular for lithium preparations.

Monoamine oxidase (MAO) inhibitors: See CONTRAINDICATIONS.

Drug/Laboratory Test Interactions

Methyldopa may interfere with measurement of: urinary uric acid by the phosphotungstate method, serum creatinine by the alkaline picrate method, and SGOT by colorimetric methods. Interference with spectrophotometric methods for SGOT analysis has not been reported.

Since methyldopa causes fluorescence in urine samples at the same wave lengths as catecholamines, falsely high levels of urinary catecholamines may be reported. This will interfere with the diagnosis of pheochromocytoma. It is important to recognize this phenomenon before a patient with a possible pheochromocytoma is subjected to surgery. Methyldopa does not interfere with measurement of VMA (vanillylmandelic acid), a test for pheochromocytoma, by those methods which convert VMA to vanillin. Methyldopa is not recommended for the treatment of patients with pheochromocytoma. Rarely, when urine is exposed to air after voiding, it may darken because of breakdown of methyldopa or its metabolites.

Carcinogenesis, Mutagenesis, Impairment of Fertility

No evidence of a tumorigenic effect was seen when methyldopa was given for two years to mice at doses up to 1800 mg/kg/day or to rats at doses up to 240 mg/kg/day (30 and 4 times the maximum recommended human dose in mice and rats, respectively, when compared on the basis of body weight; 2.5 and 0.6 times the maximum recommended human dose in mice and rats, respectively, when compared on the basis of body surface area; calculations assume a patient weight of 50 kg).

Methyldopa was not mutagenic in the Ames Test and did not increase chromosomal aberration or sister chromatid exchanges in Chinese hamster ovary cells. These *in vitro* studies were carried out both with and without exogenous metabolic activation.

Fertility was unaffected when methyldopa was given to male and female rats at 100 mg/kg/day (1.7 times the maximum daily human dose when compared on the basis of body weight; 0.2 times the maximum daily human dose when compared on the basis of body surface area). Methyldopa decreased sperm count, sperm motility, the number of late spermatids and the male fertility index when given to male rats at 200 and 400 mg/kg/day (3.3 and 6.7 times the maximum daily human dose when compared on the basis of body weight; 0.5 and 1 times the maximum daily human dose when compared on the basis of body surface area).

Long-term studies in animals have not been performed to evaluate the carcinogenic potential of methyldopate hydrochloride; nor have evaluations of this ester's mutagenic potential or potential to affect fertility been carried out.

Pregnancy

Pregnancy Category C. Animal reproduction studies have not been conducted with ALDOMET Ester Hydrochloride. It is also not known whether ALDOMET Ester Hydrochloride can affect reproduction capacity or can cause fetal harm when given to a pregnant woman. ALDOMET Ester Hydrochloride should be given to a pregnant woman only if clearly needed.

Nursing Mothers

Methyldopa appears in breast milk. Therefore, caution should be exercised when methyldopa is given to a nursing woman.

Pediatric Use

There are no well-controlled clinical trials in pediatric patients. Information on dosing in pediatric patients is supported by evidence from published literature regarding the treatment of hypertension in pediatric patients. (See DOSAGE AND ADMINISTRATION.)

ADVERSE REACTIONS

Sedation, usually transient, may occur during the initial period of therapy or whenever the dose is increased. Headache, asthenia, or weakness may be noted as early and transient symptoms. However, significant adverse effects due to methyldopa have been infrequent and this agent usually is well tolerated.

The following adverse reactions have been reported and, within each category, are listed in order of decreasing severity.

Cardiovascular: Aggravation of angina pectoris, congestive heart failure, prolonged carotid sinus hypersensitivity, paradoxical pressor response with intravenous use, orthostatic hypotension (decrease daily dosage), edema or weight gain, bradycardia.

Digestive: Pancreatitis, colitis, vomiting, diarrhea, sialadenitis, sore or "black" tongue, nausea, constipation, distension, flatus, dryness of mouth.

Endocrine: Hyperprolactinemia.

Hematologic: Bone marrow depression, leukopenia, granulocytopenia, thrombocytopenia, hemolytic anemia; positive tests for antinuclear antibody, LE cells, and rheumatoid factor, positive Coombs tests.

Hepatic: Liver disorders including hepatitis, jaundice, abnormal liver function tests (see WARNINGS).

Hypersensitivity: Myocarditis, pericarditis, vasculitis, lupus-like syndrome, drug-related fever, eosinophilia.

Nervous System/Psychiatric: Parkinsonism, Bell's palsy, decreased mental acuity, involuntary choreoathetotic movements, symptoms of cerebrovascular insufficiency, psychic disturbances including nightmares and reversible mild psychoses or depression, headache, sedation, asthenia or weakness, dizziness, lightheadedness, paresthesias.

Metabolic: Rise in BUN.

Musculoskeletal: Arthralgia, with or without joint swelling; myalgia.

Respiratory: Nasal stuffiness.

Skin: Toxic epidermal necrolysis, rash.

Urogenital: Amenorrhea, breast enlargement, gynecomastia, lactation, impotence, decreased libido.

OVERDOSAGE

Acute overdosage may produce acute hypotension with other responses attributable to brain and gastrointestinal

malfunction (excessive sedation, weakness, bradycardia, dizziness, lightheadedness, constipation, distention, flatus, diarrhea, nausea, vomiting).
In the event of overdosage, symptomatic and supportive measures should be employed. Management includes special attention to cardiac rate and output, blood volume, electrolyte balance, paralytic ileus, urinary function and cerebral activity.
Sympathomimetic drugs [e.g. levarterenol, epinephrine, ARAMINE* (Metaraminol Bitartrate)] may be indicated.
The acute intravenous LD_{50} of ALDOMET Ester Hydrochloride in the mouse is 321 mg/kg.

*Registered trademark of MERCK & CO., INC.

DOSAGE AND ADMINISTRATION

Injection ALDOMET Ester Hydrochloride, when given intravenously in effective doses, causes a decline in blood pressure that may begin in four to six hours and last 10 to 16 hours after injection.
Add the desired dose of Injection ALDOMET Ester Hydrochloride to 100 mL of 5 percent Dextrose Injection USP. Alternatively the desired dose may be given in 5% dextrose in water in a concentration of 100 mg / 10 mL. Give this intravenous infusion slowly over a period of 30 to 60 minutes.
The vial containing Injection ALDOMET Ester Hydrochloride should be inspected visually for particulate matter and discoloration before use whenever solution and container permit.

ADULTS

The usual adult dosage intravenously is 250 to 500 mg at six hour intervals as required. The maximum recommended intravenous dose is 1 g every six hours.
When control has been obtained, oral therapy with Tablets ALDOMET (Methyldopa) may be substituted for intravenous therapy, starting with the same dosage schedule used for the parenteral route. The effectiveness and anticipated responses are described in the circular for Tablets ALDOMET (Methyldopa).
Since methyldopa has a relatively short duration of action, withdrawal is followed by return of hypertension usually within 48 hours. This is not complicated by an overshoot of blood pressure.
Occasionally tolerance may occur, usually between the second and third month of therapy. Adding a diuretic or increasing the dosage of methyldopa frequently will restore effective control of blood pressure. A thiazide may be added at any time during methyldopa therapy and is recommended if therapy has not been started with a thiazide or if effective control of blood pressure cannot be maintained on 2 g of methyldopa daily.
Methyldopa is largely excreted by the kidney and patients with impaired renal function may respond to smaller doses. Syncope in older patients may be related to an increased sensitivity and advanced arteriosclerotic vascular disease. This may be avoided by lower doses.

PEDIATRIC PATIENTS

The recommended daily dosage is 20 to 40 mg/kg of body weight in divided doses every six hours. The maximum dosage is 65 mg/kg or 3 g daily, whichever is less. When the blood pressure is under control, continue with oral therapy using Tablets ALDOMET (Methyldopa) in the same dosage as for the parenteral route. (See PRECAUTIONS, *Pediatric Use*.)

HOW SUPPLIED

No. 3293—Injection ALDOMET Ester Hydrochloride, 250 mg per 5 mL, is a clear, colorless solution and is supplied as follows:
NDC 0006-3293-05 in 5 mL vials
(6505-01-096-2735, 5 mL vial).
Storage
Store below 30°C (86°F).
Protect from freezing.
7900438 Issued February 1997

ALDORIL® Tablets ℞
(Methyldopa-Hydrochlorothiazide)

WARNING

This fixed combination drug is not indicated for initial therapy of hypertension. Hypertension requires therapy titrated to the individual patient. If the fixed combination represents the dosage so determined, its use may be more convenient in patient management. The treatment of hypertension is not static, but must be reevaluated as conditions in each patient warrant.

DESCRIPTION

ALDORIL* (Methyldopa-Hydrochlorothiazide) combines two antihypertensives: methyldopa and hydrochlorothiazide.
Methyldopa
Methyldopa is an antihypertensive and is the *L* -isomer of alphamethyldopa. It is levo-3-(3,4-dihydroxyphenyl)-2-methylalanine. Its empirical formula is $C_{10}H_{13}NO_4$, with a molecular weight of 211.22, and its structural formula is:

HO, HO, $CH_2-C(CH_3)(NH_2)-CO_2H$

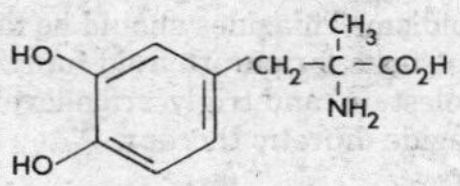

Methyldopa is a white to yellowish white, odorless fine powder, and is soluble in water.
Hydrochlorothiazide
Hydrochlorothiazide is a diuretic and antihypertensive. It is the 3,4-dihydro derivative of chlorothiazide. Its chemical name is 6-chloro-3,4-dihydro-2*H* -1,2,4-benzothiadiazine-7-sulfonamide 1,1-dioxide. Its empirical formula is $C_7H_8ClN_3O_4S_2$ and its structural formula is:

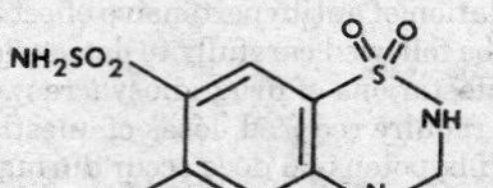

NH_2SO_2, Cl, SO_2, NH, N H

Hydrochlorothiazide is a white, or practically white, crystalline powder with a molecular weight of 297.74, which is slightly soluble in water, but freely soluble in sodium hydroxide solution.
ALDORIL is supplied as tablets in four strengths for oral use:
ALDORIL 15, contains 250 mg of methyldopa and 15 mg of hydrochlorothiazide.
ALDORIL 25, contains 250 mg of methyldopa and 25 mg of hydrochlorothiazide.
ALDORIL D30, contains 500 mg of methyldopa and 30 mg of hydrochlorothiazide.
ALDORIL D50, contains 500 mg of methyldopa and 50 mg of hydrochlorothiazide.
Each tablet contains the following inactive ingredients: calcium disodium edetate, calcium phosphate, cellulose, citric acid, colloidal silicon dioxide, ethylcellulose, guar gum, hydroxypropyl methylcellulose, magnesium stearate, propylene glycol, talc, and titanium dioxide. ALDORIL 15 and ALDORIL D30 also contain iron oxide.

*Registered trademark of MERCK & CO., INC.

CLINICAL PHARMACOLOGY

Methyldopa
Methyldopa is an aromatic-amino-acid decarboxylase inhibitor in animals and in man. Although the mechanism of action has yet to be conclusively demonstrated, the antihypertensive effect of methyldopa probably is due to its metabolism to alpha-methylnorepinephrine, which then lowers arterial pressure by stimulation of central inhibitory alpha-adrenergic receptors, false neurotransmission, and/or reduction of plasma renin activity. Methyldopa has been shown to cause a net reduction in the tissue concentration of serotonin, dopamine, norepinephrine, and epinephrine.
Only methyldopa, the *L* -isomer of alpha-methyldopa, has the ability to inhibit dopa decarboxylase and to deplete animal tissues of norepinephrine. In man, the antihypertensive activity appears to be due solely to the *L*-isomer. About twice the dose of the racemate (*DL* -alpha-methyldopa) is required for equal antihypertensive effect.
Methyldopa has no direct effect on cardiac function and usually does not reduce glomerular filtration rate, renal blood flow, or filtration fraction. Cardiac output usually is maintained without cardiac acceleration. In some patients the heart rate is slowed.
Normal or elevated plasma renin activity may decrease in the course of methyldopa therapy.
Methyldopa reduces both supine and standing blood pressure. It usually produces highly effective lowering of the supine pressure with infrequent symptomatic postural hypotension. Exercise hypotension and diurnal blood pressure variations rarely occur.
Hydrochlorothiazide
The mechanism of the antihypertensive effect of thiazides is unknown. Hydrochlorothiazide does not usually affect normal blood pressure.
Hydrochlorothiazide affects the distal renal tubular mechanism of electrolyte reabsorption. At maximal therapeutic dosage all thiazides are approximately equal in their diuretic efficacy.
Hydrochlorothiazide increases excretion of sodium and chloride in approximately equivalent amounts. Natriuresis may be accompanied by some loss of potassium and bicarbonate.
After oral use diuresis begins within 2 hours, peaks in about 4 hours and lasts about 6 to 12 hours.
Pharmacokinetics and Metabolism
Methyldopa
The maximum decrease in blood pressure occurs four to six hours after oral dosage. Once an effective dosage level is attained, a smooth blood pressure response occurs in most patients in 12 to 24 hours. After withdrawal, blood pressure usually returns to pretreatment levels within 24–48 hours.
Methyldopa is extensively metabolized. The known urinary metabolites are: α-methyldopa mono-0-sulfate; 3-0-methyl-α-methyldopa; 3,4-dihydroxyphenylacetone; α-methyldopamine; 3-0-methyl-α-methyldopamine and their conjugates.
Approximately 70 percent of the drug which is absorbed is excreted in the urine as methyldopa and its mono-0-sulfate conjugate. The renal clearance is about 130 mL/min in normal subjects and is diminished in renal insufficiency. The plasma half-life of methyldopa is 105 minutes. After oral doses, excretion is essentially complete in 36 hours.
Methyldopa crosses the placental barrier, appears in cord blood, and appears in breast milk.
Hydrochlorothiazide
Hydrochlorothiazide is not metabolized but is eliminated rapidly by the kidney. When plasma levels have been followed for at least 24 hours, the plasma half-life has been observed to vary between 5.6 and 14.8 hours. At least 61 percent of the oral dose is eliminated unchanged within 24 hours. Hydrochlorothiazide crosses the placental but not the blood-brain barrier and is excreted in breast milk.

INDICATION AND USAGE

Hypertension (see box warning).

CONTRAINDICATIONS

ALDORIL is contraindicated in patients:
— with active hepatic disease, such as acute hepatitis and active cirrhosis
— with liver disorders previously associated with methyldopa therapy (see WARNINGS)
— with anuria
— with hypersensitivity to methyldopa, or to hydrochlorothiazide or other sulfonamide-derived drugs
— on therapy with monoamine oxidase (MAO) inhibitors.

WARNINGS

Methyldopa
It is important to recognize that a positive Coombs test, hemolytic anemia, and liver disorders may occur with methyldopa therapy. The rare occurrences of hemolytic anemia or liver disorders could lead to potentially fatal complications unless properly recognized and managed. Read this section carefully to understand these reactions.
With prolonged methyldopa therapy, 10 to 20 percent of patients develop a positive direct Coombs test which usually occurs between 6 and 12 months of methyldopa therapy. Lowest incidence is at daily dosage of 1 g or less. This on rare occasions may be associated with hemolytic anemia, which could lead to potentially fatal complications. One cannot predict which patients with a positive direct Coombs test may develop hemolytic anemia.
Prior existence or development of a positive direct Coombs test is not in itself a contraindication to use of methyldopa. If a positive Coombs test develops during methyldopa therapy, the physician should determine whether hemolytic anemia exists and whether the positive Coombs test may be a problem. For example, in addition to a positive direct Coombs test there is less often a positive indirect Coombs test which may interfere with cross matching of blood.
Before treatment is started it is desirable to do a blood count (hematocrit, hemoglobin, or red cell count) for a baseline or to establish whether there is anemia. Periodic blood counts should be done during therapy to detect hemolytic anemia. It may be useful to do a direct Coombs test before therapy and at 6 and 12 months after the start of therapy.
If Coombs-positive hemolytic anemia occurs, the cause may be methyldopa and the drug should be discontinued. Usually the anemia remits promptly. If not, corticosteroids may be given and other causes of anemia should be considered. If the hemolytic anemia is related to methyldopa, the drug should not be reinstituted.
When methyldopa causes Coombs positivity alone or with hemolytic anemia, the red cell is usually coated with gamma globulin of the IgG (gamma G) class only. The positive Coombs test may not revert to normal until weeks to months after methyldopa is stopped.
Should the need for transfusion arise in a patient receiving methyldopa, both a direct and an indirect Coombs test should be performed. In the absence of hemolytic anemia, usually only the direct Coombs test will be positive. A positive direct Coombs test alone will not interfere with typing or cross matching. If the indirect Coombs test is also positive, problems may arise in the major cross match and the assistance of a hematologist or transfusion expert will be needed.
Occasionally, fever has occurred within the first three weeks of methyldopa therapy, associated in some cases with eosinophilia or abnormalities in one or more liver function tests, such as serum alkaline phosphatase, serum transaminases (SGOT, SGPT), bilirubin, and prothrombin time. Jaundice, with or without fever, may occur with onset usually within the first two to three months of therapy. In some patients the findings are consistent with those of cholestasis. In others the findings are consistent with hepatitis and hepatocellular injury.

Continued on next page

Information on the Merck & Co., Inc. products listed on these pages is the full prescribing information from product circulars in use September 30, 2000. For information, please call 1-800-NSC MERCK [1-800-672-6372].

Aldoril Tablets—Cont.

Rarely, fatal hepatic necrosis has been reported after use of methyldopa. These hepatic changes may represent hypersensitivity reactions. Periodic determination of hepatic function should be done particularly during the first 6 to 12 weeks of therapy or whenever an unexplained fever occurs. If fever, abnormalities in liver function tests, or jaundice appear, stop therapy with methyldopa. If caused by methyldopa, the temperature and abnormalities in liver function characteristically have reverted to normal when the drug was discontinued. Methyldopa should not be reinstituted in such patients.

Rarely, a reversible reduction of the white blood cell count with a primary effect on the granulocytes has been seen. The granulocyte count returned promptly to normal on discontinuance of the drug. Rare cases of granulocytopenia have been reported. In each instance, upon stopping the drug, the white cell count returned to normal. Reversible thrombocytopenia has occurred rarely.

Hydrochlorothiazide

Use with caution in severe renal disease. In patients with renal disease, thiazides may precipitate azotemia. Cumulative effects of the drug may develop in patients with impaired renal function.

Thiazides should be used with caution in patients with impaired hepatic function or progressive liver disease, since minor alterations of fluid and electrolyte balance may precipitate hepatic coma.

Thiazides may add to or potentiate the action of other antihypertensive drugs.

Sensitivity reactions may occur in patients with or without a history of allergy or bronchial asthma.

The possibility of exacerbation or activation of systemic lupus erythematosus has been reported.

Lithium generally should not be given with diuretics (see PRECAUTIONS, *Drug Interactions*).

PRECAUTIONS

General

Methyldopa

Methyldopa should be used with caution in patients with a history of previous liver disease or dysfunction (see WARNINGS).

Some patients taking methyldopa experience clinical edema or weight gain which may be controlled by use of a diuretic. Methyldopa should not be continued if edema progresses or signs of heart failure appear.

Hypertension has recurred occasionally after dialysis in patients given methyldopa because the drug is removed by this procedure.

Rarely, involuntary choreoathetotic movements have been observed during therapy with methyldopa in patients with severe bilateral cerebrovascular disease. Should these movements occur, stop therapy.

Hydrochlorothiazide

All patients receiving diuretic therapy should be observed for evidence of fluid or electrolyte imbalance: namely; hyponatremia, hypochloremic alkalosis, and hypokalemia. Serum and urine electrolyte determinations are particularly important when the patient is vomiting excessively or receiving parenteral fluids. Warning signs or symptoms of fluid and electrolyte imbalance, irrespective of cause, include dryness of mouth, thirst, weakness, lethargy, drowsiness, restlessness, confusion, seizures, muscle pains or cramps, muscular fatigue, hypotension, oliguria, tachycardia, and gastrointestinal disturbances such as nausea and vomiting.

Hypokalemia may develop especially after prolonged therapy or when severe cirrhosis is present (see CONTRAINDICATIONS and WARNINGS).

Interference with adequate oral electrolyte intake will also contribute to hypokalemia. Hypokalemia may cause cardiac arrhythmia and may also sensitize or exaggerate the response of the heart to the toxic effects of digitalis (e.g., increased ventricular irritability). Hypokalemia may be avoided or treated by use of potassium sparing diuretics or potassium supplements such as foods with a high potassium content.

Although any chloride deficit is generally mild and usually does not require specific treatment except under extraordinary circumstances (as in liver disease or renal disease), chloride replacement may be required in the treatment of metabolic alkalosis.

Dilutional hyponatremia may occur in edematous patients in hot weather; appropriate therapy is water restriction, rather than administration of salt, except in rare instances when the hyponatremia is life threatening. In actual salt depletion, appropriate replacement is the therapy of choice.

Hyperuricemia may occur or acute gout may be precipitated in certain patients receiving thiazides.

In diabetic patients dosage adjustment of insulin or oral hypoglycemic agents may be required. Hyperglycemia may occur with thiazide diuretics. Thus latent diabetes mellitus may become manifest during thiazide therapy.

The antihypertensive effects of the drug may be enhanced in the postsympathectomy patient.

If progressive renal impairment becomes evident, consider withholding or discontinuing diuretic therapy.

Thiazides have been shown to increase the urinary excretion of magnesium; this may result in hypomagnesemia.

Thiazides may decrease urinary calcium excretion. Thiazides may cause intermittent and slight elevation of serum calcium in the absence of known disorders of calcium metabolism. Marked hypercalcemia may be evidence of hidden hyperparathyroidism. Thiazides should be discontinued before carrying out tests for parathyroid function.

Increases in cholesterol and triglyceride levels may be associated with thiazide diuretic therapy.

Laboratory Tests

Methyldopa

Blood count, Coombs test and liver function test, are recommended before initiating therapy and at periodic intervals (see WARNINGS).

Hydrochlorothiazide

Periodic determination of serum electrolytes to detect possible electrolyte imbalance should be done at appropriate intervals.

Drug Interactions

Methyldopa

When methyldopa is used with other antihypertensive drugs, potentiation of antihypertensive effect may occur. Patients should be followed carefully to detect side reactions or unusual manifestations of drug idiosyncrasy.

Patients may require reduced doses of anesthetics when on methyldopa. If hypotension does occur during anesthesia, it usually can be controlled by vasopressors. The adrenergic receptors remain sensitive during treatment with methyldopa.

When methyldopa and lithium are given concomitantly the patient should be carefully monitored for symptoms of lithium toxicity. Read the prescribing information for lithium preparations.

Several studies demonstrate a decrease in the bioavailability of methyldopa when it is ingested with ferrous sulfate or ferrous gluconate. This may adversely affect blood pressure control in patients treated with methyldopa. Coadministration of methyldopa with ferrous sulfate or ferrous gluconate is not recommended.

Monoamine oxidase (MAO) inhibitors: see CONTRAINDICATIONS.

Hydrochlorothiazide

When given concurrently the following drugs may interact with thiazide diuretics.

Alcohol, barbiturates, or narcotics —potentiation of orthostatic hypotension may occur.

Antidiabetic drugs (oral agents and insulin) —dosage adjustment of the antidiabetic drug may be required.

Other antihypertensive drugs —additive effect or potentiation.

Cholestyramine and colestipol resins—Absorption of hydrochlorothiazide is impaired in the presence of anionic exchange resins. Single doses of either cholestyramine or colestipol resins bind the hydrochlorothiazide and reduce its absorption from the gastrointestinal tract by up to 85 and 43 percent, respectively.

Corticosteroids, ACTH —intensified electrolyte depletion, particularly hypokalemia.

Pressor amines (e.g., norepinephrine) —possible decreased response to pressor amines but not sufficient to preclude their use.

Skeletal muscle relaxants, nondepolarizing (e.g., tubocurarine) —possible increased responsiveness to the muscle relaxant.

Lithium —generally should not be given with diuretics. Diuretic agents reduce the renal clearance of lithium and add a high risk of lithium toxicity. Refer to the package insert for lithium preparations before use of such preparations with ALDORIL.

Non-steroidal Anti-inflammatory Drugs —In some patients, the administration of a non-steroidal anti-inflammatory agent can reduce the diuretic, natriuretic, and antihypertensive effects of loop, potassium-sparing and thiazide diuretics. Therefore, when ALDORIL and non-steroidal anti-inflammatory agents are used concomitantly, the patient should be observed closely to determine if the desired effect of the diuretic is obtained.

Drug/Laboratory Test Interactions

Methyldopa

Methyldopa may interfere with measurement of: urinary uric acid by the phosphotungstate method, serum creatinine by the alkaline picrate method, and SGOT by colorimetric methods. Interference with spectrophotometric methods for SGOT analysis has not been reported.

Since methyldopa causes fluorescence in urine samples at the same wave lengths as catecholamines, falsely high levels of urinary catecholamines may be reported. This will interfere with the diagnosis of pheochromocytoma. It is important to recognize this phenomenon before a patient with a possible pheochromocytoma is subjected to surgery. Methyldopa does not interfere with measurement of VMA (vanillylmandelic acid), a test for pheochromocytoma, by those methods which convert VMA to vanillin. Methyldopa is not recommended for the treatment of patients with pheochromocytoma. Rarely, when urine is exposed to air after voiding, it may darken because of breakdown of methyldopa or its metabolites.

Hydrochlorothiazide

Thiazides should be discontinued before carrying out tests for parathyroid function (see PRECAUTIONS, *General).*

Carcinogenesis, Mutagenesis, Impairment of Fertility

Long-term studies in animals have not been performed to evaluate the effects upon fertility, mutagenic or carcinogenic potential of the combination.

Methyldopa

No evidence of a tumorigenic effect was seen when methyldopa was given for two years to mice at doses up to 1800 mg/kg/day or to rats at doses up to 240 mg/kg/day (30 and 4 times the maximum recommended human dose in mice and rats, respectively, when compared on the basis of body weight; 2.5 and 0.6 times the maximum recommended human dose in mice and rats, respectively, when compared on the basis of body surface area; calculations assume a patient weight of 50 kg).

Methyldopa was not mutagenic in the Ames Test and did not increase chromosomal aberration or sister chromatid exchanges in Chinese hamster ovary cells. These *in vitro* studies were carried out both with and without exogenous metabolic activation.

Fertility was unaffected when methyldopa was given to male and female rats at 100 mg/kg/day (1.7 times the maximum daily human dose when compared on the basis of body weight; 0.2 times the maximum daily human dose when compared on the basis of body surface area). Methyldopa decreased sperm count, sperm motility, the number of late spermatids and the male fertility index when given to male rats at 200 and 400 mg/kg/day (3.3 and 6.7 times the maximum daily human dose when compared on the basis of body weight; 0.5 and 1 times the maximum daily human dose when compared on the basis of body surface area).

Hydrochlorothiazide

Two-year feeding studies in mice and rats conducted under the auspices of the National Toxicology Program (NTP) uncovered no evidence of a carcinogenic potential of hydrochlorothiazide in female mice (at doses of up to approximately 600 mg/kg/day) or in male and female rats (at doses of up to approximately 100 mg/kg/day). The NTP, however, found equivocal evidence for hepatocarcinogenicity in male mice.

Hydrochlorothiazide was not genotoxic *in vitro* in the Ames mutagenicity assay of *Salmonella typhimurium* strains TA 98, TA 100, TA 1535, TA 1537, and TA 1538 and in the Chinese Hamster Ovary (CHO) test for chromosomal aberrations, or *in vivo* in assays using mouse germinal cell chromosomes, Chinese hamster bone marrow chromosomes, and the *Drosophila* sex-linked recessive lethal trait gene. Positive test results were obtained only in the *in vitro* CHO Sister Chromatid Exchange (clastogenicity) and in the Mouse Lymphoma Cell (mutagenicity) assays, using concentrations of hydrochlorothiazide from 43 to 1300 μg/mL, and in the *Aspergillus nidulans* non-disjunction assay at an unspecified concentration.

Hydrochlorothiazide had no adverse effects on the fertility of mice and rats of either sex in studies wherein these species were exposed, via their diet, to doses of up to 100 and 4 mg/kg, respectively, prior to conception and throughout gestation.

Pregnancy

Use of diuretics during normal pregnancy is inappropriate and exposes mother and fetus to unnecessary hazard. Diuretics do not prevent development of toxemia of pregnancy and there is no satisfactory evidence that they are useful in the treatment of toxemia.

Teratogenic Effects—Pregnancy Category C: Animal reproduction studies have not been conducted with ALDORIL. It is also not known whether ALDORIL can affect reproduction capacity or can cause fetal harm when given to a pregnant woman. ALDORIL should be given to a pregnant woman only if clearly needed.

Hydrochlorothiazide: Studies in which hydrochlorothiazide was orally administered to pregnant mice and rats during their respective periods of major organogenesis at doses up to 3000 and 1000 mg hydrochlorothiazide/kg, respectively, provided no evidence of harm to the fetus. There are, however, no adequate and well-controlled studies in pregnant women.

Methyldopa: Reproduction studies performed with methyldopa at oral doses up to 1000 mg/kg in mice, 200 mg/kg in rabbits and 100 mg/kg in rats revealed no evidence of harm to the fetus. These doses are 16.6 times, 3.3 times and 1.7 times, respectively, the maximum daily human dose when compared on the basis of body weight; 1.4 times, 1.1 times and 0.2 times, respectively, when compared on the basis of body surface area; calculations assume a patient weight of 50 kg. There are, however, no adequate and well-controlled studies in pregnant women in the first trimester of pregnancy. Because animal reproduction studies are not always predictive of human response, methyldopa should be used during pregnancy only if clearly needed.

Published reports of the use of methyldopa during all trimesters indicate that if this drug is used during pregnancy the possibility of fetal harm appears remote. In five studies, three of which were controlled, involving 332 pregnant hypertensive women, treatment with methyldopa was associated with an improved fetal outcome. The majority of these women were in the third trimester when methyldopa therapy was begun.

In one study, women who had begun methyldopa treatment between weeks 16 and 20 of pregnancy gave birth to infants whose average head circumference was reduced by a small amount (34.2 ± 1.7 cm vs. 34.6 ± 1.3 cm [mean ± 1 S.D.]). Long term follow-up of 195 (97.5%) of the children born to methyldopa-treated pregnant women (including those who began treatment between weeks 16 and 20) failed to uncover any significant adverse effect on the children. At four years of age, the developmental delay commonly seen in children born to hypertensive mothers was less evident in those whose mothers were treated with methyldopa during pregnancy than those whose mothers were untreated. The children of the treated group scored consistently higher than the children of the untreated group on five major indices of intellectual and motor development. At age 7 and one-half developmental scores and intelligence indices showed no significant differences in children of treated or untreated hypertensive women.

Nonteratogenic Effects: Thiazides cross the placental barrier and appear in cord blood. There is a risk of fetal or neonatal jaundice, thrombocytopenia, and possibly other adverse reactions that have occurred in adults.

Nursing Mothers

Methyldopa and thiazides appear in breast milk. Therefore, because of the potential for serious adverse reactions in nursing infants from hydrochlorothiazide, a decision should be made whether to discontinue nursing or to discontinue the drug, taking into account the importance of the drug to the mother.

Pediatric Use

Safety and effectiveness of ALDORIL in pediatric patients have not been established.

ADVERSE REACTIONS

The following adverse reactions have been reported and, within each category, are listed in order of decreasing severity.

Methyldopa

Sedation, usually transient, may occur during the initial period of therapy or whenever the dose is increased. Headache, asthenia, or weakness may be noted as early and transient symptoms. However, significant adverse effects due to methyldopa have been infrequent and this agent usually is well tolerated.

Cardiovascular: Aggravation of angina pectoris, congestive heart failure, prolonged carotid sinus hypersensitivity, orthostatic hypotension (decrease daily dosage), edema or weight gain, bradycardia.

Digestive: Pancreatitis, colitis, vomiting, diarrhea, sialadenitis, sore or "black" tongue, nausea, constipation, distention, flatus, dryness of mouth.

Endocrine: Hyperprolactinemia.

Hematologic: Bone marrow depression, leukopenia, granulocytopenia, thrombocytopenia, hemolytic anemia; positive tests for antinuclear antibody, LE cells, and rheumatoid factor, positive Coombs test.

Hepatic: Liver disorders including hepatitis, jaundice, abnormal liver function tests (see WARNINGS).

Hypersensitivity: Myocarditis, pericarditis, vasculitis, lupus-like syndrome, drug-related fever, eosinophilia.

Nervous System/Psychiatric: Parkinsonism, Bell's palsy, decreased mental acuity, involuntary choreoathetotic movements, symptoms of cerebrovascular insufficiency, psychic disturbances including nightmares and reversible mild psychoses or depression, headache, sedation, asthenia or weakness, dizziness, lightheadedness, paresthesias.

Metabolic: Rise in BUN.

Musculoskeletal: Arthralgia, with or without joint swelling; myalgia.

Respiratory: Nasal stuffiness.

Skin: Toxic epidermal necrolysis, rash.

Urogenital: Amenorrhea, breast enlargement, gynecomastia, lactation, impotence, decreased libido.

Hydrochlorothiazide

Body as a Whole: Weakness.

Cardiovascular: Hypotension including orthostatic hypotension (may be aggravated by alcohol, barbiturates, narcotics or antihypertensive drugs).

Digestive: Pancreatitis, jaundice (intrahepatic cholestatic jaundice), diarrhea, vomiting, sialadenitis, cramping, constipation, gastric irritation, nausea, anorexia.

Hematologic: Aplastic anemia, agranulocytosis, leukopenia, hemolytic anemia, thrombocytopenia.

Hypersensitivity: Anaphylactic reactions, necrotizing angiitis (vasculitis and cutaneous vasculitis), respiratory distress including pneumonitis and pulmonary edema, photosensitivity, fever, urticaria, rash, purpura.

Metabolic: Electrolyte imbalance (see PRECAUTIONS), hyperglycemia, glycosuria, hyperuricemia.

Musculoskeletal: Muscle spasm.

Nervous System/Psychiatric: Vertigo, paresthesias, dizziness, headache, restlessness.

Renal: Renal failure, renal dysfunction, interstitial nephritis. (See WARNINGS.)

Skin: Erythema multiforme including Stevens-Johnson syndrome, exfoliative dermatitis including toxic epidermal necrolysis, alopecia.

Special Senses: Transient blurred vision, xanthopsia.

Urogenital: Impotence.

OVERDOSAGE

Acute overdosage may produce acute hypotension with other responses attributable to brain and gastrointestinal malfunction (excessive sedation, weakness, bradycardia, dizziness, lightheadedness, constipation, distention, flatus, diarrhea, nausea, vomiting).

In the event of overdosage, symptomatic and supportive measures should be employed. When ingestion is recent, gastric lavage or emesis may reduce absorption. When ingestion has been earlier, infusions may be helpful to promote urinary excretion. Otherwise, management includes special attention to cardiac rate and output, blood volume, electrolyte balance, paralytic ileus, urinary function and cerebral activity.

Sympathomimetic drugs [e.g., levarterenol, epinephrine, ARAMINE* (Metaraminol Bitartrate)] may be indicated. Methyldopa is dialyzable. The degree to which hydrochlorothiazide is removed by hemodialysis has not been established.

The oral LD_{50} of methyldopa is greater than 1.5 g/kg in both the mouse and the rat. The oral LD_{50} of hydrochlorothiazide is greater than 10 g/kg in the mouse and rat.

*Registered trademark of MERCK & CO., INC.

DOSAGE AND ADMINISTRATION

DOSAGE MUST BE INDIVIDUALIZED, AS DETERMINED BY TITRATION OF THE INDIVIDUAL COMPONENTS (see box warning). Once the patient has been successfully titrated, ALDORIL may be substituted if the previously determined titrated doses are the same as in the combination. The usual starting dosage is one tablet of ALDORIL 15 two or three times a day or one tablet of ALDORIL 25 two times a day. Alternatively, one tablet of ALDORIL D30 or ALDORIL D50 once daily may be used. Hydrochlorothiazide doses greater than 50 mg daily should be avoided.

Hydrochlorothiazide can be given at doses of 12.5 to 50 mg per day when used alone. The usual daily dosage of methyldopa is 500 mg to 2 g. To minimize the sedation associated with methyldopa, start dosage increases in the evening. The maximum recommended daily dose of methyldopa is 3 g.

Occasionally tolerance to methyldopa may occur, usually between the second and third month of therapy. Additional separate doses of methyldopa or replacement of ALDORIL with single entity agents is necessary until the new effective dose ratio is re-established by titration.

If ALDORIL does not adequately control blood pressure, additional doses of other agents may be given. When ALDORIL is given with antihypertensives other than thiazides, the initial dosage of methyldopa should be limited to 500 mg daily in divided doses and the dose of these other agents may need to be adjusted to effect a smooth transition.

Since both components of ALDORIL have a relatively short duration of action, withdrawal is followed by return of hypertension usually within 48 hours. This is not complicated by an overshoot of blood pressure.

Since methyldopa is largely excreted by the kidney, patients with impaired renal function may respond to smaller doses. Syncope in older patients may be related to an increased sensitivity and advanced arteriosclerotic vascular disease. This may be avoided by lower doses.

HOW SUPPLIED

No. 3294—Tablets ALDORIL 15 are salmon, round, film coated tablets, coded MSD 423 on one side and ALDORIL on the other. Each tablet contains 250 mg of methyldopa and 15 mg of hydrochlorothiazide. They are supplied as follows:

NDC 0006-0423-68 bottles of 100

Shown in Product Identification Guide, page 323

No. 3295—Tablets ALDORIL 25 are white, round, film coated tablets, coded MSD 456 on one side and ALDORIL on the other. Each tablet contains 250 mg of methyldopa and 25 mg of hydrochlorothiazide. They are supplied as follows:

NDC 0006-0456-68 bottles of 100

NDC 0006-0456-82 bottles of 1000.

Shown in Product Identification Guide, page 323

No. 3362—Tablets ALDORIL D30 are salmon, oval, film coated tablets, coded MSD 694 on one side and ALDORIL on the other. Each tablet contains 500 mg of methyldopa and 30 mg of hydrochlorothiazide. They are supplied as follows:

NDC 0006-0694-68 bottles of 100.

Shown in Product Identification Guide, page 323

No. 3363—Tablets ALDORIL D50 are white, oval, film coated tablets, coded MSD 935 on one side and ALDORIL on the other. Each tablet contains 500 mg of methyldopa and 50 mg of hydrochlorothiazide. They are supplied as follows:

NDC 0006-0935-68 bottles of 100.

Shown in Product Identification Guide, page 323

Storage

Keep container tightly closed. Protect from light, moisture, freezing, −20°C (−4°F) and store at controlled room temperature, 15–30°C (59–86°F).

7843554 Issued March 1999

AMINOHIPPURATE SODIUM "PAH" ℞

Injection

DESCRIPTION

Aminohippurate sodium* is an agent to measure effective renal plasma flow (ERPF). It is the sodium salt of para-aminohippuric acid, commonly abbreviated "PAH."It is water soluble, lipid-insoluble, and has a pKa of 3.83. The empirical formula of the anhydrous salt is $C_9H_9N_2NaO_3$ and its structural formula is:

H_2N–C_6H_4–$CONHCH_2COONa$

It is provided as a sterile, non-preserved 20 percent aqueous solution for injection, with a pH of 6.7 to 7.6. Each 10 mL contains: Aminohippurate sodium 2 g. Inactive ingredients: Sodium hydroxide to adjust pH, water for injection, q.s.

*Formerly referred to as Sodium para-Aminohippurate.

CLINICAL PHARMACOLOGY

PAH is filtered by the glomeruli and is actively secreted by the proximal tubules. At low plasma concentrations (1.0 to 2.0 mg/100 mL), an average of 90 percent of PAH is cleared by the kidneys from the renal blood stream in a single circulation. It is ideally suited for measurement of ERPF since it has a high clearance, is essentially nontoxic at the plasma concentrations reached with recommended doses and its analytical determination is relatively simple and accurate.

PAH is also used to measure the functional capacity of the renal tubular secretory mechanism or transport maximum (Tm_{PAH}). This is accomplished by elevating the plasma concentration to levels (40–60 mg/100 mL) sufficient to saturate the maximal capacity of the tubular cells to secrete PAH.

Inulin clearance is generally measured during Tm_{PAH} determinations since glomerular filtration rate (GFR) must be known before calculations of secretory Tm measurements can be done (See *Calculations*).

INDICATIONS AND USAGE

Estimation of effective renal plasma flow.

Measurement of the functional capacity of the renal tubular secretory mechanism.

CONTRAINDICATIONS

Hypersensitivity to this product or to its components.

PRECAUTIONS

General

Intravenous solutions must be given with caution to patients with low cardiac reserve, since a rapid increase in plasma volume can precipitate congestive heart failure.

For measurement of ERPF, small doses of PAH are used. However, in research procedures to measure Tm_{PAH}, high plasma levels are required to saturate the capacity of the tubular cells. During these procedures the intravenous administration of PAH solutions should be carried out slowly and with caution. The patient should be continuously observed for any adverse reactions.

Drug Interactions

Renal clearance measurements of PAH cannot be made with any significant accuracy in patients receiving sulfonamides, procaine, or thiazolesulfone. These compounds interfere with chemical color development essential to the analytical procedures.

Probenecid depresses tubular secretion of certain weak acids such as PAH. Therefore, patients receiving probenecid will have erroneously low ERPF and Tm_{PAH} values.

Carcinogenesis, Mutagenesis, Impairment of Fertility

Long-term studies in animals have not been done to evaluate any effects upon fertility or carcinogenic potential of PAH.

Pregnancy

Pregnancy Category C. Animal reproduction studies have not been done with PAH. It is also not known whether PAH can cause fetal harm when given to a pregnant woman or can affect reproduction capacity. PAH should be given to a pregnant woman only if clearly needed.

Nursing Mothers

It is not known whether this drug is excreted in human milk. Because many drugs are excreted in human milk, caution should be exercised when PAH is administered to a nursing woman.

Pediatric Use

Safety and effectiveness in pediatric patients have not been established.

Geriatric Use

Clinical studies of PAH did not include sufficient numbers of subjects aged 65 and over to determine whether they respond differently from younger subjects. Other reported clinical experience has not identified differences in responses between the elderly and younger patients.

ADVERSE REACTIONS

Hypersensitivity reactions, vasomotor disturbances, flushing, tingling, nausea, vomiting, and cramps may occur.

Patients may have a sensation of warmth or the desire to defecate or urinate during or shortly following initiation of infusion.

OVERDOSAGE

The intravenous LD_{50} in female mice is 7.22 g/kg.

DOSAGE AND ADMINISTRATION

For intravenous use only

Clearance measurements using single injection technics are generally inaccurate, particularly in the measurement of

Continued on next page

Information on the Merck & Co., Inc. products listed on these pages is the full prescribing information from product circulars in use September 30, 2000. For information, please call 1-800-NSC MERCK [1-800-672-6372].

Aminohippurate Sodium—Cont.

ERPF. For this reason, intravenous infusions at fixed rates are used to sustain the plasma PAH concentration at the desired level.
To measure ERPF, the concentration of PAH in the plasma should be maintained at 2 mg per 100 mL, which can be achieved with a priming dose of 6 to 10 mg/kg and an infusion dose of 10 to 24 mg/min.
As a research procedure for the measurement of Tm_{PAH}, the plasma level of PAH must be sufficient to saturate the capacity of the tubular secretory cells. Concentrations of from 40 to 60 mg per 100 mL are usually necessary.
Technical details of these tests may be found in Smith[1]; Wesson[2]; Bauer[3]; Pitts[4]; and Schnurr.[5]
Parenteral drug products should be inspected visually for particulate matter and discoloration prior to use, whenever solution and container permit. NOTE: The normal color range for this product is a colorless to yellow/brown solution. The efficacy is not affected by color changes within this range.
Calculations
Effective Renal Plasma Flow (ERPF)
The clearance of PAH, which is extracted almost completely from the plasma during its passage through the renal circulation, constitutes a measure of ERPF. Hence:

$$ERPF \quad \frac{U_{PAH}V}{P_{PAH}}$$

Where U_{PAH} = concentration of PAH (mg/mL) in the urine
V = rate of urine excretion (mL/min), and
P_{PAH} = plasma concentration of PAH (mg/mL).

Example: U_{PAH} = 8.0 mg/mL
V = 1.5 mL/min
P_{PAH} = 0.02 mg/mL

$$ERPF = \frac{8.0 \times 1.5}{0.02} = 600 \text{ mL/min.}$$

Based on PAH clearance studies, the normal values for ERPF are:

men	675 ± 150 mL/min
women	595 ± 125 mL/min.

Maximum Tubular Secretory Mechanism (Tm_{PAH})
The quantity of PAH, secreted by the tubules (Tm_{PAH}) is given by the difference between the total rate of excretion ($U_{PAH}V$) and the quantity filtered by the glomeruli (GFR × P_{PAH}). Hence:

$$Tm_{PAH} = U_{PAH}V - (GFR \times P_{PAH} \times 0.83)$$

The factor, 0.83, corrects for that portion of PAH which is bound to plasma protein and hence is unfilterable.

Example: U_{PAH} = 9.55 mg/mL
V = 16.68 mL/min
GFR = 120 mL/min
P_{PAH} = 0.60 mg/mL

Then $Tm_{PAH} = 9.55 \times 16.68 - (120 \times 0.60 \times 0.83) = 100$ mg/min.
Average normal values of Tm_{PAH} are 80–90 mg/min.
The value of the expression $U_{PAH}V$, used in calculations of ERPF and Tm_{PAH}, may be found by determining the amount of PAH in a measured volume of urine excreted within a specific period of time.
These calculations are based on a body surface area of 1.73 m^2. Corrections for variations in surface area are made by multiplying the values obtained for ERPF and Tm_{PAH} by 1.73/A, where A is the subject surface area.

HOW SUPPLIED

No. 95—Aminohippurate Sodium, 20 percent sterile solution for intravenous injection, is supplied as follows:
NDC 0006-3395-11 in 10 mL vials.
Storage
Avoid storage at temperatures below −20°C (−4°F) and above 40°C (104°F).

REFERENCES

1. Smith, H. W.: Lectures on the kidney, University Extension Division, University of Kansas, Lawrence, Kansas, 1943.
2. Wesson, L. G., Jr.: "Physiology of the Human Kidney," New York, Grune & Stratton, 1969, pp. 632–655.
3. Bauer, J. D.; Ackermann, P. G.; Toro, G.: "Brays Clinical Laboratory Methods," ed. 7, St. Louis, Mosby, 1968.
4. Pitts, R. F.: "Physiology of the Kidney and Body Fluids," ed. 2, Chicago, Year Book Medical Publishers, 1968.
5. Schnurr, E., Lahme, W., Kuppers, H.: Measurement of renal clearance of inulin and PAH in the steady state without urine collection; Clinical Nephrology, *13* (1): (26–29), 1980.

9051022 Issued September 1998

ANTIVENIN ℞
(Latrodectus mactans)
(Black Widow Spider Antivenin)
Equine Origin

DESCRIPTION

Antivenin (Latrodectus mactans) is a sterile, non-pyrogenic preparation derived by drying a frozen solution of specific venom-neutralizing globulins obtained from the blood serum of healthy horses immunized against venom of black widow spiders (Latrodectus mactans). It is standardized by biological assay on mice, in terms of one dose of antivenin neutralizing the venom in not less than 6000 mouse LD_{50} of Latrodectus mactans. Thimerosal (mercury derivative) 1:10,000 is added as a preservative. When constituted as specified, it is opalescent, ranging in color from light (straw) to very dark (iced tea), and contains not more than 20.0 percent of solids.
Each vial contains not less than 6000 Antivenin units. One unit of Antivenin will neutralize one average mouse lethal dose of black widow spider venom when the Antivenin and the venom are injected simultaneously in mice under suitable conditions.

CLINICAL PHARMACOLOGY

The pharmacological mode of action is unknown and metabolic and pharmacokinetic data in humans are unavailable.

INDICATIONS AND USAGE

Antivenin (Latrodectus mactans) is used to treat patients with symptoms due to bites by the black widow spider (Latrodectus mactans). Early use of the Antivenin is emphasized for prompt relief.
Local muscular cramps begin from 15 minutes to several hours after the bite which usually produces a sharp pain similar to that caused by puncture with a needle. The exact sequence of symptoms depends somewhat on the location of the bite. The venom acts on the myoneural junctions or on the nerve endings, causing an ascending motor paralysis or destruction of the peripheral nerve endings. The groups of muscles most frequently affected at first are those of the thigh, shoulder, and back. After a varying length of time, the pain becomes more severe, spreading to the abdomen, and weakness and tremor usually develop. The abdominal muscles assume a boardlike rigidity, but tenderness is slight. Respiration is thoracic. The patient is restless and anxious. Feeble pulse, cold, clammy skin, labored breathing and speech, light stupor, and delirium may occur. Convulsions also may occur, particularly in small children. The temperature may be normal or slightly elevated. Urinary retention, shock, cyanosis, nausea and vomiting, insomnia, and cold sweats also have been reported. The syndrome following the bite of the black widow spider may be confused easily with any medical or surgical condition with acute abdominal symptoms.
The symptoms of black widow spider bite increase in severity for several hours, perhaps a day, and then very slowly become less severe, gradually passing off in the course of two or three days except in fatal cases. Residual symptoms such as general weakness, tingling, nervousness, and transient muscle spasm may persist for weeks or months after recovery from the acute stage.
If possible, the patient should be hospitalized. Other additional measures giving greatest relief are prolonged warm baths and intravenous injection of 10 mL of 10 percent solution of calcium gluconate repeated as necessary to control muscle pain. Morphine also may be required to control pain. Barbiturates may be used for extreme restlessness. However, as the venom is a neurotoxin, it can cause respiratory paralysis. This must be borne in mind when considering use of morphine or a barbiturate. Adrenocorticosteroids have been used with varying degrees of success. Supportive therapy is indicated by the condition of the patient. Local treatment of the site of the bite is of no value. Nothing is gained by applying a tourniquet or by attempting to remove venom from the site of the bite by incision and suction.
In otherwise healthy individuals between the ages of 16 and 60, the use of Antivenin may be deferred and treatment with muscle relaxants may be considered.

WARNINGS

Prior to treatment with any product prepared from horse serum, a careful review of the patient's history should be taken emphasizing prior exposure to horse serum or any allergies. Serious sickness and even death could result from the use of horse serum in a sensitive patient. A skin or conjunctival test should be performed prior to administration of Antivenin.
Skin test: Inject into (not under) the skin not more than 0.02 mL of the test material (1:10 dilution of normal horse serum in physiologic saline). Evaluate result in 10 minutes. A positive reaction is an urticarial wheal surrounded by a zone of erythema. A control test using Sodium Chloride Injection facilitates interpretation of the results.
Conjunctival test: For adults instill into the conjunctival sac one drop of a 1:10 dilution of horse serum and for children one drop of 1:100 dilution. Itching of the eye and reddening of the conjunctiva indicate a positive reaction, usually within 10 minutes.
Patients should be observed for serum sickness for an average of 8 to 12 days following administration of Antivenin.
Desensitization should be attempted only when the administration of Antivenin is considered necessary to save life. Epinephrine must be available in case of untoward reaction.
Desensitization: If the history is positive or the results of the sensitivity tests are mildly or quetionably positive, Antivenin should be administered as follows to reduce the risk of an immediate severe allergic reaction:

1. In separate sterile vials or syringes prepare 1:10 or 1:100 dilutions of Antivenin in Sodium Chloride for Injection.
2. Allow at least 15 but preferably 30 minutes between injections and only proceed with the next dose if no reactions occurred following the previous dose.
3. Using a tuberculin syringe, inject subcutaneously 0.1, 0.2 and 0.5 mL of the 1:100 dilution at 15 or 30 minute intervals; repeat with the 1:10 dilution, and finally the undiluted Antivenin.
4. If there is a reaction after any of the injections, place a tourniquet proximal to the sites of injection and administer epinephrine, 1:1000 (0.3 to 1.0 mL subcutaneously, 0.05 to 0.1 mL intravenously), proximal to the tourniquet or into another extremity. Wait at least 30 minutes before giving another injection of Antivenin, the amount of which should be the same as the last one not evoking a reaction.
5. If no reaction has occurred after 0.5 mL of undiluted Antivenin has been given, it is probably safe to continue the dose at 15 minute intervals until the entire dose has been injected.

PRECAUTIONS

Carcinogenesis, Mutagenesis, Impairment of Fertility
No long term studies in animals have been performed to evaluate the potential for carcinogenesis, mutagenesis, or impairment of fertility.
Pregnancy
Pregnancy Category C. Animal reproduction studies have not been conducted with Black Widow Spider Antivenin. It is also not known whether Black Widow Spider Antivenin can cause fetal harm when administered to a pregnant woman or can affect reproduction capacity. Black Widow Spider Antivenin should be given to a pregnant woman only if clearly needed.
Nursing Mothers
It is not known whether this drug is excreted in human milk. Because many drugs are excreted in human milk, caution should be exercised when Black Widow Spider Antivenin is administered to a nursing woman.
Pediatric Use
Controlled clinical studies for safety and effectiveness in children have not been conducted; however, there have been virtually no adverse effects reported in those children who have received the product.

ADVERSE REACTIONS

Anaphylaxis and serum sickness have been reported following use of Antivenin.

DOSAGE AND ADMINISTRATION

Using a sterile syringe, remove from the accompanying vial 2.5 mL of Sterile Diluent for Antivenin and inject into the vial of Antivenin. With the needle still in the rubber stopper, shake the vial to dissolve the contents completely.
Parenteral drug products should be inspected visually for particulate matter prior to administration, whenever solution and container permit (see DESCRIPTION).
The dose for adults and children is the entire contents of a restored vial (2.5 mL) of Antivenin. It may be given intramuscularly, preferably in the region of the anterolateral thigh so that a tourniquet may be applied in the event of a systemic reaction. Symptoms usually subside in 1 to 3 hours. Although one dose of Antivenin usually is adequate, a second dose may be necessary in some cases.
Antivenin also may be given intravenously in 10 to 50 mL of saline solution over a 15 minute period. It is the preferred route in severe cases, or when the patient is under 12, or in shock. One restored vial usually is enough.

HOW SUPPLIED

No. 4084—Antivenin (Latrodectus mactans) equine origin is a white to grey crystalline powder, each vial containing not less than 6000 Antivenin units. Thimerosal (mercury derivative) 1:10,000 is added as preservative, **NDC** 0006-4084-00. A 2.5 mL vial of Sterile Diluent for Antivenin is included. Also supplied is a 1 mL vial of normal horse serum (1:10 dilution) for sensitivity testing. Thimerosal (mercury derivative) 1:10,000 is added as preservative.
Storage
Antivenin must be stored and shipped at 2–8°C (36–46°F). When reconstituted as directed, the color of Antivenin ranges from light (straw) to very dark (iced tea), but the color has no effect on potency. *Do not freeze.*
A.H.F.S. Category: 80:04
7972114 Issued March 1995

AquaMEPHYTON® Injection ℞
(Phytonadione)
Aqueous Colloidal Solution of Vitamin K_1

WARNING—INTRAVENOUS USE
Severe reactions, including fatalities, have occurred during and immediately after INTRAVENOUS injection of AquaMEPHYTON* (Phytonadione), even when precautions have been taken to dilute the AquaMEPHYTON and to avoid rapid infusion. Typically these severe reactions have resembled hypersensitivity or anaphylaxis, including shock and cardiac and/or respiratory arrest. Some patients have exhibited these severe reactions on receiving AquaMEPHYTON for the first time. Therefore the INTRAVENOUS route should be restricted to those situations where other routes are not feasible and the serious risk involved is considered justified.

*Registered trademark of MERCK & CO., INC.

DESCRIPTION

Phytonadione is a vitamin, which is a clear, yellow to amber, viscous, odorless or nearly odorless liquid. It is insoluble in water, soluble in chloroform and slightly soluble in ethanol. It has a molecular weight of 450.70.
Phytonadione is 2-methyl-3-phytyl-1,4-naphthoquinone. Its empirical formula is $C_{31}H_{46}O_2$ and its structural formula is:

$$-CH_2CH{=}C(CH_3)(CH_2)_3CH(CH_3)(CH_2)_3CH(CH_3)(CH_2)_3CHCH_3(CH_3)$$

AquaMEPHYTON injection is a yellow, sterile, aqueous colloidal solution of vitamin K_1, with a pH of 5.0 to 7.0, available for injection by the intravenous, intramuscular, and subcutaneous routes. Each milliliter contains:
Phytonadione .... 2 mg or 10 mg
Inactive ingredients:
Polyoxyethylated fatty acid derivative .... 70 mg
Dextrose .... 37.5 mg
Water for Injection, q.s. .... 1 mL
Added as preservative:
Benzyl alcohol 0.9%

CLINICAL PHARMACOLOGY

AquaMEPHYTON aqueous colloidal solution of vitamin K_1 for parenteral injection, possesses the same type and degree of activity as does naturally-occurring vitamin K, which is necessary for the production via the liver of active prothrombin (factor II), proconvertin (factor VII), plasma thromboplastin component (factor IX), and Stuart factor (factor X). The prothrombin test is sensitive to the levels of three of these four factors—II, VII, and X. Vitamin K is an essential cofactor for a microsomal enzyme that catalyzes the post-translational carboxylation of multiple, specific, peptide-bound glutamic acid residues in inactive hepatic precursors of factors II, VII, IX, and X. The resulting gamma-carboxyglutamic acid residues convert the precursors into active coagulation factors that are subsequently secreted by liver cells into the blood.
Phytonadione is readily absorbed following intramuscular administration. After absorption, phytonadione is initially concentrated in the liver, but the concentration declines rapidly. Very little vitamin K accumulates in tissues. Little is known about the metabolic fate of vitamin K. Almost no free unmetabolized vitamin K appears in bile or urine.
In normal animals and humans, phytonadione is virtually devoid of pharmacodynamic activity. However, in animals and humans deficient in vitamin K, the pharmacological action of vitamin K is related to its normal physiological function, that is, to promote the hepatic biosynthesis of vitamin K dependent clotting factors.
The action of the aqueous colloidal solution, when administered intravenously, is generally detectable within an hour or two and hemorrhage is usually controlled within 3 to 6 hours. A normal prothrombin level may often be obtained in 12 to 14 hours.
In the prophylaxis and treatment of hemorrhagic disease of the newborn, phytonadione has demonstrated a greater margin of safety than that of the water-soluble vitamin K analogues.

INDICATIONS AND USAGE

AquaMEPHYTON is indicated in the following coagulation disorders which are due to faulty formation of factors II, VII, IX and X when caused by vitamin K deficiency or interference with vitamin K activity.
AquaMEPHYTON injection is indicated in:
— anticoagulant-induced prothrombin deficiency caused by coumarin or indanedione derivatives;
— prophylaxis and therapy of hemorrhagic disease of the newborn;
— hypoprothrombinemia due to antibacterial therapy;
— hypoprothrombinemia secondary to factors limiting absorption or synthesis of vitamin K, e.g., obstructive jaundice, biliary fistula, sprue, ulcerative colitis, celiac disease, intestinal resection, cystic fibrosis of the pancreas, and regional enteritis;
— other drug-induced hypoprothrombinemia where it is definitely shown that the result is due to interference with vitamin K metabolism, e.g., salicylates.

CONTRAINDICATION

Hypersensitivity to any component of this medication.

WARNINGS

Benzyl alcohol as a preservative in Bacteriostatic Sodium Chloride Injection has been associated with toxicity in newborns. Data are unavailable on the toxicity of other preservatives in this age group. There is no evidence to suggest that the small amount of benzyl alcohol contained in AquaMEPHYTON, when used as recommended, is associated with toxicity.
An immediate coagulant effect should not be expected after administration of phytonadione. It takes a minimum of 1 to 2 hours for measurable improvement in the prothrombin time. Whole blood or component therapy may also be necessary if bleeding is severe.
Phytonadione will not counteract the anticoagulant action of heparin.
When vitamin K_1 is used to correct excessive anticoagulant-induced hypoprothrombinemia, anticoagulant therapy still being indicated, the patient is again faced with the clotting hazards existing prior to starting the anticoagulant therapy. Phytonadione is not a clotting agent, but overzealous therapy with vitamin K_1 may restore conditions which originally permitted thromboembolic phenomena. Dosage should be kept as low as possible, and prothrombin time should be checked regularly as clinical conditions indicate.
Repeated large doses of vitamin K are not warranted in liver disease if the response to initial use of the vitamin is unsatisfactory. Failure to respond to vitamin K may indicate that the condition being treated is inherently unresponsive to vitamin K.

PRECAUTIONS

Drug Interactions
Temporary resistance to prothrombin-depressing anticoagulants may result, especially when larger doses of phytonadione are used. If relatively large doses have been employed, it may be necessary when reinstituting anticoagulant therapy to use somewhat larger doses of the prothrombin-depressing anticoagulant, or to use one which acts on a different principle, such as heparin sodium.
Laboratory Tests
Prothrombin time should be checked regularly as clinical conditions indicate.
Carcinogenesis, Mutagenesis, Impairment of Fertility
Studies of carcinogenicity, mutagenesis or impairment of fertility have not been conducted with AquaMEPHYTON.
Pregnancy
Pregnancy Category C: Animal reproduction studies have not been conducted with AquaMEPHYTON. It is also not known whether AquaMEPHYTON can cause fetal harm when administered to a pregnant woman or can affect reproduction capacity. AquaMEPHYTON should be given to a pregnant woman only if clearly needed.
Nursing Mothers
It is not known whether this drug is excreted in human milk. Because many drugs are excreted in human milk, caution should be exercised when AquaMEPHYTON is administered to a nursing woman.
Pediatric Use
Hemolysis, jaundice, and hyperbilirubinemia in newborns, particularly in premature infants, may be related to the dose of AquaMEPHYTON. Therefore, the recommended dose should not be exceeded (see ADVERSE REACTIONS and DOSAGE AND ADMINISTRATION).

AquaMEPHYTON
Summary of Dosage Guidelines
(See circular text for details)

Newborns	Dosage
Hemorrhagic Disease of the Newborn	
Prophylaxis	0.5–1 mg IM within 1 hour of birth
Treatment	1 mg SC or IM (Higher doses may be necessary if the mother has been receiving oral anticoagulants)
Adults	**Initial Dosage**
Anticoagulant-Induced Prothrombin Deficiency (caused by coumarin or indanedione derivatives)	2.5 mg–10 mg or up to 25 mg (rarely 50 mg)
Hypoprothrombinemia due to other causes (Antibiotics; Salicylates or other drugs; Factors limiting absorption or synthesis)	2.5 mg–25 mg or more (rarely up to 50 mg)

ADVERSE REACTIONS

Deaths have occurred after intravenous administration. (See Box Warning at beginning of circular.)
Transient "flushing sensations" and "peculiar" sensations of taste have been observed, as well as rare instances of dizziness, rapid and weak pulse, profuse sweating, brief hypotension, dyspnea, and cyanosis.
Pain, swelling, and tenderness at the injection site may occur.
The possibility of allergic sensitivity, including an anaphylactoid reaction, should be kept in mind.
Infrequently, usually after repeated injection, erythematous, indurated, pruritic plaques have occurred; rarely, these have progressed to sclerodermalike lesions that have persisted for long periods. In other cases, these lesions have resembled erythema perstans.
Hyperbilirubinemia has been observed in the newborn following administration of phytonadione. This has occurred rarely and primarily with doses above those recommended. (See PRECAUTIONS, *Pediatric Use.*)

OVERDOSAGE

The intravenous LD_{50} of AquaMEPHYTON in the mouse is 41.5 and 52 mL/kg for the 0.2% and 1% concentrations respectively.

DOSAGE AND ADMINISTRATION

Whenever possible, AquaMEPHYTON should be given by the subcutaneous or intramuscular route. When intravenous administration is considered unavoidable, the drug should be injected very slowly, not exceeding 1 mg per minute.
Protect from light at all times.
Parenteral drug products should be inspected visually for particulate matter and discoloration prior to administration, whenever solution and container permit.
Directions for Dilution
AquaMEPHYTON may be diluted with 0.9% Sodium Chloride Injection, 5% Dextrose Injection, or 5% Dextrose and Sodium Chloride Injection. Benzyl alcohol as a preservative has been associated with toxicity in newborns. *Therefore, all of the above diluents should be preservative-free* (see WARNINGS). *Other diluents should not be used.* When dilutions are indicated, administration should be started immediately after mixture with the diluent, and unused portions of the dilution should be discarded, as well as unused contents of the ampul.
Prophylaxis of Hemorrhagic Disease of the Newborn
The American Academy of Pediatrics recommends that vitamin K_1 be given to the newborn. A single intramuscular dose of AquaMEPHYTON 0.5 to 1 mg within one hour of birth is recommended.
Treatment of Hemorrhagic Disease of the Newborn
Empiric administration of vitamin K_1 should not replace proper laboratory evaluation of the coagulation mechanism. A prompt response (shortening of the prothrombin time in 2 to 4 hours) following administration of vitamin K_1 is usually diagnostic of hemorrhagic disease of the newborn, and failure to respond indicates another diagnosis or coagulation disorder.
AquaMEPHYTON 1 mg should be given either subcutaneously or intramuscularly. Higher doses may be necessary if the mother has been receiving oral anticoagulants.
[See table above]
Whole blood or component therapy may be indicated if bleeding is excessive. This therapy, however, does not correct the underlying disorder and AquaMEPHYTON should be given concurrently.

Continued on next page

Information on the Merck & Co., Inc. products listed on these pages is the full prescribing information from product circulars in use September 30, 2000. For information, please call 1-800-NSC MERCK [1-800-672-6372].

AquaMephyton—Cont.

Anticoagulant-Induced Prothrombin Deficiency in Adults
To correct excessively prolonged prothrombin time caused by oral anticoagulant therapy—2.5 to 10 mg or up to 25 mg initially is recommended. In rare instances 50 mg may be required. Frequency and amount of subsequent doses should be determined by prothrombin time response or clinical condition (see WARNINGS). If in 6 to 8 hours after parenteral administration the prothrombin time has not been shortened satisfactorily, the dose should be repeated.
In the event of shock or excessive blood loss, the use of whole blood or component therapy is indicated.
Hypoprothrombinemia Due to Other Causes in Adults
A dosage of 2.5 to 25 mg or more (rarely up to 50 mg) is recommended, the amount and route of administration depending upon the severity of the condition and response obtained.
If possible, discontinuation or reduction of the dosage of drugs interfering with coagulation mechanisms (such as salicylates, antibiotics) is suggested as an alternative to administering concurrent AquaMEPHYTON. The severity of the coagulation disorder should determine whether the immediate administration of AquaMEPHYTON is required in addition to discontinuation or reduction of interfering drugs.

HOW SUPPLIED

Injection AquaMEPHYTON is a yellow, sterile, aqueous colloidal solution and is supplied in the following concentrations:
No. 7780—10 mg of vitamin K_1 per mL
NDC 0006-7780-64 boxes of 6 × 1 mL ampuls
(6505-00-854-2499 10 mg 1 mL 6's)
NDC 0006-7780-66 boxes of 25 × 1 mL ampuls.
No. 7782—10 mg of vitamin K_1 per mL
NDC 0006-7782-30 in 2.5 mL multiple dose vials
NDC 0006-7782-03 in 5 mL multiple dose vials.
No. 7784—1 mg of vitamin K_1 per 0.5 mL
NDC 0006-7784-33 boxes of 25 × 0.5 mL ampuls
(6505-00-180-6372 1 mg 0.5 mL 25's).
Storage
Store in a dark place.
9073021 Issued September 1997

ARAMINE® Injection ℞
(Metaraminol Bitartrate)

DESCRIPTION

Metaraminol bitartrate is a potent sympathomimetic amine that increases both systolic and diastolic blood pressure.
Metaraminol bitartrate is [*R*-(*R**,*S**)]-α-(1-aminoethyl)-3-hydroxybenzenemethanol [*R*-(*R**,*R**)]-2,3-dihydroxybutanedioate (1:1) (salt), which is levorotatory. Its empirical formula is $C_9H_{13}NO_2 \cdot C_4H_6O_6$ and its structural formula is:

OH NH₂ — C—C—CH₃ · HCOH / HOCH — H H — HO — COOH / COOH

Metaraminol bitartrate is a white, crystalline powder with a molecular weight of 317.29, is freely soluble in water, slightly soluble in alcohol, and practically insoluble in chloroform and in ether.
Injection ARAMINE* (Metaraminol Bitartrate) is a sterile solution. Each mL contains:
Metaraminol bitartrate equivalent to
metaraminol .... 10 mg
Inactive ingredients:
Sodium chloride .... 4.4 mg
Water for Injection q.s. ad .... 1 mL
Methylparaben 0.15%, propylparaben 0.02%, and sodium bisulfite 0.2% added as preservatives.

*Registered trademark of MERCK & CO., INC.

CLINICAL PHARMACOLOGY

The pressor effect of ARAMINE begins in 1 to 2 minutes after intravenous infusion, in about 10 minutes after intramuscular injection, and in 5 to 20 minutes after subcutaneous injection. The effect lasts from about 20 minutes to one hour. ARAMINE has a positive inotropic effect on the heart and a peripheral vasoconstrictor action.
Renal, coronary, and cerebral blood flow are a function of perfusion pressure and regional resistance. In patients with insufficient or failing vasoconstriction, there is additional advantage to the peripheral action of ARAMINE, but in most patients with shock, vasoconstriction is adequate and any further increase is unnecessary. Blood flow to vital organs may decrease with ARAMINE if regional resistance increases excessively.
The pressor effect of ARAMINE is decreased but not reversed by alpha-adrenergic blocking agents. Primary or secondary fall in blood pressure and tachyphylactic response to repeated use are uncommon.

INDICATIONS AND USAGE

ARAMINE is indicated for prevention and treatment of the acute hypotensive state occurring with spinal anesthesia. It is also indicated as adjunctive treatment of hypotension due to hemorrhage, reactions to medications, surgical complications, and shock associated with brain damage due to trauma or tumor.

CONTRAINDICATIONS

Use of ARAMINE with cyclopropane or halothane anesthesia should be avoided, unless clinical circumstances demand such use.
Hypersensitivity to any component of this product, including sulfites (see WARNINGS).

WARNINGS

Use of sympathomimetic amines with monoamine oxidase inhibitors or tricyclic antidepressants may result in potentiation of the pressor effect. (See PRECAUTIONS, *Drug Interactions.*)
ARAMINE contains sodium bisulfite, a sulfite that may cause allergic-type reactions including anaphylactic symptoms and life-threatening or less severe asthmatic episodes in certain susceptible people. The overall prevalence of sulfite sensitivity in the general population is unknown and probably low. Sulfite sensitivity is seen more frequently in asthmatic than in nonasthmatic people.

PRECAUTIONS

General
Caution should be used to avoid excessive blood pressure response. Rapidly induced hypertensive responses have been reported to cause acute pulmonary edema, arrhythmias, cerebral hemorrhage, or cardiac arrest.
Patients with cirrhosis should be treated with caution, with adequate restoration of electrolytes if diuresis ensues. Fatal ventricular arrhythmia was reported in one patient with Laennec's cirrhosis while receiving metaraminol bitartrate. In several instances, ventricular extrasystoles that appeared during infusion of this vasopressor subsided promptly when the rate of infusion was reduced.
With the prolonged action of ARAMINE, a cumulative effect is possible. If there is an excessive vasopressor response there may be a prolonged elevation of blood pressure even after discontinuation of therapy.
When vasopressor amines are used for long periods, the resulting vasoconstriction may prevent adequate expansion of circulating volume and may cause perpetuation of shock. There is evidence that plasma volume may be reduced in all types of shock, and that the measurement of central venous pressure is useful in assessing the adequacy of the circulating blood volume. Therefore, blood or plasma volume expanders should be used when the principal reason for hypotension or shock is decreased circulating volume.
Because of its vasoconstrictor effect ARAMINE should be given with caution in heart or thyroid disease, hypertension, or diabetes. Sympathomimetic amines may provoke a relapse in patients with a history of malaria.
Drug Interactions
ARAMINE should be used with caution in digitalized patients, since the combination of digitalis and sympathomimetic amines may cause ectopic arrhythmias.
Monoamine oxidase inhibitors or tricyclic antidepressants may potentiate the action of sympathomimetic amines. Therefore, when initiating pressor therapy in patients receiving these drugs, the initial dose should be small and given with caution. (See WARNINGS.)
Carcinogenesis, Mutagenesis, Impairment of Fertility
Studies in animals have not been performed to evaluate the mutagenic or carcinogenic potential of ARAMINE or its potential to affect fertility.
Pregnancy
Pregnancy Category C. Animal reproduction studies have not been conducted with ARAMINE. It is not known whether ARAMINE can cause fetal harm when given to a pregnant woman or can affect reproduction capacity. ARAMINE should be given to a pregnant woman only if clearly needed.
Nursing Mothers
It is not known whether this drug is secreted in human milk. Because many drugs are secreted in human milk, caution should be exercised when ARAMINE is given to a nursing woman.
Pediatric Use
Safety and effectiveness in pediatric patients have not been established.

ADVERSE REACTIONS

Sympathomimetic amines, including ARAMINE, may cause sinus or ventricular tachycardia, or other arrhythmias, especially in patients with myocardial infarction. (See PRECAUTIONS.)
In patients with a history of malaria, these compounds may provoke a relapse.
Abscess formation, tissue necrosis, or sloughing rarely may follow the use of ARAMINE. In choosing the site of injection, it is important to avoid those areas recognized as *not* suitable for use of any pressor agent and to discontinue the infusion immediately if infiltration or thrombosis occurs. Although the physician may be forced by the urgent nature of the patient's condition to choose injection sites that are not recognized as suitable, he should, when possible, use the preferred areas of injection. The larger veins of the antecubital fossa or the thigh are preferred to veins in the dorsum of the hand or ankle veins, particularly in patients with peripheral vascular disease, diabetes mellitus, Buerger's disease, or conditions with coexistent hypercoagulability.

OVERDOSAGE

Overdosage may result in severe hypertension accompanied by headache, constricting sensation in the chest, nausea, vomiting, euphoria, diaphoresis, pulmonary edema, tachycardia, bradycardia, sinus arrhythmia, atrial or ventricular arrhythmias, cerebral hemorrhage, myocardial infarction, cardiac arrest or convulsions.
Should an excessive elevation of blood pressure occur, it may be immediately relieved by a sympatholytic agent, e.g. phentolamine. An appropriate antiarrhythmic agent may also be required.
The oral LD_{50} in the rat and mouse is 240 mg/kg and 99 mg/kg, respectively.

DOSAGE AND ADMINISTRATION

ARAMINE may be given intramuscularly, subcutaneously, or intravenously, the route depending on the nature and severity of the indication.
Parenteral drug products should be inspected visually for particulate matter and discoloration prior to use, whenever solution and container permit.
Allow at least 10 minutes to elapse before increasing the dose because the maximum effect is not immediately apparent. When the vasopressor is discontinued, observe the patient carefully as the effect of the drug tapers off, so that therapy can be reinitiated promptly if the blood pressure falls too rapidly. The response to vasopressors may be poor in patients with coexistent shock and acidosis. When indicated, established methods of shock management should be used, such as blood or fluid replacement.
Intramuscular or Subcutaneous Injection (for prevention of hypotension—see INDICATIONS): The recommended dose is 2 to 10 mg (0.2 to 1 mL). As with other agents given subcutaneously, only the preferred sites of injection, as set forth in standard texts, should be used.
Intravenous Infusion (for adjunctive treatment of hypotension—see INDICATIONS): The recommended dose is 15 to 100 mg (1.5 to 10 mL) in 500 mL of Sodium Chloride Injection or 5% Dextrose Injection, adjusting the rate of infusion to maintain the blood pressure at the desired level. Higher concentrations of ARAMINE, 150 to 500 mg per 500 mL of infusion fluid, have been used.
If the patient needs more saline or dextrose solution at a rate of flow that would provide an excessive dose of the vasopressor, the recommended volume of infusion fluid (500 mL) should be increased accordingly. ARAMINE may also be added to *less* than 500 mL of infusion fluid if a smaller volume is desired.
Compatibility Information
In addition to Sodium Chloride Injection and Dextrose Injection 5%, the following infusion solutions were found physically and chemically compatible with Injection ARAMINE when 5 mL of Injection ARAMINE, 10 mg/mL (metaraminol equivalent), was added to 500 mL of infusion solution: Ringer's Injection, Lactated Ringer's Injection, Dextran 6% in Saline**, Normosol®-R pH 7.4**, and Normosol®-M in D5-W**.
When Injection ARAMINE is mixed with an infusion solution, sterile precautions should be observed. Since infusion solutions generally do not contain preservatives, mixtures should be used within 24 hours.
Direct Intravenous Injection: In severe shock, when time is of great importance, this agent should be given by direct intravenous injection. The suggested dose is 0.5 to 5 mg (0.05 to 0.5 mL), followed by an infusion of 15 to 100 mg (1.5 to 10 mL) in 500 mL of infusion fluid as described previously.
Vials may be sterilized by autoclaving or by immersion in a sterilizing solution.

**Product of Abbott Laboratories

HOW SUPPLIED

No. 3222X—Injection ARAMINE 1%, containing metaraminol bitartrate equivalent to 10 mg of metaraminol per mL, is a clear, colorless solution and is supplied as follows:
NDC 0006-3222-10 in 10 mL vials
(6505-00-753-9601 10 mL vial).
Storage
Protect from light. Store container in carton until contents have been used.
Avoid storage at temperatures below -20°C (-4°F) and above 40°C (104°F).
7348524 Issued September 1996

ATTENUVAX® ℞
(Measles Virus Vaccine Live)

DESCRIPTION
ATTENUVAX* (Measles Virus Vaccine Live) is a live virus vaccine for vaccination against measles (rubeola).

ATTENUVAX is a sterile lyophilized preparation of a more attenuated line of measles virus derived from Enders' attenuated Edmonston strain and propagated in chick embryo cell culture.
The growth medium for measles is Medium 199 (a buffered salt solution containing vitamins and amino acids and supplemented with fetal bovine serum) containing SPGA (sucrose, phosphate, glutamate, and human albumin) as stabilizer and neomycin.
The cells, virus pools, fetal bovine serum, and human albumin are all screened for the absence of adventitious agents. Human albumin is processed using the Cohn cold ethanol fractionation procedure.
The reconstituted vaccine is for subcutaneous administration. Each 0.5 mL dose contains not less than 1,000 $TCID_{50}$ (tissue culture infectious doses) of measles virus. Each dose of the vaccine is calculated to contain sorbitol (14.5 mg), sodium phosphate, sucrose (1.9 mg), sodium chloride, hydrolyzed gelatin (14.5 mg), human albumin (0.3 mg), fetal bovine serum (<1 ppm), other buffer and media ingredients and approximately 25 mcg of neomycin. The product contains no preservative.
Before reconstitution, the lyophilized vaccine is a light yellow compact crystalline plug. ATTENUVAX, when reconstituted as directed, is clear yellow.

*Registered trademark of MERCK & CO., Inc.

CLINICAL PHARMACOLOGY

Measles is a common childhood disease, caused by measles virus (paramyxovirus), that may be associated with serious complications and/or death. For example, pneumonia and encephalitis are caused by measles.
The impact of measles vaccination on the natural history of each disease in the United States can be quantified by comparing the maximum number of measles cases reported in a given year prior to vaccine use to the number of cases of each disease reported in 1995. A total of 894,134 cases reported in 1941 compared to 288 cases reported in 1995 resulted in a 99.97% decrease in reported cases of measles.
Extensive clinical trials have demonstrated that ATTENUVAX is highly immunogenic and generally well tolerated. A single injection of the vaccine has been shown to induce measles hemagglutination-inhibition (HI) antibodies in 97% or more of susceptible persons. However, a small percentage (1–5%) of vaccinees may fail to seroconvert after the primary dose (see also INDICATIONS AND USAGE, *Recommended Vaccination Schedule*).
A study of 6 month old and 15 month old infants born to vaccine-immunized mothers demonstrated that, following vaccination with ATTENUVAX, 74% of the 6 month old infants developed detectable neutralizing antibody (NT) titers while 100% of the 15 month old infants developed NT. This rate of seroconversion is higher than that previously reported for 6 month old infants born to naturally immune mothers tested by HI assay. When the 6 month old infants of immunized mothers were revaccinated at 15 months, they developed antibody titers equivalent to the 15 month old vaccinees. The lower seroconversion rate in 6 month olds has two possible explanations: 1) Due to the limit of the detection level of the assays (NT and enzyme immunoassay [EIA]), the presence of trace amounts of undetectable maternal antibody might interfere with the seroconversion of infants; or 2) the immune system of 6 month olds is not always capable of mounting a response to measles vaccine as measured by the two antibody assays.
There is some evidence to suggest that infants who are born to mothers who had natural measles and who are vaccinated at less than one year of age may not develop sustained antibody levels when later revaccinated. The advantage of early protection must be weighed against the chance for failure to respond adequately on reimmunization.
Efficacy of measles vaccine was established in a series of double-blind controlled field trials which demonstrated a high degree of protective efficacy. These studies also established that seroconversion in response to measles vaccination paralleled protection from these diseases.
Following vaccination, antibodies associated with protection can be measured by neutralization assays, HI, or ELISA (enzyme linked immunosorbent assay) tests. Neutralizing and ELISA antibodies to measles virus are still detectable in most individuals 11–13 years after primary vaccination.

INDICATIONS AND USAGE

Recommended Vaccination Schedule
ATTENUVAX is indicated for vaccination against measles in persons 12 months of age or older.
Individuals first vaccinated with ATTENUVAX at 12 months of age or older should be revaccinated with M-M-R* II (Measles, Mumps, and Rubella Virus Vaccine Live) prior to elementary school entry. Revaccination may seroconvert primary failures or boost antibody titers of those individuals whose titers have declined. The Advisory Committee on Immunization Practices (ACIP) recommends administration of the first dose of M-M-R II at 12–15 months of age and administration of the second dose of M-M-R II at 4–6 years of age. In addition, some public health jurisdictions mandate the age for revaccination. Consult the complete text of applicable guidelines regarding routine revaccination including that of high-risk adult populations.

Measles Outbreak Schedule
Infants Between 6–12 Months of Age
Local health authorities may recommend measles vaccination of infants between 6–12 months of age in outbreak situations. This population may fail to respond to the measles component of the vaccine. The younger the infant, the lower the likelihood of seroconversion (see CLINICAL PHARMACOLOGY). Such infants should receive a second dose of M-M-R II between 12 to 15 months of age followed by revaccination prior to elementary school entry.
Unnecessary doses of a vaccine are best avoided by ensuring that written documentation of vaccination is preserved and a copy given to each vaccinee's parent or guardian.
Other Vaccination Considerations
Other Populations
Individuals planning travel outside the United States, if not immune, can acquire measles, mumps or rubella and import these diseases into the United States. Therefore, prior to international travel, individuals known to be susceptible to one or more of these diseases can receive either a monovalent vaccine (measles, mumps or rubella), or a combination vaccine as appropriate. However, M-M-R II is preferred for persons likely to be susceptible to mumps and rubella; and if monovalent measles vaccine is not readily available, travelers should receive M-M-R II regardless of their immune status to mumps or rubella.
Vaccination is recommended for susceptible individuals in high-risk groups such as college students, health-care workers, and military personnel.
According to ACIP recommendations, most persons born in 1956 or earlier are likely to have been infected with measles naturally and generally need not be considered susceptible. All children, adolescents, and adults born after 1956 are considered susceptible and should be vaccinated, if there are no contraindications. This includes persons who may be immune to measles but who lack adequate documentation of immunity such as: (1) physician-diagnosed measles, (2) laboratory evidence of measles immunity, or (3) adequate immunization with live measles vaccine on or after the first birthday.
The ACIP recommends that "Persons vaccinated with inactivated vaccine followed within 3 months by live vaccine should be revaccinated with two doses of live vaccine. Revaccination is particularly important when the risk of exposure to natural measles virus is increased, as may occur during international travel."
Post-Exposure Vaccination
ATTENUVAX given immediately after exposure to natural measles may provide some protection if the vaccine can be administered within 72 hours of exposure. If, however, the vaccine is given a few days before exposure, substantial protection may be provided.
Use With Other Vaccines
See DOSAGE AND ADMINISTRATION, *Use With Other Vaccines*.

CONTRAINDICATIONS

Hypersensitivity to any component of the vaccine, including gelatin.
Do not give ATTENUVAX to pregnant females; the possible effects of the vaccine on fetal development are unknown at this time. If vaccination of postpubertal females is undertaken, pregnancy should be avoided for 3 months following vaccination (see PRECAUTIONS, *Pregnancy*).
Anaphylactic or anaphylactoid reactions to neomycin (each dose of reconstituted vaccine contains approximately 25 mcg of neomycin).
Febrile respiratory illness or other active febrile infection. However, the ACIP has recommended that all vaccines can be administered to persons with minor illnesses such as diarrhea, mild upper respiratory infection with or without low-grade fever, or other low-grade febrile illness.
Patients receiving immunosuppressive therapy. This contraindication does not apply to patients who are receiving corticosteroids as replacement therapy, e.g., for Addison's disease.
Individuals with blood dyscrasias, leukemia, lymphomas of any type, or other malignant neoplasms affecting the bone marrow or lymphatic systems.
Primary and acquired immunodeficiency states, including patients who are immunosuppressed in association with AIDS or other clinical manifestations of infection with human immunodeficiency viruses; cellular immune deficiencies; and hypogammaglobulinemic and dysgammaglobulinemic states. Measles inclusion body encephalitis (MIBE), pneumonitis and death as a direct consequence of disseminated measles vaccine virus infection has been reported in immunocompromised individuals inadvertently vaccinated with measles-containing vaccine.
Individuals with a family history of congenital or hereditary immunodeficiency, until the immune competence of the potential vaccine recipient is demonstrated.

WARNINGS

Due caution should be employed in administration of ATTENUVAX to persons with a history of cerebral injury, individual or family histories of convulsions, or any other condition in which stress due to fever should be avoided. The physician should be alert to the temperature elevation which may occur following vaccination (see ADVERSE REACTIONS).

Hypersensitivity To Eggs
Live measles vaccine is produced in chick embryo cell culture. Persons with a history of anaphylactic, anaphylactoid or other immediate reactions (e.g., hives, swelling of the mouth and throat, difficulty breathing, hypotension and shock) subsequent to egg ingestion may be at an enhanced risk of immediate-type hypersensitivity reactions after receiving vaccines containing traces of chick embryo antigen. The potential risk to benefit ratio should be carefully evaluated before considering vaccination in such cases. Such individuals may be vaccinated with extreme caution, having adequate treatment on hand should a reaction occur (see PRECAUTIONS).
However, the AAP has stated, "Most children with a history of anaphylactic reactions to eggs have no untoward reactions to measles or MMR vaccine. Persons are not at increased risk if they have egg allergies that are not anaphylactic, and they should be vaccinated in the usual manner. In addition, skin testing of egg-allergic children with vaccine has not been predictive of which children will have an immediate hypersensitivity reaction...Persons with allergies to chickens or chicken feathers are not at increased risk of reaction to the vaccine."
Hypersensitivity to Neomycin
The AAP states, "Persons who have experienced anaphylactic reactions to topically or systemically administered neomycin should not receive measles vaccine. Most often, however, neomycin allergy manifests as a contact dermatitis, which is a delayed-type (cell-mediated) immune response rather than anaphylaxis. In such persons, an adverse reaction to neomycin in the vaccine would be an erythematous, pruritic nodule or papule, 48 to 96 hours after vaccination. A history of contact dermatitis to neomycin is not a contraindication to receiving measles vaccine."
Thrombocytopenia
Individuals with current thrombocytopenia may develop more severe thrombocytopenia following vaccination. In addition, individuals who experienced thrombocytopenia with the first dose of M-M-R II (or its component vaccines) may develop thrombocytopenia with repeat doses. Serologic status may be evaluated to determine whether or not additional doses of vaccine are needed. The potential risk to benefit ratio should be carefully evaluated before considering vaccination in such cases (see ADVERSE REACTIONS).

PRECAUTIONS

General
Adequate treatment provisions including epinephrine injection (1:1000), should be available for immediate use should an anaphylactic or anaphylactoid reaction occur.
Special care should be taken to ensure that the injection does not enter a blood vessel.
Children and young adults who are known to be infected with human immunodeficiency viruses and are not immunosuppressed may be vaccinated. However, vaccinees who are infected with HIV should be monitored closely for vaccine-preventable diseases because immunization may be less effective than for uninfected persons (see CONTRAINDICATIONS).
Vaccination should be deferred for 3 months or longer following blood or plasma transfusions, or administration of immune globulin (human).
There are no reports of transmission of live attenuated measles virus from vaccinees to susceptible contacts.
It has been reported that attenuated measles virus vaccine live may result in a temporary depression of tuberculin skin sensitivity. Therefore, if a tuberculin test is to be done, it should be administered either before or simultaneously with ATTENUVAX.
Children under treatment for tuberculosis have not experienced exacerbation of the disease when immunized with live meaels virus vaccine; no studies have been reported to date of the effect of measles virus vaccines on untreated tuberculous children. However, individuals with active untreated tuberculosis should not be vaccinated.
As for any vaccine, vaccination with ATTENUVAX may not result in protection in 100% of vaccinees.
The health-care provider should determine the current health status and previous vaccination history of the vaccinee.
The health-care provider should question the patient, parent, or guardian about reactions to a previous dose of ATTENUVAX or other measles-containing vaccines.
Drug Interactions
See DOSAGE AND ADMINISTRATION, *Use With Other Vaccines*.
Information For Patients
The health-care provider should provide the vaccine information required to be given with each vaccination to the patient, parent or guardian.
The health-care provider should inform the patient, parent or guardian of the benefits and risks associated with vaccination. For risks associated with vaccination see WARNINGS, PRECAUTIONS, ADVERSE REACTIONS.

Continued on next page

Information on the Merck & Co., Inc. products listed on these pages is the full prescribing information from product circulars in use September 30, 2000. For information, please call 1-800-NSC MERCK [1-800-672-6372].

Attenuvax—Cont.

Patients, parents or guardians should be instructed to report any serious adverse reactions to their health-care provider who in turn should report such events to the U.S. Department of Health and Human Services through the Vaccine Adverse Event Reporting System (VAERS), 1-800-822-7967.
Pregnancy should be avoided for 3 months following vaccination.
Immunosuppressive Therapy
The immune status of patients about to undergo immunosuppressive therapy should be evaluated so that the physician can consider whether vaccination prior to the initiation of treatment is indicated (see CONTRAINDICATIONS and PRECAUTIONS).
The ACIP has stated that "patients with leukemia in remission who have not received chemotherapy for at least 3 months may receive live-virus vaccines. Short-term (<2 weeks), low- to moderate-dose systemic corticosteroid therapy, topical steroid therapy (e.g., nasal, skin), long-term alternate-day treatment with low to moderate doses of short-acting systemic steroid, and intra-articular, bursal, or tendon injection of corticosteroids are not immunosuppressive in their usual doses and do not contraindicate the administration of measles vaccine."
Immune Globulin
Administration of immune globulins concurrently with ATTENUVAX may interfere with the expected immune response.
See also PRECAUTIONS, *General*.
Carcinogenesis, Mutagenesis, Impairment of Fertility
ATTENUVAX has not been evaluated for carcinogenic or mutagenic potential, or potential to impair fertility.
Pregnancy
Pregnancy Category C
Animal reproduction studies have not been conducted with ATTENUVAX. It is also not known whether ATTENUVAX can cause fetal harm when administered to a pregnant woman or can affect reproduction capacity. Therefore, the vaccine should not be administered to pregnant females; furthermore, pregnancy should be avoided for 3 months following vaccination (see CONTRAINDICATIONS).
In counseling women who are inadvertently vaccinated when pregnant or who become pregnant within 3 months of vaccination, the physician should be aware that reports have indicated that contracting natural measles during pregnancy enhances fetal risk. Increased rates of spontaneous abortion, stillbirth, congenital defects and prematurity have been observed subsequent to natural measles during pregnancy. There are no adequate studies of the attenuated (vaccine) strain of measles virus in pregnancy. However, it would be prudent to assume that the vaccine strain of virus is also capable of inducing adverse fetal effects.
Nursing Mothers
It is not known whether measles vaccine virus is secreted in human milk. Therefore, because many drugs are excreted in human milk, caution should be exercised when ATTENUVAX is administered to a nursing woman.
Pediatric Use
Safety and effectiveness in infants below the age of 6 months have not been established (see also CLINICAL PHARMACOLOGY).

ADVERSE REACTIONS

The following adverse reactions are listed in decreasing order of severity, without regard to causality, within each body system category and have been reported during clinical trials, with use of the marketed vaccine, or with use of polyvalent vaccine containing measles:
Body as a Whole
Panniculitis; atypical measles; fever; syncope; headache; dizziness; malaise; irritability.
Cardiovascular System
Vasculitis.
Digestive System
Diarrhea.
Hemic and Lymphatic System
Thrombocytopenia (see WARNINGS, *Thrombocytopenia*); purpura; lymphadenopathy; leukocytosis.
Immune System
Anaphylaxis and anaphylactoid reactions have been reported as well as related phenomena such as angioneurotic edema (including peripheral or facial edema) and bronchial spasm.
Nervous System
Encephalitis; encephalopathy; measles inclusion body encephalitis (MIBE) (see CONTRAINDICATIONS); subacute sclerosing panencephalitis (SSPE); Guillain-Barré Syndrome (GBS); febrile convulsions; afebrile convulsions or seizures; ataxia; ocular palsies.
Experience from more than 80 million doses of all live measles vaccines given in the U.S. through 1975 indicates that significant central nervous system reactions such as encephalitis and encephalopathy, occurring within 30 days after vaccination, have been temporally associated with measles vaccine very rarely. In no case has it been shown that reactions were actually caused by vaccine. The Centers for Disease Control and Prevention has pointed out that "a certain number of cases of encephalitis may be expected to occur in a large childhood population in a defined period of time even when no vaccines are administered". However, the data suggest the possibility that some of these cases may have been caused by measles vaccines. The risk of such serious neurological disorders following live measles virus vaccine administration remains far less than that for encephalitis and encephalopathy with natural measles (one per two thousand reported cases).
Post-marketing surveillance of the more than 200 million doses of M-M-R and M-M-R II that have been distributed worldwide over 25 years (1971–1996) indicates that serious adverse events such as encephalitis and encephalopathy continue to be rarely reported.
There have been reports of subacute sclerosing panencephalitis (SSPE) in children who did not have a history of natural measles but did receive measles vaccine. Some of these cases may have resulted from unrecognized measles in the first year of life or possibly from the measles vaccination. Based on estimated nationwide measles vaccine distribution, the association of SSPE cases to measles vaccination is about one case per million vaccine doses distributed. This is far less than the association with natural measles, 6–22 cases of SSPE per million cases of measles. The results of a retrospective case-controlled study conducted by the Centers for Disease Control and Prevention suggest that the overall effect of measles vaccine has been to protect against SSPE by preventing measles with its inherent higher risk of SSPE.
Respiratory System
Pneumonitis (see CONTRAINDICATIONS); cough; rhinitis.
Skin
Stevens-Johnson Syndrome; erythema multiforme; urticaria; rash.
Local reactions including burning/stinging at injection site; wheal and flare; redness (erythema); swelling; vesiculation at injection site.
Special Senses—Ear
Nerve deafness; otitis media.
Special Senses—Eye
Retinitis; optic neuritis; papillitis; retrobulbar neuritis; conjunctivitis.
Other
Death from various, and in some cases unknown, causes has been reported rarely following vaccination with measles, mumps, and rubella vaccines; however, a causal relationship has not been established. No deaths or permanent sequelae were reported in a published post-marketing surveillance study in Finland involving 1.5 million children and adults who were vaccinated with M-M-R II during 1982–1993.
Under the National Childhood Vaccine Injury Act of 1986, health-care providers and manufacturers are required to record and report certain suspected adverse events occurring within specific time periods after vaccination. However, the U.S. Department of Health and Human Services (DHHS) has established a Vaccine Adverse Event Reporting System (VAERS) which will accept all reports of suspected events. A VAERS report form as well as information regarding reporting requirements can be obtained by calling VAERS 1-800-822-7967.

DOSAGE AND ADMINISTRATION

FOR SUBCUTANEOUS ADMINISTRATION
Do not inject intravenously.
The dose for any age is 0.5 mL administered subcutaneously, preferably into the outer aspect of the upper arm.
The recommended age for primary vaccination is 12 to 15 months.
Revaccination with M-M-R II is recommended prior to elementary school entry. See also INDICATIONS AND USAGE, *Recommended Vaccination Schedule.*
Children first vaccinated when younger than 12 months of age should receive another dose between 12 to 15 months of age followed by revaccination prior to elementary school entry. See also INDICATIONS AND USAGE, *Measles Outbreak Schedule.*
Immune Globulin (IG) is not to be given concurrently with ATTENUVAX.
CAUTION: A sterile syringe free of preservatives, antiseptics, and detergents should be used for each injection and/or reconstitution of the vaccine because these substances may inactivate the live virus vaccine. A 25 gauge, 5/8″ needle is recommended.
To reconstitute, use only the diluent supplied, since it is free of preservatives or other antiviral substances which might inactivate the vaccine.
Single Dose Vial—First withdraw the entire volume of diluent into the syringe to be used for reconstitution. Inject all the diluent in the syringe into the vial of lyophilized vaccine, and agitate to mix thoroughly. If the lyophilized vaccine cannot be dissolved, discard. Withdraw the entire contents into a syringe and inject the total volume of restored vaccine subcutaneously.
It is important to use a separate sterile syringe and needle for each individual patient to prevent transmission of hepatitis B and other infectious agents from one person to another.
50 Dose Vial (available only to government agencies/institutions)—Withdraw the entire contents (30 mL) of diluent vial into the sterile syringe to be used for reconstitution and introduce into the 50 dose vial of lyophilized vaccine. Agitate to ensure thorough mixing. If the lyophilized vaccine cannot be dissolved, discard. With full aseptic precautions, attach the vial to the sterilized multidose jet injector apparatus. Use 0.5 mL of the reconstituted vaccine for subcutaneous injection.
Parenteral drug products should be inspected visually for particulate matter and discoloration prior to administration whenever solution and container permit. ATTENUVAX, when reconstituted, is clear yellow.
Use With Other Vaccines
ATTENUVAX should not be given less than one month before or after administration of other live viral vaccines.
M-M-R II has been administered concurrently with VARIVAX* [Varicella Virus Vaccine Live (Oka/Merck)], and PedvaxHIB* [Haemophilus b Conjugate Vaccine (Meningococcal Protein Conjugate)] using separate sites and syringes. No impairment of immune response to individual tested vaccine antigens was demonstrated. The type, frequency, and severity of adverse experiences observed with M-M-R II were similar to those seen when each vaccine was given alone.
Routine administration of DTP (diphtheria, tetanus, pertussis) and/or OPV (oral poliovirus vaccine) concurrently with measles, mumps and rubella vaccines is not recommended because there are limited data relating to the simultaneous administration of these antigens.
However, other schedules have been used. The ACIP has stated "Although data are limited concerning the simultaneous administration of the entire recommended vaccine series (i.e., DTP, OPV, MMR, and Hib vaccines, with or without hepatitis B vaccine), data from numerous studies have indicated no interference between routinely recommended childhood vaccines (either live, attenuated, or killed). These findings support the simultaneous use of all vaccines as recommended."

HOW SUPPLIED

No. 4709—ATTENUVAX is supplied as a single-dose vial of lyophilized vaccine, **NDC** 0006-4709-00, and a vial of diluent.
No. 4589X/4309—ATTENUVAX is supplied as follows: (1) a box of 10 single-dose vials of lyophilized vaccine (package A), **NDC** 0006-4589-00; and (2) a box of 10 vials of diluent (package B). To conserve refrigerator space, the diluent may be stored separately at room temperature.
Storage
During shipment, to ensure that there is no loss of potency, the vaccine must be maintained at a temperature of 10°C (50°F) or colder. Freezing during shipment will not affect potency.
Protect the vaccine from light at all times, since such exposure may inactivate the virus.
Before reconstitution, store the vial of lyophilized vaccine at 2–8°C (36–46°F) or colder. The diluent may be stored in the refrigerator with the lyophilized vaccine or separately at room temperature.
It is recommended that the vaccine be used as soon as possible after reconstitution. Store reconstituted vaccine in the vaccine vial in a dark place at 2–8°C (36–46°F) and discard if not used within 8 hours.
924320 Issued February 2000

BIAVAX®$_{II}$ ℞
(Rubella and Mumps Virus Vaccine Live)

DESCRIPTION

BIAVAX* II (Rubella and Mumps Virus Vaccine Live) is a live virus vaccine for immunization against rubella (German measles) and mumps.
BIAVAX II is a sterile lyophilized preparation of the Wistar RA 27/3 strain of live attenuated rubella virus grown in human diploid cell (WI-38) culture; and the Jeryl Lynn (B level) strain of mumps virus grown in cell cultures of chick embryo. The vaccine viruses are the same as those used in the manufacture of MERUVAX* II (Rubella Virus Vaccine Live) and MUMPSVAX* (Mumps Virus Vaccine Live). The two viruses are mixed before being lyophilized.
The reconstituted vaccine is for subcutaneous administration. When reconstituted as directed, the dose for injection is 0.5 mL and contains not less than the equivalent of 1,000 $TCID_{50}$ of the U.S. Reference Rubella Virus and 20,000 $TCID_{50}$ of the U.S. Reference Mumps Virus. Each dose contains approximately 25 mcg of neomycin. The product contains no preservative. Sorbitol and hydrolized gelatin are added as stabilizers.

*Registered trademark of MERCK & CO., Inc.

CLINICAL PHARMACOLOGY

Clinical studies of 73 double seronegative children 12 months to 2 years of age demonstrated that BIAVAX II is highly immunogenic and generally well tolerated. In these studies, a single injection of the vaccine induced rubella hemagglutination-inhibition (HI) antibodies in 100 percent, and mumps neutralizing antibodies in 97 percent of the susceptible children.
The RA 27/3 rubella strain in BIAVAX II elicits higher immediate post-vaccination HI, complement-fixing and neutralizing antibody levels than other strains of rubella vaccine and has been shown to induce a broader profile of cir-

culating antibodies including anti-theta and anti-iota precipitating antibodies. The RA 27/3 rubella strain immunologically simulates natural infection more closely than other rubella vaccine viruses. The increased levels and broader profile of antibodies produced by RA 27/3 strain rubella virus vaccine appear to correlate with greater resistance to subclinical reinfection with the wild virus, and provide greater confidence for lasting immunity.
Vaccine induced antibody levels following administration of BIAVAX II have been shown to persist for at least two years without substantial decline. Antibody levels after immunization with BIAVAX (Rubella and Mumps Virus Vaccine Live), containing the HPV-77 strain of rubella, have persisted for 10.5 years without substantial decline. If the present pattern continues, it will provide a basis for the expectation that immunity following vaccination will be permanent. However, continued surveillance will be required to demonstrate this point.

INDICATIONS AND USAGE

BIAVAX II is indicated for simultaneous immunization against rubella and mumps in persons 12 months of age or older. A booster is not needed.
The vaccine is not recommended for infants younger than 12 months because they may retain maternal rubella and mumps neutralizing antibodies which may interfere with the immune response.
Previously unimmunized children of susceptible pregnant women should receive live attenuated rubella vaccine, because an immunized child will be less likely to acquire natural rubella and introduce the virus into the household.
Individuals planning travel outside the United States, if not immune, can acquire measles, mumps or rubella and import these diseases to the United States. Therefore, prior to International travel, individuals known to be susceptible to one or more of these diseases can receive either a single antigen vaccine (measles, mumps, or rubella), or a combined antigen vaccine as appropriate. However, M-M-R* II (Measles, Mumps, and Rubella Virus Vaccine Live) is preferred for persons likely to be susceptible to mumps and rubella; and if single-antigen measles vaccine is not readily available, travelers should receive M-M-R II (Measles, Mumps, and Rubella Virus Vaccine Live) regardless of their immune status to mumps or rubella.
Non-Pregnant Adolescent and Adult Females
Immunization of susceptible non-pregnant adolescent and adult females of childbearing age with live attenuated rubella virus vaccine is indicated if certain precautions are observed (see below and PRECAUTIONS). Vaccinating susceptible postpubertal females confers individual protection against subsequently acquiring rubella infection during pregnancy, which in turn prevents infection of the fetus and consequent congenital rubella injury.
Women of childbearing age should be advised not to become pregnant for three months after vaccination and should be informed of the reasons for this precaution.**
It is recommended that rubella susceptibility be determined by serologic testing prior to immunization.***
If immune, as evidenced by a specific rubella antibody titer of 1:8 or greater (hemagglutination-inhibition test), vaccination is unnecessary. Congenital malformations do occur in up to seven percent of all live births. Their chance appearance after vaccination could lead to misinterpretation of the cause, particularly if the prior rubella-immune status of vaccinees is unknown.
Postpubertal females should be informed of the frequent occurrence of generally self-limited arthralgia and/or arthritis beginning 2 to 4 weeks after vaccination (see ADVERSE REACTIONS).
Postpartum Women
It has been found convenient in many instances to vaccinate rubella-susceptible women in the immediate postpartum period. (See *Nursing Mothers*).
Revaccination: Children vaccinated when younger than 12 months of age should be revaccinated. Based on available evidence, there is no reason to routinely revaccinate persons who were vaccinated originally when 12 months of age or older. However, persons should be revaccinated if there is evidence to suggest that initial immunization was ineffective.
Use with other Vaccines
Routine administration of DTP (diphtheria, tetanus, pertussis) and/or OPV (oral poliovirus vaccine) concomitantly with measles, mumps and rubella vaccines is not recommended because there are insufficient data relating to the simultaneous administration of these antigens. However, the American Academy of Pediatrics has noted that in some circumstances, particularly when the patient may not return, some practitioners prefer to administer all these antigens on a single day. If done, separate sites and syringes should be used for DTP and BIAVAX II.
BIAVAX II should not be given less than one month before or after administration of other virus vaccines.

* Registered trademark of MERCK & CO., INC.
** NOTE: The Immunization Practices Advisory Committee (ACIP) has recommended "In view of the importance of protecting this age group against rubella, reasonable precautions in a rubella immunization program include asking females if they are pregnant, excluding those who say they are, and explaining the theoretical risks to the others."
*** NOTE: The Immunization Practices Advisory Committee (ACIP) has stated "When practical, and when reliable laboratory services are available, potential vaccinees of childbearing age can have serologic tests to determine susceptibility to rubella. . . . However, routinely performing serologic tests for all females of childbearing age to determine susceptibility so that vaccine is given only to proven susceptibles is expensive and has been ineffective in some areas. Accordingly, the ACIP believes that rubella vaccination of a woman who is not known to be pregnant and has no history of vaccination is justifiable without serologic testing."

CONTRAINDICATIONS

Do not give BIAVAX II to pregnant females; the possible effects of the vaccine on fetal development are unknown at this time. If vaccination of postpubertal females is undertaken, pregnancy should be avoided for three months following vaccination. (See PRECAUTIONS, *Pregnancy*).
Anaphylactic or anaphylactoid reactions to neomycin (each dose of reconstituted vaccine contains approximately 25 mcg of neomycin).
History of anaphylactic or anaphylactoid reactions to eggs (see HYPERSENSITIVITY TO EGGS below).
Any febrile respiratory illness or other active febrile infection.
Active untreated tuberculosis.
Patients receiving immunosuppressive therapy. This contraindication does not apply to patients who are receiving corticosteroids as replacement therapy, e.g., for Addison's disease.
Individuals with blood dyscrasias, leukemia, lymphomas of any type, or other malignant neoplasms affecting the bone marrow or lymphatic systems.
Primary and acquired immunodeficiency states, including patients who are immunosuppressed in association with AIDS or other clinical manifestations of infection with human immunodeficiency viruses; cellular immune deficiencies; and hypogammaglobulinemic and dysgammaglobulinemic states.
Individuals with a family history of congenital or hereditary immunodeficiency, until the immune competence of the potential vaccine recipient is demonstrated.

HYPERSENSITIVITY TO EGGS

Live mumps vaccine is produced in chick embryo cell culture. Persons with a history of anaphylactic, anaphylactoid, or other immediate reactions (e.g., hives, swelling of the mouth and throat, difficulty breathing, hypotension, or shock) subsequent to egg ingestion should not be vaccinated. Evidence indicates that persons are not at increased risk if they have egg allergies that are not anaphylactic or anaphylactoid in nature. Such persons may be vaccinated in the usual manner. There is no evidence to indicate that persons with allergies to chickens or feathers are at increased risk of reaction to the vaccine.

PRECAUTIONS

General
Adequate treatment provisions including epinephrine, should be available for immediate use should an anaphylactic or anaphylactoid reaction occur.
Children and young adults who are known to be infected with human immunodeficiency viruses but without overt clinical manifestations of immunosuppression may be vaccinated; however, the vaccinees should be monitored closely for vaccine-preventable diseases because immunization may be less effective than for uninfected persons.
Vaccination should be deferred for at least 3 months following blood or plasma transfusions, or administration of human immune serum globulin.
Excretion of small amounts of the live attenuated rubella virus from the nose and throat has occurred in the majority of susceptible individuals 7–28 days after vaccination. There is no confirmed evidence to indicate that such virus is transmitted to susceptible persons who are in contact with the vaccinated individuals. Consequently, transmission through close personal contact, while accepted as a theoretical possibility, is not regarded as a significant risk. However, transmission of the rubella vaccine virus to infants via breast milk has been documented (see *Nursing Mothers*).
There are no reports of transmission of live attenuated mumps virus from vaccinees to susceptible contacts.
It has been reported that live attenuated rubella and mumps virus vaccines given individually may result in a temporary depression of tuberculin skin sensitivity. Therefore, if a tuberculin test is to be done, it should be administered either before or simultaneously with BIAVAX II.
As for any vaccine, vaccination with BIAVAX II may not result in seroconversion in 100% of susceptible persons given the vaccine.
Pregnancy
Pregnancy Category C
Animal reproduction studies have not been conducted with BIAVAX II. It is also not known whether BIAVAX II can cause fetal harm when administered to a pregnant woman or can affect reproduction capacity. Therefore, the vaccine should not be administered to pregnant females; furthermore, pregnancy should be avoided for three months following vaccination (see CONTRAINDICATIONS).
In counseling women who are inadvertently vaccinated when pregnant or who become pregnant within 3 months of vaccination, the physician should be aware of the following: (1) In a 10 year survey involving over 700 pregnant women who received rubella vaccine within 3 months before or after conception, (of whom 189 received the Wistar RA 27/3 strain) none of the newborns had abnormalities compatible with congenital rubella syndrome; and (2) although mumps virus is capable of infecting the placenta and fetus, there is no good evidence that it causes congenital malformations in humans. Mumps vaccine virus also has been shown to infect the placenta, but the virus has not been isolated from the fetal tissues from susceptible women who were vaccinated and underwent elective abortions.
Nursing Mothers
It is not known whether mumps vaccine virus is secreted in human milk. Recent studies have shown that lactating postpartum women immunized with live attenuated rubella vaccine may secrete the virus in breast milk and transmit it to breast-fed infants. In the infants with serological evidence of rubella infection, none exhibited severe disease; however, one exhibited mild clinical illness typical of acquired rubella. Caution should be exercised when BIAVAX II is administered to a nursing woman.

ADVERSE REACTIONS

Burning and/or stinging of short duration at the injection site have been reported.
The adverse clinical reactions associated with the use of BIAVAX II are those expected to follow administration of the monovalent vaccines given separately. These may include malaise, sore throat, cough, rhinitis, headache, dizziness, fever, rash, nausea, vomiting or diarrhea; mild local reactions such as erythema, induration, tenderness and regional lymphadenopathy; parotitis, orchitis, nerve deafness, thrombocytopenia and purpura; allergic reactions such as wheal and flare at the injection site or urticaria; polyneuritis; and arthralgia and/or arthritis (usually transient and rarely chronic).
Anaphylaxis and anaphylactoid reactions have been reported.
Vasculitis has been reported rarely.
Moderate fever [101–102.9°F (38.3–39.4°C)] occurs occasionally, and high fever [above 103°F (39.4°C)] occurs less commonly. On rare occasions, children developing fever may exhibit febrile convulsions. Syncope, particularly at the time of mass vaccination, has been reported. Rash occurs infrequently and is usually minimal, but rarely may be generalized. Erythema multiforme has also been reported rarely.
Forms of optic neuritis, including retrobulbar neuritis and papillitis may infrequently follow viral infections, and have been reported to occur 1 to 3 weeks following inoculation with some live virus vaccines.
Isolated reports of polyneuropathy including Guillain-Barré syndrome have been reported after immunization with rubella-containing vaccines.
Clinical experience with live attenuated rubella and mumps virus vaccines given individually indicates that encephalitis and other nervous system reactions have occurred very rarely. These might occur also with BIAVAX II.
Arthralgia and/or arthritis (usually transient and rarely chronic), and polyneuritis are features of natural rubella and vary in frequency and severity with age and sex, being greatest in adult females and least in prepubertal children. This type of involvement as well as myalgia and paresthesia have also been reported following administration of MERUVAX II (Rubella Virus Vaccine Live).
Chronic arthritis has been associated with natural rubella infection and has been related to persistent virus and/or viral antigen isolated from body tissues. Only rarely have vaccine recipients developed chronic joint symptoms.
Following vaccination in children, reactions in joints are uncommon and generally of brief duration. In women, incidence rates for arthritis and arthralgia are generally higher than those seen in children (children: 0–3%; women: 12–20%), and the reactions tend to be more marked and of longer duration. Symptoms may persist for a matter of months or on rare occasions for years. In adolescent girls, the reactions appear to be intermediate in incidence between those seen in children and in adult women. Even in older women (35–45 years), these reactions are generally well tolerated and rarely interfere with normal activities.

DOSAGE AND ADMINISTRATION

FOR SUBCUTANEOUS ADMINISTRATION
Do not inject intravenously.
The dosage of vaccine is the same for all persons. Inject the total volume (about 0.5 mL) of reconstituted vaccine subcutaneously, preferably into the outer aspect of upper arm. *Do not give immune globulin (IG) concurrently with* BIAVAX II.
During shipment, to insure that there is no loss of potency, the vaccine must be maintained at a temperature of 10°C (50°F) or less.
Before reconstitution, store BIAVAX II at 2–8°C (36–46°F). *Protect from light.*

Continued on next page

Information on the Merck & Co., Inc. products listed on these pages is the full prescribing information from product circulars in use September 30, 2000. For information, please call 1-800-NSC MERCK [1-800-672-6372].

Biavox II—Cont.

CAUTION: A sterile syringe free of preservatives, antiseptics, and detergents should be used for each injection of the vaccine because these substances may inactivate the live virus vaccine. A 25 gauge, $^5/_8$" needle is recommended.
To reconstitute, use only the diluent supplied, since it is free of preservatives or other antiviral substances which might inactivate the vaccine. First withdraw the entire volume of diluent into the syringe to be used for reconstitution. Inject all the diluent in the syringe into the vial of lyophilized vaccine, and agitate to mix thoroughly. Withdraw the entire contents into a syringe and inject the total volume of restored vaccine subcutaneously.
It is important to use a separate sterile syringe and needle for each individual patient to prevent transmission of hepatitis B virus and other infectious agents from one person to another.
Each dose of BIAVAX II contains not less than the equivalent of 1,000 $TCID_{50}$ of the U.S. Reference Rubella Virus and 20,000 $TCID_{50}$ of the U.S. Reference Mumps Virus.
Parenteral drug products should be inspected visually for particulate matter and discoloration prior to administration. BIAVAX II, when reconstituted, is clear yellow.

HOW SUPPLIED

No. 4746—BIAVAX II is supplied as a single-dose vial of lyophilized vaccine, **NDC** 0006-4746-00, and a vial of diluent.
No. 4669/4309—BIAVAX II is supplied as follows: (1) a box of 10 single-dose vials of lyophilized vaccine (package A), **NDC** 0006-4669-00; and (2) a box of 10 vials of diluent (package B). To conserve refrigerator space, the diluent may be stored separately at room temperature.
Storage
It is recommended that the vaccine be used as soon as possible after reconstitution. Protect the vaccine from light at all times, since such exposure may inactivate the virus. Store reconstituted vaccine in the vaccine vial in a dark place at 2–8°C (36–46°F) and discard if not used within eight hours.

A.H.F.S. Category: 80:12
7680116 Issued March 1995

BLOCADREN® Tablets ℞
(Timolol Maleate)

DESCRIPTION

BLOCADREN* (Timolol Maleate) is a non-selective beta-adrenergic receptor blocking agent. The chemical name for timolol maleate is (*S*)-1-[(1,1-dimethylethyl)amino] -3-[[4-(4-morpholinyl)-1,2,5-thiadiazol-3-yl]oxy]-2-propanol (*Z*)-2-butenedioate (1:1) salt. It possesses an asymmetric carbon atom in its structure and is provided as the levo isomer. Its empirical formula is $C_{13}H_{24}N_4O_3S{\cdot}C_4H_4O_4$ and its structural formula is:

Timolol maleate has a molecular weight of 432.50. It is a white, odorless, crystalline powder which is soluble in water, methanol, and alcohol.
BLOCADREN is supplied as tablets in three strengths containing 5 mg, 10 mg or 20 mg timolol maleate for oral administration. Inactive ingredients are cellulose, FD&C Blue 2, magnesium stearate, and starch.

*Registered trademark of MERCK & CO., INC.

CLINICAL PHARMACOLOGY

BLOCADREN is a $beta_1$ and $beta_2$ (non-selective) adrenergic receptor blocking agent that does not have significant intrinsic sympathomimetic, direct myocardial depressant, or local anesthetic activity.
Pharmacodynamics
Clinical pharmacology studies have confirmed the beta-adrenergic blocking activity as shown by (1) changes in resting heart rate and response of heart rate to changes in posture; (2) inhibition of isoproterenol-induced tachycardia; (3) alteration of the response to the Valsalva maneuver and amyl nitrite administration; and (4) reduction of heart rate and blood pressure changes on exercise.
BLOCADREN decreases the positive chronotropic, positive inotropic, bronchodilator, and vasodilator responses caused by beta-adrenergic receptor agonists. The magnitude of this decreased response is proportional to the existing sympathetic tone and the concentration of BLOCADREN at receptor sites.
In normal volunteers, the reduction in heart rate response to a standard exercise was dose dependent over the test range of 0.5 to 20 mg, with a peak reduction at 2 hours of approximately 30% at higher doses.
Beta-adrenergic receptor blockade reduces cardiac output in both healthy subjects and patients with heart disease. In patients with severe impairment of myocardial function beta-adrenergic receptor blockade may inhibit the stimulatory effect of the sympathetic nervous system necessary to maintain adequate cardiac function.
Beta-adrenergic receptor blockade in the bronchi and bronchioles results in increased airway resistance from unopposed parasympathetic activity. Such an effect in patients with asthma or other bronchospastic conditions is potentially dangerous.
Clinical studies indicate that BLOCADREN at a dosage of 20–60 mg/day reduces blood pressure without causing postural hypotension in most patients with essential hypertension. Administration of BLOCADREN to patients with hypertension results initially in a decrease in cardiac output, little immediate change in blood pressure, and an increase in calculated peripheral resistance. With continued administration of BLOCADREN, blood pressure decreases within a few days, cardiac output usually remains reduced, and peripheral resistance falls toward pretreatment levels. Plasma volume may decrease or remain unchanged during therapy with BLOCADREN. In the majority of patients with hypertension BLOCADREN also decreases plasma renin activity. Dosage adjustment to achieve optimal antihypertensive effect may require a few weeks. When therapy with BLOCADREN is discontinued, the blood pressure tends to return to pretreatment levels gradually. In most patients the antihypertensive activity of BLOCADREN is maintained with long-term therapy and is well tolerated.
The mechanism of the antihypertensive effects of beta-adrenergic receptor blocking agents is not established at this time. Possible mechanisms of action include reduction in cardiac output, reduction in plasma renin activity, and a central nervous system sympatholytic action.
A Norwegian multi-center, double-blind study compared the effects of timolol maleate with placebo in 1,884 patients who had survived the acute phase of a myocardial infarction. Patients with systolic blood pressure below 100 mm Hg, sick sinus syndrome and contraindications to beta blockers, including uncontrolled heart failure, second or third degree AV block and bradycardia (<50 beats per minute), were excluded from the multi-center trial. Therapy with BLOCADREN, begun 7 to 28 days following infarction, was shown to reduce overall mortality; this was primarily attributable to a reduction in cardiovascular mortality. BLOCADREN significantly reduced the incidence of sudden deaths (deaths occurring without symptoms or within 24 hours of the onset of symptoms), including those occurring within one hour, and particularly instantaneous deaths (those occurring without preceding symptoms). The protective effect of BLOCADREN was consistent regardless of age, sex or site of infarction. The effect was clearest in patients with a first infarction who were considered at a high risk of dying, defined as those with one or more of the following characteristics during the acute phase: transient left ventricular failure, cardiomegaly, newly appearing atrial fibrillation or flutter, systolic hypotension, or SGOT (ASAT) levels greater than four times the upper limit of normal. Therapy with BLOCADREN also reduced the incidence of non-fatal reinfarction. The mechanism of the protective effect of BLOCADREN is unknown.
BLOCADREN was studied for the prophylactic treatment of migraine headache in placebo-controlled clinical trials involving 400 patients, mostly women between the ages of 18 and 66 years. Common migraine was the most frequent diagnosis. All patients had at least two headaches per month at baseline. Approximately 50 percent of patients who received BLOCADREN had a reduction in the frequency of migraine headache of at least 50 percent, compared to a similar decrease in frequency in 30 percent of patients receiving placebo. The most common cardiovascular adverse effect was bradycardia (5%).
Pharmacokinetics and Metabolism
BLOCADREN is rapidly and nearly completely absorbed (about 90%) following oral ingestion. Detectable plasma levels of timolol occur within one-half hour and peak plasma levels occur in about one to two hours. The drug half-life in plasma is approximately 4 hours and this is essentially unchanged in patients with moderate renal insufficiency. Timolol is partially metabolized by the liver and timolol and its metabolites are excreted by the kidney. Timolol is not extensively bound to plasma proteins; i.e., <10% by equilibrium dialysis and approximately 60% by ultrafiltration. An *in vitro* hemodialysis study, using ^{14}C timolol added to human plasma or whole blood, showed that timolol was readily dialyzed from these fluids; however, a study of patients with renal failure showed that timolol did not dialyze readily. Plasma levels following oral administration are about half those following intravenous administration indicating approximately 50% first pass metabolism. The level of beta sympathetic activity varies widely among individuals, and no simple correlation exists between the dose or plasma level of timolol maleate and its therapeutic activity. Therefore, objective clinical measurements such as reduction of heart rate and/or blood pressure should be used as guides in determining the optimal dosage for each patient.

INDICATIONS AND USAGE

Hypertension
BLOCADREN is indicated for the treatment of hypertension. It may be used alone or in combination with other antihypertensive agents, especially thiazide-type diuretics.
Myocardial Infarction
BLOCADREN is indicated in patients who have survived the acute phase of a myocardial infarction, and are clinically stable, to reduce cardiovascular mortality and the risk of reinfarction.
Migraine
BLOCADREN is indicated for the prophylaxis of migraine headache.

CONTRAINDICATIONS

BLOCADREN is contraindicated in patients with bronchial asthma or with a history of bronchial asthma, or severe chronic obstructive pulmonary disease (see WARNINGS); sinus bradycardia; second and third degree atrioventricular block; overt cardiac failure (see WARNINGS); cardiogenic shock; hypersensitivity to this product.

WARNINGS

Cardiac Failure
Sympathetic stimulation may be essential for support of the circulation in individuals with diminished myocardial contractility, and its inhibition by beta-adrenergic receptor blockade may precipitate more severe failure. Although beta blockers should be avoided in overt congestive heart failure, they can be used, if necessary, with caution in patients with a history of failure who are well-compensated, usually with digitalis and diuretics. Both digitalis and timolol maleate slow AV conduction. If cardiac failure persists, therapy with BLOCADREN should be withdrawn.
In Patients Without a History of Cardiac Failure continued depression of the myocardium with beta-blocking agents over a period of time can, in some cases, lead to cardiac failure. At the first sign or symptom of cardiac failure, patients receiving BLOCADREN should be digitalized and/or be given a diuretic, and the response observed closely. If cardiac failure continues, despite adequate digitalization and diuretic therapy, BLOCADREN should be withdrawn.

> *Exacerbation of Ischemic Heart Disease Following Abrupt Withdrawal* —Hypersensitivity to catecholamines has been observed in patients withdrawn from beta blocker therapy; exacerbation of angina and, in some cases, myocardial infarction have occurred after *abrupt* discontinuation of such therapy. When discontinuing chronically administered timolol maleate, particularly in patients with ischemic heart disease, the dosage should be gradually reduced over a period of one to two weeks and the patient should be carefully monitored. If angina markedly worsens or acute coronary insufficiency develops, timolol maleate administration should be reinstituted promptly, at least temporarily, and other measures appropriate for the management of unstable angina should be taken. Patients should be warned against interruption or discontinuation of therapy without the physician's advice. Because coronary artery disease is common and may be unrecognized, it may be prudent not to discontinue timolol maleate therapy abruptly even in patients treated only for hypertension.

Obstructive Pulmonary Disease
PATIENTS WITH CHRONIC OBSTRUCTIVE PULMONARY DISEASE (e.g., CHRONIC BRONCHITIS, EMPHYSEMA) OF MILD OR MODERATE SEVERITY, BRONCHOSPASTIC DISEASE OR A HISTORY OF BRONCHOSPASTIC DISEASE (OTHER THAN BRONCHIAL ASTHMA OR A HISTORY OF BRONCHIAL ASTHMA, IN WHICH 'BLOCADREN' IS CONTRAINDICATED, see CONTRAINDICATIONS), SHOULD IN GENERAL NOT RECEIVE BETA BLOCKERS, INCLUDING 'BLOCADREN'. However, if BLOCADREN is necessary in such patients, then the drug should be administered with caution since it may block bronchodilation produced by endogenous and exogenous catecholamine stimulation of $beta_2$ receptors.
Major Surgery
The necessity or desirability of withdrawal of beta-blocking therapy prior to major surgery is controversial. Beta-adrenergic receptor blockade impairs the ability of the heart to respond to beta-adrenergically mediated reflex stimuli. This may augment the risk of general anesthesia in surgical procedures. Some patients receiving beta-adrenergic receptor blocking agents have been subject to protracted severe hypotension during anesthesia. Difficulty in restarting and maintaining the heartbeat has also been reported. For these reasons, in patients undergoing elective surgery, some authorities recommend gradual withdrawal of beta-adrenergic receptor blocking agents.
If necessary during surgery, the effects of beta-adrenergic blocking agents may be reversed by sufficient doses of such agonists as isoproterenol, dopamine, dobutamine or levarterenol (see OVERDOSAGE).
Diabetes Mellitus
BLOCADREN should be administered with caution in patients subject to spontaneous hypoglycemia or to diabetic patients (especially those with labile diabetes) who are receiving insulin or oral hypoglycemic agents. Beta-adrenergic receptor blocking agents may mask the signs and symptoms of acute hypoglycemia.
Thyrotoxicosis
Beta-adrenergic blockade may mask certain clinical signs (e.g., tachycardia) of hyperthyroidism. Patients suspected of

developing thyrotoxicosis should be managed carefully to avoid abrupt withdrawal of beta blockade which might precipitate a thyroid storm.

PRECAUTIONS

General

Impaired Hepatic or Renal Function: Since BLOCADREN is partially metabolized in the liver and excreted mainly by the kidneys, dosage reductions may be necessary when hepatic and/or renal insufficiency is present.

Dosing in the Presence of Marked Renal Failure: Although the pharmacokinetics of BLOCADREN are not greatly altered by renal impairment, marked hypotensive responses have been seen in patients with marked renal impairment undergoing dialysis after 20 mg doses. Dosing in such patients should therefore be especially cautious.

Muscle Weakness: Beta-adrenergic blockade has been reported to potentiate muscle weakness consistent with certain myasthenic symptoms (e.g., diplopia, ptosis, and generalized weakness). Timolol has been reported rarely to increase muscle weakness in some patients with myasthenia gravis or myasthenic symptoms.

Cerebrovascular Insufficiency: Because of potential effects of beta-adrenergic blocking agents relative to blood pressure and pulse, these agents should be used with caution in patients with cerebrovascular insufficiency. If signs or symptoms suggesting reduced cerebral blood flow are observed, consideration should be given to discontinuing these agents.

Drug Interactions

Catecholamine-depleting drugs: Close observation of the patient is recommended when BLOCADREN is administered to patients receiving catecholamine-depleting drugs such as reserpine, because of possible additive effects and the production of hypotension and/or marked bradycardia, which may produce vertigo, syncope, or postural hypotension.

Non-steroidal anti-inflammatory drugs: Blunting of the antihypertensive effect of beta-adrenoceptor blocking agents by non-steroidal anti-inflammatory drugs has been reported. When using these agents concomitantly, patients should be observed carefully to confirm that the desired therapeutic effect has been obtained.

Calcium antagonists: Literature reports suggest that oral calcium antagonists may be used in combination with beta-adrenergic blocking agents when heart function is normal, but should be avoided in patients with impaired cardiac function. Hypotension, AV conduction disturbances, and left ventricular failure have been reported in some patients receiving beta-adrenergic blocking agents when an oral calcium antagonist was added to the treatment regimen. Hypotension was more likely to occur if the calcium antagonist were a dihydropyridine derivative, e.g., nifedipine, while left ventricular failure and AV conduction disturbances were more likely to occur with either verapamil or diltiazem.

Intravenous calcium antagonists should be used with caution in patients receiving beta-adrenergic blocking agents.

Digitalis and either diltiazem or verapamil: The concomitant use of beta-adrenergic blocking agents with digitalis and either diltiazem or verapamil may have additive effects in prolonging AV conduction time.

Quinidine: Potentiated systemic beta-blockade (e.g., decreased heart rate) has been reported during combined treatment with quinidine and timolol, possibly because quinidine inhibits the metabolism of timolol via the P-450 enzyme, CYP2D6.

Clonidine: Beta adrenergic blocking agents may exacerbate the rebound hypertension which can follow the withdrawal of clonidine. If the two drugs are coadministered, the beta adrenergic blocking agent should be withdrawn several days before the gradual withdrawal of clonidine. If replacing clonidine by beta-blocker therapy, the introduction of beta adrenergic blocking agents should be delayed for several days after clonidine administration has stopped.

Risk from Anaphylactic Reaction: While taking beta-blockers, patients with a history of atopy or a history of severe anaphylactic reaction to a variety of allergens may be more reactive to repeated accidental, diagnostic, or therapeutic challenge with such allergens. Such patients may be unresponsive to the usual doses of epinephrine used to treat anaphylactic reactions.

Carcinogenesis, Mutagenesis, Impairment of Fertility

In a two-year study of timolol maleate in rats, there was a statistically significant increase in the incidence of adrenal pheochromocytomas in male rats administered 300 mg/kg/day (250 times** the maximum recommended human dose). Similar differences were not observed in rats administered doses equivalent to approximately 20 or 80 times** the maximum recommended human dose.

In a lifetime study in mice, there were statistically significant increases in the incidence of benign and malignant pulmonary tumors, benign uterine polyps and mammary adenocarcinoma in female mice at 500 mg/kg/day (approximately 400 times** the maximum recommended human dose), but not at 5 or 50 mg/kg/day. In a subsequent study in female mice, in which post-mortem examinations were limited to uterus and lungs, a statistically significant increase in the incidence of pulmonary tumors was again observed at 500 mg/kg/day.

The increased occurrence of mammary adenocarcinoma was associated with elevations in serum prolactin that occurred in female mice administered timolol at 500 mg/kg/day, but not at doses of 5 or 50 mg/kg/day. An increased incidence of mammary adenocarcinomas in rodents has been associated with administration of several other therapeutic agents which elevate serum prolactin, but no correlation between serum prolactin levels and mammary tumors has been established in man. Furthermore, in adult human female subjects who received oral dosages of up to 60 mg of timolol maleate, the maximum recommended human oral dosage, there were no clinically meaningful changes in serum prolactin.

Timolol maleate was devoid of mutagenic potential when evaluated *in vivo* (mouse) in the micronucleus test and cytogenetic assay (doses up to 800 mg/kg) and *in vitro* in a neoplastic cell transformation assay (up to 100 µg/mL). In Ames tests the highest concentrations of timolol employed, 5000 or 10,000 µg/plate, were associated with statistically significant elevations of revertants observed with tester strain TA100 (in seven replicate assays), but not in three additional strains. In the assays with tester strain TA100, no consistent dose response relationship was observed, nor did the ratio of test to control revertants reach 2. A ratio of 2 is usually considered the criterion for a positive Ames test.

Reproduction and fertility studies in rats showed no adverse effect on male or female fertility at doses up to 125 times** the maximum recommended human dose.

**Based on patient weight of 50 kg

Pregnancy

Pregnancy Category C. Teratogenicity studies with timolol in mice, rats and rabbits at doses up to 50 mg/kg/day (approximately 40 times** the maximum recommended daily human dose) showed no evidence of fetal malformations. Although delayed fetal ossification was observed at this dose in rats, there were no adverse effects on postnatal development of offspring. Doses of 1000 mg/kg/day (approximately 830 times** the maximum recommended daily human dose) were maternotoxic in mice and resulted in an increased number of fetal resorptions. Increased fetal resorptions were also seen in rabbits at doses of approximately 40 times** the maximum recommended daily human dose, in this case without apparent maternotoxicity. There are no adequate and well-controlled studies in pregnant women. BLOCADREN should be used during pregnancy only if the potential benefit justifies the potential risk to the fetus.

**Based on patient weight of 50 kg

Nursing Mothers

Timolol maleate has been detected in human milk.

Because of the potential for serious adverse reactions from timolol in nursing infants, a decision should be made whether to discontinue nursing or to discontinue the drug, taking into account the importance of the drug to the mother.

Pediatric Use

Safety and effectiveness in pediatric patients have not been established.

ADVERSE REACTIONS

BLOCADREN is usually well tolerated in properly selected patients. Most adverse effects have been mild and transient.

In a multicenter (12-week) clinical trial comparing timolol maleate and placebo in hypertensive patients, the following adverse reactions were reported spontaneously and considered to be causally related to timolol maleate:

	Timolol Maleate (n = 176) %	Placebo (n = 168) %
BODY AS A WHOLE		
fatigue/tiredness	3.4	0.6
headache	1.7	1.8
chest pain	0.6	0
asthenia	0.6	0
CARDIOVASCULAR		
bradycardia	9.1	0
arrhythmia	1.1	0.6
syncope	0.6	0
edema	0.6	1.2
DIGESTIVE		
dyspepsia	0.6	0.6
nausea	0.6	0
SKIN		
pruritus	1.1	0
NERVOUS SYSTEM		
dizziness	2.3	1.2
vertigo	0.6	0
paresthesia	0.6	0
PSYCHIATRIC		
decreased libido	0.6	0
RESPIRATORY		
dyspnea	1.7	0.6
bronchial spasm	0.6	0
rales	0.6	0
SPECIAL SENSES		
eye irritation	1.1	0.6
tinnitus	0.6	0

These data are representative of the incidence of adverse effects that may be observed in properly selected patients treated with BLOCADREN, i.e., excluding patients with bronchospastic disease, congestive heart failure or other contraindications to beta blocker therapy.

In patients with migraine the incidence of bradycardia was 5 percent.

In a coronary artery disease population studied in the Norwegian multi-center trial (see CLINICAL PHARMACOLOGY), the frequency of the principal adverse reactions and the frequency with which these resulted in discontinuation of therapy in the timolol and placebo groups were:

[See first table above]

BLOCADREN	Adverse Reaction*** Timolol (n = 945) %	Adverse Reaction*** Placebo (n = 939) %	Withdrawal† Timolol (n = 945) %	Withdrawal† Placebo (n = 939) %
Asthenia or Fatigue	5	1	<1	<1
Heart Rate <40 beats/minute	5	<1	4	<1
Cardiac Failure—Nonfatal	8	7	3	2
Hypotension	3	2	3	1
Pulmonary Edema—Nonfatal	2	<1	<1	<1
Claudication	3	3	1	<1
AV Block 2nd or 3rd degree	<1	<1	<1	<1
Sinoatrial Block	<1	<1	<1	<1
Cold Hands and Feet	8	<1	<1	0
Nausea or Digestive Disorders	8	6	1	<1
Dizziness	6	4	1	0
Bronchial Obstruction	2	<1	1	<1

***When an adverse reaction recurred in a patient, it is listed only once.
†Only principal reason for withdrawal in each patient is listed.
These adverse reactions can also occur in patients treated for hypertension.

The following additional adverse effects have been reported in clinical experience with the drug: *Body as a Whole:* extremity pain, decreased exercise tolerance, weight loss, fever; *Cardiovascular:* cardiac arrest, cardiac failure, cerebrovascular accident, worsening of angina pectoris, worsening of arterial insufficiency, Raynaud's phenomenon, palpitations, vasodilatation; *Digestive:* gastrointestinal pain, hepatomegaly, vomiting, diarrhea, dyspepsia; *Hematologic:* nonthrombocytopenic purpura; *Endocrine:* hyperglycemia, hypoglycemia; *Skin:* rash, skin irritation, increased pigmentation, sweating, alopecia; *Musculoskeletal:* arthralgia; *Nervous System:* local weakness, increase in signs and symptoms of myasthenia gravis; *Psychiatric:* depression, nightmares, somnolence, insomnia, nervousness, diminished concentration, hallucinations; *Respiratory:* cough; *Special Senses:* visual disturbances, diplopia, ptosis, dry eyes; *Urogenital:* impotence, urination difficulties.

There have been reports of retroperitoneal fibrosis in patients receiving timolol maleate and in patients receiving other beta-adrenergic blocking agents. A causal relationship between this condition and therapy with beta-adrenergic blocking agents has not been established.

Potential Adverse Effects: In addition, a variety of adverse effects not observed in clinical trials with BLOCADREN, but reported with other beta-adrenergic blocking agents, should be considered potential adverse effects of BLOCADREN: *Nervous System:* Reversible mental depression progressing to catatonia; an acute reversible syndrome characterized by disorientation for time and place, short-term memory loss, emotional lability, slightly clouded sensorium, and decreased performance on neuropsychometrics; *Cardiovascular:* Intensification of AV block (see CONTRAINDICATIONS); *Digestive:* Mesenteric arterial thrombosis, ischemic colitis; *Hematologic:* Agranulocytosis, thrombocytopenic purpura; *Allergic:* Erythematous rash, fever combined with aching and sore throat, laryngospasm with respiratory distress; *Miscellaneous:* Peyronie's disease.

There have been reports of a syndrome comprising psoriasiform skin rash, conjunctivitis sicca, otitis, and sclerosing se-

Continued on next page

Information on the Merck & Co., Inc. products listed on these pages is the full prescribing information from product circulars in use September 30, 2000. For information, please call 1-800-NSC MERCK [1-800-672-6372].

Blocadren—Cont.

rositis attributed to the beta-adrenergic receptor blocking agent, practolol. This syndrome has not been reported with BLOCADREN.
Clinical Laboratory Test Findings: Clinically important changes in standard laboratory parameters were rarely associated with the administration of BLOCADREN. Slight increases in blood urea nitrogen, serum potassium, uric acid, and triglycerides, and slight decreases in hemoglobin, hematocrit and HDL cholesterol occurred, but were not progressive or associated with clinical manifestations. Increases in liver function tests have been reported.

OVERDOSAGE

Overdosage has been reported with Tablets BLOCADREN. A 30-year-old female ingested 650 mg of BLOCADREN (maximum recommended daily dose—60 mg) and experienced second and third degree heart block. She recovered without treatment but approximately two months later developed irregular heartbeat, hypertension, dizziness, tinnitus, faintness, increased pulse rate and borderline first degree heart block.
The oral LD_{50} of the drug is 1190 and 900 mg/kg in female mice and female rats, respectively.
An *in vitro* hemodialysis study, using ^{14}C timolol added to human plasma or whole blood, showed that timolol was readily dialyzed from these fluids; however, a study of patients with renal failure showed that timolol did not dialyze readily.
The most common signs and symptoms to be expected with overdosage with a beta-adrenergic receptor blocking agent are symptomatic bradycardia, hypotension, bronchospasm, and acute cardiac failure. Therapy with BLOCADREN should be discontinued and the patient observed closely. The following additional therapeutic measures should be considered:

(1) *Gastric lavage*
(2) *Symptomatic bradycardia:* Use atropine sulfate intravenously in a dosage of 0.25 mg to 2 mg to induce vagal blockade. If bradycardia persists, intravenous isoproterenol hydrochloride should be administered cautiously. In refractory cases the use of a transvenous cardiac pacemaker may be considered.
(3) *Hypotension:* Use sympathomimetic pressor drug therapy, such as dopamine, dobutamine or levarterenol. In refractory cases the use of glucagon hydrochloride has been reported to be useful.
(4) *Bronchospasm:* Use isoproterenol hydrochloride. Additional therapy with aminophylline may be considered.
(5) *Acute cardiac failure:* Conventional therapy with digitalis, diuretics, and oxygen should be instituted immediately. In refractory cases the use of intravenous aminophylline is suggested. This may be followed if necessary by glucagon hydrochloride which has been reported to be useful.
(6) *Heart block (second or third degree):* Use isoproterenol hydrochloride or a transvenous cardiac pacemaker.

DOSAGE AND ADMINISTRATION

Hypertension
The usual initial dosage of BLOCADREN is 10 mg twice a day, whether used alone or added to diuretic therapy. Dosage may be increased or decreased depending on heart rate and blood pressure response. The usual total maintenance dosage is 20–40 mg per day. Increases in dosage to a maximum of 60 mg per day divided into two doses may be necessary. There should be an interval of at least seven days between increases in dosages.
BLOCADREN may be used with a thiazide diuretic or with other antihypertensive agents. Patients should be observed carefully during initiation of such concomitant therapy.
Myocardial Infarction
The recommended dosage for long-term prophylactic use in patients who have survived the acute phase of a myocardial infarction is 10 mg given twice daily (see CLINICAL PHARMACOLOGY).
Migraine
The usual initial dosage of BLOCADREN is 10 mg twice a day. During maintenance therapy the 20 mg daily dosage may be administered as a single dose. Total daily dosage may be increased to a maximum of 30 mg, given in divided doses, or decreased to 10 mg once per day, depending on clinical response and tolerability. If a satisfactory response is not obtained after 6-8 weeks use of the maximum daily dosage, therapy with BLOCADREN should be discontinued.

HOW SUPPLIED

No. 3343—Tablets BLOCADREN, 5 mg, are light blue, round, compressed tablets, with code MSD 59 on one side and BLOCADREN on the other. They are supplied as follows:
NDC 0006-0059-68 bottles of 100.
Shown in Product Identification Guide, page 323
No. 3344—Tablets BLOCADREN, 10 mg, are light blue, round, scored, compressed tablets, with code MSD 136 on one side and BLOCADREN on the other. They are supplied as follows:
NDC 0006-0136-68 bottles of 100.
(6505-01-132-0651, 10 mg 100's)
Shown in Product Identification Guide, page 323
No. 3371—Tablets BLOCADREN, 20 mg, are light blue, capsule shaped, scored, compressed tablets, with code MSD 437 on one side and BLOCADREN on the other. They are supplied as follows:
NDC 0006-0437-68 bottles of 100
(6505-01-132-0652, 20 mg 100's).
Shown in Product Identification Guide, page 323
Storage
Store at controlled room temperature. 15–30°C (59–86°F). Keep container tightly closed. Protect from light.
7901231 Issued November 1997

CHIBROXIN® ℞
(norfloxacin ophthalmic solution)
Sterile Ophthalmic Solution

DESCRIPTION

CHIBROXIN* (norfloxacin ophthalmic solution) is a synthetic broad-spectrum antibacterial agent supplied as a sterile isotonic solution for topical ophthalmic use. Norfloxacin, a fluoroquinolone, is 1-ethyl-6-fluoro-1,4-dihydro-4-oxo-7-(1-piperazinyl) -3- quinoline-carboxylic acid. Its empirical formula is $C_{16}H_{18}FN_3O_3$ and the structural formula is:

Norfloxacin is a white to pale yellow crystalline powder with a molecular weight of 319.34 and a melting point of about 221°C. It is freely soluble in glacial acetic acid and very slightly soluble in ethanol, methanol and water.
CHIBROXIN Ophthalmic Solution 0.3% is supplied as a sterile isotonic solution. Each mL contains 3 mg norfloxacin. Inactive ingredients: disodium edetate, sodium acetate, sodium chloride, hydrochloric acid (to adjust pH) and water for injection, Benzalkonium chloride 0.0025% is added as preservative. The pH of CHIBROXIN is approximately 5.2 and the osmolarity is approximately 285 m0smol/liter.
Norfloxacin, a fluoroquinolone, differs from quinolones by having a fluorine atom at the 6 position and a piperazine moiety at the 7 position.

*Registered trademark of MERCK & CO., INC.

CLINICAL PHARMACOLOGY

Microbiology
Norfloxacin has *in vitro* activity against a broad spectrum of gram-positive and gram-negative aerobic bacteria. The fluorine atom at the 6 position provides increased potency against gram-negative organisms and the piperazine moiety at the 7 position is responsible for anti-pseudomonal activity.
Norfloxacin inhibits bacterial deoxyribonucleic acid synthesis and is bactericidal. At the molecular level three specific events are attributed to CHIBROXIN in *E. coli* cells:
1) inhibition of the ATP-dependent DNA supercoiling reaction catalyzed by DNA gyrase;
2) inhibition of the relaxation of supercoiled DNA;
3) promotion of double-stranded DNA breakage.
There is generally no cross-resistance between norfloxacin and other classes of antibacterial agents. Therefore, norfloxacin generally demonstrates activity against indicated organisms resistant to some other antimicrobial agents. When such cross-resistance does occur, it is probably due to decreased entry of the drugs into the bacterial cells. Antagonism has been demonstrated *in vitro* between norfloxacin and nitrofurantoin.
Norfloxacin has been shown to be active against most strains of the following organisms both *in vitro* and clinically in ophthalmic infections (see INDICATIONS AND USAGE):
Gram-positive bacteria including:
Staphylococcus aureus
Staphylococcus epidermidis
Staphylococcus warnerii
Streptococcus pneumoniae
Gram-negative bacteria including:
Acinetobacter calcoaceticus
Aeromonas hydrophila
Haemophilus influenzae
Proteus mirabilis
Pseudomonas aeruginosa
Serratia marcescens
Norfloxacin has been shown to be active *in vitro* against most strains of the following organisms; however, *the clinical significance of these data in ophthalmic infections is unknown.*
Gram-positive bacteria:
Bacillus cereus
Enterococcus faecalis (formerly *Streptococcus faecalis*)
Staphylococcus saprophyticus
Gram-negative bacteria:
Citrobacter diversus
Citrobacter freundii
Edwardsiella tarda
Enterobacter aerogenes
Enterobacter cloacae
Escherichia coli
Hafnia alvei
Haemophilus aegyptius (Koch-Weeks bacillus)
Klebsiella oxytoca
Klebsiella pneumoniae
Klebsiella rhinoscleromatis
Morganella morganii
Neisseria gonorrhoeae
Proteus vulgaris
Providencia alcalifaciens
Providencia rettgeri
Providencia stuartii
Salmonella typhi
Vibrio cholerae
Vibrio parahemolyticus
Yersinia enterocolitica
Other:
Ureaplasma urealyticum
Norfloxacin is not active against obligate anaerobes.
Clinical Studies
Clinical studies were conducted comparing CHIBROXIN Ophthalmic Solution (n=152) with ophthalmic solutions of tobramycin, gentamicin, and chloramphenicol (n=158) in patients with conjunctivitis and positive bacterial cultures. After seven days of therapy with CHIBROXIN Ophthalmic Solution, 72 percent of patients were clinically cured. Of those cured, 85 percent had all their pathogens eradicated. Eradication was also achieved in 62 percent (23/37) of patients whose clinical outcome was not completely cured by day seven. These results were similar among all treatment groups.
Another clinical study compared CHIBROXIN Ophthalmic Solution with placebo in patients with conjunctivitis and positive bacterial cultures. Placebo in this study was the liquid vehicle for CHIBROXIN Ophthalmic Solution and contained the preservative. After five days of therapy, 64 percent (36/56) of patients on CHIBROXIN Ophthalmic Solution were clinically cured compared to 50 percent (23/46) of patients receiving placebo. Of those cured, 78 percent had all their pathogens eradicated. Eradication was also achieved in 50 percent (10/20) of patients whose clinical outcome was not completely cured. The response to CHIBROXIN Ophthalmic Solution was statistically significantly better than the response to placebo.

INDICATIONS AND USAGE

CHIBROXIN Ophthalmic Solution is indicated for the treatment of conjunctivitis when caused by susceptible strains of the following bacteria:
*Acinetobacter calcoaceticus***
*Aeromonas hydrophila***
Haemophilus influenzae
*Proteus mirabilis***
*Pseudomonas aeruginosa***
*Serratia marcescens***
Staphylococcus aureus
Staphylococcus epidermidis
*Staphylococcus warnerii***
Streptococcus pneumoniae
Appropriate monitoring of bacterial response to topical antibiotic therapy should accompany the use of CHIBROXIN Ophthalmic Solution.

**Efficacy for this organism was studied in fewer than 10 infections.

CONTRAINDICATIONS

CHIBROXIN Ophthalmic Solution is contraindicated in patients with a history of hypersensitivity to norfloxacin, or the other members of the quinolone group of antibacterial agents or any other component of this medication.

WARNINGS

NOT FOR INJECTION INTO THE EYE.
Serious and occasionally fatal hypersensitivity (anaphylactoid or anaphylactic) reactions, some following the first dose, have been reported in patients receiving systemic quinolone therapy. Some reactions were accompanied by cardiovascular collapse, loss of consciousness, tingling, pharyngeal or facial edema, dyspnea, urticaria, and itching. Only a few patients had a history of hypersensitivity reactions. Serious anaphylactoid or anaphylactic reactions require immediate emergency treatment with epinephrine. Oxygen, intravenous steroids and airway management, including intubation, should be administered as indicated.

PRECAUTIONS

General
As with other antibiotic preparations, prolonged use may result in overgrowth of nonsusceptible organisms, including fungi. If superinfection occurs, appropriate measures should be initiated. Whenever clinical judgment dictates, the patient should be examined with the aid of magnification, such as slit lamp biomicroscopy and, where appropriate, fluorescein staining.
There have been reports of bacterial keratitis associated with the use of multiple dose containers of topical ophthal-

mic products. These containers have been inadvertently contaminated by patients who, in most cases, had a concurrent corneal disease or a disruption of the ocular epithelial surface. (See PRECAUTIONS, *Information for Patients*.)

Information For Patients

Patients should be instructed to avoid allowing the tip of the dispensing container to contact the eye or surrounding structures.

Patients should also be instructed that ocular preparations, if handled improperly or if the tip of the dispensing container contacts the eye or surrounding structures, can become contaminated by common bacteria known to cause ocular infections. Serious damage to the eye and subsequent loss of vision may result from using contaminated preparations (see PRECAUTIONS, *General*). If redness, irritation, swelling, or pain persists or becomes aggravated, the patient should be advised to consult a physician.

Patients should also be advised that if they have ocular surgery or develop an intercurrent ocular condition (e.g., trauma or infection), they should immediately seek their physician's advice concerning the continued use of the present multidose container.

Patients should be advised that norfloxacin may be associated with hypersensitivity reactions, even following a single dose, and to discontinue the drug at the first sign of a skin rash or other allergic reaction.

Patients should be advised not to wear contact lenses if they have signs and symptoms of bacterial conjunctivitis.

Drug Interactions

Specific drug interaction studies have not been conducted with norfloxacin ophthalmic solution. However, the systemic administration of some quinolones has been shown to elevate plasma concentrations of theophylline, interfere with the metabolism of caffeine, and enhance the effects of the oral anticoagulant warfarin and its derivatives. Elevated serum levels of cyclosporine have been reported with concomitant use of cyclosporine with norfloxacin. Therefore, cyclosporine serum levels should be monitored and appropriate cyclosporine dosage adjustments made when these drugs are used concomitantly.

Carcinogenesis, Mutagenesis, Impairment of Fertility

No increase in neoplastic changes was observed with norfloxacin as compared to controls in a study in rats, lasting up to 96 weeks at doses eight to nine times the usual human oral dose***.

Norfloxacin was tested for mutagenic activity in a number of *in vivo* and *in vitro* tests. Norfloxacin had no mutagenic effect in the dominant lethal test in mice and did not cause chromosomal aberrations in hamsters or rats at doses 30 to 60 times the usual oral dose***. Norfloxacin had no mutagenic activity *in vitro* in the Ames microbial mutagen test, Chinese hamster fibroblasts and V-79 mammalian cell assay. Although norfloxacin was weakly positive in the Rec-assay for DNA repair, all other mutagenic assays were negative including a more sensitive test (V-79).

Norfloxacin did not adversely affect the fertility of male and female mice at oral doses up to 33 times the usual human oral dose***.

Pregnancy

Teratogenic Effects—Pregnancy Category C. Norfloxacin has been shown to produce embryonic loss in monkeys when given in doses 10 times the maximum human oral dose*** (400 mg b.i.d.), with peak plasma levels that are two to three times those obtained in humans. There has been no evidence of a teratogenic effect in any of the animal species tested (rat, rabbit, mouse, monkey) at 6 to 50 times the human oral dose. There are no adequate and well-controlled studies in pregnant women. CHIBROXIN Ophthalmic Solution should be used during pregnancy only if the potential benefit justifies the potential risk to the fetus.

Nursing Mothers

It is not known whether norfloxacin is excreted in human milk following ocular administration. Because many drugs are excreted in human milk, and because of the potential for serious adverse reactions in nursing infants from norfloxacin, a decision should be made to discontinue nursing or to discontinue the drug, taking into account the importance of the drug to the mother (see ANIMAL PHARMACOLOGY).

Pediatric Use

Safety and effectiveness in infants below the age of one year have not been established.

Although quinolones including norfloxacin have been shown to cause arthropathy in immature animals after oral administration, topical ocular administration of other quinolones to immature animals has not shown any arthropathy and there is no evidence that the ophthalmic dosage form of those quinolones has any effects on the weight-bearing joints.

Geriatric Use

No overall differences in safety or effectiveness have been observed between elderly and young patients.

*** All factors are based on a standard patient weight of 50 kg. The usual oral dose of norfloxacin is 800 mg daily. One drop of CHIBROXIN Ophthalmic Solution 0.3% contains about 1/6,666 of this dose (0.12 mg).

ADVERSE REACTIONS

In clinical trials, the most frequently reported drug-related adverse reaction was local burning or discomfort. Other drug-related adverse reactions were conjunctival hyperemia, chemosis, photophobia and a bitter taste following instillation.

DOSAGE AND ADMINISTRATION

The recommended dose in adults and pediatric patients (one year and older) is one or two drops of CHIBROXIN Ophthalmic Solution applied topically to the affected eye(s) four times daily for up to seven days. Depending on the severity of the infection, the dosage for the first day of therapy may be one or two drops every two hours during the waking hours.

HOW SUPPLIED

CHIBROXIN Ophthalmic Solution is a clear, colorless to light yellow solution.

No. 3526—CHIBROXIN Ophthalmic Solution 0.3% is supplied in a white, opaque, plastic OCUMETER* ophthalmic dispenser with a controlled drop tip as follows:

NDC 0006-3526-03, 5 mL.

Storage

Store CHIBROXIN Ophthalmic Solution at room temperature, 15°–30°C (59°–86°F). Protect from light.

*Registered trademark of MERCK & CO., INC.

ANIMAL PHARMACOLOGY

The oral administration of single doses of norfloxacin, six times the recommended human oral dose***, caused lameness in immature dogs. Histologic examination of the weight-bearing joints of these dogs revealed permanent lesions of the cartilage. Related drugs also produced erosions of the cartilage in weight-bearing joints and other signs of arthropathy in immature animals of various species.

*** All factors are based on a standard patient weight of 50 kg. The usual oral dose of norfloxacin is 800 mg daily. One drop of CHIBROXIN Ophthalmic Solution 0.3% contains about 1/6,666 of this dose (0.12 mg).

ADDITIONAL CAUTIONARY INFORMATION

Norfloxacin is available as an oral dosage form in addition to the ophthalmic dosage form. The following adverse effects, while they have not been reported with the ophthalmic dosage form, have been reported with the oral dosage form. However, it should be noted that the usual dosage of oral norfloxacin (800 mg/day) contains 6,666 times the amount in one drop of CHIBROXIN Ophthalmic Solution 0.3% (0.12 mg).

Convulsions have been reported in patients receiving oral norfloxacin. Convulsions, increased intracranial pressure, and toxic psychoses have been reported with other drugs in this class. Orally administered quinolones may also cause central nervous system (CNS) stimulation which may lead to tremors, restlessness, lightheadedness, confusion and hallucinations. If these reactions occur in patients receiving norfloxacin, the drug should be discontinued and appropriate measures instituted.

The effects of norfloxacin on brain function or on the electrical activity of the brain have not been tested. Therefore, as with the oral formulation, norfloxacin should be used with caution in patients with known or suspected CNS disorders, such as severe cerebral arteriosclerosis, epilepsy, and other factors which predispose to seizures.

The following adverse effects have been reported with Tablets NOROXON* (norfloxacin tablets).

Hypersensitivity Reactions: Hypersensitivity reactions including anaphylactoid reactions, angioedema, arthralgia, arthritis, dyspnea, myalgia, urticaria, vasculitis; *Gastrointestinal:* Hepatitis, jaundice, including cholestatic jaundice, pancreatitis, pseudomembranous colitis; *Hematologic:* Hemolytic anemia, sometimes associated with glucose-6-phosphate dehydrogenase deficiency, leukopenia, neutropenia, thrombocytopenia; *Musculoskeletal:* Possible exacerbation of myasthenia gravis, tendinitis, tendon rupture; *Nervous System/Psychiatric:* Ataxia, CNS effects characterized as generalized seizures and myoclonus, Guillain-Barré syndrome, paresthesia, peripheral neuropathy, psychic disturbances including confusion, depression, psychotic reactions; *Renal:* Interstitial nephritis, renal failure; *Skin:* Erythema multiforme and Stevens-Johnson syndrome, exfoliative dermatitis, photosensitivity, rash, toxic epidermal necrolysis; *Special Senses:* Diplopia, tinnitus, transient hearing loss.

Abnormal laboratory values observed with oral norfloxacin included elevation of ALT (SGPT) and AST (SGOT), alkaline phosphatase, BUN, serum creatinine, and LDH.

Please consult the package circular for Tablets NOROXIN (norfloxacin tablets) for additional information concerning these and other adverse effects and other cautionary information.

*Registered trademark of MERCK & CO., INC.

9011207 Issued October 1999

CLINORIL® Tablets ℞
(Sulindac)

DESCRIPTION

Sulindac is a non-steroidal, anti-inflammatory indene derivative designated chemically as (Z)- 5-fluoro-2-methyl - 1 - [[*p* - (methylsulfinyl) phenyl]methylene]-1*H*-indene-3-acetic acid. It is not a salicylate, pyrazolone or propionic acid derivative. Its empirical formula is $C_{20}H_{17}FO_3S$, with a molecular weight of 356.42. Sulindac, a yellow crystalline compound, is a weak organic acid practically insoluble in water below pH 4.5, but very soluble as the sodium salt or in buffers of pH 6 or higher.

CLINORIL* (Sulindac) is available in 150 and 200 mg tablets for oral administration. Each tablet contains the following inactive ingredients: cellulose, magnesium stearate, starch.

Following absorption, sulindac undergoes two major biotransformations—reversible reduction to the sulfide metabolite, and irreversible oxidation to the sulfone metabolite. Available evidence indicates that the biological activity resides with the sulfide metabolite.

The structural formulas of sulindac and its metabolites are:

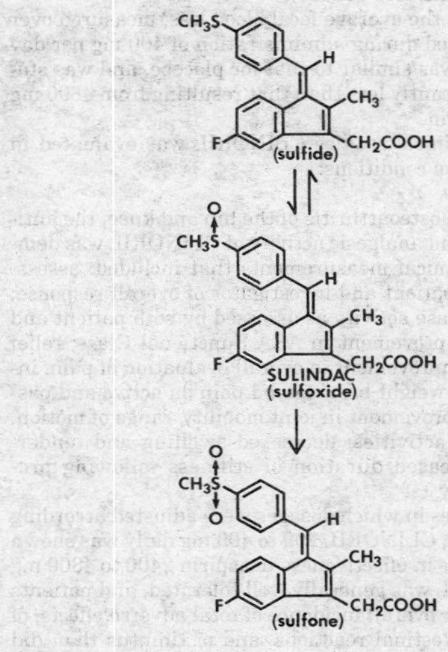

(sulfide)

SULINDAC (sulfoxide)

(sulfone)

*Registered trademark of MERCK & CO., INC.

CLINICAL PHARMACOLOGY

CLINORIL is a non-steroidal anti-inflammatory drug, also possessing analgesic and antipyretic activities. Its mode of action, like that of other non-steroidal anti-inflammatory agents, is not known; however, its therapeutic action is not due to pituitary-adrenal stimulation. Inhibition of prostaglandin synthesis by the sulfide metabolite may be involved in the anti-inflammatory action of CLINORIL.

Sulindac is approximately 90% absorbed in man after oral administration. The peak plasma concentrations of the biologically active sulfide metabolite are achieved in about two hours when sulindac is administered in the fasting state, and in about three to four hours when sulindac is administered with food. The mean half-life of sulindac is 7.8 hours while the mean half-life of the sulfide metabolite is 16.4 hours. Sustained plasma levels of the sulfide metabolite are consistent with a prolonged anti-inflammatory action which is the rationale for a twice per day dosage schedule.

Sulindac and its sulfone metabolite undergo extensive enterohepatic circulation relative to the sulfide metabolite in animals. Studies in man have also demonstrated that recirculation of the parent drug, sulindac, and its sulfone metabolite, is more extensive than that of the active sulfide metabolite. The active sulfide metabolite accounts for less than six percent of the total intestinal exposure to sulindac and its metabolites.

The primary route of excretion in man is via the urine as both sulindac and its sulfone metabolite (free and glucuronide conjugates). Approximately 50% of the administered dose is excreted in the urine, with the conjugated sulfone metabolite accounting for the major portion. Less than 1% of the administered dose of sulindac appears in the urine as the sulfide metabolite. Approximately 25% is found in the feces, primarily as the sulfone and sulfide metabolites.

The bioavailability of sulindac, as assessed by urinary excretion, was not changed by concomitant administration of an antacid containing magnesium hydroxide 200 mg and aluminum hydroxide 225 mg per 5 mL.

Because CLINORIL is excreted in the urine primarily as biologically inactive forms, it may possibly affect renal function to a lesser extent than other non-steroidal anti-inflammatory drugs, however, renal adverse experiences have been reported with CLINORIL (see ADVERSE REACTIONS). In a study of patients with chronic glomerular disease treated with therapeutic doses of CLINORIL, no effect

Continued on next page

Information on the Merck & Co., Inc. products listed on these pages is the full prescribing information from product circulars in use September 30, 2000. For information, please call 1-800-NSC MERCK [1-800-672-6372].

Clinoril—Cont.

was demonstrated on renal blood flow, glomerular filtration rate, or urinary excretion of prostaglandin E_2 and the primary metabolite of prostacyclin, 6-keto-PGF$_1\alpha$. However, in other studies in healthy volunteers and patients with liver disease, CLINORIL was found to blunt the renal responses to intravenous furosemide, i.e., the diuresis, natriuresis, increments in plasma renin activity and urinary excretion of prostaglandins. These observations may represent a differentiation of the effects of CLINORIL on renal functions based on differences in pathogenesis of the renal prostaglandin dependence associated with differing dose-response relationships of different NSAIDs to the various renal functions influenced by prostaglandins. These observations need further clarification and in the interim, sulindac should be used with caution in patients whose renal function may be impaired (see PRECAUTIONS).

In healthy men, the average fecal blood loss, measured over a two-week period during administration of 400 mg per day of CLINORIL, was similar to that for placebo, and was statistically significantly less than that resulting from 4800 mg per day of aspirin.

In controlled clinical studies CLINORIL was evaluated in the following five conditions:

1. *Osteoarthritis*

In patients with osteoarthritis of the hip and knee, the anti-inflammatory and analgesic activity of CLINORIL was demonstrated by clinical measurements that included: assessments by both patient and investigator of overall response; decrease in disease activity as assessed by both patient and investigator; improvement in ARA Functional Class; relief of night pain; improvement in overall evaluation of pain, including pain on weight bearing and pain on active and passive motion; improvement in joint mobility, range of motion, and functional activities; decreased swelling and tenderness; and decreased duration of stiffness following prolonged inactivity.

In clinical studies in which dosages were adjusted according to patient needs, CLINORIL 200 to 400 mg daily was shown to be comparable in effectiveness to aspirin 2400 to 4800 mg daily. CLINORIL was generally well tolerated, and patients on it had a lower overall incidence of total adverse effects, of milder gastrointestinal reactions, and of tinnitus than did patients on aspirin. (See ADVERSE REACTIONS.)

2. *Rheumatoid Arthritis*

In patients with rheumatoid arthritis, the anti-inflammatory and analgesic activity of CLINORIL was demonstrated by clinical measurements that included: assessments by both patient and investigator of overall response; decrease in disease activity as assessed by both patient and investigator; reduction in overall joint pain; reduction in duration and severity of morning stiffness; reduction in day and night pain; decrease in time required to walk 50 feet; decrease in general pain as measured on a visual analog scale; improvement in the Ritchie articular index; decrease in proximal interphalangeal joint size; improvement in ARA Functional Class; increase in grip strength; reduction in painful joint count and score; reduction in swollen joint count and score; and increased flexion and extension of the wrist.

In clinical studies in which dosages were adjusted according to patient needs, CLINORIL 300 to 400 mg daily was shown to be comparable in effectiveness to aspirin 3600 to 4800 mg daily. CLINORIL was generally well tolerated, and patients on it had a lower overall incidence of total adverse effects, of milder gastrointestinal reactions, and of tinnitus than did patients on aspirin. (See ADVERSE REACTIONS.)

In patients with rheumatoid arthritis, CLINORIL may be used in combination with gold salts at usual dosage levels. In clinical studies, CLINORIL added to the regimen of gold salts usually resulted in additional symptomatic relief but did not alter the course of the underlying disease.

3. *Ankylosing spondylitis*

In patients with ankylosing spondylitis, the anti-inflammatory and analgesic activity of CLINORIL was demonstrated by clinical measurements that included: assessments by both patient and investigator of overall response; decrease in disease activity as assessed by both patient and investigator; improvement in ARA Functional Class; improvement in patient and investigator evaluation of spinal pain, tenderness and/or spasm; reduction in the duration of morning stiffness; increase in the time to onset of fatigue; relief of night pain; increase in chest expansion; and increase in spinal mobility evaluated by fingers-to-floor distance, occiput to wall distance, the Schober Test, and the Wright Modification of the Schober Test. In a clinical study in which dosages were adjusted according to patient need, CLINORIL 200 to 400 mg daily was as effective as indomethacin 75 to 150 mg daily. In a second study, CLINORIL 300 to 400 mg daily was comparable in effectiveness to phenylbutazone 400 to 600 mg daily. CLINORIL was better tolerated than phenylbutazone. (See ADVERSE REACTIONS.)

4. *Acute painful shoulder (Acute subacromial bursitis/supraspinatus tendinitis)*

In patients with acute painful shoulder (acute subacromial bursitis/supraspinatus tendinitis), the anti-inflammatory and analgesic activity of CLINORIL was demonstrated by clinical measurements that included: assessments by both patient and investigator of overall response; relief of night pain, spontaneous pain, and pain on active motion; decrease in local tenderness; and improvement in range of motion measured by abduction, and internal and external rotation.

In clinical studies in acute painful shoulder, CLINORIL 300 to 400 mg daily and oxyphenbutazone 400 to 600 mg daily were shown to be equally effective and well tolerated.

5. *Acute gouty arthritis*

In patients with acute gouty arthritis, the anti-inflammatory and analgesic activity of CLINORIL was demonstrated by clinical measurements that included: assessments by both the patient and investigator of overall response; relief of weight-bearing pain; relief of pain at rest and on active and passive motion; decrease in tenderness; reduction in warmth and swelling; increase in range of motion; and improvement in ability to function. In clinical studies, CLINORIL at 400 mg daily and phenylbutazone at 600 mg daily were shown to be equally effective. In these short-term studies in which reduction of dosage was permitted according to response, both drugs were equally well tolerated.

INDICATIONS AND USAGE

CLINORIL is indicated for acute or long-term use in the relief of signs and symptoms of the following:

1. Osteoarthritis
2. Rheumatoid arthritis**
3. Ankylosing spondylitis
4. Acute painful shoulder (Acute subacromial bursitis/supraspinatus tendinitis)
5. Acute gouty arthritis

**The safety and effectiveness of CLINORIL have not been established in rheumatoid arthritis patients who are designated in the American Rheumatism Association classification as Functional Class IV (incapacitated, largely or wholly bedridden, or confined to wheelchair; little or no self-care).

CONTRAINDICATIONS

CLINORIL should not be used in:

Patients who are hypersensitive to this product.

Patients in whom acute asthmatic attacks, urticaria, or rhinitis are precipitated by aspirin or other non-steroidal anti-inflammatory agents.

WARNINGS

Gastrointestinal Effects

Peptic ulceration and gastrointestinal bleeding have been reported in patients receiving CLINORIL. Fatalities have occurred. Gastrointestinal bleeding is associated with higher morbidity and mortality in patients acutely ill with other conditions, the elderly and patients with hemorrhagic disorders. In patients with active gastrointestinal bleeding or an active peptic ulcer, an appropriate ulcer regimen should be instituted, and the physician must weigh the benefits of therapy with CLINORIL against possible hazards, and carefully monitor the patient's progress. When CLINORIL is given to patients with a history of either upper or lower gastrointestinal tract disease, it should be given under close supervision and only after consulting the ADVERSE REACTIONS section.

Risk of GI Ulcerations, Bleeding and Perforation with NSAID Therapy

Serious gastrointestinal toxicity such as bleeding, ulceration, and perforation can occur at any time, with or without warning symptoms, in patients treated chronically with NSAID therapy. Although minor upper gastrointestinal problems, such as dyspepsia, are common, usually developing early in therapy, physicians should remain alert for ulceration and bleeding in patients treated chronically with NSAIDs even in the absence of previous GI tract symptoms. In patients observed in clinical trials of several months to two years duration, symptomatic upper GI ulcers, gross bleeding or perforation appear to occur in approximately 1% of patients treated for 3-6 months, and in about 2-4% of patients treated for one year. Physicians should inform patients about the signs and/or symptoms of serious GI toxicity and what steps to take if they occur.

Studies to date have not identified any subset of patients not at risk of developing peptic ulceration and bleeding. Except for a prior history of serious GI events and other risk factors known to be associated with peptic ulcer disease, such as alcoholism, smoking, etc., no risk factors (e.g., age, sex) have been associated with increased risk. Elderly or debilitated patients seem to tolerate ulceration or bleeding less well than other individuals and most spontaneous reports of fatal GI events are in this population. Studies to date are inconclusive concerning the relative risk of various NSAIDs in causing such reactions. High doses of any NSAID probably carry a greater risk of these reactions, although controlled clinical trials showing this do not exist in most cases. In considering the use of relatively large doses (within the recommended dosage range), sufficient benefit should be anticipated to offset the potential increased risk of GI toxicity.

Hypersensitivity

Rarely, fever and other evidence of hypersensitivity (see ADVERSE REACTIONS) including abnormalities in one or more liver function tests and severe skin reactions have occurred during therapy with CLINORIL. Fatalities have occurred in these patients. Hepatitis, jaundice, or both, with or without fever, may occur usually within the first one to three months of therapy. Determinations of liver function should be considered whenever a patient on therapy with CLINORIL develops unexplained fever, rash or other dermatologic reactions or constitutional symptoms. If unexplained fever or other evidence of hypersensitivity occurs, therapy with CLINORIL should be discontinued. The elevated temperature and abnormalities in liver function caused by CLINORIL characteristically have reverted to normal after discontinuation of therapy. Administration of CLINORIL should not be reinstituted in such patients.

Hepatic Effects

In addition to hypersensitivity reactions involving the liver, in some patients the findings are consistent with those of cholestatic hepatitis. As with other non-steroidal anti-inflammatory drugs, borderline elevations of one or more liver tests without any other signs and symptoms may occur in up to 15% of patients. These abnormalities may progress, may remain essentially unchanged, or may be transient with continued therapy. The SGPT (ALT) test is probably the most sensitive indicator of liver dysfunction. Meaningful (3 times the upper limit of normal) elevations of SGPT or SGOT (AST) occurred in controlled clinical trials in less than 1% of patients. A patient with symptoms and/or signs suggesting liver dysfunction, or in whom an abnormal liver test has occurred, should be evaluated for evidence of the development of more severe hepatic reaction while on therapy with CLINORIL. Although such reactions as described above are rare, if abnormal liver tests persist or worsen, if clinical signs and symptoms consistent with liver disease develop, or if systemic manifestations occur (e.g. eosinophilia, rash, etc.), CLINORIL should be discontinued.

In clinical trials with CLINORIL, the use of doses of 600 mg/ day has been associated with an increased incidence of mild liver test abnormalities (see DOSAGE AND ADMINISTRATION for maximum dosage recommendation).

PRECAUTIONS

General

Non-steroidal anti-inflammatory drugs, including CLINORIL, may mask the usual signs and symptoms of infection. Therefore, the physician must be continually on the alert for this and should use the drug with extra care in the presence of existing infection.

Although CLINORIL has less effect on platelet function and bleeding time than aspirin, it is an inhibitor of platelet function; therefore, patients who may be adversely affected should be carefully observed when CLINORIL is administered.

Pancreatitis has been reported in patients receiving CLINORIL (see ADVERSE REACTIONS). Should pancreatitis be suspected, the drug should be discontinued and not restarted, supportive medical therapy instituted, and the patient monitored closely with appropriate laboratory studies (e.g., serum and urine amylase, amylase/creatinine clearance ratio, electrolytes, serum calcium, glucose, lipase, etc.). A search for other causes of pancreatitis as well as those conditions which mimic pancreatitis should be conducted.

Because of reports of adverse eye findings with non-steroidal anti-inflammatory agents, it is recommended that patients who develop eye complaints during treatment with CLINORIL have ophthalmologic studies.

In patients with poor liver function, delayed, elevated and prolonged circulating levels of the sulfide and sulfone metabolites may occur. Such patients should be monitored closely; a reduction of daily dosage may be required.

Edema has been observed in some patients taking CLINORIL. Therefore, as with other non-steroidal anti-inflammatory drugs, CLINORIL should be used with caution in patients with compromised cardiac function, hypertension, or other conditions predisposing to fluid retention.

CLINORIL may allow a reduction in dosage or the elimination of chronic corticosteroid therapy in some patients with rheumatoid arthritis. However, it is generally necessary to reduce corticosteroids gradually over several months in order to avoid an exacerbation of disease or signs and symptoms of adrenal insufficiency. Abrupt withdrawal of chronic corticosteroid treatment is generally not recommended even when patients have had a serious complication of chronic corticosteroid therapy.

Renal Effects

As with other non-steroidal anti-inflammatory drugs, long-term administration of sulindac to animals has resulted in renal papillary necrosis and other abnormal renal pathology. In humans, there have been reports of acute interstitial nephritis with hematuria, proteinuria, and occasionally nephrotic syndrome.

A second form of renal toxicity has been seen in patients with prerenal and renal conditions leading to a reduction in renal blood flow or blood volume, where the renal prostaglandins have a supportive role in the maintenance of renal perfusion. In these patients, administration of an NSAID may cause a dose dependent reduction in prostaglandin formation and may precipitate overt renal decompensation. CLINORIL may affect renal function less than other NSAIDs in patients with chronic glomerular renal disease (see CLINICAL PHARMACOLOGY). Until these observations are better understood and clarified, however, and because renal adverse experiences have been reported with CLINORIL (see ADVERSE REACTIONS), caution should be exercised when administering the drug to patients with conditions associated with increased risk of the effects of non-steroidal anti-inflammatory drugs on renal function, such as those with renal or hepatic dysfunction, diabetes mellitus, advanced age, extracellular volume depletion from any cause, congestive heart failure, septicemia, pyelonephritis, or concomitant use of any nephrotoxic drug. Discontinuation of NSAID therapy is typically followed by recovery to the pretreatment state.

Since CLINORIL is eliminated primarily by the kidneys, patients with significantly impaired renal function should be closely monitored; a lower daily dosage should be anticipated to avoid excessive drug accumulation.

Sulindac metabolites have been reported rarely as the major or a minor component in renal stones in association with other calculus components. CLINORIL should be used with caution in patients with a history of renal lithiasis, and they should be kept well hydrated while receiving CLINORIL.

Information for Patients

CLINORIL, like other drugs of its class, is not free of side effects. The side effects of these drugs can cause discomfort and, rarely, there are more serious side effects such as gastrointestinal bleeding, which may result in hospitalization and even fatal outcomes.

NSAIDs (Non-steroidal Anti-inflammatory Drugs) are often essential agents in the management of arthritis, but they also may be commonly employed for conditions which are less serious.

Physicians may wish to discuss with their patients the potential risks (see WARNINGS, PRECAUTIONS and ADVERSE REACTIONS) and likely benefits of NSAID treatment, particularly when the drugs are used for less serious conditions where treatment without NSAIDs may represent an acceptable alternative to both the patient and physician.

Laboratory Tests

Because serious GI tract ulceration and bleeding can occur without warning symptoms, physicians should follow chronically treated patients for the signs and symptoms of ulceration and bleeding and should inform them of the importance of this follow-up (see WARNINGS, *Risk of GI Ulcerations, Bleeding and Perforation with NSAID Therapy).*

Use in Pregnancy

CLINORIL is not recommended for use in pregnant women, since safety for use has not been established. The known effects of drugs of this class on the human fetus during the third trimester of pregnancy include: constriction of the ductus arteriosus prenatally, tricuspid incompetence, and pulmonary hypertension; non-closure of the ductus arteriosus postnatally which may be resistant to medical management; myocardial degenerative changes, platelet dysfunction with resultant bleeding, intracranial bleeding, renal dysfunction or failure, renal injury/dysgenesis which may result in prolonged or permanent renal failure, oligohydramnios, gastrointestinal bleeding or perforation, and increased risk of necrotizing enterocolitis.

In reproduction studies in the rat, a decrease in average fetal weight and an increase in numbers of dead pups were observed on the first day of the postpartum period at dosage levels of 20 and 40 mg/kg/day ($2^1/_2$ and 5 times the usual maximum daily dose in humans), although there was no adverse effect on the survival and growth during the remainder of the postpartum period. CLINORIL prolongs the duration of gestation in rats, as do other compounds of this class which also may cause dystocia and delayed parturition in pregnant animals. Visceral and skeletal malformations observed in low incidence among rabbits in some teratology studies did not occur at the same dosage levels in repeat studies, nor at a higher dosage level in the same species.

Nursing Mothers

Nursing should not be undertaken while a patient is on CLINORIL. It is not known whether sulindac is secreted in human milk; however, it is secreted in the milk of lactating rats.

Pediatric Use

Safety and effectiveness in pediatric patients have not been established.

Geriatric Use

As with any NSAID, caution should be exercised in treating the elderly (65 years and older) since advancing age appears to increase the possibility of adverse reactions. Elderly patients seem to tolerate ulceration or bleeding less well than other individuals and many spontaneous reports of fatal GI events are in this population (see WARNINGS, *Gastrointestinal Effects* and *Risk of GI Ulcerations, Bleeding and Perforation with NSAID Therapy*).

This drug is known to be substantially excreted by the kidney and the risk of toxic reactions to this drug may be greater in patients with impaired renal function. Because elderly patients are more likely to have decreased renal function, care should be taken in dose selection and it may be useful to monitor renal function (see PRECAUTIONS, *Renal Effects*).

Drug Interactions

DMSO should not be used with sulindac. Concomitant administration has been reported to reduce the plasma levels of the active sulfide metabolite and potentially reduce efficacy. In addition, this combination has been reported to cause peripheral neuropathy.

Although sulindac and its sulfide metabolite are highly bound to protein, studies, in which CLINORIL was given at a dose of 400 mg daily, have shown no clinically significant interaction with oral anticoagulants or oral hypoglycemic agents. However, patients should be monitored carefully until it is certain that no change in their anticoagulant or hypoglycemic dosage is required. Special attention should be paid to patients taking higher doses than those recommended and to patients with renal impairment or other metabolic defects that might increase sulindac blood levels.

The concomitant administration of aspirin with sulindac significantly depressed the plasma levels of the active sulfide metabolite. A double-blind study compared the safety and efficacy of CLINORIL 300 or 400 mg daily given alone or with aspirin 2.4 g/day for the treatment of osteoarthritis. The addition of aspirin did not alter the types of clinical or laboratory adverse experiences for CLINORIL; however, the combination showed an increase in the incidence of gastrointestinal adverse experiences. Since the addition of aspirin did not have a favorable effect on the therapeutic response to CLINORIL, the combination is not recommended.

The concomitant use of CLINORIL with other NSAIDs is not recommended due to the increased possibility of gastrointestinal toxicity, with little or no increase in efficacy.

Caution should be used if CLINORIL is administered concomitantly with methotrexate. Nonsteroidal anti-inflammatory drugs have been reported to decrease the tubular secretion of methotrexate and to potentiate its toxicity.

Administration of non-steroidal anti-inflammatory drugs concomitantly with cyclosporine has been associated with an increase in cyclosporine-induced toxicity, possibly due to decreased synthesis of renal prostacyclin. NSAIDs should be used with caution in patients taking cyclosporine, and renal function should be carefully monitored.

The concomitant administration of CLINORIL and diflunisal in normal volunteers resulted in lowering of the plasma levels of the active sulindac sulfide metabolite by approximately one-third.

Probenecid given concomitantly with sulindac had only a slight effect on plasma sulfide levels, while plasma levels of sulindac and sulfone were increased. Sulindac was shown to produce a modest reduction in the uricosuric action of probenecid, which probably is not significant under most circumstances.

Neither propoxyphene hydrochloride nor acetaminophen had any effect on the plasma levels of sulindac or its sulfide metabolite.

ADVERSE REACTIONS

The following adverse reactions were reported in clinical trials or have been reported since the drug was marketed. The probability exists of a causal relationship between CLINORIL and these adverse reactions. The adverse reactions which have been observed in clinical trials encompass observations in 1,865 patients, including 232 observed for at least 48 weeks.

Incidence Greater Than 1%

Gastrointestinal

The most frequent types of adverse reactions occurring with CLINORIL are gastrointestinal; these include gastrointestinal pain (10%), dyspepsia***, nausea*** with or without vomiting, diarrhea***, constipation***, flatulence, anorexia and gastrointestinal cramps.

Dermatologic

Rash***, pruritus.

Central Nervous System

Dizziness***, headache***, nervousness.

Special Senses

Tinnitus.

Miscellaneous

Edema (see PRECAUTIONS).

***Incidence between 3% and 9%. Those reactions occurring in 1% to 3% of patients are not marked with an asterisk.

Incidence Less Than 1 in 100

Gastrointestinal

Gastritis, gastroenteritis or colitis. Peptic ulcer and gastrointestinal bleeding have been reported. GI perforation and intestinal strictures (diaphragms) have been reported rarely.

Liver function abnormalities; jaundice, sometimes with fever; cholestasis; hepatitis; hepatic failure.

There have been rare reports of sulindac metabolites in common bile duct "sludge" and in biliary calculi in patients with symptoms of cholecystitis who underwent a cholecystectomy.

Pancreatitis (see PRECAUTIONS).

Ageusia; glossitis.

Dermatologic

Stomatitis, sore or dry mucous membranes, alopecia, photosensitivity.

Erythema multiforme, toxic epidermal necrolysis, Stevens-Johnson syndrome, and exfoliative dermatitis have been reported.

Cardiovascular

Congestive heart failure, especially in patients with marginal cardiac function; palpitation; hypertension.

Hematologic

Thrombocytopenia; ecchymosis; purpura; leukopenia; agranulocytosis; neutropenia; bone marrow depression, including aplastic anemia; hemolytic anemia; increased prothrombin time in patients on oral anticoagulants (see PRECAUTIONS).

Genitourinary

Urine discoloration; dysuria; vaginal bleeding; hematuria; proteinuria; crystalluria; renal impairment, including renal failure; interstitial nephritis; nephrotic syndrome.

Renal calculi containing sulindac metabolites have been observed rarely.

Metabolic

Hyperkalemia.

Musculoskeletal

Muscle weakness.

Psychiatric

Depression; psychic disturbances including acute psychosis.

Nervous System

Vertigo; insomnia; somnolence; paresthesia; convulsions; syncope; aseptic meningitis.

Special Senses

Blurred vision; visual disturbances; decreased hearing; metallic or bitter taste.

Respiratory

Epistaxis.

Hypersensitivity Reactions

Anaphylaxis; angioneurotic edema; bronchial spasm; dyspnea.

Hypersensitivity vasculitis.

A potentially fatal apparent hypersensitivity syndrome has been reported. This syndrome may include constitutional symptoms (fever, chills, diaphoresis, flushing), cutaneous findings (rash or other dermatologic reactions—see above), conjunctivitis, involvement of major organs (changes in liver function including hepatic failure, jaundice, pancreatitis, pneumonitis with or without pleural effusion, leukopenia, leukocytosis, eosinophilia, disseminated intravascular coagulation, anemia, renal impairment, including renal failure), and other less specific findings (adenitis, arthralgia, arthritis, myalgia, fatigue, malaise, hypotension, chest pain, tachycardia).

Causal Relationship Unknown

A rare occurrence of fulminant necrotizing fasciitis, particularly in association with Group A β-hemolytic streptococcus, has been described in persons treated with non-steroidal anti-inflammatory agents, sometimes with fatal outcome (see also PRECAUTIONS, *General).*

Other reactions have been reported in clinical trials or since the drug was marketed, but occurred under circumstances where a causal relationship could not be established. However, in these rarely reported events, that possibility cannot be excluded. Therefore, these observations are listed to serve as alerting information to physicians.

Cardiovascular

Arrhythmia.

Metabolic

Hyperglycemia.

Nervous System

Neuritis.

Special Senses

Disturbances of the retina and its vasculature.

Miscellaneous

Gynecomastia.

MANAGEMENT OF OVERDOSAGE

Cases of overdosage have been reported and rarely, deaths have occurred. The following signs and symptoms may be observed following overdosage: stupor, coma, diminished urine output and hypotension.

In the event of overdosage, the stomach should be emptied by inducing vomiting or by gastric lavage, and the patient carefully observed and given symptomatic and supportive treatment.

Animal studies show that absorption is decreased by the prompt administration of activated charcoal and excretion is enhanced by alkalinization of the urine.

DOSAGE AND ADMINISTRATION

CLINORIL should be administered orally twice a day with food. The maximum dosage is 400 mg per day. Dosages above 400 mg per day are not recommended.

In osteoarthritis, rheumatoid arthritis, and ankylosing spondylitis, the recommended starting dosage is 150 mg twice a day. The dosage may be lowered or raised depending on the response.

A prompt response (within one week) can be expected in about one-half of patients with osteoarthritis, ankylosing spondylitis, and rheumatoid arthritis. Others may require longer to respond.

In acute painful shoulder (acute subacromial bursitis/supraspinatus tendinitis) and acute gouty arthritis, the recommended dosage is 200 mg twice a day. After a satisfactory response has been achieved, the dosage may be reduced according to the response. In acute painful shoulder, therapy for 7–14 days is usually adequate. In acute gouty arthritis, therapy for 7 days is usually adequate.

HOW SUPPLIED

No. 3360—Tablets CLINORIL 150 mg are bright yellow, hexagon-shaped, compressed tablets, coded MSD 941 on one side and CLINORIL on the other. They are supplied as follows:

NDC 0006-0941-68 in bottles of 100
(6505-01-071-5559, 150 mg 100's).

Shown in Product Identification Guide, page 323

Continued on next page

Information on the Merck & Co., Inc. products listed on these pages is the full prescribing information from product circulars in use September 30, 2000. For information, please call 1-800-NSC MERCK [1-800-672-6372].

Clinoril—Cont.

No. 3353—Tablets CLINORIL 200 mg are bright yellow, hexagon-shaped, scored, compressed tablets, coded MSD 942 on one side and CLINORIL on the other. They are supplied as follows:
NDC 0006-0942-68 in bottles of 100
(6505-01-072-3426, 200 mg 100's).
Shown in Product Identification Guide, page 323
7858637 Issued July 1998

COGENTIN® Tablets ℞
(Benztropine Mesylate)
COGENTIN® Injection ℞
(Benztropine Mesylate)

DESCRIPTION

Benztropine mesylate is a synthetic compound containing structural features found in atropine and diphenhydramine. It is designated chemically as 8-azabicyclo[3.2.1] octane, 3-(diphenylmethoxy)-,*endo,* methanesulfonate. Its empirical formula is $C_{21}H_{25}NO \cdot CH_4O_3S$, and its structural formula is:

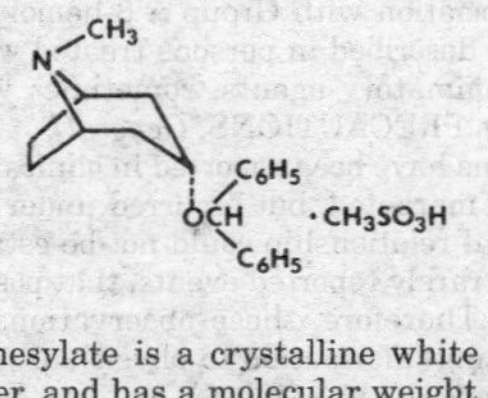

N—CH_3 ... C_6H_5 OCH C_6H_5 $\cdot CH_3SO_3H$

Benztropine mesylate is a crystalline white powder, very soluble in water, and has a molecular weight of 403.54.
COGENTIN* (Benztropine Mesylate) is supplied as tablets in three strengths (0.5 mg, 1 mg, and 2 mg per tablet), and as a sterile injection for intravenous and intramuscular use.
Tablets COGENTIN contain 0.5, 1 or 2 mg of benztropine mesylate. Each tablet contains the following inactive ingredients: calcium phosphate, cellulose, lactose, magnesium stearate and starch.
Each milliliter of the injection contains:

Benztropine mesylate	1 mg
Sodium chloride	9 mg
Water for Injection q.s.	1 mL

*Registered trademark of MERCK & CO., INC.

ACTIONS

COGENTIN possesses both anticholinergic and antihistaminic effects, although only the former have been established as therapeutically significant in the management of parkinsonism.
In the isolated guinea pig ileum, the anticholinergic activity of this drug is about equal to that of atropine; however, when administered orally to unanesthetized cats, it is only about half as active as atropine.
In laboratory animals, its antihistaminic activity and duration of action approach those of pyrilamine maleate.

INDICATIONS

For use as an adjunct in the therapy of all forms of parkinsonism.
Useful also in the control of extrapyramidal disorders (except tardive dyskinesia—see PRECAUTIONS) due to neuroleptic drugs (e.g., phenothiazines).

CONTRAINDICATIONS

Hypersensitivity to COGENTIN tablets or to any component of COGENTIN injection.
Because of its atropine-like side effects, this drug is contraindicated in pediatric patients under three years of age, and should be used with caution in older pediatric patients.

WARNINGS

Safe use in pregnancy has not been established.
COGENTIN may impair mental and/or physical abilities required for performance of hazardous tasks, such as operating machinery or driving a motor vehicle.
When COGENTIN is given concomitantly with phenothiazines, haloperidol, or other drugs with anticholinergic or antidopaminergic activity, patients should be advised to report gastrointestinal complaints, fever or heat intolerance promptly. Paralytic ileus, hyperthermia and heat stroke, all of which have sometimes been fatal, have occurred in patients taking anticholinergic-type antiparkinsonism drugs, including COGENTIN, in combination with phenothiazines and/or tricyclic antidepressants.
Since COGENTIN contains structural features of atropine, it may produce anhidrosis. For this reason, it should be administered with caution during hot weather, especially when given concomitantly with other atropine-like drugs to the chronically ill, the alcoholic, those who have central nervous system disease, and those who do manual labor in a hot environment. Anhidrosis may occur more readily when some disturbance of sweating already exists. If there is evidence of anhidrosis, the possibility of hyperthermia should be considered. Dosage should be decreased at the discretion of the physician so that the ability to maintain body heat equilibrium by perspiration is not impaired. Severe anhidrosis and fatal hyperthermia have occurred.

PRECAUTIONS

General
Since COGENTIN has cumulative action, continued supervision is advisable. Patients with a tendency to tachycardia and patients with prostatic hypertrophy should be observed closely during treatment.
Dysuria may occur, but rarely becomes a problem. Urinary retention has been reported with COGENTIN.
The drug may cause complaints of weakness and inability to move particular muscle groups, especially in large doses. For example, if the neck has been rigid and suddenly relaxes, it may feel weak, causing some concern. In this event, dosage adjustment is required.
Mental confusion and excitement may occur with large doses, or in susceptible patients. Visual hallucinations have been reported occasionally. Furthermore, in the treatment of extrapyramidal disorders due to neuroleptic drugs (e.g., phenothiazines), in patients with mental disorders, occasionally there may be intensification of mental symptoms. In such cases, antiparkinsonian drugs can precipitate a toxic psychosis. Patients with mental disorders should be kept under careful observation, especially at the beginning of treatment or if dosage is increased.
Tardive dyskinesia may appear in some patients on long-term therapy with phenothiazines and related agents, or may occur after therapy with these drugs has been discontinued. Antiparkinsonism agents do not alleviate the symptoms of tardive dyskinesia, and in some instances may aggravate them. COGENTIN is not recommended for use in patients with tardive dyskinesia.
The physician should be aware of the possible occurrence of glaucoma. Although the drug does not appear to have any adverse effect on simple glaucoma, it probably should not be used in angle-closure glaucoma.
Drug Interactions
Antipsychotic drugs such as phenothiazines or haloperidol; tricyclic antidepressants (see WARNINGS).
Pediatric use
Because of the atropine-like side effects, COGENTIN should be used with caution in pediatric patients over three years of age (see CONTRAINDICATIONS).

ADVERSE REACTIONS

The adverse reactions below, most of which are anticholinergic in nature, have been reported and within each category are listed in order of decreasing severity.
Cardiovascular
Tachycardia.
Digestive
Paralytic ileus, constipation, vomiting, nausea, dry mouth.
If dry mouth is so severe that there is difficulty in swallowing or speaking, or loss of appetite and weight, reduce dosage, or discontinue the drug temporarily.
Slight reduction in dosage may control nausea and still give sufficient relief of symptoms. Vomiting may be controlled by temporary discontinuation, followed by resumption at a lower dosage.
Nervous System
Toxic psychosis, including confusion, disorientation, memory impairment, visual hallucinations; exacerbation of pre-existing psychotic symptoms; nervousness; depression; listlessness; numbness of fingers.
Special Senses
Blurred vision, dilated pupils.
Urogenital
Urinary retention, dysuria.
Metabolic/Immune or Skin
Occasionally, an allergic reaction, e.g., skin rash, develops. If this can not be controlled by dosage reduction, the medication should be discontinued.
Other
Heat stroke, hyperthermia, fever.

DOSAGE AND ADMINISTRATION

COGENTIN tablets should be used when patients are able to take oral medication.
The injection is especially useful for psychotic patients with acute dystonic reactions or other reactions that make oral medication difficult or impossible. It is recommended also when a more rapid response is desired than can be obtained with the tablets.
Since there is no significant difference in onset of effect after intravenous or intramuscular injection, usually there is no need to use the intravenous route. The drug is quickly effective after either route, with improvement sometimes noticeable a few minutes after injection. In emergency situations, when the condition of the patient is alarming, 1 to 2 mL of the injection normally will provide quick relief. If the parkinsonian effect begins to return, the dose can be repeated.
Because of cumulative action, therapy should be initiated with a low dose which is increased gradually at five or six-day intervals to the smallest amount necessary for optimal relief. Increases should be made in increments of 0.5 mg, to a maximum of 6 mg, or until optimal results are obtained without excessive adverse reactions.
Postencephalitic and
Idiopathic Parkinsonism—
The usual daily dose is 1 to 2 mg, with a range of 0.5 to 6 mg orally or parenterally.
As with any agent used in parkinsonism, dosage must be individualized according to age and weight, and the type of parkinsonism being treated. Generally, older patients and thin patients cannot tolerate large doses. Most patients with postencephalitic parkinsonism need fairly large doses and tolerate them well. Patients with a poor mental outlook are usually poor candidates for therapy.
In idiopathic parkinsonism, therapy may be initiated with a single daily dose of 0.5 to 1 mg at bedtime. In some patients, this will be adequate; in others 4 to 6 mg a day may be required.
In postencephalitic parkinsonism, therapy may be initiated in most patients with 2 mg a day in one or more doses. In highly sensitive patients, therapy may be initiated with 0.5 mg at bedtime, and increased as necessary.
Some patients experience greatest relief by taking the entire dose at bedtime; others react more favorably to divided doses, two to four times a day. Frequently, one dose a day is sufficient, and divided doses may be unnecessary or undesirable.
The long duration of action of this drug makes it particularly suitable for bedtime medication when its effects may last throughout the night, enabling patients to turn in bed during the night more easily, and to rise in the morning.
When COGENTIN is started, do not terminate therapy with other antiparkinsonian agents abruptly. If the other agents are to be reduced or discontinued, it must be done gradually. Many patients obtain greatest relief with combination therapy.
COGENTIN may be used concomitantly with SINEMET* (Carbidopa-Levodopa), or with levodopa, in which case periodic dosage adjustment may be required in order to maintain optimum response.
*Drug-Induced Extrapyramidal Disorders—*In treating extrapyramidal disorders due to neuroleptic drugs (e.g., phenothiazines), the recommended dosage is 1 to 4 mg once or twice a day orally or parenterally. Dosage must be individualized according to the need of the patient. Some patients require more than recommended; others do not need as much.
In acute dystonic reactions, 1 to 2 mL of the injection usually relieves the condition quickly. After that, the tablets, 1 to 2 mg twice a day, usually prevent recurrence.
When extrapyramidal disorders develop soon after initiation of treatment with neuroleptic drugs (e.g., phenothiazines), they are likely to be transient. One to 2 mg of COGENTIN tablets two or three times a day usually provides relief within one or two days. After one or two weeks, the drug should be withdrawn to determine the continued need for it. If such disorders recur, COGENTIN can be reinstituted.
Certain drug-induced extrapyramidal disorders that develop slowly may not respond to COGENTIN.

*Registered trademark of MERCK & CO., INC.

OVERDOSAGE

Manifestations—May be any of those seen in atropine poisoning or antihistamine overdosage: CNS depression, preceded or followed by stimulation; confusion; nervousness; listlessness; intensification of mental symptoms or toxic psychosis in patients with mental illness being treated with neuroleptic drugs (e.g., phenothiazines); hallucinations (especially visual); dizziness; muscle weakness; ataxia; dry mouth; mydriasis; blurred vision; palpitations; tachycardia; elevated blood pressure; nausea; vomiting; dysuria; numbness of fingers; dysphagia; allergic reactions, e.g., skin rash; headache; hot, dry, flushed skin; delirium; coma; shock; convulsions; respiratory arrest; anhidrosis; hyperthermia; glaucoma; constipation.
Treatment —Physostigmine salicylate, 1 to 2 mg, SC or IV, reportedly will reverse symptoms of anticholinergic intoxication.** A second injection may be given after 2 hours if required. Otherwise treatment is symptomatic and supportive. Induce emesis or perform gastric lavage (contraindicated in precomatose, convulsive, or psychotic states). Maintain respiration. A short-acting barbiturate may be used for CNS excitement, but with caution to avoid subsequent depression; supportive care for depression (avoid convulsant stimulants such as picrotoxin, pentylenetetrazol, or bemegride); artificial respiration for severe respiratory depression; a local miotic for mydriasis and cycloplegia; ice bags or other cold applications and alcohol sponges for hyperpyrexia, a vasopressor and fluids for circulatory collapse. Darken room for photophobia.

**Duvoisin, R.C.; Katz, R.J.; Amer. Med. Ass. *206* :1963–1965, Nov. 25, 1968.

HOW SUPPLIED

No. 3297—Tablets COGENTIN, 0.5 mg, are white, round, scored, compressed tablets, coded MSD 21 on one side and COGENTIN on the other. They are supplied as follows:
NDC 0006-0021-68 in bottles of 100.
Shown in Product Identification Guide, page 323

No. 3334—Tablets COGENTIN, 1 mg, are white, oval shaped, scored, compressed tablets, coded MSD 635 on one side and COGENTIN on the other. They are supplied as follows:

NDC 0006-0635-68 in bottles of 100.

Shown in Product Identification Guide, page 323

No. 3172—Tablets COGENTIN, 2 mg, are white, round, scored, compressed tablets, coded MSD 60 on one side and COGENTIN on the other. They are supplied as follows:

NDC 0006-0060-68 in bottles of 100
(6505-01-230-8726, 2 mg 100's).

Shown in Product Identification Guide, page 323

No. 3275—Injection COGENTIN, 1 mg per mL, is a clear, colorless solution and is supplied as follows:

NDC 0006-3275-16 in boxes of 6×2 mL ampuls
(6505-00-785-0307, tray of 6×2 mL ampuls).

7924121 Issued July 1996

COMVAX® ℞

[Haemophilus b conjugate (meningococcal protein conjugate) and hepatitis B (recombinant) vaccine]

DESCRIPTION

COMVAX* [Haemophilus b Conjugate (Meningococcal Protein Conjugate) and Hepatitis B (Recombinant) Vaccine] is a sterile bivalent vaccine made of the antigenic components used in producing PedvaxHIB* [Haemophilus b Conjugate Vaccine (Meningococcal Protein Conjugate)] and RECOMBIVAX HB* [Hepatitis B Vaccine (Recombinant)]. These components are the *Haemophilus influenzae* type b capsular polysaccharide (PRP) that is covalently bound to an outer membrane protein complex (OMPC) of *Neisseria meningitidis* and hepatitis B surface antigen (HBsAg) from recombinant yeast cultures.

Haemophilus influenzae type b and *Neisseria meningitidis* serogroup B are grown in complex fermentation media. The PRP is purified from the culture broth by purification procedures which include ethanol fractionation, enzyme digestion, phenol extraction and diafiltration. The OMPC from *Neisseria meningitidis* is purified by detergent extraction, ultracentrifugation, diafiltration and sterile filtration.

The PRP-OMPC conjugate is prepared by the chemical coupling of the highly purified PRP (polyribosylribitol phosphate) of *Haemophilus influenzae* type b (Haemophilus b, Ross strain) to an OMPC of the B11 strain of *Neisseria meningitidis* serogroup B. The coupling of the PRP to the OMPC, which is necessary for enhanced immunogenicity of the PRP, is confirmed by analysis of the conjugate's components following chemical treatment which yields a unique amino acid. After conjugation, the aqueous bulk is then adsorbed onto an aluminum hydroxide adjuvant.

HBsAg is produced in recombinant yeast cells. A portion of the hepatitis B virus gene, coding for HBsAg, is cloned into yeast, and the vaccine for hepatitis B is produced from cultures of this recombinant yeast strain according to methods developed in the Merck Research Laboratories. The antigen is harvested and purified from fermentation cultures of a recombinant strain of the yeast *Saccharomyces cerevisiae* containing the gene for the *adw* subtype of HBsAg. The HBsAg protein is released from the yeast cells by cell disruption and purified by a series of physical and chemical methods. The vaccine contains no detectable yeast DNA but may contain not more than 1% yeast protein. The aqueous bulk is treated with formaldehyde and then adsorbed onto an aluminum hydroxide adjuvant.

After each PRP-OMPC and HBsAg aqueous bulk is adsorbed onto the aluminum hydroxide adjuvant, they are then combined to produce COMVAX. Each 0.5 mL dose of COMVAX is formulated to contain 7.5 mcg of Haemophilus b PRP, 125 mcg of *Neisseria meningitidis* OMPC, 5 mcg of HBsAg, approximately 225 mcg of aluminum as aluminum hydroxide, and 35 mcg sodium borate (decahydrate) as a pH stabilizer, in 0.9% sodium chloride.

The product contains no preservative.

COMVAX is a sterile suspension for intramuscular injection.

*Registered trademark of MERCK & CO., Inc.

CLINICAL PHARMACOLOGY

Haemophilus influenzae type b Disease

Prior to the introduction of *Haemophilus b* conjugate vaccines, *Haemophilus influenzae* type b (Hib) was the most frequent cause of bacterial meningitis and a leading cause of serious, systemic bacterial disease in young children worldwide.

Hib disease occurred primarily in children under 5 years of age, and in the United States prior to the initiation of a vaccine program was estimated to account for nearly 20,000 cases of invasive infections annually, approximately 12,000 of which were meningitis. The mortality rate from Hib meningitis is about 5%. In addition, up to 35% of survivors develop neurologic sequelae including seizures, deafness, and mental retardation. Other invasive diseases caused by this bacterium include cellulitis, epiglottitis, sepsis, pneumonia, septic arthritis, osteomyelitis, and pericarditis.

Prior to the introduction of the vaccine, it was estimated that 17% of all cases of Hib disease occurred in infants less than 6 months of age. The peak incidence of Hib meningitis occurred between 6 to 11 months of age. Forty-seven percent of all cases occurred by one year of age with the remaining 53% of cases occurring over the next four years.

Among children under 5 years of age, the risk of invasive Hib disease is increased in certain populations including the following

- Daycare attendees
- Lower socio-economic groups
- Blacks (especially those who lack the Km(1) immunoglobulin allotype)
- Caucasians who lack the G2m(23) immunoglobulin allotype)
- Native Americans
- Household contacts of cases
- Individuals with asplenia, sickle cell disease, or antibody deficiency syndromes.

An important virulence factor of the Hib bacterium is its polysaccharide capsule (PRP). Antibody to PRP (anti-PRP) has been shown to correlate with protection against Hib disease. While the anti-PRP level associated with protection using conjugated vaccines has not yet been determined, the level of anti-PRP associated with protection in studies using bacterial polysaccharide immune globulin or nonconjugated PRP vaccines ranged from ≥0.15 to ≥1.0 mcg/mL.

Nonconjugated PRP vaccines are capable of stimulating B-lymphocytes to produce antibody without the help of T-lymphocytes (T-independent). The responses to many other antigens are augmented by helper T-lymphocytes (T-dependent). PedvaxHIB is a PRP-conjugate vaccine in which the PRP is covalently bound to the OMPC carrier producing an antigen which is postulated to convert the T-independent antigen (PRP alone) into a T-dependent antigen resulting in both an enhanced antibody response and immunologic memory.

The protective efficacy of the PRP-OMPC component of COMVAX was demonstrated in a randomized, double-blind, placebo-controlled study involving 3486 Native American (Navajo) infants (The Protective Efficacy Study) who completed the primary two-dose regimen for lyophilized PedvaxHIB. This population has a much higher incidence of Hib disease than the United States population as a whole and also has a lower antibody response to Haemophilus b conjugate vaccines, including PedvaxHIB.

Each infant in this study received two doses of either placebo or lyophilized PedvaxHIB (15 mcg Haemophilus b PRP) with the first dose administered at a mean of 8 weeks of age and the second administered approximately two months later; DTP and OPV were administered concomitantly. In a subset of 416 subjects, lyophilized PedvaxHIB (15 mcg Haemophilus b PRP) induced anti-PRP levels >0.15 mcg/mL in 88% and >1.0 mcg/mL in 52% with a geometric mean titer (GMT) of 0.95 mcg/mL one to three months after the first dose; the corresponding anti-PRP levels one to three months following the second dose were 91% and 60%, respectively, with a GMT of 1.43 mcg/mL. These antibody responses were associated with a high level of protection.

Most subjects were initially followed until 15 to 18 months of age. During this time, 22 cases of invasive Haemophilus b disease occurred in the placebo group (8 cases after the first dose and 14 cases after the second dose) and only 1 case in the vaccine group (none after the first dose and 1 after the second dose). Following the primary two-dose regimen, the protective efficacy of lyophilized PedvaxHIB was calculated to be 93% with a 95% confidence interval of 57-98%. In the two months between the first and second doses, the difference in number of cases of disease between placebo and vaccine recipients (8 vs 0 cases, respectively) was statistically significant (p=0.008). At termination of the study, placebo recipients were offered vaccine. All original participants were then followed two years and nine months from termination of the study. During this extended follow-up, invasive haemophilus b disease occurred in an additional 7 of the original placebo recipients prior to receiving vaccine and in 1 of the original vaccine recipients (who had received only 1 dose of vaccine). No cases of invasive haemophilus b disease were observed in placebo recipients after they received at least one dose of vaccine. Efficacy for this follow-up period, estimated from person-days at risk, was 96.6% (95 C.I., 72.2-99.9%) in children under 18 months of age and 100% (95 C.I., 23.5-100%) in children over 18 months of age.

Thus, in this study, a protective efficacy of 93% was achieved with an anti-PRP level of >1.0 mcg/mL in 60% of vaccinees and a GMT of 1.43 mcg/mL one to three months after the second dose. In a randomized, multicenter study comparing COMVAX (7.5 mcg Haemophilus b PRP; 5 mcg HBsAg) to concurrent administration of monovalent liquid PedvaxHIB and monovalent RECOMBIVAX HB, anti-PRP levels were measured in 576 of 645 infants who received two doses of COMVAX. In these infants, COMVAX induced anti-PRP levels >0.15 mcg/mL in 95% and >1.0 mcg/mL in 72% with a GMT of 2.5 mcg/mL, approximately two months after the second dose (see Table 1). Because the PRP-OMPC component of COMVAX induces a comparable anti-PRP response (see Table 1), the efficacy of COMVAX is expected to be similar to that obtained with monovalent lyophilized PedvaxHIB in the Protective Efficacy Trial in the prevention of invasive Hib disease.

Hepatitis B Disease

Hepatitis B virus is an important cause of viral hepatitis. There is no specific treatment for this disease. The incubation period for hepatitis B is relatively long; six weeks to six months may elapse between exposure and the onset of clinical symptoms. The prognosis following infection with hepatitis B virus is variable and dependent on at least three factors: (1) Age—infants and younger children usually experience milder initial disease than older persons but are much more likely to remain persistently infected and become at risk of developing serious chronic liver disease; (2) Dose of virus—the higher the dose, the more likely acute icteric hepatitis B will result; and, (3) Severity of associated underlying disease—underlying malignancy or pre-existing hepatic disease predisposes to increased mortality and morbidity.

Hepatitis B infection fails to resolve and progresses to a chronic carrier state in 5 to 10% of older children and adults and in up to 90% of infants; chronic infection also occurs more frequently after initial anicteric hepatitis B than after initial icteric disease. Consequently, carriers of HBsAg frequently give no history of having had recognized acute hepatitis. It has been estimated that more than 285 million people in the world today are persistently infected with hepatitis B virus. The Centers for Disease Control (CDC) estimates that there are approximately 0.75 to 1 million chronic carriers of hepatitis B virus in the USA. Chronic carriers represent the largest human reservoir of hepatitis B virus.

A serious complication of acute hepatitis B virus infection is massive hepatic necrosis while sequelae of chronic hepatitis B include cirrhosis of the liver, chronic active hepatitis, and hepatocellular carcinoma. Chronic carriers of HBsAg appear to be at increased risk of developing hepatocellular carcinoma. Although a number of etiologic factors are associated with development of hepatocellular carcinoma, the single most important etiologic factor appears to be chronic infection with hepatitis B virus.

The vehicles for transmission of the virus are most often blood and blood products but the viral antigen has also been found in tears, saliva, breast milk, urine, semen, and vaginal secretions. Hepatitis B virus is capable of surviving for days on environmental surfaces exposed to body fluids containing hepatitis B virus. Infection may occur when hepatitis B virus, transmitted by infected body fluids, is implanted via mucous surfaces or percutaneously introduced through accidental or deliberate breaks in the skin. Transmission of hepatitis B virus infection is often associated with close interpersonal contact with an infected individual and with crowded living conditions.

Hepatitis B is endemic throughout the world and is a serious medical problem in population groups at increased risk. Because vaccination limited to high-risk individuals has failed to substantially lower the overall incidence of hepatitis B infection, both the Advisory Committee on Immunization Practices (ACIP) and the Committee on Infectious Diseases of the American Academy of Pediatrics (AAP) have also endorsed universal infant immunization as part of a comprehensive strategy for the control of hepatitis B infection.

Multiple clinical studies have defined a protective antibody (anti-HBs) level as 1) 10 or more sample ratio units (SRU or S/N) as determined by radioimmunoassay or 2) a positive result as determined by enzyme immunoassay. Note: 10 SRU is comparable to 10 mIU/mL of antibody. The ACIP and an international group of hepatitis B experts consider an anti-HBs titer ≥10 mIU/mL an adequate response to a complete course of hepatitis B vaccine and protective against clinically significant infection (antigenemia with or without clinical disease).

In clinical studies, 99% of 125 infants under 1 year of age born of non-carrier mothers developed a protective level of antibody (anti-HBs ≥10 mIU/mL) after receiving three 2.5-mcg doses of RECOMBIVAX HB at intervals of 0, 1, and 6 months.

In another clinical study, protective levels of antibody were achieved in 98% of 52 healthy infants after receiving 2.5 mcg of RECOMBIVAX HB at 2, 4, and 12 months of age. Protective anti-HBs levels were achieved in 100% of an additional 50 infants who also received three 2.5-mcg doses of RECOMBIVAX HB but at 2, 4, and 15 months of age.

The protective efficacy of three 5-mcg doses of RECOMBIVAX HB has been demonstrated in neonates born of mothers positive for both HBsAg and HBeAg (a core-associated antigenic complex which correlates with high infectivity). In a clinical study of infants who received one dose of Hepatitis B Immune Globulin at birth followed by the recommended three-dose regimen of RECOMBIVAX HB, chronic infection had not occurred in 96% of 130 infants after nine months of follow-up. The estimated efficacy in prevention of chronic hepatitis B infection was 95% as compared to the infection rate in untreated historical controls.

In a randomized, multicenter study comparing COMVAX to liquid PedvaxHIB and RECOMBIVAX HB, anti-HBs levels were measured in 571 of 598 infants who received 3 doses of COMVAX. In these infants, COMVAX induced protective anti-HBs levels (≥10 mIU/mL) in 98%. Because the HBs component of COMVAX induces a comparable anti-HBs response to that obtained with RECOMBIVAX HB, the efficacy of COMVAX is expected to be similar (Table 1).

COMVAX

The safety and immunogenicity of COMVAX (7.5 mcg Haemophilus b PRP, 5 mcg HBsAg) were compared with those of the component monovalent vaccines, liquid PedvaxHIB (7.5 mcg Haemophilus b PRP) and RECOMBIVAX HB (5 mcg

Continued on next page

Information on the Merck & Co., Inc. products listed on these pages is the full prescribing information from product circulars in use September 30, 2000. For information, please call 1-800-NSC MERCK [1-800-672-6372].

Comvax—Cont.

HBsAg) given concurrently at separate sites, in combined clinical trials involving 1216 healthy infants. Each infant received a three-dose regimen of either COMVAX (n=856) or liquid PedvaxHIB and RECOMBIVAX HB administered either concomitantly (n=290) or one month apart (n=70) beginning at approximately 2 months of age; other standard pediatric vaccines (M-M-R†II [Measles, Mumps, and Rubella Virus Vaccine Live], DTP [diphtheria, tetanus, pertussis] or DTaP [diphtheria, tetanus, acellular pertussis] or OPV [oral poliovirus vaccine]) were administered concomitantly to most subjects. Antibody responses following the recommended three-dose regimen of COMVAX were similar to those following concurrent administration of the monovalent vaccines according to the same schedule. Table 1 summarizes antibody responses in a subset of infants from one multicenter, randomized, open-label study. These infants received a three-dose regimen of either COMVAX or liquid PedvaxHIB plus RECOMBIVAX HB at approximately 2, 4, and 12–15 months of age.

The anti-HBs GMT associated with the use of COMVAX was 4467.5 mIU/mL and the anti-HBs GMT associated with the concomitant use of monovalent PedvaxHIB plus monovalent RECOMBIVAX HB was 6943.9 mIU/mL. Although the difference is statistically significant (p=0.011), both values are much greater than the level of 10 mIU/mL previously established as marking a protective response to hepatitis B. These GMTs are also higher than those reported in a number of studies wherein healthy neonates or young infants received the currently licensed regimen of RECOMBIVAX HB consisting of 2.5 mcg doses administered on the standard 0, 1 and 6-month schedule. In those studies, the infants developed GMTs of 216–1269 mIU/mL. Another study has shown that infants given 2.5 mcg doses of RECOMBIVAX HB according to the schedule used for COMVAX (2, 4, and 12–15 months of age) developed GMTs of 1356–3424 mIU/mL. While a difference in the GMT between two vaccination regimens may result in differential retention of ≥10 mIU/mL of anti-HBs after a number of years, this is of no apparent clinical significance because of immunologic memory.

[See table 1 below]

Data are currently available for 38 infants in a study in which COMVAX was administered concomitantly with DTaP and IPV at 2 and 4 months of age. Two months after the second dose, 100% of the infants had ≥0.15 mcg/mL of anti-PRP, 84% had ≥1.0 mcg/mL of anti-PRP, 74% had ≥10 mIU/mL of anti-HBs (100% after 3 doses of COMVAX, n=19), and 100% possessed detectable antibody to all three types of poliovirus.

An additional 1756 infants were involved in clinical trials where COMVAX was administered concomitantly with either an investigational pneumococcal polysaccharide protein conjugate vaccine or an investigational preparation of diphtheria, tetanus, pertussis, and enhanced inactivated poliovirus vaccine. The serious adverse experience information for these subjects is provided in this circular (see ADVERSE REACTIONS).

Interchangeability of COMVAX and Licensed Haemophilus b Conjugate Vaccines or Recombinant Hepatitis B Vaccines

One multicenter study has shown similar safety profiles and similar anti-PRP and anti-HBs responses among children vaccinated with a three-dose course of COMVAX or a three-dose course of monovalent PedvaxHIB and monovalent RECOMBIVAX HB. Therefore, it is expected that responses would be comparable if COMVAX were used as a component of a mixed Haemophilus b conjugate vaccine series involving PedvaxHIB or a mixed hepatitis B vaccine series involving RECOMBIVAX HB. Published studies presenting limited clinical data have examined the interchangeability of other licensed Haemophilus b conjugate vaccines and PedvaxHIB. In addition, a clinical study has shown that in healthy neonates a regimen of hepatitis B vaccine can be initiated with another currently licensed hepatitis B vaccine and completed with RECOMBIVAX HB.

INDICATIONS AND USAGE

COMVAX is indicated for vaccination against invasive disease caused by *Haemophilus influenzae* type b and against infection caused by all known subtypes of hepatitis B virus in infants 6 weeks to 15 months of age born of HBsAg negative mothers. Infants born of HBsAg positive mothers should receive Hepatitis B Immune Globulin and Hepatitis B Vaccine (Recombinant) at birth and should complete the hepatitis B vaccination series given according to a particular schedule (see manufacturer's circular for Hepatitis B Vaccine [Recombinant]).

Infants born of mothers of unknown HBsAg status should receive Hepatitis B Vaccine (Recombinant) at birth and should complete the hepatitis B vaccination series given according to a particular schedule (see manufacturer's circular for Hepatitis B Vaccine [Recombinant]).

Vaccination with COMVAX should ideally begin at approximately 2 months of age or as soon thereafter as possible. In order to complete the three-dose regimen of COMVAX, vaccination should be initiated no later than 10 months of age. Infants in whom vaccination with a PRP-OMPC-containing product (i.e., PedvaxHIB, COMVAX) is not initiated until 11 months of age do not require three doses of PRP-OMPC; however, three doses of an HBsAg-containing product are required for complete vaccination against hepatitis B, regardless of age. For infants and children not vaccinated according to the recommended schedule see DOSAGE AND ADMINISTRATION.

Use With Other Vaccines

Results from clinical studies indicate that COMVAX can be administered concomitantly with DTP, OPV, eIPV (enhanced inactivated poliovirus vaccine), VARIVAX* [Varicella Virus Vaccine Live (Oka/Merck)], and M-M-R* II, and with a booster dose of DTaP at approximately 15 months of age, using separate sites and syringes for injectable vaccines (see CLINICAL PHARMACOLOGY, *COMVAX*). No impairment of immune response to these individually tested vaccine antigens was demonstrated.

COMVAX has been administered concomitantly with the primary series of DTaP to a limited number of infants. No serious vaccine-related adverse events were reported. Immune response data are satisfactory for COMVAX but are currently unavailable for DTaP (see CLINICAL PHARMACOLOGY, *COMVAX*).

COMVAX SHOULD NOT BE USED IN INFANTS YOUNGER THAN 6 WEEKS OF AGE (see PRECAUTIONS).

CONTRAINDICATIONS

Hypersensitivity to any component of the vaccine.

WARNINGS

If COMVAX is used in persons with malignancies or those receiving immunosuppressive therapy or who are otherwise immunocompromised, the expected immune response may not be obtained.

Patients who develop symptoms suggestive of hypersensitivity after an injection should not receive further injections of the vaccine (see CONTRAINDICATIONS).

PRECAUTIONS

General

COMVAX will not protect against invasive disease caused by *Haemophilus influenzae* other than type b or against invasive disease (such as meningitis or sepsis) caused by other microorganisms. COMVAX will not prevent hepatitis by other viruses known to infect the liver. Because of the long incubation period for hepatitis B, it is possible for unrecognized infection to be present at the time the vaccine is given. The vaccine may not prevent hepatitis B in such patients.

As for any vaccine, adequate treatment provisions, including epinephrine, should be available for immediate use should an anaphylactic or anaphylactoid reaction occur.

As with other vaccines, COMVAX may not induce protective antibody levels immediately following vaccination and may not result in a protective antibody response in all individuals given the vaccine.

As reported with Haemophilus b Polysaccharide Vaccine and another Haemophilus b Conjugate Vaccine, cases of Haemophilus b disease may occur in the week after vaccination, prior to the onset of the protective effects of the vaccines.

The decision to administer or delay vaccination because of current or recent febrile illness depends on the severity of symptoms and on the etiology of the disease. The ACIP has recommended that immunization should be delayed during the course of an acute febrile illness. All vaccines can be administered to persons with minor illnesses such as diarrhea, mild upper-respiratory infection with or without low-grade fever, or other low-grade febrile illness. Persons with moderate or severe febrile illness should be vaccinated as soon as they have recovered from the acute phase of the illness.

Instructions to Health-care Provider

The health-care provider should determine the current health status and previous vaccination history of the vaccinee.

The health-care provider should question the patient, parent, or guardian about reactions to a previous dose of COMVAX, PedvaxHIB or other Haemophilus b conjugate vaccines or RECOMBIVAX HB or other hepatitis B vaccines.

Information for Patients

The health-care provider should provide the vaccine information required to be given with each vaccination to the patient, parent or guardian.

The health-care provider should inform the patient, parent or guardian of the benefits and risks associated with vaccination. For risks associated with vaccination, see WARNINGS, PRECAUTIONS, and ADVERSE REACTIONS.

Patients, parents and guardians should be instructed to report any serious adverse reactions to their health-care provider who in turn should report such events to the U.S. Department of Health and Human Services through the Vaccine Adverse Event Reporting System (VAERS), 1-800-822-7967.

Laboratory Test Interactions

Sensitive tests (e.g., Latex Agglutination Kits) may detect PRP derived from the vaccine in the urine of some vaccinees for at least 30 days following vaccination with lyophilized PedvaxHIB; in clinical studies with lyophilized PedvaxHIB, such children demonstrated a normal immune response to the vaccine. It is not known whether antigenuria will occur after vaccination with COMVAX.

Carcinogenesis, Mutagenesis, Impairment of Fertility

COMVAX has not been evaluated for its carcinogenic or mutagenic potential, or its potential to impair fertility.

Pregnancy

Pregnancy Category C: Animal reproduction studies have not been conducted with COMVAX. It is also not known whether COMVAX can cause fetal harm when administered to a pregnant woman or can affect reproduction capacity. COMVAX is not recommended for use in women of childbearing age.

Pediatric Use

COMVAX has been shown to be generally well tolerated and highly immunogenic in infants 6 weeks to 15 months of age. See DOSAGE AND ADMINISTRATION for recommended dosage schedules.

Safety and effectiveness of COMVAX in infants below the age of 6 weeks and above the age of 15 months have not been established. However, studies have demonstrated that PedvaxHIB is safe and immunogenic when administered to infants and children up to the age of 71 months and RECOMBIVAX HB is safe and immunogenic in persons of all ages.

COMVAX should not be used in infants younger than 6 weeks of age because this will lead to a reduced anti-PRP response and may lead to immune tolerance (impaired ability to respond to subsequent exposure to the PRP antigen).

Infants born of HBsAg-positive mothers should not receive COMVAX but instead should receive Hepatitis B Immune Globulin and Hepatitis B Vaccine (Recombinant) at birth and should complete the hepatitis B vaccination series given according to a particular schedule (see manufacturer's circular for Hepatitis B Vaccine [Recombinant]). (See DOSAGE AND ADMINISTRATION.)

ADVERSE REACTIONS

In clinical trials involving the administration of 6705 doses of COMVAX to 2612 healthy infants 6 weeks to 15 months of age, COMVAX was generally well tolerated. Of these infants, 856 were involved in clinical trials (730 infants in controlled, randomized trials) in which most received COMVAX concomitantly with other licensed pediatric vaccines. These 856 infants were monitored for both serious and non-serious adverse experiences. The remaining 1756 infants were involved in trials where COMVAX was administered concomitantly with either an investigational pneumococcal polysaccharide protein conjugate vaccine or an investigational preparation of diphtheria, tetanus, pertussis, and inactivated poliovirus vaccine and were under surveillance for serious adverse experiences. The serious adverse experiences for these subjects are described following Table 2.

Adverse experiences observed within a five-day period following each dose of COMVAX were generally similar in type and frequency to those observed in infants who received concurrent injections of liquid PedvaxHIB and RECOMBIVAX HB at separate sites.

As judged by the investigators, no serious vaccine-related adverse experiences were observed during clinical trials.

Table 2 summarizes the local reactions and systemic complaints within five days of vaccination that were reported to occur among ≥1.0% of children given a three-dose course of COMVAX as well as the frequencies of these events among children in the study given concomitant injections of monovalent PedvaxHIB and RECOMBIVAX HB. In this randomized, multicenter study, 882 infants were assigned in a 3:1

Table 1
Antibody Responses to COMVAX, liquid PedvaxHIB, and RECOMBIVAX HB

Vaccine	Age (months)	Time	N	Anti-PRP % Subjects with >0.15 mcg/mL	Anti-PRP % Subjects with >1.0 mcg/mL	Anti-PRP GMT (mcg/mL)	N	% Subjects ≥10 mIU/mL Anti-HBs	Anti-HBs GMT
COMVAX		Prevaccination	633	34.4	4.7	0.1	603	10.6	0.6
(7.5 mcg PRP,	2	Dose 1*	620	88.9	51.5	1.0	595	34.3	4.2
5 mcg HBsAg)	4	Dose 2*	576	94.8	72.4	2.5	571	92.1	113.9
	12/15	Dose 3**	570	99.3	92.6	9.5	571	98.4	4467.5
Liquid PedvaxHIB		Prevaccination	208	33.7	5.8	0.1	196	7.1	0.5
(7.5 mcg PRP)	2	Dose 1*	202	90.1	53.5	1.1	198	41.9	5.3
+	4	Dose 2*	186	95.2	76.3	2.8	185	98.4	255.7
RECOMBIVAX HB	12/15	Dose 3**	181	98.9	92.3	10.2	179	100.0	6943.9
(5 mcg HBsAg)									

*Postvaccination responses were determined approximately two months after doses 1 and 2.
**Postvaccination responses were determined approximately one month after administration of dose 3.

ratio to receive either COMVAX or PedvaxHIB plus RECOMBIVAX HB at 2, 4, and 12–15 months of age, with the children monitored daily for five days after each injection for local reactions and systemic complaints.
[See table 2 above]

Table 2
Local Reactions and Systemic Complaints Within 5 Days After Injection Reported to Occur in ≥1.0%† of Children Given a 3-Dose Course of COMVAX Compared to These Events in Children Given Concomitant Injections of PedvaxHIB and RECOMBIVAX HB

	Injection 1‡		Injection 2‡		Injection 3	
Event	COMVAX (N=660) %	PedvaxHIB and RECOMBIVAX HB*** (N=221) %	COMVAX (N=645) %	PedvaxHIB and RECOMBIVAX HB*** (N=213) %	COMVAX (N=593) %	PedvaxHIB and RECOMBIVAX HB*** (N=193) %
Injection Site Reactions						
Pain/Soreness*	34.5	37.6	24.3	25.8	23.9	21.2
Erythema (>1 in.)*	22.4 (2.7)	25.8 (2.7)	25.7 (1.4)	23.5 (3.3)	27.2 (3.0)	24.4 (1.6)
Swelling/Induration (>1 in.)*	27.6 (3.0)	33.5 (4.1)	30.4 (2.9)	31.0 (3.8)	27.2 (3.2)	29.5 (4.1)
Systemic Complaints						
Irritability*	57.0	46.6	50.7	44.1	32.2	29.0
Somnolence*	49.5	47.1	37.4	31.9	21.1	22.3
Crying—						
unusual, high pitched*	10.6	8.6	6.7	2.3	2.9	3.6
not otherwise specified	2.3	2.3	1.4	2.3	0.7	1.6
prolonged (>4 hrs.)*	2.4	2.3	0.8	1.4	0.2	0
Anorexia	3.9	2.3	2.0	0.9	0.8	0.5
Vomiting	2.1	1.8	2.5	0.9	1.0	1.6
Otitis media	0.5	0	2.0	1.4	2.7	1.6
Fever (°F, rectal equiv.)**						
101.0–102.9	14.2	11.9	13.8	12.2	10.5	6.4
≥103.0	0.8	0	1.6	1.4	2.7	4.3
Diarrhea	1.7	1.8	0.8	0.9	2.2	0.5
Upper respiratory infection	0.5	0.5	1.1	0.9	1.3	0.5
Rash	0.8	0	0.9	0	0.8	0.5
Rhinorrhea	0.2	0	1.1	0.9	1.3	2.1
Respiratory congestion	0.6	0.5	1.2	0.9	0.3	0.5
Cough	0.2	0	0.9	0.5	0.2	1.0
Candidiasis, oral	0.3	0.5	0.8	0	0.2	0
Rash, diaper	0.5	0.5	0.5	0.9	0.2	0

†Overall frequency of each event listed above is ≥1% even though the frequency after a given dose may be <1%.
‡Most children received DTP and OPV concomitantly with the first two doses of COMVAX or PedvaxHIB and RECOMBIVAX HB.
*Events prompted for on Vaccination Report Card given to parents/guardians of vaccinees.
**N for injections 1, 2, and 3 equals 655, 639, and 588, respectively, for COMVAX; N for injections 1, 2, and 3 equals 218, 213, and 187, respectively, for PedvaxHIB and RECOMBIVAX HB.
***Injection site reactions for PedvaxHIB and RECOMBIVAX HB based on occurrence with either of the monovalent components.

Among 856 infants from combined clinical trials who were monitored for both serious and non-serious adverse experiences, the following serious events were reported to occur in 13 infants during a 14-day period following vaccination with COMVAX (usually coadministered with other pediatric vaccines). These adverse experiences are grouped by case: viral infection; febrile seizure; asthma; diarrhea, vomiting, acidosis, dehydration, hypoglycemia, and seizure disorder; bacterial infection; bronchiolitis and reflux esophagitis; dehydration and fever; asthma, respiratory congestion, and tachypnea; asthma and upper respiratory infection; urinary tract infection and vomiting; pneumonia and asthma; apnea and reflux esophagitis; and vitreous hemorrhage. A causal relationship to the vaccine is unknown; however, these serious adverse events were judged not to be related to vaccination with COMVAX by the investigator.
Among 1756 infants who received COMVAX concomitantly with either an investigational pneumococcal polysaccharide protein conjugate vaccine or an investigational preparation of diphtheria, tetanus, pertussis, and inactivated poliovirus vaccine, the following serious events were reported to occur in 9 infants during a 14-day period following vaccination with COMVAX. These adverse experiences are grouped by case: respiratory syncytial virus; respiratory distress and otitis media; bronchiolitis in two vaccinees; viral gastroenteritis; skull fracture; bronchiolitis, respiratory syncytial virus, and pneumonia; respiratory syncytial virus and bronchiolitis; and upper respiratory infection, viral (see CLINICAL PHARMACOLOGY). A causal relationship to the vaccine is unknown; however, these serious events were judged not to be related to vaccination with COMVAX by the investigator.
In a group of infants (n=126) given a three-dose course of COMVAX after previously receiving a dose of Hepatitis B Vaccine (Recombinant) at or shortly after birth, the type, frequency, and severity of adverse experiences did not appear to be greater or different from those observed in infants given only COMVAX.
Post-Marketing Experience
As with any vaccine, there is the possibility that broad use of COMVAX could reveal adverse experiences not observed in clinical trials. The following additional adverse reaction has been reported with use of the marketed vaccine.
Hypersensitivity
Angioedema
Potential Adverse Effects
In addition, a variety of adverse effects have been reported with marketed use of either PedvaxHIB or RECOMBIVAX HB in infants and children through 71 months of age. These adverse effects are listed below.
PedvaxHIB
Hematologic/Lymphatic
Lymphadenopathy
Nervous System
Febrile seizures
Skin
Sterile injection-site abscess; pain at the injection site
RECOMBIVAX HB
Hypersensitivity
Anaphylaxis and symptoms of hypersensitivity including reports of rash, pruritus, urticaria, edema, arthralgia, dyspnea, hypotension, erythema multiforme, and ecchymoses
Cardiovascular System
Tachycardia; syncope
Digestive System
Elevation of liver enzymes
Hematologic
Increased erythrocyte sedimentation rate; thrombocytopenia
Musculoskeletal System
Arthritis
Nervous System
Bell's Palsy; Guillain-Barré Syndrome
Psychiatric/Behavioral
Agitation; somnolence; irritability
Skin
Stevens-Johnson Syndrome; alopecia.
Special Senses
Conjunctivitis; visual disturbances

DOSAGE AND ADMINISTRATION

FOR INTRAMUSCULAR ADMINISTRATION
Do not inject intravenously, intradermally, or subcutaneously.
Recommended Schedule
Infants born of HBsAg negative mothers should be vaccinated with three 0.5 mL doses of COMVAX, ideally at 2, 4, and 12-15 months of age. If the recommended schedule cannot be followed exactly, the interval between the first two doses should be at least two months and the interval between the second and third dose should be as close as possible to eight to eleven months.
Infants born of HBsAg-positive mothers should receive Hepatitis B Immune Globulin and Hepatitis B Vaccine (Recombinant) at birth and should complete the hepatitis B vaccination series given according to a particular schedule (see manufacturer's circular for Hepatitis B Vaccine [Recombinant]).
Infants born of mothers of unknown HBsAg status should receive Hepatitis B Vaccine (Recombinant) at birth and should complete the hepatitis B vaccination series given according to a particular schedule (see manufacturer's circular for Hepatitis B Vaccine [Recombinant]).
The subsequent administration of COMVAX for completion of the hepatitis B vaccination series in infants who were born of HBsAg positive mothers and received HBIG or infants born of mothers of unknown status has not been studied.
COMVAX should not be administered to any infant before the age of 6 weeks.
Modified Schedules
Children previously vaccinated with one or more doses of either hepatitis B vaccine or Haemophilus b conjugate vaccine
Children who receive one dose of hepatitis B vaccine at or shortly after birth may be administered COMVAX on the schedule of 2, 4, and 12–15 months of age. There are no data to support the use of a three-dose series of COMVAX in infants who have previously received more than one dose of hepatitis B vaccine. However, COMVAX may be administered to children otherwise scheduled to receive concurrent RECOMBIVAX HB and PedvaxHIB.
Children not vaccinated according to recommended schedule
Vaccination schedules for children not vaccinated according to the recommended schedule should be considered on an individual basis. The number of doses of a PRP-OMPC-containing product (i.e., COMVAX, PedvaxHIB) depends on the age that vaccination is begun. An infant 2 to 10 months of age should receive three doses of a product containing PRP-OMPC. An infant 11 to 14 months of age should receive two doses of a product containing PRP-OMPC. A child 15 to 71 months of age should receive one dose of a product containing PRP-OMPC. Infants and children, regardless of age, should receive three doses of an HBsAg-containing product.
COMVAX is for intramuscular injection. The *anterolateral thigh* is the recommended site for intramuscular injection in infants. Data suggests that injections given in the buttocks frequently are given into fatty tissue instead of into muscle. Such injections have resulted in a lower seroconversion rate (for hepatitis B vaccine) than was expected.
Injection must be accomplished with a needle long enough to ensure intramuscular deposition of the vaccine. The ACIP has recommended that for intramuscular injections, the needle should be of sufficient length to reach the muscle mass itself. In a clinical trial with COMVAX (see CLINICAL PHARMACOLOGY, *COMVAX,* Table 1) vaccination was accomplished with a needle length of 5/8 inches in accordance with ACIP recommendations in effect at that time. ACIP currently recommends that needles of longer length (7/8 to 1 inch) be used.
The vaccine should be used as supplied; no reconstitution is necessary.
Shake well before withdrawal and use. Thorough agitation is necessary to maintain suspension of the vaccine.
Parenteral drug products should be inspected visually for extraneous particulate matter and discoloration prior to administration whenever solution and container permit. After thorough agitation, COMVAX is a slightly opaque, white suspension.
It is important to use a separate sterile syringe and needle for each patient to prevent transmission of infectious agents from one person to another.

HOW SUPPLIED

No. 4843—COMVAX is supplied as 7.5 mcg Haemophilus b PRP and 5 mcg HBsAg/0.5 mL in a 0.5 mL single dose vial.
NDC 0006-4843-00.
No. 4898—COMVAX is supplied as 7.5 mcg Haemophilus b PRP and 5 mcg HBsAg/0.5 mL in a 0.5 mL single dose vial, in a box of 10 single dose vials.
NDC 0006-4898-00.
Storage
Store vaccine at 2–8°C (36–46°F). Storage above or below the recommended temperature may reduce potency.
DO NOT FREEZE since freezing destroys potency.
9024702 Issued September 1999

CORTONE® Acetate Injectable Suspension ℞
(Cortisone Acetate)
(Formerly called Sterile Suspension CORTONE® Acetate)

For intramuscular injection only
NOT FOR INTRAVENOUS USE

DESCRIPTION

Cortisone acetate, a synthetic adrenocortical steroid, is a white or practically white, odorless, crystalline powder. It is stable in air. It is insoluble in water. The molecular weight is 402.49. It is designated chemically as 21-(acetyloxy)-17-

Continued on next page

Information on the Merck & Co., Inc. products listed on these pages is the full prescribing information from product circulars in use September 30, 2000. For information, please call 1-800-NSC MERCK [1-800-672-6372].

Cortone Acetate Injectable—Cont.

hydroxypregn-4-ene-3,11,20-trione. The empirical formula is $C_{23}H_{30}O_6$ and the structural formula is:

O
CH2OCCH3
C=O
CH3 ---OH
O
CH3
O

CORTONE* Acetate (Cortisone Acetate) Injectable Suspension is a sterile suspension containing 50 mg per milliliter of cortisone acetate in an aqueous medium (pH 5.0 to 7.0). Inactive ingredients per mL: sodium chloride, 9 mg; polysorbate 80, 4 mg; sodium carboxymethylcellulose, 5 mg; Water for Injection q.s. 1 mL. Benzyl alcohol, 9 mg, added as preservative.
No attempt should be made to alter CORTONE Acetate Injectable Suspension. Diluting it or mixing it with other substances may affect the state of suspension or change the rate of absorption and reduce its effectiveness.

---

*Registered trademark of MERCK & CO., INC.

ACTIONS

CORTONE Acetate Injectable Suspension has a slow onset but long duration of action when compared with more soluble preparations. When daily corticosteroid therapy is required and oral therapy is not feasible, the required daily dosage may be given in a single intramuscular injection of this preparation.
Naturally occurring glucocorticoids (hydrocortisone and cortisone), which also have salt-retaining properties, are used as replacement therapy in adrenocortical deficiency states. They are also used for their potent anti-inflammatory effects in disorders of many organ systems.
Glucocorticoids cause profound and varied metabolic effects. In addition, they modify the body's immune responses to diverse stimuli.

INDICATIONS

When oral therapy is not feasible:
1. *Endocrine disorders*
Primary or secondary adrenocortical insufficiency (hydrocortisone or cortisone is the drug of choice; synthetic analogs may be used in conjunction with mineralocorticoids where applicable; in infancy, mineralocorticoid supplementation is of particular importance)
Acute adrenocortical insufficiency (hydrocortisone or cortisone is the drug of choice; mineralocorticoid supplementation may be necessary, particularly when synthetic analogs are used)
Preoperatively, and in the event of serious trauma or illness, in patients with known adrenal insufficiency or when adrenocortical reserve is doubtful
Shock unresponsive to conventional therapy if adrenocortical insufficiency exists or is suspected
  Congenital adrenal hyperplasia
  Nonsuppurative thyroiditis
  Hypercalcemia associated with cancer
2. *Rheumatic disorders*
As adjunctive therapy for short-term administration (to tide the patient over an acute episode or exacerbation) in:
  Post-traumatic osteoarthritis
  Synovitis of osteoarthritis
  Rheumatoid arthritis, including juvenile rheumatoid arthritis (selected cases may require low-dose maintenance therapy)
  Acute and subacute bursitis
  Epicondylitis
  Acute nonspecific tenosynovitis
  Acute gouty arthritis
  Psoriatic arthritis
  Ankylosing spondylitis
3. *Collagen diseases*
During an exacerbation or as maintenance therapy in selected cases of:
  Systemic lupus erythematosus
  Acute rheumatic carditis
  Systemic dermatomyositis (polymyositis)
4. *Dermatologic diseases*
  Pemphigus
  Severe erythema multiforme (Stevens-Johnson syndrome)
  Exfoliative dermatitis
  Bullous dermatitis herpetiformis
  Severe seborrheic dermatitis
  Severe psoriasis
  Mycosis fungoides
5. *Allergic states*
Control of severe or incapacitating allergic conditions intractable to adequate trials of conventional treatment in:
  Bronchial asthma
  Contact dermatitis
  Atopic dermatitis
  Serum sickness
  Seasonal or perennial allergic rhinitis
  Drug hypersensitivity reactions
  Urticarial transfusion reactions
  Acute noninfectious laryngeal edema (epinephrine is the drug of first choice)
6. *Ophthalmic diseases*
Severe acute and chronic allergic and inflammatory processes involving the eye, such as:
  Herpes zoster ophthalmicus
  Iritis, iridocyclitis
  Chorioretinitis
  Diffuse posterior uveitis and choroiditis
  Optic neuritis
  Sympathetic ophthalmia
  Anterior segment inflammation
  Allergic conjunctivitis
  Keratitis
  Allergic corneal marginal ulcers
7. *Gastrointestinal diseases*
To tide the patient over a critical period of the disease in:
  Ulcerative colitis (Systemic therapy)
  Regional enteritis (Systemic therapy)
8. *Respiratory diseases*
  Symptomatic sarcoidosis
  Berylliosis
  Fulminating or disseminated pulmonary tuberculosis when used concurrently with appropriate antituberculous chemotherapy
  Loeffler's syndrome not manageable by other means
  Aspiration pneumonitis
9. *Hematologic disorders*
  Acquired (autoimmune) hemolytic anemia
  Erythroblastopenia (RBC anemia)
  Congenital (erythroid) hypoplastic anemia
10. *Neoplastic diseases*
  For palliative management of:
  Leukemias and lymphomas in adults
  Acute leukemia of childhood
11. *Edematous states*
  To induce diuresis or remission of proteinuria in the nephrotic syndrome, without uremia, of the idiopathic type, or that due to lupus erythematosus
12. *Miscellaneous*
  Tuberculous meningitis with subarachnoid block or impending block when used concurrently with appropriate antituberculous chemotherapy
  Trichinosis with neurologic or myocardial involvement.

CONTRAINDICATIONS

Systemic fungal infections
Hypersensitivity to any component of this product

WARNINGS

Because rare instances of anaphylactoid reactions have occurred in patients receiving parenteral corticosteroid therapy, appropriate precautionary measures should be taken prior to administration, especially when the patient has a history of allergy to any drug. Anaphylactoid and hypersensitivity reactions have been reported for CORTONE Acetate Injectable Suspension (see ADVERSE REACTIONS).
In patients on corticosteroid therapy subjected to any unusual stress, increased dosage of rapidly acting corticosteroids before, during, and after the stressful situation is indicated.
Drug-induced secondary adrenocortical insufficiency may result from too rapid withdrawal of corticosteroids and may be minimized by gradual reduction of dosage. This type of relative insufficiency may persist for months after discontinuation of therapy; therefore, in any situation of stress occurring during that period, hormone therapy should be reinstituted. If the patient is receiving steroids already, dosage may have to be increased. Since mineralocorticoid secretion may be impaired, salt and/or a mineralocorticoid should be administered concurrently.
Corticosteroids may mask some signs of infection, and new infections may appear during their use. There may be decreased resistance and inability to localize infection when corticosteroids are used. Moreover, corticosteroids may affect the nitroblue-tetrazolium test for bacterial infection and produce false negative results.
In cerebral malaria, a double-blind trial has shown that the use of corticosteroids is associated with prolongation of coma and a higher incidence of pneumonia and gastrointestinal bleeding.
Corticosteroids may activate latent amebiasis. Therefore, it is recommended that latent or active amebiasis be ruled out before initiating corticosteroid therapy in any patient who has spent time in the tropics or any patient with unexplained diarrhea.
Prolonged use of corticosteroids may produce posterior subcapsular cataracts, glaucoma with possible damage to the optic nerves, and may enhance the establishment of secondary ocular infections due to fungi or viruses.
Usage in pregnancy. Since adequate human reproduction studies have not been done with corticosteroids, use of these drugs in pregnancy or in women of childbearing potential requires that the anticipated benefits be weighed against the possible hazards to the mother and embryo or fetus. Infants born of mothers who have received substantial doses of corticosteroids during pregnancy should be carefully observed for signs of hypoadrenalism.
Corticosteroids appear in breast milk and could suppress growth, interfere with endogenous corticosteroid production, or cause other unwanted effects. Mothers taking pharmacologic doses of corticosteroids should be advised not to nurse.
Average and large doses of cortisone or hydrocortisone can cause elevation of blood pressure, salt and water retention, and increased excretion of potassium. These effects are less likely to occur with the synthetic derivatives except when used in large doses. Dietary salt restriction and potassium supplementation may be necessary. All corticosteroids increase calcium excretion.
Administration of live virus vaccines, including smallpox, is contraindicated in individuals receiving immunosuppressive doses of corticosteroids. If inactivated viral or bacterial vaccines are administered to individuals receiving immunosuppressive doses of corticosteroids, the expected serum antibody response may not be obtained.
Patients who are on drugs which suppress the immune system are more susceptible to infections than healthy individuals. Chickenpox and measles, for example, can have a more serious or even fatal course in non-immune patients on corticosteroids. In such patients who have not had these diseases, particular care should be taken to avoid exposure. The risk of developing a disseminated infection varies among individuals and can be related to the dose, route and duration of corticosteroid administration as well as to the underlying disease. If exposed to chickenpox, prophylaxis with varicella zoster immune globulin (VZIG) may be indicated. If chickenpox develops, treatment with antiviral agents may be considered. If exposed to measles, prophylaxis with immune globulin (IG) may be indicated. (See the respective package inserts for VZIG and IG for complete prescribing information.)
Similarly, corticosteroids should be used with great care in patients with known or suspected Strongyloides (threadworm) infestation. In such patients, corticosteroid-induced immunosuppression may lead to Strongyloides hyperinfection and dissemination with widespread larval migration, often accompanied by severe enterocolitis and potentially fatal gram-negative septicemia.
The use of CORTONE Acetate Injectable Suspension in active tuberculosis should be restricted to those cases of fulminating or disseminated tuberculosis in which the corticosteroid is used for the management of the disease in conjunction with an appropriate antituberculous regimen.
If corticosteroids are indicated in patients with latent tuberculosis or tuberculin reactivity, close observation is necessary as reactivation of the disease may occur. During prolonged corticosteroid therapy, these patients should receive chemoprophylaxis.
Literature reports suggest an apparent association between use of corticosteroids and left ventricular free wall rupture after a recent myocardial infarction; therefore, therapy with corticosteroids should be used with great caution in these patients.

PRECAUTIONS

CORTONE Acetate Injectable Suspension, like many other steroid formulations, is sensitive to heat. Therefore, it should not be autoclaved when it is desirable to sterilize the exterior of the vial.
Following prolonged therapy, withdrawal of corticosteroids may result in symptoms of the corticosteroid withdrawal syndrome including fever, myalgia, arthralgia, and malaise. This may occur in patients even without evidence of adrenal insufficiency.
There is an enhanced effect of corticosteroids in patients with hypothyroidism and in those with cirrhosis.
Corticosteroids should be used cautiously in patients with ocular herpes simplex for fear of corneal perforation.
The lowest possible dose of corticosteroid should be used to control the condition under treatment, and when reduction in dosage is possible, the reduction must be gradual.
Psychic derangements may appear when corticosteroids are used, ranging from euphoria, insomnia, mood swings, personality changes, and severe depression to frank psychotic manifestations. Also, existing emotional instability or psychotic tendencies may be aggravated by corticosteroids.
Aspirin should be used cautiously in conjunction with corticosteroids in hypoprothrombinemia.
Steroids should be used with caution in nonspecific ulcerative colitis, if there is a probability of impending perforation, abscess, or other pyogenic infection, also in diverticulitis, fresh intestinal anastomoses, active or latent peptic ulcer, renal insufficiency, hypertension, osteoporosis, and myasthenia gravis. Signs of peritoneal irritation following gastrointestinal perforation in patients receiving large doses of corticosteroids may be minimal or absent. Fat embolism has been reported as a possible complication of hypercortisonism.
When large doses are given, some authorities advise that antacids be administered between meals to help to prevent peptic ulcer.
Steroids may increase or decrease motility and number of spermatozoa in some patients.
Phenytoin, phenobarbital, ephedrine, and rifampin may enhance the metabolic clearance of corticosteroids, resulting in decreased blood levels and lessened physiologic activity, thus requiring adjustment in corticosteroid dosage.

The prothrombin time should be checked frequently in patients who are receiving corticosteroids and coumarin anticoagulants at the same time because of reports that corticosteroids have altered the response to these anticoagulants. Studies have shown that the usual effect produced by adding corticosteroids is inhibition of response to coumarins, although there have been some conflicting reports of potentiation not substantiated by studies.
When corticosteroids are administered concomitantly with potassium-depleting diuretics, patients should be observed closely for development of hypokalemia.
Injection of a steroid into an infected site is to be avoided.
Information for Patients
Susceptible patients who are on immunosuppressant doses of corticosteroids should be warned to avoid exposure to chickenpox or measles. Patients should also be advised that if they are exposed, medical advice should be sought without delay.
Pediatric Use
Growth and development of pediatric patients on prolonged corticosteroid therapy should be carefully followed.

ADVERSE REACTIONS

Fluid and electrolyte disturbances
Sodium retention
Fluid retention
Congestive heart failure in susceptible patients
Potassium loss
Hypokalemic alkalosis
Hypertension
Musculoskeletal
Muscle weakness
Steroid myopathy
Loss of muscle mass
Osteoporosis
Vertebral compression fractures
Aseptic necrosis of femoral and humeral heads
Pathologic fracture of long bones
Tendon rupture
Gastrointestinal
Peptic ulcer with possible subsequent perforation and hemorrhage
Perforation of the small and large bowel, particularly in patients with inflammatory bowel disease
Pancreatitis
Abdominal distention
Ulcerative esophagitis
Dermatologic
Impaired wound healing
Thin fragile skin
Petechiae and ecchymoses
Erythema
Increased sweating
May suppress reactions to skin tests
Other cutaneous reactions, such as allergic dermatitis, urticaria, angioneurotic edema
Neurologic
Convulsions
Increased intracranial pressure with papilledema (pseudotumor cerebri) usually after treatment
Vertigo
Headache
Psychic disturbances
Endocrine
Menstrual irregularities
Development of cushingoid state
Suppression of growth in children
Secondary adrenocortical and pituitary unresponsiveness, particularly in times of stress, as in trauma, surgery, or illness
Decreased carbohydrate tolerance
Manifestations of latent diabetes mellitus
Increased requirements for insulin or oral hypoglycemic agents in diabetics
Hirsutism
Ophthalmic
Posterior subcapsular cataracts
Increased intraocular pressure
Glaucoma
Exophthalmos
Metabolic
Negative nitrogen balance due to protein catabolism
Cardiovascular
Myocardial rupture following recent myocardial infarction (see WARNINGS)
Other
Anaphylactoid or hypersensitivity reactions
Thromboembolism
Weight gain
Increased appetite
Nausea
Malaise
The following *additional* adverse reactions are related to parenteral corticosteroid therapy:
Rare instances of blindness associated with intralesional therapy around the face and head
Hyperpigmentation or hypopigmentation
Subcutaneous and cutaneous atrophy
Sterile abscess

OVERDOSAGE

Reports of acute toxicity and/or death following overdosage of glucocorticoids are rare. In the event of overdosage, no specific antidote is available; treatment is supportive and symptomatic.
The intraperitoneal LD_{50} of cortisone acetate in female mice was 1405 mg/kg.

DOSAGE AND ADMINISTRATION

NOT FOR INTRAVENOUS USE
For intramuscular injection only
DOSAGE REQUIREMENTS ARE VARIABLE AND MUST BE INDIVIDUALIZED ON THE BASIS OF THE DISEASE AND THE RESPONSE OF THE PATIENT.
The initial dosage varies from 20 to 300 mg a day depending on the disease being treated. In less severe diseases doses lower than 20 mg may suffice, while in severe diseases doses higher than 300 mg may be required. The initial dosage should be maintained or adjusted until the patient's response is satisfactory. If a satisfactory clinical response does not occur after a reasonable period of time, discontinue CORTONE Acetate Injectable Suspension and transfer the patient to other therapy.
After a favorable initial response, the proper maintenance dosage should be determined by decreasing the initial dosage in small amounts to the lowest dosage that maintains an adequate clinical response.
Patients should be observed closely for signs that might require dosage adjustment, including changes in clinical status resulting from remissions or exacerbations of the disease, individual drug responsiveness, and the effect of stress (e.g., surgery, infection, trauma). During stress it may be necessary to increase dosage temporarily.
If the drug is to be stopped after more than a few days of treatment, it usually should be withdrawn gradually.

HOW SUPPLIED

No. 7069—CORTONE Acetate Injectable Suspension is a white, mobile suspension, each mL containing 50 mg cortisone acetate, and is supplied as follows:
NDC 0006-7069-10 in 10 mL vials.
Storage
Sensitive to heat. Do not autoclave.
Protect from freezing.
7411918 Issued February 1997

CORTONE® Acetate Tablets ℞
(Cortisone Acetate)

DESCRIPTION

Glucocorticoids are adrenocortical steroids, both naturally occurring and synthetic, which are readily absorbed from the gastrointestinal tract.
Cortisone acetate is a white or practically white, odorless, crystalline powder. It is stable in air. It is insoluble in water. The molecular weight is 402.49. It is designated chemically as 21-(acetyloxy)-17-hydroxypregn-4-ene-3,11,20-trione. The empirical formula is $C_{23}H_{30}O_6$ and the structural formula is:

CH₂OCCH₃ ... C=O ... CH₃ ---OH ... CH₃

CORTONE* Acetate (Cortisone Acetate) tablets contain 25 mg of cortisone acetate in each tablet.
Inactive ingredients are lactose, magnesium stearate, and starch.

*Registered trademark of MERCK & CO., INC.

ACTIONS

Naturally occurring glucocorticoids (hydrocortisone and cortisone), which also have salt-retaining properties, are used as replacement therapy in adrenocortical deficiency states. They are also used for their potent anti-inflammatory effects in disorders of many organ systems.
Glucocorticoids cause profound and varied metabolic effects. In addition, they modify the body's immune responses to diverse stimuli.

INDICATIONS
1. *Endocrine Disorders*
Primary or secondary adrenocortical insufficiency (hydrocortisone or cortisone is the first choice; synthetic analogs may be used in conjunction with mineralocorticoids where applicable; in infancy mineralocorticoid supplementation is of particular importance).
Congenital adrenal hyperplasia
Nonsuppurative thyroiditis
Hypercalcemia associated with cancer
2. *Rheumatic Disorders*
As adjunctive therapy for short-term administration (to tide the patient over an acute episode or exacerbation) in:
Psoriatic arthritis
Rheumatoid arthritis, including juvenile rheumatoid arthritis (selected cases may require low-dose maintenance therapy)
Ankylosing spondylitis
Acute and subacute bursitis
Acute nonspecific tenosynovitis
Acute gouty arthritis
Post-traumatic osteoarthritis
Synovitis of osteoarthritis
Epicondylitis
3. *Collagen Diseases*
During an exacerbation or as maintenance therapy in selected cases of—
Systemic lupus erythematosus
Acute rheumatic carditis
Systemic dermatomyositis (polymyositis)
4. *Dermatologic Diseases*
Pemphigus
Bullous dermatitis herpetiformis
Severe erythema multiforme (Stevens-Johnson syndrome)
Exfoliative dermatitis
Mycosis fungoides
Severe psoriasis
Severe seborrheic dermatitis
5. *Allergic States*
Control of severe or incapacitating allergic conditions intractable to adequate trials of conventional treatment:
Seasonal or perennial allergic rhinitis
Bronchial asthma
Contact dermatitis
Atopic dermatitis
Serum sickness
Drug hypersensitivity reactions
6. *Ophthalmic Diseases*
Severe acute and chronic allergic and inflammatory processes involving the eye and its adnexa, such as—
Allergic conjunctivitis
Keratitis
Allergic corneal marginal ulcers
Herpes zoster ophthalmicus
Iritis and iridocyclitis
Chorioretinitis
Anterior segment inflammation
Diffuse posterior uveitis and choroiditis
Optic neuritis
Sympathetic ophthalmia
7. *Respiratory Diseases*
Symptomatic sarcoidosis
Loeffler's syndrome not manageable by other means
Berylliosis
Fulminating or disseminated pulmonary tuberculosis when used concurrently with appropriate antituberculous chemotherapy
Aspiration pneumonitis
8. *Hematologic Disorders*
Idiopathic thrombocytopenic purpura in adults
Secondary thrombocytopenia in adults
Acquired (autoimmune) hemolytic anemia
Erythroblastopenia (RBC anemia)
Congenital (erythroid) hypoplastic anemia
9. *Neoplastic Diseases*
For palliative management of:
Leukemias and lymphomas in adults
Acute leukemia of childhood
10. *Edematous States*
To induce a diuresis or remission of proteinuria in the nephrotic syndrome, without uremia, of the idiopathic type or that due to lupus erythematosus
11. *Gastrointestinal Diseases*
To tide the patient over a critical period of the disease in:
Ulcerative colitis
Regional enteritis
12. *Miscellaneous*
Tuberculous meningitis with subarachnoid block or impending block when used concurrently with appropriate antituberculous chemotherapy
Trichinosis with neurologic or myocardial involvement

CONTRAINDICATIONS

Systemic fungal infections
Hypersensitivity to this product

WARNINGS

In patients on corticosteroid therapy subjected to unusual stress, increased dosage of rapidly acting corticosteroids before, during, and after the stressful situation is indicated.

Continued on next page

Information on the Merck & Co., Inc. products listed on these pages is the full prescribing information from product circulars in use September 30, 2000. For information, please call 1-800-NSC MERCK [1-800-672-6372].

Cortone Acetate Tablets—Cont.

Drug-induced secondary adrenocortical insufficiency may result from too rapid withdrawal of corticosteroids and may be minimized by gradual reduction of dosage. This type of relative insufficiency may persist for months after discontinuation of therapy; therefore, in any situation of stress occurring during that period, hormone therapy should be reinstituted. If the patient is receiving steroids already, dosage may have to be increased. Since mineralocorticoid secretion may be impaired, salt and/or a mineralocorticoid should be administered concurrently.
Corticosteroids may mask some signs of infection, and new infections may appear during their use. There may be decreased resistance and inability to localize infection when corticosteroids are used. Moreover, corticosteroids may affect the nitroblue-tetrazolium test for bacterial infection and produce false negative results.
In cerebral malaria, a double-blind trial has shown that the use of corticosteroids is associated with prolongation of coma and a higher incidence of pneumonia and gastrointestinal bleeding.
Corticosteroids may activate latent amebiasis. Therefore, it is recommended that latent or active amebiasis be ruled out before initiating corticosteroid therapy in any patient who has spent time in the tropics or any patient with unexplained diarrhea.
Prolonged use of corticosteroids may produce posterior subcapsular cataracts, glaucoma with possible damage to the optic nerves, and may enhance the establishment of secondary ocular infections due to fungi or viruses.
Usage in pregnancy: Since adequate human reproduction studies have not been done with corticosteroids, use of these drugs in pregnancy or in women of childbearing potential requires that the anticipated benefits be weighed against the possible hazards to the mother and embryo or fetus. Infants born of mothers who have received substantial doses of corticosteroids during pregnancy should be carefully observed for signs of hypoadrenalism.
Corticosteroids appear in breast milk and could suppress growth, interefere with endogenous corticosteroid production, or cause other unwanted effects. Mothers taking pharmacologic doses of corticosteroids should be advised not to nurse.
Average and large doses of hydrocortisone or cortisone can cause elevation of blood pressure, salt and water retention, and increased excretion of potassium. These effects are less likely to occur with the synthetic derivatives except when used in large doses. Dietary salt restriction and potassium supplementation may be necessary. All corticosteroids increase calcium excretion.
Administration of live virus vaccines, including smallpox, is contraindicated in individuals receiving immunosuppressive doses of corticosteroids. If inactivated viral or bacterial vaccines are administered to individuals receiving immunosuppressive doses of corticosteroids, the expected serum antibody response may not be obtained. However, immunization procedures may be undertaken in patients who are receiving corticosteroids as replacement therapy, e.g., for Addison's disease.
Patients who are on drugs which suppress the immune system are more susceptible to infections than healthy individuals. Chickenpox and measles, for example, can have a more serious or even fatal course in non-immune patients on corticosteroids. In such patients who have not had these diseases, particular care should be taken to avoid exposure. The risk of developing a disseminated infection varies among individuals and can be related to the dose, route and duration of corticosteroid administration as well as to the underlying disease. If exposed to chickenpox, prophylaxis with varicella zoster immune globulin (VZIG) may be indicated. If chickenpox develops, treatment with antiviral agents may be considered. If exposed to measles, prophylaxis with immune globulin (IG) may be indicated. (See the respective package inserts for VZIG and IG for complete prescribing information.)
Similarly, corticosteroids should be used with great care in patients with known or suspected Strongyloides (threadworm) infestation. In such patients, corticosteroid-induced immunosuppression may lead to Strongyloides hyperinfection and dissemination with widespread larval migration, often accompanied by severe enterocolitis and potentially fatal gram-negative septicemia.
The use of CORTONE Acetate tablets in active tuberculosis should be restricted to those cases of fulminating or disseminated tuberculosis in which the corticosteroid is used for the management of the disease in conjunction with an appropriate antituberculous regimen.
If corticosteroids are indicated in patients with latent tuberculosis or tuberculin reactivity, close observation is necessary as reactivation of the disease may occur. During prolonged corticosteroid therapy, these patients should receive chemoprophylaxis.
Literature reports suggest an apparent association between use of corticosteroids and left ventricular free wall rupture after a recent myocardial infarction; therefore, therapy with corticosteroids should be used with great caution in these patients.

PRECAUTIONS

Following prolonged therapy, withdrawal of corticosteroids may result in symptoms of the corticosteroid withdrawal syndrome including fever, myalgia, arthralgia, and malaise. This may occur in patients even without evidence of adrenal insufficiency.
There is an enhanced effect of corticosteroids in patients with hypothyroidism and in those with cirrhosis.
Corticosteroids should be used cautiously in patients with ocular herpes simplex because of possible corneal perforation.
The lowest possible dose of corticosteroid should be used to control the condition under treatment, and when reduction in dosage is possible, the reduction should be gradual.
Psychic derangements may appear when corticosteroids are used, ranging from euphoria, insomnia, mood swings, personality changes, and severe depression, to frank psychotic manifestations. Also, existing emotional instability or psychotic tendencies may be aggravated by corticosteroids.
Aspirin should be used cautiously in conjunction with corticosteroids in hypoprothrombinemia.
Steroids should be used with caution in nonspecific ulcerative colitis, if there is a probability of impending perforation, abscess, or other pyogenic infection, diverticulitis, fresh intestinal anastomoses, active or latent peptic ulcer, renal insufficiency, hypertension, osteoporosis, and myasthenia gravis. Signs of peritoneal irritation following gastrointestinal perforation in patients receiving large doses of corticosteroids may be minimal or absent. Fat embolism has been reported as a possible complication of hypercortisonism.
When large doses are given, some authorities advise that corticosteroids be taken with meals and antacids taken between meals to help to prevent peptic ulcer.
Steroids may increase or decrease motility and number of spermatozoa in some patients.
Phenytoin, phenobarbital, ephedrine, and rifampin may enhance the metabolic clearance of corticosteroids, resulting in decreased blood levels and lessened physiologic activity, thus requiring adjustment in corticosteroid dosage.
The prothrombin time should be checked frequently in patients who are receiving corticosteroids and coumarin anticoagulants at the same time because of reports that corticosteroids have altered the response to these anticoagulants. Studies have shown that the usual effect produced by adding corticosteroids is inhibition of response to coumarins, although there have been some conflicting reports of potentiation not substantiated by studies.
When corticosteroids are administered concomitantly with potassium-depleting diuretics, patients should be observed closely for development of hypokalemia.
Information for Patients
Susceptible patients who are on immunosuppressant doses of corticosteroids should be warned to avoid exposure to chickenpox or measles. Patients should also be advised that if they are exposed, medical advice should be sought without delay.
Pediatric Use
Growth and development of pediatric patients on prolonged corticosteroid therapy should be carefully followed.

ADVERSE REACTIONS

Fluid and Electrolyte Disturbances
Sodium retention
Fluid retention
Congestive heart failure in susceptible patients
Potassium loss
Hypokalemic alkalosis
Hypertension
Musculoskeletal
Muscle weakness
Steroid myopathy
Loss of muscle mass
Osteoporosis
Vertebral compression fractures
Aseptic necrosis of femoral and humeral heads
Pathologic fracture of long bones
Tendon rupture
Gastrointestinal
Peptic ulcer with possible perforation and hemorrhage
Perforation of the small and large bowel, particularly in patients with inflammatory bowel disease
Pancreatitis
Abdominal distention
Ulcerative esophagitis
Dermatologic
Impaired wound healing
Thin fragile skin
Petechiae and ecchymoses
Erythema
Increased sweating
May suppress reactions to skin tests
Other cutaneous reactions, such as allergic dermatitis, urticaria, angioneurotic edema
Neurologic
Convulsions
Increased intracranial pressure with papilledema (pseudotumor cerebri), usually after treatment
Vertigo
Headache
Psychic disturbances
Endocrine
Menstrual irregularities
Development of cushingoid state
Suppression of growth in children
Secondary adrenocortical and pituitary unresponsiveness, particularly in times of stress, as in trauma, surgery, or illness
Decreased carbohydrate tolerance
Manifestations of latent diabetes mellitus
Increased requirements for insulin or oral hypoglycemic agents in diabetics
Hirsutism
Ophthalmic
Posterior subcapsular cataracts
Increased intraocular pressure
Glaucoma
Exophthalmos
Metabolic
Negative nitrogen balance due to protein catabolism
Cardiovascular
Myocardial rupture following recent myocardial infarction (see WARNINGS)
Other
Hypersensitivity
Thromboembolism
Weight gain
Increased appetite
Nausea
Malaise

OVERDOSAGE

Reports of acute toxicity and/or death following overdosage of glucocorticoids are rare. In the event of overdosage, no specific antidote is available; treatment is supportive and symptomatic.
The intraperitoneal LD_{50} of cortisone acetate in female mice was 1405 mg/kg.

DOSAGE AND ADMINISTRATION

For oral administration
DOSAGE REQUIREMENTS ARE VARIABLE AND MUST BE INDIVIDUALIZED ON THE BASIS OF THE DISEASE AND THE RESPONSE OF THE PATIENT.
The initial dosage varies from 25 to 300 mg a day depending on the disease being treated. In less severe diseases doses lower than 25 mg may suffice, while in severe diseases doses higher than 300 mg may be required. The initial dosage should be maintained or adjusted until the patient's response is satisfactory. If satisfactory clinical response does not occur after a reasonable period of time, discontinue CORTONE Acetate tablets and transfer the patient to other therapy.
After a favorable initial response, the proper maintenance dosage should be determined by decreasing the initial dosage in small amounts to the lowest dosage that maintains an adequate clinical response.
Patients should be observed closely for signs that might require dosage adjustment, including changes in clinical status resulting from remissions or exacerbations of the disease, individual drug responsiveness, and the effect of stress (e.g., surgery, infection, trauma). During stress it may be necessary to increase dosage temporarily.
If the drug is to be stopped after more than a few days of treatment, it usually should be withdrawn gradually.

HOW SUPPLIED

No. 7063—Tablets Cortone Acetate, 25 mg each, are white, round, scored, compressed tablets, coded MSD 219 on one side and CORTONE on the other. They are supplied as follows:
NDC 0006-0219-68 in bottles of 100.

Shown in Product Identification Guide, page 323

7930632 Issued February 1997

COSMEGEN® for Injection ℞
(Dactinomycin for Injection)
(Actinomycin D)

WARNING

Dactinomycin is extremely corrosive to soft tissue. If extravasation occurs during intravenous use, severe damage to soft tissues will occur. In at least one instance, this has led to contracture of the arms.

DOSAGE

The dosage of COSMEGEN* (Dactinomycin for Injection) is calculated in micrograms (mcg). The usual adult dosage is 500 micrograms (0.5 mg) daily intravenously for a maximum of five days. The dosage for adults or children should not exceed 15 mcg/kg or 400–600 mcg/square meter of body surface daily intravenously for five days. Calculation of the dosage for obese or edematous patients should be on the basis of surface area in an effort to relate dosage to lean body mass.

*Registered trademark of MERCK & CO., INC.

DESCRIPTION

Dactinomycin is one of the actinomycins, a group of antibiotics produced by various species of *Streptomyces.* Dactinomycin is the principal component of the mixture of actinomycins produced by *Streptomyces parvullus*. Unlike other species of *Streptomyces*, this organism yields an essentially pure substance that contains only traces of similar compounds differing in the amino acid content of the peptide side chains. The empirical formula is $C_{62}H_{86}N_{12}O_{16}$ and the structural formula is:

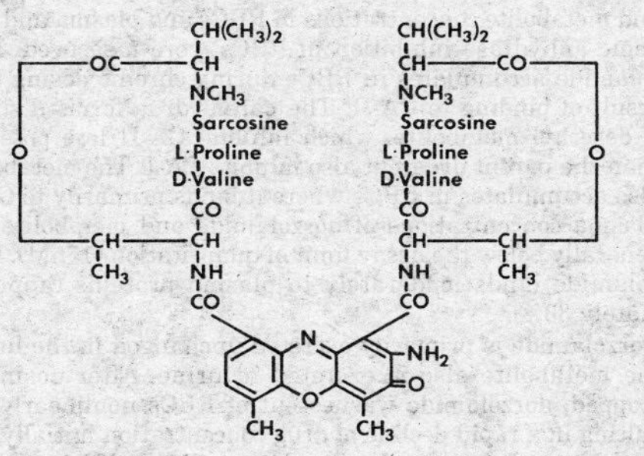

CH(CH3)2 CH(CH3)2
OC—CH CH—CO
NCH3 NCH3
Sarcosine Sarcosine
O L-Proline L-Proline O
D-Valine D-Valine
CO CO
CH—CH CH—CH
CH3 NH NH CH3
CO CO
N NH2
O
CH3 O CH3

COSMEGEN is a sterile, yellow lyophilized powder for injection by the intravenous route or by regional perfusion after reconstitution. Each vial contains 0.5 mg (500 mcg) of dactinomycin and 20.0 mg of mannitol.

CLINICAL PHARMACOLOGY

Action

Generally, the actinomycins exert an inhibitory effect on gram-positive and gram-negative bacteria and on some fungi. However, the toxic properties of the actinomycins (including dactinomycin) in relation to antibacterial activity are such as to preclude their use as antibiotics in the treatment of infectious diseases.

Because the actinomycins are cytotoxic, they have an antineoplastic effect which has been demonstrated in experimental animals with various types of tumor implant. This cytotoxic action is the basis for their use in the palliative treatment of certain types of cancer.

Pharmacokinetics and Metabolism

Results of a study in patients with malignant melanoma indicate that dactinomycin (^3H actinomycin D) is minimally metabolized, is concentrated in nucleated cells, and does not penetrate the blood-brain barrier. Approximately 30% of the dose was recovered in urine and feces in one week. The terminal plasma half-life for radioactivity was approximately 36 hours.

INDICATIONS AND USAGE

Wilms' Tumor

The neoplasm responding most frequently to COSMEGEN is Wilms' tumor. With low doses of both dactinomycin and radiotherapy, temporary objective improvement may be as good as and may last longer than with higher doses of each given alone. In the National Wilms' Tumor study, combination therapy with dactinomycin and vincristine together with surgery and radiotherapy, was shown to have significantly improved the prognosis of patients in groups II and III. Dactinomycin and vincristine were given for a total of seven cycles, so that maintenance therapy continued for approximately 15 months.

Postoperative radiotherapy in group I patients and optimal combination chemotherapy for those in group IV are unsettled issues. About 70 percent of lung metastases have disappeared with an appropriate combination of radiation, dactinomycin and vincristine.

Rhabdomyosarcoma

Temporary regression of the tumor and beneficial subjective results have occurred with dactinomycin in rhabdomyosarcoma which, like most soft tissue sarcomas, is comparatively radio-resistant.

Several groups have reported successful use of cyclophosphamide, vincristine, dactinomycin and doxorubicin hydrochloride in various combinations. Effective combinations have included vincristine and dactinomycin; vincristine, dactinomycin and cyclophosphamide (VAC therapy) and all four drugs in sequence. At present, the most effective treatment for children with inoperable or metastatic rhabdomyosarcoma has been VAC chemotherapy. Two-thirds of these children were doing well without evidence of disease at a median time of three years after diagnosis.

Carcinoma of Testis and Uterus

The sequential use of dactinomycin and methotrexate, along with meticulous monitoring of human chorionic gonadotropin levels until normal, has resulted in survival in the majority of women with metastatic choriocarcinoma. Sequential therapy is used if there is:

1. Stability in gonadotropin titers following two successive courses of an agent.
2. Rising gonadotropin titers during treatment.
3. Severe toxicity preventing adequate therapy.

In patients with nonmetastatic choriocarcinoma, dactinomycin or methotrexate or both, have been used successfully, with or without surgery.

Dactinomycin has been beneficial as a single agent in the treatment of metastatic nonseminomatour testicular carcinoma when used in cycles of 500 mcg/day for five consecutive days, every 6–8 weeks for periods of four months or longer.

Other Neoplasms

Dactinomycin has been given intravenously or by regional perfusion, either alone or with other antineoplastic compounds or x-ray therapy, in the palliative treatment of Ewing's sarcoma and sarcoma botryoides. For nonmetastatic Ewing's sarcoma, promising results were obtained when dactinomycin (45 mcg/m^2) and cyclophosphamide (1200 mg/m^2) were given sequentially and with radiotherapy, over an 18 month period. Those with metastatic disease remain the subject of continued investigation with a more aggressive chemotherapeutic regimen employed initially.

Temporary objective improvement and relief of pain and discomfort have followed the use of dactinomycin usually in conjunction with radiotherapy for sarcoma botryoides. This palliative effect ranges from transitory inhibition of tumor growth to a considerable but temporary regression in tumor size.

COSMEGEN (Dactinomycin for Injection) and Radiation Therapy

Much evidence suggests that dactinomycin potentiates the effects of x-ray therapy. The converse also appears likely; i.e., dactinomycin may be more effective when radiation therapy also is given.

With combined dactinomycin-radiation therapy, the normal skin, as well as the buccal and pharyngeal mucosa, show early erythema. A smaller than usual x-ray dose when given with dactinomycin causes erythema and vesiculation, which progress more rapidly through the stages of tanning and desquamation. Healing may occur in four to six weeks rather than two to three months. Erythema from previous x-ray therapy may be reactivated by dactinomycin alone, even when irradiation occurred many months earlier, and especially when the interval between the two forms of therapy is brief. This potentiation of radiation effect represents a special problem when the irradiation treatment area includes the mucous membrane. When irradiation is directed toward the nasopharynx, the combination may produce severe oropharyngeal mucositis. *Severe reactions may ensue if high doses of both dactinomycin and radiation therapy are used or if the patient is particularly sensitive to such combined therapy.*

Because of this potentiating effect, dactinomycin may be tried in radio-sensitive tumors not responding to doses of x-ray therapy that can be tolerated. Objective improvement in tumor size and activity may be observed when lower, better tolerated doses of both types of therapy are employed.

COSMEGEN (Dactinomycin for Injection) and Perfusion Technic

Dactinomycin alone or with other antineoplastic agents has also been given by the isolation-perfusion technic, either as palliative treatment or as an adjunct to resection of a tumor. Some tumors considered resistant to chemotherapy and radiation therapy may respond when the drug is given by the perfusion technic. Neoplasms in which dactinomycin has been tried by this technic include various types of sarcoma, carcinoma, and adenocarcinoma.

In some instances tumors regressed, pain was relieved for variable periods, and surgery made possible. On other occasions, however, the outcome has been less favorable. Nevertheless, in selected cases, the drug by perfusion may provide more effective palliation than when given systemically.

Dactinomycin by the isolation-perfusion technic offers certain advantages, provided leakage of the drug through the general circulation into other areas of the body is minimal. By this technic the drug is in continuous contact with the tumor for the duration of treatment. The dose may be increased well over that used by the systemic route, usually without adding to the danger of toxic effects. If the agent is confined to an isolated part, it should not interfere with the patient's defense mechanism. Systemic absorption of toxic products from neoplastic tissue can be minimized by removing the perfusate when the procedure is finished.

CONTRAINDICATIONS

If dactinomycin is given at or about the time of infection with chicken pox or herpes zoster, a severe generalized disease, which may result in death, may occur.

PRECAUTIONS

General

COSMEGEN should be administered only under the supervision of a physician who is experienced in the use of cancer chemotherapeutic agents.

This drug is highly toxic and both powder and solution must be handled and administered with care. Inhalation of dust or vapors and contact with skin or mucous membranes, especially those of the eyes, must be avoided. Should accidental eye contact occur, copious irrigation with water should be instituted immediately, followed by prompt ophthalmologic consultation. Should accidental skin contact occur, the affected part must be irrigated immediately with copious amounts of water for at least 15 minutes.

As with all antineoplastic agents, dactinomycin is a toxic drug and very careful and frequent observation of the patient for adverse reactions is necessary. These reactions may involve any tissue of the body. The possibility of an anaphylactoid reaction should be borne in mind.

Increased incidence of gastrointestinal toxicity and marrow suppression has been reported when dactinomycin was given with x-ray therapy.

Particular caution is necessary when administering dactinomycin within two months of irradiation for the treatment of right-sided Wilms' tumor, since hepatomegaly and elevated SGOT levels have been noted.

Nausea and vomiting due to dactinomycin make it necessary to give this drug intermittently. It is extremely important to observe the patient daily for toxic side effects when multiple chemotherapy is employed, since a full course of therapy occasionally is not tolerated. If stomatitis, diarrhea, or severe hemopoietic depression appear during therapy, these drugs should be discontinued until the patient has recovered.

Recent reports indicate an increased incidence of second primary tumors following treatment with radiation and antineoplastic agents, such as dactinomycin. Multi-modal therapy creates the need for careful, long-term observation of cancer survivors.

Laboratory Tests

Many abnormalities of renal, hepatic, and bone marrow function have been reported in patients with neoplastic disease and receiving dactinomycin. It is advisable to check renal, hepatic, and bone marrow functions frequently.

Drug/Laboratory Test Interactions

It has been reported that dactinomycin may interfere with bioassay procedures for the determination of antibacterial drug levels.

Carcinogenesis, Mutagenesis, Impairment of Fertility

The International Agency on Research on Cancer has judged that dactinomycin is a positive carcinogen in animals. Local sarcomas were produced in mice and rats after repeated subcutaneous or intraperitoneal injection. Mesenchymal tumors occurred in male F344 rats given intraperitoneal injections of 0.05 mg/kg, 2 to 5 times per week for 18 weeks. The first tumor appeared at 23 weeks.

Dactinomycin has been shown to be mutagenic in a number of test systems *in vitro* and *in vivo* including human fibroblasts and leucocytes, and HELA cells. DNA damage and cytogenetic effects have been demonstrated in the mouse and the rat.

Adequate fertility studies have not been reported.

Pregnancy

Pregnancy Category C.

COSMEGEN has been shown to cause malformations and embryotoxicity in the rat, rabbit and hamster when given in doses of 50–100 mcg/kg intravenously (3–7 times the maximum recommended human dose). There are no adequate and well-controlled studies in pregnant women. COSMEGEN should be used during pregnancy only if the potential benefit justifies the potential risk to the fetus.

Nursing Mothers

It is not known whether this drug is excreted in human milk. Because many drugs are excreted in human milk and because of the potential for serious adverse reactions in nursing infants from COSMEGEN, a decision should be made whether to discontinue nursing or to discontinue the drug, taking into account the importance of the drug to the mother.

Pediatric Use

The greater frequency of toxic effects of dactinomycin in infants suggest that this drug should be given to infants only over the age of 6 to 12 months.

ADVERSE REACTIONS

Toxic effects (excepting nausea and vomiting) usually do not become apparent until two to four days after a course of therapy is stopped, and may not be maximal before one to two weeks have elapsed. Deaths have been reported. However, adverse reactions are usually reversible on discontinuance of therapy. They include the following:

Miscellaneous: malaise, fatigue, lethargy, fever, myalgia, proctitis, hypocalcemia.

Oral: cheilitis, dysphagia, esophagitis, ulcerative stomatitis, pharyngitis.

Gastrointestinal: anorexia, nausea, vomiting, abdominal pain, diarrhea, gastrointestinal ulceration, liver toxicity including ascites, hepatomegaly, hepatitis, and liver function test abnormalities. Nausea and vomiting, which occur early during the first few hours after administration, may be alleviated by giving antiemetics.

Hematologic: anemia, even to the point of aplastic anemia, agranulocytosis, leukopenia, thrombopenia, pancytopenia, reticulopenia. Platelet and white cell counts should be done *daily* to detect severe hemopoietic depression. If either count markedly decreases, the drug should be withheld to allow marrow recovery. This often takes up to three weeks.

Dermatologic: alopecia, skin eruptions, acne, flare-up of erythema or increased pigmentation of previously irradiated skin.

Soft tissues. Dactinomycin is extremely corrosive. If extravasation occurs during intravenous use, severe damage to soft tissues will occur. In at least one instance, this has led to contracture of the arms.

Continued on next page

Information on the Merck & Co., Inc. products listed on these pages is the full prescribing information from product circulars in use September 30, 2000. For information, please call 1-800-NSC MERCK [1-800-672-6372].

Cosmegen—Cont.

OVERDOSAGE

The intravenous LD_{50} of COSMEGEN in the rat is 460 mcg/kg.

DOSAGE AND ADMINISTRATION

Toxic reactions due to dactinomycin are frequent and may be severe (see ADVERSE REACTIONS), thus limiting in many instances the amount that may be given. However, the severity of toxicity varies markedly and is only partly dependent on the dose employed. The drug must be given in short courses.

Intravenous Use

The dosage of dactinomycin varies depending on the tolerance of the patient, the size and location of the neoplasm, and the use of other forms of therapy. It may be necessary to decrease the usual dosages suggested below when other chemotherapy or x-ray therapy is used concomitantly or has been used previously.

The dosage for adults or children should not exceed 15 mcg/kg or 400–600 mcg/square meter of body surface daily intravenously for five days. Calculation of the dosage for obese or edematous patients should be on the basis of surface area in an effort to relate dosage to lean body mass.

Adults: The usual adult dosage is 500 mcg (0.5 mg) daily intravenously for a maximum of five days.

Children: In children 15 mcg (0.015 mg) per kilogram of body weight is given intravenously daily for five days. An alternative schedule is a total dosage of 2500 mcg (2.5 mg) per square meter of body surface given intravenously over a one week period.

In both adults and children, a second course may be given after at least three weeks have elapsed, provided all signs of toxicity have disappeared.

Reconstitute COSMEGEN by adding 1.1 ml of **Sterile Water for Injection (without preservative)** using aseptic precautions. The resulting solution of dactinomycin will contain approximately 500 mcg (0.5 mg) per mL.

Parenteral drug products should be inspected visually for particulate matter and discoloration prior to administration, whenever solution and container permit. When reconstituted, COSMEGEN is a clear, gold-colored solution.

Once reconstituted, the solution of dactinomycin can be added to infusion solutions of Dextrose Injection 5 percent or Sodium Chloride Injection either directly or to the tubing of a running intravenous infusion.

Although reconstituted COSMEGEN is chemically stable, the product does not contain a preservative and accidental microbial contamination might result. Any unused portion should be discarded. Use of water containing preservatives (benzyl alcohol or parabens) to reconstitute COSMEGEN for Injection, results in the formation of a precipitate.

Partial removal of dactinomycin from intravenous solutions by cellulose ester membrane filters used in some intravenous in-line filters has been reported.

Since dactinomycin is extremely corrosive to soft tissue, precautions for materials of this nature should be observed.

If the drug is given directly into the vein without the use of an infusion, the "two-needle technic" should be used. Reconstitute and withdraw the calculated dose from the vial with one sterile needle. Use another sterile needle for direct injection into the vein.

Discard any unused portion of the dactinomycin solution.

Isolation-Perfusion Technic

The dosage schedules and the technic itself vary from one investigator to another; the published literature, therefore, should be consulted for details. In general, the following doses are suggested:

50 mcg (0.05 mg) per kilogram of body weight for lower extremity or pelvis.

35 mcg (0.035 mg) per kilogram of body weight for upper extremity.

It may be advisable to use lower doses in obese patients, or when previous chemotherapy or radiation therapy has been employed.

Complications of the perfusion technic are related mainly to the amount of drug that escapes into the systemic circulation and may consist of hemopoietic depression, absorption of toxic products from massive destruction of neoplastic tissue, increased susceptibility to infection, impaired wound healing, and superficial ulceration of the gastric mucosa. Other side effects may include edema of the extremity involved, damage to soft tissues of the perfused area, and (potentially) venous thrombosis.

HOW SUPPLIED

No. 3298—COSMEGEN for Injection is a lyophilized powder. In the dry form the compound is an amorphous yellow powder. The solution is clear and gold-colored. COSMEGEN for Injection is supplied as follows:

NDC 0006-3298-22 in vials containing 0.5 mg (500 micrograms) of dactinomycin and 20.0 mg of mannitol (6505-00-902-1222, 0.5 mg).

Storage

Store at controlled room temperature, 15–30°C (59–86°F). Protect from light, humidity, and excessive heat.

Special Handling

Due to the drug's toxic and mutagenic properties, appropriate precautions including the use of appropriate safety equipment are recommended for the preparation of COSMEGEN for parenteral administration. The National Institutes of Health presently recommends that the preparation of injectable antineoplastic drugs should be performed in a Class II laminar flow biological safety cabinet and that personnel preparing drugs of this class should wear surgical gloves and a closed front surgical-type gown with knit cuffs.

9000829 Issued February 1997

COSOPT® Sterile Ophthalmic Solution ℞
(dorzolamide hydrochloride-timolol maleate ophthalmic solution)

DESCRIPTION

COSOPT* (dorzolamide hydrochloride-timolol maleate ophthalmic solution) is the combination of a topical carbonic anhydrase inhibitor and a topical beta-adrenergic receptor blocking agent.

Dorzolamide hydrochloride is described chemically as: (4*S-trans*)-4-(ethylamino)-5,6-dihydro-6-methyl-4*H*-thieno[2,3-*b*]thiopyran-2-sulfonamide 7,7-dioxide monohydrochloride. Dorzolamide hydrochloride is optically active. The specific rotation is:

$[\alpha]$ 25°C / 405 nm (C=1, water)=~-17°.

Its empirical formula is $C_{10}H_{16}N_2O_4S_3 \bullet HCl$ and its structural formula is:

Dorzolamide hydrochloride has a molecular weight of 360.91. It is a white to off-white, crystalline powder, which is soluble in water and slightly soluble in methanol and ethanol.

Timolol maleate is described chemically as: (-)-1-(*tert*-butylamino)-3-[(4-morpholino-1,2,5-thiadiazol-3-yl)oxy]-2-propanol maleate (1:1) (salt). Timolol maleate possesses an asymmetric carbon atom in its structure and is provided as the levo-isomer. The nominal optical rotation of timolol maleate is:

$[\alpha]$ 25°C / 405 nm in 1N HCl (C=5)=-12.2° (-11.7° to -12.5°).

Its molecular formula is $C_{13}H_{24}N_4O_3S \bullet C_4H_4O_4$ and its structural formula is:

Timolol maleate has a molecular weight of 432.50. It is a white, odorless, crystalline powder which is soluble in water, methanol, and alcohol. Timolol maleate is stable at room temperature.

COSOPT is supplied as a sterile, isotonic, buffered, slightly viscous, aqueous solution. The pH of the solution is approximately 5.65, and the osmolarity is 242-323 mOsM. Each mL of COSOPT contains 20 mg dorzolamide (22.26 mg of dorzolamide hydrochloride) and 5 mg timolol (6.83 mg timolol maleate). Inactive ingredients are sodium citrate, hydroxyethyl cellulose, sodium hydroxide, mannitol, and water for injection. Benzalkonium chloride 0.0075% is added as a preservative.

*Registered trademark of MERCK & CO., Inc.

CLINICAL PHARMACOLOGY

Mechanism of Action

COSOPT is comprised of two components: dorzolamide hydrochloride and timolol maleate. Each of these two components decreases elevated intraocular pressure, whether or not associated with glaucoma, by reducing aqueous humor secretion. Elevated intraocular pressure is a major risk factor in the pathogenesis of optic nerve damage and glaucomatous visual field loss. The higher the level of intraocular pressure, the greater the likelihood of glaucomatous field loss and optic nerve damage.

Dorzolamide hydrochloride is an inhibitor of human carbonic anhydrase II. Inhibition of carbonic anhydrase in the ciliary processes of the eye decreases aqueous humor secretion, presumably by slowing the formation of bicarbonate ions with subsequent reduction in sodium and fluid transport. Timolol maleate is a $beta_1$ and $beta_2$ (non-selective) adrenergic receptor blocking agent that does not have significant intrinsic sympathomimetic, direct myocardial depressant, or local anesthetic (membrane-stabilizing) activity.

The combined effect of these two agents administered as COSOPT b.i.d. results in additional intraocular pressure reduction compared to either component administered alone, but the reduction is not as much as when dorzolamide t.i.d. and timolol b.i.d. are administered concomitantly (see *Clinical Studies*).

Pharmacokinetics/Pharmacodynamics

Dorzolamide Hydrochloride

When topically applied, dorzolamide reaches the systemic circulation. To assess the potential for systemic carbonic anhydrase inhibition following topical administration, drug and metabolite concentrations in RBCs and plasma and carbonic anhydrase inhibition in RBCs were measured. Dorzolamide accumulates in RBCs during chronic dosing as a result of binding to CA-II. The parent drug forms a single N-desethyl metabolite, which inhibits CA-II less potently than the parent drug but also inhibits CA-I. The metabolite also accumulates in RBCs where it binds primarily to CA-I. Plasma concentrations of dorzolamide and metabolite are generally below the assay limit of quantitation (15nM). Dorzolamide binds moderately to plasma proteins (approximately 33%).

Dorzolamide is primarily excreted unchanged in the urine; the metabolite also is excreted in urine. After dosing is stopped, dorzolamide washes out of RBCs nonlinearly, resulting in a rapid decline of drug concentration initially, followed by a slower elimination phase with a half-life of about four months.

To simulate the systemic exposure after long-term topical ocular administration, dorzolamide was given orally to eight healthy subjects for up to 20 weeks. The oral dose of 2 mg b.i.d. closely approximates the amount of drug delivered by topical ocular administration of dorzolamide 2% t.i.d. Steady state was reached within 8 weeks. The inhibition of CA-II and total carbonic anhydrase activities was below the degree of inhibition anticipated to be necessary for a pharmacological effect on renal function and respiration in healthy individuals.

Timolol Maleate

In a study of plasma drug concentrations in six subjects, the systemic exposure to timolol was determined following twice daily topical administration of timolol maleate ophthalmic solution 0.5%. The mean peak plasma concentration following morning dosing was 0.46 ng/mL.

Clinical Studies

Clinical studies of 3 to 15 months duration were conducted to compare the IOP-lowering effect over the course of the day of COSOPT b.i.d. (dosed morning and bedtime) to individually- and concomitantly-administered 0.5% timolol (b.i.d.) and 2.0% dorzolamide (b.i.d. and t.i.d.). The IOP-lowering effect of COSOPT b.i.d. was greater (1-3 mmHg) than that of monotherapy with either 2.0% dorzolamide t.i.d. or 0.5% timolol b.i.d. The IOP-lowering effect of COSOPT b.i.d. was approximately 1 mmHg less than that of concomitant therapy with 2.0% dorzolamide t.i.d. and 0.5% timolol b.i.d.

Open-label extensions of two studies were conducted for up to 12 months. During this period, the IOP-lowering effect of COSOPT b.i.d. was consistent during the 12 month follow-up period.

INDICATIONS AND USAGE

COSOPT is indicated for the reduction of elevated intraocular pressure in patients with open-angle glaucoma or ocular hypertension who are insufficiently responsive to beta-blockers (failed to achieve target IOP determined after multiple measurements over time). The IOP-lowering of COSOPT b.i.d. was slightly less than that seen with the concomitant administration of 0.5% timolol b.i.d. and 2.0% dorzolamide t.i.d. (see CLINICAL PHARMACOLOGY, *Clinical Studies*).

CONTRAINDICATIONS

COSOPT is contraindicated in patients with (1) bronchial asthma; (2) a history of bronchial asthma; (3) severe chronic obstructive pulmonary disease (see WARNINGS); (4) sinus bradycardia; (5) second or third degree atrioventricular block; (6) overt cardiac failure (see WARNINGS); (7) cardiogenic shock; or (8) hypersensitivity to any component of this product.

WARNINGS

Systemic Exposure

COSOPT contains dorzolamide, a sulfonamide, and timolol maleate, a beta-adrenergic blocking agent; and although administered topically, is absorbed systemically. Therefore, the same types of adverse reactions that are attributable to sulfonamides and/or systemic administration of beta-adrenergic blocking agents may occur with topical administration. For example, severe respiratory reactions and cardiac reactions, including death due to bronchospasm in patients with asthma, and rarely death in association with cardiac failure, have been reported following systemic ophthalmic administration of timolol maleate (see CONTRAINDICATIONS). Fatalities have occurred, although rarely, due to severe reactions to sulfonamides including Stevens-Johnson syndrome, toxic epidermal necrolysis, fulminant hepatic necrosis, agranulocytosis, aplastic anemia, and other blood dyscrasias. Sensitization may recur when a sulfonamide is readministered irrespective of the route of administration. If signs of serious reactions or hypersensitivity occur, discontinue the use of this preparation.

Cardiac Failure
Sympathetic stimulation may be essential for support of the circulation in individuals with diminished myocardial contractility, and its inhibition by beta-adrenergic receptor blockade may precipitate more severe failure.
In Patients Without a History of Cardiac Failure continued depression of the myocardium with beta-blocking agents over a period of time can, in some cases, lead to cardiac failure. At the first sign or symptom of cardiac failure, COSOPT should be discontinued.
Obstructive Pulmonary Disease
Patients with chronic obstructive pulmonary disease (e.g., chronic bronchitis, emphysema) of mild or moderate severity, bronchospastic disease, or a history of bronchospastic disease (other than bronchial asthma or a history of bronchial asthma, in which COSOPT is contraindicated [see CONTRAINDICATIONS]) should, in general, not receive beta-blocking agents, including COSOPT.
Major Surgery
The necessity or desirability of withdrawal of beta-adrenergic blocking agents prior to major surgery is controversial. Beta-adrenergic receptor blockade impairs the ability of the heart to respond to beta-adrenergically mediated reflex stimuli. This may augment the risk of general anesthesia in surgical procedures. Some patients receiving beta-adrenergic receptor blocking agents have experienced protracted severe hypotension during anesthesia. Difficulty in restarting and maintaining the heartbeat has also been reported. For these reasons, in patients undergoing elective surgery, some authorities recommend gradual withdrawal of beta-adrenergic receptor blocking agents.
If necessary during surgery, the effects of beta-adrenergic blocking agents may be reversed by sufficient doses of adrenergic agonists.
Diabetes Mellitus
Beta-adrenergic blocking agents should be administered with caution in patients subject to spontaneous hypoglycemia or to diabetic patients (especially those with labile diabetes) who are receiving insulin or oral hypoglycemic agents. Beta-adrenergic receptor blocking agents may mask the signs and symptoms of acute hypoglycemia.
Thyrotoxicosis
Beta-adrenergic blocking agents may mask certain clinical signs (e.g., tachycardia) of hyperthyroidism. Patients suspected of developing thyrotoxicosis should be managed carefully to avoid abrupt withdrawal of beta-adrenergic blocking agents that might precipitate a thyroid storm.

PRECAUTIONS

General
Dorzolamide has not been studied in patients with severe renal impairment (CrCl < 30 mL/min). Because dorzolamide and its metabolite are excreted predominantly by the kidney, COSOPT is not recommended in such patients.
Dorzolamide has not been studied in patients with hepatic impairment and should therefore be used with caution in such patients.
While taking beta-blockers, patients with a history of atopy or a history of severe anaphylactic reactions to a variety of allergens may be more reactive to repeated accidental, diagnostic, or therapeutic challenge with such allergens. Such patients may be unresponsive to the usual doses of epinephrine used to treat anaphylactic reactions.
In clinical studies, local ocular adverse effects, primarily conjunctivitis and lid reactions, were reported with chronic administration of COSOPT. Many of these reactions had the clinical appearance and course of an allergic-type reaction that resolved upon discontinuation of drug therapy. If such reactions are observed, COSOPT should be discontinued and the patient evaluated before considering restarting the drug. (See ADVERSE REACTIONS.)
The management of patients with acute angle-closure glaucoma requires therapeutic interventions in addition to ocular hypotensive agents. COSOPT has not been studied in patients with acute angle-closure glaucoma.
Choroidal detachment after filtration procedures has been reported with the administration of aqueous suppressant therapy (e.g., timolol).
Beta-adrenergic blockade has been reported to potentiate muscle weakness consistent with certain myasthenic symptoms (e.g., diplopia, ptosis, and generalized weakness). Timolol has been reported rarely to increase muscle weakness in some patients with myasthenia gravis or myasthenic symptoms.
There have been reports of bacterial keratitis associated with the use of multiple dose containers of topical ophthalmic products. These containers had been inadvertently contaminated by patients who, in most cases, had a concurrent corneal disease or a disruption of the ocular epithelial surface. (See PRECAUTIONS, *Information for Patients.*)
Information for Patients
Patients with bronchial asthma, a history of bronchial asthma, severe chronic obstructive pulmonary disease, sinus bradycardia, second or third degree atrioventricular block, or cardiac failure should be advised not to take this product. (See CONTRAINDICATIONS.)
COSOPT contains dorzolamide (which is a sulfonamide) and although administered topically is absorbed systemically. Therefore the same types of adverse reactions that are attributable to sulfonamides may occur with topical administration. Patients should be advised that if serious or unusual reactions or signs of hypersensitivity occur, they should discontinue the use of the product (see WARNINGS).
Patients should be advised that if they develop any ocular reactions, particularly conjunctivitis and lid reactions, they should discontinue use and seek their physician's advice.
Patients should be instructed to avoid allowing the tip of the dispensing container to contact the eye or surrounding structures.
Patients should also be instructed that ocular solutions, if handled improperly or if the tip of the dispensing container contacts the eye or surrounding structures, can become contaminated by common bacteria known to cause ocular infections. Serious damage to the eye and subsequent loss of vision may result from using contaminated solutions. (See PRECAUTIONS, *General.*)
Patients also should be advised that if they have ocular surgery or develop an intercurrent ocular condition (e.g., trauma or infection), they should immediately seek their physician's advice concerning the continued use of the present multidose container.
If more than one topical ophthalmic drug is being used, the drugs should be administered at least ten minutes apart.
Patients should be advised that COSOPT contains benzalkonium chloride which may be absorbed by soft contact lenses. Contact lenses should be removed prior to administration of the solution. Lenses may be reinserted 15 minutes following administration of COSOPT.
Drug Interactions
Carbonic anhydrase inhibitors: There is a potential for an additive effect on the known systemic effects of carbonic anhydrase inhibition in patients receiving an oral carbonic anhydrase inhibitor and COSOPT. The concomitant administration of COSOPT and oral carbonic anhydrase inhibitors is not recommended.
Acid-base disturbances: Although acid-base and electrolyte disturbances were not reported in the clinical trials with dorzolamide hydrochloride ophthalmic solution, these disturbances have been reported with oral carbonic anhydrase inhibitors and have, in some instances, resulted in drug interactions (e.g., toxicity associated with high-dose salicylate therapy). Therefore, the potential for such drug interactions should be considered in patients receiving COSOPT.
Beta-adrenergic blocking agents: Patients who are receiving a beta-adrenergic blocking agent orally and COSOPT should be observed for potential additive effects of beta-blockade, both systemic and on intraocular pressure. The concomitant use of two topical beta-adrenergic blocking agents is not recommended.
Calcium antagonists: Caution should be used in the coadministration of beta-adrenergic blocking agents, such as COSOPT, and oral or intravenous calcium antagonists because of possible atrioventricular conduction disturbances, left ventricular failure, and hypotension. In patients with impaired cardiac function, coadministration should be avoided.
Catecholamine-depleting drugs: Close observation of the patient is recommended when a beta-blocker is administered to patients receiving catecholamine-depleting drugs such as reserpine, because of possible additive effects and the production of hypotension and/or marked bradycardia, which may result in vertigo, syncope, or postural hypotension.
Digitalis and calcium antagonists: The concomitant use of beta-adrenergic blocking agents with digitalis and calcium antagonists may have additive effects in prolonging atrioventricular conduction time.
Quinidine: Potentiated systemic beta-blockade (e.g., decreased heart rate) has been reported during combined treatment with quinidine and timolol, possibly because quinidine inhibits the metabolism of timolol via the P-450 enzyme, CYP2D6.
Clonidine: Oral beta-adrenergic blocking agents may exacerbate the rebound hypertension which can follow the withdrawal of clonidine. There have been no reports of exacerbation of rebound hypertension with ophthalmic timolol maleate.
Injectable Epinephrine: (See PRECAUTIONS, *General, Anaphylaxis.)*
Carcinogenesis, Mutagenesis, Impairment of Fertility
In a two-year study of dorzolamide hydrochloride administered orally to male and female Sprague-Dawley rats, urinary bladder papillomas were seen in male rats in the highest dosage group of 20 mg/kg/day (250 times the recommended human ophthalmic dose). Papillomas were not seen in rats given oral doses equivalent to approximately 12 times the recommended human ophthalmic dose. No treatment-related tumors were seen in a 21-month study in female and male mice given oral doses up to 75 mg/kg/day (~900 times the recommended human ophthalmic dose).
The increased incidence of urinary bladder papillomas seen in the high-dose male rats is a class-effect of carbonic anhydrase inhibitors in rats. Rats are particularly prone to developing papillomas in response to foreign bodies, compounds causing crystalluria, and diverse sodium salts.
No changes in bladder urothelium were seen in dogs given oral dorzolamide hydrochloride for one year at 2 mg/kg/day (25 times the recommended human ophthalmic dose) or monkeys dosed topically to the eye at 0.4 mg/kg/day (~5 times the recommended human ophthalmic dose) for one year.
In a two-year study of timolol maleate administered orally to rats, there was a statistically significant increase in the incidence of adrenal pheochromocytomas in male rats administered 300 mg/kg/day (approximately 42,000 times the systemic exposure following the maximum recommended human ophthalmic dose). Similar differences were not observed in rats administered oral doses equivalent to approximately 14,000 times the maximum recommended human ophthalmic dose.
In a lifetime oral study of timolol maleate in mice, there were statistically significant increases in the incidence of benign and malignant pulmonary tumors, benign uterine polyps and mammary adenocarcinomas in female mice at 500 mg/kg/day, (approximately 71,000 times the systemic exposure following the maximum recommended human ophthalmic dose), but not at 5 or 50 mg/kg/day (approximately 700 or 7,000, respectively, times the systemic exposure following the maximum recommended human ophthalmic dose). In a subsequent study in female mice, in which post-mortem examinations were limited to the uterus and the lungs, a statistically significant increase in the incidence of pulmonary tumors was again observed at 500 mg/kg/day.
The increased occurrence of mammary adenocarcinomas was associated with elevations in serum prolactin which occurred in female mice administered oral timolol at 500 mg/kg/day, but not at doses of 5 or 50 mg/kg/day. An increased incidence of mammary adenocarcinomas in rodents has been associated with administration of several other therapeutic agents that elevate serum prolactin, but no correlation between serum prolactin levels and mammary tumors has been established in humans. Furthermore, in adult human female subjects who received oral dosages of up to 60 mg of timolol maleate (the maximum recommended human oral dosage), there were no clinically meaningful changes in serum prolactin.
The following tests for mutagenic potential were negative for dorzolamide: (1) *in vivo* (mouse) cytogenetic assay; (2) *in vitro* chromosomal aberration assay; (3) alkaline elution assay; (4) V-79 assay; and (5) Ames test.
Timolol maleate was devoid of mutagenic potential when tested *in vivo* (mouse) in the micronucleus test and cytogenetic assay (doses up to 800 mg/kg) and *in vitro* in a neoplastic cell transformation assay (up to 100 µg/mL). In Ames tests the highest concentrations of timolol employed, 5,000 or 10,000 µg/plate, were associated with statistically significant elevations of revertants observed with tester strain TA100 (in seven replicate assays), but not in the remaining three strains. In the assays with tester strain TA100, no consistent dose response relationship was observed, and the ratio of test to control revertants did not reach 2. A ratio of 2 is usually considered the criterion for a positive Ames test.
Reproduction and fertility studies in rats with either timolol maleate or dorzolamide hydrochloride demonstrated no adverse effect on male or female fertility at doses up to approximately 100 times the systemic exposure following the maximum recommended human ophthalmic dose.
Pregnancy
Teratogenic Effects. Pregnancy Category C. Developmental toxicity studies with dorzolamide hydrochloride in rabbits at oral doses of ≥ 2.5 mg/kg/day (31 times the recommended human ophthalmic dose) revealed malformations of the vertebral bodies. These malformations occurred at doses that caused metabolic acidosis with decreased body weight gain in dams and decreased fetal weights. No treatment-related malformations were seen at 1.0 mg/kg/day (13 times the recommended human ophthalmic dose).
Teratogenicity studies with timolol in mice, rats, and rabbits at oral doses up to 50 mg/kg/day (7,000 times the systemic exposure following the maximum recommended human ophthalmic dose) demonstrated no evidence of fetal malformations. Although delayed fetal ossification was observed at this dose in rats, there were no adverse effects on postnatal development of offspring. Doses of 1000 mg/kg/day (142,000 times the systemic exposure following the maximum recommended human ophthalmic dose) were maternotoxic in mice and resulted in an increased number of fetal resorptions. Increased fetal resorptions were also seen in rabbits at doses of 14,000 times the systemic exposure following the maximum recommended human ophthalmic dose, in this case without apparent maternotoxicity.
There are no adequate and well-controlled studies in pregnant women. COSOPT should be used during pregnancy only if the potential benefit justifies the potential risk to the fetus.
Nursing Mothers
It is not known whether dorzolamide is excreted in human milk. Timolol maleate has been detected in human milk following oral and ophthalmic drug administration. Because of the potential for serious adverse reactions from COSOPT in nursing infants, a decision should be made whether to discontinue nursing or to discontinue the drug, taking into account the importance of the drug to the mother.
Pediatric Use
Safety and effectiveness in pediatric patients have not been established.
Geriatric Use
No overall differences in safety and effectiveness have been observed between elderly and younger patients.

Continued on next page

Information on the Merck & Co., Inc. products listed on these pages is the full prescribing information from product circulars in use September 30, 2000. For information, please call 1-800-NSC MERCK [1-800-672-6372].

Cosopt—Cont.

ADVERSE REACTIONS

COSOPT was evaluated for safety in 1035 patients with elevated intraocular pressure treated for open-angle-glaucoma or ocular hypertension. Approximately 5% of all patients discontinued therapy with COSOPT because of adverse reactions. The most frequently reported adverse events were taste perversion (bitter, sour, or unusual taste) or ocular burning and/or stinging in up to 30% of patients. Conjunctival hyperemia, blurred vision, superficial punctate keratitis or eye itching were reported between 5-15% of patients. The following adverse events were reported in 1-5% of patients: abdominal pain, back pain, blepharitis, bronchitis, cloudy vision, conjunctival discharge, conjunctival edema, conjunctival follicles, conjunctival injection, conjunctivitis, corneal erosion, corneal staining, cortical lens opacity, cough, dizziness, dryness of eyes, dyspepsia, eye debris, eye discharge, eye pain, eye tearing, eyelid edema, eyelid erythema, eyelid exudate/scales, eyelid pain or discomfort, foreign body sensation, glaucomatous cupping, headache, hypertension, influenza, lens nucleus coloration, lens opacity, nausea, nuclear lens opacity, pharyngitis, post-subcapsular cataract, sinusitis, upper respiratory infection, urinary tract infection, visual field defect, vitreous detachment.

The following adverse events have occurred either at low incidence (<1%) during clinical trials or have been reported during the use of COSOPT in clinical practice where these events were reported voluntarily from a population of unknown size and frequency of occurrence cannot be determined precisely. They have been chosen for inclusion based on factors such as seriousness, frequency of reporting, possible causal connection to COSOPT, or a combination of these factors: bradycardia, cardiac failure, cerebral vascular accident, chest pain, depression, diarrhea, dry mouth, dyspnea, hypotension, iridocyclitis, myocardial infarction, nasal congestion, paresthesia, photophobia, respiratory failure, skin rashes, urolithiasis, and vomiting.

Other adverse reactions that have been reported with the individual components are listed below:

Dorzolamide—Allergic/Hypersensitivity: Signs and symptoms of local reactions including palpebral reactions and systemic allergic reactions including angioedema, bronchospasm, pruritus, urticaria; *Body as a Whole:* Asthenia/fatigue; *Skin/Mucous Membranes:* Contact dermatitis, throat irritation; *Special Senses:* Eyelid crusting, signs and symptoms of ocular allergic reactions, and transient myopia.

Timolol (ocular administration)—Body as a Whole: Asthenia/fatigue; *Cardiovascular:* Arrhythmia, syncope, heart block, cerebral ischemia, worsening of angina pectoris, palpitation, cardiac arrest, pulmonary edema, edema, claudication, Raynaud's phenomenon, and cold hands and feet; *Digestive:* Anorexia; *Immunologic:* Systemic lupus erythematosus; *Nervous System/Psychiatric:* Increase in signs and symptoms of myasthenia gravis, somnolence, insomnia, nightmares, behavioral changes and psychic disturbances including confusion, hallucinations, anxiety, disorientation, nervousness, and memory loss; *Skin:* Alopecia, psoriasiform rash or exacerbation of psoriasis; *Hypersensitivity:* Signs and symptoms of systemic allergic reactions, including angioedema, urticaria, and localized and generalized rash; *Respiratory:* Bronchospasm (predominantly in patients with pre-existing bronchospastic disease); *Endocrine:* Masked symptoms of hypoglycemia in diabetic patients (see WARNINGS); *Special Senses:* Ptosis; decreased corneal sensitivity; cystoid macular edema; visual disturbances including refractive changes and diplopia; pseudopemphigoid; choroidal detachment following filtration surgery (see PRECAUTIONS, *General*); and tinnitus; *Urogenital:* Retroperitoneal fibrosis, decreased libido, impotence, and Peyronie's disease.

The following additional adverse effects have been reported in clinical experience with ORAL timolol maleate or other ORAL beta-blocking agents and may be considered potential effects of ophthalmic timolol maleate: *Allergic:* Erythematous rash, fever combined with aching and sore throat, laryngospasm with respiratory distress; *Body as a Whole:* Extremity pain, decreased exercise tolerance, weight loss; *Cardiovascular:* Worsening of arterial insufficiency, vasodilatation; *Digestive:* Gastrointestinal pain, hepatomegaly, mesenteric arterial thrombosis, ischemic colitis; *Hematologic:* Nonthrombocytopenic purpura; thrombocytopenic purpura, agranulocytosis; *Endocrine:* Hyperglycemia, hypoglycemia; *Skin:* Pruritus, skin irritation, increased pigmentation, sweating; *Musculoskeletal:* Arthralgia; *Nervous System/Psychiatric:* Vertigo, local weakness, diminished concentration, reversible mental depression progressing to catatonia, an acute reversible syndrome characterized by disorientation for time and place, emotional lability, slightly clouded sensorium, and decreased performance on neuropsychometrics; *Respiratory:* Rales, bronchial obstruction; *Urogenital:* Urination difficulties.

OVERDOSAGE

There are no human data available on overdosage with COSOPT.

Symptoms consistent with systemic administration of beta-blockers or carbonic anhydrase inhibitors may occur, including electrolyte imbalance, development of an acidotic state, dizziness, headache, shortness of breath, bradycardia, bronchospasm, cardiac arrest and possible central nervous system effects. Serum electrolyte levels (particularly potassium) and blood pH levels should be monitored (see also ADVERSE REACTIONS).

A study of patients with renal failure showed that timolol did not dialyze readily.

DOSAGE AND ADMINISTRATION

The dose is one drop of COSOPT in the affected eye(s) two times daily.

If more than one topical ophthalmic drug is being used, the drugs should be administered at least ten minutes apart (see also PRECAUTIONS, *Drug Interactions*).

HOW SUPPLIED

COSOPT Ophthalmic Solution is a clear, colorless to nearly colorless, slightly viscous solution.

No. 3628 — COSOPT Ophthalmic Solution is supplied in an OCUMETER®*, a white, opaque, plastic ophthalmic dispenser with a controlled drop tip as follows:

NDC 0006-3628-03, 5 mL

NDC 0006-3628-10, 10 mL.

Storage

Store COSOPT between 15 and 25°C (59–77°F). Protect from light.

9098904 Issued April 2000

COZAAR® ℞
(losartan potassium tablets)

> **USE IN PREGNANCY**
> **When used in pregnancy during the second and third trimesters, drugs that act directly on the renin-angiotensin system can cause injury and even death to the developing fetus.** When pregnancy is detected, COZAAR should be discontinued as soon as possible. See WARNINGS: *Fetal/Neonatal Morbidity and Mortality.*

DESCRIPTION

COZAAR* (losartan potassium), the first of a new class of antihypertensives, is an angiotensin II receptor (type AT_1) antagonist.

Losartan potassium, a non-peptide molecule, is chemically describedas2-butyl-4-chloro-1-[*p*-(*o*-1*H*-tetrazol-5-ylphenyl)-benzyl]imidazole-5-methanol monopotassium salt.

Its empirical formula is $C_{22}H_{22}ClKN_6O$, and its structural formula is:

Losartan potassium is a white to off-white free-flowing crystalline powder with a molecular weight of 461.01. It is freely soluble in water, soluble in alcohols, and slightly soluble in common organic solvents, such as acetonitrile and methyl ethyl ketone. Oxidation of the 5-hydroxymethyl group on the imidazole ring results in the active metabolite of losartan.

COZAAR is available as tablets for oral administration containing either 25 mg, 50 mg or 100 mg of losartan potassium and the following inactive ingredients: microcrystalline cellulose, lactose hydrous, pregelatinized starch, magnesium stearate, hydroxypropyl cellulose, hydroxypropyl methylcellulose, titanium dioxide, D&C yellow No. 10 aluminum lake and FD&C blue No. 2 aluminum lake.

COZAAR 25 mg, 50 mg and 100 mg tablets contain potassium in the following amounts: 2.12 mg (0.054 mEq), 4.24 mg (0.108 mEq) and 8.48 mg (0.216 mEq), respectively.

*Registered trademark of E. I. du Pont de Nemours and Company, Wilmington, Delaware, USA

CLINICAL PHARMACOLOGY

Mechanism of Action

Angiotensin II [formed from angiotensin I in a reaction catalyzed by angiotensin converting enzyme (ACE, kininase II)], is a potent vasoconstrictor, the primary vasoactive hormone of the renin-angiotensin system and an important component in the pathophysiology of hypertension. It also stimulates aldosterone secretion by the adrenal cortex. Losartan and its principal active metabolite block the vasoconstrictor and aldosterone-secreting effects of angiotensin II by selectively blocking the binding of angiotensin II to the AT_1 receptor found in many tissues, (e.g., vascular smooth muscle, adrenal gland). There is also an AT_2 receptor found in many tissues but it is not known to be associated with cardiovascular homeostatis. Both losartan and its principal active metabolite do not exhibit any partial agonist activity at the AT_1 receptor and have much greater affinity (about 1000-fold) for the AT_1 receptor than for the AT_2 receptor. *In vitro* binding studies indicate that losartan is a reversible, competitive inhibitor of the AT_1 receptor. The active metabolite is 10 to 40 times more potent by weight than losartan and appears to be a reversible, non-competitive inhibitor of the AT_1 receptor.

Neither losartan nor its active metabolite inhibits ACE (kininase II, the enzyme that converts angiotensin I to angiotensin II and degrades bradykinin); nor do they bind to or block other hormone receptors or ion channels known to be important in cardiovascular regulation.

Pharmacokinetics

General

Losartan is an orally active agent that undergoes substantial first-pass metabolism by cytochrome P450 enzymes. It is converted, in part, to an active carboxylic acid metabolite that is responsible for most of the angiotensin II receptor antagonism that follows losartan treatment. The terminal half-life of losartan is about 2 hours and of the metabolite is about 6–9 hours. The pharmacokinetics of losartan and its active metabolite are linear with oral losartan doses up to 200 mg and do not change over time. Neither losartan nor its metabolite accumulate in plasma upon repeated once-daily dosing.

Following oral administration, losartan is well absorbed (based on absorption of radiolabeled losartan) and undergoes substantial first-pass metabolism; the systemic bioavailability of losartan is approximately 33%. About 14% of an orally-administered dose of losartan is converted to the active metabolite. Mean peak concentrations of losartan and its active metabolite are reached in 1 hour and in 3–4 hours, respectively. While maximum plasma concentrations of losartan and its active metabolite are approximately equal, the AUC of the metabolite is about 4 times as great as that of losartan. A meal slows absorption of losartan and decreases its C_{max} but has only minor effects on losartan AUC or on the AUC of the metabolite (about 10% decreased).

Both losartan and its active metabolite are highly bound to plasma proteins, primarily albumin, with plasma free fractions of 1.3% and 0.2% respectively. Plasma protein binding is constant over the concentration range achieved with recommended doses. Studies in rats indicate that losartan crosses the blood-brain barrier poorly, if at all.

Losartan metabolites have been identified in human plasma and urine. In addition to the active carboxylic acid metabolite, several inactive metabolites are formed. Following oral and intravenous administration of ^{14}C-labeled losartan potassium, circulating plasma radioactivity is primarily attributed to losartan and its active metabolite. *In vitro* studies indicate that cytochrome P450 2C9 and 3A4 are involved in the biotransformation of losartan to its metabolites. Minimal conversion of losartan to the active metabolite (less than 1% of the dose compared to 14% of the dose in normal subjects) was seen in about one percent of individuals studied.

The volume of distribution of losartan is about 34 liters and of the active metabolite is about 12 liters. Total plasma clearance of losartan and the active metabolite is about 600 mL/min and 50 mL/min, respectively, with renal clearance of about 75 mL/min and 25 mL/min, respectively. When losartan is administered orally, about 4% of the dose is excreted unchanged in the urine and about 6% is excreted in urine as active metabolite. Biliary excretion contributes to the elimination of losartan and its metabolites. Following oral ^{14}C-labeled losartan, about 35% of radioactivity is recovered in the urine and about 60% in the feces. Following an intravenous dose of ^{14}C-labeled losartan, about 45% of radioactivity is recovered in the urine and 50% in the feces.

Special Populations

Pediatric: Losartan pharmacokinetics have not been investigated in patients <18 years of age.

Geriatric and Gender: Losartan pharmacokinetics have been investigated in the elderly (65–75 years) and in both genders. Plasma concentrations of losartan and its active metabolite are similar in elderly and young hypertensives. Plasma concentrations of losartan were about twice as high in female hypertensives as male hypertensives, but concentrations of the active metabolite were similar in males and females. No dosage adjustment is necessary (see DOSAGE AND ADMINISTRATION).

Race: Pharmacokinetic differences due to race have not been studied.

Renal Insufficiency: Plasma concentrations of losartan are not altered in patients with creatinine clearance above 30 mL/min. In patients with lower creatinine clearance, AUCs are about 50% greater and they are doubled in hemodialysis patients. Plasma concentrations of the active metabolite are not significantly altered in patients with renal impairment or in hemodialysis patients. Neither losartan nor its active metabolite can be removed by hemodialysis. No dosage adjustment is necessary for patients with renal impairment unless they are volume-depleted (see WARNINGS, *Hypotension—Volume-Depleted Patients* and DOSAGE AND ADMINISTRATION).

Hepatic Insufficiency: Following oral administration in patients with mild to moderate alcoholic cirrhosis of the liver, plasma concentrations of losartan and its active metabolite were, respectively, 5-times and about 1.7-times those in young male volunteers. Compared to normal subjects the total plasma clearance of losartan in patients with hepatic insufficiency was about 50% lower and the oral bioavailability was about 2-times higher. A lower starting dose is recommended for patients with a history of hepatic impairment (see DOSAGE AND ADMINISTRATION).

Drug Interactions

Losartan, administered for 12 days, did not affect the pharmacokinetics or pharmacodynamics of a single dose of warfarin. Losartan did not affect the pharmacokinetics of oral or intravenous digoxin. Coadministration of losartan and cimetidine led to an increase of about 18% in AUC of losartan but did not affect the pharmacokinetics of its active metabolite. Coadministration of losartan and phenobarbital led to a reduction of about 20% in the AUC of losartan and that of its active metabolite. Conversion of losartan to its active metabolite after intravenous administration is not affected by ketoconazole, an inhibitor of P450 3A4. There is no pharmacokinetic interaction between losartan and hydrochlorothiazide.

Pharmacodynamics and Clinical Effects

Losartan inhibits the pressor effect of angiotensin II (as well as angiotensin I) infusions. A dose of 100 mg inhibits the pressor effect by about 85% at peak with 25–40% inhibition persisting for 24 hours. Removal of the negative feedback of angiotensin II causes a 2–3 fold rise in plasma renin activity and consequent rise in angiotensin II plasma concentration in hypertensive patients. Losartan does not affect the response to bradykinin, whereas ACE inhibitors increase the response to bradykinin. Aldosterone plasma concentrations fall following losartan administration. In spite of the effect of losartan on aldosterone secretion, very little effect on serum potassium was observed.

In a single-dose study in normal volunteers, losartan had no effects on glomerular filtration rate, renal plasma flow or filtration fraction. In multiple dose studies in hypertensive patients, there were no notable effects on systemic or renal prostaglandin concentrations, fasting triglycerides, total cholesterol or HDL-cholesterol or fasting glucose concentrations. There was a small uricosuric effect leading to a minimal decrease in serum uric acid (mean decrease <0.4 mg/dL) during chronic oral administration.

The antihypertensive effects of COZAAR were demonstrated principally in 4 placebo-controlled 6–12 week trials of dosages from 10 to 150 mg per day in patients with baseline diastolic blood pressures of 95–115. The studies allowed comparisons of two doses (50–100 mg/day) as once-daily or twice-daily regimens, comparisons of peak and trough effects, and comparisons of response by gender, age, and race. Three additional studies examined the antihypertensive effects of losartan and hydrochlorothiazide in combination.

The 4 studies of losartan monotherapy included a total of 1075 patients randomized to several doses of losartan and 334 to placebo. The 10 and 25 mg doses produced some effect at peak (6 hours after dosing) but small and inconsistent trough (24 hour) responses. Doses of 50, 100 and 150 mg once daily gave statistically significant systolic/diastolic mean decreases in blood pressure, compared to placebo in the range of 5.5–10.5/3.5–7.5 mmHg, with the 150 mg dose giving no greater effect than 50–100 mg. Twice-daily dosing at 50–100 mg/day gave consistently larger trough responses than once-daily dosing at the same total dose. Peak (6 hour) effects were uniformly, but moderately, larger than trough effects, with the trough-to-peak ratio for systolic and diastolic responses 50–95% and 60–90%, respectively.

Addition of a low dose of hydrochlorothiazide (12.5 mg) to losartan 50 mg once daily resulted in placebo-adjusted blood pressure reductions of 15.5/9.2 mmHg.

Analysis of age, gender, and race subgroups of patients showed that men and women, and patients over and under 65, had generally similar responses. COZAAR was effective in reducing blood pressure regardless of race, although the effect was somewhat less in black patients (usually a low-renin population).

The effect of losartan is substantially present within one week but in some studies the maximal effect occurred in 3–6 weeks. In long-term follow-up studies (without placebo control) the effect of losartan appeared to be maintained for up to a year. There is no apparent rebound effect after abrupt withdrawal of losartan. There was essentially no change in average heart rate in losartan-treated patients in controlled trials.

INDICATIONS AND USAGE

COZAAR is indicated for the treatment of hypertension. It may be used alone or in combination with other antihypertensive agents.

CONTRAINDICATIONS

COZAAR is contraindicated in patients who are hypersensitive to any component of this product.

WARNINGS

Fetal/Neonatal Morbidity and Mortality

Drugs that act directly on the renin-angiotensin system can cause fetal and neonatal morbidity and death when administered to pregnant women. Several dozen cases have been reported in the world literature in patients who were taking angiotensin converting enzyme inhibitors. When pregnancy is detected, COZAAR should be discontinued as soon as possible.

The use of drugs that act directly on the renin-angiotensin system during the second and third trimesters of pregnancy has been associated with fetal and neonatal injury, including hypotension, neonatal skull hypoplasia, anuria, reversible or irreversible renal failure, and death. Oligohydramnios has also been reported, presumably resulting from decreased fetal renal function; oligohydramnios in this setting has been associated with fetal limb contractures, craniofacial deformation, and hypoplastic lung development. Prematurity, intrauterine growth retardation, and patent ductus arteriosus have also been reported, although it is not clear whether these occurrences were due to exposure to the drug.

These adverse effects do not appear to have resulted from intrauterine drug exposure that has been limited to the first trimester.

Mothers whose embryos and fetuses are exposed to an angiotensin II receptor antagonist only during the first trimester should be so informed. Nonetheless, when patients become pregnant, physicians should have the patient discontinue the use of COZAAR as soon as possible.

Rarely (probably less often than once in every thousand pregnancies), no alternative to an angiotensin II receptor antagonist will be found. In these rare cases, the mothers should be apprised of the potential hazards to their fetuses, and serial ultrasound examinations should be performed to assess the intraamniotic environment.

If oligohydramnios is observed, COZAAR should be discontinued unless it is considered life-saving for the mother. Contraction stress testing (CST), a non-stress test (NST), or biophysical profiling (BPP) may be appropriate, depending upon the week of pregnancy. Patients and physicians should be aware, however, that oligohydramnios may not appear until after the fetus has sustained irreversible injury.

Infants with histories of *in utero* exposure to an angiotensin II receptor antagonist should be closely observed for hypotension, oliguria, and hyperkalemia. If oliguria occurs, attention should be directed toward support of blood pressure and renal perfusion. Exchange transfusion or dialysis may be required as means of reversing hypotension and/or substituting for disordered renal function.

Losartan potassium has been shown to produce adverse effects in rat fetuses and neonates, including decreased body weight, delayed physical and behavioral development, mortality and renal toxicity. With the exception of neonatal weight gain (which was affected at doses as low as 10 mg/kg/day), doses associated with these effects exceeded 25 mg/kg/day (approximately three times the maximum recommended human dose of 100 mg on a mg/m^2 basis). These findings are attributed to drug exposure in late gestation and during lactation. Significant levels of losartan and its active metabolite were shown to be present in rat fetal plasma during late gestation and in rat milk.

Hypotension—Volume-Depleted Patients

In patients who are intravascularly volume-depleted (e.g., those treated with diuretics), symptomatic hypotension may occur after initiation of therapy with COZAAR. These conditions should be corrected prior to administration of COZAAR, or a lower starting dose should be used (see DOSAGE AND ADMINISTRATION).

PRECAUTIONS

General

Hypersensitivity: Angioedema. See ADVERSE REACTIONS, *Post-Marketing Experience.*

Impaired Hepatic Function

Based on pharmacokinetic data which demonstrate significantly increased plasma concentrations of losartan in cirrhotic patients, a lower dose should be considered for patients with impaired liver function (see DOSAGE AND ADMINISTRATION and CLINICAL PHARMACOLOGY, *Pharmacokinetics*).

Impaired Renal Function

As a consequence of inhibiting the renin-angiotensin-aldosterone system, changes in renal function have been reported in susceptible individuals treated with COZAAR; in some patients, these changes in renal function were reversible upon discontinuation of therapy.

In patients whose renal function may depend on the activity of the renin-angiotensin-aldosterone system (e.g., patients with severe congestive heart failure), treatment with angiotensin converting enzyme inhibitors has been associated with oliguria and/or progressive azotemia and (rarely) with acute renal failure and/or death. Similar outcomes have been reported with COZAAR.

In studies of ACE inhibitors in patients with unilateral or bilateral renal artery stenosis, increases in serum creatinine or BUN have been reported. Similar effects have been reported with COZAAR; in some patients, these effects were reversible upon discontinuation of therapy.

Information for Patients

Pregnancy: Female patients of childbearing age should be told about the consequences of second- and third-trimester exposure to drugs that act on the renin-angiotensin system, and they should also be told that these consequences do not appear to have resulted from intrauterine drug exposure that has been limited to the first trimester. These patients should be asked to report pregnancies to their physicians as soon as possible.

Potassium Supplements: A patient receiving COZAAR should be told not to use potassium supplements or salt substitutes containing potassium without consulting the prescribing physician (see PRECAUTIONS, *Drug Interactions*).

Drug Interactions

No significant drug-drug pharmacokinetic interactions have been found in interaction studies with hydrochlorothiazide, digoxin, warfarin, cimetidine and phenobarbital. (See CLINICAL PHARMACOLOGY, *Drug Interactions.*) Potent inhibitors of cytochrome P450 3A4 and 2C9 have not been studied clinically but *in vitro* studies show significant inhibition of the formation of the active metabolite by inhibitors of P450 3A4 (ketoconazole, troleandomycin, gestodene), or P450 2C9 (sulfaphenazole) and nearly complete inhibition by the combination of sulfaphenazole and ketoconazole. In humans, ketoconazole, an inhibitor of P450 3A4, did not affect the conversion of losartan to the active metabolite after intravenous administration of losartan. Inhibitors of cytochrome P450 2C9 have not been studied clinically. The pharmacodynamic consequences of concomitant use of losartan and inhibitors of P450 2C9 have not been examined.

As with other drugs that block angiotensin II or its effects, concomitant use of potassium-sparing diuretics (e.g., spironolactone, triamterene, amiloride), potassium supplements, or salt substitutes containing potassium may lead to increases in serum potassium.

Carcinogenesis, Mutagenesis, Impairment of Fertility

Losartan potassium was not carcinogenic when administered at maximally tolerated dosages to rats and mice for 105 and 92 weeks, respectively. Female rats given the highest dose (270 mg/kg/day) had a slightly higher incidence of pancreatic acinar adenoma. The maximally tolerated dosages (270 mg/kg/day in rats, 200 mg/kg/day in mice) provided systemic exposures for losartan and its pharmacologically active metabolite that were approximately 160- and 90-times (rats) and 30- and 15-times (mice) the exposure of a 50 kg human given 100 mg per day.

Losartan potassium was negative in the microbial mutagenesis and V-79 mammalian cell mutagenesis assays and in the *in vitro* alkaline elution and *in vitro* and *in vivo* chromosomal aberration assays. In addition, the active metabolite showed no evidence of genotoxicity in the microbial mutagenesis, *in vitro* alkaline elution, and *in vitro* chromosomal aberration assays.

Fertility and reproductive performance were not affected in studies with male rats given oral doses of losartan potassium up to approximately 150 mg/kg/day. The administration of toxic dosage levels in females (300/200 mg/kg/day) was associated with a significant ($p<0.05$) decrease in the number of corpora lutea/female, implants/female, and live fetuses/female at C-section. At 100 mg/kg/day only a decrease in the number of corpora lutea/female was observed. The relationship of these findings to drug-treatment is uncertain since there was no effect at these dosage levels on implants/pregnant female, percent post-implantation loss, or live animals/litter at parturition. In nonpregnant rats dosed at 135 mg/kg/day for 7 days, systemic exposure (AUCs) for losartan and its active metabolite were approximately 66 and 26 times the exposure achieved in man at the maximum recommended human daily dosage (100 mg).

Pregnancy

Pregnancy Categories C (first trimester) and D (second and third trimesters). See WARNINGS, *Fetal/Neonatal Morbidity and Mortality.*

Nursing Mothers

It is not known whether losartan is excreted in human milk, but significant levels of losartan and its active metabolite were shown to be present in rat milk. Because of the potential for adverse effects on the nursing infant, a decision should be made whether to discontinue nursing or discontinue the drug, taking into account the importance of the drug to the mother.

Pediatric Use

Safety and effectiveness in pediatric patients have not been established.

Use in the Elderly

Of the total number of patients receiving COZAAR in controlled clinical studies, 391 patients (19%) were 65 years and over, while 37 patients (2%) were 75 years and over. No overall differences in effectiveness or safety were observed between these patients and younger patients, but greater sensitivity of some older individuals cannot be ruled out.

ADVERSE REACTIONS

COZAAR has been evaluated for safety in more than 3300 patients treated for essential hypertension and 4058 patients/subjects overall. Over 1200 patients were treated for over 6 months and more than 800 for over one year. In general, treatment with COZAAR was well-tolerated. The overall incidence of adverse experiences reported with COZAAR was similar to placebo.

In controlled clinical trials, discontinuation of therapy due to clinical adverse experiences was required in 2.3 percent of patients treated with COZAAR and 3.7 percent of patients given placebo.

The following table of adverse events is based on four 6–12 week placebo controlled trials involving over 1000 patients on various doses (10–150 mg) of losartan and over 300 patients given placebo. All doses of losartan are grouped be-

Continued on next page

Information on the Merck & Co., Inc. products listed on these pages is the full prescribing information from product circulars in use September 30, 2000. For information, please call 1-800-NSC MERCK [1-800-672-6372].

Cozaar—Cont.

cause none of the adverse events appeared to have a dose-related frequency. The table includes all adverse events, whether or not attributed to the treatment, occurring in at least 1% of patients treated with losartan and that were more frequent on losartan than placebo.

	Losartan (n=1075) Incidence	Placebo (n=334) Incidence
Digestive		
Diarrhea	2.4	2.1
Dyspepsia	1.3	1.2
Musculoskeletal		
Cramp, muscle	1.1	0.3
Myalgia	1.0	0.9
Pain, back	1.8	1.2
Pain, leg	1.0	0.0
Nervous System/Psychiatric		
Dizziness	3.5	2.1
Insomnia	1.4	0.6
Respiratory		
Congestion, nasal	2.0	1.2
Cough	3.4	3.3
Infection, upper respiratory	7.9	6.9
Sinus disorder	1.5	1.2
Sinusitis	1.0	0.3

The following adverse events were also reported at a rate of 1% or greater in patients treated with losartan, but were as, or more frequent, in the placebo group: asthenia/fatigue, edema/swelling, abdominal pain, chest pain, nausea, headache, pharyngitis.

Adverse events occurred at about the same rates in men and women, older and younger patients, and black and non-black patients.

A patient with known hypersensitivity to aspirin and penicillin, when treated with COZAAR, was withdrawn from study due to swelling of the lips and eyelids and facial rash, reported as angioedema, which returned to normal 5 days after therapy was discontinued.

Superficial peeling of palms and hemolysis was reported in one subject.

In addition to the adverse events above, potentially important events that occurred in at least two patients/subjects exposed to losartan or other adverse events that occurred in <1% of patients in clinical studies are listed below. It cannot be determined whether these events were causally related to losartan: *Body as a Whole:* facial edema, fever, orthostatic effects, syncope; *Cardiovascular:* angina pectoris, second degree AV block, CVA, hypotension, myocardial infarction, arrhythmias including atrial fibrillation, palpitation, sinus bradycardia, tachycardia, ventricular tachycardia, ventricular fibrillation; *Digestive:* anorexia, constipation, dental pain, dry mouth, flatulence, gastritis, vomiting; *Hematologic:* anemia; *Metabolic:* gout; *Musculoskeletal:* arm pain, hip pain, joint swelling, knee pain, musculoskeletal pain, shoulder pain, stiffness, arthralgia, arthritis, fibromyalgia, muscle weakness; *Nervous System/ Psychiatric:* anxiety, anxiety disorder, ataxia, confusion, depression, dream abnormality, hypesthesia, decreased libido, memory impairment, migraine, nervousness, paresthesia, peripheral neuropathy, panic disorder, sleep disorder, somnolence, tremor, vertigo; *Respiratory:* dyspnea, bronchitis, pharyngeal discomfort, epistaxis, rhinitis, respiratory congestion; *Skin:* alopecia, dermatitis, dry skin, ecchymosis, erythema, flushing, photosensitivity, pruritus, rash, sweating, urticaria; *Special Senses:* blurred vision, burning/stinging in the eye, conjunctivitis, taste perversion, tinnitus, decrease in visual acuity; *Urogenital:* impotence, nocturia, urinary frequency, urinary tract infection.

Persistent dry cough (with an incidence of a few percent) has been associated with ACE inhibitor use and in practice can be a cause of discontinuation of ACE inhibitor therapy. Two prospective, parallel-group, double-blind, randomized, controlled trials were conducted to assess the effects of losartan on the incidence of cough in hypertensive patients who had experienced cough while receiving ACE inhibitor therapy. Patients who had typical ACE inhibitor cough when challenged with lisinopril, whose cough disappeared on placebo, were randomized to losartan 50 mg, lisinopril 20 mg, or either placebo (one study, n=97) or 25 mg hydrochlorothiazide (n=135). The double-blind treatment period lasted up to 8 weeks. The incidence of cough is shown below.

Study 1†	HCTZ	Losartan	Lisinopril
Cough	25%	17%	69%
Study 2††	Placebo	Losartan	Lisinopril
Cough	35%	29%	62%

†Demographics = (89% caucasian, 64% female)
††Demographics = (90% caucasian, 51% female)

These studies demonstrate that the incidence of cough associated with losartan therapy, in a population that all had cough associated with ACE inhibitor therapy, is similar to that associated with hydrochlorothiazide or placebo therapy.

Cases of cough, including positive re-challenges, have been reported with the use of losartan in post-marketing experience.

Post-Marketing Experience

The following additional adverse reactions have been reported in post-marketing experience:

Hypersensitivity: Angioedema, including swelling of the larynx and glottis, causing airway obstruction and/or swelling of the face, lips, pharynx, and/or tongue has been reported rarely in patients treated with losartan; some of these patients previously experienced angioedema with other drugs including ACE inhibitors. Anaphylactic reactions have been reported.

Digestive: Hepatitis (reported rarely).

Respiratory: Dry cough (see above).

Hyperkalemia and hyponatremia have been reported.

Laboratory Test Findings

In controlled clinical trials, clinically important changes in standard laboratory parameters were rarely associated with administration of COZAAR.

Creatinine, Blood Urea Nitrogen: Minor increases in blood urea nitrogen (BUN) or serum creatinine were observed in less than 0.1 percent of patients with essential hypertension treated with COZAAR alone (see PRECAUTIONS, *Impaired Renal Function*).

Hemoglobin and Hematocrit: Small decreases in hemoglobin and hematocrit (mean decreases of approximately 0.11 grams percent and 0.09 volume percent, respectively) occurred frequently in patients treated with COZAAR alone, but were rarely of clinical importance. No patients were discontinued due to anemia.

Liver Function Tests: Occasional elevations of liver enzymes and/or serum bilirubin have occurred. In patients with essential hypertension treated with COZAAR alone, one patient (<0.1%) was discontinued due to these laboratory adverse experiences.

OVERDOSAGE

Significant lethality was observed in mice and rats after oral administration of 1000 mg/kg and 2000 mg/kg, respectively, about 44 and 170 times the maximum recommended human dose on a mg/m^2 basis.

Limited data are available in regard to overdosage in humans. The most likely manifestation of overdosage would be hypotension and tachycardia; bradycardia could occur from parasympathetic (vagal) stimulation. If symptomatic hypotension should occur, supportive treatment should be instituted.

Neither losartan nor its active metabolite can be removed by hemodialysis.

DOSAGE AND ADMINISTRATION

The usual starting dose of COZAAR is 50 mg once daily, with 25 mg used in patients with possible depletion of intravascular volume (e.g., patients treated with diuretics) (see WARNINGS, *Hypotension—Volume-Depleted Patients*) and patients with a history of hepatic impairment (see PRECAUTIONS, *General*). COZAAR can be administered once or twice daily with total daily doses ranging from 25 mg to 100 mg.

If the antihypertensive effect measured at trough using once-a-day dosing is inadequate, a twice-a-day regimen at the same total daily dose or an increase in dose may give a more satisfactory response.

If blood pressure is not controlled by COZAAR alone, a low dose of a diuretic may be added. Hydrochlorothiazide has been shown to have an additive effect (see CLINICAL PHARMACOLOGY, *Pharmacodynamics and Clinical Effects*).

No initial dosage adjustment is necessary for elderly patients or for patients with renal impairment, including patients on dialysis.

COZAAR may be administered with other antihypertensive agents.

COZAAR may be administered with or without food.

HOW SUPPLIED

No. 3612—Tablets COZAAR, 25 mg, are light green, teardrop-shaped, film-coated tablets with code MRK on one side and 951 on the other. They are supplied as follows:

NDC 0006-0951-54 unit of use bottles of 90
NDC 0006-0951-58 unit of use bottles of 100
NDC 0006-0951-28 unit dose packages of 100

Shown in Product Identification Guide, page 323

No. 3613—Tablets COZAAR, 50 mg, are green, teardrop-shaped, film-coated tablets with code MRK 952 on one side and COZAAR on the other. They are supplied as follows:

NDC 0006-0952-31 unit of use bottles of 30
NDC 0006-0952-54 unit of use bottles of 90
NDC 0006-0952-58 unit of use bottles of 100
NDC 0006-0952-28 unit dose packages of 100
NDC 0006-0952-82 bottles of 1,000.

Shown in Product Identification Guide, page 323

No. 6536—Tablets COZAAR, 100 mg, are dark green, teardrop-shaped, film-coated tablets with code 960 on one side and MRK on the other. They are supplied as follows:

NDC 0006-0960-31 unit of use bottles of 30
NDC 0006-0960-58 unit of use bottles of 100
NDC 0006-0960-28 unit dose packages of 100.

Shown in Product Identification Guide, page 323

Storage

Store at 25°C (77°F); excursions permitted to 15–30°C (59–86°F) [see USP Controlled Room Temperature]. Keep container tightly closed. Protect from light.

Manufactured for:
MERCK & CO., INC., West Point, PA 19486, USA
by:
DuPont Pharma, Wilmington, DE 19880 USA
7882914 Issued December 1999

CRIXIVAN® Capsules ℞
(indinavir sulfate)

DESCRIPTION

CRIXIVAN* (indinavir sulfate) is an inhibitor of the human immunodeficiency virus (HIV) protease. CRIXIVAN Capsules are formulated as a sulfate salt and are available for oral administration in strengths of 200, 333, and 400 mg of indinavir (corresponding to 250, 416.3, and 500 mg indinavir sulfate, respectively). Each capsule also contains the inactive ingredients anhydrous lactose and magnesium stearate. The capsule shell has the following inactive ingredients and dyes: gelatin, titanium dioxide, silicon dioxide and sodium lauryl sulfate.

The chemical name for indinavir sulfate is [1(1*S*,2*R*),5(*S*)]-2,3,5-trideoxy-*N*-(2,3-dihydro-2-hydroxy-1 *H*-inden-1-yl)-5-[2-[[(1,1-dimethylethyl)amino]carbonyl]-4-(3-pyridinylmethyl)-1-piperazinyl] -2 -(phenylmethyl)-D-*erythro*-pentonamide sulfate (1:1) salt. Indinavir sulfate has the following structural formula:

OH OH • H_2SO_4 NHC(CH_3)$_3$

Indinavir sulfate is a white to off-white, hygroscopic, crystalline powder with the molecular formula $C_{36}H_{47}N_5O_4 \bullet H_2SO_4$ and a molecular weight of 711.88. It is very soluble in water and in methanol.

*Registered trademark of MERCK & CO., Inc.

MICROBIOLOGY

Mechanism of Action: HIV protease is an enzyme required for the proteolytic cleavage of the viral polyprotein precursors into the individual functional proteins found in infectious HIV. Indinavir binds to the protease active site and inhibits the activity of the enzyme. This inhibition prevents cleavage of the viral polyproteins resulting in the formation of immature noninfectious viral particles.

Antiretroviral Activity In Vitro: The relationship between *in vitro* susceptibility of HIV to indinavir and inhibition of HIV replication in humans has not been established. The *in vitro* activity of indinavir was assessed in cell lines of lymphoblastic and monocytic origin and in peripheral blood lymphocytes. HIV variants used to infect the different cell types include laboratory-adapted variants, primary clinical isolates and clinical isolates resistant to nucleoside analogue and nonnucleoside inhibitors of the HIV reverse transcriptase. The IC_{95} (95% inhibitory concentration) of indinavir in these test systems was in the range of 25 to 100 nM. In drug combination studies with the nucleoside analogues zidovudine and didanosine, as well as with an investigational nonnucleoside (L-697,661), indinavir showed synergistic activity in cell culture.

Drug Resistance: Isolates of HIV with reduced susceptibility to the drug have been recovered from some patients treated with indinavir. Viral resistance was correlated with the accumulation of mutations that resulted in the expression of amino acid substitutions in the viral protease. Eleven amino acid residue positions, at which substitutions are associated with resistance, have been identified. Resistance was mediated by the co-expression of multiple and variable substitutions at these positions. In general, higher levels of resistance were associated with the co-expression of greater numbers of substitutions.

Cross-Resistance to Other Antiviral Agents: Cross-resistance was noted between indinavir and the protease inhibitor ritonavir. Varying degrees of cross-resistance have been observed between indinavir and other HIV-protease inhibitors.

CLINICAL PHARMACOLOGY

Pharmacokinetics

Absorption: Indinavir was rapidly absorbed in the fasted state with a time to peak plasma concentration (T_{max}) of 0.8 ± 0.3 hours (mean ± S.D.) (n=11). A greater than dose-proportional increase in indinavir plasma concentrations was observed over the 200–1000 mg dose range. At a dosing regimen of 800 mg every 8 hours, steady-state area under the plasma concentration time curve (AUC) was 30,691 ± 11,407 nM·hour (n=16), peak plasma concentration (C_{max}) was 12,617 ± 4037 nM (n=16), and plasma concentration eight hours post dose (trough) was 251 ± 178 nM (n=16).

Effect of Food on Oral Absorption: Administration of indinavir with a meal high in calories, fat, and protein (784 kcal, 48.6 g fat, 31.3 g protein) resulted in a 77% ± 8% reduction in AUC and an 84% ± 7% reduction in C_{max} (n=10). Administration with lighter meals (e.g., a meal of dry toast with jelly, apple juice, and coffee with skim milk and sugar or a meal of corn flakes, skim milk and sugar) resulted in little or no change in AUC, C_{max} or trough concentration.

Distribution: Indinavir was approximately 60% bound to human plasma proteins over a concentration range of 81 nM to 16,300 nM.

Metabolism: Following a 400-mg dose of ^{14}C-indinavir, 83 ± 1% (n=4) and 19 ± 3% (n=6) of the total radioactivity was recovered in feces and urine, respectively; radioactivity due to parent drug in feces and urine was 19.1% and 9.4%, respectively. Seven metabolites have been identified, one glucuronide conjugate and six oxidative metabolites. *In vitro* studies indicate that cytochrome P-450 3A4 (CYP3A4) is the major enzyme responsible for formation of the oxidative metabolites.

Elimination: Less than 20% of indinavir is excreted unchanged in the urine. Mean urinary excretion of unchanged drug was 10.4 ± 4.9% (n=10) and 12.0 ± 4.9% (n=10) following a single 700-mg and 1000-mg dose, respectively. Indinavir was rapidly eliminated with a half-life of 1.8 ± 0.4 hours (n=10). Significant accumulation was not observed after multiple dosing at 800 mg every 8 hours.

Special Populations

Hepatic Insufficiency: Patients with mild to moderate hepatic insufficiency and clinical evidence of cirrhosis had evidence of decreased metabolism of indinavir resulting in approximately 60% higher mean AUC following a single 400-mg dose (n=12). The half-life of indinavir increased to 2.8 ± 0.5 hours. Indinavir pharmacokinetics have not been studied in patients with severe hepatic insufficiency (see DOSAGE AND ADMINISTRATION, *Hepatic Insufficiency*).

Renal Insufficiency: The pharmacokinetics of indinavir have not been studied in patients with renal insufficiency.

Gender: Pharmacokinetics of indinavir appear to be comparable in men and women based on pharmacokinetic studies including 32 women (15 HIV-positive).

Race: Pharmacokinetics of indinavir appear to be comparable in Caucasians and Blacks based on pharmacokinetic studies including 42 Caucasians (26 HIV-positive) and 16 Blacks (4 HIV-positive).

Drug Interactions (also see PRECAUTIONS, *Drug Interactions*)

Specific drug interaction studies were performed with indinavir and a number of drugs.

Drugs That Should Not Be Coadministered With CRIXIVAN

Administration of indinavir (800 mg every 8 hours) with rifampin (600 mg once daily) for one week resulted in an 89% ± 9% decrease in indinavir AUC.

In a published study, eight HIV-negative volunteers received indinavir 800 mg every eight hours for four doses prior to and at the end of a 14-day course of St. John's wort (*Hypericum perforatum*, standardized to 0.3% hypericin) 300 mg three times daily. Indinavir plasma pharmacokinetics were determined following the fourth dose of indinavir prior to and following St. John's wort. Following the course of St. John's wort, the AUC_{0-8h} of indinavir was decreased 57% ± 19% and the C_{8h} of indinavir was decreased 81% ± 16% compared to when indinavir was taken alone. All subjects demonstrated a decrease in AUC_{0-8h} (range 36 to 79%) and a decrease in C_{8h} (range 49 to 99%).

Drugs Requiring Dose Modification

Delavirdine: Preliminary date (n=14) indicate that delavirdine inhibits the metabolism of indinavir such that coadministration of a 400-mg single dose of indinavir with delavirdine (400 mg three times a day) resulted in indinavir AUC values slightly less than those observed following administration of an 800-mg dose of indinavir alone. Also, coadministration of a 600-mg dose of indinavir with delavirdine (400 mg three times a day) resulted in indinavir AUC values approximately 40% greater than those observed following administration of an 800-mg dose of indinavir alone. Indinavir had no effect on delavirdine pharmacokinetics (see DOSAGE AND ADMINISTRATION, *Concomitant Therapy, Delavirdine*).

Efavirenz: When indinavir (800 mg every 8 hours) was given with efavirenz (200 mg once daily) for two weeks, the indinavir AUC and C_{max} were decreased by approximately 31% and 16%, respectively, as a result of enzyme induction. (See DOSAGE AND ADMINISTRATION, *Concomitant Therapy, Efavirenz.*)

Itraconazole: In a multiple-dose study, administration in the fasted state of itraconazole capsules 200 mg twice daily with indinavir 600 mg every 8 hours resulted in an indinavir AUC similar to that observed during administration of indinavir 800 mg every 8 hours alone for one week (see DOSAGE AND ADMINISTRATION, *Concomitant Therapy, Itraconazole*).

Ketoconazole: In a single-dose study, administration of a 400-mg dose of ketoconazole with a 400-mg dose of indinavir resulted in a 68% ± 48% increase in indinavir AUC compared to a 400-mg dose of indinavir alone. In a multiple-dose study, administration of ketoconazole 400 mg once daily with indinavir 600 mg every 8 hours resulted in an 18% ± 17% decrease in indinavir AUC compared to an 800-mg dose of indinavir alone every 8 hours (see DOSAGE AND ADMINISTRATION, *Concomitant Therapy, Ketoconazole*).

Rifabutin: The coadministration of indinavir 800 mg every 8 hours with rifabutin either 300 mg once daily or 150 mg once daily was evaluated in two separate clinical studies. The results of these studies showed a decrease in indinavir AUC (32% ± 19% and 31% ± 15%, respectively) vs. indinavir 800 mg every 8 hours alone and an increase in rifabutin AUC (204% ± 142% and 60% ± 47%, respectively) vs. rifabutin 300 mg once daily alone (See DOSAGE AND ADMINISTRATION, *Concomitant Therapy, Rifabutin*).

Drugs Not Requiring Dose Modification

Cimetidine, Quinidine, Grapefruit Juice: Administration of a single 400-mg dose of indinavir following six days of cimetidine (600 mg every 12 hours) did not affect indinavir AUC. Administration of a single 400-mg dose of indinavir with 8 oz. of grapefruit juice resulted in a decrease in indinavir AUC (26% ± 18%). Administration of a single 400-mg dose of indinavir with 200 mg of quinidine sulfate resulted in a 10% ± 26% increase in indinavir AUC.

Methadone: Administration of indinavir (800 mg every 8 hours) with methadone (20 mg to 60 mg daily) for one week resulted in no change in methadone AUC and little or no change in indinavir AUC.

Nucleoside analogue antiretroviral agents: Administration of indinavir (1000 mg every 8 hours) with zidovudine (200 mg every 8 hours) for one week resulted in a 13% ± 48% increase in indinavir AUC and a 17% ± 23% increase in zidovudine AUC. In another study, administration of indinavir (800 mg every 8 hours) with zidovudine (200 mg every 8 hours) in combination with lamivudine (150 mg twice daily) for one week resulted in no change in indinavir AUC, a 36% increase in zidovudine AUC, and a 6% decrease in lamivudine AUC. Administration of indinavir (800 mg every 8 hours) in combination with stavudine (40 mg every 12 hours) for one week resulted in no change in indinavir AUC and a 25% ± 26% increase in stavudine AUC.

*ORTHO-NOVUM 1/35:*** Administration of indinavir (800 mg every 8 hours) with ORTHO-NOVUM 1/35 for one week resulted in a 24% ± 17% increase in ethinyl estradiol AUC and a 26% ± 14% increase in norethindrone AUC.

Trimethoprim/Sulfamethoxazole, Fluconazole, Isoniazid, Clarithromycin: Administration of indinavir (400 mg every 6 hours) with trimethroprim/sulfamethoxazole (one double strength tablet every 12 hours) for one week resulted in no change in indinavir AUC, a 19% ± 31% increase in trimethoprim AUC, and no change in sulfamethoxazole AUC. Administration of indinavir (1000 mg every 8 hours) with fluconazole (400 mg once daily) for one week resulted in a 19% ± 33% decrease in indinavir AUC and no change in fluconazole AUC. Administration of indinavir (800 mg every 8 hours) with isoniazid (300 mg once daily) for one week resulted in no change in indinavir AUC and a 13% ± 15% increase in isoniazid AUC. Administration of indinavir (800 mg every 8 hours) with clarithromycin (500 mg every 12 hours) for one week resulted in a 29% ± 42% increase in indinavir AUC and a 53% ± 36% increase in clarithromycin AUC.

**Registered trademark of Ortho Pharmaceutical Corporation

INDICATIONS AND USAGE

CRIXIVAN in combination with antiretroviral agents is indicated for the treatment of HIV infection.

This indication is based on two clinical trials of approximately 1 year duration that demonstrated: 1) a reduction in the risk of AIDS defining illnesses or death; 2) a prolonged suppression of HIV RNA.

Description of Studies

In all clinical studies, with the exception of ACTG 320, the AMPLICOR HIV MONITOR assay was used to determine the level of circulating HIV RNA in serum. This is an experimental use of the assay. HIV RNA results should not be directly compared to results from other trials using different HIV RNA assays or using other sample sources.

Study ACTG 320 was a multicenter, randomized, double-blind clinical endpoint trial to compare the effect of CRIXIVAN in combination with zidovudine and lamivudine with that of zidovudine plus lamivudine on the progression to an AIDS-defining illness (ADI) or death. Patients were protease inhibitor and lamivudine naive and zidovudine experienced, with CD4 cell counts of ≤200 cells/mm^3. The study enrolled 1156 HIV-infected patients (17% female, 28% Black, 18% Hispanic, mean age 39 years). The mean baseline CD4 cell count was 87 cells/mm^3. The mean baseline HIV RNA for a subset of 190 patients was 4.98 $\log_{10}$ copies/mL (95,432 copies/mL). The study was terminated after a planned interim analysis, resulting in a median follow-up of 38 weeks and a maximum follow-up of 52 weeks. Results are shown in Table 1 and Figures 1 & 2.

Table 1
ACTG 320

Endpoint	Number (%) of Patients with AIDS-defining Illness or Death IDV+ZDV+L (n=577)	ZDV+L (n=579)
HIV Progression or Death	35 (6.1)	63 (10.9)
Death*	10 (1.7)	19 (3.3)

*The number of deaths is inadequate to assess the impact of Indinavir on survival.

IDV = Indinavir, ZDV = Zidovudine, L = Lamivudine

Study ACTG 320: Figure 1

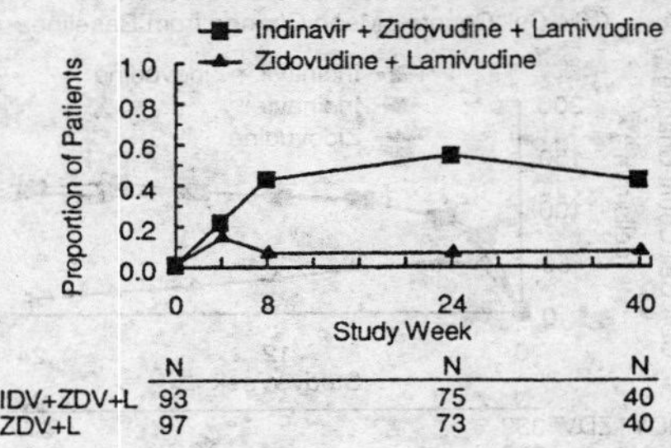

Study ACTG 320: Figure 2

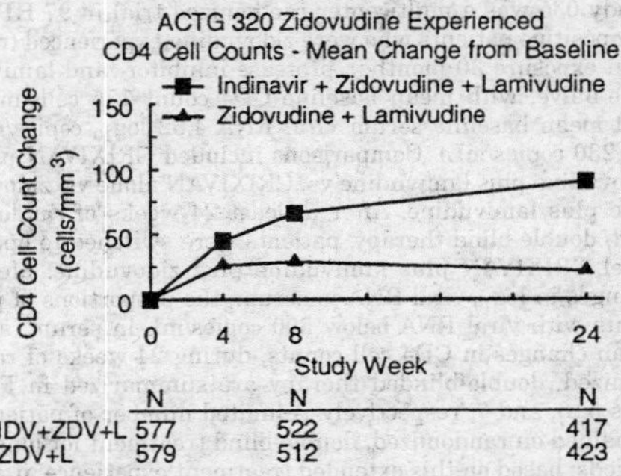

Study 028, a double-blind, multicenter, randomized, clinical endpoint trial conducted in Brazil, compared the effects of CRIXIVAN plus zidovudine with those of CRIXIVAN alone or zidovudine alone on the progression to an ADI or death, and on surrogate marker responses. All patients were antiretroviral naive with CD4 cell counts of 50 to 250 cells/mm^3. The study enrolled 996 HIV-1 seropositive patients [28% female, 11% Black, 1% Asian/Other, median age 33 years, mean baseline CD4 cell count of 152 cells/mm^3, mean serum viral RNA of 4.44 $\log_{10}$ copies/mL (27,824 copies/mL)]. Treatment regimens containing zidovudine were modified in a blinded manner with the optional addition of lamivudine (median time: week 40). The median length of follow-up was 56 weeks with a maximum of 97 weeks. The study was terminated after a planned interim analysis, resulting in a median follow-up of 56 weeks and a maximum follow-up of 97 weeks. Results are shown in Table 2 and Figures 3 and 4.

Table 2
Protocol 028

Endpoint	Number (%) of Patients with AIDS-defining Illness or Death IDV+ZDV (n=332)	IDV (n=332)	ZDV (n=332)
HIV Progression or Death	21 (6.3)	27 (8.1)	62 (18.7)
Death*	8 (2.4)	5 (1.5)	11 (3.3)

*The number of deaths is inadequate to assess the impact of Indinavir on survival.

Study 028: Figure 3

Indinavir Protocol 028 Zidovudine Naive
Viral RNA - Proportions Below 500 Copies/mL in Serum

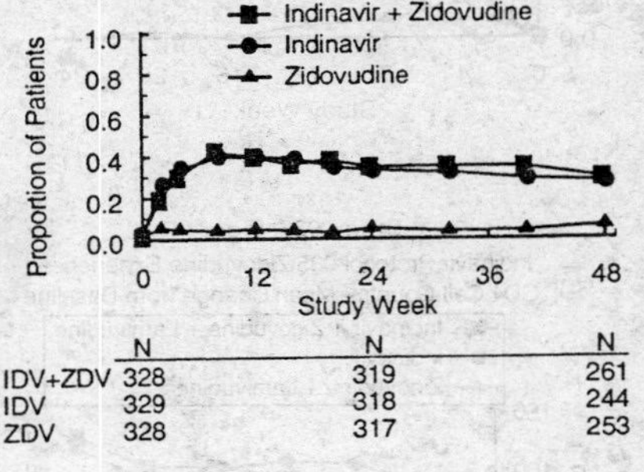

[See figure 4 at top of next page]

Continued on next page

Crixivan—Cont.

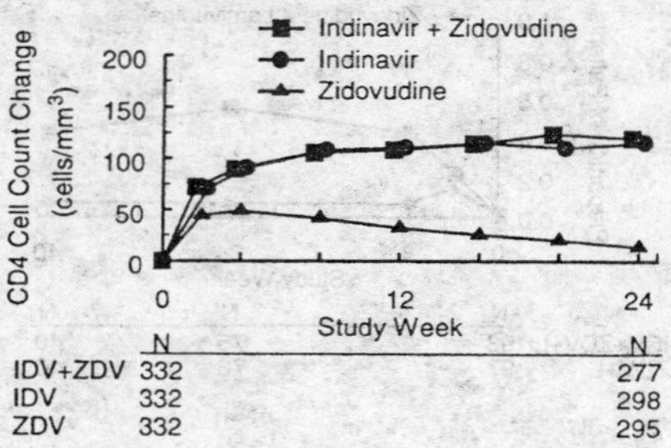

Study 035 was a multicenter randomized trial in 97 HIV-1 seropositive patients who were zidovudine-experienced (median exposure 30 months), protease-inhibitor- and lamivudine-naive, with mean baseline CD4 count 175 cells/mm^3 and mean baseline serum viral RNA 4.62 $\log_{10}$ copies/mL (41,230 copies/mL). Comparisons included CRIXIVAN plus zidovudine plus lamivudine vs. CRIXIVAN alone vs. zidovudine plus lamivudine. After at least 24 weeks of randomized, double-blind therapy, patients were switched to open-label CRIXIVAN plus lamivudine plus zidovudine. Mean changes in $\log_{10}$ viral RNA in serum, the proportions of patients with viral RNA below 500 copies/mL in serum, and mean changes in CD4 cell counts, during 24 weeks of randomized, double-blinded therapy are summarized in Figures 5, 6, and 7, respectively. A limited number of patients remained on randomized, double-blind treatment for longer periods; based on this extended treatment experience, it appears that a greater number of subjects randomized to CRIXIVAN plus zidovudine plus lamivudine demonstrated HIV RNA levels below 500 copies/mL during one year of therapy as compared to those in other treatment groups.

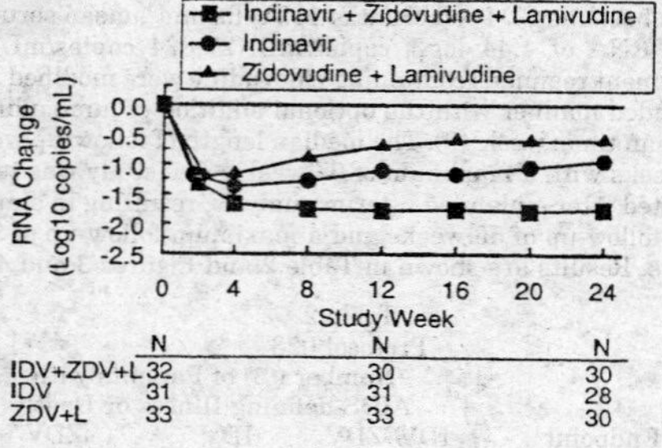

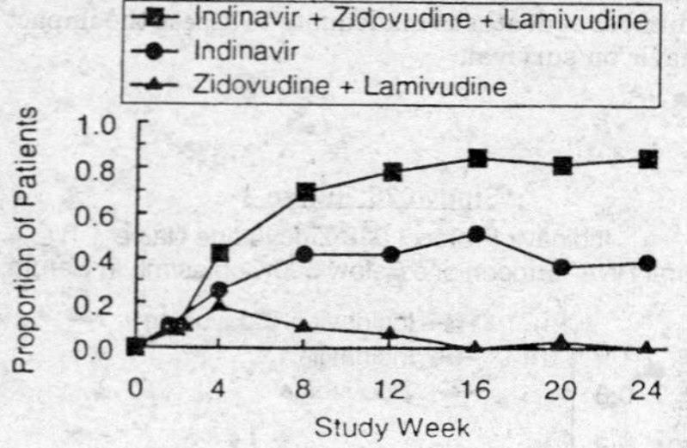

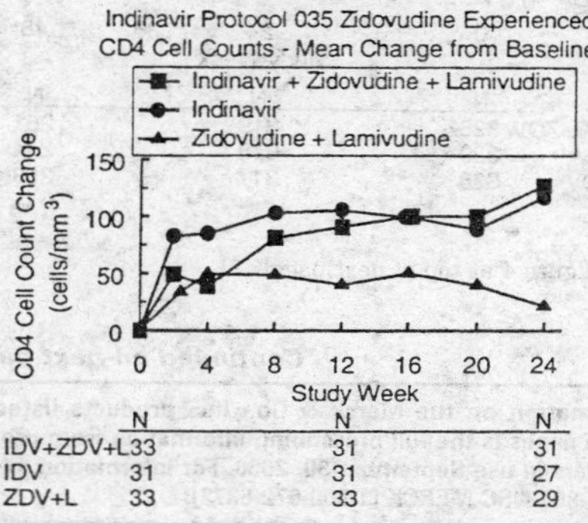

Genotypic Resistance in Clinical Studies
Study 006 (10/15/93–10/12/94) was a dose-ranging study in which patients were initially treated with CRIXIVAN at a dose of <2.4 g/day followed by 2.4 g/day. Study 019 (6/23/94–4/10/95) was a randomized comparison of CRIXIVAN 600 mg every 6 hours, CRIXIVAN plus zidovudine, and zidovudine alone. Table 3 shows the incidence of genotypic resistance at 24 weeks in these studies.

Table 3
Genotypic Resistance at 24 Weeks

Treatment Group	Resistance to IDV n/N*	Resistance to ZDV n/N*
IDV	—	—
<2.4 g/day	31/37 (84%)	—
2.4 g/day	9/21 (43%)	1/17 (6%)
IDV/ZDV	4/22 (18%)	1/22 (5%)
ZDV	1/18 (6%)	11/17 (65%)

*N – includes patients with non-amplifiable virus at 24 weeks who had amplifiable virus at week 0.

CONTRAINDICATIONS

CRIXIVAN is contraindicated in patients with clinically significant hypersensitivity to any of its components.
CRIXIVAN should not be administered concurrently with terfenadine, cisapride, astemizole, triazolam, midazolam, pimozide, or ergot derivatives. Inhibition of CYP3A4 by CRIXIVAN could result in elevated plasma concentrations of these drugs, potentially causing serious or life-threatening reactions.

WARNINGS

Nephrolithiasis/Urolithiasis
Nephrolithiasis/urolithiasis has occurred with CRIXIVAN therapy. In some cases, nephrolithiasis has been associated with renal insufficiency or acute renal failure. If signs or symptoms of nephrolithiasis/urolithiasis occur, (including flank pain, with or without hematuria or microscopic hematuria), temporary interruption (e.g., 1–3 days) or discontinuation of therapy may be considered. **Adequate hydration is recommended in all patients treated with CRIXIVAN. (See ADVERSE REACTIONS, *Post-Marketing Experience* and DOSAGE AND ADMINISTRATION, *Nephrolithiasis/Urolithiasis*.)**
Hemolytic Anemia
Acute hemolytic anemia, including cases resulting in death, has been reported in patients treated with CRIXIVAN. Once a diagnosis is apparent, appropriate measures for the treatment of hemolytic anemia should be instituted, including discontinuation of CRIXIVAN.
Hepatitis
Hepatitis including cases resulting in hepatic failure and death has been reported in patients treated with CRIXIVAN. Because the majority of these patients had confounding medical conditions and/or were receiving concomitant therapy(ies), a causal relationship between CRIXIVAN and these events has not been established.
Hyperglycemia
New onset diabetes mellitus, exacerbation of pre-existing diabetes mellitus and hyperglycemia have been reported during post-marketing surveillance in HIV-infected patients receiving protease inhibitor therapy. Some patients required either initiation or dose adjustments of insulin or oral hypoglycemic agents for treatment of these events. In some cases, diabetic ketoacidosis has occurred. In those patients who discontinued protease inhibitor therapy, hyperglycemia persisted in some cases. Because these events have been reported voluntarily during clinical practice, estimates of frequency cannot be made and a causal relationship between protease inhibitor therapy and these events has not been established.
Drug Interactions
Concomitant use of CRIXIVAN with lovastatin or simvastatin is not recommended. Caution should be exercised if HIV protease inhibitors, including CRIXIVAN, are used concurrently with other HMG-CoA reductase inhibitors that are also metabolized by the CYP3A4 pathway (e.g., atorvastatin or cerivastatin). The risk of myopathy including rhabdomyolysis may be increased when HIV protease inhibitors, including CRIXIVAN, are used in combination with these drugs.
Concomitant use of CRIXIVAN and St. John's wort (*Hypericum perforatum*) or products containing St. John's wort is not recommended. Coadministration of CRIXIVAN and St. John's wort has been shown to substantially decrease indinavir concentrations (see CLINICAL PHARMACOLOGY, *Pharmacokinetics, Drugs That Should Not Be Coadministered With CRIXIVAN*) and may lead to loss of virologic response and possible resistance to CRIXIVAN or to the class of protease inhibitors.

PRECAUTIONS

General
Indirect hyperbilirubinemia has occurred frequently during treatment with CRIXIVAN and has infrequently been associated with increases in serum transaminases (see also ADVERSE REACTIONS, *Clinical Trials* and *Post-Marketing Experience*). It is not known whether CRIXIVAN will exacerbate the physiologic hyperbilirubinemia seen in neonates. (See *Pregnancy*)
Coexisting Conditions
Patients with hemophilia: There have been reports of spontaneous bleeding in patients with hemophilia A and B treated with protease inhibitors. In some patients, additional factor VIII was required. In many of the reported cases, treatment with protease inhibitors was continued or restarted. A causal relationship between protease inhibitor therapy and these episodes has not been established. (See ADVERSE REACTIONS, *Post-Marketing Experience*).
Patients with hepatic insufficiency due to cirrhosis: In these patients, the dosage of CRIXIVAN should be lowered because of decreased metabolism of CRIXIVAN (see DOSAGE AND ADMINISTRATION).
Patients with renal insufficiency: Patients with renal insufficiency have not been studied.
Fat Redistribution
Redistribution/accumulation of body fat including central obesity, dorsocervical fat enlargement (buffalo hump), peripheral wasting, breast enlargement, and "cushingoid appearance" have been observed in patients receiving protease inhibitors. The mechanism and long-term consequences of these events are currently unknown. A causal relationship has not been established.
Information for Patients
CRIXIVAN is not a cure for HIV infection and patients may continue to develop opportunistic infections and other complications associated with HIV disease. The long-term effects of CRIXIVAN unknown at this time. CRIXIVAN has not been shown to reduce the risk of transmission of HIV to others through sexual contact or blood contamination.
Patients should be advised to remain under the care of a physician when using CRIXIVAN and should not modify or discontinue treatment without first consulting the physician. Therefore, if a dose is missed, patients should take the next dose at the regularly scheduled time and should not double this dose. Therapy with CRIXIVAN should be initiated and maintained at the recommended dosage.
CRIXIVAN may interact with some drugs; therefore, patients should be advised to report to their doctor the use of any other prescription, non-prescription medication or herbal products, particularly St. John's wort.
For optimal absorption, CRIXIVAN should be administered without food but with water 1 hour before or 2 hours after a meal. Alternatively, CRIXIVAN may be administered with other liquids such as skim milk, juice, coffee, or tea, or with a light meal, e.g., dry toast with jelly, juice, and coffee with skim milk and sugar; or corn flakes, skim milk and sugar (see CLINICAL PHARMACOLOGY, *Effect of Food on Oral Absorption* and DOSAGE AND ADMINISTRATION). Ingestion of CRIXIVAN with a meal high in calories, fat, and protein reduces the absorption of indinavir.
Patients should be informed that redistribution or accumulation of body fat may occur in patients receiving protease inhibitors and that the cause and long-term health effects of these conditions are not known at this time.
CRIXIVAN Capsules are sensitive to moisture. Patients should be informed that CRIXIVAN should be stored and used in the original container and the desiccant should remain in the bottle.
Drug Interactions
Delavirdine
Due to an increase in indinavir plasma concentrations (preliminary results), a dosage reduction of indinavir should be considered when CRIXIVAN and delavirdine are coadministered. (See DOSAGE AND ADMINISTRATION, *Concomitant Therapy, Delavirdine*; CLINICAL PHARMACOLOGY, *Drug Interactions, Drugs Requiring Dose Modification, Delavirdine.*)
Efavirenz
Due to a decrease in the plasma concentrations of indinavir, a dosage increase of indinavir is recommended when CRIXIVAN and efavirenz are coadministered. No adjustment of the dose of efavirenz is necessary when given with indinavir. (See DOSAGE AND ADMINISTRATION, *Concomitant Therapy, Efavirenz*; CLINICAL PHARMACOLOGY, *Drug Interactions, Drugs Requiring Dose Modification, Efavirenz.*)
Itraconazole
Itraconazole is an inhibitor of P-450 3A4 that increases plasma concentrations of indinavir. Therefore, a dosage reduction of indinavir is recommended when CRIXIVAN and itraconazole are coadministered (see DOSAGE AND ADMINISTRATION, *Concomitant Therapy, Itraconazole*; CLINICAL PHARMACOLOGY, *Drug Interactions, Drugs Requiring Dose Modification, Itraconazole*).
Ketoconazole
Ketoconazole is an inhibitor of P-450 3A4 that increases plasma concentrations of indinavir. Therefore, a dosage reduction of indinavir is recommended when CRIXIVAN and ketoconazole are coadministered (see DOSAGE AND ADMINISTRATION, *Concomitant Therapy, Ketoconazole*; CLINICAL PHARMACOLOGY, *Drug Interactions, Drugs Requiring Dose Modification, Ketoconazole*).
Rifabutin
When rifabutin and CRIXIVAN are coadministered, there is an increase in the plasma concentrations of rifabutin and a decrease in the plasma concentrations of indinavir. A dosage reduction of rifabutin and a dosage increase of CRIXIVAN are necessary when rifabutin is coadministered with CRIXIVAN. The suggested dose adjustments are expected to result in rifabutin concentrations at least 50% higher than typically observed when rifabutin is administered alone at its usual dose (300 mg/day) and indinavir concentrations which may be slightly less than typically observed

when indinavir is administered alone at its usual dose (800 mg every 8 hours). (See DOSAGE AND ADMINISTRATION, *Concomitant Therapy, Rifabutin*; CLINICAL PHARMACOLOGY, *Drug Interactions, Drugs Requiring Dose Modification, Rifabutin*).

Rifampin

Rifampin is a potent inducer of P-450 3A4 that markedly diminishes plasma concentrations of indinavir. Therefore, CRIXIVAN and rifampin should not be coadministered (see CLINICAL PHARMACOLOGY, *Drugs That Should Not Be Coadministered With CRIXIVAN*).

Other

If CRIXIVAN and didanosine are administered concomitantly, they should be administered at least one hour apart on an empty stomach; a normal (acidic) gastric pH may be necessary for optimum absorption of indinavir, whereas acid rapidly degrades didanosine which is formulated with buffering agents to increase pH (consult the manufacturer's product circular for didanosine).

Interactions between indinavir and less potent CYP3A4 inducers than rifampin, such as phenobarbital, phenytoin, carbamazepine, and dexamethasone have not been studied. These agents should be used with caution if administered concomitantly with indinavir because decreased indinavir plasma concentrations may result.

Carcinogenesis, Mutagenesis, Impairment of Fertility

Carcinogenicity studies were conducted in mice and rats. In mice, no increased incidence of any tumor type was observed. The highest dose tested in rats was 640 mg/kg/day; at this dose a statistically significant increased incidence of thyroid adenomas was seen only in male rats. At that dose, daily systemic exposure in rats was approximately 1.3 times higher than daily systemic exposure in humans. No evidence of mutagenicity or genotoxicity was observed in *in vitro* microbial mutagenesis (Ames) tests, *in vitro* alkaline elution assays for DNA breakage, *in vitro* and *in vivo* chromosomal aberration studies, and *in vitro* mammalian cell mutagenesis assays. No treatment-related effects on mating, fertility, or embryo survival were seen in female rats and no treatment-related effects on mating performance were seen in male rats at doses providing systemic exposure comparable to or slightly higher than that with the clinical dose. In addition, no treatment-related effects were observed in fecundity or fertility of untreated females mated to treated males.

Pregnancy

Pregnancy Category C: Developmental toxicity studies were performed in rabbits (at doses up to 240 mg/kg/day), dogs (at doses up to 80 mg/kg/day), and rats (at doses up to 640 mg/kg/day). The highest doses in these studies produced systemic exposures in these species comparable to or slightly greater than human exposure. No treatment-related external, visceral, or skeletal changes were observed in rabbits or dogs. No treatment-related external or visceral changes were observed in rats. Treatment-related increases over controls in the incidence of supernumerary ribs (at exposures at or below those in humans) and of cervical ribs (at exposures comparable to or slightly greater than those in humans) were seen in rats. In all three species, no treatment-related effects on embryonic/fetal survival or fetal weights were observed.

In rabbits, at a maternal dose of 240 mg/kg/day, no drug was detected in fetal plasma 1 hour after dosing. Fetal plasma drug levels 2 hours after dosing were approximately 3% of maternal plasma drug levels. In dogs, at a maternal dose of 80 mg/kg/day, fetal plasma drug levels were approximately 50% of maternal plasma drug levels both 1 and 2 hours after dosing. In rats, at maternal doses of 40 and 640 mg/kg/day, fetal plasma drug levels were approximately 10 to 15% and 10 to 20% of maternal plasma drug levels 1 and 2 hours after dosing, respectively.

Indinavir was administered to Rhesus monkeys during the third trimester of pregnancy (at doses up to 160 mg/kg twice daily) and to neonatal Rhesus monkeys (at doses up to 160 mg/kg twice daily). When administered to neonates, indinavir caused an exacerbation of the transient physiologic hyperbilirubinemia seen in this species after birth; serum bilirubin values were approximately fourfold above controls at 160 mg/kg twice daily. A similar exacerbation did not occur in neonates after *in utero* exposure to indinavir during the third trimester of pregnancy. In Rhesus monkeys, fetal plasma drug levels were approximately 1 to 2% of maternal plasma drug levels approximately 1 hour after maternal dosing at 40, 80, or 160 mg/kg twice daily.

Hyperbilirubinemia has occurred during treatment with CRIXIVAN (see PRECAUTIONS and ADVERSE REACTIONS). It is unknown whether CRIXIVAN administered to the mother in the perinatal period will exacerbate physiologic hyperbilirubinemia in neonates.

There are no adequate and well-controlled studies in pregnant women. CRIXIVAN should be used during pregnancy only if the potential benefit justifies the potential risk to the fetus.

Antiviral Pregnancy Registry

To monitor maternal-fetal outcomes of pregnant women exposed to CRIXIVAN, an Antiretroviral Pregnancy Registry has been established. Physicians are encouraged to register patients by calling 1-800-258-4263.

Nursing Mothers

Studies in lactating rats have demonstrated that indinavir is excreted in milk. Although it is not known whether CRIXIVAN is excreted in human milk, there exists the potential for adverse effects from indinavir in nursing infants. Mothers should be instructed to discontinue nursing if they are receiving CRIXIVAN. This is consistent with the recommendation by the U.S. Public Health Service Centers for Disease Control and Prevention that HIV-infected mothers not breast-feed their infants to avoid risking postnatal transmission of HIV.

Table 4
Clinical Adverse Experiences Reported in ≥2% of Patients

	Study 028 Considered Drug-Related and of Moderate or Severe Intensity		Study ACTG 320 of Unknown Drug Relationship and of Severe or Life-threatening Intensity		
Adverse Experience	CRIXIVAN Percent (n=332)	CRIXIVAN plus Zidovudine Percent (n=332)	Zidovudine Percent (n=332)	CRIXIVAN plus Zidovudine plus Lamivudine Percent (n=571)	Zidovudine plus Lamivudine Percent (n=575)
Body as a Whole					
Abdominal pain	16.6	16.0	12.0	1.9	0.7
Asthenia/fatigue	2.1	14.2	3.6	2.4	4.5
Fever	1.5	1.5	2.1	3.8	3.0
Malaise	2.1	2.7	1.8	0	0
Digestive System					
Nausea	11.7	31.9	19.6	2.8	1.4
Diarrhea	3.3	3.0	2.4	0.9	1.2
Vomiting	8.4	17.8	9.0	1.4	1.4
Acid regurgitation	2.7	5.4	1.8	0.4	0
Anorexia	2.7	5.4	3.0	0.5	0.2
Appetite increase	2.1	1.5	1.2	0	0
Dyspepsia	1.5	2.7	0.9	0	0
Jaundice	1.5	2.1	0.3	0	0
Hemic and Lymphatic System					
Anemia	0.6	1.2	2.1	2.4	3.5
Musculoskeletal System					
Back pain	8.4	4.5	1.5	0.9	0.7
Nervous System / Psychiatric					
Headache	5.4	9.6	6.0	2.4	2.8
Dizziness	3.0	3.9	0.9	0.5	0.7
Somnolence	2.4	3.3	3.3	0	0
Skin and Skin Appendage					
Pruritus	4.2	2.4	1.8	0.5	0
Rash	1.2	0.6	2.4	1.1	0.5
Respiratory System					
Cough	1.5	0.3	0.6	1.6	1.0
Difficulty breathing/ dyspnea/shortness of breath	0	0.6	0.3	1.8	1.0
Urogenital System					
Nephrolithiasis/ urolithiasis*	8.7	7.8	2.1	2.6	0.3
Dysuria	1.5	2.4	0.3	0.4	0.2
Special Senses					
Taste perversion	2.7	8.4	1.2	0.2	0

* Including renal colic, and flank pain with and without hematuria

Pediatric Use

Safety and effectiveness in pediatric patients have not been established.

ADVERSE REACTIONS

Clinical Trials

Nephrolithiasis/urolithiasis, including flank pain with or without hematuria (including microscopic hematuria), has been reported in approximately 9.3% (193/2071) of patients receiving CRIXIVAN in clinical trials at the recommended dose, compared to 1.8% in the control arms. Of the patients treated with CRIXIVAN who developed nephrolithiasis/urolithiasis, 3.1% (6/193) were reported to develop hydronephrosis and 3.1% (6/193) underwent stent placement. Following the acute episode, 3.6% (7/193) of patients discontinued therapy. (See WARNINGS and DOSAGE AND ADMINISTRATION, *Nephrolithiasis / Urolithiasis*.)

Asymptomatic hyperbilirubinemia (total bilirubin ≥2.5 mg/dL), reported predominantly as elevated indirect bilirubin, has occurred in approximately 14% of patients treated with CRIXIVAN. In <1% this was associated with elevations in ALT or AST.

Hyperbilirubinemia and nephrolithiasis/urolithiasis occurred more frequently at doses exceeding 2.4 g/day compared to doses ≤2.4 g/day.

Clinical adverse experiences reported in ≥2% of patients treated with CRIXIVAN alone, CRIXIVAN in combination with zidovudine or zidovudine plus lamivudine, zidovudine alone, or zidovudine plus lamivudine are presented in Table 4.

[See table 4 above]

In Phase I and II controlled trials, the following adverse events were reported significantly more frequently by those randomized to the arms containing CRIXIVAN than by those randomized to nucleoside analogues: rash, upper respiratory infection, dry skin, pharyngitis, taste perversion.

Selected laboratory abnormalities of severe or life-threatening intensity reported in patients treated with CRIXIVAN alone, CRIXIVAN in combination with zidovudine or zidovudine plus lamivudine, zidovudine alone, or zidovudine plus lamivudine are presented in Table 5.

[See table 5 at top of next page]

Post-Marketing Experience

Body As A Whole: redistribution/accumulation of body fat (see PRECAUTIONS, *Fat Redistribution*).

Cardiovascular System: cardiovascular disorders including myocardial infarction and angina pectoris.

Digestive System: liver function abnormalities; hepatitis including reports of hepatic failure (see WARNINGS); pancreatitis; jaundice; abdominal distention; dyspepsia.

Hematologic: increased spontaneous bleeding in patients with hemophilia (see PRECAUTIONS); acute hemolytic anemia (see WARNINGS).

Endocrine / Metabolic: new onset diabetes mellitus, exacerbation of pre-existing diabetes mellitus, hyperglycemia (see WARNINGS).

Hypersensitivity: anaphylactoid reactions; urticaria.

Musculoskeletal System: arthralgia.

Nervous System / Psychiatric: oral paresthesia; depression.

Skin and Skin Appendage: rash including erythema multiforme and Stevens-Johnson Syndrome; hyperpigmentation; alopecia; ingrown toenails and/or paronychia; pruritus.

Urogenital System: nephrolithiasis/urolithiasis; in some cases resulting in renal insufficiency or acute renal failure (see WARNINGS); interstitial nephritis sometimes with indinavir crystal deposits; in some patients, the interstitial nephritis did not resolve following discontinuation of CRIXIVAN; crystalluria; dysuria.

Laboratory Abnormalities

Increased serum triglycerides, increased serum cholesterol.

OVERDOSAGE

There have been more than 60 reports of acute or chronic human overdosage (up to 23 times the recommended total

Continued on next page

Information on the Merck & Co., Inc. products listed on these pages is the full prescribing information from product circulars in use September 30, 2000. For information, please call 1-800-NSC MERCK [1-800-672-6372].

Crixivan—Cont.

daily dose of 2400 mg) with CRIXIVAN. The most commonly reported symptoms were renal (e.g., nephrolithiasis/urolithiasis, flank pain, hematuria) and gastrointestinal (e.g., nausea, vomiting, diarrhea).
It is not known whether CRIXIVAN is dialyzable by peritoneal or hemodialysis.

DOSAGE AND ADMINISTRATION

The recommended dosage of CRIXIVAN is 800 mg (**two** 400-mg capsules) orally every 8 hours. The dosage is the same whether CRIXIVAN is used alone or in combination with other antiretroviral agents.
CRIXIVAN must be taken at intervals of 8 hours. For optimal absorption, CRIXIVAN should be administered without food but with water 1 hour before or 2 hours after a meal. Alternatively, CRIXIVAN may be administered with other liquids such as skim milk, juice, coffee, or tea, or with a light meal, e.g., dry toast with jelly, juice, and coffee with skim milk and sugar; or corn flakes, skim milk and sugar. (See CLINICAL PHARMACOLOGY, *Effect of Food on Oral Absorption.*)
To ensure adequate hydration, it is recommended that the patient drink at least 1.5 liters (approximately 48 ounces) of liquids during the course of 24 hours.
Concomitant Therapy (See CLINICAL PHARMACOLOGY, *Drug Interactions*, and/or PRECAUTIONS, *Drug Interactions.*)
Delavirdine
Dose reduction of CRIXIVAN to 600 mg every 8 hours should be considered when administering delavirdine 400 mg three times a day.
Didanosine
If indinavir and didanosine are administered concomitantly, they should be administered at least one hour apart on an empty stomach (consult the manufacturer's product circular for didanosine).
Efavirenz
Dose increase of CRIXIVAN to 1000 mg every 8 hours is recommended when administering efavirenz concurrently (consult the manufacturer's product circular for efavirenz).
Itraconazole
Dose reduction of CRIXIVAN to 600 mg every 8 hours is recommended when administering itraconazole 200 mg twice daily concurrently.
Ketoconazole
Dose reduction of CRIXIVAN to 600 mg every 8 hours is recommended when administering ketoconazole concurrently.
Rifabutin
Dose reduction of rifabutin to half the standard dose (consult the manufacturer's product circular for rifabutin) and a dose increase of CRIXIVAN to 1000 mg (**three** 333-mg capsules) every 8 hours are recommended when rifabutin and CRIXIVAN are coadministered.
Hepatic Insufficiency
The dosage of CRIXIVAN should be reduced to 600 mg every 8 hours in patients with mild-to-moderate hepatic insufficiency due to cirrhosis.
Nephrolithiasis/Urolithiasis
In addition to adequate hydration, medical management in patients who experience nephrolithiasis/urolithiasis may include temporary interruption (e.g., 1–3 days) or discontinuation of therapy.

HOW SUPPLIED

CRIXIVAN Capsules are supplied as follows:
No. 3756—200 mg capsules: semi-translucent white capsules coded **"CRIXIVAN™ 200 mg"** in blue. Available as:
NDC 0006-0571-42 unit-of-use bottles of 270 (with desiccant)
NDC 0006-0571-43 unit-of-use bottles of 360 (with desiccant).
Shown in Product Identification Guide, page 323
No. 3802—333 mg capsules: semi-translucent white capsules coded **"CRIXIVAN™ 333 mg"** in red and a radial red band on the body. Available as:
NDC 0006-0574-65 unit-of-use bottles of 135 (with desicant).
Shown in Product Identification Guide, page 323
No. 3758—400 mg capsules: semi-translucent white capsules coded **"CRIXIVAN™ 400 mg"** in green. Available as:
NDC 0006-0573-42 unit-dose packages of 42
NDC 0006-0573-62 unit-of-use bottles of 180 (with desiccant)
NDC 0006-0573-54 unit-of-use bottles of 90 (with desiccant).
NDC 0006-0573-18 unit-of-use bottles of 18 (with desiccant).
Shown in Product Identification Guide, page 323
Storage
Bottles: Store in a tightly-closed container at room temperature, 15–30°C (59–86°F). Protect from moisture.
CRIXIVAN Capsules are sensitive to moisture. CRIXIVAN should be dispensed and stored in the original container. The desiccant should remain in the original bottle.
Unit-Dose Packages: Store at room temperature, 15–30°C (59–86°F). Protect from moisture.
7979816 Issued May 2000

Table 5
Selected Laboratory Abnormalities of Severe or Life-threatening Intensity
Reported in Studies 028 and ACTG 320

	Study 028			Study ACTG 320	
	CRIXIVAN Percent (n=329)	CRIXIVAN plus Zidovudine Percent (n=320)	Zidovudine Percent (n=330)	CRIXIVAN plus Zidovudine plus Lamivudine Percent (n=571)	Zidovudine plus Lamivudine Percent (n=575)
Hematology					
Decreased hemoglobin <7.0 g/dL	0.6	0.9	3.3	2.4	3.5
Decreased platelet count <50 THS/mm^3	0.9	0.9	1.8	0.2	0.9
Decreased neutrophils <0.75 THS/mm^3	2.4	2.2	6.7	5.1	14.6
Blood chemistry					
Increased ALT >500% ULN*	4.9	4.1	3.0	2.6	2.6
Increased AST >500% ULN	3.7	2.8	2.7	3.3	2.8
Total serum bilirubin >250% ULN	11.9	9.7	0.6	6.1	1.4
Increased serum amylase >200% ULN	2.1	1.9	1.8	0.9	0.3
Increased glucose >250 mg/dL	0.9	0.9	0.6	1.6	1.9
Increased creatinine >300% ULN	0	0	0.6	0.2	0

* Upper limit of the normal range.

Patient Information about

CRIXIVAN® (KRIK-sih-van)
for HIV (Human Immunodeficiency Virus) Infection
Generic name: indinavir (in-DIH-nuh-veer) sulfate

Please read this information before you start taking CRIXIVAN*. Also, read the leaflet each time you renew your prescription, just in case anything has changed. Remember, this leaflet does not take the place of careful discussions with your doctor. You and your doctor should discuss CRIXIVAN when you start taking your medication and at regular checkups. You should remain under a doctor's care when using CRIXIVAN and should not change or stop treatment without first talking with your doctor.

*Registered trademark of MERCK & CO., Inc.

What is CRIXIVAN?
CRIXIVAN is an oral capsule used for the treatment of HIV (Human Immunodeficiency Virus). HIV is the virus that causes AIDS (acquired immune deficiency syndrome). CRIXIVAN is a type of HIV drug called a protease (PRO-tee-ase) inhibitor.

How does CRIXIVAN work?
CRIXIVAN is a protease inhibitor that fights HIV. CRIXIVAN can help reduce your chances of getting illnesses associated with HIV. CRIXIVAN can also help lower the amount of HIV in your body (called "viral load") and raise your CD4 (T) cell count. CRIXIVAN may not have these effects in all patients.
CRIXIVAN is usually prescribed with other anti-HIV drugs such as ZDV (also called AZT), 3TC, ddI, ddC, or d4T. CRIXIVAN works differently from these other anti-HIV drugs. Talk with your doctor about how you should take CRIXIVAN.
CRIXIVAN has been studied in adults. The safety and effectiveness of CRIXIVAN in children and adolescents have not been established.

How should I take CRIXIVAN?
There are six important things you must do to help you benefit from CRIXIVAN:

1. **Take CRIXIVAN capsules every day as prescribed by your doctor.** Continue taking CRIXIVAN unless your doctor tells you to stop. Take the exact amount of CRIXIVAN that your doctor tells you to take, right from the very start. To help make sure you will benefit from CRIXIVAN, you must not skip doses or take "drug holidays". If you don't take CRIXIVAN as prescribed, the activity of CRIXIVAN may be reduced (due to resistance).
2. **Take CRIXIVAN capsules every 8 hours around the clock, *every day*.** It may be easier to remember to take CRIXIVAN if you take it at the same time every day. If you have questions about when to take CRIXIVAN, your doctor or health care provider can help you decide what schedule works for you.
3. **If you miss a dose by more than 2 hours, wait and then take the next dose at the regularly scheduled time.** However, if you miss a dose by less than 2 hours, take your missed dose immediately. Then take your next dose at the regularly scheduled time. Do not take more or less than your prescribed dose of CRIXIVAN at any one time.
4. **Take CRIXIVAN with water.** You can also take CRIXIVAN with other beverages such as skim or non-fat milk, juice, coffee, or tea.
5. **Ideally, take each dose of CRIXIVAN without food but with water at least one hour before or two hours after a meal.** Or you can take CRIXIVAN with a light meal. Examples of light meals include:
   dry toast with jelly, juice, and coffee (with skim or non-fat milk and sugar if you want)
   cornflakes with skim or non-fat milk and sugar

   Do not take CRIXIVAN at the same time as any meals that are high in calories, fat, and protein (for example—a bacon and egg breakfast). When taken at the same time as CRIXIVAN, these foods can interfere with CRIXIVAN being absorbed into your bloodstream and may lessen its effect.
6. **It is critical that you drink at least six 8-ounce glasses of liquids (preferably water) throughout the day, every day. CRIXIVAN can cause kidney stones.** Having enough fluids in your body should help reduce the chances of forming a kidney stone. Call your doctor or other health care provider if you develop kidney pains (middle to lower stomach or back pain) or blood in the urine.

Does CRIXIVAN cure HIV or AIDS?
CRIXIVAN is not a cure for HIV or AIDS. People taking CRIXIVAN may still develop infections or other conditions associated with HIV. Because of this, it is very important for you to remain under the care of a doctor. Although CRIXIVAN is not a cure for HIV or AIDS, CRIXIVAN can help reduce your chances of getting illnesses, including death, associated with HIV. CRIXIVAN may not have these effects in all patients.

Does CRIXIVAN reduce the risk of passing HIV to others?
CRIXIVAN has not been shown to reduce the risk of passing HIV to others through sexual contact or blood contamination.

Who should not take CRIXIVAN?
Do not take CRIXIVAN if you have had a serious allergic reaction to CRIXIVAN or any of its components.

What other medical problems or conditions should I discuss with my doctor?
Talk to your doctor if:
- You are pregnant or if you become pregnant while you are taking CRIXIVAN.
  We do not yet know how CRIXIVAN affects pregnant women or their developing babies.
- You are breast-feeding. You should stop breast-feeding if you are taking CRIXIVAN.

Also talk to your doctor if you have:
- Problems with your liver, especially if you have mild or moderate liver disease caused by cirrhosis.
- Problems with your kidneys.
- Diabetes
- Hemophilia
- High cholesterol and you are taking cholesterol-lowering medicines called "statins".

Tell your doctor about any medicines you are taking or plan to take, including non-prescription medicines, herbal products including St. John's wort (*Hypericum perforatum*), or dietary supplements.

Can CRIXIVAN be taken with other medications?**
Drugs you should not take with CRIXIVAN:
SELDANE®
(terfenadine)
VERSED®
(midazolam)
ORAP®
(pimozide)
PROPULSID®
(cisapride)
HISMANAL®
(astemizole)
HALCION®
(triazolam)
Ergot medications

(e.g., Wigraine® and Cafergot®)
Taking CRIXIVAN with the above medications could result in serious or life-threatening problems (such as irregular heartbeat or excessive sleepiness).
In addition, you should not take CRIXIVAN with the following:
Rifampin, known as RIFADIN®, RIFAMATE®, RIFATER®, or RIMACTANE®.
It is not recommended to take CRIXIVAN with the cholesterol-lowering drugs MEVACOR* (lovastatin) or ZOCOR* (simvastatin) because of possible drug interactions. There is also an increased risk of drug interactions between CRIXIVAN and LIPITOR® (atorvastatin) and BAYCOL® (cerivastatin); talk to your doctor before you take any of these cholesterol-lowering drugs with CRIXIVAN.
Taking CRIXIVAN with St. John's wort (*Hypericum perforatum*), an herbal product sold as a dietary supplement, or products containing St. John's wort is not recommended. Taking St. John's wort has been shown to decrease CRIXIVAN levels and may lead to increased viral load and possible resistance to CRIXIVAN or cross resistance to other antiretroviral drugs.
Drugs you can take with CRIXIVAN include:
RETROVIR®
(zidovudine, ZDV
also called AZT)
ZERIT®
(stavudine, d4T)
BACTRIM®/SEPTRA®
(trimethoprim/sulfamethoxazole)
BIAXIN®
(clarithromycin)
TAGAMET®
(cimetidine)
EPIVIR™
(lamivudine, 3TC)
isoniazid
(INH)
DIFLUCAN®
(fluconazole)
ORTHO-NOVUM 1/35®
(oral contraceptive)
Methadone
VIDEX® (didanosine, ddI)—If you take CRIXIVAN with VIDEX®, take them at least one hour apart.
MYCOBUTIN® (rifabutin)—If you take CRIXIVAN with MYCOBUTIN®, your doctor may adjust both the dose of MYCOBUTIN and the dose of CRIXIVAN.
NIZORAL® (ketoconazole)—If you take CRIXIVAN with NIZORAL®, your doctor may adjust the dose of CRIXIVAN.
RESCRIPTOR® (delavirdine)—If you take CRIXIVAN with RESCRIPTOR®, your doctor may adjust the dose of CRIXIVAN.
SPORANOX® (itraconazole)—If you take CRIXIVAN with SPORANOX®, your doctor may adjust the dose of CRIXIVAN.
SUSTIVA™ (efavirenz)—If you take CRIXIVAN with SUSTIVA™, your doctor may adjust the dose of CRIXIVAN.
Talk to your doctor about any medications you are taking.

**The brands listed are the registered trademarks of their respective owners and are not trademarks of Merck & Co., Inc.

What are the possible side effects of CRIXIVAN?
Like all prescription drugs, CRIXIVAN can cause side effects. The following is **not** a complete list of side effects reported with CRIXIVAN when taken either alone or with other anti-HIV drugs. Do not rely on this leaflet alone for information about side effects. Your doctor can discuss with you a more complete list of side effects.
Some patients treated with CRIXIVAN developed kidney stones. In some of these patients this led to more severe kidney problems, including kidney failure or inflammation of the kidneys. Drinking at least six 8-ounce glasses of liquid (preferably water) each day should help reduce the chances of forming a kidney stone. Call your doctor or other health care provider if you develop kidney pains (middle to lower stomach or back pain) or blood in the urine.
Some patients treated with CRIXIVAN have had rapid breakdown of red blood cells (hemolytic anemia) which in some cases was severe or resulted in death.
Some patients treated with CRIXIVAN have had liver problems including liver failure and death. Some patients had other illnesses or were taking other drugs. It is uncertain if CRIXIVAN caused these liver problems.
Diabetes and high blood sugar (hyperglycemia) have occurred in patients taking protease inhibitors. In some of these patients, this led to ketoacidosis, a serious condition caused by poorly controlled blood sugar. Some patients had diabetes before starting protease inhibitors, others did not. Some patients required adjustments to their diabetes medication. Others needed new diabetes medication.
In some patients with hemophilia, increased bleeding has been reported.
Severe muscle pain and weakness have occurred in patients taking protease inhibitors, including CRIXIVAN, together with some of the cholesterol-lowering medicines called "statins." Call your doctor if you develop severe muscle pain or weakness.
Changes in body fat have been seen in some patients taking protease inhibitors. These changes may include increased amount of fat in the upper back and neck ("buffalo hump"), breast, and around the trunk. Loss of fat from the legs and arms may also happen. The cause and long term health effects of these conditions are not known at this time.
Clinical Studies
Increases in bilirubin (one laboratory test of liver function) have been reported in approximately 10% of patients. Usually, this finding has not been associated with liver problems. However, on rare occasions, a person may develop yellowing of the skin and/or eyes.
Side effects occurring in 2% or more of patients included: abdominal pain, fatigue or weakness, low red blood cell count, flank pain, painful urination, feeling unwell, nausea, upset stomach, diarrhea, vomiting, acid regurgitation, increased or decreased appetite, back pain, headache, dizziness, taste changes, rash, itchy skin, yellowing of the skin and/or eyes, upper respiratory infection, dry skin, and sore throat.
Swollen kidneys due to blocked urine flow occurred rarely.
Marketing Experience
Other side effects reported since CRIXIVAN has been marketed include: allergic reactions; severe skin reactions; yellowing of the skin and/or eyes; heart problems including heart attack; abdominal swelling; indigestion; inflammation of the kidneys; inflammation of the pancreas; joint pain; depression; itching; hives; change in skin color; hair loss, ingrown toenails with or without infection; crystals in the urine; painful urination; and numbness of the mouth.
Tell your doctor promptly about these or any other unusual symptoms. If the condition persists or worsens, seek medical attention.
How should I store CRIXIVAN capsules?
- Keep CRIXIVAN capsules in the bottle they came in and at room temperature (59°–86°F).
- Keep CRIXIVAN capsules dry by leaving the small desiccant "pillow" in the bottle. Keep the bottle closed.

This medication was prescribed for your particular condition. Do not use it for any other condition or give it to anybody else. Keep CRIXIVAN and all medicines out of the reach of children. If you suspect that more than the prescribed dose of this medicine has been taken, contact your local poison control center or emergency room immediately.
This leaflet provides a summary of information about CRIXIVAN. If you have any questions or concerns about either CRIXIVAN or HIV, talk to your doctor.
9024512 Issued May 2000

CUPRIMINE® Capsules (Penicillamine) ℞

> Physicians planning to use penicillamine should thoroughly familiarize themselves with its toxicity, special dosage considerations, and therapeutic benefits. Penicillamine should never be used casually. Each patient should remain constantly under the close supervision of the physician. Patients should be warned to report promptly any symptoms suggesting toxicity.

DESCRIPTION

Penicillamine is a chelating agent used in the treatment of Wilson's disease. It is also used to reduce cystine excretion in cystinuria and to treat patients with severe, active rheumatoid arthritis unresponsive to conventional therapy (see INDICATIONS). It is 3-mercapto-D-valine. It is a white or practically white, crystalline powder, freely soluble in water, slightly soluble in alcohol, and insoluble in ether, acetone, benzene, and carbon tetrachloride. Although its configuration is D, it is levorotatory as usually measured:

$$[\alpha]^{25°}_{D} = -62.5° \pm 2° \text{ (c = 1, 1N NaOH)},$$

calculated on a dried basis.
The empirical formula is $C_5H_{11}NO_2S$, giving it a molecular weight of 149.21. The structural formula is:

$$(CH_3)_2C(SH)-CH(NH_2)COOH$$

It reacts readily with formaldehyde or acetone to form a thiazolidine-carboxylic acid.
Capsules CUPRIMINE* (Penicillamine) for oral administration contain either 125 mg or 250 mg of penicillamine. Each capsule contains the following inactive ingredients: D & C Yellow 10, gelatin, lactose, magnesium stearate, and titanium dioxide. The 125 mg capsule also contains iron oxide.

*Registered trademark of MERCK & CO., INC.

CLINICAL PHARMACOLOGY

Penicillamine is a chelating agent recommended for the removal of excess copper in patients with Wilson's disease. From *in vitro* studies which indicate that one atom of copper combines with two molecules of penicillamine, it would appear that one gram of penicillamine should be followed by the excretion of about 200 milligrams of copper; however, the actual amount excreted is about one percent of this.
Penicillamine also reduces excess cystine excretion in cystinuria. This is done, at least in part, by disulfide interchange between penicillamine and cystine, resulting in formation of penicillamine-cysteine disulfide, a substance that is much more soluble than cystine and is excreted readily.
Penicillamine interferes with the formation of cross-links between tropocollagen molecules and cleaves them when newly formed.
The mechanism of action of penicillamine in rheumatoid arthritis is unknown although it appears to suppress disease activity. Unlike cytotoxic immunosuppressants, penicillamine markedly lowers IgM rheumatoid factor but produces no significant depression in absolute levels of serum immunoglobulins. Also unlike cytotoxic immunosuppressants which act on both, penicillamine *in vitro* depresses T-cell activity but not B-cell activity.
In vitro, penicillamine dissociates macroglobulins (rheumatoid factor) although the relationship of the activity to its effect in rheumatoid arthritis is not known.
In rheumatoid arthritis, the onset of therapeutic response to CUPRIMINE may not be seen for two or three months. In those patients who respond, however, the first evidence of suppression of symptoms such as pain, tenderness, and swelling is generally apparent within three months. The optimum duration of therapy has not been determined. If remissions occur, they may last from months to years, but usually require continued treatment (see DOSAGE AND ADMINISTRATION).
In all patients receiving penicillamine, it is important that CUPRIMINE be given on an empty stomach, at least one hour before meals or two hours after meals, and at least one hour apart from any other drug, food, or milk. This permits maximum absorption and reduces the likelihood of inactivation by metal binding in the gastrointestinal tract.
Methodology for determining the bioavailability of penicillamine is not available; however, penicillamine is known to be a very soluble substance.

INDICATIONS

CUPRIMINE is indicated in the treatment of Wilson's disease, cystinuria, and in patients with severe, active rheumatoid arthritis who have failed to respond to an adequate trial of conventional therapy. Available evidence suggests that CUPRIMINE is not of value in ankylosing spondylitis.
Wilson's Disease—Wilson's disease (hepatolenticular degeneration) results from the interaction of an inherited defect and an abnormality in copper metabolism. The metabolic defect, which is the consequence of the autosomal inheritance of one abnormal gene from each parent, manifests itself in a greater positive copper balance than normal. As a result, copper is deposited in several organs and appears eventually to produce pathologic effects most prominently seen in the brain, where degeneration is widespread; in the liver, where fatty infiltration, inflammation, and hepatocellular damage progress to postnecrotic cirrhosis; in the kidney, where tubular and glomerular dysfunction results; and in the eye, where characteristic corneal copper deposits are known as Kayser-Fleischer rings.
Two types of patients require treatment for Wilson's disease: (1) the symptomatic, and (2) the asymptomatic in whom it can be assumed the disease will develop in the future if the patient is not treated.
Diagnosis, suspected on the basis of family or individual history, physical examination, or a low serum concentration of ceruloplasmin**, is confirmed by the demonstration of Kayser-Fleischer rings or, particularly in the asymptomatic patient, by the quantitative demonstration in a liver biopsy specimen of a concentration of copper in excess of 250 mcg/g dry weight.
Treatment has two objectives:
(1) to minimize dietary intake and absorption of copper.
(2) to promote excretion of copper deposited in tissues.
The first objective is attained by a daily diet that contains no more than one or two milligrams of copper. Such a diet should exclude, most importantly, chocolate, nuts, shellfish, mushrooms, liver, molasses, broccoli, and cereals enriched with copper, and be composed to as great an extent as possible of foods with a low copper content. Distilled or demineralized water should be used if the patient's drinking water contains more than 0.1 mg of copper per liter.
For the second objective, a copper chelating agent is used. In symptomatic patients this treatment usually produces marked neurologic improvement, fading of Kayser-Fleischer rings, and gradual amelioration of hepatic dysfunction and psychic disturbances.
Clinical experience to date suggests that life is prolonged with the above regimen.
Noticeable improvement may not occur for one to three months. Occasionally, neurologic symptoms become worse during initiation of therapy with CUPRIMINE. Despite this, the drug should not be discontinued permanently. Although temporary interruption may result in clinical im-

Continued on next page

Information on the Merck & Co., Inc. products listed on these pages is the full prescribing information from product circulars in use September 30, 2000. For information, please call 1-800-NSC MERCK [1-800-672-6372].

Cuprimine—Cont.

provement of the neurological symptoms, it carries an increased risk of developing a sensitivity reaction upon resumption of therapy. (See WARNINGS.)

Treatment of asymptomatic patients has been carried out for over ten years. Symptoms and signs of the disease appear to be prevented indefinitely if daily treatment with CUPRIMINE can be continued.

Cystinuria—Cystinuria is characterized by excessive urinary excretion of the dibasic amino acids, arginine, lysine, ornithine, and cystine, and the mixed disulfide of cysteine and homocysteine. The metabolic defect that leads to cystinuria is inherited as an autosomal, recessive trait. Metabolism of the affected amino acids is influenced by at least two abnormal factors: (1) defective gastrointestinal absorption and (2) renal tubular dysfunction.

Arginine, lysine, ornithine, and cysteine are soluble substances, readily excreted. There is no apparent pathology connected with their excretion in excessive quantities.

Cystine, however, is so slightly soluble at the usual range of urinary pH that it is not excreted readily, and so crystallizes and forms stones in the urinary tract. Stone formation is the only known pathology in cystinuria.

Normal daily output of cystine is 40 to 80 mg. In cystinuria, output is greatly increased and may exceed 1 g/day. At 500 to 600 mg/day, stone formation is almost certain. When it is more than 300 mg/day, treatment is indicated.

Conventional treatment is directed at keeping urinary cystine diluted enough to prevent stone formation, keeping the urine alkaline enough to dissolve as much cystine as possible, and minimizing cystine production by a diet low in methionine (the major dietary precursor of cystine). Patients must drink enough fluid to keep urine specific gravity below 1.010, take enough alkali to keep urinary pH at 7.5 to 8, and maintain a diet low in methionine. This diet is not recommended in growing children and probably is contraindicated in pregnancy because of its low protein content (see PRECAUTIONS).

When these measures are inadequate to control recurrent stone formation, CUPRIMINE may be used as additional therapy. When patients refuse to adhere to conventional treatment, CUPRIMINE may be a useful substitute. It is capable of keeping cystine excretion to near normal values, thereby hindering stone formation and the serious consequences of pyelonephritis and impaired renal function that develop in some patients.

Bartter and colleagues depict the process by which penicillamine interacts with cystine to form penicillamine-cysteine mixed disulfide as:

CSSC + PS′ ⇄ CS′ + CSSP
PSSP + CS′ ⇄ PS′ + CSSP
CSSC + PSSP ⇄ 2 CSSP
CSSC = cystine
CS′ = deprotonated cysteine
PSSP = penicillamine
PS′ = deprotonated penicillamine sulfhydryl
CSSP = penicillamine-cysteine mixed disulfide

In this process, it is assumed that the deprotonated form of penicillamine, PS′, is the active factor in bringing about the disulfide interchange.

Rheumatoid Arthritis —Because CUPRIMINE can cause severe adverse reactions, its use in rheumatoid arthritis should be restricted to patients who have severe, active disease and who have failed to respond to an adequate trial of conventional therapy. Even then, benefit-to-risk ratio should be carefully considered. Other measures, such as rest, physiotherapy, salicylates, and corticosteroids should be used, when indicated, in conjunction with CUPRIMINE (see PRECAUTIONS).

**For quantitative test for serum ceruloplasmin see: Morell, A.G.; Windsor, J.; Sternlieb, I.; Scheinberg, I.H.: Measurement of the concentration of ceruloplasmin in serum by determination of its oxidase activity, in "Laboratory Diagnosis of Liver Disease", F.W. Sunderman; F.W. Sunderman, Jr. (eds.), St. Louis, Warren H. Green, Inc., 1968, pp. 193-195.

CONTRAINDICATIONS

Except for the treatment of Wilson's disease or certain cases of cystinuria, use of penicillamine during pregnancy is contraindicated (see WARNINGS).

Although breast milk studies have not been reported in animals or humans, mothers on therapy with penicillamine should not nurse their infants.

Patients with a history of penicillamine-related aplastic anemia or agranulocytosis should not be restarted on penicillamine (see WARNINGS and ADVERSE REACTIONS).

Because of its potential for causing renal damage, penicillamine should not be administered to rheumatoid arthritis patients with a history or other evidence of renal insufficiency.

WARNINGS

The use of penicillamine has been associated with fatalities due to certain diseases such as aplastic anemia, agranulocytosis, thrombocytopenia, Goodpasture's syndrome, and myasthenia gravis.

Because of the potential for serious hematological and renal adverse reactions to occur at any time, routine urinalysis, white and differential blood cell count, hemoglobin determination, and direct platelet count must be done every two weeks for at least the first six months of penicillamine therapy and monthly thereafter. Patients should be instructed to report promptly the development of signs and symptoms of granulocytopenia and/or thrombocytopenia such as fever, sore throat, chills, bruising or bleeding. The above laboratory studies should then be promptly repeated.

Leukopenia and thrombocytopenia have been reported to occur in up to five percent of patients during penicillamine therapy. Leukopenia is of the granulocytic series and may or may not be associated with an increase in eosinophils. A confirmed reduction in WBC below 3500/mm^3 mandates discontinuance of penicillamine therapy. Thrombocytopenia may be on an idiosyncratic basis, with decreased or absent megakaryocytes in the marrow, when it is part of an aplastic anemia. In other cases the thrombocytopenia is presumably on an immune basis since the number of megakaryocytes in the marrow has been reported to be normal or sometimes increased. The development of a platelet count below 100,000/mm^3, even in the absence of clinical bleeding, requires at least temporary cessation of penicillamine therapy. A progressive fall in either platelet count or WBC in three successive determinations, even though values are still within the normal range, likewise requires at least temporary cessation.

Proteinuria and/or hematuria may develop during therapy and may be warning signs of membranous glomerulopathy which can progress to a nephrotic syndrome. Close observation of these patients is essential. In some patients the proteinuria disappears with continued therapy; in others, penicillamine must be discontinued. When a patient develops proteinuria or hematuria the physician must ascertain whether it is a sign of drug-induced glomerulopathy or is unrelated to penicillamine.

Rheumatoid arthritis patients who develop moderate degrees of proteinuria may be continued cautiously on penicillamine therapy, provided that quantitative 24-hour urinary protein determinations are obtained at intervals of one to two weeks. Penicillamine dosage should not be increased under these circumstances. Proteinuria which exceeds 1 g/24 hours, or proteinuria which is progressively increasing, requires either discontinuance of the drug or a reduction in the dosage. In some patients, proteinuria has been reported to clear following reduction in dosage.

In rheumatoid arthritis patients, penicillamine should be discontinued if unexplained gross hematuria or persistent microscopic hematuria develops.

In patients with Wilson's disease or cystinuria the risks of continued penicillamine therapy in patients manifesting potentially serious urinary abnormalities must be weighed against the expected therapeutic benefits.

When penicillamine is used in cystinuria, an annual x-ray for renal stones is advised. Cystine stones form rapidly, sometimes in six months.

Up to one year or more may be required for any urinary abnormalities to disappear after penicillamine has been discontinued.

Because of rare reports of intrahepatic cholestasis and toxic hepatitis, liver function tests are recommended every six months for the duration of therapy.

Goodpasture's syndrome has occurred rarely. The development of abnormal urinary findings associated with hemoptysis and pulmonary infiltrates on x-ray requires immediate cessation of penicillamine.

Obliterative bronchiolitis has been reported rarely. The patient should be cautioned to report immediately pulmonary symptoms such as exertional dyspnea, unexplained cough or wheezing. Pulmonary function studies should be considered at that time.

Onset of new neurologic symptoms has been reported with CUPRIMINE (see ADVERSE REACTIONS). Occasionally, neurologic symptoms become worse during initiation of therapy with CUPRIMINE (see INDICATIONS). Myasthenic syndrome sometimes progressing to myasthenia gravis has been reported. Ptosis and diplopia, with weakness of the extraocular muscles, are often early signs of myasthenia. In the majority of cases, symptoms of myasthenia have receded after withdrawal of penicillamine.

Most of the various forms of pemphigus have occurred during treatment with penicillamine. Pemphigus vulgaris and pemphigus foliaceus are reported most frequently, usually as a late complication of therapy. The seborrhea-like characteristics of pemphigus foliaceus may obscure an early diagnosis. When pemphigus is suspected, CUPRIMINE should be discontinued. Treatment has consisted of high doses of corticosteroids alone or, in some cases, concomitantly with an immunosuppressant. Treatment may be required for only a few weeks or months, but may need to be continued for more than a year.

Once instituted for Wilson's disease or cystinuria, treatment with penicillamine should, as a rule, be continued on a daily basis. Interruptions for even a few days have been followed by sensitivity reactions after reinstitution of therapy.

Pregnancy

Penicillamine has been shown to be teratogenic in rats when given in doses 6 times higher than the highest dose recommended for human use. Skeletal defects, cleft palates and fetal toxicity (resorptions) have been reported.

There are no controlled studies on the use of penicillamine in pregnant women. Although normal outcomes have been reported, characteristic congenital cutis laxa and associated birth defects have been reported in infants born of mothers who received therapy with penicillamine during pregnancy. Penicillamine should be used in women of childbearing potential only when the expected benefits outweigh the possible hazards. Women on therapy with penicillamine who are of childbearing potential should be apprised of this risk, advised to report promptly any missed menstrual periods or other indications of possible pregnancy, and followed closely for early recognition of pregnancy.

Wilson's Disease—Reported experience*** shows that continued treatment with penicillamine throughout pregnancy protects the mother against relapse of the Wilson's disease, and that discontinuation of penicillamine has deleterious effects on the mother.

If penicillamine is administered during pregnancy to patients with Wilson's disease, it is recommended that the daily dosage be limited to 1 g. If cesarean section is planned, the daily dosage should be limited to 250 mg during the last six weeks of pregnancy and postoperatively until wound healing is complete.

Cystinuria —If possible, penicillamine should not be given during pregnancy to women with cystinuria (see CONTRAINDICATIONS). There are reports of women with cystinuria on therapy with penicillamine who gave birth to infants with generalized connective tissue defects who died following abdominal surgery. If stones continue to form in these patients, the benefits of therapy to the mother must be evaluated against the risk to the fetus.

Rheumatoid Arthritis—Penicillamine should not be administered to rheumatoid arthritis patients who are pregnant (see CONTRAINDICATIONS) and should be discontinued promptly in patients in whom pregnancy is suspected or diagnosed.

There is a report that a woman with rheumatoid arthritis treated with less than one gram a day of penicillamine during pregnancy gave birth (cesarean delivery) to an infant with growth retardation, flattened face with broad nasal bridge, low set ears, short neck with loose skin folds, and unusually lax body skin.

***Scheinberg, I.H., Sternlieb, I.: N. Engl. J. Med. *293* : 1300-1302, Dec. 18, 1975.

PRECAUTIONS

Some patients may experience drug fever, a marked febrile response to penicillamine, usually in the second to third week following initiation of therapy. Drug fever may sometimes be accompanied by a macular cutaneous eruption.

In the case of drug fever in patients with Wilson's disease or cystinuria, penicillamine should be temporarily discontinued until the reaction subsides. Then penicillamine should be reinstituted with a small dose that is gradually increased until the desired dosage is attained. Systemic steroid therapy may be necessary, and is usually helpful, in such patients in whom toxic reactions develop a second or third time.

In the case of drug fever in rheumatoid arthritis patients, because other treatments are available, penicillamine should be discontinued and another therapeutic alternative tried since experience indicates that the febrile reaction will recur in a very high percentage of patients upon readministration of penicillamine.

The skin and mucous membranes should be observed for allergic reactions. Early and late rashes have occurred. Early rash occurs during the first few months of treatment and is more common. It is usually a generalized pruritic, erythematous, maculopapular or morbilliform rash and resembles the allergic rash seen with other drugs. Early rash usually disappears within days after stopping penicillamine and seldom recurs when the drug is restarted at a lower dosage. Pruritus and early rash may often be controlled by the concomitant administration of antihistamines. Less commonly, a late rash may be seen, usually after six months or more of treatment, and requires discontinuation of penicillamine. It is usually on the trunk, is accompanied by intense pruritus, and is usually unresponsive to topical corticosteroid therapy. Late rash may take weeks to disappear after penicillamine is stopped and usually recurs if the drug is restarted.

The appearance of a drug eruption accompanied by fever, arthralgia, lymphadenopathy or other allergic manifestations usually requires discontinuation of penicillamine.

Certain patients will develop a positive antinuclear antibody (ANA) test and some of these may show a lupus erythematosus-like syndrome similar to drug-induced lupus associated with other drugs. The lupus erythematosus-like syndrome is not associated with hypocomplementemia and may be present without nephropathy. The development of a positive ANA test does not mandate discontinuance of the drug; however, the physician should be alerted to the possibility that a lupus erythematosus-like syndrome may develop in the future.

Some patients may develop oral ulcerations which in some cases have the appearance of aphthous stomatitis. The stomatitis usually recurs on rechallenge but often clears on a lower dosage. Although rare, cheilosis, glossitis and gingivostomatitis have also been reported. These oral lesions are frequently dose-related and may preclude further increase in penicillamine dosage or require discontinuation of the drug.

Hypogeusia (a blunting or diminution in taste perception) has occurred in some patients. This may last two to three months or more and may develop into a total loss of taste;

however, it is usually self-limited despite continued penicillamine treatment. Such taste impairment is rare in patients with Wilson's disease.
Penicillamine should not be used in patients who are receiving concurrently gold therapy, antimalarial or cytotoxic drugs, oxyphenbutazone or phenylbutazone because these drugs are also associated with similar serious hematologic and renal adverse reactions. Patients who have had gold salt therapy discontinued due to a major toxic reaction may be at greater risk of serious adverse reactions with penicillamine but not necessarily of the same type.
Patients who are allergic to penicillin may theoretically have cross-sensitivity to penicillamine. The possibility of reactions from contamination of penicillamine by trace amounts of penicillin has been eliminated now that penicillamine is being produced synthetically rather than as a degradation product of penicillin.
Because of their dietary restrictions, patients with Wilson's disease and cystinuria should be given 25 mg/day of pyridoxine during therapy, since penicillamine increases the requirement for this vitamin. Patients also may receive benefit from a multivitamin preparation, although there is no evidence that deficiency of any vitamin other than pyridoxine is associated with penicillamine. In Wilson's disease, multivitamin preparations must be copper-free.
Rheumatoid arthritis patients whose nutrition is impaired should also be given a daily supplement of pyridoxine. Mineral supplements should not be given, since they may block the response to penicillamine.
Iron deficiency may develop, especially in pediatric patients and in menstruating women. In Wilson's disease, this may be a result of adding the effects of the low copper diet, which is probably also low in iron, and the penicillamine to the effects of blood loss or growth. In cystinuria, a low methionine diet may contribute to iron deficiency, since it is necessarily low in protein. If necessary, iron may be given in short courses, but a period of two hours should elapse between administration of penicillamine and iron, since orally administered iron has been shown to reduce the effects of penicillamine.
Penicillamine causes an increase in the amount of soluble collagen. In the rat this results in inhibition of normal healing and also a decrease in tensile strength of intact skin. In man this may be the cause of increased skin friability at sites especially subject to pressure or trauma, such as shoulders, elbows, knees, toes, and buttocks. Extravasations of blood may occur and may appear as purpuric areas, with external bleeding if the skin is broken, or as vesicles containing dark blood. Neither type is progressive. There is no apparent association with bleeding elsewhere in the body and no associated coagulation defect has been found. Therapy with penicillamine may be continued in the presence of these lesions. They may not recur if dosage is reduced. Other reported effects probably due to the action of penicillamine on collagen are excessive wrinkling of the skin and development of small, white papules at venipuncture and surgical sites.
The effects of penicillamine on collagen and elastin make it advisable to consider a reduction in dosage to 250 mg/day, when surgery is contemplated. Reinstitution of full therapy should be delayed until wound healing is complete.
Carcinogenesis
Long-term animal carcinogenicity studies have not been done with penicillamine. There is a report that five of ten autoimmune disease-prone NZB hybrid mice developed lymphocytic leukemia after 6 months' intraperitoneal treatment with a dose of 400 mg/kg penicillamine 5 days per week.
Nursing Mothers
See CONTRAINDICATIONS.
Pediatric Use
The efficacy of CUPRIMINE in juvenile rheumatoid arthritis has not been established.

ADVERSE REACTIONS

Penicillamine is a drug with a high incidence of untoward reactions, some of which are potentially fatal. Therefore, it is mandatory that patients receiving penicillamine therapy remain under close medical supervision throughout the period of drug administration (see WARNINGS and PRECAUTIONS).
Reported incidences (%) for the most commonly occurring adverse reactions in rheumatoid arthritis patients are noted, based on 17 representative clinical trials reported in the literature (1270 patients).
Allergic—Generalized pruritus, early and late rashes (5%), pemphigus (see WARNINGS), and drug eruptions which may be accompanied by fever, arthralgia, or lymphadenopathy have occurred (see WARNINGS and PRECAUTIONS). Some patients may show a lupus erythematosus-like syndrome similar to drug-induced lupus produced by other pharmacological agents (see PRECAUTIONS).
Urticaria and exfoliative dermatitis have occurred.
Thyroiditis has been reported; hypoglycemia in association with anti-insulin antibodies has been reported. These reactions are extremely rare.
Some patients may develop a migratory polyarthralgia, often with objective synovitis (see DOSAGE AND ADMINISTRATION).
Gastrointestinal—Anorexia, epigastric pain, nausea, vomiting, or occasional diarrhea may occur (17%).
Isolated cases of reactivated peptic ulcer have occurred, as have hepatic dysfunction and pancreatitis. Intrahepatic cholestasis and toxic hepatitis have been reported rarely. There have been a few reports of increased serum alkaline phosphatase, lactic dehydrogenase, and positive cephalin flocculation and thymol turbidity tests.
Some patients may report a blunting, diminution, or total loss of taste perception (12%); or may develop oral ulcerations. Although rare, cheilosis, glossitis, and gingivostomatitis have been reported (see PRECAUTIONS).
Gastrointestinal side effects are usually reversible following cessation of therapy.
Hematological—Penicillamine can cause bone marrow depression (see WARNINGS). Leukopenia (2%) and thrombocytopenia (4%) have occurred. Fatalities have been reported as a result of thrombocytopenia, agranulocytosis, aplastic anemia, and sideroblastic anemia.
Thrombotic thrombocytopenic purpura, hemolytic anemia, red cell aplasia, monocytosis, leukocytosis, eosinophilia, and thrombocytosis have also been reported.
Renal—Patients on penicillamine therapy may develop proteinuria (6%) and/or hematuria which, in some, may progress to the development of the nephrotic syndrome as a result of an immune complex membranous glomerulopathy (see WARNINGS).
Central Nervous System—Tinnitus, optic neuritis and peripheral sensory and motor neuropathies (including polyradiculoneuropathy, i.e., Guillain-Barre syndrome) have been reported. Muscular weakness may or may not occur with the peripheral neuropathies. Visual and psychic disturbances; mental disorders; and agitation and anxiety have been reported.
Neuromuscular—Myasthenia gravis (see WARNINGS); dystonia.
Other—Adverse reactions that have been reported rarely include thrombophlebitis; hyperpyrexia (see PRECAUTIONS); falling hair or alopecia; lichen planus; polymyositis; dermatomyositis; mammary hyperplasia; elastosis perforans serpiginosa; toxic epidermal necrolysis; anetoderma (cutaneous macular atrophy); and Goodpasture's syndrome, a severe and ultimately fatal glomerulonephritis associated with intra-alveolar hemorrhage (see WARNINGS). Fatal renal vasculitis has also been reported. Allergic alveolitis, obliterative bronchiolitis, interstitial pneumonitis and pulmonary fibrosis have been reported in patients with severe rheumatoid arthritis, some of whom were receiving penicillamine. Bronchial asthma also has been reported.
Increased skin friability, excessive wrinkling of skin, and development of small white papules at venipuncture and surgical sites have been reported (see PRECAUTIONS).
The chelating action of the drug may cause increased excretion of other heavy metals such as zinc, mercury and lead.
There have been reports associating penicillamine with leukemia. However, circumstances involved in these reports are such that a cause and effect relationship to the drug has not been established.

DOSAGE AND ADMINISTRATION

In all patients receiving penicillamine, it is important that CUPRIMINE be given on an empty stomach, at least one hour before meals or two hours after meals, and at least one hour apart from any other drug, food, or milk. Because penicillamine increases the requirement for pyridoxine, patients may require a daily supplement of pyridoxine (see PRECAUTIONS).
Wilson's Disease— Optimal dosage can be determined by measurement of urinary copper excretion and the determination of free copper in the serum. The urine must be collected in copper-free glassware, and should be quantitatively analyzed for copper before and soon after initiation of therapy with CUPRIMINE.
Determination of 24-hour urinary copper excretion is of greatest value in the first week of therapy with penicillamine. In the absence of any drug reaction, a dose between 0.75 and 1.5 g that results in an initial 24-hour cupriuresis of over 2 mg should be continued for about three months, by which time the most reliable method of monitoring maintenance treatment is the determination of free copper in the serum. This equals the difference between quantitatively determined total copper and ceruloplasmin-copper. Adequately treated patients will usually have less than 10 mcg free copper/dL of serum. It is seldom necessary to exceed a dosage of 2 g/day. If the patient is intolerant to therapy with CUPRIMINE, alternative treatment is trientine hydrochloride.
In patients who cannot tolerate as much as 1 g/day initially, initiating dosage with 250 mg/day, and increasing gradually to the requisite amount, gives closer control of the effects of the drug and may help to reduce the incidence of adverse reactions.
Cystinuria—It is recommended that CUPRIMINE be used along with conventional therapy. By reducing urinary cystine, it decreases crystalluria and stone formation. In some instances, it has been reported to decrease the size of, and even to dissolve, stones already formed.
The usual dosage of CUPRIMINE in the treatment of cystinuria is 2 g/day for adults, with a range of 1 to 4 g/day. For pediatric patients, dosage can be based on 30 mg/kg/day. The total daily amount should be divided into four doses. If four equal doses are not feasible, give the larger portion at bedtime. If adverse reactions necessitate a reduction in dosage, it is important to retain the bedtime dose.
Initiating dosage with 250 mg/day, and increasing gradually to the requisite amount, gives closer control of the effects of the drug and may help to reduce the incidence of adverse reactions.
In addition to taking CUPRIMINE, patients should drink copiously. It is especially important to drink about a pint of fluid at bedtime and another pint once during the night when urine is more concentrated and more acid than during the day. The greater the fluid intake, the lower the required dosage of CUPRIMINE.
Dosage must be individualized to an amount that limits cystine excretion to 100–200 mg/day in those with no history of stones, and below 100 mg/day in those who have had stone formation and/or pain. Thus, in determining dosage, the inherent tubular defect, the patient's size, age, and rate of growth, and his diet and water intake all must be taken into consideration.
The standard nitroprusside cyanide test has been reported useful as a qualitative measure of the effective dose†: Add 2 mL of freshly prepared 5 percent sodium cyanide to 5 mL of a 24-hour aliquot of protein-free urine and let stand ten minutes. Add 5 drops of freshly prepared 5 percent sodium nitroprusside and mix. Cystine will turn the mixture magenta. If the result is negative, it can be assumed that cystine excretion is less than 100 mg/g creatinine.
Although penicillamine is rarely excreted unchanged, it also will turn the mixture magenta. If there is any question as to which substance is causing the reaction, a ferric chloride test can be done to eliminate doubt: Add 3 percent ferric chloride dropwise to the urine. Penicillamine will turn the urine an immediate and quickly fading blue. Cystine will not produce any change in appearance.

†Lotz, M., Potts, J.T. and Bartter, F.C.: Brit. Med. J. *2* :521, Aug. 28, 1965 (in Medical Memoranda).

Rheumatoid Arthritis—The principal rule of treatment with CUPRIMINE in rheumatoid arthritis is patience. The onset of therapeutic response is typically delayed. Two or three months may be required before the first evidence of a clinical response is noted (see CLINICAL PHARMACOLOGY).
When treatment with CUPRIMINE has been interrupted because of adverse reactions or other reasons, the drug should be reintroduced cautiously by starting with a lower dosage and increasing slowly.
Initial Therapy—The currently recommended dosage regimen in rheumatoid arthritis begins with a single daily dose of 125 mg or 250 mg which is thereafter increased at one to three month intervals, by 125 mg or 250 mg/day, as patient response and tolerance indicate. If a satisfactory remission of symptoms is achieved, the dose associated with the remission should be continued (see *Maintenance Therapy*). If there is no improvement and there are no signs of potentially serious toxicity after two to three months of treatment with doses of 500–750 mg/day, increases of 250 mg/day at two to three month intervals may be continued until a satisfactory remission occurs (see *Maintenance Therapy*) or signs of toxicity develop (see WARNINGS and PRECAUTIONS). If there is no discernible improvement after three to four months of treatment with 1000 to 1500 mg of penicillamine/day, it may be assumed the patient will not respond and CUPRIMINE should be discontinued.
Maintenance Therapy—The maintenance dosage of CUPRIMINE must be individualized, and may require adjustment during the course of treatment. Many patients respond satisfactorily to a dosage within the 500–750 mg/day range. Some need less.
Changes in maintenance dosage levels may not be reflected clinically or in the erythrocyte sedimentation rate for two to three months after each dosage adjustment.
Some patients will subsequently require an increase in the maintenance dosage to achieve maximal disease suppression. In those patients who do respond, but who evidence incomplete suppression of their disease after the first six to nine months of treatment, the daily dosage of CUPRIMINE may be increased by 125 mg or 250 mg/day at three-month intervals. It is unusual in current practice to employ a dosage in excess of 1 g/day, but up to 1.5 g/day has sometimes been required.
Management of Exacerbations—During the course of treatment some patients may experience an exacerbation of disease activity following an initial good response. These may be self-limited and can subside within twelve weeks. They are usually controlled by the addition of non-steroidal anti-inflammatory drugs, and only if the patient has demonstrated a true "escape" phenomenon (as evidenced by failure of the flare to subside within this time period) should an increase in the maintenance dose ordinarily be considered.
In the rheumatoid patient, migratory polyarthralgia due to penicillamine is extremely difficult to differentiate from an exacerbation of the rheumatoid arthritis. Discontinuance or a substantial reduction in dosage of CUPRIMINE for up to several weeks will usually determine which of these processes is responsible for the arthralgia.
Duration of Therapy—The optimum duration of therapy with CUPRIMINE in rheumatoid arthritis has not been determined. If the patient has been in remission for six months or more, a gradual, stepwise dosage reduction in decrements of 125 mg or 250 mg/day at approximately three month intervals may be attempted.

Continued on next page

Information on the Merck & Co., Inc. products listed on these pages is the full prescribing information from product circulars in use September 30, 2000. For information, please call 1-800-NSC MERCK [1-800-672-6372].

Cuprimine—Cont.

Concomitant Drug Therapy—CUPRIMINE should not be used in patients who are receiving gold therapy, antimalarial or cytotoxic drugs, oxyphenbutazone, or phenylbutazone (see PRECAUTIONS). Other measures, such as salicylates, other non-steroidal anti-inflammatory drugs, or systemic corticosteroids, may be continued when penicillamine is initiated. After improvement commences, analgesic and anti-inflammatory drugs may be slowly discontinued as symptoms permit. Steroid withdrawal must be done gradually, and many months of treatment with CUPRIMINE may be required before steroids can be completely eliminated.
Dosage Frequency—Based on clinical experience dosages up to 500 mg/day can be given as a single daily dose. Dosages in excess of 500 mg/day should be administered in divided doses.

HOW SUPPLIED

No. 3299—Capsules CUPRIMINE, 250 mg, are ivory-colored capsules containing a white or nearly white powder, and are coded CUPRIMINE and MSD 602. They are supplied as follows:
NDC 0006-0602-68 in bottles of 100
(6505-01-049-9494, 250 mg 100's).
Shown in Product Identification Guide, page 323
No. 3350—Capsules CUPRIMINE, 125 mg, are opaque ivory and gray capsules containing a white or nearly white powder, and are coded CUPRIMINE and MSD 672. They are supplied as follows:
NDC 0006-0672-68 in bottles of 100
(6505-01-097-1232, 125 mg 100's).
Shown in Product Identification Guide, page 323
Storage
Keep container tightly closed.
7873241 Issued May 1999

DARANIDE® Tablets (Dichlorphenamide) ℞

DESCRIPTION

DARANIDE* (Dichlorphenamide) is an oral carbonic anhydrase inhibitor. Dichlorphenamide, a dichlorinated benzenedisulfonamide, is known chemically as 4,5-dichloro-1,3-benzenedisulfonamide. Its empirical formula is $C_6H_6Cl_2N_2O_4S_2$ and its structural formula is:

SO_2NH_2 Cl SO_2NH_2 Cl

Dichlorphenamide is a white or practically white, crystalline compound with a molecular weight of 305.16. It is very slightly soluble in water but soluble in dilute solutions of sodium carbonate and sodium hydroxide. Dilute alkaline solutions of dichlorphenamide are stable at room temperature.
DARANIDE is supplied as tablets, for oral administration, each containing 50 mg dichlorphenamide. Inactive ingredients are D&C Yellow 10, lactose, magnesium stearate, and starch.

*Registered trademark of MERCK & CO., INC.

CLINICAL PHARMACOLOGY

Carbonic anhydrase inhibitors reduce intraocular pressure by partially suppressing the secretion of aqueous humor (inflow), although the mechanism by which they do this is not fully understood. Evidence suggests that HCO_3^- ions are produced in the ciliary body by hydration of carbon dioxide under the influence of carbonic anhydrase and diffuse into the posterior chamber with Na^+ ions. The aqueous fluid contains more Na^+ and HCO_3^- ions than does plasma and consequently is hypertonic. Water is attracted to the posterior chamber by osmosis. Systemic administration of a carbonic anhydrase inhibitor has been shown to inactivate carbonic anhydrase in the ciliary body of the rabbit's eye and to reduce the high concentration of HCO_3^- ions in ocular fluids. As is the case with all carbonic anhydrase inhibitors, DARANIDE in high doses causes some decrease in renal blood flow and glomerular filtration rate.
In man, DARANIDE begins to act within an hour and maximal effect is observed in two to four hours. The lowered intraocular tension may be maintained for approximately 6 to 12 hours.

INDICATIONS AND USAGE

For adjunctive treatment of: chronic simple (open-angle) glaucoma, secondary glaucoma, and preoperatively in acute angle-closure glaucoma where delay of surgery is desired in order to lower intraocular pressure.

CONTRAINDICATIONS

DARANIDE is contraindicated in hepatic insufficiency, renal failure, adrenocortical insufficiency, hyperchloremic acidosis, or in conditions in which serum levels of sodium or potassium are depressed. DARANIDE should not be used in patients with severe pulmonary obstruction who are unable to increase their alveolar ventilation since their acidosis may be increased.
DARANIDE is contraindicated in patients who are hypersensitive to this product.

PRECAUTIONS

General
Potassium excretion is increased by DARANIDE and hypokalemia may develop with brisk diuresis, when severe cirrhosis is present, or during concomitant use of steroids or ACTH.
Interference with adequate oral electrolyte intake will also contribute to hypokalemia. Hypokalemia can sensitize or exaggerate the response of the heart to the toxic effects of digitalis (e.g., increased ventricular irritability). Hypokalemia may be avoided or treated by use of potassium supplements such as foods with a high potassium content. DARANIDE should be used with caution in patients with respiratory acidosis.
Drug Interactions
Caution is advised in patients receiving concomitant high-dose aspirin and carbonic anhydrase inhibitors, as anorexia, tachypnea, lethargy and coma have been rarely reported due to a possible drug interaction.
Carcinogenesis, Mutagenesis, Impairment of Fertility
Long-term studies in animals have not been performed to evaluate the effects upon fertility or carcinogenic potential of DARANIDE.
Pregnancy
Pregnancy Category C. Diclorphenamide has been shown to be teratogenic in the rat (skeletal anomalies) when given in doses 100 times the human dose. There are no adequate and well-controlled studies in pregnant women. DARANIDE should not be used in women of childbearing age or in pregnancy, especially during the first trimester, unless the potential benefits outweigh the potential risks.
Nursing Mothers
It is not known whether diclorphenamide is excreted in human milk. Because many drugs are excreted in human milk, caution should be exercised when diclorphenamide is administered to a nursing woman.
Pediatric Use
Safety and effectiveness in pediatric patients have not been established.

ADVERSE REACTIONS

Certain side effects characteristic of carbonic anhydrase inhibitors may occur with DARANIDE, particularly with increasing doses.
The most common effects include gastrointestinal disturbances (anorexia, nausea, and vomiting), drowsiness and paresthesias.
Included in the listing which follows are some adverse reactions which have not been reported with DARANIDE. However, pharmacological similarities among the carbonic anhydrase inhibitors make it advisable to consider the following reactions when diclorphenamide is administered.
Central Nervous System/Psychiatric: ataxia, tremor, tinnitus, headache, weakness, nervousness, globus hystericus, lassitude, depression, confusion, disorientation, dizziness;
Gastrointestinal: constipation, hepatic insufficiency;
Metabolic: loss of weight, metabolic acidosis, electrolyte imbalance (hypokalemia, hyperchloremia), hyperuricemia;
Hypersensitivity: skin eruptions, pruritus, fever;
Hematologic: leukopenia, agranulocytosis, thrombocytopenia;
Genitourinary: urinary frequency, renal colic, renal calculi, phosphaturia.

OVERDOSAGE

The oral LD_{50} of DARANIDE is 1710 and 2600 mg/kg in the mouse and rat respectively.
Symptoms of overdosage or toxicity may include drowsiness, anorexia, nausea, vomiting, dizziness, paresthesias, ataxia, tremor and tinnitus.
In the event of overdosage, induce emesis or perform gastric lavage. The electrolyte disturbance most likely to be encountered from overdosage is hyperchloremic acidosis that may respond to bicarbonate administration. Potassium supplementation may be required. The patient should be carefully observed and given supportive treatment.

DOSAGE AND ADMINISTRATION

DARANIDE is usually given in conjunction with topical ocular hypotensive agents. In acute angle-closure glaucoma, it may be used together with miotics and osmotic agents in an attempt to reduce intraocular tension rapidly. If this is not quickly relieved, surgery may be mandatory.
Dosage must be adjusted carefully to meet the requirements of the individual patient. A priming dose of 100 to 200 mg of DARANIDE (2 to 4 tablets) is suggested for adults, followed by 100 mg (2 tablets) every 12 hours until the desired response has been obtained. The recommended maintenance dosage for adults is 25 to 50 mg ($^1/_2$ to 1 tablet) once to three times daily.

HOW SUPPLIED

No. 3256—Tablets DARANIDE, 50 mg each, are yellow, round, scored, compressed tablets, coded MSD 49 on one side and DARANIDE on the other. They are supplied as follows:
NDC 0006-0049-68 bottles of 100.
7870319 Issued October 1996

DECADRON® Elixir (Dexamethasone) ℞

DESCRIPTION

Glucocorticoids are adrenocortical steroids, both naturally occurring and synthetic, which are readily absorbed from the gastrointestinal tract.
Dexamethasone, a synthetic adrenocortical steroid, is a white to practically white, odorless, crystalline powder. It is stable in air. It is practically insoluble in water. The molecular weight is 392.47. It is designated chemically as 9-fluoro-11β,17,21-trihydroxy-16α-methylpregna -1, 4- diene-3,20-dione. The empirical formula is $C_{22}H_{29}FO_5$ and the structural formula is:

CH_2OH C=O HO CH_3 OH CH_3 CH_3 F O

DECADRON* (Dexamethasone) elixir contains 0.5 mg of dexamethasone in each 5 mL. Benzoic acid, 0.1%, is added as a preservative. It also contains alcohol 5%. Inactive ingredients are FD&C Red 40, flavors, glycerin, purified water, and sodium saccharin.

*Registered trademark of MERCK & CO., INC.

ACTIONS

Naturally occurring glucocorticoids (hydrocortisone and cortisone), which also have salt-retaining properties, are used as replacement therapy in adrenocortical deficiency states. Their synthetic analogs, including dexamethasone, are primarily used for their potent anti-inflammatory effects in disorders of many organ systems.
Glucocorticoids cause profound and varied metabolic effects. In addition, they modify the body's immune responses to diverse stimuli.
At equipotent anti-inflammatory doses, dexamethasone almost completely lacks the sodium-retaining property of hydrocortisone and closely related derivatives of hydrocortisone.

INDICATIONS

1. *Endocrine Disorders*
Primary or secondary adrenocortical insufficiency (hydrocortisone or cortisone is the first choice; synthetic analogs may be used in conjunction with mineralocorticoids where applicable; in infancy mineralocorticoid supplementation is of particular importance)
Congenital adrenal hyperplasia
Nonsuppurative thyroiditis
Hypercalcemia associated with cancer
2. *Rheumatic Disorders*
As adjunctive therapy for short-term administration (to tide the patient over an acute episode or exacerbation) in:
Psoriatic arthritis
Rheumatoid arthritis, including juvenile rheumatoid arthritis (selected cases may require low-dose maintenance therapy)
Ankylosing spondylitis
Acute and subacute bursitis
Acute nonspecific tenosynovitis
Acute gouty arthritis
Post-traumatic osteoarthritis
Synovitis of osteoarthritis
Epicondylitis
3. *Collagen Diseases*
During an exacerbation or as maintenance therapy in selected cases of—
Systemic lupus erythematosus
Acute rheumatic carditis
4. *Dermatologic Diseases*
Pemphigus
Bullous dermatitis herpetiformis
Severe erythema multiforme (Stevens-Johnson syndrome)
Exfoliative dermatitis
Mycosis fungoides

Severe psoriasis
Severe seborrheic dermatitis

5. *Allergic States*
Control of severe or incapacitating allergic conditions intractable to adequate trials of conventional treatment:
Seasonal or perennial allergic rhinitis
Bronchial asthma
Contact dermatitis
Atopic dermatitis
Serum sickness
Drug hypersensitivity reactions

6. *Ophthalmic Diseases*
Severe acute and chronic allergic and inflammatory processes involving the eye and its adnexa, such as—
Allergic conjunctivitis
Keratitis
Allergic corneal marginal ulcers
Herpes zoster ophthalmicus
Iritis and iridocyclitis
Chorioretinitis
Anterior segment inflammation
Diffuse posterior uveitis and choroiditis
Optic neuritis
Sympathetic ophthalmia

7. *Respiratory Diseases*
Symptomatic sarcoidosis
Loeffler's syndrome not manageable by other means
Berylliosis
Fulminating or disseminated pulmonary tuberculosis when used concurrently with appropriate antituberculous chemotherapy
Aspiration pneumonitis

8. *Hematologic Disorders*
Idiopathic thrombocytopenic purpura in adults
Secondary thrombocytopenia in adults
Acquired (autoimmune) hemolytic anemia
Erythroblastopenia (RBC anemia)
Congenital (erythroid) hypoplastic anemia

9. *Neoplastic Diseases*
For palliative management of:
Leukemias and lymphomas in adults
Acute leukemia of childhood

10. *Edematous States*
To induce a diuresis or remission of proteinuria in the nephrotic syndrome, without uremia, of the idiopathic type or that due to lupus erythematosus

11. *Gastrointestinal Diseases*
To tide the patient over a critical period of the disease in:
Ulcerative colitis
Regional enteritis

12. *Miscellaneous*
Tuberculous meningitis with subarachnoid block or impending block when used concurrently with appropriate antituberculous chemotherapy
Trichinosis with neurologic or myocardial involvement

13. *Diagnostic testing of adrenocortical hyperfunction.*

CONTRAINDICATIONS

Systemic fungal infections
Hypersensitivity to this product

WARNINGS

In patients on corticosteroid therapy subjected to unusual stress, increased dosage of rapidly acting corticosteroids before, during, and after the stressful situation is indicated.
Drug-induced secondary adrenocortical insufficiency may result from too rapid withdrawal of corticosteroids and may be minimized by gradual reduction of dosage. This type of relative insufficiency may persist for months after discontinuation of therapy; therefore, in any situation of stress occurring during that period, hormone therapy should be reinstituted. If the patient is receiving steroids already, dosage may have to be increased. Since mineralocorticoid secretion may be impaired, salt and/or a mineralocorticoid should be administered concurrently.
Corticosteroids may mask some signs of infection, and new infections may appear during their use. There may be decreased resistance and inability to localize infection when corticosteroids are used. Moreover, corticosteroids may affect the nitroblue-tetrazolium test for bacterial infection and produce false negative results.
In cerebral malaria, a double-blind trial has shown that the use of corticosteroids is associated with prolongation of coma and a higher incidence of pneumonia and gastrointestinal bleeding.
Corticosteroids may activate latent amebiasis. Therefore, it is recommended that latent or active amebiasis be ruled out before initiating corticosteroid therapy in any patient who has spent time in the tropics or any patient with unexplained diarrhea.
Prolonged use of corticosteroids may produce posterior subcapsular cataracts, glaucoma with possible damage to the optic nerves, and may enhance the establishment of secondary ocular infections due to fungi or viruses.
Usage in pregnancy: Since adequate human reproduction studies have not been done with corticosteroids, use of these drugs in pregnancy or in women of childbearing potential requires that the anticipated benefits be weighed against the possible hazards to the mother and embryo or fetus. Infants born of mothers who have received substantial doses of corticosteroids during pregnancy should be carefully observed for signs of hypoadrenalism.
Corticosteroids appear in breast milk and could suppress growth, interfere with endogenous corticosteroid production, or cause other unwanted effects. Mothers taking pharmacologic doses of corticosteroids should be advised not to nurse.
Average and large doses of hydrocortisone or cortisone can cause elevation of blood pressure, salt and water retention, and increased excretion of potassium. These effects are less likely to occur with the synthetic derivatives except when used in large doses. Dietary salt restriction and potassium supplementation may be necessary. All corticosteroids increase calcium excretion.
Administration of live virus vaccines, including smallpox, is contraindicated in individuals receiving immunosuppressive doses of corticosteroids. If inactivated viral or bacterial vaccines are administered to individuals receiving immunosuppressive doses of corticosteroids, the expected serum antibody response may not be obtained. However, immunization procedures may be undertaken in patients who are receiving corticosteroids as replacement therapy, e.g., for Addison's disease.
Patients who are on drugs which suppress the immune system are more susceptible to infections than healthy individuals. Chickenpox and measles, for example, can have a more serious or even fatal course in non-immune patients on corticosteroids. In such patients who have not had these diseases, particular care should be taken to avoid exposure. The risk of developing a disseminated infection varies among individuals and can be related to the dose, route and duration of corticosteroid administration as well as to the underlying disease. If exposed to chickenpox, prophylaxis with varicella zoster immune globulin (VZIG) may be indicated. If chickenpox develops, treatment with antiviral agents may be considered. If exposed to measles, prophylaxis with immune globulin (IG) may be indicated. (See the respective package inserts for VZIG and IG for complete prescribing information.)
Similarly, corticosteroids should be used with great care in patients with known or suspected Strongyloides (threadworm) infestation. In such patients, corticosteroid-induced immunosuppression may lead to Strongyloides hyperinfection and dissemination with widespread larval migration, often accompanied by severe enterocolitis and potentially fatal gram-negative septicemia.
The use of DECADRON elixir in active tuberculosis should be restricted to those cases of fulminating or disseminated tuberculosis in which the corticosteroid is used for the management of the disease in conjunction with an appropriate antituberculous regimen.
If corticosteroids are indicated in patients with latent tuberculosis or tuberculin reactivity, close observation is necessary as reactivation of the disease may occur. During prolonged corticosteroid therapy, these patients should receive chemoprophylaxis.
Literature reports suggest an apparent association between use of corticosteroids and left ventricular free wall rupture after a recent myocardial infarction; therefore, therapy with corticosteroids should be used with great caution in these patients.

PRECAUTIONS

Following prolonged therapy, withdrawal of corticosteroids may result in symptoms of the corticosteroid withdrawal syndrome including fever, myalgia, arthralgia, and malaise. This may occur in patients even without evidence of adrenal insufficiency.
There is an enhanced effect of corticosteroids in patients with hypothyroidism and in those with cirrhosis.
Corticosteroids should be used cautiously in patients with ocular herpes simplex because of possible corneal perforation.
The lowest possible dose of corticosteroid should be used to control the condition under treatment, and when reduction in dosage is possible, the reduction should be gradual.
Psychic derangements may appear when corticosteroids are used, ranging from euphoria, insomnia, mood swings, personality changes, and severe depression, to frank psychotic manifestations. Also, existing emotional instability or psychotic tendencies may be aggravated by corticosteroids.
Aspirin should be used cautiously in conjunction with corticosteroids in hypoprothrombinemia.
Steroids should be used with caution in nonspecific ulcerative colitis, if there is a probability of impending perforation, abscess, or other pyogenic infection, diverticulitis, fresh intestinal anastomoses, active or latent peptic ulcer, renal insufficiency, hypertension, osteoporosis, and myasthenia gravis. Signs of peritoneal irritation following gastrointestinal perforation in patients receiving large doses of corticosteroids may be minimal or absent. Fat embolism has been reported as a possible complication of hypercortisonism.
When large doses are given, some authorities advise that corticosteroids be taken with meals and antacids taken between meals to help to prevent peptic ulcer.
Steroids may increase or decrease motility and number of spermatozoa in some patients.
Phenytoin, phenobarbital, ephedrine, and rifampin may enhance the metabolic clearance of corticosteroids, resulting in decreased blood levels and lessened physiologic activity, thus requiring adjustment in corticosteroid dosage. These interactions may interfere with dexamethasone suppression tests which should be interpreted with caution during administration of these drugs.
False-negative results in the dexamethasone suppression test (DST) in patients being treated with indomethacin have been reported. Thus, results of the DST should be interpreted with caution in these patients.
The prothrombin time should be checked frequently in patients who are receiving corticosteroids and coumarin anticoagulants at the same time because of reports that corticosteroids have altered the response to these anticoagulants. Studies have shown that the usual effect produced by adding corticosteroids is inhibition of response to coumarins, although there have been some conflicting reports of potentiation not substantiated by studies.
When corticosteroids are administered concomitantly with potassium-depleting diuretics, patients should be observed closely for development of hypokalemia.

Information for Patients
Susceptible patients who are on immunosuppressant doses of corticosteroids should be warned to avoid exposure to chickenpox or measles. Patients should also be advised that if they are exposed, medical advice should be sought without delay.

Pediatric Use
Growth and development of pediatric patients on prolonged corticosteroid therapy should be carefully followed.

ADVERSE REACTIONS

Fluid and Electrolyte Disturbances
Sodium retention
Fluid retention
Congestive heart failure in susceptible patients
Potassium loss
Hypokalemic alkalosis
Hypertension

Musculoskeletal
Muscle weakness
Steroid myopathy
Loss of muscle mass
Osteoporosis
Vertebral compression fractures
Aseptic necrosis of femoral and humeral heads
Pathologic fracture of long bones
Tendon rupture

Gastrointestinal
Peptic ulcer with possible perforation and hemorrhage
Perforation of the small and large bowel, particularly in patients with inflammatory bowel disease
Pancreatitis
Abdominal distention
Ulcerative esophagitis

Dermatologic
Impaired wound healing
Thin fragile skin
Petechiae and ecchymoses
Erythema
Increased sweating
May suppress reactions to skin tests
Other cutaneous reactions, such as allergic dermatitis, urticaria, angioneurotic edema

Neurologic
Convulsions
Increased intracranial pressure with papilledema (pseudotumor cerebri) usually after treatment
Vertigo
Headache
Psychic disturbances

Endocrine
Menstrual irregularities
Development of cushingoid state
Suppression of growth in children
Secondary adrenocortical and pituitary unresponsiveness, particularly in times of stress, as in trauma, surgery, or illness
Decreased carbohydrate tolerance
Manifestations of latent diabetes mellitus
Increased requirements for insulin or oral hypoglycemic agents in diabetics
Hirsutism

Ophthalmic
Posterior subcapsular cataracts
Increased intraocular pressure
Glaucoma
Exophthalmos

Metabolic
Negative nitrogen balance due to protein catabolism

Cardiovascular
Myocardial rupture following recent myocardial infarction (see WARNINGS)

Other
Hypersensitivity
Thromboembolism
Weight gain
Increased appetite
Nausea
Malaise
Hiccups

Continued on next page

Information on the Merck & Co., Inc. products listed on these pages is the full prescribing information from product circulars in use September 30, 2000. For information, please call 1-800-NSC MERCK [1-800-672-6372].

Decadron Elixir—Cont.

OVERDOSAGE

Reports of acute toxicity and/or death following overdosage of glucocorticoids are rare. In the event of overdosage, no specific antidote is available; treatment is supportive and symptomatic.
The oral LD_{50} of dexamethasone in female mice was 6.5 g/kg.

DOSAGE AND ADMINISTRATION

For oral administration
DOSAGE REQUIREMENTS ARE VARIABLE AND MUST BE INDIVIDUALIZED ON THE BASIS OF THE DISEASE AND THE RESPONSE OF THE PATIENT.
The initial dosage varies from 0.75 to 9 mg a day depending on the disease being treated. In less severe diseases doses lower than 0.75 mg may suffice, while in severe diseases doses higher than 9 mg may be required. The initial dosage should be maintained or adjusted until the patient's response is satisfactory. If satisfactory clinical response does not occur after a reasonable period of time, discontinue DECADRON elixir and transfer the patient to other therapy.
After a favorable initial response, the proper maintenance dosage should be determined by decreasing the initial dosage in small amounts to the lowest dosage that maintains an adequate clinical response.
Patients should be observed closely for signs that might require dosage adjustment, including changes in clinical status resulting from remissions or exacerbations of the disease, individual drug responsiveness, and the effect of stress (e.g., surgery, infection, trauma). During stress it may be necessary to increase dosage temporarily.
If the drug is to be stopped after more than a few days of treatment, it usually should be withdrawn gradually.
The following milligram equivalents facilitate changing to DECADRON from other glucocorticoids:

DECADRON	Methylprednisolone and Triamcinolone	Prednisolone and Prednisone	Hydrocortisone	Cortisone
0.75 mg =	4 mg =	5 mg =	20 mg =	25 mg

Dexamethasone suppression tests
1. Tests for Cushing's syndrome
   Give 1.0 mg of DECADRON orally at 11:00 p.m. Blood is drawn for plasma cortisol determination at 8:00 a.m. the following morning.
   For greater accuracy, give 0.5 mg of DECADRON orally every 6 hours for 48 hours. Twenty-four hour urine collections are made for determination of 17-hydroxycorticosteroid excretion.
2. Test to distinguish Cushing's syndrome due to pituitary ACTH excess from Cushing's syndrome due to other causes
   Give 2.0 mg of DECADRON orally every 6 hours for 48 hours. Twenty-four hour urine collections are made for determination of 17-hydroxycorticosteroid excretion.

HOW SUPPLIED

No. 7622—Elixir DECADRON, 0.5 mg dexamethasone per 5 mL, is a clear, red liquid and is supplied as follows:
NDC 0006-7622-55 bottles of 100 mL with calibrated dropper assembly.
NDC 0006-7622-66 bottles of 237 mL without dropper assembly.
(6505-01-137-8465, 237 mL).
Storage
Keep container tightly closed.
7412730 Issued February 1997

DECADRON® Tablets ℞
(Dexamethasone)

DESCRIPTION

Glucocorticoids are adrenocortical steroids, both naturally occurring and synthetic, which are readily absorbed from the gastrointestinal tract.
Dexamethasone, a synthetic adrenocortical steroid, is a white to practically white, odorless, crystalline powder. It is stable in air. It is practically insoluble in water. The molecular weight is 392.47. It is designated chemically as 9-fluoro-11β, 17, 21-trihydroxy-16α-methylpregna-1, 4-diene-3,20-dione. The empirical formula is $C_{22}H_{29}FO_5$ and the structural formula is:

DECADRON* (Dexamethasone) tablets are supplied in three potencies, 0.5 mg, 0.75 mg, and 4 mg. Inactive ingredients are calcium phosphate, lactose, magnesium stearate, and starch. Tablets DECADRON 0.5 mg also contain D&C Yellow 10 and FD&C Yellow 6. Tablets DECADRON 0.75 mg also contain FD&C Blue 1.

*Registered trademark of MERCK & CO., INC.

ACTIONS

Naturally occurring glucocorticoids (hydrocortisone and cortisone), which also have salt-retaining properties, are used as replacement therapy in adrenocortical deficiency states. Their synthetic analogs including dexamethasone are primarily used for their potent anti-inflammatory effects in disorders of many organ systems.
Glucocorticoids cause profound and varied metabolic effects. In addition, they modify the body's immune responses to diverse stimuli.
At equipotent anti-inflammatory doses, dexamethasone almost completely lacks the sodium-retaining property of hydrocortisone and closely related derivatives of hydrocortisone.

INDICATIONS

1. *Endocrine Disorders*
   Primary or secondary adrenocortical insufficiency (hydrocortisone or cortisone is the first choice; synthetic analogs may be used in conjunction with mineralocorticoids where applicable; in infancy mineralocorticoid supplementation is of particular importance)
   Congenital adrenal hyperplasia
   Nonsuppurative thyroiditis
   Hypercalcemia associated with cancer
2. *Rheumatic Disorders*
   As adjunctive therapy for short-term administration (to tide the patient over an acute episode or exacerbation) in:
   Psoriatic arthritis
   Rheumatoid arthritis, including juvenile rheumatoid arthritis (selected cases may require low-dose maintenance therapy)
   Ankylosing spondylitis
   Acute and subacute bursitis
   Acute nonspecific tenosynovitis
   Acute gouty arthritis
   Post-traumatic osteoarthritis
   Synovitis of osteoarthritis
   Epicondylitis
3. *Collagen Diseases*
   During an exacerbation or as maintenance therapy in selected cases of—
   Systemic lupus erythematosus
   Acute rheumatic carditis
4. *Dermatologic Diseases*
   Pemphigus
   Bullous dermatitis herpetiformis
   Severe erythema multiforme (Stevens-Johnson syndrome)
   Exfoliative dermatitis
   Mycosis fungoides
   Severe psoriasis
   Severe seborrheic dermatitis
5. *Allergic States*
   Control of severe or incapacitating allergic conditions intractable to adequate trials of conventional treatment:
   Seasonal or perennial allergic rhinitis
   Bronchial asthma
   Contact dermatitis
   Atopic dermatitis
   Serum sickness
   Drug hypersensitivity reactions
6. *Ophthalmic Diseases*
   Severe acute and chronic allergic and inflammatory processes involving the eye and its adnexa, such as—
   Allergic conjunctivitis
   Keratitis
   Allergic corneal marginal ulcers
   Herpes zoster ophthalmicus
   Iritis and iridocyclitis
   Chorioretinitis
   Anterior segment inflammation
   Diffuse posterior uveitis and choroiditis
   Optic neuritis
   Sympathetic ophthalmia
7. *Respiratory Diseases*
   Symptomatic sarcoidosis
   Loeffler's syndrome not manageable by other means
   Berylliosis
   Fulminating or disseminated pulmonary tuberculosis when used concurrently with appropriate antituberculous chemotherapy
   Aspiration pneumonitis
8. *Hematologic Disorders*
   Idiopathic thrombocytopenic purpura in adults
   Secondary thrombocytopenia in adults
   Acquired (autoimmune) hemolytic anemia
   Erythroblastopenia (RBC anemia)
   Congenital (erythroid) hypoplastic anemia
9. *Neoplastic Diseases*
   For palliative management of:
   Leukemias and lymphomas in adults
   Acute leukemia of childhood
10. *Edematous States*
   To induce a diuresis or remission of proteinuria in the nephrotic syndrome, without uremia, of the idiopathic type or that due to lupus erythematosus
11. *Gastrointestinal Diseases*
   To tide the patient over a critical period of the disease in:
   Ulcerative colitis
   Regional enteritis
12. *Cerebral Edema* associated with primary or metastatic brain tumor, craniotomy, or head injury. Use in cerebral edema is not a substitute for careful neurosurgical evaluation and definitive management such as neurosurgery or other specific therapy.
13. *Miscellaneous*
   Tuberculous meningitis with subarachnoid block or impending block when used concurrently with appropriate antituberculous chemotherapy
   Trichinosis with neurologic or myocardial involvement
14. *Diagnostic testing of adrenocortical hyperfunction.*

CONTRAINDICATIONS

Systemic fungal infections
Hypersensitivity to this drug

WARNINGS

In patients on corticosteroid therapy subjected to unusual stress, increased dosage of rapidly acting corticosteroids before, during, and after the stressful situation is indicated.
Drug-induced secondary adrenocortical insufficiency may result from too rapid withdrawal of corticosteroids and may be minimized by gradual reduction of dosage. This type of relative insufficiency may persist for months after discontinuation of therapy; therefore, in any situation of stress occurring during that period, hormone therapy should be reinstituted. If the patient is receiving steroids already, dosage may have to be increased. Since mineralocorticoid secretion may be impaired, salt and/or a mineralocorticoid should be administered concurrently.
Corticosteroids may mask some signs of infection, and new infections may appear during their use. There may be decreased resistance and inability to localize infection when corticosteroids are used. Moreover, corticosteroids may affect the nitroblue-tetrazolium test for bacterial infection and produce false negative results.
In cerebral malaria, a double-blind trial has shown that the use of corticosteroids is associated with prolongation of coma and a higher incidence of pneumonia and gastrointestinal bleeding.
Corticosteroids may activate latent amebiasis. Therefore, it is recommended that latent or active amebiasis be ruled out before initiating corticosteroid therapy in any patient who has spent time in the tropics or any patient with unexplained diarrhea.
Prolonged use of corticosteroids may produce posterior subcapsular cataracts, glaucoma with possible damage to the optic nerves, and may enhance the establishment of secondary ocular infections due to fungi or viruses.
Usage in pregnancy: Since adequate human reproduction studies have not been done with corticosteroids, use of these drugs in pregnancy or in women of childbearing potential requires that the anticipated benefits be weighed against the possible hazards to the mother and embryo or fetus. Infants born of mothers who have received substantial doses of corticosteroids during pregnancy should be carefully observed for signs of hypoadrenalism.
Corticosteroids appear in breast milk and could suppress growth, interfere with endogenous corticosteroid production, or cause other unwanted effects. Mothers taking pharmacologic doses of corticosteroids should be advised not to nurse.
Average and large doses of hydrocortisone or cortisone can cause elevation of blood pressure, salt and water retention, and increased excretion of potassium. These effects are less likely to occur with the synthetic derivatives except when used in large doses. Dietary salt restriction and potassium supplementation may be necessary. All corticosteroids increase calcium excretion.
Administration of live virus vaccines, including smallpox, is contraindicated in individuals receiving immunosuppressive doses of corticosteroids. If inactivated viral or bacterial vaccines are administered to individuals receiving immunosuppressive doses of corticosteroid the expected serum antibody response may not be obtained. However, immunization procedures may be undertaken in patients who are receiving corticosteroids as replacement therapy, e.g., for Addison's disease.
Patients who are on drugs which suppress the immune system are more susceptible to infections than healthy individuals. Chickenpox and measles, for example, can have a more serious or even fatal course in non-immune patients on corticosteroids. In such patients who have not had these

diseases, particular care should be taken to avoid exposure. The risk of developing a disseminated infection varies among individuals and can be related to the dose, route and duration of corticosteroid administration as well as to the underlying disease. If exposed to chickenpox, prophylaxis with varicella zoster immune globulin (VZIG) may be indicated. If chickenpox develops, treatment with antiviral agents may be considered. If exposed to measles, prophylaxis with immune globulin (IG) may be indicated. (See the respective package inserts for VZIG and IG for complete prescribing information.)

Similarly, corticosteroids should be used with great care in patients with known or suspected Strongyloides (threadworm) infestation. In such patients, corticosteroid-induced immunosuppression may lead to Strongyloides hyperinfection and dissemination with widespread larval migration, often accompanied by severe enterocolitis and potentially fatal gram-negative septicemia.

The use of DECADRON tablets in active tuberculosis should be restricted to those cases of fulminating or disseminated tuberculosis in which the corticosteroid is used for the management of the disease in conjunction with an appropriate antituberculous regimen.

If corticosteroids are indicated in patients with latent tuberculosis or tuberculin reactivity, close observation is necessary as reactivation of the disease may occur. During prolonged corticosteroid therapy, these patients should receive chemoprophylaxis.

Literature reports suggest an apparent association between use of corticosteroids and left ventricular free wall rupture after a recent myocardial infarction; therefore, therapy with corticosteroids should be used with great caution in these patients.

PRECAUTIONS

Following prolonged therapy, withdrawal of corticosteroids may result in symptoms of the corticosteroid withdrawal syndrome including fever, myalgia, arthralgia, and malaise. This may occur in patients even without evidence of adrenal insufficiency.

There is an enhanced effect of corticosteroids in patients with hypothyroidism and in those with cirrhosis.

Corticosteroids should be used cautiously in patients with ocular herpes simplex because of possible corneal perforation.

The lowest possible dose of corticosteroids should be used to control the condition under treatment, and when reduction in dosage is possible, the reduction should be gradual.

Psychic derangements may appear when corticosteroids are used, ranging from euphoria, insomnia, mood swings, personality changes, and severe depression, to frank psychotic manifestations. Also, existing emotional instability or psychotic tendencies may be aggravated by corticosteroids.

Aspirin should be used cautiously in conjunction with corticosteroids in hypoprothrombinemia.

Steroids should be used with caution in nonspecific ulcerative colitis, if there is a probability of impending perforation, abscess, or other pyogenic infection, diverticulitis, fresh intestinal anastomoses, active or latent peptic ulcer, renal insufficiency, hypertension, osteoporosis, and myasthenia gravis. Signs of peritoneal irritation following gastrointestinal perforation in patients receiving large doses of corticosteroids may be minimal or absent. Fat embolism has been reported as a possible complication of hypercortisonism.

When large doses are given, some authorities advise that corticosteroids be taken with meals and antacids taken between meals to help to prevent peptic ulcer.

Steroids may increase or decrease motility and number of spermatozoa in some patients.

Phenytoin, phenobarbital, ephedrine, and rifampin may enhance the metabolic clearance of corticosteroids, resulting in decreased blood levels and lessened physiologic activity, thus requiring adjustment in corticosteroid dosage. These interactions may interfere with dexamethasone suppression tests which should be interpreted with caution during administration of these drugs.

False-negative results in the dexamethasone suppression test (DST) in patients being treated with indomethacin have been reported. Thus, results of the DST should be interpreted with caution in these patients.

The prothrombin time should be checked frequently in patients who are receiving corticosteroids and coumarin anticoagulants at the same time because of reports that corticosteroids have altered the response to these anticoagulants. Studies have shown that the usual effect produced by adding corticosteroids is inhibition of response to coumarins, although there have been some conflicting reports of potentiation not substantiated by studies.

When corticosteroids are administered concomitantly with potassium-depleting diuretics, patients should be observed closely for development of hypokalemia.

Information for Patients

Susceptible patients who are on immunosuppressant doses of corticosteroids should be warned to avoid exposure to chickenpox or measles. Patients should also be advised that if they are exposed, medical advice should be sought without delay.

Pediatric Use

Growth and development of pediatric patients on prolonged corticosteroid therapy should be carefully followed.

ADVERSE REACTIONS

Fluid and Electrolyte Disturbances

Sodium retention
Fluid retention
Congestive heart failure in susceptible patients
Potassium loss
Hypokalemic alkalosis
Hypertension

Musculoskeletal

Muscle weakness
Steroid myopathy
Loss of muscle mass
Osteoporosis
Vertebral compression fractures
Aseptic necrosis of femoral and humeral heads
Pathologic fracture of long bones
Tendon rupture

Gastrointestinal

Peptic ulcer with possible perforation and hemorrhage
Perforation of the small and large bowel, particularly in patients with inflammatory bowel disease
Pancreatitis
Abdominal distention
Ulcerative esophagitis

Dermatologic

Impaired wound healing
Thin fragile skin
Petechiae and ecchymoses
Erythema
Increased sweating
May suppress reactions to skin tests
Other cutaneous reactions, such as allergic dermatitis, urticaria, angioneurotic edema

Neurologic

Convulsions
Increased intracranial pressure with papilledema (pseudotumor cerebri) usually after treatment
Vertigo
Headache
Psychic disturbances

Endocrine

Menstrual irregularities
Development of cushingoid state
Suppression of growth in children
Secondary adrenocortical and pituitary unresponsiveness, particularly in times of stress, as in trauma, surgery, or illness
Decreased carbohydrate tolerance
Manifestations of latent diabetes mellitus
Increased requirements for insulin or oral hypoglycemic agents in diabetics
Hirsutism

Ophthalmic

Posterior subcapsular cataracts
Increased intraocular pressure
Glaucoma
Exophthalmos

Metabolic

Negative nitrogen balance due to protein catabolism

Cardiovascular

Myocardial rupture following recent myocardial infarction (see WARNINGS)

Other

Hypersensitivity
Thromboembolism
Weight gain
Increased appetite
Nausea
Malaise
Hiccups

OVERDOSAGE

Reports of acute toxicity and/or death following overdosage of glucocorticoids are rare. In the event of overdosage, no specific antidote is available; treatment is supportive and symptomatic.

The oral LD_{50} of dexamethasone in female mice was 6.5 g/kg.

DOSAGE AND ADMINISTRATION

For oral administration

DOSAGE REQUIREMENTS ARE VARIABLE AND MUST BE INDIVIDUALIZED ON THE BASIS OF THE DISEASE AND THE RESPONSE OF THE PATIENT.

The initial dosage varies from 0.75 to 9 mg a day depending on the disease being treated. In less severe diseases doses lower than 0.75 mg may suffice, while in severe diseases doses higher than 9 mg may be required. The initial dosage should be maintained or adjusted until the patient's response is satisfactory. If satisfactory clinical response does not occur after a reasonable period of time, discontinue DECADRON tablets and transfer the patient to other therapy.

After a favorable initial response, the proper maintenance dosage should be determined by decreasing the initial dosage in small amounts to the lowest dosage that maintains an adequate clinical response.

Patients should be observed closely for signs that might require dosage adjustment, including changes in clinical status resulting from remissions or exacerbations of the disease, individual drug responsiveness, and the effect of stress (e.g., surgery, infection, trauma). During stress it may be necessary to increase dosage temporarily.

If the drug is to be stopped after more than a few days of treatment, it usually should be withdrawn gradually.

The following milligram equivalents facilitate changing to DECADRON from other glucocorticoids:

DECADRON	Methylprednisolone and Triamcinolone	Prednisolone and Prednisone	Hydrocortisone	Cortisone
0.75 mg =	4 mg =	5 mg =	20 mg =	25 =

In *acute, self-limited allergic disorders or acute exacerbations of chronic allergic disorders,* the following dosage schedule combining parenteral and oral therapy is suggested:

DECADRON* Phosphate (Dexamethasone Sodium Phosphate) injection, 4 mg per mL:

First Day
1 or 2 mL, intramuscularly

DECADRON tablets, 0.75 mg:

Second Day
4 tablets in two divided doses

Third Day
4 tablets in two divided doses

Fourth Day
2 tablets in two divided doses

Fifth Day
1 tablet

Sixth Day
1 tablet

Seventh Day
No treatment

Eighth Day
Follow-up visit

This schedule is designed to ensure adequate therapy during acute episodes, while minimizing the risk of overdosage in chronic cases.

In *cerebral edema,* DECADRON Phosphate (Dexamethasone Sodium Phosphate) injection is generally administered initially in a dosage of 10 mg intravenously followed by 4 mg every six hours intramuscularly until the symptoms of cerebral edema subside. Response is usually noted within 12 to 24 hours and dosage may be reduced after two to four days and gradually discontinued over a period of five to seven days. For palliative management of patients with recurrent or inoperable brain tumors, maintenance therapy with either DECADRON Phosphate (Dexamethasone Sodium Phosphate) injection or DECADRON tablets in a dosage of two mg two or three times daily may be effective.

Dexamethasone suppression tests

1. Tests for Cushing's syndrome
   Give 1.0 mg of DECADRON orally at 11:00 p.m. Blood is drawn for plasma cortisol determination at 8:00 a.m. the following morning.
   For greater accuracy, give 0.5 mg of DECADRON orally every 6 hours for 48 hours. Twenty-four hour urine collections are made for determination of 17-hydroxycorticosteroid excretion.
2. Test to distinguish Cushing's syndrome due to pituitary ACTH excess from Cushing's syndrome due to other causes
   Give 2.0 mg of DECADRON orally every 6 hours for 48 hours. Twenty-four hour urine collections are made for determination of 17-hydroxycorticosteroid excretion.

*Registered trademark of MERCK & CO., INC.

HOW SUPPLIED

Tablets DECADRON are compressed, pentagonal-shaped tablets, colored to distinguish potency. They are scored and coded on one side and embossed with DECADRON on the other. They are available as follows:

No. 7645—4 mg, white in color and coded MSD 97.
NDC 0006-0097-50 bottles of 50
Shown in Product Identification Guide, page 323

No. 7601—0.75 mg, bluish-green in color and coded MSD 63.
NDC 0006-0063-12 5-12 PAK* (package of 12)
NDC 0006-0063-68 bottles of 100.
Shown in Product Identification Guide, page 323

No. 7598—0.5 mg, yellow in color and coded MSD 41.
NDC 0006-0041-68 bottles of 100.
Shown in Product Identification Guide, page 323

*Registered trademark of MERCK & CO., INC.
7921148 Issued February 1997

Continued on next page

Information on the Merck & Co., Inc. products listed on these pages is the full prescribing information from product circulars in use September 30, 2000. For information, please call 1-800-NSC MERCK [1-800-672-6372].

DECADRON® Phosphate Injection ℞
(Dexamethasone Sodium Phosphate)

DESCRIPTION

Dexamethasone sodium phosphate, a synthetic adrenocortical steroid, is a white or slightly yellow, crystalline powder. It is freely soluble in water and is exceedingly hygroscopic. The molecular weight is 516.41. It is designated chemically as 9-fluoro-11β, 17-dihydroxy-16α-methyl-21-(phosphonooxy)pregna-1, 4-diene-3, 20-dione disodium salt. The empirical formula is $C_{22}H_{28}FNa_2O_8P$ and the structural formula is:

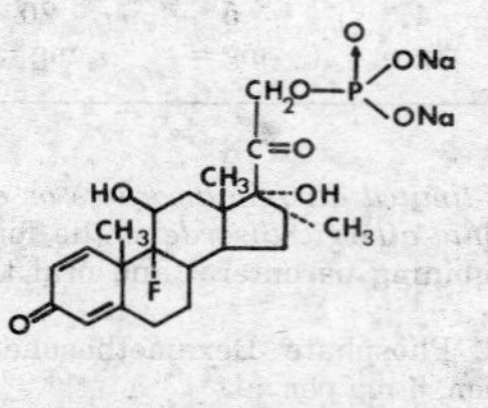

DECADRON* Phosphate (Dexamethasone Sodium Phosphate) injection is a sterile solution (pH 7.0 to 8.5) of dexamethasone sodium phosphate, sealed under nitrogen, and is supplied in two concentrations: 4 mg/mL and 24 mg/mL. The 24 mg/mL concentration offers the advantage of less volume in indications where high doses of corticosteroids by the intravenous route are needed.

Each milliliter of DECADRON Phosphate injection, 4 mg/mL, contains dexamethasone sodium phosphate equivalent to 4 mg dexamethasone phosphate or 3.33 mg dexamethasone. Inactive ingredients per mL: 8 mg creatinine, 10 mg sodium citrate, sodium hydroxide to adjust pH, and Water for Injection q.s., with 1 mg sodium bisulfite, 1.5 mg methylparaben, and 0.2 mg propylparaben added as preservatives.

Each milliliter of DECADRON Phosphate injection, 24 mg/mL, contains dexamethasone sodium phosphate equivalent to 24 mg dexamethasone phosphate or 20 mg dexamethasone. Inactive ingredients per mL: 8 mg creatinine, 10 mg sodium citrate, 0.5 mg disodium edetate, sodium hydroxide to adjust pH, and Water for Injection q.s., with 1 mg sodium bisulfite, 1.5 mg methylparaben, and 0.2 mg propylparaben added as preservatives.

*Registered trademark of MERCK & CO., INC.

ACTIONS

DECADRON Phosphate injection has a rapid onset but short duration of action when compared with less soluble preparations. Because of this, it is suitable for the treatment of acute disorders responsive to adrenocortical steroid therapy.

Naturally occurring glucocorticoids (hydrocortisone and cortisone), which also have salt-retaining properties, are used as replacement therapy in adrenocortical deficiency states. Their synthetic analogs, including dexamethasone, are primarily used for their potent anti-inflammatory effects in disorders of many organ systems.

Glucocorticoids cause profound and varied metabolic effects. In addition, they modify the body's immune responses to diverse stimuli.

At equipotent anti-inflammatory doses, dexamethasone almost completely lacks the sodium-retaining property of hydrocortisone and closely related derivatives of hydrocortisone.

INDICATIONS

A. By intravenous or intramuscular injection when oral therapy is not feasible:

1. *Endocrine disorders*

Primary or secondary adrenocortical insufficiency (hydrocortisone or cortisone is the drug of choice; synthetic analogs may be used in conjunction with mineralocorticoids where applicable; in infancy, mineralocorticoid supplementation is of particular importance)

Acute adrenocortical insufficiency (hydrocortisone or cortisone is the drug of choice; mineralocorticoid supplementation may be necessary, particularly when synthetic analogs are used)

Preoperatively, and in the event of serious trauma or illness, in patients with known adrenal insufficiency or when adrenocortical reserve is doubtful

Shock unresponsive to conventional therapy if adrenocortical insufficiency exists or is suspected

Congenital adrenal hyperplasia

Nonsuppurative thyroiditis

Hypercalcemia associated with cancer

2. *Rheumatic disorders*

As adjunctive therapy for short-term administration (to tide the patient over an acute episode or exacerbation) in:

Post-traumatic osteoarthritis

Synovitis of osteoarthritis

Rheumatoid arthritis, including juvenile rheumatoid arthritis (selected cases may require low-dose maintenance therapy)

Acute and subacute bursitis

Epicondylitis

Acute nonspecific tenosynovitis

Acute gouty arthritis

Psoriatic arthritis

Ankylosing spondylitis

3. *Collagen diseases*

During an exacerbation or as maintenance therapy in selected cases of:

Systemic lupus erythematosus

Acute rheumatic carditis

4. *Dermatologic diseases*

Pemphigus

Severe erythema multiforme (Stevens-Johnson syndrome)

Exfoliative dermatitis

Bullous dermatitis herpetiformis

Severe seborrheic dermatitis

Severe psoriasis

Mycosis fungoides

5. *Allergic states*

Control of severe or incapacitating allergic conditions intractable to adequate trials of conventional treatment in:

Bronchial asthma

Contact dermatitis

Atopic dermatitis

Serum sickness

Seasonal or perennial allergic rhinitis

Drug hypersensitivity reactions

Urticarial transfusion reactions

Acute noninfectious laryngeal edema (epinephrine is the drug of first choice)

6. *Ophthalmic diseases*

Severe acute and chronic allergic and inflammatory processes involving the eye, such as:

Herpes zoster ophthalmicus

Iritis, iridocyclitis

Chorioretinitis

Diffuse posterior uveitis and choroiditis

Optic neuritis

Sympathetic ophthalmia

Anterior segment inflammation

Allergic conjunctivitis

Keratitis

Allergic corneal marginal ulcers

7. *Gastrointestinal diseases*

To tide the patient over a critical period of the disease in:

Ulcerative colitis (Systemic therapy)

Regional enteritis (Systemic therapy)

8. *Respiratory diseases*

Symptomatic sarcoidosis

Berylliosis

Fulminating or disseminated pulmonary tuberculosis when used concurrently with appropriate antituberculous chemotherapy

Loeffler's syndrome not manageable by other means

Aspiration pneumonitis

9. *Hematologic disorders*

Acquired (autoimmune) hemolytic anemia

Idiopathic thrombocytopenic purpura in adults (I.V. only; I.M. administration is contraindicated)

Secondary thrombocytopenia in adults

Erythroblastopenia (RBC anemia)

Congenital (erythroid) hypoplastic anemia

10. *Neoplastic diseases*

For palliative management of:

Leukemias and lymphomas in adults

Acute leukemia of childhood

11. *Edematous states*

To induce diuresis or remission of proteinuria in the nephrotic syndrome, without uremia, of the idiopathic type, or that due to lupus erythematosus

12. *Miscellaneous*

Tuberculous meningitis with subarachnoid block or impending block when used concurrently with appropriate antituberculous chemotherapy

Trichinosis with neurologic or myocardial involvement

13. *Diagnostic testing of adrenocortical hyperfunction*

14. *Cerebral Edema* associated with primary or metastatic brain tumor, craniotomy, or head injury. Use in cerebral edema is not a substitute for careful neurosurgical evaluation and definitive management such as neurosurgery or other specific therapy.

B. By intra-articular or soft tissue injection:

As adjunctive therapy for short-term administration (to tide the patient over an acute episode or exacerbation) in:

Synovitis of osteoarthritis

Rheumatoid arthritis

Acute and subacute bursitis

Acute gouty arthritis

Epicondylitis

Acute nonspecific tenosynovitis

Post-traumatic osteoarthritis.

C. By intralesional injection:

Keloids

Localized hypertrophic, infiltrated, inflammatory lesions of: lichen planus, psoriatic plaques, granuloma annulare, and lichen simplex chronicus (neurodermatitis)

Discoid lupus erythematosus

Necrobiosis lipoidica diabeticorum

Alopecia areata

May also be useful in cystic tumors of an aponeurosis or tendon (ganglia).

CONTRAINDICATIONS

Systemic fungal infections. (See WARNINGS regarding amphotericin B).

Hypersensitivity to any component of this product, including sulfites (see WARNINGS).

WARNINGS

Because rare instances of anaphylactoid reactions have occurred in patients receiving parenteral corticosteroid therapy, appropriate precautionary measures should be taken prior to administration, especially when the patient has a history of allergy to any drug. Anaphylactoid and hypersensitivity reactions have been reported for Injection DECADRON Phosphate (see ADVERSE REACTIONS).

Injection DECADRON Phosphate contains sodium bisulfite, a sulfite that may cause allergic-type reactions including anaphylactic symptoms and life-threatening or less severe asthmatic episodes in certain susceptible people. The overall prevalence of sulfite sensitivity in the general population is unknown and probably low. Sulfite sensitivity is seen more frequently in asthmatic than in nonasthmatic people.

Corticosteroids may exacerbate systemic fungal infections and therefore should not be used in the presence of such infections unless they are needed to control drug reactions due to amphotericin B. Moreover, there have been cases reported in which concomitant use of amphotericin B and hydrocortisone was followed by cardiac enlargement and congestive failure.

In patients on corticosteroid therapy subjected to any unusual stress, increased dosage of rapidly acting corticosteroids before, during, and after the stressful situation is indicated.

Drug-induced secondary adrenocortical insufficiency may result from too rapid withdrawal of corticosteroids and may be minimized by gradual reduction of dosage. This type of relative insufficiency may persist for months after discontinuation of therapy; therefore, in any situation of stress occurring during that period, hormone therapy should be reinstituted. If the patient is receiving steroids already, dosage may have to be increased. Since mineralocorticoid secretion may be impaired, salt and/or a mineralocorticoid should be administered concurrently.

Corticosteroids may mask some signs of infection, and new infections may appear during their use. There may be decreased resistance and inability to localize infection when corticosteroids are used. Moreover, corticosteroids may affect the nitroblue-tetrazolium test for bacterial infection and produce false negative results.

In cerebral malaria, a double-blind trial has shown that the use of corticosteroids is associated with prolongation of coma and a higher incidence of pneumonia and gastrointestinal bleeding.

Corticosteroids may activate latent amebiasis. Therefore, it is recommended that latent or active amebiasis be ruled out before initiating corticosteroid therapy in any patient who has spent time in the tropics or any patient with unexplained diarrhea.

Prolonged use of corticosteroids may produce posterior subcapsular cataracts, glaucoma with possible damage to the optic nerves, and may enhance the establishment of secondary ocular infections due to fungi or viruses.

Usage in pregnancy. Since adequate human reproduction studies have not been done with corticosteroids, use of these drugs in pregnancy or in women of childbearing potential requires that the anticipated benefits be weighed against the possible hazards to the mother and embryo or fetus. Infants born of mothers who have received substantial doses of corticosteroids during pregnancy should be carefully observed for signs of hypoadrenalism.

Corticosteroids appear in breast milk and could suppress growth, interfere with endogenous corticosteroid production, or cause other unwanted effects. Mothers taking pharmacologic doses of corticosteroids should be advised not to nurse.

Average and large doses of cortisone or hydrocortisone can cause elevation of blood pressure, salt and water retention, and increased excretion of potassium. These effects are less likely to occur with the synthetic derivatives except when used in large doses. Dietary salt restriction and potassium supplementation may be necessary. All corticosteroids increase calcium excretion.

Administration of live virus vaccines, including smallpox, is contraindicated in individuals receiving immunosuppressive doses of corticosteroids. If inactivated viral or bacterial vaccines are administered to individuals receiving immunosuppressive doses of corticosteroids, the expected serum antibody response may not be obtained. However, immunization procedures may be undertaken in patients who are receiving corticosteroids as replacement therapy, e.g., for Addison's disease.

Patients who are on drugs which suppress the immune system are more susceptible to infections than healthy individuals. Chickenpox and measles, for example, can have a more serious or even fatal course in non-immune patients on corticosteroids. In such patients who have not had these diseases, particular care should be taken to avoid exposure. The risk of developing a disseminated infection varies among individuals and can be related to the dose, route and duration of corticosteroid administration as well as to the underlying disease. If exposed to chickenpox, prophylaxis with varicella zoster immune globulin (VZIG) may be indicated. If chickenpox develops, treatment with antiviral

agents may be considered. If exposed to measles, prophylaxis with immune globulin (IG) may be indicated. (See the respective package inserts for VZIG and IG for complete prescribing information.)
Similarly, corticosteroids should be used with great care in patients with known or suspected Strongyloides (threadworm) infestation. In such patients, corticosteroid-induced immunosuppression may lead to Strongyloides hyperinfection and dissemination with widespread larval migration, often accompanied by severe enterocolitis and potentially fatal gram-negative septicemia.
The use of DECADRON Phosphate injection in active tuberculosis should be restricted to those cases of fulminating or disseminated tuberculosis in which the corticosteroid is used for the management of the disease in conjunction with an appropriate antituberculous regimen.
If corticosteroids are indicated in patients with latent tuberculosis or tuberculin reactivity, close observation is necessary as reactivation of the disease may occur. During prolonged corticosteroid therapy, these patients should receive chemoprophylaxis.
Literature reports suggest an apparent association between use of corticosteroids and left ventricular free wall rupture after a recent myocardial infarction; therefore, therapy with corticosteroids should be used with great caution in these patients.

PRECAUTIONS

This product, like many other steroid formulations, is sensitive to heat. Therefore, it should not be autoclaved when it is desirable to sterilize the exterior of the vial.
Following prolonged therapy, withdrawal of corticosteroids may result in symptoms of the corticosteroid withdrawal syndrome including fever, myalgia, arthralgia, and malaise. This may occur in patients even without evidence of adrenal insufficiency.
There is an enhanced effect of corticosteroids in patients with hypothyroidism and in those with cirrhosis.
Corticosteroids should be used cautiously in patients with ocular herpes simplex for fear of corneal perforation.
The lowest possible dose of corticosteroid should be used to control the condition under treatment, and when reduction in dosage is possible, the reduction must be gradual.
Psychic derangements may appear when corticosteroids are used, ranging from euphoria, insomnia, mood swings, personality changes, and severe depression to frank psychotic manifestations. Also, existing emotional instability or psychotic tendencies may be aggravated by corticosteroids.
Aspirin should be used cautiously in conjunction with corticosteroids in hypoprothrombinemia.
Steroids should be used with caution in nonspecific ulcerative colitis, if there is a probability of impending perforation, abscess, or other pyogenic infection, also in diverticulitis, fresh intestinal anastomoses, active or latent peptic ulcer, renal insufficiency, hypertension, osteoporosis, and myasthenia gravis. Signs of peritoneal irritation following gastrointestinal perforation in patients receiving large doses of corticosteroids may be minimal or absent. Fat embolism has been reported as a possible complication of hypercortisonism.
When large doses are given, some authorities advise that antacids be administered between meals to help to prevent peptic ulcer.
Steroids may increase or decrease motility and number of spermatozoa in some patients.
Phenytoin, phenobarbital, ephedrine, and rifampin may enhance the metabolic clearance of corticosteroids resulting in decreased blood levels and lessened physiologic activity, thus requiring adjustment in corticosteroid dosage. These interactions may interfere with dexamethasone suppression tests which should be interpreted with caution during administration of these drugs.
False negative results in the dexamethasone suppression test (DST) in patients being treated with indomethacin have been reported. Thus, results of the DST should be interpreted with caution in these patients.
The prothrombin time should be checked frequently in patients who are receiving corticosteroids and coumarin anticoagulants at the same time because of reports that corticosteroids have altered the response to these anticoagulants. Studies have shown that the usual effect produced by adding corticosteroids is inhibition of response to coumarins, although there have been some conflicting reports of potentiation not substantiated by studies.
When corticosteroids are administered concomitantly with potassium-depleting diuretics, patients should be observed closely for development of hypokalemia.
Intra-articular injection of a corticosteroid may produce systemic as well as local effects.
Appropriate examination of any joint fluid present is necessary to exclude a septic process.
A marked increase in pain accompanied by local swelling, further restriction of joint motion, fever, and malaise is suggestive of septic arthritis. If this complication occurs and the diagnosis of sepsis is confirmed, appropriate antimicrobial therapy should be instituted.
Injection of a steroid into an infected site is to be avoided.
Corticosteroids should not be injected into unstable joints.
Patients should be impressed strongly with the importance of not overusing joints in which symptomatic benefit has been obtained as long as the inflammatory process remains active.
Frequent intra-articular injection may result in damage to joint tissues.
The slower rate of absorption by intramuscular administration should be recognized.
Information for Patients
Susceptible patients who are on immunosuppressant doses of corticosteroids should be warned to avoid exposure to chickenpox or measles. Patients should also be advised that if they are exposed, medical advice should be sought without delay.
Pediatric Use
Growth and development of pediatric patients on prolonged corticosteroid therapy should be carefully followed.

ADVERSE REACTIONS

Fluid and electrolyte disturbances
Sodium retention
Fluid retention
Congestive heart failure in susceptible patients
Potassium loss
Hypokalemic alkalosis
Hypertension
Musculoskeletal
Muscle weakness
Steroid myopathy
Loss of muscle mass
Osteoporosis
Vertebral compression fractures
Aseptic necrosis of femoral and humeral heads
Pathologic fracture of long bones
Tendon rupture
Gastrointestinal
Peptic ulcer with possible subsequent perforation and hemorrhage
Perforation of the small and large bowel, particularly in patients with inflammatory bowel disease
Pancreatitis
Abdominal distention
Ulcerative esophagitis
Dermatologic
Impaired wound healing
Thin fragile skin
Petechiae and ecchymoses
Erythema
Increased sweating
May suppress reactions to skin tests
Burning or tingling, especially in the perineal area (after I.V. injection)
Other cutaneous reactions, such as allergic dermatitis, urticaria, angioneurotic edema
Neurologic
Convulsions
Increased intracranial pressure with papilledema (pseudotumor cerebri) usually after treatment
Vertigo
Headache
Psychic disturbances
Endocrine
Menstrual irregularities
Development of cushingoid state
Suppression of growth in pediatric patients
Secondary adrenocortical and pituitary unresponsiveness, particularly in times of stress, as in trauma, surgery, or illness
Decreased carbohydrate tolerance
Manifestations of latent diabetes mellitus
Increased requirements for insulin or oral hypoglycemic agents in diabetics
Hirsutism
Ophthalmic
Posterior subcapsular cataracts
Increased intraocular pressure
Glaucoma
Exophthalmos
Retinopathy of prematurity
Metabolic
Negative nitrogen balance due to protein catabolism
Cardiovascular
Myocardial rupture following recent myocardial infarction (see WARNINGS)
Hypertrophic cardiomyopathy in low birth weight infants
Other
Anaphylactoid or hypersensitivity reactions
Thromboembolism
Weight gain
Increased appetite
Nausea
Malaise
Hiccups
The following *additional* adverse reactions are related to parenteral corticosteroid therapy:
Rare instances of blindness associated with intralesional therapy around the face and head
Hyperpigmentation or hypopigmentation
Subcutaneous and cutaneous atrophy
Sterile abscess
Postinjection flare (following intra-articular use)
Charcot-like arthropathy

OVERDOSAGE

Reports of acute toxicity and/or death following overdosage of glucocorticoids are rare. In the event of overdosage, no specific antidote is available; treatment is supportive and symptomatic.
Significant lethality was observed in female mice at single oral doses of 3630 mg/m^2 (1210 mg/kg) and single intravenous doses of 2382 mg/m^2 (794 mg/kg).

DOSAGE AND ADMINISTRATION

DECADRON Phosphate injection, 4 mg/mL—*For intravenous, intramuscular, intra-articular, intralesional, and soft tissue injection.*
DECADRON Phosphate injection, 24 mg/mL—*For intravenous injection only.*
DECADRON Phosphate injection can be given directly from the vial, or it can be added to Sodium Chloride Injection or Dextrose Injection and administered by intravenous drip.
Solutions used for intravenous administration or further dilution of this product should be preservative-free when used in the neonate, especially the premature infant.
When it is mixed with an infusion solution, sterile precautions should be observed. Since infusion solutions generally do not contain preservatives, mixtures should be used within 24 hours.
Parenteral drug products should be inspected visually for particulate matter and discoloration prior to administration, whenever solution and container permit.
DOSAGE REQUIREMENTS ARE VARIABLE AND MUST BE INDIVIDUALIZED ON THE BASIS OF THE DISEASE AND THE RESPONSE OF THE PATIENT.

Intravenous and Intramuscular Injection

The initial dosage of DECADRON Phosphate injection varies from 0.5 to 9 mg a day depending on the disease being treated. In less severe diseases doses lower than 0.5 mg may suffice, while in severe diseases doses higher than 9 mg may be required.
The initial dosage should be maintained or adjusted until the patient's response is satisfactory. If a satisfactory clinical response does not occur after a reasonable period of time, discontinue DECADRON Phosphate injection and transfer the patient to other therapy.
After a favorable initial response, the proper maintenance dosage should be determined by decreasing the initial dosage in small amounts to the lowest dosage that maintains an adequate clinical response.
Patients should be observed closely for signs that might require dosage adjustment, including changes in clinical status resulting from remissions or exacerbations of the disease, individual drug responsiveness, and the effect of stress (e.g., surgery, infection, trauma). During stress it may be necessary to increase dosage temporarily.
If the drug is to be stopped after more than a few days of treatment, it usually should be withdrawn gradually.
When the intravenous route of administration is used, dosage usually should be the same as the oral dosage. In certain overwhelming, acute, life-threatening situations, however, administration in dosages exceeding the usual dosages may be justified and may be in multiples of the oral dosages.
The slower rate of absorption by intramuscular administration should be recognized.
Shock
There is a tendency in current medical practice to use high (pharmacologic) doses of corticosteroids for the treatment of unresponsive shock. The following dosages of DECADRON phosphate injection have been suggested by various authors:

*Author***	*Dosage*
Cavanagh[1]	3 mg/kg of body weight per 24 hours by constant intravenous infusion after an initial intravenous injection of 20 mg
Dietzman[2]	2 to 6 mg/kg of body weight as a single intravenous injection
Frank[3]	40 mg initially followed by repeat intravenous injection every 4 to 6 hours while shock persists
Oaks[4]	40 mg initially followed by repeat intravenous injection every 2 to 6 hours while shock persists
Schumer[5]	1 mg/kg of body weight as a single intravenous injection

Administration of high dose corticosteroid therapy should be continued only until the patient's condition has stabilized and usually not longer than 48 to 72 hours.
Although adverse reactions associated with high dose, short term corticosteroid therapy are uncommon, peptic ulceration may occur.

**1. Cavanagh, D.; Singh, K. B.: Endotoxin shock in pregnancy and abortion, in "Corticosteroids in the Treatment of Shock", Schumer, W.; Nyhus, L. M., Editors, Urbana, University of Illinois Press, 1970, pp. 86-96.

Continued on next page

Information on the Merck & Co., Inc. products listed on these pages is the full prescribing information from product circulars in use September 30, 2000. For information, please call 1-800-NSC MERCK [1-800-672-6372].

Decadron Phosphate Inj.—Cont.

2. Dietzman, R. H.; Ersek, R. A.; Bloch, J. M.; Lillehei, R. C.: High-output, low-resistance gram-negative septic shock in man, Angiology *20:* 691-700, Dec. 1969.
3. Frank, E.: Clinical observations in shock and management (In: Shields, T. F., ed.: Symposium on current concepts and management of shock), J. Maine Med. Ass. *59:* 195-200, Oct. 1968.
4. Oaks, W. W.; Cohen, H. E.: Endotoxin shock in the geriatric patient, Geriat. *22:* 120-130, Mar. 1967.
5. Schumer, W.; Nyhus, L. M.: Corticosteroid effect on biochemical parameters of human oligemic shock, Arch. Surg. *100:* 405-408, Apr. 1970.

Cerebral Edema

DECADRON Phosphate injection is generally administered initially in a dosage of 10 mg intravenously followed by 4 mg every six hours intramuscularly until the symptoms of cerebral edema subside. Response is usually noted within 12 to 24 hours and dosage may be reduced after two to four days and gradually discontinued over a period of five to seven days. For palliative management of patients with recurrent or inoperable brain tumors, maintenance therapy with two mg two or three times a day may be effective.

Acute Allergic Disorders

In acute, self-limited allergic disorders or acute exacerbations of chronic allergic disorders, the following dosage schedule combining parenteral and oral therapy is suggested:

DECADRON Phosphate injection, 4 mg/mL: *first day,* 1 or 2 mL (4 or 8 mg), intramuscularly.

DECADRON (Dexamethasone) tablets, 0.75 mg: *second and third days,* 4 tablets in two divided doses each day; *fourth day,* 2 tablets in two divided doses; *fifth and sixth days,* 1 tablet each day; *seventh day,* no treatment; *eighth day,* follow-up visit.

This schedule is designed to ensure adequate therapy during acute episodes, while minimizing the risk of overdosage in chronic cases.

Intra-articular, Intralesional, and Soft Tissue Injection

Intra-articular, intralesional, and soft tissue injections are generally employed when the affected joints or areas are limited to one or two sites. Dosage and frequency of injection varies depending on the condition and the site of injection. The usual dose is from 0.2 to 6 mg. The frequency usually ranges from once every three to five days to once every two to three weeks. Frequent intra-articular injection may result in damage to joint tissues.

Some of the usual single doses are:

Site of Injection	Amount of Dexamethasone Phosphate (mg)
Large Joints (e.g., Knee)	2 to 4
Small Joints (e.g., Interphalangeal, Temporomandibular)	0.8 to 1
Bursae	2 to 3
Tendon Sheaths	0.4 to 1
Soft Tissue Infiltration	2 to 6
Ganglia	1 to 2

DECADRON Phosphate injection is particularly recommended for use in conjunction with one of the less soluble, longer-acting steroids for intra-articular and soft tissue injection.

HOW SUPPLIED

No 7628X—Injection DECADRON Phosphate, 4 mg per mL, is a clear, colorless solution, and is available in 5 mL and 25 mL vials as follows:

NDC 0006-7628-03, 5 mL vial
(6505-00-963-5355, 5 mL vial)
NDC 0006-7628-25, 25 mL vial.

FOR INTRAVENOUS USE ONLY:

No. 7646—Injection DECADRON Phosphate, 24 mg per mL, is a clear, colorless to light yellow solution and is available in 5 mL vials as follows:

NDC 0006-7646-03, 5 mL vial
(6505-01-153-3524, 5 mL vial).

Storage

Store at 25°C (77°F), excursions permitted to 15–30°C (59–86°F) [See USP Controlled Room Temperature].

Sensitive to heat. Do not autoclave.

Protect from freezing.

Protect from light. Store container in carton until contents have been used.

9051532 Issued July 1999

DECADRON® Phosphate ℞
(Dexamethasone Sodium Phosphate)
0.05% Dexamethasone Phosphate Equivalent
Sterile Ophthalmic Ointment

DESCRIPTION

Dexamethasone sodium phosphate is 9-fluoro-11β,17-dihydroxy-16α -methyl-21- (phosphonooxy) pregna-1,4-diene-3,20-dione disodium salt. Its empirical formula is $C_{22}H_{28}FNa_2O_8P$ and its structural formula is:

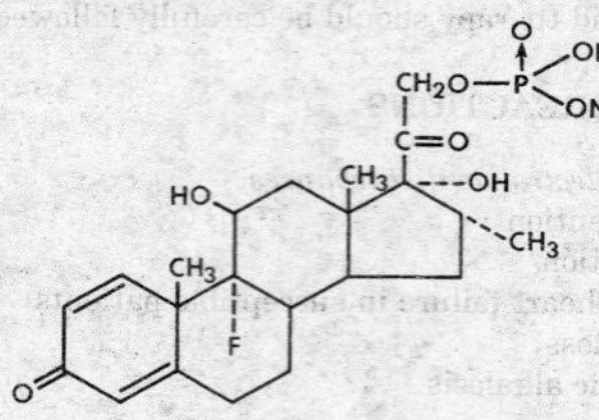

Glucocorticoids are adrenocortical steroids, both naturally occurring and synthetic. Dexamethasone is a synthetic analog of naturally occurring glucocorticoids (hydrocortisone and cortisone). Dexamethasone sodium phosphate is a water soluble, inorganic ester of dexamethasone. Its molecular weight is 516.41.

Sterile Ophthalmic Ointment DECADRON* Phosphate (Dexamethasone Sodium Phosphate) is a topical steroid ointment containing dexamethasone sodium phosphate equivalent to 0.5 mg (0.05%) dexamethasone phosphate in each gram. Inactive ingredients: white petrolatum and mineral oil.

Dexamethasone sodium phosphate is an inorganic ester of dexamethasone.

*Registered trademark of MERCK & CO., INC.

CLINICAL PHARMACOLOGY

Dexamethasone sodium phosphate suppresses the inflammatory response to a variety of agents and it probably delays or slows healing. No generally accepted explanation of these steroid properties has been advanced.

INDICATIONS AND USAGE

For the treatment of the following conditions:

Steroid responsive inflammatory conditions of the palpebral and bulbar conjunctiva, cornea, and anterior segment of the globe, such as allergic conjunctivitis, acne rosacea, superficial punctate keratitis, herpes zoster keratitis, iritis, cyclitis, selected infective conjunctivitis when the inherent hazard of steroid use is accepted to obtain an advisable diminution in edema and inflammation; corneal injury from chemical or thermal burns, or penetration of foreign bodies.

CONTRAINDICATIONS

Epithelial herpes simplex keratitis (dendritic keratitis).
Acute infectious stages of vaccinia, varicella, and many other viral diseases of the cornea and conjunctiva.
Mycobacterial infection of the eye.
Fungal diseases of ocular structures.
Hypersensitivity to a component of the medication.

WARNINGS

Prolonged use may result in ocular hypertension and/or glaucoma, with damage to the optic nerve, defects in visual acuity and fields of vision, and posterior subcapsular cataract formation. Prolonged use may suppress the host response and thus increase the hazard of secondary ocular infections. In those diseases causing thinning of the cornea or sclera, perforations have been known to occur with the use of topical corticosteroids. In acute purulent conditions of the eye, corticosteroids may mask infection or enhance existing infection. If these products are used for 10 days or longer, intraocular pressure should be routinely monitored even though it may be difficult in children and uncooperative patients.

Employment of corticosteroid medication in the treatment of herpes simplex other than epithelial herpes simplex keratitis, in which it is contraindicated, requires great caution; periodic slit-lamp microscopy is essential.

PRECAUTIONS

General

The possibility of persistent fungal infections of the cornea should be considered after prolonged corticosteroid dosing. There have been reports of bacterial keratitis associated with the use of multiple dose containers of topical ophthalmic products. These containers had been inadvertently contaminated by patients who, in most cases, had a concurrent corneal disease or a disruption of the ocular epithelial surface. (See PRECAUTIONS, *Information for Patients.*)

Information for Patients

Patients should be instructed to avoid allowing the tip of the dispensing container to contact the eye or surrounding structures.

Patients should also be instructed that ocular preparations, if handled improperly, can become contaminated by common bacteria known to cause ocular infections. Serious damage to the eye and subsequent loss of vision may result from using contaminated preparations. (See PRECAUTIONS, *General.*)

Patients should also be advised that if they develop an intercurrent ocular condition (e.g., trauma, ocular surgery or infection), they should immediately seek their physician's advice concerning the continued use of the present multidose container.

Carcinogenesis, Mutagenesis, Impairment of Fertility

Long-term animal studies have not been performed to evaluate the carcinogenic potential or the effect on fertility of Ophthalmic Ointment DECADRON Phosphate.

Pregnancy

Pregnancy Category C. Dexamethasone has been shown to be teratogenic in mice and rabbits following topical ophthalmic application in multiples of the therapeutic dose.

In the mouse, corticosteroids produce fetal resorptions and a specific abnormality, cleft palate. In the rabbit, corticosteroids have produced fetal resorptions and multiple abnormalities involving the head, ears, limbs, palate, etc.

There are no adequate or well-controlled studies in pregnant women. Ophthalmic Ointment DECADRON Phosphate should be used during pregnancy only if the potential benefit to the mother justifies the potential risk to the embryo or fetus. Infants born of mothers who have received substantial doses of corticosteroids during pregnancy should be observed carefully for signs of hypoadrenalism.

Nursing Mothers

Topically applied steroids are absorbed systemically. Therefore, because of the potential for serious adverse reactions in nursing infants from dexamethasone sodium phosphate, a decision should be made whether to discontinue nursing or discontinue the drug, taking into account the importance of the drug to the mother.

Pediatric Use

Safety and effectiveness in pediatric patients have not been established.

ADVERSE REACTIONS

Glaucoma with optic nerve damage, visual acuity and field defects, posterior subcapsular cataract formation, secondary ocular infection from pathogens including herpes simplex, perforation of the globe.

Rarely, filtering blebs have been reported when topical steroids have been used following cataract surgery.

Rarely, stinging or burning may occur.

DOSAGE AND ADMINISTRATION

The duration of treatment will vary with the type of lesion and may extend from a few days to several weeks, according to therapeutic response. Relapses, more common in chronic active lesions than in self-limited conditions, usually respond to retreatment.

Apply a thin coating of ointment three or four times a day. When a favorable response is observed, reduce the number of daily applications to two, and later to one a day as a maintenance dose if this is sufficient to control symptoms.

Ophthalmic Ointment DECADRON Phosphate is particularly convenient when an eye pad is used. It may also be the preparation of choice for patients in whom therapeutic benefit depends on prolonged contact of the active ingredients with ocular tissues.

HOW SUPPLIED

No. 7615—0.05% Sterile Ophthalmic Ointment DECADRON Phosphate is a clear unctuous ointment and is supplied as follows:

NDC 0006-7615-04 in 3.5 g tubes
(6505-00-961-5508 0.05% 3.5 g).

7612332 Issued October 1996

DECADRON® Phosphate ℞
(Dexamethasone Sodium Phosphate)
0.1% Dexamethasone Phosphate Equivalent
Sterile Ophthalmic Solution

DESCRIPTION

Dexamethasone sodium phosphate is 9-fluoro-11β,17-dihydroxy-16α -methyl-21- (phosphonooxy) pregna-1,4-diene-3,20-dione disodium salt. Its empirical formula is $C_{22}H_{28}FNa_2O_8P$ and its structural formula is:

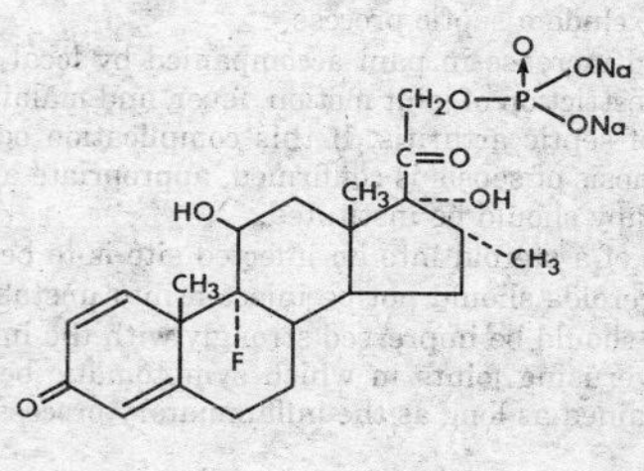

Glucocorticoids are adrenocortical steroids, both naturally occurring and synthetic. Dexamethasone is a synthetic analog of naturally occurring glucocorticoids (hydrocortisone and cortisone). Dexamethasone sodium phosphate is a water soluble, inorganic ester of dexamethasone. It is approximately three thousand times more soluble in water at 25°C than hydrocortisone. Its molecular weight is 516.41.
Ophthalmic Solution DECADRON* Phosphate (Dexamethasone Sodium Phosphate) in the 5 mL OCUMETER* ophthalmic dispenser is a topical steroid solution containing dexamethasone sodium phosphate equivalent to 1 mg (0.1%) dexamethasone phosphate in each milliliter of buffered solution. Inactive ingredients: creatinine, sodium citrate, sodium borate, polysorbate 80, disodium edetate, hydrochloric acid to adjust pH, and water for injection. Sodium bisulfite 0.1%, phenylethanol 0.25% and benzalkonium chloride 0.02% added as preservatives.

*Registered trademark of MERCK & CO., INC.

CLINICAL PHARMACOLOGY

Dexamethasone sodium phosphate suppresses the inflammatory response to a variety of agents and it probably delays or slows healing. No generally accepted explanation of these steroid properties has been advanced.

INDICATIONS AND USAGE

For the treatment of the following conditions:
Ophthalmic:
Steroid responsive inflammatory conditions of the palpebral and bulbar conjunctiva, cornea, and anterior segment of the globe, such as allergic conjunctivitis, acne rosacea, superficial punctate keratitis, herpes zoster keratitis, iritis, cyclitis, selected infective conjunctivitis when the inherent hazard of steroid use is accepted to obtain an advisable diminution in edema and inflammation; corneal injury from chemical or thermal burns, or penetration of foreign bodies.
Otic:
Steroid responsive inflammatory conditions of the external auditory meatus, such as allergic otitis externa, selected purulent and nonpurulent infective otitis externa when the hazard of steroid use is accepted to obtain an advisable diminution in edema and inflammation.

CONTRAINDICATIONS

Epithelial herpes simplex keratitis (dendritic keratitis).
Acute infectious stages of vaccinia, varicella, and many other viral diseases of the cornea and conjunctiva.
Mycobacterial infection of the eye.
Fungal diseases of ocular or auricular structures.
Hypersensitivity to any component of this product, including sulfites (see WARNINGS).
Perforation of a drum membrane.

WARNINGS

Prolonged use may result in ocular hypertension and/or glaucoma, with damage to the optic nerve, defects in visual acuity and fields of vision, and posterior subcapsular cataract formation. Prolonged use may suppress the host response and thus increase the hazard of secondary ocular infections. In those diseases causing thinning of the cornea or sclera, perforations have been known to occur with the use of topical corticosteroids. In acute purulent conditions of the eye or ear, corticosteroids may mask infection or enhance existing infection. If these products are used for 10 days or longer, intraocular pressure should be routinely monitored even though it may be difficult in children and uncooperative patients.
Employment of corticosteroid medication in the treatment of herpes simplex other than epithelial herpes simplex keratitis, in which it is contraindicated, requires great caution; periodic slit-lamp microscopy is essential.
Ophthalmic Solution DECADRON Phosphate contains sodium bisulfite, a sulfite that may cause allergic-type reactions including anaphylactic symptoms and life-threatening or less severe asthmatic episodes in certain susceptible people. The overall prevalence of sulfite sensitivity in the general population is unknown and probably low. Sulfite sensitivity is seen more frequently in asthmatic than in nonasthmatic people.

PRECAUTIONS

General
The possibility of persistent fungal infections of the cornea should be considered after prolonged corticosteroid dosing.
There have been reports of bacterial keratitis associated with the use of multiple dose containers of topical ophthalmic products. These containers had been inadvertently contaminated by patients who, in most cases, had a concurrent corneal disease or a disruption of the ocular epithelial surface. (See PRECAUTIONS, *Information for Patients.*)
Information for Patients
Patients should be instructed to avoid allowing the tip of the dispensing container to contact the eye or surrounding structures.
Patients should also be instructed that ocular solutions, if handled improperly, can become contaminated by common bacteria known to cause ocular infections. Serious damage to the eye and subsequent loss of vision may result from using contaminated solutions. (See PRECAUTIONS, *General.*)
Patients should also be advised that if they develop an intercurrent ocular condition (e.g., trauma, ocular surgery or infection), they should immediately seek their physician's advice concerning the continued use of the present multidose container.
One of the preservatives in Ophthalmic Solution DECADRON Phosphate, benzalkonium chloride, may be absorbed by soft contact lenses. Patients wearing soft contact lenses should be instructed to wait at least 15 minutes after instilling Ophthalmic Solution DECADRON Phosphate before they insert their lenses.
Carcinogenesis, Mutagenesis, Impairment of Fertility
Long-term animal studies have not been performed to evaluate the carcinogenic potential or the effect on fertility of Ophthalmic Solution DECADRON Phosphate.
Pregnancy
Pregnancy Category C. Dexamethasone has been shown to be teratogenic in mice and rabbits following topical ophthalmic application in multiples of the therapeutic dose.
In the mouse, corticosteroids produce fetal resorptions and a specific abnormality, cleft palate. In the rabbit, corticosteroids have produced fetal resorptions and multiple abnormalities involving the head, ears, limbs, palate, etc.
There are no adequate or well-controlled studies in pregnant women. Ophthalmic Solution DECADRON Phosphate should be used during pregnancy only if the potential benefit to the mother justifies the potential risk to the embryo or fetus. Infants born of mothers who have received substantial doses of corticosteroids during pregnancy should be observed carefully for signs of hypoadrenalism.
Nursing Mothers
Topically applied steroids are absorbed systemically. Therefore, because of the potential for serious adverse reactions in nursing infants from dexamethasone sodium phosphate, a decision should be made whether to discontinue nursing or discontinue the drug, taking into account the importance of the drug to the mother.
Pediatric Use
Safety and effectiveness in pediatric patients have not been established.

ADVERSE REACTIONS

Glaucoma with optic nerve damage, visual acuity and field defects, posterior subcapsular cataract formation, secondary ocular infection from pathogens including herpes simplex, perforation of the globe.
Rarely, filtering blebs have been reported when topical steroids have been used following cataract surgery.
Rarely, stinging or burning may occur.

DOSAGE AND ADMINISTRATION

The duration of treatment will vary with the type of lesion and may extend from a few days to several weeks, according to therapeutic response. Relapses, more common in chronic active lesions than in self-limited conditions, usually respond to retreatment.
Eye—Instill one or two drops of solution into the conjunctival sac every hour during the day and every two hours during the night as initial therapy. When a favorable response is observed, reduce dosage to one drop every four hours. Later, further reduction in dosage to one drop three or four times daily may suffice to control symptoms.
Ear—Clean the aural canal thoroughly and sponge dry. Instill the solution directly into the aural canal. A suggested initial dosage is three or four drops two or three times a day. When a favorable response is obtained, reduce dosage gradually and eventually discontinue.
If preferred, the aural canal may be packed with a gauze wick saturated with solution. Keep the wick moist with the preparation and remove from the ear after 12 to 24 hours. Treatment may be repeated as often as necessary at the discretion of the physician.

HOW SUPPLIED

Sterile Ophthalmic Solution DECADRON Phosphate is a clear, colorless to pale yellow solution.
No. 7643—Ophthalmic Solution DECADRON Phosphate is supplied as follows:
NDC 0006-7643-03 in 5 mL white, opaque, plastic OCUMETER ophthalmic dispenser with a controlled drop tip.
(6505-00-007-4536 0.1% 5 mL).
9011622 Issued September 1996

DEMSER® Capsules ℞
(Metyrosine)

DESCRIPTION

DEMSER* (Metyrosine) is (−)-α-methyl-*L* -tyrosine or (α-MPT). It has the following structural formula:
[See chemical structure at top of next column]
Metyrosine is a white, crystalline compound of molecular weight 195. It is very slightly soluble in water, acetone, and methanol, and insoluble in chloroform and benzene. It is soluble in acidic aqueous solutions. It is also soluble in alkaline aqueous solutions, but is subject to oxidative degradation under these conditions.

$$HO-C_6H_4-CH_2-C(CH_3)(NH_2)-COOH$$

DEMSER is supplied as capsules, for oral administration. Each capsule contains 250 mg metyrosine. Inactive ingredients are colloidal silicon dioxide, gelatin, hydroxypropyl cellulose, magnesium stearate, and titanium dioxide. The capsules may also contain any combination of D&C Red 33, D&C Yellow 10, FD&C Blue 1, and FD&C Blue 2.

*Registered trademark of MERCK & CO., INC.

CLINICAL PHARMACOLOGY

DEMSER inhibits tyrosine hydroxylase, which catalyzes the first transformation in catecholamine biosynthesis, i.e., the conversion of tyrosine to dihydroxyphenylalanine (DOPA). Because the first step is also the rate-limiting step, blockade of tyrosine hydroxylase activity results in decreased endogenous levels of catecholamines, usually measured as decreased urinary excretion of catecholamines and their metabolites.
In patients with pheochromocytoma, who produce excessive amounts of norepinephrine and epinephrine, administration of one to four grams of DEMSER per day has reduced catecholamine biosynthesis from about 35 to 80 percent as measured by the total excretion of catecholamines and their metabolites (metanephrine and vanillylmandelic acid). The maximum biochemical effect usually occurs within two to three days, and the urinary concentration of catecholamines and their metabolites usually returns to pretreatment levels within three to four days after DEMSER is discontinued. In some patients the total excretion of catecholamines and catecholamine metabolites may be lowered to normal or near normal levels (less than 10 mg/24 hours). In most patients the duration of treatment has been two to eight weeks, but several patients have received DEMSER for periods of one to 10 years.
Most patients with pheochromocytoma treated with DEMSER experience decreased frequency and severity of hypertensive attacks with their associated headache, nausea, sweating, and tachycardia. In patients who respond, blood pressure decreases progressively during the first two days of therapy with DEMSER; after withdrawal, blood pressure usually increases gradually to pretreatment values within two to three days.
Metyrosine is well absorbed from the gastrointestinal tract. From 53 to 88 percent (mean 69 percent) was recovered in the urine as unchanged drug following maintenance oral doses of 600 to 4000 mg/24 hours in patients with pheochromocytoma or essential hypertension. Less than 1% of the dose was recovered as catechol metabolites. These metabolites are probably not present in sufficient amounts to contribute to the biochemical effects of metyrosine. The quantities excreted, however, are sufficient to interfere with accurate determination of urinary catecholamines determined by routine techniques.
Plasma half-life of metyrosine determined over an 8-hour period after single oral doses was 3.4–3.7 hours in three patients.
For further information, refer to: Sjoerdsma, A.; Engelman, K.; Waldman, T. A.; Cooperman, L. H.; Hammond, W. G.: Pheochromocytoma: Current concepts of diagnosis and treatment, Ann. Intern. Med. *65:* 1302–1326, Dec. 1966.

INDICATIONS AND USAGE

DEMSER is indicated in the treatment of patients with pheochromocytoma for:
1. Preoperative preparation of patients for surgery
2. Management of patients when surgery is contraindicated
3. Chronic treatment of patients with malignant pheochromocytoma.

DEMSER is not recommended for the control of essential hypertension.

CONTRAINDICATIONS

DEMSER is contraindicated in persons known to be hypersensitive to this compound.

WARNINGS

Maintain Fluid Volume During and After Surgery
When DEMSER is used preoperatively, alone or especially in combination with alpha-adrenergic blocking drugs, adequate intravascular volume must be maintained intraoperatively (especially after tumor removal) and postoperatively to avoid hypotension and decreased perfusion of vital organs resulting from vasodilatation and expanded volume capacity. Following tumor removal, large volumes of plasma may be needed to maintain blood pressure and central venous pressure within the normal range.

Continued on next page

Information on the Merck & Co., Inc. products listed on these pages is the full prescribing information from product circulars in use September 30, 2000. For information, please call 1-800-NSC MERCK [1-800-672-6372].

Demser—Cont.

In addition, life-threatening arrhythmias may occur during anesthesia and surgery, and may require treatment with a beta blocker or lidocaine. During surgery, patients should have continuous monitoring of blood pressure and electrocardiogram.

Intraoperative Effects

While the preoperative use of DEMSER in patients with pheochromocytoma is thought to decrease intraoperative problems with blood pressure control, DEMSER does not eliminate the danger of hypertensive crises or arrhythmias during manipulation of the tumor, and the alpha-adrenergic blocking drug, phentolamine, may be needed.

Interaction with Alcohol

DEMSER may add to the sedative effects of alcohol and other CNS depressants, e.g., hypnotics, sedatives, and tranquilizers. (See PRECAUTIONS, *Information for Patients and Drug Interactions.*)

PRECAUTIONS

General

Metyrosine Crystalluria: **Crystalluria and urolithiasis have been found in dogs treated with DEMSER (Metyrosine) at doses similar to those used in humans, and crystalluria has also been observed in a few patients. To minimize the risk of crystalluria, patients should be urged to maintain water intake sufficient to achieve a daily urine volume of 2000 mL or more, particularly when doses greater than 2 g per day are given. Routine examination of the urine should be carried out. Metyrosine will crystallize as needles or rods. If metyrosine crystalluria occurs, fluid intake should be increased further. If crystalluria persists, the dosage should be reduced or the drug discontinued.**

Relatively Little Data Regarding Long-term Use: The total human experience with the drug is quite limited and few patients have been studied long-term. Chronic animal studies have not been carried out. Therefore, suitable laboratory tests should be carried out periodically in patients requiring prolonged use of DEMSER and caution should be observed in patients with impaired hepatic or renal function.

Information for Patients

When receiving DEMSER, patients should be warned about engaging in activities requiring mental alertness and motor coordination, such as driving a motor vehicle or operating machinery. DEMSER may have additive sedative effects with alcohol and other CNS depressants, e.g., hypnotics, sedatives, and tranquilizers.

Patients should be advised to maintain a liberal fluid intake. (See PRECAUTIONS, *General.*)

Drug Interactions

Caution should be observed in administering DEMSER to patients receiving phenothiazines or haloperidol because the extrapyramidal effects of these drugs can be expected to be potentiated by inhibition of catecholamine synthesis.

Concurrent use of DEMSER with alcohol or other CNS depressants can increase their sedative effects. (See WARNINGS and PRECAUTIONS, *Information for Patients.*)

Laboratory Test Interference

Spurious increases in urinary catecholamines may be observed in patients receiving DEMSER due to the presence of metabolites of the drug.

Carcinogenesis, Mutagenesis, Impairment of Fertility

Long-term carcinogenic studies in animals and studies on mutagenesis and impairment of fertility have not been performed with metyrosine.

Pregnancy

Pregnancy Category C. Animal reproduction studies have not been conducted with DEMSER. It is also not known whether DEMSER can cause fetal harm when administered to a pregnant woman or can affect reproduction capacity. DEMSER should be given to a pregnant woman only if clearly needed.

Nursing Mothers

It is not known whether DEMSER is excreted in human milk. Because many drugs are excreted in human milk, caution should be exercised when DEMSER is administered to a nursing woman.

Pediatric Use

Safety and effectiveness in pediatric patients below the age of 12 years have not been established.

ADVERSE REACTIONS

Central Nervous System

Sedation: The most common adverse reaction to DEMSER is moderate to severe sedation, which has been observed in almost all patients. It occurs at both low and high dosages. Sedative effects begin within the first 24 hours of therapy, are maximal after two to three days, and tend to wane during the next few days. Sedation usually is not obvious after one week unless the dosage is increased, but at dosages greater than 2000 mg/day some degree of sedation or fatigue may persist.

In most patients who experience sedation, temporary changes in sleep pattern occur following withdrawal of the drug. Changes consist of insomnia that may last for two or three days and feelings of increased alertness and ambition. Even patients who do not experience sedation while on DEMSER may report symptoms of psychic stimulation when the drug is discontinued.

Extrapyramidal Signs: Extrapyramidal signs such as drooling, speech difficulty, and tremor have been reported in approximately 10 percent of patients. These occasionally have been accompanied by trismus and frank parkinsonism.

Anxiety and Psychic Disturbances: Anxiety and psychic disturbances such as depression, hallucinations, disorientation, and confusion may occur. These effects seem to be dose-dependent and may disappear with reduction of dosage.

Diarrhea

Diarrhea occurs in about 10 percent of patients and may be severe. Anti-diarrheal agents may be required if continuation of DEMSER is necessary.

Miscellaneous

Infrequently, slight swelling of the breast, galactorrhea, nasal stuffiness, decreased salivation, dry mouth, headache, nausea, vomiting, abdominal pain, and impotence or failure of ejaculation may occur. Crystalluria (see PRECAUTIONS) and transient dysuria and hematuria have been observed in a few patients. Hematologic disorders (including eosinophilia, anemia, thrombocytopenia, and thrombocytosis), increased SGOT levels, peripheral edema, and hypersensitivity reactions such as urticaria and pharyngeal edema have been reported rarely.

OVERDOSAGE

Signs of metyrosine overdosage include those central nervous system effects observed in some patients even at low dosages.

At doses exceeding 2000 mg/day, some degree of sedation or feeling of fatigue may persist. Doses of 2000–4000 mg/day can result in anxiety or agitated depression, neuromuscular effects (including fine tremor of the hands, gross tremor of the trunk, tightening of the jaw with trismus), diarrhea, and decreased salivation with dry mouth.

Reduction of drug dose or cessation of treatment results in the disappearance of these symptoms.

The acute toxicity of metyrosine was 442 mg/kg and 752 mg/kg in the female mouse and rat respectively.

DOSAGE AND ADMINISTRATION

The recommended initial dosage of DEMSER for adults and children 12 years of age and older is 250 mg orally four times daily. This may be increased by 250 mg to 500 mg every day to a maximum of 4.0 g/day in divided doses. When used for preoperative preparation, the optimally effective dosage of DEMSER should be given for at least five to seven days.

Optimally effective dosages of DEMSER usually are between 2.0 and 3.0 g/day, and the dose should be titrated by monitoring clinical symptoms and catecholamine excretion. In patients who are hypertensive, dosage should be titrated to achieve normalization of blood pressure and control of clinical symptoms. In patients who are usually normotensive, dosage should be titrated to the amount that will reduce urinary metanephrines and/or vanillylmandelic acid by 50 percent or more.

If patients are not adequately controlled by the use of DEMSER, an alpha-adrenergic blocking agent (phenoxybenzamine) should be added.

Use of DEMSER in children under 12 years of age has been limited and a dosage schedule for this age group cannot be given.

HOW SUPPLIED

No. 3355—Capsules DEMSER, 250 mg, are opaque, two-toned blue capsules coded MSD 690 on one side and DEMSER on the other. They are supplied as follows:

NDC 0006-0690-68 bottles of 100.

Shown in Product Identification Guide, page 323

7900807 Issued July 1996

DIURIL® Sodium Intravenous (Chlorothiazide Sodium) ℞

DESCRIPTION

Intravenous Sodium DIURIL* (Chlorothiazide Sodium) is a diuretic and antihypertensive. It is 6-chloro-2*H* -1,2,4-benzothiadiazine-7-sulfonamide 1,1-dioxide monosodium salt and its molecular weight is 317.71. Its empirical formula is $C_7H_5ClN_3NaO_4S_2$ and its structural formula is:

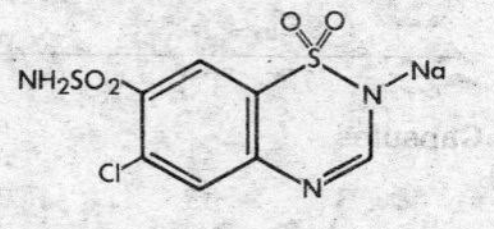

Intravenous Sodium DIURIL is a sterile lyophilized white powder and is supplied in a vial containing:

Chlorothiazide sodium equivalent to chlorothiazide	0.5 g
Inactive ingredients:	
Mannitol	0.25 g
Sodium hydroxide to adjust pH.	

DIURIL* (Chlorothiazide) is a diuretic and antihypertensive. It is 6-chloro-2*H* -1,2,4-benzothiadiazine-7-sulfonamide 1,1-dioxide. Its empirical formula is $C_7H_6ClN_3O_4S_2$ and its structural formula is:

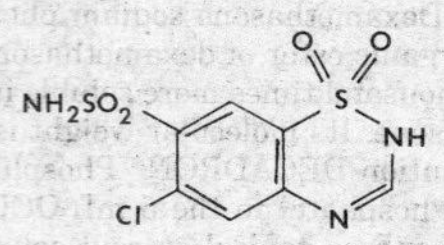

It is a white, or practically white, crystalline powder with a molecular weight of 295.72, which is very slightly soluble in water, but readily soluble in dilute aqueous sodium hydroxide. It is soluble in urine to the extent of about 150 mg per 100 mL at pH 7.

*Registered trademark of MERCK & CO., INC.

CLINICAL PHARMACOLOGY

The mechanism of the antihypertensive effect of thiazides is unknown. DIURIL (Chlorothiazide) does not usually affect normal blood pressure.

DIURIL (Chlorothiazide) affects the distal renal tubular mechanism of electrolyte reabsorption. At maximal therapeutic dosage all thiazides are approximately equal in their diuretic efficacy.

DIURIL (Chlorothiazide) increases excretion of sodium and chloride in approximately equivalent amounts. Natriuresis may be accompanied by some loss of potassium and bicarbonate.

After oral use diuresis begins within 2 hours, peaks in about 4 hours and lasts about 6 to 12 hours. Following intravenous use of Sodium DIURIL, onset of the diuretic action occurs in 15 minutes and the maximal action in 30 minutes.

Pharmacokinetics and Metabolism

DIURIL is not metabolized but is eliminated rapidly by the kidney; 96 percent of an intravenous dose is excreted unchanged in the urine within 23 hours. The plasma half-life of chlorothiazide is 45–120 minutes. Chlorothiazide crosses the placental but not the blood-brain barrier and is excreted in breast milk.

INDICATIONS AND USAGE

Intravenous Sodium DIURIL is indicated as adjunctive therapy in edema associated with congestive heart failure, hepatic cirrhosis, and corticosteroid and estrogen therapy.

Intravenous Sodium DIURIL has also been found useful in edema due to various forms of renal dysfunction such as nephrotic syndrome, acute glomerulonephritis, and chronic renal failure.

Use in Pregnancy. Routine use of diuretics during normal pregnancy is inappropriate and exposes mother and fetus to unnecessary hazard. Diuretics do not prevent development of toxemia of pregnancy and there is no satisfactory evidence that they are useful in the treatment of toxemia.

Edema during pregnancy may arise from pathologic causes or from the physiologic and mechanical consequences of pregnancy. Thiazides are indicated in pregnancy when edema is due to pathologic causes, just as they are in the absence of pregnancy (see PRECAUTIONS, *Pregnancy*). Dependent edema in pregnancy, resulting from restriction of venous return by the gravid uterus, is properly treated through elevation of the lower extremities and use of support stockings. Use of diuretics to lower intravascular volume in this instance is illogical and unnecessary. During normal pregnancy there is hypervolemia which is not harmful to the fetus or the mother in the absence of cardiovascular disease. However, it may be associated with edema, rarely generalized edema. If such edema causes discomfort, increased recumbency will often provide relief. Rarely this edema may cause extreme discomfort which is not relieved by rest. In these instances, a short course of diuretic therapy may provide relief and be appropriate.

CONTRAINDICATIONS

Anuria.

Hypersensitivity to any component of this product or to other sulfonamide-derived drugs.

WARNINGS

Intravenous use in infants and children has been limited and is not generally recommended.

Use with caution in severe renal disease. In patients with renal disease, thiazides may precipitate azotemia. Cumulative effects of the drug may develop in patients with impaired renal function.

Thiazides should be used with caution in patients with impaired hepatic function or progressive liver disease, since minor alterations of fluid and electrolyte balance may precipitate hepatic coma.

Thiazides may add to or potentiate the action of other antihypertensive drugs.

Sensitivity reactions may occur in patients with or without a history of allergy or bronchial asthma.

The possibility of exacerbation or activation of systemic lupus erythematosus has been reported.

Lithium generally should not be given with diuretics (see PRECAUTIONS, *Drug Interactions*).

PRECAUTIONS

General

All patients receiving diuretic therapy should be observed for evidence of fluid or electrolyte imbalance: namely, hyponatremia, hypochloremic alkalosis, and hypokalemia. Serum and urine electrolyte determinations are particularly important when the patient is vomiting excessively or receiving parenteral fluids. Warning signs or symptoms of fluid and electrolyte imbalance, irrespective of cause, include dryness of mouth, thirst, weakness, lethargy, drowsiness, restlessness, confusion, seizures, muscle pains or cramps, muscular fatigue, hypotension, oliguria, tachycardia, and gastrointestinal disturbances such as nausea and vomiting.

Hypokalemia may develop especially with brisk diuresis, when severe cirrhosis is present or after prolonged therapy. Interference with adequate oral electrolyte intake will also contribute to hypokalemia. Hypokalemia may cause cardiac arrhythmias and may also sensitize or exaggerate the response of the heart to the toxic effects of digitalis (e.g., increased ventricular irritability). Hypokalemia may be avoided or treated by use of potassium sparing diuretics or potassium supplements such as foods with a high potassium content.

Although any chloride deficit is generally mild and usually does not require specific treatment except under extraordinary circumstances (as in liver disease or renal disease), chloride replacement may be required in the treatment of metabolic alkalosis.

Dilutional hyponatremia may occur in edematous patients in hot weather; appropriate therapy is water restriction, rather than administration of salt, except in rare instances when the hyponatremia is life threatening. In actual salt depletion, appropriate replacement is the therapy of choice.

Hyperuricemia may occur or acute gout may be precipitated in certain patients receiving thiazides.

In diabetic patients dosage adjustments of insulin or oral hypoglycemic agents may be required. Hyperglycemia may occur with thiazide diuretics. Thus latent diabetes mellitus may become manifest during thiazide therapy.

The antihypertensive effects of the drug may be enhanced in the postsympathectomy patient.

If progressive renal impairment becomes evident, consider withholding or discontinuing diuretic therapy.

Thiazides have been shown to increase the urinary excretion of magnesium; this may result in hypomagnesemia.

Thiazides may decrease urinary calcium excretion. Thiazides may cause intermittent and slight elevation of serum calcium in the absence of known disorders of calcium metabolism. Marked hypercalcemia may be evidence of hidden hyperparathyroidism. Thiazides should be discontinued before carrying out tests for parathyroid function.

Increases in cholesterol and triglyceride levels may be associated with thiazide diuretic therapy.

Laboratory Tests

Periodic determination of serum electrolytes to detect possible electrolyte imbalance should be done at appropriate intervals.

Drug Interactions

When given concurrently the following drugs may interact with thiazide diuretics.

Alcohol, barbiturates, or narcotics —potentiation of orthostatic hypotension may occur.

Antidiabetic drugs —(oral agents and insulin)—dosage adjustment of the antidiabetic drug may be required.

Other antihypertensive drugs —additive effect or potentiation.

Corticosteroids, ACTH —intensified electrolyte depletion, particularly hypokalemia.

Pressor amines (e.g., norepinephrine) —possible decreased response to pressor amines but not sufficient to preclude their use.

Skeletal muscle relaxants, nondepolarizing (e.g., tubocurarine) —possible increased responsiveness to the muscle relaxant.

Lithium —generally should not be given with diuretics. Diuretic agents reduce the renal clearance of lithium and add a high risk of lithium toxicity. Refer to the package insert for lithium preparations before use of such preparations with Sodium DIURIL.

Non-steroidal Anti-inflammatory Drugs —In some patients, the administration of a non-steroidal anti-inflammatory agent can reduce the diuretic, natriuretic, and antihypertensive effects of loop, potassium-sparing and thiazide diuretics. Therefore, when Sodium DIURIL and non-steroidal anti-inflammatory agents are used concomitantly, the patient should be observed closely to determine if the desired effect of the diuretic is obtained.

Drug/Laboratory Test Interactions

Thiazides should be discontinued before carrying out tests for parathyroid function (see PRECAUTIONS, *General*).

Carcinogenesis, Mutagenesis, Impairment of Fertility

Carcinogenicity studies have not been conducted with chlorothiazide.

Chlorothiazide was not mutagenic *in vitro* in the Ames microbial mutagen test (using a maximum concentration of 5 mg/plate and *Salmonella typhimurium* strains TA98 and TA100) and was not mutagenic and did not induce mitotic nondisjunction in diploid-strains of *Aspergillus nidulans*.

Chlorothiazide had no adverse effects on fertility in female rats at doses up to 60 mg/kg/day and no adverse effects on fertility in male rats at doses up to 40 mg/kg/day. These doses are 1.5 and 1.0 times* the recommended maximum human dose, respectively, when compared on a body weight basis.

*Calculations based on a human body weight of 50 kg

Pregnancy

Teratogenic Effects—Pregnancy Category C: Although reproduction studies performed with chlorothiazide doses of 50 mg/kg/day in rabbits, 60 mg/kg/day in rats and 500 mg/kg/day in mice revealed no external abnormalities of the fetus or impairment of growth and survival of the fetus due to chlorothiazide, such studies did not include complete examinations for visceral and skeletal abnormalities. It is not known whether chlorothiazide can cause fetal harm when administered to a pregnant woman; however, thiazides cross the placental barrier and appear in cord blood. DIURIL should be used during pregnancy only if clearly needed (see INDICATIONS AND USAGE).

Nonteratogenic Effects: Chlorothiazide may cause fetal or neonatal jaundice, thrombocytopenia, and possibly other adverse reactions which have occurred in the adult.

Nursing Mothers

Because of the potential for serious adverse reactions in nursing infants from Intravenous Sodium DIURIL, a decision should be made whether to discontinue nursing or to discontinue the drug, taking into account the importance of the drug to the mother.

Pediatric Use

Safety and effectiveness of Intravenous Sodium DIURIL in pediatric patients have not been established.

ADVERSE REACTIONS

The following adverse reactions have been reported and, within each category, are listed in order of decreasing severity.

Body as a Whole: Weakness.

Cardiovascular: Hypotension including orthostatic hypotension (may be aggravated by alcohol, barbiturates, narcotics or antihypertensive drugs).

Digestive: Pancreatitis, jaundice (intrahepatic cholestatic jaundice), diarrhea, vomiting, sialadenitis, cramping, constipation, gastric irritation, nausea, anorexia.

Hematologic: Aplastic anemia, agranulocytosis, leukopenia, hemolytic anemia, thrombocytopenia.

Hypersensitivity: Anaphylactic reactions, necrotizing angiitis (vasculitis and cutaneous vasculitis), respiratory distress including pneumonitis and pulmonary edema, photosensitivity, fever, urticaria, rash, purpura.

Metabolic: Electrolyte imbalance (see PRECAUTIONS), hyperglycemia, glycosuria, hyperuricemia.

Musculoskeletal: Muscle spasm.

Nervous System/Psychiatric: Vertigo, paresthesias, dizziness, headache, restlessness.

Skin: Erythema multiforme including Stevens-Johnson syndrome, exfoliative dermatitis including toxic epidermal necrolysis, alopecia.

Special Senses: Transient blurred vision, xanthopsia.

Renal: Renal failure, renal dysfunction, interstitial nephritis (see WARNINGS); hematuria (following intravenous use).

Urogenital: Impotence.

Whenever adverse reactions are moderate or severe, thiazide dosage should be reduced or therapy withdrawn.

OVERDOSAGE

The most common signs and symptoms observed are those caused by electrolyte depletion (hypokalemia, hypochloremia, hyponatremia) and dehydration resulting from excessive diuresis. If digitalis has also been administered, hypokalemia may accentuate cardiac arrhythmias.

In the event of overdosage, symptomatic and supportive measures should be employed. Correct dehydration, electrolyte imbalance, hepatic coma and hypotension by established procedures. If required, give oxygen or artificial respiration for respiratory impairment.

The degree to which chlorothiazide sodium is removed by hemodialysis has not been established.

The intravenous LD_{50} of chlorothiazide in the mouse is 1.1 g/kg.

DOSAGE AND ADMINISTRATION

Intravenous Sodium DIURIL should be reserved for patients unable to take oral medication or for emergency situations.

Therapy should be individualized according to patient response. Use the smallest dosage necessary to achieve the required response.

Intravenous use in infants and children has been limited and is not generally recommended.

When medication can be taken orally, therapy with DIURIL tablets or oral suspension may be substituted for intravenous therapy, using the same dosage schedule as for the parenteral route.

Intravenous Sodium DIURIL may be given slowly by direct intravenous injection or by intravenous infusion.

Add 18 mL of Sterile Water for Injection to the vial to form an isotonic solution for intravenous injection. Never add less than 18 mL. When reconstituted with 18 mL of Sterile Water, the final concentration of Intravenous Sodium DIURIL is 28 mg/mL. Parenteral drug products should be inspected visually for particulate matter and discoloration prior to use whenever solution and container permit. The solution is compatible with dextrose or sodium chloride solutions for intravenous infusion. Avoid simultaneous administration of solutions of chlorothiazide with whole blood or its derivatives.

Extravasation must be rigidly avoided. Do not give subcutaneously or intramuscularly.

The usual adult dosage is 0.5 to 1.0 g once or twice a day. Many patients with edema respond to intermittent therapy, i.e., administration on alternate days or on three to five days each week. With an intermittent schedule, excessive response and the resulting undesirable electrolyte imbalance are less likely to occur.

HOW SUPPLIED

No. 3619—Intravenous Sodium DIURIL is a dry, sterile lyophilized white powder usually in plug form, supplied in vials containing chlorothiazide sodium equivalent to 0.5 g of chlorothiazide.

NDC 0006-3619-32.

Storage

Store lyophilized powder between 2–25°C (36–77°F).

For single dose only. Discard unused portion of the reconstituted solution.

9273236 Issued September 1999

DIURIL® Tablets ℞
(Chlorothiazide)
DIURIL® Oral Suspension ℞
(Chlorothiazide)

DESCRIPTION

DIURIL* (Chlorothiazide) is a diuretic and antihypertensive. It is 6-chloro-2*H* -1,2,4 -benzothiadiazine-7-sulfonamide 1,1-dioxide. Its empirical formula is $C_7H_6ClN_3O_4S_2$ and its structural formula is:

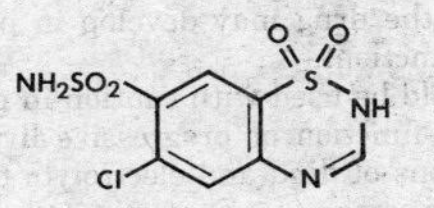

It is a white, or practically white, crystalline powder with a molecular weight of 295.73, which is very slightly soluble in water, but readily soluble in dilute aqueous sodium hydroxide. It is soluble in urine to the extent of about 150 mg per 100 mL at pH 7.

DIURIL is supplied as 250 mg and 500 mg tablets, for oral use. Each tablet contains the following inactive ingredients: gelatin, magnesium stearate, starch and talc. The 250 mg tablet also contains lactose.

Oral Suspension DIURIL contains 250 mg of chlorothiazide per 5 mL, alcohol 0.5 percent, with methylparaben 0.12 percent, propylparaben 0.02 percent, and benzoic acid 0.1 percent added as preservatives. The inactive ingredients are D&C Yellow 10, flavors, glycerin, purified water, sodium saccharin, sucrose and tragacanth.

*Registered trademark of MERCK & CO., INC.

CLINICAL PHARMACOLOGY

The mechanism of the antihypertensive effect of thiazides is unknown. DIURIL does not usually affect normal blood pressure.

DIURIL affects the distal renal tubular mechanism of electrolyte reabsorption. At maximal therapeutic dosage all thiazides are approximately equal in their diuretic efficacy.

DIURIL increases excretion of sodium and chloride in approximately equivalent amounts. Natriuresis may be accompanied by some loss of potassium and bicarbonate.

After oral use diuresis begins within 2 hours, peaks in about 4 hours and lasts about 6 to 12 hours.

Pharmacokinetics and Metabolism

DIURIL is not metabolized but is eliminated rapidly by the kidney. The plasma half-life of chlorothiazide is 45–120 minutes. After oral doses, 10–15 percent of the dose is excreted unchanged in the urine. Chlorothiazide crosses the placental but not the blood-brain barrier and is excreted in breast milk.

INDICATIONS AND USAGE

DIURIL is indicated as adjunctive therapy in edema associated with congestive heart failure, hepatic cirrhosis, and corticosteroid and estrogen therapy.

Continued on next page

Information on the Merck & Co., Inc. products listed on these pages is the full prescribing information from product circulars in use September 30, 2000. For information, please call 1-800-NSC MERCK [1-800-672-6372].

Diuril Tablets—Cont.

DIURIL has also been found useful in edema due to various forms of renal dysfunction such as nephrotic syndrome, acute glomerulonephritis, and chronic renal failure.
DIURIL is indicated in the management of hypertension either as the sole therapeutic agent or to enhance the effectiveness of other antihypertensive drugs in the more severe forms of hypertension.
Use in Pregnancy. Routine use of diuretics during normal pregnancy is inappropriate and exposes mother and fetus to unnecessary hazard. Diuretics do not prevent development of toxemia of pregnancy and there is no satisfactory evidence that they are useful in the treatment of toxemia.
Edema during pregnancy may arise from pathologic causes or from the physiologic and mechanical consequences of pregnancy. Thiazides are indicated in pregnancy when edema is due to pathologic causes, just as they are in the absence of pregnancy (see PRECAUTIONS, *Pregnancy*). Dependent edema in pregnancy, resulting from restriction of venous return by the gravid uterus, is properly treated through elevation of the lower extremities and use of support stockings. Use of diuretics to lower intravascular volume in this instance is illogical and unnecessary. During normal pregnancy there is hypervolemia which is not harmful to the fetus or the mother in the absence of cardiovascular disease. However, it may be associated with edema, rarely generalized edema. If such edema causes discomfort, increased recumbency will often provide relief. Rarely this edema may cause extreme discomfort which is not relieved by rest. In these instances, a short course of diuretic therapy may provide relief and be appropriate.

CONTRAINDICATIONS

Anuria.
Hypersensitivity to this product or to other sulfonamide-derived drugs.

WARNINGS

Use with caution in severe renal disease. In patients with renal disease, thiazides may precipitate azotemia. Cumulative effects of the drug may develop in patients with impaired renal function.
Thiazides should be used with caution in patients with impaired hepatic function or progressive liver disease, since minor alterations of fluid and electrolyte balance may precipitate hepatic coma.
Thiazides may add to or potentiate the action of other antihypertensive drugs.
Sensitivity reactions may occur in patients with or without a history of allergy or bronchial asthma.
The possibility of exacerbation or activation of systemic lupus erythematosus has been reported.
Lithium generally should not be given with diuretics (see PRECAUTIONS, *Drug Interactions*).

PRECAUTIONS

General
All patients receiving diuretic therapy should be observed for evidence of fluid or electrolyte imbalance: namely, hyponatremia, hypochloremic alkalosis, and hypokalemia. Serum and urine electrolyte determinations are particularly important when the patient is vomiting excessively or receiving parenteral fluids. Warning signs or symptoms of fluid and electrolyte imbalance, irrespective of cause, include dryness of mouth, thirst, weakness, lethargy, drowsiness, restlessness, confusion, seizures, muscle pains or cramps, muscular fatigue, hypotension, oliguria, tachycardia, and gastrointestinal disturbances such as nausea and vomiting.
Hypokalemia may develop, especially with brisk diuresis, when severe cirrhosis is present or after prolonged therapy. Interference with adequate oral electrolyte intake will also contribute to hypokalemia. Hypokalemia may cause cardiac arrhythmias and may also sensitize or exaggerate the response of the heart to the toxic effects of digitalis (e.g., increased ventricular irritability). Hypokalemia may be avoided or treated by use of potassium sparing diuretics or potassium supplements such as foods with a high potassium content.
Although any chloride deficit is generally mild and usually does not require specific treatment except under extraordinary circumstances (as in liver disease or renal disease), chloride replacement may be required in the treatment of metabolic alkalosis.
Dilutional hyponatremia may occur in edematous patients in hot weather; appropriate therapy is water restriction, rather than administration of salt, except in rare instances when the hyponatremia is life-threatening. In actual salt depletion, appropriate replacement is the therapy of choice.
Hyperuricemia may occur or acute gout may be precipitated in certain patients receiving thiazides.
In diabetic patients dosage adjustments of insulin or oral hypoglycemic agents may be required. Hyperglycemia may occur with thiazide diuretics. Thus latent diabetes mellitus may become manifest during thiazide therapy.
The antihypertensive effects of the drug may be enhanced in the post-sympathectomy patient.
If progressive renal impairment becomes evident, consider withholding or discontinuing diuretic therapy.
Thiazides have been shown to increase the urinary excretion of magnesium; this may result in hypomagnesemia.
Thiazides may decrease urinary calcium excretion. Thiazides may cause intermittent and slight elevation of serum calcium in the absence of known disorders of calcium metabolism. Marked hypercalcemia may be evidence of hidden hyperparathyroidism. Thiazides should be discontinued before carrying out tests for parathyroid function.
Increases in cholesterol and triglyceride levels may be associated with thiazide diuretic therapy.
Laboratory Tests
Periodic determination of serum electrolytes to detect possible electrolyte imbalance should be done at appropriate intervals.
Drug Interactions
When given concurrently the following drugs may interact with thiazide diuretics.
Alcohol, barbiturates, or narcotics —potentiation of orthostatic hypotension may occur.
Antidiabetic drugs (oral agents and insulin)—dosage adjustment of the antidiabetic drug may be required.
Other antihypertensive drugs —additive effect or potentiation.
Cholestyramine and colestipol resins—Both cholestyramine and colestipol resins have the potential of binding thiazide diuretics and reducing diuretic absorption from the gastrointestinal tract.
Corticosteroids, ACTH —intensified electrolyte depletion, particularly hypokalemia.
Pressor amines (e.g., norepinephrine) —possible decreased response to pressor amines but not sufficient to preclude their use.
Skeletal muscle relaxants, nondepolarizing (e.g., tubocurarine) —possible increased responsiveness to the muscle relaxant.
Lithium —generally should not be given with diuretics. Diuretic agents reduce the renal clearance of lithium and add a high risk of lithium toxicity. Refer to the package insert for lithium preparations before use of such preparations with DIURIL.
Non-steroidal Anti-inflammatory Drugs —In some patients, the administration of a non-steroidal anti-inflammatory agent can reduce the diuretic, natriuretic, and antihypertensive effects of loop, potassium-sparing and thiazide diuretics. Therefore, when DIURIL and non-steroidal anti-inflammatory agents are used concomitantly, the patient should be observed closely to determine if the desired effect of the diuretic is obtained.
Drug/Laboratory Test Interactions
Thiazides should be discontinued before carrying out tests for parathyroid function (see PRECAUTIONS, *General*).
Carcinogenesis, Mutagenesis, Impairment of Fertility
Carcinogenicity studies have not been conducted with chlorothiazide.
Chlorothiazide was not mutagenic *in vitro* in the Ames microbial mutagen test (using a maximum concentration of 5 mg/plate and *Salmonella typhimurium* strains TA98 and TA100) and was not mutagenic and did not induce mitotic nondisjunction in diploid-strains of *Aspergillus nidulans*.
Chlorothiazide had no adverse effects on fertility in female rats at doses up to 60 mg/kg/day and no adverse effects on fertility in male rats at doses up to 40 mg/kg/day. These doses are 1.5 and 1.0 times** the recommended maximum human dose, respectively, when compared on a body weight basis.

**Calculations based on a human body weight of 50 kg

Pregnancy
Teratogenic Effects —Pregnancy Category C: Although reproduction studies performed with chlorothiazide doses of 50 mg/kg/day in rabbits, 60 mg/kg/day in rats and 500 mg/kg/day in mice revealed no external abnormalities of the fetus or impairment of growth and survival of the fetus due to chlorothiazide, such studies did not include complete examinations for visceral and skeletal abnormalities. It is not known whether chlorothiazide can cause fetal harm when administered to a pregnant woman; however, thiazides cross the placental barrier and appear in cord blood. DIURIL should be used during pregnancy only if clearly needed (see INDICATIONS AND USAGE).
Nonteratogenic Effects: Chlorothiazide may cause fetal or neonatal jaundice, thrombocytopenia, and possibly other adverse reactions which have occurred in the adult.
Nursing Mothers
Because of the potential for serious adverse reactions in nursing infants from DIURIL, a decision should be made whether to discontinue nursing or to discontinue the drug, taking into account the importance of the drug to the mother.
Pediatric Use
There are no well-controlled clinical trials in pediatric patients. Information on dosing in this age group is supported by evidence from empiric use in pediatric patients and published literature regarding the treatment of hypertension in such patients. (See DOSAGE AND ADMINISTRATION, *Infants and Children*.)

ADVERSE REACTIONS

The following adverse reactions have been reported and, within each category, are listed in order of decreasing severity.
Body as a Whole: Weakness.
Cardiovascular: Hypotension including orthostatic hypotension (may be aggravated by alcohol, barbiturates, narcotics or antihypertensive drugs).
Digestive: Pancreatitis, jaundice (intrahepatic cholestatic jaundice), diarrhea, vomiting, sialadenitis, cramping, constipation, gastric irritation, nausea, anorexia.
Hematologic: Aplastic anemia, agranulocytosis, leukopenia, hemolytic anemia, thrombocytopenia.
Hypersensitivity: Anaphylactic reactions, necrotizing angiitis (vasculitis and cutaneous vasculitis), respiratory distress including pneumonitis and pulmonary edema, photosensitivity, fever, urticaria, rash, purpura.
Metabolic: Electrolyte imbalance (see PRECAUTIONS), hyperglycemia, glycosuria, hyperuricemia.
Musculoskeletal: Muscle spasm.
Nervous System/Psychiatric: Vertigo, paresthesias, dizziness, headache, restlessness.
Renal: Renal failure, renal dysfunction, interstitial nephritis. (See WARNINGS.)
Skin: Erythema multiforme including Stevens-Johnson syndrome, exfoliative dermatitis including toxic epidermal necrolysis, alopecia.
Special Senses: Transient blurred vision, xanthopsia.
Urogenital: Impotence.
Whenever adverse reactions are moderate or severe, thiazide dosage should be reduced or therapy withdrawn.

OVERDOSAGE

The most common signs and symptoms observed are those caused by electrolyte depletion (hypokalemia, hypochloremia, hyponatremia) and dehydration resulting from excessive diuresis. If digitalis has also been administered, hypokalemia may accentuate cardiac arrhythmias.
In the event of overdosage, symptomatic and supportive measures should be employed. Emesis should be induced or gastric lavage performed. Correct dehydration, electrolyte imbalance, hepatic coma and hypotension by established procedures. If required, give oxygen or artificial respiration for respiratory impairment.
The degree to which chlorothiazide sodium is removed by hemodialysis has not been established.
The oral LD_{50} of chlorothiazide is 8.5 g/kg, greater than 10 g/kg, and greater than 1 g/kg, in the mouse, rat and dog respectively.

DOSAGE AND ADMINISTRATION

Therapy should be individualized according to patient response. Use the smallest dosage necessary to achieve the required response.

Adults

For Edema
The usual adult dosage is 0.5 to 1.0 g once or twice a day. Many patients with edema respond to intermittent therapy, i.e., administration on alternate days or on three to five days each week. With an intermittent schedule, excessive response and the resulting undesirable electrolyte imbalance are less likely to occur.
For Control of Hypertension
The usual adult starting dosage is 0.5 or 1.0 g a day as a single or divided dose. Dosage is increased or decreased according to blood pressure response. Rarely some patients may require up to 2.0 g a day in divided doses.

Infants and Children

For Diuresis and For Control of Hypertension
The usual pediatric dosage is 5 to 10 mg per pound (10 to 20 mg/kg) per day in single or two divided doses, not to exceed 375 mg per day (2.5 to 7.5 mL or $^1/_2$ to $1^1/_2$ teaspoonfuls of the oral suspension daily) in infants up to 2 years of age or 1 g per day in children 2 to 12 years of age. In infants less than 6 months of age, doses up to 15 mg per pound (30 mg/kg) per day in two divided doses may be required. (See PRECAUTIONS, *Pediatric Use*.)

HOW SUPPLIED

No. 3244—Tablets DIURIL, 250 mg, are white, round, scored, compressed tablets, coded MSD 214 on one side and DIURIL on the other. They are supplied as follows:
NDC 0006-0214-68 bottles of 100
Shown in Product Identification Guide, page 323
No. 3245—Tablets DIURIL, 500 mg, are white, round, scored, compressed tablets, coded MSD 432 on one side and DIURIL on the other. They are supplied as follows:
NDC 0006-0432-68 bottles of 100
Shown in Product Identification Guide, page 323
No. 3239—Oral Suspension DIURIL, 250 mg of chlorothiazide per 5 mL, is a yellow, creamy suspension, and is supplied as follows:
NDC 0006-3239-66 bottles of 237 mL
(6505-01-156-1600, 250 mg/5 mL, 237 mL).
Storage
Tablets DIURIL: Keep container tightly closed. Protect from moisture, freezing, -20°C (-4°F) and store at room temperature, 15–30°C (59–86°F).
Oral Suspension DIURIL: Keep container tightly closed. Protect from freezing, -20°C (-4°F) and store at room temperature, 15–30°C (59–86°F).
7897959 Issued June 1998

DOLOBID® Tablets ℞
(Diflunisal)

DESCRIPTION

Diflunisal is 2′, 4′-difluoro-4-hydroxy-3-biphenylcarboxylic acid. Its empirical formula is $C_{13}H_8F_2O_3$ and its structural formula is:

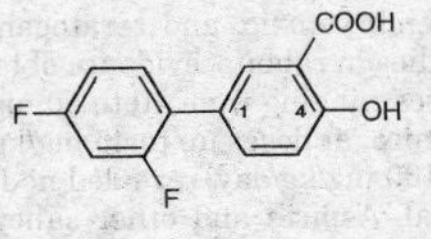

Diflunisal has a molecular weight of 250.20. It is a stable, white, crystalline compound with a melting point of 211–213°C. It is practically insoluble in water at neutral or acidic pH. Because it is an organic acid, it dissolves readily in dilute alkali to give a moderately stable solution at room temperature. It is soluble in most organic solvents including ethanol, methanol, and acetone.

DOLOBID* (Diflunisal) is available in 250 and 500 mg tablets for oral administration. Tablets DOLOBID contain the following inactive ingredients: cellulose, FD&C Yellow 6 hydroxypropyl cellulose, hydroxypropyl methylcellulose, magnesium stearate, starch, talc, and titanium dioxide.

*Registered trademark of MERCK & CO., INC.

CLINICAL PHARMACOLOGY

Action

DOLOBID is a non-steroidal drug with analgesic, anti-inflammatory and antipyretic properties. It is a peripherally-acting non-narcotic analgesic drug. Habituation, tolerance and addiction have not been reported.

Diflunisal is a difluorophenyl derivative of salicylic acid. Chemically, diflunisal differs from aspirin (acetylsalicylic acid) in two respects. The first of these two is the presence of a difluorophenyl substituent at carbon 1. The second difference is the removal of the 0-acetyl group from the carbon 4 position. Diflunisal is not metabolized to salicylic acid, and the fluorine atoms are not displaced from the difluorophenyl ring structure.

The precise mechanism of the analgesic and anti-inflammatory actions of diflunisal is not known. Diflunisal is a prostaglandin synthetase inhibitor. In animals, prostaglandins sensitize afferent nerves and potentiate the action of bradykinin in inducing pain. Since prostaglandins are known to be among the mediators of pain and inflammation, the mode of action of diflunisal may be due to a decrease of prostaglandins in peripheral tissues.

Pharmacokinetics and Metabolism

DOLOBID is rapidly and completely absorbed following oral administration with peak plasma concentrations occurring between 2 to 3 hours. The drug is excreted in the urine as two soluble glucuronide conjugates accounting for about 90% of the administered dose. Little or no diflunisal is excreted in the feces. Diflunisal appears in human milk in concentrations of 2–7% of those in plasma. More than 99% of diflunisal in plasma is bound to proteins.

As is the case with salicylic acid, concentration-dependent pharmacokinetics prevail when DOLOBID is administered; a doubling of dosage produces a greater than doubling of drug accumulation. The effect becomes more apparent with repetitive doses. Following single doses, peak plasma concentrations of 41 ± 11 µg/mL (mean ± S.D.) were observed following 250 mg doses, 87 ± 17 µg/mL were observed following 500 mg and 124 ± 11 µg/mL following single 1000 mg doses. However, following administration of 250 mg b.i.d., a mean peak level of 56 ± 14 µg/mL was observed on day 8, while the mean peak level after 500 mg b.i.d. for 11 days was 190 ± 33 µg/mL. In contrast to salicylic acid which has a plasma half-life of $2^1/_2$ hours, the plasma half-life of diflunisal is 3 to 4 times longer (8 to 12 hours), because of a difluorophenyl substituent at carbon 1. Because of its long half-life and nonlinear pharmacokinetics, several days are required for diflunisal plasma levels to reach steady state following multiple doses. For this reason, an initial loading dose is necessary to shorten the time to reach steady state levels, and 2 to 3 days of observation are necessary for evaluating changes in treatment regimens if a loading dose is not used.

Studies in baboons to determine passage across the blood-brain barrier have shown that only small quantities of diflunisal, under normal or acidotic conditions are transported into the cerebrospinal fluid (CSF). The ratio of blood/CSF concentrations after intravenous doses of 50 mg/kg or oral doses of 100 mg/kg of diflunisal was 100:1. In contrast, oral doses of 500 mg/kg of aspirin resulted in a blood/CSF ratio of 5:1.

Mild to Moderate Pain

DOLOBID is a peripherally-acting analgesic agent with a long duration of action. DOLOBID produces significant analgesia within 1 hour and maximum analgesia within 2 to 3 hours.

Consistent with its long half-life, clinical effects of DOLOBID mirror its pharmacokinetic behavior, which is the basis for recommending a loading dose when instituting therapy. Patients treated with DOLOBID, on the first dose, tend to have a slower onset of pain relief when compared with drugs achieving comparable peak effects. However, DOLOBID produces longer-lasting responses than the comparative agents.

Comparative single dose clinical studies have established the analgesic efficacy of DOLOBID at various dose levels relative to other analgesics. Analgesic effect measurements were derived from hourly evaluations by patients during eight and twelve-hour postdosing observation periods. The following information may serve as a guide for prescribing DOLOBID.

DOLOBID 500 mg was comparable in analgesic efficacy to aspirin 650 mg, acetaminophen 600 mg or 650 mg, and acetaminophen 650 mg with propoxyphene napsylate 100 mg. Patients treated with DOLOBID had longer lasting responses than the patients treated with the comparative analgesics.

DOLOBID 1000 mg was comparable in analgesic efficacy to acetaminophen 600 mg with codeine 60 mg. Patients treated with DOLOBID had longer lasting responses than the patients who received acetaminophen with codeine.

A loading dose of 1000 mg provides faster onset of pain relief, shorter time to peak analgesic effect, and greater peak analgesic effect than an initial 500 mg dose.

In contrast to the comparative analgesics, a significantly greater proportion of patients treated with DOLOBID did not remedicate and continued to have a good analgesic effect eight to twelve hours after dosing. Seventy-five percent (75%) of patients treated with DOLOBID continued to have a good analgesic response at four hours. When patients having a good analgesic response at four hours were followed, 78% of these patients continued to have a good analgesic response at eight hours and 64% at twelve hours.

Chronic Anti-inflammatory Therapy in Osteoarthritis and Rheumatoid Arthritis

In the controlled, double-blind clinical trials in which DOLOBID (500 mg to 1000 mg a day) was compared with anti-inflammatory doses of aspirin (2–4 grams a day), patients treated with DOLOBID had a significantly lower incidence of tinnitus and of adverse effects involving the gastrointestinal system than patients treated with aspirin. (See also *Effect on Fecal Blood Loss*).

Osteoarthritis

The effectiveness of DOLOBID for the treatment of osteoarthritis was studied in patients with osteoarthritis of the hip and/or knee. The activity of DOLOBID was demonstrated by clinical improvement in the signs and symptoms of disease activity.

In a double-blind multicenter study of 12 weeks' duration in which dosages were adjusted according to patient response, DOLOBID, 500 or 750 mg daily, was shown to be comparable in effectiveness to aspirin, 2000 or 3000 mg daily. In open-label extensions of this study to 24 or 48 weeks, DOLOBID continued to show similar effectiveness and generally was well tolerated.

Rheumatoid Arthritis

In controlled clinical trials, the effectiveness of DOLOBID was established for both acute exacerbations and long-term management of rheumatoid arthritis. The activity of DOLOBID was demonstrated by clinical improvement in the signs and symptoms of disease activity.

In a double-blind multicenter study of 12 weeks' duration in which dosages were adjusted according to patient response, DOLOBID 500 or 750 mg daily was comparable in effectiveness to aspirin 2,600 or 3,900 mg daily. In open-label extensions of this study to 52 weeks, DOLOBID continued to be effective and was generally well tolerated.

DOLOBID 500, 750, or 1000 mg daily was compared with aspirin 2000, 3000, or 4000 mg daily in a multicenter study of 8 weeks' duration in which dosages were adjusted according to patient response. In this study, DOLOBID was comparable in efficacy to aspirin.

In a double-blind multicenter study of 12 weeks' duration in which dosages were adjusted according to patient needs, DOLOBID 500 or 750 mg daily and ibuprofen 1600 or 2400 mg daily were comparable in effectiveness and tolerability.

In a double-blind multicenter study of 12 weeks' duration, DOLOBID 750 mg daily was comparable in efficacy to naproxen 750 mg daily. The incidence of gastrointestinal adverse effects and tinnitus was comparable for both drugs. This study was extended to 48 weeks on an open-label basis. DOLOBID continued to be effective and generally well tolerated.

In patients with rheumatoid arthritis, DOLOBID and gold salts may be used in combination at their usual dosage levels. In clinical studies, DOLOBID added to the regimen of gold salts usually resulted in additional symptomatic relief but did not alter the course of the underlying disease.

Antipyretic Activity

DOLOBID is not recommended for use as an antipyretic agent. In single 250 mg, 500 mg, or 750 mg doses, DOLOBID produced measurable but not clinically useful decreases in temperature in patients with fever; however, the possibility that it may mask fever in some patients, particularly with chronic or high doses, should be considered.

Uricosuric Effect

In normal volunteers, an increase in the renal clearance of uric acid and a decrease in serum uric acid was observed when DOLOBID was administered at 500 mg or 750 mg daily in divided doses. Patients on long-term therapy taking DOLOBID at 500 mg to 1000 mg daily in divided doses showed a prompt and consistent reduction across studies in mean serum uric acid levels, which were lowered as much as 1.4 mg%. It is not known whether DOLOBID interferes with the activity of other uricosuric agents.

Effect on Platelet Function

As an inhibitor of prostaglandin synthetase, DOLOBID has a dose-related effect on platelet function and bleeding time. In normal volunteers, 250 mg b.i.d. for 8 days had no effect on platelet function, and 500 mg b.i.d., the usual recommended dose, had a slight effect. At 1000 mg b.i.d., which exceeds the maximum recommended dosage, however, DOLOBID inhibited platelet function. In contrast to aspirin, these effects of DOLOBID were reversible, because of the absence of the chemically labile and biologically reactive 0-acetyl group at the carbon 4 position. Bleeding time was not altered by a dose of 250 mg b.i.d., and was only slightly increased at 500 mg b.i.d. At 1000 mg b.i.d., a greater increase occurred, but was not statistically significantly different from the change in the placebo group.

Effect on Fecal Blood Loss

When DOLOBID was given to normal volunteers at the usual recommended dose of 500 mg twice daily, fecal blood loss was not significantly different from placebo. Aspirin at 1000 mg four times daily produced the expected increase in fecal blood loss. DOLOBID at 1000 mg twice daily (NOTE: exceeds the recommended dosage) caused a statistically significant increase in fecal blood loss, but this increase was only one-half as large as that associated with aspirin 1300 mg twice daily.

Effect on Blood Glucose

DOLOBID did not affect fasting blood sugar in diabetic patients who were receiving tolbutamide or placebo.

INDICATIONS AND USAGE

DOLOBID is indicated for acute or long-term use for symptomatic treatment of the following:

1. Mild to moderate pain
2. Osteoarthritis
3. Rheumatoid arthritis

CONTRAINDICATIONS

Patients who are hypersensitive to this product.

Patients in whom acute asthmatic attacks, urticaria, or rhinitis are precipitated by aspirin or other non-steroidal anti-inflammatory drugs.

WARNINGS

Peptic ulceration and gastrointestinal bleeding have been reported in patients receiving DOLOBID. Fatalities have occurred rarely. Gastrointestinal bleeding is associated with higher morbidity and mortality in patients acutely ill with other conditions, the elderly and patients with hemorrhagic disorders. In patients with active gastrointestinal bleeding or an active peptic ulcer, the physician must weigh the benefits of therapy with DOLOBID against possible hazards, institute an appropriate ulcer regimen, and carefully monitor the patient's progress. When DOLOBID is given to patients with a history of either upper or lower gastrointestinal tract disease, it should be given only after consulting the ADVERSE REACTIONS section and under close supervision.

Risk of GI Ulcerations, Bleeding and Perforation with NSAID Therapy

Serious gastrointestinal toxicity such as bleeding, ulceration, and perforation, can occur at any time, with or without warning symptoms, in patients treated chronically with NSAID therapy. Although minor upper gastrointestinal problems, such as dyspepsia, are common, usually developing early in therapy, physicians should remain alert for ulceration and bleeding in patients treated chronically with NSAIDs even in the absence of previous GI tract symptoms. In patients observed in clinical trials of several months to two years duration, symptomatic upper GI ulcers, gross bleeding or perforation appear to occur in approximately 1% of patients treated for 3–6 months, and in about 2–4% of patients treated for one year. Physicians should inform patients about the signs and/or symptoms of serious GI toxicity and what steps to take if they occur.

Studies to date have not identified any subset of patients not at risk of developing peptic ulceration and bleeding. Except for a prior history of serious GI events and other risk factors known to be associated with peptic ulcer disease, such as alcoholism, smoking, etc., no risk factors (e.g., age, sex) have been associated with increased risk. Elderly or debilitated patients seem to tolerate ulceration or bleeding less well than other individuals and most spontaneous reports of fatal GI events are in this population. Studies to date are inconclusive concerning the relative risk of various NSAIDs in causing such reactions. High doses of any NSAID probably carry a greater risk of these reactions, although controlled clinical trials showing this do not exist in most cases. In considering the use of relatively large doses (within the recommended dosage range), sufficient benefit should be anticipated to offset the potential increased risk of GI toxicity.

Continued on next page

Information on the Merck & Co., Inc. products listed on these pages is the full prescribing information from product circulars in use September 30, 2000. For information, please call 1-800-NSC MERCK [1-800-672-6372].

Dolobid—Cont.

PRECAUTIONS

General
Non-steroidal anti-inflammatory drugs, including DOLOBID, may mask the usual signs and symptoms of infection. Therefore, the physician must be continually on the alert for this and should use the drug with extra care in the presence of existing infection.
Although DOLOBID has less effect on platelet function and bleeding time than aspirin, at higher doses it is an inhibitor of platelet function; therefore, patients who may be adversely affected should be carefully observed when DOLOBID is administered (see CLINICAL PHARMACOLOGY).
Because of reports of adverse eye findings with agents of this class, it is recommended that patients who develop eye complaints during treatment with DOLOBID have ophthalmologic studies.
Peripheral edema has been observed in some patients taking DOLOBID. Therefore, as with other drugs in this class, DOLOBID should be used with caution in patients with compromised cardiac function, hypertension, or other conditions predisposing to fluid retention.
Acetylsalicylic acid has been associated with Reye syndrome. Because diflunisal is a derivative of salicylic acid, the possibility of its association with Reye syndrome cannot be excluded.
Hypersensitivity Syndrome
A potentially life-threatening, apparent hypersensitivity syndrome has been reported. This multisystem syndrome includes constitutional symptoms (fever, chills), and cutaneous findings (see ADVERSE REACTIONS, *Dermatologic*). It may also include involvement of major organs (changes in liver function, jaundice, leukopenia, thrombocytopenia, eosinophilia, disseminated intravascular coagulation, renal impairment, including renal failure), and less specific findings (adenitis, arthralgia, myalgia, arthritis, malaise, anorexia, disorientation). If evidence of hypersensitivity occurs, therapy with DOLOBID should be discontinued.
Renal Effects
As with other non-steroidal anti-inflammatory drugs, long term administration of diflunisal to animals has resulted in renal papillary necrosis and other abnormal renal pathology. In humans, there have been reports of acute interstitial nephritis with hematuria and proteinuria and occasionally nephrotic syndrome.
A second form of renal toxicity has been seen in patients with prerenal and renal conditions leading to a reduction in renal blood flow or blood volume, where the renal prostaglandins have a supportive role in the maintenance of renal perfusion. In these patients administration of an NSAID may cause a dose dependent reduction in prostaglandin formation and may precipitate overt renal decompensation. Patients at greatest risk of this reaction are those with conditions such as renal or hepatic dysfunction, diabetes mellitus, advanced age, extracellular volume depletion from any cause, congestive heart failure, septicemia, pyelonephritis, or concomitant use of any nephrotoxic drug. DOLOBID or other NSAIDs should be given with caution and renal function should be monitored in any patient who may have reduced renal reserve. Discontinuation of NSAID therapy is typically followed by recovery to the pretreatment state.
Since DOLOBID is eliminated primarily by the kidneys, patients with significantly impaired renal function should be closely monitored; a lower daily dosage should be anticipated to avoid excessive drug accumulation.
Information for Patients
DOLOBID, like other drugs of its class, is not free of side effects. The side effects of these drugs can cause discomfort and, rarely, there are more serious side effects such as gastrointestinal bleeding, which may result in hospitalization and even fatal outcomes.
NSAIDs (Non-steroidal Anti-inflammatory Drugs) are often essential agents in the management of arthritis and have a major role in the treatment of pain, but they also may be commonly employed for conditions which are less serious.
Physicians may wish to discuss with their patients the potential risks (see WARNINGS, PRECAUTIONS and ADVERSE REACTIONS) and likely benefits of NSAID treatment, particularly when the drugs are used for less serious conditions where treatment without NSAIDs may represent an acceptable alternative to both the patient and physician.
Laboratory Tests
Liver Function Tests: As with other non-steroidal anti-inflammatory drugs, borderline elevations of one or more liver tests may occur in up to 15% of patients. These abnormalities may progress, may remain essentially unchanged, or may be transient with continued therapy. The SGPT (ALT) test is probably the most sensitive indicator of liver dysfunction. Meaningful (3 times the upper limit of normal) elevations of SGPT or SGOT (AST) occurred in controlled clinical trials in less than 1% of patients. A patient with symptoms and/or signs suggesting liver dysfunction, or in whom an abnormal liver test has occurred, should be evaluated for evidence of the development of more severe hepatic reactions while on therapy with DOLOBID. Severe hepatic reactions, including jaundice, have been reported with DOLOBID as well as with other non-steroidal anti-inflammatory drugs. Although such reactions are rare, if abnormal liver tests persist or worsen, if clinical signs and symptoms consistent with liver disease develop, or if systemic manifestations occur (e.g., eosinophilia, rash, etc.), DOLOBID should be discontinued, since liver reactions can be fatal.
Gastrointestinal: Because serious GI tract ulceration and bleeding can occur without warning symptoms, physicians should follow chronically treated patients for the signs and symptoms of ulceration and bleeding and should inform them of the importance of this follow-up (see WARNINGS, *Risk of GI Ulcerations, Bleeding and Perforation with NSAID Therapy*).
Drug Interactions
Oral Anticoagulants: In some normal volunteers, the concomitant administration of DOLOBID and warfarin, acenocoumarol, or phenprocoumon resulted in prolongation of prothrombin time. This may occur because diflunisal competitively displaces coumarins from protein binding sites. Accordingly, when DOLOBID is administered with oral anticoagulants, the prothrombin time should be closely monitored during and for several days after concomitant drug administration. Adjustment of dosage of oral anticoagulants may be required.
Tolbutamide: In diabetic patients receiving DOLOBID and tolbutamide, no significant effects were seen on tolbutamide plasma levels or fasting blood glucose.
Hydrochlorothiazide: In normal volunteers, concomitant administration of DOLOBID and hydrochlorothiazide resulted in significantly increased plasma levels of hydrochlorothiazide. DOLOBID decreased the hyperuricemic effect of hydrochlorothiazide.
Furosemide: In normal volunteers, the concomitant administration of DOLOBID and furosemide had no effect on the diuretic activity of furosemide. DOLOBID decreased the hyperuricemic effect of furosemide.
Antacids: Concomitant administration of antacids may reduce plasma levels of DOLOBID. This effect is small with occasional doses of antacids, but may be clinically significant when antacids are used on a continuous schedule.
Acetaminophen: In normal volunteers, concomitant administration of DOLOBID and acetaminophen resulted in an approximate 50% increase in plasma levels of acetaminophen. Acetaminophen had no effect on plasma levels of DOLOBID. Since acetaminophen in high doses has been associated with hepatotoxicity, concomitant administration of DOLOBID and acetaminophen should be used cautiously, with careful monitoring of patients.
Concomitant administration of DOLOBID and acetaminophen in dogs, but not in rats, at approximately 2 times the recommended maximum human therapeutic dose of each (40-52 mg/kg/day of DOLOBID/acetaminophen), resulted in greater gastrointestinal toxicity than when either drug was administered alone. The clinical significance of these findings has not been established.
Methotrexate: Caution should be used if DOLOBID is administered concomitantly with methotrexate. Non-steroidal anti-inflammatory drugs have been reported to decrease the tubular secretion of methotrexate and to potentiate its toxicity.
Cyclosporine: Administration of non-steroidal anti-inflammatory drugs concomitantly with cyclosporine has been associated with an increase in cyclosporine-induced toxicity, possibly due to decreased synthesis of renal prostacyclin. NSAIDs should be used with caution in patients taking cyclosporine, and renal function should be carefully monitored.
Drug Interactions: Non-steroidal Anti-inflammatory Drugs
The administration of diflunisal to normal volunteers receiving indomethacin decreased the renal clearance and significantly increased the plasma levels of indomethacin. In some patients the combined use of indomethacin and DOLOBID has been associated with fatal gastrointestinal hemorrhage. Therefore, indomethacin and DOLOBID should not be used concomitantly.
The concomitant use of DOLOBID and other NSAIDs is not recommended due to the increased possibility of gastrointestinal toxicity, with little or no increase in efficacy. The following information was obtained from studies in normal volunteers.
Aspirin: In normal volunteers, a small decrease in diflunisal levels was observed when multiple doses of DOLOBID and aspirin were administered concomitantly.
Sulindac: The concomitant administration of DOLOBID and sulindac in normal volunteers resulted in lowering of the plasma levels of the active sulindac sulfide metabolite by approximately one-third.
Naproxen: The concomitant administration of DOLOBID and naproxen in normal volunteers had no effect on the plasma levels of naproxen, but significantly decreased the urinary excretion of naproxen and its glucuronide metabolite. Naproxen had no effect on plasma levels of DOLOBID.
Drug/Laboratory Test Interactions
Serum Salicylate Assays: Caution should be used in interpreting the results of serum salicylate assays when diflunisal is present. Salicylate levels have been found to be falsely elevated with some assay methods.
Carcinogenesis, Mutagenesis, Impairment of Fertility
Diflunisal did not affect the type or incidence of neoplasia in a 105-week study in the rat given doses up to 40 mg/kg/day (equivalent to approximately 1.3 times the maximum recommended human dose), or in long-term carcinogenic studies in mice given diflunisal at doses up to 80 mg/kg/day (equivalent to approximately 2.7 times the maximum recommended human dose). It was concluded that there was no carcinogenic potential for DOLOBID.
Diflunisal passes the placental barrier to a minor degree in the rat. Diflunisal had no mutagenic activity after oral administration in the dominant lethal assay, in the Ames microbial mutagen test or in the V-79 Chinese hamster lung cell assay.
No evidence of impaired fertility was found in reproduction studies in rats at doses up to 50 mg/kg/day.
Pregnancy
Pregnancy Category C. A dose of 60 mg/kg/day of diflunisal (equivalent to two times the maximum human dose) was maternotoxic, embryotoxic, and teratogenic in rabbits. In three of six studies in rabbits, evidence of teratogenicity was observed at doses ranging from 40 to 50 mg/kg/day. Teratology studies in mice, at doses up to 45 mg/kg/day, and in rats at doses up to 100 mg/kg/day, revealed no harm to the fetus due to diflunisal. Aspirin and other salicylates have been shown to be teratogenic in a wide variety of species, including the rat and rabbit, at doses ranging from 50 to 400 mg/kg/day (approximately one to eight times the human dose). There are no adequate and well controlled studies with diflunisal in pregnant women. DOLOBID should be used during the first two trimesters of pregnancy only if the potential benefit justifies the potential risk to the fetus. The known effects of drugs of this class on the human fetus during the third trimester of pregnancy include: constriction of the ductus arteriosus prenatally, tricuspid incompetence, and pulmonary hypertension; non-closure of the ductus arteriosus postnatally which may be resistant to medical management; myocardial degenerative changes, platelet dysfunction with resultant bleeding, intracranial bleeding, renal dysfunction or failure, renal injury/dysgenesis which may result in prolonged or permanent renal failure, oligohydramnios, gastrointestinal bleeding or perforation, and increased risk of necrotizing enterocolitis. Use during the third trimester of pregnancy is not recommended.
In rats at a dose of one and one-half times the maximum human dose, there was an increase in the average length of gestation. Similar increases in the length of gestation have been observed with aspirin, indomethacin, and phenylbutazone, and may be related to inhibition of prostaglandin synthetase. Drugs of this class may cause dystocia and delayed parturition in pregnant animals.
Nursing Mothers
Diflunisal is excreted in human milk in concentrations of 2–7% of those in plasma. Because of the potential for serious adverse reactions in nursing infants from DOLOBID, a decision should be made whether to discontinue nursing or to discontinue the drug, taking into account the importance of the drug to the mother.
Pediatric Use
Safety and effectiveness of DOLOBID in pediatric patients have not been established. Use of DOLOBID in pediatric patients below the age of 12 years is not recommended.
The adverse effects observed following diflunisal administration to neonatal animals appear to be species, age, and dose-dependent. At dose levels approximately 3 times the usual human therapeutic dose, both aspirin (200 to 400 mg/kg/ day) and diflunisal (80 mg/kg/day) resulted in death, leukocytosis, weight loss, and bilateral cataracts in neonatal (4 to 5-day-old) beagle puppies after 2 to 10 doses. Administration of an 80 mg/kg/day dose of diflunisal to 25-day-old puppies resulted in lower mortality, and did not produce cataracts. In newborn rats, a 400 mg/kg/day dose of aspirin resulted in increased mortality and some cataracts, whereas the effects of diflunisal administration at doses up to 140 mg/kg/day were limited to a decrease in average body weight gain.
Geriatric Use
As with any NSAID, caution should be exercised in treating the elderly (65 years and older) since advancing age appears to increase the possibility of adverse reactions. Elderly patients seem to tolerate ulceration or bleeding less well than other individuals and many spontaneous reports of fatal GI events are in this population (see WARNINGS, *Risk of GI Ulcerations, Bleeding and Perforation with NSAID Therapy*).
This drug is known to be substantially excreted by the kidney and the risk of toxic reactions to this drug may be greater in patients with impaired renal function. Because elderly patients are more likely to have decreased renal function, care should be taken in dose selection and it may be useful to monitor renal function (see PRECAUTIONS, *Renal Effects*).

ADVERSE REACTIONS

The adverse reactions observed in controlled clinical trials encompass observations in 2,427 patients.
Listed below are the adverse reactions reported in the 1,314 of these patients who received treatment in studies of two weeks or longer. Five hundred thirteen patients were treated for at least 24 weeks, 255 patients were treated for at least 48 weeks, and 46 patients were treated for 96 weeks. In general, the adverse reactions listed below were 2 to 14 times less frequent in the 1,113 patients who received short-term treatment for mild to moderate pain.
Incidence Greater Than 1%
Gastrointestinal
The most frequent types of adverse reactions occurring with DOLOBID are gastrointestinal: these include nausea**, vomiting, dyspepsia**, gastrointestinal pain**, diarrhea**, constipation, and flatulence.
Psychiatric
Somnolence, insomnia.

Central Nervous System
Dizziness.
Special Senses
Tinnitus.
Dermatologic
Rash**.
Miscellaneous
Headache**, fatigue/tiredness.

Incidence Less Than 1 in 100

The following adverse reactions, occurring less frequently than 1 in 100, were reported in clinical trials or since the drug was marketed. The probability exists of a causal relationship between DOLOBID and these adverse reactions.
Dermatologic
Erythema multiforme, exfoliative dermatitis, Stevens-Johnson syndrome, toxic epidermal necrolysis, urticaria, pruritus, sweating, dry mucous membranes, stomatitis, photosensitivity.
Gastrointestinal
Peptic ulcer, gastrointestinal bleeding, anorexia, eructation, gastrointestinal perforation, gastritis.
Liver function abnormalities; jaundice, sometimes with fever; cholestasis; hepatitis.
Hematologic
Thrombocytopenia; agranulocytosis; hemolytic anemia.
Genitourinary
Dysuria; renal impairment, including renal failure; interstitial nephritis; hematuria; proteinuria.
Psychiatric
Nervousness, depression, hallucinations, confusion, disorientation.
Central Nervous System
Vertigo; light-headedness; paresthesias.
Special Senses
Transient visual disturbances including blurred vision.
Hypersensitivity Reactions
Acute anaphylactic reaction with bronchospasm; angioedema; flushing.
Hypersensitivity vasculitis.
Hypersensitivity syndrome (see PRECAUTIONS).
Miscellaneous
Asthenia, edema.

Causal Relationship Unknown

Other reactions have been reported in clinical trials or since the drug was marketed, but occurred under circumstances where a causal relationship could not be established. However, in these rarely reported events, that possibility cannot be excluded. Therefore, these observations are listed to serve as alerting information to physicians.
Respiratory
Dyspnea.
Cardiovascular
Palpitation, syncope.
Musculoskeletal
Muscle cramps.
Genitourinary
Nephrotic syndrome.
Special Senses
Hearing loss.
Miscellaneous
Chest pain.

A rare occurrence of fulminant necrotizing fasciitis, particularly in association with Group A β-hemolytic streptococcus, has been described in persons treated with non-steroidal anti-inflammatory agents, including diflunisal, sometimes with fatal outcome (see also PRECAUTIONS, *General*).

Potential Adverse Effects

In addition, a variety of adverse effects not observed with DOLOBID in clinical trials or in marketing experience, but reported with other non-steroidal analgesic/anti-inflammatory agents, should be considered potential adverse effects of DOLOBID.

**Incidence between 3% and 9%. Those reactions occurring in 1% to 3% are not marked with an asterisk.

OVERDOSAGE

Cases of overdosage have occurred and deaths have been reported. Most patients recovered without evidence of permanent sequelae. The most common signs and symptoms observed with overdosage were drowsiness, vomiting, nausea, diarrhea, hyperventilation, tachycardia, sweating, tinnitus, disorientation, stupor and coma. Diminished urine output and cardiorespiratory arrest have also been reported. The lowest dosage of DOLOBID at which a death has been reported was 15 grams without the presence of other drugs. In a mixed drug overdose, ingestion of 7.5 grams of DOLOBID resulted in death.

In the event of overdosage, the stomach should be emptied by inducing vomiting or by gastric lavage, and the patient carefully observed and given symptomatic and supportive treatment. Because of the high degree of protein binding, hemodialysis may not be effective.

The oral LD_{50} of the drug is 500 mg/kg and 826 mg/kg in female mice and female rats respectively.

DOSAGE AND ADMINISTRATION

Concentration-dependent pharmacokinetics prevail when DOLOBID is administered; a doubling of dosage produces a greater than doubling of drug accumulation. The effect becomes more apparent with repetitive doses.

For mild to moderate pain, an initial dose of 1000 mg followed by 500 mg every 12 hours is recommended for most patients. Following the initial dose, some patients may require 500 mg every 8 hours.

A lower dosage may be appropriate depending on such factors as pain severity, patient response, weight, or advanced age; for example, 500 mg initially, followed by 250 mg every 8–12 hours.

For osteoarthritis and rheumatoid arthritis, the suggested dosage range is 500 mg to 1000 mg daily in two divided doses. The dosage of DOLOBID may be increased or decreased according to patient response.

Maintenance doses higher than 1500 mg a day are not recommended.

DOLOBID may be administered with water, milk or meals. Tablets should be swallowed whole, not crushed or chewed.

HOW SUPPLIED

Tablets DOLOBID are capsule-shaped, film-coated tablets supplied as follows:

No. 3390—250 mg peach colored, coded DOLOBID on one side and MSD 675 on the other.
NDC 0006-0675-61 unit of use bottles of 60
(6505-01-164-0501, 250 mg 60's).

Shown in Product Identification Guide, page 323

No. 3392—500 mg orange colored, coded DOLOBID on one side and MSD 697 on the other.
NDC 0006-0697-61 unit of use bottles of 60
(6505-01-144-9724, 500 mg 60's).

Shown in Product Identification Guide, page 323

7928833 Issued July 1998

EDECRIN® Tablets ℞
(Ethacrynic Acid)

Intravenous
SODIUM EDECRIN® ℞
(Ethacrynate Sodium)

EDECRIN* (Ethacrynic Acid) is a potent diuretic which, if given in excessive amounts, may lead to profound diuresis with water and electrolyte depletion. Therefore, careful medical supervision is required, and dose and dose schedule must be adjusted to the individual patient's needs (see DOSAGE AND ADMINISTRATION).

DESCRIPTION

Ethacrynic acid is an unsaturated ketone derivative of an aryloxyacetic acid. It is designated chemically as [2,3-dichloro-4-(2-methylene-1-oxobutyl)phenoxy] acetic acid, and has a molecular weight of 303.14. Ethacrynic acid is a white, or practically white, crystalline powder, very slightly soluble in water, but soluble in most organic solvents such as alcohols, chloroform, and benzene. Its empirical formula is $C_{13}H_{12}Cl_2O_4$ and its structural formula is:

OCH_2COOH / Cl / Cl / $COCCH_2CH_3$ / CH_2

Ethacrynate sodium, the sodium salt of ethacrynic acid, is soluble in water at 25°C to the extent of about 7 percent. Solutions of the sodium salt are relatively stable at about pH 7 at room temperature for short periods, but as the pH or temperature increases the solutions are less stable. The molecular weight of ethacrynate sodium is 325.12. Its empirical formula is $C_{13}H_{11}Cl_2NaO_4$ and its structural formula is:

OCH_2COONa / Cl / Cl / $COCCH_2CH_3$ / CH_2

EDECRIN is supplied as 25 mg and 50 mg tablets for oral use. Each tablet contains the following inactive ingredients: colloidal silicon dioxide, lactose, magnesium stearate, starch and talc. The 50 mg tablet also contains D&C Yellow 10, FD&C Blue 1 and FD&C Yellow 6. Intravenous SODIUM EDECRIN* (Ethacrynate Sodium) is a sterile freeze-dried powder and is supplied in a vial containing:

Ethacrynate sodium equivalent to ethacrynic acid .... 50.0 mg

Inactive ingredients:
Mannitol .... 62.5 mg

*Registered trademark of MERCK & CO., INC.

CLINICAL PHARMACOLOGY

Pharmacokinetics and Metabolism

EDECRIN acts on the ascending limb of the loop of Henle and on the proximal and distal tubules. Urinary output is usually dose dependent and related to the magnitude of fluid accumulation. Water and electrolyte excretion may be increased several times over that observed with thiazide diuretics, since EDECRIN inhibits reabsorption of a much greater proportion of filtered sodium than most other diuretic agents. Therefore, EDECRIN is effective in many patients who have significant degrees of renal insufficiency (see WARNINGS concerning deafness). EDECRIN has little or no effect on glomerular filtration or on renal blood flow, except following pronounced reductions in plasma volume when associated with rapid diuresis.

The electrolyte excretion pattern of ethacrynic acid varies from that of the thiazides and mercurial diuretics. Initial sodium and chloride excretion is usually substantial and chloride loss exceeds that of sodium. With prolonged administration, chloride excretion declines, and potassium and hydrogen ion excretion may increase. EDECRIN is effective whether or not there is clinical acidosis or alkalosis.

Although EDECRIN, in carefully controlled studies in animals and experimental subjects, produces a more favorable sodium/potassium excretion ratio than the thiazides, in patients with increased diuresis excessive amounts of potassium may be excreted.

Onset of action is rapid, usually within 30 minutes after an oral dose of EDECRIN or within 5 minutes after an intravenous injection of SODIUM EDECRIN. After oral use, diuresis peaks in about 2 hours and lasts about 6 to 8 hours. The sulfhydryl binding propensity of ethacrynic acid differs somewhat from that of the organomercurials. Its mode of action is not by carbonic anhydrase inhibition.

Ethacrynic acid does not cross the blood-brain barrier.

INDICATIONS AND USAGE

EDECRIN is indicated for treatment of edema when an agent with greater diuretic potential than those commonly employed is required.

1. Treatment of the edema associated with congestive heart failure, cirrhosis of the liver, and renal disease, including the nephrotic syndrome.
2. Short-term management of ascites due to malignancy, idiopathic edema, and lymphedema.
3. Short-term management of hospitalized pediatric patients, other than infants, with congenital heart disease or the nephrotic syndrome.
4. Intravenous SODIUM EDECRIN is indicated when a rapid onset of diuresis is desired, e.g., in acute pulmonary edema, or when gastrointestinal absorption is impaired or oral medication is not practicable.

CONTRAINDICATIONS

All diuretics, including ethacrynic acid, are contraindicated in anuria. If increasing electrolyte imbalance, azotemia, and/or oliguria occur during treatment of severe, progressive renal disease, the diuretic should be discontinued.

In a few patients this diuretic has produced severe, watery diarrhea. If this occurs, it should be discontinued and not used again.

Until further experience in infants is accumulated, therapy with oral and parenteral EDECRIN is contraindicated.

Hypersensitivity to any component of this product.

WARNINGS

The effects of EDECRIN on electrolytes are related to its renal pharmacologic activity and are dose dependent. The possibility of profound electrolyte and water loss may be avoided by weighing the patient throughout the treatment period, by careful adjustment of dosage, by initiating treatment with small doses, and by using the drug on an intermittent schedule when possible. When excessive diuresis occurs, the drug should be withdrawn until homeostasis is restored. When excessive electrolyte loss occurs, the dosage should be reduced or the drug temporarily withdrawn.

Initiation of diuretic therapy with EDECRIN in the cirrhotic patient with ascites is best carried out in the hospital. When maintenance therapy has been established, the individual can be satisfactorily followed as an outpatient.

EDECRIN should be given with caution to patients with advanced cirrhosis of the liver, particularly those with a history of previous episodes of electrolyte imbalance or hepatic encephalopathy. Like other diuretics it may precipitate hepatic coma and death.

Too vigorous a diuresis, as evidenced by rapid and excessive weight loss, may induce an acute hypotensive episode. In elderly cardiac patients, rapid contraction of plasma volume

Continued on next page

Information on the Merck & Co., Inc. products listed on these pages is the full prescribing information from product circulars in use September 30, 2000. For information, please call 1-800-NSC MERCK [1-800-672-6372].

Edecrin—Cont.

and the resultant hemoconcentration should be avoided to prevent the development of thromboembolic episodes, such as cerebral vascular thromboses and pulmonary emboli which may be fatal. Excessive loss of potassium in patients receiving digitalis glycosides may precipitate digitalis toxicity. Care should also be exercised in patients receiving potassium-depleting steroids.

A number of possibly drug-related deaths have occurred in critically ill patients refractory to other diuretics. These generally have fallen into two categories: (1) patients with severe myocardial disease who have been receiving digitalis and presumably developed acute hypokalemia with fatal arrhythmia; (2) patients with severely decompensated hepatic cirrhosis with ascites, with or without accompanying encephalopathy, who were in electrolyte imbalance and died because of intensification of the electrolyte defect.

Deafness, tinnitus, and vertigo with a sense of fullness in the ears have occurred, most frequently in patients with severe impairment of renal function. These symptoms have been associated most often with intravenous administration and with doses in excess of those recommended. The deafness has usually been reversible and of short duration (one to 24 hours). However, in some patients the hearing loss has been permanent. A number of these patients were also receiving drugs known to be ototoxic. EDECRIN may increase the ototoxic potential of other drugs (see PRECAUTIONS, subsection *Drug Interactions*).

Lithium generally should not be given with diuretics (see PRECAUTIONS, subsection *Drug Interactions*).

PRECAUTIONS

General

Weakness, muscle cramps, paresthesias, thirst, anorexia, and signs of hyponatremia, hypokalemia, and/or hypochloremic alkalosis may occur following vigorous or excessive diuresis and these may be accentuated by rigid salt restriction. Rarely tetany has been reported following vigorous diuresis. *During therapy with ethacrynic acid, liberalization of salt intake and supplementary potassium chloride are often necessary.*

When a metabolic alkalosis may be anticipated, e.g., in cirrhosis with ascites, the use of potassium chloride or a potassium-sparing agent before and during therapy with EDECRIN may mitigate or prevent the hypokalemia.

Loop diuretics have been shown to increase the urinary excretion of magnesium; this may result in hypomagnesemia.

The safety and efficacy of ethacrynic acid in hypertension have not been established. However, the dosage of coadministered antihypertensive agents may require adjustment.

Orthostatic hypotension may occur in patients receiving other antihypertensive agents when given ethacrynic acid.

EDECRIN has little or no effect on glomerular filtration or on renal blood flow, except following pronounced reductions in plasma volume when associated with rapid diuresis. A transient increase in serum urea nitrogen may occur. Usually, this is readily reversible when the drug is discontinued.

As with other diuretics used in the treatment of renal edema, hypoproteinemia may reduce responsiveness to ethacrynic acid and the use of salt-poor albumin should be considered.

A number of drugs, including ethacrynic acid, have been shown to displace warfarin from plasma protein; a reduction in the usual anticoagulant dosage may be required in patients receiving both drugs.

EDECRIN may increase the risk of gastric hemorrhage associated with corticosteroid treatment.

Laboratory Tests

Frequent serum electrolyte, CO_2 and BUN determinations should be performed early in therapy and periodically thereafter during active diuresis. Any electrolyte abnormalities should be corrected or the drug temporarily withdrawn.

Increases in blood glucose and alterations in glucose tolerance tests have been observed in patients receiving EDECRIN.

Drug Interactions

Lithium generally should not be given with diuretics because they reduce its renal clearance and add a high risk of lithium toxicity. Read circulars for lithium preparations before use of such concomitant therapy.

EDECRIN may increase the ototoxic potential of other drugs such as aminoglycoside and some cephalosporin antibiotics. Their concurrent use should be avoided.

A number of drugs, including ethacrynic acid, have been shown to displace warfarin from plasma protein; a reduction in the usual anticoagulant dosage may be required in patients receiving both drugs.

In some patients, the administration of a non-steroidal anti-inflammatory agent can reduce the diuretic, natriuretic, and antihypertensive effects of loop, potassium-sparing and thiazide diuretics. Therefore, when EDECRIN and non-steroidal anti-inflammatory agents are used concomitantly, the patient should be observed closely to determine if the desired effect of the diuretic is obtained.

Carcinogenesis, Mutagenesis, Impairment of Fertility

There was no evidence of a tumorigenic effect in a 79-week oral chronic toxicity study in rats at doses up to 45 times the human dose.

Ethacrynic acid had no effect on fertility in a two-litter study in rats or a two-generation study in mice at 10 times the human dose.

Pregnancy

Pregnancy Category B: Reproduction studies in the mouse and rabbit at doses up to 50 times the human dose showed no evidence of external abnormalities of the fetus due to EDECRIN.

In a two-litter study in the dog and rat, oral doses of 5 or 20 mg/kg/day ($2^1/_2$ or 10 times the human dose), respectively, did not interfere with pregnancy or with growth and development of the pups. Although there was reduction in the mean body weights of the fetuses in a teratogenic study in the rat at a dose level of 100 mg/kg (50 times the human dose), there was no effect on mortality or postnatal development. Functional and morphologic abnormalities were not observed.

There are, however, no adequate and well-controlled studies in pregnant women. Since animal reproduction studies are not always predictive of human response, EDECRIN should be used during pregnancy only if clearly needed.

Nursing Mothers

It is not known whether this drug is excreted in human milk. Because many drugs are excreted in human milk and because of the potential for serious adverse reactions in nursing infants from EDECRIN, a decision should be made whether to discontinue nursing or to discontinue the drug, taking into account the importance of the drug to the mother.

Pediatric Use

There are no well-controlled clinical trials in pediatric patients. The information on oral dosing in pediatric patients, other than infants, is supported by evidence from empiric use in this age group.

For information on oral use in pediatric patients, other than infants, see INDICATIONS AND USAGE and DOSAGE AND ADMINISTRATION.

Safety and effectiveness of oral and parenteral use in infants have not been established (see CONTRAINDICATIONS).

Safety and effectiveness of intravenous use in pediatric patients have not been established (see DOSAGE AND ADMINISTRATION, *Intravenous Use*).

ADVERSE REACTIONS

Gastrointestinal

Anorexia, malaise, abdominal discomfort or pain, dysphagia, nausea, vomiting, and diarrhea have occurred. These are more frequent with large doses or after one to three months of continuous therapy. A few patients have had sudden onset of profuse, watery diarrhea. Discontinue EDECRIN if diarrhea is severe and do not give it again. Gastrointestinal bleeding has occurred in some patients. Rarely, acute pancreatitis has been reported.

Metabolic

Reversible hyperuricemia and acute gout have been reported. Acute symptomatic hypoglycemia with convulsions occurred in two uremic patients who received doses above those recommended. Hyperglycemia has been reported. Rarely, jaundice and abnormal liver function tests have been reported in seriously ill patients receiving multiple drug therapy, including EDECRIN.

Hematologic

Agranulocytosis or severe neutropenia has been reported in a few critically ill patients also receiving agents known to produce this effect. Thrombocytopenia has been reported rarely. Henoch-Schönlein purpura has been reported rarely in patients with rheumatic heart disease receiving multiple drug therapy, including EDECRIN.

Special Senses (See WARNINGS)

Deafness, tinnitus and vertigo with a sense of fullness in the ears, and blurred vision have occurred.

Central Nervous System

Headache, fatigue, apprehension, confusion.

Miscellaneous

Skin rash, fever, chills, hematuria.

SODIUM EDECRIN occasionally has caused local irritation and pain after intravenous use.

OVERDOSAGE

Overdosage may lead to excessive diuresis with electrolyte depletion and dehydration.

In the event of overdosage, symptomatic and supportive measures should be employed. Emesis should be induced or gastric lavage performed. Correct dehydration, electrolyte imbalance, hepatic coma, and hypotension by established procedures. If required, give oxygen or artificial respiration for respiratory impairment.

In the mouse, the oral LD_{50} of ethacrynic acid is 627 mg/kg and the intravenous LD_{50} of ethacrynate sodium is 175 mg/kg.

DOSAGE AND ADMINISTRATION

Dosage must be regulated carefully to prevent a more rapid or substantial loss of fluid or electrolyte than is indicated or necessary. The magnitude of diuresis and natriuresis is largely dependent on the degree of fluid accumulation present in the patient. Similarly, the extent of potassium excretion is determined in large measure by the presence and magnitude of aldosteronism.

Oral Use

EDECRIN is available for oral use as 25 mg and 50 mg tablets.

Dosage: To Initiate Diuresis

In Adults: The smallest dose required to produce gradual weight loss (about 1 to 2 pounds per day) is recommended. Onset of diuresis usually occurs at 50 to 100 mg for adults. After diuresis has been achieved, the minimally effective dose (usually from 50 to 200 mg daily) may be given on a continuous or intermittent dosage schedule. Dosage adjustments are usually in 25 to 50 mg increments to avoid derangement of water and electrolyte excretion.

The patient should be weighed under standard conditions before and during the institution of diuretic therapy with this compound. Small alterations in dose should effectively prevent a massive diuretic response. The following schedule may be helpful in determining the smallest effective dose.

Day 1— 50 mg (single dose) after a meal

Day 2— 50 mg twice daily after meals, if necessary

Day 3— 100 mg in the morning and 50 to 100 mg following the afternoon or evening meal, depending upon response to the morning dose

A few patients may require initial and maintenance doses as high as 200 mg twice daily. These higher doses, which should be achieved gradually, are most often required in patients with severe, refractory edema.

In Pediatric Patients (excluding infants, see CONTRAINDICATIONS): The initial dose should be 25 mg. Careful stepwise increments in dosage of 25 mg should be made to achieve effective maintenance.

Maintenance Therapy

It is usually possible to reduce the dosage and frequency of administration once dry weight has been achieved.

EDECRIN (Ethacrynic Acid) may be given intermittently after an effective diuresis is obtained with the regimen outlined above. Dosage may be on an alternate daily schedule or more prolonged periods of diuretic therapy may be interspersed with rest periods. Such an intermittent dosage schedule allows time for correction of any electrolyte imbalance and may provide a more efficient diuretic response.

The chloruretic effect of this agent may give rise to retention of bicarbonate and a metabolic alkalosis. This may be corrected by giving chloride (ammonium chloride or arginine chloride). Ammonium chloride should not be given to cirrhotic patients.

EDECRIN has additive effects when used with other diuretics. For example, a patient who is on maintenance dosage of an oral diuretic may require additional intermittent diuretic therapy, such as an organomercurial, for the maintenance of basal weight. The intermittent use of EDECRIN orally may eliminate the need for injections of organomercurials. Small doses of EDECRIN may be added to existing diuretic regimens to maintain basal weight. This drug may potentiate the action of carbonic anhydrase inhibitors, with augmentation of natriuresis and kaliuresis. Therefore, when adding EDECRIN the initial dose and changes of dose should be in 25 mg increments, to avoid electrolyte depletion. Rarely, patients who failed to respond to ethacrynic acid have responded to older established agents.

While many patients do not require supplemental potassium, the use of potassium chloride or potassium-sparing agents, or both, during treatment with EDECRIN is advisable, especially in cirrhotic or nephrotic patients and in patients receiving digitalis.

Salt liberalization usually prevents the development of hyponatremia and hypochloremia. During treatment with EDECRIN, salt may be liberalized to a greater extent than with other diuretics. Cirrhotic patients, however, usually require at least moderate salt restriction concomitant with diuretic therapy.

Intravenous Use

Intravenous SODIUM EDECRIN is for intravenous use when oral intake is impractical or in urgent conditions, such as acute pulmonary edema.

The usual intravenous dose for the average sized adult is 50 mg, or 0.5 to 1.0 mg per kg of body weight. Usually only one dose has been necessary; occasionally a second dose at a new injection site, to avoid possible thrombophlebitis, may be required. A single intravenous dose not exceeding 100 mg has been used in critical situations.

Insufficient pediatric experience precludes recommendation for this age group.

To reconstitute the dry material, add 50 mL of 5 percent Dextrose Injection, or Sodium Chloride Injection to the vial. Occasionally, some 5 percent Dextrose Injection solutions may have a low pH (below 5). The resulting solution with such a diluent may be hazy or opalescent. Intravenous use of such a solution is not recommended. Inspect the vial containing Intravenous SODIUM EDECRIN for particulate matter and discoloration before use.

The solution may be given slowly through the tubing of a running infusion or by direct intravenous injection over a period of several minutes. Do not mix this solution with whole blood or its derivatives. Discard unused reconstituted solution after 24 hours.

SODIUM EDECRIN should not be given subcutaneously or intramuscularly because of local pain and irritation.

HOW SUPPLIED

No. 3321—Tablets EDECRIN, 25 mg, are white, capsule shaped, scored tablets, coded MSD 65 on one side and EDECRIN on the other. They are supplied as follows:

NDC 0006-0065-68 in bottles of 100.

Shown in Product Identification Guide, page 323

No. 3322—Tablets EDECRIN, 50 mg, are green, capsule shaped, scored tablets, coded MSD 90 on one side and EDECRIN on the other. They are supplied as follows:
NDC 0006-0090-68 in bottles of 100
(6505-00-834-0473, 50 mg bottles of 100).
Shown in Product Identification Guide, page 323
No. 3620—Intravenous SODIUM EDECRIN is a dry white material either in a plug form or as a powder. It is supplied in vials containing ethacrynate sodium equivalent to 50 mg of ethacrynic acid, **NDC** 0006-3620-50.
Storage:
Store in a tightly closed container at 25°C (77°F); excursions permitted to 15–30°C (59–86°F). [see USP Controlled Room Temperature]
7901428 Issued April 1998

ELSPAR® ℞
(Asparaginase)

WARNINGS
It is recommended that asparaginase be administered to patients only in a hospital setting under the supervision of a physician who is qualified by training and experience to administer cancer chemotherapeutic agents, because of the possibility of severe reactions, including anaphylaxis and sudden death. The physician must be prepared to treat anaphylaxis at each administration of the drug. In the treatment of each patient the physician must weigh carefully the possibility of achieving therapeutic benefit versus the risk of toxicity.
This drug has various toxic properties, therefore, both powder and solution must be handled and administered with care. Inhalation of dust or vapors and contact with skin or mucous membranes, especially those of the eyes, must be avoided. Special handling procedures should be reviewed prior to handling and followed diligently.
The following data should be thoroughly reviewed before administering the compound.

DESCRIPTION

ELSPAR* (Asparaginase) contains the enzyme L-asparagine amidohydrolase, type EC-2, derived from *Escherichia coli.* It is a white crystalline powder that is freely soluble in water and practically insoluble in methanol, acetone and chloroform. Its activity is expressed in terms of International Units (I.U.) according to the recommendation of the International Union of Biochemistry. The specific activity of ELSPAR is at least 225 I.U. per milligram of protein and each vial contains 10,000 I.U. of asparaginase and 80 mg of mannitol, an inactive ingredient, as a sterile, white lyophilized plug or powder for intravenous or intramuscular injection after reconstitution.

*Registered trademark of MERCK & CO., INC.

CLINICAL PHARMACOLOGY

Action
In a significant number of patients with acute leukemia, particularly lymphocytic, the malignant cells are dependent on an exogenous source of asparagine for survival. Normal cells, however, are able to synthesize asparagine and thus are affected less by the rapid depletion produced by treatment with the enzyme asparaginase. This is a unique approach to therapy based on a metabolic defect in asparagine synthesis of some malignant cells. ELSPAR, derived from *Escherichia coli,* is effective in inducing remissions in some patients with acute lymphocytic leukemia.
Asparagine Dependence Test
An asparagine dependence test has been utilized during the investigational studies. In this test leukemic cells obtained from some marrow cultures could be shown to require asparagine in *vitro,* suggesting sensitivity to asparaginase therapy in *vivo.* However, present data indicate that the correlation between asparagine dependence in such tests and the final response to therapy is sufficiently poor that the test is not recommended as a basis for selection of patients for treatment.
Pharmacokinetics and Metabolism
In a study in patients with metastatic cancer and leukemia, initial plasma levels of L-asparaginase following intravenous administration were correlated to dose. Daily administration resulted in a cumulative increase in plasma levels. Plasma half-life varied from 8 to 30 hours; it did not appear to be influenced by dosage, either single or repetitive, and could not be correlated with age, sex, surface area, renal or hepatic function, diagnosis or extent of disease. Apparent volume of distribution was approximately 70–80% of estimated plasma volume. There was some slow movement of asparaginase from vascular to extravascular, extracellular space. L-asparaginase was detected in the lymph. Cerebrospinal fluid levels were less than 1% of concurrent plasma levels. Only trace amounts appeared in the urine.
In a study in which patients with leukemia and metastatic cancer received intramuscular L-asparaginase, peak plasma levels of asparaginase were reached 14 to 24 hours after dosing. Plasma half-life was 39 to 49 hours. No asparaginase was detected in the urine.

INDICATIONS AND USAGE

ELSPAR is indicated in the therapy of patients with acute lymphocytic leukemia. This agent is useful primarily in combination with other chemotherapeutic agents in the induction of remissions of the disease in pediatric patients. ELSPAR should not be used as the sole induction agent unless combination therapy is deemed inappropriate. ELSPAR is not recommended for maintenance therapy.

CONTRAINDICATIONS

ELSPAR is contraindicated in patients with pancreatitis or a history of pancreatitis. Acute hemorrhagic pancreatitis, in some instances fatal, has been reported following asparaginase administration. Asparaginase is also contraindicated in patients who have had previous anaphylactic reactions to it.

WARNINGS

Allergic reactions to asparaginase are frequent and may occur during the primary course of therapy. They are not completely predictable on the basis of the intradermal skin test. Anaphylaxis and death have occurred even in a hospital setting with experienced observers.
Once a patient has received ELSPAR as part of a treatment regimen, retreatment with this agent at a later time is associated with increased risk of hypersensitivity reactions. In patients found by skin testing to be hypersensitive to asparaginase, and in any patient who has received a previous course of therapy with asparaginase, therapy with this agent should be instituted or reinstituted only after successful desensitization, and then only if in the judgement of the physician the possible benefit is greater than the increased risk. Desensitization itself may be hazardous. (See DOSAGE AND ADMINISTRATION, *Intradermal Skin Test.*)
In view of the unpredictability of the adverse reactions to asparaginase, it is recommended that this product be used in a hospital setting. Asparaginase has an adverse effect on liver function in the majority of patients. Therapy with asparaginase may increase pre-existing liver impairment caused by prior therapy or the underlying disease. Because of this there is a possibility that asparaginase may increase the toxicity of other medications.
The administration of ELSPAR *intravenously concurrently with or immediately before* a course of vincristine and prednisone may be associated with increased toxicity. (See DOSAGE AND ADMINISTRATION, *Recommended Induction Regimens.*)

PRECAUTIONS

General
This drug has various toxic properties, therefore, both powder and solution must be handled and administered with care. (See boxed warning and DIRECTIONS FOR RECONSTITUTION, *Special Handling.*) ELSPAR may be irritating to eyes, skin, and the upper respiratory tract. Inhalation of dust or vapors and contact with skin or mucous membranes, especially those of the eyes, must be avoided. Appropriate protective equipment should be worn when handling ELSPAR. Should accidental eye contact occur, copious irrigation for at least 15 minutes with water, normal saline or a balanced salt ophthalmic irrigating solution should be instituted immediately followed by prompt ophthalmologic consultation. Should accidental skin contact occur, the affected part should be washed immediately with soap and water. Medical attention should be sought. If inhaled, remove from exposure and seek medical attention. (See DIRECTIONS FOR RECONSTITUTION, *Special Handling.*)
Asparaginase has been reported to have immunosuppressive activity in animal experiments. Accordingly, the possibility that use of the drug in man may predispose to infection should be considered.
Asparaginase toxicity is reported to be greater in adults than in pediatric patients.
Laboratory Tests
The fall in circulating lymphoblasts often is quite marked; normal or below normal leukocyte counts are noted frequently within the first several days after initiating therapy. This may be accompanied by a marked rise in serum uric acid. The possible development of uric acid nephropathy should be borne in mind. Appropriate preventive measures should be taken, e.g., allopurinol, increased fluid intake, alkalization of urine. As a guide to the effects of therapy, the patient's peripheral blood count and bone marrow should be monitored frequently.
Frequent serum amylase determinations should be obtained to detect early evidence of pancreatitis. If pancreatitis occurs, therapy should be stopped and not reinstituted. Blood sugar should be monitored during therapy with ELSPAR because hyperglycemia may occur.
Drug Interactions
Tissue culture and animal studies indicate that ELSPAR can diminish or abolish the effect of methotrexate on malignant cells. This effect on methotrexate activity persists as long as plasma asparagine levels are suppressed. These results would seem to dictate against the clinical use of methotrexate with ELSPAR, or during the period following ELSPAR therapy when plasma asparagine levels are below normal.
Drug/Laboratory Test Interactions
L-asparaginase has been reported to interfere with the interpretation of thyroid function tests by producing a rapid and marked reduction in serum concentrations of thyroxine-binding globulin within two days after the first dose. Serum concentrations of thyroxine-binding globulin returned to pretreatment values within four weeks of the last dose of L-asparaginase.
Animal Toxicology
A one-month intravenous toxicity study of ELSPAR in dogs at doses of 250, 1000, and 2000 I.U./kg/day revealed reduced serum total protein and albumin with loss of body weight at the highest dose level and anorexia, emesis, and diarrhea at all dosage levels. A similar study in monkeys at doses of 100, 300, and 1000 I.U./kg/day also revealed reduction of serum total protein and albumin and body weight loss at all dosage levels. Bromsulfalein retention and fatty changes in the liver were noted in monkeys that were given 300 and 1000 I.U./kg/day. The rabbit was unusually sensitive to ELSPAR since a single intravenous dose of 1000 I.U./kg caused hypocalcemia associated with necrosis of the parathyroid cells, convulsions, and death in about one third of the animals. Some rabbits that died showed small thymic and lymph node hemorrhages and necrosis of the germinal centers in the lymph nodes and spleen. The intravenous administration of calcium gluconate alleviated or prevented the adverse effects.
Changes in the pancreatic islets (not pancreatitis) ranging from edema to necrosis were observed in the rabbits in the acute intravenous toxicity studies (doses of 12,500 to 50,000 I.U./kg) but not in rabbits that received 1000 I.U./kg. The anatomical changes and the hypocalcemia found in the rabbits were not observed in the subacute intravenous studies in the dogs and monkeys.
Carcinogenesis, Mutagenesis, Impairment of Fertility
The intraperitoneal injection of 2500 I.U./kg/ day for 4 days in newborn Swiss mice resulted in a small increase in pulmonary adenomas; lymphatic leukemia was not increased. L-asparaginase at concentrations of 152-909 I.U./plate was not mutagenic in the Ames microbial mutagen test with or without metabolic activation.
There are no adequate studies on the effects of asparaginase on fertility.
Pregnancy
Pregnancy Category C. In mice and rats ELSPAR has been shown to retard the weight gain of mothers and fetuses when given in doses of more than 1000 I.U./kg (the recommended human dose). Resorptions, gross abnormalities and skeletal abnormalities were observed. The intravenous administration of 50 or 100 I.U./kg (one-twentieth or one-tenth of the human dose) to pregnant rabbits on Day 8 and 9 of gestation resulted in dose dependent embryotoxicity and gross abnormalities. There are no adequate and well-controlled studies in pregnant women. ELSPAR should be used during pregnancy only if the potential benefit justifies the potential risk to the fetus.
Nursing Mothers
It is not known whether this drug is secreted in human milk. Because many drugs are secreted in human milk and because of the potential for serious adverse reactions in nursing infants from ELSPAR, a decision should be made whether to discontinue nursing or to discontinue the drug, taking into account the importance of the drug to the mother.
Pediatric Use
Asparaginase toxicity is reported to be greater in adults than in pediatric patients.

ADVERSE REACTIONS

Allergic reactions, including skin rashes, urticaria, arthralgia, respiratory distress, and acute anaphylaxis have been reported. (See WARNINGS.) Acute reactions have occurred in the absence of a positive skin test and during continued maintenance of therapeutic serum levels of ELSPAR.
In pediatric patients with advanced leukemia, a lower incidence of anaphylaxis has been reported with intramuscular administration, although there was a higher incidence of milder hypersensitivity reactions than with intravenous administration.
Fatal hyperthermia has been reported.
Pancreatitis, sometimes fulminant and fatal, has occurred during or following therapy with ELSPAR.
Hyperglycemia with glucosuria and polyuria has been reported in low incidence. Serum and urine acetone usually have been absent or negligible in these patients; this syndrome thus resembles hyperosmolar, nonketotic, hyperglycemia induced by a variety of other agents. This complication usually responds to discontinuance of ELSPAR, judicious use of intravenous fluid, and insulin, but may be fatal on occasion.
In addition to hypofibrinogenemia, depression of various other clotting factors has been reported. Most marked has been a decrease in plasma levels of factors V and VIII with a variable decrease in factors VII and IX. A decrease in circulating platelets has occurred in low incidence which, together with the increased levels of fibrin degradation products in the serum, may indicate development of a consumption coagulopathy. Bleeding has been a problem in only a

Continued on next page

Information on the Merck & Co., Inc. products listed on these pages is the full prescribing information from product circulars in use September 30, 2000. For information, please call 1-800-NSC MERCK [1-800-672-6372].

Elspar—Cont.

minority of patients with demonstrable coagulopathy. However, intracranial hemorrhage and fatal bleeding associated with low fibrinogen levels have been reported. Increased fibrinolytic activity, apparently compensatory in nature, also has occurred.
Some patients have shown central nervous system effects consisting of depression, somnolence, fatigue, coma, confusion, agitation, and hallucinations varying from mild to severe. Rarely, a Parkinson-like syndrome has occurred, with tremor and a progressive increase in muscular tone. These side effects usually have reversed spontaneously after treatment was stopped. Therapy with ELSPAR is associated with an increase in blood ammonia during the conversion of asparagine to aspartic acid by the enzyme. No clear correlation exists between the degree of elevation of blood ammonia levels and the appearance of CNS changes. Chills, fever, nausea, vomiting, anorexia, abdominal cramps, weight loss, headache, and irritability may occur and usually are mild. Azotemia, usually pre-renal, occurs frequently. Acute renal shut down and fatal renal insufficiency have been reported during treatment. Proteinuria has occurred infrequently.
A variety of liver function abnormalities have been reported, including elevations of AST (SGOT), ALT (SGPT), alkaline phosphatase, bilirubin (direct and indirect), and depression of serum albumin, cholesterol (total and esters), and plasma fibrinogen. Increases and decreases of total lipids have occurred. Marked hypoalbuminemia associated with peripheral edema has been reported. However, these abnormalities usually are reversible on discontinuance of therapy and some reversal may occur during the course of therapy. Fatty changes in the liver have been documented by biopsy. Malabsorption syndrome has been reported.
Rarely, transient bone marrow depression has been observed, as evidenced by a delay in return of hemoglobin or hematocrit levels to normal in patients undergoing hematologic remission of leukemia. Marked leukopenia has been reported.

OVERDOSAGE

The acute intravenous LD_{50} of ELSPAR for mice was about 500,000 I.U./kg and for rabbits about 22,000 I.U./kg.

DOSAGE AND ADMINISTRATION

This drug has various toxic properties, therefore, both powder and solution must be handled and administered with care. Special handling procedures should be reviewed prior to handling and followed diligently. Inhalation of dust or vapors and contact with skin or mucous membranes, especially those of the eyes, must be avoided. Appropriate protective equipment should be worn when handling ELSPAR. Should accidental eye contact occur, copious irrigation for at least 15 minutes with water, normal saline or a balanced salt ophthalmic irrigating solution should be instituted immediately, followed by prompt ophthalmologic consultation. Should accidental skin contact occur, the affected part should be washed immediately with soap and water. Medical attention should be sought. If inhaled, remove from exposure and seek medical attention. (See DIRECTIONS FOR RECONSTITUTION, *Special Handling*.)
As a component of selected multiple agent induction regimens, ELSPAR may be administered by either the intravenous or the intramuscular route. When administered intravenously this enzyme should be given over a period of not less than thirty minutes through the side arm of an already running infusion of Sodium Chloride Injection or Dextrose Injection 5% (D_5W). ELSPAR has little tendency to cause phlebitis when given intravenously. Anaphylactic reactions require the immediate use of epinephrine, oxygen, and intravenous steroids.
When administering ELSPAR intramuscularly, the volume at a single injection site should be limited to 2 ml. If a volume greater than 2 ml is to be administered, two injection sites should be used.
Unfavorable interactions of ELSPAR with some antitumor agents have been demonstrated. It is recommended therefore, that ELSPAR be used in combination regimens only by physicians familiar with the benefits and risks of a given regimen. During the period of its inhibition of protein synthesis and cell replication ELSPAR may interfere with the action of drugs such as methotrexate which require cell replication for their lethal effect. ELSPAR may interfere with the enzymatic detoxification of other drugs, particularly in the liver.
Recommended Induction Regimens:
When using chemotherapeutic agents in combination for the induction of remissions in patients with acute lymphocytic leukemia, regimens are sought which provide maximum chance of success while avoiding excessive cumulative toxicity or negative drug interactions.
One of the following combination regimens incorporating ELSPAR is recommended for acute lymphocytic leukemia in pediatric patients:
In the regimens below, Day 1 is considered to be the first day of therapy.
Regimen I
Prednisone 40 mg/square meter of body surface area per day orally in three divided doses for 15 days, followed by tapering of the dosage as follows: 20 mg/square meter for 2 days, 10 mg/square meter for 2 days, 5 mg/square meter for 2 days, 2.5 mg/square meter for 2 days and then discontinue.
Vincristine sulfate 2 mg/square meter of body surface area intravenously once weekly on Days 1, 8, and 15 of the treatment period. The maximum single dose should not exceed 2.0 mg.
Asparaginase 1,000 I.U./kg/day intravenously for ten successive days beginning on Day 22 of the treatment period.
Regimen II
Prednisone 40 mg/square meter of body surface area per day orally in three divided doses for 28 days (the total daily dose should be to the nearest 2.5 mg), following which the dosage of prednisone should be discontinued gradually over a 14 day period.
Vincristine sulfate 1.5 mg/square meter of body surface area intravenously weekly for four doses, on Days 1, 8, 15, and 22 of the treatment period. The maximum single dose should not exceed 2.0 mg.
Asparaginase 6,000 I.U./square meter of body surface area intramuscularly on Days 4, 7, 10, 13, 16, 19, 22, 25, and 28 of the treatment period. When a remission is obtained with either of the above regimens, appropriate maintenance therapy must be instituted. ELSPAR should not be used as part of a maintenance regimen. The above regimens do not preclude a need for special therapy directed toward the prevention of central nervous system leukemia.
It should be noted that ELSPAR has been used in combination regimens other than those recommended above. It is important to keep in mind that ELSPAR administered intravenously concurrently with or immediately before a course of vincristine and prednisone may be associated with increased toxicity. Physicians using a given regimen should be thoroughly familiar with its benefits and risks. Clinical data are insufficient for a recommendation concerning the use of combination regimens in adults. Asparaginase toxicity is reported to be greater in adults than in pediatric patients.
Use of ELSPAR as the sole induction agent should be undertaken only in an unusual situation when a combined regimen is inappropriate because of toxicity or other specific patient-related factors, or in cases refractory to other therapy. When ELSPAR is to be used as the sole induction agent for pediatric patients or adults the recommended dosage regimen is 200 I.U./kg/ day intravenously for 28 days. When complete remissions were obtained with this regimen, they were of short duration, 1 to 3 months. ELSPAR has been used as the sole induction agent in other regimens. Physicians using a given regimen should be thoroughly familiar with its benefits and risks.
Patients undergoing induction therapy must be carefully monitored and the therapeutic regimen adjusted according to response and toxicity.
Such adjustments should always involve decreasing dosages of one or more agents or discontinuation depending on the degree of toxicity. Patients who have received a course of ELSPAR, if retreated, have an increased risk of hypersensitivity reactions. Therefore, retreatment should be undertaken only when the benefit of such therapy is weighed against the increased risk.
Intradermal Skin Test:
Because of the occurrence of allergic reactions, an intradermal skin test should be performed prior to the initial administration of ELSPAR and when ELSPAR is given after an interval of a week or more has elapsed between doses. The skin test solution may be prepared as follows: Reconstitute the contents of a 10,000 I.U. vial with 5.0 ml of diluent. From this solution (2,000 I.U./ml) withdraw 0.1 ml and inject it into another vial containing 9.9 ml of diluent, yielding a skin test solution of approximately 20.0 I.U./ml. Use 0.1 ml of this solution (about 2.0 I.U.) for the intradermal skin test. The skin test site should be observed for at least one hour for the appearance of a wheal or erythema either of which indicates a positive reaction. An allergic reaction even to the skin test dose in certain sensitized individuals may rarely occur. A negative skin test reaction does not preclude the possibility of the development of an allergic reaction.

Desensitization:
Desensitization should be performed before administering the first dose of ELSPAR on initiation of therapy in positive reactors, and on retreatment of any patient in whom such therapy is deemed necessary after carefully weighing the increased risk of hypersensitivity reactions. Rapid desensitization of the patient may be attempted with progressively increasing amounts of intravenously administered ELSPAR provided adequate precautions are taken to treat an acute allergic reaction should it occur. One reported schedule begins with a total of 1 I.U. given intravenously and doubles the dose every 10 minutes, provided no reaction has occurred, until the accumulated total amount given equals the planned doses for that day.
For convenience the following table is included to calculate the number of doses necessary to reach the patient's total dose for that day:

Injection Number	ELSPAR Dose in I.U.	Accumulated Total Dose
1	1	1
2	2	3
3	4	7
4	8	15
5	16	31
6	32	63
7	64	127
8	128	255
9	256	511
10	512	1023
11	1024	2047
12	2048	4095
13	4096	8191
14	8192	16383
15	16384	32767
16	32768	65535
17	65536	131071
18	131072	262143

For example: A patient weighing 20 kg who is to receive 200 I.U./kg (total dose 4000 I.U.) would receive injections 1 through 12 during desensitization.

DIRECTIONS FOR RECONSTITUTION

This drug has various toxic properties, therefore, both powder and solution must be handled and administered with care. (See *Special Handling*.) Inhalation of dust or vapors and contact with skin or mucous membranes, especially those of the eyes, must be avoided. Appropriate protective equipment should be worn when handling ELSPAR. (See *Special Handling*.)
Parenteral drug products should be inspected visually for particulate matter and discoloration prior to administration whenever solution and container permit. When reconstituted, ELSPAR should be a clear, colorless solution. If the solution becomes cloudy, discard.
For Intravenous Use
Reconstitute with Sterile Water for Injection or with Sodium Chloride Injection. The volume recommended for reconstitution is 5 ml for the 10,000 unit vials. Ordinary shaking during reconstitution does not inactivate the enzyme. This solution may be used for direct intravenous administration within an eight hour period following restoration. For administration by infusion, solutions should be diluted with the isotonic solutions, Sodium Chloride Injection or Dextrose Injection 5%. These solutions should be infused within eight hours and only if clear.
Occasionally, a very small number of gelatinous fiber-like particles may develop on standing. Filtration through a 5.0 micron filter during administration will remove the particles with no resultant loss in potency. Some loss of potency has been observed with the use of a 0.2 micron filter.
For Intramuscular Use
When ELSPAR is administered intramuscularly according to the schedule cited in the induction regimen, reconstitution is carried out by adding 2 ml Sodium Chloride Injection to the 10,000 unit vial. The resulting solution should be used within eight hours and only if clear.
Special Handling
L-asparaginase may be irritating to eyes, skin and the upper respiratory tract. It has also been shown to be embryotoxic and teratogenic by the intravenous route in animal studies. Due to the drug's toxic properties, appropriate precautions including the use of appropriate safety equipment are recommended for the preparation of ELSPAR for administration. Inhalation of dust or vapors and contact with skin or mucous membranes, especially those of the eyes, must be avoided. The National Institutes of Health presently recommends that the preparation of injectable anti-neoplastic drugs should be performed in a Class II laminar flow biological safety cabinet. Personnel preparing drugs of this class should wear chemical resistant, impervious gloves, safety goggles, outer garments and shoe covers. Additional body garments should be used based upon the task being performed (e.g., sleevelets, apron, gauntlets, disposable suits) to avoid exposed skin surfaces and inhalation of vapors and dust. Appropriate techniques should be used to remove potentially contaminated clothing.
Several other guidelines for proper handling and disposal of antineoplastic drugs have been published and should be considered.
Accidental Contact Measures
Should accidental eye contact occur, copious irrigation for at least 15 minutes with water, normal saline or a balanced salt ophthalmic irrigating solution should be instituted immediately, followed by prompt ophthalmologic consultation. Should accidental skin contact occur, the affected part should be washed immediately with soap and water. Medical attention should be sought. If inhaled, remove from exposure and seek medical attention. (See PRECAUTIONS, *General* and DOSAGE AND ADMINISTRATION.)

HOW SUPPLIED

No. 4612 — ELSPAR is a white lyophilized plug or powder supplied as follows:
NDC 0006-4612-00 in a sterile 10 ml vial containing 10,000 I.U. of asparaginase and 80 mg mannitol, an inactive ingredient.
(6505-01-153-9650 10 mL vial).
Storage
Store at 2–8°C (36–46°F). ELSPAR does not contain a preservative. Unused, reconstituted solution should be stored at 2 to 8°C (36 to 46°F) and discarded after eight hours, or sooner if it becomes cloudy.

FLEXERIL® Tablets ℞
(Cyclobenzaprine HCl)

DESCRIPTION

Cyclobenzaprine hydrochloride is a white, crystalline tricyclic amine salt with the empirical formula $C_{20}H_{21}N{\cdot}HCl$ and a molecular weight of 311.9. It has a melting point of 217°C, and a pK_a of 8.47 at 25°C. It is freely soluble in water and alcohol, sparingly soluble in isopropanol, and insoluble in hydrocarbon solvents. If aqueous solutions are made alkaline, the free base separates. Cyclobenzaprine HCl is designated chemically as 3-(5*H* -dibenzo[*a,d*]cyclohepten-5-ylidene)-*N, N* -dimethyl-1-propanamine hydrochloride, and has the following structural formula:

$HCCH_2CH_2N(CH_3)_2 \cdot HCl$

FLEXERIL* (Cyclobenzaprine HCl) is supplied as 10 mg tablets for oral administration.
Tablets FLEXERIL contain the following inactive ingredients: hydroxypropyl cellulose, hydroxypropyl methylcellulose, iron oxide, lactose, magnesium stearate, starch, and titanium dioxide.

*Registered trademark of MERCK & CO., INC.

CLINICAL PHARMACOLOGY

Cyclobenzaprine HCl relieves skeletal muscle spasm of local origin without interfering with muscle function. It is ineffective in muscle spasm due to central nervous system disease.
Cyclobenzaprine reduced or abolished skeletal muscle hyperactivity in several animal models. Animal studies indicate that cyclobenzaprine does not act at the neuromuscular junction or directly on skeletal muscle. Such studies show that cyclobenzaprine acts primarily within the central nervous system at brain stem as opposed to spinal cord levels, although its action on the latter may contribute to its overall skeletal muscle relaxant activity. Evidence suggests that the net effect of cyclobenzaprine is a reduction of tonic somatic motor activity, influencing both gamma (γ) and alpha (α) motor systems.
Pharmacological studies in animals showed a similarity between the effects of cyclobenzaprine and the structurally related tricyclic antidepressants, including reserpine antagonism, norepinephrine potentiation, potent peripheral and central anticholinergic effects, and sedation. Cyclobenzaprine caused slight to moderate increase in heart rate in animals.
Cyclobenzaprine is well absorbed after oral administration, but there is a large intersubject variation in plasma levels. Cyclobenzaprine is eliminated quite slowly with a half-life as long as one to three days. It is highly bound to plasma proteins, is extensively metabolized primarily to glucuronide-like conjugates, and is excreted primarily via the kidneys.
No significant effect on plasma levels or bioavailability of FLEXERIL or aspirin was noted when single or multiple doses of the two drugs were administered concomitantly. Concomitant administration of FLEXERIL and aspirin is usually well tolerated and no unexpected or serious clinical or laboratory adverse effects have been observed. No studies have been performed to indicate whether FLEXERIL enhances the clinical effect of aspirin or other analgesics, or whether analgesics enhance the clinical effect of FLEXERIL in acute musculoskeletal conditions.
Clinical Studies
Controlled clinical studies show that FLEXERIL significantly improves the signs and symptoms of skeletal muscle spasm as compared with placebo. The clinical responses include improvement in muscle spasm as determined by palpation, reduction in local pain and tenderness, increased range of motion, and less restriction in activities of daily living. When daily observations were made, clinical improvement was observed as early as the first day of therapy.
Eight double-blind controlled clinical studies were performed in 642 patients comparing FLEXERIL, diazepam**, and placebo. Muscle spasm, local pain and tenderness, limitation of motion, and restriction in activities of daily living were evaluated. In three of these studies there was a significantly greater improvement with FLEXERIL than with diazepam, while in the other studies the improvement following both treatments was comparable.
Although the frequency and severity of adverse reactions observed in patients treated with FLEXERIL were comparable to those observed in patients treated with diazepam, dry mouth was observed more frequently in patients treated with FLEXERIL and dizziness more frequently in those treated with diazepam. The incidence of drowsiness, the most frequent adverse reaction, was similar with both drugs.
Analysis of the data from controlled studies shows that FLEXERIL produces clinical improvement whether or not sedation occurs.

**VALIUM® (diazepam, Roche)

Surveillance Program
A post-marketing surveillance program was carried out in 7607 patients with acute musculoskeletal disorders, and included 297 patients treated for 30 days or longer. The overall effectiveness of FLEXERIL was similar to that observed in the double-blind controlled studies; the overall incidence of adverse effects was less (see ADVERSE REACTIONS).

INDICATIONS AND USAGE

FLEXERIL is indicated as an adjunct to rest and physical therapy for relief of muscle spasm associated with acute, painful musculoskeletal conditions.
Improvement is manifested by relief of muscle spasm and its associated signs and symptoms, namely, pain, tenderness, limitation of motion, and restriction in activities of daily living.
FLEXERIL (Cyclobenzaprine HCl) should be used only for short periods (up to two or three weeks) because adequate evidence of effectiveness for more prolonged use is not available and because muscle spasm associated with acute, painful musculoskeletal conditions is generally of short duration and specific therapy for longer periods is seldom warranted.
FLEXERIL has not been found effective in the treatment of spasticity associated with cerebral or spinal cord disease, or in children with cerebral palsy.

CONTRAINDICATIONS

Hypersensitivity to the drug.
Concomitant use of monoamine oxidase inhibitors or within 14 days after their discontinuation.
Acute recovery phase of myocardial infarction, and patients with arrhythmias, heart block or conduction disturbances, or congestive heart failure.
Hyperthyroidism.

WARNINGS

Cyclobenzaprine is closely related to the tricyclic antidepressants, e.g., amitriptyline and imipramine. In short term studies for indications other than muscle spasm associated with acute musculoskeletal conditions, and usually at doses somewhat greater than those recommended for skeletal muscle spasm, some of the more serious central nervous system reactions noted with the tricyclic antidepressants have occurred (see WARNINGS, below, and ADVERSE REACTIONS).
FLEXERIL may interact with monoamine oxidase (MAO) inhibitors. Hyperpyretic crisis, severe convulsions, and deaths have occurred in patients receiving tricyclic antidepressants and MAO inhibitor drugs.
Tricyclic antidepressants have been reported to produce arrhythmias, sinus tachycardia, prolongation of the conduction time leading to myocardial infarction and stroke.
FLEXERIL may enhance the effects of alcohol, barbiturates, and other CNS depressants.

PRECAUTIONS

General
Because of its atropine-like action, FLEXERIL should be used with caution in patients with a history of urinary retention, angle-closure glaucoma, increased intraocular pressure, and in patients taking anticholinergic medication.
The elderly may be more at risk for CNS adverse effects such as hallucinations and confusion.
Information for Patients
FLEXERIL may impair mental and/or physical abilities required for performance of hazardous tasks, such as operating machinery or driving a motor vehicle.
Drug Interactions
FLEXERIL may enhance the effects of alcohol, barbiturates, and other CNS depressants.
Tricyclic antidepressants may block the antihypertensive action of guanethidine and similarly acting compounds.
Tricyclic antidepressants may enhance the seizure risk in patients taking tramadol.†

†ULTRAM® (tramadol HCl tablets, Ortho-McNeil Pharmaceutical)

Carcinogenesis, Mutagenesis, Impairment of Fertility
In rats treated with FLEXERIL for up to 67 weeks at doses of approximately 5 to 40 times the maximum recommended human dose, pale, sometimes enlarged, livers were noted and there was a dose-related hepatocyte vacuolation with lipidosis. In the higher dose groups this microscopic change was seen after 26 weeks and even earlier in rats which died prior to 26 weeks; at lower doses, the change was not seen until after 26 weeks.
Cyclobenzaprine did not affect the onset, incidence or distribution of neoplasia in an 81-week study in the mouse or in a 105-week study in the rat.
At oral doses of up to 10 times the human dose, cyclobenzaprine did not adversely affect the reproductive performance or fertility of male or female rats. Cyclobenzaprine did not demonstrate mutagenic activity in the male mouse at dose levels of up to 20 times the human dose.

Pregnancy
Pregnancy Category B: Reproduction studies have been performed in rats, mice and rabbits at doses up to 20 times the human dose, and have revealed no evidence of impaired fertility or harm to the fetus due to FLEXERIL. There are, however, no adequate and well-controlled studies in pregnant women. Because animal reproduction studies are not always predictive of human response, this drug should be used during pregnancy only if clearly needed.
Nursing Mothers
It is not known whether this drug is excreted in human milk. Because cyclobenzaprine is closely related to the tricyclic antidepressants, some of which are known to be excreted in human milk, caution should be exercised when FLEXERIL is administered to a nursing woman.
Pediatric Use
Safety and effectiveness of FLEXERIL in pediatric patients below 15 years of age have not been established.

ADVERSE REACTIONS

The following list of adverse reactions is based on the experience in 473 patients treated with FLEXERIL in controlled clinical studies, 7607 patients in the post-marketing surveillance program, and reports received since the drug was marketed. The overall incidence of adverse reactions among patients in the surveillance program was less than the incidence in the controlled clinical studies.
The adverse reactions reported most frequently with FLEXERIL were drowsiness, dry mouth and dizziness. The incidence of these common adverse reactions was lower in the surveillance program than in the controlled clinical studies:

	Clinical Studies	*Surveillance Program*
drowsiness	39%	16%
dry mouth	27%	7%
dizziness	11%	3%

Among the less frequent adverse reactions, there was no appreciable difference in incidence in controlled clinical studies or in the surveillance program. Adverse reactions which were reported in 1% to 3% of the patients were: fatigue/tiredness, asthenia, nausea, constipation, dyspepsia, unpleasant taste, blurred vision, headache, nervousness, and confusion.

Incidence Less Than 1 in 100

The following adverse reactions have been reported at an incidence of less than 1 in 100:
Body as a Whole: Syncope; malaise.
Cardiovascular: Tachycardia; arrhythmia; vasodilatation; palpitation; hypotension.
Digestive: Vomiting; anorexia; diarrhea; gastrointestinal pain; gastritis; thirst; flatulence; edema of the tongue; abnormal liver function and rare reports of hepatitis, jaundice and cholestasis.
Hypersensitivity: Anaphylaxis; angioedema; pruritus; facial edema; urticaria; rash.
Musculoskeletal: Local weakness.
Nervous System and Psychiatric: Ataxia; vertigo; dysarthria; tremors; hypertonia; convulsions; muscle twitching; disorientation; insomnia; depressed mood; abnormal sensations; anxiety; agitation; abnormal thinking and dreaming; hallucinations; excitement; paresthesia; diplopia.
Skin: Sweating.
Special Senses: Ageusia; tinnitus.
Urogenital: Urinary frequency and/or retention.

Causal Relationship Unknown

Other reactions, reported rarely for FLEXERIL under circumstances where a causal relationship could not be established or reported for other tricyclic drugs, are listed to serve as alerting information to physicians:
Body as a Whole: Chest pain; edema.
Cardiovascular: Hypertension; myocardial infarction; heart block; stroke.
Digestive: Paralytic ileus; tongue discoloration; stomatitis; parotid swelling.
Endocrine: Inappropriate ADH syndrome.
Hematic and Lymphatic: Purpura; bone marrow depression; leukopenia; eosinophilia; thrombocytopenia.
Metabolic, Nutritional and Immune: Elevation and lowering of blood sugar levels; weight gain or loss.
Musculoskeletal: Myalgia.
Nervous System and Psychiatric: Decreased or increased libido; abnormal gait; delusions; aggressive behavior; paranoia; peripheral neuropathy; Bell's palsy; alteration in EEG patterns; extrapyramidal symptoms.
Respiratory: Dyspnea.
Skin: Photosensitization; alopecia.
Urogenital: Impaired urination; dilatation of urinary tract; impotence; testicular swelling; gynecomastia; breast enlargement; galactorrhea.

DRUG ABUSE AND DEPENDENCE

Pharmacologic similarities among the tricyclic drugs require that certain withdrawal symptoms be considered

Continued on next page

Information on the Merck & Co., Inc. products listed on these pages is the full prescribing information from product circulars in use September 30, 2000. For information, please call 1-800-NSC MERCK [1-800-672-6372].

Flexeril—Cont.

when FLEXERIL is administered, even though they have not been reported to occur with this drug. Abrupt cessation of treatment after prolonged administration may produce nausea, headache, and malaise. These are not indicative of addiction.

OVERDOSAGE

Manifestations: High doses may cause temporary confusion, disturbed concentration, transient visual hallucinations, agitation, hyperactive reflexes, muscle rigidity, vomiting, or hyperpyrexia, in addition to anything listed under ADVERSE REACTIONS. Based on the known pharmacologic actions of the drug, overdosage may cause drowsiness, hypothermia, tachycardia and other cardiac rhythm abnormalities such as bundle branch block, ECG evidence of impaired conduction, and congestive heart failure. Other manifestations may be dilated pupils, convulsions, severe hypotension, stupor, and coma.
The acute oral LD_{50} of FLEXERIL is approximately 338 and 425 mg/kg in mice and rats, respectively.
Treatment: Treatment is symptomatic and supportive. Empty the stomach as quickly as possible by emesis, followed by gastric lavage. After gastric lavage, activated charcoal may be administered. Twenty to 30 g of activated charcoal may be given every four to six hours during the first 24 to 48 hours after ingestion. An ECG should be taken and close monitoring of cardiac function must be instituted if there is any evidence of dysrhythmia. Maintenance of an open airway, adequate fluid intake, and regulation of body temperature are necessary.
The intravenous administration of 1-3 mg of physostigmine salicylate is reported to reverse symptoms of poisoning by atropine and other drugs with anticholinergic activity. Physostigmine may be helpful in the treatment of cyclobenzaprine overdose. Because physostigmine is rapidly metabolized, the dosage of physostigmine should be repeated as required, particularly if life-threatening signs such as arrhythmias, convulsions, and deep coma recur or persist after the initial dosage of physostigmine. Because physostigmine itself may be toxic, it is not recommended for routine use.
Standard medical measures should be used to manage circulatory shock and metabolic acidosis. Cardiac arrhythmias may be treated with neostigmine, pyridostigmine, or propranolol. When signs of cardiac failure occur, the use of a short-acting digitalis preparation should be considered. Close monitoring of cardiac function for not less than five days is advisable.
Anticonvulsants may be given to control seizures.
Dialysis is probably of no value because of low plasma concentrations of the drug.
Since overdosage is often deliberate, patients may attempt suicide by other means during the recovery phase. Deaths by deliberate or accidental overdosage have occurred with this class of drugs.

DOSAGE AND ADMINISTRATION

The usual dosage of FLEXERIL is 10 mg three times a day, with a range of 20 to 40 mg a day in divided doses. Dosage should not exceed 60 mg a day. Use of FLEXERIL for periods longer than two or three weeks is not recommended. (See INDICATIONS AND USAGE.)

HOW SUPPLIED

No. 3358—Tablets FLEXERIL, 10 mg, are butterscotch yellow, 5-sided D-shaped, film coated tablets, coded MSD 931 on one side and FLEXERIL on the other. They are supplied as follows:
NDC 0006-0931-68 in bottles of 100
NDC 0006-0931-28 unit dose packages of 100.
Shown in Product Identification Guide, page 323
7897216 Issued December 1999

FOSAMAX® Tablets ℞
(alendronate sodium tablets)

DESCRIPTION

FOSAMAX* (alendronate sodium) is a bisphosphonate that acts as a specific inhibitor of osteoclast-mediated bone resorption. Bisphosphonates are synthetic analogs of pyrophosphate that bind to the hydroxyapatite found in bone.
Alendronate sodium is chemically described as (4-amino-1-hydroxybutylidene) bisphosphonic acid monosodium salt trihydrate.
The empirical formula of alendronate sodium is $C_4H_{12}NNaO_7P_2 \cdot 3H_2O$ and its formula weight is 325.12. The structural formula is:
[See chemical structure at top of next column]
Alendronate sodium is a white, crystalline, nonhygroscopic powder. It is soluble in water, very slightly soluble in alcohol, and practically insoluble in chloroform.
Tablets FOSAMAX for oral administration contain 6.53, 13.05 or 52.21 mg of alendronate monosodium salt trihydrate, which is the molar equivalent of 5.0, 10.0 and 40.0 mg, respectively, of free acid, and the following inactive ingredients: microcrystalline cellulose, anhydrous lactose, croscarmellose sodium, and magnesium stearate. Tablets FOSAMAX 10 mg also contain carnauba wax.

```
              NH2
              |
              CH2
              |
              CH2
        O     |     O
        ||    CH2   ||
HO —    P  —  C  —  P — ONa • 3H2O
        |     |     |
        OH    OH    OH
```

*Registered trademark of MERCK & CO., Inc.

CLINICAL PHARMACOLOGY

Mechanism of Action
Animal studies have indicated the following mode of action. At the cellular level, alendronate shows preferential localization to sites of bone resorption, specifically under osteoclasts. The osteoclasts adhere normally to the bone surface but lack the ruffled border that is indicative of active resorption. Alendronate does not interfere with osteoclast recruitment or attachment, but it does inhibit osteoclast activity. Studies in mice on the localization of radioactive [^{3}H]alendronate in bone showed about 10-fold higher uptake on osteoclast surfaces than on osteoblast surfaces. Bones examined 6 and 49 days after [^{3}H]alendronate administration in rats and mice, respectively, showed that normal bone was formed on top of the alendronate, which was incorporated inside the matrix. While incorporated in bone matrix, alendronate is not pharmacologically active. Thus, alendronate must be continuously administered to suppress osteoclasts on newly formed resorption surfaces. Histomorphometry in baboons and rats showed that alendronate treatment reduces bone turnover (i.e., the number of sites at which bone is remodeled). In addition, bone formation exceeds bone resorption at these remodeling sites, leading to progressive gains in bone mass.
Pharmacokinetics
Absorption
Relative to an intravenous (IV) reference dose, the mean oral bioavailability of alendronate in women was 0.7% for doses ranging from 5 to 40 mg when administered after an overnight fast and two hours before a standardized breakfast. Oral bioavailability of the 10 mg tablet in men (0.59%) was similar to that in women (0.78%) when administered after an overnight fast and 2 hours before breakfast.
A study examining the effect of timing of a meal on the bioavailability of alendronate was performed in 49 postmenopausal women. Bioavailability was decreased (by approximately 40%) when 10 mg alendronate was administered either 0.5 or 1 hour before a standardized breakfast, when compared to dosing 2 hours before eating. In studies of treatment and prevention of osteoporosis, alendronate was effective when administered at least 30 minutes before breakfast.
Bioavailability was negligible whether alendronate was administered with or up to two hours after a standardized breakfast. Concomitant administration of alendronate with coffee or orange juice reduced bioavailability by approximately 60%.
Distribution
Preclinical studies (in male rats) show that alendronate transiently distributes to soft tissues following 1 mg/kg IV administration but is then rapidly redistributed to bone or excreted in the urine. The mean steady-state volume of distribution, exclusive of bone, is at least 28 L in humans. Concentrations of drug in plasma following therapeutic oral doses are too low (less than 5 ng/mL) for analytical detection. Protein binding in human plasma is approximately 78%.
Metabolism
There is no evidence that alendronate is metabolized in animals or humans.
Excretion
Following a single IV dose of [^{14}C]alendronate, approximately 50% of the radioactivity was excreted in the urine within 72 hours and little or no radioactivity was recovered in the feces. Following a single 10 mg IV dose, the renal clearance of alendronate was 71 mL/min, and systemic clearance did not exceed 200 mL/min. Plasma concentrations fell by more than 95% within 6 hours following IV administration. The terminal half-life in humans is estimated to exceed 10 years, probably reflecting release of alendronate from the skeleton. Based on the above, it is estimated that after 10 years of oral treatment with FOSAMAX (10 mg daily) the amount of alendronate released daily from the skeleton is approximately 25% of that absorbed from the gastrointestinal tract.
Special Populations
Pediatric: Alendronate pharmacokinetics have not been investigated in patients <18 years of age.
Gender: Bioavailability and the fraction of an IV dose excreted in urine were similar in men and women.
Geriatric: Bioavailability and disposition (urinary excretion) were similar in elderly (≥65 years of age) and younger patients. No dosage adjustment is necessary (see DOSAGE AND ADMINISTRATION).
Race: Pharmacokinetic differences due to race have not been studied.
Renal Insufficiency: Preclinical studies show that, in rats with kidney failure, increasing amounts of drug are present in plasma, kidney, spleen, and tibia. In healthy controls, drug that is not deposited in bone is rapidly excreted in the urine. No evidence of saturation of bone uptake was found after 3 weeks dosing with cumulative IV doses of 35 mg/kg in young male rats. Although no clinical information is available, it is likely that, as in animals, elimination of alendronate via the kidney will be reduced in patients with impaired renal function. Therefore, somewhat greater accumulation of alendronate in bone might be expected in patients with impaired renal function.
No dosage adjustment is necessary for patients with mild-to-moderate renal insufficiency (creatinine clearance 35 to 60 mL/min). **FOSAMAX is not recommended for patients with more severe renal insufficiency (creatinine clearance <35 mL/min) due to lack of experience.**
Hepatic Insufficiency: As there is evidence that alendronate is not metabolized or excreted in the bile, no studies were conducted in patients with hepatic insufficiency. No dosage adjustment is necessary.
Drug Interactions (also see PRECAUTIONS, *Drug Interactions*)
Intravenous ranitidine was shown to double the bioavailability of oral alendronate. The clinical significance of this increased bioavailability and whether similar increases will occur in patients given oral H_2-antagonists is unknown.
In healthy subjects, oral prednisone (20 mg three times daily for five days) did not produce a clinically meaningful change in the oral bioavailability of alendronate (a mean increase ranging from 20 to 44%).
Products containing calcium and other multivalent cations are likely to interfere with absorption of alendronate.
[See table below]
Pharmacodynamics
Osteoporosis in postmenopausal women
Osteoporosis is characterized by low bone mass that leads to an increased risk of fracture. The diagnosis can be confirmed by the finding of low bone mass, evidence of fracture on x-ray, a history of osteoporotic fracture, or height loss or kyphosis, indicative of vertebral (spinal) fracture. Osteoporosis occurs in both males and females but is most common among women following the menopause, when bone turnover increases and the rate of bone resorption exceeds that of bone formation. These changes result in progressive bone loss and lead to osteoporosis in a significant proportion of women over age 50. Fractures, usually of the spine, hip, and wrist, are the common consequences. From age 50 to age 90, the risk of hip fracture in white women increases 50-fold and the risk of vertebral fracture 15- to 30-fold. It is estimated that approximately 40% of 50-year-old women will sustain one or more osteoporosis-related fractures of the spine, hip, or wrist during their remaining lifetimes. Hip fractures, in particular, are associated with substantial morbidity, disability, and mortality.
Alendronate is a bisphosphonate that binds to bone hydroxyapatite and specifically inhibits the activity of osteoclasts, the bone-resorbing cells. Alendronate reduces bone resorption with no direct effect on bone formation although the latter process is ultimately reduced because bone re-

Summary of Pharmacokinetic Parameters in the Normal Population

	Mean	90% Confidence Interval
Absolute bioavailability of 5 mg tablet, taken 2 hours before first meal of the day	0.63% (females)	(0.48, 0.83)
Absolute bioavailability of 10 mg tablet, taken 2 hours before first meal of the day	0.78% (females)	(0.61, 1.04)
	0.59% (males)	(0.43, 0.81)
Absolute bioavailability of 40 mg tablet, taken 2 hours before first meal of the day	0.60% (females)	(0.46, 0.78)
Renal Clearance (mL/min) (n=6)	71	(64, 78)

sorption and formation are coupled during bone turnover. Alendronate thus reduces the elevated rate of bone turnover observed in postmenopausal women to approximate more closely that in premenopausal women. Alendronate is not an estrogen and does not have the benefits and risks of estrogen replacement therapy.
Daily oral doses of alendronate (5, 20, and 40 mg for six weeks) in postmenopausal women produced biochemical changes indicative of dose-dependent inhibition of bone resorption, including decreases in urinary calcium and urinary markers of bone collagen degradation (such as deoxypyridinoline and cross-linked N-talopeptides of type I collagen). These biochemical changes tended to return toward baseline values as early as 3 weeks following the discontinuation of therapy with alendronate and did not differ from placebo after 7 months.
Long-term treatment of osteoporosis with FOSAMAX 10 mg/day (for up to five years) reduced urinary excretion of markers of bone resportion, deoxypyridinoline and cross-linked N-talopeptides of type I collagen, by approximately 50% and 70%, respectively, to reach levels similar to those seen in healthy premenopausal women. Similar decreases were seen in patients in osteoporosis prevention studies who received FOSAMAX 5 mg/day. The decrease in the rate of bone resorption indicated by these markers was evident as early as one month and at three to six months reached a plateau that was maintained for the entire duration of treatment with FOSAMAX. In osteoporosis treatment studies FOXAMAX 10 mg/day decreased the markers of bone formation, osteocalcin and bone specific alkaline phosphatase by approximately 50%, and total serum alkaline phosphatase, by approximately 25 to 30% to reach a plateau after 6 to 12 months. In osteoporosis prevention studies FOSAMAX 5 mg/day decreased osteocalcin and total serum alkaline phosphatase by approximately 40% and 15%, respectively. These data indicate that the rate of bone turnover reached a new steady-state, despite the progressive increase in the total amount of alendronate deposited within bone.
As a result of inhibition of bone resorption, asymptomatic reductions in serum calcium and phosphate concentrations were also observed following treatment with FOSAMAX. In the long-term studies, reductions from baseline in serum calcium (approximately 2%) and phosphate (approximately 4 to 6%) were evident the first month after the initiation of FOSAMAX 10 mg. No further decreases in serum calcium were observed for the five-year duration of treatment, however, serum phosphate returned toward prestudy levels during years three through five. Similar reductions were observed with FOSAMAX 5 mg/day. The reduction in serum phosphate may reflect not only the positive bone mineral balance due to FOSAMAX but also a decrease in renal phosphate reabsorption.

Glucocorticoid-induced Osteoporosis

Sustained use of glucocorticoids is commonly associated with development of osteoporosis and resulting fractions (especially vertebral, hip, and rib). It occurs both in males and females of all ages. Osteoporosis occurs as a result of inhibited bone formation and increased bone resorption resulting in net bone loss. Alendronate decreases bone resorption without directly inhibiting bone formation.
In clinical studies of up to two years' duration, FOSAMAX 5 and 10 mg/day reduced cross-linked N-telopeptides of type 1 collagen (a marker of bone resorption) by approximately 60% and reduced bone-specific alkaline phosphatase and total serum alkaline phosphatase (markers of bone formation) by approximatley 15 to 30% and 8 to 18%, respectively. As a result of inhibition of bone resorption, FOSAMAX 5 and 10 mg/day induced asymptomatic decreases in serum calcium (approximately 1 to 2%) and serum phosphate (approximately 1 to 8%).

Paget's disease of bone

Paget's disease of bone is a chronic, focal skeletal disorder characterized by greatly increased and disorderly bone remodeling. Excessive osteoclastic bone resorption is followed by osteoclastic new bone formation, leading to the replacement of the normal bone architecture by disorganized, enlarged, and weakened bone structure.
Clinical manifestations of Paget's disease range from no symptoms to severe morbidity due to bone pain, bone deformity, pathological fractures, and neurological and other complications. Serum alkaline phosphatase, the most frequently used biochemical index of disease activity, provides an objective measure of disease severity and response to therapy.
FOSAMAX decreases the rate of bone resorption directly, which leads to an indirect decrease in bone formation. In clinical trials, FOSAMAX 40 mg once daily for six months produced highly significant decreases in serum alkaline phosphatase as well as in urinary markers of bone collagen degradation. As a result of the inhibition of bone resorption, FOSAMAX induced generally mild, transient, and asymptomatic decreases in serum calcium and phosphate.

Clinical Studies

Treatment of osteoporosis in postmenopausal women

Effect on bone mineral density

The efficacy of FOSAMAX 10 mg once daily in postmenopausal women, 44 to 84 years of age, with osteoporosis (lumbar spine bone mineral density [BMD] of at least 2 standard deviations below the premenopausal mean) was demonstrated in four double-blind, placebo-controlled clinical studies of two or three years' duration. These included two three-year, multicenter studies of virtually identical design, one performed in the United States (U.S.) and the other in 15 different countries (Multinational), which enrolled 478 and 516 patients, respectively. The following graph shows the mean increases in BMD of the lumbar spine, femoral neck, and trochanter in patients receiving FOSAMAX 10 mg/day relative to placebo-treated patients at three years for each of these studies.

Osteoporosis Treatment Studies in Postmenopausal Women

Increase in BMD
FOSAMAX 10 mg/day at Three Years

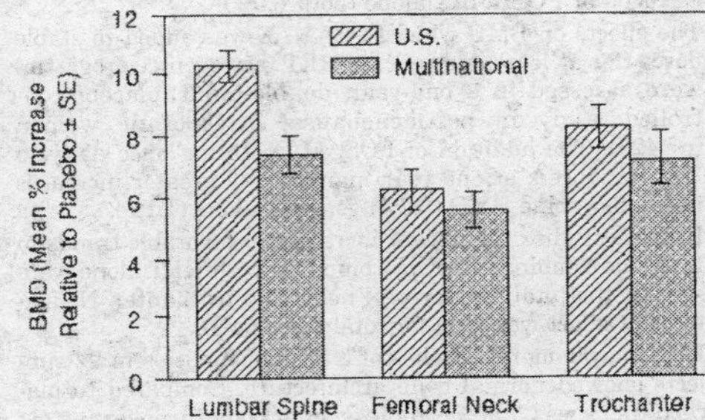

At three years highly significant increases in BMD, relative both to baseline and placebo, were ween at each measurement site in each study in patients who received FOSAMAX 10 mg/day. Total body BMD also increased significantly in each study, suggesting that the increases in bone mass of the spine and hip did not occur at the expense of other skeletal sites. Increases in BMD were evident as early as three months and continued throughout the three years of treatment. (See figures below for lumbar spine results.) In the two-year extension of these studies, treatment of 147 patients with FOSAMAX 10 mg/day resulted in continued increases in BMD at the lumbar spine and trochanter (absolute additional increases between years 3 and 5: lumbar spine, 0.94%; trochanter, 0.88%). BMD at the femoral neck, forearm and total body were maintained. FOSAMAX was similarly effective regardless of age, race, baseline rate of bone turnover, and baseline BMD in the range studied (at least 2 standard deviations below the premenopausal mean). Thus, overall FOSAMAX reverses the loss of bone mineral density, a central factor in the progression of osteoporosis.
[See graphic at top of page]
In patients with postmenopausal osteoporosis treated with FOSAMAX for one or two years, the effects of treatment withdrawal were assessed. Following discontinuation, there were no further increases in bone mass and the rates of bone loss were similar to those of the placebo groups. These data indicate that continuous daily treatment with FOSAMAX is required to maintain the effect of the drug.

Effect on fracture incidence

Data on the effects of FOSAMAX on fracture incidence are derived from three clinical studies: 1) U.S. and Multinational combined: a study of patients with a BMD "T" score at or below minus 2.5 with or without a prior vertebral fracture, 2) Three-Year Study of the Fracture Intervention Trial (FIT): a study of patients with at least one baseline vertebral fracture, and 3) Four-Year Study of FIT: a study of patients with low bone mass but without a baseline vertebral fracture.
To assess the effects of FOSAMAX on the incidence of vertebral fractures (detected by digitized radiography; approximately one third of these were clinically symptomatic), the U.S. and Multinational studies were combined in an analysis that compared placebo to the pooled dosage groups of FOSAMAX (5 or 10 mg for three years or 20 mg for two years followed by 5 mg for one year). There was a statistically significant reduction in the proportion of patients treated with FOSAMAX experiencing one or more new vertebral fractures relative to those treated with placebo (3.2% vs. 6.2%; a 48% relative risk reduction). A reduction in the total number of new vertebral fractures (4.2 vs. 11.3 per 100 patients) was also observed. In the pooled analysis, patients who received FOSAMAX had a loss in stature that was statistically significantly less than was observed in those who received placebo (−3.0 mm vs. −4.6 mm).
The Fracture Intervention Trial (FIT) consisted of two studies in postmenopausal women: the Three-Year Study of patients who had at least one baseline radiographic vertebral fracture and the Four-Year Study of patients with low bone mass but without a baseline vertebral fracture. In both studies of FIT, 96% of randomized patients completed the studies (i.e. had a closeout visit at the scheduled end of the study); approximately 80% of patients were still taking study medication upon completion.

Fracture Intervention Trial: Three-Year Study (patients with at least one baseline radiographic vertebral fracture)

This randomized, double-blind, placebo-controlled, 2027-patient study (FOSAMAX, n=1022; placebo, n=1005) demonstrated that treatment with FOSAMAX resulted in statistically significant reductions in fracture incidence at three years as shown in the table below.
[See table above]

Osteoporosis Treatment Studies in Postmenopausal Women

Time Course of Effect of FOSAMAX 10 mg/day Versus Placebo:
Lumbar Spine BMD Percent Change From Baseline

U.S. Study

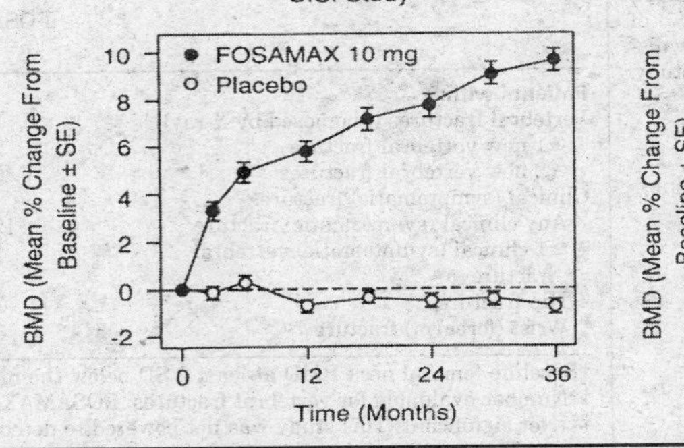

Multinational Study

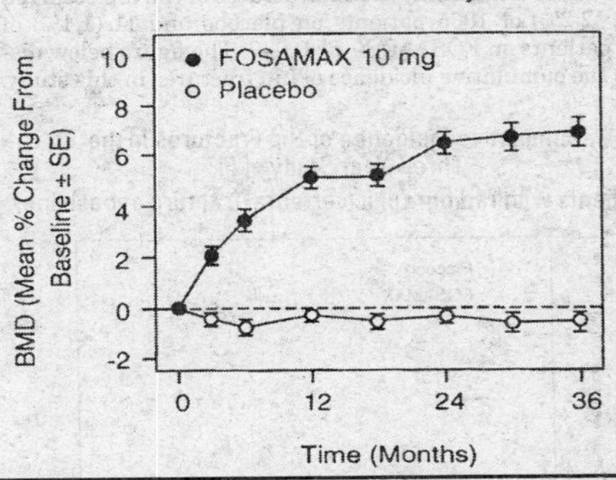

Effect of FOSAMAX on Fracture Incidence in the Three-Year Study of FIT
(patients with vertebral fracture at baseline)

	Percent of Patients		Absolute Reduction in Fracture Incidence	Relative Reduction in Fracture Risk %
	FOSAMAX (n=1022)	Placebo (n=1005)		
Patients with:				
Vertebral fractures (diagnosed by X-ray)†				
≥1 new vertebral fracture	7.9	15.0	7.1	47***
≥2 new vertebral fractures	0.5	4.9	4.4	90***
Clinical (symptomatic) fractures				
Any clinical (symptomatic) fracture	13.8	18.1	4.3	26‡
≥1 clinical (symptomatic) vertebral fracture	2.3	5.0	2.7	54**
Hip fracture	1.1	2.2	1.1	51*
Wrist (forearm) fracture	2.2	4.1	1.9	48*

†Number evaluable for vertebral fractures: FOSAMAX, n=984; placebo, n=966
*$p<0.05$, **$p<0.01$, ***$p<0.001$, ‡$p=0.007$

Continued on next page

Information on the Merck & Co., Inc. products listed on these pages is the full prescribing information from product circulars in use September 30, 2000. For information, please call 1-800-NSC MERCK [1-800-672-6372].

Fosamax—Cont.

Furthermore, in this population of patients with baseline vertebral fracture, treatment with FOSAMAX significantly reduced the incidence of hospitalizations (25.0% vs. 30.7%). In the Three-Year Study of FIT, fractures of the hip occurred in 22 (2.2%) of 1005 patients on placebo and 11 (1.1%) of 1022 patients on FOSAMAX, p=0.047. The figure below displays the cumulative incidence of hip fractures in this study.

Cumulative Incidence of Hip Fractures in the Three-Year Study of FIT (patients with radiographic vertebral fracture at baseline)

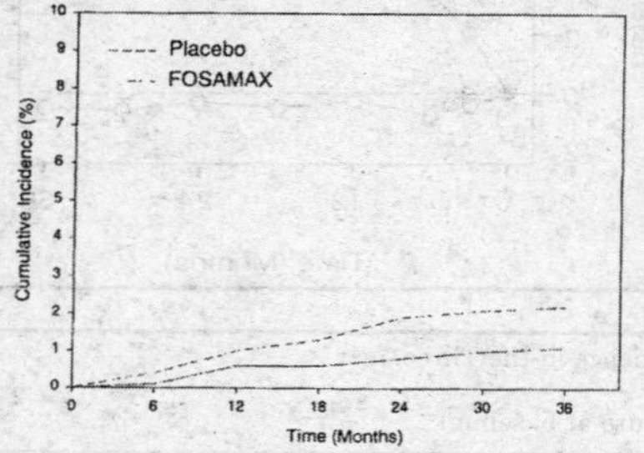

Fracture Intervention trial: Four-Year Study (patients with low bone mass but without a baseline radiographic vertebral fracture)

This randomized, double-blind, placebo-controlled, 4432-patient study (FOSAMAX, n=2214; placebo, n=2218) further investigated the reduction in fracture incidence due to FOSAMAX. The intent of the study was to recruit women with osteoporosis, defined as a baseline femoral neck BMD at least two standard deviations below the mean for young adult women. However, due to subsequent revisions to the normative values for femoral neck BMD, 31% of patients were found not to meet this entry criterion and thus this study included both osteoporotic and non-osteoporotic women. The results are shown in the table below for the patients with osteoporosis.

[See table above]

Fracture results across studies

In the Three-Year Study of FIT, FOSAMAX reduced the percentage of women experiencing at least one new radiographic vertebral fracture from 15.0% to 7.9% (47% relative risk reduction, p<0.001); in the Four-Year Study of FIT, the percentage was reduced from 3.8% to 2.1% (44% relative risk reduction, p=0.001); and in the combined U.S./Multinational studies, from 6.2% to 3.2% (48% relative risk reduction, p=0.034).

FOSAMAX reduced the percentage of women experiencing multiple (two or more) new vertebral fractures from 4.2% to 0.6% (87% relative risk reduction, p<0.001) in the combined U.S./Multinational studies and from 4.9% to 0.5% (90% relative risk reduction, p<0.001) in the Three-Year Study of FIT. In the Four-Year Study of FIT, FOSAMAX reduced the percentage of osteoporotic women experiencing multiple vertebral fractures from 0.6% to 0.1% (78% relative risk reduction, p=0.035).

Thus, FOSAMAX reduced the incidence of radiographic vertebral fractures in osteoporotic women whether or not they had a previous radiographic vertebral fracture.

FOSAMAX, over a three- or four-year period, was associated with statistically significant reductions in loss of height vs. placebo in patients with and without baseline radiographic vertebral fractures. At the end of the FIT studies the between-treatment group differences were 3.2 mm in the Three-Year Study and 1.3 mm in the Four-Year Study.

Bone histology

Bone histology in 270 postmenopausal patients with osteoporosis treated with FOSAMAX at doses ranging from 1 to 20 mg/day for one, two, or three years revealed normal mineralization and structure, as well as the expected decrease in bone turnover relative to placebo. These data, together with the normal bone histology and increased bone strength observed in rats and baboons exposed to long-term alendronate treatment, support the conclusion that bone formed during therapy with FOSAMAX is of normal quality.

Prevention of osteoporosis in postmenopausal women

Prevention of bone loss was demonstrated in two double-blind, placebo-controlled studies of postmenopausal women 40–60 years of age. One thousand six hundred nine patients (FOSAMAX 5 mg/day; n = 498) who were at least six months postmenopausal were entered into a two-year study without regard to their baseline BMD. In the other study, 447 patients (FOSAMAX 5 mg/day; n = 88), who were between six months and three years postmenopause, were treated for up to three years. In the placebo-treated patients BMD losses of approximately 1% per year were seen at the spine, hip (femoral neck and trochanter) and total body. In contrast, FOSAMAX 5 mg/day prevented bone loss in the majority of patients and induced significant increases in mean bone mass at each of these sites (see figures below). In addition, FOSAMAX 5 mg/day reduced the rate of bone loss at the forearm by approximately half relative to placebo. FOSAMAX 5 mg/day was similarly effective in this population regardless of age, time since menopause, race and baseline rate of bone turnover.

[See graphic above]

Effect of FOSAMAX on Fracture Incidence in Osteoporotic† Patients in the Four-Year Study of FIT (patients without vertebral fracture at baseline)

	Percent of Patients			
	FOSAMAX (n=1545)	Placebo (n=1521)	Absolute Reduction in Fracture Incidence	Relative Reduction in Fracture Risk %
Patients with:				
Vertebral fractures (diagnosed by X-ray)††				
≥1 new vertebral fracture	2.5	4.8	2.3	48***
≥2 new vertebral fractures	0.1	0.6	0.5	78*
Clinical (symptomatic) fractures				
Any clinical (symptomatic) fracture	12.9	16.2	3.3	22**
≥1 clinical (symptomatic) vertebral fracture	1.0	1.6	0.6	41 (NS)†††
Hip fracture	1.0	1.4	0.4	29 (NS)†††
Wrist (forearm) fracture	3.9	3.8	−0.1	NS†††

†Baseline femoral neck BMD at least 2 SD below the mean for young adult women
††Number evaluable for vertebral fractures: FOSAMAX, n=1426; placebo, n=1428
†††Not significant. This study was not powered to detect differences at these sites.
*p=0.035, **p=0.01, ***p<0.001

Osteoporosis Prevention Studies in Postmenopausal Women

Change in BMD from Baseline
2 - Year Study

Fosamax 5mg/day
Placebo
BMD (Mean % Change ± SE)
Lumbar Spine, Femoral Neck, Trochanter, Total Body

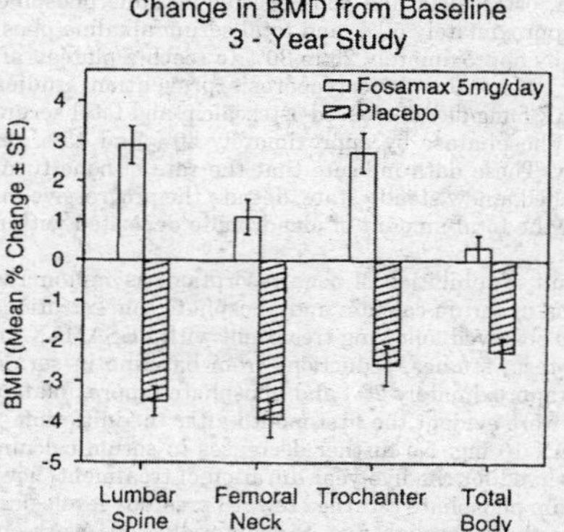

Bone histology was normal in the 28 patients biopsied at the end of three years who received FOSAMAX at doses of up to 10 mg/day.

Concomitant use with estrogen/hormone replacement therapy (HRT)

The effects on BMD of treatment with FOSAMAX 10 mg once daily and conjugated estrogen (0.625 mg/day) either alone or in combination were assessed in a two-year, double-blind, placebo-controlled study of hysterectomized postmenopausal osteoporotic women (n=425). At two years, the increases in lumbar spine BMD from baseline were significantly greater with the combination (8.3%) than with either estrogen or FOSAMAX alone (both 6.0%).

The effects on BMD when FOSAMAX was added to stable doses (for at least one year) of HRT (estrogen ± progestin) were assessed in a one-year, double-blind, placebo-controlled study in postmenopausal osteoporotic women (n=428). The addition of FOSAMAX 10 mg once daily to HRT produced, at one year, significantly greater increases in lumbar spine BMD (3.7%) vs. HRT alone (1.1%).

In these studies, significant increases or favorable trends in BMD for combined therapy compared with HRT alone were seen at the total hip, femoral neck, and trochanter. No significant effect was seen for total body BMD.

Histomorphometric studies of transiliac biopsies in 92 subjects showed normal bone architecture. Compared to placebo there was a 98% suppression of bone turnover (as assessed by mineralizing surface) after 18 months of combined treatment with FOSAMAX and HRT, 94% on FOSAMAX alone, and 78% on HRT alone. The long-term effects of combined FOSAMAX and HRT on fracture occurrence and fracture healing have not been studied.

Glucocorticoid-induced osteoporosis

The efficacy of FOSAMAX 5 and 10 mg once daily in men and women receiving glucocorticoids (at least 7.5 mg/day of prednisone or equivalent) was demonstrated in two, one-year, double-blind, randomized, placebo-controlled, multicenter studies of virtually identical design, one performed in the United States and the other is 15 different countries (Multinational [which also included FOSAMAX 2.5 mg/day]). These studies enrolled 232 and 328 patients, respectively, between the ages of 17 and 83 with a variety of glucocorticoid-requiring diseases. Patients received supplemental calcium and vitamin D. The following figure shows the mean increases relative to placebo in BMD of the lumbar spine, femoral neck, and trochanter in patients receiving FOSAMAX 5 mg/day for each study.

[See figure at top of next column]

After one year, significant increases relative to placebo in BMD were seen in the combined studies at each of these sites in patients who received FOSAMAX 5 mg/day. In the placebo-treated patients, a significant decrease in BMD occurred at the femoral neck (−1.2%), and smaller decreases were seen at the lumbar spine and trochanter. Total body BMD was maintained with FOSAMAX 5 mg/day. The increases in BMD with FOSAMAX 10 mg/day were similar to those with FOSAMAX 5 mg/day in all patients except for postmenopausal women not receiving estrogen therapy. In these women, the increases (relative to placebo) with FOSAMAX 10 mg/day were greater than those with FOSAMAX 5 mg/day at the lumbar spine (4.1% vs. 1.6%) and trochanter (2.8 vs. 1.7%), but not at other sites. FOSAMAX was effective regardless of dose or duration of glucocorticoid use. In addition, FOSAMAX was similarly effective regardless of age (<65 vs. ≥65 years), race (Caucasian vs. other races), gender, underlying disease, baseline BMD, baseline bone turnover, and use with a variety of common medications.

Studies in Glucocorticoid - Treated Patients
Increase in BMD
FOSAMAX 5 mg/day at One Year

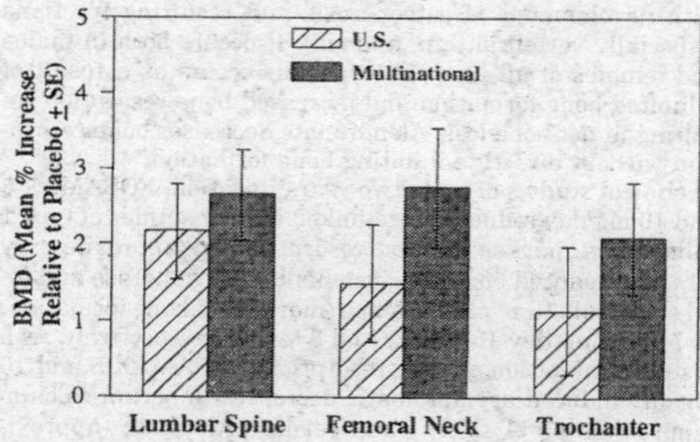

Bone histology was normal in the 49 patients biopsied at the end of one year who received FOSAMAX at doses of up to 10 mg/day.

Of the original 560 patients in these studies, 208 patients who remained on at least 7.5 mg/day of prednisone or equivalent continued into a one-year double-blind extension. After two years of treatment, spine BMD increased by 3.7% and 5.0% relative to placebo with FOSAMAX 5 and 10 mg/day, respectively. Significant increases in BMD (relative to placebo) were also observed at the femoral neck, trochanter, and total body.

After one year, 2.3% of patients treated with FOSAMAX 5 or 10 mg/day (pooled) vs. 3.7% of those treated with placebo experienced a new vertebral fracture (not significant). However, in the population studied for two years, treatment with FOSAMAX (pooled dosage groups: 5 or 10 mg for two years or 2.5 mg for one year followed by 10 mg for one year) significantly reduced the incidence of patients with a new vertebral fracture (FOSAMAX 0.7% vs. placebo 6.8%).

Paget's disease of bone
The efficacy of FOSAMAX 40 mg once daily for six months was demonstrated in two double-blind clinical studies of male and female patients with moderate to severe Paget's disease (alkaline phosphatase at least twice the upper limit of normal): a placebo-controlled multinational study and a U.S. comparative study with etidronate disodium 400 mg/day. The following figure shows the mean percent changes from baseline in serum alkaline phosphatase for up to six months of randomized treatment.

Studies in Paget's Disease of Bone
Effect on Serum Alkaline Phosphatase of FOSAMAX 40 mg/day Versus Placebo or Etidronate 400 mg/day

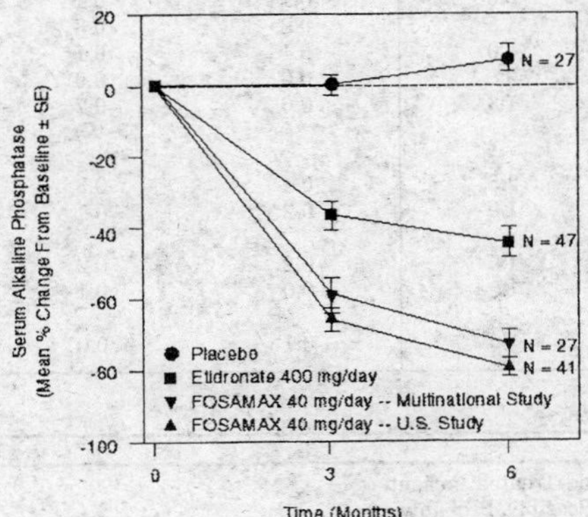

At six months the suppression in alkaline phosphatase in patients treated with FOSAMAX was significantly greater than that achieved with etidronate and contrasted with the complete lack of response in placebo-treated patients. Response (defined as either normalization of serum alkaline phosphatase or decrease from baseline ≥60%) occurred in approximately 85% of patients treated with FOSAMAX in the combined studies vs. 30% in the etidronate group and 0% in the placebo group. FOSAMAX was similarly effective irrespective of age, gender, race, prior use of other bisphosphonates, or baseline alkaline phosphatase within the range studied (at least twice the upper limit of normal).
Bone histology was evaluated in 33 patients with Paget's disease treated with FOSAMAX 40 mg/day for 6 months. As in patients treated for osteoporosis (see *Clinical Studies, Treatment of osteoporosis in postmenopausal women, Bone histology*), FOSAMAX did not impair mineralization, and the expected decrease in the rate of bone turnover was observed. Normal lamellar bone was produced during treatment with FOSAMAX, even where preexisting bone was woven and disorganized. Overall, bone histology data support the conclusion that bone formed during treatment with FOSAMAX is of normal quality.

ANIMAL PHARMACOLOGY

The relative inhibitory activities on bone resorption and mineralization of alendronate and etidronate were compared in the Schenk assay, which is based on histological examination of the epiphyses of growing rats. In this assay, the lowest dose of alendronate that interfered with bone mineralization (leading to osteomalacia) was 6000-fold the antiresorptive dose. The corresponding ratio for etidronate was one to one. These data suggest that alendronate administered in therapeutic doses is highly unlikely to induce osteomalacia.

INDICATIONS AND USAGE

FOSAMAX is indicated for:
- Treatment and prevention of osteoporosis in postmenopausal women
  - For the treatment of osteoporosis, FOSAMAX increases bone mass and reduces the incidence of fractures, including those of the hip and spine (vertebral compression fractures). Osteoporosis may be confirmed by the finding of low bone mass (for example, at least 2 standard deviations below the premenopausal mean) or by the presence or history of osteoporotic fracture. (See CLINICAL PHARMACOLOGY, *Pharmacodynamics*.)
  - For the prevention of osteoporosis, FOSAMAX may be considered in postmenopausal women who are at risk of developing osteoporosis and for whom the desired clinical outcome is to maintain bone mass and to reduce the risk of future fracture.
  Bone loss is particularly rapid in postmenopausal women younger than age 60. Risk factors often associated with the development of postmenopausal osteoporosis include early menopause; moderately low bone mass (for example, at least 1 standard deviation below the mean for healthy young adult women); thin body build; Caucasian or Asian race; and family history of osteoporosis. The presence of such risk factors may be important when considering the use of FOSAMAX for prevention of osteoporosis.
- Treatment of glucorticoid-induced osteoporosis in men and women receiving glucocorticoids in a daily dosage equivalent to 7.5 mg or greater of prednisone and who have low bone mineral density (see PRECAUTIONS, *Glucocorticoid-induced osteoporosis*). Patients treated with glucocorticoids should receive adequate amounts of calcium and vitamin D.
- Treatment of Paget's disease of bone in men and women
  - Treatment is indicated in patients with Paget's disease of bone having alkaline phosphatase at least two times the upper limit of normal, or those who are symptomatic, or those at risk for future complications from their disease.

CONTRAINDICATIONS
- Abnormalities of the esophagus which delay esophageal emptying such as stricture or achalasia
- Inability to stand or sit upright for at least 30 minutes
- Hypersensitivity to any component of this product
- Hypocalcemia (see PRECAUTIONS, *General*)

WARNINGS

FOSAMAX, like other bisphosphonates, may cause local irritation of the upper gastrointestinal mucosa.
Esophageal adverse experiences, such as esophagitis, esophageal ulcers and esophageal erosions, occasionally with bleeding and rarely followed by esophageal stricture, have been reported in patients receiving treatment with FOSAMAX. In some cases these have been severe and required hospitalization. Physicians should therefore be alert to any signs or symptoms signaling a possible esophageal reaction and patients should be instructed to discontinue FOSAMAX and seek medical attention if they develop dysphagia, odynophagia, retrosternal pain or new or worsening heartburn.
The risk of severe esophageal adverse experiences appears to be greater in patients who lie down after taking FOSAMAX and/or who fail to swallow it with a full glass (6–8 oz) of water, and/or who continue to take FOSAMAX after developing symptoms suggestive of esophageal irritation. Therefore, it is very important that the full dosing instructions are provided to, and understood by, the patient (see DOSAGE AND ADMINISTRATION). In patients who cannot comply with dosing instructions due to mental disability, therapy with FOSAMAX should be used under appropriate supervision.
Because of possible irritant effects of FOSAMAX on the upper gastrointestinal mucosa and a potential for worsening of the underlying disease, caution should be used when FOSAMAX is given to patients with active upper gastrointestinal problems, (such as dysphagia, esophageal diseases, gastritis, duodenitis, or ulcers).
There have been post-marketing reports of gastric and duodenal ulcers, some severe and with complications, although no increased risk was observed in controlled clinical trials.

PRECAUTIONS

General
Causes of osteoporosis other than estrogen deficiency, aging, and glucocorticoid use should be considered.
Hypocalcemia must be corrected before initiating therapy with FOSAMAX (see CONTRAINDICATIONS). Other disturbances of mineral metabolism (such as vitamin D deficiency) should also be effectively treated. Presumably due to the effects of FOSAMAX on increasing bone mineral, small, asymptomatic decreases in serum calcium and phosphate may occur, especially in patients with Paget's disease, in whom the pretreatment rate of bone turnover may be greatly elevated and in patients receiving glucocorticoids, in whom calcium absorption may be decreased.
Ensuring adequate calcium and vitamin D intake is especially important in patients with Paget's disease of bone and in patients receiving glucocorticoids.
Renal Insufficiency
FOSAMAX is not recommended for patients with renal insufficiency (creatinine clearance <35 mL/min). (See DOSAGE AND ADMINISTRATION.)
Glucocorticoid-induced osteoporosis
The risk versus benefit of FOSAMAX for treatment at daily dosages of glucocorticoids less than 7.5 mg of prenisone or equivalent has not been established (see INDICATIONS AND USAGE). Before initiating treatment, the hormonal status of both men and women should be ascertained and appropriate replacement considered.
A bone mineral density measurement should be made at the initiation of therapy and repeated after 6 to 12 months of combined FOSAMAX and glucocorticoid treatment.
The efficacy of FOSAMAX for the treatment of glucocorticoid-induced osteoporosis has been shown in patients with a median bone mineral density which was 1.2 standard deviations below the mean for healthy young adults.
The efficacy of FOSAMAX has been established in studies of two years' duration. The greatest increase in bone mineral density occurred in the first year with maintenance or smaller gains during the second year. Efficacy of FOSAMAX beyond two years has not been studied.
The efficacy of FOSAMAX in respect to fracture prevention has been demonstrated for vertebral fractures. However, this finding was based on very few fractures that occurred primarily in postmenopausal women. The efficacy for prevention of non-vertebral fractures has not been demonstrated.
Information for Patients
General
Physicians should instruct their patients to read the patient package insert before starting therapy with FOSAMAX and to reread it each time the prescription is renewed.
Patients should be instructed to take supplemental calcium and vitamin D, if daily dietary intake is inadequate. Weight-bearing exercise should be considered along with the modification of certain behavioral factors, such as cigarette smoking and/or excessive alcohol consumption, if these factors exist.
Dosing Instructions
Patients should be instructed that the expected benefits of FOSAMAX may only be obtained when each tablet is swallowed with plain water the first thing upon arising for the day at least 30 minutes before the first food, beverage, or medication of the day. Even dosing with orange juice or coffee has been shown to markedly reduce the absorption of FOSAMAX (see CLINICAL PHARMACOLOGY, *Pharmacokinetics, Absorption*).
To facilitate delivery to the stomach and thus reduce the potential for esophageal irritation patients should be instructed to swallow FOSAMAX with a full glass of water (6–8 oz) and not to lie down for at least 30 minutes and until after their first food of the day. Patients should not chew or suck on the tablet because of a potential for oropharyngeal ulceration. Patients should be specifically instructed not to take FOSAMAX at bedtime or before arising for the day. Patients should be informed that failure to follow these instructions may increase their risk of esophageal problems. Patients should be instructed that if they develop symptoms of esophageal disease (such as difficulty or pain upon swallowing, retrosternal pain or new or worsening heartburn) they should stop taking FOSAMAX and consult their physician.
Drug Interactions (also see CLINICAL PHARMACOLOGY, *Pharmacokinetics, Drug Interactions*)
Estrogen/hormone replacement therapy (HRT)
Concomitant use of HRT (estrogen ± progestin) and FOSAMAX was assessed in two clinical studies of one or two years' duration in postmenopausal osteoporotic women. In these studies, the safety and tolerability profile of the combination was consistent with those of the individual treatments; however, the degree of suppression of bone turnover (as assessed by mineralizing surface) was significantly greater with the combination than with either component alone. The long-term effects of combined FOSAMAX and HRT on fracture occurrence have not been studied (see CLINICAL PHARMACOLOGY, *Clinical Studies, Concomitant use with estrogen/hormone replacement therapy (HRT)* and ADVERSE REACTIONS, *Clinical Studies, Concomitant use with estrogen/hormone replacement therapy*).
Calcium Supplements/Antacids
It is likely that calcium supplements, antacids, and some oral medications will interfere with absorption of FOSAMAX. Therefore, patients must wait at least one-half hour after taking FOSAMAX before taking any other oral medications.
Aspirin
In clinical studies, the incidence of upper gastrointestinal adverse events was increased in patients receiving concomitant therapy with doses of FOSAMAX greater than 10 mg/day and aspirin-containing products.
Nonsteroidal Anti-Inflammatory Drugs (NSAIDs)
FOSAMAX may be administered to patients taking NSAIDs. In a 3-year, controlled, clinical study (n = 2207) during which a majority of patients received concomitant NSAIDs, the incidence of upper gastrointestinal adverse events was similar in patients taking FOSAMAX 5 or 10 mg compared to those taking placebo. However, since NSAID use is associated with gastrointestinal irritation, caution should be used during concomitant use with FOSAMAX.
Carcinogenesis, Mutagenesis, Impairment of Fertility
Harderian gland (a retro-orbital gland not present in humans) adenomas were increased in high-dose female mice (p=0.003) in a 92-week carcinogenicity study at doses of alendronate of 1, 3, and 10 mg/kg/day (males) or 1, 2, and 5 mg/kg/day (females). These doses are equivalent to 0.5 to 4 times the 10 mg human dose based on surface area, mg/m^2. The relevance of this finding to humans is unknown.
Parafollicular cell (thyroid) adenomas were increased in high-dose male rats (p=0.003) in a 2-year carcinogenicity study at doses of 1 and 3.75 mg/kg body weight. These doses are equivalent to 1 and 3 times the 10 mg human dose based on surface area. The relevance of this finding to humans is unknown.
Alendronate was not genotoxic in the *in vitro* microbial mutagenesis assay with and without metabolic activation, in an *in vitro* mammalian cell mutagenesis assay, in an *in vitro* alkaline elution assay in rat hepatocytes, and in an *in vivo* chromosomal aberration assay in mice. In an *in vitro* chro-

Continued on next page

Information on the Merck & Co., Inc. products listed on these pages is the full prescribing information from product circulars in use September 30, 2000. For information, please call 1-800-NSC MERCK [1-800-672-6372].

Fosamax—Cont.

mosomal aberration assay in Chinese hamster ovary cells, however, alendronate was weakly positive at concentrations ≥5 mM in the presence of cytotoxicity.
Alendronate had no effect on fertility (male or female) in rats at oral doses up to 5 mg/kg/day (four times the 10 mg human dose based on surface area).

Pregnancy

Pregnancy Category C:

Reproduction studies in rats showed decreased postimplantation survival at 2 mg/kg/day and decreased body weight gain in normal pups at 1 mg/kg/day. Sites of incomplete fetal ossification were statistically significantly increased in rats beginning at 10 mg/kg/day in vertebral (cervical, thoracic, and lumbar), skull, and sternebral bones. The above doses ranged from 1 times (1 mg/kg) to 9 times (10 mg/kg) the 10 mg human dose based on surface area, mg/m^2. No similar fetal effects were seen when pregnant rabbits were treated at doses up to 35 mg/kg/day (50 times the 10 mg human dose based on surface area, mg/m^2).
Both total and ionized calcium decreased in pregnant rats at 15 mg/kg/day (13 times the 10 mg human dose based on surface area) resulting in delays and failures of delivery. Protracted parturition due to maternal hypocalcemia occurred in rats at doses as low as 0.5 mg/kg/day (0.5 times the recommended human dose) when rats were treated from before mating through gestation. Maternotoxicity (late pregnancy deaths) occurred in the female rats treated with 15 mg/kg/day for varying periods of time ranging from treatment only during pre-mating to treatment only during early, middle, or late gestation; these deaths were lessened but not eliminated by cessation of treatment. Calcium supplementation either in the drinking water or by minipump could not ameliorate the hypocalcemia or prevent maternal and neonatal deaths due to delays in delivery; calcium supplementation IV prevented maternal, but not fetal deaths.
There are no studies in pregnant women. FOSAMAX should be used during pregnancy only if the potential benefit justifies the potential risk to the mother and fetus.

Nursing Mothers

It is not known whether alendronate is excreted in human milk. Because many drugs are excreted in human milk, caution should be exercised when FOSAMAX is administered to nursing women.

Pediatric Use

Safety and effectiveness in pediatric patients have not been established.

Use in the Elderly

Of the patients receiving FOSAMAX in the two large osteoporosis treatment studies, glucocorticoid-induced osteoporosis studies, and Paget's disease studies (see CLINICAL PHARMACOLOGY, *Clinical Studies*), 45%, 37% and 70%, respectively, were 65 years of age or over. No overall differences in efficacy or safety were observed between these patients and younger patients but greater sensitivity of some older individuals cannot be ruled out.

Use in Men

Safety and effectiveness have been demonstrated in clinical studies in men receiving FOSAMAX both for Paget's disease of bone and for treatment of glucocorticoid-induced osteoporosis. However, the safety and effectiveness in men for osteoporosis due to other causes have not been established.

ADVERSE REACTIONS

Clinical Studies

In clinical studies of up to five years in duration adverse experiences associated with FOSAMAX usually were mild, and generally did not require discontinuation of therapy.
FOSAMAX has been evaluated for safety in approximately 6000 postmenopausal women in clinical studies.

Treatment of osteoporosis

In two identically designed, three-year, placebo-controlled, double-blind, multicenter studies (United States and Multinational; n=994), discontinuation of therapy due to any clinical adverse experience occurred in 4.1% of 196 patients treated with FOSAMAX 10 mg/day and 6.0% of 397 patients treated with placebo. In the Fracture Intervention Trial (n=6459), discontinuation of therapy due to any clinical adverse experience occurred in 9.1% of 3236 patients treated with FOSAMAX 5 mg/day for 2 years and 10 mg/day for either one or two additional years and 10.1% of 3223 patients treated with placebo. Discontinuations due to upper gastrointestinal adverse experiences were: FOSAMAX, 3.2%; placebo, 2.7%. In these study populations, 49–54% had a history of gastrointestinal disorders at baseline and 54–89% used nonsteroidal anti-inflammatory drugs or aspirin at some time during the studies. Adverse experiences from these studies considered by the investigators as possibly, probably, or definitely drug related in ≥1% of patients treated with either FOSAMAX or placebo are presented in the following table.
[See first table above]
Rarely, rash and erythema have occurred.
One patient treated with FOSAMAX (10 mg/day), who had a history of peptic ulcer disease and gastrectomy and who was taking concomitant aspirin developed an anastomotic ulcer with mild hemorrhage, which was considered drug related. Aspirin and FOSAMAX were discontinued and the patient recovered.
The adverse experience profile was similar for the 401 patients treated with either 5 or 20 mg doses of FOSAMAX in the United States and Multinational studies. The adverse experience profile for the 296 patients who received continued treatment with either 5 or 10 mg doses of FOSAMAX in the two-year extension of these studies (treatment years 4 and 5) was similar to that observed during the three-year placebo-controlled period. During the extension period, of the 151 patients treated with FOSAMAX 10 mg/day, the proportion of patients who discontinued therapy due to any clinical adverse experience was similar to that during the first three years of the study.

Osteoporosis Treatment Studies in Postmenopausal Women—Adverse Experiences Considered Possibly, Probably, or Definitely Drug Related by the Investigators and Reported in ≥1% of Patients

	United States/Multinational Studies		Fracture Intervention Trial	
	FOSAMAX* % (n = 196)	Placebo % (n = 397)	FOSAMAX** % (n = 3236)	Placebo % (n = 3223)
Gastrointestinal				
abdominal pain	6.6	4.8	1.5	1.5
nausea	3.6	4.0	1.1	1.5
dyspepsia	3.6	3.5	1.1	1.2
constipation	3.1	1.8	0.0	0.2
diarrhea	3.1	1.8	0.6	0.3
flatulence	2.6	0.5	0.2	0.3
acid regurgitation	2.0	4.3	1.1	0.9
esophageal ulcer	1.5	0.0	0.1	0.1
vomiting	1.0	1.5	0.2	0.3
dysphagia	1.0	0.0	0.1	0.1
abdominal distention	1.0	0.8	0.0	0.0
gastritis	0.5	1.3	0.6	0.7
Musculoskeletal				
musculoskeletal (bone, muscle or joint) pain	4.1	2.5	0.4	0.3
muscle cramp	0.0	1.0	0.2	0.1
Nervous System/Psychiatric				
headache	2.6	1.5	0.2	0.2
dizziness	0.0	1.0	0.0	0.1
Special Senses				
taste perversion	0.5	1.0	0.1	0.0

*10 mg/day for three years
**5 mg/day for 2 years and 10 mg/day for either 1 or 2 additional years

One-Year Studies in Glucocorticoid-Treated Patients Adverse Experiences Considered Possibly, Probably, or Definitely Drug Related by the Investigators and Reported in ≥1% of Patients

	FOSAMAX 10 mg/day % (n = 157)	FOSAMAX 5 mg/day % (n = 161)	Placebo % (n = 159)
Gastrointestinal			
abdominal pain	3.2	1.9	0.0
acid regurgitation	2.5	1.9	1.3
constipation	1.3	0.6	0.0
melena	1.3	0.0	0.0
nausea	0.6	1.2	0.6
diarrhea	0.0	0.0	1.3
Nervous System/Psychiatric			
headache	0.6	0.0	1.3

Prevention of osteoporosis

The safety of FOSAMAX in postmenopausal women 40–60 years of age has been evaluated in three double-blind, placebo-controlled studies involving over 1,400 patients randomized to receive FOSAMAX for either two or three years. In these studies the overall safety profiles of FOSAMAX 5 mg/day and placebo were similar. Discontinuation of therapy due to any clinical adverse experience occurred in 7.5% of 642 patients treated with FOSAMAX 5 mg/day and 5.7% of 648 patients treated with placebo. The adverse experiences considered by the investigators as possibly, probably or definitely drug related in ≥1% of patients treated with either FOSAMAX 5 mg/day or placebo are presented in the following table.

Osteoporosis Prevention Studies in Postmenopausal Women
Adverse Experiences Considered Possibly, Probably, or Definitely Drug Related by the Investigators and Reported in ≥1% of Patients

	FOSAMAX 5mg/day % (n=642)	Placebo % (n=648)
Gastrointestinal		
abdominal pain	1.7	3.4
acid regurgitation	1.4	2.5
diarrhea	1.1	1.7
dyspepsia	1.9	1.7
nausea	1.4	1.4

Concomitant use with estrogen/hormone replacement therapy

In two studies (of one and two years' duration) of postmenopausal osteoporotic women (total: n=853), the safety and tolerability profile of combined treatment with FOSAMAX 10 mg once daily and estrogen ± progestin (n=354) was consistent with those of the individual treatments.

Treatment of glucocorticoid-induced osteoporosis

In two, one-year, placebo-controlled, double-blind, multicenter studies in patients receiving glucocorticoid treatment, the overall safety and tolerability profiles of FOSAMAX 5 and 10 mg/day were generally similar to that of placebo. The adverse experiences considered by the investigators as possibly, probably, or definitely drug related in ≥1% of patients treated with either FOSAMAX 5 or 10 mg/day or placebo are presented in the following table.
[See second table above]
The overall safety and tolerability profile in the glucocorticoid-induced osteoporosis population that continued therapy for the second year of the studies (FOSAMAX: n=147) was consistent with that observed in the first year.

Paget's disease of the bone

In clinical studies (osteoporosis and Paget's disease) adverse experiences reported in 175 patients taking FOSAMAX 40 mg/day for 3–12 months were similar to those in postmenopausal women treated with FOSAMAX 10 mg/day. However, there was an apparent increased incidence of upper gastrointestinal adverse experiences in patients taking FOSAMAX 40 mg/day (17.7% FOSAMAX vs. 10.2% placebo). One case of esophagitis and two cases of gastritis resulted in discontinuation of treatment.
Additionally, musculoskeletal (bone, muscle or joint) pain, which has been described in patients with Paget's disease treated with other bisphosphonates, was considered by the investigators as possibly, probably, or definitely drug related in approximately 6% of patients treated with FOSAMAX 40 mg/day versus approximately 1% of patients treated with placebo, but rarely resulted in discontinuation of therapy. Discontinuation of therapy due to any clinical adverse experience occurred in 6.4% of patients with Paget's disease treated with FOSAMAX 40 mg day and 2.4% of patients treated with placebo.

Laboratory Test Findings

In double-blind, multicenter, controlled studies, asymptomatic, mild, and transient decreases in serum calcium and phosphate were observed in approximately 18% and 10%, respectively, of patients taking FOSAMAX versus approximately 12% and 3% of those taking placebo. However, the incidences of decreases in serum calcium to <8.0 mg/dL (2.0 mM) and serum phosphate to ≤2.0 mg/dL (0.65 mM) were similar in both treatment groups.

Post-Marketing Experience

The following adverse reactions have been reported in post-marketing use:
Body as a Whole: hypersensitivity reactions including urticaria and rarely angioedema.

Gastrointestinal: esophagitis, esophageal erosions, esophageal ulcers, rarely esophageal stricture, and oropharyngeal ulceration. Gastric or duodenal ulcers, some severe and with complications have been reported (see WARNINGS, PRECAUTIONS, *Information for Patients*, and DOSAGE AND ADMINISTRATION).
Skin: rash (occasionally with photosensitivity).
Special Senses: rarely uveitis.

OVERDOSAGE

Significant lethality after single oral doses was seen in female rats and mice at 552 mg/kg (3256 mg/m^2) and 966 mg/kg (2898 mg/m^2), respectively. In males, these values were slightly higher, 626 and 1280 mg/kg, respectively. There was no lethality in dogs at oral doses up to 200 mg/kg (4000 mg/m^2).
No specific information is available on the treatment of overdosage with FOSAMAX. Hypocalcemia, hypophosphatemia, and upper gastrointestinal adverse events, such as upset stomach, heartburn, esophagitis, gastritis, or ulcer, may result from oral overdosage. Milk or antacids should be given to bind alendronate. Due to the risk of esophageal irritation, vomiting should not be induced and the patient should remain fully upright.
Dialysis would not be beneficial.

DOSAGE AND ADMINISTRATION

FOSAMAX must be taken *at least* one-half hour before the first food, beverage, or medication of the day with plain water only (see PRECAUTIONS, *Information for Patients*). Other beverages (including mineral water), food, and some medications are likely to reduce the absorption of FOSAMAX (see PRECAUTIONS, *Drug Interactions*). Waiting less than 30 minutes, or taking FOSAMAX with food, beverages (other than plain water) or other medications will lessen the effect of FOSAMAX by decreasing its absorption into the body.
To facilitate delivery to the stomach and thus reduce the potential for esophageal irritation, FOSOMAX should only be swallowed upon arising for the day with a full glass of water (6–8 oz) and patients should not lie down for at least 30 minutes and until after their first food of the day. FOSAMAX should not be taken at bedtime or before arising for the day. Failure to follow these instructions may increase the risk of esophageal adverse experiences (see WARNINGS, PRECAUTIONS, *Information for Patients*).
Patients should receive supplemental calcium and vitamin D, if dietary intake is inadequate (see PRECAUTIONS, *General*).
No dosage adjustment is necessary for the elderly or for patients with mild-to-moderate renal insufficiency (creatinine clearance 35 to 60 mL/min). FOSAMAX is not recommended for patients with more severe renal insufficiency (creatinine clearance <35 mL/min) due to lack of experience.
Treatment of osteoporosis in postmenopausal women (see INDICATIONS AND USAGE)
The recommended dosage is 10 mg once a day.
Prevention of osteoporosis in postmenopausal women (see INDICATIONS AND USAGE)
The recommended dosage is 5 mg once a day.
Safety of treatment or prevention of osteoporosis with FOSAMAX for longer than four years has not been studied; extension studies are ongoing.
Treatment of glucocorticoid-induced osteoporosis in men and women
The recommended dosage is 5 mg once a day, except for postmenopausal women not receiving estrogen, for whom the recommended dosage is 10 mg once a day.
Paget's disease of bone in men and women
The recommended treatment regimen is 40 mg once a day for six months.
Retreatment of Paget's disease
In clinical studies in which patients were followed every six months, relapses during the 12 months following therapy occurred in 9% (3 out of 32) of patients who responded to treatment with FOSAMAX. Specific retreatment data are not available, although responses to FOSAMAX were similar in patients who had received prior bisphosphonate therapy and those who had not. Retreatment with FOSAMAX may be considered, following a six-month post-treatment evaluation period in patients who have relapsed, based on increases in serum alkaline phosphatase, which should be measured periodically. Retreatment may also be considered in those who failed to normalize their serum alkaline phosphatase.

HOW SUPPLIED

No. 3759—Tablets FOSAMAX, 5 mg, are white, round, uncoated tablets with an outline of a bone image on one side and code MRK 925 on the other. They are supplied as follows:
NDC 0006-0925-31 unit-of-use bottles of 30
NDC 0006-0925-58 unit-of-use bottles of 100.
Shown in Product Identification Guide, page 323
No. 3797—Tablets FOSAMAX, 10 mg, are white, oval, wax-polished tablets with code MRK on one side and 936 on the other. They are supplied as follows:
NDC 0006-0936-31 unit-of-use bottles of 30
NDC 0006-0936-58 unit-of-use bottles of 100
NDC 0006-0936-28 unit dose packages of 100
NDC 0006-0936-82 bottles of 1000
NDC 0006-0936-72 carton of 25 UNIBLISTER™ cards of 31 tablets each.
Shown in Product Identification Guide, page 323
No. 3592—Tablets FOSAMAX, 40 mg, are white, triangular-shaped, uncoated tablets with code MRK 212 on one side and FOSAMAX on the other. They are supplied as follows:
NDC 0006-0212-31 unit-of-use bottles of 30.
Storage
Store in a well-closed container at room temperature, 15–30°C (59–86°F).
7957015 Issued November 1999

Patient Information about
FOSAMAX® (FOSS-ah-max) for Osteoporosis
Generic name: alendronate sodium (a-LEN-dro-nate)

Please read this information before you start taking FOSAMAX*. Also, read the leaflet each time you renew your prescription, just in case anything has changed. Remember, this leaflet does not take the place of careful discussions with your doctor. You and your doctor should discuss FOSAMAX when you start taking your medication and at regular checkups.

* Registered trademark of MERCK & CO., Inc.

How should I take FOSAMAX?
These are the important things you must do to help make sure you will benefit from FOSAMAX:
1. **After getting up for the day, swallow your FOSAMAX tablet with a full glass (6–8 oz) of plain water only.**
   Not mineral water
   Not coffee or tea
   Not juice
2. **After swallowing your FOSAMAX tablet do not lie down—stay fully upright (sitting or standing) for at least 30 minutes and until after your first food of the day. Do not chew or suck on a tablet of FOSAMAX.** This will help the FOSAMAX tablet reach your stomach quickly and help reduce the potential for irritation of your esophagus (the tube that connects your mouth with your stomach).
3. **After swallowing your FOSAMAX tablet, wait at least 30 minutes before taking your first food, beverage, or other medication of the day,** including antacids, calcium supplements and vitamins. FOSAMAX is effective only if taken when your stomach is empty.
4. **Do not take FOSAMAX at bedtime or before getting up for the day.**
5. **If you have difficulty or pain upon swallowing, chest pain, or new or worsening heartburn, stop taking FOSAMAX and call your doctor.**
6. Take one FOSAMAX tablet once a day, every day.
7. It is important that you continue taking FOSAMAX for as long as your doctor prescribes it. FOSAMAX can treat your osteoporosis or help you from getting osteoporosis only if you continue to take it.
8. If you miss a dose do not take it later in the day. Continue your usual schedule of 1 tablet once a day the next morning.

What is FOSAMAX?
FOSAMAX is for the treatment or prevention of osteoporosis (thinning of bone) in women after menopause. It reduces the chance of having a hip or spinal fracture.
FOSAMAX is also for the treatment of osteoporosis in both men and women receiving corticosteroid medications (for example, prednisone).
You will find more information about osteoporosis at the end of this leaflet.

How does FOSAMAX work?
FOSAMAX works by:
- Reducing the activity of the cells that cause bone loss
- Decreasing the faster rate of bone loss that occurs after menopause or with use of corticosteroid medications
- Increasing the amount of bone in most patients

These effects are seen as soon as three months after therapy with FOSAMAX has begun. These effects continue as long as you keep taking FOSAMAX. The density of bone is maintained or increased and the bone is less likely to fracture.

Who should not take FOSAMAX?
Patients with:
- Certain disorders of the esophagus (the tube that connects your mouth with your stomach)
- Inability to stand or sit upright for at least 30 minutes
- Low levels of calcium in their blood
- Severe kidney disease
- Allergy to FOSAMAX

Patients who are:
- Pregnant or Nursing
  If you are pregnant or nursing, you should not be taking FOSAMAX. Talk to your doctor.

What other medical problems should I discuss with my doctor?
Talk to your doctor about any:
- Problems with swallowing
- Stomach or digestive problems
- Other medical problems you have or have had in the past

What are the possible side effects of FOSAMAX?
Some patients may develop severe digestive reactions including irritation, inflammation or ulceration (occasionally with bleeding) of the esophagus (the tube that connects your mouth with your stomach). These reactions can cause chest pain, heartburn or difficulty or pain upon swallowing. This may occur especially if patients do not drink a full glass of water with FOSAMAX and/or if they lie down in less than 30 minutes or before their first food of the day. Esophageal reactions may worsen if patients continue to take FOSAMAX after developing symptoms suggesting irritation of the esophagus.
Like all prescription drugs, FOSAMAX may cause side effects. Side effects usually have been mild. They generally have not caused patients to stop taking FOSAMAX. Some patients treated with FOSAMAX experienced abdominal (stomach) pain. This is the most commonly reported side effect. Less frequently reported side effects are:
Nausea, heartburn, irritation or pain of the esophagus (the tube that connects your mouth with your stomach), vomiting, difficulty swallowing, a full or bloated feeling in the stomach, constipation, diarrhea, black and/or bloody stools, stomach or other peptic ulcers (some severe), and gas.
Bone, muscle or joint pain, headache, or an altered sense of taste were also experienced by some patients. Rarely, a rash (occasionally made worse by sunlight) or eye pain have occurred. Allergic reactions such as hives or, rarely, swelling of the face, lips, tongue and/or throat which may cause difficulty in breathing or swallowing have also been reported. Mouth ulcers have occurred when the tablet was chewed or dissolved in the mouth.
Anytime you have a medical problem you think may be related to FOSAMAX, talk to your doctor.

What should I know about osteoporosis?
Normally your bones are being rebuilt all the time. First, old bone is removed (resorbed). Then a similar amount of new bone is formed. This balanced process keeps your skeleton healthy and strong.
Osteoporosis is a thinning and weakening of the bones. It is common in women after menopause. It may also be caused by certain medications called corticosteroids in both men and women. At the start osteoporosis usually has no symptoms, but it can result in fractures (broken bones). Fractures usually cause pain. Fractures of the bones of the spine may not be painful, but over time they cause height loss. Eventually the spine becomes curved and the body becomes bent over. Fractures may happen during normal, everyday activity, such as lifting, or from minor injury that would normally not cause bone to break. Fractures most often occur at the hip, spine, or wrist. This can lead to pain, severe disability, or loss of mobility.

Osteoporosis in women after menopause
Menopause happens when the ovaries stop producing the female hormone, estrogen, or are removed (which may occur, for example, at the time of a hysterectomy). After menopause, bone is removed faster than it is formed, so bone loss occurs and bones become weaker. Therefore, maintaining bone mass is important to keep your bones healthy.

Osteoporosis in men and women caused by corticosteroids
Corticosteroids can cause bone to be removed faster than it is formed, so bone loss occurs and bones become weaker. Therefore, maintaining bone mass is important to keep your bones healthy. It is important to take your corticosteroid medication as recommended by your doctor.

How can osteoporosis be treated or prevented?
- **Medication.**
  Your doctor has prescribed FOSAMAX. FOSAMAX acts specifically on your bones. FOSAMAX is not a hormone and does not have the benefits and risks of estrogen (hormone replacement therapy used in postmenopausal women) elsewhere in your body. In postmenopausal women, either FOSAMAX or estrogen may be used to treat or prevent osteoporosis. You may want to talk to your doctor about these options.
- **Lifestyle changes.**
  In addition to FOSAMAX, your doctor may recommend one or more of the following lifestyle changes:
  - **Stop smoking.** Smoking appears to increase the risk of osteoporosis.
  - **Reduce the use of alcohol.** Too much alcohol appears to increase the risk of osteoporosis and injuries that may cause fractures.
  - **Exercise regularly.** Like muscles, bones need exercise to stay strong and healthy. Exercise must be safe to prevent injuries including fractures. You should consult your doctor before you begin any exercise program.
  - **Eat a balanced diet.** Adequate dietary calcium is important. Your doctor can advise you whether you need to change your diet or take any dietary supplements such as calcium or vitamin D.

This medication was prescribed for your particular condition. Do not use if for another condition or give the drug to others. Keep FOSAMAX and all medicines out of the reach

Continued on next page

Information on the Merck & Co., Inc. products listed on these pages is the full prescribing information from product circulars in use September 30, 2000. For information, please call 1-800-NSC MERCK [1-800-672-6372].

Fosamax—Cont.

of children. If you suspect that more than the prescribed dose of this medicine has been taken, drink a full glass of milk and contact your local poison control center or emergency room immediately. Do not induce vomiting. Do not lie down.

This leaflet provides a summary of information about FOSAMAX. If you have any questions or concerns about either FOSAMAX or osteoporosis, talk to your doctor. In addition, talk to your pharmacist or other health care provider.

7969408 Issued November 1999

HUMORSOL® Sterile Ophthalmic Solution ℞
(Demecarium Bromide)
For Topical Application into the Conjunctival Sac Only

DESCRIPTION

Ophthalmic Solution HUMORSOL* (Demecarium Bromide) is a sterile solution supplied in two dosage strengths: 0.125 percent and 0.25 percent. The inactive ingredients are sodium chloride and water for injection; benzalkonium chloride 1:5000 is added as preservative. Demecarium bromide is a quaternary ammonium compound with a molecular weight of 716.60. Its chemical name is 3,3'-[1,10-decanediylbis [(methylimino)carbonyloxy]] bis [*N,N,N*-trimethylbenzenaminium] dibromide. Its empirical formula is $C_{32}H_{52}Br_2N_4O_4$ and its structural formula is:

*Registered trademark of MERCK & CO., INC.

CLINICAL PHARMACOLOGY

HUMORSOL is a cholinesterase inhibitor with sustained activity. It acts mainly on true (erythrocyte) cholinesterase. Application of HUMORSOL to the eye produces intense miosis and ciliary muscle contraction due to inhibition of cholinesterase, allowing acetylcholine to accumulate at sites of cholinergic transmission. These effects are accompanied by increased capillary permeability of the ciliary body and iris, increased permeability of the blood-aqueous barrier, and vasodilation. Myopia may be induced or, if present, may be augmented by the increased refractive power of the lens that results from the accommodative effect of the drug. HUMORSOL indirectly produces some of the muscarinic and nicotinic effects of acetylcholine as quantities of the latter accumulate.

INDICATIONS AND USAGE

Open-angle glaucoma (HUMORSOL should be used in glaucoma only when shorter-acting miotics have proved inadequate.)
Conditions obstructing aqueous outflow, such as synechial formation, that are amenable to miotic therapy
Following iridectomy
Accommodative esotropia (accommodative convergent strabismus)

CONTRAINDICATIONS

Hypersensitivity to any component of this product.
Because of the toxicity of cholinesterase inhibitors in general, HUMORSOL is contraindicated in women who are or who may become pregnant. If this drug is used during pregnancy, or if the patient becomes pregnant while taking this drug, the patient should be apprised of the potential hazard to the fetus.
Because miotics may aggravate inflammation, HUMORSOL should not be used in active uveal inflammation and/or glaucoma associated with iridocyclitis.

WARNINGS

In patients receiving cholinesterase inhibitors such as HUMORSOL, succinylcholine should be administered with extreme caution before and during general anesthesia.
Because of possible adverse additive effects, HUMORSOL should be administered only with extreme caution to patients with myasthenia gravis who are receiving systemic anticholinesterase therapy; conversely, extreme caution should be exercised in the use of an anticholinesterase drug for the treatment of myasthenia gravis patients who are already undergoing topical therapy with cholinesterase inhibitors.

PRECAUTIONS

General
Gonioscopy is recommended prior to medication with HUMORSOL.
HUMORSOL should be used with caution in patients with chronic angle-closure (narrow-angle) glaucoma or in patients with narrow angles, because of the possibility of producing pupillary block and increasing angle blockage.
When an intraocular inflammatory process is present, the intensity and persistence of miosis and ciliary muscle contraction that result from anticholinesterase therapy require abstention from, or cautious use of, HUMORSOL.
Systemic effects are infrequent when HUMORSOL is instilled carefully. Compression of the lacrimal duct for several seconds immediately following instillation minimizes drainage into the nasal chamber with its extensive absorption surface. Wash the hands immediately after instillation.
Discontinue HUMORSOL if salivation, urinary incontinence, diarrhea, profuse sweating, muscle weakness, respiratory difficulties, shock, or cardiac irregularities occur.
Persons receiving cholinesterase inhibitors who are exposed to organophosphate-type insecticides and pesticides (gardeners, organophosphate plant or warehouse workers, farmers, residents of communities which are undergoing insecticide spraying or dusting, etc.) should be warned of the added systemic effects possible from absorption through the respiratory tract or skin. Wearing of respiratory masks, frequent washing, and clothing changes may be advisable.
Anticholinesterase drugs should be used with extreme caution, if at all, in patients with marked vagotonia, bronchial asthma, spastic gastrointesinal disturbances, peptic ulcer, pronounced bradycardia and hypotension, recent myocardial infarction, epilepsy, parkinsonism, and other disorders that may respond adversely to vagotonic effects.
After long-term use of HUMORSOL, dilation of blood vessels and resulting greater permeability increase the possibility of hyphema during ophthalmic surgery. Therefore, this drug should be discontinued before surgery.
Despite observance of all precautions and the use of only the recommended dose, there is some evidence that repeated administration may cause depression of the concentration of cholinesterase in the serum and erythrocytes, with resultant systemic effects.
There have been reports of bacterial keratitis associated with the use of multiple dose containers of topical ophthalmic products. These containers had been inadvertently contaminated by patients who, in most cases, had a concurrent corneal disease or a disruption of the ocular epithelial surface. (See PRECAUTIONS, *Information for Patients*.)
Information for Patients
Patients should be instructed to avoid allowing the tip of the dispensing container to contact the eye or surrounding structures.
Patients should also be instructed that ocular solutions, if handled improperly, can become contaminated by common bacteria known to cause ocular infections. Serious damage to the eye and subsequent loss of vision may result from using contaminated solutions. (See PRECAUTIONS, *General*.)
Patients should also be advised that if they develop an intercurrent ocular condition (e.g., trauma, ocular surgery or infection), they should immediately seek their physician's advice concerning the continued use of the present multidose container.
The preservative in HUMORSOL, benzalkonium chloride, may be absorbed by soft contact lenses. Patients wearing soft contact lenses should be instructed to wait at least 15 minutes after instilling HUMORSOL before they insert their lenses.
Drug Interactions
See WARNINGS regarding possible drug interactions of HUMORSOL with succinylcholine or with other anticholinesterase agents.
Carcinogenesis, Mutagenesis, Impairment of Fertility
Long-term studies in animals have not been performed to evaluate the effects of HUMORSOL on fertility or carcinogenic potential.
Pregnancy
Pregnancy Category X: See CONTRAINDICATIONS.
Nursing Mothers
It is not known whether this drug is excreted in human milk. Because of the potential for serious adverse reactions in nursing infants from HUMORSOL, a decision should be made whether to discontinue nursing or to discontinue the drug, taking into account the importance of the drug to the mother.
Pediatric Use
The occurrence of iris cysts is more frequent in pediatric patients. (See ADVERSE REACTIONS and DOSAGE AND ADMINISTRATION.)
Extreme caution should be exercised in pediatric patients receiving HUMORSOL who may require general anesthesia (see WARNINGS).
Since HUMORSOL is a potent cholinesterase inhibitor it should be kept out of the reach of children.

ADVERSE REACTIONS

Stinging, burning, lacrimation, lid muscle twitching, conjunctival and ciliary redness, brow ache, headache, and induced myopia with visual blurring may occur.
Activation of latent iritis or uveitis may occur.
As with all miotic therapy, retinal detachment has been reported occasionally.
Iris cysts may form, enlarge, and obscure vision. Occurrence is more frequent in children. The iris cyst usually shrinks upon discontinuance of the miotic. Rarely, the cyst may rupture or break free into the aqueous. Frequent examination for this occurrence is advised.
Lens opacities have been reported in patients on miotic therapy. Routine slit-lamp examinations, including the lens, should accompany prolonged use.
Paradoxical increase in intraocular pressure may follow anticholinesterase instillation. This may be alleviated by pupil-dilating medication.
Prolonged use may cause conjunctival thickening and obstruction of nasolacrimal canals.
Systemic effects, which occur rarely, are suggestive of increased cholinergic activity. Such effects may include nausea, vomiting, abdominal cramps, diarrhea, urinary incontinence, salivation, sweating, difficulty in breathing, bradycardia, or cardiac irregularities. Medical management of systemic effects may be indicated (see TREATMENT OF ADVERSE EFFECTS).

TREATMENT OF ADVERSE EFFECTS

If HUMORSOL is taken systemically by accident, or if systemic effects occur after topical application in the eye or from accidental skin contact, administer atropine sulfate parenterally (intravenously if necessary) in a dose (for adults) of 0.4 to 0.6 mg or more. The recommended dosage of atropine in infants and children up to 12 years of age is 0.01 mg/kg repeated every two hours as needed until the desired effect is obtained, or adverse effects of atropine preclude further usage. The maximum single dose should not exceed 0.4 mg.
The use of much larger doses of atropine in treating anticholinesterase intoxication in adults has been reported in the literature. Initially 2 to 6 mg may be given followed by 2 mg every hour or more often, as long as muscarinic effects continue. The greater possibility of atropinization with large doses, particularly in sensitive individuals, should be borne in mind.
Pralidoxime** chloride has been reported to be useful in treating systemic effects due to cholinesterase inhibitors. However, its use is recommended in addition to and not as substitute for atropine.
A short-acting barbiturate is indicated if convulsions occur that are not entirely relieved by atropine. Barbiturate dosage should be carefully adjusted to avoid central respiratory depression. Marked weakness or paralysis of muscles of respiration should be treated promptly by artificial respiration and maintenance of a clear airway.
The oral LD_{50} of HUMORSOL is 2.96 mg/kg in the mouse.

**PROTOPAM® Chloride (Pralidoxime Chloride). Ayerst Laboratories

DOSAGE AND ADMINISTRATION

HUMORSOL *is intended solely for topical use in the conjunctival sac.*
As HUMORSOL is an extremely potent drug, the physician should thoroughly familiarize himself with its use and the technic of instillation.
The required dose is applied in the conjunctival sac, with the patient supine, care being taken not to touch the cornea with the tip of the OCUMETER* ophthalmic dispenser. *The patient or person administering the medication should apply continuous gentle pressure on the lacrimal duct with the index finger for several seconds immediately following instillation of the drops. This is to prevent drainage overflow of solution into the nasal and pharyngeal spaces, which might cause systemic absorption. Wash the hands immediately after administration.*
HUMORSOL *should not be used more often than directed. Caution is necessary to avoid overdosage.*
Initial titration and dosage adjustments with HUMORSOL must be individualized to obtain maximal therapeutic effect. The patient must be closely observed during the initial period. If the response is not adequate within the first 24 hours, other measures should be considered.
Keep frequency of use to a minimum in all patients, but especially in children, to reduce the chance of iris cyst development (see ADVERSE REACTIONS).
Glaucoma
For initial therapy with HUMORSOL (0.125 percent or 0.25 percent) place 1 drop (children) or 1 or 2 drops (adults) in the glaucomatous eye. A decrease in intraocular pressure should occur within a few hours. During this period, keep the patient under supervision and make tonometric examinations at least hourly for 3 or 4 hours to be sure that no immediate rise in pressure occurs (see ADVERSE REACTIONS).
Duration of effect varies with the individual. The usual dosage can vary from as much as 1 or 2 drops twice a day to as little as 1 or 2 drops twice a week. The 0.125 percent strength used twice a day usually results in smooth control of the physiologic diurnal variation in intraocular pressure. This is probably the preferred dosage for most wide (open) angle glaucoma patients.
Strabismus
Essentially equal visual acuity of both eyes is a prerequisite to the successful treatment of esotropia with HUMORSOL. For initial evaluation it may be used as a diagnostic aid to determine if an accommodative factor exists. This is especially useful preoperatively in young children and in pa-

tients with normal hypermetropic refractive errors. One drop is given daily for 2 weeks, then 1 drop every 2 days for 2 to 3 weeks. If the eyes become straighter, an accommodative factor is demonstrated. This technic may supplement or complement standard testing with atropine and trial with glasses for the accommodative factor.
In esotropia uncomplicated by amblyopia or anisometropia, HUMORSOL may be instilled in both eyes, *not more than 1 drop at a time every day for 2 to 3 weeks,* as too severe a degree of miosis may interfere with vision. Then reduce the dosage to 1 drop every other day for 3 to 4 weeks and re-evaluate the patient's status.
HUMORSOL may be continued in a dosage of 1 drop every 2 days to 1 drop twice a week. (The latter dosage may be maintained for several months.) Evaluate the patient's condition every 4 to 12 weeks. If improvement continues, change the schedule to 1 drop once a week and eventually to a trial without medication. However, if after 4 months, control of the condition still requires 1 drop every 2 days, therapy with HUMORSOL should be stopped.

*Registered trademark of MERCK & CO., INC.

HOW SUPPLIED

Sterile Ophthalmic Solution HUMORSOL is a clear, colorless, aqueous solution and is supplied in a 5 mL white, opaque, plastic OCUMETER ophthalmic dispenser with a controlled-drop tip:
No. 3255—0.125 percent solution.
NDC 0006-3255-03.
No. 3267—0.25 percent solution.
NDC 0006-3267-03.
Storage
Protect from freezing and excessive heat.
7414315 Issued September 1996

HYDROCORTONE® Acetate ℞

Injectable Suspension
(Hydrocortisone Acetate)
(Formerly called Sterile Suspension HYDROCORTONE® Acetate)

For intra-articular, intralesional, and soft tissue injection only.

NOT FOR INTRAVENOUS USE

DESCRIPTION

Hydrocortisone acetate, a synthetic adrenocortical steroid, is a white to practically white, odorless, crystalline powder. It is insoluble in water and slightly soluble in alcohol and chloroform. The molecular weight is 404.50. It is designated chemically as 21-(acetyloxy)-11β,17-dihydroxypregn-4-ene-3,20-dione. The empirical formula is $C_{23}H_{32}O_6$ and the structural formula is:

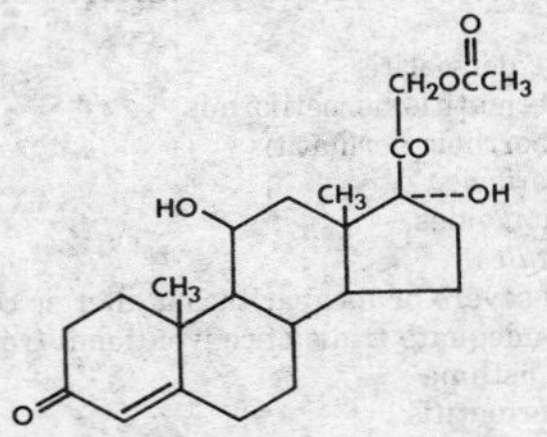

HYDROCORTONE* Acetate (Hydrocortisone Acetate) Injectable Suspension is a sterile suspension containing 50 mg per milliliter of hydrocortisone acetate in a suitable aqueous medium (pH -5.0 to 7.0). Inactive ingredients per mL: sodium chloride, 9 mg; polysorbate 80, 4 mg; sodium carboxymethylcellulose, 5 mg; and Water for Injection, q.s., 1 mL. Benzyl alcohol, 9 mg, added as preservative.

*Registered trademark of MERCK & CO., INC.

ACTIONS

HYDROCORTONE Acetate Injectable Suspension has a slow onset but long duration of action when compared with more soluble preparations. Because of its insolubility, it is suitable for intra-articular, intralesional, and soft tissue injection where its anti-inflammatory effects are confined mainly to the area in which it has been injected, although it is capable of producing systemic hormonal effects.
Naturally occurring glucocorticoids (hydrocortisone and cortisone), which also have salt-retaining properties, are used as replacement therapy in adrenocortical deficiency states. They are also used for their potent anti-inflammatory effect in disorders of many organ systems.
Glucocorticoids cause profound and varied metabolic effects. In addition, they modify the body's immune responses to diverse stimuli.

INDICATIONS

A. By intra-articular or soft tissue injection:
As adjunctive therapy for short-term administration (to tide the patient over an acute episode or exacerbation) in:
Synovitis of osteoarthritis
Rheumatoid arthritis
Acute and subacute bursitis
Acute gouty arthritis
Epicondylitis
Acute nonspecific tenosynovitis
Post-traumatic osteoarthritis
B. By intralesional injection:
Keloids
Localized hypertrophic, infiltrated, inflammatory lesions of: lichen planus, psoriatic plaques, granuloma annulare, and lichen simplex chronicus (neurodermatitis)
Discoid lupus erythematosus
Necrobiosis lipoidica diabeticorum
Alopecia areata
May also be useful in cystic tumors of an aponeurosis or tendon (ganglia).

CONTRAINDICATIONS

Systemic fungal infections
Hypersensitivity to any component of this product

WARNINGS

Because rare instances of anaphylactoid reactions have occurred in patients receiving parenteral corticosteroid therapy, appropriate precautionary measures should be taken prior to administration, especially when the patient has a history of allergy to any drug.
In patients on corticosteroid therapy subjected to any unusual stress, increased dosage of rapidly acting corticosteroids before, during, and after the stressful situation is indicated.
Drug-induced secondary adrenocortical insufficiency may result from too rapid withdrawal of corticosteroids and may be minimized by gradual reduction of dosage. This type of relative insufficiency may persist for months after discontinuation of therapy; therefore, in any situation of stress occurring during that period, hormone therapy should be reinstituted. If the patient is receiving steroids already, dosage may have to be increased. Since mineralocorticoid secretion may be impaired, salt and/or a mineralocorticoid should be administered concurrently.
Corticosteroids may mask some signs of infection, and new infections may appear during their use. There may be decreased resistance and inability to localize infection when corticosteroids are used. Moreover, corticosteroids may affect the nitroblue-tetrazolium test for bacterial infection and produce false negative results.
In cerebral malaria, a double-blind trial has shown that the use of corticosteroids is associated with prolongation of coma and a higher incidence of pneumonia and gastrointestinal bleeding.
Corticosteroids may activate latent amebiasis. Therefore, it is recommended that latent or active amebiasis be ruled out before initiating corticosteroid therapy in any patient who has spent time in the tropics or any patient with unexplained diarrhea.
Prolonged use of corticosteroids may produce posterior subcapsular cataracts, glaucoma with possible damage to the optic nerves, and may enhance the establishment of secondary ocular infections due to fungi or viruses.
Usage in pregnancy: Since adequate human reproduction studies have not been done with corticosteroids, use of these drugs in pregnancy or in women of childbearing potential requires that the anticipated benefits be weighed against the possible hazards to the mother and embryo or fetus. Infants born of mothers who have received substantial doses of corticosteroids during pregnancy should be carefully observed for signs of hypoadrenalism.
Corticosteroids appear in breast milk and could suppress growth, interfere with endogenous corticosteroid production, or cause other unwanted effects. Mothers taking pharmacologic doses of corticosteroids should be advised not to nurse.
Average and large doses of cortisone or hydrocortisone can cause elevation of blood pressure, salt and water retention, and increased excretion of potassium. These effects are less likely to occur with the synthetic derivatives except when used in large doses. Dietary salt restriction and potassium supplementation may be necessary. All corticosteroids increase calcium excretion.
Administration of live virus vaccines, including smallpox, is contraindicated in individuals receiving immunosuppressive doses of corticosteroids. If inactivated viral or bacterial vaccines are administered to individuals receiving immunosuppressive doses of corticosteroids, the expected serum antibody response may not be obtained.
Patients who are on drugs which suppress the immune system are more susceptible to infections than healthy individuals. Chickenpox and measles, for example, can have a more serious or even fatal course in non-immune patients on corticosteroids. In such patients who have not had these diseases, particular care should be taken to avoid exposure. The risk of developing a disseminated infection varies among individuals and can be related to the dose, route and duration of corticosteroid administration as well as to the underlying disease. If exposed to chickenpox, prophylaxis with varicella zoster immune globulin (VZIG) may be indicated. If chickenpox develops, treatment with antiviral agents may be considered. If exposed to measles, prophylaxis with immune globulin (IG) may be indicated. (See the respective package inserts for VZIG and IG for complete prescribing information.)
Similarly, corticosteroids should be used with great care in patients with known or suspected Strongyloides (threadworm) infestation. In such patients, corticosteroid-induced immunosuppression may lead to Strongyloides hyperinfection and dissemination with widespread larval migration, often accompanied by severe enterocolitis and potentially fatal gram-negative septicemia.
If corticosteroids are indicated in patients with latent tuberculosis or tuberculin reactivity, close observation is necessary as reactivation of the disease may occur. During prolonged corticosteroid therapy, these patients should receive chemoprophylaxis.
Literature reports suggest an apparent association between use of corticosteroids and left ventricular free wall rupture after a recent myocardial infarction; therefore, therapy with corticosteroids should be used with great caution in these patients.

PRECAUTIONS

This product, like many other steroid formulations, is sensitive to heat. Therefore, it should not be autoclaved when it is desirable to sterilize the exterior of the vial.
Following prolonged therapy, withdrawal of corticosteroids may result in symptoms of the corticosteroid withdrawal syndrome including fever, myalgia, arthralgia, and malaise. This may occur in patients even without evidence of adrenal insufficiency.
There is an enhanced effect of corticosteroids in patients with hypothyroidism and in those with cirrhosis.
Corticosteroids should be used cautiously in patients with ocular herpes simplex for fear of corneal perforation.
Psychic derangements may appear when corticosteroids are used, ranging from euphoria, insomnia, mood swings, personality changes, and severe depression to frank psychotic manifestations. Also, existing emotional instability or psychotic tendencies may be aggravated by corticosteroids.
Aspirin should be used cautiously in conjunction with corticosteroids in hypoprothrombinemia.
Steroids should be used with caution in nonspecific ulcerative colitis, if there is a probability of impending perforation, abscess, or other pyogenic infection, also in diverticulitis, fresh intestinal anastomoses, active or latent peptic ulcer, renal insufficiency, hypertension, osteoporosis, and myasthenia gravis. Signs of peritoneal irritation following gastrointestinal perforation in patients receiving large doses of corticosteroids may be minimal or absent. Fat embolism has been reported as a possible complication of hypercortisonism.
When large doses are given, some authorities advise that antacids be administered between meals to help to prevent peptic ulcer.
Steroids may increase or decrease motility and number of spermatozoa in some patients.
Phenytoin, phenobarbital, ephedrine, and rifampin may enhance the metabolic clearance of corticosteroids resulting in decreased blood levels and lessened physiologic activity, thus requiring adjustment in corticosteroid dosage.
The prothrombin time should be checked frequently in patients who are receiving corticosteroids and coumarin anticoagulants at the same time because of reports that corticosteroids have altered the response to these anticoagulants. Studies have shown that the usual effect produced by adding corticosteroids is inhibition of response to coumarins, although there have been some conflicting reports of potentiation not substantiated by studies.
When corticosteroids are administered concomitantly with potassium-depleting diuretics, patients should be observed closely for development of hypokalemia.
Intra-articular injection of a corticosteroid may produce systemic as well as local effects.
Appropriate examination of any joint fluid present is necessary to exclude a septic process.
A marked increase in pain accompanied by local swelling, further restriction of joint motion, fever, and malaise is suggestive of septic arthritis. If this complication occurs and the diagnosis of sepsis is confirmed, appropriate antimicrobial therapy should be instituted.
Injection of a steroid into an infected site is to be avoided.
Corticosteroids should not be injected into unstable joints.
Patients should be impressed strongly with the importance of not overusing joints in which symptomatic benefit has been obtained as long as the inflammatory process remains active.
Frequent intra-articular injection may result in damage to joint tissues.
Information for Patients
Susceptible patients who are on immunosuppressant doses of corticosteroids should be warned to avoid exposure to chickenpox or measles. Patients should also be advised that if they are exposed, medical advice should be sought without delay.

Continued on next page

Information on the Merck & Co., Inc. products listed on these pages is the full prescribing information from product circulars in use September 30, 2000. For information, please call 1-800-NSC MERCK [1-800-672-6372].

Hydrocortone Acetate—Cont.

Pediatric Use
Growth and development of pediatric patients on prolonged corticosteroid therapy should be carefully followed.

ADVERSE REACTIONS

Fluid and electrolyte disturbances
Sodium retention
Fluid retention
Congestive heart failure in susceptible patients
Potassium loss
Hypokalemic alkalosis
Hypertension

Musculoskeletal
Muscle weakness
Steroid myopathy
Loss of muscle mass
Osteoporosis
Vertebral compression fractures
Aseptic necrosis of femoral and humeral heads
Pathologic fracture of long bones
Tendon rupture

Gastrointestinal
Peptic ulcer with possible subsequent perforation and hemorrhage
Perforation of the small and large bowel, particularly in patients with inflammatory bowel disease
Pancreatitis
Abdominal distention
Ulcerative esophagitis

Dermatologic
Impaired wound healing
Thin fragile skin
Petechiae and ecchymoses
Erythema
Increased sweating
May suppress reactions to skin tests
Other cutaneous reactions, such as allergic dermatitis, urticaria, angioneurotic edema

Neurologic
Convulsions
Increased intracranial pressure with papilledema (pseudotumor cerebri) usually after treatment
Vertigo
Headache
Psychic disturbances

Endocrine
Menstrual irregularities
Development of cushingoid state
Suppression of growth in children
Secondary adrenocortical and pituitary unresponsiveness, particularly in times of stress, as in trauma, surgery, or illness
Decreased carbohydrate tolerance
Manifestations of latent diabetes mellitus
Increased requirements for insulin or oral hypoglycemic agents in diabetics
Hirsutism

Ophthalmic
Posterior subcapsular cataracts
Increased intraocular pressure
Glaucoma
Exophthalmos

Metabolic
Negative nitrogen balance due to protein catabolism

Cardiovascular
Myocardial rupture following recent myocardial infarction (see WARNINGS)

Other
Anaphylactoid or hypersensitivity reactions
Thromboembolism
Weight gain
Increased appetite
Nausea
Malaise

The following *additional* adverse reactions are related to injection of corticosteroids:
Rare instances of blindness associated with intralesional therapy around the face and head
Hyperpigmentation or hypopigmentation
Subcutaneous and cutaneous atrophy
Sterile abscess
Postinjection flare (following intra-articular use)
Charcot-like arthropathy.

OVERDOSAGE

Reports of acute toxicity and/or death following overdosage of glucocorticoids are rare. In the event of overdosage, no specific antidote is available; treatment is supportive and symptomatic.

DOSAGE AND ADMINISTRATION

NOT FOR INTRAVENOUS USE

For intra-articular, intralesional, and soft tissue injection only

DOSAGE AND FREQUENCY OF INJECTION ARE VARIABLE AND MUST BE INDIVIDUALIZED ON THE BASIS OF THE DISEASE AND THE RESPONSE OF THE PATIENT.

The initial dose varies from 5 to 75 mg depending on the disease being treated and the size of the area to be injected. Frequency of injection depends on symptomatic response, and usually is once every two or three weeks. Severe conditions may require injection once a week. Frequent intra-articular injection may result in damage to joint tissues. If satisfactory clinical response does not occur after a reasonable period of time, discontinue HYDROCORTONE Acetate Injectable Suspension and transfer the patient to other therapy.

Patients should be observed closely for signs that might require dosage adjustment, including changes in clinical status resulting from remissions or exacerbations of the disease, and individual drug responsiveness.

Some of the usual single doses are:

Large Joints (e.g., Knee)	25 mg, occasionally 37.5 mg. Doses over 50 mg not recommended
Small Joints (e.g, Interphalangeal, Temporomandibular)	10 to 25 mg
Bursae	25 to 37.5 mg
Tendon Sheaths	5 to 12.5 mg
Soft Tissue Infiltration	25 to 50 mg, occasionally 75 mg
Ganglia	12.5 to 25 mg

For rapid onset of action, a soluble adrenocortical hormone preparation, such as DECADRON* Phosphate (Dexamethasone Sodium Phosphate) injection or HYDELTRASOL* (Prednisolone Sodium Phosphate) injection, may be given with HYDROCORTONE Acetate Injectable Suspension.

If desired, a local anesthetic may be used, and may be injected before HYDROCORTONE Acetate Injectable Suspension or mixed in a syringe with HYDROCORTONE Acetate Injectable Suspension and given simultaneously.

If used prior to intra-articular injection of the steroid, inject most of the anesthetic into the soft tissues of the surrounding area and instill a small amount into the joint.

If given together, mixing should be done in the injection syringe by drawing the steroid in *first*, then the anesthetic. In this way, the anesthetic will not be introduced inadvertently into the vial of steroid. *The mixture must be used immediately and any unused portion discarded.*

*Registered trademark of MERCK & CO., INC.

HOW SUPPLIED

No. 7519—HYDROCORTONE Acetate Injectable Suspension is a white, mobile suspension, containing 50 mg hydrocortisone acetate in each mL, and is supplied as follows:
NDC 0006-7519-03 in 5 mL vials.

Storage
Sensitive to heat. Do not autoclave.
Protect from freezing.

7348729 Issued February 1997

HYDROCORTONE® Phosphate Injection, Sterile (Hydrocortisone Sodium Phosphate) ℞

DESCRIPTION

Hydrocortisone sodium phosphate, a synthetic adrenocortical steroid, is a white to light yellow, odorless or practically odorless powder. It is freely soluble in water and is exceedingly hygroscopic. The molecular weight is 486.41. It is designated chemically as 11β,17-dihydroxy-21-(phosphonooxy)-pregn-4-ene-3,20-dione disodium salt. The empirical formula is $C_{21}H_{29}Na_2O_8P$ and the structural formula is:

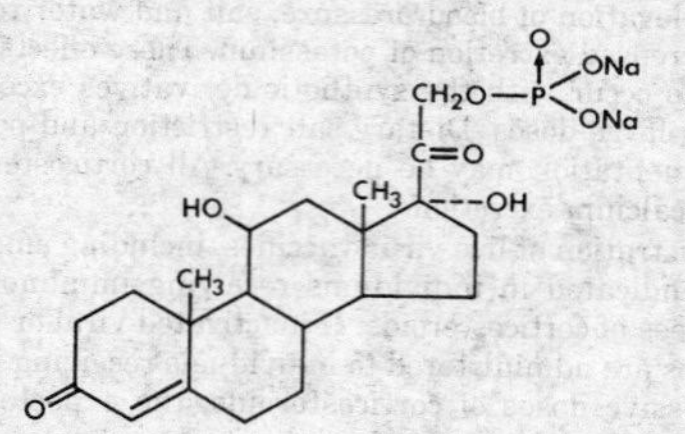

HYDROCORTONE* Phosphate (Hydrocortisone Sodium Phosphate) injection is a sterile solution (pH 7.5 to 8.5), sealed under nitrogen, for intravenous, intramuscular, and subcutaneous administration.

Each milliliter contains hydrocortisone sodium phosphate equivalent to 50 mg hydrocortisone. Inactive ingredients per mL: 8 mg creatinine, 10 mg sodium citrate, sodium hydroxide to adjust pH, and Water for Injection, q.s. 1 mL, with 3.2 mg sodium bisulfite, 1.5 mg methylparaben, and 0.2 mg propylparaben added as preservatives.

*Registered trademark of MERCK & CO., INC.

ACTIONS

HYDROCORTONE Phosphate injection has a rapid onset but short duration of action when compared with less soluble preparations. Because of this, it is suitable for the treatment of acute disorders responsive to adrenocortical steroid therapy.

Naturally occurring glucocorticoids (hydrocortisone and cortisone), which also have salt-retaining properties, are used as replacement therapy in adrenocortical deficiency states. They are also used for their potent anti-inflammatory effects in disorders of many organ systems.

Glucocorticoids cause profound and varied metabolic effects. In addition, they modify the body's immune responses to diverse stimuli.

INDICATIONS

When oral therapy is not feasible:

1. *Endocrine disorders*
Primary or secondary adrenocortical insufficiency (hydrocortisone or cortisone is the drug of choice; synthetic analogs may be used in conjunction with mineralocorticoids where applicable; in infancy, mineralocorticoid supplementation is of particular importance)
Acute adrenocortical insufficiency (hydrocortisone or cortisone is the drug of choice; mineralocorticoid supplementation may be necessary, particularly when synthetic analogs are used)
Preoperatively, and in the event of serious trauma or illness, in patients with known adrenal insufficiency or when adrenocortical reserve is doubtful
Shock unresponsive to conventional therapy if adrenocortical insufficiency exists or is suspected
Congenital adrenal hyperplasia
Nonsuppurative thyroiditis
Hypercalcemia associated with cancer

2. *Rheumatic disorders*
As adjunctive therapy for short-term administration (to tide the patient over an acute episode or exacerbation) in:
Post-traumatic osteoarthritis
Synovitis of osteoarthritis
Rheumatoid arthritis, including juvenile rheumatoid arthritis (selected cases may require low-dose maintenance therapy)
Acute and subacute bursitis
Epicondylitis
Acute nonspecific tenosynovitis
Acute gouty arthritis
Psoriatic arthritis
Ankylosing spondylitis

3. *Collagen diseases*
During an exacerbation or as maintenance therapy in selected cases of:
Systemic lupus erythematosus
Acute rheumatic carditis
Systemic dermatomyositis (polymyositis)

4. *Dermatologic diseases*
Pemphigus
Severe erythema multiforme (Stevens-Johnson syndrome)
Exfoliative dermatitis
Bullous dermatitis herpetiformis
Severe seborrheic dermatitis
Severe psoriasis
Mycosis fungoides

5. *Allergic states*
Control of severe or incapacitating allergic conditions intractable to adequate trials of conventional treatment in:
Bronchial asthma
Contact dermatitis
Atopic dermatitis
Serum sickness
Seasonal or perennial allergic rhinitis
Drug hypersensitivity reactions
Urticarial transfusion reactions
Acute noninfectious laryngeal edema (epinephrine is the drug of first choice)

6. *Ophthalmic diseases*
Severe acute and chronic allergic and inflammatory processes involving the eye, such as:
Herpes zoster ophthalmicus
Iritis, iridocyclitis
Chorioretinitis
Diffuse posterior uveitis and choroiditis
Optic neuritis
Sympathetic ophthalmia
Anterior segment inflammation
Allergic conjunctivitis
Keratitis
Allergic corneal marginal ulcers

7. *Gastrointestinal diseases*
To tide the patient over a critical period of the disease in:
Ulcerative colitis (Systemic therapy)
Regional enteritis (Systemic therapy)

8. *Respiratory diseases*
Symptomatic sarcoidosis
Berylliosis
Fulminating or disseminated pulmonary tuberculosis when used concurrently with appropriate antituberculous chemotherapy
Loeffler's syndrome not manageable by other means
Aspiration pneumonitis

9. *Hematologic disorders*
   Acquired (autoimmune) hemolytic anemia
   Idiopathic thrombocytopenic purpura in adults (I.V. only; I.M. administration is contraindicated)
   Secondary thrombocytopenia in adults
   Erythroblastopenia (RBC anemia)
   Congenital (erythroid) hypoplastic anemia
10. *Neoplastic diseases*
   For palliative management of:
   Leukemias and lymphomas in adults
   Acute leukemia of childhood
11. *Edematous states*
   To induce diuresis or remission of proteinuria in the nephrotic syndrome, without uremia, of the idiopathic type, or that due to lupus erythematosus
12. *Miscellaneous*
   Tuberculous meningitis with subarachnoid block or impending block when used concurrently with appropriate antituberculous chemotherapy
   Trichinosis with neurologic or myocardial involvement

CONTRAINDICATIONS

Systemic fungal infections (see WARNINGS regarding amphotericin B)
Hypersensitivity to any component of this product, including sulfites (see WARNINGS).

WARNINGS

Because rare instances of anaphylactoid reactions have occurred in patients receiving parenteral corticosteroid therapy, appropriate precautionary measures should be taken prior to administration, especially when the patient has a history of allergy to any drug. Anaphylactoid and hypersensitivity reactions have been reported for Injection HYDROCORTONE Phosphate (see ADVERSE REACTIONS).
Injection HYDROCORTONE Phosphate contains sodium bisulfite, a sulfite that may cause allergic-type reactions including anaphylactic symptoms and life-threatening or less severe asthmatic episodes in certain susceptible people. The overall prevalence of sulfite sensitivity in the general population is unknown and probably low. Sulfite sensitivity is seen more frequently in asthmatic than in nonasthmatic people.
Corticosteroids may exacerbate systemic fungal infections and therefore should not be used in the presence of such infections unless they are needed to control drug reactions due to amphotericin B. Moreover, there have been cases reported in which concomitant use of amphotericin B and hydrocortisone was followed by cardiac enlargement and congestive failure.
In patients on corticosteroid therapy subjected to any unusual stress, increased dosage of rapidly acting corticosteroids before, during, and after the stressful situation is indicated.
Drug-induced secondary adrenocortical insufficiency may result from too rapid withdrawal of corticosteroids and may be minimized by gradual reduction of dosage. This type of relative insufficiency may persist for months after discontinuation of therapy; therefore, in any situation of stress occurring during that period, hormone therapy should be reinstituted. If the patient is receiving steroids already, dosage may have to be increased. Since mineralocorticoid secretion may be impaired, salt and/or a mineralocorticoid should be administered concurrently.
Corticosteroids may mask some signs of infection, and new infections may appear during their use. There may be decreased resistance and inability to localize infection when corticosteroids are used. Moreover, corticosteroids may affect the nitroblue-tetrazolium test for bacterial infection and produce false negative results.
In cerebral malaria, a double-blind trial has shown that the use of corticosteroids is associated with prolongation of coma and a higher incidence of pneumonia and gastrointestinal bleeding.
Corticosteroids may activate latent amebiasis. Therefore, it is recommended that latent or active amebiasis be ruled out before initiating corticosteroid therapy in any patient who has spent time in the tropics or any patient with unexplained diarrhea.
Prolonged use of corticosteroids may produce posterior subcapsular cataracts, glaucoma with possible damage to the optic nerves, and may enhance the establishment of secondary ocular infections due to fungi or viruses.
Usage in pregnancy. Since adequate human reproduction studies have not been done with corticosteroids, use of these drugs in pregnancy or in women of childbearing potential requires that the anticipated benefits be weighed against the possible hazards to the mother and embryo or fetus. Infants born of mothers who have received substantial doses of corticosteroids during pregnancy should be carefully observed for signs of hypoadrenalism.
Corticosteroids appear in breast milk and could suppress growth, interfere with endogenous corticosteroid production, or cause other unwanted effects. Mothers taking pharmacologic doses of corticosteroids should be advised not to nurse.
Average and large doses of cortisone or hydrocortisone can cause elevation of blood pressure, salt and water retention, and increased excretion of potassium. These effects are less likely to occur with the synthetic derivatives except when used in large doses. Dietary salt restriction and potassium supplementation may be necessary. All corticosteroids increase calcium excretion.
Administration of live virus vaccines, including smallpox, is contraindicated in individuals receiving immunosuppressive doses of corticosteroids. If inactivated viral or bacterial vaccines are administered to individuals receiving immunosuppressive doses of corticosteroids, the expected serum antibody response may not be obtained. However, immunization procedures may be undertaken in patients who are receiving corticosteroids as replacement therapy, e.g., for Addison's disease.
Patients who are on drugs which suppress the immune system are more susceptible to infections than healthy individuals. Chickenpox and measles, for example, can have a more serious or even fatal course in non-immune patients on corticosteroids. In such patients who have not had these diseases, particular care should be taken to avoid exposure. The risk of developing a disseminated infection varies among individuals and can be related to the dose, route and duration of corticosteroid administration as well as to the underlying disease. If exposed to chickenpox, prophylaxis with varicella zoster immune globulin (VZIG) may be indicated. If chickenpox develops, treatment with antiviral agents may be considered. If exposed to measles, prophylaxis with immune globulin (IG) may be indicated. (See the respective package inserts for VZIG and IG for complete prescribing information.)
Similarly, corticosteroids should be used with great care in patients with known or suspected Strongyloides (threadworm) infestation. In such patients, corticosteroid-induced immunosuppression may lead to Strongyloides hyperinfection and dissemination with widespread larval migration, often accompanied by severe enterocolitis and potentially fatal gram-negative septicemia.
The use of HYDROCORTONE Phosphate injection in active tuberculosis should be restricted to those cases of fulminating or disseminated tuberculosis in which the corticosteroid is used for the management of the disease in conjunction with an appropriate antituberculous regimen.
If corticosteroids are indicated in patients with latent tuberculosis or tuberculin reactivity, close observation is necessary as reactivation of the disease may occur. During prolonged corticosteroid therapy, these patients should receive chemoprophylaxis.
Literature reports suggest an apparent association between use of corticosteroids and left ventricular free wall rupture after a recent myocardial infarction; therefore, therapy with corticosteroids should be used with great caution in these patients.

PRECAUTIONS

This product, like many other steroid formulations, is sensitive to heat. Therefore, it should not be autoclaved when it is desirable to sterilize the exterior of the vial.
Following prolonged therapy, withdrawal of corticosteroids may result in symptoms of the corticosteroid withdrawal syndrome including fever, myalgia, arthralgia, and malaise. This may occur in patients even without evidence of adrenal insufficiency.
There is an enhanced effect of corticosteroids in patients with hypothyroidism and in those with cirrhosis.
Corticosteroids should be used cautiously in patients with ocular herpes simplex for fear of corneal perforation.
The lowest possible dose of corticosteroid should be used to control the condition under treatment, and when reduction in dosage is possible, the reduction must be gradual.
Psychic derangements may appear when corticosteroids are used, ranging from euphoria, insomnia, mood swings, personality changes, and severe depression to frank psychotic manifestations. Also, existing emotional instability or psychotic tendencies may be aggravated by corticosteroids.
Aspirin should be used cautiously in conjunction with corticosteroids in hypoprothrombinemia.
Steroids should be used with caution in nonspecific ulcerative colitis, if there is a probability of impending perforation, abscess, or other pyogenic infection, also in diverticulitis, fresh intestinal anastomoses, active or latent peptic ulcer, renal insufficiency, hypertension, osteoporosis, and myasthenia gravis. Signs of peritoneal irritation following gastrointestinal perforation in patients receiving large doses of corticosteroids may be minimal or absent. Fat embolism has been reported as a possible complication of hypercortisonism.
When large doses are given, some authorities advise that antacids be administered between meals to help to prevent peptic ulcer.
Steroids may increase or decrease motility and number of spermatozoa in some patients.
Phenytoin, phenobarbital, ephedrine, and rifampin may enhance the metabolic clearance of corticosteroids, resulting in decreased blood levels and lessened physiologic activity, thus requiring adjustment in corticosteroid dosage.
The prothrombin time should be checked frequently in patients who are receiving corticosteroids and coumarin anticoagulants at the same time because of reports that corticosteroids have altered the response to these anticoagulants. Studies have shown that the usual effect produced by adding corticosteroids is inhibition of response to coumarins, although there have been some conflicting reports of potentiation not substantiated by studies.
When corticosteroids are administered concomitantly with potassium-depleting diuretics, patients should be observed closely for development of hypokalemia.
Injection of a steroid into an infected site is to be avoided.
The slower rate of absorption by intramuscular administration should be recognized.
Information for Patients
Susceptible patients who are on immunosuppressant doses of corticosteroids should be warned to avoid exposure to chickenpox or measles. Patients should also be advised that if they are exposed, medical advice should be sought without delay.
Pediatric Use
Growth and development of pediatric patients on prolonged corticosteroid therapy should be carefully followed.

ADVERSE REACTIONS

Fluid and electrolyte disturbances
   Sodium retention
   Fluid retention
   Congestive heart failure in susceptible patients
   Potassium loss
   Hypokalemic alkalosis
   Hypertension
Musculoskeletal
   Muscle weakness
   Steroid myopathy
   Loss of muscle mass
   Osteoporosis
   Vertebral compression fractures
   Aseptic necrosis of femoral and humeral heads
   Pathologic fracture of long bones
   Tendon rupture
Gastrointestinal
   Peptic ulcer with possible subsequent perforation and hemorrhage
   Perforation of the small and large bowel, particularly in patients with inflammatory bowel disease
   Pancreatitis
   Abdominal distention
   Ulcerative esophagitis
Dermatologic
   Impaired wound healing
   Thin fragile skin
   Petechiae and ecchymoses
   Erythema
   Increased sweating
   May suppress reactions to skin tests
   Burning or tingling, especially in the perineal area (after I.V. injection)
   Other cutaneous reactions, such as allergic dermatitis, urticaria, angioneurotic edema
Neurologic
   Convulsions
   Increased intracranial pressure with papilledema (pseudotumor cerebri) usually after treatment
   Vertigo
   Headache
   Psychic disturbances
Endocrine
   Menstrual irregularities
   Development of cushingoid state
   Suppression of growth in children
   Secondary adrenocortical and pituitary unresponsiveness, particularly in times of stress, as in trauma, surgery, or illness
   Decreased carbohydrate tolerance
   Manifestations of latent diabetes mellitus
   Increased requirements for insulin or oral hypoglycemic agents in diabetics
   Hirsutism
Ophthalmic
   Posterior subcapsular cataracts
   Increased intraocular pressure
   Glaucoma
   Exophthalmos
Metabolic
   Negative nitrogen balance due to protein catabolism
Cardiovascular
   Myocardial rupture following recent myocardial infarction (see WARNINGS)
Other
   Anaphylactoid or hypersensitivity reactions
   Thromboembolism
   Weight gain
   Increased appetite
   Nausea
   Malaise
The following *additional* adverse reactions are related to parenteral corticosteroid therapy:
   Rare instances of blindness associated with intralesional therapy around the face and head
   Hyperpigmentation or hypopigmentation
   Subcutaneous and cutaneous atrophy
   Sterile abscess

Continued on next page

Information on the Merck & Co., Inc. products listed on these pages is the full prescribing information from product circulars in use September 30, 2000. For information, please call 1-800-NSC MERCK [1-800-672-6372].

Hydrocortone Phosphate—Cont.

OVERDOSAGE

Reports of acute toxicity and/or death following overdosage of glucocorticoids are rare. In the event of overdosage, no specific antidote is available; treatment is supportive and symptomatic.
The intraperitoneal LD_{50} of hydrocortisone in female mice was 1740 mg/kg.

DOSAGE AND ADMINISTRATION

For intravenous, intramuscular, and subcutaneous injection. For single dose use only. Maintenance of sterility cannot be assured when used as a multiple dose vial.
HYDROCORTONE Phosphate injection can be given directly from the vial, or it can be added to Sodium Chloride Injection or Dextrose Injection and administered by intravenous drip.
Benzyl alcohol as a preservative has been associated with toxicity in premature infants. Solutions used for intravenous administration or further dilution of this product should be preservative-free when used in the neonate, especially the premature infant.
When it is mixed with an infusion solution, sterile precautions should be observed. Since infusion solutions generally do not contain preservatives, mixtures should be used within 24 hours.
DOSAGE REQUIREMENTS ARE VARIABLE AND MUST BE INDIVIDUALIZED ON THE BASIS OF THE DISEASE AND THE RESPONSE OF THE PATIENT.
The initial dosage varies from 15 to 240 mg a day depending on the disease being treated. In less severe diseases doses lower than 15 mg may suffice, while in severe diseases doses higher than 240 mg may be required. Usually the parenteral dosage ranges are one-third to one-half the oral dose given every 12 hours. However, in certain overwhelming, acute, life-threatening situations, administration in dosages exceeding the usual dosages may be justified and may be in multiples of the oral dosages.
The initial dosage should be maintained or adjusted until the patient's response is satisfactory. If a satisfactory clinical response does not occur after a reasonable period of time, discontinue HYDROCORTONE Phosphate injection and transfer the patient to other therapy.
After a favorable initial response, the proper maintenance dosage should be determined by decreasing the initial dosage in small amounts to the lowest dosage that maintains an adequate clinical response.
Patients should be observed closely for signs that might require dosage adjustment, including changes in clinical status resulting from remissions or exacerbations of the disease, individual drug responsiveness, and the effect of stress (e.g., surgery, infection, trauma). During stress it may be necessary to increase dosage temporarily.
If the drug is to be stopped after more than a few days of treatment, it usually should be withdrawn gradually.

HOW SUPPLIED

No. 7633—Injection HYDROCORTONE Phosphate, 50 mg hydrocortisone equivalent per mL, is a clear, light yellow solution, and is supplied as follows:
NDC 0006-7633-04 in 2 mL single dose vials.
Storage
Sensitive to heat. Do not autoclave.
9024029 Issued February 1997

HYDROCORTONE® Tablets (Hydrocortisone) ℞

DESCRIPTION

Glucocorticoids are adrenocortical steroids, both naturally occurring and synthetic, which are readily absorbed from the gastrointestinal tract.
Hydrocortisone is a white to practically white, odorless, crystalline powder, very slightly soluble in water. The molecular weight is 362.47. It is designated chemically as 11β,17,21-trihydroxypregn-4-ene-3,20-dione. The empirical formula is $C_{21}H_{30}O_5$ and the structural formula is:

Hydrocortisone is believed to be the principal hormone secreted by the adrenal cortex.
HYDROCORTONE* (Hydrocortisone) tablets contain 10 mg of hydrocortisone in each tablet.
Inactive ingredients are lactose, magnesium stearate, and starch.

*Registered trademark of MERCK & CO., INC.

ACTIONS

Naturally occurring glucocorticoids (hydrocortisone and cortisone), which also have salt-retaining properties, are used as replacement therapy in adrenocortical deficiency states. They are also used for their potent anti-inflammatory effects in disorders of many organ systems.
Glucocorticoids cause profound and varied metabolic effects. In addition, they modify the body's immune responses to diverse stimuli.

INDICATIONS

1. *Endocrine Disorders*
Primary or secondary adrenocortical insufficiency (hydrocortisone or cortisone is the first choice; synthetic analogs may be used in conjunction with mineralocorticoids where applicable; in infancy mineralocorticoid supplementation is of particular importance)
Congenital adrenal hyperplasia
Nonsuppurative thyroiditis
Hypercalcemia associated with cancer
2. *Rheumatic Disorders*
As adjunctive therapy for short-term administration (to tide the patient over an acute episode or exacerbation) in:
Psoriatic arthritis
Rheumatoid arthritis, including juvenile rheumatoid arthritis (selected cases may require low-dose maintenance therapy)
Ankylosing spondylitis
Acute and subacute bursitis
Acute nonspecific tenosynovitis
Acute gouty arthritis
Post-traumatic osteoarthritis
Synovitis of osteoarthritis
Epicondylitis
3. *Collagen Diseases*
During an exacerbation or as maintenance therapy in selected cases of—
Systemic lupus erythematosus
Acute rheumatic carditis
Systemic dermatomyositis (polymyositis)
4. *Dermatologic Diseases*
Pemphigus
Bullous dermatitis herpetiformis
Severe erythema multiforme (Stevens-Johnson syndrome)
Exfoliative dermatitis
Mycosis fungoides
Severe psoriasis
Severe seborrheic dermatitis
5. *Allergic States*
Control of severe or incapacitating allergic conditions intractable to adequate trials of conventional treatment:
Seasonal or perennial allergic rhinitis
Bronchial asthma
Contact dermatitis
Atopic dermatitis
Serum sickness
Drug hypersensitivity reactions
6. *Ophthalmic Diseases*
Severe acute and chronic allergic and inflammatory processes involving the eye and its adnexa, such as—
Allergic conjunctivitis
Keratitis
Allergic corneal marginal ulcers
Herpes zoster ophthalmicus
Iritis and iridocyclitis
Chorioretinitis
Anterior segment inflammation
Diffuse posterior uveitis and choroiditis
Optic neuritis
Sympathetic ophthalmia
7. *Respiratory Diseases*
Symptomatic sarcoidosis
Loeffler's syndrome not manageable by other means
Berylliosis
Fulminating or disseminated pulmonary tuberculosis when used concurrently with appropriate antituberculous chemotherapy
Aspiration pneumonitis
8. *Hematologic Disorders*
Idiopathic thrombocytopenic purpura in adults
Secondary thrombocytopenia in adults
Acquired (autoimmune) hemolytic anemia
Erythroblastopenia (RBC anemia)
Congenital (erythroid) hypoplastic anemia
9. *Neoplastic Diseases*
For palliative management of:
Leukemias and lymphomas in adults
Acute leukemia of childhood
10. *Edematous States*
To induce a diuresis or remission of proteinuria in the nephrotic syndrome, without uremia, of the idiopathic type or that due to lupus erythematosus
11. *Gastrointestinal Diseases*
To tide the patient over a critical period of the disease in:
Ulcerative colitis
Regional enteritis
12. *Miscellaneous*
Tuberculous meningitis with subarachnoid block or impending block when used concurrently with appropriate antituberculous chemotherapy
Trichinosis with neurologic or myocardial involvement

CONTRAINDICATIONS

Systemic fungal infections
Hypersensitivity to this product

WARNINGS

In patients on corticosteroid therapy subjected to unusual stress, increased dosage of rapidly acting corticosteroids before, during, and after the stressful situation is indicated.
Drug-induced secondary adrenocortical insufficiency may result from too rapid wthdrawal of corticosteroids and may be minimized by gradual reduction of dosage. This type of relative insufficiency may persist for months after discontinuation of therapy; therefore, in any situation of stress occurring during that period, hormone therapy should be reinstituted. If the patient is receiving steroids already, dosage may have to be increased. Since mineralocorticoid secretion may be impaired, salt and/or a mineralocorticoid should be administered concurrently.
Corticosteroids may mask some signs of infection, and new infections may appear during their use. There may be decreased resistance and inability to localize infection when corticosteroids are used. Moreover, corticosteroids may affect the nitroblue-tetrazolium test for bacterial infection and produce false negative results.
In cerebral malaria, a double-blind trial has shown that the use of corticosteroids is associated with prolongation of coma and a higher incidence of pneumonia and gastrointestinal bleeding.
Corticosteroids may activate latent amebiasis. Therefore, it is recommended that latent or active amebiasis be ruled out before initiating corticosteroid therapy in any patient who has spent time in the tropics or any patient with unexplained diarrhea.
Prolonged use of corticosteroids may produce posterior subcapsular cataracts, glaucoma with possible damage to the optic nerves, and may enhance the establishment of secondary ocular infections due to fungi or viruses.
Usage in pregnancy: Since adequate human reproduction studies have not been done with corticosteroids, use of these drugs in pregnancy or in women of childbearing potential requires that the anticipated benefits be weighed against the possible hazards to the mother and embryo or fetus. Infants born of mothers who have received substantial doses of corticosteroids during pregnancy should be carefully observed for signs of hypoadrenalism.
Corticosteroids appear in breast milk and could suppress growth, interfere with endogenous corticosteroid production, or cause other unwanted effects. Mothers taking pharmacologic doses of corticosteroids should be advised not to nurse.
Average and large doses of hydrocortisone or cortisone can cause elevation of blood pressure, salt and water retention, and increased excretion of potassium. These effects are less likely to occur with the synthetic derivatives except when used in large doses. Dietary salt restriction and potassium supplementation may be necessary. All corticosteroids increase calcium excretion.
Administration of live virus vaccines, including smallpox, is contraindicated in individuals receiving immunosuppressive doses of corticosteroids. If inactivated viral or bacterial vaccines are administered to individuals receiving immunosuppressive doses of corticosteroids, the expected serum antibody response may not be obtained. However, immunization procedures may be undertaken in patients who are receiving corticosteroids as replacement therapy, e.g., for Addison's disease.
Patients who are on drugs which suppress the immune system are more susceptible to infections than healthy individuals. Chickenpox and measles, for example, can have a more serious or even fatal course in non-immune patients on corticosteroids. In such patients who have not had these diseases, particular care should be taken to avoid exposure. The risk of developing a disseminated infection varies among individuals and can be related to the dose, route and duration of corticosteroid administration as well as to the underlying disease. If exposed to chickenpox, prophylaxis with varicella zoster immune globulin (VZIG) may be indicated. If chickenpox develops, treatment with antiviral agents may be considered. If exposed to measles, prophylaxis with immune globulin (IG) may be indicated. (See the respective package inserts for VZIG and IG for complete prescribing information.)
Similarly, corticosteroids should be used with great care in patients with known or suspected Strongyloides (threadworm) infestation. In such patients, corticosteroid-induced immunosuppression may lead to Strongyloides hyperinfection and dissemination with widespread larval migration, often accompanied by severe enterocolitis and potentially fatal gram-negative septicemia.
The use of HYDROCORTONE tablets in active tuberculosis should be restricted to those cases of fulminating or disseminated tuberculosis in which the corticosteroid is used for the management of the disease in conjunction with an appropriate antituberculous regimen.
If corticosteroids are indicated in patients with latent tuberculosis or tuberculin reactivity, close observation is neces-

sary as reactivation of the disease may occur. During prolonged corticosteroid therapy, these patients should receive chemoprophylaxis.
Literature reports suggest an apparent association between use of corticosteroids and left ventricular free wall rupture after a recent myocardial infarction; therefore, therapy with corticosteroids should be used with great caution in these patients.

PRECAUTIONS

Following prolonged therapy, withdrawal of corticosteroids may result in symptoms of the corticosteroid withdrawal syndrome including fever, myalgia, arthralgia, and malaise. This may occur in patients even without evidence of adrenal insufficiency.
There is an enhanced effect of corticosteroids in patients with hypothyroidism and in those with cirrhosis.
Corticosteroids should be used cautiously in patients with ocular herpes simplex because of possible corneal perforation.
The lowest possible dose of corticosteroid should be used to control the condition under treatment, and when reduction in dosage is possible, the reduction should be gradual.
Psychic derangements may appear when corticosteroids are used, ranging from euphoria, insomnia, mood swings, personality changes, and severe depression, to frank psychotic manifestations. Also, existing emotional instability or psychotic tendencies may be aggravated by corticosteroids.
Aspirin should be used cautiously in conjunction with corticosteroids in hypoprothrombinemia.
Steroids should be used with caution in nonspecific ulcerative colitis, if there is a probability of impending perforation, abscess, or other pyogenic infection, diverticulitis, fresh intestinal anastomoses, active or latent peptic ulcer, renal insufficiency, hypertension, osteoporosis, and myasthenia gravis. Signs of peritoneal irritation following gastrointestinal perforation in patients receiving large doses of corticosteroids may be minimal or absent. Fat embolism has been reported as a possible complication of hypercortisonism.
When large doses are given, some authorities advise that corticosteroids be taken with meals and antacids taken between meals to help to prevent peptic ulcer.
Steroids may increase or decrease motility and number of spermatozoa in some patients.
Phenytoin, phenobarbital, ephedrine, and rifampin may enhance the metabolic clearance of corticosteroids, resulting in decreased blood levels and lessened physiologic activity, thus requiring adjustment in corticosteroid dosage.
The prothrombin time should be checked frequently in patients who are receiving corticosteroids and coumarin anticoagulants at the same time because of reports that corticosteroids have altered the response to these anticoagulants. Studies have shown that the usual effect produced by adding corticosteroids is inhibition of response to coumarins, although there have been some conflicting reports of potentiation not substantiated by studies.
When corticosteroids are administered concomitantly with potassium-depleting diuretics, patients should be observed closely for development of hypokalemia.
Information for Patients
Susceptible patients who are on immunosuppressant doses of corticosteroids should be warned to avoid exposure to chickenpox or measles. Patients should also be advised that if they are exposed, medical advice should be sought without delay.
Pediatric Use
Growth and development of pediatric patients on prolonged corticosteroid therapy should be carefully followed.

ADVERSE REACTIONS

Fluid and Electrolyte Disturbances
Sodium retention
Fluid retention
Congestive heart failure in susceptible patients
Potassium loss
Hypokalemic alkalosis
Hypertension
Musculoskeletal
Muscle weakness
Steroid myopathy
Loss of muscle mass
Osteoporosis
Vertebral compression fractures
Aseptic necrosis of femoral and humeral heads
Pathologic fracture of long bones
Tendon rupture
Gastrointestinal
Peptic ulcer with possible perforation and hemorrhage
Perforation of the small and large bowel, particularly in patients with inflammatory bowel disease
Pancreatitis
Abdominal distention
Ulcerative esophagitis
Dermatologic
Impaired wound healing
Thin fragile skin
Petechiae and ecchymoses
Erythema
Increased sweating
May suppress reactions to skin tests
Other cutaneous reactions, such as allergic dermatitis, urticaria, angioneurotic edema
Neurologic
Convulsions
Increased intracranial pressure with papilledema (pseudotumor cerebri) usually after treatment
Vertigo
Headache
Psychic disturbances
Endocrine
Menstrual irregularities
Development of cushingoid state
Suppression of growth in children
Secondary adrenocortical and pituitary unresponsiveness, particularly in times of stress, as in trauma, surgery, or illness
Decreased carbohydrate tolerance
Manifestations of latent diabetes mellitus
Increased requirements for insulin or oral hypoglycemic agents in diabetics
Hirsutism
Ophthalmic
Posterior subcapsular cataracts
Increased intraocular pressure
Glaucoma
Exophthalmos
Metabolic
Negative nitrogen balance due to protein catabolism
Cardiovascular
Myocardial rupture following recent myocardial infarction (see WARNINGS)
Other
Hypersensitivity
Thromboembolism
Weight gain
Increased appetite
Nausea
Malaise

OVERDOSAGE

Reports of acute toxicity and/or death following overdosage of glucocorticoids are rare. In the event of overdosage, no specific antidote is available; treatment is supportive and symptomatic.
The intraperitoneal LD_{50} of hydrocortisone in female mice was 1740 mg/kg.

DOSAGE AND ADMINISTRATION

For oral administration
DOSAGE REQUIREMENTS ARE VARIABLE AND MUST BE INDIVIDUALIZED ON THE BASIS OF THE DISEASE AND THE RESPONSE OF THE PATIENT.
The initial dosage varies from 20 to 240 mg a day depending on the disease being treated. In less severe diseases doses lower than 20 mg may suffice, while in severe diseases doses higher than 240 mg may be required. The initial dosage should be maintained or adjusted until the patient's response is satisfactory. If satisfactory clinical response does not occur after a reasonable period of time, discontinue HYDROCORTONE tablets and transfer the patient to other therapy.
After a favorable initial response, the proper maintenance dosage should be determined by decreasing the initial dosage in small amounts to the lowest dosage that maintains an adequate clinical response.
Patients should be observed closely for signs that might require dosage adjustment, including changes in clinical status resulting from remissions or exacerbations of the disease, individual drug responsiveness, and the effect of stress (e.g, surgery, infection, trauma). During stress it may be necessary to increase dosage temporarily.
If the drug is to be stopped after more than a few days of treatment, it usually should be withdrawn gradually.

HOW SUPPLIED

No. 7604—Tablets HYDROCORTONE, 10 mg each, are white, oval shaped compressed tablets, scored on one side, coded MSD 619, and are supplied as follows:
NDC 0006-0619-68 in bottles of 100.
Shown in Product Identification Guide, page 323
7920528 Issued February 1997

HydroDIURIL® Tablets
(Hydrochlorothiazide) ℞

DESCRIPTION

HydroDIURIL* (Hydrochlorothiazide) is a diuretic and antihypertensive. It is the 3,4-dihydro derivative of chlorothiazide. Its chemical name is 6-chloro-3,4-dihydro-2*H* -1,2,4-benzothiadiazine-7-sulfonamide 1,1-dioxide. Its empirical formula is $C_7H_8ClN_3O_4S_2$ and its structural formula is:
[See chemical structure at top of next column]
It is a white, or practically white, crystalline powder with a molecular weight of 297.74, which is slightly soluble in water, but freely soluble in sodium hydroxide solution.
HydroDIURIL is supplied as 25 mg and 50 mg tablets for oral use. Each tablet contains the following inactive ingredients: calcium phosphate, FD&C Yellow 6, gelatin, lactose, magnesium stearate, starch and talc.

*Registered trademark of MERCK & CO., INC.

CLINICAL PHARMACOLOGY

The mechanism of the antihypertensive effect of thiazides is unknown. HydroDIURIL does not usually affect normal blood pressure.
HydroDIURIL affects the distal renal tubular mechanism of electrolyte reabsorption. At maximal therapeutic dosage all thiazides are approximately equal in their diuretic efficacy.
HydroDIURIL increases excretion of sodium and chloride in approximately equivalent amounts. Natriuresis may be accompanied by some loss of potassium and bicarbonate.
After oral use diuresis begins within 2 hours, peaks in about 4 hours and lasts about 6 to 12 hours.
Pharmacokinetics and Metabolism
HydroDIURIL is not metabolized but is eliminated rapidly by the kidney. When plasma levels have been followed for at least 24 hours, the plasma half-life has been observed to vary between 5.6 and 14.8 hours. At least 61 percent of the oral dose is eliminated unchanged within 24 hours. Hydrochlorothiazide crosses the placental but not the blood-brain barrier and is excreted in breast milk.

INDICATIONS AND USAGE

HydroDIURIL is indicated as adjunctive therapy in edema associated with congestive heart failure, hepatic cirrhosis, and corticosteroid and estrogen therapy.
HydroDIURIL has also been found useful in edema due to various forms of renal dysfunction such as nephrotic syndrome, acute glomerulonephritis, and chronic renal failure.
HydroDIURIL is indicated in the management of hypertension either as the sole therapeutic agent or to enhance the effectiveness of other antihypertensive drugs in the more severe forms of hypertension.
Use in Pregnancy. Routine use of diuretics during normal pregnancy is inappropriate and exposes mother and fetus to unnecessary hazard. Diuretics do not prevent development of toxemia of pregnancy and there is no satisfactory evidence that they are useful in the treatment of toxemia.
Edema during pregnancy may arise from pathologic causes or from the physiologic and mechanical consequences of pregnancy. Thiazides are indicated in pregnancy when edema is due to pathologic causes, just as they are in the absence of pregnancy (see PRECAUTIONS, *Pregnancy*). Dependent edema in pregnancy, resulting from restriction of venous return by the gravid uterus, is properly treated through elevation of the lower extremities and use of support stockings. Use of diuretics to lower intravascular volume in this instance is illogical and unnecessary. During normal pregnancy there is hypervolemia which is not harmful to the fetus or the mother in the absence of cardiovascular disease. However, it may be associated with edema, rarely generalized edema. If such edema causes discomfort, increased recumbency will often provide relief. Rarely this edema may cause extreme discomfort which is not relieved by rest. In these instances, a short course of diuretic therapy may provide relief and be appropriate.

CONTRAINDICATIONS

Anuria.
Hypersensitivity to this product or to other sulfonamide-derived drugs.

WARNINGS

Use with caution in severe renal disease. In patients with renal disease, thiazides may precipitate azotemia. Cumulative effects of the drug may develop in patients with impaired renal function.
Thiazides should be used with caution in patients with impaired hepatic function or progressive liver disease, since minor alterations of fluid and electrolyte balance may precipitate hepatic coma.
Thiazides may add to or potentiate the action of other antihypertensive drugs.
Sensitivity reactions may occur in patients with or without a history of allergy or bronchial asthma.
The possibility of exacerbation or activation of systemic lupus erythematosus has been reported.
Lithium generally should not be given with diuretics (see PRECAUTIONS, *Drug Interactions*).

PRECAUTIONS

General
All patients receiving diuretic therapy should be observed for evidence of fluid or electrolyte imbalance: namely, hypo-

Continued on next page

Information on the Merck & Co., Inc. products listed on these pages is the full prescribing information from product circulars in use September 30, 2000. For information, please call 1-800-NSC MERCK [1-800-672-6372].

HydroDiuril—Cont.

natremia, hypochloremic alkalosis, and hypokalemia. Serum and urine electrolyte determinations are particularly important when the patient is vomiting excessively or receiving parenteral fluids. Warning signs or symptoms of fluid and electrolyte imbalance, irrespective of cause, include dryness of mouth, thirst, weakness, lethargy, drowsiness, restlessness, confusion, seizures, muscle pains or cramps, muscular fatigue, hypotension, oliguria, tachycardia, and gastrointestinal disturbances such as nausea and vomiting.
Hypokalemia may develop, especially with brisk diuresis, when severe cirrhosis is present or after prolonged therapy. Interference with adequate oral electrolyte intake will also contribute to hypokalemia. Hypokalemia may cause cardiac arrhythmia and may also sensitize or exaggerate the response of the heart to the toxic effects of digitalis (e.g., increased ventricular irritability). Hypokalemia may be avoided or treated by use of potassium sparing diuretics or potassium supplements such as foods with a high potassium content.
Although any chloride deficit is generally mild and usually does not require specific treatment except under extraordinary circumstances (as in liver disease or renal disease), chloride replacement may be required in the treatment of metabolic alkalosis.
Dilutional hyponatremia may occur in edematous patients in hot weather; appropriate therapy is water restriction, rather than administration of salt, except in rare instances when the hyponatremia is life threatening. In actual salt depletion, appropriate replacement is the therapy of choice.
Hyperuricemia may occur or acute gout may be precipitated in certain patients receiving thiazides.
In diabetic patients dosage adjustments of insulin or oral hypoglycemic agents may be required. Hyperglycemia may occur with thiazide diuretics. Thus latent diabetes mellitus may become manifest during thiazide therapy.
The antihypertensive effects of the drug may be enhanced in the post-sympathectomy patient.
If progressive renal impairment becomes evident, consider withholding or discontinuing diuretic therapy.
Thiazides have been shown to increase the urinary excretion of magnesium; this may result in hypomagnesemia.
Thiazides may decrease urinary calcium excretion. Thiazides may cause intermittent and slight elevation of serum calcium in the absence of known disorders of calcium metabolism. Marked hypercalcemia may be evidence of hidden hyperparathyroidism. Thiazides should be discontinued before carrying out tests for parathyroid function.
Increases in cholesterol and triglyceride levels may be associated with thiazide diuretic therapy.

Laboratory Tests
Periodic determination of serum electrolytes to detect possible electrolyte imbalance should be done at appropriate intervals.

Drug Interactions
When given concurrently the following drugs may interact with thiazide diuretics.
Alcohol, barbiturates, or narcotics —potentiation of orthostatic hypotension may occur.
Antidiabetic drugs —(oral agents and insulin)—dosage adjustment of the antidiabetic drug may be required.
Other antihypertensive drugs —additive effect or potentiation.
Cholestyramine and colestipol resins—Absorption of hydrochlorothiazide is impaired in the presence of anionic exchange resins. Single doses of either cholestyramine or colestipol resins bind the hydrochlorothiazide and reduce its absorption from the gastrointestinal tract by up to 85 and 43 percent, respectively.
Corticosteroids, ACTH —intensified electrolyte depletion, particularly hypokalemia.
Pressor amines (e.g., norepinephrine) —possible decreased response to pressor amines but not sufficient to preclude their use.
Skeletal muscle relaxants, nondepolarizing (e.g., tubocurarine) —possible increased responsiveness to the muscle relaxant.
Lithium —generally should not be given with diuretics. Diuretic agents reduce the renal clearance of lithium and add a high risk of lithium toxicity. Refer to the package insert for lithium preparations before use of such preparations with HydroDIURIL.
Non-steroidal Anti-inflammatory Drugs —In some patients, the administration of a non-steroidal anti-inflammatory agent can reduce the diuretic, natriuretic, and antihypertensive effects of loop, potassium-sparing and thiazide diuretics. Therefore, when HydroDIURIL and non-steroidal anti-inflammatory agents are used concomitantly, the patient should be observed closely to determine if the desired effect of the diuretic is obtained.

Drug/Laboratory Test Interactions
Thiazides should be discontinued before carrying out tests for parathyroid function (see PRECAUTIONS, *General*).

Carcinogenesis, Mutagenesis, Impairment of Fertility
Two-year feeding studies in mice and rats conducted under the auspices of the National Toxicology Program (NTP) uncovered no evidence of a carcinogenic potential of hydrochlorothiazide in female mice (at doses of up to approximately 600 mg/kg/day) or in male and female rats (at doses of up to approximately 100 mg/kg/day). The NTP, however, found equivocal evidence for hepatocarcinogenicity in male mice.
Hydrochlorothiazide was not genotoxic *in vitro* in the Ames mutagenicity assay of *Salmonella typhimurium* strains TA 98, TA 100, TA 1535, TA 1537, and TA 1538 and in the Chinese Hamster Ovary (CHO) test for chromosomal aberrations, or *in vivo* in assays using mouse germinal cell chromosomes, Chinese hamster bone marrow chromosomes, and the *Drosophila* sex-linked recessive lethal trait gene. Positive test results were obtained only in the *in vitro* CHO Sister Chromatid Exchange (clastogenicity) and in the Mouse Lymphoma Cell (mutagenicity) assays, using concentrations of hydrochlorothiazide from 43 to 1300 μg/mL, and in the *Aspergillus nidulans* non-disjunction assay at an unspecified concentration.
Hydrochlorothiazide had no adverse effects on the fertility of mice and rats of either sex in studies wherein these species were exposed, via their diet, to doses of up to 100 and 4 mg/kg, respectively, prior to conception and throughout gestation.

Pregnancy
Teratogenic Effects—Pregnancy Category B: Studies in which hydrochlorothiazide was orally administered to pregnant mice and rats during their respective periods of major organogenesis at doses up to 3000 and 1000 mg hydrochlorothiazide/kg, respectively, provided no evidence of harm to the fetus.
There are, however, no adequate and well-controlled studies in pregnant women. Because animal reproduction studies are not always predictice of human response, this drug should be used during pregnancy only if clearly needed.
Nonteratogenic Effects: Thiazides cross the placental barrier and appear in cord blood. There is a risk of fetal or neonatal jaundice, thrombocytopenia, and possibly other adverse reactions that have occurred in adults.

Nursing Mothers
Thiazides are excreted in breast milk. Because of the potential for serious adverse reactions in nursing infants, a decision should be made whether to discontinue nursing or to discontinue hydrochlorothiazide, taking into account the importance of the drug to the mother.

Pediatric Use
There are no well-controlled clinical trials in pediatric patients. Information on dosing in this age group is supported by evidence from empiric use in pediatric patients and published literature regarding the treatment of hypertension in such patients. (See DOSAGE AND ADMINISTRATION, *Infants and Children.*)

ADVERSE REACTIONS

The following adverse reactions have been reported and, within each category, are listed in order of decreasing severity.
Body as a Whole: Weakness.
Cardiovascular: Hypotension including orthostatic hypotension (may be aggravated by alcohol, barbiturates, narcotics or antihypertensive drugs).
Digestive: Pancreatitis, jaundice (intrahepatic cholestatic jaundice), diarrhea, vomiting, sialadenitis, cramping, constipation, gastric irritation, nausea, anorexia.
Hematologic: Aplastic anemia, agranulocytosis, leukopenia, hemolytic anemia, thrombocytopenia.
Hypersensitivity: Anaphylactic reactions, necrotizing angiitis (vasculitis and cutaneous vasculitis), respiratory distress including pneumonitis and pulmonary edema, photosensitivity, fever, urticaria, rash, purpura.
Metabolic: Electrolyte imbalance (see PRECAUTIONS), hyperglycemia, glycosuria, hyperuricemia.
Musculoskeletal: Muscle spasm.
Nervous System/Psychiatric: Vertigo, paresthesias, dizziness, headache, restlessness.
Renal: Renal failure, renal dysfunction, interstitial nephritis. (See WARNINGS.)
Skin: Erythema multiforme including Stevens-Johnson syndrome, exfoliative dermatitis including toxic epidermal necrolysis, alopecia.
Special Senses: Transient blurred vision, xanthopsia.
Urogenital: Impotence.
Whenever adverse reactions are moderate or severe, thiazide dosage should be reduced or therapy withdrawn.

OVERDOSAGE

The most common signs and symptoms observed are those caused by electrolyte depletion (hypokalemia, hypochloremia, hyponatremia) and dehydration resulting from excessive diuresis. If digitalis has also been administered, hypokalemia may accentuate cardiac arrhythmias.
In the event of overdosage, symptomatic and supportive measures should be employed. Emesis should be induced or gastric lavage performed. Correct dehydration, electrolyte imbalance, hepatic coma and hypotension by established procedures. If required, give oxygen or artificial respiration for respiratory impairment. The degree to which hydrochlorothiazide is removed by hemodialysis has not been established.
The oral LD_{50} of hydrochlorothiazide is greater than 10 g/kg in the mouse and rat.

DOSAGE AND ADMINISTRATION

Therapy should be individualized according to patient response. Use the smallest dosage necessary to achieve the required response.

Adults
For Edema
The usual adult dosage is 25 to 100 mg daily as a single or divided dose. Many patients with edema respond to intermittent therapy, i.e., administration on alternate days or on three to five days each week. With an intermittent schedule, excessive response and the resulting undesirable electrolyte imbalance are less likely to occur.
For Control of Hypertension
The usual initial dose in adults is 25 mg daily given as a single dose. The dose may be increased to 50 mg daily, given as a single or two divided doses. Doses above 50 mg are often associated with marked reductions in serum potassium (see also PRECAUTIONS).
Patients usually do not require doses in excess of 50 mg of hydrochlorothiazide daily when used concomitantly with other antihypertensive agents.

Infants and Children
For Diuresis and For Control of Hypertension
The usual pediatric dosage is 0.5 to 1 mg per pound (1 to 2 mg/kg) per day in single or two divided doses, not to exceed 37.5 mg per day in infants up to 2 years of age or 100 mg per day in children 2 to 12 years of age. In infants less than 6 months of age, doses up to 1.5 mg per pound (3 mg/kg) per day in two divided doses may be required. (See PRECAUTIONS, *Pediatric Use.*)

HOW SUPPLIED

No. 3263—Tablets HydroDIURIL, 25 mg, are peach-colored, round, scored, compressed tablets, coded MSD 42 on one side and HydroDIURIL on the other. They are supplied as follows:
NDC 0006-0042-68 bottles of 100
NDC 0006-0042-82 bottles of 1000.
Shown in Product Identification Guide, page 323
No. 3264—Tablets HydroDIURIL, 50 mg, are peach-colored, round, scored, compressed tablets, coded MSD 105 on one side and HydroDIURIL on the other. They are supplied as follows:
NDC 0006-0105-68 bottles of 100
NDC 0006-0105-86 bottles of 5000.

Storage
Keep container tightly closed. Protect from light, moisture, freezing, −20°C (−4°F) and store at room temperature, 15–30°C (59–86°F).

7897450 Issued June 1998

HYZAAR® 50-12.5 ℞
(losartan potassium-hydrochlorothiazide tablets)

HYZAAR® 100-25 ℞
(losartan potassium-hydrochlorothiazide tablets)

USE IN PREGNANCY
When used in pregnancy during the second and third trimesters, drugs that act directly on the renin-angiotensin system can cause injury and even death to the developing fetus. When pregnancy is detected, HYZAAR should be discontinued as soon as possible. See WARNINGS: *Fetal/Neonatal Morbidity and Mortality.*

DESCRIPTION

HYZAAR* 50-12.5 (losartan potassium-hydrochlorothiazide) and HYZAAR* 100-25 (losartan potassium-hydrochlorothiazide), combines an angiotensin II receptor (type AT_1) antagonist and a diuretic, hydrochlorothiazide.
Losartan potassium, a non-peptide molecule, is chemically described as 2-butyl-4-chloro-1-[*p*-(*o*-1*H*-tetrazol-5-ylphenyl)benzyl]imidazole-5-methanol monopotassium salt. Its empirical formula is $C_{22}H_{22}ClKN_6O$, and its structural formula is:

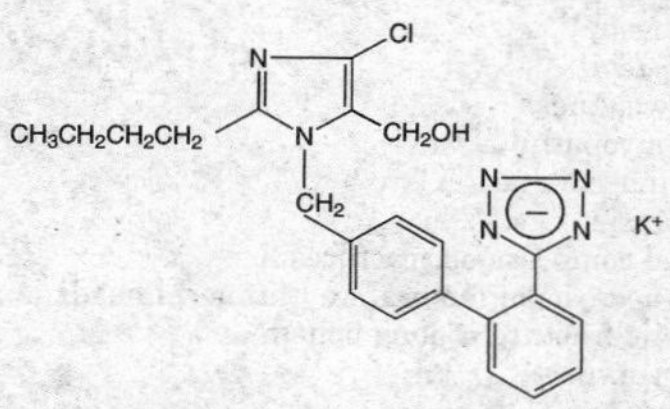

Losartan potassium is a white to off-white free-flowing crystalline powder with a molecular weight of 461.01. It is freely soluble in water, soluble in alcohols, and slightly soluble in common organic solvents, such as acetonitrile and methyl ethyl ketone.
Oxidation of the 5-hydroxymethyl group on the imidazole ring results in the active metabolite of losartan.
Hydrochlorothiazide is 6-chloro-3,4-dihydro-2*H*-1,2,4-benzothiadiazine-7-sulfonamide 1,1-dioxide. Its empirical formula is $C_7H_8ClN_3O_4S_2$ and its structural formula is:
[See chemical structure at top of next column]
Hydrochlorothiazide is a white, or practically white, crystalline powder with a molecular weight of 297.74, which is slightly soluble in water, but freely soluble in sodium hydroxide solution.

HYZAAR is available for oral administration in two tablet combinations of losartan and hydrochlorothiazide. HYZAAR 50-12.5 contains 50 mg of losartan potassium and 12.5 mg of hydrochlorothiazide. HYZAAR 100-25 contains 100 mg of losartan potassium and 25 mg of hydrochlorothiazide. Inactive ingredients are microcrystalline cellulose, lactose hydrous, pregelatinized starch, magnesium stearate, hydroxypropyl cellulose, hydroxypropyl methylcellulose, titanium dioxide and D&C yellow No. 10 aluminum lake.
HYZAAR 50-12.5 contains 4.24 mg (0.108 mEq) of potassium and HYZAAR 100-25 contains 8.48 mg (0.216 mEq) of potassium.

*Registered trademark of E.I. du Pont de Nemours and Company, Wilmington, Delaware, USA

CLINICAL PHARMACOLOGY

Mechanism of Action
Angiotensin II [formed from angiotensin I in a reaction catalyzed by angiotensin converting enzyme (ACE, kininase II)], is a potent vasoconstrictor, the primary vasoactive hormone of the renin-angiotensin system and an important component in the pathophysiology of hypertension. It also stimulates aldosterone secretion by the adrenal cortex. Losartan and its principal active metabolite block the vasoconstrictor and aldosterone-secreting effects of angiotensin II by selectively blocking the binding of angiotensin II to the AT_1 receptor found in many tissues, (e.g., vascular smooth muscle, adrenal gland). There is also an AT_2 receptor found in many tissues but it is not known to be associated with cardiovascular homeostasis. Both losartan and its principal active metabolite do not exhibit any partial agonist activity at the AT_1 receptor and have much greater affinity (about 1000-fold) for the AT_1 receptor than for the AT_2 receptor. *In vitro* binding studies indicate that losartan is a reversible, competitive inhibitor of the AT_1 receptor. The active metabolite is 10 to 40 times more potent by weight than losartan and appears to be a reversible, non-competitive inhibitor of the AT_1 receptor.
Neither losartan nor its active metabolite inhibits ACE (kininase II, the enzyme that converts angiotensin I to angiotensin II and degrades bradykinin); nor do they bind to or block other hormone receptors or ion channels known to be important in cardiovascular regulation.
Hydrochlorothiazide is a thiazide diuretic. Thiazides affect the renal tubular mechanisms of electrolyte reabsorption, directly increasing excretion of sodium and chloride in approximately equivalent amounts. Indirectly, the diuretic action of hydrochlorothiazide reduces plasma volume, with consequent increases in plasma renin activity, increases in aldosterone secretion, increases in urinary potassium loss, and decreases in serum potassium. The renin-aldosterone link is mediated by angiotensin II, so coadministration of an angiotensin II receptor antagonist tends to reverse the potassium loss associated with these diuretics.
The mechanism of the antihypertensive effect of thiazides is unknown.
Pharmacokinetics
General
Losartan Potassium
Losartan is an orally active agent that undergoes substantial first-pass metabolism by cytochrome P450 enzymes. It is converted, in part, to an active carboxylic acid metabolite that is responsible for most of the angiotensin II receptor antagonism that follows losartan treatment. The terminal half-life of losartan is about 2 hours and of the metabolite is about 6–9 hours. The pharmacokinetics of losartan and its active metabolite are linear with oral losartan doses up to 200 mg and do not change over time. Neither losartan nor its metabolite accumulate in plasma upon repeated once-daily dosing.
Following oral administration, losartan is well absorbed (based on absorption of radiolabeled losartan) and undergoes substantial first-pass metabolism; the systemic bioavailability of losartan is approximately 33%. About 14% of an orally-administered dose of losartan is converted to the active metabolite. Mean peak concentrations of losartan and its active metabolite are reached in 1 hour and in 3–4 hours, respectively. While maximum plasma concentrations of losartan and its active metabolite are approximately equal, the AUC of the metabolite is about 4 times as great as that of losartan. A meal slows absorption of losartan and decreases its C_{max} but has only minor effects on losartan AUC or on the AUC of the metabolite (about 10% decreased).
Both losartan and its active metabolite are highly bound to plasma proteins, primarily albumin, with plasma free fractions of 1.3% and 0.2% respectively. Plasma protein binding is constant over the concentration range achieved with recommended doses. Studies in rats indicate that losartan crosses the blood-brain barrier poorly, if at all.
Losartan metabolites have been identified in human plasma and urine. In addition to the active carboxylic acid metabolite, several inactive metabolites are formed. Following oral and intravenous administration of ^{14}C-labeled losartan potassium, circulating plasma radioactivity is primarily attributed to losartan and its active metabolite. *In vitro* studies indicate that cytochrome P450 2C9 and 3A4 are involved in the biotransformation of losartan to its metabolites. Minimal conversion of losartan to the active metabolite (less than 1% of the dose compared to 14% of the dose in normal subjects) was seen in about one percent of individuals studied.
The volume of distribution of losartan is about 34 liters and of the active metabolite is about 12 liters. Total plasma clearance of losartan and the active metabolite is about 600 mL/min and 50 mL/min, respectively, with renal clearance of about 75 mL/min and 25 mL/min, respectively. When losartan is administered orally, about 4% of the dose is excreted unchanged in the urine and about 6% is excreted in urine as active metabolite. Biliary excretion contributes to the elimination of losartan and its metabolites. Following oral ^{14}C-labeled losartan, about 35% of radioactivity is recovered in the urine and about 60% in the feces. Following an intravenous dose of ^{14}C-labeled losartan, about 45% of radioactivity is recovered in the urine and 50% in the feces.
Special Populations
Pediatric: Losartan pharmacokinetics have not been investigated in patients <18 years of age.
Geriatric and Gender: Losartan pharmacokinetics have been investigated in the elderly (65–75 years) and in both genders. Plasma concentrations of losartan and its active metabolite are similar in elderly and young hypertensives. Plasma concentrations of losartan were about twice as high in female hypertensives as male hypertensives, but concentrations of the active metabolite were similar in males and females.
Race: Pharmacokinetic differences due to race have not been studied.
Renal Insufficiency: Plasma concentrations of losartan are not altered in patients with creatinine clearance above 30 mL/min. In patients with lower creatinine clearance, AUCs are about 50% greater and are doubled in hemodialysis patients. Plasma concentrations of the active metabolite are not significantly altered in patients with renal impairment or in hemodialysis patients. Neither losartan nor its active metabolite can be removed by hemodialysis.
Hepatic Insufficiency: Following oral administration in patients with mild to moderate alcoholic cirrhosis of the liver, plasma concentrations of losartan and its active metabolite were, respectively, 5 times and about 1.7 times those in young male volunteers. Compared to normal subjects the total plasma clearance of losartan in patients with hepatic insufficiency was about 50% lower and the oral bioavailability was about 2-times higher. The lower starting dose of losartan recommended for use in patients with hepatic impairment cannot be given using HYZAAR. Its use in such patients as a means of losartan titration is, therefore, not recommended (see DOSAGE AND ADMINISTRATION).
Drug Interactions
Losartan Potassium
Losartan, administered for 12 days, did not affect the pharmacokinetics or pharmacodynamics of a single dose of warfarin. Losartan did not affect the pharmacokinetics of oral or intravenous digoxin. Coadministration of losartan and cimetidine led to an increase of about 18% in AUC of losartan but did not affect the pharmacokinetics of its active metabolite. Coadministration of losartan and phenobarbital led to a reduction of about 20% in the AUC of losartan and that of its active metabolite. Conversion of losartan to its active metabolite after intravenous administration is not affected by ketoconazole, an inhibitor of P450 3A4. There is no pharmacokinetic interaction between losartan and hydrochlorothiazide.
Hydrochlorothiazide
After oral administration of hydrochlorothiazide, diuresis begins within 2 hours, peaks in about 4 hours and lasts about 6 to 12 hours.
Hydrochlorothiazide is not metabolized but is eliminated rapidly by the kidney. When plasma levels have been followed for at least 24 hours, the plasma half-life has been observed to vary between 5.6 and 14.8 hours. At least 61 percent of the oral dose is eliminated unchanged within 24 hours. Hydrochlorothiazide crosses the placental but not the blood-brain barrier and is excreted in breast milk.
Pharmacodynamics and Clinical Effects
Losartan Potassium
Losartan inhibits the pressor effect of angiotensin II (as well as angiotensin I) infusions. A dose of 100 mg inhibits the pressor effect by about 85% at peak with 25–40% inhibition persisting for 24 hours. Removal of the negative feedback of angiotensin II causes a 2–3 fold rise in plasma renin activity and consequent rise in angiotensin II plasma concentration in hypertensive patients. Losartan does not affect the response to bradykinin, whereas ACE inhibitors increase the response to bradykinin. Aldosterone plasma concentrations fall following losartan administration. In spite of the effect of losartan on aldosterone secretion, very little effect on serum potassium was observed.
In a single-dose study in normal volunteers, losartan had no effects on glomerular filtration rate, renal plasma flow or filtration fraction. In multiple dose studies in hypertensive patients, there were no notable effects on systemic or renal prostaglandin concentrations, fasting triglycerides, total cholesterol or HDL-cholesterol or fasting glucose concentrations. There was a small uricosuric effect leading to a minimal decrease in serum uric acid (mean decrease <0.4 mg/dL) during chronic oral administration.
The antihypertensive effects of losartan were demonstrated principally in 4 placebo-controlled 6–12 week trials of dosages from 10 to 150 mg per day in patients with baseline diastolic blood pressures of 95–115. The studies allowed comparisons of two doses (50–100 mg/day) as once-daily or twice-daily regimens, comparisons of peak and trough effects, and comparisons of response by gender, age, and race. Three additional studies examined the antihypertensive effects of losartan and hydrochlorothiazide in combination.
The 4 studies of losartan monotherapy included a total of 1075 patients randomized to several doses of losartan and 334 to placebo. The 10 and 25 mg doses produced some effect at peak (6 hours after dosing) but small and inconsistent trough (24 hour) responses. Doses of 50, 100, and 150 mg once daily gave statistically significant systolic/diastolic mean decreases in blood pressure, compared to placebo in the range of 5.5–10.5/3.5–7.5 mmHg, with the 150 mg dose giving no greater effect than 50–100 mg. Twice-daily dosing at 50–100 mg/day gave consistently larger trough responses than once daily dosing at the same total dose. Peak (6 hour) effects were uniformly, but moderately larger than trough effects, with the trough to peak ratio for systolic and diastolic responses 50–95% and 60–90% respectively.
Analysis of age, gender, and race subgroups of patients showed that men and women, and patients over and under 65, had generally similar responses. Losartan was effective in reducing blood pressure regardless of race, although the effect was somewhat less in black patients (usually a low-renin population).
The effect of losartan is substantially present within one week but in some studies the maximal effect occurred in 3–6 weeks. In long-term follow-up studies (without placebo control) the effect of losartan appeared to be maintained for up to a year. There is no apparent rebound effect after abrupt withdrawal of losartan. There was essentially no change in average heart rate in losartan-treated patients in controlled trials.
Losartan Potassium-Hydrochlorothiazide
The 3 controlled studies of losartan and hydrochlorothiazide included over 1300 patients assessing the antihypertensive efficacy of various doses of losartan (25, 50 and 100 mg) and concomitant hydrochlorothiazide (6.25, 12.5 and 25 mg). A factorial study compared the combination of losartan/hydrochlorothiazide 50/12.5 mg with its components and placebo. The combination of losartan/hydrochlorothiazide 50/12.5 mg resulted in an approximately additive placebo-adjusted systolic/diastolic response (15.5/9.0 mmHg for the combination compared to 8.5/5.0 mmHg for losartan alone and 7.0/3.0 mmHg for hydrochlorothiazide alone). Another study investigated the dose-response relationship of various doses of hydrochlorothiazide (6.25, 12.5 and 25 mg) or placebo on a background of losartan (50 mg) in patients not adequately controlled (SiDBP 93–120 mmHg) on losartan (50 mg) alone. The third study investigated the dose-response relationship of various doses of losartan (25, 50 and 100 mg) or placebo on a background of hydrochlorothiazide (25 mg) in patients not adequately controlled (SiDBP 93–120 mmHg) on hydrochlorothiazide (25 mg) alone. These studies showed an added antihypertensive response at trough (24 hours post-dosing) of hydrochlorothiazide 12.5 or 25 mg added to losartan 50 mg of 5.5/3.5 and 10.0/6.0 mmHg, respectively. Similarly, there was an added antihypertensive response at trough when losartan 50 or 100 mg was added to hydrochlorothiazide 25 mg of 9.0/5.5 and 12.5/6.5 mmHg, respectively. There was no significant effect on heart rate.
There was no difference in response for men and women or in patients over or under 65 years of age.
Black patients had a larger response to hydrochlorothiazide than non-black patients and a smaller response to losartan. The overall response to the combination was similar for black and non-black patients.

INDICATIONS AND USAGE

HYZAAR is indicated for the treatment of hypertension. This fixed dose combination is not indicated for initial therapy (see DOSAGE AND ADMINISTRATION).

CONTRAINDICATIONS

HYZAAR is contraindicated in patients who are hypersensitive to any component of this product.
Because of the hydrochlorothiazide component, this product is contraindicated in patients with anuria or hypersensitivity to other sulfonamide-derived drugs.

WARNINGS

Fetal/Neonatal Morbidity and Mortality
Drugs that act directly on the renin-angiotensin system can cause fetal and neonatal morbidity and death when administered to pregnant women. Several dozen cases have been reported in the world literature in patients who were taking angiotensin converting enzyme inhibitors. When pregnancy is detected, HYZAAR should be discontinued as soon as possible.
The use of drugs that act directly on the renin-angiotensin system during the second and third trimesters of pregnancy

Continued on next page

Hyzaar—Cont.

has been associated with fetal and neonatal injury, including hypotension, neonatal skull hypoplasia, anuria, reversible or irreversible renal failure, and death. Oligohydramnios has also been reported, presumably resulting from decreased fetal renal function; oligohydramnios in this setting has been associated with fetal limb contractures, craniofacial deformation, and hypoplastic lung development. Prematurity, intrauterine growth retardation, and patent ductus arteriosus have also been reported, although it is not clear whether these occurrences were due to exposure to the drug.

These adverse effects do not appear to have resulted from intrauterine drug exposure that has been limited to the first trimester.

Mothers whose embryos and fetuses are exposed to an angiotensin II receptor antagonist only during the first trimester should be so informed. Nonetheless, when patients become pregnant, physicians should have the patient discontinue the use of HYZAAR as soon as possible.

Rarely (probably less often than once in every thousand pregnancies), no alternative to an angiotensin II receptor antagonist will be found. In these rare cases, the mothers should be apprised of the potential hazards to their fetuses, and serial ultrasound examinations should be performed to assess the intra-amniotic environment.

If oligohydramnios is observed, HYZAAR should be discontinued unless it is considered life-saving for the mother. Contraction stress testing (CST), a non-stress test (NST), or biophysical profiling (BPP) may be appropriate, depending upon the week of pregnancy. Patients and physicians should be aware, however, that oligohydramnios may not appear until after the fetus has sustained irreversible injury.

Infants with histories of *in utero* exposure to an angiotensin II receptor antagonist should be closely observed for hypotension, oliguria, and hyperkalemia. If oliguria occurs, attention should be directed toward support of blood pressure and renal perfusion. Exchange transfusion or dialysis may be required as means of reversing hypotension and/or substituting for disordered renal function.

There was no evidence of teratogenicity in rats or rabbits treated with a maximum losartan potassium dose of 10 mg/kg/day in combination with 2.5 mg/kg/day of hydrochlorothiazide. At these dosages, respective exposures (AUCs) of losartan, its active metabolite, and hydrochlorothiazide in rabbits were approximately 5-, 1.5-, and 1.0-times those achieved in humans with 100 mg losartan in combination with 25 mg hydrochlorothiazide. AUC values for losartan, its active metabolite and hydrochlorothiazide, extrapolated from data obtained with losartan administered to rats at a dose of 50 mg/kg/day in combination with 12.5 mg/kg/day of hydrochlorothiazide, were approximately 6, 2, and 2 times greater than those achieved in humans with 100 mg of losartan in combination with 25 mg of hydrochlorothiazide.

Fetal toxicity in rats, as evidenced by a slight increase in supernumerary ribs, was observed when females were treated prior to and throughout gestation with 10 mg/kg/day losartan in combination with 2.5 mg/kg/day hydrochlorothiazide. As also observed in studies with losartan alone, adverse fetal and neonatal effects, including decreased body weight, renal toxicity, and mortality, occurred when pregnant rats were treated during late gestation and/or lactation with 50 mg/kg/day losartan in combination with 12.5 mg/kg/day hydrochlorothiazide. Respective AUCs for losartan, its active metabolite and hydrochlorothiazide at these dosages in rats were approximately 35, 10 and 10 times greater than those achieved in humans with the administration of 100 mg of losartan in combination with 25 mg hydrochlorothiazide. When hydrochlorothiazide was administered without losartan to pregnant mice and rats during their respective periods of major organogenesis, at doses up to 3000 and 1000 mg/kg/day, respectively, there was no evidence of harm to the fetus.

Thiazides cross the placental barrier and appear in cord blood. There is a risk of fetal or neonatal jaundice, thrombocytopenia, and possibly other adverse reactions that have occurred in adults.

Hypotension—Volume-Depleted Patients

In patients who are intravascularly volume-depleted (e.g., those treated with diuretics), symptomatic hypotension may occur after initiation of therapy with HYZAAR. This condition should be corrected prior to administration of HYZAAR (see DOSAGE AND ADMINISTRATION).

Impaired Hepatic Function

Losartan Potassium-Hydrochlorothiazide

HYZAAR is not recommended for patients with hepatic impairment who require titration with losartan. The lower starting dose of losartan recommended for use in patients with hepatic impairment cannot be given using HYZAAR.

Hydrochlorothiazide

Thiazides should be used with caution in patients with impaired hepatic function or progressive liver disease, since minor alterations of fluid and electrolyte balance may precipitate hepatic coma.

Hypersensitivity Reaction

Hypersensitivity reactions to hydrochlorothiazide may occur in patients with or without a history of allergy or bronchial asthma, but are more likely in patients with such a history.

Systemic Lupus Erythematosus

Thiazide diuretics have been reported to cause exacerbation or activation of systemic lupus erythematosus.

Lithium Interaction

Lithium generally should not be given with thiazides (see PRECAUTIONS, *Drug Interactions, Hydrocholorothiazide, Lithium*).

PRECAUTIONS

General

Hypersensitivity. Angioedema. See ADVERSE REACTIONS, *Post-Marketing Experience.*

Losartan Potassium-Hydrochlorothiazide

In double-blind clinical trials of various doses of losartan potassium and hydrochlorothiazide, the incidence of hypertensive patients who developed hypokalemia (serum potassium <3.5 mEq/L) was 6.7% versus 3.5% for placebo; the incidence of hyperkalemia (serum potassium >5.7 mEq/L) was 0.4%. No patient discontinued due to increases or decreases in serum potassium. The mean decrease in serum potassium in patients treated with various doses of losartan and hydrochlorothiazide was 0.123 mEq/L. In patients treated with various doses of losartan and hydrochlorothiazide, there was also a dose-related decrease in the hypokalemic response to hydrochlorothiazide as the dose of losartan was increased, as well as a dose-related decrease in serum uric acid with increasing doses of losartan.

Hydrochlorothiazide

Periodic determination of serum electrolytes to detect possible electrolyte imbalance should be performed at appropriate intervals.

All patients receiving thiazide therapy should be observed for clinical signs of fluid or electrolyte imbalance: hyponatremia, hypochloremic alkalosis, and hypokalemia. Serum and urine electrolyte determinations are particularly important when the patient is vomiting excessively or receiving parenteral fluids. Warning signs or symptoms of fluid and electrolyte imbalance, irrespective of cause, include dryness of mouth, thirst, weakness, lethargy, drowsiness, restlessness, confusion, seizures, muscle pains or cramps, muscular fatigue, hypotension, oliguria, tachycardia, and gastrointestinal disturbances such as nausea and vomiting.

Hypokalemia may develop, especially with brisk diuresis, when severe cirrhosis is present, or after prolonged therapy. Interference with adequate oral electrolyte intake will also contribute to hypokalemia. Hypokalemia may cause cardiac arrhythmia and may also sensitize or exaggerate the response of the heart to the toxic effects of digitalis (e.g., increased ventricular irritability).

Although any chloride deficit is generally mild and usually does not require specific treatment except under extraordinary circumstances (as in liver disease or renal disease), chloride replacement may be required in the treatment of metabolic alkalosis.

Dilutional hyponatremia may occur in edematous patients in hot weather; appropriate therapy is water restriction, rather than administration of salt except in rare instances when the hyponatremia is life-threatening. In actual salt depletion, appropriate replacement is the therapy of choice.

Hyperuricemia may occur or frank gout may be precipitated in certain patients receiving thiazide therapy. Because losartan decreases uric acid, losartan in combination with hydrochlorothiazide attenuates the diuretic-induced hyperuricemia.

In diabetic patients dosage adjustments of insulin or oral hypoglycemic agents may be required. Hyperglycemia may occur with thiazide diuretics. Thus latent diabetes mellitus may become manifest during thiazide therapy.

The antihypertensive effects of the drug may be enhanced in the postsympathectomy patient.

If progressive renal impairment becomes evident consider withholding or discontinuing diuretic therapy.

Thiazides have been shown to increase the urinary excretion of magnesium; this may result in hypomagnesemia.

Thiazides may decrease urinary calcium excretion. Thiazides may cause intermittent and slight elevation of serum calcium in the absence of known disorders of calcium metabolism. Marked hypercalcemia may be evidence of hidden hyperparathyroidism. Thiazides should be discontinued before carrying out tests for parathyroid function.

Increases in cholesterol and triglyceride levels may be associated with thiazide diuretic therapy.

Impaired Renal Function

As a consequence of inhibiting the renin-angiotensin-aldosterone system, changes in renal function have been reported in susceptible individuals treated with losartan; in some patients, these changes in renal function were reversible upon discontinuation of therapy.

In patients whose renal function may depend on the activity of the renin-angiotensin-aldosterone system (e.g., patients with severe congestive heart failure), treatment with angiotensin converting enzyme inhibitors has been associated with oliguria and/or progressive azotemia and (rarely) with acute renal failure and/or death. Similar outcomes have been reported with losartan.

In studies of ACE inhibitors in patients with unilateral or bilateral renal artery stenosis, increases in serum creatinine or BUN have been reported. Similar effects have been reported with losartan; in some patients, these effects were reversible upon discontinuation of therapy.

Thiazides should be used with caution in severe renal disease. In patients with renal disease, thiazides may precipitate azotemia. Cumulative effects of the drug may develop in patients with impaired renal function.

Information for Patients

Pregnancy: Female patients of childbearing age should be told about the consequences of second- and third-trimester exposure to drugs that act on the renin-angiotensin system, and they should also be told that these consequences do not appear to have resulted from intrauterine drug exposure that has been limited to the first trimester. These patients should be asked to report pregnancies to their physicians as soon as possible.

Symptomatic Hypotension: A patient receiving HYZAAR should be cautioned that lightheadedness can occur, especially during the first days of therapy, and that it should be reported to the prescribing physician. The patients should be told that if syncope occurs, HYZAAR should be discontinued until the physician has been consulted.

All patients should be cautioned that inadequate fluid intake, excessive perspiration, diarrhea, or vomiting can lead to an excessive fall in blood pressure, with the same consequences of lightheadedness and possible syncope.

Potassium Supplements: A patient receiving HYZAAR should be told not to use potassium supplements or salt substitutes containing potassium without consulting the prescribing physician (see PRECAUTIONS, *Drug Interactions, Losartan Potassium*).

Drug Interactions

Losartan Potassium

No significant drug-drug pharmacokinetic interactions have been found in interaction studies with hydrochlorothiazide, digoxin, warfarin, cimetidine and phenobarbital. (See CLINICAL PHARMACOLOGY, *Drug Interactions.*) Potent inhibitors of cytochrome P450 3A4 and 2C9 have not been studied clinically but *in vitro* studies show significant inhibition of the formation of the active metabolite by inhibitors of P450 3A4 (ketoconazole, troleandomycin, gestodene), or P450 2C9 (sulfaphenazole) and nearly complete inhibition by the combination of sulfaphenazole and ketoconazole. In humans, ketoconazole, an inhibitor of P450 3A4, did not affect the conversion of losartan to the active metabolite after intravenous administration of losartan. Inhibitors of cytochrome P450 2C9 have not been studied clinically. The pharmacodynamic consequences of concomitant use of losartan and inhibitors of P450 2C9 have not been examined.

As with other drugs that block angiotensin II or its effects, concomitant use of potassium-sparing diuretics (e.g., spironolactone, triamterene, amiloride), potassium supplements, or salt substitutes containing potassium may lead to increases in serum potassium (see PRECAUTIONS, *Information for Patients, Potassium Supplements*).

Hydrochlorothiazide

When administered concurrently the following drugs may interact with thiazide diuretics:

Alcohol, barbiturates, or narcotics—potentiation of orthostatic hypotension may occur.

Antidiabetic drugs (oral agents and insulin)—dosage adjustment of the antidiabetic drug may be required.

Other antihypertensive drugs—additive effect or potentiation.

Cholestyramine and colestipol resins—Absorption of hydrochlorothiazide is impaired in the presence of anionic exchange resins. Single doses of either cholestyramine or colestipol resins bind the hydrochlorothiazide and reduce its absorption from the gastrointestinal tract by up to 85 and 43 percent, respectively.

Corticosteroids, ACTH—intensified electrolyte depletion, particularly hypokalemia.

Pressor amines (e.g., norepinephrine)—possible decreased response to pressor amines but not sufficient to preclude their use.

Skeletal muscle relaxants, nondepolarizing (e.g., tubocurarine)—possible increased responsiveness to the muscle relaxant.

Lithium—should not generally be given with diuretics. Diuretic agents reduce the renal clearance of lithium and add a high risk of lithium toxicity. Refer to the package insert for lithium preparations before use of such preparations with HYZAAR.

Non-steroidal Anti-inflammatory Drugs—In some patients, the administration of a non-steroidal anti-inflammatory agent can reduce the diuretic, natriuretic, and antihypertensive effects of loop, potassium-sparing and thiazide diuretics. Therefore, when HYZAAR and non-steroidal anti-inflammatory agents are used concomitantly, the patient should be observed closely to determine if the desired effect of the diuretic is obtained.

Carcinogenesis, Mutagenesis, Impairment of Fertility

Losartan Potassium-Hydrochlorothiazide

No carcinogenicity studies have been conducted with the losartan potassium-hydrochlorothiazide combination.

Losartan potassium-hydrochlorothiazide when tested at a weight ratio of 4:1, was negative in the Ames microbial mutagenesis assay and the V-79 Chinese hamster lung cell mutagenesis assay. In addition, there was no evidence of direct genotoxicity in the *in vitro* alkaline elution assay in rat hepatocytes and *in vitro* chromosomal aberration assay in Chinese hamster ovary cells at noncytotoxic concentrations.

Losartan potassium, coadministered with hydrochlorothiazide, had no effect on the fertility or mating behavior of male rats of dosages up to 135 mg/kg/day of losartan and 33.75 mg/kg/day of hydrochlorothiazide. These dosages have been shown to provide respective systemic exposures (AUCs) for losartan, its active metabolite and hydrochlorothiazide that are approximately 60, 60 and 30 times greater than those achieved in humans with 100 mg of losartan potassium in combination with 25 mg of hydrochlorothiazide.

In female rats, however, the coadministration of doses as low as 10 mg/kg/day of losartan and 2.5 mg/kg/day of hydrochlorothiazide was associated with slight but statistically significant decreases in fecundity and fertility indices. AUC values for losartan, its active metabolite and hydrochlorothiazide, extrapolated from data obtained with losartan administered to rats at a dose of 50 mg/kg/day in combination with 12.5 mg/kg/day of hydrochlorothiazide, were approximately 6, 2, and 2 times greater than those achieved in humans with 100 mg of losartan in combination with 25 mg of hydrochlorothiazide.

Losartan Potassium

Losartan potassium was not carcinogenic when administered at maximally tolerated dosages to rats and mice for 105 and 92 weeks, respectively. Female rats given the highest dose (270 mg/kg/day) had a slightly higher incidence of pancreatic acinar adenoma. The maximally tolerated dosages (270 mg/kg/day in rats, 200 mg/kg/day in mice) provided systemic exposures for losartan and its pharmacologically active metabolite that were approximately 160 and 90 times (rats) and 30 and 15 times (mice) the exposure of a 50 kg human given 100 mg per day.

Losartan potassium was negative in the microbial mutagenesis and V-79 mammalian cell mutagenesis assays and in the *in vitro* alkaline elution and *in vitro* and *in vivo* chromosomal aberration assays. In addition, the active metabolite showed no evidence of genotoxicity in the microbial mutagenesis, *in vitro* alkaline elution, and *in vitro* chromosomal aberration assays.

Fertility and reproductive performance were not affected in studies with male rats given oral doses of losartan potassium up to approximately 150 mg/kg/day. The administration of toxic dosage levels in females (300/200 mg/kg/day) was associated with a significant ($p<0.05$) decrease in the number of corpora lutea/female, implants/female, and live fetuses/female at C-section. At 100 mg/kg/day only a decrease in the number of corpora lutea/female was observed. The relationship of these findings to drug-treatment is uncertain since there was no effect at these dosage levels on implants/pregnant female, percent post-implantation loss, or live animals/litter at parturition. In nonpregnant rats dosed at 135 mg/kg/day for 7 days, systemic exposure (AUCs) for losartan and its active metabolite were approximately 66 and 26 times the exposure achieved in man at the maximum recommended human daily dosage (100 mg).

Hydrochlorothiazide

Two-year feeding studies in mice and rats conducted under the auspices of the National Toxicology Program (NTP) uncovered no evidence of a carcinogenic potential of hydrochlorothiazide in female mice (at doses of up to approximately 600 mg/kg/day) or in male and female rats (at doses of up to approximately 100 mg/kg/day). The NTP, however, found equivocal evidence for hepatocarcinogenicity in male mice.

Hydrochlorothiazide was not genotoxic *in vitro* in the Ames mutagenicity assay of *Salmonella typhimurium* strains TA 98, TA 100, TA 1535, TA 1537, and TA 1538 and in the Chinese Hamster Ovary (CHO) test for chromosomal aberrations, or *in vivo* in assays using mouse germinal cell chromosomes, Chinese hamster bone marrow chromosomes, and the *Drosophila* sex-linked recessive lethal trait gene. Positive test results were obtained only in the *in vitro* CHO Sister Chromatid Exchange (clastogenicity) and in the Mouse Lymphoma Cell (mutagenicity) assays, using concentrations of hydrochlorothiazide from 43 to 1300 µg/mL, and in the *Aspergillus nidulans* non-disjunction assay at an unspecified concentration.

Hydrochlorothiazide had no adverse effects on the fertility of mice and rats of either sex in studies wherein these species were exposed, via their diet, to doses of up to 100 and 4 mg/kg, respectively, prior to mating and throughout gestation.

Pregnancy

Pregnancy Categories C (first trimester) and D (second and third trimesters). See WARNINGS, *Fetal/Neonatal Morbidity and Mortality*.

Nursing Mothers

It is not known whether losartan is excreted in human milk, but significant levels of losartan and its active metabolite were shown to be present in rat milk. Thiazides appear in human milk. Because of the potential for adverse effects on the nursing infant, a decision should be made whether to discontinue nursing or discontinue the drug, taking into account the importance of the drug to the mother.

Pediatric Use

Safety and effectiveness in pediatric patients have not been established.

Use in the Elderly

Of the total number of patients in controlled clinical studies of hypertension with HYZAAR, 107 patients (12.5%) were 65 years and over, while 9 patients (1.0%) were 75 years and over. No overall differences in effectiveness or safety were observed between these patients and younger patients, but greater sensitivity of some older individuals cannot be ruled out.

ADVERSE REACTIONS

Losartan potassium-hydrochlorothiazide has been evaluated for safety in 858 patients treated for essential hypertension. In clinical trials with losartan potassium-hydrochlorothiazide, no adverse experiences peculiar to this combination have been observed. Adverse experiences have been limited to those that were reported previously with losartan potassium and/or hydrochlorothiazide. The overall incidence of adverse experiences reported with the combination was comparable to placebo.

In general, treatment with losartan potassium-hydrochlorothiazide was well tolerated. For the most part, adverse experiences have been mild and transient in nature and have not required discontinuation of therapy. In controlled clinical trials, discontinuation of therapy due to clinical adverse experiences was required in only 2.8% and 2.3% of patients treated with the combination and placebo, respectively.

In these double-blind controlled clinical trials, the following adverse experiences reported with losartan-hydrochlorothiazide occurred in ≥1 percent of patients, and more often on drug than placebo, regardless of drug relationship:

	Losartan Potassium-Hydrochlorothiazide (n=858)	Placebo (n=173)
Body as a Whole		
Abdominal pain	1.2	0.6
Edema/swelling	1.3	1.2
Cardiovascular		
Palpitation	1.4	0.0
Musculoskeletal		
Back pain	2.1	0.6
Nervous/Psychiatric		
Dizziness	5.7	2.9
Respiratory		
Cough	2.6	2.3
Sinusitis	1.2	0.6
Upper respiratory infection	6.1	4.6
Skin		
Rash	1.4	0.0

The following adverse events were also reported at a rate of 1% or greater, but were as, or more, common in the placebo group: asthenia/fatigue, diarrhea, nausea, headache, bronchitis, pharyngitis.

Adverse events occurred at about the same rates in men and women, older and younger patients, and black and non-black patients.

A patient with known hypersensitivity to aspirin and penicillin, when treated with losartan potassium, was withdrawn from study due to swelling of the lips and eyelids and facial rash, reported as angioedema, which returned to normal 5 days after therapy was discontinued.

Superficial peeling of palms and hemolysis was reported in one subject treated with losartan potassium.

Losartan Potassium

Other adverse experiences that have been reported with losartan, without regard to causality, are listed below:

Body as a Whole: chest pain, facial edema, fever, orthostatic effects, syncope; *Cardiovascular:* angina pectoris, arrhythmias including atrial fibrillation, sinus bradycardia, tachycardia, ventricular tachycardia and ventricular fibrillation, CVA, hypotension, myocardial infarction, second degree AV block; *Digestive:* anorexia, constipation, dental pain, dry mouth, dyspepsia, flatulence, gastritis, vomiting; *Hematologic:* anemia; *Metabolic:* gout; *Musculoskeletal:* arm pain, arthralgia, arthritis, fibromyalgia, hip pain, joint swelling, knee pain, leg pain, muscle cramps, muscle weakness, musculoskeletal pain, myalgia, shoulder pain, stiffness; *Nervous System/Psychiatric:* anxiety, anxiety disorder, ataxia, confusion, depression, dream abnormality, hypesthesia, insomnia, libido decreased, memory impairment, migraine, nervousness, panic disorder, paresthesia, peripheral neuropathy, sleep disorder, somnolence, tremor, vertigo; *Respiratory:* dyspnea, epistaxis, nasal congestion, pharyngeal discomfort, respiratory congestion, rhinitis, sinus disorder; *Skin:* alopecia, dermatitis, dry skin, ecchymosis, erythema, flushing, photosensitivity, pruritus, sweating, urticaria; *Special Senses:* blurred vision, burning/stinging in the eye, conjunctivitis, decrease in visual acuity, taste perversion, tinnitus; *Urogenital:* impotence, nocturia, urinary frequency, urinary tract infection.

Hydrochlorothiazide

Other adverse experiences that have been reported with hydrochlorothiazide, without regard to causality, are listed below:

Body as a Whole: weakness; *Digestive:* pancreatitis, jaundice (intrahepatic cholestatic jaundice), sialadenitis, cramping, gastric irritation; *Hematologic:* aplastic anemia, agranulocytosis, leukopenia, hemolytic anemia, thrombocytopenia; *Hypersensitivity:* purpura, photosensitivity, urticaria, necrotizing angiitis (vasculitis and cutaneous vasculitis), fever, respiratory distress including pneumonitis and pulmonary edema, anaphylactic reactions; *Metabolic:* hyperglycemia, glycosuria, hyperuricemia; *Musculoskeletal:* muscle spasm; *Nervous System/Psychiatric:* restlessness; *Renal:* renal failure, renal dysfunction, interstitial nephritis; *Skin:* erythema multiforme including Stevens-Johnson syndrome, exfoliative dermatitis including toxic epidermal necrolysis; *Special Senses:* transient blurred vision, xanthopsia.

Persistent dry cough (with an incidence of a few percent) has been associated with ACE inhibitor use and in practice can be a cause of discontinuation of ACE inhibitor therapy. Two prospective, parallel-group, double-blind, randomized, controlled trials were conducted to assess the effects of losartan on the incidence of cough in hypertensive patients who had experienced cough while receiving ACE inhibitor therapy. Patients who had typical ACE inhibitor cough when challenged with lisinopril, whose cough disappeared on placebo, were randomized to losartan 50 mg, lisinopril 20 mg, or either placebo (one study, n=97) or 25 mg hydrochlorothiazide (n=135). The double-blind treatment period lasted up to 8 weeks. The incidence of cough is shown below.

Study 1†	HCTZ	Losartan	Lisinopril
Cough	25%	17%	69%
Study 2††	**Placebo**	**Losartan**	**Lisinopril**
Cough	35%	29%	62%

†Demographics = (89% caucasian, 64% female)
††Demographics = (90% caucasian, 51% female)

These studies demonstrate that the incidence of cough associated with losartan therapy, in a population that all had cough associated with ACE inhibitor therapy, is similar to that associated with hydrochlorothiazide or placebo therapy.

Cases of cough, including positive re-challenges, have been reported with the use of losartan in post-marketing experience.

Post-Marketing Experience

The following additional adverse reactions have been reported in post-marketing experience:

Hypersensitivity: Angioedema, including swelling of the larynx and glottis, causing airway obstruction and/or swelling of the face, lips, pharynx, and/or tongue has been reported rarely in patients treated with losartan; some of these patients previously experienced angioedema with other drugs including ACE inhibitors. Anaphylactic reactions have been reported.

Digestive: Hepatitis has been reported rarely in patients treated with losartan.

Respiratory: Dry cough (see above) has been reported with losartan.

Hyperkalemia and hyponatremia have been reported with losartan.

Laboratory Test Findings

In controlled clinical trials, clinically important changes in standard laboratory parameters were rarely associated with administration of HYZAAR.

Creatinine, Blood Urea Nitrogen: Minor increases in blood urea nitrogen (BUN) or serum creatinine were observed in 0.6 and 0.8 percent, respectively, of patients with essential hypertension treated with HYZAAR alone. No patient discontinued taking HYZAAR due to increased BUN. One patient discontinued taking HYZAAR due to a minor increase in serum creatinine.

Hemoglobin and Hematocrit: Small decreases in hemoglobin and hematocrit (mean decreases of approximately 0.14 grams percent and 0.72 volume percent, respectively) occurred frequently in patients treated with HYZAAR alone, but were rarely of clinical importance. No patients were discontinued due to anemia.

Liver Function Tests: Occasional elevations of liver enzymes and/or serum bilirubin have occurred. In patients with essential hypertension treated with HYZAAR alone, no patients were discontinued due to these laboratory adverse experiences.

Serum Electrolytes: See PRECAUTIONS.

OVERDOSAGE

Losartan Potassium

Significant lethality was observed in mice and rats after oral administration of 1000 mg/kg and 2000 mg/kg, respectively, about 44 and 170 times the maximum recommended human dose on a mg/m^2 basis.

Limited data are available in regard to overdosage in humans. The most likely manifestation of overdosage would be hypotension and tachycardia; bradycardia could occur from parasympathetic (vagal) stimulation. If symptomatic hypotension should occur, supportive treatment should be instituted.

Neither losartan nor its active metabolite can be removed by hemodialysis.

Hydrochlorothiazide

The oral LD_{50} of hydrochlorothiazide is greater than 10 g/kg in both mice and rats. The most common signs and symptoms observed are those caused by electrolyte depletion (hypokalemia, hypochloremia, hyponatremia) and dehydration resulting from excessive diuresis. If digitalis has also been administered, hypokalemia may accentuate cardiac arrhythmias. The degree to which hydrochlorothiazide is removed by hemodialysis has not been established.

DOSAGE AND ADMINISTRATION

The usual starting dose of losartan is 50 mg once daily, with 25 mg recommended for patients with intravascular volume depletion (e.g., patients treated with diuretics) (see WARNINGS, *Hypotension—Volume-Depleted Patients*) and pa-

Continued on next page

Information on the Merck & Co., Inc. products listed on these pages is the full prescribing information from product circulars in use September 30, 2000. For information, please call 1-800-NSC MERCK [1-800-672-6372].

Hyzaar—Cont.

tients with a history of hepatic impairment (see WARNINGS, *Impaired Hepatic Function*). Losartan can be administered once or twice daily at total daily doses of 25 to 100 mg. If the antihypertensive effect measured at trough using once-a-day dosing is inadequate, a twice-a-day regimen at the same total daily dose or an increase in dose may give a more satisfactory response.
Hydrochlorothiazide is effective in doses of 12.5 to 50 mg once daily and can be given at doses of 12.5 to 25 mg as HYZAAR.
To minimize dose-independent side effects, it is usually appropriate to begin combination therapy only after a patient has failed to achieve the desired effect with monotherapy.
The side effects (see WARNINGS) of losartan are generally rare and apparently independent of dose; those of hydrochlorothiazide are a mixture of dose-dependent (primarily hypokalemia) and dose-independent phenomena (e.g., pancreatitis), the former much more common than the latter. Therapy with any combination of losartan and hydrochlorothiazide will be associated with both sets of dose-independent side effects.
Replacement Therapy: The combination may be substituted for the titrated components.
Dose Titration by Clinical Effect: A patient whose blood pressure is not adequately controlled with losartan monotherapy (see above) may be switched to HYZAAR 50-12.5 (losartan 50 mg/hydrochlorothiazide 12.5 mg) once daily. If blood pressure remains uncontrolled after about 3 weeks of therapy, the dose may be increased to two tablets of HYZAAR 50-12.5 once daily or one tablet of HYZAAR 100-25 (losartan 100 mg/hydrochlorothiazide 25 mg) once daily.
A patient whose blood pressure is inadequately controlled by 25 mg once daily of hydrochlorothiazide, or is controlled but who experiences hypokalemia with this regimen, may be switched to HYZAAR 50-12.5 (losartan 50 mg/hydrochlorothiazide 12.5 mg) once daily, reducing the dose of hydrochlorothiazide without reducing the overall expected antihypertensive response. The clinical response to HYZAAR 50-12.5 should be subsequently evaluated and if blood pressure remains uncontrolled after about 3 weeks of therapy, the dose may be increased to two tablets of HYZAAR 50-12.5 once daily or one tablet of HYZAAR 100-25 (losartan 100 mg/hydrochlorothiazide 25 mg) once daily.
The usual dose of HYZAAR is one tablet of HYZAAR 50-12.5 once daily. More than two tablets of HYZAAR 50-12.5 once daily or more than one tablet of HYZAAR 100-25 once daily is not recommended. The maximal antihypertensive effect is attained about 3 weeks after initiation of therapy.
Use in Patients with Renal Impairment: The usual regimens of therapy with HYZAAR may be followed as long as the patient's creatinine clearance is >30 mL/min. In patients with more severe renal impairment, loop diuretics are preferred to thiazides, so HYZAAR is not recommended.
Patients with Hepatic Impairment: HYZAAR is not recommended for titration in patients with hepatic impairment (see WARNINGS, *Impaired Hepatic Function*) because the appropriate 25 mg starting dose of losartan cannot be given.
HYZAAR may be administered with other antihypertensive agents.
HYZAAR may be administered with or without food.

HOW SUPPLIED

No. 3502—Tablets HYZAAR, 50-12.5 are yellow, teardrop shaped, film-coated tablets, coded MRK 717 on one side and HYZAAR on the other. Each tablet contains 50 mg of losartan potassium and 12.5 mg of hydrochlorothiazide. They are supplied as follows:
NDC 0006-0717-31 unit of use bottles of 30
NDC 0006-0717-54 unit of use bottles of 90
NDC 0006-0717-58 unit of use bottles of 100.
NDC 0006-0717-28 unit dose packages of 100
NDC 0006-0717-82 unit of use bottles of 1,000.
Shown in Product Identification Guide, page 323
No. 3793—Tablets HYZAAR 100-25 are light yellow, teardrop shaped, film-coated tablets, coded MRK 747 on one side and HYZAAR on the other. Each tablet contains 100 mg of losartan potassium and 25 mg of hydrochlorothiazide. They are supplied as follows:
NDC 0006-0747-31 unit of use bottles of 30
NDC 0006-0747-58 unit of use bottles of 100
NDC 0006-0747-28 unit dose packages of 100.
Shown in Product Identification Guide, page 323
Storage
Store at 25°C (77°F); excursions permitted to 15–30°C (59–86°F) [see USP Controlled Room Temperature]. Keep container tightly closed. Protect from light.
Manufactured for:
MERCK & CO., INC., West Point, PA 19486, USA
by:
DuPont Pharma, Wilmington, DE 19880 USA
7892813 Issued December 1999

INDOCIN® Capsules, Oral Suspension and Suppositories (Indomethacin) ℞

DESCRIPTION

INDOCIN* (Indomethacin) cannot be considered a simple analgesic and should not be used in conditions other than those recommended under INDICATIONS.
INDOCIN is supplied in three dosage forms. Capsules INDOCIN for oral administration contain either 25 mg or 50 mg of indomethacin and the following inactive ingredients: colloidal silicon dioxide, FD & C Blue 1, FD & C Red 3, gelatin, lactose, lecithin, magnesium stearate, and titanium dioxide. Suspension INDOCIN for oral use contains 25 mg of indomethacin per 5 mL, alcohol 1%, and sorbic acid 0.1% added as a preservative and the following inactive ingredients: antifoam AF emulsion, flavors, purified water, sodium hydroxide or hydrochloric acid to adjust pH, sorbitol solution, tragacanth. Suppositories INDOCIN for rectal use contain 50 mg of indomethacin and the following inactive ingredients: butylated hydroxyanisole, butylated hydroxytoluene, edetic acid, glycerin, polyethylene glycol 3350, polyethylene glycol 8000 and sodium chloride. Indomethacin is a non-steroidal anti-inflammatory indole derivative designated chemically as 1-(4-chlorobenzoyl)-5-methoxy-2-methyl-1*H* -indole-3-acetic acid. Indomethacin is practically insoluble in water and sparingly soluble in alcohol. It has a pKa of 4.5 and is stable in neutral or slightly acidic media and decomposes in strong alkali. The suspension has a pH of 4.0–5.0. The structural formula is:

CO, Cl, N, CH_3, CH_3O, CH_2COOH

*Registered trademark of MERCK & CO., INC.

CLINICAL PHARMACOLOGY

INDOCIN is a non-steroidal drug with anti-inflammatory, antipyretic and analgesic properties. Its mode of action, like that of other anti-inflammatory drugs, is not known. However, its therapeutic action is not due to pituitary-adrenal stimulation.
INDOCIN is a potent inhibitor of prostaglandin synthesis *in vitro*. Concentrations are reached during therapy which have been demonstrated to have an effect *in vivo* as well. Prostaglandins sensitize afferent nerves and potentiate the action of bradykinin in inducing pain in animal models. Moreover, prostaglandins are known to be among the mediators of inflammation. Since indomethacin is an inhibitor of prostaglandin synthesis, its mode of action may be due to a decrease of prostaglandins in peripheral tissues.
INDOCIN has been shown to be an effective anti-inflammatory agent, appropriate for long-term use in rheumatoid arthritis, ankylosing spondylitis, and osteoarthritis.
INDOCIN affords relief of symptoms; it does not alter the progressive course of the underlying disease.
INDOCIN suppresses inflammation in rheumatoid arthritis as demonstrated by relief of pain, and reduction of fever, swelling and tenderness. Improvement in patients treated with INDOCIN for rheumatoid arthritis has been demonstrated by a reduction in joint swelling, average number of joints involved, and morning stiffness; by increased mobility as demonstrated by a decrease in walking time; and by improved functional capability as demonstrated by an increase in grip strength.
Indomethacin has been reported to diminish basal and CO_2 stimulated cerebral blood flow in healthy volunteers following acute oral and intravenous administration. In one study after one week of treatment with orally administered indomethacin, this effect on basal cerebral blood flow had disappeared. The clinical significance of this effect has not been established.
Capsules INDOCIN have been found effective in relieving the pain, reducing the fever, swelling, redness, and tenderness of acute gouty arthritis—see INDICATIONS.
Following single oral doses of Capsules INDOCIN 25 mg or 50 mg, indomethacin is readily absorbed, attaining peak plasma concentrations of about 1 and 2 mcg/mL, respectively, at about 2 hours. Orally administered Capsules INDOCIN are virtually 100% bioavailable, with 90% of the dose absorbed within 4 hours. A single 50 mg dose of Oral Suspension INDOCIN was found to be bioequivalent to a 50 mg INDOCIN capsule when each was administered with food.
Indomethacin is eliminated via renal excretion, metabolism, and biliary excretion. Indomethacin undergoes appreciable enterohepatic circulation. The mean half-life of indomethacin is estimated to be about 4.5 hours. With a typical therapeutic regimen of 25 or 50 mg t.i.d., the steady-state plasma concentrations of indomethacin are an average 1.4 times those following the first dose.
The rate of absorption is more rapid from the rectal suppository than from Capsules INDOCIN. Ordinarily, therefore, the total amount absorbed from the suppository would be expected to be at least equivalent to the capsule. In controlled clinical trials, however, the amount of indomethacin absorbed was found to be somewhat less (80–90%) than that absorbed from Capsules INDOCIN. This is probably because some subjects did not retain the material from the suppository for the one hour necessary to assure complete absorption. Since the suppository dissolves rather quickly rather than melting slowly, it is seldom recovered in recognizable form if the patient retains the suppository for more than a few minutes.
Indomethacin exists in the plasma as the parent drug and its desmethyl, desbenzoyl, and desmethyl-desbenzoyl metabolites, all in the unconjugated form. About 60 percent of an oral dosage is recovered in urine as drug and metabolites (26 percent as indomethacin and its glucuronide), and 33 percent is recovered in feces (1.5 percent as indomethacin).
About 99% of indomethacin is bound to protein in plasma over the expected range of therapeutic plasma concentrations. Indomethacin has been found to cross the blood-brain barrier and the placenta.
In a gastroscopic study in 45 healthy subjects, the number of gastric mucosal abnormalities was significantly higher in the group receiving Capsules INDOCIN than in the group taking Suppositories INDOCIN or placebo.
In a double-blind comparative clinical study involving 175 patients with rheumatoid arthritis, however, the incidence of upper gastrointestinal adverse effects with Suppositories or Capsules INDOCIN was comparable. The incidence of lower gastrointestinal adverse effects was greater in the suppository group.

INDICATIONS

Indomethacin has been found effective in active stages of the following:
1. Moderate to severe rheumatoid arthritis including acute flares of chronic disease.
2. Moderate to severe ankylosing spondylitis.
3. Moderate to severe osteoarthritis.
4. Acute painful shoulder (bursitis and/or tendinitis).
5. Acute gouty arthritis.

INDOCIN may enable the reduction of steroid dosage in patients receiving steroids for the more severe forms of rheumatoid arthritis. In such instances the steroid dosage should be reduced slowly and the patients followed very closely for any possible adverse effects.
The use of INDOCIN in conjunction with aspirin or other salicylates is not recommended. Controlled clinical studies have shown that the combined use of INDOCIN and aspirin does not produce any greater therapeutic effect than the use of INDOCIN alone. Furthermore, in one of these clinical studies, the incidence of gastrointestinal side effects was significantly increased with combined therapy (see DRUG INTERACTIONS).

CONTRAINDICATIONS

INDOCIN should not be used in:
Patients who are hypersensitive to this product.
Patients in whom acute asthmatic attacks, urticaria, or rhinitis are precipitated by aspirin or other non-steroidal anti-inflammatory agents.
Suppositories INDOCIN are contraindicated in patients with a history of proctitis or recent rectal bleeding.

WARNINGS

General:
Because of the variability of the potential of INDOCIN to cause adverse reactions in the individual patient, the following are strongly recommended:
1. The lowest possible effective dose for the individual patient should be prescribed. Increased dosage tends to increase adverse effects, particularly in doses over 150–200 mg/day, without corresponding increase in clinical benefits.
2. Careful instructions to, and observations of, the individual patient are essential to the prevention of serious adverse reactions. As advancing years appear to increase the possibility of adverse reactions, INDOCIN should be used with greater care in the elderly.
3. Effectiveness of INDOCIN in pediatric patients has not been established. INDOCIN should not be prescribed for pediatric patients 14 years of age and younger unless toxicity or lack of efficacy associated with other drugs warrants the risk.
In experience with more than 900 pediatric patients reported in the literature or to the manufacturer who were treated with Capsules INDOCIN, side effects in pediatric patients were comparable to those reported in adults. Experience in pediatric patients has been confined to the use of Capsules INDOCIN.
If a decision is made to use indomethacin for pediatric patients two years of age or older, such patients should be monitored closely and periodic assessment of liver function is recommended. There have been cases of hepatotoxicity reported in pediatric patients with juvenile rheumatoid arthritis, including fatalities. If indomethacin treatment is instituted, a suggested starting dose is 2 mg/kg/day given in divided doses. Maximum daily dosage should not exceed 4 mg/kg/day or 150–200 mg/day, whichever is less. As symptoms subside, the total daily dosage should be reduced to the lowest level required to control symptoms, or the drug should be discontinued.

Gastrointestinal Effects:
Single or multiple ulcerations, including perforation and hemorrhage of the esophagus, stomach, duodenum or small and large intestine, have been reported to occur with INDOCIN. Fatalities have been reported in some instances. Rarely, intestinal ulceration has been associated with stenosis and obstruction.
Gastrointestinal bleeding without obvious ulcer formation and perforation of pre-existing sigmoid lesions (diverticulum, carcinoma, etc.) have occurred. Increased abdominal

Incidence greater than 1%	*Incidence less than 1%*	
GASTROINTESTINAL		
nausea* with or without vomiting dyspepsia* (including indigestion, heartburn and epigastric pain) diarrhea abdominal distress or pain constipation	anorexia bloating (includes distention) flatulence peptic ulcer gastroenteritis rectal bleeding proctitis single or multiple ulcerations, including perforation and hemorrhage of the esophagus, stomach, duodenum or small and large intestines intestinal ulceration associated with stenosis and obstruction	gastrointestinal bleeding without obvious ulcer formation and perforation of pre-existing sigmoid lesions (diverticulum, carcinoma, etc.) development of ulcerative colitis and regional ileitis ulcerative stomatitis toxic hepatitis and jaundice (some fatal cases have been reported) intestinal strictures (diaphragms)
CENTRAL NERVOUS SYSTEM		
headache (11.7%) dizziness* vertigo somnolence depression and fatigue (including malaise and listlessness)	anxiety (includes nervousness) muscle weakness involuntary muscle movements insomnia muzziness psychic disturbances including psychotic episodes mental confusion drowsiness	light-headedness syncope paresthesia aggravation of epilepsy and parkinsonism depersonalization coma peripheral neuropathy convulsions dysarthria
SPECIAL SENSES		
tinnitus	ocular—corneal deposits and retinal disturbances, including those of the macula, have been reported in some patients on prolonged therapy with INDOCIN	blurred vision diplopia hearing disturbances, deafness

pain in ulcerative colitis patients or the development of ulcerative colitis and regional ileitis have been reported to occur rarely.

Because of the occurrence, and at times severity, of gastrointestinal reactions to INDOCIN, the prescribing physician must be continuously alert for any sign or symptom signaling a possible gastrointestinal reaction. The risks of continuing therapy with INDOCIN in the face of such symptoms must be weighed against the possible benefits to the individual patient.

INDOCIN should not be given to patients with active gastrointestinal lesions or with a history of recurrent gastrointestinal lesions except under circumstances which warrant the very high risk and where patients can be monitored very closely.

The gastrointestinal effects may be reduced by giving Capsules INDOCIN immediately after meals, with food, or with antacids.

Risk of GI Ulcerations, Bleeding and Perforation with NSAID Therapy

Serious gastrointestinal toxicity such as bleeding, ulceration, and perforation, can occur at any time, with or without warning symptoms, in patients treated chronically with NSAID therapy. Although minor upper gastrointestinal problems, such as dyspepsia, are common, usually developing early in therapy, physicians should remain alert for ulceration and bleeding in patients treated chronically with NSAIDs even in the absence of previous GI tract symptoms. In patients observed in clinical trials of several months to two years duration, symptomatic upper GI ulcers, gross bleeding or perforation appear to occur in approximately 1% of patients treated for 3–6 months, and in about 2–4% of patients treated for one year. Physicians should inform patients about the signs and/or symptoms of serious GI toxicity and what steps to take if they occur.

Studies to date have not identified any subset of patients not at risk of developing peptic ulceration and bleeding. Except for a prior history of serious GI events and other risk factors known to be associated with peptic ulcer disease, such as alcoholism, smoking, etc., no risk factors (e.g., age, sex) have been associated with increased risk. Elderly or debilitated patients seem to tolerate ulceration or bleeding less well than other individuals and most spontaneous reports of fatal GI events are in this population. Studies to date are inconclusive concerning the relative risk of various NSAIDs in causing such reactions. High doses of any NSAID probably carry a greater risk of these reactions, although controlled clinical trials showing this do not exist in most cases. In considering the use of relatively large doses (within the recommended dosage range), sufficient benefit should be anticipated to offset the potential increased risk of GI toxicity.

Renal Effects:

As with other non-steroidal anti-inflammatory drugs, long term administration of indomethacin to animals has resulted in renal papillary necrosis and other abnormal renal pathology. In humans, there have been reports of acute interstitial nephritis with hematuria, proteinuria, and occasionally nephrotic syndrome.

A second form of renal toxicity has been seen in patients with prerenal and renal conditions leading to a reduction in renal blood flow or blood volume, where the renal prostaglandins have a supportive role in the maintenance of renal perfusion. In these patients administration of an NSAID may cause a dose dependent reduction in prostaglandin formation and may precipitate overt renal decompensation. Patients at greatest risk of this reaction are those with conditions such as renal or hepatic dysfunction, diabetes mellitus, advanced age, extracellular volume depletion from any cause, congestive heart failure, septicemia, pyelonephritis, or concomitant use of any nephrotoxic drug. INDOCIN or other NSAIDs should be given with caution and renal function should be monitored in any patient who may have reduced renal reserve. Discontinuation of NSAID therapy is typically followed by recovery to the pretreatment state.

Increases in serum potassium concentration, including hyperkalemia, have been reported, even in some patients without renal impairment. In patients with normal renal function, these effects have been attributed to a hyporeninemic-hypoaldosteronism state (see PRECAUTIONS, *Drug Interactions*).

Since INDOCIN is eliminated primarily by the kidneys, patients with significantly impaired renal function should be closely monitored; a lower daily dosage should be anticipated to avoid excessive drug accumulation.

Ocular Effects:

Corneal deposits and retinal disturbances, including those of the macula, have been observed in some patients who had received prolonged therapy with INDOCIN. The prescribing physician should be alert to the possible association between the changes noted and INDOCIN. It is advisable to discontinue therapy if such changes are observed. Blurred vision may be a significant symptom and warrants a thorough ophthalmological examination. Since these changes may be asymptomatic, ophthalmologic examination at periodic intervals is desirable in patients where therapy is prolonged.

Central Nervous System Effects:

INDOCIN may aggravate depression or other psychiatric disturbances, epilepsy, and parkinsonism, and should be used with considerable caution in patients with these conditions. If severe CNS adverse reactions develop, INDOCIN should be discontinued.

INDOCIN may cause drowsiness; therefore, patients should be cautioned about engaging in activities requiring mental alertness and motor coordination, such as driving a car. INDOCIN may also cause headache. Headache which persists despite dosage reduction requires cessation of therapy with INDOCIN.

Use in Pregnancy and the Neonatal Period

INDOCIN is not recommended for use in pregnant women, since safety for use has not been established. The known effects of indomethacin and other drugs of this class on the human fetus during the third trimester of pregnancy include: constriction of the ductus arteriosus prenatally, tricuspid incompetence, and pulmonary hypertension; nonclosure of the ductus arteriosus postnatally which may be resistant to medical management; myocardial degenerative changes, platelet dysfunction with resultant bleeding, intracranial bleeding, renal dysfunction or failure, renal injury/dysgenesis which may result in prolonged or permanent renal failure, oligohydramnios, gastrointestinal bleeding or perforation, and increased risk of necrotizing enterocolitis.

Teratogenic studies were conducted in mice and rats at dosages of 0.5, 1.0, 2.0, and 4.0 mg/kg/day. Except for retarded fetal ossification at 4 mg/kg/day considered secondary to the decreased average fetal weights, no increase in fetal malformations was observed as compared with control groups. Other studies in mice reported in the literature using higher doses (5 to 15 mg/kg/day) have described maternal toxicity and death, increased fetal resorptions, and fetal malformations. Comparable studies in rodents using high doses of aspirin have shown similar maternal and fetal effects.

As with other non-steroidal anti-inflammatory agents which inhibit prostaglandin synthesis, indomethacin has been found to delay parturition in rats.

In rats and mice, 4.0 mg/kg/day given during the last three days of gestation caused a decrease in maternal weight gain and some maternal and fetal deaths. An increased incidence of neuronal necrosis in the diencephalon in the live-born fetuses was observed. At 2.0 mg/kg/day, no increase in neuronal necrosis was observed as compared to the control groups. Administration of 0.5 or 4.0 mg/kg/day during the first three days of life did not cause an increase in neuronal necrosis at either dose level.

Use in Nursing Mothers

INDOCIN is excreted in the milk of lactating mothers. INDOCIN is not recommended for use in nursing mothers.

PRECAUTIONS

General

Non-steroidal anti-inflammatory drugs, including INDOCIN, may mask the usual signs and symptoms of infection. Therefore, the physician must be continually on the alert for this and should use the drug with extra care in the presence of existing infection.

Fluid retention and peripheral edema have been observed in some patients taking INDOCIN. Therefore, as with other non-steroidal anti-inflammatory drugs, INDOCIN should be used with caution in patients with cardiac dysfunction, hypertension, or other conditions predisposing to fluid retention.

In a study of patients with severe heart failure and hyponatremia, INDOCIN was associated with significant deterioration of circulatory hemodynamics, presumably due to inhibition of prostaglandin dependent compensatory mechanisms.

INDOCIN, like other non-steroidal anti-inflammatory agents, can inhibit platelet aggregation. This effect is of shorter duration than that seen with aspirin and usually disappears within 24 hours after discontinuation of INDOCIN. INDOCIN has been shown to prolong bleeding time (but within the normal range) in normal subjects. Because this effect may be exaggerated in patients with underlying hemostatic defects, INDOCIN should be used with caution in persons with coagulation defects.

As with other non-steroidal anti-inflammatory drugs, borderline elevations of one or more liver tests may occur in up to 15% of patients. These abnormalities may progress, may remain essentially unchanged, or may be transient with continued therapy. The SGPT (ALT) test is probably the most sensitive indicator of liver dysfunction. Meaningful (3 times the upper limit of normal) elevations of SGPT or SGOT (AST) occurred in controlled clinical trials in less than 1% of patients. A patient with symptoms and/or signs suggesting liver dysfunction, or in whom an abnormal liver test has occurred, should be evaluated for evidence of the development of more severe hepatic reaction while on therapy with INDOCIN. Severe hepatic reactions, including jaundice and cases of fatal hepatitis, have been reported with INDOCIN as with other non-steroidal anti-inflammatory drugs. Although such reactions are rare, if abnormal liver tests persist or worsen, if clinical signs and symptoms consistent with liver disease develop, or if systemic manifestations occur (e.g., eosinophilia, rash, etc.), INDOCIN should be discontinued.

Information for Patients

INDOCIN, like other drugs of its class, is not free of side effects. The side effects of these drugs can cause discomfort and, rarely, there are more serious side effects such as gastrointestinal bleeding, which may result in hospitalization and even fatal outcomes.

Continued on next page

Information on the Merck & Co., Inc. products listed on these pages is the full prescribing information from product circulars in use September 30, 2000. For information, please call 1-800-NSC MERCK [1-800-672-6372].

Indocin—Cont.

NSAIDs (Non-steroidal Anti-inflammatory Drugs) are often essential agents in the management of arthritis; but they also may be commonly employed for conditions which are less serious.

Physicians may wish to discuss with their patients the potential risks (see WARNINGS, PRECAUTIONS and ADVERSE REACTIONS) and likely benefits of NSAID treatment, particularly when the drugs are used for less serious conditions where treatment without NSAIDs may represent an acceptable alternative to both the patient and physician.

Laboratory Tests

Because serious GI tract ulceration and bleeding can occur without warning symptoms, physicians should follow chronically treated patients for the signs and symptoms of ulceration and bleeding and should inform them of the importance of this follow-up (see WARNINGS, *Risk of GI Ulcerations, Bleeding and Perforation with NSAID Therapy*).

Carcinogenesis, Mutagenesis, Impairment of Fertility

In an 81-week chronic oral toxicity study in the rat at doses up to 1 mg/kg/day, indomethacin had no tumorigenic effect. Indomethacin produced no neoplastic or hyperplastic changes related to treatment in carcinogenic studies in the rat (dosing period 73–110 weeks) and the mouse (dosing period 62–88 weeks) at doses up to 1.5 mg/kg/day.

Indomethacin did not have any mutagenic effect in *in vitro* bacterial tests (Ames test and *E. coli* with or without metabolic activation) and a series of *in vivo* tests including the host-mediated assay, sex-linked recessive lethals in *Drosophila*, and the micronucleus test in mice.

Indomethacin at dosage levels up to 0.5 mg/kg/day had no effect on fertility in mice in a two generation reproduction study or a two litter reproduction study in rats.

Drug Interactions

In normal volunteers receiving indomethacin, the administration of diflunisal decreased the renal clearance and significantly increased the plasma levels of indomethacin. In some patients, combined use of INDOCIN and diflunisal has been associated with fatal gastrointestinal hemorrhage. Therefore, diflunisal and INDOCIN should not be used concomitantly.

In a study in normal volunteers, it was found that chronic concurrent administration of 3.6 g of aspirin per day decreases indomethacin blood levels approximately 20%.

The concomitant use of INDOCIN with other NSAIDs is not recommended due to the increased possibility of gastrointestinal toxicity, with little or no increase in efficacy.

Clinical studies have shown that INDOCIN does not influence the hypoprothrombinemia produced by anticoagulants. However, when any additional drug, including INDOCIN, is added to the treatment of patients on anticoagulant therapy, the patients should be observed for alterations of the prothrombin time.

When INDOCIN is given to patients receiving probenecid, the plasma levels of indomethacin are likely to be increased. Therefore, a lower total daily dosage of INDOCIN may produce a satisfactory therapeutic effect. When increases in the dose of INDOCIN are made, they should be made carefully and in small increments.

Caution should be used if INDOCIN is administered simultaneously with methotrexate. INDOCIN has been reported to decrease the tubular secretion of methotrexate and to potentiate its toxicity.

Administration of non-steroidal anti-inflammatory drugs concomitantly with cyclosporine has been associated with an increase in cyclosporine-induced toxicity, possibly due to decreased synthesis of renal prostacyclin. NSAIDs should be used with caution in patients taking cyclosporine, and renal function should be monitored.

Capsules INDOCIN 50 mg t.i.d. produced a clinically relevant elevation of plasma lithium and reduction in renal lithium clearance in psychiatric patients and normal subjects with steady state plasma lithium concentrations. This effect has been attributed to inhibition of prostaglandin synthesis. As a consequence, when INDOCIN and lithium are given concomitantly, the patient should be carefully observed for signs of lithium toxicity. (Read circulars for lithium preparations before use of such concomitant therapy.) In addition, the frequency of monitoring serum lithium concentration should be increased at the outset of such combination drug treatment.

INDOCIN given concomitantly with digoxin has been reported to increase the serum concentration and prolong the half-life of digoxin. Therefore, when INDOCIN and digoxin are used concomitantly, serum digoxin levels should be closely monitored.

In some patients, the administration of INDOCIN can reduce the diuretic, natriuretic, and, antihypertensive effects of loop, potassium-sparing, and thiazide diuretics. Therefore, when INDOCIN and diuretics are used concomitantly, the patient should be observed closely to determine if the desired effect of the diuretic is obtained.

INDOCIN reduces basal plasma renin activity (PRA), as well as those elevations of PRA induced by furosemide administration, or salt or volume depletion. These facts should be considered when evaluating plasma renin activity in hypertensive patients.

It has been reported that the addition of triamterene to a maintenance schedule of INDOCIN resulted in reversible acute renal failure in two of four healthy volunteers. INDOCIN and triamterene should not be administered together.

	Incidence greater than 1%	*Incidence less than 1%*	
CARDIOVASCULAR	none	hypertension hypotension tachycardia chest pain	congestive heart failure arrhythmia; palpitations
METABOLIC	none	edema weight gain fluid retention flushing or sweating	hyperglycemia glycosuria hyperkalemia
INTEGUMENTARY	none	pruritus rash; urticaria petechiae or ecchymosis	exfoliative dermatitis erythema nodosum loss of hair Stevens-Johnson syndrome erythema multiforme toxic epidermal necrolysis
HEMATOLOGIC	none	leukopenia bone marrow depression anemia secondary to obvious or occult gastrointestinal bleeding	aplastic anemia hemolytic anemia agranulocytosis thrombocytopenic purpura disseminated intravascular coagulation
HYPERSENSITIVITY	none	acute anaphylaxis acute respiratory distress rapid fall in blood pressure resembling a shock-like state angioedema	dyspnea asthma purpura angiitis pulmonary edema fever
GENITOURINARY	none	hematuria vaginal bleeding proteinuria nephrotic syndrome interstitial nephritis	BUN elevation renal insufficiency, including renal failure
MISCELLANEOUS	none	epistaxis breast changes, including enlargement and tenderness, or gynecomastia	

* Reactions occurring in 3% to 9% of patients treated with INDOCIN. (Those reactions occurring in less than 3% of the patients are unmarked.)

INDOCIN and potassium-sparing diuretics each may be associated with increased serum potassium levels. The potential effects of INDOCIN and potassium-sparing diuretics on potassium kinetics and renal function should be considered when these agents are administered concurrently.

Most of the above effects concerning diuretics have been attributed, at least in part, to mechanisms involving inhibition of prostaglandin synthesis by INDOCIN.

Blunting of the antihypertensive effect of beta-adrenoceptor blocking agents by non-steroidal anti-inflammatory drugs including INDOCIN has been reported. Therefore, when using these blocking agents to treat hypertension, patients should be observed carefully in order to confirm that the desired therapeutic effect has been obtained. There are reports that INDOCIN can reduce the antihypertensive effect of captopril in some patients.

False-negative results in the dexamethasone suppression test (DST) in patients being treated with INDOCIN have been reported. Thus, results of the DST should be interpreted with caution in these patients.

Pediatric Use

Effectiveness in pediatric patients 14 years of age and younger has not been established (see WARNINGS).

Geriatric Use

As with any NSAID, caution should be exercised in treating the elderly (65 years and older) since advancing age appears to increase the possibility of adverse reactions (see WARNINGS, *General*; and DOSAGE AND ADMINISTRATION). Elderly patients seem to tolerate ulceration or bleeding less well than other individuals and many spontaneous reports of fatal GI events are in this population (see WARNINGS, *Risk of GI Ulcerations, Bleeding and Perforation with NSAID Therapy*).

Indomethacin may cause confusion or, rarely, psychosis (see ADVERSE REACTIONS); physicians should remain alert to the possibility of such adverse effects in the elderly.

This drug is known to be substantially excreted by the kidney and the risk of toxic reactions to this drug may be greater in patients with impaired renal function. Because elderly patients are more likely to have decreased renal function, care should be taken in dose selection and it may be useful to monitor renal function (see WARNINGS, *Renal Effects*).

ADVERSE REACTIONS

The adverse reactions for Capsules INDOCIN listed in the following table have been arranged into two groups: (1) incidence greater than 1%; and (2) incidence less than 1%. The incidence for group (1) was obtained from 33 double-blind controlled clinical trials reported in the literature (1,092 patients). The incidence for group (2) was based on reports in clinical trials, in the literature, and on voluntary reports since marketing. The probability of a causal relationship exists between INDOCIN and these adverse reactions, some of which have been reported only rarely.

The adverse reactions reported with Capsules INDOCIN may occur with use of the suppositories. In addition, rectal irritation and tenesmus have been reported in patients who have received the suppositories.

The adverse reactions reported with Capsules INDOCIN may also occur with use of the suspension.

[See table at top of previous page]
[See table above]

Causal relationship unknown: Other reactions have been reported but occurred under circumstances where a causal relationship could not be established. However, in these rarely reported events, the possibility cannot be excluded. Therefore, these observations are being listed to serve as alerting information to physicians:

Cardiovascular: Thrombophlebitis

Hematologic: Although there have been several reports of leukemia, the supporting information is weak.

Genitourinary: Urinary frequency.

A rare occurrence of fulminant necrotizing fasciitis, particularly in association with Group A β-hemolytic streptococcus, has been described in persons treated with non-steroidal anti-inflammatory agents, including indomethacin, sometimes with fatal outcome (see also PRECAUTIONS, *General*).

OVERDOSAGE

The following symptoms may be observed following overdosage: nausea, vomiting, intense headache, dizziness, mental confusion, disorientation, or lethargy. There have been reports of paresthesias, numbness, and convulsions.

Treatment is symptomatic and supportive. The stomach should be emptied as quickly as possible if the ingestion is recent. If vomiting has not occurred spontaneously, the patient should be induced to vomit with syrup of ipecac. If the patient is unable to vomit, gastric lavage should be performed. Once the stomach has been emptied, 25 or 50 g of activated charcoal may be given. Depending on the condition of the patient, close medical observation and nursing

care may be required. The patient should be followed for several days because gastrointestinal ulceration and hemorrhage have been reported as adverse reactions of indomethacin. Use of antacids may be helpful.
The oral LD_{50} of indomethacin in mice and rats (based on 14 day mortality response) was 50 and 12 mg/kg, respectively.

DOSAGE AND ADMINISTRATION

INDOCIN is available as 25 and 50 mg Capsules INDOCIN, Oral Suspension INDOCIN, containing 25 mg of indomethacin per 5 mL, and 50 mg Suppositories INDOCIN for rectal use.
Adverse reactions appear to correlate with the size of the dose of INDOCIN in most patients but not all. Therefore, every effort should be made to determine the smallest effective dosage for the individual patient.
Always give Capsules INDOCIN or Oral Suspension INDOCIN with food, immediately after meals, or with antacids to reduce gastric irritation.
Pediatric Use
INDOCIN ordinarily should not be prescribed for pediatric patients 14 years of age and under (see WARNINGS).
Adult Use
Dosage Recommendations for Active Stages of the Following:

1. Moderate to severe rheumatoid arthritis including acute flares of chronic disease; moderate to severe ankylosing spondylitis; and moderate to severe osteoarthritis.
   Suggested Dosage:
   Capsules INDOCIN 25 mg b.i.d. or t.i.d. If this is well tolerated, increase the daily dosage by 25 or by 50 mg, if required by continuing symptoms, at weekly intervals until a satisfactory response is obtained or until a total daily dose of 150–200 mg is reached. DOSES ABOVE THIS AMOUNT GENERALLY DO NOT INCREASE THE EFFECTIVENESS OF THE DRUG.

In patients who have persistent night pain and/or morning stiffness, the giving of a large portion, up to a maximum of 100 mg, of the total daily dose at bedtime, either orally or by rectal suppositories, may be helpful in affording relief. The total daily dose should not exceed 200 mg. In acute flares of chronic rheumatoid arthritis, it may be necessary to increase the dosage by 25 mg or, if required, by 50 mg daily.
If minor adverse effects develop as the dosage is increased, reduce the dosage rapidly to a tolerated dose and OBSERVE THE PATIENT CLOSELY.
If severe adverse reactions occur, STOP THE DRUG. After the acute phase of the disease is under control, an attempt to reduce the daily dose should be made repeatedly until the patient is receiving the smallest effective dose or the drug is discontinued.
Careful instructions to, and observations of, the individual patient are essential to the prevention of serious, irreversible, including fatal, adverse reactions.
As advancing years appear to increase the possibility of adverse reactions, INDOCIN should be used with greater care in the elderly (see PRECAUTIONS, *Geriatric Use*).

2. Acute painful shoulder (bursitis and/or tendinitis).
   Initial Dose:
   75–150 mg daily in 3 or 4 divided doses.
   The drug should be discontinued after the signs and symptoms of inflammation have been controlled for several days. The usual course of therapy is 7–14 days.
3. Acute gouty arthritis.
   Suggested Dosage:
   Capsules INDOCIN 50 mg t.i.d. until pain is tolerable. The dose should then be rapidly reduced to complete cessation of the drug. Definite relief of pain has been reported within 2 to 4 hours. Tenderness and heat usually subside in 24 to 36 hours, and swelling gradually disappears in 3 to 5 days.

HOW SUPPLIED

No. 3316—Capsules INDOCIN, 25 mg are opaque blue and white capsules, coded INDOCIN and MSD 25. They are supplied as follows:
NDC 0006-0025-68 bottles of 100
NDC 0006-0025-82 bottles of 1000
Shown in Product Identification Guide, page 323
No. 3317—Capsules INDOCIN, 50 mg are opaque blue and white capsules, coded INDOCIN and MSD 50. They are supplied as follows:
NDC 0006-0050-68 bottles of 100
No. 3376—Oral Suspension INDOCIN, 25 mg per 5 mL, is an off-white suspension with a pineapple coconut mint flavor. It is supplied as follows:
NDC 0006-3376-66 in bottles of 237 mL.
No. 3354—Suppositories INDOCIN, 50 mg each, are white, opaque, rectal suppositories and are supplied as follows:
NDC 0006-0150-30, boxes of 30
Shown in Product Identification Guide, page 323 & 324
Storage
Store Oral Suspension INDOCIN below 30°C (86°F). Avoid temperatures above 50°C (122°F). Protect from freezing.
Store Suppositories INDOCIN below 30°C (86°F). Avoid transient temperatures above 40°C (104°F).

Suppositories INDOCIN are distributed by:
MERCK SHARP & DOHME, Division of Merck & Co., INC.
West Point, Pa. 19486
Manufactured by:
MERCK SHARP & DOHME
(Italia) S.p.A.
27100—Pavia, Italy
Capsules and Oral Suspension INDOCIN® are distributed and manufactured by:
MERCK SHARP & DOHME, Division of Merck & Co., INC.
West Point, Pa. 19486
7873327 Issued October 1999

INDOCIN® I.V. ℞
(Indomethacin Sodium Trihydrate)

DESCRIPTION

Sterile INDOCIN* I.V. (Indomethacin Sodium Trihydrate) for intravenous administration is lyophilized indomethacin sodium trihydrate. Each vial contains indomethacin sodium trihydrate equivalent to 1 mg indomethacin as a white to yellow lyophilized powder or plug. Variations in the size of the lyophilized plug and the intensity of color have no relationship to the quality or amount of indomethacin present in the vial.
Indomethacin sodium trihydrate is designated chemically as 1-(4-chlorobenzoyl) -5- methoxy-2-methyl-1*H* -indole-3-acetic acid, sodium salt, trihydrate. Its molecular weight is 433.82. Its empirical formula is $C_{19}H_{15}ClNNaO_4 \cdot 3H_2O$ and its structural formula is:

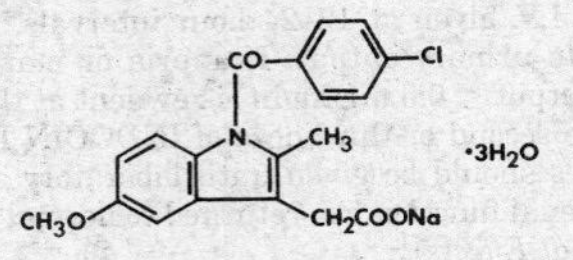

*Registered trademark of MERCK & CO., INC.

CLINICAL PHARMACOLOGY

Although the exact mechanism of action through which indomethacin causes closure of a patent ductus arteriosus is not known, it is believed to be through inhibition of prostaglandin synthesis. Indomethacin has been shown to be a potent inhibitor of prostaglandin synthesis, both *in vitro* and *in vivo*. In human newborns with certain congenital heart malformations, PGE 1 dilates the ductus arteriosus. In fetal and newborn lambs, E type prostaglandins have also been shown to maintain the patency of the ductus, and as in human newborns, indomethacin causes its constriction.
Studies in healthy young animals and in premature infants with patent ductus arteriosus indicated that, after the first dose of intravenous indomethacin, there was a transient reduction in cerebral blood flow velocity and cerebral blood flow. Similar decreases in mesenteric blood flow and velocity have been observed. The clinical significance of these effects has not been established.
In double-blind placebo-controlled studies of INDOCIN I.V. in 460 small pre-term infants, weighing 1750 g or less, the neonates treated with placebo had a ductus closure rate after 48 hours of 25 to 30 percent, whereas those treated with INDOCIN I.V. had a 75 to 80 percent closure rate. In one of these studies, a multicenter study, involving 405 pre-term infants, later re-opening of the ductus arteriosus occurred in 26 percent of neonates treated with INDOCIN I.V., however, 70 percent of these closed subsequently without the need for surgery or additional indomethacin.
Pharmacokinetics and Metabolism
The disposition of indomethacin following intravenous administration (0.2 mg/kg) in pre-term neonates with patent ductus arteriosus has not been extensively evaluated. Even though the plasma half-life of indomethacin was variable among premature infants, it was shown to vary inversely with postnatal age and weight. In one study, of 28 neonates who could be evaluated, the plasma half-life in those less than 7 days old averaged 20 hours (range: 3–60 hours, n = 18). In neonates older than 7 days, the mean plasma half-life of indomethacin was 12 hours (range: 4–38 hours, n = 10). Grouping the neonates by weight, mean plasma half-life in those weighing less than 1000 g was 21 hours (range: 9–60 hours, n = 10); in those neonates weighing more than 1000 g, the mean plasma half-life was 15 hours (range: 3–52 hours, n = 18).
Following intravenous administration in adults, indomethacin is eliminated via renal excretion, metabolism, and biliary excretion. Indomethacin undergoes appreciable enterohepatic circulation. The mean plasma half-life of indomethacin is 4.5 hours. In the absence of enterohepatic circulation, it is 90 minutes. Indomethacin has been found to cross the blood-brain barrier and the placenta.
In adults, about 99 percent of indomethacin is bound to protein in plasma over the expected range of therapeutic plasma concentrations. The percent bound in neonates has not been studied. In controlled trials in premature infants, however, no evidence of bilirubin displacement has been observed as evidenced by increased incidence of bilirubin encephalopathy (kernicterus).

INDICATIONS AND USAGE

INDOCIN I.V. is indicated to close a hemodynamically significant patent ductus arteriosus in premature infants weighing between 500 and 1750 g when after 48 hours usual medical management (e.g., fluid restriction, diuretics, digitalis, respiratory support, etc.) is ineffective. Clear-cut clinical evidence of a hemodynamically significant patent ductus arteriosus should be present, such as respiratory distress, a continuous murmur, a hyperactive precordium, cardiomegaly and pulmonary plethora on chest x-ray.

CONTRAINDICATIONS

INDOCIN I.V. is contraindicated in: neonates with proven or suspected infection that is untreated; neonates who are bleeding, especially those with active intracranial hemorrhage or gastrointestinal bleeding; neonates with thrombocytopenia; neonates with coagulation defects; neonates with or who are suspected of having necrotizing enterocolitis; neonates with significant impairment of renal function; neonates with congenital heart disease in whom patency of the ductus arteriosus is necessary for satisfactory pulmonary or systemic blood flow (e.g., pulmonary atresia, severe tetralogy of Fallot, severe coarctation of the aorta).

WARNINGS

Gastrointestinal Effects:
In the collaborative study, major gastrointestinal bleeding was no more common in those neonates receiving indomethacin than in those neonates on placebo. However, minor gastrointestinal bleeding (i.e., chemical detection of blood in the stool) was more commonly noted in those neonates treated with indomethacin. Severe gastrointestinal effects have been reported in adults with various arthritic disorders treated chronically with oral indomethacin. [For further information, see package circular for Capsules INDOCIN* (Indomethacin)].
Central Nervous System Effects:
Prematurity per se, is associated with an increased incidence of spontaneous intraventricular hemorrhage. Because indomethacin may inhibit platelet aggregation, the potential for intraventricular bleeding may be increased. However, in the large multi-center study of INDOCIN I.V. (see CLINICAL PHARMACOLOGY), the incidence of intraventricular hemorrhage in neonates treated with INDOCIN I.V. was not significantly higher than in the control neonates.
Renal Effects:
INDOCIN I.V. may cause significant reduction in urine output (50 percent or more) with concomitant elevations of blood urea nitrogen and creatinine, and reductions in glomerular filtration rate and creatinine clearance. These effects in most neonates are transient, disappearing with cessation of therapy with INDOCIN I.V. However, because adequate renal function can depend upon renal prostaglandin synthesis, INDOCIN I.V. may precipitate renal insufficiency, including acute renal failure, especially in neonates with other conditions that may adversely affect renal function (e.g., extracellular volume depletion from any cause, congestive heart failure, sepsis, concomitant use of any nephrotoxic drug, hepatic dysfunction). When significant suppression of urine volume occurs after a dose of INDOCIN I.V., no additional dose should be given until the urine output returns to normal levels.
INDOCIN I.V. in pre-term infants may suppress water excretion to a greater extent than sodium excretion. When this occurs, a significant reduction in serum sodium values (i.e., hyponatremia) may result. Neonates should have serum electrolyte determinations done during therapy with INDOCIN I.V. Renal function and serum electrolytes should be monitored (see PRECAUTIONS, *Drug Interactions* and DOSAGE AND ADMINISTRATION).

* Registered trademark of MERCK & CO., INC.

PRECAUTIONS

General
INDOCIN (Indomethacin) may mask the usual signs and symptoms of infection. Therefore, the physician must be continually on the alert for this and should use the drug with extra care in the presence of existing controlled infection.
Severe hepatic reactions have been reported in adults treated chronically with oral indomethacin for arthritic disorders. [For further information, see package circular for Capsules INDOCIN (Indomethacin)]. If clinical signs and symptoms consistent with liver disease develop in the neonate, or if systemic manifestations occur, INDOCIN I.V. should be discontinued.
INDOCIN I.V. may inhibit platelet aggregation. In one small study, platelet aggregation was grossly abnormal after indomethacin therapy (given orally to premature infants to close the ductus arteriosus). Platelet aggregation returned to normal by the tenth day. Premature infants should be observed for signs of bleeding.

Continued on next page

Information on the Merck & Co., Inc. products listed on these pages is the full prescribing information from product circulars in use September 30, 2000. For information, please call 1-800-NSC MERCK [1-800-672-6372].

Indocin I.V.—Cont.

The drug should be administered carefully to avoid extravascular injection or leakage as the solution may be irritating to tissue.

Drug Interactions

Since renal function may be reduced by INDOCIN I.V., consideration should be given to reduction in dosage of those medications that rely on adequate renal function for their elimination. Because the half-life of digitalis (given frequently to pre-term infants with patent ductus arteriosus and associated cardiac failure) may be prolonged when given concomitantly with indomethacin, the neonate should be observed closely; frequent ECGs and serum digitalis levels may be required to prevent or detect digitalis toxicity early. Furthermore, in one study of premature infants treated with INDOCIN I.V. and also receiving either gentamicin or amikacin, both peak and trough levels of these aminoglycosides were significantly elevated.

Therapy with indomethacin may blunt the natriuretic effect of furosemide. This response has been attributed to inhibition of prostaglandin synthesis by non-steroidal anti-inflammatory drugs. In a study of 19 premature infants with patent ductus arteriosus treated with either INDOCIN I.V. alone or a combination of INDOCIN I.V. and furosemide, results showed that neonates receiving both INDOCIN I.V. and furosemide had significantly higher urinary output, higher levels of sodium and chloride excretion, and higher glomerular filtration rates than did those receiving INDOCIN I.V. alone. In this study, the data suggested that therapy with furosemide helped to maintain renal function in the premature infant when INDOCIN I.V. was added to the treatment of patent ductus arteriosus.

Neonatal Effects

In rats and mice, oral indomethacin 4.0 mg/kg/day given during the last three days of gestation caused a decrease in maternal weight gain and some maternal and fetal deaths. An increased incidence of neuronal necrosis in the diencephalon in the live-born fetuses was observed. At 2.0 mg/kg/day, no increase in neuronal necrosis was observed as compared to the control groups. Administration of 0.5 or 4.0 mg/kg/day during the first three days of life did not cause an increase in neuronal necrosis at either dose level.

Pregnant rats, given 2.0 mg/kg/day and 4.0 mg/kg/day during the last trimester of gestation, delivered offspring whose pulmonary blood vessels were both reduced in number and excessively muscularized. These findings are similar to those observed in the syndrome of persistent pulmonary hypertension of the neonate.

ADVERSE REACTIONS

In a double-blind placebo-controlled trial of 405 premature infants weighing less than or equal to 1750 g with evidence of large ductal shunting, in those neonates treated with indomethacin (n = 206), there was a statistically significantly greater incidence of bleeding problems, including gross or microscopic bleeding into the gastrointestinal tract, oozing from the skin after needle stick, pulmonary hemorrhage, and disseminated intravascular coagulopathy. There was no statistically significant difference between treatment groups with reference to intracranial hemorrhage.

The neonates treated with indomethacin sodium trihydrate also had a significantly higher incidence of transient oliguria and elevations of serum creatinine (greater than or equal to 1.8 mg/dL) than did the neonates treated with placebo.

The incidences of retrolental fibroplasia (grades III and IV) and pneumothorax in neonates treated with INDOCIN I.V. were no greater than in placebo controls and were statistically significantly lower than in surgically-treated neonates.

The following additional adverse reactions in neonates have been reported from the collaborative study, anecdotal case reports, from other studies using rectal, oral, or intravenous indomethacin for treatment of patent ductus arteriosus or in marketed use. The rates are calculated from a database which contains experience of 849 indomethacin-treated neonates reported in the medical literature, regardless of the route of administration. One year follow-up is available on 175 neonates and shows no long-term sequelae which could be attributed to indomethacin. In controlled clinical studies, only electrolyte imbalance and renal dysfunction (of the reactions listed below) occurred statistically significantly more frequently after INDOCIN I.V. than after placebo. Reactions marked with a single asterick (*) occurred in 3–9 percent of indomethacin-treated neonates: those marked with a double asterisk (**) occurred in 3–9 percent of both indomethacin- and placebo-treated neonates. Unmarked reactions occurred in less than 3 percent of neonates.

Renal: renal dysfunction in 41 percent of neonates, including one or more of the following: reduced urinary output; reduced urine sodium, chloride, or potassium urine osmolality, free water clearance, or glomerular filtration, rate; elevated serum creatinine or BUN; uremia.

Cardiovascular: intracranial bleeding**, pulmonary hypertension.

Gastrointestinal: gastrointestinal bleeding*, vomiting, abdominal distention, transient ileus, localized perforation(s) of the small and/or large intestine.

Metabolic: hyponatremia*, elevated serum potassium*, reduction in blood sugar, including hypoglycemia, increased weight gain (fluid retention).

Coagulation: decreased platelet aggregation (see PRECAUTIONS).

The following adverse reactions have also been reported in neonates treated with indomethacin, however, a causal relationship to therapy with INDOCIN I.V. has not been established:

Cardiovascular: bradycardia.

Respiratory: apnea, exacerbation of pre-existing pulmonary infection.

Metabolic: acidosis/alkalosis.

Hematologic: disseminated intravascular coagulation.

Gastrointestinal: necrotizing enterocolitis.

Ophthalmic: retrolental fibroplasia.**

A variety of additional adverse experiences have been reported in adults treated with oral indomethacin for moderate to severe rheumatoid arthritis, osteoarthritis, ankylosing spondylitis, acute painful shoulder and acute gouty arthritis (see section ADDITIONAL ADVERSE REACTIONS—ADULTS). Their relevance to the pre-term infant receiving indomethacin for patent ductus arteriosus is unknown, however, the possibility exists that these experiences may be associated with the use of INDOCIN I.V. in pre-term infants.

DOSAGE AND ADMINISTRATION

FOR INTRAVENOUS ADMINISTRATION ONLY.

Dosage recommendations for closure of the ductus arteriosus depends on the age of the infant at the time of therapy. A course of therapy is defined as three intravenous doses of INDOCIN I.V. given at 12–24 hour intervals, with careful attention to urinary output. If anuria or marked oliguria (urinary output < 0.6 mL/kg/hr) is evident at the scheduled time of the second or third dose of INDOCIN I.V., no additional doses should be given until laboratory studies indicate that renal function has returned to normal (see WARNINGS, *Renal Effects*).

Dosage according to age is as follows:

AGE at 1st dose	DOSAGE (mg/kg)		
	1st	2nd	3rd
Less than 48 hours	0.2	0.1	0.1
2–7 days	0.2	0.2	0.2
over 7 days	0.2	0.25	0.25

If the ductus arteriosus closes or is significantly reduced in size after an interval of 48 hours or more from completion of the first course of INDOCIN I.V., no further doses are necessary. If the ductus arteriosus re-opens, a second course of 1–3 doses may be given, each dose separated by a 12–24 hour interval as described above.

If the infant remains unresponsive to therapy with INDOCIN I.V. after 2 courses, surgery may be necessary for closure of the ductus arteriosus. If severe adverse reactions occur, STOP THE DRUG.

Directions for Use

Parenteral drug products should be inspected visually for particulate matter and discoloration prior to administration whenever solution and container permit.

The solution should be prepared only with 1 to 2 mL of preservative-free sterile Sodium Chloride Injection, 0.9 percent or preservative-free Sterile Water for Injection. Benzyl alcohol as a preservative has been associated with toxicity in neonates. Therefore, all diluents should be preservative-free. If 1 mL of diluent is used, the concentration of indomethacin in the solution will equal approximately 0.1 mg/0.1 mL; if 2 mL of diluent are used, the concentration of the solution will equal approximately 0.05 mg/0.1 mL. Any unused portion of the solution should be discarded because there is no preservative contained in the vial. A fresh solution should be prepared just prior to each administration. Once reconstituted, the indomethacin solution may be injected intravenously. While the optimal rate of injection has not been established, published literature suggests an infusion rate over 20–30 minutes.

Further dilution with intravenous infusion solutions is not recommended. INDOCIN I.V. is not buffered, and reconstitution with solutions at pH values below 6.0 may result in precipitation of the insoluble indomethacin free acid moiety.

HOW SUPPLIED

No. 3406—Sterile INDOCIN I.V. is a lyophilized white to yellow powder or plug supplied as single dose vials containing indomethacin sodium trihydrate, equivalent to 1 mg indomethacin.

NDC 0006-3406-17
(6505-01-209-1192, 3 single dose vials).

Storage

Store below 30°C (86°F). *Protect from light.* Store container in carton until contents have been used.

ADDITIONAL ADVERSE REACTIONS—ADULTS

The following adverse reactions have been reported in adults treated with oral indomethacin for moderate to severe rheumatoid arthritis, osteoarthritis, ankylosing spondylitis, acute painful shoulder and acute gouty arthritis. Complaints not of relevance in the treatment of the premature infant, such as anorexia, psychic disturbances, and blurred vision, are not listed.

Incidence 1% to 3%	*Incidence less than 1%*	
GASTROINTESTINAL		
diarrhea constipation	bloating (includes distention) flatulence peptic ulcer gastroenteritis rectal bleeding proctitis single or multiple ulcerations, including perforation and hemorrhage of the esophagus, stomach, duodenum or small and large intestines intestinal ulceration associated with stenosis and obstruction	gastrointestinal bleeding without obvious ulcer formation and perforation of pre-existing sigmoid lesions development of ulcerative stomatitis toxic hepatitis and jaundice (some fatal cases have been reported) intestinal strictures (diaphragms)
CENTRAL NERVOUS SYSTEM		
none	involuntary muscle movements	aggravation of epilepsy coma peripheral neuropathy convulsions
SPECIAL SENSES		
none	hearing disturbances, deafness	
CARDIOVASCULAR		
none	hypertension hypotension tachycardia	arrhythmia congestive heart failure thrombophlebitis
METABOLIC		
none	edema weight gain flushing	hyperglycemia glycosuria hyperkalemia
INTEGUMENTARY		
none	rash; urticaria petechiae or ecchymosis	exfoliative dermatitis erythema nodosum loss of hair Stevens-Johnson syndrome erythema multiforme toxic epidermal necrolysis
HEMATOLOGIC		
none	leukopenia bone marrow depression anemia secondary to obvious or occult gastrointestinal bleeding	aplastic anemia hemolytic anemia agranulocytosis thrombocytopenic purpura
HYPERSENSITIVITY		
none	acute anaphylaxis acute respiratory distress rapid fall in blood pressure resembling a shock-like state	dyspnea asthma purpura angiitis pulmonary edema
GENITOURINARY		
none	hematuria vaginal bleeding	renal insufficiency, including renal failure
MISCELLANEOUS		
none	epistaxis breast changes, including enlargement and tenderness, or gynecomastia	

See package circular for Capsules INDOCIN (Indomethacin) for additional information concerning adverse reactions and other cautionary statements.

9293616 Issued February 2000

INVERSINE® Tablets (Mecamylamine HCl) ℞

DESCRIPTION

INVERSINE* (Mecamylamine HCl) is a potent, oral antihypertensive agent and ganglion blocker, and is a secondary amine. It is *N*, 2,3,3-tetramethylbicyclo[2.2.1] heptan-2-amine hydrochloride. Its empirical formula is $C_{11}H_{21}N \cdot HCl$ and its structural formula is:

It is a white, odorless, or practically odorless, crystalline powder, is highly stable, soluble in water and has a molecular weight of 203.75.

INVERSINE is supplied as tablets for oral use, each containing 2.5 mg mecamylamine HCl. Inactive ingredients are acacia, calcium phosphate, D&C Yellow 10, FD&C Yellow 6, lactose, magnesium stearate, starch, and talc.

*Registered trademark of MERCK & CO., INC.

CLINICAL PHARMACOLOGY

Mecamylamine reduces blood pressure in both normotensive and hypertensive individuals. It has a gradual onset of action (1/2 to 2 hours) and a long-lasting effect (usually 6 to 12 hours or more). A small oral dosage often produces a smooth and predictable reduction of blood pressure. Although this antihypertensive effect is predominantly orthostatic, the supine blood pressure is also significantly reduced.

Pharmacokinetics and Metabolism

Mecamylamine is almost completely absorbed from the gastrointestinal tract, resulting in consistent lowering of blood pressure in most patients with hypertensive cardiovascular disease. Mecamylamine is excreted slowly in the urine in the unchanged form. The rate of its renal elimination is influenced markedly by urinary pH. Alkalinization of the urine reduces, and acidification promotes, renal excretion of mecamylamine.

Mecamylamine crosses the blood-brain and placental barriers.

INDICATIONS AND USAGE

For the management of moderately severe to severe essential hypertension and in uncomplicated cases of malignant hypertension.

CONTRAINDICATIONS

INVERSINE should not be used in mild, moderate, labile hypertension and may prove unsuitable in uncooperative patients. It is contraindicated in coronary insufficiency or recent myocardial infarction.

INVERSINE should be given with great discretion, if at all, when renal insufficiency is manifested by a rising or elevated BUN. The drug is contraindicated in uremia. Patients receiving antibiotics and sulfonamides should generally not be treated with ganglion blockers. Other contraindications are glaucoma, organic pyloric stenosis or hypersensitivity to the product.

WARNINGS

Mecamylamine, a secondary amine, readily penetrates into the brain and thus may produce central nervous sytem effects. Tremor, choreiform movements, mental aberrations, and convulsions may occur rarely. These have occurred most often when large doses of INVERSINE were used, especially in patients with cerebral or renal insufficiency.

When ganglion blockers or other potent antihypertensive drugs are discontinued suddenly, hypertensive levels return. In patients with malignant hypertension and others, this may occur abruptly and may cause fatal cerebral vascular accidents or acute congestive heart failure. When INVERSINE is withdrawn, this should be done gradually and other antihypertensive therapy usually must be substituted. On the other hand, the effects of INVERSINE sometimes may last from hours to days after therapy is discontinued.

PRECAUTIONS

General

The patient's condition should be evaluated carefully, particularly as to renal and cardiovascular function. When renal, cerebral, or coronary blood flow is deficient, any additional impairment, which might result from added hypotension, must be avoided. The use of INVERSINE in patients with marked cerebral and coronary arteriosclerosis or after a recent cerebral accident requires caution.

The action of INVERSINE may be potentiated by excessive heat, fever, infection, hemorrhage, pregnancy, anesthesia, surgery, vigorous exercise, other antihypertensive drugs, alcohol, and salt depletion as a result of diminished intake or increased excretion due to diarrhea, vomiting, excessive sweating, or diuretics.

During therapy with INVERSINE, sodium intake should not be restricted but, if necessary, the dosage of the ganglion blocker must be adjusted.

Since urinary retention may occur in patients on ganglion blockers, caution is required in patients with prostatic hypertrophy, bladder neck obstruction, and urethral stricture.

Frequent loose bowel movements with abdominal distention and decreased borborygmi may be the first signs of paralytic ileus. If these are present, INVERSINE should be discontinued immediately and remedial steps taken.

Information for Patients

INVERSINE may cause dizziness, lightheadedness, or fainting, especially when rising from a lying or sitting position. This effect may be increased by alcoholic beverages, exercise, or during hot weather. Getting up slowly may help alleviate such a reaction.

Drug Interactions

Patients receiving antibiotics and sulfonamides generally should not be treated with ganglion blockers.

The action of INVERSINE may be potentiated by anesthesia, other antihypertensive drugs and alcohol.

Carcinogenesis, Mutagenesis, Impairment of Fertility

Long-term studies in animals have not been performed to evaluate the effects upon fertility, mutagenic or carcinogenic potential of INVERSINE.

Pregnancy

Pregnancy Category C. Animal reproduction studies have not been conducted with INVERSINE. It is not known whether INVERSINE can cause fetal harm when given to a pregnant woman or can affect reproductive capacity. INVERSINE should be given to a pregnant woman only if clearly needed.

Nursing Mothers

Because of the potential for serious adverse reactions in nursing infants from INVERSINE, a decision should be made whether to discontinue nursing or to discontinue the drug, taking into account the importance of the drug to the mother.

Pediatric Use

Safety and effectiveness in pediatric patients have not been established.

ADVERSE REACTIONS

The following adverse reactions have been reported and within each category are listed in order of decreasing severity.

Gastrointestinal: Ileus, constipation (sometimes preceded by small, frequent liquid stools), vomiting, nausea, anorexia, glossitis and dryness of mouth.

Cardiovascular: Orthostatic dizziness and syncope, postural hypotension.

Nervous System/Psychiatric: Convulsions, choreiform movements, mental aberrations, tremor, and paresthesias (see WARNINGS).

Respiratory: Interstitial pulmonary edema and fibrosis.

Urogenital: Urinary retention, impotence, decreased libido.

Special Senses: Blurred vision, dilated pupils.

Miscellaneous: Weakness, fatigue, sedation.

OVERDOSAGE

Signs of overdosage include: hypotension (which may progress to peripheral vascular collapse), postural hypotension, nausea, vomiting, diarrhea, constipation, paralytic ileus, urinary retention, dizziness, anxiety, dry mouth, mydriasis, blurred vision, or palpitations. A rise in intraocular pressure may occur.

Pressor amines may be used to counteract excessive hypotension. Since patients being treated with ganglion blockers are more than normally reactive to pressor amines, small doses of the latter are recommended to avoid excessive response.

The oral LD_{50} of mecamylamine in the mouse is 92 mg/kg.

DOSAGE AND ADMINISTRATION

Therapy is usually started with one 2.5 mg tablet of INVERSINE twice a day. This initial dosage should be modified by increments of one 2.5 mg tablet at intervals of not less than 2 days until the desired blood pressure response occurs (the criterion being a dosage just under that which causes signs of mild postural hypotension).

The average total daily dosage of INVERSINE is 25 mg, usually in three divided doses. However, as little as 2.5 mg daily may be sufficient to control hypertension in some patients. A range of two to four or even more doses may be required in severe cases when smooth control is difficult to obtain. In severe or urgent cases, larger increments at smaller intervals may be needed. Partial tolerance may develop in certain patients, requiring an increase in the daily dosage of INVERSINE.

Administration of INVERSINE after meals may cause a more gradual absorption and smoother control of excessively high blood pressure. The timing of doses in relation to meals should be consistent. Since the blood pressure response to antihypertensive drugs is increased in the early morning, the larger dose should be given at noontime and perhaps in the evening. The morning dose, as a rule, should be relatively small and in some instances may even be omitted.

The *initial regulation of dosage* should be determined by blood pressure readings in the erect position at the time of maximal effect of the drug, as well as by other signs and symptoms of orthostatic hypotension.

The *effective maintenance dosage* should be regulated by blood pressure readings in the erect position and by limitation of dosage to that which causes slight faintness or dizziness in this position. If the patient or a relative can use a sphygmomanometer, instructions may be given to reduce or omit a dose if readings fall below a designated level or if faintness or lightheadedness occurs. *However, no change should be instituted without the knowledge of the physician.*

Close supervision and education of the patient, as well as critical adjustment of dosage, are essential to successful therapy.

Other Antihypertensive Agents

When INVERSINE is given with other antihypertensive drugs, the dosage of these other agents, as well as that of INVERSINE, should be reduced to avoid excessive hypotension. However, thiazides should be continued in their usual dosage, while that of INVERSINE is decreased by at least 50 percent.

HOW SUPPLIED

No. 3219—Tablets INVERSINE, 2.5 mg, are yellow, round, scored, compressed tablets, coded MSD 52 on one side and INVERSINE on the other. They are supplied as follows:

NDC 0006-0052-68 in bottles of 100.

Shown in Product Identification Guide, page 324

7898723 Issued September 1996

LACRISERT® Sterile Ophthalmic Insert ℞

(hydroxypropyl cellulose ophthalmic insert)

DESCRIPTION

LACRISERT* (hydroxypropyl cellulose ophthalmic insert) is a sterile, translucent, rod-shaped, water soluble, ophthalmic insert made of hydroxypropyl cellulose, for administration into the inferior cul-de-sac of the eye.

The chemical name for hydroxypropyl cellulose is cellulose, 2-hydroxypropyl ether. It is an ether of cellulose in which hydroxypropyl groups ($-CH_2CHOHCH_3$) are attached to the hydroxyls present in the anhydroglucose rings of cellulose by ether linkages. A representative structure of the monomer is:

$R=CH_2CH(OH)CH_3$

The molecular weight is typically 1×10^6.

Hydroxypropyl cellulose is an off-white, odorless, tasteless powder. It is soluble in water below 38°C, and in many polar organic solvents such as ethanol, propylene glycol, dioxane, methanol, isopropyl alcohol (95%), dimethyl sulfoxide, and dimethyl formamide.

Each LACRISERT is 5 mg of hydroxypropyl cellulose. LACRISERT contains no preservatives or other ingredients. It is about 1.27 mm in diameter by about 3.5 mm long.

LACRISERT is supplied in packages of 60 units, together with illustrated instructions and a special applicator for removing LACRISERT from the unit dose blister and inserting it into the eye. A spare applicator is included in each package.

*Registered trademark of MERCK & CO., INC.

CLINICAL PHARMACOLOGY

Pharmacodynamics

LACRISERT acts to stabilize and thicken the precorneal tear film and prolong the tear film breakup time which is usually accelerated in patients with dry eye states. LACRISERT also acts to lubricate and protect the eye.

LACRISERT usually reduces the signs and symptoms resulting from moderate to severe dry eye syndromes, such as conjunctival hyperemia, corneal and conjunctival staining with rose bengal, exudation, itching, burning, foreign body sensation, smarting, photophobia, dryness and blurred or cloudy vision. Progressive visual deterioration which occurs in some patients may be retarded, halted, or sometimes reversed.

In a multicenter crossover study the 5 mg LACRISERT administered once a day during the waking hours was compared to artificial tears used four or more times daily. There was a prolongation of tear film breakup time and a decrease in foreign body sensation associated with dry eye syndrome in patients during treatment with inserts as compared to artificial tears; these findings were statistically significantly different between the treatment groups. Improvement, as measured by amelioration of symptoms, by slit-lamp examination and by rose bengal staining of the cornea and conjunctiva, was greater in most patients with moderate to severe symptoms during treatment with LACRISERT. Patient comfort was usually better with LACRISERT than with artificial tears solution, and most patients preferred LACRISERT.

In most patients treated with LACRISERT for over one year, improvement was observed as evidenced by amelioration of symptoms generally associated with keratoconjunctivitis sicca such as burning, tearing, foreign body sensation, itching, photophobia and blurred or cloudy vision.

During studies in healthy volunteers, a thickened precorneal tear film was usually observed through the slit-lamp while LACRISERT was present in the conjunctival sac.

Continued on next page

Information on the Merck & Co., Inc. products listed on these pages is the full prescribing information from product circulars in use September 30, 2000. For information, please call 1-800-NSC MERCK [1-800-672-6372].

Lacrisert—Cont.

Pharmacokinetics and Metabolism
Hydroxypropyl cellulose is a physiologically inert substance. In a study of rats fed hydroxypropyl cellulose or unmodified cellulose at levels up to 5% of their diet, it was found that the two were biologically equivalent in that neither was metabolized.
Studies conducted in rats fed ^{14}C-labeled hydroxypropyl cellulose demonstrated that when orally administered, hydroxypropyl cellulose is not absorbed from the gastrointestinal tract and is quantitatively excreted in the feces.
Dissolution studies in rabbits showed that hydroxypropyl cellulose inserts became softer within 1 hour after they were placed in the conjunctival sac. Most of the inserts dissolved completely in 14 to 18 hours; with a single exception, all had disappeared by 24 hours after insertion. Similar dissolution of the inserts was observed during prolonged administration (up to 54 weeks).

INDICATIONS AND USAGE

LACRISERT is indicated in patients with moderate to severe dry eye syndromes, including keratoconjunctivitis sicca. LACRISERT is indicated especially in patients who remain symptomatic after an adequate trial of therapy with artificial tear solutions.
LACRISERT is also indicated for patients with:
- Exposure keratitis
- Decreased corneal sensitivity
- Recurrent corneal erosions

CONTRAINDICATIONS

LACRISERT is contraindicated in patients who are hypersensitive to hydroxypropyl cellulose.

WARNINGS

Instructions for inserting and removing LACRISERT should be carefully followed.

PRECAUTIONS

General
If improperly placed, LACRISERT may result in corneal abrasion (see DOSAGE AND ADMINISTRATION).
Information for Patients
Patients should be advised to follow the instructions for using LACRISERT which accompany the package.
Because this product may produce transient blurring of vision, patients should be instructed to exercise caution when operating hazardous machinery or driving a motor vehicle.
Drug Interactions
Application of hydroxypropyl cellulose ophthalmic inserts to the eyes of unanesthetized rabbits immediately prior to or two hours before instilling pilocarpine, proparacaine HCl (0.5%), or phenylephrine (5%) did not markedly alter the magnitude and/or duration of the miotic, local corneal anesthetic, or mydriatic activity, respectively, of these agents.
Under various treatment schedules, the anti-inflammatory effect of ocularly instilled dexamethasone (0.1%) in unanesthetized rabbits with primary uveitis was not affected by the presence of hydroxypropyl cellulose inserts.
Carcinogenesis, Mutagenesis, Impairment of Fertility
Feeding of hydroxypropyl cellulose to rats at levels up to 5% of their diet produced no gross or histopathologic changes or other deleterious effects.
Pediatric Use
Safety and effectiveness in pediatric patients have not been established.

ADVERSE REACTIONS

The following adverse reactions have been reported in patients treated with LACRISERT, but were in most instances mild and transient:
- Transient blurring of vision (See PRECAUTIONS)
- Ocular discomfort or irritation
- Matting or stickiness of eyelashes
- Photophobia
- Hypersensitivity
- Edema of the eyelids
- Hyperemia

DOSAGE AND ADMINISTRATION

One LACRISERT ophthalmic insert in each eye once daily is usually sufficient to relieve the symptoms associated with moderate to severe dry eye syndromes. Individual patients may require more flexibility in the use of LACRISERT; some patients may require twice daily use for optimal results.
Clinical experience with LACRISERT indicates that in some patients several weeks may be required before satisfactory improvement of symptoms is achieved.
LACRISERT is inserted into the inferior cul-de-sac of the eye beneath the base of the tarsus, not in apposition to the cornea, nor beneath the eyelid at the level of the tarsal plate. If not properly positioned, it will be expelled into the interpalpebral fissure, and may cause symptoms of a foreign body. Illustrated instructions are included in each package. While in the licensed practitioner's office, the patient should read the instructions, then practice insertion and removal of LACRISERT until proficiency is achieved.
NOTE: Occasionally LACRISERT is inadvertently expelled from the eye, especially in patients with shallow conjunctival fornices. The patient should be cautioned against rubbing the eye(s) containing LACRISERT, especially upon awakening, so as not to dislodge or expel the insert. If required, another LACRISERT ophthalmic insert may be inserted. If experience indicates that transient blurred vision develops in an individual patient, the patient may want to remove LACRISERT a few hours after insertion to avoid this. Another LACRISERT ophthalmic insert may be inserted if needed.
If LACRISERT causes worsening of symptoms, the patient should be instructed to inspect the conjunctival sac to make certain LACRISERT is in the proper location, deep in the inferior cul-de-sac of the eye beneath the base of the tarsus. If these symptoms persist, LACRISERT should be removed and the patient should contact the practitioner.

HOW SUPPLIED

No. 3380—LACRISERT, a sterile, translucent, rod-shaped, water soluble, ophthalmic insert made of hydroxypropyl cellulose, 5 mg, is supplied as follows:
NDC 0006-3380-60 in packages containing 60 unit doses, two reusable applicators and a storage container.
(6505-01-153-4360, 5 mg 60's).
Storage
Store below 30°C (86°F).
7415111 Issued October 1997

M-M-R®$_{II}$ ℞
(Measles, Mumps, and Rubella Virus Vaccine Live)

DESCRIPTION

M-M-R* II (Measles, Mumps, and Rubella Virus Vaccine Live) is a live virus vaccine for vaccination against measles (rubeola), mumps and rubella (German measles).
M-M-R II is a sterile lyophilized preparation of (1) ATTENUVAX* (Measles Virus Vaccine Live), a more attenuated line of measles virus, derived from Enders' attenuated Edmonston strain and propagated in chick embryo cell culture; (2) MUMPSVAX* (Mumps Virus Vaccine Live), the Jeryl Lynn** (B level) strain of mumps virus propagated in chick embryo cell culture; and (3) MERUVAX* II (Rubella Virus Vaccine Live), the Wistar RA 27/3 strain of live attenuated rubella virus propagated in WI-38 human diploid lung fibroblasts.
The growth medium for measles and mumps is Medium 199 (a buffered salt solution containing vitamins and amino acids and supplemented with fetal bovine serum) containing SPGA (sucrose, phosphate, glutamate, and human albumin) as stabilizer and neomycin.
The growth medium for rubella is Minimum Essential Medium (MEM) [a buffered salt solution containing vitamins and amino acids and supplemented with fetal bovine serum] containing human serum albumin and neomycin. Sorbitol and hydrolyzed gelatin stabilizer are added to the individual virus harvests.
The cells, virus pools, fetal bovine serum, and human albumin are all screened for the absence of adventitious agents. Human albumin is processed using the Cohn cold ethanol fractionation procedure.
The reconstituted vaccine is for subcutaneous administration. Each 0.5 mL dose contains not less than 1,000 $TCID_{50}$ (tissue culture infectious doses) of measles virus; 20,000 $TCID_{50}$ of mumps virus; and 1,000 $TCID_{50}$ of rubella virus. Each dose of the vaccine is calculated to contain sorbitol (14.5 mg), sodium phosphate, sucrose (1.9 mg), sodium chloride, hydrolyzed gelatin (14.5 mg), human albumin (0.3 mg), fetal bovine serum (<1 ppm), other buffer and media ingredients and approximately 25 mcg of neomycin. The product contains no preservative.
Before reconstitution, the lyophilized vaccine is a light yellow compact crystalline plug. M-M-R II, when reconstituted as directed, is clear yellow.

---
*Registered trademark of MERCK & CO., Inc.
**Trademark of MERCK & CO., Inc.

CLINICAL PHARMACOLOGY

Measles, mumps, and rubella are three common childhood diseases, caused by measles virus, mumps virus (paramyxoviruses), and rubella virus (togavirus), respectively, that may be associated with serious complications and/or death. For example, pneumonia and encephalitis are caused by measles. Mumps is associated with aseptic meningitis, deafness and orchitis; and rubella during pregnancy may cause congenital rubella syndrome in the infants of infected mothers.
The impact of measles, mumps, and rubella vaccination on the natural history of each disease in the United States can be quantified by comparing the maximum number of measles, mumps, and rubella cases reported in a given year prior to vaccine use to the number of cases of each disease reported in 1995. For measles, 894,134 cases reported in 1941 compared to 288 cases reported in 1995 resulted in a 99.97% decrease in reported cases; for mumps, 152,209 cases reported in 1968 compared to 840 cases reported in 1995 resulted in a 99.45% decrease in reported cases; and for rubella, 57,686 cases reported in 1969 compared to 200 cases reported in 1995 resulted in a 99.65% decrease.
Clinical studies of 279 triple seronegative children, 11 months to 7 years of age, demonstrated that M-M-R II is highly immunogenic and generally well tolerated. In these studies, a single injection of the vaccine induced measles hemagglutination-inhibition (HI) antibodies in 95%, mumps neutralizing antibodies in 96%, and rubella HI antibodies in 99% of susceptible persons. However, a small percentage (1–5%) of vaccines may fail to seroconvert after the primary dose (see also INDICATIONS AND USAGE, *Recommended Vaccination Schedule*).
A study of 6 month old and 15 month old infants born to vaccine-immunized mothers demonstrated that, following vaccination with ATTENUVAX, 74% of the 6 month old infants developed detectable neutralizing antibody (NT) titers while 100% of the 15 month old infants developed NT. This rate of seroconversion is higher than that previously reported for 6 month old infants born to naturally immune mothers tested by HI assay. When the 6 month old infants of immunized mothers were revaccinated at 15 months, they developed antibody titers equivalent to the 15 month old vaccinees. The lower seroconversion rate in 6 month olds has two possible explanations: 1) Due to the limit of the detection level of the assays (NT and enzyme immunoassay [EIA]), the presence of trace amounts of undetectable maternal antibody might interfere with the seroconversion of infants; or 2) the immune system of 6 month olds is not always capable of mounting a response to measles vaccine as measured by the two antibody assays.
There is some evidence to suggest that infants who are born to mothers who had natural measles and who are vaccinated at less than one year of age may not develop sustained antibody levels when later revaccinated. The advantage of early protection must be weighed against the chance for failure to respond adequately on reimmunization.
Efficacy of measles, mumps and rubella vaccine was established in a series of double-blind controlled field trials which demonstrated a high degree of protective efficacy afforded by the individual vaccine components. These studies also established that seroconversion in response to vaccination against measles, mumps, and rubella paralleled protection from these diseases.
Following vaccination, antibodies associated with protection can be measured by neutralization assays, HI, or ELISA (enzyme linked immunosorbent assay) tests. Neutralizing and ELISA antibodies to measles, mumps, and rubella viruses are still detectable in most individuals 11–13 years after primary vaccination. See INDICATIONS AND USAGE, *Non-Pregnant Adolescents and Adult Females*, for Rubella Susceptibility Testing.
The RA 27/3 rubella strain in M-M-R II elicits higher immediate post-vaccination HI, complement-fixing and neutralizing antibody levels than other strains of rubella vaccine and has been shown to induce a broader profile of circulating antibodies including anti-theta and anti-iota precipitating antibodies. The RA 27/3 rubella strain immunologically simulates natural infection more closely than other rubella vaccine viruses. The increased levels and broader profile of antibodies produced by RA 27/3 strain rubella virus vaccine appear to correlate with greater resistance to subclinical reinfection with the wild virus, and provide greater confidence for lasting immunity.

INDICATIONS AND USAGE

Recommended Vaccination Schedule
M-M-R II is indicated for simultaneous vaccination against measles, mumps, and rubella in individuals 12 months of age or older.
Individuals first vaccinated at 12 months of age or older should be revaccinated prior to elementary school entry. Revaccination may seroconvert primary failures or boost antibody titers of previously vaccinated individuals whose titers have declined. The Advisory Committee on Immunization Practices (ACIP) recommends administration of the first dose of M-M-R II at 12–15 months of age and administration of the second dose of M-M-R II at 4–6 years of age. In addition, some public health jurisdictions mandate the age for revaccination. Consult the complete text of applicable guidelines regarding routine revaccination including that of high-risk adult populations.
Measles Outbreak Schedule
Infants Between 6–12 Months of Age
Local health authorities may recommend measles vaccination of infants between 6–12 months of age in outbreak situations. This population may fail to respond to the components of the vaccine. Safety and effectiveness of mumps and rubella vaccine in infants less than 12 months of age have not been established. The younger the infant, the lower the likelihood of seroconversion (see CLINICAL PHARMACOLOGY). Such infants should receive a second dose of M-M-R II between 12 to 15 months of age followed by revaccination at elementary school entry.
Unnecessary doses of a vaccine are best avoided by ensuring that written documentation of vaccination is preserved and a copy given to each vaccinee's parent or guardian.
Other Vaccination Considerations
Non-Pregnant Adolescent and Adult Females
Immunization of susceptible non-pregnant adolescent and adult females of childbearing age with live attenuated ru-

bella virus vaccine is indicated if certain precautions are observed (see below and PRECAUTIONS). Vaccinating susceptible postpubertal females confers individual protection against subsequently acquiring rubella infection during pregnancy, which in turn prevents infection of the fetus and consequent congenital rubella injury.
Women of childbearing age should be advised not to become pregnant for 3 months after vaccination and should be informed of the reasons for this precaution.***
The ACIP has stated "If it is practical and if reliable laboratory services are available, women of childbearing age who are potential candidates for vaccination can have serologic tests to determine susceptibility to rubella. However, with the exception of premarital and prenatal screening, routinely performing serologic tests for all women of childbearing age to determine susceptibility (so that vaccine is given only to proven susceptible women) can be effective but is expensive. Also, 2 visits to the health-care provider would be necessary—one for screening and one for vaccination. Accordingly, rubella vaccination of a woman who is not known to be pregnant and has no history of vaccination is justifiable without serologic testing—and may be preferable, particularly when costs of serology are high and follow-up of identified susceptible women for vaccination is not assured."
Postpubertal females should be informed of the frequent occurrence of generally self-limited arthralgia and/or arthritis beginning 2 to 4 weeks after vaccination (see ADVERSE REACTIONS).
Postpartum Women
It has been found convenient in many instances to vaccinate rubella-susceptible women in the immediate postpartum period (see PRECAUTIONS, *Nursing Mothers*).
Other Populations
Previously unvaccinated children older than 12 months who are in contact with susceptible pregnant women should receive live attenuated rubella vaccine (such as that contained in monovalent rubella vaccine or in M-M-R II) to reduce the risk of exposure of the pregnant woman.
Individuals planning travel outside the United States, if not immune, can acquire measles, mumps or rubella and import these diseases into the United States. Therefore, prior to international travel, individuals known to be susceptible to one or more of these diseases can receive either a monovalent vaccine (measles, mumps or rubella), or a combination vaccine as appropriate. However, M-M-R II is preferred for persons likely to be susceptible to mumps and rubella; and if monovalent measles vaccine is not readily available, travelers should receive M-M-R II regardless of their immune status to mumps or rubella.
Vaccination is recommended for susceptible individuals in high-risk groups such as college students, health-care workers, and military personnel.
According to ACIP recommendations, most persons born in 1956 or earlier are likely to have been infected with measles naturally and generally need not be considered susceptible. All children, adolescents, and adults born after 1956 are considered susceptible and should be vaccinated, if there are no contraindications. This includes persons who may be immune to measles but who lack adequate documentation of immunity such as: (1) physician-diagnosed measles, (2) laboratory evidence of measles immunity, or (3) adequate immunization with live measles vaccine on or after the first birthday.
The ACIP recommends that "Persons vaccinated with inactivated vaccine followed within 3 months by live vaccine should be revaccinated with two doses of live vaccine. Revaccination is particularly important when the risk of exposure to natural measles virus is increased, as may occur during international travel."
Post-Exposure Vaccination
Vaccination of individuals exposed to natural measles may provide some protection if the vaccine can be administered within 72 hours of exposure. If, however, vaccine is given a few days before exposure, substantial protection may be afforded. There is no conclusive evidence that vaccination of individuals recently exposed to natural mumps or natural rubella will provide protection.
Use With Other Vaccines
See DOSAGE AND ADMINISTRATION, *Use With Other Vaccines.*

*** NOTE: The ACIP has recommended "In view of the importance of protecting this age group against rubella, reasonable practices in a rubella immunization program include a) asking women if they are pregnant, b) excluding those who say they are, c) explaining the concern about risk for the fetus to the others, and d) explaining the importance of not becoming pregnant during the 3 months following vaccination."

CONTRAINDICATIONS

Hypersensitivity to any component of the vaccine, including gelatin.
Do not give M-M-R II to pregnant females; the possible effects of the vaccine on fetal development are unknown at this time. If vaccination of postpubertal females is undertaken, pregnancy should be avoided for three months following vaccination (see PRECAUTIONS, *Pregnancy*).
Anaphylactic or anaphylactoid reactions to neomycin (each dose of reconstituted vaccine contains approximately 25 mcg of neomycin).
Febrile respiratory illness or other active febrile infection. However, the ACIP has recommended that all vaccines can be administered to persons with minor illnesses such as diarrhea, mild upper respiratory infection with or without low-grade fever, or other low-grade febrile illness.
Patients receiving immunosuppressive therapy. This contraindication does not apply to patients who are receiving corticosteroids as replacement therapy, e.g., for Addison's disease.
Individuals with blood dyscrasias, leukemia, lymphomas of any type, or other malignant neoplasms affecting the bone marrow or lymphatic systems.
Primary and acquired immunodeficiency states, including patients who are immunosuppressed in association with AIDS or other clinical manifestations of infection with human immunodeficiency viruses; cellular immune deficiencies; and hypogammaglobulinemic and dysgammaglobulinemic states. Measles inclusion body encephalitis (MIBE), pneumonitis and death as a direct consequence of disseminated measles vaccine virus infection has been reported in immunocompromised individuals inadvertently vaccinated with measles-containing vaccine.
Individuals with a family history of congenital or hereditary immunodeficiency, until the immune competence of the potential vaccine recipient is demonstrated.

WARNINGS

Due caution should be employed in administration of M-M-R II to persons with a history of cerebral injury, individual or family histories of convulsions, or any other condition in which stress due to fever should be avoided. The physician should be alert to the temperature elevation which may occur following vaccination (see ADVERSE REACTIONS).
Hypersensitivity To Eggs
Live measles vaccine and live mumps vaccine are produced in chick embryo cell culture. Persons with a history of anaphylactic, anaphylactoid, or other immediate reactions (e.g., hives, swelling of the mouth and throat, difficulty breathing, hypotension, or shock) subsequent to egg ingestion may be at an enhanced risk of immediate-type hypersensitivity reactions after receiving vaccines containing traces of chick embryo antigen. The potential risk to benefit ratio should be carefully evaluated before considering vaccination in such cases. Such individuals may be vaccinated with extreme caution, having adequate treatment on hand should a reaction occur (see PRECAUTIONS).
However, the AAP has stated, "Most children with a history of anaphylactic reactions to eggs have no untoward reactions to measles or MMR vaccine. Persons are not at increased risk if they have egg allergies that are not anaphylactic, and they should be vaccinated in the usual manner. In addition, skin testing of egg-allergic children with vaccine has not been predictive of which children will have an immediate hypersensitivity reaction…Persons with allergies to chickens or chicken feathers are not at increased risk of reaction to the vaccine."
Hypersensitivity to Neomycin
The AAP states, "Persons who have experienced anaphylactic reactions to topically or systemically administered neomycin should not receive measles vaccine. Most often, however, neomycin allergy manifests as a contact dermatitis, which is a delayed-type (cell-mediated) immune response rather than anaphylaxis. In such persons, an adverse reaction to neomycin in the vaccine would be an erythematous, pruritic nodule or papule, 48 to 96 hours after vaccination. A history of contact dermatitis to neomycin is not a contraindication to receiving measles vaccine."
Thrombocytopenia
Individuals with current thrombocytopenia may develop more severe thrombocytopenia following vaccination. In addition, individuals who experienced thrombocytopenia with the first dose of M-M-R II (or its component vaccines) may develop thrombocytopenia with repeat doses. Serologic status may be evaluated to determine whether or not additional doses of vaccine are needed. The potential risk to benefit ratio should be carefully evaluated before considering vaccination in such cases (see ADVERSE REACTIONS).

PRECAUTIONS

General
Adequate treatment provisions including epinephrine injection (1:1000), should be available for immediate use should an anaphylactic or anaphylactoid reaction occur.
Special care should be taken to ensure that the injection does not enter a blood vessel.
Children and young adults who are known to be infected with human immunodeficiency viruses and are not immunosuppressed may be vaccinated. However, vaccinees who are infected with HIV should be monitored closely for vaccine-preventable diseases because immunization may be less effective than for uninfected persons (see CONTRAINDICATIONS).
Vaccination should be deferred for 3 months or longer following blood or plasma transfusions, or administration of immune globulin (human).
Excretion of small amounts of the live attenuated rubella virus from the nose or throat has occurred in the majority of susceptible individuals 7–28 days after vaccination. There is no confirmed evidence to indicate that such virus is transmitted to susceptible persons who are in contact with the vaccinated individuals. Consequently, transmission through close personal contact, while accepted as a theoretical possibility, is not regarded as a significant risk. However, transmission of the rubella vaccine virus to infants via breast milk has been documented (see *Nursing Mothers*).
There are no reports of transmission of live attenuated measles or mumps viruses from vaccinees to susceptible contacts.
It has been reported that live attenuated measles, mumps and rubella virus vaccines given individually may result in a temporary depression of tuberculin skin sensitivity. Therefore, if a tuberculin test is to be done, it should be administered either before or simultaneously with M-M-R II. Children under treatment for tuberculosis have not experienced exacerbation of the disease when immunized with live measles virus vaccine; no studies have been reported to date of the effect of measles virus vaccines on untreated tuberculous children. However, individuals with active untreated tuberculosis should not be vaccinated.
As for any vaccine, vaccination with M-M-R II may not result in protection in 100% of vaccinees.
The health-care provider should determine the current health status and previous vaccination history of the vaccinee.
The health-care provider should question the patient, parent, or guardian about reactions to a previous dose of M-M-R II or other measles-, mumps-, or rubella-containing vaccines.
Information for Patients
The health-care provider should provide the vaccine information required to be given with each vaccination to the patient, parent or guardian.
The health-care provider should inform the patient, parent or guardian of the benefits and risks associated with vaccination. For risks associated with vaccination see WARNINGS, PRECAUTIONS, ADVERSE REACTIONS.
Patients, parents or guardians should be instructed to report any serious adverse reactions to their health-care provider who in turn should report such events to the U.S. Department of Health and Human Services through the Vaccine Adverse Event Reporting System (VAERS), 1-800-822-7967.
Pregnancy should be avoided for 3 months following vaccination.
Laboratory Tests
See INDICATIONS AND USAGE, *Non-Pregnant Adolescents and Adult Females,* for Rubella Susceptibility Testing, and CLINICAL PHARMACOLOGY.
Drug Interactions
See DOSAGE AND ADMINISTRATION, *Use With Other Vaccines.*
Immunosuppressive Therapy
The immune status of patients about to undergo immunosuppressive therapy should be evaluated so that the physician can consider whether vaccination prior to the initiation of treatment is indicated. (see CONTRAINDICATIONS and PRECAUTIONS)
The ACIP has stated that "patients with leukemia in remission who have not received chemotherapy for at least 3 months may receive live-virus vaccines. Short-term (<2 weeks), low- to moderate-dose systemic corticosteroid therapy, topical steroid therapy (e.g. nasal, skin), long-term alternate-day treatment with low to moderate doses of short-acting systemic steroid, and intra-articular, bursal, or tendon injection of corticosteroids are not immunosuppressive in their usual doses and do not contraindicate the administration of [measles, mumps or rubella vaccine]."
Immune Globulin
Administration of immune globulins concurrently with M-M-R II may interfere with the expected immune response.
See also PRECAUTIONS, *General.*
Carcinogenesis, Mutagenesis, Impairment of Fertility
M-M-R II has not been evaluated for carcinogenic or mutagenic potential, or potential to impair fertility.
Pregnancy
Pregnancy Category C
Animal reproduction studies have not been conducted with M-M-R II. It is also not known whether M-M-R II can cause fetal harm when administered to a pregnant woman or can affect reproduction capacity. Therefore, the vaccine should not be administered to pregnant females; furthermore, pregnancy should be avoided for 3 months following vaccination (see CONTRAINDICATIONS).
In counseling women who are inadvertently vaccinated when pregnant or who become pregnant within 3 months of vaccination, the physician should be aware of the following: (1) In a 10 year survey involving over 700 pregnant women who received rubella vaccine within 3 months before or after conception (of whom 189 received the Wistar RA 27/3 strain), none of the newborns had abnormalities compatible with congenital rubella syndrome; (2) Mumps infection during the first trimester of pregnancy may increase the rate of spontaneous abortion. Although mumps vaccine virus has been shown to infect the placenta and fetus, there is no evidence that it causes congenital malformations in humans; and (3) Reports have indicated that contracting natural

Continued on next page

Information on the Merck & Co., Inc. products listed on these pages is the full prescribing information from product circulars in use September 30, 2000. For information, please call 1-800-NSC MERCK [1-800-672-6372].

M-M-R II—Cont.

measles during pregnancy enhances fetal risk. Increased rates of spontaneous abortion, stillbirth, congenital defects and prematurity have been observed subsequent to natural measles during pregnancy. There are no adequate studies of the attenuated (vaccine) strain of measles virus in pregnancy. However, it would be prudent to assume that the vaccine strain of virus is also capable of inducing adverse fetal effects.

Nursing Mothers

It is not known whether measles or mumps vaccine virus is secreted in human milk. Recent studies have shown that lactating postpartum women immunized with live attenuated rubella vaccine may secrete the virus in breast milk and transmit it to breast-fed infants. In the infants with serological evidence of rubella infection, none exhibited severe disease; however, one exhibited mild clinical illness typical of acquired rubella. Caution should be exercised when M-M-R II is administered to a nursing woman.

Pediatric Use

Safety and effectiveness of measles vaccine in infants below the age of 6 months have not been established (see also CLINICAL PHARMACOLOGY). Safety and effectiveness of mumps and rubella vaccine in infants less than 12 months of age have not been established.

ADVERSE REACTIONS

The following adverse reactions are listed in decreasing order of severity, without regard to causality, within each body system category and have been reported during clinical trials, with use of the marketed vaccine, or with use of monovalent or bivalent vaccine containing measles, mumps, or rubella:

Body as a Whole

Panniculitis; atypical measles; fever; syncope, headache; dizziness; malaise; irritability.

Cardiovascular System

Vasculitis.

Digestive System

Pancreatitis; diarrhea; vomiting; parotitis; nausea.

Endocrine System

Diabetes mellitus.

Hemic and Lymphatic System

Thrombocytopenia (see WARNINGS, *Thrombocytopenia*); purpura; regional lymphadenopathy; leukocytosis.

Immune System

Anaphylaxis and anaphylactoid reactions have been reported as well as related phenomena such as angioneurotic edema (including peripheral or facial edema) and bronchial spasm.

Musculoskeletal System

Arthritis; arthralgia; myalgia.

Arthralgia and/or arthritis (usually transient and rarely chronic), and polyneuritis are features of natural rubella and vary in frequency and severity with age and sex, being greatest in adult females and least in prepubertal children. This type of involvement as well as myalgia and paresthesia, have also been reported following administration of MERUVAX II.

Chronic arthritis has been associated with natural rubella infection and has been related to persistent virus and/or viral antigen isolated from body tissues. Only rarely have vaccine recipients developed chronic joint symptoms.

Following vaccination in children, reactions in joints are uncommon and generally of brief duration. In women, incidence rates for arthritis and arthralgia are generally higher than those seen in children (children: 0–3%; women: 12–26%), and the reactions tend to be more marked and of longer duration. Symptoms may persist for a matter of months or on rare occasions for years. In adolescent girls, the reactions appear to be intermediate in incidence between those seen in children and in adult women. Even in women older than 35 years, these reactions are generally well tolerated and rarely interfere with normal activities.

Nervous System

Encephalitis; encephalopathy; measles inclusion body encephalitis (MIBE) (see CONTRAINDICATIONS); subacute sclerosing panencephalitis (SSPE); Guillain-Barré Syndrome (GBS); febrile convulsions; afebrile convulsions or seizures; ataxia; polyneuritis; polyneuropathy; ocular palsies; paresthesia.

Experience from more than 80 million doses of all live measles vaccines given in the U.S. through 1975 indicates that significant central nervous system reactions such as encephalitis and encephalopathy, occurring within 30 days after vaccination, have been temporally associated with measles vaccine very rarely. In no case has it been shown that reactions were actually caused by vaccine. The Centers for Disease Control and Prevention has pointed out that "a certain number of cases of encephalitis may be expected to occur in a large childhood population in a defined period of time even when no vaccines are administered". However, the data suggest the possibility that some of these cases may have been caused by measles vaccines. The risk of such serious neurological disorders following live measles virus vaccine administration remains far less than that for encephalitis and encephalopathy with natural measles (one per two thousand reported cases).

Post-marketing surveillance of the more than 200 million doses of M-M-R and M-M-R II that have been distributed worldwide over 25 years (1971–1996) indicates that serious adverse events such as encephalitis and encephalopathy continue to be rarely reported.

There have been reports of subacute sclerosing panencephalitis (SSPE) in children who did not have a history of natural measles but did receive measles vaccine. Some of these cases may have resulted from unrecognized measles in the first year of life or possibly from the measles vaccination. Based on estimated nationwide measles vaccine distribution, the association of SSPE cases to measles vaccination is about one case per million vaccine doses distributed. This is far less than the association with natural measles, 6–22 cases of SSPE per million cases of measles. The results of a retrospective case-controlled study conducted by the Centers for Disease Control and Prevention suggest that the overall effect of measles vaccine has been to protect against SSPE by preventing measles with its inherent higher risk of SSPE.

Cases of aseptic meningitis have been reported to VAERS following measles, mumps, and rubella vaccination. Although a causal relationship between the Urabe strain of mumps vaccine and aseptic meningitis has been shown, there are no data to link Jeryl Lynn mumps vaccine to aseptic meningitis.

Respiratory System

Pneumonitis (see CONTRAINDICATIONS); sore throat; cough; rhinitis.

Skin

Stevens-Johnson Syndrome; erythema multiforme; urticaria; rash.

Local reactions including burning/stinging at injection site; wheal and flare; redness (erythema); swelling; induration; tenderness; vesiculation at injection site.

Special Senses—Ear

Nerve deafness; otitis media.

Special Senses—Eye

Retinitis; optic neuritis; papillitis; retrobulbar neuritis; conjunctivitis.

Urogenital System

Orchitis.

Other

Death from various, and in some cases unknown, causes has been reported rarely following vaccination with measles, mumps, and rubella vaccines; however, a causal relationship has not been established. No deaths or permanent sequelae were reported in a published post-marketing surveillance study in Finland involving 1.5 million children and adults who were vaccinated with M-M-R II during 1982–1993.

Under the National Childhood Vaccine Injury Act of 1986, health-care providers and manufacturers are required to record and report certain suspected adverse events occurring within specific time periods after vaccination. However, the U.S. Department of Health and Human Services (DHHS) has established a Vaccine Adverse Event Reporting System (VAERS) which will accept all reports of suspected events. A VAERS report form as well as information regarding reporting requirements can be obtained by calling VAERS 1-800-822-7967.

DOSAGE AND ADMINISTRATION

FOR SUBCUTANEOUS ADMINISTRATION

Do not inject intravenously

The dose for any age is 0.5 mL administered subcutaneously, preferably into the outer aspect of the upper arm.

The recommended age for primary vaccination is 12 to 15 months.

Revaccination with M-M-R II is recommended prior to elementary school entry. See also INDICATIONS AND USAGE, *Recommended Vaccination Schedule.*

Children first vaccinated when younger than 12 months of age should receive another dose between 12 to 15 months of age followed by revaccination prior to elementary school entry. See also INDICATIONS AND USAGE, *Measles Outbreak Schedule.*

Immune Globulin (IG) is not to be given concurrently with M-M-R II.

CAUTION: A sterile syringe free of preservatives, antiseptics, and detergents should be used for each injection and/or reconstitution of the vaccine because these substances may inactivate the live virus vaccine. A 25 gauge, 5/8" needle is recommended.

To reconstitute, use only the diluent supplied, since it is free of preservatives or other antiviral substances which might inactivate the vaccine.

Single Dose Vial—First withdraw the entire volume of diluent into the syringe to be used for reconstitution. Inject all the diluent in the syringe into the vial of lyophilized vaccine, and agitate to mix thoroughly. If the lyophilized vaccine cannot be dissolved, discard. Withdraw the entire contents into a syringe and inject the total volume of restored vaccine subcutaneously.

It is important to use a separate sterile syringe and needle for each individual patient to prevent transmission of hepatitis B and other infectious agents from one person to another.

10 Dose Vial (available only to government agencies/institutions)—Withdraw the entire contents (7 mL) of the diluent vial into the sterile syringe to be used for reconstitution, and introduce into the 10 dose vial of lyophilized vaccine. Agitate to ensure thorough mixing. If the lyophilized vaccine cannot be dissolved, discard. The outer labeling suggests "For Jet Injector or Syringe Use." Use with separate sterile syringes is permitted for containers of 10 doses or less. The vaccine and diluent do not contain preservatives; therefore, the user must recognize the potential contamination hazards and exercise special precautions to protect the sterility and potency of the product. The use of aseptic techniques and proper storage prior to and after restoration of the vaccine and subsequent withdrawal of the individual doses is essential. Use 0.5 mL of the reconstituted vaccine for subcutaneous injection.

It is important to use a separate sterile syringe and needle for each individual patient to prevent transmission of hepatitis B and other infectious agents from one person to another.

Parenteral drug products should be inspected visually for particulate matter and discoloration prior to administration whenever solution and container permit. M-M-R II, when reconstituted, is clear yellow.

Use With Other Vaccines

M-M-R II should be given one month before or after administration of other live viral vaccines.

M-M-R II has been administered concurrently with VARIVAX* [Varicella Virus Vaccine Live (Oka/Merck)], and PedvaxHIB* [Haemophilus b Conjugate Vaccine (Meningococcal Protein Conjugate)] using separate sites and syringes. No impairment of immune response to individual tested vaccine antigens was demonstrated. The type, frequency, and severity of adverse experiences observed with M-M-R II were similar to those seen when each vaccine was given alone.

Routine administration of DTP (diphtheria, tetanus, pertussis) and/or OPV (oral poliovirus vaccine) concurrently with measles, mumps and rubella vaccines is not recommended because there are limited data relating to the simultaneous administration of these antigens.

However, other schedules have been used. The ACIP has stated "Although data are limited concerning the simultaneous administration of the entire recommended vaccine series (i.e., DTP, OPV, MMR, and Hib vaccines, with or without hepatitis B vaccine), data from numerous studies have indicated no interference between routinely recommended childhood vaccines (either live, attenuated, or killed). These findings support the simultaneous use of all vaccines as recommended."

HOW SUPPLIED

No. 4749—M-M-R II is supplied as a single-dose vial of lyophilized vaccine, **NDC** 0006-4749-00, and a vial of diluent.

No. 4681/4309—M-M-R II is supplied as follows: (1) a box of 10 single-dose vials of lyophilized vaccine (package A), **NDC** 0006-4681-00; and (2) a box of 10 vials of diluent (package B). To conserve refrigerator space, the diluent may be stored separately at room temperature.

Available only to government agencies/institutions:

No. 4682X—M-M-R II is supplied as one 10 dose vial of lyophilized vaccine.

NDC 0006-4682-00, and one 7 mL vial of diluent.

Storage

During shipment, to ensure that there is no loss of potency, the vaccine must be maintained at a temperature of 10°C (50°F) or colder. Freezing during shipment will not affect potency.

Protect the vaccine from light at all times, since such exposure may inactivate the virus.

Before reconstitution, store the vial of lyophilized vaccine at 2–8°C (36–46°F) or colder. The diluent may be stored in the refrigerator with the lyophilized vaccine or separately at room temperature.

It is recommended that the vaccine be used as soon as possible after reconstitution. Store reconstituted vaccine in the vaccine vial in a dark place at 2–8°C (36–46°F) and discard if not used within 8 hours.

9265201 Issued February 2000

M-R-VAX®II ℞
(Measles and Rubella Virus Vaccine Live)

DESCRIPTION

M-R-VAX* II (Measles and Rubella Virus Vaccine Live), is a live virus vaccine for immunization against measles (rubeola) and rubella (German measles).

M-R-VAX II is a sterile lyophilized preparation of (1) ATTENUVAX* (Measles Virus Vaccine Live), a more attenuated line of measles virus, derived from Enders' attenuated Edmonston strain and grown in cell cultures of chick embryo; and (2) MERUVAX* II (Rubella Virus Vaccine Live), the Wistar RA 27/3 strain of live attenuated rubella virus grown in human diploid cell (WI-38) culture. The vaccine viruses are the same as those used in the manufacture of ATTENUVAX (Measles Virus Vaccine Live) and MERUVAX II (Rubella Virus Vaccine Live). The two viruses are mixed before being lyophilized. The product contains no preservative.

The reconstituted vaccine is for subcutaneous administration. When reconstituted as directed, the dose for injection is 0.5 mL and contains not less than the equivalent of 1,000 $TCID_{50}$ (tissue culture infectious doses) of the U.S. Reference Measles Virus; and 1,000 $TCID_{50}$ of the U.S. Reference

Rubella Virus. Each dose contains approximately 25 mcg of neomycin. The product contains no preservative. Sorbitol and hydrolized gelatin are added as stabilizers.

*Registered trademark of MERCK & CO., INC.

CLINICAL PHARMACOLOGY

Clinical studies of 237 double seronegative children, 10 months to 10 years of age, demonstrated that M-R-VAX II is highly immunogenic and generally well tolerated. In these studies, a single injection of the vaccine induced measles hemagglutination-inhibition (HI) antibodies in 95 percent and rubella HI antibodies in 99 percent of susceptible persons.

The RA 27/3 rubella strain in M-R-VAX II elicits higher immediate post-vaccination HI, complement-fixing and neutralizing antibody levels than other strains of rubella vaccine and has been shown to induce a broader profile of circulating antibodies including anti-theta and anti-iota precipitating antibodies. The RA 27/3 rubella strain immunologically simulates natural infection more closely than other rubella vaccine viruses. The increased levels and broader profile of antibodies produced by RA 27/3 strain rubella virus vaccine appear to correlate with greater resistance to subclinical reinfection with the wild virus, and provide greater confidence for lasting immunity.

Vaccine induced antibody levels following administration of M-R-VAX II have been shown to persist up to 11 years without substantial decline. Continued surveillance will be necessary to determine further duration of antibody persistence.

INDICATIONS AND USAGE

M-R-VAX II is indicated for simultaneous immunization against measles and rubella in persons 15 months of age or older. A second dose of M-R-VAX II or monovalent measles vaccine is recommended (see *Revaccination*).

Infants who are less than 15 months of age may fail to respond to the measles component of the vaccine due to presence in the circulation of residual measles antibody of maternal origin; the younger the infant, the lower the likelihood of seroconversion. In geographically isolated or other relatively inaccessible populations for whom immunization programs are logistically difficult, and in population groups in which natural measles infection may occur in a significant proportion of infants before 15 months of age, it may be desirable to give the vaccine to infants at an earlier age. Infants vaccinated under these conditions at less than 12 months of age should be revaccinated after reaching 15 months of age. There is some evidence to suggest that infants immunized at less than one year of age may not develop sustained antibody levels when later reimmunized. The advantage of early protection must be weighed against the chance for failure to respond adequately on reimmunization.

Previously unimmunized children of susceptible pregnant women should receive live attenuated rubella vaccine, because an immunized child will be less likely to acquire natural rubella and introduce the virus into the household.

Individuals planning travel outside the United States, if not immune, can acquire measles, mumps or rubella and import these diseases to the United States. Therefore, prior to International travel, individuals known to be susceptible to one or more of these diseases can receive either a single antigen vaccine (measles, mumps, or rubella), or a combined antigen vaccine as appropriate. However, M-M-R* II (Measles, Mumps, and Rubella Virus Vaccine Live) is preferred for persons likely to be susceptible to mumps and rubella; and if a single-antigen measles vaccine is not readily available, travelers should receive M-M-R II (Measles, Mumps, and Rubella Virus Vaccine Live) regardless of their immune status to mumps or rubella.

Non-Pregnant Adolescent and Adult Females

Immunization of susceptible non-pregnant adolescent and adult females of childbearing age with live attenuated rubella virus vaccine is indicated if certain precautions are observed (see below and PRECAUTIONS). Vaccinating susceptible postpubertal females confers individual protection against subsequently acquiring rubella infection during pregnancy, which in turn prevents infection of the fetus and consequent congenital rubella injury.

Women of childbearing age should be advised not to become pregnant for three months after vaccination and should be informed of the reason for this precaution.**

It is recommended that rubella susceptibility be determined by serologic testing prior to immunization.*** If immune, as evidenced by a specific rubella antibody titer of 1:8 or greater (hemagglutination-inhibition test), vaccination is unnecessary. Congenital malformations do occur in up to seven percent of all live births. Their chance appearance after vaccination could lead to misinterpretation of the cause, particularly if the prior rubella-immune status of vaccinees is unknown.

Postpubertal females should be informed of the frequent occurrence of generally self-limited arthralgia and/or arthritis beginning 2 to 4 weeks after vaccination (see ADVERSE REACTIONS).

Postpartum Women

It has been found convenient in many instances to vaccinate rubella-susceptible women in the immediate postpartum period. (See *Nursing Mothers*).

Revaccination: Children first vaccinated when younger than 12 months of age should be revaccinated at 15 months of age.

The American Academy of Pediatrics (AAP), the Immunization Practices Advisory Committee (ACIP), and some state and local health agencies have recommended guidelines for routine measles revaccination and to help control measles outbreaks.†

Vaccines available for revaccination include monovalent measles vaccine [ATTENUVAX (Measles Virus Vaccine Live)] and polyvalent vaccines containing measles [e.g., M-M-R II (Measles, Mumps, and Rubella Virus Vaccine Live), M-R-VAX II]. If the prevention of sporadic measles outbreaks is the sole objective, revaccination with a monovalent measles vaccine should be considered (see appropriate product circular). If concern also exists about immune status regarding mumps or rubella, revaccination with appropriate monovalent or polyvalent vaccines should be considered after consulting the appropriate product circulars. Unnecessary doses of a vaccine are best avoided by ensuring that written documentation of vaccination is preserved and a copy given to each vaccinee's parent or guardian.

Use with other Vaccines

Routine administration of DTP (diphtheria, tetanus, pertussis) and/or OPV (oral poliovirus vaccine) concomitantly with measles, mumps and rubella vaccines is not recommended because there are insufficient data relating to the simultaneous administration of these antigens. However, the American Academy of Pediatrics has noted that in some circumstances, particularly when the patient may not return, some practitioners prefer to administer all these antigens on a single day. If done, separate sites and syringes should be used for DTP and M-R-VAX II.

M-R-VAX II should not be given less than one month before or after administration of other virus vaccines.

*Registered trademark of MERCK & CO., INC.

**NOTE: The Immunization Practices Advisory Committee (ACIP) has recommended "In view of the importance of protecting this age group against rubella, reasonable precautions in a rubella immunization program include asking females if they are pregnant, excluding those who say they are, and explaining the theoretical risks to the others."

***NOTE: The Immunization Practices Advisory Committee (ACIP) has stated "When practical, and when reliable laboratory services are available, potential vaccinees of childbearing age can have serologic tests to determine susceptibility to rubella. . . . However, routinely performing serologic tests for all females of childbearing age to determine susceptibility so that vaccine is given only to proven susceptibles is expensive and has been ineffective in some areas. Accordingly, the ACIP believes that rubella vaccination of a woman who is not known to be pregnant and has no history of vaccination is justifiable without serologic testing."

†NOTE: A primary difference among these recommendations is the timing of revaccination: the ACIP recommends routine revaccination at entry into Kindergarten or first grade, whereas the AAP recommends routine revaccination at entrance to middle school or junior high school. In addition, some public health jurisdictions mandate the age for revaccination. The complete text of applicable guidelines should be consulted.

CONTRAINDICATIONS

Do not give M-R-VAX II to pregnant females; the possible effects of the vaccine on fetal development are unknown at this time. If vaccination of postpubertal females is undertaken, pregnancy should be avoided for three months following vaccination. (See PRECAUTIONS, *Pregnancy*).

Anaphylactic or anaphylactoid reactions to neomycin (each dose of reconstituted vaccine contains approximately 25 mcg of neomycin).

History of anaphylactic or anaphylactoid reactions to eggs (see HYPERSENSITIVITY TO EGGS below).

Any febrile respiratory illness or other active febrile infection.

Active untreated tuberculosis.

Patients receiving immunosuppressive therapy. This contraindication does not apply to patients who are receiving corticosteroids as replacement therapy, e.g., for Addison's disease.

Individuals with blood dyscrasias, leukemia, lymphomas of any type, or other malignant neoplasms affecting the bone marrow or lymphatic systems.

Primary and acquired immunodeficiency states, including patients who are immunosuppressed in association with AIDS or other clinical manifestations of infection with human immunodeficiency viruses; cellular immune deficiencies; and hypogammaglobulinemic and dysgammaglobulinemic states.

Individuals with a family history of congenital or hereditary immunodeficiency, until the immune competence of the potential vaccine recipient is demonstrated.

HYPERSENSITIVITY TO EGGS

Live measles vaccine is produced in chick embryo cell culture. Persons with a history of anaphylactic, anaphylactoid, or other immediate reactions (e.g., hives, swelling of the mouth and throat, difficulty breathing, hypotension, or shock) subsequent to egg ingestion should not be vaccinated. Evidence indicates that persons are not at increased risk if they have egg allergies that are not anaphylactic or anaphylactoid in nature. Such persons may be vaccinated in the usual manner. There is no evidence to indicate that persons with allergies to chickens or feathers are at increased risk of reaction to the vaccine.

PRECAUTIONS

General

Adequate treatment provisions including epinephrine, should be available for immediate use should an anaphylactic or anaphylactoid reaction occur.

Due caution should be employed in administration of M-R-VAX II to persons with a history of cerebral injury, individual or family histories of convulsions, or any other condition in which stress due to fever should be avoided. The physician should be alert to the temperature elevation which may occur following vaccination. (See ADVERSE REACTIONS.)

Children and young adults who are known to be infected with human immunodeficiency viruses but without overt clinical manifestations of immunosuppression may be vaccinated; however, the vaccinees should be monitored closely for vaccine-preventable diseases because immunization may be less effective than for uninfected persons.

Vaccination should be deferred for at least 3 months following blood or plasma transfusions, or administration of human immune serum globulin.

Excretion of small amounts of the live attenuated rubella virus from the nose or throat has occurred in the majority of susceptible individuals 7–28 days after vaccination. There is no confirmed evidence to indicate that such virus is transmitted to susceptible persons who are in contact with the vaccinated individuals. Consequently, transmission through close personal contact, while accepted as a theoretical possibility, is not regarded as a significant risk. However, transmission of the rubella vaccine virus to infants via breast milk has been documented (see *Nursing Mothers*).

There are no reports of transmission of live attenuated measles virus from vaccinees to susceptible contacts.

It has been reported that live attenuated measles and rubella virus vaccines given individually may result in a temporary depression of tuberculin skin sensitivity. Therefore, if a tuberculin test is to be done, it should be administered either before or simultaneously with M-R-VAX II.

Children under treatment for tuberculosis have not experienced exacerbation of the disease when immunized with live measles virus vaccine; no studies have been reported to date of the effect of measles virus vaccines on untreated tuberculous children.

As for any vaccine, vaccination with M-R-VAX II may not result in seroconversion in 100% of susceptible persons given the vaccine.

Pregnancy

Pregnancy Category C

Animal reproduction studies have not been conducted with M-R-VAX II. It is also not known whether M-R-VAX II can cause fetal harm when administered to a pregnant woman or can affect reproduction capacity. Therefore, the vaccine should not be administered to pregnant females; futhermore, pregnancy should be avoided for three months following vaccination (see CONTRAINDICATIONS).

In counseling women who are inadvertently vaccinated when pregnant or who become pregnant within 3 months of vaccination, the physician should be aware of the following: (1) In a 10 year survey involving over 700 pregnant women who received rubella vaccine within 3 months before or after conception, (of whom 189 received the Wistar RA 27/3 strain), none of the newborns had abnormalities compatible with congenital rubella syndrome; (2) Reports have indicated that contracting of natural measles during pregnancy enhances fetal risk. Increased rates of spontaneous abortion, stillbirth, congenital defects and prematurity have been observed subsequent to natural measles during pregnancy. There are no adequate studies of the attenuated (vaccine) strain of measles virus in pregnancy. However, it would be prudent to assume that the vaccine strain of virus is also capable of inducing adverse fetal effects.

Nursing Mothers

It is not known whether measles vaccine virus is secreted in human milk. Recent studies have shown that lactating postpartum women immunized with live attenuated rubella vaccine may secrete the virus in breast milk and transmit it to breast-fed infants. In the infants with serological evidence of rubella infection, none exhibited severe disease; however, one exhibited mild clinical illness typical of acquired rubella. Caution should be exercised when M-R-VAX II is administered to a nursing woman.

ADVERSE REACTIONS

Burning and/or stinging of short duration at the injection site have been reported.

The adverse clinical reactions associated with the use of M-R-VAX II are those expected to follow administration of the monovalent vaccines given separately. These may include

Continued on next page

Information on the Merck & Co., Inc. products listed on these pages is the full prescribing information from product circulars in use September 30, 2000. For information, please call 1-800-NSC MERCK [1-800-672-6372].

M-R-Vax II—Cont.

malaise, sore throat, cough, rhinitis, headache, dizziness, fever, rash, nausea, vomiting or diarrhea; mild local reactions such as erythema, induration, tenderness and regional lymphadenopathy; thrombocytopenia and purpura; allergic reactions such as wheal and flare at the injection site or urticaria; polyneuritis, and arthralgia and/or arthritis (usually transient and rarely chronic).

Anaphylaxis and anaphylactoid reactions have been reported.

Vasculitis has been reported rarely.

Moderate fever [101–102.9°F (38.3–39.4°C)] occurs occasionally, and high fever [above 103°F (39.4°C)] occurs less commonly. On rare occasions, children developing fever may exhibit febrile convulsions. Afebrile convulsions or seizures have occurred rarely following vaccination with live attenuated measles vaccine. Syncope, particularly at the time of mass vaccination, has been reported. Rash occurs infrequently and is usually minimal, but rarely may be generalized. Erythema multiforme has also been reported rarely.

Forms of optic neuritis, including retrobulbar neuritis, papillitis, and retinitis may infrequently follow viral infections, and have been reported to occur 1 to 3 weeks following inoculation with some live virus vaccines.

Clinical experience with live attenuated measles and rubella virus vaccines given individually indicates that encephalitis and other nervous system reactions have occurred very rarely. These might occur also with M-R-VAX II. Experience from more than 80 million doses of all live measles vaccines given in the U.S. through 1975 indicates that significant central nervous system reactions such as encephalitis and encephalopathy, occurring within 30 days after vaccination, have been temporally associated with measles vaccine very rarely. In no case has it been shown that reactions were actually caused by vaccine. The Center for Disease Control has pointed out that "a certain number of cases of encephalitis may be expected to occur in a large childhood population in a defined period of time even when no vaccines are administered". However, the data suggest the possibility that some of these cases may have been caused by measles vaccines. The risk of such serious neurological disorders following live measles virus vaccine administration remains far less than that for encephalitis and encephalopathy with natural measles (one per two thousand reported cases).

There have been rare reports of ocular palsies, Guillain-Barré syndrome, or ataxia occurring after immunization with vaccines containing live attenuated measles virus. The ocular palsies have occurred approximately 3–24 days following vaccination. No definite causal relationship has been established between these events and vaccination. Isolated reports of polyneuropathy including Guillain-Barré syndrome have also been reported after immunization with rubella-containing vaccines.

There have been reports of subacute sclerosing panencephalitis (SSPE) in children who did not have a history of natural measles but did receive measles vaccine. Some of these cases may have resulted from unrecognized measles in the first year of life or possibly from the measles vaccination. Based on estimated nationwide measles vaccine distribution, the association of SSPE cases to measles vaccination is about one case per million vaccine doses distributed. This is far less than the association with natural measles, 6–22 cases of SSPE per million cases of measles. The results of a retrospective case-controlled study conducted by the Center for Disease Control suggest that the overall effect of measles vaccine has been to protect against SSPE by preventing measles with its inherent higher risk of SSPE.

Local reactions characterized by marked swelling, redness and vesiculation at the injection site of attenuated live measles virus vaccines, and systemic reactions including atypical measles, have occurred in persons who received killed measles vaccine previously. M-R-VAX II was not given under this condition in clinical trials. Rarely, more severe reactions that require hospitalization, including prolonged high fevers and extensive local reactions, have been reported. Panniculitis has been reported rarely following administration of measles vaccine.

Arthralgia and/or arthritis (usually transient and rarely chronic), and polyneuritis are features of natural rubella and vary in frequency and severity with age and sex, being greatest in adult females and least in prepubertal children. This type of involvement as well as myalgia and paresthesia have also been reported following administration of MERUVAX II (Rubella Virus Vaccine Live).

Chronic arthritis has been associated with natural rubella infection and has been related to persistent virus and/or viral antigen isolated from body tissues. Only rarely have vaccine recipients developed chronic joint symptoms.

Following vaccination in children, reactions in joints are uncommon and generally of brief duration. In women, incidence rates for arthritis and arthralgia are generally higher than those seen in children (children: 0–3%; women: 12–20%), and the reactions tend to be more marked and of longer duration. Symptoms may persist for a matter of months or on rare occasions for years. In adolescent girls, the reactions appear to be intermediate in incidence between those seen in children and in adult women. Even in older women (35–45 years), these reactions are generally well tolerated and rarely interfere with normal activities.

DOSAGE AND ADMINISTRATION

FOR SUBCUTANEOUS ADMINISTRATION
Do not inject intravenously

The dosage of vaccine is the same for all persons. Inject the total volume of the single dose vial (about 0.5 mL) or 0.5 mL of the multiple dose vial of reconstituted vaccine subcutaneously, preferably into the outer aspect of upper arm. *Do not give immune globulin (IG) concurrently with* M-R-VAX II.

During shipment, to insure that there is no loss of potency, the vaccine must be maintained at a temperature of 10°C (50°F) or less.

Before reconstitution, store M-R-VAX II at 2–8°C (36–46°F). *Protect from light.*

CAUTION: A sterile syringe free of preservatives, antiseptics, and detergents should be used for each injection and/or reconstitution of the vaccine because these substances may inactivate the live virus vaccine. A 25 gauge, 5/8" needle is recommended.

To reconstitute, use only the diluent supplied, since it is free of preservatives or other antiviral substances which might inactivate the vaccine.

Single Dose Vial —First withdraw the entire volume of diluent into the syringe to be used for reconstitution. Inject all the diluent in the syringe into the vial of lyophilized vaccine, and agitate to mix thoroughly. Withdraw the entire contents into a syringe and inject the total volume of restored vaccine subcutaneously.

It is important to use a separate sterile syringe and needle for each individual patient to prevent transmission of hepatitis B and other infectious agents from one person to another.

10 Dose Vial (available only to government agencies/institutions) —Withdraw the entire contents (7 mL) of the diluent vial into the sterile syringe to be used for reconstitution, and introduce into the 10 dose vial of lyophilized vaccine. Agitate to ensure thorough mixing. The outer labeling suggests "For Jet Injector or Syringe Use". Use with separate sterile syringes is permitted for containers of 10 doses or less. The vaccine and diluent do not contain preservatives; therefore, the user must recognize the potential contamination hazards and exercise special precautions to protect the sterility and potency of the product. The use of aseptic techniques and proper storage prior to and after restoration of the vaccine and subsequent withdrawal of the individual doses is essential. Use 0.5 mL of the reconstituted vaccine for subcutaneous injection.

It is important to use a separate sterile syringe and needle for each individual patient to prevent transmission of hepatitis B and other infectious agents from one person to another.

50 Dose Vial (available only to government agencies/institutions) —Withdraw the entire contents (30 mL) of diluent vial into the sterile syringe to be used for reconstitution and introduce into the 50 dose vial of lyophilized vaccine. Agitate to ensure thorough mixing. With full aseptic precautions, attach the vial to the sterilized multidose jet injector apparatus. Use 0.5 mL of the reconstituted vaccine for subcutaneous injection.

Each dose contains not less than the equivalent of 1,000 $TCID_{50}$ of the U.S. Reference Measles Virus and 1,000 $TCID_{50}$ of the U.S. Reference Rubella Virus.

Parenteral drug products should be inspected visually for particulate matter and discoloration prior to administration. M-R-VAX II, when reconstituted, is clear yellow.

HOW SUPPLIED

No. 4751—M-R-VAX II is supplied as a single-dose vial of lyophilized vaccine, **NDC** 0006-4751-00, and a vial of diluent.

No. 4677/4309—M-R-VAX II is supplied as follows: (1) a box of 10 single-dose vials of lyophilized vaccine (package A), **NDC** 0006-4677-00; and (2) a box of 10 vials of diluent (package B). To conserve refrigerator space, the diluent may be stored separately at room temperature (6505-01-098-8004, Ten Pack).

Available only to government agencies/institutions:

No. 4678—M-R-VAX II is supplied as one 10 dose vial of lyophilized vaccine, **NDC** 0006-4678-00, and one 7 mL vial of diluent.

No. 4679—M-R-VAX II is supplied as one 50 dose vial of lyophilized vaccine, **NDC** 0006-4679-00, and one 30 mL vial of diluent (6505-01-098-8005, 50 dose).

Storage

It is recommended that the vaccine be used as soon as possible after reconstitution. Protect vaccine from light at all times, since such exposure may inactivate the virus. Store reconstituted vaccine in the vaccine vial in a dark place at 2–8°C (36–46°F) and discard if not used within 8 hours.

A.H.F.S. Category: 80:12
7680217 Issued March 1995

MAXALT® ℞
(RIZATRIPTAN BENZOATE)
TABLETS
MAXALT-MLT™ ℞
(RIZATRIPTAN BENZOATE)
ORALLY DISINTEGRATING TABLETS

DESCRIPTION

MAXALT* contains rizatriptan benzoate, a selective 5-hydroxytryptamine$_{1B/1D}$ ($5\text{-}HT_{1B/1D}$) receptor agonist.

Rizatriptan benzoate is described chemically as: *N,N*-dimethyl-5-(1*H*-1,2,4-triazol-1-ylmethyl)-1*H*-indole-3-ethanamine monobenzoate and its structural formula is:

Its empirical formula is $C_{15}H_{19}N_5 \bullet C_7H_6O_2$, representing a molecular weight of the free base of 269.4. Rizatriptan benzoate is a white to off-white, crystalline solid that is soluble in water at about 42 mg per mL (expressed as free base) at 25°C.

MAXALT Tablets and MAXALT-MLT** Orally Disintegrating Tablets are available for oral administration in strengths of 5 and 10 mg (corresponding to 7.265 mg or 14.53 mg of the benzoate salt, respectively). Each compressed tablet contains the following inactive ingredients: lactose monohydrate, microcrystalline cellulose, pregelatinized starch, ferric oxide (red), and magnesium stearate.

Each lyophilized orally disintegrating tablet contains the following inactive ingredients: gelatin, mannitol, glycine, aspartame, and peppermint flavor.

* Registered trademark of MERCK & CO., Inc.
**Trademark of MERCK & CO., Inc.

CLINICAL PHARMACOLOGY

Mechanism of Action

Rizatriptan binds with high affinity to human cloned $5\text{-}HT_{1B}$ and $5\text{-}HT_{1D}$ receptors. Rizatriptan has weak affinity for other $5\text{-}HT_1$ receptor subtypes ($5\text{-}HT_{1A}$, $5\text{-}HT_{1E}$, $5\text{-}HT_{1F}$) and the $5\text{-}HT_7$ receptor, but has no significant activity at $5\text{-}HT_2$, $5\text{-}HT_3$, alpha- and beta-adrenergic, dopaminergic, histaminergic, muscarinic or benzodiazepine receptors.

Current theories on the etiology of migraine headache suggest that symptoms are due to local cranial vasodilatation and/or to the release of vasoactive and pro-inflammatory peptides from sensory nerve endings in an activated trigeminal system. The therapeutic activity of rizatriptan in migraine can most likely be attributed to agonist effects at $5\text{-}HT_{1B/1D}$ receptors on the extracerebral, intracranial blood vessels that become dilated during a migraine attack and on nerve terminals in the trigeminal system. Activation of these receptors results in cranial vessel constriction, inhibition of neuropeptide release and reduced transmission in trigeminal pain pathways.

Pharmacokinetics

Rizatriptan is completely absorbed following oral administration. The mean oral absolute bioavailability of the MAXALT Tablet is about 45%, and mean peak plasma concentrations (C_{max}) are reached in approximately 1–1.5 hours (T_{max}). The presence of a migraine headache did not appear to affect the absorption or pharmacokinetics of rizatriptan. Food has no significant effect on the bioavailability of rizatriptan but delays the time to reach peak concentration by an hour. In clinical trials, MAXALT was administered without regard to food. The plasma half-life of rizatriptan in males and females averages 2–3 hours.

The bioavailability and C_{max} of rizatriptan were similar following administration of MAXALT Tablets and MAXALT-MLT Orally Disintegrating Tablets, but the rate of absorption is somewhat slower with MAXALT-MLT, with T_{max} averaging 1.6–2.5 hours. AUC of rizatriptan is approximately 30% higher in females than in males. No accumulation occurred on multiple dosing.

The mean volume of distribution is approximately 140 liters in male subjects and 110 liters in female subjects. Rizatriptan is minimally bound (14%) to plasma proteins.

The primary route of rizatriptan metabolism is via oxidative deamination by monoamine oxidase-A (MAO-A) to the indole acetic acid metabolite, which is not active at the $5\text{-}HT_{1B/1D}$ receptor. N-monodesmethyl-rizatriptan, a metabolite with activity similar to that of parent compound at the $5\text{-}HT_{1B/1D}$ receptor, is formed to a minor degree. Plasma concentrations of N-monodesmethyl-rizatriptan are approximately 14% of those of parent compound, and it is eliminated at a similar rate. Other minor metabolites the N-oxide, the 6-hydroxy compound, and the sulfate conjugate of the 6-hydroxy metabolite are not active at the $5\text{-}HT_{1B/1D}$ receptor.

The total radioactivity of the administered dose recovered over 120 hours in urine and feces was 82% and 12%, respectively, following a single 10 mg oral administration of ^{14}C-rizatriptan. Following oral administration of ^{14}C-rizatriptan, rizatriptan accounted for about 17% of circulating plasma radioactivity. Approximately 14% of an oral dose is excreted in urine as unchanged rizatriptan while 51% is excreted as indole acetic acid metabolite, indicating substantial first pass metabolism.

Cytochrome P450 Isoforms: Rizatriptan is not an inhibitor of the activities of human liver cytochrome P450 isoforms 3A4/5, 1A2, 2C9, 2C19, or 2E1; rizatriptan is a competitive inhibitor (Ki=1400 nM) of cytochrome P450 2D6, but only at high, clinically irrelevant concentrations.

Special Populations

Age: Rizatriptan pharmacokinetics in healthy elderly non-migraineur volunteers (age 65–77 years) were similar to those in younger non-migraineur volunteers (age 18–45 years).

Gender: The mean $AUC_{0-\infty}$ and C_{max} of rizatriptan (10 mg orally) were about 30% and 11% higher in females as compared to males, respectively, while T_{max} occurred at approximately the same time.
Hepatic impairment: Following oral administration in patients with hepatic impairment caused by mild to moderate alcoholic cirrhosis of the liver, plasma concentrations of rizatriptan were similar in patients with mild hepatic insufficiency compared to a control group of healthy subjects; plasma concentrations of rizatriptan were approximately 30% greater in patients with moderate hepatic insufficiency. (See PRECAUTIONS.)
Renal impairment: In patients with renal impairment (creatinine clearance 10–60 mL/min/1.73 m^2), the $AUC_{0-\infty}$ of rizatriptan was not significantly different from that in healthy subjects. In hemodialysis patients, (creatinine clearance < 2 mL/min/1.73 m^2), however, the AUC for rizatriptan was approximately 44% greater than that in patients with normal renal function. (See PRECAUTIONS.)
Race: Pharmacokinetic data revealed no significant differences between African American and Caucasian subjects.
Drug Interactions (See also PRECAUTIONS, *Drug Interactions.*)
Monoamine oxidase inhibitors: Rizatriptan is principally metabolized via monoamine oxidase, 'A' subtype (MAO-A). Plasma concentrations of rizatriptan may be increased by drugs that are selective MAO-A inhibitors (e.g., moclobemide) or nonselective MAO inhibitors [type A and B] (e.g., isocarboxazid, phenelzine, tranylcypromine, and pargyline). In a drug interaction study, when MAXALT 10 mg was administered to subjects (n=12) receiving concomitant therapy with the selective, reversible MAO-A inhibitor, moclobemide 150 mg t.i.d., there were mean increases in rizatriptan AUC and C_{max} of 119% and 41% respectively; and the AUC of the active N-monodesmethyl metabolite of rizatriptan was increased more than 400%. The interaction would be expected to be greater with irreversible MAO inhibitors. No pharmacokinetic interaction is anticipated in patients receiving selective MAO-B inhibitors. (See CONTRAINDICATIONS; PRECAUTIONS, *Drug Interactions.*)
Propranolol: In a study of concurrent administration of propranolol 240 mg/day and a single dose of rizatriptan 10 mg in healthy subjects (n=11), mean plasma AUC for rizatriptan was increased by 70% during propranolol administration, and a fourfold increase was observed in one subject. The AUC of the active N-monodesmethyl metabolite of rizatriptan was not affected by propranolol. (See PRECAUTIONS; DOSAGE AND ADMINISTRATION.)
Nadolol/Metoprolol: In a drug interactions study, effects of multiple doses of nadolol 80 mg or metoprolol 100 mg every 12 hours on the pharmacokinetics of a single dose of 10 mg rizatriptan were evaluated in healthy subjects (n=12). No pharmacokinetic interactions were observed.
Paroxetine: In a study of the interaction between the selective serotonin reuptake inhibitor (SSRI) paroxetine 20 mg/day for two weeks and a single dose of MAXALT 10 mg in healthy subjects (n=12), neither the plasma concentrations of rizatriptan nor its safety profile were affected by paroxetine.
Oral contraceptives: In a study of concurrent administration of an oral contraceptive during 6 days of administration of MAXALT (10–30 mg/day) in healthy female volunteers (n=18), rizatriptan did not affect plasma concentrations of ethinyl estradiol or norethindrone.
Clinical Studies
The efficacy of MAXALT Tablets was established in four multicenter, randomized, placebo-controlled trials. Patients enrolled in these studies were primarily female (84%) and Caucasian (88%), with a mean age of 40 years (range of 18 to 71). Patients were instructed to treat a moderate to severe headache. Headache response, defined as a reduction of moderate or severe headache pain to no or mild headache pain, was assessed for up to 2 hours (Study 1) or up to 4 hours after dosing (Studies 2, 3 and 4). Associated symptoms of nausea, photophobia, and phonophobia and maintenance of response up to 24 hours postdose were evaluated. A second dose of MAXALT Tablets was allowed 2 to 24 hours after dosing for treatment of recurrent headache in Studies 1 and 2. Additional analgesics and/or antiemetics were allowed 2 hours after initial treatment for rescue in all four studies.
In all studies, the percentage of patients achieving headache response 2 hours after treatment was significantly greater in patients who received either MAXALT 5 or 10 mg compared to those who received placebo. In a separate study, doses of 2.5 mg were not different from placebo. Doses greater than 10 mg were associated with an increased incidence of adverse effects. The results from the 4 controlled studies using the marketed formulation are summarized in Table 1.

Table 1
Response Rates 2 Hours Following Treatment of Initial Headache

Study	Placebo	MAXALT Tablets 5 mg	MAXALT Tablets 10 mg
1	35% (n=304)	62%* (n=458)	71%*,** (n=456)
2†	37% (n=82)	—	77%* (n=320)
3	23% (n=80)	63%* (n=352)	—
4	40% (n=159)	60%* (n=164)	67%* (n=385)

*p value <0.05 in comparison with placebo
**p value <0.05 in comparison with 5 mg
†Results for initial headache only.

Comparisons of drug performance based upon results obtained in different clinical trials are never reliable. Because studies are conducted at different times, with different samples of patients, by different investigators, employing different criteria and/or different interpretations of the same criteria, under different conditions (dose, dosing regimen, etc.), quantitative estimates of treatment response and the timing of response may be expected to vary considerably from study to study.
The estimated probability of achieving an initial headache response within 2 hours following treatment is depicted in Figure 1.

Figure 1: Estimated Probability of Achieving an Initial Headache Response by 2 Hours††

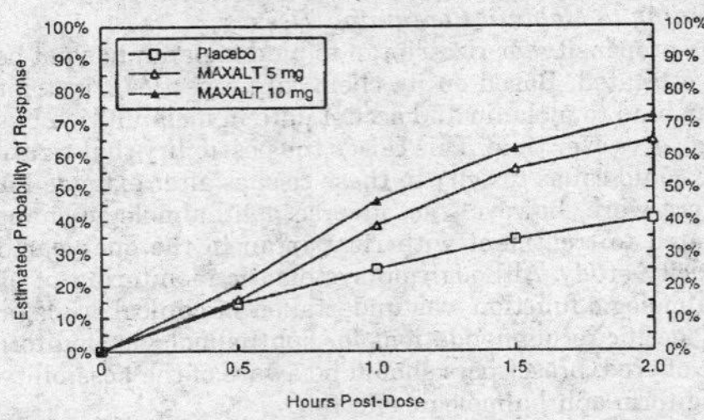

†† Figure 1 shows the Kaplan-Meier plot of the probability over time of obtaining headache response (no or mild pain) following treatment with rizatriptan or placebo. The averages displayed are based on pooled data from 4 placebo-controlled, outpatient trials providing evidence of efficacy (Studies 1, 2, 3, and 4). Patients taking additional treatment or not achieving headache response prior to 2 hours were censored at 2 hours.

For patients with migraine-associated photophobia, phonophobia, and nausea at baseline, there was a decreased incidence of these symptoms following administration of MAXALT compared to placebo.
Two to 24 hours following the initial dose of study treatment, patients were allowed to use additional treatment for pain response in the form of a second dose of study treatment or other medication. The estimated probability of patients taking a second dose or other medication for migraine over the 24 hours following the initial dose of study treatment is summarized in Figure 2.

Figure 2: Estimated Probability of Patients Taking a Second Dose of MAXALT Tablets or Other Medication for Migraines Over the 24 Hours Following the Initial Dose of Study Treatment†††

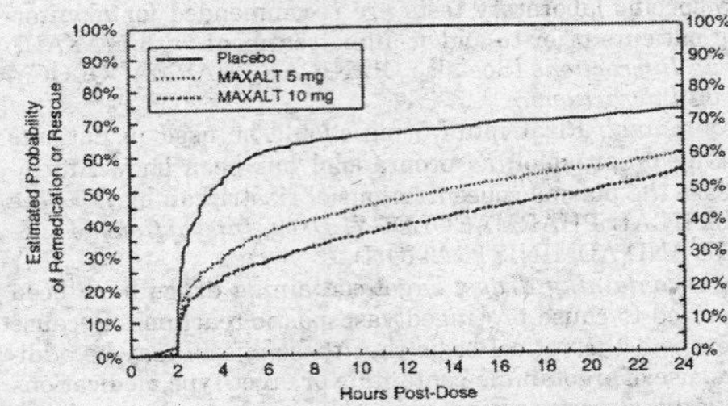

††† This Kaplan-Meier plot is based on data obtained in 4 placebo-controlled outpatient clinical trials (Studies 1, 2, 3, and 4). Patients not using additional treatments were censored at 24 hours. The plot includes both patients who had headache response at 2 hours and those who had no response to the initial dose. Remedication was not allowed within 2 hours post-dose.

Efficacy was unaffected by the presence of aura; by the gender, or age of the patient; or by concomitant use of common migraine prophylactic drugs (e.g., beta-blockers, calcium channel blockers, tricyclic antidepressants) or oral contraceptives. There were insufficient data to assess the impact of race on efficacy.
MAXALT-MLT Orally Disintegrating Tablets
The efficacy of MAXALT-MLT was established in two multicenter, randomized, placebo-controlled trials that were similar in design to the trials of MAXALT Tablets. Patients were instructed to treat a moderate to severe headache. Patients treated in these studies were primarily female (88%) and Caucasian (95%), with a mean age of 42 years (range 18–72).
In both studies, the percentage of patients achieving headache response 2 hours after treatment was significantly greater in patients who received either MAXALT-MLT 5 or 10 mg compared to those who received placebo. The results from the 2 controlled studies using the marketed formulation are summarized in Table 2.

Table 2
Response Rates 2 Hours Following Treatment of Initial Headache

Study	Placebo	MAXALT-MLT 5 mg	MAXALT-MLT 10 mg
1	47% (n=98)	66%* (n=100)	66%* (n=113)
2	28% (n=180)	59%* (n=181)	74%*,** (n=186)

*p value <0.01 in comparison with placebo
**p value <0.01 in comparison with 5 mg

The estimated probability of achieving an initial headache response by 2 hours following treatment with MAXALT-MLT is depicted in Figure 3.

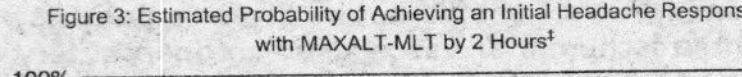
Figure 3: Estimated Probability of Achieving an Initial Headache Response with MAXALT-MLT by 2 Hours‡

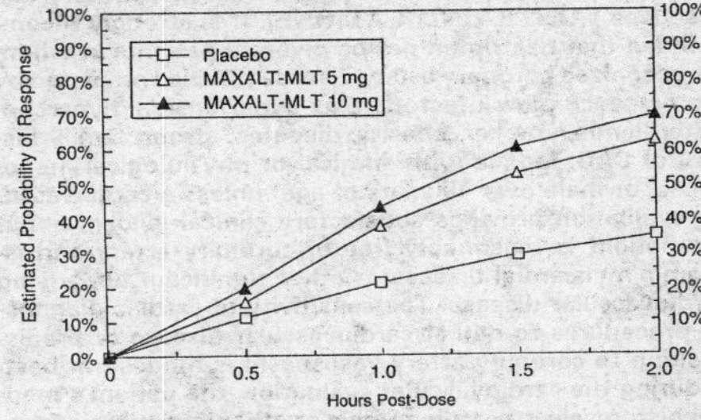

‡Figure 3 shows the Kaplan-Meier plot of the probability over time of obtaining headache response (no or mild pain) following treatment with MAXALT-MLT or placebo. The averages displayed are based on pooled data from 2 placebo-controlled, outpatient trials providing evidence of efficacy (Studies 1 and 2). Patients taking additional treatment or not achieving headache response prior to 2 hours were censored at 2 hours.

For patients with migraine-associated photophobia and phonophobia at baseline, there was a decreased incidence of these symptoms following administration of MAXALT-MLT as compared to placebo.
Two to 24 hours following the initial dose of study treatment, patients were allowed to use additional treatment for pain response in the form of a second dose of study treatment or other medication. The estimated probability of patients taking a second dose or other medication for migraine over the 24 hours following the initial dose of study treatment is summarized in Figure 4.

Figure 4: Estimated Probability of Patients Taking a Second Dose of MAXALT-MLT or Other Medication for Migraines Over the 24 Hours Following the Initial Dose of Study Treatment‡‡

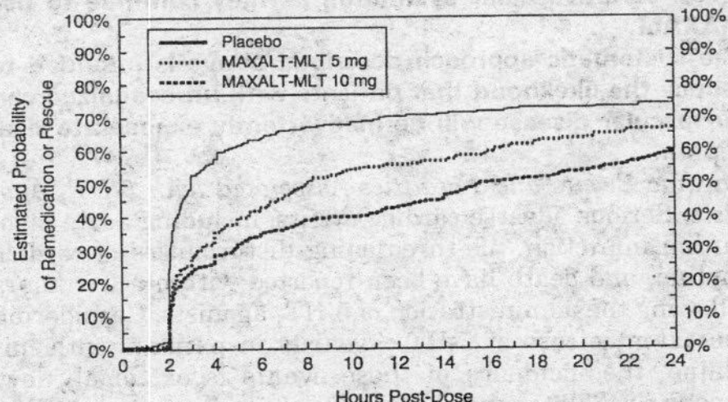

‡‡ This Kaplan-Meier plot is based on data obtained in 2 placebo-controlled outpatient clinical trials (Studies 1 and 2). Patients not using additional treatments were censored at 24 hours. The plot includes both patients who had headache response at 2 hours and those who had no response to the initial dose. Remedication was not allowed within 2 hours post-dose.

INDICATIONS AND USAGE

MAXALT is indicated for the acute treatment of migraine attacks with or without aura in adults.
MAXALT is not intended for the prophylactic therapy of migraine or for use in the management of hemiplegic or basilar migraine (see CONTRAINDICATIONS). Safety and effectiveness of MAXALT has not been established for cluster headache, which is present in an older, predominantly male population.

CONTRAINDICATIONS

MAXALT should not be given to patients with ischemic heart disease (e.g., angina pectoris, history of myocardial infarction, or documented silent ischemia) or to patients who have symptoms or findings consistent with ischemic heart disease, coronary artery vasospasm, including Prinzmetal's variant angina, or other significant underlying cardiovascular disease (see WARNINGS).
Because MAXALT may increase blood pressure, it should not be given to patients with uncontrolled hypertension (see WARNINGS).
MAXALT should not be used within 24 hours of treatment with another 5-HT_1 agonist, or an ergotamine-containing or ergot-type medication like dihydroergotamine or methysergide.
MAXALT should not be administered to patients with hemiplegic or basilar migraine.
Concurrent administration of MAO inhibitors or use of rizatriptan within 2 weeks of discontinuation of MAO inhibitor therapy is contraindicated (see CLINICAL PHARMACOLOGY, *Drug Interactions* and PRECAUTIONS, *Drug Interactions*).
MAXALT is contraindicated in patients who are hypersensitive to rizatriptan or any of its inactive ingredients.

WARNINGS

MAXALT should only be used where a clear diagnosis of migraine has been established.
***Risk of Myocardial Ischemia and/or Infarction and Other Adverse Cardiac Events:* Because of the potential of this**

Continued on next page

Information on the Merck & Co., Inc. products listed on these pages is the full prescribing information from product circulars in use September 30, 2000. For information, please call 1-800-NSC MERCK [1-800-672-6372].

Maxalt—Cont.

class of compounds (5-$HT_{1B/1D}$ agonists) to cause coronary vasospasm, MAXALT should not be given to patients with documented ischemic or vasospastic coronary artery disease (see CONTRAINDICATIONS). It is strongly recommended that rizatriptan not be given to patients in whom unrecognized coronary artery disease (CAD) is predicted by the presence of risk factors (e.g., hypertension, hypercholesterolemia, smoker, obesity, diabetes, strong family history of CAD, female with surgical or physiological menopause, or male over 40 years of age) unless a cardiovascular evaluation provides satisfactory clinical evidence that the patient is reasonably free of coronary artery and ischemic myocardial disease or other significant underlying cardiovascular disease. The sensitivity of cardiac diagnostic procedures to detect cardiovascular disease or predisposition to coronary artery vasospasm is modest, at best. If, during the cardiovascular evaluation, the patient's medical history, electrocardiographic or other investigations reveal findings indicative of, or consistent with, coronary artery vasospasm or myocardial ischemia, rizatriptan should not be administered (see CONTRAINDICATIONS).

For patients with risk factors predictive of CAD, who are determined to have a satisfactory cardiovascular evaluation, it is strongly recommended that administration of the first dose of rizatriptan take place in the setting of a physician's office or similar medically staffed and equipped facility unless the patient has previously received rizatriptan. Because cardiac ischemia can occur in the absence of clinical symptoms, consideration should be given to obtaining on the first occasion of use an electrocardiogram (ECG) during the interval immediately following MAXALT, in these patients with risk factors.

It is recommended that patients who are intermittent long-term users of MAXALT and who have or acquire risk factors predictive of CAD, as described above, undergo periodic interval cardiovascular evaluation as they continue to use MAXALT.

The systematic approach described above is intended to reduce the likelihood that patients with unrecognized cardiovascular disease will be inadvertently exposed to rizatriptan.

Cardiac Events and Fatalities Associated with 5-HT_1 Agonists: Serious adverse cardiac events, including acute myocardial infarction, life-threatening disturbances of cardiac rhythm, and death have been reported within a few hours following the administration of 5-HT_1 agonists. Considering the extent of use of 5-HT_1 agonists in patients with migraine, the incidence of these events is extremely low. Among the 3700 patients with migraine who participated in premarketing clinical trials of MAXALT, one patient was reported to have chest pain with possible ischemic ECG changes following a single dose of 10 mg.

Cerebrovascular Events and Fatalities Associated with 5-HT_1 Agonists: Cerebral hemorrhage, subarachnoid hemorrhage, stroke, and other cerebrovascular events have been reported in patients treated with 5-HT_1 agonists; and some have resulted in fatalities. In a number of cases, it appears possible that the cerebrovascular events were primary, the agonist having been administered in the incorrect belief that the symptoms experienced were a consequence of migraine, when they were not. It should be noted that patients with migraine may be at increased risk of certain cerebrovascular events (e.g., stroke, hemorrhage, transient ischemic attack).

Other Vasospasm-Related Events: 5-HT_1 agonists may cause vasospastic reactions other than coronary artery vasospasm. Both peripheral vascular ischemia and colonic ischemia with abdominal pain and bloody diarrhea have been reported with 5-HT_1 agonists.

Increase in Blood Pressure: Significant elevation in blood pressure, including hypertensive crisis, has been reported on rare occasions in patients receiving 5-HT_1 agonists with and without a history of hypertension. In healthy young male and female subjects who received maximal doses of MAXALT (10 mg every 2 hours for 3 doses), slight increases in blood pressure (approximately 2–3 mmHg) were observed. Rizatriptan is contraindicated in patients with uncontrolled hypertension (see CONTRAINDICATIONS).

An 18% increase in mean pulmonary artery pressure was seen following dosing with another 5-HT_1 agonist in a study evaluating subjects undergoing cardiac catheterization.

PRECAUTIONS

General

As with other 5-$HT_{1B/1D}$ agonists, sensations of tightness, pain, pressure, and heaviness have been reported after treatment with MAXALT in the precordium, throat, neck and jaw. These events have not been associated with arrhythmias or definite ischemic ECG changes in clinical trials (one patient experienced chest pain with possible ischemic ECG changes). Because drugs in this class may cause coronary artery vasospasm, patients who experience signs or symptoms suggestive of angina following dosing should be evaluated for the presence of CAD or a predisposition to Prinzmetal's variant angina before receiving additional doses of medication, and should be monitored electrocardiographically if dosing is resumed and similar symptoms recur. Similarly, patients who experience other symptoms or signs suggestive of decreased arterial flow, such as ischemic bowel syndrome or Raynaud's syndrome following the use of any 5-HT_1 agonist are candidates for further evaluation (see WARNINGS).

Rizatriptan should also be administered with caution to patients with diseases that may alter the absorption, metabolism, or excretion of drugs (see CLINICAL PHARMACOLOGY, *Special Populations*).

Renally Impaired Patients: Rizatriptan should be used with caution in dialysis patients due to a decrease in the clearance of rizatriptan (see CLINICAL PHARMACOLOGY, *Special Populations*).

Hepatically Impaired Patients: Rizatriptan should be used with caution in patients with moderate hepatic insufficiency due to an increase in plasma concentrations of approximately 30% (see CLINICAL PHARMACOLOGY, *Special Populations*).

For a given attack, if a patient has no response to the first dose of rizatriptan, the diagnosis of migraine should be reconsidered before administration of a second dose.

Binding to Melanin-Containing Tissues

The propensity for rizatriptan to bind melanin has not been investigated. Based on its chemical properties, rizatriptan may bind to melanin and accumulate in melanin rich tissue (e.g., eye) over time. This raises the possibility that rizatriptan could cause toxicity in these tissues after extended use. There were, however, no adverse ophthalmologic changes related to treatment with rizatriptan in the one year dog toxicity study. Although no systematic monitoring of ophthalmologic function was undertaken in clinical trials, and no specific recommendations for ophthalmologic monitoring are offered, prescribers should be aware of the possibility of long-term ophthalmologic effects.

Phenylketonurics

Phenylketonuric patients should be informed that MAXALT-MLT Orally Disintegrating Tablets contain phenylalanine (a component of aspartame). Each 5-mg orally disintegrating tablet contains 1.05 mg phenylalanine, and each 10-mg orally disintegrating tablet contains 2.10 mg phenylalanine.

Information for Patients

Migraine or treatment with MAXALT may cause somnolence in some patients. Dizziness has also been reported in some patients receiving MAXALT. Patients should, therefore, evaluate their ability to perform complex tasks during migraine attacks and after administration of MAXALT.

Physicians should instruct their patients to read the patient package insert before taking MAXALT. See the accompanying PATIENT INFORMATION leaflet.

MAXALT-MLT Orally Disintegrating Tablets

Patients should be instructed not to remove the blister from the outer pouch until just prior to dosing. The blister pack should then be peeled open with dry hands and the orally disintegrating tablet placed on the tongue, where it will dissolve and be swallowed with the saliva.

Laboratory Tests

No specific laboratory tests are recommended for monitoring patients prior to and/or after treatment with MAXALT.

Drug Interactions (See also CLINICAL PHARMACOLOGY, *Drug Interactions*.)

Propranolol: Rizatriptan 5 mg should be used in patients taking propranolol, as propranolol has been shown to increase the plasma concentrations of rizatriptan by 70% (see CLINICAL PHARMACOLOGY, *Drug Interactions*; DOSAGE AND ADMINISTRATION).

Ergot-containing drugs: Ergot-containing drugs have been reported to cause prolonged vasospastic reactions. Because there is a theoretical basis that these effects may be additive, use of ergotamine-containing or ergot-type medications (like dihydroergotamine or methysergide) and rizatriptan within 24 hours is contraindicated (see CONTRAINDICATIONS).

Other 5-HT_1 agonists: The administration of rizatriptan with other 5-HT_1 agonists has not been evaluated in migraine patients. Because their vasospastic effects may be additive, coadministration of rizatriptan and other 5-HT_1 agonists within 24 hours of each other is not recommended (see CONTRAINDICATIONS).

Selective serotonin reuptake inhibitors (SSRIs): SSRIs (e.g., fluoxetine, fluvoxamine, paroxetine, sertraline) have been reported, rarely, to cause weakness, hyperreflexia, and incoordination when coadministered with 5-HT_1 agonists. If concomitant treatment with rizatriptan and an SSRI is clinically warranted, appropriate observation of the patient is advised. No clinical or pharmacokinetic interactions were observed when MAXALT 10 mg was administered with paroxetine.

Monoamine oxidase inhibitors: Rizatriptan should not be administered to patients taking MAO-A inhibitors and non-selective MAO inhibitors; it has been shown that moclobemide (a specific MAO-A inhibitor) increased the systemic exposure of rizatriptan and its metabolite (see CLINICAL PHARMACOLOGY, *Drug Interactions*; CONTRAINDICATIONS).

Drug/Laboratory Test Interactions

MAXALT is not known to interfere with commonly employed clinical laboratory tests.

Carcinogenesis, Mutagenesis, Impairment of Fertility

Carcinogenesis: The lifetime carcinogenic potential of rizatriptan was evaluated in a 100-week study in mice and a 106-week study in rats at oral gavage doses of up to 125 mg/kg/day. Exposure data were not obtained in those studies, but plasma AUC's of parent drug measured in other studies after 5 and 21 weeks of oral dosing in mice and rats, respectively, indicate that the exposures to parent drug at the highest dose level in the carcinogenicity studies would have been approximately 150 times (mice) and 240 times (rats) average AUC's measured in humans after three 10 mg doses, the maximum recommended total daily dose. There was no evidence of an increase in tumor incidence related to rizatriptan in either species.

Mutagenesis: Rizatriptan, with and without metabolic activation, was neither mutagenic, nor clastogenic in a battery of *in vitro* and *in vivo* genetic toxicity studies, including: the microbial mutagenesis (Ames) assay, the *in vitro* mammalian cell mutagenesis assay in V-79 Chinese hamster lung cells, the *in vitro* alkaline elution assay in rat hepatocytes, the *in vitro* chromosomal aberration assay in Chinese hamster ovary cells and the *in vivo* chromosomal aberration assay in mouse bone marrow.

Impairment of Fertility: In a fertility study in rats, altered estrus cyclicity and delays in time to mating were observed in females treated orally with 100 mg/kg/day rizatriptan. Plasma drug exposure (AUC) at this dose was approximately 225 times the exposure in humans receiving the maximum recommended daily dose (MRDD) of 30 mg. The no-effect dose was 10 mg/kg/day (approximately 15 times the human exposure at the MRDD). There were no other fertility-related effects in the female rats. There was no impairment of fertility or reproductive performance in male rats treated with up to 250 mg/kg/day (approximately 550 times the human exposure at the MRDD).

Pregnancy: Pregnancy Category C

In a reproduction study in rats, birth weights and pre- and post-weaning weight gain were reduced in the offspring of females treated prior to and during mating and throughout gestation and lactation with doses of 10 and 100 mg/kg/day. Maternal plasma drug exposures (AUC) at these doses were approximately 15 and 225 times, respectively, the exposure in humans receiving the maximum recommended daily dose (MRDD) of 30 mg. The effects on offspring growth occurred in the absence of any apparent maternal toxicity in this study. The developmental no-effect dose was 2 mg/kg/day (maternal exposure approximately 1.5 times human exposure at the MRDD). The full spectrum of developmental toxicity is not known because adequately high doses, i.e., those producing some maternal toxicity, were not evaluated in the reproduction study. When higher, maternally toxic doses (250 mg/kg/day or greater) were evaluated over the same period of development in a rat dose range-finding study, pup mortality was increased.

In embryofetal development studies, no teratogenic effects were observed when pregnant rats and rabbits were administered doses of 100 and 50 mg/kg/day, respectively, during organogenesis. Fetal weights were decreased in conjunction with decreased maternal weight gain at the highest doses (maternal exposures approximately 225 and 115 times the human exposure at the MRDD in rats and rabbits, respectively). The developmental no-effect dose in these studies was 10 mg/kg/day in both rats and rabbits (maternal exposures approximately 15 times human exposure at the MRDD). Toxicokinetic studies demonstrated placental transfer of drug in both species.

There are no adequate and well-controlled studies in pregnant women; therefore, rizatriptan should be used during pregnancy only if the potential benefit justifies the potential risk to the fetus.

Merck & Co., Inc. maintains a registry to monitor the pregnancy outcomes of women exposed to MAXALT while pregnant. Healthcare providers are encouraged to report any prenatal exposure to MAXALT by calling the Pregnancy Registry at (800) 986-8999.

Nursing Mothers

It is not known whether this drug is excreted in human milk. Because many drugs are excreted in human milk, caution should be exercised when MAXALT is administered to women who are breast-feeding. Rizatriptan is extensively excreted in rat milk, at a level of 5-fold or greater than maternal plasma levels.

Pediatric Use

Safety and effectiveness of rizatriptan in pediatric patients have not been established; therefore, MAXALT is not recommended for use in patients under 18 years of age.

Geriatric Use

The pharmacokinetics of rizatriptan were similar in elderly (aged ≥ 65 years) and in younger adults. Because migraine occurs infrequently in the elderly, clinical experience with MAXALT is limited in such patients. In clinical trials, there were no apparent differences in efficacy or in overall adverse experience rates between patients under 65 years of age and those 65 and above (n=17).

ADVERSE REACTIONS

Serious cardiac events, including some that have been fatal, have occurred following use of 5-HT_1 agonists. These events are extremely rare and most have been reported in patients with risk factors predictive of CAD. Events reported have included coronary artery vasospasm, transient myocardial ischemia, myocardial infarction, ventricular tachycardia, and ventricular fibrillation (see CONTRAINDICATIONS, WARNINGS, and PRECAUTIONS).

Incidence in Controlled Clinical Trials: Adverse experiences to rizatriptan were assessed in controlled clinical trials that included over 3700 patients who received single or multiple doses of MAXALT Tablets. The most common adverse events during treatment with MAXALT were asthenia/fatigue, somnolence, pain/pressure sensation and dizziness. These events appeared to be dose related. In long term extension studies where patients were allowed to treat multiple attacks for up to 1 year, 4% (59 out of 1525 patients) withdrew because of adverse experiences.

Table 2 lists the adverse events regardless of drug relationship (incidence ≥2% and greater than placebo) after a single dose of MAXALT. The events cited reflect experience gained under closely monitored conditions of clinical trials in a highly selected patient population. In actual clinical practice or in other clinical trials, these frequency estimates may not apply, as the conditions of use, reporting behavior, and the kinds of patients treated may differ.

Table 2
Incidence (≥ 2% and Greater than Placebo) of Adverse Experiences After a Single Dose of MAXALT Tablets or Placebo

	% of Patients		
Adverse Experiences	MAXALT 5 mg (N=977)	MAXALT 10 mg (N=1167)	Placebo (N=627)
Atypical Sensations	4	5	4
Paresthesia	3	4	<2
Pain and other Pressure Sensations	6	9	3
Chest Pain: tightness/pressure and/or heaviness	<2	3	1
Neck/throat/jaw: pain/tightness/pressure	<2	2	1
Regional Pain: tightness/pressure/ heaviness	<1	2	0
Pain, location unspecified	3	3	<2
Digestive	9	13	8
Dry Mouth	3	3	1
Nausea	4	6	4
Neurological	14	20	11
Dizziness	4	9	5
Headache	<2	2	<1
Somnolence	4	8	4
Other			
Asthenia/fatigue	4	7	2

MAXALT was generally well-tolerated. Adverse experiences were typically mild in intensity and were transient. The frequencies of adverse experiences in clinical trials did not increase when up to three doses were taken within 24 hours. Adverse event frequencies were also unchanged by concomitant use of drugs commonly taken for migraine prophylaxis (including propranolol), oral contraceptives, or analgesics. The incidences of adverse experiences were not affected by age or gender. There were insufficient data to assess the impact of race on the incidence of adverse events.

Other Events Observed in Association with the Administration of MAXALT: In the section that follows, the frequencies of less commonly reported adverse clinical events are presented. Because the reports include events observed in open studies, the role of MAXALT in their causation cannot be reliably determined. Furthermore, variability associated with adverse event reporting, the terminology used to describe adverse events, etc., limit the value of the quantitative frequency estimates provided. Event frequencies are calculated as the number of patients who used MAXALT (N=3716) and reported an event divided by the total number of patients exposed to MAXALT. All reported events are included, except those already listed in the previous table, those too general to be informative, and those not reasonably associated with the use of the drug. Events are further classified within body system categories and enumerated in order of decreasing frequency using the following definitions: frequent adverse events are those defined as those occurring in at least (>)1/100 patients; infrequent adverse experiences are those occurring in 1/100 to 1/1000 patients; and rare adverse experiences are those occurring in fewer than 1/1000 patients.

General: Infrequent were chills, heat sensitivity, facial edema, hangover effect, and abdominal distention. Rare were fever, orthostatic effects, syncope and edema/swelling.

Atypical Sensations: Frequent were warm/cold sensations.

Cardiovascular: Frequent was palpitation. Infrequent were tachycardia, cold extremities, hypertension, arrhythmia, and bradycardia. Rare was angina pectoris.

Digestive: Frequent were diarrhea and vomiting. Infrequent were dyspepsia, thirst, acid regurgitation, dysphagia, constipation, flatulence, and tongue edema. Rare were anorexia, appetite increase, gastritis, paralysis (tongue), and eructation.

Metabolic: Infrequent was dehydration.

Musculoskeletal: Infrequent were muscle weakness, stiffness, myalgia, muscle cramp, musculoskeletal pain, arthralgia, and muscle spasm.

Neurological/Psychiatric: Frequent were hypesthesia, mental acuity decreased, euphoria and tremor. Infrequent were nervousness, vertigo, insomnia, anxiety, depression, disorientation, ataxia, dysarthria, confusion, dream abnormality, gait abnormality, irritability, memory impairment, agitation and hyperesthesia. Rare were: dysesthesia, depersonalization, akinesia/bradykinesia, apprehension, hyperkinesia, hypersomnia, and hyporeflexia.

Respiratory: Frequent was dyspnea. Infrequent were pharyngitis, irritation (nasal), congestion (nasal), dry throat, upper respiratory infection, yawning, respiratory congestion (nasal), dry nose, epistaxis, and sinus disorder. Rare were cough, hiccups, hoarseness, rhinorrhea, sneezing, tachypnea, and pharyngeal edema.

Special Senses: Infrequent were blurred vision, tinnitus, dry eyes, burning eye, eye pain, eye irritation, ear pain, and tearing. Rare were hyperacusis, smell perversion, photophobia, photopsia, itching eye, and eye swelling.

Skin and Skin Appendage: Frequent was flushing. Infrequent were sweating, pruritus, rash, and urticaria. Rare were erythema, acne, and photosensitivity.

Urogenital system: Frequent was hot flashes. Infrequent were urinary frequency, polyuria, and menstruation disorder. Rare was dysuria.

The adverse experience profile seen with MAXALT-MLT Orally Disintegrating Tablets was similar to that seen with MAXALT Tablets.

Post-Marketing Experience

The following additional adverse reactions have been reported very rarely and most have been reported in patients with risk factors predictive of CAD: myocardial ischemia or infarction, cerebrovascular accident.

The following adverse reaction has also been reported:

Special Senses: Dysgeusia.

DRUG ABUSE AND DEPENDENCE

Although the abuse potential of MAXALT has not been specifically assessed, no abuse of, tolerance to, withdrawal from, or drug-seeking behavior was observed in patients who received MAXALT in clinical trials or their extensions. The 5-$HT_{1B/1D}$ agonists, as a class, have not been associated with drug abuse.

OVERDOSAGE

No overdoses of MAXALT were reported during clinical trials.

Rizatriptan 40 mg (administered as either a single dose or as two doses with a 2-hour interdose interval) was generally well tolerated in over 300 patients; dizziness and somnolence were the most common drug-related adverse effects.

In a clinical pharmacology study in which 12 subjects received rizatriptan, at total cumulative doses of 80 mg (given within four hours), two subjects experienced syncope and/or bradycardia. One subject, a female aged 29 years, developed vomiting, bradycardia, and dizziness beginning three hours after receiving a total of 80 mg rizatriptan (administered over two hours); a third degree AV block, responsive to atropine, was observed an hour after the onset of the other symptoms. The second subject, a 25 year old male, experienced transient dizziness, syncope, incontinence, and a 5-second systolic pause (on ECG monitor) immediately after a painful venipuncture. The venipuncture occurred two hours after the subject had received a total of 80 mg rizatriptan (administered over four hours).

In addition, based on the pharmacology of rizatriptan, hypertension or other more serious cardiovascular symptoms could occur after overdosage. Gastrointestinal decontamination, (i.e., gastric lavage followed by activated charcoal) should be considered in patients suspected of an overdose with MAXALT. Clinical and electrocardiographic monitoring should be continued for at least 12 hours, even if clinical symptoms are not observed.

The effects of hemo- or peritoneal dialysis on serum concentrations of rizatriptan are unknown.

DOSAGE AND ADMINISTRATION

In controlled clinical trials, single doses of 5 and 10 mg of MAXALT Tablets or MAXALT-MLT were effective for the acute treatment of migraines in adults. There is evidence that the 10-mg dose may provide a greater effect than the 5-mg dose (see *Clinical Studies*). Individuals may vary in response to doses of MAXALT Tablets. The choice of dose should therefore be made on an individual basis, weighing the possible benefit of the 10-mg dose with the potential risk for increased adverse events.

Redosing: Doses should be separated by at least 2 hours; no more than 30 mg should be taken in any 24-hour period.

The safety of treating, on average, more than four headaches in a 30-day period has not been established.

Patients receiving propranolol: In patients receiving propranolol, the 5-mg dose of MAXALT should be used, up to a maximum of 3 doses in any 24-hour period. (See CLINICAL PHARMACOLOGY, *Drug Interactions.*)

For MAXALT-MLT Orally Disintegrating Tablets, administration with liquid is not necessary. The orally disintegrating tablet is packaged in a blister within an outer aluminum pouch. Patients should be instructed not to remove the blister from the outer pouch until just prior to dosing. The blister pack should then be peeled open with dry hands and the orally disintegrating tablet placed on the tongue, where it will dissolve and be swallowed with the saliva.

HOW SUPPLIED

No. 3732—MAXALT Tablets, 5 mg, are pale pink, capsule-shaped, compressed tablets coded MRK on one side and 266 on the other. They are supplied as follows:

NDC 0006-0266-06, unit of use carrying case of 6 tablets.

Shown in Product Identification Guide, page 324

No. 3733—MAXALT Tablets, 10 mg, are pale pink, capsule-shaped, compressed tablets coded MAXALT on one side and MRK 267 on the other. They are supplied as follows:

NDC 0006-0267-06, unit of use carrying case of 6 tablets.

Shown in Product Identification Guide, page 324

No. 3800—MAXALT-MLT Orally Disintegrating Tablets, 5 mg, are white to off-white, round lyophilized orally disintegrating tablets debossed with a modified triangle on one side, and measuring 10.0–11.5 mm (side-to-side) with a peppermint flavor. Each orally disintegrating tablet is individually packaged in a blister inside an aluminum pouch (sachet). They are supplied as follows:

NDC 0006-3800-06, 2 × unit of use carrying case of 3 orally disintegrating tablets (6 tablets total).

Shown in Product Identification Guide, page 324

No. 3801—MAXALT-MLT Orally Disintegrating Tablets, 10 mg, are white to off-white, round lyophilized orally disintegrating tablets debossed with a modified square on one side, and measuring 12.0–13.8 mm (side-to-side) with a peppermint flavor. Each orally disintegrating tablet is individually packaged in a blister inside an aluminum pouch (sachet). They are supplied as follows:

NDC 0006-3801-06, 2 × unit of use carrying case of 3 orally disintegrating tablets (6 tablets total).

Shown in Product Identification Guide, page 324

Storage

Store MAXALT Tablets at room temperature, 15–30°C (59–86°F). Dispense in a tight container, if product is subdivided.

Store MAXALT-MLT Orally Disintegrating Tablets at room temperature, 15–30°C (59–86°F). The patient should be instructed not to remove the blister from the outer aluminum pouch until the patient is ready to consume the orally disintegrating tablet inside.

MAXALT Tablets are manufactured for:
MERCK & CO., INC., West Point, PA 19486, USA
By:
MSD, Ltd. Cramlington
Northumberland, NE23 9JU, UK
MAXALT-MLT Orally Disintegrating Tablets are manufactured for:
MERCK & CO., INC., West Point, PA 19486, USA
By:
Scherer DDS, Ltd.
Swindon, Wiltshire, SN5 8RU, UK

9122105 Issued November 1999

Patient Information about
MAXALT® (max-awlt) and MAXALT-MLT™
for Migraine
Generic name: rizatriptan benzoate

Please read this information before you start taking MAXALT*. Also, read the leaflet each time you renew your prescription, just in case anything has changed. Remember, this leaflet does not take the place of careful discussions with your doctor. You and your doctor should discuss MAXALT when you start taking your medication and at regular checkups.

What is MAXALT and what is it used for?

MAXALT is a medication used for the treatment of migraine attacks in adults. MAXALT is a member of a class of drugs called selective 5-$HT_{1B/1D}$ receptor agonists.

It is available as a traditional tablet (MAXALT) and as an orally disintegrating tablet (MAXALT-MLT**). Unless otherwise stated, the information contained in this leaflet applies both to MAXALT Tablets and to MAXALT-MLT orally disintegrating tablets.

Tell your doctor about your symptoms. Your doctor will decide if you have migraine. Use MAXALT only for a migraine attack. MAXALT should not be used to treat headaches that might be caused by other, more serious conditions.

You will find more information about migraine at the end of this leaflet.

* Registered trademark of MERCK & CO., Inc.
**Trademark of MERCK & CO., Inc.

How should I take MAXALT?

Your doctor has prescribed either a 5 mg or 10 mg dosage of MAXALT or MAXALT-MLT for your migraine attack. When you have a migraine headache, take your medication as directed by your doctor.

MAXALT Tablets

If you are using MAXALT Tablets, swallow the tablet whole with liquid.

MAXALT-MLT Orally Disintegrating Tablets

If you are using MAXALT-MLT, leave the orally disintegrating tablet in its package until you are ready to take it. Remove the blister from the foil pouch. Do not push the tablet through the blister; rather, peel open the blister pack with dry hands and place the tablet on your tongue. The tablet will dissolve rapidly and be swallowed with your saliva. No liquid is needed to take the orally disintegrating tablet.

If your headache comes back after your initial dose, a second dose may be taken anytime after 2 hours of administering the first dose. For any attack where you have no response to the first dose, do not take a second dose without first consulting with your doctor. Do not take more than 30 mg of MAXALT in a 24-hour period, (for example, do not take more than three 10-mg tablets in a 24-hour period).

If you are receiving propranolol, you should use the 5-mg dose of MAXALT or MAXALT-MLT, up to a maximum of 3 doses (15 mg total) in a 24-hour period.

If your condition worsens, seek medical attention.

Continued on next page

Information on the Merck & Co., Inc. products listed on these pages is the full prescribing information from product circulars in use September 30, 2000. For information, please call 1-800-NSC MERCK [1-800-672-6372].

Maxalt—Cont.

Who should not take MAXALT?
Do not take MAXALT if you:
- have had a serious allergic reaction to MAXALT or any of its ingredients
- have uncontrolled high blood pressure
- have heart disease or history of heart disease
- are currently taking monoamine oxidase (MAO) inhibitors*** such as phenelzine sulfate (NARDIL®) or tranylcypromine sulfate (PARNATE®) for mental depression, or have taken MAO inhibitors within the last two weeks.

MAXALT should not be used within 24 hours of treatment with another 5-HT_1 agonist*** such as sumatriptan (IMITREX®), naratriptan (AMERGE™) or zolmitriptan (ZOMIG™); or ergotamine-type medications such as ergotamine (BELLERGAL-S®, CAFERGOT®, ERGOMAR®, WIGRAINE®), dihydro-ergotamine (D.H.E. 45®), or methysergide (SANSERT®).

*** The brands listed are the trademarks of their respective owners and are not trademarks of Merck & Co., Inc.

What should I tell my doctor before and during treatment with MAXALT?
Tell your doctor:
- about any past or present medical problems
- about any history of high blood pressure, chest pain, shortness of breath, heart disease, or stroke
- about any risk factors for heart disease or blood vessel disease
  - high blood pressure or diabetes
  - high cholesterol
  - obesity
  - smoking
  - family history of heart disease or blood vessel disease
  - post menopausal
  - male over 40
- about any allergies you have or have had
- if you are pregnant or plan to become pregnant
- if you are breast-feeding or plan to breast-feed
- about all drugs you are taking or plan to take, including those obtained without a prescription, and those you normally take for a migraine.

What if I am pregnant?
Do not use MAXALT if you are pregnant, think you might be pregnant, are trying to become pregnant, or are not using adequate contraception, unless you have discussed this with your doctor.

Can I take MAXALT with other medications*?**
Do not take MAXALT with any other drug in the same class within 24 hours, such as sumatriptan (IMITREX®), naratriptan (AMERGE™) or zolmitriptan (ZOMIG™).
Do not take MAXALT within 24 hours of taking ergotamine-type medications such as ergotamine (BELLERGAL-S®, CAFERGOT®, ERGOMAR®, WIGRAINE®), dihydro-ergotamine (D.H.E. 45®) or methysergide (SANSERT®) to treat your migraine.
Do not take MAXALT when you are taking monoamine oxidase (MAO) inhibitors, such as phenelzine sulfate (NARDIL®) or tranylcypromine sulfate (PARNATE®) for mental depression, or if it has been less than two weeks since you stopped taking an MAO inhibitor.
Ask your doctor for instructions about taking MAXALT if you are now taking propranolol (INDERAL®). (See **How should I take MAXALT?** section.)

What are the possible side effects of MAXALT?
Like all prescription drugs, MAXALT can cause side effects. In studies, MAXALT was generally well-tolerated. The side effects were usually mild and temporary. The following is **not** a complete list of side effects reported with MAXALT. Do not rely on this leaflet alone for information about side effects. Ask your doctor to discuss with you the more complete list of side effects.
In studies, the **most common** side effects reported were:
- **dizziness**
- **sleepiness, tiredness, fatigue**
- **pain or pressure sensation (e.g., in the chest or throat)**

If you experience dizziness, sleepiness, tiredness or fatigue, you should evaluate your ability to perform complex tasks such as driving or operating heavy machinery.
Other, **less common** side effects were related to the:
Heart and blood vessels – Alterations in heartbeat, increased blood pressure and cold extremities.
Muscles – Muscle weakness, stiffness, and spasm; and muscle and bone pain.
Nervous system – Nervousness, decreased mental sharpness, tremor, headache, abnormal sensation, vertigo, sleep disturbance, mood and personality changes, alterations in speech and movement, memory impairment, confusion and dream abnormality.
Digestive system – Stomach upset, diarrhea, dry mouth, constipation, gas, thirst, acid reflux, difficulty swallowing, tongue swelling, changes in appetite, burping and inability of the tongue to move.
Skin – Flushing (redness of the face lasting a short time), hot flashes, sweating, itching, rash, hives, acne and skin reaction to sunlight.
Respiratory – Difficult or rapid breathing, dryness or discomfort of the throat or nose, nose bleed, yawning and sinus disorder, cold-like symptoms, cough, hiccups and swelling of the throat.
Special Senses – Visual disturbances, ringing in the ears, ear pain, eye discomfort, swelling or tearing; alterations in hearing and smelling and visual intolerance to light.
Miscellaneous – Chills, heat sensitivity, swelling, bloating, hangover effect, fever, fainting, dizziness on standing up, warm/cold sensations, dehydration and changes in urination and menstruation.
In addition, bad taste has occurred.
As with other drugs in this class, there have been very rare reports of heart attack and stroke generally occurring in patients with risk factors for heart and blood vessel disease (see **What should I tell my doctor before and during treatment with MAXALT?**).
Tell your doctor about these or any other symptoms. If the symptoms persist or worsen, seek medical attention promptly. In addition, tell your doctor if you experience any symptoms that suggest an allergic reaction (such as a rash or itching) after taking MAXALT.

What should I do if I take an overdose?
If you take more medication than you have been told to take, you should contact your doctor, hospital emergency department, or nearest poison control center immediately.

What is migraine and how does it differ from other headaches?
Migraine is an intense, throbbing, typically one-sided headache that often includes nausea, vomiting, sensitivity to light, and sensitivity to sound. According to many migraine sufferers, the pain and symptoms from a migraine headache are more intense than the pain and symptoms of a common headache.
Some people may have visual symptoms before the headache, such as flashing lights or wavy lines, called an aura. Migraine attacks typically last for hours or, rarely, for more than a day, and they can return frequently. The severity and frequency of migraine attacks may vary.
Based on your symptoms, your doctor will decide whether you have migraine.

Who gets migraine?
Migraine headaches tend to occur in members of the same family. Both men and women get migraine, but it is more common in women.

What may trigger a migraine attack?
Certain things are thought to trigger migraine attacks in some people. Some of these triggers are:
- certain foods or beverages (e.g., cheese, chocolate, citrus fruit, caffeine, alcohol)
- stress
- change in a behavior (e.g., under/oversleeping; missing a meal; change in diet)
- hormonal changes in women (e.g., menstruation)

You may be able to prevent migraine attacks or diminish their frequency if you understand what specifically triggers your attacks. Keeping a headache diary may help you identify and monitor the possible migraine triggers you encounter. Once the triggers are identified, you and your doctor can modify your treatment and lifestyle appropriately.

How does MAXALT work during a migraine attack?
Treatment with MAXALT:
1. Reduces swelling of blood vessels surrounding the brain. This swelling results in the headache pain of a migraine attack.
2. Blocks the release of substances from nerve endings that cause more pain and other symptoms of migraine.
3. Interrupts the sending of specific pain signals to your brain.

It is thought that each of these actions contributes to relief of your symptoms by MAXALT.

How should I store MAXALT?
Keep your medicine in a safe place where children cannot reach it. It may be harmful to children. Store your medication away from heat, light, moisture, and at a controlled room temperature 59°–86°F (15°–30°C). If your medication has expired, throw it away as instructed. If your doctor decides to stop your treatment, do not keep any leftover medicine unless your doctor tells you to do so. Throw away your medicine as instructed. Be sure that the discarded tablets are out of the reach of children.
If you are storing MAXALT-MLT, do not remove the blister from the outer aluminum pouch until you are ready to take the medication inside.
This leaflet provides a summary of information about MAXALT. If you have any questions or concerns about either MAXALT or migraine, talk to your doctor. In addition, talk to your pharmacist or other health care provider.

9122201 Issued August 1999

MEFOXIN® ℞
(Cefoxitin for Injection)

DESCRIPTION

MEFOXIN† (Cefoxitin for Injection) is a semi-synthetic, broad-spectrum cepha antibiotic sealed under nitrogen for intravenous administration. It is derived from cephamycin C, which is produced by *Streptomyces lactamdurans*. Its chemical name is sodium (6*R*, 7*S*)-3-(hydroxymethyl)-7-methoxy-8-oxo-7-[2-(2-thienyl)acetamido]-5-thia-1-azabicyclo[4.2.0]oct-2-ene-2-carboxylate carbamate (ester).
The empirical formula is $C_{16}H_{16}N_3NaO_7S_2$, and the structural formula is:

MEFOXIN contains approximately 53.8 mg (2.3 milliequivalents) of sodium per gram of cefoxitin activity. Solutions of MEFOXIN range from colorless to light amber in color. The pH of freshly constituted solutions usually ranges from 4.2 to 7.0.

† Registered trademark of MERCK & CO., Inc.

CLINICAL PHARMACOLOGY

Clinical Pharmacology
Following an intravenous dose of 1 gram, serum concentrations were 110 mcg/mL at 5 minutes, declining to less than 1 mcg/mL at 4 hours. The half-life after an intravenous dose is 41 to 59 minutes. Approximately 85 percent of cefoxitin is excreted unchanged by the kidneys over a 6-hour period, resulting in high urinary concentrations. Probenecid slows tubular excretion and produces higher serum levels and increases the duration of measurable serum concentrations.
Cefoxitin passes into pleural and joint fluids and is detectable in antibacterial concentrations in bile.
Microbiology
The bactericidal action of cefoxitin results from inhibition of cell wall synthesis. Cefoxitin has *in vitro* activity against a wide range of gram-positive and gram-negative organisms. The methoxy group in the 7α position provides MEFOXIN with a high degree of stability in the presence of beta-lactamases, both penicillinases and cephalosporinases, of gram-negative bacteria. While *in vitro* studies have demonstrated the susceptibility of most strains of the following organisms, clinical efficacy for infections other than those included in the INDICATIONS AND USAGE section is unknown.
Gram-positive
Staphylococcus aureus, including penicillinase and non-penicillinase producing strains.
Staphylococcus epidermidis
Beta-hemolytic and other streptococci (most strains of enterococci, e.g., *Enterococcus faecalis* [formerly *Streptococcus faecalis*], are resistant)
Streptococcus pneumoniae
Gram-negative
Eikenella corrodens (beta-lactamase negative strains)
Escherichia coli
Klebsiella species (including *K. pneumoniae*)
Haemophilus influenzae
Neisseria gonorrhoeae, including penicillinase and non-penicillinase producing strains
Proteus mirabilis
Morganella morganii
Proteus vulgaris
Providencia species, including *Providencia rettgeri*
Anaerobic organisms
Peptococcus niger
Peptostreptococcus species
Clostridium species
Bacteroides species, including the *B. fragilis* group (includes *B. fragilis, B. distasonis, B. ovatus, B. thetaiotaomicron*)
MEFOXIN is inactive *in vitro* against most strains of *Pseudomonas aeruginosa* and enterococci and many strains of *Enterobacter cloacae*.
Methicillin-resistant staphylococci are almost uniformly resistant to MEFOXIN.
Susceptibility Tests
For fast-growing aerobic organisms, quantitative methods that require measurements of zone diameters give the most precise estimates of antibiotic susceptibility. One such procedure* has been recommended for use with discs to test susceptibility to cefoxitin. Interpretation involves correlation of the diameters obtained in the disc test with minimal inhibitory concentration (MIC) values for cefoxitin.
Reports from the laboratory giving results of the standardized single disc susceptibility test* using a 30 mcg cefoxitin disc should be interpreted according to the following criteria:
Organisms producing zones of 18 mm or greater are considered susceptible, indicating that the tested organism is likely to respond to therapy.
Organisms of intermediate susceptibility produce zones of 15 to 17 mm, indicating that the tested organism would be susceptible if high dosage is used or if the infection is confined to tissues and fluids (e.g., urine) in which high antibiotic levels are attained.
Resistant organisms produce zones of 14 mm or less, indicating that other therapy should be selected.
The cefoxitin disc should be used for testing cefoxitin susceptibility.
Cefoxitin has been shown by *in vitro* tests to have activity against certain strains of *Enterobacteriaceae* found resistant when tested with the cephalosporin class disc. For this reason, the cefoxitin disc should not be used for testing susceptibility to cephalosporins, and cephalosporin discs should not be used for testing susceptibility to cefoxitin.

Dilution methods, preferably the agar plate dilution procedure, are most accurate for susceptibility testing of obligate anaerobes.
A bacterial isolate may be considered susceptible if the MIC value for cefoxitin** is not more than 16 mcg/mL. Organisms are considered resistant if the MIC is greater than 32 mcg/mL.

* Bauer, A. W.; Kirby, W. M. M.; Sherris, J. C.; Turck, M.: Antibiotic susceptibility testing by a standardized single disc method, Amer. J. Clin. Path. *45* : 493–496, Apr. 1966. Standardized disc susceptibility test, Federal Register *37* : 20527–20529, 1972. National Committee for Clinical Laboratory Standards: Performance Standards for Antimicrobial Disc Susceptibility Tests–Fifth Edition; Approved Standard, NCCLS Document M2-A5, Vol 13, No. 24,
NCCLS, Villanova, PA, December 1993.

** Determined by the ICS agar dilution method (Ericsson and Sherris, Acta Path. Microbiol. Scand. (B) Suppl. No. 217, 1971) or any other method that has been shown to give equivalent results.

INDICATIONS AND USAGE

Treatment
MEFOXIN is indicated for the treatment of serious infections caused by susceptible strains of the designated microorganisms in the diseases listed below.
(1) Lower respiratory tract infections, including pneumonia and lung abscess, caused by *Streptococcus pneumoniae,* other streptococci (excluding enterococci, e.g., *Enterococcus faecalis* [formerly *Streptococcus faecalis*]), *Staphylococcus aureus* (penicillinase and non-penicillinase producing), *Escherichia coli, Klebsiella* species, *Haemophilus influenzae,* and *Bacteroides* species.
(2) Urinary tract infections caused by *Escherichia coli, Klebsiella* species, *Proteus mirabilis, Morganella morganii, Proteus vulgaris* and *Providencia* species (including *P. rettgeri*).
(3) Intra-abdominal infections, including peritonitis and intra-abdominal abscess, caused by *Escherichia coli, Klebsiella* species, *Bacteroides* species including the *Bacteroides fragilis* group***, and *Clostridium* species.
(4) Gynecological infections, including endometritis, pelvic cellulitis, and pelvic inflammatory disease caused by *Escherichia coli, Neisseria gonorrhoeae* (penicillinase and non-penicillinase producing), *Bacteroides* species including *B. fragilis, Clostridium* species, *Peptococcus niger, Peptostreptococcus* species, and Group B streptococci. MEFOXIN, like cephalosporins, has no activity against *Chlamydia trachomatis.* Therefore, when MEFOXIN is used in the treatment of patients with pelvic inflammatory disease and *C. trachomatis* is one of the suspected pathogens, appropriate antichlamydial coverage should be added.
(5) Septicemia caused by *Streptococcus pneumoniae, Staphylococcus aureus* (penicillinase and non-penicillinase producing), *Escherichia coli, Klebsiella* species, and *Bacteroides* species including *B. fragilis.*
(6) Bone and joint infections caused by *Staphylococcus aureus* (penicillinase and non-penicillinase producing).
(7) Skin and skin structure infections caused by *Staphylococcus aureus* (penicillinase and non-penicillinase producing), *Staphylococcus epidermidis,* streptococci (excluding enterococci, e.g., *Enterococcus faecalis* [formerly *Streptococcus faecalis*]), *Escherichia coli, Proteus mirabilis, Klebsiella* species, *Bacteroides* species including *B. fragilis, Clostridium* species, *Peptococcus niger,* and *Peptostreptococcus* species.
Appropriate culture and susceptibility studies should be performed to determine the susceptibility of the causative organisms to MEFOXIN. Therapy may be started while awaiting the results of these studies.
In randomized comparative studies, MEFOXIN and cephalothin were comparably safe and effective in the management of infections caused by gram-positive cocci and gram-negative rods susceptible to the cephalosporins. MEFOXIN has a high degree of stability in the presence of bacterial beta-lactamases, both penicillinases and cephalosporinases. Many infections caused by aerobic and anaerobic gram-negative bacteria resistant to some cephalosporins respond to MEFOXIN. Similarly, many infections caused by aerobic and anaerobic bacteria resistant to some penicillin antibiotics (ampicillin, carbenicillin, penicillin G) respond to treatment with MEFOXIN. Many infections caused by mixtures of susceptible aerobic and anaerobic bacteria respond to treatment with MEFOXIN.
Prevention
MEFOXIN is indicated for the prophylaxis of infection in patients undergoing uncontaminated gastrointestinal surgery, vaginal hysterectomy, abdominal hysterectomy, or cesarean section.
If there are signs of infection, specimens for culture should be obtained for identification of the causative organism so that appropriate treatment may be instituted.

****B. fragilis, B. distasonis, B. ovatus, B. thetaiotaomicron.*

CONTRAINDICATIONS

MEFOXIN is contraindicated in patients who have shown hypersensitivity to cefoxitin and the cephalosporin group of antibiotics.

WARNINGS

BEFORE THERAPY WITH 'MEFOXIN' IS INSTITUTED, CAREFUL INQUIRY SHOULD BE MADE TO DETERMINE WHETHER THE PATIENT HAS HAD PREVIOUS HYPERSENSITIVITY REACTIONS TO CEFOXITIN, CEPHALOSPORINS, PENICILLINS, OR OTHER DRUGS. THIS PRODUCT SHOULD BE GIVEN WITH CAUTION TO PENICILLIN-SENSITIVE PATIENTS. ANTIBIOTICS SHOULD BE ADMINISTERED WITH CAUTION TO ANY PATIENT WHO HAS DEMONSTRATED SOME FORM OF ALLERGY, PARTICULARLY TO DRUGS. IF AN ALLERGIC REACTION TO 'MEFOXIN' OCCURS, DISCONTINUE THE DRUG. SERIOUS HYPERSENSITIVITY REACTIONS MAY REQUIRE EPINEPHRINE AND OTHER EMERGENCY MEASURES.
Pseudomembranous colitis has been reported with nearly all antibacterial agents, including cefoxitin, and may range in severity from mild to life threatening. Therefore, it is important to consider this diagnosis in patients who present with diarrhea subsequent to the administration of antibacterial agents.
Treatment with antibacterial agents alters the normal flora of the colon and my permit overgrowth of clostridia. Studies indicate that a toxin produced by *Clostridium difficile* is one primary cause of "antibiotic-associated colitis."
After the diagnosis of pseudomembranous colitis has been established, appropriate therapeutic measures should be initiated. Mild cases of pseudomembranous colitis usually respond to drug discontinuation alone. In moderate to severe cases, consideration should be given to management with fluids and electrolytes, protein supplementation, and treatment with an antibacterial drug clinically effective against *Clostridium difficile* colitis.

PRECAUTIONS

General
The total daily dose should be reduced when MEFOXIN is administered to patients with transient or persistent reduction of urinary output due to renal insufficiency (see DOSAGE AND ADMINISTRATION), because high and prolonged serum antibiotic concentrations can occur in such individuals from usual doses.
Antibiotics (including cephalosporins) should be prescribed with caution in individuals with a history of gastrointestinal disease, particularly colitis.
As with other antibiotics, prolonged use of MEFOXIN may result in overgrowth of nonsusceptible organisms. Repeated evaluation of the patient's condition is essential. If superinfection occurs during therapy, appropriate measures should be taken.
Laboratory Tests
As with any potent antibacterial agent, periodic assessment of organ system functions, including renal, hepatic, and hematopoietic, is advisable during prolonged therapy.
Drug Interactions
Increased nephrotoxicity has been reported following concomitant administration of cephalosporins and aminoglycoside antibiotics.
Drug/Laboratory Test Interactions
As with cephalothin, high concentrations of cefoxitin (>100 micrograms/mL) may interfere with measurement of serum and urine creatinine levels by the Jaffé reaction, and produce false increases of modest degree in the levels of creatinine reported. Serum samples from patients treated with cefoxitin should not be analyzed for creatinine if withdrawn within 2 hours of drug administration.
High concentrations of cefoxitin in the urine may interfere with measurement of urinary 17-hydroxy-corticosteroids by the Porter-Silber reaction, and produce false increases of modest degree in the levels reported.
A false-positive reaction for glucose in the urine may occur. This has been observed with CLINITEST[††] reagent tablets.
Carcinogenesis, Mutagenesis, Impairment of Fertility
Long-term studies in animals have not been performed with cefoxitin to evaluate carcinogenic or mutagenic potential. Studies in rats treated intravenously with 400 mg/kg of cefoxitin (approximately three times the maximum recommended human dose) revealed no effects on fertility or mating ability.
Pregnancy
Pregnancy Category B. Reproduction studies performed in rats and mice at parenteral doses of approximately one to seven and one-half times the maximum recommended human dose did not reveal teratogenic or fetal toxic effects, although a slight decrease in fetal weight was observed.
There are, however, no adequate and well-controlled studies in pregnant women. Because animal reproduction studies are not always predictive of human response, this drug should be used during pregnancy only if clearly needed.
In the rabbit, cefoxitin was associated with a high incidence of abortion and maternal death. This was not considered to be a teratogenic effect but an expected consequence of the rabbit's unusual sensitivity to antibiotic-induced changes in the population of the microflora of the intestine.
Nursing Mothers
MEFOXIN is excreted in human milk in low concentrations. Caution should be exercised when MEFOXIN is administered to a nursing woman.
Pediatric Use
Safety and efficacy in pediatric patients from birth to three months of age have not yet been established. In pediatric patients three months of age and older, higher doses of MEFOXIN have been associated with an increased incidence of eosinophilia and elevated SGOT.

†† Registered trademark of Ames Company, Division of Miles Laboratories, Inc.

ADVERSE REACTIONS

MEFOXIN is generally well tolerated. The most common adverse reactions have been local reactions following intravenous injection. Other adverse reactions have been encountered infrequently.
Local Reactions
Thrombophlebitis has occurred with intravenous administration.
Allergic Reactions
Rash (including exfoliative dermatitis and toxic epidermal necrolysis), pruritus, eosinophilia, fever, dyspnea, and other allergic reactions including anaphylaxis, interstitial nephritis and angioedema have been noted.
Cardiovascular
Hypotension
Gastrointestinal
Diarrhea, including documented pseudomembranous colitis which can appear during or after antibiotic treatment. Nausea and vomiting have been reported rarely.
Neuromuscular
Possible exacerbation of myasthenia gravis
Blood
Eosinophilia, leukopenia, including granulocytopenia, neutropenia, anemia, including hemolytic anemia, thrombocytopenia, and bone marrow depression. A positive direct Coombs test may develop in some individuals, especially those with azotemia.
Liver Function
Transient elevations in SGOT, SGPT, serum LDH, serum alkaline phosphatase; and jaundice have been reported.
Renal Function
Elevations in serum creatinine and/or blood urea nitrogen levels have been observed. As with the cephalosporins, acute renal failure has been reported rarely. The role of MEFOXIN in changes in renal function tests is difficult to assess, since factors predisposing to prerenal azotemia or to impaired renal function usually have been present.
In addition to the adverse reactions listed above which have been observed in patients treated with MEFOXIN, the following adverse reactions and altered laboratory test results have been reported for cephalosporin class antibiotics:
Urticaria, erythema multiforme, Stevens-Johnson syndrome, serum sickness-like reactions, abdominal pain, colitis, renal dysfunction, toxic nephropathy, false-positive test for urinary glucose, hepatic dysfunction including cholestasis, elevated bilirubin, aplastic anemia, hemorrhage, prolonged prothrombin time, pancytopenia, agranulocytosis, superinfection, vaginitis including vaginal candidiasis.
Several cephalosporins have been implicated in triggering seizures, particularly in patients with renal impairment when the dosage was not reduced. (See DOSAGE AND ADMINISTRATION.) If seizures associated with drug therapy occur, the drug should be discontinued. Anticonvulsant therapy can be given if clinically indicated.

OVERDOSAGE

The acute intravenous LD_{50} in the adult female mouse and rabbit was about 8.0 g/kg and greater than 1.0 g/kg respectively. The acute intraperitoneal LD_{50} in the adult rat was greater than 10.0 g/kg.

DOSAGE AND ADMINISTRATION

TREATMENT
Adults
The usual adult dosage range is 1 gram to 2 grams every six to eight hours. Dosage should be determined by susceptibility of the causative organisms, severity of infection, and the condition of the patient (see Table 1 for dosage guidelines).
If *C. trachomatis* is a suspected pathogen, appropriate antichlamydial coverage should be added, because cefoxitin sodium has no activity against this organism.
[See table 1 at top of next page]
MEFOXIN may be used in patients with reduced renal function with the following dosage adjustments:
In adults with renal insufficiency, an initial loading dose of 1 gram to 2 grams may be given. After a loading dose, the recommendations for *maintenance dosage* (Table 2) may be used as a guide.
[See table 2 at top of next page]
When only the serum creatinine level is available, the following formula (based on sex, weight, and age of the patient) may be used to convert this value into creatinine

Continued on next page

Information on the Merck & Co., Inc. products listed on these pages is the full prescribing information from product circulars in use September 30, 2000. For information, please call 1-800-NSC MERCK [1-800-672-6372].

Mefoxin—Cont.

clearance. The serum creatinine should represent a steady state of renal function.

Males: $\frac{\text{Weight (kg)} \times (140 - \text{age})}{72 \times \text{serum creatinine (mg/100 mL)}}$

Females: 0.85 × above value

In patients undergoing hemodialysis, the loading dose of 1 to 2 grams should be given after each hemodialysis, and the maintenance dose should be given as indicated in Table 2.

Antibiotic therapy for group A beta-hemolytic streptococcal infections should be maintained for at least 10 days to guard against the risk of rheumatic fever or glomerulonephritis. In staphylococcal and other infections involving a collection of pus, surgical drainage should be carried out where indicated.

Pediatric Patients

The recommended dosage in pediatric patients three months of age and older is 80 to 160 mg/kg of body weight per day divided into four to six equal doses. The higher dosages should be used for more severe or serious infections. The total daily dosage should not exceed 12 grams.

At this time no recommendation is made for pediatric patients from birth to three months of age (see PRECAUTIONS).

In pediatric patients with renal insufficiency, the dosage and frequency of dosage should be modified consistent with the recommendations for adults (see Table 2).

PREVENTION

Effective prophylactic use depends on the time of administration. MEFOXIN usually should be given one-half to one hour before the operation, which is sufficient time to achieve effective levels in the wound during the procedure. Prophylactic administration should usually be stopped within 24 hours since continuing administration of any antibiotic increases the possibility of adverse reactions but, in the majority of surgical procedures, does not reduce the incidence of subsequent infection.

For prophylactic use in uncontaminated gastrointestinal surgery, vaginal hysterectomy, or abdominal hysterectomy, the following doses are recommended:

Adults:

2 grams administered intravenously just prior to surgery (approximately one-half to one hour before the initial incision) followed by 2 grams every 6 hours after the first dose for no more than 24 hours.

Pediatric Patients (3 months and older):

30 to 40 mg/kg doses may be given at the times designated above.

Cesarean section patients:

For patients undergoing cesarean section, either a single 2 gram dose administered intravenously as soon as the umbilical cord is clamped OR a 3-dose regimen consisting of 2 grams given intravenously as soon as the umbilical cord is clamped followed by 2 grams 4 and 8 hours after the initial dose is recommended. (See CLINICAL STUDIES.)

PREPARATION OF SOLUTION

Table 3 is provided for convenience in constituting MEFOXIN for intravenous administration.

For Vials

One gram should be constituted with at least 10 mL, and 2 grams with 10 or 20 mL, of Sterile Water for Injection, Bacteriostatic Water for Injection, 0.9 percent Sodium Chloride Injection, or 5 percent Dextrose Injection. These primary solutions may be further diluted in 50 to 1000 mL of the diluents listed under the *Vials and Bulk Packages* portion of the *COMPATIBILITY AND STABILITY* section.

For Bulk Packages

The 10 gram bulk packages should be constituted with 43 or 93 mL of Sterile Water for Injection, Bacteriostatic Water for Injection, 0.9 percent Sodium Chloride Injection, or 5 percent Dextrose Injection. CAUTION: THE 10 GRAM BULK STOCK SOLUTION IS NOT FOR DIRECT INFUSION. These primary solutions may be further diluted in 50 to 1000 mL of the diluents listed under the *Vials and Bulk Packages* portion of the *COMPATIBILITY AND STABILITY* section.

Benzyl alcohol as a preservative has been associated with toxicity in neonates. While toxicity has not been demonstrated in pediatric patients greater than three months of age, in whom use of MEFOXIN may be indicated, small pediatric patients in this age range may also be at risk for benzyl alcohol toxicity. Therefore, diluent containing benzyl alcohol should not be used when MEFOXIN is constituted for administration to pediatric patients in this age range.

For Infusion Bottles

One or 2 grams of MEFOXIN for infusion may be constituted with 50 or 100 mL of 0.9 percent Sodium Chloride Injection, or 5 percent or 10 percent Dextrose Injection.

For ADD-Vantage®[†††] Vials

See separate INSTRUCTIONS FOR USE OF MEFOXIN IN ADD-Vantage® VIALS. MEFOXIN in ADD-Vantage® vials should be constituted with ADD-Vantage® diluent containers containing 50 mL or 100 mL of either 0.9 percent Sodium Chloride Injection or 5 percent Dextrose Injection. MEFOXIN in ADD-Vantage® vials is for IV use only.

[See table 3 above]

[†††]Registered trademark of Abbott Laboratories.

ADMINISTRATION

MEFOXIN may be administered intravenously after constitution.

Table 1—Guidelines for Dosage of MEFOXIN

Type of Infection	Daily Dosage	Frequency and Route
Uncomplicated forms* of infections such as pneumonia, urinary tract infection, cutaneous infection	3–4 grams	1 gram every 6–8 hours IV
Moderately severe or severe infections	6–8 grams	1 gram every 4 hours *or* 2 grams every 6–8 hours IV
Infections commonly needing antibiotics in higher dosage (e.g., gas gangrene)	12 grams	2 grams every 4 hours *or* 3 grams every 6 hours IV

*Including patients in whom bacteremia is absent or unlikely

Table 2—Maintenance Dosage of MEFOXIN in Adults with Reduced Renal Function

Renal Function	Creatinine Clearance (mL/min)	Dose (grams)	Frequency
Mild impairment	50–30	1–2	every 8–12 hours
Moderate impairment	29–10	1–2	every 12–24 hours
Severe impairment	9–5	0.5–1	every 12–24 hours
Essentially no function	<5	0.5–1	every 24–48 hours

Table 3—Preparation of Solution

MEFOXIN

Strength	Amount of Diluent to be Added (mL)[++]	Approximate Withdrawable Volume (mL)	Approximate Average Concentration (mg/mL)
1 gram Vial	10	10.5	95
2 gram Vial	10 or 20	11.1 or 21.0	180 or 95
1 gram Infusion Bottle	50 or 100	50 or 100	20 or 10
2 gram Infusion Bottle	50 or 100	50 or 100	40 or 20
10 gram Bulk	43 or 93	49 or 98.5	200 or 100

[++]Shake to dissolve and let stand until clear.

Parenteral drug products should be inspected visually for particulate matter and discoloration prior to administration whenever solution and container permit.

Intravenous Administration

The intravenous route is preferable for patients with bacteremia, bacterial septicemia, or other severe or life-threatening infections, or for patients who may be poor risks because of lowered resistance resulting from such debilitating conditions as malnutrition, trauma, surgery, diabetes, heart failure, or malignancy, particularly if shock is present or impending.

For intermittent intravenous administration, a solution containing 1 gram or 2 grams in 10 mL of Sterile Water for Injection can be injected over a period of three to five minutes. Using an infusion system, it may also be given over a longer period of time through the tubing system by which the patient may be receiving other intravenous solutions. However, during infusion of the solution containing MEFOXIN, it is advisable to temporarily discontinue administration of any other solutions at the same site.

For the administration of higher doses by continuous intravenous infusion, a solution of MEFOXIN may be added to an intravenous bottle containing 5 percent Dextrose Injection, 0.9 percent Sodium Chloride Injection, or 5 percent Dextrose and 0.9 percent Sodium Chloride Injection. BUTTERFLY[†††] or scalp vein-type needles are preferred for this type of infusion.

Solutions of MEFOXIN, like those of most beta-lactam antibiotics, should not be added to aminoglycoside solutions (e.g., gentamicin sulfate, tobramycin sulfate, amikacin sulfate) because of potential interaction. However, MEFOXIN and aminoglycosides may be administered separately to the same patient.

[†††] Registered trademark of Abbott Laboratories.

COMPATIBILITY AND STABILITY

Vials and Bulk Packages

MEFOXIN, as supplied in vials or the bulk package and constituted to 1 gram/10 mL with Sterile Water for Injection, Bacteriostatic Water for Injection (see *PREPARATION OF SOLUTION*), 0.9 percent Sodium Chloride Injection, or 5 percent Dextrose Injection, maintains satisfactory potency for 6 hours at room temperature or for one week under refrigeration (below 5°C).

These primary solutions may be further diluted in 50 to 1000 mL of the following diluents and maintain potency for an additional 18 hours at room temperature or an additional 48 hours under refrigeration:

- 0.9 percent Sodium Chloride Injection
- 5 percent or 10 percent Dextrose Injection
- 5 percent Dextrose and 0.9 percent Sodium Chloride Injection
- 5 percent Dextrose Injection with 0.2 percent or 0.45 percent saline solution
- Lactated Ringer's Injection
- 5 percent Dextrose in Lactated Ringer's Injection
- 10 percent invert sugar in water
- 10 percent invert sugar in saline solution
- 5 percent Sodium Bicarbonate Injection
- M/6 sodium lactate solution
- Mannitol 5% and 10%

Infusion Bottles

MEFOXIN, as supplied in infusion bottles and constituted with 50 to 100 mL of 0.9 percent Sodium Chloride Injection, or 5 percent or 10 percent Dextrose Injection, maintains satisfactory potency for 24 hours at room temperature or for 1 week under refrigeration (below 5°C).

ADD-Vantage® Vials

MEFOXIN is supplied in single dose ADD-Vantage® vials and should be prepared as directed in the accompanying INSTRUCTIONS FOR USE OF MEFOXIN IN ADD-Vantage® VIALS using ADD-Vantage® diluent containers containing 50 mL or 100 mL of either 0.9 percent Sodium Chloride Injection or 5 percent Dextrose Injection. When prepared with either of these diluents, MEFOXIN maintains satisfactory potency for 24 hours at room temperature.

After the periods mentioned above, any unused solutions should be discarded.

HOW SUPPLIED

Sterile MEFOXIN is a dry white to off-white powder supplied in vials and infusion bottles containing cefoxitin sodium as follows:

No. 3356—1 gram cefoxitin equivalent
NDC 0006-3356-45 in trays of 25 vials
(6505-01-119-6005, 1 g 25's).

No. 3368—1 gram cefoxitin equivalent
NDC 0006-3368-71 in trays of 10 infusion bottles
(6505-01-195-0649, 1 g infusion bottle 10's).

No. 3357—2 gram cefoxitin equivalent
NDC 0006-3357-53 in trays of 25 vials
(6505-01-104-6393, 2 g 25's).

No. 3369—2 gram cefoxitin equivalent
NDC 0006-3369-73 in trays of 10 infusion bottles
(6505-01-185-2624, 2 g infusion bottle 10's).

No. 3388—10 gram cefoxitin equivalent
NDC 0006-3388-67 in trays of 6 bulk bottles
(6505-01-263-0730, 10 g 6's).

No. 3548—1 gram cefoxitin equivalent
NDC 0006-3548-45 in trays of 25 ADD-Vantage® vials.
(6505-01-262-9509, 1 g ADD-Vantage® 25's).

No. 3549—2 gram cefoxitin equivalent
NDC 0006-3549-53 in trays of 25 ADD-Vantage® vials.
(6505-01-263-4531, 2 g ADD-Vantage® 25's).

Special storage instructions

MEFOXIN in the dry state should be stored between 2–25°C (36–77°F). Avoid exposure to temperatures above 50°C. The dry material as well as solutions tend to darken, depending on storage conditions; product potency, however, is not adversely affected.

CLINICAL STUDIES

A prospective, randomized, double-blind, placebo-controlled clinical trial was conducted to determine the efficacy of short-term prophylaxis with MEFOXIN in patients undergoing cesarean section who were at high risk for subsequent endometritis because of ruptured membranes. Patients were randomized to receive either three doses of placebo (n=58), a single dose of MEFOXIN (2 g) followed by two doses of placebo (n=64), or a three-dose regimen of MEFOXIN (each dose consisting of 2 g) (n=60), given intravenously, usually beginning at the time of clamping of the umbilical cord, with the second and third doses given 4 and 8 hours post-operatively. Endometritis occurred in 16/58 (27.6%) patients given placebo, 5/63 (7.9%) patients given a single dose of MEFOXIN, and 3/58 (5.2%) patients given three doses of MEFOXIN. The differences between the two groups treated with MEFOXIN and placebo with respect to endometritis were statistically significant ($p<0.01$) in favor of MEFOXIN. The differences between the one-dose and three-dose regimens of MEFOXIN were not statistically significant.

Two double-blind, randomized studies compared the efficacy of a single 2 gram intravenous dose of MEFOXIN to a single 2 gram dose of cefotetan in the prevention of surgical site-related infection (major morbidity) and non-site-related infections (minor morbidity) in patients following cesarean section. In the first study, 82/98 (83.7%) patients treated with MEFOXIN and 71/95 (74.7%) patients treated with cefotetan experienced no major or minor morbidity. The difference in the outcomes in this study (95% CI: −0.03, +0.21) was not statistically significant. In the second study, 65/75 (86.7%) patients treated with MEFOXIN and 62/76 (81.6%) patients treated with cefotetan experienced no major or minor morbidity. The difference in the outcomes in this study (95% CI: −0.08, +0.18) was not statistically significant.

In clinical trials of patients with intra-abdominal infections due to *Bacteroides fragilis* group microorganisms, eradication rates at 1 to 2 weeks posttreatment for isolates were in the range of 70% to 80%. Eradication rates for individual species are listed below:

Bacteroides distasonis	7/10	(70%)
Bacteroides fragilis	26/33	(79%)
Bacteroides ovatus	10/13	(77%)
B. thetaiotaomicron	13/18	(72%)

7882337 Issued October 1996

MEFOXIN®
Premixed Intravenous Solution ℞
(Cefoxitin Injection)

DESCRIPTION

Cefoxitin sodium is a semi-synthetic, broad-spectrum cepha antibiotic for intravenous administration. It is derived from cephamycin C, which is produced by *Streptomyces lactamdurans.* Its chemical name is sodium (6*R*,7*S*)-3-(hydroxymethyl)-7-methoxy-8-oxo-7-[2- (2-thienyl)acetamido]-5-thia-1-azabicyclo [4.2.0]oct-2-ene-2-carboxylate carbamate (ester). The empirical formula is $C_{16}H_{16}N_3NaO_7S_2$, and the molecular weight is 449.44. The structural formula is:

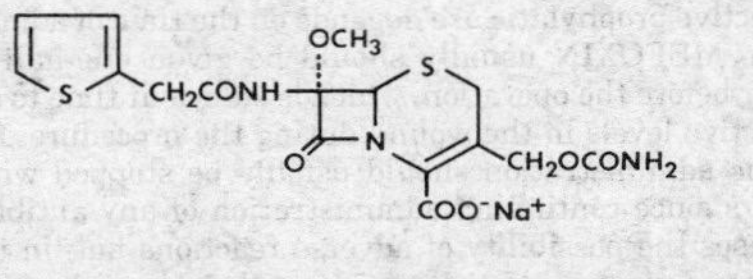

Cefoxitin sodium contains approximately 53.8 mg (2.3 milliequivalents) of sodium per gram of cefoxitin activity.

Premixed Intravenous Solution MEFOXIN* (Cefoxitin Sodium Injection) is supplied as a sterile, nonpyrogenic, frozen, iso-osmotic solution of cefoxitin sodium. Each 50 mL contains cefoxitin sodium equivalent to either 1 gram or 2 grams cefoxitin. Dextrose hydrous USP has been added to the above dosages to adjust osmolality (approximately 2 grams and 1.1 grams to 1 gram and 2 gram dosages, respectively). The pH is adjusted with sodium bicarbonate and may have been adjusted with hydrochloric acid. The pH is approximately 6.5. After thawing, the solution is intended for intravenous use only. Solutions of MEFOXIN range from colorless to light amber.

The plastic container is fabricated from a specially designed multilayer plastic (PL 2040). Solutions are in contact with the polyethylene layer of this container and can leach out certain chemical components of the plastic in very small amounts within the expiration period. The suitability and safety of the plastic have been confirmed in tests in animals according to the USP biological tests for plastic containers, as well as by tissue culture toxicity studies.

*Registered trademark of MERCK & CO., INC.

CLINICAL PHARMACOLOGY

Clinical Pharmacology

Following an intravenous dose of 1 gram of cefoxitin, serum concentrations were 110 mcg/mL at 5 minutes, declining to less than 1 mcg/mL at 4 hours. The half-life after an intravenous dose is 41 to 59 minutes. Approximately 85 percent of cefoxitin is excreted unchanged by the kidneys over a 6-hour period, resulting in high urinary concentrations. Probenecid slows tubular excretion and produces higher serum levels and increases the duration of measurable serum concentrations.

Cefoxitin passes into pleural and joint fluids and is detectable in antibacterial concentrations in bile.

Microbiology

The bactericidal action of cefoxitin results from inhibition of cell wall synthesis. Cefoxitin has *in vitro* activity against a wide range of gram-positive and gram-negative organisms. The methoxy group in the 7α position provides MEFOXIN with a high degree of stability in the presence of beta-lactamases, both penicillinases and cephalosporinases, of gram-negative bacteria. While *in vitro* studies have demonstrated the susceptibility of most strains of the following organisms, clinical efficacy for infections other than those included in the INDICATIONS AND USAGE section is unknown.

Gram-positive

Staphylococcus aureus, including penicillinase and non-penicillinase producing strains
Staphylococcus epidermidis
Beta-hemolytic and other streptococci (most strains of enterococci, e.g., *Enterococcus faecalis* [formerly *Streptococcus faecalis*], are resistant)
Streptococcus pneumoniae

Gram-negative

Eikenella corrodens (beta-lactamase negative strains)
Escherichia coli
Klebsiella species (including *K. pneumoniae*)
Haemophilus influenzae
Neisseria gonorrhoeae, including penicillinase and non-penicillinase producing strains
Proteus mirabilis
Morganella morganii
Proteus vulgaris
Providencia species, including *Providencia rettgeri*

Anaerobic organisms

Peptococcus niger
Peptostreptococcus species
Clostridium species
Bacteroides species, including the *B. fragilis* group (includes *B. fragilis, B. distasonis, B. ovatus, B. thetaiotaomicron*)

MEFOXIN is inactive *in vitro* against most strains of *Pseudomonas aeruginosa* and enterococci and many strains of *Enterobacter cloacae.*

Methicillin-resistant staphylococci are almost uniformly resistant to MEFOXIN.

Susceptibility Tests

For fast-growing aerobic organisms, quantitative methods that require measurements of zone diameters give the most precise estimates of antibiotic susceptibility. One such procedure** has been recommended for use with discs to test susceptibility to cefoxitin. Interpretation involves correlation of the diameters obtained in the disc test with minimal inhibitory concentration (MIC) values for cefoxitin.

Reports from the laboratory giving results of the standardized single disc susceptibility test** using a 30 mcg cefoxitin disc should be interpreted according to the following criteria:

Organisms producing zones of 18 mm or greater are considered susceptible, indicating that the tested organism is likely to respond to therapy.

Organisms of intermediate susceptibility produce zones of 15 to 17 mm, indicating that the tested organism would be susceptible if high dosage is used or if the infection is confined to tissues and fluids (e.g., urine) in which high antibiotic levels are attained.

Resistant organisms produce zones of 14 mm or less, indicating that other therapy should be selected.

The cefoxitin disc should be used for testing cefoxitin susceptibility.

Cefoxitin has been shown by *in vitro* tests to have activity against certain strains of *Enterobacteriaceae* found resistant when tested with the cephalosporin class disc. For this reason, the cefoxitin disc should not be used for testing susceptibility to cephalosporins, and cephalosporin discs should not be used for testing susceptibility to cefoxitin.

Dilution methods, preferably the agar plate dilution procedure, are most accurate for susceptibility testing of obligate anaerobes.

A bacterial isolate may be considered susceptible if the MIC value for cefoxitin*** is not more than 16 mcg/mL. Organisms are considered resistant if the MIC is greater than 32 mcg/mL.

** Bauer, A. W.; Kirby, W. M. M.; Sherris, J. C.; Turck, M.: Antibiotic susceptibility testing by a standardized single disc method, Amer. J. Clin. Path. *45* : 493–496, Apr. 1966. Standardized disc susceptibility test, Federal Register *37* : 20527–20529, 1972. National Committee for Clinical Laboratory Standards: Performance Standards for Antimicrobial Disc Susceptibility Tests—Fifth Edition; Approved Standard, NCCLS Document M2-A5, Vol 13, No. 24, NCCLS, Villanova, PA, December 1993.

*** Determined by the ICS agar dilution method (Ericsson and Sherris, Acta Path. Microbiol. Scand. [B] Suppl. No. 217, 1971) or any other method that has been shown to give equivalent results.

INDICATIONS AND USAGE

MEFOXIN, supplied as a premixed solution in plastic containers, is intended for intravenous use only.

Treatment

MEFOXIN is indicated for the treatment of serious infections caused by susceptible strains of the designated microorganisms in the diseases listed below.

(1) **Lower respiratory tract infections,** including pneumonia and lung abscess, caused by *Streptococcus pneumoniae,* other streptococci (excluding enterococci, e.g., *Enterococcus faecalis* [formerly *Streptococcus faecalis*]), *Staphylococcus aureus* (penicillinase and non-penicillinase producing), *Escherichia coli, Klebsiella* species, *Haemophilus influenzae,* and *Bacteroides* species.

(2) **Urinary tract infections** caused by *Escherichia coli, Klebsiella* species, *Proteus mirabilis, Morganella morganii, Proteus vulgaris* and *Providencia* species (including *P. rettgeri*).

(3) **Intra-abdominal infections,** including peritonitis and intra-abdominal abscess, caused by *Escherichia coli, Klebsiella* species, *Bacteroides* species including the *Bacteroides fragilis* group[†], and *Clostridium* species.

(4) **Gynecological infections,** including endometritis, pelvic cellulitis, and pelvic inflammatory disease caused by *Escherichia coli, Neisseria gonorrhoeae* (penicillinase and non-penicillinase producing), *Bacteroides* species including *B. fragilis, Clostridium* species, *Peptococcus niger, Peptostreptococcus* species, and Group B streptococci. MEFOXIN, like cephalosporins, has no activity against *Chlamydia trachomatis.* Therefore, when MEFOXIN is used in the treatment of patients with pelvic inflammatory disease and *C. trachomatis* is one of the suspected pathogens, appropriate anti-chlamydial coverage should be added.

(5) **Septicemia** caused by *Streptococcus pneumoniae, Staphylococcus aureus* (penicillinase and non-penicillinase producing), *Escherichia coli, Klebsiella* species, and *Bacteroides* species including *B. fragilis.*

(6) **Bone and joint infections** caused by *Staphylococcus aureus* (penicillinase and non-penicillinase producing).

(7) **Skin and skin structure infections** caused by *Staphylococcus aureus* (penicillinase and non-penicillinase producing), *Staphylococcus epidermidis,* streptococci (excluding enterococci, e.g., *Enterococcus faecalis* [formerly *Streptococcus faecalis*]), *Escherichia coli, Proteus mirabilis, Klebsiella* species, *Bacteroides* species including *B. fragilis, Clostridium* species, *Peptococcus niger,* and *Peptostreptococcus* species.

Appropriate culture and susceptibility studies should be performed to determine the susceptibility of the causative organisms to MEFOXIN. Therapy may be started while awaiting the results of these studies.

In randomized comparative studies, cefoxitin and cephalothin were comparably safe and effective in the management of infections caused by gram-positive cocci and gram-negative rods susceptible to the cephalosporins. MEFOXIN has a high degree of stability in the presence of bacterial beta-lactamases, both penicillinases and cephalosporinases.

Many infections caused by aerobic and anaerobic gram-negative bacteria resistant to some cephalosporins respond to MEFOXIN. Similarly, many infections caused by aerobic and anaerobic bacteria resistant to some penicillin antibiotics (ampicillin, carbenicillin, penicillin G) respond to treatment with MEFOXIN. Many infections caused by mixtures of susceptible aerobic and anaerobic bacteria respond to treatment with MEFOXIN.

Prevention

MEFOXIN is indicated for the prophylaxis of infection in patients undergoing uncontaminated gastrointestinal surgery, vaginal hysterectomy, abdominal hysterectomy, or cesarean section.

If there are signs of infection, specimens for culture should be obtained for identification of the causative organism so that appropriate treatment may be instituted.

† *B. fragilis, B. distasonis, B. ovatus, B. thetaiotaomicron.*

CONTRAINDICATIONS

MEFOXIN is contraindicated in patients who have shown hypersensitivity to cefoxitin and the cephalosporin group of antibiotics.

WARNINGS

BEFORE THERAPY WITH 'MEFOXIN' IS INSTITUTED, CAREFUL INQUIRY SHOULD BE MADE TO DETERMINE WHETHER THE PATIENT HAS HAD PREVIOUS HYPERSENSITIVITY REACTIONS TO CEFOXITIN, CEPHALOSPORINS, PENICILLINS, OR OTHER DRUGS. THIS PRODUCT SHOULD BE GIVEN WITH CAUTION TO PENICILLIN-SENSITIVE PATIENTS. ANTIBIOTICS SHOULD BE ADMINISTERED WITH CAUTION TO ANY PATIENT WHO HAS DEMONSTRATED SOME FORM OF ALLERGY, PARTICULARLY TO DRUGS. IF AN ALLERGIC REACTION TO 'MEFOXIN' OCCURS, DISCONTINUE THE DRUG. SERIOUS HYPERSENSITIVITY REACTIONS MAY REQUIRE EPINEPHRINE AND OTHER EMERGENCY MEASURES.

Continued on next page

Information on the Merck & Co., Inc. products listed on these pages is the full prescribing information from product circulars in use September 30, 2000. For information, please call 1-800-NSC MERCK [1-800-672-6372].

Mefoxin Premixed—Cont.

Pseudomembranous colitis has been reported with nearly all antibacterial agents, including cefoxitin, and may range in severity from mild to life threatening. Therefore, it is important to consider this diagnosis in patients who present with diarrhea subsequent to the administration of antibacterial agents.

Treatment with antibacterial agents alters the normal flora of the colon and may permit overgrowth of clostridia. Studies indicate that a toxin produced by *Clostridium difficile* is one primary cause of "antibiotic-associated colitis."

After the diagnosis of pseudomembranous colitis has been established, appropriate therapeutic measures should be initiated. Mild cases of pseudomembranous colitis usually respond to drug discontinuation alone. In moderate to severe cases, consideration should be given to management with fluids and electrolytes, protein supplementation, and treatment with an antibacterial drug clinically effective against *Clostridium difficile* colitis.

PRECAUTIONS

General

The total daily dose should be reduced when MEFOXIN is administered to patients with transient or persistent reduction of urinary output due to renal insufficiency (see DOSAGE AND ADMINISTRATION, *TREATMENT*), because high and prolonged serum antibiotic concentrations can occur in such individuals from usual doses.

Antibiotics (including cephalosporins) should be prescribed with caution in individuals with a history of gastrointestinal disease, particularly colitis.

As with other antibiotics, prolonged use of MEFOXIN may result in overgrowth of nonsusceptible organisms. Repeated evaluation of the patient's condition is essential. If superinfection occurs during therapy, appropriate measures should be taken.

Do not use unless solution is clear and seal is intact.

Laboratory Tests

As with any potent antibacterial agent, periodic assessment of organ system functions, including renal, hepatic, and hematopoietic, is advisable during prolonged therapy.

Drug Interactions

Increased nephrotoxicity has been reported following concomitant administration of cephalosporins and aminoglycoside antibiotics.

Drug/Laboratory Test Interactions

As with cephalothin, high concentrations of cefoxitin (>100 micrograms/mL) may interfere with measurement of serum and urine creatinine levels by the Jaffé reaction, and produce false increases of modest degree in the levels of creatinine reported. Serum samples from patients treated with cefoxitin should not be analyzed for creatinine if withdrawn within 2 hours of drug administration.

High concentrations of cefoxitin in the urine may interfere with measurement of urinary 17-hydroxy-corticosteroids by the Porter-Silber reaction, and produce false increases of modest degree in the levels reported.

A false-positive reaction for glucose in the urine may occur. This has been observed with CLINITEST[††] reagent tablets.

[††]Registered trademark of Ames Company, Division of Miles Laboratories, Inc.

Carcinogenesis, Mutagenesis, Impairment of Fertility

Long term studies in animals have not been performed with cefoxitin to evaluate carcinogenic or mutagenic potential. Studies in rats treated intravenously with 400 mg/kg of cefoxitin (approximately three times the maximum recommended human dose) revealed no effects on fertility or mating ability.

Pregnancy

Pregnancy Category B. Reproduction studies performed in rats and mice at parenteral doses of approximately one to seven and one-half times the maximum recommended human dose did not reveal teratogenic or fetal toxic effects, although a slight decrease in fetal weight was observed.

There are, however, no adequate and well-controlled studies in pregnant women. Because animal reproduction studies are not always predictive of human response, this drug should be used during pregnancy only if clearly needed.

In the rabbit, cefoxitin was associated with a high incidence of abortion and maternal death. This was not considered to be a teratogenic effect but an expected consequence of the rabbit's unusual sensitivity to antibiotic-induced changes in the population of the microflora of the intestine.

Nursing Mothers

Cefoxitin is excreted in human milk in low concentrations. Caution should be exercised when MEFOXIN is administered to a nursing woman.

Pediatric Use

Safety and efficacy in pediatric patients from birth to three months of age have not yet been established. In pediatric patients three months of age and older, higher doses of cefoxitin have been associated with an increased incidence of eosinophilia and elevated SGOT.

The potential for toxic effects in pediatric patients from chemicals that may leach from the single-dose I.V. preparation in plastic has not been determined.

ADVERSE REACTIONS

Cefoxitin is generally well tolerated. The most common adverse reactions have been local reactions following intravenous injection. Other adverse reactions have been encountered infrequently.

Table 1—Guidelines for Dosage of MEFOXIN

Type of Infection	Daily Dosage	Frequency and Route
Uncomplicated forms‡ of infections such as pneumonia, urinary tract infection, cutaneous infection	3–4 grams	1 gram every 6–8 hours IV
Moderately severe or severe infections	6–8 grams	1 gram every 4 hours *or* 2 grams every 6–8 hours IV
Infections commonly needing antibiotics in higher dosage (e.g., gas gangrene)	12 grams	2 grams every 4 hours *or* 3 grams every 6 hours IV

‡ Including patients in whom bacteremia is absent or unlikely.

Table 2—Maintenance Dosage of MEFOXIN in Adults with Reduced Renal Function

Renal Function	Creatinine Clearance (mL/min)	Dose (grams)	Frequency
Mild impairment	50–30	1–2	every 8–12 hours
Moderate impairment	29–10	1–2	every 12–24 hours
Severe impairment	9–5	0.5–1	every 12–24 hours
Essentially no function	<5	0.5–1	every 24–48 hours

Local Reactions

Thrombophlebitis has occurred with intravenous administration.

Allergic Reactions

Rash (including exfoliative dermatitis and toxic epidermal necrolysis), pruritus, eosinophilia, fever, dyspnea, and other allergic reactions including anaphylaxis, interstitial nephritis and angioedema have been noted.

Cardiovascular

Hypotension

Gastrointestinal

Diarrhea, including documented pseudomembranous colitis which can appear during or after antibiotic treatment. Nausea and vomiting have been reported rarely.

Neuromuscular

Possible exacerbation of myasthenia gravis.

Blood

Eosinophilia, leukopenia including granulocytopenia, neutropenia, anemia, including hemolytic anemia, thrombocytopenia, and bone marrow depression. A positive direct Coombs test may develop in some individuals, especially those with azotemia.

Liver Function

Transient elevations in SGOT, SGPT, serum LDH, and serum alkaline phosphatase; and jaundice have been reported.

Renal Function

Elevations in serum creatinine and/or blood urea nitrogen levels have been observed. As with the cephalosporins, acute renal failure has been reported rarely. The role of MEFOXIN in changes in renal function tests is difficult to assess, since factors predisposing to prerenal azotemia or to impaired renal function usually have been present.

In addition to the adverse reactions listed above which have been observed in patients treated with MEFOXIN, the following adverse reactions and altered laboratory test results have been reported for cephalosporin class antibiotics: Urticaria, erythema multiforme, Stevens-Johnson syndrome, serum sickness-like reactions, abdominal pain, colitis, renal dysfunction, toxic nephropathy, false-positive test for urinary glucose, hepatic dysfunction including cholestasis, elevated bilirubin, aplastic anemia, hemorrhage, prolonged prothrombin time, pancytopenia, agranulocytosis, superinfection, vaginitis including vaginal candidiasis.

Several cephalosporins have been implicated in triggering seizures, particularly in patients with renal impairment when the dosage was not reduced. (See DOSAGE AND ADMINISTRATION.) If seizures associated with drug therapy occur, the drug should be discontinued. Anticonvulsant therapy can be given if clinically indicated.

OVERDOSAGE

The acute intravenous LD_{50} in the adult female mouse and rabbit was about 8.0 g/kg and greater than 1.0 g/kg respectively. The acute intraperitoneal LD_{50} in the adult rat was greater than 10.0 g/kg.

DOSAGE AND ADMINISTRATION

NOTE: MEFOXIN® in Galaxy[†††] container is for intravenous infusion only.

TREATMENT

Adults

The usual adult dosage range is 1 gram to 2 grams every six to eight hours. Dosage should be determined by susceptibility of the causative organisms, severity of infection, and the condition of the patient (see Table 1 for dosage guidelines).

If *C. trachomatis* is a suspected pathogen, appropriate antichlamydial coverage should be added, because cefoxitin sodium has no activity against this organism.

MEFOXIN may be used in patients with reduced renal function with the following dosage adjustments:

In adults with renal insufficiency, an initial loading dose of 1 gram to 2 grams may be given. After a loading dose, the recommendations for *maintenance dosage* (Table 2) may be used as a guide.

When only the serum creatinine level is available, the following formula (based on sex, weight, and age of the patient) may be used to convert this value into creatinine clearance. The serum creatinine should represent a steady state of renal function.

$$\text{Males: } \frac{\text{Weight (kg)} \times (140 - \text{age})}{72 \times \text{serum creatinine (mg/100 mL)}}$$

$$\text{Females: } 0.85 \times \text{male value}$$

In patients undergoing hemodialysis, the loading dose of 1 to 2 grams should be given after each hemodialysis, and the maintenance dose should be given as indicated in Table 2.

Antibiotic therapy for group A beta-hemolytic streptococcal infections should be maintained for at least 10 days to guard against the risk of rheumatic fever or glomerulonephritis. In staphylococcal and other infections involving a collection of pus, surgical drainage should be carried out where indicated.

Pediatric Patients

The recommended dosage in pediatric patients three months of age and older is 80 to 160 mg/kg of body weight per day divided into four to six equal doses. The higher dosages should be used for more severe or serious infections. The total daily dosage should not exceed 12 grams.

At this time no recommendation is made for pediatric patients from birth to three months of age (see PRECAUTIONS).

In pediatric patients with renal insufficiency, the dosage and frequency of dosage should be modified consistent with the recommendations for adults (see Table 2).

PREVENTION

Effective prophylatic use depends on the time of administration. MEFOXIN usually should be given one-half to one hour before the operation, which is sufficient time to achieve effective levels in the wound during the procedure. Prophylactic administration should usually be stopped within 24 hours since continuing administration of any antibiotic increases the possibility of adverse reactions but, in the majority of surgical procedures, does not reduce the incidence of subsequent infection.

For prophylactic use in uncontaminated gastrointestinal surgery, vaginal hysterectomy, or abdominal hysterectomy, the following doses are recommended:

Adults:

2 grams administered intravenously just prior to surgery (approximately one-half to one hour before the initial incision) followed by 2 grams every 6 hours after the first dose for no more than 24 hours.

Pediatric Patients (3 months and older):

30 to 40 mg/kg doses may be given at the times designated above.

Cesarean section patients:

For patients undergoing cesarean section, either a single 2 gram dose administered intravenously as soon as the umbilical cord is clamped OR a 3-dose regimen consisting of 2 grams given intravenously as soon as the umbilical cord is clamped followed by 2 grams 4 and 8 hours after the initial dose is recommended. (See CLINICAL STUDIES.)

[See tables 1 & 2 above]

ADMINISTRATION

This premixed solution is for intravenous use only. Premixed Intravenous Solution MEFOXIN in Galaxy® containers (PL 2040 Plastic) is to be administered either as a continuous or intermittent infusion using sterile equipment. Scalp vein-type needles are preferred for this type of infusion. It is recommended that the intravenous administration apparatus be replaced at least once every 48 hours.

The intravenous route is preferred for patients with bacteremia, bacterial septicemia, or other severe or life-threatening infections, or for patients who may be poor risks because of lowered resistance resulting from such debilitating conditions as malnutrition, trauma, surgery, diabetes, heart failure, or malignancy, particularly if shock is present or impending.

Directions for Use of Galaxy® Containers (PL 2040 Plastic)
Thaw frozen container at room temperature, 25°C (77°F), or under refrigeration, 2–8°C (36–46°F). DO NOT FORCE THAW BY IMMERSION IN WATER BATHS OR BY MICROWAVE IRRADIATION.
After thawing, check for minute leaks by squeezing container firmly. If leaks are detected, discard solution as sterility may be impaired.
The container should be visually inspected for particulate matter and discoloration prior to administration. Components of the solution may precipitate in the frozen state and will dissolve upon reaching room temperature with little or no agitation. Agitate after solution has reached room temperature.
Do not use if the solution is cloudy or a precipitate has formed. If any seals or outlet ports are not intact, the container should be discarded. Solutions of MEFOXIN tend to darken depending on storage conditions; product potency, however, is not adversely affected.
Additives should not be introduced into this solution.
CAUTION: Do not use plastic containers in series connections. Such use would result in air embolism due to residual air being drawn from the primary container before administration of the fluid from the secondary container is complete.
Preparation for Intravenous Administration:
1. Suspend container from eyelet support.
2. Remove plastic protector from outlet port at bottom of container.
3. Attach administration set. Refer to complete directions accompanying set.

MEFOXIN may be administered through the tubing system by which the patient may be receiving other intravenous solutions. However, during infusion of the solution containing MEFOXIN, it is advisable to temporarily discontinue administration of any other solutions at the same site.
Solutions of MEFOXIN, like those of most beta-lactam antibiotics, should not be added to aminoglycoside solutions (e.g., gentamicin sulfate, tobramycin sulfate, amikacin sulfate) because of potential interaction. However, MEFOXIN and aminoglycosides may be administered separately to the same patient.
STABILITY
MEFOXIN, supplied as frozen, premixed, iso-osmotic solution in Galaxy® containers (PL 2040 Plastic), maintains satisfactory potency after thawing for 24 hours at a room temperature of 25°C (77°F) or 21 days under refrigeration, 2–8°C (36–46°F). After these periods, any unused solutions should be discarded.
DO NOT REFREEZE.

†††Galaxy® is a registered trademark of Baxter International Inc.

HOW SUPPLIED

Premixed Intravenous Solution MEFOXIN is supplied in single dose Galaxy® containers (PL 2040 Plastic) containing cefoxitin sodium as follows:
No. 2G3506—1 gram cefoxitin equivalent, iso-osmotic in 50 mL diluent containing approximately 2 grams dextrose hydrous USP
NDC 0006-3545-24 in boxes of 24
(6505-01-380-3410, 1 g 24's).
No. 2G3507—2 gram cefoxitin equivalent, iso-osmotic in 50 mL diluent containing approximately 1.1 grams dextrose hydrous USP
NDC 0006-3547-25 in boxes of 24
(6505-01-379-9245, 2 g 24's).
Special storage instructions
Store at or below −20°C (−4°F). [See Directions for Use of Galaxy® container (PL 2040 Plastic)].
MEFOXIN is also available in dry powder form in vials and infusion bottles containing sterile cefoxitin sodium equivalent to either 1 gram or 2 grams of cefoxitin, and in vials for pharmacy bulk use containing sterile cefoxitin sodium equivalent to 10 grams of cefoxitin, for constitution and intravenous administration (see appropriate product circular).

CLINICAL STUDIES

A prospective, randomized, double-blind, placebo-controlled clinical trial was conducted to determine the efficacy of short-term prophylaxis with MEFOXIN in patients undergoing cesarean section who were at high risk for subsequent endometritis because of ruptured membranes. Patients were randomized to receive either three doses of placebo (n=58), a single dose of MEFOXIN (2 g) followed by two doses of placebo (n=64), or a three-dose regimen of MEFOXIN (each dose consisting of 2 g) (n=60), given intravenously, usually beginning at the time of clamping of the umbilical cord, with the second and third doses given 4 and 8 hours post-operatively. Endometritis occurred in 16/58 (27.6%) patients given placebo, 5/63 (7.9%) patients given a single dose of MEFOXIN, and 3/58 (5.2%) patients given three doses of MEFOXIN. The differences between the two groups treated with MEFOXIN and placebo with respect to endometritis were statistically significant ($p<0.01$) in favor of MEFOXIN. The differences between the one-dose and three-dose regimens of MEFOXIN were not statistically significant.
Two double-blind, randomized studies compared the efficacy of a single 2 gram intravenous dose of MEFOXIN to a single 2 gram dose of cefotetan in the prevention of surgical site-related infection (major morbidity) and non-site-related infections (minor morbidity) in patients following cesarean section. In the first study, 82/98 (83.7%) patients treated with MEFOXIN and 71/95 (74.7%) patients treated with cefotetan experienced no major or minor morbidity. The difference in the outcomes in this study (95% CI: −0.03, +0.21) was not statistically significant. In the second study, 65/75 (86.7%) patients treated with MEFOXIN and 62/76 (81.6%) patients treated with cefotetan experienced no major or minor morbidity. The difference in the outcomes in this study (95% CI: −0.08, +0.18) was not statistically significant.
In clinical trials of patients with intra-abdominal infections due to *Bacteroides fragilis* group microorganisms, eradication rates at 1 to 2 weeks posttreatment for isolates were in the range of 70% to 80%. Eradication rates for individual species are listed below:

Bacteroides distasonis	7/10	(70%)
Bacteroides fragilis	26/33	(79%)
Bacteroides ovatus	10/13	(77%)
B. thetaiotaomicron	13/18	(72%)

Manufactured for:
MERCK & CO., INC., WEST POINT, PA 19486, USA
By:
BAXTER HEALTHCARE CORPORATION
Deerfield, Illinois 60015, USA
7948521 Issued October 1996

MEPHYTON® Tablets ℞
(Phytonadione)
Vitamin K_1

DESCRIPTION

Phytonadione is a vitamin which is a clear, yellow to amber, viscous, and nearly odorless liquid. It is insoluble in water, soluble in chloroform and slightly soluble in ethanol. It has a molecular weight of 450.70.
Phytonadione is 2-methyl-3-phytyl-1, 4-naphthoquinone. Its empirical formula is $C_{31}H_{46}O_2$ and its structural formula is:

MEPHYTON* (Phytonadione) tablets containing 5 mg of phytonadione are yellow, compressed tablets, scored on one side. Inactive ingredients are acacia, calcium phosphate, colloidal silicon dioxide, lactose, magnesium stearate, starch, and talc.

*Registered trademark of MERCK & CO., INC.

CLINICAL PHARMACOLOGY

MEPHYTON tablets possess the same type and degree of activity as does naturally-occurring vitamin K, which is necessary for the production via the liver of active prothrombin (factor II), proconvertin (factor VII), plasma thromboplastin component (factor IX), and Stuart factor (factor X). The prothrombin test is sensitive to the levels of three of these four factors—II, VII, and X. Vitamin K is an essential cofactor for a microsomal enzyme that catalyzes the post-translational carboxylation of multiple, specific, peptide-bound glutamic acid residues in inactive hepatic precursors of factors II, VII, IX, and X. The resulting gamma-carboxyglutamic acid residues convert the precursors into active coagulation factors that are subsequently secreted by liver cells into the blood.
Oral phytonadione is adequately absorbed from the gastrointestinal tract only if bile salts are present. After absorption, phytonadione is initially concentrated in the liver, but the concentration declines rapidly. Very little vitamin K accumulates in tissues. Little is known about the metabolic fate of vitamin K. Almost no free unmetabolized vitamin K appears in bile or urine.
In normal animals and humans, phytonadione is virtually devoid of pharmacodynamic activity. However, in animals and humans deficient in vitamin K, the pharmacological action of vitamin K is related to its normal physiological function; that is, to promote the hepatic biosynthesis of vitamin K-dependent clotting factors.
MEPHYTON tablets generally exert their effect within 6 to 10 hours.

INDICATIONS AND USAGE

MEPHYTON is indicated in the following coagulation disorders which are due to faulty formation of factors II, VII, IX and X when caused by vitamin K deficiency or interference with vitamin K activity.
MEPHYTON tablets are indicated in:
— anticoagulant-induced prothrombin deficiency caused by coumarin or indanedione derivatives;
— hypoprothrombinemia secondary to antibacterial therapy;
— hypoprothrombinemia secondary to administration of salicylates;
— hypoprothrombinemia secondary to obstructive jaundice or biliary fistulas but only if bile salts are administered concurrently, since otherwise the oral vitamin K will not be absorbed.

CONTRAINDICATION

Hypersensitivity to any component of this medication.

WARNINGS

An immediate coagulant effect should not be expected after administration of phytonadione.
Phytonadione will not counteract the anticoagulant action of heparin.
When vitamin K_1 is used to correct excessive anticoagulant-induced hypoprothrombinemia, anticoagulant therapy still being indicated, the patient is again faced with the clotting hazards existing prior to starting the anticoagulant therapy. Phytonadione is not a clotting agent, but overzealous therapy with vitamin K_1 may restore conditions which originally permitted thromboembolic phenomena. Dosage should be kept as low as possible, and prothrombin time should be checked regularly as clinical conditions indicate.
Repeated large doses of vitamin K are not warranted in liver disease if the response to initial use of the vitamin is unsatisfactory. Failure to respond to vitamin K may indicate a congenital coagulation defect or that the condition being treated is unresponsive to vitamin K.

PRECAUTIONS

General
Temporary resistance to prothrombin-depressing anticoagulants may result, especially when larger doses of phytonadione are used. If relatively large doses have been employed, it may be necessary when reinstituting anticoagulant therapy to use somewhat larger doses of the prothrombin-depressing anticoagulant, or to use one which acts on a different principle, such as heparin sodium.
Laboratory Tests
Prothrombin time should be checked regularly as clinical conditions indicate.
Carcinogenesis, Mutagenesis, Impairment of Fertility
Studies of carcinogenicity or impairment of fertility have not been performed with MEPHYTON. MEPHYTON at concentrations up to 2000 mcg/plate with or without metabolic activation, was negative in the Ames microbial mutagen test.
Pregnancy
Pregnancy Category C: Animal reproduction studies have not been conducted with MEPHYTON. It is also not known whether MEPHYTON can cause fetal harm when administered to a pregnant woman or can affect reproduction capacity. MEPHYTON should be given to a pregnant woman only if clearly needed.
Pediatric Use
Safety and effectiveness in pediatric patients have not been established with MEPHYTON. Hemolysis, jaundice, and hyperbilirubinemia in newborns, particularly in premature infants, have been reported with vitamin K.
Nursing Mothers
It is not known whether this drug is excreted in human milk. Because many drugs are excreted in human milk, caution should be exercised when MEPHYTON is administered to a nursing woman.

ADVERSE REACTIONS

Transient "flushing sensations" and "peculiar" sensations of taste have been observed with parenteral phytonadione, as well as rare instances of dizziness, rapid and weak pulse, profuse sweating, brief hypotension, dyspnea, and cyanosis. Hyperbilirubinemia has been observed in the newborn following administration of parenteral phytonadione. This has occurred rarely and primarily with doses above those recommended.

OVERDOSAGE

The intravenous and oral LD_{50}s in the mouse are approximately 1.17 g/kg and greater than 24.18 g/kg, respectively.

Continued on next page

Information on the Merck & Co., Inc. products listed on these pages is the full prescribing information from product circulars in use September 30, 2000. For information, please call 1-800-NSC MERCK [1-800-672-6372].

Mephyton—Cont.

DOSAGE AND ADMINISTRATION

MEPHYTON
Summary of Dosage Guidelines
(See circular text for details)

Adults	Initial Dosage
Anticoagulant-Induced Prothrombin Deficiency (caused by coumarin or indanedione derivatives)	2.5 mg–10 mg or up to 25 mg (rarely 50 mg)
Hypoprothrombinemia due to other causes (Antibiotics; Salicylates or other drugs; Factors limiting absorption or synthesis)	2.5 mg–25 mg or more (rarely up to 50 mg)

Anticoagulant-Induced Prothrombin Deficiency in Adults
To correct excessively prolonged prothrombin times caused by oral anticoagulant therapy—2.5 to 10 mg or up to 25 mg initially is recommended. In rare instances 50 mg may be required. Frequency and amount of subsequent doses should be determined by prothrombin time response or clinical condition. (See WARNINGS.) If, in 12 to 48 hours after oral administration, the prothrombin time has not been shortened satisfactorily, the dose should be repeated.
Hypoprothrombinemia Due to Other Causes in Adults
If possible, discontinuation or reduction of the dosage of drugs interfering with coagulation mechanisms (such as salicylates, antibiotics) is suggested as an alternative to administering concurrent MEPHYTON. The severity of the coagulation disorder should determine whether the immediate administration of MEPHYTON is required in addition to discontinuation or reduction of interfering drugs.
A dosage of 2.5 to 25 mg or more (rarely up to 50 mg) is recommended, the amount and route of administration depending upon the severity of the condition and response obtained.
The oral route should be avoided when the clinical disorder would prevent proper absorption. Bile salts must be given with the tablets when the endogenous supply of bile to the gastrointestinal tract is deficient.

HOW SUPPLIED

No. 7776—Tablets MEPHYTON, 5 mg vitamin K_1, are yellow, round, scored, compressed tablets, coded MSD 43 on one side and MEPHYTON on the other. They are supplied as follows:
NDC 0006-0043-68 bottles of 100
(6505-00-660-0460, 5 mg 100's).
Shown in Product Identification Guide, page 324
Storage:
Store in a tightly closed container at 25°C (77°F); excursions permitted to 15–30°C (59–86°F) [See USP Controlled Room Temperature]. Protect from light. Store container in carton until contents have been used.
7918716 Issued August 1998

MERUVAX®$_{II}$ ℞
(Rubella Virus Vaccine Live)
Wistar RA 27/3 Strain

DESCRIPTION

MERUVAX* II (Rubella Virus Vaccine Live) is a live virus vaccine for vaccination against rubella (German measles).
MERUVAX II is a sterile lyophilized preparation of the Wistar Institute RA 27/3 strain of live attenuated rubella virus. The virus was adapted to and propagated in WI-38 human diploid lung fibroblasts.
The growth medium is Minimum Essential Medium (MEM) [a buffered salt solution containing vitamins and amino acids and supplemented with fetal bovine serum] containing human serum albumin and neomycin. Sorbitol and hydrolyzed gelatin stabilizer is added to the individual virus harvests.
The cells, virus pools, fetal bovine serum, and human albumin are all screened for the absence of adventitious agents. Human albumin is processed using the Cohn cold ethanol fractionation procedure.
The reconstituted vaccine is for subcutaneous administration. Each 0.5 mL dose contains not less than 1,000 $TCID_{50}$ (tissue culture infectious doses) of rubella virus. Each dose of the vaccine is calculated to contain sorbitol (14.5 mg), sodium phosphate, sucrose (1.9 mg), sodium chloride, hydrolyzed gelatin (14.5 mg), human albumin (0.3 mg), fetal bovine serum (<1 ppm), other buffer and media ingredients and approximately 25 mcg of neomycin. The product contains no preservative.
Before reconstitution, the lyophilized vaccine is a light yellow compact crystalline plug. MERUVAX II, when reconstituted as directed, is clear yellow.

---
* Registered trademark of MERCK & CO., Inc.

CLINICAL PHARMACOLOGY

Rubella is a common childhood disease, caused by rubella virus (togavirus), that may be associated with serious complications and/or death. For example, rubella during pregnancy may cause congenital rubella syndrome in the infants of infected mothers.
The impact of measles, mumps, and rubella vaccination on the natural history of each disease in the United States can be quantified by comparing the maximum number of rubella cases reported in a given year prior to vaccine use to the number of cases of each disease reported in 1995. For rubella, 57,686 cases reported in 1969 compared to 200 cases reported in 1995 resulted in a 99.65% decrease.
Extensive clinical trials of rubella virus vaccines, prepared using RA 27/3 strain rubella virus, have been carried out in more than 28,000 human subjects (approximately 11,000 with MERUVAX II) in the U.S.A. and more than 20 additional countries. A single injection of the vaccine has been shown to induce rubella hemagglutination-inhibition (HI) antibodies in 97% or more of susceptible persons. However, a small percentage (1–5%) of vaccinees may fail to seroconvert after the primary dose (see also INDICATIONS AND USAGE, *Recommended Vaccination Schedule).*
Efficacy of rubella vaccine was established in a series of double-blind controlled field trials which demonstrated a high degree of protective efficacy. These studies also established that seroconversion in response to rubella vaccination paralleled protection from this disease.
Following vaccination, antibodies associated with protection can be measured by neutralization assays, HI, or ELISA (enzyme linked immunosorbent assay) tests. Neutralizing and ELISA antibodies to rubella virus are still detectable in most individuals 11–13 years after primary vaccination. See INDICATIONS AND USAGE, *Non-Pregnant Adolescents and Adult Females*, for Rubella Susceptibility Testing.
The RA 27/3 rubella strain elicits higher immediate postvaccination HI, complement-fixing and neutralizing antibody levels than other strains of rubella vaccine and has been shown to induce a broader profile of circulating antibodies including anti-theta and anti-iota precipitating antibodies. The RA 27/3 rubella strain immunologically simulates natural infection more closely than other rubella vaccine viruses. The increased levels and broader profile of antibodies produced by RA 27/3 strain rubella virus vaccine appear to correlate with greater resistance to subclinical reinfection with the wild virus, and provide greater confidence for lasting immunity.

INDICATIONS AND USAGE

Recommended Vaccination Schedule
MERUVAX II is indicated for vaccination against rubella in persons 12 months of age or older.
It is not recommended for infants younger than 12 months because they may retain maternal rubella neutralizing antibodies that may interfere with the immune response.
Children in kindergarten and the first grades of elementary school deserve priority for vaccination because often they are epidemiologically the major source of virus dissemination in the community. A history of rubella illness is usually not reliable enough to exclude children from immunization.
Previously unimmunized children of susceptible pregnant women should receive live attenuated rubella vaccine, because an immunized child will be less likely to acquire natural rubella and introduce the virus into the household.
Individuals first vaccinated with MERUVAX II at 12 months of age or older should be revaccinated with M-M-R* II (Measles, Mumps, and Rubella Virus Vaccine Live) prior to elementary school entry. Revaccination may seroconvert primary failures or boost antibody titers of those individuals whose titers have declined. The Advisory Committee on Immunization Practices (ACIP) recommends administration of the first dose of M-M-R II at 12–15 months of age and administration of the second dose of M-M-R II at 4–6 years of age. In addition, some public health jurisdictions mandate the age for revaccination. Consult the complete text of applicable guidelines regarding routine revaccination including that of high-risk adult populations.
Unnecessary doses of a vaccine are best avoided by ensuring that written documentation of vaccination is preserved and a copy given to each vaccinee's parent or guardian.
Other Vaccination Considerations
Adolescent and Adult Males
Vaccination of adolescent or adult males may be a useful procedure in preventing or controlling outbreaks of rubella in circumscribed population groups (e.g., military bases and schools).
Non-Pregnant Adolescent and Adult Females
Immunization of susceptible non-pregnant adolescent and adult females of childbearing age with live attenuated rubella virus vaccine is indicated if certain precautions are observed (see below and PRECAUTIONS). Vaccinating susceptible postpubertal females confers individual protection against subsequently acquiring rubella infection during pregnancy, which in turn prevents infection of the fetus and consequent congenital rubella injury.
Women of childbearing age should be advised not to become pregnant for 3 months after vaccination and should be informed of the reason for this precaution.**
The ACIP has stated "If it is practical and if reliable laboratory services are available, women of childbearing age who are potential candidates for vaccination can have serologic tests to determine susceptibility to rubella. However, with the exception of premarital and prenatal screening, routinely performing serologic tests for all women of childbearing age to determine susceptibility (so that vaccine is given only to proven susceptible women) can be effective but is expensive. Also, 2 visits to the health-care provider would be necessary—one for screening and one for vaccination. Accordingly, rubella vaccination of a woman who is not known to be pregnant and has no history of vaccination is justifiable without serologic testing—and may be preferable, particularly when costs of serology are high and follow-up of identified susceptible women for vaccination is not assured."
Postpubertal females should be informed of the frequent occurrence of generally self-limited arthralgia and/or arthritis beginning 2 to 4 weeks after vaccination (see ADVERSE REACTIONS).
Other Populations
Previously unvaccinated children in contact with susceptible pregnant women should receive live attenuated rubella vaccine (such as that contained in MERUVAX II) to reduce the risk of exposure of the pregnant woman.
Individuals planning travel outside the United States, if not immune, can acquire measles, mumps or rubella and import these diseases into the United States. Therefore, prior to international travel, individuals known to be susceptible to one or more of these diseases can receive either a monovalent vaccine (measles, mumps or rubella), or a combination vaccine as appropriate. However, M-M-R II is preferred for persons likely to be susceptible to mumps and rubella; and if monovalent measles vaccine is not readily available, travelers should receive M-M-R II regardless or their immune status to mumps or rubella.
Vaccination is recommended for susceptible individuals in high-risk groups such as college students, health-care workers, and military personnel.
Postpartum Women
It has been found convenient in many instances to vaccinate rubella-susceptible women in the immediate postpartum period (see PRECAUTIONS, *Nursing Mothers).*
Post-Exposure Vaccination
There is no conclusive evidence that vaccination of individuals recently exposed to natural rubella will provide protection. There is, however, no contraindication to vaccinating children already exposed to natural rubella.
Use With Other Vaccines
See DOSAGE AND ADMINISTRATION, *Use With Other Vaccines.*

** NOTE: The ACIP has recommended "In view of the importance of protecting this age group against rubella, reasonable practices in a rubella immunization program include a) asking women if they are pregnant, b) excluding those who say they are, c) explaining the concern about risk for the fetus to the others, and d) explaining the importance of not becoming pregnant during the 3 months following vaccination."

CONTRAINDICATIONS

Hypersensitivity to any component of the vaccine, including gelatin.
Do not give MERUVAX II to pregnant females; the possible effects of the vaccine on fetal development are unknown at this time. If vaccination of postpubertal females is undertaken, pregnancy should be avoided for three months following vaccination (see PRECAUTIONS, *Pregnancy).*
Anaphylactic or anaphylactoid reactions to neomycin (each dose of reconstituted vaccine contains approximately 25 mcg of neomycin).
Febrile respiratory illness or other active febrile infection. However, the ACIP has recommended that all vaccines can be administered to persons with minor illnesses such as diarrhea, mild upper respiratory infection with or without low-grade fever, or other low-grade febrile illness.
Patients receiving immunosuppressive therapy. This contraindication does not apply to patients who are receiving corticosteroids as replacement therapy, e.g., for Addison's disease.
Individuals with blood dyscrasias, leukemia, lymphomas of any type, or other malignant neoplasms affecting the bone marrow or lymphatic systems.
Primary and acquired immunodeficiency states, including patients who are immunosuppressed in association with AIDS or other clinical manifestations of infection with human immunodeficiency viruses; cellular immune deficiencies; and hypogammaglobulinemic and dysgammaglobulinemic states.
Individuals with a family history of congenital or hereditary immunodeficiency, until the immune competence of the potential vaccine recipient is demonstrated.

WARNINGS

The physician should be alert to the temperature elevation which may occur following vaccination (see ADVERSE REACTIONS).
Hypersensitivity to Neomycin
The AAP states, "Persons who have experienced anaphylactic reactions to topically or systemically administered neomycin should not receive measles vaccine. Most often, however, neomycin allergy manifests as a contact dermatitis, which is a delayed-type (cell-mediated) immune response rather than anaphylaxis. In such persons, an adverse reac-

tion to neomycin in the vaccine would be an erythematous, pruritic nodule or papule, 48 to 96 hours after vaccination. A history of contact dermatitis to neomycin is not a contraindication to receiving measles vaccine."

Thrombocytopenia

Individuals with current thrombocytopenia may develop more severe thrombocytopenia following vaccination. In addition, individuals who experienced thrombocytopenia with the first dose of M-M-R II (or its component vaccines) may develop thrombocytopenia with repeat doses. Serologic status may be evaluated to determine whether or not additional doses of vaccine are needed. The potential risk to benefit ratio should be carefully evaluated before considering vaccination in such cases (see ADVERSE REACTIONS).

PRECAUTIONS

General

Adequate treatment provisions including epinephrine injection (1:1000), should be available for immediate use should an anaphylactic or anaphylactoid reaction occur.

Special care should be taken to ensure that the injection does not enter a blood vessel.

Excretion of small amounts of the live attenuated rubella virus from the nose or throat has occurred in the majority of susceptible individuals 7–28 days after vaccination. There is no confirmed evidence to indicate that such virus is transmitted to susceptible persons who are in contact with the vaccinated individuals. Consequently, transmission through close personal contact, while accepted as a theoretical possibility, is not regarded as a significant risk. However, transmission of the vaccine virus to infants via breast milk has been documented (see *Nursing Mothers*).

Children and young adults who are known to be infected with human immunodeficiency viruses and are not immunosuppressed may be vaccinated. However, vaccinees who are infected with HIV should be monitored closely for vaccine-preventable diseases because immunization may be less effective than for uninfected persons (see CONTRAINDICATIONS).

Vaccination should be deferred for 3 months or longer following blood or plasma transfusions, or administration of immune globulin (human). However, susceptible postpartum patients who received blood products may receive MERUVAX II prior to discharge provided that a repeat HI titer is drawn 6–8 weeks after vaccination to insure seroconversion. Similarly, although studies with other live rubella virus vaccines suggest that MERUVAX II may be given in the immediate postpartum period to those nonimmune women who have received anti-Rho (D) globulin (human) without interfering with vaccine effectiveness, a follow-up post-vaccination HI titer should also be determined.

It has been reported that attenuated rubella virus vaccine, live, may result in a temporary depression of tuberculin skin sensitivity. Therefore, if a tuberculin test is to be done, it should be administered either before or simultaneously with MERUVAX II.

Individuals with active untreated tuberculosis should not be vaccinated.

As for any vaccine, vaccination with MERUVAX II may not result in protection in 100% of vaccinees.

The health-care provider should determine the current health status and previous vaccination history of the vaccinee.

The health-care provider should question the patient, parent, or guardian about reactions to a previous dose of MERUVAX II or other measles-, mumps-, or rubella-containing vaccines.

Information For Patients

The health-care provider should provide the vaccine information required to be given with each vaccination to the patient, parent or guardian.

The health-care provider should inform the patient, parent or guardian of the benefits and risks associated with vaccination. For risks associated with vaccination see WARNINGS, PRECAUTIONS, ADVERSE REACTIONS.

Patients, parents or guardians should be instructed to report any serious adverse reactions to their health-care provider who in turn should report such events to the U.S. Department of Health and Human Services through the Vaccine Adverse Event Reporting System (VAERS), 1-800-822-7967.

Pregnancy should be avoided for three months following vaccination.

Laboratory Tests

See INDICATIONS AND USAGE, *Non-Pregnant Adolescents and Adult Females*, for Rubella Susceptibility Testing, and CLINICAL PHARMACOLOGY.

Immunosuppressive Therapy

The immune status of patients about to undergo immunosuppressive therapy should be evaluated so that the physician can consider whether vaccination prior to the initiation of treatment is indicated. (see CONTRAINDICATIONS and PRECAUTIONS).

The ACIP has stated that "patients with leukemia in remission who have not received chemotherapy for at least 3 months may receive live-virus vaccines. Short-term (<2 weeks), low- to moderate-dose systemic corticosteroid therapy, topical steroid therapy (e.g., nasal, skin), long-term alternate-day treatment with low to moderate doses of short-acting systemic steroid, and intra-articular, bursal, or tendon injection of corticosteroids are not immunosuppressive in their usual doses and do not contraindicate the administration of rubella vaccine."

Immune Globulin

Administration of immune globulins concurrently with MERUVAX II may interfere with the expected immune response.

See also PRECAUTIONS, *General*.

Carcinogenesis, Mutagenesis, Impairment of Fertility

MERUVAX II has not been evaluated for carcinogenic or mutagenic potential, or potential to impair fertility.

Pregnancy

Pregnancy Category C

Animal reproduction studies have not been conducted with MERUVAX II. It is also not known whether MERUVAX II can cause fetal harm when administered to a pregnant woman or can affect reproduction capacity. There is evidence suggesting transmission of rubella vaccine viruses to products of conception. Therefore, rubella vaccine should not be administered to pregnant females (see CONTRAINDICATIONS).

In counseling women who are inadvertently vaccinated when pregnant or who become pregnant within 3 months of vaccination, the physician should be aware of the following: In a 10 year survey involving over 700 pregnant women who received rubella vaccine within 3 months before or after conception, (of whom 189 received the Wistar RA 27/3 strain) none of the newborns had abnormalities compatible with congenital rubella syndrome.

Nursing Mothers

Recent studies have shown that lactating postpartum women immunized with live attenuated rubella vaccine may secrete the virus in breast milk and transmit it to breast-fed infants. In the infants with serological evidence of rubella infection, none exhibited severe disease; however, one exhibited mild clinical illness typical of acquired rubella. Caution should be exercised when MERUVAX II is administered to a nursing woman.

Pediatric Use

Safety and effectiveness in infants below the age of 12 months have not been established (see INDICATIONS AND USAGE, *Recommended Vaccination Schedule*).

ADVERSE REACTIONS

The following adverse reactions are listed in decreasing order of severity, without regard to causality, within each body system category and have been reported during clinical trials, with use of the marketed vaccine, or with use of polyvalent vaccine containing rubella:

Body as a Whole

Fever; syncope; headache; dizziness; malaise; irritability.

Cardiovascular System

Vasculitis.

Digestive System

Diarrhea; vomiting; nausea.

Hemic and Lymphatic System

Thrombocytopenia (see WARNINGS, *Thrombocytopenia*); purpura; regional lymphadenopathy; leukocytosis.

Immune System

Anaphylaxis and anaphylactoid reactions have been reported as well as related phenomena such as angioneurotic edema (including peripheral or facial edema) and bronchial spasm.

Musculoskeletal System

Arthritis; arthralgia; myalgia.

Chronic arthritis has been associated with natural rubella infection and has been related to persistent virus and/or viral antigen isolated from body tissues. Only rarely have vaccine recipients developed chronic joint symptoms.

Following vaccination in children, reactions in joints are uncommon and generally of brief duration. In women, incidence rates for arthritis and arthralgia are generally higher than those seen in children (children: 0–3%; women: 12–26%) and the reactions tend to be more marked and of longer duration. Symptoms may persist for a matter of months or on rare occasions for years. In adolescent girls, the reactions appear to be intermediate in incidence between those seen in children and in adult women. Even in women older than 35 years, these reactions are generally well tolerated and rarely interfere with normal activities.

Myalgia and paresthesia have been reported rarely after administration of MERUVAX II.

Nervous System

Encephalitis; Guillain-Barré Syndrome (GBS); polyneuritis; polyneuropathy; paresthesia.

Respiratory System

Sore throat; cough; rhinitis.

Skin

Stevens-Johnson Syndrome; erythema multiforme; urticaria; rash.

Local reactions including burning/stinging at injection site; wheal and flare; redness (erythema); pain; induration.

Special Senses–Ear

Nerve deafness; otitis media.

Special Senses–Eye

Optic neuritis; papillitis; retrobulbar neuritis; conjunctivitis.

Other

Death from various, and in some cases unknown, causes has been reported rarely following vaccination with measles, mumps, and rubella vaccines; however, a causal relationship has not been established. No deaths or permanent sequelae were reported in a published post-marketing surveillance study in Finland involving 1.5 million children and adults who were vaccinated with M-M-R II during 1982–1993.

Under the National Childhood Vaccine Injury Act of 1986, health-care providers and manufacturers are required to record and report certain suspected adverse events occurring within specific time periods after vaccination. However, the U.S. Department of Health and Human Services (DHHS) has established a Vaccine Adverse Event Reporting System (VAERS) which will accept all reports of suspected events. A VAERS report form as well as information regarding reporting requirements can be obtained by calling VAERS 1-800-822-7967.

DOSAGE AND ADMINISTRATION

FOR SUBCUTANEOUS ADMINISTRATION

Do not inject intravenously

The dose for any age is 0.5 mL administered subcutaneously, preferably into the outer aspect of the upper arm.

The recommended age for primary vaccination is 12 to 15 months.

Revaccination with M-M-R II is recommended prior to elementary school entry. See also INDICATIONS AND USAGE, *Recommended Vaccination Schedule*.

Immune Globulin (IG) is not to be given concurrently with MERUVAX II.

CAUTION: A sterile syringe free of perservatives, antiseptics, and detergents should be used for each injection and/or reconstitution of the vaccine because these substances may inactivate the live virus vaccine. A 25 gauge, 5/8" needle is recommended.

To reconstitute, use only the diluent supplied, since it is free of preservatives or other antiviral substances which might inactivate the vaccine.

Single Dose Vial–First withdraw the entire volume of diluent into the syringe to be used for reconstitution. Inject all the diluent in the syringe into the vial of lyophilized vaccine, and agitate to mix thoroughly. If the lyophilized vaccine cannot be dissolved, discard. Withdraw the entire contents into a syringe and inject the total volume of restored vaccine subcutaneously.

It is important to use a separate sterile syringe and needle for each individual patient to prevent transmission of hepatitis B and other infectious agents from one person to another.

Parenteral drug products should be inspected visually for particulate matter and discoloration prior to administration whenever solution and container permit. MERUVAX II, when reconstituted, is clear yellow.

Use With Other Vaccines

MERUVAX II should not be given less than one month before or after administration of other live viral vaccines.

M-M-R II has been administered concurrently with VARIVAX* [Varicella Virus Vaccine Live (Oka/Merck)], and PedvaxHIB* [Haemophilus b Conjugate Vaccine (Meningococcal Protein Conjugate)] using separate sites and syringes. No impairment of immune response to individual tested vaccine antigens was demonstrated. The type, frequency, and severity of adverse experiences observed in these studies with M-M-R II were similar to those seen when each vaccine was given alone.

Routine administration of DTP (diphtheria, tetanus, pertussis) and/or OPV (oral poliovirus vaccine) concurrently with measles, mumps and rubella vaccines is not recommended because there are limited data relating to the simultaneous administration of these antigens.

However, other schedules have been used. The ACIP has stated "Although data are limited concerning the simultaneous administration of the entire recommended vaccine series (i.e., DTP, OPV, MMR, and Hib vaccines, with or without hepatitis B vaccine), data from numerous studies have indicated no interference between routinely recommended childhood vaccines (either live, attenuated, or killed). These findings support the simultaneous use of all vaccines as recommended."

HOW SUPPLIED

No. 4747–MERUVAX II is supplied as a single-dose vial of lyophilized vaccine

NDC 0006-4747-00, and a vial of diluent.

No. 4673/4309–MERUVAX II is supplied as follows: (1) a box of 10 single-dose vials of lyophilized vaccine (package A) **NDC** 0006-4673-00; and (2) a box of 10 vials of diluent (package B). To conserve refrigerator space, the diluent may be stored separately at room temperature

(6505-00-145-0180, Ten Pack).

Storage

During shipment, to ensure that there is no loss of potency, the vaccine must be maintained at a temperature of 10°C (50°F) or colder. Freezing during shipment will not affect potency.

Protect the vaccine from light at all times, since such exposure may inactivate the virus.

Continued on next page

Information on the Merck & Co., Inc. products listed on these pages is the full prescribing information from product circulars in use September 30, 2000. For information, please call 1-800-NSC MERCK [1-800-672-6372].

Meruvax II—Cont.

Before reconstitution, store the vial of lyophilized vaccine at 2–8°C (36–46°F) or colder. The diluent may be stored in the refrigerator with the lyophilized vaccine or separately at room temperature.
It is recommended that the vaccine be used as soon as possible after reconstitution. Store reconstituted vaccine in the vaccine vial in a dark place at 2–8°C (36–46°F) and discard if not used within 8 hours.
9243400 Issued April 1999

MEVACOR® Tablets ℞
(Lovastatin)

DESCRIPTION

MEVACOR* (Lovastatin), is a cholesterol lowering agent isolated from a strain of *Aspergillus terreus*. After oral ingestion, lovastatin, which is an inactive lactone, is hydrolyzed to the corresponding β-hydroxyacid form. This is a principal metabolite and an inhibitor of 3-hydroxy-3-methylglutaryl-coenzyme A (HMG-CoA) reductase. This enzyme catalyzes the conversion of HMG-CoA to mevalonate, which is an early and rate limiting step in the biosynthesis of cholesterol.
Lovastatin is [1*S* -[1α(*R* *),3α,7β,8β(2*S* *,4*S* *),8aβ]]-1,2,3,7,8,8a-hexahydro-3,7-dimethyl-8-[2-(tetrahydro-4-hydroxy-6-oxo-2*H*-pyran-2-yl)ethyl]-1-naphthalenyl 2-methylbutanoate. The empirical formula of lovastatin is $C_{24}H_{36}O_5$ and its molecular weight is 404.55. Its structural formula is:

Lovastatin is a white, nonhygroscopic crystalline powder that is insoluble in water and sparingly soluble in ethanol, methanol, and acetonitrile.
Tablets MEVACOR are supplied as 10 mg, 20 mg and 40 mg tablets for oral administration. In addition to the active ingredient lovastatin, each tablet contains the following inactive ingredients: cellulose, lactose, magnesium stearate, and starch. Butylated hydroxyanisole (BHA) is added as a preservative. Tablets MEVACOR 10 mg also contain red ferric oxide and yellow ferric oxide. Tablets MEVACOR 20 mg also contain FD&C Blue 2. Tablets MEVACOR 40 mg also contain D&C Yellow 10 and FD&C Blue 2.

*Registered trademark of MERCK & CO., INC.

CLINICAL PHARMACOLOGY

The involvement of low-density lipoprotein cholesterol (LDL-C) in atherogenesis has been well-documented in clinical and pathological studies, as well as in many animal experiments. Epidemiological and clinical studies have established that high LDL-C and low high-density lipoprotein cholesterol (HDL-C) are both associated with coronary heart disease. However, the risk of developing coronary heart disease is continuous and graded over the range of cholesterol levels and many coronary events do occur in patients with total cholesterol (total-C) and LDL-C in the lower end of this range.
MEVACOR has been shown to reduce both normal and elevated LDL-C concentrations. LDL is formed from very low-density lipoprotein (VLDL) and is catabolized predominantly by the high affinity LDL receptor. The mechanism of the LDL-lowering effect of MEVACOR may involve both reduction of VLDL-C concentration, and induction of the LDL receptor, leading to reduced production and/or increased catabolism of LDL-C. Apolipoprotein B also falls substantially during treatment with MEVACOR. Since each LDL particle contains one molecule of apolipoprotein B, and since little apolipoprotein B is found in other lipoproteins, this strongly suggests that MEVACOR does not merely cause cholesterol to be lost from LDL, but also reduces the concentration of circulating LDL particles. In addition, MEVACOR can produce increases of variable magnitude in HDL-C, and modestly reduces VLDL-C and plasma triglycerides (TG) (see Tables I–III under *Clinical Studies*). The effects of MEVACOR on Lp(a), fibrinogen, and certain other independent biochemical risk markers for coronary heart disease are unknown.
MEVACOR is a specific inhibitor of HMG-CoA reductase, the enzyme which catalyzes the conversion of HMG-CoA to mevalonate. The conversion of HMG-CoA to mevalonate is an early step in the biosynthetic pathway for cholesterol.

TABLE I
MEVACOR vs Placebo
(Mean Percent Change from Baseline After 6 Weeks)

DOSAGE	N	TOTAL-C	LDL-C	HDL-C	LDL-C/ HDL-C	TOTAL-C/ HDL/C	TRIG.
Placebo	33	−2	−1	−1	0	+1	+9
MEVACOR							
10 mg q.p.m.	33	−16	−21	+5	−24	−19	−10
20 mg q.p.m.	33	−19	−27	+6	−30	−23	+9
10 mg b.i.d.	32	−19	−28	+8	−33	−25	−7
40 mg q.p.m.	33	−22	−31	+5	−33	−25	−8
20 mg b.i.d.	36	−24	−32	+2	−32	−24	−6

TABLE II
MEVACOR vs. Cholestyramine
(Percent Change from Baseline After 12 Weeks)

TREATMENT	N	TOTAL-C (mean)	LDL-C (mean)	HDL-C (mean)	LDL-C/ HDL-C (mean)	TOTAL-C/ HDL-C (mean)	VLDL-C (median)	TRIG. (median)
MEVACOR								
20 mg b.i.d.	85	−27	−32	+9	−36	−31	−34	−21
40 mg b.i.d.	88	−34	−42	+8	−44	−37	−31	−27
Cholestyramine								
12 g b.i.d.	88	−17	−23	+8	−27	−21	+2	+11

TABLE III
MEVACOR vs. Placebo
(Percent Change from Baseline—
Average Values Between Weeks 12 and 48)

DOSAGE	N**	TOTAL-C (mean)	LDL-C (mean)	HDL-C (mean)	LDL-C/ HDL-C (mean)	TOTAL-C/ HDL-C (mean)	TRIG. (median)
Placebo	1663	+0.7	+0.4	+2.0	+0.2	+0.6	+4
MEVACOR							
20 mg q.p.m.	1642	−17	−24	+6.6	−27	−21	−10
40 mg q.p.m.	1645	−22	−30	+7.2	−34	−26	−14
20 mg b.i.d.	1646	−24	−34	+8.6	−38	−29	−16
40 mg b.i.d.	1649	−29	−40	+9.5	−44	−34	−19

**Patients enrolled

Pharmacokinetics
Lovastatin is a lactone which is readily hydrolyzed *in vivo* to the corresponding β-hydroxyacid, a potent inhibitor of HMG-CoA reductase. Inhibition of HMG-CoA reductase is the basis for an assay in pharmacokinetic studies of the β-hydroxyacid metabolites (active inhibitors) and, following base hydrolysis, active plus latent inhibitors (total inhibitors) in plasma following administration of lovastatin.
Following an oral dose of ^{14}C-labeled lovastatin in man, 10% of the dose was excreted in urine and 83% in feces. The latter represents absorbed drug equivalents excreted in bile, as well as any unabsorbed drug. Plasma concentrations of total radioactivity (lovastatin plus ^{14}C-metabolites) peaked at 2 hours and declined rapidly to about 10% of peak by 24 hours postdose. Absorption of lovastatin, estimated relative to an intravenous reference dose, in each of four animal species tested, averaged about 30% of an oral dose. In animal studies, after oral dosing, lovastatin had high selectivity for the liver, where it achieved substantially higher concentrations than in non-target tissues. Lovastatin undergoes extensive first-pass extraction in the liver, its primary site of action, with subsequent excretion of drug equivalents in the bile. As a consequence of extensive hepatic extraction of lovastatin, the availability of drug to the general circulation is low and variable. In a single dose study in four hypercholesterolemic patients, it was estimated that less than 5% of an oral dose of lovastatin reaches the general circulation as active inhibitors. Following administration of lovastatin tablets the coefficient of variation, based on between-subject variability, was approximately 40% for the area under the curve (AUC) of total inhibitory activity in the general circulation.
Both lovastatin and its β-hydroxyacid metabolite are highly bound (>95%) to human plasma proteins. Animal studies demonstrated that lovastatin crosses the blood-brain and placental barriers.
The major active metabolites present in human plasma are the β-hydroxyacid of lovastatin, its 6′-hydroxy derivative, and two additional metabolites. Peak plasma concentrations of both active and total inhibitors were attained within 2 to 4 hours of dose administration. While the recommended therapeutic dose range is 10 to 80 mg/day, linearity of inhibitory activity in the general circulation was established by a single dose study employing lovastatin tablet dosages from 60 to as high as 120 mg. With a once-a-day dosing regimen, plasma concentrations of total inhibitors over a dosing interval achieved a steady state between the second and third days of therapy and were about 1.5 times those following a single dose. When lovastatin was given under fasting conditions, plasma concentrations of total inhibitors were on average about two-thirds those found when lovastatin was administered immediately after a standard test meal.
In a study of patients with severe renal insufficiency (creatinine clearance 10–30 mL/min), the plasma concentrations of total inhibitors after a single dose of lovastatin were approximately two-fold higher than those in healthy volunteers.

Clinical Studies
MEVACOR has been shown to be highly effective in reducing total-C and LDL-C in heterozygous familial and non-familial forms of primary hypercholesterolemia and in mixed hyperlipidemia. A marked response was seen within 2 weeks, and the maximum therapeutic response occurred within 4–6 weeks. The response was maintained during continuation of therapy. Single daily doses given in the evening were more effective than the same dose given in the morning, perhaps because cholesterol is synthesized mainly at night.
In multicenter, double-blind studies in patients with familial or non-familial hypercholesterolemia, MEVACOR, administered in doses ranging from 10 mg q.p.m. to 40 mg b.i.d., was compared to placebo. MEVACOR consistently and significantly decreased plasma total-C, LDL-C, total-C/HDL-C ratio and LDL-C/HDL-C ratio. In addition, MEVACOR produced increases of variable magnitude in HDL-C, and modestly decreased VLDL-C and plasma TG (see Tables I through III for dose response results).
The results of a study in patients with primary hypercholesterolemia are presented in Table I.
[See table I above]
MEVACOR was compared to cholestyramine in a randomized open parallel study. The study was performed with patients with hypercholesterolemia who were at high risk of myocardial infarction. Summary results are presented in Table II.
[See table II above]
MEVACOR was studied in controlled trials in hypercholesterolemic patients with well-controlled non-insulin dependent diabetes mellitus with normal renal function. The effect of MEVACOR on lipids and lipoproteins and the safety profile of MEVACOR were similar to that demonstrated in studies in nondiabetics. MEVACOR had no clinically important effect on glycemic control or on the dose requirement of oral hypoglycemic agents.
Expanded Clinical Evaluation of Lovastatin (EXCEL) Study
MEVACOR was compared to placebo in 8,245 patients with hypercholesterolemia (total-C 240–300 mg/dL [6.2 mmol/L–7.6 mmol/L], LDL-C >160 mg/dL [4.1 mmol/L]) in the randomized, double-blind, parallel, 48-week EXCEL study. All changes in the lipid measurements (Table III) in MEVACOR treated patients were dose-related and significantly different from placebo (p ≤0.001). These results were sustained throughout the study.
[See table III above]
Air Force/Texas Coronary Atherosclerosis Prevention Study (AFCAPS/TexCAPS)
The Air Force/Texas Coronary Atherosclerosis Prevention Study (AFCAPS/TexCAPS), a double-blind, randomized, placebo-controlled, primary prevention study, demonstrated that treatment with MEVACOR decreased the rate of acute major coronary events (composite endpoint of myocardial infarction, unstable angina, and sudden cardiac death) compared with placebo during a median of 5.1 years of follow-up. Participants were middle-aged and elderly men (ages 45–73) and women (ages 55–73) without symptomatic cardiovascular disease with average to moderately elevated to-

tal-C and LDL-C, below average HDL-C, and who were at high risk based on elevated total-C/HDL-C. In addition to age, 63% of the participants had at least one other risk factor (baseline HDL-C <35 mg/dL, hypertension, family history, smoking and diabetes).

AFCAPS/TexCaps enrolled 6,605 participants (5,608 men, 997 women) based on the following lipid entry criteria: total-C range of 180–264 mg/dL, LDL-C range of 130–190 mg/dL, HDL-C of ≤45 mg/dL for men and ≤47 mg/dL for women, and TG of ≤400 mg/dL. Participants were treated with standard care, including diet, and either MEVACOR 20–40 mg daily (n= 3,304) or placebo (n= 3,301). Approximately 50% of the participants treated with MEVACOR were titrated to 40 mg daily when their LDL-C remained >110 mg/dL at the 20-mg starting dose.

MEVACOR reduced the risk of a first acute major coronary event, the primary efficacy endpoint, by 37% (MEVACOR 3.5%, placebo 5.5%; p<0.001; Figure 1). A first acute major coronary event was defined as myocardial infarction (54 participants on MEVACOR, 94 on placebo) or unstable angina (54 vs. 80) or sudden cardiac death (8 vs. 9). Furthermore, among the secondary endpoints, MEVACOR reduced the risk of unstable angina by 32% (1.8 vs. 2.6%; p=0.023), of myocardial infarction by 40% (1.7 vs. 2.9%; p=0.002), and of undergoing coronary revascularization procedures (e.g., coronary artery bypass grafting or percutaneous transluminal coronary angioplasty) by 33% (3.2 vs. 4.8%; p=0.001). Trends in risk reduction associated with treatment with MEVACOR were consistent across men and women, smokers and non-smokers, hypertensives and non-hypertensives, and older and younger participants. Participants with ≥2 risk factors had risk reductions (RR) in both acute major coronary events (RR 43%) and coronary revascularization procedures (RR 37%). Because there were too few events among those participants with age as their only risk factor in this study, the effect of MEVACOR on outcomes could not be adequately assessed in this subgroup.

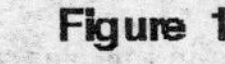
Figure 1

Acute Major Coronary Events (Primary Endpoint)

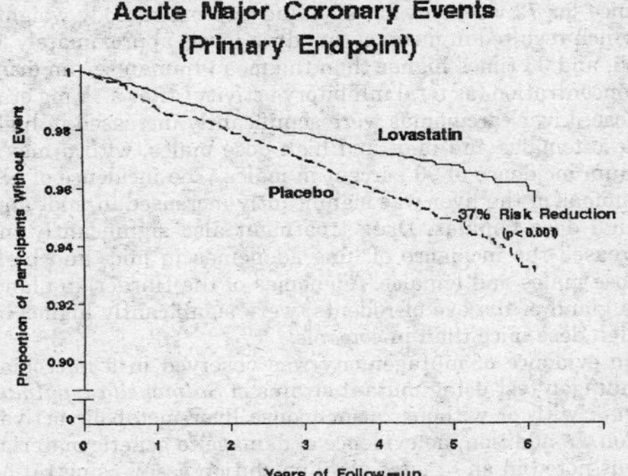

Atherosclerosis

In the Canadian Coronary Atherosclerosis Intervention Trial (CCAIT), the effect of therapy with lovastatin on coronary atherosclerosis was assessed by coronary angiography in hyperlipidemic patients. In this randomized, double-blind, controlled clinical trial, patients were treated with conventional measures (usually diet and 325 mg of aspirin every other day) and either lovastatin 20–80 mg daily or placebo. Angiograms were evaluated at baseline and at two years by computerized quantitative coronary angiography (QCA). Lovastatin significantly slowed the progression of lesions as measured by the mean change per-patient in minimum lumen diameter (the primary endpoint) and percent diameter stenosis, and decreased the proportions of patients categorized with disease progression (33% vs. 50%) and with new lesions (16% vs. 32%).

In a similarly designed trial, the Monitored Atherosclerosis Regression Study (MARS), patients were treated with diet and either lovastatin 80 mg daily or placebo. No statistically significant difference between lovastatin and placebo was seen for the primary endpoint (mean change per patient in percent diameter stenosis of all lesions), or for most secondary QCA endpoints. Visual assessment by angiographers who formed a consensus opinion of overall angiographic change (Global Change Score) was also a secondary endpoint. By this endpoint, significant slowing of disease was seen, with regression in 23% of patients treated with lovastatin compared to 11% of placebo patients.

In the Familial Atherosclerosis Treatment Study (FATS), either lovastatin or niacin in combination with a bile acid sequestrant for 2.5 years in hyperlipidemic subjects significantly reduced the frequency of progression and increased the frequency of regression of coronary atherosclerotic lesions by QCA compared to diet and, in some cases, low-dose resin.

The effect of lovastatin on the progression of atherosclerosis in the coronary arteries has been corroborated by similar findings in another vasculature. In the Asymptomatic Carotid Artery Progression Study (ACAPS), the effect of therapy with lovastatin on carotid atherosclerosis was assessed by B-mode ultrasonography in hyperlipidemic patients with early carotid lesions and without known coronary heart disease at baseline. In this double-blind, controlled clinical trial, 919 patients were randomized in a 2 x 2 factorial design to placebo, lovastatin 10–40 mg daily and/or warfarin. Ultrasonograms of the carotid walls were used to determine the change per patient from baseline to three years in mean maximum intimal-medial thickness (IMT) of 12 measured segments. There was a significant regression of carotid lesions in patients receiving lovastatin alone compared to those receiving placebo alone (p=0.001). The predictive value of changes in IMT for stroke has not yet been established. In the lovastatin group there was a significant reduction in the number of patients with major cardiovascular events relative to the placebo group (5 vs. 14) and a significant reduction in all-cause mortality (1 vs. 8).

Eye

There was a high prevalence of baseline lenticular opacities in the patient population included in the early clinical trials with lovastatin. During these trials the appearance of new opacities was noted in both the lovastatin and placebo groups. There was no clinically significant change in visual acuity in the patients who had new opacities reported nor was any patient, including those with opacities noted at baseline, discontinued from therapy because of a decrease in visual acuity.

A three-year, double-blind, placebo-controlled study in hypercholesterolemic patients to assess the effect of lovastatin on the human lens demonstrated that there were no clinically or statistically significant differences between the lovastatin and placebo groups in the incidence, type or progression of lenticular opacities. There are no controlled clinical data assessing the lens available for treatment beyond three years.

INDICATIONS AND USAGE

Therapy with MEVACOR should be a component of multiple risk factor intervention in those individuals with dyslipidemia at risk for atherosclerotic vascular disease. MEVACOR should be used in addition to a diet restricted in saturated fat and cholesterol as part of a treatment strategy to lower total-C and LDL-C to target levels when the response to diet and other nonpharmacological measures alone has been inadequate to reduce risk.

Primary Prevention of Coronary Heart Disease

In individuals without symptomatic cardiovascular disease, average to moderately elevated total-C and LDL-C, and below average HDL-C, MEVACOR is indicated to reduce the risk of:

— Myocardial infarction
— Unstable angina
— Coronary revascularization procedures

(See CLINICAL PHARMACOLOGY, *Clinical Studies.*)

Coronary Heart Disease

MEVACOR is indicated to slow the progression of coronary atherosclerosis in patients with coronary heart disease as part of a treatment strategy to lower total-C and LDL-C to target levels.

Hypercholesterolemia

Therapy with lipid-altering agents should be a component of multiple risk factor intervention in those individuals at significantly increased risk for artherosclerotic vascular disease due to hypercholesterolemia. MEVACOR is indicated as an adjunct to diet for the reduction of elevated total-C and LDL-C levels in patients with primary hypercholesterolemia (Types IIa and IIb***), when the response to diet restricted in saturated fat and cholesterol and to other nonpharmacological measures alone has been inadequate.

General Recommendations

Prior to initiating therapy with lovastatin, secondary causes for hypercholesterolemia (e.g., poorly controlled diabetes mellitus, hypothyroidism, nephrotic syndrome, dysproteinemias, obstructive liver disease, other drug therapy, alcoholism) should be excluded, and a lipid profile performed to measure total-C, HDL-C, and TG. For patients with TG less than 400 mg/dL (<4.5 mmol/L), LDL-C can be estimated using the following equation:

LDL-C = total-C − [0.2 × (TG) + HDL-C]

For TG levels >400 mg/dL (>4.5 mmol/L), this equation is less accurate and LDL-C concentrations should be determined by ultracentrifugation. In hypertriglyceridemic patients, LDL-C may be low or normal despite elevated total-C. In such cases, MEVACOR is not indicated.

The National Cholesterol Education Program (NCEP) Treatment Guidelines are summarized below:

Definite Atherosclerotic Disease†	Two or More Other Risk Factors††	LDL-Cholesterol mg/dL (mmol/L) Initiation Level	Goal
NO	NO	≥190 (≥4.9)	<160 (<4.1)
NO	YES	≥160 (≥4.1)	<130 (<3.4)
YES	YES or NO	≥130††† (≥3.4)	≤100 (≤2.6)

† Coronary heart disease or peripheral vascular disease (including symptomatic carotid artery disease).

†† Other risk factors for coronary heart disease (CHD) include: age (males: ≥45 years; females: ≥55 years of premature menopause without estrogen replacement therapy); family history of premature CHD; current cigarette smoking; hypertension; confirmed HDL-C <35 mg/dL (<0.91 mmol/L); and diabetes mellitus. Subtract one risk factor if HDL-C is ≥60 mg/dL (≥1.6 mmol/L).

††† In CHD patients with LDL-C levels 100–129 mg/dL, the physician should exercise clinical judgment in deciding whether to initiate drug treatment.

At the time of hospitalization for an acute coronary event, consideration can be given to initiating drug therapy at discharge if the LDL-C is ≥130 mg/dL (see NCEP Guidelines above).

Since the goal of treatment is to lower LDL-C, the NCEP recommends that LDL-C levels be used to initiate and assess treatment response. Only if LDL-C levels are not available, should the total-C be used to monitor therapy.

Although MEVACOR may be useful to reduce elevated LDL-C levels in patients with combined hypercholesterolemia and hypertriglyceridemia where hypercholesterolemia is the major abnormality (Type IIb hyperlipoproteinemia), it has not been studied in conditions where the major abnormality is elevation of chylomicrons, VLDL or IDL (i.e., hyperlipoproteinemia types I, III, IV, or V).***

***Classification of Hyperlipoproteinemias

Type	Lipoproteins elevated	Lipid Elevations major	minor
I (rare)	chylomicrons	TG	→C
IIa	LDL	C	—
IIb	LDL, VLDL	C	TG
III (rare)	IDL	C/TG	—
IV	VLDL	TG	→C
V (rare)	chylomicrons, VLDL	TG	→C

IDL = intermediate-density lipoprotein.

CONTRAINDICATIONS

Hypersensitivity to any component of this medication.

Active liver disease or unexplained persistent elevations of serum transaminases (see WARNINGS).

Pregnancy and lactation. Atherosclerosis is a chronic process and the discontinuation of lipid-lowering drugs during pregnancy should have little impact on the outcome of long-term therapy of primary hypercholesterolemia. Moreover, cholesterol and other products of the cholesterol biosynthesis pathway are essential components for fetal development, including synthesis of steroids and cell membranes. Because of the ability of inhibitors of HMG-CoA reductase such as MEVACOR to decrease the synthesis of cholesterol and possibly other products of the cholesterol biosynthesis pathway, MEVACOR is contraindicated during pregnancy and in nursing mothers. **MEVACOR should be administered to women of childbearing age only when such patients are highly unlikely to conceive.** If the patient becomes pregnant while taking this drug, MEVACOR should be discontinued immediately and the patient should be apprised of the potential hazard to the fetus (see PRECAUTIONS, *Pregnancy*).

WARNINGS

Skeletal Muscle

Lovastatin and other inhibitors of HMG-CoA reductase occasionally cause myopathy, which is manifested as muscle pain or weakness associated with grossly elevated creatine kinase (>10× the upper limit of normal [ULN]). **Rhabdomyolysis, with or without acute renal failure secondary to myoglobinuria, has been reported rarely and can occur at any time.** In the EXCEL study, there was one case of myopathy among 4933 patients randomized to lovastatin 20–40 mg daily for 48 weeks, and 4 among 1649 patients randomized to 80 mg daily. When drug treatment was interrupted or discontinued in these patients, muscle symptoms and creatine kinase (CK) increases promptly resolved. The risk of myopathy is increased by concomitant therapy with certain drugs, some of which were excluded by the EXCEL study design.

Myopathy caused by drug interactions.

The incidence and severity of myopathy are increased by concomitant administration of HMG-CoA reductase inhibitors with drugs that can cause myopathy when given alone, such as gemfibrozil and other fibrates, and lipid-lowering doses (≥ 1 g/day) of niacin (nicotonic acid).

In addition, the risk of myopathy appears to be increased by high levels of HMG-CoA reductase inhibitory activity in plasma. Lovastatin is metabolized by the cytochrome P450 isoform 3A4. Certain drugs which share this metabolic pathway can raise the plasma levels of lovastatin and may increase the risk of myopathy. These include cyclosporine, itraconazole, ketoconazole and other antifungal azoles, the macrolide antibiotics erythromycin and clarithromycin, HIV protease inhibitors, and the antidepressant nefazodone.

Reducing the risk of myopathy.

1. General measures. Patients starting therapy with lovastatin should be advised of the risk of myopathy, and told to

Continued on next page

Information on the Merck & Co., Inc. products listed on these pages is the full prescribing information from product circulars in use September 30, 2000. For information, please call 1-800-NSC MERCK [1-800-672-6372].

Mevacor—Cont.

report promptly unexplained muscle pain, tenderness or weakness. A creatine kinase (CK) level above 10× ULN in a patient with unexplained muscle symptoms indicates myopathy. **Lovastatin therapy should be discontinued if myopathy is diagnosed or suspected.** In most cases, when patients were promptly discontinued from treatment, muscle symptoms and CK increases resolved.

Of the patients with rhabdomyolysis, many had complicated medical histories. Some had preexisting renal insufficiency, usually as a consequence of long-standing diabetes. In such patients, dose escalation requires caution. Also, as there are no known adverse consequences of brief interruption of therapy, treatment with lovastatin should be stopped a few days before elective major surgery and when any major acute medical or surgical condition supervenes.

2. Measures to reduce the risk of myopathy caused by drug interactions (see above and PRECAUTIONS, *Drug Interactions*). Physicians contemplating combined therapy with lovastatin and any of the interacting drugs should weigh the potential benefits and risks, and should carefully monitor patients for any signs and symptoms of muscle pain, tenderness, or weakness, particularly during the initial months of therapy and during any periods of upward dosage titration of either drug. Periodic CK determinations may be considered in such situations, but there is no assurance that such monitoring will prevent myopathy.

The combined use of lovastatin with fibrates or niacin should be avoided unless the benefit of further alteration in lipid levels is likely to outweigh the increased risk of this drug combination. Combinations of fibrates or niacin with low doses of lovastatin have been used without myopathy in small, short-term clinical trials with careful monitoring. Addition of these drugs to lovastatin typically provides little additional reduction in LDL cholesterol, but further reductions of triglycerides and further increases in HDL cholesterol may be obtained. If one of these drugs must be used with lovastatin, clinical experience suggests that the risk of myopathy is less with niacin than with the fibrates.

In patients taking concomitant cyclosporine, fibrates or niacin, the dose of lovastatin should generally not exceed 20 mg (see DOSAGE AND ADMINISTRATION and DOSAGE AND ADMINISTRATION, *Concomitant Lipid-Lowering Therapy*), as the risk of myopathy increases substantially at higher doses. Interruption of lovastatin therapy during a course of treatment with a systemic antifungal azole or a macrolide antibiotic should be considered.

Liver Dysfunction

Persistent increases (to more than 3 times the upper limit of normal) in serum transaminases occurred in 1.9% of adult patients who received lovastatin for at least one year in early clinical trials (see ADVERSE REACTIONS). When the drug was interrupted or discontinued in these patients, the transaminase levels usually fell slowly to pretreatment levels. The increases usually appeared 3 to 12 months after the start of therapy with lovastatin, and were not associated with jaundice or other clinical signs or symptoms. There was no evidence of hypersensitivity. In the EXCEL study (see CLINICAL PHARMACOLOGY, *Clinical Studies*), the incidence of persistent increases in serum transaminases over 48 weeks was 0.1% for placebo, 0.1% at 20 mg/day, 0.9% at 40 mg/day, and 1.5% at 80 mg/day in patients on lovastatin. However, in post-marketing experience with MEVACOR, symptomatic liver disease has been reported rarely at all dosages (see ADVERSE REACTIONS).

In AFCAPS/TexCAPS, the number of participants with consecutive elevations of either alanine aminotransferase (ALT) or aspartate aminotransferase (AST) (> 3 times the upper limit of normal), over a median of 5.1 years of follow-up, was not significantly different between the MEVACOR and placebo groups (18 [0.6%] vs. 11 [0.3%]). The starting dose of MEVACOR was 20 mg/day; 50% of the MEVACOR treated participants were titrated to 40 mg/day at Week 18. Of the 18 participants on MEVACOR with consecutive elevations of either ALT or AST, 11 (0.7%) elevations occurred in participants taking 20 mg/day, while 7 (0.4%) elevations occurred in participants titrated to 40 mg/day. Elevated transaminases resulted in discontinuation of 6 (0.2%) participants from therapy in the MEVACOR group (n=3,304) and 4 (0.1%) in the placebo group (n=3,301).

It is recommended that liver function tests be performed before the initiation of treatment, at 6 and 12 weeks after initiation of therapy or elevation of dose, and periodically thereafter (e.g., semiannually). Patients who develop increased transaminase levels should be monitored with a second liver function evaluation to confirm the finding and be followed thereafter with frequent liver function tests until the abnormality(ies) return to normal. Should an increase in AST or ALT of three times the upper limit of normal or greater persist, withdrawal of therapy with MEVACOR is recommended.

The drug should be used with caution in patients who consume substantial quantities of alcohol and/or have a past history of liver disease. Active liver disease or unexplained transaminase elevations are contraindications to the use of lovastatin.

As with other lipid-lowering agents, moderate (less than three times the upper limit of normal) elevations of serum transaminases have been reported following therapy with MEVACOR (see ADVERSE REACTIONS). These changes appeared soon after initiation of therapy with MEVACOR, were often transient, were not accompanied by any symptoms and interruption of treatment was not required.

PRECAUTIONS

General

Lovastatin may elevate creatine phosphokinase and transaminase levels (see WARNINGS and ADVERSE REACTIONS). This should be considered in the differential diagnosis of chest pain in a patient on therapy with lovastatin.

Homozygous Familial Hypercholesterolemia

MEVACOR is less effective in patients with the rare homozygous familial hypercholesterolemia, possibly because these patients have no functional LDL receptors. MEVACOR appears to be more likely to raise serum transaminases (see ADVERSE REACTIONS) in these homozygous patients.

Information for Patients

Patients should be advised to report promptly unexplained muscle pain, tenderness or weakness (see WARNINGS, *Skeletal Muscle*).

Drug Interactions

Cyclosporine, Itraconazole, Ketoconazole, Gemfibrozil, Niacin (Nicotinic Acid), Erythromycin, Clarithromycin, HIV protease inhibitors, Nefazodone: see WARNINGS, *Skeletal Muscle*.

Coumarin Anticoagulants: In a small clinical trial in which lovastatin was administered to warfarin treated patients, no effect on prothrombin time was detected. However, another HMG-CoA reductase inhibitor has been found to produce a less than two seconds increase in prothrombin time in healthy volunteers receiving low doses of warfarin. Also, bleeding and/or increased prothrombin time have been reported in a few patients taking coumarin anticoagulants concomitantly with lovastatin. It is recommended that in patients taking anticoagulants, prothrombin time be determined before starting lovastatin and frequently enough during early therapy to insure that no significant alteration of prothrombin time occurs. Once a stable prothrombin time has been documented, prothrombin times can be monitored at the intervals usually recommended for patients on coumarin anticoagulants. If the dose of lovastatin is changed, the same procedure should be repeated. Lovastatin therapy has not been associated with bleeding or with changes in prothrombin time in patients not taking anticoagulants.

Antipyrine: Lovastatin had no effect on the pharmacokinetics of antipyrine or its metabolites. However, since lovastatin is metabolized by the cytochrome P450 isoform 3A4, this does not preclude an interaction with other drugs metabolized by the same isoform (see WARNINGS, *Skeletal Muscle*).

Propranolol: In normal volunteers, there was no clinically significant pharmacokinetic or pharmacodynamic interaction with concomitant administration of single doses of lovastatin and propranolol.

Digoxin: In patients with hypercholesterolemia, concomitant administration of lovastatin and digoxin resulted in no effect on digoxin plasma concentrations.

Oral Hypoglycemic Agents: In pharmacokinetic studies of MEVACOR in hypercholesterolemic non-insulin dependent diabetic patients, there was no drug interaction with glipizide or with chlorpropamide (see CLINICAL PHARMACOLOGY, *Clinical Studies*).

Endocrine Function

HMG-CoA reductase inhibitors interfere with cholesterol synthesis and as such might theoretically blunt adrenal and/or gonadal steroid production. Results of clinical trials with drugs in this class have been inconsistent with regard to drug effects on basal and reserve steroid levels. However, clinical studies have shown that lovastatin does not reduce basal plasma cortisol concentration or impair adrenal reserve, and does not reduce basal plasma testosterone concentration. Another HMG-CoA reductase inhibitor has been shown to reduce the plasma testosterone response to HCG. In the same study, the mean testosterone response to HCG was slightly but not significantly reduced after treatment with lovastatin 40 mg daily for 16 weeks in 21 men. The effects of HMG-CoA reductase inhibitors on male fertility have not been studied in adequate numbers of male patients. The effects, if any, on the pituitary-gonadal axis in premenopausal women are unknown. Patients treated with lovastatin who develop clinical evidence of endocrine dysfunction should be evaluated appropriately. Caution should also be exercised if an HMG-CoA reductase inhibitor or other agent used to lower cholesterol levels is administered to patients also receiving other drugs (e.g., ketoconazole, spironolactone, cimetidine) that may decrease the levels or activity of endogenous steroid hormones.

CNS Toxicity

Lovastatin produced optic nerve degeneration (Wallerian degeneration of retinogeniculate fibers) in clinically normal dogs in a dose-dependent fashion starting at 60 mg/kg/day, a dose that produced mean plasma drug levels about 30 times higher than the mean drug level in humans taking the highest recommended dose (as measured by total enzyme inhibitory activity). Vestibulocochlear Wallerian-like degeneration and retinal ganglion cell chromatolysis were also seen in dogs treated for 14 weeks at 180 mg/kg/day, a dose which resulted in a mean plasma drug level (C_{max}) similar to that seen with the 60 mg/kg/day dose.

CNS vascular lesions, characterized by perivascular hemorrhage and edema, mononuclear cell infiltration of perivascular spaces, perivascular fibrin deposits and necrosis of small vessels, were seen in dogs treated with lovastatin at a dose of 180 mg/kg/day, a dose which produced plasma drug levels (C_{max}) which were about 30 times higher than the mean values in humans taking 80 mg/day.

Similar optic nerve and CNS vascular lesions have been observed with other drugs of this class.

Cataracts were seen in dogs treated for 11 and 28 weeks at 180 mg/kg/day and 1 year at 60 mg/kg/day.

Carcinogenesis, Mutagenesis, Impairment of Fertility

In a 21-month carcinogenic study in mice, there was a statistically significant increase in the incidence of hepatocellular carcinomas and adenomas in both males and females at 500 mg/kg/day. This dose produced a total plasma drug exposure 3 to 4 times that of humans given the highest recommended dose of lovastatin (drug exposure was measured as total HMG-CoA reductase inhibitory activity in extracted plasma). Tumor increases were not seen at 20 and 100 mg/kg/day, doses that produced drug exposures of 0.3 to 2 times that of humans at the 80 mg/day dose. A statistically significant increase in pulmonary adenomas was seen in female mice at approximately 4 times the human drug exposure. (Although mice were given 300 times the human dose [HD] on a mg/kg body weight basis, plasma levels of total inhibitory activity were only 4 times higher in mice than in humans given 80 mg of MEVACOR.)

There was an increase in incidence of papilloma in the non-glandular mucosa of the stomach of mice beginning at exposures of 1 to 2 times that of humans. The glandular mucosa was not affected. The human stomach contains only glandular mucosa.

In a 24-month carcinogenicity study in rats, there was a positive dose response relationship for hepatocellular carcinogenicity in males at drug exposures between 2–7 times that of human exposure at 80 mg/day (doses in rats were 5, 30 and 180 mg/kg/day).

An increased incidence of thyroid neoplasms in rats appears to be a response that has been seen with other HMG-CoA reductase inhibitors.

A chemically similar drug in this class was administered to mice for 72 weeks at 25, 100, and 400 mg/kg body weight, which resulted in mean serum drug levels approximately 3, 15, and 33 times higher than the mean human serum drug concentration (as total inhibitory activity) after a 40 mg oral dose. Liver carcinomas were significantly increased in high dose females and mid- and high dose males, with a maximum incidence of 90 percent in males. The incidence of adenomas of the liver was significantly increased in mid- and high dose females. Drug treatment also significantly increased the incidence of lung adenomas in mid- and high dose males and females. Adenomas of the Harderian gland (a gland of the eye of rodents) were significantly higher in high dose mice than in controls.

No evidence of mutagenicity was observed in a microbial mutagen test using mutant strains of *Salmonella typhimurium* with or without rat or mouse liver metabolic activation. In addition, no evidence of damage to genetic material was noted in an *in vitro* alkaline elution assay using rat or mouse hepatocytes, a V-79 mammalian cell forward mutation study, an *in vitro* chromosome aberration study in CHO cells, or an *in vivo* chromosomal aberration assay in mouse bone marrow.

Drug-related testicular atrophy, decreased spermatogenesis, spermatocytic degeneration and giant cell formation were seen in dogs starting at 20 mg/kg/day. Similar findings were seen with another drug in this class. No drug-related effects on fertility were found in studies with lovastatin in rats. However, in studies with a similar drug in this class, there was decreased fertility in male rats treated for 34 weeks at 25 mg/kg body weight, although this effect was not observed in a subsequent fertility study when this same dose was administered for 11 weeks (the entire cycle of spermatogenesis, including epididymal maturation). In rats treated with this same reductase inhibitor at 180 mg/kg/day, seminiferous tubule degeneration (necrosis and loss of spermatogenic epithelium) was observed. No microscopic changes were observed in the testes from rats of either study. The clinical significance of these findings is unclear.

Pregnancy

Pregnancy Category X

See CONTRAINDICATIONS.

Safety in pregnant women has not been established.

Lovastatin has been shown to produce skeletal malformations at plasma levels 40 times the human exposure (for mouse fetus) and 80 times the human exposure (for rat fetus) based on mg/m^2 surface area (doses were 800 mg/kg/day). No drug-induced changes were seen in either species at multiples of 8 times (rat) or 4 times (mouse) based on surface area. No evidence of malformations was noted in rabbits at exposures up to 3 times the human exposure (dose of 15 mg/kg/day, highest tolerated dose).

Rare reports of congenital anomalies have been received following intrauterine exposure to HMG-CoA reductase inhibitors. In a review[†] of approximately 100 prospectively followed pregnancies in women exposed to MEVACOR or another structurally related HMG-CoA reductase inhibitor, the incidences of congenital anomalies, spontaneous abortions and fetal deaths/stillbirths did not exceed what would be expected in the general population. The number of cases is adequate only to exclude a 3 to 4-fold increase in congenital anomalies over the background incidence. In 89% of the prospectively followed pregnancies, drug treatment was initiated prior to pregnancy and was discontinued at some point in the first trimester when pregnancy was identified. As safety in pregnant women has not been established and there is no apparent benefit to therapy with MEVACOR during pregnancy (see CONTRAINDICATIONS), treatment should be immediately discontinued as soon as pregnancy is recognized. MEVACOR should be administered to women of child-bearing potential only when such patients are highly unlikely to conceive and have been informed of the potential hazard.

Nursing Mothers

It is not known whether lovastatin is excreted in human milk. Because a small amount of another drug in this class is excreted in human breast milk and because of the potential for serious adverse reactions in nursing infants, women taking MEVACOR should not nurse their infants (see CONTRAINDICATIONS).

Pediatric Use

Safety and effectiveness in pediatric patients have not been established. Because pediatric patients are not likely to benefit from cholesterol lowering for at least a decade and because experience with this drug is limited (no studies in subjects below the age of 20 years), treatment of pediatric patients with lovastatin is not recommended at this time.

†Manson, J.M., Freyssinges, C., Ducrocq, M.B., Stephenson, W.P., Postmarketing Surveillance of Lovastatin and Simvastatin Exposure During Pregnancy. *Reproductive Toxicology.* 10(6):439-446. 1996.

ADVERSE REACTIONS

MEVACOR is generally well tolerated; adverse reactions usually have been mild and transient.

Phase III Clinical Studies

In Phase III controlled clinical studies involving 613 patients treated with MEVACOR, the adverse experience profile was similar to that shown below for the 8,245-patient EXCEL study (see *Expanded Clinical Evaluation of Lovastatin [EXCEL] Study*).

Persistent increases of serum transaminases have been noted (see WARNINGS, *Liver Dysfunction*). About 11% of patients had elevations of CK levels of at least twice the normal value on one or more occasions. The corresponding values for the control agent cholestyramine was 9 percent. This was attributable to the noncardiac fraction of CK. Large increases in CK have sometimes been reported (see WARNINGS, *Skeletal Muscle*).

Expanded Clinical Evaluation of Lovastatin (EXCEL) Study

MEVACOR was compared to placebo in 8,245 patients with hypercholesterolemia (total-C 240–300 mg/dL [6.2–7.8 mmol/L]) in the randomized, double-blind, parallel, 48-week EXCEL study. Clinical adverse experiences reported as possibly, probably or definitely drug-related in ≥1% in any treatment group are shown in the table below. For no event was the incidence on drug and placebo statistically different.

	Placebo (N=1663) %	MEVACOR 20 mg q.p.m. (N=1642) %	MEVACOR 40 mg q.p.m. (N=1645) %	MEVACOR 20 mg b.i.d. (N=1646) %	MEVACOR 40 mg b.i.d. (N=1649) %
Body As a Whole					
Asthenia	1.4	1.7	1.4	1.5	1.2
Gastrointestinal					
Abdominal pain	1.6	2.0	2.0	2.2	2.5
Constipation	1.9	2.0	3.2	3.2	3.5
Diarrhea	2.3	2.6	2.4	2.2	2.6
Dyspepsia	1.9	1.3	1.3	1.0	1.6
Flatulence	4.2	3.7	4.3	3.9	4.5
Nausea	2.5	1.9	2.5	2.2	2.2
Musculoskeletal					
Muscle cramps	0.5	0.6	0.8	1.1	1.0
Myalgia	1.7	2.6	1.8	2.2	3.0
Nervous System / Psychiatric					
Dizziness	0.7	0.7	1.2	0.5	0.5
Headache	2.7	2.6	2.8	2.1	3.2
Skin					
Rash	0.7	0.8	1.0	1.2	1.3
Special Senses					
Blurred vision	0.8	1.1	0.9	0.9	1.2

[See table above]

Other clinical adverse experiences reported as possibly, probably or definitely drug-related in 0.5 to 1.0 percent of patients in any drug-treated group are listed below. In all these cases the incidence on drug and placebo was not statistically different. *Body as a Whole:* chest pain; *Gastrointestinal:* acid regurgitation, dry mouth, vomiting; *Musculoskeletal:* leg pain, shoulder pain, arthralgia; *Nervous System / Psychiatric:* insomnia, paresthesia; *Skin:* alopecia, pruritus; *Special Senses:* eye irritation.

In the EXCEL study (see CLINICAL PHARMACOLOGY, *Clinical Studies*), 4.6% of the patients treated up to 48 weeks were discontinued due to clinical or laboratory adverse experiences which were rated by the investigator as possibly, probably or definitely related to therapy with MEVACOR. The value for the placebo group was 2.5%.

Air Force / Texas Coronary Atherosclerosis Prevention Study (AFCAPS / TexCAPS)

In AFCAPS/TexCAPS (see CLINICAL PHARMACOLOGY, *Clinical Studies*) involving 6,605 participants treated with 20–40 mg/day of MEVACOR (n=3,304) or placebo (n=3,301), the safety and tolerability profile of the group treated with MEVACOR was comparable to that of the group treated with placebo during a median of 5.1 years of follow-up. The adverse experiences reported in AFCAPS/TexCAPS were similar to those reported in EXCEL (see ADVERSE REACTIONS, *Expanded Clinical Evaluation of Lovastatin (EXCEL) Study*).

Concomitant Therapy

In controlled clinical studies in which lovastatin was administered concomitantly with cholestyramine, no adverse reactions peculiar to this concomitant treatment were observed. The adverse reactions that occurred were limited to those reported previously with lovastatin or cholestyramine. Other lipid-lowering agents were not administered concomitantly with lovastatin during controlled clinical studies. Preliminary data suggests that the addition of gemfibrozil to therapy with lovastatin is not associated with greater reduction in LDL-C than that achieved with lovastatin alone. In uncontrolled clinical studies, most of the patients who have developed myopathy were receiving concomitant therapy with cyclosporine, gemfibrozil or niacin (nicotinic acid) (see WARNINGS, *Skeletal Muscle*).

The following effects have been reported with drugs in this class. Not all the effects listed below have necessarily been associated with lovastatin therapy.

Skeletal: muscle cramps, myalgia, myopathy, rhabdomyolysis, arthralgias.

Neurological: dysfunction of certain cranial nerves (including alteration of taste, impairment of extra-ocular movement, facial paresis), tremor, dizziness, vertigo, memory loss, paresthesia, peripheral neuropathy, peripheral nerve palsy, psychic disturbances, anxiety, insomnia, depression.

Hypersensitivity Reactions: An apparent hypersensitivity syndrome has been reported rarely which has included one or more of the following features: anaphylaxis, angioedema, lupus erythematous-like syndrome, polymyalgia rheumatica, vasculitis, purpura, thrombocytopenia, leukopenia, hemolytic anemia, positive ANA, ESR increase, eosinophilia, arthritis, arthralgia, urticaria, asthenia, photosensitivity, fever, chills, flushing, malaise, dyspnea, toxic epidermal necrolysis, erythema multiforme, including Stevens-Johnson syndrome.

Gastrointestinal: pancreatitis, hepatitis, including chronic active hepatitis, cholestatic jaundice, fatty change in liver; and rarely, cirrhosis, fulminant hepatic necrosis, and hepatoma; anorexia, vomiting.

Skin: alopecia, pruritus. A variety of skin changes (e.g., nodules, discoloration, dryness of skin/mucous membranes, changes to hair/nails) have been reported.

Reproductive: gynecomastia, loss of libido, erectile dysfunction.

Eye: progression of cataracts (lens opacities), ophthalmoplegia.

Laboratory Abnormalities: elevated transaminases, alkaline phosphatase, γ-glutamyl transpeptidase, and bilirubin; thyroid function abnormalities.

OVERDOSAGE

After oral administration of MEVACOR to mice the median lethal dose observed was >15 g/m^2.

Five healthy human volunteers have received up to 200 mg of lovastatin as a single dose without clinically significant adverse experiences. A few cases of accidental overdosage have been reported; no patients had any specific symptoms, and all patients recovered without sequelae. The maximum dose taken was 5–6 g.

Until further experience is obtained, no specific treatment of overdosage with MEVACOR can be recommended.

The dialyzability of lovastatin and its metabolites in man is not known at present.

DOSAGE AND ADMINISTRATION

The patient should be placed on a standard cholesterol-lowering diet before receiving MEVACOR and should continue on this diet during treatment with MEVACOR (see NCEP Treatment Guidelines for details on dietary therapy). MEVACOR should be given with meals.

The usual recommended starting dose is 20 mg once a day given with the evening meal. The recommended dosing range is 10–80 mg/day in single or two divided doses; the maximum recommended dose is 80 mg/day. Doses should be individualized according to the recommended goal of therapy (see NCEP Guidelines and CLINICAL PHARMACOLOGY). Patients requiring reductions in LDL-C of 20% or more to achieve their goal (see INDICATIONS AND USAGE) should be started on 20 mg/day of MEVACOR. A starting dose of 10 mg may be considered for patients requiring smaller reductions. Adjustments should be made at intervals of 4 weeks or more.

In patients taking cyclosporine concomitantly with lovastatin (see WARNINGS, *Skeletal Muscle*), therapy should begin with 10 mg of MEVACOR and should not exceed 20 mg/day. Cholesterol levels should be monitored periodically and consideration should be given to reducing the dosage of MEVACOR if cholesterol levels fall significantly below the targeted range.

Concomitant Lipid-Lowering Therapy

MEVCOR is effective alone or when used concomitantly with bile-acid sequestrants. Use of MEVACOR with fibrates or niacin should generally be avoided. However, if MEVACOR is used in combination with fibrates or niacin, the dose of MEVACOR should not exceed 20 mg (see WARNINGS, *Skeletal Muscle*).

Dosage in Patients with Renal Insufficiency

In patients with severe renal insufficiency (creatinine clearance <30 mL/min), dosage increases above 20 mg/day should be carefully considered and, if deemed necessary, implemented cautiously (see CLINICAL PHARMACOLOGY and WARNINGS, *Skeletal Muscle*).

HOW SUPPLIED

No. 3560—Tablets MEVACOR 10 mg are peach, octagonal tablets, coded MSD 730 on one side and MEVACOR on the other. They are supplied as follows:

NDC 0006-0730-61 unit of use bottles of 60.

Shown in Product Identification Guide, page 324

No. 3561—Tablets MEVACOR 20 mg are light blue, octagonal tablets, coded MSD 731 on one side and MEVACOR on the other. They are supplied as follows:

NDC 0006-0731-61 unit of use bottles of 60
(6505-01-267-2497, 20 mg 60's)
NDC 0006-0731-94 unit of use bottles of 90
NDC 0006-0731-28 unit dose packages of 100
(6505-01-267-7925, 20 mg 100's)
NDC 0006-0731-82 bottles of 1,000
(6505-01-359-1865, 20 mg 1,000's)
NDC 0006-0731-87 bottles of 10,000
(6505-01-379-7905, 20 mg 10,000's).

Shown in Product Identification Guide, page 324

No. 3562—Tablets MEVACOR 40 mg are green, octagonal tablets, coded MSD 732 on one side and MEVACOR on the other. They are supplied as follows:

NDC 0006-0732-61 unit of use bottles of 60
(6505-01-310-0615, 40 mg 60's)
NDC 0006-0732-94 unit of use bottles of 90
NDC 0006-0732-82 bottles of 1,000
NDC 0006-0732-87 bottles of 10,000
(6505-01-379-7903, 40 mg 10,000's).

Shown in Product Identification Guide, page 324

Storage

Store between 5–30°C (41–86°F). Tablets MEVACOR must be protected from light and stored in a well-closed, light-resistant container.

7825346 Issued March 1999

MIDAMOR® Tablets ℞
(Amiloride HCl)

DESCRIPTION

Amiloride HCl, an antikaliuretic-diuretic agent, is a pyrazine-carbonyl-guanidine that is unrelated chemically to other known antikaliuretic or diuretic agents. It is the salt of a moderately strong base (pKa 8.7). It is designated chemically as 3,5-diamino-6-chloro-*N*-(diaminomethylene) pyrazinecarboxamide monohydrochloride, dihydrate and has a molecular weight of 302.12. Its empirical formula is $C_6H_8ClN_7O \cdot HCl \cdot 2H_2O$ and its structural formula is:

[See chemical structure at top of next column]

MIDAMOR* (Amiloride HCl) is available for oral use as tablets containing 5 mg of anhydrous amiloride HCl. Each tab-

Continued on next page

Information on the Merck & Co., Inc. products listed on these pages is the full prescribing information from product circulars in use September 30, 2000. For information, please call 1-800-NSC MERCK [1-800-672-6372].

Midamor—Cont.

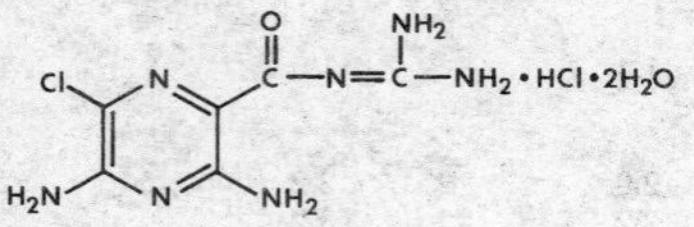

let contains the following inactive ingredients: calcium phosphate, D&C Yellow 10, iron oxide, lactose, magnesium stearate and starch.

---

*Registered trademark of MERCK & CO., INC.

CLINICAL PHARMACOLOGY

MIDAMOR is a potassium-conserving (antikaliuretic) drug that possesses weak (compared with thiazide diuretics) natriuretic, diuretic, and antihypertensive activity. These effects have been partially additive to the effects of thiazide diuretics in some clinical studies. When administered with a thiazide or loop diuretic, MIDAMOR has been shown to decrease the enhanced urinary excretion of magnesium which occurs when a thiazide or loop diuretic is used alone. MIDAMOR has potassium-conserving activity in patients receiving kaliuretic-diuretic agents.

MIDAMOR is not an aldosterone antagonist and its effects are seen even in the absence of aldosterone.

MIDAMOR exerts its potassium sparing effect through the inhibition of sodium reabsorption at the distal convoluted tubule, cortical collecting tubule and collecting duct; this decreases the net negative potential of the tubular lumen and reduces both potassium and hydrogen secretion and their subsequent excretion. This mechanism accounts in large part for the potassium sparing action of amiloride.

MIDAMOR usually begins to act within 2 hours after an oral dose. Its effect on electrolyte excretion reaches a peak between 6 and 10 hours and lasts about 24 hours. Peak plasma levels are obtained in 3 to 4 hours and the plasma half-life varies from 6 to 9 hours. Effects on electrolytes increase with single doses of amiloride HCl up to approximately 15 mg.

Amiloride HCl is not metabolized by the liver but is excreted unchanged by the kidneys. About 50 percent of a 20 mg dose of MIDAMOR is excreted in the urine and 40 percent in the stool within 72 hours. MIDAMOR has little effect on glomerular filtration rate or renal blood flow. Because amiloride HCl is not metabolized by the liver, drug accumulation is not anticipated in patients with hepatic dysfunction, but accumulation can occur if the hepatorenal syndrome develops.

INDICATIONS AND USAGE

MIDAMOR is indicated as adjunctive treatment with thiazide diuretics or other kaliuretic-diuretic agents in congestive heart failure or hypertension to:

a. help restore normal serum potassium levels in patients who develop hypokalemia on the kaliuretic diuretic
b. prevent development of hypokalemia in patients who would be exposed to particular risk if hypokalemia were to develop, e.g., digitalized patients or patients with significant cardiac arrhythmias.

The use of potassium-conserving agents is often unnecessary in patients receiving diuretics for uncomplicated essential hypertension when such patients have a normal diet. MIDAMOR has little additive diuretic or antihypertensive effect when added to a thiazide diuretic.

MIDAMOR should rarely be used alone. It has weak (compared with thiazides) diuretic and antihypertensive effects. Used as single agents, potassium sparing diuretics, including MIDAMOR, result in an increased risk of hyperkalemia (approximately 10% with amiloride). MIDAMOR should be used alone only when persistent hypokalemia has been documented and only with careful titration of the dose and close monitoring of serum electrolytes.

CONTRAINDICATIONS

Hyperkalemia

MIDAMOR should not be used in the presence of elevated serum potassium levels (greater than 5.5 mEq per liter).

Antikaliuretic Therapy or Potassium Supplementation

MIDAMOR should not be given to patients receiving other potassium-conserving agents, such as spironolactone or triamterene. Potassium supplementation in the form of medication, potassium-containing salt substitutes or a potassium-rich diet should not be used with MIDAMOR except in severe and/or refractory cases of hypokalemia. Such concomitant therapy can be associated with rapid increases in serum potassium levels. If potassium supplementation is used, careful monitoring of the serum potassium level is necessary.

Impaired Renal Function

Anuria, acute or chronic renal insufficiency, and evidence of diabetic nephropathy are contraindications to the use of MIDAMOR. Patients with evidence of renal functional impairment (blood urea nitrogen [BUN] levels over 30 mg per 100 mL or serum creatinine levels over 1.5 mg per 100 mL) or diabetes mellitus should not receive the drug without careful, frequent and continuing monitoring of serum electrolytes, creatinine, and BUN levels. Potassium retention associated with the use of an antikaliuretic agent is accentuated in the presence of renal impairment and may result in the rapid development of hyperkalemia.

Hypersensitivity

MIDAMOR is contraindicated in patients who are hypersensitive to this product.

WARNINGS

Hyperkalemia

> Like other potassium-conserving agents, amiloride may cause hyperkalemia (serum potassium levels greater than 5.5 mEq per liter) which, if uncorrected, is potentially fatal. Hyperkalemia occurs commonly (about 10%) when amiloride is used without a kaliuretic diuretic. This incidence is greater in patients with renal impairment, diabetes mellitus (with or without recognized renal insufficiency), and in the elderly. When MIDAMOR is used concomitantly with a thiazide diuretic in patients without these complications, the risk of hyperkalemia is reduced to about 1–2 percent. It is thus essential to monitor serum potassium levels carefully in any patient receiving amiloride, particularly when it is first introduced, at the time of diuretic dosage adjustments, and during any illness that could affect renal function.

The risk of hyperkalemia may be increased when potassium-conserving agents, including MIDAMOR, are administered concomitantly with an angiotensin-converting enzyme inhibitor. (See PRECAUTIONS, *Drug Interactions.*) Warning signs or symptoms of hyperkalemia include paresthesias, muscular weakness, fatigue, flaccid paralysis of the extremities, bradycardia, shock, and ECG abnormalities. Monitoring of the serum potassium level is essential because mild hyperkalemia is not usually associated with an abnormal ECG.

When abnormal, the ECG in hyperkalemia is characterized primarily by tall, peaked T waves or elevations from previous tracings. There may also be lowering of the R wave and increased depth of the S wave, widening and even disappearance of the P wave, progressive widening of the QRS complex, prolongation of the PR interval, and ST depression.

Treatment of hyperkalemia: If hyperkalemia occurs in patients taking MIDAMOR, the drug should be discontinued immediately. If the serum potassium level exceeds 6.5 mEq per liter, active measures should be taken to reduce it. Such measures include the intravenous administration of sodium bicarbonate solution or oral or parenteral glucose with a rapid-acting insulin preparation. If needed, a cation exchange resin such as sodium polystyrene sulfonate may be given orally or by enema. Patients with persistent hyperkalemia may require dialysis.

Diabetes Mellitus

In diabetic patients, hyperkalemia has been reported with the use of all potassium-conserving diuretics, including MIDAMOR, even in patients without evidence of diabetic nephropathy. Therefore, MIDAMOR should be avoided, if possible, in diabetic patients and, if it is used, serum electrolytes and renal function must be monitored frequently.

MIDAMOR should be discontinued at least three days before glucose tolerance testing.

Metabolic or Respiratory Acidosis

Antikaliuretic therapy should be instituted only with caution in severely ill patients in whom respiratory or metabolic acidosis may occur, such as patients with cardiopulmonary disease or poorly controlled diabetes. If MIDAMOR is given to these patients, frequent monitoring of acid-base balance is necessary. Shifts in acid-base balance alter the ratio of extracellular/intracellular potassium, and the development of acidosis may be associated with rapid increases in serum potassium levels.

PRECAUTIONS

General

Electrolyte Imbalance and BUN Increases

Hyponatremia and hypochloremia may occur when MIDAMOR is used with other diuretics and increases in BUN levels have been reported. These increases usually have accompanied vigorous fluid elimination, especially when diuretic therapy was used in seriously ill patients, such as those who had hepatic cirrhosis with ascites and metabolic alkalosis, or those with resistant edema. Therefore, when MIDAMOR is given with other diuretics to such patients, careful monitoring of serum electrolytes and BUN levels is important. In patients with pre-existing severe liver disease, hepatic encephalopathy, manifested by tremors, confusion, and coma, and increased jaundice, have been reported in association with diuretics, including amiloride HCl.

Drug Interactions

When amiloride HCl is administered concomitantly with an angiotensin-converting enzyme inhibitor, the risk of hyperkalemia may be increased. Therefore, if concomitant use of these agents is indicated because of demonstrated hypokalemia, they should be used with caution and with frequent monitoring of serum potassium. (See WARNINGS.)

Lithium generally should not be given with diuretics because they reduce its renal clearance and add a high risk of lithium toxicity. Read circulars for lithium preparations before use of such concomitant therapy.

In some patients, the administration of a non-steroidal anti-inflammatory agent can reduce the diuretic, natriuretic, and antihypertensive effects of loop, potassium-sparing and thiazide diuretics. Therefore, when MIDAMOR and non-steroidal anti-inflammatory agents are used concomitantly, the patient should be observed closely to determine if the desired effect of the diuretic is obtained. Since indomethacin and potassium-sparing diuretics, including MIDAMOR, may each be associated with increased serum potassium levels, the potential effects on potassium kinetics and renal function should be considered when these agents are administered concurrently.

Carcinogenicity, Mutagenicity, Impairment of Fertility

There was no evidence of a tumorigenic effect when amiloride HCl was administered for 92 weeks to mice at doses up to 10 mg/kg/day (25 times the maximum daily human dose). Amiloride HCl has also been administered for 104 weeks to male and female rats at doses up to 6 and 8 mg/kg/day (15 and 20 times the maximum daily dose for humans, respectively) and showed no evidence of carcinogenicity.

Amiloride HCl was devoid of mutagenic activity in various strains of *Salmonella typhimurium* with or without a mammalian liver microsomal activation system (Ames test).

Pregnancy

Pregnancy Category B. Teratogenicity studies with amiloride HCl in rabbits and mice given 20 and 25 times the maximum human dose, respectively, revealed no evidence of harm to the fetus, although studies showed that the drug crossed the placenta in modest amounts. Reproduction studies in rats at 20 times the expected maximum daily dose for humans showed no evidence of impaired fertility. At approximately 5 or more times the expected maximum daily dose for humans, some toxicity was seen in adult rats and rabbits and a decrease in rat pup growth and survival occurred.

There are, however, no adequate and well-controlled studies in pregnant women. Because animal reproduction studies are not always predictive of human response, this drug should be used during pregnancy only if clearly needed.

Nursing Mothers

Studies in rats have shown that amiloride is excreted in milk in concentrations higher than those found in blood, but it is not known whether MIDAMOR is excreted in human milk. Because many drugs are excreted in human milk and because of the potential for serious adverse reactions in nursing infants from MIDAMOR, a decision should be made whether to discontinue nursing or to discontinue the drug, taking into account the importance of the drug to the mother.

Pediatric Use

Safety and effectiveness in pediatric patients have not been established.

ADVERSE REACTIONS

MIDAMOR is usually well tolerated and, except for hyperkalemia (serum potassium levels greater than 5.5 mEq per liter—see WARNINGS), significant adverse effects have been reported infrequently. Minor adverse reactions were reported relatively frequently (about 20%) but the relationship of many of the reports to amiloride HCl is uncertain and the overall frequency was similar in hydrochlorothiazide treated groups. Nausea/anorexia, abdominal pain, flatulence, and mild skin rash have been reported and probably are related to amiloride. Other adverse experiences that have been reported with amiloride are generally those known to be associated with diuresis, or with the underlying disease being treated.

The adverse reactions for MIDAMOR listed in the following table have been arranged into two groups: (1) incidence greater than one percent; and (2) incidence one percent or less. The incidence for group (1) was determined from clinical studies conducted in the United States (837 patients treated with MIDAMOR). The adverse effects listed in group (2) include reports from the same clinical studies and voluntary reports since marketing. The probability of a causal relationship exists between MIDAMOR and these adverse reactions, some of which have been reported only rarely.

Incidence > 1%	Incidence ≤ 1%
Body as a Whole	
Headache**	Back pain
Weakness	Chest pain
Fatigability	Neck/shoulder ache
	Pain, extremeties
Cardiovascular	
None	Angina pectoris
	Orthostatic hypotension
	Arrhythmia
	Palpitation
Digestive	
Nausea/anorexia**	Jaundice
Diarrhea**	GI bleeding
Vomiting**	Abdominal fullness
Abdominal pain	GI disturbance
Gas pain	Thirst
Appetite changes	Heartburn
Constipation	Flatulence
	Dyspepsia
Metabolic	
Elevated serum potassium levels (> 5.5 mEq per liter)***	None
Skin	
None	Skin rash
	Itching

	Dryness of mouth
	Pruritus
	Alopecia
Musculoskeletal	
Muscle cramps	Joint pain
	Leg ache
Nervous	
Dizziness	Paresthesia
Encephalopathy	Tremors
	Vertigo
Psychiatric	
None	Nervousness
	Mental confusion
	Insomnia
	Decreased libido
	Depression
	Somnolence
Respiratory	
Cough	Shortness of breath
Dyspnea	
Special Senses	
None	Visual disturbances
	Nasal congestion
	Tinnitus
	Increased intraocular pressure
Urogenital	
Impotence	Polyuria
	Dysuria
	Urinary frequency
	Bladder spasms
	Gynecomastia

** Reactions occurring in 3% to 8% of patients treated with MIDAMOR. (Those reactions occurring in less than 3% of the patients are unmarked.)

*** See WARNINGS.

Causal Relationship Unknown
Other reactions have been reported but occurred under circumstances where a causal relationship could not be established. However, in these rarely reported events, that possibility cannot be excluded. Therefore, these observations are listed to serve as alerting information to physicians.
Activation of probable pre-existing peptic ulcer
Aplastic anemia
Neutropenia
Abnormal liver function

OVERDOSAGE

No data are available in regard to overdosage in humans.
The oral LD_{50} of amiloride hydrochloride (calculated as the base) is 56 mg/kg in mice and 36 to 85 mg/kg in rats, depending on the strain.
It is not known whether the drug is dialyzable.
The most likely signs and symptoms to be expected with overdosage are dehydration and electrolyte imbalance. These can be treated by established procedures. Therapy with MIDAMOR should be discontinued and the patient observed closely. There is no specific antidote. Emesis should be induced or gastric lavage performed. Treatment is symptomatic and supportive. If hyperkalemia occurs, active measures should be taken to reduce the serum potassium levels.

DOSAGE AND ADMINISTRATION

MIDAMOR should be administered with food.
MIDAMOR, one 5 mg tablet daily, should be added to the usual antihypertensive or diuretic dosage of a kaliuretic diuretic. The dosage may be increased to 10 mg per day, if necessary. More than two 5 mg tablets of MIDAMOR daily usually are not needed, and there is little controlled experience with such doses. If persistent hypokalemia is documented with 10 mg, the dose can be increased to 15 mg, then 20 mg, with careful monitoring of electrolytes.
In treating patients with congestive heart failure after an initial diuresis has been achieved, potassium loss may also decrease and the need for MIDAMOR should be reevaluated. Dosage adjustment may be necessary. Maintenance therapy may be on an intermittent basis.
If it is necessary to use MIDAMOR alone (see INDICATIONS), the starting dosage should be one 5 mg tablet daily. This dosage may be increased to 10 mg per day, if necessary. More than two 5 mg tablets usually are not needed, and there is little controlled experience with such doses. If persistent hypokalemia is documented with 10 mg, the dose can be increased to 15 mg, then 20 mg, with careful monitoring of electrolytes.

HOW SUPPLIED

No. 3381—Tablets MIDAMOR, 5 mg, are yellow, diamond-shaped, compressed tablets, coded MSD 92 on one side and MIDAMOR on the other. They are supplied as follows:
NDC 0006-0092-68 bottles of 100
(6505-01-127-8721 5 mg, 100's).

Shown in Product Identification Guide, page 324

Storage
Protect from moisture, freezing and excessive heat.
7905116 Issued August 1996

MINTEZOL® Chewable Tablets (Thiabendazole) ℞
MINTEZOL® Suspension (Thiabendazole) ℞

DESCRIPTION

MINTEZOL* (Thiabendazole) is an anthelmintic provided as 500 mg chewable tablets, and as a suspension, containing 500 mg thiabendazole per 5 mL. The suspension also contains sorbic acid 0.1% added as a preservative. Inactive ingredients in the tablets are acacia, calcium phosphate, flavors, lactose, magnesium stearate, mannitol, methylcellulose, and sodium saccharin. Inactive ingredients in the suspension are an antifoam agent, flavors, polysorbate, purified water, sorbitol solution, and tragacanth.
Thiabendazole is a white to off-white odorless powder with a molecular weight of 201.26, which is practically insoluble in water but readily soluble in dilute acid and alkali. Its chemical name is 2-(4-thiazolyl)-1*H*-benzimidazole. The empirical formula is $C_{10}H_7N_3S$ and the structural formula is:

*Registered trademark of MERCK & CO., INC.

CLINICAL PHARMACOLOGY

In man, thiabendazole is rapidly absorbed and peak plasma concentration is reached within 1 to 2 hours after the oral administration of a suspension. It is metabolized almost completely to the 5-hydroxy form which appears in the urine as glucuronide or sulfate conjugates. In 48 hours, about 5% of the administered dose is recovered from the feces and about 90% from the urine. Most is excreted in the first 24 hours.

Mechanism of Action
The precise mode of action of thiabendazole on the parasite is unknown, but it may inhibit the helminth-specific enzyme fumarate reductase.
Thiabendazole is vermicidal and/or vermifugal against *Ascaris lumbricoides* ("common roundworm"), *Strongyloides stercoralis* (threadworm), *Necator americanus*, and *Ancylostoma duodenale* (hookworm), *Trichuris trichiura* (whipworm), *Ancylostoma braziliense* (dog and cat hookworm), *Toxocara canis* and *Toxocara cati* (ascarids), and *Enterobius vermicularis* (pinworm).
Its effect on larvae of *Trichinella spiralis* that have migrated to muscle is questionable.
Thiabendazole also suppresses egg and/or larval production and may inhibit the subsequent development of those eggs or larvae which are passed in the feces.

INDICATIONS AND USAGE

MINTEZOL is indicated for the treatment of:
Strongyloidiasis (threadworm)
Cutaneous larva migrans (creeping eruption)
Visceral larva migrans
Trichinosis: Relief of symptoms and fever and a reduction of eosinophilia have followed the use of MINTEZOL during the invasion stage of the disease.
Thiabendazole is usually inappropriate as first line therapy for enterobiasis (pinworm). However, when enterobiasis occurs with any of the conditions listed above, additional therapy is not required for most patients.
MINTEZOL should be used only in the following infestations when more specific therapy is not available or cannot be used or when further therapy with a second agent is desirable: Uncinariasis (hookworm: *Necator americanus* and *Ancylostoma duodenale*); Trichuriasis (whipworm); Ascariasis (large roundworm).

CONTRAINDICATION

Hypersensitivity to this product.
Thiabendazole is contraindicated as prophylactic treatment for pinworm infestation.

WARNINGS

If hypersensitivity reactions occur, the drug should be discontinued immediately and not be resumed. Erythema multiforme has been associated with thiabendazole therapy; in severe cases (Stevens-Johnson syndrome), fatalities have occurred.
Because CNS side effects may occur quite frequently, activities requiring mental alertness should be avoided.
Jaundice, cholestasis, and parenchymal liver damage have been reported in patients treated with MINTEZOL. In rare cases, liver damage has been severe and has led to irreversible hepatic failure. (See **ADVERSE REACTIONS.**)
Abnormal sensation in eyes, xanthopsia, blurred vision, drying of mucous membranes, and SICCA syndrome have been reported in patients treated with MINTEZOL. These adverse effects of the eye were in some cases persistent for prolonged intervals which have exceeded one year. (See **ADVERSE REACTIONS.**)
Thiabendazole should not usually be used as first line therapy for the treatment of enterobiasis. It should be reserved for use in patients who have experienced allergic reactions, or resistance to other treatments.

PRECAUTIONS

General
MINTEZOL is not suitable for the treatment of mixed infections with ascaris because it may cause these worms to migrate.
Ideally, supportive therapy is indicated for anemic, dehydrated or malnourished patients prior to initiation of the anthelmintic therapy.
In the presence of hepatic or renal dysfunction, patients should be carefully monitored.
MINTEZOL should be used only in patients in whom susceptible worm infestation has been diagnosed and should not be used prophylactically.

Information for Patients
Because CNS side effects may occur quite frequently, activities requiring mental alertness should be avoided.

Laboratory Tests
Rarely, a transient rise in liver function tests has occurred in patients receiving MINTEZOL.

Drug Interactions
Thiabendazole may compete with other drugs, such as theophylline, for sites of metabolism in the liver, thus elevating the serum levels of such compounds to potentially toxic levels. Therefore, when concomitant use of thiabendazole and xanthine derivatives is anticipated, it may be necessary to monitor blood levels and/or reduce the dosage of such compounds. Such concomitant use should be administered under careful medical supervision.

Carcinogenesis, Mutagenesis, Impairment of Fertility
Thiabendazole has been used in numerous short- and long-term studies in animals at doses up to 15 times the usual human dose and was without carcinogenic effects. It did not adversely affect fertility in the mouse at $2^1/_2$ times the usual human dose or in the rat at a dose equivalent to the usual human dose. Thiabendazole had no mutagenic activity in *in vitro* microbial mutagen test, the micronucleus test and the host mediated assay *in vivo*.

Pregnancy
Pregnancy Category C: Reproduction and teratogenic studies done in the rabbit at a dose up to 15 times the usual human dose, in the rat at a dose equivalent to the human dose, and in the mouse at a dose up to $2^1/_2$ times the usual human dose, revealed no evidence of harm to the fetus. In an additional study in the mouse, no defects were observed when thiabendazole was given in an aqueous suspension, at a dose 10 times the usual human dose; however, cleft palate and axial skeletal defects were observed when thiabendazole was suspended in olive oil and given at the same dose. There are no adequate and well controlled studies in pregnant women. MINTEZOL should be used during pregnancy only if the potential benefit justifies the potential risk to the fetus.

Nursing Mothers
It is not known whether this drug is excreted in human milk. Because of the potential for serious adverse reactions in nursing infants from MINTEZOL, a decision should be made whether to discontinue nursing or to discontinue the drug, taking into account the importance of the drug to the mother.

Pediatric Use
The safety and effectiveness of thiabendazole for the treatment of Strongyloidiasis, Ascariasis, Uncinariasis, Trichuriasis and Trichinosis in pediatric patients weighing less than 30 lbs has been limited.

ADVERSE REACTIONS

Gastrointestinal: anorexia, nausea, vomiting, diarrhea, epigastric distress, abdominal pain, jaundice, cholestasis, parenchymal liver damage and hepatic failure. (See **WARNINGS.**)
Central Nervous System: dizziness, weariness, drowsiness, giddiness, headache, numbness, hyperirritability, convulsions, collapse, confusion, depression, floating sensation, weakness and lack of coordination.
Special Senses: tinnitus, abnormal sensation in eyes, xanthopsia, blurred vision, reduced vision, drying of mucous membranes (mouth, eyes, etc.), SICCA syndrome. (See **WARNINGS.**)
Cardiovascular: hypotension.
Metabolic: hyperglycemia.
Hematologic: transient leukopenia.
Genitourinary: hematuria, enuresis, malodor of the urine, crystalluria.
Hypersensitivity: pruritus, fever, facial flush, chills, conjunctival injection, angioedema, anaphylaxis, skin rashes (including perianal), erythema multiforme (including Stevens-Johnson syndrome), and lymphadenopathy.
Miscellaneous: appearance of live Ascaris in the mouth and nose.

Continued on next page

Information on the Merck & Co., Inc. products listed on these pages is the full prescribing information from product circulars in use September 30, 2000. For information, please call 1-800-NSC MERCK [1-800-672-6372].

Mintezol—Cont.

OVERDOSAGE

Overdosage may be associated with transient disturbances of vision and psychic alterations.
There is no specific antidote in the event of overdosage. Therefore, symptomatic and supportive measures should be employed. Emesis should be induced or gastric lavage performed carefully.
The oral LD_{50} of MINTEZOL is 3.6 g/kg, 3.1 g/kg and 3.8 g/kg in the mouse, rat, and rabbit respectively.

DOSAGE AND ADMINISTRATION

The recommended maximum daily dose of MINTEZOL *is 3 grams.*
MINTEZOL should be given after meals if possible. Tablets MINTEZOL should be chewed before swallowing. Dietary restriction, complementary medications and cleansing enemas are not needed.
The usual dosage schedule for all conditions is two doses per day. The dosage is determined by the patient's weight.
A weight-dose chart follows:

Weight	Each Dose g	Each Dose mL
30 lb	0.25 (½ tablet)	2.5 (½ teaspoon)
50 lb	0.5 (1 tablet)	5.0 (1 teaspoon)
75 lb	0.75 (1½ tablets)	7.5 (1½ teaspoons)
100 lb	1.0 (2 tablets)	10.0 (2 teaspoons)
125 lb	1.25 (2½ tablets)	12.5 (2½ teaspoons)
150 lb & over	1.5 (3 tablets)	15.0 (3 teaspoons)

The regimen for each indication follows:
[See table below]

HOW SUPPLIED

No. 3331 — MINTEZOL Suspension, 500 mg per 5 mL, is white to off-white and is supplied as follows:
NDC 0006-3331-60 in bottles of 120 mL
(6505-00-935-5835, 0.5 g/5 mL, 120 mL).
Storage
Store in a well-closed container at controlled room temperature [15–30°C (59–86°F)]. Protect from freezing.
No. 3332 — MINTEZOL Chewable Tablets, 500 mg, are white to off-white, orange-flavored, round, scored, compressed tablets, coded MSD 907 on one side and MINTEZOL on the other.
They are supplied as follows:
NDC 0006-0907-36 unit dose packages of 36
(6505-01-226-9909, 500 mg chewable, individually sealed 36's).
Shown in Product Identification Guide, page 324
Storage
Store in a well-closed container at controlled room temperature [15–30°C (59–86°F)].
7930814 Issued January 1998

Therapeutic Regimens

Indication	*Regimen*	*Comments*
**STRONGYLOIDIASIS	2 doses per day for 2 successive days.	A single dose of 20 mg/lb or 50 mg/kg may be employed as an alternative schedule, but a higher incidence of side effects should be expected.
CUTANEOUS LARVA MIGRANS (Creeping Eruption)	2 doses per day for 2 successive days.	If active lesions are still present 2 days after completion of therapy, a second course is recommended.
VISCERAL LARVA MIGRANS	2 doses per day for 7 successive days.	Safety and efficacy data on the seven-day treatment course are limited.
**TRICHINOSIS	2 doses per day for 2–4 successive days according to the response of the patient.	The optimal dosage for the treatment of trichinosis has not been established.
Other Indications		
** Intestinal roundworms (including Ascariasis, Uncinariasis and Trichuriasis)	2 doses per day for 2 successive days.	A single dose of 20 mg/lb or 50 mg/kg may be employed as an alternative schedule, but a higher incidence of side effects should be expected.

** Clinical experience with thiabendazole for treatment of each of these conditions in pediatric patients weighing less than 30 lbs has been limited.

MODURETIC® Tablets ℞
(Amiloride HCl-Hydrochlorothiazide)

DESCRIPTION

MODURETIC* (Amiloride HCl-Hydrochlorothiazide) combines the potassium-conserving action of amiloride HCl with the natriuretic action of hydrochlorothiazide.
Amiloride HCl is designated chemically as 3,5-diamino-6-chloro-*N*- (diaminomethylene) pyrazinecarboxamide monohydrochloride, dihydrate and has a molecular weight of 302.12. Its empirical formula is $C_6H_8ClN_7O{\cdot}HCl{\cdot}2H_2O$ and its structural formula is:

Hydrochlorothiazide is designated chemically as 6-chloro-3,4-dihydro-2*H*-1,2,4-benzothiadiazine-7-sulfonamide 1,1-dioxide. Its empirical formula is $C_7H_8ClN_3O_4S_2$ and its structural formula is:

It is a white, or practically white, crystalline powder with a molecular weight of 297.74, which is slightly soluble in water, but freely soluble in sodium hydroxide solution.
MODURETIC is available for oral use as tablets containing 5 mg of anhydrous amiloride HCl and 50 mg of hydrochlorothiazide. Each tablet contains the following inactive ingredients: calcium phosphate, FD&C Yellow 6, guar gum, lactose, magnesium stearate and starch.

*Registered trademark of MERCK & CO., INC.

CLINICAL PHARMACOLOGY

MODURETIC provides diuretic and antihypertensive activity (principally due to the hydrochlorothiazide component), while acting through the amiloride component to prevent the excessive potassium loss that may occur in patients receiving a thiazide diuretic. Due to its amiloride component, the urinary excretion of magnesium is less with MODURETIC than with a thiazide or loop diuretic used alone (see PRECAUTIONS). The onset of the diuretic action of MODURETIC is within 1 to 2 hours and this action appears to be sustained for approximately 24 hours.
Amiloride HCl
Amiloride HCl is a potassium-conserving (antikaliuretic) drug that possesses weak (compared with thiazide diuretics) natriuretic, diuretic, and antihypertensive activity. These effects have been partially additive to the effects of thiazide diuretics in some clinical studies. Amiloride HCl has potassium-conserving activity in patients receiving kaliuretic-diuretic agents.
Amiloride HCl is not an aldosterone antagonist and its effects are seen even in the absence of aldosterone.
Amiloride HCl exerts its postassium sparing effect through the inhibition of sodium reabsorption at the distal convoluted tubule, cortical collecting tubule and collecting duct; this decreases the net negative potential of the tubular lumen and reduces both potassium and hydrogen secretion and their subsequent excretion. This mechanism accounts in large part for the potassium sparing action of amiloride.
Amiloride HCl usually begins to act within 2 hours after an oral dose. Its effect on electrolyte excretion reaches a peak between 6 and 10 hours and lasts about 24 hours. Peak plasma levels are obtained in 3 to 4 hours and the plasma half-life varies from 6 to 9 hours. Effects on electrolytes increase with single doses of amiloride HCl up to approximately 15 mg.
Amiloride HCl is not metabolized by the liver but is excreted unchanged by the kidneys. About 50 percent of a 20 mg dose of amiloride HCl is excreted in the urine and 40 percent in the stool within 72 hours. Amiloride HCl has little effect on glomerular filtration rate or renal blood flow. Because amiloride HCl is not metabolized by the liver, drug accumulation is not anticipated in patients with hepatic dysfunction, but accumulation can occur if the hepatorenal syndrome develops.
Hydrochlorothiazide
The mechanism of the antihypertensive effect of thiazides is unknown. Thiazides do not usually affect normal blood pressure.
Hydrochlorothiazide is a diuretic and antihypertensive. It affects the distal renal tubular mechanism of electrolyte reabsorption. Hydrochlorothiazide increases excretion of sodium and chloride in approximately equivalent amounts. Natriuresis may be accompanied by some loss of potassium and bicarbonate.
After oral use diuresis begins within two hours, peaks in about four hours and lasts about 6 to 12 hours.
Hydrochlorothiazide is not metabolized but is eliminated rapidly by the kidney. When plasma levels have been followed for at least 24 hours, the plasma half-life has been observed to vary between 5.6 and 14.8 hours. At least 61 percent of the oral dose is eliminated unchanged within 24 hours. Hydrochlorothiazide crosses the placental but not the blood-brain barrier and is excreted in breast milk.

INDICATIONS AND USAGE

MODURETIC is indicated in those patients with hypertension or with congestive heart failure who develop hypokalemia when thiazides or other kaliuretic diuretics are used alone, or in whom maintenance of normal serum potassium levels is considered to be clinically important, e.g., digitalized patients, or patients with significant cardiac arrhythmias.
The use of potassium-conserving agents is often unnecessary in patients receiving diuretics for uncomplicated essential hypertension when such patients have a normal diet.
MODURETIC may be used alone or as an adjunct to other antihypertensive drugs, such as methyldopa or beta blockers. Since MODURETIC enhances the action of these agents, dosage adjustments may be necessary to avoid an excessive fall in blood pressure and other unwanted side effects.
This fixed combination drug is not indicated for the initial therapy of edema or hypertension except in individuals in whom the development of hypokalemia cannot be risked.

CONTRAINDICATIONS

Hyperkalemia
MODURETIC should not be used in the presence of elevated serum potassium levels (greater than 5.5 mEq per liter).
Antikaliuretic Therapy or Potassium Supplementation
MODURETIC should not be given to patients receiving other potassium-conserving agents, such as spironolactone or triamterene. Potassium supplementation in the form of medication, potassium-containing salt substitutes or a potassium-rich diet should not be used with MODURETIC except in severe and/or refractory cases of hypokalemia. Such concomitant therapy can be associated with rapid increases in serum potassium levels. If potassium supplementation is used, careful monitoring of the serum potassium level is necessary.
Impaired Renal Function
Anuria, acute or chronic renal insufficiency, and evidence of diabetic nephropathy are contraindications to the use of MODURETIC. Patients with evidence of renal functional impairment (blood urea nitrogen [BUN] levels over 30 mg per 100 mL or serum creatinine levels over 1.5 mg per 100 mL) or diabetes mellitus should not receive the drug without careful, frequent and continuing monitoring of serum electrolytes, creatinine, and BUN levels. Potassium retention associated with the use of an antikaliuretic agent is accentuated in the presence of renal impairment and may result in the rapid development of hyperkalemia.
Hypersensitivity
MODURETIC is contraindicated in patients who are hypersensitive to this product, or to other sulfonamide-derived drugs.

WARNINGS

Hyperkalemia

Like other potassium-conserving diuretic combinations, MODURETIC may cause hyperkalemia (serum potassium levels greater than 5.5 mEq per liter). In patients without renal impairment or diabetes mellitus, the risk of hyperkalemia with MODURETIC is about 1-2 percent. This risk is higher in patients with renal impairment or diabetes mellitus (even without recognized diabetic nephropathy). Since hyperkalemia, if uncorrected, is potentially fatal, it is essential to monitor serum potassium levels carefully in any patient receiving MODURETIC, particularly when it is first introduced, at the time of dosage adjustments, and during any illness that could affect renal function.

The risk of hyperkalemia may be increased when potassium-conserving agents, including MODURETIC, are administered concomitantly with an angiotensin-converting enzyme inhibitor. (See PRECAUTIONS, *Drug Interactions.*) Warning signs or symptoms of hyperkalemia include paresthesias, muscular weakness, fatigue, flaccid paralysis of the extremities, bradycardia, shock, and ECG abnormalities. Monitoring of the serum potassium level is essential because mild hyperkalemia is not usually associated with an abnormal ECG.

When abnormal, the ECG in hyperkalemia is characterized primarily by tall, peaked T waves or elevations from previous tracings. There may also be lowering of the R wave and increased depth of the S wave, widening and even disappearance of the P wave, progressive widening of the QRS complex, prolongation of the PR interval, and ST depression.

Treatment of hyperkalemia: If hyperkalemia occurs in patients taking MODURETIC, the drug should be discontinued immediately. If the serum potassium level exceeds 6.5 mEq per liter, active measures should be taken to reduce it. Such measures include the intravenous administration of sodium bicarbonate solution or oral or parenteral glucose with a rapid-acting insulin preparation. If needed, a cation exchange resin such as sodium polystyrene sulfonate may be given orally or by enema. Patients with persistent hyperkalemia may require dialysis.

Diabetes Mellitus

In diabetic patients, hyperkalemia has been reported with the use of all potassium-conserving diuretics, including amiloride HCl, even in patients without evidence of diabetic nephropathy. Therefore, MODURETIC should be avoided, if possible, in diabetic patients and, if it is used, serum electrolytes and renal function must be monitored frequently. MODURETIC should be discontinued at least three days before glucose tolerance testing.

Metabolic or Respiratory Acidosis

Antikaliuretic therapy should be instituted only with caution in severely ill patients in whom respiratory or metabolic acidosis may occur, such as patients with cardiopulmonary disease or poorly controlled diabetes. If MODURETIC is given to these patients, frequent monitoring of acid-base balance is necessary. Shifts in acid-base balance alter the ratio of extracellular/intracellular potassium, and the development of acidosis may be associated with rapid increases in serum potassium levels.

PRECAUTIONS

General

Electrolyte Imbalance and BUN Increases

Determination of serum electrolytes to detect possible electrolyte imbalance should be performed at appropriate intervals.

Patients should be observed for clinical signs of fluid or electrolyte imbalance: i.e., hyponatremia, hypochloremic alkalosis, and hypokalemia. Serum and urine electrolyte determinations are particularly important when the patient is vomiting excessively or receiving parenteral fluids. Warning signs or symptoms of fluid and electrolyte imbalance, irrespective of cause, include dryness of mouth, thirst, weakness, lethargy, drowsiness, restlessness, confusion, seizures, muscle pains or cramps, muscular fatigue, hypotension, oliguria, tachycardia, and gastrointestinal disturbances such as nausea and vomiting.

Hyponatremia and hypochloremia may occur during the use of thiazides and other diuretics. Any chloride deficit during thiazide therapy is generally mild and may be lessened by the amiloride HCl component of MODURETIC. Hypochloremia usually does not require specific treatment except under extraordinary circumstances (as in liver disease or renal disease). Dilutional hyponatremia may occur in edematous patients in hot weather; appropriate therapy is water restriction, rather than administration of salt, except in rare instances when the hyponatremia is life-threatening. In actual salt depletion, appropriate replacement is the therapy of choice.

Hypokalemia may develop during thiazide therapy, especially with brisk diuresis, when severe cirrhosis is present, during concomitant use of corticosteroids or ACTH, or after prolonged therapy. However, this usually is prevented by the amiloride HCl component of MODURETIC.

Interference with adequate oral electrolyte intake will also contribute to hypokalemia. Hypokalemia may cause cardiac arrhythmia and may also sensitize or exaggerate the response of the heart to the toxic effects of digitalis (e.g., increased ventricular irritability).

Thiazides have been shown to increase the urinary excretion of magnesium; this may result in hypomagnesemia. Amiloride HCl, a component of MODURETIC, has been shown to decrease the enhanced urinary excretion of magnesium which occurs when a thiazide or loop diuretic is used alone.

Increases in BUN levels have been reported with amiloride HCl and with hydrochlorothiazide. These increases usually have accompanied vigorous fluid elimination, especially when diuretic therapy was used in seriously ill patients, such as those who had hepatic cirrhosis with ascites and metabolic alkalosis, or those with resistant edema. Therefore, when MODURETIC is given to such patients, careful monitoring of serum electrolyte and BUN levels is important. In patients with pre-existing severe liver disease, hepatic encephalopathy, manifested by tremors, confusion, and coma, and increased jaundice, have been reported in association with diuretic therapy including amiloride HCl and hydrochlorothiazide.

In patients with renal disease, diuretics may precipitate azotemia. Cumulative effects of the components of MODURETIC may develop in patients with impaired renal function. If renal impairment becomes evident, MODURETIC should be discontinued (see CONTRAINDICATIONS and WARNINGS).

Drug Interactions

In some patients, the administration of a non-steroidal anti-inflammatory agent can reduce the diuretic, natriuretic, and antihypertensive effects of loop, potassium-sparing and thiazide diuretics. Therefore, when MODURETIC and non-steroidal anti-inflammatory agents are used concomitantly, the patient should be observed closely to determine if the desired effect of the diuretic is obtained. Since indomethacin and potassium-sparing diuretics, including MODURETIC, may each be associated with increased serum potassium levels, the potential effects on potassium kinetics and renal function should be considered when these agents are administered concurrently.

Amiloride HCl

When amiloride HCl is administered concomitantly with an angiotensin-converting enzyme inhibitor, the risk of hyperkalemia may be increased. Therefore, if concomitant use of these agents in indicated because of demonstrated hypokalemia, they should be used with caution and with frequent monitoring of serum potassium. (See WARNINGS.)

Hydrochlorothiazide

When given concurrently the following drugs may interact with thiazide diuretics.

Alcohol, barbiturates, or narcotics —potentiation of orthostatic hypotension may occur.

Antidiabetic drugs (oral agents and insulin)—dosage adjustment of the antidiabetic drug may be required.

Other antihypertensive drugs —additive effect or potentiation.

Cholestyramine and colestipol resins—Absorption of hydrochlorothiazide is impaired in the presence of anionic exchange resins. Single doses of either cholestyramine or colestipol resins bind the hydrochlorothiazide and reduce its absorption from the gastrointestinal tract by up to 85 and 43 percent, respectively.

Corticosteroids, ACTH —intensified electrolyte depletion, particularly hypokalemia.

Pressor amines (e.g., norepinephrine) —possible decreased response to pressor amines but not sufficient to preclude their use.

Skeletal muscle relaxants, nondepolarizing (e.g., tubocurarine) —possible increased responsiveness to the muscle relaxant.

Lithium —generally should not be given with diuretics. Diuretic agents reduce the renal clearance of lithium and add a high risk of lithium toxicity. Refer to the package insert for lithium preparations before use of such preparations with MODURETIC.

Metabolic and Endocrine Effects

In diabetic patients, insulin requirements may be increased, decreased, or unchanged due to the hydrochlorothiazide component. Diabetes mellitus that has been latent may become manifest during administration of thiazide diuretics.

Because calcium excretion is decreased by thiazides, MODURETIC should be discontinued before carrying out tests for parathyroid function. Pathologic changes in the parathyroid glands, with hypercalcemia and hypophosphatemia have been observed in a few patients on prolonged thiazide therapy; however, the common complications of hyperparathyroidism such as renal lithiasis, bone resorption, and peptic ulceration have not been seen.

Hyperuricemia may occur or acute gout may be precipitated in certain patients receiving thiazide therapy.

Other Precautions

In patients receiving thiazides, sensitivity reactions may occur with or without a history of allergy or bronchial asthma. The possibility of exacerbation or activation of systemic lupus erythematosus has been reported with the use of thiazides.

Increases in cholesterol and triglyceride levels may be associated with thiazide diuretic therapy.

Carcinogenicity, Mutagenicity, Impairment of Fertility

Long-term studies in animals have not been performed to evaluate the effects upon fertility, mutagenicity or carcinogenic potential of MODURETIC.

Amiloride HCl

There was no evidence of a tumorigenic effect when amiloride HCl was administered for 92 weeks to mice at doses up to 10 mg/kg/day (25 times the maximum daily human dose). Amiloride HCl has also been administered for 104 weeks to male and female rats at doses up to 6 and 8 mg/kg/day (15 and 20 times the maximum daily dose for humans, respectively) and showed no evidence of carcinogenicity.

Amiloride HCl was devoid of mutagenic activity in various strains of *Salmonella typhimurium* with or without a mammalian liver microsomal activation system (Ames test).

Hydrochlorothiazide

Two-year feeding studies in mice and rats conducted under the auspices of the National Toxicology Program (NTP) uncovered no evidence of a carcinogenic potential of hydrochlorothiazide in female mice (at doses of up to approximately 600 mg/kg/day) or in male and female rats (at doses of up to approximately 100 mg/kg/day). The NTP, however, found equivocal evidence for hepatocarcinogenicity in male mice. Hydrochlorothiazide was not genotoxic *in vitro* in the Ames mutagenicity assay of *Salmonella typhimurium* strains TA 98, TA 100, TA 1535, TA 1537, and TA 1538 and in the Chinese Hamster Ovary (CHO) test for chromosomal aberrations, or *in vivo* in assays using mouse germinal cell chromosomes, Chinese hamster bone marrow chromosomes, and the *Drosophila* sex-linked recessive lethal trait gene. Positive test results were obtained only in the *in vitro* CHO Sister Chromatid Exchange (clastogenicity) and in the Mouse Lymphoma Cell (mutagenicity) assays, using concentrations of hydrochlorothiazide from 43 to 1300 µg/mL, and in the *Asperigillus nidulans* non-disjunction assay at an unspecified concentration.

Hydrochlorothiazide had no adverse effects on the fertility of mice and rats of either sex in studies wherein these species were exposed, via their diet, to doses of up to 100 and 4 mg/kg, respectively, prior to conception and throughout gestation.

Pregnancy

Pregnancy Category B. Teratogenicity studies have been performed with combinations of amiloride HCl and hydrochlorothiazide in rabbits and mice at doses up to 25 times the expected maximum daily dose for humans and have revealed no evidence of harm to the fetus. No evidence of impaired fertility in rats was apparent at dosage levels up to 25 times the expected maximum human daily dose. A perinatal and postnatal study in rats showed a reduction in maternal body weight gain during and after gestation at a daily dose of 25 times the expected maximum daily dose for humans. The body weights of alive pups at birth and at weaning were also reduced at this dose level. There are no adequate and well-controlled studies in pregnant women. Because animal reproduction studies are not always predictive of human responses, and because of the data listed below with the individual components, this drug should be used during pregnancy only if clearly needed.

Amiloride HCl

Teratogenicity studies with amiloride HCl in rabbits and mice given 20 and 25 times the maximum human dose, respectively, revealed no evidence of harm to the fetus, although studies showed that the drug crossed the placenta in modest amounts. Reproduction studies in rats at 20 times the expected maximum daily dose for humans showed no evidence of impaired fertility. At approximately 5 or more times the expected maximum daily dose for humans, some toxicity was seen in adult rats and rabbits and a decrease in rat pup growth and survival occurred.

Hydrochlorothiazide

Teratogenic Effects: Studies in which hydrochlorothiazide was orally administered to pregnant mice and rats during their respective periods of major organogenesis at doses up to 3000 and 1000 mg hydrochlorothiazide/kg, respectively, provided no evidence of harm to the fetus. There are, however, no adequate and well-controlled studies in pregnant women.

Nonteratogenic Effects: Thiazides cross the placental barrier and appear in cord blood. There is a risk of fetal or neonatal jaundice, thrombocytopenia, and possibly other adverse reactions that have occurred in adults.

Nursing Mothers

Studies in rats have shown that amiloride is excreted in milk in concentrations higher than those found in blood, but it is not known whether amiloride HCl is excreted in human milk. However, thiazides appear in breast milk. Because of the potential for serious adverse reactions in nursing infants, a decision should be made whether to discontinue nursing or to discontinue the drug, taking into account the importance of the drug to the mother.

Pediatric Use

Safety and effectiveness in pediatric patients have not been established.

ADVERSE REACTIONS

MODURETIC is usually well tolerated and significant clinical adverse effects have been reported infrequently. The risk of hyperkalemia (serum potassium levels greater than 5.5 mEq per liter) with MODURETIC is about 1–2 percent in patients without renal impairment or diabetes mellitus (see WARNINGS). Minor adverse reactions to amiloride HCl have been reported relatively frequently (about 20%) but the relationship of many of the reports to amiloride HCl is uncertain and the overall frequency was similar in hydrochlorothiazide treated groups. Nausea/anorexia, abdominal pain, flatulence, and mild skin rash have been reported and

Continued on next page

Information on the Merck & Co., Inc. products listed on these pages is the full prescribing information from product circulars in use September 30, 2000. For information, please call 1-800-NSC MERCK [1-800-672-6372].

Moduretic—Cont.

probably are related to amiloride. Other adverse experiences that have been reported with MODURETIC are generally those known to be associated with diuresis, thiazide therapy, or with the underlying disease being treated. Clinical trials have not demonstrated that combining amiloride and hydrochlorothiazide increases the risk of adverse reactions over those seen with the individual components.
The adverse reactions for MODURETIC listed in the following table have been arranged into two groups: (1) incidence greater than one percent; and (2) incidence one percent or less. The incidence for group (1) was determined from clinical studies conducted in the United States (607 patients treated with MODURETIC). The adverse effects listed in group (2) include reports from the same clinical studies and voluntary reports since marketing. The probability of a causal relationship exists between MODURETIC and these adverse reactions, some of which have been reported only rarely.

Incidence > 1%	*Incidence ≤ 1%*
Body as a Whole	
Headache**	Malaise
Weakness**	Chest pain
Fatigue/tiredness	Back pain
	Syncope
Cardiovascular	
Arryhthmia	Tachycardia
	Digitalis toxicity
	Orthostatic hypotension
	Angina pectoris
Digestive	
Nausea/anorexia**	Constipation
Diarrhea	GI bleeding
Gastrointestinal pain	GI disturbance
	Appetite changes
Abdominal pain	Abdominal fullness
	Hiccups
	Thirst
	Vomiting
	Anorexia
	Flatulence
Metabolic	
Elevated serum potassium levels (>5.5 mEq per liter)***	Gout
	Dehydration
	Symptomatic hyponatremia†
Musculoskeletal	
Leg ache	Muscle cramps/spasm
	Joint pain
Nervous	
Dizziness**	Paraesthesia/numbness
	Stupor
	Vertigo
Psychiatric	
None	Insomnia
	Nervousness
	Depression
	Sleepiness
	Mental confusion
Respiratory	
Dyspnea	None
Skin	
Rash**	Flushing
Pruritus	Diaphoresis
	Erythema multiforme including Stevens-Johnson syndrome
	Exfoliative dermatitis including toxic epidermal necrolysis
	Alopecia
Special Senses	
None	Bad taste
	Visual disturbance
	Nasal congestion
Urogenital	
None	Impotence
	Nocturia
	Dysuria
	Incontinence
	Renal dysfunction including renal failure
	Gynecomastia

** Reactions occurring in 3% to 8% of patients treated with MODURETIC. (Those reactions occurring in less than 3% of the patients are unmarked.)
*** See WARNINGS.
† See PRECAUTIONS.

Other adverse reactions that have been reported with the individual components and within each category are listed in order of decreasing severity:
Amiloride —Body as a Whole: Painful extremities, neck/shoulder ache, fatigability; *Cardiovascular:* Palpitation; *Digestive:* Activation of probable pre-existing peptic ulcer, abnormal liver function, jaundice, dyspepsia, heartburn; *Hematologic:* Aplastic anemia, neutropenia; *Integumentary:* Alopecia, itching, dry mouth; *Nervous System/Psychiatric:* Encephalopathy, tremors, decreased libido; *Respiratory:* Shortness of breath, cough; *Special Senses:* Increased intraocular pressure, tinnitus; *Urogenital:* Bladder spasms, polyuria, urinary frequency.
Hydrochlorothiazide —Digestive: Pancreatitis, jaundice (intrahepatic cholestatic jaundice), sialadenitis, cramping, gastric irritation; *Hematologic:* Aplastic anemia, agranulocytosis, leukopenia, hemolytic anemia, thrombocytopenia; *Hypersensitivity:* Anaphylactic reactions, necrotizing angiitis (vasculitis, cutaneous vasculitis), respiratory distress including pneumonitis and pulmonary edema, photosensitivity, fever, urticaria, purpura; *Metabolic:* Electrolyte imbalance (see PRECAUTIONS), hyperglycemia, glycosuria, hyperuricemia; *Nervous System/Psychiatric:* Restlessness; *Special Senses:* Transient blurred vision, xanthopsia; *Urogenital:* Interstitial nephritis (see WARNINGS).

OVERDOSAGE

No data are available in regard to overdosage in humans.
The oral LD_{50} of the combination drug is 189 and 422 mg/kg for female mice and female rats, respectively.
It is not known whether the drug is dialyzable.
No specific information is available on the treatment of overdosage with MODURETIC, and no specific antidote is available. Treatment is symptomatic and supportive. Therapy with MODURETIC should be discontinued and the patient observed closely. Suggested measures include induction of emesis and/or gastric lavage.
Amiloride HCl: No data are available in regard to overdosage in humans.
The oral LD_{50} of amiloride HCl (calculated as the base) is 56 mg/kg in mice and 36 to 85 mg/kg in rats, depending on the strain.
The most common signs and symptoms to be expected with overdosage are dehydration and electrolyte imbalance. If hyperkalemia occurs, active measures should be taken to reduce the serum potassium levels.
Hydrochlorothiazide: The oral LD_{50} of hydrochlorothiazide is greater than 10.0 g/kg in both mice and rats.
The most common signs and symptoms observed are those caused by electrolyte depletion (hypokalemia, hypochloremia, hyponatremia) and dehydration resulting from excessive diuresis. If digitalis has also been administered, hypokalemia may accentuate cardiac arrhythmias.

DOSAGE AND ADMINISTRATION

MODURETIC should be administered with food.
The usual starting dosage is 1 tablet a day. The dosage may be increased to 2 tablets a day, if necessary. More than 2 tablets of MODURETIC daily usually are not needed and there is no controlled experience with such doses. Hydrochlorothiazide can be given at doses of 12.5 to 50 mg per day when used alone. Patients usually do not require doses of hydrochlorothiazide in excess of 50 mg daily when combined with other antihypertensive agents.
The daily dose is usually given as a single dose but may be given in divided doses. Once an initial diuresis has been achieved, dosage adjustment may be necessary. Maintenance therapy may be on an intermittent basis.

HOW SUPPLIED

No. 3385—Tablets MODURETIC are peach-colored, diamond-shaped, scored, compressed tablets, coded MSD 917 on one side and M on the other. Each tablet contains 5 mg of anhydrous amiloride HCl and 50 mg of hydrochlorothiazide.
They are supplied as follows:
NDC 0006-0917-68 in bottles of 100
(6505-01-139-1498 100's).
Shown in Product Identification Guide, page 324
Storage
Keep container tightly closed. Protect from light, moisture, freezing, –20°C (–4°F) and store at room temperature, 15–30°C (59–86°F).
7887326 Issued April 1998

MUMPSVAX® ℞
(Mumps Virus Vaccine Live)
Jeryl Lynn Strain

DESCRIPTION

MUMPSVAX* (Mumps Virus Vaccine Live) is a live virus vaccine for vaccination against mumps.
MUMPSVAX is a sterile lyophilized preparation of the Jeryl Lynn** (B level) strain of mumps virus. The virus was adapted to and propagated in chick embryo cell culture.
The growth medium for mumps is Medium 199 (a buffered salt solution containing vitamins and amino acids and supplemented with fetal bovine serum) containing SPGA (sucrose, phosphate, glutamate, and human albumin) as stabilizer and neomycin.
The cells, virus pools, fetal bovine serum, and human albumin are all screened for the absence of adventitious agents. Human albumin is processed using the Cohn cold ethanol fractionation procedure.
The reconstituted vaccine is for subcutaneous administration. Each 0.5 mL dose contains not less than 20,000 $TCID_{50}$ (tissue culture infectious doses) of mumps virus. Each dose of the vaccine is calculated to contain sorbitol (14.5 mg), sodium phosphate, sucrose (1.9 mg), sodium chloride, hydrolyzed gelatin (14.5 mg), human albumin (0.3 mg), fetal bovine serum (<1 ppm), other buffer and media ingredients and approximately 25 mcg of neomycin. The product contains no preservative.
Before reconstitution, the lyophilized vaccine is a light yellow compact crystalline plug. MUMPSVAX, when reconstituted as directed, is clear yellow.

*Registered trademark of MERCK & CO., Inc.
**Trademark of MERCK & CO., Inc.

CLINICAL PHARMACOLOGY

Mumps is a common childhood disease, caused by mumps virus (paramyxovirus), that may be associated with serious complications and/or death. For example, mumps is associated with aseptic meningitis, deafness and orchitis.
The impact of mumps vaccination on the natural history of each disease in the United States can be quantified by comparing the maximum number of mumps cases reported in a given year prior to vaccine use to the number of cases of each disease reported in 1995. For mumps, 152,209 cases reported in 1968 compared to 840 cases reported in 1995 resulted in a 99.45% decrease in reported cases.
Extensive clinical trials have demonstrated that MUMPSVAX is highly immunogenic and well tolerated. A single injection of the vaccine has been shown to induce mumps neutralizing antibodies in approximately 97% of susceptible children and approximately 93% of susceptible adults. The pattern of antibody response closely resembles that observed for natural mumps. Although the antibody level is significantly lower than that following natural infection; it is protective and long lasting. However, a small percentage (1–5%) of vaccinees may fail to seroconvert after the primary dose (see also INDICATIONS AND USAGE, *Recommended Vaccination Schedule*).
Efficacy of mumps vaccine was established in a series of double-blind controlled field trials which demonstrated a high degree of protective efficacy. These studies also established that seroconversion in response to mumps vaccination paralleled protection from these diseases.
Following vaccination, antibodies associated with protection can be measured by neutralization assays, hemagglutination-inhibition (HI), or ELISA (enzyme linked immunosorbent assay) tests. Neutralizing and ELISA antibodies to mumps virus are still detectable in most individuals 11–13 years after primary vaccination.

INDICATIONS AND USAGE

Recommended Vaccination Schedule
MUMPSVAX is indicated for vaccination against mumps in persons 12 months of age or older.
It is not recommended for infants younger than 12 months because they may retain maternal mumps neutralizing antibodies which may interfere with the immune response.
Individuals first vaccinated with MUMPSVAX at 12 months of age or older should be revaccinated with M-M-R* II (Measles, Mumps, and Rubella Virus Vaccine Live) prior to elementary school entry. Revaccination may seroconvert primary failures or boost antibody titers of those individuals whose titers have declined. The Advisory Committee on Immunization Practices (ACIP) recommends administration of the first dose of M-M-R II at 12–15 months of age and administration of the second dose of M-M-R II at 4–6 years of age. In addition, some public health jurisdictions mandate the age for revaccination. Consult the complete text of applicable guidelines regarding routine revaccination including that of high-risk adult populations.
Unnecessary doses of a vaccine are best avoided by ensuring that written documentation of vaccination is preserved and a copy given to each vaccinee's parent or guardian.
Other Vaccination Considerations
Other Populations
Individuals planning travel outside the United States, if not immune, can acquire measles, mumps or rubella and import these diseases into the United States. Therefore, prior to international travel, individuals known to be susceptible to one or more of these diseases can receive either a monovalent vaccine (measles, mumps or rubella), or a combination vaccine as appropriate. However, M-M-R II is preferred for persons likely to be susceptible to mumps and rebella; and if monovalent measles vaccine is not readily available, travelers should receive M-M-R II regardless of their immune status to mumps or rubella.
Vaccination is recommended for susceptible individuals in high-risk groups such as college students, health-care workers, and military personnel.
Post Exposure Vaccination
There is no conclusive evidence that vaccination of individuals recently exposed to natural mumps will provide protection.
Use With Other Vaccines
See DOSAGE AND ADMINISTRATION, *Use With Other Vaccines*

CONTRAINDICATIONS

Hypersensitivity to any component of the vaccine, including gelatin.
Do not give MUMPSVAX to pregnant females; the possible effects of the vaccine on fetal development are unknown at this time. If vaccination of postpubertal females is undertaken, pregnancy should be avoided for 3 months following vaccination (see PRECAUTIONS, *Pregnancy*).

Anaphylactic or anaphylactoid reactions to neomycin (each dose of reconstituted vaccine contains approximately 25 mcg of neomycin).
Any febrile respiratory illness or other active febrile infection. However, the ACIP has recommended that all vaccines can be administered to persons with minor illnesses such as diarrhea, mild upper respiratory infection with or without low-grade fever, or other low-grade febrile illness.
Patients receiving immunosuppressive therapy. This contraindication does not apply to patients who are receiving corticosteroids as replacement therapy, e.g., for Addison's disease.
Individuals with blood dyscrasias, leukemia, lymphomas of any type, or other malignant neoplasms affecting the bone marrow or lymphatic systems.
Primary and acquired immunodeficiency states, including patients who are immunosuppressed in association with AIDS or other clinical manifestations of infection with human immunodeficiency viruses; cellular immune deficiencies; and hypogammaglobulinemic and dysgammaglobulinemic states.
Individuals with a family history of congenital or hereditary immunodeficiency, until the immune competence of the potential vaccine recipient is demonstrated.

WARNINGS

The physician should be alert to the temperature elevation which may occur following vaccination (see ADVERSE REACTIONS).
Hypersensitivity to Eggs
Live mumps vaccine is produced in chick embryo cell culture. Persons with a history of anaphylactic, anaphylactoid, or other immediate reactions (e.g., hives, swelling of the mouth and throat, difficulty breathing, hypotension, or shock) subsequent to egg ingestion may be at an enhanced risk of immediate-type hypersensitivity reactions after receiving vaccines containing traces of chick embryo antigen. The potential risk to benefit ratio should be carefully evaluated before considering vaccination in such cases. Such individuals may be vaccinated with extreme caution, having adequate treatment on hand should a reaction occur (see PRECAUTIONS).
However, the AAP has stated, "Most children with a history of anaphylactic reactions to eggs have no untoward reactions to measles or MMR vaccine. Persons are not at increased risk if they have egg allergies that are not anaphylactic, and they should be vaccinated in the usual manner. In addition, skin testing of egg-allergic children with vaccine has not been predictive of which children will have an immediate hypersensitivity reaction...Persons with allergies to chickens or chicken feathers are not at increased risk of reaction to the vaccine."
Hypersensitivity to Neomycin
The AAP states, "Persons who have experienced anaphylactic reactions to topically or systemically administered neomycin should not receive measles vaccine. Most often, however, neomycin allergy manifests as a contact dermatitis, which is a delayed-type (cell-mediated) immune response rather than anaphylaxis. In such persons, an adverse reaction to neomycin in the vaccine would be an erythematous, pruritic nodule or papule, 48 to 96 hours after vaccination. A history of contact dermatitis to neomycin is not a contraindication to receiving measles vaccine."
Thrombocytopenia
Individuals with current thrombocytopenia may develop more severe thrombocytopenia following vaccination. In addition, individuals who experienced thrombocytopenia with the first dose of M-M-R II (or its component vaccines) may develop thrombocytopenia with repeat doses. Serologic status may be evaluated to determine whether or not additional doses of vaccine are needed. The potential risk to benefit ratio should be carefully evaluated before considering vaccination in such cases.

PRECAUTIONS

General
Adequate treatment provisions including epinephrine injection (1:1000), should be available for immediate use should an anaphylactic or anaphylactoid reaction occur.
Special care should be taken to ensure that the injection does not enter a blood vessel.
Children and young adults who are known to be infected with human immunodeficiency viruses and are not immunosuppressed may be vaccinated. However, vaccinees who are infected with HIV should be monitored closely for vaccine-preventable diseases because immunization may be less effective than for uninfected persons (see CONTRAINDICATIONS).
Vaccination should be deferred for 3 months or longer following blood or plasma transfusions, or administration of immune globulin (human).
There are no reports of transmission of live mumps virus from vaccinees to susceptible contacts.
It has been reported that mumps virus vaccine live may result in a temporary depression of tuberculin skin sensitivity. Therefore, if a tuberculin test is to be done, it should be administered either before or simultaneously with MUMPSVAX.
Individuals with active untreated tuberculosis should not be vaccinated.
As for any vaccine, vaccination with MUMPSVAX may not result in protection in 100% of vaccinees.
The health-care provider should determine the current health status and previous vaccination history of the vaccinee.
The health-care provider should question the patient, parent, or guardian about reactions to a previous dose of MUMPSVAX or other mumps-containing vaccines.
Drug Interactions
See DOSAGE AND ADMINISTRATION, *Use With Other Vaccines*.
Information for Patients
The health-care provider should provide the vaccine information required to be given with each vaccination to the patient, parent or guardian.
The health-care provider should inform the patient, parent or guardian of the benefits and risks associated with vaccination. For risks associated with vaccination see WARNINGS, PRECAUTIONS, ADVERSE REACTIONS.
Patients, parents or guardians should be instructed to report any serious adverse reactions to their health-care provider who in turn should report such events to the U.S. Department of Health and Human Services through the Vaccine Adverse Event Reporting System (VAERS), 1-800-822-7967.
Pregnancy should be avoided for 3 months following vaccination.
Immunosuppressive Therapy
The immune status of patients about to undergo immunosuppressive therapy should be evaluated so that the physician can consider whether vaccination prior to the initiation of treatment is indicated (see CONTRAINDICATIONS and PRECAUTIONS).
The ACIP has indicated that patients with leukemia in remission who have not received chemotherapy for at least 3 months may receive live virus vaccines. Short-term (<2 weeks), low- to moderate-dose systemic corticosteroid therapy, topical steroid therapy (e.g., nasal, skin), long-term alternate-day treatment with low to moderate doses of short-acting systemic steroid, and intra-articular, bursal, or tendon injection of corticosteroids are not immunosuppressive in their usual doses and do not contraindicate the administration of mumps vaccine.
Immune Globulin
Administration of immune globulins concurrently with MUMPSVAX may interfere with the expected immune response.
See also PRECAUTIONS, *General*.
Carcinogenesis, Mutagenesis, Impairment of Fertility
MUMPSVAX has not been evaluated for carcinogenic or mutagenic potential, or potential to impair fertility.
Pregnancy
Pregnancy Category C
Animal reproduction studies have not been conducted with MUMPSVAX. It is also not known whether MUMPSVAX can cause fetal harm when administered to a pregnant woman or can affect reproduction capacity. Therefore, mumps virus vaccine should not be given to persons known to be pregnant; furthermore, pregnancy should be avoided for 3 months following vaccination (see CONTRAINDICATIONS).
In counseling women who are inadvertently vaccinated when pregnant or who become pregnant within 3 months of vaccination, the physician should be aware that mumps infection during the first trimester of pregnancy may increase the rate of spontaneous abortion. Although mumps vaccine virus has been shown to infect the placenta and fetus, there is no evidence that it causes congenital malformations in humans.
Nursing Mothers
It is not known whether mumps vaccine virus is secreted in human milk. Therefore, because many drugs are excreted in human milk, caution should be exercised when MUMPSVAX is administered to a nursing woman.
Pediatric Use
Safety and effectiveness in infants below the age of 12 months have not been established (see INDICATIONS AND USAGE, *Recommended Vaccination Schedule*).

ADVERSE REACTIONS

The following adverse reactions are listed in decreasing order of severity, without regard to causality, within each body system category and have been reported during clinical trials, with use of the marketed vaccine, or with use of polyvalent vaccine containing mumps:
Body as a Whole
Fever; syncope; irritability.
Cardiovascular System
Vasculitis.
Digestive System
Pancreatitis; diarrhea; parotitis.
Endocrine System
Diabetes mellitus.
Hemic and Lymphatic System
Thrombocytopenia; purpura; lymphadenopathy; leukocytosis.
Immune System
Anaphylaxis and anaphylactoid reactions have been reported as well as related phenomena such as angioneurotic edema (including peripheral or facial edema) and bronchial spasm.
Nervous System
Encephalitis; Guillain-Barré Syndrome (GBS); febrile seizures; ocular palsies.
Cases of aseptic meningitis have been reported to VAERS following measles, mumps, and rubella vaccination. Although a causal relationship between the Urabe strain of mumps vaccine and aseptic meningitis has been shown, there are no data to link Jeryl Lynn mumps vaccine to aseptic meningitis.
Respiratory System
Cough; rhinitis.
Skin
Stevens-Johnson Syndrome; erythema multiforme; urticaria.
Local reactions including burning/stinging at injection site; wheal and flare.
Special Senses—Ear
Nerve deafness; otitis media.
Special Senses—Eye
Optic neuritis; papillitis; retrobulbar neuritis; conjunctivitis.
Urogenital System
Orchitis.
Other
Death from various, and in some cases unknown, causes has been reported rarely following vaccination with measles, mumps, and rubella vaccines; however, a causal relationship has not been established. No deaths or permanent sequelae were reported in a published post-marketing surveillance study in Finland involving 1.5 million children and adults who were vaccinated with M-M-R II during 1982–1993.
Under the National Childhood Vaccine Injury Act of 1986, health-care providers and manufacturers are required to record and report certain suspected adverse events occurring within specific time periods after vaccination. However, the U.S. Department of Health and Human Services (DHHS) has established a Vaccine Adverse Event Reporting System (VAERS) which will accept all reports of suspected events. A VAERS report form as well as information regarding reporting requirements can be obtained by calling VAERS 1-800-822-7967.

DOSAGE AND ADMINISTRATION

FOR SUBCUTANEOUS ADMINISTRATION
Do not inject intravenously
The dose for any age is 0.5 mL administered subcutaneously, preferably into the outer aspect of the upper arm.
The recommended age for primary vaccination is 12 to 15 months.
Revaccination with M-M-R II is recommended prior to elementary school entry. See also INDICATIONS AND USAGE, *Recommended Vaccination Schedule*.
Immune Globulin (IG) is not to be given concurrently with MUMPSVAX.
CAUTION: A sterile syringe free of preservatives, antiseptics, and detergents should be used for each injection and/or reconstitution of the vaccine because these substances may inactivate the live virus vaccine. A 25 gauge, 5/8″ needle is recommended.
To reconstitute, use only the diluent supplied, since it is free of preservatives or other antiviral substances which might inactivate the vaccine.
Single Dose Vial—First withdraw the entire volume of diluent into the syringe to be used for reconstitution. Inject all the diluent in the syringe into the vial of lyophilized vaccine, and agitate to mix thoroughly. If the lyophilized vaccine cannot be dissolved, discard. Withdraw the entire contents into a syringe and inject the total volume of restored vaccine subcutaneously.
It is important to use a separate sterile syringe and needle for each individual patient to prevent transmission of hepatitis B and other infectious agents from one person to another.
10 Dose Vial (available only to government agencies/institutions)—Withdraw the entire contents (7 mL) of the diluent vial into the sterile syringe to be used for reconstitution, and introduce into the 10 dose vial of lyophilized vaccine. Agitate to ensure thorough mixing. If the lyophilized vaccine cannot be dissolved, discard. The outer labeling suggests "For Jet Injector or Syringe Use". Use with separate sterile syringes is permitted for containers of 10 doses or less. The vaccine and diluent do not contain preservatives; therefore, the user must recognize the potential contamination hazards and exercise special precautions to protect the sterility and potency of the product. The use of aseptic techniques and proper storage prior to and after restoration of the vaccine and subsequent withdrawal of the individual doses is essential. Use 0.5 mL of the reconstituted vaccine for subcutaneous injection.
It is important to use a separate sterile syringe and needle for each individual patient to prevent transmission of hepatitis B and other infectious agents from one person to another.
50 Dose Vial (available only to government agencies/institutions)—Withdraw the entire contents (30 mL) of the diluent vial into the sterile syringe to be used for reconstitution and introduce into the 50 dose vial of lyophilized vaccine. Agi-

Continued on next page

Information on the Merck & Co., Inc. products listed on these pages is the full prescribing information from product circulars in use September 30, 2000. For information, please call 1-800-NSC MERCK [1-800-672-6372].

Mumpsvax—Cont.

tate to ensure thorough mixing. If the lyophilized vaccine cannot be dissolved, discard. With full aseptic precautions, attach the vial to the sterilized multidose jet injector apparatus. Use 0.5 mL of the reconstituted vaccine for subcutaneous injection.
Parenteral drug products should be inspected visually for particulate matter and discoloration prior to administration whenever solution and container permit. MUMPSVAX, when reconstituted, is clear yellow.
Use With Other Vaccines
MUMPSVAX should not be given less than one month before or after administration of other live viral vaccines.
M-M-R II has been administered concurrently with VARIVAX* [Varicella Virus Vaccine Live (Oka/Merck)], and PedvaxHIB* [Haemophilus b Conjugate Vaccine (Meningococcal Protein Conjugate)] using separate sites and syringes. No impairment of immune response to individual tested vaccine antigens was demonstrated. The type, frequency, and severity of adverse experiences observed with M-M-R II were similar to those seen when each vaccine was given alone.
Routine administration of DTP (diphtheria, tetanus, pertussis) and/or OPV (oral poliovirus vaccine) concurrently with measles, mumps and rubella vaccines is not recommended because there are limited data relating to the simultaneous administration of these antigens.
However, other schedules have been used. The ACIP has stated "Although data are limited concerning the simultaneous administration of the entire recommended vaccine series (i.e., DTP, OPV, MMR, and Hib vaccines, with or without hepatitis B vaccine), data from numerous studies have indicated no interference between routinely recommended childhood vaccines (either live, attenuated, or killed). These findings support the simultaneous use of all vaccines as recommended."

HOW SUPPLIED

No. 4753—MUMPSVAX is supplied as a single-dose vial of lyophilized vaccine, **NDC** 0006-4753-00, and a vial of diluent.
No. 4584X/4309—MUMPSVAX is supplied as follows: (1) a box of 10 single-dose vials of lyophilized vaccine (package A), **NDC** 0006-4584-00; and (2) a box of 10 vials of diluent (package B). To conserve refrigerator space, the diluent may be stored separately at room temperature (6505-01-037-6792, Ten Pack).
Storage
During shipment, to ensure that there is not loss of potency, the vaccine must be maintained at a temperature of 10°C (50°F) or colder. Freezing during shipment will not affect potency.
Protect the vaccine from light at all times, since such exposure may inactivate the virus.
Before reconstitution, store the vial of lyophilized vaccine at 2–8°C (36–46°F) or colder. The diluent may be stored in the refrigerator with the lyophilized vaccine or separately at room temperature.
It is recommended that the vaccine be used as soon as possible after reconstitution. Store reconstituted vaccine in the vaccine vial in a dark place at 2–8°C (36–46°F) and discard if not used within 8 hours.
9243500 Issued April 1999

MUSTARGEN®, Trituration of (Mechlorethamine HCl for Injection) ℞

WARNINGS
MUSTARGEN* (Mechlorethamine HCl) should be administered only under the supervision of a physician who is experienced in the use of cancer chemotherapeutic agents.
This drug is **HIGHLY TOXIC** and both powder and solution must be handled and administered with care. Inhalation of dust or vapors and contact with skin or mucous membranes, especially those of the eyes, must be avoided. Due to the toxic properties of mechlorethamine (e.g., corrosivity, carcinogenicity, mutagenicity, teratogenicity), special handling procedures should be reviewed prior to handling and followed diligently.
Extravasation of the drug into subcutaneous tissues results in a painful inflammation. The area usually becomes indurated and sloughing may occur. If leakage of drug is obvious, prompt infiltration of the area with sterile isotonic sodium thiosulfate (1/6 molar) and application of an ice compress for 6 to 12 hours may minimize the local reaction. For 1/6 molar solution of sodium thiosulfate, use 4.14 g of sodium thiosulfate per 100 mL of Sterile Water for Injection or 2.64 g of anhydrous sodium thiosulfate per 100 mL or dilute 4 mL of Sodium Thiosulfate Injection (10%) with 6 mL of Sterile Water for Injection.

DESCRIPTION

MUSTARGEN, an antineoplastic nitrogen mustard also known as HN2 hydrochloride, is a nitrogen analog of sulfur mustard. It is a light yellow brown, crystalline, hygroscopic powder that is very soluble in water and also soluble in alcohol.
Mechlorethamine hydrochloride is designated chemically as 2-chloro-*N*-(2-chloroethyl)-*N*-methylethanamine hydrochloride. The molecular weight is 192.52 and the melting point is 108–111°C. The empirical formula is $C_5H_{11}Cl_2N \cdot HCl$, and the structural formula is: $CH_3N(CH_2CH_2Cl)_2 \cdot HCl$.
Trituration of MUSTARGEN is a sterile, light yellow brown crystalline powder for injection by the intravenous or intracavitary routes after dissolution. Each vial of MUSTARGEN contains 10 mg of mechlorethamine hydrochloride triturated with sodium chloride q.s. 100 mg. When dissolved with 10 mL Sterile Water for Injection or 0.9% Sodium Chloride Injection, the resulting solution has a pH of 3–5 at a concentration of 1 mg mechlorethamine HCl per mL.

*Registered trademark of MERCK & CO., Inc.

CLINICAL PHARMACOLOGY

Mechlorethamine, a biologic alkylating agent, has a cytotoxic action which inhibits rapidly proliferating cells.
Pharmacokinetics and Metabolism
In water or body fluids, mechlorethamine undergoes rapid chemical transformation and combines with water or reactive compounds of cells, so that the drug is no longer present in active form a few minutes after administration.

INDICATIONS AND USAGE

Before using MUSTARGEN *see CONTRAINDICATIONS, WARNINGS, PRECAUTIONS, ADVERSE REACTIONS, DOSAGE AND ADMINISTRATION, and HOW SUPPLIED, Special Handling.*
MUSTARGEN, administered intravenously, is indicated for the palliative treatment of Hodgkin's disease (Stages III and IV), lymphosarcoma, chronic myelocytic or chronic lymphocytic leukemia, polycythemia vera, mycosis fungoides, and bronchogenic carcinoma.
MUSTARGEN, administered intrapleurally, intraperitoneally, or intrapericardially, is indicated for the palliative treatment of metastatic carcinoma resulting in effusion.

CONTRAINDICATIONS

The use of MUSTARGEN is contraindicated in the presence of known infectious diseases and in patients who have had previous anaphylactic reactions to MUSTARGEN.

WARNINGS

Before using MUSTARGEN, *an accurate histologic diagnosis of the disease, a knowledge of its natural course, and an adequate clinical history are important. The hematologic status of the patient must first be determined. It is essential to understand the hazards and therapeutic effects to be expected. Careful clinical judgment must be exercised in selecting patients. If the indication for its use is not clear, the drug should not be used.*
As nitrogen mustard therapy may contribute to extensive and rapid development of amyloidosis, it should be used only if foci of acute and chronic suppurative inflammation are absent.
Usage in Pregnancy
Mechlorethamine hydrochloride can cause fetal harm when administered to a pregnant woman. MUSTARGEN has been shown to produce fetal malformations in the rat and ferret when given as single subcutaneous injections of 1 mg/kg (2–3 times the maximum recommended human dose). There are no adequate and well controlled studies in pregnant women. If this drug is used during pregnancy, or if the patient becomes pregnant while taking this drug, the patient should be apprised of the potential hazard to the fetus. Women of childbearing potential should be advised to avoid becoming pregnant.

PRECAUTIONS

General
This drug is **HIGHLY TOXIC** and both powder and solution must be handled and administered with care. (See boxed warning and DOSAGE AND ADMINISTRATION, *Special Handling.*) Since MUSTARGEN is a powerful vesicant, it is intended primarily for intravenous use, and in most cases is given by this route. Inhalation of dust or vapors and contact with skin or mucous membranes, especially those of the eyes, must be avoided. Appropriate protective equipment should be worn when handling MUSTARGEN. Should accidental eye contact occur, copious irrigation for at least 15 minutes with water, normal saline or a balanced salt ophthalmic irrigating solution should be instituted immediately, followed by prompt ophthalmologic consultation. Should accidental skin contact occur, the affected part must be irrigated immediately with copious amounts of water, for at least 15 minutes while removing contaminated clothing and shoes, followed by 2% sodium thiosulfate solution. Medical attention should be sought immediately. Contaminated clothing should be destroyed. (See DOSAGE AND ADMINISTRATION, *Special Handling.*)
Because of the toxicity of MUSTARGEN, and the unpleasant side effects following its use, the potential risk and discomfort from the use of this drug in patients with inoperable neoplasms or in the terminal stage of the disease must be balanced against the limited gain obtainable. These gains will vary with the nature and the status of the disease under treatment. The routine use of MUSTARGEN in all cases of widely disseminated neoplasms is to be discouraged.
The use of MUSTARGEN in patients with leukopenia, thrombocytopenia, and anemia, due to invasion of the bone marrow by tumor carries a greater risk. In such patients a good response to treatment with disappearance of the tumor from the bone marrow may be associated with improvement of bone marrow function. However, in the absence of a good response or in patients who have been previously treated with chemotherapeutic agents, hematopoiesis may be further compromised, and leukopenia, thrombocytopenia and anemia may become more severe and lead to the demise of the patient.
Tumors of bone and nervous tissue have responded poorly to therapy. Results are unpredictable in disseminated and malignant tumors of different types.
Precautions must be observed with the use of MUSTARGEN and x-ray therapy or other chemotherapy in alternating courses. Hematopoietic function is characteristically depressed by either form of therapy, and neither MUSTARGEN following x-ray therapy nor x-ray therapy subsequent to the drug should be given until bone marrow function has recovered. In particular, irradiation of such areas as sternum, ribs, and vertebrae shortly after a course of nitrogen mustard may lead to hematologic complications.
MUSTARGEN has been reported to have immunosuppressive activity. Therefore, it should be borne in mind that use of the drug may predispose the patient to bacterial, viral or fungal infection.
Hyperuricemia may develop during therapy with MUSTARGEN. The problem of urate precipitation should be anticipated, particularly in the treatment of the lymphomas, and adequate methods for control of hyperuricemia should be instituted and careful attention directed toward adequate fluid intake before treatment.
Since drug toxicity, especially sensitivity to bone marrow failure, seems to be more common in chronic lymphatic leukemia than in other conditions, the drug should be given in this condition with great caution, if at all.
Extreme caution must be used in exceeding the average recommended dose. (See OVERDOSAGE.)
Laboratory Tests
Many abnormalities of renal, hepatic, and bone marrow function have been reported in patients with neoplastic disease and receiving mechlorethamine. It is advisable to check renal, hepatic, and bone marrow functions frequently.
Carcinogenesis, Mutagenesis, Impairment of Fertility
Therapy with alkylating agents such as MUSTARGEN may be associated with an increased incidence of a second malignant tumor, especially when such therapy is combined with other antineoplastic agents or radiation therapy.
The International Agency on Research on Cancer has judged that mechlorethamine is a probable carcinogen in humans. This is supported by limited evidence of carcinogenicity in humans and sufficient evidence of carcinogenicity in animals. Young-adult female RF mice were injected intravenously with four doses of 2.4 mg/kg of mechlorethamine (0.1% solution) at 2-week intervals with observations for up to 2 years. An increased incidence of thymic lymphomas and pulmonary adenomas was observed. Painting mechlorethamine on the skin of mice for periods up to 33 weeks resulted in squamous cell tumors in 9 of 33 mice.
Mechlorethamine induced mutations in the Ames test, in *E. coli*, and *Neurospora crassa*. Mechlorethamine caused chromosome aberrations in a variety of plant and mammalian cells. Dominant lethal mutations were produced in ICR/Ha Swiss mice.
Mechlorethamine impaired fertility in the rat at a daily dose of 500 mg/kg intravenously for two weeks.
Pregnancy
Pregnancy Category D. See WARNINGS.
Nursing Mothers
It is not known whether this drug is excreted in human milk. Because many drugs are excreted in human milk and because of the potential for serious adverse reactions in nursing infants from MUSTARGEN, a decision should be made whether to discontinue nursing or to discontinue the drug, taking into account the importance of the drug to the mother.
Pediatric Use
Safety and effectiveness in pediatric patients have not been established by well-controlled studies. Use of MUSTARGEN in pediatric patients has been quite limited. MUSTARGEN has been used in Hodgkin's disease, stages III and IV, in combination with other oncolytic agents (MOPP schedule). The MOPP chemotherapy combination includes mechlorethamine, vincristine, procarbazine, and prednisone or prednisolone.

ADVERSE REACTIONS

Clinical use of MUSTARGEN *usually is accompanied by toxic manifestations.*
Local Toxicity
Thrombosis and thrombophlebitis may result from direct contact of the drug with the intima of the injected vein. Avoid high concentration and prolonged contact with the

drug, especially in cases of elevated pressure in the antebrachial vein (e.g., in mediastinal tumor compression from severe vena cava syndrome).

Systemic Toxicity

General: Hypersensitivity reactions, including anaphylaxis, have been reported. Nausea, vomiting and depression of formed elements in the circulating blood are dose-limiting side effects and usually occur with the use of full doses of MUSTARGEN. Jaundice, alopecia, vertigo, tinnitus and diminished hearing may occur infrequently. Rarely, hemolytic anemia associated with such diseases as the lymphomas and chronic lymphocytic leukemia may be precipitated by treatment with alkylating agents including MUSTARGEN. Also, various chromosomal abnormalities have been reported in association with nitrogen mustard therapy.

MUSTARGEN is given preferably at night in case sedation for side effects is required. Nausea and vomiting usually occur 1 to 3 hours after use of the drug. Emesis may disappear in the first 8 hours, but nausea may persist for 24 hours. Nausea and vomiting may be so severe as to precipitate vascular accidents in patients with a hemorrhagic tendency. Premedication with antiemetics, in addition to sedatives, may help control severe nausea and vomiting. Anorexia, weakness and diarrhea may also occur.

Hematologic: The usual course of MUSTARGEN (total dose of 0.4 mg/kg either given as a single intravenous dose or divided into two or four daily doses of 0.2 or 0.1 mg/kg respectively) generally produces a lymphocytopenia within 24 hours after the first injection; significant granulocytopenia occurs within 6 to 8 days and lasts for 10 days to 3 weeks. Agranulocytosis appears to be relatively infrequent and recovery from leukopenia in most cases is complete within two weeks of the maximum reduction. Thrombocytopenia is variable but the time course of the appearance and recovery from reduced platelet counts generally parallels the sequence of granulocyte levels. In some cases severe thrombocytopenia may lead to bleeding from the gums and gastrointestinal tract, petechiae, and small subcutaneous hemorrhages; these symptoms appear to be transient and in most cases disappear with return to a normal platelet count. However, a severe and even uncontrollable depression of the hematopoietic system occasionally may follow the usual dose of MUSTARGEN, particularly in patients with widespread disease and debility and in patients previously treated with other antineoplastic agents or x-ray. Persistent pancytopenia has been reported. In rare instances, hemorrhagic complications may be due to hyperheparinemia. Erythrocyte and hemoglobin levels may decline during the first 2 weeks after therapy but rarely significantly. Depression of the hematopoietic system may be found up to 50 days or more after starting therapy.

Integumentary: Occasionally, a maculopapular skin eruption occurs, but this may be idiosyncratic and does not necessarily recur with subsequent courses of the drug. Erythema multiforme has been observed. Herpes zoster, a common complicating infection in patients with lymphomas, may first appear after therapy is instituted and on occasion may be precipitated by treatment. Further treatment should be discontinued during the acute phase of this illness to avoid progression to generalized herpes zoster.

Reproductive: Since the gonads are susceptible to MUSTARGEN, treatment may be followed by delayed catamenia, oligomenorrhea, or temporary or permanent amenorrhea. Impaired spermatogenesis, azoospermia, and total germinal aplasia have been reported in male patients treated with alkylating agents, especially in combination with other drugs. In some instances spermatogenesis may return in patients in remission, but this may occur only several years after intensive chemotherapy has been discontinued. Patients should be warned of the potential risk to their reproductive capacity.

OVERDOSAGE

With total doses exceeding 0.4 mg/kg of body weight for a single course, severe leukopenia, anemia, thrombocytopenia and a hemorrhagic diathesis with subsequent delayed bleeding may develop. Death may follow. The only treatment in instances of excessive dosage appears to be repeated blood product transfusions, antibiotic treatment of complicating infections and general supportive measures.

The intravenous LD_{50} of MUSTARGEN is 2 mg/kg and 1.6 mg/kg in the mouse and rat, respectively.

DOSAGE AND ADMINISTRATION

Intravenous Administration

The dosage of MUSTARGEN varies with the clinical situation, the therapeutic response and the magnitude of hematologic depression. A total dose of 0.4 mg/kg of body weight for each course usually is given either as a single dose or in divided doses of 0.1 to 0.2 mg/kg per day. Dosage should be based on ideal dry body weight. The presence of edema or ascites must be considered so that dosage will be based on actual weight unaugmented by these conditions.

The margin of safety in therapy with MUSTARGEN *is narrow and considerable care must be exercised in the matter of dosage.* Repeated examinations of blood are *mandatory* as a guide to subsequent therapy. (See OVERDOSAGE.)

Within a few minutes after intravenous injection, MUSTARGEN undergoes chemical transformation, combines with reactive compounds, and is no longer present in its active form in the blood stream. Subsequent courses should not be given until the patient has recovered hematologically from the previous course; this is best determined by repeated studies of the peripheral blood elements awaiting their return to normal levels. It is often possible to give repeated courses of MUSTARGEN as early as three weeks after treatment.

Preparation of Solution for Intravenous Administration

This drug is **HIGHLY TOXIC** and both powder and solution must be handled and administered with care. (See boxed warning and DOSAGE AND ADMINISTRATION, *Special Handling*.) Since MUSTARGEN is a powerful vesicant, it is intended primarily for intravenous use, and in most cases is given by this route. Inhalation of dust or vapors and contact with skin or mucous membranes, especially those of the eyes, must be avoided. Appropriate protective equipment should be worn when handling MUSTARGEN. Should accidental eye contact occur, copious irrigation for at least 15 minutes with water, normal saline or a balanced salt ophthalmic irrigating solution should be instituted immediately, followed by prompt ophthalmologic consultation. Should accidental skin contact occur, the affected part must be irrigated immediately with copious amounts of water, for at least 15 minutes while removing contaminated clothing and shoes, followed by 2% sodium thiosulfate solution. Medical attention should be sought immediately. Contaminated clothing should be destroyed. (See DOSAGE AND ADMINISTRATION, *Special Handling*).

Each vial of MUSTARGEN contains 10 mg of mechlorethamine hydrochloride triturated with sodium chloride q.s. 100 mg. In neutral or alkaline aqueous solution it undergoes rapid chemical transformation and is highly unstable. Although solutions prepared according to instructions are acidic and do not decompose as rapidly, they should be prepared immediately before each injection since they will decompose on standing. When reconstituted, MUSTARGEN is a clear colorless solution. *Do not use if the solution is discolored or if droplets of water are visible within the vial prior to reconstitution.*

Using a sterile 10 mL syringe, inject 10 mL of Sterile Water for Injection or 10 mL Sodium Chloride Injection into a vial of MUSTARGEN. With the needle (syringe attached) still in the rubber stopper, shake the vial several times to dissolve the drug completely. The resultant solution contains 1 mg of mechlorethamine hydrochloride per mL.

Parenteral drug products should be inspected visually for particulate matter and discoloration prior to administration whenever solution and container permit.

Special Handling

Animal studies have shown mechlorethamine to be corrosive to skin and eyes, a powerful vesicant, irritating to the mucous membranes of the respiratory tract and highly toxic by the oral route. It has also been shown to be carcinogenic, mutagenic and teratogenic. Due to the drug's toxic properties, appropriate precautions including the use of appropriate safety equipment are recommended for the preparation of MUSTARGEN for parenteral administration. Inhalation of dust or vapors and contact with skin or mucous membranes, especially those of the eyes, must be avoided. The National Institutes of Health presently recommends that the preparation of injectable anti-neoplastic drugs should be performed in a Class II laminar flow biological safety cabinet. Personnel preparing drugs of this class should wear chemical resistant, impervious gloves, safety goggles, outer garments and shoe covers. Additional body garments should be used based upon the task being performed (e.g., sleevelets, apron, gauntlets, disposable suits) to avoid exposed skin surfaces and inhalation of vapors and dust. Appropriate techniques should be used to remove potentially contaminated clothing.

Several other guidelines for proper handling and disposal of antineoplastic drugs have been published and should be considered.

Accidental Contact Measures

Should accidental eye contact occur, copious irrigation for at least 15 minutes with water, normal saline or a balanced salt ophthalmic irrigating solution should be instituted immediately, followed by prompt ophthalmologic consultation. Should accidental skin contact occur, the affected part must be irrigated immediately with copious amounts of water, for at least 15 minutes while removing contaminated clothing and shoes, followed by 2% sodium thiosulfate solution. Medical attention should be sought immediately. Contaminated clothing should be destroyed. (See PRECAUTIONS, *General* and DOSAGE AND ADMINISTRATION, *Preparation of Solution for Intravenous Administration*.)

Technique for Intravenous Administration

Withdraw into the syringe the calculated volume of solution required for a single injection. *Dispose of any remaining solution after neutralization* (see below). Although the drug may be injected directly into any suitable vein, it is injected preferably into the rubber or plastic tubing of a flowing intravenous infusion set. This reduces the possibility of severe local reactions due to extravasation or high concentration of the drug. Injecting the drug into the tubing rather than adding it to the entire volume of the infusion fluid minimizes a chemical reaction between the drug and the solution. The rate of injection apparently is not critical provided it is completed within a few minutes.

Intracavitary Administration

Nitrogen mustard has been used by intracavitary administration with varying success in certain malignant conditions for the control of pleural, peritoneal, and pericardial effusions caused by malignant cells.

The technique and the dose used by any of these routes varies. Therefore, if MUSTARGEN is given by the intracavitary route, the published articles concerning such use should be consulted. *Because of the inherent risks involved, the physician should be experienced in the appropriate injection techniques, and be thoroughly aware of the indications, dosages, hazards, and precautions as set forth in the published literature. When using* MUSTARGEN *by the intracavitary route, the general precautions concerning this agent should be borne in mind.*

As a general guide, reference is made especially to the techniques of Weisberger et al. Intracavitary use is indicated in the presence of pleural, peritoneal, or pericardial effusion due to metastatic tumors. Local therapy with nitrogen mustard is used only when malignant cells are demonstrated in the effusion. Intracavitary injection is not recommended when the accumulated fluid is chylous in nature, since results are likely to be poor.

Paracentesis is first performed with most of the fluid being removed from the pleural or peritoneal cavity. The intracavitary use of MUSTARGEN may exert at least some of its effect through production of a chemical poudrage. Therefore, the removal of excess fluid allows the drug to more easily contact the peritoneal and pleural linings. For intrapleural or intrapericardial injection nitrogen mustard is introduced directly through the thoracentesis needle. For intraperitoneal injection it is given through a rubber catheter inserted into the trocar used for paracentesis or through a No. 18 gauge needle inserted at another site. This drug should be injected slowly, with frequent aspiration to ensure that a free flow of fluid is present. If fluid cannot be aspirated, pain and necrosis due to injection of solution outside the cavity may occur. Free flow of fluid also is necessary to prevent injection into a loculated pocket and to ensure adequate dissemination of nitrogen mustard.

The usual dose of nitrogen mustard for intracavitary injection is 0.4 mg/kg of body weight, though 0.2 mg/kg (or 10 to 20 mg) has been used by the intrapericardial route. The solution is prepared, as previously described for intravenous injection, by adding 10 mL of Sterile Water for Injection or 10 mL of Sodium Chloride Injection to the vial containing 10 mg of mechlorethamine hydrochloride. (Amounts of diluent of 50 to 100 mL of normal saline have also been used.) The position of the patient should be changed every 5 to 10 minutes for an hour after injection to obtain more uniform distribution of the drug throughout the serous cavity. The remaining fluid may be removed from the pleural or peritoneal cavity by paracentesis 24 to 36 hours later. The patient should be followed carefully by clinical and x-ray examination to detect reaccumulation of fluid.

Pain occurs rarely with intrapleural use; it is common with intraperitoneal injection and is often associated with nausea, vomiting, and diarrhea of 2 to 3 days duration. Transient cardiac irregularities may occur with intrapericardial injection. Death, possibly accelerated by nitrogen mustard, has been reported following the use of this agent by the intracavitary route. Although absorption of MUSTARGEN when given by the intracavitary route is probably not complete because of its rapid deactivation by body fluids, the systemic effect is unpredictable. The acute side effects such as nausea and vomiting are usually mild. Bone marrow depression is generally milder than when the drug is given intravenously. Care should be taken to avoid use by the intracavitary route when other agents which may suppress bone marrow function are being used systemically.

Neutralization of Equipment and Unused Solution

To clean rubber gloves, tubing, glassware, etc., after giving MUSTARGEN, soak them in an aqueous solution containing equal volumes of sodium thiosulfate (5%) and sodium bicarbonate (5%) for 45 minutes. Excess reagents and reaction products are washed away easily with water. Any unused injection solution should be neutralized by mixing with an equal volume of sodium thiosulfate/sodium bicarbonate solution. Allow the mixture to stand for 45 minutes. Vials that have contained MUSTARGEN should be treated in the same way with thiosulfate/bicarbonate solution before disposal.

HOW SUPPLIED

No. 7753—Trituration of MUSTARGEN is a light yellow brown crystalline powder, each vial containing 10 mg mechlorethamine hydrochloride with sodium chloride q.s. 100 mg, and is supplied as follows:

NDC 0006-7753-31 in treatment sets of 4 vials.

Storage

Store at controlled room temperature 15–30°C (59–86°F). Protect from light and humidity. Solutions of mechlorethamine HCl decompose on standing; therefore, solutions of the drug should be prepared immediately before use.

7417932 Issued March 1999

Continued on next page

Information on the Merck & Co., Inc. products listed on these pages is the full prescribing information from product circulars in use September 30, 2000. For information, please call 1-800-NSC MERCK [1-800-672-6372].

MYOCHRYSINE® Injection ℞
(Gold Sodium Thiomalate)

Physicians planning to use MYOCHRYSINE* *(Gold Sodium Thiomalate) should thoroughly familiarize themselves with its toxicity and its benefits. The possibility of toxic reactions should always be explained to the patient before starting therapy. Patients should be warned to report promptly any symptoms suggesting toxicity. Before each injection of* MYOCHRYSINE, *the physician should review the results of laboratory work, and see the patient to determine the presence or absence of adverse reactions since some of these can be severe or even fatal.*

*Registered trademark of MERCK & CO., INC.

DESCRIPTION

MYOCHRYSINE is a sterile aqueous solution of gold sodium thiomalate. It contains 0.5 percent benzyl alcohol added as a preservative. The pH of the product is 5.8–6.5. Gold sodium thiomalate is a mixture of the mono- and disodium salts of gold thiomalic acid. The structural formula is:

$$\begin{array}{l} \quad\quad CH_2COO^- \\ \quad\quad | \\ Au{-}S{-}CHCOO^- \end{array} \cdot xNa^+ \cdot (2-x)H^+$$

mercaptobutanedioic acid, monogold (1+) sodium salt

The molecular weight for $C_4H_3AuNa_2O_4S$ (the disodium salt) is 390.07 and for $C_4H_4AuNaO_4S$ (the monosodium salt) is 368.09.
MYOCHRYSINE is supplied as a solution for intramuscular injection containing 50 mg of gold sodium thiomalate per mL.

CLINICAL PHARMACOLOGY

The mode of action of gold sodium thiomalate is unknown. The predominant action appears to be a suppressive effect on the synovitis of active rheumatoid disease.

INDICATIONS AND USAGE

MYOCHRYSINE is indicated in the treatment of selected cases of active rheumatoid arthritis— both adult and juvenile type. The greatest benefit occurs in the early active stage. In late stages of the illness when cartilage and bone damage have occurred, gold can only check the progression of rheumatoid arthritis and prevent further structural damage to joints. It cannot repair damage caused by previously active disease.
MYOCHRYSINE should be used only as *one part* of a complete program of therapy; alone it is not a complete treatment.

CONTRAINDICATIONS

Hypersensitivity to any component of this product.
Severe toxicity resulting from previous exposure to gold or other heavy metals.
Severe debilitation.
Systemic lupus erythematosus.

WARNINGS

Before treatment is started, the patient's hemoglobin, erythrocyte, white blood cell, differential and platelet counts should be determined, and urinalysis should be done to serve as basic reference. Urine should be analyzed for protein and sediment changes prior to each injection. Complete blood counts including platelet estimation should be made before every second injection throughout treatment. The occurrence of purpura or ecchymoses at any time always requires a platelet count.
Danger signals of possible gold toxicity include: rapid reduction of hemoglobin, leukopenia below 4000 WBC/mm^3, eosinophilia above 5 percent, platelet decrease below 100,000/mm^3, albuminuria, hematuria, pruritus, skin eruption, stomatitis, or persistent diarrhea. No additional injections of MYOCHRYSINE should be given unless further studies show these abnormalities to be caused by conditions other than gold toxicity.

PRECAUTIONS

General
Gold salts should not be used concomitantly with penicillamine.
The safety of coadministration with cytotoxic drugs has not been established.
Caution is indicated in the use of MYOCHRYSINE in patients with the following:
1. a history of blood dyscrasias such as granulocytopenia or anemia caused by drug sensitivity,
2. allergy or hypersensitivity to medications,
3. skin rash,
4. previous kidney or liver disease,
5. marked hypertension,
6. compromised cerebral or cardiovascular circulation.
Diabetes mellitus or congestive heart failure should be under control before gold therapy is instituted.
Carcinogenicity
Renal adenomas have been reported in long-term toxicity studies of rats receiving MYOCHRYSINE at high dose levels (2 mg/kg weekly for 45 weeks, followed by 6 mg/kg daily for 47 weeks), approximately 2 to 42 times the usual human dose. These adenomas are histologically similar to those produced in rats by chronic administration of experimental gold compounds and other heavy metals, such as lead. No reports have been received of renal adenomas in man in association with the use of MYOCHRYSINE.
Pregnancy
Pregnancy Category C.
MYOCHRYSINE has been shown to be teratogenic during the organogenetic period in rats and rabbits when given in doses, respectively, of 140 and 175 times the usual human dose. Hydrocephaly and microphthalmia were the malformations observed in rats when MYOCHRYSINE was administered subcutaneously at a dose of 25 mg/kg/day from day 6 through day 15 of gestation. In rabbits, limb malformations and gastroschisis were the malformations observed when MYOCHRYSINE was administered subcutaneously at doses of 20–45 mg/kg/day from day 6 through day 18 of gestation.
There are no adequate and well-controlled studies in pregnant women. MYOCHRYSINE should be used during pregnancy only if the potential benefit to the mother justifies the potential risk to the fetus.
Nursing Mothers
The presence of gold has been demonstrated in the milk of lactating mothers. In addition, gold has been found in the serum and red blood cells of a nursing infant. In view of the above findings and because of the potential for serious adverse reactions in nursing infants from MYOCHRYSINE, a decision should be made whether to discontinue nursing or to discontinue the drug, taking into account the importance of the drug to the mother. The slow excretion and persistence of gold in the mother, even after therapy is discontinued, must also be kept in mind.

ADVERSE REACTIONS

A variety of adverse reactions may develop during the initial phase (weekly injections) of therapy or during maintenance treatment. Adverse reactions are observed most frequently when the cumulative dose of MYOCHRYSINE administered is between 400 and 800 mg. Very uncommonly, complications occur days to months after cessation of treatment.
Cutaneous reactions: Dermatitis is the most common reaction. *Any eruption, especially if pruritic, that develops during treatment with* MYOCHRYSINE *should be considered a reaction to gold until proven otherwise.* Pruritus often exists before dermatitis becomes apparent, and therefore should be considered a warning signal of impending cutaneous reaction. The most serious form of cutaneous reaction is generalized exfoliative dermatitis which may lead to alopecia and shedding of nails. Gold dermatitis may be aggravated by exposure to sunlight or an actinic rash may develop.
Mucous membrane reactions: Stomatitis is the second most common adverse reaction. Shallow ulcers on the buccal membranes, on the borders of the tongue, and on the palate or in the pharynx may occur as the only adverse reaction, or along with dermatitis. Sometimes diffuse glossitis or gingivitis develops. A metallic taste may precede these oral mucous membrane reactions and should be considered a warning signal.
Conjunctivitis is a rare reaction.
Renal reactions: Gold may be toxic to the kidney and produce a nephrotic syndrome or glomerulitis with hematuria. These renal reactions are usually relatively mild and subside completely if recognized early and treatment is discontinued. They may become severe and chronic if treatment is continued after onset of the reaction. Therefore, it is important to perform a *urinalysis before every injection,* and to discontinue treatment promptly if proteinuria or hematuria develops.
Hematologic reactions: Blood dyscrasia due to gold toxicity is rare, but because of the potential serious consequences it must be constantly watched for and recognized early by frequent blood examinations done throughout treatment. Granulocytopenia; thrombocytopenia, with or without purpura; hypoplastic and aplastic anemia; and eosinophilia have all been reported. These hematologic disorders may occur separately or in combinations.
Nitritoid and allergic reactions: Reactions of the "nitritoid type" which may resemble anaphylactoid effects have been reported. Flushing, fainting, dizziness and sweating are most frequently reported. Other symptoms that may occur include: nausea, vomiting, malaise, headache, and weakness.
More severe, but less common effects include: anaphylactic shock, syncope, bradycardia, thickening of the tongue, difficulty in swallowing and breathing, and angioneurotic edema. These effects may occur almost immediately after injection or as late as 10 minutes following injection. They may occur at any time during the course of therapy and if observed, treatment with MYOCHRYSINE should be discontinued.
Miscellaneous reactions: Gastrointestinal reactions have been reported, including nausea, vomiting, anorexia, abdominal cramps and diarrhea. Ulcerative enterocolitis, which can be severe or even fatal, has been reported rarely.
There have been rare reports of reactions involving the eye such as iritis, corneal ulcers, and gold deposits in ocular tissues. Peripheral and central nervous system complications have been reported rarely. Peripheral neuropathy, with or without fasciculations, sensorimotor effects (including Guillain-Barré syndrome) and elevated spinal fluid protein have been reported. Central nervous system complications have included confusion, hallucinations and seizures. Usually these signs and symptoms cleared upon discontinuation of gold therapy.
Hepatitis, jaundice, with or without cholestasis, gold bronchitis, pulmonary injury manifested by interstitial pneumonitis and fibrosis, partial or complete hair loss and fever have also been reported.
Sometimes arthralgia occurs for a day or two after an injection of MYOCHRYSINE; this reaction usually subsides after the first few injections.

MANAGEMENT OF ADVERSE REACTIONS

Treatment with MYOCHRYSINE should be discontinued immediately when toxic reactions occur. Minor complications such as localized dermatitis, mild stomatitis, or slight proteinuria generally require no other therapy and resolve spontaneously with suspension of MYOCHRYSINE. Moderately severe skin and mucous membrane reactions often benefit from topical corticosteroids, oral antihistaminics, and soothing or anesthetic lotions.
If stomatitis or dermatitis becomes severe or more generalized, systemic corticosteroids (generally, prednisone 10 to 40 mg daily in divided doses) may provide symptomatic relief. For serious renal, hematologic, pulmonary, and enterocolitic complications, high doses of systemic corticosteroids (prednisone 40 to 100 mg daily in divided doses) are recommended. The optimum duration of corticosteroid treatment varies with the response of the individual patient. Therapy may be required for many months when adverse effects are unusually severe or progressive.
In patients whose complications do not improve with high-dose corticosteroid treatment, or who develop significant steroid-related adverse reactions, a chelating agent may be given to enhance gold excretion. Dimercaprol (BAL) has been used successfully, but patients must be monitored carefully as numerous untoward reactions may attend its use. Corticosteroids and a chelating agent may be used concomitantly.
MYOCHRYSINE *should not be reinstituted after severe or idiosyncratic reactions.*
MYOCHRYSINE may be readministered following resolution of mild reactions, using a reduced dosage schedule. If an initial test dose of 5 mg MYOCHRYSINE is well-tolerated, progressively larger doses (5 to 10 mg increments) may be given at weekly to monthly intervals until a dose of 25 to 50 mg is reached.

DOSAGE AND ADMINISTRATION

MYOCHRYSINE should be administered only by intramuscular injection, preferably intragluteally. It should be given with the patient lying down. He should remain recumbent for approximately 10 minutes after the injection.
Therapeutic effects from MYOCHRYSINE occur slowly. Early improvement, often limited to a reduction in morning stiffness, may begin after six to eight weeks of treatment, but beneficial effects may not be observed until after months of therapy.
Parenteral drug products should be inspected visually for particulate matter and discoloration prior to administration. Do not use if material has darkened. Color should not exceed pale yellow.
For the adult of average size the following dosage schedule is suggested:

Weekly Injections	
1st injection	10 mg
2nd injection	25 mg

3rd and subsequent injections, 25 to 50 mg until there is toxicity or major clinical improvement, or, in the absence of either of these, the cumulative dose of MYOCHRYSINE reaches one gram.
MYOCHRYSINE is continued until the cumulative dose reaches one gram unless toxicity or major clinical improvement occurs. If significant clinical improvement occurs before a cumulative dose of one gram has been administered, the dose may be decreased or the interval between injections increased as with maintenance therapy. Maintenance doses of 25 to 50 mg every other week for two to 20 weeks are recommended. If the clinical course remains stable, injections of 25 to 50 mg may be given every third and subsequently every fourth week indefinitely. Some patients may require maintenance treatment at intervals of one to three weeks. Should the arthritis exacerbate during maintenance therapy, weekly injections may be resumed temporarily until disease activity is suppressed.
Should a patient fail to improve during initial therapy (cumulative dose of one gram), several options are available:
1— the patient may be considered to be unresponsive and MYOCHRYSINE is discontinued
2— the same dose (25 to 50 mg) of MYOCHRYSINE may be continued for approximately ten additional weeks
3— the dose of MYOCHRYSINE may be increased by increments of 10 mg every one to four weeks, not to exceed 100 mg in a single injection.

If significant clinical improvement occurs using option 2 or 3, the maintenance schedule described above should be initiated. If there is no significant improvement or if toxicity occurs, therapy with MYOCHRYSINE should be stopped. The higher the individual dose of MYOCHRYSINE, the greater the risk of gold toxicity. Selection of one of these options for chrysotherapy should be based upon a number of factors, including the physician's experience with gold salt therapy, the course of the patient's condition, the choice of alternative treatments, and the availability of the patient for the close supervision required.

Juvenile Rheumatoid Arthritis

The pediatric dose of MYOCHRYSINE is proportional to the adult dose on a weight basis. After the initial test dose of 10 mg, the recommended dose for children is one mg per kilogram body weight, not to exceed 50 mg for a single injection. Otherwise, the guidelines given above for administration to adults also apply to children.

Concomitant Drug Therapy—Gold salts should not be used concomitantly with penicillamine.

The safety of coadministration with cytotoxic drugs has not been established. Other measures, such as salicylates, other non-steroidal anti-inflammatory drugs, or systemic corticosteroids, may be continued when MYOCHRYSINE is initiated. After improvement commences, analgesic and anti-inflammatory drugs may be discontinued slowly as symptoms permit.

HOW SUPPLIED

Injection MYOCHRYSINE is a light yellow to yellow solution which must be protected from light. It is supplied as follows:

No. 7762—50 mg of gold sodium thiomalate per mL as

NDC 0006-7762-64 in boxes of 6 x 1 mL ampuls

NDC 0006-7762-10 in 10 mL vials

(6505-00-973-8579, 10 mL vial).

Storage

Protect from light.

Store container in carton until contents have been used.

7594528 Issued April 1994

NEODECADRON® ℞

Sterile Ophthalmic Ointment
(Neomycin Sulfate-Dexamethasone Sodium Phosphate)

DESCRIPTION

Sterile Ophthalmic Ointment NEODECADRON* (Neomycin Sulfate-Dexamethasone Sodium Phosphate) is a topical corticosteroid-antibiotic ointment for ophthalmic use.

Dexamethasone sodium phosphate is 9-fluoro-11β, 17-dihydroxy-16α-methyl-21-(phosphonooxy)pregna-1, 4-diene-3, 20- dione disodium salt. Its empirical formula is $C_{22}H_{28}FNa_2O_8P$ and its structural formula is:

Dexamethasone is a synthetic analog of naturally occurring glucocorticoids (hydrocortisone and cortisone).

Dexamethasone sodium phosphate is a water soluble, inorganic ester of dexamethasone. Its molecular weight is 516.41.

Neomycin sulfate, an antibiotic of the aminoglycoside group, is a mixture of the sulfate salts of neomycin, produced by the growth of *Streptomyces fradiae* Waksman (Fam. Streptomycetaceae). Neomycin is a complex typically containing 8–13% neomycin C, less than 0.2% neomycin A, and the rest, neomycin B. The empirical formula for both neomycin B and neomycin C is $C_{23}H_{46}N_6O_{13}$, and the molecular weight for each is 614.65. Neomycin A (also referred to as neamine) has an empirical formula of $C_{12}H_{26}N_4O_6$ and a molecular weight of 322.36. The structural formulae for neomycin sulfate are:

[See chemical structure at top of next column]

Neomycin B	Neomycin C
R_1=H, R_2=CH_2NH_2	R_1=CH_2NH_2, R_2=H

Ophthalmic Ointment NEODECADRON contains in each gram: dexamethasone sodium phosphate equivalent to 0.5 mg (0.05%) dexamethasone phosphate and neomycin sulfate equivalent to 3.5 mg neomycin base. Inactive ingredients: white petrolatum and mineral oil.

*Registered trademark of MERCK & CO., INC.

CLINICAL PHARMACOLOGY

Corticosteroids suppress the inflammatory response to a variety of agents, and they probably delay or slow healing.

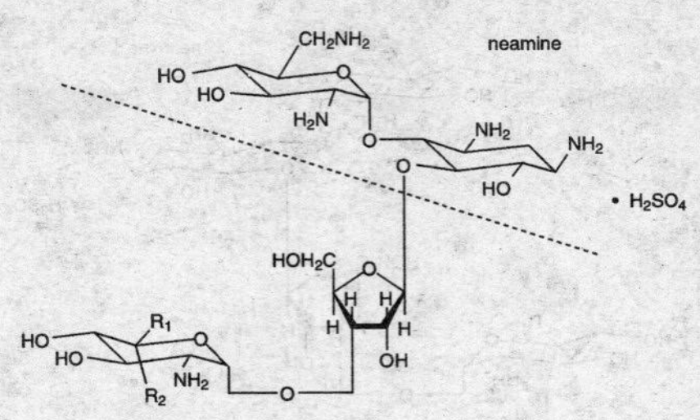

Since corticosteroids may inhibit the body's defense mechanism against infection, a concomitant antimicrobial drug may be used when this inhibition is considered to be clinically significant in a particular case.

When a decision to administer both a corticosteroid and an antimicrobial is made, the administration of such drugs in combination has the advantage of greater patient compliance and convenience, with the added assurance that the appropriate dosage of both drugs is administered, plus assured compatibility of ingredients when both types of drug are in the same formulation and, particularly, that the correct volume of drug is delivered and retained.

The relative potency of corticosteroids depends on the molecular structure, concentration, and release from the vehicle.

Microbiology

The anti-infective component in Ophthalmic Ointment NEODECADRON is included to provide action against specific organisms susceptible to it. Neomycin sulfate is active *in vitro* against susceptible strains of the following microorganisms: *Staphylococcus aureus, Escherichia coli, Haemophilus influenzae, Klebsiella/Enterobacter* species, and *Neisseria* species. The product does not provide adequate coverage against: *Pseudomonas aeruginosa, Serratia marcescens,* and streptococci, including *Streptococcus pneumoniae.* (See INDICATIONS AND USAGE.)

INDICATIONS AND USAGE

For steroid-responsive inflammatory ocular conditions for which a corticosteroid is indicated and where bacterial infection or a risk of bacterial ocular infection exists.

Ocular steroids are indicated in inflammatory conditions of the palpebral and bulbar conjunctiva, cornea, and anterior segment of the globe where the inherent risk of steroid use in certain infective conjunctivitides is accepted to obtain a diminution in edema and inflammation. They are also indicated in chronic anterior uveitis and corneal injury from chemical, radiation, or thermal burns, or penetration of foreign bodies.

The use of a combination drug with an anti-infective component is indicated where the risk of infection is high or where there is an expectation that potentially dangerous numbers of bacteria will be present in the eye.

The particular anti-infective drug in this product is active against the following common bacterial eye pathogens:

Staphylococcus aureus
Escherichia coli
Haemophilus influenzae
Klebsiella/Enterobacter species
Neisseria species

The product does not provide adequate coverage against:

Pseudomonas aeruginosa
Serratia marcescens
Streptococci, including *Streptococcus pneumoniae*

CONTRAINDICATIONS

NEODECADRON is contraindicated in most viral diseases of the cornea and conjunctiva including epithelial herpes simplex keratitis (dendritic keratitis), vaccinia varicella, and also in mycobacterial infection of the eye and fungal diseases of ocular structures. NEODECADRON is also contraindicated in individuals with known or suspected hypersensitivity to any of the ingredients of this preparation and to other corticosteroids (see WARNINGS). Hypersensitivity to the antibiotic component occurs at a higher rate than for other components.

WARNINGS

NOT FOR INJECTION INTO THE EYE

Prolonged use of corticosteroids may result in ocular hypertension and/or glaucoma with damage to the optic nerve, defects in visual acuity and fields of vision, and in posterior subcapsular cataract formation.

Prolonged use of corticosteroids may suppress the host response and thus increase the hazard of secondary ocular infections. In those diseases causing thinning of the cornea or sclera, perforations have been known to occur with the use of topical corticosteroids. In acute purulent conditions of the eye, corticosteroids may mask infection or enhance existing infection.

If this product is used for 10 days or longer, intraocular pressure should be routinely monitored even though it may be difficult in children and uncooperative patients. Corticosteroids should be used with caution in the presence of ocular hypertension and/or glaucoma. Intraocular pressure should be checked frequently.

The use of corticosteroids after cataract surgery may delay healing and increase the incidence of filtering blebs.

Use of ocular corticosteroids may prolong the course and may exacerbate the severity of many viral infections of the eye (including herpes simplex). Employment of a corticosteroid medication in the treatment of patients with a history of herpes simplex requires great caution; periodic slit lamp microscopy is essential. (See CONTRAINDICATIONS.)

Neomycin sulfate may occasionally cause cutaneous sensitization. If any reaction indicating such sensitivity is observed, discontinue use.

PRECAUTIONS

General

The initial prescription and renewal of the medication order beyond 8 grams should be made by a physician only after examination of the patient with the aid of magnification, such as slit-lamp biomicroscopy and, where appropriate, fluorescein staining. If signs and symptoms fail to improve after two days, the patient should be re-evaluated.

The possibility of fungal infections of the cornea should be considered after prolonged corticosteroid dosing. Fungal cultures should be taken when appropriate.

If this product is used for 10 days or longer, intraocular pressure should be monitored (see WARNINGS).

There have been reports of bacterial keratitis associated with the use of multiple dose containers of topical ophthalmic products. These containers had been inadvertently contaminated by patients who, in most cases, had a concurrent corneal disease or a disruption of the ocular epithelial surface. (See PRECAUTIONS, *Information for Patients.*)

Information for Patients

Patients should be instructed to avoid allowing the tip of the dispensing container to contact the eye, eyelid, fingers, or any other surface. The use of this product by more than one person may spread infection. Keep tightly closed when not in use.

Patients should also be instructed that ocular preparations, if handled improperly, can become contaminated by common bacteria known to cause ocular infections. Serious damage to the eye and subsequent loss of vision may result from using contaminated preparations. (See PRECAUTIONS, *General.*)

If redness, irritation, swelling or pain persists or becomes aggravated, the patient should be advised to consult a physician. Patients should also be advised that if they have ocular surgery or develop an intercurrent ocular condition (e.g., trauma or infection), they should immediately seek their physician's advice.

Keep out of the reach of children.

Carcinogenesis, Mutagenesis, Impairment of Fertility

Long term animal studies have not been performed to evaluate the carcinogenic potential or the effect on fertility of Ophthalmic Ointment NEODECADRON. Treatment of human lymphocytes *in-vitro* with neomycin increased the frequency of chromosome aberrations at the highest concentration (80μg/mL) tested; however, the effects of neomycin on carcinogenesis and mutagenesis in humans are unknown.

Pregnancy

Teratogenic effects

Pregnancy Category C

Corticosteroids have been found to be teratogenic in animal studies. Ocular administration of 0.1% dexamethasone resulted in 15.6% and 32.3% incidence of fetal anomalies in two groups of pregnant rabbits. Fetal growth retardation and increased mortality rates have been observed in rats with chronic dexamethasone therapy. There are no adequate and well-controlled studies in pregnant women. Ophthalmic Ointment NEODECADRON should be used during pregnancy only if the potential benefit justifies the potential risk to the fetus. Infants born of mothers who have received substantial doses of corticosteroids during pregnancy should be observed carefully for signs of hypoadrenalism.

Nursing Mothers

It is not known whether topical administration of corticosteroids could result in sufficient systemic absorption to produce detectable quantities in human milk. Systemically-administered corticosteroids appear in human milk and could suppress growth, interfere with endogenous corticosteroid production, or cause other untoward effects. Because of the potential for serious adverse reactions in nursing infants from Ophthalmic Ointment NEODECADRON, a decision should be made whether to discontinue nursing or to discontinue the drug, taking into account the importance of the drug to the mother.

Pediatric Use

Safety and effectiveness in pediatric patients have not been established.

ADVERSE REACTIONS

Adverse reactions have occurred with corticosteroid/anti-infective combination drugs which can be attributed to the

Continued on next page

Information on the Merck & Co., Inc. products listed on these pages is the full prescribing information from product circulars in use September 30, 2000. For information, please call 1-800-NSC MERCK [1-800-672-6372].

Neodecadron Ointment—Cont.

corticosteroid component, the anti-infective component, or the combination. Exact incidence figures are not available since no denominator of treated patients is available.
Reactions occurring most often from the presence of the anti-infective ingredient are allergic sensitizations. The reactions due to the corticosteroid component in decreasing order of frequency are: elevation of intraocular pressure (IOP) with possible development of glaucoma, and infrequent optic nerve damage; posterior subcapsular cataract formation; and delayed wound healing.
Secondary Infection: The development of secondary infection has occurred after use of combinations containing corticosteroids and antimicrobials. Fungal and viral infections of the cornea are particularly prone to develop coincidentally with long-term applications of a corticosteroid. The possibility of fungal invasion must be considered in any persistent corneal ulceration where corticosteroid treatment has been used.

DOSAGE AND ADMINISTRATION

NOT FOR INJECTION INTO THE EYE
The duration of treatment will vary with the type of lesion and may extend from a few days to several weeks, according to therapeutic response.
Apply a thin coating of Ophthalmic Ointment NEODECADRON three or four times a day. When a favorable response is observed, reduce the number of daily applications to two, and later to one a day as maintenance dose if this is sufficient to control symptoms.
Not more than 8 grams should be prescribed initially and the prescription should not be refilled without further evaluation as outlined in PRECAUTIONS above.

HOW SUPPLIED

No. 7617—Sterile Ophthalmic Ointment NEODECADRON is a clear, unctuous ointment, and is supplied as follows:
NDC 0006-7617-04 in 3.5 g tubes
(6505-00-982-0291 0.05% 3.5 g)
Storage
Store at controlled room temperature, 15°–30°C (59°–86°F).
7612628 Issued December 1995

NEODECADRON® ℞
Sterile Ophthalmic Solution
(Neomycin Sulfate-Dexamethasone Sodium Phosphate)

DESCRIPTION

Ophthalmic Solution NEODECADRON* (Neomycin Sulfate-Dexamethasone Sodium Phosphate) is a topical corticosteroid-antibiotic solution for ophthalmic use.
Dexamethasone sodium phosphate is 9-fluoro-11β, 17-dihydroxy-16α-methyl-21-(phosphonooxy)pregna-1, 4-diene-3, 20-dione disodium salt. Its empirical formula is $C_{22}H_{28}FNa_2O_8P$ and its structural formula is:

Dexamethasone is a synthetic analog of naturally occurring glucocorticoids (hydrocortisone and cortisone).
Dexamethasone sodium phosphate is a water soluble, inorganic ester of dexamethasone. Its molecular weight is 516.41.
Neomycin sulfate, an antibiotic of the aminoglucoside group, is a mixture of the sulfate salts of neomycin, produced by the growth of *Streptomyces fradiae* Waksman (Fam. Stretomycetaceae). Neomycin is a complex typically containing 8–13% neomycin C, less than 0.2% neomycin A, and the rest, neomycin B. The empirical formula for both neomycin B and neomycin C is $C_{23}H_{46}N_6O_{13}$, and the molecular weight for each is 614.65. Neomycin A (also referred to as neamine) has an empirical formula of $C_{12}H_{26}N_4O_6$ and a molecular weight of 322.36. The structural formulae for neomycin sulfate are:
[See chemical structure at top of next column]

Neomycin B	Neomycin C
R_1=H, R_2=CH_2NH_2	R_1=CH_2NH_2, R_2=H

Each milliliter of buffered Ophthalmic Solution NEODECADRON in the OCUMETER* ophthalmic dispenser contains: dexamethasone sodium phosphate equivalent to 1 mg (0.1%) dexamethasone phosphate, and neomycin sulfate equivalent to 3.5 mg neomycin base. Inactive ingredients:

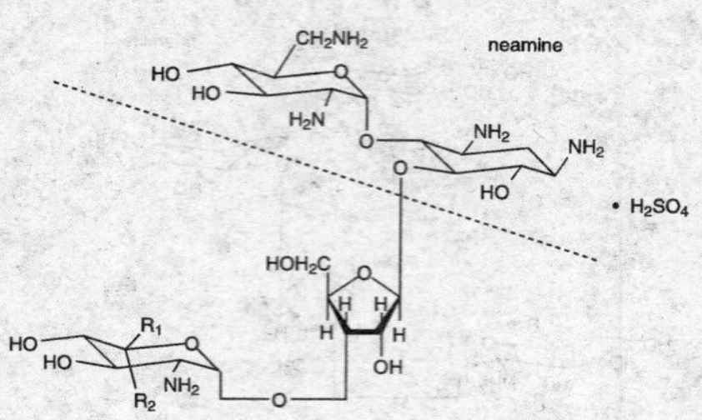

creatinine, sodium citrate, sodium borate, polysorbate 80, disodium edetate, hydrochloric acid to adjust pH to 6.6–7.2, and water for injection. Benzalkonium chloride 0.02% and sodium bisulfite 0.1% added as preservatives.

* Registered trademark of MERCK & CO., Inc.

CLINICAL PHARMACOLOGY

Corticosteroids suppress the inflammatory response to a variety of agents, and they probably delay or slow healing. Since corticosteroids may inhibit the body's defense mechanism against infection, a concomitant antimicrobial drug may be used when this inhibition is considered to be clinically significant in a particular case.
When a decision to administer both a corticosteroid and an antimicrobial is made, the administration of such drugs in combination has the advantage of greater patient compliance and convenience, with the added assurance that the appropriate dosage of both drugs is administered, plus assured compatibility of ingredients when both types of drug are in the same formulation and, particularly, that the correct volume of drug is delivered and retained.
The relative potency of corticosteroids depends on the molecular structure, concentration, and release from the vehicle.
Microbiology
The anti-infective component in Ophthalmic Solution NEODECADRON is included to provide action against specific organisms susceptible to it. Neomycin sulfate is active *in vitro* against susceptible strains of the following microorganisms: *Staphylococcus aureus, Escherichia coli, Haemophilus influenzae, Klebsiella/Enterobacter* species, and *Neisseria* species. The product does not provide adequate coverage against: *Pseudomonas aeruginosa, Serratia marcescens,* and streptococci, including *Streptococcus pneumoniae*. (See INDICATIONS AND USAGE.)

INDICATIONS AND USAGE

For steroid-responsive inflammatory ocular conditions for which a corticosteroid is indicated and where bacterial infection a risk of bacterial ocular infection exists.
Ocular steroids are indicated in inflammatory conditions of the palpebral and bulbar conjunctiva, cornea, and anterior segment of the globe where the inherent risk of steroid use in certain infective conjunctivitides is accepted to obtain a diminution in edema and inflammation. They are also indicated in chronic anterior uveitis and corneal injury from chemical, radiation, or thermal burns, or penetration of foreign bodies.
The use of a combination drug with an anti-infective component is indicated where the risk of infection is high or where there is an expectation that potentially dangerous numbers of bacteria will be present in the eye.
The particular anti-infective drug in this product is active against the following common bacterial eye pathogens:
Staphylococcus aureus
Escherichia coli
Haemophilus influenzae
Klebsiella/Enterobacter species
Neisseria species
The product does not provide adequate coverage against:
Pseudomonas aeruginosa
Serratia marcescens
Streptococci, including *Streptococcus pneumoniae*

CONTRAINDICATIONS

NEODECADRON is contraindicated in most viral diseases of the cornea and conjunctiva including epithelial herpes simplex keratitis (dendritic keratitis), vaccinia, varicella, and also in mycobacterial infection of the eye and fungal diseases of ocular structures. NEODECADRON is also contraindicated in individuals with known or suspected hypersensitivity to any of the ingredients of this preparation, including sulfites, and to other corticosteroids (see WARNINGS). (Hypersensitivity to the antibiotic component occurs at a higher rate than for other components.)

WARNINGS

NOT FOR INJECTION INTO THE EYE
Prolonged use of corticosteroids may result in ocular hypertension and/or glaucoma with damage to the optic nerve, defects in visual acuity and fields of vision, and in posterior subcapsular cataract formation.
Prolonged use of corticosteroids may suppress the host response and thus increase the hazard of secondary ocular infections. In those diseases causing thinning of the cornea or sclera, perforations have been known to occur with the use of topical corticosteroids. In acute purulent conditions of the eye, corticosteroids may mask infection or enhance existing infection.
If this product is used for 10 days or longer, intraocular pressure should be routinely monitored even though it may be difficult in children and uncooperative patients. Corticosteroids should be used with caution in the presence of ocular hypertension and/or glaucoma. Intraocular pressure should be checked frequently.
The use of corticosteroids after cataract surgery may delay healing and increase the incidence of filtering blebs.
Use of ocular corticosteroids may prolong the course and may exacerbate the severity of many viral infections of the eye (including herpes simplex). Employment of a corticosteroid medication in the treatment of patients with a history of herpes simplex requires great caution; periodic slit lamp microscopy is essential. (See CONTRAINDICATIONS.)
Neomycin sulfate may occasionally cause cutaneous sensitization. If any reaction indicating such sensitivity is observed, discontinue use.
Ophthalmic Solution NEODECADRON contains sodium bisulfite, a sulfite that may cause allergic-type reactions including anaphylactic symptoms and life-threatening or less severe asthmatic episodes in certain susceptible people. The overall prevalence of sulfite sensitivity in the general population is unknown and probably low. Sulfite sensitivity is seen more frequently in asthmatic than in nonasthmatic people.

PRECAUTIONS

General
The initial prescription and renewal of the medication order beyond 20 milliliters should be made by a physician only after examination of the patient with the aid of magnification, such as slit lamp biomicroscopy and, where appropriate, fluorescein staining. If signs and symptoms fail to improve after two days, the patient should be re-evaluated.
The possibility of fungal infections of the cornea should be considered after prolonged corticosteroid dosing. Fungal cultures should be taken when appropriate.
If this product is used for 10 days or longer, intraocular pressure should be monitored (see WARNINGS).
There have been reports of bacterial keratitis associated with the use of multiple dose containers of topical ophthalmic products. These containers had been inadvertently contaminated by patients who, in most cases, had a concurrent corneal disease or a disruption of the ocular epithelial surface. (See PRECAUTIONS, *Information for Patients.*)
Information for Patients
Patients should be instructed to avoid allowing the tip of the dispensing container to contact the eye, eyelid, fingers, or any other surface. The use of this product by more than one person may spread infection. Keep tightly closed when not in use.
Patients should also be instructed that ocular preparations, if handled improperly, can become contaminated by common bacteria known to cause ocular infections. Serious damage to the eye and subsequent loss of vision may result from using contaminated preparations (see PRECAUTIONS, *General*).
If redness, irritation, swelling or pain persists or becomes aggravated, the patient should be advised to consult a physician. Patients should also be advised that if they have ocular surgery or develop an intercurrent ocular condition (e.g., trauma or infection), they should immediately seek their physician's advice.
One of the preservatives in Ophthalmic Solution NEODECADRON, benzalkonium chloride, may be absobed by soft contact lenses. Patients wearing soft contact lenses should be instructed to wait at least 15 minutes after instilling Ophthalmic Solution NEODECADRON before they insert their lenses.
Keep out of the reach of children.
Carcinogenesis, Mutagenesis, Impairment of Fertility
Long term animal studies have not been performed to evaluate the carcinogenic potential or the effect on fertility of Ophthalmic Solution NEODECADRON. Treatment of human lymphocytes *in-vitro* with neomycin increased the frequency of chromosome aberrations at the highest concentration (80 µg/mL) tested; however, the effects of neomycin on carcinogenesis and mutagenesis in humans are unknown.
Pregnancy
Teratogenic effects
Pregnancy Category C.
Corticosteroids have been found to be teratogenic in animal studies. Ocular administration of 0.1% dexamethasone resulted in 15.6% and 32.3% incidence of fetal anomalies in two groups of pregnant rabbits. Fetal growth retardation and increased mortality rates have been observed in rats with chronic dexamethasone therapy. There are no adequate and well-controlled studies in pregnant women. Ophthalmic Solution NEODECADRON should be used during pregnancy only if the potential benefit justifies the potential risk to the fetus. Infants born of mothers who have received substantial doses of corticosteroids during pregnancy should be observed carefully for signs of hypoadrenalism.
Nursing Mothers
It is not known whether topical administration of corticosteroids could result in sufficient systemic absorption to produce detectable quantities in human milk. Systemically-

administered corticosteroids appear in human milk and could suppress growth, interfere with endogenous corticosteroid production, or cause other untoward effects. Because of the potential for serious adverse reactions in nursing infants from Ophthalmic Solution NEODECADRON, a decision should be made whether to discontinue nursing or to discontinue the drug, taking into account the importance of the drug to the mother.

Pediatric Use

Safety and effectiveness in pediatric patients have not been established.

ADVERSE REACTIONS

Adverse reactions have occurred with corticosteroid/anti-infective combination drugs which can be attributed to the corticosteroid component, the anti-infective component, the combination, or any other component of the product. Exact incidence figures are not available since no denominator of treated patients is available.

Reactions occurring most often from the presence of the anti-infective ingredient are allergic sensitizations. The reactions due to the corticosteroid component in decreasing order of frequency are: elevation of intraocular pressure (IOP) with possible development of glaucoma, and infrequent optic nerve damage; posterior subcapsular cataract formation; and delayed wound healing.

Secondary Infection: The development of secondary infection has occurred after use of combinations containing corticosteroids and antimicrobials. Fungal and viral infections of the cornea are particularly prone to develop coincidentally with long-term applications of a corticosteroid. The possibility of fungal invasion must be considered in any persistent corneal ulceration where corticosteroid treatment has been used.

DOSAGE AND ADMINISTRATION

The duration of treatment will vary with the type of lesion and may extend from a few days to several weeks, according to therapeutic response.

Instill one or two drops of Ophthalmic Solution NEODECADRON into the conjunctival sac every hour during the day and every two hours during the night as initial therapy. When a favorable response is observed, reduce dosage to one drop every four hours. Later, further reduction in dosage to one drop three or four times daily may suffice to control symptoms.

Not more than 20 milliliters should be prescribed initially and the prescription should not be refilled without further evaluation as outlined in PRECAUTIONS above.

HOW SUPPLIED

Sterile Ophthalmic Solution NEODECADRON is a clear, colorless to pale yellow solution.

No. 7639—Ophthalmic Solution NEODECADRON is supplied as follows:

NDC 0006-7639-03 in 5 mL white opaque, plastic OCUMETER ophthalmic dispenser with a controlled drop tip.
(6505-01-039-4352 0.1% 5 mL).

Storage

Store at controlled room temperature, 15°–30°C (59°–86°F). Protect from light.

7261326 Issued December 1995

NOROXIN® Tablets ℞
(Norfloxacin)

DESCRIPTION

NOROXIN† (Norfloxacin) is a synthetic, broad-spectrum antibacterial agent for oral administration. Norfloxacin, a fluoroquinolone, is 1-ethyl-6-fluoro-1,4-dihydro-4-oxo-7-(1-piperazinyl)-3-quinolinecarboxylic acid. Its empirical formula is $C_{16}H_{18}FN_3O_3$ and the structural formula is:

Norfloxacin is a white to pale yellow crystalline powder with a molecular weight of 319.34 and a melting point of about 221°C. It is freely soluble in glacial acetic acid, and very slightly soluble in ethanol, methanol and water.

NOROXIN is available in 400-mg tablets. Each tablet contains the following inactive ingredients: cellulose, croscarmellose sodium, hydroxypropyl cellulose, hydroxypropyl methylcellulose, iron oxide, magnesium stearate, and titanium dioxide.

Norfloxacin, a fluoroquinolone, differs from non-fluorinated quinolones by having a fluorine atom at the 6 position and a piperazine moiety at the 7 position.

†Registered trademark of MERCK & CO., INC.

CLINICAL PHARMACOLOGY

In fasting healthy volunteers, at least 30–40% of an oral dose of NOROXIN is absorbed. Absorption is rapid following single doses of 200 mg, 400 mg and 800 mg. At the respective doses, mean peak serum and plasma concentrations of 0.8, 1.5 and 2.4 µg/mL are attained approximately one hour after dosing. The presence of food and/or dairy products may decrease absorption. The effective half-life of norfloxacin in serum and plasma is 3–4 hours. Steady-state concentrations of norfloxacin will be attained within two days of dosing.

In healthy elderly volunteers (65–75 years of age with normal renal function for their age), norfloxacin is eliminated more slowly because of their slightly decreased renal function. Drug absorption appears unaffected. However, the effective half-life of norfloxacin in these elderly subjects is 4 hours.

The disposition of norfloxacin in patients with creatinine clearance rates greater than 30 mL/min/1.73m^2 is similar to that in healthy volunteers. In patients with creatinine clearance rates equal to or less than 30 mL/min/1.73m^2, the renal elimination of norfloxacin decreases so that the effective serum half-life is 6.5 hours. In these patients, alteration of dosage is necessary (see DOSAGE AND ADMINISTRATION). Drug absorption appears unaffected by decreasing renal function.

Norfloxacin is eliminated through metabolism, biliary excretion, and renal excretion. After a single 400-mg dose of NOROXIN, mean antimicrobial activities equivalent to 278, 773, and 82 µg of norfloxacin/g of feces were obtained at 12, 24, and 48 hours, respectively. Renal excretion occurs by both glomerular filtration and tubular secretion as evidenced by the high rate of renal clearance (approximately 275 mL/min). Within 24 hours of drug administration, 26 to 32% of the administered dose is recovered in the urine as norfloxacin with an additional 5–8% being recovered in the urine as six active metabolites of lesser antimicrobial potency. Only a small percentage (less than 1%) of the dose is recovered thereafter. Fecal recovery accounts for another 30% of the administered dose.

Two to three hours after a single 400-mg dose, urinary concentrations of 200 µg/mL or more are attained in the urine. In healthy volunteers, mean urinary concentrations of norfloxacin remain above 30 µg/mL for at least 12 hours following a 400-mg dose. The urinary pH may affect the solubility of norfloxacin. Norfloxacin is least soluble at urinary pH of 7.5 with greater solubility occurring at pHs above and below this value. The serum protein binding of norfloxacin is between 10 and 15%.

The following are mean concentrations of norfloxacin in various fluids and tissues measured 1 to 4 hours post-dose after two 400-mg doses, unless otherwise indicated:

Renal Parenchyma	7.3 µg/g
Prostate	2.5 µg/g
Seminal Fluid	2.7 µg/mL
Testicle	1.6 µg/g
Uterus/Cervix	3.0 µg/g
Vagina	4.3 µg/g
Fallopian Tube	1.9 µg/g
Bile	6.9 µg/mL (after two 200-mg doses)

Microbiology

Norfloxacin has *in vitro* activity against a broad range of gram-positive and gram-negative aerobic bacteria. The fluorine atom at the 6 position provides increased potency against gram-negative organisms, and the piperazine moiety at the 7 position is responsible for anti-pseudomonal activity.

Norfloxacin inhibits bacterial deoxyribonucleic acid synthesis and is bactericidal. At the molecular level, three specific events are attributed to norfloxacin in *E. coli* cells:

1) inhibition of the ATP-dependent DNA supercoiling reaction catalyzed by DNA gyrase,
2) inhibition of the relaxation of supercoiled DNA,
3) promotion of double-stranded DNA breakage.

Resistance to norfloxacin due to spontaneous mutation *in vitro* is a rare occurrence (range: 10^{-9} to 10^{-12} cells). Resistant organisms have emerged during therapy with norfloxacin in less than 1% of patients treated. Organisms in which development of resistance is greatest are the following:

Pseudomonas aeruginosa
Klebsiella pneumoniae
Acinetobacter spp.
Enterococcus spp.

For this reason, when there is a lack of satisfactory clinical response, repeat culture and susceptibility testing should be done. Nalidixic acid-resistant organisms are generally susceptible to norfloxacin *in vitro;* however, these organisms may have higher minimum inhibitory concentrations (MICs) to norfloxacin than nalidixic acid-susceptible strains. There is generally no cross-resistance between norfloxacin and other classes of antibacterial agents. Therefore, norfloxacin may demonstrate activity against indicated organisms resistant to some other antimicrobial agents including the aminoglycosides, penicillins, cephalosporins, tetracyclines, macrolides, and sulfonamides, including combinations of sulfamethoxazole and trimethoprim. Antagonism has been demonstrated *in vitro* between norfloxacin and nitrofurantoin.

Norfloxacin has been shown to be active against most strains of the following microorganisms both *in vitro* and in clinical infections as described in the **INDICATIONS AND USAGE** section.

Gram-positive aerobes:
Enterococcus faecalis
Staphylococcus aureus
Staphylococcus epidermidis
Staphylococcus saprophyticus
Streptococcus agalactiae

Gram-negative aerobes:
Citrobacter freundii
Enterobacter aerogenes
Enterobacter cloacae
Escherichia coli
Klebsiella pneumoniae
Neisseria gonorrhoeae
Proteus mirabilis
Proteus vulgaris
Pseudomonas aeruginosa
Serratia marcescens

The following *in vitro* data are available, **but their clinical significance is unknown.**

Norfloxacin exhibits *in vitro* minimal inhibitory concentrations (MIC's) of ≤4 µg/mL against most (≥90%) strains of the following microorganisms; however, the safety and effectiveness of norfloxacin in treating clinical infections due to these microorganisms have not been established in adequate and well-controlled clinical trials.

Gram-negative aerobes:
Citrobacter diversus
Edwardsiella tarda
Enterobacter agglomerans
Haemophilus ducreyi
Klebsiella oxytoca
Morganella morganii
Providencia alcalifaciens
Providencia rettgeri
Providencia stuartii
Pseudomonas fluorescens
Pseudomonas stutzeri

Other:
Ureaplasma urealyticum

NOROXIN is not generally active against obligate anaerobes.

Norfloxacin has not been shown to be active against *Treponema pallidum.* (See WARNINGS.)

Susceptibility Tests

Dilution Techniques:

Quantitative methods are used to determine antimicrobial minimal inhibitory concentrations (MIC's). These MIC's provide estimates of the susceptibility of bacteria to antimicrobial compounds. The MIC's should be determined using a standardized procedure. Standardized procedures are based on a dilution method[1] (broth, agar, or microdilution) or equivalent with standardized inoculum concentrations and standardized concentrations of norfloxacin powder. The MIC values should be interpreted according to the following criteria*:

MIC (µg/mL)	Interpretation
≤4	Susceptible (S)
8	Intermediate (I)
≥16	Resistant (R)

A report of "Susceptible" indicates that the pathogen is likely to be inhibited if the antimicrobial compound in the blood reaches the concentrations usually achievable. A report of "Intermediate" indicates that the result should be considered equivocal, and, if the microorganism is not fully susceptible to alternative, clinically feasible drugs, the test should be repeated. This category implies possible clinical applicability in body sites where the drug is physiologically concentrated or in situations where high dosage of drug can be used. This category also provides a buffer zone which prevents small uncontrolled technical factors from causing major discrepancies in interpretation. A report of "Resistant" indicates that the pathogen is not likely to be inhibited if the antimicrobial compound in the blood reaches the concentrations usually achievable; other therapy should be selected.

Standardized susceptibility test procedures require the use of laboratory control microorganisms to control the technical aspects of the laboratory procedures. Standard norfloxacin powder should provide the following MIC values:

Organism	MIC range (µg/mL)
E. coli ATCC 25922	0.03–0.12
E. faecalis ATCC 29212	2–8
P. aeruginosa ATCC 27853	1–4
S. aureus ATCC 29213	0.5–2

Diffusion Techniques:

Quantitative methods that require measurement of zone diameters also provide reproducible estimates of the susceptibility of bacteria to antimicrobial compounds. One such standardized procedure[2] requires the use of standardized inoculum concentrations. This procedure uses paper disks impregnated with 10-µg norfloxacin to test the susceptibility of microorganisms to norfloxacin. Reports from the lab-

Continued on next page

Information on the Merck & Co., Inc. products listed on these pages is the full prescribing information from product circulars in use September 30, 2000. For information, please call 1-800-NSC MERCK [1-800-672-6372].

Noroxin—Cont.

oratory providing results of the standard single-disk susceptibility test with a 10-μg norfloxacin disk should be interpreted according to the following criteria*:

Zone diameter (mm)	Interpretation
≥17	Susceptible (S)
13–16	Intermediate (I)
≤12	Resistant (R)

Interpretation should be as stated above for results using dilution techniques. Interpretation involves correlation of the diameter obtained in the disk test with the MIC for norfloxacin.

As with standard dilution techniques, diffusion methods require the use of laboratory control microorganisms that are used to control the technical aspects of the laboratory procedures. For the diffusion techniques, the 10-μg norfloxacin disk should provide the following zone diameters in these laboratory test quality control strains:

Organism	Zone Diameter (mm)
E. coli ATCC 25922	28–35
P. aeruginosa ATCC 27853	22–29
S. aureus ATCC 25923	17–28

*These interpretive criteria apply only to isolates from urinary tract infections. There are no established norfloxacin interpretive criteria for *Neisseria gonorrhoeae* or organisms isolated from other infection sites.

INDICATIONS AND USAGE

NOROXIN is indicated for the treatment of adults with the following infections caused by susceptible strains of the designated microorganisms:

Urinary tract infections:

Uncomplicated urinary tract infections (including cystitis) due to *Enterococcus faecalis, Escherichia coli, Klebsiella pneumoniae, Proteus mirabilis, Pseudomonas aeruginosa, Staphylococcus epidermidis, Staphylococcus saprophyticus, Citrobacter freundii**, Enterobacter aerogenes**, Enterobacter cloacae**, Proteus vulgaris**, Staphylococcus aureus***, or *Streptococcus agalactiae***.

Complicated urinary tract infections due to *Enterococcus faecalis, Escherichia coli, Klebsiella pneumoniae, Proteus mirabilis, Pseudomonas aeruginosa*, or *Serratia marcescens***.

Sexually transmitted diseases (See WARNINGS.):

Uncomplicated urethral and cervical gonorrhea due to *Neisseria gonorrhoeae*.

Prostatitis:

Prostatitis due to *Escherichia coli*.

(See DOSAGE AND ADMINISTRATION for appropriate dosing instructions.)

Penicillinase production should have no effect on norfloxacin activity.

Appropriate culture and susceptibility tests should be performed before treatment in order to isolate and identify organisms causing the infection and to determine their susceptibility to norfloxacin. Therapy with norfloxacin may be initiated before results of these tests are known; once results become available, appropriate therapy should be given. Repeat culture and susceptibility testing performed periodically during therapy will provide information not only on the therapeutic effect of the antimicrobial agents but also on the possible emergence of bacterial resistance.

**Efficacy for this organism in this organ system was studied in fewer than 10 infections.

CONTRAINDICATIONS

NOROXIN (norfloxacin) is contraindicated in persons with a history of hypersensitivity, tendinitis, or tendon rupture associated with the use of norfloxacin or any member of the quinolone group of antimicrobial agents.

WARNINGS

THE SAFETY AND EFFICACY OF ORAL NORFLOXACIN IN PEDIATRIC PATIENTS, ADOLESCENTS (UNDER THE AGE OF 18), PREGNANT WOMEN, AND NURSING MOTHERS HAVE NOT BEEN ESTABLISHED. (See PRECAUTIONS, *Pediatric Use, Pregnancy,* and *Nursing Mothers* subsections.)

The oral administration of single doses of norfloxacin, 6 times*** the recommended human clinical dose (on a mg/kg basis), caused lameness in immature dogs. Histologic examination of the weight-bearing joints of these dogs revealed permanent lesions of the cartilage. Other quinolones also produced erosions of the cartilage in weight-bearing joints and other signs of arthropathy in immature animals of various species. (See ANIMAL PHARMACOLOGY.)

Convulsions have been reported in patients receiving norfloxacin. Convulsions, increased intracranial pressure, and toxic psychoses have been reported in patients receiving drugs in this class. Quinolones may also cause central nervous system (CNS) stimulation which may lead to tremors, restlessness, lightheadedness, confusion, and hallucinations. If these reactions occur in patients receiving norfloxacin, the drug should be discontinued and appropriate measures instituted.

The effects of norfloxacin on brain function or on the electrical activity of the brain have not been tested. Therefore, until more information becomes available, norfloxacin, like all other quinolones, should be used with caution in patients with known or suspected CNS disorders, such as severe cerebral arteriosclerosis, epilepsy, and other factors which predispose to seizures. (See ADVERSE REACTIONS.)

Serious and occasionally fatal hypersensitivity (anaphylactoid or anaphylactic) reactions, some following the first dose, have been reported in patients receiving quinolone therapy. Some reactions were accompanied by cardiovascular collapse, loss of consciousness, tingling, pharyngeal or facial edema, dyspnea, urticaria and itching. Only a few patients had a history of hypersensitivity reactions. If an allergic reaction to norfloxacin occurs, discontinue the drug. Serious acute hypersensitivity reactions may require immediate emergency treatment with epinephrine. Oxygen, intravenous fluids, antihistamines, corticosteroids, pressor amines, and airway management, including intubation, should be administered as indicated.

Pseudomembranous colitis has been reported with nearly all antibacterial agents, including norfloxacin, and may range in severity from mild to life-threatening. Therefore, it is important to consider this diagnosis in patients who present with diarrhea subsequent to the administration of antibacterial agents.

Treatment with antibacterial agents alters the normal flora of the colon and may permit overgrowth of clostridia. Studies indicate that a toxin produced by *Clostridium difficile* is one primary cause of "antibiotic-associated colitis."

After the diagnosis of pseudomembranous colitis has been established, therapeutic measures should be initiated. Mild cases of pseudomembranous colitis usually respond to drug discontinuation alone. In moderate to severe cases, consideration should be given to management with fluids and electrolytes, protein supplementation, and treatment with an antibacterial drug clinically effective against *C. difficile* colitis.

Ruptures of the shoulder, hand, and Achilles tendons that required surgical repair or resulted in prolonged disability have been reported with norfloxacin. Norfloxacin should be discontinued if the patient experiences pain, inflammation, or rupture of a tendon. Patients should rest and refrain from exercise until the diagnosis of tendinitis or tendon rupture has been confidently excluded. Tendon rupture can occur at any time during or after therapy with norfloxacin.

Norfloxacin has not been shown to be effective in the treatment of syphilis. Antimicrobial agents used in high doses for short periods of time to treat gonorrhea may mask or delay the symptoms of incubating syphilis. All patients with gonorrhea should have a serologic test for syphilis at the time of diagnosis. Patients treated with norfloxacin should have a follow-up serologic test for syphilis after three months.

***Based on a patient weight of 50 kg.

PRECAUTIONS

General:

Needle-shaped crystals were found in the urine of some volunteers who received either placebo, 800 mg norfloxacin, or 1600 mg norfloxacin (at or twice the recommended daily dose, respectively) while participating in a double-blind, crossover study comparing single doses of norfloxacin with placebo. While crystalluria is not expected to occur under usual conditions with a dosage regimen of 400 mg b.i.d., as a precaution, the daily recommended dosage should not be exceeded and the patient should drink sufficient fluids to ensure a proper state of hydration and adequate urinary output.

Alteration in dosage regimen is necessary for patients with impaired renal function (see DOSAGE AND ADMINISTRATION).

Moderate to severe phototoxicity reactions have been observed in patients who are exposed to excessive sunlight while receiving some members of this drug class. Excessive sunlight should be avoided. Therapy should be discontinued if phototoxicity occurs.

Rarely, hemolytic reactions have been reported in patients with latent or actual defects in glucose-6-phosphate dehydrogenase activity who take quinolone antibacterial agents, including norfloxacin. (See ADVERSE REACTIONS.)

Quinolones, including norfloxacin, may exacerbate the signs of myasthenia gravis and lead to life threatening weakness of the respiratory muscles. Caution should be exercised when using quinolones, including NOROXIN, in patients with myasthenia gravis (see ADVERSE REACTIONS).

Information for Patients

Patients should be advised:

— to drink fluids liberally.

— that norfloxacin should be taken at least one hour before or at least two hours after a meal or ingestion of milk and/or other dairy products.

— that multivitamins or other products containing iron or zinc, antacids or Videx®‡ (Didanosine), chewable/buffered tablets or the pediatric powder for oral solution, should not be taken within the two-hour period before or within the two-hour period after taking norfloxacin. (See PRECAUTIONS, *Drug Interactions.*)

— that norfloxacin can cause dizziness and lightheadedness and, therefore, patients should know how they react to norfloxacin before they operate an automobile or machinery or engage in activities requiring mental alertness and coordination.

— to discontinue treatment and inform their physician if they experience pain, inflammation, or rupture of a tendon, and to rest and refrain from exercise until the diagnosis of tendinitis or tendon rupture has been confidently excluded.

— that norfloxacin may be associated with hypersensitivity reactions, even following the first dose, and to discontinue the drug at the first sign of a skin rash or other allergic reaction.

— to avoid undue exposure to excessive sunlight while receiving norfloxacin and to discontinue therapy if phototoxicity occurs.

— that some quinolones may increase the effects of theophylline and/or caffeine. (See PRECAUTIONS, *Drug Interactions.*)

— that convulsions have been reported in patients taking quinolones, including norfloxacin, and to notify their physician before taking this drug if there is a history of this condition.

Laboratory Tests

As with any potent antibacterial agent, periodic assessment of organ system functions, including renal, hepatic, and hematopoietic, is advisable during prolonged therapy.

Drug Interactions

Elevated plasma levels of theophylline have been reported with concomitant quinolone use. There have been reports of theophylline-related side effects in patients on concomitant therapy with norfloxacin and theophylline. Therefore, monitoring of theophylline plasma levels should be considered and dosage of theophylline adjusted as required.

Elevated serum levels of cyclosporine have been reported with concomitant use of cyclosporine with norfloxacin. Therefore cyclosporine serum levels should be monitored and appropriate cyclosporine dosage adjustments made when these drugs are used concomitantly.

Quinolones, including norfloxacin, may enhance the effects of the oral anticoagulant warfarin or its derivatives. When these products are administered concomitantly, prothrombin time or other suitable coagulation tests should be closely monitored.

Diminished urinary excretion of norfloxacin has been reported during the concomitant administration of probenecid and norfloxacin.

The concomitant use of nitrofurantoin is not recommended since nitrofurantoin may antagonize the antibacterial effect of NOROXIN in the urinary tract.

Multivitamins, or other products containing iron or zinc, antacids or sucralfate should not be administered concomitantly with, or within 2 hours of, the administration of norfloxacin, because they may interfere with absorption resulting in lower serum and urine levels of norfloxacin.

Videx® (Didanosine) chewable/buffered tablets or the pediatric powder for oral solution should not be administered concomitantly with, or within 2 hours of, the administration of norfloxacin, because these products may interfere with absorption resulting in lower serum and urine levels of norfloxacin.

Some quinolones have also been shown to interfere with the metabolism of caffeine. This may lead to reduced clearance of caffeine and a prolongation of its plasma half-life.

Carcinogenesis, Mutagenesis, Impairment of Fertility

No increase in neoplastic changes was observed with norfloxacin as compared to controls in a study in rats, lasting up to 96 weeks at doses 8–9 times*** the usual human dose (on a mg/kg basis).

Norfloxacin was tested for mutagenic activity in a number of *in vivo* and *in vitro* tests. Norfloxacin had no mutagenic effect in the dominant lethal test in mice and did not cause chromosomal aberrations in hamsters or rats at doses 30–60 times*** the usual human dose (on a mg/kg basis). Norfloxacin had no mutagenic activity *in vitro* in the Ames microbial mutagen test, Chinese hamster fibroblasts and V-79 mammalian cell assay. Although norfloxacin was weakly positive in the Rec-assay for DNA repair, all other mutagenic assays were negative including a more sensitive test (V-79).

Norfloxacin did not adversely affect the fertility of male and female mice at oral doses up to 30 times*** the usual human dose (on a mg/kg basis).

Pregnancy

Teratogenic Effects. Pregnancy Category C. Norfloxacin has been shown to produce embryonic loss in monkeys when given in doses 10 times*** the maximum daily total human dose (on a mg/kg basis). At this dose, peak plasma levels obtained in monkeys were approximately 2 times those obtained in humans. There has been no evidence of a teratogenic effect in any of the animal species tested (rat, rabbit, mouse, monkey) at 6–50 times*** the maximum daily human dose (on a mg/kg basis). There are, however, no adequate and well controlled studies in pregnant women. Norfloxacin should be used during pregnancy only if the potential benefit justifies the potential risk to the fetus.

Nursing Mothers

It is not known whether norfloxacin is excreted in human milk.

When a 200-mg dose of NOROXIN was administered to nursing mothers, norfloxacin was not detected in human milk. However, because the dose studied was low, because other drugs in this class are secreted in human milk, and because of the potential for serious adverse reactions from norfloxacin in nursing infants, a decision should be made to discontinue nursing or to discontinue the drug, taking into account the importance of the drug to the mother.

Pediatric Use
The safety and effectiveness of oral norfloxacin in pediatric patients and adolescents below the age of 18 years have not been established. Norfloxacin causes arthropathy in juvenile animals of several animal species. (See WARNINGS and ANIMAL PHARMACOLOGY.)

‡Registered trademark of Bristol-Myers Squibb Company.
***Based on a patient weight of 50 kg.

ADVERSE REACTIONS

Single-Dose Studies
In clinical trials involving 82 healthy subjects and 228 patients with gonorrhea, treated with a single dose of norfloxacin, 6.5% reported drug-related adverse experiences. However, the following incidence figures were calculated without reference to drug relationship.
The most common adverse experiences (>1.0%) were: dizziness (2.6%), nausea (2.6%), headache (2.0%), and abdominal cramping (1.6%).
Additional reactions (0.3%–1.0%) were: anorexia, diarrhea, hyperhidrosis, asthenia, anal/rectal pain, constipation, dyspepsia, flatulence, tingling of the fingers, and vomiting.
Laboratory adverse changes considered drug-related were reported in 4.5% of patients/subjects. These laboratory changes were: increased AST (SGOT) (1.6%), decreased WBC (1.3%), decreased platelet count (1.0%), increased urine protein (1.0%), decreased hematocrit and hemoglobin (0.6%), and increased eosinophils (0.6%).
Multiple-Dose Studies
In clinical trials involving 52 healthy subjects and 1980 patients with urinary tract infections or prostatitis, treated with multiple doses of norfloxacin, 3.6% reported drug-related adverse experiences. However, the incidence figures below were calculated without reference to drug relationship.
The most common adverse experiences (>1.0%) were: nausea (4.2%), headache (2.8%), dizziness (1.7%), and asthenia (1.3%).
Additional reactions (0.3%–1.0%) were: abdominal pain, back pain, constipation, diarrhea, dry mouth, dyspepsia/heartburn, fever, flatulence, hyperhidrosis, loose stools, pruritus, rash, somnolence, and vomiting.
Less frequent reactions (0.1%–0.2%) included: abdominal swelling, allergies, anorexia, anxiety, bitter taste, blurred vision, bursitis, chest pain, chills, depression, dysmenorrhea, edema, erythema, foot or hand swelling, insomnia, mouth ulcer, myocardial infarction, palpitation, pruritus ani, renal colic, sleep disturbances, and urticaria.
Abnormal laboratory values observed in these patients/subjects were: eosinophilia (1.5%), elevation of ALT (SGPT) (1.4%), decreased WBC and/or neutrophil count (1.4%), elevation of AST (SGOT) (1.4%), and increased alkaline phosphatase (1.1%). Those occurring less frequently included increased BUN, increased LDH, increased serum creatinine, decreased hematocrit, and glycosuria.
Post Marketing
The most frequently reported adverse reaction in post-marketing experience is rash.
CNS effects characterized as generalized seizures, myoclonus and tremors have been reported with NOROXIN (see WARNINGS). Visual disturbances have been reported with drugs in this class.
The following additional adverse reactions have been reported since the drug was marketed:
Hypersensitivity Reactions
Hypersensitivity reactions have been reported including anaphylactoid reactions, angioedema, dyspnea, vasculitis, urticaria, arthritis, arthralgia and myalgia (see WARNINGS).
Skin
Toxic epidermal necrolysis, Stevens-Johnson syndrome and erythema multiforme, exfoliative dermatitis, photosensitivity
Gastrointestinal
Pseudomembranous colitis, hepatitis, jaundice including cholestatic jaundice and elevated liver function tests, pancreatitis (rare), stomatitis. The onset of pseudomembranous colitis symptoms may occur during or after antibacterial treatment. (See WARNINGS.)
Renal
Interstitial nephritis, renal failure
Nervous System/Psychiatric
Peripheral neuropathy, Guillain-Barré syndrome, ataxia, paresthesia; psychic disturbances including psychotic reactions and confusion
Musculoskeletal
Tendinitis, tendon rupture, exacerbation of myasthenia gravis (see PRECAUTIONS)
Hematologic
Neutropenia, leukopenia, hemolytic anemia, sometimes associated with glucose-6-phosphate dehydrogenase deficiency; thrombocytopenia
Special Senses
Transient hearing loss (rare), tinnitus, diplopia, dysgeusia

Other adverse events reported with quinolones include: agranulocytosis, albuminuria, candiduria, crystalluria, cylindruria, dysphagia, elevation of blood glucose, elevation of serum cholesterol, elevation of serum potassium, elevation of serum triglycerides, hematuria, hepatic necrosis, symptomatic hypoglycemia, nystagmus, postural hypotension, prolongation of prothrombin time, and vaginal candidiasis.

Infection	Description	Unit Dose	Frequency	Duration	Daily Dose
Urinary Tract	Uncomplicated UTI's (crystitis) due to *E. coli, K. pneumoniae*, or *P. mirabilis*	400 mg	q12h	3 days	800 mg
	Uncomplicated UTI's due to other indicated organisms	400 mg	q12h	7–10 days	800 mg
	Complicated UTI's	400 mg	q12h	10–21 days	800 mg
Sexually Transmitted Diseases	Uncomplicated Gonorrhea	800 mg	single dose	1 day	800 mg
Prostatitis	Acute or Chronic	400 mg	q12h	28 days	800 mg

OVERDOSAGE

No significant lethality was observed in male and female mice and rats at single oral doses up to 4 g/kg.
In the event of acute overdosage, the stomach should be emptied by inducing vomiting or by gastric lavage, and the patient carefully observed and given symptomatic and supportive treatment. Adequate hydration must be maintained.

DOSAGE AND ADMINISTRATION

Tablets NOROXIN should be taken at least one hour before or at least two hours after a meal or ingestion of milk and/or other dairy products. Multivitamins, other products containing iron or zinc, antacids containing magnesium and aluminum, sucralfate, or Videx® (Didanosine), chewable/buffered tablets or the pediatric powder for oral solution, should not be taken within 2 hours of administration of norfloxacin. Tablets NOROXIN should be taken with a glass of water. Patients receiving NOROXIN should be well hydrated (see PRECAUTIONS).
Normal Renal Function
The recommended daily dose of NOROXIN is as described in the following chart:
[See table above]
Renal Impairment
NOROXIN may be used for the treatment of urinary tract infections in patients with renal insufficiency. In patients with a creatinine clearance rate of 30 mL/min/1.73m^2 or less, the recommended dosage is one 400-mg tablet once daily for the duration given above. At this dosage, the urinary concentration exceeds the MICs for most urinary pathogens susceptible to norfloxacin, even when the creatinine clearance is less than 10 mL/min/1.73m^2.
When only the serum creatinine level is available, the following formula (based on sex, weight, and age of the patient) may be used to convert this value into creatinine clearance. The serum creatinine should represent a steady state of renal function.

$$\text{Males: } \frac{(\text{weight in kg}) \times (140 - \text{age})}{(72) \times \text{serum creatinine (mg/100 mL)}}$$

$$\text{Females: } (0.85) \times (\text{above value})$$

Elderly
Elderly patients being treated for urinary tract infections who have a creatinine clearance of greater than 30 mL/min/1.73m^2 should receive the dosages recommended under *Normal Renal Function.*
Elderly patients being treated for urinary tract infections who have a creatinine clearance of 30 mL/min/1.73m^2 or less should receive 400 mg once daily as recommended under *Renal Impairment.*

HOW SUPPLIED

No. 3522—Tablets NOROXIN 400 mg are dark pink, oval shaped, film-coated tablets, coded MSD 705 on one side and NOROXIN on the other. They are supplied as follows:
NDC 0006-0705-68 bottles of 100
NDC 0006-0705-20 unit of use bottles of 20
NDC 0006-0705-28 unit dose packages of 100.
Storage
Store at 25°C (77°F); excursions permitted to 15–30°C (59–86°F) [see USP Controlled Room Temperature]. Keep container tightly closed.

ANIMAL PHARMACOLOGY

Norfloxacin and related drugs have been shown to cause arthropathy in immature animals of most species tested (see WARNINGS).
Crystalluria has occurred in laboratory animals tested with norfloxacin. In dogs, needle-shaped drug crystals were seen in the urine at doses of 50 mg/kg/day. In rats, crystals were reported following doses of 200 mg/kg/day.
Embryo lethality and slight maternotoxicity (vomiting and anorexia) were observed in cynomolgus monkeys at doses of 150 mg/kg/day or higher.
Ocular toxicity, seen with some related drugs, was not observed in any norfloxacin-treated animals.

REFERENCES

1. National Committee for Clinical Laboratory Standards, Methods for dilution antimicrobial susceptibility tests for bacteria that grow aerobically – 3rd ed., Approved Standard NCCLS Document M7–A3, Vol. 13, No. 25, NCCLS, Villanova, PA, 1993.
2. National Committee for Clinical Laboratory Standards, Performance standards for antimicrobial disk susceptibility tests – 5th ed., Approved Standard NCCLS Document M2–A5, Vol. 13, No. 24, NCCLS, Villanova, PA, 1993.

7898528 Issued September 1999

Shown in Product Identification Guide, page 324

Liquid PedvaxHIB® ℞
[Haemophilus b Conjugate Vaccine (Meningococcal Protein Conjugate)]

DESCRIPTION

PedvaxHIB* [Haemophilus b Conjugate Vaccine (Meningococcal Protein Conjugate)] is a highly purified capsular polysaccharide (polyribosylribitol phosphate or PRP) of *Haemophilus influenzae* type b (Haemophilus b, Ross strain) that is covalently bound to an outer membrane protein complex (OMPC) of the B11 strain of *Neisseria meningitidis* serogroup B. The covalent bonding of the PRP to the OMPC which is necessary for enhanced immunogenicity of the PRP is confirmed by quantitative analysis of the conjugate's components following chemical treatment which yields a unique amino acid. The potency of PedvaxHIB is determined by assay of PRP.
Haemophilus influenzae type b and *Neisseria meningitidis* serogroup B are grown in complex fermentation media. The PRP is purified from the culture broth by purification procedures which include ethanol fractionation, enzyme digestion, phenol extraction and diafiltration. The OMPC from *Neisseria meningitidis* is purified by detergent extraction, ultracentrifugation, diafiltration and sterile filtration.
Liquid PedvaxHIB is ready to use and does not require a diluent. Each 0.5 mL dose of Liquid PedvaxHIB is a sterile product formulated to contain: 7.5 mcg of Haemophilus b PRP, 125 mcg of *Neisseria meningitidis* OMPC and 225 mcg of aluminum as aluminum hydroxide, in 0.9% sodium chloride, but does not contain lactose or thimerosal.
Liquid PedvaxHIB is a slightly opaque white suspension.
This vaccine is for intramuscular administration and not for intravenous injection. (See DOSAGE AND ADMINISTRATION.)

* Registered trademark of MERCK & CO., Inc.

CLINICAL PHARMACOLOGY

Prior to the introduction of Haemophilus b Conjugate Vaccines, *Haemophilus influenzae* type b (Hib) was the most frequent cause of bacterial meningitis and a leading cause of serious, systemic bacterial disease in young children worldwide.
Hib disease occurred primarily in children under 5 years of age in the United States prior to the initiation of a vaccine program and was estimated to account for nearly 20,000 cases of invasive infections annually, approximately 12,000 of which were meningitis. The mortality rate from Hib meningitis is about 5%. In addition, up to 35% of survivors develop neurologic sequelae including seizures, deafness, and mental retardation. Other invasive diseases caused by this bacterium include cellulitis, epiglottitis, sepsis, pneumonia, septic arthritis, osteomyelitis and pericarditis.
Prior to the introduction of the vaccine, it was estimated that 17% of all cases of Hib disease occurred in infants less than 6 months of age. The peak incidence of Hib meningitis occurs between 6 to 11 months of age. Forty-seven percent of all cases occur by one year of age with the remaining 53% of cases occurring over the next four years.

Continued on next page

Information on the Merck & Co., Inc. products listed on these pages is the full prescribing information from product circulars in use September 30, 2000. For information, please call 1-800-NSC MERCK [1-800-672-6372].

PedvaxHIB—Cont.

Among children under 5 years of age, the risk of invasive Hib disease is increased in certain populations including the following:

- Daycare attendees
- Lower socio-economic groups
- Blacks (especially those who lack the Km(1) immunoglobulin allotype)
- Caucasians who lack the G2m (n or 23) immunoglobulin allotype
- Native Americans
- Household contacts of cases
- Individuals with asplenia, sickle cell disease, or antibody deficiency syndromes

An important virulence factor of the Hib bacterium is its polysaccharide capsule (PRP). Antibody to PRP (anti-PRP) has been shown to correlate with protection against Hib disease. While the anti-PRP level associated with protection using conjugated vaccines has not yet been determined, the level of anti-PRP associated with protection in studies using bacterial polysaccharide immune globulin or nonconjugated PRP vaccines ranged from >0.15 to >1.0 mcg/mL.

Nonconjugated PRP vaccines are capable of stimulating B-lymphocytes to produce antibody without the help of T-lymphocytes (T-independent). The responses to many other antigens are augmented by helper T-lymphocytes (T-dependent). PedvaxHIB is a PRP-conjugate vaccine in which the PRP is covalently bound to the OMPC carrier producing an antigen which is postulated to convert the T-independent antigen (PRP alone) into a T-dependent antigen resulting in both an enhanced antibody response and immunologic memory.

Clinical Evaluation of PedvaxHIB

PedvaxHIB, in a lyophilized formulation (lyophilized PedvaxHIB), was initially evaluated in 3,486 Native American (Navajo) infants, who completed the primary two-dose regimen in a randomized, double-blind, placebo-controlled study (The Protective Efficacy Study). At the time of the study, this population had a much higher incidence of Hib disease than the United States population as a whole and also had a lower antibody response to Haemophilus b Conjugate Vaccines, including PedvaxHIB.

Each infant in this study received two doses of either placebo or lyophilized PedvaxHIB with the first dose administered at a mean of 8 weeks of age and the second administered approximately two months later; DTP and OPV were administered concomitantly. Antibody levels were measured in a subset of each group (TABLE 1).

[See table 1 above]

Most subjects were initially followed until 15 to 18 months of age. During this time, 22 cases of invasive Hib disease occurred in the placebo group (8 cases after the first dose and 14 cases after the second dose) and only 1 case in the vaccine group (none after the first dose and 1 after the second dose). Following the primary two-dose regimen, the protective efficacy of lyophilized PedvaxHIB was calculated to be 93% with a 95% confidence interval of 57%–98% (p=0.001, two-tailed). In the two months between the first and second doses, the difference in number of cases of disease between placebo and vaccine recipients (8 vs. 0 cases, respectively) was statistically significant (p=0.008, two-tailed); however, a primary two-dose regimen is required for infants 2–14 months of age.

At termination of the study, placebo recipients were offered vaccine. All original participants were then followed two years and nine months from termination of the study. During this extended follow-up, invasive Hib disease occurred in an additional seven of the original placebo recipients prior to receiving vaccine and in one of the original vaccine recipients (who had received only one dose of vaccine). No cases of invasive Hib disease were observed in placebo recipients after they received at least one dose of vaccine. Efficacy for this follow-up period, estimated from person-days at risk, was 96.6% (95 C.I., 72.2–99.9%) in children under 18 months of age and 100% (95 C.I., 23.5–100%) in children over 18 months of age.

Since protective efficacy with lyophilized PedvaxHIB was demonstrated in such a high risk population, it would be expected to be predictive of efficacy in other populations.

The safety and immunogenicity of lyophilized PedvaxHIB were evaluated in infants and children in other clinical studies that were conducted in various locations throughout the United States. PedvaxHIB was highly immunogenic in all age groups studied.

Lyophilized PedvaxHIB induced antibody levels greater than 1.0 mcg/mL in children who were poor responders to nonconjugated PRP vaccines. In a study involving such a subpopulation, 34 children ranging in age from 27 to 61 months who developed invasive Hib disease despite previous vaccination with nonconjugated PRP vaccines were randomly assigned to 2 groups. One group (n=14) was vaccinated with lyophilized PedvaxHIB and the other group (n=20) with a nonconjugated PRP vaccine at a mean interval of approximately 12 months after recovery from disease. All 14 children vaccinated with lyophilized PedvaxHIB but only 6 of 20 children re-vaccinated with a nonconjugated PRP vaccine achieved an antibody level of >1.0 mcg/mL. The 14 children who had not responded to revaccination with the nonconjugated PRP vaccine were then vaccinated with a single dose of lyophilized PedvaxHIB; following this vaccination, all achieved antibody levels of >1.0 mcg/mL.

TABLE 1
Antibody Responses in Navajo Infants

Vaccine	No. of Subjects	Time	% Subjects with >0.15 mcg/mL	% Subjects with >1.0 mcg/mL	Anti-PRP GMT (mcg/mL)
Lyophilized	416**	Pre-Vaccination	44	10	0.16
PedvaxHIB*	416	Post-Dose 1	88	52	0.95
	416	Post-Dose 2	91	60	1.43
Placebo*	461**	Pre-Vaccination	44	9	0.16
	461	Post-Dose 1	21	2	0.09
	461	Post-Dose 2	14	1	0.08
Lyophilized	27†	Prebooster	70	33	0.51
PedvaxHIB	27	Postbooster††	100	89	8.39

*Post-Vaccination values obtained approximately 1–3 months after each dose.
**The Protective Efficacy Study
†Immunogenicity Trial[34]
††Booster given at 12 months of age; Post-Vaccination values obtained 1 month after administration of booster dose.

TABLE 2
Antibody Responses to Liquid and Lyophilized PedvaxHIB in Infants From the General U.S. Population

Formulation	Age (Months)	Time	No. of Subjects	% Subjects with anti-PRP >0.15 mcg/mL	% Subjects with anti-PRP >1.0 mcg/mL	Anti-PRP GMT (mcg/mL)
		Pre-Vaccination	487	32	7	0.12
Liquid	2–3	Post-Dose 1*	480	94	64	1.55
PedvaxHIB		Post-Dose 2**	393	97	80	3.22
(7.5 mcg PRP)	12–15	Prebooster	284	80	30	0.49
		Postbooster**	284	99	95	10.23
	24†	Persistence	94	97	55	1.29
		Pre-Vaccination	171	37	6	0.13
Lyophilized	2–3	Post-Dose 1*	169	97	72	1.88
PedvaxHIB		Post-Dose 2**	133	99	81	2.69
(15 mcg PRP)	12–15	Prebooster	87	71	28	0.39
		Postbooster**	87	99	91	7.64
	24†	Persistence	37	97	54	1.10

*Approximately two months Post-Vaccination
**Approximately one month Post-Vaccination
†Approximately

TABLE 3
Antibody Responses*
After Two Doses of Lyophilized PedvaxHIB Among Infants Initially Vaccinated at 2–3 Months of Age By Racial/Ethnic Group

LYOPHILIZED

Racial/Ethnic Groups	No. of Subjects	% Subjects With Anti-PRP >0.15 mcg/mL	% Subjects With Anti-PRP >1.0 mcg/mL	Anti-PRP GMT (mcg/mL)
Native American†	54	96	70	2.47
Caucasian	201	99	82	3.52
Hispanic	76	99	88	3.54
Black	23	100	96	5.40

* One month after the second dose
† Apache and Navajo

TABLE 4
Antibody Responses*
After Two Doses of Liquid PedvaxHIB Among Infants Initially Vaccinated at 2–3 Months of Age By Racial/Ethnic Group

LIQUID

Racial/Ethnic Groups	No. of Subjects	% Subjects with Anti-PRP >0.15 mcg/mL	% Subjects with Anti-PRP >1.0 mcg/mL	Anti-PRP GMT (mcg/mL)
Native American**	90	97	78	2.76
Caucasian	143	94	72	2.16
Hispanic	184	98	85	4.34
Black	18	100	94	7.58

* One month after the second dose
**Apache and Navajo

In addition, lyophilized PedvaxHIB has been studied in children at high risk of Hib disease because of genetically-related deficiencies [Blacks who were Km(1) allotype negative and Caucasians who were G2m(23) allotype negative] and are considered hyporesponsive to nonconjugated PRP vaccines on this basis. The hyporesponsive children had anti-PRP responses comparable to those of allotype positive children of similar age range when vaccinated with lyophilized PedvaxHIB. All children achieved anti-PRP levels of >1.0 mcg/mL.

The safety and immunogenicity of Liquid PedvaxHIB were compared with those of lyophilized PedvaxHIB is a randomized clinical study involving 903 infants 2 to 6 months of age from the general U.S. population. DTP and OPV were administered concomitantly to most subjects. The antibody responses induced by each formulation of PedvaxHIB were similar. TABLE 2 shows antibody responses from this clinical study in subjects who received their first dose at 2 to 3 months of age.

[See table 2 above]

A booster dose of PedvaxHIB is required in infants who complete the primary two-dose regimen before 12 months of age. This booster dose will help maintain antibody levels during the first two years of life when children are at highest risk for invasive Hib disease. (See TABLE 2 and DOSAGE AND ADMINISTRATION.)

In four United States studies, antibody responses to lyophilized PedvaxHIB were evaluated in several subpopulations of infants initially vaccinated between 2 to 3 months of age. (See TABLE 3.)

[See table 3 above]

In two United States studies, antibody responses to Liquid PedvaxHIB were evaluated in several subpopulations of infants initially vaccinated between 2 to 3 months of age. (See TABLE 4.)

[See table 4 above]

Antibodies to the OMPC of *N. meningitidis* have been demonstrated in vaccinee sera, but the clinical relevance of these antibodies has not been established.

Interchangeability of Licensed Haemophilus b Conjugate Vaccines and PedvaxHIB

Published studies have examined the interchangeability of other licensed Haemophilus b Conjugate Vaccines and PedvaxHIB. According to the American Academy of Pediatrics, excellent immune responses have been achieved when different vaccines have been interchanged in the primary series. If PedvaxHIB is given in a series with one of the other products licensed for infants, the recommended number of doses to complete the series is determined by the other product and not by PedvaxHIB. PedvaxHIB may be interchanged with other licensed Haemophilus b Conjugate Vaccines for the booster dose.

Use with Other Vaccines
Results from clinical studies indicate that Liquid PedvaxHIB can be administered concomitantly with DTP, OPV, eIPV (enhanced inactivated poliovirus vaccine), VARIVAX* [Varicella Virus Vaccine Live (Oka/Merck)], M-M-R* II (Measles, Mumps, and Rubella Virus Vaccine Live) or RECOMBIVAX HB* [Hepatitis B Vaccine (Recombinant)]. No impairment of immune response to individual tested vaccine antigens was demonstrated.
The type, frequency and severity of adverse experiences observed in these studies with PedvaxHIB were similar to those seen when the other vaccines were given alone.
In addition, a PRP-OMPC-containing product, COMVAX* [Haemophilus b Conjugate (Meningococcal Protein Conjugate) and Hepatitis B (Recombinant) Vaccine], was given concomitantly with a booster dose of DTaP [diphtheria, tetanus, acellular pertussis] at approximately 15 months of age, using separate sites and syringes for injectable vaccines. No impairment of immune response to these individually tested vaccine antigens was demonstrated. COMVAX has also been administered concomitantly with the primary series of DTaP to a limited number of infants. PRP antibody responses are satisfactory for COMVAX, but immune responses are currently unavailable for DTaP (see Manufacturer's Product Circular for COMVAX). No serious vaccine-related adverse events were reported.

INDICATIONS AND USAGE

Liquid PedvaxHIB is indicated for routine vaccination against invasive disease caused by *Haemophilus influenzae* type b in infants and children 2 to 71 months of age.
Liquid PedvaxHIB will not protect against disease caused by *Haemophilus influenzae* other than type b or against other microorganisms that cause invasive disease such as meningitis or sepsis. As with any vaccine, vaccination with Liquid PedvaxHIB may not result in a protective antibody response in all individuals given the vaccine.
BECAUSE OF THE POTENTIAL FOR IMMUNE TOLERANCE, Liquid PedvaxHIB IS NOT RECOMMENDED FOR USE IN INFANTS YOUNGER THAN 6 WEEKS OF AGE. (See PRECAUTIONS.)
Revaccination
Infants completing the primary two-dose regimen before 12 months of age should receive a booster dose (see DOSAGE AND ADMINISTRATION).

CONTRAINDICATIONS

Hypersensitivity to any component of the vaccine or the diluent.
Persons who develop symptoms suggestive of hypersensitivity after an injection should not receive further injections of the vaccine.

PRECAUTIONS

General
As for any vaccine, adequate treatment provisions, including epinephrine, should be available for immediate use should an anaphylactoid reaction occur.
Special care should be taken to ensure that the injection does not enter a blood vessel.
It is important to use a separate sterile syringe and needle for each patient to prevent transmission of hepatitis B or other infectious agents from one person to another.
As with other vaccines, Liquid PedvaxHIB may not induce protective antibody levels immediately following vaccination.
As reported with Haemophilus b Polysaccharide Vaccine and another Haemophilus b Conjugate Vaccine, cases of Hib disease may occur in the week after vaccination, prior to the onset of the protective effects of the vaccines.
There is insufficient evidence that Liquid PedvaxHIB given immediately after exposure to natural *Haemophilus influenzae* type b will prevent illness.
The decision to administer or delay vaccination because of current or recent febrile illness depends on the severity of symptoms and on the etiology of the disease. The Advisory Committee on Immunization Practices (ACIP) has recommended that vaccination should be delayed during the course of an acute febrile illness. All vaccines can be administered to persons with minor illnesses such as diarrhea, mild upper-respiratory infection with or without low-grade fever, or other low-grade febrile illness. Persons with moderate or severe febrile illness should be vaccinated as soon as they have recovered from the acute phase of the illness.
If PedvaxHIB is used in persons with malignancies or those receiving immunosuppressive therapy or who are otherwise immunocompromised, the expected immune response may not be obtained.
Instructions to Healthcare Provider
The healthcare provider should determine the current health status and previous vaccination history of the vaccinee.
The healthcare provider should question the patient, parent, or guardian about reactions to a previous dose of PedvaxHIB or other Haemophilus b Conjugate Vaccines.
Information for Patients
The healthcare provider should provide the vaccine information required to be given with each vaccination to the patient, parent, or guardian.

TABLE 5
Fever or Local Reactions in Subjects First Vaccinated at 2 to 6 Months of Age with Liquid PedvaxHIB*

Reaction	No. of Subjects Evaluated	Post-Dose 1 (hr) 6	24	48	No. of Subjects Evaluated	Post-Dose 2 (hr) 6	24	48
		Percentage				Percentage		
Fever** >38.3°C (≥101°F) Rectal	222	18.1	4.4	0.5	206	14.1	9.4	2.8
Erythema >2.5 cm diameter	674	2.2	1.0	0.5	562	1.6	1.1	0.4
Swelling >2.5 cm diameter	674	2.5	1.9	0.9	562	0.9	0.9	1.3

*DTP and OPV were administered concomitantly to most subjects.
**Fever was also measured by another method or reported as normal for an additional 345 infants after dose 1 and for an additional 249 infants after dose 2; however, these data are not included in this table.

The healthcare provider should inform the patient, parent, or guardian of the benefits and risks associated with vaccination. For risks associated with vaccination, see ADVERSE REACTIONS.
Patients, parents, and guardians should be instructed to report any serious adverse reactions to their healthcare provider who in turn should report such events to the U.S. Department of Health and Human Services through the Vaccine Adverse Event Reporting System (VAERS), 1-800-822-7967.
Laboratory Test Interactions
Sensitive tests (e.g., Latex Agglutination Kits) may detect PRP derived from the vaccine in urine of some vaccinees for at least 30 days following vaccination with lyophilized PedvaxHIB; in clinical studies with lyophilized PedvaxHIB, such children demonstrated normal immune response to the vaccine.
Carcinogenesis, Mutagenesis, Impairment of Fertility
Liquid PedvaxHIB has not been evaluated for carcinogenic or mutagenic potential, or potential to impair fertility.
Pregnancy
Pregnancy Category C: Animal reproduction studies have not been conducted with PedvaxHIB. Liquid PedvaxHIB is not recommended for use in individuals 6 years of age and older.
Pediatric Use
Safety and effectiveness in infants below the age of 2 months and in children 6 years of age and older have not been established. In addition, Liquid PedvaxHIB should not be used in infants younger than 6 weeks of age because this will lead to a reduced anti-PRP response and may lead to immune tolerance (impaired ability to respond to subsequent exposure to the PRP antigen). Liquid PedvaxHIB is not recommended for use in individuals 6 years of age and older because they are generally not a risk of Hib disease.

ADVERSE REACTIONS

Liquid PedvaxHIB
In a multicenter clinical study (n=903) comparing the effects of Liquid PedvaxHIB with those of lyophilized PedvaxHIB, 1,699 doses of Liquid PedvaxHIB were administered to 678 healthy infants 2 to 6 months of age from the general U.S. population. DTP and OPV were administered concomitantly to most subjects. Both formulations of PedvaxHIB were generally well tolerated and no serious vaccine-related adverse reactions were reported.
During a three-day period following primary vaccination with Liquid PedvaxHIB in these infants, the most frequently reported (>1%) adverse reactions, without regard to causality, excluding those shown in TABLE 5, in decreasing order of frequency, were: irritability, sleepiness, injection site pain/soreness, injection site erythema (≤2.5 cm diameter, see also TABLE 5), injection site swelling/induration (≤2.5 cm diameter, see also TABLE 5), unusual high-pitched crying, prolonged crying (>4 hr), diarrhea, vomiting, crying, pain, otitis media, rash, and upper respiratory infection.
Selected objective observations reported by parents over a 48-hour period in these infants following primary vaccination with Liquid PedvaxHIB are summarized in TABLE 5. [See table 5 above]
Adverse reactions during a three-day period following administration of the booster dose were generally similar in type and frequency to those seen following primary vaccination.
Lyophilized PedvaxHIB
In The Protective Efficacy Study (see CLINICAL PHARMACOLOGY), 4,459 healthy Navajo infants 6 to 12 weeks of age received lyophilized PedvaxHIB or placebo. Most of these infants received DTP/OPV concomitantly. No differences were seen in the type and frequency of serious health problems expected in this Navajo population or in serious adverse experiences reported among those who received lyophilized PedvaxHIB and those who received placebo, and none was reported to be related to lyophilized PedvaxHIB. Only one serious reaction (tracheitis) was reported as possibly related to lyophilized PedvaxHIB and only one (diarrhea) as possibly related to placebo. Seizures occurred infrequently in both groups (9 occurred in vaccine recipients, 8 of whom also received DTP; 8 occurred in placebo recipients, 7 of whom also received DTP) and were not reported to be related to lyophilized PedvaxHIB.
In early clinical studies involving the administration of 8,086 doses of lyophilized PedvaxHIB alone to 5,027 healthy infants and children 2 months to 71 months of age, lyophilized PedvaxHIB was generally well tolerated. No serious adverse reactions were reported. In a subset of these infants, urticaria was reported in two children, and thrombocytopenia was seen in one child. A cause and effect relationship between these side effects and the vaccination has not been established.
Potential Adverse Reactions
The use of Haemophilus b Polysaccharide Vaccines and another Haemophilus b Conjugate Vaccine has been associated with the following additional adverse effects: early onset Hib disease and Guillain-Barré syndrome. A cause and effect relationship between these side effects and the vaccination was not established.
Post-Marketing Adverse Reactions
The following additional adverse reactions have been reported with the use of the lyophilized and liquid formulations of PedvaxHIB:
Hemic and Lymphatic System
Lymphadenopathy
Hypersensitivity
Rarely, angioedema
Nervous System
Febrile seizures
Skin
Sterile injection site abscess

DOSAGE AND ADMINISTRATION

Liquid PedvaxHIB
FOR INTRAMUSCULAR ADMINISTRATION
DO NOT INJECT INTRAVENOUSLY
If there is an interruption or delay between doses in the primary series, there is no need to repeat the series, but dosing should be continued at the next clinic visit. (See CONTRAINDICATIONS and PRECAUTIONS.)
2 to 14 Months of Age
Infants 2 to 14 months of age should receive a 0.5 mL dose of vaccine ideally beginning at 2 months of age followed by a 0.5 mL dose 2 months later (or as soon as possible thereafter). When the primary two-dose regimen is completed before 12 months of age, a booster dose is required (see below and TABLE 6). Infants born prematurely, regardless of birth weight, should be vaccinated at the same chronological age and according to the same schedule and precautions as full-term infants and children.
15 Months of Age and Older
Children 15 months of age and older previously unvaccinated against Hib disease should receive a single 0.5 mL dose of vaccine.
Booster Dose
In infants completing the primary two-dose regimen before 12 months of age, a booster dose (0.5 mL) should be administered at 12 to 15 months of age, but not earlier than 2 months after the second dose.
Vaccination regimens for Liquid PedvaxHIB by age group are outlined in TABLE 6.

Continued on next page

Information on the Merck & Co., Inc. products listed on these pages is the full prescribing information from product circulars in use September 30, 2000. For information, please call 1-800-NSC MERCK [1-800-672-6372].

PedvaxHIB—Cont.

TABLE 6
Vaccination Regimens for Liquid PedvaxHIB
By Age Groups

Age (Months) at First Dose	Primary	Age (Months) at Booster Dose
2–10	2 doses, 2 mo. apart	12–15
11–14	2 doses, 2 mo. apart	—
15–71	1 dose	—

Interchangeability
PedvaxHIB may be interchanged with other licensed Haemophilus b Conjugate Vaccines for the primary and booster doses. (See CLINICAL PHARMACOLOGY.)
Use with Other Vaccines
Results from clinical studies indicate that Liquid PedvaxHIB can be administered concomitantly with DTP, OPV, eIPV (enhanced inactivated poliovirus vaccine), VARIVAX [Varicella Virus Vaccine Live (Oka/Merck)], M-M-R II (Measles, Mumps, and Rubella Virus Vaccine Live) or RECOMBIVAX HB [Hepatitis B Vaccine (Recombinant)]. No impairment of immune response to these individually tested vaccine antigens was demonstrated.
The type, frequency and severity of adverse experiences observed in these studies with PedvaxHIB were similar to those seen with other vaccines when given alone. (See CLINICAL PHARMACOLOGY.)
In addition, a PRP-OMPC-containing product, COMVAX [Haemophilus b Conjugate (Meningococcal Protein Conjugate) and Hepatitis B (Recombinant) Vaccine], was given concomitantly with a booster dose of DTaP [diphtheria, tetanus, acellular pertussis] at approximately 15 months of age, using separate sites and syringes for injectable vaccines. No impairment of immune response to these individually tested vaccine antigens was demonstrated. COMVAX has also been administered concomitantly with the primary series of DTaP to a limited number of infants. PRP antibody responses are satisfactory for COMVAX, but immune responses are currently unavailable for DTaP (see Manufacturer's Product Circular for COMVAX). No serious vaccine-related adverse events were reported.
Parenteral drug products should be inspected visually for extraneous particulate matter and discoloration prior to administration whenever solution and container permit.
Liquid PedvaxHIB is a slightly opaque white suspension. (See DESCRIPTION.)
The vaccine should be used as supplied; no reconstitution is necessary.
Shake well before withdrawal and use. Thorough agitation is necessary to maintain suspension of the vaccine.
Inject 0.5 mL intramuscularly, preferably into the anterolateral thigh or the outer aspect of the upper arm. The buttocks should not be used for active vaccination of infants and children, because of the potential risk of injury to the sciatic nerve.

HOW SUPPLIED

Liquid PedvaxHIB is supplied as follows:
No. 4877—A single-dose vial of liquid vaccine, **NDC** 0006-4877-00.
No. 4897—A box of 10 single-dose vials of liquid vaccine, **NDC** 0006-4897-00.
Storage
Store vaccine at 2–8°C (34–46°F).
DO NOT FREEZE.
9018901 Issued March 1998

PEPCID® Tablets ℞
(famotidine)
PEPCID® for Oral Suspension ℞
(famotidine)
PEPCID RPD® Orally Disintegrating Tablets ℞
(famotidine)

DESCRIPTION

The active ingredient in PEPCID* (Famotidine), is a histamine H_2-receptor antagonist. Famotidine is *N*′-(aminosulfonyl) -3- [[[2-[(diaminomethylene)amino] -4- thiazolyl] methyl]thio]propanimidamide. The empirical formula of famotidine is $C_8H_{15}N_7O_2S_3$ and its molecular weight is 337.43. Its structural formula is:

Famotidine is a white to pale yellow crystalline compound that is freely soluble in glacial acetic acid, slightly soluble in methanol, very slightly soluble in water, and practically insoluble in ethanol.
Each tablet for oral administration contains either 20 mg or 40 mg of famotidine and the following inactive ingredients: hydroxypropyl cellulose, hydroxypropyl methylcellulose, iron oxides, magnesium stearate, microcrystalline cellulose, corn starch, talc, titanium dioxide.
Each PEPCID Orally Disintegrating Tablet for oral administration contains either 20 mg or 40 mg of famotidine and the following inactive ingredients: aspartame, mint flavor, gelatin, mannitol, red ferric oxide, and xanthan gum.
Each 5 mL of the oral suspension when prepared as directed contains 40 mg of famotidine and the following inactive ingredients: citric acid, flavors, microcrystalline cellulose and carboxymethylcellulose sodium, sucrose and xanthan gum. Added as preservatives are sodium benzoate 0.1%, sodium methylparaben 0.1%, and sodium propylparaben 0.02%.

*Registered trademark of MERCK & CO., Inc.

CLINICAL PHARMACOLOGY IN ADULTS

GI Effects
PEPCID is a competitive inhibitor of histamine H_2-receptors. The primary clinically important pharmacologic activity of PEPCID is inhibition of gastric secretion. Both the acid concentration and volume of gastric secretion are suppressed by PEPCID, while changes in pepsin secretion are proportional to volume output.
In normal volunteers and hypersecretors, PEPCID inhibited basal and nocturnal gastric secretion, as well as secretion stimulated by food and pentagastrin. After oral administration, the onset of the antisecretory effect occurred within one hour; the maximum effect was dose-dependent, occurring within one to three hours. Duration of inhibition of secretion by doses of 20 and 40 mg was 10 to 12 hours.
Single evening oral doses of 20 and 40 mg inhibited basal and nocturnal acid secretion in all subjects; mean nocturnal gastric acid secretion was inhibited by 86% and 94%, respectively, for a period of at least 10 hours. The same doses given in the morning suppressed food-stimulated acid secretion in all subjects. The mean suppression was 76% and 84% respectively 3 to 5 hours after administration, and 25% and 30% respectively 8 to 10 hours after administration. In some subjects who received the 20 mg dose, however, the antisecretory effect was dissipated within 6–8 hours. There was no cumulative effect with repeated doses. The nocturnal intragastric pH was raised by evening doses of 20 and 40 mg of PEPCID to mean values of 5.0 and 6.4, respectively. When PEPCID was given after breakfast, the basal daytime interdigestive pH at 3 and 8 hours after 20 or 40 mg of PEPCID was raised to about 5.
PEPCID had little or no effect on fasting or postprandial serum gastrin levels. Gastric emptying and exocrine pancreatic function were not affected by PEPCID.
Other Effects
Systemic effects of PEPCID in the CNS, cardiovascular, respiratory or endocrine systems were not noted in clinical pharmacology studies. Also, no antiandrogenic effects were noted. (See ADVERSE REACTIONS.) Serum hormone levels, including prolactin, cortisol, thyroxine (T_4), and testosterone, were not altered after treatment with PEPCID.
Pharmacokinetics
PEPCID is incompletely absorbed. The bioavailability of oral doses is 40–45%. PEPCID Tablets, PEPCID for Oral Suspension and PEPCID RPD Orally Disintegrating Tablets are bioequivalent. Bioavailability may be slightly increased by food, or slightly decreased by antacids; however, these effects are of no clinical consequence. PEPCID undergoes minimal first-pass metabolism. After oral doses, peak plasma levels occur in 1–3 hours. Plasma levels after multiple doses are similar to those after single doses. Fifteen to 20% of PEPCID in plasma is protein bound. PEPCID has an elimination half-life of 2.5–3.5 hours. PEPCID is eliminated by renal (65–70%) and metabolic (30–35%) routes. Renal clearance is 250–450 mL/min, indicating some tubular excretion. Twenty-five to 30% of an oral dose and 65–70% of an intravenous dose are recovered in the urine as unchanged compound. The only metabolite identified in man is the S-oxide.
There is a close relationship between creatinine clearance values and the elimination half-life of PEPCID. In patients with severe renal insufficiency, i.e., creatinine clearance less than 10 mL/min, the elimination half-life of PEPCID may exceed 20 hours and adjustment of dose or dosing intervals may be necessary (see PRECAUTIONS, DOSAGE AND ADMINISTRATION).
In elderly patients, there are no clinically significant age-related changes in the pharmacokinetics of PEPCID.
Clinical Studies
Duodenal Ulcer
In a U.S. multicenter, double-blind study in outpatients with endoscopically confirmed duodenal ulcer, orally administered PEPCID was compared to placebo. As shown in Table 1, 70% of patients treated with PEPCID 40 mg h.s. were healed by week 4.

Table 1
Outpatients with Endoscopically
Confirmed Healed Duodenal Ulcers

	PEPCID 40 mg h.s. (N=89)	PEPCID 20 mg b.i.d. (N=84)	Placebo h.s. (N=97)
Week 2	**32%	**38%	17%
Week 4	**70%	**67%	31%

** Statistically significantly different than placebo ($p < 0.001$)

Patients not healed by week 4 were continued in the study. By week 8, 83% of patients treated with PEPCID had healed versus 45% of patients treated with placebo. The incidence of ulcer healing with PEPCID was significantly higher than with placebo at each time point based on proportion of endoscopically confirmed healed ulcers.
In this study, time to relief of daytime and nocturnal pain was significantly shorter for patients receiving PEPCID than for patients receiving placebo; patients receiving PEPCID also took less antacid than the patients receiving placebo.
Long-Term Maintenance
Treatment of Duodenal Ulcers
PEPCID, 20 mg p.o. h.s. was compared to placebo h.s. as maintenance therapy in two double-blind, multicenter studies of patients with endoscopically confirmed healed duodenal ulcers. In the U.S. study the observed ulcer incidence within 12 months in patients treated with placebo was 2.4 times greater than in the patients treated with PEPCID. The 89 patients treated with PEPCID had a cumulative observed ulcer incidence of 23.4% compared to an observed ulcer incidence of 56.6% in the 89 patients receiving placebo ($p<0.01$). These results were confirmed in an international study where the cumulative observed ulcer incidence within 12 months in the 307 patients treated with PEPCID was 35.7%, compared to an incidence of 75.5% in the 325 patients treated with placebo ($p<0.01$).
Gastric Ulcer
In both a U.S. and an international multicenter, double-blind study in patients with endoscopically confirmed active benign gastric ulcer, orally administered PEPCID, 40 mg h.s., was compared to placebo h.s. Antacids were permitted during the studies, but consumption was not significantly different between the PEPCID and placebo groups. As shown in Table 2, the incidence of ulcer healing (dropouts counted as unhealed) with PEPCID was statistically significantly better than placebo at weeks 6 and 8 in the U.S. study, and at weeks 4, 6 and 8 in the international study, based on the number of ulcers that healed, confirmed by endoscopy.

Table 2
Patients with Endoscopically
Confirmed Healed Gastric Ulcers

	U.S. Study		International Study	
	PEPCID 40 mg h.s. (N=74)	Placebo h.s. (N=75)	PEPCID 40 mg h.s. (N=149)	Placebo h.s. (N=145)
Week 4	45%	39%	†47%	31%
Week 6	†66%	44%	†65%	46%
Week 8	***78%	64%	†80%	54%

***,† Statistically significantly better than placebo ($p \leq 0.05$, $p \leq 0.01$ respectively)

Time to complete relief of daytime and nighttime pain was statistically significantly shorter for patients receiving PEPCID than for patients receiving placebo; however, in neither study was there a statistically significant difference in the proportion of patients whose pain was relieved by the end of the study (week 8).
Gastroesophageal Reflux Disease (GERD)
Orally administered PEPCID was compared to placebo in a U.S. study that enrolled patients with symptoms of GERD and without endoscopic evidence of erosion or ulceration of the esophagus. PEPCID 20 mg b.i.d. was statistically significantly superior to 40 mg h.s. and to placebo in providing a successful symptomatic outcome, defined as moderate or excellent improvement of symptoms (Table 3).

Table 3
% Successful Symptomatic Outcome

	PEPCID 20 mg b.i.d. (N=154)	PEPCID 40 mg h.s. (N=149)	Placebo (N=73)
Week 6	82††	69	62

†† $p \leq 0.01$) vs Placebo

By two weeks of treatment, symptomatic success was observed in a greater percentage of patients taking PEPCID 20 mg b.i.d. compared to placebo ($p \leq 0.01$).
Symptomatic improvement and healing of endoscopically verified erosion and ulceration were studied in two additional trials. Healing was defined as complete resolution of all erosions or ulcerations visible with endoscopy. The U.S. study comparing PEPCID 40 mg p.o. b.i.d. to placebo and PEPCID 20 mg p.o. b.i.d. showed a significantly greater percentage of healing for PEPCID 40 mg b.i.d. at weeks 6 and 12 (Table 4).

Table 4
% Endoscopic Healing—U.S. Study

	PEPCID 40 mg b.i.d. (N=127)	PEPCID 20 mg b.i.d. (N=125)	Placebo (N=66)
Week 6	48†††,‡‡	32	18
Week 12	69†††,‡	54†††	29

††† $p \leq 0.01$ vs Placebo
‡ $p \leq 0.05$ vs PEPCID 20 mg b.i.d.
‡‡ $p \leq 0.01$ vs PEPCID 20 mg b.i.d.

As compared to placebo, patients who received PEPCID had faster relief of daytime and nighttime heartburn and a greater percentage of patients experienced complete relief of nighttime heartburn. These differences were statistically significant.

In the international study, when PEPCID 40 mg p.o. b.i.d. was compared to ranitidine 150 mg p.o. b.i.d., a statistically significantly greater percentage of healing was observed with PEPCID 40 mg b.i.d. at week 12 (Table 5). There was, however, no significant difference among treatments in symptom relief.

Table 5

% Endoscopic Healing—International Study

	PEPCID 40 mg b.i.d. (N=175)	PEPCID 20 mg b.i.d. (N=93)	Ranitidine 150 mg b.i.d. (N=172)
Week 6	48	52	42
Week 12	71‡‡‡	68	60

‡‡‡ $p \leq 0.05$ vs Ranitidine 150 mg b.i.d.

Pathological Hypersecretory Conditions (e.g., Zollinger-Ellison Syndrome, Multiple Endocrine Adenomas)

In studies of patients with pathological hypersecretory conditions such as Zollinger-Ellison Syndrome with or without multiple endocrine adenomas, PEPCID significantly inhibited gastric acid secretion and controlled associated symptoms. Orally administered doses from 20 to 160 mg q 6 h maintained basal acid secretion below 10 mEq/hr; initial doses were titrated to the individual patient need and subsequent adjustments were necessary with time in some patients. PEPCID was well tolerated at these high dose levels for prolonged periods (greater than 12 months) in eight patients, and there were no cases reported of gynecomastia, increased prolactin levels, or impotence which were considered to be due to the drug.

CLINICAL PHARMACOLOGY IN PEDIATRIC PATIENTS

Pharmacokinetics

Table 6 presents pharmacokinetic data from published studies of small numbers of pediatric patients given famotidine intravenously. Areas under the curve (AUCs) are normalized to a dose of 0.5 mg/kg I.V. for pediatric patients and compared with an extrapolated 40 mg intravenous dose in adults (extrapolation based on results obtained with a 20 mg I.V. adult dose).

[See table 6 above]

Values of pharmacokinetic parameters for pediatric patients, ages 1–15 years, are comparable to those obtained for adults.

Bioavailability studies of 8 pediatric patients (11–15 years of age) showed a mean oral bioavailability of 0.5 compared to adult values of 0.42 to 0.49. Oral doses of 0.5 mg/kg achieved an AUC of 580 ± 60 ng-hr/mL in pediatric patients 11–15 years of age compared to 482 ± 181 ng-hr/mL in adults treated with 40 mg orally.

Pharmacodynamics

Pharmacodynamics of famotidine were evaluated in 5 pediatric patients 2–13 years of age using the sigmoid E_{max} model. These data suggest that the relationship between serum concentration of famotidine and gastric acid suppression is similar to that observed in one study of adults (Table 7).

[See table 7 above]

Four published studies (Table 8) examined the effect of famotidine on gastric pH and duration of acid suppression in pediatric patients. While each study had a different design, acid suppression data over time are summarized as follows:

[See table 8 above]

INDICATIONS AND USAGE

PEPCID is indicated in:

1. *Short term treatment of active duodenal ulcer.* Most adult patients heal within 4 weeks; there is rarely reason to use PEPCID at full dosage for longer than 6 to 8 weeks. Studies have not assessed the safety of famotidine in uncomplicated active duodenal ulcer for periods of more than eight weeks.
2. *Maintenance therapy for duodenal ulcer patients at reduced dosage after healing of an active ulcer.* Controlled studies in adults have not extended beyond one year.
3. *Short term treatment of active benign gastric ulcer.* Most adult patients heal within 6 weeks. Studies have not assessed the safety or efficacy of famotidine in uncomplicated active benign gastric ulcer for periods of more than 8 weeks.
4. *Short term treatment of gastroesophageal reflux disease (GERD).* PEPCID is indicated for short term treatment of patients with symptoms of GERD (see CLINICAL PHARMACOLOGY IN ADULTS, *Clinical Studies*).
   PEPCID is also indicated for the short term treatment of esophagitis due to GERD including erosive or ulcerative disease diagnosed by endoscopy (see CLINICAL PHARMACOLOGY IN ADULTS, *Clinical Studies*).
5. *Treatment of pathological hypersecretory conditions (e.g., Zollinger-Ellison Syndrome, multiple endocrine adenomas)* (see CLINICAL PHARMACOLOGY IN ADULTS, *Clinical Studies*).

Table 6

Pharmacokinetic Parameters[a] of Intravenous Famotidine

Age (N=number of patients)	Area Under the Curve (AUC) (ng-hr/mL)	Total Clearance (Cl) (L/hr/kg)	Volume of Distribution (V_d) (L/kg)	Elimination Half-life ($T_{1/2}$) (hours)
1–11 yrs (N=20)	1089 ± 834	0.54 ± 0.34	2.07 ± 1.49	3.38 ± 2.60
11–15 yrs (N=6)	1140 ± 320	0.48 ± 0.14	1.5 ± 0.4	2.3 ± 0.4
Adults (N=16)	1726[b]	0.39 ± 0.14	1.3 ± 0.2	2.83 ± 0.99

[a]Values are presented as means ± SD unless indicated otherwise.
[b]Mean value only.

Table 7

Pharmacodynamics of famotidine using the sigmoid E_{max} model

Pediatric Patients	EC_{50} (ng/mL)*
	26 ± 13
Data from one study	
a) healthy adult subjects	26.5 ± 10.3
b) adult patients with upper GI bleeding	18.7 ± 10.8

*Serum concentration of famotidine associated with 50% maximum gastric acid reduction. Values are presented as means ± SD.

Table 8

Dosage	Route	Effect[a]	Number of Patients
0.3 mg/kg, single dose	I.V.	gastric pH >3.5 for 8.7 ± 4.7[b] hours	6
0.4–0.8 mg/kg	I.V.	gastric pH >4 for 6–9 hours	18
0.5 mg/kg, single dose	I.V.	a >2 pH unit increase above baseline gastric pH for >8 hours	9
0.5 mg/kg b.i.d.	I.V.	gastric pH >5 for 13.5 ± 1.8[b] hours	4
0.5 mg/kg b.i.d.	oral	gastric pH >5 for 5.0 ± 1.1[b] hours	4

[a]Values reported in published literature.
[b]Means ± SD.

CONTRAINDICATIONS

Hypersensitivity to any component of these products. Cross sensitivity in this class of compounds has been observed. Therefore, PEPCID should not be administered to patients with a history of hypersensitivity to other H_2-receptor antagonists.

PRECAUTIONS

General

Symptomatic response to therapy with PEPCID does not preclude the presence of gastric malignancy.

Patients with Severe Renal Insufficiency

Longer intervals between doses or lower doses may need to be used in patients with severe renal insufficiency (creatinine clearance <10 mL/min) to adjust for the longer elimination half-life of famotidine. (See CLINICAL PHARMACOLOGY IN ADULTS and DOSAGE AND ADMINISTRATION.) However, currently, no drug-related toxicity has been found with high plasma concentrations of famotidine.

Information for Patients

The patient should be instructed to shake the oral suspension vigorously for 5–10 seconds prior to each use. Unused constituted oral suspension should be discarded after 30 days.

Patients should be instructed to leave the PEPCID RPD Orally Disintegrating Tablet in the unopened package until the time of use. Patients should then open the tablet blister pack with dry hands, place the tablet on the tongue to dissolve and be swallowed with saliva. No water is needed for taking the tablet.

Phenylketonurics: Phenylketonuric patients should be informed that PEPCID RPD contains phenylalanine 1.05 mg per 20 mg orally disintegrating tablet and 2.10 mg per 40 mg orally disintegrating tablet.

Drug Interactions

No drug interactions have been identified. Studies with famotidine in man, in animal models, and *in vitro* have shown no significant interference with the disposition of compounds metabolized by the hepatic microsomal enzymes, e.g., cytochrome P450 system. Compounds tested in man include warfarin, theophylline, phenytoin, diazepam, aminopyrine and antipyrine. Indocyanine green as an index of hepatic drug extraction has been tested and no significant effects have been found.

Carcinogenesis, Mutagenesis, Impairment of Fertility

In a 106 week study in rats and a 92 week study in mice given oral doses of up to 2000 mg/kg/day (approximately 2500 times the recommended human dose for active duodenal ulcer), there was no evidence of carcinogenic potential for PEPCID.

Famotidine was negative in the microbial mutagen test (Ames test) using *Salmonella typhimurium* and *Escherichia coli* with or without rat liver enzyme activation at concentrations up to 10,000 mcg/plate. In *in vivo* studies in mice, with a micronucleus test and a chromosomal aberration test, no evidence of a mutagenic effect was observed.

In studies with rats given oral doses of up to 2000 mg/kg/day or intravenous doses of up to 200 mg/kg/day, fertility and reproductive performance were not affected.

Pregnancy

Pregnancy Category B

Reproductive studies have been performed in rats and rabbits at oral doses of up to 2000 and 500 mg/kg/day respectively and in both species at I.V. doses of up to 200 mg/kg/day, and have revealed no significant evidence of impaired fertility or harm to the fetus due to PEPCID. While no direct fetotoxic effects have been observed, sporadic abortions occurring only in mothers displaying marked decreased food intake were seen in some rabbits at oral doses of 200 mg/kg/day (250 times the usual human dose) or higher. There are, however, no adequate or well-controlled studies in pregnant women. Because animal reproductive studies are not always predictive of human response, this drug should be used during pregnancy only if clearly needed.

Nursing Mothers

Studies performed in lactating rats have shown that famotidine is secreted into breast milk. Transient growth depression was observed in young rats suckling from mothers treated with maternotoxic doses of at least 600 times the usual human dose. Famotidine is detectable in human milk. Because of the potential for serious adverse reactions in nursing infants from PEPCID, a decision should be made whether to discontinue nursing or discontinue the drug, taking into account the importance of the drug to the mother.

Pediatric Patients

Use of PEPCID in pediatric patients 1–16 years of age is supported by evidence from adequate and well-controlled studies of PEPCID in adults, and by the following studies in pediatric patients: In published studies in small numbers of pediatric patients 1–15 years of age, clearance of famotidine was similar to that seen in adults. In pediatric patients 11–15 years of age, oral doses of 0.5 mg/kg were associated with a mean area under the curve (AUC) similar to that seen in adults treated orally with 40 mg. Similarly, in pediatric patients 1–15 years of age, intravenous doses of 0.5 mg/kg were associated with a mean AUC similar to that seen in adults treated intravenously with 40 mg. Limited published studies also suggest that the relationship between serum concentration and acid suppression is similar in pediatric patients 1–15 years of age as compared with adults. These studies suggest a starting dose for pediatric patients 1–16 years of age as follows:

Peptic ulcer—0.5 mg/kg/day p.o. at bedtime or divided b.i.d. up to 40 mg/day.

Gastroesophageal Reflux Disease with or without esophagitis including erosions and ulcerations—1.0 mg/kg/day p.o. divided b.i.d. up to 40 mg b.i.d.

While published uncontrolled studies suggest effectiveness of famotidine in the treatment of gastroesophageal reflux disease and peptic ulcer, data in pediatric patients are in-

Continued on next page

Information on the Merck & Co., Inc. products listed on these pages is the full prescribing information from product circulars in use September 30, 2000. For information, please call 1-800-NSC MERCK [1-800-672-6372].

Pepcid—Cont.

sufficient to establish percent response with dose and duration of therapy. Therefore, treatment duration (initially based on adult duration recommendations) and dose should be individualized based on clinical response and/or pH determination (gastric or esophageal) and endoscopy. Published uncontrolled clinical studies in pediatric patients have employed doses up to 1 mg/kg/day for peptic ulcer and 2 mg/kg/day for GERD with or without esophagitis including erosions and ulcerations.
No pharmacokinetic or pharmacodynamic data are available on pediatric patients under 1 year of age.
Use in Elderly Patients
No dosage adjustment is required based on age (see CLINICAL PHARMACOLOGY IN ADULTS, *Pharmacokinetics*). Dosage adjustment in the case of severe renal impairment may be necessary.

ADVERSE REACTIONS

The adverse reactions listed below have been reported during domestic and international clinical trials in approximately 2500 patients. In those controlled clinical trials in which PEPCID Tablets were compared to placebo, the incidence of adverse experiences in the group which received PEPCID Tablets, 40 mg at bedtime, was similar to that in the placebo group.
The following adverse reactions have been reported to occur in more than 1% of patients on therapy with PEPCID in controlled clinical trials, and may be causally related to the drug: headache (4.7%), dizziness (1.3%), constipation (1.2%) and diarrhea (1.7%).
The following other adverse reactions have been reported infrequently in clinical trials or since the drug was marketed. The relationship to therapy with PEPCID has been unclear in many cases. Within each category the adverse reactions are listed in order of decreasing severity:
Body as a Whole: fever, asthenia, fatigue
Cardiovascular: arrhythmia, AV block, palpitation
Gastrointestinal: cholestatic jaundice, liver enzyme abnormalities, vomiting, nausea, abdominal discomfort, anorexia, dry mouth
Hematologic: rare cases of agranulocytosis, pancytopenia, leukopenia, thrombocytopenia
Hypersensitivity: anaphylaxis, angioedema, orbital or facial edema, urticaria, rash, conjunctival injection
Musculoskeletal: musculoskeletal pain including muscle cramps, arthralgia
Nervous System/Psychiatric: grand mal seizure; psychic disturbances, which were reversible in cases for which follow-up was obtained, including hallucinations, confusion, agitation, depression, anxiety, decreased libido; paresthesia; insomnia; somnolence
Respiratory: bronchospasm
Skin: toxic epidermal necrolysis (very rare), alopecia, acne, pruritus, dry skin, flushing
Special Senses: tinnitus, taste disorder
Other: rare cases of impotence and rare cases of gynecomastia have been reported; however, in controlled clinical trials, the incidences were not greater than those seen with placebo.
The adverse reactions reported for PEPCID Tablets may also occur with PEPCID for Oral Suspension and PEPCID RPD Orally Disintegrating Tablets.

OVERDOSAGE

There is no experience to date with deliberate overdosage. Oral doses of up to 640 mg/day have been given to adult patients with pathological hypersecretory conditions with no serious adverse effects. In the event of overdosage, treatment should be symptomatic and supportive. Unabsorbed material should be removed from the gastrointestinal tract, the patient should be monitored, and supportive therapy should be employed.
The oral LD_{50} of famotidine in male and female rats and mice was greater than 3000 mg/kg and the minimum lethal acute oral dose in dogs exceeded 2000 mg/kg. Famotidine did not produce overt effects at high oral doses in mice, rats, cats and dogs, but induced significant anorexia and growth depression in rabbits starting with 200 mg/kg/day orally. The intravenous LD_{50} of famotidine for mice and rats ranged from 254–563 mg/kg and the minimum lethal single I.V. dose in dogs was approximately 300 mg/kg. Signs of acute intoxication in I.V. treated dogs were emesis, restlessness, pallor of mucous membranes or redness of mouth and ears, hypotension, tachycardia and collapse.

DOSAGE AND ADMINISTRATION

Duodenal Ulcer
Acute Therapy: The recommended adult oral dosage for active duodenal ulcer is 40 mg once a day at bedtime. Most patients heal within 4 weeks; there is rarely reason to use PEPCID at full dosage for longer than 6 to 8 weeks. A regimen of 20 mg b.i.d. is also effective.
Maintenance Therapy: The recommended adult oral dose is 20 mg once a day at bedtime.
Benign Gastric Ulcer
Acute Therapy: The recommended adult oral dosage for active benign gastric ulcer is 40 mg once a day at bedtime.
Gastroesophageal Reflux Disease (GERD)
The recommended oral dosage for treatment of adult patients with symptoms of GERD is 20 mg b.i.d. for up to 6 weeks. The recommended oral dosage for the treatment of adult patients with esophagitis including erosions and ulcerations and accompanying symptoms due to GERD is 20 or 40 mg b.i.d. for up to 12 weeks (see CLINICAL PHARMACOLOGY IN ADULTS, *Clinical Studies*).
Dosage for Pediatric Patients
See PRECAUTIONS, *Pediatric Patients*.
The studies described in PRECAUTIONS, *Pediatric Patients* suggest the following starting doses in pediatric patients 1–16 years of age:
Peptic ulcer—0.5 mg/kg/day p.o. at bedtime or divided b.i.d. up to 40 mg/day.
Gastroesophageal Reflux Disease with or without esophagitis including erosions and ulcerations—1.0 mg/kg/day p.o. divided b.i.d. up to 40 mg b.i.d.
While published uncontrolled studies suggest effectiveness of famotidine in the treatment of gastroesophageal reflux disease and peptic ulcer, data in pediatric patients are insufficient to establish percent response with dose and duration of therapy. Therefore, treatment duration (initially based on adult duration recommendations) and dose should be individualized based on clinical response and/or pH determination (gastric or esophageal) and endoscopy. Published uncontrolled clinical studies in pediatric patients have employed doses up to 1 mg/kg/day for peptic ulcer and 2 mg/kg/day for GERD with or without esophagitis including erosions and ulcerations.
No pharmacokinetic or pharmacodynamic data are available on pediatric patients under 1 year of age.
Pathological Hypersecretory Conditions (e.g., Zollinger-Ellison Syndrome, Multiple Endocrine Adenomas)
The dosage of PEPCID in patients with pathological hypersecretory conditions varies with the individual patient. The recommended adult oral starting dose for pathological hypersecretory conditions is 20 mg q 6 h. In some patients, a higher starting dose may be required. Doses should be adjusted to individual patient needs and should continue as long as clinically indicated. Doses up to 160 mg q 6 h have been administered to some adult patients with severe Zollinger-Ellison Syndrome.
Oral Suspension
PEPCID Oral Suspension may be substituted for PEPCID Tablets in any of the above indications. Each five mL contains 40 mg of famotidine after constitution of the powder with 46 mL of Purified Water as directed.
Directions for Preparing PEPCID Oral Suspension
Prepare suspension at time of dispensing. Slowly add 46 mL of Purified Water. Shake vigorously for 5–10 seconds immediately after adding the water and immediately before use.
Stability of PEPCID for Oral Suspension
Unused constituted oral suspension should be discarded after 30 days.
Orally Disintegrating Tablets
PEPCID RPD Orally Disintegrating Tablets may be substituted for PEPCID Tablets in any of the above indications at the same recommended dosages.
PEPCID RPD Orally Disintegrating Tablets rapidly disintegrate on the tongue. No water is needed for taking the tablet. Patients should be instructed to open the tablet blister pack with dry hands, place the tablet on the tongue to disintegrate and be swallowed with saliva.
Concomitant Use of Antacids
Antacids may be given concomitantly if needed.
Dosage Adjustment for Patients with Severe Renal Insufficiency
In adult patients with severe renal insufficiency, i.e., with a creatinine clearance less than 10 mL/min, the elimination half-life of PEPCID may exceed 20 hours, reaching approximately 24 hours in anuric patients. Although no relationship of adverse effects to high plasma levels has been established, to avoid excess accumulation of the drug, the dose of PEPCID may be reduced to 20 mg h.s. or the dosing interval may be prolonged to 36–48 hours as indicated by the patient's clinical response.
Based on the comparison of pharmacokinetic parameters for PEPCID in adults and pediatric patients, dosage adjustment in pediatric patients with severe renal insufficiency should be considered.

HOW SUPPLIED

No. 3535—PEPCID Tablets, 20 mg, are beige colored, U-shaped, film-coated tablets coded MSD 963 on one side and PEPCID on the other. They are supplied as follows:
NDC 0006-0963-31 unit of use bottles of 30
(6505-01-260-0902, 20 mg 30's)
NDC 0006-0963-94 unit of use bottles of 90
NDC 0006-0963-58 unit of use bottles of 100
NDC 0006-0963-28 unit dose package of 100
NDC 0006-0963-82 bottles of 1,000
NDC 0006-0963-87 bottles of 10,000
NDC 0006-0963-72 carton of 25
UNIBLISTER™ cards of 31 tablets each.
Shown in Product Identification Guide, page 324
No. 3536—PEPCID Tablets, 40 mg, are light brownish-orange, U-shaped, film-coated tablets coded MSD 964 on one side and PEPCID on the other. They are supplied as follows:
NDC 0006-0964-31 unit of use bottles of 30
(6505-01-257-3164, 40 mg 30's)
NDC 0006-0964-94 unit of use bottles of 90
NDC 0006-0964-58 unit of use bottles of 100
NDC 0006-0964-28 unit dose package of 100
(6505-01-318-0464, 40 mg individually sealed 100's)
NDC 0006-0964-82 bottles of 1,000
NDC 0006-0964-87 bottles of 10,000
NDC 0006-0964-72 carton of 25
UNIBLISTER™ cards of 31 tablets each.
Shown in Product Identification Guide, page 324
No. 3553—PEPCID RPD Orally Disintegrating Tablets, 20 mg, are pale rose colored, hexagonal-shaped, lyophilized tablets measuring 13.1 mm (side to side) and 15.2 mm (point to point), with a mint flavor. They are supplied as follows:
NDC 0006-3553-31 unit dose package of 30
NDC 0006-3553-48 unit dose package of 100
NDC 0006-3553-28 unit dose package of 100.
Shown in Product Identification Guide, page 324
No. 3554—PEPCID RPD Orally Disintegrating Tablets, 40 mg, are pale rose colored, hexagonal-shaped, lyophilized tablets measuring 15.9 mm (side to side) and 18.4 mm (point to point), with a mint flavor. They are supplied as follows:
NDC 0006-3554-31 unit dose package of 30
NDC 0006-3554-48 unit dose package of 100.
Shown in Product Identification Guide, page 324
No. 3538—Oral Suspension PEPCID is a white to off-white powder containing 400 mg of famotidine for constitution. When constituted as directed, PEPCID Oral Suspension is a smooth, mobile, off-white, homogeneous suspension with a cherry-banana-mint flavor, containing 40 mg of famotidine per 5 mL.
NDC 0006-3538-92, bottles containing 400 mg famotidine.
Storage
Avoid storage of PEPCID Tablets at temperatures above 40°C (104°F).
Store PEPCID RPD Orally Disintegrating Tablets below 30°C (86°F).
Avoid storage of the powder for oral suspension at temperatures above 40°C (104°F). After constitution store the suspension below 30°C (86°F). Do not freeze. Discard unused suspension after 30 days.
7825032 Issued November 1998

PEPCID® Injection Premixed (Famotidine) ℞
PEPCID® Injection (Famotidine) ℞

DESCRIPTION

The active ingredient in PEPCID* (Famotidine) Injection Premixed and PEPCID (famotidine) Injection is a histamine H_2-receptor antagonist. Famotidine is *N*′-(aminosulfonyl)-3-[[[2-[(diaminomethylene)amino]-4-thiazolyl]methyl]thio]-propanimidamide. The empirical formula of famotidine is $C_8H_{15}N_7O_2S_3$ and its molecular weight is 337.43. Its structural formula is:

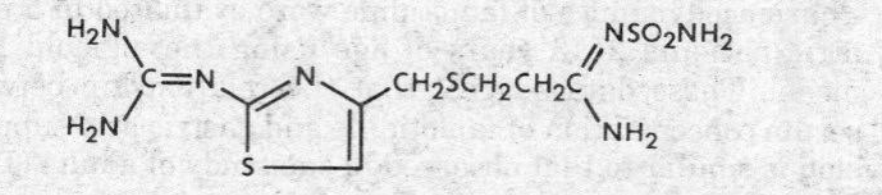

Famotidine is a white to pale yellow crystalline compound that is freely soluble in glacial acetic acid, slightly soluble in methanol, very slightly soluble in water, and practically insoluble in ethanol.
PEPCID Injection Premixed is supplied as a sterile solution, for intravenous use only, in plastic single dose containers. Each 50 mL of the premixed, iso-osmotic intravenous injection contains 20 mg famotidine, USP, and the following inactive ingredients: L-aspartic acid 6.8 mg, sodium chloride, USP, 450 mg, and Water for Injection. The pH ranges from 5.7 to 6.4 and may have been adjusted with additional L-aspartic acid or with sodium hydroxide.
The plastic container is fabricated from a specially designed multi-layer plastic (PL 2501). Solutions are in contact with the polyethylene layer of the container and can leach out certain chemical components of the plastic in very small amounts within the expiration period. The suitability and safety of the plastic have been confirmed in tests in animals according to the USP biological tests for plastic containers, as well as by tissue culture toxicity studies.
PEPCID (famotidine) Injection is supplied as a sterile concentrated solution for intravenous injection. Each mL of the solution contains 10 mg of famotidine and the following inactive ingredients: L-aspartic acid 4 mg, mannitol 20 mg, and Water for Injection q.s. 1 mL. The multidose injection also contains benzyl alcohol 0.9% added as preservative.

*Registered trademark of MERCK & CO., INC.

CLINICAL PHARMACOLOGY IN ADULTS

GI Effects
PEPCID is a competitive inhibitor of histamine H_2-receptors. The primary clinically important pharmacologic activity of PEPCID is inhibition of gastric secretion. Both the acid concentration and volume of gastric secretion are suppressed by PEPCID, while changes in pepsin secretion are proportional to volume output.

In normal volunteers and hypersecretors, PEPCID inhibited basal and nocturnal gastric secretion, as well as secretion stimulated by food and pentagastrin. After oral administration, the onset of the antisecretory effect occurred within one hour; the maximum effect was dose-dependent, occurring within one to three hours. Duration of inhibition of secretion by doses of 20 and 40 mg was 10 to 12 hours. After intravenous administration, the maximum effect was achieved within 30 minutes. Single intravenous doses of 10 and 20 mg inhibited nocturnal secretion for a period of 10 to 12 hours. The 20 mg dose was associated with the longest duration of action in most subjects.
Single evening oral doses of 20 and 40 mg inhibited basal and nocturnal acid secretion in all subjects; mean nocturnal gastric acid secretion was inhibited by 86% and 94%, respectively, for a period of at least 10 hours. The same doses given in the morning suppressed food-stimulated acid secretion in all subjects. The mean suppression was 76% and 84% respectively, 3 to 5 hours after administration, and 25% and 30%, respectively, 8 to 10 hours after administration. In some subjects who received the 20 mg dose, however, the antisecretory effect was dissipated within 6–8 hours. There was no cumulative effect with repeated doses. The nocturnal intragastric pH was raised by evening doses of 20 and 40 mg of PEPCID to mean values of 5.0 and 6.4, respectively. When PEPCID was given after breakfast, the basal daytime interdigestive pH at 3 and 8 hours after 20 or 40 mg of PEPCID was raised to about 5.
PEPCID had little or no effect on fasting or postprandial serum gastrin levels. Gastric emptying and exocrine pancreatic function were not affected by PEPCID.

Other Effects
Systemic effects of PEPCID in the CNS, cardiovascular, respiratory or endocrine systems were not noted in clinical pharmacology studies. Also, no antiandrogenic effects were noted. (See ADVERSE REACTIONS.) Serum hormone levels, including prolactin, cortisol, thyroxine (T_4), and testosterone, were not altered after treatment with PEPCID.

Pharmacokinetics
Orally administered PEPCID is incompletely absorbed and its bioavailability is 40–45%. PEPCID undergoes minimal first-pass metabolism. After oral doses, peak plasma levels occur in 1–3 hours. Plasma levels after multiple doses are similar to those after single doses. Fifteen to 20% of PEPCID in plasma is protein bound. PEPCID has an elimination half-life of 2.5–3.5 hours. PEPCID is eliminated by renal (65–70%) and metabolic (30–35%) routes. Renal clearance is 250–450 mL/min, indicating some tubular excretion. Twenty-five to 30% of an oral dose and 65–70% of an intravenous dose are recovered in the urine as unchanged compound. The only metabolite identified in man is the S-oxide. There is a close relationship between creatinine clearance values and the elimination half-life of PEPCID. In patients with severe renal insufficiency, i.e., creatinine clearance less than 10 mL/min, the elimination half-life of PEPCID may exceed 20 hours and adjustment of dose or dosing intervals may be necessary (see PRECAUTIONS, DOSAGE AND ADMINISTRATION).
In elderly patients, there are no clinically significant age-related changes in the pharmacokinetics of PEPCID.

Clinical Studies
The majority of clinical study experience involved oral administration of PEPCID Tablets, and is provided herein for reference.

Duodenal Ulcer
In a U.S. multicenter, double-blind study in outpatients with endoscopically confirmed duodenal ulcer, orally administered PEPCID was compared to placebo. As shown in Table 1, 70% of patients treated with PEPCID 40 mg h.s. were healed by week 4.

Table 1
Outpatients with Endoscopically Confirmed Healed Duodenal Ulcers

	PEPCID 40 mg h.s. (N=89)	PEPCID 20 mg b.i.d. (N=84)	Placebo h.s. (N=97)
Week 2	**32%	**38%	17%
Week 4	**70%	**67%	31%

** Statistically significantly different than placebo ($p < 0.001$)

Patients not healed by week 4 were continued in the study. By week 8, 83% of patients treated with PEPCID had healed versus 45% of patients treated with placebo. The incidence of ulcer healing with PEPCID was significantly higher than with placebo at each time point based on proportion of endoscopically confirmed healed ulcers.
In this study, time to relief of daytime and nocturnal pain was significantly shorter for patients receiving PEPCID than for patients receiving placebo; patients receiving PEPCID also took less antacid than the patients receiving placebo.

Long-Term Maintenance
Treatment of Duodenal Ulcers
PEPCID, 20 mg p.o. h.s. was compared to placebo h.s. as maintenance therapy in two double-blind, multicenter studies of patients with endoscopically confirmed healed duodenal ulcers. In the U.S. study the observed ulcer incidence within 12 months in patients treated with placebo was 2.4 times greater than in the patients treated with PEPCID. The 89 patients treated with PEPCID had a cumulative observed ulcer incidence of 23.4% compared to an observed ulcer incidence of 56.6% in the 89 patients receiving placebo ($p<0.01$). These results were confirmed in an international study where the cumulative observed ulcer incidence within 12 months in the 307 patients treated with PEPCID was 35.7%, compared to an incidence of 75.5% in the 325 patients treated with placebo ($p<0.01$).

Table 6
Pharmacokinetic Parameters[a] of Intravenous Famotidine

Age (N=number of patients)	Age Under the Curve (AUC) (ng-hr/mL)	Total Clearance (Cl) (L/hr/kg)	Volume of Distribution (Vd) (L/kg)	Elimination Half-Life (T½) (hours)
1–11 years (N=20)	1089 ± 834	0.54 ± 0.34	2.07 ± 1.49	3.38 ± 2.60
11–15 years (N=6)	1140 ± 320	0.48 ± 0.14	1.5 ± 0.4	2.3 ± 0.4
Adult (N=16)	1726[b]	0.39 ± 0.14	1.3 ± 0.2	2.83 ± 0.99

[a]Values are presented as means ± SD unless indicated otherwise.
[b]Mean value only.

Gastric Ulcer
In both a U.S. and an international multicenter, double-blind study in patients with endoscopically confirmed active benign gastric ulcer, orally administered PEPCID, 40 mg h.s., was compared to placebo h.s. Antacids were permitted during the studies, but consumption was not significantly different between the PEPCID and placebo groups. As shown in Table 2, the incidence of ulcer healing (dropouts counted as unhealed) with PEPCID was statistically significantly better than placebo at weeks 6 and 8 in the U.S. study, and at weeks 4, 6 and 8 in the international study, based on the number of ulcers that healed, confirmed by endoscopy.

Table 2
Patients with Endoscopically Confirmed Healed Gastric Ulcers

	U.S. Study		International Study	
	PEPCID 40 mg h.s. (N=74)	Placebo h.s. (N=75)	PEPCID 40 mg h.s. (N=149)	Placebo h.s. (N=145)
Week 4	45%	39%	†47%	31%
Week 6	†66%	44%	†65%	46%
Week 8	***78%	64%	†80%	54%

***,† Statistically significantly better than placebo ($p \leq 0.05$, $p \leq 0.01$ respectively)

Time to complete relief of daytime and nighttime pain was statistically significantly shorter for patients receiving PEPCID than for patients receiving placebo; however, in neither study was there a statistically significant difference in the proportion of patients whose pain was relieved by the end of the study (week 8).

Gastroesophageal Reflux Disease (GERD)
Orally administered PEPCID was compared to placebo in a U.S. study that enrolled patients with symptoms of GERD and without endoscopic evidence of erosion or ulceration of the esophagus. PEPCID 20 mg b.i.d. was statistically significantly superior to 40 mg h.s. and to placebo in providing a successful symptomatic outcome, defined as moderate or excellent improvement of symptoms (Table 3).

Table 3
% Successful Symptomatic Outcome

	PEPCID 20 mg b.i.d. (N=154)	PEPCID 40 mg h.s. (N=49)	Placebo (N=73)
Week 6	82††	69	62

†† $p \leq 0.01$ vs Placebo

By two weeks of treatment, symptomatic success was observed in a greater percentage of patients taking PEPCID 20 mg b.i.d. compared to placebo ($p \leq 0.01$).
Symptomatic improvement and healing of endoscopically verified erosion and ulceration were studied in two additional trials. Healing was defined as complete resolution of all erosions or ulcerations visible with endoscopy. The U.S. study comparing PEPCID 40 mg p.o. b.i.d. to placebo and PEPCID 20 mg p.o. b.i.d., showed a significantly greater percentage of healing for PEPCID 40 mg b.i.d. at weeks 6 and 12 (Table 4).

Table 4
% Endoscopic Healing—U.S. Study

	PEPCID 40 mg b.i.d. (N=127)	PEPCID 20 mg b.i.d. (N=125)	Placebo (N=66)
Week 6	48†††,‡‡	32	18
Week 12	69†††,‡	54†††	29

††† $p \leq 0.01$ vs Placebo
‡ $p \leq 0.05$ vs PEPCID 20 mg b.i.d.
‡‡ $p \leq 0.01$ vs PEPCID 20 mg b.i.d.

As compared to placebo, patients who received PEPCID had faster relief of daytime and nighttime heartburn and a greater percentage of patients experienced complete relief of nighttime heartburn. These differences were statistically significant.

In the international study, when PEPCID 40 mg p.o. b.i.d. was compared to ranitidine 150 mg p.o. b.i.d., a statistically significantly greater percentage of healing was observed with PEPCID 40 mg b.i.d. at week 12 (Table 5). There was, however, no significant difference among treatments in symptom relief.

Table 5
% Endoscopic Healing—International Study

	PEPCID 40 mg b.i.d. (N=175)	PEPCID 20 mg b.i.d. (N=93)	Ranitidine 150 mg b.i.d. (N=172)
Week 6	48	52	42
Week 12	71‡‡‡	68	60

‡‡‡ $p \leq 0.05$ vs Ranitidine 150 mg b.i.d.

Pathological Hypersecretory Conditions (e.g., Zollinger-Ellison Syndrome, Multiple Endocrine Adenomas)
In studies of patients with pathological hypersecretory conditions such as Zollinger-Ellison Syndrome with or without multiple endocrine adenomas, PEPCID significantly inhibited gastric acid secretion and controlled associated symptoms. Orally administered doses from 20 to 160 mg q 6 h maintained basal acid secretion below 10 mEq/hr; initial doses were titrated to the individual patient need and subsequent adjustments were necessary with time in some patients. PEPCID was well tolerated at these high dose levels for prolonged periods (greater than 12 months) in eight patients, and there were no cases reported of gynecomastia, increased prolactin levels, or impotence which were considered to be due to the drug.

CLINICAL PHARMACOLOGY IN PEDIATRIC PATIENTS

Pharmacokinetics
Table 6 presents pharmacokinetic data from published studies of small numbers of pediatric patients given famotidine intravenously. Areas under the curve (AUCs) are normalized to a dose of 0.5 mg/kg I.V. for pediatric patients and compared with an extrapolated 40 mg intravenous dose in adults (extrapolation based on results obtained with a 20 mg I.V. adult dose).
[See table 6 above]
Values of pharmacokinetic parameters for pediatric patients, ages 1–15 years, are comparable to those obtained for adults.
Bioavailability studies of 8 pediatric patients (11–15 years of age) showed a mean oral bioavailability of 0.5 compared to adult values of 0.42 to 0.49. Oral doses of 0.5 mg/kg achieved an AUC of 580 ± 60 ng-hr/mL in pediatric patients 11–15 years of age compared to 482 ± 181 ng-hr/mL in adults treated with 40 mg orally.

Pharmacodynamics
Pharmacodynamics of famotidine were evaluated in 5 pediatric patients 2–13 years of age using the sigmoid E_{max} model. These data suggest that the relationship between serum concentration of famotidine and gastric acid suppression is similar to that observed in one study of adults (Table 7).

Table 7
Pharmacodynamics of famotidine using the sigmoid E_{max} model

	EC_{50} (ng/mL)*
Pediatric Patients	26 ± 13
Data from one study	
a) healthy adult subjects	26.5 ± 10.3
b) adult patients with upper GI bleeding	18.7 ± 10.8

* Serum concentration of famotidine associated with 50% maximum gastric acid reduction. Values are presented as means ± SD.

Four published studies (Table 8) examined the effect of famotidine on gastric pH and duration of acid suppression in pediatric patients. While each study had a different design, acid suppression data over time are summarized as follows:
[See table 8 at bottom of next page]

Continued on next page

Information on the Merck & Co., Inc. products listed on these pages is the full prescribing information from product circulars in use September 30, 2000. For information, please call 1-800-NSC MERCK [1-800-672-6372].

Pepcid Injection—Cont.

INDICATIONS AND USAGE

PEPCID Injection Premixed, supplied as a premixed solution in plastic containers (PL 2501 Plastic), and PEPCID Injection, supplied as a concentrated solution for intravenous injection, are intended for intravenous use only. PEPCID Injection Premixed and PEPCID Injection are indicated in some hospitalized patients with pathological hypersecretory conditions or intractable ulcers, or as an alternative to the oral dosage forms for short term use in patients who are unable to take oral medication for the following conditions:
1. *Short term treatment of active duodenal ulcer.* Most adult patients heal within 4 weeks; there is rarely reason to use PEPCID at full dosage for longer than 6 to 8 weeks. Studies have not assessed the safety of famotidine in uncomplicated active duodenal ulcer for periods of more than eight weeks.
2. *Maintenance therapy for duodenal ulcer patients at reduced dosage after healing of an active ulcer.* Controlled studies in adults have not extended beyond one year.
3. *Short term treatment of active benign gastric ulcer.* Most adult patients heal within 6 weeks. Studies have not assessed the safety or efficacy of famotidine in uncomplicated active benign gastric ulcer for periods of more than 8 weeks.
4. *Short term treatment of gastroesophageal reflux disease (GERD).* PEPCID is indicated for short term treatment of patients with symptoms of GERD (see CLINICAL PHARMACOLOGY IN ADULTS, *Clinical Studies*).
PEPCID is also indicated for the short term treatment of esophagitis due to GERD including erosive or ulcerative disease diagnosed by endoscopy (see CLINICAL PHARMACOLOGY IN ADULTS, *Clinical Studies*).
5. *Treatment of pathological hypersecretory conditions (e.g., Zollinger-Ellison Syndrome, multiple endocrine adenomas)* (see CLINICAL PHARMACOLOGY IN ADULTS, *Clinical Studies*).

CONTRAINDICATIONS

Hypersensitivity to any component of these products. Cross sensitivity in this class of compounds has been observed. Therefore, PEPCID should not be administered to patients with a history of hypersensitivity to other H_2-receptor antagonists.

PRECAUTIONS

General
Symptomatic response to therapy with PEPCID does not preclude the presence of gastric malignancy.
Patients with Severe Renal Insufficiency
Longer intervals between doses or lower doses may need to be used in patients with severe renal insufficiency (creatinine clearance <10 mL/min) to adjust for the longer elimination half-life of famotidine. (See CLINICAL PHARMACOLOGY IN ADULTS, DOSAGE AND ADMINISTRATION.) However, currently, no drug-related toxicity has been found with high plasma concentrations of famotidine.
Drug Interactions
No drug interactions have been identified. Studies with famotidine in man, in animal models, and *in vitro* have shown no significant interference with the disposition of compounds metabolized by the hepatic microsomal enzymes, e.g., cytochrome P450 system. Compounds tested in man include warfarin, theophylline, phenytoin, diazepam, aminopyrine and antipyrine. Indocyanine green as an index of hepatic drug extraction has been tested and no significant effects have been found.
Carcinogenesis, Mutagenesis, Impairment of Fertility
In a 106 week study in rats and a 92 week study in mice given oral doses of up to 2000 mg/kg/day (approximately 2500 times the recommended human dose for active duodenal ulcer), there was no evidence of carcinogenic potential for PEPCID.
Famotidine was negative in the microbial mutagen test (Ames test) using *Salmonella typhimurium* and *Escherichia coli* with or without rat liver enzyme activation at concentrations up to 10,000 mcg/plate. In *in vivo* studies in mice, with a micronucleus test and a chromosomal aberration test, no evidence of a mutagenic effect was observed.
In studies with rats given oral doses of up to 2000 mg/kg/day or intravenous doses of up to 200 mg/kg/day fertility and reproductive performance were not affected.
Pregnancy
Pregnancy Category B
Reproductive studies have been performed in rats and rabbits at oral doses of up to 2000 and 500 mg/kg/day, respectively, and in both species at I.V. doses of up to 200 mg/kg/day, and have revealed no significant evidence of impaired fertility or harm to the fetus due to PEPCID. While no direct fetotoxic effects have been observed, sporadic abortions occurring only in mothers displaying marked decreased food intake were seen in some rabbits at oral doses of 200 mg/kg/day (250 times the usual human dose) or higher. There are, however, no adequate or well-controlled studies in pregnant women. Because animal reproductive studies are not always predictive of human response, this drug should be used during pregnancy only if clearly needed.
Nursing Mothers
Studies performed in lactating rats have shown that famotidine is secreted into breast milk. Transient growth depression was observed in young rats suckling from mothers treated with maternotoxic doses of at least 600 times the usual human dose. Famotidine is detectable in human milk. Because of the potential for serious adverse reactions in nursing infants from PEPCID, a decision should be made whether to discontinue nursing or discontinue the drug, taking into account the importance of the drug to the mother.
Pediatric Patients
Use of PEPCID in pediatric patients 1–16 years of age is supported by evidence from adequate and well-controlled studies of PEPCID in adults, and by the following studies in pediatric patients: In published studies in small numbers of pediatric patients 1–15 years of age, clearance of famotidine was similar to that seen in adults. In pediatric patients 11–15 years of age, oral doses of 0.5 mg/kg were associated with a mean area under the curve (AUC) similar to that seen in adults treated orally with 40 mg. Similarly, in pediatric patients 1–15 years of age, intravenous doses of 0.5 mg/kg were associated with a mean AUC similar to that seen in adults treated intravenously with 40 mg. Limited published studies also suggest that the relationship between serum concentration and acid suppression is similar in pediatric patients 1–15 years of age as compared with adults. These studies suggest that the starting dose for pediatric patients 1–16 years of age is 0.25 mg/kg intravenously (injected over a period of not less than two minutes or as a 15 minute infusion) q 12 h up to 40 mg/day.
While published uncontrolled clinical studies suggest effectiveness of famotidine in the treatment of peptic ulcer, data in pediatric patients are insufficient to establish percent response with dose and duration of therapy. Therefore, treatment duration (initially based on adult duration recommendations) and dose should be individualized based on clinical response and/or gastric pH determination and endoscopy. Published uncontrolled studies in pediatric patients have demonstrated gastric acid suppression with doses up to 0.5 mg/kg intravenously q 12 h.
No pharmacokinetic or pharmacodynamic data are available on pediatric patients under 1 year of age.
Use in Elderly Patients
No dosage adjustment is required based on age (see CLINICAL PHARMACOLOGY IN ADULTS, *Pharmacokinetics*). Dosage adjustment in the case of severe renal impairment may be necessary.

ADVERSE REACTIONS

The adverse reactions listed below have been reported during domestic and international clinical trials in approximately 2500 patients. In those controlled clinical trials in which PEPCID Tablets were compared to placebo, the incidence of adverse experiences in the group which received PEPCID Tablets, 40 mg at bedtime, was similar to that in the placebo group.
The following adverse reactions have been reported to occur in more than 1% of patients on therapy with PEPCID in controlled clinical trials, and may be causally related to the drug: headache (4.7%), dizziness (1.3%), constipation (1.2%) and diarrhea (1.7%).
The following other adverse reactions have been reported infrequently in clinical trials or since the drug was marketed. The relationship to therapy with PEPCID has been unclear in many cases. Within each category the adverse reactions are listed in order of decreasing severity:
Body as a Whole: fever, asthenia, fatigue
Cardiovascular: arrhythmia, AV block, palpitation
Gastrointestinal: cholestatic jaundice, liver enzyme abnormalities, vomiting, nausea, abdominal discomfort, anorexia, dry mouth
Hematologic: rare cases of agranulocytosis, pancytopenia, leukopenia, thrombocytopenia
Hypersensitivity: anaphylaxis, angioedema, orbital or facial edema, urticaria, rash, conjunctival injection
Musculoskeletal: musculoskeletal pain including muscle cramps, arthralgia
Nervous System/Psychiatric: grand mal seizure; psychic disturbances, which were reversible in cases for which follow-up was obtained, including hallucinations, confusion, agitation, depression, anxiety, decreased libido; paresthesia; insomnia; somnolence
Respiratory: bronchospasm
Skin: toxic epidermal necrolysis (very rare), alopecia, acne, pruritus, dry skin, flushing
Special Senses: tinnitus, taste disorder
Other: rare cases of impotence and rare cases of gynecomastia have been reported; however, in controlled clinical trials, the incidences were not greater than those seen with placebo.
The adverse reactions reported for PEPCID Tablets may also occur with PEPCID for Oral Suspension, PEPCID RPD Orally Disintegrating Tablets, PEPCID Injection Premixed or PEPCID Injection. In addition, transient irritation at the injection site has been observed with PEPCID Injection.

OVERDOSAGE

There is no experience to date with deliberate overdosage. Oral doses of up to 640 mg/day have been given to adult patients with pathological hypersecretory conditions with no serious adverse effects. In the event of overdosage, treatment should be symptomatic and supportive. Unabsorbed material should be removed from the gastrointestinal tract, the patient should be monitored, and supportive therapy should be employed.
The intravenous LD_{50} of famotidine for mice and rats ranged from 254–563 mg/kg and the minimum lethal single I.V. dose in dogs was approximately 300 mg/kg. Signs of acute intoxication in I.V. treated dogs were emesis, restlessness, pallor of mucous membranes or redness of mouth and ears, hypotension, tachycardia and collapse. The oral LD_{50} of famotidine in male and female rats and mice was greater than 3000 mg/kg and the minimum lethal acute oral dose in dogs exceeded 2000 mg/kg. Famotidine did not produce overt effects at high oral doses in mice, rats, cats and dogs, but induced significant anorexia and growth depression in rabbits starting with 200 mg/kg/day orally.

DOSAGE AND ADMINISTRATION

In some hospitalized patients with pathological hypersecretory conditions or intractable ulcers, or in patients who are unable to take oral medication, PEPCID Injection Premixed or PEPCID Injection may be administered until oral therapy can be instituted.
The recommended dosage for PEPCID Injection Premixed and PEPCID Injection in adult patients is 20 mg intravenously q 12 h.
The doses and regimen for parenteral administration in patients with GERD have not been established.
Dosage for Pediatric Patients
See PRECAUTIONS, *Pediatric Patients.*
The studies described in PRECAUTIONS, *Pediatric Patients* suggest that the starting dose in pediatric patients 1–16 years of age is 0.25 mg/kg intravenously (injected over a period of not less than two minutes or as a 15 minute infusion) q 12 h up to 40 mg/day.
While published uncontrolled clinical studies suggest effectiveness of famotidine in the treatment of peptic ulcer, data in pediatric patients are insufficient to establish percent response with dose and duration of therapy. Therefore, treatment duration (initially based on adult duration recommendations) and dose should be individualized based on clinical response and/or gastric pH determination and endoscopy. Published uncontrolled studies in pediatric patients have demonstrated gastric acid suppression with doses up to 0.5 mg/kg intravenously q 12 h.
No pharmacokinetic or pharmacodynamic data are available on pediatric patients under 1 year of age.
Dosage Adjustments for Patients with Severe Renal Insufficiency
In adult patients with severe renal insufficiency, i.e., with a creatinine clearance less than 10 mL/min, the elimination half-life of PEPCID may exceed 20 hours, reaching approximately 24 hours in anuric patients. Although no relationship of adverse effects to high plasma levels has been established, to avoid excess accumulation of the drug, the dose of PEPCID Injection Premixed or PEPCID Injection may be reduced to 20 mg h.s. or the dosing interval may be prolonged to 36–48 hours as indicated by the patient's clinical response.
Based on the comparison of pharmacokinetic parameters for PEPCID in adults and pediatric patients, dosage adjustment in pediatric patients with severe renal insufficiency should be considered.
Pathological Hypersecretory Conditions (e.g., Zollinger-Ellison Syndrome, Multiple Endocrine Adenomas)
The dosage of PEPCID in patients with pathological hypersecretory conditions varies with the individual patient. The recommended adult intravenous dose is 20 mg q 12 h. Doses should be adjusted to individual patient needs and should continue as long as clinically indicated. In some patients, a higher starting dose may be required. Oral doses up to 160 mg q 6 h have been administered to some adult patients with severe Zollinger-Ellison Syndrome.
PEPCID Injection Premixed
PEPCID Injection Premixed, supplied in Galaxy§ containers (PL 2501 Plastic), is a 50 mL iso-osmotic solution premixed

Table 8

Dosage	Route	Effect[a]	Number of Patients
0.3 mg/kg, single dose	I.V.	gastric pH >3.5 for 8.7 ± 4.7[b] hours	6
0.4–0.8 mg/kg	I.V.	gastric pH >4 for 6–9 hours	18
0.5 mg/kg, single dose	I.V.	a >2 pH unit increase above baseline in gastric pH for >8 hours	9
0.5 mg/kg b.i.d.	I.V.	gastric pH >5 for 13.5 ± 1.8[b] hours	4
0.5 mg/kg b.i.d.	oral	gastric pH >5 for 5.0 ± 1.1[b] hours	4

[a]Values reported in published literature.
[b]Means ± SD.

with 0.9% sodium chloride for administration as an infusion over a 15–30 minute period. *This premixed solution is for intravenous use only using sterile equipment.*

Directions for Use of Galaxy® Containers

Check the container for minute leaks prior to use by squeezing the bag firmly. If leaks are found, discard solution as sterility may be impaired. Do not add supplementary medication. Do not use unless solution is clear and seal is intact.

CAUTION: Do not use plastic containers in series connections. Such use could result in air embolism due to residual air being drawn from the primary container before administration of the fluid from the secondary container is complete.

Preparation for administration:

1. Suspend container from eyelet support.
2. Remove plastic protector from outlet port at bottom of container.
3. Attach administration set. Refer to complete directions accompanying set.

To prepare PEPCID intravenous solutions, aseptically dilute 2 mL of PEPCID Injection (solution containing 10 mg/mL) with 0.9% Sodium Chloride Injection or other compatible intravenous solution (see *Stability, PEPCID Injection*) to a total volume of either 5 mL or 10 mL and inject over a period of not less than 2 minutes.

To prepare PEPCID intravenous infusion solutions, aseptically dilute 2 mL of PEPCID Injection with 100 mL of 5% dextrose or other compatible solution (see *Stability, PEPCID Injection*), and infuse over a 15–30 minute period.

Concomitant Use of Antacids

Antacids may be given concomitantly if needed.

Stability

Parenteral drug products should be inspected visually for particulate matter and discoloration prior to administration whenever solution and container permit.

PEPCID Injection Premixed

PEPCID Injection Premixed, as supplied premixed in 0.9% sodium chloride in Galaxy® containers (PL 2501 Plastic), is stable through the labeled expiration date when stored under the recommended conditions. (See HOW SUPPLIED, *Storage*).

PEPCID Injection

When added to or diluted with most commonly used intravenous solutions, e.g., Water for Injection, 0.9% Sodium Chloride Injection, 5% and 10% Dextrose Injection, or Lactated Ringer's Injection, diluted PEPCID Injection is physically and chemically stable (i.e., maintains at least 90% of initial potency) for 7 days at room temperature—see HOW SUPPLIED, *Storage.*

When added to or diluted with Sodium Bicarbonate Injection, 5%, PEPCID Injection at a concentration of 0.2 mg/mL (the recommended concentration of PEPCID intravenous infusion solutions) is physically and chemically stable (i.e., maintains at least 90% of initial potency) for 7 days at room temperature—see HOW SUPPLIED, *Storage*. However, a precipitate may form at higher concentrations of PEPCID Injection (>0.2 mg/mL) in Sodium Bicarbonate Injection, 5%.

§ Galaxy® is a registered trademark of Baxter International Inc.

HOW SUPPLIED

FOR INTRAVENOUS USE ONLY

No. 3537—PEPCID (famotidine) Injection Premixed 20 mg per 50 mL is a clear, non-preserved, sterile solution premixed in a vehicle made iso-osmotic with Sodium Chloride, and is supplied as follows:

NDC 0006-3537-50, 50 mL single dose Galaxy® containers (PL 2501 Plastic).

No. 3539—PEPCID Injection 10 mg per 1 mL, is a non-preserved, clear, colorless solution and is supplied as follows:

NDC 0006-3539-04, 10 × 2 mL single dose vials

No. 3541—PEPCID Injection 10 mg per 1 mL, is a clear, colorless solution and is supplied as follows:

NDC 0006-3541-14, 4 mL vials

NDC 0006–3541–20, 20 mL vials

NDC 0006–3541–49, 10 ×20 mL vials.

Storage

Store PEPCID Injection Premixed in Galaxy® containers (PL 2501 Plastic) at room temperature (25°C, 77°F). Exposure of the premixed product to excessive heat should be avoided. Brief exposure to temperatures up to 35°C (95°F) does not adversely affect the product.

Store PEPCID Injection at 2–8°C (36–46°F). If solution freezes, bring to room temperature; allow sufficient time to solubilize all the components.

Although diluted PEPCID Injection has been shown to be physically and chemically stable for 7 days at room temperature, there are no data on the maintenance of sterility after dilution. Therefore, it is recommended that if not used immediately after preparation, diluted solutions of PEPCID Injection should be refrigerated and used within 48 hours (see DOSAGE AND ADMINISTRATION).

PEPCID (famotidine) Injection Premixed is manufactured for:

MERCK & CO., INC., West Point, PA 19486, USA

By:

BAXTER HEALTHCARE CORPORATION

Deerfield, Illinois 60015 USA

PEPCID (famotidine) Injection is manufactured by:

MERCK & CO., INC., West Point, PA 19486, USA

9042508 Issued November 1998

PERIACTIN® Tablets ℞
(Cyproheptadine HCl)

DESCRIPTION

PERIACTIN* (Cyproheptadine HCl) is an antihistaminic and antiserotonergic agent.

Cyproheptadine hydrochloride is a white to slightly yellowish, crystalline solid, with a molecular weight of 350.89, which is soluble in water, freely soluble in methanol, sparingly soluble in ethanol, soluble in chloroform, and practically insoluble in ether. It is the sesquihydrate of 4-(5*H*-dibenzo[*a,d*]cyclohepten-5-ylidene)-1-methylpiperidine hydrochloride. The empirical formula of the anhydrous salt is $C_{21}H_{21}N{\cdot}HCl$ and the structural formula of the anhydrous salt is:

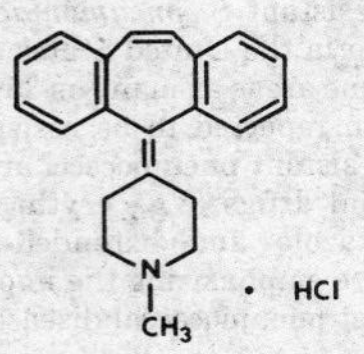

PERIACTIN is available in tablets, containing 4 mg of cyproheptadine hydrochloride.

The tablets also contain the following inactive ingredients: calcium phosphate, lactose, magnesium stearate, and starch.

*Registered trademark of MERCK & CO., INC.

CLINICAL PHARMACOLOGY

PERIACTIN is a serotonin and histamine antagonist with anticholinergic and sedative effects. Antiserotonin and antihistamine drugs appear to compete with serotonin and histamine, respectively, for receptor sites.

Pharmacokinetics and Metabolism

After a single 4 mg oral dose of ^{14}C-labelled cyproheptadine HCl in normal subjects, given as tablets, 2-20% of the radioactivity was excreted in the stools. Only about 34% of the stool radioactivity was unchanged drug, corresponding to less than 5.7% of the dose. At least 40% of the administered radioactivity was excreted in the urine. No detectable amounts of unchanged drug were present in the urine of patients on chronic 12-20 mg daily doses. The principal metabolite found in human urine has been identified as a quaternary ammonium glucuronide conjugate of cyproheptadine. Elimination is diminished in renal insufficiency.

INDICATIONS AND USAGE

Perennial and seasonal allergic rhinitis

Vasomotor rhinitis

Allergic conjunctivitis due to inhalant allergens and foods

Mild, uncomplicated allergic skin manifestations of urticaria and angioedema

Amelioration of allergic reactions to blood or plasma

Cold urticaria

Dermatographism

As therapy for anaphylactic reactions *adjunctive* to epinephrine and other standard measures after the acute manifestations have been controlled.

CONTRAINDICATIONS

Newborn or Premature Infants

This drug should *not* be used in newborn or premature infants.

Nursing Mothers

Because of the higher risk of antihistamines for infants generally and for newborns and prematures in particular, antihistamine therapy is contraindicated in nursing mothers.

Other Conditions

Hypersensitivity to cyproheptadine and other drugs of similar chemical structure:

Monoamine oxidase inhibitor therapy (see DRUG INTERACTIONS)
Angle-closure glaucoma
Stenosing peptic ulcer
Symptomatic prostatic hypertrophy
Bladder neck obstruction
Pyloroduodenal obstruction
Elderly, debilitated patients

WARNINGS

Pediatric Patients

Overdosage of antihistamines, particularly in infants and young children, may produce hallucinations, central nervous system depression, convulsions, respiratory and cardiac arrest, and death.

Antihistamines may diminish mental alertness; conversely, particularly, in the young child, they may occasionally produce excitation.

CNS Depressants

Antihistamines may have additive effects with alcohol and other CNS depressants, e.g., hypnotics, sedatives, tranquilizers, antianxiety agents.

Activities Requiring Mental Alertness

Patients should be warned about engaging in activities requiring mental alertness and motor coordination, such as driving a car or operating machinery.

Antihistamines are more likely to cause dizziness, sedation, and hypotension in elderly patients (see PRECAUTIONS, *Geriatric Use*).

PRECAUTIONS

General

Cyproheptadine has an atropine-like action and, therefore, should be used with caution in patients with:

History of bronchial asthma
Increased intraocular pressure
Hyperthyroidism
Cardiovascular disease
Hypertension

Information for Patients

Antihistamines may diminish mental alertness; conversely, particularly, in the young child, they may occasionally produce excitation.

Patients should be warned about engaging in activities requiring mental alertness and motor coordination, such as driving a car or operating machinery.

Drug Interactions

MAO inhibitors prolong and intensify the anticholinergic effects of antihistamines.

Antihistamines may have additive effects with alcohol and other CNS depressants, e.g., hypnotics, sedatives, tranquilizers, antianxiety agents.

Carcinogenesis, Mutagenesis, Impairment of Fertility

Long-term carcinogenic studies have not been done with cyproheptadine.

Cyproheptadine had no effect on fertility in a two-litter study in rats or a two generation study in mice at about 10 times the human dose.

Cyproheptadine did not produce chromosome damage in human lymphocytes or fibroblasts *in vitro;* high doses (10^{-4} M) were cytotoxic. Cyproheptadine did not have any mutagenic effect in the Ames microbial mutagen test; concentrations of above 500 mcg/plate inhibited bacterial growth.

Pregnancy

Pregnancy Category B: Reproduction studies have been performed in rabbits, mice, and rats at oral or subcutaneous doses up to 32 times the maximum recommended human oral dose and have revealed no evidence of impaired fertility or harm to the fetus due to cyproheptadine. Cyproheptadine has been shown to be fetotoxic in rats when given by intraperitoneal injection in doses four times the maximum recommended human oral dose. Two studies in pregnant women, however, have not shown that cyproheptadine increases the risk of abnormalities when administered during the first, second and third trimesters of pregnancy. No teratogenic effects were observed in any of the newborns. Nevertheless, because the studies in humans cannot rule out the possibility of harm, cyproheptadine should be used during pregnancy only if clearly needed.

Nursing Mothers

It is not known whether this drug is excreted in human milk. Because many drugs are excreted in human milk, and because of the potential for serious adverse reactions in nursing infants from PERIACTIN, a decision should be made whether to discontinue nursing or to discontinue the drug, taking into account the importance of the drug to the mother (see CONTRAINDICATIONS).

Pediatric Use

Safety and effectiveness in pediatric patients below the age of two have not been established. See CONTRAINDICATIONS, *Newborn or Premature Infants,* and WARNINGS, *Pediatric Patients.*

Geriatric Use

Clinical studies of PERIACTIN Tablets did not include sufficient numbers of subjects aged 65 and over to determine whether they respond differently from younger subjects. Other reported clinical experience has not identified differences in responses between the elderly and younger patients. In general, dose selection for an elderly patient should be cautious, usually starting at the low end of the dosing range, reflecting the greater frequency of decreased hepatic, renal, or cardiac function, and of concomitant disease or other drug therapy (see WARNINGS, *Activities Requiring Mental Alertness*).

ADVERSE REACTIONS

Adverse reactions which have been reported with the use of antihistamines are as follows:

Central Nervous System: Sedation and sleepiness (often transient), dizziness, disturbed coordination, confusion,

Continued on next page

Information on the Merck & Co., Inc. products listed on these pages is the full prescribing information from product circulars in use September 30, 2000. For information, please call 1-800-NSC MERCK [1-800-672-6372].

Periactin—Cont.

restlessness, excitation, nervousness, tremor, irritability, insomnia, paresthesias, neuritis, convulsions, euphoria, hallucinations, hysteria, faintness.
Integumentary: Allergic manifestation of rash and edema, excessive perspiration, urticaria, photosensitivity.
Special Senses: Acute labyrinthitis, blurred vision, diplopia, vertigo, tinnitus.
Cardiovascular: Hypotension, palpitation, tachycardia, extrasystoles, anaphylactic shock.
Hematologic: Hemolytic anemia, leukopenia, agranulocytosis, thrombocytopenia.
Digestive System: Cholestasis, hepatic failure, hepatitis, hepatic function abnormality, dryness of mouth, epigastric distress, anorexia, nausea, vomiting, diarrhea, constipation, jaundice.
Genitourinary: Urinary frequency, difficult urination, urinary retention, early menses.
Respiratory: Dryness of nose and throat, thickening of bronchial secretions, tightness of chest and wheezing, nasal stuffiness.
Miscellaneous: Fatigue, chills, headache, increased appetite/weight gain.

OVERDOSAGE

Antihistamine overdosage reactions may vary from central nervous system depression to stimulation especially in pediatric patients. Also, atropine-like signs and symptoms (dry mouth; fixed, dilated pupils; flushing, etc.) as well as gastrointestinal symptoms may occur.
If vomiting has not occurred spontaneously the patient should be induced to vomit with syrup of ipecac.
If the patient is unable to vomit, perform gastric lavage followed by activated charcoal. Isotonic or $^1/_2$ isotonic saline is the lavage of choice. Precautions against aspiration must be taken especially in infants and children.
When life threatening CNS signs and symptoms are present, intravenous physostigmine salicylate may be considered. Dosage and frequency of administration are dependent on age, clinical response, and recurrence after response. (See package circulars for physostigmine products.)
Saline cathartics, as milk of magnesia, by osmosis draw water into the bowel and, therefore, are valuable for their action in rapid dilution of bowel content.
Stimulants should *not* be used.
Vasopressors may be used to treat hypotension.
The oral LD_{50} of cyproheptadine is 123 mg/kg, and 295 mg/kg in the mouse and rat, respectively.

DOSAGE AND ADMINISTRATION

DOSAGE SHOULD BE INDIVIDUALIZED ACCORDING TO THE NEEDS AND THE RESPONSE OF THE PATIENT.
Each PERIACTIN tablet contains 4 mg of cyproheptadine hydrochloride.
Pediatric Patients
Age 2 to 6 years
The total daily dosage for pediatric patients may be calculated on the basis of body weight or body area using approximately 0.25 mg/kg/day or 8 mg per square meter of body surface (8 mg/m^2).
The usual dose is 2 mg ($^1/_2$ tablet) two or three times a day, adjusted as necessary to the size and response of the patient. The dose is not to exceed 12 mg a day.
Age 7 to 14 years
The usual dose is 4 mg (1 tablet) two or three times a day, adjusted as necessary to the size and response of the patient. The dose is not to exceed 16 mg a day.
Adults
The total daily dose for adults should not exceed 0.5 mg/kg/day.
The therapeutic range is 4 to 20 mg a day, with the majority of patients requiring 12 to 16 mg a day. An occasional patient may require as much as 32 mg a day for adequate relief. It is suggested that dosage be initiated with 4 mg (1 tablet) three times a day and adjusted according to the size and response of the patient.

HOW SUPPLIED

No. 3276—Tablets PERIACTIN, containing 4 mg of cyproheptadine hydrochloride each, are white, round, scored, compressed tablets, coded MSD 62 on one side and PERIACTIN on the other. They are supplied as follows:
NDC 0006-0062-68 bottles of 100.
Shown in Product Identification Guide, page 324
Storage
Store Tablets PERIACTIN at controlled room temperature, 15–30°C (59–86°F), in a well-closed container.
7926423 Issued September 1999

PNEUMOVAX® 23 ℞
(PNEUMOCOCCAL VACCINE POLYVALENT)

DESCRIPTION

PNEUMOVAX* 23 (Pneumococcal Vaccine Polyvalent), is a sterile, liquid vaccine for intramuscular or subcutaneous injection. It consists of a mixture of highly purified capsular polysaccharides from the 23 most prevalent or invasive pneumococcal types of *Streptococcus pneumoniae,* including the six serotypes that most frequently cause invasive drug-resistant pneumococcal infections among children and adults in the United States. (See Table 1.) The 23-valent vaccine accounts for at least 90% of pneumococcal blood isolates and at least 85% of all pneumococcal isolates from sites which are generally sterile as determined by ongoing surveillance of U.S. data.
PNEUMOVAX 23 is manufactured according to methods developed by the MERCK Research Laboratories. Each 0.5 mL dose of vaccine contains 25 µg of each polysaccharide type dissolved in isotonic saline solution containing 0.25% phenol as preservative.
[See table below]

*Registered trademark of MERCK & CO., Inc.

CLINICAL PHARMACOLOGY

Pneumococcal infection is a leading cause of death throughout the world and a major cause of pneumonia, bacteremia, meningitis, and otitis media.
Strains of drug-resistant *S. pneumoniae* have become increasingly common in the United States and in other parts of the world. In some areas as many as 35% of pneumococcal isolates have been reported to be resistant to penicillin. Many penicillin-resistant pneumococci are also resistant to other antimicrobial drugs (e.g., erythromycin, trimethoprim-sulfamethoxazole and extended-spectrum cephalosporins); therefore emphasizing the importance of vaccine prophylaxis against pneumococcal disease.
Epidemiology
Pneumococcal infection causes approximately 40,000 deaths annually in the United States.
At least 500,000 cases of pneumococcal pneumonia are estimated to occur annually in the United States; *S. pneumoniae* accounts for approximately 25–35% of cases of community-acquired bacterial pneumonia in persons who require hospitalization.
Pneumococcal disease accounts for an estimated 50,000 cases of pneumococcal bacteremia annually in the United States. Some studies suggest the overall annual incidence of bacteremia to be approximately 15 to 30 cases/100,000 population with 50 to 83 cases/100,000 for persons 65 years of age and older and 160 cases/100,000 for children less than two years of age.
The incidence of pneumococcal bacteremia is as high as 1% (940 cases/100,000 population) among persons with acquired immunodeficiency syndrome (AIDS).
In the United States, the risk of acquiring bacteremia is lower among whites than among persons in some other racial/ethnic groups (i.e., blacks, Alaskan Natives, and American Indians).
Despite appropriate antimicrobial therapy and intensive medical care, the overall case-fatality rate for pneumococcal bacteremia is 15–20% among adults, and among elderly patients this rate is approximately 30–40%. An overall case-fatality rate of 36% was documented for adult inner-city residents who were hospitalized for pneumococcal bacteremia.
In the United States, pneumococcal disease accounts for an estimated 3,000 cases of meningitis annually. The estimated overall annual incidence of pneumococcal meningitis is approximately 1 to 2 cases per 100,000 population. The incidence of pneumococcal meningitis is highest among children six to 24 months and persons aged ≥ 65 years; rates for blacks are twice as high as those for whites or Hispanics. Recurrent pneumococcal meningitis may occur in patients who have chronic cerebrospinal fluid leakage resulting from congenital lesions, skull fractures, or neurosurgical procedures.
Invasive pneumococcal disease (e.g., bacteremia or meningitis) and pneumonia cause high morbidity and mortality in spite of effective antimicrobial control by antibiotics. These effects of pneumococcal disease appear due to irreversible physiologic damage caused by the bacteria during the first 5 days following onset of illness, and occur irrespective of antimicrobial therapy. Vaccination offers an effective means of further reducing the mortality and morbidity of this disease.
Risk Factors
In addition to the very young and persons 65 years of age or older, patients with certain chronic conditions are at increased risk of developing pneumococcal infection and severe pneumococcal illness.
Patients with chronic cardiovascular diseases (e.g., congestive heart failure or cardiomyopathy), chronic pulmonary diseases (e.g., chronic obstructive pulmonary disease or emphysema), or chronic liver diseases (e.g., cirrhosis), diabetes mellitus, alcoholism or asthma (when it occurs with chronic bronchitis, emphysema, or long-term use of systemic corticosteroids) have an increased risk of pneumococcal disease. In adults, this population is generally immunocompetent.
Patients at high risk are those who have a decreased responsiveness to polysaccharide antigen or an increased rate of decline in serum antibody concentrations as a result of: immunosuppressive conditions (congenital immunodeficiency, human immunodeficiency virus [HIV] infection, leukemia, lymphoma, multiple myeloma, Hodgkin's disease, or generalized malignancy); organ or bone marrow transplantation; therapy with alkylating agents, antimetabolites, or systemic corticosteroids; chronic renal failure or nephrotic syndrome.
Patients at the highest risk of pneumococcal infection are those with functional or anatomic asplenia (e.g., sickle cell disease or splenectomy), because this condition leads to reduced clearance of encapsulated bacteria from the bloodstream. Children who have sickle cell disease or have had a splenectomy are at increased risk for fulminant pneumococcal sepsis associated with high mortality.
Immunogenicity
It has been established that the purified pneumococcal capsular polysaccharides induce antibody production and that such antibody is effective in preventing pneumococcal disease. Clinical studies have demonstrated the immunogenicity of each of the 23 capsular types when tested in polyvalent vaccines.
Studies with 12-, 14-, and 23-valent pneumococcal vaccines in children two years of age and older and in adults of all ages showed immunogenic responses. Protective capsular type-specific antibody levels generally develop by the third week following vaccination.
Bacterial capsular polysaccharides induce antibodies primarily by T-cell-independent mechanisms. Therefore, antibody response to most pneumococcal capsular types is generally poor or inconsistent in children aged < 2 years whose immune systems are immature.
Efficacy
The protective efficacy of pneumococcal vaccines containing 6 or 12 capsular polysaccharides was investigated in two controlled studies of young, healthy gold miners in South Africa, in whom there was a high attack rate for pneumococcal pneumonia and bacteremia. Capsular type-specific attack rates for pneumococcal pneumonia were observed for the period from 2 weeks through about 1 year after vaccination. Protective efficacy was 76% and 92%, respectively, in the two studies for the capsular types represented.
In similar studies carried out by Dr. R. Austrian and associates, using similar pneumococcal vaccines prepared for the National Institute of Allergy and Infectious Diseases, the reduction in pneumonia caused by the capsular types contained in the vaccines was 79%. Reduction in type-specific pneumococcal bacteremia was 82%.
A prospective study in France found pneumococcal vaccine to be 77% effective in reducing the incidence of pneumonia among nursing home residents.
In the United States, two postlicensure randomized controlled trials, in the elderly or patients with chronic medical conditions, who received a multivalent polysaccharide vaccine, did not support the efficacy of the vaccine for nonbacteremic pneumonia. However, these studies may have lacked sufficient statistical power to detect a difference in the incidence of laboratory-confirmed, nonbacteremic pneumococcal pneumonia between the vaccinated and nonvaccinated study groups.
A meta-analysis of nine randomized controlled trials of pneumococcal vaccine concluded that pneumococcal vaccine is efficacious in reducing the frequency of nonbacteremic pneumococcal pneumonia among adults in low risk groups but not in high-risk groups. These studies may have been limited because of the lack of specific and sensitive diagnostic tests for nonbacteremic pneumococcal pneumonia. The pneumococcal polysaccharide vaccine is not effective for the prevention of common upper respiratory disease in children.
More recently, multiple, case-control studies have shown pneumococcal vaccine is effective in the prevention of serious pneumococcal disease, with point estimates of efficacy ranging from 56% to 81% in immunocompetent persons.
Only one case-control study did not document effectiveness against bacteremic disease possibly due to study limitations, including small sample size and incomplete ascertainment of vaccination status in patients. In addition, case-patients and persons who served as controls may not have been comparable regarding the severity of their underlying medical conditions, potentially creating a biased underestimate of vaccine effectiveness.
A serotype prevalence study, based on the Centers for Disease Control pneumococcal surveillance system, demonstrated 57% overall protective effectiveness against invasive infections caused by serotypes included in the vaccine in persons ≥ 6 years of age, 65–84% effectiveness among specific patient groups (e.g., persons with diabetes mellitus, coronary vascular disease, congestive heart failure, chronic pulmonary disease, and anatomic asplenia) and 75% effectiveness in immunocompetent persons aged ≥ 65 years of age. Vaccine effectiveness could not be confirmed for certain

Table 1
23 Pneumococcal Capsular Types Included in
PNEUMOVAX 23

Nomenclature	Pneumococcal Types
Danish	1 2 3 4 5 6B** 7F 8 9N 9V** 10A 11A 12F 14** 15B 17F 18C 19F** 19A** 20 22F 23F** 33F

**These serotypes most frequently cause drug-resistant pneumococcal infections

groups of immunocompromised patients; however, the study could not recruit sufficient numbers of unvaccinated patients from each disease group.

In an early study, vaccinated children and yound adults aged 2 to 25 years who had sickle cell disease, congenital asplenia, or undergone a splenectomy experienced significantly less bacteremic pneumococcal disease than patients who were not vaccinated.

Duration of Immunity

Following pneumococcal vaccination, serotype-specific antibody levels decline after 5–10 years. A more rapid decline in antibody levels may occur in some groups (e.g., children). Limited published data suggest that antibody levels may decline in the elderly > 60 years of age.

The Advisory Committee on Immunization Practices (ACIP) states that these findings indicate that revaccination may be needed to provide continued protection. (See INDICATIONS AND USAGE, *Revaccination.*)

The results from one epidemiologic study suggest that vaccination may provide protection for at least nine years after receipt of the initial dose. Decreasing estimates of effectiveness with increasing interval since vaccination, particularly among the very elderly (persons aged ≥ 85 years) have been reported.

INDICATIONS AND USAGE

PNEUMOVAX 23 is indicated for vaccination against pneumococcal disease caused by those pneumococcal types included in the vaccine. Effectiveness of the vaccine in the prevention of pneumococcal pneumonia and pneumococcal bacteremia has been demonstrated in controlled trials in South Africa, France and in case-control studies.

PNEUMOVAX 23 will not prevent disease caused by capsular types of pneumococcus other than those contained in the vaccine.

If it is known that a person has not received any pneumococcal vaccine or if earlier pneumococcal vaccination status is unknown, then persons in the categories listed below should be administered pneumococcal vaccine; however, if a person has received a primary dose of pneumococcal vaccine, before administering an additional dose of vaccine, please refer to the Revaccination section.

Vaccination with PNEUMOVAX 23 is recommended for selected individuals as follows:

Immunocompetent persons:

— routine vaccination for persons 50 years of age or older†

— persons aged ≥ 2 years with chronic cardiovascular disease (including congestive heart failure and cardiomyopathies), chronic pulmonary disease (including chronic obstructive pulmonary disease and emphysema), or diabetes mellitus

— persons aged ≥ 2 years with alcoholism, chronic liver disease (including cirrhosis) or cerebrospinal fluid leaks

— persons aged ≥ 2 years with functional or anatomic asplenia (including sickle cell disease and splenectomy)

— persons aged ≥ 2 years living in special environments or social settings (including Alaskan Natives and certain American Indian populations)

Immunocompromised persons:

— persons aged ≥ 2 years, including those with HIV infection, leukemia, lymphoma, Hodgkin's disease, multiple myeloma, generalized malignancy, chronic renal failure or nephrotic syndrome; those receiving immunosuppressive chemotherapy (including corticosteroids); and those who have received an organ or bone marrow transplant.

†NOTE: The ACIP recommends routine vaccination for immunocompetent persons 65 years of age and older.

Timing of Vaccination

Pneumococcal vaccine should be given at least two weeks before elective splenectomy, if possible.

For planning cancer chemotherapy or other immunosuppressive therapy (e.g., for patients with Hodgkin's disease or those who undergo organ or bone marrow transplantation), pneumococcal vaccination should be administered at least two weeks prior to the initiation of immunosuppressive therapy. Vaccination during chemotherapy or radiation therapy should be avoided. Based on literature reports, pneumococcal vaccine may be given as early as several months following completion of chemotherapy or radiation therapy for neoplastic disease. In Hodgkin's disease, immune response to vaccination may be impaired for two years or longer after intensive chemotherapy (with or without radiation). During the two years following the completion of chemotherapy or other immunosuppressive therapy, antibody responses improve in some patients as the interval between the end of treatment and pneumococcal vaccination increases.

Persons with asymptomatic or symptomatic HIV infection should be vaccinated as soon as possible after their diagnosis is confirmed.

Use With Other Vaccines

The ACIP states that pneumococcal vaccine may be administered at the same time as influenza vaccine (by separate injection in the other arm) without an increase in side effects or decreased antibody response to either vaccine. In contrast to pneumococcal vaccine, influenza vaccine is recommended annually, for appropriate populations.

Revaccination

Early studies have indicated that local reactions (i.e., arthus-type reactions) among adults receiving the second dose of 14–valent vaccine within 2 years after the first dose are more severe than those occurring after initial vaccination. However, subsequent studies have suggested that revaccination after intervals of ≥ 4 years is not associated with an increased incidence of adverse side effects.

Routine revaccination of immunocompetent persons previously vaccinated with 23–valent polysaccharide vaccine is not recommended. However, revaccination once is recommended for persons ≥ 2 years of age who are at highest risk of serious pneumococcal infection and those likely to have a rapid decline in pneumococcal antibody levels, provided that at least five years have passed since receipt of a first dose of pneumococcal vaccine.

The highest risk group includes persons with functional or anatomic asplenia (e.g., sickle cell disease or splenectomy), HIV infection, leukemia, lymphoma, Hodgkin's disease, multiple myeloma, generalized malignancy, chronic renal failure, nephrotic syndrome, or other conditions associated with immunosupression (e.g., organ or bone marrow transplantation), and those receiving immunosuppressive chemotherapy (including long-term systemic corticosteroids).

For children ≤ 10 years of age at revaccination and at highest risk of severe pneumococcal infection (e.g., children with functional or anatomic asplenia, including sickle cell disease or splenectomy or conditions associated with rapid antibody decline after initial vaccination including nephrotic syndrome, renal failure or renal transplantation), the ACIP recommends that revaccination may be considered three years after the previous dose.

If prior vaccination status is unknown for patients in the high risk group, patients should be given pneumococcal vaccine.

All persons ≥ 65 years of age who have not received vaccine within 5 years (and were < 65 years of age at the time of vaccination) should receive another dose of vaccine.

Because data are insufficient concerning the safety of pneumococcal vaccine when administered three or more times, revaccination following a second dose is not routinely recommended.

CONTRAINDICATIONS

Hypersensitivity to any component of the vaccine. Epinephrine injection (1:1000) must be immediately available should an acute anaphylactoid reaction occur due to any component of the vaccine.

WARNINGS

For planning cancer chemotherapy or other immunosuppressive therapy (e.g., for patients with Hodgkin's disease or those who undergo organ or bone marrow transplantation), the timing of the vaccination is critical. (See INDICATIONS AND USAGE, *Timing of Vaccination.*)

If the vaccine is used in persons receiving immunosuppressive therapy, the expected serum antibody response may not be obtained and potential impairment of future immune responses to pneumococcal antigens may occur. (See INDICATIONS AND USAGE, *Timing of Vaccination.*)

Intradermal administration may cause severe local reactions.

PRECAUTIONS

General

Caution and appropriate care should be exercised in administering PNEUMOVAX 23 to individuals with severely compromised cardiovascular and/or pulmonary function in whom a systemic reaction would pose a significant risk.

Any febrile respiratory illness or other active infection is reason for delaying use of PNEUMOVAX 23, except when, in the opinion of the physician, withholding the agent entails even greater risk.

In patients who require penicillin (or other antibiotic) prophylaxis against pneumococcal infection, such prophylaxis should not be discontinued after vaccination with PNEUMOVAX 23.

PNEUMOVAX 23 may not be effective in preventing pneumococcal meningitis in patients who have chronic cerebrospinal fluid (CSF) leakage resulting from congenital lesions, skull fractures, or neurosurgical procedures.

Routine revaccination of immunocompetent persons previously vaccinated with a 23–valent vaccine is not recommended. However, revaccination once is recommended for persons aged ≥ 2 years who are at highest risk for serious pneumococcal infections and those likely to have a rapid decline in pneumococcal antibody levels. (See INDICATIONS AND USAGE, *Revaccination.*)

Instructions to Healthcare Provider

The healthcare provider should determine the current health status and previous vaccination history of the vaccinee. (See INDICATIONS AND USAGE, *Revaccination.*)

The healthcare provider should question the patient, parent or guardian about reactions to a previous dose of PNEUMOVAX 23 or other pneumococcal vaccine.

Information for Patients

The healthcare provider should inform the patient, parent or guardian of the benefits and risks associated with vaccination. For risks associated with vaccination, see WARNINGS, PRECAUTIONS, and ADVERSE REACTIONS.

Patients, parents, and guardians should be instructed to report any serious adverse reactions to their healthcare provider who in turn should report such events to the vaccine manufacturer or the U.S. Department of Health and Human Services through the Vaccine Adverse Event Reporting System (VAERS), 1-800-822-7967.

Pregnancy

Pregnancy Category C: Animal reproduction studies have not been conducted with PNEUMOVAX 23. It is also not known whether PNEUMOVAX 23 can cause fetal harm when administered to a pregnant woman or can affect reproduction capacity. PNEUMOVAX 23 should be given to a pregnant woman only if clearly needed.

Nursing Mothers

It is not known whether this drug is excreted in human milk. Because many drugs are excreted in human milk, caution should be excercised when PNEUMOVAX 23 is administered to a nursing woman.

Pediatric Use

In general, children less than 2 years of age respond poorly to the capsular types of PNEUMOVAX 23 that are most often the cause of pneumococcal disease in this age group. (See CLINICAL PHARMACOLOGY, *Immunogenicity.*) Safety and effectiveness in children below the age of 2 years have not been established. Accordingly, PNEUMOVAX 23 is not recommended in this age group.

ADVERSE REACTIONS

The following adverse experiences have been reported with PNEUMOVAX 23 in clinical trials and post-marketing experience:

The most common adverse experiences reported in clinical trials were:

Local reactions at injection site including soreness, warmth, erythema, swelling and induration

Fever ≤ 102°F.

Other adverse experiences reported in clinical trials and in post-marketing experience include:

Body as a Whole

Asthenia

Malaise

Fever (>102°F)

Digestive System

Nausea

Vomiting

Hematologic / Lymphatic

Lymphadenitis

Thrombocytopenia in patients with stabilized idiopathic thrombocytopenic purpura

Hemolytic anemia in patients who have had other hematologic disorders

Hypersensitivity

Anaphylactoid reactions

Serum Sickness

Musculoskeletal System

Arthralgia

Arthritis

Myalgia

Nervous System

Headache

Paresthesia

Radiculoneuropathy

Guillain-Barré Syndrome

Skin

Rash

Urticaria.

DOSAGE AND ADMINISTRATION

Do not inject intravenously or intradermally.

For Vial and Pre-filled Single-Dose Syringe, parenteral drug products should be inspected visually for particulate matter and discoloration prior to administration, whenever solution and container permit. PNEUMOVAX 23 is a clear, colorless solution. The vaccine is used directly as supplied. No dilution or reconstitution is necessary. Phenol 0.25% has been added as a preservative.

It is important to use a separate sterile syringe and needle for each individual patient to prevent transmission of infectious agents from one person to another.

For the Vial, withdraw 0.5 mL from the vial using a sterile needle and syringe free of preservatives, antiseptics, and detergents.

Administer a single 0.5 mL dose of PNEUMOVAX 23 subcutaneously or intramuscularly (preferably in the deltoid muscle or lateral mid-thigh), with appropriate precautions to avoid intravascular administration.

Store unopened and opened vials and pre-filled single-dose syringes at 2–8°C (36–46°F). All vaccines must be discarded after the expiration date.

Use With Other Vaccines

The ACIP states that pneumococcal vaccine may be administered at the same time as influenza vaccine (by separate injection in the other arm) without an increase in side effects or decreased antibody response to either vaccine. In contrast to pneumococcal vaccine, influenza vaccine is recommended annually, for appropriate populations.

HOW SUPPLIED

No. 4739 — PNEUMOVAX 23 is supplied as one 5-dose vial of liquid vaccine, color coded with a purple cap and stripe on the vial labels and cartons, **NDC** 0006-4739-00.

For use with syringe only (6505-01-092-0391).

No. 4943 — PNEUMOVAX 23 is supplied as a single-dose vial of liquid vaccine, in a box of 10 single-dose vials, color coded with a purple cap and sripe on the vial labels and cartons, **NDC** 0006-4943-00.

Continued on next page

Information on the Merck & Co., Inc. products listed on these pages is the full prescribing information from product circulars in use September 30, 2000. For information, please call 1-800-NSC MERCK [1-800-672-6372].

Pneumovax 23—Cont.

No. 4894 — PNEUMOVAX 23 is supplied as liquid vaccine in a pre-filled single-dose glass syringe with a 1 inch needle, in a box of 5 single-dose syringes with 1 inch needles, color coded with a purple plunger rod and stripe on the syringe labels and cartons, **NDC** 0006-4894-00.

7999816 Issued March 1999

PRIMAXIN® I.M. ℞

(Imipenem and Cilastatin for Injectable Suspension)

For Intramuscular Injection Only

DESCRIPTION

PRIMAXIN† I.M. (Imipenem and Cilastatin for Injectable Suspension) is a formulation of imipenem (a thienamycin antibiotic) and cilastatin sodium (the inhibitor of the renal dipeptidase, dehydropeptidase I). PRIMAXIN I.M. is a potent broad spectrum antibacterial agent for intramuscular administration.

Imipenem (N-formimidoylthienamycin monohydrate) is a crystalline derivative of thienamycin, which is produced by *Streptomyces cattleya*. Its chemical name is [5*R* -[5α, 6α (*R* *)]]-6-(1-hydroxyethyl)-3-[[2-[(iminomethyl)amino] ethyl]thio]-7-oxo-1-azabicyclo [3.2.0] hept-2-ene-2-carboxylic acid monohydrate. It is an off-white, nonhygroscopic crystalline compound with a molecular weight of 317.37. It is sparingly soluble in water, and slightly soluble in methanol. Its empirical formula is $C_{12}H_{17}N_3O_4S{\cdot}H_2O$, and its structural formula is:

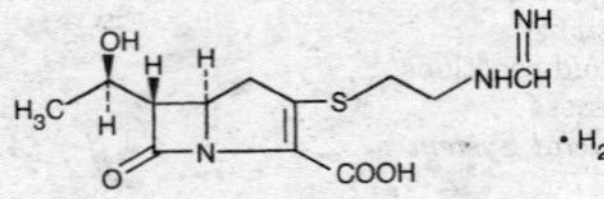

Cilastatin sodium is the sodium salt of a derivatized heptenoic acid. Its chemical name is [*R*- [*R**,*S**- (*Z*)]]-7-[(2-amino-2-carboxyethyl)thio]-2-[[(2, 2-dimethylcyclopropyl) carbonyl]amino]-2-heptenoic acid, monosodium salt. It is an off-white to yellowish-white, hygroscopic, amorphous compound with a molecular weight of 380.43. It is very soluble in water and in methanol. Its empirical formula is $C_{16}H_{25}N_2O_5SNa$, and its structural formula is:

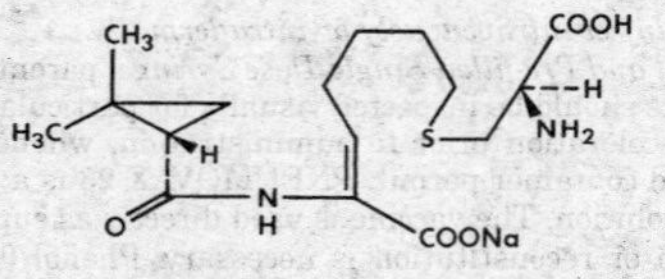

PRIMAXIN I.M. 500 contains 32 mg of sodium (1.4 mEq) and PRIMAXIN I.M. 750 contains 48 mg of sodium (2.1 mEq). Prepared PRIMAXIN I.M. suspensions are white to light tan in color. Variations of color within this range do not affect the potency of the product.

† Registered trademark of MERCK & CO., INC.

CLINICAL PHARMACOLOGY

Following intramuscular administrations of 500 or 750 mg doses of imipenem-cilastatin sodium in a 1:1 ratio with 1% lidocaine, peak plasma levels of imipenem antimicrobial activity occur within 2 hours and average 10 and 12 µg/mL, respectively. For cilastatin, peak plasma levels average 24 and 33 µg/mL, respectively, and occur within 1 hour. When compared to intravenous administration of imipenem-cilastatin sodium, imipenem is approximately 75% bioavailable following intramuscular administration while cilastatin is approximately 95% bioavailable. The absorption of imipenem from the IM injection site continues for 6 to 8 hours while that for cilastatin is essentially complete within 4 hours. This prolonged absorption of imipenem following the administration of the intramuscular formulation of imipenem-cilastatin sodium results in an effective plasma half-life of imipenem of approximately 2 to 3 hours and plasma levels of the antibiotic which remain above 2 µg/mL for at least 6 or 8 hours, following a 500 mg or 750 mg dose, respectively. This plasma profile for imipenem permits IM administration of the intramuscular formulation of imipenem-cilastatin sodium every 12 hours with no accumulation of cilastatin and only slight accumulation of imipenem.

A comparison of plasma levels of imipenem after a single dose of 500 mg or 750 mg of imipenem-cilastatin sodium (intravenous formulation) administered intravenously or of imipenem-cilastatin sodium (intramuscular formulation) diluted with 1% lidocaine and administered intramuscularly is as follows:

PLASMA CONCENTRATIONS OF IMIPENEM (µg/mL)

	500 MG		750 MG	
TIME	I.V.	I.M.	I.V.	I.M.
25 min	45.1	6.0	57.0	6.7
1 hr	21.6	9.4	28.1	10.0
2 hr	10.0	9.9	12.0	11.4
4 hr	2.6	5.6	3.4	7.3
6 hr	0.6	2.5	1.1	3.8
12 hr	ND†	0.5	ND**	0.8

** ND: Not Detectable (<0.3 µg/mL)

Imipenem urine levels remain above 10 µg/mL for the 12 hour dosing interval following the administration of 500 mg or 750 mg doses of the intramuscular formulation of imipenem-cilastatin sodium. Total urinary excretion of imipenem averages 50% while that for cilastatin averages 75% following either dose of the intramuscular formulation of imipenem-cilastatin sodium.

Imipenem, when administered alone, is metabolized in the kidneys by dehydropeptidase I resulting in relatively low levels in urine. Cilastatin sodium, an inhibitor of this enzyme, effectively prevents renal metabolism of imipenem so that when imipenem and cilastatin sodium are given concomitantly, increased levels of imipenem are achieved in the urine. The binding of imipenem to human serum proteins is approximately 20% and that of cilastatin is approximately 40%.

In a clinical study in which a 500 mg dose of the intramuscular formulation of imipenem-cilastatin sodium was administered to healthy subjects, the average peak level of imipenem in interstitial fluid (skin blister fluid) was approximately 5.0 µg/mL within 3.5 hours after administration.

Imipenem-cilastatin sodium is hemodialyzable. However, usefulness of this procedure in the overdosage setting is questionable. (See **OVERDOSAGE**.)

Microbiology

The bactericidal activity of imipenem results from the inhibition of cell wall synthesis. Its greatest affinity is for penicillin-binding proteins (PBPs) 1A, 1B, 2, 4, 5 and 6 of *Escherichia coli*, and 1A, 1B, 2, 4 and 5 of *Pseudomonas aeruginosa*. The lethal effect is related to binding to PBP 2 and PBP 1B.

Imipenem has a high degree of stability in the presence of beta-lactamases, including penicillinases and cephalosporinases produced by gram-negative and gram-positive bacteria. It is a potent inhibitor of beta-lactamases from certain gram-negative bacteria which are inherently resistant to many beta-lactam antibiotics, e.g., *Pseudomonas aeruginosa, Serratia* spp. and *Enterobacter* spp.

Imipenem has *in vitro* activity against a wide range of gram-positive and gram-negative organisms. Imipenem has been shown to be active against most strains of the following microorganisms, both *in vitro* and in clinical infections treated with the intramuscular formulation of imipenem-cilastatin sodium as described in the INDICATIONS AND USAGE section.

Gram-positive aerobes:
- *Staphylococcus aureus* including penicillinase-producing strains
  - (NOTE: Methicillin-resistant staphylococci should be reported as resistant to imipenem.)
- Group D streptococcus including *Enterococcus faecalis* (formerly *S. faecalis*)
  - (NOTE: Imipenem is inactive *in vitro* against *Enterococcus faecium* [formerly *S. faecium*].)
- *Streptococcus pneumoniae*
- *Streptococcus pyogenes* (Group A streptococci)
- *Streptococcus viridans* group

Gram-negative aerobes:
- *Acinetobacter* spp., including *A. calcoaceticus*
- *Citrobacter* spp.
- *Enterobacter cloacae*
- *Escherichia coli*
- *Haemophilus influenzae*
- *Klebsiella pneumoniae*
- *Pseudomonas aeruginosa*
  - (NOTE: Imipenem is inactive *in vitro* against *Xanthomonas (Pseudomonas) maltophilia* and *P. cepacia.*)

Gram-positive anaerobes:
- *Peptostreptococcus* spp.

Gram-negative anaerobes:
- *Bacteroides* spp., including
  - *Bacteroides distasonis*
  - *Bacteroides intermedius* (formerly *B. melaninogenicus intermedius)*
  - *Bacteroides fragilis*
  - *Bacteroides thetaiotaomicron*
- *Fusobacterium* spp.

Imipenem exhibits *in vitro* minimal inhibitory concentrations (MICs) of 4 µg/mL or less against most (≥90%) strains of the following microorganisms; however, the safety and effectiveness of imipenem in treating clinical infections due to these microorganisms have not been established in adequate and well-controlled clinical trials.

Gram-positive aerobes:
- *Bacillus* spp.
- *Listeria monocytogenes*
- *Nocardia* spp.
- Group C streptococci
- Group G streptococci

Gram-negative aerobes:
- *Aeromonas hydrophila*
- *Alcaligenes* spp.
- *Capnocytophaga* spp.
- *Enterobacter agglomerans*
- *Haemophilus ducreyi*
- *Klebsiella oxytoca*
- *Neisseria gonorrhoeae* including penicillinase-producing strains
- *Pasteurella* spp.
- *Proteus mirabilis*
- *Providencia stuartii*

Gram-positive anaerobes:
- *Clostridium perfringens*

Gram-negative anaerobes:
- *Prevotella bivia*
- *Prevotella disiens*
- *Prevotella melaninogenica*
- *Veillonella* spp.

In vitro tests show imipenem to act synergistically with aminoglycoside antibiotics against some isolates of *Pseudomonas aeruginosa.*

Susceptibility Tests:

Dilution techniques:

Use a standardized dilution method[1] (broth, agar, microdilution) or equivalent with imipenem powder. The MIC values obtained should be interpreted according to the following criteria:

MIC (µg/mL)	Interpretation
≤4	Susceptible
8	Moderately Susceptible
≥16	Resistant

A report of "susceptible" indicates that the pathogen is likely to be inhibited by generally achievable blood levels. A report of "moderately susceptible" suggests that the organism would be susceptible if high dosage is used or if the infection is confined to tissues and fluids in which high antibiotic levels are attained. A report of "resistant" indicates that achievable concentrations are unlikely to be inhibitory and other therapy should be selected.

Standardized susceptibility test procedures require the use of laboratory control organisms. Standard imipenem powder should provide the following MIC values:

Organism	MIC (µg/mL)
E. coli ATCC 25922	0.06–0.25
S. aureus ATCC 29213	0.015–0.06
E. faecalis ATCC 29212	0.5–2.0
P. aeruginosa ATCC 27853	1.0–4.0

Diffusion techniques:

Quantitative methods that require measurement of zone diameters give the most precise estimate of antibiotic susceptibility. One such standard procedure[2], which has been recommended for use with disks to test susceptibility of organisms to imipenem, uses the 10-µg imipenem disk. Interpretation involves the correlation of the diameters obtained in the disk test with the minimum inhibitory concentration (MIC) for imipenem.

Reports from the laboratory giving results of the standard single-disk susceptibility test with a 10-µg imipenem disk should be interpreted according to the following criteria:

Zone Diameter (mm)	Interpretation
≥16	Susceptible
14–15	Moderately Susceptible
≤13	Resistant

Standardized procedures require the use of laboratory control organisms. The 10-µg imipenem disk should give the following zone diameters:

Organism	Zone Diameter (mm)
E. coli ATCC 25922	26–32
P. aeruginosa ATCC 27853	20–28

For anaerobic bacteria, the MIC of imipenem can be determined by agar or broth dilution (including microdilution) techniques.[3]

The MIC values obtained should be interpreted according to the following criteria:

MIC (µg/mL)	Interpretation
≤4	Susceptible
8	Moderately Susceptible
≥16	Resistant

INDICATIONS AND USAGE

PRIMAXIN I.M. is indicated for the treatment of serious infections (listed below) of mild to moderate severity for which intramuscular therapy is appropriate. **PRIMAXIN I.M. is not intended for the therapy of severe or life-threatening infections, including bacterial sepsis or endocarditis, or in instances of major physiological impairments such as shock.**

PRIMAXIN I.M. is indicated for the treatment of infections caused by susceptible strains of the designated microorganisms in the conditions listed below:

(1) **Lower respiratory tract infections,** including pneumonia and bronchitis as an exacerbation of COPD, caused by *Streptococcus pneumoniae* and *Haemophilus influenzae.*

(2) **Intra-abdominal infections,** including acute gangrenous or perforated appendicitis and appendicitis with peritonitis, caused by Group D streptococcus including *Enterococcus faecalis*; Streptococcus viridans* group*; *Escherichia coli; Klebsiella pneumoniae*; Pseudomonas aeruginosa*; Bacteroides* species including *B. fragilis, B. distasonis*, B. intermedius** and *B. thetaiotaomicron*; Fusobacterium* species and *Peptostreptococcus** species.
(3) **Skin and skin structure infections,** including abscesses, cellulitis, infected skin ulcers and wound infections caused by *Staphylococcus aureus* including penicillinase-producing strains; *Streptococcus pyogenes**; Group D streptococcus including *Enterococcus faecalis; Acinetobacter* species* including *A. calcoaceticus*; Citrobacter* species*; *Escherichia coli; Enterobacter cloacae; Klebsiella pneumoniae*; Pseudomonas aeruginosa** and *Bacteroides* species* including *B. fragilis**.
(4) **Gynecologic infections,** including postpartum endomyometritis, caused by Group D streptococcus including *Enterococcus faecalis*; Escherichia coli; Klebsiella pneumoniae*; Bacteroides intermedius**; and *Peptostreptococcus* species*.

As with other beta-lactam antibiotics, some strains of *Pseudomonas aeruginosa* may develop resistance fairly rapidly during treatment with PRIMAXIN I.M. During therapy of *Pseudomonas aeruginosa* infections, periodic susceptibility testing should be done when clinically appropriate.

*Efficacy for this organism in this organ system was studied in fewer than 10 infections.

CONTRAINDICATIONS

PRIMAXIN I.M. is contraindicated in patients who have shown hypersensitivity to any component of this product. Due to the use of lidocaine hydrochloride diluent, this product is contraindicated in patients with a known hypersensitivity to local anesthetics of the amide type and in patients with severe shock or heart block. (Refer to the package circular for lidocaine hydrochloride).

WARNINGS

SERIOUS AND OCCASIONALLY FATAL HYPERSENSITIVITY (anaphylactic) REACTIONS HAVE BEEN REPORTED IN PATIENTS RECEIVING THERAPY WITH BETA-LACTAMS. THESE REACTIONS ARE MORE LIKELY TO OCCUR IN INDIVIDUALS WITH A HISTORY OF SENSITIVITY TO MULTIPLE ALLERGENS. THERE HAVE BEEN REPORTS OF INDIVIDUALS WITH A HISTORY OF PENICILLIN HYPERSENSITIVITY WHO HAVE EXPERIENCED SEVERE REACTIONS WHEN TREATED WITH ANOTHER BETA-LACTAM. BEFORE INITIATING THERAPY WITH PRIMAXIN® I.M., CAREFUL INQUIRY SHOULD BE MADE CONCERNING PREVIOUS HYPERSENSITIVITY REACTIONS TO PENICILLINS, CEPHALOSPORINS, OTHER BETA-LACTAMS, AND OTHER ALLERGENS. IF AN ALLERGIC REACTION OCCURS, PRIMAXIN® SHOULD BE DISCONTINUED. **SERIOUS ANAPHYLACTIC REACTIONS REQUIRE IMMEDIATE EMERGENCY TREATMENT WITH EPINEPHRINE. OXYGEN, INTRAVENOUS STEROIDS, AND AIRWAY MANAGEMENT, INCLUDING INTUBATION, MAY ALSO BE ADMINISTERED AS INDICATED.**

Pseudomembranous colitis has been reported with nearly all antibacterial agents, including PRIMAXIN, and may range in severity from mild to life-threatening. Therefore, it is important to consider this diagnosis in patients who present with diarrhea subsequent to the administration of antibacterial agents.

Treatment with antibacterial agents alters the normal flora of the colon and may permit overgrowth of clostridia. Studies indicate that a toxin produced by *Clostridium difficile* is one primary cause of "antibiotic-associated colitis".

After the diagnosis of pseudomembranous colitis has been established, therapeutic measures should be initiated. Mild cases of pseudomembranous colitis usually respond to drug discontinuation alone. In moderate to severe cases, consideration should be given to management with fluids and electrolytes, protein supplementation and treatment with an antibacterial drug clinically effective against *C. difficile* colitis.

Lidocaine HCl —Refer to the package circular for lidocaine HCl.

PRECAUTIONS

General

CNS adverse experiences such as myoclonic activity, confusional states, or seizures have been reported with PRIMAXIN I.V. (Imipenem and Cilastatin for Injection). These experiences have occurred most commonly in patients with CNS disorders (e.g., brain lesions or history of seizures) who also have compromised renal function. However, there were reports in which there was no recognized or documented underlying CNS disorder. These adverse CNS effects have not been seen with PRIMAXIN I.M.; however, should they occur during treatment, PRIMAXIN I.M. should be discontinued. Anticonvulsant therapy should be continued in patients with a known seizure disorder.

As with other antibiotics, prolonged use of PRIMAXIN I.M. may result in overgrowth of nonsusceptible organisms. Repeated evaluation of the patient's condition is essential. If superinfection occurs during therapy, appropriate measures should be taken.

DOSAGE GUIDELINES

Type††/Location of Infection	Severity	Dosage Regimen
Lower respiratory tract Skin and skin structure Gynecologic	Mild/Moderate	500 or 750 mg q 12 h depending on the severity of infection
Intra-abdominal	Mild/Moderate	750 mg q 12 h

†† See INDICATIONS AND USAGE section.

Caution should be taken to avoid inadvertent injection into a blood vessel. (See DOSAGE AND ADMINISTRATION.) For additional precautions, refer to the package circular for lidocaine HCl.

Drug Interactions

Since concomitant administration of PRIMAXIN (Imipenem-Cilastatin Sodium) and probenecid results in only minimal increases in plasma levels of imipenem and plasma half-life, it is not recommended that probenecid be given with PRIMAXIN I.M.

PRIMAXIN I.M. should not be mixed with or physically added to other antibiotics. However, PRIMAXIN I.M. may be administered concomitantly with other antibiotics, such as aminoglycosides.

Carcinogenesis, Mutagenesis, Impairment of Fertility

Long term studies in animals have not been performed to evaluate carcinogenic potential of imipenem-cilastatin. Genetic toxicity studies were performed in a variety of bacterial and mammalian tests *in vivo* and *in vitro.* The tests used were: V79 mammalian cell mutagenesis assay (imipenem-cilastatin sodium alone and imipenem alone), Ames test (cilastatin sodium alone and imipenem alone), unscheduled DNA synthesis assay (imipenem-cilastatin sodium) and *in vivo* mouse cytogenetics test (imipenem-cilastatin sodium). None of these tests showed any evidence of genetic alterations.

Reproductive tests in male and female rats were performed with imipenem-cilastatin sodium at dosage levels up to 11 times*** the maximum daily recommended human dose of the intramuscular formulation (on a mg/kg basis). Slight decreases in live fetal body weight were restricted to the highest dosage level. No other adverse effects were observed on fertility, reproductive performance, fetal viability, growth or postnatal development of pups. Similarly, no adverse effects on the fetus or on lactation were observed when imipenem-cilastatin sodium was administered to rats late in gestation.

Pregnancy: Teratogenic Effects

Pregnancy Category C: Teratology studies with cilastatin sodium in rabbits and rats at 10 and 33 times*** the maximum recommended daily human dose of the intramuscular formulation (30 mg/kg/day) of PRIMAXIN, respectively, showed no evidence of adverse effects on the fetus. No evidence of teratogenicity was observed in rabbits and rats given imipenem at doses up to 2 and 30 times*** the maximum recommended daily human dose of the intramuscular formulation of PRIMAXIN, respectively.

Teratology studies with imipenem-cilastatin sodium at doses up to 11 times*** the maximum recommended human dose in pregnant mice and rats during the period of major organogenesis revealed no evidence of teratogenicity.

Imipenem-cilastatin sodium, when administered to pregnant rabbits at dosages above the usual human dose of the intramuscular formulation (1000–1500 mg/day), caused body weight loss, diarrhea, and maternal deaths. When comparable doses of imipenem-cilastatin sodium were given to nonpregnant rabbits, body weight loss, diarrhea, and deaths were also observed. This intolerance is not unlike that seen with other beta-lactam antibiotics in this species and is probably due to alteration of gut flora.

A teratology study in pregnant cynomolgus monkeys given imipenem-cilastatin sodium at doses of 40 mg/kg/day (bolus intravenous injection) or 160 mg/kg/day (subcutaneous injection) resulted in maternal toxicity including emesis, inappetence, body weight loss, diarrhea, abortion and death in some cases. In contrast, no significant toxicity was observed when nonpregnant cynomolgus monkeys were given doses of imipenem-cilastatin sodium up to 180 mg/kg/day (subcutaneous injection). When doses of imipenem-cilastatin sodium (approximately 100 mg/kg/day or approximately 3 times*** the maximum daily recommended human dose of the intramuscular formulation) were administered to pregnant cynomolgus monkeys at an intraveous infusion rate which mimics human clinical use, there was minimal maternal intolerance (occasional emesis), no maternal deaths, no evidence of teratogenicity, but an increase in embryonic loss relative to the control groups.

There are, however, no adequate and well-controlled studies in pregnant women. PRIMAXIN I.M. should be used during pregnancy only if the potential benefit justifies the potential risk to the mother and fetus.

Nursing Mothers

It is not known whether imipenem-cilastatin sodium or lidocaine HCl (diluent) is excreted in human milk. Because many drugs are excreted in human milk, caution should be exercised when PRIMAXIN I.M. is administered to a nursing woman.

Pediatric Use

Safety and effectiveness in pediatric patients below the age of 12 years have not been established.

*** Based on patient weight of 50 kg.

ADVERSE REACTIONS

PRIMAXIN I.M.

In 686 patients in multiple dose clinical trials of PRIMAXIN I.M., the following adverse reactions were reported:

Local Adverse Reactions

The most frequent adverse local clinical reaction that was reported as possibly, probably or definitely related to therapy with PRIMAXIN I.M. was pain at the injection site (1.2%).

Systemic Adverse Reactions

The most frequently reported systemic adverse clinical reactions that were reported as possibly, probably, or definitely related to PRIMAXIN I.M. were nausea (0.6%), diarrhea (0.6%), vomiting (0.3%) and rash (0.4%).

Adverse Laboratory Changes

Adverse laboratory changes without regard to drug relationship that were reported during clinical trials were:

Hemic: decreased hemoglobin and hematocrit, eosinophilia, increased and decreased WBC, increased and decreased platelets, decreased erythrocytes, and increased prothrombin time.

Hepatic: increased AST, ALT, alkaline phosphatase, and bilirubin.

Renal: increased BUN and creatinine.

Urinalysis: presence of red blood cells, white blood cells, casts, and bacteria in the urine.

Potential ADVERSE EFFECTS:

In addition, a variety of adverse effects, not observed in clinical trials with PRIMAXIN I.M., have been reported with intravenous administration of PRIMAXIN I.V. (Imipenem and Cilastatin for Injection). Those listed below are to serve as alerting information to physicians.

Systemic Adverse Reactions

The most frequently reported systemic adverse clinical reactions that were reported as possibly, probably, or definitely related to PRIMAXIN I.V. (Imipenem and Cilastatin for Injection) were fever, hypotension, seizures (see PRECAUTIONS), dizziness, pruritus, urticaria, and somnolence.

Additional adverse systemic clinical reactions reported possibly, probably, or definitely drug related or reported since the drug was marketed are listed within each body system in order of decreasing severity: *Gastrointestinal:* pseudomembranous colitis (the onset of pseudomembranous colitis symptoms may occur during or after antibiotic treatment, see WARNINGS), hemorrhagic colitis, hepatitis, jaundice, gastroenteritis, abdominal pain, glossitis, tongue papillar hypertrophy, staining of the teeth and/or tongue, heartburn, pharyngeal pain, increased salivation; *Hematologic:* pancytopenia, bone marrow depression, thrombocytopenia, neutropenia, leukopenia, hemolytic anemia; *CNS:* encephalopathy, tremor, confusion, myoclonus, paresthesia, vertigo, headache, psychic disturbances including hallucinations; *Special Senses:* hearing loss, tinnitus, taste perversion; *Respiratory:* chest discomfort, dyspnea, hyperventilation, thoracic spine pain; *Cardiovascular:* palpitations, tachycardia; *Renal:* acute renal failure, oliguria/anuria, polyuria, urine discoloration; *Skin:* toxic epidermal necrolysis, Stevens-Johnson syndrome, erythema multiforme, angioneurotic edema, flushing, cyanosis, hyperhidrosis, skin texture changes, candidiasis, pruritus vulvae; *Body as a whole:* polyarthralgia, asthenia/weakness, drug fever.

Adverse Laboratory Changes

Adverse laboratory changes without regard to drug relationship that were reported during clinical trials or reported since the drug was marketed were:

Hepatic: increased LDH; *Hemic:* positive Coombs test, decreased neutrophils, agranulocytosis, increased monocytes, abnormal prothrombin time, increased lymphocytes, increased basophils; *Electrolytes:* decreased serum sodium, increased potassium, increased chloride; *Urinalysis:* presence of urine protein, urine bilirubin, and urine urobilinogen.

Lidocaine HCl —Refer to the package circular for lidocaine HCl.

OVERDOSAGE

The acute intravenous toxicity of imipenem-cilastatin sodium in a ratio of 1:1 was studied in mice at doses of 751 to 1359 mg/kg. Following drug administration, ataxia was rapidly produced and clonic convulsions were noted in about 45 minutes. Deaths occurred within 4–56 minutes at all doses.

Continued on next page

Information on the Merck & Co., Inc. products listed on these pages is the full prescribing information from product circulars in use September 30, 2000. For information, please call 1-800-NSC MERCK [1-800-672-6372].

Primaxin I.M.—Cont.

The acute intravenous toxicity of imipenem-cilastatin sodium was produced within 5–10 minutes in rats at doses of 771 to 1583 mg/kg. In all dosage groups, females had decreased activity, bradypnea and ptosis with clonic convulsions preceding death; in males, ptosis was seen at all dose levels while tremors and clonic convulsions were seen at all but the lowest dose (771 mg/kg). In another rat study, female rats showed ataxia, bradypnea and decreased activity in all but the lowest dose (550 mg/kg); deaths were preceded by clonic convulsions. Male rats showed tremors at all doses and clonic convulsions and ptosis were seen at the two highest doses (1130 and 1734 mg/kg). Deaths occurred between 6 and 88 minutes with doses of 771 to 1734 mg/kg.
In the case of overdosage, discontinue PRIMAXIN I.M., treat symptomatically, and institute supportive measures as required. Imipenem-cilastatin sodium is hemodialyzable. However, usefulness of this procedure in the overdosage setting is questionable.

DOSAGE AND ADMINISTRATION

PRIMAXIN I.M. is for intramuscular use only.
The dosage recommendations for PRIMAXIN I.M. represent the quantity of imipenem to be administered. An equivalent amount of cilastatin is also present.
Patients with lower respiratory tract infections, skin and skin structure infections, and gynecologic infections of mild to moderate severity may be treated with 500 mg or 750 mg administered every 12 hours depending on the severity of the infection.
Intra-abdominal infection may be treated with 750 mg every 12 hours.
[See table at top of previous page]
Total daily IM dosages greater than 1500 mg per day are not recommended.
The dosage for any particular patient should be based on the location of and severity of the infection, the susceptibility of the infecting pathogen(s), and renal function.
The duration of therapy depends upon the type and severity of the infection. Generally, PRIMAXIN I.M. should be continued for at least two days after the signs and symptoms of infection have resolved. Safety and efficacy of treatment beyond fourteen days have not been established.
PRIMAXIN I.M. should be administered by deep intramuscular injection into a large muscle mass (such as the gluteal muscles or lateral part of the thigh) with a 21 gauge 2″ needle. Aspiration is necessary to avoid inadvertent injection into a blood vessel.

ADULTS WITH IMPAIRED RENAL FUNCTION
The safety and efficacy of PRIMAXIN I.M. have not been studied in patients with creatinine clearance of less than 20 mL/ min/1.73m². Serum creatinine alone may not be a sufficiently accurate measure of renal function. Creatinine clearance (T_{cc}) may be estimated from the following equation:

$$T_{cc}\text{ (Males)} = \frac{(\text{wt. in kg})\,(140-\text{age})}{(72)\,(\text{creatinine in mg/dL})}$$

$$T_{cc}\text{ (Females)} = 0.85 \times \text{above value}$$

PREPARATION FOR ADMINISTRATION

PRIMAXIN I.M. should be prepared for use with 1.0% lidocaine HCl solution††† (without epinephrine). PRIMAXIN I.M. 500 should be prepared with 2 mL and PRIMAXIN I.M. 750 with 3 mL of lidocaine HCl. Agitate to form a suspension then withdraw and inject the entire contents of vial intramuscularly. The suspension of PRIMAXIN I.M. in lidocaine HCl should be used within one hour after preparation.
Note: The IM formulation is not for IV use.

††† Refer to the package circular for lidocaine HCl for detailed information concerning CONTRAINDICATIONS, WARNINGS, PRECAUTIONS, and ADVERSE REACTIONS.

COMPATIBILITY AND STABILITY

Before reconstitution:
The dry powder should be stored at a temperature below 25°C (77°F).
Suspensions for IM Administration
Suspensions of PRIMAXIN I.M. are white to light tan in color. Variations of color within this range do not affect the potency of the product.
The suspension of PRIMAXIN I.M. in lidocaine HCl should be used within one hour after preparation.
PRIMAXIN I.M. should not be mixed with or physically added to other antibiotics. However, PRIMAXIN I.M. may be administered concomitantly but at separate sites with other antibiotics, such as aminoglycosides.

HOW SUPPLIED

PRIMAXIN I.M. is supplied as a sterile powder mixture in vials for IM administration as follows:
No. 3582—500 mg imipenem equivalent and 500 mg cilastatin equivalent
NDC 0006-3582-75 in trays of 10 vials
(6505-01-337-3131 500 mg, 10's).
No. 3583—750 mg imipenem equivalent and 750 mg cilastatin equivalent
NDC 0006-3583-76 in trays of 10 vials
(6505-01-337-3130 750 mg, 10's).

REFERENCES

1. National Committee for Clinical Laboratory Standards, Methods for Dilution Antimicrobial Susceptibility Tests for Bacteria that Grow Aerobically—Fourth Edition. Approved Standard NCCLS Document M7-A4, Vol. 17, No. 2 NCCLS, Villanova, PA, 1997.
2. National Committee for Clinical Laboratory Standards, Performance Standards for Antimicrobial Disk Susceptibility Tests—Sixth Edition. Approved Standard NCCLS Document M2-A6, Vol. 17, No. 1 NCCLS, Villanova, PA, 1997.
3. National Committee for Clinical Laboratory Standards, Method for Antimicrobial Susceptibility Testing of Anaerobic Bacteria—Third Edition. Approved Standard NCCLS Document M11-A3, Vol. 13, No. 26 NCCLS, Villanova, PA, 1993.

7632908 Issued February 1999

PRIMAXIN® I.V. ℞
(Imipenem and Cilastatin for Injection)
For Intravenous Injection Only

DESCRIPTION

PRIMAXIN† I.V. (Imipenem and Cilastatin for Injection) is a sterile formulation of imipenem (a thienamycin antibiotic) and cilastatin sodium (the inhibitor of the renal dipeptidase, dehydropeptidase I), with sodium bicarbonate added as a buffer. PRIMAXIN I.V. is a potent broad spectrum antibacterial agent for intravenous administration.
Imipenem (N-formimidoylthienamycin monohydrate) is a crystalline derivative of thienamycin, which is produced by *Streptomyces cattleya.* Its chemical name is (5*R* ,6*S*)-3-[[2-(formimidoylamino)ethyl]thio]-6-[(*R*)-1-hydroxyethyl]-7-oxo-1-azabicyclo[3.2.0]hept-2-ene-2-carboxylic acid monohydrate. It is an off-white, nonhygroscopic crystalline compound with a molecular weight of 317.37. It is sparingly soluble in water and slightly soluble in methanol. Its empirical formula is $C_{12}H_{17}N_3O_4S \cdot H_2O$, and its structural formula is:

Cilastatin sodium is the sodium salt of a derivatized heptenoic acid. Its chemical name is sodium (*Z*)-7-[[(*R*)-2-amino-2-carboxyethyl]thio] -2- [(*S*) - 2,2- dimethylcyclopropanecarboxamido]-2-heptenoate. It is an off-white to yellowish-white, hygroscopic, amorphous compound with a molecular weight of 380.43. It is very soluble in water and in methanol. Its empirical formula is $C_{16}H_{25}N_2O_5S$ Na, and its structural formula is:

PRIMAXIN I.V. is buffered to provide solutions in the pH range of 6.5 to 8.5. There is no significant change in pH when solutions are prepared and used as directed. (See **COMPATIBILITY AND STABILITY.**) PRIMAXIN I.V. 250 contains 18.8 mg of sodium (0.8 mEq) and PRIMAXIN I.V. 500 contains 37.5 mg of sodium (1.6 mEq). Solutions of PRIMAXIN I.V. range from colorless to yellow. Variations of color within this range do not affect the potency of the product.

† Registered trademark of MERCK & CO., INC.

CLINICAL PHARMACOLOGY

Adults
Intravenous Administration
Intravenous infusion of PRIMAXIN I.V. over 20 minutes results in peak plasma levels of imipenem antimicrobial activity that range from 14 to 24 µg/mL for the 250 mg dose, from 21 to 58 µg/mL for the 500 mg dose, and from 41 to 83 µg/mL for the 1000 mg dose. At these doses, plasma levels of imipenem antimicrobial activity decline to below 1 µg/mL or less in 4 to 6 hours. Peak plasma levels of cilastatin following a 20-minute intravenous infusion of PRIMAXIN I.V., range from 15 to 25 µg/mL for the 250 mg dose, from 31 to 49 µg/mL for the 500 mg dose, and from 56 to 88 µg/mL for the 1000 mg dose.
The plasma half-life of each component is approximately 1 hour. The binding of imipenem to human serum proteins is approximately 20% and that of cilastatin is approximately 40%. Approximately, 70% of the administered imipenem is recovered in the urine within 10 hours after which no further urinary excretion is detectable. Urine concentrations of imipenem in excess of 10 µg/mL can be maintained for up to 8 hours with PRIMAXIN I.V. at the 500-mg dose. Approximately, 70% of the cilastatin sodium dose is recovered in the urine within 10 hours of administration of PRIMAXIN I.V.
No accumulation of imipenem/cilastastin in plasma or urine is observed with regimens administered as frequently as every 6 hours in patients with normal renal function.
Imipenem, when administered alone, is metabolized in the kidneys by dehydropeptidase I resulting in relatively low levels in urine. Cilastatin sodium, an inhibitor of this enzyme, effectively prevents renal metabolism of imipenem so that when imipenem and cilastatin sodium are given concomitantly, fully adequate antibacterial levels of imipenem are achieved in the urine.
After a 1 gram dose of PRIMAXIN I.V., the following average levels of imipenem were measured (usually at 1 hour post-dose except where indicated) in the tissues and fluids listed:
[See table below]
Imipenem-cilastatin sodium is hemodialyzable. However, usefulness of this procedure in the overdosage setting is questionable. (See **OVERDOSAGE.**)
Microbiology
The bactericidal activity of imipenem results from the inhibition of cell wall synthesis. Its greatest affinity is for penicillin binding proteins (PBPs) 1A, 1B, 2, 4, 5 and 6 of *Escherichia coli,* and 1A, 1B, 2, 4 and 5 of *Pseudomonas aeruginosa.* The lethal effect is related to binding to PBP 2 and PBP 1B.
Imipenem has a high degree of stability in the presence of beta-lactamases, both penicillinases and cephalosporinases produced by gram-negative and gram-positive bacteria. It is a potent inhibitor of beta-lactamases from certain gram-negative bacteria which are inherently resistant to most beta-lactam antibiotics, e.g., *Pseudomonas aeruginosa, Serratia* spp., and *Enterobacter* spp.
Imipenem has *in vitro* activity against a wide range of gram-positive and gram-negative organisms. Imipenem has been shown to be active against most strains of the following microorganisms, both *in vitro* and in clinical infections treated with the intravenous formulation of imipenem-cilastatin sodium as described in the **INDICATIONS AND USAGE** section.
Gram-positive aerobes:
Enterococcus faecalis (formerly *S. faecalis*)
(NOTE: Imipenem is inactive *in vitro* against *Enterococcus faecium* [formerly *S. faecium*].)
Staphylococcus aureus including penicillinase-producing strains
Staphylococcus epidermidis including penicillinase-producing strains
(NOTE: Methicillin-resistant staphylococci should be reported as resistant to imipenem.)
Streptococcus agalactiae (Group B streptococci)
Streptococcus pneumoniae
Streptococcus pyogenes

Tissue or Fluid	n	Imipenem Level µg/mL or µg/g	Range
Vitreous Humor	3	3.4 (3.5 hours post dose)	2.88–3.6
Aqueous Humor	5	2.99 (2 hours post dose)	2.4–3.9
Lung Tissue	8	5.6 (median)	3.5–15.5
Sputum	1	2.1	—
Pleural	1	22.0	—
Peritoneal	12	23.9 S.D. ±5.3 (2 hours post dose)	—
Bile	2	5.3 (2.25 hours post dose)	4.6 to 6.0
CSF (uninflamed)	5	1.0 (4 hours post dose)	0.26–2.0
CSF (inflamed)	7	2.6 (2 hours post dose)	0.5–5.5
Fallopian Tubes	1	13.6	—
Endometrium	1	11.1	—
Myometrium	1	5.0	—
Bone	10	2.6	0.4–5.4
Interstitial Fluid	12	16.4	10.0–22.6
Skin	12	4.4	NA
Fascia	12	4.4	NA

Gram-negative aerobes:
Acinetobacter spp.
Citrobacter spp.
Enterobacter spp.
Escherichia coli
Gardnerella vaginalis
Haemophilus influenzae
Haemophilus parainfluenzae
Klebsiella spp.
Morganella morganii
Proteus vulgaris
Providencia rettgeri
Pseudomonas aeruginosa
(NOTE: Imipenem is inactive *in vitro* against *Xanthomonas (Pseudomonas) maltophilia* and some strains of *P. cepacia.*)
Serratia spp., including *S. marcescens*
Gram-positive anaerobes:
Bifidobacterium spp.
Clostridium spp.
Eubacterium spp.
Peptococcus spp.
Peptostreptococcus spp.
Propionibacterium spp.
Gram-negative anaerobes:
Bacteroides spp., including *B. fragilis*
Fusobacterium spp.

The following *in vitro* data are available, **but their clinical significance is unknown.**
Imipenem exhibits *in vitro* minimum inhibitory concentrations (MICs) of 4 μg/mL or less against most (≥90%) strains of the following microorganisms; however, the safety and effectiveness of imipenem in treating clinical infections due to these microorganisms have not been established in adequate and well-controlled clinical trials.
Gram-positive aerobes:
Bacillus spp.
Listeria monocytogenes
Nocardia spp.
Staphylococcus saprophyticus
Group C streptococci
Group G streptococci
Viridans group streptococci
Gram-negative aerobes:
Aeromonas hydrophila
Alcaligenes spp.
Capnocytophaga spp.
Haemophilus ducreyi
Neisseria gonorrhoeae including penicillinase-producing strains
Pasteurella spp.
Providencia stuartii
Gram-negative anaerobes:
Prevotella bivia
Prevotella disiens
Prevotella melaninogenica
Veillonella spp.

In vitro tests show imipenem to act synergistically with aminoglycoside antibiotics against some isolates of *Pseudomonas aeruginosa.*
Susceptibility Tests:
Measurement of MIC or minimum bactericidal concentration (MBC) and achieved antimicrobial compound concentrations may be appropriate to guide therapy in some infections. (See **CLINICAL PHARMACOLOGY** section for further information on drug concentrations achieved in infected body sites and other pharmacokinetic properties of this antimicrobial drug product.)
Dilution Techniques:
Quantitative methods that are used to determine MICs provide reproducible estimates of the susceptibility of bacteria to antimicrobial compounds. One such procedure uses a standardized dilution method[1] (broth, agar, or microdilution) or equivalent with imipenem powder.
The MIC values obtained should be interpreted according to the following criteria:

MIC (μg/mL)	Interpretation
≤4	Susceptible (S)
8	Intermediate (I)
≥16	Resistant (R)

A report of "Susceptible" indicates that the pathogen is likely to be inhibited by usually achievable concentrations of the antimicrobial compound in blood. A report of "Intermediate" indicates that the result should be considered equivocal, and, if the microorganism is not fully susceptible to alternative, clinically feasible drugs, the test should be repeated. This category implies possible clinical applicability in body sites where the drug is physiologically concentrated or in situations where high dosage of drug can be used. This category also provides a buffer zone that prevents small uncontrolled technical factors from causing major discrepancies in interpretation. A report of "Resistant" indicates that usually achievable concentrations of the antimicrobial compound in the blood are unlikely to be inhibitory and that other therapy should be selected.
Standardized susceptibility test procedures require the use of laboratory control microorganisms. Standard imipenem powder should provide the following MIC values:

Microorganism	MIC (μg/mL)
E. coli ATCC 25922	0.06–0.25
S. aureus ATCC 29213	0.015–0.06
E. faecalis ATCC 29212	0.5–2.0
P. aeruginosa ATCC 27853	1.0–4.0

Diffusion Techniques:
Quantitative methods that require measurement of zone diameters provide reproducible estimates of the susceptibility of bacteria to antimicrobial compounds. One such standardized procedure[2] that has been recommended for use with disks to test the susceptibility of microorganisms to imipenem uses the 10-μg imipenem disk. Interpretation involves correlation of the diameter obtained in the disk test with the MIC for imipenem.
Reports from the laboratory providing results of the standard single-disk susceptibility test with a 10-μg imipenem disk should be interpreted according to the following criteria:

Zone Diameter (mm)	Interpretation
≥16	Susceptible (S)
14–15	Intermediate (I)
≤13	Resistant (R)

Interpretation should be as stated above for results using dilution techniques.
Standardized susceptibility test procedures require the use of laboratory control microorganisms. The 10-μg imipenem disk should provide the following diameters in these laboratory test quality control strains:

Microorganism	Zone Diameter (mm)
E. coli ATCC 25922	26–32
P. aeruginosa ATCC 27853	20–28

Anaerobic techniques:
For anaerobic bacteria, the susceptibility to imipenem can be determined by the reference agar dilution method or by alternate standardized test methods.[3]
The MIC values obtained should be interpreted according to the following criteria:

MIC (μg/mL)	Interpretation
≤4	Susceptible (S)
8	Intermediate (I)
≥16	Resistant (R)

As with other susceptibility techniques, the use of laboratory control microorganisms is required. Standard imipenem powder should provide the following MIC values:
Reference Agar Dilution Testing:

Microorganism	MIC (μg/mL)
B. fragilis ATCC 25285	0.03–0.12
B. thetaiotaomicron ATCC 29741	0.06–0.25
E. lentum ATCC 43055	0.25–1.0

Broth Microdilution Testing:

Microorganism	MIC (μg/mL)
B. thetaiotaomicron ATCC 29741	0.06–0.25
E. lentum ATCC 43055	0.12–0.5

INDICATIONS AND USAGE

PRIMAXIN I.V. is indicated for the treatment of serious infections caused by susceptible strains of the designated microorganisms in the conditions listed below:
(1) **Lower respiratory tract infections.** *Staphylococcus aureus* (penicillinase-producing strains), *Acinetobacter* species, *Enterobacter* species, *Escherichia coli, Haemophilus influenzae, Haemophilus parainfluenzae*, Klebsiella* species, *Serratia marcescens*
(2) **Urinary tract infections** (complicated and uncomplicated). *Enterococcus faecalis, Staphylococcus aureus* (penicillinase-producing strains)*, *Enterobacter* species, *Escherichia coli, Klebsiella* species, *Morganella morganii*, Proteus vulgaris*, Providencia rettgeri*, Pseudomonas aeruginosa*
(3) **Intra-abdominal infections.** *Enterococcus faecalis, Staphylococcus aureus* (penicillinase-producing strains)*, *Staphylococcus epidermidis, Citrobacter* species, *Enterobacter* species, *Escherichia coli, Klebsiella* species, *Morganella morganii*, Proteus* species, *Pseudomonas aeruginosa, Bifidobacterium* species, *Clostridium* species, *Eubacterium* species, *Peptococcus* species, *Peptostreptococcus* species, *Propionibacterium* species*, *Bacteroides* species including *B. fragilis, Fusobacterium* species
(4) **Gynecologic infections.** *Enterococcus faecalis, Staphylococcus aureus* (penicillinase-producing strains)*, *Staphylococcus epidermidis, Streptococcus agalactiae* (Group B streptococci), *Enterobacter* species*, *Escherichia coli, Gardnerella vaginalis, Klebsiella* species*, *Proteus* species, *Bifidobacterium* species*, *Peptococcus* species*, *Peptostreptococcus* species, *Propionibacterium* species*, *Bacteroides* species including *B. fragilis**
(5) **Bacterial septicemia.** *Enterococcus faecalis, Staphylococcus aureus* (penicillinase-producing strains), *Enterobacter* species, *Escherichia coli, Klebsiella* species, *Pseudomonas aeruginosa, Serratia* species*, *Bacteroides* species including *B. fragilis**
(6) **Bone and joint infections.** *Enterococcus faecalis, Staphylococcus aureus* (penicillinase-producing strains), *Staphylococcus epidermidis, Enterobacter* species, *Pseudomonas aeruginosa*
(7) **Skin and skin structure infections.** *Enterococcus faecalis, Staphylococcus aureus* (penicillinase-producing strains), *Staphylococcus epidermidis, Acinetobacter* species, *Citrobacter* species, *Enterobacter* species, *Escherichia coli, Klebsiella* species, *Morganella morganii, Proteus vulgaris, Providencia rettgeri*, Pseudomonas aeruginosa, Serratia* species, *Peptococcus* species, *Peptostreptococcus* species, *Bacteroides* species including *B. fragilis, Fusobacterium* species*
(8) **Endocarditis.** *Staphylococcus aureus* (penicillinase-producing strains)
(9) **Polymicrobic infections.** PRIMAXIN I.V. is indicated for polymicrobic infections including those in which *S. pneumoniae* (pneumonia, septicemia), *S. pyogenes* (skin and skin structure), or nonpenicillinase-producing *S. aureus* is one of the causative organisms. However, monobacterial infections due to these organisms are usually treated with narrower spectrum antibiotics, such as penicillin G.

PRIMAXIN I.V. is not indicated in patients with meningitis because safety and efficacy have not been established.
For Pediatric Use information, See **PRECAUTIONS**, *Pediatric Use*, and **DOSAGE AND ADMINISTRATION** sections.
Because of its broad spectrum of bactericidal activity against gram-positive and gram-negative aerobic and anaerobic bacteria, PRIMAXIN I.V. is useful for the treatment of mixed infections and as presumptive therapy prior to the identification of the causative organisms.
Although clinical improvement has been observed in patients with cystic fibrosis, chronic pulmonary disease, and lower respiratory tract infections caused by *Pseudomonas aeruginosa,* bacterial eradication may not necessarily be achieved.
As with other beta-lactam antibiotics, some strains of *Pseudomonas aeruginosa* may develop resistance fairly rapidly during treatment with PRIMAXIN I.V. During therapy of *Pseudomonas aeruginosa* infections, periodic susceptibility testing should be done when clinically appropriate.
Infections resistant to other antibiotics, for example, cephalosporins, penicillin, and aminoglycosides, have been shown to respond to treatment with PRIMAXIN I.V.

*Efficacy for this organism in this organ system was studied in fewer than 10 infections.

CONTRAINDICATIONS

PRIMAXIN I.V. is contraindicated in patients who have shown hypersensitivity to any component of this product.

WARNINGS

SERIOUS AND OCCASIONALLY FATAL HYPERSENSITIVITY (ANAPHYLACTIC) REACTIONS HAVE BEEN REPORTED IN PATIENTS RECEIVING THERAPY WITH BETA-LACTAMS. THESE REACTIONS ARE MORE APT TO OCCUR IN PERSONS WITH A HISTORY OF SENSITIVITY TO MULTIPLE ALLERGENS.
THERE HAVE BEEN REPORTS OF PATIENTS WITH A HISTORY OF PENICILLIN HYPERSENSITIVITY WHO HAVE EXPERIENCED SEVERE HYPERSENSITIVITY REACTIONS WHEN TREATED WITH ANOTHER BETA-LACTAM. BEFORE INITIATING THERAPY WITH PRIMAXIN I.V., CAREFUL INQUIRY SHOULD BE MADE CONCERNING PREVIOUS HYPERSENSITIVITY REACTIONS TO PENICILLINS, CEPHALOSPORINS, OTHER BETA-LACTAMS, AND OTHER ALLERGENS. IF AN ALLERGIC REACTION OCCURS, PRIMAXIN SHOULD BE DISCONTINUED.
SERIOUS ANAPHYLACTIC REACTIONS REQUIRE IMMEDIATE EMERGENCY TREATMENT WITH EPINEPHRINE. OXYGEN, INTRAVENOUS STEROIDS, AND AIRWAY MANAGEMENT, INCLUDING INTUBATION, MAY ALSO BE ADMINISTERED AS INDICATED.
Seizures and other CNS adverse experiences, such as confusional states and myoclonic activity, have been reported during treatment with PRIMAXIN I.V. (See **PRECAUTIONS.**)
Pseudomembranous colitis has been reported with nearly all antibacterial agents, including imipenem-cilastatin sodium, and may range in severity from mild to life threatening. Therefore, it is important to consider this diagnosis in patients who present with diarrhea subsequent to the administration of antibacterial agents.
Treatment with antibacterial agents alters the normal flora of the colon and may permit overgrowth of clostridia. Studies indicate that a toxin produced by *Clostridium difficile* is one primary cause of "antibiotic-associated colitis".
After the diagnosis of pseudomembranous colitis has been established, therapeutic measures should be initiated. Mild cases of pseudomembranous colitis usually respond to drug discontinuation alone. In moderate to severe cases, consideration should be given to management with fluids and electrolytes, protein supplementation and treatment with an antibacterial drug clinically effective against *C. difficile* colitis.

Continued on next page

Information on the Merck & Co., Inc. products listed on these pages is the full prescribing information from product circulars in use September 30, 2000. For information, please call 1-800-NSC MERCK [1-800-672-6372].

Primaxin I.V.—Cont.

PRECAUTIONS

General

CNS adverse experiences such as confusional states, myoclonic activity, and seizures have been reported during treatment with PRIMAXIN I.V., especially when recommended dosages were exceeded. These experiences have occurred most commonly in patients with CNS disorders (e.g., brain lesions or history of seizures) and/or compromised renal function. However, there have been reports of CNS adverse experiences in patients who had no recognized or documented underlying CNS disorder or compromised renal function.

When recommended doses were exceeded, adult patients with creatinine clearances of ≤20 mL/min/1.73 m^2, whether or not undergoing hemodialysis, had a higher risk of seizure activity than those without impairment of renal function. Therefore, close adherence to the dosing guidelines for these patients is recommended. (See **DOSAGE AND ADMINISTRATION**.)

Patients with creatinine clearances of ≤5 mL/min/1.73 m^2 should not receive PRIMAXIN I.V. unless hemodialysis is instituted within 48 hours.

For patients on hemodialysis, PRIMAXIN I.V. is recommended only when the benefit outweighs the potential risk of seizures.

Close adherence to the recommended dosage and dosage schedules is urged, especially in patients with known factors that predispose to convulsive activity. Anticonvulsant therapy should be continued in patients with known seizure disorders. If focal tremors, myoclonus, or seizures occur, patients should be evaluated neurologically, placed on anticonvulsant therapy if not already instituted, and the dosage of PRIMAXIN I.V. re-examined to determine whether it should be decreased or the antibiotic discontinued.

As with other antibiotics, prolonged use of PRIMAXIN I.V. may result in overgrowth of nonsusceptible organisms. Repeated evaluation of the patient's condition is essential. If superinfection occurs during therapy, appropriate measures should be taken.

Laboratory Tests

While PRIMAXIN I.V. possesses the characteristic low toxicity of the beta-lactam group of antibiotics, periodic assessment of organ system functions, including renal, hepatic, and hematopoietic, is advisable during prolonged therapy.

Drug Interactions

Generalized seizures have been reported in patients who received ganciclovir and PRIMAXIN. These drugs should not be used concomitantly unless the potential benefits outweigh the risks.

Since concomitant administration of PRIMAXIN and probenecid results in only minimal increases in plasma levels of imipenem and plasma half-life, it is not recommended that probenecid be given with PRIMAXIN.

PRIMAXIN should not be mixed with or physically added to other antibiotics. However, PRIMAXIN may be administered concomitantly with other antibiotics, such as aminoglycosides.

Carcinogenesis, Mutagenesis, Impairment of Fertility

Long term studies in animals have not been performed to evaluate carcinogenic potential of imipenem-cilastatin. Genetic toxicity studies were performed in a variety of bacterial and mammalian tests in *in vivo* and *in vitro*. The tests used were: V79 mammalian cell mutagenesis assay (imipenem-cilastatin sodium alone and imipenem alone), Ames test (cilastatin sodium alone and imipenem alone), unscheduled DNA synthesis assay (imipenem-cilastatin sodium) and *in vivo* mouse cytogenetics test (imipenem-cilastatin sodium). None of these tests showed any evidence of genetic alterations.

Reproductive tests in male and female rats were performed with imipenem-cilastatin sodium at dosage levels up to 11 times†† the usual human dose of the intravenous formulation (on a mg/kg basis). Slight decreases in live fetal body weight were restricted to the highest dosage level. No other adverse effects were observed on fertility, reproductive performance, fetal viability, growth or postnatal development of pups. Similarly, no adverse effects on the fetus or on lactation were observed when imipenem-cilastatin sodium was administered to rats late in gestation.

Pregnancy: Teratogenic Effects

Pregnancy Category C: Teratology studies with cilastatin sodium in rabbits and rats at 6 and 20 times†† the maximum recommended human dose of the intravenous formulation of imipenem-cilastatin sodium (50 mg/kg/day††), respectively, showed no evidence of adverse effect on the fetus. No evidence of teratogenicity was observed in rabbits and rats given imipenem at doses up to 1 and 18 times†† the maximum recommended daily human dose of the intravenous formulation of imipenem-cilastatin sodium, respectively.

Teratology studies with imipenem-cilastatin sodium at doses up to 11 times†† the usual recommended human dose of the intravenous formulation (30 mg/kg/day††) in pregnant mice and rats during the period of major organogenesis revealed no evidence of teratogenicity.

Imipenem-cilastatin sodium, when administered to pregnant rabbits at dosages equivalent to the usual human dose of the intravenous formulation and higher, caused body weight loss, diarrhea, and maternal deaths. When comparable doses of imipenem-cilastatin sodium were given to non-pregnant rabbits, body weight loss, diarrhea, and deaths were also observed. This intolerance is not unlike that seen with other beta-lactam antibiotics in this species and is probably due to alteration of gut flora.

A teratology study in pregnant cynomolgus monkeys given imipenem-cilastatin sodium at doses of 40 mg/kg/day (bolus intravenous injection) or 160 mg/kg/day (subcutaneous injection) resulted in maternal toxicity including emesis, inappetence, body weight loss, diarrhea, abortion, and death in some cases. In contrast, no significant toxicity was observed when non-pregnant cynomolgus monkeys were given doses of imipenem-cilastatin sodium up to 180 mg/kg/day (subcutaneous injection). When doses of imipenem-cilastatin sodium (approximately 100 mg/kg/day or approximately 2 times†† the maximum recommended daily human dose of the intravenous formulation) were administered to pregnant cynomolgus monkeys at an intravenous infusion rate which mimics human clinical use, there was minimal maternal intolerance (occasional emesis), no maternal deaths, no evidence of teratogenicity, but an increase in embryonic loss relative to control groups.

There are, however, no adequate and well-controlled studies in pregnant women. PRIMAXIN I.V. should be used during pregnancy only if the potential benefit justifies the potential risk to the mother and fetus.

Nursing Mothers

It is not known whether imipenem-cilastatin sodium is excreted in human milk. Because many drugs are excreted in human milk, caution should be exercised when PRIMAXIN I.V. is administered to a nursing woman.

Pediatric Use

Use of PRIMAXIN I.V. in pediatric patients, neonates to 16 years of age, is supported by evidence from adequate and well-controlled studies of PRIMAXIN I.V. in adults and by the following clinical studies and published literature in pediatric patients: Based on published studies of 178** pediatric patients ≥3 months of age (with non-CNS infections), the recommended dose of PRIMAXIN I.V. is 15–25 mg/kg/dose administered every six hours. Doses of 25 mg/kg/dose in patients 3 months to <3 years of age, and 15 mg/kg/dose in patients 3–12 years of age were associated with mean trough plasma concentrations of imipenem of 1.1±0.4 µg/mL and 0.6±0.2 µg/mL following multiple 60-minute infusions, respectively; trough urinary concentrations of imipenem were in excess of 10 µg/mL for both doses. These doses have provided adequate plasma and urine concentrations for the treatment of non-CNS infections. Based on studies in adults, the maximum daily dose for treatment of infections with fully susceptible organisms is 2.0 g per day, and of infections with moderately susceptible organisms (primarily some strains of *P. aeruginosa*) is 4.0 g/day. (See Table 1, **DOSAGE AND ADMINISTRATION**.) Higher doses (up to 90 mg/kg/day in older children) have been used in patients with cystic fibrosis. (See **DOSAGE AND ADMINISTRATION**.)

Based on studies of 135*** pediatric patients ≤3 months of age (weighing ≥1,500 gms), the following dosage schedule is recommended for non-CNS infections:

<1 wk of age: 25 mg/kg every 12 hrs
1–4 wks of age: 25 mg/kg every 8 hrs
4 wks-3 mos. of age: 25 mg/kg every 6 hrs.

In a published dose-ranging study of smaller premature infants (670–1,890 gms) in the first week of life, a dose of 20 mg/kg q12h by 15–30 minutes infusion was associated with mean peak and trough plasma imipenem concentrations of 43 µg/mL and 1.7 µg/mL after multiple doses, respectively. However, moderate accumulation of cilastatin in neonates may occur following multiple doses of PRIMAXIN I.V. The safety of this accumulation is unknown.

PRIMAXIN I.V. is not recommended in pediatric patients with CNS infections because of the risk of seizures.

PRIMAXIN I.V. is not recommended in pediatric patients <30 kg with impaired renal function, as no data are available.

†† Based on patient weight of 70 kg.
** Two patients were less than 3 months of age.
*** One patient was greater than 3 months of age.

ADVERSE REACTIONS

Adults

PRIMAXIN I.V. is generally well tolerated. Many of the 1,723 patients treated in clinical trials were severely ill and had multiple background diseases and physiological impairments, making it difficult to determine causal relationship of adverse experiences to therapy with PRIMAXIN I.V.

Local Adverse Reactions

Adverse local clinical reactions that were reported as possibly, probably or definitely related to therapy with PRIMAXIN I.V. were:

Phlebitis/thrombophlebitis—3.1%
Pain at the injection site—0.7%
Erythema at the injection site—0.4%
Vein induration—0.2%
Infused vein infection—0.1%

Systemic Adverse Reactions

The most frequently reported systemic adverse clinical reactions that were reported as possibly, probably, or definitely related to PRIMAXIN I.V. were nausea (2.0%), diarrhea (1.8%), vomiting (1.5%), rash (0.9%), fever (0.5%), hypotension (0.4%), seizures (0.4%) (see **PRECAUTIONS**), dizziness (0.3%), pruritus (0.3%), urticaria (0.2%), somnolence (0.2%).

Additional adverse systemic clinical reactions reported as possibly, probably or definitely drug related occurring in less than 0.2% of the patients or reported since the drug was marketed are listed within each body system in order of decreasing severity: *Gastrointestinal* —pseudomembranous colitis (the onset of pseudomembranous colitis symptoms may occur during or after antibacterial treatment, see **WARNINGS**), hemorrhagic colitis, hepatitis, jaundice, gastroenteritis, abdominal pain, glossitis, tongue papillar hypertrophy, staining of the teeth and/or tongue, heartburn, pharyngeal pain, increased salivation; *Hematologic* —pancytopenia, bone marrow depression, thrombocytopenia, neutropenia, leukopenia, hemolytic anemia; *CNS* —encephalopathy, tremor, confusion, myoclonus, paresthesia, vertigo, headache, psychic disturbances including hallucinations; *Special Senses* —hearing loss, tinnitus, taste perversion; *Respiratory* —chest discomfort, dyspnea, hyperventilation, thoracic spine pain; *Cardiovascular* —palpitations, tachycardia; *Skin* —Stevens-Johnson syndrome, toxic epidermal necrolysis, erythema multiforme, angioneurotic edema, flushing, cyanosis, hyperhidrosis, skin texture changes, candidiasis, pruritus vulvae; *Body as a whole* —polyarthralgia, asthenia/weakness, drug fever; *Renal* —acute renal failure, oliguria/anuria, polyuria, urine discoloration. The role of PRIMAXIN I.V. in changes in renal function is difficult to assess, since factors predisposing to pre-renal azotemia or to impaired renal function usually have been present.

Adverse Laboratory Changes

Adverse laboratory changes without regard to drug relationship that were reported during clinical trials or reported since the drug was marketed were:

Hepatic: Increased ALT (SGPT), AST (SGOT), alkaline phosphatase, bilirubin and LDH

Hemic: Increased eosinophils, positive Coombs test, increased WBC, increased platelets, decreased hemoglobin and hematocrit, agranulocytosis, increased monocytes, abnormal prothrombin time, increased lymphocytes, increased basophils

Electrolytes: Decreased serum sodium, increased potassium, increased chloride

Renal: Increased BUN, creatinine

Urinalysis: Presence of urine protein, urine red blood cells, urine white blood cells, urine casts, urine bilirubin, and urine urobilinogen

Pediatric Patients

In studies of 178 pediatric patients ≥3 months of age, the following adverse events were noted:

The Most Common Clinical Adverse Experiences Without Regard to Drug Relationship
(Patient Incidence >1%)

Adverse Experience	No. of Patients (%)
Digestive System	
Diarrhea	7* (3.9)
Gastroenteritis	2 (1.1)
Vomiting	2* (1.1)
Skin	
Rash	4 (2.2)
Irritation, I.V. site	2 (1.1)
Urogenital System	
Urine discoloration	2 (1.1)
Cardiovascular System	
Phlebitis	4 (2.2)

*One patient had both vomiting and diarrhea and is counted in each category.

In studies of 135 patients (newborn to 3 months of age), the following adverse events were noted:

The Most Common Clinical Adverse Experiences Without Regard to Drug Relationship
(Patient Incidence >1%)

Adverse Experience	No. of Patients (%)
Digestive System	
Diarrhea	4 (3.0%)
Oral Candidiasis	2 (1.5%)
Skin	
Rash	2 (1.5%)
Urogenital System	
Oliguria/anuria	3 (2.2%)
Cardiovascular System	
Tachycardia	2 (1.5%)
Nervous System	
Convulsions	8 (5.9%)

[See first table at top of next page]

Patients (<3 Months of Age) With Normal Pretherapy but Abnormal During Therapy Laboratory Values

Laboratory Parameter	No. of Patients With Abnormalities* (%)
Eosinophil Count ↑	11 (9.0%)
Hematocrit ↓	3 (2.0%)
Hematocrit ↑	1 (1.0%)
Platelet Count ↑	5 (4.0%)
Platelet Count ↓	2 (2.0%)
Serum Creatinine ↑	5 (5.0%)
Bilirubin ↑	3 (3.0%)
Bilirubin ↓	1 (1.0%)
AST (SGOT) ↑	5 (6.0%)
ALT (SGPT) ↑	3 (3.0%)
Serum Alkaline Phosphate ↑	2 (3.0%)

*The denominator used for percentages was the number of patients for whom the test was performed during or post-treatment and, therefore, varies by test.

Examination of published literature and spontaneous adverse event reports suggested a similar spectrum of adverse events in adult and pediatric patients.

OVERDOSAGE

The acute intravenous toxicity of imipenem-cilastatin sodium in a ratio of 1:1 was studied in mice at doses of 751 to 1359 mg/kg. Following drug administration, ataxia was rapidly produced and clonic convulsions were noted in about 45 minutes. Deaths occurred within 4–56 minutes at all doses. The acute intravenous toxicity of imipenem-cilastatin sodium was produced within 5–10 minutes in rats at doses of 771 to 1583 mg/kg. In all dosage groups, females had decreased activity, bradypnea, and ptosis with clonic convulsions preceding death; in males, ptosis was seen at all dose levels while tremors and clonic convulsions were seen at all but the lowest dose (771 mg/kg). In another rat study, female rats showed ataxia, bradypnea, and decreased activity in all but the lowest dose (550 mg/kg); deaths were preceded by clonic convulsions. Male rats showed tremors at all doses and clonic convulsions, and ptosis were seen at the two highest doses (1130 and 1734 mg/kg). Deaths occurred between 6 and 88 minutes with doses of 771 to 1734 mg/kg. In the case of overdosage, discontinue PRIMAXIN I.V., treat symptomatically, and institute supportive measures as required. Imipenem-cilastatin sodium is hemodialyzable. However, usefulness of this procedure in the overdosage setting is questionable.

DOSAGE AND ADMINISTRATION

Adults

The dosage recommendations for PRIMAXIN I.V. represent the quantity of imipenem to be administered. An equivalent amount of cilastatin is also present in the solution. Each 125 mg, 250 mg, or 500 mg dose should be given by intravenous administration over 20 to 30 minutes. Each 750 mg or 1000 mg dose should be infused over 40 to 60 minutes. In patients who develop nausea during the infusion, the rate of infusion may be slowed.

The total daily dosage for PRIMAXIN I.V. should be based on the type or severity of infection and given in equally divided doses based on consideration of degree of susceptibility of the pathogen(s), renal function, and body weight. Adult patients with impaired renal function, as judged by creatinine clearance ≤ 70 mL/min/1.73 m^2, require adjustment of dosage as described in the succeeding section of these guidelines.

Intravenous Dosage Schedule for Adults with Normal Renal Function and Body Weight ≥70 kg

Doses cited in Table I are based on a patient with normal renal function and a body weight of 70 kg. These doses should be used for a patient with a creatinine clearance of ≥71 mL/min/1.73 m^2 and a body weight of ≥70 kg. A reduction in dose must be made for a patient with a creatinine clearance ≤70 mL/min/1.73 m^2 and/or a body weight less than 70 kg. (See Tables II and III.)

Dosage regimens in column A of Table I are recommended for infections caused by fully susceptible organisms which represent the majority of pathogenic species. Dosage regimens in column B of Table I are recommended for infections caused by organisms with moderate susceptibility to imipenem, primarily some strains of *P. aeruginosa.*

TABLE I
INTRAVENOUS DOSAGE SCHEDULE FOR ADULTS WITH NORMAL RENAL FUNCTION AND BODY WEIGHT ≥ 70 kg

Type or Severity of Infection	A Fully susceptible organisms including gram-positive and gram-negative aerobes and anaerobes	B Moderately susceptible organisms, primarily some strains of *P. aeruginosa*
Mild	250 mg q6h (TOTAL DAILY DOSE=1.0g)	500 mg q6h (TOTAL DAILY DOSE=2.0g)
Moderate	500 mg q8h (TOTAL DAILY DOSE =1.5g) or 500 mg q6h (TOTAL DAILY DOSE=2.0g)	500 mg q6h (TOTAL DAILY DOSE=2.0g) or 1 g q8h (TOTAL DAILY DOSE=3.0g)
Severe, life threatening only	500 mg q6h (TOTAL DAILY DOSE=2.0g)	1 g q8h (TOTAL DAILY DOSE=3.0g) or 1 g q6h (TOTAL DAILY DOSE=4.0g)
Uncomplicated urinary tract infection	250 mg q6h (TOTAL DAILY DOSE=1.0g)	250 mg q6h (TOTAL DAILY DOSE=1.0g)
Complicated urinary tract infection	500 mg q6h (TOTAL DAILY DOSE=2.0g)	500 mg q6h (TOTAL DAILY DOSE=2.0g)

Patients ≥3 Months of Age With Normal Pretherapy but Abnormal During Therapy Laboratory Values

Laboratory Parameter	Abnormality		No. of Patients With Abnormalities/ No. of Patients With Lab Done	(%)
Hemoglobin	Age <5 mos.:	<10 gm %	19/129	(14.7)
	6 mos.-12 yrs.:	<11.5 gm%		
Hematocrit	Age <5 mos.:	<30 vol%	23/129	(17.8)
	6 mos.-12 yrs.:	<34.5 vol %		
Neutrophils	≤1000/mm^3 (absolute)		4/123	(3.3)
Eosinophils	≥7%		15/117	(12.8)
Platelet Count	≥500 ths/mm^3		16/119	(13.4)
Urine Protein	≥1		8/97	(8.2)
Serum Creatinine	>1.2 mg/dL		0/105	(0)
BUN	>22 mg/dL		0/108	(0)
AST (SGOT)	>36 IU/L		14/78	(17.9)
ALT (SGPT)	>30 IU/L		10/93	(10.8)

TABLE II
REDUCED INTRAVENOUS DOSAGE OF PRIMAXIN I.V. IN ADULT PATIENTS WITH IMPAIRED RENAL FUNCTION AND/OR BODY WEIGHT <70 kg

If TOTAL DAILY DOSE from TABLE I is: 1.0 g/day; 1.5 g/day; 2.0 g/day — and creatinine clearance ($mL/min/1.73m^2$) is: — then the reduced dosage regimen (mg) is:

and Body Weight (kg) is:	1.0 g/day ≥71	1.0 g/day 41–70	1.0 g/day 21–40	1.0 g/day 6–20	1.5 g/day ≥71	1.5 g/day 41–70	1.5 g/day 21–40	1.5 g/day 6–20	2.0 g/day ≥71	2.0 g/day 41–70	2.0 g/day 21–40	2.0 g/day 6–20
≥70	250 q6h	250 q8h	250 q12h	250 q12h	500 q8h	250 q6h	250 q8h	250 q12h	500 q6h	500 q8h	250 q6h	250 q12h
60	250 q8h	125 q6h	250 q12h	125 q12h	250 q6h	250 q8h	250 q8h	250 q12h	500 q8h	250 q6h	250 q8h	250 q12h
50	125 q6h	125 q6h	125 q8h	125 q12h	250 q6h	250 q8h	250 q12h	250 q12h	250 q6h	250 q6h	250 q8h	250 q12h
40	125 q6h	125 q8h	125 q12h	125 q12h	250 q8h	125 q6h	125 q8h	125 q12h	250 q6h	250 q8h	250 q12h	250 q12h
30	125 q8h	125 q8h	125 q12h	125 q12h	125 q6h	125 q8h	125 q8h	125 q12h	250 q8h	125 q6h	125 q8h	125 q12h

TABLE III
REDUCED INTRAVENOUS DOSAGE OF PRIMAXIN I.V. IN ADULT PATIENTS WITH IMPAIRED RENAL FUNCTION AND/OR BODY WEIGHT <70 kg

If TOTAL DAILY DOSE from TABLE I is: 3.0 g/day; 4.0 g/day — and creatinine clearance ($mL/min/1.73m^2$) is: — then the reduced dosage regimen (mg) is:

and Body Weight (kg) is:	3.0 g/day ≥71	3.0 g/day 41–70	3.0 g/day 21–40	3.0 g/day 6–20	4.0 g/day ≥71	4.0 g/day 41–70	4.0 g/day 21–40	4.0 g/day 6–20
≥70	1000 q8h	500 q6h	500 q8h	500 q12h	1000 q6h	750 q8h	500 q6h	500 q12h
60	750 q8h	500 q8h	500 q8h	500 q12h	1000 q8h	750 q8h	500 q8h	500 q12h
50	500 q6h	500 q8h	250 q6h	250 q12h	750 q8h	500 q6h	500 q8h	500 q12h
40	500 q8h	250 q6h	250 q8h	250 q12h	500 q6h	500 q8h	250 q6h	250 q12h
30	250 q6h	250 q8h	250 q8h	250 q12h	500 q8h	250 q6h	250 q8h	250 q12h

Due to the high antimicrobial activity of PRIMAXIN I.V., it is recommended that the maximum total daily dosage not exceed 50 mg/kg/day or 4.0 g/day, whichever is lower. There is no evidence that higher doses provide greater efficacy. However, patients over twelve years of age with cystic fibrosis and normal renal function have been treated with PRIMAXIN I.V. at doses up to 90 mg/kg/day in divided doses, not exceeding 4.0 g/day.

Reduced Intravenous Dosage Schedule for Adults with Impaired Renal Function and/or Body Weight <70 kg

Patients with creatinine clearance of ≤ 70 mL/min/1.73 m^2 and/or body weight less than 70 kg require dosage reduction of PRIMAXIN I.V. as indicated in the tables below. Creatinine clearance may be calculated from serum creatinine concentration by the following equation:

$$T_{cc}\ (\text{Males}) = \frac{(\text{wt. in kg})\ (140 - \text{age})}{(72)\ (\text{creatinine in mg/dL})}$$

$$T_{cc}\ (\text{Females}) = 0.85 \times \text{above value}$$

To determine the dose for adults with impaired renal function and/or reduced body weight:

1. Choose a total daily dose from Table I based on infection characteristics.
2. a) If the total daily dose is 1.0 g, 1.5 g, or 2.0 g, use the appropriate subsection of Table II and continue with step 3.
   b) If the total daily dose is 3.0 g or 4.0 g, use the appropriate subsection of Table III and continue with step 3.
3. From Table II or III:
   a) Select the body weight on the far left which is closest to the patient's body weight (kg).
   b) Select the patient's creatinine clearance category.
   c) Where the row and column intersect is the reduced dosage regimen.

[See table II above]
[See table III above]

Patients with creatinine clearances of 6 to 20 mL/min/1.73 m^2 should be treated with PRIMAXIN I.V. 125 mg or 250 mg every 12 hours for most pathogens. There may be an increased risk of seizures when doses of 500 mg every 12 hours are administered to these patients.

Patients with creatinine clearance ≤5 mL/min/1.73 m^2 should not receive PRIMAXIN I.V. unless hemodialysis is

Continued on next page

Information on the Merck & Co., Inc. products listed on these pages is the full prescribing information from product circulars in use September 30, 2000. For information, please call 1-800-NSC MERCK [1-800-672-6372].

Primaxin I.V.—Cont.

instituted within 48 hours. There is inadequate information to recommend usage of PRIMAXIN I.V. for patients undergoing peritoneal dialysis.

Hemodialysis

When treating patients with creatinine clearances of ≤5 mL/min/1.73 m² who are undergoing hemodialysis, use the dosage recommendations for patients with creatinine clearances of 6–20 mL/min/1.73 m². (See *Reduced Intravenous Dosage Schedule for Adults with Impaired Renal Function and/or Body Weight <70 kg.*) Both imipenem and cilastatin are cleared from the circulation during hemodialysis. The patient should receive PRIMAXIN I.V. after hemodialysis and at 12 hour intervals timed from the end of that hemodialysis session. Dialysis patients, especially those with background CNS disease, should be carefully monitored; for patients on hemodialysis, PRIMAXIN I.V. is recommended only when the benefit outweighs the potential risk of seizures. (See **PRECAUTIONS**.)

Pediatric Patients

See **PRECAUTIONS**, *Pediatric Patients*.

For pediatric patients ≥3 months of age, the recommended dose for non-CNS infections is 15–25 mg/kg/dose administered every six hours. Based on studies in adults, the maximum daily dose for treatment of infections with fully susceptible organisms is 2.0 g per day, and of infections with moderately susceptible organisms (primarily some strains of *P. aeruginosa*) is 4.0 g/day. Higher doses (up to 90 mg/kg/day in older children) have been used in patients with cystic fibrosis.

For pediatric patients ≤3 months of age (weighing ≥1,500 gms), the following dosage schedule is recommended for non-CNS infections:

<1 wk of age: 25 mg/kg every 12 hrs
1–4 wks of age: 25 mg/kg every 8 hrs
4 wks–3 mos. of age: 25 mg/kg every 6 hrs.

Doses less than or equal to 500 mg should be given by intravenous infusion over 15 to 30 minutes. Doses greater than 500 mg should be given by intravenous infusion over 40 to 60 minutes.

PRIMAXIN I.V. is not recommended in pediatric patients with CNS infections because of the risk of seizures.

PRIMAXIN I.V. is not recommended in pediatric patients <30 kg with impaired renal function, as no data are available.

PREPARATION OF SOLUTION

Infusion Bottles

Contents of the infusion bottles of PRIMAXIN I.V. Powder should be restored with 100 mL of diluent (see list of diluents under **COMPATIBILITY AND STABILITY**) and shaken until a clear solution is obtained.

Vials

Contents of the vials must be suspended and transferred to 100 mL of an appropriate infusion solution.

A suggested procedure is to add approximately 10 mL from the appropriate infusion solution (see list of diluents under **COMPATIBILITY AND STABILITY**) to the vial. Shake well and transfer the resulting suspension to the infusion solution container.

Benzyl alcohol as a preservative has been associated with toxicity in neonates. While toxicity has not been demonstrated in pediatric patients greater than three months of age, small pediatric patients in this age range may also be at risk for benzyl alcohol toxicity. Therefore, diluents containing benzyl alcohol should not be used when PRIMAXIN I.V. is constituted for administration to pediatric patients in this age range.

CAUTION: THE SUSPENSION IS NOT FOR DIRECT INFUSION.

Repeat with an additional 10 mL of infusion solution to ensure complete transfer of vial contents to the infusion solution. **The resulting mixture should be agitated until clear.**

ADD-Vantage ®††† Vials

See separate INSTRUCTIONS FOR USE OF 'PRIMAXIN I.V.' IN ADD-Vantage® VIALS. PRIMAXIN I.V. in ADD-Vantage® vials should be reconstituted with ADD-Vantage® diluent containers containing 100 mL of either 0.9% Sodium Chloride Injection or 100 mL 5% Dextrose Injection.

MONOVIAL ®‡ Vials

See separate INSTRUCTIONS FOR USE OF 'PRIMAXIN I.V.' in MONOVIAL® VIALS. PRIMAXIN I.V. in MONOVIAL® vials should be reconstituted using an appropriate diluent in an infusion bag, with a maximum port length of 14 mm.

The MONOVIAL vial is not compatible with the ADD-Vantage® diluent bags.

††† Registered trademark of Abbott Laboratories, Inc.
‡ Registered trademark of Becton Dickinson and Company.

COMPATIBILITY AND STABILITY

Before reconstitution:

The dry powder should be stored at a temperature below 25°C (77°F).

Reconstituted solutions:

Solutions of PRIMAXIN I.V. range from colorless to yellow. Variations of color within this range do not affect the potency of the product.

PRIMAXIN I.V., as supplied in single use infusion bottles, vials and MONOVIAL® vials and reconstituted with the following diluents (See **PREPARATION OF SOLUTION**), maintains satisfactory potency for 4 hours at room temperature or for 24 hours under refrigeration (5°C). Solutions of PRIMAXIN I.V. should not be frozen.

0.9% Sodium Chloride Injection
5% or 10% Dextrose Injection
5% Dextrose and 0.9% Sodium Chloride Injection
5% Dextrose Injection with 0.225% or 0.45% saline solution
5% Dextrose Injection with 0.15% potassium chloride solution
Mannitol 5% and 10%

PRIMAXIN I.V., as supplied in single dose ADD-Vantage® vials and reconstituted with the following diluents (See **PREPARATION OF SOLUTION**), maintains satisfactory potency for 4 hours at room temperature.

0.9% Sodium Chloride Injection
5% Dextrose Injection

PRIMAXIN I.V. should not be mixed with or physically added to other antibiotics. However, PRIMAXIN I.V. may be administered concomitantly with other antibiotics, such as aminoglycosides.

HOW SUPPLIED

PRIMAXIN I.V. is supplied as a sterile powder mixture in single dose containers including vials, infusion bottles, ADD-Vantage® vials, and MONOVIAL® vials containing imipenem (anhydrous equivalent) and cilastatin sodium as follows:

No. 3514—250 mg imipenem equivalent and 250 mg cilastatin equivalent and 10 mg sodium bicarbonate as a buffer
NDC 0006-3514-58 in trays of 25 vials
(6505-01-332-4793 250 mg, 25's).

No. 3516—500 mg imipenem equivalent and 500 mg cilastatin equivalent and 20 mg sodium bicarbonate as a buffer
NDC 0006-3516-59 in trays of 25 vials
(6505-01-332-4794 500 mg, 25's).

No. 3517—500 mg imipenem equivalent and 500 mg cilastatin equivalent and 20 mg sodium bicarbonate as a buffer
NDC 0006-3517-75 in trays of 10 infusion bottles
(6505-01-234-0240 infusion bottle, 10's).

No. 3551 —250 mg imipenem equivalent and 250 mg cilastatin equivalent and 10 mg sodium bicarbonate as a buffer
NDC 0006-3551-58 in trays of 25 ADD-Vantage® vials.

No. 3552 —500 mg imipenem equivalent and 500 mg cilastatin equivalent and 20 mg sodium bicarbonate as a buffer
NDC 0006-3552-59 in trays of 25 ADD-Vantage® vials
(6505-01-279-9627 500 mg ADD-Vantage®, 25's).

No. 3666 —500 mg imipenem equivalent and 500 mg cilastatin equivalent and 20 mg sodium bicarbonate as a buffer
NDC 0006-3666-59 in trays of 25 MONOVIAL® vials.

REFERENCES

1. National Committee for Clinical Laboratory Standards, Methods for Dilution Antimicrobial Susceptibility Tests for Bacteria that Grow Aerobically—Fourth Edition. Approved Standard NCCLS Document M7–A4, Vol. 17, No. 2 NCCLS, Villanova, PA, 1997.
2. National Committee for Clinical Laboratory Standards, Performance Standards for Antimicrobial Disk Susceptibility Tests—Sixth Edition. Approved Standard NCCLS Document M2–A6, Vol. 17, No. 1 NCCLS, Villanova, PA, 1997.
3. National Committee for Clinical Laboratory Standards, Method for Antimicrobial Susceptibility Testing of Anaerobic Bacteria—Third Edition. Approved Standard NCCLS Document M11-A3, Vol. 13, No. 26 NCCLS, Villanova, PA, 1993.

7882125 Issued February 1999

PRINIVIL® Tablets ℞
(Lisinopril)

> **USE IN PREGNANCY**
> **When used in pregnancy during the second and third trimesters, ACE inhibitors can cause injury and even death to the developing fetus.** When pregnancy is detected, PRINIVIL should be discontinued as soon as possible. See WARNINGS, *Fetal/Neonatal Morbidity and Mortality.*

DESCRIPTION

PRINIVIL* (Lisinopril), a synthetic peptide derivative, is an oral long-acting angiotensin converting enzyme inhibitor. Lisinopril is chemically described as (*S*)-1-[N^2-(1-carboxy-3-phenylpropyl)-L-lysyl]-L-proline dihydrate. Its empirical formula is $C_{21}H_{31}N_3O_5 \cdot 2H_2O$ and its structural formula is:

[See chemical structure at top of next column]

Lisinopril is a white to off-white, crystalline powder, with a molecular weight of 441.52. It is soluble in water and sparingly soluble in methanol and practically insoluble in ethanol.

PRINIVIL is supplied as 2.5 mg, 5 mg, 10 mg, 20 mg and 40 mg tablets for oral administration. In addition to the active ingredient lisinopril, each tablet contains the following inactive ingredients: calcium phosphate, mannitol, magnesium stearate, and starch. The 10 mg, 20 mg and 40 mg tablets also contain iron oxide.

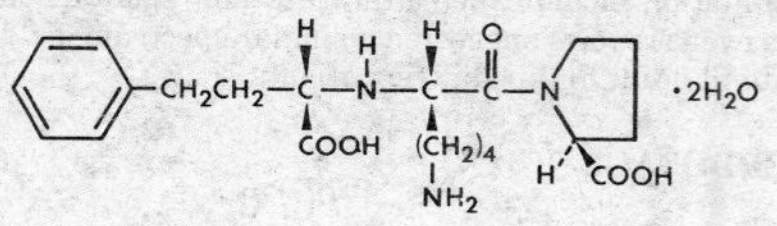

*Registered trademark of MERCK & CO., INC.

CLINICAL PHARMACOLOGY

Mechanism of Action

Lisinopril inhibits angiotensin converting enzyme (ACE) in human subjects and animals. ACE is a peptidyl dipeptidase that catalyzes the conversion of angiotensin I to the vasoconstrictor substance, angiotensin II. Angiotensin II also stimulates aldosterone secretion by the adrenal cortex. The beneficial effects of lisinopril in hypertension and heart failure appear to result primarily from suppression of the renin-angiotensin-aldosterone system. Inhibition of ACE results in decreased plasma angiotensin II which leads to decreased vasopressor activity and to decreased aldosterone secretion. The latter decrease may result in a small increase of serum potassium. In hypertensive patients with normal renal function treated with PRINIVIL alone for up to 24 weeks, the mean increase in serum potassium was approximately 0.1 mEq/L; however, approximately 15 percent of patients had increases greater than 0.5 mEq/L and approximately six percent had a decrease greater than 0.5 mEq/L. In the same study, patients treated with PRINIVIL and hydrochlorothiazide for up to 24 weeks had a mean decrease in serum potassium of 0.1 mEq/L; approximately 4 percent of patients had increases greater than 0.5 mEq/L and approximately 12 percent had a decrease greater than 0.5 mEq/L. (See PRECAUTIONS.) Removal of angiotensin II negative feedback on renin secretion leads to increased plasma renin activity.

ACE is identical to kininase, an enzyme that degrades bradykinin. Whether increased levels of bradykinin, a potent vasodepressor peptide, play a role in the therapeutic effects of PRINIVIL remains to be elucidated.

While the mechanism through which PRINIVIL lowers blood pressure is believed to be primarily suppression of the renin-angiotensin-aldosterone system, PRINIVIL is antihypertensive even in patients with low-renin hypertension. Although PRINIVIL was antihypertensive in all races studied, black hypertensive patients (usually a low-renin hypertensive population) had a smaller average response to monotherapy than non-black patients.

Concomitant administration of PRINIVIL and hydrochlorothiazide further reduced blood pressure in black and non-black patients and any racial difference in blood pressure response was no longer evident.

Pharmacokinetics and Metabolism

Following oral administration of PRINIVIL, peak serum concentrations of lisinopril occur within about 7 hours, although there was a trend to a small delay in time taken to reach peak serum concentrations in acute myocardial infarction patients. Declining serum concentrations exhibit a prolonged terminal phase which does not contribute to drug accumulation. This terminal phase probably represents saturable binding to ACE and is not proportional to dose. Lisinopril does not appear to be bound to other serum proteins. Lisinopril does not undergo metabolism and is excreted unchanged entirely in the urine. Based on urinary recovery, the mean extent of absorption of lisinopril is approximately 25 percent, with large intersubject variability (6–60 percent) at all doses tested (5–80 mg). Lisinopril absorption is not influenced by the presence of food in the gastrointestinal tract. The absolute bioavailability of lisinopril is reduced to about 16% in patients with stable NYHA Class II-IV congestive heart failure, and the volume of distribution appears to be slightly smaller than that in normal subjects.

The oral bioavailability of lisinopril in patients with acute myocardial infarction is similar to that in healthy volunteers.

Upon multiple dosing, lisinopril exhibits an effective half-life of accumulation of 12 hours.

Impaired renal function decreases elimination of lisinopril, which is excreted principally through the kidneys, but this decrease becomes clinically important only when the glomerular filtration rate is below 30 mL/min. Above this glomerular filtration rate, the elimination half-life is little changed. With greater impairment, however, peak and trough lisinopril levels increase, time to peak concentration increases and time to attain steady state is prolonged. Older patients, on average, have (approximately doubled) higher blood levels and area under the plasma concentration time curve (AUC) than younger patients. (See DOSAGE AND ADMINISTRATION.) Lisinopril can be removed by hemodialysis.

Studies in rats indicate that lisinopril crosses the blood-brain barrier poorly. Multiple doses of lisinopril in rats do not result in accumulation in any tissues. Milk of lactating rats contains radioactivity following administration of ^{14}C lisinopril. By whole body autoradiography, radioactivity was found in the placenta following administration of labeled drug to pregnant rats, but none was found in the fetuses.

Pharmacodynamics and Clinical Effects

Hypertension: Administration of PRINIVIL to patients with hypertension results in a reduction of supine and standing blood pressure to about the same extent with no compensatory tachycardia. Symptomatic postural hypotension is usually not observed although it can occur and should be anticipated in volume and/or salt-depleted patients. (See WARNINGS.) When given together with thiazide-type diuretics, the blood pressure lowering effects of the two drugs are approximately additive.

In most patients studied, onset of antihypertensive activity was seen at one hour after oral administration of an individual dose of PRINIVIL, with peak reduction of blood pressure achieved by six hours. Although an antihypertensive effect was observed 24 hours after dosing with recommended single daily doses, the effect was more consistent and the mean effect was considerably larger in some studies with doses of 20 mg or more than with lower doses. However, at all doses studied, the mean antihypertensive effect was substantially smaller 24 hours after dosing than it was six hours after dosing.

In some patients achievement of optimal blood pressure reduction may require two to four weeks of therapy.

The antihypertensive effects of PRINIVIL are maintained during long-term therapy. Abrupt withdrawal of PRINIVIL has not been associated with a rapid increase in blood pressure or a significant increase in blood pressure compared to pretreatment levels.

Two dose-response studies utilizing a once daily regimen were conducted in 438 mild to moderate hypertensive patients not on a diuretic. Blood pressure was measured 24 hours after dosing. An antihypertensive effect of PRINIVIL was seen with 5 mg in some patients. However, in both studies blood pressure reduction occurred sooner and was greater in patients treated with 10, 20, or 80 mg of PRINIVIL. In controlled clinical studies, PRINIVIL 20–80 mg has been compared in patients with mild to moderate hypertension to hydrochlorothiazide 12.5–50 mg and with atenolol 50–200 mg; and in patients with moderate to severe hypertension to metoprolol 100–200 mg. It was superior to hydrochlorothiazide in effects on systolic and diastolic blood pressure in a population that was $^3/_4$ caucasian. PRINIVIL was approximately equivalent to atenolol and metoprolol in effects on diastolic blood pressure and had somewhat greater effects on systolic blood pressure.

PRINIVIL had similar effectiveness and adverse effects in younger and older (>65 years) patients. It was less effective in blacks than in caucasians.

In hemodynamic studies in patients with essential hypertension, blood pressure reduction was accompanied by a reduction in peripheral arterial resistance with little or no change in cardiac output and in heart rate. In a study in nine hypertensive patients, following administration of PRINIVIL, there was an increase in mean renal blood flow that was not significant. Data from several small studies are inconsistent with respect to the effect of PRINIVIL on glomerular filtration rate in hypertensive patients with normal renal function, but suggest that changes, if any, are not large.

In patients with renovascular hypertension PRINIVIL has been shown to be well tolerated and effective in controlling blood pressure (see PRECAUTIONS).

Heart Failure: During baseline-controlled clinical studies, in patients receiving digitalis and diuretics, single doses of PRINIVIL resulted in decreases in pulmonary capillary wedge pressure, systemic vascular resistance and blood pressure accompanied by an increase in cardiac output and no change in heart rate.

In two placebo controlled, 12-week clinical studies, PRINIVIL as adjunctive therapy to digitalis and diuretics improved the following signs and symptoms due to congestive heart failure: edema, rales, paroxysmal nocturnal dyspnea and jugular venous distention. In one of the studies beneficial response was also noted for: orthopnea, presence of third heart sound and the number of patients classified as NYHA Class III and IV. Exercise tolerance was also improved in this study. The effect of lisinopril on mortality in patients with heart failure has not been evaluated.

The once daily dosage for the treatment of congestive heart failure was the only dosage regimen used during clinical trial development and was determined by the measurement of hemodynamic responses.

Acute Myocardial Infarction: The Gruppo Italiano per lo Studio della Sopravvienza nell'Infarto Miocardico (GISSI-3) study was a multicenter, controlled, randomized, unblinded clinical trial conducted in 19,394 patients with acute myocardial infarction admitted to a coronary care unit. It was designed to examine the effects of short-term (6 week) treatment with lisinopril, nitrates, their combination, or no therapy on short-term (6 week) mortality and on long-term death and markedly impaired cardiac function. Patients presenting within 24 hours of the onset of symptoms who were hemodynamically stable were randomized, in a 2 × 2 factorial design, to six weeks of either

1) PRINIVIL alone (n = 4841),
2) nitrates alone (n = 4869),
3) PRINIVIL plus nitrates (n = 4841), or
4) open control (n = 4843).

All patients received routine therapies, including thrombolytics (72%), aspirin (84%), and a beta-blocker (31%), as appropriate, normally utilized in acute myocardial infarction (MI) patients.

The protocol excluded patients with hypotension (systolic blood pressure ≤100 mmHg), severe heart failure, cardiogenic shock and renal dysfunction (serum creatinine >2 mg/dL and/or proteinuria >500 mg/24 h). Doses of PRINIVIL were adjusted as necessary according to protocol. (See DOSAGE AND ADMINISTRATION.)

Study treatment was withdrawn at six weeks except where clinical conditions indicated continuation of treatment.

The primary outcomes of the trial were the overall mortality at six weeks and a combined endpoint at six months after the myocardial infarction, consisting of the number of patients who died, had late (day 4) clinical congestive heart failure, or had extensive left ventricular damage defined as ejection fraction ≤35%, or an akinetic-dyskinetic [A-D] score ≥45%. Patients receiving PRINIVIL (n = 9646) alone or with nitrates, had an 11 percent lower risk of death (2p [two-tailed] = 0.04) compared to patients receiving no PRINIVIL (n = 9672) (6.4 percent versus 7.2 percent, respectively) at six weeks. Although patients randomized to receive PRINIVIL for up to six weeks also fared numerically better on the combined endpoint at 6 months, the open nature of the assessment of heart failure, substantial loss of follow-up echocardiography, and substantial excess use of lisinopril between 6 weeks and 6 months in the group randomized to 6 weeks of lisinopril, preclude any conclusion about this endpoint.

Patients with acute myocardial infarction, treated with PRINIVIL had a higher (9.0 percent versus 3.7 percent, respectively) incidence of persistent hypotension (systolic blood pressure <90 mmHg for more than 1 hour) and renal dysfunction (2.4 percent versus 1.1 percent) in-hospital and at six weeks (increasing creatinine concentration to over 3 mg/dL or a doubling or more of the baseline serum creatinine concentration). See ADVERSE REACTIONS, *ACUTE MYOCARDIAL INFARCTION.*

INDICATIONS AND USAGE

Hypertension

PRINIVIL is indicated for the treatment of hypertension. It may be used alone as initial therapy or concomitantly with other classes of antihypertensive agents.

Heart Failure

PRINIVIL is indicated as adjunctive therapy in the management of heart failure in patients who are not responding adequately to diuretics and digitalis.

Acute Myocardial Infarction

PRINIVIL is indicated for the treatment of hemodynamically stable patients within 24 hours of acute myocardial infarction, to improve survival. Patients should receive, as appropriate, the standard recommended treatments such as thrombolytics, aspirin and beta-blockers.

In using PRINIVIL, consideration should be given to the fact that another angiotensin converting enzyme inhibitor, captopril, has caused agranulocytosis, particularly in patients with renal impairment or collagen vascular disease, and that available data are insufficient to show that PRINIVIL does not have a similar risk. (See WARNINGS.)

In considering use of PRINIVIL, it should be noted that in controlled clinical trials ACE inhibitors have an effect on blood pressure that is less in black patients than in non-blacks. In addition, it should be noted that black patients receiving ACE inhibitors have been reported to have a higher incidence of angioedema compared to non-blacks.

CONTRAINDICATIONS

PRINIVIL is contraindicated in patients who are hypersensitive to this product and in patients with a history of angioedema related to previous treatment with an angiotensin converting enzyme inhibitor and in patients with hereditary or idiopathic angioedema.

WARNINGS

Anaphylactoid and Possibly Related Reactions

Presumably because angiotensin converting enzyme inhibitors affect the metabolism of eicosanoids and polypeptides, including endogenous bradykinin, patients receiving ACE inhibitors (including PRINIVIL) may be subject to a variety of adverse reactions, some of them serious.

Angioedema: Angioedema of the face, extremities, lips, tongue, glottis and/or larynx has been reported in patients treated with angiotensin converting enzyme inhibitors, including PRINIVIL. This may occur at any time during treatment. In such cases PRINIVIL should be promptly discontinued and appropriate therapy and monitoring should be provided until complete and sustained resolution of signs and symptoms has occurred. In instances where swelling has been confined to the face and lips the condition has generally resolved without treatment, although antihistamines have been useful in relieving symptoms. Angioedema associated with laryngeal edema may be fatal. **Where there is involvement of the tongue, glottis or larynx, likely to cause airway obstruction, appropriate therapy, e.g., subcutaneous epinephrine solution 1:1000 (0.3 mL to 0.5 mL) and/or measures necessary to ensure a patent airway, should be promptly provided.** (See ADVERSE REACTIONS.)

Patients with a history of angioedema unrelated to ACE inhibitor therapy may be at increased risk of angioedema while receiving an ACE inhibitor (see also INDICATIONS AND USAGE and CONTRAINDICATIONS).

Anaphylactoid reactions during desensitization: Two patients undergoing desensitizing treatment with hymenoptera venom while receiving ACE inhibitors sustained life-threatening anaphylactoid reactions. In the same patients, these reactions were avoided when ACE inhibitors were temporarily withheld, but they reappeared upon inadvertent rechallenge.

Anaphylactoid reactions during membrane exposure: Anaphylactoid reactions have been reported in patients dialyzed with high-flux membranes and treated concomitantly with an ACE inhibitor. Anaphylactoid reactions have also been reported in patients undergoing low-density lipoprotein apheresis with dextran sulfate absorption.

Hypotension

Excessive hypotension is rare in patients with uncomplicated hypertension treated with PRINIVIL alone.

Patients with heart failure given PRINIVIL commonly have some reduction in blood pressure with peak blood pressure reduction occurring 6 to 8 hours post dose, but discontinuation of therapy because of continuing symptomatic hypotension usually is not necessary when dosing instructions are followed; caution should be observed when initiating therapy. (See DOSAGE AND ADMINISTRATION.)

Patients at risk of excessive hypotension, sometimes associated with oliguria and/or progressive azotemia, and rarely with acute renal failure and/or death, include those with the following conditions or characteristics: heart failure with systolic blood pressure below 100 mmHg, hyponatremia, high dose diuretic therapy, recent intensive diuresis or increase in diuretic dose, renal dialysis, or severe volume and/or salt depletion of any etiology. It may be advisable to eliminate the diuretic (except in patients with heart failure), reduce the diuretic dose or increase salt intake cautiously before initiating therapy with PRINIVIL in patients at risk for excessive hypotension who are able to tolerate such adjustments. (See PRECAUTIONS, *Drug Interactions,* and ADVERSE REACTIONS.)

Patients with acute myocardial infarction in the GISSI-3 study had a higher (9.0 versus 3.7 percent) incidence of persistent hypotension (systolic blood pressure <90 mmHg for more than 1 hour) when treated with PRINIVIL. Treatment with PRINIVIL must not be initiated in acute myocardial infarction patients at risk of further serious hemodynamic deterioration after treatment with a vasodilator (e.g., systolic blood pressure of 100 mmHg or lower) or cardiogenic shock.

In patients at risk of excessive hypotension, therapy should be started under very close medical supervision and such patients should be followed closely for the first two weeks of treatment and whenever the dose of PRINIVIL and/or diuretic is increased. Similar considerations may apply to patients with ischemic heart or cerebrovascular disease, or in patients with acute myocardial infarction, in whom an excessive fall in blood pressure could result in a myocardial infarction or cerebrovascular accident.

If excessive hypotension occurs, the patient should be placed in the supine position and, if necessary, receive an intravenous infusion of normal saline. A transient hypotensive response is not a contraindication to further doses of PRINIVIL which usually can be given without difficulty once the blood pressure has stabilized. If symptomatic hypotension develops, a dose reduction or discontinuation of PRINIVIL or concomitant diuretic may be necessary.

Neutropenia/Agranulocytosis

Another angiotensin converting enzyme inhibitor, captopril, has been shown to cause agranulocytosis and bone marrow depression, rarely in uncomplicated patients but more frequently in patients with renal impairment especially if they also have a collagen vascular disease. Available data from clinical trials of PRINIVIL are insufficient to show that PRINIVIL does not cause agranulocytosis at similar rates. Marketing experience has revealed rare cases of neutropenia and bone marrow depression in which a causal relationship to lisinopril cannot be excluded. Periodic monitoring of white blood cell counts in patients with collagen vascular disease and renal disease should be considered.

Hepatic Failure: Rarely, ACE inhibitors have been associated with a syndrome that starts with cholestatic jaundice and progresses to fulminant hepatic necrosis, and (sometimes) death. The mechanism of this syndrome is not understood. Patients receiving ACE inhibitors who develop jaundice or marked elevations of hepatic enzymes should discontinue the ACE inhibitor and receive appropriate medical follow-up.

Fetal/Neonatal Morbidity and Mortality

ACE inhibitors can cause fetal and neonatal morbidity and death when administered to pregnant women. Several dozen cases have been reported in the world literature. When pregnancy is detected, ACE inhibitors should be discontinued as soon as possible.

The use of ACE inhibitors during the second and third trimesters of pregnancy has been associated with fetal and neonatal injury, including hypotension, neonatal skull hypoplasia, anuria, reversible or irreversible renal failure, and death. Oligohydramnios has also been reported, presumably resulting from decreased fetal renal function; oligohydramnios in this setting has been associated with fetal limb contractures, craniofacial deformation, and hypoplastic lung development. Prematurity, intrauterine growth retardation,

Continued on next page

Prinivil—Cont.

and patent ductus arteriosus have also been reported, although it is not clear whether these occurrences were due to the ACE-inhibitor exposure.

These adverse effects do not appear to have resulted from intrauterine ACE-inhibitor exposure that has been limited to the first trimester. Mothers whose embryos and fetuses are exposed to ACE inhibitors only during the first trimester should be so informed. Nonetheless, when patients become pregnant, physicians should make every effort to discontinue the use of PRINIVIL as soon as possible.

Rarely (probably less often than once in every thousand pregnancies), no alternative to ACE inhibitors will be found. In these rare cases, the mothers should be apprised of the potential hazards to their fetuses, and serial ultrasound examinations should be performed to assess the intraamniotic environment.

If oligohydramnios is observed, PRINIVIL should be discontinued unless it is considered lifesaving for the mother. Contraction stress testing (CST), a non-stress test (NST), or biophysical profiling (BPP) may be appropriate, depending upon the week of pregnancy. Patients and physicians should be aware, however, that oligohydramnios may not appear until after the fetus has sustained irreversible injury.

Infants with histories of *in utero* exposure to ACE inhibitors should be closely observed for hypotension, oliguria, and hyperkalemia. If oliguria occurs, attention should be directed toward support of blood pressure and renal perfusion. Exchange transfusion or dialysis may be required as means of reversing hypotension and/or substituting for disordered renal function. Lisinopril, which crosses the placenta, has been removed from neonatal circulation by peritoneal dialysis with some clinical benefit, and theoretically may be removed by exchange transfusion, although there is no experience with the latter procedure.

No teratogenic effects of lisinopril were seen in studies of pregnant mice, rats, and rabbits. On a body surface area basis, the doses used were up to 55 times, 33 times, and 0.15 times, respectively, the maximum recommended human daily dose (MRHDD).

PRECAUTIONS

General

Aortic Stenosis/Hypertrophic Cardiomyopathy: As with all vasodilators, lisinopril should be given with caution to patients with obstruction in the outflow tract of the left ventricle.

Impaired Renal Function: As a consequence of inhibiting the renin-angiotensin-aldosterone system, changes in renal function may be anticipated in susceptible individuals. In patients with severe congestive heart failure whose renal function may depend on the activity of the renin-angiotensin-aldosterone system, treatment with angiotensin converting enzyme inhibitors, including PRINIVIL, may be associated with oliguria and/or progressive azotemia and rarely with acute renal failure and/or death.

In hypertensive patients with unilateral or bilateral renal artery stenosis, increases in blood urea nitrogen and serum creatinine may occur. Experience with another angiotensin converting enzyme inhibitor suggests that these increases are usually reversible upon discontinuation of PRINIVIL and/or diuretic therapy. In such patients renal function should be monitored during the first few weeks of therapy.

Some patients with hypertension or heart failure with no apparent pre-existing renal vascular disease have developed increases in blood urea nitrogen and serum creatinine, usually minor and transient, especially when PRINIVIL has been given concomitantly with a diuretic. This is more likely to occur in patients with pre-existing renal impairment. Dosage reduction and/or discontinuation of the diuretic and/or PRINIVIL may be required.

Patients with acute myocardial infarction in the GISSI-3 study, treated with PRINIVIL, had a higher (2.4 percent versus 1.1 percent) incidence of renal dysfunction in-hospital and at six weeks (increasing creatinine concentration to over 3 mg/dL or a doubling or more of the baseline serum creatinine concentration). In acute myocardial infarction, treatment with PRINIVIL should be initiated with caution in patients with evidence of renal dysfunction, defined as serum creatinine concentration exceeding 2 mg/dL. If renal dysfunction develops during treatment with PRINIVIL (serum creatinine concentration exceeding 3 mg/dL or a doubling from the pre-treatment value) then the physician should consider withdrawal of PRINIVIL.

Evaluation of patients with hypertension, heart failure, or myocardial infarction should always include assessment of renal function. (See DOSAGE AND ADMINISTRATION.)

Hyperkalemia: In clinical trials hyperkalemia (serum potassium greater than 5.7 mEq/L) occurred in approximately 2.2 percent of hypertensive patients and 4.8 percent of patients with heart failure. In most cases these were isolated values which resolved despite continued therapy. Hyperkalemia was a cause of discontinuation of therapy in approximately 0.1 percent of hypertensive patients, 0.6 percent of patients with heart failure and 0.1 percent of patients with myocardial infarction. Risk factors for the development of hyperkalemia include renal insufficiency, diabetes mellitus, and the concomitant use of potassium-sparing diuretics, potassium supplements and/or potassium-containing salt substitutes, which should be used cautiously, if at all, with PRINIVIL. (See *Drug Interactions.*)

Cough: Presumably due to the inhibition of the degradation of endogenous bradykinin, persistent nonproductive cough has been reported with all ACE inhibitors, always resolving after discontinuation of therapy. ACE inhibitor-induced cough should be considered in the differential diagnosis of cough.

Surgery/Anesthesia: In patients undergoing major surgery or during anesthesia with agents that produce hypotension, PRINIVIL may block angiotensin II formation secondary to compensatory renin release. If hypotension occurs and is considered to be due to this mechanism, it can be corrected by volume expansion.

Information for Patients

Angioedema: Angioedema, including laryngeal edema, may occur at any time during treatment with angiotensin converting enzyme inhibitors, including lisinopril. Patients should be so advised and told to report immediately any signs or symptoms suggesting angioedema (swelling of face, extremities, eyes, lips, tongue, difficulty in swallowing or breathing) and to take no more drug until they have consulted with the prescribing physician.

Symptomatic Hypotension: Patients should be cautioned to report lightheadedness especially during the first few days of therapy. If actual syncope occurs, the patients should be told to discontinue the drug until they have consulted with the prescribing physician.

All patients should be cautioned that excessive perspiration and dehydration may lead to an excessive fall in blood pressure because of reduction in fluid volume. Other causes of volume depletion such as vomiting or diarrhea may also lead to a fall in blood pressure; patients should be advised to consult with their physician.

Hyperkalemia: Patients should be told not to use salt substitutes containing potassium without consulting their physician.

Neutropenia: Patients should be told to report promptly any indication of infection (e.g., sore throat, fever) which may be a sign of neutropenia.

Pregnancy: Female patients of childbearing age should be told about the consequences of second- and third-trimester exposure to ACE inhibitors, and they should also be told that these consequences do not appear to have resulted from intrauterine ACE-inhibitor exposure that has been limited to the first trimester. These patients should be asked to report pregnancies to their physicians as soon as possible.

NOTE: As with many other drugs, certain advice to patients being treated with PRINIVIL is warranted. This information is intended to aid in the safe and effective use of this medication. It is not a disclosure of all possible adverse or intended effects.

Drug Interactions

Hypotension—Patients on Diuretic Therapy: Patients on diuretics, and especially those in whom diuretic therapy was recently instituted, may occasionally experience an excessive reduction of blood pressure after initiation of therapy with PRINIVIL. The possibility of hypotensive effects with PRINIVIL can be minimized by either discontinuing the diuretic or increasing the salt intake prior to initiation of treatment with PRINIVIL. If it is necessary to continue the diuretic, initiate therapy with PRINIVIL at a dose of 5 mg daily, and provide close medical supervision after the initial dose until blood pressure has stabilized. (See WARNINGS, and DOSAGE AND ADMINISTRATION.) When a diuretic is added to the therapy of a patient receiving PRINIVIL, an additional antihypertensive effect is usually observed. Studies with ACE inhibitors in combination with diuretics indicate that the dose of the ACE inhibitor can be reduced when it is given with a diuretic. (See DOSAGE AND ADMINISTRATION.)

Non-steroidal Anti-inflammatory Agents: In some patients with compromised renal function who are being treated with non-steroidal anti-inflammatory drugs, the co-administration of lisinopril may result in a further deterioration of renal function. These effects are usually reversible. In a study in 36 patients with mild to moderate hypertension where the antihypertensive effects of PRINIVIL alone were compared to PRINIVIL given concomitantly with indomethacin, the use of indomethacin was associated with a reduced effect, although the difference between the two regimens was not significant.

Other Agents: PRINIVIL has been used concomitantly with nitrates and/or digoxin without evidence of clinically significant adverse interactions. This included post myocardial infarction patients who were receiving intravenous or transdermal nitroglycerin. No clinically important pharmacokinetic interactions occurred when PRINIVIL was used concomitantly with propranolol or hydrochlorothiazide. The presence of food in the stomach does not alter the bioavailability of PRINIVIL.

Agents Increasing Serum Potassium: PRINIVIL attenuates potassium loss caused by thiazide-type diuretics. Use of PRINIVIL with potassium-sparing diuretics (e.g., spironolactone, triamterene, or amiloride), potassium supplements, or potassium-containing salt substitutes may lead to significant increases in serum potassium. Therefore, if concomitant use of these agents is indicated because of demonstrated hypokalemia, they should be used with caution and with frequent monitoring of serum potassium. Potassium sparing agents should generally not be used in patients with heart failure who are receiving PRINIVIL.

Lithium: Lithium toxicity has been reported in patients receiving lithium concomitantly with drugs which cause elimination of sodium, including ACE inhibitors. Lithium toxicity was usually reversible upon discontinuation of lithium and the ACE inhibitor. It is recommended that serum lithium levels be monitored frequently if PRINIVIL is administered concomitantly with lithium.

Carcinogenesis, Mutagenesis, Impairment of Fertility

There was no evidence of a tumorigenic effect when lisinopril was administered orally for 105 weeks to male and female rats at doses up to 90 mg/kg/day or for 92 weeks to male and female mice at doses up to 135 mg/kg/day. These doses are 10 times and 7 times, respectively, the maximum recommended human daily dose (MRHDD) when compared on a body surface area basis.

Lisinopril was not mutagenic in the Ames microbial mutagen test with or without metabolic activation. It was also negative in a forward mutation assay using Chinese hamster lung cells. Lisinopril did not produce single strand DNA breaks in an *in vitro* alkaline elution rat hepatocyte assay. In addition, lisinopril did not produce increases in chromosomal aberrations in an *in vitro* test in Chinese hamster ovary cells or in an *in vivo* study in mouse bone marrow.

There were no adverse effects on reproductive performance in male and female rats treated with up to 300 mg/kg/day of lisinopril (33 times the MRHDD when compared on a body surface area basis).

Pregnancy

Pregnancy Categories C (first trimester) *and D* (second and third trimesters). See WARNINGS, *Fetal/Neonatal Morbidity and Mortality.*

Nursing Mothers

Milk of lactating rats contains radioactivity following administration of ^{14}C lisinopril. It is not known whether this drug is secreted in human milk. Because many drugs are secreted in human milk, and because of the potential for serious adverse reactions in nursing infants from ACE inhibitors, a decision should be made whether to discontinue PRINIVIL, taking into account the importance of the drug to the mother.

Pediatric Use

Safety and effectiveness in pediatric patients have not been established.

ADVERSE REACTIONS

PRINIVIL has been found to be generally well tolerated in controlled clinical trials involving 1969 patients with hypertension or heart failure. For the most part, adverse experiences were mild and transient.

HYPERTENSION

In clinical trials in patients with hypertension treated with PRINIVIL, discontinuation of therapy due to clinical adverse experiences occurred in 5.7 percent of patients. The overall frequency of adverse experiences could not be related to total daily dosage within the recommended therapeutic dosage range.

For adverse experiences occurring in greater than one percent of patients with hypertension treated with PRINIVIL or PRINIVIL plus hydrochlorothiazide in controlled clinical trials and more frequently with PRINIVIL and/or PRINIVIL plus hydrochlorothiazide than placebo, comparative incidence data are listed in the table below:

[See table at bottom of next page]

Chest pain and back pain were also seen but were more common on placebo than PRINIVIL.

HEART FAILURE

In patients with heart failure treated with PRINIVIL for up to four years, discontinuation of therapy due to clinical adverse experiences occurred in 11.0 percent of patients. In controlled studies in patients with heart failure, therapy was discontinued in 8.1 percent of patients treated with PRINIVIL for up to 12 weeks, compared to 7.7 percent of patients treated with placebo for 12 weeks.

The following table lists those adverse experiences which occurred in greater than one percent of patients with heart failure treated with PRINIVIL or placebo for up to 12 weeks in controlled clinical trials and more frequently on PRINIVIL than placebo.

	Controlled Trials	
	PRINIVIL (n=407) Incidence (discontinuation) 12 weeks	Placebo (n=155) Incidence (discontinuation) 12 weeks
Body As A Whole		
Chest Pain	3.4 (0.2)	1.3 (0.0)
Abdominal Pain	2.2 (0.7)	1.9 (0.0)
Cardiovascular		
Hypotension	4.4 (1.7)	0.6 (0.6)
Digestive		
Diarrhea	3.7 (0.5)	1.9 (0.0)
Nervous/Psychiatric		
Dizziness	11.8 (1.2)	4.5 (1.3)
Headache	4.4 (0.2)	3.9 (0.0)
Respiratory		
Upper Respiratory Infection	1.5 (0.0)	1.3 (0.0)
Skin		
Rash	1.7 (0.5)	0.6 (0.6)

Also observed at >1% with PRINIVIL but more frequent or as frequent on placebo than PRINIVIL in controlled trials were asthenia, angina pectoris, nausea, dyspnea, cough and pruritus.

Worsening of heart failure, anorexia, increased salivation, muscle cramps, back pain, myalgia, depression, chest sound abnormalities and pulmonary edema were also seen in controlled clinical trials, but were more common on placebo than PRINIVIL.

ACUTE MYOCARDIAL INFARCTION

In the GISSI-3 trial, in patients treated with PRINIVIL for six weeks following acute myocardial infarction, discontinuation of therapy occurred in 17.6 percent of patients.

Patients treated with PRINIVIL had a significantly higher incidence of hypotension and renal dysfunction compared with patients not taking PRINIVIL.

In the GISSI-3 trial, hypotension (9.7 percent), renal dysfunction (2.0 percent), cough (0.5 percent), post-infarction angina (0.3 percent), skin rash and generalized edema (0.01 percent), and angioedema (0.01 percent) resulted in withdrawal of treatment. In elderly patients treated with PRINIVIL, discontinuation due to renal dysfunction was 4.2 percent.

Other clinical adverse experiences occurring in 0.3 to 1.0 percent of patients with hypertension or heart failure treated with PRINIVIL in controlled trials and rarer, serious, possibly drug-related events reported in uncontrolled studies or marketing experience are listed below, and within each category, are in order of decreasing severity:

Body as a Whole: Anaphylactoid reactions (see WARNINGS, *Anaphylactoid and Possible Related Reactions*), syncope, orthostatic effects, chest discomfort, pain, pelvic pain, flank pain, edema, facial edema, virus infection, fever, chills, malaise.

Cardiovascular: Cardiac arrest; myocardial infarction or cerebrovascular accident, possibly secondary to excessive hypotension in high risk patients (see WARNINGS, *Hypotension*); pulmonary embolism and infarction, arrhythmias (including ventricular tachycardia, atrial tachycardia, atrial fibrillation, bradycardia and premature ventricular contractions), palpitations, transient ischemic attacks, paroxysmal nocturnal dyspnea, orthostatic hypotension, decreased blood pressure, peripheral edema, vasculitis.

Digestive: Pancreatitis, hepatitis (hepatocellular or cholestatic jaundice) (see WARNINGS, *Hepatic Failure*), vomiting, gastritis, dyspepsia, heartburn, gastrointestinal cramps, constipation, flatulence, dry mouth.

Hematologic: Rare cases of bone marrow depression, neutropenia, and thrombocytopenia.

Endocrine: Diabetes mellitus.

Metabolic: Weight loss, dehydration, fluid overload, gout, weight gain.

Musculoskeletal: Arthritis, arthralgia, neck pain, hip pain, low back pain, joint pain, leg pain, knee pain, shoulder pain, arm pain, lumbago.

Nervous System/Psychiatric: Stroke, ataxia, memory impairment, tremor, peripheral neuropathy (e.g., dysesthesia) spasm, paresthesia, confusion, insomnia, somnolence, hypersomnia, irritability, and nervousness.

Respiratory System: Malignant lung neoplasms, hemoptysis, pulmonary infiltrates, eosinophilic pneumonitis, bronchospasm, asthma, pleural effusion, pneumonia, bronchitis, wheezing, orthopnea, painful respiration, epistaxis, laryngitis, sinusitis, pharyngeal pain, pharyngitis, rhinitis, rhinorrhea.

Skin: Urticaria, alopecia, herpes zoster, photosensitivity, skin lesions, skin infections, pemphigus, erythema, flushing, diaphoresis. Other severe skin reactions (including toxic epidermal necrolysis and Stevens-Johnson syndrome) have been reported rarely; causal relationship has not been established.

Special Senses: Visual loss, diplopia, blurred vision, tinnitus, photophobia, taste disturbances.

Urogenital System: Acute renal failure, oliguria, anuria, uremia, progressive azotemia, renal dysfunction (see PRECAUTIONS and DOSAGE AND ADMINISTRATION), pyelonephritis, dysuria, urinary tract infection, breast pain.

Miscellaneous: A symptom complex has been reported which may include a positive ANA, an elevated erythrocyte sedimentation rate, arthralgia/arthritis, myalgia, fever, vasculitis, leukocytosis, eosinophilia, photosensitivity, rash, and other dermatological manifestations.

Angioedema: Angioedema has been reported in patients receiving PRINIVIL with an incidence higher in black than in non-black patients. Angioedema associated with laryngeal edema may be fatal. If angioedema of the face, extremities, lips, tongue, glottis and/or larynx occurs, treatment with PRINIVIL should be discontinued and appropriate therapy instituted immediately. (See WARNINGS.)

Hypotension: In hypertensive patients, hypotension occurred in 1.2 percent and syncope occurred in 0.1 percent of patients. Hypotension or syncope was a cause for discontinuation of therapy in 0.5 percent of hypertensive patients. In patients with heart failure, hypotension occurred in 5.3 percent and syncope occurred in 1.8 percent of patients. These adverse experiences were causes for discontinuation of therapy in 1.8 percent of these patients. In patients treated with PRINIVIL for six weeks after acute myocardial infarction, hypotension (systolic blood pressure $\leq$ 100 mmHg) resulted in discontinuation of therapy in 9.7 percent of the patients. (See WARNINGS.)

Fetal/Neonatal Morbidity and Mortality: See WARNINGS, *Fetal/Neonatal Morbidity and Mortality.*

Cough: See PRECAUTIONS, *Cough.*

Clinical Laboratory Test Findings

Serum Electrolytes: Hyperkalemia (see PRECAUTIONS), hyponatremia.

Creatinine, Blood Urea Nitrogen: Minor increases in blood urea nitrogen and serum creatinine, reversible upon discontinuation of therapy, were observed in about 2.0 percent of patients with essential hypertension treated with PRINIVIL alone. Increases were more common in patients receiving concomitant diuretics and in patients with renal artery stenosis. (See PRECAUTIONS.) Reversible minor increases in blood urea nitrogen and serum creatinine were observed in approximately 11.6 percent of patients with heart failure on concomitant diuretic therapy. Frequently, these abnormalities resolved when the dosage of the diuretic was decreased.

Hemoglobin and Hematocrit: Small decreases in hemoglobin and hematocrit (mean decreases of approximately 0.4 g percent and 1.3 vol percent, respectively) occurred frequently in patients treated with PRINIVIL but were rarely of clinical importance in patients without some other cause of anemia. In clinical trials, less than 0.1 percent of patients discontinued therapy due to anemia. Hemolytic anemia has been reported; a causal relationship to lisinopril cannot be excluded.

Liver Function Tests: Rarely, elevations of liver enzymes and/or serum bilirubin have occurred (see WARNINGS, *Hepatic Failure*).

	Percent of Patients in Controlled Studies		
	PRINIVIL (n = 1349) Incidence (discontinuation)	PRINIVIL/ Hydrochlorothiazide (n = 629) Incidence (discontinuation)	Placebo (n =207) Incidence (discontinuation)
Body As A Whole			
Fatigue	2.5 (0.3)	4.0 (0.5)	1.0 (0.0)
Asthenia	1.3 (0.5)	2.1 (0.2)	1.0 (0.0)
Orthostatic Effects	1.2 (0.0)	3.5 (0.2)	1.0 (0.0)
Cardiovascular			
Hypotension	1.2 (0.5)	1.6 (0.5)	0.5 (0.5)
Digestive			
Diarrhea	2.7 (0.2)	2.7 (0.3)	2.4 (0.0)
Nausea	2.0 (0.4)	2.5 (0.2)	2.4 (0.0)
Vomiting	1.1 (0.2)	1.4 (0.1)	0.5 (0.0)
Dyspepsia	0.9 (0.0)	1.9 (0.0)	0.0 (0.0)
Musculoskeletal			
Muscle Cramps	0.5 (0.0)	2.9 (0.8)	0.5 (0.0)
Nervous/Psychiatric			
Headache	5.7 (0.2)	4.5 (0.5)	1.9 (0.0)
Dizziness	5.4 (0.4)	9.2 (1.0)	1.9 (0.0)
Paresthesia	0.8 (0.1)	2.1 (0.2)	0.0 (0.0)
Decreased Libido	0.4 (0.1)	1.3 (0.1)	0.0 (0.0)
Vertigo	0.2 (0.1)	1.1 (0.2)	0.0 (0.0)
Respiratory			
Cough	3.5 (0.7)	4.6 (0.8)	1.0 (0.0)
Upper Respiratory Infection	2.1 (0.1)	2.7 (0.1)	0.0 (0.0)
Common Cold	1.1 (0.1)	1.3 (0.1)	0.0 (0.0)
Nasal Congestion	0.4 (0.1)	1.3 (0.1)	0.0 (0.0)
Influenza	0.3 (0.1)	1.1 (0.1)	0.0 (0.0)
Skin			
Rash	1.3 (0.4)	1.6 (0.2)	0.5 (0.5)
Urogenital			
Impotence	1.0 (0.4)	1.6 (0.5)	0.0 (0.0)

In hypertensive patients, 2.0 percent discontinued therapy due to laboratory adverse experiences, principally elevations in blood urea nitrogen (0.6 percent), serum creatinine (0.5 percent) and serum potassium (0.4 percent). In the heart failure trials, 3.4 percent of patients discontinued therapy due to laboratory adverse experiences, 1.8 percent due to elevations in blood urea nitrogen and/or creatinine and 0.6 percent due to elevations in serum potassium. In the myocardial infarction trial, 2.0 percent of patients receiving PRINIVIL discontinued therapy due to renal dysfunction (increasing creatinine concentration to over 3 mg/dL or a doubling or more of the baseline serum creatinine concentration); less than 1.0 percent of patients discontinued therapy due to other laboratory adverse experiences: 0.1 percent with hyperkalemia and less than 0.1 percent with hepatic enzyme alterations.

OVERDOSAGE

Following a single oral dose of 20 g/kg, no lethality occurred in rats and death occurred in one of 20 mice receiving the same dose. The most likely manifestation of overdosage would be hypotension, for which the usual treatment would be intravenous infusion of normal saline solution.

Lisinopril can be removed by hemodialysis. (See WARNINGS, *Anaphylactoid reactions during membrane exposure.*)

DOSAGE AND ADMINISTRATION

Hypertension

Initial Therapy: In patients with uncomplicated essential hypertension not on diuretic therapy, the recommended initial dose is 10 mg once a day. Dosage should be adjusted according to blood pressure response. The usual dosage range is 20 to 40 mg per day administered in a single daily dose. The antihypertensive effect may diminish toward the end of the dosing interval regardless of the administered dose, but most commonly with a dose of 10 mg daily. This can be evaluated by measuring blood pressure just prior to dosing to determine whether satisfactory control is being maintained for 24 hours. If it is not, an increase in dose should be considered. Doses up to 80 mg have been used but do not appear to give a greater effect. If blood pressure is not controlled with PRINIVIL alone, a low dose of a diuretic may be added. Hydrochlorothiazide 12.5 mg has been shown to provide an additive effect. After the addition of a diuretic, it may be possible to reduce the dose of PRINIVIL.

Diuretic Treated Patients: In hypertensive patients who are currently being treated with a diuretic, symptomatic hypotension may occur occasionally following the initial dose of PRINIVIL. The diuretic should be discontinued, if possible, for two to three days before beginning therapy with PRINIVIL to reduce the likelihood of hypotension. (See WARNINGS.) The dosage of PRINIVIL should be adjusted according to blood pressure response. If the patient's blood pressure is not controlled with PRINIVIL alone, diuretic therapy may be resumed as described above.

If the diuretic cannot be discontinued, an initial dose of 5 mg should be used under medical supervision for at least two hours and until blood pressure has stabilized for at least an additional hour. (See WARNINGS and PRECAUTIONS, *Drug Interactions.*)

Concomitant administration of PRINIVIL with potassium supplements, potassium salt substitutes, or potassium-sparing diuretics may lead to increases of serum potassium (see PRECAUTIONS).

Dosage Adjustment in Renal Impairment: The usual dose of PRINIVIL (10 mg) is recommended for patients with a creatinine clearance $>$ 30 mL/min (serum creatinine of up to approximately 3 mg/dL). For patients with creatinine clearance $\geq$ 10 mL/min $\leq$ 30 mL/min (serum creatinine $\geq$ 3 mg/dL), the first dose is 5 mg once daily. For patients with creatinine clearance $<$ 10 mL/min (usually on hemodialysis) the recommended initial dose is 2.5 mg. The dosage may be titrated upward until blood pressure is controlled or to a maximum of 40 mg daily.

Renal Status	Creatinine-Clearance mL/min	Initial Dose mg/day
Normal Renal Function to Mild Impairment	$>$ 30 mL/min	10 mg
Moderate to Severe Impairment	$\geq 10 \leq 30$ mL/min	5 mg
Dialysis Patients**	$<$ 10 mL/min	2.5 mg ***

** See WARNINGS, *Anaphylactoid reactions during membrane exposure.*

*** *Dosage or dosing interval should be adjusted depending on the blood pressure response.*

Continued on next page

Information on the Merck & Co., Inc. products listed on these pages is the full prescribing information from product circulars in use September 30, 2000. For information, please call 1-800-NSC MERCK [1-800-672-6372].

Prinivil—Cont.

Heart Failure
PRINIVIL is indicated as adjunctive therapy with diuretics and digitalis. The recommended starting dose is 5 mg once a day.
When initiating treatment with lisinopril in patients with heart failure, the initial dose should be administered under medical observation, especially in those patients with low blood pressure (systolic blood pressure below 100 mmHg). The mean peak blood pressure lowering occurs six to eight hours after dosing. Observation should continue until blood pressure is stable. The concomitant diuretic dose should be reduced, if possible, to help minimize hypovolemia which may contribute to hypotension. (See WARNINGS and PRECAUTIONS, *Drug Interactions.*) The appearance of hypotension after the initial dose of PRINIVIL does not preclude subsequent careful dose titration with the drug, following effective management of the hypotension.
The usual effective dosage range is 5 to 20 mg per day administered as a single daily dose.
Dosage Adjustment in Patients with Heart Failure and Renal Impairment or Hyponatremia: In patients with heart failure who have hyponatremia (serum sodium $<$130 mEq/L) or moderate to severe renal impairment (creatinine clearance $\leq$30 mL/min or serum creatinine $>$3 mg/dL), therapy with PRINIVIL should be initiated at a dose of 2.5 mg once a day under close medical supervision. (See WARNINGS and PRECAUTIONS, *Drug Interactions.*)
Acute Myocardial Infarction
In hemodynamically stable patients within 24 hours of the onset of acute myocardial infarction, the first dose of PRINIVIL is 5 mg given orally, followed by 5 mg after 24 hours, 10 mg after 48 hours and then 10 mg of PRINIVIL once daily. Dosing should continue for six weeks. Patients should receive, as appropriate, the standard recommended treatments such as thrombolytics, aspirin and beta-blockers. Patients with a low systolic blood pressure ($\leq$120 mmHg) when treatment is started or during the first 3 days after the infarct should be given a lower 2.5 mg oral dose of PRINIVIL (see WARNINGS). If hypotension occurs (systolic blood pressure $\leq$100 mmHg) a daily maintenance dose of 5 mg may be given with temporary reductions to 2.5 mg if needed. If prolonged hypotension occurs (systolic blood pressure $<$90 mmHg for more than 1 hour) PRINIVIL should be withdrawn. For patients who develop symptoms of heart failure, see DOSAGE AND ADMINISTRATION, *Heart Failure.*
Dosage Adjustment in Patients with Myocardial Infarction with Renal Impairment: In acute myocardial infarction, treatment with PRINIVIL should be initiated with caution in patients with evidence of renal dysfunction, defined as serum creatinine concentration exceeding 2 mg/dL. No evaluation of dosage adjustment in myocardial infarction patients with severe renal impairment has been performed.
Use in Elderly: In general, blood pressure response and adverse experiences were similar in younger and older patients given similar doses of PRINIVIL. Pharmacokinetic studies, however, indicate that maximum blood levels and area under the plasma concentration time curve (AUC) are doubled in older patients so that dosage adjustments should be made with particular caution.

HOW SUPPLIED

No. 3658—Tablets PRINIVIL, 2.5 mg, are white, round flat-faced beveled edged compressed tablets, coded MSD on one side and 15 on the other. They are supplied as follows:
NDC 0006-0015-28 unit dose packages of 100
NDC 0006-0015-31 unit of use bottles of 30
NDC 0006-0015-58 unit of use bottles of 100
NDC 0006-0015-72 carton of 25 UNIBLISTER™ cards of 31 tablets each.
Shown in Product Identification Guide, page 324
No. 3577—Tablets PRINIVIL, 5 mg, are white, shield shaped, scored, compressed tablets, with code MSD 19 on one side and PRINIVIL on the other. They are supplied as follows:
NDC 0006-0019-28 unit dose packages of 100
NDC 0006-0019-58 unit of use bottles of 100
(6505-01-281-2771, 5 mg 100's)
NDC 0006-0019-94 unit of use bottles of 90
NDC 0006-0019-82 bottles of 1,000
NDC 0006-0019-86 bottles of 5,000
(6505-01-367-8874, 5 mg 5,000's)
NDC 0006-0019-87 bottles of 10,000
(6505-01-377-8061, 5 mg 10,000's)
NDC 0006-0019-72 carton of 25 UNIBLISTER™ cards of 31 tablets each.
Shown in Product Identification Guide, page 324
No. 3578—Tablets PRINIVIL, 10 mg, are light yellow, shield shaped, compressed tablets, with code MSD 106 on one side and PRINIVIL on the other. They are supplied as follows:
NDC 0006-0106-28 unit dose packages of 100
(6505-01-342-4861, 10 mg individually sealed 100's
NDC 0006-0106-31 unit of use bottles of 30
NDC 0006-0106-58 unit of use bottles of 100
(6505-01-275-0061, 10 mg 100's)
NDC 0006-0106-94 unit of use bottles of 90
NDC 0006-0106-82 bottles of 1,000
NDC 0006-0106-86 bottles of 5,000
(6505-01-368-6604, 10 mg 5,000's)
NDC 0006-0106-87 bottles of 10,000
(6505-01-377-8064, 10 mg 10,000's)
NDC 0006-0106-72 carton of 25 UNIBLISTER™ cards of 31 tablets each.
Shown in Product Identification Guide, page 324
No. 3579—Tablets PRINIVIL, 20 mg, are peach, shield shaped, compressed tablets, with code MSD 207 on one side and PRINIVIL on the other. They are supplied as follows:
NDC 0006-0207-28 unit dose packages of 100
NDC 0006-0207-31 unit of use bottles of 30
NDC 0006-0207-58 unit of use bottles of 100
(6505-01-282-6327, 20 mg 100's)
NDC 0006-0207-94 unit of use bottles of 90
NDC 0006-0207-82 bottles of 1,000
NDC 0006-0207-86 bottles of 5,000
(6505-01-368-2704, 20 mg 5,000's)
NDC 0006-0207-87 bottles of 10,000
(6505-01-8066, 20 mg 10,000's)
NDC 0006-0207-72 carton of 25 UNIBLISTER™ cards of 31 tablets each.
Shown in Product Identification Guide, page 324
No. 3580—Tablets PRINIVIL, 40 mg, are rose red, shield shaped, compressed tablets, with code MSD 237 on one side and PRINIVIL on the other. They are supplied as follows:
NDC 0006-0237-58 unit of use bottles of 100.
Shown in Product Identification Guide, page 324
Storage
Store at controlled room temperature, 15–30°C (59–86°F), and protect from moisture.
Dispense in a tight container, if product package is subdivided.

7825243 Issued June 1999

PRINZIDE® Tablets ℞
(Lisinopril-Hydrochlorothiazide)

> **USE IN PREGNANCY**
> **When used in pregnancy during the second and third trimesters, ACE inhibitors can cause injury and even death to the developing fetus.** When pregnancy is detected, PRINZIDE should be discontinued as soon as possible. See WARNINGS, *Pregnancy, Lisinopril, Fetal/Neonatal Morbidity and Mortality.*

DESCRIPTION

PRINZIDE* (Lisinopril-Hydrochlorothiazide) combines an angiotensin converting enzyme inhibitor, lisinopril, and a diuretic, hydrochlorothiazide.
Lisinopril, a synthetic peptide derivative, is an oral long-acting angiotensin converting enzyme inhibitor. It is chemically described as (*S*)-1-[N^2-(1-carboxy-3-phenylpropyl)-L-lysyl]-L-proline dihydrate. Its empirical formula is $C_{21}H_{31}N_3O_5 \cdot 2H_2O$ and its structural formula is:

Lisinopril is a white to off-white, crystalline powder, with a molecular weight of 441.52. It is soluble in water, sparingly soluble in methanol, and practically insoluble in ethanol.
Hydrochlorothiazide is 6-chloro-3,4-dihydro-2*H*-1,2,4-benzothiadiazine-7-sulfonamide 1,1-dioxide. Its empirical formula is $C_7H_8ClN_3O_4S_2$ and its structural formula is:

Hydrochlorothiazide is a white, or practically white, crystalline powder with a molecular weight of 297.73, which is slightly soluble in water, but freely soluble in sodium hydroxide solution.
PRINZIDE is available for oral use in three tablet combinations of lisinopril with hydrochlorothiazide: PRINZIDE 10-12.5, containing 10 mg lisinopril and 12.5 mg hydrochlorothiazide. PRINZIDE 20-12.5, containing 20 mg lisinopril and 12.5 mg hydrochlorothiazide and PRINZIDE 20-25, containing 20 mg lisinopril and 25 mg hydrochlorothiazide. Inactive ingredients are calcium phosphate, magnesium stearate, mannitol, and starch. PRINZIDE 10-12.5 also contains FD&C Blue #2 aluminum lake. PRINZIDE 20-12.5 and PRINZIDE 20-25 also contain iron oxide.

*Registered trademark of MERCK & CO., INC.

CLINICAL PHARMACOLOGY

Lisinopril-Hydrochlorothiazide
As a result of its diuretic effects, hydrochlorothiazide increases plasma renin activity, increases aldosterone secretion, and decreases serum potassium. Administration of lisinopril blocks the renin-angiotensin-aldosterone axis and tends to reverse the potassium loss associated with the diuretic.
In clinical studies, the extent of blood pressure reduction seen with the combination of lisinopril and hydrochlorothiazide was approximately additive. The PRINZIDE 10-12.5 combination worked equally well in black and white patients. The PRINZIDE 20-12.5 and PRINZIDE 20-25 combinations appeared somewhat less effective in black patients, but relatively few black patients were studied. In most patients, the antihypertensive effect of PRINZIDE was sustained for at least 24 hours.
In a randomized, controlled comparison, the main antihypertensive effects of PRINZIDE 20-12.5 and PRINZIDE 20-25 were similar, suggesting that many patients who respond adequately to the latter combination may be controlled with PRINZIDE 20-12.5. (See DOSAGE AND ADMINISTRATION.)
Concomitant administration of lisinopril and hydrochlorothiazide has little or no effect on the bioavailability of either drug. The combination tablet is bioequivalent to concomitant administration of the separate entities.
Lisinopril
Mechanism of Action
Lisinopril inhibits angiotensin-converting enzyme (ACE) in human subjects and animals. ACE is a peptidyl dipeptidase that catalyzes the conversion of angiotensin I to the vasoconstrictor substance, angiotensin II. Angiotensin II also stimulates aldosterone secretion by the adrenal cortex. Inhibition of ACE results in decreased plasma angiotensin II which leads to decreased vasopressor activity and to decreased aldosterone secretion. The latter decrease may result in a small increase of serum potassium. Removal of angiotensin II negative feedback on renin secretion leads to increased plasma renin activity. In hypertensive patients with normal renal function treated with lisinopril alone for up to 24 weeks, the mean increase in serum potassium was less than 0.1 mEq/L; however, approximately 15 percent of patients had increases greater than 0.5 mEq/L and approximately six percent had a decrease greater than 0.5 mEq/L. In the same study, patients treated with lisinopril plus a thiazide diuretic showed essentially no change in serum potassium. (See PRECAUTIONS.)
ACE is identical to kininase, an enzyme that degrades bradykinin. Whether increased levels of bradykinin, a potent vasodepressor peptide, play a role in the therapeutic effects of lisinopril remains to be elucidated.
While the mechanism through which lisinopril lowers blood pressure is believed to be primarily suppression of the renin-angiotensin-aldosterone system, lisinopril is antihypertensive even in patients with low-renin hypertension. Although lisinopril was antihypertensive in all races studied, black hypertensive patients (usually a low-renin hypertensive population) had a smaller average response to lisinopril monotherapy than non-black patients.
Pharmacokinetics and Metabolism
Following oral administration of lisinopril, peak serum concentrations occur within about 7 hours. Declining serum concentrations exhibit a prolonged terminal phase which does not contribute to drug accumulation. This terminal phase probably represents saturable binding to ACE and is not proportional to dose. Lisinopril does not appear to be bound to other serum proteins.
Lisinopril does not undergo metabolism and is excreted unchanged entirely in the urine. Based on urinary recovery, the mean extent of absorption of lisinopril is approximately 25 percent, with large intersubject variability (6–60 percent) at all doses tested (5–80 mg). Lisinopril absorption is not influenced by the presence of food in the gastrointestinal tract.
Upon multiple dosing, lisinopril exhibits an effective half-life of accumulation of 12 hours.
Impaired renal function decreases elimination of lisinopril, which is excreted principally through the kidneys, but this decrease becomes clinically important only when the glomerular filtration rate is below 30 mL/min. Above this glomerular filtration rate, the elimination half-life is little changed. With greater impairment, however, peak and trough lisinopril levels increase, time to peak concentration increases and time to attain steady state is prolonged. Older patients, on average, have (approximately doubled) higher blood levels and area under the plasma concentration time curve (AUC) than younger patients. (See DOSAGE AND ADMINISTRATION.) Lisinopril can be removed by hemodialysis.
Studies in rats indicate that lisinopril crosses the blood-brain barrier poorly. Multiple doses of lisinopril in rats do not result in accumulation in any tissues. However, milk of lactating rats contains radioactivity following administration of ^{14}C lisinopril. By whole body autoradiography, radioactivity was found in the placenta following administration of labeled drug to pregnant rats, but none was found in the fetuses.
Pharmacodynamics
Administration of lisinopril to patients with hypertension results in a reduction of supine and standing blood pressure to about the same extent with no compensatory tachycardia. Symptomatic postural hypotension is usually not observed although it can occur and should be anticipated in volume and/or salt-depleted patients. (See WARNINGS.)
In most patients studied, onset of antihypertensive activity was seen at one hour after oral administration of an individual dose of lisinopril, with peak reduction of blood pressure achieved by six hours.

In some patients achievement of optimal blood pressure reduction may require two to four weeks of therapy.
At recommended single daily doses, antihypertensive effects have been maintained for at least 24 hours after dosing, although the effect at 24 hours was substantially smaller than the effect six hours after dosing.
The antihypertensive effects of lisinopril have continued during long-term therapy. Abrupt withdrawal of lisinopril has not been associated with a rapid increase in blood pressure; nor with a significant overshoot of pretreatment blood pressure.
In hemodynamic studies in patients with essential hypertension, blood pressure reduction was accompanied by a reduction in peripheral arterial resistance with little or no change in cardiac output and in heart rate. In a study in nine hypertensive patients, following administration of lisinopril, there was an increase in mean renal blood flow that was not significant. Data from several small studies are inconsistent with respect to the effect of lisinopril on glomerular filtration rate in hypertensive patients with normal renal function, but suggest that changes, if any, are not large.
In patients with renovascular hypertension lisinopril has been shown to be well tolerated and effective in controlling blood pressure (see PRECAUTIONS).
Hydrochlorothiazide
The mechanism of the antihypertensive effect of thiazides is unknown. Thiazides do not usually affect normal blood pressure.
Hydrochlorothiazide is a diuretic and antihypertensive. It affects the distal renal tubular mechanism of electrolyte reabsorption. Hydrochlorothiazide increases excretion of sodium and chloride in approximately equivalent amounts. Natriuresis may be accompanied by some loss of potassium and bicarbonate.
After oral use diuresis begins within two hours, peaks in about four hours and lasts about 6 to 12 hours.
Hydrochlorothiazide is not metabolized but is eliminated rapidly by the kidney. When plasma levels have been followed for at least 24 hours, the plasma half-life has been observed to vary between 5.6 and 14.8 hours. At least 61 percent of the oral dose is eliminated unchanged within 24 hours. Hydrochlorothiazide crosses the placental but not the blood-brain barrier.

INDICATIONS AND USAGE

PRINZIDE is indicated for the treatment of hypertension.
These fixed-dose combinations are not indicated for initial therapy (see DOSAGE AND ADMINISTRATION).
In using PRINZIDE, consideration should be given to the fact that an angiotensin converting enzyme inhibitor, captopril, has caused agranulocytosis, particularly in patients with renal impairment or collagen vascular disease, and that available data are insufficient to show that lisinopril does not have a similar risk. (See WARNINGS.)
In considering use of PRINZIDE, it should be noted that black patients receiving ACE inhibitors have been reported to have a higher incidence of angioedema compared to nonblacks. (See WARNINGS, *Angioedema.*)

CONTRAINDICATIONS

PRINZIDE is contraindicated in patients who are hypersensitive to any component of this product and in patients with a history of angioedema related to previous treatment with an angiotensin converting enzyme inhibitor and in patients with hereditary or idiopathic angioedema. Because of the hydrochlorothiazide component, this product is contraindicated in patients with anuria or hypersensitivity to other sulfonamide-derived drugs.

WARNINGS

General
Lisinopril
Anaphylactoid and Possibly Related Reactions:
Presumably because angiotensin-converting enzyme inhibitors affect the metabolism of eicosanoids and polypeptides, including endogenous bradykinin, patients receiving ACE inhibitors (including PRINZIDE) may be subject to a variety of adverse reactions, some of them serious.
Angioedema: Angioedema of the face, extremities, lips, tongue, glottis and/or larynx has been reported rarely in patients treated with angiotensin converting enzyme inhibitors, including lisinopril. This may occur at any time during treatment. In such cases PRINZIDE should be promptly discontinued and appropriate therapy and monitoring should be provided until complete and sustained resolution of signs and symptoms has occurred. In instances where swelling has been confined to the face and lips the condition has generally resolved without treatment, although antihistamines have been useful in relieving symptoms. Angioedema associated with laryngeal edema may be fatal. **Where there is involvement of the tongue, glottis or larynx, likely to cause airway obstruction, subcutaneous epinephrine solution 1:1000 (0.3 mL to 0.5 mL) and/or measures necessary to ensure a patent airway, should be promptly provided.** (See ADVERSE REACTIONS.)
Patients with a history of angioedema unrelated to ACE inhibitor therapy may be at increased risk of angioedema while receiving an ACE inhibitor (see also INDICATIONS AND USAGE and CONTRAINDICATIONS).
Anaphylactoid reactions during desensitization: Two patients undergoing desensitizing treatment with hymenoptera venom while receiving ACE inhibitors sustained life-threatening anaphylactoid reactions. In the same patients, these reactions were avoided when ACE inhibitors were temporarily withheld, but they reappeared upon inadvertent rechallenge.
Anaphylactoid reactions during membrane exposure: Anaphylactoid reactions have been reported in patients dialyzed with high-flux membranes and treated concomitantly with an ACE inhibitor. Anaphylactoid reactions have also been reported in patients undergoing low-density lipoprotein apheresis with dextran sulfate absorption.
Hypotension and Related Effects:
Excessive hypotension was rarely seen in uncomplicated hypertensive patients but is a possible consequence of lisinopril use in salt/volume-depleted persons, such as those treated vigorously with diuretics or patients on dialysis. (See PRECAUTIONS, *Drug Interactions* and ADVERSE REACTIONS.)
Syncope has been reported in 0.8 percent of patients receiving PRINZIDE. In patients with hypertension receiving lisinopril alone, the incidence of syncope was 0.1 percent. The overall incidence of syncope may be reduced by proper titration of the individual components. (See PRECAUTIONS, *Drug Interactions,* ADVERSE REACTIONS and DOSAGE AND ADMINISTRATION.)
In patients with severe congestive heart failure, with or without associated renal insufficiency, excessive hypotension has been observed and may be associated with oliguria and/or progressive azotemia, and rarely with acute renal failure and/or death. Because of the potential fall in blood pressure in these patients, therapy should be started under very close medical supervision. Such patients should be followed closely for the first two weeks of treatment and whenever the dose of lisinopril and/or diuretic is increased. Similar considerations apply to patients with ischemic heart or cerebrovascular disease in whom an excessive fall in blood pressure could result in a myocardial infarction or cerebrovascular accident.
If hypotension occurs, the patient should be placed in supine position and, if necessary, receive an intravenous infusion of normal saline. A transient hypotensive response is not a contraindication to further doses which usually can be given without difficulty once the blood pressure has increased after volume expansion.
Neutropenia/Agranulocytosis:
Another angiotensin converting enzyme inhibitor, captopril, has been shown to cause agranulocytosis and bone marrow depression, rarely in uncomplicated patients but more frequently in patients with renal impairment, especially if they also have a collagen vascular disease. Available data from clinical trials of lisinopril are insufficient to show that lisinopril does not cause agranulocytosis at similar rates. Marketing experience has revealed rare cases of neutropenia and bone marrow depression in which a causal relationship to lisinopril cannot be excluded. Periodic monitoring of white blood cell counts in patients with collagen vascular disease and renal disease should be considered.
Hepatic Failure:
Rarely, ACE inhibitors have been associated with a syndrome that starts with cholestatic jaundice and progresses to fulminant hepatic necrosis, and (sometimes) death. The mechanism of this syndrome is not understood. Patients receiving ACE inhibitors who develop jaundice or marked elevations of hepatic enzymes should discontinue the ACE inhibitor and receive appropriate medical follow-up.
Hydrochlorothiazide
Thiazides should be used with caution in severe renal disease. In patients with renal disease, thiazides may precipitate azotemia. Cumulative effects of the drug may develop in patients with impaired renal function.
Thiazides should be used with caution in patients with impaired hepatic function or progressive liver disease, since minor alterations of fluid and electrolyte balance may precipitate hepatic coma.
Sensitivity reactions may occur in patients with or without a history of allergy or bronchial asthma.
The possibility of exacerbation or activation of systemic lupus erythematosus has been reported.
Lithium generally should not be given with thiazides (see PRECAUTIONS, *Drug Interactions, Lisinopril* and *Hydrochlorothiazide*).
Pregnancy
Lisinopril-Hydrochlorothiazide
Teratogenicity studies were conducted in mice and rats with up to 90 mg/kg/day of lisinopril in combination with 10 mg/kg/day of hydrochlorothiazide. This dose of lisinopril is 5 times (in mice) and 10 times (in rats) the maximum recommended human daily dose (MRHDD) when compared on a body surface area basis (mg/m^2); the dose of hydrochlorothiazide is 0.9 times (in mice) and 1.8 times (in rats) the MRHDD. Maternal or fetotoxic effects were not seen in mice with the combination. In rats decreased maternal weight gain and decreased fetal weight occurred down to 3/10 mg/kg/day (the lowest dose tested). Associated with the decreased fetal weight was a delay in fetal ossification. The decreased fetal weight and delay in fetal ossification were not seen in saline-supplemented animals given 90/10 mg/kg/day.
When used in pregnancy during the second and third trimesters, ACE inhibitors can cause injury and even death to the developing fetus. When pregnancy is detected, PRINZIDE should be discontinued as soon as possible. (See *Lisinopril, Fetal/Neonatal Morbidity and Mortality,* below.)
Lisinopril
Fetal/Neonatal Morbidity and Mortality: ACE inhibitors can cause fetal and neonatal morbidity and death when administered to pregnant women. Several dozen cases have been reported in the world literature. When pregnancy is detected, ACE inhibitors should be discontinued as soon as possible.
The use of ACE inhibitors during the second and third trimesters of pregnancy has been associated with fetal and neonatal injury, including hypotension, neonatal skull hypoplasia, anuria, reversible or irreversible renal failure, and death. Oligohydramnios has also been reported, presumably resulting from decreased fetal renal function; oligohydramnios in this setting has been associated with fetal limb contractures, craniofacial deformation, and hypoplastic lung development. Prematurity, intrauterine growth retardation, and patent ductus arteriosus have also been reported, although it is not clear whether these occurrences were due to the ACE-inhibitor exposure.
These adverse effects do not appear to have resulted from intrauterine ACE-inhibitor exposure that has been limited to the first trimester. Mothers whose embryos and fetuses are exposed to ACE inhibitors only during the first trimester should be so informed. Nonetheless, when patients become pregnant, physicians should make every effort to discontinue the use of PRINZIDE as soon as possible.
Rarely (probably less often than once in every thousand pregnancies), no alternative to ACE inhibitors will be found. In these rare cases, the mothers should be apprised of the potential hazards to their fetuses, and serial ultrasound examinations should be performed to assess the intraamniotic environment.
If oligohydramnios is observed, PRINZIDE should be discontinued unless it is considered lifesaving for the mother. Contraction stress testing (CST), a non-stress test (NST), or biophysical profiling (BPP) may be appropriate, depending upon the week of pregnancy. Patients and physicians should be aware, however, that oligohydramnios may not appear until after the fetus has sustained irreversible injury.
Infants with histories of *in utero* exposure to ACE inhibitors should be closely observed for hypotension, oliguria, and hyperkalemia. If oliguria occurs, attention should be directed toward support of blood pressure and renal perfusion. Exchange transfusion or dialysis may be required as means of reversing hypotension and/or substituting for disordered renal function. Lisinopril, which crosses the placenta, has been removed from neonatal circulation by peritoneal dialysis with some clinical benefit, and theoretically may be removed by exchange transfusion, although there is no experience with the latter procedure.
No teratogenic effects of lisinopril were seen in studies of pregnant mice, rats, and rabbits. On a body surface area basis, the doses used were up to 55 times, 33 times, and 0.15 times, respectively, the MRHDD.
Hydrochlorothiazide
Studies in which hydrochlorothiazide was orally administered to pregnant mice and rats during their respective periods of major organogenesis at doses up to 3000 and 1000 mg/kg/day, respectively, provided no evidence of harm to the fetus. These doses are more than 150 times the MRHDD on a body surface area basis. Thiazides cross the placental barrier and appear in cord blood. There is a risk of fetal or neonatal jaundice, thrombocytopenia and possibly other adverse reactions that have occurred in adults.

PRECAUTIONS

General
Lisinopril
Aortic Stenosis/Hypertrophic Cardiomyopathy: As with all vasodilators, lisinopril should be given with caution to patients with obstruction in the outflow tract of the left ventricle.
Impaired Renal Function: As a consequence of inhibiting the renin-angiotensin-aldosterone system, changes in renal function may be anticipated in susceptible individuals. In patients with severe congestive heart failure whose renal function may depend on the activity of the renin-angiotensin-aldosterone system, treatment with angiotensin converting enzyme inhibitors, including lisinopril, may be associated with oliguria and/or progressive azotemia and rarely with acute renal failure and/or death.
In hypertensive patients with unilateral or bilateral renal artery stenosis, increases in blood urea nitrogen and serum creatinine may occur. Experience with another angiotensin converting enzyme inhibitor suggests that these increases are usually reversible upon discontinuation of lisinopril and/ or diuretic therapy. In such patients renal function should be monitored during the first few weeks of therapy.
Some hypertensive patients with no apparent pre-existing renal vascular disease have developed increases in blood urea and serum creatinine, usually minor and transient, especially when lisinopril has been given concomitantly with a diuretic. This is more likely to occur in patients with pre-existing renal impairment. Dosage reduction of lisinopril and/or discontinuation of the diuretic may be required.

Continued on next page

Information on the Merck & Co., Inc. products listed on these pages is the full prescribing information from product circulars in use September 30, 2000. For information, please call 1-800-NSC MERCK [1-800-672-6372].

Prinzide—Cont.

Evaluation of the hypertensive patient should always include assessment of renal function. (See DOSAGE AND ADMINISTRATION.)

Hyperkalemia: In clinical trials hyperkalemia (serum potassium greater than 5.7 mEq/L) occurred in approximately 1.4 percent of hypertensive patients treated with lisinopril plus hydrochlorothiazide. In most cases these were isolated values which resolved despite continued therapy. Hyperkalemia was not a cause of discontinuation of therapy. Risk factors for the development of hyperkalemia include renal insufficiency, diabetes mellitus, and the concomitant use of potassium-sparing diuretics, potassium supplements and/or potassium-containing salt substitutes, which should be used cautiously if at all with PRINZIDE. (See *Drug Interactions.*)

Cough: Presumably due to the inhibition of the degradation of endogenous bradykinin, persistent nonproductive cough has been reported with all ACE inhibitors, always resolving after discontinuation of therapy. ACE inhibitor-induced cough should be considered in the differential diagnosis of cough.

Surgery/Anesthesia: In patients undergoing major surgery or during anesthesia with agents that produce hypotension, lisinopril may block angiotensin II formation secondary to compensatory renin release. If hypotension occurs and is considered to be due to this mechanism, it can be corrected by volume expansion.

Hydrochlorothiazide

Periodic determination of serum electrolytes to detect possible electrolyte imbalance should be performed at appropriate intervals.

All patients receiving thiazide therapy should be observed for clinical signs of fluid or electrolyte imbalance: namely, hyponatremia, hypochloremic alkalosis, and hypokalemia. Serum and urine electrolyte determinations are particularly important when the patient is vomiting excessively or receiving parenteral fluids. Warning signs or symptoms of fluid and electrolyte imbalance, irrespective of cause, include dryness of mouth, thirst, weakness, lethargy, drowsiness, restlessness, confusion, seizures, muscle pains or cramps, muscular fatigue, hypotension, oliguria, tachycardia, and gastrointestinal disturbances such as nausea and vomiting.

Hypokalemia may develop, especially with brisk diuresis, when severe cirrhosis is present, or after prolonged therapy. Interference with adequate oral electrolyte intake will also contribute to hypokalemia. Hypokalemia may cause cardiac arrhythmia and may also sensitize or exaggerate the response of the heart to the toxic effects of digitalis (e.g., increased ventricular irritability). Because lisinopril reduces the production of aldosterone, concomitant therapy with lisinopril attenuates the diuretic-induced potassium loss (see *Drug Interactions, Agents Increasing Serum Potassium*).

Although any chloride deficit is generally mild and usually does not require specific treatment, except under extraordinary circumstances (as in liver disease or renal disease), chloride replacement may be required in the treatment of metabolic alkalosis.

Dilutional hyponatremia may occur in edematous patients in hot weather; appropriate therapy is water restriction, rather than administration of salt except in rare instances when the hyponatremia is life-threatening. In actual salt depletion, appropriate replacement is the therapy of choice.

Hyperuricemia may occur or frank gout may be precipitated in certain patients receiving thiazide therapy.

In diabetic patients dosage adjustments of insulin or oral hypoglycemic agents may be required. Hyperglycemia may occur with thiazide diuretics. Thus latent diabetes mellitus may become manifest during thiazide therapy.

The antihypertensive effects of the drug may be enhanced in the postsympathectomy patient.

If progressive renal impairment becomes evident consider withholding or discontinuing diuretic therapy.

Thiazides have been shown to increase the urinary excretion of magnesium; this may result in hypomagnesemia.

Thiazides may decrease urinary calcium excretion. Thiazides may cause intermittent and slight elevation of serum calcium in the absence of known disorders of calcium metabolism. Marked hypercalcemia may be evidence of hidden hyperparathyroidism. Thiazides should be discontinued before carrying out tests for parathyroid function.

Increases in cholesterol and triglyceride levels may be associated with thiazide diuretic therapy.

Information for Patients

Angioedema: Angioedema, including laryngeal edema, may occur at any time during treatment with angiotensin converting enzyme inhibitors, including lisinopril. Patients should be so advised and told to report immediately any signs or symptoms suggesting angioedema (swelling of face, extremities, eyes, lips, tongue, difficulty in swallowing or breathing) and to take no more drug until they have consulted with the prescribing physician.

Symptomatic Hypotension: Patients should be cautioned to report lightheadedness especially during the first few days of therapy. If actual syncope occurs, the patients should be told to discontinue the drug until they have consulted with the prescribing physician.

All patients should be cautioned that excessive perspiration and dehydration may lead to an excessive fall in blood pressure because of reduction in fluid volume. Other causes of volume depletion such as vomiting or diarrhea may also lead to a fall in blood pressure; patients should be advised to consult with their physician.

Hyperkalemia: Patients should be told not to use salt substitutes containing potassium without consulting their physician.

Neutropenia: Patients should be told to report promptly any indication of infection (e.g., sore throat, fever) which may be a sign of neutropenia.

Pregnancy: Female patients of childbearing age should be told about the consequences of second- and third-trimester exposure to ACE inhibitors, and they should also be told that these consequences do not appear to have resulted from intrauterine ACE-inhibitor exposure that has been limited to the first trimester. These patients should be asked to report pregnancies to their physicians as soon as possible.

NOTE: As with many other drugs, certain advice to patients being treated with PRINZIDE is warranted. This information is intended to aid in the safe and effective use of this medication. It is not a disclosure of all possible adverse or intended effects.

Drug Interactions

Lisinopril

Hypotension —Patients on Diuretic Therapy: Patients on diuretics, and especially those in whom diuretic therapy was recently instituted, may occasionally experience an excessive reduction of blood pressure after initiation of therapy with lisinopril. The possibility of hypotensive effects with lisinopril can be minimized by either discontinuing the diuretic or increasing the salt intake prior to initiation of treatment with lisinopril. If it is necessary to continue the diuretic, initiate therapy with lisinopril at a dose of 5 mg daily, and provide close medical supervision after the initial dose for at least two hours and until blood pressure has stabilized for at least an additional hour. (See WARNINGS and DOSAGE AND ADMINISTRATION.) When a diuretic is added to the therapy of a patient receiving lisinopril, an additional antihypertensive effect is usually observed. (See DOSAGE AND ADMINISTRATION.)

Non-steroidal Anti-inflammatory Agents: In some patients with compromised renal function who are being treated with non-steroidal anti-inflammatory drugs, the co-administration of lisinopril may result in a further deterioration of renal function. These effects are usually reversible. In a study in 36 patients with mild to moderate hypertension where the antihypertensive effects of lisinopril alone were compared to lisinopril given concomitantly with indomethacin, the use of indomethacin was associated with a reduced effect, although the difference between the two regimens was not significant.

Other Agents: Lisinopril has been used concomitantly with nitrates and/or digoxin without evidence of clinically significant adverse interactions. No meaningful clinically important pharmacokinetic interactions occurred when lisinopril was used concomitantly with propranolol, digoxin, or hydrochlorothiazide. The presence of food in the stomach does not alter the bioavailability of lisinopril.

Agents Increasing Serum Potassium: Lisinopril attenuates potassium loss caused by thiazide-type diuretics. Use of lisinopril with potassium-sparing diuretics (e.g., spironolactone, triamterene, or amiloride), potassium supplements, or potassium-containing salt substitutes may lead to significant increases in serum potassium. Therefore, if concomitant use of these agents is indicated, because of demonstrated hypokalemia, they should be used with caution and with frequent monitoring of serum potassium.

Lithium: Lithium toxicity has been reported in patients receiving lithium concomitantly with drugs which cause elimination of sodium, including ACE inhibitors. Lithium toxicity was usually reversible upon discontinuation of lithium and the ACE inhibitor. It is recommended that serum lithium levels be monitored frequently if lisinopril is administered concomitantly with lithium.

Hydrochlorothiazide

When administered concurrently the following drugs may interact with thiazide diuretics.

Alcohol, barbiturates, or narcotics —potentiation of orthostatic hypotension may occur.

Antidiabetic drugs (oral agents and insulin)—dosage adjustment of the antidiabetic drug may be required.

Other antihypertensive drugs —additive effect or potentiation.

Cholestyramine and colestipol resins —Absorption of hydrochlorothiazide is impaired in the presence of anionic exchange resins. Single doses of either cholestyramine or colestipol resins bind the hydrochlorothiazide and reduce its absorption from the gastrointestinal tract by up to 85 and 43 percent, respectively.

Corticosteroids, ACTH —intensified electrolyte depletion, particularly hypokalemia.

Pressor amines (e.g., norepinephrine) —possible decreased response to pressor amines but not sufficient to preclude their use.

Skeletal muscle relaxants, nondepolarizing (e.g., tubocurarine) —possible increased responsiveness to the muscle relaxant.

Lithium —should not generally be given with diuretics. Diuretic agents reduce the renal clearance of lithium and add a high risk of lithium toxicity. Refer to the package insert for lithium preparations before use of such preparations with PRINZIDE.

Non-steroidal Anti-inflammatory Drugs —In some patients, the administration of a non-steroidal anti-inflammatory agent can reduce the diuretic, natriuretic, and antihypertensive effects of loop, potassium-sparing and thiazide diuretics. Therefore, when PRINZIDE and non-steroidal anti-inflammatory agents are used concomitantly, the patient should be observed closely to determine if the desired effect of PRINZIDE is obtained.

Carcinogenesis, Mutagenesis, Impairment of Fertility

Lisinopril-Hydrochlorothiazide

Lisinopril in combination with hydrochlorothiazide was not mutagenic in a microbial mutagen test using *Salmonella typhimurium* (Ames test) or *Escherichia coli* with or without metabolic activation or in a forward mutation assay using Chinese hamster lung cells. Lisinopril-hydrochlorothiazide did not produce DNA single strand breaks in an *in vitro* alkaline elution rat hepatocyte assay. In addition, it did not produce increases in chromosomal aberrations in an *in vitro* test in Chinese hamster ovary cells or in an *in vivo* study in mouse bone marrow.

Lisinopril

There was no evidence of a tumorigenic effect when lisinopril was administered orally for 105 weeks to male and female rats at doses up to 90 mg/kg/day or for 92 weeks to male and female mice at doses up to 135 mg/kg/day. These doses are 10 times and 7 times, respectively, the maximum recommended human daily dose (MRHDD) when compared on a body surface area basis.

Lisinopril was not mutagenic in the Ames microbial mutagen test with or without metabolic activation. It was also negative in a forward mutation assay using Chinese hamster lung cells. Lisinopril did not produce single strand DNA breaks in an *in vitro* alkaline elution rat hepatocyte assay. In addition, lisinopril did not produce increases in chromosomal aberrations in an *in vitro* test in Chinese hamster ovary cells or in an *in vivo* study in mouse bone marrow.

There were no adverse effects on reproductive performance in male and female rats treated with up to 300 mg/kg/day of lisinopril (33 times the MRHDD when compared on a body surface area basis).

Hydrochlorothiazide

Two-year feeding studies in mice and rats conducted under the auspices of the National Toxicology Program (NTP) uncovered no evidence of a carcinogenic potential of hydrochlorothiazide in female mice at doses of up to approximately 600 mg/kg/day (53 times the MRHDD when compared on a body surface area basis) or in male and female rats at doses of up to approximately 100 mg/kg/day (18 times the MRHDD when compared on a body surface area basis). The NTP, however, found equivocal evidence for hepatocarcinogenicity in male mice.

Hydrochlorothiazide was not genotoxic *in vitro* in the Ames mutagenicity assay of *Salmonella typhimurium* strains TA 98, TA 100, TA 1535, TA 1537, and TA 1538 and in the Chinese Hamster Ovary (CHO) test for chromosomal aberrations, or *in vivo* in assays using mouse germinal cell chromosomes, Chinese hamster bone marrow chromosomes, and the *Drosophila* sex-linked recessive lethal trait gene. Positive test results were obtained only in the *in vitro* CHO Sister Chromatid Exchange (clastogenicity) and in the Mouse Lymphoma Cell (mutagenicity) assays, using concentrations of hydrochlorothiazide from 43 to 1300 μg/mL, and in the *Aspergillus nidulans* non-disjunction assay at an unspecified concentration.

Hydrochlorothiazide had no adverse effects on the fertility of mice and rats of either sex in studies wherein these species were exposed, via their diet, to doses of up to 100 and 4 mg/kg, respectively, prior to conception and throughout gestation. In mice and rats these doses are 9 times and 0.7 times, respectively, the MRHDD when compared on a body surface area basis.

Pregnancy

Pregnancy Categories C (first trimester) *and D* (second and third trimesters). See WARNINGS, *Pregnancy, Lisinopril, Fetal/Neonatal Morbidity and Mortality.*

Nursing Mothers

It is not known whether lisinopril is secreted in human milk. However, milk of lactating rats contains radioactivity following administration of ^{14}C lisinopril. In another study, lisinopril was present in rat milk at levels similar to plasma levels in the dams. Thiazides do appear in human milk. Because of the potential for serious reactions in nursing infants from ACE inhibitors and hydrochlorothiazide, a decision should be made whether to discontinue nursing or to discontinue PRINZIDE, taking into account the importance of the drug to the mother.

Pediatric Use

Safety and effectiveness in pediatric patients have not been established.

ADVERSE REACTIONS

PRINZIDE has been evaluated for safety in 930 patients, including 100 patients treated for 50 weeks or more.

In clinical trials with PRINZIDE no adverse experiences peculiar to this combination drug have been observed. Adverse experiences that have occurred have been limited to those that have been previously reported with lisinopril or hydrochlorothiazide.

The most frequent clinical adverse experiences in controlled trials (including open label extensions) with any combination of lisinopril and hydrochlorothiazide were: dizziness (7.5 percent), headache (5.2 percent), cough (3.9 percent), fatigue (3.7 percent) and orthostatic effects (3.2 percent), all of which were more common than in placebo-treated patients. Generally, adverse experiences were mild and transient in

nature; but see WARNINGS regarding angioedema and excessive hypotension or syncope. Discontinuation of therapy due to adverse effects was required in 4.4 percent of patients, principally because of dizziness, cough, fatigue and muscle cramps.
Adverse experiences occurring in greater than one percent of patients treated with lisinopril plus hydrochlorothiazide in controlled clinical trials are shown below.
[See table above]

	Percent of Patients in Controlled Studies	
	Lisinopril-Hydrochlorothiazide (n=930) Incidence (discontinuation)	Placebo (n=207) Incidence
Dizziness	7.5 (0.8)	1.9
Headache	5.2 (0.3)	1.9
Cough	3.9 (0.6)	1.0
Fatigue	3.7 (0.4)	1.0
Orthostatic Effects	3.2 (0.1)	1.0
Diarrhea	2.5 (0.2)	2.4
Nausea	2.2 (0.1)	2.4
Upper Respiratory Infection	2.2 (0.0)	0.0
Muscle Cramps	2.0 (0.4)	0.5
Asthenia	1.8 (0.2)	1.0
Paresthesia	1.5 (0.1)	0.0
Hypotension	1.4 (0.3)	0.5
Vomiting	1.4 (0.1)	0.5
Dyspepsia	1.3 (0.0)	0.0
Rash	1.2 (0.1)	0.5
Impotence	1.2 (0.3)	0.0

Clinical adverse experiences occurring in 0.3 to 1.0 percent of patients in controlled trials included: *Body as a Whole:* Chest pain, abdominal pain, syncope, chest discomfort, fever, trauma, virus infection. *Cardiovascular:* Palpitation, orthostatic hypotension. *Digestive:* Gastrointestinal cramps, dry mouth, constipation, heartburn. *Musculoskeletal:* Back pain, shoulder pain, knee pain, back strain, myalgia, foot pain. *Nervous/Psychiatric:* Decreased libido, vertigo, depression, somnolence. *Respiratory:* Common cold, nasal congestion, influenza, bronchitis, pharyngeal pain, dyspnea, pulmonary congestion, chronic sinusitis, allergic rhinitis, pharyngeal discomfort. *Skin:* Flushing, pruritus, skin inflammation, diaphoresis. *Special Senses:* Blurred vision, tinnitus, otalgia. *Urogenital:* Urinary tract infection.
Angioedema: Angioedema has been reported in patients receiving PRINZIDE, with an incidence higher in black than in non-black patients. Angioedema associated with laryngeal edema may be fatal. If angioedema of the face, extremities, lips, tongue, glottis and/or larynx occurs, treatment with PRINZIDE should be discontinued and appropriate therapy instituted immediately. (See WARNINGS.)
Hypotension: In clinical trials, adverse effects relating to hypotension occurred as follows: hypotension (1.4), orthostatic hypotension (0.5), other orthostatic effects (3.2). In addition syncope occurred in 0.8 percent of patients. (See WARNINGS.)
Cough: See PRECAUTIONS, *Cough.*
Clinical Laboratory Test Findings
Serum Electrolytes: See PRECAUTIONS.
Creatinine, Blood Urea Nitrogen: Minor reversible increases in blood urea nitrogen and serum creatinine were observed in patients with essential hypertension treated with PRINZIDE. More marked increases have also been reported and were more likely to occur in patients with renal artery stenosis. (See PRECAUTIONS.)
Serum Uric Acid, Glucose, Magnesium, Cholesterol, Triglycerides and Calcium: See PRECAUTIONS.
Hemoglobin and Hematocrit: Small decreases in hemoglobin and hematocrit (mean decreases of approximately 0.5 g percent and 1.5 vol percent, respectively) occurred frequently in hypertensive patients treated with PRINZIDE but were rarely of clinical importance unless another cause of anemia coexisted. In clinical trials, 0.4 percent of patients discontinued therapy due to anemia.
Liver Function Tests: Rarely, elevations of liver enzymes and/or serum bilirubin have occurred (see WARNINGS, *Hepatic Failure*).

Other adverse reactions that have been reported with the individual components are listed below:
Lisinopril —In clinical trials adverse reactions which occurred with lisinopril were also seen with PRINZIDE. In addition, and since lisinopril has been marketed, the following adverse reactions have been reported with lisinopril and should be considered potential adverse reactions for PRINZIDE: *Body as a Whole:* Anaphylactoid reactions (see WARNINGS, *Anaphylactoid and Possibly Related Reactions*), malaise, edema, facial edema, pain, pelvic pain, flank pain, chills; *Cardiovascular:* Cardiac arrest, myocardial infarction or cerebrovascular accident, possibly secondary to excessive hypotension in high risk patients (see WARNINGS, *Hypotension*), pulmonary embolism and infarction, worsening of heart failure, arrhythmias (including tachycardia, ventricular tachycardia, atrial tachycardia, atrial fibrillation, bradycardia, and premature ventricular contractions), angina pectoris, transient ischemic attacks, paroxysmal nocturnal dyspnea, decreased blood pressure, peripheral edema, vasculitis; *Digestive:* Pancreatitis, hepatitis (hepatocellular or cholestatic jaundice) (see WARNINGS, *Hepatic Failure*), gastritis, anorexia, flatulence, increased salivation; *Endocrine:* Diabetes mellitus; *Hematologic:* Rare cases of neutropenia, thrombocytopenia, and bone marrow depression have been reported. Hemolytic anemia has been reported; a causal relationship to lisinopril cannot be excluded; *Metabolic:* Gout, weight loss, dehydration, fluid overload, weight gain; *Musculoskeletal:* Arthritis, arthralgia, neck pain, hip pain, joint pain, leg pain, arm pain, lumbago; *Nervous System/Psychiatric:* Ataxia, memory impairment, tremor, insomnia, stroke, nervousness, confusion, peripheral neuropathy (e.g., paresthesia, dysesthesia), spasm, hypersomnia, irritability; *Respiratory:* Malignant lung neoplasms, hemoptysis, pulmonary edema, pulmonary infiltrates, eosinophilic pneumonitis, bronchospasm, asthma, pleural effusion, pneumonia, wheezing, orthopnea, painful respiration, epistaxis, laryngitis, sinusitis, pharyngitis, rhinitis, rhinorrhea, chest sound abnormalities; *Skin:* Urticaria, alopecia, herpes zoster, photosensitivity, skin lesions, skin infections, pemphigus, erythema. Other severe skin reactions (including toxic epidermal necrolysis and Stevens-Johnson syndrome) have been reported rarely; causal relationship has not been established; *Special Senses:* Visual loss, diplopia, photophobia, taste disturbances; *Urogenital:* Acute renal failure, oliguria, anuria, uremia, progressive azotemia, renal dysfunction (see PRECAUTIONS and DOSAGE AND ADMINISTRATION), pyelonephritis, dysuria, breast pain.

Miscellaneous: A symptom complex has been reported which may include a positive ANA, an elevated erythrocyte sedimentation rate, arthralgia/arthritis, myalgia, fever, vasculitis, leukocytosis, eosinophilia, photosensitivity, rash, and other dermatological manifestations.
Fetal/Neonatal Morbidity and Mortality: See WARNINGS, *Pregnancy, Lisinopril, Fetal/Neonatal Morbidity and Mortality.*
Hydrochlorothiazide —Body as a Whole: Weakness; *Digestive:* Anorexia, gastric irritation, cramping, jaundice (intrahepatic cholestatic jaundice), pancreatitis, sialadenitis, constipation; *Hematologic:* Leukopenia, agranulocytosis, thrombocytopenia, aplastic anemia, hemolytic anemia; *Musculoskeletal:* Muscle spasm; *Nervous System/Psychiatric:* Restlessness; *Renal:* Renal failure, renal dysfunction, interstitial nephritis (see WARNINGS); *Skin:* Erythema multiforme including Stevens-Johnson syndrome, exfoliative dermatitis including toxic epidermal necrolysis, alopecia; *Special Senses:* Xanthopsia; *Hypersensitivity:* Purpura, photosensitivity, urticaria, necrotizing angiitis (vasculitis and cutaneous vasculitis), respiratory distress including pneumonitis and pulmonary edema, anaphylactic reactions.

OVERDOSAGE

No specific information is available on the treatment of overdosage with PRINZIDE. Treatment is symptomatic and supportive. Therapy with PRINZIDE should be discontinued and the patient observed closely. Suggested measures include induction of emesis and/or gastric lavage, and correction of dehydration, electrolyte imbalance and hypotension by established procedures.
Lisinopril
Following a single oral dose of 20 mg/kg, no lethality occurred in rats and death occurred in one of 20 mice receiving the same dose. The most likely manifestation of overdosage would be hypotension, for which the usual treatment would be intravenous infusion of normal saline solution.
Lisinopril can be removed by hemodialysis. (See WARNINGS, *Anaphylactoid reactions during membrane exposure.*)
Hydrochlorothiazide
Oral administration of a single oral dose of 10 mg/kg to mice and rats was not lethal. The most common signs and symptoms observed are those caused by electrolyte depletion (hypokalemia, hypochloremia, hyponatremia) and dehydration resulting from excessive diuresis. If digitalis has also been administered, hypokalemia may accentuate cardiac arrhythmias.

DOSAGE AND ADMINISTRATION

Lisinopril is an effective treatment of hypertension in once-daily doses of 10–80 mg, while hydrochlorothiazide is effective in doses of 12.5–50 mg. In clinical trials of lisinopril/hydrochlorothiazide combination therapy using lisinopril doses of 10–80 mg and hydrochlorothiazide doses of 6.25–50 mg, the antihypertensive response rates generally increased with increasing dose of either component.
The side effects (see WARNINGS) of lisinopril are generally rare and apparently independent of dose; those of hydrochlorothiazide are a mixture of dose-dependent phenomena (primarily hypokalemia) and dose-independent phenomena (e.g., pancreatitis), the former much more common than the latter. Therapy with any combination of lisinopril and hydrochlorothiazide will be associated with both sets of dose-independent side effects, but addition of lisinopril in clinical trials blunted the hypokalemia normally seen with diuretics.
To minimize dose-independent side effects, it is usually appropriate to begin combination therapy only after a patient has failed to achieve the desired effect with monotherapy.
Dose Titration Guided by Clinical Effect
A patient whose blood pressure is not adequately controlled with either lisinopril or hydrochlorothiazide monotherapy may be switched to PRINZIDE 10/12.5 or PRINZIDE 20/12.5. Further increases of either or both components could depend on clinical response. The hydrochlorothiazide dose should generally not be increased until 2–3 weeks have elapsed. Patients whose blood pressures are adequately controlled with 25 mg of daily hydrochlorothiazide, but who experience significant potassium loss with this regimen, may achieve similar or greater blood pressure control with less potassium loss if they are switched to PRINZIDE 10/12.5.
Replacement Therapy
The combination may be substituted for the titrated individual components.
Use in Renal Impairment
The usual regimens of therapy with PRINZIDE need not be adjusted as long as the patient's creatinine clearance is >30 mL /min/1.73 m^2 (serum creatinine approximately ≤3 mg/dL or 265 μmol/L. In patients with more severe renal impairment, loop diuretics are preferred to thiazides, so PRINZIDE is not recommended (see WARNINGS, *Anaphylactoid reactions during membrane exposure*).
Use in Elderly In general, blood pressure response and adverse experiences were similar in younger and older patients given PRINZIDE. However, in a multiple dose pharmacokinetic study in elderly versus young patients using the lisinopril/hydrochlorothiazide combination, area under the plasma concentration time curve (AUC) increased approximately 120% for lisinopril and approximately 80% for hydrochlorothiazide in older patients. Therefore, dosage adjustments in elderly patients should be made with particular caution.

HOW SUPPLIED

No. 3616—Tablets PRINZIDE 10-12.5 are blue hexagon-shaped tablets, coded MSD 145 on one side and PRINZIDE on the other. Each tablet contains 10 mg of lisinopril and 12.5 mg of hydrochlorothiazide. They are supplied as follows:
NDC 0006-0145-31 unit of use bottles of 30.
NDC 0006-0145-58 unit of use bottles of 100.
Shown in Product Identification Guide, page 324
No. 3594—Tablets PRINZIDE 20-12.5 are yellow, round, fluted-edge tablets, coded MSD 140 on one side and PRINZIDE on the other. Each tablet contains 20 mg of lisinopril and 12.5 mg of hydrochlorothiazide. They are supplied as follows:
NDC 0006-0140-31 unit of use bottles of 30
NDC 0006-0140-58 unit of use bottles of 100.
Shown in Product Identification Guide, page 324
No. 3595—Tablets PRINZIDE 20-25 are peach, round, fluted-edge tablets, coded MSD 142 on one side and PRINZIDE on the other. Each tablet contains 20 mg of lisinopril and 25 mg of hydrochlorothiazide. They are supplied as follows:
NDC 0006-0142-31 unit of use bottles of 30
NDC 0006-0142-58 unit of use bottles of 100.
Shown in Product Identification Guide, page 324
Storage
Store at controlled room temperature. 15–30°C (59–86°F).
Protect from excessive light and humidity.
Dispense in a well-closed container, if product package is subdivided.

7836332 Issued June 1999

PROPECIA® ℞
(Finasteride)
Tablets, 1 mg

DESCRIPTION

PROPECIA* (finasteride), a synthetic 4-azasteroid compound, is a specific inhibitor of steroid Type II 5α-reductase, an intracellular enzyme that converts the androgen testosterone into 5α-dihydrotestosterone (DHT).
Finasteride is 4-azaandrost-1-ene-17-carboxamide,*N*-(1,1-dimethylethyl)-3-oxo-,(5α,17β)-. The empirical formula of

Continued on next page

Information on the Merck & Co., Inc. products listed on these pages is the full prescribing information from product circulars in use September 30, 2000. For information, please call 1-800-NSC MERCK [1-800-672-6372].

Propecia—Cont.

finasteride is $C_{23}H_{36}N_2O_2$ and its molecular weight is 372.55. Its structural formula is:

Finasteride is a white crystalline powder with a melting point near 250°C. It is freely soluble in chloroform and in lower alcohol solvents but is practically insoluble in water.

PROPECIA tablets for oral administration are film-coated tablets that contain 1 mg of finasteride and the following inactive ingredients: lactose monohydrate, microcrystalline cellulose, pregelatinized starch, sodium starch glycolate, docusate sodium, magnesium stearate, hydroxypropyl methylcellulose 2910, hydroxypropyl cellulose, titanium dioxide, talc, yellow ferric oxide, and red ferric oxide.

*Registered trademark of MERCK & CO., INC.

CLINICAL PHARMACOLOGY

Finasteride is a competitive and specific inhibitor of Type II 5α-reductase, an intracellular enzyme that converts the androgen testosterone into DHT. Two distinct isozymes are found in mice, rats, monkeys, and humans: Type I and II. Each of these isozymes is differentially expressed in tissues and developmental stages. In humans, Type I 5α-reductase is predominant in the sebaceous glands of most regions of skin, including scalp, and liver. Type I 5α-reductase is responsible for approximately one-third of circulating DHT. The Type II 5α-reductase isozyme is primarily found in prostate, seminal vesicles, epididymides, and hair follicles as well as liver, and is responsible for two-thirds of circulating DHT.

In humans, the mechanism of action of finasteride is based on its preferential inhibition of the Type II isozyme. Using native tissues (scalp and prostate), *in vitro* binding studies examining the potential of finasteride to inhibit either isozyme revealed a 100-fold selectivity for the human Type II 5α-reductase over Type I isozyme (IC_{50}=500 and 4.2 nM for Type I and II, respectively). For both isozymes, the inhibition by finasteride is accompanied by reduction of the inhibitor to dihydrofinasteride and adduct formation with NADP+. The turnover for the enzyme complex is slow ($t_{1/2}$ approximately 30 days for the Type II enzyme complex and 14 days for the Type I complex).

Finasteride has no affinity for the androgen receptor and has no androgenic, antiandrogenic, estrogenic, antiestrogenic, or progestational effects. Inhibition of Type II 5α-reductase blocks the peripheral conversion of testosterone to DHT, resulting in significant decreases in serum and tissue DHT concentrations. Finasteride produces a rapid reduction in serum DHT concentration, reaching 65% suppression within 24 hours of oral dosing with a 1-mg tablet.

In men with male pattern hair loss (androgenetic alopecia), the balding scalp contains miniaturized hair follicles and increased amounts of DHT compared with hairy scalp. Administration of finasteride decreases scalp and serum DHT concentrations in these men. The relative contributions of these reductions to the treatment effect of finasteride have not been defined. By this mechanism, finasteride appears to interrupt a key factor in the development of androgenetic alopecia in those patients genetically predisposed.

Finasteride had no effect on circulating levels of cortisol, thyroid-stimulating hormone, or thyroxine, nor did it affect the plasma lipid profile (e.g., total cholesterol, low-density lipoproteins, high-density lipoproteins and triglycerides) or bone mineral density. In studies with finasteride, no clinically meaningful changes in luteinizing hormone (LH) or follicle-stimulating hormone (FSH) were detected. In healthy volunteers, treatment with finasteride did not alter the response of LH and FSH to gonadotropin-releasing hormone, indicating that the hypothalamic-pituitary-testicular axis was not affected. Mean circulating levels of testosterone and estradiol were increased by approximately 15% as compared to baseline, but these remained within the physiologic range.

Pharmacokinetics

Following an oral dose of ^{14}C-finasteride in man, a mean of 39% (range, 32–46%) of the dose was excreted in the urine in the form of metabolites; 57% (range, 51–64%) was excreted in the feces. The major compound isolated from urine was the monocarboxylic acid metabolite; virtually no unchanged drug was recovered. The t-butyl side chain monohydroxylated metabolite has been isolated from plasma. These metabolites possessed no more than 20% of the 5α-reductase inhibitory activity of finasteride.

In a study in 15 healthy male subjects, the mean bioavailability of finasteride 1-mg tablets was 65% (range 26–170%), based on the ratio of AUC relative to a 5-mg intravenous dose infused over 60 minutes. Following intravenous infusion, mean plasma clearance was 165 mL/min (range, 70–279 mL/min) and mean steady-state volume of distribution was 76 liters (range, 44–96 liters). In a separate study, the bioavailability of finasteride was not affected by food.

Approximately 90% of circulating finasteride is bound to plasma proteins. Finasteride has been found to cross the blood-brain barrier.

There is a slow accumulation phase for finasteride after multiple dosing. At steady state following dosing with 1 mg/day, maximum finasteride plasma concentration averaged 9.2 ng/mL (range, 4.9–13.7 ng/mL) and was reached 1 to 2 hours postdose; $AUC_{(0-24\ hr)}$ was 53 ng·hr/mL (range, 20–154 ng·hr/mL) and mean terminal half-life of elimination was 4.8 hours (range, 3.3–13.4 hours).

Semen levels have been measured in 35 men taking finasteride 1 mg daily for 6 weeks. In 60% (21 of 35) of the samples, finasteride levels were undetectable. The mean finasteride level was 0.26 ng/mL and the highest level measured was 1.52 ng/mL. Using this highest semen level measured and assuming 100% absorption from a 5-mL ejaculate per day, human exposure through vaginal absorption would be up to 7.6 ng per day, which is 750 times lower than the exposure from the no-effect dose for developmental abnormalities in Rhesus monkeys (see PRECAUTIONS, *Pregnancy*).

The elimination rate of finasteride decreases somewhat with age. Mean terminal half-life is approximately 5–6 hours in men 18–60 years of age and 8 hours in men more than 70 years of age. These findings are of no clinical significance, and a reduction in dosage in the elderly is not warranted.

No dosage adjustment is necessary in patients with renal insufficiency. In patients with chronic renal impairment (creatinine clearance ranging from 9.0 to 55 mL/min), the values for AUC, maximum plasma concentration, half-life, and protein binding after a single dose of ^{14}C-finasteride were similar to those obtained in healthy volunteers. Urinary excretion of metabolites was decreased in patients with renal impairment. This decrease was associated with an increase in fecal excretion of metabolites. Plasma concentrations of metabolites were significantly higher in patients with renal impairment (based on a 60% increase in total radioactivity AUC). Furthermore, finasteride has been well tolerated in men with normal renal function receiving up to 80 mg/day for 12 weeks where exposure of these patients to metabolites would presumably be much greater.

Clinical Studies

The efficacy of PROPECIA was demonstrated in men (88% Caucasian) with mild to moderate androgenetic alopecia (male pattern hair loss) between 18 and 41 years of age. In order to prevent seborrheic dermatitis which might confound the assessment of hair growth in these studies (controlled phase and extensions), all men, whether treated with finasteride or placebo, were instructed to use a specified, medicated, tar-based shampoo (Neutrogena T/Gel®** Shampoo).

There were three double-blind, randomized, placebo-controlled studies of 12-month duration. The two primary endpoints were hair count and patient self-assessment; the two secondary endpoints were investigator assessment and ratings of photographs. The three studies were conducted in 1,879 men with mild to moderate, but not complete, hair loss. Two of the studies enrolled men with predominantly mild to moderate vertex hair loss (n=1,553). The third enrolled men having mild to moderate hair loss in the anterior midscalp area with or without vertex balding (n=326).

Two studies on Vertex Baldness

Of the men who completed the first 12 months of the two vertex baldness trials, 1,215 elected to continue in double-blind, placebo-controlled, 12-month extension studies. There were 547 men receiving PROPECIA for both the initial and extension periods (up to 24 months) and 60 men receiving placebo for the same periods. In addition, there were 65 men who received PROPECIA for the initial 12 months followed by placebo in the 12-month extension period, and 543 men who received placebo for the initial 12 months followed by PROPECIA in the 12-month extension period (See Figure below).

Hair counts were assessed by photographic enlargements of a representative area of active hair loss. In these two studies in men with vertex baldness, significant increases in hair count were demonstrated at 6 and 12 months in men treated with PROPECIA, while significant hair loss from baseline was demonstrated in those treated with placebo. At 12 months there was a 107-hair difference from placebo ($p<0.001$, PROPECIA [n=679 evaluable men] vs placebo [n=672 evaluable men]) within a 1-inch diameter circle (5.1 cm^2). Hair count was maintained in those men taking PROPECIA (n=433 evaluable men) for up to 24 months, while the placebo group (n=47 evaluable men) continued to show progressive hair loss. At 24 months, this resulted in a 138-hair difference between treatment groups ($p<0.001$) within the same area. Patients who switched from placebo to PROPECIA (n=426 evaluable men) at the end of the initial 12 months had an increase in hair count at 24 months. A change of treatment from PROPECIA to placebo (n=48 evaluable men) at the end of the initial 12 months resulted in reversal of the increase in hair count 12 months later, at 24 months. See figure below for combined study results.

At 12 months, 14% of men treated with PROPECIA had hair loss (defined as any decrease in hair count from baseline) compared with 58% of men in the placebo group. In men treated for up to 24 months, 17% of those treated with PROPECIA demonstrated hair loss compared with 72% of those in the placebo group.

[See graphic below]

Patient self-assessment was obtained at each clinic visit from a self-administered questionnaire, which included questions on their perception of hair growth, hair loss, and appearance. This self-assessment demonstrated an increase in amount of hair, a decrease in hair loss, and improvement in appearance in men treated with PROPECIA. Overall improvement compared with placebo was seen as early as 3 months ($p<0.05$), with continued improvement over 24 months.

Investigator assessment was based on a 7-point scale evaluating increases or decreases in scalp hair at each patient visit. This assessment showed significantly greater increases in hair growth in men treated with PROPECIA compared with placebo as early as 3 months ($p<0.001$). At 12 months, the investigators rated 65% of men treated with PROPECIA as having increased hair growth compared with 37% in the placebo group. At 24 months, the investigators rated 80% of men treated with PROPECIA as having increased hair growth compared with 47% of men treated with placebo.

Standardized photographs of the head were assessed in a blinded fashion, at the beginning of the study and at 6, 12, 18 and 24 months. An independent panel rated increases or decreases in scalp hair on the same 7-point scale as the investigator assessment. At 12 months, 48% of men treated with PROPECIA had an increase as compared with 7% of men treated with placebo. At 24 months, an increase in hair growth was demonstrated in 66% of men treated with PROPECIA compared with 7% of men treated with placebo. Based on this assessment, continued treatment with PROPECIA resulted in further improvement. These results were observed in the context of no further increase in hair count between month 12 and month 24.

In one of the two vertex baldness studies, patients were questioned on non-scalp body hair growth. PROPECIA did not appear to affect non-scalp body hair.

Study on Hair Loss in the Anterior Mid-Scalp Area

A third study of 12-month duration, designed to assess the efficacy of PROPECIA in men with hair loss in the anterior mid-scalp area, also demonstrated significant increases in hair count compared with placebo. Increases in hair count were accompanied by improvements in patient self-assess-

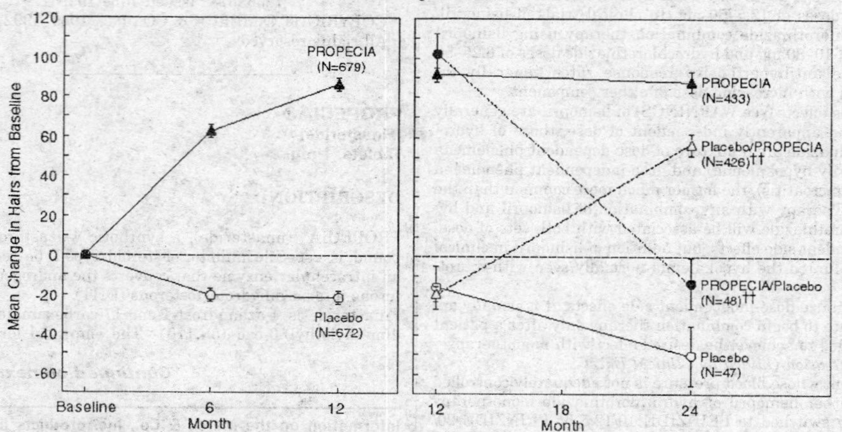

† Pooled data from vertex hair loss studies (mean baseline hair count = 876)

†† At the end of initial 12-month period, treatment switched from PROPECIA to placebo (———— PROPECIA/Placebo) or from placebo to PROPECIA (------------ Placebo/PROPECIA).

ment, investigator assessment, and ratings based on standardized photographs. Hair counts were obtained in the anterior mid-scalp area, and did not include the area of bitemporal recession or the anterior hairline.

Summary of Clinical Studies

Clinical studies were conducted in men aged 18 to 41 with mild to moderate degrees of androgenetic alopecia. All men treated with PROPECIA or placebo received a tar-based shampoo (Neutrogena T/Gel®** Shampoo). Clinical improvement was seen as early as 3 months in the patients treated with PROPECIA and led to a net increase in scalp hair count and hair regrowth. In addition, clinical studies demonstrated slowing of hair loss with PROPECIA by patient self-assessment. These effects were maintained through the second year of treatment. Maintenance of or improvement in clinical efficacy has also been demonstrated in controlled and open-extension studies for up to 3 years.

Ethnic Analysis of Clinical Data

In a combined analysis of the two studies on vertex baldness, mean hair count changes from baseline were 91 vs –19 hairs (PROPECIA vs placebo) among Caucasians (n=1,185), 49 vs 27 hairs among Blacks (n=84), 53 vs –38 hairs among Asians (n=17), 67 vs 5 hairs among Hispanics (n=45) and 67 vs −15 hairs among other ethnic groups (n=20). Patient self-assessment showed improvement across racial groups with PROPECIA treatment, except for satisfaction of the frontal hairline and vertex in Black men, who were satisfied overall.

A sexual function questionnaire was self-administered by patients participating in the two vertex baldness trials to detect more subtle changes in sexual function. At Month 12, statistically significant differences in favor of placebo were found in 3 of 4 domains (sexual interest, erections, and perception of sexual problems). However, no significant difference was seen in the question on overall satisfaction with sex life.

**Registered trademark of Johnson & Johnson

INDICATIONS AND USAGE

PROPECIA is indicated for the treatment of male pattern hair loss (androgenetic alopecia) in **MEN ONLY**. Safety and efficacy were demonstrated in men between 18 to 41 years of age with mild to moderate hair loss of the vertex and anterior mid-scalp area (See CLINICAL PHARMACOLOGY, *Clinical Studies*).

Efficacy in bitemporal recession has not been established.

PROPECIA is not indicated in women (see CONTRAINDICATIONS).

PROPECIA is not indicated in children (see PRECAUTIONS, *Pediatric Use*).

CONTRAINDICATIONS

PROPECIA is contraindicated in the following:

Pregnancy. Finasteride use is contraindicated in women when they are or may potentially be pregnant. Because of the ability of 5α-reductase inhibitors to inhibit the conversion of testosterone to DHT, finasteride may cause abnormalities of the external genitalia of a male fetus of a pregnant woman who receives finasteride. If this drug is used during pregnancy, or if pregnancy occurs while taking this drug, the pregnant woman should be apprised of the potential hazard to the male fetus. (See also WARNINGS, EXPOSURE OF WOMEN - RISK TO MALE FETUS; and PRECAUTIONS, *Information for Patients* and *Pregnancy*.) In female rats, low doses of finasteride administered during pregnancy have produced abnormalities of the external genitalia in male offspring.

Hypersensitivity to any component of this medication.

WARNINGS

PROPECIA is not indicated for use in pediatric patients (See INDICATIONS AND USAGE; and PRECAUTIONS, *Pediatric Use*) or women (See also PRECAUTIONS, *Information for Patients* and *Pregnancy*; and HOW SUPPLIED, *Storage and Handling*.)

EXPOSURE OF WOMEN - RISK TO MALE FETUS

Women should not handle crushed or broken PROPECIA tablets when they are pregnant or may potentially be pregnant because of the possibility of absorption of finasteride and the subsequent potential risk to a male fetus. PROPECIA tablets are coated and will prevent contact with the active ingredient during normal handling, provided that the tablets have not been broken or crushed. (See also CONTRAINDICATIONS; PRECAUTIONS, *Information for Patients* and *Pregnancy*; and HOW SUPPLIED, *Storage and Handling*.)

PRECAUTIONS

General

Caution should be used in the administration of PROPECIA in patients with liver function abnormalities, as finasteride is metabolized extensively in the liver.

Information for Patients

Women should not handle crushed or broken PROPECIA tablets when they are pregnant or may potentially be pregnant because of the possibility of absorption of finasteride and the subsequent potential risk to a male fetus. PROPECIA tablets are coated and will prevent contact with the active ingredient during normal handling, provided that the tablets have not been broken or crushed. (See also CONTRAINDICATIONS; WARNINGS, EXPOSURE OF WOMEN - RISK TO MALE FETUS; PRECAUTIONS, *Pregnancy*; and HOW SUPPLIED, *Storage and Handling*.)

See also Patient Package Insert.

Drug/Laboratory Test Interactions

In clinical studies with PROPECIA in men 18–41 years of age, the mean value of serum prostate-specific antigen (PSA) decreased from 0.7 ng/mL at baseline to 0.5 ng/mL at Month 12. When finasteride is used in older men who have benign prostatic hyperplasia (BPH), PSA levels are decreased by approximately 50%. Until further information is gathered in men >41 years of age without BPH, consideration should be given to doubling the PSA level in men undergoing this test while taking PROPECIA.

Drug Interactions

No drug interactions of clinical importance have been identified. Finasteride does not appear to affect the cytochrome P450-linked drug metabolizing enzyme system. Compounds that have been tested in man include antipyrine, digoxin, propranolol, theophylline, and warfarin and no interactions were found.

Other concomitant therapy: Although specific interaction studies were not performed, finasteride doses of 1 mg or more were concomitantly used in clinical studies with acetaminophen, α-blockers, analgesics, angiotensin-converting enzyme (ACE) inhibitors, anticonvulsants, benzodiazepines, beta blockers, calcium-channel blockers, cardiac nitrates, diuretics, H_2 antagonists, HMG-CoA reductase inhibitors, prostaglandin synthetase inhibitors (NSAIDs), and quinolone anti-infectives without evidence of clinically significant adverse interactions.

Carcinogenesis, Mutagenesis, Impairment of Fertility

No evidence of a tumorigenic effect was observed in a 24-month study in Sprague-Dawley rats receiving doses of finasteride up to 160 mg/kg/day in males and 320 mg/kg/day in females. These doses produced respective systemic exposure in rats of 888 and 2,192 times those observed in man receiving the recommended human dose of 1 mg/day. All exposure calculations were based on calculated $AUC_{(0-24\ hr)}$ for animals and mean $AUC_{(0-24\ hr)}$ for man (0.05 μg·hr/mL).

In a 19-month carcinogenicity study in CD-1 mice, a statistically significant ($p \leq 0.05$) increase in the incidence of testicular Leydig cell adenomas was observed at a dose of 250 mg/kg/day (1,824 times the human exposure). In mice at a dose of 25 mg/kg/day (184 times the human exposure, estimated) and in rats at a dose of ≥40 mg/kg/day (312 times the human exposure) an increase in the incidence of Leydig cell hyperplasia was observed. A positive correlation between the proliferative changes in the Leydig cells and an increase in serum LH levels (2–3 fold above control) has been demonstrated in both rodent species treated with high doses of finasteride. No drug-related Leydig cell changes were seen in either rats or dogs treated with finasteride for 1 year at doses of 20 mg/kg/day and 45 mg/kg/day (240 and 2,800 times, respectively, the human exposure) or in mice treated for 19 months at a dose of 2.5 mg/kg/day (18.4 times the human exposure).

No evidence of mutagenicity was observed in an *in vitro* bacterial mutagenesis assay, a mammalian cell mutagenesis assay, or in an *in vitro* alkaline elution assay. In an *in vitro* chromosome aberration assay, when Chinese hamster ovary cells were treated with high concentrations (450–550 μmol) of finasteride, there was a slight increase in chromosome aberrations. These concentrations correspond to 18,000–22,000 times the peak plasma levels in man given a total dose of 1 mg. Further, the concentrations (450–550 μmol) used in *in vitro* studies are not achievable in a biological system. In an *in vivo* chromosome aberration assay in mice, no treatment-related increase in chromosome aberration was observed with finasteride at the maximum tolerated dose of 250 mg/kg/day (1,824 times the human exposure, estimated) as determined in the carcinogenicity studies.

In sexually mature male rabbits treated with finasteride at 80 mg/kg/day (4,344 times the estimated human exposure) for up to 12 weeks, no effect on fertility, sperm count, or ejaculate volume was seen. In sexually mature male rats treated with 80 mg/kg/day of finasteride (488 times the estimated human exposure), there were no significant effects on fertility after 6 or 12 weeks of treatment; however, when treatment was continued for up to 24 or 30 weeks, there was an apparent decrease in fertility, fecundity, and an associated significant decrease in the weights of the seminal vesicles and prostate. All these effects were reversible within 6 weeks of discontinuation of treatment. No drug-related effect on testes or on mating performance has been seen in rats or rabbits. This decrease in fertility in finasteride-treated rats is secondary to its effect on accessory sex organs (prostate and seminal vesicles) resulting in failure to form a seminal plug. The seminal plug is essential for normal fertility in rats but is not relevant in man.

Pregnancy

Teratogenic Effects: Pregnancy Category X

See CONTRAINDICATIONS.

PROPECIA is not indicated for use in women.

Administration of finasteride to pregnant rats at doses ranging from 100 μg/kg/day to 100 mg/kg/day (5–5,000 times the recommended human dose of 1 mg/day) resulted in dose-dependent development of hypospadias in 3.6 to 100% of male offspring. Pregnant rats produced male offspring with decreased prostatic and seminal vesicular weights, delayed preputial separation, and transient nipple development when given finasteride at ≥30 μg/kg/day (≥ 1.5 times the recommended human dose of 1 mg/day) and decreased anogenital distance when given finasteride at ≥3 μg/kg/day (one-fifth the recommended human dose of 1 mg/day). The critical period during which these effects can be induced in male rats has been defined to be days 16–17 of gestation. The changes described above are expected pharmacological effects of drugs belonging to the class of Type II 5α-reductase inhibitors and are similar to those reported in male infants with a genetic deficiency of Type II 5α-reductase. No abnormalities were observed in female offspring exposed to any dose of finasteride *in utero*.

No developmental abnormalities have been observed in first filial generation (F_1) male or female offspring resulting from mating finasteride-treated male rats (80 mg/kg/day; 488 times the human exposure) with untreated females. Administration of finasteride at 3 mg/kg/day (150 times the recommended human dose of 1 mg/day) during the late gestation and lactation period resulted in slightly decreased fertility in F_1 male offspring. No effects were seen in female offspring. No evidence of malformations has been observed in rabbit fetuses exposed to finasteride *in utero* from days 6–18 of gestation at doses up to 100 mg/kg/day (5000 times the recommended human dose of 1 mg/day). However, effects on male genitalia would not be expected since the rabbits were not exposed during the critical period of genital system development.

The *in utero* effects of finasteride exposure during the period of embryonic and fetal development were evaluated in the rhesus monkey (gestation days 20–100), a species more predictive of human development than rats or rabbits. Intravenous administration of finasteride to pregnant monkeys at doses as high as 800 ng/day (at least 750 times the highest estimated exposure of pregnant women to finasteride from semen of men taking 1 mg/day) resulted in no abnormalities in male fetuses. In confirmation of the relevance of the rhesus model for human fetal development, oral administration of a very high dose of finasteride (2 mg/kg/day; 100 times the recommended human dose of 1 mg/day or approximately 12 million times the highest estimated exposure to finasteride from semen of men taking 1 mg/day) to pregnant monkeys resulted in external genital abnormalities in male fetuses. No other abnormalities were observed in male fetuses and no finasteride-related abnormalities were observed in female fetuses at any dose.

Nursing Mothers

PROPECIA is not indicated for use in women.

It is not known whether finasteride is excreted in human milk.

Pediatric Use

PROPECIA is not indicated for use in pediatric patients.

Safety and effectiveness in pediatric patients have not been established.

Geriatric Use

Clinical efficacy studies with PROPECIA did not include subjects aged 65 and over. Based on pharmacokinetics, no dosage adjustment is necessary in the elderly (see CLINICAL PHARMACOLOGY, *Pharmacokinetics*).

ADVERSE REACTIONS

Clinical Studies for PROPECIA (finasteride 1 mg) in the Treatment of Male Pattern Hair Loss

In controlled clinical trials for PROPECIA of 12-month duration, 1.4% of the patients were discontinued due to adverse experiences that were considered to be possibly, probably or definitely drug-related (1.6% for placebo); 1.2% of patients on PROPECIA and 0.9% of patients on placebo discontinued therapy because of a drug-related sexual adverse experience. The following clinical adverse reactions were reported as possibly, probably or definitely drug-related in ≥1% of patients treated for 12 months with PROPECIA or placebo, respectively: decreased libido (1.8%, 1.3%), erectile dysfunction (1.3%, 0.7%) and ejaculation disorder (1.2%, 0.7%; primarily decreased volume of ejaculate:[0.8%, 0.4%]). Integrated analysis of clinical adverse experiences showed that during treatment with PROPECIA, 36 (3.8%) of 945 men had reported one or more of these adverse experiences as compared to 20 (2.1%) of 934 men treated with placebo (p=0.04). Resolution occurred in all men who discontinued therapy with PROPECIA due to these side effects and in 58% of those who continued therapy.

In a study of finasteride 1 mg daily in healthy men, a median decrease in ejaculate volume of 0.3 mL (-11%) compared with 0.2 mL (−8%) for placebo was observed after 48 weeks of treatment. Two other studies showed that finasteride at 5 times the dosage of PROPECIA (5 mg daily) produced significant median decreases of approximately 0.5 mL (-25%) compared to placebo in ejaculate volume but this was reversible after discontinuation of treatment.

In the clinical studies with PROPECIA, the incidences for breast tenderness and enlargement, hypersensitivity reactions, and testicular pain in finasteride-treated patients were not different from those in patients treated with placebo.

Continued on next page

Information on the Merck & Co., Inc. products listed on these pages is the full prescribing information from product circulars in use September 30, 2000. For information, please call 1-800-NSC MERCK [1-800-672-6372].

Propecia—Cont.

Postmarketing Experience for PROPECIA (finasteride 1 mg)
Breast tenderness and enlargement; hypersensitivity reactions including rash, pruritus, urticaria, and swelling of the lips and face; and testicular pain.
Controlled Clinical Trials and Long-Term Open Extension Studies for PROSCAR (finasteride 5 mg) in the Treatment of Benign Prostatic Hyperplasia*
In controlled clinical trials for PROSCAR of 12-month duration, 1.3% of the patients were discontinued due to adverse experiences that were considered to be possibly, probably or definitely drug-related (0.9% for placebo); only one patient on PROSCAR (0.2%) and one patient on placebo (0.2%) discontinued therapy because of a drug-related sexual adverse experience. The following clinical adverse reactions were reported as possibly, probably or definitely drug-related in ≥1% of patients treated for 12 months with PROSCAR or placebo, respectively: erectile dysfunction (3.7%, 1.1%), decreased libido (3.3%, 1.6%) and decreased volume of ejaculate (2.8%, 0.9%). The adverse experience profiles for patients treated with finasteride 1 mg/day for 12 months and those maintained on PROSCAR for 24 to 48 months were similar to that observed in the 12-month controlled studies with PROSCAR. Sexual adverse experiences resolved with continued treatment in over 60% of patients who reported them.

OVERDOSAGE

In clinical studies, single doses of finasteride up to 400 mg and multiple doses of finasteride up to 80 mg/day for three months did not result in adverse reactions. Until further experience is obtained, no specific treatment for an overdose with finasteride can be recommended.
Significant lethality was observed in male and female mice at single oral doses of 1,500 mg/m^2 (500 mg/kg) and in female and male rats at single oral doses of 2,360 mg/m^2 (400 mg/kg) and 5,900 mg/m^2 (1,000 mg/kg), respectively.

DOSAGE AND ADMINISTRATION

The recommended dosage is 1 mg once a day.
PROPECIA may be administered with or without meals.
In general, daily use for three months or more is necessary before benefit is observed. Continued use is recommended to sustain benefit. Withdrawal of treatment leads to reversal of effect within 12 months.

HOW SUPPLIED

No. 6642—PROPECIA tablets, 1 mg, are tan, octagonal, film-coated convex tablets with "stylized P" on one side and PROPECIA on the other. They are supplied as follows:
NDC 0006-0071-31 unit of use bottles of 30
NDC 0006-0071-61 ProPak®***- carton of 3 unit of use bottles of 30.

Shown in Product Identification Guide, page 324

Storage and Handling
Store at room temperature, 15–30°C (59–86°F). Keep container closed and protect from moisture.
Women should not handle crushed or broken PROPECIA tablets when they are pregnant or may potentially be pregnant because of the possibility of absorption of finasteride and the subsequent potential risk to a male fetus. PROPECIA tablets are coated and will prevent contact with the active ingredient during normal handling, provided that the tablets are not broken or crushed. (See WARNINGS, EXPOSURE OF WOMEN - RISK TO MALE FETUS; and PRECAUTIONS, *Information for Patients* and *Pregnancy*.)

*** Registered trademark of MERCK & CO., Inc.
9328500 Issued May 2000

Patient Information about
PROPECIA® (Pro-pee-sha)
Generic name: finasteride
(fin-AS-tur-eyed)

PROPECIA is for use by MEN ONLY.**
Please read this leaflet before you start taking PROPECIA. Also, read the information included with PROPECIA each time you renew your prescription, just in case anything has changed. Remember, this leaflet does not take the place of careful discussions with your doctor. You and your doctor should discuss PROPECIA when you start taking your medication and at regular checkups.

** Registered trademark of MERCK & CO., Inc.

What is PROPECIA used for?
PROPECIA is used for the treatment of male pattern hair loss on the vertex and the anterior mid-scalp area.
PROPECIA is for use by **MEN ONLY** and should **NOT** be used by women or children.
What is male pattern hair loss?
Male pattern hair loss is a common condition in which men experience thinning of the hair on the scalp. Often, this results in a receding hairline and/or balding on the top of the head. These changes typically begin gradually in men in their 20s.
Doctors believe male pattern hair loss is due to heredity and is dependent on hormonal effects. Doctors refer to this type of hair loss as androgenetic alopecia.
Results of clinical studies:
For 12 months, doctors studied over 1800 men aged 18 to 41 with mild to moderate amounts of ongoing hair loss. All men, whether receiving PROPECIA or placebo (a pill containing no medication) were given a medicated shampoo (Neutrogena T/Gel®*** Shampoo). Of these men, approximately 1200 with hair loss at the top of the head were studied for an additional 12 months. In general, men who took PROPECIA maintained or increased the number of visible scalp hairs and noticed improvement in their hair in the first year, with the effect maintained in the second year. Hair counts in men who did not take PROPECIA continued to decrease.
In one study, patients were questioned on the growth of body hair. PROPECIA did not appear to affect hair in places other than the scalp.

*** Registered trademark of Johnson & Johnson

Will PROPECIA work for me?
For most men, PROPECIA increases the number of scalp hairs, helping to fill in thin or balding areas of the scalp. Men taking PROPECIA noted a slowing of hair loss during two years of use. Although results will vary, generally you will not be able to grow back all of the hair you have lost. There is not sufficient evidence that PROPECIA works in the treatment of receding hairline in the temporal area on both sides of the head.
Male pattern hair loss occurs gradually over time. On average, healthy hair grows only about half an inch each month. Therefore, it will take time to see any effect.
You may need to take PROPECIA daily for three months or more before you see a benefit from taking PROPECIA. PROPECIA can only work over the long term if you continue taking it. If the drug has not worked for you in twelve months, further treatment is unlikely to be of benefit. If you stop taking PROPECIA, you will likely lose the hair you have gained within 12 months of stopping treatment. You should discuss this with your doctor.
How should I take PROPECIA?
Follow your doctor's instructions.
- Take one tablet by mouth each day.
- You may take PROPECIA with or without food.
- If you forget to take PROPECIA, do not take an extra tablet. Just take the next tablet as usual.

PROPECIA will not work faster or better if you take it more than once a day.
Who should NOT take PROPECIA?
- PROPECIA is for the treatment of male pattern hair loss in **MEN ONLY** and should not be taken by women or children.
- Anyone allergic to any of the ingredients.

A warning about PROPECIA and pregnancy.
- **Women who are or may potentially be pregnant:**
  - **— must not use PROPECIA**
  - **— should not handle crushed or broken tablets of PROPECIA.**

If a woman who is pregnant with a male baby absorbs the active ingredient in PROPECIA, either by swallowing or through the skin, it may cause abnormalities of a male baby's sex organs. If a woman who is pregnant comes into contact with the active ingredient in PROPECIA, a doctor should be consulted. PROPECIA tablets are coated and will prevent contact with the active ingredient during normal handling, provided that the tablets are not broken or crushed.
What are the possible side effects of PROPECIA?
Like all prescription products, PROPECIA may cause side effects. In clinical studies, side effects from PROPECIA were uncommon and did not affect most men. A small number of men experienced certain sexual side effects. These men reported one or more of the following: less desire for sex; difficulty in achieving an erection; and, a decrease in the amount of semen. Each of these side effects occurred in less than 2% of men. These side effects went away in men who stopped taking PROPECIA. They also disappeared in most men who continued taking PROPECIA.
In general use, the following have been reported infrequently: allergic reactions including rash, itching, hives and swelling of the lips and face; problems with ejaculation; breast tenderness and enlargement; and testicular pain.
Tell your doctor promptly about these or any other unusual effects.
- **PROPECIA can affect a blood test called PSA (Prostate-Specific Antigen) for the screening of prostate cancer. If you have a PSA test done, you should tell your doctor that you are taking PROPECIA.**

Storage and handling.
Keep PROPECIA in the original container and keep the container closed. Store it in a dry place at room temperature.
PROPECIA tablets are coated and will prevent contact with the active ingredient during normal handling, provided that the tablets are not broken or crushed.
Do not give your PROPECIA tablets to anyone else. It has been prescribed only for you. Keep PROPECIA and all medications out of the reach of children.
THIS LEAFLET PROVIDES A SUMMARY OF INFORMATION ABOUT PROPECIA. IF AFTER READING THIS LEAFLET YOU HAVE ANY QUESTIONS OR ARE NOT SURE ABOUT ANYTHING, ASK YOUR DOCTOR.
1-888-637-2522, Monday through Friday, 8:30 A.M. TO 7:00 P.M. (ET).
www.propecia.com
9329300 Issued May 2000

PROSCAR® ℞
(FINASTERIDE)
Tablets

DESCRIPTION

PROSCAR* (finasteride), a synthetic 4-azasteroid compound, is a specific inhibitor of steroid Type II 5α-reductase, an intracellular enzyme that converts the androgen testosterone into 5α-dihydrotestosterone (DHT).
Finasteride is 4-azaandrost-1-ene-17-carboxamide, *N*-(1,1-dimethylethyl)-3-oxo-,(5α,17β)-. The empirical formula of finasteride is $C_{23}H_{36}N_2O_2$ and its molecular weight is 372.55. Its structural formula is:

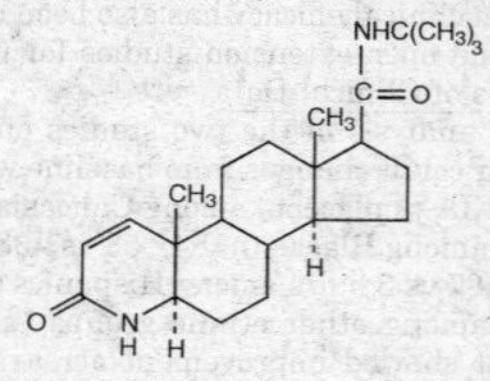

Finasteride is a white crystalline powder with a melting point near 250°C. It is freely soluble in chloroform and in lower alcohol solvents, but is practically insoluble in water.
PROSCAR (finasteride) tablets for oral administration are film-coated tablets that contain 5 mg of finasteride and the following inactive ingredients: hydrous lactose, microcrystalline cellulose, pregelatinized starch, sodium starch glycolate, hydroxypropyl cellulose LF, hydroxypropylmethyl cellulose, titanium dioxide, magnesium stearate, talc, docusate sodium, FD&C Blue 2 aluminum lake and yellow iron oxide.

*Registered trademark of MERCK & CO., Inc.

CLINICAL PHARMACOLOGY

The development and enlargement of the prostate gland is dependent on the potent androgen, 5α-dihydrotestosterone (DHT). Type II 5α-reductase metabolizes testosterone to DHT in the prostate gland, liver and skin. DHT induces androgenic effects by binding to androgen receptors in the cell nuclei of these organs.
Finasteride is a competitive and specific inhibitor of Type II 5α-reductase with which it slowly forms a stable enzyme complex. Turnover from this complex is extremely slow ($t_{1/2}$ ~ 30 days). This has been demonstrated both *in vivo* and *in vitro*. Finasteride has no affinity for the androgen receptor. In man, the 5α-reduced steroid metabolites in blood and urine are decreased after administration of finasteride.
In man, a single 5-mg oral dose of PROSCAR produces a rapid reduction in serum DHT concentration, with the maximum effect observed 8 hours after the first dose. The suppression of DHT is maintained throughout the 24-hour dosing interval and with continued treatment. Daily dosing of PROSCAR at 5 mg/day for up to 4 years has been shown to reduce the serum DHT concentration by approximately 70%. The median circulating level of testosterone increased by approximately 10–20% but remained within the physiologic range.
Adult males with genetically inherited Type II 5α-reductase deficiency also have decreased levels of DHT. Except for the associated urogenital defects present at birth, no other clinical abnormalities related to Type II 5α-reductase deficiency have been observed in these individuals. These individuals have a small prostate gland throughout life and do not develop BPH.
In patients with BPH treated with finasteride (1–100 mg/day) for 7–10 days prior to prostatectomy, an approximate 80% lower DHT content was measured in prostatic tissue removed at surgery, compared to placebo; testosterone tissue concentration was increased up to 10 times over pretreatment levels, relative to placebo. Intraprostatic content of prostate-specific antigen (PSA) was also decreased.
In healthy male volunteers treated with PROSCAR for 14 days, discontinuation of therapy resulted in a return of DHT levels to pretreatment levels in approximately 2 weeks. In patients treated for three months, prostate volume, which declined by approximately 20%, returned to close to baseline value after approximately three months of discontinuation of therapy.
Pharmacokinetics
Absorption
In a study of 15 healthy young subjects, the mean bioavailability of finasteride 5-mg tablets was 63% (range 34–108%), based on the ratio of area under the curve (AUC) relative to an intravenous (IV) reference dose. Maximum finasteride plasma concentration averaged 37 ng/mL (range, 27–49 ng/mL) and was reached 1–2 hours postdose. Bioavailability of finasteride was not affected by food.
Distribution
Mean steady-state volume of distribution was 76 liters (range, 44–96 liters). Approximately 90% of circulating finasteride is bound to plasma proteins. There is a slow accumulation phase for finasteride after multiple dosing. After dosing with 5 mg/day of finasteride for 17 days, plasma concentrations of finasteride were 47 and 54% higher than after the first dose in men 45–60 years old (n=12) and ≥70 years old (n=12), respectively. Mean trough concentrations after 17 days of dosing were 6.2 ng/mL (range, 2.4–9.8 ng/

mL) and 8.1 ng/mL (range, 1.8–19.7 ng/mL), respectively, in the two age groups. Although steady state was not reached in this study, mean trough plasma concentration in another study in patients with BPH (mean age, 65 years) receiving 5 mg/day was 9.4 ng/mL (range, 7.1–13.3 ng/mL; n=22) after over a year of dosing.

Finasteride has been shown to cross the blood brain barrier but does not appear to distribute preferentially to the CSF. In 2 studies of healthy subjects (n=69) receiving PROSCAR 5 mg/day for 6–24 weeks, finasteride concentrations in semen ranged from undetectable (<0.1 ng/mL) to 10.54 ng/mL. In an earlier study using a less sensitive assay, finasteride concentrations in the semen of 16 subjects receiving PROSCAR 5 mg/day ranged from undetectable (<1.0 ng/mL) to 21 ng/mL. Thus, based on a 5-mL ejaculate volume, the amount of finasteride in semen was estimated to be 50- to 100-fold less than the dose of finasteride (5 µg) that had no effect on circulating DHT levels in men (see also PRECAUTIONS, Pregnancy).

Metabolism

Finasteride is extensively metabolized in the liver, primarily via the cytochrome P450 3A4 enzyme subfamily. Two metabolites, the t-butyl side chain monohydroxylated and monocarboxylic acid metabolites, have been identified that possess no more than 20% of the 5α-reductase inhibitory activity of finasteride

Excretion

In healthy young subjects (n=15), mean plasma clearance of finasteride was 165 mL/min (range, 70–279 mL/min) and mean elimination half-life in plasma was 6 hours (range, 3–16 hours). Following an oral dose of ^{14}C-finasteride in man (n=6), a mean of 39% (range, 32–46%) of the dose was excreted in the urine in the form of metabolites; 57% (range, 51–64%) was excreted in the feces.

The mean terminal half-life of finasteride in subjects ≥ 70 years of age was approximately 8 hours (range, 6–15 hours; n=12), compared with 6 hours (range, 4–12 hours; n=12) in subjects 45–60 years of age. As a result, mean AUC (0–24 hr) after 17 days of dosing was 15% higher in subjects ≥ 70 years of age than in subjects 45–60 years of age (p=0.02).

Special Populations

Pediatric: Finasteride pharmacokinetics have not been investigated in patients <18 years of age.

Gender: Finasteride pharmacokinetics in women are not available.

Geriatric: No dosage adjustment is necessary in the elderly. Although the elimination rate of finasteride is decreased in the elderly, these findings are of no clinical significance. See also *Pharmacokinetics*, *Excretion* and DOSAGE AND ADMINISTRATION.

Race: The effect of race on finasteride pharmacokinetics has not been studied.

Renal Insufficiency: No dosage adjustment is necessary in patients with renal insufficiency. In patients with chronic renal impairment, with creatinine clearances ranging from 9.0 to 55 mL/min, AUC, maximum plasma concentration, half-life, and protein binding after a single dose of ^{14}C-finasteride were similar to values obtained in healthy volunteers. Urinary excretion of metabolites was decreased in patients with renal impairment. This decrease was associated with an increase in fecal excretion of metabolites. Plasma concentrations of metabolites were significantly higher in patients with renal impairment (based on a 60% increase in total radioactivity AUC). However, finasteride has been well tolerated in BPH patients with normal renal function receiving up to 80 mg/day for 12 weeks, where exposure of these patients to metabolites would presumably be much greater.

Hepatic Insufficiency: The effect of hepatic insufficiency on finasteride pharmacokinetics has not been studied. Caution should be used in the administration of PROSCAR in those patients with liver function abnormalities, as finasteride is metabolized extensively in the liver.

Drug Interactions (also see PRECAUTIONS, *Drug Interactions*)

No drug interactions of clinical importance have been identified. Finasteride does not appear to affect the cytochrome P450-linked drug metabolism enzyme system. Compounds that have been tested in man have included antipyrine, digoxin, propranolol, theophylline, and warfarin, and no clinically meaningful interactions were found.

Mean (SD) Pharmacokinetic Parameters in Healthy Young Subjects (n=15)

	Mean (± SD)
Bioavailability	63% (34–108%)*
Clearance (mL/min)	165 (55)
Volume of Distribution (L)	76 (14)
Half-Life (hours)	6.2 (2.1)

*Range

[See first table above]

Clinical Studies

PROSCAR 5 mg/day was initially evaluated in patients with symptoms of BPH and enlarged prostates by digital rectal examination in two 1-year, placebo-controlled, randomized, double-blind, studies and their 5-year open extensions.

Mean (SD) Noncompartmental Pharmacokinetic Parameters After Multiple Doses of 5 mg/day in Older Men

	Mean (± SD)	
	45–60 years old (n=12)	≥70 years old (n=12)
AUC (ng•hr/mL)	389 (98)	463 (186)
Peak Concentration (ng/mL)	46.2 (8.7)	48.4 (14.7)
Time to Peak (hours)	1.8 (0.7)	1.8 (0.6)
Half-Life (hours)*	6.0 (1.5)	8.2 (2.5)

*First-dose values; all other parameters are last-dose values

Table 1
All Treatment Failures in PLESS

Event	Patients (%) *		Relative Risk**	95% CI	P Value**
	Placebo N=1503	Finasteride N=1513			
All Treatment Failures	37.1	26.2	0.68	(0.57 to 0.79)	<0.001
Surgical Interventions for BPH	10.1	4.6	0.45	(0.32 to 0.63)	<0.001
Acute Urinary Retention Requiring Catheterization	6.6	2.8	0.43	(0.28 to 0.66)	<0.001
Two consecutive symptoms scores ≥20	9.2	6.7			
Bladder Stone	0.4	0.5			
Incontinence	2.1	1.7			
Renal Failure	0.5	0.6			
UTI	5.7	4.9			
Discontinuation due to worsening of BPH, lack of improvement, or to receive other medical treatment	21.8	13.3			

*patients with multiple events may be counted more than once for each type of event
**Hazard ratio based on log rank test

PROSCAR was further evaluated in the PROSCAR Long-Term Efficacy and Safety Study (PLESS), a double-blind randomized, placebo-controlled, 4-year multicenter study. 3040 patients between the ages of 45 and 78, with moderate to severe symptoms of BPH and an enlarged prostate upon digital rectal examination, were randomized into the study (1524 to finasteride, 1516 to placebo) and 3016 patients were evaluable for efficacy. 1883 patients completed the 4-year study (1000 in the finasteride group, 883 in the placebo group).

Effect on Symptom Score

Symptoms were quantified using a score similar to the American Urological Association Symptom Score, which evaluated both obstructive symptoms (impairment of size and force of stream, sensation of incomplete bladder emptying, delayed or interrupted urination) and irritative symptoms (nocturia, daytime frequency, need to strain or push the flow of urine) by rating on a 0 to 5 scale for six symptoms and a 0 to 4 scale for one symptom, for a total possible score of 34.

Patients in PLESS, had moderate to severe symptoms at baseline (mean of approximately 15 points on a 0–34 point scale). Patients randomized to PROSCAR who remained on therapy for 4 years had a mean (± 1 SD) decrease in symptom score of 3.3 (± 5.8) points compared with 1.3 (± 5.6) points in the placebo group. (See Figure 1.) A statistically significant improvement in symptom score was evident at 1 year in patients treated with PROSCAR vs placebo (–2.3 vs –1.6), and this improvement continued through Year 4.

[See figure 1 at top of next column]

Results seen in earlier studies were comparable to those seen in PLESS. Although an early improvement in urinary symptoms was seen in some patients, a therapeutic trial of at least 6 months was generally necessary to assess whether a beneficial response in symptom relief had been achieved. The improvement in BPH symptoms was seen during the first year and maintained throughout an additional 5 years of open extension studies.

Effect on Acute Urinary Retention and the Need for Surgery

In PLESS, efficacy was also assessed by evaluating treatment failures. Treatment failure was prospectively defined as BPH-related urological events or clinical deterioration, lack of improvement and/or the need for alternative therapy. BPH-related urological events were defined as urological surgical intervention and acute urinary retention requiring catheterization. Complete event information was available for 92% of the patients. The following table (Table 1) summarizes the results.

[See table 1 above]

Figure 1
Symptom Score in PLESS

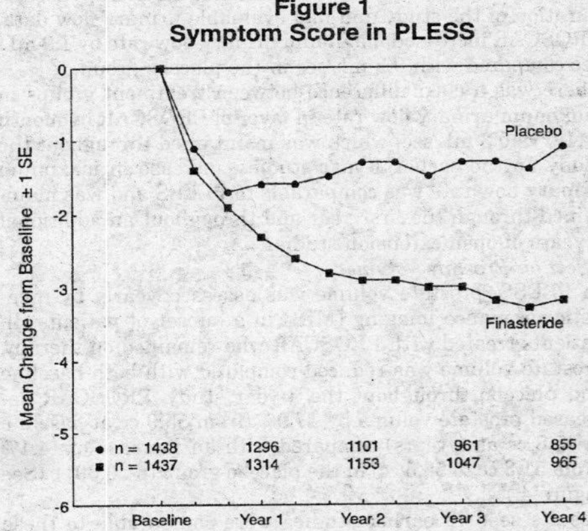

Compared with placebo, PROSCAR was associated with a significantly lower risk for acute urinary retention or the need for BPH-related surgery [13.2% for placebo vs 6.6% for PROSCAR; 51% reduction in risk, 95% CI: (34 to 63%)]. Compared with placebo, PROSCAR was associated with a significantly lower risk for surgery [10.1% for placebo vs 4.6% for PROSCAR; 55% reduction in risk, 95% CI: (37 to 68%)] and with a significantly lower risk of acute urinary

Continued on next page

Information on the Merck & Co., Inc. products listed on these pages is the full prescribing information from product circulars in use September 30, 2000. For information, please call 1-800-NSC MERCK [1-800-672-6372].

Proscar—Cont.

retention [6.6% for placebo vs 2.8% for PROSCAR; 57% reduction in risk, 95% CI: (34 to 72%)]; See Figures 2 and 3.

Figure 2
Percent of Patients Having Surgery for BPH, Including TURP

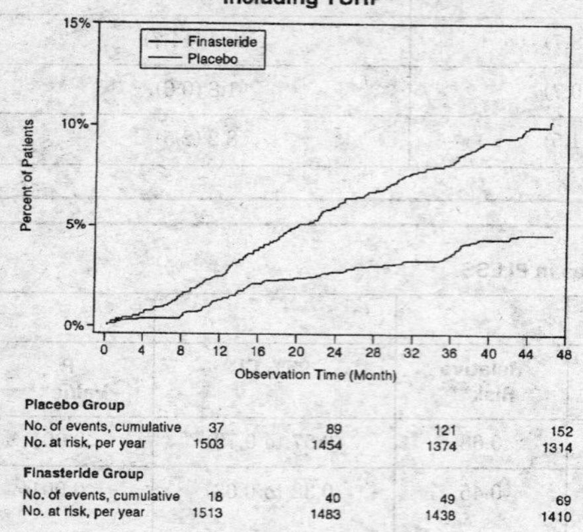

Figure 3
Percent of Patients Developing Acute Urinary Retention (Spontaneous and Precipitated)

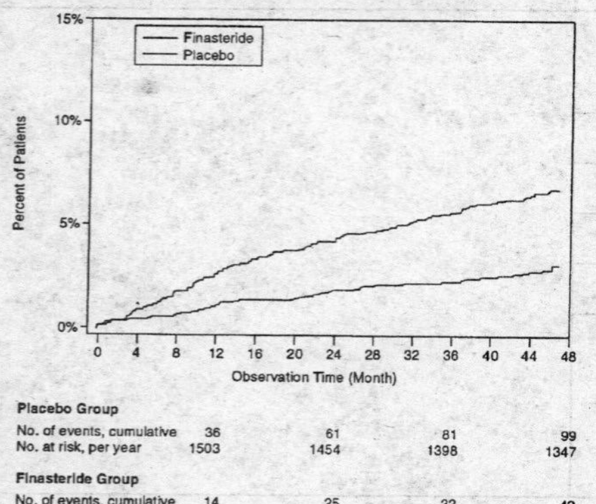

Effect on Maximum Urinary Flow Rate
In the patients in PLESS who remained on therapy for the duration of the study and had evaluable urinary flow data, PROSCAR increased maximum urinary flow rate by 1.9 mL/sec compared with 0.2 mL/sec in the placebo group.
There was a clear difference between treatment groups in maximum urinary flow rate in favor of PROSCAR by month 4 (1.0 vs 0.3 mL/sec) which was maintained throughout the study. In the earlier 1-year studies, increase in maximum urinary flow rate was comparable to PLESS and was maintained through the first year and throughout an additional 5 years of open extension studies.
Effect on Prostate Volume
In PLESS, prostate volume was assessed yearly by magnetic resonance imaging (MRI) in a subset of patients. In patients treated with PROSCAR who remained on therapy, prostate volume was reduced compared with both baseline and placebo throughout the 4-year study. PROSCAR decreased prostate volume by 17.9% (from 55.9 cc at baseline to 45.8 cc at 4 years) compared with an increase of 14.1% (from 51.3 cc to 58.5 cc) in the placebo group (p<0.001). (See Figure 4.)
Results seen in earlier studies were comparable to those seen in PLESS. Mean prostate volume at baseline ranged between 40-50 cc. The reduction in prostate volume was seen during the first year and maintained throughout an additional five years of open extension studies.

Figure 4
Prostate Volume in PLESS

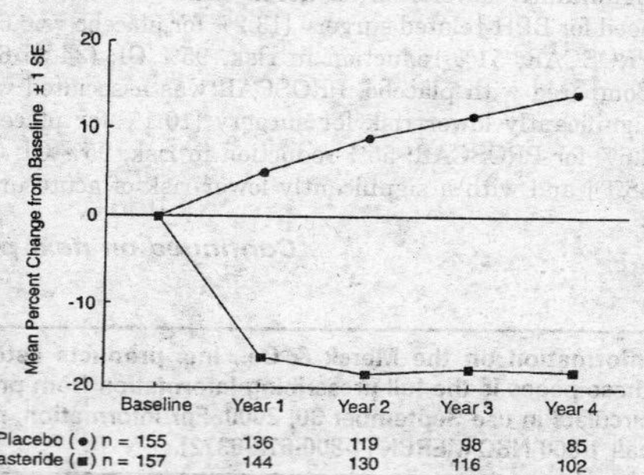

Prostate Volume as a Predictor of Therapeutic Response
A meta-analysis combining 1-year data from seven double-blind, placebo-controlled studies of similar design, including 4491 patients with symptomatic BPH, demonstrated that, in patients treated with PROSCAR, the magnitude of symptom response and degree of improvement in maximum urinary flow rate were greater in patients with an enlarged prostate at baseline.
Summary of Clinical Studies
The data from these studies, showing improvement in BPH-related symptoms, reduction in treatment failure (BPH-related urological events), increased maximum urinary flow rates, and decreasing prostate volume, suggest that PROSCAR arrests the disease process of BPH in men with an enlarged prostate.

INDICATIONS AND USAGE

PROSCAR is indicated for the treatment of symptomatic benign prostatic hyperplasia (BPH) in men with an enlarged prostate to:
- Improve symptoms
- Reduce the risk of acute urinary retention
- Reduce the risk of the need for surgery including transurethral resection of the prostate (TURP) and prostatectomy.

CONTRAINDICATIONS

PROSCAR is contraindicated in the following:
Hypersensitivity to any component of this medication.
Pregnancy. Finasteride use is contraindicated in women when they are or may potentially be pregnant. Because of the ability of Type II 5α-reductase inhibitors to inhibit the conversion of testosterone to DHT, finasteride may cause abnormalities of the external genitalia of a male fetus of a pregnant woman who receives finasteride. If this drug is used during pregnancy, or if pregnancy occurs while taking this drug, the pregnant woman should be apprised of the potential hazard to the male fetus. (See also WARNINGS, EXPOSURE OF WOMEN—RISK TO MALE FETUS and PRECAUTIONS, *Information for Patients* and *Pregnancy*.) In female rats, low doses of finasteride administered during pregnancy have produced abnormalities of the external genitalia in male offspring.

WARNINGS

PROSCAR is not indicated for use in pediatric patients (see PRECAUTIONS, *Pediatric Use*) or women (see also WARNINGS, EXPOSURE OF WOMEN—RISK TO MALE FETUS; PRECAUTIONS, *Information for Patients* and *Pregnancy*, and HOW SUPPLIED).
EXPOSURE OF WOMEN—RISK TO MALE FETUS
Women should not handle crushed or broken PROSCAR tablets when they are pregnant or may potentially be pregnant because of the possibility of absorption of finasteride and the subsequent potential risk to a male fetus. PROSCAR tablets are coated and will prevent contact with the active ingredient during normal handling, provided that the tablets have not been broken or crushed. (See CONTRAINDICATIONS; PRECAUTIONS, *Information for Patients* and *Pregnancy*, and HOW SUPPLIED).

PRECAUTIONS

General
Prior to initiating therapy with PROSCAR, appropriate evaluation should be performed to identify other conditions such as infection, prostate cancer, stricture disease, hypotonic bladder or other neurogenic disorders that might mimic BPH.
Patients with large residual urinary volume and/or severely diminished urinary flow should be carefully monitored for obstructive uropathy. These patients may not be candidates for finasteride therapy.
Caution should be used in the administration of PROSCAR in those patients with liver function abnormalities, as finasteride is metabolized extensively in the liver.
Effects on PSA and Prostate Cancer Detection
No clinical benefit has been demonstrated in patients with prostate cancer treated with PROSCAR. Patients with BPH and elevated PSA were monitored in controlled clinical studies with serial PSAs and prostate biopsies. In these studies, PROSCAR did not appear to alter the rate of prostate cancer detection. The overall incidence of prostate cancer was not significantly different in patients treated with PROSCAR or placebo.
PROSCAR causes a decrease in serum PSA levels by approximately 50% in patients with BPH, even in the presence of prostate cancer. This decrease is predictable over the entire range of PSA values, although it may vary in individual patients. Analysis of PSA data from over 3000 patients in PLESS confirmed that in typical patients treated with PROSCAR for six months or more, PSA values should be doubled for comparison with normal ranges in untreated men. This adjustment preserves the sensitivity and specificity of the PSA assay and maintains its ability to detect prostate cancer.
Any sustained increases in PSA levels while on PROSCAR should be carefully evaluated, including consideration of non-compliance to therapy with PROSCAR.
Percent free PSA (free to total PSA ratio) is not significantly decreased by PROSCAR. The ratio of free to total PSA remains constant even under the influence of PROSCAR. If clinicians elect to use percent free PSA as an aid in the detection of prostate cancer in men undergoing finasteride therapy, no adjustment to its value appears necessary.

Information for Patients
Women should not handle crushed or broken PROSCAR tablets when they are pregnant or may potentially be pregnant because of the possibility of absorption of finasteride and the subsequent potential risk to the male fetus (see CONTRAINDICATIONS; WARNINGS, EXPOSURE OF WOMEN—RISK TO MALE FETUS; PRECAUTIONS, *Pregnancy* and HOW SUPPLIED).
Physicians should inform patients that the volume of ejaculate may be decreased in some patients during treatment with PROSCAR. This decrease does not appear to interfere with normal sexual function. However, impotence and decreased libido may occur in patients treated with PROSCAR (see ADVERSE REACTIONS).
Physicians should instruct their patients to read the patient package insert before starting therapy with PROSCAR and to reread it each time the prescription is renewed so that they are aware of current information for patients regarding PROSCAR.
Drug/Laboratory Test Interactions
In patients with BPH, PROSCAR has no effect on circulating levels of cortisol, estradiol, prolactin, thyroid-stimulating hormone, or thyroxine. No clinically meaningful effect was observed on the plasma lipid profile (i.e., total cholesterol, low density lipoproteins, high density lipoproteins and triglycerides) or bone mineral density. Increases of about 10% were observed in luteinizing hormone (LH) and follicle-stimulating hormone (FSH) in patients receiving PROSCAR, but levels remained within the normal range. In healthy volunteers, treatment with PROSCAR did not alter the response of LH and FSH to gonadotropin-releasing hormone indicating that the hypothalamic-pituitary-testicular axis was not affected.
Treatment with PROSCAR for 24 weeks to evaluate semen parameters in healthy male volunteers revealed no clinically meaningful effects on sperm concentration, mobility, morphology, or pH. A 0.6 mL (22.1%) median decrease in ejaculate volume with a concomitant reduction in total sperm per ejaculate, was observed. These parameters remained within the normal range and were reversible upon discontinuation of therapy with an average time to return to baseline of 84 weeks.
Drug Interactions
No drug interactions of clinical importance have been identified. Finasteride does not appear to affect the cytochrome P450-linked drug metabolizing enzyme system. Compounds that have been tested in man have included antipyrine, digoxin, propranolol, theophylline, and warfarin and no clinically meaningful interactions were found.
Other Concomitant Therapy: Although specific interaction studies were not performed, PROSCAR was concomitantly used in clinical studies with acetaminophen, acetylsalicylic acid, α-blockers, angiotensin-converting enzyme (ACE) inhibitors, analgesics, anti-convulsants, beta-adrenergic blocking agents, diuretics, calcium channel blockers, cardiac nitrates, HMG-CoA reductase inhibitors, nonsteroidal anti-inflammatory drugs (NSAIDSs), benzodiazepines, H_2 antagonists and quinolone anti-infectives without evidence of clinically significant adverse interactions.
Carcinogenesis, Mutagenesis, Impairment of Fertility
No evidence of a tumorigenic effect was observed in a 24-month study in Sprague-Dawley rats receiving doses of finasteride up to 160 mg/kg/day in males and 320 mg/kg/day in females. These doses produced respective systemic exposure in rats of 111 and 274 times those observed in man receiving the recommended human dose of 5 mg/day. All exposure calculations were based on calculated AUC (0–24hr) for animals and mean AUC (0–24 hr) for man (0.4 μg • hr/mL).
In a 19-month carcinogenicity study in CD-1 mice, a statistically significant (p≤0.05) increase in the incidence of testicular Leydig cell adenomas was observed at a dose of 250 mg/kg/day (228 times the human exposure). In mice at a dose of 25 mg/kg/day (23 times the human exposure, estimated) and in rats at a dose of ≥40 mg/kg/day (39 times the human exposure) an increase in the incidence of Leydig cell hyperplasia was observed. A positive correlation between the proliferative changes in the Leydig cells and an increase in serum LH levels (2–3 fold above control) has been demonstrated in both rodent species treated with high doses of finasteride. No drug-related Leydig cell changes were seen in either rats or dogs treated with finasteride for 1 year at doses of 20 mg/kg/day and 45 mg/kg/day (30 and 350 times, respectively, the human exposure) or in mice treated for 19 months at a dose of 2.5 mg/kg/day (2.3 times the human exposure, estimated).
No evidence of mutagenicity was observed in an *in vitro* bacterial mutagenesis assay, a mammalian cell mutagenesis assay, or in an *in vitro* alkaline elution assay. In an *in vitro* chromosome aberration assay, using Chinese hamster ovary cells, there was a slight increase in chromosome aberrations. These concentrations correspond to 4000–5000 times the peak plasma levels in man given a total dose of 5 mg. In an *in vivo* chromosome aberration assay in mice, no treatment-related increase in chromosome aberration was observed with finasteride at the maximum tolerated dose of 250 mg/kg/day (228 times the human exposure) as determined in the carcinogenicity studies.
In sexually mature male rabbits treated with finasteride at 80 mg/kg/day (543 times the human exposure) for up to 12 weeks, no effect on fertility, sperm count, or ejaculate volume was seen. In sexually mature male rats treated with 80 mg/kg/day of finasteride (61 times the human exposure), there were no significant effects on fertility after 6 or 12 weeks of treatment; however, when treatment was contin-

ued for up to 24 or 30 weeks, there was an apparent decrease in fertility, fecundity and an associated significant decrease in the weights of the seminal vesicles and prostate. All these effects were reversible within 6 weeks of discontinuation of treatment. No drug-related effect on testes or on mating performance has been seen in rats or rabbits. This decrease in fertility in finasteride-treated rats is secondary to its effect on accessory sex organs (prostate and seminal vesicles) resulting in failure to form a seminal plug. The seminal plug is essential for normal fertility in rats and is not relevant in man.

Pregnancy

Pregnancy Category X

See CONTRAINDICATIONS.

PROSCAR is not indicated for use in women.

Administration of finasteride to pregnant rats at doses ranging from 100 µg/kg/day to 100 mg/kg/day (1–1000 times the recommended human dose of 5 mg/day) resulted in dose-dependent development of hypospadias in 3.6 to 100% of male offspring. Pregnant rats produced male offspring with decreased prostatic and seminal vesicular weights, delayed preputial separation and transient nipple development when given finasteride at ≥30 µg/kg/day (≥3/10 of the recommended human dose of 5 mg/day) and decreased anogenital distance when given finasteride at ≥3 µg/kg/day (≥3/100 of the recommended human dose of 5 mg/day). The critical period during which these effects can be induced in male rats has been defined to be days 16–17 of gestation. The changes described above are expected pharmacological effects of drugs belonging to the class of Type II 5α-reductase inhibitors and are similar to those reported in male infants with a genetic deficiency of Type II 5α-reductase. No abnormalities were observed in female offspring exposed to any dose of finasteride *in utero*.

No developmental abnormalities have been observed in first filial generation (F_1) male or female offspring resulting from mating finasteride-treated male rats (80 mg/kg/day; 61 times the human exposure) with untreated females. Administration of finasteride at 3 mg/kg/day (30 times the recommended human dose of 5 mg/day) during the late gestation and lactation period resulted in slightly decreased fertility in F_1 male offspring. No effects were seen in female offspring. No evidence of malformations has been observed in rabbit fetuses exposed to finasteride *in utero* from days 6–18 of gestation at doses up to 100 mg/kg/day (1000 times the recommended human dose of 5 mg/day). However, effects on male genitalia would not be expected since the rabbits were not exposed during the critical period of genital system development.

The *in utero* effects of finasteride exposure during the period of embryonic and fetal development were evaluated in the rhesus monkey (gestation days 20–100), a species more predictive of human development than rats or rabbits. Intravenous administration of finasteride to pregnant monkeys at doses as high as 800 ng/day (at least 60 to 120 times the highest estimated exposure of pregnant women to finasteride from semen of men taking 5 mg/day) resulted in no abnormalities in male fetuses. In confirmation of the relevance of the rhesus model for human fetal development, oral administration of a dose of finasteride (2 mg/kg/day; 20 times the recommended human dose of 5 mg/day or approximately 1–2 million times the highest estimated exposure to finasteride from semen of men taking 5 mg/day) to pregnant monkeys resulted in external genital abnormalities in male fetuses. No other abnormalities were observed in male fetuses and no finasteride-related abnormalities were observed in female fetuses at any dose.

Nursing Mothers

PROSCAR is not indicated for use in women.

It is not known whether finasteride is excreted in human milk.

Pediatric Use

PROSCAR is not indicated for use in pediatric patients.

Safety and effectiveness in pediatric patients have not been established.

ADVERSE REACTIONS

PROSCAR is generally well tolerated; adverse reactions usually have been mild and transient.

4-Year Placebo-Controlled Study

In PLESS, 1524 patients treated with PROSCAR and 1516 patients treated with placebo were evaluated for safety over a period of 4 years. The most frequently reported adverse reactions were related to sexual function. 3.7% (57 patients) treated with PROSCAR and 2.1% (32 patients) treated with placebo discontinued therapy as a result of adverse reactions related to sexual function, which are the most frequently reported adverse reactions.

Table 2 presents the only clinical adverse reactions considered possibly, probably or definitely drug related by the investigator, for which the incidence on PROSCAR was ≥1% and greater than placebo over the 4 years of the study. In years 2–4 of the study, there was no significant difference between treatment groups in the incidences of impotence, decreased libido and ejaculation disorder.

[See table 2 above]

Phase III Studies and 5-Year Open Extensions

The adverse experience profile in the 1-year, placebo-controlled, Phase III studies, the 5-year open extensions, and PLESS were similar.

There is no evidence of increased adverse experiences with increased duration of treatment with PROSCAR. New reports of drug-related sexual adverse experiences decreased with duration of therapy.

TABLE 2
Drug-Related Adverse Experiences

	Year 1 (%)		Years 2, 3 and 4* (%)	
	Finasteride	Placebo	Finasteride	Placebo
Impotence	8.1	3.7	5.1	5.1
Decreased Libido	6.4	3.4	2.6	2.6
Decreased Volume of Ejaculate	3.7	0.8	1.5	0.5
Ejaculation Disorder	0.8	0.1	0.2	0.1
Breast Enlargement	0.5	0.1	1.8	1.1
Breast Tenderness	0.4	0.1	0.7	0.3
Rash	0.5	0.2	0.5	0.1

*Combined Years 2–4

N = 1524 and 1516, finasteride vs placebo, respectively

The following additional adverse effects have been reported in post-marketing experience:

—hypersensitivity reactions, including pruritus, urticaria, and swelling of the lips and face

—testicular pain.

OVERDOSAGE

Patients have received single doses of PROSCAR up to 400 mg and multiple doses of PROSCAR up to 80 mg/day for three months without adverse effects. Until further experience is obtained, no specific treatment for an overdose with PROSCAR can be recommended.

Significant lethality was observed in male and female mice at single oral doses of 1500 mg/m^2 (500 mg/kg) and in female and male rats at single oral doses of 2360 mg/m^2 (400 mg/kg) and 5900 mg/m^2 (1000 mg/kg), respectively.

DOSAGE AND ADMINISTRATION

The recommended dose is 5 mg orally once a day.

PROSCAR may be administered with or without meals.

No dosage adjustment is necessary for patients with renal impairment or for the elderly (see CLINICAL PHARMACOLOGY, *Pharmacokinetics*).

HOW SUPPLIED

No. 3094—PROSCAR tablets 5 mg are blue, modified apple-shaped, film-coated tablets, with the code MSD 72 on one side and PROSCAR on the other. They are supplied as follow:

NDC 0006-0072-31 unit of use bottles of 30

NDC 0006-0072-58 unit of use bottles of 100

NDC 0006-0072-28 unit dose packages of 100.

Shown in Product Identification Guide, page 324

Storage and Handling

Store at room temperatures below 30°C (86°F). Protect from light and keep container tightly closed.

Women should not handle crushed or broken PROSCAR tablets when they are pregnant or may potentially be pregnant because of the possibility of absorption of finasteride and the subsequent potential risk to a male fetus (see WARNINGS, EXPOSURE OF WOMEN—RISK TO MALE FETUS, and PRECAUTIONS, *Information for Patients* and *Pregnancy*).

9132102 Issued August 1999

Patient Information about

PROSCAR® (Prahs-car)

Generic name: finasteride

(fin-AS-tur-eyed)

PROSCAR* is for use by men only.

Please read this leaflet before you start taking PROSCAR. Also, read it each time you renew your prescription, just in case anything has changed. Remember, this leaflet does not take the place of careful discussions with your doctor. You and your doctor should discuss PROSCAR when you start taking your medication and at regular checkups.

*Registered trademark of MERCK & CO., INC.

Why your doctor has prescribed PROSCAR

Your doctor has prescribed PROSCAR because you have a medical condition called benign prostatic hyperplasia or BPH. This occurs only in men.

What is BPH?

BPH is an enlargement of the prostate gland. After age 50, most men develop enlarged prostates. The prostate is located below the bladder. As the prostate enlarges, it may slowly restrict the flow of urine. This can lead to symptoms such as:

- a weak or interrupted urinary stream
- a feeling that you cannot empty your bladder completely
- a feeling of delay or hesitation when you start to urinate
- a need to urinate often, especially at night
- a feeling that you must urinate right away.

In some men, BPH can lead to serious problems, including urinary tract infections, a sudden inability to pass urine (acute urinary retention), as well as the need for surgery.

Treatment options for BPH

There are three main treatment options for symptoms of BPH:

- **Program of monitoring or "Watchful Waiting".** If a man has an enlarged prostate gland and no symptoms or if his symptoms do not bother him, he and his doctor may decide on a program of monitoring which would include regular checkups, instead of medication or surgery.
- **Medication.** Your doctor may prescribe PROSCAR for BPH. See **"What PROSCAR does"** below.
- **Surgery.** Some patients may need surgery. Your doctor can suggest several different surgical procedures for BPH. Which procedure is best depends on your symptoms and medical condition.

There are two main treatment options to reduce the risk of serious problems due to BPH:

- **Medication.** Your doctor may prescribe PROSCAR for BPH. See **"What PROSCAR does"** below.
- **Surgery.** Some patients may need surgery. Your doctor can suggest several different surgical procedures for BPH. Which procedure is best depends on your symptoms and medical condition.

What PROSCAR does

PROSCAR lowers levels of a key hormone called DHT (dihydrotestosterone), which is a major cause of prostate growth. Lowering DHT leads to shrinkage of the enlarged prostate gland in most men. This can lead to gradual improvement in urine flow and symptoms over the next several months. PROSCAR will help reduce the risk of developing a sudden inability to pass urine and the need for surgery. However, since each case of BPH is different, you should know that:

- Even though the prostate shrinks, you may NOT notice an improvement in urine flow or symptoms.
- You may need to take PROSCAR for six (6) months or more to see whether it improves your symptoms.
- Therapy with PROSCAR may reduce your risk for a sudden inability to pass urine and the need for surgery.

What you need to know while taking PROSCAR

- **You must see your doctor regularly.** While taking PROSCAR, you must have regular checkups. Follow your doctor's advice about when to have these checkups.
- **About side effects.** Like all prescription drugs, PROSCAR may cause side effects. Side effects due to PROSCAR may include impotence (an inability to have an erection) or less desire for sex.

  Some men taking PROSCAR may have changes or problems with ejaculation, such as a decrease in the amount of semen released during sex. This decrease in the amount of semen does not appear to interfere with normal sexual function. In some cases these side effects went away while the patient continued to take PROSCAR.

  In addition, some men may have breast swelling and/or tenderness. Some men have reported allergic reactions such as rash, itching, hives, and swelling of the lips and face. Rarely, testicular pain has been reported.

You should discuss side effects with your doctor before taking PROSCAR and anytime you think you are having a side effect.

- **Checking for prostate cancer.** Your doctor has prescribed PROSCAR for symptomatic BPH and not for cancer—but a man can have BPH and prostate cancer at the same

Continued on next page

Information on the Merck & Co., Inc. products listed on these pages is the full prescribing information from product circulars in use September 30, 2000. For information, please call 1-800-NSC MERCK [1-800-672-6372].

Proscar—Cont.

time. Doctors usually recommend that men be checked for prostate cancer once a year when they turn 50 (or 40 if a family member has had prostate cancer). These checks should continue while you take PROSCAR. PROSCAR is not a treatment for prostate cancer.

- **About Prostate-Specific Antigen (PSA).**
  Your doctor may have done a blood test called PSA. PROSCAR can alter PSA values. For more information, talk to your doctor.
- **A warning about PROSCAR and pregnancy.**
  PROSCAR is for use by MEN only.
  Women who are or may potentially be pregnant must not use PROSCAR. They should also not handle crushed or broken tablets of PROSCAR.
  If a woman who is pregnant with a male baby absorbs the active ingredient in PROSCAR after oral use or through the skin, it may cause the male baby to be born with abnormalities of the sex organs.
  PROSCAR tablets are coated and will prevent contact with the active ingredient during normal handling, provided that the tablets are not broken or crushed.

If a woman who is pregnant comes into contact with the active ingredient in PROSCAR, a doctor should be consulted. Remember, these warnings apply only when the woman is pregnant or could potentially be pregnant.

How to take PROSCAR

Follow your doctor's advice about how to take PROSCAR. You must take it every day. You may take it with or between meals. To avoid forgetting to take PROSCAR, it may be helpful to take it at the same time every day.

Do not share PROSCAR with anyone else; it was prescribed only for you.

Keep PROSCAR and all medicines out of the reach of children.

FOR MORE INFORMATION ABOUT 'PROSCAR' AND BPH, TALK WITH YOUR DOCTOR. IN ADDITION, TALK TO YOUR PHARMACIST OR OTHER HEALTH CARE PROVIDER.

7819307 Issued August 1999

RECOMBIVAX HB® ℞
Hepatitis B Vaccine (Recombinant)

DESCRIPTION

RECOMBIVAX HB* Hepatitis B Vaccine (Recombinant) is a non-infectious subunit viral vaccine derived from Hepatitis B surface antigen (HBsAg) produced in yeast cells. A portion of the hepatitis B virus gene, coding for HBsAg, is cloned into yeast, and the vaccine for hepatitis B is produced from cultures of this recombinant yeast strain according to methods developed in the Merck Research Laboratories.

The antigen is harvested and purified from fermentation cultures of a recombinant strain of the yeast *Saccharomyces cerevisiae* containing the gene for the *adw* subtype of HBsAg. The HBsAg protein is released from the yeast cells by cell disruption and purified by a series of physical and chemical methods. The vaccine contains no detectable yeast DNA but may contain not more than 1% yeast protein. The vaccine produced by the Merck method has been shown to be comparable to the plasma-derived vaccine in terms of animal potency (mouse, monkey, and chimpanzee) and protective efficacy (chimpanzee and human).

The vaccine against hepatitis B, prepared from recombinant yeast cultures, is free of association with human blood or blood products.

Each lot of hepatitis B vaccine is tested for safety, in mice and guinea pigs, and for sterility.

RECOMBIVAX HB is a sterile suspension for intramuscular injection. However, for persons at risk of hemorrhage following intramuscular injection, the vaccine may be administered subcutaneously. (See DOSAGE AND ADMINISTRATION).

RECOMBIVAX HB Hepatitis B Vaccine (Recombinant) is supplied in three formulations. (See HOW SUPPLIED,)

Pediatric/Adolescent Formulation (With and Without Preservative), 10 mcg/mL: each 0.5 mL dose contains 5 mcg of hepatitis B surface antigen.

Adult Formulation, 10 mcg/mL: each 1 mL dose contains 10 mcg of hepatitis B surface antigen.

Dialysis Formulation, 40 mcg/mL: each 1 mL dose contains 40 mcg of hepatitis B surface antigen.

Formulations that contain a preservative include thimerosal, a mercury derivative, at 1:20,000 or 50 mcg/mL. All formulations have been treated with formaldehyde prior to adsorption onto aluminum hydroxide. In each formulation, hepatitis B surface antigen is adsorbed onto approximately 0.5 mg of aluminum (provided as aluminum hydroxide) per mL of vaccine. The vaccine is of the *adw* subtype. RECOMBIVAX HB is indicated for vaccination of persons at risk of infection from hepatitis B virus including all known subtypes. RECOMBIVAX HB Dialysis Formulation is indicated for vaccination of adult predialysis and dialysis patients against infection caused by all known subtypes of hepatitis B virus.

*Registered trademark of MERCK & CO., INC.

CLINICAL PHARMACOLOGY

Hepatitis B virus is one of several hepatitis viruses that cause a systemic infection, with a major pathology in the liver. These include hepatitis A virus, hepatitis D virus, and hepatitis C and E viruses, previously referred to as non-A, non-B hepatitis viruses.

Hepatitis B virus is an important cause of viral hepatitis. There is no specific treatment for this disease. The incubation period for hepatitis B is relatively long; six weeks to six months may elapse between exposure and the onset of clinical symptoms. The prognosis following infection with hepatitis B virus is variable and dependent on at least three factors: (1) Age—Infants and younger children usually experience milder initial disease than older persons; (2) Dose of virus—The higher the dose, the more likely acute icteric hepatitis B will result; and, (3) Severity of associated underlying disease —underlying malignancy or pre-existing hepatic disease predisposes to increased morbidity and mortality.

Persistence of viral infection (the chronic hepatitis B virus carrier state) occurs in 5–10% of persons following acute hepatitis B, and occurs more frequently after initial anicteric hepatitis B than after initial icteric disease. Consequently, carriers of hepatitis B surface antigen (HBsAg) frequently give no history of having had recognized acute hepatitis. The Centers for Disease Control and Prevention (CDC) estimates that there are approximately 200–300 million chronic carriers worldwide and 1.25 million chronic carriers of hepatitis B virus in the USA. Chronic carriers represent the largest human reservoir of hepatitis B virus.

The serious complications and sequelae of hepatitis B virus infection include massive hepatic necrosis, cirrhosis of the liver, chronic active hepatitis, and hepatocellular carcinoma. It is the cause of up to 80% of hepatocellular carcinomas. More than 250,000 people worldwide die each year of hepatitis B-associated acute and chronic liver disease. In the United States, hepatitis B-virus-related acute and chronic liver disease causes approximately 4-5000 deaths annually.

There is also evidence that several diseases other than hepatitis have been associated with hepatitis B virus infection through an immunologic mechanism involving antigen-antibody complexes. Such diseases include a syndrome with rash, urticaria, and arthralgia resembling serum sickness; periarteritis nodosa; membranous glomerulonephritis; and infantile papular acrodermatitis.

Although the vehicles for transmission of the virus are often blood and blood products, viral antigen has also been found in tears, saliva, breast milk, urine, semen and vaginal secretions. Hepatitis B virus is capable of surviving at least a month on environmental surfaces exposed to body fluids containing hepatitis B virus. Infection may occur when hepatitis B virus, transmitted by infected body fluids, is implanted via mucous surfaces or percutaneously introduced through accidental or deliberate breaks in the skin.

Transmission of hepatitis B virus infection is often associated with close interpersonal contact with an infected individual and with crowded living conditions. In such circumstances, transmission by inoculation via routes other than overt percutaneous ones may be quite common. Perinatal transmission of hepatitis B infection from infected mother to child, at or shortly after birth, can occur if the mother is a hepatitis B surface antigen (HBsAg) carrier or if the mother has an acute hepatitis B infection in the third trimester. Infection in infancy by the hepatitis B virus usually leads to the chronic carrier state. Without prophylaxis, infants born to women whose sera are positive for both the hepatitis B surface antigen and the e antigen have an 85–90% likelihood of being infected and becoming a chronic carrier. Well-controlled studies have shown that administration of three 0.5 mL doses of Hepatitis B Immune Globulin (Human)-HBIG starting at birth is 75% effective in preventing establishment of the chronic carrier state in these infants during the first year of life. However, the protective effect of HBIG is transient.

Hepatitis B is endemic throughout the world and is a serious medical problem in population groups at increased risk. Because vaccination limited to high-risk individuals has failed to substantially lower the overall incidence of hepatitis B infection, both the Advisory Committee on Immunization Practices (ACIP) and the Committee on Infectious Diseases of the American Academy of Pediatrics (AAP) have also endorsed universal infant immunization as part of a comprehensive strategy for the control of hepatitis B infection. In addition, the ACIP also recommends hepatitis B vaccination for all infants and children born after November 21, 1991 and catch-up vaccination of children at high risk of infection (children <11 years of age in households of Pacific Islander ethnicity or of first generation immigrants/refugees from countries with an intermediate or high endemicity of infection). These advisory groups further recommend broad-based vaccination of adolescents. The ACIP recommends that all individuals not previously vaccinated with hepatitis B vaccine be vaccinated at 11–12 years of age with the age-appropriate dose of vaccine and that the vaccination schedule take into account the feasibility of delivering three doses of vaccine to this age group. In addition, older unvaccinated adolescents with identified risk factors for hepatitis B virus infection should also be vaccinated. Similarly, the AAP recommends that universal immunization of all adolescents should be implemented when resources permit with emphasis on those individuals in high-risk settings. (Refer to INDICATIONS AND USAGE.)

Numerous epidemiological studies have shown that persons who develop anti-HBs following active infection with the hepatitis B virus are protected against the disease on reexposure to the virus.

Clinical studies have shown that RECOMBIVAX HB when injected into the deltoid muscle induced protective levels of antibody in 96% of 1213 healthy adults who received the recommended 3-dose regimen. Antibody responses varied with age; a protective level of antibody was induced in 98% of 787 young adults 20–29 years of age, 94% of 249 adults 30–39 years of age and in 89% of 177 adults ≥ 40 years of age. Studies with hepatitis B vaccine derived from plasma have shown that a lower response rate (81%) to vaccine may be obtained if the vaccine is administered as a buttock injection. Seroconversion rates and geometric mean antibody titers were measured 1 to 2 months after the third dose. Multiple clinical studies have defined a protective antibody (anti-HBs) level as 1) 10 or more sample ratio units (SRU) as determined by radioimmunoassay or 2) a positive result as determined by enzyme immunoassay. Note: 10 SRU is comparable to 10 mIU/mL of antibody.

RECOMBIVAX HB was shown to be highly immunogenic in clinical studies involving infants, children, and adolescents. Three 5 mcg doses of vaccine induced a protective level of antibody in 100% of 92 infants, 99% of 129 children, and in 99% of 112 adolescents (see DOSAGE AND ADMINISTRATION).

The protective efficacy of three 5 mcg doses of RECOMBIVAX HB has been demonstrated in neonates born of mothers positive for both HBsAg and HBeAg (a core-associated antigenic complex which correlates with high infectivity). In a clinical study of infants who received one dose of HBIG at birth followed by the recommended three dose regimen of RECOMBIVAX HB, chronic infection had not occurred in 96% of 130 infants after nine months of follow-up. The estimated efficacy in prevention of chronic hepatitis B infection was 95% as compared to the infection rate in untreated historical controls. Significantly fewer neonates became chronically infected when given one dose of HBIG at birth followed by the recommended three dose regimen of RECOMBIVAX HB when compared to historical controls who received only a single dose of HBIG. Testing for HBsAg and anti-HBs is recommended at 12–15 months of age. If HBsAg is not detectable, and anti-HBs is present, the child has been protected.

As demonstrated in the above study, HBIG, when administered simultaneously with RECOMBIVAX HB at separate body sites, did not interfere with the induction of protective antibodies against hepatitis B virus elicited by the vaccine.

For adolescents (11 to 15 years of age), the immunogenicity of a two-dose regimen (10 mcg at 0 and 4–6 months) was compared with that of the standard three-dose regimen (5 mcg at 0, 1 and 6 months) in an open, randomized, multicenter study. The proportion of adolescents receiving the two-dose regimen who developed a protective level of antibody one month after the last dose (99% of 255 subjects) appears similar to that among adolescents who received the three-dose regimen (98% of 121 subjects). After adolescents (11 to 15 years of age) received the first 10-mcg dose of the two-dose regimen, the proportion who developed a protective level of antibody was approximately 72%.

As with other hepatitis B vaccines, the duration of the protective effect of RECOMBIVAX HB in healthy vaccinees is unknown at present, and the need for booster doses is not yet defined. However, long-term follow-up (5 to 9 years) of approximately 3000 high-risk vaccinees (infants of carrier mothers, male homosexuals, Alaskan Natives) who developed an anti-HBs titer of ≥10 mIU/mL when given a similar plasma-derived vaccine at intervals of 0, 1, and 6 months showed that no subjects developed clinically apparent hepatitis B infection and that 5 subjects developed antigenemia, even though up to half of the subjects failed to maintain a titer at this level. Persistence of vaccine-induced immunologic memory among healthy vaccinees who responded to a primary course of plasma-derived or recombinant hepatitis B vaccine has been demonstrated by an anamnestic antibody response to a booster dose of RECOMBIVAX HB given 5–12 years later.

Predialysis and Dialysis Patients

Predialysis and dialysis adult patients respond less well to hepatitis B vaccines than do healthy individuals; however, vaccination of adult patients early in the course of their renal disease produces higher seroconversion rates than vaccination after dialysis has been initiated. In addition, the responses to these vaccines may be lower if the vaccine is administered as a buttock injection. When 40 mcg of Hepatitis B Vaccine (Recombinant) was administered in the deltoid muscle, 89% of 28 participants developed anti-HBs with 86% achieving levels ≥ 10 mIU/mL. However, when the same dosage of this vaccine was administered inappropriately either in the buttock or a combination of buttock and deltoid, 62% of 47 participants developed anti-HBs with 55% achieving levels of ≥ 10 mIU/mL.

A booster dose or revaccination with RECOMBIVAX HB Dialysis Formulation may be considered in predialysis/dialysis patients if the anti-HBs level is less than 10 mIU/mL.

Reports in the literature describe a more virulent form of hepatitis B associated with superinfections or coinfections by delta virus, an imcomplete RNA virus. Delta virus can only infect and cause illness in persons infected with hepatitis B virus since the delta agent requires a coat of HBsAg in order to become infectious. Therefore, persons immune to hepatitis B virus infection should also be immune to delta virus infection.

Interchangeability of Plasma-Derived and Recombinant Hepatitis B Vaccines
Although there have been no clinical studies in which a three-dose vaccine series was initiated with HEPTAVAX-B* (Hepatitis B Vaccine) and completed with RECOMBIVAX HB, or vice versa, extensive *in vitro* and *in vivo* studies have demonstrated that two vaccines are immunologically comparable.

*Registered trademark of MERCK & CO., INC.

INDICATIONS AND USAGE

RECOMBIVAX HB is indicated for vaccination against infection caused by all known subtypes of hepatitis B virus. **RECOMBIVAX HB Dialysis Formulation** is indicated for vaccination of adult predialysis and dialysis patients against infection caused by all known subtypes of hepatitis B virus.
Vaccination with RECOMBIVAX HB is recommended for:
1) Infants including those born to HBsAg positive mothers (high-risk infants).
2) Children born after November 21, 1991.
3) Adolescents (see CLINICAL PHARMACOLOGY).
4) Other persons of all ages in areas of high prevalence or those who are or may be at increased risk of infection with hepatitis B virus, such as:

- *Health Care Personnel*
  Dentists and oral surgeons.
  Physicians and surgeons.
  Nurses.
  Paramedical personnel and custodial staff who may be exposed to the virus via blood or other patient specimens.
  Dental hygienists and dental nurses.
  Laboratory personnel handling blood, blood products, and other patient specimens.
  Dental, medical and nursing students.
- *Selected Patients and Patient Contacts*
  Staff in hemodialysis units and hematology/oncology units.
  Hemodialysis patients and patients with early renal failure before they require hemodialysis.
  Patients requiring frequent and/or large volume blood transfusions or clotting factor concentrates (e.g., persons with hemophilia, thalassemia).
  Clients (residents) and staff of institutions for the mentally handicapped.
  Classroom contacts of deinstitutionalized mentally handicapped persons who have persistent hepatitis B surface antigenemia and who show aggressive behavior.
  Household and other intimate contacts of persons with persistent hepatitis B surface antigenemia.
- *Sub-populations with a known high incidence of the disease,* such as:
  Alaskan Natives.
  Pacific Islanders.
  Refugees from areas where hepatitis B virus infection is endemic.
  Adoptees from countries where hepatitis B virus infection is endemic.
- *International Travelers*
- *Military Personnel identified as being at increased risk*
- *Morticians and Embalmers*
- *Blood bank and plasma fractionation workers*
- *Persons at Increased Risk of the Disease Due to Their Sexual Practices,* such as:
  Persons who have heterosexual activity with multiple partners.
  Persons who repeatedly contract sexually transmitted diseases.
  Homosexual and bisexual adolescent and adult men.
  Female prostitutes.
- *Prisoners*
- *Injection drug users*

Neither dosage strength will prevent hepatitis caused by other agents, such as hepatitis A virus, hepatitis C virus, hepatitis E virus, or other viruses known to infect the liver.
Revaccination
See CLINICAL PHARMACOLOGY
Use with Other Vaccines
Results from clinical studies indicate that RECOMBIVAX HB can be administered concomitantly with DTP (Diphtheria, Tetanus and whole cell Pertussis), OPV (oral Poliomyelitis vaccine), M-M-R* II (Measles, Mumps, and Rubella Virus Vaccine Live), Liquid PedvaxHIB* [Haemophilus b Conjugate Vaccine (Meningococcal Protein Conjugate)] or a booster dose of DTaP [Diphtheria, Tetanus, acellular Pertussis], using separate sites and syringes for injectable vaccines. No impairment of immune response to individual tested vaccine antigens was demonstrated.
The type, frequency and severity of adverse experiences observed in these studies with RECOMBIVAX HB were similar to those seen when the other vaccines were given alone.
In addition, a HBsAg-containing product, COMVAX* [Haemophilus b Conjugate (Meningococcal Protein Conjugate) and Hepatitis B (Recombinant) Vaccine], was given concomitantly with eIPV (enhanced inactivated Poliovirus vaccine) or VARIVAX* [Varicella Virus Vaccine Live (Oka/Merck)], using separate sites and syringes for injectable vaccines. No impairment of immune response to these individually tested vaccine antigens was demonstrated. No serious vaccine-related adverse events were reported.
COMVAX has also been administered concomitantly with the primary series of DTaP to a limited number of infants. No serious vaccine-related adverse events were reported.

*Registered trademark of MERCK & CO., INC.

CONTRAINDICATIONS

Hypersensitivity to yeast or any component of the vaccine.

WARNINGS

Patients who develop symptoms suggestive of hypersensitivity after an injection should not receive further injections of the vaccine (see CONTRAINDICATIONS).
Because of the long incubation period for hepatitis B, it is possible for unrecognized infection to be present at the time the vaccine is given. The vaccine may not prevent hepatitis B in such patients.

PRECAUTIONS

General
As with any percutaneous vaccine, epinephrine (1:1000) should be available for immediate use should an anaphylactoid reaction occur.
Any serious active infection including febrile illness is reason for delaying use of the vaccine except when in the opinion of the physician, withholding the vaccine entails a greater risk.
Caution and appropriate care should be exercised in administering the vaccine to individuals with severely compromised cardiopulmonary status or to others in whom a febrile or systemic reaction could pose a significant risk.
Instructions to Healthcare Provider
The healthcare provider should determine the current health status and previous vaccination history of the vaccinee.
The healthcare provider should question the patient, parent or guardian about reactions to a previous dose of RECOMBIVAX HB or other hepatitis B vaccines.
The healthcare provider must record in the patient's permanent record: the manufacturer, lot number, date of administration, and the name and address of the person administering the vaccine.
Injection of a blood vessel should be avoided.
Information for Vaccine Recipients and Parents/Guardians
The healthcare provider should provide the vaccine information required to be given with each vaccination to the patient, parent or guardian.
The healthcare provider should inform the patient, parent or guardian of the benefits and risks associated with vaccination, as well as the importance of completing the immunization series. For risks associated with vaccination, see WARNINGS, PRECAUTIONS, and ADVERSE REACTIONS.
Patients, parents and guardians should be instructed to report any serious adverse reactions to their healthcare provider, who in turn should report such events to the U.S. Department of Health and Human Services through the Vaccine Adverse Event Reporting System (VAERS), 1-800-822-7967. The healthcare provider should inform the parent or guardian of the National Vaccine Injury Compensation Program (NVICP), 1-888-338-2382 or http://www.hrsa.dhhs.gov/bhpr/vicp.
Drug Interactions
There are no known drug interactions. (See INDICATIONS AND USAGE, *Use with Other Vaccines.*)
Pregnancy
Pregnancy Category C: Animal reproduction studies have not been conducted with the vaccine. It is also not known whether the vaccine can cause fetal harm when administered to a pregnant woman or can affect reproduction capacity. The vaccine should be given to a pregnant woman only if clearly needed.
Nursing Mothers
It is not known whether the vaccine is excreted in human milk. Because many drugs are excreted in human milk, cautions should be exercised when the vaccine is administered to a nursing woman.
Pediatric Use
RECOMBIVAX HB has been shown to be usually well-tolerated and highly immunogenic in infants and children of all ages. Newborns also respond well; maternally transferred antibodies do not interfere with the active immune response to the vaccine. See DOSAGE AND ADMINISTRATION for recommended pediatric dosage and for recommended dosage for infants born to HBsAg positive mothers.
The safety and effectiveness of RECOMBIVAX HB Dialysis Formulation in children have not been established.
Carcinogenesis, Mutagenesis, Impairment of Fertility
RECOMBIVAX HB has not been evaluated for its carcinogenic or mutagenic potential, or its potential to impair fertility.

ADVERSE REACTIONS

RECOMBIVAX HB and RECOMBIVAX HB Dialysis Formulation are generally well-tolerated. No serious adverse reactions attributable to the vaccine have been reported during the course of clinical trials. No adverse experiences were reported during clinical trials which could be related to changes in the titers of antibodies to yeast. As with any vaccine, there is the possibility that broad use of the vaccine could reveal adverse reactions not observed in clinical trials.
In three clinical studies, 434 doses of RECOMBIVAX HB, 5 mcg, were administered to 147 healthy infants and children (up to 10 years of age) who were monitored for 5 days after each dose. Injection site reactions and systemic complaints were reported following 0.2% and 10.4% of the injections, respectively. The most frequently reported systemic adverse reactions (>1% injections), in decreasing order of frequency, were irritability, fever (≥101°F oral equivalent), diarrhea, fatigue/weakness, diminished appetite, and rhinitis.
In a study that compared the three-dose regimen (5 mcg) with the two-dose regimen (10 mcg) of RECOMBIVAX HB in adolescents, the overall frequency of adverse reactions was generally similar.
In a group of studies, 3258 doses of RECOMBIVAX HB, 10 mcg, were administered to 1252 healthy adults who were monitored for 5 days after each dose. Injection site reactions and systemic complaints were reported following 17% and 15% of the injections, respectively. The following adverse reactions were reported:

Incidence Equal to or Greater Than 1% of Injections
LOCAL REACTION (INJECTION SITE)
Injection site reactions consisting principally of soreness, and including pain, tenderness, pruritus, erythema, ecchymosis, swelling, warmth, and nodule formation.
BODY AS A WHOLE
The most frequent systemic complaints include fatigue/weakness; headache; fever (≥100°F); and malaise.
DIGESTIVE SYSTEM
Nausea; and diarrhea
RESPIRATORY SYSTEM
Pharyngitis; and upper respiratory infection

Incidence Less than 1% of Injections
BODY AS A WHOLE
Sweating; achiness; sensation of warmth; lightheadedness; chills; and flushing
DIGESTIVE SYSTEM
Vomiting; abdominal pains/cramps; dyspepsia; and diminished appetite
RESPIRATORY SYSTEM
Rhinitis; influenza; and cough
NERVOUS SYSTEM
Vertigo/dizziness; and paresthesia
INTEGUMENTARY SYSTEM
Pruritus; rash (non-specified); angioedema; and urticaria
MUSCULOSKELETAL SYSTEM
Arthralgia including monoarticular; myalgia; back pain; neck pain; shoulder pain; and neck stiffness
HEMIC/LYMPHATIC SYSTEM
Lymphadenopathy
PSYCHIATRIC/BEHAVIORAL
Insomnia/Disturbed sleep
SPECIAL SENSES
Earache
UROGENITAL SYSTEM
Dysuria
CARDIOVASCULAR SYSTEM
Hypotension
Marketed Experience
The following additional adverse reactions have been reported with use of the marketed vaccine. In many instances, the relationship to the vaccine was unclear.
Hypersensitivity
Anaphylaxis and symptoms of immediate hypersensitivity reactions including rash, pruritus, urticaria, edema, angioedema, dyspnea, chest discomfort, bronchial spasm, palpitation, or symptoms consistent with a hypotensive episode have been reported within the first few hours after vaccination. An apparent hypersensitivity syndrome (serum-sickness-like) of delayed onset has been reported days to weeks after vaccination, including: arthralgia/arthritis (usually transient), fever, and dermatologic reactions such as urticaria, erythema multiforme, ecchymoses and erythema nodosum (See WARNINGS and PRECAUTIONS).
Digestive System
Elevation of liver enzymes; constipation
Nervous System
Guillain-Barré Syndrome; multiple sclerosis; myelitis including transverse myelitis; peripheral neuropathy including Bell's Palsy; radiculopathy; herpes zoster; migraine; muscle weakness; hypesthesia; encephalitis
Integumentary System
Stevens-Johnson Syndrome; petechiae
Musculoskeletal System
Arthritis
Hematologic
Increased erythrocyte sedimentation rate; thrombocytopenia
Immune System
Systemic lupus erythematosus (SLE); lupus-like syndrome; vasculitis
Psychiatric/Behavioral
Irritability; agitation; somnolence
Special Senses
Optic neuritis; tinnitus; conjunctivitis; visual disturbances
Cardiovascular System
Syncope; tachycardia.

Continued on next page

Information on the Merck & Co., Inc. products listed on these pages is the full prescribing information from product circulars in use September 30, 2000. For information, please call 1-800-NSC MERCK [1-800-672-6372].

Recombivax HB—Cont.

The following adverse reaction has been reported with another Heaptitis B Vaccine (Recombinant) but not with RECOMBIVAX HB: keratitis.

Patients, parents and guardians should be instructed to report any serious adverse reactions to their healthcare provider, who in turn should report such events to the U.S. Department of Health and Human Services through the Vaccine Adverse Event Reporting System (VAERS), 1-800-822-7967.

DOSAGE AND ADMINISTRATION

Do not inject intravenously or intradermally.

RECOMBIVAX HB Hepatitis B Vaccine (Recombinant) DIALYSIS FORMULATION (40 mcg/mL) IS INTENDED ONLY FOR ADULT PREDIALYSIS/DIALYSIS PATIENTS.

RECOMBIVAX HB Hepatitis B Vaccine (Recombinant) PEDIATRIC/ADOLESCENT (WITH AND WITHOUT PRESERVATIVE) and ADULT FORMULATIONS ARE NOT INTENDED FOR USE IN PREDIALYSIS/DIALYSIS PATIENTS.

RECOMBIVAX HB Hepatitis B Vaccine (Recombinant) PEDIATRIC/ADOLESCENT FORMULATION (WITHOUT PRESERVATIVE) IS AVAILABLE FOR USE IN INDIVIDUALS FOR WHOM A THIMEROSAL-FREE VACCINE IS ADVISABLE (e.g., INFANTS 0 TO 6 MONTHS OF AGE WHO MAY RECEIVE OTHER VACCINES CONTAINING THIMEROSAL).

Three-Dose Regimen

The vaccination regimen for each population consists of 3 doses of vaccine given according to the following schedule:

First dose: at elected date

Second dose: 1 month later

Third dose: 6 months after the first dose

For infants born of mothers who are HBsAg positive or mothers of unknown HBsAg status, treatment recommendations are described in the subsection titled: *Guidelines For Treatment of Infants Born of HBsAg Positive Mothers or Mothers of Unknown HBsAg Status.*

Two-Dose Regimen—Adolescents (11–15 years of age)

An alternate two-dose regimen is available for routine vaccination of adolescents (11 to 15 years of age). The regimen consists of two doses of vaccine (10 mcg) given according to the following schedule:

First injection: at elected date

Second dose: 4–6 months later

Table 1 summarizes the dose and formulation of RECOMBIVAX HB for specific populations, regardless of the risk of infection with hepatitis B virus.

[See table 1 below]

RECOMBIVAX HB is for intramuscular injection. The *deltoid muscle* is the preferred site for intramuscular injection in adults. Data suggests that injections given in the buttocks frequently are given into fatty tissue instead of into muscle. Such injections have resulted in a lower seroconversion rate than was expected. The *anterolateral thigh* is the recommended site for intramuscular injection in infants and young children.

For persons at risk of hemorrhage following intramuscular injection, RECOMBIVAX HB may be administered subcutaneously. However, when other aluminum-adsorbed vaccines have been administered subcutaneously, an increased incidence of local reactions including subcutaneous nodules has been observed. Therefore, subcutaneous administration should be used only in persons (e.g., hemophiliacs) who are at risk of hemorrhage following intramuscular injections.

The vaccine should be used as supplied; no dilution or reconstitution is necessary. The full recommended dose of the vaccine should be used.

For the Pediatric/Adolescent Formulation (Without Preservative): Once the single-dose vial has been penetrated, the withdrawn vaccine should be used promptly, and the vial must be discarded.

For Vial and Pre-filled Single Dose Syringe: Shake well before use. Thorough agitation at the time of administration is necessary to maintain suspension of the vaccine.

Parenteral drug products should be inspected visually for particulate matter and discoloration prior to administration. After thorough agitation, the vaccine is a slightly opaque, white suspension.

For Vial: Withdraw the recommended dose from the vial using a sterile needle and syringe free of preservatives, antiseptics, and detergents.

It is important to use a separate sterile syringe and needle for each individual patient to prevent transmission of hepatitis and other infectious agents from one person to another. Needles should be disposed of properly and should not be recapped.

Injection must be accomplished with a needle long enough to ensure intramuscular deposition of the vaccine.

Guidelines For Treatment of Infants Born of HBsAg Positive Mothers or Mothers of Unknown HBsAg Status

Each infant should receive three 5 mcg doses of RECOMBIVAX HB irrespective of the mother's HBsAg status (see Table 1). The ACIP recommends that if the mother is determined to be HBsAg positive within 7 days of delivery, the infant also should be given a dose of HBIG (0.5 mL) immediately. The first dose of RECOMBIVAX HB may be given at the same time as HBIG, but it should be administered in the opposite anterolateral thigh.

Revaccination

The duration of the protective effect of RECOMBIVAX HB in healthy vaccinees is unknown at present and the need for booster doses is not yet defined (see CLINICAL PHARMACOLOGY).

A booster dose or revaccination with RECOMBIVAX HB Dialysis Formulation (blue color code) may be considered in predialysis/dialysis patients if the anti-HBs level is less than 10 MIU/mL 1 to 2 months after the third dose. The ACIP recommends that the need for booster doses of vaccine should be assessed by annual antibody testing and a booster dose given when antibody levels decline to $<$10 mIU/mL.

Known or Presumed Exposure to HBsAg

There are no prospective studies directly testing the efficacy of a combination of HBIG and RECOMBIVAX HB in preventing clinical hepatitis B following percutaneous, ocular or mucous membrane exposure to hepatitis B virus. However, since most persons with such exposures (e.g., healthcare workers) are candidates for RECOMBIVAX HB and since combined HBIG plus vaccine is more efficacious than HBIG alone in perinatal exposures, the following guidelines are recommended for persons who have been exposed to hepatitis B virus such as through (1) percutaneous (needlestick), ocular, mucous membrane exposure to blood known or presumed to contain HBsAg, (2) human bites by known or presumed HBsAg carriers, that penetrate the skin, or (3) following intimate sexual contact with known or presumed HBsAg carriers:

HBIG (0.06 mL/kg) should be given intramuscularly as soon as possible after exposure and within 24 hours if possible. RECOMBIVAX HB (see dosage recommendation) should be given intramuscularly at a separate site within 7 days of exposure and second and third doses given one and six months, respectively, after the first dose.

HOW SUPPLIED

PEDIATRIC/ADOLESCENT FORMULATION (PRESERVATIVE-FREE)

No. 4980—RECOMBIVAX HB for use in infants, children, and adolescents is supplied as 5 mcg/0.5 mL of HBsAg in a 0.5 mL single-dose vial, color coded with a yellow cap and stripe on the vial labels and cartons, **NDC** 0006-4980-00.

No. 4981—RECOMBIVAX HB for use in infants, children, and adolescents is supplied as 5 mcg/0.5 mL of HBsAg in a 0.5 mL single-dose vial, in a box of 10 single-dose vials, color coded with a yellow cap and stripe on the vial labels and cartons, **NDC** 0006-4981-00.

PEDIATRIC/ADOLESCENT FORMULATION

No. 4769—RECOMBIVAX HB for use in infants, children, and adolescents is supplied as 5 mcg/0.5 mL of HBsAg in a 0.5 mL single-dose vial, color coded with a yellow cap and stripe on the vial labels and cartons, **NDC** 0006-4769-00.

No. 4876—RECOMBIVAX HB for use in infants, children, and adolescents is supplied as 5 mcg/0.5 mL of HBsAg in a 0.5 mL single-dose vial, in a box of 10 single-dose vials, color coded with a yellow cap and stripe on the vial labels and cartons, **NDC** 0006-4876-00.

No. 4849—RECOMBIVAX HB for use in infants, children, and adolescents is supplied as 5 mcg/0.5 mL of HBsAg in a 0.5 mL pre-filled single-dose glass syringe with a 1 inch, 23 gauge needle, in a box of 5 pre-filled single-dose syringes with 1 inch, 23 gauge needles, color coded with a yellow plunger rod and stripe on the syringe labels and cartons, **NDC** 0006-4849-00.

No. 4969—RECOMBIVAX HB for use in infants, children, and adolescents is supplied as 5 mcg/0.5 mL of HBsAg in a 0.5 mL pre-filled single-dose glass syringe with a 5/8 inch, 25 gauge needle, in a box of 5 pre-filled single-dose syringes with 5/8 inch, 25 gauge needles, color coded with a yellow plunger rod and stripe on the syringe labels and cartons, **NDC** 0006-4969-00.

ADULT FORMULATION

No. 4775—RECOMBIVAX HB for use in adults and adolescents (11 to 15 years of age) is supplied as 10 mcg/mL of HBsAg in a 1 mL single-dose vial, color coded with a green cap and stripe on the vial labels and cartons, **NDC** 0006-4775-00.

No. 4773—RECOMBIVAX HB for use in adults and adolescents (11 to 15 years of age) is supplied as 10 mcg/mL of HBsAg in a 3 mL multiple-dose vial, color coded with a green cap and stripe on the vial labels and cartons, **NDC** 0006-4773-00.

No. 4872—RECOMBIVAX HB for use in adults and adolescents (11 to 15 years of age) is supplied as 10 mcg/mL of HBsAg in a 1 mL single-dose vial, in a box of 10 single-dose vials, color coded with a green cap and stripe on the vial labels and cartons, **NDC** 0006-4872-00.

No.4873—RECOMBIVAX HB for use in adults and adolescents (11 to 15 years of age) is supplied as 10 mcg/mL of HBsAg in a 3 mL multiple-dose vial, in a box of 10 multi-dose vials, color coded with a green cap and stripe on the vial labels and cartons, **NDC** 0006-4873-00.

No. 4848—RECOMBIVAX HB for use in adults and adolescents (11 to 15 years of age) is supplied as 10 mcg/mL of HBsAg in a 1 mL pre-filled single-dose glass syringe, with a 1 inch, 23 gauge needle, in a box of 5 pre-filled single-dose syringes with 1 inch, 23 gauge needles, color coded with a green plunger rod and stripe on the syringe labels and cartons, **NDC** 0006-4848-00.

DIALYSIS FORMULATION

No. 4776—RECOMBIVAX HB Dialysis Formulation is supplied as 40 mcg/mL of HBsAg in a 1 mL single-dose vial, color coded with a blue cap and stripe on the vial labels and cartons, **NDC** 0006-4776-00.

Storage

Store vials and syringes at 2–8°C (36°–46°F). Storage above or below the recommended temperature may reduce potency.

Do not freeze since freezing destroys potency.

7994319 Issued February 2000

Table 1

Group	Dose/Regimen**	Formulation	Color Code
Infants, Children, and Adolescents 0–19 years of age	5 mcg (0.5 mL) 3 × 5 mcg	Pediatric/Adolescent	Yellow
Adolescents◆ 11–15 years of age	10 mcg (1.0 mL) 2 × 10 mcg	Adult	Green
Adults ≥20 years of age	10 mcg (1.0 mL) 3 × 10 mcg	Adult	Green
Predialysis and Dialysis Patients†	40 mcg (1.0 mL) 3 × 40 mcg	Dialysis	Blue

** If the suggested formulation is not available, the appropriate dosage can be achieved from another formulation provided that the total volume of vaccine administered does not exceed 1 mL (see text above regarding use of the Pediatric/Adolescent Formulation Without Preservative). However, the Dialysis Formulation may be used only for adult predialysis/dialysis patients.

◆ Adolescents (11 to 15 years of age) may receive either regimen: the 3 × 5 mcg (Pediatric/Adolescent Formulation) or the 2 × 10 mcg (Adult Formulation).

† See also recommendations for revaccination of predialysis and dialysis patients in DOSAGE AND ADMINISTRATION, *Revaccination.*

SINGULAIR® Tablets and Chewable Tablets ℞
(montelukast sodium)

DESCRIPTION

Montelukast sodium, the active ingredient in SINGULAIR*, is a selective and orally active leukotriene receptor antagonist that inhibits the cysteinyl leukotriene CysLT$_1$ receptor.

Montelukast sodium is described chemically as [R-(E)]-1-[[[1-[3-[2-(7-chloro-2-quinolinyl)ethenyl]phenyl]-3-[2-(1-hydroxy-1-methylethyl)phenyl]propyl]thio]methyl]cyclopropaneacetic acid, monosodium salt.

The empirical formula is $C_{35}H_{35}ClNNaO_3S$, and its molecular weight is 608.18. The structural formula is:

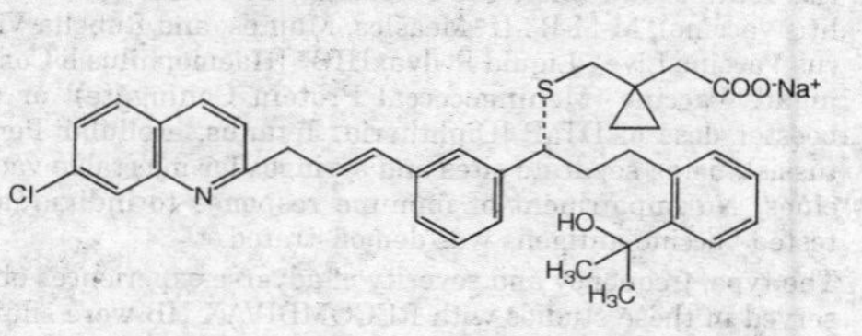

Montelukast sodium is a hygroscopic, optically active, white to off-white powder. Montelukast sodium is freely soluble in ethanol, methanol, and water and practically insoluble in acetonitrile.

Each 10-mg film-coated SINGULAIR tablet contains 10.4 mg montelukast sodium, which is the molar equivalent to 10.0 mg of free acid, and the following inactive ingredients: microcrystalline cellulose, lactose monohydrate, croscarmellose sodium, hydroxypropyl cellulose, and magnesium stea-

rate. The film coating consists of: hydroxypropyl methylcellulose, hydroxypropyl cellulose, titanium dioxide, red ferric oxide, yellow ferric oxide, and carnauba wax.
Each 4-mg and 5-mg chewable SINGULAIR tablet for oral administration contains 4.2 and 5.2 mg montelukast sodium, respectively, which are the molar equivalents to 4.0 and 5.0 mg of free acid, respectively. Both chewable tablets contain the following inactive ingredients: mannitol, microcrystalline cellulose, hydroxypropyl cellulose, red ferric oxide, croscarmellose sodium, cherry flavor, aspartame, and magnesium stearate.

* Registered trademark of MERCK & CO., Inc.

CLINICAL PHARMACOLOGY

Mechanism of Action
The cysteinyl leukotrienes (LTC_4, LTD_4, LTE_4) are products of arachidonic acid metabolism and are released from various cells, including mast cells and eosinophils. These eicosanoids bind to cysteinyl leukotriene receptors (CysLT) found in the human airway. Cysteinyl leukotrienes and leukotriene receptor occupation have been correlated with the pathophysiology of asthma, including airway edema, smooth muscle contraction, and altered cellular activity associated with the inflammatory process, which contribute to the signs and symptoms of asthma.
Montelukast is an orally active compound that binds with high affinity and selectivity to the $CysLT_1$ receptor (in preference to other pharmacologically important airway receptors, such as the prostanoid, cholinergic, or β-adrenergic receptor). Montelukast inhibits physiologic actions of LTD_4 at the $CysLT_1$ receptor without any agonist activity.
Pharmacokinetics
Absorption
Montelukast is rapidly absorbed following oral administration. After administration of the 10-mg film-coated tablet to fasted adults, the mean peak montelukast plasma concentration (C_{max}) is achieved in 3 to 4 hours (T_{max}). The mean oral bioavailability is 64%. The oral bioavailability and C_{max} are not influenced by a standard meal in the morning.
For the 5-mg chewable tablet, the mean C_{max} is achieved in 2 to 2.5 hours after administration to adults in the fasted state. The mean oral bioavailability is 73% in the fasted state versus 63% when administered with a standard meal in the morning.
For the 4-mg chewable tablet, the mean C_{max} is achieved 2 hours after administration in pediatric patients 2 to 5 years of age in the fasted state.
The safety and efficacy of SINGULAIR were demonstrated in clinical trials in which the 10-mg and 5-mg formulations were administered in the evening without regard to the timing of food ingestion.
The comparative pharmacokinetics of montelukast when administered as two 5-mg chewable tablets versus one 10-mg film-coated tablet have not been evaluated.
Distribution
Montelukast is more than 99% bound to plasma proteins. The steady-state volume of distribution of montelukast averages 8 to 11 liters. Studies in rats with radiolabeled montelukast indicate minimal distribution across the blood-brain barrier. In addition, concentrations of radiolabeled material at 24 hours postdose were minimal in all other tissues.
Metabolism
Montelukast is extensively metabolized. In studies with therapeutic doses, plasma concentrations of metabolites of montelukast are undetectable at steady state in adults and pediatric patients.
In vitro studies using human liver microsomes indicate that cytochromes P450 3A4 and 2C9 are involved in the metabolism of montelukast. Clinical studies investigating the effect of known inhibitors of cytochromes P450 3A4 (e.g., ketoconazole, erythromycin) or 2C9 (e.g., fluconazole) on montelukast pharmacokinetics have not been conducted. Based on further *in vitro* results in human liver microsomes, therapeutic plasma concentrations of montelukast do not inhibit cytochromes P450 3A4, 2C9, 1A2, 2A6, 2C19, or 2D6 (see *Drug Interactions*).
Elimination
The plasma clearance of montelukast averages 45 mL/min in healthy adults. Following an oral dose of radiolabeled montelukast, 86% of the radioactivity was recovered in 5-day fecal collections and <0.2% was recovered in urine. Coupled with estimates of montelukast oral bioavailability, this indicates that montelukast and its metabolites are excreted almost exclusively via the bile.
In several studies, the mean plasma half-life of montelukast ranged from 2.7 to 5.5 hours in healthy young adults. The pharmacokinetics of montelukast are nearly linear for oral doses up to 50 mg. During once-daily dosing with 10-mg montelukast, there is little accumulation of the parent drug in plasma (~14%).
Special Populations
Gender: The pharmacokinetics of montelukast are similar in males and females.
Elderly: The pharmacokinetic profile and the oral bioavailability of a single 10-mg oral dose of montelukast are similar in elderly and younger adults. The plasma half-life of montelukast is slightly longer in the elderly. No dosage adjustment in the elderly is required.
Race: Pharmacokinetic differences due to race have not been studied.

TABLE 1
Effect of SINGULAIR on Primary and Secondary Endpoints in Placebo-controlled Trials
(Combined Analyses - U.S. and Multinational Trials)

	SINGULAIR		Placebo	
Endpoint	Baseline	Mean Change from Baseline	Baseline	Mean Change from Baseline
Daytime Asthma Symptoms (0 to 6 scale)	2.43	-0.45*	2.45	-0.22
β-agonist (puffs per day)	5.38	-1.56*	5.55	-0.41
AM PEFR (L/min)	361.3	24.5*	364.9	3.3
PM PEFR (L/min)	385.2	17.9*	389.3	2.0
Nocturnal Awakenings (#/week)	5.37	-1.84*	5.44	-0.79

* p<0.001, compared with placebo

Hepatic Insufficiency: Patients with mild-to-moderate hepatic insufficiency and clinical evidence of cirrhosis had evidence of decreased metabolism of montelukast resulting in 41% (90% CI=7%, 85%) higher mean montelukast area under the plasma concentration curve (AUC) following a single 10-mg dose. The elimination of montelukast was slightly prolonged compared with that in healthy subjects (mean half-life, 7.4 hours). No dosage adjustment is required in patients with mild-to-moderate hepatic insufficiency. The pharmacokinetics of SINGULAIR in patients with more severe hepatic impairment or with hepatitis have not been evaluated.
Renal Insufficiency: Since montelukast and its metabolites are not excreted in the urine, the pharmacokinetics of montelukast were not evaluated in patients with renal insufficiency. No dosage adjustment is recommended in these patients.
Adolescents and Pediatric Patients: The plasma concentration profile of montelukast following administration of the 10-mg film-coated tablet is similar in adolescents ≥15 years of age and young adults. The 10-mg film-coated tablet is recommended for use in patients ≥15 years of age.
Pharmacokinetic studies show that the mean systemic exposure (in terms of AUC) of the 5-mg chewable tablet in pediatric patients 6 to 14 years of age is similar to that of the 10-mg film-coated tablet in adults. In a pharmacokinetic study in pediatric patients 2 to 5 years of age, the mean systemic exposure (AUC) of the 4-mg chewable tablet is also similar to that of the 10-mg film-coated tablet in adults. The 5-mg chewable tablet should be used in pediatric patients 6 to 14 years of age and the 4-mg chewable tablet should be used in pediatric patients 2 to 5 years of age.
Drug Interactions
Montelukast at a dose of 10 mg once daily dosed to pharmacokinetic steady state:
- did not cause clinically significant changes in the kinetics of a single intravenous dose of theophylline (predominantly a cytochrome P450 1A2 substrate).
- did not change the pharmacokinetic profile of warfarin (a substrate of cytochromes P450 2A6 and 2C9) or influence the effect of a single 30-mg oral dose of warfarin on prothrombin time or the INR (International Normalized Ratio).
- did not change the pharmacokinetic profile or urinary excretion of immunoreactive digoxin.
- did not change the plasma concentration profile of terfenadine (a substrate of cytochrome P450 3A4) or fexofenadine, its carboxylated metabolite, and did not prolong the QTc interval following coadministration with terfenadine 60 mg twice daily.

Montelukast at doses of ≥100 mg daily dosed to pharmacokinetic steady state:
- did not significantly alter the plasma concentrations of either component of an oral contraceptive containing norethindrone 1 mg/ethinyl estradiol 35 mcg.
- did not cause any clinically significant change in plasma profiles of prednisone or prednisolone following administration of either oral prednisone or intravenous prednisolone.

Phenobarbital, which induces hepatic metabolism, decreased the AUC of montelukast approximately 40% following a single 10-mg dose of montelukast. No dosage adjustment for SINGULAIR is recommended. It is reasonable to employ appropriate clinical monitoring when potent cytochrome P450 enzyme inducers, such as phenobarbital or rifampin, are co-administered with SINGULAIR.
Pharmacodynamics
Montelukast causes inhibition of airway cysteinyl leukotriene receptors as demonstrated by the ability to inhibit bronchoconstriction due to inhaled LTD_4 in asthmatics. Doses as low as 5 mg cause substantial blockage of LTD_4-induced bronchoconstriction. In a placebo-controlled, crossover study (n=12), SINGULAIR inhibited early- and late-phase bronchoconstriction due to antigen challenge by 75% and 57%, respectively.
The effect of SINGULAIR on eosinophils in the peripheral blood was examined in clinical trials in adults and pediatric asthmatic patients. SINGULAIR decreased mean peripheral blood eosinophils approximately 13 to 15% from baseline compared with placebo over the double-blind treatment periods. The relationship between this observation and the clinical benefits noted in the clinical trials is not known (see CLINICAL PHARMACOLOGY, *Clinical Studies*).
Clinical Studies
GENERAL
There have been no clinical trials evaluating the relative efficacy of morning versus evening dosing. Although the pharmacokinetics of montelukast are similar whether dosed in the morning or the evening, efficacy was demonstrated in clinical trials in adults and pediatric patients in which montelukast was administered in the evening without regard to the time of food ingestion.
ADOLESCENTS AND ADULTS 15 YEARS OF AGE AND OLDER
Clinical trials in adolescents and adults 15 years of age and older demonstrated there is no additional clinical benefit to montelukast doses above 10 mg once daily. This was shown in two chronic asthma trials using doses up to 200 mg once daily and in one exercise challenge study using doses up to 50 mg, evaluated at the end of the once-daily dosing interval.
The efficacy of SINGULAIR for the chronic treatment of asthma in adolescents and adults 15 years of age and older was demonstrated in two (U.S. and Multinational) similarly designed, randomized, 12-week, double-blind, placebo-controlled trials in 1576 patients (795 treated with SINGULAIR, 530 treated with placebo, and 251 treated with active control). The patients studied were mild and moderate, non-smoking asthmatics who required approximately 5 puffs of inhaled β-agonist per day on an "as-needed" basis. The patients had a mean baseline percent of predicted forced expiratory volume in 1 second (FEV_1) of 66% (approximate range, 40 to 90%). The co-primary endpoints in these trials were FEV_1 and daytime asthma symptoms. Secondary endpoints included morning and evening peak expiratory flow rates (AM PEFR, PM PEFR), rescue β-agonist requirements, nocturnal awakening due to asthma, and other asthma-related outcomes. In both studies after 12 weeks, a random subset of patients receiving SINGULAIR was switched to placebo for an additional 3 weeks of double-blind treatment to evaluate for possible rebound effects. The results of the U.S. trial on the primary endpoint, FEV_1, expressed as mean percent change from baseline, are shown in FIGURE 1.

FIGURE 1
FEV_1 Mean Percent Change from Baseline
(U.S. Trial)

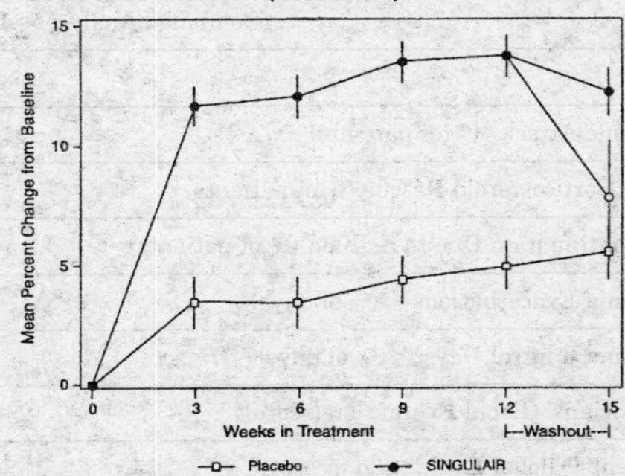

The effect of SINGULAIR on other primary and secondary endpoints is shown in TABLE 1 as combined analyses of the U.S. and Multinational trials.
[See table 1 above]

Continued on next page

Information on the Merck & Co., Inc. products listed on these pages is the full prescribing information from product circulars in use September 30, 2000. For information, please call 1-800-NSC MERCK [1-800-672-6372].

Singulair—Cont.

In adult patients, SINGULAIR reduced "as-needed" β-agonist use by 26.1% from baseline compared with 4.6% for placebo. In patients with nocturnal awakenings of at least 2 nights per week, SINGULAIR reduced the nocturnal awakenings by 34% from baseline, compared with 15% for placebo (combined analysis).

SINGULAIR, compared with placebo, significantly improved other protocol-defined, asthma-related outcome measurements (see TABLE 2).

[See table 2 below]

In one of these trials, a non-U.S. formulation of inhaled beclomethasone dipropionate dosed at 200 mcg (two puffs of 100 mcg ex-valve) twice daily with a spacer device was included as an active control. Over the 12-week treatment period, the mean percentage change in FEV_1 over baseline for SINGULAIR and beclomethasone were 7.49% vs 13.3% ($p<0.001$) respectively, see FIGURE 2; and the change in daytime symptom scores was -0.49 vs -0.70 on a 0 to 6 scale ($p<0.001$) for SINGULAIR and beclomethasone, respectively. The percentages of individual patients treated with SINGULAIR or beclomethasone achieving any given percentage change in FEV_1 from baseline are shown in FIGURE 3.

FIGURE 2
FEV_1
Mean Percent Change From Baseline
(Multinational Trial)

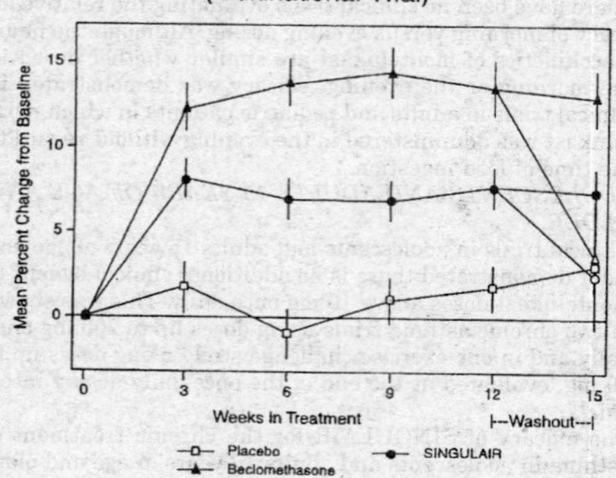

[See figure 3 at top of next column]

Onset of Action and Maintenance of Benefits

In each placebo-controlled trial in adults, the treatment effect of SINGULAIR, measured by daily diary card parameters, including symptom scores, "as-needed" β-agonist use, and PEFR measurements, was achieved after the first dose and was maintained throughout the dosing interval (24 hours). No significant change in treatment effect was observed during continuous once-daily evening administration in non-placebo-controlled extension trials for up to one year. Withdrawal of SINGULAIR in asthmatic patients after 12 weeks of continuous use did not cause rebound worsening of asthma.

PEDIATRIC PATIENTS 6 TO 14 YEARS OF AGE

The efficacy of SINGULAIR in pediatric patients 6 to 14 years of age was demonstrated in one 8-week double-blind, placebo-controlled trial in 336 patients (201 treated with SINGULAIR and 135 treated with placebo) using an inhaled β-agonist on an "as-needed" basis. The patients had a mean baseline percent predicted FEV_1 of 72% (approximate range, 45 to 90%) and a mean daily inhaled β-agonist requirement of 3.4 puffs of albuterol. Approximately 36% of the patients were on inhaled corticosteroids.

FIGURE 3
FEV_1
Distribution of Individual Patient Response
(Multinational Trial)

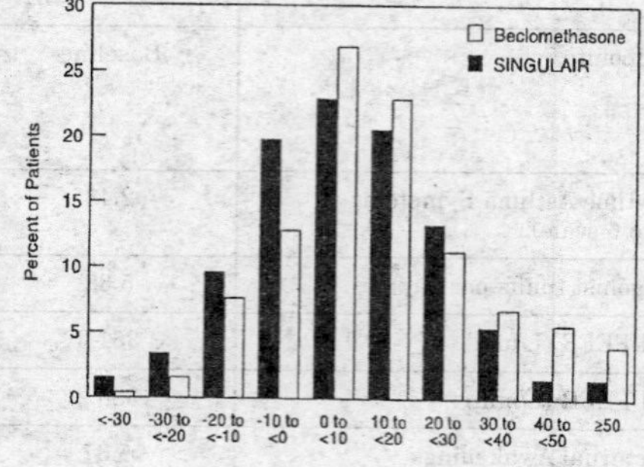

Compared with placebo, treatment with one 5-mg SINGULAIR chewable tablet daily, resulted in a significant improvement in mean morning FEV_1 percent change from baseline (8.7% in the group treated with SINGULAIR vs 4.2% change from baseline in the placebo group, $p<0.001$). There was a significant decrease in the mean percentage change in daily "as-needed" inhaled β-agonist use (11.7% decrease from baseline in the group treated with SINGULAIR vs 8.2% increase from baseline in the placebo group, $p<0.05$). This effect represents a mean decrease from baseline of 0.56 and 0.23 puffs per day for the montelukast and placebo groups, respectively. Subgroup analyses indicated that younger pediatric patients aged 6 to 11 had efficacy results comparable to those of the older pediatric patients aged 12 to 14.

SINGULAIR, one 5-mg chewable tablet daily at bedtime, significantly decreased the percent of days asthma exacerbations occurred (SINGULAIR 20.6% vs placebo 25.7%, $p\leq0.05$). (See TABLE 2 for definition of asthma exacerbation.) Parents' global asthma evaluations (parental evaluations of the patients' asthma, see TABLE 2 for definition of score) were significantly better with SINGULAIR compared with placebo (SINGULAIR 1.34 vs placebo 1.69, $p\leq0.05$).

Similar to the adult studies, no significant change in the treatment effect was observed during continuous once-daily administration in one open-label extension trial without a concurrent placebo group for up to 6 months.

EFFECTS IN PATIENTS ON CONCOMITANT INHALED CORTICOSTEROIDS

Separate trials in adults evaluated the ability of SINGULAIR to add to the clinical effect of inhaled corticosteroids and to allow inhaled corticosteroid tapering when used concomitantly.

One randomized, placebo-controlled, parallel-group trial (n=226) enrolled stable asthmatic adults with a mean FEV_1 of approximately 84% of predicted who were previously maintained on various inhaled corticosteroids (delivered by metered-dose aerosol or dry powder inhalers). The types of inhaled corticosteroids and their mean baseline requirements included beclomethasone dipropionate (mean dose, 1203 mcg/day), triamcinolone acetonide (mean dose, 2004 mcg/day), flunisolide (mean dose, 1971 mcg/day), fluticasone propionate (mean dose, 1083 mcg/day), or budesonide (mean dose, 1192 mcg/day). Some of these inhaled corticosteroids were non-U.S.-approved formulations, and doses expressed may not be ex-actuator. The pre-study inhaled corticosteroid requirements were reduced by approximately 37% during a 5- to 7-week placebo run-in period designed to titrate patients toward their lowest effective inhaled corticosteroid dose. Treatment with SINGULAIR resulted in a further 47% reduction in mean inhaled corticosteroid dose compared with a mean reduction of 30% in the placebo group over the 12-week active treatment period ($p\leq0.05$). Approximately 40% of the montelukast-treated patients and 29% of the placebo-treated patients could be tapered off inhaled corticosteroids and remained off inhaled corticosteroids at the conclusion of the study (p=NS). It is not known whether the results of this study are generalizable to asthmatics who require higher doses of inhaled corticosteroids or systemic corticosteroids.

In another randomized, placebo-controlled, parallel-group trial (n=642) in a similar population of adult patients previously maintained, but not adequately controlled, on inhaled corticosteroids (beclomethasone 336 mcg/day), the addition of SINGULAIR to beclomethasone resulted in statistically significant improvements in FEV_1 compared with those patients who were continued on beclomethasone alone or those patients who were withdrawn from beclomethasone and treated with montelukast or placebo alone over the last 10 weeks of the 16-week, blinded treatment period. Patients who were randomized to treatment arms containing beclomethasone had statistically significantly better asthma control than those patients randomized to SINGULAIR alone or placebo alone as indicated by FEV_1, daytime asthma symptoms, PEFR, nocturnal awakenings due to asthma, and "as-needed" β-agonist requirements.

In adult asthmatic patients with documented aspirin sensitivity, nearly all of whom were receiving concomitant inhaled and/or oral corticosteroids, a 4-week randomized, parallel-group trial (n=80) demonstrated that SINGULAIR, compared with placebo, resulted in significant improvement in parameters of asthma control. The magnitude of effect of SINGULAIR in aspirin-sensitive patients was similar to the effect observed in the general population of asthmatic patients studied. The effect of SINGULAIR on the bronchoconstrictor response to aspirin or other non-steroidal anti-inflammatory drugs in aspirin-sensitive asthmatic patients has not been evaluated (see PRECAUTIONS, *General*).

EFFECTS ON EXERCISE-INDUCED BRONCHOCONSTRICTION (ADULTS AND PEDIATRIC PATIENTS)

In a 12-week, randomized, double-blind, parallel group study of 110 adolescent and adult asthmatics 15 years of age and older, with a mean baseline FEV_1 percent of predicted of 83% and with documented exercise-induced exacerbation of asthma, treatment with SINGULAIR, 10 mg, once daily in the evening, resulted in a statistically significant reduction in mean maximal percent fall in FEV_1 and mean time to recovery to within 5% of the pre-exercise FEV_1. Exercise challenge was conducted at the end of the dosing interval (i.e., 20 to 24 hours after the preceding dose). This effect was maintained throughout the 12-week treatment period indicating that tolerance did not occur. SINGULAIR did not, however, prevent clinically significant deterioration in maximal percent fall in FEV_1 after exercise (i.e., ≥20% decrease from pre-exercise baseline) in 52% of patients studied. In a separate crossover study in adults, a similar effect was observed after two once-daily 10-mg doses of SINGULAIR.

In pediatric patients 6 to 14 years of age, using the 5-mg chewable tablet, a 2-day crossover study demonstrated effects similar to those observed in adults when exercise challenge was conducted at the end of the dosing interval (i.e., 20 to 24 hours after the preceding dose).

SINGULAIR should not be used as monotherapy for the treatment and management of exercise-induced bronchospasm. Patients who have exacerbations of asthma after exercise should continue to use their usual regimen of inhaled β-agonists as prophylaxis and have available for rescue a short-acting inhaled β-agonist (see PRECAUTIONS, *General* and *Information for Patients*).

TABLE 2
Effect of SINGULAIR on Asthma-Related Outcome Measurements
(Combined Analyses - U.S. and Multinational Trials)

	SINGULAIR	Placebo
Asthma Attack* (% of patients)	11.6†	18.4
Oral Corticosteroid Rescue (% of patients)	10.7†	17.5
Discontinuation Due to Asthma (% of patients)	1.4‡	4.0
Asthma Exacerbations **(% of days)	12.8†	20.5
Asthma Control Days***(% of days)	38.5†	27.2
Physicians' Global Evaluation (score)§	1.77†	2.43
Patients' Global Evaluation (score)§§	1.60†	2.15
† $p<0.001$, compared with placebo ‡ $p<0.01$, compared with placebo		

* Asthma Attack defined as utilization of health-care resources such as an unscheduled visit to a doctor's office, emergency room, or hospital; or treatment with oral, intravenous, or intramuscular corticosteroid.

** Asthma Exacerbation defined by specific clinically important decreases in PEFR, increase in β-agonist use, increases in day or nighttime symptoms, or the occurrence of an asthma attack.

*** An Asthma Control Day defined as a day without any of the following: nocturnal awakening, use of more than 2 puffs of β-agonist, or an asthma attack.

§ Physicians' evaluation of the patient's asthma, ranging from 0 to 6 ("very much better" through "very much worse," respectively).

§§ Patients' evaluation of asthma, ranging from 0 to 6 ("very much better" through "very much worse," respectively).

INDICATIONS AND USAGE

SINGULAIR is indicated for the prophylaxis and chronic treatment of asthma in adults and pediatric patients 2 years of age and older.

CONTRAINDICATIONS

Hypersensitivity to any component of this product.

PRECAUTIONS

General

SINGULAIR is not indicated for use in the reversal of bronchospasm in acute asthma attacks, including status asthmaticus.

Patients should be advised to have appropriate rescue medication available. Therapy with SINGULAIR can be continued during acute exacerbations of asthma.

While the dose of inhaled corticosteroid may be reduced gradually under medical supervision, SINGULAIR should not be abruptly substituted for inhaled or oral corticosteroids.

SINGULAIR should not be used as monotherapy for the treatment and management of exercise-induced bronchospasm. Patients who have exacerbations of asthma after exercise should continue to use their usual regimen of inhaled β-agonists as prophylaxis and have available for rescue a short-acting inhaled β-agonist.

Patients with known aspirin sensitivity should continue avoidance of aspirin or non-steroidal anti-inflammatory agents while taking SINGULAIR. Although SINGULAIR is effective in improving airway function in asthmatics with documented aspirin sensitivity, it has not been shown to truncate bronchoconstrictor response to aspirin and other non-steroidal anti-inflammatory drugs in aspirin-sensitive asthmatic patients (see CLINICAL PHARMACOLOGY, *Clinical Studies*).

Eosinophilic Conditions

In rare cases, patients on therapy with SINGULAIR may present with systemic eosinophilia, sometimes presenting with clinical features of vasculitis consistent with Churg-Strauss syndrome, a condition which is often treated with systemic corticosteroid therapy. These events usually, but not always, have been associated with the reduction of oral corticosteroid therapy. Physicians should be alert to eosinophilia, vasculitic rash, worsening pulmonary symptoms, cardiac complications, and/or neuropathy presenting in their patients. A causal association between SINGULAIR and these underlying conditions has not been established (see ADVERSE REACTIONS).

Information for Patients

- Patients should be advised to take SINGULAIR daily as prescribed, even when they are asymptomatic, as well as during periods of worsening asthma, and to contact their physicians if their asthma is not well controlled.
- Patients should be advised that oral tablets of SINGULAIR are not for the treatment of acute asthma attacks. They should have appropriate short-acting inhaled β-agonist medication available to treat asthma exacerbations.
- Patients should be advised that, while using SINGULAIR, medical attention should be sought if short-acting inhaled bronchodilators are needed more often than usual, or if more than the maximum number of inhalations of short-acting bronchodilator treatment prescribed for 24-hour period are needed.
- Patients receiving SINGULAIR should be instructed not to decrease the dose or stop taking any other antiasthma medications unless instructed by a physician.
- Patients who have exacerbations of asthma after exercise should be instructed to continue to use their usual regimen of inhaled β-agonists as prophylaxis unless otherwise instructed by their physician. All patients should have available for rescue a short-acting inhaled β-agonist.
- Patients with known aspirin sensitivity should be advised to continue avoidance of aspirin or non-steroidal anti-inflammatory agents while taking SINGULAIR.

Chewable Tablets

- *Phenylketonurics:* Phenylketonuric patients should be informed that the 4-mg and 5-mg chewable tablets contain phenylalanine (a component of aspartame), 0.674 and 0.842 mg per 4-mg and 5-mg chewable tablet, respectively.

Drug Interactions

SINGULAIR has been administered with other therapies routinely used in the prophylaxis and chronic treatment of asthma with no apparent increase in adverse reactions. In drug-interaction studies, the recommended clinical dose of montelukast did not have clinically important effects on the pharmacokinetics of the following drugs: theophylline, prednisone, prednisolone, oral contraceptives (norethindrone 1 mg/ethinyl estradiol 35 mcg), terfenadine, digoxin, and warfarin.

Although additional specific interaction studies were not performed, SINGULAIR was used concomitantly with a wide range of commonly prescribed drugs in clinical studies without evidence of clinical adverse interactions. These medications included thyroid hormones, sedative hypnotics, non-steroidal anti-inflammatory agents, benzodiazepines, and decongestants.

Phenobarbital, which induces hepatic metabolism, decreased the AUC of montelukast approximately 40% following a single 10-mg dose of montelukast. No dosage adjustment for SINGULAIR is recommended. It is reasonable to employ appropriate clinical monitoring when potent cytochrome P450 enzyme inducers, such as phenobarbital or rifampin, are co-administered with SINGULAIR.

Carcinogenesis, Mutagenesis, Impairment of Fertility

No evidence of tumorigenicity was seen in either a 2-year carcinogenicity study in Sprague-Dawley rats at oral (gavage) doses up to 200 mg/kg/day (estimated exposure was approximately 120 times the area under the plasma concentration versus time curve (AUC) for adults and children at the maximum recommended daily oral dose) or in a 92-week carcinogenicity study in mice at oral (gavage) doses up to 100 mg/kg/day (estimated exposure was approximately 45 times the AUC for adults and children at the maximum recommended daily oral dose.

Montelukast demonstrated no evidence of mutagenic or clastogenic activity in the following assays: the microbial mutagenesis assay, the V-79 mammalian cell mutagenesis assay, the alkaline elution assay in rat hepatocytes, the chromosomal aberration assay in Chinese hamster ovary cells, and in the *in vivo* mouse bone marrow chromosomal aberration assay.

In fertility studies in female rats, montelukast produced reductions in fertility and fecundity indices at an oral dose of 200 mg/kg (estimated exposure was approximately 70 times the AUC for adults at the maximum recommended daily oral dose). No effects on female fertility or fecundity were observed at an oral dose of 100 mg/kg (estimated exposure was approximately 20 times the AUC for adults at the maximum recommended daily oral dose). Montelukast had no effects on fertility in male rats at oral doses up to 800 mg/kg (estimated exposure was approximately 160 times the AUC for adults at the maximum recommended daily oral dose).

Pregnancy, Teratogenic Effects

Pregnancy Category B:

No teratogenicity was observed in rats at oral doses up to 400 mg/kg/day (estimated exposure was approximately 100 times the AUC for adults at the maximum recommended daily oral dose) and in rabbits at oral doses up to 300 mg/kg/day (estimated exposure was approximately 110 times the AUC for adults at the maximum recommended daily oral dose). Montelukast crosses the placenta following oral dosing in rats and rabbits. There are, however, no adequate and well-controlled studies in pregnant women. Because animal reproduction studies are not always predictive of human response, SINGULAIR should be used during pregnancy only if clearly needed.

Merck & Co., Inc. maintains a registry to monitor the pregnancy outcomes of women exposed to SINGULAIR while pregnant. Healthcare providers are encouraged to report any prenatal exposure to SINGULAIR by calling the Pregnancy Registry at (800) 986-8999.

Nursing Mothers

Studies in rats have shown that montelukast is excreted in milk. It is not known if montelukast is excreted in human milk. Because many drugs are excreted in human milk, caution should be exercised when SINGULAIR is given to a nursing mother.

Pediatric Use

Safety and efficacy of SINGULAIR have been established in adequate and well-controlled studies in pediatric patients 6 to 14 years of age. Safety and efficacy profiles in this age group are similar to those seen in adults. (See *Clinical Studies* and ADVERSE REACTIONS.)

The safety of SINGULAIR 4-mg chewable tablets in pediatric patients 2 to 5 years of age has been demonstrated in an interim analysis of 314 pediatric patients in a 12-week double-blind, placebo-controlled study in approximately 650 patients (see ADVERSE REACTIONS). Efficacy of SINGULAIR in this age group is extrapolated from the demonstrated efficacy in adolescent and adult patients 15 years of age and older and pediatric patients 6 to 14 years of age with asthma based on similar mean systemic exposure (AUC), and that the disease course, pathophysiology and the drug's effect are substantially similar among these populations.

The safety and effectiveness in pediatric patients below the age of 2 years have not been established. Long-term trials evaluating the effect of chronic administration of SINGULAIR on linear growth in pediatric patients have not been conducted.

Geriatric Use

Of the total number of subjects in clinical studies of montelukast, 3.5% were 65 years of age and over and 0.4% were 75 years of age and over. No overall differences in safety or effectiveness were observed between these subjects and younger subjects, and other reported clinical experience has not identified differences in responses between the elderly and younger patients, but greater sensitivity of some older individuals cannot be ruled out.

ADVERSE REACTIONS

Adolescents and Adults 15 Years of Age and Older

SINGULAIR has been evaluated for safety in approximately 2600 adolescent and adult patients 15 years of age and older in clinical trials. In placebo-controlled clinical trials, the following adverse experiences reported with SINGULAIR occurred in greater than or equal to 1% of patients and at an incidence greater than that in patients treated with placebo, regardless of causality assessment:

[See table above]

Adverse Experiences Occurring in ≥1% of Patients with an Incidence Greater than that in Patients Treated with Placebo, Regardless of Causality Assessment

	SINGULAIR 10 mg/day (%) (n=1955)	Placebo (%) (n=1180)
Body As A Whole		
Asthenia/fatigue	1.8	1.2
Fever	1.5	0.9
Pain, abdominal	2.9	2.5
Trauma	1.0	0.8
Digestive System Disorders		
Dyspepsia	2.1	1.1
Gastroenteritis, infectious	1.5	0.5
Pain, dental	1.7	1.0
Nervous System / Psychiatric		
Dizziness	1.9	1.4
Headache	18.4	18.1
Respiratory System Disorders		
Congestion, nasal	1.6	1.3
Cough	2.7	2.4
Influenza	4.2	3.9
Skin / Skin Appendages Disorder		
Rash	1.6	1.2
*Laboratory Adverse Experiences**		
ALT increased	2.1	2.0
AST increased	1.6	1.2
Pyuria	1.0	0.9

*Number of patients tested (SINGULAIR and placebo, respectively): ALT and AST, 1935, 1170; pyuria, 1924, 1159.

The frequency of less common adverse events was comparable between SINGULAIR and placebo.

Cumulatively, 569 patients were treated with SINGULAIR for at least 6 months, 480 for one year, and 49 for two years in clinical trials. With prolonged treatment, the adverse experience profile did not significantly change.

Pediatric Patients 6 to 14 Years of Age

SINGULAIR has also been evaluated for safety in approximately 320 pediatric patients 6 to 14 years of age. Cumulatively, 169 pediatric patients were treated with SINGULAIR for at least 6 months, and 121 for one year or longer in clinical trials. The safety profile of SINGULAIR versus placebo in the double-blind, 8-week, pediatric efficacy trial was generally similar to the adult safety profile with the exception of the adverse events listed below. In pediatric patients 6 to 14 years of age receiving SINGULAIR, the following events occurred with a frequency ≥2% and more frequently than in pediatric patients who received placebo, regardless of causality assessment: diarrhea, laryngitis, pharyngitis, nausea, otitis, sinusitis, and viral infection. The frequency of less common adverse events was comparable between SINGULAIR and placebo. With prolonged treatment, the adverse experience profile did not significantly change.

Pediatric Patients 2 to 5 Years of Age

Safety data for SINGULAIR in pediatric patients 2 to 5 years of age are available from an interim analysis of 314 pediatric patients from a 12-week, double-blind, placebo-controlled clinical study in approximately 650 patients. The safety profile of SINGULAIR in this interim analysis of patients who received SINGULAIR for at least 6 weeks was generally similar to the safety profile in pediatric patients 6 to 14 years of age. In pediatric patients 2 to 5 years of age receiving SINGULAIR, the following events occurred with a frequency ≥2% and more frequently than in pediatric patients who received placebo, regardless of causality assessment: rhinorrhea, otitis, ear pain, bronchitis, leg pain, thirst, sneezing, rash and urticaria.

Post-Marketing Experience

The following additional adverse reactions have been reported in post-marketing use: hypersensitivity reactions (including anaphylaxis, angioedema, pruritus, urticaria, and very rarely, hepatic eosinophilic infiltration), dream abnormalities, drowsiness, irritability, restlessness, insomnia, nausea, vomiting, dyspepsia and diarrhea.

In rare cases, patients on therapy with SINGULAIR may present with systemic eosinophilia, sometimes presenting with clinical features of vasculitis consistent with Churg-Strauss syndrome, a condition which is often treated with systemic corticosteroid therapy. These events usually, but not always, have been associated with the reduction of oral corticosteroid therapy. Physicians should be alert to eosinophilia, vasculitic rash, worsening pulmonary symptoms, cardiac complications, and/or neuropathy presenting in their patients. A causal association between SINGULAIR and these underlying conditions has not been established (see PRECAUTIONS, *Eosinophilic Conditions*).

Continued on next page

Information on the Merck & Co., Inc. products listed on these pages is the full prescribing information from product circulars in use September 30, 2000. For information, please call 1-800-NSC MERCK [1-800-672-6372].

Singulair—Cont.

OVERDOSAGE

No mortality occurred following single oral doses of montelukast up to 5000 mg/kg in mice (estimated exposure was approximately 340 times the AUC for adults and children at the maximum recommended daily oral dose) and rats (estimated exposure was approximately 230 times the AUC for adults and children at the maximum recommended daily oral dose).

No specific information is available on the treatment of overdosage with SINGULAIR. In chronic asthma studies, montelukast has been administered at doses up to 200 mg/day to patients for 22 weeks and, in short-term studies, up to 900 mg/day to patients for approximately a week without clinically important adverse experiences. In the event of overdose, it is reasonable to employ the usual supportive measures; e.g., remove unabsorbed material from the gastrointestinal tract, employ clinical monitoring, and institute supportive therapy, if required.

There have been reports of acute overdosage in pediatric patients in post-marketing experience and clinical studies of up to at least 150 mg/day with SINGULAIR. The clinical and laboratory findings observed were consistent with the safety profile in adults and older pediatric patients. There were no adverse experiences reported in the majority of overdosage reports. The most frequent adverse experiences observed were thirst, somnolence, mydriasis, hyperkinesia, and abdominal pain.

It is not known whether montelukast is removed by peritoneal dialysis or hemodialysis.

DOSAGE AND ADMINISTRATION

General Information:

Adolescents and Adults 15 Years of Age and Older

The dosage for adolescents and adults 15 years of age and older is one 10-mg tablet daily to be taken in the evening.

Pediatric Patients 6 to 14 Years of Age

The dosage for pediatric patients 6 to 14 years of age is one 5-mg chewable tablet daily to be taken in the evening. No dosage adjustment within this age group is necessary.

Pediatric Patients 2 to 5 Years of Age

The dosage for pediatric patients 2 to 5 years of age is one 4-mg chewable tablet daily to be taken in the evening. Safety and effectiveness in pediatric patients younger than 2 years of age have not been established.

The safety and efficacy of SINGULAIR was demonstrated in clinical trials where it was administered in the evening without regard to the time of food ingestion. There have been no clinical trials evaluating the relative efficacy of morning versus evening dosing.

HOW SUPPLIED

No. 3796—SINGULAIR Tablets, 4 mg, are pink, oval biconvex-shaped chewable tablets, with code MRK 711 on one side and SINGULAIR on the other. They are supplied as follows:

NDC 0006-0711-31 unit of use high-density polyethylene (HDPE) bottles of 30 with a polypropylene child-resistant cap, an aluminum foil induction seal, and a silica gel desiccant canister

NDC 0006-0711-54 unit of use high-density polyethylene (HDPE) bottles of 90 with a polypropylene child-resistant cap, an aluminum foil induction seal, and a silica gel desiccant canister

NDC 0006-0711-68 high-density polyethylene (HDPE) bulk bottles of 100 with a polypropylene non-child-resistant cap, an aluminum foil induction seal, and a silica gel desiccant canister

NDC 0006-0711-74 high-density polyethylene (HDPE) bulk bottles of 500 with a polypropylene non-child-resistant cap, an aluminum foil induction seal, and three silica gel desiccant canisters

NDC 0006-0711-28 unit dose paper and aluminum foil-backed aluminum foil peelable blister packs of 100.

Shown in Product Identification Guide, page 324

No. 3760—SINGULAIR Tablets, 5 mg, are pink, round, biconvex-shaped chewable tablets, with code MRK 275 on one side and SINGULAIR on the other. They are supplied as follows:

NDC 0006-0275-31 unit of use high-density polyethylene (HDPE) bottles of 30 with a polypropylene child-resistant cap, an aluminum foil induction seal, and a silica gel desiccant canister

NDC 0006-0275-54 unit of use high-density polyethylene (HDPE) bottles of 90 with a polypropylene child-resistant cap, an aluminum foil induction seal, and a silica gel desiccant canister

NDC 0006-0275-28 unit dose paper and aluminum foil-backed aluminum foil peelable blister packs of 100.

Shown in Product Identification Guide, page 324

No. 3761—SINGULAIR Tablets, 10 mg, are beige, rounded square-shaped, film-coated tablets, with code MRK 117 on one side and SINGULAIR on the other. They are supplied as follows:

NDC 0006-0117-31 unit of use high-density polyethylene (HDPE) bottles of 30 with a polypropylene child-resistant cap, an aluminum foil induction seal, and a silica gel desiccant canister

NDC 0006-0117-54 unit of use high-density polyethylene (HDPE) bottles of 90 with a polypropylene child-resistant cap, an aluminum foil induction seal, and a silica gel desiccant canister

NDC 0006-0117-28 unit dose paper and aluminum foil-backed aluminum foil peelable blister pack of 100.

Shown in Product Identification Guide, page 324

Storage

Store the 4-mg chewable tablets, the 5-mg chewable tablets and the 10-mg film-coated tablets at room temperature 15–30°C (59–86°F), protected from moisture and light.

9088807 Issued March 2000

Patient Information about
SINGULAIR® (SING-u-lair)
Generic name: montelukast (mon-te-LOO-kast) sodium

Read this information before you start taking SINGULAIR®. Also, read the leaflet each time you renew your prescription, in case anything has changed. This leaflet does not take the place of complete discussions with your doctor. You and your doctor should discuss SINGULAIR when you start taking your medicine and at regular checkups.

What is SINGULAIR*?

- Your doctor has prescribed SINGULAIR once a day for the long-term treatment of your (or your child's) asthma.
- SINGULAIR is a medicine called a leukotriene receptor antagonist. It works by blocking substances in the body called leukotrienes. Blocking leukotrienes improves asthma symptoms. SINGULAIR is not a steroid.
- SINGULAIR comes in 3 forms:
  1. A 10-mg tablet that you swallow whole (for adults and children above age 14).
  2. A 5-mg chewable tablet (for children ages 6–14).
  3. A 4-mg chewable tablet (for children ages 2–5).
- **SINGULAIR should NOT be used for the fast relief of asthma attacks.** If you get an asthma attack, you should follow the instructions your doctor has given you for treating asthma attacks.

* Registered trademark of MERCK & CO., Inc.

What is asthma?

- Asthma is a continuing (chronic) lung disease. It cannot be cured, but it can be controlled.
- Symptoms of asthma include:
  - coughing
  - wheezing
  - chest tightness
- In some patients, symptoms worsen during the night or after exercise.

Who should not take SINGULAIR?

Patients with allergies to any components of SINGULAIR should not take SINGULAIR. The active ingredient in SINGULAIR is montelukast sodium. The inactive ingredients are listed at the end of this leaflet.

The safety and efficacy of SINGULAIR has not been established in children younger than age 2.

What should I tell my doctor before taking SINGULAIR?

Tell your doctor:

- If you are pregnant or plan to become pregnant. SINGULAIR may not be right for you.
- If you are breast-feeding. SINGULAIR may be passed in your milk to your baby.
- About any medical problems or allergies you have now or have had.
- About all medicines that you are taking or plan to take, including those you can get without a prescription.

How should I take SINGULAIR?

- Take SINGULAIR once a day in the evening.
- Take SINGULAIR daily for as long as your doctor prescribes it, even if you have no symptoms.
- You may take SINGULAIR with or without food.
- Children who are prescribed SINGULAIR should take it under the supervision of an adult.
- If your symptoms get worse, of if you need to increase the use of your inhaled rescue medicine for asthma attacks, contact your doctor at once.
- **Do NOT take SINGULAIR to stop an asthma attack.** If an attack occurs, follow the instructions your doctor gave you for asthma attacks.
- It is very important that you continue taking your other asthma medicines unless your doctor tells you to stop. In addition, do not lower the dose of any of your asthma medicines unless you are told to do so by your doctor. Your doctor may decide to reduce the amount you use of your current asthma medicine.
- If your asthma is made worse by exercise, continue to use the medicines your doctor prescribed for you to use before exercise, unless your doctor tells you otherwise. Always have your inhaled rescue medicine for asthma attacks with you in case you need it.

The dose for adults and adolescents 15 years and older is one 10-mg tablet daily. The dose for children 6 to 14 years old is one 5-mg chewable tablet daily. The dose for children 2 to 5 years old is one 4-mg chewable tablet daily.

What should I avoid while taking SINGULAIR?

- If your asthma is made worse by aspirin, you should continue to avoid aspirin or other non-steroidal anti-inflammatory drugs, such as ibuprofen and naproxen.

What are the possible side effects of SINGULAIR?

The side effects of SINGULAIR are usually mild.

- The side effects in patients treated with SINGULAIR were similar in type and frequency to side effects in patients who were given a placebo (a pill containing no medication).

The list below is NOT a complete list of side effects reported with SINGULAIR. Your doctor can discuss with you a more complete list of side effects. The most common side effects are listed below.

tiredness
fever
abdominal (stomach) pain
stomach or intestinal upset (gastroenteritis)
heartburn
dizziness
headache
rash
cough
flu
stuffy nose

Less common side effects included the following

- allergic reactions including
  - swelling of the face, lips, tongue, and/or throat, which may cause difficulty in breathing or swallowing
  - hives
  - itching
- bad/vivid dreams
- irritability
- restlessness
- insomnia
- nausea
- vomiting
- dyspepsia
- diarrhea

Rarely, patients taking SINGULAIR have experienced a condition that includes a combination of certain symptoms that do not go away or that get worse. These symptoms may include:

- a flu-like illness
- rash
- a feeling of pins and needles or numbness of arms or legs
- severe inflammation (pain and swelling) of the sinuses (sinusitus)

These have occurred usually, but not always, in patients who were taking oral corticosteroid pills for asthma and those corticosteroids were being slowly lowered or stopped. Although SINGULAIR has not been shown to cause this condition, you must tell your doctor right away if you develop one or more of these symptoms.

Remember, anytime you have a medical problem you think may be related to SINGULAIR, talk to your doctor.

Other Information

Do not share SINGULAIR with anyone else; it was prescribed only for you. Do not use it for a condition for which it was not prescribed.

Keep SINGULAIR and all medicines out of the reach of children.

Phenylketonurics: SINGULAIR 4-mg and 5-mg chewable tablets contain 0.674 and 0.842 mg phenylalanine, respectively.

This leaflet provides a summary of information about SINGULAIR. If you have any questions or concerns about either SINGULAIR or asthma, talk to your doctor. In addition, you can talk to your pharmacist or other health care provider. Your doctor or pharmacist can give you an additional leaflet that is written for health professionals.

Inactive ingredients:

4-mg and 5-mg chewable tablets: mannitol, microcrystalline cellulose, hydroxypropyl cellulose, red ferric oxide, croscarmellose sodium, cherry flavor, aspartame, and magnesium stearate.

10-mg tablet: microcrystalline cellulose, lactose monohydrate, croscarmellose sodium, hydroxypropyl cellulose, magnesium stearate, hydroxypropyl methylcellulose, titanium dioxide, red ferric oxide, yellow ferric oxide, and carnauba wax.

9094207 Issued March 2000

STROMECTOL® Tablets ℞
(ivermectin)

DESCRIPTION

STROMECTOL* (Ivermectin) is a semisynthetic, anthelmintic agent for oral administration. Ivermectin is derived from the avermectins, a class of highly active broad-spectrum anti-parasitic agents isolated from the fermentation products of *Streptomyces avermitilis.* Ivermectin is a mixture containing at least 90% 5-*O*-demethyl-22,23-dihydroavermectin A_{1a} and less than 10% 5-*O*-demethyl-25-de(1-methylpropyl)-22,23-dihydro-25-(1-methylethyl)avermectin A_{1a}, generally referred to as 22,23-dihydroavermectin B_{1a} and B_{1b}, H_2B_{1a} and H_2B_{1b}, respectively. The respective empirical formulas are $C_{48}H_{74}O_{14}$ and $C_{47}H_{72}O_{14}$, with molecular weights of 875.10 and 861.07, respectively. The structural formulas are:

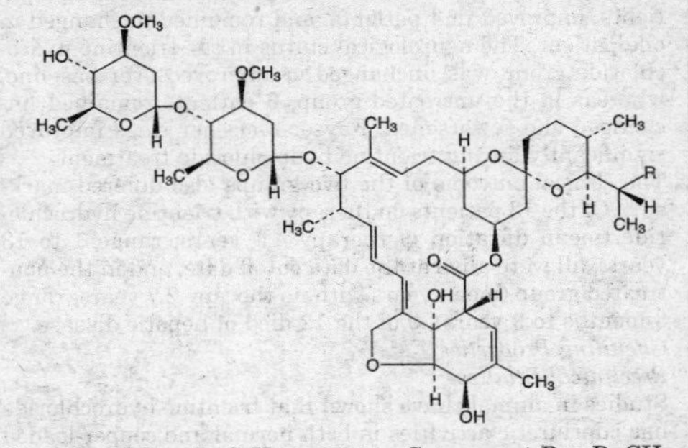

Component B_{1a}, $R=C_2H_5$ Component B_{1b}, $R=CH_3$

Ivermectin is a white to yellowish-white, nonhygroscopic, crystalline powder with a melting point of about 155°C. It is insoluble in water but is freely soluble in methanol and soluble in 95% ethanol.

STROMECTOL is available in 3-mg tablets and 6-mg scored tablets. Each tablet contains the following inactive ingredients: microcrystalline cellulose, pregelatinized starch, magnesium stearate, butylated hydroxyanisole, and citric acid powder (anhydrous).

* Registered trademark of MERCK & CO., Inc.

CLINICAL PHARMACOLOGY

Pharmacokinetics

Following oral administration of ivermectin, plasma concentrations are approximately proportional to the dose. In two studies, after single 12-mg doses of STROMECTOL (2×6 mg) in fasting healthy volunteers (representing a mean dose of 165 µg/kg), the mean peak plasma concentrations of the major component (H_2B_{1a}) were 46.6 (±21.9) (range: 16.4–101.1) and 30.6 (±15.6) (range: 13.9–68.4) ng/mL respectively at approximately 4 hours after dosing. Ivermectin is metabolized in the liver, and ivermectin and/or its metabolites are excreted almost exclusively in the feces over an estimated 12 days, with less than 1% of the administered dose excreted in the urine. The apparent plasma half-life of ivermectin is approximately at least 16 hours following oral administration.

The effect(s) of food on the systemic availability of ivermectin has not been studied.

Microbiology

Ivermectin is a member of the avermectin class of broad-spectrum antiparasitic agents which have a unique mode of action. Compounds of the class bind selectively and with high affinity to glutamate-gated chloride ion channels which occur in invertebrate nerve and muscle cells. This leads to an increase in the permeability of the cell membrane to chloride ions with hyperpolarization of the nerve or muscle cell, resulting in paralysis and death of the parasite. Compounds of this class may also interact with other ligand-gated chloride channels, such as those gated by the neurotransmitter gamma-aminobutyric acid (GABA).

The selective activity of compounds of this class is attributable to the facts that some mammals do not have glutamate-gated chloride channels and that the avermectins have a low affinity for mammalian ligand-gated chloride channels. In addition, ivermectin does not readily cross the blood-brain barrier in humans.

Ivermectin is active against various life-cycle stages of many but not all nematodes. It is active against the tissue microfilariae of *Onchocerca volvulus* but not against the adult form. Its activity against *Strongyloides stercoralis* is limited to the intestinal stages.

Clinical Studies

Strongyloidiasis

Two controlled clinical studies using albendazole as the comparative agent were carried out in international sites where albendazole is approved for the treatment of strongyloidiasis of the gastrointestinal tract, and three controlled studies were carried out in the US and internationally using thiabendazole as the comparative agent. Efficacy, as measured by cure rate, was defined as the absence of larvae in at least two follow-up stool examinations 3 to 4 weeks post-therapy. Based on this criterion, efficacy was significantly greater for STROMECTOL (a single dose of 170 to 200 µg/kg) than for albendazole (200 mg b.i.d. for 3 days). STROMECTOL administered as a single dose of 200 µg/kg for 1 day was as efficacious as thiabendazole administered at 25 mg/kg b.i.d. for 3 days.

Summary of Cure Rates for Ivermectin Versus Comparative Agents in the Treatment of Strongyloidiasis

	Cure Rate* (%)	
	Ivermectin**	Comparative Agent
Albendazole *** Comparative		
International Study	24/26 (92)	12/22 (55)
WHO Study	126/152 (83)	67/149 (45)
Thiabendazole† Comparative		
International Study	9/14 (64)	13/15 (87)
US Studies	14/14 (100)	16/17 (94)

* Number and % of evaluable patients
** 170–200 µg/kg
*** 200 mg b.i.d. for 3 days
† 25 mg/kg b.i.d. for 3 days

In one study conducted in France, a non-endemic area where there was no possibility of reinfection, several patients were observed to have recrudescence of *Strongyloides* larvae in their stool as long as 106 days following ivermectin therapy. Therefore, at least three stool examinations should be conducted over the three months following treatment to ensure eradication. If recrudescence of larvae is observed, retreatment with ivermectin is indicated. Concentration techniques (such as using a Baermann apparatus) should be employed when performing these stool examinations, as the number of *Strongyloides* larvae per gram of feces may be very low.

Onchocerciasis

The evaluation of STROMECTOL in the treatment of onchocerciasis is based on the results of clinical studies involving 1278 patients. In a double-blind, placebo-controlled study involving adult patients with moderate to severe onchocercal infection, patients who received a single dose of 150 µg/kg STROMECTOL experienced an 83.2% and 99.5% decrease in skin microfilariae count (geometric mean) 3 days and 3 months after the dose, respectively. A marked reduction of > 90% was maintained for up to 12 months after the single dose. As with other microfilaricidal drugs, there was an increase in the microfilariae count in the anterior chamber of the eye at day 3 after treatment in some patients. However, at 3 and 6 months after the dose, a significantly greater percentage of patients treated with STROMECTOL had decreases in microfilariae count in the anterior chamber than patients treated with placebo.

In a separate open study involving pediatric patients ages 6 to 13 (n=103; weight range: 17–41 kg), similar decreases in skin microfilariae counts were observed for up to 12 months after dosing.

INDICATIONS AND USAGE

STROMECTOL is indicated for the treatment of the following infections:

Strongyloidiasis of the intestinal tract. STROMECTOL is indicated for the treatment of intestinal (i.e. nondisseminated) strongyloidiasis due to the nematode parasite *Strongyloides stercoralis.*

This indication is based on clinical studies of both comparative and open-label designs, in which from 64–100% of infected patients were cured following a single 200-µg/kg dose of ivermectin. (See *Clinical Studies.*)

Onchocerciasis. STROMECTOL is indicated for the treatment of onchocerciasis due to the nematode parasite *Onchocerca volvulus.*

This indication is based on randomized, double-blind, placebo-controlled and comparative studies conducted in 1427 patients in onchocerciasis-endemic areas of West Africa. The comparative studies used diethylcarbamazine citrate (DEC-C).

NOTE: STROMECTOL has no activity against adult *Onchocerca volvulus* parasites. The adult parasites reside in subcutaneous nodules which are infrequently palpable. Surgical excision of these nodules (nodulectomy) may be considered in the management of patients with onchocerciasis, since this procedure will eliminate the microfilariae-producing adult parasites.

CONTRAINDICATIONS

STROMECTOL is contraindicated in patients who are hypersensitive to any component of this product.

WARNINGS

Historical data have shown that microfilaricidal drugs, such as diethylcarbamazine citrate (DEC-C), might cause cutaneous and/or systemic reactions of varying severity (the Mazzotti reaction) and ophthalmological reactions in patients with onchocerciasis. These reactions are probably due to allergic and inflammatory responses to the death of microfilariae. Patients treated with STROMECTOL for onchocerciasis may experience these reactions in addition to clinical adverse reactions possibly, probably, or definitely related to the drug itself. (See ADVERSE REACTIONS, *Onchocerciasis.*)

The treatment of severe Mazzotti reactions has not been subjected to controlled clinical trials. Oral hydration, recumbency, intravenous normal saline, and/or parenteral corticosteroids have been used to treat postural hypotension. Antihistamines and/or aspirin have been used for most mild to moderate cases.

PRECAUTIONS

General

After treatment with microfilaricidal drugs, patients with hyperreactive onchodermatitis (sowda) may be more likely than others to experience severe advserse reactions, especially edema and aggravation of onchodermatitis.

Carcinogenesis, Mutagenesis, Impairment of Fertility

Long-term studies in animals have not been performed to evaluate the carcinogenic potential of ivermectin.

Ivermectin was not genotoxic *in vitro* in the Ames microbial mutagenicity assay of *Salmonella typhimurium* strains TA 1535, TA 1537, TA98, and TA100 with and without rat liver enzyme activation, the Mouse Lymphoma Cell Line L5178Y (cytotoxicity and mutagenicity) assays, or the unscheduled DNA synthesis assay in human fibroblasts.

Ivermectin had no adverse effects on the fertility in rats in studies at repeated doses of up to 3 times the maximum recommended human dose of 200 µg/kg (on a mg/m^2/day basis).

Information for Patients

STROMECTOL should be taken with water.

Strongyloidiasis: The patient should be reminded of the need for repeated stool examinations to document clearance of infection with *Strongyloides stercoralis.*

Onchocerciasis: The patient should be reminded that treatment with STROMECTOL does not kill the adult *Onchocerca* parasites, and therefore repeated follow-up and retreatment is usually required.

Pregnancy, Teratogenic Effects

Pregnancy Category C

Ivermectin has been shown to be teratogenic in mice, rats, and rabbits when given in repeated doses of 0.2, 8.1 and 4.5 times the maximum recommended human dose, respectively (on a mg/m^2/day basis). Teratogenicity was characterized in the three species tested by cleft palate; clubbed forepaws were additionally observed in rabbits. These development effects were found only at or near doses that were maternotoxic to the pregnant female. Therefore, ivermectin does not appear to be selectively fetotoxic to the developing fetus. There are, however, no adequate and well-controlled studies in pregnant women. Ivermectin should not be used during pregnancy since safety in pregnancy has not been established.

Nursing Mothers

STROMECTOL is excreted in human milk in low concentrations. Treatment of mothers who intend to breast feed should only be undertaken when the risk of delayed treatment to the mother outweighs the possible risk to the newborn.

Pediatric Use

Safety and effectiveness in pediatric patients weighing less than 15 kg have not been established.

Strongyloidiasis in Immunocompromised Hosts

In immunocompromised (including HIV-infected) patients being treated for intestinal strongyloidiasis, repeated courses of therapy may be required. Adequate and well-controlled clinical studies have not been conducted in such patients to determine the optimal dosing regimen. Several treatments, i.e., at 2 week intervals, may be required, and cure may not be achievable. Control of extra-intestinal strongyloidiasis in these patients is difficult, and suppressive therapy, i.e., once per month may be helpful.

ADVERSE REACTIONS

Strongyloidiasis

In four clinical studies involving a total of 109 patients given either one or two doses of 170–200 µg/kg of STROMECTOL, the following adverse reactions were reported as possibly, probably, or definitely related to STROMECTOL:

Body as a whole: asthenia/fatigue (0.9%), abdominal pain (0.9%)

Gastrointestinal: anorexia (0.9%), constipation (0.9%), diarrhea (1.8%), nausea (1.8%), vomiting (0.9%)

Nervous System/Psychiatric: dizziness (2.8%), somnolence (0.9%), vertigo (0.9%), tremor (0.9%)

Skin: pruritus (2.8%), rash (0.9%), and urticaria (0.9%)

In comparative trials, patients treated with STROMECTOL experienced more abdominal distention and chest discomfort than patients treated with albendazole. However, STROMECTOL was better tolerated than thiabendazole in comparative studies involving 37 patients treated with thiabendazole.

The Mazzotti-type and ophthalmologic reactions associated with the treatment of onchocerciasis or the disease itself would not be expected to occur in strongyloidiasis patients treated with STROMECTOL. (See ADVERSE REACTIONS, *Onchocerciasis.*)

Laboratory Test Findings

In clinical trials involving 109 patients given either one or two doses of 170–200 µg/kg STROMECTOL, the following laboratory abnormalities were seen irrespective of drug relationship: elevation in ALT and/or AST (2%), decrease in leukocyte count (3%). Leukopenia and anemia were seen in one patient.

Onchocerciasis

In clinical trials involving 963 adult patients treated with 100 to 200 µg/kg STROMECTOL, worsening of the following Mazzotti reactions during the first 4 days post-treatment were reported: arthralgia/synovitis (9.3%), axillary lymph node enlargement and tenderness (11.0% and 4.4%, respectively), cervical lymph node enlargement and tenderness (5.3% and 1.2%, respectively), inguinal lymph node enlargement and tenderness (12.6% and 13.9%, respectively), other lymph node enlargement and tenderness (3.0% and 1.9%,

Continued on next page

Information on the Merck & Co., Inc. products listed on these pages is the full prescribing information from product circulars in use September 30, 2000. For information, please call 1-800-NSC MERCK [1-800-672-6372].

Stromectol—Cont.

respectively), pruritus (27.5%), skin involvement including edema, papular and pustular or frank urticarial rash (22.7%), and fever (22.6%). (See WARNINGS.)
In clinical trials, ophthalmological conditions were examined in 963 adult patients before treatment, at day 3, and months 3 and 6 after treatment with 100 to 200 µg/kg STROMECTOL. Changes observed were primarily deterioration from baseline 3 days post-treatment. Most changes either returned to baseline condition or improved over baseline severity at the month 3 and 6 visits. The percentages of patients with worsening of the following conditions at day 3, month 3 and 6, respectively, were: limbitis: 5.5%, 4.8%, and 3.5% and punctate opacity: 1.8%, 1.8%, and 1.4%. The corresponding percentages for patients treated with placebo were: limbitis: 6.2%, 9.9% and 9.4% and punctate opacity: 2.0%, 6.4% and 7.2%. (See WARNINGS.)
In clinical trials involving 963 adult patients who received 100 to 200 µg/kg STROMECTOL, the following clinical adverse reactions were reported as possibly, probably, or definitely related to the drug in $\geq$ 1% of the patients: facial edema (1.2%), peripheral edema (3.2%), orthostatic hypotension (1.1%), and tachycardia (3.5%). Drug-related headache and myalgia occurred in $<$ 1% of patients (0.2%, and 0.4%, respectively). However, these were the most common adverse experiences reported overall during these trials regardless of causality (22.3% and 19.7%, respectively).
A similar safety profile was observed in an open study in pediatric patients ages 6 to 13.
Additionally, hypotension (mainly orthostatic hypotension) and worsening of bronchial asthma have been reported since the drug was registered overseas.
The following ophthalmological side effects do occur due to the disease itself but have also been reported after treatment with STROMECTOL: abnormal sensation in the eyes, eyelid edema, anterior uveitis, conjunctivitis, limbitis, keratitis, and chorioretinitis or choroiditis. These have rarely been severe or associated with loss of vision and have generally resolved without corticosteroid treatment.
Laboratory Test Findings
In controlled clinical trials, the following laboratory adverse experiences were reported as possibly, probably, or definitely related to the drug in $\geq$ 1% of the patients: eosinophilia (3%) and hemoglobin increase (1%).

OVERDOSAGE

Significant lethality was observed in mice and rats after single oral doses of 25 to 50 mg/kg and 40 to 50 mg/kg, respectively. No significant lethality was observed in dogs after single oral doses of up to 10 mg/kg. At these doses, the treatment related signs that were observed in these animals include ataxia, bradypnea, tremors, ptosis, decreased activity, emesis, and mydriasis.
In accidental intoxication with or significant exposure to unknown quantities of veterinary formulations of ivermectin in humans, either by ingestion, inhalation, injection, or exposure to body surfaces, the following adverse effects have been reported most frequently: rash, edema, headache, dizziness, asthenia, nausea, vomiting, and diarrhea. Other adverse effects that have been reported include: seizure, ataxia, dyspnea, abdominal pain, paresthesia, and urticaria.
In case of accidental poisoning, supportive therapy, if indicated, should include parenteral fluids and electrolytes, respiratory support (oxygen and mechanical ventilation if necessary) and pressor agents if clinically significant hypotension is present. Induction of emesis and/or gastric lavage as soon as possible, followed by purgatives and other routine anti-poison measures, may be indicated if needed to prevent absorption of ingested material.

DOSAGE AND ADMINISTRATION

Strongyloidiasis
The recommended dosage of STROMECTOL for the treatment of strongyloidiasis is a single oral dose designed to provide approximately 200 µg of ivermectin per kg of body weight. See Table 1 for dosage guidelines. Patients should take tablets with water. In general, additional doses are not necessary. However, follow-up stool examinations should be performed to verify eradication of infection (see *Clinical Studies*.)

Table 1
Dosage Guidelines for
STROMECTOL for Strongyloidiasis

Body Weight (kg)	Single Oral Dose Number of 3-mg Tablets	Number of 6-mg Tablets
15–24	1 tablet	1/2 tablet
25–35	2 tablets	1 tablet
36–50	3 tablets	1 1/2 tablets
51–65	4 tablets	2 tablets
66–79	5 tablets	2 1/2 tablets
≥80	200 µg/kg	200 µg/kg

Onchocerciasis
The recommended dosage of STROMECTOL for the treatment of onchocerciasis is a single oral dose designed to provide approximately 150 µg of ivermectin per kg of body weight. See Table 2 for dosage guidelines. Patients should take tablets with water. In mass distribution campaigns in international treatment programs, the most commonly used dose interval is 12 months. For the treatment of individual patients, retreatment may be considered at intervals as short as 3 months.

Table 2
Dosage Guidelines for
STROMECTOL for Onchocerciasis

Body Weight (kg)	Single Oral Dose Number of 3-mg Tablets	Number of 6-mg Tablets
15–25	1 tablet	1/2 tablet
26–44	2 tablets	1 tablet
45–64	3 tablets	1 1/2 tablets
65–84	4 tablets	2 tablets
≥85	150 µg/kg	150 µg/kg

HOW SUPPLIED

No. 8107—Tablets STROMECTOL 6 mg are white, scored, round, flat, beveled-edged tablets coded MSD 139 on one side and scored on the other. They are supplied as follows:
NDC 0006-0139-10 unit dose packages of 10.
Shown in Product Identification Guide, page 324
No. 8495—Tablets STROMECTOL 3 mg are white, round, flat, bevel-edged tablets coded MSD on one side and 32 on the other. They are supplied as follows:
NDC 0006–0032–20 unit dose packages of 20.
Shown in Product Identification Guide, page 324
Storage
Store at temperatures below 30°C (86°F).
9032301 Issued October 1998

SYPRINE® Capsules (Trientine Hydrochloride) ℞

DESCRIPTION

Trientine hydrochloride is *N,N′* -bis (2-aminoethyl)-1,2-ethanediamine dihydrochloride. It is a white to pale yellow crystalline hygroscopic powder. It is freely soluble in water, soluble in methanol, slightly soluble in ethanol, and insoluble in chloroform and ether.
The empirical formula is $C_6H_{18}N_4{\cdot}2HCl$ with a molecular weight of 219.2. The structural formula is:

$$NH_2(CH_2)_2NH(CH_2)_2NH(CH_2)_2NH_2{\cdot}2HCl$$

Trientine hydrochloride is a chelating compound for removal of excess copper from the body. SYPRINE* (Trientine Hydrochloride) is available as 250 mg capsules for oral administration. Capsules SYPRINE contain gelatin, iron oxides, stearic acid, and titanium dioxide as inactive ingredients.

*Registered trademark of MERCK & CO., INC.

CLINICAL PHARMACOLOGY

Introduction
Wilson's disease (hepatolenticular degeneration) is an autosomal inherited metabolic defect resulting in an inability to maintain a near-zero balance of copper. Excess copper accumulates possibly because the liver lacks the mechanism to excrete free copper into the bile. Hepatocytes store excess copper but when their capacity is exceeded copper is released into the blood and is taken up into extrahepatic sites. This condition is treated with a low copper diet and the use of chelating agents that bind copper to facilitate its excretion from the body.
Clinical Summary
Forty-one patients (18 male and 23 female) between the ages of 6 and 54 with a diagnosis of Wilson's disease and who were intolerant of d-penicillamine were treated in two separate studies with trientine hydrochloride. The dosage varied from 450 to 2400 mg per day. The average dosage required to achieve an optimal clinical response varied between 1000 mg and 2000 mg per day. The mean duration of trientine hydrochloride therapy was 48.7 months (range 2–164 months). Thirty-four of the 41 patients improved, 4 had no change in clinical global response, 2 were lost to follow-up and one showed deterioration in clinical condition. One of the patients who improved while on therapy with trientine hydrochloride experienced a recurrence of the symptoms of systemic lupus erythematosus which had appeared originally during therapy with penicillamine. Therapy with trientine hydrochloride was discontinued. No other adverse reactions, except iron deficiency, were noted among any of these 41 patients.
One investigator treated 13 patients with trientine hydrochloride following their development of intolerance to d-penicillamine. Retrospectively, he compared these patients to an additional group of 12 patients with Wilson's disease who were both tolerant of and controlled with d-penicillamine therapy, but who failed to continue any copper chelation therapy. The mean age at onset of disease of the latter group was 12 years as compared to 21 years for the former group. The trientine hydrochloride group received d-penicillamine for an average of 4 years as compared to an average of 10 years for the non-treated group.
Various laboratory parameters showed changes in favor of the patients treated with trientine hydrochloride. Free and total serum copper, SGOT, and serum bilirubin all showed mean increases over baseline in the untreated group which were significantly larger than with the patients treated with trientine hydrochloride. In the 13 patients treated with trientine hydrochloride, previous symptoms and signs relating to d-penicillamine intolerance disappeared in 8 patients, improved in 4 patients, and remained unchanged in one patient. The neurological status in the trientine hydrochloride group was unchanged or improved over baseline, whereas in the untreated group, 6 patients remained unchanged and 6 worsened. Kayser-Fleischer rings improved significantly during trientine hydrochloride treatment.
The clinical outcome of the two groups also differed markedly. Of the 13 patients on therapy with trientine hydrochloride (mean duration of therapy 4.1 years; range 1 to 13 years), all were alive at the data cutoff date, and in the non-treated group (mean years with no therapy 2.7 years; range 3 months to 9 years), 9 of the 12 died of hepatic disease.
Chelating Properties
Preclinical Studies
Studies in animals have shown that trientine hydrochloride has cupriuretic activities in both normal and copper-loaded rats. In general, the effects of trientine hydrochloride on urinary copper excretion are similar to those of equimolar doses of penicillamine, although in one study they were significantly smaller.
Human Studies
Renal clearance studies were carried out with penicillamine and trientine hydrochloride on separate occasions in selected patients treated with penicillamine for at least one year. Six-hour excretion rates of copper were determined off treatment and after a single dose of 500 mg of penicillamine or 1.2 g of trientine hydrochloride. The mean urinary excretion rates of copper were as follows:

No. of Patients	Single Dose Treatment	Basal Excretion Rate (µg Cu^{++}/6hr)	Test-dose Excretion Rate (µ Cu^{++}/6hr)
6	Trientine, 1.2 g	19	234
4	Penicillamine, 500 mg	17	320

In patients *not* previously treated with chelating agents, a similar comparison was made:

No. of Patients	Single Dose Treatment	Basal Excretion Rate (µ Cu^{++}/6hr)	Test-dose Excretion Rate (µ Cu++/6hr)
8	Trientine, 1.2 g	71	1326
7	Penicillamine, 500 mg	68	1074

These results demonstrate that SYPRINE is effective as a cupriuretic agent in patients with Wilson's disease although on a molar basis it appears to be less potent or less effective than penicillamine. Evidence from a radio-labelled copper study indicates that the different cupriuretic effect between these two drugs could be due to a difference in selectivity of the drugs for different copper pools within the body.
Pharmacokinetics
Data on the pharmacokinetics of trientine hydrochloride are not available. Dosage adjustment recommendations are based upon clinical use of the drug (see DOSAGE AND ADMINISTRATION).

INDICATIONS AND USAGE

SYPRINE is indicated in the treatment of patients with Wilson's disease who are intolerant of penicillamine. Clinical experience with SYPRINE is limited and alternate dosing regimens have not been well-characterized; all endpoints in determining an individual patient's dose have not been well defined. SYPRINE and penicillamine cannot be considered interchangeable. SYPRINE should be used when continued treatment with penicillamine is no longer possible because of intolerable or life endangering side effects.
Unlike penicillamine, SYPRINE is not recommended in cystinuria or rheumatoid arthritis. The absence of a sulfhydryl moiety renders it incapable of binding cystine and, therefore, it is of no use in cystinuria. In 15 patients with rheumatoid arthritis, SYPRINE was reported not to be effective in improving any clinical or biochemical parameter after 12 weeks of treatment.
SYPRINE is not indicated for treatment of biliary cirrhosis.

CONTRAINDICATIONS

Hypersensitivity to this product.

WARNINGS

Patient experience with trientine hydrochloride is limited (see CLINICAL PHARMACOLOGY). Patients receiving SYPRINE should remain under regular medical supervision throughout the period of drug administration. Patients (especially women) should be closely monitored for evidence of iron deficiency anemia.

PRECAUTIONS

General
There are no reports of hypersensitivity in patients who have been administered trientine hydrochloride for Wilson's

disease. However, there have been reports of asthma, bronchitis and dermatitis occurring after prolonged environmental exposure in workers who use trientine hydrochloride as a hardener of epoxy resins. Patients should be observed closely for signs of possible hypersensitivity.

Information for Patients

Patients should be directed to take SYPRINE on an empty stomach, at least one hour before meals or two hours after meals and at least one hour apart from any other drug, food, or milk. The capsules should be swallowed whole with water and should not be opened or chewed. Because of the potential for contact dermatitis, any site of exposure to the capsule contents should be washed with water promptly. For the first month of treatment, the patient should have his temperature taken nightly, and he should be asked to report any symptom such as fever or skin eruption.

Laboratory Tests

The most reliable index for monitoring treatment is the determination of free copper in the serum, which equals the difference between quantitatively determined total copper and ceruloplasmin-copper. Adequately treated patients will usually have less than 10 mcg free copper/dL of serum.

Therapy may be monitored with a 24 hour urinary copper analysis periodically (i.e., every 6–12 months). Urine must be collected in copper-free glassware. Since a low copper diet should keep copper absorption down to less than one milligram a day, the patient probably will be in the desired state of negative copper balance if 0.5 to 1.0 milligram of copper is present in a 24-hour collection of urine.

Drug Interactions

In general, mineral supplements should not be given since they may block the absorption of SYPRINE. However, iron deficiency may develop, especially in children and menstruating or pregnant women, or as a result of the low copper diet recommended for Wilson's disease. If necessary, iron may be given in short courses, but since iron and SYPRINE each inhibit absorption of the other, two hours should elapse between administration of SYPRINE and iron.

It is important that SYPRINE be taken on an empty stomach, at least one hour before meals or two hours after meals and at least one hour apart from any other drug, food, or milk. This permits maximum absorption and reduces the likelihood of inactivation of the drug by metal binding in the gastrointestinal tract.

Carcinogenesis, Mutagenesis, Impairment of Fertility

Data on carcinogenesis, mutagenesis, and impairment of fertility are not available.

Pregnancy

Pregnancy Category C. Trientine hydrochloride was teratogenic in rats at doses similar to the human dose. The frequencies of both resorptions and fetal abnormalities, including hemorrhage and edema, increased while fetal copper levels decreased when trientine hydrochloride was given in the maternal diets of rats. There are no adequate and well-controlled studies in pregnant women. SYPRINE should be used during pregnancy only if the potential benefit justifies the potential risk to the fetus.

Nursing Mothers

It is not known whether this drug is excreted in human milk. Because many drugs are excreted in human milk, caution should be exercised when SYPRINE is administered to a nursing mother.

Pediatric Use

Controlled studies of the safety and effectiveness of SYPRINE in pediatric patients have not been conducted. It has been used clinically in pediatric patients as young as 6 years with no reported adverse experiences.

ADVERSE REACTIONS

Clinical experience with SPYRINE has been limited. The following adverse reactions have been reported in a clinical study in patients with Wilson's disease who were on therapy with trientine hydrochloride: iron deficiency, systemic lupus erythematosus (see CLINICAL PHARMACOLOGY). In addition, the following adverse reactions have been reported in marketed use: dystonia, muscular spasm, myasthenia gravis.

SYPRINE is not indicated for treatment of biliary cirrhosis, but in one study of 4 patients treated with trientine hydrochloride for primary biliary cirrhosis, the following adverse reactions were reported: heartburn; epigastric pain and tenderness; thickening, fissuring and flaking of the skin; hypochromic microcytic anemia; acute gastritis; aphthoid ulcers; abdominal pain; melena; anorexia; malaise; cramps; muscle pain; weakness; rhabdomyolysis. A causal relationship of these reactions to drug therapy could not be rejected or established.

OVERDOSAGE

There is a report of an adult woman who ingested 30 grams of trientine hydrochloride without apparent ill effects. No other data on overdosage are available.

DOSAGE AND ADMINISTRATION

Systemic evaluation of dose and/or interval between dose has not been done. However, on limited clinical experience, the recommended initial dose of SYPRINE is 500–750 mg/day for pediatric patients and 750–1250 mg/day for adults given in divided doses two, three or four times daily. This may be increased to a maximum of 2000 mg/day for adults or 1500 mg/day for pediatric patients age 12 or under. The daily dose of SYPRINE should be increased only when the clinical response is not adequate or the concentration of free serum copper is persistently above 20 mcg/dL. Optimal long-term maintenance dosage should be determined at 6–12 month intervals (see PRECAUTIONS, *Laboratory Tests*).

It is important that SYPRINE be given on an empty stomach, at least one hour before meals or two hours after meals and at least one hour apart from any other drug, food, or milk. The capsules should be swallowed whole with water and should not be opened or chewed.

HOW SUPPLIED

No. 3408—Capsules SYPRINE, 250 mg, are light brown opaque capsules and are coded SYPRINE and MSD 661. They are supplied as follows:

NDC 0006-0661-68 in bottles of 100.

Shown in Product Identification Guide, page 324

Storage

Keep container tightly closed.

Store at 2°–8°C (36°–46°F).

7664603 Issued May 1999

TIMOLIDE® Tablets ℞
(Timolol Maleate-Hydrochlorothiazide)

DESCRIPTION

TIMOLIDE* (Timolol Maleate-Hydrochlorothiazide) is for the treatment of hypertension. It combines the antihypertensive activity of two agents: a non-selective beta-adrenergic receptor blocking agent (timolol maleate) and a diuretic (hydrochlorothiazide).

Timolol maleate is (*S*)-1-[(1, 1-dimethylethyl) amino]-3-[[4-(4-morpholinyl)-1, 2, 5-thiadiazol -3- yl] oxy]-2-propanol (*Z*)-2-butenedioate (1:1) salt. Its empirical formula is $C_{13}H_{24}N_4O_3S{\cdot}C_4H_4O_4$ and its structural formula is:

[structural formula: OCH₂CCH₂NHC—CH₃ with OH, H, CH₃, CH₃ substituents; • HC – COOH ‖ HC – COOH]

Timolol maleate has a molecular weight of 432.50. It is a white, odorless, crystalline powder which is soluble in water, methanol, and alcohol.

Hydrochlorothiazide is 6-chloro-3,4-dihydro-2*H*-1,2,4-benzothiadiazine-7-sulfonamide 1, 1- dioxide. Its empirical formula is $C_7H_8ClN_3O_4S_2$ and its structural formula is:

[structural formula: NH_2SO_2, Cl, NH, N H, S with O O]

Hydrochlorothiazide has a molecular weight of 297.73. It is a white, or practically white, crystalline powder which is slightly soluble in water, but freely soluble in sodium hydroxide solution.

TIMOLIDE is supplied as tablets containing 10 mg of timolol maleate and 25 mg of hydrochlorothiazide for oral administration. Inactive ingredients are cellulose, FD&C Blue 2, magnesium stearate, and starch.

*Registered trademark of MERCK & CO., INC.

CLINICAL PHARMACOLOGY

TIMOLIDE

Timolol maleate and hydrochlorothiazide have been used singly and concomitantly for the treatment of hypertension. The antihypertensive effects of these agents are additive. The two components of TIMOLIDE have similar dosage schedules, and studies have shown that there is no interference with bioavailability when these agents are given together in the single combination tablet. Therefore, this combination provides a convenient formulation for the concomitant administration of these two entities.

In controlled clinical trials with TIMOLIDE in selected patients with mild to moderate essential hypertension, about 90 percent had a good to excellent response. In patients with more severe hypertension, TIMOLIDE may be administered with other antihypertensives such as ALDOMET* (Methyldopa) or a vasodilator.

Although the mechanisms of action of timolol maleate and hydrochlorothiazide in the treatment of hypertension have not been established, they are thought to be different; for example, hydrochlorothiazide increases plasma renin activity while timolol maleate reduces plasma renin activity.

Timolol Maleate

Timolol maleate is a $beta_1$ and $beta_2$ (non-selective) adrenergic receptor blocking agent that does not have significant intrinsic sympathomimetic, direct myocardial depressant, or local anesthetic activity.

Pharmacodynamics

Clinical pharmacology studies have confirmed the beta-adrenergic blocking activity as shown by (1) changes in resting heart rate and response of heart rate to changes in posture; (2) inhibition of isoproterenol-induced tachycardia; (3) alteration of the response to the Valsalva maneuver and amyl nitrite administration; and (4) reduction of heart rate and blood pressure changes on exercise.

Timolol maleate decreases the positive chronotropic, positive inotropic, bronchodilator, and vasodilator responses caused by beta-adrenergic receptor agonists. The magnitude of this decreased response is proportional to the existing sympathetic tone and the concentration of timolol maleate at receptor sites.

In normal volunteers, the reduction in heart rate response to a standard exercise was dose dependent over the test range of 0.5 to 20 mg, with a peak reduction at 2 hours of approximately 30% at higher doses.

Beta-adrenergic receptor blockade reduces cardiac output in both healthy subjects and patients with heart disease. In patients with severe impairment of myocardial function beta-adrenergic receptor blockade may inhibit the stimulatory effect of the sympathetic nervous system necessary to maintain adequate cardiac function.

Beta-adrenergic receptor blockade in the bronchi and bronchioles results in increased airway resistance from unopposed parasympathetic activity. Such an effect in patients with asthma or other bronchospastic conditions is potentially dangerous.

Clinical studies indicate that timolol maleate at a dosage of 20–60 mg/day reduces blood pressure without causing postural hypotension in most patients with essential hypertension. Administration of timolol maleate to patients with hypertension results initially in a decrease in cardiac output, little immediate change in blood pressure, and an increase in calculated peripheral resistance. With continued administration of timolol maleate blood pressure decreases within a few days, cardiac output usually remains reduced, and peripheral resistance falls toward pretreatment levels. Plasma volume may decrease or remain unchanged during therapy with timolol maleate. In the majority of patients with hypertension, timolol maleate also decreases plasma renin activity. Dosage adjustment to achieve optimal antihypertensive effect may require a few weeks. When therapy with timolol maleate is discontinued, the blood pressure tends to return to pretreatment levels gradually. In most patients the antihypertensive activity of timolol maleate is maintained with long-term therapy and is well tolerated.

The mechanism of the antihypertensive effects of beta-adrenergic receptor blocking agents is not established at this time. Possible mechanisms of action include reduction in cardiac output, reduction in plasma renin activity, and a central nervous system sympatholytic action.

Pharmacokinetics and Metabolism

Timolol maleate is rapidly and nearly completely absorbed (about 90%) following oral ingestion. Detectable plasma levels of timolol occur within one-half hour and peak plasma levels occur in about one to two hours. The drug half-life in plasma is approximately 4 hours and this is essentially unchanged in patients with moderate renal insufficiency. Timolol is partially metabolized by the liver and timolol and its metabolites are excreted by the kidney. Timolol is not extensively bound to plasma proteins; i.e., $<10\%$ by equilibrium dialysis and approximately 60% by ultrafiltration. An *in vitro* hemodialysis study, using ^{14}C timolol added to human plasma or whole blood, showed that timolol was readily dialyzed from these fluids; however, a study of patients with renal failure showed that timolol did not dialyze readily.

Plasma levels following oral administration are about half those following intravenous administration indicating approximately 50% first pass metabolism. The level of beta sympathetic activity varies widely among individuals, and no simple correlation exists between the dose or plasma level of timolol maleate and its therapeutic activity. Therefore, objective clinical measurements such as reduction of heart rate and/or blood pressure should be used as guides in determining the optimal dosage for each patient.

Hydrochlorothiazide

Hydrochlorothiazide is a diuretic and antihypertensive agent. It affects the renal tubular mechanism of electrolyte reabsorption. Hydrochlorothiazide increases excretion of sodium and chloride in approximately equivalent amounts. Natriuresis may be accompanied by some loss of potassium and bicarbonate. The mechanism of the antihypertensive effect of thiazides may be related to the excretion and redistribution of body sodium. Hydrochlorothiazide usually does not cause clinically important changes in normal blood pressure.

*Registered trademark of MERCK & CO., INC.

INDICATIONS AND USAGE

TIMOLIDE is indicated for the treatment of hypertension.

Continued on next page

Information on the Merck & Co., Inc. products listed on these pages is the full prescribing information from product circulars in use September 30, 2000. For information, please call 1-800-NSC MERCK [1-800-672-6372].

Timolide—Cont.

This fixed combination drug is not indicated for initial therapy of hypertension. If the fixed combination represents the dose titrated to an individual patient's needs, it may be more convenient than the separate components.

CONTRAINDICATIONS

TIMOLIDE is contraindicated in patients with bronchial asthma or with a history of bronchial asthma, or severe chronic obstructive pulmonary disease (see WARNINGS); sinus bradycardia; second and third degree atrioventricular block; overt cardiac failure (see WARNINGS); cardiogenic shock; anuria; hypersensitivity to this product or to sulfonamide-derived drugs.

WARNINGS

Cardiac Failure
Sympathetic stimulation may be essential for support of the circulation in individuals with diminished myocardial contractility, and its inhibition by beta-adrenergic receptor blockade may precipitate more severe failure. Although beta blockers should be avoided in overt congestive heart failure, they can be used, if necessary, with caution in patients with a history of failure who are well-compensated, usually with digitalis and diuretics. Both digitalis and timolol maleate slow AV conduction. If cardiac failure persists, therapy with TIMOLIDE should be withdrawn.

In Patients Without a History of Cardiac Failure continued depression of the myocardium with beta-blocking agents over a period of time can, in some cases, lead to cardiac failure. At the first sign or symptom of cardiac failure, patients receiving TIMOLIDE should be digitalized and/or be given additional diuretic therapy. Observe the patient closely. If cardiac failure continues, despite adequate digitalization and diuretic therapy, TIMOLIDE should be withdrawn.

Renal and Hepatic Disease and Electrolyte Disturbances
Since timolol maleate is partially metabolized in the liver and excreted mainly by the kidneys, dosage reductions may be necessary when hepatic and/or renal insufficiency is present.

Although the pharmacokinetics of timolol maleate are not greatly altered by renal impairment, marked hypotensive responses have been seen in patients with marked renal impairment undergoing dialysis after 20 mg doses. Dosing in such patients should therefore be especially cautious.

In patients with renal disease, thiazides may precipitate azotemia, and cumulative effects may develop in the presence of impaired renal function. If progressive renal impairment becomes evident, TIMOLIDE should be discontinued.

In patients with impaired hepatic function or progressive liver disease, even minor alterations in fluid and electrolyte balance may precipitate hepatic coma. Hepatic encephalopathy, manifested by tremors, confusion, and coma, has been reported in association with diuretic therapy including hydrochlorothiazide.

Exacerbation of Ischemic Heart Disease Following Abrupt Withdrawal —Hypersensitivity to catecholamines has been observed in patients withdrawn from beta blocker therapy; exacerbation of angina and, in some cases, myocardial infarction have occurred after *abrupt* discontinuation of such therapy. When discontinuing chronically administered timolol maleate, particularly in patients with ischemic heart disease, the dosage should be gradually reduced over a period of one to two weeks and the patient should be carefully monitored. If angina markedly worsens or acute coronary insufficiency develops, timolol maleate administration should be reinstituted promptly, at least temporarily, and other measures appropriate for the management of unstable angina should be taken. Patients should be warned against interruption or discontinuation of therapy without the physician's advice. Because coronary artery disease is common and may be unrecognized, it may be prudent not to discontinue timolol maleate therapy abruptly even in patients treated only for hypertension.

Obstructive Pulmonary Disease
PATIENTS WITH CHRONIC OBSTRUCTIVE PULMONARY DISEASE (e.g., CHRONIC BRONCHITIS, EMPHYSEMA) OF MILD OR MODERATE SEVERITY, BRONCHOSPASTIC DISEASE OR A HISTORY OF BRONCHOSPASTIC DISEASE (OTHER THAN BRONCHIAL ASTHMA OR A HISTORY OF BRONCHIAL ASTHMA, IN WHICH 'TIMOLIDE' IS CONTRAINDICATED, see CONTRAINDICATIONS), SHOULD IN GENERAL NOT RECEIVE BETA BLOCKERS, INCLUDING 'TIMOLIDE'. However, if TIMOLIDE is necessary in such patients, then the drug should be administered with caution since it may block bronchodilation produced by endogenous and exogenous catecholamine stimulation of $beta_2$ receptors.

Major Surgery
The necessity or desirability of withdrawal of beta-blocking therapy prior to major surgery is controversial. Beta-adrenergic receptor blockade impairs the ability of the heart to respond to beta-adrenergically mediated reflex stimuli. This may augment the risk of general anesthesia in surgical procedures. Some patients receiving beta-adrenergic receptor blocking agents have been subject to protracted severe hypotension during anesthesia. Difficulty in restarting and maintaining the heartbeat has also been reported. For these reasons, in patients undergoing elective surgery, some authorities recommend gradual withdrawal of beta-adrenergic receptor blocking agents.

If necessary during surgery, the effects of beta-adrenergic blocking agents may be reversed by sufficient doses of such agonists as isoproterenol, dopamine, dobutamine or levarterenol (see OVERDOSAGE).

Metabolic and Endocrine Effects
Beta-adrenergic blockade may mask certain clinical signs (e.g., tachycardia) of hyperthyroidism. Patients suspected of developing thyrotoxicosis should be managed carefully to avoid abrupt withdrawal of beta blockade which might precipitate a thyroid storm. Thiazides may decrease serum PBI levels without signs of thyroid disturbance.

Beta-adrenergic receptor blocking agents may mask the signs and symptoms of acute hypoglycemia. Therefore, TIMOLIDE should be administered with caution to patients subject to spontaneous hypoglycemia, or to diabetic patients (especially those with labile diabetes) who are receiving insulin or oral hypoglycemic agents. Insulin requirements in diabetic patients may be increased, decreased, or unchanged by thiazides. Diabetes mellitus which has been latent may become manifest during administration of thiazide diuretics.

Because calcium excretion is decreased by thiazides, TIMOLIDE should be discontinued before carrying out tests for parathyroid function. Pathologic changes in the parathyroid glands, with hypercalcemia and hypophosphatemia, have been observed in a few patients on prolonged thiazide therapy; however, the common complications of hyperparathyroidism such as renal lithiasis, bone resorption, and peptic ulceration have not been seen.

Hyperuricemia may occur or acute gout may be precipitated in certain patients receiving thiazide therapy.

PRECAUTIONS

General
Electrolyte and Fluid Balance Status: Periodic determination of serum electrolytes to detect possible electrolyte imbalance should be performed at appropriate intervals.

Patients should be observed for clinical signs of fluid or electrolyte imbalance, i.e., hyponatremia, hypochloremic alkalosis, and hypokalemia. Serum and urine electrolyte determinations are particularly important when the patient is vomiting excessively or receiving parenteral fluids. Warning signs or symptoms of fluid and electrolyte imbalance, irrespective of cause, include dryness of the mouth, thirst, weakness, lethargy, drowsiness, restlessness, confusion, seizures, muscle pains or cramps, muscular fatigue, hypotension, oliguria, tachycardia, and gastrointestinal disturbances such as nausea and vomiting.

Hypokalemia may develop, especially with brisk diuresis, when severe cirrhosis is present, or during concomitant use of corticosteroids or ACTH.

Interference with adequate oral electrolyte intake will also contribute to hypokalemia. Hypokalemia may cause cardiac arrhythmia and may also sensitize or exaggerate the response of the heart to the toxic effects of digitalis (e.g., increased ventricular irritability). Hypokalemia may be avoided or treated by use of potassium sparing diuretics or potassium supplements such as foods with a high potassium content.

Any chloride deficit during thiazide therapy is generally mild and usually does not require specific treatment except under extraordinary circumstances (as in liver disease or renal disease). Dilutional hyponatremia may occur in edematous patients in hot weather; appropriate therapy is water restriction rather than administration of salt except in rare instances when the hyponatremia is life threatening. In actual salt depletion, appropriate replacement is the therapy of choice.

Thiazides have been shown to increase urinary excretion of magnesium, which may result in hypomagnesemia.

Effects on Cholesterol and Triglyceride Levels:
Increases in cholesterol and triglyceride levels may be associated with thiazide diuretic therapy.

Muscle Weakness: Beta-adrenergic blockade has been reported to potentiate muscle weakness consistent with certain myasthenic symptoms (e.g., diplopia, ptosis, and generalized weakness). Timolol has been reported rarely to increase muscle weakness in some patients with myasthenia gravis or myasthenic symptoms.

Cerebrovascular Insufficiency: Because of potential effects of beta-adrenergic blocking agents relative to blood pressure and pulse, these agents should be used with caution in patients with cerebrovascular insufficiency. If signs or symptoms suggesting reduced cerebral blood flow are observed, consideration should be given to discontinuing these agents.

Drug Interactions
TIMOLIDE may potentiate the action of other antihypertensive agents used concomitantly. Close observation of the patient is recommended when TIMOLIDE is administered to patients receiving catecholamine-depleting drugs such as reserpine, because of possible additive effects and the production of hypotension and/or marked bradycardia, which may produce vertigo, syncope, or postural hypotension.

Blunting of the antihypertensive effect of beta-adrenoceptor blocking agents by non-steroidal anti-inflammatory drugs has been reported. In some patients, the administration of a non-steroidal anti-inflammatory agent can reduce the diuretic, natriuretic, and antihypertensive effects of loop, potassium-sparing and thiazide diuretics. Therefore, when TIMOLIDE and non-steroidal anti-inflammatory agents are used concomitantly, the patient should be observed closely to determine if the desired therapeutic effect has been obtained.

Literature reports suggest that oral calcium antagonists may be used in combination with beta-adrenergic blocking agents when heart function is normal, but should be avoided in patients with impaired cardiac function. Hypotension, AV conduction disturbances, and left ventricular failure have been reported in some patients receiving beta-adrenergic blocking agents when an oral calcium antagonist was added to the treatment regimen. Hypotension was more likely to occur if the calcium antagonist were a dihydropyridine derivative, e.g., nifedipine, while left ventricular failure and AV conduction disturbances were more likely to occur with either verapamil or diltiazem.

Intravenous calcium antagonists should be used with caution in patients receiving beta-adrenergic blocking agents.

The concomitant use of beta-adrenergic blocking agents with digitalis and either diltiazem or verapamil may have additive effects in prolonging AV conduction time.

Potentiated systemic beta-blockade (e.g., decreased heart rate) has been reported during combined treatment with quinidine and timolol, possibly because quinidine inhibits the metabolism of timolol via the P-450 enzyme, CYP2D6.

Beta adrenergic blocking agents may exacerbate the rebound hypertension which can follow the withdrawal of clonidine. If the two drugs are coadministered, the beta adrenergic blocking agent should be withdrawn several days before the gradual withdrawal of clonidine. If replacing clonidine by beta-blocker therapy, the introduction of beta adrenergic blocking agents should be delayed for several days after clonidine administration has stopped.

Risk from Anaphylactic Reaction: While taking beta-blockers, patients with a history of atopy or a history of severe anaphylactic reaction to a variety of allergens may be more reactive to repeated accidental, diagnostic, or therapeutic challenge with such allergens. Such patients may be unresponsive to the usual doses of epinephrine used to treat anaphylactic reactions.

In patients receiving thiazides, sensitivity reactions may occur with or without a history of allergy or bronchial asthma. The possible exacerbation or activation of systemic lupus erythematosus has been reported. The antihypertensive effects of thiazides may be enhanced in the post-sympathectomy patient.

Thiazides may decrease arterial responsiveness to norepinephrine. This diminution is not sufficient to preclude the therapeutic effectiveness of norepinephrine. Thiazides may increase the responsiveness to tubocurarine.

Lithium generally should not be given with diuretics because they reduce its renal clearance and add a high risk of lithium toxicity. Read circulars for lithium preparations before use of such preparations with TIMOLIDE.

Absorption of hydrochlorothiazide is impaired in the presence of anionic exchange resins. Single doses of either cholestyramine or colestipol resins bind the hydrochlorothiazide and reduce its absorption from the gastrointestinal tract by up to 85 and 43 percent, respectively.

Carcinogenesis, Mutagenesis, Impairment of Fertility
Carcinogenicity, mutagenicity, and fertility studies have not been conducted in animals with TIMOLIDE.

Timolol maleate: In a two-year study of timolol maleate in rats, there was a statistically significant increase in the incidence of adrenal pheochromocytomas in male rats administered 300 mg/kg/day (250 times** the maximum recommended daily human dose). Similar differences were not observed in rats administered doses equivalent to approximately 20 or 80 times** the maximum recommended daily human dose.

In a lifetime study in mice, there were statistically significant increases in the incidence of benign and malignant pulmonary tumors, benign uterine polyps and mammary adenocarcinoma in female mice at 500 mg/kg/day (approximately 400 times** the maximum recommended daily human dose), but not at 5 or 50 mg/kg/day. In a subsequent study in female mice, in which post-mortem examinations were limited to uterus and lungs, a statistically significant increase in the incidence of pulmonary tumors was again observed at 500 mg/kg/day.

The increased occurrence of mammary adenocarcinoma was associated with elevations of serum prolactin that occurred in female mice administered timolol at 500 mg/kg/day, but not at doses of 5 or 50 mg/kg/day. An increased incidence of mammary adenocarcinomas in rodents has been associated with administration of several other therapeutic agents which elevate serum prolactin, but no correlation between serum prolactin levels and mammary tumors has been established in man. Furthermore, in adult human female subjects who received oral dosages of up to 60 mg of timolol maleate, the maximum recommended daily human oral dosage, there were no clinically meaningful changes in serum prolactin.

Timolol maleate was devoid of mutagenic potential when evaluated *in vivo* (mouse) in the micronucleus test and cytogenetic assay (doses up to 800 mg/kg) and *in vitro* in a neoplastic cell transformation assay (up to 100 µg/mL). In Ames tests the highest concentrations of timolol employed, 5000 or 10,000 µg/plate, were associated with statistically significant elevations of revertants observed with tester strain TA100 (in seven replicate assays), but not in three additional strains. In the assays with tester strain TA100, no consistent dose response relationship was observed, nor did the ratio of test to control revertants reach 2. A ratio of 2 is usually considered the criterion for a positive Ames test. Reproduction and fertility studies in rats showed no adverse effect on male or female fertility at doses up to 125 times** the maximum recommended daily human dose.

Hydrochlorothiazide: Two-year feeding studies in mice and rats conducted under the auspices of the National Toxicology Program (NTP) uncovered no evidence of a carcinogenic potential of hydrochlorothiazide in female mice (at doses of up to approximately 600 mg/kg/day) or in male and female rats (at doses of up to approximately 100 mg/kg/day). The NTP, however, found equivocal evidence for hepatocarcinogenicity in male mice.

Hydrochlorothiazide was not genotoxic *in vitro* in the Ames mutagenicity assay of *Salmonella typhimurium* strains TA 98, TA 100, TA 1535, TA 1537, and TA 1538 and in the Chinese Hamster Ovary (CHO) test for chromosomal aberrations, or *in vivo* in assays using mouse germinal cell chromosomes, Chinese hamster bone marrow chromosomes, and the *Drosophila* sex-linked recessive lethal trait gene. Positive test results were obtained only in the *in vitro* CHO Sister Chromatid Exchange (clastogenicity) and in the Mouse Lymphoma Cell (mutagenicity) assay, using concentrations of hydrochlorothiazide from 43 to 1300 μg/mL, and in the *Aspergillus nidulans* nondisjunction assay at an unspecified concentration.

Hydrochlorothiazide had no adverse effects on the fertility of mice and rats of either sex in studies wherein these species were exposed, via their diet, to doses of up to 100 and 4 mg/kg, respectively, prior to conception and throughout gestation.

** Based on patient weight of 50 kg

Pregnancy

Teratogenic Effects—Pregnancy Category C. Combinations of timolol maleate and hydrochlorothiazide were studied for teratogenic potential in the mouse and rabbit. The timolol maleate/hydrochlorothiazide combinations were administered orally to pregnant mice and pregnant rabbits at dosage levels of 1/2.5, 4/10, or 8/10 mg/kg/day. No teratogenic, embryotoxic, fetotoxic, or maternotoxic effects attributable to treatment were observed in either species. There are no adequate and well-controlled studies in pregnant women with TIMOLIDE. Because of the data listed below with the individual components, TIMOLIDE should be used during pregnancy only if the potential benefit justifies the potential risk to the fetus.

Timolol Maleate: Teratogenicity studies with timolol maleate in mice, rats and rabbits at doses up to 50 mg/kg/day (approximately 40 times** the maximum recommended daily human dose) showed no evidence of fetal malformations. Although delayed fetal ossification was observed at this dose in rats, there were no adverse effects on postnatal development of offspring. Doses of 1000 mg/kg/day (approximately 830 times** the maximum recommended daily human dose) were maternotoxic in mice and resulted in an increased number of fetal resorptions. Increased fetal resorptions were also seen in rabbits at doses of approximately 40 times** the maximum recommended daily human dose, in this case without apparent maternotoxicity.

Hydrochlorothiazide: Studies in which hydrochlorothiazide was orally administered to pregnant mice and rats during their respecitve periods of major organogenesis at doses up to 3000 and 1000 mg hydrochlorothiazide/kg, respectively, provided no evidence of harm to the fetus.

Nonteratogenic Effects.

Hydrochlorothiazide: TIMOLIDE contains hydrochlorothiazide. Thiazides cross the placental barrier and appear in cord blood. The possible hazards to the fetus include fetal or neonatal jaundice, thrombocytopenia, and possibly other adverse reactions which have occurred in the adult.

** Based on patient weight of 50 kg

Nursing Mothers

Timolol maleate and thiazides have been detected in human milk. Because of the potential for serious adverse reactions from timolol and hydrochlorothiazide in nursing infants, a decision should be made whether to discontinue nursing or to discontinue the drug, taking into account the importance of the drug to the mother.

Pediatric Use

Safety and effectiveness in pediatric patients have not been established.

ADVERSE REACTIONS

TIMOLIDE is usually well tolerated in properly selected patients. Most adverse effects have been mild and transient. The adverse reactions listed in the following table were spontaneously reported and have been arranged into two groups; (1) incidence greater than 1%; and (2) incidence less than 1%. The incidence was obtained from clinical studies conducted in the United States (257 patients treated with TIMOLIDE).

Incidence Greater Than 1%	*Incidence Less Than 1%*
BODY AS A WHOLE	
fatigue/tiredness (1.9%)	chest pain
	headache
asthenia (1.95)	
CARDIOVASCULAR	
hypotension (1.6%)	arrhythmia
bradycardia (1.2%)	syncope
	cardiac failure
DIGESTIVE SYSTEM	
none	diarrhea
	dyspepsia
	nausea
	gastrointestinal pain
	constipation
INTEGUMENTARY	
none	rash
	increased pigmentation
	dry mucous membranes
MUSCULOSKELETAL	
none	myalgia
NERVOUS SYSTEM	
dizziness (1.2%)	none
PSYCHIATRIC	
none	insomnia
	decreased libido
	nervousness
	confusion
	trouble concentrating
	somnolence
RESPIRATORY	
bronchial spasm (1.6%)	rales
dyspnea (1.2%)	
UROGENITAL	
none	renal colic

The following additional adverse effects have been reported in clinical experience with the drug: cerebral ischemia, cerebral vascular accident, gout, muscle cramps, oculogyric crisis, worsening of chronic obstructive pulmonary disease, earache, and impotence.

Other adverse reactions that have been reported with the individual components are listed below:

Timolol Maleate —Body as a Whole: extremity pain, decreased exercise tolerance, weight loss, fever; *Cardiovascular:* cardiac arrest, cerebral vascular accident, worsening of angina pectoris, sinoatrial block, AV block, worsening of arterial insufficiency, Raynaud's phenomenon, claudication, palpitations, vasodilatation, cold hands and feet, edema; *Digestive:* hepatomegaly, elevated liver function tests, vomiting; *Hematologic:* nonthrombocytopenic purpura; *Endocrine:* hyperglycemia, hypoglycemia; *Skin:* skin irritation, pruritus, sweating, alopecia; *Musculoskeletal:* arthralgia; *Nervous System:* local weakness, vertigo, paresthesia, increase in signs and symptoms of myasthenia gravis; *Psychiatric:* depression, nightmares, hallucinations; *Respiratory:* cough; *Special Senses:* visual disturbances, diplopia, ptosis, eye irritation, dry eyes, tinnitus; *Urogenital:* urination difficulties.

There have been reports of retroperitoneal fibrosis in patients receiving timolol maleate and in patients receiving other beta-adrenergic blocking agents. A causal relationship between this condition and therapy with beta-adrenergic blocking agents has not been established.

Hydrochlorothiazide —Body as a Whole: weakness; *Digestive:* anorexia, gastric irritation, vomiting, cramping, jaundice (intrahepatic cholestatic jaundice), pancreatitis, sialadenitis; *Nervous System / Psychiatric:* vertigo, paresthesias, restlessness; *Hematologic:* leukopenia, agranulocytosis, thrombocytopenia, aplastic anemia, hemolytic anemia; *Cardiovascular:* hypotension including orthostatic hypotension (may be aggravated by alcohol, barbiturates, narcotics or antihypertensive drugs); *Hypersensitivity:* purpura, photosensitivity, urticaria, necrotizing angiitis (vasculitis, cutaneous vasculitis), fever, respiratory distress including pneumonitis and pulmonary edema, anaphylactic reactions; *Metabolic:* hyperglycemia, glycosuria, hyperuricemia, electrolyte imbalance (see PRECAUTIONS); *Musculoskeletal:* muscle spasm; *Renal:* renal failure, renal dysfunction, interstitial nephritis (See WARNINGS); *Skin:* erythema multiforme including Stevens-Johnson syndrome, exfoliative dermatitis including toxic epidermal necrolysis, alopecia; *Special Senses:* transient blurred vision, xanthopsia.

Potential Adverse Effects: In addition, a variety of adverse effects not observed in clinical trials with timolol maleate, but reported with other beta-adrenergic blocking agents, should be considered potential adverse effects of timolol maleate: *Nervous System:* reversible mental depression progressing to catatonia; an acute reversible syndrome characterized by disorientation for time and place, short-term memory loss, emotional lability, slightly clouded sensorium, and decreased performance on neuropsychometrics; *Cardiovascular:* intensification of AV block (see CONTRAINDICATIONS); *Digestive:* mesenteric arterial thrombosis, ischemic colitis; *Hematologic:* agranulocytosis, thrombocytopenic purpura; *Allergic:* erythematous rash, fever combined with aching and sore throat, laryngospasm with respiratory distress; *Miscellaneous:* Peyronie's disease.

There have been reports of a syndrome comprising psoriasiform skin rash, conjunctivitis sicca, otitis, and sclerosing serositis attributed to the beta-adrenergic receptor blocking agent, practolol. This syndrome has not been reported with TIMOLIDE or BLOCADREN* (timolol maleate).

Clinical Laboratory Test Findings: Clinically important changes in standard laboratory parameters were rarely associated with the administration of TIMOLIDE. The changes in laboratory parameters were not progressive and usually were not associated with clinical manifestations. The most common changes were increases in serum triglycerides and uric acid and decreases in serum potassium and chloride. Decreases in HDL cholesterol have been reported.

*Registered trademark of MERCK & CO., Inc.

OVERDOSAGE

No data are available with regard to overdosage with TIMOLIDE in humans.

Pretreatment of mice with hydrochlorothiazide (5 mg/kg) did not alter the LD_{50} of timolol (1320 mg/kg compared to 1300 mg/kg without pretreatment).

No specific information is available on the treatment of overdosage with TIMOLIDE, and no specific antidote is available. Treatment is symptomatic and supportive. Therapy with TIMOLIDE should be discontinued and the patient observed closely. Suggested measures include induction of emesis and/or gastric lavage, and correction of dehydration, electrolyte imbalance, and hypotension by established procedures.

Timolol Maleate

Overdosage has been reported with Tablets BLOCADREN* (timolol maleate). A 30-year-old female ingested 650 mg of BLOCADREN (maximum recommended daily dose—60 mg) and experienced second and third degree heart block. She recovered without treatment but approximately two months later developed irregular heartbeat, hypertension, dizziness, tinnitus, faintness, increased pulse rate and borderline first degree heart block.

The oral LD_{50} of the drug is 1190 and 900 mg/kg in female mice and female rats, respectively.

An *in vitro* hemodialysis study, using ^{14}C timolol added to human plasma or whole blood, showed that timolol was readily dialyzed from these fluids; however, a study of patients with renal failure showed that timolol did not dialyze readily.

The most common signs and symptoms to be expected with overdosage with a beta-adrenergic receptor blocking agent are symptomatic bradycardia, hypotension, bronchospasm, and acute cardiac failure. If overdosage occurs the following therapeutic measures should be considered:

(1) *Gastric lavage.*

(2) *Symptomatic bradycardia:* Use atropine sulfate intravenously in a dosage of 0.25 mg to 2 mg to induce vagal blockade. If bradycardia persists, intravenous isoproterenol hydrochloride should be administered cautiously. In refractory cases the use of a transvenous cardiac pacemaker may be considered.

(3) *Hypotension:* Use sympathomimetic pressor drug therapy, such as dopamine, dobutamine or levarterenol. In refractory cases the use of glucagon hydrochloride has been reported to be useful.

(4) *Bronchospasm:* Use isoproterenol hydrochloride. Additional therapy with aminophylline may be considered.

(5) *Acute cardiac failure:* Conventional therapy with digitalis, diuretics, and oxygen should be instituted immediately. In refractory cases the use of intravenous aminophylline is suggested. This may be followed, if necessary, by glucagon hydrochloride which has been reported to be useful.

(6) *Heart block (second or third degree):* Use isoproterenol hydrochloride or a transvenous cardiac pacemaker.

Hydrochlorothiazide

The most common signs and symptoms observed with hydrochlorothiazide overdosage are those caused by electrolyte depletion (hypokalemia, hypochloremia, hyponatremia) and dehydration resulting from excessive diuresis. If digitalis has also been administered, hypokalemia may accentuate cardiac arrhythmias.

*Registered trademark of MERCK & CO., Inc.

DOSAGE AND ADMINISTRATION

The recommended starting and maintenance dosage is 1 tablet twice a day or 2 tablets once a day. Hydrochlorothiazide can be given at doses of 12.5 to 50 mg per day when used alone. If the antihypertensive response is not satisfactory, another nondiuretic antihypertensive agent may be added.

HOW SUPPLIED

No. 3373—Tablets TIMOLIDE 10-25 are light blue, flat, hexagonal-shaped, compressed tablets, with code MSD 67 on one side and TIMOLIDE on the other. Each tablet contains 10 mg of timolol maleate and 25 mg of hydrochlorothiazide. They are supplied as follows:

NDC 0006-0067-68 bottles of 100.

Shown in Product Identification Guide, page 324

Storage

Store at controlled room temperature, 15–30°C (59–86°F). Keep container tightly closed. Protect from light.

7928433 Issued June 1998

Continued on next page

Information on the Merck & Co., Inc. products listed on these pages is the full prescribing information from product circulars in use September 30, 2000. For information, please call 1-800-NSC MERCK [1-800-672-6372].

TIMOPTIC® Sterile Ophthalmic Solution 0.25% and 0.5% ℞
(Timolol Maleate Ophthalmic Solution)

DESCRIPTION

TIMOPTIC* (timolol maleate ophthalmic solution) is a non-selective beta-adrenergic receptor blocking agent. Its chemical name is (-)-1-(*tert*-butylamino)-3-[(4-morpholino-1,2,5-thiadiazol-3-yl)oxy]-2-propanol maleate (1:1) (salt). Timolol maleate possesses an asymmetric carbon atom in its structure and is provided as the levo-isomer. The optical rotation of timolol maleate is:

$[\alpha]^{25°}_{405\ nm}$ in 1.0N HCl (C = 5%) = −12.2° (−11.7° to −12.5°).

Its molecular formula is $C_{13}H_{24}N_4O_3S{\cdot}C_4H_4O_4$ and its structural formula is:

Timolol maleate has a molecular weight of 432.50. It is a white, odorless, crystalline powder which is soluble in water, methanol, and alcohol. TIMOPTIC is stable at room temperature.
TIMOPTIC Ophthalmic Solution is supplied as a sterile, isotonic, buffered, aqueous solution of timolol maleate in two dosage strengths: Each mL of TIMOPTIC 0.25% contains 2.5 mg of timolol (3.4 mg of timolol maleate). Each mL of TIMOPTIC 0.5% contains 5 mg of timolol (6.8 mg of timolol maleate). Inactive ingredients: monobasic and dibasic sodium phosphate, sodium hydroxide to adjust pH, and water for injection. Benzalkonium chloride 0.01% is added as preservative.

*Registered trademark of MERCK & CO., INC.

CLINICAL PHARMACOLOGY

Mechanism of Action

Timolol maleate is a $beta_1$ and $beta_2$ (non-selective) adrenergic receptor blocking agent that does not have significant intrinsic sympathomimetic, direct myocardial depressant, or local anesthetic (membrane-stabilizing) activity.
Beta-adrenergic receptor blockade reduces cardiac output in both healthy subjects and patients with heart disease. In patients with severe impairment of myocardial infarction, beta-adrenergic receptor blockade may inhibit the stimulatory effect of the sympathetic nervous system necessary to maintain adequate cardiac function.
Beta-adrenergic receptor blockade in the bronchi and bronchioles results in increased airway resistance from unopposed parasympathetic activity. Such an effect in patients with asthma or other bronchospastic conditions is potentially dangerous.
TIMOPTIC Ophthalmic Solution, when applied topically on the eye, has the action of reducing elevated as well as normal intraocular pressure, whether or not accompanied by glaucoma. Elevated intraocular pressure is a major risk factor in the pathogenesis of glaucomatous visual field loss. The higher the level of intraocular pressure, the greater the likelihood of glaucomatous visual field loss and optic nerve damage.
The onset of reduction in intraocular pressure following administration of TIMOPTIC can usually be detected within one-half hour after a single dose. The maximum effect usually occurs in one to two hours and significant lowering of intraocular pressure can be maintained for periods as long as 24 hours with a single dose. Repeated observations over a period of one year indicate that the intraocular pressure-lowering effect of TIMOPTIC is well maintained.
The precise mechanism of the ocular hypotensive action of TIMOPTIC is not clearly established at this time. Tonography and fluorophotometry studies in man suggest that its predominant action may be related to reduced aqueous formation. However, in some studies a slight increase in outflow facility was also observed.
Pharmacokinetics
In a study of plasma drug concentration in six subjects, the systemic exposure to timolol was determined following twice daily administration of TIMOPTIC 0.5%. The mean peak plasma concentration following morning dosing was 0.46 ng/mL and following afternoon dosing was 0.35 ng/mL.
Clinical Studies
In controlled multiclinic studies in patients with untreated intraocular pressures of 22 mmHg or greater, TIMOPTIC 0.25 percent or 0.5 percent administered twice a day produced a greater reduction in intraocular pressure than 1, 2, 3, or 4 percent pilocarpine solution administered four times a day or 0.5, 1, or 2 percent epinephrine hydrochloride solution administered twice a day.
In these studies, TIMOPTIC was generally well tolerated and produced fewer and less severe side effects than either pilocarpine or epinephrine. A slight reduction of resting heart rate in some patients receiving TIMOPTIC (mean reduction 2.9 beats/minute standard deviation 10.2) was observed.

INDICATIONS AND USAGE

TIMOPTIC Ophthalmic Solution is indicated in the treatment of elevated intraocular pressure in patients with ocular hypertension or open-angle glaucoma.

CONTRAINDICATIONS

TIMOPTIC is contraindicated in patients with (1) bronchial asthma; (2) a history of bronchial asthma; (3) severe chronic obstructive pulmonary disease (see WARNINGS); (4) sinus bradycardia; (5) second or third degree atrioventricular block; (6) overt cardiac failure (see WARNINGS); (7) cardiogenic shock; or (8) hypersensitivity to any component of this product.

WARNINGS

As with many topically applied ophthalmic drugs, this drug is absorbed systemically.
The same adverse reactions found with systemic administration of beta-adrenergic blocking agents may occur with topical administration. For example, severe respiratory reactions and cardiac reactions, including death due to bronchospasm in patients with asthma, and rarely death in association with cardiac failure, have been reported following systemic or ophthalmic administration of timolol maleate (see CONTRAINDICATIONS).
Cardiac Failure
Sympathetic stimulation may be essential for support of the circulation in individuals with diminished myocardial contractility, and its inhibition by beta-adrenergic receptor blockade may precipitate more severe failure.
In Patients Without a History of Cardiac Failure continued depression of the myocardium with beta-blocking agents over a period of time can, in some cases, lead to cardiac failure. At the first sign or symptom of cardiac failure TIMOPTIC should be discontinued.
Obstructive Pulmonary Disease
Patients with chronic obstructive pulmonary disease (e.g., chronic bronchitis, emphysema) of mild or moderate severity, bronchospastic disease, or a history of bronchospastic disease (other than bronchial asthma or a history of bronchial asthma, in which TIMOPTIC is contraindicated [see CONTRAINDICATIONS]) should, in general, not receive beta-blockers, including TIMOPTIC.
Major Surgery
The necessity or desirability of withdrawal of beta-adrenergic blocking agents prior to major surgery is controversial. Beta-adrenergic receptor blockade impairs the ability of the heart to respond to beta-adrenergically mediated reflex stimuli. This may augment the risk of general anesthesia in surgical procedures. Some patients receiving beta-adrenergic receptor blocking agents have experienced protracted severe hypotension during anesthesia. Difficulty in restarting and maintaining the heartbeat has also been reported. For these reasons, in patients undergoing elective surgery, some authorities recommend gradual withdrawal of beta-adrenergic receptor blocking agents.
If necessary during surgery, the effects of beta-adrenergic blocking agents may be reversed by sufficient doses of adrenergic agonists.
Diabetes Mellitus
Beta-adrenergic blocking agents should be administered with caution in patients subject to spontaneous hypoglycemia or to diabetic patients (especially those with labile diabetes) who are receiving insulin or oral hypoglycemic agents. Beta-adrenergic receptor blocking agents may mask the signs and symptoms of acute hypoglycemia.
Thyrotoxicosis
Beta-adrenergic blocking agents may mask certain clinical signs (e.g., tachycardia) of hyperthyroidism. Patients suspected of developing thyrotoxicosis should be managed carefully to avoid abrupt withdrawal of beta-adrenergic blocking agents that might precipitate a thyroid storm.

PRECAUTIONS

General
Because of potential effects of beta-adrenergic blocking agents on blood pressure and pulse, these agents should be used with caution in patients with cerebrovascular insufficiency. If signs or symptoms suggesting reduced cerebral blood flow develop following initiation of therapy with TIMOPTIC, alternative therapy should be considered.
There have been reports of bacterial keratitis associated with the use of multiple dose containers of topical ophthalmic products. These containers had been inadvertently contaminated by patients who, in most cases, had a concurrent corneal disease or a disruption of the ocular epithelial surface. (See PRECAUTIONS, *Information for Patients.*)
Choroidal detachment after filtration procedures has been reported with the administration of aqueous suppressant therapy (e.g. timolol).
Angle-closure glaucoma: In patients with angle-closure glaucoma, the immediate objective of treatment is to reopen the angle. This requires constricting the pupil. Timolol maleate has little or no effect on the pupil. TIMOPTIC should not be used alone in the treatment of angle-closure glaucoma.
Anaphylaxis: While taking beta-blockers, patients with a history of atopy or a history of severe anaphylactic reactions to a variety of allergens may be more reactive to repeated accidental, diagnostic, or therapeutic challenge with such allergens. Such patients may be unresponsive to the usual doses of epinephrine used to treat anaphylactic reactions.
Muscle Weakness: Beta-adrenergic blockade has been reported to potentiate muscle weakness consistent with certain myasthenic symptoms (e.g., diplopia, ptosis, and generalized weakness). Timolol has been reported rarely to increase muscle weakness in some patients with myasthenia gravis or myasthenic symptoms.
Information for Patients
Patients should be instructed to avoid allowing the tip of the dispensing container to contact the eye or surrounding structures.
Patients should also be instructed that ocular solutions, if handled improperly, can become contaminated by common bacteria known to cause ocular infections. Serious damage to the eye and subsequent loss of vision may result from using contaminated solutions. (See PRECAUTIONS, *General.*)
Patients should also be advised that if they have ocular surgery or develop an intercurrent ocular condition (e.g., trauma or infection), they should immediately seek their physician's advice concerning the use of the present multidose container.
Patients with bronchial asthma, a history of bronchial asthma, severe chronic obstructive pulmonary disease, sinus bradycardia, second or third degree atrioventricular block, or cardiac failure should be advised not to take this product. (See CONTRAINDICATIONS.)
Patients should be advised that TIMOPTIC contains benzalkonium chloride which may be absorbed by soft contact lenses. Contact lenses should be removed prior to administration of the solution. Lenses may be reinserted 15 minutes following TIMOPTIC administration.
Drug Interactions
Although TIMOPTIC used alone has little or no effect on pupil size, mydriasis resulting from concomitant therapy with TIMOPTIC and epinephrine has been reported occasionally.
Beta-adrenergic blocking agents: Patients who are receiving a beta-adrenergic blocking agent orally and TIMOPTIC should be observed for potential additive effects of beta-blockade, both systemic and on intraocular pressure. The concomitant use of two topical beta-adrenergic blocking agents is not recommended.
Calcium antagonists: Caution should be used in the coadministration of beta-adrenergic blocking agents, such as TIMOPTIC, and oral or intravenous calcium antagonists because of possible atrioventricular conduction disturbances, left ventricular failure, and hypotension. In patients with impaired cardiac function, coadministration should be avoided.
Catecholamine-depleting drugs: Close observation of the patient is recommended when a beta blocker is administered to patients receiving catecholamine-depleting drugs such as reserpine, because of possible additive effects and the production of hypotension and/or marked bradycardia, which may result in vertigo, syncope, or postural hypotension.
Digitalis and calcium antagonists: The concomitant use of beta-adrenergic blocking agents with digitalis and calcium antagonists may have additive effects in prolonging atrioventricular conduction time.
Quinidine: Potentiated systemic beta-blockade (e.g., decreased heart rate) has been reported during combined treatment with quinidine and timolol, possibly because quinidine inhibits the metabolism of timolol via the P-450 enzyme, CYP2D6.
Clonidine: Oral beta-adrenergic blocking agents may exacerbate the rebound hypertension which can follow the withdrawal of clonidine. There have been no reports of exacerbation of rebound hypertension with ophthalmic timolol maleate.
Injectable epinephrine: (See PRECAUTIONS, *General, Anaphylaxis*)
Carcinogenesis, Mutagenesis, Impairment of Fertility
In a two-year oral study of timolol maleate administered orally to rats, there was a statistically significant increase in the incidence of adrenal pheochromocytomas in male rats administered 300 mg/kg/day (approximately 42,000 times the systemic exposure following the maximum recommended human ophthalmic dose). Similar differences were not observed in rats administered oral doses equivalent to approximately 14,000 times the maximum recommended human ophthalmic dose.
In a lifetime oral study in mice, there were statistically significant increases in the incidence of benign and malignant pulmonary tumors, benign uterine polyps and mammary adenocarcinomas in female mice at 500 mg/kg/day (approximately 71,000 times the systemic exposure following the maximum recommended human ophthalmic dose), but not at 5 or 50 mg/kg/day (approximately 700 or 7,000, respectively, times the systemic exposure following the maximum recommended human ophthalmic dose). In a subsequent study in female mice, in which post-mortem examinations were limited to the uterus and the lungs, a statistically significant increase in the incidence of pulmonary tumors was again observed at 500 mg/kg/day.
The increased occurrence of mammary adenocarcinomas was associated with elevations in serum prolactin which occurred in female mice administered oral timolol at 500 mg/kg/day, but not at doses of 5 or 50 mg/kg/day. An increased incidence of mammary adenocarcinomas in rodents has been associated with administration of several other therapeutic agents that elevate serum prolactin, but no correlation between serum prolactin levels and mammary tumors

has been established in humans. Furthermore, in adult human female subjects who received oral dosages of up to 60 mg of timolol maleate (the maximum recommended human oral dosage), there were no clinically meaningful changes in serum prolactin.

Timolol maleate was devoid of mutagenic potential when tested *in vivo* (mouse) in the micronucleus test and cytogenetic assay (doses up to 800 mg/kg) and *in vitro* in a neoplastic cell transformation assay (up to 100 mcg/mL). In Ames tests the highest concentrations of timolol employed, 5000 or 10,000 mcg/plate, were associated with statistically significant elevations of revertants observed with tester strain TA100 (in seven replicate assays), but not in the remaining three strains. In the assays with tester strain TA100, no consistent dose response relationship was observed, and the ratio of test to control revertants did not reach 2. A ratio of 2 is usually considered the criterion for a positive Ames test.

Reproduction and fertility studies in rats demonstrated no adverse effect on male or female fertility at doses up to 21,000 times the systemic exposure following the maximum recommended human ophthalmic dose.

Pregnancy:

Teratogenic Effects—Pregnancy Category C. Teratogenicity studies with timolol in mice, rats, and rabbits at oral doses up to 50 mg/kg/day (7,000 times the systemic exposure following the maximum recommended human ophthalmic dose) demonstrated no evidence of fetal malformations. Although delayed fetal ossification was observed at this dose in rats, there were no adverse effects on postnatal development of offspring. Doses of 1000 mg/kg/day (142,000 times the systemic exposure following the maximum recommended human ophthalmic dose) were maternotoxic in mice and resulted in an increased number of fetal resorptions. Increased fetal resorptions were also seen in rabbits at doses of 14,000 times the systemic exposure following the maximum recommended human ophthalmic dose, in this case without apparent maternotoxicity.

There are no adequate and well-controlled studies in pregnant women. TIMOPTIC should be used during pregnancy only if the potential benefit justifies the potential risk to the fetus.

Nursing Mothers

Timolol maleate has been detected in human milk following oral and ophthalmic drug administration. Because of the potential for serious adverse reactions from TIMOPTIC in nursing infants, a decision should be made whether to discontinue nursing or to discontinue the drug, taking into account the importance of the drug to the mother.

Pediatric Use

Safety and effectiveness in pediatric patients have not been established.

ADVERSE REACTIONS

The most frequently reported adverse experiences have been burning and stinging upon instillation (approximately one in eight patients).

The following additional adverse experiences have been reported less frequently with ocular administration of this or other timolol maleate formulations:

BODY AS A WHOLE

Headache, asthenia/fatigue, and chest pain.

CARDIOVASCULAR

Bradycardia, arrhythmia, hypotension, hypertension, syncope, heart block, cerebral vascular accident, cerebral ischemia, cardiac failure, worsening of angina pectoris, palpitation, cardiac arrest, pulmonary edema, edema, claudication, Raynaud's phenomenon, and cold hands and feet.

DIGESTIVE

Nausea, diarrhea, dyspepsia, anorexia, and dry mouth.

IMMUNOLOGIC

Systemic lupus erythematosus.

NERVOUS SYSTEM/PSYCHIATRIC

Dizziness, increase in signs and symptoms of myasthenia gravis, paresthesia, somnolence, insomnia, nightmares, behavioral changes and psychic disturbances including depression, confusion, hallucinations, anxiety, disorientation, nervousness, and memory loss.

SKIN

Alopecia and psoriasiform rash or exacerbation of psoriasis.

HYPERSENSITIVITY

Signs and symptoms of systemic allergic reactions, including angioedema, urticaria, and localized and generalized rash.

RESPIRATORY

Bronchospasm (predominantly in patients with pre-existing bronchospastic disease), respiratory failure, dyspnea, nasal congestion, cough and upper respiratory infections.

ENDOCRINE

Masked symptoms of hypoglycemia in diabetic patients (see WARNINGS).

SPECIAL SENSES

Signs and symptoms of ocular irritation including conjunctivitis, blepharitis, keratitis, ocular pain, discharge (e.g., crusting), foreign body sensation, itching and tearing, and dry eyes; ptosis; decreased corneal sensitivity; cystoid macular edema; visual disturbances including refractive changes and diplopia; pseudopemphigoid; choroidal detachment following filtration surgery (see PRECAUTIONS, *General*); and tinnitus.

UROGENITAL

Retroperitoneal fibrosis, decreased libido, impotence, and Peyronie's disease.

The following additional adverse effects have been reported in clinical experience with ORAL timolol maleate or other ORAL beta-blocking agents and may be considered potential effects of ophthalmic timolol maleate: *Allergic:* Erythematous rash, fever combined with aching and sore throat, laryngospasm with respiratory distress; *Body as a Whole:* Extremity pain, decreased exercise tolerance, weight loss; *Cardiovascular:* Worsening of arterial insufficiency, vasodilatation; *Digestive:* Gastrointestinal pain, hepatomegaly, vomiting, mesenteric arterial thrombosis, ischemic colitis; *Hematologic:* Nonthrombocytopenic purpura; thrombocytopenic purpura, agranulocytosis; *Endocrine:* Hyperglycemia, hypoglycemia; *Skin:* Pruritus, skin irritation, increased pigmentation, sweating; *Musculoskeletal:* Arthralgia; *Nervous System/Psychiatric:* Vertigo, local weakness, diminished concentration, reversible mental depression progressing to catatonia, an acute reversible syndrome characterized by disorientation for time and place, emotional lability, slightly clouded sensorium, and decreased performance on neuropsychometrics; *Respiratory:* Rales, bronchial obstruction; *Urogenital:* Urination difficulties.

OVERDOSAGE

There have been reports of inadvertent overdosage with TIMOPTIC Ophthalmic Solution resulting in systemic effects similar to those seen with systemic beta-adrenergic blocking agents such as dizziness, headache, shortness of breath, bradycardia, bronchospasm, and cardiac arrest (see also ADVERSE REACTIONS).

Overdosage has been reported with Tablets BLOCADREN* (timolol maleate tablets). A 30 year old female ingested 650 mg of BLOCADREN (maximum recommended oral daily dose is 60 mg) and experienced second and third degree heart block. She recovered without treatment but approximately two months later developed irregular heartbeat, hypertension, dizziness, tinnitus, faintness, increased pulse rate, and borderline first degree heart block.

An *in vitro* hemodialysis study, using^{14}C timolol added to human plasma or whole blood, showed that timolol was readily dialyzed from these fluids; however, a study of patients with renal failure showed that timolol did not dialyze readily.

* Registered trademark of MERCK & CO., INC.

DOSAGE AND ADMINISTRATION

TIMOPTIC Ophthalmic Solution is available in concentrations of 0.25 and 0.5 percent. The usual starting dose is one drop of 0.25 percent TIMOPTIC in the affected eye(s) twice a day. If the clinical response is not adequate, the dosage may be changed to one drop of 0.5 percent solution in the affected eye(s) twice a day.

Since in some patients the pressure-lowering response to TIMOPTIC may require a few weeks to stabilize, evaluation should include a determination of intraocular pressure after approximately 4 weeks of treatment with TIMOPTIC.

If the intraocular pressure is maintained at satisfactory levels, the dosage schedule may be changed to one drop once a day in the affected eye(s). Because of diurnal variations in intraocular pressure, satisfactory response to the once-a-day dose is best determined by measuring the intraocular pressure at different times during the day.

Dosages above one drop of 0.5 percent TIMOPTIC twice a day generally have not been shown to produce further reduction in intraocular pressure. If the patient's intraocular pressure is still not at a satisfactory level on this regimen, concomitant therapy with other agent(s) for lowering intraocular pressure can be instituted. The concomitant use of two topical beta-adrenergic blocking agents is not recommended. (See PRECAUTIONS, *Drug Interactions, Beta-adrenergic blocking agents.*)

HOW SUPPLIED

Sterile Ophthalmic Solution TIMOPTIC is a clear, colorless to light yellow solution.

No. 3366—TIMOPTIC Ophthalmic Solution, 0.25% timolol equivalent, is supplied in a white, opaque, plastic OCUMETER* ophthalmic dispenser with a controlled drop tip as follows:

NDC 0006-3366-32, 2.5 mL
NDC 0006-3366-03, 5 mL
NDC 0006-3366-10, 10 mL
NDC 0006-3366-12, 15 mL.

No. 3367—TIMOPTIC Ophthalmic Solution, 0.5% timolol equivalent, is supplied in a white, opaque, plastic OCUMETER ophthalmic dispenser with a controlled drop tip as follows:

NDC 0006-3367-32, 2.5 mL
NDC 0006-3367-03, 5 mL
NDC 0006-3367-10, 10 mL
NDC 0006-3367-12, 15 mL.

Storage

Store at room temperature, 15–30°C (59–86°F).
Protect from freezing. Protect from light.

*Registered trademark of MERCK & CO., INC.

9010842 Issued April 2000

TIMOPTIC® ℞
0.25% and 0.5%
(Timolol Maleate Ophthalmic Solution)
in OCUDOSE® (Dispenser)
Preservative-Free Sterile Ophthalmic Solution
in a Sterile Ophthalmic Unit Dose Dispenser

DESCRIPTION

Timolol maleate is a non-selective beta-adrenergic receptor blocking agent. Its chemical name is (-)-1-(*tert*-butylamino)-3-[(4-morpholino-1,2,5-thiadiazol-3-yl)oxy]-2-propanol maleate (1:1) (salt). Timolol maleate possesses an asymmetric carbon atom in its structure and is provided as the levo-isomer. The nominal optical rotation of timolol maleate is

$$[\alpha]^{25°}_{405\ nm} \text{ in 1.0N HCl (C = 5\%) } = -12.2° \ (-11.7° \text{ to } -12.5°).$$

Its molecular formula is $C_{13}H_{24}N_4O_3S{\cdot}C_4H_4O_4$ and its structural formula is:

Timolol maleate has a molecular weight of 432.50. It is a white, odorless, crystalline powder which is soluble in water, methanol, and alcohol. Timolol maleate is stable at room temperature.

Timolol maleate ophthalmic solution is supplied in two formulations: Ophthalmic Solution TIMOPTIC* (timolol maleate ophthalmic solution), which contains the preservative benzalkonium chloride; and Ophthalmic Solution TIMOPTIC* (timolol maleate ophthalmic solution), the preservative-free formulation.

Preservative-free Ophthalmic Solution TIMOPTIC is supplied in OCUDOSE*, a unit dose container, as a sterile, isotonic, buffered, aqueous solution of timolol maleate in two dosage strengths: Each mL of Preservative-free TIMOPTIC in OCUDOSE 0.25% contains 2.5 mg of timolol (3.4 mg of timolol maleate). Each mL of Preservative-free TIMOPTIC in OCUDOSE 0.5% contains 5 mg of timolol (6.8 mg of timolol maleate). Inactive ingredients: monobasic and dibasic sodium phosphate, sodium hydroxide to adjust pH, and water for injection.

*Registered trademark of MERCK & CO., INC.

CLINICAL PHARMACOLOGY

Mechanism of Action

Timolol maleate is a $beta_1$ and $beta_2$ (non-selective) adrenergic receptor blocking agent that does not have significant intrinsic sympathomimetic, direct myocardial depressant, or local anesthetic (membrane-stabilizing) activity.

Beta-adrenergic receptor blockade reduces cardiac output in both healthy subjects and patients with heart disease. In patients with severe impairment of myocardial function beta-adrenergic receptor blockade may inhibit the stimulatory effect of the sympathetic nervous system necessary to maintain adequate cardiac function.

Beta-adrenergic receptor blockade in the bronchi and bronchioles results in increased airway resistance from unopposed parasympathetic activity. Such an effect in patients with asthma or other bronchospastic conditions is potentially dangerous.

TIMOPTIC (timolol maleate ophthalmic solution), when applied topically on the eye, has the action of reducing elevated as well as normal intraocular pressure, whether or not accompanied by glaucoma. Elevated intraocular pressure is a major risk factor in the pathogenesis of glaucomatous visual field loss. The higher the level of intraocular pressure, the greater the likelihood of glaucomatous visual field loss and optic nerve damage.

The onset of reduction in intraocular pressure following administration of TIMOPTIC (timolol maleate ophthalmic solution) can usually be detected within one-half hour after a single dose. The maximum effect usually occurs in one to two hours and significant lowering of intraocular pressure can be maintained for periods as long as 24 hours with a single dose. Repeated observations over a period of one year indicate that the intraocular pressure-lowering effect of TIMOPTIC (timolol maleate ophthalmic solution) is well maintained.

The precise mechanism of the ocular hypotensive action of TIMOPTIC (timolol maleate ophthalmic solution) is not clearly established at this time. Tonography and fluorophotometry studies in man suggest that its predominant action may be related to reduced aqueous formation. However, in some studies a slight increase in outflow facility was also observed.

Continued on next page

Information on the Merck & Co., Inc. products listed on these pages is the full prescribing information from product circulars in use September 30, 2000. For information, please call 1-800-NSC MERCK [1-800-672-6372].

Timoptic in Ocudose—Cont.

Pharmacokinetics
In a study of plasma drug concentration in six subjects, the systemic exposure to timolol was determined following twice daily administration of TIMOPTIC 0.5%. The mean peak plasma concentration following morning dosing was 0.46 ng/mL and following afternoon dosing was 0.35 ng/mL.
Clinical Studies
In controlled multiclinic studies in patients with untreated intraocular pressures of 22 mmHg or greater, TIMOPTIC (timolol maleate ophthalmic solution) 0.25 percent or 0.5 percent administered twice a day produced a greater reduction in intraocular pressure than 1,2,3, or 4 percent pilocarpine solution administered four times a day or 0.5, 1, or 2 percent epinephrine hydrochloride solution administered twice a day.
In these studies, TIMOPTIC (timolol maleate ophthalmic solution) was generally well tolerated and produced fewer and less severe side effects than either pilocarpine or epinephrine. A slight reduction of resting heart rate in some patients receiving TIMOPTIC (timolol maleate ophthalmic solution) (mean reduction 2.9 beats/minute standard deviation 10.2) was observed.

INDICATIONS AND USAGE

Preservative-free TIMOPTIC in OCUDOSE is indicated in the treatment of elevated intraocular pressure in patients with ocular hypertension or open-angle glaucoma.
Preservative-free TIMOPTIC in OCUDOSE may be used when a patient is sensitive to the preservative in TIMOPTIC (timolol maleate ophthalmic solution), benzalkonium chloride, or when use of a preservative-free topical medication is advisable.

CONTRAINDICATIONS

Preservative-free TIMOPTIC in OCUDOSE is contraindicated in patients with (1) bronchial asthma; (2) a history of bronchial asthma; (3) severe chronic obstructive pulmonary disease (see WARNINGS); (4) sinus bradycardia; (5) second or third degree atrioventricular block; (6) overt cardiac failure (see WARNINGS); (7) cardiogenic shock; or (8) hypersensitivity to any component of this product.

WARNINGS

As with many topically applied ophthalmic drugs, this drug is absorbed systemically.
The same adverse reactions found with systemic administration of beta-adrenergic blocking agents may occur with topical administration. For example, severe respiratory reactions and cardiac reactions, including death due to bronchospasm in patients with asthma, and rarely death in association with cardiac failure, have been reported following systemic or ophthalmic administration of timolol maleate (see CONTRAINDICATIONS).
Cardiac Failure
Sympathetic stimulation may be essential for support of the circulation in individuals with diminished myocardial contractility, and its inhibition by beta-adrenergic receptor blockade may precipitate more severe failure.
In Patients Without a History of Cardiac Failure continued depression of the myocardium with beta-blocking agents over a period of time can, in some cases, lead to cardiac failure. At the first sign or symptom of cardiac failure Preservative-free TIMOPTIC in OCUDOSE should be discontinued.
Obstructive Pulmonary Disease
Patients with chronic obstructive pulmonary disease (e.g., chronic bronchitis, emphysema) of mild or moderate severity, bronchospastic disease, or a history of bronchospastic disease (other than bronchial asthma or a history of bronchial asthma, in which TIMOPTIC in OCUDOSE is contraindicated [see CONTRAINDICATIONS]) should, in general, not receive beta-blockers, including Preservative-free TIMOPTIC in OCUDOSE.
Major Surgery
The necessity or desirability of withdrawal of beta-adrenergic blocking agents prior to major surgery is controversial. Beta-adrenergic receptor blockade impairs the ability of the heart to respond to beta-adrenergically mediated reflex stimuli. This may augment the risk of general anesthesia in surgical procedures. Some patients receiving beta-adrenergic receptor blocking agents have experienced protracted severe hypotension during anesthesia. Difficulty in restarting and maintaining the heartbeat has also been reported. For these reasons, in patients undergoing elective surgery, some authorities recommend gradual withdrawal of beta-adrenergic receptor blocking agents.
If necessary during surgery, the effects of beta-adrenergic blocking agents may be reversed by sufficient doses of adrenergic agonists.
Diabetes Mellitus
Beta-adrenergic blocking agents should be administered with caution in patients subject to spontaneous hypoglycemia or to diabetic patients (especially those with labile diabetes) who are receiving insulin or oral hypoglycemic agents. Beta-adrenergic receptor blocking agents may mask the signs and symptoms of acute hypoglycemia.
Thyrotoxicosis
Beta-adrenergic blocking agents may mask certain clinical signs (e.g., tachycardia) of hyperthyroidism. Patients suspected of developing thyrotoxicosis should be managed carefully to avoid abrupt withdrawal of beta-adrenergic blocking agents that might precipitate a thyroid storm.

PRECAUTIONS

General
Because of potential effects of beta-adrenergic blocking agents on blood pressure and pulse, these agents should be used with caution in patients with cerebrovascular insufficiency. If signs or symptoms suggesting reduced cerebral blood flow develop following initiation of therapy with Preservative-free TIMOPTIC in OCUDOSE, alternative therapy should be considered.
Choroidal detachment after filtration procedures has been reported with the administration of aqueous suppressant therapy (e.g. timolol).
Angle-closure glaucoma: In patients with angle-closure glaucoma, the immediate objective of treatment is to reopen the angle. This requires constricting the pupil. Timolol maleate has little or no effect on the pupil. TIMOPTIC in OCUDOSE should not be used alone in the treatment of angle-closure glaucoma.
Anaphylaxis: While taking beta-blockers, patients with a history of atopy or a history of severe anaphylactic reactions to a variety of allergens may be more reactive to repeated accidental, diagnostic, or therapeutic challenge with such allergens. Such patients may be unresponsive to the usual doses of epinephrine used to treat anaphylactic reactions.
Muscle Weakness: Beta-adrenergic blockade has been reported to potentiate muscle weakness consistent with certain myasthenic symptoms (e.g., diplopia, ptosis, and generalized weakness). Timolol has been reported rarely to increase muscle weakness in some patients with myasthenia gravis or myasthenic symptoms.
Information for Patients
Patients should be instructed about the use of Preservative-free TIMOPTIC in OCUDOSE.
Since sterility cannot be maintained after the individual unit is opened, patients should be instructed to use the product immediately after opening, and to discard the individual unit and any remaining contents immediately after use.
Patients with bronchial asthma, a history of bronchial asthma, severe chronic obstructive pulmonary disease, sinus bradycardia, second or third degree atrioventricular block, or cardiac failure should be advised not to take this product. (See CONTRAINDICATIONS.)
Drug Interactions
Although TIMOPTIC (timolol maleate ophthalmic solution) used alone has little or no effect on pupil size, mydriasis resulting from concomitant therapy with TIMOPTIC (timolol maleate ophthalmic solution) and epinephrine has been reported occasionally.
Beta-adrenergic blocking agents: Patients who are receiving a beta-adrenergic blocking agent orally and Preservative-free TIMOPTIC in OCUDOSE should be observed for potential additive effects of beta-blockade, both systemic and on intraocular pressure. The concomitant use of two topical beta-adrenergic blocking agents is not recommended.
Calcium antagonists: Caution should be used in the coadministration of beta-adrenergic blocking agents, such as Preservative-free TIMOPTIC in OCUDOSE, and oral or intravenous calcium antagonists, because of possible atrioventricular conduction disturbances, left ventricular failure, and hypotension. In patients with impaired cardiac function, coadministration should be avoided.
Catecholamine-depleting drugs: Close observation of the patient is recommended when a beta blocker is administered to patients receiving catecholamine-depleting drugs such as reserpine, because of possible additive effects and the production of hyotension and/or marked bradycardia, which may result in vertigo, syncope, or postural hypotension.
Digitalis and calcium antagonists: The concomitant use of beta-adrenergic blocking agents with digitalis and calcium antagonists may have additive effects in prolonging atrioventricular conduction time.
Quinidine: Potentiated systemic beta-blockade (e.g., decreased heart rate) has been reported during combined treatment with quinidine and timolol, possibly because quinidine inhibits the metabolism of timolol via the P-450 enzyme, CYP2D6.
Clonidine: Oral beta-adrenergic blocking agents may exacerbate the rebound hypertension which can follow the withdrawal of clonidine. There have been no reports of exacerbation of rebound hypertension with ophthalmic timolol maleate.
Injectable epinephrine: (See PRECAUTIONS, *General, Anaphylaxis*)
Carcinogenesis, Mutagenesis, Impairment of Fertility
In a two-year oral study of timolol maleate administered orally to rats, there was a statistically significant increase in the incidence of adrenal pheochromocytomas in male rats administered 300 mg/kg/day (approximately 42,000 times the systemic exposure following the maximum recommended human ophthalmic dose). Similar differences were not observed in rats administered oral doses equivalent to approximately 14,000 times the maximum recommended human ophthalmic dose.
In a lifetime oral study in mice, there were statistically significant increases in the incidence of benign and malignant pulmonary tumors, benign uterine polyps and mammary adenocarcinomas in female mice at 500 mg/kg/day (approximately 71,000 times the systemic exposure following the maximum recommended human ophthalmic dose), but not at 5 or 50 mg/kg/day (approximately 700 or 7,000 times, respectively, the systemic exposure following the maximum recommended human ophthalmic dose). In a subsequent study in female mice, in which post-mortem examinations were limited to the uterus and the lungs, a statistically significant increase in the incidence of pulmonary tumors was again observed at 500 mg/kg/day.
The increased occurrence of mammary adenocarcinomas was associated with elevations in serum prolactin which occurred in female mice administered oral timolol at 500 mg/kg/day, but not at doses of 5 or 50 mg/kg/day. An increased incidence of mammary adenocarcinomas in rodents has been associated with administration of several other therapeutic agents that elevate serum prolactin, but no correlation between serum prolactin levels and mammary tumors has been established in humans. Furthermore, in adult human female subjects who received oral dosages of up to 60 mg of timolol maleate (the maximum recommended human oral dosage), there were no clinically meaningful changes in serum prolactin.
Timolol maleate was devoid of mutagenic potential when tested *in vivo* (mouse) in the micronucleus test and cytogenetic assay (doses up to 800 mg/kg) and *in vitro* in a neoplastic cell transformation assay (up to 100 mcg/mL). In Ames tests the highest concentrations of timolol employed, 5000 or 10,000 mcg/plate, were associated with statistically significant elevations of revertants observed with tester strain TA 100 (in seven replicate assays), but not in the remaining three strains. In the assays with tester strain TA 100, no consistent dose response relationship was observed, and the ratio of test to control revertants did not reach 2. A ratio of 2 is usually considered the criterion for a positive Ames test.
Reproduction and fertility studies in rats demonstrated no adverse effect on male or female fertility at doses up to 21,000 times the systemic exposure following the maximum recommended human ophthalmic dose.
Pregnancy:
Teratogenic Effects—Pregnancy Category C. Teratogenicity studies with timolol in mice, rats and rabbits at oral doses up to 50 mg/kg/day (7,000 times the systemic exposure following the maximum recommended human ophthalmic dose) demonstrated no evidence of fetal malformations. Although delayed fetal ossification was observed at this dose in rats, there were no adverse effects on postnatal development of offspring. Doses of 1000 mg/kg/day (142,000 times the systemic exposure following the maximum recommended human ophthalmic dose) were maternotoxic in mice and resulted in an increased number of fetal resorptions. Increased fetal resorptions were also seen in rabbits at doses of 14,000 times the systemic exposure following the maximum recommended human ophthalmic dose, in this case without apparent maternotoxicity.
There are no adequate and well-controlled studies in pregnant women. Preservative-free TIMOPTIC in OCUDOSE should be used during pregnancy only if the potential benefit justifies the potential risk to the fetus.
Nursing Mothers
Timolol maleate has been detected in human milk following oral and ophthalmic drug administration. Because of the potential for serious adverse reactions from timolol in nursing infants, a decision should be made whether to discontinue nursing or to discontinue the drug, taking into account the importance of the drug to the mother.
Pediatric Use
Safety and effectiveness in pediatric patients have not been established.

ADVERSE REACTIONS

The most frequently reported adverse experiences have been burning and stinging upon instillation (approximately one in eight patients).
The following additional adverse experiences have been reported less frequently with ocular administration of this or other timolol maleate formulations:
BODY AS A WHOLE
Headache, asthenia/fatigue, and chest pain.
CARDIOVASCULAR
Bradycardia, arrhythmia, hypotension, hypertension, syncope, heart block, cerebral vascular accident, cerebral ischemia, cardiac failure, worsening of angina pectoris, palpitation, cardiac arrest, pulmonary edema, edema, claudication, Raynaud's phenomenon, and cold hands and feet.
DIGESTIVE
Nausea, diarrhea, dyspepsia, anorexia, and dry mouth.
IMMUNOLOGIC
Systemic lupus erythematosus.
NERVOUS SYSTEM/PSYCHIATRIC
Dizziness, increase in signs and symptoms of myasthenia gravis, paresthesia, somnolence, insomnia, nightmares, behavioral changes and psychic disturbances including depression, confusion, hallucinations, anxiety, disorientation, nervousness, and memory loss.
SKIN
Alopecia and psoriasiform rash or exacerbation of psoriasis.
HYPERSENSITIVITY
Signs and symptoms of systemic allergic reactions, including angioedema, urticaria, and localized and generalized rash.

RESPIRATORY
Bronchospasm (predominantly in patients with pre-existing bronchospastic disease), respiratory failure, dyspnea, nasal congestion, cough and upper respiratory infections.
ENDOCRINE
Masked symptoms of hypoglycemia in diabetic patients (see **WARNINGS**).
SPECIAL SENSES
Signs and symptoms of ocular irritation including conjunctivitis, blepharitis, keratitis, ocular pain, discharge (e.g., crusting), foreign body sensation, itching and tearing, and dry eyes; ptosis; decreased corneal sensitivity; cystoid macular edema; visual disturbances including refractive changes and diplopia; pseudopemphigoid; choroidal detachment following filtration surgery (see PRECAUTIONS, *General*); and tinnitus.
UROGENITAL
Retroperitoneal fibrosis, decreased libido, impotence, and Peyronie's disease.
The following additional adverse effects have been reported in clinical experience with ORAL timolol maleate or other ORAL beta blocking agents, and may be considered potential effects of ophthalmic timolol maleate: *Allergic:* Erythematous rash, fever combined with aching and sore throat, laryngospasm with respiratory distress; *Body as a Whole:* Extremity pain, decreased exercise tolerance, weight loss; *Cardiovascular:* Worsening of arterial insufficiency, vasodilatation; *Digestive:* Gastrointestinal pain, hepatomegaly, vomiting, mesenteric arterial thrombosis, ischemic colitis; *Hematologic:* Nonthrombocytopenic purpura; thrombocytopenic purpura; agranulocytosis; *Endocrine:* Hyperglycemia, hypoglycemia; *Skin:* Pruritus, skin irritation, increased pigmentation, sweating; *Musculoskeletal:* Arthralgia; *Nervous System/Psychiatric:* Vertigo, local weakness, diminished concentration, reversible mental depression progressing to catatonia, an acute reversible syndrome characterized by disorientation for time and place, emotional lability, slightly clouded sensorium, and decreased performance on neuropsychometrics; *Respiratory:* Rales, bronchial obstruction; *Urogenital:* Urination difficulties.

OVERDOSAGE

There have been reports of inadvertent overdosage with Ophthalmic Solution TIMOPTIC (timolol maleate ophthalmic solution) resulting in systemic effects similar to those seen with systemic beta-adrenergic blocking agents such as dizziness, headache, shortness of breath, bradycardia, bronchospasm, and cardiac arrest (see also **ADVERSE REACTIONS**).
Overdosage has been reported with Tablets BLOCADREN* (timolol maleate tablets). A 30 year old female ingested 650 mg of BLOCADREN (maximum recommended oral daily dose is 60 mg) and experienced second and third degree heart block. She recovered without treatment but approximately two months later developed irregular heartbeat, hypertension, dizziness, tinnitus, faintness, increased pulse rate, and borderline first degree heart block.
An *in vitro* hemodialysis study, using ^{14}C timolol added to human plasma or whole blood, showed that timolol was readily dialyzed from these fluids; however, a study of patients with renal failure showed that timolol did not dialyze readily.

*Registered trademark of MERCK & CO., Inc.

DOSAGE AND ADMINISTRATION

Preservative-free TIMOPTIC in OCUDOSE is a sterile solution that does not contain a preservative. The solution from one individual unit is to be used immediately after opening for administration to one or both eyes. Since sterility cannot be guaranteed after the individual unit is opened, the remaining contents should be discarded immediately after administration.
Preservative-free TIMOPTIC in OCUDOSE is available in concentrations of 0.25 and 0.5 percent. The usual starting dose is one drop of 0.25 percent Preservative-free TIMOPTIC in OCUDOSE in the affected eye(s) administered twice a day. Apply enough gentle pressure on the individual container to obtain a single drop of solution. If the clinical response is not adequate, the dosage may be changed to one drop of 0.5 percent solution in the affected eye(s) administered twice a day.
Since in some patients the pressure-lowering response to Preservative-free TIMOPTIC in OCUDOSE may require a few weeks to stabilize, evaluation should include a determination of intraocular pressure after approximately 4 weeks of treatment with Preservative-free TIMOPTIC in OCUDOSE.
If the intraocular pressure is maintained at satisfactory levels, the dosage schedule may be changed to one drop once a day in the affected eye(s). Because of diurnal variations in intraocular pressure, satisfactory response to the once-a-day dose is best determined by measuring the intraocular pressure at different times during the day.
Dosages above one drop of 0.5 percent TIMOPTIC (timolol maleate ophthalmic solution) twice a day generally have not been shown to produce further reduction in intraocular pressure. If the patient's intraocular pressure is still not at a satisfactory level on this regimen, concomitant therapy with other agent(s) for lowering intraocular pressure can be instituted taking into consideration that the preparation(s) used concomitantly may contain one or more preservatives.
The concomitant use of two topical beta-adrenergic blocking agents is not recommended. (See PRECAUTIONS, *Drug Interactions, Beta-adrenergic blocking agents.*)

HOW SUPPLIED

Preservative-free Sterile Ophthalmic Solution TIMOPTIC in OCUDOSE is a clear, colorless to light yellow solution.
No. 9689—Preservative-free TIMOPTIC, 0.25% timolol equivalent, is supplied in OCUDOSE, a clear low density polyethylene unit dose container. Each individual unit contains 0.2 mL of solution, and is available in a foil laminate overwrapped pouch as follows:
NDC 0006-9689-60; 60 Individual Unit Doses
(6505-01-316-8791, 0.25% 60 Individual Unit Doses).
No. 9690—Preservative-free TIMOPTIC, 0.5% timolol equivalent, is supplied in OCUDOSE, a clear low density polyethylene unit dose container. Each individual unit contains 0.2 mL of solution, and is available in a foil laminate overwrapped pouch as follows:
NDC 0006-9690-60; 60 Individual Unit Doses
(6505-01-284-5154, 0.5% 60 Individual Unit Doses).
Storage
Store at room temperature, 15-30°C (59-86°F). Protect from freezing. Protect from light.
Because evaporation can occur through the unprotected polyethylene unit dose container and prolonged exposure to direct light can modify the product, the unit dose container should be kept in the protective foil overwrap and used within one month after the foil package has been opened.
9288801 Issued March 2000

TIMOPTIC-XE® ℞
0.25% and 0.5%
Sterile Ophthalmic Gel Forming Solution
(timolol maleate ophthalmic gel forming solution)

DESCRIPTION

TIMOPTIC-XE* (timolol maleate ophthalmic gel forming solution) is a non-selective beta-adrenergic receptor blocking agent. Its chemical name is (-)-1-(*tert*-butyl-amino)-3-[(4-morpholino-1,2,5-thiadiazol-3-yl)oxy]-2-propanol maleate (1:1) (salt). Timolol maleate possesses an asymmetric carbon atom in its structure and is provided as the levo-isomer. The nominal optical rotation of timolol maleate is:

$$[\alpha]^{25°}_{405\ nm} \quad \text{in 1.0N HCl (C = 5\%)} = -12.2° \quad (-11.7° \text{ to } -12.5°).$$

Its molecular formula is $C_{13}H_{24}N_4O_3S{\cdot}C_4H_4O_4$ and its structural formula is:

Timolol maleate has a molecular weight of 432.50. It is a white, odorless, crystalline powder which is soluble in water, methanol, and alcohol.
TIMOPTIC-XE Sterile Ophthalmic Gel Forming Solution is supplied as a sterile, isotonic, buffered, aqueous solution of timolol maleate in two dosage strengths. Each mL of TIMOPTIC-XE 0.25% contains 2.5 mg of timolol (3.4 mg of timolol maleate). Each mL of TIMOPTIC-XE 0.5% contains 5 mg of timolol (6.8 mg of timolol maleate). Inactive ingredients: GELRITE* gellan gum, tromethamine, mannitol, and water for injection. Preservative: benzododecinium bromide 0.012%.
GELRITE is a purified anionic heteropolysaccharide derived from gellan gum. An aqueous solution of GELRITE, in the presence of a cation, has the ability to gel. Upon contact with the precorneal tear film, TIMOPTIC-XE forms a gel that is subsequently removed by the flow of tears.

* Registered trademark of Merck & Co., Inc.

CLINICAL PHARMACOLOGY

Mechanism of Action
Timolol maleate is a $beta_1$ and $beta_2$ (non-selective) adrenergic receptor blocking agent that does not have significant intrinsic sympathomimetic, direct myocardial depressant, or local anesthetic (membrane-stabilizing) activity.
TIMOPTIC-XE, when applied topically on the eye, has the action of reducing elevated, as well as normal intraocular pressure, whether or not accompanied by glaucoma. Elevated intraocular pressure is a major risk factor in the pathogenesis of glaucomatous visual field loss and optic nerve damage.
The precise mechanism of the ocular hypotensive action of TIMOPTIC-XE is not clearly established at this time. Tonography and fluorophotometry studies of TIMOPTIC* (timolol maleate ophthalmic solution) in man suggest that its predominant action may be related to reduced aqueous formation. However, in some studies, a slight increase in outflow facility was also observed.
Beta-adrenergic receptor blockade reduces cardiac output in both healthy subjects and patients with heart disease. In patients with severe impairment of myocardial function beta-adrenergic receptor blockade may inhibit the stimulatory effect of the sympathetic nervous system necessary to maintain adequate cardiac function.
Beta-adrenergic receptor blockade in the bronchi and bronchioles results in increased airway resistance from unopposed parasympathetic activity. Such an effect in patients with asthma or other bronchospastic conditions is potentially dangerous.
Pharmacokinetics
In a study of plasma drug concentration in six subjects, the systemic exposure to timolol was determined following once daily administration of TIMOPTIC-XE 0.5% in the morning. The mean peak plasma concentration following this morning dose was 0.28 ng/mL.
Clinical Studies
In controlled, double-masked, multicenter clinical studies, comparing TIMOPTIC-XE 0.25% to TIMOPTIC 0.25% and TIMOPTIC-XE 0.5% to TIMOPTIC 0.5%, TIMOPTIC-XE administered once a day was shown to be equally effective in lowering intraocular pressure as the equivalent concentration of TIMOPTIC administered twice a day. The effect of timolol in lowering intraocular pressure was evident for 24 hours with a single dose of TIMOPTIC-XE. Repeated observations over a period of six months indicate that the intraocular pressure-lowering effect of TIMOPTIC-XE was consistent. The results from the largest U.S. and international clinical trials comparing TIMOPTIC-XE 0.5% to TIMOPTIC 0.5% are shown in Figure 1.

Figure 1

Mean IOP and Std Deviation (mm Hg) by Treatment Group

U.S. Study

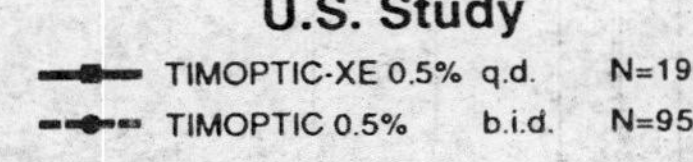

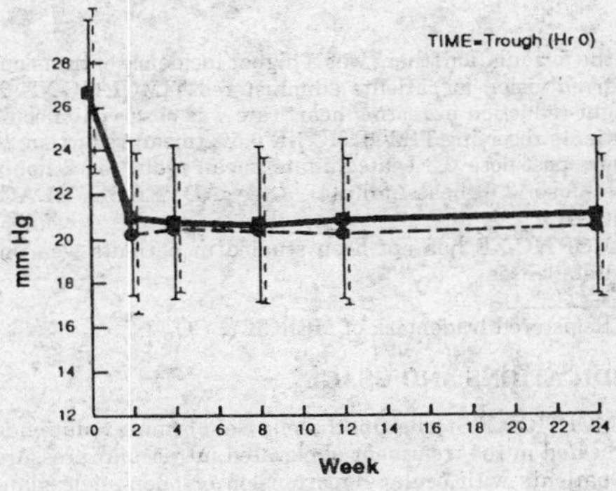

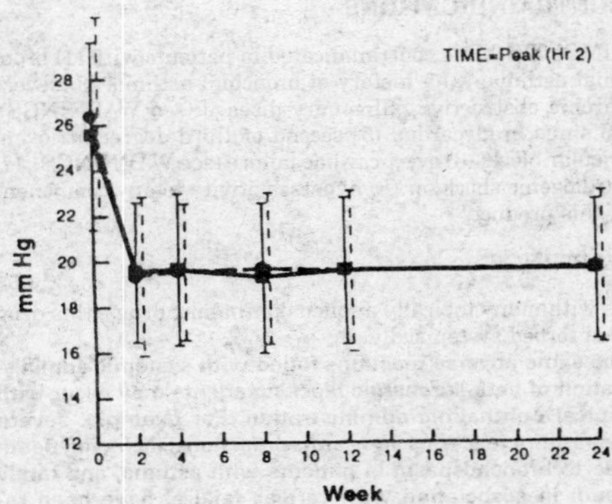

[See figure at top of next column]
TIMOPTIC-XE administered once daily had a safety profile similar to that of an equivalent concentration of TIMOPTIC administered twice daily. Due to the physical characteristics

Continued on next page

Information on the Merck & Co., Inc. products listed on these pages is the full prescribing information from product circulars in use September 30, 2000. For information, please call 1-800-NSC MERCK [1-800-672-6372].

Timoptic-XE—Cont.

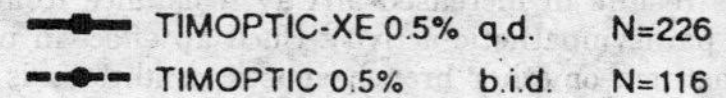

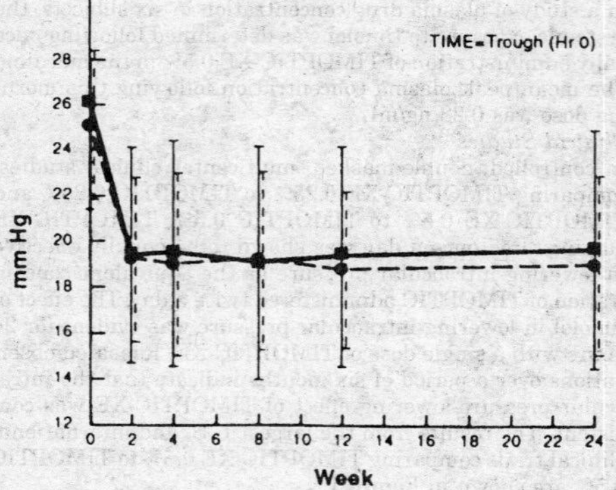

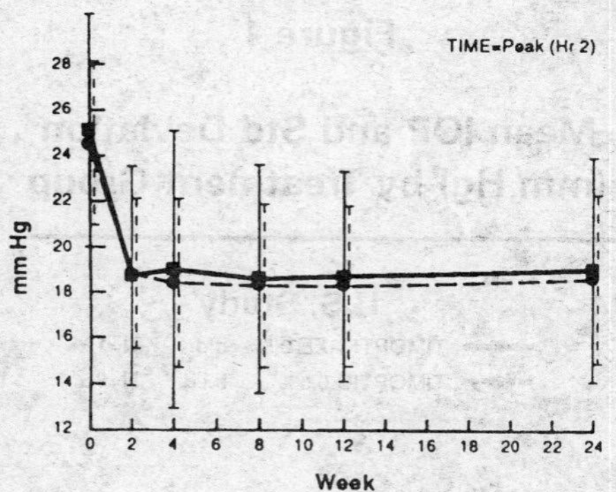

of the formulation, there was a higher incidence of transient blurred vision in patients administered TIMOPTIC-XE. A slight reduction in resting heart rate was observed in some patients receiving TIMOPTIC-XE 0.5% (mean reduction 24 hours post-dose 0.8 beats/minute, mean reduction 2 hours post-dose 3.8 beats/minute). (See **ADVERSE REACTIONS.**)

TIMOPTIC-XE has not been studied in patients wearing contact lenses.

* Registered trademark of MERCK & CO., INC.

INDICATIONS AND USAGE

TIMOPTIC-XE Sterile Ophthalmic Gel Forming Solution is indicated in the treatment of elevated intraocular pressure in patients with ocular hypertension or open-angle glaucoma.

CONTRAINDICATIONS

TIMOPTIC-XE is contraindicated in patients with (1) bronchial asthma; (2) a history of bronchial asthma; (3) severe chronic obstructive pulmonary disease (see WARNINGS); (4) sinus bradycardia; (5) second or third degree atrioventricular block; (6) overt cardiac failure (see WARNINGS); (7) cardiogenic shock; or (8) hypersensitivity to any component of this product.

WARNINGS

As with many topically applied ophthalmic drugs, this drug is absorbed systemically.

The same adverse reactions found with systemic administration of beta-adrenergic blocking agents may occur with topical ophthalmic administration. For example, severe respiratory reactions and cardiac reactions, including death due to bronchospasm in patients with asthma, and rarely death in association with cardiac failure, have been reported following systemic or ophthalmic administration of timolol maleate. (See CONTRAINDICATIONS.)

Cardiac Failure

Sympathetic stimulation may be essential for support of the circulation in individuals with diminished myocardial contractility, and its inhibition by beta-adrenergic receptor blockade may precipitate more severe failure.

In Patients Without a History of Cardiac Failure, continued depression of the myocardium with beta-blocking agents over a period of time can, in some cases, lead to cardiac failure. At the first sign or symptom of cardiac failure, TIMOPTIC-XE should be discontinued.

Obstructive Pulmonary Disease

Patients with chronic obstructive pulmonary disease (e.g., chronic bronchitis, emphysema) of mild or moderate severity, bronchospastic disease, or a history of bronchospastic disease (other than bronchial asthma or a history of bronchial asthma, in which TIMOPTIC-XE is contraindicated [see CONTRAINDICATIONS]) should, in general, not receive beta-blockers, including TIMOPTIC-XE.

Major Surgery

The necessity or desirability of withdrawal of beta-adrenergic blocking agents prior to major surgery is controversial. Beta-adrenergic receptor blockade impairs the ability of the heart to respond to beta-adrenergically mediated reflex stimuli. This may augment the risk of general anesthesia in surgical procedures. Some patients receiving beta-adrenergic receptor blocking agents have experienced protracted, severe hypotension during anesthesia. Difficulty in restarting and maintaining the heartbeat has also been reported. For these reasons, in patients undergoing elective surgery, some authorities recommend gradual withdrawal of beta-adrenergic receptor blocking agents.

If necessary during surgery, the effects of beta-adrenergic blocking agents may be reversed by sufficient doses of adrenergic agonists.

Diabetes Mellitus

Beta-adrenergic blocking agents should be administered with caution in patients subject to spontaneous hypoglycemia or to diabetic patients (especially those with labile diabetes) who are receiving insulin or oral hypoglycemic agents. Beta-adrenergic receptor blocking agents may mask the signs and symptoms of acute hypoglycemia.

Thyrotoxicosis

Beta-adrenergic blocking agents may mask certain clinical signs (e.g., tachycardia) of hyperthyroidism. Patients suspected of developing thyrotoxicosis should be managed carefully to avoid abrupt withdrawal of beta-adrenergic blocking agents that might precipitate a thyroid storm.

PRECAUTIONS

General

Because of potential effects of beta-adrenergic blocking agents on blood pressure and pulse, these agents should be used with caution in patients with cerebrovascular insufficiency. If signs or symptoms suggesting reduced cerebral blood flow develop following initiation of therapy with TIMOPTIC-XE, alternative therapy should be considered.

There have been reports of bacterial keratitis associated with the use of multiple dose containers of topical ophthalmic products. These containers had been inadvertently contaminated by patients who, in most cases, had a concurrent corneal disease or a disruption of the ocular epithelial surface. (See PRECAUTIONS, *Information for Patients.*)

Choroidal detachment after filtration procedures has been reported with the administration of aqueous suppressant therapy (e.g. timolol).

Angle-closure glaucoma: In patients with angle-closure glaucoma, the immediate objective of treatment is to reopen the angle. This may require constricting the pupil. Timolol maleate has little or no effect on the pupil. TIMOPTIC-XE should not be used alone in the treatment of angle-closure glaucoma.

Anaphylaxis: While taking beta-blockers, patients with a history of atopy or a history of severe anaphylactic reactions to a variety of allergens may be more reactive to repeated accidental, diagnostic, or therapeutic challenge with such allergens. Such patients may be unresponsive to the usual doses of epinephrine used to treat anaphylactic reactions.

Muscle Weakness: Beta-adrenergic blockade has been reported to potentiate muscle weakness consistent with certain myasthenic symptoms (e.g., diplopia, ptosis, and generalized weakness). Timolol has been reported rarely to increase muscle weakness in some patients with myasthenia gravis or myasthenic symptoms.

Information for Patients

Patients should be instructed to avoid allowing the tip of the dispensing container to contact the eye or surrounding structures.

Patients should also be instructed that ocular solutions, if handled improperly or if the tip of the dispensing container contacts the eye or surrounding structures, can become contaminated by common bacteria known to cause ocular infections. Serious damage to the eye and subsequent loss of vision may result from using contaminated solutions. (See PRECAUTIONS, *General.*)

Patients should also be advised that if they have ocular surgery or develop an intercurrent ocular condition (e.g., trauma or infection), they should immediately seek their physician's advice concerning the continued use of the present multidose container.

Patients should be instructed to invert the closed container and shake once before each use. It is not necessary to shake the container more than once.

Patients requiring concomitant topical ophthalmic medications should be instructed to administer these at least 10 minutes before instilling TIMOPTIC-XE.

Patients with bronchial asthma, a history of bronchial asthma, severe chronic obstructive pulmonary disease, sinus bradycardia, second or third degree atrioventricular block, or cardiac failure should be advised not to take this product. (See CONTRAINDICATIONS.)

Transient blurred vision, generally lasting from 30 seconds to 5 minutes, following instillation, and potential visual disturbances may impair the ability to perform hazardous tasks such as operating machinery or driving a motor vehicle.

Drug Interactions

Beta-adrenergic blocking agents: Patients who are receiving a beta-adrenergic blocking agent orally and TIMOPTIC-XE should be observed for potential additive effects of beta-blockade, both systemic and on intraocular pressure. The concomitant use of two topical beta-adrenergic blocking agents is not recommended.

Calcium antagonists: Caution should be used in the coadministration of beta-adrenergic blocking agents, such as TIMOPTIC-XE, and oral or intravenous calcium antagonists because of possible atrioventricular conduction disturbances, left ventricular failure, or hypotension. In patients with impaired cardiac function, coadministration should be avoided.

Catecholamine-depleting drugs: Close observation of the patient is recommended when a beta blocker is administered to patients receiving catecholamine-depleting drugs such as reserpine, because of possible additive effects and the production of hypotension and/or marked bradycardia, which may result in vertigo, syncope, or postural hypotension.

Digitalis and calcium antagonists: The concomitant use of beta-adrenergic blocking agents with digitalis and calcium antagonists may have additive effects in prolonging atrioventricular conduction time.

Quinidine: Potentiated systemic beta-blockade (e.g., decreased heart rate) has been reported during combined treatment with quinidine and timolol, possibly because quinidine inhibits the metabolism of timolol via the P-450 enzyme, CYP2D6.

Clonidine: Oral beta-adrenergic blocking agents may exacerbate the rebound hypertension which can follow the withdrawal of clonidine. There have been no reports of exacerbation of rebound hypertension with ophthalmic timolol maleate.

Injectable epinephrine: (See PRECAUTIONS, *General, Anaphylaxis:)*

Carcinogenesis, Mutagenesis, Impairment of Fertility

In a two-year study of timolol maleate administered orally to rats, there was a statistically significant increase in the incidence of adrenal pheochromocytomas in male rats administered 300 mg/kg/day (approximately 42,000 times the systemic exposure following the maximum recommended human ophthalmic dose). Similar differences were not observed in rats administered oral doses equivalent to approximately 14,000 times the maximum recommended human ophthalmic dose.

In a lifetime oral study in mice, there were statistically significant increases in the incidence of benign and malignant pulmonary tumors, benign uterine polyps, and mammary adenocarcinomas in female mice at 500 mg/kg/day (approximately 71,000 times the systemic exposure following the maximum recommended human ophthalmic dose), but not at 5 or 50 mg/kg/day (approximately 700 or 7,000, respectively, times the systemic exposure following the maximum recommended human ophthalmic dose). In a subsequent study in female mice, in which post-mortem examinations were limited to the uterus and the lungs, a statistically significant increase in the incidence of pulmonary tumors was again observed at 500 mg/kg/day.

The increased occurrence of mammary adenocarcinomas was associated with elevations in serum prolactin, which occurred in female mice administered oral timolol at 500 mg/kg/day, but not at oral doses of 5 or 50 mg/kg/day. An increased incidence of mammary adenocarcinomas in rodents has been associated with administration of several other therapeutic agents that elevate serum prolactin, but no correlation between serum prolactin levels and mammary tumors has been established in humans. Furthermore, in adult human female subjects who received oral dosages of up to 60 mg of timolol maleate (the maximum recommended human oral dosage), there were no clinically meaningful changes in serum prolactin.

Timolol maleate was devoid of mutagenic potential when tested *in vivo* (mouse) in the micronucleus test and cytogenetic assay (doses up to 800 mg) and *in vitro* in a neoplastic cell transformation assay (up to 100 mcg/mL). In Ames tests, the highest concentrations of timolol employed, 5,000 or 10,000 mcg/plate, were associated with statistically significant elevations of revertants observed with tester strain TA100 (in seven replicate assays), but not in the remaining three strains. In the assays with tester strain TA100, no consistent dose response relationship was observed, and the ratio of test to control revertants did not reach 2. A ratio of 2 is usually considered the criterion for a positive Ames test.

Reproduction and fertility studies in rats demonstrated no adverse effect on male or female fertility at doses up to 21,000 times the systemic exposure following the maximum recommended human ophthalmic dose.

Pregnancy:

Teratogenic Effects—Pregnancy Category C. Teratogenicity studies with timolol in mice and rabbits at oral doses up to 50 mg/kg/day (7,000 times the systemic exposure following the maximum recommended human ophthalmic dose) demonstrated no evidence of fetal malformations. Although delayed fetal ossification was observed at this dose in rats, there were no adverse effects on postnatal development of offspring. Doses of 1000 mg/kg/day (142,000 times the systemic exposure following the maximum recommended human ophthalmic dose) were maternotoxic in mice and resulted in an increased number of fetal resorptions. Increased fetal resorptions were also seen in rabbits at doses of 14,000 times the systemic exposure following the maximum recommended human ophthalmic dose, in this case without apparent maternotoxicity.

There are no adequate and well-controlled studies in pregnant women. TIMOPTIC-XE should be used during pregnancy only if the potential benefit justifies the potential risk to the fetus.

Nursing Mothers

Timolol maleate has been detected in human milk following oral and ophthalmic drug administration. Because of the potential for serious adverse reactions from TIMOPTIC-XE in nursing infants, a decision should be made whether to discontinue nursing or to discontinue the drug, taking into account the importance of the drug to the mother.

Pediatric Use

Safety and effectiveness in pediatric patients have not been established.

Geriatric Use

No overall differences in safety or effectiveness have been observed between elderly and younger patients.

ADVERSE REACTIONS

In clinical trials, transient blurred vision upon instillation of the drop was reported in approximately one in three patients (lasting from 30 seconds to 5 minutes). Less than 1% of patients discontinued from the studies due to blurred vision. The frequency of patients reporting burning and stinging upon instillation was comparable between TIMOPTIC-XE and TIMOPTIC (approximately one in eight patients).

Adverse experiences reported in 1–5% of patients were:

Ocular: Pain, conjunctivitis, discharge (e.g. crusting), foreign body sensation, itching and tearing;

Systemic: Headache, dizziness, and upper respiratory infections.

The following additional adverse experiences have been reported with the ocular administration of this or other timolol maleate formulations:

BODY AS A WHOLE

Asthenia/fatigue, and chest pain.

CARDIOVASCULAR

Bradycardia, arrhythmia, hypotension, hypertension, syncope, heart block, cerebral vascular accident, cerebral ischemia, cardiac failure, worsening of angina pectoris, palpitation, cardiac arrest, pulmonary edema, edema, claudication, Raynaud's phenomenon, and cold hands and feet.

DIGESTIVE

Nausea, diarrhea, dyspepsia, anorexia, and dry mouth.

IMMUNOLOGIC

Systemic lupus erythematosus.

NERVOUS SYSTEM/PSYCHIATRIC

Increase in signs and symptoms of myasthenia gravis, paresthesia, somnolence, insomnia, nightmares, behavioral changes and psychic disturbances including depression, confusion, hallucinations, anxiety, disorientation, nervousness, and memory loss.

SKIN

Alopecia and psoriasiform rash or exacerbation of psoriasis.

HYPERSENSITIVITY

Signs and symptoms of systemic allergic reactions, including angioedema, urticaria, and localized and generalized rash.

RESPIRATORY

Bronchospasm (predominantly in patients with preexisting bronchospastic disease), respiratory failure, dyspnea, nasal congestion, and cough.

ENDOCRINE

Masked symptoms of hypoglycemia in diabetic patients (see WARNINGS).

SPECIAL SENSES

Signs and symptoms of ocular irritation including blepharitis, keratitis, and dry eyes; ptosis; decreased corneal sensitivity; cystoid macular edema; visual disturbances including refractive changes and diplopia; pseudopemphigoid; choroidal detachment following filtration surgery (see PRECAUTIONS, *General*); and tinnitus.

UROGENITAL

Retroperitoneal fibrosis, decreased libido, impotence, and Peyronie's disease.

The following additional adverse effects have been reported in clinical experience with ORAL timolol maleate or other ORAL beta-blocking agents and may be considered potential effects of ophthalmic timolol maleate: *Allergic:* Erythematous rash, fever combined with aching and sore throat, laryngospasm with respiratory distress; *Body as a Whole:* Extremity pain, decreased exercise tolerance, weight loss; *Cardiovascular:* Worsening of arterial insufficiency, vasodilatation; *Digestive:* Gastrointestinal pain, hepatomegaly, vomiting, mesenteric arterial thrombosis, ischemic colitis; *Hematologic:* Nonthrombocytopenic purpura, thrombocytopenic purpura, agranulocytosis; *Endocrine:* Hyperglycemia, hypoglycemia; *Skin:* Pruritus, skin irritation, increased pigmentation, sweating; *Musculoskeletal:* Arthralgia; *Nervous System/Psychiatric:* Vertigo, local weakness, diminished concentration, reversible mental depression progressing to catatonia, an acute reversible syndrome characterized by disorientation for time and place, emotional lability, slightly clouded sensorium, and decreased performance on neuropsychometrics; *Respiratory:* Rales, bronchial obstruction; *Urogenital:* Urination difficulties.

OVERDOSAGE

No data are available in regard to human overdosage with or accidental oral ingestion of TIMOPTIC-XE.

There have been reports of inadvertent overdosage with TIMOPTIC Ophthalmic Solution resulting in systemic effects similar to those seen with systemic beta-adrenergic blocking agents such as dizziness, headache, shortness of breath, bradycardia, bronchospasm, and cardiac arrest (see also ADVERSE REACTIONS).

Overdosage has been reported with Tablets BLOCADREN* (timolol maleate tablets). A 30 year old female ingested 650 mg of BLOCADREN (maximum recommended oral daily dose is 60 mg) and experienced second and third degree heart block. She recovered without treatment but approximately two months later developed irregular heartbeat, hypertension, dizziness, tinnitus, faintness, increased pulse rate, and borderline first degree heart block.

An *in vitro* hemodialysis study, using ^{14}C timolol added to human plasma or whole blood, showed that timolol was readily dialyzed from these fluids; however, a study of patients with renal failure showed that timolol did not dialyze readily.

*Registered trademark of MERCK & CO., Inc.

DOSAGE AND ADMINISTRATION

Patients should be instructed to invert the closed container and shake once before each use. It is not necessary to shake the container more than once. Other topically applied ophthalmic medications should be administered at least 10 minutes before TIMOPTIC-XE. (See PRECAUTIONS, *Information for Patients* and accompanying INSTRUCTIONS FOR USE.)

TIMOPTIC-XE Sterile Ophthalmic Gel Forming Solution is available in concentrations of 0.25% and 0.5%. The dose is one drop of TIMOPTIC-XE (either 0.25% or 0.5%) in the affected eye(s) once a day.

Because in some patients the pressure-lowering response to TIMOPTIC-XE may require a few weeks to stabilize, evaluation should include a determination of intraocular pressure after approximately 4 weeks of treatment with TIMOPTIC-XE.

Dosages higher than one drop of 0.5% TIMOPTIC-XE once a day have not been studied. If the patient's intraocular pressure is still not at a satisfactory level on this regimen, concomitant therapy can be considered. The concomitant use of two topical beta-adrenergic blocking agents is not recommended. (See PRECAUTIONS, *Drug Interactions, Beta-adrenergic blocking agents.*)

When patients have been switched from therapy with TIMOPTIC administered twice daily to TIMOPTIC-XE administered once daily, the ocular hypotensive effect has remained consistent.

HOW SUPPLIED

TIMOPTIC-XE Sterile Ophthalmic Gel Forming Solution is a colorless to nearly colorless, slightly opalescent, and slightly viscous solution.

No. 3557—TIMOPTIC-XE Sterile Ophthalmic Gel Forming Solution, 0.25% timolol equivalent, is supplied in OCUMETER*, a white, opaque, plastic, ophthalmic dispenser with a controlled drop tip as follows:

NDC 0006-3557-32, 2.5 mL

NDC 0006-3557-03, 5 mL.

No. 3558—TIMOPTIC-XE Sterile Ophthalmic Gel Forming Solution, 0.5% timolol equivalent, is supplied in OCUMETER, a white, opaque, plastic, ophthalmic dispenser with a controlled drop tip as follows:

NDC 0006-3558-32, 2.5 mL

NDC 0006-3558-03, 5 mL.

Storage

Store between 15° and 25°C (59° and 77°F). **AVOID FREEZING.** Protect from light.

TIMOPTIC-XE®
0.25% and 0.5%
(timolol maleate ophthalmic gel forming solution)

INSTRUCTIONS FOR USE

Please follow these instructions carefully when using TIMOPTIC-XE*. Use TIMOPTIC-XE as prescribed by your doctor.

1. If you use other topically applied ophthalmic medications, they should be administered at least 10 minutes before TIMOPTIC-XE.
2. Wash hands before each use.
3. Invert the closed bottle and shake ONCE before each use. (It is not necessary to shake the bottle more than once.) [See first figure at top of next column]
4. Remove the cap from the bottle carefully so that the dispenser tip does not touch anything. Place the cap in a clean, dry area.
5. Hold the bottle between the thumb and index finger. Use the index finger of the other hand to pull down the lower eyelid to form a pocket for the eye drop. Tilt your head back.
[See second figure at top of next column]
6. Place the dispenser tip close to your eye and gently squeeze the bottle to administer one drop. Remove pressure after a single drop has been released. If instructed, repeat steps 5 and 6 in the other eye.

DO NOT ALLOW THE DISPENSER TIP TO TOUCH THE EYE OR SURROUNDING AREAS.

Ophthalmic medications, if handled improperly, can become contaminated by common bacteria known to cause eye infections. Serious damage to the eye and subsequent loss of vision may result from using contaminated ophthalmic medications. If you think your medication may be

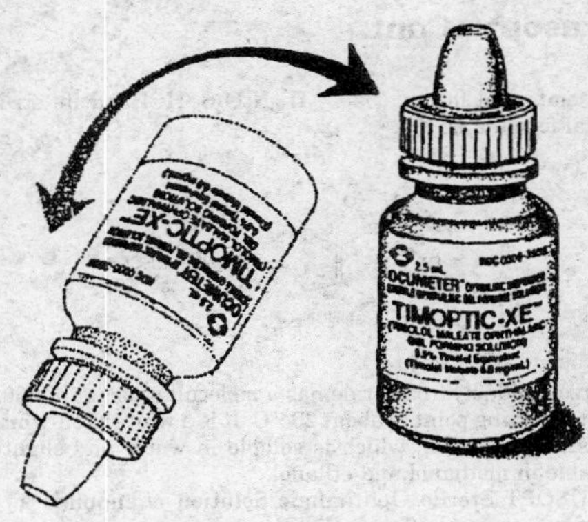

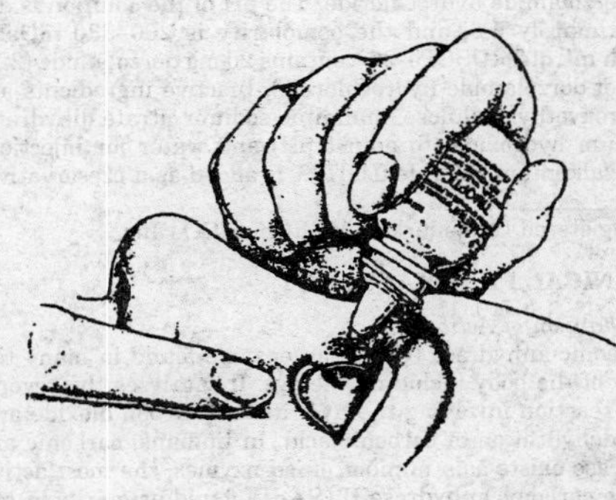

contaminated, or you develop an eye infection, contact your doctor immediately concerning continued use of this bottle.

7. Replace the cap. Store the bottle at room temperature in an upright position in a clean area.
8. The dispenser tip is designed to provide a pre-measured drop; therefore, do NOT enlarge the hole of the dispenser.
9. Do NOT wash the tip of the dispenser with water, soap, or any other cleaner.

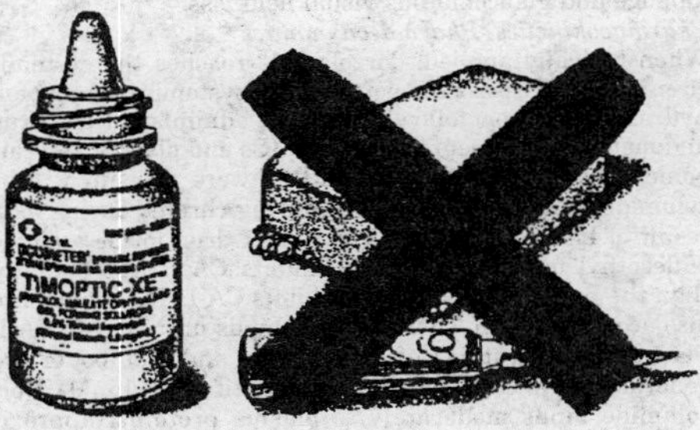

WARNING: Keep out of reach of children.
If you have any questions about the use of TIMOPTIC-XE, please consult your doctor.

* Registered trademark of MERCK & CO., INC.

9028711 Issued April 2000

MERCK & CO., Inc.
West Point, PA 19486, USA

TRUSOPT® Sterile Ophthalmic Solution 2% ℞
(dorzolamide hydrochloride ophthalmic solution)

DESCRIPTION

TRUSOPT* (dorzolamide hydrochloride ophthalmic solution) is a carbonic anhydrase inhibitor formulated for topical ophthalmic use.

Dorzolamide hydrochloride is described chemically as: (4*S*-*trans*)-4-(ethylamino)-5,6-dihydro-6-methyl-4*H*-thieno [2,3-*b*]thiopyran-2-sulfonamide 7,7-dioxide monohydrochloride. Dorzolamide hydrochloride is optically active. The specific rotation is

$$\alpha^{25°}_{405} \text{ (C =1, water) = -17 °.}$$

Continued on next page

Information on the Merck & Co., Inc. products listed on these pages is the full prescribing information from product circulars in use September 30, 2000. For information, please call 1-800-NSC MERCK [1-800-672-6372].

Trusopt—Cont.

Its empirical formula is $C_{10}H_{16}N_2O_4S_3 \cdot HCl$ and its structural formula is:

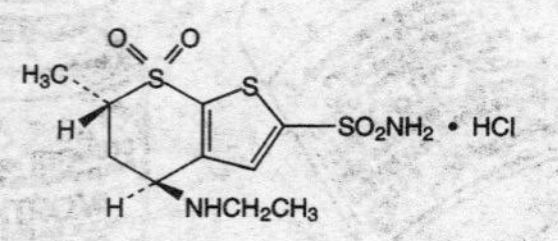

Dorzolamide hydrochloride has a molecular weight of 360.9 and a melting point of about 264°C. It is a white to off-white, crystalline powder, which is soluble in water and slightly soluble in methanol and ethanol.
TRUSOPT Sterile Ophthalmic Solution is supplied as a sterile, isotonic, buffered, slightly viscous, aqueous solution of dorzolamide hydrochloride. The pH of the solution is approximately 5.6, and the osmolarity is 260–330 mOsM. Each mL of TRUSOPT 2% contains 20 mg dorzolamide (22.3 mg of dorzolamide hydrochloride). Inactive ingredients are hydroxyethyl cellulose, mannitol, sodium citrate dihydrate, sodium hydroxide (to adjust pH) and water for injection. Benzalkonium chloride 0.0075% is added as a preservative.

* Registered trademark of MERCK & CO., Inc.

CLINICAL PHARMACOLOGY

Mechanism of Action
Carbonic anhydrase (CA) is an enzyme found in many tissues of the body including the eye. It catalyzes the reversible reaction involving the hydration of carbon dioxide and the dehydration of carbonic acid. In humans, carbonic anhydrase exists as a number of isoenzymes, the most active being carbonic anhydrase II (CA-II), found primarily in red blood cells (RBCs), but also in other tissues. Inhibition of carbonic anhydrase in the ciliary processes of the eye decreases aqueous humor secretion, presumably by slowing the formation of bicarbonate ions with subsequent reduction in sodium and fluid transport. The result is a reduction in intraocular pressure (IOP).
TRUSOPT Ophthalmic Solution contains dorzolamide hydrochloride, an inhibitor of human carbonic anhydrase II. Following topical ocular administration, TRUSOPT reduces elevated intraocular pressure. Elevated intraocular pressure is a major risk factor in the pathogenesis of optic nerve damage and glaucomatous visual field loss.
Pharmacokinetics/Pharmacodynamics
When topically applied, dorzolamide reaches the systemic circulation. To assess the potential for systemic carbonic anhydrase inhibition following topical administration, drug and metabolite concentrations in RBCs and plasma and carbonic anhydrase inhibition in RBCs were measured. Dorzolamide accumulates in RBCs during chronic dosing as a result of binding to CA-II. The parent drug forms a single N-desethyl metabolite, which inhibits CA-II less potently than the parent drug but also inhibits CA-I. The metabolite also accumulates in RBCs where it binds primarily to CA-I. Plasma concentrations of dorzolamide and metabolite are generally below the assay limit of quantitation (15nM). Dorzolamide binds moderately to plasma proteins (approximately 33%). Dorzolamide is primarily excreted unchanged in the urine; the metabolite also is excreted in urine. After dosing is stopped, dorzolamide washes out of RBCs nonlinearly, resulting in a rapid decline of drug concentration initially, followed by a slower elimination phase with a half-life of about four months.
To simulate the systemic exposure after long-term topical ocular administration, dorzolamide was given orally to eight healthy subjects for up to 20 weeks. The oral dose of 2 mg b.i.d. closely approximates the amount of drug delivered by topical ocular administration of TRUSOPT 2% t.i.d. Steady state was reached within 8 weeks. The inhibition of CA-II and total carbonic anhydrase activities was below the degree of inhibition anticipated to be necessary for a pharmacological effect on renal function and respiration in healthy individuals.
Clinical Studies
The efficacy of TRUSOPT was demonstrated in clinical studies in the treatment of elevated intraocular pressure in patients with glaucoma or ocular hypertension (baseline IOP ≥23 mmHg). The IOP-lowering effect of TRUSOPT was approximately 3 to 5 mmHg throughout the day and this was consistent in clinical studies of up to one year duration. The efficacy of TRUSOPT when dosed less frequently than three times a day (alone or in combination with other products) has not been established.
In a one year clinical study, the effect of TRUSOPT 2% t.i.d. on the corneal endothelium was compared to that of betaxolol ophthalmic solution b.i.d. and timolol maleate ophthalmic solution 0.5% b.i.d. There were no statistically significant differences between groups in corneal endothelial cell counts or in corneal thickness measurements. There was a mean loss of approximately 4% in the endothelial cell counts for each group over the one year period.

INDICATIONS AND USAGE

TRUSOPT Ophthalmic Solution is indicated in the treatment of elevated intraocular pressure in patients with ocular hypertension or open-angle glaucoma.

CONTRAINDICATIONS

TRUSOPT is contraindicated in patients who are hypersensitive to any component of this product.

WARNINGS

TRUSOPT is a sulfonamide and although administered topically is absorbed systemically. Therefore, the same types of adverse reactions that are attributable to sulfonamides may occur with topical administration with TRUSOPT. Fatalities have occurred, although rarely, due to severe reactions to sulfonamides including Stevens-Johnson syndrome, toxic epidermal necrolysis, fulminant hepatic necrosis, agranulocytosis, aplastic anemia, and other blood dyscrasias. Sensitization may recur when a sulfonamide is readministered irrespective of the route of administration. If signs of serious reactions or hypersensitivity occur, discontinue the use of this preparation.

PRECAUTIONS

General
The management of patients with acute angle-closure glaucoma requires therapeutic interventions in addition to ocular hypotensive agents. TRUSOPT has not been studied in patients with acute angle-closure glaucoma.
TRUSOPT has not been studied in patients with severe renal impairment (CrCl < 30 mL/min). Because TRUSOPT and its metabolite are excreted predominantly by the kidney, TRUSOPT is not recommended in such patients.
TRUSOPT has not been studied in patients with hepatic impairment and should therefore be used with caution in such patients.
In clinical studies, local ocular adverse effects, primarily conjunctivitis and lid reactions, were reported with chronic administration of TRUSOPT. Many of these reactions had the clinical appearance and course of an allergic-type reaction that resolved upon discontinuation of drug therapy. If such reactions are observed, TRUSOPT should be discontinued and the patient evaluated before considering restarting the drug. (See ADVERSE REACTIONS.)
There is a potential for an additive effect on the known systemic effects of carbonic anhydrase inhibition in patients receiving an oral carbonic anhydrase inhibitor and TRUSOPT. The concomitant administration of TRUSOPT and oral carbonic anhydrase inhibitors is not recommended.
There have been reports of bacterial keratitis associated with the use of multiple dose containers of topical ophthalmic products. These containers had been inadvertently contaminated by patients who, in most cases, had a concurrent corneal disease or a disruption of the ocular epithelial surface.
Information for Patients
TRUSOPT is a sulfonamide and although administered topically is absorbed systemically. Therefore the same types of adverse reactions that are attributable to sulfonamides may occur with topical administration. Patients should be advised that if serious or unusual reactions or signs of hypersensitivity occur, they should discontinue the use of the product (see WARNINGS).
Patients should be advised that if they develop any ocular reactions, particularly conjunctivitis and lid reactions, they should discontinue use and seek their physician's advice.
Patients should be instructed to avoid allowing the tip of the dispensing container to contact the eye or surrounding structures.
Patients should also be instructed that ocular solutions, if handled improperly or if the tip of the dispensing container contacts the eye or surrounding structures, can become contaminated by common bacteria known to cause ocular infections. Serious damage to the eye and subsequent loss of vision may result from using contaminated solutions.
Patients also should be advised that if they have ocular surgery or develop an intercurrent ocular condition (e.g., trauma or infection), they should immediately seek their physician's advice concerning the continued use of the present multidose container.
If more than one topical ophthalmic drug is being used, the drugs should be administered at least ten minutes apart.
Patients should be advised that TRUSOPT contains benzalkonium chloride which may be absorbed by soft contact lenses. Contact lenses should be removed prior to administration of the solution. Lenses may be reinserted 15 minutes following TRUSOPT administration.
Drug Interactions
Although acid-base and electrolyte disturbances were not reported in the clinical trials with TRUSOPT, these disturbances have been reported with oral carbonic anhydrase inhibitors and have, in some instances, resulted in drug interactions (e.g., toxicity associated with high-dose salicylate therapy). Therefore, the potential for such drug interactions should be considered in patients receiving TRUSOPT.
Carcinogenesis, Mutagenesis, Impairment of Fertility
In a two-year study of dorzolamide hydrochloride administered orally to male and female Sprague-Dawley rats, urinary bladder papillomas were seen in male rats in the highest dosage group of 20 mg/kg/day (250 times the recommended human ophthalmic dose). Papillomas were not seen in rats given oral doses equivalent to approximately 12 times the recommended human ophthalmic dose. No treatment-related tumors were seen in a 21-month study in female and male mice given oral doses up to 75 mg/kg/day (900 times the recommended human ophthalmic dose).
The increased incidence of urinary bladder papillomas seen in the high-dose male rats is a class-effect of carbonic anhydrase inhibitors in rats. Rats are particularly prone to developing papillomas in response to foreign bodies, compounds causing crystalluria, and diverse sodium salts.
No changes in bladder urothelium were seen in dogs given oral dorzolamide hydrochloride for one year at 2 mg/kg/day (25 times the recommended human ophthalmic dose) or monkeys dosed topically to the eye at 0.4 mg/kg/day (5 times the recommended human ophthalmic dose) for one year.
The following tests for mutagenic potential were negative: (1) *in vivo* (mouse) cytogenetic assay; (2) *in vitro* chromosomal aberration assay; (3) alkaline elution assay; (4) V-79 assay; and (5) Ames test.
In reproduction studies of dorzolamide hydrochloride in rats, there were no adverse effects on the reproductive capacity of males or females at doses up to 188 or 94 times, respectively, the recommended human ophthalmic dose.
Pregnancy
Teratogenic Effects. Pregnancy Category C. Developmental toxicity studies with dorzolamide hydrochloride in rabbits at oral doses of ≥2.5 mg/kg/day (31 times the recommended human ophthalmic dose) revealed malformations of the vertebral bodies. These malformations occurred at doses that caused metabolic acidosis with decreased body weight gain in dams and decreased fetal weights. No treatment-related malformations were seen at 1.0 mg/kg/day (13 times the recommended human ophthalmic dose). There are no adequate and well-controlled studies in pregnant women. TRUSOPT should be used during pregnancy only if the potential benefit justifies the potential risk to the fetus.
Nursing Mothers
In a study of dorzolamide hydrochloride in lactating rats, decreases in body weight gain of 5 to 7% in offspring at an oral dose of 7.5 mg/kg/day (94 times the recommended human ophthalmic dose) were seen during lactation. A slight delay in postnatal development (incisor eruption, vaginal canalization and eye openings), secondary to lower fetal body weight, was noted.
It is not known whether this drug is excreted in human milk. Because many drugs are excreted in human milk and because of the potential for serious adverse reactions in nursing infants from TRUSOPT, a decision should be made whether to discontinue nursing or to discontinue the drug, taking into account the importance of the drug to the mother.
Pediatric Use
Safety and effectiveness in pediatric patients have not been established.
Geriatric Use
No overall differences in safety and effectiveness have been observed between elderly and younger patients.

ADVERSE REACTIONS

Controlled clinical trials: The most frequent adverse events associated with TRUSOPT were ocular burning, stinging, or discomfort immediately following ocular administration (approximately one-third of patients). Approximately one-quarter of patients noted a bitter taste following administration. Superficial punctate keratitis occurred in 10–15% of patients and signs and symptoms of ocular allergic reaction in approximately 10%. Events occurring in approximately 1–5% of patients were conjunctivitis and lid reactions (see PRECAUTIONS, *General*), blurred vision, eye redness, tearing, dryness, and photophobia. Other ocular events and systemic events were reported infrequently, including headache, nausea, asthenia/fatigue; and, rarely, skin rashes, urolithiasis, and iridocyclitis.
Clinical practice: The following adverse events have occurred either at low incidence (<1%) during clinical trials or have been reported during the use of TRUSOPT in clinical practice where these events were reported voluntarily from a population of unknown size and frequency of occurrence cannot be determined precisely. They have been chosen for inclusion based on factors such as seriousness, frequency of reporting, possible causal connection to TRUSOPT, or a combination of these factors: signs and symptoms of systemic allergic reactions including angioedema, bronchospasm, pruritus, and urticaria; dizziness, paresthesia; ocular pain, transient myopia, eyelid crusting; dyspnea; contact dermatitis, dry mouth and throat irritation.

OVERDOSAGE

Electrolyte imbalance, development of an acidotic state, and possible central nervous system effects may occur. Serum electrolyte levels (particularly potassium) and blood pH levels should be monitored.

DOSAGE AND ADMINISTRATION

The dose is one drop of TRUSOPT Ophthalmic Solution in the affected eye(s) three times daily.
TRUSOPT may be used concomitantly with other topical ophthalmic drug products to lower intraocular pressure. If more than one topical ophthalmic drug is being used, the drugs should be administered at least ten minutes apart.

HOW SUPPLIED

TRUSOPT Ophthalmic Solution is a slightly opalescent, nearly colorless, slightly viscous solution.
No. 3519—TRUSOPT Ophthalmic Solution 2% is supplied in OCUMETER®*, a white, opaque, plastic ophthalmic dispenser with a controlled drop tip as follows:

NDC 0006-3519-03, 5 mL
NDC 0006-3519-10, 10 mL.
Storage
Store TRUSOPT Ophthalmic Solution at 15–30°C (59–86°F). Protect from light.

* Registered trademark of MERCK & CO., Inc.
9010009 Issued July 1999

URECHOLINE® Tablets ℞
(Bethanechol Chloride)

URECHOLINE® Injection ℞
(Bethanechol Chloride)

DESCRIPTION

URECHOLINE* (Bethanechol Chloride), a cholinergic agent, is a synthetic ester which is structurally and pharmacologically related to acetylcholine.
It is designated chemically as 2-[(aminocarbonyl)oxy]-*N, N, N-* trimethyl-1-propanaminium chloride. Its empirical formula is $C_7H_{17}ClN_2O_2$ and its structural formula is:

$$\left[\begin{array}{l}CH_3CH-CH_2N^+(CH_3)_3\\ \quad\;|\\ \quad OCONH_2\end{array}\right]Cl^-$$

It is a white, hygroscopic crystalline compound having a slight amine-like odor, freely soluble in water, and has a molecular weight of 196.68.
URECHOLINE is supplied as 5 mg, 10 mg, 25 mg, and 50 mg tablets for oral use. Inactive ingredients in the tablets are calcium phosphate, lactose, magnesium stearate, and starch. Tablets URECHOLINE 10 mg also contain FD&C Red 3 and FD&C Red 40. Tablets URECHOLINE 25 mg and 50 mg also contain D&C Yellow 10 and FD&C Yellow 6.
URECHOLINE is also supplied as a sterile solution **for subcutaneous use only.** The sterile solution is essentially neutral. Each milliliter contains bethanechol chloride, 5.15 mg, and Water for Injection, q.s., 1 mL. It may be autoclaved at 120° C for 20 minutes without discoloration or loss of potency.

*Registered trademark of MERCK & CO., INC.

CLINICAL PHARMACOLOGY

Bethanechol chloride acts principally by producing the effects of stimulation of the parasympathetic nervous system. It increases the tone of the detrusor urinae muscle, usually producing a contraction sufficiently strong to initiate micturition and empty the bladder. It stimulates gastric motility, increases gastric tone, and often restores impaired rhythmic peristalsis.
Stimulation of the parasympathetic nervous system releases acetylcholine at the nerve endings. When spontaneous stimulation is reduced and therapeutic intervention is required, acetylcholine can be given, but it is rapidly hydrolyzed by cholinesterase, and its effects are transient. Bethanechol chloride is not destroyed by cholinesterase and its effects are more prolonged than those of acetylcholine.
Effects on the GI and urinary tracts sometimes appear within 30 minutes after oral administration of bethanechol chloride, but more often 60–90 minutes are required to reach maximum effectiveness. Following oral administration, the usual duration of action of bethanechol is one hour, although large doses (300–400 mg) have been reported to produce effects for up to six hours. Subcutaneous injection produces a more intense action on bladder muscle than does oral administration of the drug.
Because of the selective action of bethanechol, nicotinic symptoms of cholinergic stimulation are usually absent or minimal when orally or subcutaneously administered in therapeutic doses, while muscarinic effects are prominent. Muscarinic effects usually occur within 5–15 minutes after subcutaneous injection, reach a maximum in 15–30 minutes, and disappear within two hours. Doses that stimulate micturition and defecation and increase peristalsis do not ordinarily stimulate ganglia or voluntary muscles. Therapeutic test doses in normal human subjects have little effect on heart rate, blood pressure, or peripheral circulation.
Bethanechol chloride does not cross the blood-brain barrier because of its charged quaternary amine moiety. The metabolic fate and mode of excretion of the drug have not been elucidated.
A clinical study** was conducted on the relative effectiveness of oral and subcutaneous doses of bethanechol chloride on the stretch response of bladder muscle in patients with urinary retention. Results showed that 5 mg of the drug given subcutaneously stimulated a response that was more rapid in onset and of larger magnitude than an oral dose of 50 mg, 100 mg, or 200 mg. All the oral doses, however, had a longer duration of effect than the subcutaneous dose. Although the 50 mg oral dose caused little change in intravesical pressure in this study, this dose has been found in other studies to be clinically effective in the rehabilitation of patients with decompensated bladders.

**Diokno, A. C.; Lapides, J., Urol. *10:* 23–24, July 1977.

INDICATIONS AND USAGE

For the treatment of acute postoperative and postpartum nonobstructive (functional) urinary retention and for neurogenic atony of the urinary bladder with retention.

CONTRAINDICATIONS

Hypersensitivity to URECHOLINE tablets or to any component of URECHOLINE injection, hyperthyroidism, peptic ulcer, latent or active bronchial asthma, pronounced bradycardia or hypotension, vasomotor instability, coronary artery disease, epilepsy, and parkinsonism.
URECHOLINE should not be employed when the strength or integrity of the gastrointestinal or bladder wall is in question, or in the presence of mechanical obstruction; when increased muscular activity of the gastrointestinal tract or urinary bladder might prove harmful, as following recent urinary bladder surgery, gastrointestinal resection and anastomosis, or when there is possible gastrointestinal obstruction; in bladder neck obstruction, spastic gastrointestinal disturbances, acute inflammatory lesions of the gastrointestinal tract, or peritonitis; or in marked vagotonia.

WARNING

The sterile solution is for subcutaneous use only. It should never be given intramuscularly or intravenously. Violent symptoms of cholinergic over-stimulation, such as circulatory collapse, fall in blood pressure, abdominal cramps, bloody diarrhea, shock, or sudden cardiac arrest are likely to occur if the drug is given by either of these routes. Although rare, these same symptoms have occurred after subcutaneous injection, and may occur in cases of hypersensitivity or overdosage.

PRECAUTIONS

General
In urinary retention, if the sphincter fails to relax as URECHOLINE contracts the bladder, urine may be forced up the ureter into the kidney pelvis. If there is bacteriuria, this may cause reflux infection.
Information for Patients
URECHOLINE tablets should preferably be taken one hour before or two hours after meals to avoid nausea or vomiting. Dizziness, lightheadedness or fainting may occur, especially when getting up from a lying or sitting position.
Drug Interactions
Special care is required if this drug is given to patients receiving ganglion blocking compounds because a critical fall in blood pressure may occur. Usually, severe abdominal symptoms appear before there is such a fall in the blood pressure.
Carcinogenesis, Mutagenesis, Impairment of Fertility
Long-term studies in animals have not been performed to evaluate the effects upon fertility, mutagenic or carcinogenic potential of URECHOLINE.
Pregnancy
Pregnancy Category C. Animal reproduction studies have not been conducted with URECHOLINE. It is also not known whether URECHOLINE can cause fetal harm when administered to a pregnant woman or can affect reproduction capacity. URECHOLINE should be given to a pregnant woman only if clearly needed.
Nursing Mothers
It is not known whether this drug is secreted in human milk. Because many drugs are secreted in human milk and because of the potential for serious adverse reactions from URECHOLINE in nursing infants, a decision should be made whether to discontinue nursing or to discontinue the drug, taking into account the importance of the drug to the mother.
Pediatric Use
Safety and effectiveness in pediatric patients have not been established.

ADVERSE REACTIONS

Adverse reactions are rare following oral administration of bethanechol, but are more common following subcutaneous injection. Adverse reactions are more likely to occur when dosage is increased.
The following adverse reactions have been observed: *Body as a Whole:* malaise; *Digestive:* abdominal cramps or discomfort, colicky pain, nausea and belching, diarrhea, borborygmi, salivation; *Renal:* urinary urgency; *Nervous System:* headache; *Cardiovascular:* a fall in blood pressure with reflex tachycardia, vasomotor response; *Skin:* flushing producing a feeling of warmth, sensation of heat about the face, sweating; *Respiratory:* bronchial constriction, asthmatic attacks; *Special Senses:* lacrimation, miosis.
Causal Relationship Unknown: The following adverse reactions have been reported, and a causal relationship to therapy with URECHOLINE has not been established: *Body as a Whole:* hypothermia: *Nervous System:* seizures.

OVERDOSAGE

Early signs of overdosage are abdominal discomfort, salivation, flushing of the skin ("hot feeling"), sweating, nausea and vomiting.
Atropine is a specific antidote. The recommended dose for adults is 0.6 mg (1/100 grain). Repeat doses can be given every two hours, according to clinical response. The recommended dosage in infants and children up to 12 years of age is 0.01 mg/kg (to a maximum single dose of 0.4 mg) repeated every two hours as needed until the desired effect is obtained, or adverse effects of atropine preclude further usage. Subcutaneous injection of atropine is preferred except in emergencies when the intravenous route may be employed.
When URECHOLINE is administered subcutaneously, a syringe containing a dose of atropine sulfate should always be available to treat symptoms of toxicity.
The oral LD_{50} of bethanechol chloride is 1510 mg/kg in the mouse.

DOSAGE AND ADMINISTRATION

Dosage and route of administration must be individualized, depending on the type and severity of the condition to be treated.
Preferably give the drug when the stomach is empty. If taken soon after eating, nausea and vomiting may occur.
Oral—The usual adult dosage is 10 to 50 mg three or four times a day. The minimum effective dose is determined by giving 5 or 10 mg initially and repeating the same amount at hourly intervals until satisfactory response occurs or until a maximum of 50 mg has been given. The effects of the drug sometimes appear within 30 minutes and usually within 60 to 90 minutes. They persist for about an hour.
Subcutaneous—The usual dose is 1 mL (5.15 mg), although some patients respond satisfactorily to as little as 0.5 mL (2.575 mg). The minimum effective dose is determined by injecting 0.5 mL (2.575 mg) initially and repeating the same amount at 15 to 30 minute intervals to a maximum of four doses until satisfactory response is obtained, unless disturbing reactions appear. The minimum effective dose may be repeated thereafter three or four times a day as required.
Rarely, single doses up to 2 mL (10.30 mg) may be required. Such large doses may cause severe reactions and should be used only after adequate trial of single doses of 0.5 to 1 mL (2.575 to 5.15 mg) has established that smaller doses are not sufficient.
URECHOLINE is usually effective in 5 to 15 minutes after subcutaneous injection.
If necessary, the effects of the drug can be abolished promptly by atropine (see OVERDOSAGE).
Parenteral drug products should be inspected visually for particulate matter and discoloration prior to administration, whenever solution and container permit.

HOW SUPPLIED

Tablets URECHOLINE are round, compressed tablets, scored on one side. They are supplied as follows:
No. 7785—5 mg, white in color, coded MSD 403 on one side and URECHOLINE on the other.
NDC 0006-0403-68 in bottles of 100.
Shown in Product Identification Guide, page 324
No. 7787—10 mg, pink in color, coded MSD 412 on one side and URECHOLINE on the other.
NDC 0006-0412-68 in bottles of 100
(6505-00-616-7856 10 mg 100's).
Shown in Product Identification Guide, page 324
No. 7788—25 mg, yellow in color, coded MSD 457 on one side and URECHOLINE on the other.
NDC 0006-0457-68 in bottles of 100
(6505-00-912-7440 25 mg, 100's).
Shown in Product Identification Guide, page 324
No. 7790 — 50 mg, yellow in color, coded MSD 460 on one side and URECHOLINE on the other.
NDC 0006-0460-68 in bottles of 100.
Shown in Product Identification Guide, page 324
No. 7786—Injection URECHOLINE, 5.15 mg per mL, is a clear, colorless solution, and is supplied as follows:
NDC 0006-7786-29 in box of 6 × 1 mL vials
(6505-00-616-8947 in box of 6 × 1 mL vials).
Storage
Store Tablets URECHOLINE in a tightly-closed container.
Avoid storage at temperatures above 40°C (104°F).
Avoid storage of Injection URECHOLINE at temperatures below −20°C (−4°F) and above 40°C (104°F).
7875834 Issued August 1997

Continued on next page

Information on the Merck & Co., Inc. products listed on these pages is the full prescribing information from product circulars in use September 30, 2000. For information, please call 1-800-NSC MERCK [1-800-672-6372].

VAQTA® ℞
(Hepatitis A Vaccine, Inactivated)

DESCRIPTION

VAQTA* [Hepatitis A Vaccine, Inactivated] is an inactivated whole virus vaccine derived from hepatitis A virus (HAV) grown in cell culture in human MRC-5 diploid fibroblasts. It contains inactivated virus of a strain which was originally derived by further serial passage of a proven attenuated strain. The virus is grown, harvested, purified by a combination of physical and high performance liquid chromatographic techniques developed at the Merck Research Laboratories, formalin inactivated, and then adsorbed onto aluminum hydroxide. One milliliter of the vaccine contains approximately 50 units (U) of hepatitis A virus antigen, which is purified and formulated without a preservative. Within the limits of current assay variability, the 50U dose of VAQTA contains less than 0.1 mcg of non-viral protein, less than 4×10^{-6} mcg of DNA, less than 10^{-4} mcg of bovine albumin, and less than 0.8 mcg of formaldehyde. Other process chemical residuals are less than 10 parts per billion (ppb).

VAQTA is a sterile suspension for intramuscular injection. VAQTA is supplied in two formulations:

Pediatric/Adolescent Formulation: each 0.5 mL dose contains approximately 25U of hepatitis A virus antigen adsorbed onto approximately 0.225 mg of aluminum provided as aluminum hydroxide, and 35 mcg of sodium borate as a pH stabilizer, in 0.9% sodium chloride.

Adult Formulation: each 1 mL dose contains approximately 50U of hepatitis A virus antigen adsorbed onto approximately 0.45 mg of aluminum provided as aluminum hydroxide, and 70 mcg of sodium borate as a pH stabilizer, in 0.9% sodium chloride.

*Registered trademark of MERCK & CO., Inc.

CLINICAL PHARMACOLOGY

Hepatitis A Disease

Hepatitis A virus is one of several hepatitis viruses that cause a systemic infection with pathology in the liver. The incubation period ranges from approximately 20 to 50 days. While the course of the disease is generally benign and does not result in chronic hepatitis, infection with hepatitis A virus remains an important cause of morbidity and occasional fulminant hepatitis and death.

Hepatitis A is transmitted most often by the fecal-oral route, with infection occurring primarily within private households. Common-source outbreaks due to contaminated food and water supplies have occurred following consumption of certain foods such as raw shellfish, and uncooked foods prepared by an infected food-handler or otherwise contaminated prior to ingestion (salads, sandwiches, frozen raspberries, etc.) Bloodborne transmission, while uncommon, is possible via blood transfusion, contaminated blood products, or from needles shared with an infected viremic individual. Sexual transmission has also been reported.

The disease burden due to hepatitis A in the United States has been estimated to be approximately 143,000 infections per year, of which 75,800 result in clinical hepatitis A disease, 11,400 hospitalizations, and 80 deaths due to fulminant hepatitis. Worldwide, it has been estimated that 1.4 million cases are reported annually. The clinical manifestations of hepatitis A infection often pass unrecognized in children ≤2 years of age whereas overt hepatitis A develops in the majority of infected older children and adults. Symptoms and signs of hepatitis A infection are similar to those associated with other types of viral hepatitis and include anorexia, nausea, fever/chills, jaundice, dark urine, light-colored stools, abdominal pain, malaise, and fatigue.

Clinical Trials

Clinical trials conducted worldwide with several formulations of the vaccine in 9181 healthy individuals ranging from 2 to 85 years of age have demonstrated that VAQTA is highly immunogenic and generally well tolerated.

Protection from hepatitis A disease has been shown to be related to the presence of antibody; an anamnestic antibody response occurs in healthy individuals with a history of infection who are subsequently re-exposed to hepatitis A virus. Similarly, protection after vaccination with VAQTA has been associated with the onset of seroconversion (≥10 mIU/mL of hepatitis A antibody, measured by a modification of the HAVAB** radioimmunoassay [RIA]) and with an anamnestic antibody response following booster vaccination with VAQTA.

Immunology

In combined clinical studies, 97% of 1214 healthy children and adolescents 2 through 17 years of age seroconverted with a geometric mean titer (GMT) of 43 mIU/mL within 4 weeks after a single ~25U/0.5 mL intramuscular dose of VAQTA. Similarly, 95% of 1428 adults ≥18 years of age seroconverted with a GMT of 37 mIU/mL within 4 weeks after a single ~50U/1.0 mL intramuscular dose of VAQTA. Furthermore, at 2 weeks post-vaccination, 69% (n=744) of adults seroconverted with a GMT of 16 mIU/mL after a single dose of VAQTA. Immune memory was demonstrated by an anamnestic antibody response in individuals who received a booster dose (see *Persistence*).

While a study evaluating VAQTA alone in a post-exposure setting has not been conducted, the concurrent use of VAQTA (~50U) and immune globulin (IG, 0.06 mL/kg) was evaluated in a clinical study involving healthy adults 18 to 39 years of age. Table 1 provides seroconversion rates and GMT at 4 and 24 weeks after the first dose in each treatment group and at one month after a booster dose of VAQTA (administered at 24 weeks).

Table 1
Seroconversion Rates (%) and Geometric Mean Titers (GMT) after Vaccination with VAQTA plus IG, VAQTA Alone, and IG Alone

Weeks	VAQTA plus IG	VAQTA	IG
	Seroconversion Rate GMT (mIU/mL)		
4	100% 42 (n=129)	96% 38 (n=135)	87% 19 (n=30)
24	92% 83 (n=125)	97%* 137* (n=132)	0% 5 (n=28)
28	100% 4872 (n=114)	100% 6498 (n=128)	N/A

* The seroconversion rate and the GMT in the group receiving VAQTA alone were significantly higher than in the group receiving VAQTA plus IG (p=0.05, p<0.001, respectively).

N/A=Not Applicable

Efficacy

A very high degree of protection has been demonstrated after a single dose of VAQTA in children and adolescents. The protective efficacy, immunogenicity and safety of VAQTA were evaluated in a randomized, double-blind, placebo-controlled study involving 1037 susceptible healthy children and adolescents 2 through 16 years of age in a U.S. community with recurrent outbreaks of hepatitis A (The Monroe Efficacy Study). Each child received an intramuscular dose of VAQTA (~25U) or placebo. Among those individuals who were initially seronegative (by modified HAVAB), seroconversion was achieved in >99% of vaccine recipients within 4 weeks after vaccination. The onset of seroconversion following a single dose of VAQTA was shown to parallel the onset of protection against clinical hepatitis A disease.

Because of the long incubation period of the disease (approximately 20 to 50 days, or longer in children), the primary endpoint was based on clinically confirmed cases*** of hepatitis A occurring ≥50 days after vaccination in order to exclude any children incubating the infection before vaccination. In subjects who were initially seronegative, the protective efficacy of a single dose of VAQTA was observed to be 100% with 21 cases of clinically confirmed hepatitis A occurring in the placebo group and none in the vaccine group (p<0.001). A secondary endpoint was pre-defined as the number of clinically confirmed cases of hepatitis A ≥30 days. With this secondary endpoint, 28 cases of clinically confirmed hepatitis A occurred in the placebo group while none occurred in the vaccine group ≥30 days after vaccination. In addition, it was observed in this trial that no cases of clinically confirmed hepatitis A occurred in the vaccine group after day 16.† Following demonstration of protection with a single dose and termination of the study, a booster dose was administered to a subset of vaccinees 6, 12, or 18 months after the primary dose.

Persistence

The total duration of the protective effect of VAQTA in healthy vaccinees is unknown at present. However, seropositivity was shown to persist up to 18 months after a single ~25U dose in a cohort of 35 out of 39 children and adolescents who participated in the Monroe Efficacy Study; 95% of this cohort responded anamnestically following a booster at 18 months. To date, no cases of clinically confirmed hepatitis A disease ≥50 days after vaccination have occurred in those vaccinees from The Monroe Efficacy Study monitored for up to 4 years.

The effectiveness of VAQTA for use in community outbreak control has been demonstrated by the fact that, although cases of imported infection have occurred, the study community has remained free of outbreaks. In contrast, three nearby sister communities to Monroe have continued to experience outbreaks.

In adults, seropositivity has been shown to persist up to 6 months after a single ~50U dose. Studies are ongoing to evaluate longer-term persistence and the need, if any, for additional booster doses. Persistence of immunologic memory was demonstrated with an anamnestic antibody response to a booster dose of ~25U given 6 to 18 months after the primary dose in children and adolescents (Table 2), and to a booster dose of ~50U given 6 months after the primary dose to adults (Table 3).

Table 2
Children/Adolescents
Seroconversion Rates (%) and Geometric Mean Titers (GMT) for Cohorts of Initially Seronegative Vaccinees at the Time of the Booster (~25U) and 4 Weeks Later

Weeks Following Initial ~25U Dose	Cohort* (n=949) 0 and 6 Months	Cohort* (n=35) 0 and 12 Months	Cohort* (n=39) 0 and 18 Months
	Seroconversion Rate GMT (mIU/mL)		
24	97% 109	—	—
28	100% 10609	—	—
52	—	91% 48	—
56	—	100% 12308	—
78	—	—	90% 50
82	—	—	100% 9591

*Blood samples taken at both time points.

Table 3
Adults
Seroconversion Rates (%) and Geometric Mean Titers (GMT) for a Cohort of Vaccinees After a Booster Dose (~50U) of VAQTA Administered at 6 Months

Weeks Following Initial ~50U Dose	Cohort (n=1152) 0 and 6 Months
	Seroconversion Rate GMT (mIU/mL)
24	98% 134
28	100% 6010

** Trademark of Abbott Laboratories

*** The clinical case definition included all of the following occurring at the same time: 1) one or more typical clinical signs or symptoms of hepatitis A (e.g., jaundice, malaise, fever ≥ 38.3°C), 2) elevation of hepatitis A IgM antibody (HAVAB-M), 3) elevation of alanine transferase (ALT) ≥2 times the upper limit of normal.

† One vaccinee did not meet the pre-defined criteria for clinically confirmed hepatitis A but did have positive hepatitis A IgM and borderline liver enzyme (ALT) elevations on days 34, 50, and 58 after vaccination with mild clinical symptoms observed on days 49 and 50.

INDICATIONS AND USAGE

VAQTA is indicated for active pre-exposure prophylaxis against disease caused by hepatitis A virus in persons 2 years of age and older. Primary immunization should be given at least 2 weeks prior to expected exposure to HAV.

Individuals who are or will be at increased risk of infection by HAV include:

TRAVELERS

Persons traveling to areas of higher endemicity for hepatitis A. These areas include, but are not limited to, Africa, Asia (except Japan), the Mediterranean basin, Eastern Europe, the Middle East, Central and South America, Mexico, and parts of the Caribbean. Current CDC (Centers for Disease Control and Prevention) advisories should be consulted with regard to specific locales.

MILITARY PERSONNEL

PEOPLE LIVING IN, OR RELOCATING TO, AREAS OF HIGH ENDEMICITY

CERTAIN ETHNIC AND GEOGRAPHIC POPULATIONS THAT EXPERIENCE CYCLIC HEPATITIS A EPIDEMICS SUCH AS:

Native peoples of Alaska and the Americas.

OTHERS

Persons engaging in high-risk sexual activity (such as homosexually active males); users of illicit injectable drugs; residents of a community experiencing an outbreak of hepatitis A.

Hemophiliacs and other recipients of therapeutic blood products (see PRECAUTIONS and DOSAGE AND ADmap edit MINISTRATION).

Although the epidemiology of hepatitis A does not permit the identification of other specific populations at high risk of disease, outbreaks of hepatitis A or exposure to hepatitis A virus have been described in a variety of populations in which VAQTA may be useful:

— Certain institutional workers (e.g., caretakers for the developmentally challenged)
— Employees of child day-care centers
— Laboratory workers who handle live hepatitis A virus
— Handlers of primate animals that may be harboring HAV

PEOPLE EXPOSED TO HEPATITIS A
For those requiring both immediate and long-term protection, VAQTA may be administered concomitantly with IG.
Revaccination
See DOSAGE AND ADMINISTRATION, *DOSAGE.*
Use With Other Vaccines
Data to recommend concurrent use with other vaccines are limited.
Use With Immune Globulin
For individuals requiring either post-exposure prophylaxis or combined immediate and longer-term protection (e.g., travelers departing on short notice to endemic areas), VAQTA may be administered concomitantly with IG using separate sites and syringes (see CLINICAL PHARMACOLOGY and DOSAGE AND ADMINISTRATION).
VAQTA IS NOT RECOMMENDED FOR USE IN INFANTS YOUNGER THAN 2 YEARS OF AGE SINCE DATA ON USE IN THIS AGE GROUP ARE NOT CURRENTLY AVAILABLE.

CONTRAINDICATIONS

Hypersensitivity to any component of the vaccine.

WARNINGS

Individuals who develop symptoms suggestive of hypersensitivity after an injection of VAQTA should not receive further injections of the vaccine (see CONTRAINDICATIONS).
If VAQTA is used in individuals with malignancies or those receiving immunosuppressive therapy or who are otherwise immunocompromised, the expected immune response may not be obtained.

PRECAUTIONS

General
VAQTA will not prevent hepatitis caused by infectious agents other than hepatitis A virus. Because of the long incubation period (approximately 20 to 50 days) for hepatitis A, it is possible for unrecognized hepatitis A infection to be present at the time the vaccine is given. The vaccine may not prevent hepatitis A in such individuals.
As with any vaccine, adequate treatment provisions, including epinephrine, should be available for immediate use should an anaphylactic or anaphylactoid reaction occur.
VAQTA should be administered with caution to people with bleeding disorders who are at risk of hemorrhage following intramuscular injection (see DOSAGE AND ADMINISTRATION).
As with any vaccine, vaccination with VAQTA may not result in a protective response in all susceptible vaccinees.
An acute infection or febrile illness may be reason for delaying use of VAQTA except when, in the opinion of the physician, withholding the vaccine entails a greater risk.
Carcinogenesis, Mutagenesis, Impairment of Fertility
VAQTA has not been evaluated for its carcinogenic or mutagenic potential, or its potential to impair fertility.
Pregnancy
Pregnancy Category C: Animal reproduction studies have not been conducted with VAQTA. It is also not known whether VAQTA can cause fetal harm when administered to a pregnant woman or can affect reproduction capacity. VAQTA should be given to a pregnant woman only if clearly needed.
Nursing Mothers
It is not known whether VAQTA is excreted in human milk. Because many drugs are excreted in human milk, caution should be exercised when VAQTA is administered to a woman who is breast feeding.
Pediatric Use
VAQTA has been shown to be generally well tolerated and highly immunogenic in individuals 2 through 17 years of age. See DOSAGE AND ADMINISTRATION for the recommended dosage schedule.
Safety and effectiveness in infants below 2 years of age have not been established.

ADVERSE REACTIONS

In combined clinical trials, 16,252 doses of VAQTA were administered to 9181 healthy children, adolescents, and adults. VAQTA was generally well tolerated.
No serious vaccine-related adverse experiences were observed during clinical trials.
The Monroe Efficacy Study
In this study, 1037 healthy children and adolescents, 2 through 16 years of age, received a primary dose of ~25U of hepatitis A vaccine and a booster 6, 12, or 18 months later, or placebo. Subjects were observed during a 5-day period for fever and local complaints and during a 14-day period for systemic complaints. Injection-site complaints, generally mild and transient, were the most frequently reported complaints. Table 4 summarizes the local and systemic complaints (≥1%) reported in this study, without regard to causality. There were no significant differences in the rates of any complaints between vaccine and placebo recipients after Dose 1.
[See table above]

Table 4
Local and Systemic Complaints (≥1%) in Healthy Children and Adolescents from The Monroe Efficacy Study

Reaction	VAQTA Dose 1*	VAQTA Booster	Placebo*†
Injection-Site Complaints			
Pain	6.4% (33/515)	3.4% (16/475)	6.3% (32/510)
Tenderness	4.9% (25/515)	1.7% (8/475)	6.1% (31/510
Erythema	1.9% (10/515)	0.8% (4/475)	1.8% (9/510)
Swelling	1.7% (9/515)	1.5% (7/475)	1.6% (8/510)
Warmth	1.7% (9/515)	0.6% (3/475)	1.6% (8/510)
Systemic Complaints			
Abdominal Pain	1.2% (6/519)	1.1% (5/475)	1.0% (5/518)
Pharyngitis	1.2% (6/519)	0% (0/475)	0.8% (4/518)
Headache	0.4% (2/519)	0.8% (4/475)	1.0% (5/518)

* No statistically significant differences between the two groups.
† Second injection of placebo not administered because code for the trial was broken.

Children/Adolescents — 2 through 17 Years of Age
In combined clinical trials (including Monroe Efficacy Study participants) involving 2595 healthy children and adolescents who received one or more ~25U doses of hepatitis A vaccine, fever and local complaints were observed during a 5-day period following vaccination and systemic complaints during a 14-day period following vaccination. Injection-site complaints, generally mild and transient, were the most frequently reported complaints. Listed below are the complaints (≥1%) reported, without regard to causality, in decreasing order of frequency within each body system.
LOCALIZED INJECTION-SITE REACTIONS (generally mild and transient)
Pain (18.7%); tenderness (16.8%); warmth (8.6%); erythema (7.5%); swelling (7.3%); ecchymosis (1.3%).
BODY AS A WHOLE
Fever (≥102°F, Oral) (3.1%); abdominal pain (1.6%).
DIGESTIVE SYSTEM
Diarrhea (1.0%); vomiting (1.0%).
NERVOUS SYSTEM/PSYCHIATRIC
Headache (2.3%).
RESPIRATORY SYSTEM
Pharyngitis (1.5%); upper respiratory infection (1.1%); cough (1.0%).
LABORATORY FINDINGS
Very few laboratory abnormalities were reported and included isolated reports of elevated liver function tests, eosinophilia, and increased urine protein.
Adults—18 Years of Age and Older
In combined clinical trials involving 1529 healthy adults who received one or more ~50U doses of hepatitis A vaccine, fever and local complaints were observed during a 5-day period following vaccination and systemic complaints during a 14-day period following vaccination. Injection-site complaints, generally mild and transient, were the most frequently reported complaints. Listed below are the complaints (≥1%) reported, without regard to causality, in decreasing order of frequency within each body system.
LOCALIZED INJECTION-SITE REACTIONS (generally mild and transient)
Tenderness (52.6%); pain (51.1%); warmth (17.3%); swelling (13.6%); erythema (12.9%); ecchymosis (1.5%); pain/soreness (1.2%).
BODY AS A WHOLE
Asthenia/fatigue (3.9%); fever (≥101°F, Oral) (2.6%); abdominal pain (1.3%).
DIGESTIVE SYSTEM
Diarrhea (2.4%); nausea (2.3%).
MUSCULOSKELETAL SYSTEM
Myalgia (2.0%); arm pain (1.3%); back pain (1.1%); stiffness (1.0%).
NERVOUS SYSTEM/PSYCHIATRIC
Headache (16.1%).
RESPIRATORY SYSTEM
Pharyngitis (2.7%); upper respiratory infection (2.8%); nasal congestion (1.1%).
UROGENITAL SYSTEM
Menstruation disorder (1.1%).
Allergic Reactions
Local and/or systemic allergic reactions that occurred in <1% of children/adolescents or adults in clinical trials regardless of causality included:
LOCAL
Injection site pruritus and/or rash.
SYSTEMIC
Bronchial constriction; asthma; wheezing; edema/swelling; rash; generalized erythema; urticaria; pruritus; eye irritation/itching; dermatitis. (See CONTRAINDICATIONS and WARNINGS.)
As with any vaccine, there is the possibility that use of VAQTA in very large populations might reveal adverse experiences not observed in clinical trials.

DOSAGE AND ADMINISTRATION

Do not inject intravenously, intradermally, or subcutaneously.
VAQTA is for intramuscular injection. The *deltoid muscle* is the preferred site for intramuscular injection.
DOSAGE
The vaccination regimen consists of one primary dose and one booster dose for healthy children, adolescents, and adults, as follows:
Pediatric/Adolescent
Individuals 2 through 17 years of age should receive a single 0.5 mL (~25U) dose of vaccine at elected date and a booster dose of 0.5 mL (~25U) 6 to 18 months later.
Adult
Adults 18 years of age and older should receive a single 1.0 mL (~50U) dose of vaccine at elected date and a booster dose of 1.0 mL (~50U) 6 months later.
Use With Immune Globulin
VAQTA may be administered concomitantly with IG using separate sites and syringes. The vaccination regimen for VAQTA should be followed as stated above. Consult the manufacturer's product circular for the appropriate dosage of IG. A booster dose of VAQTA should be administered at the appropriate time as outlined above.
ADMINISTRATION
Known or Presumed Exposure to HAV/Travel to Endemic Areas
For individuals requiring either post-exposure prophylaxis or combined immediate and longer term protection (e.g., travelers departing on short notice to endemic areas), VAQTA may be administered concomitantly with IG using separate sites and syringes (see CLINICAL PHARMACOLOGY and DOSAGE AND ADMINISTRATION, *Use With Immune Globulin*).
Injection must be accomplished with a needle long enough to ensure intramuscular deposition of the vaccine. The Advisory Committee on Immunization Practices (ACIP) has recommended that "For all intramuscular injections, the needle should be long enough to reach the muscle mass and prevent vaccine from seeping into subcutaneous tissue, but not so long as to endanger underlying neurovascular structures or bone." For toddlers and older children they further state that "...the deltoid may be used if the muscle mass is adequate. The needle size can range from 22 to 25 gauge and from 5/8 to $1^1/_4$ inches, based on the size of the muscle...the anterolateral thigh may be used, but the needle should be longer—generally ranging from 7/8 to $1^1/_4$ inches." For adults they state that "...the deltoid is recommended for routine intramuscular vaccination among adults...The suggested needle size is 1 to $1^1/_2$ inches and 20 to 25 gauge."
For individuals with bleeding disorders who are at risk of hemorrhage following intramuscular injection, the ACIP recommends that when any intramuscular vaccine is indicated for such patients, "...it should be administered intramuscularly if, in the opinion of a physician familiar with the patient's bleeding risk, the vaccine can be administered with reasonable safety by this route. If the patient receives antihemophilia or other similar therapy, intramuscular vaccination can be scheduled shortly after such therapy is administered. A fine needle (≤23 gauge) can be used for the vaccination and firm pressure applied to the site (without rubbing) for at least two minutes. The patient or family should be instructed concerning the risk of hematoma from the injection."
The vaccine should be used as supplied; no reconstitution is necessary.
Shake well before withdrawal and use. Thorough agitation is necessary to maintain suspension of the vaccine. Discard if the suspension does not appear homogenous.
Parenteral drug products should be inspected visually for extraneous particulate matter and discoloration prior to administration whenever solution and container permit. After thorough agitation, VAQTA is a slightly opaque, white suspension.
It is important to use a separate sterile syringe and needle for each individual to prevent transmission of infectious agents from one person to another.

Continued on next page

Information on the Merck & Co., Inc. products listed on these pages is the full prescribing information from product circulars in use September 30, 2000. For information, please call 1-800-NSC MERCK [1-800-672-6372].

Vaqta—Cont.

HOW SUPPLIED

PEDIATRIC/ADOLESCENT FORMULATION

Vials

No. 4831—VAQTA for pediatric/adolescent use is supplied as 25U/0.5 mL of hepatitis A virus protein in a 0.5 mL single-dose vial, **NDC** 0006-4831-00.

No. 4831—VAQTA for pediatric/adolescent use is supplied as 25U/0.5 mL of hepatitis A virus protein in a 0.5 mL single-dose vial, in a box of 5 single-dose vials, **NDC** 0006-4831-38.

Syringes

No. 4845—VAQTA for pediatric/adolescent use is supplied as 25U/0.5 mL of hepatitis A virus protein in a 0.5 mL single-dose prefilled syringe, **NDC** 0006-4845-00.

No. 4845—VAQTA for pediatric/adolescent use is supplied as 25U/0.5 mL of hepatitis A virus protein in a 0.5 mL single-dose prefilled syringe, in a box of 5 single-dose prefilled syringes, **NDC** 0006-4845-38.

ADULT FORMULATION

Vials

No. 4841—VAQTA for adult use is supplied as 50U/1 mL of hepatitis A virus protein in a 1 mL single-dose vial, **NDC** 0006-4841-00.

No. 4841—VAQTA for adult use is supplied as 50U/1 mL of hepatitis A virus protein in a 1 mL single-dose vial, in a box of 5 single-dose vials, **NDC** 0006-4841-38.

Syringes

No. 4844—VAQTA for adult use is supplied as 50U/1 mL of hepatitis A virus protein in a 1 mL single-dose prefilled syringe, **NDC** 0006-4844-00.

No. 4844—VAQTA for adult use is supplied as 50U/1 mL of hepatitis A virus protein in a 1 mL single-dose prefilled syringe, in a box of 5 single-dose, prefilled syringes, **NDC** 0006-4844-38.

Storage

Store vaccine at 2–8°C (36–46°F).

DO NOT FREEZE since freezing destroys potency.

Syringes of VAQTA are also filled by:

Evans Medical Ltd.

Gaskill Road, Speke, Liverpool L24 9GR, England

7977500 Issued March 1996

VARIVAX® ℞
[Varicella Virus Vaccine Live (Oka/Merck)]

DESCRIPTION

VARIVAX* [Varicella Virus Vaccine Live (Oka/Merck)] is a preparation of the Oka/Merck strain of live, attenuated varicella virus. The virus was initially obtained from a child with natural varicella, then introduced into human embryonic lung cell cultures, adapted to and propagated in embryonic guinea pig cell cultures and finally propagated in human diploid cell cultures (WI-38). Further passage of the virus for varicella vaccine was performed at Merck Research Laboratories (MRL) in human diploid cell cultures (MRC-5) that were free of adventitious agents. This live, attenuated varicella vaccine is a lyophilized preparation containing sucrose, phosphate, glutamate, and processed gelatin as stabilizers.

VARIVAX, when reconstituted as directed, is a sterile preparation for subcutaneous administration. Each 0.5 mL dose contains the following: a minimum of 1350 PFU (plaque forming units) of Oka/Merck varicella virus when reconstituted and stored at room temperature for 30 minutes, approximately 25 mg of sucrose, 12.5 mg hydrolyzed gelatin, 3.2 mg sodium chloride, 0.5 mg monosodium L-glutamate, 0.45 mg of sodium phosphate dibasic, 0.08 mg of potassium phosphate monobasic, 0.08 mg of potassium chloride; residual components of MRC-5 cells including DNA and protein; and trace quantities of sodium phosphate monobasic, EDTA, neomycin, and fetal bovine serum. The product contains no preservative.

To maintain potency, the lyophilized vaccine must be kept frozen at an average temperature of −15°C (+5°F) or colder and must be used before the expiration date (see HOW SUPPLIED, *Stability* and *Storage*). Storage in any freezer (e.g., chest, frost-free) that reliably maintains an average temperature of −15°C (+5°F) or colder and has a separate sealed freezer door is acceptable.

*Registered trademark of MERCK & CO., Inc.

CLINICAL PHARMACOLOGY

Varicella is a highly communicable disease in children, adolescents, and adults caused by the varicella-zoster virus. The disease usually consists of 300 to 500 maculopapular and/or vesicular lesions accompanied by a fever (oral temperature ≥100°F) in up to 70% of individuals. Approximately 3.5 million cases of varicella occurred annually from 1980–1994 in the United States with the peak incidence occurring in children five to nine years of age. The incidence rate of chickenpox is 8.3–9.1% per year in children 1–9 years of age. The attack rate of natural varicella following household exposure among healthy susceptible children was shown to be 87%. Although it is generally a benign, self-limiting disease, varicella may be associated with serious complications (e.g., bacterial superinfection, pneumonia, encephalitis, Reye's Syndrome), and/or death.

Evaluation of Clinical Efficacy Afforded by VARIVAX

Clinical Data in Children

In combined clinical trials of VARIVAX at doses ranging from 1,000–17,000 PFU, the majority of subjects who received VARIVAX and were exposed to wild-type virus were either completely protected from chickenpox or developed a milder form (for clinical description see below) of the disease. The protective efficacy of VARIVAX was evaluated in three different ways: 1) by comparing chickenpox rates in vaccinees versus historical controls, 2) by assessment of protection from disease following household exposure, and 3) by a placebo-controlled, double-blind clinical trial.

In early clinical trials, a total of 4142 children received 1000–1625 PFU of attenuated virus per dose of VARIVAX and have been followed for up to six years post single-dose vaccination. In this group there was considerable variation in chickenpox rates among studies and study sites, and much of the reported data were acquired by passive follow-up. It was observed that 2.1%–3.6% of vaccinees per year reported chickenpox (called breakthrough cases). This represents an approximate 67% (57–77%) decrease from the total number of cases expected based on attack rates in children aged 1–9 over this same period (8.3–9.1%). In those who developed breakthrough chickenpox postvaccination, the majority experienced mild disease (median number of lesions <50). In one study, a total of 47% (27/58) of breakthrough cases had <50 lesions compared with 8% (7/92) in unvaccinated individuals, and 7% (4/58) of breakthrough cases had >300 lesions compared with 50% (46/92) in unvaccinated individuals. In studies of vaccinated children who contracted chickenpox after a household exposure, 57% (31/54) of the cases reported <50 lesions, while 1.9% (1/54) reported >300 lesions with an oral temperature above 100°F.

In later clinical trials with the current vaccine, a total of 1164 children received 2900–9000 PFU of attenuated virus per dose of VARIVAX and have been followed for up to three years post single-dose vaccination. It was observed that 0.2%–1.0% of vaccinees per year reported breakthrough chickenpox for up to three years post single-dose vaccination. This represents an approximate 93% decrease from the total number of cases expected based on attack rates in children aged 1–9 over this same period (8.3%–9.1%). In those who developed breakthrough chickenpox postvaccination, the majority experienced mild disease.

Among a subset of vaccinees who were actively followed, 259 were exposed to an individual with chickenpox in a household setting. There were no reports of breakthrough chickenpox in 80% of exposed children; 20% reported a mild form of chickenpox. This represents a 77% reduction in the expected number of cases when compared to the historical attack rate of varicella following household exposure to chickenpox of 87% in unvaccinated individuals.

Although no placebo-controlled trial was carried out with VARIVAX using the current vaccine, a placebo-controlled trial was conducted using a formulation containing 17,000 PFU per dose. In this trial, a single dose of VARIVAX protected 96–100% of children against chickenpox over a two-year period. The study enrolled healthy individuals 1 to 14 years of age (n=491 vaccine, n=465 placebo). In the first year, 8.5% of placebo recipients contracted chickenpox, while no vaccine recipient did, for a calculated protection rate of 100% during the first varicella season. In the second year, when only a subset of individuals agreed to remain in the blinded study (n=163 vaccine, n=161 placebo), 96% protective efficacy was calculated for the vaccine group as compared to placebo.

There are insufficient data to assess the rate of protection against the complications of chickenpox (e.g., encephalitis, hepatitis, pneumonia) in children.

Clinical Data in Adolescents and Adults

Although no placebo-controlled trial was carried out in adolescents and adults, efficacy was determined by evaluation of protection when vaccinees received 2 doses of VARIVAX 4 or 8 weeks apart and were subsequently exposed to chickenpox in a household setting. In up to two years of active follow-up, 17 of 64 (27%) vaccinees reported breakthrough chickenpox following household exposure; of the 17 cases, 12 (71%) reported <50 lesions, 5 reported 50–300 lesions, and none reported >300 lesions with an oral temperature above 100°F. In combined clinical studies of adolescents and adults (n=1019) who received two doses of VARIVAX and later developed breakthrough chickenpox and reported numbers of lesions (42 of 1019), 25 of 42 (60%) reported <50 lesions, 16 of 42 (38%) reported 50–300 lesions, and 1 of 42 (2%) reported >300 lesions and an oral temperature above 100°F.

The attack rate of unvaccinated adults exposed to a single contact in a household has not been previously studied. When compared to the previously reported attack rate of natural varicella of 87% following household exposure among unvaccinated children, this represents an approximate 70% reduction in the expected number of cases in the household setting.

There are insufficient data to assess the rate of protection of VARIVAX against the serious complications of chickenpox in adults (e.g., encephalitis, hepatitis, pneumonitis) and during pregnancy (congenital varicella syndrome).

Immunogenicity of VARIVAX

Clinical trials with several formulations of the vaccine containing attenuated virus ranging from 1000 to 17,000 PFU per dose have demonstrated that VARIVAX induces detectable immune responses in a high proportion of individuals and is generally well tolerated in healthy individuals ranging from 12 months to 55 years of age.

Seroconversion as defined by the acquisition of any detectable varicella antibodies (gpELISA >0.3, a highly sensitive assay which is not commercially available) was observed in 97% of vaccinees at approximately 4–6 weeks postvaccination in 6889 susceptible children 12 months to 12 years of age. Rates of breakthrough disease were significantly lower among children with varicella antibody titers ≥5 compared to children with titers <5. Titers ≥5 were induced in approximately 76% of children vaccinated with a single dose of vaccine at 1000–17,000 PFU per dose. In a multicenter study involving susceptible adolescents and adults 13 years of age and older, two doses of VARIVAX administered four to eight weeks apart induced a seroconversion rate (gpELISA >0.3) of approximately 75% in 539 individuals four weeks after the first dose and of 99% in 479 individuals four weeks after the second dose. The average antibody response in vaccinees who received the second dose eight weeks after the first dose was higher than that in those, who received the second dose four weeks after the first dose. In another multicenter study involving adolescents and adults, two doses of VARIVAX administered eight weeks apart induced a seroconversion rate (gpELISA >0.3) of 94% in 142 individuals six weeks after the first dose and 99% in 122 individuals six weeks after the second dose.

VARIVAX also induces cell-mediated immune responses in vaccinees. The relative contributions of humoral immunity and cell-mediated immunity to protection from chickenpox are unknown.

Persistence of Immune Response

Studies in vaccinees examining chickenpox breakthrough rates over 5 years showed the lowest rates (0.2–2.9%) in the first two years postvaccination, with somewhat higher but stable rates in the third through fifth year. The severity of reported breakthrough chickenpox, as measured by number of lesions and maximum temperature, appeared not to increase with time since vaccination.

In clinical studies involving healthy children who received 1 dose of vaccine, detectable varicella antibodies (gpELISA >0.3) were present in 98.8% (3775/3822) at 1 year, 98.9% (1057/1069) at 2 years, 97.5% (548/562) at 3 years, and 99.5% (220/221) at 4 years postvaccination. Antibody levels were present at least one year in 97.2% (423/435) of healthy adolescents and adults who received two doses of live varicella vaccine separated by 4 to 8 weeks. A boost in antibody levels has been observed in vaccinees following exposure to natural varicella which could account for the apparent long-term persistence of antibody levels after vaccination in these studies. The duration of protection from varicella obtained using VARIVAX in the absence of wild-type boosting is unknown. VARIVAX also induces cell-mediated immune responses in vaccinees. The relative contributions of humoral immunity and cell-mediated immunity to protection from chickenpox are unknown.

Transmission

In the placebo-controlled trial, transmission of vaccine virus was assessed in household settings (during the 8-week post-vaccination period) in 416 susceptible placebo recipients who were household contacts of 445 vaccine recipients. Of the 416 placebo recipients, three developed chickenpox and seroconverted, nine reported a varicella-like rash and did not seroconvert, and six had no rash but seroconverted. If vaccine virus transmission occurred, it did so at a very low rate and possibly without recognizable clinical disease in contacts. These cases may represent either natural varicella from community contacts or a low incidence of transmission of vaccine virus from vaccinated contacts (see PRECAUTIONS, *Transmission*). Post-marketing experience suggests that transmission of vaccine virus may occur rarely between healthy vaccinees who develop a varicella-like rash and healthy susceptible contacts. Transmission of vaccine virus from vaccinees without a varicella-like rash has been reported but has not been confirmed.

Herpes Zoster

Overall, 9454 healthy children (12 months to 12 years of age) and 1648 adolescents and adults (13 years of age and older) have been vaccinated with Oka/Merck live attenuated varicella vaccine in clinical trials. Eight cases of herpes zoster have been reported in children during 42,556 person years of follow-up in clinical trials, resulting in a calculated incidence of at least 18.8 cases per 100,000 person years. The completeness of this reporting has not been determined. One case of herpes zoster has been reported in the adolescent and adult age group during 5410 person years of follow-up in clinical trials resulting in a calculated incidence of 18.5 cases per 100,000 person years.

All nine cases were mild and without sequelae. Two cultures (one child and one adult) obtained from vesicles were positive for wild-type varicella zoster virus as confirmed by restriction endonuclease analysis. The long-term effect of VARIVAX on the incidence of herpes zoster, particularly in those vaccinees exposed to natural varicella, is unknown at present.

In children, the reported rate of zoster in vaccine recipients appears not to exceed that previously determined in a population-based study of healthy children who had experienced natural varicella. The incidence of zoster in adults who have had natural varicella infection is higher than that in children.

Reye's Syndrome
Reye's Syndrome has occurred in children and adolescents following natural varicella infection, the majority of whom had received salicylates. In clinical studies in healthy children and adolescents in the United States, physicians advised varicella vaccine recipients not to use salicylates for six weeks after vaccination. There were no reports of Reye's Syndrome in varicella vaccine recipients during these studies.
Studies with Other Vaccines
In combined clinical studies involving 1080 children 12 to 36 months of age, 653 received VARIVAX and M-M-R*II (Measles, Mumps, and Rubella Virus Vaccine Live) concomitantly at separate sites and 427 received the vaccines six weeks apart. Seroconversion rates and antibody levels were comparable between the two groups at approximately six weeks postvaccination to each of the virus vaccine components. No differences were noted in adverse reactions reported in those who received VARIVAX concomitantly with M-M-R II (Measles, Mumps, and Rubella Virus Vaccine Live) at separate sites and those who received VARIVAX and M-M-R II (Measles, Mumps, and Rubella Virus Vaccine Live) at different times (see PRECAUTIONS, *Drug Interactions, Use with Other Vaccines*).
In a clinical study involving 318 children 12 months to 42 months of age, 160 received an investigational vaccine (a formulation combining measles, mumps, rubella, and varicella in one syringe) concomitantly with booster doses of DTaP (diphtheria, tetanus, acellular pertussis) and OPV (oral poliovirus vaccine) while 144 received M-M-R II (Measles, Mumps, and Rubella Virus Vaccine Live) concomitantly with booster doses of DTaP and OPV followed by VARIVAX 6 weeks later. At six weeks postvaccination, seroconversion rates for measles, mumps, rubella, and varicella and the percentage of vaccinees whose titers were boosted for diphtheria, tetanus, pertussis, and polio were comparable between the two groups, but anti-varicella levels were decreased when the investigational vaccine containing varicella was administered concomitantly with DTaP. No clinically significant differences were noted in adverse reactions between the two groups.
In another clinical study involving 307 children 12 to 18 months of age, 150 received an investigational vaccine (a formulation combining measles, mumps, rubella, and varicella in one syringe) concomitantly with a booster dose of PedvaxHIB* [Haemophilus b Conjugate Vaccine (Meningococcal Protein Conjugate)] while 130 received M-M-R II (Measles, Mumps, and Rubella Virus Vaccine Live) concomitantly with a booster dose of PedvaxHIB followed by VARIVAX 6 weeks later. At six weeks postvaccination, seroconversion rates for measles, mumps, rubella, and varicella, and geometric mean titers for PedvaxHIB were comparable between the two groups, but anti-varicella levels were decreased when the investigational vaccine containing varicella was administered concomitantly with PedvaxHIB. No clinically significant differences in adverse reactions were seen between the two groups.
VARIVAX is recommended for subcutaneous administration. However, during clinical trials, some children received VARIVAX intramuscularly resulting in seroconversion rates similar to those in children who received the vaccine by the subcutaneous route. Persistence of antibody and efficacy in those receiving intramuscular injections have not been defined.

* Registered trademark of MERCK & Co., Inc.

INDICATIONS AND USAGE

VARIVAX is indicated for vaccination against varicella in individuals 12 months of age and older.
Revaccination
The duration of protection of VARIVAX is unknown at present and the need for booster doses is not defined. However, a boost in antibody levels has been observed in vaccinees following exposure to natural varicella as well as following a booster dose of VARIVAX administered four to six years postvaccination.
In a highly vaccinated population, immunity for some individuals may wane due to lack of exposure to natural varicella as a result of shifting epidemiology. Post-marketing surveillance studies are ongoing to evaluate the need and timing for booster vaccination.
Vaccination with VARIVAX may not result in protection of all healthy, susceptible children, adolescents, and adults (see CLINICAL PHARMACOLOGY).

CONTRAINDICATIONS

A history of hypersensitivity to any component of the vaccine, including gelatin.
A history of anaphylactoid reaction to neomycin (each dose of reconstituted vaccine contains trace quantities of neomycin).
Individuals with blood dyscrasias, leukemia, lymphomas of any type, or other malignant neoplasms affecting the bone marrow or lymphatic systems.
Individuals receiving immunosuppressive therapy. Individuals who are on immunosuppressant drugs are more susceptible to infections than healthy individuals. Vaccination with live attenuated varicella vaccine can result in a more extensive vaccine-associated rash or disseminated disease in individuals on immunosuppressant doses of corticosteroids.

Table 1
Fever, Local Reactions, or Rashes (%) in Children 0 to 42 Days Postvaccination

Reaction	N	Post dose 1	Peak Occurrence in Postvaccination Days
Fever ≥102°F (39°C) Oral	8827	14.7%	0-42
Injection-site complaints (pain/soreness, swelling and/or erythema, rash, pruritus, hematoma, induration, stiffness)	8916	19.3%	0–2
Varicella-like rash (injection site) Median number of lesions	8916	3.4% 2	8–19
Varicella-like rash (generalized) Median number of lesions	8916	3.8% 5	5–26

Individuals with primary and acquired immunodeficiency states, including those who are immunosuppressed in association with AIDS or other clinical manifestations of infection with human immunodeficiency virus; cellular immune deficiencies; and hypogammaglobulinemic and dysgammaglobulinemic states.
A family history of congenital or hereditary immunodeficiency, unless the immune competence of the potential vaccine recipient is demonstrated.
Active untreated tuberculosis.
Any febrile respiratory illness or other active febrile infection.
Pregnancy; the possible effects of the vaccine on fetal development are unknown at this time. However, natural varicella is known to sometimes cause fetal harm. If vaccination of postpubertal females is undertaken, pregnancy should be avoided for three months following vaccination. (See PRECAUTIONS, *Pregnancy*).

WARNINGS

Children and adolescents with acute lymphoblastic leukemia (ALL) in remission can receive the vaccine under an investigational protocol. More information is available by contacting the VARIVAX coordinating center, IBAH, Inc., 4 Valley Square, Blue Bell, PA 19422 (215) 283-0897.

PRECAUTIONS

General
Adequate treatment provisions, including epinephrine injection (1:1000), should be available for immediate use should an anaphylactoid reaction occur.
The duration of protection from varicella infection after vaccination with VARIVAX is unknown.
It is not known whether VARIVAX given immediately after exposure to natural varicella virus will prevent illness.
Vaccination should be deferred for at least 5 months following blood or plasma transfusions, or administration of immune globulin or varicella zoster immune globulin (VZIG).
Following administration of VARIVAX, any immune globulin including VZIG should not be given for 2 months thereafter unless its use outweighs the benefits of vaccination.
Vaccine recipients should avoid use of salicylates for 6 weeks after vaccination with VARIVAX as Reye's Syndrome has been reported following the use of salicylates during natural varicella infection (see CLINICAL PHARMACOLOGY, *Reye's Syndrome*).
The safety and efficacy of VARIVAX have not been established in children and young adults who are known to be infected with human immunodeficiency viruses with and without evidence of immunosuppression (see also CONTRAINDICATIONS).
Care is to be taken by the health care provider for safe and effective use of VARIVAX.
The health care provider should question the patient, parent, or guardian about reactions to a previous dose of VARIVAX or a similar product.
The health care provider should obtain the previous immunization history of the vaccinee.
VARIVAX should not be injected into a blood vessel.
Vaccination should be deferred in patients with a family history of congenital or hereditary immunodeficiency until the patient's own immune system has been evaluated.
A separate sterile needle and syringe should be used for administration of each dose of VARIVAX to prevent transfer of infectious diseases.
Needles should be disposed of properly and should not be recapped.
Transmission
Post-marketing experience suggests that transmission of vaccine virus may occur rarely between healthy vaccinees who develop a varicella-like rash and healthy susceptible contacts. Transmission of vaccine virus from vaccinees without a varicella-like rash has been reported but has not been confirmed.
Therefore, vaccine recipients should attempt to avoid, whenever possible, close association with susceptible high-risk individuals for up to six weeks. In circumstances where contact with high-risk individuals is unavoidable, the potential risk of transmission of vaccine virus should be weighed against the risk of acquiring and transmitting natural varicella virus. Susceptible high-risk individuals include:

- immunocompromised individuals
- pregnant women without documented history of chickenpox or laboratory evidence of prior infection
- newborn infants of mothers without documented history of chickenpox or laboratory evidence of prior infection

Information for Patients
The health care provider should inform the patient, parent or guardian of the benefits and risks of VARIVAX.
Patients, parents, or guardians should be instructed to report any adverse reactions to the health care provider.
The U.S. Department of Health and Human Services has established a Vaccine Adverse Event Reporting System (VAERS) to accept all reports of suspected adverse events after the administration of any vaccine, including but not limited to the reporting of events required by the National Childhood Vaccine Injury Act of 1986. The VAERS toll-free number for VAERS forms and information is 1-800-822-7967.
Pregnancy should be avoided for three months following vaccination.
Drug Interactions
See PRECAUTIONS, *General*, regarding the administration of immune globulins, salicylates, and transfusions.
Drug Interactions, Use with Other Vaccines
Results from clinical studies indicate that VARIVAX can be administered concomitantly with M-M-R II (Measles, Mumps, and Rubella Virus Vaccine Live).
Limited data from an experimental product containing varicella vaccine suggest that VARIVAX can be administered concomitantly with DTaP (diphtheria, tetanus, acellular pertussis) and PedvaxHIB using separate sites and syringes (see CLINICAL PHARMACOLOGY, *Studies with Other Vaccines*). However, there are no data relating to simultaneous administration of VARIVAX with DTP or OPV.
Carcinogenesis, Mutagenesis, Impairment of Fertility
VARIVAX has not been evaluated for its carcinogenic or mutagenic potential, or its potential to impair fertility.
Pregnancy
Pregnancy Category C: Animal reproduction studies have not been conducted with VARIVAX. It is also not known whether VARIVAX can cause fetal harm when administered to a pregnant woman or can affect reproduction capacity. Therefore, VARIVAX should not be administered to pregnant females; furthermore, pregnancy should be avoided for three months following vaccination (see CONTRAINDICATIONS).
Merck & Co., Inc. maintains a Pregnancy Registry to monitor fetal outcomes of pregnant women exposed to VARIVAX. Patients and healthcare providers are encouraged to report any exposure to VARIVAX during pregnancy by calling (800) 986-8999.
Nursing Mothers
It is not known whether varicella vaccine virus is secreted in human milk. Therefore, because some viruses are secreted in human milk, caution should be exercised if VARIVAX is administered to a nursing woman.
Geriatric Use
Clinical studies of VARIVAX did not include sufficient numbers of seronegative subjects aged 65 and over to determine whether they respond differently from younger subjects. Other reported clinical experience has not identified differences in responses between the elderly and younger subjects.
Pediatric Use
No clinical data are available on safety or efficacy of VARIVAX in children less than one year of age and administration to infants under twelve months of age is not recommended.

ADVERSE REACTIONS

In clinical trials, VARIVAX was administered to 11,102 healthy children, adolescents, and adults. VARIVAX was generally well tolerated.
In a double-blind placebo controlled study among 914 healthy children and adolescents who were serologically

Continued on next page

Information on the Merck & Co., Inc. products listed on these pages is the full prescribing information from product circulars in use September 30, 2000. For information, please call 1-800-NSC MERCK [1-800-672-6372].

Varivax—Cont.

confirmed to be susceptible to varicella, the only adverse reactions that occurred at a significantly ($p<0.05$) greater rate in vaccine recipients than in placebo recipients were pain and redness at the injection site.

Children 1 to 12 Years of Age

In clinical trials involving healthy children monitored for up to 42 days after a single dose of VARIVAX, the frequency of fever, injection-site complaints, or rashes were reported as follows:

[See table 1 at top of previous page]

In addition, the most frequently (≥1%) reported adverse experiences, without regard to causality, are listed in decreasing order of frequency: upper respiratory illness, cough, irritability/nervousness, fatigue, disturbed sleep, diarrhea, loss of appetite, vomiting, otitis, diaper rash/contact rash, headache, teething, malaise, abdominal pain, other rash, nausea, eye complaints, chills, lymphadenopathy, myalgia, lower respiratory illness, allergic reactions (including allergic rash, hives), stiff neck, heat rash/prickly heat, arthralgia, eczema/dry skin/dermatitis, constipation, itching.

Pneumonitis has been reported rarely (<1%) in children vaccinated with VARIVAX; a causal relationship has not been established.

Febrile seizures have occurred rarely (<0.1%) in children vaccinated with VARIVAX; a causal relationship has not been established.

Adolescents and Adults 13 Years of Age and Older

In clinical trials involving healthy adolescents and adults, the majority of whom received two doses of VARIVAX and were monitored for up to 42 days after any dose, the frequency of fever, injection-site complaints, or rashes were reported as follows:

[See table 2 above]

In addition, the most frequently (≥1%) reported adverse experiences, without regard to causality, are listed in decreasing order of frequency: upper respiratory illness, headache, fatigue, cough, myalgia, disturbed sleep, nausea, malaise, diarrhea, stiff neck, irritability/nervousness, lymphadenopathy, chills, eye complaints, abdominal pain, loss of appetite, arthralgia, otitis, itching, vomiting, other rashes, constipation, lower respiratory illness, allergic reactions (including allergic rash, hives), contact rash, cold/canker sore.

As with any vaccine, there is the possibility that broad use of the vaccine could reveal adverse reactions not observed in clinical trials.

The following additional adverse reactions have been reported since the vaccine has been marketed:

Body As A Whole

Anaphylaxis.

Hemic and Lymphatic System

Thrombocytopenia.

Nervous/Psychiatric

Encephalitis; non-febrile seizures; Guillain-Barré syndrome; transverse myelitis; Bell's palsy; ataxia; dizziness; paresthesia.

Respiratory

Pharyngitis.

Skin

Stevens-Johnson syndrome; erythema multiforme; Henoch-Schönlein purpura; secondary bacterial infections of skin and soft tissue, including impetigo and cellulitis; herpes zoster.

DOSAGE AND ADMINISTRATION

FOR SUBCUTANEOUS ADMINISTRATION

Do not inject intravenously

Children 12 months to 12 years of age should receive a single 0.5 mL dose administered subcutaneously.

Adolescents and adults 13 years of age and older should receive a 0.5 mL dose administered subcutaneously at elected date and a second 0.5 mL dose 4 to 8 weeks later.

VARIVAX is for subcutaneous administration. The outer aspect of the upper arm (deltoid) is the preferred site of injection.

VARIVAX **SHOULD BE STORED FROZEN** at an average temperature of −15°C (+5°F) or colder until it is reconstituted for injection (see HOW SUPPLIED, *Storage*). Any freezer (e.g. chest, frost-free) that reliably maintains an average temperature of −15°C and has a separate sealed freezer door is acceptable for storing VARIVAX. The diluent should be stored separately at room temperature or in the refrigerator. To reconstitute the vaccine, first withdraw 0.7 mL of diluent into the syringe to be used for reconstitution. Inject all the diluent in the syringe into the vial of lyophilized vaccine and gently agitate to mix thoroughly. Withdraw the entire contents into a syringe and inject the total volume (about 0.5 mL) of reconstituted vaccine subcutaneously, preferably into the outer aspect of the upper arm (deltoid) or the anterolateral thigh. **IT IS RECOMMENDED THAT THE VACCINE BE ADMINISTERED IMMEDIATELY AFTER RECONSTITUTION, TO MINIMIZE LOSS OF POTENCY. DISCARD IF RECONSTITUTED VACCINE IS NOT USED WITHIN 30 MINUTES.**

CAUTION: A sterile syringe free of preservatives, antiseptics, and detergents should be used for each injection and/or reconstitution of VARIVAX because these substances may inactivate the vaccine virus.

It is important to use a separate sterile syringe and needle for each patient to prevent transmission of infectious agents from one individual to another.

Table 2
Fever, Local Reactions, or Rashes (%) in Adolescents and Adults
0 to 42 Days Postvaccination

Reaction	N	Post Dose 1	Peak Occurrence in Postvaccination Days	N	Post Dose 2	Peak Occurrence in Postvaccination Days
Fever ≥100°F (37.7°C) Oral	1584	10.2%	14-27	956	9.5%	0-42
Injection-site complaints (soreness, erythema, swelling, rash, pruritus, pyrexia, hematoma, induration, numbness)	1606	24.4%	0–2	955	32.5%	0–2
Varicella-like rash (injection site)	1606	3%	6–20	955	1%	0–6
Median number of lesions		2			2	
Varicella-like rash (generalized)	1606	5.5%	7–21	955	0.9%	0–23
Median number of lesions		5			5.5	

To reconstitute the vaccine, use only the Merck sterile diluent supplied with VARIVAX, M-M-R II, or the component vaccines of M-M-R II, since it is free of preservatives or other anti-viral substances which might inactivate the vaccine virus.

Do not freeze reconstituted vaccine.

Do not give immune globulin including Varicella Zoster Immune Globulin concurrently with VARIVAX (see also PRECAUTIONS).

Parenteral drug products should be inspected visually for particulate matter and discoloration prior to administration, whenever solution and container permit. VARIVAX when reconstituted is a clear, colorless to pale yellow liquid.

HOW SUPPLIED

No. 4826/4309—VARIVAX is supplied as follows: (1) a single-dose vial of lyophilized vaccine, **NDC** 0006-4826-00 (package A); and (2) a box of 10 vials of diluent (package B).

No. 4827/4309—VARIVAX is supplied as follows: (1) a box of 10 single-dose vials of lyophilized vaccine (package A), **NDC** 0006-4827-00; and (2) a box of 10 vials of diluent (package B).

Stability

VARIVAX retains a potency level of 1500 PFU or higher per dose for at least 24 months in a frost-free freezer with an average temperature of −15°C (+5°F) or colder.

VARIVAX has a minimum potency level of approximately 1350 PFU 30 minutes after reconstitution at room temperature (20-25°C, 68-77°F).

Prior to reconstitution, VARIVAX retains potency when stored for up to 72 continuous hours at refrigerator temperature (2-8°C, 36-46°F).

For information regarding stability under conditions other than those recommended, call 1-800-9-VARIVAX.

Storage

During shipment, to ensure that there is no loss of potency, the vaccine must be maintained at a temperature of −20°C (−4°F) or colder.

Before reconstitution, store the lyophilized vaccine in a freezer at an average temperature of −15°C (+5°F) or colder. Any freezer (e.g. chest, frost-free) that reliably maintains an average temperature of −15°C and has a separate sealed freezer door is acceptable for storing VARIVAX.

VARIVAX may be stored at refrigerator temperature (2-8°C, 36-46°F) for up to 72 continuous hours prior to reconstitution. Vaccine stored at 2-8°C which is not used within 72 hours of removal from −15°C storage should be discarded.

Before reconstitution, protect from light.

The diluent should be stored separately at room temperature (20-25°C, 68-77°F), or in the refrigerator.

7999909 Issued February 2000

VASERETIC® Tablets ℞
(Enalapril Maleate-Hydrochlorothiazide)

USE IN PREGNANCY

When used in pregnancy during the second and third trimesters, ACE inhibitors can cause injury and even death to the developing fetus. When pregnancy is detected, VASERETIC should be discontinued as soon as possible. See WARNINGS, *Pregnancy, Enalapril Maleate, Fetal/Neonatal Morbidity and Mortality.*

DESCRIPTION

VASERETIC* (Enalapril Maleate-Hydrochlorothiazide) combines an angiotensin converting enzyme inhibitor, enalapril maleate, and a diuretic, hydrochlorothiazide.

Enalapril maleate is the maleate salt of enalapril, the ethyl ester of a long-acting angiotensin converting enzyme inhibitor, enalaprilat. Enalapril maleate is chemically described as (*S*)-1-[*N*-[1-(ethoxycarbonyl)-3-phenylpropyl]-L-alanyl]-L-proline, (*Z*)-2-butenedioate salt (1:1). Its empirical formula is $C_{20}H_{28}N_2O_5 \cdot C_4H_4O_4$, and its structural formula is:

Enalapril maleate is a white to off-white crystalline powder with a molecular weight of 492.53. It is sparingly soluble in water, soluble in ethanol, and freely soluble in methanol.

Enalapril is a pro-drug; following oral administration, it is bioactivated by hydrolysis of the ethyl ester to enalaprilat, which is the active angiotensin converting enzyme inhibitor.

Hydrochlorothiazide is 6-chloro-3,4-dihydro-2*H*-1,2,4-benzothiadiazine-7-sulfonamide 1,1-dioxide. Its empirical formula is $C_7H_8ClN_3O_4S_2$ and its structural formula is:

It is a white, or practically white, crystalline powder with a molecular weight of 297.74, which is slightly soluble in water, but freely soluble in sodium hydroxide solution.

VASERETIC is available in two tablet combinations of enalapril maleate with hydrochlorothiazide: VASERETIC 5–12.5, containing 5 mg enalapril maleate and 12.5 mg hydrochlorothiazide and VASERETIC 10–25, containing 10 mg enalapril maleate and 25 mg hydrochlorothiazide. Inactive ingredients are: iron oxides, lactose, magnesium stearate, starch and other ingredients.

*Registered trademark of MERCK & CO., Inc.

CLINICAL PHARMACOLOGY

As a result of its diuretic effects, hydrochlorothiazide increases plasma renin activity, increases aldosterone secretion, and decreases serum potassium. Administration of enalapril maleate blocks the renin-angiotensin-aldosterone axis and tends to reverse the potassium loss associated with the diuretic.

In clinical studies, the extent of blood pressure reduction seen with the combination of enalapril maleate and hydrochlorothiazide was approximately additive. The antihypertensive effect of VASERETIC was usually sustained for at least 24 hours.

Concomitant administration of enalapril maleate and hydrochlorothiazide has little, or no effect on the bioavailability of either drug. The combination tablet is bioequivalent to concomitant administration of the separate entities.

Enalapril Maleate

Mechanism of Action: Enalapril, after hydrolysis to enalaprilat, inhibits angiotensin-converting enzyme (ACE) in human subjects and animals. ACE is a peptidyl dipeptidase that catalyzes the conversion of angiotensin I to the vasoconstrictor substance, angiotensin II. Angiotensin II also stimulates aldosterone secretion by the adrenal cortex. Inhibition of ACE results in decreased plasma angiotensin II, which leads to decreased vasopressor activity and to decreased aldosterone secretion. Although the latter decrease is small, it results in small increases of serum potassium. In hypertensive patients treated with enalapril maleate alone for up to 48 weeks, mean increases in serum potassium of approximately 0.2 mEq/L were observed. In patients treated with enalapril maleate plus a thiazide diuretic, there was essentially no change in serum potassium. (See PRECAUTIONS.) Removal of angiotensin II negative feedback on renin secretion leads to increased plasma renin activity.

ACE is identical to kininase, an enzyme that degrades bradykinin. Whether increased levels of bradykinin, a potent vasodepressor peptide, play a role in the therapeutic effects of enalapril remains to be elucidated.

While the mechanism through which enalapril lowers blood pressure is believed to be primarily suppression of the renin-angiotensin-aldosterone system, enalapril is antihypertensive even in patients with low-renin hypertension. Although enalapril was antihypertensive in all races studied, black hypertensive patients (usually a low-renin hypertensive population) had a smaller average response to enalapril maleate monotherapy than non-black patients. In contrast, hydrochlorothiazide was more effective in black patients than enalapril. Concomitant administration of enalapril maleate and hydrochlorothiazide was equally effective in black and non-black patients.

Pharmacokinetics and Metabolism: Following oral administration of enalapril maleate, peak serum concentrations of enalapril occur within about one hour. Based on urinary recovery, the extent of absorption of enalapril is approximately 60 percent. Enalapril absorption is not influenced by the presence of food in the gastrointestinal tract. Following absorption, enalapril is hydrolyzed to enalaprilat, which is a more potent angiotensin converting enzyme inhibitor than enalapril; enalaprilat is poorly absorbed when administered orally. Peak serum concentrations of enalaprilat occur three to four hours after an oral dose of enalapril maleate. Excretion of enalaprilat and enalapril is primarily renal. Approximately 94 percent of the dose is recovered in the urine and feces as enalaprilat or enalapril. The principal components in urine are enalaprilat, accounting for about 40 percent of the dose, and intact enalapril. There is no evidence of metabolites of enalapril, other than enalaprilat.

The serum concentration profile of enalaprilat exhibits a prolonged terminal phase, apparently representing a small fraction of the administered dose that has been bound to ACE. The amount bound does not increase with dose, indicating a saturable site of binding. The effective half-life for accumulation of enalaprilat following multiple doses of enalapril maleate is 11 hours.

The disposition of enalapril and enalaprilat in patients with renal insufficiency is similar to that in patients with normal renal function until the glomerular filtration rate is 30 mL/min or less. With glomerular filtration rate ≤30 mL/min, peak and trough enalaprilat levels increase, time to peak concentration increases and time to steady state may be delayed. The effective half-life of enalaprilat following multiple doses of enalapril maleate is prolonged at this level of renal insufficiency. Enalaprilat is dialyzable at the rate of 62 mL/min.

Studies in dogs indicate that enalapril crosses the blood-brain barrier poorly, if at all; enalaprilat does not enter the brain. Multiple doses of enalapril maleate in rats do not result in accumulation in any tissues. Milk of lactating rats contains radioactivity following administration of ^{14}C enalapril maleate. Radioactivity was found to cross the placenta following administration of labeled drug to pregnant hamsters.

Pharmacodynamics: Administration of enalapril maleate to patients with hypertension of severity ranging from mild to severe results in a reduction of both supine and standing blood pressure usually with no orthostatic component. Symptomatic postural hypotension is infrequent with enalapril alone but it can be anticipated in volume-depleted patients, such as patients treated with diuretics. In clinical trials with enalapril and hydrochlorothiazide administered concurrently, syncope occurred in 1.3 percent of patients. (See WARNINGS and DOSAGE AND ADMINISTRATION.)

In most patients studied, after oral administration of a single dose of enalapril maleate, onset of antihypertensive activity was seen at one hour with peak reduction of blood pressure achieved by four to six hours.

At recommended doses, antihypertensive effects of enalapril maleate monotherapy have been maintained for at least 24 hours. In some patients the effects may diminish toward the end of the dosing interval; this was less frequently observed with concomitant administration of enalapril maleate and hydrochlorothiazide.

Achievement of optimal blood pressure reduction may require several weeks of enalapril therapy in some patients. The antihypertensive effects of enalapril have continued during long term therapy. Abrupt withdrawal of enalapril has not been associated with a rapid increase in blood pressure.

In hemodynamic studies in patients with essential hypertension, blood pressure reduction produced by enalapril was accompanied by a reduction in peripheral arterial resistance with an increase in cardiac output and little or no change in heart rate. Following administration of enalapril maleate, there is an increase in renal blood flow; glomerular filtration rate is usually unchanged. The effects appear to be similar in patients with renovascular hypertension.

In a clinical pharmacology study, indomethacin or sulindac was administered to hypertensive patients receiving enalapril maleate. In this study there was no evidence of a blunting of the antihypertensive action of enalapril maleate.

Hydrochlorothiazide

The mechanism of the antihypertensive effect of thiazides is unknown. Thiazides do not usually affect normal blood pressure. Hydrochlorothiazide is a diuretic and antihypertensive. It affects the distal renal tubular mechanism of electrolyte reabsorption. Hydrochlorothiazide increases excretion of sodium and chloride in approximately equivalent amounts. Natriuresis may be accompanied by some loss of potassium and bicarbonate. After oral use diuresis begins within two hours, peaks in about four hours and lasts about 6 to 12 hours. Hydrochlorothiazide is not metabolized but is eliminated rapidly by the kidney. When plasma levels have been followed for at least 24 hours, the plasma half-life has been observed to vary between 5.6 and 14.8 hours. At least 61 percent of the oral dose is eliminated unchanged within 24 hours. Hydrochlorothiazide crosses the placental but not the blood-brain barrier.

INDICATIONS AND USAGE

VASERETIC is indicated for the treatment of hypertension. These fixed dose combinations are not indicated for initial treatment (see DOSAGE AND ADMINISTRATION).

In using VASERETIC, consideration should be given to the fact that another angiotensin converting enzyme inhibitor, captopril, has caused agranulocytosis, particularly in patients with renal impairment or collagen vascular disease, and that available data are insufficient to show that enalapril does not have a similar risk. (See WARNINGS.)

In considering use of VASERETIC, it should be noted that black patients receiving ACE inhibitors have been reported to have a higher incidence of angioedema compared to non-blacks. (See WARNINGS, *Angioedema.*)

CONTRAINDICATIONS

VASERETIC is contraindicated in patients who are hypersensitive to any component of this product and in patients with a history of angioedema related to previous treatment with an angiotensin converting enzyme inhibitor and in patients with hereditary or idiopathic angioedema. Because of the hydrochlorothiazide component, this product is contraindicated in patients with anuria or hypersensitivity to other sulfonamide-derived drugs.

WARNINGS

General

Enalapril Maleate

Hypotension: Excessive hypotension was rarely seen in uncomplicated hypertensive patients but is a possible consequence of enalapril use in severely salt/volume depleted persons such as those treated vigorously with diuretics or patients on dialysis.

Syncope has been reported in 1.3 percent of patients receiving VASERETIC. In patients receiving enalapril alone, the incidence of syncope is 0.5 percent. The overall incidence of syncope may be reduced by proper titration of the individual components. (See PRECAUTIONS, *Drug Interactions,* ADVERSE REACTIONS and DOSAGE AND ADMINISTRATION.)

In patients with severe congestive heart failure, with or without associated renal insufficiency, excessive hypotension has been observed and may be associated with oliguria and/or progressive azotemia, and rarely with acute renal failure and/or death. Because of the potential fall in blood pressure in these patients, therapy should be started under very close medical supervision. Such patients should be followed closely for the first two weeks of treatment and whenever the dose of enalapril and/or diuretic is increased. Similar considerations may apply to patients with ischemic heart or cerebrovascular disease, in whom an excessive fall in blood pressure could result in a myocardial infarction or cerebrovascular accident.

If hypotension occurs, the patient should be placed in the supine position and, if necessary, receive an intravenous infusion of normal saline. A transient hypotensive response is not a contraindication to further doses, which usually can be given without difficulty once the blood pressure has increased after volume expansion.

Anaphylactoid and Possibly Related Reactions:

Presumably because angiotensin-converting enzyme inhibitors affect the metabolism of eicosanoids and polypeptides, including endogenous bradykinin, patients receiving ACE inhibitors (including VASERETIC) may be subject to a variety of adverse reactions, some of them serious.

Angioedema: Angioedema of the face, extremities, lips, tongue, glottis and/or larynx has been reported in patients treated with angiotensin converting enzyme inhibitors, including enalapril. This may occur at any time during treatment. In such cases VASERETIC should be promptly discontinued and appropriate therapy and monitoring should be provided until complete and sustained resolution of signs and symptoms has occurred. In instances where swelling has been confined to the face and lips the condition has generally resolved without treatment, although antihistamines have been useful in relieving symptoms. Angioedema associated with laryngeal edema may be fatal. **Where there is involvement of the tongue, glottis or larynx, likely to cause airway obstruction, appropriate therapy, e.g., subcutaneous epinephrine solution 1:1000 (0.3 mL to 0.5 mL) and/or measures necessary to ensure a patent airway, should be promptly provided.** (See ADVERSE REACTIONS.)

Patients with a history of angioedema unrelated to ACE inhibitor therapy may be at increased risk of angioedema while receiving an ACE inhibitor (see also INDICATIONS AND USAGE and CONTRAINDICATIONS).

Anaphylactoid reactions during desensitization: Two patients undergoing desensitizing treatment with hymenoptera venom while receiving ACE inhibitors sustained life-threatening anaphylactoid reactions. In the same patients, these reactions were avoided when ACE inhibitors were temporarily withheld, but they reappeared upon inadvertent rechallenge.

Anaphylactoid reactions during membrane exposure: Anaphylactoid reactions have been reported in patients dialyzed with high-flux membranes and treated concomitantly with an ACE inhibitor. Anaphylactoid reactions have also been reported in patients undergoing low-density lipoprotein apheresis with dextran sulfate absorption.

Neutropenia/Agranulocytosis: Another angiotensin converting enzyme inhibitor, captopril, has been shown to cause agranulocytosis and bone marrow depression, rarely in uncomplicated patients but more frequently in patients with renal impairment especially if they also have a collagen vascular disease. Available data from clinical trials of enalapril are insufficient to show that enalapril does not cause agranulocytosis at similar rates. Marketing experience has revealed cases of neutropenia or agranulocytosis in which a causal relationship to enalapril cannot be excluded. Periodic monitoring of white blood cell counts in patients with collagen vascular disease and renal disease should be considered.

Hepatic Failure: Rarely, ACE inhibitors have been associated with a syndrome that starts with cholestatic jaundice and progresses to fulminant hepatic necrosis, and (sometimes) death. The mechanism of this syndrome is not understood. Patients receiving ACE inhibitors who develop jaundice or marked elevations of hepatic enzymes should discontinue the ACE inhibitor and receive appropriate medical follow-up.

Hydrochlorothiazide

Thiazides should be used with caution in severe renal disease. In patients with renal disease, thiazides may precipitate azotemia. Cumulative effects of the drug may develop in patients with impaired renal function.

Thiazides should be used with caution in patients with impaired hepatic function or progressive liver disease, since minor alterations of fluid and electrolyte balance may precipitate hepatic coma.

Sensitivity reactions may occur in patients with or without a history of allergy or bronchial asthma.

The possibility of exacerbation or activation of systemic lupus erythematosus has been reported.

Lithium generally should not be given with thiazides (see PRECAUTIONS, *Drug Interactions, Enalapril Maleate* and *Hydrochlorothiazide*).

Pregnancy

Enalapril-Hydrochlorothiazide

There was no teratogenicity in mice given up to 30 mg/kg/day or in rats given up to 90 mg/kg/day of enalapril in combination with 10 mg/kg/day of hydrochlorothiazide. These doses of enalapril are 4.3 and 26 times (mice and rats, respectively) the maximum recommended human daily dose (MRHDD) when compared on a body surface area basis (mg/m^2); the dose of hydrochlorothiazide is 0.8 times (in mice) and 1.6 times (in rats) the MRHDD. At these doses, fetotoxicity expressed as a decrease in average fetal weight occurred in both species. No fetotoxicity occurred at lower doses; 30/10 mg/kg/day of enalapril-hydrochlorothiazide in rats and 10/10 mg/kg/day of enalapril-hydrochlorothiazide in mice.

When used in pregnancy during the second and third trimesters, ACE inhibitors can cause injury and even death to the developng fetus. When pregnancy is detected, VASERETIC should be discontinued as soon as possible. (See *Enalapril Maleate, Fetal/Neonatal Morbidity and Mortality,* below.)

Enalapril Maleate

Fetal/Neonatal Morbidity and Mortality: ACE inhibitors can cause fetal and neonatal morbidity and death when administered to pregnant women. Several dozen cases have been reported in the world literature. When pregnancy is detected, ACE inhibitors should be discontinued as soon as possible.

The use of ACE inhibitors during the second and third trimesters of pregnancy has been associated with fetal and neonatal injury, including hypotension, neonatal skull hypoplasia, anuria, reversible or irreversible renal failure, and death. Oligohydramnios has also been reported, presumably resulting from decreased fetal renal function; oligohydramnios in this setting has been associated with fetal limb contractures, craniofacial deformation, and hypoplastic lung development. Prematurity, intrauterine growth retardation, and patent ductus arteriosus have also been reported, although it is not clear whether these occurrences were due to the ACE-inhibitor exposure.

These adverse effects do not appear to have resulted from intrauterine ACE-inhibitor exposure that has been limited to the first trimester. Mothers whose embryos and fetuses are exposed to ACE inhibitors only during the first trimester should be so informed. Nonetheless, when patients become pregnant, physicians should make every effort to discontinue the use of VASERETIC as soon as possible.

Rarely (probably less often than once in every thousand pregnancies), no alternative to ACE inhibitors will be found. In these rare cases, the mothers should be apprised of the potential hazards to their fetuses, and serial ultrasound examinations should be performed to assess the intraamniotic environment.

Continued on next page

Information on the Merck & Co., Inc. products listed on these pages is the full prescribing information from product circulars in use September 30, 2000. For information, please call 1-800-NSC MERCK [1-800-672-6372].

Vaseretic—Cont.

If oligohydramnios is observed, VASERETIC should be discontinued unless it is considered lifesaving for the mother. Contraction stress testing (CST), a non-stress test (NST), or biophysical profiling (BPP) may be appropriate, depending upon the week of pregnancy. Patients and physicians should be aware, however, that oligohydramnios may not appear until after the fetus has sustained irreversible injury.
Infants with histories of *in utero* exposure to ACE inhibitors should be closely observed for hypotension, oliguria, and hyperkalemia. If oliguria occurs, attention should be directed toward support of blood pressure and renal perfusion. Exchange transfusion or dialysis may be required as means of reversing hypotension and/or substituting for disordered renal functon. Enalapril, which crosses the placenta, has been removed from neonatal circulation by peritoneal dialysis with some clinical benefit, and theoretically may be removed by exchange transfusion, although there is no experience with the latter procedure.
No teratogenic effects of enalapril were seen in studies of pregnant rats and rabbits. On a body surface area basis, the doses were 57 times and 12 times, respectively, the MRHDD.
Hydrochlorothiazide
Studies in which hydrochlorothiazide was orally administered to pregnant mice and rats during their respective periods of major organogenesis at doses up to 3000 and 1000 mg/kg/day, respectively, provided no evidence of harm to the fetus. These doses are more than 150 times the MRHDD on a body surface area basis. Thiazides cross the placental barrier and appear in cord blood. There is a risk of fetal or neonatal jaundice, thrombocytopenia, and possibly other adverse reactions that have occurred in adults.

PRECAUTIONS

General
Enalapril Maleate
Aortic Stenosis/Hypertrophic Cardiomyopathy: As with all vasodilators, enalapril should be given with caution to patients with obstruction in the outflow tract of the left ventricle.
Impaired Renal Function: As a consequence of inhibiting the renin-angiotensin-aldosterone system, changes in renal function may be anticipated in susceptible individuals. In patients with severe congestive heart failure whose renal function may depend on the activity of the renin-angiotensin-aldosterone system, treatment with angiotensin converting enzyme inhibitors, including enalapril, may be associated with oliguria and/or progressive azotemia and rarely with acute renal failure and/or death.
In clinical studies in hypertensive patients with unilateral or bilateral renal artery stenosis, increases in blood urea nitrogen and serum creatinine were observed in 20 percent of patients. These increases were almost always reversible upon discontinuation of enalapril and/or diuretic therapy. In such patients renal function should be monitored during the first few weeks of therapy.
Some patients with hypertension or heart failure with no apparent pre-existing renal vascular disease have developed increases in blood urea and serum creatinine, usually minor and transient, especially when enalapril has been given concomitantly with a diuretic. This is more likely to occur in patients with pre-existing renal impairment. Dosage reduction of enalapril and/or discontinuation of the diuretic may be required.
Evaluation of the hypertensive patient should always include assessment of renal function.
Hyperkalemia: Elevated serum potassium (greater than 5.7 mEq/L) was observed in approximately one percent of hypertensive patients in clinical trials treated with enalapril alone. In most cases these were isolated values which resolved despite continued therapy, although hyperkalemia was a cause of discontinuation of therapy in 0.28 percent of hypertensive patients. Hyperkalemia was less frequent (approximately 0.1 percent) in patients treated with enalapril plus hydrochlorothiazide. Risk factors for the development of hyperkalemia include renal insufficiency, diabetes mellitus, and the concomitant use of potassium-sparing diuretics, potassium supplements and/or potassium-containing salt substitutes, which should be used cautiously, if at all, with enalapril. (See *Drug Interactions.*)
Cough: Presumably due to the inhibition of the degradation of endogenous bradykinin, persistent nonproductive cough has been reported with all ACE inhibitors, always resolving after discontinuation of therapy. ACE inhibitor-induced cough should be considered in the differential diagnosis of cough.
Surgery/Anesthesia: In patients undergoing major surgery or during anesthesia with agents that produce hypotension, enalapril may block angiotensin II formation secondary to compensatory renin release. If hypotension occurs and is considered to be due to this mechanism, it can be corrected by volume expansion.
Hydrochlorothiazide
Periodic determination of serum electrolytes to detect possible electrolyte imbalance should be performed at appropriate intervals. All patients receiving thiazide therapy should be observed for clinical signs of fluid or electrolyte imbalance: namely hyponatremia, hypochloremic alkalosis, and hypokalemia. Serum and urine electrolyte determinations are particularly important when the patient is vomiting excessively or receiving parenteral fluids. Warning signs or symptoms of fluid and electrolyte imbalance, irrespective of cause, include dryness of mouth, thirst, weakness, lethargy, drowsiness, restlessness, confusion, seizures, muscle pains or cramps, muscular fatigue, hypotension, oliguria, tachycardia, and gastrointestinal disturbances such as nausea and vomiting.
Hypokalemia may develop, especially with brisk diuresis, when severe cirrhosis is present, or after prolonged therapy. Interference with adequate oral electrolyte intake will also contribute to hypokalemia. Hypokalemia may cause cardiac arrhythmia and may also sensitize or exaggerate the response of the heart to the toxic effects of digitalis (e.g., increased ventricular irritability). Because enalapril reduces the production of aldosterone, concomitant therapy with enalapril attenuates the diuretic-induced potassium loss (see *Drug Interactions, Agents Increasing Serum Potassium*).
Although any chloride deficit is generally mild and usually does not require specific treatment except under extraordinary circumstances (as in liver disease or renal disease), chloride replacement may be required in the treatment of metabolic alkalosis.
Dilutional hyponatremia may occur in edematous patients in hot weather; appropriate therapy is water restriction, rather than administration of salt except in rare instances when the hyponatremia is life-threatening. In actual salt depletion, appropriate replacement is the therapy of choice.
Hyperuricemia may occur or frank gout may be precipitated in certain patients receiving thiazide therapy.
In diabetic patients dosage adjustments of insulin or oral hypoglycemic agents may be required. Hyperglycemia may occur with thiazide diuretics. Thus latent diabetes mellitus may become manifest during thiazide therapy.
The antihypertensive effects of the drug may be enhanced in the postsympathectomy patient.
If progressive renal impairment becomes evident consider withholding or discontinuing diuretic therapy.
Thiazides have been shown to increase the urinary excretion of magnesium; this may result in hypomagnesemia.
Thiazides may decrease urinary calcium excretion. Thiazides may cause intermittent and slight elevation of serum calcium in the absence of known disorders of calcium metabolism. Marked hypercalcemia may be evidence of hidden hyperparathyroidism. Thiazides should be discontinued before carrying out tests for parathyroid function.
Increases in cholesterol and triglyceride levels may be associated with thiazide diuretic therapy.
Information for Patients
Angioedema: Angioedema, including laryngeal edema, may occur at any time during treatment with angiotensin converting enzyme inhibitors, including enalapril. Patients should be so advised and told to report immediately any signs or symptoms suggesting angioedema (swelling of face, extremities, eyes, lips, tongue, difficulty in swallowing or breathing) and to take no more drug until they have consulted with the prescribing physician.
Hypotension: Patients should be cautioned to report lightheadedness especially during the first few days of therapy. If actual syncope occurs, the patients should be told to discontinue the drug until they have consulted with the prescribing physician.
All patients should be cautioned that excessive perspiration and dehydration may lead to an excessive fall in blood pressure because of reduction in fluid volume. Other causes of volume depletion such as vomiting or diarrhea may also lead to a fall in blood pressure; patients should be advised to consult with the physician.
Hyperkalemia: Patients should be told not to use salt substitutes containing potassium without consulting their physician.
Neutropenia: Patients should be told to report promptly any indication of infection (e.g., sore throat, fever) which may be a sign of neutropenia.
Pregnancy: Female patients of childbearing age should be told about the consequences of second- and third-trimester exposure to ACE inhibitors, and they should also be told that these consequences do not appear to have resulted from intrauterine ACE-inhibitor exposure that has been limited to the first trimester. These patients should be asked to report pregnancies to their physicians as soon as possible.
NOTE: As with many other drugs, certain advice to patients being treated with VASERETIC is warranted. This information is intended to aid in the safe and effective use of this medication. It is not a disclosure of all possible adverse or intended effects.
Drug Interactions
Enalapril Maleate
Hypotension —Patients on Diuretic Therapy: Patients on diuretics and especially those in whom diuretic therapy was recently instituted, may occasionally experience an excessive reduction of blood pressure after initiation of therapy with enalapril. The possibility of hypotensive effects with enalapril can be minimized by either discontinuing the diuretic or increasing the salt intake prior to initiation of treatment with enalapril. If it is necessary to continue the diuretic, provide medical supervision for at least two hours and until blood pressure has stabilized for at least an additional hour. (See WARNINGS, and DOSAGE AND ADMINISTRATION.)
Agents Causing Renin Release: The antihypertensive effect of enalapril is augmented by antihypertensive agents that cause renin release (e.g., diuretics).
Non-steroidal Anti-inflammatory Agents: In some patients with compromised renal function who are being treated with non-steroidal anti-inflammatory drugs, the coadministration of enalapril may result in a further deterioration of renal function. These effects are usually reversible.
Other Cardiovascular Agents: Enalapril has been used concomitantly with beta adrenergic-blocking agents, methyldopa, nitrates, calcium-blocking agents, hydralazine and prazosin without evidence of clinically significant adverse interactions.
Agents Increasing Serum Potassium: Enalapril attenuates diuretic-induced potassium loss. Potassium-sparing diuretics (e.g., spironolactone, triamterene, or amiloride), potassium supplements, or potassium-containing salt substitutes may lead to significant increases in serum potassium. Therefore, if concomitant use of these agents is indicated because of demonstrated hypokalemia they should be used with caution and with frequent monitoring of serum potassium.
Lithium: Lithium toxicity has been reported in patients receiving lithium concomitantly with drugs which cause elimination of sodium, including ACE inhibitors. A few cases of lithium toxicity have been reported in patients receiving concomitant enalapril and lithium and were reversible upon discontinuation of both drugs. It is recommended that serum lithium levels be monitored frequently if enalapril is administered concomitantly with lithium.
Hydrochlorothiazide
When administered concurrently the following drugs may interact with thiazide diuretics:
Alcohol, barbiturates, or narcotics —potentiation of orthostatic hypotension may occur.
Antidiabetic drugs (oral agents and insulin)—dosage adjustment of the antidiabetic drug may be required.
Other antihypertensive drugs —additive effect or potentiation.
Cholestyramine and colestipol resins —Absorption of hydrochlorothiazide is impaired in the presence of anionic exchange resins. Single doses of either cholestyramine or colestipol resins bind the hydrochlorothiazide and reduce its absorption from the gastrointestinal tract by up to 85 and 43 percent, respectively.
Corticosteroids, ACTH —intensified electrolyte depletion, particularly hypokalemia.
Pressor amines (e.g., norepinephrine) —possible decreased response to pressor amines but not sufficient to preclude their use.
Skeletal muscle relaxants, nondepolarizing (e.g., tubocurarine) —possible increased responsiveness to the muscle relaxant.
Lithium —should not generally be given with diuretics. Diuretic agents reduce the renal clearance of lithium and add a high risk of lithium toxicity. Refer to the package insert for lithium preparations before use of such preparations with VASERETIC.
Non-steroidal Anti-inflammatory Drugs —In some patients, the administration of a non-steroidal anti-inflammatory agent can reduce the diuretic, natriuretic, and antihypertensive effects of loop, potassium-sparing and thiazide diuretics. Therefore, when VASERETIC and non-steroidal anti-inflammatory agents are used concomitantly, the patient should be observed closely to determine if the desired effect of the diuretic is obtained.
Carcinogenesis, Mutagenesis, Impairment of Fertility
Enalapril in combination with hydrochlorothiazide was not mutagenic in the Ames microbial mutagen test with or without metabolic activation. Enalapril-hydrochlorothiazide did not produce DNA single strand breaks in an *in vitro* alkaline elution assay in rat hepatocytes or chromosomal aberrations in an *in vivo* mouse bone marrow assay.
Enalapril Maleate
There was no evidence of a tumorigenic effect when enalapril was administered for 106 weeks to male and female rats at doses up to 90 mg/kg/day or for 94 weeks to male and female mice at doses up to 90 and 180 mg/kg/day, respectively. These doses are 26 times (in rats and female mice) and 13 times (in male mice) the maximum recommended human daily dose (MRHDD) when compared on a body surface area basis.
Neither enalapril maleate nor the active diacid was mutagenic in the Ames microbial mutagen test with or without metabolic activation. Enalapril was also negative in the following genotoxicity studies: rec-assay, reverse mutation assay with *E. coli,* sister chromatid exchange with cultured mammalian cells, and the micronucleus test with mice, as well as in an *in vivo* cytogenic study using mouse bone marrow.
There were no adverse effects on reproductive performance of male and female rats treated with up to 90 mg/kg/day of enalapril (26 times the MRHDD when compared on a body surface area basis).
Hydrochlorothiazide
Two year feeding studies in mice and rats conducted under the auspices of the National Toxicology Program (NTP) uncovered no evidence of a carcinogenic potential of hydrochlorothiazide in female mice at doses up to approximately 600 mg/kg/day (53 times the MRHDD when compared on a body surface area basis) or in male and female rats at doses up to approximately 100 mg/kg/day (18 times the MRHDD when compared on a body surface area basis). The NTP, however, found equivocal evidence for hepatocarcinogenicity in male mice.
Hydrochlorothiazide was not genotoxic *in vitro* in the Ames mutagenicity assay of *Salmonella typhimurium* strains TA

98, TA 100, TA 1535, TA 1537, and TA 1538 and in the Chinese Hamster Ovary (CHO) test for chromosomal aberrations, or *in vivo* in assays using mouse germinal cell chromosomes, Chinese hamster bone marrow chromosomes, and the *Drosophila* sex-linked recessive lethal trait gene. Positive test results were obtained only in the *in vitro* CHO Sister Chromatid Exchange (clastogenicity) and in the Mouse Lymphoma Cell (mutagenicity) assays, using concentrations of hydrochlorothiazide from 43 to 1300 μg/mL, and in the *Aspergillus nidulans* non-disjunction assay at an unspecified concentration.

Hydrochlorothiazide had no adverse effects on the fertility of mice and rats of either sex in studies wherein these species were exposed, via their diet, to doses of up to 100 and 4 mg/kg, respectively, prior to mating and throughout gestation. In mice and rats these doses are 9 times and 0.7 times, respectively, the MRHDD when compared on a body surface area basis.

Pregnancy

Pregnancy Categories C (first trimester) *and D* (second and third trimesters). See WARNINGS, *Pregnancy, Enalapril Maleate, Fetal/Neonatal Morbidity and Mortality.*

Nursing Mothers

Enalapril, enalaprilat, and hydrochlorothiazide have been detected in human breast milk. Because of the potential for serious reactions in nursing infants from either drug, a decision should be made whether to discontinue nursing or to discontinue VASERETIC, taking into account the importance of the drug to the mother.

Pediatric Use

Safety and effectiveness in pediatric patients have not been established.

ADVERSE REACTIONS

VASERETIC has been evaluated for safety in more than 1500 patients, including over 300 patients treated for one year or more. In clinical trials with VASERETIC no adverse experiences peculiar to this combination drug have been observed. Adverse experiences that have occurred, have been limited to those that have been previously reported with enalapril or hydrochlorothiazide.

The most frequent clinical adverse experiences in controlled trials were: dizziness (8.6 percent), headache (5.5 percent), fatigue (3.9 percent) and cough (3.5 percent). Generally, adverse experiences were mild and transient in nature. Adverse experiences occurring in greater than two percent of patients treated with VASERETIC in controlled clinical trials are shown below.

	Percent of Patients in Controlled Studies	
	VASERETIC (n=1580) Incidence (discontinuation)	Placebo (n=230) Incidence
Dizziness	8.6 (0.7)	4.3
Headache	5.5 (0.4)	9.1
Fatigue	3.9 (0.8)	2.6
Cough	3.5 (0.4)	0.9
Muscle Cramps	2.7 (0.2)	0.9
Nausea	2.5 (0.4)	1.7
Asthenia	2.4 (0.3)	0.9
Orthostatic Effects	2.3 (<0.1)	0.0
Impotence	2.2 (0.5)	0.5
Diarrhea	2.1 (<0.1)	1.7

Clinical adverse experiences occurring in 0.5 to 2.0 percent of patients in controlled trials included: *Body As A Whole:* Syncope, chest pain, abdominal pain; *Cardiovascular:* Orthostatic hypotension, palpitation, tachycardia; *Digestive:* Vomiting, dyspepsia, constipation, flatulence, dry mouth; *Nervous/Psychiatric:* Insomnia, nervousness, paresthesia, somnolence, vertigo; *Skin:* Pruritus, rash; *Other:* Dyspnea, gout, back pain, arthralgia, diaphoresis, decreased libido, tinnitus, urinary tract infection.

Angioedema: Angioedema has been reported in patients receiving VASERETIC, with an incidence higher in black than in non-black patients. Angioedema associated with laryngeal edema may be fatal. If angioedema of the face, extremities, lips, tongue, glottis and/or larynx occurs, treatment with VASERETIC should be discontinued and appropriate therapy instituted immediately. (See WARNINGS.)

Hypotension: In clinical trials, adverse effects relating to hypotension occurred as follows: hypotension (0.9 percent), orthostatic hypotension (1.5 percent), other orthostatic effects (2.3 percent). In addition syncope occurred in 1.3 percent of patients. (See WARNINGS.)

Cough: See PRECAUTIONS, *Cough.*

Clinical Laboratory Test Findings

Serum Electrolytes: See PRECAUTIONS.

Creatinine, Blood Urea Nitrogen: In controlled clinical trials minor increases in blood urea nitrogen and serum creatinine, reversible upon discontinuation of therapy, were observed in about 0.6 percent of patients with essential hypertension treated with VASERETIC. More marked increases have been reported in other enalapril experience. Increases are more likely to occur in patients with renal artery stenosis. (See PRECAUTIONS.)

Serum Uric Acid, Glucose, Magnesium, and Calcium: See PRECAUTIONS.

Hemoglobin and Hematocrit: Small decreases in hemoglobin and hematocrit (mean decreases of approximately 0.3 g percent and 1.0 vol percent, respectively) occur frequently in hypertensive patients treated with VASERETIC but are rarely of clinical importance unless another cause of anemia coexists. In clinical trials, less than 0.1 percent of patients discontinued therapy due to anemia.

Liver Function Tests: Rarely, elevations of liver enzymes and/or serum bilirubin have occurred (see WARNINGS, *Hepatic Failure*).

Other adverse reactions that have been reported with the individual components are listed below and, within each category, are in order of decreasing severity.

Enalapril Maleate —Enalapril has been evaluated for safety in more than 10,000 patients. In clinical trials adverse reactions which occurred with enalapril were also seen with VASERETIC. However, since enalapril has been marketed, the following adverse reactions have been reported: *Body As A Whole:* Anaphylactoid reactions (see WARNINGS, *Anaphylactoid reactions during membrane exposure*); *Cardiovascular:* Cardiac arrest; myocardial infarction or cerebrovascular accident, possibly secondary to excessive hypotension in high risk patients (see WARNINGS, *Hypotension*); pulmonary embolism and infarction; pulmonary edema; rhythm disturbances including atrial tachycardia and bradycardia, atrial fibrillation; hypotension; angina pectoris, Raynaud's phenomenon; *Digestive:* Ileus, pancreatitis, hepatic failure, hepatitis (hepatocellular [proven on rechallenge] or cholestatic jaundice) (see WARNINGS, *Hepatic Failure*), melena, anorexia, glossitis, stomatitis, dry mouth; *Hematologic:* Rare cases of neutropenia, thrombocytopenia and bone marrow depression. Hemolytic anemia, including cases of hemolysis in patients with G-6-PD deficiency, has been reported; a causal relationship to enalapril cannot be excluded. *Nervous System/Psychiatric:* Depression, confusion, ataxia, peripheral neuropathy (e.g., paresthesia, dysesthesia), dream abnormality; *Urogenital:* Renal failure, oliguria, renal dysfunction, (see PRECAUTION-Sand DOSAGE AND ADMINISTRATION), flank pain, gynecomastia; *Respiratory:* Pulmonary infiltrates, eosinophilic pneumonitis, bronchospasm, pneumonia, bronchitis, rhinorrhea, sore throat and hoarseness, asthma, upper respiratory infection; *Skin:* Exfoliative dermatitis, toxic epidermal necrolysis, Stevens-Johnson syndrome, herpes zoster, erythema multiforme, urticaria, pemphigus, alopecia, flushing, photosensitivity; *Special Senses:* Blurred vision, taste alteration, anosmia, conjunctivitis, dry eyes, tearing.

Miscellaneous: A symptom complex has been reported which may include some or all of the following: a positive ANA, an elevated erythrocyte sedimentation rate, arthralgia/arthritis, myalgia/myositis, fever, serositis, vasculitis, leukocytosis, eosinophilia, photosensitivity, rash and other dermatologic manifestations.

Fetal/Neonatal Morbidity and Mortality: See WARNINGS, *Pregnancy, Enalapril Maleate, Fetal/Neonatal Morbidity and Mortality.*

Hydrochlorothiazide—Body as a Whole: Weakness; *Digestive:* Pancreatitis, jaundice (intrahepatic cholestatic jaundice), sialadenitis, cramping, gastric irritation, anorexia); *Hematologic:* Aplastic anemia, agranulocytosis, leukopenia, hemolytic anemia, thrombocytopenia; *Hypersensitivity:* Purpura, photosensitivity, urticaria, necrotizing angiitis (vasculitis and cutaneous vasculitis), fever, respiratory distress including pneumonitis and pulmonary edema, anaphylactic reactions; *Musculoskeletal:* Muscle spasm; *Nervous system/Psychiatric:* Restlessness; *Renal:* Renal failure, renal dysfunction, interstitial nephritis (see WARNINGS); *Skin:* Erythema multiforme including Stevens-Johnson syndrome, exfoliative dermatitis including toxic epidermal necrolysis, alopecia; *Special Senses:* Transient blurred vision, xanthopsia.

OVERDOSAGE

No specific information is available on the treatment of overdosage with VASERETIC. Treatment is symptomatic and supportive. Therapy with VASERETIC should be discontinued and the patient observed closely. Suggested measures include induction of emesis and/or gastric lavage, and correction of dehydration, electrolyte imbalance and hypotension by established procedures.

Enalapril Maleate —Single oral doses of enalapril above 1,000 mg/kg and ≥1,775 mg/kg were associated with lethality in mice and rats, respectively. The most likely manifestation of overdosage would be hypotension, for which the usual treatment would be intravenous infusion of normal saline solution. Enalaprilat may be removed from general circulation by hemodialysis and has been removed from neonatal circulation by peritoneal dialysis. (See WARNINGS, *Anaphylactoid reactions during membrane exposure.*)

Hydrochlorothiazide —Lethality was not observed after administration of an oral dose of 10 g/kg to mice and rats. The most common signs and symptoms observed are those caused by electrolyte depletion (hypokalemia, hypochloremia, hyponatremia) and dehydration resulting from excessive diuresis. If digitalis has also been administered, hypokalemia may accentuate cardiac arrhythmias.

DOSAGE AND ADMINISTRATION

Enalapril and hydrochlorothiazide are effective treatments for hypertension. The usual dosage range of enalapril is 10 to 40 mg per day administered in a single or two divided doses; hydrochlorothiazide is effective in doses of 12.5 to 50 mg daily. The side effects (see WARNINGS) of enalapril are generally rare and apparently independent of dose; those of hydrochlorothiazide are a mixture of dose-dependent phenomena (primarily hypokalemia) and dose-independent phenomena (e.g., pancreatitis), the former much more common than the latter. Therapy with any combination of enalapril and hydrochlorothiazide will be associated with both sets of dose-independent side effects but the addition of enalapril in clinicial trials blunted the hypokalemia normally seen with diuretics. To minimize dose-independent side effects, it is usually appropriate to begin combination therapy only after a patient has failed to achieve the desired effect with monotherapy.

Dose Titration Guided by Clinical Effect: A patient whose blood pressure is not adequately controlled with either enalapril or hydrochlorothiazide monotherapy may be given VASERETIC 5–12.5 or VASERETIC 10–25. Further increases of enalapril, hydrochlorothiazide or both depend on clinical response. The hydrochlorothiazide dose should generally not be increased until 2–3 weeks have elapsed. In general, patients do not require doses in excess of 20 mg of enalapril or 50 mg of hydrochlorothiazide. The daily dosage should not exceed four tablets of VASERETIC 5–12.5 or two tablets of VASERETIC 10–25.

Replacement Therapy: The combination may be substituted for the titrated components.

Use in Renal Impairment: The usual regimens of therapy with VASERETIC need not be adjusted as long as the patient's creatinine clearance is >30 mL/min/1.73 m^2 (serum creatinine approximately ≤3 mg/dL or 265 μmol/L). In patients with more severe renal impairment, loop diuretics are preferred to thiazides, so enalapril maleate-hydrochlorothiazide is not recommended (see WARNINGS, *Anaphylactoid reactions during membrane exposure*).

Use in Elderly: Clinical studies in VASERETIC did not include sufficient numbers of patients aged 65 and over to determine whether they respond differently from younger patients. In general, dose selection for an elderly patient should be cautious, usually starting at the low end of the dosing range.

HOW SUPPLIED

No. 3644—Tablets VASERETIC 5-12.5 are green, squared capsule-shaped compressed tablets, coded MSD on one side and 173 on the other. Each tablet contains 5 mg of enalapril maleate and 12.5 mg of hydrochlorothiazide. They are supplied as follows:

NDC 0006-0173-68 bottles of 100 (with desiccant).

Shown in Product Identification Guide, page 324

No. 3418—Tablets VASERETIC 10-25, are rust, squared capsule-shaped, compressed tablets, coded MSD 720 on one side and VASERETIC on the other. Each tablet contains 10 mg of enalapril maleate and 25 mg of hydrochlorothiazide. They are supplied as follows:

NDC 0006-0720-68 bottles of 100 (with desiccant).

Shown in Product Identification Guide, page 324

Storage

Store below 30°C (86°F) and avoid transient temperatures above 50°C (122°F). Keep container tightly closed. Protect from moisture.

Dispense in a tight container, if product package is subdivided.

7843634 Issued October 1998

VASOTEC® I.V. Injection ℞
(Enalaprilat)

USE IN PREGNANCY

When used in pregnancy during the second and third trimesters, ACE inhibitors can cause injury and even death to the developing fetus. When pregnancy is detected, VASOTEC I.V. should be discontinued as soon as possible. See WARNINGS, *Fetal/Neonatal Morbidity and Mortality.*

DESCRIPTION

VASOTEC* I.V. (Enalaprilat) is a sterile aqueous solution for intravenous administration. Enalaprilat is an angiotensin converting enzyme inhibitor. It is chemically described as (*S*)-1-[*N*-(1-carboxy-3-phenylpropyl)-L-alanyl]-L-proline dihydrate. Its empirical formula is $C_{18}H_{24}N_2O_5 \cdot 2H_2O$ and its structural formula is:

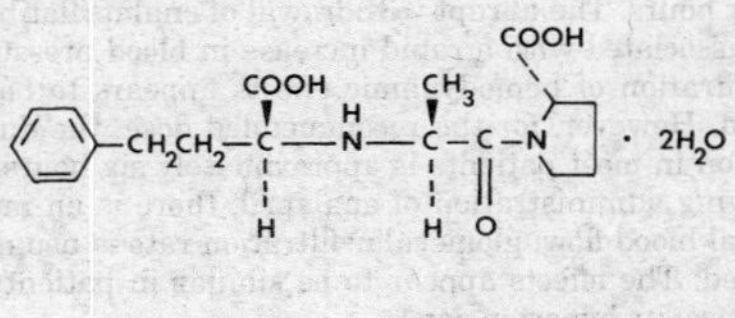

$\cdot\ 2H_2O$

Continued on next page

Information on the Merck & Co., Inc. products listed on these pages is the full prescribing information from product circulars in use September 30, 2000. For information, please call 1-800-NSC MERCK [1-800-672-6372].

Vasotec I.V.—Cont.

Enalaprilat is a white to off-white, crystalline powder with a molecular weight of 384.43. It is sparingly soluble in methanol and slightly soluble in water.
Each milliliter of VASOTEC I.V. contains 1.25 mg enalaprilat (anhydrous equivalent); sodium chloride to adjust tonicity; sodium hydroxide to adjust pH; water for injection, q.s.; with benzyl alcohol, 9 mg, added as a preservative.

*Registered trademark of MERCK & CO., INC.

CLINICAL PHARMACOLOGY

Enalaprilat, an angiotensin-converting enzyme (ACE) inhibitor when administered intravenously, is the active metabolite of the orally administered pro-drug, enalapril maleate. Enalaprilat is poorly absorbed orally.
Mechanism of Action
Intravenous enalaprilat, or oral enalapril, after hydrolysis to enalaprilat, inhibits ACE in human subjects and animals. ACE is a peptidyl dipeptidase that catalyzes the conversion of angiotensin I to the vasoconstrictor substance, angiotensin II. Angiotensin II also stimulates aldosterone secretion by the adrenal cortex. Inhibition of ACE results in decreased plasma angiotensin II, which leads to decreased vasopressor activity and to decreased aldosterone secretion. Although the latter decrease is small, it results in small increases of serum potassium. In hypertensive patients treated with enalapril alone for up to 48 weeks, mean increases in serum potassium of approximately 0.2 mEq/L were observed. In patients treated with enalapril plus a thiazide diuretic, there was essentially no change in serum potassium. (See PRECAUTIONS.) Removal of angiotensin II negative feedback on renin secretion leads to increased plasma renin activity.
ACE is identical to kininase, an enzyme that degrades bradykinin. Whether increased levels of bradykinin, a potent vasodepressor peptide, play a role in the therapeutic effects of enalaprilat remains to be elucidated.
While the mechanism through which enalaprilat lowers blood pressure is believed to be primarily suppression of the renin-angiotensin-aldosterone system, enalaprilat has antihypertensive activity even in patients with low-renin hypertension. In clinical studies, black hypertensive patients (usually a low-renin hypertensive population) had a smaller average response to enalaprilat monotherapy than non-black patients.
Pharmacokinetics and Metabolism
Following intravenous administration of a single dose, the serum concentration profile of enalaprilat is polyexponential with a prolonged terminal phase, apparently representing a small fraction of the administered dose that has been bound to ACE. The amount bound does not increase with dose, indicating a saturable site of binding. The effective half-life for accumulation of enalaprilat, as determined from oral administration of multiple doses of enalapril maleate, is approximately 11 hours. Excretion of enalaprilat is primarily renal with more than 90 percent of an administered dose recovered in the urine as unchanged drug within 24 hours. Enalaprilat is poorly absorbed following oral administration.
The disposition of enalaprilat in patients with renal insufficiency is similar to that in patients with normal renal function until the glomerular filtration rate is 30 mL/min or less. With glomerular filtration rate ≤30 mL/min, peak and trough enalaprilat levels increase, time to peak concentration increases and time to steady state may be delayed. The effective half-life of enalaprilat is prolonged at this level of renal insufficiency. (See DOSAGE AND ADMINISTRATION.) Enalaprilat is dialyzable at the rate of 62 mL/min. Studies in dogs indicate that enalaprilat does not enter the brain, and that enalapril crosses the blood-brain barrier poorly, if at all. Multiple doses of enalapril maleate in rats do not result in accumulation in any tissues. Milk in lactating rats contains radioactivity following administration of ^{14}C enalapril maleate. Radioactivity was found to cross the placenta following administration of labeled drug to pregnant hamsters.
Pharmacodynamics
VASOTEC I.V. results in the reduction of both supine and standing systolic and diastolic blood pressure, usually with no orthostatic component. Symptomatic postural hypotension is therefore infrequent, although it might be anticipated in volume-depleted patients (see WARNINGS). The onset of action usually occurs within fifteen minutes of administration with the maximum effect occurring within one to four hours. The abrupt withdrawal of enalaprilat has not been associated with a rapid increase in blood pressure.
The duration of hemodynamic effects appears to be dose-related. However, for the recommended dose, the duration of action in most patients is approximately six hours.
Following administration of enalapril, there is an increase in renal blood flow; glomerular filtration rate is usually unchanged. The effects appear to be similar in patients with renovascular hypertension.

INDICATIONS AND USAGE

VASOTEC I.V. is indicated for the treatment of hypertension when oral therapy is not practical.
VASOTEC I.V. has been studied with only one other antihypertensive agent, furosemide, which showed approximately additive effects on blood pressure. Enalapril, the pro-drug of enalaprilat, has been used extensively with a variety of other antihypertensive agents, without apparent difficulty except for occasional hypotension.
In using VASOTEC I.V., consideration should be given to the fact that another angiotensin converting enzyme inhibitor, captopril, has caused agranulocytosis, particularly in patients with renal impairment or collagen vascular disease, and that available data are insufficient to show that VASOTEC I.V. does not have a similar risk. (See WARNINGS.)
In considering use of VASOTEC I.V., it should be noted that in controlled clinical trials ACE inhibitors have an effect on blood pressure that is less in black patients than in non-blacks. In addition, it should be noted that black patients receiving ACE inhibitors have been reported to have a higher incidence of angioedema compared to non-blacks. (See WARNINGS, *Angioedema*.)

CONTRAINDICATIONS

VASOTEC I.V. is contraindicated in patients who are hypersensitive to any component of this product and in patients with a history of angioedema related to previous treatment with an angiotensin converting enzyme inhibitor and in patients with hereditary or idiopathic angioedema.

WARNINGS

Hypotension
Excessive hypotension is rare in uncomplicated hypertensive patients but is a possible consequence of the use of enalaprilat especially in severely salt/volume depleted persons such as those treated vigorously with diuretics or patients on dialysis. Patients at risk for excessive hypotension, sometimes associated with oliguria and/or progressive azotemia, and rarely with acute renal failure and/or death, include those with the following conditions or characteristics: heart failure, hyponatremia, high dose diuretic therapy, recent intensive diuresis or increase in diuretic dose, renal dialysis, or severe volume and/or salt depletion of any etiology. It may be advisable to eliminate the diuretic, reduce the diuretic dose or increase salt intake cautiously before initiating therapy with VASOTEC I.V. in patients at risk for excessive hypotension who are able to tolerate such adjustment. (See PRECAUTIONS, *Drug Interactions*, ADVERSE REACTIONS, and DOSAGE AND ADMINISTRATION.) In patients with heart failure, with or without associated renal insufficiency, excessive hypotension has been observed and may be associated with oliguria and/or progressive azotemia, and rarely with acute renal failure and/or death. Because of the potential for an excessive fall in blood pressure especially in these patients, therapy should be followed closely whenever the dose of enalaprilat is adjusted and/or diuretic is increased. Similar consideration may apply to patients with ischemic heart or cerebrovascular disease, in whom an excessive fall in blood pressure could result in a myocardial infarction or cerebrovascular accident.
If hypotension occurs, the patient should be placed in the supine position and, if necessary, receive an intravenous infusion of normal saline. A transient hypotensive response is not a contraindication to further doses, which usually can be given without difficulty once the blood pressure has increased after volume expansion.
Anaphylactoid and Possibly Related Reactions
Presumably because angiotensin-converting enzyme inhibitors affect the metabolism of eicosanoids and polypeptides, including endogenous bradykinin, patients receiving ACE inhibitors (including VASOTEC I.V.) may be subject to a variety of adverse reactions, some of them serious.
Angioedema: Angioedema of the face, extremities, lips, tongue, glottis and/or larynx has been reported in patients treated with angiotensin converting enzyme inhibitors, including enalaprilat. This may occur at any time during treatment. In such cases VASOTEC I.V. should be promptly discontinued and appropriate therapy and monitoring should be provided until complete and sustained resolution of signs and symptoms has occurred. In instances where swelling has been confined to the face and lips the condition has generally resolved without treatment, although antihistamines have been useful in relieving symptoms. Angioedema associated with laryngeal edema may be fatal. **Where there is involvement of the tongue, glottis or larynx, likely to cause airway obstruction, appropriate therapy, e.g., subcutaneous epinephrine solution 1:1000 (0.3 mL to 0.5 mL) and/or measures necessary to ensure a patent airway, should be promptly provided.** (See ADVERSE REACTIONS.)
Patients with a history of angioedema unrelated to ACE inhibitor therapy may be at increased risk of angioedema while receiving an ACE inhibitor (see also INDICATIONS AND USAGE and CONTRAINDICATIONS).
Anaphylactoid reactions during desensitization: Two patients undergoing desensitizing treatment with hymenoptera venom while receiving ACE inhibitors sustained life-threatening anaphylactoid reactions. In the same patients, these reactions were avoided when ACE inhibitors were temporarily withheld, but they reappeared upon inadvertent rechallenge.
Anaphylactoid reactions during membrane exposure: Anaphylactoid reactions have been reported in patients dialyzed with high-flux membranes and treated concomitantly with an ACE inhibitor. Anaphylactoid reactions have also been reported in patients undergoing low-density lipoprotein apheresis with dextran sulfate absorption.
Neutropenia/Agranulocytosis
Another angiotensin converting enzyme inhibitor, captopril, has been shown to cause agranulocytosis and bone marrow depression, rarely in uncomplicated patients but more frequently in patients with renal impairment especially if they also have a collagen vascular disease. Available data from clinical trials of enalapril are insufficient to show that enalapril does not cause agranulocytosis in similar rates. Marketing experience has revealed cases of neutropenia, or agranulocytosis in which a causal relationship to enalapril cannot be excluded. Periodic monitoring of white blood cell counts in patients with collagen vascular disease and renal disease should be considered.
Hepatic Failure
Rarely, ACE inhibitors have been associated with a syndrome that starts with cholestatic jaundice and progresses to fulminant hepatic necrosis, and (sometimes) death. The mechanism of this syndrome is not understood. Patients receiving ACE inhibitors who develop jaundice or marked elevations of hepatic enzymes should discontinue the ACE inhibitor and receive appropriate medical follow-up.
Fetal/Neonatal Morbidity and Mortality
ACE inhibitors can cause fetal and neonatal morbidity and death when administered to pregnant women. Several dozen cases have been reported in the world literature. When pregnancy is detected, ACE inhibitors should be discontinued as soon as possible.
The use of ACE inhibitors during the second and third trimesters of pregnancy has been associated with fetal and neonatal injury, including hypotension, neonatal skull hypoplasia, anuria, reversible or irreversible renal failure, and death. Oligohydramnios has also bee reported, presumably resulting from decreased fetal renal function: oligohydramnois in this setting has been associated with fetal limb contractures, craniofacial deformation, and hypoplastic lung development. Prematurity, intrauterine growth retardation, and patent ductus arteriosus have also been reported, although it is not clear whether these occurrences were due to the ACE-inhibitor exposure.
These adverse effects do not appear to have resulted from intrauterine ACE-inhibitor exposure that has been limited to the first trimester. Mothers whose embryos and fetuses are exposed to ACE inhibitors only during the first trimester should be so informed. Nonetheless, when patients become pregnant, physicians should make every effort to discontinue the use of VASOTEC I.V. as soon as possible.
Rarely (probably less often than once in every thousand pregnancies), no alternative to ACE inhibitors will be found. In these rare cases, the mothers should be apprised of the potential hazards to their fetuses, and serial ultrasound examinations should be performed to assess the intraamniotic environment.
If oligohydramnois is observed, VASOTEC I.V. should be discontinued unless it is considered lifesaving for the mother. Contraction stress testing (CST), a non-stress test (NST), or biophysical profiling (BPP) may be appropriate, depending upon the week of pregnancy. Patients and physicians should be aware, however, that oligohydramnois may not appear until after the fetus has sustained irreversible injury.
Infants with histories of *in utero* exposure to ACE inhibitors should be closely observed for hypotension, oliguria, and hyperkalemia. If oliguria occurs, attention should be directed toward support of blood pressure and renal perfusion. Exchange transfusion or dialysis may be required as means of reversing hypotension and/or substituting for disordered renal function. Enalapril, which crosses the placenta, has been removed from neonatal circulation by peritoneal dialysis with some clinical benefit, and theoretically may be removed by exchange transfusion, although there is no experience with the latter procedure.
No teratogenic effects of oral enalapril were seen in studies of pregnant rats and rabbits. On a body surface area basis, the doses used were 57 times and 12 times, respectively, the maximum recommended human daily dose (MRHDD).

PRECAUTIONS

General
Aortic Stenosis/Hypertrophic Cardiomyopathy: As with all vasodilators, enalapril should be given with caution to patients with obstruction in the outflow tract of the left ventricle.
Impaired Renal Function: As a consequence of inhibiting the renin-angiotensin-aldosterone system, changes in renal function may be anticipated in susceptible individuals. In patients with severe heart failure whose renal function may depend on the activity of the renin-angiotensin-aldosterone system, treatment with angiotensin converting enzyme inhibitors, including enalapril or enalaprilat, may be associated with oliguria and/or progressive azotemia and rarely with acute renal failure and/or death.
In clinical studies in hypertensive patients with unilateral or bilateral renal artery stenosis, increases in blood urea nitrogen and serum creatinine were observed in 20 percent of patients receiving enalapril. These increases were almost always reversible upon discontinuation of enalapril or enalaprilat and/or diuretic therapy. In such patients renal function should be monitored during the first few weeks of therapy.
Some hypertensive patients with no apparent pre-existing renal vascular disease have developed increases in blood urea and serum creatinine, usually minor and transient, especially when enalaprilat has been given concomitantly

with a diuretic. This is more likely to occur in patients with pre-existing renal impairment. Dosage reduction of enalaprilat and/or discontinuation of the diuretic may be required.

Evaluation of the hypertensive patient should always include assessment of renal function. (See DOSAGE AND ADMINISTRATION.)

Hyperkalemia: Elevated serum potassium (greater than 5.7 mEq/L) was observed in approximately one percent of hypertensive patients in clinical trials receiving enalapril. In most cases these were isolated values which resolved despite continued therapy. Hyperkalemia was a cause of discontinuation of therapy in 0.28 percent of hypertensive patients. Risk factors for the development of hyperkalemia include renal insufficiency, diabetes mellitus, and the concomitant use of potassium-sparing agents or potassium supplements, which should be used cautiously, if at all, with VASOTEC I.V. (See *Drug Interactions.*)

Cough: Presumably due to the inhibition of the degradation of endogenous bradykinin, persistent nonproductive cough has been reported with all ACE inhibitors, always resolving after discontinuation of therapy. ACE inhibitor-induced cough should be considered in the differential diagnosis of cough.

Surgery/Anesthesia: In patients undergoing major surgery or during anesthesia with agents that produce hypotension, enalapril may block angiotensin II formation secondary to compensatory renin release. If hypotension occurs and is considered to be due to this mechanism, it can be corrected by volume expansion.

Drug Interactions

Hypotension—Patients on Diuretic Therapy: Patients on diuretics and especially those in whom diuretic therapy was recently instituted, may occasionally experience an excessive reduction of blood pressure after initiation of therapy with enalaprilat. The possibility of hypotensive effects with enalaprilat can be minimized by administration of an intravenous infusion of normal saline, discontinuing the diuretic or increasing the salt intake prior to initiation of treatment with enalaprilat. If it is necessary to continue the diuretic, provide close medical supervision for at least one hour after the initial dose of enalaprilat. (See WARNINGS.)

Agents Causing Renin Release: The antihyertensive effect of VASOTEC I.V. appears to be augmented by antihypertensive agents that cause renin release (e.g., diuretics.)

Non-steroidal Anti-inflammatory Agents: In some patients with compromised renal function who are being treated with non-steroidal anti-inflammatory drugs, the co-administration of enalapril may result in a further deterioration of renal function. These effects are usually reversible.

Other Cardiovascular Agents: VASOTEC I.V. has been used concomitantly with digitalis, beta adrenergic-blocking agents, methyldopa, nitrates, calcium-blocking agents, hydralazine and prazosin without evidence of clinically significant adverse interactions.

Agents Increasing Serum Potassium: VASOTEC I.V. attenuates potassium loss caused by thiazide-type diuretics. Potassium-sparing diuretics (e.g., spironolactone, triamterene, or amiloride), potassium supplements, or potassium-containing salt substitutes may lead to significant increases in serum potassium. Therefore, if concomitant use of these agents is indicated because of demonstrated hypokalemia, they should be used with caution and with frequent monitoring of serum potassium.

Lithium: Lithium toxicity has been reported in patients receiving lithium concomitantly with drugs which cause elimination of sodium, including ACE inhibitors. A few cases of lithium toxicity have been reported in patients receiving concomitant enalapril and lithium and were reversible upon discontinuation of both drugs. It is recommended that serum lithium levels be monitored frequently if enalapril is administered concomitantly with lithium.

Carcinogenesis, Mutagenesis, Impairment of Fertility

Carcinogenicity studies have not been done with VASOTEC I.V.

VASOTEC I.V. is the bioactive form of its ethyl ester, enalapril maleate. There was no evidence of a tumorigenic effect when enalapril was administered for 106 weeks to male and female rats at doses up to 90 mg/kg/day or for 94 weeks to male and female mice at doses up to 90 and 180 mg/kg/day, respectively. These doses are 26 times (in rats and female mice) and 13 times (in male mice) the maximum recommended human daily dose (MRHDD) when compared on a body surface area basis.

VASOTEC I.V. was not mutagenic in the Ames microbial mutagen test with or without metabolic activation. Enalapril showed no drug-related changes in the following genotoxicity studies: rec-assay, reverse mutation assay with *E. coli*, sister chromatid exchange with cultured mammalian cells, the micronucleus test with mice, and in an *in vivo* cytogenic study using mouse bone marrow. There were no adverse effects on reproductive performance of male and female rats treated with up to 90 mg/kg/day of enalapril (26 times the MRHDD when compared on a body surface area basis).

Pregnancy

Pregnancy Categories C (first trimester) and *D* (second and third trimesters). See WARNINGS, *Fetal/Neonatal Morbidity and Mortality.*

Nursing Mothers

Enalapril and enalaprilat have been detected in human breast milk. Because of the potential for serious adverse reactions in nursing infants from enalapril, a decision should be made whether to discontinue nursing or to discontinue VASOTEC I.V., taking into account the importance of the drug to the mother.

Pediatric Use

Safety and effectiveness in pediatric patients have not been established.

ADVERSE REACTIONS

VASOTEC I.V. has been found to be generally well tolerated in controlled clinical trials involving 349 patients (168 with hypertension, 153 with congestive heart failure and 28 with coronary artery disease). The most frequent clinically significant adverse experience was hypotension (3.4 percent), occurring in eight patients (5.2 percent) with congestive heart failure, three (1.8 percent) with hypertension and one with coronary artery disease. Other adverse experiences occurring in greater than one percent of patients were: headache (2.9 percent) and nausea (1.1 percent).

Adverse experiences occurring in 0.5 to 1.0 percent of patients in controlled clinical trials included: myocardial infarction, fatigue, dizziness, fever, rash and constipation.

Angioedema: Angioedema has been reported in patients receiving enalaprilat, with an incidence higher in black than in non-black patients. Angioedema associated with laryngeal edema may be fatal. If angioedema of the face, extremities, lips, tongue, glottis and/or larynx occurs, treatment with enalaprilat should be discontinued and appropriate therapy instituted immediately. (See WARNINGS.)

Cough: See PRECAUTIONS, *Cough.*

Enalapril Maleate

Since enalapril is converted to enalaprilat, those adverse experiences associated with enalapril might also be expected to occur with VASOTEC I.V.

The following adverse experiences have been reported with enalapril and, within each category, are listed in order of decreasing severity.

Body As A Whole: Syncope, orthostatic effects, anaphylactoid reactions (see WARNINGS, *Anaphylactoid reactions during membrane exposure*), chest pain, abdominal pain, asthenia.

Cardiovascular: Cardiac arrest; myocardial infarction or cerebrovascular accident, possibly secondary to excessive hypotension in high risk patients (see WARNINGS, *Hypotension*); pulmonary embolism and infarction; pulmonary edema; rhythm disturbances including atrial tachycardia and bradycardia; atrial fibrillation; orthostatic hypotension; angina pectoris; palpitation, Raynaud's phenomenon.

Digestive: Ileus, pancreatitis, hepatic failure, hepatitis (hepatocellular [proven on rechallenge] or cholestatic jaundice) (see WARNINGS, *Hepatic Failure*), melena, diarrhea, vomiting, dyspepsia, anorexia, glossitis, stomatitis, dry mouth.

Hematologic: Rare cases of neutropenia, thrombocytopenia and bone marrow depression.

Musculoskeletal: Muscle cramps.

Nervous/Psychiatric: Depression, vertigo, confusion, ataxia, somnolence, insomnia, nervousness, peripheral neuropathy (e.g. paresthesia, dysesthesia), dream abnormality.

Respiratory: Bronchospasm, dyspnea, pneumonia, bronchitis, cough, rhinorrhea, sore throat and hoarseness, asthma, upper respiratory infection, pulmonary infiltrates, eosinophilic pneumonitis.

Skin: Exfoliative dermatitis, toxic epidermal necrolysis, Stevens-Johnson syndrome, pemphigus, herpes zoster, erythema multiforme, urticaria, pruritus, alopecia, flushing, diaphoresis, photosensitivity.

Special Senses: Blurred vision, taste alteration, anosmia, tinnitus, conjunctivitis, dry eyes, tearing.

Urogenital: Renal failure, oliguria, renal dysfunction (see PRECAUTIONS and DOSAGE AND ADMINISTRATION), urinary tract infection, flank pain, gynecomastia, impotence.

Miscellaneous: A symptom complex has been reported which may include some or all of the following: a positive ANA, an elevated erythrocyte sedimentation rate, arthralgia/arthritis, myalgia/myositis, fever, serositis, vasculitis, leukocytosis, eosinophilia, photosensitivity, rash and other dermatologic manifestations.

Hypotension: Combining the results of clinical trials in patients with hypertension or congestive heart failure, hypotension (including postural hypotension, and other orthostatic effects) was reported in 2.3 percent of patients following the initial dose of enalapril or during extended therapy. In the hypertensive patients, hypotension occurred in 0.9 percent and syncope occurred in 0.5 percent of patients. Hypotension or syncope was a cause for discontinuation of therapy in 0.1 percent of hypertensive patients. (See WARNINGS.)

Fetal/Neonatal Morbidity and Mortality: See WARNINGS, *Fetal/Neonatal Morbidity and Mortality.*

Clinical Laboratory Test Findings

Serum Electrolytes: Hyperkalemia (see PRECAUTIONS), hyponatremia.

Creatinine, Blood Urea Nitrogen: In controlled clinical trials minor increases in blood urea nitrogen and serum creatinine, reversible upon discontinuation of therapy, were observed in about 0.2 percent of patients with essential hypertension treated with enalapril alone. Increases are more likely to occur in patients receiving concomitant diuretics or in patients with renal artery stenosis. (See PRECAUTIONS.)

Hematology: Small decreases in hemoglobin and hematocrit (mean decreases of approximately 0.3 g percent and 1.0 vol percent, respectively) occur frequently in hypertensive patients treated with enalapril but are rarely of clinical importance unless another cause of anemia coexists. In clinical trials, less than 0.1 percent of patients discontinued therapy due to anemia. Hemolytic anemia, including cases of hemolysis in patients with G-6-PD deficiency, has been reported; a causal relationship to enalapril cannot be excluded.

Liver Function Tests: Elevations of liver enzymes and/or serum bilirubin have occurred (see WARNINGS, *Hepatic Failure*).

OVERDOSAGE

In clinical studies, some hypertensive patients received a maximum dose of 80 mg of enalaprilat intravenously over a fifteen minute period. At this high dose, no adverse effects beyond those as associated with the recommended dosages were observed.

A single intravenous dose of ≤ 4167 mg/kg of enalaprilat was associated with lethality in female mice. No lethality occurred after an intravenous dose of 3472 mg/kg.

The most likely manifestation of overdosage would be hypotension, for which the usual treatment would be intravenous infusion of normal saline solution.

Enalaprilat may be removed from general circulation by hemodialysis and has been removed from neonatal circulation by peritoneal dialysis. (See WARNINGS, *Anaphylactoid reactions during membrane exposure.*)

DOSAGE AND ADMINISTRATION

FOR INTRAVENOUS ADMINISTRATION ONLY

The dose in hypertension is 1.25 mg every six hours administered intravenously over a five minute period. A clinical response is usually seen within 15 minutes. Peak effects after the first dose may not occur for up to four hours after dosing. The peak effects of the second and subsequent doses may exceed those of the first.

No dosage regimen for VASOTEC I.V. has been clearly demonstrated to be more effective in treating hypertension than 1.25 mg every six hours. However, in controlled clinical studies in hypertension, doses as high as 5 mg every six hours were well tolerated for up to 36 hours. There has been inadequate experience with doses greater than 20 mg per day.

In studies of patients with hypertension, VASOTEC I.V. has not been administered for periods longer than 48 hours. In other studies, patients have received VASOTEC I.V. for as long as seven days.

The dose for patients being converted to VASOTEC I.V. from oral therapy for hypertension with enalapril maleate is 1.25 mg every six hours. For conversion from intravenous to oral therapy, the recommended initial dose of Tablets VASOTEC (Enalapril Maleate) is 5 mg once a day with subsequent dosage adjustments as necessary.

Patients on Diuretic Therapy

For patients on diuretic therapy the recommended starting dose for hypertension is 0.625 mg administered intravenously over a five minute period. A clinical response is usually seen within 15 minutes. Peak effects after the first dose may not occur for up to four hours after dosing, although most of the effect is usually apparent within the first hour. If after one hour there is an inadequate clinical response, the 0.625 mg dose may be repeated. Additional doses of 1.25 mg may be administered at six hour intervals.

For conversion from intravenous to oral therapy, the recommended initial dose of Tablets VASOTEC (Enalapril Maleate) for patients who have responded to 0.625 mg of enalaprilat every six hours is 2.5 mg once a day with subsequent dosage adjustment as necessary.

Dosage Adjustment in Renal Impairment

The usual dose of 1.25 mg of enalaprilat every six hours is recommended for patients with a creatinine clearance >30 mL/min (serum creatinine of up to approximately 3 mg/dL). For patients with creatinine clearance ≤30 mL/min (serum creatinine ≥3 mg/dL), the initial dose is 0.625 mg. (See WARNINGS.)

If after one hour there is an inadequate clinical response, the 0.625 mg dose may be repeated. Additional doses of 1.25 mg may be administered at six hour intervals.

For dialysis patients, see below, *Patients at Risk of Excessive Hypotension.*

For conversion from intravenous to oral therapy, the recommended initial dose of Tablets VASOTEC (Enalapril Maleate) is 5 mg once a day for patients with creatinine clearance >30 mL/min and 2.5 mg once daily for patients with creatinine clearance ≤30 mL/min. Dosage should then be adjusted according to blood pressure response.

Patients at Risk of Excessive Hypotension

Hypertensive patients at risk of excessive hypotension include those with the following concurrent conditions or characteristics: heart failure, hyponatremia, high dose diuretic therapy, recent intensive diuresis or increase in diuretic dose, renal dialysis, or severe volume and/or salt depletion of any etiology (see WARNINGS). Single doses of enalaprilat as low as 0.2 mg have produced excessive hypo-

Continued on next page

Information on the Merck & Co., Inc. products listed on these pages is the full prescribing information from product circulars in use September 30, 2000. For information, please call 1-800-NSC MERCK [1-800-672-6372].

Vasotec I.V.—Cont.

tension in normotensive patients with these diagnoses. Because of the potential for an extreme hypotensive response in these patients, therapy should be started under very close medical supervision. The starting dose should be no greater than 0.625 mg administered intravenously over a period of no less than five minutes and preferably longer (up to one hour).

Patients should be followed closely whenever the dose of enalaprilat is adjusted and/or diuretic is increased.

Administration

VASOTEC I.V. should be administered as a slow intravenous infusion, as indicated above, over at least five minutes. It may be administered as provided or diluted with up to 50 mL of a compatible diluent.

Parenteral drug products should be inspected visually for particulate matter and discoloration prior to use whenever solution and container permit.

Compatibility and Stability

VASOTEC I.V. as supplied and mixed with the following intravenous diluents has been found to maintain full activity for 24 hours at room temperature:

5 percent Dextrose Injection
0.9 percent Sodium Chloride Injection
0.9 percent Sodium Chloride Injection in 5 percent Dextrose
5 percent Dextrose in Lactated Ringer's Injection
McGaw ISOLYTE* E.

* Registered trademark of American Hospital Supply Corporation.

HOW SUPPLIED

No. 3508—VASOTEC I.V., 1.25 mg per mL, is a clear, colorless solution and is supplied in vials containing 1 mL and 2 mL.

NDC 0006-3508-01, 1 mL vials
(6505-01-356-8505, 1 mL vial)
NDC 0006-3508-04, 2 mL vials
(6505-01-305-6988, 2 mL vial).

Storage

Store below 30°C (86°F).

7875729 Issued January 1998

VASOTEC® Tablets ℞
(Enalapril Maleate)

USE IN PREGNANCY

When used in pregnancy during the second and third trimesters, ACE inhibitors can cause injury and even death to the developing fetus. When pregnancy is detected, VASOTEC should be discontinued as soon as possible. See WARNINGS, *Fetal/Neonatal Morbidity and Mortality*.

DESCRIPTION

VASOTEC* (Enalapril Maleate) is the maleate salt of enalapril, the ethyl ester of a long-acting angiotensin converting enzyme inhibitor, enalaprilat. Enalapril maleate is chemically described as (*S*)-1-[*N*-[1-(ethoxycarbonyl)-3- phenylpropyl]-L-alanyl]-L-proline, (*Z*)-2-butenedioate salt (1:1). Its empirical formula is $C_{20}H_{28}N_2O_5 \cdot C_4H_4O_4$, and its structural formula is:

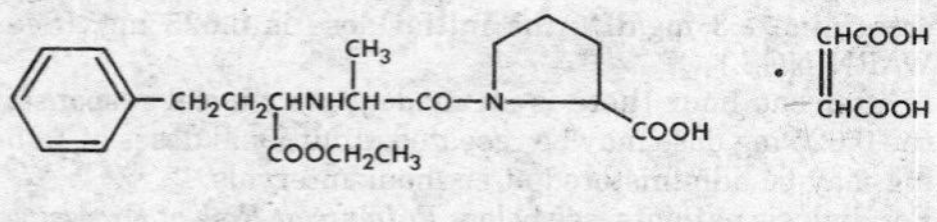

Enalapril maleate is a white to off-white, crystalline powder with a molecular weight of 492.53. It is sparingly soluble in water, soluble in ethanol, and freely soluble in methanol.

Enalapril is a pro-drug; following oral administration, it is bioactivated by hydrolysis of the ethyl ester to enalaprilat, which is the active angiotensin converting enzyme inhibitor.

Enalapril maleate is supplied as 2.5 mg, 5 mg, 10 mg, and 20 mg tablets for oral administration. In addition to the active ingredient enalapril maleate, each tablet contains the following inactive ingredients: lactose, magnesium stearate, starch, and other ingredients. The 2.5 mg, 10 mg and 20 mg tablets also contain iron oxides.

* Registered trademark of MERCK & CO., INC.

CLINICAL PHARMACOLOGY

Mechanism of Action

Enalapril, after hydrolysis to enalaprilat, inhibits angiotensin-converting enzyme (ACE) in human subjects and animals. ACE is a peptidyl dipeptidase that catalyzes the conversion of angiotensin I to the vasoconstrictor substance, angiotensin II. Angiotensin II also stimulates aldosterone secretion by the adrenal cortex. The beneficial effects of enalapril in hypertension and heart failure appear to result primarily from suppression of the renin-angiotensin-aldosterone system. Inhibition of ACE results in decreased plasma angiotensin II, which leads to decreased vasopressor activity and to decreased aldosterone secretion. Although the latter decrease is small, it results in small increases of serum potassium. In hypertensive patients treated with VASOTEC alone for up to 48 weeks, mean increases in serum potassium of approximately 0.2 mEq/L were observed. In patients treated with VASOTEC plus a thiazide diuretic, there was essentially no change in serum potassium. (See PRECAUTIONS.) Removal of angiotensin II negative feedback on renin secretion leads to increased plasma renin activity.

ACE is identical to kininase, an enzyme that degrades bradykinin. Whether increased levels of bradykinin, a potent vasodepressor peptide, play a role in the therapeutic effects of VASOTEC remains to be elucidated.

While the mechanism through which VASOTEC lowers blood pressure is believed to be primarily suppression of the renin-angiotensin-aldosterone system, VASOTEC is antihypertensive even in patients with low-renin hypertension. Although VASOTEC was antihypertensive in all races studied, black hypertensive patients (usually a low-renin hypertensive population) had a smaller average response to enalapril monotherapy than non-black patients.

Pharmacokinetics and Metabolism

Following oral administration of VASOTEC, peak serum concentrations of enalapril occur within about one hour. Based on urinary recovery, the extent of absorption of enalapril is approximately 60 percent. Enalapril absorption is not influenced by the presence of food in the gastrointestinal tract. Following absorption, enalapril is hydrolyzed to enalaprilat, which is a more potent angiotensin converting enzyme inhibitor than enalapril; enalaprilat is poorly absorbed when administered orally. Peak serum concentrations of enalaprilat occur three to four hours after an oral dose of enalapril maleate. Excretion of VASOTEC is primarily renal. Approximately 94 percent of the dose is recovered in the urine and feces as enalaprilat or enalapril. The principal components in urine are enalaprilat, accounting for about 40 percent of the dose, and intact enalapril. There is no evidence of metabolites of enalapril, other than enalaprilat.

The serum concentration profile of enalaprilat exhibits a prolonged terminal phase, apparently representing a small fraction of the administered dose that has been bound to ACE. The amount bound does not increase with dose, indicating a saturable site of binding. The effective half-life for accumulation of enalaprilat following multiple doses of enalapril maleate is 11 hours.

The disposition of enalapril and enalaprilat in patients with renal insufficiency is similar to that in patients with normal renal function until the glomerular filtration rate is 30 mL/min or less. With glomerular filtration rate ≤30 mL/min, peak and trough enalaprilat levels increase, time to peak concentration increases and time to steady state may be delayed. The effective half-life of enalaprilat following multiple doses of enalapril maleate is prolonged at this level of renal insufficiency. (See DOSAGE AND ADMINISTRATION.) Enalaprilat is dialyzable at the rate of 62 mL/min.

Studies in dogs indicate that enalapril crosses the blood-brain barrier poorly, if at all; enalaprilat does not enter the brain. Multiple doses of enalapril maleate in rats do not result in accumulation in any tissues. Milk of lactating rats contains radioactivity following administration of ^{14}C enalapril maleate. Radioactivity was found to cross the placenta following administration of labeled drug to pregnant hamsters.

Pharmacodynamics and Clinical Effects

Hypertension: Administration of VASOTEC to patients with hypertension of severity ranging from mild to severe results in a reduction of both supine and standing blood pressure usually with no orthostatic component. Symptomatic postural hypotension is therefore infrequent, although it might be anticipated in volume-depleted patients. (See WARNINGS.)

In most patients studied, after oral administration of a single dose of enalapril, onset of antihypertensive activity was seen at one hour with peak reduction of blood pressure achieved by four to six hours.

At recommended doses, antihypertensive effects have been maintained for at least 24 hours. In some patients the effects may diminish toward the end of the dosing interval (see DOSAGE AND ADMINISTRATION).

In some patients achievement of optimal blood pressure reduction may require several weeks of therapy.

The antihypertensive effects of VASOTEC have continued during long term therapy. Abrupt withdrawal of VASOTEC has not been associated with a rapid increase in blood pressure.

In hemodynamic studies in patients with essential hypertension, blood pressure reduction was accompanied by a reduction in peripheral arterial resistance with an increase in cardiac output and little or no change in heart rate. Following administration of VASOTEC, there is an increase in renal blood flow; glomerular filtration rate is usually unchanged. The effects appear to be similar in patients with renovascular hypertension.

When given together with thiazide-type diuretics, the blood pressure lowering effects of VASOTEC are approximately additive.

In a clinical pharmacology study, indomethacin or sulindac was administered to hypertensive patients receiving VASOTEC. In this study there was no evidence of a blunting of the antihypertensive action of VASOTEC.

Heart Failure: In trials in patients treated with digitalis and diuretics, treatment with enalapril resulted in decreased systemic vascular resistance, blood pressure, pulmonary capillary wedge pressure and heart size, and increased cardiac output and exercise tolerance. Heart rate was unchanged or slightly reduced, and mean ejection fraction was unchanged or increased. There was a beneficial effect on severity of heart failure as measured by the New York Heart Association (NYHA) classification and on symptoms of dyspnea and fatigue. Hemodynamic effects were observed after the first dose, and appeared to be maintained in uncontrolled studies lasting as long as four months. Effects on exercise tolerance, heart size, and severity and symptoms of heart failure were observed in placebo-controlled studies lasting from eight weeks to over one year.

Heart Failure, Mortality Trials: In a multicenter, placebo-controlled clinical trial, 2,569 patients with all degrees of symptomatic heart failure and ejection fraction ≤35 percent were randomized to placebo or enalapril and followed for up to 55 months (SOLVD-Treatment). Use of enalapril was associated with an 11 percent reduction in all-cause mortality and a 30 percent reduction in hospitalization for heart failure. Diseases that excluded patients from enrollment in the study included severe stable angina (>2 attacks/day), hemodynamically significant valvular or outflow tract obstruction, renal failure (creatinine >2.5 mg/dL), cerebral vascular disease (e.g., significant carotid artery disease), advanced pulmonary disease, malignancies, active myocarditis and constrictive pericarditis. The mortality benefit associated with enalapril does not appear to depend upon digitalis being present.

A second multicenter trial used the SOLVD protocol for study of asymptomatic or minimally symptomatic patients. SOLVD-Prevention patients, who had left ventricular ejection fraction ≤35% and no history of symptomatic heart failure, were randomized to placebo (n=2117) or enalapril (n=2111) and followed for up to 5 years. The majority of patients in the SOLVD-Prevention trial had a history of ischemic heart disease. A history of myocardial infarction was present in 80 percent of patients, current angina pectoris in 34 percent, and a history of hypertension in 37 percent. No statistically significant mortality effect was demonstrated in this population. Enalapril-treated subjects had 32% fewer first hospitalizations for heart failure, and 32% fewer total heart failure hospitalizations. Compared to placebo, 32 percent fewer patients receiving enalapril developed symptoms of overt heart failure. Hospitalizations for cardiovascular reasons were also reduced. There was an insignificant reduction in hospitalizations for any cause in the enalapril treatment group (for enalapril vs. placebo, respectively, 1166 vs. 1201 first hospitalizations, 2649 vs. 2840 total hospitalizations), although the study was not powered to look for such an effect.

The SOLVD-Prevention trial was not designed to determine whether treatment of asymptomatic patients with low ejection fraction would be superior, with respect to preventing hospitalization, to closer follow-up and use of enalapril at the earliest sign of heart failure. However, under the conditions of follow-up in the SOLVD-Prevention trial (every 4 months at the study clinic; personal physician as needed), 68% of patients on placebo who were hospitalized for heart failure had no prior symptoms recorded which would have signaled initiation of treatment.

The SOLVD-Prevention trial was also not designed to show whether enalapril modified the progression of underlying heart disease.

In another multicenter, placebo-controlled trial (CONSENSUS) limited to patients with NYHA class IV congestive heart failure and radiographic evidence of cardiomegaly, use of enalapril was associated with improved survival. The results are shown in the following table.

	SURVIVAL (%)	
	Six Months	One Year
VASOTEC (n=127)	74	64
Placebo (n=126)	56	48

In both CONSENSUS and SOLVD-Treatment trials, patients were also usually receiving digitalis, diuretics or both.

INDICATIONS AND USAGE

Hypertension

VASOTEC is indicated for the treatment of hypertension.

VASOTEC is effective alone or in combination with other antihypertensive agents, especially thiazide-type diuretics. The blood pressure lowering effects of VASOTEC and thiazides are approximately additive.

Heart Failure

VASOTEC is indicated for the treatment of symptomatic congestive heart failure, usually in combination with diuretics and digitalis. In these patients VASOTEC improves symptoms, increases survival, and decreases the frequency of hospitalization (see CLINICAL PHARMACOLOGY, *Heart Failure, Mortality Trials* for details and limitations of survival trials).

Asymptomatic Left Ventricular Dysfunction

In clinically stable asymptomatic patients with left ventricular dysfunction (ejection fraction ≤35 percent), VASOTEC decreases the rate of development of overt heart failure and

decreases the incidence of hospitalization for heart failure. (See CLINICAL PHARMACOLOGY, *Heart Failure, Mortality Trials* for details and limitations of survival trials.)
In using VASOTEC consideration should be given to the fact that another angiotensin converting enzyme inhibitor, captopril, has caused agranulocytosis, particularly in patients with renal impairment or collagen vascular disease, and that available data are insufficient to show that VASOTEC does not have a similar risk. (See WARNINGS.)
In considering use of VASOTEC, it should be noted that in controlled clinical trials ACE inhibitors have an effect on blood pressure that is less in black patients than in non-blacks. In addition, it should be noted that black patients receiving ACE inhibitors have been reported to have a higher incidence of angioedema compared to non-blacks. (See WARNINGS, *Angioedema*.)

CONTRAINDICATIONS

VASOTEC is contraindicated in patients who are hypersensitive to this product and in patients with a history of angioedema related to previous treatment with an angiotensin converting enzyme inhibitor and in patients with hereditary or idiopathic angioedema.

WARNINGS

Anaphylactoid and Possibly Related Reactions
Presumably because angiotensin-converting enzyme inhibitors affect the metabolism of eicosanoids and polypeptides, including endogenous bradykinin, patients receiving ACE inhibitors (including VASOTEC) may be subject to a variety of adverse reactions, some of them serious.
Angioedema: Angioedema of the face, extremities, lips, tongue, glottis and/or larynx has been reported in patients treated with angiotensin converting enzyme inhibitors, including VASOTEC. This may occur at any time during treatment. In such cases VASOTEC should be promptly discontinued and appropriate therapy and monitoring should be provided until complete and sustained resolution of signs and symptoms has occurred. In instances where swelling has been confined to the face and lips the condition has generally resolved without treatment, although antihistamines have been useful in relieving symptoms. Angioedema associated with laryngeal edema may be fatal. **Where there is involvement of the tongue, glottis or larynx, likely to cause airway obstruction, appropriate therapy, e.g., subcutaneous epinephrine solution 1:1000 (0.3 mL to 0.5 mL) and/or measures necessary to ensure a patent airway, should be promptly provided.** (See ADVERSE REACTIONS.)
Patients with a history of angioedema unrelated to ACE inhibitor therapy may be at increased risk of angioedema while receiving an ACE inhibitor (see also INDICATIONS AND USAGE and CONTRAINDICATIONS).
Anaphylactoid reactions during desensitization: Two patients undergoing desensitizing treatment with hymenoptera venom while receiving ACE inhibitors sustained life-threatening anaphylactoid reactions. In the same patients, these reactions were avoided when ACE inhibitors were temporarily withheld, but they reappeared upon inadvertent rechallenge.
Anaphylactoid reactions during membrane exposure: Anaphylactoid reactions have been reported in patients dialyzed with high-flux membranes and treated concomitantly with an ACE inhibitor. Anaphylactoid reactions have also been reported in patients undergoing low-density lipoprotein apheresis with dextran sulfate absorption.
Hypotension
Excessive hypotension is rare in uncomplicated hypertensive patients treated with VASOTEC alone. Patients with heart failure given VASOTEC commonly have some reduction in blood pressure, especially with the first dose, but discontinuation of therapy for continuing symptomatic hypotension usually is not necessary when dosing instructions are followed; caution should be observed when initiating therapy. (See DOSAGE AND ADMINISTRATION.) Patients at risk for excessive hypotension, sometimes associated with oliguria and/or progressive azotemia, and rarely with acute renal failure and/or death, include those with the following conditions or characteristics: heart failure, hyponatremia, high dose diuretic therapy, recent intensive diuresis or increase in diuretic dose, renal dialysis, or severe volume and/or salt depletion of any etiology. It may be advisable to eliminate the diuretic (except in patients with heart failure), reduce the diuretic dose or increase salt intake cautiously before initiating therapy with VASOTEC in patients at risk for excessive hypotension who are able to tolerate such adjustments. (See PRECAUTIONS, *Drug Interactions* and ADVERSE REACTIONS.) In patients at risk for excessive hypotension, therapy should be started under very close medical supervision and such patients should be followed closely for the first two weeks of treatment and whenever the dose of enalapril and/or diuretic is increased. Similar considerations may apply to patients with ischemic heart or cerebrovascular disease, in whom an excessive fall in blood pressure could result in a myocardial infarction or cerebrovascular accident.
If excessive hypotension occurs, the patient should be placed in the supine position and, if necessary, receive an intravenous infusion of normal saline. A transient hypotensive response is not a contraindication to further doses of VASOTEC, which usually can be given without difficulty once the blood pressure has stabilized. If symptomatic hypotension develops, a dose reduction or discontinuation of VASOTEC or concomitant diuretic may be necessary.
Neutropenia/Agranulocytosis
Another angiotensin converting enzyme inhibitor, captopril, has been shown to cause agranulocytosis and bone marrow depression, rarely in uncomplicated patients but more frequently in patients with renal impairment especially if they also have a collagen vascular disease. Available data from clinical trials of enalapril are insufficient to show that enalapril does not cause agranulocytosis at similar rates. Marketing experience has revealed cases of neutropenia or agranulocytosis in which a causal relationship to enalapril cannot be excluded. Periodic monitoring of white blood cell counts in patients with collagen vascular disease and renal disease should be considered.
Hepatic Failure
Rarely, ACE inhibitors have been associated with a syndrome that starts with cholestatic jaundice and progresses to fulminant hepatic necrosis, and (sometimes) death. The mechanism of this syndrome is not understood. Patients receiving ACE inhibitors who develop jaundice or marked elevations of hepatic enzymes should discontinue the ACE inhibitor and receive appropriate medical follow-up.
Fetal/Neonatal Morbidity and Mortality
ACE inhibitors can cause fetal and neonatal morbidity and death when administered to pregnant women. Several dozen cases have been reported in the world literature. When pregnancy is detected, ACE inhibitors should be discontinued as soon as possible.
The use of ACE inhibitors during the second and third trimesters of pregnancy has been associated with fetal and neonatal injury, including hypotension, neonatal skull hypoplasia, anuria, reversible or irreversible renal failure, and death. Oligohydramnios has also been reported, presumably resulting from decreased fetal renal function: oligohydramnios in this setting has been associated with fetal limb contractures, craniofacial deformation, and hypoplastic lung development. Prematurity, intrauterine growth retardation, and patent ductus arteriosus have also been reported, although it is not clear whether these occurrences were due to the ACE-inhibitor exposure.
These adverse effects do not appear to have resulted from intrauterine ACE-inhibitor exposure that has been limited to the first trimester. Mothers whose embryos and fetuses are exposed to ACE inhibitors only during the first trimester should be so informed. Nonetheless, when patients become pregnant, physicians should make every effort to discontinue the use of VASOTEC as soon as possible.
Rarely (probably less often than once in every thousand pregnancies), no alternative to ACE inhibitors will be found. In these rare cases, the mothers should be apprised of the potential hazards to their fetuses, and serial ultrasound examinations should be performed to assess the intraamniotic environment.
If oligohydramnios is observed, VASOTEC should be discontinued unless it is considered lifesaving for the mother. Contraction stress testing (CST), a non-stress test (NST), or biophysical profiling (BPP) may be appropriate, depending upon the week of pregnancy. Patients and physicians should be aware, however, that oligohydramnios may not appear until after the fetus has sustained irreversible injury.
Infants with histories of *in utero* exposure to ACE inhibitors should be closely observed for hypotension, oliguria, and hyperkalemia. If oliguria occurs, attention should be directed toward support of blood pressure and renal perfusion. Exchange transfusion or dialysis may be required as means of reversing hypotension and/or substituting for disordered renal function. Enalapril, which crosses the placenta, has been removed from neonatal circulation by peritoneal dialysis with some clinical benefit, and theoretically may be removed by exchange transfusion, although there is no experience with the latter procedure.
No teratogenic effects of enalapril were seen in studies of pregnant rats and rabbits. On a body surface area basis, the doses used were 57 times and 12 times, respectively, the maximum recommended human daily dose (MRHDD).

PRECAUTIONS

General
Aortic Stenosis/Hypertrophic Cardiomyopathy: As with all vasodilators, enalapril should be given with caution to patients with obstruction in the outflow tract of the left ventricle.
Impaired Renal Function: As a consequence of inhibiting the renin-angiotensin-aldosterone system, changes in renal function may be anticipated in susceptible individuals. In patients with severe heart failure whose renal function may depend on the activity of the renin-angiotensin-aldosterone system, treatment with angiotensin converting enzyme inhibitors, including VASOTEC, may be associated with oliguria and/or progressive azotemia and rarely with acute renal failure and/or death.
In clinical studies in hypertensive patients with unilateral or bilateral renal artery stenosis, increases in blood urea nitrogen and serum creatinine were observed in 20 percent of patients. These increases were almost always reversible upon discontinuation of enalapril and/or diuretic therapy. In such patients renal function should be monitored during the first few weeks of therapy.
Some patients with hypertension or heart failure with no apparent pre-existing renal vascular disease have developed increases in blood urea and serum creatinine, usually minor and transient, especially when VASOTEC has been given concomitantly with a diuretic. This is more likely to occur in patients with pre-existing renal impairment. Dosage reduction and/or discontinuation of the diuretic and/or VASOTEC may be required.
Evaluation of patients with hypertension or heart failure should always include assessment of renal function. (See DOSAGE AND ADMINISTRATION.)
Hyperkalemia: Elevated serum potassium (greater than 5.7 mEq/L) was observed in approximately one percent of hypertensive patients in clinical trials. In most cases these were isolated values which resolved despite continued therapy. Hyperkalemia was a cause of discontinuation of therapy in 0.28 percent of hypertensive patients. In clinical trials in heart failure, hyperkalemia was observed in 3.8 percent of patients but was not a cause for discontinuation.
Risk factors for the development of hyperkalemia include renal insufficiency, diabetes mellitus, and the concomitant use of potassium-sparing diuretics, potassium supplements and/or potassium-containing salt substitutes, which should be used cautiously, if at all, with VASOTEC. (See *Drug Interactions*.)
Cough: Presumably due to the inhibition of the degradation of endogenous bradykinin, persistent nonproductive cough has been reported with all ACE inhibitors, always resolving after discontinuation of therapy. ACE inhibitor-induced cough should be considered in the differential diagnosis of cough.
Surgery/Anesthesia: In patients undergoing major surgery or during anesthesia with agents that produce hypotension, enalapril may block angiotensin II formation secondary to compensatory renin release. If hypotension occurs and is considered to be due to this mechanism, it can be corrected by volume expansion.
Information for Patients
Angioedema: Angioedema, including laryngeal edema, may occur at any time during treatment with angiotensin converting enzyme inhibitors, including enalapril. Patients should be so advised and told to report immediately any signs or symptoms suggesting angioedema (swelling of face, extremities, eyes, lips, tongue, difficulty in swallowing or breathing) and to take no more drug until they have consulted with the prescribing physician.
Hypotension: Patients should be cautioned to report lightheadedness, especially during the first few days of therapy. If actual syncope occurs, the patients should be told to discontinue the drug until they have consulted with the prescribing physician.
All patients should be cautioned that excessive perspiration and dehydration may lead to an excessive fall in blood pressure because of reduction in fluid volume. Other causes of volume depletion such as vomiting or diarrhea may also lead to a fall in blood pressure; patients should be advised to consult with the physician.
Hyperkalemia: Patients should be told not to use salt substitutes containing potassium without consulting their physician.
Neutropenia: Patients should be told to report promptly any indication of infection (e.g., sore throat, fever) which may be a sign of neutropenia.
Pregnancy: Female patients of childbearing age should be told about the consequences of second- and third-trimester exposure to ACE inhibitors, and they should also be told that these consequences do not appear to have resulted from intrauterine ACE-inhibitor exposure that has been limited to the first trimester. These patients should be asked to report pregnancies to their physicians as soon as possible.
NOTE: As with many other drugs, certain advice to patients being treated with enalapril is warranted. This information is intended to aid in the safe and effective use of this medication. It is not a disclosure of all possible adverse or intended effects.
Drug Interactions
Hypotension—Patients on Diuretic Therapy: Patients on diuretics and especially those in whom diuretic therapy was recently instituted, may occasionally experience an excessive reduction of blood pressure after initiation of therapy with enalapril. The possibility of hypotensive effects with enalapril can be minimized by either discontinuing the diuretic or increasing the salt intake prior to initiation of treatment with enalapril. If it is necessary to continue the diuretic, provide close medical supervision after the initial dose for at least two hours and until blood pressure has stabilized for at least an additional hour. (See WARNINGS and DOSAGE AND ADMINISTRATION.)
Agents Causing Renin Release: The antihypertensive effect of VASOTEC is augmented by antihypertensive agents that cause renin release (e.g., diuretics).
Non-steroidal Anti-inflammatory Agents: In some patients with compromised renal function who are being treated with non-steroidal anti-inflammatory drugs, the co-administration of enalapril may result in a further deterioration of renal function. These effects are usually reversible.
Other Cardiovascular Agents: VASOTEC has been used concomitantly with beta adrenergic-blocking agents, methyldopa, nitrates, calcium-blocking agents, hydralazine, prazosin and digoxin without evidence of clinically significant adverse interactions.

Continued on next page

Information on the Merck & Co., Inc. products listed on these pages is the full prescribing information from product circulars in use September 30, 2000. For information, please call 1-800-NSC MERCK [1-800-672-6372].

Vasotec Tablets—Cont.

Agents Increasing Serum Potassium: VASOTEC attenuates potassium loss caused by thiazide-type diuretics. Potassium-sparing diuretics (e.g., spironolactone, triamterene, or amiloride), potassium supplements, or potassium-containing salt substitutes may lead to significant increases in serum potassium. Therefore, if concomitant use of these agents is indicated because of demonstrated hypokalemia, they should be used with caution and with frequent monitoring of serum potassium. Potassium sparing agents should generally not be used in patients with heart failure receiving VASOTEC.
Lithium: Lithium toxicity has been reported in patients receiving lithium concomitantly with drugs which cause elimination of sodium, including ACE inhibitors. A few cases of lithium toxicity have been reported in patients receiving concomitant VASOTEC and lithium and were reversible upon discontinuation of both drugs. It is recommended that serum lithium levels be monitored frequently if enalapril is administered concomitantly with lithium.
Carcinogenesis, Mutagenesis, Impairment of Fertility
There was no evidence of a tumorigenic effect when enalapril was administered for 106 weeks to male and female rats at doses up to 90 mg/kg/day or for 94 weeks to male and female mice at doses up to 90 and 180 mg/kg/day, respectively. These doses are 26 times (in rats and female mice) and 13 times (in male mice) the maximum recommended human daily dose (MRHDD) when compared on a body surface area basis.
Neither enalapril maleate nor the active diacid was mutagenic in the Ames microbial mutagen test with or without metabolic activation. Enalapril was also negative in the following genotoxicity studies: rec-assay, reverse mutation assay with *E. coli*, sister chromatid exchange with cultured mammalian cells, and the micronucleus test with mice, as well as in an *in vivo* cytogenic study using mouse bone marrow.
There were no adverse effects on reproductive performance of male and female rats treated with up to 90 mg/kg/day of enalapril (26 times the MRHDD when compared on a body surface area basis).
Pregnancy
Pregnancy Categories C (first trimester) and *D* (second and third trimesters). See WARNINGS, *Fetal/Neonatal Morbidity and Mortality.*
Nursing Mothers
Enalapril and enalaprilat have been detected in human breast milk. Because of the potential for serious adverse reactions in nursing infants from enalapril, a decision should be made whether to discontinue nursing or to discontinue VASOTEC, taking into account the importance of the drug to the mother.
Pediatric Use
Safety and effectiveness in pediatric patients have not been established.

ADVERSE REACTIONS

VASOTEC has been evaluated for safety in more than 10,000 patients, including over 1000 patients treated for one year or more. VASOTEC has been found to be generally well tolerated in controlled clinical trials involving 2987 patients.
For the most part, adverse experiences were mild and transient in nature. In clinical trials, discontinuation of therapy due to clinical adverse experiences was required in 3.3 percent of patients with hypertension and in 5.7 percent of patients with heart failure. The frequency of adverse experiences was not related to total daily dosage within the usual dosage ranges. In patients with hypertension the overall percentage of patients treated with VASOTEC reporting adverse experiences was comparable to placebo.
HYPERTENSION
Adverse experiences occurring in greater than one percent of patients with hypertension treated with VASOTEC in controlled clinical trials are shown below. In patients treated with VASOTEC, the maximum duration of therapy was three years; in placebo treated patients the maximum duration of therapy was 12 weeks.

	VASOTEC (n = 2314) Incidence (discontinuation)	Placebo (n = 230) Incidence
Body As A Whole		
Fatigue	3.0 (<0.1)	2.6
Orthostatic Effects	1.2 (<0.1)	0.0
Asthenia	1.1 (0.1)	0.9
Digestive		
Diarrhea	1.4 (<0.1)	1.7
Nausea	1.4 (0.2)	1.7
Nervous/Psychiatric		
Headache	5.2 (0.3)	9.1
Dizziness	4.3 (0.4)	4.3
Respiratory		
Cough	1.3 (0.1)	0.9
Skin		
Rash	1.4 (0.4)	0.4

HEART FAILURE
Adverse experiences occurring in greater than one percent of patients with heart failure treated with VASOTEC are shown below. The incidences represent the experiences from both controlled and uncontrolled clinical trials (maximum duration of therapy was approximately one year). In the placebo treated patients, the incidences reported are from the controlled trials (maximum duration of therapy is 12 weeks). The percentage of patients with severe heart failure (NYHA Class IV) was 29 percent and 43 percent for patients treated with VASOTEC and placebo, respectively.

	VASOTEC (n = 673) Incidence (discontinuation)	Placebo (n = 339) Incidence
Body As A Whole		
Orthostatic Effects	2.2 (0.1)	0.3
Syncope	2.2 (0.1)	0.9
Chest Pain	2.1 (0.0)	2.1
Fatigue	1.8 (0.0)	1.8
Abdominal Pain	1.6 (0.4)	2.1
Asthenia	1.6 (0.1)	0.3
Cardiovascular		
Hypotension	6.7 (1.9)	0.6
Orthostatic Hypotension	1.6 (0.1)	0.3
Angina Pectoris	1.5 (0.1)	1.8
Myocardial Infarction	1.2 (0.3)	1.8
Digestive		
Diarrhea	2.1 (0.1)	1.2
Nausea	1.3 (0.1)	0.6
Vomiting	1.3 (0.0)	0.9
Nervous/Psychiatric		
Dizziness	7.9 (0.6)	0.6
Headache	1.8 (0.1)	0.9
Vertigo	1.6 (0.1)	1.2
Respiratory		
Cough	2.2 (0.0)	0.6
Bronchitis	1.3 (0.0)	0.9
Dyspnea	1.3 (0.1)	0.4
Pneumonia	1.0 (0.0)	2.4
Skin		
Rash	1.3 (0.0)	2.4
Urogenital		
Urinary Tract Infection	1.3 (0.0)	2.4

Other serious clinical adverse experiences occurring since the drug was marketed or adverse experiences occurring in 0.5 to 1.0 percent of patients with hypertension or heart failure in clinical trials are listed below and, within each category, are in order of decreasing severity.
Body As A Whole: Anaphylactoid reactions (see WARNINGS, *Anaphylactoid and Possibly Related Reactions*).
Cardiovascular: Cardiac arrest; myocardial infarction or cerebrovascular accident, possibly secondary to excessive hypotension in high risk patients (see WARNINGS, *Hypotension*); pulmonary embolism and infarction; pulmonary edema; rhythm disturbances including atrial tachycardia and bradycardia; atrial fibrillation; palpitation, Raynaud's phenomenon.
Digestive: Ileus, pancreatitis, hepatic failure, hepatitis (hepatocellular [proven on rechallenge] or cholestatic jaundice) (see WARNINGS, *Hepatic Failure*), melena, anorexia, dyspepsia, constipation, glossitis, stomatitis, dry mouth.
Hematologic: Rare cases of neutropenia, thrombocytopenia and bone marrow depression.
Musculoskeletal: Muscle cramps.
Nervous/Psychiatric: Depression, confusion, ataxia, somnolence, insomnia, nervousness, peripheral neuropathy (e.g., paresthesia, dysesthesia), dream abnormality.
Respiratory: Bronchospasm, rhinorrhea, sore throat and hoarseness, asthma, upper respiratory infection, pulmonary infiltrates, eosinophilic pneumonitis.
Skin: Exfoliative dermatitis, toxic epidermal necrolysis, Stevens-Johnson syndrome, pemphigus, herpes zoster, erythema multiforme, urticaria, pruritus, alopecia, flushing, diaphoresis, photosensitivity.
Special Senses: Blurred vision, taste alteration, anosmia, tinnitus, conjunctivitis, dry eyes, tearing.
Urogenital: Renal failure, oliguria, renal dysfunction (see PRECAUTIONS and DOSAGE AND ADMINISTRATION), flank pain, gynecomastia, impotence.
Miscellaneous: A symptom complex has been reported which may include some or all of the following: a positive ANA, an elevated erythrocyte sedimentation rate, arthralgia/arthritis, myalgia/myositis, fever, serositis, vasculitis, leukocytosis, eosinophilia, photosensitivity, rash and other dermatologic manifestations.
Angioedema: Angioedema has been reported in patients receiving VASOTEC, with an incidence higher in black than in non-black patients. Angioedema associated with laryngeal edema may be fatal. If angioedema of the face, extremities, lips, tongue, glottis and/or larynx occurs, treatment with VASOTEC should be discontinued and appropriate therapy instituted immediately. (See WARNINGS.)
Hypotension: In the hypertensive patients, hypotension occurred in 0.9 percent and syncope occurred in 0.5 percent of patients following the initial dose or during extended therapy. Hypotension or syncope was a cause for discontinuation of therapy in 0.1 percent of hypertensive patients. In heart failure patients, hypotension occurred in 6.7 percent and syncope occurred in 2.2 percent of patients. Hypotension or syncope was a cause for discontinuation of therapy in 1.9 percent of patients with heart failure. (See WARNINGS.)
Fetal/Neonatal Morbidity and Mortality: See WARNINGS, *Fetal/Neonatal Morbidity and Mortality.*
Cough: See PRECAUTIONS, *Cough.*
Clinical Laboratory Test Findings
Serum Electrolytes: Hyperkalemia (see PRECAUTIONS), hyponatremia.
Creatinine, Blood Urea Nitrogen: In controlled clinical trials minor increases in blood urea nitrogen and serum creatinine, reversible upon discontinuation of therapy, were observed in about 0.2 percent of patients with essential hypertension treated with VASOTEC alone. Increases are more likely to occur in patients receiving concomitant diuretics or in patients with renal artery stenosis. (See PRECAUTIONS.) In patients with heart failure who were also receiving diuretics with or without digitalis increases in blood urea nitrogen or serum creatinine, usually reversible upon discontinuation of VASOTEC and/or other concomitant diuretic therapy, were observed in about 11 percent of patients. Increases in blood urea nitrogen or creatinine were a cause for discontinuation in 1.2 percent of patients.
Hematology: Small decreases in hemoglobin and hematocrit (mean decreases of approximately 0.3 g percent and 1.0 vol percent, respectively) occur frequently in either hypertension or congestive heart failure patients treated with VASOTEC but are rarely of clinical importance unless another cause of anemia coexists. In clinical trials, less than 0.1 percent of patients discontinued therapy due to anemia. Hemolytic anemia, including cases of hemolysis in patients with G-6-PD deficiency, has been reported; a causal relationship to enalapril cannot be excluded.
Liver Function Tests: Elevations of liver enzymes and/or serum bilirubin have occurred (see WARNINGS, *Hepatic Failure*).

OVERDOSAGE

Limited data are available in regard to overdosage in humans.
Single oral doses of enalapril above 1,000 mg/kg and ≥1,775 mg/kg were associated with lethality in mice and rats, respectively.
The most likely manifestation of overdosage would be hypotension, for which the usual treatment would be intravenous infusion of normal saline solution.
Enalaprilat may be removed from general circulation by hemodialysis and has been removed from neonatal circulation by peritoneal dialysis. (See WARNINGS, *Anaphylactoid reactions during membrane exposure.*)

DOSAGE AND ADMINISTRATION

Hypertension
In patients who are currently being treated with a diuretic, symptomatic hypotension occasionally may occur following the initial dose of VASOTEC. The diuretic should, if possible, be discontinued for two to three days before beginning therapy with VASOTEC to reduce the likelihood of hypotension. (See WARNINGS.) If the patient's blood pressure is not controlled with VASOTEC alone, diuretic therapy may be resumed.
If the diuretic cannot be discontinued an initial dose of 2.5 mg should be used under medical supervision for at least two hours and until blood pressure has stabilized for at least an additional hour. (See WARNINGS and PRECAUTIONS, *Drug Interactions.*)
The recommended initial dose in patients not on diuretics is 5 mg once a day. Dosage should be adjusted according to blood pressure response. The usual dosage range is 10 to 40 mg per day administered in a single dose or two divided doses. In some patients treated once daily, the antihypertensive effect may diminish toward the end of the dosing interval. In such patients, an increase in dosage or twice daily administration should be considered. If blood pressure is not controlled with VASOTEC alone, a diuretic may be added.
Concomitant administration of VASOTEC with potassium supplements, potassium salt substitutes, or potassium-sparing diuretics may lead to increases of serum potassium (see PRECAUTIONS).
Dosage Adjustment in Hypertensive Patients with Renal Impairment
The usual dose of enalapril is recommended for patients with a creatinine clearance >30 mL/min (serum creatinine of up to approximately 3 mg/dL). For patients with creatinine clearance ≤30 mL/min (serum creatinine ≥3 mg/dL), the first dose is 2.5 mg once daily. The dosage may be titrated upward until blood pressure is controlled or to a maximum of 40 mg daily.

Renal Status	Creatinine-Clearance mL/min	Initial Dose mg/day
Normal Renal Function	>80 mL/min	5 mg
Mild Impairment	≤80 >30 mL/min	5 mg
Moderate to Severe Impairment	≤30 mL/min	2.5 mg
Dialysis Patients***	—	2.5 mg on dialysis days†

*** See WARNINGS, *Anaphylactoid reactions during membrane exposure.*
† Dosage on nondialysis days should be adjusted depending on the blood pressure response.

Heart Failure
VASOTEC is indicated for the treatment of symptomatic heart failure, usually in combination with diuretics and digitalis. In the placebo-controlled studies that demonstrated improved survival, patients were titrated as tolerated up to 40 mg, administered in two divided doses.
The recommended initial dose is 2.5 mg. The recommended dosing range is 2.5 to 20 mg given twice a day. Doses should be titrated upward, as tolerated, over a period of a few days or weeks. The maximum daily dose administered in clinical trials was 40 mg in divided doses.
After the initial dose of VASOTEC, the patient should be observed under medical supervision for at least two hours and until blood pressure has stabilized for at least an additional hour. (See WARNINGS and PRECAUTIONS, *Drug Interactions.*) If possible, the dose of any concomitant diuretic should be reduced which may diminish the likelihood of hypotension. The appearance of hypotension after the initial dose of VASOTEC does not preclude subsequent careful dose titration with the drug, following effective management of the hypotension.
Asymptomatic Left Ventricular Dysfunction
In the trial that demonstrated efficacy, patients were started on 2.5 mg twice daily and were titrated as tolerated to the targeted daily dose of 20 mg (in divided doses).
After the initial dose of VASOTEC, the patient should be observed under medical supervision for at least two hours and until blood pressure has stabilized for at least an additional hour. (See WARNINGS and PRECAUTIONS, *Drug Interactions.*) If possible, the dose of any concomitant diuretic should be reduced which may diminish the likelihood of hypotension. The appearance of hypotension after the initial dose of VASOTEC does not preclude subsequent careful dose titration with the drug, following effective management of the hypotension.
Dosage Adjustment in Patients with Heart Failure and Renal Impairment or Hyponatremia
In patients with heart failure who have hyponatremia (serum sodium less than 130 mEq/L) or with serum creatinine greater than 1.6 mg/dL, therapy should be initiated at 2.5 mg daily under close medical supervision. (See DOSAGE AND ADMINISTRATION, *Heart Failure,* WARNINGS and PRECAUTIONS, *Drug Interactions.*) The dose may be increased to 2.5 mg b.i.d., then 5 mg b.i.d. and higher as needed, usually at intervals of four days or more if at the time of dosage adjustment there is not excessive hypotension or significant deterioration of renal function. The maximum daily dose is 40 mg.

HOW SUPPLIED

No. 3411—Tablets VASOTEC, 2.5 mg, are yellow, biconvex barrel shaped, scored, compressed tablets with code MSD 14 on one side and VASOTEC on the other. They are supplied as follows:
NDC 0006-0014-94 unit of use bottles of 90 (with desiccant)
NDC 0006-0014-68 bottles of 100 (with desiccant)
NDC 0006-0014-28 unit dose packages of 100
NDC 0006-0014-82 bottles of 1,000 (with desiccant)
NDC 0006-0014-87 bottles of 10,000 (with desiccant)
(6505-01-379-5607, 2.5 mg 10,000's).
Shown in Product Identification Guide, page 324
No. 3412—Tablets VASOTEC, 5 mg, are white, barrel shaped, scored, compressed tablets, with code MSD 712 on one side and VASOTEC on the other. They are supplied as follows:
NDC 0006-0712-94 unit of use bottles of 90 (with desiccant)
NDC 0006-0712-68 bottles of 100 (with desiccant)
(6505-01-236-8880, 5 mg 100's)
NDC 0006-0712-28 unit dose packages of 100
(6505-01-244-4811, 5 mg individually sealed 100's)
NDC 0006-0712-82 bottles of 1,000 (with desiccant)
NDC 0006-0712-87 bottles of 10,000 (with desiccant)
(6505-01-379-5575, 5 mg 10,000's).
Shown in Product Identification Guide, page 324
No. 3413—Tablets VASOTEC, 10 mg, are salmon, barrel shaped, compressed tablets, with code MSD 713 on one side and VASOTEC on the other. They are supplied as follows:
NDC 0006-0713-94 unit of use bottles of 90 (with desiccant)
NDC 0006-0713-68 bottles of 100 (with desiccant)
(6505-01-236-8881, 10 mg 100's)
NDC 0006-0713-28 unit dose packages of 100
(6505-01-314-6028, 10 mg individually sealed 100's)
NDC 0006-0713-82 bottles of 1,000 (with desiccant)
NDC 0006-0713-87 bottles of 10,000 (with desiccant)
(6505-01-378-8022, 10 mg 10,000's).
Shown in Product Identification Guide, page 324
No. 3414—Tablets VASOTEC, 20 mg, are peach, barrel shaped, compressed tablets, with code MSD 714 on one side and VASOTEC on the other. They are supplied as follows:
NDC 0006-0714-94 unit of use bottles of 90 (with desiccant)
NDC 0006-0714-68 bottles of 100 (with desiccant)
(6505-01-237-0545, 20 mg 100's)
NDC 0006-0714-28 unit dose packages of 100
(6505-01-318-0465, 20 mg individually sealed 100's)
NDC 0006-0714-82 bottles of 1,000 (with desiccant)
NDC 0006-0714-87 bottles of 10,000 (with desiccant)
(6505-01-378-8780, 20 mg 10,000's).
Shown in Product Identification Guide, page 324
Storage
Store below 30°C (86°F) and avoid transient temperatures above 50°C (122°F). Keep container tightly closed. Protect from moisture.
Dispense in a tight container, if product package is subdivided.

7825157 Issued June 1999

VIOXX® ℞
(rofecoxib tablets and oral suspension)

DESCRIPTION
VIOXX* (rofecoxib) is described chemically as 4-[4-(methylsulfonyl)phenyl]-3-phenyl-2(*5H*)-furanone. It has the following chemical structure:

Rofecoxib is a white to off-white to light yellow powder. It is sparingly soluble in acetone, slightly soluble in methanol and isopropyl acetate, very slightly soluble in ethanol, practically insoluble in octanol, and insoluble in water. The empirical formula for rofecoxib is $C_{17}H_{14}O_4S$, and the molecular weight is 314.36.
Each tablet of VIOXX for oral administration contains either 12.5 mg, 25 mg, or 50 mg of rofecoxib and the following inactive ingredients: croscarmellose sodium, hydroxypropyl cellulose, lactose, magnesium stearate, microcrystalline cellulose, and yellow ferric oxide. The 50 mg tablets also contain red ferric oxide.
Each 5 mL of the oral suspension contains either 12.5 or 25 mg of rofecoxib and the following inactive ingredients: citric acid (monohydrate), sodium citrate (dihydrate), sorbitol solution, strawberry flavor, xanthan gum, and purified water. Added as preservatives are sodium methylparaben 0.13% and sodium propylparaben 0.02%.

* Registered trademark of MERCK & CO., Inc., Whitehouse Station, New Jersey, USA

CLINICAL PHARMACOLOGY
Mechanism of Action
VIOXX is a nonsteroidal anti-inflammatory drug that exhibits anti-inflammatory, analgesic, and antipyretic activities in animal models. The mechanism of action of VIOXX is believed to be due to inhibition of prostaglandin synthesis, via inhibition of cyclooxygenase-2 (COX-2). At therapeutic concentrations in humans, VIOXX does not inhibit the cyclooxygenase-1 (COX-1) isoenzyme.
Pharmacokinetics
Absorption
The mean oral bioavailability of VIOXX at therapeutically recommended doses of 12.5, 25, and 50 mg is approximately 93%. The area under the curve (AUC) and peak plasma level (C_{max}) following a single 25-mg dose were 3286 (±843) ng•hr/mL and 207 (±111) ng/mL, respectively. Both C_{max} and AUC are roughly dose proportional across the clinical dose range. At doses greater than 50 mg, there is a less than proportional increase in C_{max} and AUC, which is thought to be due to the low solubility of the drug in aqueous media. The plasma concentration-time profile exhibited multiple peaks. The median time to maximal concentration (T_{max}), as assessed in nine pharmacokinetic studies, is 2 to 3 hours. Individual T_{max} values in these studies ranged between 2 to 9 hours. This may not reflect rate of absorption as T_{max} may occur as a secondary peak in some individuals. With multiple dosing, steady-state conditions are reached by Day 4. The AUC_{0-24hr} and C_{max} at steady state after multiple doses of 25 mg rofecoxib was 4018 (±1140) ng•hr/mL and 321 (±104) ng/mL, respectively. The accumulation factor based on geometric means was 1.67.
VIOXX Tablets 12.5 mg and 25 mg are bioequivalent to VIOXX Oral Suspension 12.5 mg/5 mL and 25 mg/5 mL, respectively.
Food and Antacid Effects
Food had no significant effect on either the peak plasma concentration (C_{max}) or extent of absorption (AUC) of rofecoxib when VIOXX tablets were taken with a high fat meal. The time to peak plasma concentration (T_{max}), however, was delayed by 1 to 2 hours. The food effect on the suspension formulation has not been studied. VIOXX tablets can be administered without regard to timing of meals.
There was a 13% and 8% decrease in AUC when VIOXX was administered with calcium carbonate antacid and magnesium/aluminum antacid to elderly subjects, respectively. There was an approximate 20% decrease in C_{max} of rofecoxib with either antacid.
Distribution
Rofecoxib is approximately 87% bound to human plasma protein over the range of concentrations of 0.05 to 25 mcg/mL. The apparent volume of distribution at steady state (V_{dss}) is approximately 91 L following a 12.5-dose and 86 L following a 25-mg dose.
Rofecoxib has been shown to cross the placenta in rats and rabbits, and the blood-brain barrier in rats.
Metabolism
Metabolism of rofecoxib is primarily mediated through reduction by cytosolic enzymes. The principal metabolic products are the *cis*-dihydro and *trans*-dihydro derivatives of rofecoxib, which account for nearly 56% of recovered radioactivity in the urine. An additional 8.8% of the dose was recovered as the glucuronide of the hydroxy derivative, a product of oxidative metabolism. The biotransformation of rofecoxib and this metabolite is reversible in humans to a limited extent (<5%). These metabolites are inactive as COX-1 or COX-2 inhibitors.
Cytochrome P450 plays a minor role in metabolism of rofecoxib. Inhibition of CYP 3A activity by administration of ketoconazole 400 mg daily does not affect rofecoxib disposition. However, induction of general hepatic metabolic activity by administration of the non-specific inducer rifampin 600 mg daily produces a 50% decrease in rofecoxib plasma concentrations. (Also see *Drug Interactions.*)
Excretion
Rofecoxib is eliminated predominantly by hepatic metabolism with little (<1%) unchanged drug recovered in the urine. Following a single radiolabeled dose of 125 mg, approximately 72% of the dose was excreted into the urine as metabolites and 14% in the feces as unchanged drug.
The plasma clearance after 12.5- and 25-mg doses was approximately 141 and 120 mL/min, respectively. Higher plasma clearance was observed at doses below the therapeutic range, suggesting the presence of a saturable route of metabolism (i.e., non-linear elimination). The effective half-life (based on steady-state levels) was approximately 17 hours.
Special Populations
Gender
The pharmacokinetics of rofecoxib are comparable in men and women.
Geriatric
After a single dose of 25 mg VIOXX in elderly subjects (over 65 years old) a 34% increase in AUC was observed as compared to the young subjects. Dosage adjustment in the elderly is not necessary; however, therapy with VIOXX should be initiated at the lowest recommended dose.
Pediatric
VIOXX has not been investigated in patients below 18 years of age.
Race
Meta-analysis of pharmacokinetic studies has suggested a slightly (10–15%) higher AUC of rofecoxib in Blacks and Hispanics as compared to Caucasians. No dosage adjustment is necessary on the basis of race.
Hepatic Insufficiency
A pharmacokinetic study in mild (Child-Pugh score ≤6) hepatic insufficiency patients indicated that rofecoxib AUC was similar between these patients and healthy subjects. Limited data in patients with moderate (Child-Pugh score 7–9) hepatic insufficiency suggest a trend towards higher AUC (about 69%) of rofecoxib in these patients, but more data are needed to evaluate pharmacokinetics in these patients. Patients with severe hepatic insufficiency have not been studied.
Renal Insufficiency
In a study (N=6) of patients with end stage renal disease undergoing dialysis, peak rofecoxib plasma levels and AUC declined 18% and 9%, respectively, when dialysis occurred four hours after dosing. When dialysis occurred 48 hours after dosing, the elimination profile of rofecoxib was unchanged. While renal insufficiency does not influence the pharmacokinetics of rofecoxib, use of VIOXX in advanced renal disease is not recommended at present because no safety information is available regarding the use of VIOXX in these patients.
Drug Interactions (Also see PRECAUTIONS, *Drug Interactions.*)
General
In human studies the potential for rofecoxib to inhibit or induce CYP 3A4 activity was investigated in studies using the intravenous erythromycin breath test and the oral midazolam test. No significant difference in erythromycin demethylation was observed with rofecoxib (75 mg daily) compared to placebo, indicating no induction of hepatic CYP 3A4. A 30% reduction of the AUC of midazolam was observed with rofecoxib (25 mg daily). This reduction is most likely due to increased first pass metabolism through induction of intestinal CYP 3A4 by rofecoxib. *In vitro* studies in rat hepatocytes also suggest that rofecoxib might be a mild inducer for CYP 3A4.
Drug interaction studies with rofecoxib have identified potentially significant interactions with rifampin, methotrexate and warfarin. Patients receiving these agents with VIOXX should be appropriately monitored. Drug interaction studies do not support the potential for clinically important interactions between antacids or cimetidine with rofecoxib. Similar to experience with other nonsteroidal anti-inflammatory drugs (NSAIDs), studies with rofecoxib suggest the potential for interaction with ACE inhibitors. The effects of rofecoxib on the pharmacokinetics and/or pharmacodynamics of ketoconazole, prednisone/prednisolone, oral contraceptives, and digoxin have been studied *in vivo* and clinically important interactions have not been found.

Continued on next page

Information on the Merck & Co., Inc. products listed on these pages is the full prescribing information from product circulars in use September 30, 2000. For information, please call 1-800-NSC MERCK [1-800-672-6372].

Vioxx—Cont.

CLINICAL STUDIES

Osteoarthritis (OA)

VIOXX has demonstrated significant reduction in joint pain compared to placebo. VIOXX was evaluated for the treatment of the signs and symptoms of OA of the knee and hip in placebo- and active-controlled clinical trials of 6 to 86 weeks duration that enrolled approximately 3900 patients. In patients with OA, treatment with VIOXX 12.5 mg and 25 mg once daily resulted in improvement in patient and physician global assessments and in the WOMAC (Western Ontario and McMaster Universities) osteoarthritis questionnaire, including pain, stiffness, and functional measures of OA. In six studies of pain accompanying OA flare, VIOXX provided a significant reduction in pain at the first determination (after one week in one study, after two weeks in the remaining five studies); this continued for the duration of the studies. In all OA clinical studies, once daily treatment in the morning with VIOXX 12.5 and 25 mg was associated with a significant reduction in joint stiffness upon first awakening in the morning. At doses of 12.5 and 25 mg, the effectiveness of VIOXX was shown to be comparable to ibuprofen 800 mg TID and diclofenac 50 mg TID for treatment of the signs and symptoms of OA. The ibuprofen studies were 6-week studies; the diclofenac studies were 12-month studies in which patients could receive additional arthritis medication during the last 6 months.

Analgesia, including Dysmenorrhea

In acute analgesic models of post-operative dental pain, post-orthopedic surgical pain, and primary dysmenorrhea, VIOXX relieved pain that was rated by patients as moderate to severe. The analgesic effect (including onset of action) of a single 50-mg dose of VIOXX was generally similar to 550 mg of naproxen sodium or 400 mg of ibuprofen. In single-dose post-operative dental pain studies, the onset of analgesia with a single 50-mg dose of VIOXX occurred within 45 minutes. In a multiple-dose study of post-orthopedic surgical pain in which patients received VIOXX or placebo for up to 5 days, 50 mg of VIOXX once daily was effective in reducing pain. In this study, patients on VIOXX consumed a significantly smaller amount of additional analgesic medication than patients treated with placebo (1.5 versus 2.5 doses per day of additional analgesic medication for VIOXX and placebo, respectively).

Special Studies

Upper Endoscopy in Patients with Osteoarthritis

Two identical (U.S. and Multinational) endoscopy studies in a total of 1516 patients were conducted to compare the percentage of patients who developed endoscopically detectable gastroduodenal ulcers with VIOXX 25 mg daily or 50 mg daily, ibuprofen 2400 mg daily, or placebo. Entry criteria for these studies permitted enrollment of patients with active *Helicobacter pylori* infection, baseline gastroduodenal erosions, prior history of an upper gastrointestinal perforation, ulcer, or bleed (PUB), and/or age ≥65 years. However, patients receiving aspirin (including low-dose aspirin for cardiovascular prophylaxis) were not enrolled in these studies. Patients who were 50 years of age and older with osteoarthritis and who had no ulcers at baseline were evaluated by endoscopy after weeks 6, 12, and 24 of treatment. The placebo-treatment group was discontinued at week 16 by design.

Treatment with VIOXX 25 mg daily or 50 mg daily was associated with a significantly lower percentage of patients with endoscopic gastroduodenal ulcers than treatment with ibuprofen 2400 mg daily. However, the studies cannot rule out at least some increase in the rate of endoscopic gastroduodenal ulcers when comparing VIOXX to placebo. See Figures 1 and 2 and the accompanying tables for the results of these studies.

Figure 1

COMPARISON TO IBUPROFEN

Life-Table Cumulative Incidence Rate of Gastroduodenal Ulcers ≥ 3mm (Intention-to-Treat)**

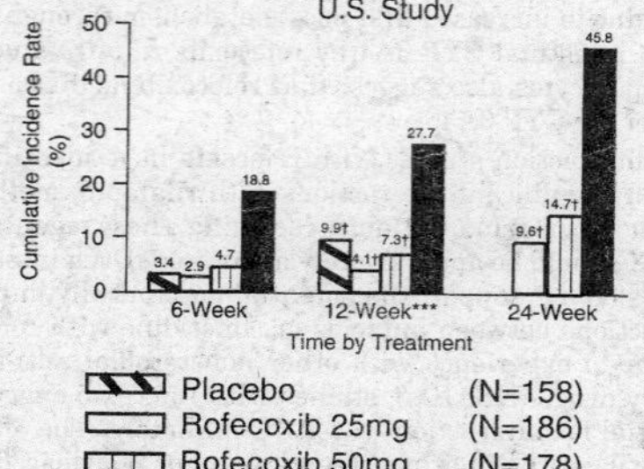

† p < 0.001 versus ibuprofen 2400 mg

** Results of analyses using a ≥ 5mm gastroduodenal ulcer endpoint were consistent.

*** The primary endpoint was the cumulative incidence of gastroduodenal ulcer at 12 weeks.

[See table 1 above]
[See figure 2 at top of next column]
[See table 2 above]

The correlation between findings of endoscopic studies, and the relative incidence of clinically serious upper GI events

TABLE 1
Endoscopic Gastroduodenal Ulcers at 12 weeks
U.S. Study

Treatment Group	Number of Patients with Ulcer/ Total Number of Patients	Cumulative Incidence Rate*	Ratio of Rates vs. Placebo	95% Cl on Ratio of Rates
Placebo	11/158	9.9%	—	—
VIOXX 25 mg	7/186	4.1%	0.41	(0.16, 1.05)
VIOXX 50 mg	12/178	7.3%	0.74	(0.33, 1.64)
Ibuprofen	42/167	27.7%	2.79	(1.47, 5.30)

*by life table analysis

TABLE 2
Endoscopic Gastroduodenal Ulcers at 12 weeks
Multinational Study

Treatment Group	Number of Patients with Ulcer/ Total Number of Patients	Cumulative Incidence Rate*	Ratio of Rates vs. Placebo	95% Cl on Ratio of Rates
Placebo	5/182	5.1%	—	—
VIOXX 25 mg	9/187	5.3%	1.04	(0.36, 3.01)
VIOXX 50 mg	15/182	8.8%	1.73	(0.65, 4.61)
Ibuprofen	49/187	29.2%	5.72	(2.36, 13.89)

*by life table analysis

Figure 2

COMPARISON TO IBUPROFEN

Life-Table Cumulative Incidence Rate of Gastroduodenal Ulcers ≥ 3mm (Intention-to-Treat)**

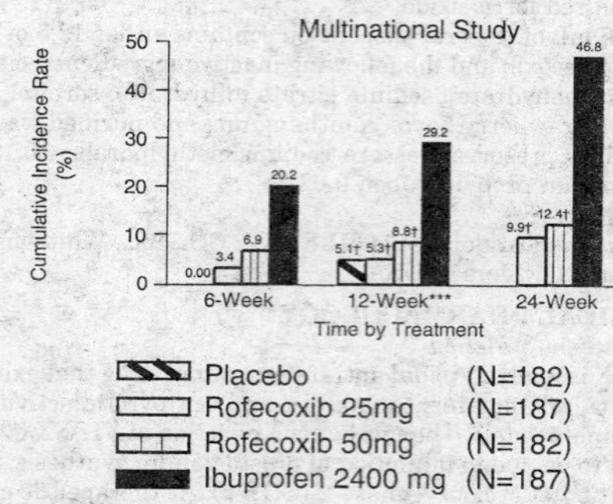

† p < 0.001 versus ibuprofen 2400 mg

** Results of analyses using a ≥ 5mm gastroduodenal ulcer endpoint were consistent.

*** The primary endpoint was the cumulative incidence of gastroduodenal ulcer at 12 weeks.

that may be observed with different products, has not been fully established. Serious clinically significant upper GI bleeding has been observed in patients receiving VIOXX in controlled trials, albeit infrequently (see WARNINGS, *Gastrointestinal (GI) Effects—Risk of GI Ulceration, Bleeding, and Perforation*). Prospective, long-term studies required to compare the incidence of serious, clinically significant upper GI adverse events in patients taking VIOXX versus comparator NSAID products have not been performed.

Assessment of Fecal Occult Blood Loss in Healthy Subjects

Occult fecal blood loss associated with VIOXX 25 mg daily, VIOXX 50 mg daily, ibuprofen 2400 mg per day, and placebo was evaluated in a study utilizing ^{51}Cr-tagged red blood cells in 67 healthy males. After 4 weeks of treatment with VIOXX 25 mg daily or VIOXX 50 mg daily, the increase in the amount of fecal blood loss was not statistically significant compared with placebo-treated subjects. In contrast, ibuprofen 2400 mg per day produced a statistically significant increase in fecal blood loss as compared with placebo-treated subjects and VIOXX-treated subjects. The clinical relevance of this finding is unknown.

Platelets

Multiple doses of VIOXX 12.5, 25, and up to 375 mg administered daily up to 12 days had no effect on bleeding time relative to placebo. Similarly, bleeding time was not altered in a single dose study with 500 or 1000 mg of VIOXX. There was no inhibition of *ex vivo* arachidonic acid- or collagen-induced platelet aggregation with 12.5, 25, and 50 mg of VIOXX.

INDICATIONS AND USAGE

VIOXX is indicated:

For relief of the signs and symptoms of osteoarthritis.

For the management of acute pain in adults (see CLINICAL STUDIES).

For the treatment of primary dysmenorrhea.

CONTRAINDICATIONS

VIOXX is contraindicated in patients with known hypersensitivity to rofecoxib or any other component of VIOXX.

VIOXX should not be given to patients who have experienced asthma, urticaria, or allergic-type reactions after taking aspirin or other NSAIDs. Severe, rarely fatal, anaphylactic-like reactions to NSAIDs have been reported in such patients (see WARNINGS, *Anaphylactoid Reactions*, and PRECAUTIONS, *Preexisting Asthma*).

WARNINGS

Gastrointestinal (GI) Effects—Risk of GI Ulceration, Bleeding, and Perforation

Serious gastrointestinal toxicity such as bleeding, ulceration, and perforation of the stomach, small intestine or large intestine, can occur at any time, with or without warning symptoms, in patients treated with nonsteroidal anti-inflammatory drugs (NSAIDs). Minor upper gastrointestinal problems, such as dyspepsia, are common and may also occur at any time during NSAID therapy. Therefore, physicians and patients should remain alert for ulceration and bleeding, even in the absence of previous GI tract symptoms. Patients should be informed about the signs and/or symptoms of serious GI toxicity and the steps to take if they occur. The utility of periodic laboratory monitoring has not been demonstrated, nor has it been adequately assessed. Only one in five patients who develop a serious upper GI adverse event on NSAID therapy is symptomatic. It has been demonstrated that upper GI ulcers, gross bleeding or perforation, caused by NSAIDs, appear to occur in approximately 1% of patients treated for 3–6 months, and in about 2–4% of patients treated for one year. These trends continue thus, increasing the likelihood of developing a serious GI event at some time during the course of therapy. However, even short-term therapy is not without risk.

It is unclear, at the present time, how the above rates apply to VIOXX (see CLINICAL STUDIES, *Special Studies, Upper Endoscopy in Patients with Osteoarthritis*). Among 3357 patients who received VIOXX in controlled clinical trials of 6-weeks to one-year duration (most were enrolled in six-month or longer studies) at a daily dose of 12.5 mg to 50 mg, a total of 4 patients experienced a serious upper GI event, using protocol-derived criteria. Two patients experienced an upper GI bleed within three months (at day 62 and 87, respectively) (0.06%). One additional patient experienced an obstruction within six months (Day 130) and the remaining patient developed an upper GI bleed within 12 months (Day 322) (0.12%). Approximately 23% of these 3357 patients were in studies that required them to be free of ulcers at study entry. It is unclear if this study population is representative of the general population. Prospective, long-term studies required to compare the incidence of serious, clinically significant upper GI adverse events in patients taking VIOXX vs comparator NSAID products have not been performed.

NSAIDs should be prescribed with extreme caution in patients with a prior history of ulcer disease or gastrointestinal bleeding. Most spontaneous reports of fatal GI events are in elderly or debilitated patients and therefore special care should be taken in treating this population. **To minimize the potential risk for an adverse GI event, the lowest effective dose should be used for the shortest possible duration.** For high risk patients, alternate therapies that do not involve NSAIDs should be considered.

Studies have shown that patients with a *prior history of peptic ulcer disease and/or gastrointestinal bleeding* and who use NSAIDs, have a greater than 10-fold higher risk for developing a GI bleed than patients with neither of these risk factors. In addition to a past history of ulcer disease, pharmacoepidemiological studies have identified several other co-therapies or co-morbid conditions that may increase the risk for GI bleeding such as: treatment with oral corticosteroids, treatment with anticoagulants, longer duration of NSAID therapy, smoking, alcoholism, older age, and poor general health status.

Anaphylactoid Reactions

As with NSAIDs in general, anaphylactoid reactions have occurred in patients without known prior exposure to VIOXX. In post-marketing experience, rare cases of anaphylactoid reactions and angioedema have been reported in patients receiving VIOXX. VIOXX should not be given to patients with the aspirin triad. This symptom complex typically occurs in asthmatic patients who experience rhinitis with or without nasal polyps, or who exhibit severe, potentially fatal bronchospasm after taking aspirin or other NSAIDs (see CONTRAINDICATIONS and PRECAUTIONS, *Preexisting Asthma*). Emergency help should be sought in cases where an anaphylactoid reaction occurs.

Advanced Renal Disease

No safety information is available regarding the use of VIOXX in patients with advanced kidney disease. Therefore, treatment with VIOXX is not recommended in these patients. If VIOXX therapy must be initiated, close monitoring of the patient's kidney function is advisable (see PRECAUTIONS, *Renal Effects*).

Pregnancy

In late pregnancy VIOXX should be avoided because it may cause premature closure of the ductus arteriosus.

PRECAUTIONS

General

VIOXX cannot be expected to substitute for corticosteroids or to treat corticosteroid insufficiency. Abrupt discontinuation of corticosteroids may lead to exacerbation of corticosteroid-responsive illness. Patients on prolonged corticosteroid therapy should have their therapy tapered slowly if a decision is made to discontinue corticosteroids.

The pharmacological activity of VIOXX in reducing inflammation, and possibly fever, may diminish the utility of these diagnostic signs in detecting infectious complications of presumed noninfectious, painful conditions.

Hepatic Effects

Borderline elevations of one or more liver tests may occur in up to 15% of patients taking NSAIDs, and notable elevations of ALT or AST (approximately three or more times the upper limit of normal) have been reported in approximately 1% of patients in clinical trials with NSAIDs. These laboratory abnormalities may progress, may remain unchanged, or may be transient with continuing therapy. Rare cases of severe hepatic reactions, including jaundice and fatal fulminant hepatitis, liver necrosis and hepatic failure (some with fatal outcome) have been reported with NSAIDs. In controlled clinical trials of VIOXX, the incidence of borderline elevations of liver tests at doses of 12.5 and 25 mg daily was comparable to the incidence observed with ibuprofen and lower than that observed with diclofenac. In placebo-controlled trials, approximately 0.5% of patients taking rofecoxib (12.5 or 25 mg QD) and 0.1% of patients taking placebo had notable elevations of ALT or AST.

A patient with symptoms and/or signs suggesting liver dysfunction, or in whom an abnormal liver test has occurred, should be monitored carefully for evidence of the development of a more severe hepatic reaction while on therapy with VIOXX. Use of VIOXX is not recommended in patients with moderate or severe hepatic insufficiency (see *Pharmacokinetics, Special Populations*). If clinical signs and symptoms consistent with liver disease develop, or if systemic manifestations occur (e.g., eosinophilia, rash, etc.), VIOXX should be discontinued.

Renal Effects

Long-term administration of NSAIDs has resulted in renal papillary necrosis and other renal injury. Renal toxicity has also been seen in patients in whom renal prostaglandins have a compensatory role in the maintenance of renal perfusion. In these patients, administration of a nonsteroidal anti-inflammatory drug may cause a dose-dependent reduction in prostaglandin formation and, secondarily, in renal blood flow, which may precipitate overt renal decompensation. Patients at greatest risk of this reaction are those with impaired renal function, heart failure, liver dysfunction, those taking diuretics and ACE inhibitors, and the elderly. Discontinuation of NSAID therapy is usually followed by recovery to the pretreatment state. Clinical trials with VIOXX at daily doses of 12.5 and 25 mg have shown renal effects (e.g., hypertension, edema) similar to those observed with comparator NSAIDs; these occur with an increased frequency with chronic use of VIOXX at doses above the 12.5 to 25 mg range. (See ADVERSE REACTIONS.)

Caution should be used when initiating treatment with VIOXX in patients with considerable dehydration. It is advisable to rehydrate patients first and then start therapy with VIOXX. Caution is also recommended in patients with pre-existing kidney disease (see WARNINGS, *Advanced Renal Disease*).

Hematological Effects

Anemia is sometimes seen in patients receiving VIOXX. In placebo-controlled trials, there were no significant differences observed between VIOXX and placebo in clinical reports of anemia. Patients on long-term treatment with VIOXX should have their hemoglobin or hematocrit checked if they exhibit any signs or symptoms of anemia or blood loss. VIOXX does not generally affect platelet counts, prothrombin time (PT), or partial thromboplastin time (PTT), and does not inhibit platelet aggregation at indicated dosages (see CLINICAL STUDIES, *Special Studies, Platelets*).

Fluid Retention and Edema

Fluid retention and edema have been observed in some patients taking VIOXX (see ADVERSE REACTIONS). VIOXX should be used with caution, and should be introduced at the lowest recommended dose in patients with fluid retention, hypertension, or heart failure.

Preexisting Asthma

Patients with asthma may have aspirin-sensitive asthma. The use of aspirin in patients with aspirin-sensitive asthma has been associated with severe bronchospasm which can be fatal. Since cross reactivity, including bronchospasm, between aspirin and other nonsteroidal anti-inflammatory drugs has been reported in such aspirin-sensitive patients, VIOXX should not be administered to patients with this form of aspirin sensitivity and should be used with caution in patients with preexisting asthma.

Information for Patients

VIOXX can cause discomfort and, rarely, more serious side effects, such as gastrointestinal bleeding, which may result in hospitalization and even fatal outcomes. Although serious GI tract ulcerations and bleeding can occur without warning symptoms, patients should be alert for the signs and symptoms of ulcerations and bleeding, and should ask for medical advice when observing any indicative signs or symptoms. Patients should be apprised of the importance of this follow-up (see WARNINGS, *Gastrointestinal (GI) Effects—Risk of GI Ulceration, Bleeding and Perforation*).

Patients should promptly report signs or symptoms of gastrointestinal ulceration or bleeding, skin rash, unexplained weight gain, or edema to their physicians.

Patients should be informed of the warning signs and symptoms of hepatotoxicity (e.g., nausea, fatigue, lethargy, pruritus, jaundice, right upper quadrant tenderness, and "flu-like" symptoms). If these occur, patients should be instructed to stop therapy and seek immediate medical therapy.

Patients should also be instructed to seek immediate emergency help in the case of an anaphylactoid reaction (see WARNINGS).

In late pregnancy VIOXX should be avoided because it may cause premature closure of the ductus arteriosus.

Laboratory Tests

Because serious GI tract ulcerations and bleeding can occur without warning symptoms, physicians should monitor for signs or symptoms of GI bleeding.

Drug Interactions

ACE inhibitors: Reports suggest that NSAIDs may diminish the antihypertensive effect of Angiotensin Converting Enzyme (ACE) inhibitors. In patients with mild to moderate hypertension, administration of 25 mg daily of VIOXX with the ACE inhibitor benazepril, 10 to 40 mg for 4 weeks, was associated with an average increase in mean arterial pressure of about 3 mm Hg compared to ACE inhibitor alone. This interaction should be given consideration in patients taking VIOXX concomitantly with ACE inhibitors.

Aspirin: Concomitant administration of low-dose aspirin with VIOXX may result in an increased rate of GI ulceration or other complications, compared to use of VIOXX alone. At steady state, VIOXX 50 mg once daily had no effect on the anti-platelet activity of low-dose (81 mg once daily) aspirin, as assessed by *ex vivo* platelet aggregation and serum TXB_2 generation in clotting blood. VIOXX is not a substitute for aspirin for cardiovascular prophylaxis.

Cimetidine: Co-administration with high doses of cimetidine [800 mg twice daily] increased the C_{max} of rofecoxib by 21%, the $AUC_{0-120hr}$ by 23% and the $t_{1/2}$ by 15%. These small changes are not clinically significant and no dose adjustment is necessary.

Digoxin: Rofecoxib 75 mg once daily for 11 days does not alter the plasma concentration profile or renal elimination of digoxin after a single 0.5 mg oral dose.

Furosemide: Clinical studies, as well as post-marketing observations, have shown that NSAIDs can reduce the natriuretic effect of furosemide and thiazides in some patients. This response has been attributed to inhibition of renal prostaglandin synthesis.

Ketoconazole: Ketoconazole 400 mg daily did not have any clinically important effect on the pharmacokinetics of rofecoxib.

Lithium: NSAIDs have produced an elevation of plasma lithium levels and a reduction in renal lithium clearance. Thus, when VIOXX and lithium are administered concurrently, subjects should be observed carefully for signs of lithium toxicity.

Methotrexate: VIOXX 75 mg administered once daily for 10 days increased plasma concentrations by 23% as measured by AUC_{0-24hr} in patients receiving methotrexate 7.5 to 15 mg/week for rheumatoid arthritis. An equivalent magnitude of reduction in methotrexate renal clearance was observed. At 24 hours postdose, a similar proportion of patients treated with methotrexate alone (94%) and subsequently treated with methotrexate co-administered with 75 mg of rofecoxib (88%) had methotrexate plasma concentrations below the measurable limit (5 ng/mL). The effects of the recommended doses for osteoarthritis (12.5 and 25 mg) of VIOXX on plasma methotrexate levels are unknown. Standard monitoring of methotrexate-related toxicity should be continued if VIOXX and methotrexate are administered concomitantly.

Oral Contraceptives: Rofecoxib did not have any clinically important effect on the pharmacokinetics of ethinyl estradiol and norethindrone.

Prednisone/prednisolone: Rofecoxib did not have any clinically important effect on the pharmacokinetics of prednisolone or prednisone.

Rifampin: Co-administration of VIOXX with rifampin 600 mg daily, a potent inducer of hepatic metabolism, produced an approximate 50% decrease in rofecoxib plasma concentrations. Therefore, a starting daily dose of 25 mg of VIOXX should be considered for the treatment of osteoarthritis when VIOXX is co-administered with potent inducers of hepatic metabolism.

Warfarin: Anticoagulant activity should be monitored, particularly in the first few days after initiating or changing VIOXX therapy in patients receiving warfarin or similar agents, since these patients are at an increased risk of bleeding complications. In single and multiple dose studies in healthy subjects receiving both warfarin and rofecoxib, prothrombin time (measured as INR) was increased by approximately 8% to 11%. In post-marketing experience, bleeding events have been reported, predominantly in the elderly, in association with increases in prothrombin time in patients receiving VIOXX concurrently with warfarin.

Carcinogenesis, Mutagenesis, Impairment of Fertility

Rofecoxib was not carcinogenic in mice given oral doses up to 30 mg/kg (male) and 60 mg/kg (female) (approximately 5- and 2-fold the human exposure at 25 and 50 mg daily based on AUC_{0-24}) and in male and female rats given oral doses up to 8 mg/kg (approximately 6- and 2-fold the human exposure at 25 and 50 mg daily based on AUC_{0-24}) for two years. Rofecoxib was not mutagenic in an Ames test or in a V-79 mammalian cell mutagenesis assay, nor clastogenic in a chromosome aberration assay in Chinese hamster ovary (CHO) cells, in an *in vitro* and an *in vivo* alkaline elution assay, or in an *in vivo* chromosomal aberration test in mouse bone marrow.

Rofecoxib did not impair male fertility in rats at oral doses up to 100 mg/kg (approximately 20- and 7-fold human exposure at 25 and 50 mg daily based on the AUC_{0-24}) and rofecoxib had no effect on fertility in female rats at doses up to 30 mg/kg (approximately 19- and 7-fold human exposure at 25 and 50 mg daily based on AUC_{0-24}).

Pregnancy

Teratogenic effects: Pregnancy Category C.

Rofecoxib was not teratogenic in rats at doses up to 50 mg/kg/day (approximately 28- and 10-fold human exposure at 25 and 50 mg daily based on AUC_{0-24}). There was a slight, non-statistically significant increase in the overall incidence of vertebral malformations only in the rabbit at doses of 50 mg/kg/day (approximately 1- or <1-fold human exposure at 25 and 50 mg daily based on AUC_{0-24}). There are no studies in pregnant women. VIOXX should be used during pregnancy only if the potential benefit justifies the potential risk to the fetus.

Nonteratogenic effects: Rofecoxib produced peri-implantation and post-implantation losses and reduced embryo/fetal survival in rats and rabbits at oral doses ≥10 and ≥75 mg/kg/day, respectively (approximately 9- and 3-fold [rats] and 2- and <1-fold [rabbits] human exposure based on the AUC_{0-24} at 25 and 50 mg daily). These changes are expected with inhibition of prostaglandin synthesis and are not the result of permanent alteration of female reproductive function. There was an increase in the incidence of postnatal pup mortality in rats at ≥5 mg/kg/day (approximately 5- and 2-fold human exposure at 25 and 50 mg daily based on AUC_{0-24}). In studies in pregnant rats administered single doses of rofecoxib, there was a treatment-related decrease in the diameter of the ductus arteriosus at all doses used (3–300 mg/kg: 3 mg/kg is approximately 2- and <1-fold human exposure at 25 or 50 mg daily based on AUC_{0-24}). As with other drugs known to inhibit prostaglandin synthesis, use of VIOXX during the third trimester of pregnancy should be avoided.

Labor and delivery

Rofecoxib produced no evidence of significantly delayed labor or parturition in females at doses 15 mg/kg in rats (approximately 10- and 3-fold human exposure as measured by the AUC_{0-24} at 25 and 50 mg). The effects of VIOXX on labor and delivery in pregnant women are unknown.

Merck & Co., Inc. maintains a registry to monitor the pregnancy outcomes of women exposed to VIOXX while pregnant. Healthcare providers are encouraged to report any prenatal exposure to VIOXX by calling the Pregnancy Registry at (800) 986-8999.

Nursing mothers

Rofecoxib is excreted in the milk of lactating rats at concentrations similar to those in plasma. There was an increase in pup mortality and a decrease in pup body weight following exposure of pups to milk from dams administered VIOXX during lactation. The dose tested represents an approximate 18- and 6-fold human exposure at 25 and 50 mg based on AUC_{0-24}. It is not known whether this drug is excreted in human milk. Because many drugs are excreted in human milk and because of the potential for serious adverse reactions in nursing infants from VIOXX, a decision should be made whether to discontinue nursing or to discontinue the drug, taking into account the importance of the drug to the mother.

Pediatric Use

Safety and effectiveness in pediatric patients below the age of 18 years have not been evaluated.

Geriatric Use

Of the patients who received VIOXX in osteoarthritis clinical trials, 1455 were 65 years of age or older (this included 460 who were 75 years or older). No substantial differences in safety and effectiveness were observed between these subjects and younger subjects. Greater sensitivity of some older individuals cannot be ruled out. Dosage adjustment in the elderly is not necessary; however, therapy with VIOXX should be initiated at the lowest recommended dose.

In one of these studies (a six-week, double-blind, randomized clinical trial), VIOXX 12.5 or 25 mg once daily was ad-

Continued on next page

Information on the Merck & Co., Inc. products listed on these pages is the full prescribing information from product circulars in use September 30, 2000. For information, please call 1-800-NSC MERCK [1-800-672-6372].

Vioxx—Cont.

ministered to 174 osteoarthritis patients ≥80 years of age. The safety profile in this elderly population was similar to that of younger patients treated with VIOXX.

ADVERSE REACTIONS

Osteoarthritis

Approximately 3600 patients with osteoarthritis were treated with VIOXX; approximately 1400 patients received VIOXX for 6 months or longer and approximately 800 patients for one year or longer. The following table of adverse experiences lists all adverse events, regardless of causality, occurring in at least 2% of patients receiving VIOXX in nine controlled studies of 6-week to 6-month duration conducted in patients with OA at the therapeutically recommended doses (12.5 and 25 mg), which included a placebo and/or positive control group.

[See table below]

The general safety profile of VIOXX 50 mg QD in OA clinical trials of up to 6 months (476 patients) was similar to that of VIOXX at the recommended OA doses of 12.5 and 25 mg QD, except for a higher incidence of gastrointestinal symptoms (abdominal pain, epigastric pain, heartburn, nausea and vomiting), lower extremity edema (6.3%) and hypertension (8.2%).

In the OA studies, the following spontaneous adverse events occurred in >0.1% to 1.9% of patients treated with VIOXX regardless of causality:

Body as a Whole: abdominal distension, abdominal tenderness, abscess, chest pain, chills, contusion, cyst, diaphragmatic hernia, fever, fluid retention, flushing, fungal infection, infection, laceration, pain, pelvic pain, peripheral edema, postoperative pain, syncope, trauma, upper extremity edema, viral syndrome.

Cardiovascular System: angina pectoris, atrial fibrillation, bradycardia, hematoma, irregular heart beat, palpitation, premature ventricular contraction, tachycardia, venous insufficiency.

Digestive System: acid reflux, aphthous stomatitis, constipation, dental caries, dental pain, digestive gas symptoms, dry mouth, duodenal disorder, dysgeusia, esophagitis, flatulence, gastric disorder, gastritis, gastroenteritis, hematochezia, hemorrhoids, infectious gastroenteritis, oral infection, oral lesion, oral ulcer, vomiting.

Eyes, Ears, Nose, and Throat: allergic rhinitis, blurred vision, cerumen impaction, conjunctivitis, dry throat, epistaxis, laryngitis, nasal congestion, nasal secretion, ophthalmic injection, otic pain, otitis, otitis media, pharyngitis, tinnitus, tonsillitis.

Immune System: allergy, hypersensitivity, insect bite reaction.

Metabolism and Nutrition: appetite change, hypercholesterolemia, weight gain.

Musculoskeletal System: ankle sprain, arm pain, arthralgia, back strain, bursitis, cartilage trauma, joint swelling, muscular cramp, muscular disorder, muscular weakness, musculoskeletal pain, musculoskeletal stiffness, myalgia, osteoarthritis, tendinitis, traumatic arthropathy, wrist fracture.

Nervous System: hypesthesia, insomnia, median nerve neuropathy, migraine, muscular spasm, paresthesia, sciatica, somnolence, vertigo.

Psychiatric: anxiety, depression, mental acuity decreased.

Respiratory System: asthma, cough, dyspnea, pneumonia, pulmonary congestion, respiratory infection.

Skin and Skin Appendages: abrasion, alopecia, atopic dermatitis, basal cell carcinoma, blister, cellulitis, contact dermatitis, herpes simplex, herpes zoster, nail unit disorder, perspiration, pruritus, rash, skin erythema, urticaria, xerosis.

Urogenital System: breast mass, cystitis, dysuria, menopausal symptoms, menstrual disorder, nocturia, urinary retention, vaginitis.

The following serious adverse events have been reported rarely (estimated <0.1%) in patients taking VIOXX, regardless of causality. Cases reported only in the post-marketing experience are indicated in italics.

Cardiovascular: cerebrovascular accident, congestive heart failure, deep venous thrombosis, myocardial infarction, pulmonary embolism, transient ischemic attack, unstable angina.

Gastrointestinal: cholecystitis, colitis, colonic malignant neoplasm, *duodenal perforation,* duodenal ulcer, *esophageal ulcer, gastric perforation, gastric ulcer,* gastrointestinal bleeding, intestinal obstruction, pancreatitis.

Hemic and lymphatic: lymphoma.

Immune System: anaphylactoid reaction, angioedema.

Nervous System: aseptic meningitis.

Psychiatric: hallucinations.

Urogenital System: acute renal failure, breast malignant neoplasm, *interstitial nephritis,* prostatic malignant neoplasm, urolithiasis, *worsening chronic renal failure.*

In 1-year controlled clinical trials and in extension studies for up to 86 weeks (approximately 800 patients treated with VIOXX for one year or longer), the adverse experience profile was qualitatively similar to that observed in studies of shorter duration.

Analgesia, including primary dysmenorrhea

Approximately one thousand patients were treated with VIOXX in analgesia studies. All patients in post-dental surgery pain studies received only a single dose of study medication. Patients in primary dysmenorrhea studies may have taken up to 3 daily doses of VIOXX, and those in the post-orthopedic surgery pain study were prescribed 5 daily doses of VIOXX.

The adverse experience profile in the analgesia studies was generally similar to those reported in the osteoarthritis studies. The following additional adverse experience, which occurred at an incidence of at least 2% of patients treated with VIOXX, was observed in the post-dental pain surgery studies: post-dental extraction alveolitis (dry socket).

In 110 patients treated with VIOXX (average age approximately 65 years) in the post-orthopedic surgery pain study, the most commonly reported adverse experiences were constipation, fever, and nausea.

OVERDOSAGE

No overdoses of VIOXX were reported during clinical trials. Administration of single doses of VIOXX 1000 mg to 6 healthy volunteers and multiple doses of 250 mg/day for 14 days to 75 healthy volunteers did not result in serious toxicity.

In the event of overdose, it is reasonable to employ the usual supportive measures, e.g., remove unabsorbed material from the gastrointestinal tract, employ clinical monitoring, and institute supportive therapy, if required.

Rofecoxib is not removed by hemodialysis; it is not known whether rofecoxib is removed by peritoneal dialysis.

Clinical Adverse Experiences occurring in ≥2.0% of Patients Treated with VIOXX

	Placebo	VIOXX 12.5 or 25 mg daily	Ibuprofen 2400 mg daily	Diclofenac 150 mg daily
	(N = 783)	(N = 2829)	(N = 847)	(N = 498)
Body As A Whole / Site Unspecified				
Abdominal Pain	4.1	3.4	4.6	5.8
Asthenia/Fatigue	1.0	2.2	2.0	2.6
Dizziness	2.2	3.0	2.7	3.4
Influenza-Like Disease	3.1	2.9	1.5	3.2
Lower Extremity Edema	1.1	3.7	3.8	3.4
Upper Respiratory Infection	7.8	8.5	5.8	8.2
Cardiovascular System				
Hypertension	1.3	3.5	3.0	1.6
Digestive System				
Diarrhea	6.8	6.5	7.1	10.6
Dyspepsia	2.7	3.5	4.7	4.0
Epigastric Discomfort	2.8	3.8	9.2	5.4
Heartburn	3.6	4.2	5.2	4.6
Nausea	2.9	5.2	7.1	7.4
Eyes, Ears, Nose, And Throat				
Sinusitis	2.0	2.7	1.8	2.4
Musculoskeletal System				
Back Pain	1.9	2.5	1.4	2.8
Nervous System				
Headache	7.5	4.7	6.1	8.0
Respiratory System				
Bronchitis	0.8	2.0	1.4	3.2
Urogenital System				
Urinary Tract Infection	2.7	2.8	2.5	3.6

DOSAGE AND ADMINISTRATION

VIOXX is administered orally. The lowest dose of VIOXX should be sought for each patient.

Osteoarthritis

The recommended starting dose of VIOXX is 12.5 mg once daily. Some patients may receive additional benefit by increasing the dose to 25 mg once daily. The maximum recommended daily dose is 25 mg.

Management of Acute Pain and Treatment of Primary Dysmenorrhea

The recommended initial dose of VIOXX is 50 mg once daily. Subsequent doses should be 50 mg once daily as needed. Use of VIOXX for more than 5 days in management of pain has not been studied (see CLINICAL STUDIES, *Analgesia, including dysmenorrhea*).

VIOXX tablets may be taken with or without food.

Oral Suspension

VIOXX Oral Suspension 12.5 mg/5 mL or 25 mg/5 mL may be substituted for VIOXX Tablets 12.5 or 25 mg, respectively, in any of the above indications. Shake before using.

HOW SUPPLIED

No. 3810—Tablets VIOXX, 12.5 mg, are cream/off-white, round, shallow cup tablets engraved MRK 74 on one side and VIOXX on the other. They are supplied as follows:

NDC 0006-0074-31 unit of use bottles of 30
NDC 0006-0074-28 unit dose packages of 100
NDC 0006-0074-68 bottles of 100
NDC 0006-0074-82 bottles of 1000
NDC 0006-0074-80 bottles of 8000.

Shown in Product Identification Guide, page 324

No. 3811—Tablets VIOXX, 25 mg, are yellow, round, tablets engraved MRK 110 on one side and VIOXX on the other. They are supplied as follows:

NDC 0006-0110-31 unit of use bottles of 30
NDC 0006-0110-28 unit dose packages of 100
NDC 0006-0110-68 bottles of 100
NDC 0006-0110-82 bottles of 1000
NDC 0006-0110-80 bottles of 8000.

Shown in Product Identification Guide, page 324

No. 3818—Tablets VIOXX, 50 mg, are orange, round, tablets engraved MRK 114 on one side and VIOXX on the other. They are supplied as follows:

NDC 0006-0114-31 unit of use bottles of 30
NDC 0006-0114-28 unit dose packages of 100
NDC 0006-0114-68 bottles of 100
NDC 0006-0114-74 bottles of 500
NDC 0006-0114-81 bottles of 4000.

Shown in Product Identification Guide, page 324

No. 3784—Oral Suspension VIOXX, 12.5 mg/5 mL is an opaque, white to faint yellow suspension with a strawberry flavor that is easily resuspended upon shaking.

NDC 0006-3784-64 unit of use bottles containing 150 mL (12.5 mg/5 mL).

No. 3785—Oral Suspension VIOXX, 25 mg/5 mL, is an opaque, white to faint yellow suspension with a strawberry flavor that is easily resuspended upon shaking.

NDC 0006-3785-64 unit of use bottles containing 150 mL (25 mg/5 mL).

Storage

VIOXX Tablets:

Store at 25°C (77°F), excursions permitted to 15–30°C (59–86°F). [See USP Controlled Room Temperature.]

VIOXX Oral Suspension:

Store at 25°C (77°F), excursions permitted to 15–30°C (59–86°F). [See USP Controlled Room Temperature.]

Rx only

9183805 Issued May 2000

Patient information about
VIOXX® (rofecoxib tablets and oral suspension)
VIOXX® (pronounced "Vi-ox")
for Osteoarthritis and Pain
Generic name: rofecoxib ("ro-fa-COX-ib")

You should read this information before you start taking VIOXX*. Also, read the leaflet each time you refill your prescription, in case any information has changed. This leaflet provides only a summary of certain information about VIOXX. Your doctor or pharmacist can give you an additional leaflet that is written for health professionals that contains more complete information. This leaflet does not take the place of careful discussions with your doctor. You and your doctor should discuss VIOXX when you start taking your medicine and at regular checkups.

*Registered trademark of MERCK & CO., Inc.

What is VIOXX?

VIOXX is a nonsteroidal anti-inflammatory drug (NSAID) that is used to reduce pain and inflammation (swelling and soreness). VIOXX is available as a tablet or a liquid that you take by mouth.

VIOXX is a medicine for:

- relief of osteoarthritis (the arthritis caused by age-related "wear and tear" on bones and joints)
- management of acute pain in adults (like the short-term pain you can get after a dental or surgical operation)
- treatment of menstrual pain (pain during women's monthly periods).

Who should not take VIOXX?
Do not take VIOXX if you:
- have had an allergic reaction such as asthma attacks, hives, or swelling of the throat and face to aspirin or other NSAIDs (for example, ibuprofen and naproxen).
- have had an allergic reaction to refecoxib, which is the active ingredient of VIOXX, or to any of its inactive ingredients. (See Inactive Ingredients at the end of this leaflet.)

What should I tell my doctor before and during treatment with VIOXX?
Tell your doctor if you are:
- pregnant or plan to become pregnant. VIOXX should not be used in late pregnancy because it may harm the fetus.
- breast-feeding or plan to breast-feed. It is not known whether VIOXX is passed through to human breast milk and what its effects could be on a nursing child.

Tell your doctor if you have:
- kidney disease
- liver disease
- heart failure
- high blood pressure
- had an allergic reaction to aspirin or other NSAIDs
- had a serious stomach problem in the past.

Tell your doctor about:
- any other medical problems or allergies you have now or have had,
- all medicines that you are taking or plan to take, even those you can get without a prescription.

Tell your doctor if you develop:
- ulcer or bleeding symptoms (for instance, stomach burning or black stools, which are signs of possible stomach bleeding).
- unexplained weight gain or swelling of the feet and/or legs.
- skin rash or allergic reactions. If you have a severe allergic reaction, get medical help right away.

How should I take VIOXX?
VIOXX should be taken once a day. Your doctor will decide what dose of VIOXX you should take and how long you should take it. You may take VIOXX with or without food.

Can I take VIOXX with other medicines?
Tell your doctor about all of the other medicines you are taking or plan to take while you are on VIOXX, even other medicines that you can get without a prescription. Your doctor may want to check that your medicines are working properly together if you are taking other medicines such as:
- methotrexate (a medicine used to suppress the immune system)
- warfarin (a blood thinner)
- rifampin (an antibiotic)
- ACE inhibitors (medicines used for high blood pressure and heart failure)

What are the possible side effects of VIOXX?
Serious but rare side effects that have been reported in patients taking VIOXX and/or related medicines have included:
- Serious stomach problems, such as stomach and intestinal bleeding, can occur with or without warning symptoms. These problems, if severe, could lead to hospitalization or death. Although this happens rarely, you should watch for signs that you may have this serious side effect and tell your doctor right away.
- Serious allergic reactions including swelling of the face, lips, tongue, and/or throat which may cause difficulty breathing or swallowing occur rarely but may require treatment right away.
- Serious kidney problems occur rarely, including acute kidney failure and worsening of chronic kidney failure.
- Severe liver problems occur rarely in patients taking NSAIDs. Tell your doctor if you develop symptoms of liver problems. These include nausea, tiredness, itching, tenderness in the upper right abdomen, and flu-like symptoms.

In addition, the following side effects have been reported: hallucinations, unusual headache with stiff neck (aseptic meningitis).
More common, but less serious side effects reported with VIOXX have included the following:
Upper and/or lower respiratory infection and/or inflammation
Headache
Dizziness
Diarrhea
Nausea and/or vomiting
Heartburn, stomach pain and upset
Swelling of the legs and/or feet
High blood pressure
Back pain
Tiredness
Urinary tract infection.
These side effects were reported in at least 2% of osteoarthritis patients receiving daily doses of VIOXX 12.5 mg to 25 mg in clinical studies.
The side effects described above do not include all of the side effects reported with VIOXX. Do not rely on this leaflet alone for information about side effects. Your doctor or pharmacist can discuss with you a more complete list of side effects. Any time you have a medical problem you think may be related to VIOXX, talk to your doctor.

What else can I do to help manage my osteoarthritis pain?
Talk to your doctor about:
- Exercise
- Controlling your weight
- Hot and cold treatments
- Using support devices.

What else should I know about VIOXX?
This leaflet provides a summary of certain information about VIOXX. If you have any questions or concerns about VIOXX, osteoarthritis or pain, talk to your health professional. Your pharmacist can give you an additional leaflet that is written for health professionals.
Do not share VIOXX with anyone else; it was prescribed only for you. It should be taken only for the condition for which it was prescribed.
Keep VIOXX and all medicines out of the reach of children:
Inactive Ingredients:
Oral suspension: citric acid (monohydrate), sodium citrate (dihydrate), sorbitol solution, strawberry flavor, xanthan gum, sodium methylparaben, sodium propylparaben.
Tablets: croscarmellose sodium, hydroxypropyl cellulose, lactose, magnesium stearate, microcrystalline cellulose, and yellow ferric oxide.
9183901 Issued March 2000

VIVACTIL® Tablets ℞
(Protriptyline HCl)

DESCRIPTION

Protriptyline HCl is *N*- methyl-5*H* -dibenzo[*a,d*]-cycloheptene-5-propanamine hydrochloride. Its empirical formula is $C_{19}H_{21}N \cdot HCl$ and its structural formula is:

H $CH_2CH_2CH_2NHCH_3 \cdot HCl$

Protriptyline HCl, a dibenzocycloheptene derivative, has a molecular weight of 299.84. It is a white to yellowish powder that is freely soluble in water and soluble in dilute HCl.
VIVACTIL* (Protriptyline HCl) is supplied as 10 mg film coated tablets. Inactive ingredients are calcium phosphate, cellulose, guar gum, hydroxypropyl cellulose, hydroxypropyl methylcellulose, lactose, magnesium stearate, starch, talc, titanium dioxide, FD&C Yellow 6, and D&C Yellow 10.

*Registered trademark of MERCK & CO., INC.

ACTIONS

VIVACTIL is an antidepressant agent. The mechanism of its antidepressant action in man is not known. It is not a monoamine oxidase inhibitor, and it does not act primarily by stimulation of the central nervous system.
VIVACTIL has been found in some studies to have a more rapid onset of action than imipramine or amitriptyline. The initial clinical effect may occur within one week. Sedative and tranquilizing properties are lacking. The rate of excretion is slow.

INDICATIONS

VIVACTIL is indicated for the treatment of symptoms of mental depression in patients who are under close medical supervision. Its activating properties make it particularly suitable for withdrawn and anergic patients.

CONTRAINDICATIONS

VIVACTIL is contraindicated in patients who have shown prior hypersensitivity to it.
It should not be given concomitantly with a monoamine oxidase inhibiting compound. Hyperpyretic crises, severe convulsions, and deaths have occurred in patients receiving tricyclic antidepressant and monoamine oxidase inhibiting drugs simultaneously. When it is desired to substitute VIVACTIL for a monoamine oxidase inhibitor, a minimum of 14 days should be allowed to elapse after the latter is discontinued. VIVACTIL should then be initiated cautiously with gradual increase in dosage until optimum response is achieved.
VIVACTIL is contraindicated in patients taking cisapride because of the possibility of adverse cardiac interactions including prolongation of the QT interval, cardiac arrhythmias and conduction system disturbances.
This drug should not be used during the acute recovery phase following myocardial infarction.

WARNINGS

VIVACTIL may block the antihypertensive effect of guanethidine or similarly acting compounds.
VIVACTIL should be used with caution in patients with a history of seizures, and, because of its autonomic activity, in patients with a tendency to urinary retention, or increased intraocular tension.
Tachycardia and postural hypotension may occur more frequently with VIVACTIL than with other antidepressant drugs. VIVACTIL should be used with caution in elderly patients and patients with cardiovascular disorders; such patients should be observed closely because of the tendency of the drug to produce tachycardia, hypotension, arrhythmias, and prolongation of the conduction time. Myocardial infarction and stroke have occurred with drugs of this class.
On rare occasions, hyperthyroid patients or those receiving thyroid medication may develop arrhythmias when this drug is given.
In patients who may use alcohol excessively, it should be borne in mind that the potentiation may increase the danger inherent in any suicide attempt or overdosage.
Pediatric Usage
The safety and effectiveness of VIVACTIL in pediatric patients have not been established.
Usage in Pregnancy
Safe use in pregnancy and lactation has not been established; therefore, use in pregnant women, nursing mothers or women who may become pregnant requires that possible benefits be weighed against possible hazards to mother and child.
In mice, rats, and rabbits, doses about ten times greater than the recommended human doses had no apparent adverse effects on reproduction.

PRECAUTIONS

General
When protriptyline HCl is used to treat the depressive component of schizophrenia, psychotic symptoms may be aggravated. Likewise, in manic-depressive psychosis, depressed patients may experience a shift toward the manic phase if they are treated with an antidepressant drug. Paranoid delusions, with or without hostility, may be exaggerated. In any of these circumstances, it may be advisable to reduce the dose of VIVACTIL or to use a major tranquilizing drug concurrently.
Symptoms, such as anxiety or agitation, may be aggravated in overactive or agitated patients.
The possibility of suicide in depressed patients remains during treatment and until significant remission occurs. This type of patient should not have access to large quantities of the drug.
Concurrent administration of VIVACTIL and electroshock therapy may increase the hazards of therapy. Such treatment should be limited to patients for whom it is essential.
Discontinue the drug several days before elective surgery, if possible.
Both elevation and lowering of blood sugar levels have been reported.
Information for Patients
While on therapy with VIVACTIL, patients should be advised as to the possible impairment of mental and/or physical abilities required for performance of hazardous tasks, such as operating machinery or driving a motor vehicle.
Drug Interactions
When VIVACTIL is given with anticholinergic agents or sympathomimetic drugs, including epinephrine combined with local anesthetics, close supervision and careful adjustment of dosages are required.
Hyperpyrexia has been reported when tricyclic antidepressants are administered with anticholinergic agents or with neuroleptic drugs, particularly during hot weather.
Cimetidine is reported to reduce hepatic metabolism of certain tricyclic antidepressants, thereby delaying elimination and increasing steady-state concentrations of these drugs. Clinically significant effects have been reported with the tricyclic antidepressants when used concomitantly with cimetidine. Increases in plasma levels of tricyclic antidepressants, and in the frequency and severity of side effects, particularly anticholinergic, have been reported when cimetidine was added to the drug regimen. Discontinuation of cimetidine in well-controlled patients receiving tricyclic antidepressants and cimetidine may decrease the plasma levels and efficacy of the antidepressants.
Tricyclic antidepressants may enhance the seizure risk in patients taking ULTRAM** (tramadol hydrochloride).
VIVACTIL may enhance the response to alcohol and the effects of barbiturates and other CNS depressants.

**Trademark of Ortho-McNeil Pharmaceutical

Drugs Metabolized by Cytochrome P450 2D6: The biochemical activity of the drug-metabolizing isozyme, cytochrome P450 2D6 (debrisoquine hydroxylase), is reduced in a subset of the Caucasian population (about 7–10% of Caucasians are so called "poor metabolizers"); reliable estimates of the prevalence of reduced P450 2D6 isozyme activity among Asian, African, and other populations are not yet available. Poor metabolizers have higher than expected plasma concentrations of tricyclic antidepressants (TCAs) when given usual doses. Depending on the fraction of drug metabolized by P450 2D6, the increase in plasma concentration may be small or quite large (8-fold increase in plasma AUC of the TCA).
In addition, certain drugs inhibit the activity of this isozyme and make normal metabolizers resemble poor metabolizers. An individual who is stable on a given dose of TCA may become abruptly toxic when given one of these inhibiting drugs as concomitant therapy. The drugs that inhibit cyto-

Continued on next page

Information on the Merck & Co., Inc. products listed on these pages is the full prescribing information from product circulars in use September 30, 2000. For information, please call 1-800-NSC MERCK [1-800-672-6372].

Vivactil—Cont.

chrome P450 2D6 include some that are not metabolized by the enzyme (quinidine; cimetidine) and many that are substrates for P450 2D6 (many other antidepressants, phenothiazines, and the Type 1C antiarrhythmics, propafenone and flecainide). While all the selective serotonin reuptake inhibitors (SSRIs), e.g., fluoxetine, sertraline, and paroxetine, inhibit P450 2D6, they may vary in the extent of inhibition. The extent to which SSRI-TCA interactions may pose clinical problems will depend on the degree of inhibition and the pharmacokinetics of the SSRI involved. Nevertheless, caution is indicated in the coadministration of TCAs with any of the SSRIs, and also in switching from one class to the other. Of particular importance, sufficient time must elapse before initiating TCA treatment in a patient being withdrawn from fluoxetine, given the long half-life of the parent and active metabolite (at least 5 weeks may be necessary).
Concomitant use of tricyclic antidepressants with drugs that can inhibit cytochrome P450 2D6 may require lower doses than usually prescribed for either the tricyclic antidepressant or the other drug. Furthermore, whenever one of these other drugs is withdrawn from co-therapy, an increased dose of tricyclic antidepressant may be required. It is desirable to monitor TCA plasma levels whenever a TCA is going to be coadministered with another drug known to be an inhibitor of P450 2D6.

Pediatric Use

The safety and effectiveness of VIVACTIL in pediatric patients have not been established.

Geriatric Use

Clinical studies of VIVACTIL did not include sufficient numbers of subjects aged 65 and over to determine whether they respond differently from younger subjects. Other reported clinical experience has not identified differences in responses between the elderly and younger patients. In general, dose selection for an elderly patient should be cautious, usually starting at the low end of the dosing range, reflecting the greater frequency of decreased hepatic, renal, or cardiac function, and of concomitant disease or other drug therapy. (See WARNINGS, DOSAGE AND ADMINISTRATION, and ADVERSE REACTIONS.)

ADVERSE REACTIONS

Within each category the following adverse reactions are listed in order of decreasing severity. Included in the listing are a few adverse reactions which have not been reported with this specific drug. However, the pharmacological similarities among the tricyclic antidepressant drugs require that each of the reactions be considered when protriptyline is administered. VIVACTIL is more likely to aggravate agitation and anxiety and produce cardiovascular reactions such as tachycardia and hypotension.

Cardiovascular: Myocardial infarction; stroke; heart block; arrhythmias; hypotension, particularly orthostatic hypotension; hypertension; tachycardia; palpitation.

Psychiatric: Confusional states (especially in the elderly) with hallucinations, disorientation, delusions, anxiety, restlessness, agitation; hypomania; exacerbation of psychosis; insomnia, panic, and nightmares.

Neurological: Seizures; incoordination; ataxia; tremors; peripheral neuropathy; numbness, tingling, and paresthesias of extremities; extrapyramidal symptoms; drowsiness; dizziness; weakness and fatigue; headache; syndrome of inappropriate ADH (antidiuretic hormone) secretion; tinnitus; alteration in EEG patterns.

Anticholinergic: Paralytic ileus; hyperpyrexia; urinary retention, delayed micturition, dilatation of the urinary tract; constipation; blurred vision, disturbance of accommodation, increased intraocular pressure, mydriasis; dry mouth and rarely associated sublingual adenitis.

Allergic: Drug fever; petechiae, skin rash, urticaria, itching, photosensitization (avoid excessive exposure to sunlight); edema (general, or of face and tongue).

Hematologic: Agranulocytosis; bone marrow depression; leukopenia; thrombocytopenia; purpura; eosinophilia.

Gastrointestinal: Nausea and vomiting; anorexia; epigastric distress; diarrhea; peculiar taste; stomatitis; abdominal cramps; black tongue.

Endocrine: Impotence, increased or decreased libido; gynecomastia in the male; breast enlargement and galactorrhea in the female; testicular swelling; elevation or depression of blood sugar levels.

Other: Jaundice (simulating obstructive); altered liver function; parotid swelling; alopecia; flushing; weight gain or loss, urinary frequency, nocturia; perspiration.

Withdrawal Symptoms: Though not indicative of addiction, abrupt cessation of treatment after prolonged therapy may produce nausea, headache, and malaise.

DOSAGE AND ADMINISTRATION

Dosage should be initiated at a low level and increased gradually, noting carefully the clinical response and any evidence of intolerance.

Usual Adult Dosage—Fifteen to 40 mg a day divided into 3 or 4 doses. If necessary, dosage may be increased to 60 mg a day. Dosages above this amount are not recommended. Increases should be made in the morning dose.

Adolescent and Elderly Patients—In general, lower dosages are recommended for these patients. Five mg 3 times a day may be given initially, and increased gradually if necessary. In elderly patients, the cardiovascular system must be monitored closely if the daily dose exceeds 20 mg.

When satisfactory improvement has been reached, dosage should be reduced to the smallest amount that will maintain relief of symptoms.

Minor adverse reactions require reduction in dosage. Major adverse reactions or evidence of hypersensitivity require prompt discontinuation of the drug.

The safety and effectiveness of VIVACTIL in pediatric patients have not been established.

OVERDOSAGE

Deaths may occur from overdosage with this class of drugs. Multiple drug ingestion (including alcohol) is common in deliberate tricyclic antidepressant overdose. As management of overdose is complex and changing, it is recommended that the physician contact a poison control center for current information on treatment. Signs and symptoms of toxicity develop rapidly after tricyclic antidepressant overdose, therefore, hospital monitoring is required as soon as possible.

MANIFESTATIONS

Critical manifestations of overdosage include: cardiac dysrhythmias, severe hypotension, convulsions, and CNS depression, including coma. Changes in the electrocardiogram, particularly in QRS axis or width, are clinically significant indicators of tricyclic antidepressant toxicity.

Other signs of overdose may include: confusion, disturbed concentration, transient visual hallucinations, dilated pupils, agitation, hyperactive reflexes, stupor, drowsiness, muscle rigidity, vomiting, hypothermia, hyperpyrexia, or any of the symptoms listed under ADVERSE REACTIONS.

MANAGEMENT

General

Obtain an ECG and immediately initiate cardiac monitoring. Protect the patient's airway, establish an intravenous line and initiate gastric decontamination. A minimum of six hours of observation with cardiac monitoring and observation for signs of CNS or respiratory depression, hypotension, cardiac dysrhythmias and/or conduction blocks, and seizures is necessary. If signs of toxicity occur at any time during this period, extended monitoring is required. There are case reports of patients succumbing to fatal dysrhythmias late after overdose. These patients had clinical evidence of significant poisoning prior to death and most received inadequate gastrointestinal decontamination. Monitoring of plasma drug levels should not guide management of the patient.

Gastrointestinal Decontamination

All patients suspected of a tricyclic antidepressant overdose should receive gastrointestinal decontamination. This should include large volume gastric lavage followed by activated charcoal. If consciousness is impaired, the airway should be secured prior to lavage. Emesis is contraindicated.

Cardiovascular

A maximal limb-lead QRS duration of ≥0.10 seconds may be the best indication of the severity of the overdose. Intravenous sodium bicarbonate should be used to maintain the serum pH in the range of 7.45 to 7.55. If the pH response is inadequate, hyperventilation may also be used. Concomitant use of hyperventilation and sodium bicarbonate should be done with extreme caution, with frequent pH monitoring. A pH >7.60 or a pCO_2 <20 mmHg is undesirable. Dysrhythmias unresponsive to sodium bicarbonate therapy/hyperventilation may respond to lidocaine, bretylium or phenytoin. Type 1A and 1C antiarrhythmics are generally contraindicated (e.g., quinidine, disopyramide, and procainamide).

In rare instances, hemoperfusion may be beneficial in acute refractory cardiovascular instability in patients with acute toxicity. However, hemodialysis, peritoneal dialysis, exchange transfusions, and forced diuresis generally have been reported as ineffective in tricyclic antidepressant poisoning.

CNS

In patients with CNS depression, early intubation is advised because of the potential for abrupt deterioration. Seizures should be controlled with benzodiazepines or, if these are ineffective, other anticonvulsants (e.g., phenobarbital, phenytoin). Physostigmine is not recommended except to treat life-threatening symptoms that have been unresponsive to other therapies, and then only in close consultation with a poison control center.

PSYCHIATRIC FOLLOW-UP

Since overdosage is often deliberate, patients may attempt suicide by other means during the recovery phase. Psychiatric referral may be appropriate.

PEDIATRIC MANAGEMENT

The principles of management of child and adult overdosages are similar. It is strongly recommended that the physician contact the local poison control center for specific pediatric treatment.

HOW SUPPLIED

No. 3314—Tablets VIVACTIL, 10 mg, are yellow, oval, film coated tablets, coded MSD 47 on one side and VIVACTIL on the other. They are supplied as follows:

NDC 0006-0047-68 bottles of 100

Shown in Product Identification Guide, page 324

Storage

Store at 25°C (77°F); excursions permitted to 15-30°C (59-86°F) [see USP Controlled Room Temperature]. Keep container tightly closed.

METABOLISM

Metabolic studies indicate that protriptyline is well absorbed from the gastrointestinal tract and is rapidly sequestered in tissues. Relatively low plasma levels are found after administration, and only a small amount of unchanged drug is excreted in the urine of dogs and rabbits. Preliminary studies indicate that demethylation of the secondary amine moiety occurs to a significant extent, and that metabolic transformation probably takes place in the liver. It penetrates the brain rapidly in mice and rats, and moreover that which is present in the brain is almost all unchanged drug.

Studies on the disposition of radioactive protriptyline in human test subjects showed significant plasma levels within 2 hours, peaking at 8 to 12 hours, then declining gradually.

Urinary excretion studies in the same subjects showed significant amounts of radioactivity in 2 hours. The rate of excretion was slow. Cumulative urinary excretion during 16 days accounted for approximately 50% of the drug. The fecal route of excretion did not seem to be important.

7904026 Issued December 1999

ZOCOR® Tablets ℞
(Simvastatin)

DESCRIPTION

ZOCOR* (simvastatin) is a lipid-lowering agent that is derived synthetically from a fermentation product of *Aspergillus terreus*. After oral ingestion, simvastatin, which is an inactive lactone, is hydrolyzed to the corresponding β-hydroxyacid form. This is an inhibitor of 3-hydroxy-3-methylglutaryl-coenzyme A (HMG-CoA) reductase. This enzyme catalyzes the conversion of HMG-CoA to mevalonate, which is an early and rate-limiting step in the biosynthesis of cholesterol.

Simvastatin is butanoic acid, 2,2-dimethyl-,1,2,3,7,8,8a-hexahydro-3,7-dimethyl-8-[2-(tetrahydro-4-hydroxy-6-oxo-2*H*-pyran-2-yl)-ethyl]-1-naphthalenyl ester, [1*S*-[1α,3α,7β,8β(2*S**,4*S**),-8aβ]]. The empirical formula of simvastatin is $C_{25}H_{38}O_5$ and its molecular weight is 418.57. Its structural formula is:

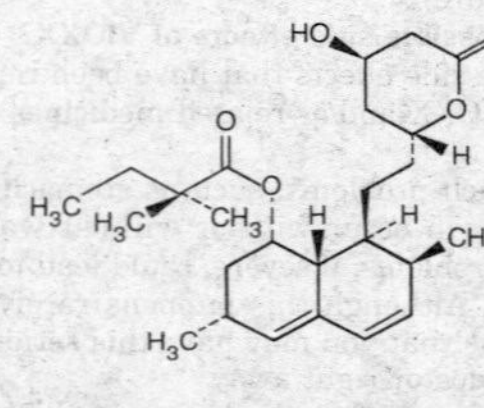

Simvastatin is a white to off-white, nonhygroscopic, crystalline powder that is practically insoluble in water, and freely soluble in chloroform, methanol and ethanol.

Tablets ZOCOR for oral administration contain either 5 mg, 10 mg, 20 mg, 40 mg or 80 mg of simvastatin and the following inactive ingredients: cellulose, hydroxypropyl cellulose, hydroxypropyl methylcellulose, iron oxides, lactose, magnesium stearate, starch, talc, titanium dioxide and other ingredients. Butylated hydroxyanisole is added as a preservative.

*Registered trademark of MERCK & CO., Inc.

CLINICAL PHARMACOLOGY

The involvement of low-density lipoprotein cholesterol (LDL-C) in atherogenesis has been well-documented in clinical and pathological studies, as well as in many animal experiments. Epidemiological studies have established that high LDL-C, low high-density lipoprotein cholesterol (HDL-C), and high plasma triglycerides (TG) are risk factors for coronary heart disease (CHD). Cholesterol-enriched TG-rich lipoproteins, including very-low-density lipoproteins (VLDL), intermediate-density lipoproteins (IDL), and remnants, can also promote atherosclerosis. Elevated plasma TG are frequently found in a triad with low HDL-C and small LDL particles, as well as in association with non-lipid metabolic risk factors for CHD. As such, total plasma TG has not consistently been shown to be an independent risk factor for CHD. Furthermore, the independent effect of raising HDL-C or lowering TG on the risk of coronary and cardiovascular morbidity and mortality has not been determined.

In the Scandinavian Simvastatin Survival Study (4S), the effect of improving lipoprotein levels with ZOCOR on total mortality was assessed in 4,444 patients with CHD and baseline total cholesterol (total-C) 212–309 mg/dL (5.5–8.0 mmol/L). The patients were followed for a median of 5.4 years. In this multicenter, randomized, double-blind, placebo-controlled study, ZOCOR significantly reduced the risk of mortality by 30% (11.5% vs 8.2%, placebo vs ZOCOR); of CHD mortality by 42% (8.5% vs 5.0%); and of having a hospital-verified non-fatal myocardial infarction by 37% (19.6%

vs 12.9%). Furthermore, ZOCOR significantly reduced the risk for undergoing myocardial revascularization procedures (coronary artery bypass grafting or percutaneous transluminal coronary angioplasty) by 37% (17.2% vs 11.4%) [see CLINICAL PHARMACOLOGY, *Clinical Studies*].

ZOCOR has been shown to reduce both normal and elevated LDL-C concentrations. LDL is formed from very-low-density lipoprotein (VLDL) and is catabolized predominantly by the high affinity LDL receptor. The mechanism of the LDL-lowering effect of ZOCOR may involve both reduction of VLDL cholesterol concentration, and induction of the LDL receptor, leading to reduced production and/or increased catabolism of LDL-C. Apolipoprotein B (Apo B) also falls substantially during treatment with ZOCOR. As each LDL particle contains one molecule of Apo B, and since in patients with predominant elevations in LDL-C (without accompanying elevation in VLDL) little Apo B is found in other lipoproteins, this strongly suggests that ZOCOR does not merely cause cholesterol to be lost from LDL, but also reduces the concentration of circulating LDL particles. In addition, ZOCOR reduces VLDL and TG and increases HDL-C. The effects of ZOCOR on Lp(a), fibrinogen, and certain other independent biochemical risk markers for CHD are unknown.

ZOCOR is a specific inhibitor of HMG-CoA reductase, the enzyme that catalyzes the conversion of HMG-CoA to mevalonate. The conversion of HMG-CoA to mevalonate is an early step in the biosynthetic pathway for cholesterol.

Pharmacokinetics

Simvastatin is a lactone that is readily hydrolyzed *in vivo* to the corresponding β-hydroxyacid, a potent inhibitor of HMG-CoA reductase. Inhibition of HMG-CoA reductase is the basis for an assay in pharmacokinetic studies of the β-hydroxyacid metabolites (active inhibitors) and, following base hydrolysis, active plus latent inhibitors (total inhibitors) in plasma following administration of simvastatin.

Following an oral dose of ^{14}C-labeled simvastatin in man, 13% of the dose was excreted in urine and 60% in feces. The latter represents absorbed drug equivalents excreted in bile, as well as any unabsorbed drug. Plasma concentrations of total radioactivity (simvastatin plus ^{14}C-metabolites) peaked at 4 hours and declined rapidly to about 10% of peak by 12 hours postdose. Absorption of simvastatin, estimated relative to an intravenous reference dose, in each of two animal species tested, averaged about 85% of an oral dose. In animal studies, after oral dosing, simvastatin achieved substantially higher concentrations in the liver than in non-target tissues. Simvastatin undergoes extensive first-pass extraction in the liver, its primary site of action, with subsequent excretion of drug equivalents in the bile. As a consequence of extensive hepatic extraction of simvastatin (estimated to be >60% in man), the availability of drug to the general circulation is low. In a single-dose study in nine healthy subjects, it was estimated that less than 5% of an oral dose of simvastatin reaches the general circulation as active inhibitors. Following administration of simvastatin tablets, the coefficient of variation, based on between-subject variability, was approximately 48% for the area under the concentration-time curve (AUC) for total inhibitory activity in the general circulation.

Both simvastatin and its β-hydroxyacid metabolite are highly bound (approximately 95%) to human plasma proteins. Animal studies have not been performed to determine whether simvastatin crosses the blood-brain and placental barriers. However, when radiolabeled simvastatin was administered to rats, simvastatin-derived radioactivity crossed the blood-brain barrier.

The major active metabolites of simvastatin present in human plasma are the β-hydroxyacid of simvastatin and its 6′-hydroxy, 6′-hydroxymethyl, and 6′-exomethylene derivatives. Peak plasma concentrations of both active and total inhibitors were attained within 1.3 to 2.4 hours postdose. While the recommended therapeutic dose range is 5 to 80 mg/day, there was no substantial deviation from linearity of AUC of inhibitors in the general circulation with an increase in dose to as high as 120 mg. Relative to the fasting state, the plasma profile of inhibitors was not affected when simvastatin was administered immediately before an American Heart Association recommended low-fat meal.

Kinetic studies with another reductase inhibitor, having a similar principal route of elimination, have suggested that for a given dose level higher systemic exposure may be achieved in patients with severe renal insufficiency (as measured by creatinine clearance).

Clinical Studies

Coronary Heart Disease

In 4S, the effect of therapy with ZOCOR on total mortality was assessed in 4,444 patients with CHD and baseline total cholesterol 212–309 mg/dL (5.5–8.0 mmol/L). In this multicenter, randomized, double blind, placebo-controlled study, patients were treated with standard care, including diet, and either ZOCOR 20–40 mg/day (n=2,221) or placebo (n=2,223) for a median duration of 5.4 years. After six weeks of treatment with ZOCOR the median (25th and 75th percentile) changes in LDL-C, TG, and HDL-C were −39% (−46, −39), −19% (−31, 0%), and 6% (−3, 17%). Over the course of the study, treatment with ZOCOR led to mean reductions in total-C, LDL-C and TG of 25%, 35%, and 10%, respectively, and a mean increase in HDL-C of 8%. ZOCOR significantly reduced the risk of mortality (Figure 1) by 30%, (p=0.0003, 182 deaths in the ZOCOR group vs 256 deaths in the placebo group). The risk of CHD mortality was significantly reduced by 42%, (p=0.00001, 111 vs 189 deaths).

Table 1
Mean Response in Patients with Primary Hypercholesterolemia and Combined (mixed) Hyperlipidemia
(Mean Percent Change from Baseline After 6 to 24 Weeks)

TREATMENT	N	TOTAL-C	LDL-C	HDL-C	TG*
Lower Dose Comparative Study (Mean % Change at Week 6)					
ZOCOR 5 mg q.p.m.	109	−19	−26	10	−12
ZOCOR 10 mg q.p.m.	110	−23	−30	12	−15
Scandinavian Simvastatin Survival Study (Mean % Change at Week 6)					
Placebo	2223	−1	−1	0	−2
ZOCOR 20 mg q.p.m.	2221	−28	−38	8	−19
Upper Dose Comparative Study (Mean % Change Averaged at Weeks 18 and 24)					
ZOCOR 40 mg q.p.m.	433	−31	−41	9	−18
ZOCOR 80 mg q.p.m.	664	−36	−47	8	−24
Multi-Center Combined Hyperlipidemia Study (Mean % Change at Week 6)					
Placebo	125	1	2	3	−4
ZOCOR 40 mg q.p.m.	123	−25	−29	13	−28
ZOCOR 80 mg q.p.m.	124	−31	−36	16	−33

* median percent change

There was no statistically significant difference between groups in non-cardiovascular mortality. ZOCOR also significantly decreased the risk of having major coronary events (CHD mortality plus hospital-verified and silent non-fatal myocardial infarction [MI]) (Figure 2) by 34%, (p<0.00001, 431 vs 622 patients with one or more events). The risk of having a hospital-verified non-fatal MI was reduced by 37%. ZOCOR significantly reduced the risk for undergoing myocardial revascularization procedures (coronary artery bypass grafting or percutaneous transluminal coronary angioplasty) by 37%, (p<0.00001, 252 vs 383 patients). Furthermore, ZOCOR significantly reduced the risk of fatal plus non-fatal cerebrovascular events (combined stroke and transient ischemic attacks) by 28% (p=0.033, 75 vs 102 patients). ZOCOR reduced the risk of major coronary events to a similar extent across the range of baseline total and LDL cholesterol levels. The risk of mortality was significantly decreased in patients ≥ 60 years of age by 27% and in patients < 60 years of age by 37%. Because there were only 53 female deaths, the effect of ZOCOR on mortality in women could not be adequately assessed. However, ZOCOR significantly lessened the risk of having major coronary events by 34% (60 vs 91 women with one or more event). The randomization was stratified by angina alone (21% of each treatment group) or a previous MI. Because there were only 57 deaths among the patients with angina alone at baseline, the effect of ZOCOR on mortality in this subgroup could not be adequately assessed. However, trends in reduced coronary mortality, major coronary events and revascularization procedures were consistent between this group and the total study cohort.

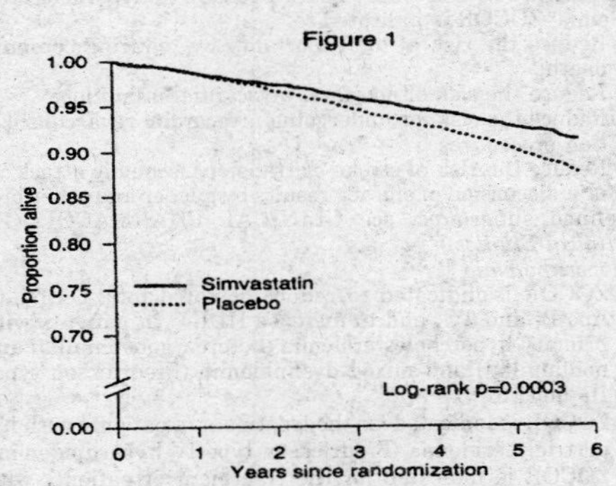

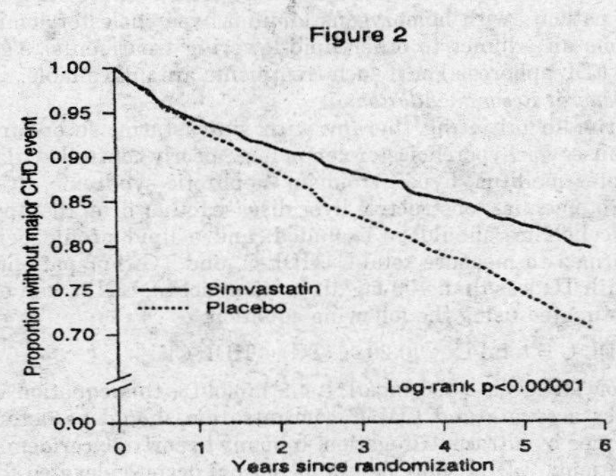

Angiographic Studies

In the Multicenter Anti-Atheroma Study, the effect of therapy with simvastatin on atherosclerosis was assessed by quantitative coronary angiography in hypercholesterolemic men and women with coronary heart disease. In this randomized, double-blind, controlled study, patients with a mean baseline total-C value of 245 mg/dL (6.4 mmol/L) and a mean baseline LDL-C value of 170 mg/dL (4.4 mmol/L) were treated with conventional measures and with simvastatin 20 mg/day or placebo. Angiograms were evaluated at baseline, two and four years. A total of 347 patients had a baseline angiogram and at least one follow-up angiogram. The co-primary endpoints of the study were mean change per-patient in minimum and mean lumen diameters, indicating focal and diffuse disease, respectively. Simvastatin significantly slowed the progression of lesions as measured in the final angiogram by both these parameters (mean changes in minimum lumen diameter: −0.04 mm with simvastatin vs −0.12 mm with placebo; mean changes in mean lumen diameter: −0.03 mm with simvastatin vs −0.08 mm with placebo), as well as by change from baseline in percent diameter stenosis (0.9% simvastatin vs 3.6% placebo). After four years, the groups also differed significantly in the proportions of patients categorized with disease progression (23% simvastatin vs 33% placebo) and disease regression (18% simvastatin vs 12% placebo). In addition, simvastatin significantly decreased the proportion of patients with new lesions (13% simvastatin vs 24% placebo) and with new total occlusions (5% vs 11%). The mean change per-patient in mean and minimum lumen diameters, calculated by comparing angiograms, in the subset of 274 patients who had matched angiographic projections at baseline, two and four years is presented below (Figures 3 and 4).

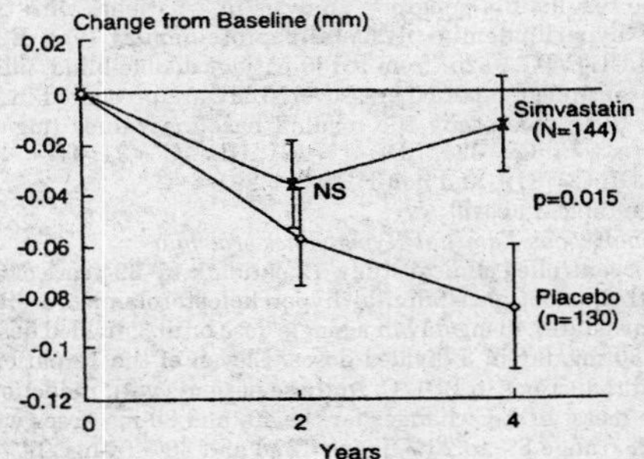

[See figure 4 at top of next column]

Primary Hypercholesterolemia (Fredrickson type IIa and IIb)

ZOCOR has been shown to be highly effective in reducing total-C and LDL-C in heterozygous familial and non-familial forms of hypercholesterolemia and in mixed hyperlipidemia. A marked response was seen within 2 weeks, and the maximum therapeutic response occurred within 4–6 weeks. The response was maintained during chronic therapy. Furthermore, improving lipoprotein levels with ZOCOR improved survival in patients with CHD and hypercholesterolemia treated with 20–40 mg/day for a median of 5.4 years. In a multicenter, double-blind, placebo-controlled, dose-response study in patients with familial or non-familial hypercholesterolemia, ZOCOR given as a single dose in the evening (the recommended dosing) was similarly effective as when given on a twice-daily basis. ZOCOR consistently

Continued on next page

Information on the Merck & Co., Inc. products listed on these pages is the full prescribing information from product circulars in use September 30, 2000. For information, please call 1-800-NSC MERCK [1-800-672-6372].

Zocor—Cont.

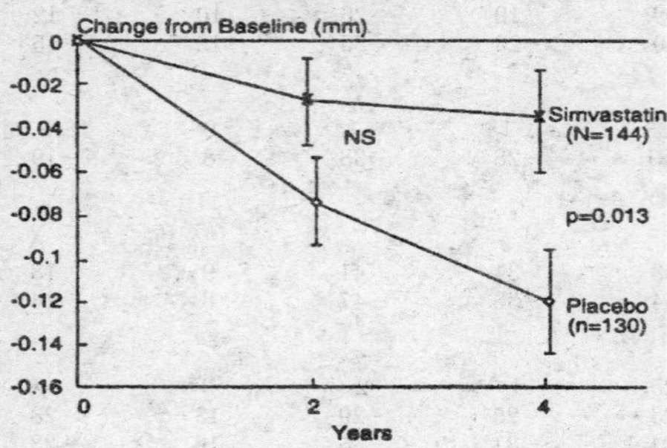

and significantly decreased total-C, LDL-C, total-C/HDL-C ratio, and LDL-C/HDL-C ratio. ZOCOR also decreased TG and increased HDL-C.

The results of studies depicting the mean response to simvastatin in patients with primary hypercholesterolemia and combined (mixed) hyperlipidemia are presented in TABLE 1.

[See table 1 at top of previous page]

In the Upper Dose Comparative Study, the mean reduction in LDL-C was 47% at the 80-mg dose. Of the 664 patients randomized to 80 mg, 475 patients with plasma TG ≤ 200 mg/dL had a median reduction in TG of 21%, while in 189 patients with TG > 200 mg/dL, the median reduction in TG was 36%. In these studies, patients with TG > 350 mg/dL were excluded.

In the Multi-Center Combined Hyperlipidemia Study, a randomized, 3-period crossover study, 130 patients with combined hyperlipidemia (LDL-C>130 mg/dL and TG: 300–700 mg/dL) were treated with placebo, ZOCOR 40, and 80 mg/day for 6 weeks. In a dose-dependent manner ZOCOR 40 and 80 mg/day, respectively, decreased mean LDL-C by 29 and 36% (placebo: +2%) and median TG levels by 28 and 33% (placebo: 4%), and increased mean HDL-C by 13 and 16% (placebo: 3%) and apolipoprotein A-1 by 8 and 11% (placebo: 4%).

Hypertriglyceridemia (Fredrickson type IV)

The results of a subgroup analysis in 74 patients with type IV hyperlipidemia from a 130-patient double-blind, placebo-controlled, 3-period crossover study are presented in Table 2. The median baseline values (mg/dL) for the patients in this study were: total-C = 254, LDL-C = 135, HDL-C = 36, TG = 404, VLDL-C = 83, and non-HDL-C = 215.

[See table 2 above]

Dysbetalipoproteinemia (Fredrickson type III)

The results of a subgroup analysis in 7 patients with type III hyperlipidemia (dysbetalipoproteinemia) (apo E2/2) (VLDL-C/TG>0.25) from a 130-patient double-blind, placebo-controlled, 3-period crossover study are presented in Table 3. In this study the median baseline values (mg/dL) were: total-C = 324, LDL-C = 121, HDL-C = 31, TG = 411, VLDL-C = 170, and non-HDL-C = 291.

[See table 3 above]

Homozygous Familial Hypercholesterolemia

In a controlled clinical study, 12 patients 15–39 years of age with homozygous familial hypercholesterolemia received simvastatin 40 mg/day in a single dose or in 3 divided doses, or 80 mg/day in 3 divided doses. Eleven of the 12 patients had reductions in LDL-C. In those patients with reductions, the mean LDL-C changes for the 40- and 80-mg doses were 14% (range 8% to 23%, mean 12%) and 30% (range 14% to 46%, median 29%), respectively. One patient had an increase of 15% in LDL-C. Another patient with absent LDL-C receptor function had an LDL-C reduction of 41% with the 80-mg dose.

Endocrine Function

In clinical studies, simvastatin did not impair adrenal reserve or significantly reduce basal plasma cortisol concentration. Small reductions from baseline in basal plasma testosterone in men were observed in clinical studies with simvastatin, an effect also observed with other inhibitors of HMG-CoA reductase and the bile acid sequestrant cholestyramine. There was no effect on plasma gonadotropin levels. In a placebo-controlled 12-week study there was no significant effect of simvastatin 80 mg on the plasma testosterone response to human chorionic gonadotropin (hCG). In another 24-week study, simvastatin 20–40 mg had no detectable effect on spermatogenesis. In 4S, in which 4,444 patients were randomized to simvastatin 20–40 mg/day or placebo for a median duration of 5.4 years, the incidence of male sexual adverse events in the two treatment groups was not significantly different. Because of these factors, the small changes in plasma testosterone are unlikely to be clinically significant. The effects, if any, on the pituitary-gonadal axis in pre-menopausal women are unknown.

INDICATIONS AND USAGE

Therapy with lipid-altering agents should be considered in those individuals at increased risk for atherosclerosis-related clinical events as a function of cholesterol level, the presence of coronary heart disease, or other risk factors. Lipid-altering agents should be used in addition to a diet restricted in saturated fat and cholesterol when the response to diet and other nonpharmacological measures alone has been inadequate (see National Cholesterol Education Program [NCEP] Treatment Guidelines, below).

Coronary Heart Disease

In patients with coronary heart disease and hypercholesterolemia, ZOCOR is indicated to:

- Reduce the risk of total mortality by reducing coronary death;
- Reduce the risk of non-fatal myocardial infarction;
- Reduce the risk for undergoing myocardial revascularization procedures.
- Reduce the risk of stroke or transient ischemic attack.

(For a discussion of efficacy results by gender and other predefined subgroups, see CLINICAL PHARMACOLOGY, *Clinical Studies*.)

Hyperlipidemia

- ZOCOR is indicated to reduce elevated total-C,LDL-C, Apo B, and TG, and to increase HDL-C in patients with primary hypercholesterolemia (heterozygous familial and nonfamilial) and mixed dyslipidemia (Fredrickson types IIa and IIb**).
- ZOCOR is indicated for the treatment of patients with hypertriglyceridemia (Fredrickson type IV hyperlipidemia).
- ZOCOR is indicated for the treatment of patients with primary dysbetalipoproteinemia (Fredrickson type III hyperlipidemia).
- ZOCOR is also indicated to reduce total-C and LDL-C in patients with homozygous familial hypercholesterolemia as an adjunct to other lipid-lowering treatments (e.g., LDL apheresis) or if such treatments are unavailable.

General Recommendations

Prior to initiating therapy with simvastatin, secondary causes for hypercholesterolemia (e.g., poorly controlled diabetes mellitus, hypothyroidism, nephrotic syndrome, dysproteinemias, obstructive liver disease, other drug therapy, alcoholism) should be excluded, and a lipid profile performed to measure total-C, HDL-C, and TG. For patients with TG less than 400 mg/dL (<4.5 mmol/L), LDL-C can be estimated using the following equation:

$$\text{LDL-C} = \text{total-C} - [0.20 \times (\text{TG}) + \text{HDL-C}]$$

For TG levels >400 mg/dL (>4.5 mmol/L), this equation is less accurate and LDL-C concentration should be determined by ultracentrifugation. In many hypertriglyceridemic patients, LDL-C may be low or normal despite elevated total-C. In such cases, ZOCOR is not indicated.

Lipid determinations should be performed at intervals of no less than four weeks and dosage adjusted according to the patient's response to therapy.

The NCEP Treatment Guidelines are summarized in Table 4:

[See table 4 above]

TABLE 2
Six-week, Lipid-lowering Effects of Simvastatin in Type IV Hyperlipidemia
Median Percent Change (25th and 75th percentile) from Baseline

TREATMENT	N	Total-C	LDL-C	HDL-C	TG	VLDL-C	Non-HDL-C
Placebo	74	+2 (−7,+7)	+1 (−8, +14)	+3 (−3, +10)	−9 (−25, +13)	−7 (−25, +11)	+1 (−9, +8)
ZOCOR 40 mg/day	74	−25 (−34, −19)	−28 (−40, −17)	+11 +5, +23)	−29 (−43, −16)	−37 (−54, −23)	−32 (−42, −23)
ZOCOR 80 mg/day	74	−32 (−38, −24)	−37 (−46, −26)	+15 +5, +23)	−34 (−45, −18)	−41 (−57, −28)	−38 (−49, −32)

TABLE 3
Six-week, Lipid-lowering Effects of Simvastatin in Type III Hyperlipidemia
Median Percent Change (min,max) from Baseline

TREATMENT	N	Total-C	LDL-C + IDL	HDL-C	TG	VLDL-C+IDL	Non-HDL-C
Placebo	7	−8 (−24,+34)	−8 (−27,+23)	−2 (−21,+16)	+4 (−22,+90)	−4 (−28,+78)	−8 (−26,−39)
ZOCOR 40 mg/day	7	−50 (−66,−39)	−50 (−60,−31)	+7 (−8,+23)	−41 (−74,−16)	−58 (−90,−37)	−57 (−72,−44)
ZOCOR 80 mg/day	7	−52 (−55,−41)	−51 (−57,−28)	+7 (−5,+29)	−38 (−58,+2)	−60 (−72,−39)	−59 (−61,−46)

Table 4
Summary of NCEP Treatment Guidelines
LDL-Cholesterol mg/dL (mmol/L)

Definite Atherosclerotic Disease†	Two or More Other Risk Factors††	Initiation Level	Goal
NO	NO	≥190 (≥4.9)	<160 (<4.1)
NO	YES	≥160 (≥4.1)	<130 (<3.4)
YES	YES OR NO	≥130††† (≥3.4)	≤100 (≤2.6)

† Coronary heart disease or peripheral vascular disease (including symptomatic carotid artery disease).

†† Other risk factors for coronary heart disease (CHD) include: age (males: ≥45 years; females: ≥55 years or premature menopause without estrogen replacement therapy); family history of premature CHD; current cigarette smoking; hypertension; confirmed HDL-C <35 mg/dL (<0.91 mmol/L); and diabetes mellitus. Subtract one risk factor if HDL-C is ≥60 mg/dL (≥1.6 mmol/L).

††† In CHD patients with LDL-C levels 100–129 mg/dL, the physician should exercise clinical judgment in deciding whether to initiate drug treatment.

At the time of hospitalization for an acute coronary event, consideration can be given to initiating drug therapy at discharge if the LDL-C is ≥ 130 mg/dL (see NCEP Guidelines, above).

Since the goal of treatment is to lower LDL-C, the NCEP recommends that LDL-C levels be used to initiate and assess treatment response. Only if LDL-C levels are not available, should the total-C be used to monitor therapy.

ZOCOR is indicated to reduce elevated LDL-C and TG levels in patients with Type IIb hyperlipidemia (where hypercholesterolemia is the major abnormality). However, it has not been studied in conditions where the major abnormality is elevation of chylomicrons (i.e., hyperlipidemia Fredrickson types I and IV).**

**Classification of Hyperlipoproteinemias

Type	Lipoproteins elevated	Lipid Elevations major	minor
I (rare)	chylomicrons	TG	↑→C
IIa	LDL	C	—
IIb	LDL, VLDL	C	TG
III (rare)	IDL	C/TG	—
IV	VLDL	TG	↑→C
V (rare)	chylomicrons, VLDL	TG	↑→C

C = cholesterol, TG = triglycerides,
LDL = low-density lipoprotein,
VLDL = very-low-density lipoprotein,
IDL = intermediate-density lipoprotein.

CONTRAINDICATIONS

Hypersensitivity to any component of this medication.

Active liver disease or unexplained persistent elevations of serum transaminases (see WARNINGS).

Pregnancy and lactation. Atherosclerosis is a chronic process and the discontinuation of lipid-lowering drugs during pregnancy should have little impact on the outcome of long-term therapy of primary hypercholesterolemia. Moreover, cholesterol and other products of the cholesterol biosynthesis pathway are essential components for fetal development, including synthesis of steroids and cell membranes. Because of the ability of inhibitors of HMG-CoA reductase such as ZOCOR to decrease the synthesis of cholesterol and possibly other products of the cholesterol biosynthesis pathway, ZOCOR is contraindicated during pregnancy and in nursing mothers. **ZOCOR should be administered to women of childbearing age only when such patients are highly unlikely to conceive.** If the patient becomes pregnant while taking this drug, ZOCOR should be discontinued immediately and the patient should be apprised of the potential hazard to the fetus (see PRECAUTIONS, *Pregnancy*).

WARNINGS

Skeletal Muscle
Simvastatin and other inhibitors of HMG-CoA reductase occasionally cause myopathy, which is manifested as muscle pain or weakness associated with grossly elevated creatine kinase (CK) (> 10X the upper limit of normal [ULN]). **Rhabdomyolysis, with or without acute renal failure secondary to myoglobinuria, has been reported rarely.** In 4S, there was one case of myopathy among 1,399 patients taking simvastatin 20 mg and no cases among 822 patients taking 40 mg/day for a median duration of 5.4 years. In two 6-month controlled clinical studies, there was one case of myopathy among 436 patients taking 40 mg and 5 cases among 669 patients taking 80 mg. The risk of myopathy is increased by concomitant therapy with certain drugs, some of which were excluded by the designs of these studies (see below).
Myopathy caused by drug interactions.
The incidence and severity of myopathy are increased by concomitant administration of HMG-CoA reductase inhibitors with drugs that can cause myopathy when given alone, such as gemfibrozil and other fibrates, and lipid-lowering doses (≥ 1 g/day) of niacin (nicotinic acid).
In addition, the risk of myopathy appears to be increased by high levels of HMG-CoA reductase inhibitory activity in plasma. Simvastatin is metabolized by the cytochrome P450 isoform 3A4. Certain drugs that are potent inhibitors of this metabolic pathway can raise the plasma levels of simvastatin and may increase the risk of myopathy. These include cyclosporine, itraconazole, ketoconazole and other antifungal azoles, the macrolide antibiotics erythromycin and clarithromycin, HIV protease inhibitors, and the antidepressant nefazodone.
Reducing the risk of myopathy.
1. General measures. Patients starting therapy with simvastatin should be advised of the risk of myopathy, and told to report promptly unexplained muscle pain, tenderness or weakness. A CK level above 10X ULN in a patient with unexplained muscle symptoms indicates myopathy. **Simvastatin therapy should be discontinued if myopathy is diagnosed or suspected.** In most cases, when patients were promptly discontinued from treatment, muscle symptoms and CK increases resolved.
Of the patients with rhabdomyolysis, many had complicated medical histories. Some had preexisting renal insufficiency, usually as a consequence of long-standing diabetes. In such patients, dose escalation requires caution. Also, as there are no known adverse consequences of brief interruption of therapy, treatment with simvastatin should be stopped a few days before elective major surgery and when any major acute medical or surgical condition supervenes.
2. Measures to reduce the risk of myopathy caused by drug interactions (see above and PRECAUTIONS, *Drug Interactions*). Physicians contemplating combined therapy with simvastatin and any of the interacting drugs should weigh the potential benefits and risks, and should carefully monitor patients for any signs and symptoms of muscle pain, tenderness, or weakness, particularly during the initial months of therapy and during any periods of upward dosage titration of either drug. Periodic CK determinations may be considered in such situations, but there is no assurance that such monitoring will prevent myopathy.
The combined use of simvastatin with fibrates or niacin should be avoided unless the benefit of further alteration in lipid levels is likely to outweigh the increased risk of this drug combination. Combinations of fibrates or niacin with low doses of simvastatin have been used without myopathy in small, short-term clinical studies with careful monitoring. Addition of these drugs to simvastatin typically provides little additional reduction in LDL-C, but further reductions of TG and further increases in HDL-C may be obtained. If one of these drugs must be used with simvastatin, clinical experience suggests that the risk of myopathy is less with niacin than with the fibrates.
In patients taking concomitant cyclosporine, fibrates or niacin, the dose of simvastatin should generally not exceed 10 mg (see DOSAGE AND ADMINISTRATION, *General Recommendations* and *Concomitant Lipid-Lowering Therapy*), as the risk of myopathy increases substantially at higher doses. Interruption of simvastatin therapy during a course of treatment with a systemic antifungal azole or a macrolide antibiotic should be considered.
Liver Dysfunction
Persistent increases (to more than 3X the ULN) in serum transaminases have occurred in approximately 1% of patients who received simvastatin in clinical studies. When drug treatment was interrupted or discontinued in these patients, the transaminase levels usually fell slowly to pretreatment levels. The increases were not associated with jaundice or other clinical signs or symptoms. There was no evidence of hypersensitivity.
In 4S (see CLINICAL PHARMACOLOGY, *Clinical Studies*), the number of patients with more than one transaminase elevation to >3X ULN, over the course of the study, was not significantly different between the simvastatin and placebo groups (14 [0.7%] vs. 12 [0.6%]). Elevated transaminases resulted in the discontinuation of 8 patients from therapy in the simvastatin group (n=2,221) and 5 in the placebo group (n=2,223). Of the 1,986 simvastatin treated patients in 4S with normal liver function tests (LFTs) at baseline, only 8 (0.4%) developed consecutive LFT elevations to >3X ULN and/or were discontinued due to transaminase elevations during the 5.4 years (median follow-up) of the study. Among these 8 patients, 5 initially developed these abnormalities within the first year. All of the patients in this study received a starting dose of 20 mg of simvastatin; 37% were titrated to 40 mg.
In 2 controlled clinical studies in 1,105 patients, the 12-month incidence of persistent hepatic transaminase elevation without regard to drug relationship was 0.9% and 2.1% at the 40- and 80-mg dose, respectively. No patients developed persistent liver function abnormalities following the initial 6 months of treatment at a given dose.
It is recommended that liver function tests be performed before the initiation of treatment, and periodically thereafter (e.g., semiannually) for the first year of treatment or until one year after the last elevation in dose. Patients titrated to the 80-mg dose should receive an additional test at 3 months. Patients who develop increased transaminase levels should be monitored with a second liver function evaluation to confirm the finding and be followed thereafter with frequent liver function tests until the abnormality(ies) return to normal. Should an increase in AST or ALT of 3X ULN or greater persist, withdrawal of therapy with ZOCOR is recommended.
The drug should be used with caution in patients who consume substantial quantities of alcohol and/or have a past history of liver disease. Active liver diseases or unexplained transaminase elevations are contraindications to the use of simvastatin.
As with other lipid-lowering agents, moderate (less than 3X ULN) elevations of serum transaminases have been reported following therapy with simvastatin. These changes appeared soon after initiation of therapy with simvastatin, were often transient, were not accompanied by any symptoms and did not require interruption of treatment.

PRECAUTIONS

General
Simvastatin may cause elevation of CK and transaminase levels (see WARNINGS and ADVERSE REACTIONS). This should be considered in the differential diagnosis of chest pain in a patient on therapy with simvastatin.
Information for Patients
Patients should be advised to report promptly unexplained muscle pain, tenderness, or weakness (see WARNINGS, *Skeletal Muscle*).
Drug Interactions
Cyclosporine, Itraconazole, Ketoconazole, Gemfibrozil, Niacin (Nicotinic Acid), Erythromycin, Clarithromycin, HIV protease inhibitors, Nefazodone (see WARNINGS, *Skeletal Muscle*).
Antipyrine: Simvastatin had no effect on the pharmacokinetics of antipyrine. However, since simvastatin is metabolized by the cytochrome P-450 isoform 3A4, this does not preclude an interaction with other drugs metabolized by the same isoform (see WARNINGS, *Skeletal Muscle*).
Propranolol: In healthy male volunteers there was a significant decrease in mean C_{max}, but no change in AUC, for simvastatin total and active inhibitors with concomitant administration of single doses of ZOCOR and propranolol. The clinical relevance of this finding is unclear. The pharmacokinetics of the enantiomers of propranolol were not affected.
Digoxin: Concomitant administration of a single dose of digoxin in healthy male volunteers receiving simvastatin resulted in a slight elevation (less than 0.3 ng/mL) in digoxin concentrations in plasma (as measured by a radioimmunoassay) compared to concomitant administration of placebo and digoxin. Patients taking digoxin should be monitored appropriately when simvastatin is initiated.
Warfarin: In two clinical studies, one in normal volunteers and the other in hypercholesterolemic patients, simvastatin 20–40 mg/day modestly potentiated the effect of coumarin anticoagulants: the prothrombin time, reported as International Normalized Ratio (INR), increased from a baseline of 1.7 to 1.8 and from 2.6 to 3.4 in the volunteer and patient studies, respectively. With other reductase inhibitors, clinically evident bleeding and/or increased prothrombin time has been reported in a few patients taking coumarin anticoagulants concomitantly. In such patients, prothrombin time should be determined before starting simvastatin and frequently enough during early therapy to insure that no significant alteration of prothrombin time occurs. Once a stable prothrombin time has been documented, prothrombin times can be monitored at the intervals usually recommended for patients on coumarin anticoagulants. If the dose of simvastatin is changed or discontinued, the same procedure should be repeated. Simvastatin therapy has not been associated with bleeding or with changes in prothrombin time in patients not taking anticoagulants.
CNS Toxicity
Optic nerve degeneration was seen in clinically normal dogs treated with simvastatin for 14 weeks at 180 mg/kg/day, a dose that produced mean plasma drug levels about 12 times higher than the mean plasma drug level in humans taking 80 mg/day.
A chemically similar drug in this class also produced optic nerve degeneration (Wallerian degeneration of retinogeniculate fibers) in clinically normal dogs in a dose-dependent fashion starting at 60 mg/kg/day, a dose that produced mean plasma drug levels about 30 times higher than the mean plasma drug level in humans taking the highest recommended dose (as measured by total enzyme inhibitory activity). This same drug also produced vestibulocochlear Wallerian-like degeneration and retinal ganglion cell chromatolysis in dogs treated for 14 weeks at 180 mg/kg/day, a dose that resulted in a mean plasma drug level similar to that seen with the 60 mg/kg/day dose.
CNS vascular lesions, characterized by perivascular hemorrhage and edema, mononuclear cell infiltration of perivascular spaces, perivascular fibrin deposits and necrosis of small vessels were seen in dogs treated with simvastatin at a dose of 360 mg/kg/day, a dose that produced mean plasma drug levels that were about 14 times higher than the mean plasma drug levels in humans taking 80 mg/day. Similar CNS vascular lesions have been observed with several other drugs of this class.
There were cataracts in female rats after two years of treatment with 50 and 100 mg/kg/day (22 and 25 times the human AUC at 80 mg/day, respectively) and in dogs after three months at 90 mg/kg/day (19 times) and at two years at 50 mg/kg/day (5 times).
Carcinogenesis, Mutagenesis, Impairment of Fertility
In a 72-week carcinogenicity study, mice were administered daily doses of simvastatin of 25, 100, and 400 mg/kg body weight, which resulted in mean plasma drug levels approximately 1, 4, and 8 times higher than the mean human plasma drug level, respectively (as total inhibitory activity based on AUC) after an 80-mg oral dose. Liver carcinomas were significantly increased in high-dose females and mid- and high-dose males with a maximum incidence of 90% in males. The incidence of adenomas of the liver was significantly increased in mid- and high-dose females. Drug treatment also significantly increased the incidence of lung adenomas in mid- and high-dose males and females. Adenomas of the Harderian gland (a gland of the eye of rodents) were significantly higher in high-dose mice than in controls. No evidence of a tumorigenic effect was observed at 25 mg/kg/day.
In a separate 92-week carcinogenicity study in mice at doses up to 25 mg/kg/day, no evidence of a tumorigenic effect was observed (mean plasma drug levels were 1 times higher than humans given 80 mg simvastatin as measured by AUC).
In a two-year study in rats at 25 mg/kg/day, there was a statistically significant increase in the incidence of thyroid follicular adenomas in female rats exposed to approximately 11 times higher levels of simvastatin than in humans given 80 mg simvastatin (as measured by AUC).
A second two-year rat carcinogenicity study with doses of 50 and 100 mg/kg/day produced hepatocellular adenomas and carcinomas (in female rats at both doses and in males at 100 mg/kg/day). Thyroid follicular cell adenomas were increased in males and females at both doses; thyroid follicular cell carcinomas were increased in females at 100 mg/kg/day. The increased incidence of thyroid neoplasms appears to be consistent with findings from other HMG-CoA reductase inhibitors. These treatment levels represented plasma drug levels (AUC) of approximately 7 and 15 times (males) and 22 and 25 times (females) the mean human plasma drug exposure after an 80 milligram daily dose.
No evidence of mutagenicity was observed in a microbial mutagenicity (Ames) test with or without rat or mouse liver metabolic activation. In addition, no evidence of damage to genetic material was noted in an *in vitro* alkaline elution assay using rat hepatocytes, a V-79 mammalian cell forward mutation study, an *in vitro* chromosome aberration study in CHO cells, or an *in vivo* chromosomal aberration assay in mouse bone marrow.
There was decreased fertility in male rats treated with simvastatin for 34 weeks at 25 mg/kg body weight (4 times the maximum human exposure level, based on AUC, in patients receiving 80 mg/day); however, this effect was not observed during a subsequent fertility study in which simvastatin was administered at this same dose level to male rats for 11 weeks (the entire cycle of spermatogenesis including epididymal maturation). No microscopic changes were observed in the testes of rats from either study. At 180 mg/kg/day, (which produces exposure levels 22 times higher than those in humans taking 80 mg/day based on surface area, mg/m^2), seminiferous tubule degeneration (necrosis and loss of spermatogenic epithelium) was observed. In dogs, there was drug-related testicular atrophy, decreased spermatogenesis, spermatocytic degeneration and giant cell formation at 10 mg/kg/day, (approximately 2 times the human exposure, based on AUC, at 80 mg/day). The clinical significance of these findings is unclear.
Pregnancy
Pregnancy Category X
See CONTRAINDICATIONS.
Safety in pregnant women has not been established.
Simvastatin was not teratogenic in rats at doses of 25 mg/kg/day or in rabbits at doses up to 10 mg/kg daily. These doses resulted in 3 times (rat) or 3 times (rabbit) the human exposure based on mg/m^2 surface area. However, in studies with another structurally-related HMG-CoA reductase inhibitor, skeletal malformations were observed in rats and mice.
Rare reports of congenital anomalies have been received following intrauterine exposure to HMG-CoA reductase inhibitors. In a review*** of approximately 100 prospectively followed pregnancies in women exposed to ZOCOR or another structurally related HMG-CoA reductase inhibitor, the inci-

Continued on next page

Information on the Merck & Co., Inc. products listed on these pages is the full prescribing information from product circulars in use September 30, 2000. For information, please call 1-800-NSC MERCK [1-800-672-6372].

Zocor—Cont.

dences of congenital anomalies, spontaneous abortions and fetal deaths/stillbirths did not exceed what would be expected in the general population. The number of cases is adequate only to exclude a 3- to 4-fold increase in congenital anomalies over the background incidence. In 89% of the prospectively followed pregnancies, drug treatment was initiated prior to pregnancy and was discontinued at some point in the first trimester when pregnancy was identified. As safety in pregnant women has not been established and there is no apparent benefit to therapy with ZOCOR during pregnancy (see CONTRAINDICATIONS), treatment should be immediately discontinued as soon as pregnancy is recognized. ZOCOR should be administered to women of childbearing potential only when such patients are highly unlikely to conceive and have been informed of the potential hazards.

Nursing Mothers

It is not known whether simvastatin is excreted in human milk. Because a small amount of another drug in this class is excreted in human milk and because of the potential for serious adverse reactions in nursing infants, women taking simvastatin should not nurse their infants (see CONTRAINDICATIONS).

Pediatric Use

Safety and effectiveness in pediatric patients have not been established. Because pediatric patients are not likely to benefit from cholesterol lowering for at least a decade and because experience with this drug is limited (no studies in subjects below the age of 20 years), treatment of pediatric patients with simvastatin is not recommended at this time.

*** Manson, J.M., Freyssinges, C., Ducrocq, M.B., Stephenson, W.P., Postmarketing Surveillance of Lovastatin and Simvastatin Exposure During Pregnancy, *Reproductive Toxicology*, 10(6):439–446, 1996.

ADVERSE REACTIONS

In the pre-marketing controlled clinical studies and their open extensions (2,423 patients with mean duration of follow-up of approximately 18 months), 1.4% of patients were discontinued due to adverse experiences attributable to ZOCOR. Adverse reactions have usually been mild and transient. ZOCOR has been evaluated for serious adverse reactions in more than 21,000 patients and is generally well-tolerated.

Clinical Adverse Experiences

Adverse experiences occurring at an incidence of 1% or greater in patients treated with ZOCOR, regardless of causality, in controlled clinical studies are shown in Table 5.

Table 5
Adverse Experiences in Clinical Studies
Incidence 1 Percent or Greater, Regardless of Causality

	ZOCOR (N = 1,583) %	Placebo (N = 157) %	Cholestyramine (N = 179) %
Body as a Whole			
Abdominal pain	3.2	3.2	8.9
Asthenia	1.6	2.5	1.1
Gastrointestinal			
Constipation	2.3	1.3	29.1
Diarrhea	1.9	2.5	7.8
Dyspepsia	1.1	—	4.5
Flatulence	1.9	1.3	14.5
Nausea	1.3	1.9	10.1
Nervous System/ Psychiatric			
Headache	3.5	5.1	4.5
Respiratory			
Upper respiratory infection	2.1	1.9	3.4

Scandinavian Simvastatin Survival Study
Clinical Adverse Experiences

In 4S (see CLINICAL PHARMACOLOGY, *Clinical Studies*) involving 4,444 patients treated with 20–40 mg/day of ZOCOR (n=2,221) or placebo (n=2,223), the safety and tolerability profiles were comparable between groups over the median 5.4 years of the study. The clinical adverse experiences reported as possibly, probably, or definitely drug-related in ≥0.5% in either treatment group are shown in Table 6.

Table 6
Drug-Related Clinical Adverse Experiences in 4S
Incidence 0.5 Percent or Greater

	ZOCOR (N = 2,221) %	Placebo (N = 2,223) %
Body as a Whole		
Abdominal pain	0.9	0.9
Gastrointestinal		
Diarrhea	0.5	0.3
Dyspepsia	0.6	0.5
Flatulence	0.9	0.7
Nausea	0.4	0.6
Musculoskeletal		
Myalgia	1.2	1.3
Skin		
Eczema	0.8	0.8
Pruritus	0.5	0.4
Rash	0.6	0.6
Special Senses		
Cataract	0.5	0.8

The following effects have been reported with drugs in this class. Not all the effects listed below have necessarily been associated with simvastatin therapy.

Skeletal: muscle cramps, myalgia, myopathy, rhabdomyolysis, arthralgias.

Neurological: dysfunction of certain cranial nerves (including alteration of taste, impairment of extra-ocular movement, facial paresis), tremor, dizziness, vertigo, memory loss, paresthesia, peripheral neuropathy, peripheral nerve palsy, psychic disturbances, anxiety, insomnia, depression.

Hypersensitivity Reactions: An apparent hypersensitivity syndrome has been reported rarely which has included one or more of the following features: anaphylaxis, angioedema, lupus erythematous-like syndrome, polymyalgia rheumatica, vasculitis, purpura, thrombocytopenia, leukopenia, hemolytic anemia, positive ANA, ESR increase, eosinophilia, arthritis, arthralgia, urticaria, asthenia, photosensitivity, fever, chills, flushing, malaise, dyspnea, toxic epidermal necrolyis, erythema multiforme, including Stevens-Johnson syndrome.

Gastrointestinal: Pancreatitis, hepatitis, including chronic active hepatitis, cholestatic jaundice, fatty change in liver, and, rarely, cirrhosis, fulminant hepatic necrosis, and hepatoma; anorexia, vomiting.

Skin: alopecia, pruritus. A variety of skin changes (e.g., nodules, discoloration, dryness of skin/mucous membranes, changes to hair/nails) have been reported.

Reproductive: gynecomastia, loss of libido, erectile dysfunction.

Eye: progression of cataracts (lens opacities), ophthalmoplegia.

Laboratory Abnormalities: elevated transaminases, alkaline phosphatase, γ-glutamyl transpeptidase, and bilurubin; thyroid function abnormalities.

Laboratory Tests

Marked persistent increases of serum transaminases have been noted (see WARNINGS, *Liver Dysfunction*). About 5% of patients had elevations of CK levels of 3 or more times the normal value on one or more occasions. This was attributable to the noncardiac fraction of CK. Muscle pain or dysfunction usually was not reported (see WARNINGS, *Skeletal Muscle*).

Concomitant Therapy

In controlled clinical studies in which simvastatin was administered concomitantly with cholestyramine, no adverse reactions peculiar to this concomitant treatment were observed. The adverse reactions that occurred were limited to those reported previously with simvastatin or cholestyramine. The combined use of simvastatin with fibrates should generally be avoided (see WARNINGS, *Skeletal Muscle*).

OVERDOSAGE

Significant lethality was observed in mice after a single oral dose of 9 g/m². No evidence of lethality was observed in rats or dogs treated with doses of 30 and 100 g/m², respectively. No specific diagnostic signs were observed in rodents. At these doses the only signs seen in dogs were emesis and mucoid stools.

A few cases of overdosage with ZOCOR have been reported; no patients had any specific symptoms, and all patients recovered without sequelae. The maximum dose taken was 450 mg. Until further experience is obtained, no specific treatment of overdosage with ZOCOR can be recommended. The dialyzability of simvastatin and its metabolites in man is not known at present.

DOSAGE AND ADMINISTRATION

The patient should be placed on a standard cholesterol-lowering diet before receiving ZOCOR and should continue on this diet during treatment with ZOCOR. The dosage should be individualized according to the baseline LDL-C level, the recommended goal of therapy (see NCEP Treatment Guidelines), and the patient's response. The dosage range is 5–80 mg/day (see below).

The recommended usual starting dose is 20 mg once a day in the evening. Patients who require a large reduction in LDL-C (more than 45%) may be started at 40 mg/day in the evening. Adjustments of dosage should be made at intervals of 4 weeks or more. See below for dosage recommendations for patients receiving concomitant therapy with cyclosporine, fibrates or niacin, and for those with renal insufficiency.

Dosage in Patients with Homozygous Familial Hypercholesterolemia

Based on the results of a controlled clinical study, the recommended dosage for patients with homozygous familial hypercholesterolemia is ZOCOR 40 mg/day in the evening or 80 mg/day in 3 divided doses of 20 mg, 20 mg, and an evening dose of 40 mg. ZOCOR should be used as an adjunct to other lipid-lowering treatments (e.g., LDL apheresis) in these patients or if such treatments are unavailable.

Dosage in Patients taking Cyclosporine

In patients taking cyclosporine concomitantly with ZOCOR (see WARNINGS, *Skeletal Muscle*), therapy should begin with 5 mg/day and should not exceed 10 mg/day.

Concomitant Lipid-Lowering Therapy

ZOCOR is effective alone or when used concomitantly with bile-acid sequestrants. Use of ZOCOR with fibrates or niacin should generally be avoided. However, if ZOCOR is used in combination with fibrates or niacin, the dose of ZOCOR should not exceed 10 mg/day (see WARNINGS, *Skeletal Muscle*).

Dosage in Patients with Renal Insufficiency

Because ZOCOR does not undergo significant renal excretion, modification of dosage should not be necessary in patients with mild to moderate renal insufficiency. However, caution should be exercised when ZOCOR is administered to patients with severe renal insufficiency; such patients should be started at 5 mg/day and be closely monitored (see CLINICAL PHARMACOLOGY, *Pharmacokinetics* and WARNINGS, *Skeletal Muscle*).

HOW SUPPLIED

No. 3588 — Tablets ZOCOR 5 mg are buff, shield-shaped, film-coated tablets, coded MSD 726 on one side and ZOCOR on the other. They are supplied as follows:
NDC 0006-0726-61 unit of use bottles of 60
NDC 0006-0726-54 unit of use bottles of 90
NDC 0006-0726-28 unit dose packages of 100.
Shown in Product Identification Guide, page 324

No. 3589 — Tablets ZOCOR 10 mg are peach, shield-shaped, film-coated tablets, coded MSD 735 on one side and ZOCOR on the other. They are supplied as follows:
NDC 0006-0735-61 unit of use bottles of 60
NDC 0006-0735-54 unit of use bottles of 90
NDC 0006-0735-28 unit dose packages of 100
NDC 0006-0735-82 bottles of 1000
NDC 0006-0735-87 bottles of 10,000.
Shown in Product Identification Guide, page 324

No. 3590 — Tablets ZOCOR 20 mg are tan, shield-shaped, film-coated tablets, coded MSD 740 on one side and ZOCOR on the other. They are supplied as follows:
NDC 0006-0740-61 unit of use bottles of 60
NDC 0006-0740-28 unit dose packages of 100
NDC 0006-0740-82 bottles of 1000
NDC 0006-0740-87 bottles of 10,000.
Shown in Product Identification Guide, page 324

No. 3591 — Tablets ZOCOR 40 mg are brick red, shield-shaped, film-coated tablets, coded MSD 749 on one side and ZOCOR on the other. They are supplied as follows:
NDC 0006-0749-61 unit of use bottles of 60.
Shown in Product Identification Guide, page 324

No. 6577 — Tablets ZOCOR 80 mg are brick red, capsule-shaped, film-coated tablets, coded 543 on one side and 80 on the other. They are supplied as follows:
NDC 0006-0543-61 unit of use bottles of 60.
Shown in Product Identification Guide, page 324

Storage

Store between 5–30°C (41–86°F).

7825437 Issued April 2000

Mericon Industries, Inc.

8819 N. PIONEER ROAD
PEORIA, IL 61615

Direct Inquiries to:
William R. Connelly
(309) 693-2150
FAX: (309) 693-2158

BIOTIN OTC

['bī-ō-tĭn]
biotin supplement–high potency

ACTIVE INGREDIENTS

Biotin 5 mg

DIRECTIONS

Take one capsule daily or as directed by your physician.

HOW SUPPLIED

Biotin is supplied as capsules in bottles of 120.
NDC 00394-0130-12

FLORICAL® OTC

[*flor ĭ cal*]
(fluoride and calcium supplement)

ACTIVE INGREDIENTS

Florical® contains 3.75 mg fluoride (as sodium fluoride), 145 mg calcium (as calcium carbonate)

DIRECTIONS

Take one tablet or capsule daily, or as recommended by physician.

HOW SUPPLIED

Florical® is supplied as tablets or capsules in bottles of 100 or 500.
NDC 00394-0102-02 (Capsules 100's)
NDC 00394-0102-05 (Capsules 500's)
NDC 00394-0100-02 (Tablets 100's)
NDC 00394-0100-05 (Tablets 500's)

MONOCAL® OTC
[mon ō cal]
(fluoride and calcium supplement)

ACTIVE INGREDIENTS
Monocal® contains 3 mg fluoride (as monofluorophosphate) and 250 mg calcium (as calcium carbonate)

DIRECTIONS
Take one tablet daily, or as recommended by physician.

HOW SUPPLIED
Monocal® is supplied as tablets in bottles of 100.
NDC 00394-0105-02

Merz Pharmaceuticals

DIVISION OF MERZ, INC.
4215 TUDOR LANE (27410)
P.O. Box 18806
GREENSBORO, NC 27419

Direct Inquiries to:
Director of Technical Operations
(336) 856-2003
FAX: (336) 856-0107

For Medical Information Contact:
In Emergencies:
Director of Technical Operations
(336) 856-2003
FAX: (336) 856-0107

ELDERTONIC® OTC

DESCRIPTION
Each 45 ml. contains: Thiamine HCl, 1.5 mg.; Riboflavin, 1.7 mg. (as Riboflavin 5′-Phosphate Sodium); Pyridoxine HCl, 2.0 mg.; Cyanocobalamin, 6.0 mcg.; Dexpanthenol, 10.0 mg.; Niacinamide, 20.0 mg.; Zinc, 15 mg. (as zinc sulfate); Manganese, 2.0 mg. (as manganese sulfate); Magnesium (minimum content as added magnesium), 2.0 mg. (as magnesium sulfate); Alcohol, 13.5%.
In a special sherry wine base.

INDICATIONS
B-complex vitamins with minerals for nutritional supplementation.

DOSAGE
Adults: one tablespoonful three times a day with meals.

WARNING
Do not exceed recommended dosage unless directed by a physician.

USAGE IN PREGNANCY
Safe use of this product in pregnancy has not been established.

CAUTION
Keep out of the reach of children.

HOW SUPPLIED
ELDERTONIC available in Pint bottles: NDC #0259-0351-16, Quart bottles: NDC #0259-0351-32.

MAY-VITA® ELIXIR ℞

DESCRIPTION
Each 45 ml. contains: Dexpanthenol, 10 mg; Niacinamide, 40 mg.; Pyridoxine HCl (B-6), 4 mg.; Cyanocobalamin (B-12), 12 mcg.; Folic Acid, 1 mg.; Iron, 36 mg. (as polysaccharide iron complex); Zinc, 15 mg. (as zinc sulfate); Manganese, 4 mg. (as manganese sulfate); Alcohol, 13%.

INDICATIONS
For vitamin and mineral replacement therapy in deficiency states and for treatment of iron deficiency anemia and/or nutritional megaloblastic anemias due to inadequate diet.

WARNINGS
Folic acid alone is improper therapy in the treatment of pernicious anemia and other megaloblastic anemias where vitamin B_{12} is deficient.

PRECAUTIONS
Folic acid, especially in doses above 0.1 mg. daily, may obscure pernicious anemia, in that hematologic remission may occur while neurological manifestations remain progressive.

ADVERSE REACTIONS
Allergic sensitization has been reported following both oral and parenteral administration of folic acid.

USE IN PREGNANCY
Safe use of this product in pregnancy has not been established.

DOSAGE
Usual adult dosage is one tablespoonful (15 ml.) three times daily with meals. Do not exceed recommended dosage unless directed by a physician.

HOW SUPPLIED
MAY-VITA ELIXIR is supplied in Pint bottles: NDC #0259-0366-16.

NAFTIN® ℞
(naftifine hydrochloride) 1%
Cream

DESCRIPTION
NAFTIN® Cream, 1% contains the synthetic, broad-spectrum, antifungal agent naftifine hydrochloride.
NAFTIN® Cream, 1% is for topical use only.
Chemical Name: (E)-N-Cinnamyl-N-methyl-1-naphthalenemethyl-amine hydrochloride. Naftifine hydrochloride has an empirical formula of $C_{21}H_{21}N{\cdot}HCl$ and a molecular weight of 323.86.
Active Ingredient: Naftifine hydrochloride 1%
Inactive Ingredients: benzyl alcohol, cetyl alcohol, cetyl esters wax, isopropyl myristate, polysorbate 60, purified water, sodium hydroxide, sorbitan monostearate, and stearyl alcohol. Hydrochloric acid may be added to adjust pH.

CLINICAL PHARMACOLOGY
Naftifine hydrochloride is a synthetic allylamine derivative. The following *in vitro* data are available, but their clinical significance is unknown. Naftifine hydrochloride has been shown to exhibit fungicidal activity *in vitro* against a broad spectrum of organisms including *Trichophyton rubrum, Trichophyton mentagrophytes, Trichophyton tonsurans, Epidermophyton floccosum, Microsporum canis, Microsporum audouini,* and *Microsporum gypseum;* and fungistatic activity against *Candida* species, including *Candida albicans.* NAFTIN® Cream, 1% has only been shown to be clinically effective against the disease entities listed in the INDICATIONS AND USAGE section.
Although the exact mechanism of action against fungi is not known, naftifine hydrochloride appears to interfere with sterol biosynthesis by inhibiting the enzyme squalene 2,3-epoxidase. This inhibition of enzyme activity results in decreased amounts of sterols, especially ergosterol, and a corresponding accumulation of squalene in the cells.
Pharmacokinetics: *In vitro* and *in vivo* bioavailability studies have demonstrated that naftifine penetrates the stratum corneum in sufficient concentration to inhibit the growth of dermatophytes.
Following a single topical application of 1% naftifine cream to the skin of healthy subjects, systemic absorption of naftifine was approximately 6% of the applied dose. Naftifine and/or its metabolites are excreted via the urine and feces with a half-life of approximately two to three days.

INDICATIONS AND USAGE
NAFTIN® Cream, 1% is indicated for topical application in the treatment of tinea pedis, tinea cruris and tinea corporis caused by the organisms *Tricophyton rubrum, Tricophyton mentagrophytes,* and *Epidermophyton floccosum.*

CONTRAINDICATIONS
NAFTIN® Cream, 1% is contraindicated in individuals who have shown hypersensitivity to any of its components.

WARNING
NAFTIN® Cream, 1% is for topical use only and not for ophthalmic use.

PRECAUTIONS
General: NAFTIN® Cream, 1% is for external use only. If irritation or sensitivity develops with the use of NAFTIN® Cream 1%, treatment should be discontinued and appropriate therapy instituted. Diagnosis of the disease should be confirmed either by direct microscopic examination of a mounting of infected tissue in a solution of potassium hydroxide or by culture on an appropriate medium.
Information for patients: The patient should be told to:
1. Avoid the use of occlusive dressings or wrappings unless otherwise directed by the physician.
2. Keep NAFTIN® Cream, 1% away from the eyes, nose, mouth and other mucous membranes.

Carcinogenesis, mutagenesis, impairment of fertility: Long-term animal studies to evaluate the carcinogenic potential of NAFTIN® Cream, 1% have not been performed. *In vitro* and animal studies have not demonstrated any mutagenic effect or effect on fertility.
Pregnancy: Teratogenic Effects: Pregnancy Category B: Reproduction studies have been performed in rats and rabbits (via oral administration) at doses 150 times or more the topical human dose and have revealed no significant evidence of impaired fertility or harm to the fetus due to naftifine. There are, however, no adequate and well-controlled studies in pregnant women. Because animal reproduction studies are not always predictive of human response, this drug should be used during pregnancy only if clearly needed.
Nursing mothers: It is not known whether this drug is excreted in human milk. Because many drugs are excreted in human milk, caution should be exercised when NAFTIN® Cream, 1% is administered to a nursing woman.
Pediatric use: Safety and effectiveness in pediatric patients have not been established.

ADVERSE REACTIONS
During clinical trials with NAFTIN® Cream 1%, the incidence of adverse reactions was as follows: burning/stinging (6%), dryness (3%), erythema (2%), itching (2%), local irritation (2%).

DOSAGE AND ADMINISTRATION
A sufficient quantity of NAFTIN® Cream, 1% should be gently massaged into the affected and surrounding skin areas once a day. The hands should be washed after application.
If no clinical improvement is seen after four weeks of treatment with NAFTIN® Cream, 1% the patient should be reevaluated.

HOW SUPPLIED
NAFTIN® (naftifine hydrochloride) 1% Cream is supplied in collapsible tubes in the following sizes.
15 g-NDC-0259-4126-15
30 g-NDC-0259-4126-30
60 g-NDC-0259-4126-60
Note: Store below 30°C (86°F).
Rx only
©Merz Pharmaceuticals L.L.C.

NAFTIN® ℞
(naftifine hydrochloride) 1%
Gel

DESCRIPTION
NAFTIN® Gel, 1% contains the synthetic, broad-spectrum, antifungal agent naftifine hydrochloride.
NAFTIN® Gel, 1% is for topical use only.
Chemical Name: (E)-N-Cinnamyl-N-methyl-1-naphthalene-methylamine hydrochloride. Naftifine hydrochloride has an empirical formula of $C_{21}H_{21}N{\cdot}HCl$ and a molecular weight of 323.86.
Contains:
Active Ingredient: Naftifine hydrochloride 1%
Inactive Ingredients: polysorbate 80, carbomer 934P, diisopropanolamine, edetate disodium, alcohol (52% v/v), and purified water.

CLINICAL PHARMACOLOGY
Naftifine hydrochloride is a synthetic allylamine derivative. The following *in vitro* data are available but their clinical significance is unknown. Naftifine hydrochloride has been shown to exhibit fungicidal activity *in vitro* against a broad spectrum of organisms including *Trichophyton rubrum, Trichophyton mentagrophytes, Trichophyton tonsurans, Epidermophyton floccosum,* and *Microsporum canis, Microsporum audouini,* and *Microsporum gypseum;* and fungistatic activity against *Candida* species including *Candida albicans.* NAFTIN® Gel, 1% has only been shown to be clinically effective against the disease entities listed in the INDICATIONS AND USAGE section.
Although the exact mechanism of action against fungi is not known, naftifine hydrochloride appears to interfere with sterol biosynthesis by inhibiting the enzyme squalene 2,3-epoxidase. This inhibition of enzyme activity results in decreased amounts of sterols, especially ergosterol, and a corresponding accumulation of squalene in the cells.
Pharmacokinetics: *In vitro* and *in vivo* bioavailability studies have demonstrated that naftifine penetrates the stratum corneum in sufficient concentration to inhibit the growth of dermatophytes.
Following single topical application of ^{3}H-labeled naftifine gel 1% to the skin of healthy subjects, up to 4.2% of the applied dose was absorbed. Naftifine and/or its metabolites are excreted via the urine and feces with a half-life of approximately two to three days.

INDICATION AND USAGE
NAFTIN® Gel, 1% is indicated for the topical treatment of tinea pedis, tinea cruris and tinea corporis caused by the organisms *Trichophyton rubrum, Trichophyton mentagrophytes, Trichophyton tonsurans** and *Epidermophyton floccosum.**
*Efficacy for this organism in this organ system was studied in fewer than 10 infections.

CONTRAINDICATIONS
NAFTIN® Gel, 1% is contraindicated in individuals who have shown hypersensitivity to any of its components.

WARNINGS
NAFTIN® Gel, 1% is for topical use only and not for ophthalmic use.

PRECAUTIONS
General: NAFTIN® Gel, 1% is for external use only. If irritation or sensitivity develop with the use of NAFTIN®

Continued on next page

Naftin Gel—Cont.

Gel, 1%, treatment should be discontinued and appropriate therapy instituted. Diagnosis of the disease should be confirmed either by direct microscopic examination of a mounting of infected tissue in a solution of potassium hydroxide or by culture on an appropriate medium.

Information for patients:
The patient should be told to:
1. Avoid the use of occlusive dressings or wrappings unless otherwise directed by the physician.
2. Keep NAFTIN® Gel, 1% away from the eyes, nose, mouth and other mucous membranes.

Carcinogenesis, mutagenesis, impairment of fertility: Long-term studies to evaluate the carcinogenic potential of NAFTIN® Gel, 1% have not been performed. *In vitro* and animal studies have not demonstrated any mutagenic effect or effect on fertility.

Pregnancy: Teratogenic Effects: Pregnancy Category B: Reproduction studies have been performed in rats and rabbits (via oral administration) at doses 150 times or more than the topical human dose and have revealed no evidence of impaired fertility or harm to the fetus due to naftifine. There are, however, no adequate and well-controlled studies in pregnant women. Because animal reproduction studies are not always predictive of human response, this drug should be used during pregnancy only if clearly needed.

Nursing mothers: It is not known whether this drug is excreted in human milk. Because many drugs are excreted in human milk, caution should be exercised when NAFTIN® Gel, 1% is administered to a nursing woman.

Pediatric use: Safety and effectiveness in pediatric patients have not been established.

ADVERSE REACTIONS

During clinical trials with NAFTIN® Gel, 1%, the incidence of adverse reactions was as follows: burning/stinging (5.0%), itching (1.0%), erythema (0.5%), rash (0.5%), skin tenderness (0.5%).

DOSAGE AND ADMINISTRATION

A sufficient quantity of NAFTIN® Gel, 1% should be gently massaged into the affected and surrounding skin areas twice a day, in the morning and evening. The hands should be washed after application.

If no clinical improvement is seen after four weeks of treatment with NAFTIN® Gel, 1%, the patient should be reevaluated.

HOW SUPPLIED

NAFTIN® (naftifine hydrochloride) is supplied in collapsible tubes in the following sizes:
20 g-NDC-0259-4770-20
40 g-NDC-0259-4770-40
60 g-NDC-0259-4770-60

Note: Store at room temperature.
Rx only

NU-IRON® 150 CAPSULES OTC
(polysaccharide-iron complex)
NU-IRON® ELIXIR (polysaccharide-iron complex)
Sugar Free Dye Free

DESCRIPTION

NU-IRON is a highly water soluble complex of iron and a low molecular weight polysaccharide.
Each NU-IRON 150 Capsule contains:
Iron (elemental) .... 150 mg.
(as Polysaccharide Iron Complex)
Each 5 ml. of NU-IRON Elixir contains:
Iron (elemental) .... 100 mg.
(as Polysaccharide Iron Complex)
Alcohol 10%

ACTION AND USES

NU-IRON is a non-ionic, easily assimilated, relatively non-toxic form of iron. Full therapeutic doses may be achieved with virtually no gastrointestinal side effects. There is no metallic aftertaste and no staining of teeth.

INDICATIONS

For treatment of uncomplicated iron deficiency anemia.

CONTRAINDICATIONS

Hemochromatosis, hemosiderosis or a known hypersensitivity to any of the ingredients.

DOSAGE

ADULTS: One or two NU-IRON 150 Capsules daily, or one or two teaspoonsful NU-IRON Elixir daily. CHILDREN; 6 to 12 years old; one teaspoonful NU-IRON Elixir daily. For younger children consult physician.

HOW SUPPLIED

NU-IRON 150 CAPSULES in blister paks of 100 (10 × 10): NDC #0259-0291-01.
NU-IRON ELIXIR in 8 oz bottles: NDC #0259-0292-08.

SEDAPAP® TABLETS ℞
(Butalbital and Acetaminophen Tablets)
50 mg/650 mg

DESCRIPTION

Butalbital and acetaminophen is supplied in tablet form for oral administration.

Butalbital (5-allyl-5-isobutylbarbituric acid), a slightly bitter, white, odorless, crystalline powder, is a short to intermediate-acting barbiturate. It has the following structural formula:

$C_{11}H_{16}N_2O_3$ MW = 224.26

Acetaminophen (4′-hydroxyacetanalide), a slightly bitter, white, odorless, crystalline powder, is a non-opiate, non-salicylate analgesic and antipyretic. It has the following structural formula:

$C_8H_9NO_2$ MW = 151.16

Each Sedapap Tablet contains:
Butalbital .... 50 mg
(Warning: May be habit forming)
Acetaminophen .... 650 mg

In addition, each tablet contains the following inactive ingredients: colloidal silicon dioxide, croscarmellose sodium, crospovidone, microcrystalline cellulose, povidone, pregelatinized starch and stearic acid.

CLINICAL PHARMACOLOGY

This combination drug product is intended as a treatment for tension headache.

It consists of a fixed combination of butalbital, and acetaminophen. The role each component plays in the relief of the complex of symptoms known as tension headache is incompletely understood.

Pharmacokinetics: The behavior of the individual components is described below.

Butalbital: Butalbital is well absorbed from the gastrointestinal tract and is expected to distribute to most tissues in the body. Barbiturates in general may appear in breast milk and readily cross the placental barrier. They are bound to plasma and tissue proteins to a varying degree and binding increases directly as a function of lipid solubility.

Elimination of butalbital is primarily via the kidney (59% to 88% of the dose) as unchanged drug or metabolites. The plasma half-life is about 35 hours. Urinary excretion products include parent drug (about 3.6% of the dose), 5-isobutyl-5-(2,3-dihydroxypropyl) barbituric acid (about 24% of the dose), 5-allyl-5(3-hydroxy-2-methyl-1-propyl) barbituric acid (about 4.8% of the dose), products with the barbituric acid ring hydrolyzed with excretion of urea (about 14% of the dose), as well as unidentified materials. Of the material excreted in the urine, 32% is conjugated.

See OVERDOSAGE for toxicity information.

Acetaminophen: Acetaminophen is rapidly absorbed from the gastrointestinal tract and is distributed throughout most body tissues. The plasma half-life is 1.25 to 3 hours, but may be increased by liver damage and following overdosage. Elimination of acetaminophen is principally by liver metabolism (conjugation) and subsequent renal excretion of metabolites. Approximately 85% of an oral dose appears in the urine within 24 hours of administration, most as the glucuronide conjugate, with small amounts of other conjugates and unchanged drug.

See OVERDOSAGE for toxicity information.

INDICATIONS AND USAGE

Butalbital and Acetaminophen Tablets are indicated for the relief of the symptom complex of tension (or muscle contraction) headache.

Evidence supporting the efficacy and safety of this combination product in the treatment of multiple recurrent headaches is unavailable. Caution in this regard is required because butalbital is habit-forming and potentially abusable.

CONTRAINDICATIONS

This product is contraindicated under the following conditions:
- Hypersensitivity or intolerance to any component of this product.
- Patients with porphyria.

WARNINGS

Butalbital is habit-forming and potentially abusable. Consequently, the extended use of this product is not recommended.

PRECAUTIONS

General: Butalbital and Acetaminophen Tablets should be prescribed with caution in certain special-risk patients, such as the elderly or debilitated, and those with severe impairment of renal or hepatic function, or acute abdominal conditions.

Information for Patients: This product may impair mental and/or physical abilities required for the performance of potentially hazardous tasks such as driving a car or operating machinery. Such tasks should be avoided while taking this product.

Alcohol and other CNS depressants may produce an additive CNS depression, when taken with this combination product, and should be avoided.

Butalbital may be habit-forming. Patients should take the drug only for as long as it is prescribed, in the amounts prescribed, and no more frequently than prescribed.

Laboratory Tests: In patients with severe hepatic or renal disease, effects of therapy should be monitored with serial liver and/or renal function tests.

Drug Interactions: The CNS effects of butalbital may be enhanced by monoamine oxidase (MAO) inhibitors.

Butalbital and acetaminophen may enhance the effects of: other narcotic analgesics, alcohol, general anesthetics, tranquilizers such as chlordiazepoxide, sedative-hypnotics, or other CNS depressants, causing increased CNS depression.

Drug/Laboratory Test Interactions: Acetaminophen may produce false-positive test results for urinary 5-hydroxyindoleacetic acid.

Carcinogenesis, Mutagenesis, Impairment of Fertility: No adequate studies have been conducted in animals to determine whether acetaminophen or butalbital have a potential for carcinogenesis, mutagenesis or impairment of fertility.

Pregnancy: *Teratogenic Effects:* Pregnancy Category C: Animal reproduction studies have not been conducted with this combination product. It is also not known whether butalbital and acetaminophen can cause fetal harm when administered to a pregnant woman or can affect reproduction capacity. This product should be given to a pregnant woman only when clearly needed.

Nonteratogenic Effects: Withdrawal seizures were reported in a two-day-old male infant whose mother had taken butalbital-containing drug during the last two months of pregnancy. Butalbital was found in the infant's serum. The infant was given phenobarbital 5 mg/kg, which was tapered without further seizure or other withdrawal symptoms.

Nursing Mothers: Barbiturates and acetaminophen are excreted in breast milk in small amounts, but the significance of their effects on nursing infants is not known. Because of potential for serious adverse reactions in nursing infants from butalbital and acetaminophen, a decision should be made whether to discontinue nursing or to discontinue the drug, taking into account the importance of the drug to the mother.

Pediatric Use: Safety and effectiveness in pediatric patients below the age of 12 have not been established.

ADVERSE REACTIONS

Frequently Observed: The most frequently reported adverse reactions are drowsiness, lightheadedness, dizziness, sedation, shortness of breath, nausea, vomiting, abdominal pain, and intoxicated feeling.

Infrequently Observed: All adverse events tabulated below are classified as infrequent.

Central Nervous: headache, shaky feeling, tingling, agitation, fainting, fatigue, heavy eyelids, high energy, hot spells, numbness, sluggishness, seizure. Mental confusion, excitement or depression can also occur due to intolerance, particularly in elderly or debilitated patients, or due to overdosage of butalbital.

Autonomic Nervous: dry mouth, hyperhidrosis.

Gastrointestinal: difficulty swallowing, heartburn, flatulence, constipation.

Cardiovascular: tachycardia.

Musculoskeletal: leg pain, muscle fatigue.

Genitourinary: diuresis.

Miscellaneous: pruritus, fever, earache, nasal congestion, tinnitus, euphoria, allergic reactions.

Several cases of dermatological reactions, including toxic epidermal necrolysis and erythema multiforme, have been reported.

The following adverse drug events may be borne in mind as a potential effect of the components of this product. Potential effects of high dosage are listed in the OVERDOSAGE section.

Acetaminophen: allergic reactions, rash, thrombocytopenia, agranulocytosis.

DRUG ABUSE AND DEPENDENCE

Abuse and Dependence: Butalbital: *Barbiturates may be habit-forming:* Tolerance, psychological dependence, and physical dependence may occur especially following prolonged use of high doses of barbiturates. The average daily dose for the barbiturate addict is usually about 1500 mg. As tolerance to barbiturates develops, the amount needed to maintain the same level of intoxication increases; tolerance to a fatal dosage, however, does not increase more than two-fold. As this occurs, the margin between an intoxication dosage and fatal dosage becomes smaller. The lethal dose of a barbiturate is far less if alcohol is also ingested. Major withdrawal symptoms (convulsions and delirium) may occur within 16 hours and last up to 5 days after abrupt cessation of these drugs. Intensity of withdrawal symptoms gradually declines over a period of approximately 15 days. Treatment of barbiturate dependence consists of cautious and gradual withdrawal of the drug. Barbiturate-dependent patients can be withdrawn by using a number of different withdrawal regimens. One method involves initiating treatment at the patient's regular dosage level and gradually decreasing the daily dosage as tolerated by the patient.

OVERDOSAGE

Following an acute overdosage of butalbital and acetaminophen, toxicity may result from the barbiturate or the acetaminophen.

Signs and Symptoms: Toxicity from barbiturate poisoning include drowsiness, confusion, and coma; respiratory depression; hypotension; and hypovolemic shock.

In acetaminophen overdosage: dose-dependent, potentially fatal hepatic necrosis is the most serious adverse effect. Renal tubular necroses, hypoglycemic coma and thrombocytopenia may also occur. Early symptoms following a potentially hepatotoxic overdose may include: nausea, vomiting, diaphoresis and general malaise. Clinical and laboratory evidence of hepatic toxicity may not be apparent until 48 to 72 hours post-ingestion. In adults hepatic toxicity has rarely been reported with acute overdoses of less than 10 grams, or fatalities with less than 15 grams.

Treatment: A single or multiple overdose with this combination product is a potentially lethal polydrug overdose, and consultation with a regional poison control center is recommended.

Immediate treatment includes support of cardiorespiratory function and measures to reduce drug absorption. Vomiting should be induced mechanically, or with syrup of ipecac, if the patient is alert (adequate pharyngeal and laryngeal reflexes). Oral activated charcoal (1 g/kg) should follow gastric emptying. The first dose should be accompanied by an appropriate cathartic. If repeated doses are used, the cathartic might be included with alternate doses as required. Hypotension is usually hypovolemic and should respond to fluids. Pressors should be avoided. A cuffed endotracheal tube should be inserted before gastric lavage of the unconscious patient and, when necessary, to provide assisted respiration. If renal function is normal, forced diuresis may aid in the elimination of the barbiturate. Alkalinization of the urine increases renal excretion of some barbiturates, especially phenobarbital.

Meticulous attention should be given to maintaining adequate pulmonary ventilation. In severe cases of intoxication, peritoneal dialysis, or preferably hemodialysis may be considered. If hypoprothrombinemia occurs due to acetaminophen overdose, vitamin K should be administered intravenously.

If the dose of acetaminophen may have exceeded 140 mg/kg, acetylcysteine should be administered as early as possible. Serum acetaminophen levels should be obtained, since levels four or more hours following ingestion help predict acetaminophen toxicity. Do not await acetaminophen assay results before initiating treatment. Hepatic enzymes should be obtained initially, and repeated at 24-hour intervals.

Methemoglobinemia over 30% should be treated with methylene blue by slow intravenous administration.

Toxic Doses (for adults):

Butalbital: toxic dose 1 g (20 tablets)
Acetaminophen: toxic dose 10 g (15 tablets)

DOSAGE AND ADMINISTRATION

Oral: One table every four hours as needed. Total daily dosage should not exceed 6 tablets.

Extended and repeated use of this product is not recommended because of the potential for physical dependence.

HOW SUPPLIED

SEDAPAP® TABLETS (Butalbital and Acetaminophen Tablets) 50 mg/650 mg are supplied in bottles of 100 tablets, NDC 0259-0392-01. Each tablet contains butalbital 50 mg (Warning: May be habit forming) and acetaminophen 650 mg. Tablets are uncoated, white, capsule-shaped and are debossed "MP" score "392" on one side.

Storage: Protect from light and moisture. Store at controlled room temperature, 15° - 30°C (59° - 86°F).

Dispense in a tight, light-resistant container with a child-resistant closure.

CAUTION: Federal law prohibits dispensing without prescription.

MFG. FOR:
MERZ PHARMACEUTICALS™
Greensboro, NC 27407

BY:
MIKART, INC.
Atlanta, GA 30318

Rev. 4/97 Code 805A00
30-1168-00

For information on over-the-counter drugs, consult **PDR For Nonprescription Drugs**.

Methapharm, Inc.

2825 UNIVERSITY DRIVE
SUITE 240
CORAL SPRINGS, FLORIDA 33065

Direct Inquiries to:
(800) 287-7686
FAX: (877) 718-9222
www.methapharm.com
sales@methapharm.com

PROVOCHOLINE® ℞

brand of
methacholine chloride
POWDER FOR INHALATION
NOT FOR INJECTION

DESCRIPTION

Provocholine® (methacholine chloride powder for inhalation) is a parasympathomimetic (cholinergic) broncho-constrictor agent to be administered in solution only, by inhalation for diagnostic purposes. Each 20 mL vial contains 100 mg of methacholine chloride powder which is to be reconstituted with 0.9% sodium chloride injection containing 0.4% phenol (pH 7.0). See DOSAGE AND ADMINISTRATION for dilution procedures, concentrations and schedule of administration.

Chemically, methacholine chloride (the active ingredient) is 1-propanaminium, 2-(acetyloxy)-*N,N,N*, -trimethyl,-chloride. It is a white to practically white deliquescant compound, soluble in water. Methacholine chloride has an empirical formula of $C_3H_2ClNO_2$, a calculated molecular weight of 195.69, and the following structural formula:

$$\left[CH_3COOCHCH_2N^+(CH_3)_3 \atop \quad | \atop \quad CH_3 \right] Cl^-$$

HOW SUPPLIED

20-mL amber vials containing 100 mg of methacholine chloride powder which is to be reconstituted with 0.9% sodium chloride injection containing 0.4% phenol (pH 7.0)—boxes of 12 (NDC 64281-100-12) or boxes of 6 (NDC 64281-100-06). Store the powder at 59° to 86°F (15° to 30°C). Refrigerate the reconstituted solutions (dilutions A-D) at 36° to 46°F (2° to 8°C) for not more than 2 weeks. Dilution E must be prepared on the day of the challenge.

MGI PHARMA, Inc.

6300 WEST OLD SHAKOPEE ROAD
SUITE 110
BLOOMINGTON, MN 55438-2318

For Medical Information Contact:
Generally:
Medical Information and Adverse Drug Experiences
(800) 644-4811
FAX: (952) 346-4800

Customer Service
(800) 562-4531
FAX: (952) 346-4800

SALAGEN® TABLETS ℞

[*sal 'ə jən*]
(pilocarpine hydrochloride)

DESCRIPTION

SALAGEN® Tablets contain pilocarpine hydrochloride, a cholinergic agonist for oral use. Pilocarpine hydrochloride is a hygroscopic, odorless, bitter tasting white crystal or powder which is soluble in water and alcohol and virtually insoluble in most non-polar solvents. Pilocarpine hydrochloride, with a chemical name of (3*S-cis*)-2(3*H*)-Furanone, 3-ethyldihydro-4-[(1-methyl-1*H*-imidazol-5-yl)methyl] monohydrochloride, has a molecular weight of 244.72.

Each SALAGEN® Tablet for oral administration contains 5 mg of pilocarpine hydrochloride. Inactive ingredients in the tablet, the tablet's film coating, polishing, and branding are: carnauba wax, hydroxypropyl methylcellulose, iron oxide, microcrystalline cellulose, stearic acid, titanium dioxide and other ingredients.

CLINICAL PHARMACOLOGY

Pharmacodynamics: Pilocarpine is a cholinergic parasympathomimetic agent exerting a broad spectrum of pharmacologic effects with predominant muscarinic action. Pilocarpine, in appropriate dosage, can increase secretion by the exocrine glands. The sweat, salivary, lacrimal, gastric, pancreatic, and intestinal glands and the mucous cells of the respiratory tract may be stimulated. When applied topically to the eye as a single dose it causes miosis, spasm of accommodation, and may cause a transitory rise in intraocular pressure followed by a more persistent fall. Dose-related smooth muscle stimulation of the intestinal tract may cause increased tone, increased motility, spasm, and tenesmus. Bronchial smooth muscle tone may increase. The tone and motility of urinary tract, gallbladder, and biliary duct smooth muscle may be enhanced. Pilocarpine may have paradoxical effects on the cardiovascular system. The expected effect of a muscarinic agonist is vasodepression, but administration of pilocarpine may produce hypertension after a brief episode of hypotension. Bradycardia and tachycardia have both been reported with use of pilocarpine.

In a study of 12 healthy male volunteers there was a dose-related increase in unstimulated salivary flow following single 5 and 10 mg oral doses of SALAGEN® Tablets. This effect of pilocarpine on salivary flow was time-related with an onset at 20 minutes and a peak effect at 1 hour with a duration of 3 to 5 hours (See **Pharmacokinetics** section).

Head and Neck Cancer Patients: In a 12 week randomized, double-blind, placebo-controlled study in 207 patients (placebo, N=65; 5 mg, N=73; 10 mg, N=69), increases from baseline (means 0.072 and 0.112 mL/min, ranges −0.690 to 0.728 and −0.380 to 1.689) of whole saliva flow for the 5 mg (63%) and 10 mg (90%) tablet, respectively, were seen 1 hour after the first dose of SALAGEN® Tablets. Increases in unstimulated parotid flow were seen following the first dose (means 0.025 and 0.046 mL/min, ranges 0 to 0.414 and −0.070 to 1.002 mL/min for the 5 and 10 mg dose, respectively). In this study, no correlation existed between the amount of increase in salivary flow and the degree of symptomatic relief.

Sjögren's Syndrome Patients: In two 12 week randomized, double-blind, placebo-controlled studies in 629 patients (placebo, n=253; 2.5 mg, n=121; 5 mg, n=255; 5-7.5 mg, n=114), the ability of SALAGEN® Tablets to stimulate saliva production was assessed. In these trials using varying doses of SALAGEN® Tablets (2.5–7.5 mg), the rate of saliva production was plotted against time. An Area Under the Curve (AUC) representing the total amount of saliva produced during the observation interval was calculated. Relative to placebo, an increase in the amount of saliva being produced was observed following the first dose of SALAGEN® Tablets and was maintained throughout the duration (12 weeks) of the trials in an approximate dose response fashion (See **Clinical Studies** section).

Pharmacokinetics: In a multiple-dose pharmacokinetic study in male volunteers following 2 days of 5 or 10 mg of oral pilocarpine hydrochloride tablets given at 8 a.m., noontime, and 6 p.m., the mean elimination half-life was 0.76 hours for the 5 mg dose and 1.35 hours for the 10 mg dose. T_{max} values were 1.25 hours and 0.85 hours. C_{max} values were 15 ng/mL and 41 ng/mL. The AUC trapezoidal values were 33 h(ng/mL) and 108 h(ng/mL), respectively, for the 5 and 10 mg doses following the last 6 hour dose.

Pharmacokinetics in elderly male volunteers (n=11) were comparable to those in younger men. In five healthy elderly female volunteers, the mean C_{max} and AUC were approximately twice that of elderly males and young normal male volunteers.

When taken with a high fat meal by 12 healthy male volunteers, there was a decrease in the rate of absorption of pilocarpine from SALAGEN® Tablets. Mean $T_{max's}$ were 1.47 and 0.87 hours, and mean $C_{max's}$ were 51.8 and 59.2 ng/mL for fed and fasted, respectively.

Limited information is available about the metabolism and elimination of pilocarpine in humans. Inactivation of pilocarpine is thought to occur at neuronal synapses and probably in plasma. Pilocarpine and its minimally active or inactive degradation products, including pilocarpic acid, are excreted in the urine. Pilocarpine does not bind to human or rat plasma proteins over a concentration range of 5 to 25,000 ng/mL. The effect of pilocarpine on plasma protein binding of other drugs has not been evaluated.

Clinical Studies: *Head & Neck Cancer Patients:* A 12 week randomized, double-blind, placebo-controlled study in 207 patients (142 men, 65 women) was conducted in patients whose mean age was 58.5 years with a range of 19 to 77; the racial distribution was Caucasian 95%, Black 4%, and other 1%. In this population, a statistically significant improvement in mouth dryness occurred in the 5 and 10 mg SALAGEN® Tablet treated patients compared to placebo treated patients. The 5 and 10 mg treated patients could not be distinguished. (See **Pharmacodynamics** section for flow study details.)

Another 12 week, double-blind, randomized, placebo-controlled study was conducted in 162 patients whose mean

Continued on next page

Salagen—Cont.

age was 57.8 years with a range of 27 to 80; the racial distribution was Caucasian 88%, Black 10%, and other 2%. The effects of placebo were compared to 2.5 mg three times a day of SALAGEN® Tablets for 4 weeks followed by titration to 5 mg three times a day and 10 mg three times a day. Lowering of the dose was necessary because of adverse events in 3 of 67 patients treated with 5 mg of SALAGEN® Tablets and in 7 of 66 patients treated with 10 mg of SALAGEN® Tablets. After 4 weeks of treatment, 2.5 mg of SALAGEN® Tablets three times a day was comparable to placebo in relieving dryness. In patients treated with 5 mg and 10 mg of SALAGEN® Tablets, the greatest improvement in dryness was noted in patients with no measurable salivary flow at baseline.

In both studies, some patients noted improvement in the global assessment of their dry mouth, speaking without liquids, and a reduced need for supplemental oral comfort agents.

In the two placebo-controlled clinical trials, the most common adverse events related to drug, and increasing in rate as dose increases, were sweating, nausea, rhinitis, diarrhea, chills, flushing, urinary frequency, dizziness, and asthenia. The most common adverse experience causing withdrawal from treatment was sweating (5 mg t.i.d. ≤ 1%; 10 mg t.i.d.=12%).

Sjögren's Syndrome Patients: Two separate studies were conducted in patients with primary or secondary Sjögren's Syndrome. In both studies, the majority of patients best fit the European criteria for having primary Sjögren's Syndrome. ["Criteria for the Classification of Sjögren's Syndrome" (Vitali C, Bombardieri S, Moutsopoulos HM, et al: Preliminary criteria for the classification of Sjögren's syndrome. Arthritis Rheum 36:340–347, 1993.)]

A 12-week, randomized, double-blind, parallel-group, placebo-controlled study was conducted in 256 patients (14 men, 242 women) whose mean age was 57 years with a range of 24 to 85 years. The racial distribution was as follows: Caucasian 91%, Black 6%, and other 3%.

The effects of placebo were compared with those of SALAGEN® Tablets 5 mg four times a day (20 mg/day) for 6 weeks. At 6 weeks, the patients' dosage was increased from 5 mg SALAGEN® Tablets q.i.d. to 7.5 mg q.i.d. The data collected during the first 6 weeks of the trial were evaluated for safety and efficacy, and the data of the second 6 weeks of the trial were used to provide additional evidence of safety. After 6 weeks of treatment, statistically significant global improvement of dry mouth was observed compared to placebo. "Global improvement" is defined as a score of 55 mm or more on a 100 mm visual analogue scale in response to the question, "Please rate your present condition of dry mouth (xerostomia) compared with your condition at the start of this study. Consider the changes to your dry mouth and other symptoms related to your dry mouth that have occurred since you have taken this medication." Patients' assessments of specific dry mouth symptoms such as severity of dry mouth, mouth discomfort, ability to speak without water, ability to sleep without drinking water, ability to swallow food without drinking, and a decreased use of saliva substitutes were found to be consistent with the significant global improvement described.

Another 12 week randomized, double-blind, parallel-group, placebo-controlled study was conducted in 373 patients (16 men, 357 women) whose mean age was 55 years with a range of 21 to 84. The racial distribution was Caucasian 80%, Oriental 14%, Black 2%, and 4% of other origin. The treatment groups were 2.5 mg pilocarpine tablets, 5 mg SALAGEN® Tablets, and placebo. All treatments were administered on a four times a day regimen.

After 12 weeks of treatment, statistically significant global improvement of dry mouth was observed at a dose of 5 mg compared with placebo. The 2.5 mg (10mg/day) group was not significantly different than placebo. However, a subgroup of patients with rheumatoid arthritis tended to improve in global assessments at both the 2.5 mg q.i.d. (9 patients) and 5 mg q.i.d. (16 patients) dose (10–20 mg/day). The clinical significance of this finding is unknown.

Patients' assessments of specific dry mouth symptoms such as severity of dry mouth, mouth discomfort, ability to sleep without drinking water, and decreased use of saliva substitutes were also found to be consistent with the significant global improvement described when measured after 6 weeks and 12 weeks of SALAGEN® Tablets use.

INDICATIONS AND USAGE

SALAGEN® Tablets are indicated for 1) the treatment of symptoms of dry mouth from salivary gland hypofunction caused by radiotherapy for cancer of the head and neck; and 2) the treatment of symptoms of dry mouth in patients with Sjögren's syndrome.

CONTRAINDICATIONS

SALAGEN® Tablets are contraindicated in patients with uncontrolled asthma, known hypersensitivity to pilocarpine, and when miosis is undesirable, e.g., in acute iritis and in narrow-angle (angle closure) glaucoma.

WARNINGS

Cardiovascular Disease: Patients with significant cardiovascular disease may be unable to compensate for transient changes in hemodynamics or rhythm induced by pilocarpine. Pulmonary edema has been reported as a complication of pilocarpine toxicity from high ocular doses given for acute angle-closure glaucoma. Pilocarpine should be administered with caution in and under close medical supervision of patients with significant cardiovascular disease.

Ocular: Ocular formulations of pilocarpine have been reported to cause visual blurring which may result in decreased visual acuity, especially at night and in patients with central lens changes, and to cause impairment of depth perception. Caution should be advised while driving at night or performing hazardous activities in reduced lighting.

Pulmonary Disease: Pilocarpine has been reported to increase airway resistance, bronchial smooth muscle tone, and bronchial secretions. Pilocarpine hydrochloride should be administered with caution to and under close medical supervision in patients with controlled asthma, chronic bronchitis, or chronic obstructive pulmonary disease requiring pharmacotherapy.

PRECAUTIONS

General: Pilocarpine toxicity is characterized by an exaggeration of its parasympathomimetic effects. These may include: headache, visual disturbance, lacrimation, sweating, respiratory distress, gastrointestinal spasm, nausea, vomiting, diarrhea, atrioventricular block, tachycardia, bradycardia, hypotension, hypertension, shock, mental confusion, cardiac arrhythmia, and tremors.

The dose-related cardiovascular pharmacologic effects of pilocarpine include hypotension, hypertension, bradycardia, and tachycardia.

Pilocarpine should be administered with caution to patients with known or suspected cholelithiasis or biliary tract disease. Contractions of the gallbladder or biliary smooth muscle could precipitate complications including cholecystitis, cholangitis, and biliary obstruction.

Pilocarpine may increase ureteral smooth muscle tone and could theoretically precipitate renal colic (or "ureteral reflux"), particularly in patients with nephrolithiasis.

Cholinergic agonists may have dose-related central nervous system effects. This should be considered when treating patients with underlying cognitive or psychiatric disturbances.

Renal Insufficiency: The pharmacokinetics of orally administered pilocarpine in patients with renal and hepatic disease is not known.

Information for Patients: Patients should be informed that pilocarpine may cause visual disturbances, especially at night, that could impair their ability to drive safely.

If a patient sweats excessively while taking pilocarpine hydrochloride and cannot drink enough liquid, the patient should consult a physician. Dehydration may develop.

Drug Interactions: Pilocarpine should be administered with caution to patients taking beta adrenergic antagonists because of the possibility of conduction disturbances. Drugs with parasympathomimetic effects administered concurrently with pilocarpine would be expected to result in additive pharmacologic effects. Pilocarpine might antagonize the anticholinergic effects of drugs used concomitantly. These effects should be considered when anticholinergic properties may be contributing to the therapeutic effect of concomitant medication (e.g., atropine, inhaled ipratropium).

While no formal drug interaction studies have been performed, the following concomitant drugs were used in at least 10% of patients in either or both Sjögren's efficacy studies: acetylsalicylic acid, artificial tears, calcium, conjugated estrogens, hydroxychloroquine sulfate, ibuprofen, levothyroxine sodium, medroxyprogesterone acetate, methotrexate, multivitamins, naproxen, omeprazole, paracetamol, and prednisone.

Carcinogenesis, Mutagenesis, Impairment of Fertility: No definitive long term animal studies have evaluated the carcinogenic potential of pilocarpine. No evidence that pilocarpine has the potential to cause genetic toxicity was obtained in a series of studies that included: 1) bacterial assays (Salmonella and E. coli) for reverse gene mutations; 2) an *in vitro* chromosome aberration assay in a Chinese hamster ovary cell line; 3) an *in vivo* chromosome aberration assay (micronucleus test) in mice; and 4) a primary DNA damage assay (unscheduled DNA synthesis) in rat hepatocyte primary cultures.

Oral administration of pilocarpine to male and female rats at a dosage of 18 mg/kg/day (approximately 5 times the maximum recommended dose for a 50 kg human when compared on the basis of body surface area (mg/m^2) estimates) resulted in impaired reproductive function, including reduced fertility, decreased sperm motility, and morphologic evidence of abnormal sperm. It is unclear whether the reduction in fertility was due to effects on male animals, female animals, or both males and females. In dogs, exposure to pilocarpine at a dosage of 3 mg/kg/day (approximately 3 times the maximum recommended dose for a 50 kg human when compared on the basis of body surface area (mg/m^2) estimates) for six months resulted in evidence of impaired spermatogenesis. The data obtained in these studies suggest that pilocarpine may impair the fertility of male and female humans.

SALAGEN® Tablets should be administered to individuals who are attempting to conceive a child only if the potential benefit justifies potential impairment of fertility.

Pregnancy: Teratogenic effects

Pregnancy Category C: Pilocarpine was associated with a reduction in the mean fetal body weight and an increase in the incidence of skeletal variations when given to pregnant rats at a dosage of 90 mg/kg/day (approximately 26 times the maximum recommended dose for a 50 kg human when compared on the basis of body surface area (mg/m^2) estimates). These effects may have been secondary to maternal toxicity. In another study, oral administration of pilocarpine to female rats during gestation and lactation at a dosage of 36 mg/kg/day (approximately 10 times the maximum recommended dose for a 50 kg human when compared on the basis of body surface area (mg/m^2) estimates) resulted in an increased incidence of stillbirths; decreased neonatal survival and reduced mean body weight of pups were observed at dosages of 18 mg/kg/day (approximately 5 times the maximum recommended dose for a 50 kg human when compared on the basis of body surface area (mg/m^2) estimates) and above. There are no adequate and well-controlled studies in pregnant women. SALAGEN® Tablets should be used during pregnancy only if the potential benefit justifies the potential risk to the fetus.

Nursing Mothers: It is not known whether this drug is excreted in human milk. Because many drugs are excreted in human milk and because of the potential for serious adverse reactions in nursing infants from SALAGEN® Tablets, a decision should be made whether to discontinue nursing or to discontinue the drug, taking into account the importance of the drug to the mother.

Pediatric Use: Safety and effectiveness in pediatric patients have not been established.

Geriatric Use: *Head and Neck Cancer Patients:* In the placebo-controlled clinical trials (see Clinical Studies section) the mean age of patients was approximately 58 years (range 19 to 80). Of these patients, 97/369 (61/217 receiving pilocarpine) were over the age of 65 years. In the healthy volunteer studies, 15/150 subjects were over the age of 65 years. In both study populations, the adverse events reported by those over 65 years and those 65 years and younger were comparable. Of the 15 elderly volunteers (5 women, 10 men), the 5 women had higher $C_{max's}$ and AUC's than the men. (See **Pharmacokinetics** section.)

Sjögren's Syndrome Patients: In the placebo-controlled clinical trials (see **Clinical Studies** section), the mean age of patients was approximately 55 years (range 21 to 85). The adverse events reported by those over 65 years and those 65 years and younger were comparable except for notable trends for urinary frequency, diarrhea, and dizziness (see **ADVERSE REACTIONS** section).

ADVERSE REACTIONS

Head & Neck Cancer Patients: In controlled studies, 217 patients received pilocarpine, of whom 68% were men and 32% were women. Race distribution was 91% Caucasian, 8% Black, and 1% of other origin. Mean age was approximately 58 years. The majority of patients were between 50 and 64 years (51%), 33% were 65 years and older and 16% were younger than 50 years of age.

The most frequent adverse experiences associated with SALAGEN® Tablets were a consequence of the expected pharmacologic effects of pilocarpine.

Adverse Event	10 mg t.i.d. (30mg/day) n=121	5 mg t.i.d. (15mg/day) n=141	Placebo (t.i.d.) n=152
Sweating	68%	29%	9%
Nausea	15	6	4
Rhinitis	14	5	7
Diarrhea	7	4	5
Chills	15	3	<1
Flushing	13	8	3
Urinary Frequency	12	9	7
Dizziness	12	5	4
Asthenia	12	6	3

In addition, the following adverse events (≥3% incidence) were reported at dosages of 15–30 mg/day in the controlled clinical trials:

Adverse Event	Pilocarpine HCl 5-10 mg t.i.d. (15-30 mg/day) n=212	Placebo (t.i.d.) n=152
Headache	11%	8%
Dyspepsia	7	5
Lacrimation	6	8
Edema	5	4
Abdominal Pain	4	4
Amblyopia	4	2
Vomiting	4	1
Pharyngitis	3	8
Hypertension	3	1

The following events were reported with treated head and neck cancer patients at incidences of 1% to 2% at dosages of 7.5 to 30 mg/day: abnormal vision, conjunctivitis, dysphagia, epistaxis, myalgias, pruritus, rash, sinusitis, tachycardia, taste perversion, tremor, voice alteration.

The following events were reported rarely in treated head and neck cancer patients (<1%): Causal relation is unknown.

Body as a whole: body odor, hypothermia, mucous membrane abnormality

Cardiovascular: bradycardia, ECG abnormality, palpitations, syncope

Digestive: anorexia, increased appetite, esophagitis, gastrointestinal disorder, tongue disorder

Hematologic: leukopenia, lymphadenopathy

Nervous: anxiety, confusion, depression, abnormal dreams, hyperkinesia, hypesthesia, nervousness, paresthesias, speech disorder, twitching
Respiratory: increased sputum, stridor, yawning
Skin: seborrhea
Special senses: deafness, eye pain, glaucoma
Urogenital: dysuria, metrorrhagia, urinary impairment
In long-term treatment were two patients with underlying cardiovascular disease of whom one experienced a myocardial infarct and another an episode of syncope. The association with drug is uncertain.
Sjögren's Syndrome Patients: In controlled studies, 376 patients received pilocarpine, of whom 5% were men and 95% were women. Race distribution was 84% Caucasian, 9% Oriental, 3% Black, and 4% of other origin. Mean age was 55 years. The majority of patients were between 40 and 69 years (70%), 16% were 70 years and older and 14% were younger than 40 years of age. Of these patients, 161/629 (89/376 receiving pilocarpine) were over the age of 65 years. The adverse events reported by those over 65 years and those 65 years and younger were comparable except for notable trends for urinary frequency, diarrhea, and dizziness. The incidences of urinary frequency and diarrhea in the elderly were about double those in the non-elderly. The incidence of dizziness was about three times as high in the elderly as in the non-elderly. These adverse experiences were not considered to be serious. In the 2 placebo-controlled studies, the most common adverse events related to drug use were sweating, urinary frequency, chills, and vasodilatation (flushing). The most commonly reported reason for patient discontinuation of treatment was sweating. Expected pharmacologic effects of pilocarpine include the following adverse experiences associated with SALAGEN® Tablets:

Adverse Event	5 mg q.i.d. (20 mg/day) n=255	Placebo (q.i.d.) n=253
Sweating	40%	7%
Urinary Frequency	10	4
Nausea	9	9
Flushing	9	2
Rhinitis	7	8
Diarrhea	6	7
Chills	4	2
Increased Salivation	3	0
Asthenia	2	2

In addition, the following adverse events (≥3% incidence) were reported at dosing of 20 mg/day in the controlled clinical trials:

Adverse Event	Pilocarpine HCl 5 mg q.i.d. (20 mg/day) n=255	Placebo (q.i.d.) n=253
Headache	13%	19%
Flu Syndrome	9	9
Dyspepsia	7	7
Dizziness	6	7
Pain	4	2
Sinusitis	4	5
Abdominal Pain	3	4
Pharyngitis	2	5
Rash	2	3
Infection	2	6

The following events were reported in Sjögren's patients at incidences of 1% to 2% at dosing of 20 mg/day: accidental injury, allergic reaction, back pain, blurred vision, constipation, increased cough, edema, epistaxis, face edema, fever, flatulence, glossitis, lab test abnormalities, including chemistry, hematology, and urinalysis, myalgia, palpitation, pruritis, somnolence, stomatitis, tachycardia, tinnitus, urinary incontinence, urinary tract infection, vaginitis, vomiting.
The following events were reported rarely in treated Sjögren's patients (<1%): Causal relation is unknown.
Body as a whole: chest pain, cyst, death, moniliasis, neck pain, neck rigidity, photosensitivity reaction
Cardiovascular: angina pectoris, arrhythmia, ECG abnormality, hypotension, hypertension, intracranial hemorrhage, migraine, myocardial infarction
Digestive: anorexia, bilirubinemia, cholelithiasis, colitis, dry mouth, eructation, gastritis, gastroenteritis, gastrointestinal disorder, gingivitis, hepatitis, abnormal liver function tests, melena, nausea & vomiting, pancreatitis, parotid gland enlargement, salivary gland enlargement, sputum increased, taste loss, tongue disorder, tooth disorder
Hematologic: hematuria, lymphadenopathy, abnormal platelets, thrombocythemia, thrombocytopenia, thrombosis, abnormal WBC
Metabolic and Nutritional: peripheral edema, hypoglycemia
Musculoskeletal: arthralgia, arthritis, bone disorder, spontaneous bone fracture, pathological fracture, myasthenia, tendon disorder, tenosynovitis
Nervous: aphasia, confusion, depression, abnormal dreams, emotional lability, hyperkinesia, hypesthesia, insomnia, leg cramps, nervousness, paresthesias, abnormal thinking, tremor
Respiratory: bronchitis, dyspnea, hiccup, laryngismus, laryngitis, pneumonia, viral infection, voice alteration
Skin: alopecia, contact dermatitis, dry skin, eczema, erythema nodosum, exfoliative dermatitis, herpes simplex, skin ulcer, vesiculobullous rash
Special senses: cataract, conjunctivitis, dry eyes, ear disorder, ear pain, eye disorder, eye hemorrhage, glaucoma, lacrimation disorder, retinal disorder, taste perversion, abnormal vision
Urogenital: breast pain, dysuria, mastitis, menorrhagia, metrorrhagia, ovarian disorder, pyuria, salpingitis, urethral pain, urinary urgency, vaginal hemorrhage, vaginal moniliasis
The following adverse experiences have been reported rarely with ocular pilocarpine: A-V block, agitation, ciliary congestion, confusion, delusion, depression, dermatitis, middle ear disturbance, eyelid twitching, malignant glaucoma, iris cysts, macular hole, shock, and visual hallucination.

MANAGEMENT OF OVERDOSE

Fatal overdosage with pilocarpine has been reported in the scientific literature at doses presumed to be greater than 100 mg in two hospitalized patients. 100 mg of pilocarpine is considered potentially fatal. Overdosage should be treated with atropine titration (0.5 mg to 1.0 mg given subcutaneously or intravenously) and supportive measures to maintain respiration and circulation. Epinephrine (0.3 mg to 1.0 mg, subcutaneously or intramuscularly) may also be of value in the presence of severe cardiovascular depression or bronchoconstriction. It is not known if pilocarpine is dialyzable.

DOSAGE AND ADMINISTRATION

Head & Neck Cancer Patients:
The recommended initial dose of SALAGEN® Tablets is one tablet (5 mg) taken three times a day. Dosage should be titrated according to therapeutic response and tolerance. The usual dosage range is up to 3–6 tablets or 15–30 mg per day. (Not to exceed 2 tablets per dose.) Although early improvement may be realized, at least 12 weeks of uninterrupted therapy with SALAGEN® Tablets may be necessary to assess whether a beneficial response will be achieved. The incidence of the most common adverse events increases with dose. The lowest dose that is tolerated and effective should be used for maintenance.
Sjögren's Syndrome Patients:
The recommended dose of SALAGEN® Tablets is one tablet (5 mg) taken four times a day. Efficacy was established by 6 weeks of use.

HOW SUPPLIED

SALAGEN® Tablets, 5 mg, are white, film coated, round tablets, coded MGI 705. Each tablet contains 5 mg pilocarpine hydrochloride. They are supplied as follows:
NDC 58063-705-10 bottles of 100
Store at Controlled Room Temperature 15°–30°C (59°–86°F).
Manufactured by:
Global Pharm Inc. Toronto, Ontario, M3B 1Y5
For: MGI PHARMA, INC., Bloomington, MN 55438-2318
 February 1998
Salagen® is a registered trademark of MGI PHARMA, INC.
Shown in Product Identification Guide, page 324

Milex Products, Inc.

4311 N. NORMANDY
CHICAGO, IL 60634-1403

Direct Inquiries to:
1-800-621-1278

AMINO-CERV™ ℞

[ah-me 'no-serv]
pH 5.5 Cervical Creme

ACTIVE INGREDIENTS

Urea 8.34%, Sodium Propionate 0.50%, Methionine 0.83%, Cystine 0.35%, Inositol 0.83%. Buffered to pH of 5.5 in a water-miscible creme base.

DESCRIPTION

An AMINO-ACID and UREA creme specifically formulated for cervical treatment: Cervicitis (mild), postpartum cervicitis, postpartum cervical tears, post surgical cervical procedures.

ADVANTAGES

METHIONINE and CYSTINE are amino-acids necessary for wound healing and forming of epithelial tissue. INOSITOL acts as an essential growth factor and promotes epithelialization.
UREA aids in debridement, dissolves the coagulum and promotes epithelialization. Its solvent action on fibroblasts prevents the formation of excessive tissue—thus preventing stenosis when used as directed.
SODIUM PROPIONATE is a topical antifungal agent.
AMINO-CERV is geared to the higher pH of the healthy cervix in contrast with pH 4 vaginal preparations. With its pH factor of 5.5 Amino-Cerv promotes faster healing of the cervix, yet will not adversely affect a healthy vagina.

DIRECTIONS

When immediate postpartum bleeding has subsided (usually from 24 to 48 hours after delivery), one Milex Jector full of AMINO-CERV creme should be applied nightly for four weeks. In mild cervicitis (not requiring cautery or cryosurgery) one applicatorful of AMINO-CERV should be injected in the vagina nightly upon retiring for 2 weeks. A small amount of AMINO-CERV should be applied immediately following a surgical cervical procedure with the exception of a cold coning procedure. One applicatorful should be injected nightly upon retiring for 2 to 4 weeks (the duration of treatment depends on extent of the surgical procedure). In each of the post surgical visits, the physician should again apply a small amount of AMINO-CERV with a probe or applicator. The canal is to be completely probed on the last visit.
After COLD CONING, one applicatorful should be injected upon retiring about 24 hours after surgery and nightly thereafter for four weeks. During the four weekly office visits following cold coning, a small amount of AMINO-CERV should be applied with a probe or applicator into the canal by the physician. The canal is to be completely probed on the last visit.
Reasons For Variation of Directions
(1) After most surgical procedures, cauterization, cryosurgery and laser surgery, immediate use of AMINO-CERV is indicated to aid in dissolving dead or burned tissue.
(2) After cold coning, there is no dead tissue to slough off. Therefore, a wait of 24 hours or longer is desirable for normal healing to take place and for some fibroblasts to be laid down before applying the AMINO-CERV (which has a solvent action on both the fibroblasts and the absorbable sutures). When NONABSORBABLE sutures are used, AMINO-CERV can be used immediately.

CONTRAINDICATIONS

Deleterious side effects have not been a problem at the doses recommended. The usual precautions against allergic reactions should be observed.

STORAGE

Store at room temperature.

PACKAGING

2³/₄ oz. tube with MILEX-JECTOR (2 weeks supply, 14 applications).

Mission Pharmacal Company

10999 IH 10 WEST
SUITE 1000
SAN ANTONIO, TX 78230-1355

Direct Inquiries to:
PO Box 786099
San Antonio, TX 78278–6099
TOLL FREE: (800) 292-7364
(210) 696-8400
FAX: (210) 696-6010
For Medical Information Contact:
In Emergencies:
George Alexandrides
(830) 249-9822
FAX: (830) 816-2545

CITRACAL® 250 MG + D

[sit 'ra-cal]
ultradense calcium citrate-Vitamin D dietary supplement

INGREDIENTS

Each tablet contains: calcium (as Ultradense™ calcium citrate) 250 mg., polyethylene glycol, citric acid, microcrystalline cellulose, HPMC, croscarmellose sodium, color added, magnesium silicate, magnesium stearate, vitamin D_3 (62.5 IU).

HOW SUPPLIED

CITRACAL® 250 MG + D is available in bottles of 150 tablets, UPC 0178-0837-15.

CITRACAL® Ⓤ

[sit 'ra-cal]
ultradense calcium citrate dietary supplement

INGREDIENTS

Calcium (as Ultradense™ calcium citrate) 200 mg., polyethylene glycol, croscarmellose sodium, HPMC, color added, magnesium silicate, magnesium stearate.

Continued on next page

Citracal Tablets—Cont.

SENSITIVE PATIENTS

CITRACAL® contains no wheat, barley, yeast or rye; is sugar, dairy and gluten free and contains no artificial colors.

ONE TABLET PROVIDES

200 mg. calcium (elemental), equaling 20% of the U.S. recommended daily allowance for adults and children 4 or more years of age.

FOUR TABLETS PROVIDE

800 mg. calcium (elemental), equaling 80% of the U.S. recommended daily allowance for adults and children 4 or more years of age.

DIRECTIONS

Take 1 to 2 tablets twice daily or as recommended by a physician, pharmacist or health professional.

HOW SUPPLIED

CITRACAL® is supplied as white, nearly oval shaped, coated tablets in bottles of 100 UPC 0178-0800-01, and bottles of 200 UPC 0178-0800-20.
Ⓤ = Kosher Parvae approved by Orthodox Union.

CITRACAL® Caplets + D

[sit 'ra-cal]
ultradense calcium citrate dietary supplement

INGREDIENTS

CITRACAL® Caplets + D are supplied in an ultra-dense caplet formulation, each containing calcium (as Ultradense™ calcium citrate) 315 mg., polyethylene glycol, croscarmellose sodium, HPMC, color added, magnesium silicate, magnesium stearate, vitamin D_3 (200IU).

HOW SUPPLIED

CITRACAL® Caplets + D are available in bottles of 60 UPC 0178-0815-60; bottles of 120 UPC 0178-0815-12, and bottles of 180 UPC 0178-0815-18.

CITRACAL® LIQUITAB® Ⓤ

[sit 'ra-cal]
calcium citrate dietary supplement

INGREDIENTS: CITRACAL® LIQUITAB® is supplied as effervescent tablets each containing calcium (as calcium citrate) 500 mg., citric acid, adipic acid, saccharin sodium, orange flavor, cellulose gum, aspartame.

This product contains NutraSweet®.
Phenylketonurics: Contains 6 mg. phenylalanine per tablet.

HOW SUPPLIED

CITRACAL® LIQUITAB® is available in bottles of 30 effervescent tablets. UPC 0178-0811-30.
Ⓤ = Kosher Parvae Approved by Orthodox Union

CITRACAL® PLUS

[sit 'ra-cal]
ultradense calcium citrate-Vitamin D-multi-mineral dietary supplement

INGREDIENTS

Each tablet contains: calcium (as Ultradense™ calcium citrate) 250 mg., polyethylene glycol, magnesium oxide, hydroxypropyl methylcellulose, povidone, croscarmellose sodium, color added, HPMC, zinc oxide, sodium borate, manganese gluconate, magnesium silicate, maltodextrin, copper gluconate, magnesium stearate, carnauba wax, vitamin D_3 (125 IU).

HOW SUPPLIED

CITRACAL® PLUS is available in bottles of 150 tablets, UPC 0178-0825-15.

CALCET®

[kăl 'sĕt]
Calcium-Vit. D Dietary Supplement
UPC-0178-0251-01

HOW SUPPLIED

CALCET® tablets are supplied as yellow, rectangular shaped, coated tablets in bottles of 100 tablets.

CALCET® PLUS

[kăl 'sĕt]
Calcium-Iron-Zinc-Multivitamin
UPC 0178-0252-60

> **WARNING:** Accidental overdose of **iron-containing** products is a leading cause of fatal poisoning in children under 6. Keep this product out of reach of children. In case of accidental overdose, call a doctor or poison control center immediately.

HOW SUPPLIED

CALCET PLUS tablets are supplied as white, elliptical shaped, coated tablets in bottles of 60's.

FOSFREE®

[fos 'frē]
Calcium—Iron—Multivitamin
UPC 0178-0031-60
UPC 0178-0031-12

> **WARNING:** Accidental overdose of **iron-containing** products is a leading cause of fatal poisoning in children under 6. Keep this product out of reach of children. In case of accidental overdose, call a doctor or poison control center immediately. If you are pregnant or nursing a baby, seek the advice of a health professional before using this product.

HOW SUPPLIED

FOSFREE® is supplied as yellow, elliptical shaped, coated tablets in bottles of either 60 or 120 tablets.

IROMIN®–G

[i 'rō-min]
Hematinic Dietary Supplement
UPC-0178-0081-01

> **WARNING:** Accidental overdose of **iron-containing** products is a leading cause of fatal poisoning in children under 6. Keep this product out of reach of children. In case of accidental overdose, call a doctor or poison control center immediately.

HOW SUPPLIED

IROMIN-G® is supplied as red rectangular shaped coated tablets in bottles of 100 tablets.

MISSION PRENATAL DIETARY SUPPLEMENT SERIES

MISSION® PRENATAL

Vitamins—Iron—Calcium—0.4 mg. Folic Acid
UPC 0178-0132-01

MISSION® PRENATAL F.A.

Vitamins—Iron—Calcium—Zinc—0.8 mg. Folic Acid
UPC 0178-0153-01

MISSION® PRENATAL H.P.

Vitamins—Iron—Calcium—0.8 mg. Folic Acid
UPC 0178-0161-01

> **WARNING:** Accidental overdose of **iron-containing** products is a leading cause of fatal poisoning in children under 6. Keep this product out of reach of children. In case of accidental overdose, call a doctor or poison control center immediately.

HOW SUPPLIED

MISSION® PRENATAL is supplied as salmon, rectangular-shaped, sugar-coated tablets in bottles of 100.
MISSION® PRENATAL F.A. is supplied as blue, rectangular-shaped, sugar coated tablets in bottles of 100.
MISSION® PRENATAL H.P. is supplied as green, rectangular-shaped, sugar-coated tablets in bottles of 100.

CITRACAL® PRENATAL Rx TABLETS ℞

[sit'ra-cal]
PRENATAL VITAMINS

DESCRIPTION

Citracal Prenatal Rx is a scored, white, oval multivitamin/multimineral tablet. The tablet is embossed "CITRACAL" on one side and "PN RX" on the other side.
Each tablet contains:

Vitamin A (Vitamin A palmitate)	2700 IU
Vitamin C (Ascorbic acid)	120 mg
Calcium (Calcium citrate)	125 mg
Iron (Carbonyl iron, Ferrous gluconate)	27 mg
Vitamin D3 (Cholecalciferol)	400 IU
Vitamin E (dl-alpha tocopheryl acetate)	30 IU
Thiamine (Vitamin B_1)	3 mg
Riboflavin (Vitamin B_2)	3.4 mg
Niacinamide (Vitamin B_3)	20 mg
Pyridoxine HCl (Vitamin B_6)	20 mg
Folic Acid	1 mg
Iodine (Potassium iodide)	150 mcg
Zinc (Zinc oxide)	25 mg
Copper (Cupric oxide)	2 mg
Docusate Sodium	50 mg

INDICATIONS

CITRACAL PRENATAL Rx is a multivitamin/multimineral prescription drug indicated for use in improving the nutritional status of women prior to conception, throughout pregnancy, and in the postnatal period for both lactating and nonlactating mothers.

CONTRAINDICATIONS

This product is contraindicated in patients with a known hypersensitivity to any of the ingredients.

> WARNING
> **Accidental overdose of iron-containing products is a leading cause of fatal poisoning in children under 6. KEEP THIS PRODUCT OUT OF THE REACH OF CHILDREN. In case of accidental overdose, call a doctor or poison control center immediately.**

Folic acid alone is improper therapy in the treatment of pernicious anemia and other megaloblastic anemias where Vitamin B_{12} is deficient.

NOTICE

Contact with moisture may produce surface discoloration or erosion of the tablet.

PRECAUTIONS

Folic acid in doses above 0.1 mg may obscure pernicious anemia in that hematologic remission can occur while neurological manifestations progress.

ADVERSE REACTIONS

Allergic sensitization has been reported following both oral and parenteral administration of folic acid.

DOSAGE AND ADMINISTRATION

One tablet daily or as directed by a physician.

HOW SUPPLIED

100's–NDC 0178-0852-01
DISPENSE IN A TIGHT, LIGHT-RESISTANT CONTAINER AS DEFINED BY THE USP/NF WITH A CHILD-RESISTANT CLOSURE.
Store at controlled room temperature.
U.S. Patent 4,814,177 Other Patent(s) pending

MISSION PHARMACAL UROLOGICALS

UROCIT®–K ℞

[yu 'ro-cit kay]
Potassium Citrate

DESCRIPTION

Urocit®-K is a citrate salt of potassium. Its empirical formula is $K_3C_6H_5O_7 \cdot H_2O$, and its structural formula is:

$$\mathrm{HO-C(CH_2-COOK)_2-COOK \cdot H_2O}$$

Potassium citrate is a white granular powder that is soluble in water at 154 g/100 ml, almost insoluble in alcohol, and insoluble in organic solvents.
Urocit®-K is supplied as wax matrix tablets, containing 5 meq (540 mg) potassium citrate and 10 meq (1080 mg) potassium citrate each, for oral administration.

CLINICAL PHARMACOLOGY

When Urocit®-K is given orally, the metabolism of absorbed citrate produces an alkaline load. The induced alkaline load in turn increases urinary pH and raises urinary citrate by augmenting citrate clearance without measurably altering ultrafilterable serum citrate. Thus, Urocit®-K therapy appears to increase urinary citrate principally by modifying the renal handling of citrate, rather than by increasing the filtered load of citrate. The increased filtered load of citrate may play some role, however, as in small comparisons of oral citrate and oral bicarbonate, citrate had a greater effect on urinary citrate.
In addition to raising urinary pH and citrate, Urocit®-K increases urinary potassium by approximately the amount contained in the medication. In some patients, Urocit®-K causes a transient reduction in urinary calcium.
The changes induced by Urocit®-K produce a urine that is less conducive to the crystallization of stone-forming salts (calcium oxalate, calcium phosphate and uric acid). Increased citrate in the urine, by complexing with calcium, decreases calcium ion activity and thus the saturation of calcium oxalate. Citrate also inhibits the spontaneous nucleation of calcium oxalate and calcium phosphate (brushite). The increase in urinary pH also decreases calcium ion activity by increasing calcium complexation to dissociated anions. The rise in urinary pH also increases the ionization of uric acid to more soluble urate ion.
Urocit®-K therapy does not alter the urinary saturation of calcium phosphate, since the effect of increased citrate com-

plexation of calcium is opposed by the rise in pH-dependent dissociation of phosphate. Calcium phosphate stones are more stable in alkaline urine.

In the setting of normal renal function, the rise in urinary citrate following a single dose begins by the first hour and lasts for 12 hours. With multiple doses the rise in citrate excretion reaches its peak by the third day and averts the normally wide circadian fluctuation in urinary citrate, thus maintaining urinary citrate at a higher, more constant level throughout the day. When the treatment is withdrawn, urinary citrate begins to decline toward the pre-treatment level on the first day.

The rise in citrate excretion is directly dependent on the Urocit®-K dosage. Following long-term treatment, Urocit®-K at a dosage of 60 meq/day raises urinary citrate by approximately 400 mg/day and increases urinary pH by approximately 0.7 units.

In patients with severe renal tubular acidosis or chronic diarrheal syndrome where urinary citrate may be very low (<100 mg/day), Urocit®-K may be relatively ineffective in raising urinary citrate. A higher dose of Urocit®-K may therefore be required to produce a satisfactory citraturic response. In patients with renal tubular acidosis in whom urinary pH may be high, Urocit®-K produces a relatively small rise in urinary pH.

INDICATIONS AND USAGE

Potassium citrate is indicated for the management of renal tubular acidosis (RTA) with calcium stones, hypocitraturic calcium oxalate nephrolithiasis of any etiology, and uric acid lithiasis with or without calcium stones.

CONTRAINDICATIONS

Urocit®-K is contraindicated in patients with hyperkalemia (or who have conditions predisposing them to hyperkalemia, as a further rise in serum potassium concentration may produce cardiac arrest. Such conditions include: chronic renal failure, uncontrolled diabetes mellitus, acute dehydration, strenuous physical exercise in unconditioned individuals, adrenal insufficiency, extensive tissue breakdown, or the administration of a potassium-sparing agent (such as triamterene, spironolactone or amiloride).

Urocit®-K is contraindicated in patients in whom there is cause for arrest or delay in tablet passage through the gastrointestinal tract, such as those suffering from delayed gastric emptying, esophageal compression, intestinal obstruction or stricture or those taking anticholinergic medication. Because of its ulcerogenic potential, Urocit®-K should not be given to patients with peptic ulcer disease.

Urocit®-K is contraindicated in patients with active urinary tract infection (with either urea-splitting or other organisms, in association with either calcium or struvite stones). The ability of Urocit®-K to increase urinary citrate may be attenuated by bacterial enzymatic degradation of citrate. Moreover, the rise in urinary pH resulting from Urocit®-K therapy might promote further bacterial growth.

Urocit®-K is contraindicated in patients with renal insufficiency (glomerular filtration rate of less than 0.7 ml/kg/min), because of the danger of soft tissue calcification and increased risk for the development of hyperkalemia.

WARNINGS

HYPERKALEMIA: In patients with impaired mechanisms for excreting potassium, Urocit®-K administration can produce hyperkalemia and cardiac arrest. Potentially fatal hyperkalemia can develop rapidly and be asymptomatic. The use of Urocit®-K in patients with chronic renal failure, or any other condition which impairs potassium excretion such as severe myocardial damage or heart failure, should be avoided.

INTERACTION WITH POTASSIUM-SPARING DIURETICS

Concomitant administration of Urocit®-K and a potassium-sparing diuretic (such as triamterene, spironolactone or amiloride) should be avoided, since the simultaneous administration of these agents can produce severe hyperkalemia.

GASTROINTESTINAL LESIONS

Because of reports of upper gastrointestinal mucosal lesions following administration of potassium chloride (wax-matrix), and endoscopic examination of the upper gastrointestinal mucosa was performed in 30 normal volunteers after they had taken glycopyrrolate 2 mg. p.o. t.i.d., Urocit®-K 95 meq/day, wax-matrix potassium chloride 96 meq/day or wax matrix placebo, in thrice daily schedule in the fasting state for one week. Urocit®-K and the wax-matrix formulation of potassium chloride were indistinguishable but both were significantly more irritating than the wax-matrix placebo. In a subsequent similar study, lesions were less severe when glycopyrrolate was omitted.

Solid dosage forms of potassium chloride have produced stenotic and/or ulcerative lesions of the small bowel and deaths. These lesions are caused by a high local concentration of potassium ions in the region of the dissolving tablets, which injured the bowel. In addition, perhaps because wax-matrix preparations are not enteric-coated and release some of their potassium content in the stomach, there have been reports of upper gastrointestinal bleeding associated with these products. The frequency of gastrointestinal lesions with wax-matrix potassium chloride products is estimated at one per 100,000 patient-years. Experience with Urocit®-K is limited, but a similar frequency of gastrointestinal lesions should be anticipated.

If there is severe vomiting, abdominal pain or gastro-intestinal bleeding, Urocit®-K should be discontinued immediately and the possibility of bowel perforation or obstruction investigated.

PRECAUTIONS

Information For Patients:

Physicians should consider reminding the patient of the following:

To take each dose without crushing, chewing or sucking the tablet.

To take this medicine only as directed. This is especially important if the patient is also taking both diuretics and digitalis preparations.

To check with physician if there is trouble swallowing tablets or if the tablet seems to stick in the throat.

To check with the doctor at once if tarry stools or other evidence of gastrointestinal bleeding is noticed.

Laboratory Tests: Regular serum potassium determinations are recommended. Careful attention should be paid to acid-base balance, other serum electrolyte levels, the electrocardiogram, and the clinical status of the patient, particularly in the presence of cardiac disease, renal disease or acidosis.

Drug Interactions: POTASSIUM-SPARING DIURETICS: See WARNINGS section.

DRUGS THAT SLOW GASTROINTESTINAL TRANSIT TIME (such as anticholinergics) can be expected to increase the gastrointestinal irritation produced by potassium salts. (See CONTRAINDICATIONS section).

Carcinogenesis, Mutagenesis, Impairment Of Fertility: Long-term carcinogenicity studies in animals have not been performed.

Pregnancy Category C: Animal reproduction studies have not been conducted with Urocit®-K. It is also not known whether Urocit®-K can cause fetal harm when administered to a pregnant woman or can affect reproduction capacity. Urocit®-K should be given to a pregnant woman only if clearly needed.

Nursing Mothers: The normal potassium ion content of human milk is about 13 meq/l. It is not known if Urocit®-K has an effect on this content. Caution should be exercised when Urocit®-K is administered to a nursing woman.

Pediatric Use: Safety and effectiveness in children have not been established.

ADVERSE REACTIONS

Some patients may develop minor gastrointestinal complaints during Urocit®-K therapy, such as abdominal discomfort, vomiting, diarrhea, loose bowel movements or nausea. These symptoms are due to the irritation of the gastrointestinal tract, and may be alleviated by taking the dose with meals or snack, or by reducing the dosage. Patients may find intact matrices in feces. (See also CONTRAINDICATIONS, WARNINGS)

OVERDOSAGE

The administration of potassium salts to persons without predisposing conditions for hyperkalemia (see CONTRAINDICATIONS) rarely causes serious hyperkalemia at recommended dosages. It is important to recognize that hyperkalemia is usually asymptomatic and may be manifested only by an increased serum potassium concentration and characteristic electrocardiographic changes (peaking of T-wave, loss of P-wave, depression of S-T segment and prolongation of the QT interval). Late manifestations include muscle paralysis and cardiovascular collapse from cardiac arrest.

Treatment measures for hyperkalemia include the following: (1) elimination of potassium-rich foods, medications containing potassium, and of potassium-sparing diuretics, (2) intravenous administration of 300–500 ml/hr of 10% dextrose solution containing 10–20 units of insulin/1000 ml, (3) correction of acidosis, if present, with intravenous sodium bicarbonate, and (4) use of exchange resins, hemodialysis or peritoneal dialysis.

In treating hyperkalemia, it should be recalled that in patients who have been stabilized on digitalis, too rapid a lowering of the serum potassium concentration can produce digitalis toxicity.

DOSAGE AND ADMINISTRATION

Treatment with Urocit®-K should be added to a regimen that limits salt intake (avoidance of foods with high salt content and of added salt at the table) and encourages high fluid intake (urine volume should be at least two liters per day). The objective of treatment with Urocit®-K is to provide Urocit®-K in sufficient dosage to restore normal urinary citrate (greater than 320 mg/day and as close to the normal mean of 640 mg/day as possible), and to increase urinary pH to a level of 6.0 to 7.0.

In patients with severe hypocitraturia (urinary citrate of less than 150 mg/day), therapy should be initiated at a dosage of 60 meq/day (20 meq three times/day or 15 meq four times/day with meals or within 30 minutes after meals or bedtime snack). In patients with mild-moderate hypocitraturia (>150 mg/day), Urocit®-K should be initiated at a dosage of 30 meq/day (10 meq three times/day with meals).

Twenty-four hour urinary citrate and/or urinary pH measurements should be used to determine the adequacy of the initial dosage and to evaluate the effectiveness of any dosage change. In addition, urinary citrate and/or pH should be measured every four months.

Doses of Urocit®-K greater than 100 meq/day have not been studied and should be avoided.

Serum electrolytes (sodium, potassium, chloride and carbon dioxide), serum creatinine, and complete blood count should be monitored every four months. Treatment should be discontinued if there is hyperkalemia, a significant rise in serum creatinine, or a significant fall in blood hematocrit or hemoglobin.

HOW SUPPLIED

Urocit®-K is available for oral administration in tablet form in the following sizes: (NDC 0178-0600-01) 5 meq potassium citrate and (NDC 0178-0610-01) 10 meq potassium citrate, packaged in bottles of 100 each.

Store in tight container.

Rev. 09980

LITHOSTAT® ℞

[lith 'o-stat]

Acetohydroxamic Acid (AHA)

DESCRIPTION

Acetohydroxamic acid (AHA) is a stable, synthetic compound derived from hydroxylamine and ethyl acetate. Its molecular structure is similar to urea:

ACETOHYDROXAMIC ACID (AHA)

AHA is weakly acidic, highly soluble in water, and chelates metals - notably iron. The molecular weight is 75.068. AHA has a pKa of 9.32 and a melting point of 89–91°C. AHA is a urease inhibitor. Available as 250 mg tablets.

HOW SUPPLIED

LITHOSTAT®, NDC 0178-0500-01, is available for oral administration as 250 mg white colored, round tablets, in unit of use packages of 100 tablets.

THIOLA™ ℞

[thi-ól-a]

Tiopronin Tablets

DESCRIPTION

THIOLA™ (Tiopronin) is a reducing and complexing thiol compound. Tiopronin is N-(2-Mercaptopropionyl) glycine and has the following structure:

CH_3–CH(SH)–CONHCH_2–COOH

Tiopronin has the empirical formula $C_5H_9NO_3S$ and a molecular weight of 163.20. In this drug product tiopronin exists as a dl racemic mixture.

Tiopronin is a white crystalline powder which is freely soluble in water.

THIOLA™ tablets are white sugar coated tablets, each containing 100 mg. of Tiopronin and are taken orally.

HOW SUPPLIED

THIOLA™ (NDC 0178-0900-01), is available for oral administration as 100 mg. round, white, sugar coated tablets in bottles of 100 tablets each.

CALCIBIND® ℞

[kal 'sĕ-bīnd]

Cellulose Sodium Phosphate Oral Powder

DESCRIPTION

Cellulose Sodium Phosphate (CSP), the active ingredient in CALCIBIND®, is a synthetic compound made by phosphorylation of cellulose and has the following structural formula:

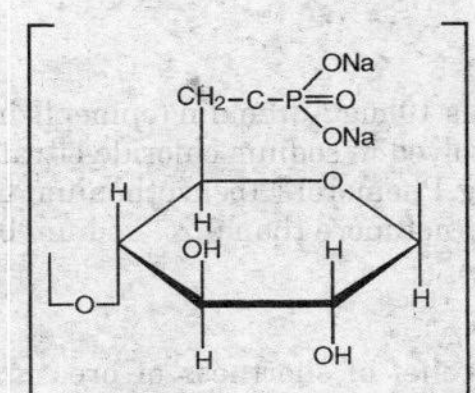

Where n indicates the degree of polymerization and has an average value of approximately 3000. The molecular weight of CSP monomer is 286.1 and the average molecular weight of the polymer is 858,000.

It has an inorganic bound phosphate of 31–36%, free phosphate of 3.5%, sodium content of approximately 11% and a

Continued on next page

Calcibind—Cont.

calcium binding capacity of 1.8 mmol of Ca per gram of the oral powder. It has excellent ion exchange properties, the sodium ion exchanging for calcium. When taken orally, CSP binds calcium, the complex of calcium and cellulose phosphate being excreted in feces. The dosage of CALCIBIND® is powder for oral administration.

HOW SUPPLIED

CALCIBIND® NDC 0178-0255-30 is available for oral administration in bottles of 300 grams of CSP bulk powder.

THERA-GESIC® OTC

[thĕr 'ə-jē-zik]
(Methyl Salicylate 15%, Menthol 1%)
TOPICAL THERAPEUTIC ANALGESIC CREME

DESCRIPTION

THERA-GESIC® contains methyl salicylate and menthol in a rapidly absorbed greaseless base containing carbomer 934, dimethicone, glycerine, methylparaben, propylparaben, sodium laurel sulfate, trolamine, water.

INDICATION

Effective temporary relief of arthritis pain and muscle soreness.

WARNINGS

FOR EXTERNAL USE ONLY. Use only as directed. Keep away from children to avoid accidental poisoning. Keep away from eyes, mucous membranes, broken or irritated skin. Do not use THERA-GESIC® if you have skin sensitive to oil of wintergreen (methyl salicylate). If skin irritation develops, if pain lasts 7 days or more, or if redness is present, discontinue use and consult a physician immediately. DO NOT SWALLOW. If swallowed induce vomiting, call a physician. Contact a physician before applying this medicine to children, including teenagers with chicken pox or flu.

DIRECTIONS

ADULTS AND CHILDREN 12 OR MORE YEARS OF AGE: An application of THERA-GESIC® is the gentle massaging of several thin layers of creme into and around the sore or painful area. The number of thin layers controls the intensity of the action. One thin layer provides a mild effect, two thin layers provide a strong effect and three thin layers provide a very strong effect. Do not apply more than 3 to 4 times daily. Once THERA-GESIC® has penetrated the skin, the area may be washed, leaving it dry, clean and fragrance-free without decreasing the effectiveness of the product. IF YOU INTEND TO WRAP, BANDAGE OR COVER THE AREA WHERE YOU HAVE APPLIED THERA-GESIC®, IT MUST BE WASHED THOROUGHLY TO AVOID EXCESSIVE IRRITATION. DO NOT USE A HEATING PAD AFTER APPLICATION OF THERA-GESIC®.

HOW SUPPLIED

NDC 0178-0320-03 3 oz. tube
NDC 0178-0320-05 5 oz. tube

Monarch Pharmaceuticals

501 FIFTH STREET
BRISTOL, TN 37620

Direct Inquiries to:
800-776-3637
FAX: 423-989-6279

Medical Emergency Contact:
Kathy Montgomery
800-546-4906
248-650-6407

ADRENALIN® CHLORIDE SOLUTION ℞

(Epinephrine Inhalation Solution, USP)
1:100 Bronchodilator

DESCRIPTION

Each mL contains 10 mg Adrenalin (epinephrine) as the hydrochloride, dissolved in sodium chloride-citrate buffer solution with 0.2 mg Phemerol® (benzethonium chloride) as a preservative and not more than 0.2% sodium bisulfite as an antioxidant.

INDICATIONS

For temporary relief of shortness of breath, tightness of chest, and wheezing due to bronchial asthma. The inhalation of Adrenalin Chloride Solution 1:100 eases breathing for asthma patients by reducing spasms of bronchial muscles.

WARNINGS

Adrenalin Chloride Solution 1:100 is supplied for use by oral (not nasal) inhalation only. Because of the relatively high concentration, Adrenalin Chloride Solution 1:100 is not suitable for hypodermic injection.

Do not use this product unless a diagnosis of asthma has been made by a physician.

Do not use this product if you have heart disease, high blood pressure, thyroid disease, or difficulty in urination due to enlargement of the prostate gland unless directed by a physician. Do not use this product if you have ever been hospitalized for asthma or if you are taking any prescription drug for asthma unless directed by a physician.

Drug interaction precaution: Do not use this product if you are presently taking a prescription drug for high blood pressure or depression without first consulting your physician.

Do not use this product more frequently or at higher doses than recommended unless directed by a physician. Excessive use may cause nervousness and rapid heart beat and, possibly, adverse effects on the heart.

Do not continue to use this product but seek medical assistance immediately if symptoms are not relieved within 20 minutes or become worse.

Do not use the inhalation solution if it is pinkish or darker than slightly yellow or if it contains a precipitate.

As with any drug, if you are pregnant or nursing a baby, seek the advice of a health professional before using this product.

DIRECTIONS

For relief of bronchial congestion in asthma, Adrenalin Chloride Solution 1:100 should be applied with a glass or plastic nebulizer capable of delivering a very fine spray, and which will work with a very small amount of solution.

Approximately 10 drops (not more) of Adrenalin Chloride Solution 1:100 are placed in the reservoir of the nebulizer, the nozzle of which is placed just inside the partially opened mouth. As the bulb is squeezed once or twice the patient inhales deeply, drawing the vaporized solution into the lungs. Treatment should be started at the first symptoms. Rinsing the mouth with water immediately after using Adrenalin Chloride Solution 1:100 will help prevent the sensation of dryness of mouth and throat which may otherwise follow.

Inhalation dosage of adults, children, and adolescents 4 years of age and older: 1 to 3 inhalations not more often than every 3 hours. The use of this product by children and adolescents should be supervised by an adult.

Pediatric patients under 4 years of age: Consult a physician.

When the nebulizer contains any liquid and is not in use, it should be stoppered and kept in an upright position. Because of oxidation, Adrenalin Chloride Solution 1:100 will turn pink to brown when exposed to air. Light, heat, alkalies, and certain metals (eg, copper, iron, zinc) will also promote deterioration. A discolored inhalation solution or one containing a precipitate should not be used.

HOW SUPPLIED

NDC 61570-301-41 Adrenalin Chloride Solution 1:100 (Epinephrine Inhalation Solution, USP), for oral inhalation use. Supplied in bottles containing 1/4 fluid ounce (7.5 mL) each.

Store between 15° and 25°C (59° and 77°F). Protect from light and freezing.

Rx only.

Distributed by: Monarch Pharmaceuticals, Inc., Bristol, TN 37620

Manufactured by: Parkedale Pharmaceuticals, Inc., Rochester, MI 48307

301G030
218

ADRENALIN® CHLORIDE SOLUTION ℞

(Epinephrine Injection, USP), 1:1000

DESCRIPTION

A sterile solution intended for subcutaneous or intramuscular injection. When diluted, it may also be administered intracardially or intravenously. Each milliliter contains 1 mg Adrenalin (epinephrine) as the hydrochloride dissolved in Water for Injection, USP, with sodium chloride added for isotonicity. The ampoules contain not more than 0.1% sodium bisulfite as an antioxidant, and the air in the ampoule has been displaced by nitrogen. The Steri-Vials® contain 0.5% Chlorobutanol (chloroform derivative) as a preservative and not more than 0.15% sodium bisulfite as an antioxidant. Epinephrine is the active principle of the adrenal medulla, chemically described as (—)-3,4-Dihydroxy-alpha-[(methylamino) methyl] benzyl alcohol, and has the following structural formula:

HO—[benzene ring]—CH-CH$_2$-NHCH$_3$ (with OH on the ring and OH on the CH)

CLINICAL PHARMACOLOGY

Adrenalin (epinephrine) is a sympathomimetic drug. It activates an adrenergic receptive mechanism on effector cells and imitates all actions of the sympathetic nervous system except those on the arteries of the face and sweat glands. Epinephrine acts on both alpha and beta receptors and is the most potent alpha receptor activator.

INDICATIONS AND USAGE

In general, the most common uses of epinephrine are to relieve respiratory distress due to bronchospasm, to provide rapid relief of hypersensitivity reactions to drugs and other allergens, and to prolong the action of infiltration anesthetics. Its cardiac effects may be of use in restoring cardiac rhythm in cardiac arrest due to various causes, but it is not used in cardiac failure or in hemorrhagic, traumatic, or cardiogenic shock.

Epinephrine is used as a hemostatic agent. It is also used in treating mucosal congestion of hay fever, rhinitis, and acute sinusitis; to relieve bronchial asthmatic paroxysms; in syncope due to complete heart block or carotid sinus hypersensitivity; for symptomatic relief of serum sickness, urticaria, angioneurotic edema; for resuscitation in cardiac arrest following anesthetic accidents; in simple (open angle) glaucoma; for relaxation of uterine musculature and to inhibit uterine contractions. Epinephrine injection can be utilized to prolong the action of intraspinal and local anesthetics (see CONTRAINDICATIONS section).

CONTRAINDICATIONS

Epinephrine is contraindicated in narrow angle (congestive) glaucoma, shock, during general anesthesia with halogenated hydrocarbons or cyclopropane and in individuals with organic brain damage. Epinephrine is also contraindicated with local anesthesia of certain areas, e.g., fingers, toes, because of the danger of vasoconstriction producing sloughing of tissue; in labor because it may delay the second stage; in cardiac dilatation and coronary insufficiency.

WARNINGS

Administer with caution to elderly people; to those with cardiovascular disease, hypertension, diabetes, or hyperthyroidism; in psychoneurotic individuals; and in pregnancy. Patients with long-standing bronchial asthma and emphysema who have developed degenerative heart disease should be administered the drug with extreme caution.

Overdosage or inadvertent intravenous injection of epinephrine may cause cerebrovascular hemorrhage resulting from the sharp rise in blood pressure.

Fatalities may also result from pulmonary edema because of the peripheral constriction and cardiac stimulation produced. Rapidly acting vasodilators, such as nitrites, or alpha blocking agents may counteract the marked pressor effects of epinephrine.

Epinephrine is the preferred treatment for serious allergic or other emergency situations even though this product contains sodium bisulfite, a sulfite that may in other products cause allergic-type reactions including anaphylactic symptoms or life-threatening or less severe asthmatic episodes in certain susceptible persons. The alternatives to using epinephrine in a life-threatening situation may not be satisfactory. The presence of a sulfite in this product should not deter administration of the drug for treatment of serious allergic or other emergency situations

PRECAUTIONS

General: Adrenalin (epinephrine injection, USP) should be protected from exposure to light. Do not remove ampoules or syringes from carton until ready to use. The solution should not be used if it is pinkish or darker than slightly yellow or if it contains a precipitate.

Epinephrine is readily destroyed by alkalies and oxidizing agents. In the latter category are oxygen, chlorine, bromine, iodine, permanganates, chromates, nitrites, and salts of easily reducible metals, especially iron.

Drug Interactions: Use of epinephrine with excessive doses of digitalis, mercurial diuretics, or other drugs that sensitize the heart to arrhythmias is not recommended. Anginal pain may be induced when coronary insufficiency is present. The effects of epinephrine may be potentiated by tricyclic antidepressants; certain antihistamines, e.g., diphenhydramine, tripelennamine, d-chlorpheniramine; and sodium l-thyroxine.

Usage in Pregnancy: Pregnancy Category C. Adrenalin (epinephrine) has been shown to be teratogenic in rats when given in doses about 25 times the human dose. There are no adequate and well-controlled studies in pregnant women. Adrenalin should be used during pregnancy only if the potential benefit justifies the potential risk to the fetus.

ADVERSE REACTIONS

Transient and minor side effects of anxiety, headache, fear, and palpitations often occur with therapeutic doses, especially in hyperthyroid individuals. Repeated local injections can result in necrosis at sites of injection from vascular constriction. "Epinephrine-fastness" can occur with prolonged use.

DOSAGE AND ADMINISTRATION

Parenteral drug products should be inspected visually for particulate matter and discoloration whenever solution and container permit.

Vial and contents must be discarded 30 days after initial use.

Subcutaneously or intramuscularly—0.2 to 1 mL (mg). Start with a small dose and increase if required.

Note: The subcutaneous is the preferred route of administration. If given intramuscularly, injection into the buttocks should be avoided.

For bronchial asthma and certain allergic manifestations, e.g., angioedema, urticaria, serum sickness, anaphylactic shock, use epinephrine subcutaneously. For bronchial asthma in pediatric patients, administer 0.01 mg/kg or 0.3 mg/m^2 to a maximum of 0.5 mg subcutaneously, repeated every four hours if required.

For cardiac resuscitation—A dose of 0.5 mL (0.5 mg) diluted to 10 mL with sodium chloride injection can be administered intravenously or intracardially to restore myocardial contrac-tility. External cardiac massage should follow intracardial administration to permit the drug to enter coronary circulation. The drug should be used secondarily to unsuccessful attempts with physical or electromechanical methods.

Ophthalmologic use (for producing conjunctival decongestion, to control hemorrhage, produce mydriasis and reduce intraocular pressure)—Use a concentration of 1:10,000 (0.1 mg/mL) to 1:1,000 (1 mg/mL).

Intraspinal use (Amp 88)—Usual dose is 0.2 to 0.4 mL (0.2 to 0.4 mg) added to anesthetic spinal fluid mixture (may prolong anesthetic action by limiting absorption). For use with local anesthetic—Epinephrine 1:100,000 (0.01 mg/mL) to 1:20,000 (0.05 mg/mL) is the usual concentration employed with local anesthetics.

HOW SUPPLIED

NDC 61570-418-81 (Amp 88) Sterile solution containing 1 mg Adrenalin (epinephrine) as the hydrochloride in each 1-mL ampoule (1:1000). For intramuscular or subcutaneous use. When diluted, it may also be administered intracardially, intravenously, or intraspinally. Supplied in packages of ten.

NDC 61570-401-11 (S.V. 11) Sterile solution containing 1 mg Adrenalin (epinephrine) as the hydrochloride (1:1000). For intramuscular or subcutaneous use. When diluted, it may also be administered intracardially or intravenously. Supplied in a 30-mL Steri-Vial® (rubber-diaphragm-capped vial).

Store between 15° and 25°C (59° and 77°F).
Protect from light and freezing.
Rx Only.
Manufactured for:
Monarch Pharmaceuticals, Inc., Bristol, TN 37620
By: Parkedale Pharmaceuticals, Inc.
Rochester, MI 48307
418G031
238

ALTACE® Capsules ℞
[ōl'tās]
(ramipril)
Prescribing Information as of February 2000

> **USE IN PREGNANCY**
> **When used in pregnancy during the second and third trimesters, ACE inhibitors can cause injury and even death to the developing fetus.** When pregnancy is detected, ALTACE® should be discontinued as soon as possible. **See WARNINGS: Fetal/neonatal morbidity and mortality.**

DESCRIPTION

Ramipril is a 2-aza-bicyclo [3.3.0]-octane-3-carboxylic acid derivative. It is a white, crystalline substance soluble in polar organic solvents and buffered aqueous solutions. Ramipril melts between 105° C and 112°C.

The CAS Registry Number is 87333-19-5. Ramipril's chemical name is (2*S*,3*aS*,6*aS*)-1[(*S*)-*N*-[(*S*)-1-Carboxy-3-phenylpropyl] alanyl]octa hydrocyclopenta [*b*]pyrrole-2-carboxylic acid, 1-ethyl ester; its structural formula is:

Its empiric formula is $C_{23}H_{32}N_2O_5$, and its molecular weight is 416.5.

Ramiprilat, the diacid metabolite of ramipril, is a non-sulfhydryl angiotensin converting enzyme inhibitor. Ramipril is converted to ramiprilat by hepatic cleavage of the ester group.

ALTACE (ramipril) is supplied as hard shell capsules for oral administration containing 1.25 mg, 2.5 mg, 5 mg, and 10 mg of ramipril. The inactive ingredients present are pregelatinized starch NF, gelatin, and titanium dioxide. The 1.25 mg capsule shell contains yellow iron oxide, the 2.5 mg capsule shell contains D&C yellow #10 and FD&C red #40, the 5 mg capsule shell contains FD&C blue #1 and FD&C red #40, and the 10 mg capsule shell contains FD&C blue #1.

CLINICAL PHARMACOLOGY

Mechanism of Action

Ramipril and ramiprilat inhibit angiotensin-converting enzyme (ACE) in human subjects and animals. ACE is a peptidyl dipeptidase that catalyzes the conversion of angiotensin I to the vasoconstrictor substance, angiotensin II. Angiotensin II also stimulates aldosterone secretion by the adrenal cortex. Inhibition of ACE results in decreased plasma angiotensin II, which leads to decreased vasopressor activity and to decreased aldosterone secretion. The latter decrease may result in a small increase of serum potassium. In hypertensive patients with normal renal function treated with ALTACE alone for up to 56 weeks, approximately 4% of patients during the trial had an abnormally high serum potassium and an increase from baseline greater than 0.75 mEq/L, and none of the patients had an abnormally low potassium and a decrease from baseline greater than 0.75 mEq/L. In the same study, approximately 2% of patients treated with ALTACE and hydrochlorothiazide for up to 56 weeks had abnormally high potassium values and an increase from baseline of 0.75 mEq/L or greater, and approximately 2% had abnormally low values and decreases from baseline of 0.75 mEq/L or greater. (See **PRECAUTIONS**.) Removal of angiotensin II negative feedback on renin secretion leads to increased plasma renin activity.

The effect of ramipril on hypertension appears to result at least in part from inhibition of both tissue and circulating ACE activity, thereby reducing angiotensin II formation in tissue and plasma.

ACE is identical to kininase, an enzyme that degrades bradykinin. Whether increased levels of bradykinin, a potent vasodepressor peptide, play a role in the therapeutic effects of ALTACE remains to be elucidated.

While the mechanism through which ALTACE lowers blood pressure is believed to be primarily suppression of the renin-angiotensin-aldosterone system, ALTACE has an antihypertensive effect even in patients with low-renin hypertension. Although ALTACE was antihypertensive in all races studied, black hypertensive patients (usually a low-renin hypertensive population) had a smaller average response to monotherapy than non-black patients.

Pharmacokinetics and Metabolism

Following oral administration of ALTACE, peak plasma concentrations of ramipril are reached within one hour. The extent of absorption is at least 50–60% and is not significantly influenced by the presence of food in the GI tract, although the rate of absorption is reduced.

In a trial in which subjects received ALTACE capsules or the contents of identical capsules dissolved in water, dissolved in apple juice, or suspended in apple sauce, serum ramiprilat levels were essentially unrelated to the use or nonuse of the concomitant liquid or food.

Cleavage of the ester group (primarily in the liver) converts ramipril to its active diacid metabolite, ramiprilat. Peak plasma concentrations of ramiprilat are reached 2–4 hours after drug intake. The serum protein binding of ramipril is about 73% and that of ramiprilat about 56%; *in vitro*, these percentages are independent of concentration over the range of 0.01 to 10μg/ml.

Ramipril is almost completely metabolized to ramiprilat, which has about 6 times the ACE inhibitory activity of ramipril, and to the diketopiperazine ester, the diketopiperazine acid, and the glucuronides of ramipril and ramiprilat, all of which are inactive. After oral administration of ramipril, about 60% of the parent drug and its metabolites is eliminated in the urine, and about 40% is found in the feces. Drug recovered in the feces may represent both biliary excretion of metabolites and/or unabsorbed drug, however the proportion of a dose eliminated by the bile has not been determined. Less than 2% of the administered dose is recovered in urine as unchanged ramipril.

Blood concentrations of ramipril and ramiprilat increase with increased dose, but are not strictly dose-proportional. The 24-hour AUC for ramiprilat, however, is dose-proportional over the 2.5–20 mg dose range. The absolute bioavailabilities of ramipril and ramiprilat were 28% and 44%, respectively, when 5 mg of oral ramipril was compared with the same dose of ramipril given intravenously.

Plasma concentrations of ramiprilat decline in a triphasic manner (initial rapid decline, apparent elimination phase, terminal elimination phase). The initial rapid decline, which represents distribution of the drug into a large peripheral compartment and subsequent binding to both plasma and tissue ACE, has a half-life of 2–4 hours. Because of its potent binding to ACE and slow dissociation from the enzyme, ramiprilat shows two elimination phases. The apparent elimination phase corresponds to the clearance of free ramiprilat and has a half-life of 9–18 hours. The terminal elimination phase has a prolonged half-life (>50 hours) and probably represents the binding/dissociation kinetics of the ramiprilat/ACE complex. It does not contribute to the accumulation of the drug. After multiple daily doses of ramipril 5-10 mg, the half-life of ramiprilat concentrations within the therapeutic range was 13–17 hours.

After once-daily dosing, steady-state plasma concentrations of ramiprilat are reached by the fourth dose. Steady-state concentrations of ramiprilat are somewhat higher than those seen after the first dose of ALTACE, especially at low doses (2.5 mg), but the difference is clinically insignificant.

In patients with creatinine clearance less than 40 ml/min/1.73m^2, peak levels of ramiprilat are approximately doubled, and trough levels may be as much as quintupled. In multiple-dose regimens, the total exposure to ramiprilat (AUC) in these patients is 3–4 times as large as it is in patients with normal renal function who receive similar doses.

The urinary excretion of ramipril, ramiprilat, and their metabolites is reduced in patients with impaired renal function. Compared to normal subjects, patients with creatinine clearance less than 40 ml/min/1.73m^2 had higher peak and trough ramiprilat levels and slightly longer times to peak concentrations. (See **DOSAGE AND ADMINISTRATION**.)

In patients with impaired liver function, the metabolism of ramipril to ramiprilat appears to be slowed, possibly because of diminished activity of hepatic esterases, and plasma ramipril levels in these patients are increased about 3-fold. Peak concentrations of ramiprilat in these patients, however, are not different from those seen in subjects with normal hepatic function, and the effect of a given dose on plasma ACE activity does not vary with hepatic function.

Pharmacodynamics

Single doses of ramipril of 2.5–20 mg produce approximately 60-80% inhibition of ACE activity 4 hours after dosing with approximately 40–60% inhibition after 24 hours. Multiple oral doses of ramipril of 2.0 mg or more cause plasma ACE activity to fall by more than 90% 4 hours after dosing, with over 80% inhibition of ACE activity remaining 24 hours after dosing. The more prolonged effect of even small multiple doses presumably reflects saturation of ACE binding sites by ramiprilat and relatively slow release from those sites.

Pharmacodynamics and Clinical Effects

Hypertension

Administration of ALTACE to patients with mild to moderate hypertension results in a reduction of both supine and standing blood pressure to about the same extent with no compensatory tachycardia. Symptomatic postural hypotension is infrequent, although it can occur in patients who are salt- and/or volume-depleted. (See **WARNINGS**.) Use of ALTACE in combination with thiazide diuretics gives a blood pressure lowering effect greater than that seen with either agent alone.

In single-dose studies, doses of 5–20 mg of ALTACE lowered blood pressure within 1–2 hours, with peak reductions achieved 3–6 hours after dosing. The antihypertensive effect of a single dose persisted for 24 hours. In longer term (4–12 weeks) controlled studies, once-daily doses of 2.5–10 mg were similar in their effect, lowering supine or standing systolic and diastolic blood pressures 24 hours after dosing by about 6/4 mm Hg more than placebo. In comparisons of peak vs. trough effect, the trough effect represented about 50–60% of the peak response. In a titration study comparing divided (bid) vs. qd treatment, the divided regimen was superior, indicating that for some patients the antihypertensive effect with once-daily dosing is not adequately maintained. (See **DOSAGE AND ADMINISTRATION**.)

In most trials, the antihypertensive effect of ALTACE increased during the first several weeks of repeated measurements. The antihypertensive effect of ALTACE has been shown to continue during long-term therapy for at least 2 years. Abrupt withdrawal of ALTACE has not resulted in a rapid increase in blood pressure.

ALTACE has been compared with other ACE inhibitors, beta-blockers, and thiazide diuretics. It was approximately as effective as other ACE inhibitors and as atenolol. In both caucasians and blacks, hydrochlorothiazide (25 or 50 mg) was significantly more effective than ramipril.

Except for thiazides, no formal interaction studies of ramipril with other antihypertensive agents have been carried out. Limited experience in controlled and uncontrolled trials combining ramipril with a calcium channel blocker, a loop diuretic, or triple therapy (beta-blocker, vasodilator, and a diuretic) indicate no unusual drug-drug interactions. Other ACE inhibitors have had less than additive effects with beta adrenergic blockers, presumably because both drugs lower blood pressure by inhibiting parts of the renin-angiotensin system.

ALTACE was less effective in blacks than in caucasians. The effectiveness of ALTACE was not influenced by age, sex, or weight.

In a baseline controlled study of 10 patients with mild essential hypertension, blood pressure reduction was accompanied by a 15% increase in renal blood flow. In healthy volunteers, glomerular filtration rate was unchanged.

Heart Failure post myocardial infarction

ALTACE was studied in the Acute Infarction Ramipril Efficacy (AIRE) trial. This was a multinational (mainly European) 161-center, 2006-patient, double-blind, randomized, parallel-group study comparing ALTACE to placebo in stable patients, 2–9 days after an acute myocardial infarction (MI), who had shown clinical signs of congestive heart failure (CHF) at any time after the MI. Patients in severe (NYHA class IV) heart failure, patients with unstable angina, patients with heart failure of congenital or valvular etiology, and patients with contraindications to ACE inhibitors were all excluded. The majority of patients had received thrombolytic therapy at the time of the index infarction, and the average time between infarction and initiation of treatment was 5 days.

Patients randomized to ramipril treatment were given an initial dose of 2.5 mg twice daily. If the initial regimen caused undue hypotension, the dose was reduced to 1.25 mg, but in either event doses were titrated upward (as tolerated) to a target regimen (achieved in 77% of patients randomized to ramipril) of 5 mg twice daily. Patients were then followed for an average of 15 months (range 6–46).

The use of ALTACE was associated with a 27% reduction (p=0.002), in the risk of death from any cause; about 90% of the deaths that occurred were cardiovascular, mainly sudden death. The risks of progression to severe heart failure and of CHF-related hospitalization were also reduced, by 23% (p=0.017) and 26% (p=0.011), respectively. The benefits of ALTACE therapy were seen in both genders, and they were not affected by the exact timing of the initiation of therapy, but older patients may have had a greater benefit than those under 65. The benefits were seen in patients on, and not on, various concomitant medications; at the time of

Continued on next page

Altace—Cont.

randomization these included aspirin (about 80% of patients), diuretics (about 60%), organic nitrates (about 55%), beta-blockers (about 20%), calcium channel blockers (about 15%), and digoxin (about 12%).

INDICATIONS AND USAGE

Hypertension

ALTACE is indicated for the treatment of hypertension. It may be used alone or in combination with thiazide diuretics.

In using ALTACE, consideration should be given to the fact that another angiotensin converting enzyme inhibitor, captopril, has caused agranulocytosis, particularly in patients with renal impairment or collagen-vascular disease. Available data are insufficient to show that ALTACE does not have a similar risk. (See **WARNINGS**.)

In considering use of ALTACE, it should be noted that in controlled trials ACE inhibitors have an effect on blood pressure that is less in black patients than in non-blacks. In addition, ACE inhibitors (for which adequate data are available) cause a higher rate of angioedema in black than in non-black patients. (See **WARNINGS, Angioedema.**)

Heart Failure post-myocardial infarction

Ramipril is indicated in stable patients who have demonstrated clinical signs of congestive heart failure within the first few days after sustaining acute myocardial infarction. Administration of ramipril to such patients has been shown to decrease the risk of death (principally cardiovascular death) and to decrease the risks of failure-related hospitalization and progression to severe/resistant heart failure. (See **CLINICAL PHARMACOLOGY, Heart Failure post-myocardial infarction** for details and limitations of the survival trial.)

CONTRAINDICATIONS

ALTACE is contraindicated in patients who are hypersensitive to this product and in patients with a history of angioedema related to previous treatment with an angiotensin converting enzyme inhibitor.

WARNINGS

Anaphylactoid and Possibly Related Reactions

Presumably because angiotensin-converting enzyme inhibitors affect the metabolism of eicosanoids and polypeptides, including endogenous bradykinin, patients receiving ACE inhibitors (including ALTACE) may be subject to a variety of adverse reactions, some of them serious.

Angioedema

Patients with a history of angioedema unrelated to ACE inhibitor therapy may be at increased risk of angioedema while receiving an ACE inhibitor. (See also **CONTRAINDICATIONS.**)

Angioedema of the face, extremities, lips, tongue, glottis, and larynx has been reported in patients treated with angiotensin converting enzyme inhibitors. Angioedema associated with laryngeal edema can be fatal. If laryngeal stridor or angioedema of the face, tongue, or glottis occurs, treatment with ALTACE should be discontinued and appropriate therapy instituted immediately. **Where there is involvement of the tongue, glottis, or larynx, likely to cause airway obstruction, appropriate therapy, e.g., subcutaneous epinephrine solution 1:1,000 (0.3 ml to 0.5 ml) should be promptly administered. (See ADVERSE REACTIONS.)**

In a large U.S. postmarketing study, angioedema (defined as reports of angio, face, larynx, tongue, or throat edema) was reported in 3/1523 (0.20%) of black patients and in 8/8680 (0.09%) of white patients. These rates were not different statistically.

Anaphylactoid reactions during desensitization: Two patients undergoing desensitizing treatment with hymenoptera venom while receiving ACE inhibitors sustained life-threatening anaphylactoid reactions. In the same patients, these reactions were avoided when ACE inhibitors were temporarily withheld, but they reappeared upon inadvertent rechallenge.

Anaphylactoid reactions during membrane exposure: Anaphylactoid reactions have been reported in patients dialyzed with high-flux membranes and treated concomitantly with an ACE inhibitor. Anaphylactoid reactions have also been reported in patients undergoing low-density lipoprotein apheresis with dextran sulfate absorption.

Hypotension

ALTACE can cause symptomatic hypotension, after either the initial dose or a later dose when the dosage has been increased. Like other ACE inhibitors, ramipril has been only rarely associated with hypotension in uncomplicated hypertensive patients. Symptomatic hypotension is most likely to occur in patients who have been volume- and/or salt-depleted as a result of prolonged diuretic therapy, dietary salt restriction, dialysis, diarrhea, or vomiting. Volume and/or salt depletion should be corrected before initiating therapy with ALTACE.

In patients with congestive heart failure, with or without associated renal insufficiency, ACE inhibitor therapy may cause excessive hypotension, which may be associated with oliguria or azotemia and, rarely, with acute renal failure and death. In such patients, ALTACE therapy should be started under close medical supervision; they should be followed closely for the first 2 weeks of treatment and whenever the dose of ramipril or diuretic is increased.

If hypotension occurs, the patient should be placed in a supine position and, if necessary, treated with intravenous infusion of physiological saline. ALTACE treatment usually can be continued following restoration of blood pressure and volume.

Hepatic Failure

Rarely, ACE inhibitors have been associated with a syndrome that starts with cholestatic jaundice and progresses to fulminant hepatic necrosis and (sometimes) death. The mechanism of this syndrome is not understood. Patients receiving ACE inhibitors who develop jaundice or marked elevations of hepatic enzymes should discontinue the ACE inhibitor and receive appropriate medical follow-up.

Neutropenia/Agranulocytosis

Another angiotensin converting enzyme inhibitor, captopril, has been shown to cause agranulocytosis and bone marrow depression, rarely in uncomplicated patients, but more frequently in patients with renal impairment, especially if they also have a collagen-vascular disease such as systemic lupus erythematosus or scleroderma. Available data from clinical trials of ramipril are insufficient to show that ramipril does not cause agranulocytosis at similar rates. Monitoring of white blood cell counts should be considered in patients with collagen-vascular disease, especially if the disease is associated with impaired renal function.

Fetal/neonatal morbidity and mortality

ACE inhibitors can cause fetal and neonatal morbidity and death when administered to pregnant women. Several dozen cases have been reported in the world literature. When pregnancy is detected, ACE inhibitors should be discontinued as soon as possible.

The use of ACE inhibitors during the second and third trimesters of pregnancy has been associated with fetal and neonatal injury, including hypotension, neonatal skull hypoplasia, anuria, reversible or irreversible renal failure, and death. Oligohydramnios has also been reported, presumably resulting from decreased fetal renal function; oligohydramnios in this setting has been associated with fetal limb contractures, craniofacial deformation, and hypoplastic lung development. Prematurity, intrauterine growth retardation, and patent ductus arteriosus have also been reported, although it is not clear whether these occurrences were due to the ACE inhibitor exposure.

These adverse effects do not appear to have resulted from intrauterine ACE inhibitor exposure that has been limited to the first trimester. Mothers whose embryos and fetuses are exposed to ACE inhibitors only during the first trimester should be so informed. Nonetheless, when patients become pregnant, physicians should make every effort to discontinue the use of ALTACE as soon as possible.

Rarely (probably less often than once in every thousand pregnancies), no alternative to ACE inhibitors will be found. In these rare cases, the mothers should be apprised of the potential hazards to their fetuses, and serial ultrasound examinations should be performed to assess the intraamniotic environment.

If oligohydramnios is observed, ALTACE should be discontinued unless it is considered life-saving for the mother. Contraction stress testing (CST), a non-stress test (NST), or biophysical profiling (BPP) may be appropriate, depending upon the week of pregnancy. Patients and physicians should be aware, however, that oligohydramnios may not appear until after the fetus has sustained irreversible injury.

Infants with histories of *in utero* exposure to ACE inhibitors should be closely observed for hypotension, oliguria, and hyperkalemia. If oliguria occurs, attention should be directed toward support of blood pressure and renal perfusion. Exchange transfusion or dialysis may be required as means of reversing hypotension and/or substituting for disordered renal function. ALTACE which crosses the placenta can be removed from the neonatal circulation by these means, but limited experience has not shown that such removal is central to the treatment of these infants.

No teratogenic effects of ALTACE were seen in studies of pregnant rats, rabbits, and cynomolgus monkeys. On a body surface area basis, the doses used were up to approximately 400 times (in rats and monkeys) and 2 times (in rabbits) the recommended human dose.

PRECAUTIONS

Impaired Renal Function: As a consequence of inhibiting the renin-angiotensin-aldosterone system, changes in renal function may be anticipated in susceptible individuals. In patients with severe congestive heart failure whose renal function may depend on the activity of the renin-angiotensin-aldosterone system, treatment with angiotensin converting enzyme inhibitors, including ALTACE, may be associated with oliguria and/or progressive azotemia and (rarely) with acute renal failure and/or death.

In hypertensive patients with unilateral or bilateral renal artery stenosis, increases in blood urea nitrogen and serum creatinine may occur. Experience with another angiotensin converting enzyme inhibitor suggests that these increases are usually reversible upon discontinuation of ALTACE and/or diuretic therapy. In such patients renal function should be monitored during the first few weeks of therapy.

Some hypertensive patients with no apparent pre-existing renal vascular disease have developed increases in blood urea nitrogen and serum creatinine, usually minor and transient, especially when ALTACE has been given concomitantly with a diuretic. This is more likely to occur in patients with pre-existing renal impairment. Dosage reduction of ALTACE and/or discontinuation of the diuretic may be required.

Evaluation of the hypertensive patient should always include assessment of renal function. (See **DOSAGE AND ADMINISTRATION.**)

Hyperkalemia: In clinical trials, hyperkalemia (serum potassium greater than 5.7 mEq/L) occurred in approximately 1% of hypertensive patients receiving ALTACE (ramipril). In most cases, these were isolated values, which resolved despite continued therapy. None of these patients was discontinued from the trials because of hyperkalemia. Risk factors for the development of hyperkalemia include renal insufficiency, diabetes mellitus, and the concomitant use of potassium-sparing diuretics, potassium supplements, and/or potassium-containing salt substitutes, which should be used cautiously, if at all, with ALTACE. (See **DRUG INTERACTIONS.**)

Cough: Presumably due to the inhibition of the degradation of endogenous bradykinin, persistent nonproductive cough has been reported with all ACE inhibitors, always resolving after discontinuation of therapy. ACE inhibitor-induced cough should be considered in the differential diagnosis of cough.

Impaired Liver Function: Since ramipril is primarily metabolized by hepatic esterases to its active moiety, ramiprilat, patients with impaired liver function could develop markedly elevated plasma levels of ramipril. No formal pharmacokinetic studies have been carried out in hypertensive patients with impaired liver function.

Surgery/Anesthesia: In patients undergoing surgery or during anesthesia with agents that produce hypotension, ramipril may block angiotensin II formation that would otherwise occur secondary to compensatory renin release. Hypotension that occurs as a result of this mechanism can be corrected by volume expansion.

Information for Patients

Pregnancy: Female patients of childbearing age should be told about the consequences of second- and third-trimester exposure to ACE inhibitors, and they should also be told that these consequences do not appear to have resulted from intrauterine ACE inhibitor exposure that has been limited to the first trimester. These patients should be asked to report pregnancies to their physicians as soon as possible.

Angioedema: Angioedema, including laryngeal edema, can occur with treatment with ACE inhibitors, especially following the first dose. Patients should be so advised and told to report immediately any signs or symptoms suggesting angioedema (swelling of face, eyes, lips, or tongue, or difficulty in breathing) and to take no more drug until they have consulted with the prescribing physician.

Symptomatic Hypotension: Patients should be cautioned that lightheadedness can occur, especially during the first days of therapy, and it should be reported. Patients should be told that if syncope occurs, ALTACE should be discontinued until the physician has been consulted.

All patients should be cautioned that inadequate fluid intake or excessive perspiration, diarrhea, or vomiting can lead to an excessive fall in blood pressure, with the same consequences of lightheadedness and possible syncope.

Hyperkalemia: Patients should be told not to use salt substitutes containing potassium without consulting their physician.

Neutropenia: Patients should be told to promptly report any indication of infection (e.g., sore throat, fever), which could be a sign of neutropenia.

Drug Interactions

With diuretics: Patients on diuretics, especially those in whom diuretic therapy was recently instituted, may occasionally experience an excessive reduction of blood pressure after initiation of therapy with ALTACE. The possibility of hypotensive effects with ALTACE can be minimized by either discontinuing the diuretic or increasing the salt intake prior to initiation of treatment with ALTACE. If this is not possible, the starting dose should be reduced. (See **DOSAGE AND ADMINISTRATION.**)

With potassium supplements and potassium-sparing diuretics: ALTACE can attenuate potassium loss caused by thiazide diuretics. Potassium-sparing diuretics (spironolactone, amiloride, triamterene, and others) or potassium supplements can increase the risk of hyperkalemia. Therefore, if concomitant use of such agents is indicated, they should be given with caution, and the patient's serum potassium should be monitored frequently.

With lithium: Increased serum lithium levels and symptoms of lithium toxicity have been reported in patients receiving ACE inhibitors during therapy with lithium. These drugs should be coadministered with caution, and frequent monitoring of serum lithium levels is recommended. If a diuretic is also used, the risk of lithium toxicity may be increased.

Other: Neither ALTACE nor its metabolites have been found to interact with food, digoxin, antacid, furosemide, cimetidine, indomethacin, and simvastatin. The combination of ALTACE and propranolol showed no adverse effects on dynamic parameters (blood pressure and heart rate). The co-administration of ALTACE and warfarin did not adversely affect the anticoagulant effects of the latter drug. Additionally, co-administration of ALTACE with phenprocoumon did not affect minimum phenprocoumon levels or interfere with the subjects' state of anti-coagulation.

Carcinogenesis, Mutagenesis, Impairment of Fertility

No evidence of a tumorigenic effect was found when ramipril was given by gavage to rats for up to 24 months at doses of up to 500 mg/kg/day or to mice for up to 18 months at doses of up to 1000 mg/kg/day. (For either species, these doses are about 200 times the maximum recommended human dose when compared on the basis of body surface area.) No mutagenic activity was detected in the Ames test in bacteria, the micronucleus test in mice, unscheduled DNA synthesis in a human cell line, or a forward gene-mutation assay in a Chinese hamster ovary cell line. Several metabolites and degradation products of ramipril were also negative in the Ames test. A study in rats with dosages as great as 500 mg/kg/day did not produce adverse effects on fertility.

Pregnancy

Pregnancy Categories C (first trimester) and D (second and third trimesters). **See WARNINGS: Fetal/neonatal morbidity and mortality.**

Nursing Mothers

Ingestion of single 10 mg oral dose of ALTACE resulted in undetectable amounts of ramipril and its metabolites in breast milk. However, because multiple doses may produce low milk concentrations that are not predictable from single doses, women receiving ALTACE should not breast feed.

Geriatric Use

Of the total number of patients who received ramipril in US clinical studies of ALTACE 11.0% were 65 and over while 0.2% were 75 and over. No overall differences in effectiveness or safety were observed between these patients and younger patients, and other reported clinical experience has not identified differences in responses between the elderly and younger patients, but greater sensitivity of some older individuals cannot be ruled out.

One pharmacokinetic study conducted in hospitalized elderly patients indicated that peak ramiprilat levels and area under the plasma concentration time curve (AUC) for ramiprilat are higher in older patients.

Pediatric Use

Safety and effectiveness in pediatric patients have not been established.

ADVERSE REACTIONS

Hypertension

ALTACE has been evaluated for safety in over 4,000 patients with hypertension; of these, 1,230 patients were studied in US controlled trials, and 1,107 were studied in foreign controlled trials. Almost 700 of these patients were treated for at least one year. The overall incidence of reported adverse events was similar in ALTACE and placebo patients. The most frequent clinical side effects (possibly or probably related to study drug) reported by patients receiving ALTACE in US placebo-controlled trials were: headache (5.4%), "dizziness" (2.2%) and fatigue or asthenia (2.0%), but only the last was more common in ALTACE patients than in patients given placebo. Generally, the side effects were mild and transient, and there was no relation to total dosage within the range of 1.25 to 20 mg. Discontinuation of therapy because of a side effect was required in approximately 3% of US patients treated with ALTACE. The most common reasons for discontinuation were: cough (1.0%), "dizziness" (0.5%), and impotence (0.4%).

The side effects considered possibly or probably related to study drug that occurred in US placebo-controlled trials in more than 1% of patients treated with ALTACE are shown below.

PATIENTS IN US PLACEBO CONTROLLED STUDIES

	ALTACE (N=651)		Placebo (N=286)	
	n	%	n	%
Headache	35	5.4	17	5.9
"Dizziness"	14	2.2	9	3.1
Asthenia (Fatigue)	13	2.0	2	0.7
Nausea/Vomiting	7	1.1	3	1.0

In placebo-controlled trials, there was also an excess of upper respiratory infection and flu syndrome in the ramipril group. As these studies were carried out before the relationship of cough to ACE inhibitors was recognized, some of these events may represent ramipril-induced cough. In a later 1-year study, increased cough was seen in almost 12% of ramipril patients, with about 4% of these patients requiring discontinuation of treatment.

Heart Failure post-myocardial infarction

Adverse reactions (except laboratory abnormalities) considered possibly/probably related to study drug that occurred in more than one percent of patients with heart failure treated with ALTACE are shown below. The incidences represent the experiences from the AIRE study. The follow-up time was between 6 and 46 months for this study.

Percentage of Patients with Adverse Events Possibly/Probably Related to Study Drug
Placebo-Controlled (AIRE) Mortality Study

Adverse Event	Ramipril (N=1004)	Placebo (N=982)
Hypotension	10.7	4.7
Cough Increased	7.6	3.7
Dizziness	4.1	3.2
Angina Pectoris	2.9	2.0
Nausea	2.2	1.4
Postural Hypotension	2.2	1.4
Syncope	2.1	1.4
Heart Failure	2.0	2.2
Severe/Resistance Heart Failure	2.0	3.0
Myocardial Infarct	1.7	1.7
Vomiting	1.6	0.5
Vertigo	1.5	0.7
Headache	1.2	0.8
Kidney Function	1.2	0.5
Abnormal Chest Pain	1.1	0.9
Diarrhea	1.1	0.4
Asthenia	0.3	0.8

Other adverse experiences reported in controlled clinical trials (in less than 1% of ramipril patients), or rarer events seen in postmarketing experience, include the following (in some, a causal relationship to drug use is uncertain):

Body As a Whole: Anaphylactoid reactions. (See **WARNINGS.**)

Cardiovascular: Symptomatic hypotension (reported in 0.5% of patients in US trials) (See **WARNINGS** and **PRECAUTIONS**), syncope (not reported in US trials), angina pectoris, arrhythmia, chest pain, palpitations, myocardial infarction, and cerebrovascular events.

Hematologic: Pancytopenia, hemolytic anemia and thrombocytopenia.

Renal: Some hypertensive patients with no apparent pre-existing renal disease have developed minor, usually transient, increases in blood urea nitrogen and serum creatinine when taking ALTACE, particularly when ALTACE was given concomitantly with a diuretic. (See **WARNINGS.**)

Angioneurotic Edema: Angioneurotic edema has been reported in 0.3% of patients in US clinical trials. (See **WARNINGS.**)

Cough: A tickling, dry, persistent, nonproductive cough has been reported with the use of ACE inhibitors. Approximately 1% of patients treated with ALTACE have required discontinuation because of cough. The cough disappears shortly after discontinuation of treatment. (See **PRECAUTIONS, Cough** subsection.)

Gastrointestinal: Pancreatitis, abdominal pain (sometimes with enzyme changes suggesting pancreatitis), anorexia, constipation, diarrhea, dry mouth, dyspepsia, dysphagia, gastroenteritis, hepatitis, nausea, increased salivation, taste disturbance, and vomiting.

Dermatologic: Apparent hypersensitivity reactions (manifested by urticaria, pruritus, or rash, with or without fever), erythema multiforme, pemphigus, photosensitivity, and purpura.

Neurologic and Psychiatric: Anxiety, amnesia, convulsions, depression, hearing loss, insomnia, nervousness, neuralgia, neuropathy, paresthesia, somnolence, tinnitus, tremor, vertigo, and vision disturbances.

Miscellaneous: As with other ACE inhibitors, a symptom complex has been reported which may include a positive ANA, an elevated erythrocyte sedimentation rate, arthralgia/arthritis, myalgia, fever, vasculitis, eosinophilia, photosensitivity, rash and other dermatologic manifestations. Additionally, as with other ACE inhibitors, eosinophilic pneumonitis has been reported.

Fetal/neonatal morbidity and mortality. **See WARNINGS: Fetal/neonatal morbidity and mortality.**

Other: arthralgia, arthritis, dyspnea, edema, epistaxis, impotence, increased sweating, malaise, myalgia, and weight gain.

Clinical Laboratory Test Findings:

Creatinine and Blood Urea Nitrogen: Increases in creatinine levels occurred in 1.2% of patients receiving ALTACE alone, and in 1.5% of patients receiving ALTACE and a diuretic. Increases in blood urea nitrogen levels occurred in 0.5% of patients receiving ALTACE alone and in 3% of patients receiving ALTACE with a diuretic. None of these increases required discontinuation of treatment. Increases in these laboratory values are more likely to occur in patients with renal insufficiency or those pretreated with a diuretic and, based on experience with other ACE inhibitors, would be expected to be especially likely in patients with renal artery stenosis. (See **WARNINGS** and **PRECAUTIONS.**)

Since ramipril decreases aldosterone secretion, elevation of serum potassium can occur. Potassium supplements and potassium-sparing diuretics should be given with caution, and the patient's serum potassium should be monitored frequently. (See **WARNINGS** and **PRECAUTIONS.**)

Hemoglobin and Hematocrit: Decreases in hemoglobin or hematocrit (a low value and a decrease of 5 g/dl or 5% respectively) were rare, occurring in 0.4% of patients receiving ALTACE alone and in 1.5% of patients receiving ALTACE plus a diuretic. No US patients discontinued treatment because of decreases in hemoglobin or hematocrit.

Other (causal relationships unknown): Clinically important changes in standard laboratory tests were rarely associated with ALTACE administration. Elevations of liver enzymes, serum bilirubin, uric acid, and blood glucose have been reported, as have cases of hyponatremia and scattered incidents of leukopenia, eosinophilia, and proteinuria. In US trials, less than 0.2% of patients discontinued treatment for laboratory abnormalities; all of these were cases of proteinuria or abnormal liver-function tests.

OVERDOSAGE

Single oral doses in rats and mice of 10–11 g/kg resulted in significant lethality. In dogs, oral doses as high as 1 g/kg induced only mild gastrointestinal distress. Limited data on human overdosage are available. The most likely clinical manifestations would be symptoms attributable to hypotension.

Laboratory determinations of serum levels of ramipril and its metabolites are not widely available, and such determinations have, in any event, no established role in the management of ramipril overdose.

No data are available to suggest physiological maneuvers (e.g., maneuvers to change the pH of the urine) that might accelerate elimination of ramipril and its metabolites. Similarly, it is not known which, if any, of these substances can be usefully removed from the body by hemodialysis.

Angiotensin II could presumably serve as a specific antagonist-antidote in the setting of ramipril overdose, but angiotensin II is essentially unavailable outside of scattered research facilities. Because the hypotensive effect of ramipril is achieved through vasodilation and effective hypovolemia, it is reasonable to treat ramipril overdose by infusion of normal saline solution.

DOSAGE AND ADMINISTRATION

Hypertension

The recommended initial dose for patients not receiving a diuretic is 2.5 mg once a day. Dosage should be adjusted according to the blood pressure response. The usual maintenance dosage range is 2.5 to 20 mg per day administered as a single dose or in two equally divided doses. In some patients treated once daily, the antihypertensive effect may diminish toward the end of the dosing interval. In such patients, an increase in dosage or twice daily administration should be considered. If blood pressure is not controlled with ALTACE alone, a diuretic can be added.

Heart Failure post myocardial infarction

For the treatment of post-infarction patients who have shown signs of congestive failure, the recommended starting dose of ALTACE is 2.5 mg twice daily. A patient who becomes hypotensive at this dose may be switched to 1.25 mg twice daily, but all patients should then be titrated (as tolerated) toward a target dose of 5 mg twice daily.

After the initial dose of ALTACE, the patient should be observed under medical supervision for at least two hours and until blood pressure has stabilized for at least an additional hour. (See **WARNINGS** and **PRECAUTIONS, Drug Interactions.**) If possible, the dose of any concomitant diuretic should be reduced which may diminish the likelihood of hypotension. The appearance of hypotension after the initial dose of ALTACE does not preclude subsequent careful dose titration with the drug, following effective management of the hypotension.

The ALTACE Capsule is usually swallowed whole. The ALTACE Capsule can also be opened and the contents sprinkled on a small amount (about 4 oz.) of apple sauce or mixed in 4 oz. (120 ml) of water or apple juice. To be sure that ramipril is not lost when such a mixture is used, the mixture should be consumed in its entirety. The described mixtures can be pre-prepared and stored for up to 24 hours at room temperature or up to 48 hours under refrigeration.

Concomitant administration of ALTACE with potassium supplements, potassium salt substitutes, or potassium-sparing diuretics can lead to increases of serum potassium. (See **PRECAUTIONS.**)

In patients who are currently being treated with a diuretic, symptomatic hypotension occasionally can occur following the initial dose of ALTACE. To reduce the likelihood of hypotension, the diuretic should, if possible, be discontinued two to three days prior to beginning therapy with ALTACE. (See **WARNINGS.**) Then, if blood pressure is not controlled with ALTACE alone, diuretic therapy should be resumed.

If the diuretic cannot be discontinued, an initial dose of 1.25 mg ALTACE should be used to avoid excess hypotension.

Dosage Adjustment in Renal Impairment

In patients with creatinine clearance <40 ml/min/1.73m^2 (serum creatinine approximately >2.5 mg/dl) doses only 25% of those normally used should be expected to induce full therapeutic levels of ramiprilat. (See **CLINICAL PHARMACOLOGY.**)

Hypertension: For patients with hypertension and renal impairment, the recommended initial dose is 1.25 mg ALTACE once daily. Dosage may be titrated upward until blood pressure is controlled or to a maximum total daily dose of 5 mg.

Heart Failure post myocardial infarction: For patients with heart failure and renal impairment, the recommended initial dose is 1.25 mg ALTACE once daily. The dose may be increased to 1.25 mg b.i.d. and up to a maximum dose of 2.5 mg b.i.d. depending upon clinical response and tolerability.

HOW SUPPLIED

ALTACE is available in potencies of 1.25 mg, 2.5 mg, 5 mg, and 10 mg in hard gelatin capsules.

ALTACE 1.25 mg capsules are supplied as yellow, hard gelatin capsules in bottles of 100 (NDC 61570-110-01), and Unit Dose packs of 100 (NDC 61570-110-56).

ALTACE 2.5 mg capsules are supplied as orange, hard gelatin capsules in bottles of 100 (NDC 61570-111-01), 500 (NDC 61570-111-05), 1000 (NDC 61570-111-10) and Unit Dose packs of 100 (NDC 61570-111-56), and Bulk pack of 5000's (NDC 61570-111-50).

ALTACE 5 mg capsules are supplied as red, hard gelatin capsules in bottles of 100 (NDC 61570-112-01), 500 (NDC 61570-112-05), 1000 (NDC 61570-112-10) and Unit Dose packs of 100 (NDC 61570-112-56), and Bulk pack of 5000's (NDC 61570-112-50).

ALTACE 10 mg capsules are supplied as Process Blue, hard gelatin capsules in bottles of 100 (NDC 61570-120-01), 500 (NDC 61570-120-05), 1000 (NDC 61570-120-10).

Dispense in well-closed container with safety closure.

Store at controlled room temperature (59 to 86° F).

Rx only.

Prescribing Information as of February 2000.

Distributed by:
Monarch Pharmaceuticals, Inc.
Bristol, TN 37620

Continued on next page

Altace—Cont.

Manufactured by:
Hoechst Marion Roussel, Inc.
Kansas City, MO 64137

000000000
Rev. 2/00

Shown in Product Identification Guide, page 324

ANUSOL-HC® 2.5% ℞
(Hydrocortisone Cream, USP)

Rx only

DESCRIPTION

The topical corticosteroids constitute a class of primarily synthetic steroids used as antiinflammatory and antipruritic agents. Anusol-HC 2.5% (Hydrocortisone Cream, USP) is a topical corticosteroid with hydrocortisone 2.5% (active ingredient) in a water-washable cream containing the following inactive ingredients: benzyl alcohol. petrolatum, stearyl alcohol, propylene glycol. isopropyl myristate, polyoxyl 40 stearate, carbomer 934, sodium lauryl sulfate, edetate disodium, sodium hydroxide to adjust the pH, and purified water.
Hydrocortisone has the chemical name Pregn-4-ene-3,20-dione, 11,17,21, trihydroxy-,(11β) and the following chemical structure:

MOLECULAR FORMULA $C_{21}H_{30}O_5$
MOLECULAR WEIGHT 362.47
CAS REGISTRY NUMBER 50-23-7

CLINICAL PHARMACOLOGY

Topical corticosteroids share antiinflammatory, antipruritic and vasoconstrictive actions.
The mechanism of antiinflammatory activity of the topical corticosteroids is unclear. Various laboratory methods, including vasoconstrictor assays, are used to compare and predict potencies and/or clinical efficacies of the topical corticosteroids. There is some evidence to suggest that a recognizable correlation exists between vasoconstrictor potency and therapeutic efficacy in man.
Pharmacokinetics: The extent of percutaneous absorption of topical corticosteroids is determined by many factors including the vehicle, the integrity of the epidermal barrier, and the use of occlusive dressings.
Topical corticosteroids can be absorbed from normal intact skin. Inflammation and/or other disease processes in the skin increase percutaneous absorption. Occlusive dressings substantially increase the percutaneous absorption of topical corticosteroids. Thus, occlusive dressings may be a valuable therapeutic adjunct for treatment of resistant dermatoses (see DOSAGE AND ADMINISTRATION).
Once absorbed through the skin, topical corticosteroids are handled through pharmacokinetic pathways similar to systemically administered corticosteroids. Corticosteroids are bound to plasma proteins in varying degrees. Corticosteroids are metabolized primarily in the liver and are then excreted by the kidneys. Some of the topical corticosteroids and their metabolites are also excreted into the bile.

INDICATIONS AND USAGE

Topical corticosteroids are indicated for the relief of the inflammatory and pruritic manifestations of corticosteroid-responsive dermatoses.

CONTRAINDICATIONS

Topical corticosteroids are contraindicated in those patients with a history of hypersensitivity to any of the components of the preparation.

PRECAUTIONS

General: Systemic absorption of topical corticosteroids has produced reversible hypothalamic-pituitary-adrenal (HPA) axis suppression, manifestations of Cushing's syndrome, hyperglycemia, and glucosuria in some patients.
Conditions which augment systemic absorption include the application of the more potent steroids, use over large surface areas, prolonged use, and the addition of occlusive dressings.
If HPA axis suppression is noted (by using the urinary free cortisol and ACTH stimulation tests) an attempt should be made to withdraw the drug or to reduce the frequency of application.
Recovery of HPA axis function is generally prompt and complete upon discontinuation of the drug. Infrequently, signs and symptoms of steroid withdrawal may occur, requiring supplemental systemic corticosteroids.
Pediatric patients may absorb proportionally larger amounts of topical corticosteroids and thus be more susceptible to systemic toxicity (see PRECAUTIONS—Use in Pediatric Patients).
If irritation develops, topical corticosteroids should be discontinued and appropriate therapy instituted. In the presence of dermatological infections, the use of an appropriate antifungal or antibacterial agent should be instituted. If a favorable response does not occur promptly, the corticosteroid should be discontinued until the infection has been adequately controlled.
Information for the Patient: Patients using topical corticosteroids should receive the following information and instructions:

1. This medication is to be used as directed by the physician. It is for external use only. Avoid contact with the eyes.
2. Patients should be advised not to use this medication for any disorder other than for which it has been prescribed.
3. The treated skin area should not be bandaged or otherwise covered or wrapped as to be occlusive unless directed by the physician.
4. Patients should report any signs of local adverse reactions especially under occlusive dressing.
5. Parents of pediatric patients should be advised not to use tight-fitting diapers or plastic pants on a child being treated in the diaper area, as these garments may constitute occlusive dressings.

Laboratory Tests: The urinary free cortisol test and the ACTH stimulation test may be helpful in evaluating the HPA axis suppression.
Carcinogenesis, Mutagenesis, and Impairment of Fertility: Long-term animal studies have not been performed to evaluate the carcinogenic potential or the effect on fertility of topical corticosteroids. Studies to determine mutagenicity with hydrocortisone have revealed negative results.
Pregnancy Category C: Corticosteroids are generally teratogenic in laboratory animals when administered systemically at relatively low dosage levels. The more potent corticosteroids have been shown to be teratogenic after dermal application in laboratory animals. There are no adequate and well-controlled studies in pregnant women on teratogenic effects from topically applied corticosteroids.
Therefore, topical corticosteroids should be used during pregnancy only if the potential benefit justifies the potential risk to the fetus. Drugs of this class should not be used extensively on pregnant patients, in large amounts, or for prolonged periods of time.
Nursing Mothers: It is not known whether topical administration of corticosteroids could result in sufficient systemic absorption to produce detectable quantities in breast milk. Systemically administered corticosteroids are secreted into breast milk in quantities not likely to have a deleterious effect on the infant. Nevertheless, caution should be exercised when topical corticosteroids are administered to a nursing woman.
Use in Pediatric Patients: PEDIATRIC PATIENTS MAY DEMONSTRATE GREATER SUSCEPTIBILITY TO TOPICAL CORTICOSTEROID-INDUCED HPA AXIS SUPPRESSION AND CUSHING'S SYNDROME THAN MATURE PATIENTS BECAUSE OF A LARGER SKIN SURFACE AREA TO BODY WEIGHT RATIO.
Hypothalamic-pituitary-adrenal (HPA) axis suppression, Cushing's syndrome, and intracranial hypertension have been reported in pediatric patients receiving topical corticosteroids. Manifestations of adrenal suppression in pediatric patients include linear growth retardation, delayed weight gain, low plasma cortisol levels, and absence of response to ACTH stimulation. Manifestations of intracranial hypertension include bulging fontanelles, headaches, and bilateral papilledema.
Administration of topical corticosteroids to pediatric patients should be limited to the least amount compatible with an effective therapeutic regimen. Chronic corticosteroid therapy may interfere with the growth and development of pediatric patients.

ADVERSE REACTIONS

The following local adverse reactions are reported infrequently with topical corticosteroids, but may occur more frequently with the use of occlusive dressings. These reactions are listed in an approximate decreasing order of occurrence:
Burning
Itching
Irritation
Dryness
Folliculitis
Hypertrichosis
Acneiform eruptions
Hypopigmentation
Perioral dermatitis
Allergic contact dermatitis
Maceration of the skin
Secondary infection
Skin atrophy
Striae
Miliaria

OVERDOSAGE

Topically applied corticosteroids can be absorbed in sufficient amounts to produce systemic effects. (See PRECAUTIONS).

DOSAGE AND ADMINISTRATION

Anusol-HC 2.5% (Hydrocortisone Cream, USP) should be applied to the affected area two to four times daily depending on the severity of the condition.
Occlusive dressings may be used for the management of psoriasis or recalcitrant conditions. If an infection develops, the use of occlusive dressings should be discontinued and appropriate antimicrobial therapy instituted.

HOW SUPPLIED

Anusol-HC 2.5% (Hydrocortisone Cream, USP) is supplied in 30 gram tubes NDC 61570-313-11.
Store at controlled room temperature 15°–30°C (59°–86°F). Store away from heat. Protect from freezing.
Revised September 1996
Manufactured by
Allergan Herbert
Skin Care Division of Allergan, Inc.
Irvine, CA 92713 USA
Distributed by: Monarch Pharmaceuticals, Inc.
Bristol, TN 37620

Shown in Product Identification Guide, page 324

ANUSOL-HC® 25-mg SUPPOSITORIES ℞
[*ăn 'ū-sŏl* ″]
(Hydrocortisone Acetate)

DESCRIPTION

Each Anusol-HC 25-mg Suppository contains 25 mg hydrocortisone acetate in a hydrogenated cocoglyceride base. Hydrocortisone acetate is a corticosteroid. Chemically, hydrocortisone acetate is pregn-4-ene-3,20-dione, 21-(acetyloxy)-11,17-dihydroxy-,(11β) with the following structural formula:

CLINICAL PHARMACOLOGY

In normal subjects, about 26 percent of hydrocortisone acetate is absorbed when the hydrocortisone acetate suppository is applied to the rectum. Absorption of hydrocortisone acetate may vary across abraded or inflamed surfaces.
Topical steroids are primarily effective because of their anti-inflammatory, antipruritic and vasoconstrictive action.

INDICATIONS AND USAGE

For use in inflamed hemorrhoids, post irradiation (factitial) proctitis, as an adjunct in the treatment of chronic ulcerative colitis, cryptitis, other inflammatory conditions of the anorectum, and pruritus ani.

CONTRAINDICATION

Anusol-HC suppositories are contraindicated in those patients with a history of hypersensitivity to any of the components.

PRECAUTIONS

Do not use unless adequate proctologic examination is made.
If irritation develops, the product should be discontinued and appropriate therapy instituted.
In the presence of an infection, the use of an appropriate antifungal or antibacterial agent should be instituted. If a favorable response does not occur promptly, the corticosteroid should be discontinued until the infection has been adequately controlled.
No long-term studies in animals have been performed to evaluate the carcinogenic potential of corticosteroid suppositories.

Information for Patients
Staining of fabric may occur with use of the suppository. Precautionary measures are recommended.

Pregnancy Category C
In laboratory animals, topical steroids have been associated with an increase in the incidence of fetal abnormalities when gestating females have been exposed to rather low dosage levels. There are no adequate and well-controlled studies in pregnant women. Anusol-HC suppositories should only be used during pregnancy if the potential benefit justifies the risk to the fetus. Drugs of this class should not be used extensively on pregnant patients, in large amounts, or for prolonged periods of time.
It is not known whether this drug is excreted in human milk, and because many drugs are excreted in human milk and because of the potential for serious adverse reactions in nursing infants from Anusol-HC suppositories, a decision should be made whether to discontinue nursing or to discontinue the drug, taking into account the importance of the drug to the mother.

ADVERSE REACTIONS

The following local adverse reactions have been reported with corticosteroid suppositories:

1. Burning
2. Itching
3. Irritation
4. Dryness
5. Folliculitis
6. Hypopigmentation
7. Allergic Contact Dermatitis
8. Secondary infection

DRUG ABUSE AND DEPENDENCE

Drug abuse and dependence have not been reported in patients treated with Anusol-HC suppositories.

OVERDOSAGE

If signs and symptoms of systemic overdosage occur discontinue use.

DOSAGE AND ADMINISTRATION

Usual dosage: One suppository in the rectum morning and night for two weeks in nonspecific proctitis. In more severe cases, one suppository three times daily; or two suppositories twice daily. In factitial proctitis, recommended therapy is six to eight weeks or less, according to response.

OPENING INSTRUCTIONS

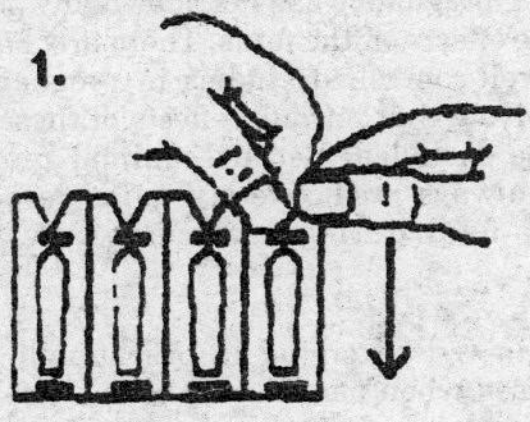

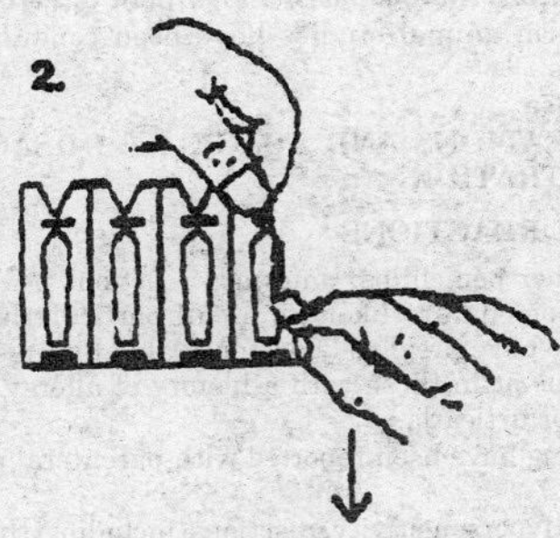

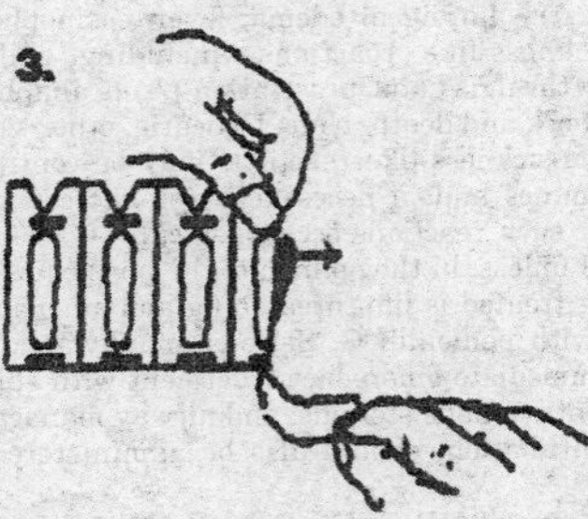

Avoid excessive handling of the suppository. It is designed to melt at body temperature.

1. Tear at the "V" cut and peel the foil in a downward motion.
2. Continue tearing downward to almost the full length of the suppository.
3. Gently remove the suppository from the foil packet.

HOW SUPPLIED

Anusol-HC 25-mg Suppositories are off-white, smooth surfaced, rod shaped with one rounded end. Package of 12 suppositories NDC 61570-172-61 and package of 24 suppositories NDC 61570-172-62.

Store below 30° C (86° F). Protect from freezing.

Revised September 1993

Rx only

Distributed by: Monarch Pharmaceuticals, Inc.
Bristol, TN 37620

Shown in Product Identification Guide, page 324

AVC™ ℞
(sulfanilamide)
Cream/Suppositories

Prescribing Information as of March 1999

DESCRIPTION

AVC™ is a preparation for vaginal administration for the treatment of *Candida albicans* infections and available in the following forms:

AVC Cream

Each tube contains:
Sulfanilamide 15.0%
in a water-miscible, non-staining base made from lactose, propylene glycol, stearic acid, diglycol stearate, methylparaben, propylparaben, trolamine, and water; buffered with lactic acid to an acid pH of approximately 4.3.

AVC Suppositories

Each suppository contains:
Sulfanilamide .... 1.05 g
with lactose, in a base made from polyethylene glycol 400, polysorbate 80, polyethylene glycol 3350, and glycerin, buffered with lactic acid to an acid pH of approximately 4.5. AVC Suppositories have an inert, white, non-staining covering, which dissolves promptly in the vagina. The covering is composed of gelatin, glycerin, water, methylparaben, propylparaben, and coloring.

Sulfanilamide is an anti-infective agent. It is *p*-amino-benzenesulfonamide with the chemical structure:

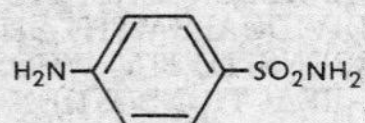

Sulfanilamide occurs as a white odorless crystalline powder with a slightly bitter taste and sweet aftertaste. It is slightly soluble in water, alcohol, acetone, glycerin, propylene glycol, hydrochloric acid, and solutions of potassium and sodium hydroxide. It is practically insoluble in chloroform, ether, benzene, and petroleum ether.

CLINICAL PHARMACOLOGY

Sulfanilamide has been a useful ingredient of vaginal formulations for about four decades. It blocks certain metabolic processes essential for the growth of susceptible bacteria. In AVC, the sulfanilamide is in a specially compounded base buffered to the pH (about 4.3) of the normal vagina to encourage the presence of the normally occurring Döderlein's bacilli of the vagina.

The use of AVC for the treatment of vulvovaginitis caused by *Candida albicans* is supported by three clinical investigations. The three studies show AVC with sulfanilamide to be significantly more effective ($p \leq 0.01$) than placebo as follows:

In Study I, the ratio of effectiveness was 71% for the AVC with sulfanilamide versus 49% for placebo with 30 days of treatment;

In Study II, the percentages were 48% and 24%, respectively, with 15 days of treatment;

In Study III, the percentages were 66% versus 33%, respectively, with 30 days of treatment.

INDICATIONS AND USAGE

For the treatment of vulvovaginitis caused by *Candida albicans*. (See CLINICAL PHARMACOLOGY.)

CONTRAINDICATIONS

AVC should not be used in patients known to be sensitive to this product or to the sulfonamides.

PRECAUTIONS

General

Because sulfonamides are absorbed from the vaginal mucosa, the usual precautions for oral sulfonamides apply. Patients should be observed for skin rash or evidence of systemic toxicity, and if these develop, the medications should be discontinued.

Deaths associated with administration of oral sulfonamides have reportedly occurred from hypersensitivity reactions, agranlocytosis, aplastic anemia, and other blood dyscrasias. Goiter production, diuresis, and hypoglycemia have reportedly occurred rarely in patients receiving oral sulfonamides. Cross-sensitivity may exist with these agents. Rats appear to be especially susceptible to the goitrogenic effects of sulfonamides, and long-term administration has reportedly produced thyroid malignancies in this species.

Vaginal applicators or inserters should be used with caution after the seventh month of pregnancy.

Information For Patients

The doctor should advise the patient that in the even unusual local itching and burning occur, or other unusual symptoms develop, medication should be discontinued and not restarted without further consultation.

Drug Interactions

Drug interactions have not been documented with AVC.

Carcinogenesis, Mutagenesis, Impairment of Fertility

No data are available on long-term potential of AVC for carcinogenicity, mutagenicity, or impairment of fertility in animals or humans.

Pregnancy.

Teratogenic Effects. Pregnancy Category C:

Animal reproductive studies have been conducted with sulfonamides, including sulfanilamide (see below). It is not known whether AVC can cause fetal harm when administered to a pregnant woman or can affect reproductive capacity. AVC should be given to a pregnant woman only if clearly needed.

Sulfonamides, including sulfanilamide, readily pass through the placenta and reach fetal circulation. The concentration in the fetus is from 50–90% of that in the maternal blood and if high enough, can cause toxic effects. The safe use of sulfonamides, including sulfanilamide, in pregnancy has not been established. The teratogenic potential of most sulfonamides has not been thoroughly investigated in either animals or humans. However, a significant increase in the incidence of cleft palate and other bony abnormalities of off-spring has been observed with certain sulfonamides of the short-, intermediate-, and long-acting types (including sulfanilamide) when given to pregnant rats and mice at high oral doses (seven to 25 times the human therapeutic oral dose).

Nursing Mothers

Sulfanilamide should be avoided in nursing mothers because absorbed sulfonamides will appear in maternal milk, and have caused kernicterus in the newborn. Because of the potential for serious adverse reactions in nursing infants from sulfonamides, a decision should be made whether to discontinue nursing or to discontinue the drug.

Pediatric Use

Safety and effectiveness of AVC in pediatric patients have not been established.

ADVERSE REACTIONS

Local sensitivity reactions such as increased discomfort or a burning sensation have occasionally been reported following the use of topical sulfonamides. With the use of AVC Cream, sensitivity reactions (only local) were reported for 0.2% of the investigational patients.

Treatment should be discontinued if either local or systemic manifestations of sulfonamide toxicity or sensitivity occur.

DRUG ABUSE AND DEPENDENCE

Tolerance, abuse, or dependence with AVC have not been reported.

OVERDOSAGE

There have been no reports of accidental overdosage with AVC.

The acute oral LD_{50} of sulfanilamide is 3700–4200 mg/kg in mice.

The minimum human lethal dose of AVC has not been established.

It is not known if AVC is dialyzable.

DOSAGE AND ADMINISTRATION

One applicatorful (about 6 g) or one suppository intravaginally once or twice daily. Improvements in symptoms should occur within a few days, but treatment should be continued for a period of 30 days.

Douching with a suitable solution before insertion may be recommended for hygienic purposes.

HOW SUPPLIED

AVC Cream

NDC 61570-103-04 4 oz tube with applicator
Store at room temperature, below 86°F. Protect from cold.
Product darkens with age. Potency is maintained throughout labeled shelf life when stored as directed.

AVC Suppositories

NDC 61570-084-16 Box of 16 white gelatin suppositories with inserter
Store at room temperature, below 86°F. Protect from excessive cold and moisture.
Prescribing Information as of February 1999
Suppositories Manufactured by:
R.P. Scherer, North America
Saint Petersburg, Florida 33716
Distributed by:
Monarch Pharmaceuticals, Inc.
Bristol, TN 37620
50007637

BICILLIN® C–R ℞
[*bī-sil 'in*]
(penicillin G benzathine and penicillin G procaine suspension)

INJECTION
FOR DEEP INTRAMUSCULAR INJECTION ONLY

DESCRIPTION

Bicillin C-R (penicillin G benzathine and penicillin G procaine suspension), contains equal amounts of the benzathine and procaine salts of penicillin G. It is available for deep intramuscular injection.

Penicillin G benzathine is prepared by the reaction of dibenzylethylene diamine with two molecules of penicillin G. It is chemically designated as (2*S*, 5*R*, 6*R*)-3,3-Dimethyl-7-oxo-6-(2-phenylacetamido)-4-thia-1-azabicyclo [3.2.0] heptane-2-carboxylic acid compound with *N,N'*-dibenzylethylenediamine (2:1), tetrahydrate. It occurs as a white, crystalline powder and is very slightly soluble in water and sparingly soluble in alcohol.

Penicillin G procaine, (2*S*, 5*R*, 6*R*)-3,3-Dimethyl-7-oxo-6-(2-phenylacetamido)-4-thia-1-azabicyclo [3.2.0] heptane-2-carboxylic acid compound with 2-(diethylamino)ethyl p-aminobenzoate (1:1) monohydrate, is an equimolar salt of procaine and penicillin G. It occurs as white crystals or a white, microcrystalline powder and is slightly soluble in water.

Bicillin C-R (penicillin G benzathine and penicillin G procaine suspension) contains in each mL the equivalent of 150,000 units of penicillin G as the benzathine salt and 150,000 units of penicillin G as the procaine salt in a stabilized aqueous suspension with sodium citrate buffer; and as w/v, approximately 0.5% lecithin, 0.55% carboxymethylcellulose, 0.55% povidone, 0.1% methylparaben, and 0.01% propylparaben.

Each disposable syringe (4 mL size) contains the equivalent of 2,400,000 units of penicillin G comprising: the equivalent of 1,200,000 units of penicillin G as the benzathine salt and the equivalent of 1,200,000 units of penicillin G as the procaine salt in a stabilized aqueous suspension with sodium citrate buffer; and as w/v, approximately 0.5% lecithin, 0.55% carboxymethylcellulose, 0.55% povidone, 0.1% methylparaben, and 0.01% propylparaben.

Each **TUBEX** cartridge (1 mL size) contains the equivalent of 600,000 units of penicillin G comprising: the equivalent of 300,000 units penicillin G as the benzathine salt and the equivalent of 300,000 units penicillin G as the procaine salt in a stabilized aqueous suspension with sodium citrate buffer; and as w/v, approximately 0.5% lecithin, 0.55% carboxymethylcellulose, 0.55% povidone, 0.1% methylparaben, and 0.01% propylparaben.

Each **TUBEX** cartridge (2 mL size) contains the equivalent of 1,200,000 units of penicillin G comprising: the equivalent

Continued on next page

Bicillin C-R—Cont.

of 600,000 units of penicillin G as the benzathine salt and the equivalent of 600,000 units of penicillin G as the procaine salt in a stabilized aqueous suspension with sodium citrate buffer; and as w/v, approximately 0.5% lecithin, 0.55% carboxymethylcellulose, 0.55% povidone, 0.1% methylparaben, and 0.01% propylparaben.
Bicillin C-R suspension in the multiple-dose-vial formulation, disposable-syringe formulation, and the **TUBEX** formulation is viscous and opaque. Read **CONTRAINDICATIONS**, **WARNINGS**, **PRECAUTIONS**, and **DOSAGE AND ADMINISTRATION** sections prior to use.

CLINICAL PHARMACOLOGY

General

Penicillin G benzathine and penicillin G procaine have a low solubility and, thus, the drugs are slowly released from intramuscular injection sites. The drugs are hydrolyzed to penicillin G. This combination of hydrolysis and slow absorption results in blood serum levels much lower but more prolonged than other parenteral penicillins.
Intramuscular administration of 600,000 units of Bicillin C-R in adults usually produces peak blood levels of 1.0 to 1.3 units per mL within 3 hours; this level falls to an average concentration of 0.32 units per mL at 12 hours, 0.19 units per mL at 24 hours, and 0.03 units per mL at seven days.
Intramuscular administration of 1,200,000 units of Bicillin C-R in adults usually produces peak blood levels of 2.1 to 2.6 units per mL within 3 hours; this level falls to an average concentration of 0.75 units per mL at 12 hours, 0.28 units per mL at 24 hours, and 0.04 units per mL at seven days.
Approximately 60% of penicillin G is bound to serum protein. The drug is distributed throughout the body tissues in widely varying amounts. Highest levels are found in the kidneys with lesser amounts in the liver, skin, and intestines. Penicillin G penetrates into all other tissues and the spinal fluid to a lesser degree. With normal kidney function, the drug is excreted rapidly by tubular excretion. In neonates and young infants and in individuals with impaired kidney function, excretion is considerably delayed.

Microbiology

Penicillin G exerts a bactericidal action against penicillin-susceptible microorganisms during the stage of active multiplication. It acts through the inhibition of biosynthesis of cell-wall mucopeptide. It is not active against the penicillinase-producing bacteria, which include many strains of staphylococci.
The following *in vitro* data are available, but their clinical significance is unknown. Penicillin G exerts high *in vitro* activity against staphylococci (except penicillinase-producing strains), streptococci (Groups A, C, G, H, L, and M), and pneumococci. Other organisms susceptible to penicillin G are *Neisseria gonorrhoeae, Corynebacterium diphtheriae, Bacillus anthracis,* Clostridia species, *Actinomyces bovis, Streptobacillus moniliformis, Listeria monocytogenes,* and Leptospira species. *Treponema pallidum* is extremely susceptible to the bactericidal action of penicillin G.
Susceptibility Test: If the Kirby-Bauer method of disc susceptibility is used, a 10-unit penicillin disc should give a zone greater than 28 mm when tested against a penicillin-susceptible bacterial strain.

INDICATIONS AND USAGE

This drug is indicated in the treatment of moderately severe infections due to penicillin-G-susceptible microorganisms that are susceptible to serum levels common to this particular dosage form. Therapy should be guided by bacteriological studies (including susceptibility testing) and by clinical response.
Bicillin C-R is indicated in the treatment of the following in adults and pediatric patients:
Moderately severe to severe infections of the upper-respiratory tract, scarlet fever, erysipelas, and skin and soft-tissue infections due to susceptible streptococci.
NOTE: Streptococci in Groups A, C, G, H, L, and M are very sensitive to penicillin G. Other groups, including Group D (enterococci), are resistant. Penicillin G sodium or potassium is recommended for streptococcal infections with bacteremia.
Moderately severe pneumonia and otitis media due to susceptible pneumococci.
NOTE: Severe pneumonia, empyema, bacteremia, pericarditis, meningitis, peritonitis, and arthritis of pneumococcal etiology are better treated with penicillin G sodium or potassium during the acute stage.
When high, sustained serum levels are required, penicillin G sodium or potassium, either IM or IV, should be used. This drug should not be used in the treatment of venereal diseases, including syphilis, gonorrhea, yaws, bejel, and pinta.

CONTRAINDICATIONS

A previous hypersensitivity reaction to any penicillin or to procaine is a contraindication.
Do not inject into or near an artery or nerve.

WARNINGS

The combination of penicillin G benzathine and penicillin G procaine should only be prescribed for the indications listed in this insert.
SERIOUS AND OCCASIONALLY FATAL HYPERSENSITIVITY (ANAPHYLACTIC) REACTIONS HAVE BEEN REPORTED IN PATIENTS ON PENICILLIN THERAPY. THESE REACTIONS ARE MORE LIKELY TO OCCUR IN INDIVIDUALS WITH A HISTORY OF PENICILLIN HYPERSENSITIVITY AND/OR A HISTORY OF SENSITIVITY TO MULTIPLE ALLERGENS. THERE HAVE BEEN REPORTS OF INDIVIDUALS WITH A HISTORY OF PENICILLIN HYPERSENSITIVITY WHO HAVE EXPERIENCED SEVERE REACTIONS WHEN TREATED WITH CEPHALOSPORINS. BEFORE INITIATING THERAPY WITH BICILLIN C-R, CAREFUL INQUIRY SHOULD BE MADE CONCERNING PREVIOUS HYPERSENSITIVITY REACTIONS TO PENICILLINS, CEPHALOSPORINS AND OTHER ALLERGENS. IF AN ALLERGIC REACTION OCCURS, BICILLIN C-R SHOULD BE DISCONTINUED AND APPROPRIATE THERAPY INSTITUTED. **SERIOUS ANAPHYLACTIC REACTIONS REQUIRE IMMEDIATE EMERGENCY TREATMENT WITH EPINEPHRINE, OXYGEN, INTRAVENOUS STEROIDS AND AIRWAY MANAGEMENT, INCLUDING INTUBATION, SHOULD ALSO BE ADMINISTERED AS INDICATED.**
Pseudomembranous colitis has been reported with nearly all antibacterial agents, including penicillin, and may range in severity from mild to life-threatening. Therefore, it is important to consider this diagnosis in patients who present with diarrhea subsequent to the administration of any antibacterial agent.
Treatment with antibacterial agents alters the normal flora of the colon and may permit overgrowth of clostridia. Studies indicate that a toxin produced by *Clostridium difficile* is one primary cause of "antibiotic-associated colitis".
After the diagnosis of pseudomembranous colitis has been established, appropriate therapeutic measures should be initiated. Mild cases of pseudomembranous colitis usually respond to drug discontinuation alone. In moderate to severe cases, consideration should be given to management with fluids and electrolytes, protein supplementation, and treatment with an antibacterial drug clinically effective against *C. difficile* colitis.
Inadvertent intravascular administration, including inadvertent direct intra-arterial injection or injection immediately adjacent to arteries, of Bicillin C-R and other penicillin preparations has resulted in severe neurovascular damage, including transverse myelitis with permanent paralysis, gangrene requiring amputation of digits and more proximal portions of extremities, and necrosis and sloughing at and surrounding the injection site. Such severe effects have been reported following injections into the buttock, thigh, and deltoid areas. Other serious complications of suspected intravascular administration which have been reported include immediate pallor, mottling or cyanosis of the extremity both distal and proximal to the injection site followed by bleb formation; severe edema requiring anterior and/or posterior compartment fasciotomy in the lower extremity. The above-described severe effects and complications have most often occurred in infants and small children. Prompt consultation with an appropriate specialist is indicated if any evidence of compromise of the blood supply occurs at, proximal to, or distal to the site of injection.[1–9] See **CONTRAINDICATIONS**, **PRECAUTIONS**, and **DOSAGE AND ADMINISTRATION** sections.
Quadriceps femoris fibrosis and atrophy have been reported following repeated intramuscular injections of penicillin preparations into the anterolateral thigh.
Injection into or near a nerve may result in permanent neurological damage.

PRECAUTIONS

General

Penicillin should be used with caution in individuals with histories of significant allergies and/or asthma.
Care should be taken to avoid intravenous or intra-arterial administration, or injection into or near major peripheral nerves or blood vessels, since such injections may produce neurovascular damage. See **CONTRAINDICATIONS**, **WARNINGS**, and **DOSAGE AND ADMINISTRATION** sections.
A small percentage of patients are sensitive to procaine. If there is a history of sensitivity, make the usual test: Inject intradermally 0.1 mL of a 1 to 2 percent procaine solution. Development of an erythema, wheal, flare, or eruption indicates procaine sensitivity. Sensitivity should be treated by the usual methods, including barbiturates, and procaine penicillin preparations should not be used. Antihistaminics appear beneficial in treatment of procaine reactions.
The use of antibiotics may result in overgrowth of nonsusceptible organisms. Constant observation of the patient is essential. If new infections due to bacteria or fungi appear during therapy, the drug should be discontinued and appropriate measures taken.
Whenever allergic reactions occur, penicillin should be withdrawn unless, in the opinion of the physician, the condition being treated is life-threatening and amenable only to penicillin therapy.
In prolonged therapy with penicillin, and particularly with high-dosage schedules, periodic evaluation of the renal and hematopoietic systems is recommended.

Laboratory Tests

In streptococcal infections, therapy must be sufficient to eliminate the organism; otherwise, the sequelae of streptococcal disease may occur. Cultures should be taken following completion of treatment to determine whether streptococci have been eradicated.

Drug Interactions

Tetracycline, a bacteriostatic antibiotic, may antagonize the bactericidal effect of penicillin, and concurrent use of these drugs should be avoided.
Concurrent administration of penicillin and probenecid increases and prolongs serum penicillin levels by decreasing the apparent volume of distribution and slowing the rate of excretion by competitively inhibiting renal tubular secretion of penicillin.

Pregnancy Category B

Reproduction studies performed in the mouse, rat, and rabbit have revealed no evidence of impaired fertility or harm to the fetus due to penicillin G. Human experience with the penicillins during pregnancy has not shown any positive evidence of adverse effects on the fetus. There are, however, no adequate and well-controlled studies in pregnant women showing conclusively that harmful effects of these drugs on the fetus can be excluded. Because animal reproduction studies are not always predictive of human response, this drug should be used during pregnancy only if clearly needed.

Nursing Mothers

Soluble penicillin G is excreted in breast milk. Caution should be exercised when penicillin G benzathine and penicillin G procaine are administered to a nursing woman.

Carcinogenesis, Mutagenesis, Impairment of Fertility

No long-term animal studies have been conducted with these drugs.

Pediatric Use

See **INDICATIONS AND USAGE** and **DOSAGE AND ADMINISTRATION**.

ADVERSE REACTIONS

As with other penicillins, untoward reactions of the sensitivity phenomena are likely to occur, particularly in individuals who have previously demonstrated hypersensitivity to penicillins or in those with a history of allergy, asthma, hay fever, or urticaria.
The following have been reported with parenteral penicillin G:
General: Hypersensitivity reactions including the following: skin eruptions (maculopapular to exfoliative dermatitis), urticaria, laryngeal edema, fever, eosinophilia; other serum-sickness-like reactions (including chills, fever, edema, arthralgia, and prostration); and anaphylaxis including shock and death. Note: Urticaria, other skin rashes, and serum-sickness-like reactions may be controlled with antihistamines and, if necessary, systemic corticosteriods. Whenever such reactions occur, penicillin G should be discontinued unless, in the opinion of the physician, the condition being treated is life-threatening and amenable only to therapy with penicillin G. Serious anaphylactic reactions require immediate emergency treatment with epinephrine. Oxygen, intravenous steroids, and airway management, including intubation, should also be administered as indicated.
Gastrointestinal: Pseudomembranous colitis. Onset of pseudomembranous colitis symptoms may occur during or after antibacterial treatment. (See **WARNINGS**).
Hematologic: Hemolytic anemia, leukopenia, thrombocytopenia.
Neurologic: Neuropathy.
Urogenital: Nephropathy.
The following adverse events have been temporally associated with parenteral administration of the penicillin G benzathine:
Body as a Whole: Hypersensitivity reactions including allergic vasculitis, pruritus, fatigue, asthenia, and pain; aggravation of existing disorder; headache.
Cardiovascular: Cardiac arrest; hypotension; tachycardia; palpitations; pulmonary hypertension; pulmonary embolism; vasodilatation; vasovagal reaction; cerebrovascular accident; syncope.
Gastrointestinal: Nausea, vomiting, blood in stool; intestinal necrosis.
Hemic and Lymphatic: Lymphadenopathy.
Injection Site: Injection site reactions including pain, inflammation, lump, abscess, necrosis, edema, hemorrhage, cellulitis, hypersensitivity, atrophy, ecchymosis, and skin ulcer. Neurovascular reactions including warmth, vasospasm, pallor, mottling, gangrene, numbness of the extremities, cyanosis of the extremities, and neurovascular damage.
Metabolic: Elevated BUN, creatinine, and SGOT.
Musculoskeletal: Joint disorder, periostitis, exacerbation of arthritis; myoglobinuria; rhabdomyolysis.
Nervous System: Nervousness; tremors; dizziness; somnolence; confusion; anxiety; euphoria; transverse myelitis; seizures; coma. A syndrome manifested by a variety of CNS symptoms such as severe agitation with confusion, visual and auditory hallucinations, and a fear of impending death (Hoigne's syndrome), has been reported after administration of penicillin G procaine and, less commonly, after injection of the combination of penicillin G benzathine and penicillin G procaine. Other symptoms associated with this syndrome, such as psychosis, seizures, dizziness, tinnitus, cyanosis, palpitations, tachycardia, and/or abnormal perception in taste, also may occur.
Respiratory: Hypoxia; apnea; dyspnea.
Skin: Diaphoresis.
Special Senses: Blurred vision; blindness.
Urogenital: Neurogenic bladder, hematuria; proteinuria; renal failure; impotence; priapism.

OVERDOSAGE

Penicillin in overdosage has the potential to cause neuromuscular hyperirritability or convulsive seizures.

DOSAGE AND ADMINISTRATION

Administer by DEEP, INTRAMUSCULAR INJECTION in the upper, outer quadrant of the buttock. In neonates, infants and small children, the midlateral aspect of the thigh may be preferable. When doses are repeated, vary the injection site.

When using the multiple-dose vial:

Shake multiple-dose vial vigorously before withdrawing the desired dose.

Due to the viscous nature of this medication, a 23 gauge or larger bore needle should be used to withdraw medication from the vial and for patient administration. A smaller bore needle, such as a 24 or 25 gauge, is not recommended.

After selection of the proper site and insertion of the needle into the selected muscle, aspirate by pulling back on the plunger. While maintaining negative pressure for 2 to 3 seconds, carefully observe the neck of the syringe immediately proximal to the needle hub for appearance of blood or any discoloration. Blood or "typical blood color" may *not* be seen if a blood vessel has been entered—only a mixture of blood and Bicillin C-R. The appearance of any discoloration is reason to withdraw the needle and discard the syringe. If it is elected to inject at another site, a new syringe and needle should be used. If no blood or discoloration appears, inject the contents of the syringe slowly. Discontinue delivery of the dose if the subject complains of severe immediate pain at the injection site or if in infants and young children symptoms or signs occur suggesting onset of severe pain.

When using the **TUBEX** cartridge:

The Wyeth-Ayerst **TUBEX®** cartridge for this product incorporates several features that are designed to facilitate the visualization of blood on aspiration if a blood vessel is inadvertently entered.

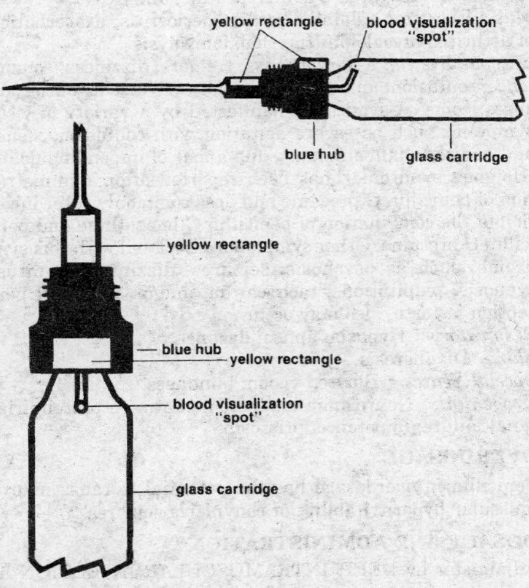

The design of this cartridge is such that blood which enters its needle will be quickly visualized as a red or dark-colored "spot." This "spot" will appear on the barrel of the glass cartridge immediately proximal to the blue hub. The **TUBEX** is designed with two orientation marks, in order to determine where the "spot" can be seen. First insert and secure the cartridge in the **TUBEX** injector in the usual fashion. Locate the yellow rectangle at the base of the blue hub. This yellow rectangle is aligned with the blood visualization "spot." An imaginary straight line, drawn from this yellow rectangle to the shoulder of the glass cartridge, will point to the area on the cartridge where the "spot" can be visualized. When the needle cover is removed, a second yellow rectangle will be visible. The second yellow rectangle is also aligned with the blood visualization "spot" to assist the operator in locating this "spot." If the 2 mL metal or plastic syringe is used, the glass cartridge should be rotated by turning the plunger of the syringe clockwise until the yellow rectangle is visualized. If the 1 mL metal syringe is used, it will not be possible to continue to rotate the glass cartridge clockwise once it is properly engaged and fully threaded; it can, however, then be rotated counterclockwise as far as necessary to properly orient the yellow rectangles and locate the observation area. (In this same area in some cartridges, a dark spot may sometimes be visualized prior to injection. This is the proximal end of the needle and does not represent a foreign body in, or other abnormality of, the suspension.)

Thus, before the needle is inserted into the selected muscle, it is important for the operator to orient the yellow rectangle so that any blood which may enter after needle insertion and during aspiration can be visualized in the area on the cartridge where it will appear and not be obscured by any obstructions.

After selection of the proper site and insertion of the needle into the selected muscle, aspirate by pulling back on the plunger. While maintaining negative pressure for 2 to 3 seconds, carefully observe the neck of the glass **TUBEX** cartridge immediately proximal to the blue plastic needle hub for appearance of blood or any discoloration. Blood or "typical blood color" may *not* be seen if a blood vessel has been entered—only a mixture of blood and Bicillin C-R. The appearance of any discoloration is reason to withdraw the needle and discard the **TUBEX**. If it is elected to inject at another site, a new **TUBEX** cartridge should be used. If no blood or discoloration appears, inject the contents of the **TUBEX** slowly. Discontinue delivery of the dose if the subject complains of severe immediate pain at the injection site or if, especially in neonates, infants and young children, symptoms or signs occur suggesting onset of severe pain.

Some **TUBEX** cartridges may contain a small air bubble which may be disregarded since it does not affect administration of the product. DO NOT clear any air bubbles from the cartridge or needle as this may interfere with the visualization of any blood or discoloration during aspiration.

Because of the high concentration of suspended material in this product, the needle may be blocked if the injection is not made at a slow, steady rate.

When using the disposable syringe:

The Wyeth-Ayerst disposable syringe for this product incorporates several new features that are designed to facilitate its use.

A single small indentation, or "dot," has been punched into the metal ring that surrounds the neck of the syringe near the base of the needle. It is important that this "dot" be placed in a position so that it can be easily visualized by the operator following the intramuscular insertion of the syringe needle.

After selection of the proper site and insertion of the needle into the selected muscle, aspirate by pulling back on the plunger. While maintaining negative pressure for 2 to 3 seconds, carefully observe the barrel of the syringe immediately proximal to the location of the "dot" for appearance of blood or any discoloration. Blood or "typical blood color" may *not* be seen if a blood vessel has been entered—only a mixture of blood and Bicillin C-R. The appearance of any discoloration is reason to withdraw the needle and discard the syringe. If it is elected to inject at another site, a new syringe should be used. If no blood or discoloration appears, inject the contents of the syringe slowly. Discontinue delivery of the dose if the subject complains of severe immediate pain at the injection site or if, especially in neonates, infants and young children symptoms or signs occur suggesting onset of severe pain.

Some disposable syringes may contain a small air bubble which may be disregarded, since it does not affect administration of the product.

Because of the high concentration of suspended material in this product, the needle may be blocked if the injection is not made at a slow, steady rate.

Streptococcal Infections Group A —Infections of the upper-respiratory tract, skin and soft-tissue infections, scarlet fever, and erysipelas.

The following doses are recommended:

Adults and pediatric patients over 60 lbs. in weight: 2,4000,000 units

Pediatric patients from 30 to 60 lbs.: 900,000 units to 1,200,000 units

Pediatric patients under 30 lbs.: 600,000 units

NOTE: Treatment with the recommended dosage is usually given at a single session using multiple IM sites when indicated. An alternative dosage schedule may be used, giving one-half ($^1/_2$) the total dose on day 1 and one-half ($^1/_2$) on day 3. This will also insure the penicillinemia required over a 10-day period; however, this alternate schedule should be used only when the physician can be assured of the patient's cooperation.

Pneumococcal Infections (Except Pneumococcal Meningitis)

600,000 units in pediatric patients and 1,200,000 units in adults, repeated every 2 or 3 days until the temperature is normal for 48 hours. Other forms of penicillin may be necessary for severe cases.

Parenteral drug products should be inspected visually for particulate matter and discoloration prior to administration whenever solution and container permit.

HOW SUPPLIED

Bicillin® C-R (penicillin G benzathine and penicillin G procaine suspension) is supplied in packages of 10 **TUBEX®** Sterile Cartridge-Needle Units as follows:

1 mL size, containing 600,000 units per **TUBEX®** (21 gauge, thin-wall 1 inch needle for pediatric use), NDC 0008-0026-37.

2 mL size, containing 1,200,000 units per **TUBEX®** (21 gauge, thin-wall 1 inch needle for pediatric use), NDC 0008-0026-36.

2 mL size, containing 1,200,000 units per **TUBEX®** (21 gauge, thin-wall 1-1/4 inch needle), NDC 0008-0026-35

Store in a refrigerator.

Keep from freezing.

Also Available

Bicillin C-R (penicillin G benzathine and penicillin G procaine suspension) is also available in packages of 10 disposable syringes as follows:

4 mL size, 2,400,000 units per syringe (18 gauge × 2 inch needle), NDC 0008-0026-22.

Bicillin C-R (penicillin G benzathine and penicillin G procaine suspension) is also available in packages of single multiple-dose vials as follows:

10 mL size, 300,000 units per mL, NDC 0008-0176-01.

Store in a refrigerator.

Keep from freezing.

Shake multiple-dose vials well before using.

REFERENCES

1. SHAW, E.: Transverse myelitis from injection of penicillin. *Am. J. Dis. Child., 111* :548, 1966.
2. KNOWLES, J.: Accidental intra-arterial injection of penicillin. *Am. J. Dis. Child., 111* :552, 1966.
3. DARBY, C., et al: Ischemia following an intragluteal injection of benzathine-procaine penicillin G mixture in a one-year-old boy. *Clin. Pediatrics, 12* :485, 1973.
4. BROWN, L. & NELSON, A.: Postinfectious intravascular thrombosis with gangrene. *Arch. Surg., 94* :652, 1967.
5. BORENSTINE, J.: Transverse myelitis and penicillin (Correspondence). *Am. J. Dis. Child., 112* :166, 1966.
6. ATKINSON, J.: Transverse myelopathy secondary to penicillin injection. *J. Pediatrics, 75* :867, 1969.
7. TALBERT, J. et al: Gangrene of the foot following intramuscular injection in the lateral thigh: A case report with recommendations for prevention. *J. Pediatrics, 70* :110, 1967.
8. FISHER, T.: Medicolegal affairs. *Canad. Med. Assoc. J., 112* :395, 1975.
9. SCHANZER, H. et al: Accidental intraarterial injection of penicillin G. *JAMA, 242* :1289, 1979.

Manufactured by:
Wyeth Laboratories
A Wyeth-Ayerst Company
Philadelphia, PA 19101
Distributed by:
Monarch Pharmaceuticals, Inc.
Bristol, TN 37620

Refer to the Tubex® Closed Injection System instructions in the Wyeth-Ayerst section of the 2001 PDR®.

BICILLIN® C-R 900/300 ℞

[*bī-sĭl 'ĭn*]

(penicillin G benzathine and penicillin G procaine suspension)

INJECTION
FOR DEEP INTRAMUSCULAR INJECTION ONLY

DESCRIPTION

Bicillin C-R 900/300 (penicillin G benzathine and penicillin G procaine suspension) contains the equivalent of 900,000 units of penicillin G as the benzathine and 300,000 units of penicillin G as the procaine salts. It is available for deep intramuscular injection.

Penicillin G benzathine is prepared by the reaction of dibenzylethylene diamine with two molecules of penicillin G. It is chemically designated as (2*S*, 5*R*, 6*R*)-3,3-Dimethyl-7-oxo-6-(2-phenylacetamido)-4-thia-1-azabicyclo[3.2.0]heptane-2-carboxylic acid compound with *N,N'*-dibenzylethylenediamine (2:1), tetrahydrate. It occurs as a white, crystalline powder and is very slightly soluble in water and sparingly soluble in alcohol.

Penicillin G procaine, (2*S*, 5*R*, 6*R*)-3,3-Dimethyl-7-oxo-6-(2-phenylacetamido)-4-thia-1-azabicyclo[3.2.0] heptane-2- carboxylic acid compound with 2-(diethylamino)ethyl *p*-aminobenzoate compound (1:1) monohydrate, is an equimolar salt of procaine and penicillin G. It occurs as white crystals or a white, microcrystalline powder and is slightly soluble in water.

Each **TUBEX®** cartridge (2 mL size) contains the equivalent to 1,200,000 units of penicillin G as follows: penicillin G benzathine equivalent to 900,000 units of penicillin G and penicillin G procaine equivalent to 300,000 units of penicillin G in a stabilized aqueous suspension with sodium citrate buffer; and as w/v, approximately 0.5% lecithin, 0.55% carboxymethylcellulose, 0.55% povidone, 0.1% methylparaben, and 0.01% propylparaben.

Bicillin C-R 900/300 suspension in **TUBEX** formulation is viscous and opaque. Read **CONTRAINDICATIONS, WARNINGS, PRECAUTIONS**, and **DOSAGE AND ADMINISTRATION** sections prior to use.

CLINICAL PHARMACOLOGY

General

Penicillin G benzathine and penicillin G procaine have a low solubility and, thus, the drugs are slowly released from intramuscular injection sites. The drugs are hydrolyzed to penicillin G. This combination of hydrolysis and slow absorption results in blood serum levels much lower but more prolonged than other parenteral penicillins. Intramuscular administration of 1,200,000 units of Bicillin C-R 900/300 in patients weighing 100 to 140 lbs. usually produces average blood levels of 0.24 units/mL at 24 hours, 0.039 units/mL at 7 days, and 0.024 units/mL at 10 days.

Approximately 60% of penicillin G is bound to serum protein. The drug is distributed throughout the body tissues in widely varying amounts. Highest levels are found in the kidneys with lesser amounts in the liver, skin, and intestines. Penicillin G penetrates into all other tissues and the spinal fluid to a lesser degree. With normal kidney function, the drug is excreted rapidly by tubular excretion. In neonates and young infants and in individuals with impaired kidney function, excretion is considerably delayed.

Microbiology

Penicillin G exerts a bactericidal action against penicillin-susceptible microorganisms during the stage of active multiplication. It acts through the inhibition of biosynthesis of

Continued on next page

Bicillin C-R 900/300—Cont.

cell-wall mucopeptide. It is not active against the penicillinase-producing bacteria, which include many strains of staphylococci.
The following *in vitro* data are available, but their clinical significance is unknown. Penicillin G exerts high *in vitro* activity against staphylococci (except penicillinase-producing strains), streptococci (Groups A, C, G, H, L, and M), and pneumococci. Other organisms susceptible to penicillin G are *Neisseria gonorrhoeae, Corynebacterium diphtheriae, Bacillus anthracis,* Clostridia species, *Actinomyces bovis, Streptobacillus moniliformis, Listeria monocytogenes,* and Leptospira species. *Treponema pallidum* is extremely susceptible to the bactericidal action of penicillin G.
Susceptibility Test: If the Kirby-Bauer method of disc susceptibility is used, a 10-unit penicillin disc should give a zone greater than 28 mm when tested against a penicillin-susceptible bacterial strain.

INDICATIONS AND USAGE

Bicillin C-R 900/300 is indicated in the treatment of infections as described below that are susceptible to serum levels characteristic of this particular dosage form. Therapy should be guided by bacteriological studies (including susceptibility testing) and by clinical response.
Bicillin C-R 900/300 is indicated in the treatment of the following in pediatric patients:
Moderately severe to severe infections of the upper-respiratory tract, scarlet fever, erysipelas, and skin and soft-tissue infections due to susceptible streptococci.
NOTE: Streptococci in Groups A, C, G, H, L, and M are very susceptible to penicillin G. Other groups, including Group D (enterococci), are resistant. Penicillin G sodium or potassium is recommended for streptococcal infections with bacteremia.
Moderately severe pneumonia and otitis media due to susceptible pneumococci.
NOTE: Severe pneumonia, empyema, bacteremia, pericarditis, meningitis, peritonitis, and arthritis of pneumococcal etiology are better treated with penicillin G sodium or potassium during the acute stage.
When high, sustained serum levels are required, penicillin G sodium or potassium, either IM or IV, should be used.
This drug should not be used in the treatment of venereal diseases, including syphilis, gonorrhea, yaws, bejel, and pinta.

CONTRAINDICATIONS

A previous hypersensitivity reaction to any penicillin or to procaine is a contraindication.
Do not inject into or near an artery or nerve.

WARNINGS

The combination of penicillin G benzathine and penicillin G procaine should only be prescribed for the indications listed in this insert.
SERIOUS AND OCCASIONALLY FATAL HYPERSENSITIVITY (ANAPHYLACTIC) REACTIONS HAVE BEEN REPORTED IN PATIENTS ON PENICILLIN THERAPY. THESE REACTIONS ARE MORE LIKELY TO OCCUR IN INDIVIDUALS WITH A HISTORY OF PENICILLIN HYPERSENSITIVITY AND/OR A HISTORY OF SENSITIVITY TO MULTIPLE ALLERGENS. THERE HAVE BEEN REPORTS OF INDIVIDUALS WITH A HISTORY OF PENICILLIN HYPERSENSITIVITY WHO HAVE EXPERIENCED SEVERE REACTIONS WHEN TREATED WITH CEPHALOSPORINS. BEFORE INITIATING THERAPY WITH BICILLIN C-R 900/300, CAREFUL INQUIRY SHOULD BE MADE CONCERNING PREVIOUS HYPERSENSITIVITY REACTIONS TO PENICILLINS, CEPHALOSPORINS AND OTHER ALLERGENS. IF AN ALLERGIC REACTION OCCURS, BICILLIN C-R 900/300 SHOULD BE DISCONTINUED AND APPROPRIATE THERAPY INSTITUTED. **SERIOUS ANAPHYLACTIC REACTIONS REQUIRE IMMEDIATE EMERGENCY TREATMENT WITH EPINEPHRINE. OXYGEN, INTRAVENOUS STEROIDS AND AIRWAY MANAGEMENT, INCLUDING INTUBATION, SHOULD ALSO BE ADMINISTERED AS INDICATED.**
Pseudomembranous colitis has been reported with nearly all antibacterial agents, including penicillin, and may range in severity from mild to life-threatening. Therefore, it is important to consider this diagnosis in patients who present with diarrhea subsequent to the administration of any antibacterial agent.
Treatment with antibacterial agents alters the normal flora of the colon and may permit overgrowth of clostridia. Studies indicate that a toxin produced by *Clostridium difficile* is one primary cause of "antibiotic colitis".
After the diagnosis of pseudomembranous colitis has been established, appropriate therapeutic measures should be initiated. Mild cases of pseudomembranous colitis usually respond to drug discontinuation alone. In moderate to severe cases, consideration should be given to management with fluids and electrolytes, protein supplementation, and treatment with an antibacterial drug clinically effective against *C. difficile* colitis.
Inadvertent intravascular administration, including inadvertent direct intra-arterial injection or injection immediately adjacent to arteries, of Bicillin C-R 900/300 and other penicillin preparations has resulted in severe neurovascular damage, including transverse myelitis with permanent paralysis, gangrene requiring amputation of digits and more proximal portions of extremities, and necrosis and sloughing at and surrounding the injection site. Such severe effects have been reported following injections into the buttock, thigh, and deltoid areas. Other serious complications of suspected intravascular administration which have been reported include immediate pallor, mottling, or cyanosis of the extremity both distal and proximal to the injection site, followed by bleb formation; severe edema requiring anterior and/or posterior compartment fasciotomy in the lower extremity. The above-described severe effects and complications have most often occurred in infants and small children. Prompt consultation with an appropriate specialist is indicated if any evidence of compromise of the blood supply occurs at, proximal to, or distal to the site of injection.[1-9] See **CONTRAINDICATIONS, PRECAUTIONS,** and **DOSAGE AND ADMINISTRATION** sections.
Quadriceps femoris fibrosis and atrophy have been reported following repeated intramuscular injections of penicillin preparations into the anterolateral thigh.
Injection into or near a nerve may result in permanent neurological damage.

PRECAUTIONS

General
Penicillin should be used with caution in individuals with histories of significant allergies and/or asthma.
Care should be taken to avoid intravenous or intra-arterial administration, or injection into or near major peripheral nerves or blood vessels, since such injections may produce neurovascular damage. See **CONTRAINDICATIONS, WARNINGS,** and **DOSAGE AND ADMINISTRATION** sections.
A small percentage of patients are sensitive to procaine. If there is a history of sensitivity, make the usual test: Inject intradermally 0.1 mL of a 1 to 2 percent procaine solution. Development of an erythema, wheal, flare, or eruption indicates procaine sensitivity. Sensitivity should be treated by the usual methods, including barbiturates, and procaine penicillin preparations should not be used. Antihistaminics appear beneficial in treatment of procaine reactions.
The use of antibiotics may result in overgrowth of nonsusceptible organisms. Constant observation of the patient is essential. If new infections due to bacteria or fungi appear during therapy, the drug should be discontinued and appropriate measures taken.
Whenever allergic reactions occur, penicillin should be withdrawn unless, in the opinion of the physician, the condition being treated is life-threatening and amenable only to penicillin therapy.
In prolonged therapy with penicillin, and particularly with high-dosage schedules, periodic evaluation of the renal and hematopoietic systems is recommended.

Laboratory Tests
In streptococcal infections, therapy must be sufficient to eliminate the organism; otherwise, the sequelae of streptococcal disease may occur. Cultures should be taken following completion of treatment to determine whether streptococci have been eradicated.

Drug Interactions
Tetracycline, a bacteriostatic antibiotic, may antagonize the bactericidal effect of penicillin, and concurrent use of these drugs should be avoided.
Concurrent administration of penicillin and probenecid increases and prolongs serum penicillin levels by decreasing the apparent volume of distribution and slowing the rate of excretion by competitively inhibiting renal tubular secretion of penicillin.

Pregnancy Category B
Reproduction studies performed in the mouse, rat, and rabbit have revealed no evidence of impaired fertility or harm to the fetus due to penicillin G. Human experience with the penicillins during pregnancy has not shown any positive evidence of adverse effects on the fetus. There are, however, no adequate and well-controlled studies in pregnant women showing conclusively that harmful effects of these drugs on the fetus can be excluded. Because animal reproduction studies are not always predictive of human response, this drug should be used during pregnancy only if clearly needed.

Nursing Mothers
Soluble penicillin G is excreted in breast milk. Caution should be exercised when penicillin G benzathine and penicillin G procaine are administered to a nursing woman.

Carcinogeneses, Mutagenesis, Impairment of Fertility
No long-term animal studies have been conducted with these drugs.

Pediatric Use
See **INDICATIONS AND USAGE** and **DOSAGE AND ADMINISTRATION.**

ADVERSE REACTIONS

As with other penicillins, untoward reactions of the sensitivity phenomena are likely to occur, particularly in individuals who have previously demonstrated hypersensitivity to penicillins or in those with a history of allergy, asthma, hay fever, or urticaria.
The following have been reported with parenteral penicillin G:
General: Hypersensitivity reactions including the following: skin eruptions (maculopapular to exfoliative dermatitis), urticaria, laryngeal edema, fever, eosinophilia; other serum-sickness-like reactions (including chills, fever, edema, arthralgia, and prostration); anaphylaxis including shock and death. NOTE: Urticaria, other skin rashes, and serum sickness-like reactions may be controlled with antihistamines and, if necessary, systemic corticosteroids.
Whenever such reactions occur, penicillin G should be discontinued unless, in the opinion of the physician, the condition being treated is life-threatening and amenable only to therapy with penicillin G. Serious anaphylactic reactions require immediate emergency treatment with epinephrine. Oxygen, intravenous steroids, and airway management, including intubation, should also be administered as indicated.
Gastrointestinal: Pseudomembranous colitis. Onset of pseudomembranous colitis symptoms may occur during or after antibacterial treatment. (See **WARNINGS.**)
Hematologic: Hemolytic anemia, leukopenia, thrombocytopenia.
Neurologic: Neuropathy.
Urogenital: Nephropathy.
The following adverse events have been temporally associated with parenteral administration of penicillin G benzathine:
Body as a Whole: Hypersensitivity reactions including allergic vasculitis, pruritus, fatigue, asthenia, and pain; aggravation of existing disorder; headache.
Cardiovascular: Cardiac arrest; hypotension; tachycardia; palpitations; pulmonary hypertension; pulmonary embolism; vasodilatation; vasovagal reaction; cerebrovascular accident; syncope.
Gastrointestinal: Nausea, vomiting; blood in stool; intestinal necrosis.
Hemic and Lymphatic: Lymphadenopathy.
Injection Site: Injection site reactions including pain, inflammation, lump, abscess, necrosis, edema, hemorrhage, cellulitis, hypersensitivity, atrophy, ecchymosis, and skin ulcer. Neurovascular reactions including warmth, vasospasm, pallor, mottling, gangrene, numbness of the extremities, cyanosis of the extremities, and neurovascular damage.
Metabolic: Elevated BUN, creatinine, and SGOT.
Musculoskeletal: Joint disorder; periostitis; exacerbation of arthritis; myoglobinuria; rhabdomyolysis.
Nervous System: Nervousness; tremors; dizziness; somnolence; confusion; anxiety; euphoria; transverse myelitis; seizures; coma. A syndrome manifested by a variety of CNS symptoms such as severe agitation with confusion, visual and auditory hallucinations, and a fear of impending death (Hoigne's syndrome), has been reported after administration of penicillin G procaine and, less commonly, after injection of the combination of penicillin G benzathine and penicillin G procaine. Other symptoms associated with this syndrome, such as psychosis, seizures, dizziness, tinnitus, cyanosis, palpitations, tachycardia, and/or abnormal perception in taste, also may occur.
Respiratory: Hypoxia; apnea; dyspnea.
Skin: Diaphoresis.
Special Senses: Blurred vision; blindness.
Urogenital: Neurogenic bladder; hematuria; proteinuria; renal failure; impotence; priapism.

OVERDOSAGE

Penicillin in overdosage has the potential to cause neuromuscular hyperirritability or convulsive seizures.

DOSAGE AND ADMINISTRATION

Administer by DEEP, INTRAMUSCULAR INJECTION in the upper, outer quadrant of the buttock. In neonates, infants and small children, the midlateral aspect of the thigh may be preferable. When doses are repeated, vary the injection site.
The Wyeth-Ayerst **TUBEX** cartridge for this product incorporates several features that are designed to facilitate the visualization of blood on aspiration if a blood vessel is inadvertently entered.

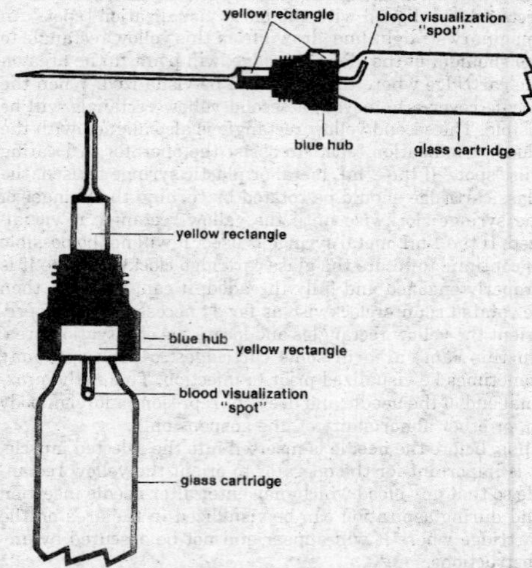

The design of this cartridge is such that blood which enters its needle will be quickly visualized as a red or dark-colored "spot." This "spot" will appear on the barrel of the glass cartridge immediately proximal to the blue hub. The **TUBEX** is designed with two orientation marks, in order to determine where the "spot" can be seen. First insert and secure the cartridge in the **TUBEX** injector in the usual fashion. Locate the yellow rectangle at the base of the blue hub. This yellow rectangle is aligned with the blood visualization "spot." An imaginary straight line, drawn from this yellow rectangle to the shoulder of the glass cartridge, will point to the area on the cartridge where the "spot" can be visualized. When the needle cover is removed, a second yellow rectangle will be visible. The second yellow rectangle is also aligned with the blood visualization "spot" to assist the operator in locating the "spot." If the 2 mL metal or plastic syringe is used, the glass cartridge should be rotated by turning the plunger of the syringe clockwise until the yellow rectangle is visualized. If the 1 mL metal syringe is used, it will not be possible to continue to rotate the glass cartridge clockwise once it is properly engaged and fully threaded; it can, however, then be rotated counterclockwise as far as necessary to properly orient the yellow rectangles and locate the observation area. (In this same area in some cartridges, a dark spot may sometimes be visualized prior to injection. This is the proximal end of the needle and does not represent a foreign body in, or other abnormality of, the suspension.)

Thus, before the needle is inserted into the selected muscle, it is important for the operator to orient the yellow rectangle so that any blood which may enter after needle insertion and during aspiration can be visualized in the area on the cartridge where it will appear and not be obscured by any obstructions.

After selection of the proper site and insertion of the needle into the selected muscle, aspirate by pulling back on the plunger. While maintaining negative pressure for 2 to 3 seconds, carefully observe the neck of the glass **TUBEX** cartridge immediately proximal to the blue plastic needle hub for appearance of blood or any discoloration.

Blood or "typical blood color" may *not* be seen if a blood vessel has been entered—only a mixture of blood and Bicillin C-R 900/300. The appearance of any discoloration is reason to withdraw the needle and discard the **TUBEX**. If it is elected to inject at another site, a new **TUBEX** cartridge should be used. If no blood or discoloration appears, inject the contents of the **TUBEX** slowly. Discontinue delivery of the dose if the subject complains of severe immediate pain at the injection site or if, especially in neonates, infants and young children, symptoms or signs occur suggesting onset of severe pain.

Some **TUBEX** cartridges may contain a small air bubble which may be disregarded, since it does not affect administration of the product. DO NOT clear any air bubbles from the cartridge or needle as this may interfere with the visualization of any blood or discoloration during aspiration.

Because of the high concentration of suspended material in this product, the needle may be blocked if the injection is not made at a slow, steady rate.

Streptococcal Infections

Group A Infections of the upper-respiratory tract, skin and soft-tissue infections, scarlet fever, and erysipelas: A single injection of Bicillin C-R 900/300 is usually sufficient for the treatment of Group A streptococcal infections in pediatric patients.

Pneumococcal Infections (except pneumococcal meningitis)

One TUBEX Bicillin C-R 900/300 repeated at 2- or 3-day intervals until the temperature is normal for 48 hours. Other forms of penicillin may be necessary for severe cases.

Parenteral drug products should be inspected visually for particulate matter and discoloration prior to administration, whenever solution and container permit.

HOW SUPPLIED

Bicillin® C-R 900/300 (penicillin G benzathine and penicillin G procaine suspension) is supplied in 2 mL size **TUBEX®** Sterile Cartridge-Needle Units in packages of 10 **TUBEX®** as follows:

1,200,000 units per **TUBEX®** (21 gauge, thin-wall 1 inch needle for pediatric use), NDC 0008-0079-36.

1,200,000 units per **TUBEX®** (21 gauge, thin-wall 1-1/4 inch needle), NDC 0008-0079-35.

Store in a refrigerator.

Keep from freezing.

REFERENCES

1. SHAW, E.: Transverse myelitis from injection of penicillin. *Am. J. Dis. Child., 111:* 548, 1966.
2. KNOWLES, J.: Accidental intra-arterial injection of penicillin. *Am. J. Dis. Child., 111:* 552, 1966.
3. DARBY, C., et al: Ischemia following an intragluteal injection of benzathine-procaine penicillin G mixture in a one-year-old boy. *Clin. Pediatrics, 12:* 485, 1973.
4. BROWN, L. & NELSON, A.: Postinfectious intravascular thrombosis with gangrene. *Arch. Surg., 94:* 652, 1967.
5. BORENSTINE, J.: Transverse myelitis and penicillin (Correspondence). *Am. J. Dis. Child., 112:* 166, 1966.
6. ATKINSON, J.: Transverse myelopathy secondary to penicillin injection. *J. Pediatrics, 75:* 867, 1969.
7. TALBERT, J. et al: Gangrene of the foot following intramuscular injection in the lateral thigh: A case report with recommendations for prevention. *J. Pediatrics, 70:* 110, 1967.
8. FISHER, T.: Medicolegal affairs. *Canad. Med. Assoc. J., 112:* 395, 1975.
9. SCHANZER, H. et al: Accidental intra-arterial injection of penicillin G. *JAMA, 242:* 1289, 1979.

Manufactured by:
Wyeth Laboratories
A Wyeth-Ayerst Company
Philadelphia, PA 19101

Distributed by:
Monarch Pharmaceuticals, Inc.
Bristol, TN 37620

Refer to the Tubex® Closed Injection System instructions in the Wyeth-Ayerst section of the 2001 PDR®.

BICILLIN® L-A ℞

[*bī-sil 'in*]

(penicillin G benzathine suspension)
INJECTION
FOR DEEP IM INJECTION ONLY

DESCRIPTION

Bicillin L-A (penicillin G benzathine suspension) is prepared by the reaction of dibenzylethylene diamine with two molecules of penicillin G. It is chemically designated as (2*S*, 5*R*, 6*R*) 3,3-Dimethyl-7-oxo -6- (2-phenylacetamido) -4-thia-1-azabicyclo[3.2.0]heptane-2-carboxylic acid compound with *N,N'*-dibenzylethylenediamine (2:1), tetrahydrate.

It is available for deep intramuscular injection. It contains penicillin G benzathine in aqueous suspension with sodium citrate buffer and, as w/v, approximately 0.5% lecithin, 0.6% carboxymethylcellulose, 0.6% povidone, 0.1% methylparaben, and 0.01% propylparaben. It occurs as a white, crystalline powder and is very slightly soluble in water and sparingly soluble in alcohol.

Bicillin L-A suspension in the multiple-dose vial formulation, disposable syringe formulation and **TUBEX** formulation is viscous and opaque. The multiple-dose vial formulation contains the equivalent of 300,000 units per mL of penicillin G as the benzathine salt. The disposable syringe formulation is available in a 4 mL size containing the equivalent of 2,400,000 units of penicillin G as the benzathine salt. The **TUBEX** formulation is available in 1 mL and 2 mL **TUBEX** Sterile Cartridge-Needle Units containing the equivalent of 600,000 units and 1,200,000 units respectively of penicillin G as the benzathine salt. Read **CONTRAINDICATIONS, WARNINGS, PRECAUTIONS,** and **DOSAGE AND ADMINISTRATION** sections prior to use.

CLINICAL PHARMACOLOGY

General

Penicillin G benzathine has an extremely low solubility and, thus, the drug is slowly released from intramuscular injection sites. The drug is hydrolyzed to penicillin G. This combination of hydrolysis and slow absorption results in blood serum levels much lower but much more prolonged than other parenteral penicillins.

Intramuscular administration of 300,000 units of penicillin G benzathine in adults results in blood levels of 0.03 to 0.05 units per mL, which are maintained for 4 to 5 days. Similar blood levels may persist for 10 days following administration of 600,000 units and for 14 days following administration of 1,200,000 units. Blood concentrations of 0.003 units per mL may still be detectable 4 weeks following administration of 1,200,000 units.

Approximately 60% of penicillin G is bound to serum protein. The drug is distributed throughout the body tissues in widely varying amounts. Highest levels are found in the kidneys with lesser amounts in the liver, skin, and intestines. Penicillin G penetrates into all other tissues and the spinal fluid to a lesser degree. With normal kidney function, the drug is excreted rapidly by tubular excretion. In neonates and young infants and in individuals with impaired kidney function, excretion is considerably delayed.

Microbiology

Penicillin G exerts a bactericidal action against penicillin-susceptible microorganisms during the stage of active multiplication. It acts through the inhibition of biosynthesis of cell-wall mucopeptide. It is not active against the penicillinase-producing bacteria, which include many strains of staphylococci.

The following *in vitro* data are available, but their clinical significance is unknown. Penicillin G exerts high *in vitro* activity against staphylococci (except penicillinase-producing strains), streptococci (Groups A, C, G, H, L, and M), and pneumococci. Other organisms susceptible to penicillin G are *Neisseria gonorrhoeae, Corynebacterium diphtheriae, Bacillus anthracis,* Clostridia species, *Actinomyces bovis, Streptobacillus moniliformis, Listeria monocytogenes,* and Leptospira species. *Treponema pallidum* is extremely susceptible to the bactericidal action of penicillin G.

Susceptibility Test: If the Kirby-Bauer method of disc susceptibility is used, a 20-unit penicillin disc should give a zone greater than 28 mm when tested against a penicillin-susceptible bacterial strain.

INDICATIONS AND USAGE

Intramuscular penicillin G benzathine is indicated in the treatment of infections due to penicillin-G-sensitive microorganisms that are susceptible to the low and very prolonged serum levels common to this particular dosage form. Therapy should be guided by bacteriological studies (including sensitivity tests) and by clinical response.

The following infections will usually respond to adequate dosage of intramuscular penicillin G benzathine:

Mild-to-moderate infections of the upper respiratory tract due to susceptible streptococci.

Venereal infections —Syphilis, yaws, bejel, and pinta.

Medical Conditions in which Penicillin G Benzathine Therapy is Indicated as Prophylaxis:

Rheumatic fever and/or chorea—Prophylaxis with penicillin G benzathine has proven effective in preventing recurrence of these conditions. It has also been used as follow-up prophylactic therapy for rheumatic heart disease and acute glomerulonephritis.

CONTRAINDICATIONS

A history of a previous hypersensitivity reaction to any of the penicillins is a contraindication.

Do not inject into or near an artery or nerve.

WARNINGS

Penicillin G benzathine should only be prescribed for the indications listed in this insert.

SERIOUS AND OCCASIONALLY FATAL HYPERSENSITIVITY (ANAPHYLACTIC) REACTIONS HAVE BEEN REPORTED IN PATIENTS ON PENICILLIN THERAPY. THESE REACTIONS ARE MORE LIKELY TO OCCUR IN INDIVIDUALS WITH A HISTORY OF PENICILLIN HYPERSENSITIVITY AND/OR A HISTORY OF SENSITIVITY TO MULTIPLE ALLERGENS. THERE HAVE BEEN REPORTS OF INDIVIDUALS WITH A HISTORY OF PENICILLIN HYPERSENSITIVITY WHO HAVE EXPERIENCED SEVERE REACTIONS WHEN TRATED WITH CEPHALOSPORINS. BEFORE INITIATING THERAPY WITH BICILLIN L-A, CAREFUL INQUIRY SHOULD BE MADE CONCERNING PREVIOUS HYPERSENSITIVITY REACTIONS TO PENICILLINS, CEPHALOSPORINS AND OTHER ALLERGENS. IF AN ALLERGIC REACTION OCCURS, BICILLIN L-A SHOULD BE DISCONTINUED AND APPROPRIATE THERAPY INSTITUTED. **SERIOUS ANAPHYLACTIC REACTIONS REQUIRE IMMEDIATE EMERGENCY TREATMENT WITH EPINEPHRINE, OXYGEN, INTRAVENOUS STEROIDS AND AIRWAY MANAGEMENT, INCLUDING INTUBATION, SHOULD ALSO BE ADMINISTERED AS INDICATED.**

Pseudomembranous colitis has been reported with nearly all antibacterial agents, including penicillin, and may range in severity from mild to life-threatening. Therefore, it is important to consider this diagnosis in patients who present with diarrhea subsequent to the administration of any antibacterial agent.

Treatment with antibacterial agents alter the normal flora of the colon and may permit overgrowth of clostridia. Studies indicate that a toxin produced by *Clostridium difficile* is one primary cause of "antibiotic-associated colitis".

After the diagnosis of pseudomembranous colitis has been established, appropriate therapeutic measures should be initiated. Mild cases of pseudomembranous colitis usually respond to drug discontinuation alone. In moderate to severe cases, consideration should be given to management with fluids and electrolytes, protein supplementation, and treatment with an antibacterial drug clinically effective against *C. difficile* colitis.

Inadvertent intravascular administration, including inadvertent direct intra-arterial injection or injection immediately adjacent to arteries, of Bicillin L-A and other penicillin preparations has resulted in severe neurovascular damage, including transverse myelitis with permanent paralysis, gangrene requiring amputation of digits and more proximal portions of extremities, and necrosis and sloughing at and surrounding the injection site. Such severe effects have been reported following injections into the buttock, thigh, and deltoid areas. Other serious complications of suspected intravascular administration which have been reported include immediate pallor, mottling, or cyanosis of the extremity both distal and proximal to the injection site, followed by bleb formation; severe edema requiring anterior and/or posterior compartment fasciotomy in the lower extremity. The above-described severe effects and complications have most often occurred in infants and small children. Prompt consultation with an appropriate specialist is indicated if any evidence of compromise of the blood supply occurs at, proximal to, or distal to the site of injection.[1-9] See **CONTRAINDICATIONS, PRECAUTIONS,** and **DOSAGE AND ADMINISTRATION** sections.

Quadriceps femoris fibrosis and atrophy have been reported following repeated intramuscular injections of penicillin preparations into the anterolateral thigh.

Injection into or near a nerve may result in permanent neurological damage.

PRECAUTIONS

General

Penicillin should be used with caution in individuals with histories of significant allergies and/or asthma.

Care should be taken to avoid intravenous or intra-arterial administration, or injection into or near major peripheral nerves or blood vessels, since such injection may produce neurovascular damage. See **CONTRAINDICATIONS, WARNINGS,** and **DOSAGE AND ADMINISTRATION** sections.

Prolonged use of antibiotics may promote the overgrowth of nonsusceptible organisms, including fungi. Should superinfection occur, appropriate measures should be taken.

Laboratory Tests

In streptococcal infections, therapy must be sufficient to eliminate the organism; otherwise, the sequelae of streptococcal disease may occur. Cultures should be taken following completion of treatment to determine whether streptococci have been eradicated.

Continued on next page

Bicillin L-A—Cont.

Drug Interactions
Tetracycline, a bacteriostatic antibiotic, may antagonize the bactericidal effect of penicillin, and concurrent use of these drugs should be avoided.
Concurrent administration of penicillin and probenecid increases and prolongs serum penicillin levels by decreasing the apparent volume of distribution and slowing the rate of excretion by competitively inhibiting renal tubular secretion of penicillin.
Pregnancy Category B
Reproduction studies performed in the mouse, rat, and rabbit have revealed no evidence of impaired fertility or harm to the fetus due to penicillin G. Human experience with the penicillins during pregnancy has not shown any positive evidence of adverse effects on the fetus. There are, however, no adequate and well-controlled studies in pregnant women showing conclusively that harmful effects of these drugs on the fetus can be excluded. Because animal reproduction studies are not always predictive of human response, this drug should be used during pregnancy only if clearly needed.
Nursing Mothers
Soluble penicillin G is excreted in breast milk. Caution should be exercised when penicillin G benzathine is administered to a nursing woman.
Carcinogenesis, Mutagenesis, Impairment Of Fertility
No long-term animal studies have been conducted with this drug.
Pediatric Use
See **INDICATIONS AND USAGE** and **DOSAGE AND ADMINISTRATION**.

ADVERSE REACTIONS

As with other penicillins, untoward reactions of the sensitivity phenomena are likely to occur, particularly in individuals who have previously demonstrated hypersensitivity to penicillins or in those with a history of allergy, asthma, hay fever, or urticaria.
As with other treatments for syphilis, the Jarisch-Herxheimer reaction has been reported.
The following have been reported with parenteral penicillin G:
General: Hypersensitivity reactions including the following: skin eruptions (maculopapular to exfoliative dermatitis), urticaria, laryngeal edema, fever, eosinophilia; other serum sickness-like reactions (including chills, fever, edema, arthralgia, and prostration); and anaphylaxis including shock and death. Note: Urticaria, other skin rashes, and serum sickness-like reactions may be controlled with antihistamines and, if necessary, systemic corticosteroids. Whenever such reactions occur, penicillin G should be discontinued unless, in the opinion of the physician, the condition being treated is life-threatening and amenable only to therapy with penicillin G. Serious anaphylactic reactions require immediate emergency treatment with epinephrine. Oxygen, intravenous steroids, and airway management, including intubation, should also be administered as indicated.
Gastrointestinal: Pseudomembranous colitis. Onset of pseudomembranous colitis symptoms may occur during or after antibacterial treatment. See **WARNINGS**.
Hematologic: Hemolytic anemia, leukopenia, thrombocytopenia.
Neurologic: Neuropathy.
Urogenital: Nephropathy.
The following adverse events have been temporally associated with parenteral administration of penicillin G benzathine:
Body as a Whole: Hypersensitivity reactions including allergic vasculitis, pruritus, fatigue, asthenia, and pain; aggravation of existing disorder; headache.
Cardiovascular: Cardiac arrest; hypotension; tachycardia; palpitations; pulmonary hypertension; pulmonary embolism; vasodilatation; vasovagal reaction; cerebrovascular accident; syncope.
Gastrointestinal: Nausea, vomiting; blood in stool; intestinal necrosis.
Hemic and Lymphatic: Lymphadenopathy.
Injection Site: Injection site reactions including pain, inflammation, lump, abscess, necrosis, edema, hemorrhage, cellulitis, hypersensitivity, atrophy, ecchymosis, and skin ulcer. Neurovascular reactions including warmth, vasospasm, pallor, mottling, gangrene, numbness of the extremities, and neurovascular damage.
Metabolic: Elevated BUN, creatinine, and SGOT.
Musculoskeletal: Joint disorder; periostitis; exacerbation of arthritis; myoglobinura; rhabdomyolysis.
Nervous System: Nervousness; tremors; dizziness; somnolence; confusion; anxiety; euphoria; transverse myelitis; seizures; coma. A syndrome manifested by a variety of CNS symptoms such as severe agitation with confusion, visual and auditory hallucinations, and a fear of impending death (Hoigne's syndrome), has been reported after administration of penicillin G procaine and, less commonly, after injection of the combination of penicillin G benzathine and penicillin G procaine. Other symptoms associated with this syndrome, such as psychosis, seizures, dizziness, tinnitus, cyanosis, palpitations, tachycardia, and/or abnormal perception in taste, also may occur.
Respiratory: Hypoxia; apnea; dyspnea.
Skin: Diaphoresis.
Special Senses: Blurred vision; blindness.
Urogenital: Neurogenic bladder; hematuria; proteinuria; renal failure; impotence; priapism.

OVERDOSAGE

Penicillin in overdosage has the potential to cause neuromuscular hyperirritability or convulsive seizures.

DOSAGE AND ADMINISTRATION

Due to the viscous nature of this medication, a 23 gauge or larger bore needle should be used to withdraw medication from the vial and for patient administration. A smaller bore needle, such as a 24 or 25 gauge, is not recommended.
Streptococcal (Group A) Upper-respiratory infections (for example, pharyngitis)
Adults—a single injection of 1,200,000 units; older pediatric patients—a single injection of 900,000 units; infants and pediatric patients under 60 lbs.—300,000 to 600,000 units.
Syphilis
Primary, secondary, and latent—2,400,000 units (1 dose).
Late (tertiary and neurosyphilis)—2,400,000 units at 7-day intervals for three doses.
Congenital—under 2 years of age: 50,000 units/kg/body weight; ages 2 to 12 years: adjust dosage based on adult dosage schedule.
Yaws, Bejel, and Pinta—1,200,000 units (1 injection).
Prophylaxis—for rheumatic fever and glomerulonephritis.
Following an acute attack, penicillin G benzathine (parenteral) may be given in doses of 1,200,000 units once a month or 600,000 units every 2 weeks.
Administer by DEEP INTRAMUSCULAR INJECTION in the upper, outer quadrant of the buttock. In neonates, infants and small children, the midlateral aspect of the thigh may be preferable. When doses are repeated, vary the injection site.
When using the multiple-dose vial:
After selection of the proper site and insertion of the needle into the selected muscle, aspirate by pulling back on the plunger. While maintaining negative pressure for 2 to 3 seconds, carefully observe the barrel of the syringe immediately proximal to the needle hub for appearance of blood or any discoloration. Blood or "typical blood color" may *not* be seen if a blood vessel has been entered—only a mixture of blood and Bicillin L-A. The appearance of any discoloration is reason to withdraw the needle and discard the syringe. If it is elected to inject at another site, a new syringe and needle should be used. If no blood or discoloration appears, inject the contents of the syringe slowly. Discontinue delivery of the dose if the subject complains of severe immediate pain at the injection site or if, especially in neonates, infants and young children symptoms or signs occur suggesting onset of severe pain.
Because of the high concentration of suspended material in this product, the needle may be blocked if the injection is not made at a slow, steady rate.
When using the **TUBEX** cartridge:
The Wyeth-Ayerst **TUBEX®** cartridge for this product incorporates several features that are designed to facilitate the visualization of blood on aspiration if a blood vessel is inadvertently entered.

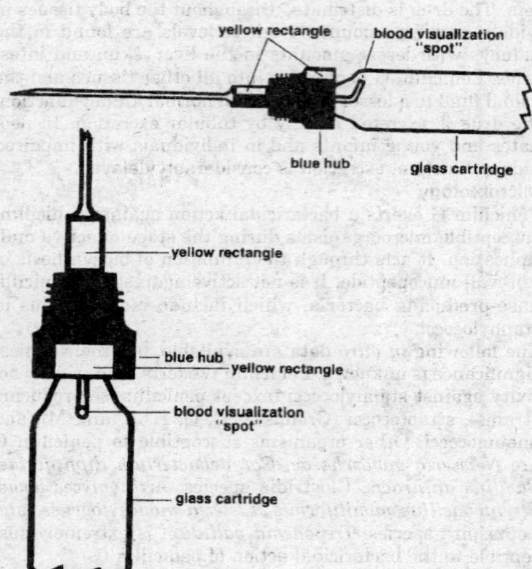

The design of this cartridge is such that blood which enters its needle will be quickly visualized as a red or dark-colored "spot." This "spot" will appear on the barrel of the glass cartridge immediately proximal to the blue hub. The **TUBEX** is designed with two orientation marks, in order to determine where the "spot" can be seen. First insert and secure the cartridge in the **TUBEX** injector in the usual fashion. Locate the yellow rectangle at the base of the blue hub. This yellow rectangle is aligned with the blood visualization "spot." An imaginary straight line, drawn from this yellow rectangle to the shoulder of the glass cartridge, will point to the area on the cartridge where the "spot" can be visualized. When the needle cover is removed, a second yellow rectangle will be visible. The second yellow rectangle is also aligned with the blood visualization "spot" to assist the operator in locating this "spot." If the 2 mL metal or plastic syringe is used, the glass cartridge should be rotated by turning the plunger of the syringe clockwise until the yellow rectangle is visualized. If the 1 mL metal syringe is used, it will not be possible to continue to rotate the glass cartridge clockwise once it is properly engaged and fully threaded; it can, however, then be rotated counterclockwise as far as necessary to properly orient the yellow rectangles and locate the observation area. (In this same area in some cartridges, a dark spot may sometimes be visualized prior to injection. This is the proximal end of the needle and does not represent a foreign body in, or other abnormality of, the suspension.)
Thus, before the needle is inserted into the selected muscle, it is important for the operator to orient the yellow rectangle so that any blood which may enter after needle insertion and during aspiration can be visualized in the area on the cartridge where it will appear and not be obscured by any obstructions.
After selection of the proper site and insertion of the needle into the selected muscle, aspirate by pulling back on the plunger. While maintaining negative pressure for 2 to 3 seconds, carefully observe the barrel of the cartridge in the area previously identified (see above) for the appearance of a red or dark-colored "spot."
Blood or "typical blood color" may not be seen if a blood vessel has been entered—only a mixture of blood and Bicillin L-A. The appearance of any discoloration is reason to withdraw the needle and discard the glass **TUBEX** cartridge. If it is elected to inject at another site, a new cartridge should be used. If no blood or discoloration appears, inject the contents of the cartridge slowly. Discontinue delivery of the dose if the subject complains of severe immediate pain at the injection site or if, especially in infants and young children, symptoms or signs occur suggesting onset of severe pain.
Some **TUBEX** cartridges may contain a small air bubble which may be disregarded, since it does not affect administration of the product.
DO NOT clear any air bubbles from the cartridge or needle as this may interfere with the visualization of any blood or discoloration during aspiration.
Because of the high concentration of suspended material in this product, the needle may be blocked if the injection is not made at a slow, steady rate.
When using the disposable syringe:
The Wyeth-Ayerst disposable syringe for this product incorporates several features that are designed to facilitate its use.
A single, small indentation, or "dot," has been punched into the metal ring that surrounds the neck of the syringe near the base of the needle. It is important that this "dot" be placed in a position so that it can be easily visualized by the operator following the intramuscular insertion of the syringe needle.
After selection of the proper site and insertion of the needle into the selected muscle, aspirate by pulling back on the plunger. While maintaining negative pressure for 2 to 3 seconds, carefully observe the barrel of the syringe immediately proximal to the location of the "dot" for appearance of blood or any discoloration. Blood or "typical blood color" may *not* be seen if a blood vessel has been entered—only a mixture of blood and Bicillin L-A. The appearance of any discoloration is reason to withdraw the needle and discard the syringe. If it is elected to inject at another site, a new syringe should be used. If no blood or discoloration appears, inject the contents of the syringe slowly. Discontinue delivery of the dose if the subject complains of severe immediate pain at the injection site or if, especially in neonates, infants and young children, symptoms or signs occur suggesting onset of severe pain.
Some disposable syringes may contain a small air bubble which may be disregarded, since it does not affect administration of the product. DO NOT clear any air bubbles from the disposable syringe or needle as this may interfere with the visualization of any blood or discoloration during aspiration.
Because of the high concentration of suspended material in this product, the needle may be blocked if the injection is not made at a slow, steady rate.
Parenteral drug products should be inspected visually for particulate matter and discoloration prior to administration whenever solution and container permit.

HOW SUPPLIED

Bicillin® L-A (penicillin G benzathine suspension) is supplied in packages of 10 **TUBEX®** Sterile Cartridge-Needle Units as follows:
1 mL size, containing 600,000 units per **TUBEX®** (21 gauge, thin-wall 1 inch needle for pediatric use), NDC 0008-0021-37.
2 mL size, containing 1,200,000 units per **TUBEX®** (21 gauge, thin-wall 1–1/4 inch needle), NDC 0008-0021-35.
Store in a refrigerator.
Keep from freezing.
ALSO AVAILABLE
Bicillin L-A (penicillin G benzathine suspension) is also available in packages of 10 disposable syringes as follows:
4 mL size, containing 2,400,000 units per syringe (18 gauge × 2 inch needle), NDC 0008-0021-12
Bicillin L-A (penicillin G benzathine suspension) is also available in packages of single multiple-dose vials as follows:
10 mL size, 300,000 units per mL, NDC 0008-0163-01.
Store in a refrigerator.
Keep from freezing.

Shake multiple-dose vials well before using.

REFERENCES

1. SHAW, E.: Transverse myelitis from injection of penicillin. *Am. J. Dis. Child., 111:* 548, 1966.
2. KNOWLES, J.: Accidental intra-arterial injection of penicillin. *Am. J. Dis. Child., 111:* 552, 1966.
3. DARBY, C., et al: Ischemia following an intragluteal injection of benzathine-procaine penicillin G mixture in a one-year-old boy. *Clin. Pediatrics, 12:* 485, 1973.
4. BROWN, L. & NELSON, A.: Postinfectious intravascular thrombosis with gangrene. *Arch. Surg., 94:* 652, 1967.
5. BORENSTINE, J.: Transverse myelitis and penicillin (Correspondence). *Am. J. Dis. Child., 112:* 166, 1966.
6. ATKINSON, J.: Transverse myelopathy secondary to penicillin injection. *J. Pediatrics, 75:* 867, 1969.
7. TALBERT, J. et al: Gangrene of the foot following intramuscular injection in the lateral thigh: A case report with recommendations for prevention. *J. Pediatrics, 70:* 110, 1967.
8. FISHER, T.: Medicolegal affairs. *Canad. Med. Assoc. J., 112:* 395, 1975.
9. SCHANZER, H. et al: Accidental intra-arterial injection of penicillin G. *JAMA, 242:* 1289, 1979.

Manufactured by:
Wyeth Laboratories
A Wyeth-Ayerst Company
Philadelphia, PA 19101
Distributed by:
Monarch Pharmaceuticals, Inc.
Bristol, TN 37620

Refer to the Tubex® Closed Injection System instructions in the Wyeth-Ayerst section of the 2001 PDR®.

COLY-MYCIN® M PARENTERAL ℞

[*cōly-mycin*]

(Sterile Colistimethate Sodium, USP)

FOR INTRAMUSCULAR AND INTRAVENOUS USE

DESCRIPTION

Coly-Mycin® M Parenteral (Sterile Colistimethate Sodium, USP) is a sterile parenteral antibiotic product which, when reconstituted (see Reconstitution), is suitable for intramuscular or intravenous administration.

Each vial contains colistimethate sodium or pentasodium colistinmethanesulfonate (150 mg colistin base activity). Colistimethate sodium is a polypeptide antibiotic with an approximate molecular weight of 1750. The empirical formula is $C_{58}H_{105}N_{16}Na_5O_{28}S_5$ and the structural formula is represented below:

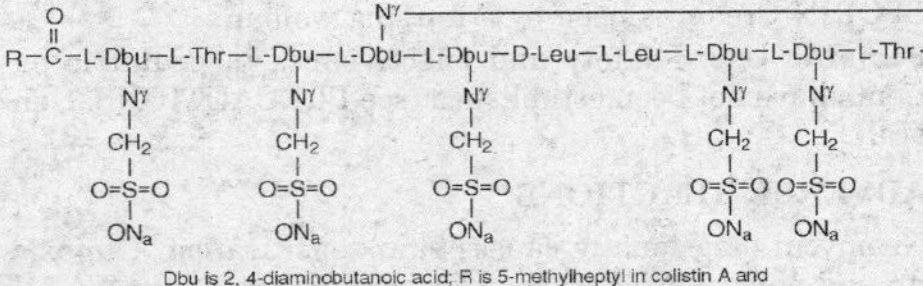

Dbu is 2, 4-diaminobutanoic acid; R is 5-methylheptyl in colistin A and 5-methylhexyl in colistin B

CLINICAL PHARMACOLOGY

Typical serum and urine levels following a single 150 mg dose of Coly-Mycin M Parenteral IM or IV in normal adult subjects are shown in Figure 1.

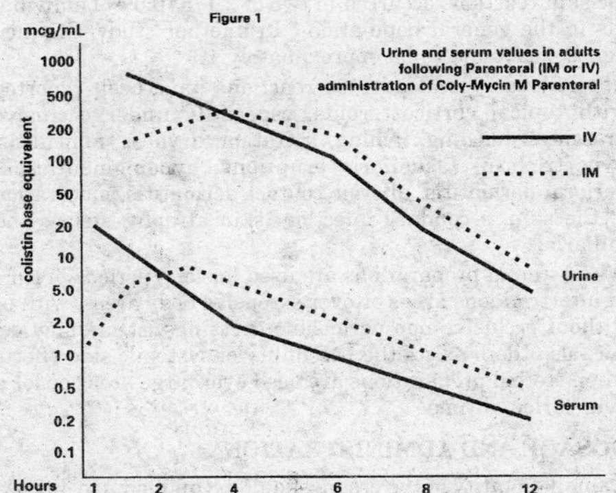

Higher serum levels were obtained at 10 minutes following IV administration. Serum concentration declined with a half-life of 2–3 hours following either intravenous or intramuscular administration in adults and in the pediatric population, including premature infants.

Average urine levels ranged from about 270 mcg/mL at 2 hours to about 15 mcg/mL at 8 hours after intravenous administration and from 200 to about 25 mcg/mL during a similar period following intramuscular administration.

Microbiology: Colistimethate sodium is a surface active agent which penetrates into and disrupts the bacterial cell membrane. It has been shown to have bactericidal activity against most strains of the following microorganisms, both *in vitro* and in clinical infections as described in the INDICATIONS AND USAGE section:

TABLE 1. Suggested Modification of Dosage Schedules of Coly-Mycin M Parenteral for Adults with Impaired Renal Function

Renal Function	Degree of Impairment			
	Normal	Mild	Moderate	Considerable
Plasma creatinine, mg/100 mL	0.7–1.2	1.3–1.5	1.6–2.5	2.6–4.0
Urea clearance, % of normal	80–100	40–70	25–40	10–25
Dosage				
Unit dose of Coly-Mycin M, mg	100–150	75–115	66–150	100–150
Frequency, times/day	4 to 2	2	2 or 1	every 36 hr
Total daily dose, mg	300	150–230	133–150	100
Approximate daily dose, mg/kg/day	5.0	2.5–3.8	2.5	1.5

Aerobic gram-negative microorganisms:
Enterobacter aerogenes, Escherichia coli, Klebsiella pneumoniae, and *Pseudomonas aeruginosa*

Susceptibility Tests: Colistimethate sodium is no longer listed as an antimicrobial for routine testing and reporting by clinical microbiology laboratories.

INDICATIONS AND USAGE

Coly-Mycin M Parenteral is indicated for the treatment of acute or chronic infections due to sensitive strains of certain gram-negative bacilli. It is particularly indicated when the infection is caused by sensitive strains of *Pseudomonas aeruginosa*. This antibiotic is not indicated for infections due to *Proteus* or *Neisseria*. Coly-Mycin M Parenteral has proven clinically effective in treatment of infections due to the following gram-negative organisms: *Enterobacter aerogenes, Escherichia coli, Klebsiella pneumoniae,* and *Pseudomonas aeruginosa*.

Coly-Mycin M Parenteral may be used to initiate therapy in serious infections that are suspected to be due to gram-negative organisms and in the treatment of infections due to susceptible gram-negative pathogenic bacilli.

CONTRAINDICATIONS

The use of Coly-Mycin M Parenteral is contraindicated for patients with a history of sensitivity to the drug or any of its components.

WARNINGS

Maximum daily dose should not exceed 5 mg/kg/day (2.3 mg/lb) with normal renal function.

Transient neurological disturbances may occur. These include circumoral paresthesia or numbness, tingling or formication of the extremities, generalized pruritus, vertigo, dizziness, and slurring of speech. For these reasons, patients should be warned not to drive vehicles or use hazardous machinery while on therapy. Reduction of dosage may alleviate symptoms. Therapy need not be discontinued, but such patients should be observed with particular care.

Nephrotoxicity can occur and is probably a dose-dependent effect of colistimethate sodium. These manifestations of nephrotoxicity are reversible following discontinuation of the antibiotic.

Overdosage can result in renal insufficiency, muscle weakness, and apnea (see OVERDOSAGE section). See PRECAUTIONS, Drug Interactions subsection for use concomitantly with other antibiotics and curariform drugs.

Respiratory arrest has been reported following intramuscular administration of colistimethate sodium. Impaired renal function increases the possibility of apnea and neuromuscular blockade following administration of colistimethate sodium. Therefore, it is important to follow recommended dosing guidelines. See DOSAGE AND ADMINISTRATION section for use in renal impairment.

Pseudomembranous colitis has been reported with nearly all antimicrobial agents, and may range in severity from mild to life-threatening. Therefore, it is important to consider this diagnosis in patients who present with diarrhea subsequent to the administration of antibacterial agents

Treatment with antibacterial agents alters the normal flora of the colon and may permit overgrowth of clostridia. Studies indicate that a toxin produced by *Clostridium difficile* is a primary cause of "antibiotic-associated colitis."

After the diagnosis of pseudomembranous colitis has been established, appropriate therapeutic measures should be initiated. Mild cases of pseudomembranous colitis usually respond to drug discontinuation alone. In moderate-to-severe cases, consideration should be given to management with fluids and electrolytes, protein supplementation, and treatment with an antibacterial drug clinically effective against *Clostridium difficile* colitis.

PRECAUTIONS

General

Since Coly-Mycin M Parenteral is eliminated mainly by renal excretion, it should be used with caution when the possibility of impaired renal function exists. The decline in renal function with advanced age should be considered.

When actual renal impairment is present, Coly-Mycin M Parenteral may be used, but the greatest caution should be exercised and the dosage should be reduced in proportion to the extent of the impairment. Administration of amounts of Coly-Mycin M Parenteral in excess of renal excretory capacity will lead to high serum levels and can result in further impairment of renal function, initiating a cycle which, if not recognized, can lead to acute renal insufficiency, renal shutdown, and further concentration of the antibiotic to toxic levels in the body. At this point, interference of nerve transmission at neuromuscular junctions may occur and result in muscle weakness and apnea (see OVERDOSAGE section).

Signs indicating the development of impaired renal function include: diminishing urine output, rising BUN and serum creatinine and decreased creatinine clearance. Therapy with Coly-Mycin M Parenteral should be discontinued immediately if signs of impaired renal function occur. However, if it is necessary to reinstate the drug, dosing should be adjusted accordingly after drug plasma levels have fallen (see DOSAGE AND ADMINISTRATION section).

Drug Interactions

Certain other antibiotics (aminoglycosides and polymyxin) have also been reported to interfere with the nerve transmission at the neuromuscular junction. Based on this reported activity, they should not be given concomitantly with Coly-Mycin M Parenteral except with the greatest caution. Curariform muscle relaxants (eg, tubocurarine) and other drugs, including ether, succinylcholine, gallamine, decamethonium and sodium citrate, potentiate the neuromuscular blocking effect and should be used with extreme caution in patients being treated with Coly-Mycin M Parenteral.

Sodium cephalothin may enhance the nephrotoxicity of Coly-Mycin M Parenteral. The concomitant use of sodium cephalothin and Coly-Mycin M Parenteral should be avoided.

Carcinogenesis, Mutagenesis, Impairment of Fertility

Long-term animal carcinogenicity studies and genetic toxicology studies have not been performed with colistimethate sodium. There were no adverse effects on fertility or reproduction in rats at doses of 9.3 mg/kg/day (0.30 times the maximum daily human dose when based on mg/mm^2).

Pregnancy - Teratogenic Effects

Pregnancy Category C: Colistimethate sodium given intramuscularly during organogenesis to rabbits at 4.15 and 9.3 mg/kg resulted in talipes varus in 2.6% and 2.9% of fetuses, respectively. These doses are 0.25 and 0.55 times the maximum daily human dose based on mg/mm^2. In addition, increased resorption occurred at 9.3 mg/kg. Colistimethate sodium was not teratogenic in rats at 4.15 or 9.3 mg/kg. These doses are 0.13 and 0.30 times the maximum daily human dose based on mg/mm^2. There are no adequate and well-controlled studies in pregnant women. Since colistimethate sodium is transferred across the placental barrier in humans, it should be used during pregnancy only if the potential benefit justifies the potential risk to the fetus.

Nursing Mothers

It is not known whether colistimethate sodium is excreted in human breast milk. However, colistin sulphate is excreted in human breast milk. Therefore, caution should be exercised when colistimethate sodium is administered to nursing women.

Pediatric Use

In clinical studies, colistimethate sodium was administered to the pediatric population (neonates, infants, children and adolescents). Although adverse reactions appear to be similar in the adult and pediatric populations, subjective symptoms of toxicity may not be reported by pediatric patients. Close clinical monitoring of pediatric patients is recommended.

ADVERSE REACTIONS

The following adverse reactions have been reported:

Gastrointestinal: gastrointestinal upset

Continued on next page

Coly-Mycin M—Cont.

Nervous System: tingling of extremities and tongue, slurred speech, dizziness, vertigo and paresthesia
Integumentary: generalized itching, urticaria and rash
Body as a Whole: fever
Laboratory Deviations: increased blood urea nitrogen (BUN), elevated creatinine and decreased creatinine clearance
Respiratory System: respiratory distress and apnea
Renal System: nephrotoxicity and decreased urine output

OVERDOSAGE

Overdosage with colistimethate sodium can cause neuromuscular blockade characterized by paresthesia, lethargy, confusion, dizziness, ataxia, nystagmus, disorders of speech and apnea. Respiratory muscle paralysis may lead to apnea, respiratory arrest and death.
Overdosage with the drug can also cause acute renal failure, manifested as decreased urine output and increases in serum concentrations of BUN and creatinine.
As in any case of overdose, colistimethate sodium therapy should be discontinued and general supportive measures should be utilized.
It is unknown whether colistimethate sodium can be removed by hemodialysis or peritoneal dialysis in overdose cases.

DOSAGE AND ADMINISTRATION

Important: Coly-Mycin M Parenteral is supplied in vials containing colistimethate sodium equivalent to 150 mg colistin base activity per vial.
Reconstitution: The **150 mg** vial should be reconstituted with **2.0 mL** Sterile Water for Injection, USP. The reconstituted solution provides colistimethate sodium at a concentration equivalent to 75 mg/mL colistin base activity.
During reconstitution swirl **gently** to avoid frothing.
Parenteral drug products should be inspected visually for particulate matter and discoloration prior to administration, whenever solution and container permit. If these conditions are observed, the product should not be used.

Dosage

Adults and pediatric patients—Intravenous or Intramuscular Administration: Coly-Mycin M Parenteral should be given in 2 to 4 divided doses at dose levels of 2.5 to 5 mg/kg per day for patients with normal renal function, depending on the severity of the infection.
In obese individuals, dosage should be based on ideal body weight.
The daily dose should be reduced in the presence of renal impairment. Modifications of dosage in the presence of renal impairment are presented in Table 1.
[See table at top of previous page]
Note: The suggested unit dose is 2.5–5 mg/kg; however, the time INTERVAL between injections should be increased in the presence of impaired renal function.

INTRAVENOUS ADMINISTRATION

1. Direct Intermittent Administration—Slowly inject one-half of the total daily dose over a period of 3 to 5 minutes every 12 hours.
2. Continuous Infusion—Slowly inject one-half of the total daily dose over 3 to 5 minutes. Add the remaining half of the total daily dose of Coly-Mycin M Parenteral to one of the following:

0.9% NaCl
5% dextrose in 0.9% NaCl
5% dextrose in water
5% dextrose in 0.45% NaCl
5% dextrose in 0.225% NaCl
Lactated Ringer's solution
10% invert sugar solution

There are not sufficient data to recommend usage of Coly-Mycin M Parenteral with other drugs or other than the above listed infusion solutions.
Administer the second half of the total daily dose by slow intravenous infusion, starting 1 to 2 hours after the initial dose, over the next 22 to 23 hours. In the presence of impaired renal function, reduce the infusion rate depending on the degree of renal impairment.
The choice of intravenous solution and the volume to be employed are dictated by the requirements of fluid and electrolyte management.
Any infusion solution containing colistimethate sodium should be freshly prepared and used for no longer than 24 hours.

HOW SUPPLIED

Coly-Mycin M Parenteral is supplied in vials containing colistimethate sodium (equivalent to 150 mg colistin base activity per vial) as a white to slightly yellow lyophilized cake and is available as one vial per carton NDC 61570-414-51
Store between 15°–30°C (59°–86°F).
Store reconstituted solution in refrigerator 2°–8°C (36°–46°F) or between 15°–30°C (59°–86°F) and use within 7 days.
Rx only.
Distributed by: Monarch Pharmaceuticals, Inc,. Bristol, TN 37620

Shown in Product Identification Guide, page 324

CORTISPORIN® Cream ℞

[*cŏr 'tĭ-spŏrin*]
(neomycin and polymyxin B sulfates and hydrocortisone acetate cream, USP)

DESCRIPTION

CORTISPORIN Cream (neomycin and polymyxin B sulfates and hydrocortisone acetate cream, USP) is a topical antibacterial cream. Each gram contains: neomycin sulfate equivalent to 3.5 mg neomycin base, polymyxin B sulfate equivalent to 10,000 polymyxin B units, and hydrocortisone acetate 5 mg (0.5%). The inactive ingredients are liquid petrolatum, white petrolatum, propylene glycol, polyoxyethylene polyoxypropylene compound, emulsifying wax, purified water, and 0.25% methylparaben added as a preservative. Sodium hydroxide or sulfuric acid may be added to adjust pH.
Neomycin sulfate is the sulfate salt of neomycin B and C, which are produced by the growth of *Streptomyces fradiae* Waksman (Fam. Streptomycetaceae). It has a potency equivalent of not less than 600 µg of neomycin standard per mg, calculated on an anhydrous basis. The structural formulae are:

• x H_2SO_4
Neomycin B (R_1=H, R_2=CH_2NH_2)
Neomycin C (R_1=CH_2NH_2, R_2=H)

Polymyxin B sulfate is the sulfate salt of polymyxin B_1 and B_2, which are produced by the growth of *Bacillus polymyxa* (Prazmowski) Migula (Fam. Bacillaceae). It has a potency of not less than 6,000 polymyxin B units per mg, calculated on an anhydrous basis. The structural formulae are:

Polymyxin B_1 (R=CH_3)
Polymyxin B_2 (R=H)
DAB=α,γ-diaminobutyric acid

Hydrocortisone acetate is the acetate ester of hydrocortisone, an anti-inflammatory hormone. Its chemical name is 21-(acetyloxy)-11β,17-dihydroxypregn-4-ene-3,20-dione. Its structural formula is:

The base is a smooth vanishing cream with a pH of approximately 5.0.

CLINICAL PHARMACOLOGY

Corticoids suppress the inflammatory response to a variety of agents and they may delay healing. Since corticoids may inhibit the body's defense mechanism against infection, a concomitant antimicrobial drug may be used when this inhibition is considered to be clinically significant in a particular case.
The anti-infective components in the combination are included to provide action against specific organisms susceptible to them. Polymyxin B sulfate and neomycin sulfate together are considered active against the following microorganisms:
Staphylococcus aureus, Escherichia coli, Haemophilus influenzae, Klebsiella-Enterobacter species, *Neisseria* species, and *Pseudomonas aeruginosa*. The product does not provide adequate coverage against *Serratia marcescens* and streptococci, including *Streptococcus pneumoniae*.
The relative potency of corticosteroids depends on the molecular structure, concentration, and release from the vehicle.
The acid pH helps restore normal cutaneous acidity. Owing to its excellent spreading and penetrating properties, the cream facilitates treatment of hairy and intertriginous areas. It may also be of value in selective cases where the lesions are moist.

INDICATIONS AND USAGE

For the treatment of corticosteroid-responsive dermatoses with secondary infection. It has not been demonstrated that this steroid-antibiotic combination provides greater benefit than the steroid component alone after 7 days of treatment (see WARNINGS).

CONTRAINDICATIONS

Not for use in the eyes or in the external ear canal if the eardrum is perforated. This product is contraindicated in tuberculous, fungal, or viral lesions of the skin (herpes simplex, vaccinia, and varicella). This product is contraindicated in those individuals who have shown hypersensitivity to any of its components.

WARNINGS

Because of the concern of nephrotoxicity and ototoxicity associated with neomycin, this combination should not be used over a wide area or for extended periods of time.

PRECAUTIONS

General: As with any antibacterial preparation, prolonged use may result in overgrowth of nonsusceptible organisms, including fungi. Appropriate measures should be taken if this occurs. Use of steroids on infected areas should be supervised with care as anti-inflammatory steroids may encourage spread of infection. If this occurs, steroid therapy should be stopped and appropriate antibacterial drugs used. Generalized dermatological conditions may require systemic corticosteroid therapy.
Signs and symptoms of exogenous hyperadrenocorticism can occur with the use of topical corticosteroids, including adrenal suppression. Systemic absorption of topically applied steroids will be increased if extensive body surface areas are treated or if occlusive dressings are used. Under these circumstances, suitable precautions should be taken when long-term use is anticipated.
Specifically, sufficient percutaneous absorption of hydrocortisone can occur in pediatric patients during prolonged use to cause cessation of growth, as well as other systemic signs and symptoms of hyperadrenocorticism.
Information for Patients: If redness, irritation, swelling or pain persists or increases, discontinue use and notify physician. Do not use in the eyes.
Laboratory Tests: Systemic effects of excessive levels of hydrocortisone may include a reduction in the number of circulating eosinophils and a decrease in urinary excretion of 17-hydroxycorticosteroids.
Carcinogenesis, Mutagenesis, Impairment of Fertility: Long-term studies in animals (rats, rabbits, mice) showed no evidence of carcinogenicity attributable to oral administration of corticosteroids.
Pregnancy: ***Teratogenic Effects:*** Pregnancy Category C. Corticosteroids have been shown to be teratogenic in rabbits when applied topically at concentrations of 0.5% on days 6 to 18 of gestation and in mice when applied topically at a concentration of 15% on days 10 to 13 of gestation. There are no adequate and well-controlled studies in pregnant women. Corticosteroids should be used during pregnancy only if the potential benefit justifies the potential risk to the fetus.
Nursing Mothers: Hydrocortisone acetate appears in human milk following oral administration of the drug. Since systemic absorption of hydrocortisone may occur when applied topically, caution should be exercised when CORTISPORIN Cream is used by a nursing woman.
Pediatric Use: Safety and effectiveness in pediatric patients have not been established (see PRECAUTIONS: General).

ADVERSE REACTIONS

Neomycin occasionally causes skin sensitization. Ototoxicity and nephrotoxicity have also been reported (see WARNINGS). Adverse reactions have occurred with topical use of antibiotic combinations including neomycin and polymyxin B. Exact incidence figures are not available since no denominator of treated patients is available. The reaction occurring most often is allergic sensitization. In one clinical study, using a 20% neomycin patch, neomycin-induced allergic skin reactions occurred in two of 2,175 (0.09%) individuals in the general population.[1] In another study, the incidence was found to be approximately 1%.[2]
The following local adverse reactions have been reported with topical corticosteroids, especially under occlusive dressings: burning, itching, irritation, dryness, folliculitis, hypertrichosis, acneiform eruptions, hypopigmentation, perioral dermatitis, allergic contact dermatitis, maceration of the skin, secondary infection, skin atrophy, striae, and miliaria.
When steroid preparations are used for long periods of time in intertriginous areas or over extensive body areas, with or without occlusive non-permeable dressings, striae may occur; also there exists the possibility of systemic side effects when steroid preparations are used over large areas or for a long period of time.

DOSAGE AND ADMINISTRATION

A small quantity of the cream should be applied 2 to 4 times daily, as required. The cream should, if conditions permit, be gently rubbed into the affected areas.

HOW SUPPLIED

Tube of 7.5 g (NDC 61570-032-75).
Store at 15° to 25°C (59° to 77°F).
Rx only

REFERENCES

1. Leyden JJ, Kligman AM. Contact dermatitis to neomycin sulfate. *JAMA.* 1979;242:1276-1278.
2. Prystowsky SD, Allen AM, Smith RW, et al. Allergic contact hypersensitivity to nickel, neomycin, ethylenediamine, and benzocaine. *Arch Dermatol.* 1979;115:959-962.

Distributed by: Monarch Pharmaceuticals, Inc., Bristol, TN 37620

Manufactured by: Catalytica Pharmaceuticals, Inc., Greenville, NC 27834

Rev. 1/98

Shown in Product Identification Guide, page 324

CORTISPORIN® Ointment ℞

[*cŏr'tĭ-spōrin*]

(neomycin and polymyxin B sulfates, bacitracin zinc, and hydrocortisone ointment, USP)

DESCRIPTION

CORTISPORIN Ointment (neomycin and polymyxin B sulfates, bacitracin zinc, and hydrocortisone ointment, USP) is a topical antibacterial ointment. Each gram contains: neomycin sulfate equivalent to 3.5 mg neomycin base, polymyxin B sulfate equivalent to 5,000 polymyxin B units, bacitracin zinc equivalent to 400 bacitracin units, hydrocortisone 10 mg (1%), and white petrolatum, qs.

Neomycin sulfate is the sulfate salt of neomycin B and C, which are produced by the growth of *Streptomyces fradiae* Waksman (Fam. Streptomycetaceae). It has a potency equivalent of not less than 600 µg of neomycin standard per mg, calculated on an anhydrous basis. The structural formulae are:

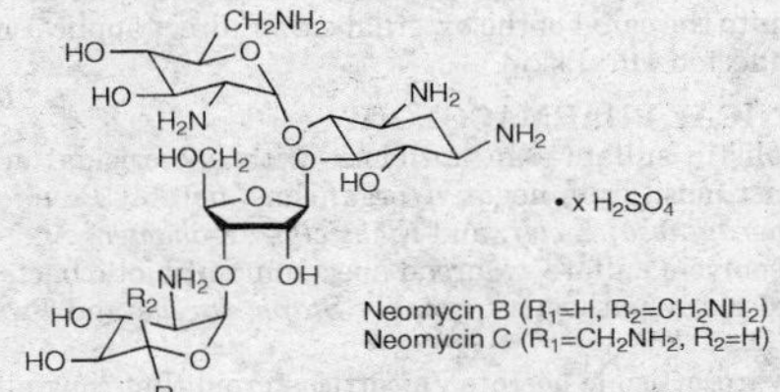

Neomycin B (R_1=H, R_2=CH_2NH_2)
Neomycin C (R_1=CH_2NH_2, R_2=H)

Polymyxin B sulfate is the sulfate salt of polymyxin B_1 and B_2, which are produced by the growth of *Bacillus polymyxa* (Prazmowski) Migula (Fam. Bacillaceae). It has a potency of not less than 6,000 polymyxin B units per mg, calculated on an anhydrous basis. The structural formulae are:

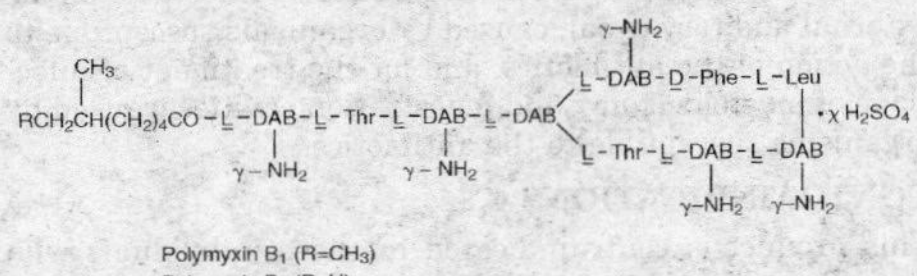

Polymyxin B_1 (R=CH_3)
Polymyxin B_2 (R=H)
DAB=α,γ-diaminobutyric acid

Bacitracin zinc is the zinc salt of bacitracin, a mixture of related cyclic polypeptides (mainly bacitracin A) produced by the growth of an organism of the *licheniformis* group of *Bacillus subtilis* (Fam. Bacillaceae). It has a potency of not less than 40 bacitracin units per mg. The structural formula is:

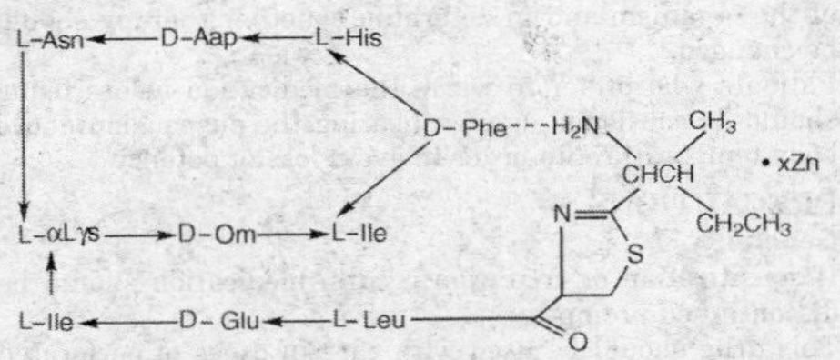

Hydrocortisone, 11β,17,21-trihydroxypregn-4-ene-3, 20-dione, is an anti-inflammatory hormone. Its structural formula is:

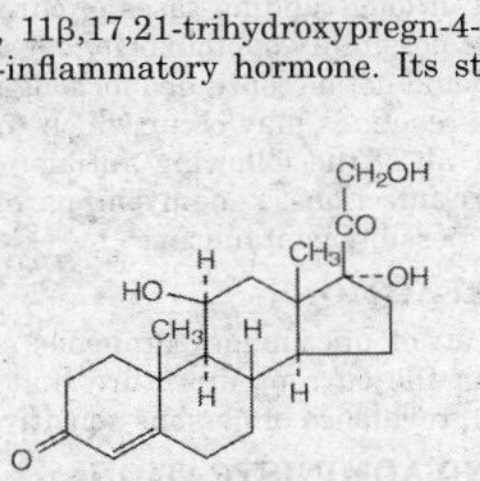

CLINICAL PHARMACOLOGY

Corticoids suppress the inflammatory response to a variety of agents and they may delay healing. Since corticoids may inhibit the body's defense mechanism against infection, a concomitant antimicrobial drug may be used when this inhibition is considered to be clinically significant in a particular case.

The anti-infective components in the combination are included to provide action against specific organisms susceptible to them. Polymyxin B sulfate, bacitracin zinc, and neomycin sulfate together are considered active against the following microorganisms: *Staphylococcus aureus*, streptococci, including *Streptococcus pneumoniae*, *Escherichia coli*, *Haemophilus influenzae*, *Klebsiella-Enterobacter* species, *Neisseria* species, and *Pseudomonas aeruginosa*.

The product does not provide adequate coverage against *Serratia marcescens*.

The relative potency of corticosteroids depends on the molecular structure, concentration, and release from the vehicle.

INDICATIONS AND USAGE

For the treatment of corticosteroid-responsive dermatoses with secondary infection. It has not been demonstrated that this steroid-antibiotic combination provides greater benefit than the steroid component alone after 7 days of treatment (see WARNINGS).

CONTRAINDICATIONS

Not for use in the eyes or in the external ear canal if the eardrum is perforated. This product is contraindicated in tuberculous, fungal, or viral lesions of the skin (herpes simplex, vaccinia, and varicella). This product is contraindicated in those individuals who have shown hypersensitivity to any of its components.

WARNINGS

Because of the concern of nephrotoxicity and ototoxicity associated with neomycin, this combination should not be used over a wide area or for extended periods of time.

PRECAUTIONS

General: As with any antibiotic preparation, prolonged use may result in the overgrowth of nonsusceptible organisms, including fungi. Appropriate measures should be taken if this occurs. Use of steroids on infected areas should be supervised with care as anti-inflammatory steroids may encourage spread of infection. If this occurs, steroid therapy should be stopped and appropriate antibacterial drugs used. Generalized dermatological conditions may require systemic corticosteroid therapy.

Signs and symptoms of exogenous hyperadrenocorticism can occur with the use of topical corticosteroids, including adrenal suppression. Systemic absorption of topically applied steroids will be increased if extensive body surface areas are treated or if occlusive dressings are used. Under these circumstances, suitable precautions should be taken when long-term use is anticipated.

Specifically, sufficient percutaneous absorption of hydrocortisone can occur in pediatric patients during prolonged use to cause cessation of growth, as well as other systemic signs and symptoms of hyperadrenocorticism.

Information for Patients: If redness, irritation, swelling, or pain persists or increases, discontinue use and notify physician. Do not use in the eyes.

Laboratory Tests: Systemic effects of excessive levels of hydrocortisone may include a reduction in the number of circulating eosinophils and a decrease in urinary excretion of 17-hydroxycorticosteroids.

Carcinogenesis, Mutagenesis, Impairment of Fertility: Long-term studies in animals (rats, rabbits, mice) showed no evidence of carcinogenicity attributable to oral administration of corticosteroids.

Pregnancy: ***Teratogenic Effects:*** Pregnancy Category C. Corticosteroids have been shown to be teratogenic in rabbits when applied topically at concentrations of 0.5% on days 6 to 18 of gestation and in mice when applied topically at a concentration of 15% on days 10 to 13 of gestation. There are no adequate and well-controlled studies in pregnant women. Corticosteroids should be used during pregnancy only if the potential benefit justifies the potential risk to the fetus.

Nursing Mothers: Hydrocortisone appears in human milk following oral administration of the drug. Since systemic absorption of hydrocortisone may occur when applied topically, caution should be exercised when CORTISPORIN Ointment is used by a nursing woman.

Pediatric Use: Safety and effectiveness in pediatric patients have not been established (see PRECAUTIONS: General).

ADVERSE REACTIONS

Neomycin occasionally causes skin sensitization. Ototoxicity and nephrotoxicity have also been reported (see WARNINGS). Adverse reactions have occurred with topical use of antibiotic combinations including neomycin, bacitracin, and polymyxin B. Exact incidence figures are not available since no denominator of treated patients is available. The reaction occurring most often is allergic sensitization. In one clinical study, using a 20% neomycin patch, neomycin-induced allergic skin reactions occurred in two of 2,175 (0.09%) individuals in the general population.[1] In another study, the incidence was found to be approximately 1%.[2]

The following local adverse reactions have been reported with topical corticosteroids, especially under occlusive dressings: burning, itching, irritation, dryness, folliculitis, hypertrichosis, acneiform eruptions, hypopigmentation, perioral dermatitis, allergic contact dermatitis, maceration of the skin, secondary infection, skin atrophy, striae, and miliaria.

When steroid preparations are used for long periods of time in intertriginous areas or over extensive body areas, with or without occlusive non-permeable dressings, striae may occur; also there exists the possibility of systemic side effects when steroid preparations are used over large areas or for a long period of time.

DOSAGE AND ADMINISTRATION

A thin film is applied 2 to 4 times daily to the affected area.

HOW SUPPLIED

Tube of ½ oz with applicator tip (NDC 61570-031-50).

Store at 15° to 25°C (59° to 77°F).

Rx only

REFERENCES

1. Leyden JJ, Kligman AM. Contact dermatitis to neomycin sulfate. *JAMA.* 1979;242:1276–1278.

2. Prystowsky SD, Allen AM, Smith RW, et al. Allergic contact hypersensitivity to nickel, neomycin, ethylenediamine, and benzocaine. *Arch Dermatol.* 1979;115:959–962.

Distributed by: Monarch Pharmaceuticals, Inc., Bristol, TN 37620

Manufactured by: Catalytica Pharmaceuticals, Inc., Greenville, NC 27834

Rev. 1/98

Shown in Product Identification Guide, page 324

CORTISPORIN® ℞
OPHTHALMIC SUSPENSION STERILE

(neomycin and polymyxin B sulfates and hydrocortisone ophthalmic suspension, USP)

DESCRIPTION

CORTISPORIN Ophthalmic Suspension (neomycin and polymyxin B sulfates and hydrocortisone ophthalmic suspension) is a sterile antimicrobial and anti-inflammatory suspension for ophthalmic use. Each mL contains: neomycin sulfate equivalent to 3.5 mg neomycin base, polymyxin B sulfate equivalent to 10,000 polymyxin B units, and hydrocortisone 10 mg (1%). The vehicle contains thimerosal 0.001% (added as a preservative) and the inactive ingredients cetyl alcohol, glyceryl monostearate, mineral oil, polyoxyl 40 stearate, propylene glycol, and Water for Injection. Sulfuric acid may be added to adjust pH.

Neomycin sulfate is the sulfate salt of neomycin B and C, which are produced by the growth of *Streptomyces fradiae* Waksman (Fam. Streptomycetaceae). It has a potency equivalent of not less than 600 µg of neomycin standard per mg, calculated on an anhydrous basis. The structural formulae are:

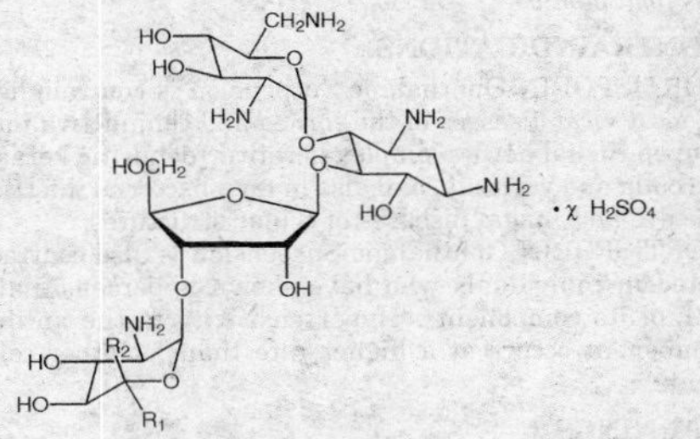

Neomycin B (R_1=H, R_2=CH_2NH_2)
Neomycin C (R_1=CH_2NH_2, R_2=H)

Polymyxin B sulfate is the sulfate salt of polymyxin B_1 and B_2, which are produced by the growth of *Bacillus polymyxa* (Prazmowski) Migula (Fam. Bacillaceae). It has a potency of not less than 6,000 polymyxin B units per mg, calculated on an anhydrous basis. The structural formulae are:

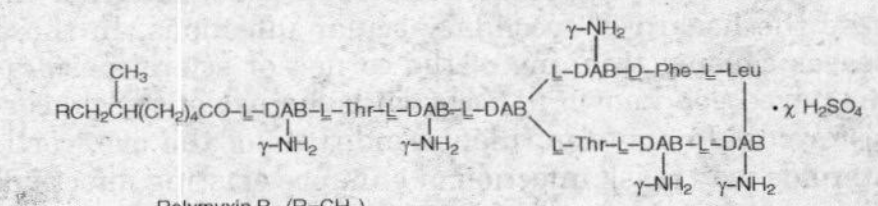

Polymyxin B_1 (R=CH_3)
Polymyxin B_2 (R=H)
DAB=α, γ-diaminobutyric acid

Hydrocortisone, 11β,17,21-trihydroxypregn-4-ene-3,20-dione, is an anti-inflammatory hormone. Its structural formula is:

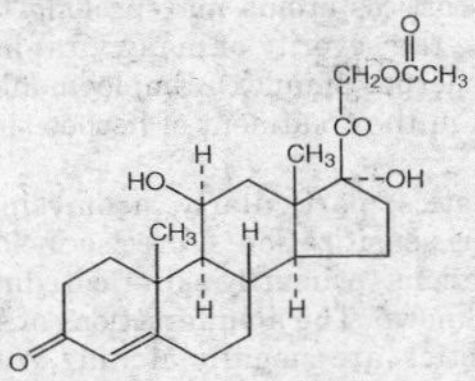

CLINICAL PHARMACOLOGY

Corticosteroids suppress the inflammatory response to a variety of agents, and they probably delay or slow healing. Since corticosteroids may inhibit the body's defense mechanism against infection, concomitant antimicrobial drugs may be used when this inhibition is considered to be clinically significant in a particular case.

When a decision to administer both a corticosteroid and antimicrobials is made, the administration of such drugs in combination has the advantage of greater patient compliance and convenience, with the added assurance that the appropriate dosage of all drugs is administered. When each type of drug is in the same formulation, compatibility of ingredients is assured and the correct volume of drug is delivered and retained.

The relative potency of corticosteroids depends on the molecular structure, concentration, and release from the vehicle.

Microbiology: The anti-infective components in CORTISPORIN Ophthalmic Suspension are included to provide action against specific organisms susceptible to it. Neomycin sulfate and polymyxin B sulfate are active in vi-

Continued on next page

Cortisporin Ophthalmic Susp.—Cont.

tro against susceptible strains of the following microorganisms: *Staphylococcus aureus, Escherichia coli, Haemophilus influenzae, Klebsiella/Enterobacter species, Neisseria species,* and *Pseudomonas aeruginosa.* The product does not provide adequate coverage against Serratia marcescens and streptococci, including Streptococcus pneumoniae (see INDICATIONS AND USAGE).

INDICATIONS AND USAGE

CORTISPORIN Ophthalmic Suspension is indicated for steroid-responsive inflammatory ocular conditions for which a corticosteroid is indicated and where bacterial infection or a risk of bacterial infection exists.
Ocular corticosteroids are indicated in inflammatory conditions of the palpebral and bulbar conjunctiva, cornea, and anterior segment of the globe where the inherent risk of corticosteroid use in certain infective conjunctivitides is accepted to obtain a diminution in edema and inflammation. They are also indicated in chronic anterior uveitis and corneal injury from chemical, radiation, or thermal burns, or penetration of foreign bodies.
The use of a combination drug with an anti-infective component is indicated where the risk of infection is high or where there is an expectation that potentially dangerous numbers of bacteria will be present in the eye (see CLINICAL PHARMACOLOGY: Microbiology).
The particular anti-infective drugs in this product are active against the following common bacterial eye pathogens: *Staphylococcus aureus, Escherichia coli, Haemophilus influenzae, Klebsiella/Enterobacter species, Neisseria species,* and *Pseudomonas aeruginosa.*
The product does not provide adequate coverage against Serratia marcescens and streptococci, including *Streptococcus pneumoniae.*

CONTRAINDICATIONS

CORTISPORIN Ophthalmic Suspension is contraindicated in most viral diseases of the cornea and conjunctiva including: epithelial herpes simplex keratitis (dendritic keratitis), vaccinia and varicella, and also in mycobacterial infection of the eye and fungal diseases of ocular structures.
CORTISPORIN Ophthalmic Suspension is also contraindicated in individuals who have shown hypersensitivity to any of its components. Hypersensitivity to the antibiotic component occurs at a higher rate than for other components.

WARNINGS

NOT FOR INJECTION INTO THE EYE. CORTISPORIN Ophthalmic Suspension should never be directly introduced into the anterior chamber of the eye.
Prolonged use of corticosteroids may result in ocular hypertension and/or glaucoma, with damage to the optic nerve, defects in visual acuity and fields of vision, and in posterior subcapsular cataract formation.
Prolonged use may suppress the host response and thus increase the hazard of secondary ocular infections. In those diseases causing thinning of the cornea or sclera, perforations have been known to occur with the use of topical corticosteroids. In acute purulent conditions of the eye, corticosteroids may mask infection or enhance existing infection.
If these products are used for 10 days or longer, intraocular pressure should be routinely monitored even though it may be difficult in uncooperative patients. Corticosteroids should be used with caution in the presence of glaucoma.
The use of corticosteroids after cataract surgery may delay healing and increase the incidence of filtering blebs.
Use of ocular corticosteroids may prolong the course and may exacerbate the severity of many viral infections of the eye (including herpes simplex). Employment of corticosteroid medication in the treatment of herpes simplex requires great caution.
Topical antibiotics, particularly, neomycin sulfate, may cause cutaneous sensitization. A precise incidence of hypersensitivity reactions (primarily skin rash) due to topical antibiotics is not known. The manifestations of sensitization to topical antibiotics are usually itching, reddening, and edema of the conjunctiva and eyelid. A sensitization reaction may manifest simply as a failure to heal. During long-term use of topical antibiotic products, periodic examination for such signs is advisable, and the patient should be told to discontinue the product if they are observed. Symptoms usually subside quickly on withdrawing the medication. Application of products containing these ingredients should be avoided for the patient thereafter (see PRECAUTIONS: General).

PRECAUTIONS

General: The initial prescription and renewal of the medication order beyond 20 milliliters should be made by a physician only after examination of the patient with the aid of magnification, such as slit lamp biomicroscopy and, where appropriate, fluorescein staining. If signs and symptoms fail to improve after 2 days, the patient should be re-evaluated.
The possibility of fungal infections of the cornea should be considered after prolonged corticosteroid dosing. Fungal cultures should be taken when appropriate.
If this product is used for 10 days or longer, intraocular pressure should be monitored (see WARNINGS).
There have been reports of bacterial keratitis associated with the use of topical ophthalmic products in multiple-dose containers which have been inadvertently contaminated by patients, most of whom had a concurrent corneal disease or a disruption of the ocular epithelial surface (see PRECAUTIONS: Information for Patients).
Allergic cross-reactions may occur which could prevent the use of any or all of the following antibiotics for the treatment of future infections: kanamycin, paromomycin, streptomycin, and possibly gentamicin.
Information for Patients: Patients should be instructed to avoid allowing the tip of the dispensing container to contact the eye, eyelid, fingers, or any other surface. The use of this product by more than one person may spread infection.
Patients should also be instructed that ocular products, if handled improperly, can become contaminated by common bacteria known to cause ocular infections. Serious damage to the eye and subsequent loss of vision may result from using contaminated products (see PRECAUTIONS: General).
If the condition persists or gets worse, or if a rash or allergic reaction develops, the patient should be advised to stop use and consult a physician. Do not use this product if you are allergic to any of the listed ingredients.
Keep tightly closed when not in use. Keep out of reach of children.
Carcinogenesis, Mutagenesis, Impairment of Fertility: Long-term studies in animals to evaluate carcinogenic or mutagenic potential have not been conducted with polymyxin B sulfate. Treatment of cultured human lymphocytes in vitro with neomycin increased the frequency of chromosome aberrations at the highest concentrations (80 mg/mL) tested; however, the effects of neomycin on carcinogenesis and mutagenesis in humans are unknown.
Long-term studies in animals (rats, rabbits, mice) showed no evidence of carcinogenicity or mutagenicity attributable to oral administration of corticosteroids. Long-term animal studies have not been performed to evaluate the carcinogenic potential of topical corticosteroids. Studies to determine mutagenicity with hydrocortisone have revealed negative results.
Polymyxin B has been reported to impair the motility of equine sperm, but its effects on male or female fertility are unknown. Long-term animal studies have not been performed to evaluate the effect on fertility of topical corticosteroids.
Pregnancy: ***Teratogenic Effects:*** Pregnancy Category C. Corticosteroids have been found to be teratogenic in rabbits when applied topically at concentrations of 0.5% on days 6 to 18 of gestation and in mice when applied topically at a concentration of 15% on days 10 to 13 of gestation. There are no adequate and well-controlled studies in pregnant women. CORTISPORIN Ophthalmic Suspension should be used during pregnancy only if the potential benefit justifies the potential risk to the fetus.
Nursing Mothers: It is not known whether topical administration of corticosteroids could result in sufficient systemic absorption to produce detectable quantities in human milk. Systemically administered corticosteroids appear in human milk and could suppress growth, interfere with endogenous corticosteroid production, or cause other untoward effects. Because of the potential for serious adverse reactions in nursing infants from CORTISPORIN Ophthalmic Suspension, a decision should be made whether to discontinue nursing or to discontinue the drug, taking into account the importance of the drug to the mother.
Pediatric Use: Safety and effectiveness in pediatric patients have not been established.

ADVERSE REACTIONS

Adverse reactions have occurred with corticosteroid/anti-infective combination drugs which can be attributed to the corticosteroid component, the anti-infective component, or the combination. The exact incidence is not known.
Reactions occurring most often from the presence of the anti-infective ingredient are allergic sensitization reactions including itching, swelling, and conjunctival erythema (see WARNINGS). More serious hypersensitivity reactions, including anaphylaxis, have been reported rarely.
The reactions due to the corticosteroid component in decreasing order of frequency are: elevation of intraocular pressure (IOP) with possible development of glaucoma, and infrequent optic nerve damage; posterior subcapsular cataract formation; and delayed wound healing.
Secondary Infection: The development of secondary infection has occurred after use of combinations containing corticosteroids and antimicrobials. Fungal and viral infections of the cornea are particularly prone to develop coincidentally with long-term applications of a corticosteroid. The possibility of fungal invasion must be considered in any persistent corneal ulceration where corticosteroid treatment has been used.
Local irritation on instillation has also been reported.

DOSAGE AND ADMINISTRATION

One or two drops in the affected eye every 3 or 4 hours, depending on the severity of the condition. The suspension may be used more frequently if necessary.
Not more than 20 milliliters should be prescribed initially and the prescription should not be refilled without further evaluation as outlined in PRECAUTIONS above.
SHAKE WELL BEFORE USING.

HOW SUPPLIED

Plastic DROP DOSE® dispenser bottle of 7.5 mL (NDC 61570-036-75).
Rx only
Store at 15° to 25°C (59° to 77°F).

Distributed by: Monarch Pharmaceuticals, Inc., Bristol, TN 37620
Manufactured By: Catalytica Pharmaceutical, Inc. Greenville, NC 27835

5/97

Shown in Product Identification Guide, page 324

CORTISPORIN®-TC Otic Suspension with Neomycin and Hydrocortisone ℞

[*cŏr 'tĭ -spŏrin*]

(colistin sulfate - neomycin sulfate - thonzonium bromide - hydrocortisone acetate otic suspension)

DESCRIPTION

Cortisporin®-TC Otic Suspension with Neomycin and Hydrocortisone (colistin sulfate—neomycin sulfate—thonzonium bromide—hydrocortisone acetate otic suspension) is a sterile aqueous suspension containing in each mL: Colistin base activity, 3mg (as the sulfate); Neomycin base activity, 3.3 mg (as the sulfate); Hydrocortisone acetate, 10 mg (1%); Thonzonium bromide, 0.5 mg (0.05%); Polysorbate 80, acetic acid, and sodium acetate in a buffered aqueous vehicle. Thimerosal (mercury derivative), 0.002%, added as a preservative. It is a nonviscous liquid, buffered at pH 5, for instillation into the canal of the external ear or direct application to the affected aural skin.

CLINICAL PHARMACOLOGY

1. Colistin sulfate - an antibiotic with bactericidal action against most gram-negative organisms, notably *Pseudomonas aeruginosa, E coli,* and *Klebsiella-Aerobacter.*
2. Neomycin sulfate - a broad-spectrum antibiotic bactericidal to many pathogens, notably *Staph aureus* and *Proteus sp.*
3. Hydrocortisone acetate - a corticosteroid that controls inflammation, edema, pruritus, and other dermal reactions.
4. Thonzonium bromide - a surface-active agent that promotes tissue contact by dispersion and penetration of the cellular debris and exudate.

INDICATIONS AND USAGE

For the treatment of superficial bacterial infections of the external auditory canal, caused by organisms susceptible to the action of the antibiotics; and for the treatment of infections of mastoidectomy and fenestration cavities, caused by organisms susceptible to the antibiotics.

CONTRAINDICATIONS

This product is contraindicated in those individuals who have shown hypersensitivity to any of its components, and in herpes simplex, vaccinia, and varicella.

WARNINGS

As with other antibiotic preparations, prolonged treatment may result in overgrowth of nonsusceptible organisms and fungi.
If the infection is not improved after one week, cultures and susceptibility tests should be repeated to verify the identity of the organism and to determine whether therapy should be changed.
Patients who prefer to warm the medication before using should be cautioned against heating the suspension above body temperature, in order to avoid loss of potency.

PRECAUTIONS

General

If sensitization or irritation occurs, medication should be discontinued promptly.
This drug should be used with care in cases of perforated eardrum and in longstanding cases of chronic otitis media because of the possibility of ototoxicity caused by neomycin.
Treatment should not be continued for longer than ten days.
Allergic cross-reactions may occur which could prevent the use of any or all of the following antibiotics for the treatment of future infections: kanamycin, paromomycin, streptomycin, and possibly gentamicin.

ADVERSE REACTIONS

Neomycin is a not uncommon cutaneous sensitizer. There are articles in the current literature that indicate an increase in the prevalence of persons sensitive to neomycin.

DOSAGE AND ADMINISTRATION

The external auditory canal should be thoroughly cleansed and dried with a sterile cotton applicator.
When using the calibrated dropper:
For adults, 5 drops of the suspension should be instilled into the affected ear 3 or 4 times daily. For pediatric patients, 4 drops are suggested because of the smaller capacity of the ear canal.
This dosage correlates to the 4 drops (for adults) and 3 drops (for pediatric patients) recommended when using the drop-per-bottle container for this product.
The patient should lie with the affected ear upward and then the drops should be instilled. This position should be maintained for 5 minutes to facilitate penetration of the drops into the ear canal. Repeat, if necessary, for the opposite ear.
If preferred, a cotton wick may be inserted into the canal and then the cotton may be saturated with the suspension. This wick should be kept moist by adding further solution every 4 hours. The wick should be replaced at least once every 24 hours.

HOW SUPPLIED

Cortisporin®-TC Otic Suspension is supplied as:
NDC 61570-090-10 .... 10-mL bottle with dropper
Each mL contains: Colistin sulfate equivalent to 3 mg of colistin base activity, Neomycin sulfate equivalent to 3.3 mg neomycin base activity, Hydrocortisone acetate 10mg (1%), Thonzonium bromide 0.5 mg (0.05%), and Polysorbate 80 in an aqueous vehicle buffered with acetic acid and sodium acetate. Thimerosal (mercury derivative) 0.002% added as a preservative.
A sterilized dropper-cap assembly for use on the bottle of suspension is included in the package.
Shake well before using.
Store at controlled room temperature 15°–30° C (59°–86° F).
Stable for 18 months at room temperature; prolonged exposure to higher temperatures should be avoided.
Rx only.
Distributed by:
Monarch Pharmaceuticals, Inc.
Bristol, TN 37620
Manufactured by:
Parkedale Pharmaceuticals, Inc.
Rochester, MI 48307

Rev. 3/98
090G030

Shown in Product Identification Guide, page 324

LORABID® ℞
[*lŏr 'ă-bĭd*]
(Loracarbef, USP)

DESCRIPTION

LORABID® (loracarbef, USP) is a synthetic β-lactam antibiotic of the carbacephem class for oral administration. Chemically, carbacephems differ from cephalosporin-class antibiotics in the dihydrothiazine ring where a methylene group has been substituted for a sulfur atom.
The chemical name for loracarbef is (6*R*, 7*S*) -7- [(*R*) -2-amino -2- phenylacetamido] -3- chloro-8-oxo-1-azabicyclo [4.2.0]oct-2-ene-2-carboxylic acid, monohydrate. It is a white to off-white solid with a molecular weight of 367.8. The empirical formula is $C_{16}H_{16}ClN_3O_4 \bullet H_2O$. The structural formula is:

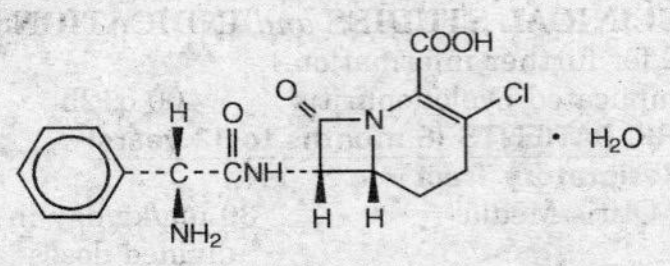

Lorabid Pulvules® (loracarbef capsules, USP) and Lorabid for Oral Suspension (loracarbef for oral suspension, USP) are intended for oral administration only.
Each Pulvule contains loracarbef equivalent to 200 mg (0.57 mmol) or 400 mg (1.14 mmol) anhydrous loracarbef activity. They also contain cornstarch, dimethicone, F D & C Blue No. 2, gelatin, iron oxides, magnesium stearate, titanium dioxide, and other inactive ingredients.
After reconstitution, each 5 mL of Lorabid for Oral Suspension contains loracarbef equivalent to 100 mg (0.286 mmol) or 200 mg (0.57 mmol) anhydrous loracarbef activity. The suspensions also contain cellulose, F D & C Red No. 40, flavors, methylparaben, propylparaben, simethicone emulsion, sodium carboxymethylcellulose, sucrose, and xanthan gum.

CLINICAL PHARMACOLOGY

Loracarbef, after oral administration, was approximately 90% absorbed from the gastrointestinal tract. When capsules were taken with food, peak plasma concentrations were 50% to 60% of those achieved when the drug was administered to fasting subjects and occurred from 30 to 60 minutes later. Total absorption, as measured by urinary recovery and area under the plasma concentration versus time curve (AUC), was unchanged. The effect of food on the rate and extent of absorption of the suspension formulation has not been studied to date.
The pharmacokinetics of loracarbef were linear over the recommended dosage range of 200 to 400 mg, with no accumulation of the drug noted when it was given twice daily.
Average peak plasma concentrations after administration of 200-mg or 400-mg single doses of loracarbef as capsules to fasting subjects were approximately 8 and 14 μg/mL, respectively, and were obtained within 1.2 hours after dosing. The average peak plasma concentration in adults following a 400-mg single dose of suspension was 17 μg/mL and was obtained within 0.8 hour after dosing (*see* Table).

Dosage (mg)	Mean Plasma Loracarbef Concentrations (μg/mL) Peak C_{max}	Time to Peak T_{max}
Capsule (single dose)		
200 mg	8	1.2 h
400 mg	14	1.2 h
Suspension (single dose)		
400 mg (adult)	17	0.8 h
7.5 mg/kg (pediatric)	13	0.8 h
15 mg/kg (pediatric)	19	0.8 h

Following administration of 7.5 and 15 mg/kg single doses of oral suspension to children, average peak plasma concentrations were 13 and 19 μg/mL, respectively, and were obtained within 40 to 60 minutes.
This increased rate of absorption (suspension > capsule) should be taken into consideration if the oral suspension is to be substituted for the capsule, and capsules should not be substituted for the oral suspension in the treatment of otitis media (*see* **DOSAGE AND ADMINISTRATION**).
The elimination half-life was an average of 1.0 h in patients with normal renal function. Concomitant administration of probenecid decreased the rate of urinary excretion and increased the half-life to 1.5 hours.
In subjects with moderate impairment of renal function (creatinine clearance 10 to 50 mL/min/1.73 m^2), following a single 400-mg dose, the plasma half-life was prolonged to approximately 5.6 hours. In subjects with severe renal impairment (creatinine clearance <10 mL/min/1.73 m^2), the half-life was increased to approximately 32 hours. During hemodialysis the half-life was approximately 4 hours. In patients with severe renal impairment, the C_{max} increased from 15.4 μg/mL to 23 μg/mL (*see* **PRECAUTIONS** *and* **DOSAGE AND ADMINISTRATION**).
In single-dose studies, plasma half-life and AUC were not significantly altered in healthy elderly subjects with normal renal function.
There is no evidence of metabolism of loracarbef in humans. Approximately 25% of circulating loracarbef is bound to plasma proteins.
Middle-ear fluid concentrations of loracarbef were approximately 48% of the plasma concentration 2 hours after drug administration in pediatric patients. The peak concentration of loracarbef in blister fluid was approximately half that obtained in plasma. Adequate data on CSF levels of loracarbef are not available.
Microbiology —Loracarbef exerts its bactericidal action by binding to essential target proteins of the bacterial cell wall, leading to inhibition of cell-wall synthesis. It is stable in the presence of some bacterial β-lactamases. Loracarbef has been shown to be active against most strains of the following organisms both *in vitro* and in clinical infections (*see* **INDICATIONS AND USAGE**):

Gram-positive aerobes:
Staphylococcus aureus (including penicillinase-producing strains)
NOTE: Loracarbef (like most β-lactam antimicrobials) is inactive against methicillin-resistant staphylococci.
Staphylococcus saprophyticus
Streptococcus pneumoniae
Streptococcus pyogenes

Gram-negative aerobes:
Escherichia coli
Haemophilus influenzae (including β-lactamase-producing strains)
Moraxella (Branhamella) catarrhalis (including β-lactamase-producing strains)

The following *in vitro* data are available: however, their clinical significance is unknown.
Loracarbef exhibits *in vitro* minimum inhibitory concentrations (MIC) of 8 μg/mL or less against most strains of the following organisms; however, the safety and efficacy of loracarbef in treating clinical infections due to these organisms have not been established in adequate and well-controlled trials.

Gram-positive aerobes:
Staphylococcus epidermidis
Streptococcus agalactiae (group B streptococci)
Streptococcus bovis
Streptococci, groups C, F, and G
viridans group streptococci

Gram-negative aerobes:
Citrobacter diversus
Haemophilus parainfluenzae
Klebsiella pneumoniae
Neisseria gonorrhoeae (including penicillinase-producing strains)
Pasteurella multocida
Proteus mirabilis
Salmonella species
Shigella species
Yersinia enterocolitica

NOTE: Loracarbef is inactive against most strains of *Acinetobacter, Enterobacter, Morganella morganii, Proteus vulgaris, Providencia, Pseudomonas,* and *Serratia.*

Anaerobic organisms:
Clostridium perfringens
Fusobacterium necrophorum
Peptococcus niger
Peptostreptococcus intermedius
Propionibacterium acnes

Susceptibility Testing
Diffusion Techniques—Quantitative methods that require measurement of zone diameters give the most precise estimate of the susceptibility of bacteria to antimicrobial agents. One such standardized method[1] has been recommended for use with the 30-μg loracarbef disk. Interpretation involves the correlation of the diameter obtained in the disk test with MIC for loracarbef.
Reports from the laboratory giving results of the standard single-disk susceptibility test with a 30-μg loracarbef disk should be interpreted according to the following criteria:

Zone Diameter (mm)	Interpretation
≥ 18	(S) Susceptible
15–17	(MS) Moderately Susceptible
≤ 14	(R) Resistant

A report of "susceptible" implies that the pathogen is likely to be inhibited by generally achievable blood concentrations. A report of "moderately susceptible" indicates that inhibitory concentrations of the antibiotic may be achieved if high dosage is used or if the infection is confined to tissues and fluids (e.g., urine) in which high antibiotic concentrations are attained. A report of "resistant" indicates that achievable concentrations of the antibiotic are unlikely to be inhibitory and other therapy should be selected.
Standardized procedures require the use of laboratory control organisms. The 30-μg loracarbef disk should give the following zone diameters with the NCCLS approved procedure:

Organism	Zone Diameter (mm)
E. coli ATCC 25922	23–29
S. aureus ATCC 25923	23–31

Dilution Techniques—Use a standardized dilution method[2] (broth, agar, or microdilution) or equivalent with loracarbef powder. The MIC values obtained should be interpreted according to the following criteria:

MIC (μg/mL)	Interpretation
≤8	(S) Susceptible
16	(MS) Moderately Susceptible
≥32	(R) Resistant

As with standard diffusion methods, dilution procedures require the use of laboratory control organisms. Standard loracarbef powder should give the following MIC values with the NCCLS approved procedure:

Organism	MIC Range (μg/mL)
E. coli ATCC 25922	0.5–2
S. aureus ATCC 29213	0.5–2

INDICATIONS AND USAGE

Lorabid is indicated in the treatment of patients with mild to moderate infections caused by susceptible strains of the designated microorganisms in the conditions listed below. (As recommended dosages, durations of therapy, and applicable patient populations vary among these infections, please see **DOSAGE AND ADMINISTRATION** for specific recommendations.)

Lower Respiratory Tract

Secondary Bacterial Infection of Acute Bronchitis caused by *S. pneumoniae, H. influenzae* (including β-lactamase-producing strains), or *M. catarrhalis* (including β-lactamase-producing strains).
Acute Bacterial Exacerbations of Chronic Bronchitis caused by *S. pneumoniae, H. influenzae* (including β-lactamase-producing strains), or *M. catarrhalis* (including β-lactamase-producing strains).
Pneumonia caused by *S. pneumoniae or H. influenzae* (non-β-lactamase-producing strains only). Data are insufficient at this time to establish efficacy in patients with pneumonia caused by β-lactamase-producing strains of *H. influenzae.*

Upper Respiratory Tract

Otitis Media† caused by *S. pneumoniae, H. influenzae* (including β-lactamase-producing strains), *M. catarrhalis* (including β-lactamase-producing strains), or *S. pyogenes.*
Acute Maxillary Sinusitis † caused by *S. pneumoniae, H. influenzae* (non-β-lactamase-producing strains only), or *M. catarrhalis* (including β-lactamase-producing strains). Data are insufficient at this time to establish efficacy in patients with acute maxillary sinusitis caused by β-lactamase-producing strains of *H. influenzae.*
†NOTE: In a patient population with significant numbers of β-lactamase-producing organisms, loracarbef's clinical cure and bacteriological eradication rates were somewhat less than those observed with a product containing a β-lactamase inhibitor. Lorabid's decreased potential for toxicity compared to products containing β-lactamase inhibitors along with the susceptibility patterns of the common microbes in a given geographic area should be taken into account when considering the use of an antimicrobial (*see* **CLINICAL STUDIES** section). For information on use in pediatric patients, *see* **PRECAUTIONS—Pediatric Use**.
Pharyngitis and Tonsillitis caused by *S. pyogenes.* (The usual drug of choice in the treatment and prevention of streptococcal infections, including the prophylaxis of rheumatic fever, is penicillin administered by the intramuscular route. Lorabid is generally effective in the eradication of *S. pyogenes* from the nasopharynx; however, data establishing the efficacy of Lorabid in the subsequent prevention of rheumatic fever are not available at present.)

Skin and Skin Structure

Uncomplicated Skin and Skin Structure Infections caused by *S. aureus* (including penicillinase-producing strains) or *S. pyogenes.* Abscesses should be surgically drained as clinically indicated.

Urinary Tract

Uncomplicated Urinary Tract Infections (cystitis) caused by *E. coli* or *S. saprophyticus**.
NOTE: In considering the use of Lorabid in the treatment of cystitis, Lorabid's lower bacterial eradication rates and lower potential for toxicity should be weighed against the increased eradica-

Continued on next page

Lorabid—Cont.

tion rates and increased potential for toxicity demonstrated by some other classes of approved agents (*see* **CLINICAL STUDIES** section).

Uncomplicated Pyelonephritis caused by *E. coli.*

* Although treatment of infections due to this organism in this organ system demonstrated a clinically acceptable overall outcome, efficacy was studied in fewer than 10 infections.

Culture and susceptibility testing should be performed when appropriate to determine the causative organism and its susceptibility to loracarbef. Therapy may be started while awaiting the results of these studies. Once these results become available, antimicrobial therapy should be adjusted accordingly.

CONTRAINDICATION

Lorabid is contraindicated in patients with known allergy to loracarbef or cephalosporin-class antibiotics.

WARNINGS

BEFORE THERAPY WITH LORABID IS INSTITUTED, CAREFUL INQUIRY SHOULD BE MADE TO DETERMINE WHETHER THE PATIENT HAS HAD PREVIOUS HYPERSENSITIVITY REACTIONS TO LORACARBEF, CEPHALOSPORINS, PENICILLINS, OR OTHER DRUGS. IF THIS PRODUCT IS TO BE GIVEN TO PENICILLIN-SENSITIVE PATIENTS, CAUTION SHOULD BE EXERCISED BECAUSE CROSS-HYPERSENSITIVITY AMONG β-LACTAM ANTIBIOTICS HAS BEEN CLEARLY DOCUMENTED AND MAY OCCUR IN UP TO 10% OF PATIENTS WITH A HISTORY OF PENICILLIN ALLERGY. IF AN ALLERGIC REACTION TO LORABID OCCURS, DISCONTINUE THE DRUG. SERIOUS ACUTE HYPERSENSITIVITY REACTIONS MAY REQUIRE THE USE OF EPINEPHRINE AND OTHER EMERGENCY MEASURES, INCLUDING OXYGEN, INTRAVENOUS FLUIDS, INTRAVENOUS ANTIHISTAMINES, CORTICOSTEROIDS, PRESSOR AMINES, AND AIRWAY MANAGEMENT, AS CLINICALLY INDICATED.

Pseudomembranous colitis has been reported with nearly all antibacterial agents and may range from mild to life-threatening. Therefore, it is important to consider this diagnosis in patients who present with diarrhea subsequent to the administration of antibacterial agents.

Treatment with broad-spectrum antibiotics alters the normal flora of the colon and may permit overgrowth of clostridia. Studies indicate that a toxin produced by *Clostridium difficile* is a primary cause of "antibiotic-associated colitis."

After the diagnosis of pseudomembranous colitis has been established, therapeutic measures should be initiated. Mild cases of pseudomembranous colitis usually respond to discontinuation of drug alone. In moderate to severe cases, consideration should be given to management with fluids and electrolytes, protein supplementation, and treatment with an antibacterial drug effective against *C. difficile*-associated colitis.

PRECAUTIONS

General —In patients with known or suspected renal impairment (*see* **DOSAGE AND ADMINISTRATION**), careful clinical observation and appropriate laboratory studies should be performed prior to and during therapy. The total daily dose of loracarbef should be reduced in these patients because high and/or prolonged plasma antibiotic concentrations can occur in such individuals administered the usual doses. Loracarbef, like cephalosporins, should be given with caution to patients receiving concurrent treatment with potent diuretics because these diuretics are suspected of adversely affecting renal function.

As with other broad-spectrum antimicrobials, prolonged use of loracarbef may result in the overgrowth of nonsusceptible organisms. Careful observation of the patient is essential. If superinfection occurs during therapy, appropriate measures should be taken.

Loracarbef, as with other broad-spectrum antimicrobials, should be prescribed with caution in individuals with a history of colitis.

Information for Patients —Lorabid should be taken either at least 1 hour prior to eating or at least 2 hours after eating a meal.

Drug Interactions —

Probenecid: As with other β-lactam antibiotics, renal excretion of loracarbef is inhibited by probenecid and resulted in an approximate 80% increase in the AUC for loracarbef (*see* **CLINICAL PHARMACOLOGY**).

Carcinogenesis, Mutagenesis, Impairment of Fertility —Although lifetime studies in animals have not been performed to evaluate carcinogenic potential, no mutagenic potential was found for loracarbef in standard tests of genotoxicity, which included bacterial mutation tests and *in vitro* and *in vivo* mammalian systems. In rats, fertility and reproductive performance were not affected by loracarbef at doses up to 33 times the maximum human exposure in mg/kg (10 times the exposure based on mg/m^2).

Usage in Pregnancy—Pregnancy Category B —Reproduction studies have been performed in mice, rats, and rabbits at doses up to 33 times the maximum human exposure in mg/kg (4, 10, and 4 times the exposure, respectively, based on mg/m^2) and have revealed no evidence of impaired fertility or harm to the fetus due to loracarbef. There are, however, no adequate and well-controlled studies in pregnant women. Because animal reproduction studies are not always predictive of human response, this drug should be used during pregnancy only if clearly needed.

Labor and Delivery —Lorabid has not been studied for use during labor and delivery. Treatment should be given only if clearly needed.

Nursing Mothers —It is not known whether this drug is excreted in human milk. Because many drugs are excreted in human milk, caution should be exercised when Lorabid is administered to a nursing woman.

Pediatric Use —The safety and efficacy of Lorabid have been established for children aged six months to twelve years for acute maxillary sinusitis based upon its approval in adults. Use of Lorabid in pediatric patients is supported by pharmacokinetic and safety data in adults and children, and by clinical and microbiologic data from adequate and well-controlled studies of the treatment of acute maxillary sinusitis in adults and of acute otitis media with effusion in children. It is also supported by post-marketing adverse events surveillance. (*See* **CLINICAL PHARMACOLOGY, INDICATIONS AND USAGE, ADVERSE REACTIONS, DOSAGE AND ADMINISTRATION,** *and* **CLINICAL STUDIES** sections).

Geriatric Use —Healthy geriatric volunteers (≥65 years old) with normal renal function who received a single 400-mg dose of loracarbef had no significant differences in AUC or clearance when compared to healthy adult volunteers 20 to 40 years of age. In clinical studies, when geriatric patients received the usual recommended adult doses, clinical efficacy and safety were comparable to results in nongeriatric adult patients. Because significant numbers of elderly patients have decreased renal function, evaluation of renal function in this population is recommended (*see* **DOSAGE AND ADMINISTRATION**).

ADVERSE REACTIONS

The nature of adverse reactions to loracarbef are similar to those observed with orally administered β-lactam antimicrobials. The majority of adverse reactions observed in clinical trials were of a mild and transient nature; 1.5% of patients discontinued therapy because of drug-related adverse reactions. No one reaction requiring discontinuation accounted for >0.03% of the total patient population; however, of those reactions resulting in discontinuation, gastrointestinal events (diarrhea and abdominal pain) and skin rashes predominated.

All Patients

The following adverse events, irrespective of relationship to drug, have been reported following the use of Lorabid in clinical trials. Incidence rates (combined for all dosing regimens and dosage forms) were less than 1% for the total patient population, except as otherwise noted:

Gastrointestinal: The most commonly observed adverse reactions were related to the gastrointestinal system. The incidence of gastrointestinal adverse reactions increased in patients treated with higher doses. Individual event rates included diarrhea, 4.1%; nausea, 1.9%; vomiting, 1.4%; abdominal pain, 1.4%; and anorexia.

Hypersensitivity: Hypersensitivity reactions including, skin rashes (1.2%), urticaria, pruritus, and erythema multiforme.

Central Nervous System: Headache (2.9%), somnolence, nervousness, insomnia, and dizziness.

Hemic and Lymphatic Systems: Transient thrombocytopenia, leukopenia, and eosinophilia.

Hepatic: Transient elevations in AST (SGOT), ALT (SGPT), and alkaline phosphatase.

Renal: Transient elevations in BUN and creatinine.

Cardiovascular System: Vasodilatation.

Genitourinary: Vaginitis (1.3%), vaginal moniliasis (1.1%).

As with other β-lactam antibiotics, the following potentially severe adverse experiences have been reported rarely with loracarbef in worldwide post-marketing surveillance: anaphylaxis, hepatic dysfunction including cholestasis, prolongation of the prothrombin time with clinical bleeding in patients taking anticoagulants, and Stevens-Johnson syndrome.

Pediatric Patients

The incidences of several adverse events, irrespective of relationship to drug, following treatment with Lorabid were significantly different in the pediatric population and the adult population as follows:

Event	Pediatric	Adult
Diarrhea	5.8%	3.6%
Headache	0.9%	3.2%
Rhinitis	6.3%	1.6%
Nausea	0.0%	2.5%
Rash	2.9%	0.7%
Vomiting	3.3%	0.5%
Somnolence	2.1%	0.4%
Anorexia	2.3%	0.3%

β-Lactam Antimicrobial Class Labeling:

The following adverse reactions and altered laboratory test results have been reported in patients treated with β-lactam antibiotics:

Adverse Reactions —Allergic reactions, aplastic anemia, hemolytic anemia, hemorrhage, agranulocytosis, toxic epidermal necrolysis, renal dysfunction, and toxic nephropathy. As with other β-lactam antibiotics, serum sickness-like reactions have been reported rarely with loracarbef.

Several β-lactam antibiotics have been implicated in triggering seizures, particularly in patients with renal impairment when the dosage was not reduced. If seizures associated with drug therapy should occur, the drug should be discontinued. Anticonvulsant therapy can be given if clinically indicated.

Altered Laboratory Tests —Increased prothrombin time, positive direct Coombs' test, elevated LDH, pancytopenia, and neutropenia.

OVERDOSAGE

Signs and Symptoms —The toxic symptoms following an overdose of β-lactams may include nausea, vomiting, epigastric distress, and diarrhea.

Loracarbef is eliminated primarily by the kidneys. Forced diuresis, peritoneal dialysis, hemodialysis, or hemoperfusion have not been established as beneficial for an overdose of loracarbef. Hemodialysis has been shown to be effective in hastening the elimination of loracarbef from plasma in patients with chronic renal failure.

DOSAGE AND ADMINISTRATION

Lorabid is administered orally either at least 1 hour prior to eating or at least 2 hours after eating. The recommended dosages, durations of treatment, and applicable patient populations are described in the following chart:

Population/Infection	Dosage (mg)	Duration (days)
ADULTS (13 years and older)		
Lower Respiratory Tract		
Secondary Bacterial Infection of Acute Bronchitis	200–400 q12h	7
Acute Bacterial Exacerbation of Chronic Bronchitis	400 q12h	7
Pneumonia	400 q12h	14
Upper Respiratory Tract		
Pharyngitis/Tonsillitis	200 q12h	10[a]
Sinusitis	400 q12h	10
(*See* **CLINICAL STUDIES** *and* **INDICATIONS AND USAGE** for further information.)		
Skin and Skin Structure		
Uncomplicated Skin and Skin Structure Infections	200 q12h	7
Urinary Tract		
Uncomplicated cystitis	200 q24h	7
(*See* **CLINICAL STUDIES** *and* **INDICATIONS AND USAGE** for further information.)		
Uncomplicated pyelonephritis	400 q12h	14
PEDIATRIC PATIENTS (6 months to 12 years)		
Upper Resipratory Tract		
Acute Otitis Media[b]	30 mg/kg/day in divided doses q12h	10
(*See* **CLINICAL STUDIES** *and* **INDICATIONS AND USAGE** for further information.)		
Acute maxillary sinusitis	30 mg/kg/day in divided doses q12h	10
(*See* **CLINICAL STUDIES** *and* **INDICATIONS AND USAGE** for further information.)		
Pharyngitis/Tonsillitis	15 mg/kg/day in divided doses q12h	10[a]
Skin and Skin Structure		
Impetigo	15 mg/kg/day in divided doses q12h	7

[a] In the treatment of infections due to *S. pyogenes,* Lorabid should be administered for at least 10 days.

[b] Otitis media should be treated with the suspension. Clinical studies of otitis media were conducted with the suspension formulation only. The suspension is more rapidly absorbed than the capsules, resulting in higher peak plasma concentrations when administered at the same dose. Therefore, the capsule should not be substituted for the suspension in the treatment of otitis media (*see* **CLINICAL PHARMACOLOGY**).

[See first table at bottom of next page]
[See second table at bottom of next page]

Renal Impairment: Lorabid may be administered to patients with impaired renal function. The usual dose and schedule may be employed in patients with creatinine clearance levels of 50 mL/min or greater. Patients with creatinine clearance between 10 and 49 mL/min may be given half of the recommended dose at the usual dosage interval, or the normal recommended dose at twice the usual dosage interval. Patients with creatinine clearance levels less than 10 mL/min may be treated with the recommended dose given every 3 to 5 days; patients on hemodialysis should receive another dose following dialysis.

When only the serum creatinine is available, the following formula (based on sex, weight, and age of the patient) may be used to convert this value into creatinine clearance (CL_{cr}, mL/min). The equation assumes the patient's renal function is stable.

$$\text{Males} = \frac{(\text{weight in kg}) \times (140 - \text{age})}{(72) \times \text{serum creatinine (mg/100 mL)}}$$

$$\text{Females} = (0.85) \times (\text{above value})$$

Reconstitution Directions for Oral Suspension

Bottle Size	Reconstitution Directions
50 mL	Add 30 mL of water in 2 portions to the dry mixture in the bottle. Shake well after each addition.
75 mL	Add 45 mL of water in 2 portions to the dry mixture in the bottle. Shake well after each addition.
100 mL	Add 60 mL of water in 2 portions to the dry mixture in the bottle. Shake well after each addition.

After mixing, the suspension may be kept at room temperature, 59° to 86°F (15° to 30°C), for 14 days without significant loss of potency. Keep tightly closed. Discard unused portion after 14 days.

HOW SUPPLIED

Pulvules:
200 mg, (blue and gray) (No. 3170) (30s) NDC 61570-170-30; (100s) NDC 61570-170-01.
400 mg, (blue and pink) (No. 3171) (30s) NDC 61570-171-30; (100s) NDC 61570-171-01.
Keep tightly closed. Store at controlled room temperature, 59° to 86°F (15° to 30°C). Protect from heat.
For Oral Suspension (strawberry bubble gum flavor):
100 mg/5 mL, (M-5135) (50-mL size) NDC 61570-135-50; (100-mL size) 61570-135-10
200 mg/5 mL, (M-5136) (50-mL size) NDC 61570-136-50; (75-mL size) NDC 61570-136-10.

Clinical Studies:

Acute Otitis Media

Study 1 In a controlled clinical study of acute otitis media performed in the United States where significant rates of β-lactamase-producing organisms were found, loracarbef was compared to an oral antimicrobial agent that contained a specific β-lactamase inhibitor. In this study, using very strict evaluability criteria and microbiologic and clinical response criteria at the 10- to 16-day post therapy follow-up, the following presumptive bacterial eradication/clinical cure outcomes (ie, clinical success) and safety results were obtained:

US Acute Otitis Media Study
Loracarbef vs β-lactamase inhibitor-containing control drug

Pathogen	% of Cases With Pathogens (n=204)	Outcome
S. pneumoniae	42.6%	Loracarbef equivalent to control
H. influenzae	30.4%	Loracarbef success rate 9% less than control
M. catarrhalis	20.6%	Loracarbef success rate 19% less than control
S. pyogenes	6.4%	Loracarbef equivalent to control
Overall	100.0%	Loracarbef success rate 12% less than control

Safety: The incidences of the following adverse events were clinically and statistically significantly higher in the control arm versus the loracarbef arm.

Event	Loracarbef	Control
Diarrhea	15%	26%
Rash*	8%	15%

*The majority of these involved the diaper area in young pediatric patients.

Study 2 In a controlled clinical study of acute otitis media performed in Europe, loracarbef was compared to amoxicillin. As expected in a European population, this study population had a lower incidence of β-lactamase-producing organisms than usually seen in US trials. In this study, using very strict evaluability criteria and microbiologic and clinical response criteria at the 10- to 16-day post therapy follow-up, the following presumptive bacterial eradication/clinical cure outcomes (ie, clinical success) were obtained:

European Acute Otitis Media Study
Loracarbef vs Amoxicillin

Efficacy:

Pathogen	% of Cases With Pathogens (n=291)	Outcome
S. pneumoniae	51.5%	Loracarbef equivalent to amoxicillin
H. influenzae	29.2%	Loracarbef success rate 14% greater than amoxicillin
M. catarrhalis	15.8%	Loracarbef success rate 31% greater than amoxicillin
S. pyogenes	3.4%	Loracarbef equivalent to amoxicillin
Overall	100.0%	Loracarbef equivalent to amoxicillin

Acute Maxilliary Sinusitis

In a controlled clinical study of acute maxillary sinusitis performed in Europe, loracarbef was compared to doxycycline. In this study, there were 210 sinus-puncture evaluable patients. As expected in a European population, this study population had a lower incidence of β-lactamase-producing organisms than usually seen in US trials. In this study, using very strict evaluability criteria and microbiologic and clinical response criteria at the 1- to 2-week post therapy follow-up, the following presumptive bacterial eradication/clinical cure outcomes (ie, clinical success) were obtained:

European Acute Maxillary Sinusitis Study
Loracarbef vs Doxycycline

Efficacy:

Pathogen	% of Cases With Pathogens (n=210)	Outcome
S. pneumoniae	47.6%	Loracarbef equivalent to doxycycline
H. influenzae	41.4%	Loracarbef equivalent to doxycycline
M. catarrhalis	11.0%	Loracarbef equivalent to doxycycline
Overall	100.0%	Loracarbef equivalent to doxycycline

CYSTITIS

Study 1 In a controlled clinical study of cystitis performed in the United States, loracarbef was compared to cefaclor. In this study, using very strict evaluability criteria and microbiologic and clinical response criteria at the 5- to 9-day post therapy follow-up, the following bacterial eradication rates were obtained:

U.S. Uncomplicated Cystitis Study
Loracarbef vs Cefaclor

Efficacy:

Pathogen	% of Cases With Pathogens (n=186)	Outcome
E. coli	77.4%	Loracarbef eradication rate 4% greater than cefaclor (loracarbef eradication rate 80%)
Other major *Enterobacteriaceae*	12.5%	Loracarbef equivalent to cefaclor (loracarbef eradication rate 61%)
S. saprophyticus	3.8%	Loracarbef equivalent to cefaclor

Study 2 In a second controlled clinical study of cystitis, performed in Europe, loracarbef was compared to an oral quinolone. In this study, using very strict evaluability criteria and microbiologic and clinical response criteria at the 5- to 9-day post therapy follow-up, the following bacterial eradication rates were obtained:

European Uncomplicated Cystitis Study
Loracarbef vs Quinolone

Efficacy:

Pathogen	% of Cases With Pathogens (n=189)	Outcome
E. coli	82.0%	Loracarbef eradication rate 7% less than quinolone (loracarbef eradication rate 81%)
Other major *Enterobacteriaceae*	10.1%	Loracarbef eradication rate 32% less than quinolone (loracarbef eradication rate 50%)

REFERENCES

1. National Committee for Clinical Laboratory Standards, M2-A4 performance standards for antimicrobial disk susceptibility tests. ed 4, Villanova, PA, April, 1990.
2. National Committee for Clinical Laboratory Standards, M7-A2 methods for dilution antimicrobial susceptibility tests for bacteria that grow aerobically. ed 2, Villanova, PA, April, 1990.

Shown in Product Identification Guide, page 321

Pulvules® is a licensed registered trademark of Eli Lilly & Co.
Rx Only.
Distributed by: Monarch Pharmaceuticals, Inc., Bristol, TN 37620
Manufactured by: Eli Lilly and Co., Indianapolis, IN 46285
Rev. 3/00

PEDIATRIC DOSAGE CHART
DAILY DOSE 15 mg/kg/day

Weight lb	Weight kg	100 mg/5 mL Suspension: Dose given twice daily mL	tsp	200 mg/5 mL Suspension: Dose given twice daily mL	tsp
15	7	2.6	0.5	—	—
29	13	4.9	1.0	2.5	0.5
44	20	7.5	1.5	3.8	0.75
57	26	9.8	2.0	4.9	1.0

PEDIATRIC DOSAGE CHART
DAILY DOSE 30 mg/kg/day

Weight lb	Weight kg	100 mg/5 mL Suspension: Dose given twice daily mL	tsp	200 mg/5 mL Suspension: Dose given twice daily mL	tsp
15	7	5.2	1.0	2.6	0.5
29	13	9.8	2.0	4.9	1.0
44	20	—	—	7.5	1.5
57	26	—	—	9.8	2.0

MENEST® ℞

[men-est']
brand of
esterified estrogens tablets, USP
PRESCRIBING INFORMATION

WARNINGS

1. ESTROGENS HAVE BEEN REPORTED TO INCREASE THE RISK OF ENDOMETRIAL CARCINOMA.

Three independent case control studies have shown an increased risk of endometrial cancer in postmenopausal women exposed to exogenous estrogens for prolonged periods.[1–3] This risk was independent of the other known risk factors for endometrial cancer. These studies are further supported by the finding that incidence rates of endometrial cancer have increased sharply since 1969 in eight different areas of the United States with population-based cancer reporting systems, an increase which may be related to the rapidly expanding use of estrogens during the last decade.[4]

The three case control studies reported that the risk of endometrial cancer in estrogen users was about 4.5 to 13.9 times greater than in nonusers. The risk appears to depend on both duration of treatment[1] and on estrogen dose.[3] In view of these findings, when estrogens are used for the treatment of menopausal symptoms, the lowest dose that will control symptoms should be utilized and medication should be discontinued as soon as possible. When prolonged treatment is medically indicated, the patient should be reassessed on at least a semiannual basis to determine the need for continued therapy. Although the evidence must be considered preliminary, one study suggests that cyclic administration of low doses of estrogen may carry less risk than continuous administration[3]; it therefore appears prudent to utilize such a regimen.

Close clinical surveillance of all women taking estrogens is important. In all cases of undiagnosed persistent or recurring abnormal vaginal bleeding, adequate diagnostic measures should be undertaken to rule out malignancy.

There is no evidence at present that "natural" estrogens are more or less hazardous than "synthetic" estrogens at equiestrogenic doses.

2. ESTROGENS SHOULD NOT BE USED DURING PREGNANCY.

The use of female sex hormones, both estrogens and progestagens, during early pregnancy may seriously damage the offspring. It has been shown that females exposed in utero to diethylstilbestrol, a nonsteroidal estrogen, have an increased risk of developing in later life a form of vaginal or cervical cancer that is ordinarily extremely rare.[5,6] The risk has been estimated as not greater than 4 per 1000 exposures.[7] Furthermore, a high percentage of such exposed women (from 30 to 90 percent) have been found to have vaginal adenosis,[8–12]

Continued on next page

Menest—Cont.

epithelial changes of the vagina and cervix. Although these changes are histologically benign, it is not known whether they are precursors of malignancy. Although similar data are not available with the use of other estrogens, it cannot be presumed they would not induce similar changes. Several reports suggest an association between intrauterine exposure to female sex hormones and congenital anomalies, including congenital heart defects and limb reduction defects.[13–15] One case control study[16] estimated a 4.7-fold increased risk of limb reduction defects in infants exposed in utero to sex hormones (oral contraceptives, hormone withdrawal tests for pregnancy, or attempted treatment for threatened abortion). Some of these exposures were very short and involved only a few days of treatment. The data suggest that the risk of limb reduction defects in exposed fetuses is somewhat less than 1 per 1000. In the past, female sex hormones have been used during pregnancy in an attempt to treat threatened or habitual abortion. There is considerable evidence that estrogens are ineffective for these indications, and there is no evidence from well-controlled studies that progestagens are effective for these uses. If Menest (esterified estrogens tablets) is used during pregnancy, or if the patient becomes pregnant while taking this drug, she should be apprised of the potential risks to the fetus, and the advisability of pregnancy continuation.

DESCRIPTION

Esterified estrogens is a mixture of the sodium salts of the sulfate esters of the estrogenic substances, principally estrone, that are of the type excreted by pregnant mares. The content of total esterified estrogens is not less than 90 percent and not more than 110 percent of the labeled amount. Esterified estrogens contain not less than 75 percent and not more than 85 percent of sodium estrone sulfate, and not less than 6 percent and not more than 15 percent of sodium equilin sulfate, in such proportion that the total of these two components is not less than 90 percent, all percentages being calculated on the basis of the total esterified estrogens content.

Inactive Ingredients: Ethyl cellulose, fragrances, hydroxypropyl cellulose, hydroxypropyl methylcellulose 2910, lactose, magnesium stearate, methylcellulose, polyethylene glycol, sodium bicarbonate, shellac, starch, stearic acid, titanium dioxide, and vanillin. Dyes in the form of aluminum lakes are contained in each tablet strength as follows: **0.3 mg Tablet:** FD&C Yellow No. 6, D&C Yellow No. 10. **0.625 mg Tablet:** FD&C Yellow No. 6, D&C Yellow No. 10. **1.25 mg Tablet:** FD&C Yellow No. 6, D&C Yellow No. 10, FD&C Blue No. 1. **2.5 mg Tablet:** D&C Red No. 30.

CLINICAL PHARMACOLOGY

Estrogens are important in the development and maintenance of the female reproductive system and secondary sex characteristics. They promote growth and development of the vagina, uterus, and fallopian tubes, and enlargement of the breasts. Indirectly, they contribute to the shaping of the skeleton, maintenance of tone and elasticity of urogenital structures, changes in the epiphyses of the long bones that allow for the pubertal growth spurt and its termination, growth of axillary and pubic hair, and pigmentation of the nipples and genitals. Decline of estrogenic activity at the end of the menstrual cycle can bring on menstruation, although the cessation of progesterone secretion is the most important factor in the mature ovulatory cycle. However, in the preovulatory or nonovulatory cycle, estrogen is the primary determinant in the onset of menstruation. Estrogens also affect the release of pituitary gonadotropins. The pharmacologic effects of esterified estrogens are similar to those of endogenous estrogens. They are soluble in water and are well absorbed from the gastrointestinal tract.

In responsive tissues (female genital organs, breasts, hypothalamus, pituitary) estrogens enter the cell and are transported into the nucleus. As a result of estrogen action, specific RNA and protein synthesis occurs. Metabolism and inactivation occur primarily in the liver. Some estrogens are excreted into the bile; however, they are reabsorbed from the intestine and returned to the liver through the portal venous system. Water soluble estrogen conjugates are strongly acidic and are ionized in body fluids, which favor excretion through the kidneys since tubular reabsorption is minimal.

INDICATIONS AND USAGE

Menest (esterified estrogens tablets) is indicated in the treatment of:

1. Moderate to severe *vasomotor* symptoms associated with the menopause. (There is no evidence that estrogens are effective for nervous symptoms or depression which might occur during menopause, and they should not be used to treat these conditions.)
2. Atrophic vaginitis.
3. Kraurosis vulvae.
4. Female hypogonadism.
5. Female castration.
6. Primary ovarian failure.
7. Breast cancer (for palliation only) in appropriately selected women and men with metastatic disease.
8. Prostatic carcinoma—palliative therapy of advanced disease.

MENEST (esterified estrogens tablets) HAS NOT BEEN SHOWN TO BE EFFECTIVE FOR ANY PURPOSE DURING PREGNANCY AND ITS USE MAY CAUSE SEVERE HARM TO THE FETUS (SEE BOXED WARNING).

CONTRAINDICATIONS

Estrogens should not be used in women (or men) with any of the following conditions:

1. Known or suspected cancer of the breast except in appropriately selected patients being treated for metastatic disease.
2. Known or suspected estrogen-dependent neoplasia.
3. Known or suspected pregnancy (See Boxed Warning).
4. Undiagnosed abnormal genital bleeding.
5. Active thrombophlebitis or thromboembolic disorders.
6. A past history of thrombophlebitis, thrombosis or thromboembolic disorders associated with previous estrogen use (except when used in treatment of breast or prostatic malignancy).

WARNINGS

1. *Induction of malignant neoplasms.* Long-term continuous administration of natural and synthetic estrogens in certain animal species increases the frequency of carcinomas of the breast, cervix, vagina, and liver. There is now evidence that estrogens increase the risk of carcinoma of the endometrium in humans. (See Boxed Warning.) At the present time there is no satisfactory evidence that estrogens given to postmenopausal women increase the risk of cancer of the breast[18] although a recent long-term followup of a single physician's practice has raised this possibility.[18A] Because of the animal data, there is a need for caution in prescribing estrogens for women with a strong family history of breast cancer or who have breast nodules, fibrocystic disease, or abnormal mammograms.
2. *Gall bladder disease.* A recent study has reported a 2- to 3-fold increase in the risk of surgically confirmed gall bladder disease in women receiving postmenopausal estrogens,[18] similar to the 2-fold increase previously noted in users of oral contraceptives.[19–24] In the case of oral contraceptives the increased risk appeared after 2 years of use.[24]
3. *Effects similar to those caused by estrogen-progestagen oral contraceptives.* There are several serious adverse effects of oral contraceptives, most of which have not, up to now, been documented as consequences of postmenopausal estrogen therapy. This may reflect the comparatively low doses of estrogen used in post-menopausal women. It would be expected that the larger doses of estrogen used to treat prostatic or breast cancer or postpartum breast engorgement are more likely to result in these adverse effects and, in fact, it has been shown that there is an increased risk of thrombosis in men receiving estrogens for prostatic cancer and women for postpartum breast engorgement.[20–23]

a. *Thromboembolic disease.* It is now well established that users of oral contraceptives have an increased risk of various thromboembolic and thrombotic vascular diseases, such as thrombophlebitis, pulmonary embolism, stroke, and myocardial infarction.[24–31] Cases of retinal thrombosis, mesenteric thrombosis, and optic neuritis have been reported in oral contraceptive users. There is evidence that the risk of several of these adverse reactions is related to the dose of the drug.[32,33] An increased risk of post-surgery thromboembolic complications has also been reported in users of oral contraceptives.[34,35] If feasible, estrogen should be discontinued at least 4 weeks before surgery of the type associated with an increased risk of thromboembolism, or during periods of prolonged immobilization.

While an increased rate of thromboembolic and thrombotic disease in postmenopausal users of estrogens has not been found,[18–36] this does not rule out the possibility that such an increase may be present or that subgroups of women who have underlying risk factors or who are receiving relatively large doses of estrogens may have increased risk.

Therefore estrogens should not be used in persons with active thrombophlebitis or thromboembolic disorders, and they should not be used (except in treatment of malignancy) in persons with a history of such disorders in association with estrogen use. They should be used with caution in patients with cerebral vascular or coronary artery disease and only for those in whom estrogens are clearly needed.

Large doses of estrogen (5 mg esterified estrogens per day), comparable to those used to treat cancer of the prostate and breast, have been shown in a large prospective clinical trial in men[37] to increase the risk of nonfatal myocardial infarction, pulmonary embolism and thrombophlebitis. When estrogen doses of this size are used, any of the thromboembolic and thrombotic adverse effects associated with oral contraceptive use should be considered a clear risk.

b. *Hepatic adenoma.* Benign hepatic adenomas appear to be associated with the use of oral contraceptives.[38–40] Although benign, and rare, these may rupture and may cause death through intra-abdominal hemorrhage. Such lesions have not yet been reported in association with other estrogen or progestagen preparations but should be considered in estrogen users having abdominal pain and tenderness, abdominal mass, or hypovolemic shock. Hepatocellular carcinoma has also been reported in women taking estrogen-containing oral contraceptives.[39] The relationship of this malignancy to these drugs is not known at this time.

c. *Elevated blood pressure.* Increased blood pressure is not uncommon in women using oral contraceptives. There is now a report that this may occur with use of estrogens in the menopause[41] and blood pressure should be monitored with estrogen use, especially if high doses are used.

d. *Glucose tolerance.* A worsening of glucose tolerance has been observed in a significant percentage of patients on estrogen-containing oral contraceptives. For this reason, diabetic patients should be carefully observed while receiving estrogen.

4. *Hypercalcemia.* Administration of estrogens may lead to severe hypercalcemia in patients with breast cancer and bone metastases. If this occurs, the drug should be stopped and appropriate measures taken to reduce the serum calcium level.

See footnotes at end of article.

PRECAUTIONS

A. *General Precautions:*

1. A complete medical and family history should be taken prior to the initiation of any estrogen therapy. The pretreatment and periodic physical examinations should include special reference to blood pressure, breast, abdomen, and pelvic organs, and should include a Papanicolau smear. As a general rule, estrogen should not be prescribed for longer than 1 year without another physical examination being performed.
2. Fluid retention—Because estrogens may cause some degree of fluid retention, conditions which might be influenced by this factor, such as epilepsy, migraine, and cardiac or renal dysfunction, require careful observation.
3. Certain patients may develop undesirable manifestations of excessive estrogenic stimulation, such as abnormal or excessive uterine bleeding, mastodynia, etc.
4. Oral contraceptives appear to be associated with an increased incidence of mental depression.[24] Although it is not clear whether this is due to the estrogenic or progestagenic component of the contraceptive, patients with a history of depression should be carefully observed.
5. Pre-existing uterine leiomyomata may increase in size during estrogen use.
6. The pathologist should be advised of estrogen therapy when relevant specimens are submitted.
7. Patients with a past history of jaundice during pregnancy have an increased risk of recurrence of jaundice while receiving estrogen-containing oral contraceptive therapy. If jaundice develops in any patient receiving estrogen, the medication should be discontinued while the cause is investigated.
8. Estrogens may be poorly metabolized in patients with impaired liver function and they should be administered with caution in such patients.
9. Because estrogens influence the metabolism of calcium and phosphorus, they should be used with caution in patients with metabolic bone diseases that are associated with hypercalcemia or in patients with renal insufficiency.
10. Because of the effects of estrogens on epiphyseal closure, they should be used judiciously in young patients in whom bone growth is not complete.
11. The lowest effective dose appropriate for the specific indication should be utilized. Studies of the addition of a progestin for 7 or more days of a cycle of estrogen administration have reported a lowered incidence of endometrial hyperplasia. Morphological and biochemical studies of endometrium suggest that 10 to 13 days of progestin are needed to provide maximal maturation of the endometrium and to eliminate any hyperplastic changes. Whether this will provide protection from endometrial carcinoma has not been clearly established. There are possible additional risks which may be associated with the inclusion of progestin in estrogen replacement regimens. The potential risks include adverse effects on carbohydrate and lipid metabolism. The choice of progestin and dosage may be important in minimizing these adverse effects.
12. Certain endocrine and liver function tests may be affected by estrogen-containing oral contraceptives. The following similar changes may be expected with larger doses of estrogen:
    a. Increased sulfobromophthalein retention.
    b. Increased prothrombin and factors VII, VIII, IX, and X; decreased antithrombin 3; increased norepinephrine-induced platelet aggregability.
    c. Increased thyroid binding globulin (TBG) leading to increased circulating total thyroid hormone, as measured by PBI, T4 by column or T4 by radioimmunoassay. Free T3 resin uptake is decreased, reflecting the elevated TBG; free T4 concentration is unaltered.
    d. Impaired glucose tolerance.
    e. Decreased pregnanediol excretion.
    f. Reduced response to metyrapone test.
    g. Reduced serum folate concentration.
    h. Increased serum triglyceride and phospholipid concentration.

B. *Information for patients:* See text which appears after PHYSICIAN REFERENCES.

C. *Pregnancy Category X*—See Contraindications and Boxed Warning.

D. *Nursing Mothers.* As a general principle, the administration of any drug to nursing mothers should be done only when clearly necessary since many drugs are excreted in human milk.

ADVERSE REACTIONS

(See Warnings regarding induction of neoplasia, adverse effects on the fetus, increased incidence of gall bladder disease, and adverse effects similar to those of oral contraceptives, including thromboembolism.) The following additional adverse reactions have been reported with estrogenic therapy, including oral contraceptives:

1. *Genitourinary system.*
   Breakthrough bleeding, spotting, change in menstrual flow.
   Dysmenorrhea.
   Premenstrual-like syndrome.
   Amenorrhea during and after treatment.
   Increase in size of uterine fibromyomata.
   Vaginal candidiasis.
   Change in cervical eversion and in degree of cervical secretion.
   Cystitis-like syndrome.
2. *Breasts.*
   Tenderness, enlargement, secretion.
3. *Gastrointestinal.*
   Nausea, vomiting.
   Abdominal cramps, bloating.
   Cholestatic jaundice.
4. *Skin.*
   Chloasma or melasma which may persist when drug is discontinued.
   Erythema multiforme.
   Erythema nodosum.
   Hemorrhagic eruption.
   Loss of scalp hair.
   Hirsutism.
5. *Eyes.*
   Steepening of corneal curvature.
   Intolerance to contact lenses.
6. *CNS.*
   Headache, migraine, dizziness.
   Mental depression.
   Chorea.
7. *Miscellaneous.*
   Increase or decrease in weight.
   Reduced carbohydrate tolerance.
   Aggravation of porphyria.
   Edema.
   Changes in libido.

ACUTE OVERDOSAGE

Numerous reports of ingestion of large doses of estrogen-containing oral contraceptives by young children indicate that serious ill effects do not occur. Overdosage of estrogen may cause nausea, and withdrawal bleeding may occur in females.

DOSAGE AND ADMINISTRATION

1. *Given cyclically for short term use only:*

For treatment of moderate to severe *vasomotor symptoms, atrophic vaginitis* or *kraurosis vulvae* associated with the menopause.

The lowest dose that will control symptoms should be chosen and medication should be discontinued as promptly as possible.

Administration should be cyclic (e.g., 3 weeks on and 1 week off).

Attempts to discontinue or taper medication should be made at 3 to 6 month intervals.

USUAL DOSAGE RANGES:

Vasomotor symptoms—1.25 mg daily. If the patient has not menstruated within the last 2 months or more, cyclic administration is started arbitrarily. If the patient is menstruating, cyclic administration is started on day 5 of bleeding.

Atrophic vaginitis and kraurosis vulvae—0.3 mg to 1.25 mg or more daily, depending upon the tissue response of the individual patient. Administer cyclically.

2. *Given cyclically:* Female hypogonadism; female castration; primary ovarian failure.

USUAL DOSAGE RANGES:

Female hypogonadism—2.5 to 7.5 mg daily, in divided doses for 20 days, followed by a rest period of 10 days' duration. If bleeding does not occur by the end of this period, the same dosage schedule is repeated. The number of courses of estrogen therapy necessary to produce bleeding may vary depending on responsiveness of the endometrium.

If bleeding occurs before the end of the 10 day period, begin a 20 day estrogen-progestin cyclic regimen with Menest (esterified estrogens tablets), 2.5 to 7.5 mg daily in divided doses, for 20 days. During the last 5 days of estrogen therapy, give an oral progestin. If bleeding occurs before this regimen is concluded, therapy is discontinued and may be resumed on the fifth day of bleeding.

Female castration and primary ovarian failure—1.25 mg daily, cyclically. Adjust dosage upward or downward according to severity of symptoms and response of the patient. For maintenance, adjust dosage to lowest level that will provide effective control.

3. *Given chronically:* Inoperable progressing prostatic cancer—1.25 to 2.5 mg three times daily. The effectiveness of therapy can be judged by phosphatase determinations as well as by symptomatic improvement of the patient.

Inoperable progressing breast cancer in appropriately selected men and postmenopausal women. (See INDICATIONS AND USAGE)—Suggested dosage is 10 mg three times daily for a period of at least 3 months.

Treated patients with an intact uterus should be monitored closely for signs of endometrial cancer and appropriate diagnostic measures should be taken to rule out malignancy in the event of persistent or recurring abnormal vaginal bleeding.

HOW SUPPLIED

Tablets:

0.3 mg yellow, film-coated oblong tablet imprinted with M72 100's: NDC 61570-072-01

0.625 mg orange, film-coated oblong tablet imprinted with M73 100's: NDC 61570-073-01

1.25 mg green, film-coated oblong tablet imprinted with M74 100's: NDC 61570-074-01

2.5 mg pink, film-coated oblong tablet imprinted with M75 50's: NDC 61570-075-50

PHYSICIAN REFERENCES

1. Ziel HK, Finkel WD: Increased Risk of Endometrial Carcinoma Among Users of Conjugated Estrogens, *New England Journal of Medicine* 293:1167–1170, 1975.
2. Smith DC, Prentic R, Thompson DJ, Hermann WL: Association of Exogenous Estrogen and Endometrial Carcinoma, *New England Journal of Medicine* 293:1164–1167, 1975.
3. Mack TM, Pike MC, Henderson BE, et al: Estrogens and Endometrial Cancer in a Retirement Community, *New England Journal of Medicine* 294:1262–1267, 1976.
4. Weiss NS, Szekely DR, Austin DF: Increasing Incidence of Endometrial Cancer in the United States, *New England Journal of Medicine* 294:1259–1262, 1976.
5. Herbst AL, Ulfelder H, Poskanzer DC: Adenocarcinoma of Vagina, *New England Journal of Medicine* 284:878–881, 1971.
6. Greenwald P, Barlow J, Nasca P, Burnett W: Vaginal Cancer After Maternal Treatment with Synthetic Estrogens, *New England Journal of Medicine* 285:390–392, 1971.
7. Lanier A, Noller K, Decker D, et al: Cancer and Stilbestrol. A Follow-up of 1719 Persons Exposed to Estrogens in Utero and Born 1943–1959, *Mayo Clinic Proceedings* 48:793–799, 1973.
8. Herbst A, Kurman R, Scully R: Vaginal and Cervical Abnormalities After Exposure to Stilbestrol In Utero, *Obstetrics and Gynecology* 40:287–298, 1972.
9. Herbst A, Robboy S, Macdonald G, Scully R: The Effects of Local Progesterone on Stilbestrol-Associated Vaginal Adenosis, *American Journal of Obstetrics and Gynecology* 118:607–615, 1974.
10. Herbst A, Poskanzer D, Robboy S, et al: Prenatal Exposure to Stilbestrol, A Prospective Comparison of Exposed Female Offspring with Unexposed Controls, *New England Journal of Medicine* 292:334–339, 1975.
11. Stafl A, Mattingly R, Foley D, Fetherston W: Clinical Diagnosis of Vaginal Adenosis, *Obstetrics and Gynecology* 43:118–128, 1974.
12. Sherman AI, Goldrath M, Berlin A, et al: Cervical-Vaginal Adenosis After *In Utero* Exposure to Synthetic Estrogens, *Obstetrics and Gynecology* 44:531–545, 1974.
13. Gal I, Kirman B, Stern J: Hormone Pregnancy Tests and Congenital Malformation, *Nature* 216:83, 1967.
14. Levy EP, Cohen A, Fraser FC: Hormone Treatment During Pregnancy and Congenital Heart Defects, *Lancet* 1:611, 1973.
15. Nora J, Nora A: Birth Defects and Oral Contraceptives, *Lancet* 1:941–942, 1973.
16. Janerich DT, Piper JM, Glebatis, DM: Oral Contraceptives and Congenital Limb-Reduction Defects, *New England Journal of Medicine* 291:697–700, 1974.
17. Estrogens for Oral or Parenteral Use, *Federal Register* 40:8212, 1975.
18. Boston Collaborative Drug Surveillance Program: Surgically Confirmed Gall Bladder Disease, Venous Thromboembolism and Breast Tumors in Relations to Post-Menopausal Estrogen Therapy, *New England Journal of Medicine* 290:15–19, 1974.

18a. Hoover R, Gray LA Sr, Cole P, MacMahon B: Menopausal Estrogens and Breast Cancer, *New England Journal of Medicine* 295:401–405, 1976.

19. Boston Collaborative Drug Surveillance Program: Oral Contraceptives and Venous Thromboembolic Disease, Surgically Confirmed Gall Bladder Disease, and Breast Tumors, *Lancet* 1:1399–1404, 1973.
20. Daniel DG, Campbell H, Turnbull AC: Puerperal Thromboembolism and Suppression of Lactation, *Lancet* 2:287–289, 1967.
21. The Veterans Administration Cooperative Urological Research Group: Carcinoma of the Prostate: Treatment Comparisons, *Journal of Urology* 98:516–522, 1967.
22. Bailar JC: Thromboembolism and Oestrogen Therapy, *Lancet* 2:560, 1967.
23. Blackard C, Doe R, Mellinger G, Byar D: Incidence of Cardiovascular Disease and Death in Patients Receiving Diethylstilbestrol for Carcinoma of the Prostate, *Cancer* 26:249–256, 1970.
24. Royal College of General Practitioners: Oral Contraception and Thromboembolic Disease, *Journal of the Royal College of General Practitioners* 13:267–279, 1967.
25. Inman WHW, Vessey MP: Investigation of Deaths from Pulmonary, Coronary and Cerebral Thrombosis and Embolism in Women of Child-Bearing Age, *British Medical Journal* 2:193–199, 1968.
26. Vessey MP, Doll R: Investigation of Relation Between Use of Oral Contraceptives and Thromboembolic Disease. A Further Report, *British Medical Journal* 2:651–657, 1969.
27. Sartwell PE, Masi AT, Arthes FG, et al: Thromboembolism and Oral Contraceptives: An Epidemiological Case Control Study, *American Journal of Epidemiology* 90: 365–380, 1969.
28. Collaborative Group for the Study of Stroke in Young Women: Oral Contraception and Increased Risk of Cerebral Ischemia or Thrombosis, *New England Journal of Medicine* 288:871–878, 1973.
29. Collaborative Group for the Study of Stroke in Young Women: Oral Contraceptives and Stroke in Young Women: Associated Risk Factors, *Journal of the American Medical Association* 231:718–722, 1975.
30. Mann JI, Inman WHW: Oral Contraceptives and Death from Myocardial Infarction, *British Medical Journal* 2:245–248, 1975.
31. Mann JI, Vessey MP, Thorogood M, Doll R: Myocardial Infarction in Young Women with Special Reference to Oral Contraceptive Practice, *British Medical Journal* 2:241–245, 1975.
32. Inman WHW, Vessey VP, Westerholm B, Engelund A: Thromboembolic Disease and the Steroidal Content of Oral Contraceptives, *British Medical Journal* 2:203–209, 1970.
33. Stolley PD, Tonascia JA, Tockman MS, et al: Thrombosis with Low-Estrogen Oral Contraceptives, *American Journal of Epidemiology* 102:197–208, 1975.
34. Vessey MP, Doll R, Fairbairn AS, Glober G: Post-Operative Thromboembolism and the Use of the Oral Contraceptives, *British Medical Journal* 3:123–126, 1970.
35. Greene GR, Sartwell PE: Oral Contraceptive Use in Patients with Thromboembolism Following Surgery, Trauma or Infection, *American Journal of Public Health* 62:680–685, 1972.
36. Rosenberg L, Armstrong MB, Jick H: Myocardial Infarction and Estrogen Therapy in Postmenopausal Women, *New England Journal of Medicine* 294:1256–1259, 1976.
37. Coronary Drug Project Research Group: The Coronary Drug Project: Initial Findings Leading to Modification of Its Research Protocol, *Journal of the American Medical Association* 214:1303–1313, 1970.
38. Baum J, Holtz F, Bookstein JJ, Klein EW: Possible Association Between Benign Hepatomas and Oral Contraceptives, *Lancet* 2:926–928, 1973.
39. Mays ET, Christopherson WM, Mahr MM, Williams HC: Hepatic Changes in Young Women Ingesting Contraceptive Steroids, Hepatic Hemorrhage and Primary Hepatic Tumors, *Journal of the American Medical Association* 235:730–782, 1976.
40. Edmondson HA, Henderson B, Benton B: Liver Cell Adenomas Associated with the Use of Oral Contraceptives, *New England Journal of Medicine* 294:470–472, 1976.
41. Pfeffer RI, Van Den Noort S: Estrogen Use and Stroke Risk in Postmenopausal Women, *American Journal of Epidemiology* 103:445–456, 1976.

PATIENT INFORMATION

WHAT YOU SHOULD KNOW ABOUT ESTROGENS

Estrogens are female hormones produced by the ovaries. The ovaries make several different kinds of estrogens. In addition, scientists have been able to make a variety of synthetic estrogens. As far as we know, all these estrogens have similar properties and therefore much the same usefulness, side effects, and risks. This leaflet is intended to help you understand what estrogens are used for the risks involved in their use, and how to use them as safely as possible.

This leaflet includes the most important information about estrogens, but not all the information. If you want to know more, you can ask your doctor or pharmacist to let you read the package inserted prepared for the doctor.

USES OF ESTROGEN

Estrogens are prescribed by doctors for a number of purposes, including:

1. To provide estrogen during a period of adjustment when a woman's ovaries no longer produce it, in order to prevent certain uncomfortable symptoms of estrogen deficiency. (All women normally stop producing estrogens, generally between the ages of 45 and 55; this is called the menopause.)
2. To prevent symptoms of estrogen deficiency when a woman's ovaries have been removed surgically before the natural menopause.
3. To prevent pregnancy. (Estrogens are given along with a progestagen, another female hormone; these combinations are called oral contraceptives or birth control pills. Patient labeling is available to women taking oral contraceptives, and they will not be discussed in this leaflet.)
4. To treat certain cancers in women and men.

THERE IS NO PROPER USE OF ESTROGENS IN A PREGNANT WOMAN.

ESTROGENS IN THE MENOPAUSE

In the natural course of their lives, all women eventually experience a decrease in estrogen production. This usually occurs between ages 45 and 55, but may occur earlier or later. Sometimes the ovaries may need to be removed before natural menopause by an operation, producing a "surgical menopause." When the amount of estrogen in the blood begins to decrease, many women may develop typical symptoms: Feelings of warmth in the face, neck, and chest or sudden intense episodes of heat and sweating throughout the body (called "hot flashes" or "hot flushes"). These symptoms are sometimes very uncomfortable. A few women eventually develop changes in the vagina (called "atrophic vaginitis") which cause discomfort, especially during and after intercourse.

Estrogens can be prescribed to treat these symptoms of the menopause. It is estimated that considerably more than

Continued on next page

Menest—Cont.

half of all women undergoing the menopause have only mild symptoms or no symptoms at all and therefore do not need estrogens. Other women may need estrogens for a few months, while their bodies adjust to lower estrogen levels. Sometimes the need will be for periods longer than 6 months. In an attempt to avoid overstimulation of the uterus (womb), estrogens are usually given cyclically during each month of use, that is 3 weeks of pills followed by 1 week without pills.

Sometimes women experience nervous symptoms or depression during menopause. There is no evidence that estrogens are effective for such symptoms and they should not be used to treat them, although other treatments may be needed.

You may have heard that taking estrogens for long periods (years) after menopause will keep your skin soft and supple and keep you feeling young. There is no evidence that this is so, however, and such long-term treatment carries important risks.

THE DANGERS OF ESTROGENS

1. *Cancer of the uterus.* If estrogens are used in the postmenopausal period for more than a year, there is an increased risk of *endometrial cancer* (cancer of the uterus). Women taking estrogens have roughly 5 to 10 times as great a chance of getting this cancer as women who take no estrogens. To put this another way, while a postmenopausal woman not taking estrogens has 1 chance in 1,000 each year of getting cancer of the uterus, a woman taking estrogens has 5 to 10 chances in 1,000 each year. For this reason *it is important to take estrogens only when you really need them.*
   The risk of this cancer is greater the longer estrogens are used and also seems to be greater when larger doses are taken. For this reason *it is important to take the lowest dose of estrogen that will control symptoms and to take it only as long as it is needed.* If estrogens are needed for longer periods of time, your doctor will want to re-evaluate your need for estrogens at least every 6 months.
   Women using estrogens should report any irregular vaginal bleeding to their doctors; such bleeding may be of no importance, but it can be an early warning of cancer of the uterus. If you have undiagnosed vaginal bleeding, you should not use estrogens until a diagnosis is made and you are certain there is no cancer of the uterus. If you have had your uterus completely removed (total hysterectomy) there is no danger of developing cancer of the uterus.
2. *Other possible cancers.* Estrogens can cause development of other tumors in animals, such as tumors of the breast, cervix, vagina, or liver, when given for a long time. At present there is no good evidence that women using estrogen in the menopause have an increased risk of such tumors, but there is no way yet to be sure they do not; and one study raises the possibility that use of estrogens in the menopause may increase risk of breast cancer many years later. This is a further reason to use estrogens only when clearly needed. While you are taking estrogens, it is important that you go to your doctor at least once a year for a physical examination. Also, if members of your family have had breast cancer or if you have breast nodules or abnormal mammograms (breast x-rays), your doctor may wish to carry out more frequent examinations of your breasts.
3. *Gall bladder disease.* Women who use estrogens after menopause are more likely to develop gall bladder disease needing surgery than women who do not use estrogens. Birth control pills have a similar effect.
4. *Abnormal blood clotting.* Oral contraceptives increase the risk of blood clotting in various parts of the body. This can result in a stroke (if the clot is in the brain), a heart attack (clot in a blood vessel of the heart), or a pulmonary embolus (a clot which forms in the legs or pelvis, then breaks off and travels to the lungs). Any of these can be fatal.
   At this time use of estrogens in the menopause is not known to cause such blood clotting, but this has not been fully studied and there could still prove to be such a risk. It is recommended that if you have had clotting in the legs or lungs or a heart attack or stroke while you were using estrogens or birth control pills, you should not use estrogens (unless they are being used to treat cancer of the breast or prostate). If you have had a stroke or heart attack or if you have angina pectoris, estrogens should be used with great caution and only if clearly needed (for example, if you have severe symptoms of the menopause).

SPECIAL WARNING ABOUT PREGNANCY

You should not receive estrogen if you are pregnant. If this should occur there is a greater than usual chance that the developing child will be born with a birth defect, although the possibility remains fairly small. A female child may have an increased risk of developing cancer of the vagina or cervix later in life (in the teens or twenties). Every possible effort should be made to avoid exposure to estrogens during pregnancy. If exposure occurs, see your doctor.

OTHER EFFECTS OF ESTROGENS

In addition to the serious known risks of estrogens described above, estrogens have the following side effects and potential risks:

1. *Nausea and vomiting.* The most common side effect of estrogen therapy is nausea. Vomiting is less common.
2. *Effects on breasts.* Estrogens may cause breast tenderness or enlargement and may cause the breasts to secrete a liquid. These effects are not dangerous.
3. *Effects on the uterus.* Estrogens may cause benign fibroid tumors of the uterus to get larger. Some women will have menstrual bleeding when estrogens are stopped. But if the bleeding occurs on days you are still taking estrogens you should report this to your doctor.
4. *Effects on liver.* Women taking oral contraceptives develop on rare occasions a tumor of the liver which can rupture and bleed into the abdomen. So far, these tumors have not been reported in women using estrogens in the menopause, but you should report any swelling or unusual pain or tenderness in the abdomen to your doctor immediately.
   Women with a past history of jaundice (yellowing of the skin and white parts of the eyes) may get jaundice again during estrogen use. If this occurs, stop taking estrogen and see your doctor.
5. *Other effects.* Estrogens may cause excess fluid to be retained in the body. This may make some conditions worse, such as epilepsy, migraine, heart disease, or kidney disease.

SUMMARY

Estrogens have important uses, but they have serious risks as well. You must decide, with your doctor, whether the risks are acceptable to you in view of the benefits of treatment. Except where your doctor has prescribed estrogens for use in special cases of cancer of the breast or prostate, you should not use estrogens if you have cancer of the breast or uterus, are pregnant, have undiagnosed abnormal vaginal bleeding, clotting in the legs or lungs, or have had a stroke, heart attack or angina, or clotting in the legs or lungs in the past while you were taking estrogens. You can use estrogens as safely as possible by understanding that your doctor will require regular physical examinations while you are taking them and will try to discontinue the drug as soon as possible and use the smallest dose possible. Be alert for signs of trouble including:

1. Abnormal bleeding from the vagina.
2. Pains in the calves or chest or sudden shortness of breath, or coughing blood (indicating possible clots in the legs, heart, or lungs).
3. Severe headache, dizziness, faintness, or changes in vision (indicating possible developing clots in the brain or eye).
4. Breast lumps (you should ask your doctor how to examine your own breasts).
5. Jaundice (yellowing of the skin).
6. Mental depression.

Based on his or her assessment of your medical needs, your doctor has prescribed this drug for you. Do not give the drug to anyone else.

Rx only.

Distributed by: Monarch Pharmaceuticals, Inc., Bristol, TN 37620

Manufactured by: King Pharmaceuticals, Inc., Bristol, TN 37620

0934041
Rev. 7/99

Shown in Product Identification Guide, page 324

NEOSPORIN® G.U. Irrigant Sterile ℞

[*nē "ō-spor 'in*]

(neomycin sulfate-polymyxin B sulfate solution for irrigation)

NOT FOR INJECTION

DESCRIPTION

NEOSPORIN G.U. Irrigant is a concentrated sterile antibiotic solution to be diluted for urinary bladder irrigation. Each mL contains neomycin sulfate equivalent to 40 mg neomycin base, 200,000 units polymyxin B sulfate, and Water for Injection. The 20-mL multiple-dose vial contains, in addition to the above, 1 mg methylparaben (0.1%) added as a preservative.

Neomycin sulfate, an antibiotic of the aminoglycoside group, is the sulfate salt of neomycin B and C produced by *Streptomyces fradiae.* It has a potency equivalent to not less than 600 μg of neomycin per mg. The structural formulae are:

Neomycin B (R_1=H, R_2=CH_2NH_2)
Neomycin C (R_1=CH_2NH_2, R_2=H)

Polymyxin B sulfate, a polypeptide antibiotic, is the sulfate salt of polymyxin B_1 and B_2 produced by the growth of *Bacillus polymyxa.* It has a potency of not less than 6,000 polymyxin B units per mg. The structural formulae are:

Polymyxin B_1 (R=CH_3)
Polymyxin B_2 (R=H)
DAB=α,γ-diaminobutyric acid

CLINICAL PHARMACOLOGY

After prophylactic irrigation of the intact urinary bladder, neomycin and polymyxin B are absorbed in clinically insignificant quantities. A neomycin serum level of 0.1 μg/mL was observed in three of 33 patients receiving the rinse solution. This level is well below that which has been associated with neomycin-induced toxicity.

When used topically, polymyxin B sulfate and neomycin are rarely irritating.

Microbiology: The prepared NEOSPORIN G.U. Irrigant Sterile solution is bactericidal. The aminoglycosides act by inhibiting normal protein synthesis in susceptible microorganisms. Polymyxins increase the permeability of bacterial cell wall membranes. The solution is active in vitro against

Escherichia coli
Staphylococcus aureus
Haemophilus influenzae
Klebsiella and *Enterobacter* species
Neisseria species, and
Pseudomonas aeruginosa.

It is not active in vitro against *Serratia marcescens* and streptococci.

Bacterial resistance may develop following the use of the antibiotics in the catheter-rinse solution.

INDICATIONS AND USAGE

NEOSPORIN G.U. Irrigant is indicated for short-term use (up to 10 days) as a continuous irrigant or rinse in the urinary bladder of abacteriuric patients to help prevent bacteriuria and gram-negative rod septicemia associated with the use of indwelling catheters.

Since organisms gain entrance to the bladder by way of, through, and around the catheter, significant bacteriuria is induced by bacterial multiplication in the bladder urine, in the mucoid film often present between catheter and urethra, and in other sites. Urinary tract infection may result from the repeated presence in the urine of large numbers of pathogenic bacteria. The use of closed systems with indwelling catheters has been shown to reduce the risk of infection. A three-way closed catheter system with constant neomycin-polymyxin B bladder rinse is indicated to prevent the development of infection while using indwelling catheters. If uropathogens are isolated, they should be identified and tested for susceptibility so that appropriate antimicrobial therapy for systemic use can be initiated.

CONTRAINDICATIONS

Hypersensitivity to neomycin, the polymyxins, or any ingredient in the solution is a contraindication to its use. A history of hypersensitivity or serious toxic reaction to an aminoglycoside may also contraindicate the use of any other aminoglycoside because of the known cross-sensitivity of patients to drugs of this class.

WARNINGS

PROPHYLACTIC BLADDER CARE WITH NEOSPORIN G.U. IRRIGANT STERILE SHOULD NOT BE GIVEN WHERE THERE IS A POSSIBILITY OF SYSTEMIC ABSORPTION. NEOSPORIN G.U. IRRIGANT STERILE SHOULD NOT BE USED FOR IRRIGATION OTHER THAN FOR THE URINARY BLADDER. Systemic absorption after topical application of neomycin to open wounds, burns, and granulating surfaces is significant and serum concentrations comparable to and often higher than those attained following oral and parenteral therapy have been reported. Absorption of neomycin from the denuded bladder surface has been reported.

However, the likelihood of toxicity following topical irrigation of the intact urinary bladder with NEOSPORIN G.U. Irrigant Sterile is low since no appreciable amounts of these antibiotics enter the systemic circulation by this route if irrigation does not exceed 10 days.

NEOSPORIN G.U. Irrigant is intended for continuous prophylactic irrigation of the lumen of the intact urinary bladder of patients with indwelling catheters. Patients should be under constant supervision by a physician. Irrigation should be avoided in patients with defects in the bladder mucosa or bladder wall, such as vesical rupture, or in association with operative procedures on the bladder wall, because of the risk of toxicity due to systemic absorption following diffusion into absorptive tissues and spaces. When absorbed, neomycin and polymyxin B are nephrotoxic antibiotics, and the nephrotoxic potentials are additive. In addition, both antibiotics, when absorbed, are neurotoxins: neomycin can destroy fibers of the acoustic nerve causing permanent bilateral deafness; neomycin and polymyxin B are additive in their neuromuscular blocking effects, not only in terms of potency and duration, but also in terms of characteristics of the blocks produced.

Aminoglycosides, when absorbed, can cause fetal harm when administered to a pregnant woman. Aminoglycoside antibiotics cross the placenta and there have been several reports of total, irreversible, bilateral, congenital deafness in children whose mothers received streptomycin during pregnancy. Although serious side effects have not been reported in the treatment of pregnant women with other aminoglycosides, the potential for harm exists. If NEOSPORIN G.U. Irrigant Sterile is used during pregnancy, the patient should be apprised of the potential hazard to the fetus (see PRECAUTIONS).

PRECAUTIONS

General: Ototoxicity, nephrotoxicity, and neuromuscular blockade may occur if NEOSPORIN G.U. Irrigant ingredients are systemically absorbed (see WARNINGS). Absorption of neomycin from the denuded bladder surface has been reported. Patients with impaired renal function, infants, dehydrated patients, elderly patients, and patients receiving high doses of prolonged treatment are especially at risk for the development of toxicity.

Irrigation of the bladder with NEOSPORIN G.U. Irrigant may result in overgrowth of nonsusceptible organisms, including fungi. Appropriate measures should be taken if this occurs. The safety and effectiveness of the preparation for use in the care of patients with recent lower urinary tract surgery have not been established.

Urine specimens should be collected during prophylactic bladder care for urinalysis, culture, and susceptibility testing. Positive cultures suggest the presence of organisms which are resistant to the bladder rinse antibiotics.

Pregnancy: *Teratogenic Effects:* Pregnancy Category D. See WARNINGS section.

Pediatric Use: Safety and effectiveness in pediatric patients have not been established.

ADVERSE REACTIONS

Neomycin occasionally causes skin sensitization when applied topically; however, topical application to mucus membranes rarely results in local or systemic hypersensitivity reactions.

Irritation of the urinary bladder mucosa has been reported. Signs of ototoxicity and nephrotoxicity have been reported following parenteral use of these drugs and following the oral and topical use of neomycin (see WARNINGS).

DOSAGE AND ADMINISTRATION

This preparation is specifically designed for use with "three-way" catheters or with other catheter systems permitting **continuous** irrigation of the urinary bladder. The usual irrigation dose is one 1-mL ampul a day for up to 10 days.

Using strict aseptic techniques, the contents of one 1-mL ampul of NEOSPORIN G.U. Irrigant Sterile (neomycin sulfate-polymyxin B sulfate solution for irrigation) should be added to a 1,000-mL container of isotonic saline solution. This container should then be connected to the inflow lumen of the "three-way" catheter which has been inserted with full aseptic precautions; use of a sterile lubricant is recommended during insertion of the catheter. The outflow lumen should be connected, via a sterile disposable plastic tube, to a disposable plastic collection bag. Stringent procedures, such as taping the inflow and outflow junction at the catheter, should be observed when necessary to insure the junctional integrity of the system.

For most patients, the inflow rate of the 1,000-mL saline solution of neomycin and polymyxin B should be adjusted to a slow drip to deliver about 1,000 mL every 24 hours. If the patient's urine output exceeds 2 liters per day, it is recommended that the inflow rate be adjusted to deliver 2,000 mL of the solution in a 24-hour period.

It is important that the rinse of the bladder be **continuous**; the inflow or rinse solution should not be interrupted for more than a few minutes.

Preparation of the irrigation solution should be performed with strict aseptic techniques. The prepared solution should be stored at 4°C, and should be used within 48 hours following preparation to reduce the risk of contamination with resistant microorganisms.

HOW SUPPLIED

1-mL ampuls, boxes of 10 (NDC 61570-047-10) and 50 ampuls (NDC 61570-047-50); 20-mL multi-dose vial (NDC 61570-048-20).

Store at 2° to 8°C (36° to 46°F).

Distributed by: Monarch Pharmaceuticals, Inc., Bristol, TN 37620

Shown in Product Identification Guide, page 325

NEOSPORIN® ℞

[*nē "ō-spor 'ĭn*]

Ophthalmic Ointment Sterile
(neomycin and polymyxin B sulfates and bacitracin zinc ophthalmic ointment, USP)

DESCRIPTION

NEOSPORIN OPHTHALMIC OINTMENT (neomycin and polymyxin B sulfates and bacitracin zinc ophthalmic ointment) is a sterile antimicrobial ointment for ophthalmic use. Each gram contains: neomycin sulfate equivalent to 3.5 mg neomycin base, polymyxin B sulfate equivalent to 10,000 polymyxin B units, bacitracin zinc equivalent to 400 bacitracin units, and white petrolatum, q.s.

Neomycin sulfate is the sulfate salt of neomycin B and C, which are produced by the growth of *Streptomyces fradiae* Waksman (Fam. Streptomycetaceae). It has a potency equivalent of not less than 600 µg of neomycin standard per mg, calculated on an anhydrous basis. The structural formulae are:

• x H_2SO_4

Neomycin B (R_1=H, R_2=CH_2NH_2)
Neomycin C (R_1=CH_2NH_2, R_2=H)

Polymyxin B sulfate is the sulfate salt of polymyxin B_1 and B_2, which are produced by the growth of *Bacillus polymyxa* (Prazmowski) Migula (Fam. Bacillaceae). It has a potency of not less than 6,000 polymyxin B units per mg, calculated on an anhydrous basis. The structural formulae are:

Polymyxin B_1 (R=CH_3)
Polymyxin B_2 (R=H)
DAB=α,γ-diaminobutyric acid

Bacitracin zinc is the zinc salt of bacitracin, a mixture of related cyclic polypeptides (mainly bacitracin A) produced by the growth of an organism of the *licheniformis* group of *Bacillus subtilis* var Tracy. It has a potency of not less than 40 bacitracin units per mg. The structural formula is:

CLINICAL PHARMACOLOGY

A wide range of antibacterial action is provided by the overlapping spectra of neomycin, polymyxin B sulfate, and bacitracin.

Neomycin is bactericidal for many gram-positive and gram-negative organisms. It is an aminoglycoside antibiotic which inhibits protein synthesis by binding with ribosomal RNA and causing misreading of the bacterial genetic code.

Polymyxin B is bactericidal for a variety of gram-negative organisms. It increases the permeability of the bacterial cell membrane by interacting with the phospholipid components of the membrane.

Bacitracin is bactericidal for a variety of gram-positive and gram-negative organisms. It interferes with bacterial cell wall synthesis by inhibition of the regeneration of phospholipid receptors involved in peptidoglycan synthesis.

Microbiology: Neomycin sulfate, polymyxin B sulfate, and bacitracin zinc together are considered active against the following microorganisms: *Staphylococcus aureus*, streptococci including *Streptococcus pneumoniae, Escherichia coli, Haemophilus influenzae, Klebsiella/Enterobacter* species, *Neisseria* species, and *Pseudomonas aeruginosa*. The product does not provide adequate coverage against *Serratia marcescens*.

INDICATIONS AND USAGE

Neosporin Ophthalmic Ointment is indicated for the topical treatment of superficial infections of the external eye and its adnexa caused by susceptible bacteria. Such infections encompass conjunctivitis, keratitis and keratoconjunctivitis, blepharitis and blepharoconjunctivitis.

CONTRAINDICATIONS

Neosporin Ophthalmic Ointment is contraindicated in individuals who have shown hypersensitivity to any of its components.

WARNINGS

NOT FOR INJECTION INTO THE EYE. NEOSPORIN OPHTHALMIC OINTMENT should never be directly introduced into the anterior chamber of the eye. Ophthalmic ointments may retard corneal wound healing.

Topical antibiotics, particularly neomycin sulfate, may cause cutaneous sensitization. A precise incidence of hypersensitivity reactions (primarily skin rash) due to topical antibiotics is not known. The manifestations of sensitization to topical antibiotics are usually itching, reddening, and edema of the conjunctiva and eyelid. A sensitization reaction may manifest simply as a failure to heal. During long-term use of topical antibiotic products, periodic examination for such signs is advisable, and the patient should be told to discontinue the product if they are observed. Symptoms usually subside quickly on withdrawing the medication. Application of products containing these ingredients should be avoided for the patient thereafter (see PRECAUTIONS: General).

PRECAUTIONS

General: As with other antibiotic preparations, prolonged use of Neosporin Ophthalmic Ointment may result in overgrowth of nonsusceptible organisms including fungi. If superinfection occurs, appropriate measures should be initiated.

Bacterial resistance to Neosporin Ophthalmic Ointment may also develop. If purulent discharge, inflammation, or pain become aggravated, the patient should discontinue use of the medication and consult a physician.

There have been reports of bacterial keratitis associated with the use of topical ophthalmic products in multiple-dose containers which have been inadvertently contaminated by patients, most of whom had a concurrent corneal disease or a disruption of the ocular epithelial surface (see PRECAUTIONS: Information for Patients).

Allergic cross-reactions may occur which could prevent the use of any or all of the following antibiotics for the treatment of future infections: kanamycin, paromomycin, streptomycin, and possibly gentamicin.

Information for Patients: Patients should be instructed to avoid allowing the tip of the dispensing container to contact the eye, eyelid, fingers, or any other surface. The use of this product by more than one person may spread infection.

Patients should also be instructed that ocular products, if handled improperly, can become contaminated by common bacteria known to cause ocular infections. Serious damage to the eye and subsequent loss of vision may result from using contaminated products (see PRECAUTIONS: General).

If the condition persists or gets worse, or if a rash or allergic reaction develops, the patient should be advised to stop use and consult a physician. Do not use this product if you are allergic to any of the listed ingredients.

Keep tightly closed when not in use. Keep out of reach of children.

Carcinogenesis, Mutagenesis, Impairment of Fertility: Long-term studies in animals to evaluate carcinogenic or mutagenic potential have not been conducted with polymyxin B sulfate or bacitracin. Treatment of cultured human lymphocytes in vitro with neomycin increased the frequency of chromosome aberrations at the highest concentration (80 µg/mL) tested; however, the effects of neomycin on carcinogenesis and mutagenesis in humans are unknown.

Polymyxin B has been reported to impair the motility of equine sperm, but its effects on male or female fertility are unknown. No adverse effects on male or female fertility, litter size or survival were observed in rabbits given bacitracin zinc 100 gm/ton of diet.

Pregnancy: *Teratogenic Effects:* Pregnancy Category C. Animal reproduction studies have not been conducted with neomycin sulfate, polymyxin B sulfate, or bacitracin. It is also not known whether NEOSPORIN® Ophthalmic Ointment can cause fetal harm when administered to a pregnant woman or can affect reproduction capacity. NEOSPORIN OPHTHALMIC OINTMENT should be given to a pregnant woman only if clearly needed.

Nursing Mothers: It is not known whether this drug is excreted in human milk. Because many drugs are excreted in human milk, caution should be exercised when NEOSPORIN OPHTHALMIC OINTMENT is administered to a nursing woman.

Pediatric Use: Safety and effectiveness in pediatric patients have not been established.

ADVERSE REACTIONS

Adverse reactions have occurred with the anti-infective components of NEOSPORIN OPHTHALMIC OINTMENT. The exact incidence is not known. Reactions occurring most often are allergic sensitization reactions including itching, swelling, and conjunctival erythema (see WARNINGS). More serious hypersensivity reactions, including anaphylaxis, have been reported rarely.

Local irritation on instillation has also been reported.

DOSAGE AND ADMINISTRATION

Apply the ointment every 3 or 4 hours for 7 to 10 days, depending on the severity of the infection.

HOW SUPPLIED

Tube of 1/8 oz (3.5 g) with ophthalmic tip (NDC 61570-046-35).

Rx only.

Store at 15° to 25°C (59° to 77°F).

Distributed by: Monarch Pharmaceuticals, Inc., Bristol, TN 37620

Shown in Product Identification Guide, page 325

NEOSPORIN® Ophthalmic Solution Sterile ℞

[*nē "ō-spor 'ĭn*]

(neomycin and polymyxin B sulfates and gramicidin ophthalmic solution, USP)

DESCRIPTION

NEOSPORIN Ophthalmic Solution (neomycin and polymyxin B sulfates and gramicidin ophthalmic solution) is a

Continued on next page

Neosporin Ophthalmic Sol.—Cont.

sterile antimicrobial solution for ophthalmic use. Each mL contains: neomycin sulfate equivalent to 1.75 mg neomycin base, polymyxin B sulfate equivalent to 10,000 polymyxin B units, and gramicidin 0.025 mg. The vehicle contains alcohol 0.5%, thimerosal 0.001% (added as a preservative), and the inactive ingredients propylene glycol, polyoxyethy lene polyoxypropylene compound, sodium chloride, and Water for Injection.
Neomycin sulfate is the sulfate salt of neomycin B and C, which are produced by the growth of *Streptomyces fradiae* Waksman (Fam. Streptomycetaceae). It has a potency equivalent of not less than 600 mg of neomycin standard per mg, calculated on an anhydrous basis. The structural formulae are:

• x H_2SO_4

Neomycin B (R_1=H, R_2=CH_2NH_2)
Neomycin C (R_1=CH_2NH_2, R_2=H)

Polymyxin B sulfate is the sulfate salt of polymyxin B_1 and B_2 which are produced by the growth of *Bacillus polymyxa* (Prazmowski) Migula (Fam. Bacillaceae). It has a potency of not less than 6,000 polymyxin B units per mg, calculated on an anhydrous basis. The structural formulae are:

Polymyxin B_1 (R=CH_3)
Polymyxin B_2 (R=H)
DAB=α,γ-diaminobutyric acid

Gramicidin (also called Gramicidin D) is a mixture of three pairs of antibacterial substances (Gramicidin A, B, and C) produced by the growth of *Bacillus brevis* Dubos (Fam. Bacillaceae). It has a potency of not less than 900 μg of standard gramicidin per mg. The structural formulae are:

Gramicidin D

HC-X-Gly-Ala-D-Leu-Ala-D-Val-Val-D-Val-Trp-D-Leu-Y-D-Leu-Trp-D-Leu-Trp-$NHCH_2CH_2OH$

	X	Y
Valine-gramicidin A	Val	Trp
Isoleucine-gramicidin A	Ile	Trp
Valine-gramicidin B	Val	Phe
Isoleucine-gramicidin B	Ile	Phe
Valine-gramicidin C	Val	Tyr
Isoleucine-gramicidin C	Ile	Tyr

CLINICAL PHARMACOLOGY

A wide range of antibacterial action is provided by the overlapping spectra of neomycin, polymyxin B sulfate, and gramicidin.
Neomycin is bactericidal for many gram-positive and gram-negative organisms. It is an aminoglycoside antibiotic which inhibits protein synthesis by binding with ribosomal RNA and causing misreading of the bacterial genetic code.
Polymyxin B is bactericidal for a variety of gram-negative organisms. It increases the permeability of the bacterial cell membrane by interacting with the phospholipid components of the membrane.
Gramicidin is bactericidal for a variety of gram-positive organisms. It increases the permeability of the bacterial cell membrane to inorganic cations by forming a network of channels through the normal lipid bilayer of the membrane.
Microbiology: Neomycin sulfate, polymyxin B sulfate, and gramicidin together are considered active against the following microorganisms: *Staphylococcus aureus*, streptococci, including *Streptococcus pneumoniae*, *Escherichia coli*, *Haemophilus influenzae*, *Klebsiella / Enterobacter* species, *Neisseria species*, and *Pseudomonas aeruginosa*. The product does not provide adequate coverage against *Serratia marcescens*.

INDICATIONS AND USAGE

NEOSPORIN Ophthalmic Solution is indicated for the topical treatment of superficial infections of the external eye and its adnexa caused by susceptible bacteria. Such infections encompass conjunctivitis, keratitis and keratoconjunctivitis, blepharitis and blepharoconjunctivitis.

CONTRAINDICATIONS

NEOSPORIN Ophthalmic Solution is contraindicated in individuals who have shown hypersensitivity to any of its components.

WARNINGS

NOT FOR INJECTION INTO THE EYE. NEOSPORIN Ophthalmic Solution should never be directly introduced into the anterior chamber of the eye or injected subconjunctivally.
Topical antibiotics, particularly neomycin sulfate, may cause cutaneous sensitization. A precise incidence of hypersensitivity reactions (primarily skin rash) due to topical antibiotics is not known. The manifestations of sensitization to topical antibiotics are usually itching, reddening, and edema of the conjunctiva and eyelid. A sensitization reaction may manifest simply as a failure to heal. During long-term use of topical antibiotic products, periodic examination for such signs is advisable, and the patient should be told to discontinue the product if they are observed. Symptoms usually subside quickly on withdrawing the medication. Application of products containing these ingredients should be avoided for the patient thereafter (see PRECAUTIONS: General).

PRECAUTIONS

General: As with other antibiotic preparations, prolonged use of NEOSPORIN Ophthalmic Solution may result in overgrowth of nonsusceptible organisms including fungi. If superinfection occurs, appropriate measures should be initiated.
Bacterial resistance to NEOSPORIN Ophthalmic Solution may also develop. If purulent discharge, inflammation, or pain becomes aggravated, the patient should discontinue use of the medication and consult a physician.
There have been reports of bacterial keratitis associated with the use of topical ophthalmic products in multiple-dose containers which have been inadvertently contaminated by patients, most of whom had a concurrent corneal disease or a disruption of the ocular epithelial surface (see PRECAUTIONS: Information for Patients).
Allergic cross-reactions may occur which could prevent the use of any or all of the following antibiotics for the treatment of future infections: kanamycin, paromomycin, streptomycin, and possibly gentamicin.
Information for Patients: Patients should be instructed to avoid allowing the tip of the dispensing container to contact the eye, eyelid, fingers, or any other surface. The use of this product by more than one person may spread infection.
Patients should also be instructed that ocular products, if handled improperly, can become contaminated by common bacteria known to cause ocular infections. Serious damage to the eye and subsequent loss of vision may result from using contaminated products (see PRECAUTIONS: General).
If the condition persists or gets worse, or if a rash or other allergic reaction develops, the patient should be advised to stop use and consult a physician. Do not use this product if you are allergic to any of the listed ingredients.
Keep tightly closed when not in use. Keep out of reach of children.
Carcinogenesis, Mutagenesis, Impairment of Fertility: Long-term studies in animals to evaluate carcinogenic or mutagenic potential have not been conducted with polymyxin B sulfate or gramicidin. Treatment of cultured human lymphocytes in vitro with neomycin increased the frequency of chromosome aberrations at the highest concentration (80 μg/mL) tested. However, the effects of neomycin on carcinogenesis and mutagenesis in humans are unknown.
Polymyxin B has been reported to impair the motility of equine sperm, but its effects on male or female fertility are unknown.
Pregnancy: ***Teratogenic Effects:*** Pregnancy Category C. Animal reproduction studies have not been conducted with neomycin sulfate, polymyxin B sulfate, or gramicidin. It is also not known whether NEOSPORIN Ophthalmic Solution can cause fetal harm when administered to a pregnant woman or can affect reproduction capacity. NEOSPORIN Ophthalmic Solution should be given to a pregnant woman only if clearly needed.
Nursing Mothers: It is not known whether this drug is excreted in human milk. Because many drugs are excreted in human milk, caution should be exercised when NEOSPORIN Ophthalmic Solution is administered to a nursing woman.
Pediatric Use: Safety and effectiveness in pediatric patients have not been established.

ADVERSE REACTIONS

Adverse reactions have occurred with the anti-infective components of NEOSPORIN Ophthalmic Solution. The exact incidence is not known. Reactions occurring most often are allergic sensitization reactions including itching, swelling, and conjunctival erythema (see WARNINGS). More serious hypersensitivity reactions, including anaphylaxis, have been reported rarely.
Local irritation on instillation has also been reported.

DOSAGE AND ADMINISTRATION

Instill one or two drops into the affected eye every 4 hours for 7 to 10 days. In severe infections, dosage may be increased to as much as two drops every hour.

HOW SUPPLIED

Drop Dose® of 10 mL (plastic dispenser bottle) (NDC 61570-045-10).
Caution: Federal law prohibits dispensing without prescription.
Store at 15° to 25°C (59° to 77°F) and protect from light.

Manufactured for: Monarch Pharmaceuticals, Inc., Bristol, TN 37620

Shown in Product Identification Guide, page 325

NORDETTE®–21 ℞

[*nŏr-dĕt* '-*21*]
TABLETS
(levonorgestrel and ethinyl estradiol tablets)

Patients should be counseled that this product does not protect against HIV infection (AIDS) and other sexually transmitted diseases.

DESCRIPTION

ORAL CONTRACEPTIVE
Each Nordette tablet contains 0.15 mg of levonorgestrel (d(-)-13 beta-ethyl-17-alpha-ethinyl-17-beta-hydroxygon-4-en-3-one), a totally synthetic progestogen, and 0.03 mg of ethinyl estradiol (19-nor-17α-pregna-1,3,5 (10)-trien-20-yne-3,17-diol). The inactive ingredients present are cellulose, FD&C Yellow 6, lactose, magnesium stearate, and polacrilin potassium.

CLINICAL PHARMACOLOGY

Combination oral contraceptives act by suppression of gonadotropins. Although the primary mechanism of this action is inhibition of ovulation, other alterations include changes in the cervical mucus (which increase the difficulty of sperm entry into the uterus) and the endometrium (which reduce the likelihood of implantation).

INDICATIONS AND USAGE

Oral contraceptives are indicated for the prevention of pregnancy in women who elect to use this product as a method of contraception.
Oral contraceptives are highly effective. Table I lists the typical accidental pregnancy rates for users of combination oral contraceptives and other methods of contraception. The efficacy of these contraceptive methods, except sterilization and the IUD, depends upon the reliability with which they are used. Correct and consistent use of methods can result in lower failure rates.

TABLE I: LOWEST EXPECTED AND TYPICAL FAILURE RATES DURING THE FIRST YEAR OF CONTINUOUS USE OF A METHOD
% of Women Experiencing an Accidental Pregnancy in the First Year of Continuous Use

Method	Lowest Expected*	Typical**
(No Contraception)	(85)	(85)
Oral contraceptives		3
combined	0.1	N/A***
progestin only	0.5	N/A***
Diaphragm with spermicidal cream or jelly	6	18
Spermicides alone (foams and vaginal suppositories)	3	21
Vaginal Sponge		
nulliparous	6	18
multiparous	9	28
DEPO-PROVERA® (injectable progestogen)	0.3	0.3
NORPLANT® SYSTEM (implants)	0.2#	0.2#
IUD		3
progesterone	2	N/A***
copper T 380A	0.8	N/A***
Condom without spermicides	2	12
Periodic abstinence (all methods)	1–9	20
Female sterilization	0.2	0.4
Male sterilization	0.1	0.15

Adapted from J. Trussell et al., Table 1, Studies in Family Planning, *21(1)*. Jan.–Feb. 1990.

* The authors' best guess of the percentage of women expected to experience an accidental pregnancy among couples who initiate a method (not necessarily for the first time) and who use it consistently and correctly during the first year if they do not stop use for any other reason.
** This term represents "typical" couples who initiate use of a method (not necessarily for the first time), who experience an accidental pregnancy during the first year if they do not stop use for any other reason.
*** N/A—Data not available
\# This data is based on NORPLANT® SYSTEM clinical trials.

CONTRAINDICATIONS

Oral contraceptives should not be used in women with any of the following conditions:
Thrombophlebitis or thromboembolic disorders.
A past history of deep-vein thrombophlebitis or thromboembolic disorders.
Cerebral-vascular or coronary-artery disease.
Known or suspected carcinoma of the breast.

Carcinoma of the endometrium or other known or suspected estrogen-dependent neoplasia.
Undiagnosed abnormal genital bleeding.
Cholestatic jaundice of pregnancy or jaundice with prior pill use.
Hepatic adenomas or carcinomas.
Known or suspected pregnancy.

WARNINGS

Cigarette smoking increases the risk of serious cardiovascular side effects from oral-contraceptive use. This risk increases with age and with heavy smoking (15 or more cigarettes per day) and is quite marked in women over 35 years of age. Women who use oral contraceptives should be strongly advised not to smoke.

The use of oral contraceptives is associated with increased risks of several serious conditions including myocardial infarction, thromboembolism, stroke, hepatic neoplasia, gallbladder disease, and hypertension, although the risk of serious morbidity or mortality is very small in healthy women without underlying risk factors. The risk of morbidity and mortality increases significantly in the presence of other underlying risk factors such as hypertension, hyperlipidemias, obesity, and diabetes.

Practitioners prescribing oral contraceptives should be familiar with the following information relating to these risks.
The information contained in this package insert is based principally on studies carried out in patients who used oral contraceptives with higher formulations of estrogens and progestogens than those in common use today. The effect of long-term use of the oral contraceptives with lower formulations of both estrogens and progestogens remains to be determined.

Throughout this labeling, epidemiological studies reported are of two types: retrospective or case control studies and prospective or cohort studies. Case control studies provide a measure of the relative risk of disease, namely, a ratio of the incidence of a disease among oral-contraceptive users to that among nonusers. The relative risk does not provide information on the actual clinical occurrence of a disease. Cohort studies provide a measure of attributable risk, which is the difference in the incidence of disease between oral-contraceptive users and nonusers. The attributable risk does provide information about the actual occurrence of a disease in the population. For further information, the reader is referred to a text on epidemiological methods.

1. THROMBOEMBOLIC DISORDERS AND OTHER VASCULAR PROBLEMS

a. *Myocardial infarction*

An increased risk of myocardial infarction has been attributed to oral-contraceptive use. This risk is primarily in smokers or women with other underlying risk factors for coronary-artery disease such as hypertension, hypercholesterolemia, morbid obesity, and diabetes. The relative risk of heart attack for current oral-contraceptive users has been estimated to be two to six. The risk is very low under the age of 30.

Smoking in combination with oral-contraceptive use has been shown to contribute substantially to the incidence of myocardial infarctions in women in their mid-thirties or older with smoking accounting for the majority of excess cases. Mortality rates associated with circulatory disease have been shown to increase substantially in smokers over the age of 35 and nonsmokers over the age of 40 (Table II) among women who use oral contraceptives.
[See Table II at top of next column]

TABLE II. (Adapted from P.M. Layde and V. Beral, Lancet. *1*:541–546, 1981.)

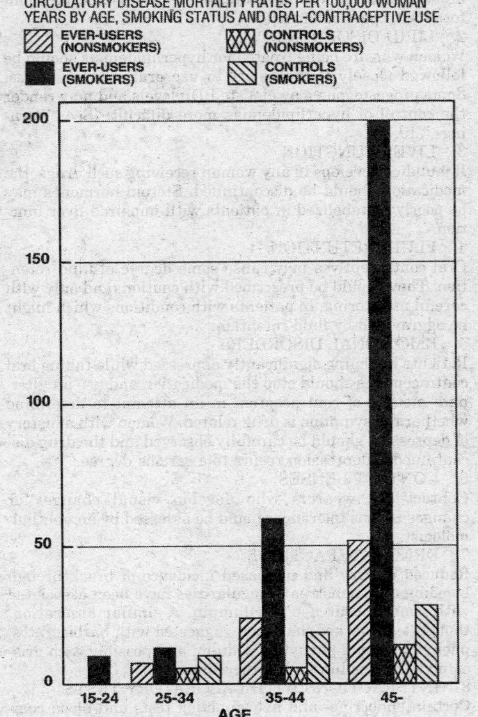

Oral contraceptives may compound the effects of well-known risk factors, such as hypertension, diabetes, hyperlipidemias, age, and obesity. In particular, some progestogens are known to decrease HDL cholesterol and cause glucose intolerance, while estrogens may create a state of hyperinsulinism. Oral contraceptives have been shown to increase blood pressure among users (see section 9 in "Warnings"). Similar effects on risk factors have been associated with an increased risk of heart disease. Oral contraceptives must be used with caution in women with cardiovascular disease risk factors.

b. *Thromboembolism*

An increased risk of thromboembolic and thrombotic disease associated with the use of oral contraceptives is well established. Case control studies have found the relative risk of users compared to nonusers to be 3 for the first episode of superficial venous thrombosis, 4 to 11 for deep-vein thrombosis or pulmonary embolism, and 1.5 to 6 for women with predisposing conditions for venous thromboembolic disease. Cohort studies have shown the relative risk to be somewhat lower, about 3 for new cases and about 4.5 for new cases requiring hospitalization. The risk of thromboembolic disease due to oral contraceptives is not related to length of use and disappears after pill use is stopped.

A two- to four-fold increase in relative risk of postoperative thromboembolic complications has been reported with the use of oral contraceptives. The relative risk of venous thrombosis in women who have predisposing conditions is twice that of women without such medical conditions. If feasible, oral contraceptives should be discontinued at least four weeks prior to and for two weeks after elective surgery of a type associated with an increase in risk of thromboembolism and during and following prolonged immobilization. Since the immediate postpartum period is also associated with an increased risk of thromboembolism, oral contraceptives should be started no earlier than four to six weeks after delivery in women who elect not to breast-feed, or a midtrimester pregnancy termination.

c. *Cerebrovascular diseases*

Oral contraceptives have been shown to increase both the relative and attributable risks of cerebrovascular events (thrombotic and hemorrhagic strokes), although, in general, the risk is greatest among older (>35 years), hypertensive women who also smoke. Hypertension was found to be a risk factor for both users and nonusers, for both types of strokes, while smoking interacted to increase the risk for hemorrhagic strokes.

In a large study, the relative risk of thrombotic strokes has been shown to range from 3 for normotensive users to 14 for users with severe hypertension. The relative risk of hemorrhagic stroke is reported to be 1.2 for nonsmokers who used oral contraceptives, 2.6 for smokers who did not use oral contraceptives, 7.6 for smokers who used oral contraceptives, 1.8 for normotensive users and 25.7 for users with severe hypertension. The attributable risk is also greater in older women.

d. *Dose-related risk of vascular disease from oral contraceptives*

A positive association has been observed between the amount of estrogen and progestogen in oral contraceptives and the risk of vascular disease. A decline in serum high-density lipoproteins (HDL) has been reported with many progestational agents. A decline in serum high-density lipoproteins has been associated with an increased incidence of ischemic heart disease. Because estrogens increase HDL cholesterol, the net effect of an oral contraceptive depends on a balance achieved between doses of estrogen and progestogen and the nature and absolute amount of progestogen used in the contraceptive. The amount of both hormones should be considered in the choice of an oral contraceptive.

Minimizing exposure to estrogen and progestogen is in keeping with good principles of therapeutics. For any particular estrogen/progestogen combination, the dosage regimen prescribed should be one which contains the least amount of estrogen and progestogen that is compatible with a low failure rate and the needs of the individual patient. New acceptors of oral-contraceptive agents should be started on preparations containing less than 50 mcg of estrogen.

e. *Persistence of risk of vascular disease*

There are two studies which have shown persistence of risk of vascular disease for ever-users of oral contraceptives. In a study in the United States, the risk of developing myocardial infarction after discontinuing oral contraceptives persists for at least 9 years for women 40 to 49 years who had used oral contraceptives for five or more years, but this increased risk was not demonstrated in other age groups. In another study in Great Britain, the risk of developing cerebrovascular disease persisted for at least 6 years after discontinuation of oral contraceptives, although excess risk was very small. However, both studies were performed with oral-contraceptive formulations containing 50 micrograms or higher of estrogens.

2. ESTIMATES OF MORTALITY FROM CONTRACEPTIVE USE

One study gathered data from a variety of sources which have estimated the mortality rate associated with different methods of contraception at different ages (Table III). These estimates include the combined risk of death associated with contraceptive methods plus the risk attributable to pregnancy in the event of method failure. Each method of contraception has its specific benefits and risks. The study concluded that with the exception of oral-contraceptive users 35 and older who smoke and 40 and older who do not smoke, mortality associated with all methods of birth control is less than that associated with childbirth. The observation of a possible increase in risk of mortality with age for oral-contraceptive users is based on data gathered in the 1970's—but not reported until 1983. However, current clinical practice involves the use of lower estrogen dose formulations combined with careful restriction of oral-contraceptive use to women who do not have the various risk factors listed in this labeling.

Because of these changes in practice and, also, because of some limited new data which suggest that the risk of cardiovascular disease with the use of oral contraceptives may now be less than previously observed, the Fertility and Maternal Health Drugs Advisory Committee was asked to review the topic in 1989. The Committee concluded that although cardiovascular-disease risks may be increased with oral-contraceptive use after age 40 in healthy nonsmoking women (even with the newer low-dose formulations), there are greater potential health risks associated with pregnancy in older women and with the alternative surgical and medical procedures which may be necessary if such women do not have access to effective and acceptable means of contraception.

Therefore, the Committee recommended that the benefits of oral-contraceptive use by healthy nonsmoking women over 40 may outweigh the possible risks. Of course, older women, as all women who take oral contraceptives, should take the lowest possible dose formulation that is effective.
[See table III above]

TABLE III—ANNUAL NUMBER OF BIRTH-RELATED OR METHOD-RELATED DEATHS ASSOCIATED WITH CONTROL OF FERTILITY PER 100,000 NONSTERILE WOMEN, BY FERTILITY-CONTROL METHOD ACCORDING TO AGE

Method of control and outcome	15–19	20–24	25–29	30–34	35–39	40–44
No fertility-control methods*	7.0	7.4	9.1	14.8	25.7	28.2
Oral contraceptives nonsmoker**	0.3	0.5	0.9	1.9	13.8	31.6
Oral contraceptives smoker**	2.2	3.4	6.6	13.5	51.1	117.2
IUD**	0.8	0.8	1.0	1.0	1.4	1.4
Condom*	1.1	1.6	0.7	0.2	0.3	0.4
Diaphragm/spermicide*	1.9	1.2	1.2	1.3	2.2	2.8
Periodic abstinence*	2.5	1.6	1.6	1.7	2.9	3.6

* Deaths are birth related
** Deaths are method related

Adapted from H.W. Ory, Family Planning Perspectives, *15*:57–63, 1983.

3. CARCINOMA OF THE REPRODUCTIVE ORGANS

Numerous epidemiological studies have been performed on the incidence of breast, endometrial, ovarian, and cervical cancer in women using oral contraceptives. The overwhelming evidence in the literature suggests that the use of oral contraceptives is not associated with an increase in the risk of developing breast cancer, regardless of the age and parity of first use or with most of the marketed brands and doses. The Cancer and Steroid Hormone (CASH) study also showed no latent effect on the risk of breast cancer for at least a decade following long-term use. A few studies have shown a slightly increased relative risk of developing breast cancer, although the methodology of these studies, which included differences in examination of users and nonusers and differences in age at start of use, has been questioned. Some studies suggest that oral-contraceptive use has been associated with an increase in the risk of cervical intraepithelial neoplasia in some populations of women. However, there continues to be controversy about the extent to which such findings may be due to differences in sexual behavior and other factors.

Continued on next page

Nordette-21—Cont.

In spite of many studies of the relationship between oral-contraceptive use and breast and cervical cancers, a cause-and-effect relationship has not been established.
4. HEPATIC NEOPLASIA
Benign hepatic adenomas are associated with oral-contraceptive use, although the incidence of benign tumors is rare in the United States. Indirect calculations have estimated the attributable risk to be in the range of 3.3 cases/100,000 for users, a risk that increases after four or more years of use. Rupture of rare, benign, hepatic adenomas may cause death through intra-abdominal hemorrhage.
Studies from Britain have shown an increased risk of developing hepatocellular carcinoma in long-term (>8 years) oral-contraceptive users. However, these cancers are extremely rare in the U.S. and the attributable risk (the excess incidence) of liver cancers in oral-contraceptive users approaches less than one per million users.
5. OCULAR LESIONS
There have been clincial case reports of retinal thrombosis associated with the use of oral contraceptives. Oral contraceptives should be discontinued if there is unexplained partial or complete loss of vision; onset of proptosis or diplopia; papilledema; or retinal vascular lesions. Appropriate diagnostic and therapeutic measures should be undertaken immediately.
6. ORAL-CONTRACEPTIVE USE BEFORE OR DURING EARLY PREGNANCY
Extensive epidemiological studies have revealed no increased risk of birth defects in women who have used oral contraceptives prior to pregnancy. Studies also do not suggest a teratogenic effect, particularly insofar as cardiac anomalies and limb-reduction defects are concerned, when taken inadvertently during early pregnancy.
The administration of oral contraceptives to induce withdrawal bleeding should not be used as a test for pregnancy. Oral contraceptives should not be used during pregnancy to treat threatened or habitual abortion.
It is recommended that for any patient who has missed two consecutive periods, pregnancy should be ruled out before continuing oral-contraceptive use. If the patient has not adhered to the prescribed schedule, the possibility of pregnancy should be considered at the time of the first missed period. Oral-contraceptive use should be discontinued if pregnancy is confirmed.
7. GALLBLADDER DISEASE
Earlier studies have reported an increased lifetime relative risk of gallbladder surgery in users of oral contraceptives and estrogens. More recent studies, however, have shown that the relative risk of developing gallbladder disease among oral-contraceptive users may be minimal. The recent findings of minimal risk may be related to the use of oral-contraceptive formulations containing lower hormonal doses of estrogens and progestogens.
8. CARBOHYDRATE AND LIPID METABOLIC EFFECTS
Oral contraceptives have been shown to cause glucose intolerance in a significant percentage of users. Oral contraceptives containing greater than 75 micrograms of estrogens cause hyperinsulinism, while lower doses of estrogen cause less glucose intolerance. Progestogens increase insulin secretion and create insulin resistance, this effect varying with different progestational agents. However, in the nondiabetic woman, oral contraceptives appear to have no effect on fasting blood glucose. Because of these demonstrated effects, prediabetic and diabetic women should be carefully observed while taking oral contraceptives.
A small proportion of women will have persistent hypertriglyceridemia while on the pill. As discussed earlier (see "Warnings" 1a and 1d), changes in serum triglycerides and lipoprotein levels have been reported in oral-contraceptive users.
9. ELEVATED BLOOD PRESSURE
An increase in blood pressure has been reported in women taking oral contraceptives, and this increase is more likely in older oral-contraceptive users and with continued use. Data from the Royal College of General Practitioners and subsequent randomized trials have shown that the incidence of hypertension increases with increasing quantities of progestogens.
Women with a history of hypertension or hypertension-related diseases, or renal disease, should be encouraged to use another method of contraception. If women with hypertension elect to use oral contraceptives, they should be monitored closely, and if significant elevation of blood pressure occurs, oral contraceptives should be discontinued. For most women, elevated blood pressure will return to normal after stopping oral contraceptives, and there is no difference in the occurrence of hypertension among ever- and never-users.
10. HEADACHE
The onset or exacerbation of migraine or development of headache with a new pattern that is recurrent, persistent, or severe requires discontinuation of oral contraceptives and evaluation of the cause.
11. BLEEDING IRREGULARITIES
Breakthrough bleeding and spotting are sometimes encountered in patients on oral contraceptives, especially during the first three months of use. The type and dose of progestogen may be important. Nonhormonal causes should be considered and adequate diagnostic measures taken to rule out malignancy or pregnancy in the event of breakthrough bleeding, as in the case of any abnormal vaginal bleeding. If pathology has been excluded, time or a change to another formulation may solve the problem. In the event of amenorrhea, pregnancy should be ruled out.
Some women may encounter post-pill amenorrhea or oligomenorrhea, especially when such a condition was preexistent.

PRECAUTIONS

Patients should be counseled that this product does not protect against HIV infection (AIDS) and other sexually transmitted diseases.
1. PHYSICAL EXAMINATION AND FOLLOW-UP
A periodic history and physical examination is appropriate for all women, including women using oral contraceptives. The physical examination, however, may be deferred until after initiation of oral contraceptives if requested by the woman and judged appropriate by the clinician. The physical examination should include special reference to blood pressure, breasts, abdomen and pelvic organs, including cervical cytology, and relevant laboratory tests. In case of undiagnosed, persistent or recurrent abnormal vaginal bleeding, appropriate measures should be conducted to rule out malignancy. Women with a strong family history of breast cancer or who have breast nodules should be monitored with particular care.
2. LIPID DISORDERS
Women who are being treated for hyperlipidemias should be followed closely if they elect to use oral contraceptives. Some progestogens may elevate LDL levels and may render the control of hyperlipidemias more difficult. (See "Warnings," 1d.)
3. LIVER FUNCTION
If jaundice develops in any woman receiving such drugs, the medication should be discontinued. Steroid hormones may be poorly metabolized in patients with impaired liver function.
4. FLUID RETENTION
Oral contraceptives may cause some degree of fluid retention. They should be prescribed with caution, and only with careful monitoring, in patients with conditions which might be aggravated by fluid retention.
5. EMOTIONAL DISORDERS
Patients becoming significantly depressed while taking oral contraceptives should stop the medication and use an alternate method of contraception in an attempt to determine whether the symptom is drug related. Women with a history of depression should be carefully observed and the drug discontinued if depression recurs to a serious degree.
6. CONTACT LENSES
Contact-lens wearers who develop visual changes or changes in lens tolerance should be assessed by an ophthalmologist.
7. DRUG INTERACTIONS
Reduced efficacy and increased incidence of breakthrough bleeding and menstrual irregularities have been associated with concomitant use of rifampin. A similar assocation, though less marked, has been suggested with barbiturates, phenylbutazone, phenytoin sodium, and possibly with griseofulvin, ampicillin and tetracyclines.
8. INTERACTIONS WITH LABORATORY TESTS
Certain endocrine- and liver-function tests and blood components may be affected by oral contraceptives:
a. Increased prothrombin and factors VII, VIII, IX, and X; decreased antithrombin 3; increased norepinephrine-induced platelet aggregability.
b. Increased thyroid-binding globulin (TBG) leading to increased circulating total thyroid hormone, as measured by protein-bound iodine (PBI), T4 by column or by radioimmunoassay. Free T3 resin uptake is decreased, reflecting the elevated TBG; free T4 concentration is unaltered.
c. Other binding proteins may be elevated in serum.
d. Sex-binding globulins are increased and result in elevated levels of total circulating sex steroids and corticoids; however, free or biologically active levels remain unchanged.
e. Triglycerides may be increased.
f. Glucose tolerance may be decreased.
g. Serum folate levels may be depressed by oral-contraceptive therapy. This may be of clinical significance if a woman becomes pregnant shortly after discontinuing oral contraceptives.
9. CARCINOGENESIS
See "Warnings" section.
10. PREGNANCY
Pregnancy Category X. See "Contraindications" and "Warnings" sections.
11. NURSING MOTHERS
Small amounts of oral-contraceptive steroids have been identified in the milk of nursing mothers, and a few adverse effects on the child have been reported, including jaundice and breast enlargement. In addition, oral contraceptives given in the postpartum period may interfere with lactation by decreasing the quantity and quality of breast milk. If possible, the nursing mother should be advised not to use oral contraceptives but to use other forms of contraception until she has completely weaned her child.

INFORMATION FOR THE PATIENT
See LO/OVRAL.

ADVERSE REACTIONS

An increased risk of the following serious adverse reactions has been associated with the use of oral contraceptives (see "Warnings" section):
Thrombophlebitis.
Arterial thromboembolism.
Pulmonary embolism.
Myocardial infarction.
Cerebral hemorrhage.
Cerebral thrombosis.
Hypertension.
Gallbladder disease.
Hepatic adenomas or benign liver tumors.
There is evidence of an association between the following conditions and the use of oral contraceptives, although additional confirmatory studies are needed:
Mesenteric thrombosis.
Retinal thrombosis
The following adverse reactions have been reported in patients receiving oral contraceptives and are believed to be drug related:
Nausea.
Vomiting.
Gastrointestinal symptoms (such as abdominal cramps and bloating).
Breakthrough bleeding.
Spotting.
Change in menstrual flow.
Amenorrhea.
Temporary infertility after discontinuation of treatment.
Edema.
Melasma which may persist.
Breast changes: tenderness, enlargement, secretion.
Change in weight (increase or decrease).
Change in cervical erosion and secretion.
Diminution in lactation when given immediately postpartum.
Cholestatic jaundice.
Migraine.
Rash (allergic).
Mental depression.
Reduced tolerance to carbohydrates.
Vaginal candidiasis.
Change in corneal curvature (steepening).
Intolerance to contact lenses.
The following adverse reactions have been reported in users of oral contraceptives, and the association has been neither confirmed nor refuted:
Congenital anomalies.
Premenstrual syndrome.
Cataracts.
Optic neuritis.
Changes in appetite.
Cystitis-like syndrome.
Headache.
Nervousness.
Dizziness.
Hirsutism.
Loss of scalp hair.
Erythema multiforme.
Erythema nodosum.
Hemorrhagic eruption.
Vaginitis.
Porphyria.
Impaired renal function.
Hemolytic uremic syndrome.
Budd-Chiari syndrome.
Acne.
Changes in libido.
Colitis.
Sickle-cell disease.
Cerebral-vascular disease with mitral valve prolapse.
Lupus-like syndromes.

OVERDOSAGE

Serious ill effects have not been reported following acute ingestion of large doses of oral contraceptives by young children. Overdosage may cause nausea, and withdrawal bleeding may occur in females.

NONCONTRACEPTIVE HEALTH BENEFITS
The following noncontraceptive health benefits related to the use of oral contraceptives are supported by epidemiological studies which largely utilized oral-contraceptive formulations containing doses exceeding 0.035 mg of ethinyl estradiol or 0.05 mg of mestranol.
Effects on menses:
Increased menstrual cycle regularity.
Decreased blood loss and decreased incidence of iron-deficiency anemia.
Decreased incidence of dysmenorrhea.
Effects related to inhibition of ovulation:
Decreased incidence of functional ovarian cysts.
Decreased incidence of ectopic pregnancies.
Effects from long-term use:
Decreased incidence of fibroadenomas and fibrocystic disease of the breast.
Decreased incidence of acute pelvic inflammatory disease.
Decreased incidence of endometrial cancer.
Decreased incidence of ovarian cancer.

DOSAGE AND ADMINISTRATION

To achieve maximum contraceptive effectiveness, Nordette-21 must be taken exactly as directed and at intervals not exceeding 24 hours.
The dosage of Nordette-21 is one tablet daily for 21 consecutive days per menstrual cycle according to prescribed schedule. Tablets are then discontinued for 7 days (three weeks on, one week off).

It is recommended that Nordette-21 tablets be taken at the same time each day, preferably after the evening meal or at bedtime.

During the first cycle of medication, the patient is instructed to take one Nordette-21 tablet daily for twenty-one consecutive days, beginning on the first day (Day 1 Start) of her menstrual cycle or on the Sunday after her period begins (Sunday Start). (The first day of menstruation is day one.) The tablets are then discontinued for one week (7 days). Withdrawal bleeding should usually occur within 3 days following discontinuation of Nordette-21. (For Day 1 Start: If Nordette-21 is first taken later than the first day of the first menstrual cycle of medication or postpartum, contraceptive reliance should not be placed on Nordette-21 until after the first seven consecutive days of administration. For Sunday Start: Contraceptive reliance should not be placed on Nordette-21 until after the first seven consecutive days of administration. The possibility of ovulation and conception prior to initiation of medication should be considered.)

The patient begins her next and all subsequent 21-day courses of Nordette-21 tablets on the same day of the week that she began her first course, following the same schedule: 21 days on—7 days off. She begins taking her tablets on the 8th day after discontinuance , regardless of whether or not a menstrual period has occurred or is still in progress. Any time a new cycle of Nordette-21 is started later than the 8th day, the patient should be protected by another means of contraception until she has taken a tablet daily for seven consecutive days.

If spotting or breakthrough bleeding occurs, the patient is instructed to continue on the same regimen. This type of bleeding is usually transient and without significance; however, if the bleeding is persistent or prolonged the patient is advised to consult her physician. Although the occurrence of pregnancy is highly unlikely if Nordette-21 is taken according to directions, if withdrawal bleeding does not occur, the possibility of pregnancy must be considered. If the patient has not adhered to the prescribed schedule (missed one or more tablets or started taking them on a day later than she should have), the probability of pregnancy should be considered at the time of the first missed period and appropriate diagnostic measures taken before the medication is resumed. If the patient has adhered to the prescribed regimen and misses two consecutive periods, pregnancy should be ruled out before continuing the contraceptive regimen.

For additional patient instructions regarding missed pills, see the "WHAT TO DO IF YOU MISS PILLS" section in the **DETAILED PATIENT LABELING** for LO/OVRAL.

Any time the patient misses two or more tablets, she should also use another method of contraception until she has taken a tablet daily for seven consecutive days. If breakthrough bleeding occurs following missed tablets, it will usually be transient and of no consequence. While there is little likelihood of ovulation occurring if only one or two tablets are missed, the possibility of ovulation increases with each successive day that scheduled tablets are missed.

In the nonlactating mother, Nordette-21 may be initiated postpartum, for contraception. When the tablets are administered in the postpartum period, the increased risk of thromboembolic disease associated with the postpartum period must be considered (see "Contraindications," "Warnings," and "Precautions" concerning thromboembolic disease). It is to be noted that early resumption of ovulation may occur if Parlodel® (bromocriptine mesylate) has been used for the prevention of lactation.

HOW SUPPLIED

Nordette®-21 Tablets (0.15 mg levonorgestrel and 0.03 mg ethinyl estradiol) are available in 6 PILPAK® dispensers with 21 tablets each as follows: NDC 0008-0075-01, light-orange, round tablet marked "WYETH" and "75".

Store at room temperature, approx. 25°C (77°F).
References available upon request.

Brief Summary Patient Package Insert: See Lo/Ovral.

DETAILED PATIENT LABELING: See Lo/Ovral.

Manufactured by:
Wyeth Laboratories
A Wyeth-Ayerst Company
Philadelphia, PA 19101
Distributed by:
Monarch Pharmaceuticals, Inc.
Bristol, TN 37620

Shown in Product Identification Guide, page 343

NORDETTE®-28 ℞

[*nŏr-dĕt ′-28*]

TABLETS

(levonorgestrel and ethinyl estradiol tablets)

Patients should be counseled that this product does not protect against HIV infection (AIDS) and other sexually transmitted diseases.

DESCRIPTION

21 light-orange Nordette tablets, each containing 0.15 mg of levonorgestrel (d (-)-13 beta-ethyl -17-alpha-ethinyl-17-beta-hydroxygon-4-en-3-one), a totally synthetic progestogen, and 0.03 mg of ethinyl estradiol (19-nor-17α-pregna-1,3,5 (10)-trien-20-yne-3,17-diol), and 7 pink inert tablets. The inactive ingredients present are cellulose, D&C Red 30, FD&C Yellow 6, lactose, magnesium stearate, and polacrilin potassium.

CLINICAL PHARMACOLOGY

See NORDETTE®-21

INDICATIONS AND USAGE

See NORDETTE-21

CONTRAINDICATIONS

See NORDETTE-21

WARNINGS

See NORDETTE-21

PRECAUTIONS

See NORDETTE-21

Drug Interactions: See NORDETTE-21
Carcinogenesis: See NORDETTE-21
Nursing Mothers: See NORDETTE-21
Information for the Patient: See LO/OVRAL.

ADVERSE REACTIONS

See NORDETTE-21

OVERDOSAGE

See NORDETTE-21

NONCONTRACEPTIVE HEALTH BENEFITS

See NORDETTE-21

DOSAGE AND ADMINISTRATION

To achieve maximum contraceptive effectiveness, Nordette-28 must be taken exactly as directed and at intervals not exceeding 24 hours.

The dosage of Nordette-28 is one light-orange tablet daily for 21 consecutive days, followed by one pink inert tablet daily for 7 consecutive days, according to prescribed schedule.

It is recommended that tablets be taken at the same time each day, preferably after the evening meal or at bedtime.

During the first cycle of medication, the patient is instructed to begin taking Nordette-28 on the first Sunday after the onset of menstruation. If menstruation begins on a Sunday, the first tablet (light-orange) is taken that day. One light-orange tablet should be taken daily for 21 consecutive days, followed by one pink inert tablet daily for 7 consecutive days. Withdrawal bleeding should usually occur within three days following discontinuation of light-orange tablets. During the first cycle, contraceptive reliance should not be placed on Nordette-28 until a light-orange tablet has been taken daily for 7 consecutive days. The possibility of ovulation and conception prior to initiation of medication should be considered.

The patient begins her next and all subsequent 28-day courses of tablets on the same day of the week (Sunday) on which she began her first course, following the same schedule: 21 days on light-orange tablets—7 days on pink inert tablets. If in any cycle the patient starts tablets later than the proper day, she should protect herself by using another method of birth control until she has taken a light-orange tablet daily for 7 consecutive days.

If spotting or breakthrough bleeding occurs, the patient is instructed to continue on the same regimen. This type of bleeding is usually transient and without significance; however, if the bleeding is persistent or prolonged, the patient is advised to consult her physician. Although the occurrence of pregnancy is highly unlikely if Nordette-28 is taken according to directions, if withdrawal bleeding does not occur, the possibility of pregnancy must be considered. If the patient has not adhered to the prescribed schedule (missed one or more tablets or started taking them on a day later than she should have), the probability of pregnancy should be considered at the time of the first missed period and appropriate diagnostic measures taken before the medication is resumed. If the patient has adhered to the prescribed regimen and misses two consecutive periods, pregnancy should be ruled out before continuing the contraceptive regimen.

For additional patient instructions regarding missed pills, see the "WHAT TO DO IF YOU MISS PILLS" section in the **DETAILED PATIENT LABELING** for LO/OVRAL.

Any time the patient misses two or more light-orange tablets, she should also use another method of contraception until she has taken a light-orange tablet daily for seven consecutive days. If the patient misses one or more pink tablets, she is still protected against pregnancy **provided** she begins taking light-orange tablets again on the proper day.

If breakthrough bleeding occurs following missed light-orange tablets, it will usually be transient and of no consequence. While there is little likelihood of ovulation occurring if only one or two light-orange tablets are missed, the possibility of ovulation increases with each successive day that scheduled light-orange tablets are missed.

In the nonlactating mother, Nordette-28 may be initiated postpartum, for contraception. When the tablets are administered in the postpartum period, the increased risk of thromboembolic disease associated with the postpartum period must be considered (see "Contraindications", "Warnings", and "Precautions" concerning thromboembolic disease). It is to be noted that early resumption of ovulation may occur if Parlodel® (bromocriptine mesylate) has been used for the prevention of lactation.

HOW SUPPLIED

Nordette®-28 Tablets (0.15 mg levonorgestrel and 0.03 mg ethinyl estradiol) are available in 6 PILPAK® dispensers, each containing 28 tablets as follows:
21 active tablets, NDC 0008-2533, light-orange, round tablet marked "WYETH" and "75".
7 inert tablets, NDC 0008-0486, pink, round tablet marked "WYETH" and "486".

ALSO AVAILABLE:
Nordette®-28 Tablets (0.15 mg levonorgestrel and 0.03 mg ethinyl estradiol) are available in packages of 12 PILPAK® dispensers for clinic use only, each containing 28 tablets as follows:
21 active tablets, NDC 0008-2533, light-orange, round tablet marked "WYETH" and "75".
7 inert tablets, NDC 0008-0486, pink, round tablet marked "WYETH" and "486".

Store at room temperature, approx. 25°C (77°F).
References available upon request.

Brief Summary Patient Package Insert: See LO/OVRAL.
DETAILED PATIENT LABELING: See LO/OVRAL.

HOW TO TAKE THE PILL
For Nordette-28 PILPAK® Dispenser, See LO/OVRAL.
For Nordette-28 Clinic Pilpak®, See below.

HOW TO TAKE THE PILL

This product (like all oral contraceptives) is intended to prevent pregnancy. It does not protect against transmission of HIV (AIDS) and other sexually transmitted diseases such as chlamydia, genital herpes, genital warts, gonorrhea, hepatitis B, and syphilis.

IMPORTANT POINTS TO REMEMBER

BEFORE YOU START TAKING YOUR PILLS:

1. BE SURE TO READ THESE DIRECTIONS:
Before you start taking your pills.
Anytime you are not sure what to do.

2. THE RIGHT WAY TO TAKE THE PILL IS TO TAKE ONE PILL EVERY DAY AT THE SAME TIME.
If you miss pills you could get pregnant. This includes starting the pack late. The more pills you miss, the more likely you are to get pregnant.

3. MANY WOMEN HAVE SPOTTING OR LIGHT BLEEDING, OR MAY FEEL SICK TO THEIR STOMACH DURING THE FIRST 1–3 PACKS OF PILLS.
If you feel sick to your stomach, do not stop taking the pill. The problem will usually go away. If it doesn't go away, check with your doctor or clinic.

4. MISSING PILLS CAN ALSO CAUSE SPOTTING OR LIGHT BLEEDING, even when you make up these pills.
On the days you take 2 pills to make up for missed pills, you could also feel a little sick to your stomach.

5. IF YOU HAVE VOMITING OR DIARRHEA, for any reason, or IF YOU TAKE SOME MEDICINES, including some antibiotics, your pills may not work as well. Use a back-up method (such as condoms or foam) until you check with your doctor or clinic.

6. IF YOU HAVE TROUBLE REMEMBERING TO TAKE THE PILL, talk to your doctor or clinic about how to make pill-taking easier or about using another method of birth control.

7. IF YOU HAVE QUESTIONS OR ARE UNSURE ABOUT THE INFORMATION IN THIS LEAFLET, call your doctor or clinic.

NORDETTE®-21, OVRAL®, LO/OVRAL®, NORDETTE®-28, OVRAL®-28, AND LO/OVRAL®-28

***BEFORE* YOU START TAKING YOUR PILLS**

---

1. DECIDE WHAT TIME OF DAY YOU WANT TO TAKE YOUR PILL
It is important to take it at about the same time every day.

2. LOOK AT YOUR PILL PACK TO SEE IF IT HAS 21 OR 28 PILLS:
The *21-pill pack* has 21 "active" white or light-orange pills (with hormones) to take for 3 weeks, followed by 1 week without pills.
The *28-pill pack* has 21 "active" white or light-orange pills (with hormones) to take for 3 weeks, followed by 1 week of reminder pink pills (without hormones).

3. ALSO FIND:
1) where on the pack to start taking the pills,
2) in what order to take the pills (follow the arrows), and
3) the week numbers as shown in the picture below.

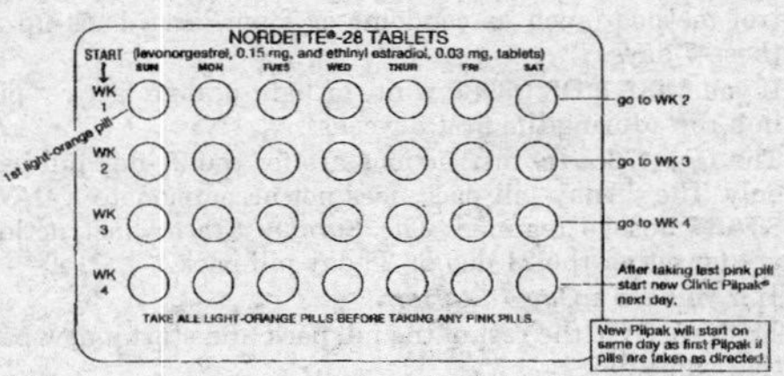

4. BE SURE YOU HAVE READY AT ALL TIMES.
ANOTHER KIND OF BIRTH CONTROL (such as condoms or foam) to use as a back-up in case you miss pills.
AND EXTRA, FULL PILL PACK

Continued on next page

Nordette-28—Cont.

WHEN YOU START THE *FIRST* PACK OF PILLS:

For the 21-day pill pack you have two choices of which day to start taking your first pack of pills. (See **DAY 1 START** or **SUNDAY START** directions below.) Decide with your doctor or clinic which is the best day for you. The 28-day pill pack accommodates a **SUNDAY START** only. For either pill pack pick a time of day which will be easy to remember.

DAY 1 START:

These instructions are for the 21-day pill pack only. The 28-day pill pack does not accommodate a **DAY 1 START** dosage regimen.

1. Take the first "active" white or light-orange pill of the first pack during the *first 24 hours of your period.*
2. You will not need to use a back-up method of birth control, since you are starting the pill at the beginning of your period.

SUNDAY START:

These instructions are for either the 21-day or the 28-day pill pack.

1. Take the first "active" white or light-orange pill of the first pack on the *Sunday after your period starts*, even if you are still bleeding. If your period begins on Sunday, start the pack that same day.
2. *Use another method of birth control* as a back-up method if you have sex anytime from the Sunday you start your first pack until the next Sunday (7 days). Condoms or foam are good back-up methods of birth control.

WHAT TO DO DURING THE MONTH:

1. **TAKE ONE PILL AT THE SAME TIME EVERY DAY UNTIL THE PACK IS EMPTY.**

Do not skip pills even if you are spotting or bleeding between monthly periods or feel sick to your stomach (nausea).

Do not skip pills even if you do not have sex very often.

2. **WHEN YOU FINISH A PACK OR SWITCH YOUR BRAND OF PILLS:**

21 pills: Wait 7 days to start the next pack. You will probably have your period during that week. Be sure that no more than 7 days pass between 21-day packs.

28 pills: Start the next pack on the day after your last "reminder" pill.

Do not wait any days between packs.

WHAT TO DO IF YOU MISS PILLS

If you **MISS 1** white or light-orange "active" pill:

1. Take it as soon as you remember. Take the next pill at your regular time. This means you take 2 pills in 1 day.
2. You do not need to use a back-up birth control method if you have sex.

If you **MISS 2** white or light-orange "active" pills in a row in **WEEK 1 OR WEEK 2** of your pack:

1. Take 2 pills on the day you remember and 2 pills the next day.
2. Then take 1 pill a day until you finish the pack.
3. You MAY BECOME PREGNANT if you have sex in the 7 *days* after you miss pills. You MUST use another birth control method (such as condoms or foam) as a back-up for those 7 days.

If you **MISS 2** white or light-orange "active" pills in a row in **THE 3rd WEEK:**

The ***Day 1 Starter*** instructions are for the 21-day pill pack only. The 28-day pill pack does not accommodate a **DAY 1 START** dosage regimen. The ***Sunday Starter*** instructions are for either the 21-day or 28-day pill pack.

1. ***If you are a Day 1 Starter:***

THROW OUT the rest of the pill pack and start a new pack that same day.

If you are a Sunday Starter:

Keep taking 1 pill every day until Sunday.

On Sunday, THROW OUT the rest of the pack and start a new pack of pills that same day.

2. You may not have your period this month but this is expected. However, if you miss your period 2 months in a row, call your doctor or clinic because you might be pregnant.
3. You MAY BECOME PREGNANT if you have sex in the 7 *days* after you miss pills. You MUST use another birth control method (such as condoms or foam) as a back-up for those 7 days.

If you **MISS 3 OR MORE** white or light-orange "active" pills in a row (during the first 3 weeks):

The ***Day 1 Starter*** instructions are for the 21-day pill pack only. The 28-day pill pack does not accommodate a **DAY 1 START** dosage regimen. The ***Sunday Starter*** instructions are for either the 21-day or 28-day pill pack.

1. ***If you are a Day 1 Starter***

THROW OUT the rest of the pill pack and start a new pack that same day.

If you are a Sunday Starter

Keep taking 1 pill every day until Sunday.

On Sunday, THROW OUT the rest of the pack and start a new pack of pills that same day.

2. You may not have your period this month but this is expected. However, if you miss your period 2 months in a row, call your doctor or clinic because you might be pregnant.
3. You MAY BECOME PREGNANT if you have sex in the 7 *days* after you miss pills. YOU MUST use another birth control method (such as condoms or foam) as back-up for those 7 days.

A REMINDER FOR THOSE ON 28-DAY PACKS:

If you forget any of the 7 pink "reminder" pills in Week 4:

THROW AWAY the pills you missed.

Keep taking 1 pill each day until the pack is empty.

You do not need a back-up method if you start your next pack on time.

FINALLY, IF YOU ARE STILL NOT SURE WHAT TO DO ABOUT THE PILLS YOU HAVE MISSED:

Use a BACK-UP METHOD anytime you have sex.

KEEP TAKING ONE PILL EACH DAY until you can reach your doctor or clinic.

OVRETTE®

Ovrette is administered on a continuous daily dosage schedule, one tablet each day, every day of the year. Take the first tablet on the first day of your menstrual period. Tablets should be taken at the same time every day, without interruption, whether bleeding occurs or not. If bleeding is prolonged (more than 8 days) or unusually heavy, you should contact your doctor.

Forgotten pills

The risk of pregnancy increases with each tablet missed. Therefore, it is very important that you take one tablet daily as directed. If you miss one tablet, take it as soon as you remember and also take your next tablet at the regular time. If you miss two tablets, take one of the missed tablets as soon as you remember, as well as your regular tablet for that day at the proper time. Furthermore, you should use another method of birth control in addition to taking Ovrette until you have taken fourteen days (2 weeks) of medication.

If more than two tablets have been missed, Ovrette should be discontinued immediately and another method of birth control used until the start of your next menstrual period. Then you may resume taking Ovrette.

Pregnancy due to pill failure

The incidence of pill failure resulting in pregnancy is approximately less than 1.0% if taken every day as directed, but more typical failure rates are less than 3.0%. If failure does occur, the risk to the fetus is minimal.

RISKS TO THE FETUS

If you do become pregnant while using oral contraceptives, the risk to the fetus is small, on the order of no more than one per thousand. You should, however, discuss the risks to the developing child with your doctor.

Pregnancy after stopping the pill

There may be some delay in becoming pregnant after you stop using oral contraceptives, especially if you had irregular menstrual cycles before you used oral contraceptives. It may be advisable to postpone conception until you begin menstruating regularly once you have stopped taking the pill and desire pregnancy.

There does not appear to be any increase in birth defects in newborn babies when pregnancy occurs soon after stopping the pill.

Overdosage

Serious ill effects have not been reported following ingestion of large doses of oral contraceptives by young children. Overdosage may cause nausea and withdrawal bleeding in females. In case of overdosage, contact your health-care provider or pharmacist.

Other information

Your health-care provider will take a medical and family history before prescibing oral contraceptives and will examine you. The physical examination may be delayed to another time if you request it and the health-care provider believes that it is appropriate to postpone it. You should be reexamined at least once a year. Be sure to inform your health-care provider if there is a family history of any of the conditions listed previously in this leaflet. Be sure to keep all appointments with your health-care provider, because this is a time to determine if there are early signs of side effects of oral-contraceptive use.

Do not use the drug for any condition other than the one for which it was prescribed. This drug has been prescribed specifically for you; do not give it to others who may want birth-control pills.

HEALTH BENEFITS FROM ORAL CONTRACEPTIVES: See LO/OVRAL.

Manufactured by:
Wyeth Laboratories
A Wyeth-Ayerst Company
Philadelphia, PA 19101
Distributed by:
Monarch Pharmaceuticals, Inc.
Bristol, TN 37620

Shown in Product Identification Guide, page 343

PEDIOTIC® SUSPENSION STERILE ℞
(neomycin and polymyxin B sulfates and hydrocortisone otic suspension, USP)

DESCRIPTION

PEDIOTIC Suspension (neomycin and polymyxin B sulfates and hydrocortisone otic suspension) is a sterile antibacterial and anti-inflammatory suspension for otic use. Each mL contains: neomycin sulfate equivalent to 3.5 mg neomycin base, polymyxin B sulfate equivalent to 10,000 polymyxin B units, and hydrocortisone 10 mg (1%). The vehicle contains thimerosal 0.001% (added as a preservative) and the inactive ingredients cetyl alcohol, glyceryl monostearate, mineral oil, polyoxyl 40 stearate, propylene glycol, and Water for Injection. Sulfuric acid may be added to adjust pH. PEDIOTIC Suspension has a minimum pH of 4.1, which is less acidic than the minimum pH of 3.0 for CORTISPORIN® Otic Suspension.

Neomycin sulfate is the sulfate salt of neomycin B and C, which are produced by the growth of *Streptomyces fradiae* Waksman (Fam. Streptomycetaceae). It has a potency equivalent of not less than 600 µg of neomycin standard per mg, calculated on an anhydrous basis. The structural formulae are:

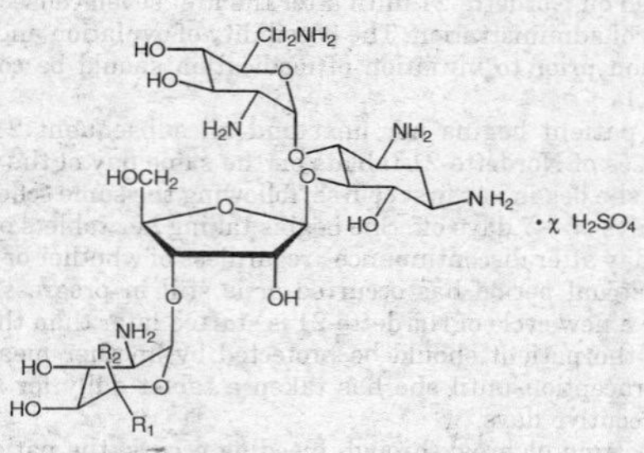

Neomycin B (R_1=H, R_2=CH_2NH_2)
Neomycin C (R_1=CH_2NH_2, R_2=H)

Polymyxin B sulfate is the sulfate salt of polymyxin B_1 and B_2, which are produced by the growth of *Bacillus polymyxa* (Prazmowski) Migula (Fam. Bacillaceae). It has a potency of not less than 6,000 polymyxin B units per mg, calculated on an anhydrous basis. The structural formulae are:

CH_3 — $RCH_2CH(CH_2)_4CO$–L–DAB–L–Thr–L–DAB–L–DAB (γ-NH_2, γ-NH_2); L–DAB–D–Phe–L–Leu (γ-NH_2); L–Thr–L–DAB–L–DAB (γ-NH_2, γ-NH_2) • χ H_2SO_4

Polymyxin B_1 (R=CH_3)
Polymyxin B_2 (R=H)
DAB=α, γ-diaminobutyric acid

Hydrocortisone, 11β, 17, 21-trihydroxypregn-4-ene-3,20-dione, is an anti-inflammatory hormone. Its structural formula is:

CLINICAL PHARMACOLOGY

Corticoids suppress the inflammatory response to a variety of agents and they may delay healing. Since corticoids may inhibit the body's defense mechanism against infection, a concomitant antimicrobial drug may be used when this inhibition is considered to be clinically significant in a particular case.

The anti-infective components in the combination are included to provide action against specific organisms susceptible to them. Neomycin sulfate and polymyxin B sulfate together are considered active against the following microorganisms: *Staphylococcus aureus, Escherichia coli, Haemophilus influenzae, Klebsiella-Enterobacter* species, *Neisseria* species, and *Pseudomonas aeruginosa.* This product does not provide adequate coverage against *Serratia marcescens* and streptococci, including *Streptococcus pneumoniae.*

The relative potency of corticosteroids depends on the molecular structure, concentration, and release from the vehicle.

INDICATIONS AND USAGE

For the treatment of superficial bacterial infections of the external auditory canal caused by organisms susceptible to the action of the antibiotics, and for the treatment of infections of mastoidectomy and fenestration cavities caused by organisms susceptible to the antibiotics.

CONTRAINDICATIONS

This product is contraindicated in those individuals who have shown hypersensitivity to any of its components, and in herpes simplex, vaccinia, and varicella infections.

WARNINGS

This product should be used with care in cases of perforated eardrum and in long-standing cases of chronic otitis media because of the possibility of ototoxicity. Neomycin sulfate may cause cutaneous sensitization. A precise incidence of hypersensitivity reactions (primarily skin rash) due to topical neomycin is not known.

When using neomycin-containing products to control secondary infection in the chronic dermatoses, such as chronic otitis externa or stasis dermatitis, it should be borne in mind that the skin in these conditions is more liable than is normal skin to become sensitized to many substances, including neomycin. The manifestation of sensitization to neomycin is usually a low-grade reddening with swelling, dry scaling, and itching; it may be manifest simply as a failure to heal. Periodic examination for such signs is advisable, and the patient should be told to discontinue the product if they are observed. These symptoms regress quickly on withdrawing the medication. Neomycin-containing applications should be avoided for the patient thereafter.

PRECAUTIONS

General: As with other antibacterial preparations, prolonged use may result in overgrowth of non-susceptible organisms, including fungi.

If the infection is not improved after 1 week, cultures and susceptibility tests should be repeated to verify the identity of the organism and to determine whether therapy should be changed.

Treatment should not be continued for longer than 10 days.

Allergic cross-reactions may occur which could prevent the use of any or all of the following antibiotics for the treatment of future infections: kanamycin, paromomycin, streptomycin, and possibly gentamicin.

Information for Patients: Avoid contaminating the dropper with material from the ear, fingers, or other source. This caution is necessary if the sterility of the drops is to be preserved.

If sensitization or irritation occurs, discontinue use immediately and contact your physician.

Do not use in the eyes.

SHAKE WELL BEFORE USING.

Laboratory Tests: Systemic effects of excessive levels of hydrocortisone may include a reduction in the number of circulating eosinophils and a decrease in urinary excretion of 17-hydroxycorticosteroids.

Carcinogenesis, Mutagenesis, Impairment of Fertility: Long-term studies in animals (rats, rabbits, mice) showed no evidence of carcinogenicity attributable to oral administration of corticosteroids.

Pregnancy: ***Teratogenic Effects:*** Pregnancy Category C. Corticosteroids have been shown to be teratogenic in rabbits when applied topically at concentrations of 0.5% on days 6 to 18 of gestation and in mice when applied topically at a concentration of 15% on days 10 to 13 of gestation. There are no adequate and well-controlled studies in pregnant women. Corticosteroids should be used during pregnancy only if the potential benefit justifies the potential risk to the fetus.

Nursing Mothers: Hydrocortisone appears in human milk following oral administration of the drug. Since systemic absorption of hydrocortisone may occur when applied topically, caution should be exercised when PEDIOTIC is used by a nursing woman.

Pediatric Use: See DOSAGE AND ADMINISTRATION.

ADVERSE REACTIONS

Neomycin occasionally causes skin sensitization. Ototoxicity and nephrotoxicity have also been reported (see WARNINGS). Adverse reactions have occurred with topical use of antibiotic combinations including neomycin and polymyxin B. Exact incidence figures are not available since no denominator of treated patients is available. The reaction occurring most often is allergic sensitization. In one clinical study, using a 20% neomycin patch, neomycin-induced allergic skin reactions occurred in two of 2,175 (0.09%) individuals in the general population.[1] In another study, the incidence was found to be approximately 1%.[2]

The following local adverse reactions have been reported with topical corticosteroids, especially under occlusive dressings: burning, itching, irritation, dryness, folliculitis, hypertrichosis, acneiform eruptions, hypopigmentation, perioral dermatitis, allergic contact dermatitis, maceration of the skin, secondary infection, skin atrophy, striae, and miliaria. Stinging and burning have been reported rarely when this drug has gained access to the middle ear.

DOSAGE AND ADMINISTRATION

The external auditory canal should be thoroughly cleansed and dried with a sterile cotton applicator.

For adults, 4 drops of the suspension should be instilled into the affected ear 3 or 4 times daily. For infants and children, 3 drops are suggested because of the smaller capacity of the ear canal.

The patient should lie with the affected ear upward and then the drops should be instilled. This position should be maintained for 5 minutes to facilitate penetration of the drops into the ear canal. Repeat, if necessary, for the opposite ear.

If preferred, a cotton wick may be inserted into the canal and then the cotton may be saturated with the suspension. This wick should be kept moist by adding further suspension every 4 hours. The wick should be replaced at least once every 24 hours.

SHAKE WELL BEFORE USING.

HOW SUPPLIED

Bottle of 7.5 mL with sterilized dropper (NDC 61570-038-75). Store at 15° to 25°C (59° to 77°F).

Rx only

REFERENCES

1. Leyden JJ, Kligman AM. Contact dermatitis to neomycin sulfate. *JAMA*. 1979;242:1276-1278.
2. Prystowsky SD, Allen AM, Smith RW, Nonomura JH, Odom RB, Akers WA. Allergic contact hypersensitivity to nickel, neomycin, ethylenediamine, and benzocaine: relationships between age, sex, history of exposure, and reactivity to standard patch tests and use tests in a general population. *Arch Dermatol*. 1979;115:959-962.

Distributed by: Monarch Pharmaceuticals, Inc.
Bristol, TN 37620
Manufactured by: Catalytica Pharmaceutical, Inc.
Greenville, NC 27835

5/97
0932683

Shown in Product Identification Guide, page 325

PROCANBID® ℞

[*prō căn 'bĭd*]

(Procainamide Hydrochloride Extended-Release Tablets*)

***Procanbid® is not USP for dissolution.**

> **WARNINGS:**
> Positive ANA Titer: The prolonged administration of procainamide often leads to the development of a positive antinuclear antibody (ANA) test, with or without symptoms of a lupus erythematosus-like syndrome. If a positive ANA titer develops, the benefits versus risks of continued procainamide therapy should be assessed.

DESCRIPTION

Procanbid® (Procainamide Hydrochloride Extended-Release Tablets), a Group 1A cardiac antiarrhythmic drug, is p-amino-N-[2-(diethylamino) ethyl]benzamide monohydrochloride, molecular weight 271.79. Its structural formula is:

$$\overset{*}{N}H_2-C_6H_4-CONHCH_2CH_2N(C_2H_5)_2 \cdot HCl$$

(*Site of acetylation to N-acetylprocainamide)

Procainamide hydrochloride differs from procaine which is the p-aminobenzoyl ester of 2-(diethylamino)-ethanol. Procainamide as the free base has a pK_a of 9.24; the monohydrochloride is very soluble in water.

Procanbid® (Procainamide Hydrochloride Extended-Release Tablets) contains 500 mg or 1000 mg of procainamide hydrochloride for oral administration. The release of procainamide hydrochloride is controlled by 2 mechanisms using patented technology. The core of the tablet consists of a wax matrix which is then coated with a polymeric, control-release layer. Both strengths of Procanbid® contain this Polymatrix™ core. Both strengths of Procanbid® contain black iron oxide; candelilla wax, FCC; carnauba wax, NF; colloidal silicon dioxide, NF; hydroxypropyl cellulose, NF; hydroxypropylmethyl cellulose; magnesium stearate, NF; polyacrylate dispersion; polyethylene glycol 3350, NF; polyethylene glycol 8000, NF; propylene glycol; simethicone emulsion, USP; talc, USP; and titanium dioxide. The 1000-mg tablet additionally contains polysorbate 80.

CLINICAL PHARMACOLOGY

Mechanism of Action: Procainamide (PA) increases the effective refractory period of the atria, and to a lesser extent the bundle of His-Purkinje system and ventricles of the heart. It reduces impulse conduction velocity in the atria, His-Purkinje fibers, and ventricular muscle, but has variable effects on the atrioventricular (A-V) node, a direct slowing action and a weaker vagolytic effect that may speed A-V conduction slightly. Myocardial excitability is reduced in the atria, Purkinje fibers, papillary muscles, and ventricles by an increase in the threshold for excitation, combined with inhibition of ectopic pacemaker activity by retardation of the slow phase of diastolic depolarization, thus decreasing automaticity especially in ectopic sites. Contractility of the undamaged heart is usually not affected by therapeutic concentrations, although slight reduction of cardiac output may occur, and may be significant in the presence of myocardial damage. Therapeutic levels of PA may exert vagolytic effects and produce slight acceleration of heart rate, while high or toxic concentrations may prolong A-V conduction time or induce A-V block, or even cause abnormal automaticity and spontaneous firing, by unknown mechanisms.

The electrocardiogram may reflect these effects by showing slight sinus tachycardia (due to the anticholinergic action) and widened QRS complexes and, less regularly, prolonged Q-T and P-R intervals (due to longer systole and slower conduction), as well as some decrease in QRS and T wave amplitude. These direct effects of PA on electrical activity, conduction, responsiveness, excitability, and automaticity are characteristic of a Group 1A antiarrhythmic agent, the prototype for which is quinidine; PA effects are very similar. However, PA has weaker vagal blocking action than does quinidine, does not induce alpha-adrenergic blockade, and is less depressing to cardiac contractility.

Pharmacokinetics and Drug Metabolism

Absorption/Bioavailability: PA is well absorbed following oral administration. The absolute bioavailability from immediate-release PA HCl capsules is approximately 85% in patients and healthy subjects. Bioavailability of Procanbid® is similar to that of PA HCl extended-release tablets, USP (Procan® SR) which have been shown to be similar to that of immediate-release PA. The Procanbid® patented delivery system is designed to control the rate of PA release such that absorption is sustained throughout a 12-hour dosing interval. After administration of Procanbid® with a high-fat meal, the extent of PA absorption was increased by about 20%. Peak, trough, and average plasma PA concentrations following twice daily administration of Procanbid® to healthy subjects are similar to those achieved when Procan® SR is administered 4 times daily. In patients with frequent ventricular premature depolarizations (VPDs), peak and steady-state average PA concentrations following administration of Procanbid® every 12 hours are bioequivalent to those following administration of an equivalent daily dose of Procan® SR. While corresponding minimum concentrations are slightly lower than those for Procan® SR, they remain within the acceptable therapeutic range of 3 to 10 mcg/mL.

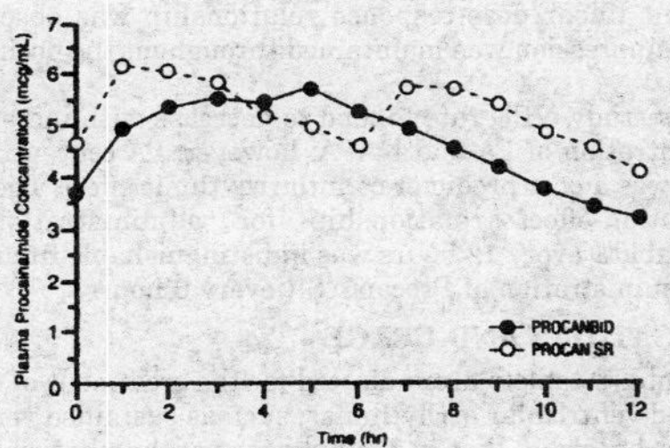

Figure 1. Mean Steady-State Plasma Concentrations Following Administration of Two 1000-mg Procanbid® Tablets Every 12 Hours or One 1000-mg Procan® SR Tablet Every 6 Hours to Patients with VPDs.

Twice-daily administration of two 1000-mg Procanbid® tablets to patients with frequent VPDs produced a mean plasma PA concentration of 4.6 mcg/mL. Average peak and trough levels are within the generally accepted therapeutic range of 3 to 10 mcg/mL. Relative proportions of PA and N-acetylprocainamide (NAPA) during administration of Procanbid® are similar to those following administration of immediate-release PA or Procan® SR.

Distribution: Plasma protein binding of PA is insignificant, approximately 20%. The apparent volume of distribution is approximately 2 L/kg. It is not known if PA crosses the placenta.

Metabolism/Excretion: The elimination half-life of PA is 3 to 4 hours in patients with normal renal function, but reduced renal function prolongs the half-life (see Special Populations). PA is mainly eliminated intact by the kidneys. The only metabolite of any significance is N-acetylprocainamide (NAPA). Renal excretion accounts for >80% of the elimination of NAPA. Approximately 16 to 21% of PA is metabolized to NAPA in "slow acetylators"; in "rapid acetylators" the range is 24 to 33%. In white and black populations the numbers of rapid and slow acetylators are about 50%. The plasma concentration of NAPA is lower than the PA concentration in most individuals. The reverse may occur in individuals forming more of the metabolite while also having reduced kidney function. NAPA has significant antiarrhythmic activity.

An average of 65% of the dose was recovered as intact drug in the urine after intravenous administration of PA. The renal clearance of PA ranged from 400 to 600 mL/min. Active renal secretion ranged from 300 to 500 mL/min, and is thus the major elimination pathway for PA. The tubular secretion utilizes the base-secreting system also responsible for secretion of metformin, cimetidine, ranitidine, triamterene, and flecainide. Thus there is a potential for drug-drug interactions at this level.

Special Populations: *Patients with Renal Disease:* Decline in renal function, such as that occurring with advancing age or renal disease, increases the PA elimination half-life which can result in relatively high plasma concentrations of PA (see WARNINGS). Accumulation of NAPA due to impaired renal function can be more extensive than accumulation of PA.

Patients with Congestive Heart Failure: PA clearance is reduced in patients with severe heart failure, in part due to decreased renal perfusion (see WARNINGS).

Age, Gender, and Race: PA clearance decreases with increasing patient age, in part due to concurrent decreases in renal function. However, the pharmacokinetics of PA and NAPA are similar in young healthy subjects (mean age 32 yr) and patients with frequent VPDs (mean age 60 yr) following administration of Procanbid® every 12 hours. Steady state plasma procainamide concentrations in women receiving Procanbid® are 30 percent higher than those seen in men receiving the same dosing regimen. When corrected for body surface area this difference is only 16 percent. Concentrations of N-acetylprocainamide are not significantly different among men and women whether corrected for body surface area or not. Procanbid® tablets produce similar PA and NAPA concentrations in black and caucasian individuals.

Pharmacodynamics: While therapeutic plasma PA concentrations have been reported to be 3 to 10 mcg/mL, patients such as those with sustained ventricular tachycardia may need higher concentrations for adequate control. This may justify an increased risk of toxicity (see OVERDOSAGE). Where programmed ventricular stimulation has been used to evaluate efficacy of PA in preventing recurring ventricular tachyarrhythmias, an average plasma PA concentration

Continued on next page

Procanbid—Cont.

of 13.6 mcg/mL was necessary for adequate control. Action of PA on the central nervous system is not prominent, but high concentrations may cause tremors.

A double-blind, placebo-controlled, dose-response, formulation-crossover study was conducted, comparing the suppression of VPDs by Procanbid® administered every 12 hours and Procan® SR administered every 6 hours. Similar VPD suppression was observed following administration of both formulations for 1 week each. Procanbid® demonstrated significant pharmacologic activity (mean percent change from baseline in VPDs) compared with placebo, and a significant linear dose-response relationship was observed. VPD suppression was maintained throughout the dosing interval.

In this study, VPD rate tended to decrease with increasing concentration of PA and NAPA; however, PA concentration alone was a poor predictor of antiarrhythmic effect. The concentration-effect relationship for administration of Procanbid® every 12 hours was indistinguishable from that for administration of Procan® SR every 6 hours.

INDICATIONS AND USAGE

Procanbid® tablets are indicated for the treatment of documented ventricular arrhythmias, such as sustained ventricular tachycardia, that in the judgment of the physician are life-threatening. Because of the proarrhythmic effects of procainamide, its use with lesser arrhythmias is generally not recommended. Treatment of patients with asymptomatic ventricular premature depolarizations should be avoided.

Initiation of procainamide treatment, as with other antiarrhythmic agents used to treat life-threatening arrhythmias, should be carried out in the hospital.

Antiarrhythmic drugs have not been shown to enhance survival in patients with ventricular arrhythmias. Because procainamide has the potential to produce serious hematologic disorders (0.5%), particularly leukopenia or agranulocytosis (sometimes fatal), its use should be reserved for patients in whom, in the opinion of the physician, the benefits of treatment clearly outweigh the risks. (See WARNINGS and Boxed Warning.)

CONTRAINDICATIONS

Complete Heart Block: Procainamide should not be administered to patients with complete heart block because of its effects in suppressing nodal or ventricular pacemakers and the hazard of asystole. It may be difficult to recognize complete heart block in patients with ventricular tachycardia, but if significant slowing of ventricular rate occurs during PA treatment without evidence of A-V conduction appearing, PA should be stopped. In cases of second degree A-V block or various types of hemiblock, PA should be avoided or discontinued because of the possibility of increased severity of block unless the ventricular rate is controlled by an electrical pacemaker.

Idiosyncratic Hypersensitivity: In patients sensitive to procaine or other ester-type local anesthetics, cross sensitivity to PA is unlikely; however, it should be borne in mind, and PA should not be used if it produces acute allergic dermatitis, asthma, or anaphylactic symptoms.

Lupus Erythematosus: An established diagnosis of systemic lupus erythematosus is a contraindication to PA therapy, since aggravation of symptoms is highly likely.

Torsades De Pointes: In the unusual ventricular arrhythmia called "les torsades de pointes" (twisting of the points), characterized by alternation of 1 or more ventricular premature beats in the directions of the QRS complexes on ECG in persons with prolonged Q-T and often enhanced U waves, Group 1A antiarrhythmic drugs are contraindicated. Administration of PA in such cases may aggravate this special type of ventricular extrasystole or tachycardia instead of suppressing it.

WARNINGS

Mortality: In the National Heart, Lung, and Blood Institute's Cardiac Arrhythmia Suppression Trial (CAST), a long-term, multi-centered, randomized, double-blind study in patients with asymptomatic non-life-threatening ventricular arrhythmias who had a myocardial infarction more than 6 days but less than 2 years previously, an excessive mortality or non-fatal cardiac arrest rate (7.7%) was seen in patients treated with encainide or flecainide compared with that seen in patients assigned to carefully matched placebo-treated groups (3.0%). The average duration of treatment with encainide or flecainide in this study was 10 months.

The applicability of the CAST results to other populations (e.g., those without recent myocardial infarction) is uncertain. Considering the known proarrhythmic properties of procainamide and the lack of evidence of improved survival for any antiarrhythmic drug in patients without life-threatening arrhythmias, the use of Procanbid® as well as other antiarrhythmic agents should be reserved for patients with life-threatening ventricular arrhythmias.

BLOOD DYSCRASIAS: Agranulocytosis, bone marrow depression, neutropenia, hypoplastic anemia, and thrombocytopenia have been reported in patients receiving procainamide hydrochloride at a rate of approximately 0.5%. Most of these patients received procainamide hydrochloride within the recommended dosage range. Fatalities have occurred (with approximately 20%–25% mortality in reported cases of agranulocytosis). Since most of these events have been noted during the first 12 weeks of therapy, it is recommended that complete blood counts including white cell, differential, and platelet counts be performed at weekly intervals for the first 3 months of therapy, and periodically thereafter. Complete blood counts should be performed promptly if the patient develops any signs of infection (such as fever, chills, sore throat, or stomatitis), bruising, or bleeding. If any of these hematologic disorders are identified, procainamide hydrochloride should be discontinued. Blood counts usually return to normal within 1 month of discontinuation. Caution should be used in patients with pre-existing marrow failure or cytopenia of any type (see ADVERSE REACTIONS).

Digitalis Intoxication: Caution should be exercised in the use of procainamide in arrhythmias associated with digitalis intoxication. Procainamide can suppress digitalis-induced arrhythmias; however, if there is concomitant marked disturbance of atrioventricular conduction, additional depression of conduction and ventricular asystole or fibrillation may result. Therefore, use of procainamide should be considered only if discontinuation of digitalis, and therapy with potassium, lidocaine, or phenytoin are ineffective.

First Degree Heart Block: Caution should be exercised also if the patient exhibits or develops first degree heart block while taking PA, and dosage reduction is advised in such cases. If the block persists despite dosage reduction, continuation of PA administration must be evaluated on the basis of current benefit versus risk of increased heart block.

Predigitalization for Atrial Flutter or Fibrillation: Patients with atrial flutter or fibrillation should be cardioverted or digitalized prior to PA administration to avoid enhancement of A-V conduction which may result in ventricular rate acceleration beyond tolerable limits. Adequate digitalization reduces but does not eliminate the possibility of sudden increase in ventricular rate as the atrial rate is slowed by PA in these arrhythmias.

Congestive Heart Failure: For patients in congestive heart failure, and those with acute ischemic heart disease or cardiomyopathy, caution should be used in PA therapy, since even slight depression of myocardial contractility may further reduce the cardiac output of the damaged heart.

Concurrent Other Antiarrhythmic Agents: Concurrent use of PA with other Group 1A antiarrhythmic agents such as quinidine or disopyramide may produce enhanced prolongation of conduction or depression of contractility and hypotension, especially in patients with cardiac decompensation. Such use should be reserved for patients with serious arrhythmias unresponsive to a single drug and employed only if close observation is possible.

Renal Insufficiency: Renal insufficiency may lead to accumulation of high plasma concentrations of PA and/or NAPA from conventional oral doses of PA, with effects similar to those of overdosage (see OVERDOSAGE), unless dosage is adjusted for the individual patient.

Myasthenia Gravis: Patients with myasthenia gravis may show worsening of symptoms from PA due to its procaine-like effect on diminishing acetylcholine release at skeletal muscle motor nerve endings, so that PA administration may be hazardous without optimal adjustment of anticholinesterase medications and other precautions.

PRECAUTIONS

General: Immediately after initiation of PA therapy, patients should be closely observed for possible hypersensitivity reactions, especially if procaine or local anesthetic sensitivity is suspected, and for muscular weakness if myasthenia gravis is a possibility.

In conversion of atrial fibrillation to normal sinus rhythm by any means, dislodgment of mural thrombi may lead to embolization, which should be kept in mind.

Based upon the approximate half-life of 3 hours for PA, pharmacokinetic steady state would be reached within 1 day. After achieving and maintaining therapeutic plasma concentrations and satisfactory electrocardiographic and clinical responses, continued frequent periodic monitoring of vital signs and electrocardiograms is advised. If evidence of QRS widening of more than 25% or marked prolongation of the Q-T interval occurs, concern for overdosage is appropriate, and reduction in dosage is advisable if a 50% increase occurs. Elevated serum creatinine or urea nitrogen, reduced creatinine clearance, or history of renal insufficiency, as well as use in older patients (over age 50), provide grounds to anticipate that less than the usual dosage may suffice, since the urinary elimination of PA and NAPA may be reduced, leading to gradual accumulation beyond normally predicted amounts. If facilities are available for measurement of plasma PA and NAPA, or acetylation capability, individual dose adjustment for optimal therapeutic concentrations may be easier, but close observation of clinical effectiveness is the most important criterion.

In the longer term, periodic complete blood counts are useful to detect possible idiosyncratic hematologic effects of PA on neutrophil, platelet, or red cell homeostasis; agranulocytosis has been reported to occur occasionally in patients on long-term PA therapy. A rising titer of serum ANA may precede clinical symptoms of the lupoid syndrome (see Boxed Warning and ADVERSE REACTIONS). If the lupus erythematosus-like syndrome develops in a patient with recurrent life-threatening arrhythmias not controlled by other agents, corticosteroid suppressive therapy may be used concomitantly with PA. Since the PA-induced lupoid syndrome rarely includes dangerous pathologic renal changes, PA therapy may not necessarily have to be stopped unless the symptoms of serositis and the possibility of further lupoid effects are of greater risk than the benefit of PA in controlling arrhythmias. Patients with rapid acetylation capability are less likely to develop the lupoid syndrome after prolonged PA therapy.

Information for Patients: The physician is advised to explain to the patient that close cooperation in adhering to the prescribed dosage schedule is of great importance in controlling the cardiac arrhythmia safely. The patient should understand clearly that more medication is not necessarily better and may be dangerous, that skipping doses or increasing intervals between doses to suit personal convenience may lead to loss of control of the heart problem, and that "making up" missed doses by doubling up later may be hazardous.

The patient should be encouraged to disclose any past history of drug sensitivity, especially to procaine or other local anesthetic agents, and to report any history of kidney disease, congestive heart failure, myasthenia gravis, liver disease, or lupus erythematosus.

The patient should be counseled to report promptly any symptoms of arthralgia, myalgia, fever, chills, skin rash, easy bruising, sore throat or sore mouth, infections, dark urine or icterus, wheezing, muscular weakness, chest or abdominal pain, palpitations, nausea, vomiting, anorexia, diarrhea, hallucinations, dizziness, or depression.

The patient should be advised not to break or chew the tablet as this would interfere with designed dissolution characteristics. The tablet matrix of Procanbid® may be seen in the stool since it does not disintegrate following release of procainamide.

Laboratory Tests: Laboratory tests such as complete blood count (CBC), electrocardiogram, and serum creatinine or urea nitrogen may be indicated, depending on the clinical situation, and periodic rechecking of the CBC and ANA may be helpful in early detection of untoward reactions.

Drug Interactions: If other antiarrhythmic drugs are being used, additive effects on the heart may occur with PA administration, and dosage reduction may be necessary (see WARNINGS). Anticholinergic drugs administered concurrently with PA may produce additive antivagal effects on A-V nodal conduction, although this is not as well documented for PA as for quinidine.

Coadministration of cimetidine decreases renal clearance of PA, potentially leading to clinically significant increases in plasma concentrations. Large (> 300 mg/day) doses of ranitidine possibly have this effect also. Plasma PA concentrations higher than those for administration of PA alone have been reported for coadministration with either amiodarone or trimethoprim. Alcohol (ethanol) consumption tends to decrease the half-life of PA in the blood through induction of its acetylation to NAPA.

Patients taking PA who require neuromuscular blocking agents such as succinylcholine may require less than usual doses of the latter, due to PA effects of reducing acetylcholine release.

Drug/Laboratory Test Interactions: Suprapharmacologic concentrations of lidocaine and meprobamate may inhibit fluorescence of PA and NAPA, and propranolol shows a native fluorescence close to the PA/NAPA peak wavelengths, so that tests which depend on fluorescence measurement may be affected.

Carcinogenesis, Mutagenesis, Impairment of Fertility: Long-term studies in animals have not been performed.

Pregnancy Category C: Animal reproduction studies have not been conducted with PA. It also is not known whether PA can cause fetal harm when administered to a pregnant woman or can affect reproduction capacity. PA should be given to a pregnant woman only if clearly needed.

Nursing Mothers: Both PA and NAPA are excreted in human milk, and absorbed by the nursing infant. Because of the potential for serious adverse reactions in nursing infants, a decision to discontinue nursing or the drug should be made, taking into account the importance of the drug to the mother.

Pediatric Use: Safety and effectiveness in pediatric patients have not been established.

Geriatric Use: Clinical studies of procainamide did not include sufficient numbers of subjects aged 65 and over to determine whether they respond differently from younger subjects. In general, dose selection for an elderly patient should be cautious, usually starting at the low end of the dosing range, reflecting the greater frequency of decreased hepatic, renal, or cardiac function, and of concomitant disease or other drug therapy. This drug is known to be substantially excreted by the kidney, and the risk of toxic reactions to the drug may be greater in patients with impaired renal function. Because elderly patients are more likely to have decreased renal function, care should be taken in dose selection, and it may be useful to monitor renal function by calculating creatinine clearance and to monitor the plasma levels of procainamide and its major metabolite, N-acetylprocainamide.

ADVERSE REACTIONS

Cardiovascular System: Hypotension following oral PA administration is rare. Hypotension and serious disturbances of cardiac rhythm such as ventricular asystole or fibrillation are more common after intravenous administration (see OVERDOSAGE, WARNINGS). Second degree heart block has been reported in 2 of almost 500 patients taking PA orally.

Multisystem Effects: A lupus erythematosus-like syndrome of arthralgia, pleural or abdominal pain, and sometimes arthritis, pleural effusion, pericarditis, fever, chills, myalgia, and possibly related hematologic or skin lesions (see below) is fairly common after prolonged PA administration, perhaps more often in patients who are slow acetylators (see Boxed Warning and PRECAUTIONS). While some studies have reported less than 1 in 500, others have reported the syndrome in up to 30% of patients on long-term oral PA therapy. If discontinuation of PA does not reverse the lupoid symptoms, corticosteroid treatment may be effective.

Hematologic System: Neutropenia, thrombocytopenia, or hemolytic anemia may rarely be encountered. Agranulocytosis has occurred after repeated use of PA, and deaths have been reported (see WARNINGS and Boxed Warning).

Skin: Angioneurotic edema, urticaria, pruritus, flushing, and maculopapular rash have also occurred occasionally.

Gastrointestinal System: Anorexia, nausea, vomiting, abdominal pain, bitter taste, or diarrhea may occur in 3 to 4 percent of patients taking oral procainamide.

Elevated Liver Enzymes: Elevations of transaminase with and without elevations of alkaline phosphatase and bilirubin have been reported in patients taking oral procainamide. Some patients have had clinical symptoms (e.g. malaise, right upper quadrant pain). Deaths from liver failure have been reported.

Nervous System: Dizziness or giddiness, weakness, mental depression, and psychosis with hallucinations have been reported occasionally.

OVERDOSAGE

Progressive widening of the QRS complex, prolonged Q-T and P-R intervals, lowering of the R and T waves, as well as increasing A-V block, may be seen with doses which are excessive for a given patient. Increased ventricular extrasystoles or even ventricular tachycardia or fibrillation may occur. After intravenous administration but seldom after oral therapy, transient high plasma concentrations of PA may induce hypotension, affecting systolic more than diastolic pressures, especially in hypertensive patients. Such high levels may also produce central nervous depression, tremor, and even respiratory depression.

Plasma levels above 10 mcg/mL are increasingly associated with toxic findings, which are seen occasionally in the 10 to 12 mcg/mL range, more often in the 12 to 15 mcg/mL range, and commonly in patients with plasma levels greater than 15 mcg/mL. A single oral dose of PA 2000 mg may produce overdosage symptoms, while 3000 mg of IR PA may be dangerous, especially if the patient is a slow acetylator, has decreased renal function, or underlying organic heart disease. Treatment of overdosage or toxic manifestations includes general supportive measures, close observation, monitoring of vital signs and possibly intravenous pressor agents, and mechanical cardiorespiratory support. If available, PA and NAPA plasma levels may be helpful in assessing the potential degree of toxicity and response to therapy. Both PA and NAPA are removed from the circulation by hemodialysis but not peritoneal dialysis. No specific antidote for PA is known.

DOSAGE AND ADMINISTRATION

The dose should be adjusted for the individual patient, based on clinical assessment of the degree of underlying myocardial disease, the patient's age, and renal function. For patients who have been receiving another formulation of procainamide, the dose of the other formulation can function as a general guide, but re-titration with Procanbid® is recommended.

As a general guide, for younger patients with normal renal function, an initial total daily oral dose of up to 50 mg/kg of body weight of Procanbid® tablets may be used, given in 2 divided doses, every 12 hours, to maintain therapeutic blood concentrations. For older patients, especially those over 50 years of age, or for patients with renal, hepatic, or cardiac insufficiency, lesser amounts or longer intervals may produce adequate blood concentrations, and decrease the probability of occurrence of dose-related adverse reactions.

CARE SHOULD BE TAKEN WHEN DISPENSING PROCANBID® TO ASSURE THE BID DOSAGE FORM HAS BEEN PRESCRIBED AND DISPENSED. Procanbid® tablets should be swallowed whole and should not be bitten or cut.

To provide up to 50 mg/kg of body weight per day*

Patients Weighing	Dose
88–110 lb (40–50 kg)	1000 mg q12 hrs
132–154 lb (60–70 kg)	1500 mg q12 hrs
176–198 lb (80–90 kg)	2000 mg q12 hrs
>220 lb (>100 kg)	2500 mg q12 hrs

*Initial dosage schedule guide only, to be adjusted for each patient individually, based on age, cardiorenal function, blood concentration (if available), and clinical response.

HOW SUPPLIED

Procanbid® tablets are supplied as follows:

500 mg: White, film-coated, elliptical tablets, coded "PROCANBID" on one side and "500" on the other.

NDC 61570-069-60 Bottles of 60
NDC 61570-069-70 Unit dose packages of 100 (10 strips of 10 tablets each).

1000 mg: Gray, film-coated, elliptical tablets, coded "PROCANBID" on one side and "1000" on the other.

NDC 61570-071-60 Bottles of 60
NDC 61570-071-70 Unit dose packages of 100 (10 strips of 10 tablets each).

Dispense in well-closed containers as defined in the USP.

Store at 20°–25°C (68°–77°F) [see USP].

Rx Only.

Distributed by: Monarch Pharmaceuticals, Inc., Bristol, TN 37620

Manufactured by: Warner-Lambert Co, Morris Plains, NJ 07950

Rev. 3/00
0562G121

Shown in Product Identification Guide, page 325

PROCTOCORT® ℞
Hydrocortisone Acetate
Rectal Suppositories, 30 mg

DESCRIPTION

Hydrocortisone Acetate is a corticosteroid designated chemically as pregn-4-ene-3, 20-dione, 21-(acetyloxy)-11, 17-dihydroxy-(11β) with the following structural formula:

$C_{23}H_{32}O_6$
MW 404.51

Each rectal suppository contains hydrocortisone acetate, USP 30 mg in a specially blended hydrogenated vegetable oil base.

CLINICAL PHARMACOLOGY

In normal subjects, about 26% of hydrocortisone acetate is absorbed when the suppository is applied to the rectum. Absorption of hydrocortisone acetate may vary across abraded or inflamed surfaces. Topical steroids are primarily effective because of their anti-inflammatory, anti-pruritic and vasoconstrictive action.

INDICATIONS AND USAGE

Proctocort® Suppositories are indicated for use in inflamed hemorrhoids, postirradiation (factitial) proctitis; as an adjunct in the treatment of chronic ulcerative colitis; cryptitis; and other inflammatory conditions of anorectum and pruritus ani.

CONTRAINDICATIONS

Proctocort® Suppositories are contraindicated in those patients having a history of hypersensitivity to hydrocortisone acetate or any of the components.

PRECAUTIONS

Do not use Proctocort® Suppositories unless adequate proctologic examination is made.

If irritation develops, the product should be discontinued and appropriate therapy instituted.

In the presence of an infection, the use of an appropriate antifungal or antibacterial agent should be instituted. If a favorable response does not occur promptly, Proctocort® Suppositories should be discontinued until the infection has been adequately controlled.

Carcinogenesis: No long term studies in animals have been performed to evaluate the carcinogenic potential of corticosteroid suppositories.

Pregnancy Category C: In laboratory animals, topical steroids have been associated with an increase in the incidence of fetal abnormalities when gestating females have been exposed to rather low dosage levels. There are no adequate and well controlled studies in pregnant women. Proctocort® Suppositories should only be used during pregnancy if the potential benefit justifies the risk to the fetus. Drugs of this class should not be used extensively on pregnant patients, in large amounts, or for prolonged periods of time.

It is not known whether this drug is excreted in human milk and because many drugs are excreted in human milk and because of the potential for serious adverse reactions in nursing infants from Proctocort® Suppositories, a decision should be made whether to discontinue nursing or to discontinue the drug, taking into account the importance of the drug to the mother.

ADVERSE REACTIONS

The following local adverse reactions have been reported with hydrocortisone acetate suppositories; burning, itching, irritation, dryness, folliculitis, hypopigmentation, allergic contact dermatitis, secondary infection.

DRUG ABUSE AND DEPENDENCE

Drug abuse and dependence have not been reported in patients treated with hydrocortisone acetate suppositories.

OVERDOSAGE

If signs and symptoms of systemic overdosage occur, discontinue use.

DOSAGE AND ADMINISTRATION

For rectal administration. Detach one suppository from strip of suppositories. Remove the foil wrapper. Avoid excessive handling of the suppository which is designed to melt at body temperature. Insert suppository into the rectum with gentle pressure, pointed end first. Insert one suppository in the rectum twice daily, morning and night for two weeks, in nonspecific proctitis. In more severe cases, one suppository three times a day or two suppositories twice daily. In factitial proctitis, the recommended duration of therapy is six to eight weeks or less, according to the response of the individual case.

HOW SUPPLIED

Box of 12 suppositories—NDC 61570-025-12
Box of 24 suppositories—NDC 61570-025-25

Rx only.

Store at controlled room temperature 15°–30°C (59°–86°F).

Distributed by: Monarch Pharmaceuticals, Inc., Bristol, TN 37620

Manufactured by: King Pharmaceuticals, Inc., Bristol, TN 37620

2/99
0932938

Shown in Product Identification Guide, page 325

PROCTOCORT® ℞
Hydrocortisone Cream USP, 1%

DESCRIPTION

PROCTOCORT® 1% Cream is a Synthetic Steroid used as anti-inflammatory and antipruritic agent. It's chemical name is Pregn-4-ene-3,20-dione, 11,17,21-trihydroxy-, (11β)-With empirical formula $C_{21}H_{30}O_5$ and molecular weight 362.47. Structural formula is:

Hydrocortisone

PROCTOCORT® 1% Cream (Each gram contains 10 mg of Hydrocortisone) in a base containing Purified Water, Propylene Glycol, Propylene Glycol Stearate, Mineral Oil and Lanolin Alcohol, Isopropyl Palmitate, Polysorbate 60, Cetyl Alcohol, Sorbitan Monostearate, Polyoxyl 40 Stearate, Sorbic Acid, Methylparaben and Propylparaben.

CLINICAL PHARMACOLOGY

Topical corticosteroids share anti-inflammatory, antipruritic and vasoconstrictive actions.

The mechanism of anti-inflammatory activity of topical corticosteroids is unclear. Various laboratory methods, including vasoconstrictor assays, are used to compare and predict potencies and/or clinical efficacies of the topical corticosteroids. There is some evidence to suggest that a recognizable correlation exists between vasoconstrictor potency and therapeutic efficacy in man.

Pharmacokinetics

The extent of percutaneous absorption of topical cortiscosteroids is determined by many factors including the vehicle, the integrity of the epidermal barrier, and the use of occlusive dressings.

Topical cortiscosteroids can be absorbed from normal intact skin. Inflammation and/or other disease processes in the skin increase percutaneous absorption. Occlusive dressings substantially increase the percutaneous absorption of topical corticosteroids. Thus, occlusive dressings may be a valuable therapeutic adjunct for treatment of resistant dermatoses. (See **DOSAGE AND ADMINISTRATION**.)

Once absorbed through the skin, topical corticosteroids are handled through pharmacokinetic pathways similar to systemically administered corticosteroids. Corticosteroids are bound to plasma proteins in varying degrees. Corticosteroids are metabolized primarily in the liver and are then excreted by the kidneys. Some of the topical corticosteroids and their metabolites are also excreted into the bile.

INDICATIONS AND USAGE

Topical corticosteroids are indicated for relief of the inflammatory and pruritic manifestations of corticosteroid-responsive dermatoses.

CONTRAINDICATIONS

Topical corticosteroids are contraindicated in those patients with a history of hypersensitivity to any of the components of the preparation.

PRECAUTIONS

General

Systemic absorption of topical corticosteroids has produced reversible hypothalamic-pituitary-adrenal (HPA) axis suppression, manifestations of Cushing's syndrome, hyperglycemia, and glucosuria in some patients.

Conditions which augment systemic absorption include the application of the more potent steroids, use over large surface areas, prolonged use, and the addition of occlusive dressings.

Continued on next page

Proctocort Cream—Cont.

Therefore, patients receiving a large dose of potent topical steroid applied to a large surface area or under an occlusive dressing should be evaluated periodically for evidence of HPA axis suppression by using the urinary free cortisol and ACTH stimulation tests. If HPA axis suppression is noted, an attempt should be made to withdraw the drug, to reduce the frequency of application, or to substitute a less potent steroid.
Recovery of HPA axis function is generally prompt and complete upon discontinuation of the drug. Infrequently, signs and symptoms of steroid withdrawal may occur, requiring supplemental systemic corticosteroids.
Children may absorb proportionally larger amounts of topical corticosteroids and thus be more susceptible to systemic toxicity. (See **PRECAUTIONS—Pediatric Use**.)
If irritation develops, topical corticosteroids should be discontinued and appropriate therapy instituted.
In the presence of dermatological infections, the use of an appropriate antifungal or antibacterial agent should be instituted. If a favorable response does not occur promptly, the corticosteroid should be discontinued until the infection has been adequately controlled.

Information for the Patient
Patients using topical corticosteroids should receive the following information and instructions:

1. This medication is to be used as directed by the physician. It is for external use only. Avoid contact with the eyes.
2. Patients should be advised not to use this medication for any disorder other than for which it was prescribed.
3. The treated skin area should not be bandaged or otherwise covered or wrapped as to be occlusive unless directed by the physician.
4. Patients should report any signs of local adverse reactions especially under occlusive dressings.
5. Parents of pediatric patients should be advised not to use tight-fitting diapers or plastic pants on a child being treated in the diaper area, as these garments may constitute occlusive dressings.

Laboratory Tests
The following tests may be helpful in evaluating the HPA axis suppression:
Urinary free cortisol test
ACTH stimulation test

Carcinogenesis, Mutagenesis, and Impairment of Fertility
Long-term animal studies have not been performed to evaluate the carcinogenic potential or the effect on fertility of topical corticosteroids.
Studies to determine mutagenicity with prednisolone and hydrocortisone have revealed negative results.

Pregnancy Category C
Corticosteroids are generally teratogenic in laboratory animals when administered systemically at relatively low dosage levels. The more potent corticosteroids have been shown to be teratogenic after dermal application in laboratory animals. There are no adequate and well-controlled studies in pregnant women on teratogenic effects from topically applied corticosteroids. Therefore, topical corticosteroids should be used during pregnancy only if the potential benefit justifies the potential risk to the fetus. Drugs of this class should not be used extensively on pregnant patients, in large amounts, or for prolonged periods of time.

Nursing Mothers
It is not known whether topical administration of corticosteroids could result in sufficient systemic absorption to produce detectable quantities in breast milk. Systemically administered corticosteroids are secreted into breast milk in quantities *not* likely to have a deleterious effect on the infant. Nevertheless, caution should be exercised when topical corticosteroids are adminstered to a nursing woman.

Pediatric Use
Pediatric patients may demonstrate greater susceptibility to topical corticosteroid-induced HPA axis suppression and Cushing's syndrome than mature patients because of a larger skin surface area to body weight ratio.
Hypothalamic-pituitary-adrenal (HPA) axis suppression, Cushing's syndrome, and intracranial hypertension have been reported in pediatric patients receiving topical corticosteroids. Manifestations of adrenal suppression in pediatric patients include linear growth retardation, delayed weight gain, low plasma cortisol levels, and absence of response to ACTH stimulation. Manifestations of intracranial hypertension include bulging fontanelles, headaches, and bilateral papilledema. Administration of topical corticosteroids to pediatric patients should be limited to the least amount compatible with an effective therapeutic regimen. Chronic corticosteroid therapy may interfere with the growth and development of pediatric patients.

ADVERSE REACTIONS

The following local adverse reactions are reported infrequently with topical corticosteroids, but may occur more frequently with the use of occlusive dressings. These reactions are listed in an approximate decreasing order of occurrence:
Burning
Itching
Irritation
Dryness
Folliculitis
Hypertrichosis
Acneiform eruptions
Hypopigmentation
Perioral dermatitis
Allergic contact dermatitis
Maceration of the skin
Secondary infection
Skin Atrophy
Striae
Miliaria

OVERDOSAGE

Topically applied corticosteroids can be absorbed in sufficient amounts to produce systemic effects (See **PRECAUTIONS**).

DOSAGE AND ADMINISTRATION

Topical corticosteroids are generally applied to the affected area as a thin film from two to four times daily depending on the severity of the condition.
Occlusive dressings may be used for the management of psoriasis or recalcitrant conditions.
If an infection develops, the use of occlusive dressings should be discontinued and appropriate antimicrobial therapy instituted.

HOW SUPPLIED

PROCTOCORT® (Hydrocortisone) 1% Cream is supplied in 1 oz (28.35 g) tubes. (NDC 61570-070-01).
Store at controlled room temperature 15°–30°C (59°–86°F).
Protect from freezing.
Rx only.
Manufactured by: Thames Pharmacal Co., Inc., Ronkonkoma, NY 11779
Distributed by: Monarch Pharmaceuticals, Inc. Bristol, TN 37620

Rev. 7/00
0934092

SEPTRA® I.V. Infusion ℞

[*sĕp 'tra*]
(trimethoprim and sulfamethoxazole)

DESCRIPTION

SEPTRA I.V. Infusion (trimethoprim and sulfamethoxazole), a sterile solution for intravenous infusion only, is a synthetic antibacterial combination product. Each mL contains 16 mg trimethoprim and 80 mg sulfamethoxazole compounded with 40% propylene glycol, 10% ethyl alcohol, and 0.3% diethanolamine; 1% benzyl alcohol and 0.1% sodium metabisulfite added as preservatives, Water for Injection, and pH adjusted to approximately 10 with sodium hydroxide.
Trimethoprim is 5-[(3,4,5-trimethoxyphenyl)methyl]-2,4-pyrimidinediamine. It is a white to light yellow, odorless, bitter compound with a molecular weight of 290.32 and the molecular formula $C_{14}H_{18}N_4O_3$. The structural formula is:

N NH₂ CH₂ N NH₂ CH₃O OCH₃ OCH₃

Sulfamethoxazole is 4-amino-*N*-(5-methyl-3-isoxazolyl)benzenesulfonamide. It is an almost white, odorless, tasteless compound with a molecular weight of 253.28 and the molecular formula $C_{10}H_{11}N_3O_3S$. The structural formula is:

H₂N SO₂NH N O CH₃

CLINICAL PHARMACOLOGY

Following a 1-hour intravenous infusion of a single dose of 160 mg trimethoprim and 800 mg sulfamethoxazole to 11 patients whose weight ranged from 105 lb to 165 lb (mean, 143 lb), the mean peak plasma concentrations of trimethoprim and sulfamethoxazole were 3.4 ± 0.3 mcg/mL and 46.3 ± 2.7 mcg/mL, respectively. Following repeated intravenous administration of the same dose at 8-hour intervals, the mean plasma concentrations just prior to and immediately after each infusion at steady-state were 5.6 ± 0.6 mcg/mL and 8.8 ± 0.9 mcg/mL for trimethoprim and 70.6 ± 7.3 mcg/mL and 105.6 ± 10.9 mcg/mL for sulfamethoxazole. The mean plasma half-life was 11.3 ± 0.7 hours for trimethoprim and 12.8 ± 1.8 hours for sulfamethoxazole. All of these 11 patients had normal renal function and their ages ranged from 17 to 78 years (median, 60 years).[1]
Pharmacokinetic studies in pediatric patients and adults suggest an age-dependent half-life of trimethoprim as indicated in the following table.[2]

Age (years)	No. of Patients	Mean TMP Half-life (hours)
<1	2	7.67
1-10	9	5.49
10-20	5	8.19
20-63	6	12.82

Patients with severely impaired renal function exhibit an increase in the half-lives of both components, requiring dosage regimen adjustment (see DOSAGE AND ADMINISTRATION).
Both trimethoprim and sulfamethoxazole exist in the blood as unbound, protein-bound, and metabolized forms; sulfamethoxazole also exists as the conjugated form. The metabolism of sulfamethoxazole occurs predominately by N_4-acetylation, although the glucuronide conjugate has been identified. The principal metabolites of trimethoprim are the 1- and 3-oxides and the 3'- and 4'-hydroxy derivatives. The free forms of trimethoprim and sulfamethoxazole are considered to be the therapeutically active forms. Approximately 44% of trimethoprim and 70% of sulfamethoxazole are bound to plasma proteins. The presence of 10 mg percent sulfamethoxazole in plasma decreases the protein binding of trimethoprim by an insignificant degree; trimethoprim does not influence the protein binding of sulfamethoxazole.
Excretion of trimethoprim and sulfamethoxazole is primarily by the kidneys through both glomerular filtration and tubular secretion. Urine concentrations of both trimethoprim and sulfamethoxazole are considerably higher than are the concentrations in the blood. The percent of dose excreted in urine over a 12-hour period following the intravenous administration of the first dose of 240 mg of trimethoprim and 1,200 mg of sulfamethoxazole on day 1 ranged from 17% to 42.4% as free trimethoprim; 7% to 12.7% as free sulfamethoxazole; and 36.7% to 56% as total (free plus the N_4-acetylated metabolite) sulfamethoxazole. When administered together as SEPTRA, neither trimethoprim nor sulfamethoxazole affects the urinary excretion pattern of the other.
Both trimethoprim and sulfamethoxazole distribute to sputum and vaginal fluid; trimethoprim also distributes to bronchial secretions, and both pass the placental barrier and are excreted in human milk.
Microbiology: Sulfamethoxazole inhibits bacterial synthesis of dihydrofolic acid by competing with *para*-aminobenzoic acid (PABA). Trimethoprim blocks the production of tetrahydrofolic acid from dihydrofolic acid by binding to and reversibly inhibiting the required enzyme, dihydrofolate reductase. Thus, SEPTRA blocks two consecutive steps in the biosynthesis of nucleic acids and proteins essential to many bacteria.
In vitro studies have shown that bacterial resistance develops more slowly with SEPTRA than with trimethoprim or sulfamethoxazole alone.
In vitro serial dilution tests have shown that the spectrum of antibacterial activity of SEPTRA includes common bacterial pathogens with the exception of *Pseudomonas aeruginosa*. The following organisms are usually susceptible: *Escherichia coli, Klebsiella* species, *Enterobacter* species, *Morganella morganii, Proteus mirabilis*, indole-positive *Proteus* species, including *Proteus vulgaris, Haemophilus influenzae* (including ampicillin-resistant strains), *Streptococcus pneumoniae, Shigella flexneri*, and *Shigella sonnei*. It should be noted, however, that there are little clinical data on the use of SEPTRA I.V. Infusion in serious systemic infections due to *Haemophilus influenzae* and *Streptococcus pneumoniae*.
[See table below]
Susceptibility Testing: The recommended quantitative disc susceptibility method may be used for estimating the sus-

Representative Minimum Inhibitory Concentration Values for Organisms Susceptible to SEPTRA (MIC-mcg/mL)

Bacteria	TMP Alone	SMX Alone	TMP/SMX (1:19)	
			TMP	SMX
Escherichia coli	0.05-1.5	1.0-245	0.05-0.5	0.95-9.5
Proteus species (indole positive)	0.5-5.0	7.35-300	0.05-1.5	0.95-28.5
Morganella morganii	0.5-5.0	7.35-300	0.05-1.5	0.95-28.5
Proteus mirabilis	0.5-1.5	7.35-30	0.05-0.15	0.95-2.85
Klebsiella species	0.15-5.0	2.45-245	0.05-1.5	0.95-28.5
Enterobacter species	0.15-5.0	2.45-245	0.05-1.5	0.95-28.5
Haemophilus influenzae	0.15-1.5	2.85-95	0.015-0.15	0.285-2.85
Streptococcus pneumoniae	0.15-1.5	7.35-24.5	0.05-0.15	0.95-2.85
*Shigella flexneri**	<0.01-0.04	<0.16->320	<0.002-0.03	0.04-0.625
*Shigella sonnei**	0.02-0.08	0.625->320	0.004-0.06	0.08-1.25

TMP = trimethoprim SMX = sulfamethoxazole
*Rudoy RC, Nelson JD, Haltalin KC. *Antimicrobial Agents and Chemotherapy.* 1974;5:439-443.

ceptibility of bacteria to SEPTRA.[3,4] With this procedure, a report from the laboratory of "Susceptible to trimethoprim and sulfamethoxazole" indicates that the infection is likely to respond to therapy with SEPTRA. If the infection is confined to the urine, a report of "Intermediate susceptibility to trimethoprim and sulfamethoxazole" also indicates that the infection is likely to respond. A report of "Resistant to trimethoprim and sulfamethoxazole" indicates that the infection is unlikely to respond to therapy with SEPTRA.

INDICATIONS AND USAGE

***Pneumocystis Carinii* Pneumonia**: SEPTRA I.V. Infusion is indicated in the treatment of *Pneumocystis carinii* pneumonia in pediatric patients and adults.

Shigellosis: SEPTRA I.V. Infusion is indicated in the treatment of enteritis caused by susceptible strains of *Shigella flexneri* and *Shigella sonnei* in pediatric patients and adults.

Urinary Tract Infections: SEPTRA I.V. Infusion is indicated in the treatment of severe or complicated urinary tract infections due to susceptible strains of *Escherichia coli*, *Klebsiella* species, *Enterobacter* species, *Morganella morganii*, and *Proteus* species when oral administration of SEPTRA is not feasible and when the organism is not susceptible to single-agent antibacterials effective in the urinary tract.

Although appropriate culture and susceptibility studies should be performed, therapy may be started while awaiting the results of these studies.

CONTRAINDICATIONS

SEPTRA is contraindicated in patients with a known hypersensitivity to trimethoprim or sulfonamides and in patients with documented megaloblastic anemia due to folate deficiency. SEPTRA is also contraindicated in pregnant patients at term and in nursing mothers, because sulfonamides pass the placenta and are excreted in the milk and may cause kernicterus. SEPTRA is contraindicated in pediatric patients less than 2 months of age.

WARNINGS

FATALITIES ASSOCIATED WITH THE ADMINISTRATION OF SULFONAMIDES, ALTHOUGH RARE, HAVE OCCURRED DUE TO SEVERE REACTIONS, INCLUDING STEVENS-JOHNSON SYNDROME, TOXIC EPIDERMAL NECROLYSIS, FULMINANT HEPATIC NECROSIS, AGRANULOCYTOSIS, APLASTIC ANEMIA, AND OTHER BLOOD DYSCRASIAS.

SULFONAMIDES, INCLUDING SULFONAMIDE-CONTAINING PRODUCTS SUCH AS TRIMETHOPRIM/SULFAMETHOXAZOLE, SHOULD BE DISCONTINUED AT THE FIRST APPEARANCE OF SKIN RASH OR ANY SIGN OF ADVERSE REACTION. In rare instances, a skin rash may be followed by a more severe reaction, such as Stevens-Johnson syndrome, toxic epidermal necrolysis, hepatic necrosis, and serious blood disorders (see PRECAUTIONS).

Clinical signs, such as rash, sore throat, fever, arthralgia, pallor, purpura, or jaundice may be early indications of serious reactions.

Cough, shortness of breath, and pulmonary infiltrates are hypersensitivity reactions of the respiratory tract that have been reported in association with sulfonamide treatment.

The sulfonamides should not be used for the treatment of group A beta-hemolytic streptococcal infections. In an established infection, they will not eradicate the streptococcus and, therefore, will not prevent sequelae such as rheumatic fever.

Pseudomembranous colitis has been reported with nearly all antibacterial agents, including trimethoprim/sulfamethoxazole, and may range in severity from mild to life-threatening. Therefore, it is important to consider this diagnosis in patients who present with diarrhea subsequent to the administration of antibacterial agents.

Treatment with antibacterial agents alters the normal flora of the colon and may permit overgrowth of clostridia. Studies indicate that a toxin produced by *Clostridium difficile* is one primary cause of "antibiotic-associated colitis."

After the diagnosis of pseudomembranous colitis has been established, therapeutic measures should be initiated. Mild cases of pseudomembranous colitis usually respond to drug discontinuation alone. In moderate to severe cases, consideration should be given to management with fluids and electrolytes, protein supplementation, and treatment with an antibacterial drug effective against *C. difficile*.

Contains sodium metabisulfite, a sulfite that may cause allergic-type reactions including anaphylactic symptoms and life-threatening or less severe asthmatic episodes in certain susceptible people. The overall prevalence of sulfite sensitivity in the general population is unknown and probably low. Sulfite sensitivity is seen more frequently in asthmatic than in nonasthmatic people.

Contains benzyl alcohol. In newborn infants, benzyl alcohol has been associated with an increased incidence of neurological and other complications which are sometimes fatal.

PRECAUTIONS

General: SEPTRA should be given with caution to patients with impaired renal or hepatic function, to those with possible folate deficiency (e.g., the elderly, chronic alcoholics, patients receiving anticonvulsant therapy, patients with malabsorption syndrome, and patients in malnutrition states), and to those with severe allergy or bronchial asthma. In glucose-6-phosphate dehydrogenase-deficient individuals, hemolysis may occur. This reaction is frequently dose-related. Adequate fluid intake must be maintained in order to prevent crystalluria and stone formation (see CLINICAL PHARMACOLOGY and DOSAGE AND ADMINISTRATION).

Local irritation and inflammation due to extravascular infiltration of the infusion has been observed with SEPTRA I.V. Infusion. If these occur, the infusion should be discontinued and restarted at another site.

Use in the Elderly: There may be an increased risk of severe adverse reactions in elderly patients, particularly when complicating conditions exist, e.g., impaired kidney and/or liver function, or concomitant use of other drugs. Severe skin reactions, or generalized bone marrow suppression (see WARNINGS and ADVERSE REACTIONS), or a specific decrease in platelets (with or without purpura) are the most frequently reported severe adverse reactions in elderly patients. In those concurrently receiving certain diuretics, primarily thiazides, an increased incidence of thrombocytopenia with purpura has been reported. Appropriate dosage adjustments should be made for patients with impaired kidney function (see DOSAGE AND ADMINISTRATION).

Use in the Treatment of *Pneumocystis carinii* Pneumonia in Patients with Acquired Immunodeficiency Syndrome (AIDS): The incidence of side effects, particularly rash, fever, leukopenia, and elevated aminotransferase (transaminase) values in AIDS patients who are being treated with SEPTRA for *Pneumocystis carinii* pneumonia has been reported to be greatly increased compared with the incidence normally associated with the use of SEPTRA in non-AIDS patients. The incidence of hyperkalemia and hyponatremia appears to be increased in AIDS patients receiving SEPTRA.

The concomitant use of leucovorin with trimethoprim-sulfamethoxazole for the acute treatment of *Pneumocystis carinii* pneumonia in patients with HIV infection was associated with increased rates of treatment failure and morbidity in a placebo-controlled study.

Laboratory Tests: Appropriate culture and susceptibility studies should be performed before and throughout treatment. Complete blood counts should be done frequently in patients receiving SEPTRA; if a significant reduction in the count of any formed blood element is noted, SEPTRA should be discontinued. Urinalyses with careful microscopic examination and renal function tests should be performed during therapy, particularly for those patients with impaired renal function.

Drug Interactions: In elderly patients concurrently receiving certain diuretics, primarily thiazides, an increased incidence of thrombocytopenia with purpura has been reported. It has been reported that SEPTRA may prolong the prothrombin time in patients who are receiving the anticoagulant warfarin. This interaction should be kept in mind when SEPTRA is given to patients already on anticoagulant therapy, and the coagulation time should be reassessed.

SEPTRA may inhibit the hepatic metabolism of phenytoin. SEPTRA, given at a common clinical dosage, increased the phenytoin half-life by 39% and decreased the phenytoin metabolic clearance rate by 27%. When administering these drugs concurrently, one should be alert for possible excessive phenytoin effect.

Sulfonamides can also displace methotrexate from plasma protein binding sites, thus increasing free methotrexate concentrations.

Drug/Laboratory Test Interactions: SEPTRA, specifically the trimethoprim component, can interfere with a serum methotrexate assay as determined by the competitive binding protein technique (CBPA) when a bacterial dihydrofolate reductase is used as the binding protein. No interference occurs, however, if methotrexate is measured by a radioimmunoassay (RIA).

The presence of trimethoprim and sulfamethoxazole may also interfere with the Jaffé alkaline picrate reaction assay for creatinine, resulting in over-estimations of about 10% in the range of normal values.

Carcinogenesis, Mutagenesis, Impairment of Fertility: ***Carcinogenesis:*** Long-term studies in animals to evaluate carcinogenic potential have not been conducted with SEPTRA I.V. Infusion.

Mutagenesis: Bacterial mutagenic studies have not been performed with sulfamethoxazole and trimethoprim in combination. Trimethoprim was demonstrated to be non-mutagenic in the Ames assay. In studies at two laboratories, no chromosomal damage was detected in cultured Chinese hamster ovary cells at concentrations approximately 500 times human plasma levels; at concentrations approximately 1,000 times human plasma levels in these same cells, a low level of chromosomal damage was induced at one of the laboratories. No chromosomal abnormalities were observed in cultured human leukocytes at concentrations of trimethoprim up to 20 times human steady-state plasma levels. No chromosomal effects were detected in peripheral lymphocytes of human subjects receiving 320 mg of trimethoprim in combination with up to 1,600 mg of sulfamethoxazole per day for as long as 112 weeks.

Impairment of Fertility: SEPTRA I.V. Infusion has not been studied in animals for evidence of impairment of fertility. However, studies in rats at oral dosages as high as 70 mg/kg trimethoprim plus 350 mg/kg sulfamethoxazole daily showed no adverse effects on fertility or general reproductive performance.

Pregnancy: ***Teratogenic Effects:*** Pregnancy Category C. In rats, oral doses of 533 mg/kg sulfamethoxazole or 200 mg/kg trimethoprim produced teratological effects manifested mainly as cleft palates. The highest dose which did not cause cleft palates in rats was 512 mg/kg sulfamethoxazole or 192 mg/kg trimethoprim when administered separately. In two studies in rats, no teratogenicity was observed when 512 mg/kg of sulfamethoxazole was used in combination with 128 mg/kg of trimethoprim. In one study, however, cleft palates were observed in one litter out of nine when 355 mg/kg of sulfamethoxazole was used in combination with 88 mg/kg of trimethoprim.

In some rabbit studies, an overall increase in fetal loss (dead and resorbed and malformed conceptuses) was associated with doses of trimethoprim six times the human therapeutic dose.

While there are no large, well-controlled studies on the use of trimethoprim and sulfamethoxazole in pregnant women, Brumfitt and Pursell,[5] in a retrospective study, reported the outcome of 186 pregnancies during which the mother received either placebo or oral trimethoprim and sulfamethoxazole. The incidence of congenital abnormalities was 4.5% (3 of 66) in those who received placebo and 3.3% (4 of 120) in those receiving trimethoprim and sulfamethoxazole. There were no abnormalities in the 10 children whose mothers received the drug during the first trimester. In a separate survey, Brumfitt and Pursell also found no congenital abnormalities in 35 children whose mothers had received oral trimethoprim and sulfamethoxazole at the time of conception or shortly thereafter.

Because trimethoprim and sulfamethoxazole may interfere with folic acid metabolism, SEPTRA I.V. Infusion should be used during pregnancy only if the potential benefit justifies the potential risk to the fetus.

Nonteratogenic Effects: See CONTRAINDICATIONS section.

Nursing Mothers: See CONTRAINDICATIONS section.

Pediatric Use: SEPTRA I.V. Infusion is not recommended for pediatric patients younger than 2 months of age (see CONTRAINDICATIONS).

ADVERSE REACTIONS

The most common adverse effects are gastrointestinal disturbances (nausea, vomiting, anorexia) and allergic skin reactions (such as rash and urticaria). **FATALITIES ASSOCIATED WITH THE ADMINISTRATION OF SULFONAMIDES, ALTHOUGH RARE, HAVE OCCURRED DUE TO SEVERE REACTIONS, INCLUDING STEVENS-JOHNSON SYNDROME, TOXIC EPIDERMAL NECROLYSIS, FULMINANT HEPATIC NECROSIS, AGRANULOCYTOSIS, APLASTIC ANEMIA, OTHER BLOOD DYSCRASIAS, AND HYPERSENSITIVITY OF THE RESPIRATORY TRACT (SEE WARNINGS).** Local reaction, pain, and slight irritation on I.V. administration are infrequent. Thrombophlebitis has rarely been observed.

Hematologic: Agranulocytosis, aplastic anemia, thrombocytopenia, leukopenia, neutropenia, hemolytic anemia, megaloblastic anemia, hypoprothrombinemia, methemoglobinemia, eosinophilia.

Allergic: Stevens-Johnson syndrome, toxic epidermal necrolysis, anaphylaxis, allergic myocarditis, erythema multiforme, exfoliative dermatitis, angioedema, drug fever, chills, Henoch-Schönlein purpura, serum sickness-like syndrome, generalized allergic reactions, generalized skin eruptions, conjunctival and scleral injection, photosensitivity, pruritus, urticaria, and rash. In addition, periarteritis nodosa and systemic lupus erythematosus have been reported.

Gastrointestinal: Hepatitis, including cholestatic jaundice and hepatic necrosis, elevation of serum transaminase and bilirubin, pseudomembranous enterocolitis, pancreatitis, stomatitis, glossitis, nausea, emesis, abdominal pain, diarrhea, anorexia.

Genitourinary: Renal failure, interstitial nephritis, BUN and serum creatinine elevation, toxic nephrosis with oliguria and anuria, and crystalluria.

Metabolic: Hyperkalemia, hyponatremia.

Neurologic: Aseptic meningitis, convulsions, peripheral neuritis, ataxia, vertigo, tinnitus, headache.

Psychiatric: Hallucinations, depression, apathy, nervousness.

Endocrine: The sulfonamides bear certain chemical similarities to some goitrogens, diuretics (acetazolamide and the thiazides), and oral hypoglycemic agents. Cross-sensitivity may exist with these agents. Diuresis and hypoglycemia have occurred rarely in patients receiving sulfonamides.

Musculoskeletal: Arthralgia and myalgia.

Respiratory System: Cough, shortness of breath, and pulmonary infiltrates (see WARNINGS).

Miscellaneous: Weakness, fatigue, insomnia.

OVERDOSAGE

Acute: Since there has been no extensive experience in humans with single doses of SEPTRA I.V. Infusion in excess of 25 mL (400 mg trimethoprim and 2,000 mg sulfamethoxazole), the maximum tolerated dose in humans is unknown. Signs and symptoms of overdosage reported with sulfonamides include anorexia, colic, nausea, vomiting, dizziness, headache, drowsiness, and unconsciousness. Pyrexia, hematuria, and crystalluria may be noted. Blood dyscrasias and jaundice are potential late manifestations of overdosage. Signs of acute overdosage with trimethoprim include nausea, vomiting, dizziness, headache, mental depression, confusion, and bone marrow depression.

General principles of treatment include the administration of intravenous fluids if urine output is low and renal function is normal. Acidification of the urine will increase renal elimination of trimethoprim.

The patient should be monitored with blood counts and appropriate blood chemistries, including electrolytes. If a significant blood dyscrasia or jaundice occurs, specific therapy

Continued on next page

Septra I.V. Infusion—Cont.

should be instituted for these complications. Peritoneal dialysis is not effective and hemodialysis is only moderately effective in eliminating trimethoprim and sulfamethoxazole.

Chronic: Use of SEPTRA I.V. Infusion at high doses and/or for extended periods of time may cause bone marrow depression manifested as thrombocytopenia, leukopenia, and/or megaloblastic anemia. If signs of bone marrow depression occur, the patient should be given leucovorin; 5 to 15 mg leucovorin daily has been recommended by some investigators.

Animal Toxicity: The LD_{50} of SEPTRA I.V. Infusion in mice is 700 mg/kg or 7.3 mL/kg; in rats and rabbits the LD_{50} is >500 mg/kg or >5.2 mL/kg. The vehicle produced the same LD_{50} in each of these species as the active drug.

The signs and symptoms noted in mice, rats, and rabbits with SEPTRA I.V. Infusion or its vehicle at the high I.V. doses used in acute toxicity studies included ataxia, decreased motor activity, loss of righting reflex, tremors or convulsions, and/or respiratory depression.

DOSAGE AND ADMINISTRATION

CONTRAINDICATED IN PEDIATRIC PATIENTS LESS THAN 2 MONTHS OF AGE. CAUTION-SEPTRA I.V. INFUSION MUST BE DILUTED IN 5% DEXTROSE IN WATER SOLUTION PRIOR TO ADMINISTRATION. DO NOT MIX SEPTRA I.V. INFUSION WITH OTHER DRUGS OR SOLUTIONS. RAPID INFUSION OR BOLUS INJECTION MUST BE AVOIDED.

Dosage: ***Pediatric Patients and Adults:***

Pneumocystis Carinii Pneumonia: Total daily dose is 15 to 20 mg/kg (based on the trimethoprim component) given in three to four equally divided doses every 6 or 8 hours for up to 14 days. One investigator noted that a total daily dose of 10 to 15 mg/kg was sufficient in 10 adult patients with normal renal function.[6]

Severe Urinary Tract Infections and Shigellosis: Total daily dose is 8 to 10 mg/kg (based on the trimethoprim component) given in two to four equally divided doses every 6, 8, or 12 hours for up to 14 days for severe urinary tract infections and 5 days for shigellosis. The maximum recommended daily dose is 60 mL per day.

For Patients with Impaired Renal Function: When renal function is impaired, a reduced dosage should be employed using the following table:

Creatinine Clearance (mL/min)	Recommended Dosage Regimen
Above 30	Use Standard Regimen
15-30	½ the Usual Regimen
Below 15	Use Not Recommended

Method of Preparation: SEPTRA I.V. Infusion must be diluted. EACH 5 mL SHOULD BE ADDED TO 125 mL OF 5% DEXTROSE IN WATER. After diluting with 5% dextrose in water, the solution should not be refrigerated and should be used within 6 hours. If a dilution of 5 mL per 100 mL of 5% dextrose in water is desired, it should be used within 4 hours. If upon visual inspection there is cloudiness or evidence of crystallization after mixing, the solution should be discarded and a fresh solution prepared.

Multiple-Dose Vial: After initial entry into the vial, the remaining contents must be used within 48 hours.

The following infusion systems have been tested and found satisfactory: unit-dose glass containers; unit-dose polyvinyl chloride and polyolefin containers. No other systems have been tested and, therefore, no others can be recommended.

Dilution: EACH 5 mL OF SEPTRA I.V. INFUSION SHOULD BE ADDED TO 125 mL OF 5% DEXTROSE IN WATER.

NOTE: **In those instances where fluid restriction is desirable,** each 5 mL may be added to 75 mL of 5% dextrose in water. Under these circumstances the solution should be mixed just prior to use and should be administered within 2 hours. If upon visual inspection there is cloudiness or evidence of crystallization after mixing, the solution should be discarded and a fresh solution prepared.

DO NOT MIX SEPTRA I.V. INFUSION-5% DEXTROSE IN WATER WITH DRUGS OR SOLUTIONS IN THE SAME CONTAINER.

Administration: The solution should be given by intravenous infusion over a period of 60 to 90 minutes. Rapid infusion or bolus injections must be avoided. SEPTRA I.V. Infusion should not be given intramuscularly.

HOW SUPPLIED

5-mL vials, containing 80 mg trimethoprim (16 mg/mL) and 400 mg sulfamethoxazole (80 mg/mL) for infusion with 5% dextrose in water. Contains benzyl alcohol (see WARNINGS). Tray of 10 (NDC 61570-056-10).

10-mL multiple-dose vials, containing 160 mg trimethoprim (16 mg/mL) and 800 mg sulfamethoxazole (80 mg/mL) for infusion with 5% dextrose in water. Contains benzyl alcohol (see WARNINGS). Tray of 10 (NDC 61570-054-10).

20-mL multiple-dose vials, containing 320 mg trimethoprim (16 mg/mL) and 1,600 mg sulfamethoxazole (80 mg/mL) for infusion with 5% dextrose in water. Contains benzyl alcohol (see WARNINGS). Tray of 10 (NDC 61570-055-10).

Store at 15° to 25°C (59° to 77°F). DO NOT REFRIGERATE.

Also available in tablets containing 80 mg trimethoprim and 400 mg sulfamethoxazole (bottle of 100); DS (double strength) tablets containing 160 mg trimethoprim and 800 mg sulfamethoxazole (bottles of 100 and 250); and oral suspension containing 40 mg trimethoprim and 200 mg sulfamethoxazole in each 5 mL (pink, cherry-flavored: bottle of 1 pint [473 mL], 100 mL–package of 6; and purple, grape-flavored: bottle of 1 pint [473 mL]).

REFERENCES

1. Grose WE, Bodey GP, Loo TL. Clinical pharmacology of intravenously administered trimethoprim-sulfamethoxazole. *Antimicrob Agents Chemother*. 1979;15:447-451.
2. Siber GR, Gorham C, Durbin W, Lesko L, Levin MJ. Pharmacology of intravenous trimethoprim-sulfamethoxazole in children and adults. In: Nelson JD, Grassi C, eds. *Current Chemotherapy of Infectious Disease*. Washington, DC: American Society for Microbiology; 1980;1:691-692.
3. Bauer AW, Kirby WMM, Sherris JC, Turck M. Antibiotic susceptibility testing by a standardized single disk method. *Am J Clin Pathol*. 1966;45:493-496.
4. National Committee for Clinical Laboratory Standards. Performance standards for antimicrobial disk susceptibility tests, 2nd ed. Villanova, PA. 1979.
5. Brumfitt W, Pursell R. Trimethoprim-sulfamethoxazole in the treatment of bacteriuria in women. *J Infect Dis*. 1973;128(suppl):S657-S663.
6. Winston DJ, Lau WK, Gale RP, Young LS. Trimethoprim-sulfamethoxazole for the treatment of *Pneumocystis carinii* pneumonia. *Ann Int Med*. 1980;92:762-769.

Distributed by: Monarch Pharmaceuticals, Inc., Bristol, TN 37620

Manufactured by: Catalytica Pharmaceuticals, Inc., Greenville, NC 27834

Rev. 1/98
595716

SEPTRA® Tablets ℞
[sĕp tra]
SEPTRA® DS (Double Strength) Tablets ℞
SEPTRA® Suspension ℞
SEPTRA® Grape Suspension ℞
(trimethoprim and sulfamethoxazole)
PRODUCT INFORMATION

DESCRIPTION

SEPTRA (trimethoprim and sulfamethoxazole) is a synthetic antibacterial combination product. Each SEPTRA Tablet contains 80 mg trimethoprim and 400 mg sulfamethoxazole and the inactive ingredients docusate sodium (0.4 mg per tablet), FD&C Red No. 40, magnesium stearate, povidone, and sodium starch glycolate.

Each SEPTRA DS (double strength) Tablet contains 160 mg trimethoprim and 800 mg sulfamethoxazole and the inactive ingredients docusate sodium (0.8 mg per tablet), FD&C Red No. 40, magnesium stearate, povidone, and sodium starch glycolate.

Each teaspoonful (5 mL) of SEPTRA Suspension contains 40 mg trimethoprim and 200 mg sulfamethoxazole and the inactive ingredients alcohol 0.26%, methylparaben 0.1% and sodium benzoate 0.1% (added as preservatives), carboxymethylcellulose sodium, citric acid, FD&C Red No. 40 and Yellow No. 6, flavor, glycerin, microcrystalline cellulose, polysorbate 80, saccharin sodium, and sorbitol. Each teaspoonful (5 mL) of SEPTRA Grape Suspension contains 40 mg trimethoprim and 200 mg sulfamethoxazole and the inactive ingredients alcohol 0.26%, methylparaben 0.1%, and sodium benzoate 0.1% (added as preservatives), carboxymethylcellulose sodium, citric acid, FD&C Red No. 40 and Blue No. 1, flavor, glycerin, microcrystalline cellulose, polysorbate 80, saccharin sodium, and sorbitol. Both tablet and suspension forms are for oral administration.

Trimethoprim is 5-[(3,4,5-trimethoxyphenyl)methyl]-2,4-pyrimidinediamine. It is a white to light yellow, odorless, bitter compound with a molecular weight of 290.32, and the molecular formula $C_{14}H_{18}N_4O_3$. The structural formula is:

N NH2 N CH2 NH2 CH3O OCH3 OCH3

Sulfamethoxazole is 4-amino-*N*-(5-methyl-3-isoxazolyl)benzenesulfonamide. It is an almost white, odorless, tasteless compound with a molecular weight of 253.28, and the molecular formula $C_{10}H_{11}N_3O_3S$. The structural formula is:

H2N— —SO2NH— N O CH3

CLINICAL PHARMACOLOGY

SEPTRA is rapidly absorbed following oral administration. Both sulfamethoxazole and trimethoprim exist in the blood as unbound, protein-bound, and metabolized forms; sulfamethoxazole also exists as the conjugated form. The metabolism of sulfamethoxazole occurs predominately by N_4-acetylation although the glucuronide conjugate has been identified. The principal metabolites of trimethoprim are the 1- and 3-oxides and the 3′- and 4′-hydroxy derivatives. The free forms of sulfamethoxazole and trimethoprim are considered to be the therapeutically active forms. Approximately 44% of trimethoprim and 70% of sulfamethoxazole are bound to plasma proteins. The presence of 10 mg percent sulfamethoxazole in plasma decreases the protein binding of trimethoprim by an insignificant degree; trimethoprim does not influence the protein binding of sulfamethoxazole.

Peak blood levels for the individual components occur 1 to 4 hours after oral administration. The mean serum half-lives of sulfamethoxazole and trimethoprim are 10 and 8 to 10 hours, respectively. However, patients with severely impaired renal function exhibit an increase in the half-lives of both components, requiring dosage regimen adjustment (see DOSAGE AND ADMINISTRATION). Detectable amounts of trimethoprim and sulfamethoxazole are present in the blood 24 hours after drug administration. During administration of 160 mg trimethoprim and 800 mg sulfamethoxazole b.i.d., the mean steady-state plasma concentration of trimethoprim was 1.72 mcg/mL. The steady-state minimal levels of free and total sulfamethoxazole were 57.4 mcg/mL and 68.0 mcg/mL, respectively. These steady-state levels were achieved after 3 days of drug administration.[1]

Excretion of sulfamethoxazole and trimethoprim is primarily by the kidneys through both glomerular filtration and tubular secretion. Urine concentrations of both sulfamethoxazole and trimethoprim are considerably higher than are the concentrations in the blood. The average percentage of the dose recovered in urine from 0 to 72 hours after a single oral dose if 84.5% for total sulfonamide and 66.8% for free trimethoprim. Thirty percent of the total sulfonamide is excreted as free sulfamethoxazole, with the remaining as N_4-acetylated metabolite.[2] When administered together as SEPTRA, neither sulfamethoxazole nor trimethoprim affects the urinary excretion pattern of the other.

Both trimethoprim and sulfamethoxazole distribute to sputum, vaginal fluid, and middle ear fluid; trimethoprim also distributes to bronchial secretions, and both pass the placental barrier and are excreted in human milk.

Microbiology: Sulfamethoxazole inhibits bacterial synthesis of dihydrofolic acid by competing with *para*-aminobenzoic acid (PABA). Trimethoprim blocks the production of tetrahydrofolic acid from dihydrofolic acid by binding to and reversibly inhibiting the required enzyme, dihydrofolate reductase. Thus, SEPTRA blocks two consecutive steps in the biosynthesis of nucleic acids and proteins essential to many bacteria.

In vitro studies have shown that bacterial resistance develops more slowly with SEPTRA than with either trimethoprim or sulfamethoxazole alone.

In vitro serial dilution tests have shown that the spectrum of antibacterial activity of SEPTRA includes the common urinary tract pathogens with the exception of *Pseudomonas aeruginosa*. The following organisms are usually susceptible: *Escherichia coli, Klebsiella* species, *Enterobacter* species, *Morganella morganii, Proteus mirabilis,* and indole-positive *Proteus* species including *Proteus vulgaris*.

The usual spectrum of antimicrobial activity of SEPTRA includes bacterial pathogens isolated from middle ear exudate and from bronchial secretions (*Haemophilus influenzae*, including ampicillin-resistant strains, and *Streptococcus pneumoniae*), and enterotoxigenic strains of *Escherichia coli* (ETEC) causing bacterial gastroenteritis. *Shigella flexneri* and *Shigella sonnei* are also usually susceptible.

[See table at bottom of next page]

Susceptibility Testing: The recommended quantitative disc susceptibility method may be used for estimating the susceptibility of bacteria of SEPTRA.[3,4] With this procedure, a report from the laboratory of "Susceptible to trimethoprim and sulfamethoxazole" indicates that the infection is likely to respond to therapy with SEPTRA. If the infection is confined to the urine, a report of "Intermediate susceptibility to trimethoprim and sulfamethoxazole" also indicates that the infection is likely to respond. A report of "Resistant to trimethoprim and sulfamethoxazole" indicates that the infection is unlikely to respond to therapy with SEPTRA.

INDICATIONS AND USAGE

Urinary Tract Infections: For the treatment of urinary tract infections due to susceptible strains of the following organisms: *Escherichia coli, Kelbsiella* species, *Enterobacter* species, *Morganella morganii, Proteus mirabilis,* and *Proteus vulgaris*. It is recommended that initial episodes of uncomplicated urinary tract infections be treated with a single effective antibacterial agent rather than the combination.

Acute Otitis Media: For the treatment of acute otitis media in pediatric patients due to susceptible strains of *Streptococcus pneumoniae* or *Haemophilus influenzae* when, in the judgment of the physician, SEPTRA offers some advantage over the use of other antimicrobial agents. To date, there are limited data on the safety of repeated use of SEPTRA in pediatric patients under two years of age. SEPTRA is not indicated for prophylactic or prolonged administration in otitis media at any age.

Acute Exacerbations of Chronic Bronchitis in Adults: For the treatment of acute exacerbations of chronic bronchitis due to susceptible strains of *Streptococcus pneumoniae* or *Haemophilus influenzae* when, in the judgment of the physician, SEPTRA offers some advantage over the use of a single antimicrobial agent.

Travelers' Diarrhea in Adults: For the treatment of travelers' diarrhea due to susceptible strains of enterotoxigenic *E. coli.* Shigellosis: For the treatment of enteritis caused by susceptible strains of *Shigella flexneri* and *Shigella sonnei* when antibacterial therapy is indicated.

***Pneumocystis Carinii* Pneumonia:** For the treatment of documented *Pneumocystis carinii* pneumonia. For prophylaxis against *Pneumocystis carinii* pneumonia in individuals who are immunosuppressed and considered to be at an increased risk of developing *Pneumocystis carinii* pneumonia.

CONTRAINDICATIONS

SEPTRA is contraindicated in patients with a known hypersensitivity to trimethoprim or sulfonamides and in patients with documented megaloblastic anemia due to folate deficiency. SEPTRA is also contraindicated in pregnant patients at term and in nursing mothers, because sulfonamides pass the placenta and are excreted in the milk and may cause kernicterus. SEPTRA is contraindicated in pediatric patients less than 2 months of age.

WARNINGS:

FATALITIES ASSOCIATED WITH THE ADMINISTRATION OF SULFONAMIDES, ALTHOUGH RARE, HAVE OCCURRED DUE TO SEVERE REACTIONS, INCLUDING STEVENS-JOHNSON SYNDROME, TOXIC EPIDERMAL NECROLYSIS, FULMINANT HEPATIC NECROSIS, AGRANULOCYTOSIS, APLASTIC ANEMIA, AND OTHER BLOOD DYSCRASIAS. SULFONAMIDES, INCLUDING SULFONAMIDE-CONTAINING PRODUCTS SUCH AS TRIMETHOPRIM/SULFAMETHOXAZOLE, SHOULD BE DISCONTINUED AT THE FIRST APPEARANCE OF SKIN RASH OR ANY SIGN OF ADVERSE REACTION. In rare instances, a skin rash may be followed by a more severe reaction, such as Stevens-Johnson syndrome, toxic epidermal necrolysis, hepatic necrosis, and serious blood disorder (see PRECAUTIONS).

Clinical signs, such as rash, sore throat, fever, arthralgia, pallor, purpura, or jaundice may be early indications of serious reactions.

Cough, shortness of breath, and pulmonary infiltrates are hypersensitivity reactions of the respiratory tract that have been reported in association with sulfonamide treatment.

The sulfonamides should not be used for the treatment of group A beta-hemolytic streptococcal infections. In an established infection, they will not eradicate the streptococcus and, therefore, will not prevent sequelae such as rheumatic fever.

Pseudomembranous colitis has been reported with nearly all antibacterial agents, including trimethoprim/sulfamethoxazole, and may range in severity from mild to life-threatening. Therefore, it is important to consider this diagnosis in patients who present with diarrhea subsequent to the administration of antibacterial agents.

Treatment with antibacterial agents alters the normal flora of the colon and may permit overgrowth of clostridia. Studies indicate that a toxin produced by Clostridium difficile is one primary cause of "antibiotic-associated colitis."

After the diagnosis of pseudomembranous colitis has been established, therapeutic measures should be initiated. Mild cases of pseudomembranous colitis usually respond to drug discontinuation alone. In moderate to severe cases, consideration should be given to management with fluids and electrolytes, protein supplementation, and treatment with an antibacterial drug effective against *C. difficile.*

PRECAUTIONS

General: SEPTRA should be given with caution to patients with impaired renal or hepatic function, to those with possible folate deficiency (e.g., the elderly, chronic alcoholics, patients receiving anticonvulsant therapy, patients with malabsorption syndrome, and patients in malnutrition states), and to those with severe allergy or bronchial asthma. In glucose-6-phosphate dehydrognase-deficient individuals, hemolysis may occur. This reaction is frequently dose-related (see CLINICAL PHARMACOLOGY and DOSAGE AND ADMINISTRATION).

Use in the Elderly: There may be an increased risk of severe adverse reactions in elderly patients, particularly when complicating conditions exist, e.g, impaired kidney and/or liver function, or concomitant use of other drugs. Severe skin reactions, or generalized bone marrow suppression (see WARNINGS and ADVERSE REACTIONS), or a specific decrease in platelets (with or without purpura) are the most frequently reported severe adverse reactions in elderly patients. In those concurrently receiving certain diuretics, primarily thiazides, an increased incidence of thrombocytopenia with purpura has been reported. Appropriate dosage adjustments should be made for patients with impaired kidney function (see DOSAGE AND ADMINISTRATION).

Use in the Treatment of and Prophylaxis for *Pneumocystis carinii* Pneumonia in Patients with Acquired Immunodeficiency Syndrome (AIDS): The incidence of side effects, particularly rash, fever, leukopenia, and elevated aminotransferase (transaminase) values in AIDS patients who are being treated with SEPTRA for *Pneumocystis carinii* pneumonia has been reported to be greatly increased compared with the incidence normally associated with the use of SEPTRA in non-AIDS patients. The incidence of hyperkalemia and hyponatremia appears to be increased in AIDS patients receiving SEPTRA. Adverse effects are generally less severe in patients receiving SEPTRA for prophylaxis. A history of mild intolerance to SEPTRA in AIDS patients does not appear to predict intolerance of subsequent secondary prophylaxis. However, if a patient develops skin rash or any sign of adverse reaction, therapy with SEPTRA should be re-evaluated (see WARNINGS).

The concomitant use of leucovorin with trimethoprim-sulfamethoxazole for the acute treatment of *Pneumocystis carinii* pneumonia in patients with HIV infection was associated with increased rates of treatment failure and morbidity in a placebo-controlled study.

Information for Patients: Patients should be instructed to maintain an adequate fluid intake in order to prevent crystalluria and stone formation.

Laboratory Tests: Complete blood counts should be done frequently in patients receiving SEPTRA; if a significant reduction in the count of any formed blood element is noted, SEPTRA should be discontinued. Urinalyses with careful microscopic examination and renal function tests should be performed during therapy, particularly for those patients with impaired renal function.

Drug Interactions: In elderly patients concurrently receiving certain diuretics, primarily thiazides, an increased incidence of thrombocytopenia with purpura has been reported. It has been reported that SEPTRA may prolong the prothrombin time in patients who are receiving the anticoagulant warfarin. This interaction should be kept in mind when SEPTRA is given to patients already on anticoagulant therapy, and the coagulation time should be reassessed.

SEPTRA may inhibit the hepatic metabolism of phenytoin. SEPTRA, given at a common clinical dosage, increased the phenytoin half-life by 39% and decreased the phenytoin metabolic clearance rate by 27%. When administering these drugs concurrently, one should be alert for possible excessive phenytoin effect.

Sulfonamides can also displace methotrexate from plasma protein binding sites, thus increasing free methotrexate concentrations.

Drug/Laboratory Test Interactions: SEPTRA, specifically the trimethoprim component, can interfere with a serum methotrexate assay as determined by the competitive binding protein technique (CBPA) when a bacterial dihydrofolate reductase is used as the binding protein. No interference occurs, however, if methotrexate is measured by a radioimmunoassay (RIA).

The presence of trimethoprim and sulfamethoxazole may also interfere with the Jaffé alkaline picrate reaction assay for creatinine, resulting in overestimations of about 10% in the range of normal values.

Carcinogenesis, Mutagenesis, Impairment of Fertility:

Carcinogenesis: Long-term studies in animals to evaluate carcinogenic potential have not been conducted with SEPTRA.

Mutagenesis: Bacterial mutagenic studies have not been performed with sulfamethoxazole and trimethoprim in combination. Trimethoprim was demonstrated to be non-mutagenic in the Ames assay. In studies at two laboratories, no chromosomal damage was detected in cultured Chinese hamster ovary cells at concentrations approximately 500 times human plasma levels; at concentrations approximately 1,000 times human plasma levels in these same cells, a low level of chromosomal damage was induced at one of the laboratories. No chormosomal abnormalities were observed in cultured human leukocytes at concentrations of trimethoprim up to 20 times human steady-state plasma levels. No chromosomal effects were detected in peripheral lympocytes of human subjects receiving 320 mg of trimethoprim in combination with up to 1,600 mg of sulfamethoxazole per day for as long as 112 weeks.

Impairment of Fertility: No adverse effects on fertility or general reproductive performance were observed in rats given oral dosages as high as 70 mg/kg/day trimethoprim plus 350 mg/kg/day sulfamethoxazole.

Pregnancy:

Teratogenic Effects: Pregnancy Category C. In rats, oral doses of 533 mg/kg sulfamethoxazole or 200 mg/kg trimethoprim produced teratological effects manifested mainly as cleft palates. The highest dose which did not cause cleft palates in rats was 512 mg/kg sulfamethoxazole or 192 mg/kg trimethoprim when administered separately. In two studies in rats, no teratogenicity was observed when 512 mg/kg of sulfamethoxazole was used in combination with 128 mg/kg of trimethoprim. In one study, however, cleft palates were observed in one litter out of nine when 355 mg/kg of sulfamethoxazole was used in combination with 88 mg/kg of trimethoprim.

In some rabbit studies, an overall increase in fetal loss (dead and resorbed and malformed conceptuses) was associated with doses of trimethoprim six times the human therapeutic dose.

While there are no large, well-controlled studies in the use of trimethoprim and sulfamethoxazole in pregnant women, Brumfitt and Pursell,[5] in a retrospective study, reported the outcome of 186 pregnancies during which the mother received either placebo or trimethoprim and sulfamethoxazole. The incidence of congenital abnormalities was 4.5% (3 of 66) in those who received placebo and 3.3% (4 of 120) in those receiving trimethoprim and sulfamethoxazole. There were no abnormalities in the 10 children whose mothers received the drug during the first trimester. In a separate survey, Brumfitt and Pursell also found no congenital abnormalities in 35 children whose mothers had received oral trimethoprim and sulfamethoxazole at the time of conception or shortly thereafter.

Because trimethoprim and sulfamethoxazole may interfere with folic acid metabolism, SEPTRA should be used during pregnancy only if the potential benefit justifies the potential risk to the fetus.

Nonteratogenic Effects: See CONTRAINDICATIONS section.

Nursing Mothers: See CONTRAINDICATIONS section.

Pediatric Use: SEPTRA is not indicated for pediatric patients younger than 2 months of age (see INDICATIONS AND USAGE and CONTRAINDICATIONS).

ADVERSE REACTIONS

The most common adverse effects are gastrointestinal disturbances (nausea, vomiting, anorexia) and allergic skin reactions (such as rash and urticaria). **FATALITIES ASSOCIATED WITH THE ADMINISTRATION OF SULFONAMIDES, ALTHOUGH RARE, HAVE OCCURRED DUE TO SEVERE REACTIONS, INCLUDING STEVENS-JOHNSON SYNDROME, TOXIC EPIDERMAL NECROLYSIS, FLUMINANT HEPATIC NECROSIS, AGRANULOCYTOSIS, APLASTIC ANEMIA, OTHER BLOOD DYSCRASIAS, AND HYPERSENSITIVITY OF THE RESPIRATORY TRACT (SEE WARNINGS).**

Hematologic: Agranulocytosis, aplastic anemia, thrombocytopenia, leukopenia, neutropenia, hemolytic anemia, megaloblastic anemia, hypoprothrombinemia, methemoglobinemia, eosinophilia.

Allergic: Stevens-Johnson syndrome, toxic epidermal necrolysis, anaphylaxis, allergic myocarditis, erythema multiforme, exfoliative dermatitis, angioedema, drug fever, chills, Henoch-Schönlein purpura, serum sickness-like syndrome, generalized allergic reactions, generalized skin eruptions, photosensitivity, conjunctival and scleral injection, pruritus, urticaria, and rash. In addition, periarteritis

REPRESENTATIVE MINIMUM INHIBITORY CONCENTRATION VALUES FOR ORGANISMS SUSCEPTIBLE TO SEPTRA (MIC-μg/mL)

Bacteria	TMP Alone	SMX Alone	TMP/SMX (1:19) TMP	TMP/SMX (1:19) SMX
Escherichia coli	0.05–1.5	1.0–245	0.05–0.5	0.95–9.5
Escherichia coli (enterotoxigenic strains)	0.015–0.15	0.285–>950	0.005–0.15	0.095–2.85
Proteus species (indole positive)	0.5–5.0	7.35–300	0.05–1.5	0.95–28.5
Morganella morganii	0.5–5.0	7.35–300	0.05–1.5	0.95–28.5
Proteus mirabilis	0.5–1.5	7.35–30	0.05–0.15	0.95–2.85
Klebsiella species	0.15–5.0	2.45–245	0.05–1.5	0.95–28.5
Enterobacter species	0.15–5.0	2.45–245	0.05–1.5	0.95–28.5
Haemophilus influenzae	0.15–1.5	2.85–95	0.015–0.15	0.285–2.85
Streptococcus pneumonia	0.15–1.5	7.35–24.5	0.05–0.15	0.95–2.85
*Shigella flexneri**	<0.01–0.04	<0.16–>320	<0.002–0.03	0.04–0.625
*Shigella sonnei**	0.02–0.08	0.625–>320	0.004–0.06	0.08–1.25

TMP=trimethoprim SMX=sulfamethoxazole

*Rudoy RC, Nelson JD, Haltalin KC. *Antimicrobial Agents and Chemotherapy.* 1974;5:439–443.

Continued on next page

Septra Tablets/Suspension—Cont.

nodosa and systemic lupus erythematosus have been reported.
Gastrointestinal: Hepatitis, including cholestatic jaundice and hepatic necrosis, elevation of serum transaminase and bilirubin, pseudomembranous enterocolitis, pancreatitis, stomatitis, glossitis, nausea, emesis, abdominal pain, diarrhea, anorexia.
Genitourinary: Renal failure, interstitial nephritis, BUN and serum creatinine elevation, toxic nephrosis with oliguria and anuria, and crystalluria.
Metabolic: Hyperkalemia, hyponatremia.
Neurologic: Aseptic meningitis, convulsions, peripheral neuritis, ataxia, vertigo, tinnitus, headache.
Psychiatric: Hallucinations, depression, apathy, nervousness.
Endocrine: The sulfonamides bear certain chemical similarities to some goitrogens, diuretics (acetazolamide and the thiazides), and oral hypoglycemic agents. Cross-sensitivity may exist with these agents. Diuresis and hypoglycemia have occurred rarely in patients receiving sulfonamides.
Musculoskeletal: Arthralgia and myalgia.
Respiratory System: Cough, shortness of breath, and pulmonary infiltrates (see WARNINGS).
Miscellaneous: Weakness, fatigue, insomnia.

OVERDOSAGE

Acute: The amount of a single dose of SEPTRA that is either associated with symptoms of overdosage or is likely to be life-threatening has not been reported. Signs and symptoms of overdosage reported with sulfonamides include anorexia, colic, nausea, vomiting, dizziness, headache, drowsiness, and unconsciousness. Pyrexia, hematuria, and crystalluria may be noted. Blood dyscrasias and jaundice are potential late manifestations of overdosage. Signs of acute overdosage with trimethoprim include nausea, vomiting, dizziness, headache, mental depression, confusion, and bone marrow depression.
General principles of treatment include the institution of gastric lavage or emesis; forcing oral fluids; and the administration of intravenous fluids if urine output is low and renal function is normal. Acidification of the urine will increase renal elimination of trimethoprim. The patient should be monitored with blood counts and appropriate blood chemistries, including electrolytes. If a significant blood dyscrasia or jaundice occurs, specific therapy should be instituted for these complications. Peritoneal dialysis is not effective and hemodialysis is only moderately effective in eliminating trimethoprim and sulfamethoxazole.
Chronic: Use of SEPTRA at high doses and/or for extended periods of time may cause bone marrow depression manifested as thrombocytopenia, leukopenia, and/or megaloblastic anemia. If signs of bone marrow depression occur, the patient should be given leucovorin; 5 to 15 mg leucovorin daily has been recommended by some investigators.

DOSAGE AND ADMINISTRATION

Contraindicated in pediatric patients less than 2 months of age.

Urinary Tract Infections And Shigellosis In Adults And Pediatric Patients and Acute Otitis Media in Pediatric Patients:

Adults: The usual adult dosage in the treatment of urinary tract infections is one SEPTRA DS (double strength) tablet, two SEPTRA tablets, or four teaspoonfuls (20 mL) SEPTRA Suspension every 12 hours for 10 to 14 days. An identical daily dosage is used for 5 days in the treatment of shigellosis.

Pediatric Patients: The recommended dose for pediatric patients with urinary tract infections or acute otitis media is 8 mg/kg trimethoprim and 40 mg/kg sulfamethoxazole per 24 hours, given in two divided doses every 12 hours for 10 days. An identical dosage is used for 5 days in the treatment of shigellosis. The following table is a guideline for the attainment of this dosage:

Pediatric Patients: Two Months of Age or Older

Weight		Dose – Every 12 Hours	
lb	kg	Teaspoonfuls	Tablets
22	10	1 (5 mL)	
44	20	2 (10 mL)	1
66	30	3 (15 mL)	$1^1/_2$
88	40	4 (20 mL)	2 (or 1 DS Tablet)

For Patients With Impaired Renal Function: When renal function is impaired, a reduced dosage should be employed using the following table:

Creatinine Clearance (mL/min)	Recommended Dosage Regimen
Above 30	Use Standard Regimen
15–30	$^1/_2$ the Usual Regimen
Below 15	Use Not Recommended

Acute Exacerbations of Chronic Bronchitis in Adults: The usual adult dosage in the treatment of acute exacerbations of chronic bronchitis is one SEPTRA DS (double strength) tablet, two SEPTRA tablets, or four teaspoonfuls (20 mL) SEPTRA Suspension every 12 hours for 14 days.
Travelers' Diarrhea in Adults: For the treatment of travelers' diarrhea, the usual adult dosage is one SEPTRA DS (double strength) tablet, two SEPTRA tablets, or four teaspoonfuls (20 mL) of SEPTRA Suspension every 12 hours for 5 days.

Pneumocystis Carinii Pneumonia: Treatment:
Adults and Pediatric Patients:
The recommended dosage for treatment of patients with documented *Pneumocystis carinii* pneumonia is 15 to 20 mg/kg trimethoprim and 75 to 100 mg/kg sulfamethoxazole per 24 hours given in equally divided doses every 6 hours for 14 to 21 days. The following table is a guideline for the upper limit of this dosage:

Weight		Dose – Every 6 Hours	
lb	kg	Teaspoonfuls	Tablets
18	8	1 (5 mL)	
35	16	2 (10 mL)	1
53	24	3 (15 mL)	$1^1/_2$
70	32	4 (20 mL)	2 (or 1 DS Tablet)
88	40	5 (25 mL)	$2^1/_2$
106	48	6 (30 mL)	3 (or $1^1/_2$ DS Tablets)
141	64	8 (40 mL)	4 (or 2 DS Tablets)
176	80	10 (50 mL)	5 (or $2^1/_2$ DS Tablets)

For the lower limit dose (15 mg/kg trimethoprim and 75 mg/kg sulfamethoxazole per 24 hours) administer 75% of the dose in the above table.

Prophylaxis:
Adults:
The recommended dosage for prophylaxis in adults is one SEPTRA DS (double strength) tablet daily.
Pediatric Patients:
For pediatric patients, the recommended dose is 150 mg/m²/day trimethoprim with 750 mg/m²/day sulfamethoxazole given orally in equally divided doses twice a day, on 3 consecutive days per week. The total daily dose should not exceed 320 mg trimethoprim and 1,600 mg sulfamethoxazole. The following table is a guideline for the attainment of this dosage in pediatric patients:

Body Surface Area (m²)	Dose – every 12 hours Teaspoonfuls	Tablets
0.26	$^1/_2$ (2.5 mL)	
0.53	1 (5 mL)	$^1/_2$
1.06	2 (10 mL)	1

HOW SUPPLIED

TABLETS (pink, scored, round-shaped) containing 80 mg trimethoprim and 400 mg sulfamethoxazole: Bottles of 100 (NDC 61570-052-01). Imprint on tablets "M052".
DS (DOUBLE STRENGTH) TABLETS (pink, scored, oval-shaped) containing 160 mg trimethoprim and 800 mg sulfamethoxazole: Bottles of 20 (NDC 61570-053-20), 100 (NDC 61570-053-01), 250 (NDC 61570-053-52) and 500 (NDC 61570-053-05). Imprint on tablets "M053".
ORAL SUSPENSIONS (pink, cherry-flavored) containing 40 mg trimethoprim and 200 mg sulfamethoxazole in each teaspoonful (5 mL): Bottle of 1 pint (473 mL) (NDC 61570-050-16) and 100 mL–package of 6 (NDC 61570-050-11); and (purple, grape-flavored) containing 40 mg trimethoprim and 200 mg sulfamethoxazole in each teaspoonful (5 mL): Bottle of 1 pint (473 mL) (NDC 61570-051-16).
Tablets should be stored at 15° to 25°C (59° to 77°F) in a dry place and protected from light.
Suspensions should be stored at 15° to 25°C (59° to 77°F) and protected from light.
Also available:
SEPTRA I.V. Infusion: 5 mL vials, containing 80 mg trimethoprim (16 mg/mL) and 400 mg sulfamethoxazole (80 mg/mL), tray of 10;
10 mL multiple dose vials containing 160 mg trimethoprim (16 mg/mL) and 800 mg sulfamethoxazole (80 mg/mL), tray of 10;
20 mL multiple dose vials containing 320 mg trimethoprim (16 mg/mL) and 1600 mg sulfamethoxazole (80 mg/mL), tray of 10.

REFERENCES

1. Kremers P, Duvivier J, Heusghem C. Pharmacokinetic studies of co-trimoxazole in man after single and repeated doses. *J Clin Pharmacol.* 1974;14:112–117.
2. Kaplan SA, Weinfeld RE, Abruzzo CW, McFaden K, Jack ML, Weissman L. Pharmacokinetic profile of trimethoprim-sulfamethoxazole in man. *J Infect Dis.* 1973;128(suppl):S547–S555.
3. Antibiotic susceptibility discs: certification procedure. *Federal Register.* 1972;37:20527–20529.
4. Bauer AW, Kirby WMM, Sherris JC, Turck M. Antibiotic susceptibility testing by standardized single disk method. *Am J Clin Pathol.* 1966;45:493–496.
5. Brumfitt W, Pursell R. Trimethoprim-sulfamethoxazole in the treatment of bacteriuria in women. *J Infect Dis.* 1973;128(suppl):S657–S663.

Manufactured for: Monarch Pharmaceuticals, Inc., Bristol, TN 37620
By: King Pharmaceuticals, Inc., Bristol, TN 37620

0934075
Rev. 2/00

SILVADENE® CREAM 1% ℞

[*sĭl vă dēn*]
(silver sulfadiazine)

DESCRIPTION

SILVADENE Cream 1% is a soft, white, water-miscible cream containing the antimicrobial agent silver sulfadiazine in micronized form, which has the following structural formula:

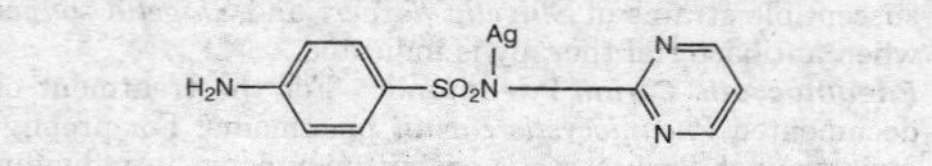

Each gram of SILVADENE Cream 1% contains 10 mg of micronized silver sulfadiazine. The cream vehicle consists of white petrolatum, stearyl alcohol, isopropyl myristate, sorbitan monooleate, polyoxyl 40 stearate, propylene glycol, and water, with methylparaben 0.3% as a preservative. SILVADENE Cream 1% (silver sulfadiazine) spreads easily and can be washed off readily with water.

CLINICAL PHARMACOLOGY

Silver sulfadiazine has broad antimicrobial activity. It is bactericidal for many gram-negative and gram-positive bacteria as well as being effective against yeast. Results from in vitro testing are listed below.
Sufficient data have been obtained to demonstrate that silver sulfadiazine will inhibit bacteria that are resistant to other antimicrobial agents and that the compound is superior to sulfadiazine.
Studies utilizing radioactive micronized silver sulfadiazine, electron microscopy, and biochemical techniques have revealed that the mechanism of action of silver sulfadiazine on bacteria differs from silver nitrate and sodium sulfadiazine. Silver sulfadiazine acts only on the cell membrane and cell wall to produce its bactericidal effect.

Results of In Vitro Testing With SILVADENE® Cream 1% (silver sulfadiazine)
Concentration of Silver Sulfadiazine
Number of Sensitive Strains/Total Number of Strains Tested

Genus & Species	50 μg/mL	100 μg/mL
Pseudomonas aeruginosa	130/130	130/130
Xanthomonas (Pseudomonas) maltophilia	7/7	7/7
Enterobacter species	48/50	50/50
Enterobacter cloacae	24/24	24/24
Klebsiella species	53/54	54/54
Escherichia coli	63/63	63/63
Serratia species	27/28	28/28
Proteus mirabilis	53/53	53/53
Morganella morganii	10/10	10/10
Providencia rettgeri	2/2	2/2
Providencia species	1/1	1/1
Proteus vulgaris	2/2	2/2
Citrobacter species	10/10	10/10
Acinetobacter calcoaceticus	10/11	11/11
Staphylococcus aureus	100/101	100/101
Staphylococcus epidermidis	51/51	51/51
B-Hemolytic *Streptococcus*	4/4	4/4
Enterococcus species	52/53	53/53
Corynebacterium diphtheriae	2/2	2/2
Clostridium perfringens	0/2	2/2
Candida albicans	43/50	50/50

Silver sulfadiazine is not a carbonic anhydrase inhibitor and may be useful in situations where such agents are contraindicated.

INDICATIONS AND USAGE

SILVADENE Cream 1% (silver sulfadiazine) is a topical antimicrobial drug indicated as an adjunct for the prevention and treatment of wound sepsis in patients with second- and third-degree burns.

CONTRAINDICATIONS

SILVADENE Cream 1% (silver sulfadiazine) is contraindicated in patients who are hypersensitive to silver sulfadiazine or any of the other ingredients in the preparation.
Because sulfonamide therapy is known to increase the possibility of kernicterus, SILVADENE Cream 1% should not be used on pregnant women approaching or at term, on premature infants, or on newborn infants during the first 2 months of life.

WARNINGS

There is potential cross-sensitvity between silver sulfadiazine and other sulfonamides. If allergic reactions attributable to treatment with silver sulfadiazine occur, continuation of therapy must be weighed against the potential hazards of the particular allergic reaction.
Fungal proliferation in and below the eschar may occur. However, the incidence of clinically reported fungal superinfection is low.
The use of SILVADENE Cream 1% (silver sulfadiazine) in some cases of glucose-6-phosphate dehydrogenase-deficient individuals may be hazardous, as hemolysis may occur.

PRECAUTIONS

General
If hepatic and renal functions become impaired and elimination of drug decreases, accumulation may occur and discontinuation of SILVADENE Cream 1% (silver sulfadiazine) should be weighed against the therapeutic benefit being achieved.

In considering the use of topical proteolytic enzymes in conjunction with SILVADENE Cream 1%, the possibility should be noted that silver may inactivate such enzymes.

Laboratory Tests

In the treatment of burn wounds involving extensive areas of the body, the serum sulfa concentrations may approach adult therapeutic levels (8 mg% to 12 mg%). Therefore, in these patients it would be advisable to monitor serum sulfa concentrations. Renal function should be carefully monitored and the urine should be checked for sulfa crystals. Absorption of the propylene glycol vehicle has been reported to affect serum osmolality, which may affect the interpretation of laboratory tests.

Carcinogenesis, Mutagenesis, Impairment of Fertility

Long-term dermal toxicity studies of 24 months' duration in rats and 18 months' in mice with concentrations of silver sulfadiazine three to ten times the concentration in SILVADENE Cream 1% revealed no evidence of carcinogenicity.

Pregnancy

Teratongenic Effects. Pregnancy Category B. A reproductive study has been performed in rabbits at doses up to three to ten times the concentration of silver sulfadiazine in SILVADENE Cream 1% and has revealed no evidence of harm to the fetus due to silver sulfadiazine. There are, however, no adequate and well-controlled studies in pregnant women. Because animal reproduction studies are not always predictive of human response, this drug should be used during pregnancy only if clearly justified, especially in pregnant women approaching or at term. (See CONTRAINDICATIONS.)

Nursing Mothers

It is not known whether silver sulfadiazine is excreted in human milk. However, sulfonamides are known to be excreted in human milk, and all sulfonamide derivatives are known to increase the possibility of kernicterus. Because of the possibility for serious adverse reactions in nursing infants from sulfonamides, a decision should be made whether to discontinue nursing or to discontinue the drug, taking into account the importance of the drug to the mother.

Pediatric Use

Safety and effectiveness in pediatric patients have not been established. (See CONTRAINDICATIONS.)

ADVERSE REACTIONS

Several cases of transient leukopenia have been reported in patients receiving silver sulfadiazine therapy.[1,2,3] Leukopenia associated with silver sulfadiazine administration is primarily characterized by decreased neutrophil count. Maximal white blood cell depression occurs within 2 to 4 days of initiation of therapy. Rebound to normal leukocyte levels follows onset within 2 to 3 days. Recovery is not influenced by continuation of silver sulfadiazine therapy. An increased incidence of leukopenia has been reported in patients treated concurrently with cimetidine.

Other infrequently occurring events include skin necrosis, erythema multiforme, skin discoloration, burning sensation, rashes, and interstitial nephritis.

Reduction in bacterial growth after application of topical antibacterial agents has been reported to permit spontaneous healing of deep partial-thickness burns by preventing conversion of the partial thickness to full thickness by sepsis. However, reduction in bacterial colonization has caused delayed separation, in some cases necessitating escharotomy in order to prevent contracture.

Absorption of silver sulfadiazine varies depending upon the percent of body surface area and the extent of the tissue damage. Although few have been reported, it is possible that any adverse reaction associated with sulfonamides may occur. Some of the reactions, which have been associated with sulfonamides, are as follows: blood dyscrasias including agranulocytosis, aplastic anemia, thrombocytopenia, leukopenia, and hemolytic anemia; dermatologic and allergic reactions, including Stevens-Johnson syndrome and exfoliative dermatitis; gastrointestinal reactions; hepatitis and hepatocellular necrosis; CNS reactions; and toxic nephrosis.

DOSAGE AND ADMINISTRATION

Prompt institution of appropriate regimens for care of the burned patient is of prime importance and includes the control of shock and pain. The burn wounds are then cleansed and debrided and SILVADENE Cream 1% (silver sulfadiazine) is applied under sterile conditions. The burn areas should be covered with SILVADENE Cream 1% at all times. The cream should be applied once to twice daily to a thickness of approximately 1/16 inch. Whenever necessary, the cream should be reapplied to any areas from which it has been removed by patient activity. Administration may be accomplished in minimal time because dressings are not required. However, if individual patient requirements make dressings necessary, they may be used.

Reapply immediately after hydrotherapy.

Treatment with SILVADENE Cream 1% should be continued until satisfactory healing has occurred, or until the burn site is ready for grafting. The drug should not be withdrawn from the therapeutic regimen while there remains the possibility of infection except if a significant adverse reaction occurs.

HOW SUPPLIED

SILVADENE Cream 1% (silver sulfadiazine) is available in jars containing 50 g (NDC 61570-131-50), 400 g (NDC 61570-131-40), and 1000 g (NDC 61570-131-98) and tubes containing 20 g (NDC 61570-131-20) and 85 g (NDC 61570-131-85).

REFERENCES

1. Caffee F, Bingham H. Leukopenia and silver sulfadiazine. *J Trauma.* 1982;22:586–587.
2. Jarret F, Ellerbe S, Demling R. Acute leukopenia during topical burn therapy with silver sulfadiazine. *Amer J Surg.* 1978;135:818–819.
3. Kiker RG, Carvajal HF, Micak RP, Larson DL. A controlled study of the effects of silver sulfadiazine on white blood cell counts in burned children. *J Trauma.* 1977;17:835–836.

Prescribing Information as of March 1999

Distributed by:
Monarch Pharmaceuticals, Inc.
Bristol, TN 37620

Manufactured by:
Hoechst Marion Roussel, Inc.
Kansas City, MO 64137

Shown in Product Identification Guide, page 325

THALITONE® ℞

[*thăl'ə-tōne*]

(chlorthalidone tablets, USP)

15 mg

Prescribing Information

DESCRIPTION

Thalitone® (chlorthalidone USP) is an antihypertensive/diuretic supplied as 15 mg tablets for oral use. It is a monosulfamyl diuretic that differs chemically from thiazide diuretics in that a double ring system is incorporated in its structure. It is a racemic mixture of 2-chloro-5-(1-hydroxy-3-oxo-1-isoindolinyl) benzenesulfonamide, with the following structural formula:

$C_{14}H_{11}ClN_2O_4S$ 338.78

Chlorthalidone is practically insoluble in water, in ether and in chloroform; soluble in methanol; slightly soluble in alcohol.

The inactive ingredients are colloidal silicon dioxide, lactose, magnesium stearate, microcrystalline cellulose, povidone, sodium starch glycolate.

CLINICAL PHARMACOLOGY

Chlorthalidone is a long-acting oral diuretic with antihypertensive activity. Its diuretic action commences a mean of 2.6 hours after dosing and continues for up to 72 hours. The drug produces diuresis with increased excretion of sodium and chloride. The diuretic effects of chlorthalidone and the benzothiadiazine (thiazide) diuretics appear to arise from similar mechanisms and the maximal effect of chlorthalidone and the thiazides appear to be similar. The site of the action appears to be the distal convoluted tubule of the nephron. The diuretic effects of chlorthalidone lead to decreased extracellular fluid volume, plasma volume, cardiac output, total exchangeable sodium, glomerular filtration rate, and renal plasma flow. Although the mechanism of action of chlorthalidone and related drugs is not wholly clear, sodium and water depletion appear to provide a basis for its antihypertensive effect. Like the thiazide diuretics, chlorthalidone produces dose-related reductions in serum potassium levels, elevations in serum uric acid and blood glucose, and it can lead to decreased sodium and chloride levels.

The mean plasma half-life of chlorthalidone is about 40 to 60 hours. It is eliminated primarily as unchanged drug in the urine. Non-renal routes of elimination have yet to be clarified. In the blood, approximately 75% of the drug is bound to plasma proteins.

Thalitone® (chlorthalidone USP) has been formulated with PVP (povidone polyvinylpyrrolidone), a bioavailability enhancer that provides 104% to 116% bioavailability relative to an oral solution of chlorthalidone. Thalitone® cannot be substituted for other formulations of chlorthalidone and likewise, other formulations of chlorthalidone cannot be substituted for Thalitone®.

INDICATIONS AND USAGE

Thalitone® (chlorthalidone USP) is indicated in the management of hypertension either alone or in combination with other antihypertensive drugs.

Chlorthalidone is indicated as adjunctive therapy in edema associated with congestive heart failure, hepatic cirrhosis, and corticosteroid and estrogen therapy.

Chlorthalidone has also been found useful in edema due to various forms of renal dysfunction such as nephrotic syndrome, acute glomerulonephritis, and chronic renal failure.

Usage in Pregnancy The routine use of diuretics in an otherwise healthy woman is inappropriate and exposes mother and fetus to unnecessary hazard. Diuretics do not prevent development of toxemia of pregnancy and there is no satisfactory evidence that they are useful in the treatment of developed toxemia.

Edema during pregnancy may arise from pathological causes or from the physiologic and mechanical consequences of pregnancy. Chlorthalidone is indicated in pregnancy when edema is due to pathologic causes just as it is in the absence of pregnancy (however, see WARNINGS below). Dependent edema in pregnancy resulting from restriction of venous return by the expanded uterus is properly treated through elevation of the lower extremities and use of support hose; use of diuretics to lower intravascular volume in this case is illogical and unnecessary. There is hypervolemia during normal pregnancy that is harmful to neither the fetus nor the mother (in the absence of cardiovascular disease) but that is associated with edema, including generalized edema, in the majority of pregnant women. If this edema produces discomfort, increased recumbency will often provide relief. In rare instances, this edema may cause extreme discomfort that is not relieved by rest. In these cases, a short course of diuretics may provide relief and may be appropriate.

CONTRAINDICATIONS

Anuria. Known hypersensitivity to chlorthalidone or other sulfonamide-derived drugs.

WARNINGS

Thalitone® (chlorthalidone USP) should be used with caution in severe renal disease. In patients with renal disease, chlorthalidone or related drugs may precipitate azotemia. Cumulative effects of the drug may develop in patients with impaired renal function.

Chlorthalidone should be used with caution in patients with impaired hepatic function or progressive liver disease, because minor alterations of fluid and electrolyte balance may precipitate hepatic coma.

Sensitivity reactions may occur in patients with a history of allergy or bronchial asthma.

The possibility of exacerbation or activation of systemic lupus erythematosus has been reported with thiazide diuretics which are structurally related to chlorthalidone. However, systemic lupus erythematosus has not been reported following chlorthalidone administration.

PRECAUTIONS

General Hypokalemia and other electrolyte abnormalities, including hyponatremia and hypochloremic alkalosis, are common in patients receiving chlorthalidone. These abnormalities are dose-related but may occur even at the lowest marketed doses of chlorthalidone. Serum electrolytes should be determined before initiating therapy and at periodic intervals during therapy. Serum and urine electrolyte determinations are particularly important when the patient is vomiting excessively or receiving parenteral fluids. All patients taking chlorthalidone should be observed for clinical signs of electrolyte imbalance, including dryness of mouth, thirst, weakness, lethargy, drowsiness, restlessness, muscle pains or cramps, muscular fatigue, hypotension, oliguria, tachycardia, palpitations and gastrointestinal disturbances, such as nausea and vomiting. Digitalis therapy may exaggerate metabolic effects of hypokalemia especially with reference to myocardial activity.

Any chloride deficit is generally mild and usually does not require specific treatment except under extraordinary circumstances (as in liver disease or renal disease). Dilutional hyponatremia may occur in edematous patients in hot weather; appropriate therapy is water restriction, rather than administration of salt, except in rare instances when the hyponatremia is life-threatening. In cases of actual salt depletion, appropriate replacement is the therapy of choice.

Thiazide-like diuretics have been shown to increase the urinary excretion of magnesium; this may result in hypomagnesemia.

Calcium excretion is decreased by thiazide-like drugs. Pathological changes in the parathyroid gland with hypercalcemia and hypophosphatemia have been observed in a few patients on thiazide therapy. The common complications of hyperparathyroidism such as renal lithiasis, bone resorption and peptic ulceration have not been seen.

Uric Acid Hyperuricemia may occur or frank gout may be precipitated in certain patients receiving chlorthalidone.

Other Increases in serum glucose may occur and latent diabetes mellitus may become manifest during chlorthalidone therapy (see PRECAUTIONS Drug Interactions). Chlorthalidone and related drugs may decrease serum PBI levels without signs of thyroid disturbance.

Information For Patients Patients should inform their doctor if they have: 1) had an allergic reaction to chlorthalidone or other diuretics or have asthma 2) kidney disease 3) liver disease 4) gout 5) systemic lupus erythematosus, or 6) been taking other drugs such as cortisone, digitalis, lithium carbonate, or drugs for diabetes.

Patients should be cautioned to contact their physician if they experience any of the following symptoms of potassium loss: excess thirst, tiredness, drowsiness, restlessness, muscle pains or cramps, nausea, vomiting or increased heart rate or pulse.

Patients should also be cautioned that taking alcohol can increase the chance of dizziness occurring.

Laboratory Tests Periodic determination of serum electrolytes to detect possible electrolyte imbalance should be performed at appropriate intervals.

All patients receiving chlorthalidone should be observed for clinical signs of fluid or electrolyte imbalance: namely, hy-

Continued on next page

Thalitone—Cont.

ponatremia, hypochloremic alkalosis and hypokalemia. Serum and urine electrolyte determinations are particularly important when the patient is vomiting excessively or receiving parenteral fluids.

Drug Interactions Chlorthalidone may add to or potentiate the action of other antihypertensive drugs.

Insulin requirements in diabetic patients may be increased, decreased or unchanged. Higher dosage of oral hypoglycemic agents may be required.

Chlorthalidone and related drugs may increase the responsiveness to tubocurarine.

Chlorthalidone and related drugs may decrease arterial responsiveness to norepinephrine. This diminution is not sufficient to preclude effectiveness of the pressor agent for therapeutic use.

Lithium renal clearance is reduced by chlorthalidone, increasing the risk of lithium toxicity.

Drug/Laboratory Test Interactions Chlorthalidone and related drugs may decrease serum PBI levels without signs of thyroid disturbance.

Carcinogenesis, Mutagenesis, Impairment of Fertility No information is available.

Pregnancy/Teratogenic Effects PREGNANCY CATEGORY B: Reproduction studies have been performed in the rat and the rabbit at doses up to 420 times the human dose and have revealed no evidence of harm to the fetus due to chlorthalidone. There are, however, no adequate and well-controlled studies in pregnant women. Because animal reproduction studies are not always predictive of human response, this drug should be used during pregnancy only if clearly needed.

Pregnancy/Non-Teratogenic Effects Thiazides cross the placental barrier and appear in cord blood. The use of chlorthalidone and related drugs in pregnant women requires that the anticipated benefits of the drug be weighed against possible hazards to the fetus. These hazards include fetal or neonatal jaundice, thrombocytopenia, and possibly other adverse reactions that have occurred in the adult.

Nursing Mothers Thiazides are excreted in human milk. Because of the potential for serious adverse reactions in nursing infants from chlorthalidone, a decision should be made whether to discontinue nursing or to discontinue the drug, taking into account the importance of the drug to the mother.

Pediatric Use Safety and effectiveness in children have not been established.

ADVERSE REACTIONS

The following adverse reactions have been observed, but there is not enough systematic collection of data to support an estimate of their frequency.

Gastrointestinal System Reactions: anorexia, gastric irritation, nausea, vomiting, cramping, diarrhea, constipation, jaundice (intrahepatic cholestatic jaundice), pancreatitis.

Central Nervous System Reactions: dizziness, vertigo, paresthesias, headache, xanthopsia.

Hematologic Reactions: leukopenia, agranulocytosis, thrombocytopenia, aplastic anemia.

Dermatologic-Hypersensitivity Reactions: purpura, photosensitivity, rash, urticaria, necrotizing angiitis (vasculitis) (cutaneous vasculitis), Lyell's syndrome (toxic epidermal necrolysis).

Cardiovascular Reaction: Orthostatic hypotension may occur and may be aggravated by alcohol, barbiturates or narcotics.

Other Adverse Reactions: hyperglycemia, glycosuria, hyperuricemia, muscle spasm, weakness, restlessness, impotence.

Whenever adverse reactions are moderate or severe, chlorthalidone dosage should be reduced or therapy withdrawn.

OVERDOSAGE

Symptoms of acute overdosage include nausea, weakness, dizziness and disturbances of electrolyte balance. The oral LD_{50} of the drug in the mouse and the rat is more than 25,000 mg/kg body weight. The minimum lethal dose (MLD) in humans has not been established. There is no specific antidote but gastric lavage is recommended, followed by supportive treatment. Where necessary, this may include intravenous dextrose-saline with potassium, administered with caution.

DOSAGE AND ADMINISTRATION

Therapy should be initiated with the lowest possible dose, then titrated according to individual patient response. A single dose given in the morning with food is recommended; divided doses are unnecessary.

Hypertension Therapy in most patients should be initiated with a single daily dose of 15 mg. If the response is insufficient after a suitable trial, the dosage may be increased to 30 mg and then to a single daily dose of 45–50 mg. If additional control is required, the addition of a second antihypertensive drug is recommended. Increases in serum uric acid and decreases in serum potassium are dose-related over the 15–50 mg/day range and beyond.

Edema INITIATION: Adults, initially 30 to 60 mg daily or 60 mg on alternate days. Some patients may require 90 to 120 mg at these intervals or up to 120 mg daily. Dosages above this level, however, do not usually produce a greater response.

MAINTENANCE: Maintenance doses may often be lower than initial doses and should be adjusted according to the individual patient. Effectiveness is well sustained during continued use.

HOW SUPPLIED

White, kidney-shaped, compressed tablets coded M/024 containing 15 mg of chlorthalidone in bottles of 100 (NDC 61570-024-01).

Storage: Store below 30°C (86°F).

Manufactured for: Monarch Pharmaceuticals, Inc., Bristol, TN 37620

Manufactured by: King Pharmaceuticals, Inc., Bristol, TN 37620

5/98
0932886

TIGAN® ℞
(trimethobenzamide hydrochloride)
Capsules, Suppositories & Injectable

DESCRIPTION

Chemically, trimethobenzamide HCl is N-[p-[2-(dimethylamino)-ethoxy]benzyl]-3,4,5-trimethoxybenzamide hydrochloride. It has a molecular weight of 424.93 and the following structural formula:

$(CH_3)_2N\text{-}CH_2CH_2O\text{-}C_6H_4\text{-}CH_2NHC(=O)\text{-}C_6H_2(OCH_3)_3 \cdot HCl$

Capsules: Each 100-mg *Tigan®* capsule for oral use contains trimethobenzamide hydrochloride equivalent to 100 mg. The capsule has an opaque blue cap marked "Tigan" and an opaque white body marked "M186". Each 250-mg *Tigan®* capsule for oral use contains trimethobenzamide hydrochloride equivalent to 250 mg. The capsule has an opaque blue cap marked "Tigan" and an opaque blue body marked "M187".

Inactive Ingredients: FD&C Blue No. 1, FD&C Red No. 3, lactose, magnesium stearate, starch and titanium dioxide.

Suppositories (200 mg): Each suppository contains 200 mg trimethobenzamide hydrochloride and 2% benzocaine in a base compounded with polysorbate 80, white beeswax and propylene glycol monostearate.

Suppositories, Pediatric (100 mg): Each suppository contains 100 mg trimethobenzamide hydrochloride and 2% benzocaine in a base compounded with polysorbate 80, white beeswax and propylene glycol monostearate.

Ampuls: Each 2-mL ampul contains 200 mg trimethobenzamide hydrochloride compounded with 0.2% parabens (methyl and propyl) as preservatives, 1 mg sodium citrate and 0.4 mg citric acid as buffers and pH adjusted to approximately 5.0 with sodium hydroxide.

Multi-Dose Vials: Each mL contains 100 mg trimethobenzamide hydrochloride compounded with 0.45% phenol as preservative, 0.5 mg sodium citrate and 0.2 mg citric acid as buffers and pH adjusted to approximately 5.0 with sodium hydroxide.

ACTIONS

The mechanism of action of *Tigan®* as determined in animals is obscure, but may be the chemoreceptor trigger zone (CTZ), an area in the medulla oblongata through which emetic impulses are conveyed to the vomiting center; direct impulses to the vomiting center apparently are not similarly inhibited. In dogs pretreated with trimethobenzamide HCl, the emetic response to apomorphine is inhibited, while little or no protection is afforded against emesis induced by intragastric copper sulfate.

INDICATIONS

Tigan® is indicated for the control of nausea and vomiting.

CONTRAINDICATIONS

The injectable form of *Tigan®* in children, the suppositories in premature or newborn infants, and use in patients with known hypersensitivity to trimethobenzamide are contraindicated. Since the suppositories contain benzocaine they should not be used in patients known to be sensitive to this or similar local anesthetics.

WARNINGS

Caution should be exercised when administering *Tigan®* to children for the treatment of vomiting. Antiemetics are not recommended for treatment of uncomplicated vomiting in children and their use should be limited to prolonged vomiting of known etiology. There are three principal reasons for caution:

1. There has been some suspicion that centrally acting antiemetics may contribute, in combination with viral illnesses (a possible cause of vomiting in children), to development of Reye's syndrome, a potentially fatal acute childhood encephalopathy with visceral fatty degeneration, especially involving the liver. Although there is no confirmation of this suspicion, caution is nevertheless recommended.
2. The extrapyramidal symptoms which can occur secondary to *Tigan®* may be confused with the central nervous system signs of an undiagnosed primary disease responsible for the vomiting, e.g., Reye's syndrome or other encephalopathy.
3. It has been suspected that drugs with hepatotoxic potential such as *Tigan®*, may unfavorably alter the course of Reye's syndrome. Such drugs should therefore be avoided in children whose signs and symptoms (vomiting) could represent Reye's syndrome. It should also be noted that salicylates and acetaminophen are hepatotoxic at large doses. Although it is not known that at usual doses they would represent a hazard in patients with the underlying hepatic disorder of Reye's syndrome, these drugs, too, should be avoided in children whose signs and symptoms could represent Reye's syndrome, unless alternative methods of controlling fever are not successful.

Tigan® may produce drowsiness. Patients should not operate motor vehicles or other dangerous machinery until their individual responses have been determined. Reye's syndrome has been associated with the use of *Tigan®* and other drugs, including antiemetics, although their contribution, if any, to the cause and course of the disease has not been established. This syndrome is characterized by an abrupt onset shortly following a non-specific febrile illness, with persistent, sever vomiting, lethargy, irrational behavior, progressive encephalopathy leading to coma, convulsions and death.

Usage in Pregnancy: Trimethobenzamide hydrochloride was studied in reproduction experiments in rats and rabbits and no teratogenicity was suggested. The only effects observed were an increased percentage of embryonic resorptions or stillborn pups in rats administered 20 mg and 100 mg/kg and increased resorptions in rabbits receiving 100 mg/kg. In each study these adverse effects were attributed to one or two dams. The relevance to humans is not known. Since there is no adequate experience in pregnant or lactating women who have received this drug, safety in pregnancy or in nursing mothers has not been established.

Usage with Alcohol: Concomitant use of alcohol with *Tigan®* may result in an adverse drug interaction.

PRECAUTIONS

During the course of acute febrile illness, encephalitides, gastroenteritis, dehydration and electrolyte imbalance, especially in children and the elderly or debilitated, CNS reactions such as opisthotonos, convulsions, coma and extrapyramidal symptoms have been reported with and without use of *Tigan®* (trimethobenzamide hydrochloride) or other antiemetic agents. In such disorders caution should be exercised in administering *Tigan®*, particularly to patients who have recently received other CNS-acting agents (phenothiazines, barbiturates, belladonna derivatives). It is recommended that severe emesis should not be treated with an antiemetic drug alone; where possible the cause of vomiting should be established. Primary emphasis should be directed toward the restoration of body fluids and electrolyte balance, the relief of fever and relief of the causative disease processes. Overhydration should be avoided since it may result in cerebral edema.

The antiemetic effects of *Tigan®* may render diagnosis more difficult in such conditions as appendicitis and obscure signs of toxicity due to overdosage of other drugs.

ADVERSE REACTIONS

There have been reports of hypersensitivity reactions and Parkinson-like symptoms. There have been instances of hypotension reported following parenteral administration to surgical patients. There have been reports of blood dyscrasias, blurring of vision, coma, convulsions, depression of mood, diarrhea, disorientation, dizziness, drowsiness, headache, jaundice, muscle cramps and opisthotonos. If these occur, the administration of the drug should be discontinued. Allergic-type skin reactions have been observed; therefore, the drug should be discontinued at the first sign of sensitization. While all symptoms will usually disappear spontaneously, symptomatic treatment may be indicated in some cases.

DOSAGE AND ADMINISTRATION

(See WARNINGS and PRECAUTIONS.)

Dosage should be adjusted according to the indication for therapy, severity of symptoms and the repsonse of the patient.

CAPSULES, 250 mg and 100 mg

Usual Adult Dosage

One 250 mg capsule t.i.d. or q.i.d.

Usual Children's Dosage

30 to 90 lbs: One or two 100 mg capsules t.i.d. or q.i.d.

SUPPOSITORIES, 200 mg (not to be used in premature or newborn infants)

Usual Adult Dosage

One suppository (200 mg) t.i.d. or q.i.d.

Usual Children's Dosage

Under 30 lbs: One-half suppository (100 mg) t.i.d. or q.i.d.

30 to 90 lbs: One-half to one suppository (100 to 200 mg) t.i.d. or q.i.d.

SUPPOSITORIES, PEDIATRIC, 10 mg (not to be used in premature or newborn infants)

Usual Children's Dosage

Under 30 lbs: One suppository (100 mg) t.i.d. or q.i.d.

30 to 90 lbs: One to two suppositories (100 to 200 mg) t.i.d. or q.i.d.

INJECTABLE, 100 mg (not for use in children)

Usual Adult Dosage

2 mL (200 mg) t.i.d. or q.i.d. intramuscularly

NOTE: The injectable form is intended for intramuscular administration only; it is not recommended for intravenous use.

Intramuscular administration may cause pain, stinging, burning, redness and swelling at the site of injection. Such effects may be minimized by deep injection into the upper outer quadrant of the gluteal region, and by avoiding the escape of solution along the route.

Rx Only.

STORAGE

Store Tigan® from 15° to 30°C (59° to 86°F).

HOW SUPPLIED

Capsules, 100 mg trimethobenzamide hydrochloride each, bottles of 100; 250 mg trimethobenzamide hydrochloride each, bottles of 100 and 500

NDC 61570-186-01 100 mg 100's
NDC 61570-187-01 250 mg 100's
NDC 61570-187-05 250 mg 500's

Suppositories, Pediatric, 100 mg, boxes of 10

Suppositories, 200 mg, boxes of 10 and 50

NDC 61570-503-10 100 mg (box of 10)
NDC 61570-504-10 200 mg (box of 10)
NDC 61570-504-50 200 mg (box of 50)

Ampuls, 2 mL, boxes of 10

NDC 61570-540-02 100 mg/mL in 2 mL ampul

Multi-Dose Vials, 20 mL

NDC 61570-541-20 100 mg/mL in 20 mL Multi-Dose Vials

Manufactured by:
King Pharmaceuticals, Inc.
Bristol, TN 37620

TUSSEND®

Syrup and Tablets Ⓒ℞

(Hydrocodone bitartrate, USP, pseudoephedrine hydrochloride, USP, chlorpheniramine hydrochloride, USP)

TUSSEND® SYRUP:

DESCRIPTION

Each teaspoonful (5 mL) contains:

Hydrocodone Bitartrate, USP	2.5 mg
Pseudoephedrine Hydrochloride, USP	30 mg
Chlorpheniramine Maleate, USP	2 mg
Alcohol, USP	5%

TUSSEND® SYRUP also contains: High Fructose Corn Syrup, Sucrose, Propylene Glycol, Flavor, Methylparaben, Saccharin Sodium, Propylparaben, FD&C Yellow No. 6, and Purified Water, USP.

TUSSEND® TABLETS:

DESCRIPTION

Each tablet contains:

Hydrocodone Bitartrate, USP	5 mg
Pseudoephedrine Hydrochloride, USP	60 mg
Chlorpheniramine Maleate, USP	4 mg

TUSSEND® TABLETS also contain: Lactose, Pregelatinized Starch, Croscarmellose Sodium, Silicon Dioxide, Magnesium Stearate and D & C Yellow #10.

Hydrocodone bitartrate is an opioid analgesic and antitussive and occurs as fine white, crystals or as crystalline powder. It is affected by light. The chemical name is 4,5α-epoxy-3-methoxy-17-methylmorphinan-6-one-tartrate (1:1) hydrate (2:5). Its structural formula is as follows:

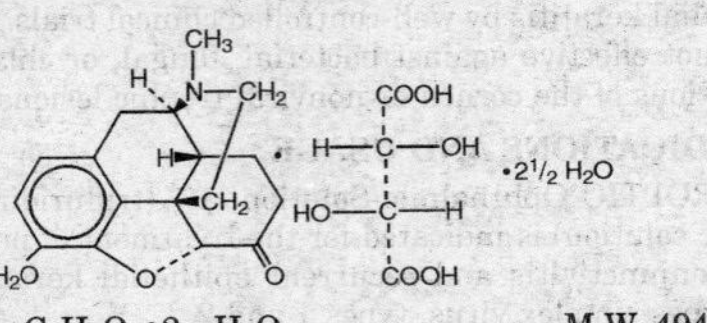

$C_{16}H_{21}NO_3 \cdot C_4H_6O_6 \cdot 2_{1/2}H_2O$ M.W. 494.50

Pseudoephedrine hydrochloride is an adrenergic (vasoconstrictor) which occurs as fine white to off-white crystals or powder, having a faint characteristic odor. It is very soluble in water, freely soluble in alcohol, and sparingly soluble in chloroform. The chemical name is benzenemethanol, α-[1-(methylamino)ethyl]- [S-(R*,R*)]-hydrochloride. Its structural formula is as follows:

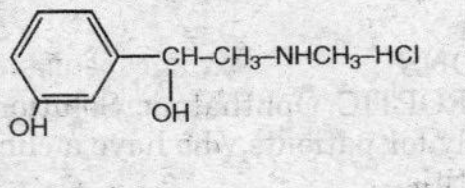

$C_{10}H_{15}NO$ HCl
M.W. 201.70

Chlorpheniramine maleate is an antihistaminic that occurs as white, odorless, crystalline powder. Its solutions have a pH between 4 and 5. It is freely soluble in water, soluble in alcohol and in chloroform, and slightly soluble in ether and benzene. The chemical name is 2-pyridinepropanamine, α-(4-chlorophenyl)-N, N-dimethyl-(Z)-2-butenedioate (1:1). Its structural formula is as follows:

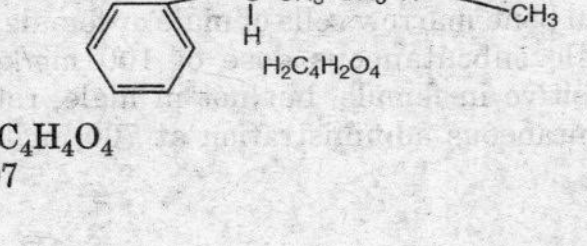

$C_{16}H_{19}CN_2C_4H_4O_4$
M.W. 300.07

CLINICAL PHARMACOLOGY

Hydrocodone is a semi-synthetic narcotic antitussive with multiple actions qualitatively similar to those of codeine. Most of these involve the central nervous system and smooth muscle. The precise mechanism of action of hydrocodone and other opiates is not known; however, hydrocodone is believed to act directly on the cough center. In excessive doses, hydrocodone, like other opium derivatives, will depress respiration. The effects of hydrocodone in therapeutic doses on the cardiovascular system are insignificant. Hydrocodone can produce miosis, euphoria, physical and physiological dependence.

Following a 10 mg oral dose of hydrocodone administered to five adult male subjects, the mean peak concentration was 23.6 +/– 5.2 ng/mL. Maximum serum levels were achieved at 1.3 +/– 0.3 hours and the half-life was determined to be 3.8 +/– 0.3 hours. Hydrocodone exhibits a complex pattern of metabolism including O-demethylation, N-demethylation and 6-keto reduction to the corresponding 6-α- and 6-β-hydroxymetabolites.

Pseudoephedrine acts as an indirect sympathomimetic agent by stimulating sympathetic (adrenergic) nerve endings to release norepinephrine. Norepinephrine in turn stimulates alpha and beta receptors throughout the body. The action of pseudoephedrine hydrochloride is apparently more specific for the blood vessels of the upper respiratory tract and less specific for the blood vessels of the systemic circulation. The vasoconstriction elicited at these sites results in the shrinkage of swollen tissues in the sinuses and nasal passages. Pseudoephedrine is rapidly and almost completely absorbed from the gastrointestinal tract. Considerable variation in half-life has been observed (from about 45 minutes to 10 hours) which is attributed to differences in absorption and excretion. Excretion rates are also altered by urine pH, increasing with acidification and decreasing with alkalinization. As a result, mean half-life falls to about 4 hours at pH 5 and increases to about 12 to 13 hours at pH 8. After administration of a 60 mg tablet, 87 to 97% of the pseudoephedrine is cleared from the body within 24 hours. The drug is distributed to body tissues and fluids, including fetal tissue, breast milk, and the central nervous system. About 55% to 75% of an administered dose is excreted unchanged in the urine; the remainder is apparently metabolized in the liver to inactive compounds by N-demethylation, parahydroxylation, and oxidative deamination.

Chlorpheniramine is an antihistamine that possesses anticholinergic and sedative effects. It is considered one of the most effective and least toxic of the histamine antagonists. Chlorpheniramine is a H_1 receptor antagonist. It antagonizes many of the pharmacologic actions of histamine. It prevents released histamine from dilating capillaries and causing edema of the respiratory mucosa. Chlorpheniramine is well absorbed and has a duration of action 4 to 6 hours. Its half-life in serum is 12 to 16 hours. Degradation products of chlorpheniramine's metabolic transformation by the liver are almost completely excreted in 24 hours.

INDICATIONS

TUSSEND® syrup and tablets are indicated for relief of cough and congestion due to colds, acute respiratory infections, laryngeal and pulmonary tuberculosis, acute and chronic bronchitis and hay fever. In addition TUSSEND® syrup and tablets helps relieve the sneezing and itching associated with hay fever.

CONTRAINDICATIONS

Hypersensitivity to any of the ingredients. Patients known to be hypersensitive to other sympathomimetic amines may exhibit cross sensitivity with pseudoephedrine. Sympathomimetic amines are contraindicated in patients with severe coronary artery disease, and patients on monoamine oxidase (MAO) inhibitor therapy.

Antihistamines are contraindicated in patients with narrow-angle glaucoma, urinary retention, peptic ulcer, during an asthmatic attack and in patients receiving MAO inhibitors.

TUSSEND® syrup and tablets should not be administered to pre-mature or full-term infants. TUSSEND® syrup and tablets are contraindicated in nursing mothers because of the higher than usual risk for infants from sympathomimetic amines.

WARNINGS

General: Sympathomimetic amines should be used with caution in patients with hypertension, ischemic heart disease, diabetes mellitus, increased intraocular pressure, hyperthyroidism, or prostatic hypertrophy. Sympathomimetics may produce central nervous system stimulation with convulsions or cardiovascular collapse with accompanying hypotension. DO NOT EXCEED RECOMMENDED DOSAGE.

Hypertensive crises can occur with concurrent use of pseudoephedrine and monoamine oxidase (MAO) inhibitors, indomethacin, or with beta blockers and methyldopa. If a hypertensive crisis occurs, these drugs should be discontinued immediately and therapy to lower blood pressure should be instituted. Fever should be managed by means of external cooling.

Chlorpheniramine has an atropine-like action and should be used with caution in patients with increased intraocular pressure, cardiovascular disease, hypertension or in patients with a history of bronchial asthma.

Head Injury and Increased Intracranial Pressure: The respiratory depressant effects of narcotics and their capacity to elevate cerebrospinal fluid pressure may be markedly exaggerated in the presence of head injury, other intracranial lesions or a pre-existing increase in intracranial pressure. Furthermore, narcotics produce adverse reactions which may obscure the clinical course of patients with head injuries.

Acute Abdominal Conditions: The administration of narcotics may obscure the diagnosis or clinical course of patients with acute abdominal conditions.

PRECAUTIONS

Special Risk Patients: As with any narcotic, TUSSEND® syrup and tablets should be used with caution in elderly or debilitated patients and those with severe impairment of hepatic or renal function, hypothyroidism, Addison's disease, prostatic hypertrophy or urethral stricture. The usual precautions should be observed and the possibility of respiratory depression should be kept in mind.

Information for Patients: Narcotics and antihistamines may impair the mental and physical abilities required for the performance of potentially hazardous tasks, such as driving a vehicle or operating machinery. Patients should also be warned about the possible additive effects with alcohol and other central nervous system depressants (hypnotics, sedatives, tranquilizers).

Drug Interactions: Patients receiving other narcotics, antipsychotics, antianxiety agents or other CNS depressants (including alcohol) concomitantly with TUSSEND® syrup and tablets may exhibit additive CNS depression. When combined therapy is contemplated, the dose of one or both agents should be reduced. The use of MAO inhibitors or tricyclic antidepressants with hydrocodone preparations may increase the effect of either the antidepressant or hydrocodone.

The concurrent use of anticholinergics with hydrocodone may produce paralytic ileus.

Beta-adrenergic blockers and MAO inhibitors may potentiate the pressor effects of pseudoephedrine. Concurrent use of digitalis glycosides may increase the possibility of cardia arrhythmias. Sympathomimetics may reduce the hypotensive effects of guanethidine, mecamylamine, methyldopa, reserpine, and veratrum alkaloids. Concurrent use of tricyclic antidepressants may antagonize the effects of pseudoephedrine.

Laboratory Test Interactions: Antihistamines may suppress the wheal and flare reactions to antigen skin testing. Considerable interindividual variation in the extent and duration of suppression have been reported, depending on the antigen and test technique, antihistamine and dosage regimen, time since the last dose and individual response to testing. In one study, usual oral dosages of chlorpheniramine suppressed the wheal response for about 2 days after the last dose. Whenever possible antihistamines should be discontinued about 4 days prior to skin testing procedures since they may prevent otherwise positive reactions to dermal reactivity indicators.

Carcinogenesis, Mutagenesis and Impairment of Fertility: No long term or reproduction studies in animals have been performed with TUSSEND® syrup or tablets to evaluate its carcinogenic, mutagenic and impairment of fertility potential.

Usage In Pregnancy: Teratogenic Effects: Pregnancy Category C. Hydrocodone has been shown to be teratogenic in hamsters when given in doses 700 times the human dose. There are no adequate and well-controlled studies in pregnant women. TUSSEND® syrup or tablets should be used during pregnancy only if the potential benefit justifies the potential risk to the fetus.

Nonteratogenic Effects: Babies born to mothers who have been taking opioids regularly prior to delivery will be physically dependent. The withdrawal signs include irritability and excessive crying, tremors, hyperactive reflexes, increased respiratory rate, increased stools, sneezing, yawning, vomiting and fever. The intensity of syndrome does not always correlate with the duration of maternal opioid use or dose. There is no consensus on the best method of managing withdrawal. Chlorpromazine 0.7–1.0 mg/kg q6h, and paregoric 2–4 drops q4h, have been used to treat withdrawal symptoms in infants. The duration of therapy is 4 to 28 days, with the dosage decreased as tolerated.

Labor and Delivery: As with all narcotics administration of TUSSEND® syrup or tablets to the mother shortly before delivery may result in some degree of respiratory depression in the newborn, especially if higher doses are used.

Nursing Mothers: TUSSEND® syrup and tablets are contraindicated in nursing mothers because of the higher than usual risk infants with sympathomimetic amines.

Pediatric Use: Antihistamines may cause excitability, especially in children. Do not exceed recommended dosage because at higher doses nervousness, dizziness or sleeplessness may occur.

In young children, as well as adults, the respiratory center is sensitive to the depressant action of narcotic cough suppressants in a dose-dependent manner. Benefit to risk ratio should be carefully considered especially in children with respiratory embarrassment (e.g., croup).

Use in the Elderly: The elderly (60 years and older) are more likely to have adverse reactions to sympathomimetics. Overdose of sympathomimetics in this age group may cause hallucinations, convulsions, CNS depression and death.

ADVERSE REACTIONS

Hydrocodone Bitartrate: The most frequently observed adverse reactions include lightheadedness, dizziness, sedation, nausea and vomiting. These effects seem to be more

Continued on next page

Tussend Syrup/Tablets—Cont.

prominent in ambulatory patients than in nonambulatory patients and some of these adverse reactions may be alleviated if the patient lies down.

Other adverse reactions include:

Central Nervous System: Drowsiness, mental clouding, lethargy, impairment of mental and physical performance, anxiety, fear, dysphoria, psychic dependence, mood changes.

Gastrointestinal System: Prolonged administration may produce constipation.

Genitourinary System: Urethral spasm, spasm of vesical sphincters and urinary retention have been reported.

Pseudoephedrine Hydrochloride: Pseudoephedrine may cause mild central nervous system stimulation, especially in those patients who are hypersensitive to sympathomimetic drugs. Nervousness, excitability, restlessness, dizziness, weakness and insomnia may also occur. Headache and drowsiness have also been reported. Large doses may cause lightheadedness, nausea and/or vomiting. Sympathomimetic drugs have also been associated with certain untoward reactions including fear, anxiety, tenseness, restlessness, tremor, weakness, pallor respiratory difficulty, dysuria, insomnia, hallucination, convulsion, CNS depression, arrhythmias and cardiovascular collapse with hypotension.

Chlorpheniramine Maleate: Slight to moderate drowsiness may occur and is the most frequent side effect.

Other possible side effects of antihistamines in general include:

General: Urticaria, drug rash, anaphylactic shock, photosensitivity, excessive perspiration, chills, dryness of the mouth, nose and throat.

Cardiovascular: Hypotension, headache, palpitation, tachycardia extrasystoles.

Hematological: Hemolytic anemia, thrombocytopenia and agranulocytosis.

CNS: Sedation, dizziness, disturbed coordination, fatigue, confusion, restlessness, excitation, nervousness, tremor, irritability, insomnia, euphoria, paresthesia, blurred vision, diplopia, vertigo, tinnitus, hysteria, neuritis, convulsion.

Gastrointestinal: Epigastric distress, anorexia, nausea, vomiting, diarrhea, constipation.

Genitourinary: Urinary frequency, difficult urination, urinary retention, early menses.

Respiratory: Thickening of bronchial secretions, tightness of chest, wheezing and nasal stuffiness.

DRUG ABUSE AND DEPENDENCE

TUSSEND® syrup and tablets are subject to the Federal Controlled Substances Act (Schedule III).

Psychic dependence and tolerance may develop upon repeated administration of narcotics; therefore, TUSSEND® syrup and tablets should be prescribed and administered with caution. However, psychic dependence is unlikely to develop when TUSSEND® syrup or tablets are used for a short time.

Physical dependence, the condition in which continued administration of the drug is required to prevent the appearance of a withdrawal syndrome, assumes clinically significant proportions only after several weeks of continued narcotic use, although some mild degree of physical dependence may develop after a few days of narcotic therapy. Tolerance, in which increasingly large doses are required to produce the same degree of effectiveness, is manifested initially by a shortened duration of effect, and subsequently by decreases in the intensity of the effect. The rate of development of tolerance varies among patients.

OVERDOSAGE

Signs and Symptoms: Hydrocodone: Serious overdosage with hydrocodone is characterized by respiratory depression (a decrease in respiratory rate and/or tidal volume, Cheyne Stokes respiration, cyanosis), extreme somnolence progressing to stupor or coma, skeletal muscle flaccidity, cold and clammy skin, and sometimes bradycardia and hypotension. In severe overdosage, apnea, circulatory collapse, cardiac arrest and death may occur.

Pseudoephedrine: Overdosage with pseudoephedrine can cause excessive central nervous system stimulation resulting in excitement, nervousness, anxiety, tremor, restlessness and insomnia. Other effects include tachycardia, hypertension, pallor, mydriasis, hyperglycemia and urinary retention. Severe overdosage may cause tachypnea, or hyperpnea, hallucinations, convulsion, or delirium, but in some individuals there may be central nervous system depression with somnolence, stupor, or respiratory depression. Arrythmias (including ventricular fibrillation) may lead to hypotension and circulatory collapse. Severe hypokalemia can occur, probably due to compartmental shift rather than depletion of potassium. No organ damage or significant metabolic arrangement is associated with pseudoephedrine overdosage. The toxic and lethal concentration in human biologic fluids are not known. Excretion rates increase with urine acidification and decrease with alkalinization. Few reports of toxicity due to pseudoephedrine have been published, and no case of fatal overdosage is known.

Chlorpheniramine: Manifestations of antihistamine overdosage may vary from central nervous system depression (sedation, apnea, cardiovascular collapse) to stimulation (insomnia, hallucinations, tremors or convulsions). Other signs and symptoms may be dizziness, tinnitus, ataxia, blurred vision and hypotension. Stimulation is particularly likely in children, as are atropine-like signs and symptoms (dry mouth, dilated pupils, flushing, hyperthermia, and gastrointestinal symptoms).

Treatment: Primary attention should be given to the reestablishment of adequate respiratory exchange through provision of a patent airway and the institution of assisted or controlled ventilation. The narcotic antagonist naloxone is a specific antidote against respiratory depression which may result from overdosage or unusual sensitivity to narcotics including hydrocodone. Therefore, an appropriate dose of naloxone hydrochloride (see package insert) should be administered, preferably by the intravenous route and simultaneously with efforts at respiratory resuscitation. Since the duration of action of hydrocodone may exceed that of the antagonist, the patient should be kept under continued surveillance and repeated doses of the antagonist should be administered as needed to maintain adequate respiration.

An antagonist should not be administered in the absence of clinically significant respiratory or cardiovascular depression. Oxygen, intravenous fluids, vasopressors and other supportive measures should be employed as indicated.

Gastric emptying may be useful in removing unabsorbed drug.

The patient should be induced to vomit even if emesis has occurred spontaneously; however, vomiting should not be induced in patients with impaired consciousness. Precautions against aspiration should be taken, especially in infants and children.

Ipecac syrup is the preferred method for inducing vomiting. The action of ipecac is facilitated by physical activity and the administration of eight to twelve fluid ounces of water. If emesis does not occur within fifteen minutes, the dose of ipecac should be repeated. Following emesis, any drug remaining in the stomach may be absorbed by activated charcoal administered as a slurry with water.

If vomiting is unsuccessful or contraindicated, gastric lavage should be performed. Isotonic and one-half isotonic saline are the lavage solution of choice. Saline cathartics, such as milk of magnesia, draw water into the bowel by osmosis and, therefore, may be valuable for their action in rapid dilution of bowel content.

Treatment of the signs and symptoms of overdosage is symptomatic and supportive. Vasopressors may be used to treat hypotension. Short-acting barbiturates diazepam or paraldehyde may be administered to control seizures.

Hyperpyrexia, especially in children, may require treatment with tepid water sponge baths or a hypothermic blanket. Apnea is treated with ventilatory support. Stimulants (analeptic agents) should not be used.

DOSAGE AND ADMINISTRATION

TUSSEND® SYRUP

ADULTS: Two teaspoonfuls (10mL) every 4–6 hours. **CHILDREN: 6–12 years:** One teaspoonful (5mL) every 4–6 hours. Do not exceed four doses in a 24 hour period.

TUSSEND® TABLETS

ADULTS: 1 tablet every 4-6 hours. **CHILDREN: 6–12 years:** 1/2 tablet every 4–6 hours. Do not exceed four doses in a 24 hour period.

HOW SUPPLIED

TUSSEND® SYRUP is supplied as a clear yellow liquid, banana-flavored, in bottles of one pint (16 fl. oz.), NDC 61570-004-16.

TUSSEND® TABLETS are yellow, scored, capsule shaped with a MPC100 identification number.

Bottles of 100 .... NDC 61570-011-01

Storage: Store at controlled room temperature, 15°–30°C (59°–86°F).

Dispense in a tight, light-resistant container as described in USP.

Rx only

A Schedule CIII Controlled Substance.

Manufactured for: Monarch Pharmaceuticals, Inc., Bristol, TN 37620

Manufactured by: King Pharmaceuticals, Inc., Bristol, TN 37620

0931880

Revised 8/96

Shown in Product Identification Guide, page 325

VIROPTIC® Ophthalmic Solution, 1% Sterile ℞
(trifluridine ophthalmic solution)

DESCRIPTION

VIROPTIC is the brand name for trifluridine (also known as trifluorothymidine, F_3TdR,F_3T), an antiviral drug for topical treatment of epithelial keratitis caused by herpes simplex virus. The chemical name of trifluridine is α,α,α-trifluorothymidine; it has the following structural formula:

[See chemical structure at top of next column]

VIROPTIC sterile ophthalmic solution contains 1% trifluridine in an aqueous solution with acetic acid and sodium acetate (buffers), sodium chloride, and thimerosal 0.001% (added as a preservative). The pH range is 5.5 to 6.0 and osmolality is approximately 283 mOsm.

CLINICAL PHARMACOLOGY

Trifluridine is a fluorinated pyrimidine nucleoside with *in vitro* and *in vivo* activity against herpes simplex virus, types 1 and 2 and vacciniavirus. Some strains of adenovirus are also inhibited *in vitro*.

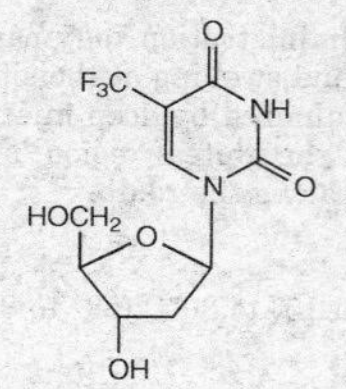

M.W. = 296.21 $C_{10}H_{11}F_3N_2O_5$

VIROPTIC is also effective in the treatment of epithelial keratitis that has not responded clinically to the topical administration of idoxuridine or when ocular toxicity or hypersensitivity to idoxuridine has occurred. In a smaller number of patients found to be resistant to topical vidarabine, VIROPTIC was also effective.

Trifluridine interferes with DNA synthesis in cultured mammalian cells. However, its antiviral mechanism of action is not completely known.

In vitro perfusion studies on excised rabbit corneas have shown that trifluridine penetrates the intact cornea as evidenced by recovery of parental drug and its major metabolite, 5-carboxy-2′-deoxyuridine, on the endothelial side of the cornea. Absence of the corneal epithelium enhances the penetration of trifluridine approximately two-fold.

Intraocular penetration of trifluridine occurs after topical instillation of VIROPTIC into human eyes. Decreased corneal integrity or stromal or uveal inflammation may enhance the penetration of trifluridine into the aqueous humor. Unlike the results of ocular penetration of trifluridine *in vitro*, 5-carboxy-2′-deoxyuridine was not found in detectable concentrations within the aqueous humor of the human eye.

Systemic absorption of trifluridine following therapeutic dosing with VIROPTIC appears to be negligible. No detectable concentrations of trifluridine or 5-carboxy-2′-deoxyuridine were found in the sera of adult healthy normal subjects who had VIROPTIC instilled into their eyes seven times daily for 14 consecutive days.

Clinical Studies: During a controlled multicenter clinical trial, 92 of 97 (95%) patients (78 of 81 with dendritic and 14 of 16 with geographic ulcers) responded to therapy with VIROPTIC as evidenced by complete corneal re-epithelialization within the 14-day therapy period. Fifty-six of 75 (75%) patients (49 of 58 with dendritic and 7 of 17 with geographic ulcers) responded to idoxuridine therapy. The mean time to corneal re-epithelialization for dendritic ulcers (6 days) and geographic ulcers (7 days) was similar for both therapies.

In other clinical studies. VIROPTIC was evaluated in the treatment of herpes simplex virus keratitis in patients who were unresponsive or intolerant to the topical administration of idoxuridine or vidarabine. VIROPTIC was effective in 138 of 150 (92%) patients (109 of 114 with dendritic and 29 of 36 with geographic ulcers) as evidenced by corneal re-epithelialization. The mean time to corneal re-epithelialization was 6 days for patients with dendritic ulcers and 12 days for patients with geographic ulcers.

The clinical efficacy of VIROPTIC in the treatment of stromal keratitis and uveitis due to herpes simplex virus or ophthalmic infections caused by vacciniavirus and adenovirus has not been established by well-controlled clinical trials. VIROPTIC has not been shown to be effective in the prophylaxis of herpes simplex virus keratoconjunctivitis and epithelial keratitis by well-controlled clinical trials. VIROPTIC is not effective against bacterial, fungal, or chlamydial infections of the cornea or nonviral trophic lesions.

INDICATIONS AND USAGE

VIROPTIC Ophthalmic Solution, 1% (trifluridine ophthalmic solution) is indicated for the treatment of primay keratoconjunctivitis and recurrent epithelial keratitis due to herpes simplex virus, types 1 and 2.

CONTRAINDICATIONS

VIROPTIC Ophthalmic Solution, 1% is contraindicated for patients who develop hypersensitivity reactions or chemical intolerance to trifluridine.

WARNINGS

The recommended dosage and frequency of administration should not be exceeded (see **DOSAGE AND ADMINISTRATION**).

PRECAUTIONS

General: VIROPTIC Ophthalmic Solution, 1% should be prescribed only for patients who have a clinical diagnosis of herpetic keratitis.

VIROPTIC may cause mild local irritation of the conjunctiva and cornea when instilled, but these effects are usually transient.

Although documented *in vitro* viral resistance to trifluridine has not been reported following multiple exposures to VIROPTIC, the possibility of the development of viral resistance exists.

Carcinogenesis, Mutagenesis, Impairment of Fertility: ***Mutagenic Potential:*** Trifluridine has been shown to exert mutagenic, DNA-damaging and cell-transforming activities in various standard *in vitro* test systems, and clastogenic activity in *Vicia faba* cells. It did not induce chromosome aberrations in bone marrow cells of male or female rats following a single subcutaneous dose of 100 mg/kg, but was weakly positive in female, but not in male, rats following daily subcutaneous administration at 700 mg/kg/day for 5 days.

Although the significance of these test results is not clear or fully understood, there exists the possibility that mutagenic agents may cause genetic damage in humans.

Oncogenic Potential: Lifetime carcinogenicity bioassays in rats and mice given daily subcutaneous doses of trifluridine have been performed. Rats tested at 1.5, 7.5, and 15 mg/kg/day had increased incidences of adenocarcinomas of the intestinal tract and mammary glands, hemangiosarcomas of the spleen and liver, carcinosarcomas of the prostate gland, and granulosa-thecal cell tumors of the ovary. Mice were tested at 1, 5, and 10 mg/kg/day; those given 10 mg/kg/day trifluridine had significantly increased incidences of adenocarcinomas of the intestinal tract and uterus. Those given 10 mg/kg/day also had a significantly increased incidence of testicular atrophy as compared to vehicle control mice.

Pregnancy: *Teratogenic Effects:* Pregnancy Category C. Trifluridine was not teratogenic at doses up to 5 mg/kg/day (23 times the estimated human exposure) when given subcutaneously to rats and rabbits. However, fetal toxicity consisting of delayed ossification of portions of the skeleton occurred at dose levels of 2.5 and 5 mg/kg/day in rats and at 2.5 resorption in rabbits. In both rats and rabbits, 1 mg/kg/day (5 times the estimated human exposure) was a no-effect level. There were no teratogenic or fetotoxic effects after topical application of VIROPTIC Ophthalmic Solution, 1% (approximately 5 times the estimated human exposure) to the eyes of rabbits on the 6th through the 18th days of pregnancy. In a non-standard test, trifluridine solution has been shown to be teratogenic when injected directly into the yolk sac of chicken eggs. There are no adequate and well-controlled studies in pregnant women. VIROPTIC Ophthalmic Solution, 1% should be used during pregnancy only if the potential benefit justifies the potential risk to the fetus.

Nursing Mothers: It is unlikely that trifluridine is excreted in human milk after ophthalmic instillation of VIROPTIC because of the relatively small dosage (≤5 mg/day), its dilution in body fluids and its extremely short half-life (approximately 12 minutes). The drug should not be prescribed for nursing mothers unless the potential benefits outweigh the potential risks.

Pediatric Use: Safety and effectiveness in pediatric patients below six years of age have not been established.

ADVERSE REACTIONS

The most frequent adverse reactions reported during controlled clinical trials were mild, transient burning or stinging upon instillation (4.6%) and palpebral edema (2.8%). Other adverse reactions in decreasing order of reported frequency were superficial punctate keratopathy, epithelial keratopathy, hypersensitivity reaction, stromal edema, irritation, keratitis sicca, hyperemia, and increased intraocular pressure.

OVERDOSAGE

Overdosage by ocular instillation is unlikely because any excess solution should be quickly expelled from the conjunctival sac.

Acute overdosage by accidental oral ingestion of VIROPTIC has not occurred. However, should such ingestion occur, the 75 mg dosage of trifluridine in a 7.5 mL bottle of VIROPTIC is not likely to produce adverse effects. Single intravenous doses of 1.5 to 30 mg/kg/day in children and adults with neoplastic disease produce reversible bone marrow depression as the only potentially serious toxic effect and only after three to five courses of therapy. The acute oral LD_{50} in the mouse and rat was 4379 mg/kg or higher.

DOSAGE AND ADMINISTRATION

Instill one drop of VIROPTIC Ophthalmic Solution, 1% onto the cornea of the affected eye every 2 hours while awake for a maximum daily dosage of nine drops until the corneal ulcer has completely re-epithelialized. Following re-epithelialization, treatment for an additional 7 days of one drop every 4 hours while awake for a minimum daily dosage of five drops is recommended.

If there are no signs of improvement after 7 days of therapy or complete re-epithelialization has not occurred after 14 days of therapy, other forms of therapy should be considered. Continuous administration of VIROPTIC for periods exceeding 21 days should be avoided because of potential ocular toxicity.

HOW SUPPLIED

VIROPTIC Ophthalmic Solution, 1% is supplied as a sterile ophthalmic solution in a plastic Drop Dose® dispenser bottle of 7.5 mL (NDC 61570-037-75).

Store under refrigeration 2° to 8°C (36° to 46°F).

ANIMAL PHARMACOLOGY AND ANIMAL TOXICOLOGY

Corneal wound healing studies in rabbits showed that VIROPTIC did not significantly retard closure of epithelial wounds. However, mild toxic changes such as intracellular edema of the basal cell layer, mild thinning of the overlying epithelium and reduced strength of stromal wounds were observed.

Whereas instillation of VIROPTIC into rabbit eyes during a subchronic toxicity study produced some degree of corneal epithelial thinning, a 12-month chronic toxicity study in rabbits in which VIROPTIC was instilled into eyes in intermittent, multiple, full-therapy courses showed no drug-related changes in the cornea.

Manufactured for: Monarch Pharmaceuticals®, Inc., Bristol, TN 37620

By: Catalytica Pharmaceutical, Inc., Greenville, NC 27835

Date of issue: 11/97
0932680

Monarch Pharmaceuticals®

Shown in Product Identification Guide, page 325

WYCILLIN® ℞

[*wi-sil 'in*]

(penicillin G procaine suspension)
INJECTION

FOR DEEP INTRAMUSCULAR INJECTION ONLY

DESCRIPTION

This product is designed to provide a stable aqueous suspension of penicillin G procaine, ready for immediate use. This eliminates the necessity for addition of any diluent, required for the usual dry formulation of injectable penicillin. Penicillin G procaine is chemically designated as (2*S*,5*R*,6*R*) -3,3-Dimethyl-7-oxo-6- (2-phenylacetamido) -4-thia-1-azabicyclo[3.2.0]heptane-2-carboxylic acid compound with 2-(diethylamino)ethyl *p*-aminobenzoate (1:1) monhydrate.

Its molecular formula is $C_{16}H_{18}N_2O_4S \bullet C_{13}H_{20}N_2O_2 \bullet H_2O$ WITH A MOLECULAR WEIGHT OF 588.72.

Each TUBEX Sterile Cartridge-Needle Unit, 1,200,000 units (2 mL size) or 600,000 units (1 mL size), or disposable syringe, 2,400,000 units (4 mL size), contains penicillin G procaine in a stabilized aqueous suspension with sodium citrate buffer; and as w/v, approximately 0.5% lecithin, 0.5% carboxymethylcellulose, 0.5% povidone, 0.1% methylparaben, and 0.01% propylparaben.

Wycillin must be stored in a refrigerator. Keep from freezing. This will prevent deterioration and assure that no significant loss of potency occurs within the expiration date.

Wycillin suspension in the TUBEX and disposable syringe formulations is viscous and opaque. Read **CONTRAINDICATIONS, WARNINGS, PRECAUTIONS,** and **DOSAGE AND ADMINISTRATION** sections prior to use.

HOW SUPPLIED

Wycillin® (penicillin G procaine suspension) is supplied in packages of 10 TUBEX® Sterile Cartridge-Needle Units (21 gauge, thin wall, $1^1/_4$ inch needle), as follows:

1 mL size, containing 600,000 units per TUBEX, NDC 0008-0018-34.

2 mL size, containing 1,200,000 units per TUBEX, NDC 0008-0018-35.

Store in a refrigerator.
Keep from freezing.

ALSO AVAILABLE:

Wycillin (penicillin G procaine suspension) is also available in packages of 10 disposable syringes as follows:

4 mL size, containing 2,400,000 units per syringe (18 gauge × 2 inch needle), NDC 0008-0018-12.

Manufactured by:
Wyeth Laboratories
A Wyeth-Ayerst Company
Philadelphia, PA 19101

For prescribing information write to Professional Service, Wyeth-Ayerst Pharmaceuticals, P.O. Box 8299, Philadelphia, PA 19101, or contact your local Wyeth-Ayerst representative.

Distributed by:
Monarch Pharmaceuticals, Inc.
Bristol, TN 37620

Refer to the Tubex® Closed Injection System instructions in the Wyeth-Ayerst section of the 2001 PDR®.

Muro Pharmaceutical, Inc.

an ASTA Medica company
890 EAST STREET
TEWKSBURY, MA 01876-1496

Direct Inquiries to:
Professional Service Department
(800) 225-0974
(978) 851-5981

BROMFED® ℞

[*brōm' fĕd*]

BROMFED-PD® ℞

℞ **only**

BROMFED® CAPSULES

A light green and clear capsule containing white beads. Extended-Release.

Each capsule contains:

Brompheniramine maleate .... 12 mg
Pseudoephedrine hydrochloride .... 120 mg

in a specially prepared base to provide prolonged action.

BROMFED-PD® CAPSULES

A dark green and clear capsule containing white beads. Extended-Release.

Each capsule contains:

Brompheniramine maleate .... 6 mg
Pseudoephedrine hydrochloride .... 60 mg

in a specially prepared base to provide prolonged action.

BROMFED® AND BROMFED-PD® CAPSULES also contain as inactive ingredients: Calcium Stearate, D&C Yellow #10, FD&C Blue #1, FD&C Yellow #6, Gelatin, Pharmaceutical Glaze, Starch, Sucrose and Talc.

BROMFED® AND BROMFED-PD® contain ingredients of the following therapeutic classes: antihistamine and decongestant.

CLINICAL PHARMACOLOGY

Brompheniramine maleate is an alkylamine-type antihistamine. This group of antihistamines are among the most active histamine antagonists and are generally effective in relatively low doses. The drugs are not so prone to produce drowsiness and are among the most suitable agents for daytime use; but again, a significant proportion of patients do experience this effect. Pseudoephedrine hydrochloride is a sympathomimetic which acts predominantly on alpha receptors and has little action on beta receptors. It therefore functions as an oral nasal decongestant with minimal central nervous system (CNS) stimulation.

INDICATIONS

For the treatment of the symptoms of seasonal and perennial allergic rhinitis, and vasomotor rhinitis, including nasal obstruction (congestion).

CONTRAINDICATIONS

Hypersensitivity to any of the ingredients. Also contraindicated in patients with severe hypertension, severe coronary artery disease, patients on monoamine oxidase (MAO) inhibitor therapy, patients with narrow-angle glaucoma, urinary retention, peptic ulcer and during an asthmatic attack.

WARNINGS

Considerable caution should be exercised in patients with hypertension, diabetes mellitus, ischemic heart disease, hyperthyroidism, increased intraocular pressure and prostatic hypertrophy. The elderly (60 years and older) are more likely to exhibit adverse reactions.

Antihistamines may cause excitability, especially in pediatric patients. At dosages higher than the recommended dose, nervousness, dizziness or sleeplessness may occur.

PRECAUTIONS

General: Caution should be exercised in patients with high blood pressure, heart disease, diabetes or thyroid disease. The antihistamine in this product may exhibit additive effects with other CNS depressants, including alcohol.

Information for Patients: Antihistamines may cause drowsiness. Ambulatory patients who operate machinery or motor vehicles should be cautioned accordingly.

Drug Interactions: MAO inhibitors and beta adrenergic blockers increase the effects of sympathomimetics. Sympathomimetics may reduce the antihypertensive effects of methyldopa, mecamylamine, reserpine and veratrum alkaloids. Concomitant use of antihistamines with alcohol and other CNS depresssants may have an additive effect.

Pregnancy

The safety or use of this product in pregnancy has not been established.

ADVERSE REACTIONS

Adverse reactions include drowsiness, lassitude, nausea, giddiness, dryness of the mouth, blurred vision, cardiac palpitations, flushing, increased irritability or excitement (especially in pediatric patients).

Pediatric Use: Antihistamines may cause excitability especially in the pediatric population. Safety and effectiveness of Bromfed® Capsules has not been established in pediatric patients less than 12 years of age, and safety and effectiveness of Bromfed-PD® Capsules has not been established in pediatric patients less than 6 years of age. See Contraindications, Warnings, and Precautions for complete information.

OVERDOSAGE

KEEP THIS AND ALL DRUGS OUT OF THE REACH OF CHILDREN. IN CASE OF SUSPECTED OVERDOSE, IMMEDIATELY CALL YOUR REGIONAL POISON CONTROL CENTER AND/OR SEEK PROFESSIONAL ASSISTANCE.

Symptoms of overdosage may be caused by pseudoephedrine. Symptoms of overdosage with pseudoephedrine include anxiety, tenseness, respiratory difficulty, headache and awareness of the slow forceful heartbeat.

Treatment of Overdose: The stomach should be emptied promptly by emetics and/or gastric lavage. The installation of activated charcoal also should be considered. Cardiac function and serum electrolytes should be monitored and treatment instituted if indicated. If convulsions or marked CNS excitement occurs, diazepam may be used.

DOSAGE AND ADMINISTRATION

BROMFED® CAPSULES

Adults and pediatric patients 12 years of age and over: 1 capsule every 12 hours.

BROMFED-PD® CAPSULES

Pediatric patients 6 to under 12 years of age: 1 capsule every 12 hours. Adults and pediatric patients 12 years of age and over: 1–2 capsules every 12 hours.

HOW SUPPLIED

BROMFED® CAPSULES

Bottle of 100
(NDC 0451-4000-50).

Continued on next page

Bromfed—Cont.

Bottle of 500
(NDC 0451-4000-60).
Each capsule is coded "BROMFED" "MURO 12-120."
BROMFED-PD® CAPSULES
Bottle of 100
(NDC 0451-4001-50).
Bottle of 500
(NDC 0451-4001-60).
Each capsule is coded "BROMFED-PD" "MURO 6-60."
Dispense in tight, child-resistant containers as defined in USP/NF. Store at controlled room temperature between 15°–30°C (59°–86°F).
Keep this and all drugs out of reach of children.
Dist. by:
MURO
Pharmaceutical, Inc.
an ASTA Medica company
Tewksbury, MA
01876-1496
Mfd. by:
PharmaFab
Grand Prairie, TX 75050
I-4000-19 PIN010801
11/99

DYNABAC® ℞

[dynă băc]
(dirithromycin tablets)

DESCRIPTION

Dynabac® (dirithromycin tablets) contains the semi-synthetic macrolide antibiotic dirithromycin for oral administration. It is a pro-drug which is converted non-enzymatically during intestinal absorption into the microbiologically active moiety erythromycylamine.

Chemically, dirithromycin is designated (9*S*)-9-Deoxo-11-deoxy-9,11-[imino[(1*R*)-2-(2-methoxyethoxy)-ethylidene]-oxy] erythromycin and has the molecular formula $C_{42}H_{78}N_2O_{14}$. Its molecular weight is 835.09. The structural formula is:

Chemically, erythromycylamine is designated 9-*(S)*-9-amino-9-deoxo-erythromycin and has a molecular formula of $C_{37}H_{70}N_2O_{12}$. Its molecular weight is 743.97. The structural formula is:

Dirithromycin is a basic compound. The free base is poorly soluble in water and readily soluble in polar organic solvents. Dirithromycin is hydrolyzed to erythromycylamine in acidic aqueous solutions; hydrolysis is virtually complete within 2 hours.

Dynabac tablets are enteric coated to protect the contents from gastric acid and to permit absorption of the antibiotic in the small intestine. Each enteric-coated tablet contains dirithromycin equivalent to 250 mg and the following inactive ingredients: benzyl alcohol, microcrystalline cellulose, croscarmellose sodium, hydroxypropyl cellulose, hydroxypropyl methylcellulose, magnesium carbonate, magnesium stearate, methacrylic acid copolymer, polyethylene glycol, propylene glycol, sodium starch glycolate, talc, titanium dioxide, and triethyl citrate.

CLINICAL PHARMACOLOGY

Pharmacokinetics: *Absorption*—Dirithromycin is rapidly absorbed and converted by nonenzymatic hydrolysis to the microbiologically active compound erythromycylamine. The absolute bioavailability of the oral formulation is approximately 10%. The pharmacokinetic parameters of erythromycylamine in plasma after single-and multiple-dose oral administration of two 250-mg Dynabac tablets once daily for 10 days in 10 fasting healthy subjects (19 to 50 years of age) were as follows:

Pharmacokinetic Parameter (n=10 subjects)	Mean (1 S.D.) Day 1		Mean (1 S.D.) Day 10	
C_{max} (µg/mL)	0.3	(0.2)	0.4	(0.2)
T_{max} (h)	3.9	(0.9)	4.1	(1.3)
AUC_{0-24h} (ug•h/mL)	0.9	(0.7)	1.8	(1.1)

[See first table above]

Distribution—The protein binding of erythromycylamine ranges from 15% to 30%. Erythromycylamine is widely distributed throughout the body with a mean apparent volume of distribution (V_{DSS}) of 800 L (504 to 1,041 L).

Rapid distribution of erythromycylamine into tissues and high concentrations within cells result in significantly higher concentrations in tissues than in plasma or serum. There are no data available on cerebrospinal fluid penetration.

Metabolism and Excretion—Erythromycylamine is primarily eliminated in the bile and undergoes little or no hepatic metabolism. Thus, the primary route of elimination is fecal/hepatic with 81% to 97% of the dose eliminated in this manner. Approximately 2% of the administered dose is eliminated through the kidney, mainly within the first 36 hours following drug administration.

The mean plasma half-life of erythromycylamine was estimated to be about 8 h (2 to 36 h), while a mean urinary terminal elimination half-life of about 44 h (16 to 65 h) and a mean apparent total body clearance of approximately 23 L/h (20 to 32 L/h) were observed in patients with normal renal function.

Food Effect on Absorption—**Dynabac tablets should be administered with food or within an hour of having eaten.** The effect of food on the bioavailability of dirithromycin was evaluated following oral administration of two 250-mg Dynabac tablets 1 or 4 hours before food and immediately after a standard breakfast. Results obtained indicated a slight increase in the absorption of erythromycylamine when dirithromycin tablets were administered after food, while a significant decrease in C_{max} (33%) and AUC (31%) occurred when administer 1 hour before food. The effects of high and low fat meals on the bioavailability of dirithromycin were also investigated. The results showed that the amount of dietary fat had little or no effect on the bioavailability of dirithromycin.

Table 1
Steady-State Tissue Concentrations
of Erythromycylamine Following Two 250-mg Tablets
(500 mg) of Dynabac Given Orally Once Daily

Tissue	Time After Last Dose (h)	Mean Tissue Concentration (µg/g or µg/10^7 cells)	Corresponding Mean Plasma or Serum Concentration (µg/mL)	Tissue/Plasma (Serum) Ratio
Tonsil	14	3.47	0.17	20.4
Healthy lung	12	3.79	0.13	29.2
Pathologic/infected lung	12	3.85	0.13	29.6
Infected bronchial secretions	48	2.15	0.31	6.9
Infected bronchial mucosa	12	1.70	0.13	13.1
	48	2.59	0.31	8.4
	72	1.74	0.33	5.3
Alveolar Macrophages	5	0.37	0.35	1.1

High tissue concentrations should not be interpreted to be quantitatively related to clinical efficacy. Erythromycylamine is concentrated in all lysosomes, which have a low organelle pH at which drug activity is reduced.

[See second table above]

Special Populations:

Hepatic Insufficiency—In patients with mild (Child's Grade A) hepatic impairment, mean peak serum concentration, AUC, and volume of distribution increased somewhat with multiple-dose administration; however, based on the magnitude of these changes, no dosage adjustment should be necessary in patients with mildly impaired hepatic function. The pharmacokinetics of dirithromycin in patients with moderate or severe impairment in hepatic function (Child's Grade B or greater) have not been studied.

Renal Insufficiency—The mean peak plasma concentration (C_{max}) and AUC tended to increase as creatinine clearance decreased; however, based on data available to date, no dosage adjustment should be necessary in patients with impaired renal function, including dialysis patients.

Geriatric Patients—In a multiple-dose study in which 19 healthy elderly subjects (65 to 83 years of age) were given two 250-mg Dynabac tablets every day for 10 days, C_{max} and AUC tended to increase with age; however, neither C_{max} nor AUC was statistically or clinically significantly altered with age. Therefore, based on these pharmacokinetic results, no dosage adjustment should be necessary in elderly patients.

Microbiology:

Erythromycylamine, the microbiologically active product of dirithromycin hydrolysis, exerts its activity by binding to the 50S ribosomal subunits of susceptible mircoorganisms resulting in inhibition of protein synthesis.

Dirithromycin/erythromycylamine has been shown to be active against most strains of the following microorganisms both *in vitro* and in clinical infections as described in the **INDICATIONS AND USAGE** section:

Aerobic gram-positive microorganisms
Staphylococcus aureus (methicillin-susceptible strains only)
Streptococcus pneumoniae
Streptococcus pyogenes

Aerobic gram-negative microorganisms
Haemophilus influenzae
Legionella pneumophila
Moraxella catarrhalis

Other microorganisms
Mycoplasma pneumoniae

The following *in vitro* data are available, **but their clinical significance is unknown.**

Dirithromycin exhibits *in vitro* minimum inhibitory concentrations (MIC's) of 0.5 µg/mL or less against most (≥ 90%) strains of streptococci and MIC's of 2 µg/mL or less against most (≥ 90%) strains of the other microorganisms in the following list; however, the safety and effectiveness of dirithromycin in treating clinical infections due to these microorganisms have not been established in adequate and well-controlled clinical trials.

Aerobic gram-positive microorganisms
Listeria monocytogenes
Streptococci, groups C, F, and G
Streptococcus agalactiae
Viridans group streptococci

Aerobic gram-negative microorganisms
Bordetella pertussis

Anaerobic microorganisms
Propionibacterium acnes

NOTE: Microorganisms that are resistant to other macrolides are cross-resistant to dirithromycin/erythromycylamine. Enterococci and most strains of methicillin-resistant staphylococci are resistant to macrolides.

Susceptibility Tests: Dilution Techniques: Quantitative methods are used to determine antimicrobial minimum inhibitory concentrations (MIC's). These MIC's provide estimates of the susceptibility of bacteria to antimicrobial compounds. The MIC's should be determined using a standardized procedure. Standardized procedures are based on a dilution method,[1] (broth or agar) or equivalent with standardized inoculum concentrations and standardized concentrations of dirithromycin powder. The MIC values should be interpreted according to the following criteria:

For testing aerobic microorganisms other than *Haemophilus influenzae* and streptococci:

MIC (µg/mL)	Interpretation
≤2	Susceptible (S)
4	Intermediate (I)
≥8	Resistant (R)

For testing *Haemophilus influenzae*[a]:

MIC (µg/mL)	Interpretation
≤8	Susceptible (S)
16	Intermediate (I)
≥32	Resistant (R)

[a]These interpretive standards are applicable only to broth microdilution susceptibility tests with *Haemophilus influenzae* using *Haemophilus* Test Medium[1] and incubated aerobically.

For testing streptococci including *Streptococcus pneumoniae*[b]:

MIC (µg/mL)	Interpretation
≤0.5	Susceptible (S)
1	Intermediate (I)
≥2	Resistant (R)

[b]These interpretive standards are applicable only to broth microdilution susceptibility tests using cation-adjusted Mueller-Hinton broth with 2–5% lysed horse blood.

A report of "Susceptible" indicates that the pathogen is likely to be inhibited if the antimicrobial compound in blood reaches the concentration usually achievable. A report of "Intermediate" indicates that the result should be considered equivocal, and, if the microorganism is not fully susceptible to alternative, clinically feasible drugs, the test should be repeated. This category implies possible clinical applicability in body sites where the drug is physiologically concentrated or in situations where high dosage of drug can be used. This category also provides a buffer zone which prevents small uncontrolled technical factors from causing major discrepancies in interpretation. A report of "Resistant" indicates that the pathogen is not likely to be inhibited if the antimicrobial compound in the blood reaches the concentration usually achievable; other therapy should be selected.

Standardized susceptibility test procedures require the use of laboratory control microorganisms to control the technical aspects of the laboratory procedures. Standard dirithromycin powder should provide the following MIC values:

[See first table above]

Diffusion Techniques: Quantitative methods that require measurement of zone diameters also provide reproducible estimates of the susceptibility of bacteria to antimicrobial compounds. One such standardized procedure[2] requires the use of standardized inoculum concentrations. This procedure uses paper disks impregnated with 15-µg dirithromycin to test the susceptibility of microorganisms to dirithromycin.

Reports from the laboratory providing results of the standard single-disk susceptibility test with a 15-µg dirithromycin disk should be interpreted according to the following criteria:

For testing aerobic microorganisms other than *Haemophilus influenzae* and streptococci:

Zone Diameter (mm)	Interpretation
≥19	Susceptible (S)
16–18	Intermediate (I)
≤15	Resistant (R)

For testing streptococci including *Streptococcus pneumoniae*[e]:

Zone Diameter (mm)	Interpretation
≥18	Susceptible (S)
14–17	Intermediate (I)
≤13	Resistant (R)

[e]These zone diameter standards for streptococci are applicable only to tests performed using Mueller-Hinton agar supplemented with 5% sheep blood incubated in 5% CO_2.

Due to lack of standardized methodology and interpretive criteria, it is impossible at present to determine if strains of *Haemophilus* are susceptible or are resistant to dirithromycin/erythromycylamine using the disk diffusion assay.

Interpretation should be as stated above for results using dilution techniques. Interpretation involves correlation of the diameter obtained in the disk test with the MIC for dirithromycin.

As with standardized dilution techniques, diffusion methods require the use of laboratory control microorganisms that are used to control the technical aspects of the laboratory procedures. For the diffusion technique, the 15-µg dirithromycin disk should provide the following zone diameters in these laboratory quality control strains:

[See second table above]

INDICATIONS AND USAGE

Dynabac (dirithromycin tablets) is indicated for the treatment of individuals age 12 years and older with mild-to-moderate infections caused by susceptible strains of the designated microorganisms in the specific conditions listed below. **Dirithromycin should not be used in patients with known, suspected, or potential bacteremias as serum levels are inadequate to provide antibacterial coverage of the blood stream.**

Acute Bacterial Exacerbations of Chronic Bronchitis due to *Haemophilus influenzae, Moraxella catarrhalis*, or *Streptococcus pneumoniae.*

Microorganism	MIC Range (µg/mL)
Haemophilus influenzae ATCC 49247[c]	8.0–32
Staphylococcus aureus ATCC 29213	1.0–4.0
Streptococcus pneumoniae ATCC 49619[d]	0.06–0.25

[c]This quality control range is applicable only to *H. influenzae* ATCC 49247 tested by a broth microdilution procedure using *Haemophilus* Test Medium (HTM)[1] and aerobically incubated.

[d]This quality control range is applicable only to *S. pneumoniae* ATCC 49619 tested by a broth microdilution procedure using cation-adjusted Mueller-Hinton broth with 2–5% lysed horse blood.

Microorganism	Zone Diameter (mm)
Staphylococcus aureus ATCC 25923	18–26
Streptococcus pneumoniae ATCC 49619[f]	18–25

[f]This quality control range is applicable only to *S. pneumoniae* ATCC 49619 tested by a disk diffusion procedure using Mueller-Hinton agar supplemented with 5% sheep blood and incubated in 5% CO_2.

Table 2
Adverse Clinical Reactions
(Incidence equal to or greater than 1%)
Clinical Trials - North America

ADVERSE REACTION	DIRITHROMYCIN		ERYTHROMYCIN	
	7–14 Day (n=1894)	5-Day (n=932)	7–14 Day (n=1894)	7-Day (n=932)
Abdominal pain	9.7%	7.1%	7.5%	6.2%
Headache	8.6%	7.7%	8.2%	7.6%
Nausea	8.3%	5.9%	7.5%	8.7%
Diarrhea	7.7%	6.7%	7.3%	9.4%
Vomiting	3.0%	1.1%	2.8%	1.3%
Dyspepsia	2.6%	4.1%	2.1%	2.7%
Dizziness/vertigo	2.3%	2.1%	2.3%	2.0%
Pain (non-specific)	2.2%	2.9%	1.6%	3.0%
Asthenia	2.0%	1.4%	1.9%	1.4%
Gastrointestinal disorder	1.6%	0	1.4%	0.2%
Increased Cough	1.5%	0.2%	2.6%	0.5%
Flatulence	1.5%	1.0%	1.5%	1.6%
Rash	1.4%	1.6%	2.6%	1.4%
Dyspnea	1.2%	1.8%	1.2%	1.6%
Pruritus/Urticaria	1.2%	0.5%	1.0%	0.6%
Insomnia	1.0%	0.9%	0.7%	1.1%
Vaginitis	0.4%	1.2%	0.6%	0.6%

Secondary Bacterial Infection of Acute Bronchitis due to *Moraxella catarrhalis* or *Streptococcus pneumoniae.*

Community-Acquired Pneumonia due to *Legionella pneumophila, Mycoplasma pneumoniae*, or *Streptococcus pneumoniae.*

Pharyngitis/Tonsilitis due to *Streptococcus pyogenes.*

NOTE: The usual drug of choice in the treatment and prevention of streptococcal infections and the prophylaxis of rheumatic fever is penicillin. Dynabac generally is effective in the eradication of *S. pyogenes* from the nasopharynx; however, data establishing the efficacy of Dynabac in the subsequent prevention of rheumatic fever are not available at present.

Uncomplicated Skin and Skin Structure Infections due to *Staphylococcus aureus* (methicillin-susceptible strains) or *Streptococcus pyogenes.* (Abscesses usually require surgical drainage.)

CONTRAINDICATIONS

Dynabac is contraindicated in patients with known hypersensitivity to dirithromycin, erythromycin, or any other macrolide antibiotic.

WARNINGS

Dirithromycin should not be used in patients with known, suspected, or potential bacteremias as serum levels are inadequate to provide antibacterial coverage of the blood stream.

Pseudomembranous colitis has been reported with nearly all antibacterial agents, including dirithromycin, and may range in severity from mild to life-threatening. Therefore, it is important to consider this diagnosis in patients who present with diarrhea subsequent to the administration of antibacterial agents.

Treatment with antibacterial agents alters the normal flora of the colon and may permit overgrowth of clostridia. Studies indicate that a toxin produced by *Clostridium difficile* is a primary cause of "antibiotic-associated colitis."

After the diagnosis of pseudomembranous colitis has been established, therapeutic measures should be initiated. Mild cases of pseudomembranous colitis usually respond to discontinuation of the drug alone. In moderate-to-severe cases, consideration should be given to management with fluids and electrolytes, protein supplementation, and treatment with an antibacterial drug clinically effective against *C. difficile* colitis.

PRECAUTIONS

Hepatic Insufficiency—Because dirithromycin/erythromycylamine is principally eliminated via the liver and because no data exist regarding the safety of administering dirithromycin to patients with Child's Grade B or greater hepatic impairment, Dynabac should be administered to such patients only when absolutely necessary. No dosage adjustment should be necessary in patients with mildly impaired hepatic function.

Information to Patients—Dynabac tablets should be taken with food or within one hour of having eaten. They should not be cut, chewed, or crushed.

Drug Interactions:

Terfenadine—In a prospective study involving six-healthy-male volunteers, dirithromycin did not affect the metabolism of terfenadine. These six volunteers received terfenadine alone (60 mg twice daily) for 8 days, followed by terfenadine in combination with dirithromycin (500 mg once daily) for 10 days. (Both drugs were thus dosed to steady state.) The pharmacokinetics of terfenadine and its acid metabolite and the electrocardiographic QT_c interval were measured during both periods: with terfenadine alone, and with terfenadine plus dirithromycin. In five men, terfenadine levels were undetectable (<5 ng/mL) throughout the study; in one man, the C_{max} of terfenadine was 8.1 ng/mL with terfenadine alone and 7.2 ng/mL with terfenadine plus dirithromycin. The mean C_{max}, T_{max}, and AUC of the acid metabolite of terfenadine were not significantly changed. The mean QT_c interval (msec) was 369 with terfenadine alone and 367 with terfenadine plus dirithromycin.

Also, *in vitro* experiments demonstrated a lack of interaction between dirithromycin and terfenadine. Thus, the interaction observed between erythromycin and terfenadine is not expected for dirithromycin.

Serious cardiac dysrhythmias, some resulting in death, have occurred in patients receiving terfenadine concomitantly with other macrolide antibiotics. In addition, most macrolides are contraindicated in patients receiving terfenadine therapy who have pre-existing cardiac abnormalities (arrhythmia, bradycardia, QT_c interval prolongation, ischemic heart disease, congestive heart failure, etc.) or electrolyte disturbances. (See terfenadine package insert.)

Theophylline—Following co-administration of two 250-mg dirithromycin tablets administered once daily with 200-mg theophylline tablets administered twice daily for 10 days to 14 healthy subjects, the steady-state plasma concentration of theophylline was not significantly altered. In general, most patients treated with dirithromycin who are receiving concomitant theophylline therapy *may* not require empiric adjustment of theophylline dosage or monitoring of theophylline plasma concentrations. However, theophylline plasma concentrations should be monitored, with dosage adjustment as appropriate, in patients whose pulmonary disease requires maintaining a given theophylline plasma concentration for optimal pulmonary function or in patients with theophylline concentrations at the higher end of the therapeutic range.

Antacids or H_2 receptor antagonists—When dirithromycin is administered immediately following antacids or H_2-receptor antagonists, the absorption of dirithromycin is slightly enhanced.

The following drug interactions have been reported with erythromycin products. It is presently not known whether

Continued on next page

Dynabac—Cont.

these same drug interactions occur with dirithromycin. **Until further data are available regarding the potential interaction of dirithromycin with these compounds, caution should be used during coadministration.**

Triazolam—Erythromycin has been reported to decrease the clearance of triazolam and, thus, may increase the pharmacologic effect of triazolam.

Digoxin—Concomitant administration of erythromycin and digoxin has been reported to result in elevated digoxin serum levels.

Anticoagulants—There have been reports of increased anticoagulant effects when erythromycin and oral anticoagulants were used concomitantly. Increased anticoagulation effects due to a drug interaction with erythromycin may be more pronounced in the elderly.

Ergotamine—Concurrent use of erythromycin and ergotamine or dihydroergotamine has been associated in some patients with acute ergot toxicity characterized by severe peripheral vasospasm and dysesthesia.

Other drugs—Drug interactions have been reported with concomitant administration of erythromycin and other medications, including cyclosporine, hexobarbital, carbamazepine, alfentanil, disopyramide, phenytoin, bromocriptine, valproate, astemizole, and lovastatin.

Carcinogenesis, Mutagenesis, Impairment of Fertility—Lifetime studies in animals to evaluate carcinogenic potential have not been performed with dirithromycin.

No mutagenic potential was demonstrated when dirithromycin was used in standard tests of genotoxicity, which included the following bacterial mutation tests *in vitro* and *in vivo* mammalian systems:

Bacterial Reverse-Mutation Test (Ames test)
DNA repair (UDS) in rat hepatocytes
Chinese hamster lung fibroblast (V79) test
Micronucleus test in mice
Sister-chromatid exchange—human lymphocytes
Sister-chromatid exchange—Chinese hamsters
Mouse Lymphoma Assay

In rats, fertility and reproductive performance were not affected when dirithromycin was administered at doses up to 21 times the maximum recommended human dose on a mg/m^2 basis.

Pregnancy: Teratogenic Effects. Pregnancy Category C—Teratology studies conducted in rats at doses up to 21 times the maximum recommended human dose on a mg/m^2 basis and in rabbits at doses up to 4 times the maximum recommended human dose on a mg/m^2 basis have revealed no evidence of impaired fertility or harm to the fetus due to dirithromycin administration. An additional teratology study in CD-1 mice demonstrated that fetal weight was significantly depressed at the 1000 mg/kg dose (8 times the maximum recommended human dose on a mg/m^2 basis), and there was an increased occurrence of incomplete ossification among these fetuses—a manifestation of retarded development. This decrease in ossification was also seen in rats given 1000 mg/kg/day for 2 weeks prior to mating, throughout the mating period, and throughout gestation.

There are no adequate and well-controlled studies in pregnant women. Dirithromycin should be used during pregnancy only if the potential benefit justifies the potential risk to the fetus.

Labor and Delivery—Dirithromycin has not been studied for use during labor and delivery. Treatment with dirithromycin should be given during labor and delivery only if clearly needed.

Nursing Mothers—It is not known whether either dirithromycin or erythromycylamine is excreted in human milk. It is known that dirithromycin is excreted in the milk of lactating rodents and that other drugs of this class are excreted in human milk. Because many drugs are excreted in human milk, caution should be exercised when dirithromycin is administered to a nursing woman.

Pediatric Use—Safety and effectiveness in pediatric patients below the age of 12 years have not been established.

Geriatric Use—In a clinical pharmacology study, 19 healthy geriatric volunteers (65 to 83 years of age) with normal renal and hepatic function had no statistically significant differences in AUC or C_{max} when compared with 10 healthy adult volunteers (19 to 50 years of age). In clinical trials in geriatric patients who received the usual recommended adult dose (500 mg q.d. P.O.), clinical efficacy and safety were comparable with results in non-geriatric adult patients.

ADVERSE REACTIONS

Clinical Trials: In clinical trials, 3299 patients were treated with dirithromycin 500 mg q.d. P.O. for approximately 7 to 14 days. There were no deaths or permanent disabilities thought related directly to drug toxicity. Eighty-seven (2.6%) patients discontinued medication due to adverse reactions. Thirty-five (40%) of the 87 patients who discontinued therapy did so because of nausea or abdominal pain.

In additional clinical trials conducted in North America, 932 patients were treated with dirithromycin 500 mg q.d. for 5 days. There were no deaths or permanent disabilities thought to be related directly to drug toxicity. Thirty-five (3.8%) patients discontinued medication due to adverse reactions. Fifteen (43%) of the 35 patients who discontinued therapy did so because of nausea or abdominal pain.

Table 3
Adverse Laboratory Reactions
(Incidence equal to or greater than 1%)
Clinical Trials - North America

ADVERSE REACTION	DIRITHROMYCIN		ERYTHROMYCIN	
	7–14 Day (n=1894)	5-Day (n=932)	7–14 Day (n=1894)	7-Day (n=932)
Platelet count *increased*	3.8%	0.7%	4.8%	1.4%
Potassium *increased*	2.6%	0	0.0%	0
Bicarbonate *decreased*	1.4%	0	2.0%	0
CPK *increased*	1.2%	0.8%	0.9%	0.7%
Eosinophils *increased*	1.2%	0.9%	0.6%	0.9%
Seg Neutrophils *increased*	1.2%	1.7%	1.3%	2.3%
Leucocytes *increased*	0.8%	1.5%	0.9%	1.2%

Table 4
Recommended Dosage Schedule for Dynabac
(12 years of age and older)

Infection (Mild to Moderate Severity)	Dose	Frequency	Duration (days)
Acute Bacterial Exacerbations of Chronic Bronchitis due to *Haemophilus influenzae, Moraxella catarrhalis*, or *Streptococcus pneumonia*	500 mg	q day	5–7
Secondary Bacterial Infection of Acute Bronchitis due to *M. catarrhalis* or *S. pneumoniae*	500 mg	q day	7
Community-Acquired Pneumonia due to *Legionella pneumophila, Mycoplasma pneumoniae*, or *S. pneumoniae*	500 mg	q day	14
Pharyngitis/Tonsillitis due to *Streptococcus pyogenes*	500 mg	q day	10
Uncomplicated Skin and Skin Structure Infections due to *Staphylococcus aureus* (methicillin-susceptible) or *S pyogenes*	500 mg	q day	5–7

The following adverse clinical and laboratory reactions were reported during the dirithromycin clinical trials conducted in North America (n=1894 patients treated for 7–14 days and 932 patients treated for 5 days). (See Tables 2 and 3.)
[See table 2 at top of previous page]

Adverse reactions occurring during all clinical trials with dirithromycin with an incidence of less than 1% but greater than 0.1% included the following (listed alphabetically): Abnormal stools, allergic reaction, amblyopia, anorexia, anxiety, constipation, dehydration, depression, dry mouth, dysmenorrhea, dysphagia, edema, epistaxis, eye disorder (not further defined), fever, flu syndrome, gastritis, gastroenteritis, hemoptysis, hyperventilation, insomnia, malaise, mouth ulceration, myalgia, myasthenia, neck pain, nervousness, palpitation, paresthesia, peripheral edema, somnolence, sweating, syncope, taste perversion, thirst, tinnitus, tremor, urinary frequency, vaginal moniliasis, vaginitis, vasodilatation.
[See table 3 above]

Adverse laboratory reactions occurring during all clinical trials with dirithromycin with an incidence of less than 1% but greater than 0.1% included the following (listed alphabetically):

Decreased: Albumin, chloride, hematocrit, hemoglobin, lymphocytes, segmented neutrophils, phosphorus, platelet count, serum alkaline phosphatase, serum uric acid, and total protein.

Increased: Alkaline phosphatase, ALT, AST, basophils, calcium, creatinine, GGT, leukocyte count, lymphocytes, hematocrit, hemoglobin, monocytes, phosphorous, total bilirubin, and uric acid.

Macrolide-class adverse reactions—Although not observed in patients treated with dirithromycin in clinical trials, the following adverse reactions and altered laboratory test results have been reported in patients treated with macrolide antibiotics:

Bullous fixed eruptions or serious allergic reactions, including anaphylaxis, have been reported. A few cases of transient deafness have been reported with high doses of oral erythromycin. Rarely, cholestatic hepatitis has been reported. In individuals with prolonged QT intervals, erythromycin has been associated, rarely, with the production of ventricular arrhythmias, including ventricular tachycardia and torsade de pointes.

OVERDOSAGE

The toxic symptoms following an overdose of a macrolide antibiotic may include nausea, vomiting, epigastric distress, and diarrhea. Forced diuresis, peritoneal dialysis, hemodialysis, or hemoperfusion have not been established as beneficial for an overdose of dirithromycin. Hemodialysis has been shown to be ineffective in hastening the elimination of erythromycylamine from plasma in patients with chronic renal failure.

DOSAGE AND ADMINISTRATION

Dynabac (dirithromycin tablets) should be administered with food or within 1 hour of having eaten. (See **CLINICAL PHARMACOLOGY**, ***Food Effect on Absorption***.) **Dynabac tablets should not be cut, crushed, or chewed.**
[See table 4 above]

HOW SUPPLIED

Dynabac® (dirithromycin tablets) are available in:

The 250 mg tablets are white, enteric-coated, elliptical-shaped, imprinted with "DYNABAC" and "UC5364." They are available as follows:

Bottles of 60 NDC 0451-0490-60 (UC5364).

Box of 3 (D5-Pak™, pack of 10) NDC 0451-0490-10 (UC5304).

Store at controlled room temperature, 15° to 30°C (59° to 86°F).

ANIMAL PHARMACOLOGY AND TOXICOLOGY

Cardiac and skeletal muscle lesions occurred in rats in studies up to three months by the intravenous route and in six-month studies in the rat and the dog by the oral route. While no target organ toxicity was identified in three-month oral studies, both cardiac and skeletal muscles were identified as target tissues after one-month intravenous studies in rats. Histologic changes from oral dosing occurred only after more than four months of treatment in rats and after six months in dogs. These findings were associated with high tissue-to-plasma concentration ratios of antimicrobial activity. The extensive drug uptake by tissues was reversible upon termination of treatment. Lesions in cardiac and skeletal muscle also were reversed upon termination of treatment. Dirithromycin and/or its microbiologically active metabolite appeared to accumulate in tissues with time. Despite the drug uptake in rat tissues at high multiples (approximately 14 times the anticipated clinical dose in mg/m^2), there were no lesions in this species until oral treatment was extended beyond four months.

REFERENCES

1. National Committee for Clinical Laboratory Standards. Methods for Dilution Antimicrobial Susceptibility Tests for Bacteria that Grow Aerobically—Fourth Edition. Approved Standard NCCLS Document M7-A4, Vol. 17, No. 2, NCCLS, Wayne, PA, January, 1997.
2. National Committee for Clinical Laboratory Standards. Performance Standards for Antimicrobial Disk Susceptibility Tests—Sixth Edition. Approved Standard NCCLS Document M2-A6, Vol. 17, No. 1, NCCLS, Wayne, PA, January, 1997.

CAUTION—Federal (USA) law prohibits dispensing without prescription.

Literature revised October 11, 1999
PV 2597 UCP [101199]

Distributed by:
Muro
Pharmaceutical, Inc.
an ASTA Medica company
Tewksbury, MA 01876

Manufactured by
Eli Lily and Company
Indianapolis, IN 46285, USA

GUAIFED® ℞
[*guă-fĕd*]
GUAIFED-PD® ℞
Rx only

GUAIFED® CAPSULES
A white opaque and clear capsule containing white beads.
Each capsule contains:
Pseudoephedrine hydrochloride .... 120 mg
in a specially prepared base to provide prolonged action.
Guaifenesin .... 250 mg
designed for immediate release to provide rapid action.
GUAIFED-PD® CAPSULES
A blue and clear capsule containing white beads.
Each capsule contains:
Pseudoephedrine hydrochloride .... 60 mg
in a specially prepared base to provide prolonged action.
Guaifenesin .... 300 mg
designed for immediate release to provide rapid action.
GUAIFED® AND GUAIFED-PD® CAPSULES also contain as inactive ingredients: Calcium Stearate, FD&C Blue #1 (Guaifed-PD® only), Gelatin, Pharmaceutical Glaze, Starch, Sucrose, Talc, and Titanium Dioxide.
GUAIFED® and GUAIFED-PD® contain ingredients of the following therapeutic classes: nasal decongestant and expectorant.

CLINICAL PHARMACOLOGY
Pseudoephedrine hydrochloride is a sympathomimetic which acts predominantly on alpha adrenergic receptors in the mucosa of the respiratory tract, producing vasoconstriction and has little action on beta receptors. It therefore functions as an oral nasal decongestant with minimal central nervous system (CNS) stimulation. Pseudoephedrine hydrochloride also increases sinus drainage and secretions. Guaifenesin is an expectorant which increases the output of phlegm (sputum) and bronchial secretions by reducing adhesiveness and surface tension. The increased flow of less viscid secretions promotes ciliary action and changes a dry, unproductive cough to one that is more productive and less frequent.

INDICATIONS
For temporary relief of nasal congestion and dry non-productive cough associated with the common cold and other respiratory allergies. Helps drainage of the bronchial tubes by thinning the mucus.

CONTRAINDICATIONS
This product is contraindicated in patients with a known hypersensitivity to any of its ingredients. Also contraindicated in patients with severe hypertension, severe coronary artery disease and patients on Monoamine Oxidase (MAO) inhibitor therapy. Should not be used during pregnancy or in nursing mothers,
Considerable caution should be exercised in patients with hypertension, diabetes mellitus, ischemic heart disease, hyperthyroidism, increased intraocular pressure and prostatic hypertrophy. The elderly (60 years or older) are more likely to exhibit adverse reactions. At dosages higher than the recommended dose, nervousness, dizziness or sleeplessness may occur.

WARNINGS
Do not take this product for persistent or chronic cough such as occurs with smoking, asthma, or emphysema, or where cough is accompanied by excessive secretions except under the advice and supervision of a physician. This medication should be taken a few hours prior to bedtime to minimize the possibility of sleeplessness. Take this medication with a glass of water after each dose, to help loosen mucus in the lungs.

PRECAUTIONS
General: Caution should be exercised in patients with high blood pressure, heart disease, diabetes or thyroid disease and in patients who exhibit difficulty in urination due to enlargement of the prostate gland. Check with a physician if symptoms do not improve within 7 days or if accompanied by high fever, rash or persistent headache.
Drug Interactions: Do not take this product if you are presently taking a prescription drug for high blood pressure or depression, without first consulting a physician. MAO inhibitors and beta adrenergic blockers may increase the effect of sympathomimetics. Sympathomimetics may reduce the antihypertensive effects of methyldopa, mecamylamine, reserpine and veratrum alkaloids. Pseudoephedrine hydrochloride may increase the possibility of cardiac arrhythmias in patients taking digitalis glycosides.
Pregnancy:
Pregnancy Category B
It has been shown that pseudoephedrine hydrochloride can cause reduced average weight, length, and rate of skeletal ossification in the animal fetus.
Nursing Mothers: Pseudoephedrine is excreted in breast milk; use by nursing mothers is not recommended because of the higher than usual risk of side effects from sympathomimetic amines for infants, especially newborn and premature infants.
Geriatrics: Pseudoephedrine should be used with caution in the elderly because they may be more sensitive to the effects of the sympathomimetics.

ADVERSE REACTIONS
Adverse reactions include nausea, cardiac palpitations, increased irritability or excitement, headache, dizziness, tachycardia, diarrhea, drowsiness, stomach pain, seizures, slowed heart rate, shortness of breath and/or troubled breathing.
Pediatric Use: Safety and effectiveness in pediatric patients less than 6 years of age has not been established for **GUAIFED-PD®**, and safety and effectiveness in pediatric patients less than 12 years of age has not been established for **GUAIFED®**. See Contraindications, Warnings, and Precautions for complete information.

OVERDOSAGE
KEEP THIS AND ALL DRUGS OUT OF THE REACH OF CHILDREN. IN CASE OF SUSPECTED OVERDOSE, IMMEDIATELY CALL YOUR REGIONAL POISON CONTROL CENTER AND/OR SEEK PROFESSIONAL ASSISTANCE.
Symptoms of overdosage may be caused by pseudoephedrine. Symptoms of overdosage with pseudoephedrine include anxiety, tenseness, respiratory difficulty, headache and awareness of the slow forceful heartbeat.
Treatment of Overdose: The stomach should be emptied promptly by emetics and/or gastric lavage. The installation of activated charcoal also should be considered. Cardiac function and serum electrolytes should be monitored and treatment instigated if indicated. If convulsions or marked CNS excitement occurs, diazepam may be used.

DOSAGE AND ADMINISTRATION
GUAIFED® CAPSULES
Adults and pediatric patients 12 years of age and over: 1 capsule every 12 hours.
GUAIFED-PD® CAPSULES
Pediatric patients 6 to under 12 years of age: 1 capsule every 12 hours. Adults and pediatric patients 12 years of age and over: 1–2 capsules every 12 hours.

HOW SUPPLIED
GUAIFED® CAPSULES
Bottles of 100
(NDC 0451-4002-50).
Bottles of 500
(NDC 0451-4002-60).
Each capsule is coded "GUAIFED" "MURO 120–250."
GUAIFED-PD® CAPSULES
Bottles of 100
(NDC 0451-4003-50).
Bottles of 500
(NDC 0451-4003-60).
Each capsule is coded "GUAIFED-PD" "MURO 60–300."
Dispense in tight, child-resistant containers as defined in USP/NF.
Store at controlled room temperature between 15°–30°C (59°–86°F).
Keep this and all drugs out of reach of children.
Dist. by:
MURO
Pharmaceutical, Inc.
an ASTA Medica company
Tewksbury, MA 01876-1496
Mfd. by:
PharmaFab
Grand Prairie, TX 75050
I-4003-12
PIN040401 11/99

OPTVAR™ ℞
[*opti-var*]
azelastine hydrochloride
ophthalmic solution, 0.05%

DESCRIPTION
OPTIVAR™ (azelastine hydrochloride ophthalmic solution) 0.05% is a sterile ophthalmic solution containing azelastine hydrochloride, a relatively selective H_1-receptor antagonist for topical administration to the eyes. Azelastine hydrochloride is a white crystalline powder with a molecular weight of 418.37. Azelastine hydrochloride is sparingly soluble in water, methanol and propylene glycol, and slightly soluble in ethanol, octanol and glycerine. Azelastine hydrochloride is a racemic mixture with a melting point of 225°C. The chemical name for azelastine hydrochloride is (±)-1-(2H)-phthalazinone,4-[(4-chlorophenyl) methyl]-2-(hexahydro-1-methyl-1H-azepin-4-yl)-, monohydrochloride and is represented by the following chemical structure:

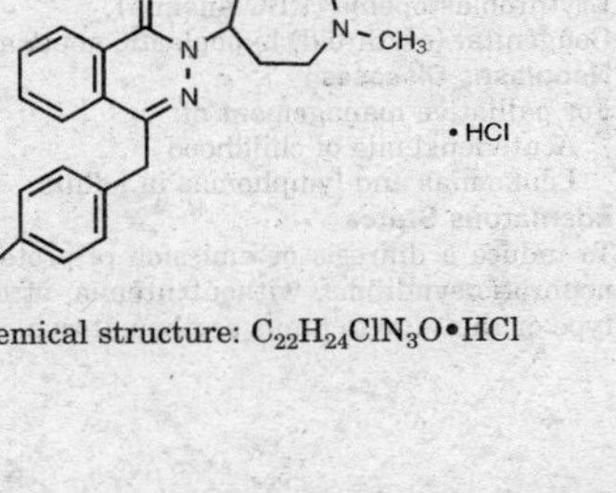

Empirical chemical structure: $C_{22}H_{24}ClN_3O \bullet HCl$

Each mL of OPTIVAR™ contains: **Active:** 0.5 mg azelastine hydrochloride, equivalent to 0.457 mg of azelastine base; **Preservative:** 0.125 mg benzalkonium chloride; **Inactives:** disodium edetate dihydrate, hydroxypropyl-methylcellulose, sorbitol solution, sodium hydroxide and water for injection. It has a pH of approximately 5.0 to 6.5 and an osmolality of approximately 271 to 312 mOsmol/L.

CLINICAL PHARMACOLOGY
Azelastine hydrochloride is a relatively selective histamine H_1 antagonist and an inhibitor of the release of histamine and other mediators from cells (e.g. mast cells) involved in the allergic response. Based on in vitro studies using human cell lines, inhibition of other mediators involved in allergic reactions (e.g. leukotrienes and PAF) has been demonstrated with azelastine hydrochloride. Decreased chemotaxis and activation of eosinophils has also been demonstrated.
Pharmacokinetics and Metabolism
Absorption of azelastine following ocular administration was relatively low. A study in symptomatic patients receiving one drop OPTIVAR™ in each eye two to four times a day (0.06 to 0.12 mg azelastine hydrochloride) demonstrated plasma concentrations of azelastine hydrochloride to generally be between 0.02 to 0.25 ng/mL after 56 days of treatment. Three of nineteen patients had quantifiable amounts of N-desmethylazelastine that ranged from 0.25–0.87 ng/mL at Day 56.
Based on intravenous and oral administration, the elimination half-life, steady-state volume of distribution and plasma clearance were 22 hours, 14.5 L/kg and 0.5 L/h/kg, respectively. Approximately 75% of an oral dose of radiolabeled azelastine hydrochloride was excreted in the feces with less than 10% as unchanged azelastine. Azelastine hydrochloride is oxidatively metabolized to the principal metabolite, N-desmethylazelastine, by the cytochrome P450 enzyme system. *In-vitro* studies in human plasma indicate that the plasma protein binding of azelastine and N-desmethylazelastine are approximately 88% and 97%, respectively.
Clinical Trials
In a conjunctival antigen challenge study, OPTIVAR™ was more effective than its vehicle in preventing itching associated with allergic conjunctivitis. OPTIVAR™ had a rapid (within 3 minutes) onset of effect and a duration of effect of approximately 8 hours for the prevention of itching.
In environmental studies, adult and pediatric, patients with seasonal allergic conjunctivitis were treated with OPTIVAR™ for two to eight weeks. In these studies, OPTIVAR™ was more effective than its vehicle in relieving itching associated with allergic conjunctivitis.

INDICATIONS AND USAGE
OPTIVAR™ is indicated for the treatment of itching of the eye associated with allergic conjunctivitis.

CONTRAINDICATIONS
OPTIVAR™ is contraindicated in persons with known or suspected hypersensitivity to any of its components.

WARNINGS
OPTIVAR™ is for ocular use only and not for injection or oral use.

PRECAUTIONS
Information for Patients:
To prevent contaminating the dropper tip and solution, care should be taken not to touch any surface, the eyelids or surrounding areas with the dropper tip of the bottle. Keep bottle tightly closed when not in use. This product is sterile when packaged.
Patients should be advised not to wear a contact lens if their eye is red. OPTIVAR™ should not be used to treat contact lens related irritation. The preservative in OPTIVAR™ , benzalkonium chloride, may be absorbed by soft contact lenses. Patients who wear soft contact lenses and **whose eyes are not red**, should be instructed to wait at least ten minutes after instilling OPTIVAR™ before they insert their contact lenses.
Carcinogenesis, Mutagenesis, Impairment of Fertility:
Azelastine hydrochloride administered orally for 24 months was not carcinogenic in rats and mice at doses up to 30 mg/kg/day and 25 mg/kg/day, respectively. Based on a 30 µl drop size, these doses were approximately 25,000 and 21,000 times higher than the maximum recommended ocular human use level of 0.001 mg/kg/day for a 50 kg adult.
Azelastine hydrochloride showed no genotoxic effects in the Ames test, DNA repair test, mouse lymphoma forward mutation assay, mouse micronucleus test, or chromosomal aberration test in rat bone marrow. Reproduction and fertility studies in rats showed no effects on male or female fertility at oral doses of up to 25,000 times the maximum recommended ocular human use level. At 68.6 mg/kg/day (57,000 times the maximum recommended ocular human use level), the duration of the estrous cycle was prolonged and copulatory activity and the number of pregnancies were decreased. The numbers of corpora lutea and implantations were decreased; however, the implantation ratio was not affected.
Pregnancy:
Teratogenic Effects: Pregnancy Category C. Azelastine hydrochloride has been shown to be embryotoxic, fetotoxic, and teratogenic (external and skeletal abnormalities) in mice at an oral dose of 68.6 mg/kg/day (57,000 times the recommended ocular human use level). At an oral dose of 30

Continued on next page

Optivar—Cont.

mg/kg/day (25,000 times the recommended ocular human use level), delayed ossification (undeveloped metacarpus) and the incidence of 14th rib were increased in rats. At 68.6 mg/kg/day (57,000 times the maximum recommended ocular human use level) azelastine hydrochloride caused resorption and fetotoxic effects in rats. The relevance to humans of these skeletal findings noted at only high drug exposure levels is unknown.

There are no adequate and well-controlled studies in pregnant women. OPTIVAR™ should be used during pregnancy only if the potential benefit justifies the potential risk to the fetus.

Nursing Mothers:

It is not known whether azelastine hydrochloride is excreted in human milk. Because many drugs are excreted in human milk, caution should be exercised when OPTIVAR™ is administered to a nursing woman.

Pediatric Use:

Safety and effectiveness in pediatric patients below the age of 3 have not been established.

Geriatric Use:

No overall differences in safety or effectiveness have been observed between elderly and younger adult patients.

ADVERSE REACTIONS:

In controlled multiple-dose studies where patients were treated for up to 56 days, the most frequently reported adverse reactions were transient eye burning/stinging (approximately 30%), headaches (approximately 15%) and bitter taste (approximately 10%). The occurrence of these events was generally mild.

The following events were reported in 1–10% of patients: asthma, conjunctivitis, dyspnea, eye pain, fatigue, influenza-like symptoms, pharyngitis, pruritus, rhinitis and temporary blurring. Some of these events were similar to the underlying disease being studied.

DOSAGE AND ADMINISTRATION

The recommended dose is one drop instilled into each affected eye twice a day.

HOW SUPPLIED

OPTIVAR™ (azelastine hydrochloride ophthalmic solution) 0.05% is supplied as follows: 6 mL solution in a translucent 10 mL HDPE container with a LDPE dropper tip, and a white HDPE screw cap.

NDC 0451-7025-06
NDC 0451-7025-00

Storage

Store UPRIGHT between 2° and 25°C (36° and 77°F)

Rx only

U.S. Patent No 5164194

Marketed by:
Muro Pharmaceutical, Inc.
an ASTA Medical Company
Tewksbury, MA 01876
Made in Germany
Issued June 2000
I-7025

PRELONE® ℞

[*prē-lonē*]
(PREDNISOLONE SYRUP, USP)
AVAILABLE IN TWO STRENGTHS
PRELONE® SYRUP **15 mg** per 5 mL **AND** PRELONE® SYRUP **5 mg** per 5 mL

DESCRIPTION

Prednisolone syrup contains prednisolone which is a glucocorticoid. Glucocorticoids are adrenocortical steroids, both naturally occurring and synthetic, which are readily absorbed from the gastrointestinal tract. Prednisolone is a white to practically white, odorless, crystalline powder. It is very slightly soluble in water, soluble in methanol and in dioxane; sparingly soluble in acetone and in alcohol, slightly soluble in chloroform.

The chemical name for Prednisolone is 11β,17,21-Trihydroxpregna-1,4-diene-3,20-dione (anhydrous). Its molecular weight is 360.45. The molecular formula is $C_{21}H_{28}O_5$, and the structural formula is:

PRELONE® Syrup 15 mg contains 15 mg of prednisolone in each 5 mL. Benzoic acid, 0.1% is added as a preservative. It also contains alcohol 5%, citric acid, edetate disodium, glycerine, propylene glycol, purified water, sodium saccharin, sucrose, artificial wild cherry flavor, FD&C blue #1 and red #40.

PRELONE® Syrup **5 mg** contains **5 mg** of prednisolone in each 5 mL. Benzoic acid, 0.1% is added as a preservative. It also contains not more than 0.4% alcohol, citric acid, edetate disodium, glycerine, propylene glycol, purified water, sodium saccharin, sorbitol and artificial wild cherry flavor.

CLINICAL PHARMACOLOGY

Naturally occurring glucocorticoids (hydrocortisone and cortisone), which also have salt-retaining properties, are used as replacement therapy in adrenocortical deficiency states. Their synthetic analogs such as prednisolone are primarily used for their potent anti-inflammatory effects in disorders of many organ systems.

Glucocorticoids such as prednisolone cause profound and varied metabolic effects. In addition, they modify the body's immune responses to diverse stimuli.

INDICATIONS

PREDNISOLONE Syrup is indicated in the following conditions:

1. Endocrine Disorders

Primary or secondary adrenocortical insufficiency (hydrocortisone or cortisone is the first choice: synthetic analogs may be used in conjunction with mineralocorticoids where applicable; in infancy mineralocorticoid supplementation is of particular importance).
- Congenital adrenal hyperplasia
- Nonsuppurative thyroiditis
- Hypercalcemia associated with cancer

2. Rheumatic Disorders

As adjunctive therapy for short-term administration (to tide the patient over an acute episode or exacerbation) in:
- Psoriatic arthritis
- Rheumatoid arthritis, including juvenile rheumatoid arthritis (selected cases may require low-dose maintenance therapy)
- Ankylosing spondylitis
- Acute and subacute bursitis
- Acute nonspecific tenosynovitis
- Acute gouty arthritis
- Post-traumatic osteoarthritis
- Synovitis of osteoarthritis
- Epicondylitis

3. Collagen Diseases

During an exacerbation or as maintenance therapy in selected cases of:
- Systemic lupus erythematosus
- Acute rheumatic carditis

4. Dermatologic Diseases

- Pemphigus
- Bullous dermatitis herpetiformis
- Severe erythema multiforme (Stevens-Johnson syndrome)
- Exfoliative dermatitis
- Mycosis fungoides
- Severe psoriasis
- Severe seborrheic dermatitis

5. Allergic States

Control of severe or incapacitating allergic conditions intractable to adequate trials of conventional treatment:
- Seasonal or perennial allergic rhinitis
- Bronchial asthma
- Contact dermatitis
- Atopic dermatitis
- Serum sickness
- Drug hypersensitivity reactions

6. Ophthalmic diseases

Severe acute and chronic allergic and inflammatory processes involving the eye and its adnexa such as:
- Allergic corneal marginal ulcers
- Herpes zoster ophthalmicus
- Anterior segment inflammation
- Diffuse posterior uveitis and choroiditis
- Sympathetic ophthalmia
- Allergic conjunctivitis
- Keratitis
- Chorioretinitis
- Optic neuritis
- Iritis and Iridocyclitis

7. Respiratory Diseases

- Symptomatic sarcoidosis
- Loeffler's syndrome not manageable by other means
- Berylliosis
- Fulminating or disseminated pulmonary tuberculosis when used concurrently with appropriate antituberculous chemotherapy
- Aspiration pneumonitis

8. Hematologic Disorders

- Idiopathic thrombocytopenic purpura in adults
- Secondary thrombocytopenia in adults
- Acquired (autoimmune) hemolytic anemia
- Erythroblastopenia (RBC anemia)
- Congenital (erythroid) hypoplastic anemia

9. Neoplastic Diseases

For palliative management of:
- Acute leukemia of childhood
- Leukemias and lymphomas in adults

10. Edematous States

To induce a diuresis or emission of proteinuria in the nephrotic syndrome, without uremia, of the idiopathic type or that due to lupus erythematosus.

11. Gastrointestinal Diseases

To tide the patient over a critical period of the disease in:
- Ulcerative colitis
- Regional enteritis

12. Miscellaneous

Tuberculous meningitis with subarachnoid block or impending block used concurrently with appropriate antituberculous chemotherapy. Trichinosis with neurologic or myocardial involvement.

In addition to the above indications ***PRELONE® Syrup*** is indicated for systemic dermatomyositis (polymyositis).

CONTRAINDICATIONS

Systemic fungal infections.

WARNINGS

In patients on corticosteroid therapy subjected to unusual stress, increased dosage of rapidly acting corticosteroids before, during, and after the stressful situation is indicated.

Corticosteroids may mask some signs of infection, and new infections may appear during their use. There may be decreased resistance and inability to localize infection when corticosteroids are used.

Prolonged use of corticosteroids may produce posterior subcapsular cataracts, glaucoma with possible damage to the optic nerves, and may enhance the establishment of secondary ocular infections due to fungi or viruses.

Average and large doses of hydrocortisone or cortisone can cause elevation of blood pressure, salt and water retention, and increased excretion of potassium. These effects are less likely to occur with the synthetic derivatives except when used in large doses. Dietary salt restriction and potassium supplementation may be necessary. All corticosteroids increase calcium excretion.

While on corticosteroid therapy, patients should not be vaccinated against smallpox. Other immunization procedures should not be undertaken in patients who are on corticosteroids, especially on high dose, because of possible hazards of neurological complications and a lack of antibody response.

Persons who are on drugs which suppress the immune system are more susceptible to infections than healthy individuals. Chickenpox and measles, for example, can have a more serious or even fatal course in non-immune children or adults on corticosteroids. In such children or adults who have not had these diseases, particular care should be taken to avoid exposure. How the dose, route and duration of corticosteroid administration affects the risk of developing a disseminated infection is not known. The contribution of the underlying disease and/or prior corticosteroid treatment to the risk is also not known. If exposed to chickenpox, prophylaxis with varicella zoster immune globulin (VZIG) may be indicated. If exposed to measles, prophylaxis with pooled intravenous immunoglobulin (IG) may be indicated. (See the respective package inserts for complete VZIG and IG prescribing information.) If chickenpox develops, treatment with antiviral agents may be considered.

The use of ***PRELONE® Syrup*** in active tuberculosis should be restricted to those cases of fulminating or disseminated tuberculosis in which the corticosteroid is used for the management of the disease in conjunction with an appropriate antituberculous regimen.

If corticosteroids are indicated in patients with latent tuberculosis or tuberculin reactivity, close observation is necessary as reactivation of the disease may occur. During prolonged corticosteroid therapy, these patients should receive chemoprophylaxis.

Use in pregnancy: Since adequate human reproduction studies have not been done with corticosteroids, the use of these drugs in pregnancy, nursing mothers or women of childbearing potential requires that the possible benefits of the drug be weighed against the potential hazards to the mother and embryo or fetus. Infants born of mothers who have received substantial doses of corticosteroids during pregnancy should be carefully observed for signs of hypoadrenalism.

PRECAUTIONS

General: Drug-induced secondary adrenocortical insufficiency may be minimized by gradual reduction of dosage. This type of relative insufficiency may persist for months after discontinuation of therapy; therefore, in any situation of stress occurring during that period hormone therapy should be reinstituted. Since mineralocorticoid secretion may be impaired, salt and/or a mineralocorticoid should be administered concurrently.

There is an enhanced effect of corticosteroids on patients with hypothyroidism and in those with cirrhosis.

Corticosteroids should be used cautiously in patients with ocular herpes simplex because of possible corneal perforation.

The lowest possible dose of corticosteroid should be used to control the condition under treatment, and when reduction in dosage is possible, the reduction should be gradual.

Psychic derangements may appear when corticosteroids are used, ranging from euphoria, insomnia, mood swings, personality changes, and severe depression, to frank psychotic manifestations. Also, existing emotional instability or psychotic tendencies may be aggravated by corticosteroids.

Aspirin should be used cautiously in conjunction with corticosteroids in hypoprothrombinemia.

Steroids should be used with caution in nonspecific ulcerative colitis, if there is a probability of impending perforation, abscess or other pyogenic infections; diverticulitis;

fresh intestinal anastomoses; active or latent peptic ulcer; renal insufficiency; hypertension; osteoporosis; and myasthenia gravis.
Growth and development of infants and children on prolonged corticosteroid therapy should be carefully observed.
Information for patients: Patients who are on immunosuppressant doses of corticosteroids should be warned to avoid exposure to chickenpox or measles. Patients should also be advised that if they are exposed, medical advice should be sought without delay.

ADVERSE REACTIONS

Fluid and Electrolyte Disturbances
- Sodium retention
- Fluid retention
- Congestive heart failure in susceptible patients
- Potassium loss
- Hypokalemic alkalosis
- Hypertension

Musculoskeletal
- Muscle weakness
- Steroid myopathy
- Loss of muscle mass
- Osteoporosis
- Vertebral compression fractures
- Aseptic necrosis of femoral and humeral heads
- Pathologic fracture of long bones

Gastrointestinal
- Peptic ulcer with possible perforation and hemorrhage
- Pancreatitis
- Abdominal distention
- Ulcerative esophagitis

Dermatologic
- Impaired wound healing
- Thin fragile skin
- Petechiae and Ecchymoses
- Facial erythema
- Increased sweating
- May suppress reactions to skin tests

Neurological
- Convulsions
- Increased intracranial pressure with papilledema (pseudo-tumor cerebri) usually after treatment
- Vertigo
- Headache

Endocrine
- Menstrual irregularities
- Development of Cushingoid state
- Suppression of growth in children
- Secondary adrenocortical and pituitary unresponsiveness, particularly in times of stress, as in trauma, surgery or illness
- Decreased carbohydrate tolerance
- Manifestations of latent diabetes mellitus
- Increased requirements for insulin or oral hypoglycemic agents in diabetics

Ophthalmic
- Posterior subcapsular cataracts
- Increased intraocular pressure
- Glaucoma
- Exophthalmos

Metabolic
- Negative nitrogen balance due to protein catabolism

DOSAGE AND ADMINISTRATION

Dosage of ***PRELONE® Syrup*** should be individualized according to the severity of the disease and the response of the patient. For infants and children, the recommended dosage should be governed by the same considerations rather than strict adherence to the ratio indicated by age or body weight.
Hormone therapy is an adjunct to and not a replacement for conventional therapy.
Dosage should be decreased or discontinued gradually when the drug has been administered for more than a few days.
The severity, prognosis, expected duration of the disease, and the reaction of the patient to medication are primary factors in determining dosage.
If a period of spontaneous remission occurs in a chronic condition, treatment should be discontinued.
Blood pressure, body weight, routine laboratory studies, including two-hour postprandial blood glucose and serum potassium, and a chest X-ray should be obtained at regular intervals during prolonged therapy. Upper GI X-rays are desirable in patients with known or suspected peptic ulcer disease.
The initial dosage of ***PRELONE® Syrup*** may vary from 5 mg to 60 mg per day depending on the specific disease entity being treated. In situations of less severity lower doses will generally suffice while in selected patients higher initial doses may be required. The initial dosage should be maintained or adjusted until a satisfactory response is noted. If after a reasonable period of time there is a lack of satisfactory clinical response, ***PRELONE® Syrup*** should be discontinued and the patient transferred to other appropriate therapy. **IT SHOULD BE EMPHASIZED THAT DOSAGE REQUIREMENTS ARE VARIABLE AND MUST BE INDIVIDUALIZED ON THE BASIS OF THE DISEASE UNDER TREATMENT AND THE RESPONSE OF THE PATIENT.**
After a favorable response is noted, the proper maintenance dosage should be determined by decreasing the initial drug dosage in small decrements at appropriate time intervals until the lowest dosage which will maintain an adequate clinical response is reached. It should be kept in mind that constant monitoring is needed in regard to drug dosage. Included in the situations which may make dosage adjustments necessary are changes in clinical status secondary to remissions or exacerbations in the disease process, the patient's individual drug responsiveness, and the effect of patient exposure to stressful situations not directly related to the disease entity under treatment. In this latter situation it may be necessary to increase the dosage of ***PRELONE® Syrup*** for a period of time consistent with the patient's condition. If after long-term therapy the drug is to be stopped, it is recommended that it be withdrawn gradually rather than abruptly.

HOW SUPPLIED

PRELONE® Syrup containing **15 mg** of Prednisolone in each 5 mL (teaspoonful) is a red cherry flavored liquid and is supplied in 240 mL bottles (NDC 0451-1500-08) and 480 mL bottles (NDC 0451-1500-16).

AND

PRELONE® Syrup containing **5 mg** of Prednisolone in each 5 mL is a dye-free, sugar free, cherry flavored clear liquid and is supplied in 120 mL bottles (NDC 0451-2201-04).
Pharmacist: Dispense 15 mg/5 mL Prelone® Syrup with suitable calibrated measuring device to assure proper measuring of dose. Dispense in tight, light-resistant and child-resistant container as defined in USP/NF.
Store at room temperature. Do not refrigerate.
Pharmacist: Dispense 5 mg/5 mL Prelone® Syrup in tight, light-resistant and child-resistant container as defined in USP/NF.
Store at controlled room temperature 15°C to 30°C (59°F to 86°F). Do not refrigerate.
Rx only

Muro
Pharmaceutical, Inc.
an ASTA Medica company
890 East Street • Tewksbury, Massachusetts 01876-1496
I-2201-1500-3 1/99

TRI-NASAL® SPRAY ℞

[trī nāsal]
(triamcinolone acetonide nasal spray, 50 mcg)
For Intranasal Use Only

DESCRIPTION

Triamcinolone acetonide, the active ingredient of **Tri-Nasal® Spray**, is a corticosteroid with the chemical name, 9α-Fluoro-11β,16α, 17, 21-tetrahydroxypregna-1,4-diene-3, 20-dione cyclic 16, 17-acetal with acetone ($C_{24}H_{31}FO_6$). Its structural formula is:

Triamcinolone acetonide, USP, is a white crystalline powder, with a molecular weight of 434.51. It is practically insoluble in water, and sparingly soluble in dehydrated alcohol, in chloroform and in methanol. It has a melting point temperature range between 292° and 294°C.
Tri-Nasal® Spray is a metered-dose manual spray pump in an amber polyethylene terephthalate (PET) bottle with 0.05% w/v triamcinolone acetonide in a solution containing citric acid, edetate disodium, polyethylene glycol 3350, propylene glycol, purified water, sodium citrate, and 0.01% benzalkonium chloride as a preservative. **Tri-Nasal® Spray** pH is 5.3.
After initial priming (three sprays) of the **Tri-Nasal® Spray** metered pump delivery system, each spray will deliver 50 mcg of triamcinolone acetonide. If the pump was not used for more than 14 days, reprime with 3 sprays or until a fine mist is observed. The majority of the droplets produced by the pump are 8 microns or greater. Each 15 mL bottle contains 7.5 mg of triamcinolone acetonide to deliver 120 metered sprays. After 120 sprays, the amount of triamcinolone acetonide delivered per spray may not be consistent and the bottle should be discarded.

CLINICAL PHARMACOLOGY

Triamcinolone acetonide is a more potent derivative of triamcinolone. Triamcinolone acetonide is approximately eight times more potent than prednisone in animal models of inflammation.
Although the precise mechanism of corticosteroid antiallergic action is unknown, corticosteroids are very effective. When allergic symptoms are very severe, local treatment with recommended doses (microgram) of available topical corticosteroids are not as effective as treatment with larger doses (milligram) of oral or parenteral formulations.
Pharmacokinetics:
Absorption: The pharmacokinetics of **Tri-Nasal® Spray** was evaluated in a single-dose study conducted in 24 patients with perennial allergic rhinitis. Following a single intranasal dose of 400 mcg of triamcinolone acetonide (twice the recommended starting dose of **Tri-Nasal® Spray**), the mean C_{max} of the drug was 1.12 ng/mL (SD = 0.38) with a median T_{max} of 0.5 hours (range: 0.08 - 1.0).
A pharmacokinetic study to demonstrate dose proportionality was conducted in patients with perennial allergic rhinitis. The C_{max} and AUC of the 200 and 400 mcg doses increased less than proportionally when compared to the 100 mcg dose. Following multiple dosing (100 or 200 or 400 mcg QD for 7 days), there was no evidence of drug accumulation.
Distribution: The volume of distribution (Vd) reported was 99.5 L (SD = 27.5).
Metabolism: In animal studies using rats and dogs, three metabolites of triamcinolone acetonide have been identified. They are 6β-hydroxytriamcinolone acetonide, 21-carboxytriamcinolone acetonide and 21-carboxy-6β-hydroxytriamcinolone acetonide. All three metabolites are expected to be substantially less active than the parent compound due to (a) the dependence of anti-inflammatory activity on the presence of a 21-hydroxyl group, (b) the decreased activity observed upon 6-hydroxylation, and (c) the markedly increased water solubility favoring rapid elimination. There appeared to be some quantitative differences in the metabolites among species. No differences were detected in metabolic pattern as a function of route of administration.
Elimination: After a single intranasal dose of 400 mcg of triamcinolone acetonide (twice the recommended starting dose of **Tri-Nasal® Spray**), the mean observed elimination half-life was 2.26 hours (SD=0.77). Based upon intravenous dosing of triamcinolone acetonide phosphate ester, the half-life of triamcinolone acetonide was reported to be 88 minutes. The reported clearance was 45.2 L/hour (SD=9.1) for triamcinolone acetonide.
Special populations
Age: The effect of age, specifically in geriatric and pediatric patients, on the pharmacokinetics of triamcinolone acetonide has not been studied.
Gender: Gender did not significantly influence the pharmacokinetics of **Tri-Nasal® Spray**.
Race: The effect of race on the pharmacokinetics of **Tri-Nasal® Spray** has not been studied.
Renal/Hepatic Insufficiency: No specific pharmacokinetic studies have been conducted in renally or hepatically impaired subjects.
Drug-Drug Interactions: No specific drug-drug interactions have been investigated.
Pharmacodynamics:
A small (approximately 5 to 7 patients per treatment group), parallel trial was conducted to assess the effect of **Tri-Nasal® Spray** on the Hypothalamic-Pituitary-Adrenal (HPA) axis. Patients with allergic rhinitis were treated for six weeks with 400 mcg, 800 mcg, or 1600 mcg total daily doses of **Tri-Nasal® Spray**, 10 mg oral prednisone once daily, or placebo. Adrenal response to a six-hour cosyntropin stimulation test suggests that intranasal **Tri-Nasal® Spray** 400 mcg/day for six weeks did not measurably affect adrenal activity. **Tri-Nasal®** treatment arms using doses of 800 and 1600 mcg/day demonstrated a trend toward dose-related suppression of HPA response. However, this decrease did not reach statistical significance, whereas 10 mg daily oral prednisone did.

CLINICAL TRIALS

The efficacy of **Tri-Nasal® Spray** has been evaluated in 746 patients with seasonal or perennial allergic rhinitis who completed 8 controlled clinical trials.
In total, 1187 patients have been treated with **Tri-Nasal® Spray** in the clinical development program. Three adequate and well controlled multi-center trials involving 541 patients with seasonal allergic rhinitis who received doses of **Tri-Nasal® Spray** ranging from 50 mcg to 400 mcg once daily were conducted. The results showed that patients who received ≥ 200 mcg daily of the active drug had statistically significant relief in the severity of nasal symptoms of seasonal allergic rhinitis including sneezing, stuffiness, discharge, and itching, compared to those receiving placebo.
In one clinical trial that examined efficacy after 2 days of 200 or 400 mcg **Tri-Nasal® Spray** treatment, only the 400 mcg dose showed statistically significant improvement over placebo in the nasal symptoms of seasonal allergic rhinitis.

INDICATIONS AND USAGE

Tri-Nasal® Spray is indicated for the treatment of the nasal symptoms of seasonal and perennial allergic rhinitis in adults and children 12 years of age or older.

CONTRAINDICATIONS

Hypersensitivity to any of the ingredients of this preparation contraindicates its use.

WARNINGS

The replacement of a systemic corticosteroid with a topical corticosteroid can be accompanied by signs of adrenal insufficiency and, in addition, some patients may experience symptoms of corticosteroid withdrawal, e.g., joint and/or muscular pain, lassitude and depression. Patients previously treated for prolonged periods with systemic corticosteroids and transferred to **Tri-Nasal® Spray** should be carefully monitored for acute adrenal insufficiency in response to stress. In those patients who have asthma or other clinical conditions which require long-term corticosteroid treatment, too rapid a decrease in systemic corticosteroid may cause a severe exacerbation of their symptoms.
Persons who are on immunosuppressant drugs are more susceptible to infections than healthy individuals. Chickenpox and measles, for example, can have a more serious or even fatal course in children or adults on immunosuppressant doses of corticosteroids. In such children or adults who have not had these diseases, particular care should be taken

Continued on next page

Tri-Nasal Spray—Cont.

to avoid exposure. If exposed, therapy with varicella zoster immune globulin (VZIG) or pooled intravenous immunoglobulin (IVIG) as appropriate, may be indicated. If chickenpox develops, treatment with antiviral agents may be considered.

PRECAUTIONS

General: Intranasal corticosteroids may cause a reduction in growth velocity when administered to pediatric patients (see **PRECAUTIONS, Pediatric Use** section).

In clinical studies with triamcinolone acetonide nasal spray, the development of localized infections of the nose and pharynx with *Candida albicans* has rarely occurred. When such an infection develops it may require treatment with appropriate local therapy and discontinuance of treatment with **Tri-Nasal® Spray**.

Tri-Nasal® Spray should be used with caution, if at all, in patients with active or quiescent tuberculous infection of the respiratory tract or in patients with untreated fungal, bacterial, or systemic viral infections or ocular herpes simplex.

Because of the inhibitory effect of corticosteroids on wound healing, in patients who have experienced recent nasal septal ulcers, nasal surgery or trauma, a corticosteroid should be used with caution until healing has occurred. As with other nasally inhaled corticosteroids, nasal septal perforations have been reported in rare instances.

When used at excessive doses, systemic corticosteroid effects such as hypercorticism and adrenal suppression may appear. If such changes occur, **Tri-Nasal® Spray** should be discontinued slowly, consistent with accepted procedures for discontinuing oral corticosteroid therapy.

Systemic Availability and HPA Axis Suppression: Triamcinolone acetonide administered intranasally as **Tri-Nasal® Spray** has been shown to be absorbed into the systemic circulation in humans. The bioavailability of triamcinolone acetonide when administered as a solution in **Tri-Nasal® Spray** is approximately 5-fold greater than when administered as a CFC aerosol suspension formulation. While **Tri-Nasal® Spray** administered to 5 patients with allergic rhinitis at 400 mcg/day for 42 days did not measurably affect adrenal response to a six-hour cosyntropin stimulation test, the 6-hour cosyntropin test is an insensitive assessment for subtle HPA effects of corticosteroids. Doses of 800 and 1600 mcg/day of **Tri-Nasal® Spray** did demonstrate a trend toward dose-related suppression of the HPA response. However, this decrease did not reach statistical significance, whereas 10 mg daily oral prednisone did. (see Clinical Pharmacology, Pharmacodynamics)

Information for Patients:

Patients being treated with **Tri-Nasal® Spray** should receive the following information and instructions:

- Patients who are on immunosuppressant doses of corticosteroids should be warned to avoid exposure to chickenpox or measles and, if exposed, to obtain medical advice.
- Patients should use **Tri-Nasal® Spray** at regular intervals since its effectiveness depends on its regular use. (See DOSAGE AND ADMINISTRATION)
- An improvement in some patient symptoms may be seen within the first two days of treatment, and generally, it takes one week of treatment to reach maximum benefit.
- The patient should take the medication as directed and should not exceed the prescribed dosage. The patient should contact the physician if symptoms do not improve after three weeks, or if the condition worsens.
- Patients who experience recurrent episodes of epistaxis (nose bleeds) or nasal septum discomfort while taking this medication should contact their physician. Transient nasal irritation and/or burning or stinging may occur upon instillation with this product. Spraying triamcinolone acetonide directly onto the nasal septum should be avoided.
- For the proper use of this unit and to attain maximum improvement, the patient should read and follow the accompanying patient instructions carefully.
- The bottle should be discarded after 120 sprays since the amount of triamcinolone acetonide delivered thereafter per spray may not be consistent.

Carcinogenesis, Mutagenesis and Impairment of Fertility: In two-year mouse and Sprague-Dawley rat studies, triamcinolone acetonide did not increase the incidence of tumors at oral doses up to 1 and 3 mcg/kg, respectively (less than the maximum recommended daily intranasal dose on a mcg/m^2 basis).

The genotoxic potential of triamcinolone acetonide has not been studied.

Triamcinolone acetonide did not impair fertility in Sprague-Dawley rats given oral doses up to 15 mcg/kg (less than the maximum recommended daily intranasal dose on a mcg/m^2 basis).

However, triamcinolone acetonide caused increased fetal resorptions and stillbirths and decreased pup weight and survival at 5 mcg/kg (less than the maximum recommended daily intranasal dose on a mcg/m^2 basis). These effects were not produced at 1 mcg/kg (less than the maximum recommended daily intranasal dose on a mcg/m^2 basis).

Pregnancy: Pregnancy Category C.

Triamcinolone acetonide induced cleft palate, internal hydrocephaly and skeletal defects in fetuses of Sprague-Dawley rats and New Zealand White rabbits treated throughout organogenesis with daily inhalation doses of 20 mcg/kg (less than the maximum recommended daily intranasal dose on a mcg/m^2 basis). Triamcinolone acetonide induced cranial malformations in fetuses of Rhesus monkeys treated throughout organogenesis with daily intramuscular doses of 500 mcg/kg and greater (approximately 20 times the maximum recommended daily intranasal dose on a mcg/m^2 basis). The 500 mcg/kg dose was the lowest dose used in this study.

There are no adequate and well-controlled studies in pregnant women. Triamcinolone acetonide should be used during pregnancy only if the potential benefits justify the potential risk to the fetus. Since their introduction, experience with oral corticosteroids in pharmacologic as opposed to physiologic doses suggests that rodents are more prone to teratogenic effects from corticosteroids than humans. In addition, because there is a natural increase in corticosteroid production during pregnancy, most women will require a lower exogenous corticosteroid dose and many will not need corticosteroid treatment during pregnancy.

Nonteratogenic Effects: Hypoadrenalism may occur in infants born of mothers receiving corticosteroids during pregnancy. Such infants should be carefully observed.

Nursing Mothers: It is not known whether triamcinolone acetonide is excreted in human breast milk. Because other corticosteroids are excreted in human milk, caution should be exercised when **Tri-Nasal® Spray** is administered to nursing women.

Pediatric Use: Controlled clinical studies have shown that intranasal corticosteroids may cause a reduction in growth velocity in pediatric patients. This effect has been observed in the absence of laboratory evidence of hypothalamic-pituitary-adrenal (HPA) axis suppression, suggesting that growth velocity is a more sensitive indicator of systemic corticosteroid exposure in pediatric patients than some commonly used tests of HPA axis function. The long-term effects of this reduction in growth velocity associated with intranasal corticosteroids, including the impact on final adult height, are unknown. The potential for "catch up" growth following discontinuation of treatment with intranasal corticosteroids has not been adequately studied. The growth of pediatric patients receiving intranasal corticosteroids, including **Tri-Nasal® Spray** should be monitored routinely (e.g. via stadiometry). The potential growth effects of prolonged treatment should be weighed against clinical benefits obtained and the availability of safe and effective noncorticosteroid treatment alternatives. To minimize the systemic effects of intranasal corticosteroids, including **Tri-Nasal® Spray**, each patient should be titrated to the lowest dose that effectively controls his/her symptoms.

ADVERSE REACTIONS

In adequate, well-controlled and uncontrolled studies, 1187 patients have received **Tri-Nasal® Spray**. The adverse reactions summarized below, are based upon seven placebo controlled clinical trials of 2–6 weeks duration in 847 patients with seasonal or perennial allergic rhinitis (504 patients received 200 mcg or 400 mcg per day of **Tri-Nasal® Spray** and 343 patients received vehicle placebo). Adverse events reported by 2% or more of patients (regardless of relationship to treatment) who received **Tri-Nasal® Spray** 200 or 400 mcg once daily and that were more common with **Tri-Nasal® Spray** than with placebo are displayed in the table below. Overall, the incidence and nature of adverse events with **Tri-Nasal®** 400 mcg was comparable to that seen with **Tri-Nasal®** 200 mcg and with vehicle placebo.

[See table below]

ADVERSE EVENTS REPORTED AT A FREQUENCY OF 2% OR GREATER AND MORE COMMON AMONG PATIENTS TREATED WITH TRI-NASAL® SPRAY THAN PLACEBO REGARDLESS OF RELATIONSHIP TO TREATMENT

ADVERSE EVENTS	200 mcg of triamcinolone acetonide once daily n = 204	400 mcg of triamcinolone acetonide once daily n = 300	Combined (200 and 400 mcg) use of triamcinolone acetonide n = 504	Vehicle Placebo n = 343
BODY AS A WHOLE				
Headache	51.0%	44.3%	47.0%	41.1%
Back Pain	7.8%	4.7%	6.0%	3.5%
RESPIRATORY SYSTEM				
Pharyngitis	13.7%	10.3%	11.7%	7.9%
Asthma	5.4%	4.3%	4.8%	2.9%
Cough Increased	2.0%	2.7%	2.4%	2.3%
DIGESTIVE SYSTEM				
Dyspepsia	4.9%	2.7%	3.6%	2.0%
Nausea	2.0%	3.0%	2.6%	0.6%
Vomiting	1.5%	2.7%	2.2%	1.5%
SPECIAL SENSES				
Taste Perversion	7.8%	5.0%	6.2%	2.9%
Conjunctivitis	4.4%	1.3%	2.6%	1.5%
MUSCULOSKELETAL SYSTEM				
Myalgia	2.5%	3.3%	3.0%	2.6%

Adverse events reported by 2% or more of patients who received **Tri-Nasal® Spray** 200 or 400 mcg once daily and that were more common with placebo than with **Tri-Nasal® Spray** included: application site reaction (e.g. transient nasal burning and stinging), rhinitis, dysmenorrhea, pain (unspecified) and allergic reaction.

The adverse effects related to the irritation of nasal mucous membranes (i.e. application site reaction) did not usually interfere with treatment. In the controlled and uncontrolled studies, approximately 0.3% of patients discontinued because of irritation of nasal mucous membranes.

In the event of accidental overdose, an increased potential for these adverse experiences may be expected, but systemic adverse experiences are unlikely.

(see OVERDOSAGE section)

Cases of growth suppression have been reported for intranasal corticosteroids. (see **PRECAUTIONS, Pediatric Use** section).

OVERDOSAGE

Like any other nasally administered corticosteroid, acute overdosage is unlikely. The acute topical application of the entire 15 mL of the bottle would most likely cause nasal irritation and headache. Significant acute systemic adverse effects are unlikely even if the entire 7.5 mg of triamcinolone acetonide is administered intranasally at one time. The intranasal median lethal dose has not been determined in animals.

Dosage and Administration

The usual recommended starting dose of **Tri-Nasal® Spray** for most patients is 200 mcg per day given as 2 sprays (approximately 50 mcg/spray) in each nostril once a day. The maximum dose should not exceed 400 mcg per day. If the 400 mcg dose is used, it may be given either as a once a day dosage (4 sprays in each nostril) or divided into two daily doses of two sprays/nostril twice a day.

The nasal spray pump must be primed before **Tri-Nasal® Spray** is used for the first time. To prime the pump, press down on the shoulder of the white nasal applicator using your forefinger and middle finger while supporting the base of the bottle with your thumb. Press down and release the pump until it sprays 3 times or until a fine mist is observed (see **DIRECTIONS FOR USE**).

INDIVIDUALIZATION OF DOSAGE

Dosing of **Tri-Nasal® Spray** should be individualized since there are many variables that determine clinical response. These variables include the degree of patient allergy and degree of pollen exposure, both of which may influence the dose required.

A starting dose of 200 mcg (2 sprays/nostril) once daily is recommended for most patients.

If the patient does not receive a satisfactory response from the initial 200 mcg/day starting dose, the dose may be increased to a maximum of 400 mcg (4 sprays/nostril) once daily. An alternative 400 mcg per day dosing regimen may be given as 200 mcg twice daily (two 50 mcg sprays in each nostril twice daily).

Some patients may obtain relief of symptoms sooner when started on a 400 mcg per day dose of **Tri-Nasal® Spray** than with 200 mcg per day. Onset of significant relief of nasal symptoms was seen within two days after starting treatment at 400 mcg once daily. A starting dose of 400 mcg per day may be considered in patients when starting therapy with **Tri-Nasal® Spray** in cases where a faster onset of relief is desirable. Generally, maximum relief of symptoms may take several days or up to one week to occur.

After symptoms have been brought under control, patients should be titrated to the minimum effective dose to reduce the possibility of adverse effects.

If relief of symptoms is not achieved after 14–21 days of **Tri-Nasal® Spray** therapy given in an adequate dose, **Tri-Nasal® Spray** should be discontinued and alternative diagnosis and therapies considered.
The maximum daily dose should not exceed 400 mcg. (see **PRECAUTIONS, WARNINGS, INFORMATION FOR PATIENTS** and **ADVERSE REACTIONS** sections).
Tri-Nasal® Spray is not recommended for use in persons under 12 years of age since its safety and effectiveness have not been established in this age group.
Directions for Use: Illustrated patient instructions for use accompany each package of **Tri-Nasal® Spray**.

HOW SUPPLIED

Each 15 mL bottle of **Tri-Nasal® Spray** (NDC# 0451-5050-15) contains 7.5 mg (0.50 mg/mL) of triamcinolone acetonide, USP and is fitted with a meter pump with white nasal applicator, teal blue dust cover and teal blue locking clip sealed in a foil pouch. The unit delivers 120 metered sprays and comes with a patient's instructions for use leaflet.
Do not spray in eyes.
Store at controlled room temperature: 20°–25°C (68°–77°F). Protect from freezing.
Use **Tri-Nasal® Spray** within 3 months after opening of the protective foil pouch or before expiration date, whichever comes first.
Rx only
Muro
Pharmaceutical, Inc.
an ASTA Medica company
Tewksbury, MA 01876
I-5050 Revision 2/2000
0000496

VOLMAX® ℞
(albuterol sulfate)
Extended-Release Tablets

DESCRIPTION

Volmax® (albuterol sulfate) Extended-Release Tablets contain albuterol sulfate, the racemic form of albuterol and a relatively selective beta$_2$-adrenergic bronchodilator, in an extended-release formulation. Albuterol sulfate has the chemical name (±), α_1-[(*tert*-butylamino)methyl]-4-hydroxy-*m*-xylene-α, α′-diol sulfate (2:1) (salt), and the following chemical structure:

[HOCH$_2$ / HO–C$_6$H$_3$–CHCH$_2$NHC(CH$_3$)$_3$ (OH)]$_2$ •H_2SO_4

Albuterol sulfate has a molecular weight of 576.7, and the molecular formula is $(C_{13}H_{21}NO_3)_2 \bullet H_2SO_4$. Albuterol sulfate is a white crystalline powder, soluble in water and slightly soluble in ethanol.
The World Health Organization recommended name for albuterol base is salbutamol.
Each Volmax® Extended-Release Tablet for oral administration contains 4 mg or 8 mg of albuterol as 4.8 mg or 9.6 mg, respectively, of albuterol sulfate in a nondeformable cellulosic material that serves as the rate-controlling membrane. Each tablet also contains the inactive ingredients cellulose acetate, croscarmellose sodium, FD&C Blue No. 1 (4 mg tablet only), hydroxypropyl cellulose (8 mg tablet only), hydroxypropyl methylcellulose, magnesium stearate, povidone, silica, sodium chloride, and titanium dioxide.

CLINICAL PHARMACOLOGY

In vitro studies and *in vivo* pharmacologic studies have demonstrated that albuterol has a preferential effect on beta$_2$-adrenergic receptors compared with isoproterenol. While it is recognized that beta$_2$-adrenergic receptors are the predominant receptors in bronchial smooth muscle, data indicate that there is a population of beta$_2$-receptors in the human heart existing in a concentration between 10% and 50%. The precise function of these receptors has not been established. (See Warnings).
The pharmacologic effects of beta-adrenergic agonist drugs, including albuterol, are at least in part attributable to stimulation through beta-adrenergic receptors on intracellular adenyl cyclase, the enzyme that catalyzes the conversion of adenosine triphosphate (ATP) to cyclic-3′, 5′-adenosine monophosphate (cyclic AMP). Increased cyclic AMP levels are associated with relaxation of bronchial smooth muscle and inhibition of release of mediators of immediate hypersensitivity from cells, especially from mast cells.
Albuterol has been shown in most controlled clinical trials to have more effect on the respiratory tract, in the form of bronchial smooth muscle relaxation, than isoproterenol at comparable doses while producing fewer cardiovascular effects.
Albuterol is longer acting than isoproterenol in most patients by any route of administration because it is not a substrate for the cellular uptake processes for catecholamines nor for catechol-*O*-methyl transferase.
Preclinical: Intravenous studies in rats with albuterol sulfate have demonstrated that albuterol crosses the blood-brain barrier and reaches brain concentrations amounting to approximately 5.0% of the plasma concentrations. In structures outside the blood-brain barrier (pineal and pituitary glands), albuterol concentrations were found to be 100 times those in the whole brain.
Studies in laboratory animals (minipigs, rodents, and dogs) have demonstrated the occurrence of cardiac arrhythmias and sudden death (with histologic evidence of myocardial necrosis) when beta-agonists and methylxanthines were administered concurrently. The clinical significance of these findings is unknown.
Pharmacokinetics and Disposition: In a single-dose study comparing one 8 mg Volmax® Extended-Release Tablet with two 4 mg immediate-release Ventolin® (albuterol sulfate, USP) Tablets in 17 normal adult volunteers, the extent of availability of Volmax® Extended-Release Tablets was shown to be about 80% of Ventolin® Tablets with or without food. In addition, lower mean peak plasma concentration and longer time to reach the peak level were observed with Volmax® Extended-Release Tablets as compared to Ventolin® Tablets. The single-dose study results also showed that food decreases the rate of absorption of albuterol from Volmax® Extended-Release Tablets without altering the extent of bioavailability. In addition, the study indicated that food causes a more gradual increase in the fraction of the available dose absorbed from the extended-release formulation as compared with the fasting condition.
In another single-dose study in adults, 8 mg and 4 mg Volmax® Extended-Release Tablets were shown to deliver dose-proportional plasma concentrations in the fasting state. Definitive studies for the effect of food on 4 mg Volmax® Extended-Release Tablets have not been conducted. However, since food lowers the rate of absorption of 8 mg Volmax® Extended-Release Tablets, it is expected that food reduces the rate of absorption of 4 mg Volmax® Extended-Release Tablets also.
Volmax® Extended-Release Tablets have been formulated to provide duration of action of up to 12 hours. In an 8-day, multiple-dose, crossover study, 15 normal adult male volunteers were given 8 mg Volmax® Extended-Release Tablets every 12 hours or 4 mg Ventolin® (albuterol sulfate, USP) Tablets every 6 hours. Each dose of Volmax® Extended-Release Tablets and the corresponding doses of Ventolin® Tablets were administered in the postprandial state. Steady-state plasma concentrations were reached within 2 days for both formulations. Fluctuations (C_{max}-C_{min}/$C_{average}$) in plasma concentrations were similar for Volmax® Extended-Release Tablets administered at 12-hour intervals and Ventolin® Tablets administered every 6 hours. In addition, the relative bioavailability of Volmax® Extended-Release Tablets was approximately 100% of the immediate-release tablet at steady state. A summary of these results is shown in the following table:
[See table above]

Mean Values at Steady State

	C_{max} (ng/mL)	C_{max} (ng/mL)	T_{max} (h)	T_{12} (h)	AUC (ng-h/mL)
VOLMAX®	13.7	8.1	6.0	9.3	134
Ventolin®	13.9	8.1	2.6	7.2	132

The mean plasma albuterol concentration versus time data at steady state after the administration of Volmax® Extended-Release Tablets 8 mg every 12 hours is displayed in the following graph:

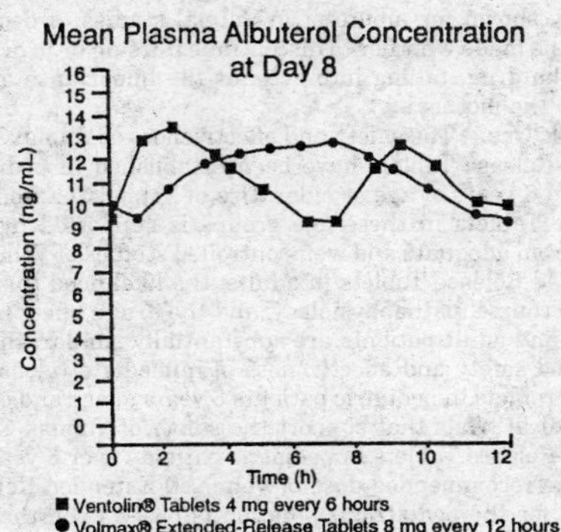

Pharmacokinetic studies of 4- and 8-mg Volmax® Extended-Release Tablets have not been conducted in pediatric patients. Bioavailability of 4- and 8-mg Volmax® Extended-Release Tablets in pediatric patients relative to 2- and 4-mg immediate release albuterol has been extrapolated from adult studies showing comparability at steady-state dosing and reduced bioavailability after single dose administration.

INDICATIONS AND USAGE

Volmax® Extended-Release Tablets are indicated for the relief of bronchospasm in adults and children 6 years of age and older with reversible obstructive airway disease.

CONTRAINDICATIONS

Volmax® Extended-Release Tablets are contraindicated in patients with a history of hypersensitivity to albuterol or any of its components.

WARNINGS

Immediate hypersensitivity reactions may occur after administration of albuterol, as demonstrated by rare cases of urticaria, angioedema, rash, bronchospasm, and oropharyngeal edema.
Cardiovascular Effects: Volmax® Extended-Release Tablets, like all other beta-adrenergic agonists, can produce a clinically significant cardiovascular effect in some patients, as measured by pulse rate, blood pressure, and/or symptoms. Although such effects are uncommon after administration of Volmax® Extended-Release Tablets at recommended doses, if they occur, the drug may need to be discontinued. In addition, beta-agonists have been reported to produce electrocardiogram (ECG) changes, such as flattening of the T wave, prolongation of the QTc interval, and ST segment depression. The clinical significance of these findings is unknown. Therefore, Volmax® Extended-Release Tablets, like all sympathomimetic amines, should be used with caution in patients with cardiovascular disorders, especially coronary insufficiency, cardiac arrhythmias, and hypertension.
Deterioration of Asthma: Asthma may deteriorate acutely over a period of hours or chronically over several days or longer. If the patient needs more doses of Volmax® Extended-Release Tablets than usual, this may be a marker of destabilization of asthma and requires reevaluation of the patient and the treatment regimen, giving special consideration to the possible need for anti-inflammatory treatment; e.g., corticosteroids.
Use of Anti-Inflammatory Agents: The use of beta adrenergic agonist bronchodilators alone may not be adequate to control asthma in many patients. Early consideration should be given to adding anti-inflammatory agents; e.g., corticosteroids.
Paradoxical Bronchospasm: Volmax® Extended-Release Tablets can produce paradoxical bronchospasm, which may be lifethreatening. If paradoxical bronchospasm occurs, Volmax® Extended-Release Tablets should be discontinued immediately and alternative therapy instituted.
Rarely, erythema multiforme and Steven-Johnson syndrome have been associated with the administration of oral albuterol in children.

PRECAUTIONS

General: Albuterol, as with all sympathomimetic amines, should be used with caution in patients with cardiovascular disorders, especially coronary insufficiency, cardiac arrhythmias, and hypertension; in patients with convulsive disorders, hyperthyroidism, or diabetes mellitus; and in patients who are unusually responsive to sympathomimetic amines. Clinically significant changes in systolic and diastolic blood pressure have been seen and could be expected to occur in some patients after use of any beta-adrenergic bronchodilator.
In controlled clinical trials in adults, patients treated with Volmax® Extended-Release Tablets had increases in selected serum chemistry values and decreases in selected hematologic values. Increases in SGPT were more frequent among patients treated with Volmax® Extended-Release Tablets (12 of 247 patients, 4.9%) than among the theophylline (6 of 188 patients, 3.2%) and placebo (1 of 138 patients, 0.7%) groups. Increases in serum glucose concentration were also more frequent among patients treated with Volmax® Extended-Release Tablets (23 of 234 patients, 9.8%) than among theothephylline (11 of 173 patients, 6.45%) and placebo (3 of 129 patients, 2.3%) groups. Increases in SGOT were also more frequent among patient treated with Volmax® Extended-Release Tablets (10 of 248 patients, 4%) and theophylline (5 of 193, 2.6%) than among patients treated with placebo. Decreases in white blood cell counts were more frequent in patients treated with Volmax® Extended-Release Tablets (10 of 247 patients, 4%) compared with patients receiving theophylline (2 of 185 patients, 1.1%) and patients receiving placebo (1 of 141 patients, 0.7%). Decreases in hemoglobin and hematocrit were more frequent in patients receiving Volmax® Extended-Release Tablets (16 of 228 patients, 7.0%, and 17 of 230 patients, 7.4%, respectively) than in patients receiving theophylline (5 of 171 patients, 2.9%, and 9 of 173 patients, 5.2%, respectively) and patients receiving placebo (5 of 129 patients, 3.9%, and 3 of 132 patients, 2.3%, respectively). The clinical significance of these results is unknown.
Large doses of intravenous albuterol have been reported to aggravate pre-existing diabetes mellitus and ketoacidosis. As with other beta-agonists, albuterol may produce significant hypokalemia in some patients, possibly through intracellular shunting, which has the potential to produce adverse cardiovascular effects. The decrease is usually transient, not requiring supplementation.
As with other nondeformable material, caution should be used when administering Volmax® Extended-Release Tablets to patients with pre-existing gastrointestinal narrowing from any cause. There have been rare reports of gastrointestinal obstruction in such patients occurring in associa-

Continued on next page

Volmax—Cont.

tion with ingestion of products containing delivery systems similar to that contained in Volmax® Extended-Release Tablets.

Information for Patients:
Each Volmax® Extended-Release Table contains a small hole that is part of the unique extended-release system. Volmax® Extended-Release Tablets must be swallowed whole with the aid of liquids. DO NOT CHEW OR CRUSH THESE TABLETS.

The outer coating of the tablet is not absorbed and is excreted in the feces; in some instances the empty outer coating may be noticeable in the stool.

The action of Volmax® Extended-Release Tablets should last up to 12 hours or longer. Volmax® Extended-Release Tablets should not be used more frequently than recommended. Do not increase the dose or frequency of Volmax® Extended-Release Tablets without consulting your physician. If you find that treatment with Volmax® Extended-Release Tablets becomes less effective for symptomatic relief, your symptoms become worse, and/or you need to use the product more frequently than usual, you should seek medical attention immediately. While you are using Volmax® Extended-Release Tablets, other inhaled drugs and asthma medications should be taken only as directed by your physician. Common adverse effects include palpitations, chest pain, rapid heart rate, tremor or nervousness. If you are pregnant or nursing, contact your physician about use of Volmax® Extended-Release Tablets. Effective and safe use of Volmax® Extended-Release Tablets includes an understanding of the way that it should be administered.

Drug Interactions: The concomitant use of Volmax® Extended-Release Tablets and other oral sympathomimetic agents is not recommended since such combined use may lead to deleterious cardiovascular effects. This recommendation does not preclude the judicious use of an aerosol bronchodilator of the adrenergic stimulant type in patients receiving Volmax® Extended-Release Tablets. Such concomitant use, however, should be individualized and not given on a routine basis. If regular coadministration is required, then alternative therapy should be considered.

Monoamine Oxidase Inhibitors or Tricyclic Antidepressants: Albuterol should be administered with extreme caution to patients being treated with monoamine oxidase inhibitors or tricyclic antidepressants, or within 2 weeks of discontinuation of such agents, because the action of albuterol on the vascular system may be potentiated.

Beta Blockers: Beta-adrenergic receptor blocking agents not only block the pulmonary effect of beta agonists, such as Volmax® Extended-Release Tablets, but may produce severe bronchospasm in asthmatic patients. Therefore, patients with asthma should not normally be treated with beta-blockers. However, under certain circumstances, e.g., as prophylaxis after myocardial infarction, there may be no acceptable alternatives to the use of beta-adrenergic blocking agents in patients with asthma. In this setting, cardioselective beta-blockers could be considered, although they should be administered with caution.

Diuretics: The ECG changes and/or hypokalemia that may result from the administration of nonpotassium-sparing diuretics (such as loop or thiazide diuretics) can be acutely worsened by beta-agonists, especially when the recommended dose of the beta-agonist is exceeded. Although the clinical significance of these effects is not known, caution is advised in the coadministration of beta-agonists with non potassium-sparing diuretics.

Digoxin: Mean decreases of 16% to 22% in serum digoxin levels were demonstrated after single dose intravenous and oral administration of albuterol, respectively, to normal volunteers who had received digoxin for 10 days. The clinical significance of these findings for patients with obstructive airway disease who are receiving albuterol and digoxin on a chronic basis is unclear. Nevertheless, it would be prudent to carefully evaluate the serum digoxin levels in patients who are currently receiving digoxin and albuterol.

CARCINOGENESIS, MUTAGENESIS, IMPAIRMENT OF FERTILITY: In a 2-year study in Sprague-Dawley rats, albuterol sulfate caused a significant dose-related increase in the incidence of benign leiomyomas of the mesovarium at dietary doses of 2.0, 10, and 50 mg/kg, (approximately 1/2, 3, and 15 times, respectively, the maximum recommended daily oral dose for adults on a mg/m^2 basis, or, approximately 2/5, 2, and 10 times, respectively, the maximum recommended daily oral dose for children on a mg/m^2 basis). In another study this effect was blocked by the coadministration of propranolol, a non-selective beta-adrenergic antagonist. In a 18 month study in CD-1 mice, albuterol sulfate showed no evidence of tumorigenicity at dietary doses of up to 500 mg/kg (approximately 65 times the maximum recommended daily oral dose for adults on a mg/m^2 basis, or, approximately 50 times the maximum recommended daily oral dose for children on a mg/m^2 basis). In a 22 month study in the Golden hamster, albuterol sulfate showed no evidence of tumorigenicity at dietary doses of 50 mg/kg. (approximately 7 times the maximum recommended daily oral dose for adults and children on a mg/m^2 basis).

Albuterol sulfate was not mutagenic in the Ames test with or without metabolic activation using tester strains *S. typhimurium* TA 1537, TA 1538, and TA98 or *E. coli* WP2, WP2uvrA, and WP67. No forward mutation was seen in yeast strain *S. cerevisiae* S9 nor any mitotic gene conversion in yeast strain *S. cerevisiae* JD1 with or without metabolic activation. Fluctuation assays in *S. typhimurium* TA98 and *E. coli* WP2, both with metabolic activation, were negative. Albuterol sulfate was not clastogenic in a human peripheral lymphocyte assay or in an AH1 strain mouse micronucleus assay at intraperitoneal doses of up to 200 mg/kg.

Reproduction studies in rats demonstrated no evidence of impaired fertility at oral doses up to 50 mg/kg, (approximately 15 times the maximum recommended daily oral dose for adults on a mg/m^2 basis).

Pregnancy: Teratogenic Effects: Pregnancy Category C: Albuterol Sulfate has been shown to be teratogenic in mice. A study in CD-1 mice at subcutaneous (SC) doses of 0.025, 0.25, and 2.5 mg/kg, (approximately 3/1000, 3/100, and 3/10 times the maximum recommended daily oral dose for adults on a mg/m^2 basis), showed cleft palate formation in 5 of 111 (4.5%) fetuses at 0.25 mg/kg and in 10 of 108 (9.3%) fetuses at 2.5 mg/kg. The drug did not induce cleft palate formation at the lowest dose, 0.025 mg/kg. Cleft palate also occurred in 22 of 72 (30.5%) fetuses of females treated with 2.5 mg/kg, of isoproterenol (positive control) subcutaneously (approximately 3/10 times the maximum recommended daily oral dose for adults on a mg/m^2 basis). A reproduction study in Stride Dutch rabbits revealed cranioschisis in 7/19 fetuses (37%) when albuterol sulfate was administered orally at a 50 mg/kg dose, (approximately 25 times the maximum recommended daily oral dose for adults on a mg/m^2 basis).

There are no adequate and well-controlled studies in pregnant women. Albuterol should be used during pregnancy only if the potential benefit justifies the potential risk to the fetus.

During worldwide marketing experience, various congenital anomalies, including cleft palate and limb defects, have been rarely reported in the offspring of patients being treated with albuterol. Some of the mothers were taking multiple medications during their pregnancies. No consistent pattern of defects can be discerned, and a relationship between albuterol use and the congenital anomalies has not been established.

Labor and Delivery: Because of the potential for beta-agonist interference with uterine contractility, use of Volmax® Extended-Release Tablets for relief of bronchospasm during labor should be restricted to those patients in whom the benefits clearly outweigh the risks.

Tocolysis: Albuterol has not been approved for the management of pre-term labor. The benefit:risk ratio when albuterol is administered for tocolysis has not been established. Serious adverse reactions, including pulmonary edema, have been reported during or following treatment of premature labor with beta$_2$-agonists, including albuterol.

Nursing Mothers: It is not known whether albuterol is excreted in human milk. Because of the potential for tumorigenicity shown for albuterol in animal studies, a decision should be made whether to discontinue nursing or to discontinue the drug, taking into account the importance of the drug to the mother.

Pediatric Use: The safety and effectiveness of Volmax® Extended-Release Tablets have been established in pediatric patients 6 years of age or older. Use of Volmax® Extended-Release Tablets in these age groups is supported by evidence from adequate and well-controlled studies of Volmax® Extended-Release Tablets in adults; the likelihood that the disease course, pathophysiology, and the drug's effect in pediatric and adult patients are substantially similar; the established safety and effectiveness of immediate release albuterol tablets in pediatric patients 6 years of age and older; and clinical trials that support the safety of Volmax ® Extended-Release Tablets in pediatric patients over 6 years of age. The recommended dose of Volmax® Extended-Release Tablets for the pediatric population is based upon the recommended pediatric dosing of immediate-release albuterol tablets and pharmacokinetic studies in adults showing comparable bioavailability at steadystate dosing and reduced bioavailability after single dose administration. Safety and effectiveness in pediatric patients below 6 years of age have not been established.

ADVERSE REACTIONS

The adverse reactions to albuterol are similar in nature to reactions to other sympathomimetic agents. The most frequent adverse reactions to albuterol are nervousness, tremor, headache, tachycardia, and palpitations. Less frequent adverse reactions are muscle cramps, insomnia, nausea, weakness, dizziness, drowsiness, flushing, restlessness, irritability, chest discomfort, and difficulty in micturition.

Rare cases of urticaria, angioedema, rash bronchospasm, and oropharyngeal edema have been reported after the use of albuterol.

In addition, albuterol, like other sympathomimetic agents, can cause adverse reactions such as hypertension, angina, vomiting, vertigo, central nervous system stimulation, unusual taste, and drying or irritation of the oropharynx.

In controlled clinical trials of adult patients conducted in the United States, the following incidence of adverse events was reported:

[See table below]

A trend was observed among patients treated with Volmax® Extended-Release Tablets toward increasing frequency of muscle cramps with increasing patient age (12–20 years, 1.2%; 21–30 years, 2.6%; 31–40 years, 6.9%; 41–50 years, 6.9%), compared with no such events in the placebo group. Also observed was an increasing frequency of tremor with increasing patient age (12–20 years, 29.4%; 21–30 years, 29.9%; 31–40 years, 27.6%; 41–50 years, 37.9%), compared to 2.9% or less in the placebo group.

The reactions are generally transient in nature, and it is usually not necessary to discontinue treatment with Volmax® Extended-Release Tablets.

OVERDOSAGE

The expected symptoms with overdosage are those of excessive beta-adrenergic stimulation and/or occurrence or exaggeration of any of the symptoms listed under ADVERSE REACTIONS; e.g., seizures, angina, hypertension or hypotension, tachycardia with rates up to 200 beats per minute, arrhythmias, nervousness, headache, tremor, dry mouth, palpitation, nausea, dizziness, fatigue, malaise, and insomnia. Hypokalemia may also occur. As with all sympathomimetic aerosol medications, cardiac arrest and even death may be associated with abuse of Volmax® Extended-Release Tablets.

Treatment consists of discontinuation of Volmax® Extended-Release Tablets together with appropriate symptomatic therapy. The judicious use of a cardioselective beta-receptor blocker may be considered, bearing in mind that such medication can produce bronchospasm. There is insufficient evidence to determine if dialysis is beneficial for overdosage of Volmax® Extended-Release Tablets.

The oral median lethal dose of albuterol sulfate in mice is greater than 2000 mg/kg, (approximately 250 times the maximum recommended daily oral dose for adults on a mg/m^2 basis, or, approximately 200 times the maximum recommended daily oral dose for chidlren on a mg/m^2 basis). In mature rats, the subcutaneous median lethal dose of albuterol sulfate is approximately 450 mg/kg (approximately 110 times the maximum recommended daily oral dose for adults on a mg/m^2 basis, or approximately 90 times the maximum recommended daily oral dose for children on a mg/m^2 basis). In small young rats, the subcutaneous median lethal dose is approximately 2000 mg/kg, (approximately 500 times the maximum recommended daily oral dose for adults on a mg/m^2 basis, or, approximately 400 times the maximum recommended daily oral dose for children on a mg/m^2 basis).

DOSAGE AND ADMINISTRATION

The following dosages of VOLMAX® Extended-Release Tablets are expressed in terms of albuterol base:

Usual Dosage:

Adults and Children over 12 years of age: The usual recommended dosage for adults and pediatric patients over 12 years of age is 8 mg every 12 hours. In some patients, 4 mg every 12 hours may be sufficient.

Children 6 to 12 years of age: The usual recommended dosage for children 6 through 12 years of age is 4 mg every 12 hours.

Dosage adjustment in Adults and Children over 12 years of age: In unusual circumstances, such as adults of low body weight, it may be desirable to use a starting dosage of 4 mg every 12 hours and progress to 8 mg every 12 hours according to response.

If control of reversible airway obstruction is not achieved with the recommended doses in patients on otherwise optimized asthma therapy, the doses may be cautiously increased stepwise under the control of the supervising physician to a maximum dose of 32 mg per day in divided doses (i.e., every 12 hours).

Dosage adjustment in Children 6 to 12 years of age: If control of reversible airway obstruction is not achieved with the recommended doses in patients on otherwise optimized asthma therapy, the doses may be cautiously increased stepwise under the control of the supervising physician to a maximum dose of 24 mg per day in divided doses (i.e., every 12 hours).

Switching from oral Ventolin® products: Patients currently maintained on Ventolin® (albuterol sulfate, USP) Tablets or Ventolin® (albuterol sulfate) Syrup can be switched to Volmax® Extended-Release Tablets. For exam-

Event(n=330)	Volmax® (n=197)	Theophylline (n=20)	Other Beta-agonists (n=178)	Placebo
Tremor	24.2%	6.1%	35.0%	1.1%
Headache	18.8%	26.9%	35.0%	20.8%
Nervousness	8.5%	5.1%	10.0%	2.8%
Nausea/Vomiting	4.2%	19.8%	5.0%	3.9%
Tachycardia	2.7%	0.5%	5.0%	0%
Muscle Cramps	2.7%	0.5%	5.0%	0.6%
Palpitations	2.4%	0.5%	0%	1.1%
Insomnia	2.4%	6.1%	0%	1.7%
Dizziness	1.5%	2.0%	0%	5.1%
Somnolence	0.3%	1.0%	0%	0.6%

ple, the administration of one 4 mg Volmax® Extended-Release Tablet every 12 hours is comparable to one 2 mg Ventolin® Tablet every 6 hours. Multiples of this regimen up to the maximum recommended daily dose also apply. **Each Volmax® Extended-Release Tablet contains a small hole that is part of the unique extended-release system. Volmax® Extended-Release Tablets must be swallowed whole with the aid of liquids. DO NOT CHEW OR CRUSH THESE TABLETS.**

HOW SUPPLIED

Volmax® Extended-Release Tablets, 4 mg of albuterol as the sulfate, are light blue, hexagonal tablets printed with "Volmax" on one side and the number "4" on the other in dark blue ink. They are supplied in HDPE bottles with child-resistant closures of 100 tablets (NDC 0451-0398-50) and HDPE bottles of 500 tablets (NDC 0451-0398-60).

Volmax® Extended-Release Tablets, 8 mg of albuterol as the sulfate, are white, hexagonal tablets printed with "Volmax" on one side and the number "8" on the other in dark blue ink. They are supplied in HDPE bottles with child-resistant closures of 100 tablets (NDC 0451-0399-50) and HDPE bottles of 500 tablets (NDC 0451-0399-60).

Store between 2° and 30° C (36° and 86° F).

Muro Pharmaceutical, Inc.
An ASTA Medica company
Marketed by: Muro Pharmaceutical, Inc.
Tewksbury, MA 01876-1496
Manufactured by: Glaxo Operations UK Ltd. England
Muro® is a registered trademark of
Muro Pharmaceutical, Inc.
*Ventolin® is a registered trademark of Glaxo-Wellcome Operations, Inc.
4/99 I-0398-0399-10

Mylan Pharmaceuticals Inc.

781 CHESTNUT RIDGE ROAD
P.O. BOX 4310
MORGANTOWN, WV 26504-4310

Direct Inquiries to:
(304) 599-2595
For Medical Information Contact:
Clinical Research Department
877-446-3679
877 4INFO-RX
Sales and Ordering:
Sales Department
(800) RX-MYLAN

The following list of Mylan products is provided to facilitate identification. It includes the color(s) and identification codes for all tablets and capsules.

PRODUCT — **IDENTIFICATION CODE**
GENERIC NAME — (Front/Back*)
Description
Color(s)

ACEBUTOLOL HYDROCHLORIDE — MYLAN 1200
Capsules, 200 mg ℞
Med. Orange & Med. Orange

ACEBUTOLOL HYDROCHLORIDE — MYLAN 1400
Capsules, 400 mg ℞
Med. Orange & Med. Orange

ACYCLOVIR — MYLAN 2200
Capsules, USP, 200 mg ℞
Lavender & Lavender

ACYCLOVIR — M253/Blank
Tablets, USP, 400 mg ℞
White

ACYCLOVIR — MYLAN/302
Tablets, USP, 800 mg ℞
White

ALBUTEROL — M255/Blank
Tablets, USP, 2 mg ℞
White

ALBUTEROL — M572/Blank
Tablets, USP, 4 mg ℞
White

ALBUTEROL SULFATE — —
Syrup, USP, 2mg/5mL ℞

ALLOPURINOL — M31/Blank
Tablets, USP, 100 mg ℞
White

ALLOPURINOL — M71/Blank
Tablets, USP, 300 mg ℞
White

ALPRAZOLAM — MYLAN A/Scored
Tablets, USP, 0.25 mg CIV/℞
White

ALPRAZOLAM — MYLAN A3/Scored
Tablets, USP, 0.5 mg CIV/℞
Peach

ALPRAZOLAM — MYLAN A1/Scored
Tablets, USP, 1 mg CIV/℞
Blue

ALPRAZOLAM — MYLAN A4/Scored
Tablets, USP, 2 mg CIV/℞
White

AMILORIDE HYDROCHLORIDE and HYDROCHLOROTHIAZIDE — M577/Blank
Tablets, USP, 5 mg/50 mg ℞
Lt. Orange

AMITRIPTYLINE HYDROCHLORIDE — M77/Blank
Tablets, USP, 10 mg ℞
White

AMITRIPTYLINE HYDROCHLORIDE — M51/Blank
Tablets, USP, 25 mg ℞
Lt. Green

AMITRIPTYLINE HYDROCHLORIDE — M36/Blank
Tablets, USP, 50 mg ℞
Brown

AMITRIPTYLINE HYDROCHLORIDE — M37/Blank
Tablets, USP, 75 mg ℞
Blue

AMITRIPTYLINE HYDROCHLORIDE — M38/Blank
Tablets, USP, 100 mg ℞
Orange

AMITRIPTYLINE HYDROCHLORIDE — M39/Blank
Tablets, USP, 150 mg ℞
Flesh

ATENOLOL — M/A2
Tablets, USP, 25 mg ℞
White

ATENOLOL — M/231
Tablets, USP, 50 mg ℞
White

ATENOLOL — M/757
Tablets, USP, 100 mg ℞
White

ATENOLOL and CHLORTHALIDONE — M63/Blank
Tablets, USP, 50 mg/25 mg ℞
White

ATENOLOL and CHLORTHALIDONE — M64/Blank
Tablets, USP, 100 mg/25 mg ℞
White

AZATHIOPRINE — AZ/Blank
Tablets, USP, 50 mg ℞
Yellow

BUMETANIDE — E128/Blank
Tablets, USP, 0.5 mg ℞
Lt. Green

BUMETANIDE — E129/Blank
Tablets, USP, 1 mg ℞
Yellow

BUMETANIDE — E130/Blank
Tablets, USP, 2 mg ℞
Peach

BUPROPION HYDROCHLORIDE — M/433
Tablets, 75 mg ℞
Peach

BUPROPION HYDROCHLORIDE — M/435
Tablets, 100 mg ℞
Lt. Blue

CAPTOPRIL — MC1/Scored
Tablets, USP, 12.5 mg ℞
White

CAPTOPRIL — MC2/Scored
Tablets, USP, 25 mg ℞
White

CAPTOPRIL — MC3/Blank
Tablets, USP, 50 mg ℞
White

CAPTOPRIL — MC4/Blank
Tablets, USP, 100 mg ℞
White

CAPTOPRIL and HYDROCHLOROTHIAZIDE — M81/Scored
Tablets, USP, 25 mg/15 mg ℞
White

CAPTOPRIL and HYDROCHLOROTHIAZIDE — M84/Scored
Tablets, USP, 50 mg/15 mg ℞
White

CAPTOPRIL and HYDROCHLOROTHIAZIDE — M83/Scored
Tablets, USP, 25 mg/25 mg ℞
Peach

CAPTOPRIL and HYDROCHLOROTHIAZIDE — M86/Scored
Tablets, USP, 50 mg/25 mg ℞
Peach

CARBIDOPA and LEVODOPA — MYLAN/88
Extended-release Tablets, 25 mg/100 mg ℞
Purple

CARBIDOPA and LEVODOPA — MYLAN/94
Extended-release Tablets, 50 mg/200 mg ℞
Purple

CEFACLOR — MYLAN 7250
Capsules, USP, 250 mg ℞
Pink & White

CEFACLOR — MYLAN 7500
Capsules, USP, 500 mg ℞
Pink & Gray

CEFACLOR — —
Powders for Oral Suspension, USP, 125 mg/5 mL ℞

CEFACLOR — —
Powders for Oral Suspension, USP, 187 mg/5 mL ℞

CEFACLOR — —
Powders for Oral Suspension, USP, 250 mg/5 mL ℞

CEFACLOR — —
Powders for Oral Suspension, USP, 375 mg/5 mL ℞

CEPHALEXIN — MYLAN 6025
Capsules, USP, 250 mg ℞
Dark Blue & White

CEPHALEXIN — MYLAN 6050
Capsules, USP, 500 mg ℞
Dark Blue & Lt. Blue

CEPHALEXIN — —
Powders for Oral Suspension, USP, 125 mg/5 mL ℞

CEPHALEXIN — —
Powders for Oral Suspension, USP, 250 mg/5 mL ℞

CHLORDIAZEPOXIDE and AMITRIPTYLINE HYDROCHLORIDE — MYLAN/211
Tablets, USP, 5 mg/12.5 mg CIV/℞
Green

CHLORDIAZEPOXIDE and AMITRIPTYLINE HYDROCHLORIDE — MYLAN/277
Tablets, USP, 10 mg/25 mg CIV/℞
White

CHLOROTHIAZIDE — M50/Blank
Tablets, USP, 250 mg ℞
White

CHLOROTHIAZIDE — MYLAN 162/Blank
Tablets, USP, 500 mg ℞
White

CHLORPROPAMIDE — MYLAN 197/100
Tablets, USP, 100 mg ℞
Green

CHLORPROPAMIDE — MYLAN 210/250
Tablets, USP, 250 mg ℞
Green

CHLORTHALIDONE — M35/Blank
Tablets, USP, 25 mg ℞
Lt. Yellow

CHLORTHALIDONE — M75/Blank
Tablets, USP, 50 mg ℞
Lt. Green

CIMETIDINE — M/53
Tablets, USP, 200 mg ℞
Green

CIMETIDINE — M/317
Tablets, USP, 300 mg ℞
Green

CIMETIDINE — M/372
Tablets, USP, 400 mg ℞
Green

CIMETIDINE — M541/Blank
Tablets, USP, 800 mg ℞
Green

CLOMIPRAMINE HYDROCHLORIDE — MYLAN 3025
Capsules, 25 mg ℞
Medium Orange & Flesh

CLOMIPRAMINE HYDROCHLORIDE — MYLAN 3050
Capsules, 50 mg ℞
Yellow & Flesh

CLOMIPRAMINE HYDROCHLORIDE — MYLAN 3075
Capsules, 75 mg ℞
Swedish Orange & Flesh

CLONAZEPAM — M/C13
Tablets, USP, 0.5 mg CIV/℞
Yellow

CLONAZEPAM — M/C14
Tablets, USP, 1 mg CIV/℞
Lt. Green

CLONAZEPAM — M/C15
Tablets, USP, 2 mg CIV/℞
White

CLONIDINE HYDROCHLORIDE — MYLAN 152/Blank
Tablets, USP, 0.1 mg ℞
White

CLONIDINE HYDROCHLORIDE — MYLAN 186/Blank
Tablets, USP, 0.2 mg ℞
White

CLONIDINE HYDROCHLORIDE — MYLAN 199/Blank
Tablets, USP, 0.3 mg ℞
White

CLORAZEPATE DIPOTASSIUM — M30/Blank
Tablets, USP, 3.75 mg CIV/℞
Blue

CLORAZEPATE DIPOTASSIUM — M40/Blank
Tablets, USP, 7.5 mg CIV/℞
Peach

CLORAZEPATE DIPOTASSIUM — M70/Blank
Tablets, USP, 15 mg CIV/℞
White

CLOZAPINE — M/C7
Tablets, 25 mg ℞
Peach

CLOZAPINE — M/C11
Tablets, 100 mg ℞
Green

CYCLOBENZAPRINE HYDROCHLORIDE — M/751
Tablets, USP, 10 mg ℞
Butterscotch-Yellow

CYSTAGON® — MYLAN/CYSTAGON 50
(Cysteamine Bitartrate)
Capsules, 50 mg ℞
White & White

CYSTAGON® — MYLAN/CYSTAGON 150
(Cysteamine Bitartrate)
Capsules, 150 mg ℞
White & White

Continued on next page

Product Listing-Mylan—Cont.

DIAZEPAM MYLAN 271/Scored
Tablets, USP, 2 mg Ⓒ/℞
White

DIAZEPAM MYLAN 345/Scored
Tablets, USP, 5 mg Ⓒ/℞
Orange

DIAZEPAM MYLAN 477/Scored
Tablets, USP, 10 mg Ⓒ/℞
Green

DICLOFENAC POTASSIUM M/D5
Tablets, 50 mg ℞
White

DICYCLOMINE HYDROCHLORIDE MYLAN 1610
Capsules, USP, 10 mg ℞
Lt. Blue & Lt. Blue

DICYCLOMINE HYDROCHLORIDE MD6/Blank
Tablets, USP, 20 mg ℞
Blue

DILTIAZEM HYDROCHLORIDE MYLAN 5220
Extended-release Capsules, USP, (once-a-day), 120 mg ℞
Lt. Pink & Flesh

DILTIAZEM HYDROCHLORIDE MYLAN 5280
Extended-release Capsules, USP, (once-a-day), 180 mg ℞
Lavender & Flesh

DILTIAZEM HYDROCHLORIDE MYLAN 5340
Extended-release Capsules, USP, (once-a-day), 240 mg ℞
Lt. Blue & Flesh

DILTIAZEM HYDROCHLORIDE MYLAN 6060
Extended-release Capsules, USP, (twice-a-day), 60 mg ℞
Coral & White

DILTIAZEM HYDROCHLORIDE MYLAN 6090
Extended-release Capsules, USP, (twice-a-day), 90 mg ℞
Coral & Ivory

DILTIAZEM HYDROCHLORIDE MYLAN 6120
Extended-release Capsules, USP, (twice-a-day), 120 mg ℞
Coral & Coral

DILTIAZEM HYDROCHLORIDE M23/Blank
Tablets, USP, 30 mg ℞
White

DILTIAZEM HYDROCHLORIDE M45/Scored
Tablets, USP, 60 mg ℞
White

DILTIAZEM HYDROCHLORIDE M135/Scored
Tablets, USP, 90 mg ℞
White

DILTIAZEM HYDROCHLORIDE M525/Scored
Tablets, USP, 120 mg ℞
White

DIPHENOXYLATE HYDROCHLORIDE and ATROPINE SULFATE M15/Blank
Tablets, USP, 2.5 mg/0.025 mg Ⓒ/℞
White

DOXEPIN HYDROCHLORIDE MYLAN 1049
Capsules, USP, 10 mg ℞
Buff & Buff

DOXEPIN HYDROCHLORIDE MYLAN 3125
Capsules, USP, 25 mg ℞
Ivory & White

DOXEPIN HYDROCHLORIDE MYLAN 4250
Capsules, USP, 50 mg ℞
Ivory & Ivory

DOXEPIN HYDROCHLORIDE MYLAN 5375
Capsules, USP, 75 mg ℞
Bright Lt. Green & Bright Lt. Green

DOXEPIN HYDROCHLORIDE MYLAN 6410
Capsules, USP, 100 mg ℞
Bright Lt. Green & White

DOXYCYCLINE HYCLATE MYLAN 145
Capsules, USP, 50 mg ℞
Aqua Blue & White

DOXYCYCLINE HYCLATE MYLAN 148
Capsules, USP, 100 mg ℞
Aqua Blue & Aqua Blue

DOXYCYCLINE HYCLATE MYLAN 167/100
Tablets, USP, 100 mg ℞
Beige

ERYTHROMYCIN ETHYLSUCCINATE M400/Blank
Tablets, USP, 400 mg ℞
Beige

ERYTHROMYCIN STEARATE MYLAN 106/250
Tablets, USP, 250 mg ℞
Yellow

ERYTHROMYCIN STEARATE MYLAN 107/500
Tablets, USP, 500 mg ℞
Yellow

ESTRADIOL M/E3
Tablets, USP, 0.5 mg ℞
White to Off-White

ESTRADIOL M/E4
Tablets, USP, 1 mg ℞
Pink

ESTRADIOL M/E5
Tablets, USP, 2 mg ℞
Pale Blue

ESTRADIOL TRANSDERMAL SYSTEM Estradiol 0.05 mg/day
Patches, 0.05 mg/day ℞
Flesh

ESTRADIOL TRANSDERMAL SYSTEM Estradiol 0.1 mg/day
Patches, 0.1 mg/day ℞
Flesh

ESTROPIPATE ME7/Blank
Tablets, USP, 0.75 mg ℞
Yellow

ESTROPIPATE ME8/Blank
Tablets, USP, 1.5 mg ℞
Peach

ESTROPIPATE ME9/Blank
Tablets, USP, 3 mg ℞
Blue

ETODOLAC MYLAN 7200
Capsules, 200 mg ℞
Brown & Brown

ETODOLAC MYLAN 7233
Capsules, 300 mg ℞
Lt. Brown & Lt. Brown

ETODOLAC MYLAN/237
Tablets, USP, 400 mg ℞
White

ETODOLAC MYLAN/242
Tablets, USP, 500 mg ℞
Pink

FENOPROFEN CALCIUM M471/Scored
Tablets, USP, 600 mg ℞
Lt. Orange

FLUPHENAZINE HYDROCHLORIDE M/4
Tablets, USP, 1 mg ℞
White

FLUPHENAZINE HYDROCHLORIDE M/9
Tablets, USP, 2.5 mg ℞
Yellow

FLUPHENAZINE HYDROCHLORIDE M/74
Tablets, USP, 5 mg ℞
Lt. Green

FLUPHENAZINE HYDROCHLORIDE M/97
Tablets, USP, 10 mg ℞
Orange

FLURAZEPAM HYDROCHLORIDE MYLAN 4415
Capsules, USP, 15 mg Ⓒ/℞
White & Powder Blue

FLURAZEPAM HYDROCHLORIDE MYLAN 4430
Capsules, USP, 30 mg Ⓒ/℞
Powder Blue & Powder Blue

FLURBIPROFEN M76/Blank
Tablets, USP, 50 mg ℞
Beige

FLURBIPROFEN M93/Blank
Tablets, USP, 100 mg ℞
Beige

FUROSEMIDE M2/Blank
Tablets, USP, 20 mg ℞
White

FUROSEMIDE MYLAN 216/40
Tablets, USP, 40 mg ℞
White

FUROSEMIDE MYLAN 232/80
Tablets, USP, 80 mg ℞
White

GEMFIBROZIL MYLAN/517
Tablets, USP, 600 mg ℞
White

GLIPIZIDE MYLAN G1/Blank
Tablets, USP, 5 mg ℞
White

GLIPIZIDE MYLAN G2/Blank
Tablets, USP, 10 mg ℞
White

GLYBURIDE M113/Blank
Tablets, USP (micronized), 1.5 mg ℞
White

GLYBURIDE M125/Blank
Tablets, USP (micronized), 3 mg ℞
Lt. Yellow

GLYBURIDE M142/Blank
Tablets, USP (micronized), 6 mg ℞
Lt. Green

GUANFACINE M/G4
Tablets, USP, 1 mg ℞
White

GUANFACINE M/G5
Tablets, USP, 2 mg ℞
Blue

HALOPERIDOL MYLAN 351/Scored
Tablets, USP, 0.5 mg ℞
Orange

HALOPERIDOL MYLAN 257/Scored
Tablets, USP, 1 mg ℞
Orange

HALOPERIDOL MYLAN 214/Scored
Tablets, USP, 2 mg ℞
Orange

HALOPERIDOL MYLAN 327/Scored
Tablets, USP, 5 mg ℞
Orange

HYDROCHLOROTHIAZIDE MYLAN 810
Capsules, 12.5 mg ℞
White

HYDROXYCHLOROQUINE SULFATE M/373
Tablets, USP, 200 mg ℞
White

IBUPROFEN MYLAN 1401/Blank
Tablets, USP, 400 mg ℞
White

IBUPROFEN MYLAN 1601/Blank
Tablets, USP, 600 mg ℞
White

IBUPROFEN MYLAN 1801/Blank
Tablets, USP, 800 mg ℞
White

INDAPAMIDE M/69
Tablets, USP, 1.25 mg ℞
Pink

INDAPAMIDE M/80
Tablets, USP, 2.5 mg ℞
White

INDOMETHACIN MYLAN 143
Capsules, USP, 25 mg ℞
Lt. Green & Lt. Green

INDOMETHACIN MYLAN 147
Capsules, USP, 50 mg ℞
Lt. Green & Lt. Green

KETOCONAZOLE M261/Blank
Tablets, USP, 200 mg ℞
White

KETOPROFEN MYLAN 4070
Capsules, 50 mg ℞
Lt. Celery & Lt. Celery

KETOPROFEN MYLAN 5750
Capsules, 75 mg ℞
Lt. Aqua & Lt. Aqua

KETOROLAC TROMETHAMINE M134
Tablets, USP, 10 mg ℞
White

LACTULOSE —
Solution, USP, 10 g/15 mL ℞

LOPERAMIDE HYDROCHLORIDE MYLAN 2100
Capsules, USP, 2 mg ℞
Lt. Brown & Lt. Brown

LORAZEPAM M/321
Tablets, USP, 0.5 mg Ⓒ/℞
White

LORAZEPAM MYLAN 457/Blank
Tablets, USP, 1 mg Ⓒ/℞
White

LORAZEPAM MYLAN 777/Blank
Tablets, USP, 2 mg Ⓒ/℞
White

MAPROTILINE HYDROCHLORIDE M/60
Tablets, USP, 25 mg ℞
White

MAPROTILINE HYDROCHLORIDE M/87
Tablets, USP, 50 mg ℞
Blue

MAPROTILINE HYDROCHLORIDE M/92
Tablets, USP, 75 mg ℞
White

MECLOFENAMATE SODIUM MYLAN 2150
Capsules, USP, 50 mg ℞
Coral & Coral

MECLOFENAMATE SODIUM MYLAN 3000
Capsules, USP, 100 mg ℞
Coral & White

METHOTREXATE M14/Blank
Tablets, USP, 2.5 mg ℞
Orange

METHYCLOTHIAZIDE M29/Blank
Tablets, USP, 5 mg ℞
Blue

METHYLDOPA MYLAN/611
Tablets, USP, 250 mg ℞
Beige

METHYLDOPA MYLAN/421
Tablets, USP, 500 mg ℞
Beige

METHYLDOPA and HYDROCHLOROTHIAZIDE MYLAN/507
Tablets, USP, 250 mg/15 mg ℞
Green

METHYLDOPA and HYDROCHLOROTHIAZIDE MYLAN/711
Tablets, USP, 250 mg/25 mg ℞
Green

METOPROLOL TARTRATE M32/Scored
Tablets, USP, 50 mg ℞
Pink

METOPROLOL TARTRATE M47/Scored
Tablets, USP, 100 mg ℞
Lt. Blue

NADOLOL M28/Blank
Tablets, USP, 20 mg ℞
Yellow

NADOLOL M171/Blank
Tablets, USP, 40 mg ℞
Yellow

NADOLOL M132/Blank
Tablets, USP, 80 mg ℞
Yellow

NAPROXEN MYLAN/377
Tablets, USP, 250 mg ℞
White

NAPROXEN MYLAN/555
Tablets, USP, 375 mg ℞
White

NAPROXEN — MYLAN/451
Tablets, USP, 500 mg ℞
White

NAPROXEN SODIUM — M/537
Tablets, USP, 275 mg ℞
Lt. Blue

NAPROXEN SODIUM — MYLAN/733
Tablets, USP, 550 mg ℞
Lt. Blue

NICARDIPINE HYDROCHLORIDE — MYLAN 1020
Capsules, 20 mg ℞
Med. Blue Green & Ivory

NICARDIPINE HYDROCHLORIDE — MYLAN 1430
Capsules, 30 mg ℞
Bluish Green & Rich Yellow

NIFEDIPINE — M475/Blank
Extended-release Tablets, 30 mg ℞
Pink

NIFEDIPINE — M482/Blank
Extended-release Tablets, 60 mg ℞
Pink

NIFEDIPINE — M495/Blank
Extended-release Tablets, 90 mg ℞
Pink

NITROFURANTOIN — MYLAN 1650
Capsules, USP, 50 mg ℞
Lt. Brown & Lt. Brown

NITROFURANTOIN — MYLAN 1700
Capsules, USP, 100 mg ℞
Gray & Gray

NITROGLYCERIN TRANSDERMAL SYSTEM — Nitroglycerin 0.1 mg/hr
Patches, 0.1 mg ℞
Translucent

NITROGLYCERIN TRANSDERMAL SYSTEM — Nitroglycerin 0.2 mg/hr
Patches, 0.2 mg ℞
Translucent

NITROGLYCERIN TRANSDERMAL SYSTEM — Nitroglycerin 0.4 mg/hr
Patches, 0.4 mg ℞
Translucent

NITROGLYCERIN TRANSDERMAL SYSTEM — Nitroglycerin 0.6 mg/hr
Patches, 0.6 mg ℞
Translucent

NORTRIPTYLINE HYDROCHLORIDE — MYLAN 1410
Capsules, USP, 10 mg ℞
Swedish Orange & Swedish Orange

NORTRIPTYLINE HYDROCHLORIDE — MYLAN 2325
Capsules, USP, 25 mg ℞
Orange & Swedish Orange

NORTRIPTYLINE HYDROCHLORIDE — MYLAN 3250
Capsules, USP, 50 mg ℞
Yellow & Swedish Orange

NORTRIPTYLINE HYDROCHLORIDE — MYLAN 4175
Capsules, USP, 75 mg ℞
Brown & Swedish Orange

ORPHENADRINE CITRATE — M/3358
Extended-release Tablets, 100 mg ℞
White

ORPHENADRINE CITRATE, ASPIRIN and CAFFEINE — M3354/Blank
Tablets, 25 mg/385 mg/30 mg ℞
White & Yellow

ORPHENADRINE CITRATE, ASPIRIN and CAFFEINE — M3356/Blank
Tablets, 50 mg/770 mg/60 mg ℞
White & Yellow

PENTOXIFYLLINE — MYLAN/357
Extended-release Tablets, 400 mg ℞
Lavender

PERPHENAZINE and AMITRIPTYLINE HYDROCHLORIDE — MYLAN/330
Tablets, USP, 2 mg/10 mg ℞
White

PERPHENAZINE and AMITRIPTYLINE HYDROCHLORIDE — MYLAN/442
Tablets, USP, 2 mg/25 mg ℞
Purple

PERPHENAZINE and AMITRIPTYLINE HYDROCHLORIDE — MYLAN/727
Tablets, USP, 4 mg/10 mg ℞
Blue

PERPHENAZINE and AMITRIPTYLINE HYDROCHLORIDE — MYLAN/574
Tablets, USP, 4 mg/25 mg ℞
Orange

PERPHENAZINE and AMITRIPTYLINE HYDROCHLORIDE — MYLAN/73
Tablets, USP, 4 mg/50 mg ℞
Purple

EXTENDED PHENYTOIN SODIUM — Bertek 560
Capsules, USP, 100 mg ℞
Lt. Lavender & White

PINDOLOL — M52/Blank
Tablets, USP, 5 mg ℞
White

PINDOLOL — M127/Blank
Tablets, USP, 10 mg ℞
White

PIROXICAM — MYLAN 1010
Capsules, USP, 10 mg ℞
Dark Green & Olive

PIROXICAM — MYLAN 2020
Capsules, USP, 20 mg ℞
Medium Green & Medium Green

PRAZOSIN HYDROCHLORIDE — MYLAN 1101
Capsules, USP, 1 mg ℞
Dark Green & Lt. Brown

PRAZOSIN HYDROCHLORIDE — MYLAN 2302
Capsules, USP, 2 mg ℞
Brown & Lt. Brown

PRAZOSIN HYDROCHLORIDE — MYLAN 3205
Capsules, USP, 5 mg ℞
Lt. Blue & Lt. Brown

PREDNISOLONE — —
Syrup, USP, 15 mg/5 mL ℞

PROBENECID — MYLAN 156/500
Tablets, USP, 500 mg ℞
Yellow

PROCHLORPERAZINE MALEATE — M/P1
Tablets, USP, 5 mg ℞
Maroon

PROCHLORPERAZINE MALEATE — M/P2
Tablets, USP, 10 mg ℞
Maroon

PROPOXYPHENE HYDROCHLORIDE, ASPIRIN and CAFFEINE — MYLAN 131
Capsules, USP, 65 mg/389 mg/32.4 mg CIV/℞
Gray & Red

PROPOXYPHENE HYDROCHLORIDE — MYLAN 129
Capsules, USP, 65 mg CIV/℞
Pink & Pink

PROPOXYPHENE HYDROCHLORIDE and ACETAMINOPHEN — MYLAN/130
Tablets, USP, 65 mg/650 mg CIV/℞
Orange

PROPOXYPHENE NAPSYLATE and ACETAMINOPHEN — MYLAN/155
Tablets, USP, 100 mg/650 mg CIV/℞
Pink

PROPOXYPHENE NAPSYLATE and ACETAMINOPHEN — MYLAN/1155
Tablets, USP, 100 mg/650 mg CIV/℞
White

PROPRANOLOL HYDROCHLORIDE — MYLAN 182/10
Tablets, USP, 10 mg ℞
Orange

PROPRANOLOL HYDROCHLORIDE — MYLAN 183/20
Tablets, USP, 20 mg ℞
Blue

PROPRANOLOL HYDROCHLORIDE — MYLAN 184/40
Tablets, USP, 40 mg ℞
Green

PROPRANOLOL HYDROCHLORIDE — MYLAN 185/80
Tablets, USP, 80 mg ℞
Yellow

PROPRANOLOL HYDROCHLORIDE and HYDROCHLOROTHIAZIDE — MYLAN 731/Scored
Tablets, USP, 40 mg/25 mg ℞
White

PROPRANOLOL HYDROCHLORIDE and HYDROCHLOROTHIAZIDE — MYLAN 347/Scored
Tablets, USP, 80 mg/25 mg ℞
White

RANITIDINE — G/00 30
Tablets, USP, 150 mg ℞
White

RANITIDINE — G/0031
Tablets, USP, 300 mg ℞
White

SPIRONOLACTONE — MYLAN 146/25
Tablets, USP, 25 mg ℞
White

SPIRONOLACTONE and HYDROCHLOROTHIAZIDE — M41/Blank
Tablets, USP, 25 mg/25 mg ℞
Ivory

SULINDAC — MYLAN/427
Tablets, USP, 150 mg ℞
Yellow-Orange

SULINDAC — MYLAN 531/Blank
Tablets, USP, 200 mg ℞
Yellow-Orange

TEMAZEPAM — MYLAN 4010
Capsules, USP, 15 mg CIV/℞
Peach & Peach

TEMAZEPAM — MYLAN 5050
Capsules, USP, 30 mg CIV/℞
Yellow & Yellow

TERAZOSIN HYDROCHLORIDE — MYLAN 2260
Capsules, USP, 1 mg ℞
Rich Yellow & Lt. Lavender

TERAZOSIN HYDROCHLORIDE — MYLAN 2264
Capsules, USP, 2 mg ℞
Black & Lt. Lavender

TERAZOSIN HYDROCHLORIDE — MYLAN 2268
Capsules, USP, 5 mg ℞
Iron Gray & Lt. Lavender

TERAZOSIN HYDROCHLORIDE — MYLAN 1570
Capsules, USP, 10 mg ℞
Lt. Lavender & Lt. Lavender

TETRACYCLINE HYDROCHLORIDE — MYLAN 101
Capsules, USP, 250 mg ℞
Med. Orange & Yellow

TETRACYCLINE HYDROCHLORIDE — MYLAN 102
Capsules, USP, 500 mg ℞
Black & Yellow

THIORIDAZINE HYDROCHLORIDE — M54/10
Tablets, USP, 10 mg ℞
Orange

THIORIDAZINE HYDROCHLORIDE — M58/25
Tablets, USP, 25 mg ℞
Orange

THIORIDAZINE HYDROCHLORIDE — M59/50
Tablets, USP, 50 mg ℞
Orange

THIORIDAZINE HYDROCHLORIDE — M61/100
Tablets, USP, 100 mg ℞
Orange

THIOTHIXENE — MYLAN 1001
Capsules, USP, 1 mg ℞
Caramel & Powder Blue

THIOTHIXENE — MYLAN 2002
Capsules, USP, 2 mg ℞
Caramel & Yellow

THIOTHIXENE — MYLAN 3005
Capsules, USP, 5 mg ℞
Caramel & White

THIOTHIXENE — MYLAN 5010
Capsules, USP, 10 mg ℞
Caramel & Peach

TIMOLOL MALEATE — M55/Blank
Tablets, USP, 5 mg ℞
Green

TIMOLOL MALEATE — M221/Blank
Tablets, USP, 10 mg ℞
Green

TIMOLOL MALEATE — M715/Blank
Tablets, USP, 20 mg ℞
Green

TOLAZAMIDE — MYLAN 217/250
Tablets, USP, 250 mg ℞
White

TOLAZAMIDE — MYLAN 551/Blank
Tablets, USP, 500 mg ℞
White

TOLBUTAMIDE — M13/Blank
Tablets, USP, 500 mg ℞
White

TOLMETIN SODIUM — MYLAN 5200
Capsules, USP, 400 mg ℞
Lt. Blue & Lt. Blue

TOLMETIN SODIUM — M313/Blank
Tablets, USP, 600 mg ℞
Beige

TRIAMTERENE and HYDROCHLOROTHIAZIDE — MYLAN 2537
Capsules, USP, 37.5 mg/25 mg ℞
Olive & Rich Yellow

TRIAMTERENE and HYDROCHLOROTHIAZIDE — MYLAN/TH1
Tablets, USP, 37.5 mg/25 mg ℞
Green

TRIAMTERENE and HYDROCHLOROTHIAZIDE — MYLAN/TH2
Tablets, USP, 75 mg/50 mg ℞
Yellow

TRIFLUOPERAZINE HYDROCHLORIDE — M/T3
Tablets, USP, 1 mg ℞
White

TRIFLUOPERAZINE HYDROCHLORIDE — M/T4
Tablets, USP, 2 mg ℞
White

TRIFLUOPERAZINE HYDROCHLORIDE — M/T5
Tablets, USP, 5 mg ℞
Lavender

TRIFLUOPERAZINE HYDROCHLORIDE — M/T6
Tablets, USP, 10 mg ℞
Lavender

VERAPAMIL HYDROCHLORIDE — MYLAN 512/Blank
Tablets, USP, 80 mg ℞
White

VERAPAMIL HYDROCHLORIDE — MYLAN 772/Blank
Tablets, USP, 120 mg ℞
White

VERAPAMIL HYDROCHLORIDE — MYLAN 6320
Extended-release Capsules, 120 mg ℞
Bluish Green & White

VERAPAMIL HYDROCHLORIDE — MYLAN 6380
Extended-release Capsules, 180 mg ℞
Bluish Green & Lt. Green

VERAPAMIL HYDROCHLORIDE — MYLAN 6440
Extended-release Capsules, 240 mg ℞
Bluish Green & Bluish Green

VERAPAMIL HYDROCHLORIDE — MYLAN/244
Extended-release Tablets, USP, 120 mg ℞
Blue

VERAPAMIL HYDROCHLORIDE — M312/Blank
Extended-release Tablets, USP, 180 mg ℞
Blue

VERAPAMIL HYDROCHLORIDE — M411/Blank
Extended-release Tablets, USP, 240 mg ℞
Blue

*Front/Back Side for Tablets or Both Cap and Body for Capsules.

Continued on next page

CAPTOPRIL TABLETS, USP ℞

12.5 mg, 25 mg, 50 mg and 100 mg
Rx only

> **USE IN PREGNANCY**
> **When used in pregnancy during the second and third trimesters, ACE inhibitors can cause injury and even death to the developing fetus.** When pregnancy is detected, captopril should be discontinued as soon as possible. **See WARNINGS: Fetal/Neonatal Morbidity and Mortality.**

DESCRIPTION

Captopril is a specific competitive inhibitor of angiotensin I-converting enzyme (ACE), the enzyme responsible for the conversion of angiotensin I to angiotensin II.

Captopril is designated chemically as 1-[(2S)-3-mercapto-2-methylpropionyl]-L-proline (MW 217.29).

Captopril is a white to off-white crystalline powder that may have a slight sulfurous odor; it is soluble in water (approx. 160 mg/mL), methanol, and ethanol and sparingly soluble in chloroform and ethyl acetate.

The structural formula is:

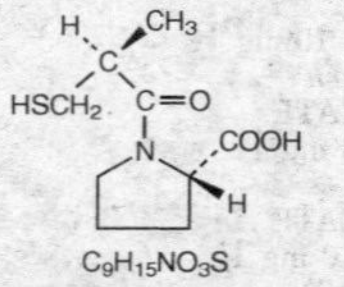

$C_9H_{15}NO_3S$

Each tablet for oral administration contains 12.5 mg, 25 mg, 50 mg or 100 mg of captopril and the following inactive ingredients: anhydrous lactose, colloidal silicon dioxide, crospovidone, microcrystalline cellulose and stearic acid.

CLINICAL PHARMACOLOGY

Mechanism of Action: The mechanism of action of captopril has not yet been fully elucidated. Its beneficial effects in hypertension and heart failure appear to result primarily from suppression of the renin-angiotensin-aldosterone system. However, there is no consistent correlation between renin levels and response to the drug. Renin, an enzyme synthesized by the kidneys, is released into the circulation where it acts on a plasma globulin substrate to produce angiotensin I, a relatively inactive decapeptide. Angiotensin I is then converted by angiotensin converting enzyme (ACE) to angiotensin II, a potent endogenous vasoconstrictor substance. Angiotensin II also stimulates aldosterone secretion from the adrenal cortex, thereby contributing to sodium and fluid retention.

Captopril prevents the conversion of angiotensin I to angiotensin II by inhibition of ACE, a peptidyldipeptide carboxy hydrolase. This inhibition has been demonstrated in both healthy human subjects and in animals by showing that the elevation of blood pressure caused by exogenously administered angiotensin I was attenuated or abolished by captopril. In animal studies, captopril did not alter the pressor responses to a number of other agents, including angiotensin II and norepinephrine, indicating specificity of action.

ACE is identical to "bradykininase", and captopril may also interfere with the degradation of the vasodepressor peptide, bradykinin. Increased concentrations of bradykinin or prostaglandin E_2 may also have a role in the therapeutic effect of captopril.

Inhibition of ACE results in decreased plasma angiotensin II and increased plasma renin activity (PRA), the latter resulting from loss of negative feedback on renin release caused by reduction in angiotensin II. The reduction of angiotensin II leads to decreased aldosterone secretion, and, as a result, small increases in serum potassium may occur along with sodium and fluid loss.

The antihypertensive effects persist for a longer period of time than does demonstrable inhibition of circulating ACE. It is not known whether the ACE present in vascular endothelium is inhibited longer than the ACE in circulating blood.

Pharmacokinetics: After oral administration of therapeutic doses of captopril, rapid absorption occurs with peak blood levels at about one hour. The presence of food in the gastrointestinal tract reduces absorption by about 30 to 40 percent; captopril therefore should be given one hour before meals. Based on carbon-14 labeling, average minimal absorption is approximately 75 percent. In a 24-hour period, over 95 percent of the absorbed dose is eliminated in the urine; 40 to 50 percent is unchanged drug; most of the remainder is the disulfide dimer of captopril and captopril-cysteine disulfide.

Approximately 25 to 30 percent of the circulating drug is bound to plasma proteins. The apparent elimination half-life for total radioactivity in blood is probably less than 3 hours. An accurate determination of half-life of unchanged captopril is not, at present, possible, but it is probably less than 2 hours. In patients with renal impairment, however, retention of captopril occurs (see DOSAGE AND ADMINISTRATION).

Pharmacodynamics: Administration of captopril results in a reduction of peripheral arterial resistance in hypertensive patients with either no change, or an increase, in cardiac output. There is an increase in renal blood flow following administration of captopril and glomerular filtration rate is usually unchanged.

Reductions of blood pressure are usually maximal 60 to 90 minutes after oral administration of an individual dose of captopril. The duration of effect is dose related. The reduction in blood pressure may be progressive, so to achieve maximal therapeutic effects, several weeks of therapy may be required. The blood pressure lowering effects of captopril and thiazide-type diuretics are additive. In contrast, captopril and beta-blockers have a less than additive effect.

Blood pressure is lowered to about the same extent in both standing and supine positions. Orthostatic effects and tachycardia are infrequent but may occur in volume-depleted patients. Abrupt withdrawal of captopril has not been associated with a rapid increase in blood pressure.

In patients with heart failure, significantly decreased peripheral (systemic vascular) resistance and blood pressure (afterload), reduced pulmonary capillary wedge pressure (preload) and pulmonary vascular resistance, increased cardiac output, and increased exercise tolerance time (ETT) have been demonstrated. These hemodynamic and clinical effects occur after the first dose and appear to persist for the duration of therapy. Placebo controlled studies of 12 weeks duration in patients who did not respond adequately to diuretics and digitalis show no tolerance to beneficial effects on ETT; open studies, with exposure up to 18 months in some cases, also indicate that ETT benefit is maintained. Clinical improvement has been observed in some patients where acute hemodynamic effects were minimal.

The Survival and Ventricular Enlargement (SAVE) study was a multicenter, randomized, double-blind, placebo-controlled trial conducted in 2,231 patients (age 21 to 79 years) who survived the acute phase of a myocardial infarction and did not have active ischemia. Patients had left ventricular dysfunction (LVD), defined as a resting left ventricular ejection fraction ≤40%, but at the time of randomization were not sufficiently symptomatic to require ACE inhibitor therapy for heart failure. About half of the patients had had symptoms of heart failure in the past. Patients were given a test dose of 6.25 mg oral captopril and were randomized within 3 to 16 days post-infarction to receive either captopril or placebo in addition to conventional therapy. Captopril was initiated at 6.25 mg or 12.5 mg tid and after two weeks titrated to a target maintenance dose of 50 mg tid. About 80% of patients were receiving the target dose at the end of the study. Patients were followed for a minimum of two years and for up to five years, with an average follow-up of 3.5 years.

Baseline blood pressure was 113/70 mm Hg and 112/70 mm Hg for the placebo and captopril groups, respectively. Blood pressure increased slightly in both treatment groups during the study and was somewhat lower in the captopril group (119/74 vs. 125/77 mm Hg at 1 yr).

Therapy with captopril improved long-term survival and clinical outcomes compared to placebo. The risk reduction for all cause mortality was 19% (P = 0.02) and for cardiovascular death was 21% (P = 0.014). Captopril treated subjects had 22% (P = 0.034) fewer first hospitalizations for heart failure. Compared to placebo, 22% fewer patients receiving captopril developed symptoms of overt heart failure. There was no significant difference between groups in total hospitalizations for all cause (2056 placebo; 2036 captopril).

In a multicenter study, a marketed brand of captopril tablets, USP were well tolerated in the presence of other therapies such as aspirin, beta blockers, nitrates, vasodilators, calcium antagonists and diuretics.

Studies in rats and cats indicate that captopril does not cross the blood-brain barrier to any significant extent.

INDICATIONS AND USAGE

Hypertension: Captopril tablets are indicated for the treatment of hypertension.

In using captopril, consideration should be given to the risk of neutropenia/agranulocytosis (see WARNINGS).

Captopril may be used as initial therapy for patients with normal renal function, in whom the risk is relatively low. In patients with impaired renal function, particularly those with collagen vascular disease, captopril should be reserved for hypertensives who have either developed unacceptable side effects on other drugs, or have failed to respond satisfactorily to drug combinations.

Captopril is effective alone and in combination with other antihypertensive agents, especially thiazide-type diuretics. The blood pressure lowering effects of captopril and thiazides are approximately additive.

Heart Failure: Captopril tablets, USP are indicated in the treatment of congestive heart failure usually in combination with diuretics and digitalis. The beneficial effect of captopril in heart failure does not require the presence of digitalis, however, most controlled clinical trial experience with captopril has been in patients receiving digitalis, as well as diuretic treatment.

Left Ventricular Dysfunction After Myocardial Infarction: Captopril tablets, USP are indicated to improve survival following myocardial infarction in clinically stable patients with left ventricular dysfunction manifested as an ejection fraction ≤ 40% and to reduce the incidence of overt heart failure and subsequent hospitalizations for congestive heart failure in these patients.

In considering use of captopril tablets, USP it should be noted that in controlled trials ACE inhibitors have an effect on blood pressure that is less in black patients than in non-blacks. In addition, ACE inhibitors (for which adequate data are available) cause a higher rate of angioedema in black than in non-black patients (see WARNINGS: Angioedema).

CONTRAINDICATIONS

Captopril tablets, USP are contraindicated in patients who are hypersensitive to this product or any other angiotensin-converting enzyme inhibitor (e.g., a patient who has experienced angioedema during therapy with any other ACE inhibitor).

WARNINGS

Anaphylactoid and Possibly Related Reactions: Presumably because angiotensin-converting enzyme inhibitors affect the metabolism of eicosanoids and polypeptides, including endogenous bradykinin, patients receiving ACE inhibitors (including captopril) may be subject to a variety of adverse reactions, some of them serious.

Angioedema: Angioedema involving the extremities, face, lips, mucous membranes, tongue, glottis or larynx has been seen in patients treated with ACE inhibitors, including captopril. If angioedema involves the tongue, glottis or larynx, airway obstruction may occur and be fatal. Emergency therapy, including but not necessarily limited to, subcutaneous administration of a 1:1000 solution of epinephrine should be promptly instituted.

Swelling confined to the face, mucous membranes of the mouth, lips and extremities has usually resolved with discontinuation of captopril; some cases required medical therapy. (See PRECAUTIONS: Information for Patients and ADVERSE REACTIONS.)

Anaphylactoid Reactions During Desensitization: Two patients undergoing desensitizing treatment with hymenoptera venom while receiving ACE inhibitors sustained life-threatening anaphylactoid reactions. In the same patients, these reactions were avoided when ACE inhibitors were temporarily withheld, but they reappeared upon inadvertent rechallenge.

Anaphylactoid Reactions During Membrane Exposure: Anaphylactoid reactions have been reported in patients dialyzed with high-flux membranes and treated concomitantly with an ACE inhibitor. Anaphylactoid reactions have also been reported in patients undergoing low-density lipoprotein apheresis with dextran sulfate absorption.

Neutropenia/Agranulocytosis: Neutropenia (< 1000/mm^3) with myeloid hypoplasia has resulted from use of captopril. About half of the neutropenic patients developed systemic or oral cavity infections or other features of the syndrome of agranulocytosis.

The risk of neutropenia is dependent on the clinical status of the patient:

In clinical trials in patients with hypertension who have normal renal function (serum creatinine less than 1.6 mg/dL and no collagen vascular disease), neutropenia has been seen in one patient out of over 8,600 exposed.

In patients with some degree of renal failure (serum creatinine at least 1.6 mg/dL) but no collagen vascular disease, the risk of neutropenia in clinical trials was about 1 per 500, a frequency over 15 times that for uncomplicated hypertension. Daily doses of captopril were relatively high in these patients, particularly in view of their diminished renal function. In foreign marketing experience in patients with renal failure, use of allopurinol concomitantly with captopril has been associated with neutropenia but this association has not appeared in U.S. reports.

In patients with collagen vascular diseases (e.g., systemic lupus erythematosus, scleroderma) and impaired renal function, neutropenia occurred in 3.7 percent of patients in clinical trials.

While none of the over 750 patients in formal clinical trials of heart failure developed neutropenia, it has occurred during the subsequent clinical experience. About half of the reported cases had serum creatinine ≥ 1.6 mg/dL and more than 75 percent were in patients also receiving procainamide. In heart failure, it appears that the same risk factors for neutropenia are present.

The neutropenia has usually been detected with in three months after captopril was started. Bone marrow examinations in patients with neutropenia consistently showed myeloid hypoplasia, frequently accompanied by erythroid hypoplasia and decreased numbers of megakaryocytes (e.g., hypoplastic bone marrow and pancytopenia); anemia and thrombocytopenia were sometimes seen.

In general, neutrophils returned to normal in about two weeks after captopril was discontinued, and serious infections were limited to clinically complex patients. About 13 percent of the cases of neutropenia have ended fatally, but almost all fatalities were in patients with serious illness, having collagen vascular disease, renal failure, heart failure or immunosuppressant therapy, or a combination of these complicating factors.

Evaluation of the hypertensive or heart failure patient should always include assessment of renal function.

If captopril is used in patients with impaired renal function, white blood cell and differential counts should be evaluated prior to starting treatment and at approximately two-week intervals for about three months, then periodically.

In patients with collagen vascular disease or who are exposed to other drugs known to affect the white cells or immune response, particularly when there is impaired renal function, captopril should be used only after an assessment of benefit and risk, and then with caution.

All patients treated with captopril should be told to report any signs of infection (e.g., sore throat, fever). If infection is suspected, white cell counts should be performed without delay.

Since discontinuation of captopril and other drugs has generally led to prompt return of the white count to normal, upon confirmation of neutropenia (neutrophil count < 1000/mm^3) the physician should withdraw captopril and closely follow the patient's course.

Proteinuria: Total urinary proteins greater than 1 g per day were seen in about 0.7 percent of patients receiving captopril. About 90 percent of affected patients had evidence of prior renal disease or received relatively high doses of captopril (in excess of 150 mg/day), or both. The nephrotic syndrome occurred in about one-fifth of proteinuric patients. In most cases, proteinuria subsided or cleared within six months whether or not captopril was continued. Parameters of renal function, such as BUN and creatinine, were seldom altered in the patients with proteinuria.

Hypotension: Excessive hypotension was rarely seen in hypertensive patients but is a possible consequence of captopril use in salt/volume depleted persons (such as those treated vigorously with diuretics), patients with heart failure or those patients undergoing renal dialysis. (See PRECAUTIONS: Drug Interactions.)

In heart failure, where the blood pressure was either normal or low, transient decreases in mean blood pressure greater than 20 percent were recorded in about half of the patients. This transient hypotension is more likely to occur after any of the first several doses and is usually well tolerated, producing either no symptoms or brief mild lightheadedness, although in rare instances it has been associated with arrhythmia or conduction defects. Hypotension was the reason for discontinuation of drug in 3.6 percent of patients with heart failure.

BECAUSE OF THE POTENTIAL FALL IN BLOOD PRESSURE IN THESE PATIENTS, THERAPY SHOULD BE STARTED UNDER VERY CLOSE MEDICAL SUPERVISION. A starting dose of 6.25 or 12.5 mg tid may minimize the hypotensive effect. Patients should be followed closely for the first two weeks of treatment and whenever the dose of captopril and/or diuretic is increased. In patients with heart failure, reducing the dose of diuretic, if feasible, may minimize the fall in blood pressure.

Hypotension is not *per se* a reason to discontinue captopril. Some decrease of systemic blood pressure is a common and desirable observation upon initiation of captopril treatment in heart failure. The magnitude of the decrease is greatest early in the course of treatment; this effect stabilizes within a week or two, and generally returns to pretreatment levels, without a decrease in therapeutic efficacy, within two months.

Fetal/Neonatal Morbidity and Mortality: ACE inhibitors can cause fetal and neonatal morbidity and death when administered to pregnant women. Several dozen cases have been reported in the world literature. When pregnancy is detected, ACE inhibitors should be discontinued as soon as possible.

The use of ACE inhibitors during the second and third trimesters of pregnancy has been associated with fetal and neonatal injury, including hypotension, neonatal skull hypoplasia, anuria, reversible or irreversible renal failure, and death. Oligohydramnios has also been reported, presumably resulting from decreased fetal renal function; oligohydramnios in this setting has been associated with fetal limb contractures, craniofacial deformation, and hypoplastic lung development. Prematurity, intrauterine growth retardation, and patent ductus arteriosus have also been reported, although it is not clear whether these occurrences were due to the ACE-inhibitor exposure.

These adverse effects do not appear to have resulted from intrauterine ACE-inhibitor exposure that has been limited to the first trimester. Mothers whose embryos and fetuses are exposed to ACE inhibitors only during the first trimester should be so informed. Nonetheless, when patients become pregnant, physicians should make every effort to discontinue the use of captopril as soon as possible.

Rarely (probably less often than once in every thousand pregnancies), no alternative to ACE inhibitors will be found. In these rare cases, the mothers should be apprised of the potential hazards to their fetuses, and serial ultrasound examinations should be performed to assess the intra-amniotic environment.

If oligohydramnios is observed, captopril should be discontinued unless it is considered life-saving for the mother. Contraction stress testing (CST), a non-stress test (NST), or biophysical profiling (BPP) may be appropriate, depending upon the week of pregnancy. Patients and physicians should be aware, however, that oligohydramnios may not appear until after the fetus has sustained irreversible injury.

Infants with histories of *in utero* exposure to ACE inhibitors should be closely observed for hypotension, oliguria, and hyperkalemia. If oliguria occurs, attention should be directed toward support of blood pressure and renal perfusion. Exchange transfusion or dialysis may be required as a means of reversing hypotension and/or substituting for disordered renal function. While captopril may be removed from the adult circulation by hemodialysis, there is inadequate data concerning the effectiveness of hemodialysis for removing it from the circulation of neonates or children. Peritoneal dialysis is not effective for removing captopril; there is no information concerning exchange transfusion for removing captopril from the general circulation.

When captopril was given to rabbits at doses about 0.8 to 70 times (on a mg/kg basis) the maximum recommended human dose, low incidences of craniofacial malformations were seen. No teratogenic effects of captopril were seen in studies of pregnant rats and hamsters. On a mg/kg basis, the doses used were up to 150 times (in hamsters) and 625 times (in rats) the maximum recommended human dose.

Hepatic Failure: Rarely, ACE inhibitors have been associated with a syndrome that starts with cholestatic jaundice and progresses to fulminant hepatic necrosis and (sometimes) death. The mechanism of this syndrome is not understood. Patients receiving ACE inhibitors who develop jaundice or marked elevations of hepatic enzymes should discontinue the ACE inhibitor and receive appropriate medical follow-up.

PRECAUTIONS

General: ***Impaired Renal Function:*** *Hypertension:* Some patients with renal disease, particularly those with severe renal artery stenosis have developed increases in BUN and serum creatinine after reduction of blood pressure with captopril. Captopril dosage reduction and/or discontinuation of diuretic may be required. For some of these patients, it may not be possible to normalize blood pressure and maintain adequate renal perfusion.

Heart Failure: About 20 percent of patients develop stable elevations of BUN and serum creatinine greater than 20 percent above normal or baseline upon long-term treatment with captopril. Less than 5 percent of patients, generally those with severe preexisting renal disease, required discontinuation of treatment due to progressively increasing creatinine; subsequent improvement probably depends upon the severity of the underlying renal disease.

See CLINICAL PHARMACOLOGY, DOSAGE AND ADMINISTRATION, ADVERSE REACTIONS: Altered Laboratory Findings.

Hyperkalemia: Elevations in serum potassium have been observed in some patients treated with ACE inhibitors, including captopril. When treated with ACE inhibitors, patients at risk for the development of hyperkalemia include those with: renal insufficiency; diabetes mellitus; and those using concomitant potassium-sparing diuretics, potassium supplements or potassium-containing salt substitutes; or other drugs associated with increases in serum potassium. (See PRECAUTIONS: Information for Patients and Drug Interactions; ADVERSE REACTIONS: Altered Laboratory Findings.)

Cough: Presumably due to the inhibition of the degradation of endogenous bradykinin, persistent nonproductive cough has been reported with all ACE inhibitors, always resolving after discontinuation of therapy. ACE inhibitor-induced cough should be considered in the differential diagnosis of cough.

Valvular Stenosis: There is concern, on theoretical grounds, that patients with aortic stenosis might be at particular risk of decreased coronary perfusion when treated with vasodilators because they do not develop as much afterload reduction as others.

Surgery/Anesthesia: In patients undergoing major surgery or during anesthesia with agents that produce hypotension, captopril will block angiotensin II formation secondary to compensatory renin release. If hypotension occurs and is considered to be due to this mechanism, it can be corrected by volume expansion.

Hemodialysis: Recent clinical observations have shown an association of hypersensitivity-like (anaphylactoid) reactions during hemodialysis with high-flux dialysis membranes (e.g., AN69) in patients receiving ACE inhibitors. In these patients, consideration should be given to using a different type of dialysis membrane or a different class of medication. (See WARNINGS: Anaphylactoid Reactions During Membrane Exposure.)

Information For Patients: Patients should be advised to immediately report to their physician any signs or symptoms suggesting angioedema (e.g., swelling of face, eyes, lips, tongue, larynx and extremities; difficulty in swallowing or breathing; hoarseness) and to discontinue therapy. (See WARNINGS: Angioedema.)

Patients should be told to report promptly any indication of infection (e.g., sore throat, fever), which may be a sign of neutropenia, or of progressive edema which might be related to proteinuria and nephrotic syndrome.

All patients should be cautioned that excessive perspiration and dehydration may lead to an excessive fall in blood pressure because of reduction in fluid volume. Other causes of volume depletion such as vomiting or diarrhea may also lead to a fall in blood pressure; patients should be advised to consult with the physician.

Patients should be advised not to use potassium-sparing diuretics, potassium supplements or potassium-containing salt substitutes without consulting their physician. (See PRECAUTIONS: General and Drug Interactions; ADVERSE REACTIONS.)

Patients should be warned against interruption or discontinuation of medication unless instructed by the physician.

Heart failure patients on captopril therapy should be cautioned against rapid increases in physical activity.

Patients should be informed that captopril should be taken one hour before meals (see DOSAGE AND ADMINISTRATION).

Pregnancy: Female patients of childbearing age should be told about the consequences of second- and third-trimester exposure to ACE inhibitors, and they should also be told that these consequences do not appear to have resulted from intrauterine ACE-inhibitor exposure that has been limited to the first trimester. These patients should be asked to report pregnancies to their physicians as soon as possible.

Drug Interactions: ***Hypotension-Patients on Diuretic Therapy:*** Patients on diuretics and especially those in whom diuretic therapy was recently instituted, as well as those on severe dietary salt restriction or dialysis, may occasionally experience a precipitous reduction of blood pressure usually within the first hour after receiving the initial dose of captopril.

The possibility of hypotensive effects with captopril can be minimized by either discontinuing the diuretic or increasing the salt intake approximately one week prior to initiation of treatment with captopril or initiating therapy with small doses (6.25 or 12.5 mg). Alternatively, provide medical supervision for at least one hour after the initial dose. If hypotension occurs, the patient should be placed in a supine position and, if necessary, receive an intravenous infusion of normal saline. This transient hypotensive response is not a contraindication to further doses which can be given without difficulty once the blood pressure has increased after volume expansion.

Agents Having Vasodilator Activity: Data on the effect of concomitant use of other vasodilators in patients receiving captopril for heart failure are not available; therefore, nitroglycerin or other nitrates (as used for management of angina) or other drugs having vasodilator activity should, if possible, be discontinued before starting captopril. If resumed during captopril therapy, such agents should be administered cautiously, and perhaps at lower dosage.

Agents Causing Renin Release: Captopril's effect will be augmented by antihypertensive agents that cause renin release. For example, diuretics (e.g., thiazides) may activate the renin-angiotensin-aldosterone system.

Agents Affecting Sympathetic Activity: The sympathetic nervous system may be especially important in supporting blood pressure in patients receiving captopril alone or with diuretics. Therefore, agents affecting sympathetic activity (e.g., ganglionic blocking agents or adrenergic neuron blocking agents) should be used with caution. Beta-adrenergic blocking drugs add some further antihypertensive effect to captopril, but the overall response is less than additive.

Agents Increasing Serum Potassium: Since captopril decreases aldosterone production, elevation of serum potassium may occur. Potassium-sparing diuretics such as spironolactone, triamterene, or amiloride, or potassium supplements should be given only for documented hypokalemia, and then with caution, since they may lead to a significant increase of serum potassium. Salt substitutes containing potassium should also be used with caution.

Inhibitors of Endogenous Prostaglandin Synthesis: It has been reported that indomethacin may reduce the antihypertensive effect of captopril, especially in cases of low renin hypertension. Other nonsteroidal anti-inflammatory agents (e.g., aspirin) may also have this effect.

Lithium: Increased serum lithium levels and symptoms of lithium toxicity have been reported in patients receiving concomitant lithium and ACE inhibitor therapy. These drugs should be co-administered with caution and frequent monitoring of serum lithium levels is recommended. If a diuretic is also used, it may increase the risk of lithium toxicity.

Cardiac Glycosides: In a study of young healthy male subjects no evidence of a direct pharmacokinetic captopril-digoxin interaction could be found.

Loop Diuretics: Furosemide administered concurrently with captopril does not alter the pharmacokinetics of captopril in renally impaired hypertensive patients.

Allopurinol: In a study of healthy male volunteers no significant pharmacokinetic interaction occurred when captopril and allopurinol were administered concomitantly for 6 days.

Drug/Laboratory Test Interactions: Captopril may cause a false-positive urine test for acetone.

Carcinogenesis, Mutagenesis and Impairment of Fertility: Two-year studies with doses of 50 to 1350 mg/kg/day in mice and rats failed to show any evidence of carcinogenic potential. The high dose in these studies is 150 times the maximum recommended human dose of 450 mg, assuming a 50 kg subject. On a body-surface-area basis, the high doses for mice and rats are 13 and 26 times the maximum recommended human dose, respectively.

Studies in rats have revealed no impairment of fertility.

Animal Toxicology: Chronic oral toxicity studies were conducted in rats (2 years), dogs (47 weeks; 1 year), mice (2 years), and monkeys (1 year). Significant drug-related toxicity included effects on hematopoiesis, renal toxicity, erosion/ulceration of the stomach, and variation of retinal blood vessels.

Reductions in hemoglobin and/or hematocrit values were seen in mice, rats, and monkeys at doses 50 to 150 times the maximum recommended human dose (MRHD) of 450 mg, assuming a 50 kg subject. On a body-surface-area basis, these doses are 5 to 25 times maximum recommended human dose (MRHD). Anemia, leukopenia, thrombocytopenia, and bone marrow suppression occurred in dogs at doses 8 to 30 times MRHD on a body-weight basis (4 to 15 times MRHD on a surface-area basis). The reductions in hemoglobin and hematocrit values in rats and mice were only significant at 1 year and returned to normal with continued dosing by the end of the study. Marked anemia was seen at all dose levels (8 to 30 times MRHD) in dogs, whereas moderate to marked leukopenia was noted only at 15 and 30 times MRHD and thrombocytopenia at 30 times MRHD. The anemia could be reversed upon discontinuation of dosing. Bone marrow suppression occurred to a varying degree, being associated only with dogs that died or were sacrificed in a moribund condition in the 1 year study. However, in the

Continued on next page

Captopril—Cont.

47-week study at a dose 30 times MRHD, bone marrow suppression was found to be reversible upon continued drug administration.
Captopril caused hyperplasia of the juxtaglomerular apparatus of the kidneys in mice and rats at doses 7 to 200 times MRHD on a body-weight basis (0.6 to 35 times MRHD on a surface-area basis); in monkeys at 20 to 60 times MRHD on a body-weight basis (7 to 20 times MRHD on a surface-area basis); and in dogs at 30 times MRHD on a body-weight basis (15 times MRHD on a surface-area basis).
Gastric erosions/ulcerations were increased in incidence in male rats at 20 to 200 times MRHD on a body-weight basis (3.5 and 35 times MRHD on a surface-area basis); in dogs at 30 times MRHD on a body-weight basis (15 times MRHD on a surface-area basis); and in monkeys at 65 times MRHD on a body-weight basis (20 times MRHD on a surface-area basis). Rabbits developed gastric and intestinal ulcers when given oral doses approximately 30 times MRHD on a body-weight basis (10 times MRHD on a surface-area basis) for only 5 to 7 days.
In the two-year rat study, irreversible and progressive variations in the caliber of retinal vessels (focal sacculations and constrictions) occurred at all dose levels (7 to 200 times MRHD) on a body-weight basis; 1 to 35 times MRHD on a surface-area basis in a dose-related fashion. The effect was first observed in the 88th week of dosing, with a progressively increased incidence thereafter, even after cessation of dosing.
Pregnancy Categories C (first trimester) and D (second and third trimesters): See WARNINGS: Fetal/Neonatal Morbidity and Mortality.
Nursing Mothers: Concentrations of captopril in human milk are approximately one percent of those in maternal blood. Because of the potential for serious adverse reactions in nursing infants from captopril, a decision should be made whether to discontinue nursing or to discontinue the drug, taking into account the importance of captopril to the mother. (See PRECAUTIONS: Pediatric Use.)
Pediatric Use: Safety and effectiveness in pediatric patients have not been established. There is limited experience reported in the literature with the use of captopril in the pediatric population; dosage, on a weight basis, was generally reported to be comparable to or less than that used in adults.
Infants, especially newborns, may be more susceptible to the adverse hemodynamic effects of captopril. Excessive, prolonged and unpredictable decreases in blood pressure and associated complications, including oliguria and seizures, have been reported.
Captopril should be used in pediatric patients only if other measures for controlling blood pressure have not been effective.

ADVERSE REACTIONS

Reported incidences are based on clinical trials involving approximately 7000 patients.
Renal: About one of 100 patients developed proteinuria (see WARNINGS).
Each of the following has been reported in approximately 1 to 2 of 1000 patients and are of uncertain relationship to drug use: renal insufficiency, renal failure, nephrotic syndrome, polyuria, oliguria, and urinary frequency.
Hematologic: Neutropenia/agranulocytosis has occurred (see WARNINGS). Cases of anemia, thrombocytopenia, and pancytopenia have been reported.
Dermatologic: Rash, often with pruritus, and sometimes with fever, arthralgia, and eosinophilia, occurred in about 4 to 7 (depending on renal status and dose) of 100 patients, usually during the first four weeks of therapy. It is usually maculopapular, and rarely urticarial. The rash is usually mild and disappears within a few days of dosage reduction, short-term treatment with an antihistaminic agent, and/or discontinuing therapy; remission may occur even if captopril is continued. Pruritus, without rash, occurs in about 2 of 100 patients. Between 7 and 10 percent of patients with skin rash have shown an eosinophilia and/or positive ANA titers. A reversible associated pemphigoid-like lesion, and photosensitivity, have also been reported.
Flushing or pallor has been reported in 2 to 5 of 1000 patients.
Cardiovascular: Hypotension may occur; see WARNINGS and PRECAUTIONS (Drug Interactions) for discussion of hypotension with captopril therapy.
Tachycardia, chest pain, and palpitations have each been observed in approximately 1 of 100 patients.
Angina pectoris, myocardial infarction, Raynaud's syndrome, and congestive heart failure have each occurred in 2 to 3 of 1000 patients.
Dysgeusia: Approximately 2 to 4 (depending on renal status and dose) of 100 patients developed a diminution or loss of taste perception. Taste impairment is reversible and usually self-limited (2 to 3 months) even with continued drug administration. Weight loss may be associated with the loss of taste.
Angioedema: Angioedema involving the extremities, face, lips, mucous membranes, tongue, glottis or larynx has been reported in approximately one in 1000 patients. Angioedema involving the upper airways has caused fatal airway obstruction. (See WARNINGS: Angioedema and PRECAUTIONS: Information for Patients.)
Cough: Cough has been reported in 0.5 to 2% of patients treated with captopril in clinical trials (see PRECAUTIONS: General: *Cough*).
The following have been reported in about 0.5 to 2 percent of patients but did not appear at increased frequency compared to placebo or other treatments used in controlled trials: gastric irritation, abdominal pain, nausea, vomiting, diarrhea, anorexia, constipation, aphthous ulcers, peptic ulcer, dizziness, headache, malaise, fatigue, insomnia, dry mouth, dyspnea, alopecia, paresthesias.
Other clinical adverse effects reported since the drug was marketed are listed below by body system. In this setting, an incidence or causal relationship cannot be accurately determined.
Body as a Whole: Anaphylactoid reactions (see WARNINGS: Anaphylactoid and Possible Related Reactions and PRECAUTIONS: Hemodialysis.)
General: Asthenia, gynecomastia.
Cardiovascular: Cardiac arrest, cerebrovascular accident/insufficiency, rhythm disturbances, orthostatic hypotension, syncope.
Dermatologic: Bullous pemphigus, erythema multiforme (including Stevens-Johnson syndrome), exfoliative dermatitis.
Gastrointestinal: Pancreatitis, glossitis, dyspepsia.
Hematologic: Anemia, including aplastic and hemolytic.
Hepatobiliary: Jaundice, hepatitis, including rare cases of necrosis, cholestasis.
Metabolic: Symptomatic hyponatremia.
Musculoskeletal: Myalgia, myasthenia.
Nervous/Psychiatric: Ataxia, confusion, depression, nervousness, somnolence.
Respiratory: Bronchospasm, eosinophilic pneumonitis, rhinitis.
Special Senses: Blurred vision.
Urogenital: Impotence.
As with other ACE inhibitors, a syndrome has been reported which may include: fever, myalgia, arthralgia, interstitial nephritis, vasculitis, rash or other dermatologic manifestations, eosinophilia and an elevated ESR.
Fetal/Neonatal Morbidity and Mortality: See WARNINGS: Fetal/Neonatal Morbidity and Mortality.
Altered Laboratory Findings: ***Serum Electrolytes:*** *Hyperkalemia:* small increases in serum potassium, especially in patients with renal impairment (see PRECAUTIONS).
Hyponatremia: particularly in patients receiving a low sodium diet or concomitant diuretics.
BUN/Serum Creatinine: Transient elevations of BUN or serum creatinine especially in volume or salt depleted patients or those with renovascular hypertension may occur. Rapid reduction of longstanding or markedly elevated blood pressure can result in decreases in the glomerular filtration rate and, in turn, lead to increases in BUN or serum creatinine.
Hematologic: A positive ANA has been reported.
Liver Function Tests: Elevations of liver transaminases, alkaline phosphatase, and serum bilirubin have occurred.

OVERDOSAGE

Correction of hypotension would be of primary concern. Volume expansion with an intravenous infusion of normal saline is the treatment of choice for restoration of blood pressure.
While captopril may be removed from the adult circulation by hemodialysis, there is inadequate data concerning the effectiveness of hemodialysis for removing it from the circulation of neonates or children. Peritoneal dialysis is not effective for removing captopril; there is no information concerning exchange transfusion for removing captopril from the general circulation.

DOSAGE AND ADMINISTRATION

Captopril should be taken one hour before meals. Dosage must be individualized.
Hypertension: Initiation of therapy requires consideration of recent antihypertensive drug treatment, the extent of blood pressure elevation, salt restriction, and other clinical circumstances. If possible, discontinue the patient's previous antihypertensive drug regimen for one week before starting captopril.
The initial dose of captopril is 25 mg bid or tid. If satisfactory reduction of blood pressure has not been achieved after one or two weeks, the dose may be increased to 50 mg bid or tid. Concomitant sodium restriction may be beneficial when captopril is used alone.
The dose of captopril in hypertension usually does not exceed 50 mg tid. Therefore, if the blood pressure has not been satisfactorily controlled after one to two weeks at this dose, (and the patient is not already receiving a diuretic), a modest dose of a thiazide-type diuretic (e.g., hydrochlorothiazide, 25 mg daily), should be added. The diuretic dose may be increased at one- to two-week intervals until its highest usual antihypertensive dose is reached.
If captopril is being started in a patient already receiving a diuretic, captopril therapy should be initiated under close medical supervision (see WARNINGS and PRECAUTIONS [Drug Interactions] regarding hypotension), with dosage and titration of captopril as noted above.
If further blood pressure reduction is required, the dose of captopril may be increased to 100 mg bid or tid and then, if necessary, to 150 mg bid or tid (while continuing the diuretic). The usual dose range is 25 to 150 mg bid or tid. A maximum daily dose of 450 mg captopril should not be exceeded.
For patients with severe hypertension (e.g., accelerated or malignant hypertension), when temporary discontinuation of current antihypertensive therapy is not practical or desirable, or when prompt titration to more normotensive blood pressure levels is indicated, diuretic should be continued but other current antihypertensive medication stopped and captopril dosage promptly initiated at 25 mg bid or tid, under close medical supervision.
When necessitated by the patient's clinical condition, the daily dose of captopril may be increased every 24 hours or less under continuous medical supervision until a satisfactory blood pressure response is obtained or the maximum dose of captopril is reached. In this regimen, addition of a more potent diuretic, e.g., furosemide, may also be indicated.
Beta-blockers may also be used in conjunction with captopril therapy (see PRECAUTIONS: Drug Interactions), but the effects of the two drugs are less than additive.
Heart Failure: Initiation of therapy requires consideration of recent diuretic therapy and the possibility of severe salt/volume depletion. In patients with either normal or low blood pressure, who have been vigorously treated with diuretics and who may be hyponatremic and/or hypovolemic, a starting dose of 6.25 or 12.5 mg tid may minimize the magnitude or duration of the hypotensive effect (see WARNINGS: Hypotension); for these patients, titration to the usual daily dosage can then occur within the next several days.
For most patients the usual initial daily dosage is 25 mg tid. After a dose of 50 mg tid is reached, further increases in dosage should be delayed, where possible, for at least two weeks to determine if a satisfactory response occurs. Most patients studied have had a satisfactory clinical improvement at 50 or 100 mg tid. A maximum daily dose of 450 mg of captopril should not be exceeded.
Captopril should generally be used in conjunction with a diuretic and digitalis. Captopril therapy must be initiated under very close medical supervision.
Left Ventricular Dysfunction After Myocardial Infarction: The recommended dose for long-term use in patients following a myocardial infarction is a target maintenance dose of 50 mg tid.
Therapy may be initiated as early as three days following a myocardial infarction. After a single dose of 6.25 mg, captopril therapy should be initiated at 12.5 mg tid. Captopril should then be increased to 25 mg tid during the next several days and to a target dose of 50 mg tid over the next several weeks as tolerated (see CLINICAL PHARMACOLOGY).
Captopril may be used in patients treated with other post-myocardial infarction therapies, e.g., thrombolytics, aspirin, beta-blockers.
Dosage Adjustment in Renal Impairment: Because captopril is excreted primarily by the kidneys, excretion rates are reduced in patients with impaired renal function. These patients will take longer to reach steady-state captopril levels and will reach higher steady-state levels for a given daily dose than patients with normal renal function. Therefore, these patients may respond to smaller or less frequent doses.
Accordingly, for patients with significant renal impairment, initial daily dosage of captopril should be reduced, and smaller increments utilized for titration, which should be quite slow (one- to two-week intervals). After the desired therapeutic effect has been achieved, the dose should be slowly back-titrated to determine the minimal effective dose. When concomitant diuretic therapy is required, a loop diuretic (e.g., furosemide), rather than a thiazide diuretic, is preferred in patients with severe renal impairment. (See WARNINGS: Anaphylactoid Reactions During Membrane Exposure and PRECAUTIONS: Hemodialysis.)

HOW SUPPLIED

Captopril tablets are available containing 12.5 mg, 25 mg, 50 mg or 100 mg of captopril.
The 12.5 mg tablets are white, partially scored (both sides), oval tablets marked with M to the left of the score and C1 to the right of the score on one side. They are available as follows:

NDC 0378-3007-01
bottles of 100 tablets
NDC 0378-3007-10
bottles of 1000 tablets

The 25 mg tablets are white, quadrisect scored, round tablets marked with M over C2 on the non-scored side. They are available as follows:

NDC 0378-3012-01
bottles of 100 tablets
NDC 0378-3012-10
bottles of 1000 tablets

The 50 mg tablets are white, scored, round tablets marked with M over C3 on the scored side. They are available as follows:

NDC 0378-3017-01
bottles of 100 tablets
NDC 0378-3017-10
bottles of 1000 tablets

The 100 mg tablets are white, scored, round tablets marked with M over C4 on the scored side. They are available as follows:

NDC 0378-3022-01
bottles of 100 tablets

Captopril tablets may exhibit a slight sulfurous odor.
Bottles contain a desiccant-charcoal canister.

STORE AT CONTROLLED ROOM TEMPERATURE 15°–30°C (59°–86°F).
PROTECT FROM MOISTURE.
Dispense in a tight container using a child-resistant closure.
Mylan Pharmaceuticals Inc.
Morgantown, WV 26505

REVISED SEPTEMBER 1999
CAPT:R8

FUROSEMIDE TABLETS, USP 20 mg, 40 mg and 80 mg ℞

WARNING: Furosemide is a potent diuretic which, if given in excessive amounts, can lead to a profound diuresis with water and electrolyte depletion. Therefore, careful medical supervision is required, and dose and dose schedule must be adjusted to the individual patient's needs. (See "DOSAGE AND ADMINISTRATION".)

DESCRIPTION

Furosemide is a diuretic which is an anthranilic acid derivative. Chemically, it is 4-chloro-*N*-furfuryl-5-sulfamoylanthranilic acid. Furosemide is a white to slightly yellow odorless, crystalline powder. It is practically insoluble in water, sparingly soluble in alcohol, freely soluble in dilute alkali solutions and insoluble in dilute acids.
The structural formula is as follows:

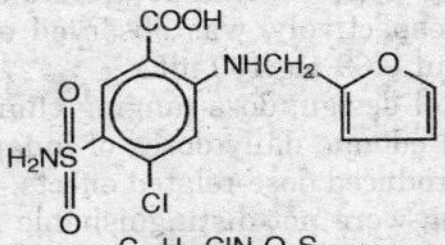

$C_{12}H_{11}ClN_2O_5S$
M.W. 330.75

Each tablet for oral administration contains 20 mg, 40 mg or 80 mg of furosemide and the following inactive ingredients: colloidal silicon dioxide, lactose monohydrate, microcrystalline cellulose, pregelatinized starch and stearic acid.
Furosemide Tablets, USP 20 mg, 40 mg and 80 mg meet *USP DISSOLUTION TEST 1.*

CLINICAL PHARMACOLOGY

Investigations into the mode of action of furosemide have utilized micropuncture studies in rats, stop flow experiments in dogs, and various clearance studies in both humans and experimental animals. It has been demonstrated that furosemide inhibits primarily the reabsorption of sodium and chloride not only in the proximal and distal tubules but also in the loop of Henle. The high degree of efficacy is largely due to this unique site of action. The action on the distal tubule is independent of any inhibitory effect on carbonic anhydrase and aldosterone.
Recent evidence suggests that furosemide glucuronide is the only or at least the major biotransformation product of furosemide in man. Furosemide is extensively bound to plasma proteins, mainly to albumin. Plasma concentrations ranging from 1 to 400 μg/mL are 91 to 99% bound in healthy individuals. The unbound fraction averages 2.3 to 4.1% at therapeutic concentrations.
The onset of diuresis following oral administration is within one hour. The peak effect occurs within the first or second hour. The duration of diuretic effect is 6 to 8 hours.
In fasted normal men, the mean bioavailability of furosemide from furosemide tablets and furosemide oral solution has been shown to be about 60% of that from an intravenous injection of the drug. Although furosemide is more rapidly absorbed from the oral solution than from the tablet, peak plasma levels and area under the plasma concentration-time curves do not differ significantly. Peak plasma concentrations of furosemide increase with increasing dose but times-to-peak do not differ among doses. The terminal half-life of furosemide is approximately 2 hours.
Significantly more furosemide is excreted in urine following the IV injection than after the tablet or oral solution. There are no significant differences between the two oral formulations in the amount of unchanged drug excreted in urine.

INDICATIONS AND USAGE

Edema: Furosemide is indicated in adults, infants, and children for the treatment of edema associated with congestive heart failure, cirrhosis of the liver, and renal disease, including the nephrotic syndrome. Furosemide is particularly useful when an agent with greater diuretic potential is desired.
Hypertension: Oral furosemide may be used in adults for the treatment of hypertension alone or in combination with other antihypertensive agents. Hypertensive patients who cannot be adequately controlled with thiazides will probably also not be adequately controlled with furosemide alone.

CONTRAINDICATIONS

Furosemide is contraindicated in patients with anuria and in patients with a history of hypersensitivity to furosemide.

WARNINGS

In patients with hepatic cirrhosis and ascites, furosemide therapy is best initiated in the hospital. In hepatic coma and in states of electrolyte depletion, therapy should not be instituted until the basic condition is improved. Sudden alteration of fluid and electrolyte balance in patients with cirrhosis may precipitate hepatic coma; therefore, strict observation is necessary during the period of diuresis. Supplemental potassium chloride and, if required, an aldosterone antagonist are helpful in preventing hypokalemia and metabolic alkalosis.
If increasing azotemia and oliguria occur during treatment of severe progressive renal disease, furosemide should be discontinued.
Cases of tinnitus and reversible or irreversible hearing impairment have been reported. Usually, reports indicate that furosemide ototoxicity is associated with rapid injection, severe renal impairment, doses exceeding several times the usual recommended dose, or concomitant therapy with aminoglycoside antibiotics, ethacrynic acid, or other ototoxic drugs. If the physician elects to use high dose parenteral therapy, controlled intravenous infusion is advisable (for adults, an infusion rate not exceeding 4 mg furosemide per minute has been used).

PRECAUTIONS

General: Excessive diuresis may cause dehydration and blood volume reduction with circulatory collapse and possible vascular thrombosis and embolism, particularly in elderly patients. As with any effective diuretic, electrolyte depletion may occur during furosemide therapy, especially in patients receiving higher doses and a restricted salt intake. Hypokalemia may develop with furosemide, especially with brisk diuresis, inadequate oral electrolyte intake, when cirrhosis is present or during concomitant use of corticosteroids or ACTH. Digitalis therapy may exaggerate metabolic effects of hypokalemia, especially myocardial effects.
All patients receiving furosemide therapy should be observed for these signs or symptoms of fluid or electrolyte imbalance (hyponatremia, hypochloremic alkalosis, hypokalemia, hypomagnesemia or hypocalcemia): dryness of mouth, thirst, weakness, lethargy, drowsiness, restlessness, muscle pains or cramps, muscular fatigue, hypotension, oliguria, tachycardia, arrhythmia, or gastrointestinal disturbances such as nausea and vomiting.
Increases in blood glucose and alterations in glucose tolerance tests (with abnormalities of the fasting and 2-hour postprandial sugar) have been observed, and rarely, precipitation of diabetes mellitus has been reported.
Asymptomatic hyperuricemia can occur and gout may rarely be precipitated.
Patients allergic to sulfonamides may also be allergic to furosemide.
The possibility exists of exacerbation or activation of systemic lupus erythematosus.
As with many other drugs, patients should be observed regularly for the possible occurrence of blood dyscrasias, liver or kidney damage or other idiosyncratic reactions.
Information for Patients: Patients receiving furosemide should be advised that they may experience symptoms from excessive fluid and/or electrolyte losses. The postural hypotension that sometimes occurs can usually be managed by getting up slowly. Potassium supplements and/or dietary measures may be needed to control or avoid hypokalemia.
Patients with diabetes mellitus should be told that furosemide may increase blood glucose levels and thereby affect urine glucose tests. The skin of some patients may be more sensitive to the effects of sunlight while taking furosemide.
Hypertensive patients should avoid medications that may increase blood pressure, including over-the-counter products for appetite suppression and cold symptoms.
Laboratory Tests: Serum electrolytes, (particularly potassium), CO_2, creatinine and BUN should be determined frequently during the first few months of furosemide therapy and periodically thereafter. Serum and urine electrolyte determinations are particularly important when the patient is vomiting profusely or receiving parenteral fluids. Abnormalities should be corrected or the drug temporarily withdrawn. Other medications may also influence serum electrolytes.
Reversible elevations of BUN may occur and are associated with dehydration which should be avoided, particularly in patients with renal insufficiency.
Urine and blood glucose should be checked periodically in diabetics receiving furosemide, even in those suspected of latent diabetes.
Furosemide may lower serum levels of calcium (rarely cases of tetany have been reported) and magnesium. Accordingly, serum levels of these electrolytes should be determined periodically.
Drug Interactions: Furosemide may increase the ototoxic potential of aminoglycoside antibiotics, especially in the presence of impaired renal function. Except in life threatening situations, avoid this combination.
Furosemide should not be used concomitantly with ethacrynic acid because of the possibility of ototoxicity.
Patients receiving high doses of salicylates concomitantly with furosemide, as in rheumatic disease, may experience salicylate toxicity at lower doses because of competitive renal excretory sites.
Furosemide has a tendency to antagonize the skeletal muscle relaxing effects of tubocurarine and may potentiate the action of succinylcholine.
Lithium generally should not be given with diuretics because they reduce lithium's renal clearance and add a high risk of lithium toxicity.
Furosemide may add to or potentiate the therapeutic effect of other antihypertensive drugs. Potentiation occurs with ganglionic or peripheral adrenergic blocking drugs.
Furosemide may decrease arterial responsiveness to norepinephrine. However, norepinephrine may still be used effectively.
Simultaneous administration of sucralfate and furosemide tablets may reduce the natriuretic and antihypertensive effects of furosemide. Patients receiving both drugs should be observed closely to determine if the desired diuretic and/or antihypertensive effect of furosemide is achieved. The intake of furosemide and sucralfate should be separated by at least two hours.
One study in six subjects demonstrated that the combination of furosemide and acetylsalicylic acid temporarily reduced creatinine clearance in patients with chronic renal insufficiency. There are case reports of patients who developed increased BUN, serum creatinine and serum potassium levels, and weight gain when furosemide was used in conjunction with NSAIDs.
Literature reports indicate that coadministration of indomethacin may reduce the natriuretic and antihypertensive effects of furosemide in some patients by inhibiting prostaglandin synthesis. Indomethacin may also affect plasma renin levels, aldosterone excretion and renin profile evaluation. Patients receiving both indomethacin and furosemide should be observed closely to determine if the desired diuretic and/or antihypertensive effect of furosemide is achieved.
Carcinogenesis, Mutagenesis, Impairment of Fertility: Furosemide was tested for carcinogenicity by oral administration in one strain of mice and one strain of rats. A small but significantly increased incidence of mammary gland carcinomas occurred in female mice at a dose 17.5 times the maximum human dose of 600 mg. There were marginal increases in uncommon tumors in male rats at a dose of 15 mg/kg (slightly greater than the maximum human dose) but not at 30 mg/kg.
Furosemide was devoid of mutagenic activity in various strains of *Salmonella typhimurium* when tested in the presence or absence of an *in vitro* metabolic activation system, and questionably positive for gene mutation in mouse lymphoma cells in the presence of rat liver S9 at the highest dose tested. Furosemide did not induce sister chromatid exchange in human cells *in vitro*, but other studies on chromosomal aberrations in human cells *in vitro* gave conflicting results. In Chinese hamster cells it induced chromosomal damage but was questionably positive for sister chromatid exchange. Studies on the induction by furosemide of chromosomal aberrations in mice were inconclusive. The urine of rats treated with this drug did not induce gene conversion in *Saccharomyces cerevisiae*.
Furosemide produced no impairment of fertility in male or female rats at 100 mg/kg/day (the maximum effective diuretic dose in the rat and 8 times the maximal human dose of 600 mg/day).
Pregnancy: ***Teratogenic Effects:*** *Pregnancy Category C:* Furosemide has been shown to cause unexplained maternal deaths and abortions in rabbits at 2, 4 and 8 times the maximal recommended human dose. There are no adequate and well-controlled studies in pregnant women. Furosemide should be used during pregnancy only if the potential benefit justifies the potential risk to the fetus.
The effects of furosemide on embryonic and fetal development and on pregnant dams were studied in mice, rats, and rabbits.
Furosemide caused unexplained maternal deaths and abortions in the rabbit at the lowest dose of 25 mg/kg (two times the maximal recommended human dose of 600 mg/day). In another study, a dose of 50 mg/kg (four times the maximal recommended human dose of 600 mg/day) also caused maternal deaths and abortions when administered to rabbits between Days 12 and 17 of gestation. In a third study, none of the pregnant rabbits survived a dose of 100 mg/kg. Data from the above studies indicate fetal lethality that can precede maternal deaths.
The results of the mouse study and one of the three rabbit studies also showed an increased incidence and severity of hydronephrosis (distention of the renal pelvis and in some cases of the ureters) in fetuses derived from the treated dams as compared with the incidence in fetuses from the control group.
Nursing Mothers: Because it appears in breast milk, caution should be exercised when furosemide is administered to a nursing mother.

ADVERSE REACTIONS

Adverse reactions are categorized below by organ system and listed by decreasing severity.

Gastrointestinal System Reactions

1. pancreatitis
2. jaundice (intrahepatic cholestatic jaundice)
3. anorexia
4. oral and gastric irritation
5. cramping
6. diarrhea
7. constipation
8. nausea
9. vomiting

Continued on next page

Furosemide—Cont.

Systemic Hypersensitivity Reactions
1. systemic vasculitis
2. interstitial nephritis
3. necrotizing angiitis

Central Nervous System Reactions
1. tinnitus and hearing loss
2. paresthesias
3. vertigo
4. dizziness
5. headache
6. blurred vision
7. xanthopsia

Hematologic Reactions
1. aplastic anemia (rare)
2. thrombocytopenia
3. agranulocytosis (rare)
4. hemolytic anemia
5. leukopenia
6. anemia

Dermatologic-Hypersensitivity Reactions
1. exfoliative dermatitis
2. erythema multiforme
3. purpura
4. photosensitivity
5. urticaria
6. rash
7. pruritus

Cardiovascular Reaction

Orthostatic hypotension may occur and may be aggravated by alcohol, barbiturates, or narcotics.

Other Reactions
1. hyperglycemia
2. glycosuria
3. hyperuricemia
4. muscle spasm
5. weakness
6. restlessness
7. urinary bladder spasm
8. thrombophlebitis
9. fever

Whenever adverse reactions are moderate or severe, furosemide dosage should be reduced or therapy withdrawn.

OVERDOSAGE

The principal signs and symptoms of overdosage with furosemide are dehydration, blood volume reduction, hypotension, electrolyte imbalance, hypokalemia and hypochloremic alkalosis, and are extensions of its diuretic action.

The acute toxicity of furosemide has been determined in mice, rats, and dogs. In all three, the oral LD_{50} exceeded 1000 mg/kg body weight while the intravenous LD_{50} ranged from 300 to 680 mg/kg. The acute intragastric toxicity in neonatal rats is 7 to 10 times that of adult rats.

The concentration of furosemide in biological fluid associated with toxicity or death is not known.

Treatment of overdosage is supportive and consists of replacement of excessive fluid and electrolyte losses. Serum electrolytes, carbon dioxide level and blood pressure should be determined frequently. Adequate drainage must be assured in patients with urinary bladder outlet obstruction (such as prostatic hypertrophy).

Hemodialysis does not accelerate furosemide elimination.

DOSAGE AND ADMINISTRATION

Edema: Therapy should be individualized according to patient response to gain maximal therapeutic response and to determine the minimal dose needed to maintain that response.

Adults: The usual initial dose of furosemide is 20 to 80 mg given as a single dose. Ordinarily a prompt diuresis ensues. If needed, the same dose can be administered 6 to 8 hours later or the dose may be increased. The dose may be raised by 20 to 40 mg and given not sooner than 6 to 8 hours after the previous dose until the desired diuretic effect has been obtained. This individually determined single dose should then be given once or twice daily (e.g., at 8 am and 2 pm). The dose of furosemide may be carefully titrated up to 600 mg/day in patients with clinically severe edematous states. Edema may be most efficiently and safely mobilized by giving furosemide on 2 to 4 consecutive days each week.

When doses exceeding 80 mg/day are given for prolonged periods, careful clinical observation and laboratory monitoring are particularly advisable. (See PRECAUTIONS: Laboratory Tests.)

Infants and Children: The usual initial dose of oral furosemide in infants and children is 2 mg/kg body weight, given as a single dose. If the diuretic response is not satisfactory after the initial dose, dosage may be increased by 1 or 2 mg/kg no sooner than 6 to 8 hours after the previous dose. Doses greater than 6 mg/kg body weight are not recommended. For maintenance therapy in infants and children, the dose should be adjusted to the minimum effective level. For ease of administration, and to allow maximum flexibility in dosing, the use of Furosemide Oral Solution is suggested.

Hypertension: Therapy should be individualized according to the patient's response to gain maximal therapeutic response and to determine the minimal dose needed to maintain that therapeutic response.

Adults: The usual initial dose of furosemide for hypertension is 80 mg, usually divided into 40 mg twice a day. Dosage should then be adjusted according to response. If response is not satisfactory, add other antihypertensive agents.

Changes in blood pressure must be carefully monitored when furosemide is used with other antihypertensive drugs, especially during initial therapy. To prevent excessive drop in blood pressure, the dosage of other agents should be reduced by at least 50 percent when furosemide is added to the regimen. As the blood pressure falls under the potentiating effect of furosemide, a further reduction in dosage or even discontinuation of other antihypertensive drugs may be necessary.

HOW SUPPLIED

The 20 mg tablets are white, round, unscored, flat-beveledged tablets marked with M2. They are available as follows:

NDC 0378-0208-01 bottles of 100 tablets
NDC 0378-0208-10 bottles of 1000 tablets

The 40 mg tablets are white, round, scored, flat-bevel-edged tablets marked with MYLAN over 216 on one side and 40 on the other side. They are available as follows:

NDC 0378-0216-01 bottles of 100 tablets
NDC 0378-0216-10 bottles of 1000 tablets

The 80 mg tablets are white, round, scored, flat-bevel-edged tablets marked with MYLAN over 232 on one side and 80 on the other side. They are available as follows:

NDC 0378-0232-01 bottles of 100 tablets
NDC 0378-0232-05 bottles of 500 tablets

STORE AT CONTROLLED ROOM TEMPERATURE 15°–30°C (59°–86°F).

PROTECT FROM LIGHT.

Dispense in a tight, light-resistant container using a child-resistant closure. Exposure to light may cause slight discoloration. Discolored tablets should not be dispensed.

MYLAN®

Mylan Pharmaceuticals Inc.
Morgantown, WV 26505

REVISED MARCH 1998
FUR:R24

INDAPAMIDE TABLETS, USP ℞

1.25 mg and 2.5 mg

DESCRIPTION

Indapamide is an oral antihypertensive/diuretic. Its molecule contains both a polar sulfamoyl chlorobenzamide moiety and a lipid-soluble methylindoline moiety. It differs chemically from the thiazides in that it does not possess the thiazide ring system and contains only one sulfonamide group. The chemical name of indapamide is 1-(4-chloro-3-sulfamoylbenzamido)-2-methylindoline, and its molecular weight is 365.83. The compound is a weak acid, pK_a=8.8, and is soluble in aqueous solutions of strong bases. It is a white to yellow-white crystalline (tetragonal) powder.

H_3C Cl CO—NH—N SO_2NH_2

$C_{16}H_{16}ClN_3O_3S$

Each tablet, for oral administration, contains 1.25 mg or 2.5 mg of indapamide and the following inactive ingredients: anhydrous lactose, colloidal silicon dioxide, hydroxypropyl methylcellulose, magnesium stearate, microcrystalline cellulose, polydextrose, polyethylene glycol, pregelatinized starch, sodium lauryl sulfate, and titanium dioxide. Additionally, the 1.25 mg product contains glyceryl triacetate and D&C Red No. 30 Aluminum Lake and the 2.5 mg product contains triacetin.

CLINICAL PHARMACOLOGY

Indapamide is the first of a new class of antihypertensive/diuretics, the indolines. It has been reported that the oral administration of 5 mg (two 2.5 mg tablets) of indapamide to healthy male subjects produced peak concentrations of approximately 260 ng/mL of the drug in the blood within two hours. A minimum of 70% of a single oral dose is eliminated by the kidneys and an additional 23% by the gastrointestinal tract, probably including the biliary route. The half-life of indapamide in whole blood is approximately 14 hours.

Indapamide is preferentially and reversibly taken up by the erythrocytes in the peripheral blood. The whole blood/plasma ratio is approximately 6:1 at the time of peak concentration and decreases to 3.5:1 at eight hours. From 71 to 79% of the indapamide in plasma is reversibly bound to plasma proteins.

Indapamide is an extensively metabolized drug, with only about 7% of the total dose administered, recovered in the urine as unchanged drug during the first 48 hours after administration. The urinary elimination of ^{14}C-labeled indapamide and metabolites is biphasic with a terminal half-life of excretion of total radioactivity of 26 hours.

In a parallel design double-blind, placebo controlled trial in hypertension, daily doses of indapamide between 1.25 mg and 10 mg produced dose-related antihypertensive effects. Doses of 5 and 10 mg were not distinguishable from each other although each was differentiated from placebo and 1.25 mg indapamide. At daily doses of 1.25 mg, 5 mg and 10 mg, a mean decrease of serum potassium of 0.28, 0.61 and 0.76 mEq/L, respectively, was observed and uric acid increased by about 0.69 mg/100 mL.

In other parallel design, dose-ranging clinical trials in hypertension and edema, daily doses of indapamide between 0.5 and 5 mg produced dose-related effects. Generally, doses of 2.5 and 5 mg were not distinguishable from each other although each was differentiated from placebo and from 0.5 or 1 mg indapamide. At daily doses of 2.5 and 5 mg a mean decrease of serum potassium of 0.5 and 0.6 mEq/Liter, respectively, was observed and uric acid increase by about 1 mg/100 mL.

At these doses, the effects of indapamide on blood pressure and edema are approximately equal to those obtained with conventional doses of other antihypertensive/diuretics.

In hypertensive patients, daily doses of 1.25, 2.5 and 5 mg of indapamide have no appreciable cardiac inotropic or chronotropic effect. The drug decreases peripheral resistance, with little or no effect on cardiac output, rate or rhythm. Chronic administration of indapamide to hypertensive patients has little or no effect on glomerular filtration rate or renal plasma flow.

Indapamide had an antihypertensive effect in patients with varying degrees of renal impairment, although in general, diuretic effects declined as renal function decreased.

In a small number of controlled studies, indapamide taken with other antihypertensive drugs such as hydralazine, propranolol, guanethidine, and methyldopa, appeared to have the additive effect typical of thiazide-type diuretics.

INDICATIONS AND USAGE

Indapamide tablets are indicated for the treatment of hypertension, alone or in combination with other antihypertensive drugs.

Indapamide tablets are also indicated for the treatment of salt and fluid retention associated with congestive heart failure.

Usage in Pregnancy: The routine use of diuretics in an otherwise healthy woman is inappropriate and exposes mother and fetus to unnecessary hazard (see PRECAUTIONS below).

Diuretics do not prevent development of toxemia of pregnancy, and there is no satisfactory evidence that they are useful in the treatment of developed toxemia.

Edema during pregnancy may arise from pathological causes or from the physiologic and mechanical consequences of pregnancy. Indapamide is indicated in pregnancy

TABLE 1: Adverse Reactions from Studies of 1.25 mg

Incidence ≥ 5%	Incidence < 5%*
BODY AS A WHOLE	
Headache	Asthenia
Infection	Flu Syndrome
Pain	Abdominal Pain
Back Pain	Chest Pain
GASTROINTESTINAL SYSTEM	
	Constipation
	Diarrhea
	Dyspepsia
	Nausea
METABOLIC SYSTEM	
	Peripheral Edema
CENTRAL NERVOUS SYSTEM	
Dizziness	Nervousness
	Hypertonia
RESPIRATORY SYSTEM	
Rhinitis	Cough
	Pharyngitis
	Sinusitis
SPECIAL SENSES	
	Conjunctivitis

*OTHER
All other clinical adverse reactions occurred at an incidence of < 1%.

when edema is due to pathologic causes, just as it is in the absence of pregnancy (however, see PRECAUTIONS below). Dependent edema in pregnancy, resulting from restriction of venous return by the expanded uterus, is properly treated through elevation of the lower extremities and use of support hose; use of diuretics to lower intravascular volume in this case is illogical and unnecessary. There is hypervolemia during normal pregnancy which is not harmful to either the fetus or the mother (in the absence of cardiovascular disease), but which is associated with edema, including generalized edema in the majority of pregnant women. If this edema produces discomfort, increased recumbency will often provide relief. In rare instances, this edema may cause extreme discomfort which is not relieved by rest. In these cases, a short course of diuretics may provide relief and may be appropriate.

CONTRAINDICATIONS

Anuria. Known hypersensitivity to indapamide or to other sulfonamide-derived drugs.

WARNINGS

Infrequent cases of severe hyponatremia, accompanied by hypokalemia, have been reported with 2.5 mg and 5 mg indapamide primarily in elderly females. Symptoms were reversed by electrolyte replenishment. Hyponatremia considered possibly clinically significant (< 125 mEq/L) has not been observed in clinical trials with the 1.25 mg dosage (see PRECAUTIONS).
Hypokalemia occurs commonly with diuretics (see ADVERSE REACTIONS, Hypokalemia), and electrolyte monitoring is essential, particularly in patients who would be at increased risk from hypokalemia, such as those with cardiac arrhythmias or who are receiving concomitant cardiac glycosides.
In general, diuretics should not be given concomitantly with lithium because they reduce its renal clearance and add a high risk of lithium toxicity. Read prescribing information for lithium preparations before use of such concomitant therapy.

PRECAUTIONS

General:

1. Hypokalemia, Hyponatremia, and Other Fluid and Electrolyte Imbalances: Periodic determinations of serum electrolytes should be performed at appropriate intervals. In addition, patients should be observed for clinical signs of fluid or electrolyte imbalance, such as hyponatremia, hypochloremic alkalosis, or hypokalemia. Warning signs include dry mouth, thirst, weakness, fatigue, lethargy, drowsiness, restlessness, muscle pains or cramps, hypotension, oliguria, tachycardia, and gastrointestinal disturbance. Electrolyte determinations are particularly important in patients who are vomiting excessively or receiving parenteral fluids, in patients subject to electrolyte imbalance (including those with heart failure, kidney disease, and cirrhosis), and in patients on a salt-restricted diet.
The risk of hypokalemia secondary to diuresis and natriuresis is increased when larger doses are used, when the diuresis is brisk, when severe cirrhosis is present and during concomitant use of corticosteroids or ACTH. Interference with adequate oral intake of electrolytes will also contribute to hypokalemia. Hypokalemia can sensitize or exaggerate the response of the heart to the toxic effects of digitalis, such as increase ventricular irritability.
Dilutional hyponatremia may occur in edematous patients; the appropriate treatment is restriction of water rather than administration of salt, except in rare instances when the hyponatremia is life threatening. However, in actual salt depletion, appropriate replacement is the treatment of choice. Any chloride deficit that may occur during treatment is generally mild and usually does not require specific treatment except in extraordinary circumstances as in liver or renal disease. Thiazide-like diuretics have been shown to increase the urinary excretion of magnesium; this may result in hypomagnesemia.

2. Hyperuricemia and Gout: Serum concentrations of uric acid increased by an average of 0.69 mg/100 mL in patients treated with indapamide 1.25 mg, and by an average of 1 mg/100 mL in patients treated with indapamide 2.5 mg and 5 mg, and frank gout may be precipitated in certain patients receiving indapamide (see ADVERSE REACTIONS below). Serum concentrations of uric acid should, therefore, be monitored periodically during treatment.

3. Renal Impairment: Indapamide, like the thiazides, should be used with caution in patients with severe renal disease, as reduced plasma volume may exacerbate or precipitate azotemia. If progressive renal impairment is observed in a patient receiving indapamide, withholding or discontinuing diuretic therapy should be considered. Renal function tests should be performed periodically during treatment with indapamide.

4. Impaired Hepatic Function: Indapamide, like the thiazides, should be used with caution in patients with impaired hepatic function or progressive liver disease, since minor alterations of fluid and electrolyte balance may precipitate hepatic coma.

5. Glucose Tolerance: Latent diabetes may become manifest and insulin requirements in diabetic patients may be altered during thiazide administration. A mean increase in glucose of 6.47 mg/dL was observed in patients treated with indapamide 1.25 mg, which was not considered clinically significant in these trials. Serum concentrations of glucose should be monitored routinely during treatment with indapamide.

TABLE 2: Adverse Reactions from Studies of 2.5 mg and 5 mg

	Incidence ≥ 5%	Incidence < 5%
CENTRAL NERVOUS SYSTEM/NEUROMUSCULAR	Headache Dizziness Fatigue, weakness, loss of energy, lethargy, tiredness, or malaise Muscle cramps or spasm, numbness of the extremities Nervousness, tension, anxiety, irritability, or agitation	Lightheadedness Drowsiness Vertigo Insomnia Depression Blurred vision
GASTROINTESTINAL SYSTEM		Constipation Nausea Vomiting Diarrhea Gastric irritation Abdominal pain or cramps Anorexia
CARDIOVASCULAR SYSTEM		Orthostatic hypotension Premature ventricular contractions Irregular heart beat Palpitations
GENITOURINARY SYSTEM		Frequency of urination Nocturia Polyuria
DERMATOLOGIC/HYPERSENSITIVITY		Rash Hives Pruritus Vasculitis
OTHER		Impotence or reduced libido Rhinorrhea Flushing Hyperuricemia Hyperglycemia Hyponatremia Hypochloremia Increase in serum urea nitrogen (BUN) or creatinine Glycosuria Weight loss Dry mouth Tingling of extremities

MEAN CHANGES FROM BASELINE AFTER 8 WEEKS OF TREATMENT
1.25 mg

	Serum Electrolytes (mEq/L)			Serum Uric Acid (mg/dL)	BUN (mg/dL)
	Potassium	Sodium	Chloride		
Indapamide 1.25 mg (n=255–257)	−0.28	−0.63	−2.60	0.69	1.46
Placebo (n=263–266)	0.00	−0.11	−0.21	0.06	0.06

MEAN CHANGES FROM BASELINE AFTER 40 WEEKS OF TREATMENT
2.5 mg and 5 mg

	Serum Electrolytes (mEq/L)			Serum Uric Acid (mg/dL)	BUN (mg/dL)
	Potassium	Sodium	Chloride		
Indapamide 2.5 mg (n=76)	−0.4	−0.6	−3.6	0.7	−0.1
Indapamide 5 mg (n=81)	−0.6	−0.7	−5.1	1.1	1.4

6. Calcium Excretion: Calcium excretion is decreased by diuretics pharmacologically related to indapamide. After six to eight weeks of indapamide 1.25 mg treatment and in long-term studies of hypertensive patients, with higher doses of indapamide, however, serum concentrations of calcium increased only slightly with indapamide. Prolonged treatment with drugs pharmacologically related to indapamide may in rare instances be associated with hypercalcemia and hypophosphatemia secondary to physiologic changes in the parathyroid gland; however, the common complications of hyperparathyroidism, such as renal lithiasis, bone resorption, and peptic ulcer, have not been seen. Treatment should be discontinued before tests for parathyroid function are performed. Like the thiazides, indapamide may decrease serum PBI levels without signs of thyroid disturbance.

7. Interaction with Systemic Lupus Erythematosus: Thiazides have exacerbated or activated systemic lupus erythematosus and this possibility should be considered with indapamide as well.

Drug Interactions:

1. Other Antihypertensives: Indapamide may add to or potentiate the action of other antihypertensive drugs. In limited controlled trials that compared the effect of indapamide combined with other antihypertensive drugs with the effect of the other drugs administered alone, there was no notable change in the nature or frequency of adverse reactions associated with the combined therapy.

2. Lithium: See WARNINGS.

3. Post-Sympathectomy Patient: The antihypertensive effect of the drug may be enhanced in the postsympathectomized patient.

4. Norepinephrine: Indapamide, like the thiazides, may decrease arterial responsiveness to norepinephrine, but this diminution is not sufficient to preclude effectiveness of the pressor agent for the therapeutic use.

Carcinogenesis, Mutagenesis, Impairment of Fertility: Both mouse and rat lifetime carcinogenicity studies were conducted. There was no significant difference in the incidence of tumors between the indapamide-treated animals and the control groups.

Pregnancy: ***Teratogenic Effects:*** Pregnancy Category B. Reproduction studies have been performed in rats, mice and rabbits at doses up to 6,250 times the therapeutic human dose and have revealed no evidence of impaired fertility or harm to the fetus due to indapamide. Postnatal development in rats and mice was unaffected by pretreatment of parent animals during gestation. There are, however, no ad-

Continued on next page

Indapamide—Cont.

equate and well-controlled studies in pregnant women. Moreover, diuretics are known to cross the placental barrier and appear in cord blood. Because animal reproduction studies are not always predictive of human response, this drug should be used during pregnancy only if clearly needed. There may be hazards associated with this use such as fetal or neonatal jaundice, thrombocytopenia, and possibly other adverse reactions that have occurred in the adult.
Nursing Mothers: It is not known whether this drug is excreted in human milk. Because most drugs are excreted in human milk, if use of this drug is deemed essential, the patient should stop nursing.

ADVERSE REACTIONS

Most adverse effects have been mild and transient.
The clinical adverse reactions listed in Table 1 represent data from Phase II/III placebo-controlled studies (306 patients given indapamide 1.25 mg). The clinical adverse reactions listed in Table 2 represent data from Phase II placebo-controlled studies and long-term controlled clinical trials (426 patients given indapamide 2.5 mg or 5 mg). The reactions are arranged into two groups: 1) a cumulative incidence equal to or greater than 5%; 2) a cumulative incidence less than 5%. Reactions are counted regardless of relation to drug.
[See table 1 at bottom of page 2122]
Approximately 4% of patients given indapamide 1.25 mg compared to 5% of the patients given placebo discontinued treatment in the trials of up to eight weeks because of adverse reactions.
In controlled clinical trials of six to eight weeks in duration, 20% of patients receiving indapamide 1.25 mg, 61% of patients receiving indapamide 5 mg, and 80% of patients receiving indapamide 10 mg had at least one potassium value below 3.4 mEq/L. In the indapamide 1.25 mg group, about 40% of those patients who reported hypokalemia as a laboratory adverse event returned to normal serum potassium values without intervention. Hypokalemia with concomitant clinical signs or symptoms occurred in 2% of patients receiving indapamide 1.25 mg.
[See table 2 at top of previous page]
Because most of these data are from long-term studies (up to 40 weeks of treatment), it is probable that many of the adverse experiences reported are due to causes other than the drug. Approximately 10% of patients given indapamide discontinued treatment in long-term trials because of reactions either related or unrelated to the drug.
Hypokalemia with concomitant clinical signs or symptoms occurred in 3% of patients receiving indapamide 2.5 mg q.d. and 7% of patients receiving indapamide 5 mg q.d. In long-term controlled clinical trials comparing the hypokalemic effects of daily doses of indapamide and hydrochlorothiazide, however, 47% of patients receiving indapamide 2.5 mg, 72% of patients receiving indapamide 5 mg, and 44% of patients receiving hydrochlorothiazide 50 mg had at least one potassium value (out of a total of 11 taken during the study) below 3.5 mEq/L. In the indapamide 2.5 mg group, over 50% of those patients returned to normal serum potassium values without intervention.
In clinical trials of six to eight weeks, the mean changes in selected values were as shown in the tables below.
See table "MEAN CHANGES FROM BASELINE AFTER 8 WEEKS OF TREATMENT, 1.25 mg"
[See second & third table on previous page]
No patients receiving indapamide 1.25 mg experienced hyponatremia considered possibly clinically significant (< 125 mEq/L).
Indapamide had no adverse effects on lipids.
See table "MEAN CHANGES FROM BASELINE AFTER 40 WEEKS OF TREATMENT, 2.5 mg and 5 mg"
[See table at bottom of previous page]
Other adverse reactions reported with antihypertensive/diuretics are jaundice (intrahepatic cholestatic jaundice), sialadenitis, xanthopsia, photosensitivity, purpura, bullous eruptions, Stevens-Johnson Syndrome, necrotizing angiitis, fever, respiratory distress (including pneumonitis), and anaphylactic reactions; also, agranulocytosis, leukopenia, thrombocytopenia, and aplastic anemia. These reactions should be considered as possible occurrences with clinical usage of indapamide.

OVERDOSAGE

Symptoms of overdosage includes nausea, vomiting, weakness, gastrointestinal disorders and disturbances of electrolyte balance. In severe instances, hypotension and depressed respiration may be observed. If this occurs, support of respiration and cardiac circulation should be instituted. There is no specific antidote. An evacuation of the stomach is recommended by emesis and gastric lavage after which the electrolyte and fluid balance should be evaluated carefully.

DOSAGE AND ADMINISTRATION

Hypertension: The adult starting indapamide dose for hypertension is 1.25 mg as a single daily dose taken in the morning. If the response to 1.25 mg is not satisfactory after four weeks, the daily dose may be increased to 2.5 mg taken once daily. If the response to 2.5 mg is not satisfactory after four weeks, the daily dose may be increased to 5 mg taken once daily, but adding another antihypertensive should be considered.
Edema of Congestive Heart Failure: The adult starting indapamide dose for edema of congestive heart failure is 2.5 mg as a single daily dose taken in the morning. If the response to 2.5 mg is not satisfactory after one week, the daily dose may be increased to 5 mg taken once daily.
If the antihypertensive response to indapamide is insufficient, indapamide may be combined with other antihypertensive drugs, with careful monitoring of blood pressure. It is recommended that the usual dose of other agents be reduced by 50% during initial combination therapy. As the blood pressure response becomes evident, further dosage adjustments may be necessary.
In general, doses of 5 mg and larger have not appeared to provide additional effects on blood pressure or heart failure, but are associated with a greater degree of hypokalemia. There is minimal clinical trial experience in patients with doses greater than 5 mg once a day.

HOW SUPPLIED

Indapamide Tablets, USP are available containing 1.25 mg and 2.5 mg of indapamide.
The 1.25 mg tablets are film-coated pink, unscored, round tablets marked with **M** on one side and **69** on the reverse side. They are available as follows:
NDC 0378-0069-01 bottles of 100 tablets
NDC 0378-0069-05 bottles of 500 tablets
The 2.5 mg tablets are film-coated white, unscored, round tablets marked with **M** on one side and **80** on the reverse side. They are available as follows:
NDC 0378-0080-01 bottles of 100 tablets
NDC 0378-0080-10 bottles of 1000 tablets
STORE AT CONTROLLED ROOM TEMPERATURE 15°–30°C (59°–86°F).
AVOID EXCESSIVE HEAT.
Dispense in a tight container as defined in the USP using a child-resistant closure.
MYLAN®
Mylan Pharmaceuticals Inc.
Morgantown, WV 26505
REVISED JULY 1998
INDAP:R3

NADOLOL TABLETS, USP ℞
20 mg, 40 mg and 80 mg

DESCRIPTION

Nadolol is a synthetic nonselective beta-adrenergic receptor blocking agent designated chemically as 1-(*tert*-butylamino)-3-[(5,6,7,8-tetrahydro-*cis*-6,7-dihydroxy-1-naphthyl)oxy]-2-propanol. Its structural formula is:

OH, H, H, OH
$OCH_2CHCH_2NHC(CH_3)_3$
OH
$C_{17}H_{27}NO_4$
M.W. 309.41

Nadolol is a white crystalline powder. It is freely soluble in ethanol, soluble in hydrochloric acid, slightly soluble in water and in chloroform, and very slightly soluble in sodium hydroxide.
Each tablet for oral administration contains 20 mg, 40 mg or 80 mg of nadolol and the following inactive ingredients: croscarmellose sodium, lactose (anhydrous), magnesium stearate, microcrystalline cellulose, sodium lauryl sulfate, and D&C Yellow #10 Aluminum Lake.

CLINICAL PHARMACOLOGY

Nadolol is a nonselective beta-adrenergic receptor blocking agent. Clinical pharmacology studies have demonstrated beta-blocking activity by showing (1) reduction in heart rate and cardiac output at rest and on exercise, (2) reduction of systolic and diastolic blood pressure at rest and on exercise, (3) inhibition of isoproterenol-induced tachycardia, and (4) reduction of reflex orthostatic tachycardia.
Nadolol specifically competes with beta-adrenergic receptor agonists for available beta receptor sites; it inhibits both the $beta_1$ receptors located chiefly in cardiac muscle and the $beta_2$ receptors located chiefly in the bronchial and vascular musculature, inhibiting the chronotropic, inotropic, and vasodilator responses to beta-adrenergic stimulation proportionately. Nadolol has no intrinsic sympathomimetic activity and, unlike some other beta-adrenergic blocking agents, nadolol has little direct myocardial depressant activity and does not have an anesthetic-like membrane-stabilizing action. Animal and human studies show that nadolol slows the sinus rate and depresses AV conduction. In dogs, only minimal amounts of nadolol were detected in the brain relative to amounts in blood and other organs and tissues. Nadolol has low lipophilicity as determined by octanol/water partition coefficient, a characteristic of certain beta-blocking agents that has been correlated with the limited extent to which these agents cross the blood-brain barrier, their low concentration in the brain, and low incidence of CNS-related side effects.
In controlled clinical studies, nadolol at doses of 40 to 320 mg/day has been shown to decrease both standing and supine blood pressure, the effect persisting for approximately 24 hours after dosing.
The mechanism of the antihypertensive effects of beta-adrenergic receptor blocking agents has not been established; however, factors that may be involved include (1) competitive antagonism of catecholamines at peripheral (non-CNS) adrenergic neuron sites (especially cardiac) leading to decreased cardiac output, (2) a central effect leading to reduced tonic-sympathetic nerve outflow to the periphery, and (3) suppression of renin secretion by blockade of the beta-adrenergic receptors responsible for renin release from the kidneys.
While cardiac output and arterial pressure are reduced by nadolol therapy, renal hemodynamics are stable, with preservation of renal blood flow and glomerular filtration rate.
By blocking catecholamine-induced increases in heart rate, velocity and extent of myocardial contraction, and blood pressure, nadolol generally reduces the oxygen requirements of the heart at any given level of effort, making it useful for many patients in the long-term management of angina pectoris. On the other hand, nadolol can increase oxygen requirements by increasing left ventricular fiber length and end diastolic pressure, particularly in patients with heart failure.
Although beta-adrenergic receptor blockade is useful in treatment of angina and hypertension, there are also situations in which sympathetic stimulation is vital. For example, in patients with severely damaged hearts, adequate ventricular function may depend on sympathetic drive. Beta-adrenergic blockade may worsen AV block by preventing the necessary facilitating effects of sympathetic activity on conduction. $Beta_2$-adrenergic blockade results in passive bronchial constriction by interfering with endogenous adrenergic bronchodilator activity in patients subject to bronchospasm and may also interfere with exogenous bronchodilators in such patients.
Absorption of nadolol after oral dosing is variable, averaging about 30%. Peak serum concentrations of nadolol usually occur in 3 to 4 hours after oral administration and the presence of food in the gastrointestinal tract does not affect the rate or extent of nadolol absorption. Approximately 30% of the nadolol present in serum is reversibly bound to plasma protein.
Unlike many other beta-adrenergic blocking agents, nadolol is not metabolized by the liver and is excreted unchanged, principally by the kidneys.
The half-life of therapeutic doses of nadolol is about 20 to 24 hours, permitting once-daily dosage. Because nadolol is excreted predominantly in the urine, its half-life increases in renal failure (see PRECAUTIONS and DOSAGE AND ADMINISTRATION). Steady-state serum concentrations of nadolol are attained in 6 to 9 days with once-daily dosage in persons with normal renal function. Because of variable absorption and different individual responsiveness, the proper dosage must be determined by titration.
Exacerbation of angina and, in some cases, myocardial infarction and ventricular dysrhythmias have been reported after abrupt discontinuation of therapy with beta-adrenergic blocking agents in patients with coronary artery disease. Abrupt withdrawal of these agents in patients without coronary artery disease has resulted in transient symptoms, including tremulousness, sweating, palpitation, headache, and malaise. Several mechanisms have been proposed to explain these phenomena, among them increased sensitivity to catecholamines because of increased numbers of beta receptors.

INDICATIONS AND USAGE

Angina Pectoris—Nadolol Tablets are indicated for the long-term management of patients with angina pectoris.
Hypertension—Nadolol Tablets are indicated in the management of hypertension; it may be used alone or in combination with other antihypertensive agents, especially thiazide-type diuretics.

CONTRAINDICATIONS

Nadolol Tablets are contraindicated in bronchial asthma, sinus bradycardia and greater than first degree conduction block, cardiogenic shock, and overt cardiac failure (see WARNINGS).

WARNINGS

Cardiac Failure—Sympathetic stimulation may be a vital component supporting circulatory function in patients with congestive heart failure, and its inhibition by beta-blockade may precipitate more severe failure. Although beta-blockers should be avoided in overt congestive heart failure, if necessary, they can be used with caution in patients with a history of failure who are well compensated, usually with digitalis and diuretics. Beta-adrenergic blocking agents do not abolish the inotropic action of digitalis on heart muscle.
IN PATIENTS WITHOUT A HISTORY OF HEART FAILURE, continued use of beta-blockers can, in some cases, lead to cardiac failure. Therefore, at the first sign or symptom of heart failure, the patient should be digitalized and/or treated with diuretics, and the response observed closely, or nadolol should be discontinued (gradually, if possible).

Exacerbation of Ischemic Heart Disease Following Abrupt Withdrawal—Hypersensitivity to catecholamines has been observed in patients withdrawn from beta-blocker therapy; exacerbation of angina and, in some cases, myocardial infarction have occurred after *abrupt* discontinuation of such therapy. When discontinuing chronically administered nadolol, particularly in patients with ischemic heart disease, the dosage should be gradually reduced over a period of 1 to 2 weeks and the patient should be carefully monitored. If angina markedly worsens or acute coronary insufficiency develops, nadolol administration should be reinstituted promptly, at least temporarily, and other measures appropriate for the management of unstable angina should be taken. Patients should be warned against interruption or discontinuation of therapy without the physician's advice. Because coronary artery disease is common and may be unrecognized, it may be prudent not to discontinue nadolol therapy abruptly even in patients treated only for hypertension.

Nonallergic Bronchospasm (e.g., chronic bronchitis, emphysema)—PATIENTS WITH BRONCHOSPASTIC DISEASES SHOULD IN GENERAL NOT RECEIVE BETA-BLOCKERS. Nadolol should be administered with caution since it may block bronchodilation produced by endogenous or exogenous catecholamine stimulation of $beta_2$ receptors.
Major Surgery—Because beta-blockade impairs the ability of the heart to respond to reflex stimuli and may increase the risks of general anesthesia and surgical procedures, resulting in protracted hypotension or low cardiac output, it has generally been suggested that such therapy should be withdrawn several days prior to surgery. Recognition of the increased sensitivity to catecholamines of patients recently withdrawn from beta-blocker therapy, however, has made this recommendation controversial. If possible, beta-blockers should be withdrawn well before surgery takes place. In the event of emergency surgery, the anesthesiologist should be informed that the patient is on beta-blocker therapy. The effects of nadolol can be reversed by administration of beta-receptor agonists such as isoproterenol, dopamine, dobutamine, or norepinephrine. Difficulty in restarting and maintaining the heart beat has also been reported with beta-adrenergic receptor blocking agents.
Diabetes and Hypoglycemia—Beta-adrenergic blockade may prevent the appearance of premonitory signs and symptoms (e.g., tachycardia and blood pressure changes) of acute hypoglycemia. This is especially important with labile diabetics. Beta-blockade also reduces the release of insulin in response to hyperglycemia; therefore, it may be necessary to adjust the dose of antidiabetic drugs.
Thyrotoxicosis—Beta-adrenergic blockade may mask certain clinical signs (e.g., tachycardia) of hyperthyroidism. Patients suspected of developing thryotoxicosis should be managed carefully to avoid abrupt withdrawal of beta-adrenergic blockade which might precipitate a thyroid storm.

PRECAUTIONS

Impaired Renal Function—Nadolol should be used with caution in patients with impaired renal function. (See DOSAGE AND ADMINISTRATION.)
Information for Patients—Patients, especially those with evidence of coronary artery insufficiency, should be warned against interruption or discontinuation of nadolol therapy without the physician's advice. Although cardiac failure rarely occurs in properly selected patients, patients being treated with beta-adrenergic blocking agents should be advised to consult the physician at the first sign or symptom of impending failure. The patient should also be advised of a proper course in the event of an inadvertently missed dose.
Drug Interactions—When administered concurrently, the following drugs may interact with beta-adrenergic receptor blocking agents:
Anesthetics, general—exaggeration of the hypotension induced by general anesthetics (see WARNINGS, Major Surgery).
Antidiabetic drugs (oral agents and insulin)—hypoglycemia or hyperglycemia; adjust dosage of antidiabetic drug accordingly (see WARNINGS, Diabetes and Hypoglycemia).
Catecholamine-depleting drugs (e.g.,reserpine)—additive effect; monitor closely for evidence of hypotension and/or excessive bradycardia (e.g., vertigo, syncope, postural hypotension).
Response to Treatment for Anaphylactic Reaction—While taking beta-blockers, patients with a history of severe anaphylactic reaction to a variety of allergens may be more reactive to repeated challenge, either accidental, diagnostic, or therapeutic. Such patients may be unresponsive to the usual doses of epinephrine used to treat allergic reaction.
Carcinogenesis, Mutagenesis, Impairment of Fertility—In chronic oral toxicologic studies (1 to 2 years) in mice, rats, and dogs, nadolol did not produce any significant toxic effects. In 2-year oral carcinogenic studies in rats and mice, nadolol did not produce any neoplastic, preneoplastic, or nonneoplastic pathologic lesions. In fertility and general reproductive performance studies in rats, nadolol caused no adverse effects.
Pregnancy Category C—In animal reproduction studies with nadolol, evidence of embryo- and fetotoxicity was found in rabbits, but not in rats or hamsters, at doses 5 to 10 times greater (on a mg/kg basis) than the maximum indicated human dose. No teratogenic potential was observed in any of these species.
There are no adequate and well-controlled studies in pregnant women. Nadolol should be used during pregnancy only if the potential benefit justifies the potential risk to the fetus. Neonates whose mothers are receiving nadolol at parturition have exhibited bradycardia, hypoglycemia, and associated symptoms.
Nursing Mothers—Nadolol is excreted in human milk. Because of the potential for adverse effects in nursing infants, a decision should be made whether to discontinue nursing or to discontinue therapy taking into account the importance of nadolol to the mother.
Pediatric Use—Safety and effectiveness in children have not been established.

ADVERSE REACTIONS

Most adverse effects have been mild and transient and have rarely required withdrawal of therapy.
Cardiovascular—Bradycardia with heart rates of less than 60 beats per minute occurs commonly, and heart rates below 40 beats per minute and/or symptomatic bradycardia were seen in about 2 of 100 patients. Symptoms of peripheral vascular insufficiency, usually of the Raynaud type, have occurred in approximately 2 of 100 patients. Cardiac failure, hypotension, and rhythm/conduction disturbances have each occurred in about 1 of 100 patients. Single instances of first degree and third degree heart block have been reported; intensification of AV block is a known effect of beta-blockers (see also CONTRAINDICATIONS, WARNINGS, and PRECAUTIONS).
Central Nervous System—Dizziness or fatigue has been reported in approximately 2 of 100 patients; paresthesias, sedation, and change in behavior have each been reported in approximately 6 of 1000 patients.
Respiratory—Bronchospasm has been reported in approximately 1 of 1000 patients (see CONTRAINDICATIONS and WARNINGS).
Gastrointestinal—Nausea, diarrhea, abdominal discomfort, constipation, vomiting, indigestion, anorexia, bloating, and flatulence have been reported in 1 to 5 of 1000 patients.
Miscellaneous—Each of the following has been reported in 1 to 5 of 1000 patients: rash; pruritus; headache; dry mouth, eyes, or skin; impotence or decreased libido; facial swelling; weight gain; slurred speech; cough; nasal stuffiness; sweating; tinnitus; blurred vision. Reversible alopecia has been reported infrequently.
The following adverse reactions have been reported in patients taking nadolol and/or other beta-adrenergic blocking agents, but no causal relationship to nadolol has been established.
Central Nervous System—Reversible mental depression progressing to catatonia; visual disturbances; hallucinations; an acute reversible syndrome characterized by disorientation for time and place, short-term memory loss, emotional lability with slightly clouded sensorium, and decreased performance on neuropsychometrics.
Gastrointestinal—Mesenteric arterial thrombosis; ischemic colitis; elevated liver enzymes.
Hematologic—Agranulocytosis; thrombocytopenic or nonthrombocytopenic purpura.
Allergic—Fever combined with aching and sore throat; laryngospasm; respiratory distress.
Miscellaneous—Pemphigoid rash; hypertensive reaction in patients with pheochromocytoma; sleep disturbances; Peyronie's disease.
The oculomucocutaneous syndrome associated with the beta-blocker practolol has not been reported with nadolol.

OVERDOSAGE

Nadolol can be removed from the general circulation by hemodialysis.
In addition to gastric lavage, the following measures should be employed, as appropriate. In determining the duration of corrective therapy, note must be taken of the long duration of the effect of nadolol.
Excessive Bradycardia—Administer atropine (0.25 to 1.0 mg). If there is no response to vagal blockade, administer isoproterenol cautiously.
Cardiac Failure—Administer a digitalis glycoside and diuretic. It has been reported that glucagon may also be useful in this situation.
Hypotension—Administer vasopressors, e.g., epinephrine or norepinephrine. (There is evidence that epinephrine may be the drug of choice.)
Bronchospasm—Administer a $beta_2$-stimulating agent and/or a theophylline derivative.

DOSAGE AND ADMINISTRATION

DOSAGE MUST BE INDIVIDUALIZED. NADOLOL MAY BE ADMINISTERED WITHOUT REGARD TO MEALS.
Angina Pectoris—The usual initial dose is 40 mg nadolol once daily. Dosage may be gradually increased in 40 to 80 mg increments at 3- to 7-day intervals until optimum clinical response is obtained or there is pronounced slowing of the heart rate. The usual maintenance dose is 40 or 80 mg administered once daily. Doses up to 160 or 240 mg administered once daily may be needed.
The usefulness and safety in angina pectoris of dosages exceeding 240 mg per day have not been established. If treatment is to be discontinued, reduce the dosage gradually over a period of one to two weeks (see WARNINGS).
Hypertension—The usual initial dose is 40 mg nadolol once daily, whether it is used alone or in addition to diuretic therapy. Dosage may be gradually increased in 40 to 80 mg increments until optimum blood pressure reduction is achieved. The usual maintenance dose is 40 or 80 mg administered once daily. Doses up to 240 or 320 mg administered once daily may be needed.
Dosage Adjustment in Renal Failure—Absorbed nadolol is excreted principally by the kidneys and, although nonrenal elimination does occur, dosage adjustments are necessary in patients with renal impairment. The following dose intervals are recommended:

Creatinine Clearance ($mL/min/1.73^2$)	Dosage Interval (hours)
>50	24
31-50	24-36
10-30	24-48
<10	40-60

HOW SUPPLIED

Nadolol tablets are available containing 20 mg, 40 mg or 80 mg of nadolol, USP.
The 20 mg tablets are yellow, round, scored tablets marked with M28. They are available as follows:
NDC 0378-0028-01 bottles of 100 tablets
The 40 mg tablets are yellow, round, scored tablets marked with M171. They are available as follows:
NDC 0378-1171-01 bottles of 100 tablets
NDC 0378-1171-10 bottles of 1000 tablets
The 80 mg tablets are yellow, round, scored tablets marked with M132. They are available as follows:
NDC 0378-1132-01 bottles of 100 tablets
NDC 0378-1132-10 bottles of 1000 tablets
STORE AT CONTROLLED ROOM TEMPERATURE 15°–30°C (59°–86°F).
PROTECT FROM LIGHT.
Dispense in a tight, light-resistant container using a child-resistant closure.
MYLAN®
Mylan Pharmaceuticals Inc.
Morgantown, WV 26505

REVISED APRIL 1998
NAD:R6

THIORIDAZINE HYDROCHLORIDE TABLETS, USP
10 mg, 25 mg, 50 mg, and 100 mg ℞

DESCRIPTION

Thioridazine hydrochloride is 10H-Phenothiazine, 10-[2-(1-methyl-2-piperidinyl)ethyl]-2-(methylthio)-, monohydrochloride. The chemical structure is:

The presence of a thiomethyl radical ($S\text{-}CH_3$) in position 2, conventionally occupied by a halogen, is unique and could account for the greater toleration obtained with recommended doses of thioridazine as well as a greater specificity of psychotherapeutic action.
Thioridazine hydrochloride is available as tablets for oral administration containing 10 mg, 25 mg, 50 mg, or 100 mg. Each tablet for oral administration contains the following inactive ingredients: colloidal silicon dioxide, croscarmellose sodium, hydroxypropyl cellulose, hydroxypropyl methylcellulose, magnesium stearate, microcrystalline cellulose, polyethylene glylcol, sodium lauryl sulfate, titanium dioxide and FD&C Yellow #6 Aluminum Lake.

CLINICAL PHARMACOLOGY

Thioridazine hydrochloride is effective in reducing excitement, hypermotility, abnormal initiative, affective tension and agitation through its inhibitory effect on psychomotor functions. Successful modification of such symptoms is the prerequisite for, and often the beginning of the process of recovery in patients exhibiting mental and emotional disturbances.
Thioridazine's basic pharmacological activity is similar to that of other phenothiazines, but certain specific qualities have come to light which support the observation that the clinical spectrum of this drug shows significant differences from those of the other agents of this class. Minimal antiemetic activity and minimal extrapyramidal stimulation, notably pseudo-parkinsonism, are distinctive features of this drug.

INDICATIONS

For the management of manifestations of psychotic disorders.
For the short-term treatment of moderate to marked depression with variable degrees of anxiety in adult patients and for the treatment of multiple symptoms such as agitation, anxiety, depressed mood, tension, sleep disturbances, and fears in geriatric patients.
For the treatment of severe behavioral problems in children marked by combativeness and/or explosive hyperexcitable behavior (out of proportion to immediate provocations), and in the short-term treatment of hyperactive children who show excessive motor activity with accompanying conduct disorders consisting of some or all of the following symptoms: impulsivity, difficulty sustaining attention, aggressivity, mood lability, and poor frustration tolerance.

CONTRAINDICATIONS

In common with other phenothiazines, thioridazine hydrochloride is contraindicated in severe central nervous system depression or comatose states from any cause. It should also be noted that hypertensive or hypotensive heart disease of extreme degree is a contraindication of phenothiazine administration.

WARNINGS

Tardive Dyskinesia: Tardive dyskinesia, a syndrome consisting of potentially irreversible, involuntary, dyskinetic movements may develop in patients treated with neuroleptic (antipsychotic) drugs. Although the prevalence of the

Continued on next page

Thioridazine HCl—Cont.

syndrome appears to be highest among the elderly, especially elderly women, it is impossible to rely upon prevalence estimates to predict, at the inception of neuroleptic treatment, which patients are likely to develop the syndrome. Whether neuroleptic drug products differ in their potential to cause tardive dyskinesia is unknown.
Both the risk of developing the syndrome and the likelihood that it will become irreversible are believed to increase as the duration of treatment and the total cumulative dose of neuroleptic drugs administered to the patients increase. However, the syndrome can develop, although much less commonly, after relatively brief treatment periods at low doses.
There is no known treatment for established cases of tardive dyskinesia, although the syndrome may remit, partially or completely, if neuroleptic treatment is withdrawn. Neuroleptic treatment, itself, however, may suppress (or partially suppress) the signs and symptoms of the syndrome and thereby may possibly mask the underlying disease process. The effect that symptomatic suppression has upon the long-term course of the syndrome is unknown.
Given these considerations, neuroleptics should be prescribed in a manner that is most likely to minimize the occurrence of tardive dyskinesia. Chronic neuroleptic treatment should generally be reserved for patients who suffer from a chronic illness that, 1) is known to respond to neuroleptic drugs, and, 2) for whom alternative, equally effective, but potentially less harmful treatments are **not** available or appropriate. In patients who do require chronic treatment, the smallest dose and the shortest duration of treatment producing a satisfactory clinical response should be sought. The need for continued treatment should be reassessed periodically.
If signs and symptoms of tardive dyskinesia appear in a patient on neuroleptics, drug discontinuation should be considered. However, some patients may require treatment despite the presence of the syndrome.
(For further information about the description of tardive dyskinesia and its clinical detection, please refer to the sections on Information for Patients and ADVERSE REACTIONS).
Neuroleptic Malignant Syndrome (NMS): A potentially fatal symptom complex sometimes referred to as Neuroleptic Malignant Syndrome (NMS) has been reported in association with antipsychotic drugs. Clinical manifestations of NMS are hyperpyrexia, muscle rigidity, altered mental status and evidence of autonomic instability (irregular pulse or blood pressure, tachycardia, diaphoresis, and cardiac dysrhythmias).
The diagnostic evaluation of patients with this syndrome is complicated. In arriving at a diagnosis, it is important to identify cases where the clinical presentation includes both serious medical illness (e.g., pneumonia, systemic infection, etc.) and untreated or inadequately treated extrapyramidal signs and symptoms (EPS). Other important considerations in the differential diagnosis include central anticholinergic toxicity, heat stroke, drug fever and primary central nervous system (CNS) pathology.
The management of NMS should include 1) immediate discontinuation of antipsychotic drugs and other drugs not essential to concurrent therapy, 2) intensive symptomatic treatment and medical monitoring, and 3) treatment of any concomitant serious medical problems for which specific treatments are available. There is no general agreement about specific pharmacological treatment regimens for uncomplicated NMS.
If the patient requires anti-psychotic drug treatment after recovery from NMS, the potential reintroduction of drug therapy should be carefully considered. The patient should be carefully monitored, since recurrences of NMS have been reported.
General: It has been suggested in regard to phenothiazines in general, that people who have demonstrated a hypersensitivity reaction (e.g., blood dyscrasias, jaundice) to one may be more prone to demonstrate a reaction to others. Attention should be paid to the fact that phenothiazines are capable of potentiating central nervous system depressants (e.g., anesthetics, opiates, alcohol, etc.) as well as atropine and phosphorus insecticides. Physicians should carefully consider benefit versus risk when treating less severe disorders.
Reproductive studies in animals and clinical experience to date have failed to show a teratogenic effect with thioridazine. However, in view of the desirability of keeping the administration of all drugs to a minimum during pregnancy, thioridazine should be given only when the benefits derived from treatment exceed the possible risks to mother and fetus.

PRECAUTIONS

Leukopenia and/or agranulocytosis and convulsive seizures have been reported but are infrequent. Thioridazine has been shown to be helpful in the treatment of behavioral disorders in epileptic patients, but anticonvulsant medication should also be maintained. Pigmentary retinopathy, which has been observed primarily in patients taking larger than recommended doses, is characterized by diminution of visual acuity, brownish coloring of vision, and impairment of night vision; examination of the fundus discloses deposits of pigment. The possibility of this complication may be reduced by remaining within the recommended limits of dosage.
Where patients are participating in activities requiring complete mental alertness (e.g., driving) it is advisable to administer the phenothiazines cautiously and to increase the dosage gradually. Female patients appear to have a greater tendency to orthostatic hypotension than male patients. The administration of epinephrine should be avoided in the treatment of drug-induced hypotension in view of the fact that phenothiazines may induce a reversed epinephrine effect on occasion. Should a vasoconstrictor be required, the most suitable are norepinephrine and phenylephrine.
Neuroleptic drugs elevate prolactin levels; the elevation persists during chronic administration. Tissue culture experiments indicate that approximately one-third of human breast cancers are prolactin dependent *in vitro*, a factor of potential importance if the prescription of these drugs is contemplated in a patient with a previously detected breast cancer. Although disturbances such as galactorrhea, amenorrhea, gynecomastia, and impotence have been reported, the clinical significance of elevated serum prolactin levels is unknown for most patients. An increase in mammary neoplasms has been found in rodents after chronic administration of neuroleptic drugs. Neither clinical studies nor epidemiologic studies conducted to date, however, have shown an association between chronic administration of these drugs and mammary tumorigenesis; the available evidence is considered too limited to be conclusive at this time.
Concurrent administration of propranolol (100 mg and 800 mg daily) has been reported to produce increases in plasma levels of thioridazine (approximately 50 to 400 percent) and its metabolites (approximately 80 to 300 percent).
It is recommended that a daily dose in excess of 300 mg be reserved for use only in severe neuropsychiatric conditions.
Information for Patients: Given the likelihood that some patients exposed chronically to neuroleptics will develop tardive dyskinesia, it is advised that all patients in whom chronic use is contemplated be given, if possible, full information about this risk. The decision to inform patients and/or their guardians must obviously take into account the clinical circumstances and the competency of the patient to understand the information provided.

ADVERSE REACTIONS

In the recommended dosage ranges with thioridazine hydrochloride most side effects are mild and transient.
Central Nervous System: Drowsiness may be encountered on occasion, especially where large doses are given early in treatment. Generally, this effect tends to subside with continued therapy or a reduction in dosage. Pseudo-parkinsonism and other extrapyramidal symptoms may occur but are infrequent. Nocturnal confusion, hyperactivity, lethargy, psychotic reactions, restlessness and headache have been reported but are extremely rare.
Autonomic Nervous System: Dryness of mouth, blurred vision, constipation, nausea, vomiting, diarrhea, nasal stuffiness and pallor have been seen.
Endocrine System: Galactorrhea, breast engorgement, amenorrhea, inhibition of ejaculation and peripheral edema have been described.
Skin: Dermatitis and skin eruptions of the urticarial type have been observed infrequently. Photosensitivity is extremely rare.
Cardiovascular System: ECG changes have been reported (see Phenothiazine Derivatives: *Cardiovascular Effects*).
Other: Rare cases described as parotid swelling have been reported following administration of thioridazine.
Phenothiazine Derivatives: It should be noted that efficacy, indications and untoward effects have varied with the different phenothiazines. It has been reported that old age lowers the tolerance for phenothiazines. The most common neurological side effects in these patients are parkinsonism and akathisia. There appears to be an increased risk of agranulocytosis and leukopenia in the geriatric population. The physician should be aware that the following have occurred with one or more phenothiazines and should be considered whenever one of these drugs is used.
Autonomic Reactions: Miosis, obstipation, anorexia, paralytic ileus.
Cutaneous Reactions: Erythema, exfoliative dermatitis, contact dermatitis.
Blood Dyscrasias: Agranulocytosis, leukopenia, eosinophilia, thrombocytopenia, anemia, aplastic anemia, pancytopenia.
Allergic Reactions: Fever, laryngeal edema, angioneurotic edema, asthma.
Hepatotoxicity: Jaundice, biliary stasis.
Cardiovascular Effects: Changes in the terminal portion of the electrocardiogram, including prolongation of the Q-T interval, lowering and inversion of the T-wave and appearance of a wave tentatively identified as a bifid T or a U wave have been observed in some patients receiving the phenothiazine tranquilizers, including thioridazine hydrochloride. To date, these appear to be due to altered repolarization and not related to myocardial damage. They appear to be reversible. While there is no evidence at present that these changes are in any way precursors of any significant disturbance of cardiac rhythm, it should be noted that several sudden and unexpected deaths apparently due to cardiac arrest have occurred in patients previously showing characteristic electrocardiographic changes while taking the drug. The use of periodic electrocardiograms has been proposed but would appear to be of questionable value as a predictive device. Hypotension, rarely resulting in cardiac arrest.
Extrapyramidal Symptoms: Akathisia, agitation, motor restlessness, dystonic reactions, trismus, torticollis, opisthotonus, oculogyric crises, tremor, muscular rigidity, akinesia.
Tardive Dyskinesia: Chronic use of neuroleptics may be associated with the development of tardive dyskinesia. The salient features of this syndrome are described in the WARNINGS section and below.
The syndrome is characterized by involuntary choreoathetoid movements which variously involve the tongue, face, mouth, lips, or jaw (e.g. protrusion of the tongue, puffing of cheeks, puckering of the mouth, chewing movements), trunk and extremities. The severity of the syndrome and the degree of impairment produced vary widely.
The syndrome may become clinically recognizable either during treatment, upon dosage reduction, or upon withdrawal of treatment. Movements may decrease in intensity and may disappear altogether if further treatment with neuroleptics is withheld. It is generally believed that reversibility is more likely after short rather than long-term neuroleptic exposure. Consequently, early detection of tardive dyskinesia is important. To increase the likelihood of detecting the syndrome at the earliest possible time, the dosage of neuroleptic drug should be reduced periodically (if clinically possible) and the patient observed for signs of the disorder. This maneuver is critical, for neuroleptic drugs may mask the signs of the syndrome.
Endocrine Disturbances: Menstrual irregularities, altered libido, gynecomastia, lactation, weight gain, edema. False positive pregnancy tests have been reported.
Urinary Disturbances: Retention, incontinence.
Others: Hyperpyrexia. Behavioral effects suggestive of a paradoxical reaction have been reported. These include excitement, bizarre dreams, aggravation of psychoses and toxic confusional states. More recently, a peculiar skin-eye syndrome has been recognized as a side effect following long-term treatment with phenothiazines. This reaction is marked by progressive pigmentation of areas of the skin or conjunctiva and/or accompanied by discoloration of the exposed sclera and cornea. Opacities of the anterior lens and cornea described as irregular or stellate in shape have also been reported. Systemic lupus erythematosus-like syndrome.

DOSAGE

Dosage must be individualized according to the degree of mental and emotional disturbance. In all cases, the smallest effective dosage should be determined for each patient.
Adults: Psychotic manifestations: The usual starting dose is 50 to 100 mg three times a day, with a gradual increment to a maximum of 800 mg daily if necessary. Once effective control of symptoms has been achieved, the dosage may be reduced gradually to determine the minimum maintenance dose. The total daily dosage ranges from 200 to 800 mg divided into two to four doses.
For the short-term treatment of moderate to marked depression with variable degrees of anxiety in adult patients and for the treatment of multiple symptoms such as agitation, anxiety, depressed mood, tension, sleep disturbances, and fears in geriatric patients:
The usual starting dose is 25 mg three times a day. Dosage ranges from 10 mg two to four times a day in milder cases to 50 mg three or four times a day for more severely disturbed patients. The total daily dosage range is from 20 mg to a maximum of 200 mg.
Children: Thioridazine is not intended for children under 2 years of age. For children aged 2 to 12 the dosage of thioridazine hydrochloride ranges from 0.5 mg to a maximum of 3 mg/kg per day. For children with moderate disorders 10 mg two or three times a day is the usual starting dose. For hospitalized, severely disturbed, or psychotic children, 25 mg two or three times daily is the usual starting dose. Dosage may be increased gradually until optimum therapeutic effect is obtained or the maximum has been reached.

HOW SUPPLIED

Thioridazine Hydrochloride Tablets, USP are available containing 10 mg, 25 mg, 50 mg, or 100 mg of thioridazine hydrochloride.
The 10 mg tablets are orange, round, unscored film coated tablets marked with M54 on one side and 10 on the other side. They are available as follows:
NDC 0378-0612-01 bottles of 100 tablets
NDC 0378-0612-10 bottles of 1000 tablets
The 25 mg tablets are orange, round, unscored film coated tablets marked with M58 on one side and 25 on the other side. They are available as follows:
NDC 0378-0614-01 bottles of 100 tablets
NDC 0378-0614-10 bottles of 1000 tablets
The 50 mg tablets are orange, round, unscored film coated tablets marked with M59 on one side and 50 on the other side. They are available as follows:
NDC 0378-0616-01 bottles of 100 tablets
NDC 0378-0616-10 bottles of 1000 tablets
The 100 mg tablets are orange, round, unscored film coated tablets marked with M61 on one side and 100 on the other side. They are available as follows:
NDC 0378-0618-01 bottles of 100 tablets
NDC 0378-0618-10 bottles of 1000 tablets
STORE AT CONTROLLED ROOM TEMPERATURE 15°–30°C (59°–86°F).
PROTECT FROM LIGHT.
Dispense in a tight, light-resistant container using a child-resistant closure.

MYLAN®
Mylan Pharmaceuticals Inc.
Morgantown, WV 26505

REVISED MARCH 1998
THIO:R7AQ

THIOTHIXENE CAPSULES, USP ℞
1 mg, 2 mg, 5 mg and 10 mg

DESCRIPTION

Thiothixene is a thioxanthene derivative. Specifically, it is the *cis* isomer of N,N-dimethyl-9-[3-(4-methyl-1-piperazinyl)-propylidene] thioxanthene-2-sulfonamide. It may be represented by the following structural formula:

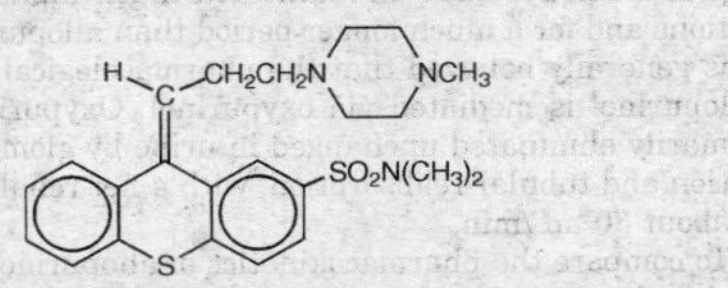

The thioxanthenes differ from the phenothiazines by the replacement of nitrogen in the central ring with a carbon-linked side chain fixed in space in a rigid structural configuration. An N,N-dimethyl sulfonamide functional group is bonded to the thioxanthene nucleus.

Each capsule contains 1 mg, 2 mg, 5 mg or 10 mg of thiothixene and the following inactive ingredients: colloidal silicon dioxide, croscarmellose sodium (Type A), gelatin, magnesium stearate, microcrystalline cellulose, powdered cellulose, pregelatinized starch, sodium lauryl sulfate, titanium dioxide and other inactive ingredients. The following coloring agents are employed:

1 mg - FD&C Blue #1, D&C Red #28, FD&C Red #40, FD&C Yellow #6

2 mg - FD&C Blue #1, FD&C Red #40, FD&C Yellow #6, D&C Yellow #10

5 mg - FD&C Blue #1, FD&C Red #40, FD&C Yellow #6

10 mg - FD&C Blue #1, FD&C Red #40, FD&C Yellow #6

CLINICAL PHARMACOLOGY

Thiothixene is a psychotropic agent of the thioxanthene series. Thiothixene possesses certain chemical and pharmacological similarities to the piperazine phenothiazines and differences from the aliphatic group of phenothiazines.

INDICATIONS AND USAGE

Thiothixene is effective in the management of manifestations of psychotic disorders. Thiothixene has not been evaluated in the management of behavioral complications in patients with mental retardation.

CONTRAINDICATIONS

Thiothixene is contraindicated in patients with circulatory collapse, comatose states, central nervous system depression due to any cause, and blood dyscrasias. Thiothixene is contraindicated in individuals who have shown hypersensitivity to the drug. It is not known whether there is a cross sensitivity between the thioxanthenes and the phenothiazine derivatives, but this possibility should be considered.

WARNINGS

Tardive Dyskinesia—Tardive dyskinesia, a syndrome consisting of potentially irreversible, involuntary, dyskinetic movements may develop in patients treated with neuroleptic (antipsychotic) drugs. Although the prevalence of the syndrome appears to be highest among the elderly, especially elderly women, it is impossible to rely upon prevalence estimates to predict, at the inception of neuroleptic treatment, which patients are likely to develop the syndrome. Whether neuroleptic drug products differ in their potential to cause tardive dyskinesia is unknown.

Both the risk of developing the syndrome and the likelihood that it will become irreversible are believed to increase as the duration and treatment and the total cumulative dose of neuroleptic drugs administered to the patient increase. However, the syndrome can develop, although much less commonly, after relatively brief treatment periods at low doses. There is no known treatment for established cases of tardive dyskinesia, although the syndrome may remit, partially or completely, if neuroleptic treatment is withdrawn. Neuroleptic treatment, itself, however, may suppress (or partially suppress) the signs and symptoms of the syndrome and thereby may possibly mask the underlying disease process. The effect that symptomatic suppression has upon the long-term course of the syndrome is unknown.

Given these considerations, neuroleptics should be prescribed in a manner that is most likely to minimize the occurrence of tardive dyskinesia. Chronic neuroleptic treatment should generally be reserved for patients who suffer from a chronic illness that, 1) is known to respond to neuroleptic drugs, and 2) for whom alternative, equally effective, but potentially less harmful treatments are *not* available or appropriate. In patients who do require chronic treatment, the smallest dose and the shortest duration of treatment producing a satisfactory clinical response should be sought. The need for continued treatment should be reassessed periodically.

If signs and symptoms of tardive dyskinesia appear in a patient on neuroleptics, drug discontinuation should be considered. However, some patients may require treatment despite the presence of the syndrome.

(For further information about the description of tardive dyskinesia and its clinical detection, please refer to Information for Patients in the PRECAUTIONS section and to the ADVERSE REACTIONS section.)

Neuroleptic Malignant Syndrome (NMS): A potentially fatal symptom complex sometimes referred to as Neuroleptic Malignant Syndrome (NMS) has been reported in association with antipsychotic drugs. Clinical manifestations of NMS are hyperpyrexia, muscle rigidity, altered mental status and evidence of autonomic instability (irregular pulse or blood pressure, tachycardia, diaphoresis, and cardiac dysrhythmias).

The diagnostic evaluation of patients with this syndrome is complicated. In arriving at a diagnosis, it is important to identify cases where the clinical presentation includes both serious medical illness (e.g., pneumonia, systemic infection, etc.) and untreated or inadequately treated extrapyramidal signs and symptoms (EPS). Other important considerations in the differential diagnosis include central anticholinergic toxicity, heat stroke, drug fever and primary central nervous system (CNS) pathology.

The management of NMS should include 1) immediate discontinuation of antipsychotic drugs and other drugs not essential to concurrent therapy, 2) intensive symptomatic treatment and medical monitoring, and 3) treatment of any concomitant serious medical problems for which specific treatments are available. There is no general agreement about specific pharmacological treatment regimens for uncomplicated NMS.

If a patient requires antipsychotic drug treatment after recovery from NMS, the potential reintroduction of drug therapy should be carefully considered. The patient should be carefully monitored, since recurrences of NMS have been reported.

Usage in Pregnancy—Safe use of thiothixene during pregnancy has not been established. Therefore, this drug should be given to pregnant patients only when, in the judgment of the physician, the expected benefits from the treatment exceed the possible risks to mother and fetus. Animal reproduction studies and clinical experience to date have not demonstrated any teratogenic effects. In the animal reproduction studies with thiothixene, there was some decrease in conception rate and litter size, and an increase in resorption rate in rats and rabbits. Similar findings have been reported with other psychotropic agents. After repeated oral administration of thiothixene to rats (5 to 15 mg/kg/day), rabbits (3 to 50 mg/kg/day), and monkeys (1 to 3 mg/kg/day) before and during gestation, no teratogenic effects were seen.

Usage in Children—The use of thiothixene in children under 12 years of age is not recommended because safe conditions for its use have not been established.

As is true with many CNS drugs, thiothixene may impair the mental and/or physical abilities required for the performance of potentially hazardous tasks such as driving a car or operating machinery, especially during the first few days of therapy. Therefore, the patient should be cautioned accordingly.

As in the case of other CNS-acting drugs, patients receiving thiothixene should be cautioned about the possible additive effects (which may include hypotension) with CNS depressants and with alcohol.

PRECAUTIONS

An antiemetic effect was observed in animal studies with thiothixene; since this effect may also occur in man, it is possible that thiothixene may mask signs of overdosage of toxic drugs and may obscure conditions such as intestinal obstruction and brain tumor.

In consideration of the known capability of thiothixene and certain other psychotropic drugs to precipitate convulsions, extreme caution should be used in patients with a history of convulsive disorders or those in a state of alcohol withdrawal, since it may lower the convulsive threshold. Although thiothixene potentiates the actions of the barbiturates, the dosage of the anticonvulsant therapy should not be reduced when thiothixene is administered concurrently.

Though exhibiting rather weak anticholinergic properties, thiothixene should be used with caution in patients who might be exposed to extreme heat or who are receiving atropine or related drugs.

Use with caution in patients with cardiovascular disease.

Caution as well as careful adjustment of the dosages is indicated when thiothixene is used in conjunction with other CNS depressants.

Also, careful observation should be made for pigmentary retinopathy, and lenticular pigmentation (fine lenticular pigmentation has been noted in a small number of patients treated with thiothixene for prolonged periods). Blood dyscrasias (agranulocytosis, pancytopenia, thrombocytopenic purpura), and liver damage (jaundice, biliary stasis), have been reported with related drugs.

Neuroleptic drugs elevate prolactin levels; the elevation persists during chronic administration. Tissue culture experiments indicate that approximately one-third of human breast cancers are prolactin dependent *in vitro*, a factor of potential importance if the prescription of these drugs is contemplated in a patient with a previously detected breast cancer. Although disturbances such as galactorrhea, amenorrhea, gynecomastia, and impotence have been reported, the clinical significance of elevated serum prolactin levels is unknown for most patients. An increase in mammary neoplasms has been found in rodents after chronic administration of neuroleptic drugs. Neither clinical studies nor epidemiologic studies conducted to date, however, have shown an association between chronic administration of these drugs and mammary tumorigenesis; the available evidence is considered too limited to be conclusive at this time.

Information for Patients: Given the likelihood that some patients exposed chronically to neuroleptics will develop tardive dyskinesia, it is advised that all patients in whom chronic use is contemplated be given, if possible, full information about this risk. The decision to inform patients and/or their guardians must obviously take into account the clinical circumstances and the competency of the patient to understand the information provided.

ADVERSE REACTIONS:

NOTE: Not all of the following adverse reactions have been reported with thiothixene. However, since thiothixene has certain chemical and pharmacologic similarities to the phenothiazines, all of the known side effects and toxicity associated with phenothiazine therapy should be borne in mind when thiothixene is used.

Cardiovascular Effects: Tachycardia, hypotension, lightheadedness, and syncope. In the event hypotension occurs, epinephrine should not be used as a pressor agent since a paradoxical further lowering of blood pressure may result. Nonspecific EKG changes have been observed in some patients receiving thiothixene. These changes are usually reversible and frequently disappear on continued thiothixene therapy. The incidence of these changes is lower than that observed with some phenothiazines. The clinical significance of these changes is not known.

CNS Effects: Drowsiness, usually mild, may occur although it usually subsides with continuation of thiothixene therapy. The incidence of sedation appears similar to that of the piperazine group of phenothiazines but less than that of certain aliphatic phenothiazines. Restlessness, agitation and insomnia have been noted with thiothixene. Seizures and paradoxical exacerbation of psychotic symptoms have occurred with thiothixene infrequently.

Hyperreflexia has been reported in infants delivered from mothers having received structurally related drugs.

In addition, phenothiazine derivatives have been associated with cerebral edema and cerebrospinal fluid abnormalities.

Extrapyramidal symptoms, such as pseudo-parkinsonism, akathisia and dystonia have been reported. Management of these extrapyramidal symptoms depends upon the type and severity. Rapid relief of acute symptoms may require the use of an injectable antiparkinson agent. More slowly emerging symptoms may be managed by reducing the dosage of thiothixene and/or administering an oral antiparkinson agent.

Persistent Tardive Dyskinesia: As with all antipsychotic agents tardive dyskinesia may appear in some patients on long term therapy or may occur after drug therapy has been discontinued. The syndrome is characterized by rhythmical involuntary movements of the tongue, face, mouth or jaw (i.e., protrusion of tongue, puffing of cheeks, puckering of mouth, chewing movements). Sometimes these may be accompanied by involuntary movements of extremities.

Since early detection of tardive dyskinesia is important, patients should be monitored on an ongoing basis. It has been reported that fine vermicular movements of the tongue may be an early sign of the syndrome. If this or any other presentation of the syndrome is observed, the clinician should consider possible discontinuation of neuroleptic medication. (See WARNINGS section.)

Hepatic Effects: Elevations of serum transaminase and alkaline phosphatase, usually transient, have been infrequently observed in some patients. No clinically confirmed cases of jaundice attributable to thiothixene have been reported.

Hematologic Effects: As is true with certain other psychotropic drugs, leukopenia and leucocytosis which are usually transient, can occur occasionally with thiothixene. Other antipsychotic drugs have been associated with agranulocytosis, eosinophilia, hemolytic anemia, thrombocytopenia and pancytopenia.

Allergic Reactions: Rash, pruritus, urticaria, photosensitivity and rare cases of anaphylaxis have been reported with thiothixene. Undue exposure to sunlight should be avoided. Although not experienced with thiothixene, exfoliative dermatitis and contact dermatitis (in nursing personnel), have been reported with certain phenothiazines.

Endocrine Disorders: Lactation, moderate breast enlargement and amenorrhea have occurred in a small percentage of females receiving thiothixene. If persistent, this may necessitate a reduction in dosage or the discontinuation of therapy. Phenothiazines have been associated with false positive pregnancy tests, gynecomastia, hypoglycemia, hyperglycemia and glycosuria.

Autonomic Effects: Dry mouth, blurred vision, nasal congestion, constipation, increased sweating, increased salivation and impotence have occurred infrequently with thiothixene therapy. Phenothiazines have been associated with miosis, mydriasis, and adynamic ileus.

Neuroleptic Malignant Syndrome (NMS): Please refer to the text regarding NMS in the WARNINGS section.

Other Adverse Reactions: Hyperpyrexia, anorexia, nausea, vomiting, diarrhea, increase in appetite and weight, weakness or fatigue, polydipsia, and peripheral edema.

Although not reported with thiothixene, evidence indicates there is a relationship between phenothiazine therapy and the occurrence of a systemic lupus erythematosus-like syndrome.

NOTE: Sudden deaths have occasionally been reported in patients who have received certain phenothiazine derivatives. In some cases the cause of death was apparently car-

Continued on next page

Thiothixene—Cont.

diac arrest or asphyxia due to failure of the cough reflex. In others, the cause could not be determined nor could it be established that death was due to phenothiazine administration.

OVERDOSAGE

Manifestations include muscular twitching, drowsiness and dizziness. Symptoms of gross overdosage may include CNS depression, rigidity, weakness, torticollis, tremor, salivation, dysphagia, hypotension, disturbances of gait, or coma.
Treatment: Essentially symptomatic and supportive. Early gastric lavage is helpful. Keep patient under careful observation and maintain an open airway, since involvement of the extrapyramidal system may produce dysphagia and respiratory difficulty in severe overdosage. If hypotension occurs, the standard measures for managing circulatory shock should be used (I.V. fluids and/or vasoconstrictors).
If a vasoconstrictor is needed, norepinephrine and phenylephrine are the most suitable drugs. Other pressor agents, including epinephrine, are not recommended, since phenothiazine derivatives may reverse the usual pressor action of these agents and cause further lowering of blood pressure. If CNS depression is marked, symptomatic treatment is indicated. Extrapyramidal symptoms may be treated with antiparkinson drugs.
There are no data on the use of peritoneal or hemodialysis, but they are known to be of little value in phenothiazine intoxication.

DOSAGE AND ADMINISTRATION

Dosage of thiothixene should be individually adjusted depending on the chronicity and severity of the condition. In general, small doses should be used initially and gradually increased to the optimal effective level, based on patient response.
Some patients have been successfully maintained on once-a-day thiothixene therapy.
The use of thiothixene in children under 12 years of age is not recommended because safe conditions for its use have not been established.
In milder conditions, an initial dose of 2 mg three times daily. If indicated, a subsequent increase to 15 mg/day total daily dose is often effective.
In more severe conditions, an initial dose of 5 mg twice daily.
The usual optimal dose is 20 to 30 mg daily. If indicated, an increase to 60 mg/day total daily dose is often effective. Exceeding a total daily dose of 60 mg rarely increases the beneficial response.

HOW SUPPLIED

Thiothixene Capsules, USP are available containing 1 mg, 2 mg, 5 mg or 10 mg of thiothixene.
The 1 mg product is a caramel and powder blue capsule marked in black ink with MYLAN 1001 on both body and cap. It is available as follows:
NDC 0378-1001-01 bottles of 100 capsules
The 2 mg product is a caramel and yellow capsule marked in black ink with MYLAN 2002 on both body and cap. It is available as follows:
NDC 0378-2002-01 bottles of 100 capsules
NDC 0378-2002-10 bottles of 1000 capsules
The 5 mg product is a caramel and white capsule marked in black ink with MYLAN 3005 on both body and cap. It is available as follows:
NDC 0378-3005-01 bottles of 100 capsules
NDC 0378-3005-10 bottles of 1000 capsules
The 10 mg product is a caramel and peach capsule marked in black ink with MYLAN 5010 on both body and cap. It is available as follows:
NDC 0378-5010-01 bottles of 100 capsules
NDC 0378-5010-10 bottles of 1000 capsules
STORE AT CONTROLLED ROOM TEMPERATURE 15°–30°C (59°–86°F).
PROTECT FROM LIGHT.
Dispense in a tight, light-resistant container using a child-resistant closure.
MYLAN®
Mylan Pharmaceuticals Inc.
Morgantown, WV 26505

REVISED JULY 1998
THTX:R14

For information on over-the-counter drugs, consult **PDR For Nonprescription Drugs**.

Nabi®

**5800 PARK OF COMMERCE BLVD., N.W.
BOCA RATON, FL 33487**

For Medical Information Contact:
Generally:
Immunotherapy Customer Service
(800) 458-4244
(305) 625-5303
(800) 4-WINRHO (494-6746)
(800) 327-7106 - AUTOPLEX
(800) 685-5579 - Medical
FAX: (305) 625-0925
In Emergencies:
Immunotherapy Customer Service
(800) 458-4244
(800) 4WINRHO (494-6746)
(800) 327-7106 AUTOPLEX
FAX: (305) 625-0925

ALOPRIM™ ℞

[al'-ō-prĭm]
(allopurinol sodium)
for Injection
For Intravenous Infusion Only

DESCRIPTION

ALOPRIM (allopurinol sodium) for Injection is the brand name for allopurinol, a xanthine oxidase inhibitor. ALOPRIM (allopurinol sodium) for Injection is a sterile solution for intravenous infusion only. It is available in vials as the sterile lyophilized sodium salt of allopurinol equivalent to 500 mg of allopurinol. ALOPRIM (allopurinol sodium) for Injection contains no preservatives.
The chemical name for allopurinol sodium is 1,5-dihydro-*4H*-pyrazolo[3,4-*d*]pyrimidin-4-one monosodium salt. It is a white amorphous mass with a molecular weight of 158.09 and molecular formula $C_5H_3N_4NaO$. The structural formula is:

The pKa of allopurinol sodium is 9.31.

CLINICAL PHARMACOLOGY

Allopurinol acts on purine catabolism without disrupting the biosynthesis of purines. It reduces the production of uric acid by inhibiting the biochemical reactions immediately preceding its formation. The degree of this decrease is dose dependent.
Allopurinol is a structural analogue of the natural purine base, hypoxanthine. It is an inhibitor of xanthine oxidase, the enzyme responsible for the conversion of hypoxanthine to xanthine and of xanthine to uric acid, the end product of purine metabolism in man. Allopurinol is metabolized to the corresponding xanthine analogue, oxypurinol (alloxanthine), which also is an inhibitor of xanthine oxidase.
Reutilization of both hypoxanthine and xanthine for nucleotide and nucleic acid synthesis is markedly enhanced when their oxidations are inhibited by allopurinol and oxypurinol. This reutilization does not disrupt normal nucleic acid anabolism, however, because feedback inhibition is an integral part of purine biosynthesis. As a result of xanthine oxidase inhibition, the serum concentration of hypoxanthine plus xanthine in patients receiving allopurinol for treatment of hyperuricemia is usually in the range of 0.3 to 0.4 mg/dL compared to a normal level of approximately 0.15 mg/dL. A maximum of 0.9 mg/dL of these oxypurines has been reported when the serum urate was lowered to less than 2 mg/dL by high doses of allopurinol. These values are far below the saturation levels, at which point their precipitation would be expected to occur (above 7 mg/dL).
The renal clearance of hypoxanthine and xanthine is at least 10 times greater than that of uric acid. The increased xanthine and hypoxanthine in the urine have not been accompanied by problems of nephrolithiasis. There are isolated case reports of xanthine crystalluria in patients who were treated with oral allopurinol.
The action of oral allopurinol differs from that of uricosuric agents, which lower the serum uric acid level by increasing urinary excretion of uric acid. Allopurinol reduces both the serum and urinary uric acid levels by inhibiting the formation of uric acid. The use of allopurinol to block the formation of urates avoids the hazard of increased renal excretion of uric acid posed by uricosuric drugs.

PHARMACOKINETICS

Following intravenous administration in six healthy male and female subjects, allopurinol was rapidly eliminated from the systemic circulation primarily via oxidative metabolism to oxypurinol, with no detectable plasma concentration of allopurinol after 5 hours post dosing. Approximately 12% of the allopurinol intravenous dose was excreted unchanged, 76% excreted as oxypurinol, and the remaining dose excreted as riboside conjugates in the urine. The rapid conversion of allopurinol to oxypurinol was not significantly different after repeated allopurinol dosing. Oxypurinol was present in systemic circulation in much higher concentrations and for a much longer period than allopurinol; thus, it is generally believed that the pharmacological action of allopurinol is mediated via oxypurinol. Oxypurinol was primarily eliminated unchanged in urine by glomerular filtration and tubular reabsorption, with a net renal clearance of about 30 mL/min.
To compare the pharmacokinetics of allopurinol and oxypurinol between intravenous (i.v.) and oral (p.o.) administration of ALOPRIM (allopurinol sodium) for Injection, a well-controlled, four-way crossover study was conducted in 16 male healthy volunteers. ALOPRIM (allopurinol sodium) for Injection was administered via an intravenous infusion over 30 minutes. Pharmacokinetic parameter estimates of allopurinol (mean ± S.D.) following single i.v. and p.o. administration of ALOPRIM (allopurinol sodium) for Injection are summarized as follows:
[See table below]
Oxypurinol was measurable in the plasma within 10 to 15 minutes following the administration of ALOPRIM (allopurinol sodium) for Injection. Pharmacokinetic parameter estimates of oxypurinol following i.v. and p.o. administration of ALOPRIM (allopurinol sodium) for Injection are shown below:
[See table at top of next page]
In general, the ratio of the area under the plasma concentration vs time curve ($AUC_{0-\infty}$) between oxypurinol and allopurinol was in the magnitude of 30 to 40. The C_{max} and $AUC_{0-\infty}$ for both allopurinol and oxypurinol following i.v. administration of ALOPRIM (allopurinol sodium) for Injection were dose proportional in the dose range of 100 to 300 mg. The half-life of allopurinol and oxypurinol was not influenced by the route of ALOPRIM (allopurinol sodium) for Injection administration. Oral and intravenous administration of ALOPRIM (allopurinol sodium) for Injection at equal doses produced nearly superimposable oxypurinol plasma concentration vs time profiles, and the relative bioavailability of oxypurinol ($F_{relative}$) was approximately 100%. Thus, the pharmacokinetics and plasma profiles of oxypurinol, the major pharmacological component derived from allopurinol, are similar after intravenous and oral administration of ALOPRIM (allopurinol sodium) for Injection.

Clinical Trials: A compassionate plea trial was conducted from 1977 through 1989 in which 718 evaluable patients with malignancies requiring treatment with cytotoxic chemotherapy, but who were unable to ingest or retain oral medication, received i.v. ALOPRIM (allopurinol sodium) for Injection in the U.S. Of these patients, 411 had established hyperuricemia and 307 had normal serum urate levels at the time that treatment was initiated. Normal serum uric acid levels were achieved in 68% (reduction of serum uric acid was documented in 93%) of the former, and were maintained throughout chemotherapy in 97% of the latter. Because of the study design, it was not possible to assess the impact of the treatment upon the clinical outcome of the patient groups.

INDICATIONS AND USAGE

ALOPRIM (allopurinol sodium) for Injection is indicated for the management of patients with leukemia, lymphoma, and solid tumor malignancies who are receiving cancer therapy which causes elevations of serum and urinary uric acid levels and who cannot tolerate oral therapy.

CONTRAINDICATIONS

Patients who have developed a severe reaction to allopurinol should not be restarted on the drug.

WARNINGS

ALLOPURINOL SHOULD BE DISCONTINUED AT THE FIRST APPEARANCE OF SKIN RASH OR OTHER SIGNS WHICH MAY INDICATE AN ALLERGIC REACTION. In

Administration of ALOPRIM™ (allopurinol sodium) for Injection

Allopurinol Parameters	100 mg i.v.	300 mg i.v.	100 mg p.o.*	300 mg p.o.
C_{max} (μg/mL)	1.58 ± 0.22	5.12 ± 0.82	0.53 ± 0.10	1.35 ± 0.49
T_{max} (hr)	0.50	0.50	1.00 ± 0.39	1.67 ± 0.96
T 1/2 (hr)	1.00 ± 0.46	1.21 ± 0.33	0.98 ± 0.43	1.32 ± 0.32
$AUC_{0-\infty}$ (hr•μg/mL)	1.99 ± 0.63	7.10 ± 1.28	1.03 ± 0.24	3.69 ± 0.96
CL (mL/min/kg)	12.2 ± 3.11	9.94 ± 2.36		
V_{SS} (L/kg)†	0.84 ± 0.13	0.87 ± 0.13		
$F_{absolute}$ (%)††			48.8 ± 19.7	52.7 ± 13.1

*n=7
†Volume of Distribution (Steady-State)
††Absolute Bioavailability

some instances with oral allopurinol, a skin rash may be followed by more severe hypersensitivity reactions such as exfoliative, urticarial, and purpuric lesions as well as Stevens-Johnson syndrome (erythema multiforme exudativum), and/or generalized vasculitis, irreversible hepatotoxicity and, on rare occasions, death.

In patients receiving mercaptopurine or azathioprine, the concomitant administration of 300 to 600 mg of ALOPRIM (allopurinol sodium) for Injection per day will require a reduction in dose to approximately one-third to one-fourth of the usual dose of mercaptopurine or azathioprine. Subsequent adjustment of doses of mercaptopurine or azathioprine should be made on the basis of therapeutic response and the appearance of toxic effects (see PRECAUTIONS: Drug Interactions).

A few cases of reversible clinical hepatotoxicity have been noted in patients taking oral allopurinol, and in some patients asymptomatic rises in serum alkaline phosphatase or serum transaminase have been observed. If anorexia, weight loss, or pruritus develop in patients on allopurinol, evaluation of liver function should be part of their diagnostic workup. In patients with pre-existing liver disease, periodic liver function tests are recommended during the early stages of therapy.

Due to the occasional occurrence of drowsiness, patients should be alerted to the need for due precaution when engaging in activites where alertness is mandatory.

The occurrence of hypersensitivity reactions to allopurinol may be increased in patients with decreased renal function receiving thiazides and allopurinol concurrently. Thus, in patients with decreased renal function, such combinations should be administered with caution.

PRECAUTIONS

General: A fluid intake sufficient to yield a daily urinary output of at least two liters in adults and the maintenance of a neutral or, preferably, slightly alkaline urine are desirable to (1) avoid the theoretical possibility of formation of xanthine calculi under the influence of allopurinol therapy and (2) help prevent renal precipitation of urates in patients receiving concomitant uricosuric agents.

A few patients with pre-existing renal disease or poor urate clearance have shown a rise in BUN during allopurinol administration, although a decrease in BUN has also been observed. In patients with hyperuricemia due to malignancy, the vast majority of changes in renal function are attributable to the underlying malignancy rather than to therapy with allopurinol. Concurrent conditions such as multiple myeloma and congestive myocardial disease were present among those patients whose renal function deteriorated after allopurinol was begun. Renal failure is rarely associated with hypersensitivity reactions to allopurinol.

Patients with decreased renal function do require lower doses of allopurinol. Patients should be carefully observed during the early stages of allopurinol administration so that the dosage can be appropriately adjusted for renal function.

In patients with severely impaired renal function or decreased urate clearance, the half-life of oxypurinol in the plasma is greatly prolonged. Patients should be treated with the lowest effective dose, in order to minimize possible side effects. The appropriate dose of ALOPRIM (allopurinol sodium) for Injection for patients with a creatinine clearance ≤10 mL/min is 100 mg per day. For patients with a creatinine clearance between 10 and 20 mL/min, a dose of 200 mg per day is recommended. With extreme renal impairment (creatinine clearance less than 3 mL/min), the interval between doses may also need to be extended.

Bone marrow suppression has been reported in patients receiving allopurinol; however, most of these patients were receiving concomitant medications with the known potential to cause such an effect. The suppression has occurred from as early as 6 weeks to as long as 6 years after the initiation of allopurinol therapy.

Laboratory Tests: The correct dosage and schedule for maintaining the serum uric acid within the normal range is best determined by using the serum uric acid as an index. In patients with pre-existing liver disease, periodic liver function tests are recommended during the early stages of therapy (see WARNINGS).

Allopurinol and its primary active metabolite, oxypurinol, are eliminated by the kidneys; therefore, changes in renal function have a profound effect on dosage. In patients with decreased renal function, or who have concurrent illnesses which can affect renal function such as hypertension and diabetes mellitus, periodic laboratory parameters of renal function, particularly BUN and serum creatinine or creatinine clearance, should be performed and the patient's allopurinol dosage reassessed.

The prothrombin time should be reassessed periodically in the patients receiving dicumarol who are given allopurinol.

Drug Interactions: The following drug interactions were observed in some patients undergoing treatment with oral allopurinol. Although the pattern of use for oral allopurinol includes longer term therapy, particularly for gout and renal calculi, the experience gained may be relevant.

Mercaptopurine/Azathioprine: Allopurinol inhibits the enzymatic oxidation of mercaptopurine and azathioprine to 6-thiouric acid. This oxidation, which is catalyzed by xanthine oxidase, inactivates mercaptopurine. Therefore, the concomitant administration of 300 to 600 mg of oral allopurinol per day will require a reduction in dose to approximately one-third to one-fourth of the usual dose of mercaptopurine or azathioprine. Subsequent adjustment of doses of mercaptopurine or azathioprine should be made on the basis of therapeutic response and the appearance of toxic effects.

Administration of ALOPRIM™ (allopurinol sodium) for Injection				
Oxypurinol Parameters	100 mg i.v.	300 mg i.v.	100 mg p.o.	300 mg p.o.
C_{max} (μg/mL)	2.20 ± 0.31	6.18 ± 0.78	2.36 ± 0.30	6.36 ± 0.83
T_{max} (hr)	3.89 ±1.41	4.16 ± 1.2	3.10 ± 1.49	4.13 ± 1.35
T 1/2 (hr)	24.1 ± 5.4	23.5 ± 4.5	24.9 ± 8.4	23.7 ± 3.4
$AUC_{0\to\infty}$ (hr•μg/mL)	80 ± 24	231 ± 54	83 ± 22	245 ± 49
$F_{relative}$ (%)*			107 ± 25	108 ± 9

*Relative Bioavailability

Drugs That are Physically Incompatible in Solution with ALOPRIM™ (alloprinol solution) for Injection	
Amikacin sulfate	Hydroxyzine HCl
Amphoterecin B	Idarubicin HCl
Carmustine	Imipenem-cilastatin sodium
Cefotaxime sodium	Mechlorethamine HCl
Chlorpromazine HCl	Meperidine HCl
Cimetidine HCl	Metoclopramide HCl
Clindamycin phosphate	Methylprednisolone sodium succinate
Cytarabine	Minocycline HCl
Dacarbazine	Nalbuphine HCl
Daunorubicin HCl	Netilmicin sulfate
Diphenhydramine HCl	Ondansetron HCl
Doxorubicin HCl	Prochlorperazine edisylate
Doxycycline hyclate	Promethiazine HCl
Droperidol	Sodium bicarbonate
Floxuridine	Streptozocin
Gentamicin sulfate	Tobramycin sulfate
Haloperidol lactate	Vinorelbine tartrate

Dicumarol: It has been reported that allopurinol prolongs the half-life of the anticoagulant, dicumarol. Consequently, prothrombin time should be reassessed periodically in patients receiving both drugs. The clinical basis of this drug interaction has not been established.

Uricosuric Agents: Since the excretion of oxypurinol is similar to that of urate, uricosuric agents, which increase the excretion of urate, are also likely to increase the excretion of oxypurinol. As a result, the concomitant administration of uricosuric agents decreases the inhibition of xanthine by oxypurinol and increases the urinary excretion of uric acid.

Thiazide Diuretics: Reports that the concomitant administration of allopurinol and thiazide diuretics contributed to increased allopurinol toxicity were reviewed; a causal mechanism or cause-and-effect relationship was not found. Renal function should be monitored in patients on thiazide diuretics and allopurinol (see WARNINGS).

Ampicillin/Amoxicillin: An increase in the frequency of skin rash has been reported among patients receiving ampicillin or amoxicillin concurrently with allopurinol compared to patients who are not receiving both drugs. The cause of this reaction has not been established.

Cytotoxic Agents: Enhanced bone marrow suppression by cyclophosphamide and other cytotoxic agents has been reported among patients with neoplastic disease, except leukemia, in the presence of allopurinol. However, in a well-controlled study of patients with lymphoma on combination therapy, allopurinol did not increase the marrow toxicity of patients treated with cyclophosphamide, doxorubicin, bleomycin, procarbazine, and/or mechlorethamine.

Chlorpropamide: The half-life of chlorpropamide in the plasma may be prolonged by allopurinol, since allopurinol and chlorpropamide may compete for excretion in the renal tubule. The risk of hypoglycemia secondary to this mechanism may be increased if allopurinol and chlorpropamide are given concomitantly in the presence of renal insufficiency.

Cyclosporin: Reports indicate that cyclosporine levels may be increased during concomitant treatment with ALOPRIM (allopurinol sodium) for Injection. Monitoring of cyclosporine levels and possible adjustment of cyclosporine dosage should be considered when these drugs are co-administered.

Drug/Laboratory Test Interactions: Allopurinol is not known to alter the accuracy of laboratory tests.

Carcinogenesis, Mutagenesis and Impairment of Fertility:

Carcinogenesis: Allopurinol was administered at doses up to 20 mg/kg/day to mice and rats for the majority of their life span. No evidence of carcinogenicity was seen in either mice or rats (at doses about 1/6 or 1/3 the recommended human dose on a mg/m^2 basis, respectively).

Mutagenesis: Allopurinol administered intravenously to rats (50 mg/kg) was not incorporated into rapidly replicating intestinal DNA. No evidence of clastogenicity was observed in an in vivo micronucleus test in rats, or in lymphocytes taken from patients treated with allopurinol (mean duration of treatment 40 months), or in an in vitro assay with human lymphocytes.

Impairment of Fertility: Allopurinol oral doses of 20 mg/kg/day had no effect on male or female fertility in rats or rabbits (about 1/3 or 1/2 the human dose on a mg/m^2 basis, respectively).

Pregnancy: ***Teratogenic Effects:*** Pregnancy Category C. There was no evidence of fetotoxicity or teratogenicity in rats or rabbits treated during the period of organogenesis with oral allopurinol at doses up to 200 mg/kg/day and up to 100 mg/kg/day, respectively (about three times the human dose on a mg/m^2 basis). However, there is a published report in pregnant mice that single intraperitoneal doses of 50 or 100 mg/kg (about 1/3 or 3/4 the human dose on a mg/m^2 basis) of allopurinol on gestation days 10 or 13 produced significant increases in fetal deaths and teratogenic effects (cleft palate, harelip, and digital defects). It is uncertain whether these findings represented a fetal effect or an effect secondary to maternal toxicity. There are, however, no adequate or well-controlled studies in pregnant women. Because animal reproduction studies are not always predictive of human response, this drug should be used during pregnant only if the potential benefit justifies the potential risk to the fetus.

Experience with allopurinol during human pregnancy has been limited partly because women of reproductive age rarely require treatment with allopurinol. Two unpublished reports and one published paper describe women giving birth to normal offspring after receiving oral allopurinol during pregnancy. There have been no pregnancies reported in patients receiving ALOPRIM (allopurinol sodium) for Injection, but it is assumed that the same risks would apply.

Nursing Mothers: Allopurinol and oxypurinol have been found in the milk of a mother who was receiving allopurinol. Since the effect of allopurinol on the nursing infant is unknown, caution should be exercised when allopurinol is administered to a nursing woman.

Pediatric Use: Clinical data are available on approximately 200 pediatric patients treated with ALOPRIM (allopurinol sodium) for Injection. The efficacy and safety profile observed in this patient population were similar to that observed in adults (see INDICATIONS and DOSAGE AND ADMINISTRATION).

Geriatric Use: Clinical studies of ALOPRIM (allopurinol sodium) for Injection did not include sufficient numbers of patients aged 65 and over to determine whether they respond differently than younger patients. Other reported clinical experience has not identified differences in responses between the elderly and younger patients. In general, dose selection for an elderly patient should be cautious, usually starting at the low end of the dosing range, reflecting the greater frequency of decreased hepatic, renal, or car-

Continued on next page

Aloprim—Cont.

diac function, and of concomitant disease or other drug therapy.

ADVERSE REACTIONS

In an uncontrolled, compassionate plea protocol, 125 of 1,378 patients reported a total of 301 adverse reactions while receiving ALOPRIM (allopurinol sodium) for Injection. Most of the patients had advanced malignancies or serious underlying diseases and were taking multiple concomitant medications. Side effects directly attributable to ALOPRIM (allopurinol sodium) for Injection were reported in 19 patients. Fifteen of these adverse experiences were allergic in nature (rash, eosinophilia, local injection site reaction). One adverse experience of severe diarrhea and one incidence of nausea were also reported as being possibly attributable to ALOPRIM (allopurinol sodium) for Injection. Two patients had serious adverse experiences (decreased renal function and generalized seizure) reported as being possibly attributable to ALOPRIM (allopurinol sodium) for Injection.

A listing of the adverse reactions regardless of causality reported from clinical trials follows:

Incidence Greater Than 1%:

Cutaneous/Dermatologic:	rash (1.5%)
Genitourinary:	renal failure/insufficiency (1.2%)
Gastrointestinal:	nausea (1.3%), vomiting (1.2%)

Incidence Less Than 1%:

Body as Whole:	fever, pain, chills, alopecia, infection, sepsis, enlarged abdomen, mucositis/pharyngitis, blast crisis, cellulitis, hypervolemia
Cardiovascular:	heart failure, cardiorespiratory arrest, hypertension, pulmonary embolus, hypotension, decreased venous pressure, flushing, headache, stroke, septic shock, cardiovascular disorder, ECG abnormality, hemorrhage, bradycardia, thrombophlebitis, ventricular fibrillation
Cutaneous/Dermatologic:	urticaria, pruritus, local injection site reaction
Gastrointestinal:	diarrhea, gastrointestinal bleeding, hyperbilirubinemia, splenomegaly, hepatomegaly, intestinal obstruction, jaundice, flatulence, constipation, liver failure, proctitis
Genitourinary:	hematuria, increased creatinine, oliguria, kidney function abnormality, urinary tract infection
Hematologic:	leukopenia, marrow aplasia, thrombocytopenia, eosinophilia, neutropenia, anemia, pancytopenia, ecchymosis, bone marrow suppression, disseminated intravascular coagulation
Metabolic:	hypocalcemia, hyperphosphatemia, hypokalemia, hyperuricemia, electrolyte abnormality, hypercalcemia, hyperglycemia, hypernatremia, hyponatremia, metabolic acidosis, edema, glycosuria, hyperkalemia, lactic acidosis, water intoxication, hypomagnesemia
Neurologic:	seizure, status epilepticus, myoclonus, twitching, agitation, mental status changes, cerebral infarction, coma, dystonia, paralysis, tremor
Pulmonary:	respiratory failure/insufficiency, ARDS, increased respiration rate, apnea
Musculoskeletal:	arthralgia
Other:	hypotonia, diaphoresis, tumor lysis syndrome

The most frequent adverse reaction to oral allopurinol is skin rash. Skin reactions can be severe and sometimes fatal. Therefore, treatment with ALOPRIM (allopurinol sodium) for Injection should be discontinued immediately if a rash develops (see WARNINGS). For further details on hypersensitivity reactions to treatment with oral allopurinol, refer to the package insert for allopurinol tablets.

OVERDOSAGE

Massive overdosing or acute poisoning by ALOPRIM (allopurinol sodium) for Injection has not been reported.

In mice, the minimal lethal dose is 45 mg/kg given intravenously or 500 mg/kg orally (about 1/3 or 4 times the usual human dose on a mg/m^2 basis). Hypoactivity was observed with these doses. In rats, the minimum lethal dose is 100 mg/kg i.v., and 5000 mg/kg orally (about 1.5 and 75 times the usual human dose on a mg/m^2 basis).

In the management of overdosage, there is no specific antidote for ALOPRIM (allopurinol sodium) for Injection. There has been no clinical experience in the management of a patient who has taken massive amounts of allopurinol.

Both allopurinol and oxypurinol are dialyzable; however, the usefulness of hemodialysis or peritoneal dialysis in the management of an overdose of ALOPRIM (allopurinol sodium) for Injection is unknown.

DOSAGE AND ADMINISTRATION

Children and Adults: The dosage of ALOPRIM (allopurinol sodium) for Injection to lower serum uric acid to normal or near-normal varies with the severity of the disease. The amount and frequency of dosage for maintaining the serum uric acid just within the normal range is best determined by using the serum uric acid level as an index. In adults, in one clinical trial, doses over 600 mg a day did not appear to be more effective. The recommended daily dose of ALOPRIM (allopurinol sodium) for Injection is as follows:

	Recommended Daily Dose
Adult:	200 to 400 mg/m^2/day Maximum 600 mg/day
Child:	Starting Dose 200 mg/m^2/day

Hydration: A fluid intake sufficient to yield a daily urinary output of at least two liters in adults and the maintenance of a neutral or, preferably, slightly alkaline urine are desirable.

Impaired Renal Function: The dose of ALOPRIM (allopurinol sodium) for Injection should be reduced in patients with impaired renal function to avoid accumulation of allopurinol and its metabolites:

Creatinine Clearance	Recommended Daily Dose
10 to 20 mL/min	200 mg/day
3 to 10 mL/min	100 mg/day
<3 mL/min	100 mg/day at extended intervals

Administration: In both adults and children, the daily dose can be given as single infusion or in equally divided infusions at 6-, 8-, or 12-hour intervals at the recommended final concentration of not greater than 6 mg/mL (see Preparation of Solution). The rate of infusion depends on the volume of infusate. Whenever possible, therapy with ALOPRIM (allopurinol sodium) for Injection should be initiated 24 to 48 hours before the start of chemotherapy known to cause tumor cell lysis (including adrenocortico steroids).

ALOPRIM (allopurinol sodium) for Injection should not be mixed with or administered through the same intravenous port with agents which are incompatible in solution with ALOPRIM (allopurinol sodium) for Injection (see Preparation of Solution).

Preparation of Solution: ALOPRIM (allopurinol sodium) for Injection must be reconstituted and diluted. The contents of each 30 mL vial should be dissolved with 25 mL of Sterile Water for Injection. Reconstitution yields a clear, almost colorless solution with no more than a slight opalescence. This concentrated solution has a pH of 11.1 to 11.8. It should be diluted to the desired concentration with 0.9% Sodium Chloride Injection of 5% Dextrose for Injection. Sodium bicarbonate-containing solutions should not be used. A final concentration of no greater than 6 mg/mL is recommended. The solution should be stored at 20° to 25°C (68° to 77°F) and administration should begin within 10 hours after reconstitution. Do not refrigerate the reconstituted and/or diluted product.

Parenteral drug products should be inspected visually for particulate matter and discoloration prior to administration, whenever solution and container permit. Do not use this product if particulate matter or discoloration is present. The following table lists drugs that are physically incompatible in solution with ALOPRIM (allopurinol sodium) for Injection.

[See second table at top of previous page]

HOW SUPPLIED

STERILE SINGLE USE VIAL FOR INTRAVENOUS INFUSION.

ALOPRIM (allopurinol sodium) for Injection, 30 mL flint glass vials with rubber stoppers each containing allopurinol sodium equivalent to 500 mg of allopurinol (white lyophilized powder), box of 1 (NDC 59730-5601-1). Store unreconstituted powder at 25°C (77°F); excursions permitted to 15°–30°C (59°–86°F) [see USP controlled room temperature].

Distributed by:
Nabi®
Boca Raton, FL 33487
Toll Free: 1-800-327-7106
Manufactured by:
Catalytica Pharmaceuticals, Inc.
Greenville, NC 27834
June 1999 650348

Shown in Product Identification Guide, page 325

AUTOPLEX® T ℞

Anti-Inhibitor Coagulant Complex
Heat Treated

Caution: This product is to be used only in patients with inhibitors to Factor VIII.

Warning: This is a potent drug with potential hazards. For maximal safety and efficacy, carefully read and follow directions below.

DESCRIPTION

Anti-Inhibitor Coagulant Complex, Heat Treated, Autoplex® T*, is a sterile product prepared from pooled human plasma with subsequent alcohol fractionation to Cohn Fraction IV_1. It contains, in concentrated form, variable amounts of activated and precursor vitamin K-dependent clotting factors. Factors of the kinin generating system are also present. The product is standardized by its ability to correct the clotting time of Factor VIII deficient plasma or Factor VIII deficient plasma which contains inhibitors to Factor VIII.

When reconstituted, this product contains a maximum of 2 units per mL of heparin and a residual amount of polyethylene glycol (2 mg per mL, maximum). It also contains 0.02 M sodium citrate and the sodium content is 177 ±15 milliequivalents per liter.

Laboratory testing of several lots of Anti-Inhibitor Coagulant Complex, Heat Treated, Autoplex® T, has shown the presence of Factor VIII coagulant antigen (VIII:CAg). Although anamnestic response to this antigen following administration of the product was not observed during the clinical trials, the possibility of such a response does exist. Each lot of Anti-Inhibitor Coagulant Complex, Heat Treated, Autoplex® T, is assayed and labeled for units of Hyland Factor VIII correctional activity. Factor VIII correctional activity may not be exclusively related to the efficacious components(s). (See **Clinical Pharmacology**.)

During the manufacturing process, this product was heated for 6 days at 60°C. This heating step is designed to reduce the risk of transmission of hepatitis and other viral diseases. However, no procedure has been shown to be totally effective in removing hepatitis infectivity from Anti-Inhibitor Coagulant Complex.

Anti-Inhibitor Coagulant Complex, Heat Treated, Autoplex® T, **must** be administered intravenously.

*This product and/or its manufacture covered by U.S. Patent Nos. 4,286,056, 4,287,180, 4,357,321, 4,382,083, 4,459,288, and 4,495,278.

CLINICAL PHARMACOLOGY

The Factor VIII correctional activity of Anti-Inhibitor Coagulant Complex, Heat Treated, Autoplex® T, is thought to be, in part, related to the Factor Xa content of the product. It is additionally hypothesized that the elevated Factor VII-VIIa content of this product is also a contributing factor in the *in vivo* reestablishment of normal hemostasis by way of Factor X activation in conjunction with tissue factor, phospholipid and ionic calcium.

Control of thrombin formation is regulated by (1) the presence of antithrombin III and other serine protease inhibitors which neutralize Factors IXa and Xa, (2) the short biological half-lives of Factors VII and VIIa and (3) the presence of the circulating Factor VIII inhibitor which additionally controls overactivation of the intrinsic coagulation system.

In work with human immunodeficiency virus (HIV), substantial reduction in viral content has been reported in a recent study of the effects of ethanol fractionation, the process by which Anti-Inhibitor Coagulant Complex, Heat Treated, Autoplex® T, is manufactured. Wells, *et al*, report 1 to 4 log reduction in each fractionation step they examined.[1] The effectiveness of the 6-day heating step in reducing viral infectivity was assessed by *in vitro* viral inactivation studies, using as markers, viruses not commonly found in plasma. When known quantities of these viruses were added to the product, the heat treatment employed inactivated the following quantities of virus:

Sindbis	10.0 Log_{10}
Vesicular stomatitis	5.0 Log_{10}
Herpes simplex	1.6 Log_{10}
HIV	4.5 Log_{10}

In separate experiments, HIV was also studied and these data are reported in the table above.

A retrospective study conducted with patients receiving unheated Anti-Inhibitor Coagulant Complex, Autoplex®, supports the effectiveness of the purification process in reducing viral burden in the product. In the study, none of the patients who received that product exclusively seroconverted for HIV antibodies, while 56% of those patients who received other treatment modalities seroconverted during the three year study.[2]

INDICATIONS AND USAGE

Anti-Inhibitor Coagulant Complex, Heat Treated, Autoplex® T, is indicated for use in patients with Factor VIII inhibitors who are bleeding or are to undergo surgery.[3-6] The intravenous administration of this preparation is intended to control bleeding episodes in such patients.

Approximately 10% of individuals with hemophilia A (classical hemophilia) have laboratory-measurable inhibitors to Factor VIII.[7] For these patients, the treatment of choice depends upon the following factors: the severity of the bleeding episode, the existing level of inhibitor and whether the patient responds to infusion of Factor VIII with increasing antibody titers (anamnestic rise of Factor VIII antibody).

The following table is presented as a guide in determining the preferred therapy with respect to the use of Anti-Inhibitor Coagulant Complex or Antihemophilic Factor (Human) in patients with Factor VIII inhibitors. Inhibitor level categories are given in the shaded areas of the table and the corresponding recommended product or products are given in the unshaded areas. Other regimens have been proposed.[8]

[See table above]

Patients whose present Factor VIII inhibitor levels are greater than 10 Bethesda Units, as well as patients whose inhibitor levels are historically known to rise to greater than 10 Bethesda Units following treatment with Antihemophilic Factor (Human), should be treated with Anti-Inhibitor Coagulant Complex.

Patients whose present Factor VIII inhibitor levels are between 2 and 10 Bethesda Units and whose inhibitor levels are historically known to remain in this range following treatment with Antihemophilic Factor (Human) may be treated with either Antihemophilic Factor (Human) or Anti-Inhibitor Coagulant Complex, depending on the patient's clinical history and the severity of the bleeding episode. Patients with Factor VIII inhibitor levels of less than 2 Bethesda Units whose inhibitor levels are historically known to remain at 2 Bethesda Units or less following treatment with Antihemophilic Factor (Human) may be treated with appropriate doses of Antihemophilic Factor (Human).

For patients who have low levels of Factor VIII inhibitor and whose history does not include adequate laboratory indications of an anamnestic response to Antihemophilic Factor (Human), the treatment of choice should be based on clinical judgement. In such patients who are having noncritical or minor bleeding episodes, the use of Anti-Inhibitor Coagulant Complex, Heat Treated, Autoplex® T, will maintain the inhibitor at a low level and allow the use of other coagulant therapeutic agents in subsequent major emergencies.

HISTORICAL MAXIMUM LEVEL OF FACTOR VIII INHIBITOR / PRESENT LEVEL OF FACTOR VIII INHIBITOR	<2 B.U.[a]	2-10 B.U.	>10 B.U.
<2 B.U.	AHF[b]	AICC[c] or AHF	AICC
2-10 B.U.	AICC or AHF	AICC or AHF	AICC
>10 B.U.	AICC	AICC	AICC

[a]B.U. designates Bethesda Units.
[b]AHF designates Antihemophilic Factor (Human).
[c]AICC designates Anti-Inhibitor Coagulant Complex.

CONTRAINDICATIONS

The use of Anti-Inhibitor Coagulant Complex, Heat Treated, Autoplex® T, is contraindicated in patients with signs of fibrinolysis and in patients with disseminated intravascular coagulation (DIC).

WARNINGS

Anti-Inhibitor Coagulant Complex, Heat Treated, Autoplex® T, is made from human plasma. Products made from human plasma may contain infectious agents, such as viruses, that can cause disease. The risk that such products will transmit an infectious agent has been reduced by screening plasma donors for prior exposure to certain viruses, by testing for the presence of certain current virus infections, and by inactivating and/or removing certain viruses (See Clinical Pharmacology). Despite these measures, such products can still potentially transmit disease. There is also the possibility that unknown infectious agents may be present in such products. ALL infections thought by a physician possibly to have been transmitted by this product should be reported by the physician or other healthcare provider to the U.S. distributor, Nabi®, at 1-800-327-7106. The physician should discuss the risks and benefits of this product with the patient. Physicians should also report adverse reactions or any disease condition which may occur concomitantly with the administration of this product to the U.S. distributor, Nabi®.

If the infusion of the concentrate occurs more than 1 hour following reconstitution, there may be increased prekallikrein activator (PKA) with consequent hypotension.

PRECAUTIONS

General

Some viruses, such as parvovirus B19 or hepatitis A, are particularly difficult to remove or inactivate at this time. Parvovirus B19 most seriously affects pregnant women, or immune-compromised individuals. Symptoms of parvovirus B19 infection include fever, drowsiness, chills, and runny nose followed about two weeks later by a rash, and joint pain. Evidence of hepatitis A may include several days to weeks of poor appetite, tiredness, and low-grade fever followed by nausea, vomiting, and pain in the belly. Dark urine and a yellowed complexion are also common symptoms. Patients should be encouraged to consult their physician if such symptoms appear.

Certain components used in the packaging of this product contain natural rubber latex.

Identification of the clotting deficiency as that caused by the presence of Factor VIII inhibitors is essential before the administration of Anti-Inhibitor Coagulant Complex, Heat Treated, Autoplex® T, is initiated.

Signs and/or symptoms of hypotension may occur with this product. In these cases, stopping the infusion allows the symptoms to disappear. With all but the most reactive individuals, the infusion may be resumed at a slower rate.

If clinical signs of intravascular coagulation occur, the infusion should be stopped promptly and the patient monitored for DIC by the appropriate laboratory tests. Symptoms of DIC include changes in blood pressure and pulse rate, respiratory distress, chest pain and cough. Laboratory indications of DIC include prolonged thrombin time, prothrombin time and partial thromboplastin time tests. Other indications of DIC are decreased fibrinogen concentration, decreased platelet count and/or the presence of fibrinogen/fibrin degradation products.

Special caution should be taken in the use of this concentrate in newborns, where a high morbidity and mortality may be associated with hepatitis, and in individuals with pre-existing liver disease.

Laboratory Tests

In some cases, laboratory tests such as the activated partial thromboplastin time test may not correlate with clinical response, in that the appearance of hemostatic improvement may occur without a reduction of partial thromboplastin time. However, the prothrombin time would be expected to be shortened.

In children, fibrinogen levels should be determined prior to the initial infusion and monitored during the course of the treatment.

Drug Interactions

Since only limited data are available on the administration of highly activated prothrombin complex products together with antifibrinolytic agents such as epsilon-aminocaproic acid (EACA) or tranexamic acid,[6] the concomitant use of Anti-Inhibitor Coagulant Complex, Heat Treated, Autoplex® T, with such agents is not recommended.

Pregnancy

Pregnancy Category C. Animal reproduction studies have not been conducted with Anti-Inhibitor Coagulant Complex, Heat Treated, Autoplex® T. It is also not known whether Anti-Inhibitor Coagulant Complex, Heat Treated, Autoplex® T, can cause fetal harm when administered to a pregnant woman or can affect reproduction capacity. Anti-Inhibitor Coagulant Complex, Heat Treated, Autoplex® T, should be given to a pregnant woman only if clearly needed.

ADVERSE REACTIONS

As with other plasma preparations, reactions manifested by fever, chills or indications of protein sensitivity may be observed with the administration of Anti-Inhibitor Coagulant Complex, Heat Treated, Autoplex® T. Signs and/or symptoms of high prekallikrein activity, such as changes in blood pressure or pulse rate may also be observed. It is advisable that appropriate medications be available for the treatment of acute allergic reactions or acute vasoactive reactions, should they occur.

A rate of infusion that is too rapid may cause headache, flushing, and changes in pulse rate and blood pressure. In such instances, stopping the infusion allows the symptoms to disappear promptly. With all but the most reactive individuals, infusion may be resumed at a slower rate.

DOSAGE AND ADMINISTRATION

Each bottle of Anti-Inhibitor Coagulant Complex, Heat Treated, Autoplex® T, is labeled with the number of Hyland Factor VIII Correctional Units that it contains. One Hyland Factor VIII Correctional Unit is that quantity of activated prothrombin complex which, upon addition to an equal volume of Factor VIII deficient or inhibitor plasma, will correct the clotting time (ellagic acid-activated partial thromboplastin time) to 35 seconds (normal).

The recommended dosage range is 25 to 100 Hyland Factor VIII Correctional Units per kg of body weight, depending upon the severity of hemorrhage. If no hemostatic improvement is observed approximately 6 hours following the initial administration, the dosage should be repeated.

Subsequent dosage and administration intervals should be adjusted according to the patient's clinical response. (See **Laboratory Tests.**)

Reconstitution: Use Aseptic Technique

1. Bring Anti-Inhibitor Coagulant Complex, Heat Treated, Autoplex® T (dry concentrate) and Sterile Water for Injection, USP, (diluent) to room temperature.
2. Remove caps from concentrate and diluent bottles to expose central portions of rubber stoppers.
3. Cleanse stoppers with germicidal solution.
4. Remove protective covering from one end of the double-ended needle and insert exposed needle through **diluent** stopper.
5. Remove protective covering from the other end of the double-ended needle. Invert diluent bottle over the upright concentrate bottle, then **rapidly** insert free end of the needle through the concentrate bottle stopper at its center. Vacuum in the concentrate bottle will draw in diluent.
6. Disconnect the two bottles by removing needle from the diluent bottle, then remove needle from concentrate bottle stopper. Swirl or rotate the concentrate bottle until all material is dissolved. Do not shake vigorously.

Parenteral drug products should be inspected visually for particulate matter and discoloration prior to administration, whenever solution and container permit.

Note: Do not refrigerate after reconstitution.

Rate of Administration

It is recommended that Anti-Inhibitor Coagulant Complex, Heat Treated, Autoplex® T, be infused initially at a rate of 2 mL/min. If infusion at this rate is well tolerated the administration rate may be gradually increased to 10 mL/min.

Administration: Use Aseptic Technique

When reconstitution of Anti-Inhibitor Coagulant Complex, Heat Treated, Autoplex® T, is complete, its infusion should commence as soon as practical; however, it must be completed within 1 hour.

The reconstituted solution should be at room temperature during infusion.

A. Intravenous Drip Infusion

When a Hyland administration set is used, follow directions for use printed on the administration set container. When an administration set from another source is used, follow directions accompanying that set where necessary. The use of a Hyland administration set is recommended as it contains a suitable filter.

B. Intravenous Syringe Injection

1. Attach filter needle to syringe and draw back plunger to admit air into the syringe.
2. Insert needle into the reconstituted Anti-Inhibitor Coagulant Complex, Heat Treated, Autoplex® T.
3. Inject air into bottle and then withdraw the reconstituted material into the syringe.
4. Remove and discard the filter needle from the syringe; attach a suitable needle and inject intravenously as instructed under **Rate of Administration**.
5. If patient is to receive more than one bottle of concentrate, the contents of two bottles may be drawn into the same syringe by drawing up each bottle through a separate used filter needle. This practice lessens the loss of concentrate. Please note: filter needles are intended to filter the contents of a single bottle of Anti-Inhibitor coagulant Complex, Heat Treated, Autoplex® T, only.

HOW SUPPLIED

Anti-Inhibitor Coagulant Complex, Heat Treated, Autoplex® T, is furnished with a suitable volume of Sterile Water for Injection, USP; a double-ended needle; a filter needle; and a package insert.

Storage

Anti-Inhibitor Coagulant Complex, Heat Treated, Autoplex® T, should be stored under ordinary refrigeration (2 – 8°C, 36 – 46°F). Avoid freezing to prevent damage to the diluent bottle.

REFERENCES

1. Wells MA, Wittek AE, Epstein JS, *et al*: Inactivation and partition of human T-cell lymphotrophic virus, type III, during ethanol fractionation. **Transfusion 26**:210-213, 1986
2. Gazengel C, Larrieu MJ: Lack of seroconversion for LAV/HTLV-III in patients exclusively given unheated activated prothrombin complex prepared with ethanol step. **Lancet 2**:1189, 1985
3. Kurczynski EM, Penner JA: Activated prothrombin concentrate for patients with factor VIII inhibitors. **New Eng J Med 291**:164-167, 1974
4. Penner JA, Kelly PE: Management of patients with factor VIII or IX inhibitors. **Semin Thromb Hemostas 1**:386-399, 1975
5. Buchanan GR, Kevy SV: Use of prothrombin complex concentrates in hemophiliacs with inhibitors: Clinical and laboratory studies. **Pediatrics 62**:767-774, 1978
6. Mannucci PM, Federici F, Vigano S, *et al*: Multiple dental extractions with a new prothrombin complex concentrate in two patients with factor VIII inhibitors. **Thromb Res 15**:359-364, 1979
7. Shapiro SS: Antibodies to blood coagulation factors. **Clinics in Haematology 8**:207-214, 1979
8. Roberts HR: Hemophiliacs with inhibitors: Therapeutic options. **New Eng J. Med 305**:757-758, 1981

BIBLIOGRAPHY

Fekete LF, Holst SL, Peetoom F, *et al*: "Auto" Factor IX Concentrate: A new therapeutic approach to treatment of hemophilia A patients with inhibitors. **Proceedings, 14th International Congress of Haematology** . Sao Paulo, Brazil, 1972

Kelly P, Penner JA: Antihemophilic factor inhibitors: Management with prothrombin complex concentrates. **JAMA 236** :2061, 1976

Seligsohn U, Kasper CK, Østerud B, *et al*: Activated factor VII. Presence in factor IX concentrates and persistence in the circulation after infusion. **Blood 53**:828, 1979

Abildgaard CF, Penner JA, Watson-Williams EJ: Anti-Inhibitor Coagulant Complex (Autoplex) for treatment of factor VIII inhibitors in hemophilia. **Blood 56**:978, 1980

NDC 59730-6059-7

Distributed by:
Nabi®
Boca Raton, FL 33487 USA

Continued on next page

Autoplex T—Cont.

Manufactured by:
Baxter Healthcare Corporation
Hyland Division
Glendale, CA 91203 USA
U.S. License No. 140
6849

Revised April 1998
Shown in Product Identification Guide, page 325

Table 1 Log Reduction of Test Viruses[5]

	Test Virus				
	HIV	**BVD**	**PRV**	**Polio**	**BPV**
Model Virus:	HIV	HCV	HBV	Hepatitis A	PVB19
Envelope/Genome:	yes/RNA	yes/RNA	yes/DNA	no/RNA	no/DNA
Manufacturing Step					
dextran sulfate	NT	NT	NT	3.32	< 1
anion-exchange	NT	NT	NT	> 3.52	> 5.34
solvent/detergent	> 4.67	> 7.43	> 5.26	2.7	> 5.81
virus filtration	> 6.02	> 7.30	> 6.77	4.25	> 4.97

BVD = Bovine Viral Diarrhea PRV = Pseudorabies Virus Polio = Poliovirus
BPV = Bovine Parvovirus PVB19 = Parvovirus B19 NT = not tested

Table 2 Recommendations for Hepatitis B Prophylaxis Following Percutaneous or Permucosal Exposure[12]

	Exposed Person	
Source	Unvaccinated	Vaccinated
HBsAg-positive	1. Hepatitis B Immune Globulin (Human) X 1 immediately* 2. Initiate HB vaccine series†	1. Test exposed person for anti-HBs 2. If inadequate antibody‡, Hepatitis B Immune Globulin (Human) X 1 immediately plus HB Vaccine booster dose
Known Source - High Risk for HBsAg-positive	1. Initiate HB vaccine series 2. Test source for HBsAg. If positive, Hepatitis B Immune Globulin (Human) X 1	1. Test source for HBsAg only if exposed is vaccine nonresponder; if source is HBsAg-positive, give Hepatitis B Immune Globulin (Human) X 1 immediately plus HB vaccine booster dose
Known Source - Low Risk for HBsAg-positive	Initiate HB vaccine series	Nothing required
Unknown Source	Initiate HB vaccine series	Nothing required

* Hepatitis B Immune Globulin (Human) dose of 0.06 mL/kg IM.
† See manufacturers' recommendation for appropriate dose.
‡ Less than 10 mIU/mL anti-HBs by radioimmunoassay, negative by enzyme immunoassay.

Nabi-HB™ ℞

Hepatitis B Immune Globulin (Human)
Solvent/Detergent Treated and Filtered

DESCRIPTION

Hepatitis B Immune Globulin (Human), Nabi-HB™, is a sterile solution of immunoglobulin (5 ± 1% protein) containing antibodies to hepatitis B surface antigen (anti-HBs). It is prepared from plasma donated by individuals with high titers of anti-HBs. The plasma is purified by an anion-exchange column chromatography method[1,2] with two added viral reduction steps described below. The product is formulated in 0.075 M sodium chloride, 0.15 M glycine, and 0.01% polysorbate 80, pH 6.25. It contains no preservative and is intended for single use by the intramuscular route only. The product appears as a clear to opalescent, nonturbid liquid.

The manufacturing steps are designed to reduce the risk of transmission of viral disease. The solvent/detergent treatment step, using tri-n-butyl phosphate and Triton® X-100, is effective in inactivating known enveloped viruses such as hepatitis B virus (HBV), hepatitis C virus (HCV), and human immunodeficiency virus (HIV).[3] Virus filtration, using a Planova® 35 nm Virus Filter, is effective in reducing some known enveloped and non-enveloped viruses.[4] The inactivation and reduction of known enveloped and non-enveloped model viruses were validated in laboratory studies as summarized in the following table:

[See table 1 above]

The product potency is expressed in international units (IU) by comparison to the World Health Organization (WHO) standard. Each vial contains greater than 312 IU/mL anti-HBs. The potency of each vial of Nabi-HB™ exceeds the potency of anti-HBs in a U.S. reference hepatitis B immune globulin (FDA). The U.S. reference has been tested by Nabi® against the WHO standard and found to be equal to 208 IU/mL.

CLINICAL PHARMACOLOGY

Hepatitis B Immune Globulin (Human) products provide passive immunization for individuals exposed to the hepatitis B virus as evidenced by a reduction in the attack rate of hepatitis B following use.[6–9]

Clinical studies conducted prior to 1983 with hepatitis B immune globulins similar to Nabi-HB™[10,11] indicate the advantage of simultaneous administration of Hepatitis B Vaccine and Hepatitis B Immune Globulin (Human). The Centers for Disease Control and Prevention Advisory Committee on Immunization Practices (ACIP) advises that the combination prophylaxis be provided based upon the increased efficacy found with that regimen in neonates.[12]

Cases of hepatitis B are rarely seen following exposure to HBV in persons with preexisting anti-HBs. However, no prospective studies have been performed on the efficacy of concurrent Hepatitis B Vaccine and Hepatitis B Immune Globulin (Human) administration following parenteral exposure, mucous membrane contact, or oral ingestion in adults.

Infants born to HBsAg-positive mothers are at risk of being infected with HBV and becoming chronic carriers.[13] The risk is especially great if the mother is also HBeAg-positive.[14] Studies conducted with hepatitis B immune globulins similar to Nabi-HB™ indicated that for an infant with perinatal exposure to an HBsAg-positive and HBeAg-positive mother, a regimen combining one dose of Hepatitis B Immune Globulin (Human) at birth with the Hepatitis B Vaccine series started soon after birth is 85–98% effective in preventing development of the HBV carrier state.[15–17] Regimens involving either multiple doses of Hepatitis B Immune Globulin (Human) alone or the vaccine series alone have a 70–90% efficacy, while a single dose of Hepatitis B Immune Globulin (Human) alone has 50% efficacy.[18]

Since infants have close contact with primary caregivers and they have a higher risk of becoming HBV carriers after acute HBV infection, prophylaxis of an infant less than 12 months of age with Hepatitis B Immune Globulin (Human) and Hepatitis B Vaccine is indicated if the mother or primary caregiver has acute HBV infection.[19]

Sexual partners of HBsAg-positive persons are at increased risk of acquiring HBV infection. A single dose of Hepatitis B Immune Globulin (Human) is 75% effective if administered within two weeks of the last sexual exposure to a person with acute hepatitis B.[19]

Pharmacokinetics

Pharmacokinetic trials[20] of Nabi-HB™, Hepatitis B Immune Globulin (Human), given intramuscularly to 48 healthy volunteers demonstrate pharmacokinetic parameters similar to those reported by Scheiermann and Kuwert.[21] The half-life for Nabi-HB™ was 24.8 ± 5.6 days. The clearance rate was 0.433 ± 0.144 L/day and the volume of distribution was 15.3 ± 6.2 L.

Maximum concentration of Nabi-HB™ was reached in 6.6 ± 3.0 days. The maximum concentration of anti-HBs achieved by Nabi-HB™ was consistent with that of another licensed Hepatitis B Immune Globulin (Human) when compared in the same pharmacokinetics trial. Comparability of pharmacokinetics between Nabi-HB™ and a commercially available hepatitis B Immunoglobulin indicate that similar efficacy of Nabi-HB™ should be inferred.

INDICATIONS AND USAGE

Nabi-HB™, Hepatitis B Immune Globulin (Human), is indicated for treatment of acute exposure to blood containing HBsAg, perinatal exposure of infants born to HBsAg-positive mothers, sexual exposure to HBsAg-positive persons and household exposure to persons with acute HBV infection in the following settings:

- Acute Exposure to Blood Containing HBsAg
  Following either parenteral exposure (needlestick, bite, sharps), direct mucous membrane contact (accidental splash), or oral ingestion (pipetting accident), involving HBsAg-positive materials such as blood, plasma or serum.
- Perinatal Exposure of Infants Born to HBsAg-positive Mothers
  Infants born to mothers positive for HBsAg with or without HBeAg.[12]
- Sexual Exposure to HBsAg-positive Persons
  Sexual partners of HBsAg-positive persons.
- Household Exposure to Persons with Acute HBV Infection
  Infants less than 12 months old whose mother or primary caregiver is positive for HBsAg. Other household contacts with an identifiable blood exposure to the index patient.

Nabi-HB™ is indicated for intramuscular use only.

CONTRAINDICATIONS

Individuals known to have had an anaphylactic or severe systemic reaction to human globulin should not receive Nabi-HB™, Hepatits B Immune Globulin (Human), or any other human immune globulin. Nabi-HB™ contains less than 40 micrograms/mL IgA. Individuals who are deficient in IgA may have the potential to develop IgA antibodies and have an anaphylactoid reaction. The physician must weigh the potential benefit of treatment with Nabi-HB™ against the potential for hypersensitivity reactions.

WARNINGS

In patients who have severe thrombocytopenia or any coagulation disorder that would contraindicate intramuscular injections, Nabi-HB™, Hepatitis B Immune Globulin (Human), should be given only if the expected benefits outweigh the potential risks.

Nabi-HB™ is made from human plasma. Products made from human plasma may carry a risk of transmitting infectious agents, e.g., viruses, and theoretically, the Creutzfeldt-Jakob disease (CJD) agent. The risk that such products can transmit an infectious agent has been reduced by screening plasma donors for prior exposure to certain viruses, by testing for the presence of certain current viral infections, and by inactivating and/or reducing certain viruses. The Nabi-HB™ manufacturing process includes a solvent/detergent treatment step (using tri-n-butyl phosphate and Triton® X-100) that is effective in inactivating known enveloped viruses such as HBV, HCV, and HIV. Nabi-HB™ is filtered using a Planova® 35 nm Virus Filter that is effective in reducing the levels of some enveloped and non-enveloped viruses. These two processes are designed to increase product safety. Despite these measures, such products can still potentially transmit disease. There is also the possibility that unknown infectious agents may be present in such products. ALL infections thought by a physician possibly to have been transmitted by this product should be reported by the physician or other health care provider to Nabi at 1-800-458-4244. The physician should discuss the risks and benefits of this product with the patient.

PRECAUTIONS

General

Nabi-HB™, Hepatitis B Immune Globulin (Human), must be administered only intramuscularly for post-exposure prophylaxis. The preferred sites for intramuscular injections are the anterolateral aspect of the upper thigh and the deltoid muscle of the upper arm. If the buttock is used due to the volume to be injected, the central region should be avoided; only the upper, outer quadrant should be used, and the needle should be directed anteriorly (i.e., not inferiorly or perpendicular to the skin) to minimize the possibility of involvement with the sciatic nerve.[22]

Drug Interactions

Vaccination with live virus vaccines should be deferred until approximately three months after administration of Nabi-HB™, Hepatitis B Immune Globulin (Human). It may be necessary to revaccinate persons who received Nabi-HB™ shortly after live virus vaccination.

There are no available data on concomitant use of Nabi-HB™ and other drugs; therefore, Nabi-HB™ should not be mixed with other drugs.

Pregnancy Category C

Animal reproduction studies have not been conducted with Nabi-HB™. It is also not known whether Nabi-HB™ can cause fetal harm when administered to a pregnant woman or can affect reproduction capacity. Nabi-HB™ should be given to a pregnant woman only if clearly indicated.

Nursing Mothers

It is not known whether this drug is excreted in human milk. Because many drugs are excreted in human milk, caution should be exercised when Nabi-HB™ is administered to a nursing mother.

Pediatric Use

Safety and effectiveness in the pediatric population have not been established for Nabi-HB™. However, the safety and effectiveness of similar Hepatitis B immune globulins have been demonstrated in infants and children.[12]

ADVERSE REACTIONS

Seventy-six male and female volunteers received Nabi-HB™, Hepatitis B Immune Globulin (Human), intramuscularly in pharmacokinetics trials.[20] The number of patients with reactions related to the administration of Nabi-HB™ included local reactions such as pain 9 (12%), ache 2 (3%), erythema 2 (3%), heat 1 (1%), and burning 2 (3%) at the injection site, as well as systemic reactions such as headache 20 (26%), malaise 4 (5%), nausea 4 (5%), diarrhea 2 (3%) and myalgia 4 (5%). The majority of reactions were reported as mild. The following adverse events were reported once each in pharmacokinetics trials and were probably related to Nabi-HB™: chills, fatigue, lightheadedness, abdominal cramping, and retching. There were no serious adverse events.

No anaphylactic reactions with Nabi-HB™ have been reported. However, these reactions, although rare, have been reported following the injection of human immune globulins.[23]

OVERDOSAGE

Although no data are available, clinical experience reported with other human immune globulins suggests that the only manifestations of overdose with Nabi-HB™, Hepatitis B Immune Globulin (Human) would be pain and tenderness at the injection site.

DOSAGE AND ADMINISTRATION

This product is for intramuscular use only. The use of this product by the intravenous route is not indicated. Parenteral drug products should be inspected visually for particulate matter and discoloration prior to administration.

It is important to use a separate vial, sterile syringe, and needle for each individual patient, in order to prevent transmission of infectious agents from one person to another. **Any vial of Nabi-HB™, Hepatitis B Immune Globulin (Human), that has been entered should be used promptly. Do not re-use or save for future use. This product contains no preservative; therefore, partially used vials should be discarded immediately.**

Hepatitis B Immune Globulin (Human) may be administered at the same time (but at a different site), or up to one month preceding hepatitis B vaccination without impairing the active immune response to Hepatitis B Vaccine.[11]

- Acute Exposure to Blood Containing HBsAg

  Table 2 summarizes prophylaxis for percutaneous (needlestick, bite, sharps), ocular, or mucous membrane exposure to blood according to the source of exposure and vaccination status of the exposed person. For greatest effectiveness, passive prophylaxis with Hepatitis B Immune Globulin (Human) should be given as soon as possible after exposure, as its value after seven days following exposure is unclear.[12] An injection of 0.06 mL/kg of body weight should be administered intramuscularly as soon as possible after exposure and within 24 hours, if possible. Consult the Hepatitis B Vaccine package insert for dosage information regarding the vaccine.

  For persons who refuse Hepatitis B Vaccine or are known non-responders to vaccine, a second dose of Hepatitis B Immune Globulin (Human) should be given one month after the first dose.[12]

[See table 2 at top of previous page]

- Prophylaxis of Infants Born to Mothers Who Are Positive for HBsAg With or Without HBeAg.

  Table 3 contains the recommended schedule of hepatitis B prophylaxis for infants born to mothers that are either known to be positive for HBsAg or have not been screened. Infants born to mothers known to be HBsAg-positive should receive 0.5 mL Hepatitis B Immune Globulin (Human) after physiologic stabilization of the infant and preferably within 12 hours of birth. The Hepatitis B Vaccine series should be initiated simultaneously, if not contraindicated, with the first dose of the vaccine given concurrently with the Hepatitis B Immune Globulin (Human), but at a different site. Subsequent doses of the vaccine should be administered in accordance with the recommendations of the manufacturer.

  Women admitted for delivery, who were not screened for HBsAg during the prenatal period, should be tested. While test results are pending, the newborn infant should receive Hepatitis B Vaccine within 12 hours of birth (see manufacturers' recommendations for dose). If the mother is later found to be HBsAg-positive, the infant should receive 0.5 mL Hepatitis B Immune Globulin (Human) as soon as possible and within seven days of birth; however, the efficacy of Hepatitis B Immune Globulin (Human) administered after 48 hours of age is not known.[10,19] Testing for HBsAg and anti-HBs is recommended at 12–15 months of age. If HBsAg is not detectable and anti-HBs is present, the child has been protected.[12]

[See table 3 above]

Table 3 Recommended Schedule of Hepatitis B Immunoprophylaxis to Prevent Perinatal Transmission of Hepatitis B Virus Infection[19]

Administer	Age of Infant	
	Infant born to mother known to be HBsAg-positive	Infant born to mother not screened for HBsAg
First Vaccination*	Birth (within 12 hours)	Birth (within 12 hours)
Hepatitis B Immune Globulin (Human)†	Birth (within 12 hours)	If mother is found to be HBsAg positive, administer dose to infant as soon as possible, not later than 1 week after birth
Second Vaccination*	1 month	1–2 months
Third Vaccination*	6 months‡	6 months‡

* See manufacturers' recommendations for appropriate dose.
† 0.5 mL administered IM at a site different from that used for the vaccine.
‡ See ACIP recommendation.

- Sexual Exposure to HBsAg-positive Persons

  All susceptible persons whose sexual partners have acute hepatitis B infection should receive a single dose of Hepatitis B Immune Globulin (Human) (0.06 mL/kg) and should begin the Hepatitis B Vaccine series, if not contraindicated, within 14 days of the last sexual contact or if sexual contact with the infected person will continue. Administering the vaccine with Hepatitis B Immune Globulin (Human) may improve the efficacy of post-exposure treatment. The vaccine has the added advantage of conferring long-lastng protection.[19]

- Household Exposure to Persons With Acute HBV Infection

  Prophylaxis of an infant less than 12 months of age with 0.5 mL Hepatitis B Immune Globulin (Human) and Hepatitis B Vaccine is indicated if the mother or primary caregiver has acute HBV infection. Prophylaxis of other household contacts of persons with acute HBV infection is not indicated unless they had an identifiable blood exposure to the index patient, such as by sharing toothbrushes or razors. Such exposures should be treated like sexual exposures. If the index patient becomes an HBV carrier, all household contacts should receive Hepatitis B Vaccine.[19]

HOW SUPPLIED

Nabi-HB™, Hepatitis B Immune Globulin (Human), is supplied as:

NDC Number	Contents
59730-4402-1	a carton containing a 1.0 mL single dose vial (>312 IU) and package insert
59730-4403-1	a carton containing a 5.0 mL single dose vial (>1560 IU) and package insert

STORAGE

Refrigerate between 2 to 8 °C (36 to 46 °F). Do not freeze. Do not use after expiration date. Use within 6 hours after the vial has been entered.

REFERENCES

1. Bowman JM, *et al.*: WinRho: Rh immune globulin prepared by ion exchange for intravenous use. *Canadian Med Assoc J* 1980; 123:1121–1125.
2. Friesen AD, *et al.*: Column ion-exchange preparation and characterization of an Rh immune globulin (WinRho) for intravenous use. *Journal of Applied Biochem* 1981; 3:164–175.
3. Horowitz B: Investigators into the application of tri(n-butyl)phosphate/detergent mixtures to blood derivatives. Morgenthaler J (ed): *Virus Inactivation in Plasma Products, Curr Stud Hematol Blood Transfus* 1989; 56: 83–96.
4. Burnouf T: Value of virus filtration as method for improving the safety of plasma products. *Vox Sang* 1996; 70:235–236.
5. Unpublished data on file, Viral Validation Study Reports, Cangene Corporation.
6. Grady GF, and Lee VA: Hepatitis B Immune globulin—prevention of hepatitis from accidental exposure among medical personnel. *N Engl J Med* 1975; 293:1067–1070.
7. Seeff LB, *et al.*: Type B hepatitis after needle-stick exposure: Prevention with hepatitis B immune globulin. *Ann Int Med* 1978; 88:285–293.
8. Krugman S, and Giles JP: Viral hepatitis, type B (MS-2-strain). Further observations on natural history and prevention. *N Engl J Med* 1973; 288:755–760.
9. Hoofnagle JH, *et al.*: Passive—active immunity from hepatitis B immune globulin. *Ann Int Med* 1979; 91: 813–818.
10. Beasley RP, *et al.*: Efficacy of hepatitis B immune globulin for prevention of perinatal transmission of the hepatitis B virus carrier state: Final report of a randomized double-blind, placebo-controlled trial. *Hepatology* 1983; 3:135–141.
11. Szmuness W, *et al.*: Passive active immunisation against hepatitis B: Immunogenicity studies in adult Americans. *Lancet* 1981; 1:575–577.
12. Centers for Disease Control: Recommendations for protection against viral hepatitis. Recommendations of the Immunization Practices Advisory Committee (ACIP). *MMWR* 1985; 34(22):313–335.
13. Shiraki Y, *et al.*: Hepatitis B surface antigen and chronic hepatitis in infants born to asymptomatic carrier mothers. *Am J Dis Child* 1977; 131:644–647.
14. Beasley RP, *et al.*: The e antigen and vertical transmission of hepatitis B surface antigen. *Am J Epidemiol* 1977; 105:94–98.
15. Wong VCW, *et al.*: Prevention of the HBsAg carrier state in newborn infants of mothers who are chronic carriers of HBsAg and HBeAg by administration of hepatitis B vaccine and hepatitis B immunoglobulin: Double-blind randomized placebo-controlled study. *Lancet* 1984; 1:921–926.
16. Poovorawan Y, *et al.*: Long term hepatitis B vaccine in infants born to hepatitis B e antigen positive mothers. *Archives of Diseases in Childhood* 1997; 77:F47–F51.
17. Stevens CE, *et al.*: Perinatal Hepatitis B virus transmission in the United States: Prevention by passive-active immunization. *JAMA* 1985; 253:1740–1745.
18. Jhaveri R, *et al.*: High titer multiple dose therapy with HBIG in newborn infants of HBsAg positive mothers. *J Pediatr* 1980; 97:305–308.
19. Centers for Disease Control: Hepatitis B virus: A comprehensive strategy for eliminating transmission in the United States through universal childhood vaccination. Recommendations of the Immunization Practices Advisory Committee (ACIP). *MMWR* 1991; 40(13):1–25.
20. Data on file, Nabi®.
21. Scheiermann N, Kuwert EK: Uptake and elimination of hepatitis B immunoglobulins after intramuscular application in man. *Develop Biol Standard* 1983; 54:347.
22. Centers for Disease Control: General recommendations on immunization. Recommendations of the Advisory Committee on Immunization Practices (ACIP). *MMWR* 1994; 1:6.
23. Ellis EF and Henney CS: Adverse reactions following administration of human gamma globulin. *J Allerg* 1969; 43:45–54.

Manufactured by:
Nabi®
Boca Raton, FL 33487
U.S. License No. 1022
Part No. 07.0210.01
June, 2000

WinRho SDF™ ℞

[*win' rō s d f*]

Rh_o (D) Immune Globulin Intravenous (Human)

DESCRIPTION

Rh_o(D) Immune Globulin Intravenous (Human) (Rh_o(D) IGIV)—WinRho SDF™—is a sterile, freeze-dried gamma globulin (IgG) fraction containing antibodies to the Rh_o(D) antigen (D antigen). WinRho SDF™ is prepared from human plasma by an anion-exchange column chromatography method.[1–3] The manufacturing process includes a solvent detergent treatment step (using tri-n-butyl phosphate and Triton X-100) that is effective in inactivating lipid enveloped viruses such as hepatitis B, hepatitis C, and HIV.[4] WinRho SDF™ is filtered using a Planova 35 nm Virus Filter which has been validated to be effective in the removal of some nonlipid enveloped viruses.[5–6] These two processes are designed to increase product safety by reducing the risk of transmission of enveloped and nonenveloped viruses, respectively.

The product potency is expressed in international units by comparison to the World Health Organization (WHO) standard. A 300 µg (1,500 International Unit [IU]*) vial contains sufficient anti-Rh_o(D) to effectively suppress the immunizing potential of approximately 17 mL of Rh_o(D) (D-positive) red blood cells (RBCs). This product contains approximately 5 µg/mL IgA per 120 µg (600 IU) vial.

The product is stabilized with 0.1 M glycine, 0.04 M sodium chloride, and 0.01% polysorbate 80. It contains no preservative.

Treatment of ITP

For use in the treatment of immune thrombocytopenic purpura (ITP), WinRho SDF™ **must be administered intravenously.**

Suppression of RH Isoimmunization

For use in the suppression of Rh isoimmunization, WinRho SDF™ may be administered either intramuscularly or intravenously.

*In the past, a full dose of Rh_o(D) Immune Globulin (Human) has traditionally been referred to as a "300 µg" dose. Potency and dosing recommendations are now expressed in IU by comparison to the WHO anti-Rh_o(D) standard. The conversion of "µg" to "IU" is 1 µg = 5 IU.

CLINICAL PHARMACOLOGY

Treatment of ITP

WinRho SDF™, Rh_o(D) Immune Globulin Intravenous (Human), has been shown to increase platelet counts in non-splenectomized, Rh_o(D) positive patients with ITP. Platelet counts usually rise within one to two days and peak within seven to 14 days after initiation of therapy. The duration of response is variable; however, the average duration is approximately 30 days. The mechanism of action is not completely understood, but is thought to be due to the formation of anti-Rh_o(D) (anti-D)-coated RBC complexes resulting in Fc receptor blockade, thus sparing antibody-coated platelets.[7–8]

Suppression of Rh Isoimmunization

WinRho SDF™ is used to suppress the immune response of non-sensitized Rh_o(D) negative individuals following exposure to Rh_o(D) positive RBCs by fetomaternal hemorrhage during delivery of an Rh_o(D) positive infant, abortion (spon-

Continued on next page

WinRho SDF—Cont.

taneous or induced), amniocentesis, abdominal trauma, or mismatched transfusion.[9–11] The mechanism of action is not completely understood.

WinRho SDF™, when administered within 72 hours of a full-term delivery of an Rh_o(D) positive infant by an Rh_o(D) negative mother, will reduce the incidence of Rh isoimmunization from 12–13% to 1–2%. The 1–2% is, for the most part, due to isoimmunization during the last trimester of pregnancy. When treatment is given both antenatally at 28 weeks gestation and postpartum, the Rh immunization rate drops to about 0.1%.[12–15]

When 120 µg (600 IU) of Rh_o(D) IGIV is administered to pregnant women, passive anti-Rh_o(D) antibodies are not detectable in the circulation for more than six weeks and therefore a dose of 300 µg (1,500 IU) should be used for antenatal administration.

In a clinical study with Rh_o(D) negative volunteers (nine males and one female), Rh_o(D) positive red cells were completely cleared from the circulation within eight hours of intravenous administration of Rh_o(D) IGIV. There was no indication of Rh isoimmunization of these subjects at six months after the clearance of the Rh_o(D) positive red cells.

Pharmacokinetics—IM versus IV Administration

In a clinical study involving Rh_o(D) negative volunteers, two subjects received 120 µg (600 IU) Rh_o(D) IGIV by intravenous (IV) administration and two subjects received this dose by intramuscular (IM) administration. Peak levels (36 to 48 ng/mL) were reached within two hours of IV administration and peak levels (18 to 19 ng/mL) were reached at five to 10 days after IM administration. The calculated areas under the curve were the same for both routes of administration. The $t_{1/2}$ for anti-Rh_o(D) was about 24 days following IV administration and about 30 days following IM administration.

INDICATIONS AND CLINICAL USE

Treatment of ITP

WinRho SDF™, Rh_o(D) Immune Globulin Intravenous (Human), is recommended for the treatment of non-splenectomized, Rh_o(D) positive

- children with chronic or acute ITP,
- adults with chronic ITP, or
- children and adults with ITP secondary to HIV infection

in clinical situations requiring an increase in platelet count to prevent excessive hemorrhage. The safety and efficacy of WinRho have not been evaluated in clinical trials for patients with non-ITP causes of thrombocytopenia or in previously splenectomized patients.

Suppression of Rh Isoimmunization

Pregnancy and Other Obstetric Conditions

WinRho SDF™ is recommended for the suppression of Rh isoimmunization in non-sensitized, Rho(D) negative (D-negative) women within 72 hours after spontaneous or induced abortions, amniocentesis, chorionic villus sampling, ruptured tubal pregnancy, abdominal trauma or transplacental hemorrhage or in the normal course of pregnancy unless the blood type of the fetus or father is known to be Rh_o(D) negative. In the case of maternal bleeding due to threatened abortion, WinRho SDF™ should be administered as soon as possible. Suppression of Rh isoimmunization reduces the likelihood of hemolytic disease in an Rh_o(D) positive fetus in present and future pregnancies.

The criteria for an Rh-incompatible pregnancy requiring administration of WinRho SDF™ at 28 weeks gestation and within 72 hours after delivery are:

- the mother must be Rh_o(D) negative,
- the mother is carrying a child whose father is either Rh_o(D) positive or Rh_o(D) unknown,
- the baby is either Rh_o(D) positive or Rh_o(D) unknown, and
- the mother must not be previously sensitized to the Rh_o(D) factor.

Transfusion

WinRho SDF™, Rh_o(D) Immune Globulin Intravenous (Human), is recommended for the suppression of Rh isoimmunization in Rh_o(D) negative female children and female adults in their childbearing years transfused with Rh_o(D) positive RBCs or blood components containing Rh_o(D) positive RBCs. Treatment should be initiated within 72 hours of exposure. Treatment should be given (without preceding exchange transfusion) only if the transfused Rh_o(D) positive blood represents less than 20% of the total circulating red cells. A 300 µg (1,500 IU) dose will suppress the immunizing potential of approximately 17 mL of Rh_o(D) positive RBCs.

CLINICAL TRIALS

Treatment of ITP

Efficacy was documented in four subgroups of patients with ITP:

Childhood Chronic ITP

In an open-label, single arm, multicenter study, 24 non-splenectomized, Rh_o(D) positive children with ITP of greater than six months duration were treated initially with 50 µg/kg (250 IU/kg) Rh_o(D) Immune Globulin Intravenous (Human) (25 µg/kg (125 IU/kg) on days 1 and 2, with subsequent doses ranging from 25 to 55 µg/kg (125 to 275 IU/kg)). Response was defined as a platelet increase to at least 50,000/mm^3 and a doubling of the baseline. Nineteen of 24 patients responded for an overall response rate of 79%, and overall mean peak platelet count of 229,400/mm^3 (range 43,300 to 456,000), and a mean duration of response of 36.5 days (range 6 to 84).[16–17]

Childhood Acute ITP

A multicenter, randomized, controlled trial comparing Rh_o(D) IGIV to high dose and low dose Immune Globulin Intravenous (Human) and prednisone was conducted in 146 non-splenectomized, Rh_o(D) positive children with acute ITP and platelet counts less than 20,000/mm^3. Of 38 patients receiving Rh_o(D) IGIV (25 µg/kg (125 IU/kg) on days 1 and 2), 32 patients (84%) responded (platelet count $\geq$ 50,000 mm^3) with a mean peak platelet count of 319,500/mm^3 (range 61,000 to 892,000), with no statistically significant differences compared to other treatment arms. The mean times to achieving $\geq$ 20,000/mm^3 or $\geq$ 50,000/mm^3 platelets for patients receiving Rho(D) IGIV were 1.9 and 2.8 days, respectively. When comparing the different therapies for time to platelet count $\geq$ 20,000/mm^3 or $\geq$ 50,000/mm^3, no statistically significant differences among treatment groups were detected, with a range of 1.3 to 1.9 days and 2.0 to 3.2 days, respectively.[18–19]

Adult Chronic ITP

Twenty-four non-splenectomized, Rh_o(D) positive adults with ITP of greater than six months duration and platelet counts < 30,000/mm^3 or requiring therapy were enrolled in a single-arm, open-label trial and treated with 20 to 75 µg/kg (100 to 375 IU/kg) Rh_o(D) IGIV (mean dose 46.2 µg/kg (231 IU/kg)). Twenty-one of 24 patients responded (increase $\geq$ 20,000/mm^3) during the first two courses of therapy for an overall response rate of 88% with a mean peak platelet count of 92,300/mm^3 (range 8,000 to 229,000).[20–21]

ITP Secondary to HIV Infection

Eleven children and 52 adults, who were non-splenectomized and Rh_o(D) positive, with all Walter Reed classes of HIV infection and ITP, with initial platelet counts of $\leq$ 30,000/mm^3 or requiring therapy, were treated with 20 to 75 µg/kg (100 to 375 IU/kg) Rh_o(D) IGIV in an open label trial. Rh_o(D) IGIV was administered for an average of 7.3 courses (range 1 to 57) over a mean period of 407 days (range 6 to 1,952). Fifty-seven of 63 patients responded (increase $\geq$ 20,000/mm^3) during the first six courses of therapy for an overall response rate of 90%. The overall mean change in platelet count for six courses was 60,900/mm^3 (range -2,000 to 565,000), and the mean peak platelet count was 81,700/mm^3 (range 16,000 to 593,000).[21–23]

Suppression of Rh Isoimmunization

The pivotal study[24] supporting this indication was conducted in 1,186 non-sensitized, Rh_o(D) negative pregnant women in cases in which the blood types of the fathers were either Rh_o(D) positive or unknown. Rh_o(D) IGIV was administered according to one of three regimens: 1) 93 women received 120 µg (600 IU) at 28 weeks; 2) 131 women received 240 µg (1200 IU) each at 28 and 34 weeks; 3) 962 women received 240 µg (1200 IU) at 28 weeks. All women received a postnatal administration of 120 µg (600 IU) if the newborn was found to be Rh_o(D) positive. Of 1,186 women who received antenatal Rh_o(D) IGIV, 806 were given Rh_o(D) IGIV postnatally following the delivery of an Rh_o(D) positive infant, of which 325 women underwent testing at six months after delivery for evidence of Rh isoimmunization. Of these 325 women, 23 would have been expected to display signs of Rh isoimmunization; however, none was observed ($p <$ 0.001 in a Chi-square test of significance of difference between observed and expected isoimmunization in the absence of Rh_o(D) IGIV).

CONTRAINDICATIONS

Treatment of ITP and Suppression of Rh Isoimmunization

Individuals known to have had an anaphylactic or severe systemic reaction to human globulin should not receive WinRho SDF™, Rh_o(D) Immune Globulin Intravenous (Human), or any other Immune Globulin (Human). WinRho SDF™ contains trace amounts of IgA (approximately 5 µg/mL per 120 µg [600 IU] vial). Individuals who are deficient in IgA may have the potential for developing IgA antibodies and have anaphylactic reactions. The physician must weigh the potential benefit of treatment with WinRho SDF™ against the potential for hypersensitivity reactions.

WARNINGS

WinRho SDF™, Rh_o(D) Immune Globulin Intravenous (Human), is made from human plasma. Products made from human plasma may carry a risk of transmitting infectious agents, e.g., viruses and theoretically, the Creutzfeldt-Jakob disease (CJD) agent. The risk that such products will transmit an infectious agent has been reduced by screening plasma donors for prior exposure to certain viruses, by testing for the presence of certain current virus infections, and by inactivating and/or removing certain viruses. The WinRho SDF™ manufacturing process includes a solvent detergent treatment step (using tri-n-butyl phosphate and Triton X-100) that is effective in inactivating lipid enveloped viruses such as hepatitis B, hepatitis C, and HIV. WinRho SDF™ is filtered using a Planova 35 nm Virus Filter that is effective in reducing the level of some non-lipid enveloped viruses such as hepatitis A. These two processes are designed to increase product safety by reducing the risk of transmission of lipid enveloped and non-lipid enveloped viruses, respectively. Despite these measures, such products can still potentially transmit disease. There is also the possibility that unknown infectious agents may be present in such products. ALL infections thought by a physician possibly to have been transmitted by this product should be reported by the physician or other healthcare provider to the distributor, Nabi® at 1-800-4WINRHO (1-800-494-6746). The physician should discuss the risks and benefits of this product with the patient.

Treatment of ITP

WinRho SDF™ **must be administered via the intravenous route** for the treatment of ITP as its efficacy has not been established by the intramuscular or subcutaneous routes. WinRho SDF™ should not be administered to Rh_o(D) negative or splenectomized individuals as its efficacy in these patients has not been demonstrated.

Suppression of Rh Isoimmunization

For the suppression of Rh isoimmunization in the mother, do not administer to the infant.

PRECAUTIONS

WinRho SDF™, Rh_o(D) Immune Globulin Intravenous (Human), should not be administered as immunoglobulin replacement therapy for immune globulin deficiency syndromes.

Treatment of ITP

Following administration of WinRho SDF™, Rh_o(D) positive ITP patients should be monitored for signs and/or symptoms of intravascular hemolysis (IVH), clinically compromising anemia, and renal insufficiency.

If patients are to be transfused, Rho(D) negative red blood cells (PRBCs) should be used so as not to exacerbate ongoing IVH. Platelet products may contain up to 5.0 mL of RBCs, thus caution should likewise be exercised if platelets from Rh_o(D) positive donors are transfused.

If the patient has a lower than normal hemoglobin level (less than 10 g/dL), a reduced dose of 25 to 40 µg/kg (125 to 200 IU/kg) should be given to minimize the risk of increasing the severity of anemia in the patient. WinRho SDF™ must be used with extreme caution in patients with a hemoglobin level that is less than 8 g/dL due to the risk of increasing the severity of the anemia (See DOSAGE AND ADMINISTRATION, Treatment of ITP).

Suppression of Rh Isoimmunization

WinRho SDF™ should not be administered to Rh_o(D) negative individuals who are Rh immunized as evidenced by an indirect antiglobulin (Coombs') test revealing the presence of anti-Rh_o(D) (anti-D) antibody.

A large fetomaternal hemorrhage late in pregnancy or following delivery may cause a weak mixed field positive D^u test result. Such an individual should be assessed for a large fetomaternal hemorrhage and the dose of WinRho SDF™ adjusted accordingly. WinRho SDF™ should be administered if there is any doubt about the mother's blood type.

Laboratory Tests

In addition to anti-D, WinRho SDF™ contains trace amounts of anti-A, anti-B, anti-C and anti-E antibodies.

Treatment of ITP

Passively acquired anti-A, anti-B, anti-C, and anti-E blood group antibodies may be detectable in direct and indirect antiglobulin (Coombs') tests obtained following WinRho SDF™, Rh_o(D) Immune Globulin Intravenous (Human), administration. Interpretation of direct and indirect antiglobulin tests must be made in the context of the patient's underlying clinical condition and supporting laboratory data.

Suppression of Rh Isoimmunization

The presence of passively administered anti-Rh_o(D) in maternal or fetal blood can lead to a positive direct antiglobulin (Coombs') test. If there is an uncertainty about the mother's Rh group or immune status, WinRho SDF™ should be administered to the mother.

Drug Interactions

Treatment of ITP and Suppression of Rh Isoimmunization

Administration of WinRho SDF™ concomitantly with other drugs has not been evaluated. Other antibodies contained in WinRho SDF™ may interfere with the response to live virus vaccines such as measles, mumps, polio or rubella. Therefore, immunization with live vaccines should not be given within 3 months after WinRho SDF™ administration.

Refer to Dosage and Administration section for information on drug compatibility.

Pregnancy Category C

Treatment of ITP and Suppression of Rh Isoimmunization

Animal reproduction studies have not been conducted with WinRho SDF™. It is not known whether WinRho SDF™ can cause fetal harm when administered to a pregnant woman or can affect reproductive capacity. WinRho SDF™ should be given to a pregnant woman only if clearly needed.

ADVERSE REACTIONS

Treatment of ITP

In clinical trials of subjects (n=161) with childhood acute ITP, adults and children with chronic ITP, and adults and children with ITP secondary to HIV, 60/848 (7%) of infusions were associated with at least one adverse event that was considered to be related to the study medication. The most common adverse events were headache (19 infusions; 2%), chills (14 infusions; <2%), and fever (nine infusions; 1%). All are expected adverse events associated with infusions of immunoglobulins.

WinRho SDF™, Rh_o(D) Immune Globulin Intravenous (Human), is administered to Rh_o(D) positive patients with ITP. Therefore, side effects related to the destruction of Rh_o(D) positive red blood cells, most notably a decreased hemoglobin, can be expected. In four clinical trials of patients treated with the recommended initial intravenous dose of 50 µg/kg (250 IU/kg), the mean maximum decrease in hemoglobin was 1.70 g/dL (range: +0.40 to -6.1 g/dL). At a reduced dose, ranging from 25 to 40 µg/kg (125 to 200 IU/kg), the mean maximum decrease in hemoglobin was 0.81 g/dL (range: +0.65 to -1.9 g/dL). Only 5/137 (3.7%) of patients had a maximum decrease in hemoglobin of greater than 4 g/dL (range 4.2 to 6.1 g/dL).

In most cases, the RBC destruction is believed to occur in the spleen. However, signs and symptoms consistent with IVH, including back pain, shaking chills, and/or hemoglobinuria, have been reported, occurring within 4 hours of WinRho administration. IVH-related complications that have been reported include death (four cases reported between May 1996 and April 1999), acute onset or exacerbation of anemia, and acute onset or exacerbation of renal insufficiency. One patient died from complications secondary to IVH-induced exacerbation of anemia after administration of WinRho for treatment of ITP. Although the primary cause of death in the other three ITP patients treated with WinRho was related to underlying disease, the extent to which IVH-related clinical complications exacerbated their conditions and contributed to their deaths in unknown.

The mean maximum decrease in hemoglobin in patients who were not transfused with PRBCs was 3.7 g/dL (range: 0.0–7.6 g/dL). Transfusions for treatment-associated anemia were administered within hours to days of the onset of IVH and consisted of between 1–6 units of PRBCs. Acute renal insufficiency was noted within 2 to 48 hours of the onset of IVH. The mean maximum increase in serum creatinine was 3.5 mg/dL (range: 0.8–10.3 mg/dL) and occurred within 2–9 days. The renal insufficiency in all surviving patients resolved with medical management, including dialysis, within 4–23 days.

The etiology of IVH following WinRho administration is unknown. No known risk factors associated with this adverse event have yet been identified from among those examined, which included age, gender, pre-treatment renal function, pretreatment hemoglobin, concomitantly administered PRBCs, or WinRho dose.

Suppression of Rh Isoimmunization

Adverse reactions to Rh_o(D) Immune Globulin Intravenous (Human) are infrequent in Rh_o(D) negative individuals. In the clinical trial[24] of 1,186 Rh_o(D) negative pregnant women, no adverse events were attributed to Rh_o(D) IGIV. Discomfort and slight swelling at the site of injection and slight elevation in temperature have been reported in a small number of cases. A post-marketing survey conducted since the Canadian licensure of Rh_o(D) IGIV in 1980 for this indication included data obtained from 31,059 injections (25,068 for routine Rh prophylaxis and 5,991 following abortions, amniocentesis, chorionic villus sampling and antepartum hemorrhage). There were 9,905 Rh_o(D) negative women who delivered Rh_o(D) positive infants, almost all of whom had received antenatal as well as postnatal prophylaxis. Of the patients followed in this survey, there were 26 reported treatment failures that resulted in the development of Rh_o(D) antibodies. There were no adverse experiences related to Rh_o(D) IGIV reported in this survey.

General Adverse Reactions

In addition to the adverse reactions described above, the following have been reported infrequently in clinical trials and/or postmarketing experience, in patients treated for ITP or the suppression of Rh isoimmunization, and are thought to be temporally associated with WinRho SDF™, Rh_o(D) Immune Globulin Intravenous (Human), use: asthenia, abdominal or back pain, hypotension, pallor, diarrhea, increased LDH, arthralgia, myalgia, dizziness, hyperkinesia, somnolence, vasodilation, pruritus, rash, and sweating. As is the case with all drugs of this nature, there is a remote chance of an idiosyncratic or anaphylactic reaction with WinRho SDF™ in individuals with hypersensitivity to blood products.

SYMPTOMS AND TREATMENT OF OVERDOSE

Treatment of ITP and Suppression of Rh Isoimmunization

There are no reports of known overdoses in patients being treated for Rh isoimmunization or ITP. In clinical studies with nonpregnant Rh_o(D) positive patients with ITP (n=141) treated with 120 to 6,500 µg (600 to 32,500 IU) of Rh_o(D) IGIV, there were no signs or symptoms that warranted medical intervention. However, these same doses were associated with a mild, transient hemolytic anemia.

DOSAGE AND ADMINISTRATION

Treatment of ITP and Suppression of Rh Isoimmunization

WinRho SDF™, Rh_o(D) Immune Globulin Intravenous (Human), should be reconstituted only with the accompanying vial of 0.9% Sodium Chloride Injection. It should not be administered concurrently with other products.

Reconstitution

Intravenous Administration

Aseptically reconstitute the product shortly before use with 2.5 mL of 0.9% Sodium Chloride Injection for 120 µg (600 IU) and 300 µg (1,500 IU) and 8.5 mL of 0.9% Sodium Chloride Injection for 1,000 µg (5,000 IU) (see the next table). Inject the diluent slowly onto the inside wall of the vial and gently swirl until dissolved. **Do not shake**.

Intramuscular Administration

Aseptically reconstitute the product shortly before use with 1.25 mL of 0.9% Sodium Chloride Injection for 120 µg (600 IU) and 300 µg (1,500 IU) and 8.5 mL of 0.9% Sodium Chloride Injection for 1,000 µg (5,000 IU) (see the next table). Inject the diluent slowly onto the inside wall of the vial and gently swirl until dissolved. **Do not shake**.

Reconstitution of WinRho SDF™

Vial Size	Volume of Diluent to be Added to Vial
Intravenous Injection	—
120 µg (600 IU)	2.5 mL
300 µg (1,500 IU)	2.5 mL
1,000 µg (5,000 IU)	8.5 mL
Intramuscular Injection	—
120 µg (600 IU)	1.25 mL
300 µg (1,500 IU)	1.25 mL
1,000 µg (5,000 IU)	8.5 mL*

* To be administered into several sites

Injection

Parenteral products such as WinRho SDF™ should be inspected for particulate matter and discoloration prior to administration. Use the product within 12 hours of reconstitution. Discard any unused portion.

Intravenous Administration

Infuse the entire dose into a suitable vein over three to five minutes. WinRho SDF™ should be administered separately from other drugs.

Intramuscular Administration

Administer into the deltoid muscle of the upper arm or the anterolateral aspects of the upper thigh. Due to the risk of sciatic nerve injury, the gluteal region should not be used as a routine injection site. If the gluteal region is used, use only the upper, outer quadrant.

Treatment of ITP

WinRho SDF™, Rh_o(D) Immune Globulin Intravenous (Human), **must be given by intravenous** administration for the treatment of ITP.

Initial Dosing: After confirming that the patient is Rh_o(D) positive, an initial dose of 50 µg/kg (250 IU/kg) body weight, given as a single injection, is recommended for the treatment of ITP. The initial dose may be administered in two divided doses given on separate days, if desired. If the patient has a hemoglobin level that is less than 10 g/dL, a reduced dose of 25 to 40 µg/kg (125 to 200 IU/kg) should be given to minimize the risk of increasing the severity of anemia in the patient. All patients should be monitored to determine clinical response by assessing platelet counts, red cell counts, hemoglobin, and reticulocyte levels (See PRECAUTIONS, *Treatment of ITP*).

Subsequent Dosing: If subsequent therapy is required to elevate platelet counts, an intravenous dose of 25 to 60 µg/kg (125 to 300 IU/kg) body weight of WinRho SDF™ is recommended. The frequency and dose used in maintenance therapy should be determined by the patient's clinical response by assessing platelet counts, red cell counts, hemoglobin, and reticulocyte levels.

If patient responded to initial dose with a satisfactory increase in platelets:

Maintenance Therapy:

Dosing (25–60 µg/kg (125–300 IU/kg)) individualized based on platelet and Hgb levels.

If patient did not respond to initial dose, administer a subsequent dose based on Hgb:

If Hgb between 8–10 g/dL, redose between 25–40 µg/kg (125–200 IU/kg).

If Hgb >10 g/dL, redose between 50–60 µg/kg (250–300 IU/kg).

If Hgb <8 g/dL, use with caution.

The following equations are provided to determine the dosage and number of vials needed for the treatment of ITP:

- weight in lbs. / 2.2083 = weight in kg
- weight in kg × selected µg (IU) dosing level = dosage
- dosage / vial size = number of vials needed

Suppression of Rh Isoimmunization

WinRho SDF™ may be given by intravenous or intramuscular administration for the suppression of Rh isoimmunization.

Pregnancy

The same dosage, as described below, is to be administered by either the intramuscular or intravenous routes.

A 300 µg (1,500 IU) dose of WinRho SDF™ should be administered at 28 weeks gestation. If WinRho SDF™ is administered early in the pregnancy, it is recommended that WinRho SDF™ be administered at 12-week intervals in order to maintain an adequate level of passively acquired anti-Rh.

A 120 µg (600 IU) dose should be administered as soon as possible after delivery of a confirmed Rh_o(D) positive baby and normally no later than 72 hours after delivery. In the event that the Rh status of the baby is not known at 72 hours, WinRho SDF™ should be administered to the mother at 72 hours after delivery. If more than 72 hours have elapsed, WinRho SDF™ should not be withheld, but administered as soon as possible up to 28 days after delivery.

Other Obstetric Conditions

The same dosage, as described below, is to be administered by either the intramuscular or intravenous routes.

A 120 µg (600 IU) dose of WinRho SDF™ should be administered immediately after abortion, amniocentesis (after 34 weeks gestation) or any other manipulation late in pregnancy (after 34 weeks gestation) associated with increased risk of Rh isoimmunization. Administration should take place within 72 hours after the event.

A 300 µg (1,500 IU) dose of WinRho SDF™ should be administered immediately after amniocentesis before 34 weeks gestation or after chorionic villus sampling. This dose should be repeated every 12 weeks while the woman is pregnant. In the case of threatened abortion, WinRho SDF™ should be administered as soon as possible.

Obstetric Indications and Recommended Dose

Indication	Dose (Administer IM or IV)
Pregnancy:	
• 28 weeks gestation	300 µg (1,500 IU)
• Postpartum (if newborn Rh positive)	120 µg (600 IU)
Obstetric Conditions:	
• Threatened abortion at any time	300 µg (1,500 IU)
• Amniocentesis and chorionic villus sampling before 34 weeks gestation	300 µg (1,500 IU)
• Abortion, amniocentesis, or any other manipulation after 34 weeks gestation	120 µg (600 IU)

Transfusion

WinRho SDF™ should be administered within 72 hours after exposure for treatment of incompatible blood transfusions or massive fetal hemorrhage.

Transfusion Indication and Recommended Dose

Route of Administration	WinRho SDF™ Dose	
	If exposed to Rh_o(D) Positive Whole Blood:	If exposed to Rh_o(D) Positive Red Blood Cells:
Intravenous	9 µg (45 IU)/ mL blood	18 µg (90 IU)/ mL cells
Intramuscular	12 µg (60 IU)/ mL blood	24 µg (120 IU)/ mL cells

Administer 600 µg (3,000 IU) **every 8 hours via the intravenous route,** until the total dose, calculated from the above table, is administered.

Administer 1,200 µg (6,000 IU) **every 12 hours via the intramuscular route,** until the total dose, calculated from the above table, is administered.

HOW SUPPLIED

WinRho SDF™, Rh_o(D) Immune Globulin Intravenous (Human), is available in packages containing:

NDC Number	Contents
60492-0021-1	A box containing a single dose vial of 120 µg (600 IU) anti-Rh_o(D) IGIV, a single dose vial of 2.5 mL 0.9% Sodium Chloride Injection, and a package insert
60492-0023-1	A box containing a single dose vial of 300 µg (1,500 IU) anti-Rh_o(D) IGIV, a single dose vial of 2.5 mL 0.9% Sodium Chloride Injection, and a package insert
60492-0024-1	A box containing a single dose vial of 1,000 µg (5,000 IU) anti-Rh_o(D) IGIV, a single dose vial of 8.5 mL 0.9% Sodium Chloride Injection, and a package insert

STORAGE

Store at 2 to 8°C (35 to 46°F). Do not freeze. Do not use after expiration date.

If the reconstituted product is not used immediately, store it at room temperature for no longer than 12 hours. Do not freeze the reconstituted product. Discard the product if not administered within 12 hours.

Rx Only

REFERENCES

1. Bowman, JM, et al.: Low protein Rh immune globulin (Rh IgG)-purity, stability, activity and prophylactic value. *Vox Sang* 1973; 24:301–316.
2. Bowman, JM, et al.: WinRho: Rh immune globulin prepared by ion exchange for intravenous use. *Can. Med. Assoc. J.* 1980; 123:1121–1125.
3. Friesen, AD, et al.: Column ion-exchange preparation and characterization of an Rh immune globulin (WinRho) for intravenous use. *J. Appl. Biochem.* 1981; 3:164–175.
4. Horowitz, B: Investigations into the application of tri(n-butyl)phosphate/detergent mixtures to blood derivatives. Morgenthaler J(ed): *Virus Inactivation in Plasma Products, Curr. Stud. Hematol. Blood. Transfus.* 1989; 56:83–96.
5. Information on file at Cangene Corporation.

Continued on next page

WinRho SD—Cont.

6. Burnouf, T: Value of virus filtration as a method for improving the safety of plasma products. *Vox Sang.* 1996; 70:235–236.
7. Ballow, M: Mechanisms of action of intravenous immunoglobulin therapy and potential use in autoimmune connective tissue diseases. *Cancer.* 1991; 68:1430–1436.
8. Kniker, WT: Immunosuppressive agents, γ-globulin, immunomodulation, immunization, and apheresis. *J. Aller. Clin. Immunol.* 1989; 84:1104–1106.
9. Chown, B, et al.: The effect of anti-D IgG on D-positive recipients. *Can. Med. Assoc. J.* 1970; 102:1161–1164.
10. Bowman, JM and Chown, B: Prevention of Rh immunization after massive Rh-positive transfusion. *Can. Med. Assoc. J.* 1968; 99:385–388.
11. Bowman, JM: Suppression of Rh isoimmunization: a review. *Obstet. & Gynec.* 1978; 52:385–393.
12. Bowman, JM, et al.: Rh isoimmunization during pregnancy: antenatal prophylaxis. *Can. Med. Assoc. J.* 1978; 118:623–627.
13. Bowman, JM, and Pollock, JM: Antenatal prophylaxis of Rh isoimmunization: 28 weeks'-gestation service program. *Can. Med. Assoc. J.* 1978; 118:627–630.
14. Bowman, JM, and Pollock, JM: Failures of intravenous Rh immune globulin prophylaxis: An analysis of the reasons for such failures. *Trans. Med. Rev.* 1987; 1:101–11
15. Bowman, JM: Antenatal suppression of Rh alloimmunization. *Clin Obstet. & Gynec.* 1991; 34:296–303.
16. Unpublished data on file, CITP Report, May 1993.
17. Andrew, M, et al.: A multicenter study of the treatment of childhood chronic idiopathic thrombocytopenic purpura with anti-D. *J Pediatrics* 120:522–527, 1992.
18. Unpublished data on file, AITP Report, May 1993.
19. Blanchette, V, et al.: Randomised trial of intravenous immunoglobulin G, intravenous anti-D, and oral prednisone in childhood acute immune thrombocytopenic purpura. *Lancet* 344:703–707, 1994.
20. Unpublished data on file, BITP-2 Report, May 1993.
21. Bussel, JB, et al.: Intravenous anti-D treatment of immune thrombocytopenic purpura: Analysis of efficacy, toxicity, and mechanism of effect. *Blood* 77:1884–1893, 1991.
22. Unpublished data on file, BITP-1 Report, May 1993.
23. Bussel, JB, et al.: IV anti-D treatment of ITP: Results in 210 cases. Abstract, *The American Society of Hematology*, Anaheim, CA, December, 1992.
24. Unpublished data on file, WR3 Report, May 1993.

Manufactured by:
Cangene Corporation
Winnipeg, Canada R3T 5Y3
U.S. License No. 1201
Distributed by:
Nabi®
Boca Raton, FL 33487
To report adverse events contact Nabi® at 1-800-327-7106
Date of Revision: 1/20/2000
Part No. 07.0205.05
Shown in Product Identification Guide, page 325

EDUCATIONAL MATERIAL

Educational Materials for WinRho SDF™
Patient Brochures
(All materials are FREE and available to physicians, pharmacists and consumers)
1) "It's About Immune Thrombocytopenic Purpura and Knowing Your Options"
Information about ITP and treatment options
2) "Immune Thrombocytopenic Purpura in Childhood" (*English or Spanish*)
Information about Pediatric ITP and treatment options
3) Patient Starter Kits (Adult and Pediatric)

Information for the Health Care Provider
(Free of Charge)
1) WinRho SDF™ Package Insert
2) WinRho SDF™ File Card
3) Patient Education Flip Chart
4) WinRho SDF™ Product Monograph
5) "Current Perspectives in Treating ITP"—series of 6 audio tapes
6) Slide Series:
"Treatment of Immune (Idiopathic) Thrombocytopenic Purpura (ITP)"

Check the **PINK** section
to find a particular **BRAND**.

Neutrogena Dermatologics

5760 WEST 96th STREET
LOS ANGELES, CA 90045

Direct Inquiries to:
Diane Foster
(310) 642-1150
FAX: (310) 337-2156
For Medical Information Contact:
In Emergencies:
Kamran Mather, Ph.D.
(310) 642-1150
FAX: (310) 216-5399

MELANEX® ℞

Topical Solution
(Hydroquinone USP, 3.0%)
FOR EXTERNAL USE ONLY

CAUTION: Federal law prohibits dispensing without prescription.

DESCRIPTION

Each milliliter of Melanex® Topical Solution contains 30 mg of hydroquinone in a hydroalcoholic base of purified water, SD Alcohol 40 (45%), Laureth-4, Isopropyl Alcohol (4%), Propylene Glycol, Ascorbic Acid.

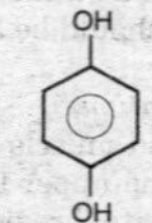

$C_6H_6O_2$ 110.11
1,4 DIHYDROXYBENZENE
Hydroquinone

CLINICAL PHARMACOLOGY

It has been suggested the primary action of hydroquinone is directed at tyrosinase.[1] The selective inhibition of the enzyme affects melanogenesis in the melanocytes resulting in cessation of melanin formation and subsequent reduction in pigmentation. Additional studies indicate hydroquinone acts on the essential subcellular metabolic processes of melanocytes with resultant cytolysis, i.e., non-enzyme-mediated depigmentation.[2]

INDICATIONS AND USAGE

Melanex® is indicated in the temporary depigmentation of hyperpigmented skin conditions such as chloasma, melasma, freckles, senile lentigines, and other forms of melanin hyperpigmentation.

DOSAGE AND ADMINISTRATION

Apply to affected areas twice daily, in the morning and before bedtime. During the day, an effective broad spectrum sunscreen like Neutrogena® Sunblock SPF 15 or SPF 30 should be used and unnecessary solar exposure avoided, or protective clothing should be worn to cover the treated area in order to prevent repigmentation from occurring.

CONTRAINDICATIONS

Melanex® is contraindicated in persons who have shown hypersensitivity to hydroquinone or any of the other ingredients. The safety of topical treatment with hydroquinone during pregnancy has not been established.

PRECAUTIONS

Concurrent use of Melanex® with peroxide products may result in transient dark staining of skin areas so treated. This is due to the oxidation of hydroquinone by the peroxide. This transient staining can be removed by discontinuing concurrent usage and normal soap cleansing.

FOR EXTERNAL USE ONLY

Hydroquinone preparations may produce skin irritation in susceptible individuals and have a slight potential to produce allergic response. Therefore, the physician should use appropriate caution. If rash or irritation develops, discontinue use and consult physician. Do not use on children under 12 years.

If no improvement is seen after two months of treatment, use of product should be discontinued. Avoid contact with eyes. In case of accidental contact, patient should rinse eyes thoroughly with water and contact physician. A bitter taste and anesthetic effect may occur if applied to lips. Keep out of reach of children. Use of Melanex® in paranasal and infraorbital areas increases the chance of irritation (see **ADVERSE REACTIONS**).

ADVERSE REACTIONS

The following have been reported: dryness and fissuring of the paranasal and infraorbital areas, erythema, and stinging. Hydroquinone has been known to produce irritation and sensitization in susceptible individuals.

HOW SUPPLIED: 1 fl. oz. (30 ML) bottle with plastic rod and Appliderm® Applicator unit.

NOTE: Slight darkening of the Melanex® solution is normal and will not affect potency. See expiration date on bottle.

[See figure at top of next column]

Store at room temperature or below. Avoid excessive heat.

(1) JIMBOW K., OBATHA H., PATHAK M., FITZPATRICK T.B. Mechanism and Depigmentation of Hydroquinone, Journal of Investigative Dermatology 1974, 62:436–449.
(2) op. cit.

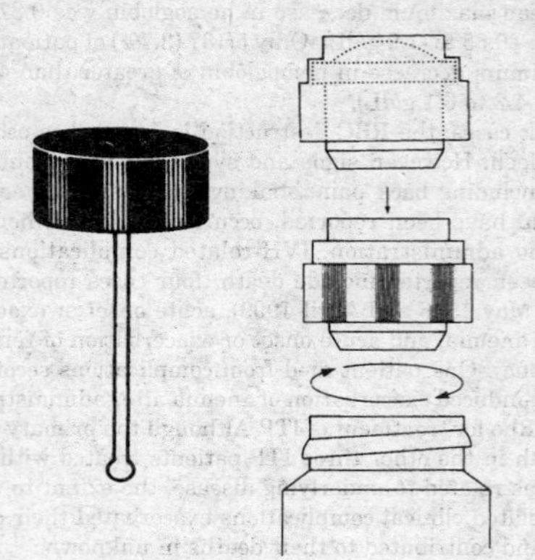

For additional information please call:
Neutrogena Technical Department toll-free (800) 421-6857; in California call (800) 649-1150.
NDC 10812-930-01
Distributed by
Neutrogena Dermatologics
5760 W. 96th St.
Los Angeles, CA 90045
Shown in Product Identification Guide, page 325

Novartis Consumer Health, Inc.

560 MORRIS AVENUE
SUMMIT, NJ 07901-1312

Direct Inquiries to:
Consumer & Professional Affairs
(800) 452-0051
FAX: (800) 635-2801
or write to 445 State Street
Fremont, MI 49423

EX-LAX® LAXATIVE Pills OTC

Regular Strength Ex-Lax,
Maximum Strength Ex-Lax
Ex-Lax Stool Softener Caplets
Ex-Lax Gentle Strength Caplets

(See PDR For Nonprescription Drugs and Dietary Supplements)

EX-LAX® Regular Strength CHOCOLATED LAXATIVE Pieces OTC

(See PDR For Nonprescription Drugs and Dietary Supplements)

GAS–X® OTC

REGULAR STRENGTH GAS-X®
ANTIGAS CHEWABLE TABLETS
EXTRA STRENGTH GAS–X®
ANTIGAS CHEWABLE TABLETS
EXTRA STRENGTH GAS–X®
ANTIGAS SOFTGELS
EXTRA STRENGTH GAS-X ANTIGAS LIQUIDS
SIMETHICONE - ANTIGAS
MAXIMUM STRENGTH GAS-X®
ANTIGAS SOFTGELS

(See PDR For Nonprescription Drugs and Dietary Supplements)

LAMISIL® AT™ OTC

LAMISIL® AT™ Cream
LAMISIL® AT™ Spray Pump
LAMISIL® AT™ Solution Dropper

(See PDR for Nonprescription Drugs and Dietary Supplements)

MAALOX® OTC

Magnesia and Alumina
Oral Suspension
Antacid

Liquids
Cooling Mint
Smooth Cherry
Refreshing Lemon

DESCRIPTION

Maalox® Antacid is used for the relief of acid indigestion, heartburn, sour stomach and upset stomach associated with these symptoms.

Active Ingredients	Maalox Suspension 5 mL teasp
Magnesium Hydroxide	200 mg
Aluminum Hydroxide (equivalent to dried gel, USP)	225 mg

INACTIVE INGREDIENTS

Cooling Mint
Calcium saccharin, flavor, guar gum, methylparaben, propylparaben, purified water, sorbitol.
Smooth Cherry and Refreshing Lemon
Calcium saccharin, flavors, methylparaben, propylparaben, purified water, sorbitol and xanthan gum.

Minimum Recommended Dosage: Maalox Suspension	
	Per 2 Tsp. (10 mL)
Acid neutralizing capacity	NLT 26.6 mEq
Sodium content	NMT 2.5 mg

DIRECTIONS FOR USE

Two to four teaspoonfuls, four times a day or as directed by a physician.

PATIENT WARNINGS

Do not take more than 16 teaspoonfuls in a 24-hour period or use the maximum dosage for more than 2 weeks or use if you have kidney disease except under the advice and supervision of a physician. Keep this and all drugs out of the reach of children.

DRUG INTERACTION PRECAUTION

Antacids may interact with certain prescription drugs. If you are presently taking a prescription drug, do not take this product without checking with your physician or other health professional.

Professional Labeling

INDICATIONS

As an antacid for symptomatic relief of hyperacidity associated with the diagnosis of peptic ulcer, gastritis, peptic esophagitis, gastric hyperacidity, heartburn, or hiatal hernia.

WARNINGS

Prolonged use of aluminum-containing antacids in patients with renal failure may result in or worsen dialysis osteomalacia. Elevated tissue aluminum levels contribute to the development of the dialysis encephalopathy and osteomalacia syndromes. Small amounts of aluminum are absorbed from the gastrointestinal tract and renal excretion of aluminum is impaired in renal failure. Aluminum is not well removed by dialysis because it is bound to albumin and transferrin, which do not cross dialysis membranes. As a result, aluminum is deposited in bone, and dialysis osteomalacia may develop when large amounts of aluminum are ingested orally by patients with impaired renal function.
Aluminum forms insoluble complexes with phosphate in the gastrointestinal tract, thus decreasing phosphate absorption. Prolonged use of aluminum-containing antacids by normophosphatemic patients may result in hypophosphatemia if phosphate intake is not adequate. In its more severe forms, hypophosphatemia can lead to anorexia, malaise, muscle weakness, and osteomalacia.

HOW SUPPLIED

Maalox® Cooling Mint Suspension is available in plastic bottles of 5 oz (0067-0330-62), 12 oz (0067-0330-71) and 26 oz (0067-0330-44).
Maalox® Smooth Cherry Suspension is available in plastic bottles of 12 oz (0067-0331-71) and 26 oz (0067-0331-44).
Maalox® Refreshing Lemon Suspension is available in plastic bottles of 12 oz (0067-0222-71) and 26 oz (0067-0222-44).

MAXIMUM STRENGTH MAALOX® ANTACID/ANTI-GAS OTC

Alumina, Magnesia and Simethicone Oral Suspensions, Antacid/Anti-Gas

- ☐ **Refreshing Lemon**
  Smooth Cherry
  Cooling Mint
- ☐ **Physician-proven Maalox® formula for antacid effectiveness.**
- ☐ **Simethicone, at a recognized clinical dose, for antiflatulent action.**

DESCRIPTION

Maximum Strength Maalox® Antacid/Anti-Gas, a balanced combination of magnesium and aluminum hydroxides plus simethicone, is a non-constipating antacid/anti-gas product to provide symptomatic relief of acid indigestion, heartburn, symptoms referred to as gas and sour stomach associated with these symptoms. Available in suspensions in Refreshing Lemon, Smooth Cherry, and Cooling Mint flavors.

COMPOSITION

To provide symptomatic relief of hyperacidity plus alleviation of gas symptoms, each teaspoonful contains:

Maximum Strength Maalox® Antacid/Anti-Gas	
Active Ingredients	Per Tsp. (5 mL)
Magnesium Hydroxide	450 mg
Aluminum Hydroxide (equivalent to dried gel, USP)	500 mg
Simethicone	40 mg

INACTIVE INGREDIENTS

Suspensions: Calcium Saccharin, FD&C Red No. 40 (Smooth Cherry only), Flavors, Guar Gum, Methylparaben, Propylparaben, Purified Water, and Sorbitol.

DIRECTIONS FOR USE

Suspensions; 2 to 4 teaspoonfuls, 4 times per day, or as directed by a physician.

PATIENT WARNINGS

Do not take more than 12 teaspoonfuls in a 24-hour period or use the maximum dosage for more than 2 weeks or use if you have kidney disease except under the advice and supervision of a physician. Keep this and all drugs out of the reach of children.

DRUG INTERACTION PRECAUTION

Antacids may interact with certain prescription drugs. If you are presently taking a prescription drug, do not take this product without checking with your physician or other health professional.
To aid in establishing proper dosage schedules, the following information is provided:

Minimum Recommended Dosage: Maximum Strength Maalox® Antacid/Anti-Gas	
	Per 2 Tsp. (10 mL)
Acid neutralizing capacity	59.6 mEq
Sodium content*	<2.5 mg

*Dietetically insignificant.

Professional Labeling

INDICATIONS

As an antacid for symptomatic relief of hyperacidity associated with the diagnosis of peptic ulcer, gastritis, peptic esophagitis, gastric hyperacidity, heartburn, or hiatal hernia. As an antiflatulent to alleviate the symptoms of gas, including postoperative gas pain.

ADVANTAGES

Among antacids, Maximum Strength Maalox® Antacid/Anti-Gas Suspension is uniquely palatable—an important feature which encourages patients to follow your dosage directions. Maximum Strength Maalox® Antacid/Anti-Gas Suspension has the time-proven, nonconstipating, very low sodium* Maalox® formula—useful for those patients suffering from the problems associated with hyperacidity. Additionally, Maximum Strength Maalox® Antacid/Anti-Gas Suspension contains simethicone to relieve symptoms referred to as gas.
*Dietetically insignificant.

WARNINGS

Prolonged use of aluminum-containing antacids in patients with renal failure may result in or worsen dialysis osteomalacia. Elevated tissue aluminum levels contribute to the development of the dialysis encephalopathy and osteomalacia syndromes. Small amounts of aluminum are absorbed from the gastrointestinal tract and renal excretion of aluminum is impaired in renal failure. Aluminum is not well removed by dialysis because it is bound to albumin and transferrin, which do not cross dialysis membranes. As a result, aluminum is deposited in bone, and dialysis osteomalacia may develop when large amounts of aluminum are ingested orally by patients with impaired renal function.
Aluminum forms insoluble complexes with phosphate in the gastrointestinal tract, thus decreasing phosphate absorption. Prolonged use of aluminum-containing antacids by normophosphatemic patients may result in hypophosphatemia if phosphate intake is not adequate. In its more severe forms, hypophosphatemia can lead to anorexia, malaise, muscle weakness, and osteomalacia.

HOW SUPPLIED

Maximum Strength Maalox® Antacid/Anti-Gas Suspensions

Available in Refreshing Lemon in the following sizes: 5 fl. oz. (148 mL) (0067-0333-62), 12 fl. oz. (355 mL) (0067-0333-71) and 26 fl. oz. (769 mL) (0067-0333-44).
Smooth Cherry is available in plastic bottles of 12 fl. oz. (355 mL) (0067-0336-71) and 26 fl. oz. (769 mL) (0067-0336-44).
Cooling Mint is available in plastic bottles of 12 fl. oz. (355 mL) (0067-0338-71) and 26 fl. oz. (769 mL) (0067-0338-44).

Quick Dissolve MAALOX® Antacid OTC
Calcium Carbonate Chewable Antacid Tablets
Regular Strength and Maximum Strength
Lemon, Wild Berry, and Wintergreen Flavors
Fast Dissolving Tablets

DESCRIPTION

Quick Dissolve Maalox® Antacid Calcium Carbonate Chewable Tablets have a unique form that dissolves quickly to relieve heartburn, acid indigestion, and sour stomach fast.

COMPOSITION

To provide symptomatic relief of hyperacidity, each Quick Dissolve Maalox® Antacid Calcium Carbonate Tablets contains:

ACTIVE INGREDIENTS

Regular Strength—600 mg Calcium Carbonate
Maximum Strength—1000 mg Calcium Carbonate
The acid neutralizing capacity (per minimum recommended dosage) for Regular Strength is 21.6 mEq; for Maximum Strength, 18 mEq.

INACTIVE INGREDIENTS

Aspartame colloidal silicon dioxide, croscarmellose sodium, dextrose, flavors, magnesium stearate, maltodextrin, mannitol, pregelatinized starch. Depending on the flavor may also contain Blue #1 lake. Red #30 lake and or Yellow #10 lake.
Sodium Content: 1 mg per tablet for Regular Strength; 2 mg per tablet for Maximum Strength.

DIRECTIONS FOR USE

Regular Strength—Chew 2 to 4 tablets as symptoms occur or as directed by a physician. Maximum Strength—Chew 1 to 2 tablets as symptoms occur or as directed by a physician.

PATIENT WARNINGS

Do not take more than 12 (8 Maximum Strength) tablets in a 24-hour period or use the maximum dosage for more than 2 weeks except under the advice and supervision of a physician.
Keep out of reach of children.
Phenylketonurics: Contains Phenylalanine .5 mg Per Tablet (.9 mg per Tablet for Maximum Strength)

DRUG INTERACTION PRECAUTION

Ask doctor before use if you are presently taking a prescription drug.

ADVANTAGES

Quick Dissolve Maalox® Calcium Carbonate Antacid Tablets have a unique form that dissolves quickly to relieve heartburn fast.

HOW SUPPLIED

Quick Dissolve Maalox® Antacid Calcium Carbonate Tablets are available in plastic bottles of 45, 85 and 145 tablets (Regular Strength) and 35, 65 and 90 tablets (Maximum Strength).
Wild Berry flavored tablets are not available in the larger sizes. Wintergreen flavored tablets are not available in the smaller sizes. Lemon flavored tablets are available in 45 and 85 tablet sizes (Regular Strength) and 35 and 65 tablet sizes (Maximum Strength.) Assorted flavored tablets are available in 45, 85 and 145 tablet sizes (Regular Strength) and 35, 65 and 90 tablet sizes (Maximum Strength). Regular Strength 3-roll packs of 30 tablets are also available in Lemon and Assorted flavors.

Fiber Therapy PERDIEM® OTC

Psyllium Fiber

DESCRIPTION

Fiber Therapy Perdiem contains a 100% natural bulk-forming fiber that gently helps relieve occasional constipation (irregularity). Fiber Therapy Perdiem contains no synthetic stimulants. Perdiem's unique form is easy to swallow and requires no mixing. Fiber Therapy Perdiem generally takes effect within 12 to 72 hours.

Continued on next page

Perdiem—Cont.

INDICATIONS

For relief of occasional constipation. This product generally produces bowel movement in 12 to 72 hours.

ACTIVE INGREDIENTS

100% psyllium (Plantago hydrocolloid).

Each rounded (6 gm) teaspoon contains:

4.03 gm psyllium, 36.1 mg potassium and 1.80 mg sodium.

Only 4 Calories

INACTIVE INGREDIENTS

Acacia, iron oxides, natural flavors, paraffin, sucrose, talc, titanium dioxide.

DIRECTIONS FOR USE

Perdiem requires no mixing in liquids for use.

TAKE THIS PRODUCT (CHILD OR ADULT DOSE) WITH AT LEAST 8 OUNCES (A FULL GLASS) OF COOL WATER OR OTHER FLUID. TAKING THIS PRODUCT WITHOUT ENOUGH LIQUID MAY CAUSE CHOKING. (SEE WARNINGS.)

Adults and Children 12 Years and Older: In the evening and/or before breakfast, 1 to 2 rounded teaspoonfuls one to two times daily should be placed in the mouth and swallowed with at least 8 oz. of cool liquid.

Children 7 to 11 Years Old: One rounded teaspoonful one to two times daily with at least 8 oz. of cool liquid. Perdiem is not intended for use in children under the age of 7 years.

For Severe Cases of Constipation: Perdiem may be taken more frequently, up to 2 rounded teaspoonfuls every 6 hours not to exceed 5 teaspoonfuls in a 24-hour period.

PERDIEM SHOULD NOT BE CHEWED.

WARNINGS

TAKING THIS PRODUCT WITHOUT ADEQUATE FLUID MAY CAUSE IT TO SWELL AND BLOCK THE THROAT OR ESOPHAGUS AND MAY CAUSE CHOKING. DO NOT TAKE THIS PRODUCT IF YOU HAVE DIFFICULTY IN SWALLOWING. IF YOU EXPERIENCE CHEST PAIN, VOMITING OR DIFFICULTY IN SWALLOWING OR BREATHING AFTER TAKING THIS PRODUCT, SEEK IMMEDIATE MEDICAL ATTENTION.

People with esophageal narrowing should not use bulk-forming agents.

If you have noticed a sudden change in bowel habits that persists over a two-week period, consult a doctor before using any laxative product.

If use of this product for constipation has produced no effect within one week or if rectal bleeding occurs after use of any bulk fiber or laxative, discontinue use and consult a doctor.

Do not use if you have a history of psyllium allergy or experience abdominal pain, nausea or vomiting unless directed by a doctor.

HOW SUPPLIED

250 gm (8.8 oz.) canisters (NDC 0067-0795-70)

Overnight Relief PERDIEM® OTC
100% Natural Bulk Fiber Plus Vegetable Laxative

DESCRIPTION

Overnight Relief Perdiem is a unique combination of natural bulk-forming psyllium fiber plus a natural senna laxative. Perdiem's unique combination of ingredients provides gentle, predictable overnight relief of constipation without synthetic laxative ingredients. Perdiem's unique form is easy to swallow, has a great mint taste and requires no mixing. Overnight Relief Perdiem generally takes effect within 12 hours, so you can depend on it to work overnight.

INDICATIONS

For relief of occasional constipation. This product generally produces bowel movement within 12 hours.

ACTIVE INGREDIENTS

82% psyllium (Plantago hydrocolloid) and 18% senna (Cassia Pod Concentrate).

Each rounded (6 gm) teaspoonful contains:

3.25 gm psyllium, 0.74 gm senna, 35.5 mg potassium and 1.8 mg sodium.

Only 4 Calories

INACTIVE INGREDIENTS

Acacia, iron oxides, natural flavors, paraffin, sucrose, talc.

DIRECTIONS FOR USE

Perdiem requires no mixing in liquids for use.

TAKE THIS PRODUCT (CHILD OR ADULT DOSE) WITH AT LEAST 8 OUNCES (A FULL GLASS) OF COOL WATER OR OTHER FLUID. TAKING THIS PRODUCT WITHOUT ENOUGH LIQUID MAY CAUSE CHOKING. (SEE WARNINGS.)

Adults and Children 12 Years and Older: In the evening and/or before breakfast, 1 to 2 rounded teaspoonfuls one to two times daily should be placed in the mouth and swallowed with at least 8 oz. of cool liquid.

Children 7 to 11 Years Old: One rounded teaspoonful one to two times daily with at least 8 oz. of cool liquid.

Perdiem is not intended for use in children under the age of 7 years.

For Severe Cases of Constipation: Perdiem may be taken more frequently, up to 2 rounded teaspoonfuls every 6 hours not to exceed 5 teaspoonfuls in a 24-hour period.

PERDIEM SHOULD NOT BE CHEWED.

PRECAUTIONS

Pregnancy category B. Results from limited animal reproduction studies have not demonstrated a risk to the fetus. However, because there are not adequate and well-controlled studies in pregnant women, this product should be used during pregnancy only if clearly needed.

WARNINGS

TAKING THIS PRODUCT WITHOUT ADEQUATE FLUID MAY CAUSE IT TO SWELL AND BLOCK THE THROAT OR ESOPHAGUS AND MAY CAUSE CHOKING. DO NOT TAKE THIS PRODUCT IF YOU HAVE DIFFICULTY IN SWALLOWING. IF YOU EXPERIENCE CHEST PAIN, VOMITING OR DIFFICULTY IN SWALLOWING OR BREATHING AFTER TAKING THIS PRODUCT, SEEK IMMEDIATE MEDICAL ATTENTION.

People with esophageal narrowing should not use bulk-forming agents.

If you have noticed a sudden change in bowel habits that persists over a two-week period, consult a doctor before using any laxative product.

If use of this product for constipation has produced no effect within one week or if rectal bleeding occurs after use of any bulk fiber or laxative, discontinue use and consult a doctor.

Do not use if you have a history of psyllium allergy or experience abdominal pain, nausea or vomiting unless directed by a doctor.

HOW SUPPLIED

400 gm (14 oz.) canisters (NDC 0067-0690-39)
250 gm (8.8 oz.) canisters (NDC 0067-0690-70)

TAVIST•D® Tablets and Caplets OTC
12 Hour Relief
Antihistamine/Nasal Decongestant

(See PDR For Nonprescription Drugs and Dietary Supplements)

TAVIST® Allergy (Formerly Tavist•1®) Tablets OTC
12 Hour Relief
Antihistamine

(See PDR for Nonprescription Drugs and Dietary Supplements)

TAVIST® Sinus Caplets OTC
Relief of Sinus Symptoms
Analgesic (Pain Reliever)/Nasal Decongestant

(See PDR for Nonprescription Drugs)

THERAFLU® OTC

- Flu and Cold *Original Formula* Hot Liquid Medicine
- Flu, Cold & Cough *Original Formula* Hot Liquid Medicine
- Maximum Strength Flu, Cold & Cough *NightTime* Hot Liquid Medicine
- Maximum Strength Flu, Cold & Cough *No Drowsiness* Hot Liquid Medicine
- Maximum Strength Flu and Cold *Sore Throat* Hot Liquid Medicine
- Maximum Strength Flu, Cold & Cough *Sore Throat & Cough* Hot Liquid Medicine
- Maximum Strength Flu, Cold & Cough *Chest Congestion and Cough* Hot Liquid Medicine
- Maximum Strength Flu, Cold & Cough *Non-Drowsy* Caplets
- Maximum Strength Flu, Cold & Cough *NightTime* Caplets

(See PDR for Nonprescription Drugs and Dietary Supplements)

TRIAMINIC® ALLERGY OTC
(formerly AM Decongestion)

(See PDR for Nonprescription Drugs and Dietary Supplements)

TRIAMINIC® CHEST CONGESTION OTC
(formerly Expectorant)

(See PDR for Nonprescription Drugs and Dietary Supplements)

TRIAMINIC COLD & ALLERGY OTC
(formerly Syrup)

(See PDR for Nonprescription Drugs and Dietary Supplements)

TRIAMINIC® COLD & COUGH OTC
(formerly Triaminicol)

(See PDR for Nonprescription Drugs and Dietary Supplements)

TRIAMINIC® COLD & NIGHTTIME COUGH OTC

(See PDR for Nonprescription Drugs and Dietary Supplements)

TRIAMINIC® COLD, COUGH & FEVER OTC
(formerly Severe Cold & Fever)

(See PDR for Nonprescription Drugs and Dietary Supplements)

TRIAMINIC® COUGH OTC
(Formerly DM)

(See PDR for Nonprescription Drugs and Dietary Supplements)

TRIAMINIC® COUGH & CONGESTION OTC
(formerly AM Cough and Decongestant)

(See PDR for Nonprescription Drugs and Dietary Supplements)

TRIAMINIC® COUGH & SORE THROAT OTC
(formerly SORE THROAT)

(See PDR for Nonprescription Drugs and Dietary Supplements)

TRIAMINIC® SOFTCHEWS COLD & ALLERGY OTC

(See PDR for Nonprescription Drugs and Dietary Supplements)

TRIAMINIC® SOFTCHEWS COLD & COUGH OTC

(See PDR for Nonprescription Drugs and Dietary Supplements)

TRIAMINIC® SOFTCHEWS COUGH OTC

(See PDR for Nonprescription Drugs and Dietary Supplements)

TRIAMINIC® SOFTCHEWS COUGH & SORE THROAT OTC

(See PDR for Nonprescription Drugs and Dietary Supplements)

TRIAMINIC VAPOR PATCH COUGH, CHERRY OTC

(See PDR for Nonprescription Drugs and Dietary Supplements)

TRIAMINIC VAPOR PATCH COUGH, MENTHOL OTC

(See PDR for Nonprescription Drugs and Dietary Supplements)

TRANSDERM SCŌP® ℞
[*trans-derm scōpe*]
scopolamine 1.5 mg

Transdermal Therapeutic System

Programmed to deliver *in-vivo* approximately 1.0 mg of scopolamine over 3 days

DESCRIPTION

The Transderm Scōp (transdermal scopolamine) system is a circular flat patch designed for continuous release of scopolamine following application to an area of intact skin on the head, behind the ear. Each system contains 1.5 mg of scopolamine base. Scopolamine is α-(hydroxymethyl) benzeneacetic acid 9-methyl-3-oxa-9-azatricyclo [3.3.1.0^{2,4}] non-7-yl ester. The empirical formula is $C_{17}H_{21}NO_4$ and its structural formula is

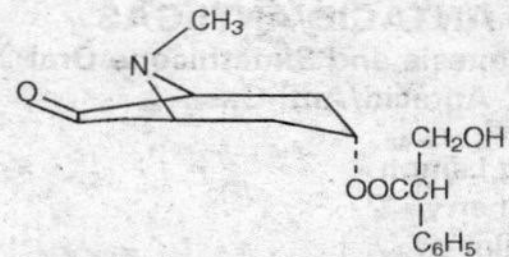

Scopolamine is a viscous liquid that has a molecular weight of 303.35 and a pKa of 7.55–7.81. The Transderm Scōp system is a film 0.2 mm thick and 2.5 cm², with four layers. Proceeding from the visible surface towards the surface attached to the skin, these layers are: (1) a backing layer of tan-colored, aluminized, polyester film; (2) a drug reservoir of scopolamine, light mineral oil, and polyisobutylene; (3) a microporous polypropylene membrane that controls the rate of delivery of scopolamine from the system to the skin surface; and (4) an adhesive formulation of mineral oil, polyisobutylene, and scopolamine. A protective peel strip of siliconized polyester, which covers the adhesive layer, is removed before the system is used. The inactive components, light mineral oil (12.4 mg) and polyisobutylene (11.4 mg), are not released from the system.

Cross section of the system:

Backing Layer
Drug Reservoir
Rate-Controlling Membrane
Contact Adhesive
Protective Peel Strip

CLINICAL PHARMACOLOGY

Pharmacology

The sole active agent of Transderm Scōp is scopolamine, a belladonna alkaloid with well-known pharmacological properties. It is an anticholinergic agent which acts: i) as a competitive inhibitor at postganglionic muscarinic receptor sites of the parasympathetic nervous system, and ii) on smooth muscles that respond to acetylcholine but lack cholinergic innervation. It has been suggested that scopolamine acts in the central nervous system (CNS) by blocking cholinergic transmission from the vestibular nuclei to higher centers in the CNS and from the reticular formation to the vomiting center[1,2]. Scopolamine can inhibit the secretion of saliva and sweat, decrease gastrointestinal secretions and motility, cause drowsiness, dilate the pupils, increase heart rate, and depress motor function[2].

Pharmacokinetics

Scopolamine's activity is due to the parent drug. The pharmacokinetics of scopolamine delivered via the system are due to the characteristics of both the drug and dosage form. The system is programmed to deliver *in-vivo* approximately 1.0 mg of scopolamine at an approximately constant rate to the systemic circulation over 3 days. Upon application to the post-auricular skin, an initial priming dose of scopolamine is released from the adhesive layer to saturate skin binding sites. The subsequent delivery of scopolamine to the blood is determined by the rate controlling membrane and is designed to produce stable plasma levels in a therapeutic range. Following removal of the used system, there is some degree of continued systemic absorption of scopolamine bound in the skin layers.

Absorption: Scopolamine is well-absorbed percutaneously. Following application to the skin behind the ear, circulating plasma levels are detected within 4 hours with peak levels being obtained, on average, within 24 hours. The average plasma concentration produced is 87 pg/mL for free scopolamine and 354 pg/mL for total scopolamine (free + conjugates).

Distribution: The distribution of scopolamine is not well characterized. It crosses the placenta and the blood brain barrier and may be reversibly bound to plasma proteins.

Metabolism: Although not well characterized, scopolamine is extensively metabolized and conjugated with less than 5% of the total dose appearing unchanged in the urine.

Elimination: The exact elimination pattern of scopolamine has not been determined. Following patch removal, plasma levels decline in a log linear fashion with an observed half-life of 9.5 hours. Less than 10% of the total dose is excreted in the urine as parent and metabolites over 108 hours.

Clinical Results: In 195 adult subjects of different racial origins who participated in clinical efficacy studies at sea or in a controlled motion environment, there was a 75% reduction in the incidence of motion-induced nausea and vomiting[3]. Transderm Scōp provided significantly greater protection than that obtained with oral dimenhydrinate.

In two pivotal clinical efficacy studies in 391 adult female patients undergoing cesarean section or gynecological surgery with anesthesia and opiate analgesia, 66% of those treated with Transderm Scōp (compared to only 46% of those receiving placebo) reported no retching/vomiting within the 24-hour period following administration of anesthesia/opiate analgesia. When the need for additional antiemetic medication was assessed during the same period, there was no need for medication in 76% of patients treated with Transderm Scōp as compared to 59% of placebo-treated patients[5,6].

INDICATIONS AND USAGE

Transderm Scōp is indicated in adults for prevention of nausea and vomiting associated with motion sickness and recovery from anesthesia and surgery. The patch should be applied only to skin in the postauricular area.

CONTRAINDICATIONS

Transderm Scōp is contraindicated in persons who are hypersensitive to the drug scopolamine or to other belladonna alkaloids, or to any ingredient or component in the formulation or delivery system, or in patients with angle-closure (narrow angle) glaucoma.

WARNINGS

Glaucoma therapy in patients with chronic open-angle (wide-angle) glaucoma should be monitored and may need to be adjusted during Transderm Scōp use, as the mydriatic effect of scopolamine may cause an increase in intraocular pressure.

Transderm Scōp should not be used in children and should be used with caution in the elderly. See PRECAUTIONS.

Since drowsiness, disorientation, and confusion may occur with the use of scopolamine, patients should be warned of the possibility and cautioned against engaging in activities that require mental alertness, such as driving a motor vehicle or operating dangerous machinery.

Rarely, idiosyncratic reactions may occur with ordinary therapeutic doses of scopolamine. The most serious of these that have been reported are: acute toxic psychosis, including confusion, agitation, rambling speech, hallucinations, paranoid behaviors, and delusions.

PRECAUTIONS

General

Scopolamine should be used with caution in patients with pyloric obstruction or urinary bladder neck obstruction. Caution should be exercised when administering and antiemetic or antimuscarinic drug to patients suspected of having intestinal obstruction.

Transderm Scōp should be used with caution in the elderly or in individuals with impaired liver or kidney functions because of the increased likelihood of CNS effects.

Caution should be exercised in patients with a history of seizures or psychosis, since scopolamine can potentially aggravate both disorders.

Information for Patients

Since scopolamine can cause temporary dilation of the pupils and blurred vision if it comes in contact with the eyes, patients should be strongly advised to wash their hands thoroughly with soap and water immediately after handling the patch. In addition, it is important that used patches be disposed of properly to avoid contact with children or pets. Patients should be advised to remove the patch immediately and promptly contact a physician in the unlikely event that they experience symptoms of acute narrow-angle glaucoma (pain and reddening of the eyes, accompanied by dilated pupils). Patients should also be instructed to remove the patch if they develop any difficulties in urinating.

Patients who expect to participate in underwater sports should be cautioned regarding the potentially disorienting effects of scopolamine. A patient brochure is available.

Drug Interactions

The absorption of oral medications may be decreased during the concurrent use of scopolamine because of decreased gastric motility and delayed gastric emptying.

Scopolamine should be used with care in patients taking other drugs that are capable of causing CNS effects such as sedatives, tranquilizers, or alcohol. Special attention should be paid to potential interactions with drugs having anticholinergic properties; e.g., other belladonna alkaloids, antihistamines (including meclizine), tricyclic antidepressants, and muscle relaxants.

Laboratory Test Interactions

Scopolamine will interfere with the gastric secretion test.

Carcinogenesis, Mutagenesis, Impairment of Fertility

No long-term studies in animals have been completed to evaluate the carcinogenic potential of scopolamine. The mutagenic potential of scopolamine has not been evaluated. Fertility studies were performed in female rats and revealed no evidence of impaired fertility or harm to the fetus due to scopolamine hydrobromide administered by daily subcutaneous injection. Maternal body weights were reduced in the highest-dose group (plasma level approximately 500 times the level achieved in humans using a transdermal system).

Pregnancy Category C

Teratogenic studies were performed in pregnant rats and rabbits with scopolamine hydrobromide administered by daily intravenous injection. No adverse effects were recorded in rats. Scopolamine hydrobromide has been shown to have a marginal embryotoxic effect in rabbits when administered by daily intravenous injection at doses producing plasma levels approximately 100 times the level achieved in humans using a transdermal system. During a clinical study among women undergoing cesarean section treated with Transderm Scōp in conjunction with epidural anesthesia and opiate analgesia, no evidence of CNS depression was found in the newborns. There are no other adequate and well-controlled studies in pregnant women. Other than in the adjunctive use for delivery by cesarean section, Transderm Scōp should be used in pregnancy only if the potential benefit justifies the potential risk to the fetus.

Nursing Mothers

Because scopolamine is excreted in human milk, caution should be exercised when Transderm Scōp is administered to a nursing woman.

Labor and Delivery

Scopolamine administered parenterally at higher doses than the dose delivered by Transderm Scōp does not increase the duration of labor, nor does it affect uterine contractions. Scopolamine does cross the placenta.

Pediatric Use

The safety and effectiveness of Transderm Scōp in children has not been established. Children are particularly susceptible to the side effects of belladonna alkaloids. Transderm Scōp should not be used in children because it is not known whether this system will release an amount of scopolamine that could produce serious adverse effects in children.

ADVERSE DRUG EXPERIENCES

The adverse reactions for Transderm Scōp are provided separately for patients with motion sickness and with post-operative nausea and vomiting.

Motion Sickness: In motion sickness clinical studies of Transderm Scōp, the most frequent adverse reaction was dryness of the mouth. This occurred in about two thirds of patients on drug. A less frequent adverse drug reaction was drowsiness, which occurred in less than one sixth of patients on drug. Transient impairment of eye accommodation, including blurred vision and dilation of the pupils, was also observed.

Post-operative Nausea and Vomiting: In a total of five clinical studies in which Transderm Scōp was administered perioperatively to a total of 461 patients and safety was assessed, dry mouth was the most frequently reported adverse drug experience, which occurred in approximately 29% of patients on drug. Dizziness was reported by approximately 12% of patients on drug[7].

Postmarketing and Other Experience: In addition to the adverse experiences reported during clinical testing of Transderm Scōp, the following are spontaneously reported adverse events from postmarketing experience. Because the reports cite events reported spontaneously from worldwide postmarketing experience, frequency of events and the role of Transderm Scōp in their causation cannot be reliably determined: acute angle-closure (narrow-angle) glaucoma; confusion; difficulty urinating; dry, itchy, or conjunctival injection of eyes; restlessness; hallucinations; memory disturbances; rashes and erythema; and transient changes in heart rate.

Drug Withdrawal/Post-Removal Symptoms: Symptoms such as dizziness, nausea, vomiting, and headache occur following abrupt discontinuation of antimuscarinics. Similar symptoms, including disturbances of equilibrium, have been reported in some patients following discontinuation of use of the Transderm Scōp system. These symptoms usually do not appear until 24 hours or more after the patch has been removed. Some symptoms may be related to adaptation from a motion environment to a motion-free environment. More serious symptoms including muscle weakness, bradycardia and hypotension may occur following discontinuation of Transderm Scōp.

OVERDOSAGE

Because strategies for the management of drug overdose continually evolve, it is strongly recommended that a poison control center be connected to obtain up-to-date information regarding the management of Transderm Scōp patch overdose. The prescriber should be mindful that antidotes used routinely in the past may no longer be considered optimal treatment. For example, physostigmine, used more or less routinely in the past, is seldom recommended for the routine management of anticholinergic syndromes.

Until up-to-date authoritative advice is obtained, routine supportive measures should be directed to maintaining adequate respiratory and cardiac function.

The signs and symptoms of anticholinergic toxicity include: lethargy, somnolence, coma, confusion, agitation, hallucinations, convulsion, visual disturbance, dry flushed skin, dry mouth, decreased bowel sounds, urinary retention, tachycardia, hypertension, and supraventricular arrhythmias.

Most cases of toxicity involving the use of the product will resolve with simple removal of the patch. Serious symptomatic cases of overdosage involving multiple patch applications and/or ingestion may be managed by initially ensuring the patient has an adequate airway, and supporting respiration and circulation. This should be rapidly followed by removal of all patches from the skin and the mouth. If there is evidence of patch ingestion, gastric lavage, endoscopic removal of swallowed patches, or administration of activated charcoal should be considered, as indicated by the clinical situation. In any case where there is serious overdosage or signs of evolving acute toxicity, continuous monitoring of vital signs and ECG, establishment of intravenous access, and administration of oxygen are all recommended. The symptoms of overdose/toxicity due to scopolamine should be carefully distinguished from the occasionally observed syndrome of withdrawal (see Drug Withdrawal/Post Removal Symptoms). Although mental confusion and dizziness may be observed with both acute toxicity and withdrawal, other characteristic findings differ: tachyarrhythmias, dry skin, and decreased bowel sounds suggest anticholinergic toxicity, while bradycardia, headache, nausea and abdominal cramps, and sweating suggest post-removal withdrawal. Obtaining a careful history is crucial to making the correct diagnosis.

DOSAGE AND ADMINISTRATION

Initiation of Therapy: To prevent the nausea and vomiting associated with motion sickness, one Transderm Scōp patch (programmed to deliver approximately 1.0 mg of scopolamine over 3 days) should be applied to the hairless area behind one ear at least 4 hours before the antiemetic effect is required. To prevent post operative nausea and vomiting, the patch should be applied the evening before scheduled surgery. To minimize exposure of the newborn baby to the drug, apply the patch one hour prior to cesarean section. Only one patch should be worn at any time. Do not cut the patch.

Handling: After the patch is applied on dry skin behind the ear, the hands should be washed thoroughly with soap and water and dried. Upon removal, the patch should be discarded. To prevent any traces of scopolamine from coming

Continued on next page

Transderm Scōp—Cont.

into direct contact with the eyes, the hands and the application site should be washed thoroughly with soap and water and dried. (A patient brochure is available).

Continuation of Therapy: Should the patch become displaced, it should be discarded, and a fresh one placed on the hairless area behind the other ear. For motion sickness, if therapy is required for longer than 3 days, the first patch should be removed and a fresh one placed on the hairless area behind the other ear. For perioperative use, the patch should be kept in place for 24 hours following surgery at which time it should be removed and discarded.

HOW SUPPLIED

The Transderm Scōp system is a tan-colored circular patch, 2.5 cm^2, on a clear, oversized, hexagonal peel strip, which is removed prior to use.

Each Transderm Scōp system contains 1.5 mg of scopolamine and is programmed to deliver *in-vivo* approximately 1.0 mg of scopolamine over 3 days. Transderm Scōp is available in packages of four patches. Each patch is foil wrapped. Patient instructions are included.

1 Package (4 patches) NDC 0067-4345-04

The system should be stored at controlled room temperature between 20°C and 25°C (68°F and 77°F).

CAUTION

Federal law prohibits dispensing without prescription.

REFERENCES

1. McEvoy, G.K. (ed.); AHSF Drug Information; American Society of Hospital Pharmacists, Bethesda, MD, pp. 608–611 (1990).
2. Gilman, A.G. et al (ed.); The pharmacological Basis of Therapeutics (8th Ed.); Pergamon Press, New York, NY, pp. 150–165 (1990).
3. Clissold, S.P. et al; "Transdermal Hyoscine (Scopolamine), A Preliminary Review of its Pharmacodynamic Properties and Therapeutic Efficacy", Drugs, 29: 189–207 (1985).
4. Pharmacokinetic clinical data on file.
5. Kotelko, D.M. et al; "Transdermal scopolamine decreases nausea and vomiting following cesarean section in patients receiving epidural morphine". Anesthesiology 71(5): 675–678 (1989).
6. Bailey, P.L. et al; "Transdermal scopolamine reduces nausea and vomiting after outpatient laparoscopy". Anesthesiology 72(6): 977–980 (1990).
7. Clinical safety data on file.

Mfd by: ALZA Corporation
Palo Alto, CA 94303-0802
Distributed by:
Novartis Consumer Health, Inc.
Summit, New Jersey 07901-1312

66659C (Rev. 4/98)

Please read this instruction sheet carefully before opening the system package.

Information for the Patient

TRANSDERM SCŌP®

Generic Name: scopolamine, pronounced skoe-POL-a-meen

Transdermal Therapeutic System

The Transderm Scōp system helps to prevent the nausea and vomiting of motion sickness for up to 3 days. It is a round adhesive patch that you place behind your ear several hours before you travel. It also helps to prevent the nausea and vomiting associated with the use of anesthesia and certain analgesics used during or after many types of surgery. If the patch is to be used in conjunction with schedule surgery, it is applied the evening before surgery. For cesarean section, the patch is applied one hour prior to surgery to minimize exposure of the unborn child to the drug. Wear only one patch at any time.

Be sure to wash your hands thoroughly with soap and water immediately after handling the patch, so that any drug that might get on your hands will not come into contact with your eyes.

Avoid drinking alcohol while using Transderm Scōp. Also, be careful about driving or operating any machinery while using the system because the drug might make you drowsy.

DO NOT USE TRANSDERM SCŌP IF YOU ARE ALLERGIC TO SCOPOLAMINE

TRANSDERM SCŌP SHOULD NOT BE USED IN CHILDREN AND SHOULD BE USED WITH CAUTION IN THE ELDERLY.

How The Transderm Scōp System Works

A group of nerve fibers deep inside the ear helps people keep their balance. For some people, the motion of ships, airplanes, trains, automobiles, and buses increases the activity of these nerve fibers. This increased activity causes the dizziness, nausea, and vomiting of motion sickness. People may have one, some, or all of these symptoms.

Transderm Scōp contains the drug scopolamine, which helps reduce the acitivity of the nerve fibers in the inner ear. When a Transderm Scōp patch is placed on the skin behind one of the ears, scopolamine passes through the skin and into the bloodstream. One patch may be kept in place for 3 days if needed.

It has been suggested that Transderm Scōp when used to reduce nausea and vomiting associated with surgical anesthesia or analgesia, acts on the same nerve fibers that are affected when the product is taken for motion sickness.

Precautions

Before using Transderm Scōp be sure to tell your doctor if you:

- Are pregnant or nursing (or plan to become pregnant)
- Have (or have had) glaucoma (increased pressure in the eyeball) or a predisposition to glaucoma
- Have (or have had) any metabolic, heart, liver, kidney, or other serious medical conditions
- Have any obstructions of the stomach or intestine
- Have any trouble urinating due to prostate enlargement or any bladder obstruction
- Have any allergy or have had a reaction such as a skin rash or redness to any drug, especially scopolamine, or chemical or food substance

Any of these conditions could make Transderm Scōp unsuitable for you. Also tell your doctor if you are taking any other medicines.

In the unlikely event that you experience pain in the eye and reddened whites of the eye while wearing the patch, which may be accompanied by widening of the pupil and blurred vision, remove the patch immediately and consult your doctor. As indicated below under **Side Effects**, widening of the pupils and blurred vision without pain or reddened whites of the eye is usually temporary and not serious.

Transderm Scōp should not be used in children. The safety of its use in children has not been determined. Children and the elderly may be particularly sensitive to the effects of scopolamine.

Side Effects

The most common side effect experienced by people using Transderm Scōp is dryness of the mouth. This occurs in about two thirds of the people. A less frequent side effect is drowsiness, which occurs in less than one sixth of the people. Temporary blurring or vision and dilation (widening) of the pupils may occur, especially if the drug is on your hands and comes in contact with the eyes. On infrequent occasions, disorientation, memory disturbances, dizziness, restlessness, hallucinations, confusion, difficulty urinating, skin rashes or redness, temporary changes in heart rate such as palpitations, dry itchy, or reddened whites of the eyes, and eye pain have been reported. If these effects do occur, remove the patch and call your doctor. Since drowsiness, disorientation, and confusion may occur with the use of scopolamine, be careful driving or operating any dangerous machinery, especially when you first start using the drug system.

In addition, if you plan to participate in underwater sports while wearing the patch, you should discuss with your doctor the potentially disorienting effects of scopolamine.

Eye Effects: Temporary blurring of vision and dilation (widening) of the pupils may occur, especially if the drug is on your fingers or hands and comes into contact with the eyes. Dry, itchy, or reddened whites of the eye and eye pain have been reported infrequently. In the unlikely event that you experience pain in the eye and reddened whites of the eye, which may be accompanied by widening of the pupil and blurred vision, remove the patch and consult your doctor promptly. Widening of the pupils and blurred vision without pain, or reddened whites of the eye, is usually temporary and not serious.

Drug Withdrawal/Post-Removal Symptoms: Symptoms such as dizziness, nausea, vomiting, headache, and disturbances of equilibrium have been reported by some people following discontinuation of use of the Transderm Scōp patch. These symptoms have occurred most often in people who have used the patches for more than 3 days, and frequently do not appear until 24 hours or more after the patch has been removed. These symptoms may be associated with adaptation from a motion environment to a motion-free environment. It is recommended that you consult with your doctor if these symptoms persist.

How to Use Transderm Scōp

Transderm Scōp should be stored at controlled room temperature between 20°C and 25°C (68°F and 77°F) until you are ready to use it.

1. For the prevention of motion sickness, plan to apply one Transderm Scōp patch at least 4 hours before you need it. If the patch is to be used in conjunction with scheduled surgery, it is applied the evening before surgery. For cesarean section, the patch is applied one hour prior to surgery to minimize exposure of the unborn child to the drug. **Wear only one patch at any time.** Do not cut the patch.
2. Select a hairless area of skin behind one ear, taking care to avoid any cuts or irritations. Wipe the area with a clean, dry tissue.
3. Peel the package open and remove the patch (Figure 1).

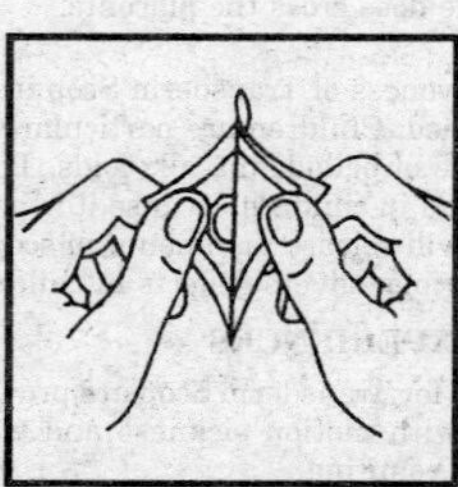

(Figure 1)

4. Remove the clear plastic six-sided backing from the round patch. Try not to touch the adhesive surface on the patch with your hands (Figure 2).

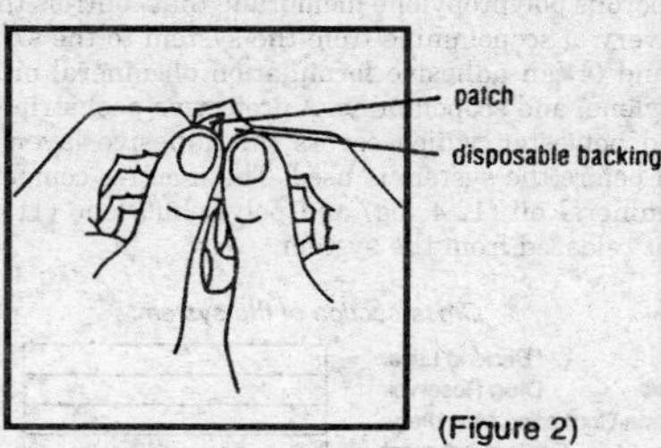

(Figure 2)

5. Firmly apply the adhesive surface (metallic side) to the dry area of skin behind the ear so that the tan-colored side is showing (Figure 3). Make good contact, especially around the edge. Once you have placed the patch behind your ear, do not move it for as long as you want to use it (e.g., up to 3 days for prevention of motion sickness).

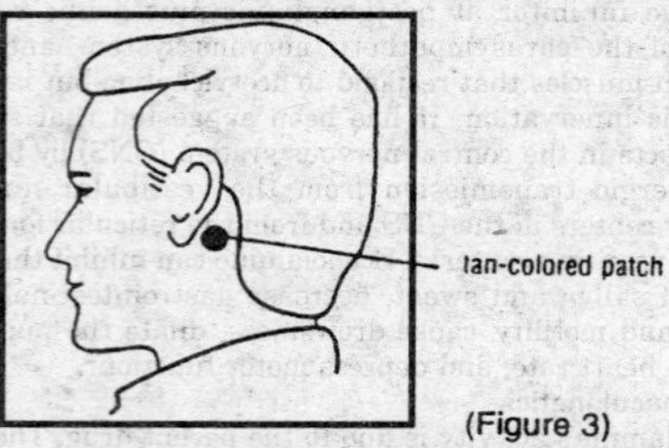

(Figure 3)

6. ***Important:* After the patch is in place, be sure to wash your hands thoroughly with soap and water to remove any scopolamine. If this drug were to come into contact with your eyes, it could cause temporary blurring of vision and dilation (widening) of the pupils (the dark circles in the center of your eyes). Unless accompanied by eye pain and reddened whites of the eyes (see Precautions), this is not serious and your pupils should return to normal.**
7. If the patch is being used to prevent the nausea and vomiting of motion sickness, remove the patch after 3 days and throw it away. (You may remove it sooner if you are no longer concerned about motion sickness). If the patch is being used to prevent nausea and vomiting associated with anesthesia or analgesia, the patch should be kept in place for 24 hours following surgery at which time it should be removed and discarded. After removing the patch, be sure to wash your hands and the area behind your ear thoroughly with soap and water. Since the patch will still contain some active ingredient after use, and to avoid accidental contact or ingestion by children or pets, fold the used patch in half with the sticky side together and dispose in the trash out of the reach of children and pets.
8. If you wish to control the nausea and vomiting of motion sickness for longer than 3 days, remove the first patch after 3 days and place a new one behind the other ear, repeating instructions 2 through 7.
9. Keep the patch dry, if possible, to prevent it from falling off. Limited contact with water, however, as in bathing or swimming, will not affect the system. In the unlikely event that the patch falls off, throw it away and put a new one behind the other ear.
10. Please inform your doctor if you are taking other medications, including over-the-counter medications.

This leaflet presents a summary of information about Transderm Scōp. If you would like more information or if you have any questions, ask your doctor or pharmacist. A more technical leaflet is available, written for your doctor. If you would like to read the leaflet, ask your pharmacist to show you a copy. You may need the help of your doctor or pharmacist to understand some of the information.

Mfd. by: ALZA Corporation
Palo Alto, CA 94303-0802
Distributed by:
Novartis Consumer Health, Inc.
Summit, NJ 07901-1312

66658C Printed in U.S.A. (Rev. 4/98)

Shown in Product Identification Guide, page 325

For information on over-the-counter drugs, consult **PDR For Nonprescription Drugs.**

Novartis Pharmaceuticals Corporation

NOVARTIS PHARMACEUTICALS CORPORATION
59 Route 10
East Hanover, NJ 07936
(for branded products)

GENEVA PHARMACEUTICALS, INC.
A NOVARTIS COMPANY
2655 West Midway Boulevard
PO Box 446
Broomfield, CO 80038-0446
(for branded generic product listing refer to Geneva Pharmaceuticals, Inc.)

For Information Contact (*branded products*):
Customer Response Department
(888) NOW-NOVARTIS [888-669-6682]

Global Internet Address:
http: //www.novartis.com

For Information Contact (*branded generic products*):
Customer Support Department
(800) 525-8747
(303) 466-2400
FAX: (303) 727-4656

APLIGRAF® ℞

[*ă-plĭ-grăf*]
(Graftskin)

The following prescribing information is based on official labeling in effect July 2000.

Caution: Federal law restricts this device to sale by or on the order of a physician (or properly licensed practitioner).

1. DEVICE DESCRIPTION

Apligraf is supplied as a living, bi-layered skin substitute: the epidermal layer is formed by human keratinocytes and has a well-differentiated stratum corneum; the dermal layer is composed of human fibroblasts in a bovine Type I collagen lattice. While matrix proteins and cytokines found in human skin are present in Apligraf, Apligraf does not contain Langerhans cells, melanocytes, macrophages, lymphocytes, blood vessels or hair follicles. In a 10 patient venous leg ulcer study to determine the longevity of Apligraf cells, 2 of 8 patients evaluated at 4 weeks demonstrated Apligraf DNA. Neither of these patients showed Apligraf DNA at 8 weeks. Apligraf is manufactured under aseptic conditions from human neonatal male foreskin tissue. The fibroblast and keratinocyte cell banks which are the source of the cells from which Apligraf is derived are tested for human and animal viruses, retroviruses, bacteria, fungi, yeast, mycoplasma, karyology, isoenzymes, and tumorigenicity. The final product is tested for morphology, cell viability, epidermal coverage, sterility, mycoplasma, and physical container integrity. Product manufacture also includes reagents derived from animal materials including bovine pituitary extract. All animal derived reagents are tested for viruses, retroviruses, bacteria, fungi, yeast, and mycoplasma before use, and all bovine material is obtained from countries free from bovine spongioform encephalopathy (BSE).

2. INTENDED USE / INDICATIONS

Apligraf is indicated for use with standard therapeutic compression for the treatment of non-infected partial and full-thickness skin ulcers due to venous insufficiency of greater than 1 month duration and which have not adequately responded to conventional ulcer therapy.

Apligraf is also indicated for use with standard diabetic foot ulcer care for the treatment of full-thickness neuropathic diabetic foot ulcers of greater than three weeks duration which have not adequately responded to conventional ulcer therapy and which extend through the dermis but without tendon, muscle, capsule or bone exposure.

3. CONTRAINDICATIONS

- Apligraf is contraindicated for use on clinically infected wounds.
- Apligraf is contraindicated in patients with known allergies to bovine collagen.
- Apligraf is contraindicated in patients with a known hypersensitivity to the components of the Apligraf agarose shipping medium (Section 8).

4. WARNINGS

Warning: DO NOT OPEN AND DO NOT USE Apligraf after the expiration date or if the pH is not within the acceptable range (6.8-7.7) as determined by the provided color chart (Section 9).

Warning: Allergic reactions to the components in the Apligraf agarose shipping medium (Section 8) and bovine collagen, (a component of Apligraf), have been reported. Discontinue product use if a patient shows evidence of an immunologic reaction. Patients should notify their physician of any symptoms of an allergic reaction. In clinical studies evaluating over 1000 patients, no allergic reactions to Apligraf were reported.

Table 1
Adverse Events Reported in Greater than 1.0% of Apligraf Patients in the Venous Leg Ulcer Study

	Apligraf (n = 161) Total	Control (n = 136) Total
Suspected wound infection[1] (study site)	47 (29.2%)	19 (14.0%)
Suspected wound infection[1] (non-study site[2])	16 (9.9%)	15 (11.0%)
Cellulitis[3] (study site)	13 (8.1%)	11 (8.1%)
Cellulitis[3] (non-study site)	12 (7.5%)	7 (5.1%)
Dermatitis (non-study site)	10 (6.2%)	10 (7.4%)
Exudate (study site)	9 (5.6%)	0 (0.0%)
Peripheral edema	8 (5.0%)	7 (5.1%)
Pain (study site)	7 (4.3%)	7 (5.1%)
Death	6 (3.7%)	6 (4.4%)
Skin ulcer (non-study site)	6 (3.7%)	5 (3.7%)
Pain (non-study site)	5 (3.1%)	4 (2.9%)
Pruritus (non-study site)	5 (3.1%)	2 (1.5%)
Skin Ulcer (study site)	5 (3.1%)	3 (2.2%)
Infection (non-wound)	4 (2.5%)	1 (0.7%)
Positive wound culture[4] (study site)	4 (2.5%)	3 (2.2%)
Rhinitis	4 (2.5%)	1 (0.7%)
Dermatitis (study site)	4 (2.5%)	2 (1.5%)
Pain (overall body)	3 (1.8%)	2 (1.5%)
Congestive heart failure	3 (1.8%)	0 (0.0%)
Accidental injury (musculoskeletal)	3 (1.8%)	0 (0.0%)
Dyspnea	3 (1.8%)	1 (0.7%)
Pharyngitis	3 (1.8%)	0 (0.0%)
Rash (study site)	3 (1.8%)	2 (1.5%)
Accidental injury (overall body)	2 (1.3%)	1 (0.7%)
Asthenia	2 (1.3%)	0 (0.0%)
Arrhythmia	2 (1.3%)	0 (0.0%)
Abscess (non-study site)	2 (1.3%)	0 (0.0%)
Arthralgia	2 (1.3%)	2 (1.5%)
Cough increased	2 (1.3%)	0 (0.0%)
Rash (non-study site)	2 (1.3%)	5 (3.7%)
Erythema (study site)	2 (1.3%)	1 (0.7%)
Kidney failure	2 (1.3%)	0 (0.0%)
Urinary tract infection	2 (1.3%)	5 (3.7%)

5. PRECAUTIONS

Caution: Do not use Apligraf if there is evidence of container damage or product contamination.

Caution: Apligraf should not be reused, frozen or sterilized after opening.

Caution: Apligraf should be kept in its tray on the shipping medium in the sealed bag under controlled temperature (20°C-31°C) until ready for use.

Caution: Apligraf should be handled using sterile technique and placed on a prepared wound bed within 15 minutes of opening the package.

Caution: Do not use cytotoxic agents, including Dakin's solution, Mafenide Acetate, Scarlet Red Dressing, Tincoban, Zinc Sulfate, Povidone-iodine solution, or Chlorhexidine with Apligraf. In *in vitro* and *in vivo* histology studies, exposure to these agents degraded Apligraf. Device exposure to Mafenide Acetate, Polymyxin/Nystatin or Dakin's Solution also reduced Apligraf cell viability.

Caution: Diagnosis of wound infection may be complicated by the white or yellow appearance of Apligraf after it becomes hydrated with wound fluid. Apligraf-treated wounds with respect to signs of suspected infection, including a change from baseline at the ulcer site for pain, edema, erythema, drainage, odor, warmth and/or unexplained fever, should be evaluated and treated according to standard practice for infection.

Caution: The persistence of Apligraf cells on the wound and the safety of this device in venous ulcer patients beyond one year and in diabetic foot ulcer patients beyond 6 months has not been evaluated. Testing to date has not revealed a tumorigenic potential of the cells contained in the device. However, the long term potential of skin cancers from these cells is unknown.

Caution: The safety and the effectiveness of Apligraf have not been established for patients receiving greater than 5 device applications.

6. ADVERSE EVENTS

A. Venous Leg Ulcers (VLU)

All reported adverse events, which occurred in the Apligraf cohort in the study evaluating Apligraf for the treatment of venous leg ulcers at an incidence of 1% or greater are listed in Table 1. The adverse events are listed in descending order according to frequency. This table lists all adverse events reported in the VLU study including those attributed and not attributed to treatment.

[See table 1 above]

Adverse events were recorded as mild, moderate, severe or life-threatening. In the venous leg ulcer study, there were 1 life-threatening and 3 severe infections reported in the Apligraf group and none in the control arm. Of the four events, two severe infections were considered related to treatment: however one occurred one month after the last application of Apligraf and the other occurred following application on a pre-existing *Pseudomonas* infection.

B. Diabetic Foot Ulcers (DFU)

All reported adverse events, which occurred in the study evaluating Apligraf for the treatment of diabetic foot ulcers at an incidence of 1% or greater in the Apligraf group are listed in Table 2. This table lists all adverse events reported in the DFU study including those attributed and not attributed to treatment.

[See table 2 at top of next page]

Table 3 lists all DFU infectious adverse events (i.e., wound infection, cellulitis, osteomyelitis, gangrene, abscess, and fungal infection) as well as resections and amputations occurring on the study limb by first occurrence.

[See table 3 at top of page 2143]

7. CLINICAL STUDIES

A. Venous Leg Ulcers (VLU)

Study Design

A prospective, randomized, controlled, multi-center, multi-specialty, unmasked study was conducted to evaluate the safety and effectiveness of Apligraf and compression therapy in comparison to an active treatment concurrent control of zinc paste gauze and compression therapy. The study population included consenting patients who were 18-89 years old, available for one year follow-up, with venous insufficiency confirmed by plethysmography (venous reflux < 20 sec.); associated with non-infected partial and/or full thickness skin loss ulcer (IAET Stage 2 or 3) of greater than one month duration and which had not adequately responded to conventional ulcer therapy. Patients were excluded for ankle brachial index < 0.65, severe rheumatoid arthritis, collagen vascular disease, pregnancy/lactation, cellulitis, osteomyelitis, ulcer with necrotic, avascular or bone/tendon/fascia exposed-bed, clinically significant wound healing impairment due to uncontrolled diabetes, or renal, hepatic, hematologic, neurologic or immune insufficiency or due to immunosuppressive agents such as corticosteroids (> 15 mg/day), radiation therapy or chemotherapy; or enrollment in studies within the past 30 days for investigational devices or within the past three months for investigational drugs related to wound healing.

Extremities with multiple ulcers were enrolled; however, only one ulcer per extremity was studied. Non-study ulcer care was not specifically defined. Study ulcer care was defined for the treatment (Apligraf and compression therapy) and control (zinc paste gauze and compression therapy), treatment groups in two phases:

1) Active Phase (0-8 weeks): All patients received: i) a non-adherent, ii) a non-occlusive, and iii) a therapeutic compression dressing on day 0, mid-week during the first week (day 3-5), and at weeks 1-8. Control treated patients also received zinc impregnated gauze at each visit. All Apligraf patients received Apligraf on day 0. At the day 3-5 and weeks 1, 2, and 3 visits, if less than 50% Apligraf take was observed, then patients received an additional application of Apligraf. Patients were not allowed to receive more than 5 Apligraf applications total.
2) Maintenance Phase (8-52 weeks): Closed-ulcer extremities received non-specified elastic compression stockings. Open-ulcer extremities continued with dressing changes.

Wound closure was defined as 100% epithelialization without drainage and assessed by clinical observation at visits on day 0, day 3-5, weekly from weeks 1-8, months 3 and 6

Continued on next page

Apligraf—Cont.

after initial treatment application or until wound closure was achieved. Additional follow-up visits were 9 and 12 months after initial treatment.

VLU Study Results

The incidence of VLU wound closure at set visits up to 6 months is presented below as the raw data results (Figure 1) and the results after adjustment for pooled center, baseline ulcer duration, and baseline area (Figure 2).

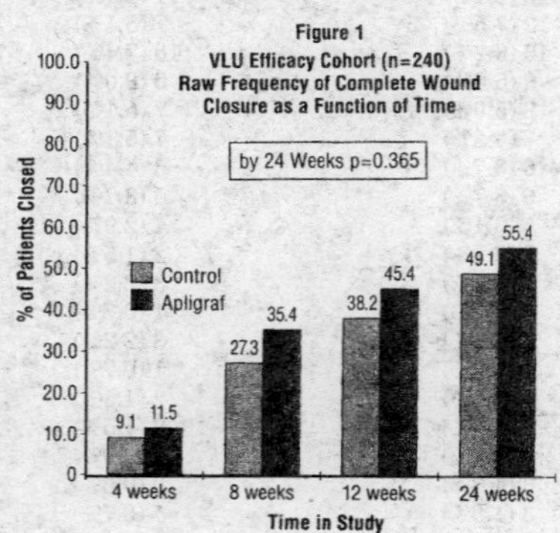

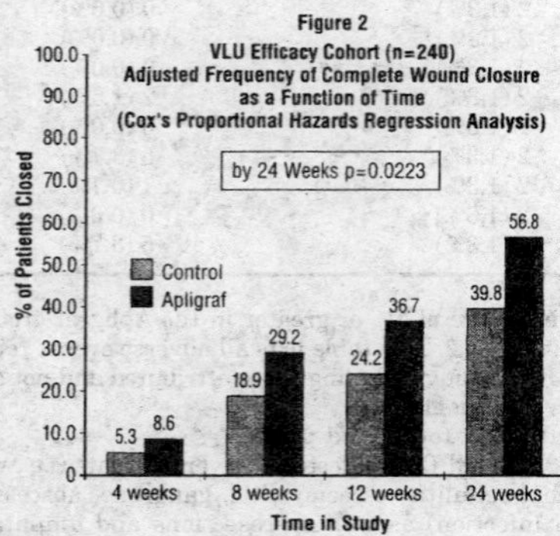

VLU Ulcer recurrence

At six months, the incidence of VLU recurrence was 8.3% (6/72) for Apligraf- and 7.4% (4/54) for control-treated patients. The incidence of VLU recurrence by 12 months was 18.1% (13/72) in the Apligraf group and 22.2% (12/54) in the control group.

VLU Suspected wound infection

In the VLU effectiveness cohort, there were 33/130 (25.4%) Apligraf-treated and 15/110 (13.6%) control-treated ulcers with suspected wound infection. While the overall incidence of wound infection was higher in the Apligraf arm, the incidence of wound closure (Figures 1 and 2) was also higher for Apligraf-treated patients.

VLU Baseline status impact on wound closure

The impact of VLU patient baseline status on wound closure was evaluated for the patient populations above and below the median values for ulcer duration and ulcer size as well as for baseline IAET Ulcer Stage, the presence of diabetes and a patient's Ankle Brachial Index. The results of these analyses are displayed in Table 4.

[See table 4 at top of next page]

VLU Secondary Endpoints

Clinical assessment (scale 1-4) of wound depth (IAET staging), erythema, edema, wound pain, fibrin, exudate, granulation tissue, and overall assessment by changes in mean score and analysis of variance from baseline to the 6 month visit indicated no differences between VLU treatment groups at 6 months.

VLU Immune response

In tests of VLU patients' sera there were no observations of antibody responses against bovine Type I collagen, bovine serum proteins or the Class I HLA antigens on human dermal fibroblasts, and human epidermal cells. T-cell specific responses were also not observed against bovine Type I collagen, human fibroblasts or human keratinocytes. There was also no clinical evidence of Apligraf rejection by any patient.

B. Diabetic Foot Ulcers (DFU)

Study Design

A prospective, randomized, controlled, multi-center unmasked study was conducted to evaluate the safety and efficacy of Apligraf in comparison to Control treatment, saline moistened gauze in the treatment of diabetic neuropathic foot ulcers. The study population included consenting patients who were between 18 and 80 years old, with a 0.4 cm^2-16.3 cm^2 full-thickness foot ulcer of neuropathic etiology of at least 2 weeks duration, located on the plantar, medial or lateral surface of the foot at least 2 cm away from any other ulcers on the same extremity. The study participants were required to be diagnosed diabetics with type 1 or type 2 diabetes, a HbA1C between 6% and 12% and available for six-month follow-up. Patients were excluded for ulcers with tracts or tunnels, a clinical infection at the study ulcer site, ABI < 0.65, active Charcot's arthropathy at the study extremity, a study ulcer that healed > 30% from post-debridement at Study Day -7 to Day 0, renal dialysis, history of alcohol or substance abuse within one year, acute or chronic hepatitis, receiving corticosteroids, immunosuppressive agents, radiation therapy or chemotherapy one month prior to study enrollment, or enrollment in clinical studies evaluating a device within the past 30 days or within the past 3 months for pharmaceuticals or biologics.

Two-hundred-seventy-seven patients were entered into the screening phase of the study. Sixty-nine patients did not meet inclusion/exclusion criteria. After randomization and screening, 208 patients were treated in the study, i.e., 112 received Apligraf and 96 received Control therapy. Patients received 12 weeks of treatment and 3 additional months of follow-up. Complete wound closure was evaluated by or on 12 weeks. Patients were evaluated weekly for the first 12 weeks with mid-week visits for dressing changes from Day 0 through Week 5 and follow-up visits at Months 4, 5 and 6. Both treatment groups received good ulcer care consisting of sharp debridement, saline moistened dressings and a non-weight bearing regimen. All patients in the Apligraf treatment group received Apligraf at Day 0. At Study Weeks 1, 2, 3 and 4, if Apligraf coverage was less than 100% and the wound was not progressing to healing then an additional Apligraf unit was applied. A maximum of 5 Apligraf applications was allowed. The Apligraf was dressed with saline-moistened non-adherent dressing, tape, dry gauze, petrolatum gauze and gauze wrap. The Control treated patients received saline-moistened non-adherent dressing, tape, saline moistened gauze, dry gauze, petrolatum gauze and gauze wrap from Day 0 through Study Week 4.

Patients in both treatment groups who did not heal by Study Week 5 were treated with saline-moistened gauze, dry gauze, petrolatum gauze and gauze wrap from Study Week 5 through Study Week 12. The patients were instructed to change this dressing two times per day.

Patients were instructed to avoid weight bearing on the affected foot throughout the duration of the study. During the first 6 weeks patients were instructed to use crutches or a wheelchair. Each patient was fitted with a customized tri-density sandal. These sandals were to be worn throughout the entire study.

In keeping with good medical practice, early detection and treatment of ulcer infection using standard procedures was advised.

DFU Study Results

The incidence of DFU wound closure at set visits is presented below (Figure 3).

[See figure 3 at top of next column]

Table 2
Adverse Events Reported in Greater than 1.0% of Apligraf Patients in the Diabetic Foot Ulcer Study

	Apligraf (n = 112)	Control (n = 96)
	Total	Total
Neuropathic ulcer (non-study site[2])	19 (17.0%)	9 (9.4%)
Suspected wound infection[1] (non-study site)	15 (13.4%)	7 (7.3%)
Non-neuropathic skin alteration (non-study site)	13 (11.6%)	11 (11.5%)
Suspected wound infection[1] (study site)	12 (10.7%)	13 (13.5%)
Cellulitis[3] (non-study site)	11 (9.8%)	4 (4.2%)
Cellulitis[3] (study site)	10 (8.9%)	8 (8.3%)
Osteomyelitis (non-study site)	10 (8.9%)	3 (3.1%)
Vesicular bullous rash (non-study site)	9 (8.0%)	5 (5.2%)
Pain (overall body)	8 (7.1%)	4 (4.2%)
Fungal infection (non-study site)	7 (6.3%)	9 (9.4%)
Hypoglycemia	7 (6.3%)	3 (3.1%)
Infection (overall body)	6 (5.4%)	4 (4.2%)
Hematoma (non-study site)	6 (5.4%)	2 (2.1%)
Deteriorating ulceration (study site)	5 (4.5%)	6 (6.3%)
Rash (non-study site)	5 (4.5%)	4 (4.2%)
Non-neuropathic skin alteration (study site)	5 (4.5%)	2 (2.1%)
Pain (non-study site)	5 (4.5%)	1 (1.0%)
Bone dislocation (non-study site)	5 (4.5%)	1 (1.0%)
Peripheral edema	4 (3.6%)	11 (11.5%)
Accidental Injury (overall body)	4 (3.6%)	8 (8.3%)
Injury Accident (non-study site)	4 (3.6%)	5 (5.2%)
Fever (overall body)	4 (3.6%)	5 (5.2%)
Hyperglycemia	4 (3.6%)	4 (4.2%)
Dry skin (non-study site)	4 (3.6%)	2 (2.1%)
Chest pain	4 (3.6%)	1 (1.0%)
Bronchitis	4 (3.6%)	0 (0.0%)
Osteomyelitis (study site)	3 (2.7%)	10 (10.4%)
Nausea	3 (2.7%)	6 (6.3%)
Pharyngitis	3 (2.7%)	6 (6.3%)
Anemia	3 (2.7%)	5 (5.2%)
Right Heart failure	3 (2.7%)	3 (3.1%)
Abscess (study site)	3 (2.7%)	3 (3.1%)
Urinary tract infection	3 (2.7%)	2 (2.1%)
Deteriorating ulceration (non-study site)	3 (2.7%)	2 (2.1%)
Gastroenteritis	3 (2.7%)	2 (2.1%)
Cataract	3 (2.7%)	2 (2.1%)
Abscess (overall body)	3 (2.7%)	0 (0.0%)
Gastritis	3 (2.7%)	0 (0.0%)
Spontaneous bone fracture	3 (2.7%)	0 (0.0%)
Diarrhea	2 (1.8%)	8 (8.3%)
Positive Wound Culture[4] (study site)	2 (1.8%)	3 (3.1%)
Arthrosis (non-study site)	2 (1.8%)	3 (3.1%)
Malaise	2 (1.8%)	2 (2.1%)
Rash (study site)	2 (1.8%)	2 (2.1%)
Hematoma (study site)	2 (1.8%)	2 (2.1%)
Gangrene (non-study site)	2 (1.8%)	2 (2.1%)
Dyspepsia	2 (1.8%)	1 (1.0%)
Injury Accident (study site)	2 (1.8%)	1 (1.0%)
Infection (non-study site)	2 (1.8%)	0 (0.0%)
Gangrene (study site)	2 (1.8%)	0 (0.0%)
Spontaneous bone fracture (non-study site)	2 (1.8%)	0 (0.0%)
Viral infection	2 (1.8%)	0 (0.0%)
Back pain	2 (1.8%)	0 (0.0%)
Angina pectoris	2 (1.8%)	0 (0.0%)
Arteriosclerosis	2 (1.8%)	0 (0.0%)
Cardiomegaly	2 (1.8%)	0 (0.0%)
Gastrointestinal carcinoma	2 (1.8%)	0 (0.0%)
Colitis	2 (1.8%)	0 (0.0%)
Rhinitis	2 (1.8%)	0 (0.0%)
Arthritis	2 (1.8%)	0 (0.0%)
Confusion	2 (1.8%)	0 (0.0%)

In the clinical trials the following definitions were used:

[1]*Suspected wound infection:* a wound with at least some clinical signs and symptoms of infection such as increased exudate, odor, redness, swelling, heat, pain, tenderness to the touch, and purulent discharge; quantitative culture was not required.

[2]*Non-study site event:* an adverse event occurring on either extremity, but not located at or involving the study ulcer.

[3]*Cellulitis:* a non-suppurative inflammation of the subcutaneous tissues extending along connective tissue planes and across intracellular spaces; widespread swelling, redness and pain without definite localization.

[4]*Positive wound culture:* reported as an adverse event, but not reported as a wound infection.

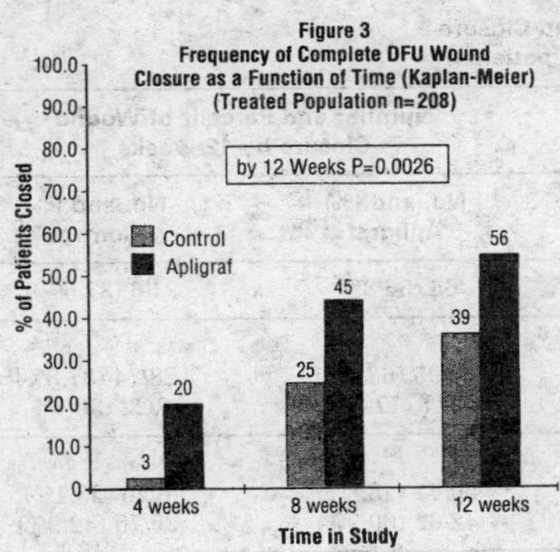

Figure 3
Frequency of Complete DFU Wound Closure as a Function of Time (Kaplan-Meier) (Treated Population n=208)

DFU Ulcer recurrence

The incidence of DFU recurrence as a function of device applications is presented in Table 5.

[See table 5 below]

DFU Baseline status impact on wound closure

The impact of DFU patient baseline status on wound closure was evaluated for patient gender, age, Charcot's status, diabetes type, number and location of ulcers on study foot as well as the patient populations above and below the median values for ulcer duration, size and HbA_{1c} level (%). The results of these analyses are displayed in Table 6.

[See table 6 at top of next page]

DFU Secondary endpoints

Between Study Day 0 and Study Week 12, both DFU Apligraf and Control groups showed statistically significant improvement in undermining, maceration, exudate, granulation, eschar and fibrin slough. At Study Week 12, Apligraf showed statistically significant improvements when compared to Control in maceration (p=0.0233), exudate (p=0.0290) and eschar (p=0.0293).

DFU Immune response

In tests of DFU patients' sera there were no observations of antibody responses against bovine Type I collagen, bovine serum proteins or Class I HLA antigens on human dermal fibroblasts, and human epidermal cells. T-cell specific responses were not observed against bovine Type I collagen, human dermal fibroblasts or human keratinocytes. In addition, there was no clinical evidence of Apligraf rejection by any patient.

8. HOW SUPPLIED

Apligraf is supplied sealed in a heavy gauge polyethylene bag with a 10% CO_2/air atmosphere and agarose nutrient medium, ready for single use. To maintain cell viability, Apligraf should be kept in the sealed bag at 20°C–31°C until use. Apligraf is supplied as a circular disk approximately 75 mm in diameter and 0.75 mm thick. The agarose shipping medium contains agarose, L-glutamine, hydrocortisone/bovine serum albumin, bovine insulin, human transferrin, triiodothyronine, ethanolamine, O-phosphorylethanolamine, adenine, selenious acid, DMEM powder, HAM's F-12 powder, sodium bicarbonate, calcium chloride, and water for injection.

To maintain cell viability, the product is aseptically manufactured, but not terminally sterilized. Apligraf is shipped following a preliminary sterility test with a 48 hour incubation to determine the absence of microbial growth. Final (14 day incubation) sterility tests results are not available at the time of application.

9. DIRECTIONS FOR USE

Apligraf is indicated for use with standard therapeutic compression for the treatment of non-infected partial and full-thickness skin ulcers due to venous insufficiency of greater than 1 month duration and which have not adequately responded to conventional ulcer therapy. Apligraf is also indicated for use in the treatment of full-thickness diabetic foot ulcers of neuropathic etiology of at least three weeks duration which have not adequately responded to conventional ulcer therapy and which extend through the dermis but without tendon, muscle, capsule or bone exposure, and are located on the plantar, medial or lateral area of the foot, excluding the heel. Apligraf consists of living cells which must be kept sealed in its nutrient medium and 10% CO_2/air atmosphere under controlled temperature (20°C-31°C) and used within 15 minutes of opening.

Preparation of the Wound Bed Prior to Apligraf Application

1. Wound Infection:

Apligraf should not be applied over infected or deteriorating wounds until the underlying condition has been resolved.

2. Bacterial Containment:

Antimicrobial agents may be used during the week prior to Apligraf application to reduce the risk of infection. Dakin's solution, Mafenide Acetate, Scarlet Red Dressing, Tincoban, Zinc Sulfate, Povidone-iodine solution, and Chlorhexidine have been determined to be cytotoxic to Apligraf.

3. Wound Bed Preparation:

Venous Leg Ulcers

Apligraf should be applied to a clean, debrided wound after thoroughly irrigating the wound with a non-cytotoxic solution. Oozing or bleeding resulting from debridement should be stopped through the use of gentle pressure.

Table 3
Infectious Adverse Events and Amputations Occurring on the Study Limb in Diabetic Foot Ulcers by Number of Apligraf Applications

# Applications	# Patients n=112	# Closed	Mean Days to Closure (range)	# First Infections on Study Limb	# Amputations and Resection on Study Limb
1	10 (8.9%)	9/10 (90.0%)	15 (7-57)	1	0
2	11 (9.8%)	8/11 (72.7%)	15 (8-36)	2	0
3	15 (13.4%)	10/15 (66.7%)	22 (22-29)	5	0
4	17 (15.2%)	9/17 (52.9%)	36 (29-78)	6	1
5	59 (52.7%)	27/59 (45.8%)	51 (36-88)	24	6
Total Apligraf	112	63 (56%)	36 (7-88)	38/112 (34%)	7
Control	96	36 (38%)	50 (15-92)	36/96 (38%)	15

Table 4
Pre-Treatment Status and Wound Closure VLU Effectiveness Cohort (n=240 patients)

	Pre-Treatment Status		Number and Percent of Wound Closure by 6 months	
Patient Condition	**No. and (%) Apligraf Pts.**	**No. and (%) Control Pts.**	**Apligraf**	**Control**
Total	130 Patients	110 Patients	72 (55.4%)	54 (49.1%)
Ulcer Duration				
≤1 year	58 (44.6%)	62 (56.3%)	38/58 (65.5%)	45/62 (72.6%)
> 1 year	72 (55.4%)	48 (43.6%)	34/72 (47.2%)	9/48 (18.8%)
***Ulcer Area**				
< 500 mm^2	65 (50.0%)	60 (54.5%)	45/65 (69.2%)	35/60 (58.3%)
> 500 mm^2	63 (48.5%)	50 (45.5%)	26/63 (41.3%)	19/50 (38.0%)
IAET Staging				
Stage II	63 (48.5%)	56 (50.9%)	34/63 (54.0%)	32/56 (57.1%)
Stage III	67 (51.5%)	54 (49.1%)	38/67 (56.7%)	22/54 (40.7%)
Diabetes				
Yes[1]	25 (19.2%)	11 (10.0%)	12/25 (48.0%)	4/11 (36.4%)
No	105 (80.8%)	99 (90.0%)	60/105 (57.1%)	50/99 (50.5%)
****Ankle Brachial Index data (ABI)**				
> 0.65 ≤ 0.8	9 (6.9%)	10 (9.1%)	4/9 (44.4%)	4/10 (40.0%)
> 0.8 < 1.0	43 (33.1%)	50 (45.5%)	26/43 (60.5%)	27/50 (54.0%)
> 1.0	75 (57.7%)	49 (44.5%)	40/75 (53.3%)	22/49 (44.9%)

*Baseline ulcer area missing for two patients in the Apligraf® group.
**ABI data are missing for 3 Apligraf and 1 control patient.
[1]This category includes both insulin-dependent and non-insulin dependent diabetes patients, because the insulin-dependence of patients was not determined in this clinical trial.

Table 5
Ulcer Recurrence in Diabetic Foot Ulcers by Number of Applications

# Applications	# Patients n=112	# Closed	# Re-opened	# Re-closed by 6 months
1	10 (8.9%)	9	4/9 (44%)	4/4
2	11 (9.8%)	8	3/8 (38%)	2/3
3	15 (13.4%)	10	4/10 (40%)	4/4
4	17 (15.2%)	9	2/9 (22%)	0/2
5	59 (52.7%)	27	12/27 (44%)	10/12
Apligraf Total*	112	63	25/63 (40%)	20/25 (80%)
Control*	96	36	16/36 (44%)	10/16 (63%)

*Three patients in each group re-opened > 4 weeks after attaining complete wound closure.

Previous ulcer treatments other than standard therapeutic compression should be discontinued.

Diabetic Foot Ulcers

Apligraf should be applied to a clean wound base. Debridement should extend to healthy, viable, bleeding tissue. Prior to Apligraf application, hemostasis must be achieved. Prior to debridement thoroughly cleanse the wound with sterile saline to remove all loose debris and necrotic tissue. Using tissue nippers, a surgical blade or curette remove all hyperkeratotic and/or necrotic tissue and debris from the wound surface. Ulcer margins should be debrided to have a saucer effect. After debridement, cleanse the wound thoroughly with sterile saline solution and gently dry with gauze. Oozing or bleeding resulting from debridement may be stopped through the use of gentle pressure.

4. Control of Heavy Exudation:

Heavy exudation may displace Apligraf and reduce adherence. Exudation should be minimized by appropriate clinical treatment. If exudation persists, Apligraf should

Continued on next page

Apligraf—Cont.

be made permeable to exudate by perforating the Apligraf to allow for drainage.

Suggested Technique for the Application of Apligraf to the Wound

1. Check expiration date. If expired, do not open or use.
2. Check product pH. If not 6.8-7.7 by the provided color pH chart, do not open or use.
3. Apligraf should be kept in its polyethylene bag at controlled temperature (20°C-31°C) until immediately prior to use.
4. Cut open the sealed polyethylene bag and transfer the plastic tray to the sterile field with aseptic technique. Apligraf should always be handled aseptically.
5. Lift off the tray lid and note epidermal and dermal layer orientation: Apligraf is packaged with the epidermal (dull, matte finish) layer facing up and the dermal (glossy) layer facing down, resting on the polycarbonate membrane.
6. Using a sterile atraumatic instrument, gently dislodge appoximately 0.5 inch of Apligraf away from the wall of the tray.
7. There should be no evidence of contamination, visible particulates or pungent odor.
8. When lifting Apligraf, be careful not to perforate or lift the polycarbonate membrane beneath Apligraf. The polycarbonate membrane should remain in the tray.
9. With sterile gloved hands, insert one index finger under the released section of Apligraf. Use the other index finger to grasp the Apligraf in a second spot along the edge of the device. Holding the Apligraf in two places lift the entire Apligraf out of the tray using a smooth, even motion. This easy motion should prevent Apligraf from bending and folding over onto itself. To minimize Apligraf damage, avoid Apligraf contact with foreign bodies and minimize handling Apligraf except by its margins.
10. Do not allow Apligraf to fold or wrinkle on itself. If excessive folding occurs, Apligraf can be floated (epidermal surface up) onto warm sterile saline solution in a sterile tray.
11. Apligraf should be placed so that the dermal layer (the glossy layer closest to the medium) is in direct contact with the wound surface. Using a saline moistened cotton applicator, smooth Apligraf onto the wound bed so there are no pockets or wrinkled edges. If there is excessive Apligraf, which is not in contact with the wound bed, it should be trimmed away or it may adhere to the dressing.
12. Dressings:

    Venous Leg Ulcers

    Secure Apligraf with a three-layer dressing so as to assure contact to wound bed:

    - Apply a non-adherent dressing over the ulcer and Apligraf, extending 0.5 inch beyond the ulcer perimeter and inflamed skin margins.
    - Apply a non-occlusive dressing such as fine mesh gauze. This may be folded or rolled as a bolster.
    - Apply a self adherent elastic wrap from metatarsals to tibial plateau so that therapeutic compression is applied to the ulcer site.

    Diabetic Foot Ulcers

    Apligraf should be dressed with non-adherent saline moistened dressing, a layer of dry gauze, a layer of petrolatum gauze and gauze wrap.

Frequency of Dressing Changes and Apligraf Applications

Venous Leg Ulcers

1. The wound should be inspected and the dressing changed at least once a week during the immediate post application period. More frequent changes may be required on highly exudative wounds.
2. Additional applications of Apligraf may be necessary. Prior to additional applications, non-adherent remnants of Apligraf should be gently removed. Healing tissue or adherent Apligraf should not be disrupted. The wound bed should be cleansed with a non-cytotoxic solution prior to additional applications of Apligraf. Additional applications of Apligraf should not be applied over areas where Apligraf is adherent.
3. The wound site should continue to be dressed with a non-adherent dressing, pressure bolster and elastic overwrap as described above.
4. Upon complete wound closure, patients should be continued with compression therapy such as support stockings.
5. The safety and the effectiveness of Apligraf have not been established for patients receiving greater than 5 device applications.

Diabetic Foot Ulcers

1. The wound should be inspected and the dressing in contact with Apligraf should be changed once a week. Outer dressings may be changed more frequently (daily).
2. Additional applications of Apligraf may be necessary. Prior to additional applications, non-adherent remnants of Apligraf should be gently removed. Additional saucerized debridement may be needed to remove non-viable tissue. Healing tissue or adherent Apligraf should not be disrupted. The wound bed should be cleansed with a non-cytotoxic solution prior to additional applications of Apligraf. Additional applications of Apligraf should not be applied over areas where Apligraf is adherent.
3. The wound site should continue to be dressed as described.
4. After healing patients should continue to wear appropriate pressure relieving footwear and utilize other ulcer preventive footcare practices.
5. The safety and the effectiveness of Apligraf have not been established for patients receiving greater than 5 device applications.

Table 6
Pre-Treatment Status and Wound Closure
DFU Treated Population (n=208 patients)

	Pre-Treatment Status		Number and Percent of Wound Closure by 12 weeks	
Patient Condition	**No. and (%) Apligraf**	**No. and (%) Control**	**No. and (%) Apligraf**	**No. and (%) Control**
Total	112 Patients	96 Patients	63 (56.3%)	36 (37.5%)
Charcot Joint Deformity				
Absent	95 (84.8%)	74 (77.1%)	60/95 (63.2%)	28/74 (37.8%)
Inactive	17 (15.2%)	22 (22.9%)	3/17 (17.6%)	8/22 (36.4%)
Diabetes*				
Type 1 (IDDM)	41 (36.6%)	26 (27.1%)	20/41 (48.8%)	6/26 (23.1%)
Type 2 (NIDDM)	69 (61.6%)	70 (72.9%)	42/69 (60.9%)	30/70 (42.9%)
Ulcer Location**				
Toes	22 (19.6%)	13 (13.5%)	14/22 (63.6%)	8/13 (61.5%)
Metatarsal heads	58 (51.8%)	49 (51.0%)	36/58 (62.1%)	20/49 (40.8%)
Midfoot	30 (26.8%)	34 (35.4%)	12/30 (40.0%)	8/34 (23.5%)
Age				
18-70 years	98 (87.5%)	91 (94.8%)	55/98 (56.1%)	34/91 (37.4%)
71-80 years	14 (12.5%)	5 (5.2%)	8/14 (57.1%)	2/5 (40.0%)
Gender				
Male	88 (78.6%)	74 (77.1%)	46/88 (52.3%)	30/74 (40.5%)
Female	24 (21.4%)	22 (22.9%)	17/24 (70.8%)	6/22 (27.2%)
Ulcer Area†				
≤ 177 (mm^2)	59 (52.7%)	45 (46.9%)	39/59 (66.1%)	20/45 (44.4%)
> 177 (mm^2)	52 (46.4%)	51 (53.1%)	23/52 (44.2%)	16/51 (31.4%)
Ulcer Duration				
≤6 months	61 (54.5%)	51 (53.1%)	38/61 (62.3%)	22/51 (43.1%)
> 6 months	51 (45.5%)	45 (46.9%)	25/51 (49.0%)	14/45 (31.1%)
Number of Ulcers on Study Foot				
Single	100 (89.3%)	90 (93.8%)	57/100 (57.0%)	33/90 (36.7%)
Multiple	12 (10.7%)	6 (6.2%)	6/12 (50.0%)	3/6 (50.0%)
HbA1c				
≤ 8.40	63 (56.3%)	42 (43.8%)	34/63 (54.0%)	12/42 (28.6%)
> 8.40	49 (43.8%)	54 (56.3%)	29/49 (59.2%)	24/54 (44.4%)

*Two patients in the Apligraf group did not have type of diabetes specified.
**Two patients in the Apligraf group had ulcers located not at the toes, metatarsal heads, or midfoot.
†One patient in the Apligraf group did not have a baseline ulcer tracing available.

10. PATIENT'S MANUAL

Venous Leg Ulcers

A brochure will be made available to:
1. Provide basic information about chronic wounds.
2. Address standard patient care while receiving Apligraf treatment.
3. Educate patients on Apligraf-related healing process.

Diabetic Foot Ulcers

A brochure will be made available to:
1. Provide basic information about diabetic foot ulcers.
2. Address standard patient care while receiving Apligraf treatment.
3. Educate patients on Apligraf-related healing process.

11. PEEL-OFF LABEL

Remove the peel-off label from the lower right corner of the Apligraf package label and place it in the patient's chart. This label bears a unique lot number and expiration date of the Apligraf.

Apligraf® (Graftskin)
Essential Prescribing Information

Numbers in parentheses ( ) refer to sections in the main part of the product labeling.

Device Description
Apligraf is supplied as a living, bi-layered skin substitute manufactured using neonatal foreskin keratinocytes and fibroblasts with bovine Type I collagen. **(1)**

Intended Use/Indications
Apligraf is indicated for use with standard therapeutic compression in the treatment of uninfected partial and/or full-thickness skin loss ulcers due to venous insufficiency of greater than 1 month duration and which have not adequately responded to conventional ulcer therapy. **(2)**
Apligraf is indicated for use with standard diabetic foot ulcer care for the treatment of full-thickness foot ulcers of neuropathic etiology of at least three weeks duration, which have not adequately responded to conventional ulcer therapy and extend through the dermis but without tendon, muscle, capsule or bone exposure. **(2)**

Contraindications
Apligraf is contraindicated for use on clinically infected wounds and in patients with known allergies to bovine collagen or hypersensitivity to the components of the shipping medium. **(3, 4, 5, 8)**

Warnings and Precautions
If the expiration date or product pH (6.8-7.7) is not within the acceptable range DO NOT OPEN AND DO NOT USE the product. A clinical determination of wound infection should be made based on all of the signs and symptoms of infection. **(4, 5)**

Adverse Events
All reported adverse events, which occurred at an incidence of greater than 1% in the clinical studies are listed in Table 1, Table 2 and Table 3. These tables list adverse events both attributed and not attributed to treatment. **(6)**

Maintaining Device Effectiveness
Apligraf has been processed under aseptic conditions and should be handled observing sterile technique. It should be kept in its tray on the medium in the sealed bag under controlled temperature (20°C-31°C) until ready for use. Apligraf should be placed on the wound bed within 15 minutes of opening the package. Handling before application to the wound site should be minimal. If there is any question that Apligraf may be contaminated or compromised, it should not be used. Apligraf should not be used beyond the listed expiration date. **(9)**

Use in Specific Populations
The safety and effectiveness of Apligraf has not been established in pregnant women, acute wounds, burns and ulcers caused by pressure.

Patient Counseling Information
VLU patients should be counseled regarding the importance of complying with compression therapy or other treatment, which may be prescribed in conjunction with Apligraf.
DFU patients should be counseled that: Apligraf is used in combination with good ulcer care including a non-weight bearing regimen and optimal metabolic control and nutrition. Once an ulcer has healed, ulcer prevention practices should be implemented including regular visits to appropriate medical providers.

Treatment of Diabetes
Apligraf does not address the underlying pathophysiology of neuropathic diabetic foot ulcers. Management of the patient's diabetes should be according to standard medical practice.

How Supplied
Apligraf is supplied sealed in a heavy gauge polyethylene bag with a 10% CO_2/air atmosphere and agarose nutrient medium, ready for single use. To maintain cell viability, Apligraf should be kept in the sealed bag at 20°C-31°C until use. Apligraf is supplied as a circular disk approximately 75 mm in diameter and 0.75 mm thick. **(8)**

Manufactured by:
Organogenesis Inc.
Canton, MA 02021
Marketed and Distributed by:
Novartis Pharmaceuticals Corporation
East Hanover, New Jersey 07936

T2000-42
USA-Z03
REV: JUNE 2000 300-111-2
Shown in Product Identification Guide, page 325

AREDIA® ℞

[ă rē dē ă]
pamidronate disodium for injection
For Intravenous Infusion

Rx only
The following prescribing information is based on official labeling in effect July 2000.
Prescribing Information

DESCRIPTION

Aredia, pamidronate disodium (APD), is a bone-resorption inhibitor available in 30-mg or 90-mg vials for intravenous administration. Each 30-mg, and 90-mg vial contains, respectively, 30 mg and 90 mg of sterile, lyophilized pamidronate disodium and 470 mg and 375 mg of mannitol, USP. The pH of a 1% solution of pamidronate disodium in distilled water is approximately 8.3. Aredia, a member of the group of chemical compounds known as bisphosphonates, is an analog of pyrophosphate. Pamidronate disodium is designated chemically as phosphonic acid (3-amino-1-hydroxypropylidene) bis-, disodium salt, pentahydrate, (APD), and its structural formula is

$$NH_2-CH_2-CH_2-C(OH)(PO_3HNa)_2 \cdot 5H_2O$$

Pamidronate disodium is a white-to-practically-white powder. It is soluble in water and in 2N sodium hydroxide, sparingly soluble in 0.1N hydrochloric acid and in 0.1N acetic acid, and practically insoluble in organic solvents. Its molecular formula is $C_3H_9NO_7P_2Na_2 \cdot 5H_2O$ and its molecular weight is 369.1.

Inactive Ingredients. Mannitol, USP, and phosphoric acid (for adjustment to pH 6.5 prior to lyophilization).

CLINICAL PHARMACOLOGY

The principal pharmacologic action of Aredia is inhibition of bone resorption. Although the mechanism of antiresorptive action is not completely understood, several factors are thought to contribute to this action. Aredia adsorbs to calcium phosphate (hydroxyapatite) crystals in bone and may directly block dissolution of this mineral component of bone. In vitro studies also suggest that inhibition of osteoclast activity contributes to inhibition of bone resorption. In animal studies, at doses recommended for the treatment of hypercalcemia, Aredia inhibits bone resorption apparently without inhibiting bone formation and mineralization. Of relevance to the treatment of hypercalcemia of malignancy is the finding that Aredia inhibits the accelerated bone resorption that results from osteoclast hyperactivity induced by various tumors in animal studies.

Pharmacokinetics

Cancer patients (n=24) who had minimal or no bony involvement were given an intravenous infusion of 30, 60, or 90 mg of Aredia over 4 hours and 90 mg of Aredia over 24 hours (Table 1).

Distribution

The mean ± SD body retention of pamidronate was calculated to be 54 ± 16% of the dose over 120 hours.

Metabolism

Pamidronate is not metabolized and is exclusively eliminated by renal excretion.

Excretion

After administration of 30, 60, and 90 mg of Aredia over 4 hours, and 90 mg of Aredia over 24 hours, an overall mean ± SD of 46 ± 16% of the drug was excreted unchanged in the urine within 120 hours. Cumulative urinary excretion was linearly related to dose. The mean ± SD elimination half-life is 28 ± 7 hours. Mean ± SD total and renal clearances of pamidronate were 107 ± 50 mL/min and 49 ± 28 mL/min, respectively. The rate of elimination from bone has not been determined.

Special Populations

There are no data available on the effects of age, gender, or race on the pharmacokinetics of pamidronate.

Pediatric

Pamidronate is not labeled for use in the pediatric population.

Renal Insufficiency

The pharmacokinetics of pamidronate were studied in cancer patients (n=19) with normal and varying degrees of renal impairment. Each patient received a single 90-mg dose of Aredia infused over 4 hours. The renal clearance of pamidronate in patients was found to closely correlate with creatinine clearance (see Figure 1). A trend toward a lower percentage of drug excreted unchanged in urine was observed in renally impaired patients. Adverse experiences noted were not found to be related to changes in renal clearance of pamidronate. Given the recommended dose, 90 mg infused over 4 hours, excessive accumulation of pamidronate in renally impaired patients is not anticipated if Aredia is administered on a monthly basis.
[See figure 1 at top of next column]

Table 1
Mean (SD, CV%) Pamidronate Pharmacokinetic Parameters in Cancer Patients
(n=6 for each group)

Dose (infusion rate)	Maximum Concentration (μg/mL)	Percent of dose excreted in urine	Total Clearance (mL/min)	Renal Clearance (mL/min)
30 mg (4 hrs)	0.73 (0.14, 19.1%)	43.9 (14.0, 31.9%)	136 (44, 32.4%)	58 (27, 46.5%)
60 mg (4 hrs)	1.44 (0.57, 39.6%)	47.4 (47.4, 54.4%)	88 (56, 63.6%)	42 (28, 66.7%)
90 mg (4 hrs)	2.61 (0.74, 28.3%)	45.3 (25.8, 56.9%)	103 (37, 35.9%)	44 (16, 36.4%)
90 mg (24 hrs)	1.38 (1.97, 142.7%)	47.5 (10.2, 21.5%)	101 (58, 57.4%)	52 (42, 80.8%)

Figure 1: Pamidronate renal clearance as a function of creatinine clearance in patients with normal and impaired renal function. The lines are the mean prediction line and 95% confidence intervals.

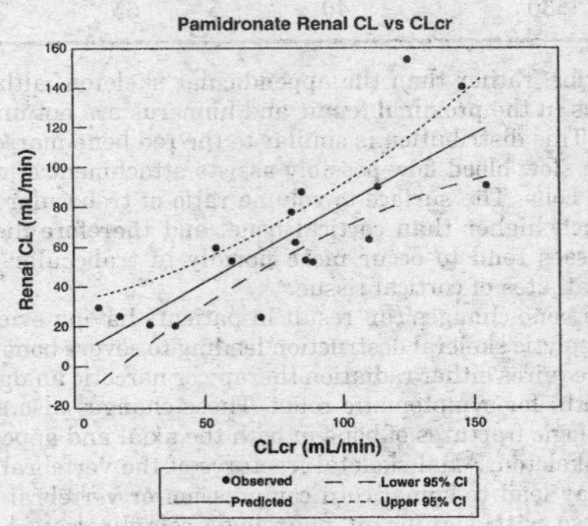

Hepatic Insufficiency

There are no human pharmacokinetic data for Aredia in patients who have hepatic insufficiency.

Drug-Drug Interactions

There are no human pharmacokinetic data for drug interactions with Aredia.
[See table 1 above]

After intravenous administration of radiolabeled pamidronate in rats, approximately 50%-60% of the compound was rapidly adsorbed by bone and slowly eliminated from the body by the kidneys. In rats given 10 mg/kg bolus injections of radiolabeled Aredia, approximately 30% of the compound was found in the liver shortly after administration and was then redistributed to bone or eliminated by the kidneys over 24-48 hours. Studies in rats injected with radiolabeled Aredia showed that the compound was rapidly cleared from the circulation and taken up mainly by bones, liver, spleen, teeth, and tracheal cartilage. Radioactivity was eliminated from most soft tissues within 1-4 days; was detectable in liver and spleen for 1 and 3 months, respectively; and remained high in bones, trachea, and teeth for 6 months after dosing. Bone uptake occurred preferentially in areas of high bone turnover. The terminal phase of elimination half-life in bone was estimated to be approximately 300 days.

Pharmacodynamics

Serum phosphate levels have been noted to decrease after administration of Aredia, presumably because of decreased release of phosphate from bone and increased renal excretion as parathyroid hormone levels, which are usually suppressed in hypercalcemia associated with malignancy, return toward normal. Phosphate therapy was administered in 30% of the patients in response to a decrease in serum phosphate levels. Phosphate levels usually returned toward normal within 7-10 days.

Urinary calcium/creatinine and urinary hydroxyproline/creatinine ratios decrease and usually return to within or below normal after treatment with Aredia. These changes occur within the first week after treatment, as do decreases in serum calcium levels, and are consistent with an antiresorptive pharmacologic action.

Hypercalcemia of Malignancy

Osteoclastic hyperactivity resulting in excessive bone resorption is the underlying pathophysiologic derangement in metastatic bone disease and hypercalcemia of malignancy. Excessive release of calcium into the blood as bone is resorbed results in polyuria and gastrointestinal disturbances, with progressive dehydration and decreasing glomerular filtration rate. This, in turn, results in increased renal resorption of calcium, setting up a cycle of worsening systemic hypercalcemia. Correction of excessive bone resorption and adequate fluid administration to correct volume deficits are therefore essential to the management of hypercalcemia.

Most cases of hypercalcemia associated with malignancy occur in patients who have breast cancer; squamous-cell tumors of the lung or head and neck; renal-cell carcinoma; and certain hematologic malignancies, such as multiple myeloma and some types of lymphomas. A few less-common malignancies, including vasoactive intestinal-peptide-producing tumors and cholangiocarcinoma, have a high incidence of hypercalcemia as a metabolic complication. Patients who have hypercalcemia of malignancy can generally be divided into two groups, according to the pathophysiologic mechanism involved.

In humoral hypercalcemia, osteoclasts are activated and bone resorption is stimulated by factors such as parathyroid-hormone-related protein, which are elaborated by the tumor and circulate systemically. Humoral hypercalcemia usually occurs in squamous-cell malignancies of the lung or head and neck or in genitourinary tumors such as renal-cell carcinoma or ovarian cancer. Skeletal metastases may be absent or minimal in these patients.

Extensive invasion of bone by tumor cells can also result in hypercalcemia due to local tumor products that stimulate bone resorption by osteoclasts. Tumors commonly associated with locally mediated hypercalcemia include breast cancer and multiple myeloma.

Total serum calcium levels in patients who have hypercalcemia of malignancy may not reflect the severity of hypercalcemia, since concomitant hypoalbuminemia is commonly present. Ideally, ionized calcium levels should be used to diagnose and follow hypercalcemic conditions; however, these are not commonly or rapidly available in many clinical situations. Therefore, adjustment of the total serum calcium value for differences in albumin levels is often used in place of measurement of ionized calcium; several nomograms are in use for this type of calculation (see DOSAGE AND ADMINISTRATION).

Clinical Trials

In one double-blind clinical trial, 52 patients who had hypercalcemia of malignancy were enrolled to receive 30 mg, 60 mg, or 90 mg of Aredia as a single 24-hour intravenous infusion if their corrected serum calcium levels were ≥12.0 mg/dL after 48 hours of saline hydration.

The mean baseline-corrected serum calcium for the 30-mg, 60-mg, and 90-mg groups were 13.8 mg/dL, 13.8 mg/dL, and 13.3 mg/dL, respectively.

The majority of patients (64%) had decreases in albumin-corrected serum calcium levels by 24 hours after initiation of treatment. Mean-corrected serum calcium levels at days 2-7 after initiation of treatment with Aredia were significantly reduced from baseline in all three dosage groups. As a result, by 7 days after initiation of treatment with Aredia, 40%, 61%, and 100% of the patients receiving 30 mg, 60 mg, and 90 mg of Aredia, respectively, had normal-corrected serum calcium levels. Many patients (33%-53%) in the 60-mg and 90-mg dosage groups continued to have normal-corrected serum calcium levels, or a partial response (≥15% decrease of corrected serum calcium from baseline), at day 14.

In a second double-blind, controlled clinical trial, 65 cancer patients who had corrected serum calcium levels of ≥12.0 mg/dL after at least 24 hours of saline hydration were randomized to receive either 60 mg of Aredia as a single 24-hour intravenous infusion or 7.5 mg/kg of Didronel (etidronate disodium) as a 2-hour intravenous infusion daily for 3 days. Thirty patients were randomized to receive Aredia and 35 to receive Didronel.

The mean baseline-corrected serum calcium for the Aredia 60-mg and Didronel groups were 14.6 mg/dL and 13.8 mg/dL, respectively.

By day 7, 70% of the patients in the Aredia group and 41% of the patients in the Didronel group had normal-corrected serum calcium levels (P<0.05). When partial responders (≥15% decrease of serum calcium from baseline) were also included, the response rates were 97% for the Aredia group and 65% for the Didronel group (P<0.01). Mean-corrected serum calcium for the Aredia and Didronel groups decreased from baseline values to 10.4 and 11.2 mg/dL, respectively, on day 7. At day 14, 43% of patients in the Aredia group and 18% of patients in the Didronel group still had normal-corrected serum calcium levels, or maintenance of a partial response. For responders in the Aredia and Didronel groups, the median duration of response was similar (7 and 5 days, respectively). The time course of effect on corrected serum calcium is summarized in the following table.
[See first table at top of next page]

In a third multicenter, randomized, parallel double-blind trial, a group of 69 cancer patients with hypercalcemia was enrolled to receive 60 mg of Aredia as a 4- or 24-hour infusion, which was compared to a saline treatment group. Patients who had a corrected serum calcium level of ≥12.0 mg/dL after 24 hours of saline hydration were eligible for this trial.

The mean baseline-corrected serum calcium levels for Aredia 60-mg 4-hour infusion, Aredia 60-mg 24-hour infusion, and saline infusion were 14.2 mg/dL, 13.7 mg/dL, and 13.7 mg/dL, respectively.

By day 7 after initiation of treatment, 78%, 61%, and 22% of the patients had normal-corrected serum calcium levels for

Continued on next page

Aredia—Cont.

the 60-mg 4-hour infusion, 60-mg 24-hour infusion, and saline infusion, respectively. At day 14, 39% of the patients in the Aredia 60-mg 4-hour infusion group and 26% of the patients in the Aredia 60-mg 24-hour infusion group had normal-corrected serum calcium levels or maintenance of a partial response.

For responders, the median duration of complete responses was 4 days and 6.5 days for Aredia 60-mg 4-hour infusion and Aredia 60-mg 24-hour infusion, respectively.

In all three trials, patients treated with Aredia had similar response rates in the presence or absence of bone metastases. Concomitant administration of furosemide did not affect response rates.

Thirty-two patients who had recurrent or refractory hypercalcemia of malignancy were given a second course of 60 mg of Aredia over a 4- or 24-hour period. Of these, 41% showed a complete response and 16% showed a partial response to the retreatment, and these responders had about a 3-mg/dL fall in mean-corrected serum calcium levels 7 days after retreatment.

Unlike Aredia 60 mg, the drug has not been investigated in a controlled clinical trial employing a 90-mg dose infused over a 4-hour period.

Paget's Disease

Paget's disease of bone (osteitis deformans) is an idiopathic disease characterized by chronic, focal areas of bone destruction complicated by concurrent excessive bone repair, affecting one or more bones. These changes result in thickened but weakened bones that may fracture or bend under stress. Signs and symptoms may be bone pain, deformity, fractures, neurological disorders resulting from cranial and spinal nerve entrapment and from spinal cord and brain stem compression, increased cardiac output to the involved bone, increased serum alkaline phosphatase levels (reflecting increased bone formation) and/or urine hydroxyproline excretion (reflecting increased bone resorption).

Clinical Trials

In one double-blind clinical trial, 64 patients with moderate to severe Paget's disease of bone were enrolled to receive 5 mg, 15 mg, or 30 mg of Aredia as a single 4-hour infusion on 3 consecutive days, for total doses of 15 mg, 45 mg, and 90 mg of Aredia.

The mean baseline serum alkaline phosphatase levels were 1409 U/L, 983 U/L, and 1085 U/L, and the mean baseline urine hydroxyproline/creatinine ratios were 0.25, 0.19, and 0.19 for the 15-mg, 45-mg, and 90-mg groups, respectively.

The effects of Aredia on serum alkaline phosphatase (SAP) and urine hydroxyproline/creatinine ratios (UOHP/C) are summarized in the following table:

[See second table above]

The median maximum percent decreases from baseline in serum alkaline phosphatase and urine hydroxyproline/creatinine ratios were 25%, 41%, and 57%, and 25%, 47%, and 61% for the 15-mg, 45-mg, and 90-mg groups, respectively. The median time to response (≥50% decrease) for serum alkaline phosphatase was approximately 1 month for the 90-mg group, and the response duration ranged from 1 to 372 days.

No statistically significant differences between treatment groups, or statistically significant changes from baseline were observed for the bone pain response, mobility, and global evaluation in the 45-mg and 90-mg groups. Improvement in radiologic lesions occurred in some patients in the 90-mg group.

Twenty-five patients who had Paget's disease were retreated with 90 mg of Aredia. Of these, 44% had a ≥50% decrease in serum alkaline phosphatase from baseline after treatment, and 39% had a ≥50% decrease in urine hydroxyproline/creatinine ratio from baseline after treatment.

Osteolytic Bone Metastases of Breast Cancer and Osteolytic Lesions of Multiple Myeloma

Osteolytic bone metastases commonly occur in patients with multiple myeloma or breast cancer. These cancers demonstrate a phenomenon known as osteotropism, meaning they possess an extraordinary affinity for bone. The distribution of osteolytic bone metastases in these cancers is predominantly in the axial skeleton, particularly the spine, pelvis, and ribs, rather than the appendicular skeleton, although lesions in the proximal femur and humerus are not uncommon. This distribution is similar to the red bone marrow in which slow blood flow possibly assists attachment of metastatic cells. The surface-to-volume ratio of trabecular bone is much higher than cortical bone, and therefore disease processes tend to occur more floridly in trabecular bone than at sites of cortical tissue.

These bone changes can result in patients having evidence of osteolytic skeletal destruction leading to severe bone pain that requires either radiation therapy or narcotic analgesics (or both) for symptomatic relief. These changes also cause pathologic fractures of bone in both the axial and appendicular skeleton. Axial skeletal fractures of the vertebral bodies may lead to spinal cord compression or vertebral body collapse with significant neurologic complications. Also, patients may experience episode(s) of hypercalcemia.

Clinical Trials

In a double-blind, randomized, placebo-controlled trial, 392 patients with advanced multiple myeloma were enrolled to receive Aredia or placebo in addition to their underlying antimyeloma therapy to determine the effect of Aredia on the occurrence of skeletal-related events (SREs). SREs were defined as episodes of pathologic fractures, radiation therapy to bone, surgery to bone, and spinal cord compression. Patients received either 90 mg of Aredia or placebo as a monthly 4-hour intravenous infusion for 9 months. Of the 392 patients, 377 were evaluable for efficacy (196 Aredia, 181 placebo). The proportion of patients developing any SRE was significantly smaller in the Aredia group (24% vs 41%, P<0.001), and the mean skeletal morbidity rate (#SRE/year) was significantly smaller for Aredia patients than for placebo patients (mean: 1.1 vs 2.1, P<.02). The times to the first SRE occurrence, pathologic fracture, and radiation to bone were significantly longer in the Aredia group (P=.001, .006, and .046, respectively). Moreover, fewer Aredia patients suffered any pathologic fracture (17% vs 30%, P=.004) or needed radiation to bone (14% vs 22%, P=.049).

In addition, decreases in pain scores from baseline occurred at the last measurement for those Aredia patients with pain at baseline (P=.026) but not in the placebo group. At the last measurement, a worsening from baseline was observed in the placebo group for the Spitzer quality of life variable (P<.001) and ECOG performance status (P<.011) while there was no significant deterioration from baseline in these parameters observed in Aredia-treated patients.*

After 21 months, the proportion of patients experiencing any skeletal event remained significantly smaller in the Aredia group than the placebo group (P=.015). In addition, the mean skeletal morbidity rate (#SRE/year) was 1.3 vs 2.2 for Aredia patients vs placebo patients (P=.008), and time to first SRE was significantly longer in the Aredia group compared to placebo (P=.016). Fewer Aredia patients suffered vertebral pathologic fractures (16% vs 27%, P=.005). Survival of all patients was not different between treatment groups.

Two double-blind, randomized, placebo-controlled trials compared the safety and efficacy of 90 mg of Aredia infused over 2 hours every 3 to 4 weeks for 24 months to that of placebo in preventing SREs in breast cancer patients with osteolytic bone metastases who had one or more predominantly lytic metastases of at least 1 cm in diameter: one in patients being treated with antineoplastic chemotherapy and the second in patients being treated with hormonal antineoplastic therapy at trial entry.

382 patients receiving chemotherapy were randomized, 185 to Aredia and 197 to placebo. 372 patients receiving hormonal therapy were randomized, 182 to Aredia and 190 to placebo. All but three patients were evaluable for efficacy. Patients were followed for 24 months of therapy or until they went off study. Median duration of follow-up was 13 months in patients receiving chemotherapy and 17 months in patients receiving hormone therapy. Twenty-five percent of the patients in the chemotherapy study and 37% of the patients in the hormone therapy study received Aredia for 24 months. The efficacy results are shown in the table below:

[See table below]

Bone lesion response was radiographically assessed at baseline and at 3, 6, and 12 months. The complete + partial response rate was 33% in Aredia patients and 18% in placebo patients treated with chemotherapy (P=.001). No difference was seen between Aredia and placebo in hormonally-treated patients.

Pain and analgesic scores, ECOG performance status and Spitzer quality of life index were measured at baseline and periodically during the trials. The changes from baseline to the last measurement carried forward are shown in the following table:

[See first table at top of next page]

INDICATIONS AND USAGE

Hypercalcemia of Malignancy

Aredia, in conjunction with adequate hydration, is indicated for the treatment of moderate or severe hypercalcemia associated with malignancy, with or without bone metastases. Patients who have either epidermoid or non-epidermoid tumors respond to treatment with Aredia. Vigorous saline hydration, an integral part of hypercalcemia therapy, should be initiated promptly and an attempt should be made to restore the urine output to about 2 L/day throughout treatment. Mild or asymptomatic hypercalcemia may be treated with conservative measures (i.e., saline hydration, with or without loop diuretics). Patients should be hydrated adequately throughout the treatment, but overhydration, especially in those patients who have cardiac failure, must be avoided. Diuretic therapy should not be employed prior to correction of hypovolemia. The safety and efficacy of Aredia in the treatment of hypercalcemia associated with hyperparathyroidism or with other non-tumor-related conditions has not been established.

Paget's Disease

Aredia is indicated for the treatment of patients with moderate to severe Paget's disease of bone. The effectiveness of

Change in Corrected Serum Calcium by Time from Initiation of Treatment

Time (hr)	Mean Change from Baseline in Corrected Serum Calcium (mg/dL) Aredia	Didronel	P-Value[1]
Baseline	14.6	13.8	
24	−0.3	−0.5	
48	−1.5	−1.1	
72	−2.6	−2.0	
96	−3.5	−2.0	<0.01
168	−4.1	−2.5	<0.01

[1]Comparison between treatment groups

Percent of Patients With Significant % Decreases in SAP and UOHP/C

	SAP			UOHP/C		
% Decrease	15 mg	45 mg	90 mg	15 mg	45 mg	90 mg
≥50	26	33	60	15	47	72
≥30	40	65	83	35	57	85

	Breast Cancer Patients Receiving Chemotherapy									Breast Cancer Patients Receiving Hormonal Therapy								
	Any SRE			Radiation			Fractures			Any SRE			Radiation			Fractures		
	A		P	A		P	A		P	A		P	A		P	A		P
N	185		195	185		195	185		195	182		189	182		189	182		189
Skeletal Morbidity Rate (#SRE/year)																		
Mean	2.5		3.7	0.8		1.3	1.6		2.2	2.4		3.6	0.6		1.2	1.6		2.2
P-Value		<.001			<.001†			.018†			.021			.013†			.040†	
Proporation of patients having an SRE	46%		65%	28%		45%	36%		49%	55%		63%	31%		40%	45%		55%
P-Value		<.001			<.001†			.014†			.094			.058†			.054†	
Median Time to SRE (months)	13.9		7.0	NR**		14.2	25.8		13.3	10.9		7.4	NR**		23.4	20.6		12.8
P-Value		<.001			<.001†			.009†			.118			.016†			.113†	

†Fractures and radiation to bone were two of several secondary endpoints. The statistical significance of these analyses may be overestimated since numerous analyses were performed.
**NR = Not Reached.

Mean Change (Δ) from Baseline at Last Measurement

	Breast Cancer Patients Receiving Chemotherapy					Breast Cancer Patients Receiving Hormonal Therapy				
	Aredia		Placebo		A vs P	Aredia		Placebo		A vs P
	N	Mean Δ	N	Mean Δ	P-Value*	N	Mean Δ	N	Mean Δ	P-Value*
Pain Score	175	+0.93	183	+1.69	.050	173	+0.50	179	+1.60	.007
Analgesic Score	175	+0.74	183	+1.55	.009	173	+0.90	179	+2.28	<.001
ECOG PS	178	+0.81	186	+1.19	.002	175	+0.95	182	+0.90	.773
Spitzer QOL	177	- 1.76	185	- 2.21	.103	173	- 1.86	181	- 2.05	.409

Decreases in pain, analgesic scores and ECOG PS, and increases in Spitzer QOL indicate an improvement from baseline.

*The statistical significance of analyses of these secondary endpoints of pain, quality of life, and performance status in all three trials may be overestimated since numerous analyses were performed.

Treatment-Related Adverse Experiences Reported in Three U.S. Controlled Clinical Trials

	Percent of Patients				
	Aredia			Didronel	Saline
	60 mg over 4 hr n=23	60 mg over 24 hr n=73	90 mg over 24 hr n=17	7.5 mg/kg × 3 days n=35	n=23
General					
Edema	0	1	0	0	0
Fatigue	0	0	12	0	0
Fever	26	19	18	9	0
Fluid overload	0	0	0	6	0
Infusion-site reaction	0	4	18	0	0
Moniliasis	0	0	6	0	0
Rigors	0	0	0	0	4
Gastrointestinal					
Abdominal pain	0	1	0	0	0
Anorexia	4	1	12	0	0
Constipation	4	0	6	3	0
Diarrhea	0	1	0	0	0
Dyspepsia	4	0	0	0	0
Gastrointestinal hemorrhage	0	0	6	0	0
Nausea	4	0	18	6	0
Stomatitis	0	1	0	3	0
Vomiting	4	0	0	0	0
Respiratory					
Dyspnea	0	0	0	3	0
Rales	0	0	6	0	0
Rhinitis	0	0	6	0	0
Upper respiratory infection	0	3	0	0	0
CNS					
Anxiety	0	0	0	0	4
Convulsions	0	0	0	3	0
Insomnia	0	1	0	0	0
Nervousness	0	0	0	0	4
Psychosis	4	0	0	0	0
Somnolence	0	1	6	0	0
Taste perversion	0	0	0	3	0
Cardiovascular					
Atrial fibrillation	0	0	6	0	4
Atrial flutter	0	1	0	0	0
Cardiac failure	0	1	0	0	0
Hypertension	0	0	6	0	4
Syncope	0	0	6	0	0
Tachycardia	0	0	6	0	4
Endocrine					
Hypothyroidism	0	0	6	0	0
Hemic and Lymphatic					
Anemia	0	0	6	0	0
Leukopenia	4	0	0	0	0
Neutropenia	0	1	0	0	0
Thrombocytopenia	0	1	0	0	0
Musculoskeletal					
Myalgia	0	1	0	0	0
Urogenital					
Uremia	4	0	0	0	0
Laboratory Abnormalities					
Hypocalcemia	0	1	12	0	0
Hypokalemia	4	4	18	0	0
Hypomagnesemia	4	10	12	3	4
Hypophosphatemia	0	9	18	3	0
Abnormal liver function	0	0	0	3	0

Aredia was demonstrated primarily in patients with serum alkaline phosphatase ≥3 times the upper limit of normal. Aredia therapy in patients with Paget's disease has been effective in reducing serum alkaline phosphatase and urinary hydroxyproline levels by ≥50% in at least 50% of patients, and by ≥30% in at least 80% of patients. Aredia therapy has also been effective in reducing these biochemical markers in patients with Paget's disease who failed to respond, or no longer responded to other treatments.

Osteolytic Bone Metastases of Breast Cancer and Osteolytic Lesions of Multiple Myeloma

Aredia is indicated, in conjunction with standard antineoplastic therapy, for the treatment of osteolytic bone metastases of breast cancer and osteolytic lesions of multiple myeloma. The Aredia treatment effect appeared to be smaller in the study of breast cancer patients receiving hormonal therapy than in the study of those receiving chemotherapy, however, overall evidence of clinical benefit has been demonstrated *(see CLINICAL PHARMACOLOGY, Osteolytic Bone Metastases of Breast Cancer and Osteolytic Lesions of Multiple Myeloma, Clinical Trials section).*

CONTRAINDICATIONS

Aredia is contraindicated in patients with clinically significant hypersensitivity to Aredia or other bisphosphonates.

WARNINGS

In both rats and dogs, nephropathy has been associated with intravenous (bolus and infusion) administration of Aredia.

Two 7-day intravenous infusion studies were conducted in the dog wherein Aredia was given for 1, 4, or 24 hours at doses of 1-20 mg/kg for up to 7 days. In the first study, the compound was well tolerated at 3 mg/kg (1.7 × highest recommended human dose [HRHD] for a single intravenous infusion) when administered for 4 or 24 hours, but renal findings such as elevated BUN and creatinine levels and renal tubular necrosis occurred when 3 mg/kg was infused for 1 hour and at doses of ≥10 mg/kg. In the second study, slight renal tubular necrosis was observed in 1 male at 1 mg/kg when infused for 4 hours. Additional findings included elevated BUN levels in several treated animals and renal tubular dilation and/or inflammation at ≥1 mg/kg after each infusion time.

Aredia was given to rats at doses of 2, 6, and 20 mg/kg and to dogs at doses of 2, 4, 6, and 20 mg/kg as a 1-hour infusion, once a week, for 3 months followed by a 1-month recovery period. In rats, nephrotoxicity was observed at ≥6 mg/kg and included increased BUN and creatinine levels and tubular degeneration and necrosis. These findings were still present at 20 mg/kg at the end of the recovery period. In dogs, moribundity/death and renal toxicity occurred at 20 mg/kg as did kidney findings of elevated BUN and creatinine levels at ≥6 mg/kg and renal tubular degeneration at ≥4 mg/kg. The kidney changes were partially reversible at 6 mg/kg. In both studies, the dose level that produced no adverse renal effects was considered to be 2 mg/kg (1.1 × HRHD for a single intravenous infusion).

Patients who receive an intravenous infusion of Aredia should have periodic evaluations of standard laboratory and clinical parameters of renal function.

Studies conducted in young rats have reported the disruption of dental dentine formation following single- and multi-dose administration of bisphosphonates. The clinical significance of these findings is unknown.

PRECAUTIONS

General

Standard hypercalcemia-related metabolic parameters, such as serum levels of calcium, phosphate, magnesium, and potassium, should be carefully monitored following initiation of therapy with Aredia. Cases of asymptomatic hypophosphatemia (12%), hypokalemia (7%), hypomagnesemia (11%), and hypocalcemia (5%-12%), were reported in Aredia-treated patients. Rare cases of symptomatic hypocalcemia (including tetany) have been reported in association with Aredia therapy. If hypocalcemia occurs, short-term calcium therapy may be necessary. In Paget's disease of bone, 17% of patients treated with 90 mg of Aredia showed serum calcium levels below 8 mg/dL.

Aredia has not been tested in patients who have class Dc renal impairment (creatinine >5.0 mg/dL), and in few multiple myeloma patients with serum creatinine ≥3.0 mg/dL. *(See also CLINICAL PHARMACOLOGY, Pharmacokinetics.)* Clinical judgment should determine whether the potential benefit outweighs the potential risk in such patients.

Laboratory Tests

Serum calcium, electrolytes, phosphate, magnesium and creatinine, and CBC, differential, and hematocrit/hemoglobin must be closely monitored in patients treated with Aredia. Patients who have preexisting anemia, leukopenia, or thrombocytopenia should be monitored carefully in the first 2 weeks following treatment.

Drug Interactions

Concomitant administration of a loop diuretic had no effect on the calcium-lowering action of Aredia.

Carcinogenesis, Mutagenesis, Impairment of Fertility

In a 104-week carcinogenicity study (daily oral administration) in rats, there was a positive dose response relationship for benign adrenal pheochromocytoma in males ($P < 0.00001$). Although this condition was also observed in females, the incidence was not statistically significant. When the dose calculations were adjusted to account for the limited oral bioavailability of Aredia in rats, the lowest daily dose associated with adrenal pheochromocytoma was similar to the intended clinical dose. Adrenal pheochromocytoma was also observed in low numbers in the control animals and is considered a relatively common spontaneous neoplasm in the rat. Aredia (daily oral administration) was not carcinogenic in an 80-week study in mice.

Aredia was nonmutagenic in six mutagenicity assays: Ames test, *Salmonella* and *Escherichia*/liver-microsome test, nucleus-anomaly test, sister-chromatid-exchange study, point-mutation test, and micronucleus test in the rat.

In rats, decreased fertility occurred in first-generation offspring of parents who had received 150 mg/kg of Aredia orally; however, this occurred only when animals were mated with members of the same dose group. Aredia has not been administered intravenously in such a study.

Pregnancy Category C

There are no adequate and well-controlled studies in pregnant women.

Bolus intravenous studies conducted in rats and rabbits determined that Aredia produces maternal toxicity and embryo/fetal effects when given during organogenesis at doses of 0.6 to 8.3 times the highest recommended human dose for a single intravenous infusion. As it has been shown that Aredia can cross the placenta in rats and has produced marked maternal and nonteratogenic embryo/fetal effects in rats and rabbits, it should not be given to women during pregnancy.

Nursing Mothers

It is not known whether Aredia is excreted in human milk. Because many drugs are excreted in human milk, caution should be exercised when Aredia is administered to a nursing woman.

Pediatric Use

Safety and effectiveness of Aredia in pediatric patients have not been established.

ADVERSE REACTIONS

Clinical Studies

Hypercalcemia of Malignancy

Transient mild elevation of temperature by at least 1°C was noted 24 to 48 hours after administration of Aredia in 34% of patients in clinical trials. In the saline trial, 18% of patients had a temperature elevation of at least 1°C 24 to 48 hours after treatment.

Drug-related local soft-tissue symptoms (redness, swelling or induration and pain on palpation) at the site of catheter insertion were most common (18%) in patients treated with

Continued on next page

Aredia—Cont.

90 mg of Aredia. When all on-therapy events are considered, that rate rises to 41%. Symptomatic treatment resulted in rapid resolution in all patients.
Rare cases of uveitis, iritis, scleritis, and episcleritis have been reported, including one case of scleritis, and one case of uveitis upon separate rechallenges.
Four of 128 patients (3%) who received Aredia during the three U.S. controlled hypercalcemia clinical studies were reported to have had seizures, 2 of whom had preexisting seizure disorders. None of the seizures were considered to be drug-related by the investigators. However, a possible relationship between the drug and the occurrence of seizures cannot be ruled out. It should be noted that in the saline arm 1 patient (4%) had a seizure.
At least 15% of patients treated with Aredia for hypercalcemia of malignancy also experienced the following adverse events during a clinical trial:

General: Fluid overload, generalized pain
Cardiovascular: Hypertension
Gastrointestinal: Abdominal pain, anorexia, constipation, nausea, vomiting
Genitourinary: Urinary tract infection
Musculoskeletal: Bone pain
Laboratory abnormality: Anemia, hypokalemia, hypomagnesemia, hypophosphatemia

Many of these adverse experiences may have been related to the underlying disease state.
The following table lists the adverse experiences considered to be treatment-related during comparative, controlled U.S. trials.
[See second table at top of previous page]

Paget's Disease

Transient mild elevation of temperature >1°C above pretreatment baseline was noted within 48 hours after completion of treatment in 21% of the patients treated with 90 mg of Aredia in clinical trials.
Drug-related musculoskeletal pain and nervous system symptoms (dizziness, headache, paresthesia, increased sweating) were more common in patients with Paget's disease treated with 90 mg of Aredia than in patients with hypercalcemia of malignancy treated with the same dose.
Adverse experiences considered to be related to trial drug, which occurred in at least 5% of patients with Paget's disease treated with 90 mg of Aredia in two U.S. clinical trials, were fever, nausea, back pain, and bone pain.
At least 10% of all Aredia-treated patients with Paget's disease also experienced the following adverse experiences during clinical trials:

Cardiovascular: Hypertension
Musculoskeletal: Arthrosis, bone pain
Nervous system: Headache

Most of these adverse experiences may have been related to the underlying disease state.

Osteolytic Bone Metastases of Breast Cancer and Osteolytic Lesions of Multiple Myeloma

The most commonly reported (>15%) adverse experiences occurred with similar frequencies in the Aredia and placebo treatment groups, and most of these adverse experiences may have been related to the underlying disease state or cancer therapy.
[See table below]
Of the toxicities commonly associated with chemotherapy, the frequency of vomiting, anorexia, and anemia were slightly more common in the Aredia patients whereas stomatitis and alopecia occurred at a frequency similar to that in placebo patients. In the breast cancer trials, mild elevations of serum creatinine occurred in 18.5% of Aredia patients and 12.3% of placebo patients. Mineral and electrolyte disturbances, including hypocalcemia, were reported rarely and in similar percentages of Aredia-treated patients compared with those in the placebo group. The reported frequencies of hypocalcemia, hypokalemia, hypophosphatemia, and hypomagnesemia for Aredia-treated patients were 3.3%, 10.5%, 1.7%, and 4.4%, respectively, and for placebo-treated patients were 1.2%, 12%, 1.7%, and 4.5%, respectively. In previous hypercalcemia of malignancy trials, patients treated with Aredia (60 or 90 mg over 24 hours) developed electrolyte abnormalities more frequently *(see ADVERSE REACTIONS, Hypercalcemia of Malignancy).*
Arthralgias and myalgias were reported slightly more frequently in the Aredia group than in the placebo group (13.6% and 26% vs 10.8% and 20.1%, respectively).
In multiple myeloma patients, there were five Aredia-related serious and unexpected adverse experiences. Four of these were reported during the 12-month extension of the multiple myeloma trial. Three of the reports were of worsening renal function developing in patients with progressive multiple myeloma or multiple myeloma-associated amyloidosis. The fourth report was the adult respiratory distress syndrome developing in a patient recovering from pneumonia and acute gangrenous cholecystitis. One Aredia-treated patient experienced an allergic reaction characterized by swollen and itchy eyes, runny nose, and scratchy throat within 24 hours after the sixth infusion.
In the breast cancer trials, there were four Aredia-related adverse experiences, all moderate in severity, that caused a patient to discontinue participation in the trial. One was due to interstitial pneumonitis, another to malaise and dyspnea. One Aredia patient discontinued the trial due to a symptomatic hypocalcemia. Another Aredia patient discontinued therapy due to severe bone pain after each infusion, which the investigator felt was trial-drug-related.

Post-Marketing Experience

Rare instances of allergic manifestations have been reported, including hypotension, dyspnea, or angioedema, and, very rarely, anaphylactic shock. Aredia is contraindicated in patients with clinically significant hypersensitivity to Aredia or other bisphosphonates *(see CONTRAINDICATIONS).*

OVERDOSAGE

There have been several cases of drug maladministration of intravenous Aredia in hypercalcemia patients with total doses of 225 mg to 300 mg given over 2 1/2 to 4 days. All of these patients survived, but they experienced hypocalcemia that required intravenous and/or oral administration of calcium.
In addition, one obese woman (95 kg) who was treated with 285 mg of Aredia/day for 3 days experienced high fever (39.5° C), hypotension (from 170/90 mmHg to 90/60 mmHg), and transient taste perversion, noted about 6 hours after the first infusion. The fever and hypotension were rapidly corrected with steroids.
If overdosage occurs, symptomatic hypocalcemia could also result; such patients should be treated with short-term intravenous calcium.

DOSAGE AND ADMINISTRATION

Hypercalcemia of Malignancy

Consideration should be given to the severity of as well as the symptoms of hypercalcemia. Vigorous saline hydration alone may be sufficient for treating mild, asymptomatic hypercalcemia. Overhydration should be avoided in patients who have potential for cardiac failure. In hypercalcemia associated with hematologic malignancies, the use of glucocorticoid therapy may be helpful.

Moderate Hypercalcemia

The recommended dose of Aredia in moderate hypercalcemia (corrected serum calcium* of approximately 12-13.5 mg/dL) is 60 to 90 mg. The 60-mg dose is given as an initial, SINGLE-DOSE, intravenous infusion over at least 4 hours. The 90-mg dose must be given by an initial, SINGLE-DOSE, intravenous infusion over 24 hours.

Severe Hypercalcemia

The recommended dose of Aredia in severe hypercalcemia (corrected serum calcium* >13.5 mg/dL) is 90 mg. The 90-mg dose must be given by an initial, SINGLE-DOSE, intravenous infusion over 24 hours.

*Albumin-corrected serum calcium (CCa,mg/dL) = serum calcium, mg/dL + 0.8 (4.0-serum albumin, g/dL).

Retreatment

A limited number of patients have received more than one treatment with Aredia for hypercalcemia. Retreatment with Aredia, in patients who show complete or partial response initially, may be carried out if serum calcium does not return to normal or remain normal after initial treatment. **It is recommended that a minimum of 7 days elapse before retreatment, to allow for full response to the initial dose.** The dose and manner of retreatment is identical to that of the initial therapy.

Paget's Disease

The recommended dose of Aredia in patients with moderate to severe Paget's disease of bone is 30 mg daily, administered as a 4-hour infusion on 3 consecutive days for a total dose of 90 mg.

Retreatment

A limited number of patients with Paget's disease have received more than one treatment of Aredia in clinical trials. When clinically indicated, patients should be retreated at the dose of initial therapy.

Osteolytic Bone Lesions of Multiple Myeloma

The recommended dose of Aredia in patients with osteolytic bone lesions of multiple myeloma is 90 mg administered as a 4-hour infusion given on a monthly basis.
Patients with marked Bence-Jones proteinuria and dehydration should receive adequate hydration prior to Aredia infusion.
Limited information is available on the use of Aredia in multiple myeloma patients with a serum creatinine ≥3.0 mg/dL.
The optimal duration of therapy is not yet known, however, in a study of patients with myeloma, final analysis after 21 months demonstrated overall benefits *(see CLINICAL TRIALS section).*

Osteolytic Bone Metastases of Breast Cancer

The recommended dose of Aredia in patients with osteolytic bone metastases is 90 mg administered over a 2-hour infusion given every 3-4 weeks.
Aredia has been frequently used with doxorubicin, fluorouracil, cyclophosphamide, methotrexate, mitoxantrone, vinblastine, dexamethasone, prednisone, melphalan, vincristine, megesterol, and tamoxifen. It has been given less frequently with etoposide, cisplatin, cytarabine, paclitaxel, and aminoglutethimide. The optimal duration of therapy is not known, however, in two breast cancer studies, final analyses performed after 24 months of therapy demonstrated overall benefits *(see CLINICAL TRIALS section).*

Preparation of Solution

Reconstitution

Aredia is reconstituted by adding 10 mL of Sterile Water for Injection, USP, to each vial, resulting in a solution of 30 mg/10 mL or 90 mg/10 mL. The pH of the reconstituted solution is 6.0-7.4. The drug should be completely dissolved before the solution is withdrawn.

Hypercalcemia of Malignancy

The daily dose must be administered as an intravenous infusion over at least 4 hours for the 60-mg dose, and over 24 hours for the 90-mg dose. The recommended dose should be diluted in 1000 mL of sterile 0.45% or 0.9% Sodium Chloride, USP, or 5% Dextrose Injection, USP. This infusion solution is stable for up to 24 hours at room temperature.

Paget's Disease

The recommended daily dose of 30 mg should be diluted in 500 mL of sterile 0.45% or 0.9% Sodium Chloride, USP, or 5% Dextrose Injection, USP, and administered over a 4-hour period for 3 consecutive days.

Osteolytic Bone Metastases of Breast Cancer

The recommended dose of 90 mg should be diluted in 250 mL of sterile 0.45% or 0.9% Sodium Chloride, USP, or 5% Dextrose Injection, USP, and administered over a 2-hour period every 3-4 weeks.

Commonly Reported Adverse Experiences in Three U.S. Controlled Clinical Trials

	Aredia 90 mg over 4 hours N=205 %	Placebo N=187 %	Aredia 90 mg over 2 hours N=367 %	Placebo N=386 %	All Aredia 90 mg N=572 %	Placebo N=573 %
General						
Asthenia	16.1	17.1	25.6	19.2	22.2	18.5
Fatigue	31.7	28.3	40.3	28.8	37.2	29.0
Fever	38.5	38.0	38.1	32.1	38.5	34.0
Metastases	1.0	3.0	31.3	24.4	20.5	17.5
Pain	13.2	11.8	15.0	18.1	14.3	16.1
Digestive System						
Anorexia	17.1	17.1	31.1	24.9	26.0	22.3
Constipation	28.3	31.7	36.0	38.6	33.2	35.1
Diarrhea	26.8	26.8	29.4	30.6	28.5	29.7
Dyspepsia	17.6	13.4	18.3	15.0	22.6	17.5
Nausea	35.6	37.4	63.5	59.1	53.5	51.8
Pain Abdominal	19.5	16.0	24.3	18.1	22.6	17.5
Vomiting	16.6	19.8	46.3	39.1	35.7	32.8
Hemic and Lymphatic						
Anemia	47.8	41.7	39.5	36.8	42.5	38.4
Granulocytopenia	20.5	15.5	19.3	20.5	19.8	18.8
Thrombocytopenia	16.6	17.1	12.5	14.0	14.0	15.0
Musculoskeletal System						
Arthralgias	10.7	7.0	15.3	12.7	13.6	10.8
Myalgia	25.4	15.0	26.4	22.5	26.0	20.1
Skeletal Pain	61.0	71.7	70.0	75.4	66.8	74.0
CNS						
Anxiety	7.8	9.1	18.0	16.8	14.3	14.3
Headache	24.4	19.8	27.2	23.6	26.2	22.3
Insomnia	17.1	17.2	25.1	19.4	22.2	19.0
Respiratory System						
Coughing	26.3	22.5	25.3	19.7	25.7	20.6
Dyspnea	22.0	21.4	35.1	24.4	30.4	23.4
Pleural Effusion	2.9	4.3	15.0	9.1	10.7	7.5
Sinusitis	14.6	16.6	16.1	10.4	15.6	12.0
Upper Respiratory Tract Infection	32.2	28.3	19.6	20.2	24.1	22.9
Urogenital System						
Urinary Tract Infection	15.6	9.1	20.2	17.6	18.5	15.6

Osteolytic Bone Lesions of Multiple Myeloma

The recommended dose of 90 mg should be diluted in 500 mL of sterile 0.45% or 0.9% Sodium Chloride, USP, or 5% Dextrose Injection, USP, and administered over a 4-hour period on a monthly basis.

Aredia must not be mixed with calcium-containing infusion solutions, such as Ringer's solution, and should be given in a single intravenous solution and line separate from all other drugs.

***Note:* Parenteral drug products should be inspected visually for particulate matter and discoloration prior to administration, whenever solution and container permit.**

Aredia reconstituted with Sterile Water for Injection may be stored under refrigeration at 36°F-46°F (2°C-8°C) for up to 24 hours.

HOW SUPPLIED

Vials - 30 mg - each contains 30 mg of sterile, lyophilized pamidronate disodium and 470 mg of mannitol, USP.

Carton of 4 vials .... NDC 0083-2601-04

Vials - 90 mg - each contains 90 mg of sterile, lyophilized pamidronate disodium and 375 mg of mannitol, USP.

Carton of 1 vial .... NDC 0083-2609-01

Do not store above 30°C (86°F).

REV: APRIL 1999 T1999-25

Shown in Product Identification Guide, page 325

BRETHINE® Tablets ℞

[breth-een']

terbutaline sulfate tablets USP

Tablets of 5 mg

Tablets of 2.5 mg

Rx only

The following prescribing information is based on official labeling in effect July 2000.

DESCRIPTION

Terbutaline sulfate USP, the active ingredient of Brethine, is a beta-adrenergic agonist bronchodilator available as tablets of 2.5 mg (2.05 mg of the free base) and 5 mg (4.1 mg of the free base) for oral administration. Terbutaline sulfate is ±-α-[(*tert*-butylamino)methyl]-3,5-dihydroxybenzyl alcohol sulfate (2:1) (salt). The empirical formula is $(C_{12}H_{19}NO_3)_2 \bullet H_2SO_4$ and the structural formula is

$$\left[\text{HO-}\underset{\text{HO}}{C_6H_3}\text{-CHCH}_2\text{NHC(CH}_3)_3 \right]_2 \cdot H_2SO_4 \quad (\text{OH on CH})$$

Terbutaline sulfate USP is a white to gray-white crystalline powder. It is odorless or has a faint odor of acetic acid. It is soluble in water and in 0.1N hydrochloric acid, slightly soluble in methanol, and insoluble in chloroform. Its molecular weight is 548.65.

Inactive Ingredients. Cellulose compounds, lactose, magnesium stearate, povidone, and corn starch.

CLINICAL PHARMACOLOGY

In vitro and in vivo pharmacologic studies have demonstrated that terbutaline exerts a preferential effect on $beta_2$-adrenergic receptors. While it is recognized that $beta_2$-adrenergic receptors are the predominant receptors in bronchial smooth muscle, data indicate that there is a population of $beta_2$-receptors in the human heart, existing in a concentration between 10%–50%. The precise function of these receptors has not been established (see WARNINGS).

In controlled clinical studies in patients given Brethine orally, proportionally greater changes occurred in pulmonary function parameters than in heart rate or blood pressure. While this suggests a relative preference for the $beta_2$-receptors in man, the usual cardiovascular effects commonly associated with other sympathomimetic agents were also observed with Brethine.

The pharmacologic effects of beta-adrenergic agonists, including terbutaline, are at least in part attributable to stimulation through beta-adrenergic receptors of intracellular adenyl cyclase, the enzyme which catalyzes the conversion of adenosine triphosphate (ATP) to cyclic 3′, 5′-adenosine monophosphate (cAMP). Increased cAMP levels are associated with relaxation of bronchial smooth muscle and inhibition of release of mediators of immediate hypersensitivity from cells, especially from mast cells.

Controlled clinical studies have shown that Brethine relieves bronchospasm in chronic obstructive pulmonary disease by significantly increasing pulmonary function (e.g., an increase of 15% or more in FEV_1 and in $FEF_{25\%-75\%}$). After administration of Brethine tablets, a measurable change in flow rate usually occurs within 30 minutes, and a clinically significant improvement in pulmonary function occurs within 60–120 minutes. The maximum effect usually occurs within 120–180 minutes. Brethine also produces a clinically significant decrease in airway and pulmonary resistance, which persists for 4 hours or longer. Significant bronchodilator action (as measured by airway resistance, $FEF_{25\%-75\%}$ or PEFR) has also been demonstrated for up to 8 hours in some studies.

In studies comparing the effectiveness of Brethine with that of ephedrine for up to 3 months, both drugs maintained a significant improvement in pulmonary function throughout this period of treatment.

Preclinical

Studies in laboratory animals (minipigs, rodents, and dogs) have demonstrated the occurrence of cardiac arrhythmias and sudden death (with histologic evidence of myocardial necrosis) when beta-agonists and methylxanthines were administered concurrently. The clinical significance of these findings is unknown.

Pharmacokinetics

Oral administration of 5-mg Brethine tablets or 5 mg terbutaline sulfate in solution in 17 healthy, adult, male subjects, resulted in mean (SD) peak plasma terbutaline concentration of 8.3 (3.9) and 8.6 (3.6) ng/mL, which were observed at median (range) times of 2 (1–3) and 1.5 (0.5–3.0) hours after dosing. The mean (SD) AUC(0–48) values were 54.6 (26.8) and 53.1 (23.5) hr•ng/mL, and corresponded to a bioavailability of 103% for the tablet relative to the solution.

After oral administration of terbutaline, 51 to 62 mcg/kg of body weight, to 3 healthy male subjects, peak serum levels of 3.1 to 6.2 ng/mL were observed 1 to 3 hours later. In the same study, after 3 days only 30%–50% of the dose was recovered from urine and the remainder from the feces, which may indicate poor absorption.

After an oral dose to asthmatic patients, the elimination half-life of terbutaline was approximately 3.4 hours.

In comparison to oral dosing, subcutaneous administration of 0.5 mg of terbutaline sulfate to 17 healthy, adult, male subjects resulted in a mean (SD) peak plasma terbutaline concentration of 9.6 (3.6) ng/mL, which was observed at a median (range) time of 0.5 (0.08–1.0) hours after dosing. The mean (SD) AUC (0–48) and total body clearance values were 29.4 (14.2) hr•ng/mL, and 311 (112) mL/min, respectively. The terminal half-life was determined in 9 of the 17 subjects and had a mean (SD) of 5.7 (2.0) hours.

About 90% of the drug was excreted in the urine at 96 hours after subcutaneous administration, with about 60% of this being unchanged drug. The sulfate conjugate is a major metabolite of terbutaline, and urinary excretion is the primary route of elimination.

There are no reports of any clinical pharmacokinetic studies investigating dose proportionality, effect of food, or special population studies with terbutaline.

INDICATIONS AND USAGE

Brethine is indicated for the prevention and reversal of bronchospasm in patients 12 years of age and older with asthma and reversible bronchospasm associated with bronchitis and emphysema.

CONTRAINDICATIONS

Brethine is contraindicated in patients known to be hypersensitive to sympathomimetic amines or any component of this drug product.

WARNINGS

Deterioration of Asthma

Asthma may deteriorate acutely over a period of hours or chronically over several days or longer. If the patient needs more doses of Brethine than usual, this may be a marker of destabilization of asthma and requires reevaluation of the patient and the treatment regimen, giving special consideration to the possible need for anti-inflammatory treatment, e.g., corticosteroids.

Use of Anti-Inflammatory Agents

The use of beta-adrenergic agonist bronchodilators alone may not be adequate to control asthma in many patients. Early consideration should be given to adding anti-inflammatory agents, e.g., corticosteroids.

Cardiovascular Effects

Brethine, like all other beta-adrenergic agonists, can produce a clinically significant cardiovascular effect in some patients as measured by pulse rate, blood pressure, and/or symptoms. Although such effects are uncommon after administration of Brethine at recommended doses, if they occur, the drug may need to be discontinued. In addition, beta-agonists have been reported to produce electrocardiogram (ECG) changes, such as flattening of the T wave, prolongation of the QTc interval, and ST segment depression. The clinical significance of these findings is unknown. Therefore, Brethine, like all sympathomimetic amines, should be used with caution in patients with cardiovascular disorders, especially coronary insufficiency, cardiac arrhythmias, and hypertension.

Seizures

There have been rare reports of seizures in patients receiving terbutaline; seizures did not recur in these patients after the drug was discontinued.

PRECAUTIONS

Tocolysis

Terbutaline sulfate has not been approved and should not be used for tocolysis. Serious adverse reactions may occur after administration of terbutaline sulfate to women in labor. In the mother, these include increased heart rate, transient hyperglycemia, hypokalemia, cardiac arrhythmias, pulmonary edema, and myocardial ischemia. Increased fetal heart rate and neonatal hypoglycemia may occur as a result of maternal administration.

General

Terbutaline, as with all sympathomimetic amines, should be used with caution in patients with cardiovascular disorders, including ischemic heart disease, hypertension, and cardiac arrhythmias; hyperthyroidism; diabetes mellitus; hypersensitivity to sympathomimetic amines; and convulsive disorders. Significant changes in systolic and diastolic blood pressure have been seen and could be expected to occur in some patients after use of any beta-adrenergic bronchodilator.

Immediate hypersensitivity reactions and exacerbation of bronchospasm have been reported after terbutaline administration.

Beta-adrenergic agonist medications may produce significant hypokalemia in some patients, possibly through intracellular shunting, which has the potential to produce adverse cardiovascular effects. The decrease is usually transient, not requiring supplementation.

Large doses of intravenous terbutaline sulfate have been reported to aggravate preexisting diabetes and ketoacidosis.

Information for Patients

The action of Brethine should last up to 6 hours or longer. Brethine should not be used more frequently than recommended. Do not increase the dose or frequency of Brethine without consulting your physician. If you find that treatment with Brethine becomes less effective for symptomatic relief, your symptoms become worse, and/or you need to use the product more frequently than usual, you should seek medical attention immediately. While taking Brethine, other inhaled drugs and asthma medications should be taken only as directed by your physician. Common adverse effects include palpitations, chest pain, rapid heart rate, tremor or nervousness. If you are pregnant or nursing, contact your physician about use of Brethine. Effective and safe use of Brethine includes an understanding of the way that it should be administered.

Drug Interactions

The concomitant use of Brethine with other sympathomimetic agents is not recommended, since the combined effect on the cardiovascular system may be deleterious to the patient. However, this does not preclude the use of an aerosol bronchodilator of the adrenergic-stimulant type for the relief of an acute bronchospasm in patients receiving chronic oral therapy with Brethine.

Monoamine Oxidase Inhibitors and Tricyclic Antidepressants

Terbutaline sulfate should be administered with extreme caution to patients being treated with monoamine oxidase inhibitors or tricyclic antidepressants, or within 2 weeks of discontinuation of such agents, since the action of terbutaline sulfate on the vascular system may be potentiated.

Beta-Blockers

Beta-adrenergic receptor blocking agents not only block the pulmonary effect of beta-agonists, such as Brethine, but may produce severe bronchospasm in asthmatic patients. Therefore, patients with asthma should not normally be treated with beta-blockers. However, under certain circumstances, e.g., as prophylaxis after myocardial infarction, there may be no acceptable alternatives to the use of beta-adrenergic blocking agents in patients with asthma. In this setting, cardioselective beta-blockers could be considered, although they should be administered with caution.

Diuretics

The ECG changes and/or hypokalemia that may result from the administration of non-potassium sparing diuretics (such as loop or thiazide diuretics) can be acutely worsened by beta-agonists, especially when the recommended dose of the beta-agonist is exceeded. Although the clinical significance of these effects is not known, caution is advised in the co-administration of beta-agonists with non-potassium sparing diuretics.

Carcinogenesis, Mutagenesis, Impairment of Fertility

In a 2-year study in Sprague-Dawley rats, terbutaline sulfate caused a significant and dose-related increase in the incidence of benign leiomyomas of the mesovarium at dietary doses of 50 mg/kg, and above (approximately 25 times the maximum recommended daily oral dose for adults on a mg/m^2 basis). In a 21-month study in CD-1 mice, terbutaline sulfate showed no evidence of tumorigenicity at dietary doses up to 200 mg/kg (approximately 55 times the maximum recommended daily oral dose for adults on a mg/m^2 basis). The mutagenicity potential of terbutaline sulfate has not been determined.

Reproduction studies in rats using terbutaline sulfate demonstrated no impairment of fertility at oral doses up to 50 mg/kg (approximately 25 times the maximum recommended daily oral dose for adults on a mg/m^2 basis).

Teratogenic Effects—Pregnancy Category B

A reproduction study in Sprague-Dawley rats revealed terbutaline sulfate was not teratogenic when administered at oral doses of 50 mg/kg (approximately 25 times the maximum recommended daily oral dose for adults on a mg/m^2 basis). A reproduction study in New Zealand white rabbits revealed terbutaline sulfate was not teratogenic when administered at oral doses up to 50 mg/kg (approximately 55 times the maximum recommended daily oral dose for adults on a mg/m^2 basis).

There are, however, no adequate and well-controlled studies in pregnant women. Because animal reproduction studies are not always predictive of human responses, this drug should be used during pregnancy only if the potential benefit justifies the potential risk to the fetus. (See PRECAUTIONS, Tocolysis).

Use in Labor and Delivery

Because of the potential for beta-agonist interference with uterine contractility, use of Brethine for relief of bronchospasm during labor should be restricted to those patients in whom the benefits clearly outweigh the risk.

Continued on next page

Brethine—Cont.

Terbutaline crosses the placenta. After single dose IV administration of terbutaline to 22 women in late pregnancy who were delivered by elective Cesarean section due to clinical reasons, umbilical blood levels of terbutaline were found to range from 11% to 48% of the maternal blood levels.

Nursing Mothers

It is not known whether this drug is excreted in human milk. Therefore, Brethine should be used during nursing only if the potential benefit justifies the possible risk to the newborn.

Pediatric Use

Brethine is not recommended for patients under the age of 12 years because of insufficient clinical data to establish safety and effectiveness (see DOSAGE AND ADMINISTRATION).

ADVERSE REACTIONS

Adverse reactions observed with Brethine are similar to those commonly seen with other sympathomimetic amines. All of these reactions are generally transient in nature and usually do not require treatment. The frequency of these side effects appears to diminish with continued therapy.

The following table lists the adverse reactions seen in 199 patients treated with terbutaline sulfate tablets during six double-blind crossover studies and four double-blind parallel studies (short- and long-term) performed in the United States.

Percent Incidence of Adverse Reactions (Total Daily Dosage Range 5–15 mg) Terbutaline N=199

Reaction	%
Nervous System	
Nervousness	35.0
Tremor	15.0
Somnolence	5.5
Dizziness	3.5
Anxiety	1.0
Insomnia	1.5
Cardiovascular	
Palpitations	5.0
Tachycardia	3.5
Extrasystoles ventricular	1.5
Vasodilations	1.0
Digestive	
Nausea	3.0
Dry mouth	1.5
Body as a Whole	
Headache	7.5
Asthenia	2.0
Skin and Appendages	
Sweating	1.0

The following adverse effects each occurred in fewer than 1% of patients: hallucinations, rash, paresthesia, hypertonia, (muscle cramps), vomiting.

There have been rare reports of elevations in liver enzymes and of hypersensitivity vasculitis.

DOSAGE AND ADMINISTRATION

Adults

The usual oral dose of Brethine for adults is 5 mg administered at approximately six-hour intervals, three times daily, during the hours the patient is usually awake. If side effects are particularly disturbing, the dose may be reduced to 2.5 mg three times daily, and still provide a clinically significant improvement in pulmonary function. The total dose within 24 hours should not exceed 15 mg.

Children

Brethine is not recommended for use in children below the age of 12 years. A dosage of 2.5 mg three times daily is recommended for children 12–15 years of age. The total dose within 24 hours should not exceed 7.5 mg.

If a previously effective dosage regimen fails to provide the usual relief, medical advice should be sought immediately as this is often a sign of seriously worsening asthma that would require reassessment of therapy.

OVERDOSAGE

The median subcutaneous lethal dose of terbutaline sulfate in mature rats is approximately 165 mg/kg (approximately 90 times the maximum recommended daily oral dose for adults on a mg/m^2 basis). The median subcutaneous lethal dose of terbutaline sulfate in young rats is approximately 2000 mg/kg (approximately 1100 times the maximum recommended daily oral dose for adults on a mg/m^2 basis).

The expected symptoms with overdosage are those of excessive beta-adrenergic stimulation and/or occurrence or exaggeration of any of the symptoms listed under ADVERSE REACTIONS, e.g., seizures, angina, hypertension or hypotension, tachycardia with rates up to 200 beats per minute, arrhythmias, nervousness, headache, tremor, dry mouth, palpitation, nausea, dizziness, fatigue, malaise, and insomnia. Hypokalemia may also occur.

There is no specific antidote. Treatment consists of discontinuation of Brethine together with appropriate symptomatic therapy. The judicious use of a cardioselective beta-receptor blocker may be considered, bearing in mind that such medication can produce bronchospasm. There is insufficient evidence to determine if dialysis is beneficial for overdosage of Brethine.

In the alert patient who has taken excessive oral medication, the stomach should be emptied by induced emesis followed by lavage. In the unconscious patient, the airway should be secured with a cuffed endotracheal tube before lavage, and emesis should not be induced. Instillation of activated charcoal slurry may help reduce absorption of terbutaline. Adequate respiratory exchange should be maintained, and cardiac and respiratory support provided as needed. The patient should be monitored until signs and symptoms of overdosage have subsided.

HOW SUPPLIED

Brethine Tablets are packaged in high density polyethylene (HDPE) bottles of 100 and 1000 tablets, and unit dose blisters. Blister packages consist of polyvinylchloride (PVC) and aluminum foil laminates. Descriptions of the 2.5 and 5 mg tablets follow:

Tablets 2.5 mg — oval, white, scored (imprinted Geigy 72)
Bottles of 100 .... NDC 0028-0072-01
Bottles of 1000 .... NDC 0028-0072-10
Unit Dose (blister pack)
Box of 100 (strips of 10) .... NDC 0028-0072-61

Tablets 5 mg — round, white, scored (imprinted Geigy 105)
Bottles of 100 .... NDC 0028-0105-01
Bottles of 1000 .... NDC 0028-0105-10
Unit Dose (blister pack)
Box of 100 (strips of 10) .... NDC 0028-0105-61

Store at controlled room temperature 15°C-30°C (59°F–86°F).

Dispense in tight, light-resistant container (USP).

REV: APRIL 1999 T1999-34

Shown in Product Identification Guide, page 325

BRETHINE® ℞

[breath-een]

terbutaline sulfate injection USP
Ampuls
A sterile aqueous solution for subcutaneous injection
Rx only

The following prescribing information is based on official labeling in effect July 2000.

DESCRIPTION

Terbutaline sulfate USP, the active ingredient of Brethine, is a beta-adrenergic agonist bronchodilator available as a sterile, nonpyrogenic, aqueous solution in ampuls, for subcutaneous administration. Each milliliter of solution contains 1 mg of terbutaline sulfate USP (0.82 mg of the free base), sodium chloride for isotonicity, and hydrochloric acid for adjustment to a target pH of 4. Terbutaline sulfate is (±)-α-[(*tert*-butylamino)methyl]-3,5-dihydroxybenzyl alcohol sulfate (2:1) (salt). The empirical formula is $(C_{12}H_{19}NO_3)_2 \bullet H_2SO_4$ and the structural formula is

[HO / HO — benzene ring — CHCH$_2$NHC(CH$_3$)$_3$ with OH]$_2$ • H$_2$SO$_4$

Terbutaline sulfate USP is a white to gray-white crystalline powder. It is odorless or has a faint odor of acetic acid. It is soluble in water and in 0.1N hydrochloric acid, slightly soluble in methanol, and insoluble in chloroform. Its molecular weight is 548.65.

CLINICAL PHARMACOLOGY

Brethine is a beta-adrenergic receptor agonist. In vitro and in vivo pharmacologic studies have demonstrated that terbutaline exerts a preferential effect on beta$_2$-adrenergic receptors. While it is recognized that beta$_2$-adrenergic receptors are the predominant receptors in bronchial smooth muscle, data indicate that there is a population of beta$_2$-receptors in the human heart, existing in a concentration between 10%–50%. The precise function of these receptors has not been established (see WARNINGS). Controlled clinical studies in patients given terbutaline subcutaneously have not revealed a preferential beta$_2$-adrenergic effect.

The pharmacologic effects of beta-adrenergic agonists, including terbutaline, are at least in part attributable to stimulation through beta-adrenergic receptors of intracellular adenyl cyclase, the enzyme which catalyzes the conversion of adenosine triphosphate (ATP) to cyclic 3′,5′-adenosine monophosphate (cAMP). Increased cAMP levels are associated with relaxation of bronchial smooth muscle and inhibition of release of mediators of immediate hypersensitivity from cells, especially from mast cells.

Controlled clinical studies have shown that Brethine relieves bronchospasm in acute and chronic obstructive pulmonary disease by significantly increasing pulmonary flow rates (e.g., an increase of 15% or more in FEV$_1$). After subcutaneous administration of 0.25 mg of Brethine, a measurable change in expiratory flow rate usually occurs within 5 minutes, and a clinically significant increase in FEV$_1$ occurs within 15 minutes. The maximum effect usually occurs within 30–60 minutes, and clinically significant bronchodilator activity may continue for 1.5 to 4 hours. The duration of clinically significant improvement is comparable to that observed with equimilligram doses of epinephrine.

Preclinical

Studies in laboratory animals (minipigs, rodents, and dogs) have demonstrated the occurrence of cardiac arrhythmias and sudden death (with histological evidence of myocardial necrosis) when beta-agonists and methylxanthines are administered concurrently. The clinical significance of these findings is unknown.

Pharmacokinetics

Subcutaneous administration of 0.5 mg of terbutaline sulfate to 17 healthy, adult, male subjects resulted in mean (SD) peak plasma terbutaline concentration of 9.6 (3.6) ng/mL, which was observed at a median (range) time of 0.5 (0.08-1.0) hours after dosing. The mean (SD) AUC (0–48) and total body clearance values were 29.4 (14.2) hr•ng/mL, and 311 (112) mL/min respectively. The terminal half-life was determined in 9 of the 17 subjects and had a mean (SD) of 5.7 (2.0) hours.

After subcutaneous administration of 0.25 mg of terbutaline sulfate to two male subjects, peak terbutaline serum concentrations of 5.2 and 5.3 ng/mL were observed at about 20 minutes after dosing.

Elimination half-life of the drug in 10 of 14 patients was approximately 2.9 hours after subcutaneous administration, but longer elimination half-lives (between 6–14 hours) were found in the other 4 patients. About 90% of the drug was excreted in the urine at 96 hours after subcutaneous administration, with about 60% of this being unchanged drug. It appears that the sulfate conjugate is a major metabolite of terbutaline and urinary excretion is the primary route of elimination.

INDICATIONS AND USAGE

Brethine is indicated for the prevention and reversal of bronchospasm in patients 12 years of age and older with asthma and reversible bronchospasm associated with bronchitis and emphysema.

CONTRAINDICATIONS

Brethine is contraindicated in patients known to be hypersensitive to sympathomimetic amines or any component of this drug product.

WARNINGS

Deterioration of Asthma

Asthma may deteriorate acutely over a period of hours or chronically over several days or longer. If the patient needs more doses of Brethine than usual, this may be a marker of destabilization of asthma and requires re-evaluation of the patient and treatment regimen, giving special consideration to the possible need for anti-inflammatory treatment, e.g., corticosteroids.

Use of Anti-Inflammatory Agents

The use of beta-adrenergic agonist bronchodilators alone may not be adequate to control asthma in many patients. Early consideration should be given to adding anti-inflammatory agents, e.g., corticosteroids.

Cardiovascular Effects

Brethine, like all other beta-adrenergic agonists, can produce a clinically significant cardiovascular effect in some patients as measured by pulse rate, blood pressure, and/or symptoms. Although such effects are uncommon after administration of Brethine at recommended doses, if they occur, the drug may need to be discontinued. In addition, beta-agonists have been reported to produce electrocardiogram (ECG) changes, such as flattening of the T wave, prolongation of the QTc interval, and ST segment depression. The clinical significance of these findings is unknown. Therefore, Brethine, like all sympathomimetic amines, should be used with caution in patients with cardiovascular disorders, especially coronary insufficiency, cardiac arrhythmias, and hypertension.

Seizures

There have been rare reports of seizures in patients receiving terbutaline; seizures did not recur in these patients after the drug was discontinued.

PRECAUTIONS

Tocolysis

Terbutaline sulfate has not been approved and should not be used for tocolysis. Serious adverse reactions may occur after administration of terbutaline sulfate to women in labor. In the mother, these include increased heart rate, transient hyperglycemia, hypokalemia, cardiac arrhythmias, pulmonary edema, and myocardial ischemia. Increased fetal heart rate and neonatal hypoglycemia may occur as a result of maternal administration.

General

Terbutaline, as with all sympathomimetic amines, should be used with caution in patients with cardiovascular disorders, including ischemic heart disease, hypertension, and cardiac arrhythmias; in patients with hyperthyroidism or diabetes mellitus; and in patients who are unusually responsive to sympathomimetic amines or who have convulsive disorders. Significant changes in systolic and diastolic blood pressure have been seen and could be expected to occur in some patients after use of any beta-adrenergic bronchodilator.

Immediate hypersensitivity reactions and exacerbations of bronchospasm have been reported after terbutaline administration.

Beta-adrenergic agonist medications may produce significant hypokalemia in some patients, possibly through intracellular shunting, which has the potential to produce adverse cardiovascular effects. The decrease is usually transient, not requiring supplementation.

Large doses of intravenous terbutaline have been reported to aggravate pre-existing diabetes mellitus and ketoacidosis.

Incidence (1%) of Adverse Reactions

	Terbutaline (%)		Epinephrine (%)	
	0.25 mg N=77	0.5 mg N=205	0.25 mg N=153	0.5 mg N=61
Reaction				
Central Nervous System				
Tremor	7.8	38.0	16.3	18.0
Nervousness	16.9	30.7	8.5	31.1
Dizziness	1.3	10.2	7.8	3.3
Headache	7.8	8.8	3.3	9.8
Drowsiness	11.7	9.8	14.4	8.2
Cardiovascular				
Palpitations	7.8	22.9	7.8	29.5
Tachycardia	1.3	1.5	2.6	0.0
Respiratory				
Dyspnea	0.0	2.0	2.0	0.0
Chest discomfort	1.3	1.5	2.6	0.0
Gastrointestinal				
Nausea/vomiting	1.3	3.9	1.3	11.5
Systemic				
Weakness	1.3	0.5	2.6	1.6
Flushed feeling	0.0	2.4	1.3	0.0
Sweating	0.0	2.4	0.0	0.0
Pain at injection site	2.6	0.5	2.6	1.6

Drug Interactions
The concomitant use of Brethine with other sympathomimetic agents is not recommended, since the combined effect on the cardiovascular system may be deleterious to the patient.
Monoamine Oxidase Inhibitors or Tricyclic Antidepressants: Terbutaline should be administered with extreme caution to patients being treated with monoamine oxidase inhibitors or tricyclic antidepressants, or within 2 weeks of discontinuation of such agents, since the action of terbutaline on the vascular system may be potentiated.
Beta-Blockers: Beta-adrenergic receptor blocking agents not only block the pulmonary effect of beta-agonists, such as Brethine, but may produce severe bronchospasm in asthmatic patients. Therefore, patients with asthma should not normally be treated with beta-blockers. However, under certain circumstances, e.g., as prophylaxis after myocardial infarction, there may be no acceptable alternatives to the use of beta-adrenergic blocking agents in patients with asthma. In this setting, cardioselective beta-blockers could be considered, although they should be administered with caution.
Diuretics: The ECG changes and/or hypokalemia that may result from the administration of nonpotassium-sparing diuretics (such as loop or thiazide diuretics) can be acutely worsened by beta-agonists, especially when the recommended dose of the beta-agonist is exceeded. Although the clinical significance of these effects is not known, caution is advised in the coadministration of beta-agonists with non-potassium-sparing diuretics.

Carcinogenesis, Mutagenesis, Impairment of Fertility
In a 2-year study in Sprague-Dawley rats, terbutaline sulfate caused a significant and dose-related increase in the incidence of benign leiomyomas of the mesovarium at dietary doses of 50 mg/kg and above (approximately 810 times the maximum recommended daily subcutaneous (sc) dose for adults on a mg/m^2 basis). In a 21-month study in CD-1 mice, terbutaline sulfate showed no evidence of tumorigenicity at dietary doses up to 200 mg/kg (approximately 1,600 times the maximum recommended daily sc dose for adults on a mg/m^2 basis). The mutagenicity potential of terbutaline sulfate has not been determined.
Reproduction studies in rats using terbutaline sulfate demonstrated no impairment of fertility at oral doses up to 50 mg/kg (approximately 810 times the maximum recommended daily sc dose for adults on a mg/m^2 basis).

Teratogenic Effects—Pregnancy Category B
A reproduction study in Sprague-Dawley rats revealed terbutaline sulfate was not teratogenic when administered orally at doses up to 50 mg/kg (approximately 810 times the maximum recommended daily sc dose for adults on a mg/m^2 basis). A reproduction study in New Zealand white rabbits revealed terbutaline sulfate was not teratogenic when administered orally at doses up to 50 mg/kg (approximately 1,600 times the maximum recommended daily sc dose for adults on a mg/m^2 basis).
There are, however, no adequate and well-controlled studies in pregnant women. Because animal reproduction studies are not always predictive of human responses, Brethine should be used during pregnancy only if the potential benefits justify the potential risk to the fetus.

Use In Labor and Delivery
Because of the potential for beta-agonist interference with uterine contractility, use of Brethine for relief of bronchospasm during labor should be restricted to those patients in whom the benefits clearly outweigh the risk.
Terbutaline crosses the placenta. After single dose IV administration of terbutaline to 22 women in late pregnancy who were delivered by elective Cesarean section due to clinical reasons, umbilical blood levels of terbutaline were found to range from 11% to 48% of the maternal blood levels.

Nursing Mothers
It is not known whether this drug is excreted in human milk. Therefore, Brethine should be used during nursing only if the potential benefit justifies the possible risk to the newborn.

Pediatric Use
Brethine is not recommended for patients under the age of 12 years because of insufficient clinical data to establish safety and effectiveness.

ADVERSE REACTIONS

Adverse reactions observed with Brethine are similar to those commonly seen with other sympathomimetic agents. All these reactions are transient in nature and usually do not require treatment.
The following table compares adverse reactions seen in patients treated with terbutaline sulfate injection (0.25 mg and 0.5 mg), with those seen in patients treated with epinephrine injection (0.25 mg and 0.5 mg), during eight double-blind crossover studies involving a total of 214 patients.
[See table above]
Note: Some patients received more than one dosage strength of terbutaline sulfate and epinephrine. In addition, there were reports of anxiety, muscle cramps, and dry mouth (<0.5%). There have been rare reports of elevations in liver enzymes and of hypersensitivity vasculitis with terbutaline administration.

OVERDOSAGE

The median sc lethal dose of terbutaline sulfate in mature rats was approximately 165 mg/kg (approximately 2,700 times the maximum recommended daily sc dose for adults on a mg/m^2 basis). The median sc lethal dose of terbutaline sulfate in young rats was approximately 2,000 mg/kg (approximately 32,000 times the maximum recommended daily sc dose for adults on a mg/m^2 basis).
The expected symptoms with overdosage are those of excessive beta-adrenergic stimulation and/or occurrence or exaggeration of any of the symptoms listed under ADVERSE REACTIONS, e.g., seizures, angina, hypertension or hypotension, tachycardia with rates up to 200 beats per minute, arrhythmias, nervousness, headache, tremor, dry mouth, palpitation, nausea, dizziness, fatigue, malaise, and insomnia. Hypokalemia may also occur. There is no specific antidote. Treatment consists of discontinuation of Brethine together with appropriate symptomatic therapy. The judicious use of a cardioselective beta-receptor blocker may be considered, bearing in mind that such medication can produce bronchospasm. There is insufficient evidence to determine if dialysis is beneficial for overdosage of Brethine.

DOSAGE AND ADMINISTRATION

Ampuls should be used only for subcutaneous administration and not intravenous infusion. Sterility and accurate dosing cannot be assured if the ampuls are not used in accordance with DOSAGE AND ADMINISTRATION.
Discard unused portion after single patient use.
The usual subcutaneous dose of Brethine is 0.25 mg injected into the lateral deltoid area. If significant clinical improvement does not occur within 15–30 minutes, a second dose of 0.25 mg may be administered. If the patient then fails to respond within another 15–30 minutes, other therapeutic measures should be considered. The total dose within 4 hours should not exceed 0.5 mg.
Note: Parenteral drug products should be inspected visually for particulate matter and discoloration prior to administration, whenever solution and container permit.

HOW SUPPLIED

Ampuls 1 mg/mL — The drug is supplied at a volume of 1 mL contained in a 2 mL clear glass ampul. Each ampul contains 1 mg of Brethine per 1 mL of solution; 0.25 mL of solution will provide the usual clinical dose of 0.25 mg. Ampuls are expiration-dated.
Box of 10 ampuls .... NDC 0028-7507-23
Box of 100 ampuls .... NDC 0028-7507-01
Keep at controlled room temperature 15°C-30°C (59°F-86°F).
Protect from light by storing ampuls in original carton until dispensed. Do not use if solution is discolored.

©2000 Novartis
REV: APRIL 2000 T2000-13
Manufactured by
Novartis Pharma AG
Basle, Switzerland for
Novartis Pharmaceuticals Corporation
East Hanover, New Jersey 07936
Shown in Product Identification Guide, page 325

CATAFLAM® ℞
diclofenac potassium
Immediate-Release Tablets
VOLTAREN® ℞
diclofenac sodium
Delayed-Release (enteric-coated) Tablets
VOLTAREN®-XR ℞
diclofenac sodium
Extended-Release Tablets
Rx only

The following prescribing information is based on official labeling in effect July 2000.

DESCRIPTION

Diclofenac, as the sodium or potassium salt, is a benzeneacetic acid derivative, designated chemically as 2-[(2,6-dichlorophenyl)amino] benzeneacetic acid, monosodium or monopotassium salt. The structural formula is shown in Figure 1.

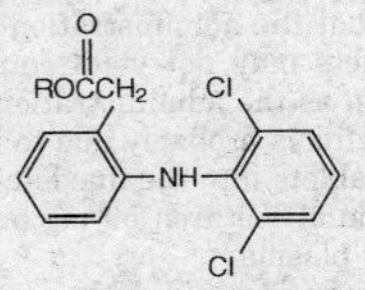

[Structural formula: ROCCH2 (C=O), Cl, NH, Cl]

Figure 1

R = K: Cataflam®, diclofenac potassium
R = Na: Voltaren® or Voltaren®-XR, diclofenac sodium
Diclofenac, as the sodium or potassium salt, is a faintly yellowish white to light beige, virtually odorless, slightly hygroscopic crystalline powder. Molecular weights of the sodium and potassium salts are 318.14 and 334.25, respectively. It is freely soluble in methanol, soluble in ethanol, and practically insoluble in chloroform and in dilute acid. Diclofenac sodium is sparingly soluble in water while diclofenac potassium is soluble in water. The n-octanol/water partition coefficient is, for both diclofenac salts, 13.4 at pH 7.4 and 1545 at pH 5.2. Both salts have a single dissociation constant (pKa) of 4.0 ± 0.2 at 25°C in water.
Diclofenac potassium is available as **Cataflam Immediate-Release Tablets** of 50 mg for oral administration.
CATAFLAM Inactive Ingredients: Calcium phosphate, colloidal silicon dioxide, iron oxides, magnesium stearate, microcrystalline cellulose, polyethylene glycol, povidone, sodium starch glycolate, starch, sucrose, talc, titanium dioxide.
Diclofenac sodium is available as **VOLTAREN Delayed-Release (enteric-coated) Tablets** of 25 mg, 50 mg, and 75 mg for oral administration, and **VOLTAREN-XR Extended-Release Tablets** of 100 mg.
VOLTAREN Inactive Ingredients: Hydroxypropyl methylcellulose, iron oxide, lactose, magnesium stearate, methacrylic acid copolymer, microcrystalline cellulose, polyethylene glycol, povidone, propylene glycol, sodium hydroxide, sodium starch glycolate, talc, titanium dioxide, D&C Yellow No. 10 Aluminum Lake (25-mg tablet only), FD&C Blue No. 1 Aluminum Lake (50-mg tablet only).
VOLTAREN-XR Inactive Ingredients: Cetyl alcohol, hydroxypropyl methylcellulose, iron oxide, magnesium stearate, polyethylene glycol, polysorbate, povidone, silicon dioxide, sucrose, talc, titanium dioxide.

CLINICAL PHARMACOLOGY

Pharmacodynamics
Diclofenac, the anion in Cataflam, Voltaren, and Voltaren-XR, is a non steroidal anti-inflammatory drug (NSAID). In pharmacologic studies, diclofenac has shown anti-inflammatory, analgesic, and antipyretic activity. As with other NSAIDs, its mode of action is not known; its ability to inhibit prostaglandin synthesis, however, may be involved in its anti-inflammatory activity, as well as contribute to its efficacy in relieving pain related to inflammation and primary dysmenorrhea. With regard to its analgesic effect, diclofenac is not a narcotic.

Pharmacokinetics
Cataflam Immediate-Release Tablets, Voltaren Delayed-Release Tablets, and Voltaren-XR Extended-Release Tablets, contain the same therapeutic moiety, diclofenac. They differ in the cationic portion of the salt (see DESCRIPTION), as well as in their release characteristics. Cataflam Immediate-Release Tablets are formulated to release diclofenac in the stomach.
Voltaren Delayed-Release (enteric-coated) Tablets are in a pharmaceutical formulation that resists dissolution in the low pH of gastric fluid but allows a rapid release of drug in the higher pH-environment of the duodenum.
Conversely, Voltaren-XR Extended-Release Tablets are formulated to release drug over a prolonged period. The primary pharmacokinetic difference between the three products is in the pattern of drug release and absorption, as described below and shown in Table 1.
[See table at top of next page]

Continued on next page

Cataflam/Voltaren—Cont.

For this reason, separate sections are provided below to describe the different absorption profiles of Cataflam Immediate-Release Tablets, Voltaren Delayed-Release Tablets, and Voltaren-XR Extended-Release Tablets.

Absorption

Under fasting condition, diclofenac is completely absorbed from the gastrointestinal tract. However, due to first-pass metabolism, only about 50% of the absorbed dose is systemically available.

Cataflam Immediate-Release Tablets: In some fasting volunteers, measurable plasma levels are observed within 10 minutes of dosing with Cataflam. Peak plasma levels are achieved in approximately 1 hour in fasting normal volunteers, with a range from 0.33 to 2 hours.

The extent of diclofenac absorption is not significantly affected when Cataflam is taken with food. However, the rate of absorption is reduced by food, as indicated by a delay in T_{max} and decrease in C_{max} values by approximately 30%. After repeated oral administration of Cataflam 50 mg t.i.d. no accumulation of diclofenac in plasma occurred.

Voltaren Delayed-Release Tablets: Peak plasma levels are achieved in 2 hours in fasting normal volunteers, with a range from 1 to 4 hours. The area-under-the-plasma-concentration curve (AUC) is dose-proportional within the range of 25 mg to 150 mg. Peak plasma levels are less than dose-proportional and are approximately 1.0, 1.5, and 2.0 µg/mL for 25-mg, 50-mg, and 75-mg doses, respectively. It should be noted that the administration of several individual Voltaren tablets may not yield equivalent results in peak concentration as the administration of one tablet of a higher strength. This is probably due to the staggered gastric emptying of tablets into the duodenum. After repeated oral administration of Voltaren 50 mg b.i.d., diclofenac did not accumulate in plasma.

When Voltaren is taken with food, there is usually a delay in the onset of absorption of 1 to 4.5 hours, with delays as long as 10 hours in some patients, and a reduction in peak plasma levels of approximately 40%. The extent of absorption of diclofenac, however, is not significantly affected by food intake.

Voltaren-XR Extended-Release Tablets: The extent of diclofenac absorption from the extended-release tablet is not significantly affected when the drug is taken with food, however, food significantly altered the absorption pattern as indicated by a delay of 1 to 2 hours in T_{max} and a two-fold increase in C_{max} values. The plasma profile of the extended-release tablet, under fasting conditions, was characterized by multiple peaks and high intersubject variability in blood profiles. In contrast, the plasma profile for the extended-release tablets under fed conditions showed a more consistent absorption pattern with a single peak usually occurring between 5 and 6 hours after the meal.

Distribution

Plasma concentrations of diclofenac decline from peak levels in a biexponential fashion, with the terminal phase having a half-life of approximately 2 hours. Clearance and volume of distribution are about 350 mL/min and 550 mL/kg, respectively. More than 99% of diclofenac is reversibly bound to human plasma albumin.

As with other NSAIDs, diclofenac diffuses into and out of the synovial fluid. Diffusion into the joint occurs when plasma levels are higher than those in the synovial fluid, after which the process reverses and synovial fluid levels are higher than plasma levels. It is not known whether diffusion into the joint plays a role in the effectiveness of diclofenac.

Metabolism and Elimination

Diclofenac is eliminated through metabolism and subsequent urinary and biliary excretion of the glucuronide and the sulfate conjugates of the metabolites. Approximately 65% of the dose is excreted in the urine, and approximately 35% in the bile.

Conjugates of unchanged diclofenac account for 5%-10% of the dose excreted in the urine and for less than 5% excreted in the bile. Little or no unchanged unconjugated drug is excreted. Conjugates of the principal metabolite account for 20%-30% of the dose excreted in the urine and for 10%-20% of the dose excreted in the bile. Conjugates of three other metabolites together account for 10%-20% of the dose excreted in the urine and for small amounts excreted in the bile. The elimination half-life values for these metabolites are shorter than those for the parent drug. Urinary excretion of an additional metabolite (half-life 80 hours) accounts for only 1.4% of the oral dose. The degree of accumulation of diclofenac metabolites is unknown. Some of the metabolites may have activity.

Special Populations

A 4-week study, comparing plasma level profiles of diclofenac (Voltaren 50 mg b.i.d.) in younger (26-46 years) versus older (66-81 years) adults, did not show differences between age groups (10 patients per age group).

Geriatric Population: An 8-day study, comparing the kinetics of diclofenac (100 mg Voltaren-XR q.d.) in osteoarthritis patients older than 65 years versus younger than 65 years showed no significant differences between the two groups with respect to peak plasma levels, time to peak levels, or AUC.

Patients with Renal and/or Hepatic Impairment: To date, no differences in the pharmacokinetics of diclofenac have been detected in studies of patients with renal (50 mg intravenously) or hepatic impairment (100-mg oral solution). In patients with renal impairment (N=5, creatinine clearance 3 to 42 mL/min), AUC values and elimination rates were comparable to those in healthy subjects. In patients with biopsy-confirmed cirrhosis or chronic active hepatitis (variably elevated transaminases and mildly elevated bilirubins, N=10), diclofenac concentrations and urinary elimination values were comparable to those in healthy subjects.

Table 1
Mean (% CV) Pharmacokinetics of Diclofenac Following Single Oral Doses of CATAFLAM, VOLTAREN Delayed-Release, and VOLTAREN-XR

Drug	Dose (mg)	AUC (ng•hr/mL)	C_{max} (ng/mL)	T_{max} (hr)
Cataflam	50	1309 (21.7%)	1312 (44.1%)	1.00 (74.6%)
Voltaren	50	1429 (38.4%)	1417 (22.4%)	2.22 (49.8%)
Voltaren-XR	100	2079 (33.7%)	417 (40.7%)	5.25 (28.3%)

Clinical Studies

Cataflam Immediate-Release Tablets in Analgesia/Primary Dysmenorrhea: The analgesic efficacy of Cataflam was demonstrated in trials of patients with postoperative pain (following gynecologic, oral, and orthopedic surgery), osteoarthritis of the knee, and primary dysmenorrhea. The effectiveness of Cataflam in studies of pain or primary dysmenorrhea showed that onset of analgesia began, in some patients, as soon as 30 minutes, and relief of pain lasted as long as 8 hours, following single 50-mg or 100-mg doses. Duration of pain relief was judged by the time at which approximately half of the patients needed remedication. The onset and duration of pain relief for either the 50-mg or 100-mg dose was essentially the same, whether patients had moderate or severe pain at baseline.

Cataflam was studied in single-dose and multiple-dose pain trials. The pain models in single-dose studies were post-dental extraction and post-gynecologic surgery: the efficacy of the 50-mg dose (N=258) and the 100-mg dose (N=255) was comparable to aspirin 650 mg in onset of pain relief, but generally provided a longer duration of analgesia than aspirin. The pain models for multiple-dose trials were post-orthopedic surgery pain as well as pain associated with primary dysmenorrhea: the efficacy of the 50-mg dose (N=101) and the 100-mg dose (N=442), followed by 50 mg every 8 hours, was comparable to naproxen sodium 550 mg followed by 275 mg every 8 hours. In one study of chronic pain, in patients with osteoarthritis (N=196), Cataflam 50 mg t.i.d. was comparable in efficacy to ibuprofen 800 mg t.i.d. and Voltaren Delayed-Release Tablets 50 mg t.i.d.

Voltaren Delayed-Release Tablets in Osteoarthritis: Voltaren was evaluated for the management of the signs and symptoms of osteoarthritis of the hip or knee in a total of 633 patients treated for up to 3 months in placebo- and active-controlled clinical trials against aspirin (N=449), and naproxen (N=92). Voltaren was given both in variable (100-150 mg/day) and fixed (150 mg/day) dosing schedules in either b.i.d. or t.i.d. dosing regimens. In these trials, Voltaren was found to be comparable to 2400 to 3600 mg/day of aspirin or 500 mg/day of naproxen. Voltaren was effective when administered as either b.i.d. or t.i.d. dosing regimens.

Voltaren Delayed-Release Tablets in Rheumatoid Arthritis: Voltaren was evaluated for managing the signs and symptoms of rheumatoid arthritis in a total of 468 patients treated for up to 3 months in placebo- and active-controlled clinical trials against aspirin (N=290), and ibuprofen (N=74). Voltaren was given in a fixed (150 or 200 mg/day) dosing schedule as either b.i.d. or t.i.d. dosing regimens. Voltaren was found to be comparable to 3600 to 4800 mg/day of aspirin, and 2400 mg/day of ibuprofen. Voltaren was used b.i.d. or t.i.d., administering 150 mg/day in most trials, but 50 mg q.i.d. (200 mg/day) was also studied.

Voltaren Delayed-Release Tablets in Ankylosing Spondylitis: Voltaren was evaluated for the management of the signs and symptoms of ankylosing spondylitis in a total of 132 patients in one active-controlled clinical trial against indomethacin (N=130). Both Voltaren and indomethacin patients were started on 25 mg t.i.d. and were permitted to increase the dose 25 mg/day each week to a maximum dose of 125 mg/day. Voltaren 75-125 mg/day was found to be comparable to indomethacin 75-125 mg/day.

Voltaren-XR Extended-Release Tablets in Osteoarthritis: The use of Voltaren-XR Tablets in controlling the signs and symptoms of osteoarthritis was assessed in two double-blind, controlled trials in which 742 patients participated and 517 patients were treated for 3 months. In one active- and placebo-controlled study, Voltaren-XR Tablets at doses of 100 mg q.d. were comparable to Voltaren Delayed-Release Tablets 50 mg b.i.d. in patients whose osteoarthritis symptoms were stabilized after 2 weeks of treatment with Voltaren Delayed-Release Tablets 75 mg b.i.d. In another study, Voltaren-XR Tablets at doses of 100 mg q.d. and 100 mg b.i.d. were compared to Voltaren Delayed-Release Tablets 50 mg q.i.d. Voltaren-XR Tablets 100 mg b.i.d. were comparable to Voltaren Delayed-Release Tablets 50 mg q.i.d. With the Voltaren-XR Tablet formulation, although there was a trend toward greater efficacy at doses of 200 mg daily than 100 mg daily, there was also an increase in side effects when 200 mg of Voltaren-XR Tablets were administered to patients with osteoarthritis.

Voltaren-XR Extended-Release Tablets in Rheumatoid Arthritis: The use of Voltaren-XR Tablets in controlling the signs and symptoms of rheumatoid arthritis was assessed in two double-blind, controlled trials in which 704 patients participated and 441 patients were treated for 3 months. In one active- and placebo-controlled study, Voltaren-XR Tablets 100 mg q.d. were comparable to Voltaren Delayed-Release Tablets 50 mg b.i.d. in patients whose rheumatoid arthritis symptoms were stabilized after 2 weeks' treatment of Voltaren Delayed-Release Tablets 75 mg b.i.d. In another study, Voltaren-XR Tablets at doses of 100 mg q.d. and 100 mg b.i.d. were compared to Voltaren Delayed-Release Tablets 50 mg q.i.d.; Voltaren-XR Tablets 100 mg b.i.d. were comparable to Voltaren Delayed-Release Tablets 50 mg q.i.d. There was a trend toward greater efficacy with doses of 200 mg daily as compared to 100 mg daily of Voltaren-XR Tablets. There was also an increase in side effects when 200 mg of Voltaren-XR Tablets were administered to patients with rheumatoid arthritis.

Special Studies *(The clinical significance of the findings outlined below is unknown.)*

G.I. Blood Loss/Endoscopy Data: G.I. blood loss and endoscopy studies were performed with Voltaren Delayed-Release (enteric-coated) Tablets that, unlike Immediate-Release Tablets, do not dissolve in the stomach where the endoscopic lesions are primarily seen; Cataflam Immediate-Release Tablets have not been similarly studied. A repeat-dose endoscopy study, in patients with rheumatoid arthritis or osteoarthritis treated with Voltaren Delayed-Release Tablets 75 mg b.i.d. (N=101), or naproxen (immediate-release tablets) 500 mg b.i.d. (N=103) for 3 months, resulted in a significantly smaller number of patients with an increase in endoscopy score from baseline and a significantly lower mean endoscopy score after treatment in the Voltaren-treated patients. Two repeat-dose endoscopic studies, in normal volunteers showed that daily doses of Voltaren Delayed-Release Tablets 75 or 100 mg (N=6 and N=14, respectively) for 1 week caused fewer gastric lesions, and those that did occur had lower scores than those observed following daily 500-mg doses of naproxen (immediate-release tablets). In healthy subjects, the daily administration of 150 mg of Voltaren (N=8) for 3 weeks resulted in a mean fecal blood loss less than that observed with 3.0 g of aspirin daily (N=8). In four repeat-dose studies, mean fecal blood loss with 150 mg of Voltaren was also less than that observed with 750 mg of naproxen (N=8 and N=6) or 150 mg of indomethacin (N=8 and N=6).

INDIVIDUALIZATION OF DOSAGE

Diclofenac, like other NSAIDs, shows interindividual differences in both pharmacokinetics and clinical response (pharmacodynamics). Consequently, the recommended strategy for initiating therapy is to use a starting dose likely to be effective for the majority of patients and to adjust dosage thereafter based on observation of diclofenac's beneficial and adverse effects.

In patients weighing less than 60 kg (132 lb), or where the severity of the disease, concomitant medication, or other diseases warrant, the maximum recommended total daily dose of Cataflam, Voltaren, or Voltaren-XR should be reduced. Experience with other NSAIDs has shown that starting therapy with maximum doses in patients at increased risk due to renal or hepatic disease, low body weight (<60 kg), advanced age, a known ulcer diathesis, or known sensitivity to NSAID effects, is likely to increase frequency of adverse reactions and is not recommended (see PRECAUTIONS).

Osteoarthritis/Rheumatoid Arthritis/Ankylosing Spondylitis: The usual starting dose of Cataflam Immediate-Release Tablets or Voltaren Delayed-Release for patients with osteoarthritis, is 100 to 150 mg/day, using a b.i.d. or t.i.d. dosing regimen. For patients with osteoarthritis, the usual starting dose of Voltaren-XR Extended-Release Tablets is 100 mg q.d. In two variable-dose clinical trials in osteoarthritis using Voltaren Delayed-Release Tablets, of 266 patients started on 100 mg/day, 176 chose to increase the dose to 150 mg/day. Dosages above 200 mg/day have not been studied in patients with osteoarthritis.

For most patients with rheumatoid arthritis, the usual starting dose of Cataflam Immediate-Release Tablets or Voltaren Delayed-Release Tablets is 150 mg/day, using a b.i.d. or t.i.d. dosing regimen. The usual starting dose of Voltaren-XR Extended-Release Tablets is 100 mg q.d. Patients requiring more relief of pain and inflammation may increase the dose to 200 mg/day. In clinical trials, patients receiving 200 mg/day were less likely to drop from the trial due to lack of efficacy than patients receiving 150 mg/day as Voltaren Delayed-Release Tablets or 100 mg/day as Voltaren-XR Extended-Release Tablets. Dosages above 225 mg/day are not recommended in patients with rheumatoid arthritis because of increased risk of adverse events.

The recommended dose of Voltaren Delayed-Release Tablets for patients with ankylosing spondylitis is 100 to 125 mg/day, using a q.i.d. dosing regimen (see DOSAGE AND AD-

MINISTRATION regarding the 125 mg/day dosing regimen). In a variable-dose clinical trial, of 132 patients started on 75 mg/day, 122 chose to increase the dose to 125 mg/day. Dosages above 125 mg/day have not been studied in patients with ankylosing spondylitis.

Analgesia/Primary Dysmenorrhea: Because of earlier absorption of diclofenac from Cataflam Immediate-Release Tablets, it is the formulation indicated for management of pain and primary dysmenorrhea when prompt onset of pain relief is desired. The results of clinical trials suggest an initial Cataflam dose of 50 mg for pain or for primary dysmenorrhea, followed by doses of 50 mg every 8 hours, as needed. With experience, some patients with recurring pain, such as dysmenorrhea, may find that an initial dose of 100 mg of Cataflam, followed by 50-mg doses, will provide better relief. After the first day, when the maximum recommended dose may be 200 mg, the total daily dose should generally not exceed 150 mg.

INDICATIONS AND USAGE

Cataflam Immediate-Release Tablets and Voltaren Delayed-Release Tablets are indicated for the acute and chronic treatment of signs and symptoms of osteoarthritis and rheumatoid arthritis. Voltaren-XR Extended-Release Tablets are indicated for chronic therapy of osteoarthritis and rheumatoid arthritis. In addition, Cataflam Immediate-Release Tablets and Voltaren Delayed-Release Tablets are indicated for the treatment of ankylosing spondylitis. Only Cataflam is indicated for the management of pain and primary dysmenorrhea, when prompt pain relief is desired, because it is formulated to provide earlier plasma concentrations of diclofenac (see CLINICAL PHARMACOLOGY, Pharmacokinetics and Clinical Studies).

CONTRAINDICATIONS

Diclofenac in all formulations, Cataflam, Voltaren, and Voltaren-XR, is contraindicated in patients with known hypersensitivity to diclofenac and diclofenac-containing products. Diclofenac should not be given to patients who have experienced asthma, urticaria, or other allergic-type reactions after taking aspirin or other NSAIDs. Severe, rarely fatal, anaphylactic-like reactions to diclofenac have been reported in such patients (see WARNINGS—Anaphylactoid Reactions, and PRECAUTIONS—Preexisting Asthma).

WARNINGS

Gastrointestinal Effects

Peptic ulceration and gastrointestinal bleeding have been reported in patients receiving diclofenac. Physicians and patients should therefore remain alert for ulceration and bleeding in patients treated chronically with diclofenac even in the absence of previous G.I. tract symptoms. It is recommended that patients be maintained on the lowest dose of diclofenac possible, consistent with achieving a satisfactory therapeutic response.

Risk of G.I. Ulcerations, Bleeding, and Perforation with NSAID Therapy: Serious gastrointestinal toxicity such as bleeding, ulceration, and perforation can occur at any time, with or without warning symptoms, in patients treated chronically with NSAID therapy. Although minor upper gastrointestinal problems, such as dyspepsia, are common, usually developing early in therapy, physicians should remain alert for ulceration and bleeding in patients treated chronically with NSAIDs even in the absence of previous G.I. tract symptoms. In patients observed in clinical trials of several months to 2 years' duration, symptomatic upper G.I. ulcers, gross bleeding, or perforation appear to occur in approximately 1% of patients for 3-6 months, and in about 2%-4% of patients treated for 1 year. Physicians should inform patients about the signs and/or symptoms of serious G.I. toxicity and what steps to take if they occur.

Studies to date have not identified any subset of patients not at risk of developing peptic ulceration and bleeding. Except for a prior history of serious G.I. events and other risk factors known to be associated with peptic ulcer disease, such as alcoholism, smoking, etc., no risk factors (e.g., age, sex) have been associated with increased risk. Elderly or debilitated patients seem to tolerate ulceration or bleeding less well than other individuals, and most spontaneous reports of fatal G.I. events are in this population. Studies to date are inconclusive concerning the relative risk of various NSAIDs in causing such reactions. High doses of any NSAID probably carry a greater risk of these reactions, although controlled clinical trials showing this do not exist in most cases. In considering the use of relatively large doses (within the recommended dosage range), sufficient benefit should be anticipated to offset the potential increased risk of G.I. toxicity.

Hepatic Effects

Elevations of one or more liver tests may occur during diclofenac therapy. These laboratory abnormalities may progress, may remain unchanged, or may be transient with continued therapy. Borderline elevations (i.e., less than 3 times the ULN [=the Upper Limit of the Normal range]), or greater elevations of transaminases occurred in about 15% of diclofenac-treated patients. Of the hepatic enzymes, ALT (SGPT) is the one recommended for the monitoring of liver injury.

In clinical trials, meaningful elevations (i.e., more than 3 times the ULN) of AST (SGOT) (ALT was not measured in all studies) occurred in about 2% of approximately 5700 patients at some time during Voltaren treatment. In a large, open, controlled trial, meaningful elevations of ALT and/or AST occurred in about 4% of 3700 patients treated for 2-6 months, including marked elevations (i.e., more than 8 times the ULN) in about 1% of the 3700 patients. In that open-label study, a higher incidence of borderline (less than 3 times the ULN), moderate (3-8 times the ULN), and marked (>8 times the ULN) elevations of ALT or AST was observed in patients receiving diclofenac when compared to other NSAIDs. Transaminase elevations were seen more frequently in patients with osteoarthritis than in those with rheumatoid arthritis (see ADVERSE REACTIONS).

In addition to enzyme elevations seen in clinical trials, postmarketing surveillance has found rare cases of severe hepatic reactions, including liver necrosis, jaundice, and fulminant fatal hepatitis with and without jaundice. Some of these rare reported cases underwent liver transplantation.

Physicians should measure transaminases periodically in patients receiving long-term therapy with diclofenac, because severe hepatotoxicity may develop without a prodrome of distinguishing symptoms. The optimum times for making the first and subsequent transaminase measurements are not known. In the largest U.S. trial (open-label) that involved 3700 patients monitored first at 8 weeks and 1200 patients monitored again at 24 weeks, almost all meaningful elevations in transaminases were detected before patients became symptomatic. In 42 of the 51 patients in all trials who developed marked transaminase elevations, abnormal tests occurred during the first 2 months of therapy with diclofenac. Postmarketing experience has shown severe hepatic reactions can occur at any time during treatment with diclofenac. Cases of drug-induced hepatotoxicity have been reported in the first month, and in some cases, the first two months of therapy. Based on these experiences, transaminases should be monitored within 4 to 8 weeks after initiating treatment with diclofenac (see PRECAUTIONS—Laboratory Tests). As with other NSAIDs, if abnormal liver tests persist or worsen, if clinical signs and/or symptoms consistent with liver disease develop, or if systemic manifestations occur (e.g., eosinophilia, rash, etc.), diclofenac should be discontinued immediately.

To minimize the possibility that hepatic injury will become severe between transaminase measurements, physicians should inform patients of the warning signs and symptoms of hepatotoxicity (e.g., nausea, fatigue, lethargy, pruritus, jaundice, right upper quadrant tenderness, and "flu-like" symptoms), and the appropriate action patients should take if these signs and symptoms appear.

Anaphylactoid Reactions

As with other NSAIDs, anaphylactoid reactions may occur in patients without prior exposure to diclofenac. Diclofenac should not be given to patients with the aspirin triad. The triad typically occurs in asthmatic patients who experience rhinitis with or without nasal polyps, or who exhibit severe, potentially fatal bronchospasm after taking aspirin or other nonsteroidal anti-inflammatory drugs. Fatal reactions have been reported in such patients (see CONTRAINDICATIONS, and PRECAUTIONS—Preexisting Asthma). Emergency help should be sought in cases where an anaphylactoid reaction occurs.

Advanced Renal Disease

In cases with advanced kidney disease, treatment with diclofenac, as with other NSAIDs, should only be initiated with close monitoring of the patient's kidney functions (see PRECAUTIONS—Renal Effects).

Pregnancy

In late pregnancy, diclofenac should, as with other NSAIDs, be avoided because it will cause premature closure of the ductus arteriosus (see PRECAUTIONS—Pregnancy, *Teratogenic Effects, Pregnancy Category B*, and Labor and Delivery).

PRECAUTIONS

General

Cataflam Immediate-Release Tablets, Voltaren Delayed-Release Tablets, and Voltaren-XR Extended-Release Tablets should not be used concomitantly with other diclofenac-containing products since they also circulate in plasma as the diclofenac anion.

Fluid Retention and Edema: Fluid retention and edema have been observed in some patients taking diclofenac. Therefore, as with other NSAIDs, diclofenac should be used with caution in patients with a history of cardiac decompensation, hypertension, or other conditions predisposing to fluid retention.

Hematologic Effects: Anemia is sometimes seen in patients receiving diclofenac or other NSAIDs. This may be due to fluid retention, G.I. blood loss, or an incompletely described effect upon erythropoiesis.

Renal Effects: As a class, NSAIDs have been associated with renal papillary necrosis and other abnormal renal pathology in long-term administration to animals. In oral diclofenac studies in animals, some evidence of renal toxicity was noted. Isolated incidents of papillary necrosis were observed in a few animals at high doses (20-120 mg/kg) in several baboon subacute studies. In patients treated with diclofenac, rare cases of interstitial nephritis and papillary necrosis have been reported (see ADVERSE REACTIONS).

A second form of renal toxicity, generally associated with NSAIDs, is seen in patients with conditions leading to a reduction in renal blood flow or blood volume, where renal prostaglandins have a supportive role in the maintenance of renal perfusion. In these patients, administration of an NSAID results in a dose-dependent decrease in prostaglandin synthesis and, secondarily, in a reduction of renal blood flow, which may precipitate overt renal failure. Patients at greatest risk of this reaction are those with impaired renal function, heart failure, liver dysfunction, those taking diuretics, and the elderly. Discontinua tion of NSAID therapy is typically followed by recovery to the pretreatment state. Cases of significant renal failure in patients receiving diclofenac have been reported from marketing experience, but were not observed in over 4000 patients in clinical trials during which serum creatinine and BUN values were followed serially. There were only 11 patients (0.3%) whose serum creatinine and concurrent serum BUN values were greater than 2.0 mg/dL and 40 mg/dL, respectively, while on diclofenac (mean rise in the 11 patients: creatinine 2.3 mg/dL and BUN 28.4 mg/dL).

Since diclofenac metabolites are eliminated primarily by the kidneys, patients with significantly impaired renal function should be more closely monitored than subjects with normal renal function.

Porphyria: The use of diclofenac in patients with hepatic porphyria should be avoided. To date, 1 patient has been described in whom diclofenac probably triggered a clinical attack of porphyria. The postulated mechanism, demonstrated in rats, for causing such attacks by diclofenac, as well as some other NSAIDs, is through stimulation of the porphyrin precursor delta-aminolevulinic acid (ALA).

Aseptic Meningitis: As with other NSAIDs, aseptic meningitis with fever and coma has been observed on rare occasions in patients on diclofenac therapy. Although it is probably more likely to occur in patients with systemic lupus erythematosus and related connective tissue diseases, it has been reported in patients who do not have an underlying chronic disease. If signs or symptoms of meningitis develop in a patient on diclofenac, the possibility of its being related to diclofenac should be considered.

Preexisting Asthma: About 10% of patients with asthma may have aspirin-sensitive asthma. The use of aspirin in patients with aspirin-sensitive asthma has been associated with severe bronchospasm which can be fatal. Since cross-reactivity, including bronchospasm, between aspirin and other nonsteroidal anti-inflammatory drugs has been reported in such aspirin-sensitive patients, diclofenac should not be administered to patients with this form of aspirin sensitivity and should be used with caution in all patients with preexisting asthma.

Other Precautions: The pharmacologic activity of diclofenac may reduce fever and inflammation, thus diminishing their utility as diagnostic signs in detecting underlying conditions.

In order to avoid exacerbation of manifestations of adrenal insufficiency, patients who have been on prolonged corticosteroid treatment should have their therapy tapered slowly rather than discontinued abruptly when diclofenac is added to the treatment program.

Blurred and/or diminished vision, scotomata, and/or changes in color vision have been reported. If a patient develops such complaints while receiving diclofenac, the drug should be discontinued and the patient should have an ophthalmologic examination which includes central visual fields and color vision testing.

Information for Patients

Diclofenac, like other drugs of its class, is not free of side effects. The side effects of these drugs can cause discomfort and, rarely, more serious side effects, such as gastrointestinal bleeding, and more rarely, liver toxicity (see WARNINGS, Hepatic Effects), which may result in hospitalization and even fatal outcomes.

NSAIDs are often essential agents in the management of arthritis and have a major role in the management of pain, but they also may be commonly employed for conditions that are less serious.

Physicians may wish to discuss with their patients the potential risks (see WARNINGS, PRECAUTIONS, and ADVERSE REACTIONS) and likely benefits of NSAID treatment, particularly when the drugs are used for less serious conditions where treatment without NSAIDs may represent an acceptable alternative to both the patient and physician.

Because serious G.I. tract ulceration and bleeding can occur without warning symptoms, physicians should follow chronically treated patients for the signs and symptoms of ulceration and bleeding and should inform them of the importance of this follow-up (see WARNINGS, Gastrointestinal Effects, *Risk of G.I. Ulcerations, Bleeding, and Perforation with NSAID Therapy*). If diclofenac is used chronically, patients should also be instructed to report any signs and symptoms that might be due to hepatotoxicity of diclofenac; these symptoms may become evident between visits when periodic liver laboratory tests are performed (see WARNINGS, Hepatic Effects, and PRECAUTIONS—Laboratory Tests).

Laboratory Tests

Hepatic Effects: Transaminases and other hepatic enzymes should be monitored in patients treated with NSAIDs. For patients on diclofenac therapy, it is recommended that a determination be made within 4 weeks of initiating therapy and at intervals thereafter. If clinical signs and symptoms consistent with liver disease develop, or if systemic manifestations occur (e.g. eosinophilia, rash, etc.) and abnormal liver tests are detected, persist or worsen, diclofenac should be discontinued immediately.

Hematologic Effects: Patients on long-term treatment with NSAIDs, including diclofenac, should have their hemoglobin or hematocrit checked periodically for signs or symp-

Continued on next page

Cataflam/Voltaren—Cont.

toms of anemia. Appropriate measures should be taken in case such signs of anemia occur.

Drug Interactions

Aspirin: Concomitant administration of diclofenac and aspirin is not recommended because diclofenac is displaced from its binding sites during the concomitant administration of aspirin, resulting in lower plasma concentrations, peak plasma levels, and AUC values.

Anticoagulants: While studies have not shown diclofenac to interact with anticoagulants of the warfarin type, caution should be exercised, nonetheless, since interactions have been seen with other NSAIDs. Because prostaglandins play an important role in hemostasis, and NSAIDs affect platelet function as well, concurrent therapy with all NSAIDs, including diclofenac, and warfarin requires close monitoring of patients to be certain that no change in their anticoagulant dosage is required.

Digoxin, Methotrexate, Cyclosporine: Diclofenac, like other NSAIDs, may affect renal prostaglandins and increase the toxicity of certain drugs. Ingestion of diclofenac may increase serum concentrations of digoxin and methotrexate and increase cyclosporine's nephrotoxicity. Patients who begin taking diclofenac or who increase their diclofenac dose or any other NSAID while taking digoxin, methotrexate, or cyclosporine may develop toxicity characteristics for these drugs. They should be observed closely, particularly if renal function is impaired. In the case of digoxin, serum levels should be monitored.

Lithium: Diclofenac decreases lithium renal clearance and increases lithium plasma levels. In patients taking diclofenac and lithium concomitantly, lithium toxicity may develop.

Oral Hypoglycemics: Diclofenac does not alter glucose metabolism in normal subjects nor does it alter the effects of oral hypoglycemic agents. There are rare reports, however, from marketing experiences, of changes in effects of insulin or oral hypoglycemic agents in the presence of diclofenac that necessitated changes in the doses of such agents. Both hypo- and hyperglycemic effects have been reported. A direct causal relationship has not been established, but physicians should consider the possibility that diclofenac may alter a diabetic patient's response to insulin or oral hypoglycemic agents.

Diuretics: Diclofenac and other NSAIDs can inhibit the activity of diuretics. Concomitant treatment with potassium-sparing diuretics may be associated with increased serum potassium levels.

Other Drugs: In small groups of patients (7-10/interaction study), the concomitant administration of azathioprine, gold, chloroquine, D-penicillamine, prednisolone, doxycycline, or digitoxin did not significantly affect the peak levels and AUC values of diclofenac. Phenobarbital toxicity has been reported to have occurred in a patient on chronic phenobarbital treatment following the initiation of diclofenac therapy.

Protein Binding

In vitro, diclofenac interferes minimally or not at all with the protein binding of salicylic acid (20% decrease in binding), tolbutamide, prednisolone (10% decrease in binding), or warfarin. Benzylpenicillin, ampicillin, oxacillin, chlortetracycline, doxycycline, cephalothin, erythromycin, and sulfamethoxazole have no influence *in vitro* on the protein binding of diclofenac in human serum.

Drug/Laboratory Test Interactions

Effect on Blood Coagulation: Diclofenac increases platelet aggregation time but does not affect bleeding time, plasma thrombin clotting time, plasma fibrinogen, or factors V and VII to XII. Statistically significant changes in prothrombin and partial thromboplastin times have been reported in normal volunteers. The mean changes were observed to be less than 1 second in both instances, however, and are unlikely to be clinically important. Diclofenac is a prostaglandin synthetase inhibitor, however, and all drugs that inhibit prostaglandin synthesis interfere with platelet function to some degree; therefore, patients who may be adversely affected by such an action should be carefully observed.

Carcinogenesis, Mutagenesis, Impairment of Fertility

Long-term carcinogenicity studies in rats given diclofenac sodium up to 2 mg/kg/day (or 12 mg/m^2/day, approximately the human dose) have revealed no significant increases in tumor incidence. There was a slight increase in benign mammary fibroadenomas in mid-dose-treated (0.5 mg/kg/day or 3 mg/m^2/day) female rats (high-dose females had excessive mortality), but the increase was not significant for this common rat tumor. A 2-year carcinogenicity study conducted in mice employing diclofenac sodium at doses up to 0.3 mg/kg/day (0.9 mg/m^2/day) in males and 1 mg/kg/day (3 mg/m^2/day) in females did not reveal any oncogenic potential. Diclofenac sodium did not show mutagenic activity in *in vitro* point mutation assays in mammalian (mouse lymphoma) and microbial (yeast, Ames) test systems and was nonmutagenic in several mammalian *in vitro* and *in vivo* tests, including dominant lethal and male germinal epithelial chromosomal studies in mice, and nucleus anomaly and chromosomal aberration studies in Chinese hamsters. Diclofenac sodium administered to male and female rats at 4 mg/kg/day (24-mg/m^2/day) did not affect fertility.

Pregnancy, Teratogenic Effects, Pregnancy Category B

Reproduction studies have been performed in mice given diclofenac sodium (up to 20 mg/kg/day or 60 mg/m^2/day) and in rats and rabbits given diclofenac sodium (up to 10 mg/kg/day or 60 mg/m^2/day for rats, and 80 mg/m^2/day for rabbits), and have revealed no evidence of teratogenicity despite the induction of maternal toxicity and fetal toxicity. In rats, maternally toxic doses were associated with dystocia, prolonged gestation, reduced fetal weights and growth, and reduced fetal survival. Diclofenac has been shown to cross the placental barrier in mice and rats. There are, however, no adequate and well-controlled studies in pregnant women. Because animal reproduction studies are not always predictive of human response, this drug should not be used during pregnancy unless the benefits to the mother justify the potential risk to the fetus. Because of the risk to the fetus resulting in premature closure of the ductus arteriosus, diclofenac should be avoided in late pregnancy.

Labor and Delivery

The effects of diclofenac on labor and delivery in pregnant women are unknown. Because of the known effects of prostaglandin-inhibiting drugs on the fetal cardiovascular system (closure of ductus arteriosus), use of diclofenac during late pregnancy should be avoided and, as with other nonsteroidal anti-inflammatory drugs, it is possible that diclofenac may inhibit uterine contractions and delay parturition.

Nursing Mothers

Because of the potential for serious adverse reactions in nursing infants from diclofenac, a decision should be made whether to discontinue nursing or to discontinue the drug, taking into account the importance of the drug to the mother.

Pediatric Use

Safety and effectiveness of diclofenac in pediatric patients have not been established.

Geriatric Use

Of the more than 6000 patients treated with diclofenac in U.S. trials, 31% were older than 65 years of age. No overall difference was observed between efficacy, adverse event, or pharmacokinetic profiles of older and younger patients. As with any NSAID, the elderly are likely to tolerate adverse reactions less well than younger patients.

ADVERSE REACTIONS

Adverse reaction information is derived from blinded, controlled, and open-label clinical trials, as well as worldwide marketing experience. In the description below, rates of more common events represent clinical study results; rarer events are derived principally from marketing experience and publications, and accurate rate estimates are generally not possible.

In 718 patients treated for shorter periods, i.e., 2 weeks or less, with Cataflam Immediate-Release Tablets, adverse reactions were reported one-half to one-tenth as frequently as by patients treated for longer periods. In a 6-month, double-blind trial comparing Cataflam Immediate-Release Tablets (N=196) versus Voltaren Delayed-Release Tablets (N=197) versus ibuprofen (N=197), adverse reactions were similar in nature and frequency. In controlled clinical trials, the incidence of adverse reactions for Voltaren Delayed-Release Tablets and Voltaren-XR Extended-Release Tablets at comparable doses were similar.

The incidence of common adverse reactions (greater than 1%) is based upon controlled clinical trials in 1543 patients treated up to 13 weeks with Voltaren Delayed-Release Tablets. By far the most common adverse effects were gastrointestinal symptoms, most of them minor, occurring in about 20%, and leading to discontinuation in about 3%, of patients. Peptic ulcer or G.I. bleeding occurred in clinical trials in 0.6% (95% confidence interval: 0.2% to 1%) of approximately 1800 patients during their first 3 months of diclofenac treatment and in 1.6% (95% confidence interval: 0.8% to 2.4%) of approximately 800 patients followed for 1 year.

Gastrointestinal symptoms were followed in frequency by central nervous system side effects such as headache (7%) and dizziness (3%).

Meaningful (exceeding 3 times the Upper Limit of Normal) elevations of ALT (SGPT) or AST (SGOT) occurred at an overall rate of approximately 2% during the first 2 months of Voltaren treatment. Unlike aspirin-related elevations, which occur more frequently in patients with rheumatoid arthritis, these elevations were more frequently observed in patients with osteoarthritis (2.6%) than in patients with rheumatoid arthritis (0.7%). Marked elevations (exceeding 8 times the ULN) were seen in 1% of patients treated for 2-6 months (see WARNINGS, Hepatic Effects).

The following adverse reactions were reported in patients treated with diclofenac:

Incidence Greater Than 1% - Causal Relationship Probable: (All derived from clinical trials.)

*Incidence, 3% to 9% (incidence of unmarked reactions is 1%-3%).

Body as a Whole: Abdominal pain or cramps,* headache,* fluid retention, abdominal distention.

Digestive: Diarrhea,* indigestion,* nausea,* constipation,* flatulence, liver test abnormalities,* PUB, i.e., peptic ulcer, with or without bleeding and/or perforation, or bleeding without ulcer (see above and also WARNINGS).

Nervous System: Dizziness.

Skin and Appendages: Rash, pruritus.

Special Senses: Tinnitus.

Incidence Less Than 1% - Causal Relationship Probable: (Adverse reactions reported only in worldwide marketing experience or in the literature, not seen in clinical trials, are considered rare and are *italicized.*)

Body as a Whole: Malaise, swelling of lips and tongue, photosensitivity, *anaphylaxis*, anaphylactoid reactions.

Cardiovascular: Hypertension, congestive heart failure.

Digestive: Vomiting, jaundice, melena, *esophageal lesions*, aphthous stomatitis, dry mouth and mucous membranes, bloody diarrhea, hepatitis, *hepatic necrosis, cirrhosis, hepatorenal syndrome*, appetite change, pancreatitis with or without concomitant hepatitis, *colitis*.

Hemic and Lymphatic: Hemoglobin decrease, leukopenia, thrombocytopenia, *eosinophilia, hemolytic anemia, aplastic anemia, agranulocytosis*, purpura, *allergic purpura*.

Metabolic and Nutritional Disorders: Azotemia.

Nervous System: Insomnia, drowsiness, depression, diplopia, anxiety, irritability, *aseptic meningitis, convulsions*.

Respiratory: Epistaxis, asthma, laryngeal edema.

Skin and Appendages: Alopecia, urticaria, eczema, dermatitis, *bullous eruption, erythema multiforme major*, angioedema, *Stevens-Johnson syndrome*.

Special Senses: Blurred vision, taste disorder, reversible and irreversible hearing loss, scotoma.

Urogenital: *Nephrotic syndrome*, proteinuria, *oliguria, interstitial nephritis, papillary necrosis, acute renal failure*.

Incidence Less Than 1% - Causal Relationship Unknown: (The following reactions have been reported in patients taking diclofenac under circumstances that do not permit a clear attribution of the reaction to diclofenac. These reactions are being included as alerting information to physicians. Adverse reactions reported only in worldwide marketing experience or in the literature, not seen in clinical trials, are considered rare and are *italicized*.)

Body as a Whole: Chest pain.

Cardiovascular: Palpitations, *flushing*, tachycardia, premature ventricular contractions, myocardial infarction, *hypotension*.

Digestive: *Intestinal perforation*.

Hemic and Lymphatic: *Bruising*.

Metabolic and Nutritional Disorders: Hypoglycemia, *weight loss*.

Nervous System: Paresthesia, memory disturbance, nightmares, tremor, tic, *abnormal coordination, disorientation, psychotic reaction*.

Respiratory: Dyspnea, hyperventilation, edema of pharynx.

Skin and Appendages: Excess perspiration, *exfoliative dermatitis*.

Special Senses: Vitreous floaters, night blindness, amblyopia.

Urogenital: Urinary frequency, nocturia, hematuria, impotence, vaginal bleeding.

OVERDOSAGE

Worldwide reports of overdosage with diclofenac cover 66 cases. In approximately one-half of these reports of overdosage, concomitant medications were also taken. The highest dose of diclofenac was 5.0 g in a 17-year-old male who suffered loss of consciousness, increased intracranial pressure, aspiration pneumonitis, and died 2 days after overdose. The next highest doses of diclofenac were 4.0 g and 3.75 g. The 24-year-old female who took 4.0 g and the 28- and 42-year-old females, each of whom took 3.75 g, did not develop any clinically significant signs or symptoms. However, there was a report of a 17-year-old female who experienced vomiting and drowsiness after an overdose of 2.37 g of diclofenac.

Animal LD_{50} values show a wide range of susceptibilities to acute overdosage, with primates being more resistant to acute toxicity than rodents (LD_{50} in mg/kg-rats, 55; dogs, 500; monkeys, 3200).

In case of acute overdosage, it is recommended that the stomach be emptied by vomiting or lavage. Forced diuresis may theoretically be bene ficial because the drug is excreted in the urine. The effect of dialysis or hemoperfusion in the elimination of diclofenac (99% protein-bound: see CLINICAL PHARMACOLOGY) remains unproven. In addition to supportive measures, the use of oral activated charcoal may help to reduce the absorption of diclofenac.

DOSAGE AND ADMINISTRATION

Diclofenac may be administered as 50-mg Cataflam Immediate-Release Tablets, as 25-mg, 50-mg, and 75-mg Voltaren Delayed-Release Tablets, or as 100-mg Voltaren-XR Extended-Release Tablets. Cataflam Immediate-Release Tablets is the formulation indicated for management of acute pain and primary dysmenorrhea when prompt onset of pain relief is desired because of earlier absorption of diclofenac. For the same reason, Voltaren-XR is not indicated for the management of acute painful conditions and should be used as chronic therapy in patients with osteoarthritis and rheumatoid arthritis.

The dosage of diclofenac should be individualized to the lowest effective dose to minimize adverse effects (see INDIVIDUALIZATION OF DOSAGE).

Osteoarthritis: The recommended dosage is 100 to 150 mg/day: Cataflam or Voltaren Delayed-Release 50 mg b.i.d. or t.i.d.; or Voltaren Delayed-Release 75 mg b.i.d. The recommended dosage for chronic therapy with Voltaren-XR is 100 mg q.d. Dosages of Voltaren-XR Extended-Release Tablets of 200 mg daily are not recommended for patients with osteoarthritis. Dosages above 200 mg/day have not been studied in patients with osteoarthritis.

Rheumatoid Arthritis: The recommended dosage is 100 to 200 mg/day: Cataflam or Voltaren Delayed-Release 50 mg t.i.d. or q.i.d.; or Voltaren Delayed-Release 75 mg b.i.d. The recommended dosage for chronic therapy with Voltaren-XR is 100 mg q.d. In the rare patient where Voltaren-XR

100 mg/day is unsatisfactory, the dose may be increased to 100 mg b.i.d. if the benefits outweigh the clinical risks. Dosages above 225 mg/day are not recommended in patients with rheumatoid arthritis.

Ankylosing Spondylitis: The recommended dosage is 100 to 125 mg/day: Voltaren 25 mg q.i.d. with an extra 25-mg dose at bedtime if necessary. Dosages above 125 mg/day have not been studied in patients with ankylosing spondylitis.

Analgesia and Primary Dysmenorrhea: The recommended starting dose of Cataflam Immediate-Release Tablets is 50 mg t.i.d. With experience, physicians may find that in some patients an initial dose of 100 mg of Cataflam, followed by 50-mg doses, will provide better relief. After the first day, when the maximum recommended dose may be 200 mg, the total daily dose should generally not exceed 150 mg.

HOW SUPPLIED

Cataflam Tablets

50 mg - light brown, round, biconvex (imprinted CATAFLAM on one side and 50 on the other side)
Bottles of 100 .... NDC 0028-0151-01
Unit Dose (blister pack)
Box of 100 (strips of 10) .... NDC 0028-0151-61

Voltaren *Delayed-Release* Tablets

25 mg - yellow, biconvex, triangular-shaped (imprinted VOLTAREN 25 on one side)
Bottles of 60 .... NDC 0028-0258-60
Bottles of 100 .... NDC 0028-0258-01
Unit Dose (blister pack)
Box of 100 (strips of 10) .... NDC 0028-0258-61

50 mg - light brown, biconvex, triangular-shaped (imprinted VOLTAREN 50 on one side)
Bottles of 60 .... NDC 0028-0262-60
Bottles of 100 .... NDC 0028-0262-01
Bottles of 1000 .... NDC 0028-0262-10
Unit Dose (blister pack)
Box of 100 (strips of 10) .... NDC 0028-0262-61

75 mg - light pink, biconvex, triangular-shaped (imprinted VOLTAREN 75 on one side)
Bottles of 60 .... NDC 0028-0264-60
Bottles of 100 .... NDC 0028-0264-01
Bottles of 1000 .... NDC 0028-0264-10
Unit Dose (blister pack)
Box of 100 (strips of 10) .... NDC 0028-0264-61

Voltaren-XR *Extended-Release* Tablets

100 mg - light pink, coated, round, biconvex with beveled edges (imprinted Voltaren-XR on one side and 100 on the other side)
Bottles of 100 .... NDC 0028-0205-01
Unit Dose (blister pack)
Box of 100 (strips of 10) .... NDC 0028-0205-61

Do not store above 30°C (86°F). Protect from moisture. Dispense in ***tight*** container (USP).

T2000-19

REV: MAY 2000

Distributed by:
Novartis Pharmaceuticals Corporation
East Hanover, New Jersey 07936

Shown in Product Identification Guide, page 325 and 326

CLOZARIL® ℞

[*klō 'ză-ril*]
(clozapine) Tablets

Rx only

The following prescribing information is based on official labeling in effect July 2000.

DESCRIPTION

CLOZARIL® (clozapine), an atypical antipsychotic drug, is a tricyclic dibenzodiazepine derivative, 8-chloro-11-(4-methyl-1-piperazinyl)-5*H*-dibenzo [*b,e*] [1,4] diazepine. The structural formula is:

$C_{18}H_{19}ClN_4$ Mol. wt. 326.83

CLOZARIL® (clozapine) is available in pale yellow tablets of 25 mg and 100 mg for oral administration.

25 mg and 100 mg Tablets

Active Ingredient: clozapine is a yellow, crystalline powder, very slightly soluble in water.

Inactive Ingredients: colloidal silicon dioxide, lactose, magnesium stearate, povidone, starch (corn), and talc.

CLINICAL PHARMACOLOGY

Pharmacodynamics

CLOZARIL® (clozapine) is classified as an 'atypical' antipsychotic drug because its profile of binding to dopamine receptors and its effects on various dopamine mediated behaviors differ from those exhibited by more typical antipsychotic drug products. In particular, although CLOZARIL® (clozapine) does interfere with the binding of dopamine at D_1, D_2, D_3 and D_5 receptors, and has a high affinity for the D_4 receptor, it does not induce catalepsy nor inhibit apomorphine-induced stereotypy. This evidence, consistent with the view that CLOZARIL® (clozapine) is preferentially more active at limbic than at striatal dopamine receptors, may explain the relative freedom of CLOZARIL® (clozapine) from extrapyramidal side effects.

CLOZARIL® (clozapine) also acts as an antagonist at adrenergic, cholinergic, histaminergic and serotonergic receptors.

Absorption, Distribution, Metabolism and Excretion

In man, CLOZARIL® (clozapine) tablets (25 mg and 100 mg) are equally bioavailable relative to a clozapine solution. Following a dosage of 100 mg b.i.d., the average steady state peak plasma concentration was 319 ng/mL (range: 102-771 ng/mL), occurring at the average of 2.5 hours (range: 1-6 hours) after dosing. The average minimum concentration at steady state was 122 ng/mL (range: 41-343 ng/mL), after 100 mg b.i.d. dosing. Food does not appear to affect the systemic bioavailability of CLOZARIL® (clozapine). Thus, CLOZARIL® (clozapine) may be administered with or without food.

Clozapine is approximately 97% bound to serum proteins. The interaction between CLOZARIL® (clozapine) and other highly protein-bound drugs has not been fully evaluated but may be important. *(See PRECAUTIONS)*

Clozapine is almost completely metabolized prior to excretion and only trace amounts of unchanged drug are detected in the urine and feces. Approximately 50% of the administered dose is excreted in the urine and 30% in the feces. The demethylated, hydroxylated and N-oxide derivatives are components in both urine and feces. Pharmacological testing has shown the desmethyl metabolite to have only limited activity, while the hydroxylated and N-oxide derivatives were inactive.

The mean elimination half-life of clozapine after a single 75 mg dose was 8 hours (range: 4-12 hours), compared to a mean elimination half-life, after achieving steady state with 100 mg b.i.d. dosing, of 12 hours (range: 4-66 hours). A comparison of single-dose and multiple-dose administration of clozapine showed that the elimination half-life increased significantly after multiple dosing relative to that after single-dose administration, suggesting the possibility of concentration dependent pharmacokinetics. However, at steady state, linearly dose-proportional changes with respect to AUC (area under the curve), peak and minimum clozapine plasma concentrations were observed after administration of 37.5 mg, 75 mg, and 150 mg b.i.d.

Human Pharmacology

In contrast to more typical antipsychotic drugs, CLOZARIL® (clozapine) therapy produces little or no prolactin elevation.

As is true of more typical antipsychotic drugs, clinical EEG studies have shown that CLOZARIL® (clozapine) increases delta and theta activity and slows dominant alpha frequencies. Enhanced synchronization occurs, and sharp wave activity and spike and wave complexes may also develop. Patients, on rare occasions, may report an intensification of dream activity during CLOZARIL® (clozapine) therapy. REM sleep was found to be increased to 85% of the total sleep time. In these patients, the onset of REM sleep occurred almost immediately after falling asleep.

INDICATIONS AND USAGE

CLOZARIL® (clozapine) is indicated for the management of severely ill schizophrenic patients who fail to respond adequately to standard antipsychotic drug treatment. Because of the significant risk of agranulocytosis and seizure associated with its use, CLOZARIL® (clozapine) should be used only in patients who have failed to respond adequately to treatment with appropriate courses of standard antipsychotic drugs, either because of insufficient effectiveness or the inability to achieve an effective dose due to intolerable adverse effects from those drugs. *(See WARNINGS)*

The effectiveness of CLOZARIL® (clozapine) in a treatment resistant schizophrenic population was demonstrated in a 6-week study comparing CLOZARIL® (clozapine) and chlorpromazine. Patients meeting DSM-III criteria for schizophrenia and having a mean BPRS total score of 61 were demonstrated to be treatment resistant by history and by open, prospective treatment with haloperidol before entering into the double-blind phase of the study. The superiority of CLOZARIL® (clozapine) to chlorpromazine was documented in statistical analyses employing both categorical and continuous measures of treatment effect.

Because of the significant risk of agranulocytosis and seizure, events which both present a continuing risk over time, the extended treatment of patients failing to show an acceptable level of clinical response should ordinarily be avoided. In addition, the need for continuing treatment in patients exhibiting beneficial clinical responses should be periodically re-evaluated.

CONTRAINDICATIONS

CLOZARIL® (clozapine) is contraindicated in patients with a previous hypersensitivity to clozapine or any other component of this drug, in patients with myeloproliferative disorders, uncontrolled epilepsy, or a history of CLOZARIL® (clozapine) induced agranulocytosis or severe granulocytopenia. As with more typical antipsychotic drugs, CLOZARIL® (clozapine) is contraindicated in severe central nervous system depression or comatose states from any cause.

CLOZARIL® (clozapine) should not be used simultaneously with other agents having a well-known potential to cause agranulocytosis or otherwise suppress bone marrow function. The mechanism of CLOZARIL® (clozapine) induced agranulocytosis is unknown; nonetheless, it is possible that causative factors may interact synergistically to increase the risk and/or severity of bone marrow suppression.

WARNINGS

General

BECAUSE OF THE SIGNIFICANT RISK OF AGRANULOCYTOSIS, A POTENTIALLY LIFE-THREATENING ADVERSE EVENT *(SEE FOLLOWING)*, CLOZARIL® (clozapine) SHOULD BE RESERVED FOR USE IN THE TREATMENT OF SEVERELY ILL SCHIZOPHRENIC PATIENTS WHO FAIL TO SHOW AN ACCEPTABLE RESPONSE TO ADEQUATE COURSES OF STANDARD ANTIPSYCHOTIC DRUG TREATMENT, EITHER BECAUSE OF INSUFFICIENT EFFECTIVENESS OR THE INABILITY TO ACHIEVE AN EFFECTIVE DOSE DUE TO INTOLERABLE ADVERSE EFFECTS FROM THOSE DRUGS. CONSEQUENTLY, BEFORE INITIATING TREATMENT WITH CLOZARIL® (clozapine), IT IS STRONGLY RECOMMENDED THAT A PATIENT BE GIVEN AT LEAST 2 TRIALS, EACH WITH A DIFFERENT STANDARD ANTIPSYCHOTIC DRUG PRODUCT, AT AN ADEQUATE DOSE, AND FOR AN ADEQUATE DURATION.

PATIENTS WHO ARE BEING TREATED WITH CLOZARIL® (clozapine) MUST HAVE A BASELINE WHITE BLOOD CELL (WBC) AND DIFFERENTIAL COUNT BEFORE INITIATION OF TREATMENT, AND A WBC COUNT EVERY WEEK FOR THE FIRST SIX MONTHS. THEREAFTER, IF ACCEPTABLE WBC COUNTS (WBC greater than or equal to 3,000/mm^3, ANC ≥1500/mm^3) HAVE BEEN MAINTAINED DURING THE FIRST 6 MONTHS OF CONTINUOUS THERAPY, WBC COUNTS CAN BE MONITORED EVERY OTHER WEEK. WBC COUNTS MUST BE MONITORED WEEKLY FOR AT LEAST 4 WEEKS AFTER THE DISCONTINUATION OF CLOZARIL® (clozapine).

CLOZARIL® (clozapine) IS AVAILABLE ONLY THROUGH A DISTRIBUTION SYSTEM THAT ENSURES MONITORING OF WBC COUNTS ACCORDING TO THE SCHEDULE DESCRIBED BELOW PRIOR TO DELIVERY OF THE NEXT SUPPLY OF MEDICATION.

Agranulocytosis

Agranulocytosis, defined as an absolute neutrophil count (ANC) of less than 500/mm^3, has been estimated to occur in association with CLOZARIL® (clozapine) use at a cumulative incidence at 1 year of approximately 1.3%, based on the occurrence of 15 US cases out of 1743 patients exposed to CLOZARIL® (clozapine) during its clinical testing prior to domestic marketing. All of these cases occurred at a time when the need for close monitoring of WBC counts was already recognized. This reaction could prove fatal if not detected early and therapy interrupted. Of the 149 cases of agranulocytosis reported worldwide in association with CLOZARIL® (clozapine) use as of December 31, 1989, 32% were fatal. However, few of these deaths occurred since 1977, at which time the knowledge of CLOZARIL® (clozapine) induced agranulocytosis became more widespread, and close monitoring of WBC counts more widely practiced. Nevertheless, it is unknown at present what the case fatality rate will be for CLOZARIL® (clozapine) induced agranulocytosis, despite strict adherence to the required frequency of monitoring. In the U.S., under a weekly WBC monitoring system with CLOZARIL® (clozapine), there have been 585 cases of agranulocytosis as of August 21, 1997; 19 were fatal. During this period 150,409 patients received CLOZARIL® (clozapine). A hematologic risk analysis was conducted based upon the available information in the Clozaril® National Registry (CNR) for U.S. patients. Based upon a cut-off date of April 30, 1995, the incidence rates of agranulocytosis based upon a weekly monitoring schedule, rose steeply during the first two months of therapy, peaking in the third month. Among Clozaril® (clozapine) patients who continued the drug beyond the third month, the weekly incidence of agranulocytosis fell to a substantial degree, so that by the sixth month the weekly incidence of agranulocytosis was reduced to 3 per 1000 person-years. After six months, the weekly incidence of agranulocytosis declines still further, however, never reaches zero. It should be noted that any type of reduction in the frequency of monitoring WBC counts may result in an increase incidence of agranulocytosis.

Because of the substantial risk for developing agranulocytosis in association with CLOZARIL® (clozapine) use, which may persist over an extended period of time, patients must have a blood sample drawn for a WBC count before initiation of treatment with CLOZARIL® (clozapine), and must have subsequent WBC counts done at least weekly for the first 6 months of continuous treatment. If WBC counts remain acceptable (WBC greater than or equal to 3000/mm^3, ANC ≥1500/mm^3) during this period, WBC counts may be monitored every other week thereafter. After the discontinuation of CLOZARIL® (clozapine), weekly WBC counts should be continued for an additional 4 weeks. If a patient is on CLOZARIL® (clozapine) therapy for less than 6 months with no abnormal blood events and

Continued on next page

Clozaril—Cont.

there is a break on therapy which is less than or equal to 1 month, then patients can continue where they left off with weekly WBC testing for 6 months. When this 6 month period has been completed, the frequency of WBC count monitoring can be reduced to every other week. If a patient is on CLOZARIL® (clozapine) therapy for less than 6 months with no abnormal blood events and there is a break on therapy which is greater than 1 month, then patients should be tested weekly for an additional 6 month period before biweekly testing is initiated. If a patient is on CLOZARIL® (clozapine) therapy for less than 6 months and experiences an abnormal blood event as described below but remains a rechallengeable patient [patients cannot be reinitiated on CLOZARIL® (clozapine) therapy if WBC counts fall below 2000/mm^3 or the ANC falls below 1000/mm^3 during CLOZARIL® (clozapine) therapy], the patient must re-start the 6 month period of weekly WBC monitoring at day 0.

If a patient is on CLOZARIL® (clozapine) therapy for 6 months or longer with no abnormal blood events and there is a break on therapy which is 1 year or less, then the patient can continue WBC count monitoring every other week if CLOZARIL® (clozapine) therapy is reinitiated. If a patient is on CLOZARIL® (clozapine) therapy for 6 months or longer with no abnormal blood events and there is a break on therapy which is greater than 1 year, then, if CLOZARIL® (clozapine) therapy is reinitiated, the patient must have WBC counts monitored weekly for an additional 6 months. If a patient on CLOZARIL® (clozapine) therapy for 6 months or longer and subsequently has an abnormal blood event, but remains a rechallengeable patient, then the patient must re-start weekly WBC count monitoring until an additional 6 months of CLOZARIL® (clozapine) therapy has been received. The distribution of CLOZARIL® (clozapine) is contingent upon performance of the required blood tests.

Treatment should not be initiated if the WBC count is less than 3500/mm^3, or if the patient has a history of a myeloproliferative disorder, or previous CLOZARIL® (clozapine) induced agranulocytosis or granulocytopenia. Patients should be advised to report immediately the appearance of lethargy, weakness, fever, sore throat or any other signs of infection. If, after the initiation of treatment, the total WBC count has dropped below 3500/mm^3 or it has dropped by a substantial amount from baseline, even if the count is above 3500/mm^3, or if immature forms are present, a repeat WBC count and a differential count should be done. A substantial drop is defined as a single drop of 3,000 or more in the WBC count or a cumulative drop of 3,000 or more within 3 weeks. If subsequent WBC counts and the differential count reveal a total WBC count between 3000 and 3500/mm^3 and an ANC above 1500/mm^3, twice weekly WBC counts and differential counts should be performed.

If the total WBC count falls below 3000/mm^3 or the ANC below 1500/mm^3, CLOZARIL® (clozapine) therapy should be interrupted, WBC count and differential should be performed daily, and patients should be carefully monitored for flu-like symptoms or other symptoms suggestive of infection. CLOZARIL® (clozapine) therapy may be resumed if no symptoms of infection develop, and if the total WBC count returns to levels above 3000/mm^3 and the ANC returns to levels above 1500/mm^3. However, in this event, twice-weekly WBC counts and differential counts should continue until total WBC counts return to levels above 3500/mm^3.

If the total WBC count falls below 2000/mm^3 or the ANC falls below 1000/mm^3, bone marrow aspiration should be considered to ascertain granulopoietic status. Protective isolation with close observation may be indicated if granulopoiesis is determined to be deficient. Should evidence of infection develop, the patient should have appropriate cultures performed and an appropriate antibiotic regimen instituted.

Patients whose total WBC counts fall below 2000/mm^3, or ANCs below 1000/mm^3 during CLOZARIL® (clozapine) therapy should have daily WBC count and differential. These patients should not be re-challenged with CLOZARIL® (clozapine). Patients discontinued from CLOZARIL® (clozapine) therapy due to significant WBC suppression have been found to develop agranulocytosis upon rechallenge, often with a shorter latency on re-exposure. To reduce the chances of rechallenge occurring in patients who have experienced significant bone marrow suppression during CLOZARIL® (clozapine) therapy, a single, national master file will be maintained confidentially.

Except for evidence of significant bone marrow suppression during initial CLOZARIL® (clozapine) therapy, there are no established risk factors, based on worldwide experience, for the development of agranulocytosis in association with CLOZARIL® (clozapine) use. However, a disproportionate number of the US cases of agranulocytosis occurred in patients of Jewish background compared to the overall proportion of such patients exposed during domestic development of CLOZARIL® (clozapine). Most of the US cases occurred within 4-10 weeks of exposure, but neither dose nor duration is a reliable predictor of this problem. No patient characteristics have been clearly linked to the development of agranulocytosis in association with CLOZARIL® (clozapine) use, but agranulocytosis associated with other antipsychotic drugs has been reported to occur with a greater frequency in women, the elderly and in patients who are cachectic or have serious underlying medical illness; such patients may also be at particular risk with CLOZARIL® (clozapine). To reduce the risk of agranulocytosis developing undetected, CLOZARIL® (clozapine) is available only through a distribution system that ensures monitoring of WBC counts according to the schedule described above prior to delivery of the next supply of medication.

Interrupted Therapy (WBC <3000/mm^3 ANC <1500/mm^3) for Bi-Weekly Monitoring

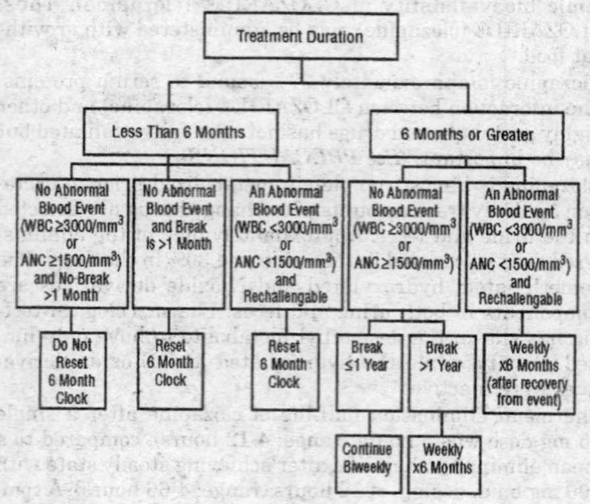

Treatment Duration

Less Than 6 Months
- No Abnormal Blood Event (WBC ≥3000/mm^3 or ANC ≥1500/mm^3) and No Break >1 Month → Do Not Reset 6 Month Clock
- No Abnormal Blood Event and Break is >1 Month → Reset 6 Month Clock
- An Abnormal Blood Event (WBC <3000/mm^3 or ANC <1500/mm^3) and Rechallengable → Reset 6 Month Clock

6 Months or Greater
- No Abnormal Blood Event (WBC ≥3000/mm^3 or ANC ≥1500/mm^3)
  - Break ≤1 Year → Continue Biweekly
  - Break >1 Year → Weekly x6 Months
- An Abnormal Blood Event (WBC <3000/mm^3 or ANC <1500/mm^3) and Rechallengable → Weekly x6 Months (after recovery from event)

Eosinophilia

In clinical trials, 1% of patients developed eosinophilia, which, in rare cases, can be substantial. If a differential count reveals a total eosinophil count above 4,000/mm^3, CLOZARIL® (clozapine) therapy should be interrupted until the eosinophil count falls below 3,000/mm^3.

Seizures

Seizure has been estimated to occur in association with CLOZARIL® (clozapine) use at a cumulative incidence at one year of approximately 5%, based on the occurrence of one or more seizures in 61 of 1743 patients exposed to CLOZARIL® (clozapine) during its clinical testing prior to domestic marketing (i.e., crude rate of 3.5%). Dose appears to be an important predictor of seizure, with a greater likelihood of seizure at the higher CLOZARIL® (clozapine) doses used.

Caution should be used in administering CLOZARIL® (clozapine) to patients having a history of seizures or other predisposing factors. Because of the substantial risk of seizure associated with CLOZARIL® (clozapine) use, patients should be advised not to engage in any activity where sudden loss of consciousness could cause serious risk to themselves or others, e.g., the operation of complex machinery, driving an automobile, swimming, climbing, etc.

Adverse Cardiovascular and Respiratory Effects

Orthostatic hypotension with or without syncope can occur with CLOZARIL® (clozapine) treatment and may represent a continuing risk in some patients. Rarely (approximately 1 case per 3,000 patients), collapse can be profound and be accompanied by respiratory and/or cardiac arrest. Orthostatic hypotension is more likely to occur during initial titration in association with rapid dose escalation and may even occur on first dose. In one report, initial doses as low as 12.5 mg were associated with collapse and respiratory arrest. When restarting patients who have had even a brief interval off CLOZARIL® (clozapine), i.e., 2 days or more since the last dose, it is recommended that treatment be reinitiated with one-half of a 25 mg tablet (12.5 mg) once or twice daily *(see DOSAGE AND ADMINISTRATION)*.

Some of the cases of collapse/respiratory arrest/ cardiac arrest during initial treatment occurred in patients who were being administered benzodiazepines; similar events have been reported in patients taking other psychotropic drugs or even CLOZARIL® (clozapine) by itself. Although it has not been established that there is an interaction between CLOZARIL® (clozapine) and benzodiazepines or other psychotropics, caution is advised when clozapine is initiated in patients taking a benzodiazepine or any other psychotropic drug.

Tachycardia, which may be sustained, has also been observed in approximately 25% of patients taking CLOZARIL® (clozapine), with patients having an average increase in pulse rate of 10-15 bpm. The sustained tachycardia is not simply a reflex response to hypotension, and is present in all positions monitored. Either tachycardia or hypotension may pose a serious risk for an individual with compromised cardiovascular function.

A minority of CLOZARIL® (clozapine) treated patients experience ECG repolarization changes similar to those seen with other antipsychotic drugs, including S-T segment depression and flattening or inversion of T waves, which all normalize after discontinuation of CLOZARIL® (clozapine). The clinical significance of these changes is unclear. However, in clinical trials with CLOZARIL® (clozapine), several patients experienced significant cardiac events, including ischemic changes, myocardial infarction, arrhythmias and sudden death. In addition there have been postmarketing reports of congestive heart failure, myocarditis, with or without eosinophilia, and pericarditis/pericardial effusions in association with CLOZARIL® (clozapine) use. Causality assessment was difficult in many of these cases because of serious preexisting cardiac disease and plausible alternative causes. Rare instances of sudden death have been reported in psychiatric patients, with or without associated antipsychotic drug treatment, and the relationship of these events to antipsychotic drug use is unknown.

CLOZARIL® (clozapine) should be used with caution in patients with known cardiovascular and/or pulmonary disease, and the recommendation for gradual titration of dose should be carefully observed.

Neuroleptic Malignant Syndrome (NMS)

A potentially fatal symptom complex sometimes referred to as Neuroleptic Malignant Syndrome (NMS) has been reported in association with antipsychotic drugs. Clinical manifestations of NMS are hyperpyrexia, muscle rigidity, altered mental status and evidence of autonomic instability (irregular pulse or blood pressure, tachycardia, diaphoresis, and cardiac dysrhythmias).

The diagnostic evaluation of patients with this syndrome is complicated. In arriving at a diagnosis, it is important to identify cases where the clinical presentation includes both serious medical illness (e.g., pneumonia, systemic infection, etc.) and untreated or inadequately treated extrapyramidal signs and symptoms (EPS). Other important considerations in the differential diagnosis include central anticholinergic toxicity, heat stroke, drug fever and primary central nervous system (CNS) pathology.

The management of NMS should include 1) immediate discontinuation of antipsychotic drugs and other drugs not essential to concurrent therapy, 2) intensive symptomatic treatment and medical monitoring, and 3) treatment of any concomitant serious medical problems for which specific treatments are available. There is no general agreement about specific pharmacological treatment regimens for uncomplicated NMS.

If a patient requires antipsychotic drug treatment after recovery from NMS, the potential reintroduction of drug therapy should be carefully considered. The patient should be carefully monitored, since recurrences of NMS have been reported.

There have been several reported cases of NMS in patients receiving CLOZARIL® (clozapine) alone or in combination with lithium or other CNS-active agents.

Tardive Dyskinesia

A syndrome consisting of potentially irreversible, involuntary, dyskinetic movements may develop in patients treated with antipsychotic drugs. Although the prevalence of the syndrome appears to be highest among the elderly, especially elderly women, it is impossible to rely upon prevalence estimates to predict, at the inception of treatment, which patients are likely to develop the syndrome.

There are several reasons for predicting that CLOZARIL® (clozapine) may be different from other antipsychotic drugs in its potential for inducing tardive dyskinesia, including the preclinical finding that it has a relatively weak dopamine blocking effect and the clinical finding of a virtual absence of certain acute extrapyramidal symptoms, e.g., dystonia. A few cases of tardive dyskinesia have been reported in patients on CLOZARIL® (clozapine) who had been previously treated with other antipsychotic agents, so that a causal relationship cannot be established. There have been no reports of tardive dyskinesia directly attributable to CLOZARIL® (clozapine) alone. Nevertheless, it cannot be concluded, without more extended experience, that CLOZARIL® (clozapine) is incapable of inducing this syndrome.

Both the risk of developing the syndrome and the likelihood that it will become irreversible are believed to increase as the duration of treatment and the total cumulative dose of antipsychotic drugs administered to the patient increase. However, the syndrome can develop, although much less commonly, after relatively brief treatment periods at low doses. There is no known treatment for established cases of tardive dyskinesia, although the syndrome may remit, partially or completely, if antipsychotic drug treatment is withdrawn. Antipsychotic drug treatment, itself, however, may suppress (or partially suppress) the signs and symptoms of the syndrome and thereby may possibly mask the underlying process. The effect that symptom suppression has upon the long-term course of the syndrome is unknown.

Given these considerations, CLOZARIL® (clozapine) should be prescribed in a manner that is most likely to minimize the occurrence of tardive dyskinesia. As with any antipsychotic drug, chronic CLOZARIL® (clozapine) use should be reserved for patients who appear to be obtaining substantial benefit from the drug. In such patients, the smallest dose and the shortest duration of treatment should be sought. The need for continued treatment should be reassessed periodically.

If signs and symptoms of tardive dyskinesia appear in a patient on CLOZARIL® (clozapine), drug discontinuation should be considered. However, some patients may require treatment with CLOZARIL® (clozapine) despite the presence of the syndrome.

PRECAUTIONS

General

Because of the significant risk of agranulocytosis and seizure, both of which present a continuing risk over time, the extended treatment of patients failing to show an acceptable level of clinical response should ordinarily be avoided. In addition, the need for continuing treatment in patients exhibiting beneficial clinical responses should be periodically re-evaluated. Although it is not known whether the risk would be increased, it is prudent either to avoid CLOZARIL® (clozapine) or use it cautiously in patients with a previous history of agranulocytosis induced by other drugs.

Fever

During CLOZARIL® (clozapine) therapy, patients may experience transient temperature elevations above 100.4°F (38°C), with the peak incidence within the first 3 weeks of treatment. While this fever is generally benign and self limiting, it may necessitate discontinuing patients from treatment. On occasion, there may be an associated increase or decrease in WBC count. Patients with fever should be carefully evaluated to rule out the possibility of an underlying infectious process or the development of agranulocytosis. In the presence of high fever, the possibility of Neuroleptic Malignant Syndrome (NMS) must be considered. There have been several reports of NMS in patients receiving CLOZARIL® (clozapine), usually in combination with lithium or other CNS-active drugs. *[See Neuroleptic Malignant Syndrome (NMS), under WARNINGS]*

Pulmonary Embolism

The possibility of pulmonary embolism should be considered in patients receiving CLOZARIL® (clozapine) who present with deep vein thrombosis, acute dyspnea, chest pain or with other respiratory signs and symptoms. As of December 31, 1993 there were 18 cases of fatal pulmonary embolism in association with CLOZARIL® (clozapine) therapy in users 10-54 years of age. Based upon the extent of use observed in the Clozaril National Registry, the mortality rate associated with pulmonary embolus was 1 death per 3450 person-years of use. This rate was about 27.5 times higher than that in the general population of a similar age and gender (95% Confidence Interval; 17.1,42.2). Deep vein thrombosis has also been observed in association with CLOZARIL® (clozapine) therapy. Whether pulmonary embolus can be attributed to CLOZARIL® (clozapine) or some characteristic(s) of its users is not clear, but the occurrence of deep vein thrombosis or respiratory symptomatology should suggest its presence.

Hyperglycemia

Severe hyperglycemia, sometimes leading to ketoacidosis, has been reported during CLOZARIL® (clozapine) treatment in patients with no prior history of hyperglycemia. While a causal relationship to CLOZARIL® (clozapine) use has not been definitively established, glucose levels normalized in most patients after discontinuation of CLOZARIL® (clozapine), and a rechallenge in one patient produced a recurrence of hyperglycemia. The effect of CLOZARIL® (clozapine) on glucose metabolism in patients with diabetes mellitus has not been studied. The possibility of impaired glucose tolerance should be considered in patients receiving CLOZARIL® (clozapine) who develop symptoms of hyperglycemia, such as polydipsia, polyuria, polyphagia, and weakness. In patients with significant treatment-emergent hyperglycemia, the discontinuation of CLOZARIL® (clozapine) should be considered.

Hepatitis

Caution is advised in patients using CLOZARIL® (clozapine) who have concurrent hepatic disease. Hepatitis has been reported in both patients with normal and pre-existing liver function abnormalities. In patients who develop nausea, vomiting, and/or anorexia during CLOZARIL® (clozapine) treatment, liver function tests should be performed immediately. If the elevation of these values is clinically relevant or if symptoms of jaundice occur, treatment with CLOZARIL® (clozapine) should be discontinued.

Anticholinergic Toxicity

CLOZARIL® (clozapine) has very potent anticholinergic effects and great care should be exercised in using this drug in the presence of prostatic enlargement or narrow angle glaucoma. In addition, CLOZARIL® (clozapine) use has been associated with varying degrees of impairment of intestinal peristalsis, ranging from constipation to intestinal obstruction, fecal impaction and paralytic ileus *(see ADVERSE REACTIONS)*. On rare occasions, these cases have been fatal. Constipation should be initially treated by ensuring adequate hydration, and use of ancillary therapy such as bulk laxatives. Consultation with a gastroenterologist is advisable in more serious cases.

Interference with Cognitive and Motor Performance

Because of initial sedation, CLOZARIL® (clozapine) may impair mental and/or physical abilities, especially during the first few days of therapy. The recommendations for gradual dose escalation should be carefully adhered to, and patients cautioned about activities requiring alertness.

Use in Patients with Concomitant Illness

Clinical experience with CLOZARIL® (clozapine) in patients with concomitant systemic diseases is limited. Nevertheless, caution is advisable in using CLOZARIL® (clozapine) in patients with renal or cardiac disease.

Use in Patients Undergoing General Anesthesia

Caution is advised in patients being administered general anesthesia because of the CNS effects of CLOZARIL® (clozapine). Check with the anesthesiologist regarding continuation of CLOZARIL® (clozapine) therapy in a patient scheduled for surgery.

Information for Patients

Physicians are advised to discuss the following issues with patients for whom they prescribe CLOZARIL® (clozapine):

— Patients who are to receive CLOZARIL® (clozapine) should be warned about the significant risk of developing agranulocytosis. They should be informed that weekly blood tests are required for the first 6 months, if acceptable WBC counts (WBC greater than or equal to 3000/mm^3, ANC $\geq$ 1500/mm^3) have been maintained during the first 6 months of continuous therapy, then WBC counts can be monitored every other week in order to monitor for the occurrence of agranulocytosis, and that CLOZARIL® (clozapine) tablets will be made available only through a special program designed to ensure the required blood monitoring. Patients should be advised to report immediately the appearance of lethargy, weakness, fever, sore throat, malaise, mucous membrane ulceration or other possible signs of infection. Particular attention should be paid to any flu-like complaints or other symptoms that might suggest infection.

— Patients should be informed of the significant risk of seizure during CLOZARIL® (clozapine) treatment, and they should be advised to avoid driving and any other potentially hazardous activity while taking CLOZARIL® (clozapine).

— Patients should be advised of the risk of orthostatic hypotension, especially during the period of initial dose titration.

— Patients should be informed that if they stop taking CLOZARIL® (clozapine) for more than 2 days, they should not restart their medication at the same dosage, but should contact their physician for dosing instructions.

— Patients should notify their physician if they are taking, or plan to take, any prescription or over-the-counter drugs or alcohol.

— Patients should notify their physician if they become pregnant or intend to become pregnant during therapy.

— Patients should not breast feed an infant if they are taking CLOZARIL® (clozapine).

Drug Interactions

The risks of using CLOZARIL® (clozapine) in combination with other drugs have not been systematically evaluated.

The mechanism of CLOZARIL® (clozapine) induced agranulocytosis is unknown; nonetheless, the possibility that causative factors may interact synergistically to increase the risk and/or severity of bone marrow suppression warrants consideration. Therefore, CLOZARIL® (clozapine) should not be used with other agents having a well-known potential to suppress bone marrow function.

Given the primary CNS effects of CLOZARIL® (clozapine), caution is advised in using it concomitantly with other CNS-active drugs or alcohol.

Orthostatic hypotension in patients taking clozapine can, in rare cases (approximately 1 case per 3,000 patients), be accompanied by profound collapse and respiratory and/or cardiac arrest. Some of the cases of collapse/respiratory arrest/cardiac arrest during initial treatment occurred in patients who were being administered benzodiazepines; similar events have been reported in patients taking other psychotropic drugs or even CLOZARIL® (clozapine) by itself. Although it has not been established that there is an interaction between CLOZARIL® (clozapine) and benzodiazepines or other psychotropics, caution is advised when clozapine is initiated in patients taking a benzodiazepine or any other psychotropic drug.

Because CLOZARIL® (clozapine) is highly bound to serum protein, the administration of CLOZARIL® (clozapine) to a patient taking another drug which is highly bound to protein (e.g., warfarin, digitoxin) may cause an increase in plasma concentrations of these drugs, potentially resulting in adverse effects. Conversely, adverse effects may result from displacement of protein-bound CLOZARIL® (clozapine) by other highly bound drugs.

Cimetidine and erythromycin may both increase plasma levels of CLOZARIL® (clozapine), potentially resulting in adverse effects. Although concomitant use of CLOZARIL® (clozapine) and carbamazepine is not recommended, it should be noted that discontinuation of concomitant carbamazepine administration may result in an increase in CLOZARIL® (clozapine) plasma levels. Phenytoin may decrease CLOZARIL® (clozapine) plasma levels, resulting in a decrease in effectiveness of a previously effective CLOZARIL® (clozapine) dose.

In a study of schizophrenic patients who received clozapine under steady state conditions, fluvoxamine or paroxetine was added in 16 and 14 patients, respectively. After 14 days of co-administration, mean trough concentrations of clozapine and its metabolites, *N*-dexmethylclozapine and clozapine *N*-oxide, were elevated with fluvoxamine by about three-fold compared to baseline concentrations. Paroxetine produced only minor changes in the levels of clozapine and its metabolites. However, other published reports describe modest elevations (less than two-fold) of clozapine and metabolite concentrations when clozapine was taken with paroxetine, fluoxetine, and sertraline. Therefore, such combined treatment should be approached with caution and patients should be monitored closely when CLOZARIL® (clozapine) is combined with these drugs, particularly fluvoxamine. A reduced CLOZARIL® (clozapine) dose should be considered.

A subset (3%-10%) of the population has reduced activity of certain drug metabolizing enzymes such as the cytochrome P450 isozyme P450 2D6. Such individuals are referred to as "poor metabolizers" of drugs such as debrisoquin, dextromethorphan, the tricyclic antidepressants, and clozapine. These individuals may develop higher than expected plasma concentrations of clozapine when given usual doses. In addition, certain drugs that are metabolized by this isozyme, including many antidepressants (clozapine, selective serotonin reuptake inhibitors, and others), may inhibit the activity of this isozyme, and thus may make normal metabolizers resemble poor metabolizers with regard to concomitant therapy with other drugs metabolized by this enzyme system, leading to drug interaction.

Concomitant use of clozapine with other drugs metabolized by cytochrome P450 2D6 may require lower doses than usually prescribed for either clozapine or the other drug. Therefore, co-administration of clozapine with other drugs that are metabolized by this isozyme, including antidepressants, phenothiazines, carbamazepine, and Type 1C antiarrhythmics (e.g., propafenone, flecainide and encainide), or that inhibit this enzyme (e.g., quinidine), should be approached with caution.

CLOZARIL® (clozapine) may also potentiate the hypotensive effects of antihypertensive drugs and the anticholinergic effects of atropine-type drugs. The administration of epinephrine should be avoided in the treatment of drug induced hypotension because of a possible reverse epinephrine effect.

Carcinogenesis, Mutagenesis, Impairment of Fertility

No carcinogenic potential was demonstrated in long-term studies in mice and rats at doses approximately 7 times the typical human dose on a mg/kg basis. Fertility in male and female rats was not adversely affected by clozapine. Clozapine did not produce genotoxic or mutagenic effects when assayed in appropriate bacterial and mammalian tests.

Pregnancy Category B

Reproduction studies have been performed in rats and rabbits at doses of approximately 2-4 times the human dose and have revealed no evidence of impaired fertility or harm to the fetus due to clozapine. There are, however, no adequate and well-controlled studies in pregnant women. Because animal reproduction studies are not always predictive of human response, and in view of the desirability of keeping the administration of all drugs to a minimum during pregnancy, this drug should be used only if clearly needed.

Nursing Mothers

Animal studies suggest that clozapine may be excreted in breast milk and have an effect on the nursing infant. Therefore, women receiving CLOZARIL® (clozapine) should not breast feed.

Pediatric Use

Safety and effectiveness in pediatric patients have not been established.

Geriatric Use

Clinical studies of clozapine did not include sufficient numbers of subjects age 65 and over to determine whether they respond differently from younger subjects.

Orthostatic hypotension can occur with CLOZARIL® (clozapine) treatment and tachycardia, which may be sustained, has been observed in about 25% of patients taking CLOZARIL® (clozapine) *(see WARNINGS, Adverse Cardiovascular and Respiratory Effects)*. Elderly patients, particularly those with compromised cardiovascular functioning, may be more susceptible to these effects.

Also, elderly patients may be particularly susceptible to the anticholinergic effects of CLOZARIL® (clozapine), such as urinary retention and constipation. *(See PRECAUTIONS, Anticholinergic Toxicity)*

Dose selection for an elderly patient should be cautious, reflecting the greater frequency of decreased hepatic, renal, or cardiac function, and of concomitant disease or other drug therapy. Other reported clinical experience does suggest that the prevalence of tardive dyskinesia appears to be highest among the elderly, especially elderly women. *(See WARNINGS, Tardive Dyskinesia)*

ADVERSE REACTIONS

Associated with Discontinuation of Treatment

Sixteen percent of 1080 patients who received CLOZARIL® (clozapine) in premarketing clinical trials discontinued treatment due to an adverse event, including both those that could be reasonably attributed to CLOZARIL® (clozapine) treatment and those that might more appropriately be considered intercurrent illness. The more common events considered to be causes of discontinuation included: CNS, primarily drowsiness/sedation, seizures, dizziness/syncope; cardiovascular, primarily tachycardia, hypotension and ECG changes; gastrointestinal, primarily nausea/vomiting; hematologic, primarily leukopenia/granulocytopenia/agranulocytosis; and fever. None of the events enumerated accounts for more than 1.7% of all discontinuations attributed to adverse clinical events.

Continued on next page

Clozaril—Cont.

Commonly Observed

Adverse events observed in association with the use of CLOZARIL® (clozapine) in clinical trials at an incidence of greater than 5% were: central nervous system complaints, including drowsiness/sedation, dizziness/vertigo, headache and tremor; autonomic nervous system complaints, including salivation, sweating, dry mouth and visual disturbances; cardiovascular findings, including tachycardia, hypotension and syncope; and gastrointestinal complaints, including constipation and nausea; and fever. Complaints of drowsiness/sedation tend to subside with continued therapy or dose reduction. Salivation may be profuse, especially during sleep, but may be diminished with dose reduction.

Incidence in Clinical Trials

The following table enumerates adverse events that occurred at a frequency of 1% or greater among CLOZARIL® (clozapine) patients who participated in clinical trials. These rates are not adjusted for duration of exposure.

Treatment-Emergent Adverse Experience Incidence Among Patients Taking CLOZARIL® (clozapine) in Clinical Trials (N = 842) (Percentage of Patients Reporting)

Body System / Adverse Event[a]	Percent
Central Nervous System	
Drowsiness/Sedation	39
Dizziness/Vertigo	19
Headache	7
Tremor	6
Syncope	6
Disturbed sleep/Nightmares	4
Restlessness	4
Hypokinesia/Akinesia	4
Agitation	4
Seizures (convulsions)	3[b]
Rigidity	3
Akasthisia	3
Confusion	3
Fatigue	2
Insomnia	2
Hyperkinesia	1
Weakness	1
Lethargy	1
Ataxia	1
Slurred speech	1
Depression	1
Epileptiform movements/Myoclonic jerks	1
Anxiety	1
Cardiovascular	
Tachycardia	25[b]
Hypotension	9
Hypertension	4
Chest pain/Angina	1
ECG change/Cardiac abnormality	1
Gastrointestinal	
Constipation	14
Nausea	5
Abdomnial discomfort/Heartburn	4
Nausea/Vomiting	3
Vomiting	3
Diarrhea	2
Liver test abnormality	1
Anorexia	1
Urogenital	
Urinary abnormalities	2
Incontinence	1
Abnormal ejaculation	1
Urinary urgency/frequency	1
Urinary retention	1
Autonomic Nervous System	
Salivation	31
Sweating	6
Dry mouth	6
Visual disturbances	5
Integumentary (Skin)	
Rash	2
Musculoskeletal	
Muscle weakness	1
Pain (back, neck, legs)	1
Muscle spasm	1
Muscle pain, ache	1
Respiratory	
Throat discomfort	1
Dyspnea, shortness of breath	1
Nasal congestion	1
Hemic/Lymphatic	
Leukopenia/Decreased WBC/Neutropenia	3
Agranulocytosis	1[b]
Eosinophilia	1
Miscellaneous	
Fever	5
Weight gain	4
Tongue numb/sore	1

[a] Events reported by at least 1% of CLOZARIL® (clozapine) patients are included.

[b] Rate based on population of approximately 1700 exposed during premarket clinical evaluation of CLOZARIL® (clozapine).

Other Events Observed During the Premarketing Evaluation of CLOZARIL® (clozapine)

This section reports additional, less frequent adverse events which occurred among the patients taking CLOZARIL® (clozapine) in clinical trials. Various adverse events were reported as part of the total experience in these clinical studies; a causal relationship to CLOZARIL® (clozapine) treatment cannot be determined in the absence of appropriate controls in some of the studies. The table above enumerates adverse events that occurred at a frequency of at least 1% of patients treated with CLOZARIL® (clozapine). The list below includes all additional adverse experiences reported as being temporally associated with the use of the drug which occurred at a frequency less than 1%, enumerated by organ system.

Central Nervous System: loss of speech, amentia, tics, poor coordination, delusions/hallucinations, involuntary movement, stuttering, dysarthria, amnesia/memory loss, histrionic movements, libido increase or decrease, paranoia, shakiness, Parkinsonism, and irritability.

Cardiovascular System: edema, palpitations, phlebitis/thrombophlebitis, cyanosis, premature ventricular contraction, bradycardia, and nose bleed.

Gastrointestinal System: abdominal distention, gastroenteritis, rectal bleeding, nervous stomach, abnormal stools, hematemesis, gastric ulcer, bitter taste, and eructation.

Urogenital System: dysmenorrhea, impotence, breast pain/discomfort, and vaginal itch/infection.

Autonomic Nervous System: numbness, polydypsia, hot flashes, dry throat, and mydriasis.

Integumentary (Skin): pruritus, pallor, eczema, erythema, bruise, dermatitis, petechiae, and urticaria.

Musculoskeletal System: twitching and joint pain.

Respiratory System: coughing, pneumonia/pneumonia-like symptoms, rhinorrhea, hyperventilation, wheezing, bronchitis, laryngitis, and sneezing.

Hemic and Lymphatic System: anemia and leukocytosis.

Miscellaneous: chills/chills with fever, malaise, appetite increase, ear disorder, hypothermia, eyelid disorder, bloodshot eyes, and nystagmus.

Postmarketing Clinical Experience

Postmarketing experience has shown an adverse experience profile similar to that presented above. Voluntary reports of adverse events temporally associated with CLOZARIL® (clozapine) not mentioned above that have been received since market introduction and that may have no causal relationship with the drug include the following:

Central Nervous System: delirium; EEG abnormal; exacerbation of psychosis; myoclonus; overdose; paresthesia; possible mild cataplexy; and status epilepticus.

Cardiovascular System: atrial or ventricular fibrillation and periorbital edema.

Gastrointestinal System: acute pancreatitis; dysphagia; fecal impaction; intestinal obstruction/paralytic ileus; and salivary gland swelling.

Hepatobiliary System: cholestasis; hepatitis; jaundice.

Hepatic System: cholestasis.

Urogenital System: acute interstitial nephritis and priapism.

Integumentary (Skin): hypersensitivity reactions: photosensitivity, vasculitis, erythema multiforme, and Stevens-Johnson Syndrome.

Musculoskeletal System: myasthenic syndrome and rhabdomyolysis.

Respiratory System: aspiration and pleural effusion.

Hemic and Lymphatic System: deep vein thrombosis; elevated hemoglobin/hematocrit; ESR increased; pulmonary embolism; sepsis; thrombocytosis; and thrombocytopenia.

Miscellaneous: CPK elevation; hyperglycemia; hyperuricemia; hyponatremia; and weight loss.

DRUG ABUSE AND DEPENDENCE

Physical and psychological dependence have not been reported or observed in patients taking CLOZARIL® (clozapine).

OVERDOSAGE

Human Experience

The most commonly reported signs and symptoms associated with CLOZARIL® (clozapine) overdose are: altered states of consciousness, including drowsiness, delirium and coma; tachycardia; hypotension; respiratory depression or failure; hypersalivation. Aspiration pneumonia and cardiac arrhythmias have also been reported. Seizures have occurred in a minority of reported cases. Fatal overdoses have been reported with CLOZARIL® (clozapine), generally at doses above 2500 mg. There have also been reports of patients recovering from overdoses well in excess of 4 g.

Management of Overdose

Establish and maintain an airway; ensure adequate oxygenation and ventilation. Activated charcoal, which may be used with sorbitol, may be as or more effective than emesis or lavage, and should be considered in treating overdosage. Cardiac and vital signs monitoring is recommended along with general symptomatic and supportive measures. Additional surveillance should be continued for several days because of the risk of delayed effects. Avoid epinephrine and derivatives when treating hypotension, and quinidine and procainamide when treating cardiac arrhythmia.

There are no specific antidotes for CLOZARIL® (clozapine). Forced diuresis, dialysis, hemoperfusion and exchange transfusion are unlikely to be of benefit.

In managing overdosage, the physician should consider the possibility of multiple drug involvement.

Up-to-date information about the treatment of overdose can often be obtained from a certified Regional Poison Control Center. Telephone numbers of certified Poison Control Centers are listed in the Physicians' Desk Reference®.*

DOSAGE AND ADMINISTRATION

Upon initiation of CLOZARIL® (clozapine) therapy, up to a 1 week supply of additional CLOZARIL® (clozapine) tablets may be provided to the patient to be held for emergencies (e.g., weather, holidays).

Initial Treatment

It is recommended that treatment with CLOZARIL® (clozapine) begin with one-half of a 25 mg tablet (12.5 mg) once or twice daily and then be continued with daily dosage increments of 25-50 mg/day, if well-tolerated, to achieve a target dose of 300-450 mg/day by the end of 2 weeks. Subsequent dosage increments should be made no more than once or twice-weekly, in increments not to exceed 100 mg. Cautious titration and a divided dosage schedule are necessary to minimize the risks of hypotension, seizure, and sedation.

In the multicenter study that provides primary support for the effectiveness of CLOZARIL® (clozapine) in patients resistant to standard antipsychotic drug treatment, patients were titrated during the first 2 weeks up to a maximum dose of 500 mg/day, on a t.i.d. basis, and were then dosed in a total daily dose range of 100-900 mg/day, on a t.i.d. basis thereafter, with clinical response and adverse effects as guides to correct dosing.

Therapeutic Dose Adjustment

Daily dosing should continue on a divided basis as an effective and tolerable dose level is sought. While many patients may respond adequately at doses between 300-600 mg/day, it may be necessary to raise the dose to the 600-900 mg/day range to obtain an acceptable response. [Note: In the multicenter study providing the primary support for the superiority of CLOZARIL® (clozapine) in treatment resistant patients, the mean and median CLOZARIL® (clozapine) doses were both approximately 600 mg/day.]

Because of the possibility of increased adverse reactions at higher doses, particularly seizures, patients should ordinarily be given adequate time to respond to a given dose level before escalation to a higher dose is contemplated.

Dosing should not exceed 900 mg/day.

Because of the significant risk of agranulocytosis and seizure, events which both present a continuing risk over time, the extended treatment of patients failing to show an acceptable level of clinical response should ordinarily be avoided.

Maintenance Treatment

While the maintenance effectiveness of CLOZARIL® (clozapine) in schizophrenia is still under study, the effectiveness of maintenance treatment is well established for many other antipsychotic drugs. It is recommended that responding patients be continued on CLOZARIL® (clozapine), but at the lowest level needed to maintain remission. Because of the significant risk associated with the use of CLOZARIL® (clozapine), patients should be periodically reassessed to determine the need for maintenance treatment.

Discontinuation of Treatment

In the event of planned termination of CLOZARIL® (clozapine) therapy, gradual reduction in dose is recommended over a 1-2 week period. However, should a patient's medical condition require abrupt discontinuation (e.g., leukopenia), the patient should be carefully observed for the recurrence of psychotic symptoms.

Reinitiation of Treatment in Patients Previously Discontinued

When restarting patients who have had even a brief interval off CLOZARIL® (clozapine), i.e., 2 days or more since the last dose, it is recommended that treatment be reinitiated with one-half of a 25 mg tablet (12.5 mg) once or twice daily *(see WARNINGS)*. If that dose is well tolerated, it may be feasible to titrate patients back to a therapeutic dose more quickly than is recommended for initial treatment. However, any patient who has previously experienced respiratory or cardiac arrest with initial dosing, but was then able to be successfully titrated to a therapeutic dose, should be re-titrated with extreme caution after even 24 hours of discontinuation.

Certain additional precautions seem prudent when reinitiating treatment. The mechanisms underlying CLOZARIL® (clozapine) induced adverse reactions are unknown. It is conceivable, however, that re-exposure of a patient might enhance the risk of an untoward event's occurrence and increase its severity. Such phenomena, for example, occur when immune mediated mechanisms are responsible. Consequently, during the reinitiation of treatment, additional caution is advised. Patients discontinued for WBC counts below 2000/mm^3 or an ANC below 1000/mm^3 must *not* be restarted on CLOZARIL® (clozapine). *(See WARNINGS)*

HOW SUPPLIED

CLOZARIL® (clozapine) is available as 25 mg and 100 mg round, pale-yellow, uncoated tablets with a facilitated score on one side.

CLOZARIL® (clozapine) Tablets

25 mg

Engraved with "CLOZARIL" once on the periphery of one side.
Engraved with a facilitated score and "25" once on the other side.
Bottle of 100 .... NDC 0078-0126-05
Bottle of 500 .... NDC 0078-0126-08
Unit dose packages of 100: 2 × 5 strips,
10 blisters per strip .... NDC 0078-0126-06

100 mg

Engraved with "CLOZARIL" once on the periphery of one side.
Engraved with a facilitated score and "100" once on the other side.
Bottle of 100 .... NDC 0078-0127-05
Bottle of 500 .... NDC 0078-0127-08
Unit dose packages of 100: 2 × 5 strips,
10 blisters per strip .... NDC 0078-0127-06

Store and Dispense

Storage temperature should not exceed 86°F (30°C). Drug dispensing should not ordinarily exceed a weekly supply. If a patient is eligible for WBC testing every other week, then a two week supply of CLOZARIL® (clozapine) can be dispensed. Dispensing should be contingent upon the results of a WBC count.

*Trademark of Medical Economics Company, Inc.

REV: SEPTEMBER 1999 T1999-62

Shown in Product Identification Guide, page 325

COMTAN® ℞

[*cŏm-tăn*]

(entacapone) Tablets

Rx only

The following prescribing information is based on official labeling in effect July, 2000.

DESCRIPTION

Comtan® (entacapone) is available as tablets containing 200-mg entacapone.

Entacapone is an inhibitor of catechol-*O*-methyltransferase (COMT), used in the treatment of Parkinson's Disease as an adjunct to levodopa/carbidopa therapy. It is a nitrocatechol-structured compound with a relative molecular mass of 305.29. The chemical name of entacapone is (E)-2-cyano-3-(3,4-dihydroxy-5-nitrophenyl)-N,N-diethyl-2-propenamide. Its empirical formula is $C_{14}H_{15}N_3O_5$ and its structural formula is:

The inactive ingredients of the Comtan tablet are microcrystalline cellulose, mannitol, croscarmellose sodium, hydrogenated vegetable oil, hydroxypropyl methylcellulose, polysorbate 80, glycerol 85%, sucrose, magnesium stearate, yellow iron oxide, red oxide, and titanium dioxide.

CLINICAL PHARMACOLOGY

Mechanism of Action

Entacapone is a selective and reversible inhibitor of catechol-*O*-methyltransferase (COMT).

In mammals, COMT is distributed throughout various organs with the highest activities in the liver and kidney. COMT also occurs in the heart, lung, smooth and skeletal muscles, intestinal tract, reproductive organs, various glands, adipose tissue, skin, blood cells, and neuronal tissues, especially in glial cells. COMT catalyzes the transfer of the methyl group of S-adenosyl-L-methionine to the phenolic group of substrates that contain a catechol structure. Physiological substrates of COMT include dopa, catecholamines (dopamine, norepinephrine, and epinephrine) and their hydroxylated metabolites. The function of COMT is the elimination of biologically active catechols and some other hydroxylated metabolites. In the presence of a decarboxylase inhibitor, COMT becomes the major metabolizing enzyme for levodopa, catalyzing the metabolism to 3-methoxy-4-hydroxy-L-phenylalanine (3-OMD) in the brain and periphery.

The mechanism of action of entacapone is believed to be through its ability to inhibit COMT and alter the plasma pharmacokinetics of levodopa. When entacapone is given in conjunction with levodopa and an aromatic amino acid decarboxylase inhibitor, such as carbidopa, plasma levels of levodopa are greater and more sustained than after administration of levodopa and an aromatic amino acid decarboxylase inhibitor alone. It is believed that at a given frequency of levodopa administration, these more sustained plasma levels of levodopa result in more constant dopaminergic stimulation in the brain, leading to greater effects on the signs and symptoms of Parkinson's Disease. The higher levodopa levels also lead to increased levodopa adverse effects, sometimes requiring a decrease in the dose of levodopa.

Table 1. Nordic Study

	Baseline	Change from Baseline at Month 6*	p-value vs. placebo
Primary Measure from Home Diary (from an 18-hour Diary Day)			
Hours of Awake Time "On"			
Placebo	9.2	+0.1	—
Comtan	9.3	+1.5	<0.001
Duration of "On" time after first AM dose (hrs)			
Placebo	2.2	0.0	—
Comtan	2.1	+0.2	<0.05
Secondary Measures from Home Diary (from an 18-hour Diary Day)			
Hours of Awake Time "Off"			
Placebo	5.3	0.0	—
Comtan	5.5	-1.3	<0.001
Proportion of Awake Time "On" * (%)**			
Placebo	63.8	+0.6	—
Comtan	62.7	+9.3	<0.001
Levodopa Total Daily Dose (mg)			
Placebo	705	+14	—
Comtan	701	-87	<0.001
Frequency of Levodopa Daily Intakes			
Placebo	6.1	+0.1	—
Comtan	6.2	-0.4	<0.001
Other Secondary Measures			
	Baseline	**Change from Baseline at Month 6**	**p-value vs. placebo**
Investigator's Global (overall) % Improved**			
Placebo	—	28	—
Comtan	—	56	<0.01
Patient's Global (overall) % Improved**			
Placebo	—	22	—
Comtan	—	39	N.S.‡
UPDRS Total			
Placebo	37.4	-1.1	—
Comtan	38.5	-4.8	<0.01
UPDRS Motor			
Placebo	24.6	-0.7	—
Comtan	25.5	-3.3	<0.05
UPDRS ADL			
Placebo	11.0	-0.4	—
Comtan	11.2	-1.8	<0.05

*Mean; the month 6 values represent the average of weeks 8, 16, and 24, by protocol-defined outcome measure.
** At least one category change at endpoint.
*** Not an endpoint for this study but primary endpoint in the North American Study.
‡ Not significant.

In animals, while entacapone enters the CNS to a minimal extent, it has been shown to inhibit central COMT activity. In humans, entacapone inhibits the COMT enzyme in peripheral tissues. The effects of entacapone on central COMT activity in humans have not been studied.

Pharmacodynamics

COMT Activity in Erythrocytes: Studies in healthy volunteers have shown that entacapone reversibly inhibits human erythrocyte catechol-*O*-methyltransferase (COMT) activity after oral administration. There was a linear correlation between entacapone dose and erythrocyte COMT inhibition, the maximum inhibition being 82% following an 800-mg single dose. With a 200-mg single dose of entacapone, maximum inhibition of erythrocyte COMT activity is on average 65% with a return to baseline level within 8 hours.

Effect on the Pharmacokinetics of Levodopa and its Metabolites

When 200 mg entacapone is administered together with levodopa/carbidopa, it increases the area under the curve (AUC) of levodopa by approximately 35% and the elimination half-life of levodopa is prolonged from 1.3 h-2.4 h. In general, the average peak levodopa plasma concentration and the time of its occurrence (T_{max} of 1 hour) are unaffected. The onset of effect occurs after the first administration and is maintained during long-term treatment. Studies in Parkinson's Disease patients suggest that the maximal effect occurs with 200-mg entacapone. Plasma levels of 3-OMD are markedly and dose-dependently decreased by entacapone when given with levodopa/carbidopa.

Pharmacokinetics of Entacapone

Entacapone pharmacokinetics are linear over the dose range of 5 mg-800 mg, and are independent of levodopa/carbidopa coadministration. The elimination of entacapone is biphasic, with an elimination half-life of 0.4 h-0.7 h based on the β-phase and 2.4 h based on the γ-phase. The γ-phase accounts for approximately 10% of the total AUC. The total body clearance after i.v. administration is 850 mL/min. After a single 200-mg dose of Comtan (entacapone), the C_{max} is approximately 1.2 μg/mL.

Absorption: Entacapone is rapidly absorbed, with a T_{max} of approximately 1 hour. The absolute bioavailability following oral administration is 35%. Food does not affect the pharmacokinetics of entacapone.

Distribution: The volume of distribution of entacapone at steady state after i.v. injection is small (20 L). Entacapone does not distribute widely into tissues due to its high plasma protein binding. Based on *in vitro* studies, the plasma protein binding of entacapone is 98% over the concentration range of 0.4-50 μg/mL. Entacapone binds mainly to serum albumin.

Metabolism and Elimination: Entacapone is almost completely metabolized prior to excretion, with only a very small amount (0.2% of dose) found unchanged in urine. The main metabolic pathway is isomerization to the *cis*-isomer, followed by direct glucuronidation of the parent and *cis*-isomer; the glucuronide conjugate is inactive. After oral administration of a ^{14}C-labeled dose of entacapone, 10% of labeled parent and metabolite is excreted in urine and 90% in feces.

Special Populations: Entacapone pharmacokinetics are independent of age. No formal gender studies have been conducted. Racial representation in clinical trials was largely limited to Caucasians (there were only 4 blacks in one US trial and no Asians in any of the clinical trials); no conclusions can therefore be reached about the effect of Comtan on groups other than Caucasian.

Hepatic Impairment: A single 200-mg dose of entacapone, without levodopa/dopa decarboxylase inhibitor coadministration, showed approximately twofold higher AUC and C_{max} values in patients with a history of alcoholism and hepatic impairment (n=10) compared to normal subjects (n=10). All patients had biopsy-proven liver cirrhosis caused by alcohol. According to Child-Pugh grading 7 patients with liver disease had mild hepatic impairment and 3 patients had moderate hepatic impairment. As only about 10% of the entacapone dose is excreted in urine as parent compound and conjugated glucuronide, biliary excretion appears to be the major route of excretion of this drug. Consequently, entacapone should be administered with care to patients with biliary obstruction.

Renal Impairment: The pharmacokinetics of entacapone have been investigated after a single 200-mg entacapone dose, without levodopa/dopa decarboxylase inhibitor coadministration, in a specific renal impairment study. There were three groups: normal subjects (n=7; creatinine clearance >1.12 mL/sec/1.73 m^2), moderate impairment (n=10; creatinine clearance ranging from 0.60-0.89 mL/sec/1.73 m^2), and severe impairment (n=7; creatinine clearance ranging from 0.20-0.44 mL/sec/1.73 m^2). No important effects of renal function on the pharmacokinetics of entacapone were found.

Drug Interactions: See PRECAUTIONS, Drug Interactions.

Continued on next page

Comtan—Cont.

Clinical Studies

The effectiveness of Comtan (entacapone) as an adjunct to levodopa in the treatment of Parkinson's Disease was established in three 24-week multicenter, randomized, double-blind placebo-controlled trials in patients with Parkinson's Disease. In two of these trials, the patients' disease was "fluctuating", i.e., was characterized by documented periods of "On" (periods of relatively good functioning) and "Off" (periods of relatively poor functioning), despite optimum levodopa therapy. There was also a withdrawal period following 6 months of treatment. In the third trial patients were not required to have been experiencing fluctuations. Prior to the controlled part of the trials, patients were stabilized on levodopa for 2-4 weeks. Comtan has not been systematically evaluated in patients who do not experience fluctuations.

In the first two studies to be described, patients were randomized to receive placebo or entacapone 200 mg administered concomitantly with each dose of levodopa/carbidopa (up to 10 times daily, but averaging 4-6 doses per day). The formal double-blind portion of both trials was 6 months long. Patients recorded the time spent in the "On" and "Off" states in home diaries periodically throughout the duration of the trial. In one study, conducted in the Nordic countries, the primary outcome measure was the total mean time spent in the "On" state during an 18-hour diary recorded day (6 AM to midnight). In the other study, the primary outcome measure was the proportion of awake time spent over 24 hours in the "On" state.

In addition to the primary outcome measure, the amount of time spent in the "Off" state was evaluated, and patients were also evaluated by subparts of the Unified Parkinson's Disease Rating Scale (UPDRS), a frequently used multi-item rating scale intended to assess mentation (Part I), activities of daily living (Part II), motor function (Part III), complications of therapy (Part IV), and disease staging (Part V & VI); an investigator's and patient's global assessment of clinical condition, a 7-point subjective scale designed to assess global functioning in Parkinson's Disease; and the change in daily levodopa/carbidopa dose.

In one of the studies, 171 patients were randomized in 16 centers in Finland, Norway, Sweden, and Denmark (Nordic study), all of whom received concomitant levodopa plus dopa-decarboxylase inhibitor (either levodopa/carbidopa or levodopa/benserazide). In the second trial, 205 patients were randomized in 17 centers in North America (US and Canada); all patients received concomitant levodopa/carbidopa.

The following tables display the results of these two trials:

[See table 1 at top of previous page]

[See table 2 above]

Table 2. North American Study

	Baseline	Change from Baseline at Month 6*	p-value vs. placebo
Primary Measure from Home Diary (for a 24-hour Diary Day)			
Percent of Awake Time "On"			
Placebo	60.8	+2.0	—
Comtan	60.0	+6.7	<0.05
Secondary Measures from Home Diary (for a 24-hour Diary Day)			
Hours of Awake Time "Off"			
Placebo	6.6	-0.3	—
Comtan	6.8	-1.2	<0.01
Hours of Awake Time "On"			
Placebo	10.3	+0.4	—
Comtan	10.2	+1.0	N.S.‡
Levodopa Total Daily Dose (mg)			
Placebo	758	+19	—
Comtan	804	-93	<0.001
Frequency of Levodopa Daily Intakes			
Placebo	6.0	+0.2	—
Comtan	6.2	0.0	N.S.‡
Other Secondary Measures			
	Baseline	**Change from Baseline at Month 6**	**p-value vs. placebo**
Investigator's Global (overall) % Improved**			
Placebo	—	21	—
Comtan	—	34	<0.05
Patient's Global (overall) % Improved**			
Placebo	—	20	—
Comtan	—	31	<0.05
UPDRS Total***			
Placebo	35.6	+2.8	—
Comtan	35.1	-0.6	<0.05
UPDRS Motor***			
Placebo	22.6	+1.2	—
Comtan	22.0	-0.9	<0.05
UPDRS ADL***			
Placebo	11.7	+1.1	—
Comtan	11.9	0.0	<0.05

*Mean; the month 6 values represent the average of weeks 8, 16, and 24, by protocol-defined outcome measure.
** At least one category change at endpoint.
*** Score change at endpoint similarly to the Nordic Study.
‡ Not significant.

Effects on "On" time did not differ by age, sex, weight, disease severity at baseline, levodopa dose and concurrent treatment with dopamine agonists or selegiline.

Withdrawal of entacapone: In the North American study, abrupt withdrawal of entacapone, without alteration of the dose of levodopa/carbidopa, resulted in a significant worsening of fluctuations, compared to placebo. In some cases, symptoms were slightly worse than at baseline, but returned to approximately baseline severity within two weeks following levodopa dose increase on average by 80 mg. In the Nordic study, similarly, a significant worsening of parkinsonian symptoms was observed after entacapone withdrawal, as assessed two weeks after drug withdrawal. At this phase, the symptoms were approximately at baseline severity following levodopa dose increase by about 50 mg.

In the third placebo controlled trial, a total of 301 patients were randomized in 32 centers in Germany and Austria. In this trial, as in the other two trials, entacapone 200 mg was administered with each dose of levodopa/dopa decarboxylase inhibitor (up to 10 times daily) and UPDRS Parts II and III and total daily "On" time were the primary measures of effectiveness. The following results were seen for the primary measures, as well as for some secondary measures:

[See table 3 at top of next page]

INDICATIONS

Comtan (entacapone) is indicated as an adjunct to levodopa/carbidopa to treat patients with idiopathic Parkinson's Disease who experience the signs and symptoms of end-of-dose "wearing-off" *(see CLINICAL PHARMACOLOGY, Clinical Studies)*.

Comtan's effectiveness has not been systematically evaluated in patients with idiopathic Parkinson's Disease who do not experience end-of-dose "wearing-off".

CONTRAINDICATIONS

Comtan (entacapone) tablets are contraindicated in patients who have demonstrated hypersensitivity to the drug or its ingredients.

WARNINGS

Monoamine oxidase (MAO) and COMT are the two major enzyme systems involved in the metabolism of catecholamines. It is theoretically possible, therefore, that the combination of Comtan (entacapone) and a non-selective MAO inhibitor (e.g., phenelzine and tranylcypromine) would result in inhibition of the majority of the pathways responsible for normal catecholamine metabolism. For this reason, patients should ordinarily not be treated concomitantly with Comtan and a non-selective MAO inhibitor.

Entacapone can be taken concomitantly with a selective MAO-B inhibitor (e.g., selegiline).

Drugs Metabolized by Catechol-*O*-methyltransferase (COMT)

When a single 400-mg dose of entacapone was given together with intravenous isoprenaline (isoproterenol) and epinephrine without coadministered levodopa/dopa decarboxylase inhibitor, the overall mean maximal changes in heart rate during infusion were about 50% and 80% higher than with placebo, for isoprenaline and epinephrine, respectively.

Therefore, drugs known to be metabolized by COMT, such as isoproterenol, epinephrine, norepinephrine, dopamine, dobutamine, alpha-methyldopa, apomorphine, isoetherine, and bitolterol should be administered with caution in patients receiving entacapone regardless of the route of administration (including inhalation), as their interaction may result in increased heart rates, possibly arrhythmias, and excessive changes in blood pressure.

Ventricular tachycardia was noted in one 32-year-old healthy male volunteer in an interaction study after epinephrine infusion and oral entacapone administration. Treatment with propranolol was required. A causal relationship to entacapone administration appears probable but cannot be attributed with certainty.

PRECAUTIONS

Hypotension/Syncope

Dopaminergic therapy in Parkinson's Disease patients has been associated with orthostatic hypotension. Entacapone enhances levodopa bioavailability and, therefore, might be expected to increase the occurrence of orthostatic hypotension. In Comtan (entacapone) clinical trials, however, no differences from placebo were seen for measured orthostasis or symptoms of orthostasis. Orthostatic hypotension was documented at least once in 2.7% and 3.0% of the patients treated with 200 mg Comtan and placebo, respectively. A total of 4.3% and 4.0% of the patients treated with 200 mg Comtan and placebo, respectively, reported orthostatic symptoms at some time during their treatment and also had at least one episode of orthostatic hypotension documented (however, the episode of orthostatic symptoms itself was not accompanied by vital sign measurements). Neither baseline treatment with dopamine agonists or selegiline, nor the presence of orthostasis at baseline, increased the risk of orthostatic hypotension in patients treated with Comtan compared to patients on placebo.

In the large controlled trials, approximately 1.2% and 0.8% of 200 mg entacapone and placebo patients, respectively, reported at least one episode of syncope. Reports of syncope were generally more frequent in patients in both treatment groups who had an episode of documented hypotension (although the episodes of syncope, obtained by history, were themselves not documented with vital sign measurement).

Diarrhea

In clinical trials, diarrhea developed in 60 of 603 (10.0%) and 16 of 400 (4.0%) of patients treated with 200 mg Comtan and placebo, respectively. In patients treated with Comtan, diarrhea was generally mild to moderate in severity (8.6%) but was regarded as severe in 1.3%. Diarrhea resulted in withdrawal in 10 of 603 (1.7%) patients, 7 (1.2%) with mild and moderate diarrhea and 3 (0.5%) with severe diarrhea. Diarrhea generally resolved after discontinuation of Comtan. Two patients with diarrhea were hospitalized. Typically, diarrhea presents within 4-12 weeks after entacapone is started, but it may appear as early as the first week and as late as many months after the initiation of treatment.

Hallucinations

Dopaminergic therapy in Parkinson's Disease patients has been associated with hallucinations. In clinical trials, hallucinations developed in approximately 4.0% of patients treated with 200 mg Comtan or placebo. Hallucinations led to drug discontinuation and premature withdrawal from clinical trials in 0.8% and 0% of patients treated with 200 mg Comtan and placebo, respectively. Hallucinations led to hospitalization in 1.0% and 0.3% of patients in the 200 mg Comtan and placebo groups, respectively.

Dyskinesia

Comtan may potentiate the dopaminergic side effects of levodopa and may cause and/or exacerbate preexisting dyskinesia. Although decreasing the dose of levodopa may ameliorate this side effect, many patients in controlled trials continued to experience frequent dyskinesias despite a reduction in their dose of levodopa. The rates of withdrawal for dyskinesia were 1.5% and 0.8% for 200 mg Comtan and placebo, respectively.

Other Events Reported With Dopaminergic Therapy

The events listed below are rare events known to be associated with the use of drugs that increase dopaminergic activity, although they are most often associated with the use of direct dopamine agonists.

Rhabdomyolysis: Cases of severe rhabdomyolysis have been reported with Comtan use. The complicated nature of these cases makes it impossible to determine what role, if any, Comtan played in their pathogenesis. Severe prolonged motor activity including dyskinesia may account for rhabdomyolysis. One case, however, included fever and alteration of consciousness. It is therefore possible that the rhabdomyolysis may be a result of the syndrome described in Hyperpyrexia and Confusion *(see PRECAUTIONS, Other Events Reported With Dopaminergic Therapy)*.

Hyperpyrexia and Confusion: Cases of a symptom complex resembling the neuroleptic malignant syndrome characterized by elevated temperature, muscular rigidity, altered consciousness, and elevated CPK have been reported in association with the rapid dose reduction or withdrawal of other dopaminergic drugs. Several cases with similar signs and symptoms have been reported in association with Comtan therapy, although no information about dose manipulation is available. The complicated nature of these cases makes it difficult to determine what role, if any, Comtan may have played in their pathogenesis. No cases have been reported following the abrupt withdrawal or dose reduction of entacapone treatment during clinical studies. Prescribers should exercise caution when discontinuing entacapone treatment. When considered necessary, withdrawal should proceed slowly. If a decision is made to discontinue treatment with Comtan, recommendations include monitoring the patient closely and adjusting other dopaminergic treatments as needed. This syndrome should be considered in the differential diagnosis for any patient who develops a high fever or severe rigidity. Tapering Comtan has not been systematically evaluated.

Fibrotic Complications: Cases of retroperitoneal fibrosis, pulmonary infiltrates, pleural effusion, and pleural thickening have been reported in some patients treated with ergot derived dopaminergic agents. These complications may resolve when the drug is discontinued, but complete resolution does not always occur. Although these adverse events are believed to be related to the ergoline structure of these compounds, whether other, nonergot derived drugs (e.g., entacapone) that increase dopaminergic activity can cause them is unknown. It should be noted that the expected incidence of fibrotic complications is so low that even if entacapone caused these complications at rates similar to those attributable to other dopaminergic therapies, it is unlikely that it would have been detected in a cohort of the size exposed to entacapone. Four cases of pulmonary fibrosis were reported during clinical development of entacapone; three of these patients were also treated with pergolide and one with bromocriptine. The duration of treatment with entacapone ranged from 7-17 months.

Renal Toxicity

In a 1 year toxicity study, entacapone (plasma exposure 20 times that in humans receiving the maximum recommended daily dose of 1600 mg) caused an increased incidence in male rats of nephrotoxicity that was characterized by regenerative tubules, thickening of basement membranes, infiltration of mononuclear cells and tubular protein casts. These effects were not associated with changes in clinical chemistry parameters, and there is no established method for monitoring for the possible occurrence of these lesions in humans. Although this toxicity could represent a species-specific effect, there is not yet evidence that this is so.

Hepatic Impairment

Patients with hepatic impairment should be treated with caution. The AUC and C_{max} of entacapone approximately doubled in patients with documented liver disease compared to controls. *(See CLINICAL PHARMACOLOGY, Pharmacokinetics of Entacapone and DOSAGE AND ADMINISTRATION).*

Information for Patients

Patients should be instructed to take Comtan only as prescribed.

Patients should be informed that hallucinations can occur.

Patients should be advised that they may develop postural (orthostatic) hypotension with or without symptoms such as dizziness, nausea, syncope, and sweating. Hypotension may occur more frequently during initial therapy. Accordingly, patients should be cautioned against rising rapidly after sitting or lying down, especially if they have been doing so for prolonged periods, and especially at the initiation of treatment with Comtan.

Patients should be advised that they should neither drive a car nor operate other complex machinery until they have gained sufficient experience on Comtan to gauge whether or not it affects their mental and/or motor performance adversely. Because of the possible additive sedative effects, caution should be used when patients are taking other CNS depressants in combination with Comtan.

Patients should be informed that nausea may occur, especially at the initiation of treatment with Comtan.

Patients should be advised of the possibility of an increase in dyskinesia.

Patients should be advised that treatment with entacapone may cause a change in the color of their urine (a brownish orange discoloration) that is not clinically relevant. In controlled trials, 10% of patients treated with Comtan reported urine discoloration compared to 0% of placebo patients.

Although Comtan has not been shown to be teratogenic in animals, it is always given in conjunction with levodopa/carbidopa, which is known to cause visceral and skeletal malformations in the rabbit. Accordingly, patients should be advised to notify their physicians if they become pregnant or intend to become pregnant during therapy *(see PRECAUTIONS, Pregnancy).*

Entacapone is excreted into maternal milk in rats. Because of the possibility that entacapone may be excreted into human maternal milk, patients should be advised to notify their physicians if they intend to breastfeed or are breastfeeding an infant.

Laboratory Tests

Comtan is a chelator of iron. The impact of entacapone on the body's iron stores is unknown; however, a tendency towards decreasing serum iron concentrations was noted in clinical trials. In a controlled clinical study serum ferritin levels (as marker of iron deficiency and subclinical anemia) were not changed with entacapone compared to placebo after one year of treatment and there was no difference in rates of anemia or decreased hemoglobin levels.

Table 3. German-Austrian Study

Primary Measures

	Baseline	Change from Baseline at Month 6	p-value vs. placebo (LOCF)
UPDRS ADL*			
Placebo	12.0	+0.5	—
Comtan	12.4	-0.4	<0.05
UPDRS Motor*			
Placebo	24.1	+0.1	—
Comtan	24.9	-2.5	<0.05
Hours of Awake Time "On" (Home diary)**			
Placebo	10.1	+0.5	—
Comtan	10.2	+1.1	N.S.‡

Secondary Measures

	Baseline	Change from Baseline at Month 6	p-value vs. placebo
UPDRS Total*			
Placebo	37.7	+0.6	—
Comtan	39.0	-3.4	<0.05
Percent of Awake Time "On" (Home diary)**			
Placebo	59.8	+3.5	—
Comtan	62.0	+6.5	N.S.‡
Hours of Awake Time "Off" (Home diary)**			
Placebo	6.8	-0.6	—
Comtan	6.3	-1.2	0.07
Levodopa Total Daily Dose (mg)*			
Placebo	572	+4	—
Comtan	566	-35	N.S.‡
Frequency of Levodopa Daily Intake*			
Placebo	5.6	+0.2	—
Comtan	5.4	0.0	<0.01
Global (overall) % Improved***			
Placebo	—	34	—
Comtan	—	38	N.S.‡

*Total population; score change at endpoint.
** Fluctuating population, with 5-10 doses; score change at endpoint.
*** Total population; at least one category change at endpoint.
‡ Not significant.

Special Populations

Patients with hepatic impairment should be treated with caution *(see INDICATIONS, DOSAGE AND ADMINISTRATION).*

Drug Interactions

In vitro studies of human CYP enzymes showed that entacapone inhibited the CYP enzymes 1A2, 2A6, 2C9, 2C19, 2D6, 2E1 and 3A only at very high concentrations (IC50 from 200 to over 1000 μM; an oral 200 mg dose achieves a highest level of approximately 5 μM in people); these enzymes would therefore not be expected to be inhibited in clinical use.

Protein Binding

Entacapone is highly protein bound (98%). *In vitro* studies have shown no binding displacement between entacapone and other highly bound drugs, such as warfarin, salicylic acid, phenylbutazone, and diazepam.

Drugs Metabolized by Catechol-*O*-methyltransferase (COMT)

See WARNINGS.

Hormone levels

Levodopa is known to depress prolactin secretion and increase growth hormone levels. Treatment with entacapone coadministered with levodopa/dopa decarboxylase inhibitor does not change these effects.

Effect of Entacapone on the Metabolism of Other Drugs

See WARNINGS regarding concomitant use of Comtan and non-selective MAO inhibitors.

No interaction was noted with the MAO-B inhibitor selegiline in two multiple-dose interaction studies when entacapone was coadministered with a levodopa/dopa decarboxylase inhibitor (n=29). More than 600 Parkinson's Disease patients in clinical trials have used selegiline in combination with entacapone and levodopa/dopa decarboxylase inhibitor.

As most entacapone excretion is via the bile, caution should be exercised when drugs known to interfere with biliary excretion, glucuronidation, and intestinal beta-glucuronidase are given concurrently with entacapone. These include probenecid, cholestyramine, and some antibiotics (e.g., erythromycin, rifampicin, ampicillin and chloramphenicol).

No interaction with the tricyclic antidepressant imipramine was shown in a single-dose study with entacapone without coadministered levodopa/dopa-decarboxylase inhibitor.

Carcinogenesis

Two-year carcinogenicity studies of entacapone were conducted in mice and rats. Rats were treated once daily by oral gavage with entacapone doses of 20, 90, or 400 mg/kg. An increased incidence of renal tubular adenomas and carcinomas was found in male rats treated with the highest dose of entacapone. Plasma exposures (AUC) associated with this dose were approximately 20 times higher than estimated plasma exposures of humans receiving the maximum recommended daily dose of entacapone (MRDD = 1600 mg). Mice were treated once daily by oral gavage with doses of 20, 100 or 600 mg/kg of entacapone (0.05, 0.3, and 2 times the MRDD for humans on a mg/m^2 basis). Because of a high incidence of premature mortality in mice receiving the highest dose of entacapone, the mouse study is not an adequate assessment of carcinogenicity. Although no treatment related tumors were observed in animals receiving the lower doses, the carcinogenic potential of entacapone has not been fully evaluated. The carcinogenic potential of entacapone administered in combination with levodopa/carbidopa has not been evaluated.

Mutagenesis

Entacapone was mutagenic and clastogenic in the *in vitro* mouse lymphoma/thymidine kinase assay in the presence and absence of metabolic activation, and was clastogenic in cultured human lymphocytes in the presence of metabolic activation. Entacapone, either alone or in combination with levodopa/carbidopa, was not clastogenic in the *in vivo* mouse micronucleus test or mutagenic in the bacterial reverse mutation assay (Ames test).

Impairment of Fertility

Entacapone did not impair fertility or general reproductive performance in rats treated with up to 700 mg/kg/day (plasma AUCs 28 times those in humans receiving the MRDD). Delayed mating, but no fertility impairment, was evident in female rats treated with 700 mg/kg/day of entacapone.

Pregnancy

Pregnancy Category C. In embryofetal development studies, entacapone was administered to pregnant animals throughout organogenesis at doses of up to 1000 mg/kg/day in rats and 300 mg/kg/day in rabbits. Increased incidences of fetal variations were evident in litters from rats treated with the highest dose, in the absence of overt signs of maternal toxicity. The maternal plasma drug exposure (AUC) associated with this dose was approximately 34 times the estimated plasma exposure in humans receiving the maximum recommended daily dose (MRDD) of 1600 mg. Increased frequencies of abortions and late/total resorptions and decreased fetal weights were observed in the litters of rabbits treated with maternotoxic doses of 100 mg/kg/day (plasma AUCs 0.4 times those in humans receiving the MRDD) or greater. There was no evidence of teratogenicity in these studies.

However, when entacapone was administered to female rats prior to mating and during early gestation, an increased incidence of fetal eye anomalies (macrophthalmia, microphthalmia, anophthalmia) was observed in the litters of dams treated with doses of 160 mg/kg/day (plasma AUCs 7 times those in humans receiving the MRDD) or greater, in the absence of maternotoxicity. Administration of up to 700 mg/kg/day (plasma AUCs 28 times those in humans receiving the MRDD) to female rats during the latter part of gestation and throughout lactation, produced no evidence of developmental impairment in the offspring.

Continued on next page

Comtan—Cont.

Entacapone is always given concomitantly with levodopa/carbidopa, which is known to cause visceral and skeletal malformations in rabbits. The teratogenic potential of entacapone in combination with levodopa/carbidopa was not assessed in animals.

There is no experience from clinical studies regarding the use of Comtan in pregnant women. Therefore, Comtan should be used during pregnancy only if the potential benefit justifies the potential risk to the fetus.

Nursing Women

In animal studies, entacapone was excreted into maternal rat milk.

It is not known whether entacapone is excreted in human milk. Because many drugs are excreted in human milk, caution should be exercised when entacapone is administered to a nursing woman.

Pediatric Use

There is no identified potential use of entacapone in pediatric patients.

ADVERSE REACTIONS

During the pre-marketing development of entacapone, 1450 patients with Parkinson's Disease were treated with entacapone. Included were patients with fluctuating symptoms, as well as those with stable responses to levodopa therapy. All patients received concomitant treatment with levodopa preparations, however, and were similar in other clinical aspects.

The most commonly observed adverse events (>5%) in the double-blind, placebo-controlled trials (N=1003) associated with the use of Comtan (entacapone) and not seen at an equivalent frequency among the placebo-treated patients were: dyskinesia/hyperkinesia, nausea, urine discoloration, diarrhea, and abdominal pain.

Approximately 14% of the 603 patients given entacapone in the double-blind, placebo-controlled trials discontinued treatment due to adverse events compared to 9% of the 400 patients who received placebo. The most frequent causes of discontinuation in decreasing order are: psychiatric reasons (2% vs. 1%), diarrhea (2% vs. 0%), dyskinesia/hyperkinesia (2% vs. 1%), nausea (2% vs. 1%), abdominal pain (1% vs. 0%), and aggravation of Parkinson's Disease symptoms (1% vs. 1%).

Adverse Event Incidence in Controlled Clinical Studies

Table 4 lists treatment emergent adverse events that occurred in at least 1% of patients treated with entacapone participating in the double-blind, placebo-controlled studies and that were numerically more common in the entacapone group, compared to placebo. In these studies, either entacapone or placebo was added to levodopa/carbidopa (or levodopa/benserazide).

[See table below]

The prescriber should be aware that these figures cannot be used to predict the incidence of adverse events in the course of usual medical practice where patient characteristics and other factors differ from those that prevailed in the clinical studies. Similarly, the cited frequencies cannot be compared with figures obtained from other clinical investigations involving different treatments, uses, and investigators. The cited figures do, however, provide the prescriber with some basis for estimating the relative contribution of drug and nondrug factors to the adverse events observed in the population studied.

Effects of gender and age on adverse reactions

No differences were noted in the rate of adverse events attributable to entacapone by age or gender.

DRUG ABUSE AND DEPENDENCE

Comtan (entacapone) is not a controlled substance. Animal studies to evaluate the drug abuse and potential dependence have not been conducted. Although clinical trials have not revealed any evidence of the potential for abuse, tolerance or physical dependence, systematic studies in humans designed to evaluate these effects have not been performed.

OVERDOSAGE

There have been no reported cases of either accidental or intentional overdose with entacapone tablets. However, COMT inhibition by entacapone treatment is dose-dependent. A massive overdose of Comtan (entacapone) may theoretically produce a 100% inhibition of the COMT enzyme in people, thereby preventing the metabolism of endogenous and exogenous catechols.

The highest single dose of entacapone administered to humans was 800 mg, resulting in a plasma concentration of 14.1 μg/mL. The highest daily dose given to humans was 2400 mg, administered in one study as 400 mg six times daily with levodopa/carbidopa for 14 days in 15 Parkinson's Disease patients, and in another study as 800 mg t.i.d. for 7 days in 8 healthy volunteers. At this daily dose, the peak plasma concentrations of entacapone averaged 2.0 μg/mL (at 45 min., compared to 1.0 and 1.2 μg/mL with 200 mg entacapone at 45 min.). Abdominal pain and loose stools were the most commonly observed adverse events during this study. Daily doses as high as 2000 mg Comtan have been administered as 200 mg 10 times daily with levodopa/carbidopa or levodopa/benserazide for at least 1 year in 10 patients, for at least 2 years in 8 patients and for at least 3 years in 7 patients. Overall, however, clinical experience with daily doses above 1600 mg is limited.

The range of lethal plasma concentrations of entacapone based on animal data was 80-130 μg/mL in mice. Respiratory difficulties, ataxia, hypoactivity, and convulsions were observed in mice after high oral (gavage) doses.

Management of Overdose

Management of Comtan overdose is symptomatic; there is no known antidote to Comtan. Hospitalization is advised, and general supportive care is indicated. There is no experience with hemodialysis or hemoperfusion, but these procedures are unlikely to be of benefit, because Comtan is highly bound to plasma proteins. An immediate gastric lavage and repeated doses of charcoal over time may hasten the elimination of Comtan by decreasing its absorption/reabsorption from the GI tract. The adequacy of the respiratory and circulatory systems should be carefully monitored and appropriate supportive measures employed. The possibility of drug interactions, especially with catechol-structured drugs, should be borne in mind.

DOSAGE AND ADMINISTRATION

The recommended dose of Comtan (entacapone) is one 200 mg tablet administered concomitantly with each levodopa/carbidopa dose to a maximum of 8 times daily (200 mg × 8 = 1600 mg per day). Clinical experience with daily doses above 1600 mg is limited.

Comtan should always be administered in association with levodopa/carbidopa. Entacapone has no antiparkinsonian effect of its own.

In clinical trials, the majority of patients required a decrease in daily levodopa dose if their daily dose of levodopa had been ≥800 mg or if patients had moderate or severe dyskinesias before beginning treatment.

To optimize an individual patient's response, reductions in daily levodopa dose or extending the interval between doses may be necessary. In clinical trials, the average reduction in daily levodopa dose was about 25% in those patients requiring a levodopa dose reduction. (More than 58% of patients with levodopa doses above 800 mg daily required such a reduction.)

Comtan can be combined with both the immediate and sustained-release formulations of levodopa/carbidopa.

Comtan may be taken with or without food *(see CLINICAL PHARMACOLOGY)*.

Patients With Impaired Hepatic Function: Patients with hepatic impairment should be treated with caution. The AUC and C_{max} of entacapone approximately doubled in patients with documented liver disease, compared to controls. However, these studies were conducted with single-dose entacapone without levodopa/dopa decarboxylase inhibitor coadministration, and therefore the effects of liver disease on the kinetics of chronically administered entacapone have not been evaluated *(see CLINICAL PHARMACOLOGY, Pharmacokinetics of Entacapone)*.

Withdrawing Patients from Comtan: Rapid withdrawal or abrupt reduction in the Comtan dose could lead to emergence of signs and symptoms of Parkinson's Disease *(see CLINICAL PHARMACOLOGY, Clinical Studies)*, and may lead to Hyperpyrexia and Confusion, a symptom complex resembling the neuroleptic malignant syndrome *(see PRECAUTIONS, Other Events Reported With Dopaminergic Therapy)*. This syndrome should be considered in the differential diagnosis for any patient who develops a high fever or severe rigidity. If a decision is made to discontinue treatment with Comtan, patients should be monitored closely and other dopaminergic treatments should be adjusted as needed. Although tapering Comtan has not been systematically evaluated, it seems prudent to withdraw patients slowly if the decision to discontinue treatment is made.

HOW SUPPLIED

Comtan (entacapone) is supplied as 200-mg film-coated tablets for oral administration. The oval-shaped tablets are brownish-orange, unscored, and embossed "COMTAN" on one side. Tablets are provided in HDPE containers as follows:

Bottles of 100 .... NDC 0078-0327-05

Store at 25°C (77°F) excursions permitted to 15°-30°C (59°-86° F).

[See USP Controlled Room Temperature.]

Comtan (entacapone) tablets are manufactured by Orion Corporation, Orion Pharma (Espoo, Finland) and marketed by Novartis Pharmaceuticals Corporation (East Hanover, N.J. 07936, U.S.A.).

REV: MARCH 2000 T2000-10

Shown in Product Identification Guide, page 325

Table 4
Summary of Patients with Adverse Events after Start of Trial Drug Administration
At least 1% in Comtan® (entacapone) group and > Placebo

SYSTEM ORGAN CLASS Preferred term	Comtan (n = 603) % of patients	Placebo (n = 400) % of patients
SKIN AND APPENDAGES DISORDERS		
Sweating increased	2	1
MUSCULOSKELETAL SYSTEM DISORDERS		
Back pain	2	1
CENTRAL & PERIPHERAL NERVOUS SYSTEM DISORDERS		
Dyskinesia	25	15
Hyperkinesia	10	5
Hypokinesia	9	8
Dizziness	8	6
SPECIAL SENSES, OTHER DISORDERS		
Taste perversion	1	0
PSYCHIATRIC DISORDERS		
Anxiety	2	1
Somnolence	2	0
Agitation	1	0
GASTROINTESTINAL SYSTEM DISORDERS		
Nausea	14	8
Diarrhea	10	4
Abdominal pain	8	4
Constipation	6	4
Vomiting	4	1
Mouth dry	3	0
Dyspepsia	2	1
Flatulence	2	0
Gastritis	1	0
Gastrointestinal disorders nos	1	0
RESPIRATORY SYSTEM DISORDERS		
Dyspnea	3	1
PLATELET, BLEEDING & CLOTTING DISORDERS		
Purpura	2	1
URINARY SYSTEM DISORDERS		
Urine discoloration	10	0
BODY AS A WHOLE – GENERAL DISORDERS		
Back pain	4	2
Fatigue	6	4
Asthenia	2	1
RESISTANCE MECHANISM DISORDERS		
Infection bacterial	1	0

DESFERAL® ℞

[des 'fer-all]

deferoxamine mesylate for injection USP
Vials
Rx only

The following prescribing information is based on official labeling in effect July 2000.

DESCRIPTION

Desferal, deferoxamine mesylate USP, is an iron-chelating agent, available in vials for intramuscular, subcutaneous, and intravenous administration. Desferal is supplied as vials containing 500 mg and 2 g of deferoxamine mesylate USP in sterile, lyophilized form. Deferoxamine mesylate is *N*-[5-[3-[(5-aminopentyl)hydroxycarbamoyl]propionamido]pentyl]-3-[[5-(*N*-hydroxyacetamido)pentyl]carbamoyl]propionohydroxamic acid monomethanesulfonate (salt), and its structural formula is

$$H_2N(CH_2)_5\underset{OH}{N}\overset{O}{C}(CH_2)_2\overset{O}{C}NH\,(CH_2)_5\underset{OH}{N}\overset{O}{C}(CH_2)_2\overset{O}{C}NH(CH_2)_5\underset{OH}{N}\overset{O}{C}CH_3 \cdot CH_3SO_3H$$

Deferoxamine mesylate USP is a white to off-white powder. It is freely soluble in water and slightly soluble in methanol. Its molecular weight is 656.79.

CLINICAL PHARMACOLOGY

Desferal chelates iron by forming a stable complex that prevents the iron from entering into further chemical reactions. It readily chelates iron from ferritin and hemosiderin but not readily from transferrin; it does not combine with the iron from cytochromes and hemoglobin. Desferal does not cause any demonstrable increase in the excretion of electrolytes or trace metals. Theoretically, 100 parts by weight of Desferal is capable of binding approximately 8.5 parts by weight of ferric iron.

Desferal is metabolized principally by plasma enzymes, but the pathways have not yet been defined. The chelate is readily soluble in water and passes easily through the kidney, giving the urine a characteristic reddish color. Some is also excreted in the feces via the bile.

INDICATIONS AND USAGE

Desferal is indicated for the treatment of acute iron intoxication and of chronic iron overload due to transfusion-dependent anemias.

Acute Iron Intoxication

Desferal is an adjunct to, and not a substitute for, standard measures used in treating acute iron intoxication, which may include the following: induction of emesis with syrup of ipecac; gastric lavage; suction and maintenance of a clear airway; control of shock with intravenous fluids, blood, oxygen, and vasopressors; and correction of acidosis.

Chronic Iron Overload

Desferal can promote iron excretion in patients with secondary iron overload from multiple transfusions (as may occur in the treatment of some chronic anemias, including thalassemia). Long-term therapy with Desferal slows accumulation of hepatic iron and retards or eliminates progression of hepatic fibrosis.

Iron mobilization with Desferal is relatively poor in patients under the age of 3 years with relatively little iron overload. The drug should ordinarily not be given to such patients unless significant iron mobilization (e.g., 1 mg or more of iron per day) can be demonstrated.

Desferal is not indicated for the treatment of primary hemochromatosis, since phlebotomy is the method of choice for removing excess iron in this disorder.

CONTRAINDICATIONS

Desferal is contraindicated in patients with severe renal disease or anuria, since the drug and the iron chelate are excreted primarily by the kidney.

WARNINGS

Ocular and auditory disturbances have been reported when Desferal was administered over prolonged periods of time, at high doses, or in patients with low ferritin levels. The ocular disturbances observed have been blurring of vision; cataracts after prolonged administration in chronic iron overload; decreased visual acuity including visual loss, visual defects, scotoma; impaired peripheral, color, and night vision; optic neuritis, cataracts, corneal opacities, and retinal pigmentary abnormalities. The auditory abnormalities reported have been tinnitus and hearing loss including high frequency sensorineural hearing loss. In most cases, both ocular and auditory disturbances were reversible upon immediate cessation of treatment (see PRECAUTIONS/Information for Patients and ADVERSE REACTIONS/Special Senses).

Visual acuity tests, slit-lamp examinations, funduscopy and audiometry are recommended periodically in patients treated for prolonged periods of time. Toxicity is more likely to be reversed if symptoms or test abnormalities are detected early.

High doses of Desferal and concomitant low ferritin levels have also been associated with growth retardation. After reduction of Desferal dose, growth velocity may partially resume to pretreatment rates (see PRECAUTIONS/Pediatric Use).

Adult respiratory distress syndrome, also reported in children, has been described following treatment with excessively high intravenous doses of Desferal in patients with acute iron intoxication or thalassemia.

PRECAUTIONS

General

Flushing of the skin, urticaria, hypotension, and shock have occurred in a few patients when Desferal was administered by rapid intravenous injection. THEREFORE, DESFERAL SHOULD BE GIVEN INTRAMUSCULARLY OR BY SLOW SUBCUTANEOUS OR INTRAVENOUS INFUSION.

Iron overload increases susceptibility of patients to *Yersinia enterocolitica* and *Yersinia pseudotuberculosis* infections. In some rare cases, treatment with Desferal has enhanced this susceptibility, resulting in generalized infections by providing this bacteria with a siderophore otherwise missing. In such cases, Desferal treatment should be discontinued until the infection is resolved.

In patients receiving Desferal, very rare cases of mucormycosis, a severe fungal infection, have been reported. If any of the suspected signs or symptoms occur, Desferal should be discontinued, mycological tests carried out and appropriate treatment instituted immediately.

Mucormycosis may also occur in patients who are not receiving Desferal, indicating that other factor determinants, such as dialysis, diabetes mellitus, disturbance of acid-base balance, hematological malignancies, immunosuppressive drugs, or a compromised immune system, may play a role in the development of this infection.

In patients with severe chronic iron overload, impairment of cardiac function has been reported following concomitant treatment with Desferal and high doses of vitamin C (more than 500 mg daily in adults). The cardiac dysfunction was reversible when vitamin C was discontinued. The following precautions should be taken when vitamin C and Desferal are to be used concomitantly:

- Vitamin C supplements should not be given to patients with cardiac failure.
- Start supplemental vitamin C only after an initial month of regular treatment with Desferal.
- Give vitamin C only if the patient is receiving Desferal regularly, ideally soon after setting up the infusion pump.
- Do not exceed a daily Vitamin C dose of 200 mg in adults, given in divided doses.
- Clinical monitoring of cardiac function is advisable during such combined therapy.

In patients with aluminum-related encephalopathy, high doses of Desferal may exacerbate neurological dysfunction (seizures), probably owing to an acute increase in circulating aluminum. Desferal may precipitate the onset of dialysis dementia. Pretreatment with clonazepam has been reported to prevent this neurological deterioration. Also, treatment with Desferal in the presence of aluminum overload may result in decreased serum calcium and aggravation of hyperparathyroidism.

Drug Interactions

Vitamin C: Patients with iron overload usually become vitamin C deficient, probably because iron oxidizes the vitamin. As an adjuvant to iron chelation therapy, vitamin C in doses up to 200 mg for adults may be given in divided doses, starting after an initial month of regular treatment with Desferal (see PRECAUTIONS). Vitamin C increases availability of iron for chelation. In general, 50 mg daily suffices for children under 10 years old and 100 mg daily for older children. Larger doses of vitamin C fail to produce any additional increase in excretion of iron complex.

Prochlorperazine: Concurrent treatment with Desferal and prochlorperazine, a phenothiazine derivative, may lead to temporary impairment of consciousness.

Gallium-67: Imaging results may be distorted because of the rapid urinary excretion of Desferal-bound gallium-67. Discontinuation of Desferal 48 hours prior to scintigraphy is advisable.

Information for Patients

Patients experiencing dizziness or other nervous system disturbances, or impairment of vision or hearing, should refrain from driving or operating potentially hazardous machines (see ADVERSE REACTIONS).

Patients should be informed that occasionally their urine may show a reddish discoloration.

Carcinogenesis, Mutagenesis, Impairment of Fertility

Long-term carcinogenicity studies in animals have not been performed with Desferal.

Cytotoxicity may occur, since Desferal has been shown to inhibit DNA synthesis in vitro.

Pregnancy Category C

Delayed ossification in mice and skeletal anomalies in rabbits were observed after Desferal was administered in daily doses up to 4.5 times the maximum daily human dose. No adverse effects were observed in similar studies in rats.

There are no adequate and well-controlled studies in pregnant women. Desferal should be used during pregnancy only if the potential benefit justifies the potential risk to the fetus.

Nursing Mothers

It is not known whether this drug is excreted in human milk. Because many drugs are excreted in human milk, caution should be exercised when Desferal is administered to a nursing woman.

Pediatric Use

Pediatric patients receiving Desferal should be monitored for body weight and growth every 3 months.

Safety and effectiveness in pediatric patients under the age of 3 years have not been established (see INDICATIONS AND USAGE, WARNINGS, PRECAUTIONS/Drug Interactions/Vitamin C, and ADVERSE REACTIONS).

ADVERSE REACTIONS

The following adverse reactions have been observed, but there are not enough data to support an estimate of their frequency.

At the Injection Site: localized irritation, pain, burning, swelling, induration, infiltration, pruritus, erythema, wheal formation, eschar, crust, vescicles, local edema. Injection site reactions may be associated with systemic allergic reactions (see Body as a Whole, below).

Hypersensitivity Reactions and Systemic Allergic Reactions: generalized rash, urticaria, anaphylactic reaction with or without shock, angioedema.

Body as a Whole: Local injection site reactions may be accompanied by systemic reactions like arthralgia, fever, headache, myalgia, nausea, vomiting, abdominal pain, or asthma.

Rare infections with *Yersinia* and *Mucormycosis* have been reported in association with Desferal use (see PRECAUTIONS).

Cardiovascular: tachycardia, hypotension, shock.

Digestive: abdominal discomfort, diarrhea, nausea, vomiting.

Hematologic: very rare blood dyscrasia (e.g., thrombocytopenia).

Musculoskeletal: Leg cramps. Growth retardation and bone changes (e.g., metaphyseal dysplasia) are common in chelated patients given doses above 60 mg/kg, especially those who begin iron chelation in the first three years of life. If doses are kept to 40 mg/kg or below, the risk is considerably reduced (see WARNINGS, PRECAUTIONS/Pediatric Use).

Nervous system: neurological disturbances including dizziness, peripheral sensory, motor, or mixed neuropathy, paresthesias; exacerbation or precipitation of aluminum-related dialysis encephalopathy (see PRECAUTIONS/Information for Patients).

Special Senses: High-frequency sensorineural hearing loss and/or tinnitus are uncommon if dosage guidelines are not exceeded and if dose is reduced when ferritin levels decline. Visual disturbances are rare if dosage guidelines are not exceeded. These may include decreased acuity, blurred vision, loss of vision, dyschromatopsia, night blindness, visual field defects, scotoma, retinopathy (pigmentary degeneration), optic neuritis, and cataracts (see WARNINGS).

Respiratory: acute respiratory distress syndrome (with dyspnea, cyanosis, and/or interstitial infiltrates) (see WARNINGS).

Skin: very rare generalized rash.

Urogenital: dysuria, impaired renal function (see CONTRAINDICATIONS).

OVERDOSAGE

Acute Toxicity

Intravenous LD_{50}s (mg/kg): mice, 287; rats, 329.

Signs and Symptoms

Inadvertent administration of an overdose or inadvertent intravenous bolus administration/rapid intravenous infusion may be associated with hypotension, tachycardia and gastrointestinal disturbances; acute but transient loss of vision, aphasia, agitation, headache, nausea, bradycardia as well as acute renal failure have been reported.

Treatment

There is no specific antidote. Desferal should be discontinued and appropriate symptomatic measures undertaken. Desferal is readily dialyzable.

DOSAGE AND ADMINISTRATION

Preparation of Solution

Desferal is preferably dissolved by adding 5 mL of Sterile Water for Injection to each 500 mg vial or 20 mL of Sterile Water for Injection to each 2 g vial, resulting in a solution of 100 mg/mL (10%). The reconstituted Desferal solution is isotonic, clear and colorless to slightly yellowish at the recommended concentration of 10%.

In clinical situations requiring a smaller volume of solution (e.g., intramuscular injection), Desferal may be dissolved by adding 2 mL of Sterile Water for Injection to each 500 mg vial or 8 mL of Sterile Water for Injection to each 2 g vial, resulting in a solution of 250 mg/mL (25%). This concentration may produce a stronger yellow-colored solution. The drug should be completely dissolved before the solution is withdrawn.

Note: **Parenteral drug products should be inspected visually for particulate matter and discoloration prior to administration, whenever solution and container permit.**

Desferal reconstituted with Sterile Water for Injection **IS FOR SINGLE USE ONLY.**

The product should be used immediately after reconstituting (commencement of treatment within 3 hours) for microbiological safety. When reconstitution is carried out under validated aseptic conditions (in a sterile laminar flow hood using aseptic technique), the product may be stored at room temperature for a maximum period of 24 hours before use. Do not refrigerate reconstituted solution. Reconstituting Desferal in solvents or under conditions other than indicated may result in precipitation. Turbid solutions should not be used.

Acute Iron Intoxication

Intramuscular Administration

This route is preferred and should be used for ALL PATIENTS NOT IN SHOCK.

Dosage. See Preparation of Solution, above. A dose of 1000 mg should be administered initially. This may be followed by 500 mg every 4 hours for two doses. Depending upon the clinical response, subsequent doses of 500 mg may be administered every 4-12 hours. The total amount administered should not exceed 6000 mg in 24 hours.

Intravenous Administration

THIS ROUTE SHOULD BE USED ONLY FOR PATIENTS IN A STATE OF CARDIOVASCULAR COLLAPSE AND THEN ONLY BY SLOW INFUSION. THE RATE OF INFUSION SHOULD NOT EXCEED 15 MG/KG/HR FOR THE FIRST 1000 MG ADMINISTERED. SUBSEQUENT IV DOSING, IF NEEDED, MUST BE AT A SLOWER RATE, NOT TO EXCEED 125 MG/HR.

Dosage. See Preparation of Solution, above. The reconstituted solution is added to physiologic saline, glucose in water, or Ringer's lactate solution.

An initial dose of 1000 mg should be administered at a rate NOT TO EXCEED 15 mg/kg/hr. This may be followed by 500 mg over 4 hours for two doses. Depending upon the clinical response, subsequent doses of 500 mg may be administered over 4-12 hours. The total amount administered should not exceed 6000 mg in 24 hours.

As soon as the clinical condition of the patient permits, intravenous administration should be discontinued and the drug should be administered intramuscularly.

Chronic Iron Overload

The more effective of the following routes of administration must be chosen on an individual basis for each patient.

Continued on next page

Desferal—Cont.

Intramuscular Administration
See Preparation of Solution, above. A daily dose of 500-1000 mg should be administered intramuscularly. In addition, 2000 mg should be administered intravenously with each unit of blood transfused; however, Desferal should be administered separately from the blood. The rate of intravenous infusion must not exceed 15 mg/kg/hr. The total daily dose should not exceed 1000 mg in the absence of a transfusion, or 6000 mg even if transfused three or more units of blood or packed red blood cells.
Subcutaneous Administration
See Preparation of Solution, above. A daily dose of 1000-2000 mg (20-40 mg/kg/day) should be administered over 8-24 hours, utilizing a small portable pump capable of providing continuous mini-infusion. The duration of infusion must be individualized. In some patients, as much iron will be excreted after a short infusion of 8-12 hours as with the same dose given over 24 hours.

HOW SUPPLIED

Vials - each containing 500 mg of sterile, lyophilized deferoxamine mesylate
Cartons of 4 vials .... NDC 0083-3801-04
Vials - each containing 2 g of sterile, lyophilized deferoxamine mesylate
Cartons of 4 vials .... NDC 0078-0347-51
Do not store above 25°C (77°F).
T2000-38

REV: JUNE 2000

NOVARTIS
Manufactured by
Novartis Pharma AG
Basle, Switzerland for
Novartis Pharmaceuticals Corporation
East Hanover, New Jersey 07936

D.H.E. 45® ℞
(dihydroergotamine mesylate)
Injection, USP

Rx only

The following prescribing information is based on official labeling in effect July 2000.

DESCRIPTION

D.H.E. 45® is ergotamine hydrogenated in the 9, 10 position as the mesylate salt. D.H.E. 45® is known chemically as ergotaman-3′, 6′, 18-trione,9,-10-dihydro-12′-hydroxy-2′-methyl-5′-(phenylmethyl)-,(5′α)-, monomethanesulfonate. Its molecular weight is 679.80 and its empirical formula is $C_{33}H_{37}N_5O_5 \bullet CH_4O_3S$).
The chemical structure is:

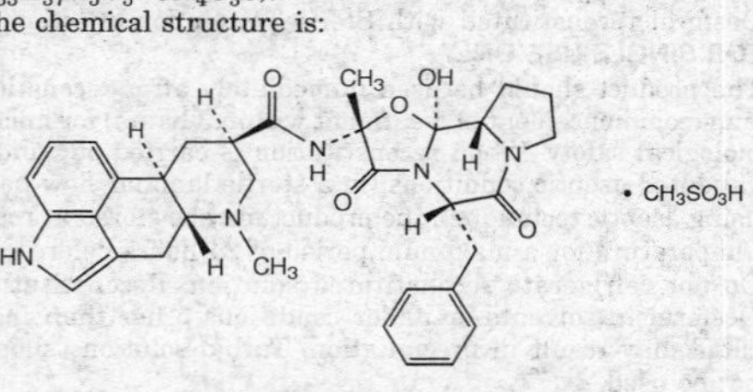

Dihydroergotamine mesylate
$C_{33}H_{37}N_5O_5 \cdot CH_4O_3S$ Mol. wt. 679.80

D.H.E. 45® (dihydroergotamine mesylate) Injection, USP is a clear, colorless solution supplied in sterile ampuls for I.V., I.M., or subcutaneous administration containing per mL:
dihydroergotamine mesylate, USP .... 1 mg
methanesulfonic acid/sodium hydroxide,
qs to .... pH 3.6 ± 0.4
alcohol, USP .... 6.1% by vol.
glycerin, USP .... 15% by wt.
water for injection, USP, qs to .... 1 mL

CLINICAL PHARMACOLOGY

Mechanism of Action
Dihydroergotamine binds with high affinity to 5-$HT_{1D\alpha}$ and 5-$HT_{1D\beta}$ receptors. It also binds with high affinity to serotonin 5-HT_{1A}, 5-HT_{2A}, and 5-HT_{2C} receptors, noradrenaline α_{2A}, α_{2B} and α, receptors, and dopamine D_{2L} and D_3 receptors.
The therapeutic activity of dihydroergotamine in migraine is generally attributed to the agonist effect at 5-HT_{1D} receptors. Two current theories have been proposed to explain the efficacy of 5-HT_{1D} receptor agonists in migraine. One theory suggests that activation of 5-HT_{1D} receptors located on intracranial blood vessels, including those on arterio-venous anastomoses, leads to vasoconstriction, which correlates with the relief of migraine headache. The alternative hypothesis suggests that activation of 5-HT_{1D} receptors on sensory nerve endings of the trigeminal system results in the inhibition of pro-inflammatory neuropeptide release.
In addition, dihydroergotamine possesses oxytocic properties. *(See CONTRAINDICATIONS)*
Pharmacokinetics
Absorption
Absolute bioavailability for the subcutaneous and intramuscular route have not been determined, however, no difference was observed in dihydroergotamine bioavailability from intramuscular and subcutaneous doses. Dihydroergotamine mesylate is poorly bioavailable following oral administration.
Distribution
Dihydroergotamine mesylate is 93% plasma protein bound. The apparent steady-state volume of distribution is approximately 800 liters.
Metabolism
Four dihydroergotamine mesylate metabolites have been identified in human plasma following oral administration. The major metabolite, 8′-β-hydroxydihydroergotamine, exhibits affinity equivalent to its parent for adrenergic and 5-HT receptors and demonstrates equivalent potency in several venoconstrictor activity models, *in vivo* and *in vitro*. The other metabolites, i.e., dihydrolysergic acid, dihydrolysergic amide, and a metabolite formed by oxidative opening of the proline ring are of minor importance. Following nasal administration, total metabolites represent only 20%-30% of plasma AUC. Quantitative pharmacokinetic characterization of the four metabolites has not been performed.
Excretion
The major excretory route of dihydroergotamine is via the bile in the feces. The total body clearance is 1.5 L/min which reflects mainly hepatic clearance. Only 6%-7% of unchanged dihydroergotamine is excreted in the urine after intramuscular injection. The renal clearance (0.1 L/min) is unaffected by the route of dihydroergotamine administration. The decline of plasma dihydroergotamine after intramuscular or intravenous administration is multi-exponential with a terminal half-life of about 9 hours.
Subpopulations
No studies have been conducted on the effect of renal or hepatic impairment, gender, race, or ethnicity on dihydroergotamine pharmacokinetics. D.H.E. 45® (dihydroergotamine mesylate) Injection, USP is contraindicated in patients with severely impaired hepatic or renal function. *(See CONTRAINDICATIONS)*
Interactions
Pharmacokinetic interactions (increased blood levels) have been reported in patients treated orally with dihydroergotamine and macrolide antibiotics, principally troleandomycin, presumably due to inhibition of cytochrome P450 3A metabolism of dihydroergotamine by troleandomycin. Dihydroergotamine has also been shown to be an inhibitor of cytochrome P450 3A catalyzed reactions. No pharmacokinetic interactions involving other cytochrome P450 isoenzymes are known.

INDICATIONS AND USAGE

D.H.E. 45® (dihydroergotamine mesylate) Injection, USP is indicated for the acute treatment of migraine headaches with or without aura and the acute treatment of cluster headache episodes.

CONTRAINDICATIONS

D.H.E. 45® (dihydroergotamine mesylate) Injection, USP should not be given to patients with ischemic heart disease (angina pectoris, history of myocardial infarction, or documented silent ischemia) or to patients who have clinical symptoms or findings consistent with coronary artery vasospasm including Prinzmetal's variant angina. *(See WARNINGS)*
Because D.H.E. 45® (dihydroergotamine mesylate) Injection, USP may increase blood pressure, it should not be given to patients with uncontrolled hypertension.
D.H.E. 45® (dihydroergotamine mesylate) Injection, USP, 5-HT_1 agonists (e.g., sumatriptan), ergotamine-containing or ergot-type medications or methysergide should not be used within 24 hours of each other.
D.H.E. 45® (dihydroergotamine mesylate) Injection, USP should not be administered to patients with hemiplegic or basilar migraine.
In addition to those conditions mentioned above, D.H.E. 45® (dihydroergotamine mesylate) Injection, USP is also contraindicated in patients with known peripheral arterial disease, sepsis, following vascular surgery and severely impaired hepatic or renal function.
D.H.E. 45® (dihydroergotamine mesylate) Injection, USP may cause fetal harm when administered to a pregnant woman. Dihydroergotamine possesses oxytocic properties and, therefore, should not be administered during pregnancy. If this drug is used during pregnancy, or if the patient becomes pregnant while taking this drug, the patient should be apprised of the potential hazard to the fetus.
There are no adequate studies of dihydroergotamine in human pregnancy, but developmental toxicity has been demonstrated in experimental animals. In embryo-fetal development studies of dihydroergotamine mesylate nasal spray, intranasal administration to pregnant rats throughout the period of organogenesis resulted in decreased fetal body weights and/or skeletal ossification at doses of 0.16 mg/day (associated with maternal plasma dihydroergotamine exposures [AUC] approximately 0.4-1.2 times the exposures in humans receiving the MRDD of 4 mg) or greater. A no effect level for embryo-fetal toxicity was not established in rats. Delayed skeletal ossification was also noted in rabbit fetuses following intranasal administration of 3.6 mg/day (maternal exposures approximately 7 times human exposures at the MRDD) during organogenesis. A no effect level was seen at 1.2 mg/day (maternal exposures approximately 2.5 times human exposures at the MRDD). When dihydroergotamine mesylate nasal spray was administered intranasally to female rats during pregnancy and lactation, decreased body weights and impaired reproductive function (decreased mating indices) were observed in the offspring at doses of 0.16 mg/day or greater. A no effect level was not established. Effects on development occurred at doses below those that produced evidence of significant maternal toxicity in these studies. Dihydroergotamine-induced intrauterine growth retardation has been attributed to reduced uteroplacental blood flow resulting from prolonged vasoconstriction of the uterine vessels and/or increased myometrial tone.
D.H.E. 45® (dihydroergotamine mesylate) Injection, USP is contraindicated in patients who have previously shown hypersensitivity to ergot alkaloids.
Dihydroergotamine mesylate should not be used by nursing mothers. *(See PRECAUTIONS)*
Dihydroergotamine mesylate should not be used with peripheral and central vasoconstrictors because the combination may result in additive or synergistic elevation of blood pressure.

WARNINGS

D.H.E. 45® (dihydroergotamine mesylate) Injection, USP should only be used where a clear diagnosis of migraine headache has been established.
Risk of Myocardial Ischemia and/or Infarction and Other Adverse Cardiac Events
D.H.E. 45® (dihydroergotamine mesylate) Injection, USP should not be used by patients with documented ischemic or vasospastic coronary artery disease. *(See CONTRAINDICATIONS.)* It is strongly recommended that D.H.E. 45® (dihydroergotamine mesylate) Injection, USP not be given to patients in whom unrecognized coronary artery disease (CAD) is predicted by the presence of risk factors (e.g., hypertension, hypercholesterolemia, smoker, obesity, diabetes, strong family history of CAD, females who are surgically or physiologically postmenopausal, or males who are over 40 years of age) unless a cardiovascular evaluation provides satisfactory clinical evidence that the patient is reasonably free of coronary artery and ischemic myocardial disease or other significant underlying cardiovascular disease. The sensitivity of cardiac diagnostic procedures to detect cardiovascular disease or predisposition to coronary artery vasospasm is modest, at best. If, during the cardiovascular evaluation, the patient's medical history or electrocardiographic investigations reveal findings indicative of or consistent with coronary artery vasospasm or myocardial ischemia, D.H.E. 45® (dihydroergotamine mesylate) Injection, USP should not be administered. *(See CONTRAINDICATIONS)*
For patients with risk factors predictive of CAD who are determined to have a satisfactory cardiovascular evaluation, it is strongly recommended that administration of the first dose of D.H.E. 45® (dihydroergotamine mesylate) Injection, USP take place in the setting of a physician's office or similar medically staffed and equipped facility unless the patient has previously received dihydroergotamine mesylate. Because cardiac ischemia can occur in the absence of clinical symptoms, consideration should be given to obtaining on the first occasion of use an electrocardiogram (ECG) during the interval immediately following D.H.E. 45® (dihydroergotamine mesylate) Injection, USP, in those patients with risk factors.
It is recommended that patients who are intermittent long-term users of D.H.E. 45® (dihydroergotamine mesylate) Injection, USP and who have or acquire risk factors predictive of CAD, as described above, undergo periodic interval cardiovascular evaluation as they continue to use D.H.E. 45® (dihydroergotamine mesylate) Injection, USP.
The systematic approach described above is currently recommended as a method to identify patients in whom D.H.E. 45® (dihydroergotamine mesylate) Injection, USP may be used to treat migraine headaches with an acceptable margin of cardiovascular safety.
Cardiac Events and Fatalities
The potential for adverse cardiac events exists. Serious adverse cardiac events, including acute myocardial infarction, life-threatening disturbances of cardiac rhythm, and death have been reported to have occurred following the administration of dihydroergotamine mesylate injection. Considering the extent of use of dihydroergotamine mesylate in patients with migraine, the incidence of these events is extremely low.
Drug-Associated Cerebrovascular Events and Fatalities
Cerebral hemorrhage, subarachnoid hemorrhage, stroke, and other cerebrovascular events have been reported in patients treated with D.H.E. 45® (dihydroergotamine mesylate) Injection, USP; and some have resulted in fatalities. In a number of cases, it appears possible that the cerebrovascular events were primary, the D.H.E. 45® (dihydroergotamine mesylate) Injection, USP having been administered in the incorrect belief that the symptoms experienced were a consequence of migraine, when they were not. It should be noted that patients with migraine may be at increased risk of certain cerebrovascular events (e.g., stroke, hemorrhage, transient ischemic attack).
Other Vasospasm Related Events
D.H.E. 45® (dihydroergotamine mesylate) Injection, USP, like other ergot alkaloids, may cause vasospastic reactions other than coronary artery vasospasm. Myocardial, peripheral vascular, and colonic ischemia have been reported with D.H.E. 45® (dihydroergotamine mesylate) Injection, USP.
D.H.E. 45® (dihydroergotamine mesylate) Injection, USP associated vasospastic phenomena may also cause muscle pains, numbness, coldness, pallor, and cyanosis of the digits. In patients with compromised circulation, persistent vaso-

spasm may result in gangrene or death. D.H.E. 45® (dihydroergotamine mesylate) Injection, USP should be discontinued immediately if signs or symptoms of vasoconstriction develop.

Increase In Blood Pressure

Significant elevation in blood pressure has been reported on rare occasions in patients with and without a history of hypertension treated with dihydroergotamine mesylate injection. D.H.E. 45® (dihydroergotamine mesylate) Injection, USP is contraindicated in patients with uncontrolled hypertension. *(See CONTRAINDICATIONS)*

An 18% increase in mean pulmonary artery pressure was seen following dosing with another 5-HT_1 agonist in a study evaluating subjects undergoing cardiac catheterization.

PRECAUTIONS

General

D.H.E. 45® (dihydroergotamine mesylate) Injection, USP may cause coronary artery vasospasm; patients who experience signs or symptoms suggestive of angina following its administration should, therefore, be evaluated for the presence of CAD or a predisposition to variant angina before receiving additional doses. Similarly, patients who experience other symptoms or signs suggestive of decreased arterial flow, such as ischemic bowel syndrome or Raynaud's syndrome following the use of any 5-HT agonist are candidates for further evaluation. *(See WARNINGS)*

Information for Patients

The text of a patient information sheet is printed at the end of this insert. To assure safe and effective use of D.H.E. 45® (dihydroergotamine mesylate) Injection, USP, the information and instructions provided in the patient information sheet should be discussed with patients.

Patients should be advised to report to the physician immediately any of the following: numbness or tingling in the fingers and toes, muscle pain in the arms and legs, weakness in the legs, pain in the chest, temporary speeding or slowing of the heart rate, swelling, or itching.

Prior to the initial use of the product by a patient, the prescriber should take steps to ensure that the patient understands how to use the product as provided. *(See Patient Information Sheet and product packaging)*

Drug Interactions

Vasoconstrictors

D.H.E. 45® (dihydroergotamine mesylate) Injection, USP should not be used with peripheral vasoconstrictors because the combination may cause synergistic elevation of blood pressure.

Sumatriptan

Sumatriptan has been reported to cause coronary artery vasospasm, and its effect could be additive with D.H.E. 45® (dihydroergotamine mesylate) Injection, USP. Sumatriptan and D.H.E. 45® (dihydroergotamine mesylate) Injection, USP should not be taken within 24 hours of each other. *(See CONTRAINDICATIONS)*

Beta Blockers

Although the results of a clinical study did not indicate a safety problem associated with the administration of D.H.E. 45® (dihydroergotamine mesylate) Injection, USP to subjects already receiving propranolol, there have been reports that propranolol may potentiate the vasoconstrictive action of ergotamine by blocking the vasodilating property of epinephrine.

Nicotine

Nicotine may provoke vasoconstriction in some patients, predisposing to a greater ischemic response to ergot therapy.

Macrolide Antibiotics (e.g., erythromycin and troleandomycin)

Agents of the ergot alkaloid class, of which D.H.E. 45® (dihydroergotamine mesylate) Injection, USP is a member, have been shown to interact with antibiotics of the macrolide class, resulting in increased plasma levels of unchanged alkaloids and peripheral vasoconstriction. Vasospastic reactions have been reported with therapeutic doses of ergotamine-containing drugs when co-administered with these antibiotics.

SSRI's

Weakness, hyperreflexia, and incoordination have been reported rarely when 5-HT_1 agonists have been co-administered with SSRI's (e.g., fluoxetine, fluvoxamine, paroxetine, sertraline). There have been no reported cases from spontaneous reports of drug interaction between SSRI's and D.H.E. 45® (dihydroergotamine mesylate) Injection, USP.

Oral Contraceptives

The effect of oral contraceptives on the pharmacokinetics of D.H.E. 45® (dihydroergotamine mesylate) Injection, USP has not been studied.

Carcinogenesis, Mutagenesis, Impairment of Fertility

Carcinogenesis

Assessment of the carcinogenic potential of dihydroergotamine mesylate in mice and rats is ongoing.

Mutagenesis

Dihydroergotamine mesylate was clastogenic in two *in vitro* chromosomal aberration assays, the V79 Chinese hamster cell assay with metabolic activation and the cultured human peripheral blood lymphocyte assay. There was no evidence of mutagenic potential when dihydroergotamine mesylate was tested in the presence or absence of metabolic activation in two gene mutation assays (the Ames test and the *in vitro* mammalian Chinese hamster V79/HGPRT assay) and in an assay for DNA damage (the rat hepatocyte unscheduled DNA synthesis test). Dihydroergotamine was not clastogenic in the *in vivo* mouse and hamster micronucleus tests.

Impairment of Fertility

Impairment of fertility was not evaluated for D.H.E. 45® (dihydroergotamine mesylate) Injection, USP. There was no evidence of impairment of fertility in rats given intranasal doses of Migranal® Nasal Spray up to 1.6 mg/day (associated with mean plasma dihydroergotamine mesylate exposures [AUC] approximately 9 to 11 times those in humans receiving the MRDD of 4 mg).

Pregnancy

Pregnancy Category X. See CONTRAINDICATIONS.

Nursing Mothers

Ergot drugs are known to inhibit prolactin. It is likely that D.H.E. 45® (dihydroergotamine mesylate) Injection, USP is excreted in human milk, but there are no data on the concentration of dihydroergotamine in human milk. It is known that ergotamine is excreted in breast milk and may cause vomiting, diarrhea, weak pulse, and unstable blood pressure in nursing infants. Because of the potential for these serious adverse events in nursing infants exposed to D.H.E. 45® (dihydroergotamine mesylate) Injection, USP, nursing should not be undertaken with the use of D.H.E. 45® (dihydroergotamine mesylate) Injection, USP. *(See CONTRAINDICATIONS)*

Pediatric Use

Safety and effectiveness in pediatric patients have not been established.

ADVERSE REACTIONS

Serious cardiac events, including some that have been fatal, have occurred following use of D.H.E. 45® (dihydroergotamine mesylate) Injection, USP, but are extremely rare. Events reported have included coronary artery vasospasm, transient myocardial ischemia, myocardial infarction, ventricular tachycardia, and ventricular fibrillation. *(See CONTRAINDICATIONS, WARNINGS, and PRECAUTIONS)*

Post-introduction Reports

The following events derived from postmarketing experience have been occasionally reported in patients receiving D.H.E. 45® (dihydroergotamine mesylate) Injection, USP: vasospasm, paraesthesia, hypertension, dizziness, anxiety, dyspnea, headache, flushing, diarrhea, rash, increased sweating, and pleural and retroperitoneal fibrosis after long-term use of dihydroergotamine. Extremely rare cases of myocardial infarction and stroke have been reported. A causal relationship has not been established.

D.H.E. 45® (dihydroergotamine mesylate) Injection, USP is not recommended for prolonged daily use. *(See DOSAGE AND ADMINISTRATION)*

DRUG ABUSE AND DEPENDENCE

Currently available data have not demonstrated drug abuse or psychological dependence with dihydroergotamine. However, cases of drug abuse and psychological dependence in patients on other forms of ergot therapy have been reported. Thus, due to the chronicity of vascular headaches, it is imperative that patients be advised not to exceed recommended dosages.

OVERDOSAGE

To date, there have been no reports of acute overdosage with this drug. Due to the risk of vascular spasm, exceeding the recommended dosages of D.H.E. 45® (dihydroergotamine mesylate) Injection, USP is to be avoided. Excessive doses of dihydroergotamine may result in peripheral signs and symptoms of ergotism. Treatment includes discontinuance of the drug, local application of warmth to the affected area, the administration of vasodilators, and nursing care to prevent tissue damage.

In general, the symptoms of an acute D.H.E. 45® (dihydroergotamine mesylate) Injection, USP overdose are similar to those of an ergotamine overdose, although there is less pronounced nausea and vomiting with D.H.E. 45® (dihydroergotamine mesylate) Injection, USP. The symptoms of an ergotamine overdose include the following: numbness, tingling, pain, and cyanosis of the extremities associated with diminished or absent peripheral pulses; respiratory depression; an increase and/or decrease in blood pressure, usually in that order; confusion, delirium, convulsions, and coma; and/or some degree of nausea, vomiting, and abdominal pain.

In laboratory animals, significant lethality occurs when dihydroergotamine is given at I.V. doses of 44 mg/kg in mice, 130 mg/kg in rats, and 37 mg/kg in rabbits.

Up-to-date information about the treatment of overdosage can often be obtained from a certified Regional Poison Control Center. Telephone numbers of certified Poison Control Centers are listed in the Physician's Desk Reference® (PDR).*

DOSAGE AND ADMINISTRATION

D.H.E. 45® (dihydroergotamine mesylate) Injection, USP should be administered in a dose of 1 mL intravenously, intramuscularly or subcutaneously. The dose can be repeated, as needed, at 1 hour intervals to a total dose of 3 mL for intramuscular or subcutaneous delivery or 2 mL for intravenous delivery in a 24 hour period. The total weekly dosage should not exceed 6 mL.

HOW SUPPLIED

D.H.E. 45® (dihydroergotamine mesylate) Injection, USP

Available as a clear, colorless, sterile solution in single 1 mL sterile ampuls containing 1 mg of dihydroergotamine mesylate per mL, in packages of 10 (NDC 0078-0041-01).

Store below 77°F (25°C), in light-resistant containers. Do not refrigerate or freeze.

To assure constant potency, protect the ampuls from light and heat. Administer only if clear and colorless.

INSTRUCTION FOR PATIENTS ON SUBCUTANEOUS SELF-INJECTION

Information for the Patient

D.H.E. 45® (dihydroergotamine mesylate) Injection, USP

Before self-injecting D.H.E. 45® (dihydroergotamine mesylate) Injection, USP by subcutaneous administration, you will need to obtain professional instruction on how to properly administer your medication. Below are some of the steps you should follow carefully. Read this leaflet completely before using this medication.

This leaflet does not contain all of the information on D.H.E. 45® (dihydroergotamine mesylate) Injection, USP. Your pharmacist and/or health care provider can provide more detailed information.

Purpose of your Medication

D.H.E. 45® (dihydroergotamine mesylate) Injection, USP is intended to treat an active migraine headache. Do not try to use it to prevent a headache if you have no symptoms. Do not use it to treat common tension headache or a headache that is not at all typical of your usual migraine headache.

Do not use D.H.E. 45® (dihydroergotamine mesylate) Injection, USP if you:

- are pregnant or nursing.
- have any disease affecting your heart, arteries, or circulation.

Important questions to consider before using D.H.E. 45® (dihydroergotamine mesylate) Injection, USP

Please answer the following questions before you use your D.H.E. 45® (dihydroergotamine mesylate) Injection, USP. If you answer YES to any of these questions or are unsure of the answer, you should talk to your doctor before using D.H.E. 45® (dihydroergotamine mesylate) Injection, USP.

- Do you have high blood pressure?
- Do you have chest pain, shortness of breath, heart disease, or have you had any surgery on your heart arteries?
- Do you have risk factors for heart disease (such as high blood pressure, high cholesterol, obesity, diabetes, smoking, strong family history of heart disease, or you are postmenopausal or a male over 40)?
- Do you have any problems with blood circulation in your arms or legs, fingers, or toes?
- Are you pregnant? Do you think you might be pregnant? Are you trying to become pregnant? Are you sexually active and not using birth control? Are you breast feeding?
- Have you ever had to stop taking this or any other medication because of an allergy or bad reaction?
- Are you taking any other migraine medications, erythromycin or other antibiotics, or medications for blood pressure prescribed by your doctor, or other medicines obtained from your drugstore without a doctor's prescription?
- Do you smoke?
- Have you had, or do you have, any disease of the liver or kidney?
- Is this headache different from your usual migraine attacks?

REMEMBER TO TELL YOUR DOCTOR IF YOU HAVE ANSWERED YES TO ANY OF THESE QUESTIONS BEFORE YOU USE D.H.E. 45® (dihydroergotamine mesylate) Injection, USP

Side Effects To Watch Out For

Although the following reactions rarely occur, they can be serious and should be reported to your physician immediately:

- Numbness or tingling in your fingers and toes.
- Pain, tightness, or discomfort in your chest.
- Muscle pain or cramps in your arms and legs.
- Weakness in your legs.
- Temporary speeding or slowing of your heart rate.
- Swelling or itching.

Dosage

Your doctor will have told you what dose to use for each migraine attack. Should you get another migraine attack in the same day as the attack you treated, you must not treat it with D.H.E. 45® (dihydroergotamine mesylate) Injection, USP unless at least 6 hours have elapsed since your last injection. No more than 6 mL of D.H.E. 45® (dihydroergotamine mesylate) Injection, USP should be injected during a one-week period.

Learn what to do in case of an Overdose

If you have used more medication than you have been instructed, contact your doctor, hospital emergency department, or nearest poison control center immediately.

How to use the D.H.E. 45® (dihydroergotamine mesylate) Injection, USP

1. Use available training materials.
   - Read and follow the instructions in the patient instruction booklet which is provided with the D.H.E. 45® (dihydroergotamine mesylate) Injection, USP package before attempting to use the product.
   - If there are any questions concerning the use of your D.H.E. 45® (dihydroergotamine mesylate) Injection, USP, ask your Doctor or pharmacist.
2. Preparing for the Injection
   - Carefully examine the ampul (glass vial) of D.H.E. 45® (dihydroergotamine mesylate) Injection, USP for any cracks or breaks, and the liquid for discoloration, cloud-

Continued on next page

D.H.E. 45—Cont.

iness, or particles. If any of these defects are present, use a new ampul, make certain it is intact, and return the defective ampul to your doctor or pharmacy. Once you open an ampul, if it is not used within an hour, it should be thrown away.

3. Locating an Injection Site
   - Administer your subcutaneous Injection in the middle of your thigh, well above the knee.
4. Drawing the Medication into the Syringe
   - Wash your hands thoroughly with soap and water.
   - Check the dose of your medication.
   - Look to see if there is any liquid at the top of the ampul. If there is, gently flick the ampul with your finger to get all the liquid into the bottom portion of the ampul.
   - Hold the bottom of the ampul in one hand. Clean the ampul neck with an alcohol wipe using your other hand. Then place the alcohol wipe around the neck of the ampul and break it open by pressing your thumb against the neck of the ampul.
   - Tilt the ampul down at a 45° angle. Insert the needle into the solution in the ampul.
   - Draw up the medication by pulling back the plunger slowly and steadily until you reach your dose.
   - Check the syringe for air bubbles. Hold it with the needle pointing upward. If there are air bubbles, tap your finger against the barrel of the syringe to get the bubbles to the top. Slowly and carefully push the plunger up so that the bubbles are pushed out through the needle and you see a drop of medication.
   - When there are no air bubbles, check the dose of the medication. If the dose is incorrect, repeat steps 6 through 8 until you draw up the right dose.
5. Preparing the Injection Site
   - With a new alcohol wipe, clean the selected injection site thoroughly with a firm, circular motion from inside to outside. Wait for the injection site to dry before injecting.
6. Administering the Injection
   - Hold the syringe/needle in your right hand.
   - With your left hand, firmly grasp about a 1-inch fold of skin at the injection site.
   - Push the needle shaft, bevel side up, all the way into the fold of skin at a 45° to 90° angle, then release the fold of skin.
   - While holding the syringe with your left hand, use your right hand to draw back slightly on the plunger.
   - If you do not see any blood coming back into the syringe, inject the medication by pushing down on the plunger. If you do see blood in the syringe, that means the needle has penetrated a vein. If this happens, pull the needle/syringe out of the skin slightly and draw back on the plunger again. If no blood is seen this time, inject the medication.
   - Use your right hand to pull the needle out of your skin quickly at the same angle you injected it. Immediately press the alcohol wipe on the injection site and rub.

Check the expiration date printed on the ampul containing medication. If the expiration date has passed, do not use it. Answers to patients' questions about D.H.E. 45® (dihydroergotamine mesylate) Injection, USP

What if I need help in using my D.H.E. 45® (dihydroergotamine mesylate) Injection, USP?

If you have any questions or if you need help in opening, putting together, or using D.H.E. 45® (dihydroergotamine mesylate) Injection, USP, speak to your doctor or pharmacist.

How much medication should I use and how often?

Your doctor will have told you what dose to use for each migraine attack. Should you get another migraine attack in the same day as the attack you treated, you must not treat it with D.H.E. 45® (dihydroergotamine mesylate) Injection, USP unless at least 6 hours have elapsed since your last injection. No more than 6 mL of D.H.E. 45® (dihydroergotamine mesylate) Injection, USP should be injected during a one-week period. Do not use more than this amount unless instructed to do so by your doctor.

If you have any other unanswered question about D.H.E. 45® (dihydroergotamine mesylate) Injection, USP, consult your doctor or pharmacist.

*Trademark of Medical Economics Company, Inc.

REV: MAY 1998 30220906

Shown in Product Identification Guide, page 325

DIOVAN® ℞

[dī-o-van]

valsartan

Capsules

Rx only

The following prescribing information is based on official labeling in effect October 2000.

USE IN PREGNANCY

When used in pregnancy during the second and third trimesters, drugs that act directly on the renin-angiotensin system can cause injury and even death to the developing fetus. When pregnancy is detected, Diovan should be discontinued as soon as possible. See **WARNINGS: Fetal/Neonatal Morbidity and Mortality.**

DESCRIPTION

Diovan (valsartan) is a nonpeptide, orally active, and specific angiotensin II antagonist acting on the AT_1 receptor subtype.

Valsartan is chemically described as *N*-(1-oxopentyl)-*N*-[[2'-(1*H*-tetrazol-5-yl) [1,1'-biphenyl]-4-yl]methyl]-L-valine. Its empirical formula is $C_{24}H_{29}N_5O_3$, its molecular weight is 435.5, and its structural formula is

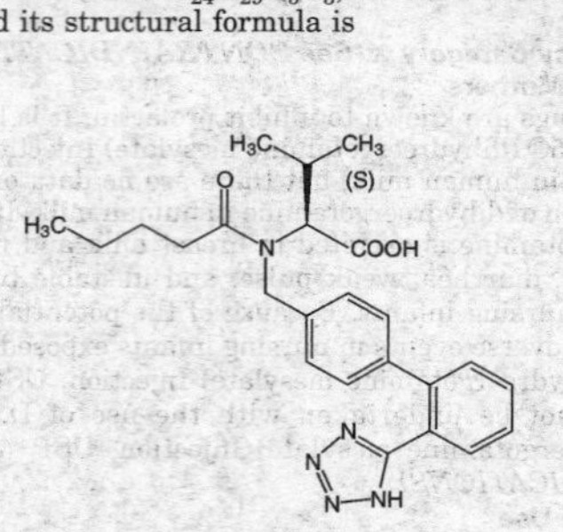

Valsartan is a white to practically white fine powder. It is soluble in ethanol and methanol and slightly soluble in water.

Diovan is available as capsules for oral administration, containing either 80 mg or 160 mg of valsartan. The inactive ingredients of the capsules are cellulose compounds, crospovidone, gelatin, iron oxides, magnesium stearate, povidone, sodium lauryl sulfate, and titanium dioxide.

CLINICAL PHARMACOLOGY

Mechanism of Action

Angiotensin II is formed from angiotensin I in a reaction catalyzed by angiotensin-converting enzyme (ACE, kininase II). Angiotensin II is the principal pressor agent of the renin-angiotensin system, with effects that include vasoconstriction, stimulation of synthesis and release of aldosterone, cardiac stimulation, and renal reabsorption of sodium. Valsartan blocks the vasoconstrictor and aldosterone-secreting effects of angiotensin II by selectively blocking the binding of angiotensin II to the AT_1 receptor in many tissues, such as vascular smooth muscle and the adrenal gland. Its action is therefore independent of the pathways for angiotensin II synthesis.

There is also an AT_2 receptor found in many tissues, but AT_2 is not known to be associated with cardiovascular homeostasis. Valsartan has much greater affinity (about 20,000-fold) for the AT_1 receptor than for the AT_2 receptor. The primary metabolite of valsartan is essentially inactive with an affinity for the AT_1 receptor about one 200th that of valsartan itself.

Blockade of the renin-angiotensin system with ACE inhibitors, which inhibit the biosynthesis of angiotensin II from angiotensin I, is widely used in the treatment of hypertension. ACE inhibitors also inhibit the degradation of bradykinin, a reaction also catalyzed by ACE. Because valsartan does not inhibit ACE (kininase II), it does not affect the response to bradykinin. Whether this difference has clinical relevance is not yet known. Valsartan does not bind to or block other hormone receptors or ion channels known to be important in cardiovascular regulation.

Blockade of the angiotensin II receptor inhibits the negative regulatory feedback of angiotensin II on renin secretion, but the resulting increased plasma renin activity and angiotensin II circulating levels do not overcome the effect of valsartan on blood pressure.

Pharmacokinetics

Valsartan peak plasma concentration is reached 2 to 4 hours after dosing. Valsartan shows bi-exponential decay kinetics following intravenous administration, with an average elimination half-life of about 6 hours. Absolute bioavailability for the capsule formulation is about 25% (range 10%-35%). Food decreases the exposure (as measured by AUC) to valsartan by about 40% and peak plasma concentration (C_{max}) by about 50%. AUC and C_{max} values of valsartan increase approximately linearly with increasing dose over the clinical dosing range. Valsartan does not accumulate appreciably in plasma following repeated administration.

Metabolism and Elimination

Valsartan, when administered as an oral solution, is primarily recovered in feces (about 83% of dose) and urine (about 13% of dose). The recovery is mainly as unchanged drug, with only about 20% of dose recovered as metabolites. The primary metabolite, accounting for about 9% of dose, is valeryl 4-hydroxy valsartan. The enzyme(s) responsible for valsartan metabolism have not been identified but do not seem to be CYP 450 isozymes.

Following intravenous administration, plasma clearance of valsartan is about 2 L/h and its renal clearance is 0.62 L/h (about 30% of total clearance).

Distribution

The steady state volume of distribution of valsartan after intravenous administration is small (17 L), indicating that valsartan does not distribute into tissues extensively. Valsartan is highly bound to serum proteins (95%), mainly serum albumin.

Special Populations

Pediatric: The pharmacokinetics of valsartan have not been investigated in patients < 18 years of age.

Geriatric: Exposure (measured by AUC) to valsartan is higher by 70% and the half-life is longer by 35% in the elderly than in the young. No dosage adjustment is necessary (see DOSAGE AND ADMINISTRATION).

Gender: Pharmacokinetics of valsartan does not differ significantly between males and females.

Renal Insufficiency: There is no apparent correlation between renal function (measured by creatinine clearance) and exposure (measured by AUC) to valsartan in patients with different degrees of renal impairment. Consequently, dose adjustment is not required in patients with mild-to-moderate renal dysfunction. No studies have been performed in patients with severe impairment of renal function (creatinine clearance < 10 mL/min). Valsartan is not removed from the plasma by hemodialysis. In the case of severe renal disease, exercise care with dosing of valsartan (see DOSAGE AND ADMINISTRATION).

Hepatic Insufficiency: On average, patients with mild-to-moderate chronic liver disease have twice the exposure (measured by AUC values) to valsartan of healthy volunteers (matched by age, sex and weight). In general, no dosage adjustment is needed in patients with mild-to-moderate liver disease. Care should be exercised in patients with liver disease (see DOSAGE AND ADMINISTRATION).

Pharmacodynamics and Clinical Effects

Valsartan inhibits the pressor effect of angiotensin II infusions. An oral dose of 80 mg inhibits the pressor effect by about 80% at peak with approximately 30% inhibition persisting for 24 hours. No information on the effect of larger doses is available.

Removal of the negative feedback of angiotensin II causes a 2- to 3-fold rise in plasma renin and consequent rise in angiotensin II plasma concentration in hypertensive patients. Minimal decreases in plasma aldosterone were observed after administration of valsartan; very little effect on serum potassium was observed.

In multiple-dose studies in hypertensive patients with stable renal insufficiency and patients with renovascular hypertension, valsartan had no clinically significant effects on glomerular filtration rate, filtration fraction, creatinine clearance, or renal plasma flow.

In multiple-dose studies in hypertensive patients, valsartan had no notable effects on total cholesterol, fasting triglycerides, fasting serum glucose, or uric acid.

The antihypertensive effects of Diovan were demonstrated principally in 7 placebo-controlled, 4- to 12-week trials (one in patients over 65) of dosages from 10 to 320 mg/day in patients with baseline diastolic blood pressures of 95-115. The studies allowed comparison of once-daily and twice-daily regimens of 160 mg/day; comparison of peak and trough effects; comparison (in pooled data) of response by gender, age, and race; and evaluation of incremental effects of hydrochlorothiazide.

Administration of valsartan to patients with essential hypertension results in a significant reduction of sitting, supine, and standing systolic and diastolic blood pressure, usually with little or no orthostatic change.

In most patients, after administration of a single oral dose, onset of antihypertensive activity occurs at approximately 2 hours, and maximum reduction of blood pressure is achieved within 6 hours. The antihypertensive effect persists for 24 hours after dosing, but there is a decrease from peak effect at lower doses (40 mg) presumably reflecting loss of inhibition of angiotensin II. At higher doses, however (160 mg), there is little difference in peak and trough effect. During repeated dosing, the reduction in blood pressure with any dose is substantially present within 2 weeks, and maximal reduction is generally attained after 4 weeks. In long-term follow-up studies (without placebo control), the effect of valsartan appeared to be maintained for up to two years. The antihypertensive effect is independent of age, gender or race. The latter finding regarding race is based on pooled data and should be viewed with caution, because antihypertensive drugs that affect the renin-angiotensin system (that is, ACE inhibitors and angiotensin-II blockers) have generally been found to be less effective in low-renin hypertensives (frequently blacks) than in high-renin hypertensives (frequently whites). In pooled, randomized, controlled trials of Diovan that included a total of 140 blacks and 830 whites, valsartan and an ACE-inhibitor control were generally at least as effective in blacks as whites. The explanation for this difference from previous findings is unclear.

Abrupt withdrawal of valsartan has not been associated with a rapid increase in blood pressure.

The blood pressure lowering effect of valsartan and thiazide-type diuretics are approximately additive.

The 7 studies of valsartan monotherapy included over 2000 patients randomized to various doses of valsartan and about 800 patients randomized to placebo. Doses below 80 mg were not consistently distinguished from those of placebo at trough, but doses of 80, 160 and 320 mg produced dose-related decreases in systolic and diastolic blood pressure, with the difference from placebo of approximately 6-9/3-5 mmHg at 80-160 mg and 9/6 mmHg at 320 mg. In a controlled trial the addition of HCTZ to valsartan 80 mg resulted in additional lowering of systolic and diastolic blood pressure by approximately 6/3 and 12/5 mmHg for 12.5 and 25 mg of HCTZ, respectively, compared to valsartan 80 mg alone.

Patients with an inadequate response to 80 mg once daily were titrated to either 160 mg once daily or 80 mg twice daily, which resulted in a comparable response in both groups.
In controlled trials, the antihypertensive effect of once-daily valsartan 80 mg was similar to that of once-daily enalapril 20 mg or once-daily lisinopril 10 mg.
There was essentially no change in heart rate in valsartan-treated patients in controlled trials.

INDICATIONS AND USAGE

Diovan is indicated for the treatment of hypertension. It may be used alone or in combination with other antihypertensive agents.

CONTRAINDICATIONS

Diovan is contraindicated in patients who are hypersensitive to any component of this product.

WARNINGS

Fetal/Neonatal Morbidity and Mortality

Drugs that act directly on the renin-angiotensin system can cause fetal and neonatal morbidity and death when administered to pregnant women. Several dozen cases have been reported in the world literature in patients who were taking angiotensin-converting enzyme inhibitors. When pregnancy is detected, Diovan should be discontinued as soon as possible.
The use of drugs that act directly on the renin-angiotensin system during the second and third trimesters of pregnancy has been associated with fetal and neonatal injury, including hypotension, neonatal skull hypoplasia, anuria, reversible or irreversible renal failure, and death. Oligohydramnios has also been reported, presumably resulting from decreased fetal renal function; oligohydramnios in this setting has been associated with fetal limb contractures, craniofacial deformation, and hypoplastic lung development. Prematurity, intrauterine growth retardation, and patent ductus arteriosus have also been reported, although it is not clear whether these occurrences were due to exposure to the drug.
These adverse effects do not appear to have resulted from intrauterine drug exposure that has been limited to the first trimester. Mothers whose embryos and fetuses are exposed to an angiotensin II receptor antagonist only during the first trimester should be so informed. Nonetheless, when patients become pregnant, physicians should advise the patient to discontinue the use of valsartan as soon as possible.
Rarely (probably less often than once in every thousand pregnancies), no alternative to a drug acting on the renin-angiotensin system will be found. In these rare cases, the mothers should be apprised of the potential hazards to their fetuses, and serial ultrasound examinations should be performed to assess the intra-amniotic environment.
If oligohydramnios is observed, valsartan should be discontinued unless it is considered life-saving for the mother. Contraction stress testing (CST), a nonstress test (NST), or biophysical profiling (BPP) may be appropriate, depending upon the week of pregnancy. Patients and physicians should be aware, however, that oligohydramnios may not appear until after the fetus has sustained irreversible injury.
Infants with histories of in utero exposure to an angiotensin II receptor antagonist should be closely observed for hypotension, oliguria, and hyperkalemia. If oliguria occurs, attention should be directed toward support of blood pressure and renal perfusion. Exchange transfusion or dialysis may be required as means of reversing hypotension and/or substituting for disordered renal function.
No teratogenic effects were observed when valsartan was administered to pregnant mice and rats at oral doses up to 600 mg/kg/day and to pregnant rabbits at oral doses up to 10 mg/kg/day. However, significant decreases in fetal weight, pup birth weight, pup survival rate, and slight delays in developmental milestones were observed in studies in which parental rats were treated with valsartan at oral, maternally toxic (reduction in body weight gain and food consumption) doses of 600 mg/kg/day during organogenesis or late gestation and lactation. In rabbits, fetotoxicity (i.e., resorptions, litter loss, abortions, and low body weight) associated with maternal toxicity (mortality) was observed at doses of 5 and 10 mg/kg/day. The no observed adverse effect doses of 600, 200 and 2 mg/kg/day in mice, rats and rabbits represent 9, 6, and 0.1 times, respectively, the maximum recommended human dose on a mg/m^2 basis. (Calculations assume an oral dose of 320 mg/day and a 60-kg patient.)

Hypotension in Volume- and/or Salt-Depleted Patients

Excessive reduction of blood pressure was rarely seen (0.1%) in patients with uncomplicated hypertension. In patients with an activated renin-angiotensin system, such as volume- and/or salt-depleted patients receiving high doses of diuretics, symptomatic hypotension may occur. This condition should be corrected prior to administration of Diovan, or the treatment should start under close medical supervision.
If hypotension occurs, the patient should be placed in the supine position and, if necessary, given an intravenous infusion of normal saline. A transient hypotensive response is not a contraindication to further treatment, which usually can be continued without difficulty once the blood pressure has stabilized.

PRECAUTIONS

General

Impaired Hepatic Function: As the majority of valsartan is eliminated in the bile, patients with mild-to-moderate hepatic impairment, including patients with biliary obstructive disorders, showed lower valsartan clearance (higher AUCs). Care should be exercised in administering Diovan to these patients.
Impaired Renal Function: As a consequence of inhibiting the renin-angiotensin-aldosterone system, changes in renal function may be anticipated in susceptible individuals. In patients whose renal function may depend on the activity of the renin-angiotensin-aldosterone system (e.g., patients with severe congestive heart failure), treatment with angiotensin-converting enzyme inhibitors and angiotensin receptor antagonists has been associated with oliguria and/or progressive azotemia and (rarely) with acute renal failure and/or death. Similar outcomes have been reported with Diovan.
In studies of ACE inhibitors in patients with unilateral or bilateral renal artery stenosis, increases in serum creatinine or blood urea nitrogen have been reported. In a 4-day trial of valsartan in 12 patients with unilateral renal artery stenosis, no significant increases in serum creatinine or blood urea nitrogen were observed. There has been no long-term use of Diovan in patients with unilateral or bilateral renal artery stenosis, but an effect similar to that seen with ACE inhibitors should be anticipated.

Information for Patients

Pregnancy: Female patients of childbearing age should be told about the consequences of second- and third-trimester exposure to drugs that act on the renin-angiotensin system, and they should also be told that these consequences do not appear to have resulted from intrauterine drug exposure that has been limited to the first trimester. These patients should be asked to report pregnancies to their physicians as soon as possible.

Drug Interactions

No clinically significant pharmacokinetic interactions were observed when valsartan was coadministered with amlodipine, atenolol, cimetidine, digoxin, furosemide, glyburide, hydrochlorothiazide, or indomethacin. The valsartan-atenolol combination was more antihypertensive than either component, but it did not lower the heart rate more than atenolol alone.
Coadministration of valsartan and warfarin did not change the pharmacokinetics of valsartan or the time-course of the anticoagulant properties of warfarin.
CYP 450 Interactions: The enzyme(s) responsible for valsartan metabolism have not been identified but do not seem to be CYP 450 isozymes. The inhibitory or induction potential of valsartan on CYP 450 is also unknown.

Carcinogenesis, Mutagenesis, Impairment of Fertility

There was no evidence of carcinogenicity when valsartan was administered in the diet to mice and rats for up to 2 years at doses up to 160 and 200 mg/kg/day, respectively. These doses in mice and rats are about 2.6 and 6 times, respectively, the maximum recommended human dose on a mg/m^2 basis. (Calculations assume an oral dose of 320 mg/day and a 60-kg patient.)
Mutagenicity assays did not reveal any valsartan-related effects at either the gene or chromosome level. These assays included bacterial mutagenicity tests with *Salmonella* (Ames) and *E coli;* a gene mutation test with Chinese hamster V79 cells; a cytogenetic test with Chinese hamster ovary cells; and a rat micronucleus test.
Valsartan had no adverse effects on the reproductive performance of male or female rats at oral doses up to 200 mg/kg/day. This dose is 6 times the maximum recommended human dose on a mg/m^2 basis. (Calculations assume an oral dose of 320 mg/day and a 60-kg patient.)

Pregnancy Categories C (first trimester) and D (second and third trimesters)

See WARNINGS, Fetal/Neonatal Morbidity and Mortality.

Nursing Mothers

It is not known whether valsartan is excreted in human milk, but valsartan was excreted in the milk of lactating rats. Because of the potential for adverse effects on the nursing infant, a decision should be made whether to discontinue nursing or discontinue the drug, taking into account the importance of the drug to the mother.

Pediatric Use

Safety and effectiveness in pediatric patients have not been established.

Geriatric Use

In the controlled clinical trials of valsartan, 1214 (36.2%) of patients treated with valsartan were ≥ 65 years and 265 (7.9%) were ≥ 75 years. No overall difference in the efficacy or safety of valsartan was observed in this patient population, but greater sensitivity of some older individuals cannot be ruled out.

ADVERSE REACTIONS

Diovan has been evaluated for safety in more than 4000 patients, including over 400 treated for over 6 months, and more than 160 for over 1 year. Adverse experiences have generally been mild and transient in nature and have only infrequently required discontinuation of therapy. The overall incidence of adverse experiences with Diovan was similar to placebo.
The overall frequency of adverse experiences was neither dose-related nor related to gender, age, race, or regimen. Discontinuation of therapy due to side effects was required in 2.3% of valsartan patients and 2.0% of placebo patients. The most common reasons for discontinuation of therapy with Diovan were headache and dizziness.
The adverse experiences that occurred in placebo-controlled clinical trials in at least 1% of patients treated with Diovan and at a higher incidence in valsartan (n=2316) than placebo (n=888) patients included viral infection (3% vs. 2%), fatigue (2% vs. 1%), and abdominal pain (2% vs. 1%).
Headache, dizziness, upper respiratory infection, cough, diarrhea, rhinitis, sinusitis, nausea, pharyngitis, edema, and arthralgia occurred at a more than 1% rate but at about the same incidence in placebo and valsartan patients.
In trials in which valsartan was compared to an ACE inhibitor with or without placebo, the incidence of dry cough was significantly greater in the ACE-inhibitor group (7.9%) than in the groups who received valsartan (2.6%) or placebo (1.5%). In a 129-patient trial limited to patients who had had dry cough when they had previously received ACE inhibitors, the incidences of cough in patients who received valsartan, HCTZ, or lisinopril were 20%, 19%, and 69% respectively ($p < 0.001$).
Dose-related orthostatic effects were seen in less than 1% of patients. An increase in the incidence of dizziness was observed in patients treated with Diovan 320 mg (8%) compared to 10 to 160 mg (2% to 4%).
Diovan has been used concomitantly with hydrochlorothiazide without evidence of clinically important adverse interactions.
Other adverse experiences that occurred in controlled clinical trials of patients treated with Diovan (> 0.2% of valsartan patients) are listed below. It cannot be determined whether these events were causally related to Diovan.
Body as a Whole: Allergic reaction and asthenia
Cardiovascular: Palpitations
Dermatologic: Pruritus and rash
Digestive: Constipation, dry mouth, dyspepsia, and flatulence
Musculoskeletal: Back pain, muscle cramps, and myalgia
Neurologic and Psychiatric: Anxiety, insomnia, paresthesia, and somnolence
Respiratory: Dyspnea
Special Senses: Vertigo
Urogenital: Impotence
Other reported events seen less frequently in clinical trials included chest pain, syncope, anorexia, vomiting, and angioedema.

Post-Marketing Experience

The following additional adverse reactions have been reported in post-marketing experience:
Hypersensitivity: There are rare reports of angioedema;
Digestive: Elevated liver enzymes and very rare reports of hepatitis;
Renal: Impaired renal function;
Clinical Laboratory Tests: Hyperkalemia;
Dermatologic: Alopecia.

Clinical Laboratory Test Findings

In controlled clinical trials, clinically important changes in standard laboratory parameters were rarely associated with administration of Diovan.
Creatinine: Minor elevations in creatinine occurred in 0.8% of patients taking Diovan and 0.6% given placebo in controlled clinical trials.
Hemoglobin and Hematocrit: Greater than 20% decreases in hemoglobin and hematocrit were observed in 0.4% and 0.8%, respectively, of Diovan patients, compared with 0.1% and 0.1% in placebo-treated patients. One valsartan patient discontinued treatment for microcytic anemia.
Liver function tests: Occasional elevations (greater than 150%) of liver chemistries occurred in Diovan-treated patients. Three patients (< 0.1%) treated with valsartan discontinued treatment for elevated liver chemistries.
Neutropenia: Neutropenia was observed in 1.9% of patients treated with Diovan and 0.8% of patients treated with placebo.
Serum Potassium: Greater than 20% increases in serum potassium were observed in 4.4% of Diovan-treated patients compared to 2.9% of placebo-treated patients.

OVERDOSAGE

Limited data are available related to overdosage in humans. The most likely manifestations of overdosage would be hypotension and tachycardia; bradycardia could occur from parasympathetic (vagal) stimulation. If symptomatic hypotension should occur, supportive treatment should be instituted.
Valsartan is not removed from the plasma by hemodialysis. Valsartan was without grossly observable adverse effects at single oral doses up to 2000 mg/kg in rats and up to 1000 mg/kg in marmosets, except for salivation and diarrhea in the rat and vomiting in the marmoset at the highest dose (60 and 37 times, respectively, the maximum recommended human dose on a mg/m^2 basis). (Calculations assume an oral dose of 320 mg/day and a 60-kg patient.)

DOSAGE AND ADMINISTRATION

The recommended starting dose of Diovan is 80 mg once daily when used as monotherapy in patients who are not volume-depleted. Diovan may be used over a dose range of 80 mg to 320 mg daily, administered once-a-day.
The antihypertensive effect is substantially present within 2 weeks and maximal reduction is generally attained after 4 weeks. If additional antihypertensive effect is required, the dosage may be increased to 160 mg or 320 mg or a diuretic may be added. Addition of a diuretic has a greater effect than dose increases beyond 80 mg.

Continued on next page

Diovan—Cont.

No initial dosage adjustment is required for elderly patients, for patients with mild or moderate renal impairment, or for patients with mild or moderate liver insufficiency. Care should be exercised with dosing of Diovan in patients with hepatic or severe renal impairment.
Diovan may be administered with other antihypertensive agents.
Diovan may be administered with or without food.

HOW SUPPLIED

Diovan is available as capsules containing valsartan 80 mg or 160 mg. Both strengths are packaged in bottles of 100 capsules and unit dose blister packages. Capsules are imprinted as follows:
80 mg Capsule - Light grey/light pink opaque, imprinted CG FZF
Bottles of 100 .... NDC 0083-4000-01
Unit Dose (blister pack) .... NDC 0083-4000-61
Box of 100 (strips of 10)
160 mg Capsule - Dark grey/light pink opaque, imprinted CG GOG
Bottles of 100 .... NDC 0083-4001-01
Unit Dose (blister pack) .... NDC 0083-4001-61
Box of 100 (strips of 10)
Store at 25°C (77°F); excursions permitted to 15°C-30°C (59°F–86°F).
Protect from moisture.
Dispense in tight container (USP).

REV: JUNE 2000 T2000-31
Shown in Product Identification Guide, page 325

DIOVAN HCT® ℞

[dī-o-van]
valsartan and hydrochlorothiazide
Combination Tablets
80 mg/12.5 mg
160 mg/12.5 mg
Rx only

The following prescribing information is based on official labeling in effect October 2000.

USE IN PREGNANCY
When used in pregnancy during the second and third trimesters, drugs that act directly on the renin-angiotensin system can cause injury and even death to the developing fetus. When pregnancy is detected, Diovan HCT should be discontinued as soon as possible. See **WARNINGS: Fetal/Neonatal Morbidity and Mortality.**

DESCRIPTION

Diovan HCT is a combination of valsartan, an orally active, specific angiotensin II antagonist acting on the AT_1 receptor subtype, and hydrochlorothiazide, a diuretic.
Valsartan, a nonpeptide molecule, is chemically described as *N*-(1-oxopentyl)-*N*-[[2′-(1*H*-tetrazol-5-yl)[1,1′-biphenyl]-4-yl]methyl]-L-Valine. Its empirical formula is $C_{24}H_{29}N_5O_3$, its molecular weight is 435.5, and its structural formula is

Valsartan is a white to practically white fine powder. It is soluble in ethanol and methanol and slightly soluble in water.
Hydrochlorothiazide USP is a white, or practically white, practically odorless, crystalline powder. It is slightly soluble in water; freely soluble in sodium hydroxide solution, in *n*-butylamine, and in dimethylformamide; sparingly soluble in methanol; and insoluble in ether, in chloroform, and in dilute mineral acids. Hydrochlorothiazide is chemically described as 6-chloro-3,4-dihydro-2*H*-1,2,4-benzothiadiazine-7-sulfonamide 1,1-dioxide. Hydrochlorothiazide is a thiazide diuretic. Its empirical formula is $C_7H_8ClN_3O_4S_2$, its molecular weight is 297.73, and its structural formula is

Diovan HCT tablets are formulated for oral administration with a combination of 80 mg or 160 mg of valsartan and 12.5 mg of hydrochlorothiazide USP. The inactive ingredients of the tablets are colloidal silicon dioxide, crospovidone, hydroxypropyl methylcellulose, iron oxides, magnesium stearate, microcrystalline cellulose, polyethylene glycol, talc, and titanium dioxide.

CLINICAL PHARMACOLOGY

Mechanism of Action
Angiotensin II is formed from angiotensin I in a reaction catalyzed by angiotensin-converting enzyme (ACE, kininase II). Angiotensin II is the principal pressor agent of the renin-angiotensin system, with effects that include vasoconstriction, stimulation of synthesis and release of aldosterone, cardiac stimulation, and renal reabsorption of sodium. Valsartan blocks the vasoconstrictor and aldosterone-secreting effects of angiotensin II by selectively blocking the binding of angiotensin II to the AT_1 receptor in many tissues, such as vascular smooth muscle and the adrenal gland. Its action is therefore independent of the pathways for angiotensin II synthesis.
There is also an AT_2 receptor found in many tissues, but AT_2 is not known to be associated with cardiovascular homeostasis. Valsartan has much greater affinity (about 20,000-fold) for the AT_1 receptor than for the AT_2 receptor. The primary metabolite of valsartan is essentially inactive with an affinity for the AT_1 receptor about one 200th that of valsartan itself.
Blockade of the renin-angiotensin system with ACE inhibitors, which inhibit the biosynthesis of angiotensin II from angiotensin I, is widely used in the treatment of hypertension. ACE inhibitors also inhibit the degradation of bradykinin, a reaction also catalyzed by ACE. Because valsartan does not inhibit ACE (kininase II) it does not affect the response to bradykinin. Whether this difference has clinical relevance is not yet known. Valsartan does not bind to or block other hormone receptors or ion channels known to be important in cardiovascular regulation.
Blockade of the angiotensin II receptor inhibits the negative regulatory feedback of angiotensin II on renin secretion, but the resulting increased plasma renin activity and angiotensin II circulating levels do not overcome the effect of valsartan on blood pressure.
Hydrochlorothiazide is a thiazide diuretic. Thiazides affect the renal tubular mechanisms of electrolyte reabsorption, directly increasing excretion of sodium and chloride in approximately equivalent amounts. Indirectly, the diuretic action of hydrochlorothiazide reduces plasma volume, with consequent increases in plasma renin activity, increases in aldosterone secretion, increases in urinary potassium loss, and decreases in serum potassium. The renin-aldosterone link is mediated by angiotensin II, so coadministration of an angiotensin II receptor antagonist tends to reverse the potassium loss associated with these diuretics.
The mechanism of the antihypertensive effect of thiazides is unknown.

Pharmacokinetics
Valsartan
Valsartan peak plasma concentration is reached 2 to 4 hours after dosing. Valsartan shows bi-exponential decay kinetics following intravenous administration, with an average elimination half-life of about 6 hours. Absolute bioavailability for the capsule formulation is about 25% (range 10%-35%). Food decreases the exposure (as measured by AUC) to valsartan by about 40% and peak plasma concentration (C_{max}) by about 50%. AUC and C_{max} values of valsartan increase approximately linearly with increasing dose over the clinical dosing range. Valsartan does not accumulate appreciably in plasma following repeated administration.

Metabolism and Elimination
Valsartan
Valsartan, when administered as an oral solution, is primarily recovered in feces (about 83% of dose) and urine (about 13% of dose). The recovery is mainly as unchanged drug, with only about 20% of dose recovered as metabolites. The primary metabolite, accounting for about 9% of dose, is valeryl 4-hydroxy valsartan. The enzyme(s) responsible for valsartan metabolism have not been identified but do not seem to be CYP 450 isozymes.
Following intravenous administration, plasma clearance of valsartan is about 2 L/h and its renal clearance is 0.62 L/h (about 30% of total clearance).
Hydrochlorothiazide
Hydrochlorothiazide is not metabolized but is eliminated rapidly by the kidney. At least 61% of the oral dose is eliminated as unchanged drug within 24 hours. The elimination half-life is between 5.8 and 18.9 hours.

Distribution
Valsartan
The steady state volume of distribution of valsartan after intravenous administration is small (17 L), indicating that valsartan does not distribute into tissues extensively. Valsartan is highly bound to serum proteins (95%), mainly serum albumin.
Hydrochlorothiazide
Hydrochlorothiazide crosses the placental but not the blood-brain barrier and is excreted in breast milk.

Special Populations
Pediatric: The pharmacokinetics of valsartan have not been investigated in patients <18 years of age.
Geriatric: Exposure (measured by AUC) to valsartan is higher by 70% and the half-life is longer by 35% in the elderly than in the young. No dosage adjustment is necessary (see DOSAGE AND ADMINISTRATION).
Gender: Pharmacokinetics of valsartan does not differ significantly between males and females.
Race: Pharmacokinetic differences due to race have not been studied.
Renal Insufficiency: There is no apparent correlation between renal function (measured by creatinine clearance) and exposure (measured by AUC) to valsartan in patients with different degrees of renal impairment. Consequently, dose adjustment is not required in patients with mild-to-moderate renal dysfunction. No studies have been performed in patients with severe impairment of renal function (creatinine clearance <10 mL/min). Valsartan is not removed from the plasma by hemodialysis. In the case of severe renal disease, exercise care with dosing of valsartan (see DOSAGE AND ADMINISTRATION).
Thiazide diuretics are eliminated by the kidney, with a terminal half-life of 5-15 hours. In a study of patients with impaired renal function (mean creatinine clearance of 19 mL/min), the half-life of hydrochlorothiazide elimination was lengthened to 21 hours.
Hepatic Insufficiency: On average, patients with mild-to-moderate chronic liver disease have twice the exposure (measured by AUC values) to valsartan of healthy volunteers (matched by age, sex and weight). In general, no dosage adjustment is needed in patients with mild-to-moderate liver disease. Care should be exercised in patients with liver disease (see DOSAGE AND ADMINISTRATION).

Pharmacodynamics and Clinical Effects
Valsartan - Hydrochlorothiazide
In controlled clinical trials including over 1500 patients, 730 patients were exposed to valsartan (80 and 160 mg) and concomitant hydrochlorothiazide (12.5 and 25 mg). A factorial trial compared the combinations of 80/12.5 mg, 80/25 mg, 160/12.5 mg and 160/25 mg with their respective components and placebo. The combination of valsartan and hydrochlorothiazide resulted in additive placebo-adjusted decreases in systolic and diastolic blood pressure at trough of 15-21/8-11 mmHg at 80/12.5 mg to 160/25 mg, compared to 7-10/4-6 mmHg for valsartan 80 mg to 160 mg and 6-10/3-5 mmHg for hydrochlorothiazide 12.5 mg to 25 mg, alone.
In another controlled trial the addition of hydrochlorothiazide to valsartan 80 mg resulted in additional lowering of systolic and diastolic blood pressure by approximately 6/3 and 12/5 mmHg for 12.5 mg and 25 mg of hydrochlorothiazide, respectively, compared to valsartan 80 mg alone.
The maximal antihypertensive effect was attained 4 weeks after the initiation of therapy, the first time point at which blood pressure was measured in these trials.
In long-term follow-up studies (without placebo control) the effect of the combination of valsartan and hydrochlorothiazide appeared to be maintained for up to two years. The antihypertensive effect is independent of age or gender. The overall response to the combination was similar for black and non-black patients.
There was essentially no change in heart rate in patients treated with the combination of valsartan and hydrochlorothiazide in controlled trials.
Valsartan
Valsartan inhibits the pressor effect of angiotensin II infusions. An oral dose of 80 mg inhibits the pressor effect by about 80% at peak with approximately 30% inhibition persisting for 24 hours. No information on the effect of larger doses is available.
Removal of the negative feedback of angiotensin II causes a 2- to 3-fold rise in plasma renin and consequent rise in angiotensin II plasma concentration in hypertensive patients. Minimal decreases in plasma aldosterone were observed after administration of valsartan; very little effect on serum potassium was observed.
In multiple-dose studies in hypertensive patients with stable renal insufficiency and patients with renovascular hypertension, valsartan had no clinically significant effects on glomerular filtration rate, filtration fraction, creatinine clearance, or renal plasma flow.
In multiple-dose studies in hypertensive patients, valsartan had no notable effects on total cholesterol, fasting triglycerides, fasting serum glucose, or uric acid.
The antihypertensive effects of valsartan were demonstrated principally in 7 placebo-controlled, 4- to 12-week trials (one in patients over 65) of dosages from 10 to 320 mg/day in patients with baseline diastolic blood pressures of 95-115. The studies allowed comparison of once-daily and twice-daily regimens of 160 mg/day; comparison of peak and trough effects; comparison (in pooled data) of response by gender, age, and race; and evaluation of incremental effects of hydrochlorothiazide.
Administration of valsartan to patients with essential hypertension results in a significant reduction of sitting, supine, and standing systolic and diastolic blood pressure, usually with little or no orthostatic change.
In most patients, after administration of a single oral dose, onset of antihypertensive activity occurs at approximately 2 hours, and maximum reduction of blood pressure is achieved within 6 hours. The antihypertensive effect persists for 24 hours after dosing, but there is a decrease from peak effect at lower doses (40 mg) presumably reflecting loss of inhibition of angiotensin II. At higher doses, however (160 mg), there is little difference in peak and trough effect. During repeated dosing, the reduction in blood pressure with any dose is substantially present within 2 weeks, and maximal reduction is generally attained after 4 weeks. In long-term follow-up studies (without placebo control) the effect of valsartan appeared to be maintained for up to two years. The antihypertensive effect is independent of age, gender or race. The latter finding regarding race is based on pooled data and should be viewed with caution, because antihypertensive drugs that affect the renin-angiotensin system (that is, ACE inhibitors and angiotensin-II blockers) have gener-

ally been found to be less effective in low-renin hypertensives (frequently blacks) than in high-renin hypertensives (frequently whites). In pooled, randomized, controlled trials of Diovan that included a total of 140 blacks and 830 whites, valsartan and an ACE-inhibitor control were generally at least as effective in blacks as whites. The explanation for this difference from previous findings is unclear.

Abrupt withdrawal of valsartan has not been associated with a rapid increase in blood pressure.

The 7 studies of valsartan monotherapy included over 2000 patients randomized to various doses of valsartan and about 800 patients randomized to placebo. Doses below 80 mg were not consistently distinguished from those of placebo at trough, but doses of 80, 160 and 320 mg produced dose-related decreases in systolic and diastolic blood pressure, with the difference from placebo of approximately 6-9/3-5 mmHg at 80-160 mg and 9/6 mmHg at 320 mg.

Patients with an inadequate response to 80 mg once daily were titrated to either 160 mg once daily or 80 mg twice daily, which resulted in a comparable response in both groups.

In controlled trials, the antihypertensive effect of once daily valsartan 80 mg was similar to that of once daily enalapril 20 mg or once daily lisinopril 10 mg.

There was essentially no change in heart rate in valsartan-treated patients in controlled trials.

Hydrochlorothiazide

After oral administration of hydrochlorothiazide, diuresis begins within 2 hours, peaks in about 4 hours and lasts about 6 to 12 hours.

INDICATIONS AND USAGE

Diovan HCT is indicated for the treatment of hypertension. This fixed dose combination is not indicated for initial therapy (see DOSAGE AND ADMINISTRATION).

CONTRAINDICATIONS

Diovan HCT is contraindicated in patients who are hypersensitive to any component of this product.

Because of the hydrochlorothiazide component, this product is contraindicated in patients with anuria or hypersensitivity to other sulfonamide-derived drugs.

WARNINGS

Fetal/Neonatal Morbidity and Mortality

Drugs that act directly on the renin-angiotensin system can cause fetal and neonatal morbidity and death when administered to pregnant women. Several dozen cases have been reported in the world literature in patients who were taking angiotensin-converting enzyme inhibitors. When pregnancy is detected, Diovan HCT should be discontinued as soon as possible.

The use of drugs that act directly on the renin-angiotensin system during the second and third trimesters of pregnancy has been associated with fetal and neonatal injury, including hypotension, neonatal skull hypoplasia, anuria, reversible or irreversible renal failure, and death. Oligohydramnios has also been reported, presumably resulting from decreased fetal renal function; oligohydramnios in this setting has been associated with fetal limb contractures, craniofacial deformation, and hypoplastic lung development. Prematurity, intrauterine growth retardation, and patent ductus arteriosus have also been reported, although it is not clear whether these occurrences were due to exposure to the drug.

These adverse effects do not appear to have resulted from intrauterine drug exposure that has been limited to the first trimester.

Mothers whose embryos and fetuses are exposed to an angiotensin II receptor antagonist only during the first trimester should be so informed. Nonetheless, when patients become pregnant, physicians should advise the patient to discontinue the use of Diovan HCT as soon as possible.

Rarely (probably less often than once in every thousand pregnancies), no alternative to a drug acting on the renin-angiotensin system will be found. In these rare cases, the mothers should be apprised of the potential hazards to their fetuses, and serial ultrasound examinations should be performed to assess the intraamniotic environment.

If oligohydramnios is observed, Diovan HCT should be discontinued unless it is considered life-saving for the mother. Contraction stress testing (CST), a nonstress test (NST), or biophysical profiling (BPP) may be appropriate, depending upon the week of pregnancy. Patients and physicians should be aware, however, that oligohydramnios may not appear until after the fetus has sustained irreversible injury.

Infants with histories of in utero exposure to an angiotensin II receptor antagonist should be closely observed for hypotension, oliguria, and hyperkalemia. If oliguria occurs, attention should be directed toward support of blood pressure and renal perfusion. Exchange transfusion or dialysis may be required as means of reversing hypotension and/or substituting for disordered renal function.

Valsartan - Hydrochlorothiazide in Animals

There was no evidence of teratogenicity in mice, rats, or rabbits treated orally with valsartan at doses up to 600, 100 and 10 mg/kg/day, respectively, in combination with hydrochlorothiazide at doses up to 188, 31 and 3 mg/kg/day. These non-teratogenic doses in mice, rats and rabbits, respectively, represent 18, 7 and 1 times the maximum recommended human dose (MRHD) of valsartan and 38, 13 and 2 times the MRHD of hydrochlorothiazide on a mg/m^2 basis. (Calculations assume an oral dose of 160 mg/day valsartan in combination with 25 mg/day hydrochlorothiazide and a 60-kg patient.)

Fetotoxicity was observed in association with maternal toxicity in rats and rabbits at valsartan doses of ≥200 and 10 mg/kg/day, respectively, in combination with hydrochlorothiazide doses of ≥63 and 3 mg/kg/day. Fetotoxicity in rats was considered to be related to decreased fetal weights and included fetal variations of sternebrae, vertebrae, ribs and/or renal papillae. Fetotoxicity in rabbits included increased numbers of late resorptions with resultant increases in total resorptions, postimplantation losses and decreased number of live fetuses. The no observed adverse effect doses in mice, rats and rabbits for valsartan were 600, 100 and 3 mg/kg/day, respectively, in combination with hydrochlorothiazide doses of 188, 31 and 1 mg/kg/day. These no adverse effect doses in mice, rats and rabbits, respectively, represent 5, 1.5 and 0.06 times the MRHD of valsartan and 38, 13 and 0.5 times the MRHD of hydrochlorothiazide on a mg/m^2 basis. (Calculations assume an oral dose of 160 mg/day valsartan in combination with 25 mg/day hydrochlorothiazide and a 60-kg patient.)

Valsartan in Animals

No teratogenic effects were observed when valsartan was administered to pregnant mice and rats at oral doses up to 600 mg/kg/day and to pregnant rabbits at oral doses up to 10 mg/kg/day. However, significant decreases in fetal weight, pup birth weight, pup survival rate, and slight delays in developmental milestones were observed in studies in which parental rats were treated with valsartan at oral, maternally toxic (reduction in body weight gain and food consumption) doses of 600 mg/kg/day during organogenesis or late gestation and lactation. In rabbits, fetotoxicity (i.e., resorptions, litter loss, abortions, and low body weight) associated with maternal toxicity (mortality) was observed at doses of 5 and 10 mg/kg/day. The no observed adverse effect doses of 600, 200 and 2 mg/kg/day in mice, rats and rabbits represent 18, 12 and 0.2 times, respectively, the maximum recommended human dose on a mg/m^2 basis. (Calculations assume an oral dose of 160 mg/day and a 60-kg patient.)

Hydrochlorothiazide in Animals

Under the auspices of the National Toxicology Program, pregnant mice and rats that received hydrochlorothiazide via gavage at doses up to 3000 and 1000 mg/kg/day, respectively, on gestation days 6 through 15 showed no evidence of teratogenicity. These doses of hydrochlorothiazide in mice and rats represent 608 and 405 times, respectively, the maximum recommended human dose on a mg/m^2 basis. (Calculations assume an oral dose of 25 mg/day and a 60-kg patient.)

Intrauterine exposure to thiazide diuretics is associated with fetal or neonatal jaundice, thrombocytopenia, and possibly other adverse reactions that have occurred in adults.

Hypotension in Volume- and/or Salt-Depleted Patients

Excessive reduction of blood pressure was rarely seen (0.5%) in patients with uncomplicated hypertension treated with Diovan HCT. In patients with an activated renin-angiotensin system, such as volume- and/or salt-depleted patients receiving high doses of diuretics, symptomatic hypotension may occur. This condition should be corrected prior to administration of Diovan HCT, or the treatment should start under close medical supervision.

If hypotension occurs, the patient should be placed in the supine position and, if necessary, given an intravenous infusion of normal saline. A transient hypotensive response is not a contraindication to further treatment, which usually can be continued without difficulty once the blood pressure has stabilized.

Hydrochlorothiazide

Impaired Hepatic Function

Thiazide diuretics should be used with caution in patients with impaired hepatic function or progressive liver disease, since minor alterations of fluid and electrolyte balance may precipitate hepatic coma.

Hypersensitivity Reaction

Hypersensitivity reactions to hydrochlorothiazide may occur in patients with or without a history of allergy or bronchial asthma, but are more likely in patients with such a history.

Systemic Lupus Erythematosus

Thiazide diuretics have been reported to cause exacerbation or activation of systemic lupus erythematosus.

Lithium Interaction

Lithium generally should not be given with thiazides (see PRECAUTIONS, Drug Interactions, Hydrochlorothiazide, Lithium).

PRECAUTIONS

Serum Electrolytes

Valsartan - Hydrochlorothiazide

In the controlled trials of various doses of the combination of valsartan and hydrochlorothiazide the incidence of hypertensive patients who developed hypokalemia (serum potassium <3.5 mEq/L) was 4.5%; the incidence of hyperkalemia (serum potassium >5.7 mEq/L) was 0.3%. Two patients (0.3%) discontinued from a trial for decreases in serum potassium.

In controlled clinical trials of Diovan HCT, the average change in serum potassium was near zero in subjects who received Diovan HCT 160/12.5 mg, but the average subject who received Diovan HCT 80/12.5 mg, 80/25 mg or 160/25 mg experienced a mild reduction in serum potassium.

In clinical trials, the opposite effects of valsartan (80 or 160 mg) and hydrochlorothiazide (12.5 mg) on serum potassium approximately balanced each other in many patients. In other patients, one or the other effect may be dominant. Periodic determinations of serum electrolytes to detect possible electrolyte imbalance should be performed at appropriate intervals.

Hydrochlorothiazide

All patients receiving thiazide therapy should be observed for clinical signs of fluid or electrolyte imbalance: hyponatremia, hypochloremic alkalosis, and hypokalemia. Serum and urine electrolyte determinations are particularly important when the patient is vomiting excessively or receiving parenteral fluids. Warning signs or symptoms of fluid and electrolyte imbalance, irrespective of cause, include dryness of mouth, thirst, weakness, lethargy, drowsiness, restlessness, confusion, seizures, muscle pains or cramps, muscular fatigue, hypotension, oliguria, tachycardia, and gastrointestinal disturbances such as nausea and vomiting.

Hypokalemia may develop, especially with brisk diuresis, when severe cirrhosis is present, or after prolonged therapy.

Interference with adequate oral electrolyte intake will also contribute to hypokalemia. Hypokalemia may cause cardiac arrhythmia and may also sensitize or exaggerate the response of the heart to the toxic effects of digitalis (e.g., increased ventricular irritability).

Although any chloride deficit is generally mild and usually does not require specific treatment except under extraordinary circumstances (as in liver disease or renal disease), chloride replacement may be required in the treatment of metabolic alkalosis.

Dilutional hyponatremia may occur in edematous patients in hot weather; appropriate therapy is water restriction, rather than administration of salt except in rare instances when the hyponatremia is life-threatening. In actual salt depletion, appropriate replacement is the therapy of choice.

Hyperuricemia may occur or frank gout may be precipitated in certain patients receiving thiazide therapy.

In diabetic patients dosage adjustments of insulin or oral hypoglycemic agents may be required. Hyperglycemia may occur with thiazide diuretics. Thus latent diabetes mellitus may become manifest during thiazide therapy.

The antihypertensive effects of the drug may be enhanced in the postsympathectomy patient.

If progressive renal impairment becomes evident, consider withholding or discontinuing diuretic therapy.

Thiazides have been shown to increase the urinary excretion of magnesium; this may result in hypomagnesemia.

Thiazides may decrease urinary calcium excretion. Thiazides may cause intermittent and slight elevation of serum calcium in the absence of known disorders of calcium metabolism. Marked hypercalcemia may be evidence of hidden hyperparathyroidism. Thiazides should be discontinued before carrying out tests for parathyroid function.

Increases in cholesterol and triglyceride levels may be associated with thiazide diuretic therapy.

Impaired Hepatic Function

Valsartan

As the majority of valsartan is eliminated in the bile, patients with mild-to-moderate hepatic impairment, including patients with biliary obstructive disorders, showed lower valsartan clearance (higher AUCs). Care should be exercised in administering valsartan to these patients.

Impaired Renal Function

Valsartan

As a consequence of inhibiting the renin-angiotensin-aldosterone system, changes in renal function may be anticipated in susceptible individuals. In patients whose renal function may depend on the activity of the renin-angiotensin-aldosterone system (e.g., patients with severe congestive heart failure), treatment with angiotensin-converting enzyme inhibitors and angiotensin receptor antagonists has been associated with oliguria and/or progressive azotemia and (rarely) with acute renal failure and/or death. Similar outcomes have been reported with Diovan.

In studies of ACE inhibitors in patients with unilateral or bilateral renal artery stenosis, increases in serum creatinine or blood urea nitrogen have been reported. In a 4-day trial of valsartan in 12 patients with unilateral renal artery stenosis, no significant increases in serum creatinine or blood urea nitrogen were observed. There has been no long-term use of valsartan in patients with unilateral or bilateral renal artery stenosis, but an effect similar to that seen with ACE inhibitors should be anticipated.

Hydrochlorothiazide

Thiazides should be used with caution in severe renal disease. In patients with renal disease, thiazides may precipitate azotemia. Cumulative effects of the drug may develop in patients with impaired renal function.

Information for Patients

Pregnancy: Female patients of childbearing age should be told about the consequences of second- and third-trimester exposure to drugs that act on the renin-angiotensin system, and they should also be told that these consequences do not appear to have resulted from intrauterine drug exposure that has been limited to the first trimester. These patients should be asked to report pregnancies to their physicians as soon as possible.

Symptomatic Hypotension: A patient receiving Diovan HCT should be cautioned that lightheadedness can occur, especially during the first days of therapy, and that it should be reported to the prescribing physician. The patients should be told that if syncope occurs, Diovan

Continued on next page

Diovan HCT—Cont.

HCT should be discontinued until the physician has been consulted.
All patients should be cautioned that inadequate fluid intake, excessive perspiration, diarrhea, or vomiting can lead to an excessive fall in blood pressure, with the same consequences of lightheadedness and possible syncope.
Potassium Supplements: A patient receiving Diovan HCT should be told not to use potassium supplements or salt substitutes containing potassium without consulting the prescribing physician.

Drug Interactions

Valsartan

No clinically significant pharmacokinetic interactions were observed when valsartan was coadministered with amlodipine, atenolol, cimetidine, digoxin, furosemide, glyburide, hydrochlorothiazide, or indomethacin. The valsartan-atenolol combination was more antihypertensive than either component, but it did not lower the heart rate more than atenolol alone.
Coadministration of valsartan and warfarin did not change the pharmacokinetics of valsartan or the time-course of the anticoagulant properties of warfarin.
CYP 450 Interactions: The enzyme(s) responsible for valsartan metabolism have not been identified but do not seem to be CYP 450 isozymes. The inhibitory or induction potential of valsartan on CYP 450 is also unknown.

Hydrochlorothiazide

When administered concurrently the following drugs may interact with thiazide diuretics:
Alcohol, barbiturates, or narcotics - Potentiation of orthostatic hypotension may occur.
Antidiabetic drugs (oral agents and insulin) - Dosage adjustment of the antidiabetic drug may be required.
Other antihypertensive drugs - Additive effect or potentiation.
Cholestyramine and colestipol resins - Absorption of hydrochlorothiazide is impaired in the presence of anionic exchange resins. Single doses of either cholestyramine or colestipol resins bind the hydrochlorothiazide and reduce its absorption from the gastrointestinal tract by up to 85% and 43% respectively.
Corticosteroids, ACTH - Intensified electrolyte depletion, particularly hypokalemia.
Pressor amines (e.g., norepinephrine) - Possible decreased response to pressor amines but not sufficient to preclude their use.
Skeletal muscle relaxants, nondepolarizing (e.g., tubocurarine) - Possible increased responsiveness to the muscle relaxant.
Lithium - Should not generally be given with diuretics. Diuretic agents reduce the renal clearance of lithium and add a high risk of lithium toxicity. Refer to the package insert for lithium preparations before use of such preparations with Diovan HCT.
Non-steroidal anti-inflammatory Drugs - In some patients, the administration of a non-steroidal anti-inflammatory agent can reduce the diuretic, natriuretic, and antihypertensive effects of loop, potassium-sparing and thiazide diuretics. Therefore, when Diovan HCT and non-steroidal anti-inflammatory agents are used concomitantly, the patient should be observed closely to determine if the desired effect of the diuretic is obtained.

Carcinogenesis, Mutagenesis, Impairment of Fertility

Valsartan - Hydrochlorothiazide

No carcinogenicity, mutagenicity or fertility studies have been conducted with the combination of valsartan and hydrochlorothiazide. However, these studies have been conducted for valsartan as well as hydrochlorothiazide alone. Based on the preclinical safety and human pharmacokinetic studies, there is no indication of any adverse interaction between valsartan and hydrochlorothiazide.

Valsartan

There was no evidence of carcinogenicity when valsartan was administered in the diet to mice and rats for up to 2 years at doses up to 160 and 200 mg/kg/day, respectively. These doses in mice and rats are about 5 and 12 times, respectively, the maximum recommended human dose on a mg/m^2 basis. (Calculations assume an oral dose of 160 mg/day and a 60-kg patient.)
Mutagenicity assays did not reveal any valsartan-related effects at either the gene or chromosome level. These assays included bacterial mutagenicity tests with *Salmonella* (Ames) and *E coli;* a gene mutation test with Chinese hamster V79 cells; a cytogenetic test with Chinese hamster ovary cells; and a rat micronucleus test.
Valsartan had no adverse effects on the reproductive performance of male or female rats at oral doses up to 200 mg/kg/day. This dose is about 12 times the maximum recommended human dose on a mg/m^2 basis. (Calculations assume an oral dose of 160 mg/day and a 60-kg patient.)

Hydrochlorothiazide

Two-year feeding studies in mice and rats conducted under the auspices of the National Toxicology Program (NTP) uncovered no evidence of a carcinogenic potential of hydrochlorothiazide in female mice (at doses of up to approximately 600 mg/kg/day) or in male and female rats (at doses of up to approximately 100 mg/kg/day). The NTP, however, found equivocal evidence for hepatocarcinogenicity in male mice.
Hydrochlorothiazide was not genotoxic In Vitro in the Ames mutagenicity assay of Salmonella Typhimurium strains TA 98, TA 100, TA 1535, TA 1537, and TA 1538 and in the Chinese Hamster Ovary (CHO) test for chromosomal aberrations, or In Vivo in assays using mouse germinal cell chromosomes, Chinese hamster bone marrow chromosomes, and the Drosophila sex-linked recessive lethal trait gene. Positive test results were obtained only in the In Vitro CHO Sister Chromatid Exchange (clastogenicity) and in the Mouse Lymphoma Cell (mutagenicity) assays, using concentrations of hydrochlorothiazide from 43 to 1300 mcgm/mL, and in the Aspergillus Nidulans non-disjunction assay at an unspecified concentration.
Hydrochlorothiazide had no adverse effects on the fertility of mice and rats of either sex in studies wherein these species were exposed, via their diet, to doses of up to 100 and 4 mg/kg, respectively, prior to mating and throughout gestation.

Pregnancy Categories C (first trimester) and D (second and third trimesters)

See WARNINGS, Fetal/Neonatal Morbidity and Mortality.

Nursing Mothers

It is not known whether valsartan is excreted in human milk, but valsartan was excreted in the milk of lactating rats. Thiazides appear in human milk. Because of the potential for adverse effects on the nursing infant, a decision should be made whether to discontinue nursing or discontinue the drug, taking into account the importance of the drug to the mother.

Pediatric Use

Safety and effectiveness in pediatric patients have not been established.

Geriatric Use

In the controlled clinical trials of Diovan HCT, 117 (16%) of patients treated with valsartan-hydrochlorothiazide were ≥65 years and 16 (2.2%) were ≥75 years. No overall difference in the efficacy or safety of valsartan-hydrochlorothiazide was observed between these patients and younger patients, but greater sensitivity of some older individuals cannot be ruled out.

ADVERSE REACTIONS

Diovan HCT has been evaluated for safety in more than 1,300 patients, including over 360 treated for over 6 months, and 170 for over 1 year. Adverse experiences have generally been mild and transient in nature and have only infrequently required discontinuation of therapy. The overall incidence of adverse experiences with Diovan HCT was comparable to placebo.
The overall frequency of adverse experiences was neither dose-related nor related to gender, age or race. In controlled clinical trials, discontinuation of therapy due to side effects was required in 3.6% of valsartan-hydrochlorothiazide patients and 4.3% of placebo patients. The most common reasons for discontinuation of therapy with Diovan HCT were headache, fatigue and dizziness.
The adverse experiences that occurred in controlled clinical trials in at least 2% of patients treated with Diovan HCT and at a higher incidence in valsartan-hydrochlorothiazide (n=730) than placebo (n=93) patients included dizziness (9% vs 7%), viral infection (3% vs 1%), fatigue (5% vs 1%), pharyngitis (3% vs 1%), coughing (3% vs 0%) and diarrhea (3% vs 0%).
Headache, upper respiratory infection, sinusitis, back pain and chest pain occurred at a more than 2% rate but at about the same incidence in placebo and valsartan-hydrochlorothiazide patients.
Dose-related orthostatic effects were seen in less than 1% of patients. A dose-related increase in the incidence of dizziness was observed in patients treated with Diovan HCT from 80/12.5 mg (6%) to 160/25 mg (16%).
Other adverse experiences that have been reported with valsartan-hydrochlorothiazide (>0.2% of valsartan-hydrochlorothiazide patients in controlled clinical trials) without regard to causality, are listed below:
Body as a Whole: Allergic reaction, anaphylaxis, asthenia, and dependent edema.
Cardiovascular: Palpitations, syncope, and tachycardia.
Dermatologic: Flushing, rash, sunburn, and increased sweating.
Digestive: Increased appetite, constipation, dyspepsia, flatulence, dry mouth, nausea, abdominal pain, and vomiting.
Metabolic: Dehydration and gout.
Musculoskeletal: Arthralgia, muscle cramps, muscle weakness, arm pain, and leg pain.
Neurologic and Psychiatric: Anxiety, depression, insomnia, decreased libido, paresthesia, and somnolence.
Respiratory: Bronchospasm, dyspnea, and epistaxis.
Special Senses: Tinnitus, vertigo, and abnormal vision.
Urogenital: Dysuria, impotence, micturition frequency, and urinary tract infection.

Valsartan

In trials in which valsartan was compared to an ACE inhibitor with or without placebo, the incidence of dry cough was significantly greater in the ACE inhibitor group (7.9%) than in the groups who received valsartan (2.6%) or placebo (1.5%). In a 129-patient trial limited to patients who had had dry cough when they had previously received ACE inhibitors, the incidences of cough in patients who received valsartan, hydrochlorothiazide, or lisinopril were 20%, 19%, 69% respectively ($p < 0.001$).
Other reported events seen less frequently in clinical trials included chest pain, syncope, anorexia, vomiting, and angioedema.

Post-Marketing Experience

The following additional adverse reactions have been reported in post-marketing experience:
Hypersensitivity: There are rare reports of angioedema;
Digestive: Elevated liver enzymes and very rare reports of hepatitis;
Renal: Impaired Renal Function;
Clinical Laboratory Tests: Hyperkalemia;
Dermatologic: Alopecia.

Hydrochlorothiazide

Other adverse experiences that have been reported with hydrochlorothiazide, without regard to causality, are listed below:
Body As A Whole: weakness;
Digestive: pancreatitis, jaundice (intrahepatic cholestatic jaundice), sialadenitis, cramping, gastric irritation;
Hematologic: aplastic anemia, agranulocytosis, leukopenia, hemolytic anemia, thrombocytopenia;
Hypersensitivity: purpura, photosensitivity, urticaria, necrotizing angiitis (vasculitis and cutaneous vasculitis), fever, respiratory distress including pneumonitis and pulmonary edema, anaphylactic reactions;
Metabolic: hyperglycemia, glycosuria, hyperuricemia;
Musculoskeletal: muscle spasm;
Nervous System/Psychiatric: restlessness;
Renal: renal failure, renal dysfunction, interstitial nephritis;
Skin: erythema multiforme including Stevens-Johnson syndrome, exfoliative dermatitis including toxic epidermal necrolysis;
Special Senses: transient blurred vision, xanthopsia.

Clinical Laboratory Test Findings

In controlled clinical trials, clinically important changes in standard laboratory parameters were rarely associated with administration of Diovan HCT.
Creatinine: Minor elevations in creatinine occurred in 1.4% of patients taking Diovan HCT and 1.1% given placebo in controlled clinical trials.
Hemoglobin and Hematocrit: Greater than 20% decreases in hemoglobin and hematocrit were observed in 0.1% and 1.0%, respectively, of Diovan HCT patients, compared with 0.0% in placebo-treated patients.
Liver function tests: Occasional elevations (greater than 150%) of liver chemistries occurred in Diovan HCT-treated patients.
Neutropenia: Neutropenia was observed in 0.6% of patients treated with Diovan HCT and 0.0% of patients treated with placebo.
Serum Electrolytes: See PRECAUTIONS.

OVERDOSAGE

Valsartan - Hydrochlorothiazide

Limited data are available related to overdosage in humans. The most likely manifestations of overdosage would be hypotension and tachycardia; bradycardia could occur from parasympathetic (vagal) stimulation. If symptomatic hypotension should occur, supportive treatment should be instituted.
Valsartan is not removed from the plasma by dialysis.
The degree to which hydrochlorothiazide is removed by hemodialysis has not been established. The most common signs and symptoms observed in patients are those caused by electrolyte depletion (hypokalemia, hypochloremia, hyponatremia) and dehydration resulting from excessive diuresis. If digitalis has also been administered, hypokalemia may accentuate cardiac arrhythmias.
In rats and marmosets, single oral doses of valsartan up to 1524 and 762 mg/kg in combination with hydrochlorothiazide at doses up to 476 and 238 mg/kg, respectively, were very well tolerated without any treatment-related effects. These no adverse effect doses in rats and marmosets, respectively, represent 93 and 56 times the maximum recommended human dose (MRHD) of valsartan and 188 and 113 times the MRHD of hydrochlorothiazide on a mg/m^2 basis. (Calculations assume an oral dose of 160 mg/day valsartan in combination with 25 mg/day hydrochlorothiazide and a 60-kg patient.)

Valsartan

Valsartan was without grossly observable adverse effects at single oral doses up to 2000 mg/kg in rats and up to 1000 mg/kg in marmosets, except for salivation and diarrhea in the rat and vomiting in the marmoset at the highest dose (31 and 18 times, respectively, the maximum recommended human dose on a mg/m^2 basis). (Calculations assume an oral dose of 160 mg/day and a 60-kg patient.)

Hydrochlorothiazide

The oral LD_{50} of hydrochlorothiazide is greater than 10 g/kg in both mice and rats, which represents 2027 and 4054 times, respectively, the maximum recommended human dose on a mg/m^2 basis. (Calculations assume an oral dose of 25 mg/day and a 60-kg patient.)

DOSAGE AND ADMINISTRATION

The recommended starting dose of valsartan is 80 mg once daily when used as monotherapy in patients who are not volume depleted. Valsartan may be used over a dose range of 80 mg to 320 mg daily, administered once-a-day. Hydrochlorothiazide is effective in doses of 12.5 to 50 mg once daily, and can be given at doses of 12.5 mg to 25 mg as Diovan HCT.
To minimize dose-independent side effects, it is usually appropriate to begin combination therapy only after a patient has failed to achieve the desired effect with monotherapy.
The side effects (see WARNINGS) of valsartan are generally rare and apparently independent of dose; those of

hydrochlorothiazide are a mixture of dose-dependent phenomena (primarily hypokalemia) and dose-independent phenomena (e.g., pancreatitis), the former much more common than the latter. Therapy with any combination of valsartan and hydrochlorothiazide will be associated with both sets of dose-independent side effects.

Replacement Therapy: The combination may be substituted for the titrated components.

Dose titration by Clinical Effect: Diovan HCT is available as tablets containing either valsartan 80 mg or 160 mg and hydrochlorothiazide 12.5 mg. A patient whose blood pressure is not adequately controlled with valsartan monotherapy (see above) may be switched to Diovan HCT, valsartan 80 mg/hydrochlorothiazide 12.5 mg once daily. If blood pressure remains uncontrolled after about 3-4 weeks of therapy, either valsartan or both components may be increased depending on clinical response. There are no studies evaluating doses of valsartan greater than 160 mg in combination with hydrochlorothiazide 25 mg.

A patient whose blood pressure is inadequately controlled by 25 mg once daily of hydrochlorothiazide, or is controlled but who experiences hypokalemia with this regimen, may be switched to Diovan HCT (valsartan 80 mg/hydrochlorothiazide 12.5 mg) once daily, reducing the dose of hydrochlorothiazide without reducing the overall expected antihypertensive response. The clinical response to Diovan HCT should be subsequently evaluated and if blood pressure remains uncontrolled after 3-4 weeks of therapy, the dose may be titrated up to valsartan 160 mg/hydrochlorothiazide 25 mg.

The maximal antihypertensive effect is attained about 4 weeks after initiation of therapy.

Patients with Renal Impairment: The usual regimens of therapy with Diovan HCT may be followed as long as the patient's creatinine clearance is >30 mL/min. In patients with more severe renal impairment, loop diuretics are preferred to thiazides, so Diovan HCT is not recommended.

Patients with Hepatic Impairment: Care should be exercised with dosing of Diovan HCT in patients with hepatic impairment.

Other: No initial dosage adjustment is required for elderly patients.

Diovan HCT may be administered with other antihypertensive agents.

Diovan HCT may be administered with or without food.

HOW SUPPLIED

Diovan HCT is available as tablets containing either valsartan 80 mg or 160 mg and hydrochlorothiazide 12.5 mg. Both strengths are packaged in bottles of 100 tablets and unit dose blister packages. Tablets are imprinted as follows:

80/12.5 mg Tablet - Light orange, imprinted CG on one side HGH on the other

Bottles of 100 .... NDC 0078-0314-05
Unit Dose (blister pack) .... NDC 0078-0314-06
Box of 100 (strips of 10)

160/12.5 mg Tablet - Dark red, imprinted CG on one side HHH on the other

Bottles of 100 .... NDC 0078-0315-05
Unit Dose (blister pack) .... NDC 0078-0315-06
Box of 100 (strips of 10)

Store at 25°C (77°F); excursions permitted to 15°C-30°C (59°F-86°F). Protect from moisture.

Dispense in tight container (USP).

REV: JUNE 2000 T2000-30

Shown in Product Identification Guide, page 325

EXELON® ℞

[ĕx ' ə-lŏn]
(rivastigmine tartrate)
Capsules
Rx only

The following prescribing information is based on official labeling in effect July 2000.

DESCRIPTION

Exelon® (rivastigmine tartrate) is a reversible cholinesterase inhibitor and is known chemically as (S)-N-Ethyl-N-methyl-3-[1-(dimethylamino)ethyl]-phenyl carbamate hydrogen-(2R,3R)-tartrate. Rivastigmine tartrate is commonly referred to in the pharmacological literature as SDZ ENA 713 or ENA 713. It has an empirical formula of $C_{14}H_{22}N_2O_2 \bullet C_4H_6O_6$ (hydrogen tartrate salt — hta salt) and a molecular weight of 400.43 (hta salt). Rivastigmine tartrate is a white to off-white, fine crystalline powder that is very soluble in water, soluble in ethanol and acetonitrile, slightly soluble in n-octanol and very slightly soluble in ethyl acetate. The distribution coefficient at 37°C in n-octanol/phosphate buffer solution pH 7 is 3.0.

O, CH_3, N, CH_2, CH_3, CH_3, N, CH_3, CH_3 • $C_4H_6O_6$

Exelon is supplied as capsules containing rivastigmine tartrate, equivalent to 1.5, 3.0, 4.5 and 6.0 mg of rivastigmine base for oral administration. Inactive ingredients are hydroxypropyl methylcellulose, magnesium stearate, microcrystalline cellulose, and silicone dioxide. Each hard-gelatin capsule contains gelatin, titanium dioxide and red and/or yellow iron oxides.

CLINICAL PHARMACOLOGY

Mechanism of Action

Pathological changes in Dementia of the Alzheimer type involve cholinergic neuronal pathways that project from the basal forebrain to the cerebral cortex and hippocampus. These pathways are thought to be intricately involved in memory, attention, learning, and other cognitive processes. While the precise mechanism of rivastigmine's action is unknown, it is postulated to exert its therapeutic effect by enhancing cholinergic function. This is accomplished by increasing the concentration of acetylcholine through reversible inhibition of its hydrolysis by cholinesterase. If this proposed mechanism is correct, Exelon's effect may lessen as the disease process advances and fewer cholinergic neurons remain functionally intact. There is no evidence that rivastigmine alters the course of the underlying dementing process. After a 6-mg dose of rivastigmine, anticholinesterase activity is present in CSF for about 10 hours, with a maximum inhibition of about 60% five hours after dosing.

Clinical Trial Data

The effectiveness of Exelon® (rivastigmine tartrate) as a treatment for Alzheimer's Disease is demonstrated by the results of two randomized, double-blind, placebo-controlled clinical investigations in patients with Alzheimer's Disease [diagnosed by NINCDS-ADRDA and DSM-IV criteria, Mini-Mental State Examination (MMSE) ≥10 and ≤26, and the Global Deterioration Scale (GDS)]. The mean age of patients participating in Exelon trials was 73 years with a range of 41-95. Approximately 59% of patients were women and 41% were men. The racial distribution was Caucasian 87%, Black 4% and Other races 9%.

Study Outcome Measures: In each study, the effectiveness of Exelon was evaluated using a dual outcome assessment strategy.

The ability of Exelon to improve cognitive performance was assessed with the cognitive subscale of the Alzheimer's Disease Assessment Scale (ADAS-cog), a multi item instrument that has been extensively validated in longitudinal cohorts of Alzheimer's Disease patients. The ADAS-cog examines selected aspects of cognitive performance including elements of memory, orientation, attention, reasoning, language and praxis. The ADAS-cog scoring range is from 0 to 70, with higher scores indicating greater cognitive impairment. Elderly normal adults may score as low as 0 or 1, but it is not unusual for non-demented adults to score slightly higher.

The patients recruited as participants in each study had mean scores on ADAS-cog of approximately 23 units, with a range from 1 to 61. Experience gained in longitudinal studies of ambulatory patients with mild to moderate Alzheimer's Disease suggest that they gain 6-12 units a year on the ADAS-cog. Lesser degrees of change, however, are seen in patients with very mild or very advanced disease because the ADAS-cog is not uniformly sensitive to change over the course of the disease. The annualized rate of decline in the placebo patients participating in Exelon trials was approximately 3-8 units per year.

The ability of Exelon to produce an overall clinical effect was assessed using a Clinician's Interview Based Impression of Change that required the use of caregiver information, the CIBIC-Plus. The CIBIC-Plus is not a single instrument and is not a standardized instrument like the ADAS-cog. Clinical trials for investigational drugs have used a variety of CIBIC formats, each different in terms of depth and structure. As such, results from a CIBIC-Plus reflect clinical experience from the trial or trials in which it was used and can not be compared directly with the results of CIBIC-Plus evaluations from other clinical trials. The CIBIC-Plus used in the Exelon trials was a structured instrument based on a comprehensive evaluation at baseline and subsequent time-points of three domains: patient cognition, behavior and functioning, including assessment of activities of daily living. It represents the assessment of a skilled clinician using validated scales based on his/her observation at interviews conducted separately with the patient and the caregiver familiar with the behavior of the patient over the interval rated. The CIBIC-Plus is scored as a seven point categorical rating, ranging from a score of 1, indicating "markedly improved," to a score of 4, indicating "no change" to a score of 7, indicating "marked worsening." The CIBIC-Plus has not been systematically compared directly to assessments not using information from caregivers (CIBIC) or other global methods.

U.S. Twenty-Six-Week Study

In a study of 26 weeks duration, 699 patients were randomized to either a dose range of 1-4 mg or 6-12 mg of Exelon per day or to placebo, each given in divided doses. The 26-week study was divided into a 12-week forced dose titration phase and a 14-week maintenance phase. The patients in the active treatment arms of the study were maintained at their highest tolerated dose within the respective range.

Effects on the ADAS-cog: Figure 1 illustrates the time course for the change from baseline in ADAS-cog scores for all three dose groups over the 26 weeks of the study. At 26 weeks of treatment, the mean differences in the ADAS-cog change scores for the Exelon-treated patients compared to the patients on placebo were 1.9 and 4.9 units for the 1-4 mg and 6-12 mg treatments, respectively. Both treatments were statistically significantly superior to placebo and the 6-12 mg/day range was significantly superior to the 1-4 mg/day range.

Figure 1: Time-course of the Change from Baseline in ADAS-cog Score for Patients Completing 26 Weeks of Treatment

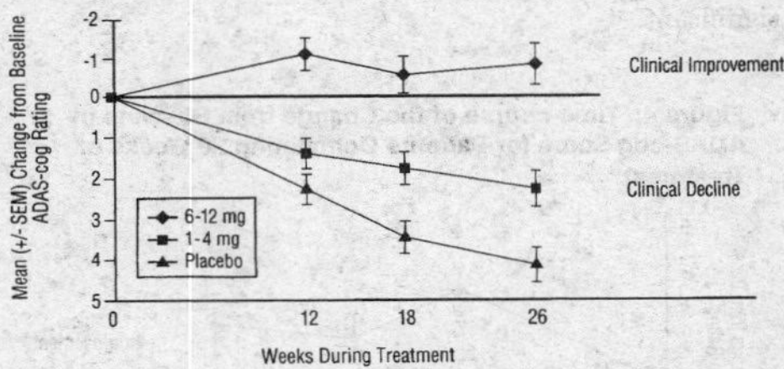

Figure 2 illustrates the cumulative percentages of patients from each of the three treatment groups who had attained at least the measure of improvement in ADAS-cog score shown on the X axis. Three change scores, (7-point and 4-point reductions from baseline or no change in score) have been identified for illustrative purposes, and the percent of patients in each group achieving that result is shown in the inset table.

The curves demonstrate that both patients assigned to Exelon and placebo have a wide range of responses, but that the Exelon groups are more likely to show the greater improvements. A curve for an effective treatment would be shifted to the left of the curve for placebo, while an ineffective or deleterious treatment would be superimposed upon, or shifted to the right of the curve for placebo, respectively.

Figure 2: Cumulative Percentage of Patients Completing 26 Weeks of Double-blind Treatment with Specified Changes from Baseline ADAS-cog Scores. The Percentages of Randomized Patients who Completed the Study were: Placebo 84%, 1-4 mg 85%, and 6-12 mg 65%.

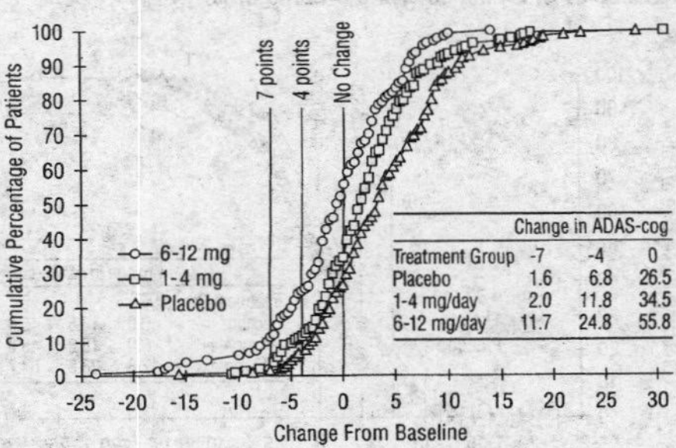

Treatment Group	Change in ADAS-cog -7	-4	0
Placebo	1.6	6.8	26.5
1-4 mg/day	2.0	11.8	34.5
6-12 mg/day	11.7	24.8	55.8

Effects on the CIBIC-Plus: Figure 3 is a histogram of the frequency distribution of CIBIC-Plus scores attained by patients assigned to each of the three treatment groups who completed 26 weeks of treatment. The mean Exelon-placebo differences for these groups of patients in the mean rating of change from baseline were 0.32 units and 0.35 units for 1-4 mg and 6-12 mg of Exelon, respectively. The mean ratings for the 6-12 mg/day and 1-4 mg/day groups were statistically significantly superior to placebo. The differences between the 6-12 mg/day and the 1-4 mg/day groups were statistically significant.

Figure 3: Frequency Distribution of CIBIC-Plus Scores at Week 26

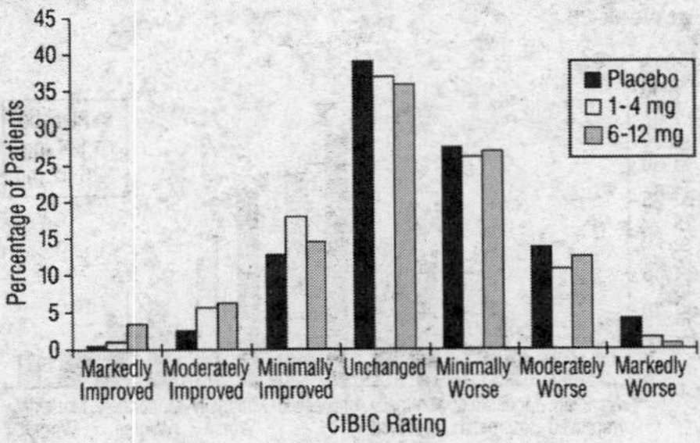

Global Twenty-Six-Week Study

In a second study of 26 weeks duration, 725 patients were randomized to either a dose range of 1-4 mg or 6-12 mg of Exelon per day or to placebo, each given in divided doses. The 26-week study was divided into a 12-week forced dose titration phase and a 14-week maintenance phase. The patients in the active treatment arms of the study were maintained at their highest tolerated dose within the respective range.

Effects on the ADAS-cog: Figure 4 illustrates the time course for the change from baseline in ADAS-cog scores for all three dose groups over the 26 weeks of the study. At 26 weeks of treatment, the mean differences in the ADAS-cog change scores for the Exelon-treated patients compared to

Continued on next page

Exelon Capsules—Cont.

the patients on placebo were 0.2 and 2.6 units for the 1-4 mg and 6-12 mg treatments, respectively. The 6-12 mg/day group was statistically significantly superior to placebo, as well as to the 1-4 mg/day group. The difference between the 1-4 mg/day group and placebo was not statistically significant.

Figure 4: Time-course of the Change from Baseline in ADAS-cog Score for Patients Completing 26 Weeks of Treatment

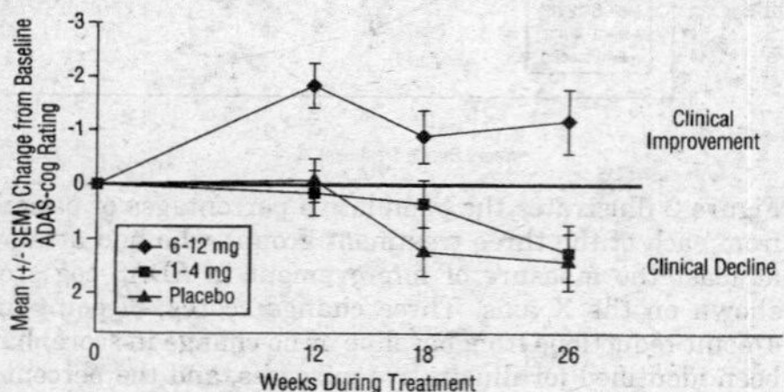

Figure 5 illustrates the cumulative percentages of patients from each of the three treatment groups who had attained at least the measure of improvement in ADAS-cog score shown on the X axis. Similar to the U.S. 26-week study, the curves demonstrate that both patients assigned to Exelon and placebo have a wide range of responses, but that the 6-12 mg/day Exelon group is more likely to show the greater improvements.

Figure 5: Cumulative Percentage of Patients Completing 26 Weeks of Double-blind Treatment with Specified Changes from Baseline ADAS- cog Scores. The Percentages of Randomized Patients who Completed the Study were: Placebo 87%, 1-4 mg 86%, and 6-12 mg 67%.

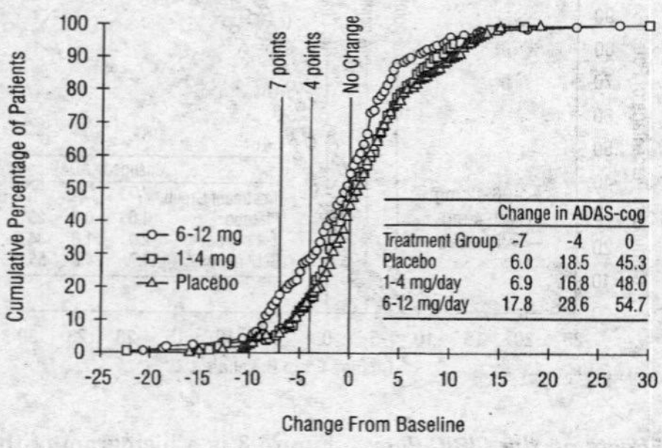

Treatment Group	-7	-4	0
Placebo	6.0	18.5	45.3
1-4 mg/day	6.9	16.8	48.0
6-12 mg/day	17.8	28.6	54.7

Effects on the CIBIC-Plus: Figure 6 is a histogram of the frequency distribution of CIBIC-Plus scores attained by patients assigned to each of the three treatment groups who completed 26 weeks of treatment. The mean Exelon-placebo differences for these groups of patients for the mean rating of change from baseline were 0.14 units and 0.41 units for 1-4 mg and 6-12 mg of Exelon, respectively. The mean ratings for the 6-12 mg/day group was statistically significantly superior to placebo. The comparison of the mean ratings for the 1-4 mg/day group and placebo group was not statistically significant.

Figure 6: Frequency Distribution of CIBIC-Plus Scores at Week 26

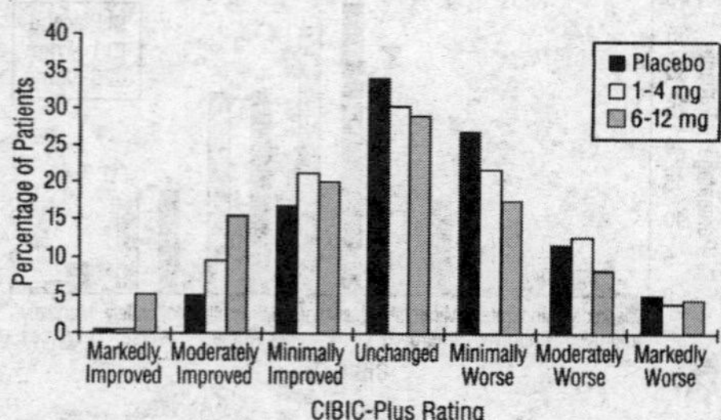

U.S. Fixed Dose Study

In a study of 26 weeks' duration, 702 patients were randomized to doses of 3, 6, or 9 mg/day of Exelon or to placebo, each given in divided doses. The fixed-dose study design, which included a 12-week forced titration phase and a 14-week maintenance phase, led to a high dropout rate in the 9 mg/day group because of poor tolerability. At 26 weeks of treatment, significant differences were observed for the ADAS-cog mean change from baseline for the 9 mg/day and 6 mg/day groups, compared to placebo. No significant differences were observed between any of the Exelon dose groups and placebo for the analysis of the CIBIC-Plus mean rating of change. Although no significant differences were observed between Exelon treatment groups, there was a trend toward numerical superiority with higher doses.

Age, Gender and Race: Patient's age, gender, or race did not predict clinical outcome to Exelon treatment.

Pharmacokinetics

Rivastigmine is well absorbed with absolute bioavailability of about 40% (3-mg dose). It shows linear pharmacokinetics up to 3 mg BID but is non-linear at higher doses. Doubling the dose from 3 to 6 mg BID results in a 3-fold increase in AUC. The elimination half-life is about 1.5 hours, with most elimination as metabolites via the urine.

Absorption: Rivastigmine is rapidly and completely absorbed. Peak plasma concentrations are reached in approximately 1 hour. Absolute bioavailability after a 3-mg dose is about 36%. Administration of Exelon with food delays absorption (t_{max}) by 90 min, lowers C_{max} by approximately 30% and increases AUC by approximately 30%.

Distribution: Rivastigmine is widely distributed throughout the body with a volume of distribution in the range of 1.8-2.7 L/kg. Rivastigmine penetrates the blood brain barrier, reaching CSF peak concentrations in 1.4-2.6 hours. Mean AUC_{1-12hr} ratio of CSF/plasma averaged 40 ± 0.5% following 1-6 mg BID doses.

Rivastigmine is about 40% bound to plasma proteins at concentrations of 1-400 ng/mL, which cover the therapeutic concentration range. Rivastigmine distributes equally between blood and plasma with a blood-to-plasma partition ratio of 0.9 at concentrations ranging from 1-400 ng/mL.

Metabolism: Rivastigmine is rapidly and extensively metabolized, primarily via cholinesterase-mediated hydrolysis to the decarbamylated metabolite. Based on evidence from *in vitro* and animal studies the major cytochrome P450 isozymes are minimally involved in rivastigmine metabolism. Consistent with these observations is the finding that no drug interactions related to cytochrome P450 have been observed in humans (see Drug-Drug Interactions).

Elimination: The major pathway of elimination is via the kidneys. Following administration of ^{14}C-rivastigmine to 6 healthy volunteers total recovery of radioactivity over 120 hours was 97% in urine and 0.4% in feces. No parent drug was detected in urine. The sulfate conjugate of the decarbamylated metabolite is the major component excreted in urine and represents 40% of the dose. Mean oral clearance of rivastigmine is 1.8 ± 0.6 L/min after 6 mg BID.

Special Populations

Hepatic Disease: Following a single 3-mg dose, mean oral clearance of rivastigmine was 60% lower in hepatically impaired patients (n=10, biopsy proven) than in healthy subjects (n=10). After multiple 6 mg BID oral dosing, the mean clearance of rivastigmine was 65% lower in mild (n=7, Child-Pugh score 5-6) and moderate (n=3, Child-Pugh score 7-9) hepatically impaired patients (biopsy proven, liver cirrhosis) than in healthy subjects (n=10). Dosage adjustment is not necessary in hepatically impaired patients as the dose of drug is individually titrated to tolerability.

Renal Disease: Following a single 3-mg dose, mean oral clearance of rivastigmine is 64% lower in moderately impaired renal patients (n=8, GFR=10-50 mL/min) than in healthy subjects (n=10, GFR≥60 mL/min); Cl/F=1.7 L/min (cv=45%) and 4.8 L/min (cv=80%), respectively. In severely impaired renal patients (n=8, GFR<10 mL/min), mean oral clearance of rivastigmine is 43% higher than in healthy subjects (n=10, GFR≥60 mL/min); Cl/F=6.9 L/min and 4.8 L/min, respectively. For unexplained reasons, the severely impaired renal patients had a higher clearance of rivastigmine than moderately impaired patients. However, dosage adjustment may not be necessary in renally impaired patients as the dose of the drug is individually titrated to tolerability.

Age: Following a single 2.5 mg oral dose to elderly volunteers (>60 years of age, n=24) and younger volunteers (n=24), mean oral clearance of rivastigmine was 30% lower in elderly (7 L/min) than in younger subjects (10 L/min).

Gender and Race: No specific pharmacokinetic study was conducted to investigate the effect of gender and race on the disposition of Exelon, but a population pharmacokinetic analysis indicates that gender (n=277 males and 348 females) and race (n=575 White, 34 Black, 4 Asian, and 12 Other) did not affect the clearance of Exelon.

Nicotine Use: Population PK analysis showed that nicotine use increases the oral clearance of rivastigmine by 23% (n=75 Smokers and 549 Nonsmokers).

Drug-Drug Interactions

Effect of Exelon on the Metabolism of Other Drugs: Rivastigmine is primarily metabolized through hydrolysis by esterases. Minimal metabolism occurs via the major cytochrome P450 isoenzymes. Based on *in vitro* studies, no pharmacokinetic drug interactions with drugs metabolized by the following isoenzyme systems are expected: CYP1A2, CYP2D6, CYP3A4/5, CYP2E1, CYP2C9, CYP2C8, or CYP2C19.

No pharmacokinetic interaction was observed between rivastigmine and digoxin, warfarin, diazepam, or fluoxetine in studies in healthy volunteers. The elevation of prothrombin time induced by warfarin is not affected by administration of Exelon.

Effect of Other Drugs on the Metabolism of Exelon: Drugs that induce or inhibit CYP450 metabolism are not expected to alter the metabolism of rivastigmine. Single dose pharmacokinetic studies demonstrated that the metabolism of rivastigmine is not significantly affected by concurrent administration of digoxin, warfarin, diazepam, or fluoxetine.

Population PK analysis with a database of 625 patients showed that the pharmacokinetics of rivastigmine were not influenced by commonly prescribed medications such as antacids (n=77), antihypertensives (n=72), β-blockers (n=42), calcium channel blockers (n=75), antidiabetics (n=21), nonsteroidal anti-inflammatory drugs (n=79), estrogens (n=70), salicylate analgesics (n=177), antianginals (n=35), and antihistamines (n=15). In addition, in clinical trials, no increased risk of clinically relevant untoward effects was observed in patients treated concomitantly with Exelon and these agents.

INDICATIONS AND USAGE

Exelon® (rivastigmine tartrate) is indicated for the treatment of mild to moderate dementia of the Alzheimer's type.

CONTRAINDICATIONS

Exelon® (rivastigmine tartrate) is contraindicated in patients with known hypersensitivity to rivastigmine, other carbamate derivatives or other components of the formulation (see DESCRIPTION).

WARNINGS

Gastrointestinal Adverse Reactions

Exelon® (rivastigmine tartrate) use is associated with significant gastrointestinal adverse reactions, including nausea and vomiting, anorexia, and weight loss.

Nausea and Vomiting: **In the controlled clinical trials, 47% of the patients treated with an Exelon dose in the therapeutic range of 6-12 mg/day (n=1189) developed nausea (compared with 12% in placebo). A total of 31% of Exelon-treated patients developed at least one episode of vomiting (compared with 6% for placebo). The rate of vomiting was higher during the titration phase (24% vs. 3% for placebo) than in the maintenance phase (14% vs. 3% for placebo). The rates were higher in women than men. Five percent of patients discontinued for vomiting, compared to less than 1% for patients on placebo. Vomiting was severe in 2% of Exelon-treated patients and was rated as mild or moderate each in 14% of patients. The rate of nausea was higher during the titration phase (43% vs. 9% for placebo) than in the maintenance phase (17% vs. 4% for placebo).**

Weight Loss: **In the controlled trials, approximately 26% of women on high doses of Exelon (greater than 9 mg/day) had weight loss of equal to or greater than 7% of their baseline weight compared to 6% in the placebo-treated patients. About 18% of the males in the high dose group experienced a similar degree of weight loss compared to 4% in placebo-treated patients. It is not clear how much of the weight loss was associated with anorexia, nausea, vomiting, and the diarrhea associated with the drug.**

Anorexia: In the controlled clinical trials, of the patients treated with an Exelon dose of 6-12 mg/day, 17% developed anorexia compared to 3% of the placebo patients. Neither the time course or the severity of the anorexia is known.

Peptic Ulcers/Gastrointestinal Bleeding: Because of their pharmacological action, cholinesterase inhibitors may be expected to increase gastric acid secretion due to increased cholinergic activity. Therefore, patients should be monitored closely for symptoms of active or occult gastrointestinal bleeding, especially those at increased risk for developing ulcers, e.g., those with a history of ulcer disease or those receiving concurrent nonsteroidal anti-inflammatory drugs (NSAIDS). Clinical studies of Exelon have shown no significant increase, relative to placebo, in the incidence of either peptic ulcer disease or gastrointestinal bleeding.

Anesthesia

Exelon as a cholinesterase inhibitor, is likely to exaggerate succinylcholine-type muscle relaxation during anesthesia.

Cardiovascular Conditions

Drugs that increase cholinergic activity may have vagotonic effects on heart rate (e.g., bradycardia). The potential for this action may be particularly important to patients with "sick sinus syndrome" or other supraventricular cardiac conduction conditions. In clinical trials, Exelon was not associated with any increased incidence of cardiovascular adverse events, heart rate or blood pressure changes, or ECG abnormalities. Syncopal episodes have been reported in 3% of patients receiving 6-12 mg/day of Exelon, compared to 2% of placebo patients.

Genitourinary

Although this was not observed in clinical trials of Exelon, drugs that increase cholinergic activity may cause urinary obstruction.

Neurological Conditions

Seizures: Drugs that increase cholinergic activity are believed to have some potential for causing seizures. However, seizure activity also may be a manifestation of Alzheimer's Disease.

Pulmonary Conditions

Like other drugs that increase cholinergic activity, Exelon should be used with care in patients with a history of asthma or obstructive pulmonary disease.

PRECAUTIONS

Information for Patients and Caregivers

Caregivers should be advised of the high incidence of nausea and vomiting associated with the use of the drug along with the possibility of anorexia and weight loss. Caregivers should be encouraged to monitor for these adverse events and inform the physician if they occur.

Drug-Drug Interactions

Effect of Exelon® (rivastigmine tartrate) on the Metabolism of Other Drugs: Rivastigmine is primarily metabolized through hydrolysis by esterases. Minimal metabolism occurs via the major cytochrome P450 isoenzymes. Based on *in vitro* studies, no pharmacokinetic drug interactions with drugs metabolized by the following isoenzyme systems are expected: CYP1A2, CYP2D6, CYP3A4/5, CYP2E1, CYP2C9, CYP2C8, or CYP2C19.

No pharmacokinetic interaction was observed between rivastigmine and digoxin, warfarin, diazepam, or fluoxetine in studies in healthy volunteers. The elevation of prothrombin time induced by warfarin is not affected by administration of Exelon.

Effect of Other Drugs on the Metabolism of Exelon: Drugs that induce or inhibit CYP450 metabolism are not expected to alter the metabolism of rivastigmine. Single dose pharmacokinetic studies demonstrated that the metabolism of rivastigmine is not significantly affected by concurrent administration of digoxin, warfarin, diazepam, or fluoxetine.

Population PK analysis with a database of 625 patients showed that the pharmacokinetics of rivastigmine were not influenced by commonly prescribed medications such as antacids (n=77), antihypertensives (n=72), β-blockers (n=42), calcium channel blockers (n=75), antidiabetics (n=21), nonsteroidal anti-inflammatory drugs (n=79), estrogens (n=70), salicylate analgesics (n=177), antianginals (n=35), and antihistamines (n=15).

Use with Anticholinergics: Because of their mechanism of action, cholinesterase inhibitors have the potential to interfere with the activity of anticholinergic medications.

Use with Cholinomimetics and Other Cholinesterase Inhibitors: A synergistic effect may be expected when cholinesterase inhibitors are given concurrently with succinylcholine, similar neuromuscular blocking agents or cholinergic agonists such as bethanechol.

Carcinogenesis, Mutagenesis, Impairment of Fertility

In carcinogenicity studies conducted at dose levels up to 1.1 mg-base/kg/day in rats and 1.6 mg-base/kg/day in mice, rivastigmine was not carcinogenic. These dose levels are approximately 0.9 times and 0.7 times the maximum recommended human daily dose of 12 mg per day on a mg/m^2 basis.

Rivastigmine was clastogenic in two *in vitro* assays in the presence, but not the absence, of metabolic activation. It caused structural chromosomal aberrations in V79 Chinese hamster lung cells and both structural and numerical (polyploidy) chromosomal aberrations in human peripheral blood lymphocytes. Rivastigmine was not genotoxic in three *in vitro* assays: the Ames test, the unscheduled DNA synthesis (UDS) test in rat hepatocytes (a test for induction of DNA repair synthesis), and the HGPRT test in V79 Chinese hamster cells. Rivastigmine was not clastogenic in the *in vivo* mouse micronucleus test.

Rivastigmine had no effect on fertility or reproductive performance in the rat at dose levels up to 1.1 mg-base/kg/day. This dose is approximately 0.9 times the maximum recommended human daily dose of 12 mg/day on a mg/m^2 basis.

Pregnancy

Pregnancy Category B: Reproduction studies conducted in pregnant rats at doses up to 2.3 mg-base/kg/day (approximately 2 times the maximum recommended human dose on a mg/m^2 basis) and in pregnant rabbits at doses up to 2.3 mg-base/kg/day (approximately 4 times the maximum recommended human dose on a mg/m^2 basis) revealed no evidence of teratogenicity. Studies in rats showed slightly decreased fetal/pup weights, usually at doses causing some maternal toxicity; decreased weights were seen at doses which were several fold lower than the maximum recommended human dose on a mg/m^2 basis. There are no adequate or well-controlled studies in pregnant women. Because animal reproduction studies are not always predictive of human response, Exelon should be used during pregnancy only if the potential benefit justifies the potential risk to the fetus.

Nursing Mothers

It is not known whether rivastigmine is excreted in human breast milk. Exelon has no indication for use in nursing mothers.

Pediatric Use

There are no adequate and well-controlled trials documenting the safety and efficacy of Exelon in any illness occurring in children.

ADVERSE REACTIONS

Adverse Events Leading to Discontinuation

The rate of discontinuation due to adverse events in controlled clinical trials of Exelon® (rivastigmine tartrate) was 15% for patients receiving 6-12 mg/day compared to 5% for patients on placebo during forced weekly dose titration. While on a maintenance dose, the rates were 6% for patients on Exelon compared to 4% for those on placebo.

The most common adverse events leading to discontinuation, defined as those occurring in at least 2% of patients and at twice the incidence seen in placebo patients, are shown in Table 1.

[See table 1 above]

Table 1. Most Frequent Adverse Events Leading to Withdrawal from Clinical Trials during Titration and Maintenance in Patients Receiving 6–12 mg/day Exelon® Using a Forced Dose Titration

Study Phase	Titration		Maintenance		Overall	
	Placebo (n=868)	Exelon ≥6-12 mg/day (n=1189)	Placebo (n=788)	Exelon ≥6-12 mg/day (n=987)	Placebo (n=868)	Exelon ≥6-12 mg/day (n=1189)
Event/% Discontinuing						
Nausea	<1	8	<1	1	1	8
Vomiting	<1	4	<1	1	<1	5
Anorexia	0	2	<1	1	<1	3
Dizziness	<1	2	<1	1	<1	2

Most Frequent Adverse Clinical Events Seen in Association with the Use of Exelon

The most common adverse events, defined as those occurring at a frequency of at least 5% and twice the placebo rate, are largely predicted by Exelon's cholinergic effects. These include nausea, vomiting, anorexia, dyspepsia, and asthenia.

Gastrointestinal Adverse Reactions

Exelon use is associated with significant nausea, vomiting, and weight loss (see WARNINGS).

Adverse Events Reported in Controlled Trials

Table 2 lists treatment emergent signs and symptoms that were reported in at least 2% of patients in placebo-controlled trials and for which the rate of occurrence was greater for patients treated with Exelon doses of 6-12 mg/day than for those treated with placebo. The prescriber should be aware that these figures cannot be used to predict the frequency of adverse events in the course of usual medical practice when patient characteristics and other factors may differ from those prevailing during clinical studies. Similarly, the cited frequencies cannot be directly compared with figures obtained from other clinical investigations involving different treatments, uses, or investigators. An inspection of these frequencies, however, does provide the prescriber with one basis by which to estimate the relative contribution of drug and non-drug factors to the adverse event incidences in the population studied.

In general, adverse reactions were less frequent later in the course of treatment.

No systematic effect of race or age could be determined on the incidence of adverse events in the controlled studies. Nausea, vomiting and weight loss were more frequent in women than men.

Table 2. Adverse Events Reported in Controlled Clinical Trials in at Least 2% of Patients Receiving Exelon® (6-12 mg/day) and at a Higher Frequency than Placebo-treated Patients

Body System/Adverse Event	Placebo (n=868)	Exelon (6-12 mg/day) (n=1189)
Percent of Patients with any Adverse Event	79	92
Autonomic Nervous System		
Sweating increased	1	4
Syncope	2	3
Body as a Whole		
Accidental Trauma	9	10
Fatigue	5	9
Asthenia	2	6
Malaise	2	5
Influenza-like Symptoms	2	3
Weight Decrease	<1	3
Cardiovascular Disorders, General		
Hypertension	2	3
Central and Peripheral Nervous System		
Dizziness	11	21
Headache	12	17
Somnolence	3	5
Tremor	1	4
Gastrointestinal System		
Nausea	12	47
Vomiting	6	31
Diarrhea	11	19
Anorexia	3	17
Abdominal Pain	6	13
Dyspepsia	4	9
Constipation	4	5
Flatulence	2	4
Eructation	1	2
Psychiatric Disorders		
Insomnia	7	9
Confusion	7	8
Depression	4	6
Anxiety	3	5
Hallucination	3	4
Aggressive Reaction	2	3
Resistance Mechanism Disorders		
Urinary Tract Infection	6	7
Respiratory System		
Rhinitis	3	4

Other adverse events observed at a rate of 2% or more on Exelon 6-12 mg/day but at a greater or equal rate on placebo were chest pain, peripheral edema, vertigo, back pain, arthralgia, pain, bone fracture, agitation, nervousness, delusion, paranoid reaction, upper respiratory tract infections, infection (general), coughing, pharyngitis, bronchitis, rash (general), urinary incontinence.

Other Adverse Events Observed During Clinical Trials

Exelon has been administered to over 5297 individuals during clinical trials worldwide. Of these, 4326 patients have been treated for at least 3 months, 3407 patients have been treated for at least 6 months, 2150 patients have been treated for 1 year, 1250 have been treated for 2 years, and 168 have been treated for over 3 years. With regard to exposure to the highest dose, 2809 patients were exposed to doses of 10-12 mg, 2615 patients treated for 3 months, 2328 patients treated for 6 months, 1378 patients treated for 1 year, 917 patients treated for 2 years, and 129 treated for over 3 years.

Treatment emergent signs and symptoms that occurred during 8 controlled clinical trials and 9 open-label trials in North America, Western Europe, Australia, South Africa, and Japan were recorded as adverse events by the clinical investigators using terminology of their own choosing. To provide an overall estimate of the proportion of individuals having similar types of events, the events were grouped into a smaller number of standardized categories using a modified WHO dictionary, and event frequencies were calculated across all studies. These categories are used in the listing below. The frequencies represent the proportion of 5297 patients from these trials who experienced that event while receiving Exelon. All adverse events occurring in at least 6 patients (approximately 0.1%) are included, except for those already listed elsewhere in labeling, WHO terms too general to be informative, relatively minor events, or events unlikely to be drug caused. Events are classified by body system and listed using the following definitions: frequent adverse events — those occurring in at least 1/100 patients; infrequent adverse events — those occurring in 1/100 to 1/1000 patients. These adverse events are not necessarily related to Exelon treatment and in most cases were observed at a similar frequency in placebo-treated patients in the controlled studies.

Autonomic Nervous System: *Infrequent:* Cold clammy skin, dry mouth, flushing, increased saliva.

Body as a Whole: *Frequent:* Accidental trauma, fever, edema, allergy, hot flushes, rigors. *Infrequent:* Edema periorbital or facial, hypothermia, edema, feeling cold, halitosis.

Cardiovascular System: *Frequent:* Hypotension, postural hypotension, cardiac failure.

Central and Peripheral Nervous System: *Frequent:* Abnormal gait, ataxia, paraesthesia, convulsions. *Infrequent:* Paresis, apraxia, aphasia, dysphonia, hyperkinesia, hyperreflexia, hypertonia, hypoesthesia, hypokinesia, migraine, neuralgia, nystagmus, peripheral neuropathy.

Endocrine System: *Infrequent:* Goitre, hypothyroidism.

Gastrointestinal System: *Frequent:* Fecal incontinence, gastritis. *Infrequent:* Dysphagia, esophagitis, gastric ulcer, gastritis, gastrosophageal reflux, GI hemorrhage, hernia, intestinal obstruction, melena, rectal hemorrhage, gastroenteritis, ulcerative stomatitis, duodenal ulcer, hematemesis, gingivitis, tenesmus, pancreatitis, colitis, glossitis.

Hearing and Vestibular Disorders: *Frequent:* Tinnitus.

Heart Rate and Rhythm Disorders: *Frequent:* Atrial fibrillation, bradycardia, palpitation. *Infrequent:* AV block, bundle branch block, sick sinus syndrome, cardiac arrest, supraventricular tachycardia, extrasystoles, tachycardia.

Liver and Biliary System Disorders: *Infrequent:* Abnormal hepatic function, cholecystitis.

Metabolic and Nutritional Disorders: *Frequent:* Dehydration, hypokalemia. *Infrequent:* Diabetes mellitus, gout, hypercholesterolemia, hyperlipemia, hypoglycemia, cachexia, thirst, hyperglycemia, hyponatremia.

Musculoskeletal Disorders: *Frequent:* Arthritis, leg cramps, myalgia. *Infrequent:* Cramps, hernia, muscle weakness.

Myo-, Endo-, Pericardial and Valve Disorders: *Frequent:* Angina pectoris, myocardial infarction.

Platelet, Bleeding, and Clotting Disorders: *Frequent:* Epistaxis. *Infrequent:* Hematoma, thrombocytopenia, purpura.

Psychiatric Disorders: *Frequent:* Paranoid reaction, confusion. *Infrequent:* Abnormal dreaming, amnesia, apathy, delirium, dementia, depersonalization, emotional lability, impaired concentration, decreased libido, personality disorder, suicide attempt, increased libido, neurosis, suicidal ideation, psychosis.

Red Blood Cell Disorders: *Frequent:* Anemia. *Infrequent:* Hypochromic anemia.

Reproductive Disorders (Female & Male): *Infrequent:* Breast pain, impotence, atrophic vaginitis.

Resistance Mechanism Disorders: *Infrequent:* Cellulitis, cystitis, herpes simplex, otitis media.

Respiratory System: *Infrequent:* Bronchospasm, laryngitis, apnea.

Skin and Appendages: *Frequent:* Rashes of various kinds (maculopapular, eczema, bullous, exfoliative, psoriaform, erythematous). *Infrequent:* Alopecia, skin ulceration, urticaria, dermatitis contact.

Special Senses: *Infrequent:* Perversion of taste, loss of taste.

Urinary System Disorders: *Frequent:* Hematuria. *Infrequent:* Albuminuria, oliguria, acute renal failure, dysuria,

Continued on next page

Exelon Capsules—Cont.

micturition urgency, nocturia, polyuria, renal calculus, urinary retention.

Vascular (extracardiac) Disorders: *Infrequent:* Hemorrhoids, peripheral ischemia, pulmonary embolism, thrombosis, thrombophlebitis deep, aneurysm, hemorrhage intracranial.

Vision Disorders: *Frequent:* Cataract. *Infrequent:* Conjunctival hemorrhage, blepharitis, diplopia, eye pain, glaucoma.

White Cell and Resistance Disorders: *Infrequent:* Lymphadenopathy, leukocytosis.

OVERDOSAGE

Because strategies for the management of overdose are continually evolving, it is advisable to contact a Poison Control Center to determine the latest recommendations for the management of an overdose of any drug.

As Exelon® (rivastigmine tartrate) has a short plasma half-life of about one hour and a moderate duration of acetylcholinesterase inhibition of 8-10 hours, it is recommended that in cases of asymptomatic overdoses, no further dose of Exelon should be administered for the next 24 hours.

As in any case of overdose, general supportive measures should be utilized. Overdosage with cholinesterase inhibitors can result in cholinergic crisis characterized by severe nausea, vomiting, salivation, sweating, bradycardia, hypotension, respiratory depression, collapse and convulsions. Increasing muscle weakness is a possibility and may result in death if respiratory muscles are involved. Atypical responses in blood pressure and heart rate have been reported with other drugs that increase cholinergic activity when co-administered with quaternary anticholinergics such as glycopyrrolate. Due to the short half-life of Exelon, dialysis (hemodialysis, peritoneal dialysis, or hemofiltration) would not be clinically indicated in the event of an overdose.

In overdoses accompanied by severe nausea and vomiting, the use of antiemetics should be considered. In a documented case of a 46 mg overdose with Exelon, the patient experienced vomiting, incontinence, hypertension, psychomotor retardation, and loss of consciousness. The patient fully recovered within 24 hours and conservative management was all that was required for treatment.

DOSAGE AND ADMINISTRATION

The dosage of Exelon® (rivastigmine tartrate) shown to be effective in controlled clinical trials is 6-12 mg/day, given as twice a day dosing (daily doses of 3 to 6 mg BID). There is evidence from the clinical trials that doses at the higher end of this range may be more beneficial.

The recommended starting dose of Exelon is 1.5 mg twice a day. If this dose is well tolerated, after a minimum of two weeks of treatment, the dose may be increased to 3 mg twice a day. Subsequent increases to 4.5 mg BID and 6 mg BID should be attempted after a minimum of 2 weeks at the previous dose. If adverse effects (e.g., nausea, vomiting, abdominal pain, loss of appetite) cause intolerance during treatment, the patient should be instructed to discontinue treatment for several doses and then restart at the same or next lower dose level. The maximum dose is 6 mg BID (12 mg/day).

Exelon should be taken with food in divided doses in the morning and evening.

HOW SUPPLIED

Exelon® (rivastigmine tartrate) capsules equivalent to 1.5 mg, 3.0 mg, 4.5 mg, or 6.0 mg of rivastigmine base are available as follows:

1.5 mg Capsule – yellow, "Exelon 1,5 mg" is printed in red on the body of the capsule.

Bottles of 60 .... NDC 0078-0323-44
Bottles of 500 .... NDC 0078-0323-08
Unit Dose (blister pack)
Box of 100 (strips of 10) .... NDC 0078-0323-06

3.0 mg Capsule – orange, "Exelon 3 mg" is printed in red on the body of the capsule.

Bottles of 60 .... NDC 0078-0324-44
Bottles of 500 .... NDC 0078-0324-08
Unit Dose (blister pack)
Box of 100 (strips of 10) .... NDC 0078-0324-06

4.5 mg Capsule – red, "Exelon 4,5 mg" is printed in white on the body of the capsule.

Bottles of 60 .... NDC 0078-0325-44
Bottles of 500 .... NDC 0078-0325-08
Unit Dose (blister pack)
Box of 100 (strips of 10) .... NDC 0078-0325-06

6.0 mg Capsule – orange and red, "Exelon 6 mg" is printed in red on the body of the capsule.

Bottles of 60 .... NDC 0078-0326-44
Bottles of 500 .... NDC 0078-0326-08
Unit Dose (blister pack)
Box of 100 (strips of 10) .... NDC 0078-0326-06

Store below 77°F (25°C) in a tight container.

APRIL 2000 T2000-11

Manufactured by
Novartis Pharma AG
Basle, Switzerland
Manufactured for
Novartis Pharmaceuticals Corporation
East Hanover, New Jersey 07936

Shown in Product Identification Guide, page 325

EXELON® ℞

[ĕx' ə-lŏn]
(rivastigmine tartrate)
Oral Solution
Rx only

The following prescribing information is based on official labeling in effect July 2000.

DESCRIPTION

Exelon® (rivastigmine tartrate) is a reversible cholinesterase inhibitor and is known chemically as (S)-N-Ethyl-N-methyl-3-[1-(dimethylamino)ethyl]-phenyl carbamate hydrogen-(2R,3R)-tartrate. Rivastigmine tartrate is commonly referred to in the pharmacological literature as SDZ ENA 713 or ENA 713. It has an empirical formula of $C_{14}H_{22}N_2O_2 \cdot C_4H_6O_6$ (hydrogen tartrate salt—hta salt) and a molecular weight of 400.43 (hta salt). Rivastigmine tartrate is a white to off-white, fine crystalline powder that is very soluble in water, soluble in ethanol and acetonitrile, slightly soluble in n-octanol and very slightly soluble in ethyl acetate. The distribution coefficient at 37°C in n-octanol/phosphate buffer solution pH 7 is 3.0.

Exelon Oral Solution is supplied as a solution containing rivastigmine tartrate, equivalent to 2 mg/mL of rivastigmine base for oral administration. Inactive ingredients are citric acid, D&C yellow #10, purified water, sodium benzoate and sodium citrate.

CLINICAL PHARMACOLOGY

Mechanism of Action

Pathological changes in Dementia of the Alzheimer type involve cholinergic neuronal pathways that project from the basal forebrain to the cerebral cortex and hippocampus. These pathways are thought to be intricately involved in memory, attention, learning, and other cognitive processes. While the precise mechanism of rivastigmine's action is unknown, it is postulated to exert its therapeutic effect by enhancing cholinergic function. This is accomplished by increasing the concentration of acetylcholine through reversible inhibition of its hydrolysis by cholinesterase. If this proposed mechanism is correct, Exelon's effect may lessen as the disease process advances and fewer cholinergic neurons remain functionally intact. There is no evidence that rivastigmine alters the course of the underlying dementing process. After a 6-mg dose of rivastigmine, anticholinesterase activity is present in CSF for about 10 hours, with a maximum inhibition of about 60% five hours after dosing.

Clinical Trial Data

The effectiveness of Exelon® (rivastigmine tartrate) as a treatment for Alzheimer's Disease is demonstrated by the results of two randomized, double-blind, placebo-controlled clinical investigations in patients with Alzheimer's Disease [diagnosed by NINCDS-ADRDA and DSM-IV criteria, Mini-Mental State Examination (MMSE) ≥10 and ≤26, and the Global Deterioration Scale (GDS)]. The mean age of patients participating in Exelon trials was 73 years with a range of 41–95. Approximately 59% of patients were women and 41% were men. The racial distribution was Caucasian 87%, Black 4% and Other races 9%.

Study Outcome Measures: In each study, the effectiveness of Exelon was evaluated using a dual outcome assessment strategy.

The ability of Exelon to improve cognitive performance was assessed with the cognitive subscale of the Alzheimer's Disease Assessment Scale (ADAS-cog), a multi-item instrument that has been extensively validated in longitudinal cohorts of Alzheimer's Disease patients. The ADAS-cog examines selected aspects of cognitive performance including elements of memory, orientation, attention, reasoning, language and praxis. The ADAS-cog scoring range is from 0 to 70, with higher scores indicating greater cognitive impairment. Elderly normal adults may score as low as 0 or 1, but it is not unusual for non-demented adults to score slightly higher.

The patients recruited as participants in each study had mean scores on ADAS-cog of approximately 23 units, with a range from 1 to 61. Experience gained in longitudinal studies of ambulatory patients with mild to moderate Alzheimer's Disease suggest that they gain 6–12 units a year on the ADAS-cog. Lesser degrees of change, however, are seen in patients with very mild or very advanced disease because the ADAS-cog is not uniformly sensitive to change over the course of the disease. The annualized rate of decline in the placebo patients participating in Exelon trials was approximately 3–8 units per year.

The ability of Exelon to produce an overall clinical effect was assessed using a Clinician's Interview Based Impression of Change that required the use of caregiver information, the CIBIC-Plus. The CIBIC-Plus is not a single instrument and is not a standardized instrument like the ADAS-cog. Clinical trials for investigational drugs have used a variety of CIBIC formats, each different in terms of depth and structure. As such, results from a CIBIC-Plus reflect clinical experience from the trial or trials in which it was used and can not be compared directly with the results of CIBIC-Plus evaluations from other clinical trials. The CIBIC-Plus used in the Exelon trials was a structured instrument based on a comprehensive evaluation at baseline and subsequent time-points of three domains: patient cognition, behavior and functioning, including assessment of activities of daily living. It represents the assessment of a skilled clinician using validated scales based on his/her observation at interviews conducted separately with the patient and the caregiver familiar with the behavior of the patient over the interval rated. The CIBIC-Plus is scored as a seven point categorical rating, ranging from a score of 1, indicating "markedly improved," to a score of 4, indicating "no change" to a score of 7, indicating "marked worsening." The CIBIC-Plus has not been systematically compared directly to assessments not using information from caregivers (CIBIC) or other global methods.

U.S. Twenty-Six-Week Study

In a study of 26 weeks duration, 699 patients were randomized to either a dose range of 1–4 mg or 6–12 mg of Exelon per day or to placebo, each given in divided doses. The 26-week study was divided into a 12-week forced dose titration phase and a 14-week maintenance phase. The patients in the active treatment arms of the study were maintained at their highest tolerated dose within the respective range.

Effects on the ADAS-cog: Figure 1 illustrates the time course for the change from baseline in ADAS-cog scores for all three dose groups over the 26 weeks of the study. At 26 weeks of treatment, the mean differences in the ADAS-cog change scores for the Exelon-treated patients compared to the patients on placebo were 1.9 and 4.9 units for the 1–4 mg and 6–12 mg treatments, respectively. Both treatments were statistically significantly superior to placebo and the 6–12 mg/day range was significantly superior to the 1–4 mg/day range.

Figure 1: Time-course of the Change from Baseline in ADAS-cog Score for Patients Completing 26 Weeks of Treatment

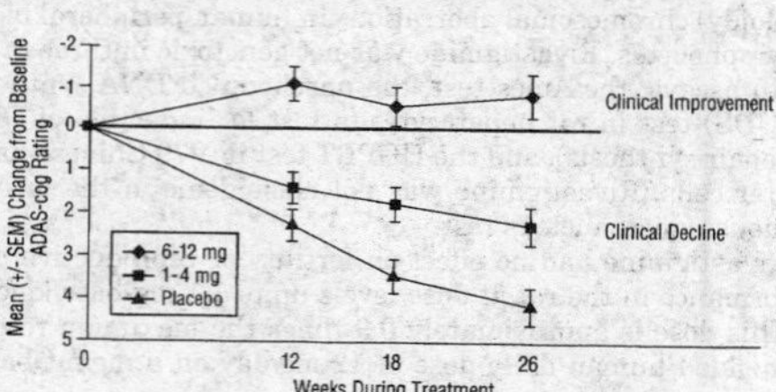

Figure 2 illustrates the cumulative percentages of patients from each of the three treatment groups who had attained at least the measure of improvement in ADAS-cog score shown on the X axis. Three change scores, (7-point and 4-point reductions from baseline or no change in score) have been identified for illustrative purposes, and the percent of patients in each group achieving that result is shown in the inset table.

The curves demonstrate that both patients assigned to Exelon and placebo have a wide range of responses, but that the Exelon groups are more likely to show the greater improvements. A curve for an effective treatment would be shifted to the left of the curve for placebo, while an ineffective or deleterious treatment would be superimposed upon, or shifted to the right of the curve for placebo, respectively.

Figure 2: Cumulative Percentage of Patients Completing 26 Weeks of Double-blind Treatment with Specified Changes from Baseline ADAS-cog Scores. The Percentages of Randomized Patients who Completed the Study were: Placebo 84%, 1-4 mg 85%, and 6-12 mg 65%.

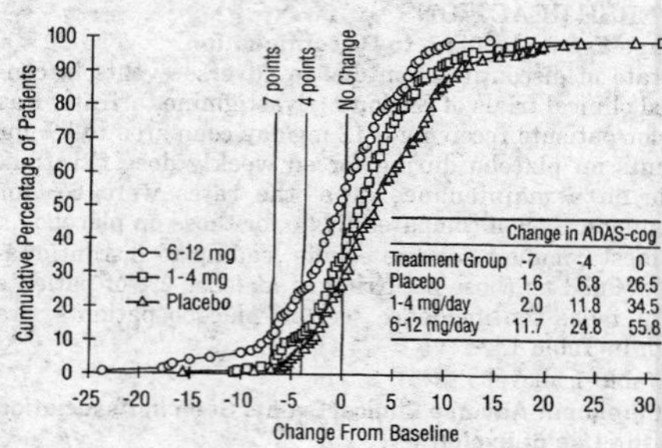

Effects on the CIBIC-Plus: Figure 3 is a histogram of the frequency distribution of CIBIC-Plus scores attained by patients assigned to each of the three treatment groups who completed 26 weeks of treatment. The mean Exelon-placebo differences for these groups of patients in the mean rating of change from baseline were 0.32 units and 0.35 units for 1–4 mg and 6–12 mg of Exelon, respectively. The mean ratings for the 6–12 mg/day and 1-4 mg/day groups were statistically significantly superior to placebo. The differences between the 6–12 mg/day and the 1–4 mg/day groups were statistically significant.

Figure 3: Frequency Distribution of CIBIC-Plus Scores at Week 26

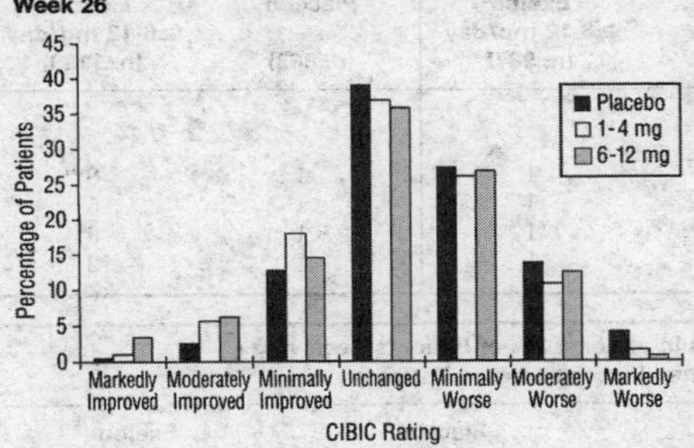

Global Twenty-Six-Week Study

In a second study of 26 weeks duration, 725 patients were randomized to either a dose range of 1–4 mg or 6–12 mg of Exelon per day or to placebo, each given in divided doses. The 26-week study was divided into a 12-week forced dose titration phase and a 14-week maintenance phase. The patients in the active treatment arms of the study were maintained at their highest tolerated dose within the respective range.

Effects on the ADAS-cog: Figure 4 illustrates the time course for the change from baseline in ADAS-cog scores for all three dose groups over the 26 weeks of the study. At 26 weeks of treatment, the mean differences in the ADAS-cog change scores for the Exelon-treated patients compared to the patients on placebo were 0.2 and 2.6 units for the 1–4 mg and 6–12 mg treatments, respectively. The 6–12 mg/day group was statistically significantly superior to placebo, as well as to the 1–4 mg/day group. The difference between the 1–4 mg/day group and placebo was not statistically significant.

Figure 4: Time-course of the Change from Baseline in ADAS-cog Score for Patients Completing 26 Weeks of Treatment

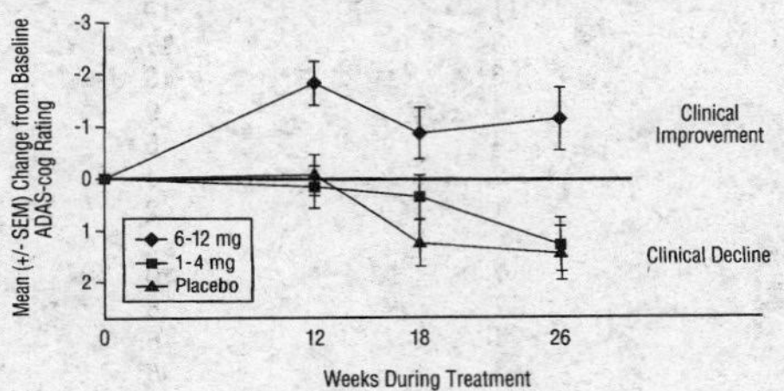

Figure 5 illustrates the cumulative percentages of patients from each of the three treatment groups who had attained at least the measure of improvement in ADAS-cog score shown on the X axis. Similar to the U.S. 26-week study, the curves demonstrate that both patients assigned to Exelon and placebo have a wide range of responses, but that the 6–12 mg/day Exelon group is more likely to show the greater improvements.

Figure 5: Cumulative Percentage of Patients Completing 26 Weeks of Double-blind Treatment with Specified Changes from Baseline ADAS-cog Scores. The Percentages of Randomized Patients who Completed the Study were: Placebo 87%, 1-4 mg 86%, and 6-12 mg 67%.

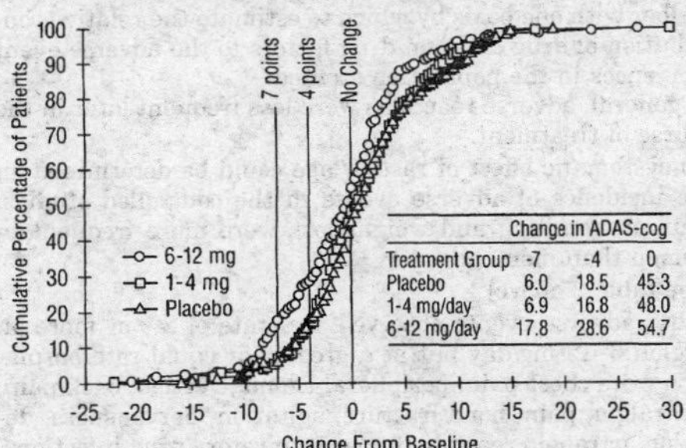

Effects on the CIBIC-Plus: Figure 6 is a histogram of the frequency distribution of CIBIC-Plus scores attained by patients assigned to each of the three treatment groups who completed 26 weeks of treatment. The mean Exelon-placebo differences for these groups of patients for the mean rating of change from baseline were 0.14 units and 0.41 units for 1–4 mg and 6–12 mg of Exelon, respectively. The mean ratings for the 6–12 mg/day group was statistically significantly superior to placebo. The comparison of the mean ratings for the 1–4 mg/day group and placebo group was not statistically significant.

[See figure at top of next column]

U.S. Fixed Dose Study

In a study of 26 weeks' duration, 702 patients were randomized to doses of 3, 6, or 9 mg/day of Exelon or to placebo, each given in divided doses. The fixed-dose study design, which included a 12-week forced titration phase and a 14-week maintenance phase, led to a high dropout rate in the 9 mg/day group because of poor tolerability. At 26 weeks of treatment, significant differences were observed for the ADAS-cog mean change from baseline for the 9 mg/day and 6 mg/day groups, compared to placebo. No significant differences were observed between any of the Exelon dose groups and placebo for the analysis of the CIBIC-Plus mean rating of change. Although no significant differences were observed between Exelon treatment groups, there was a trend toward numerical superiority with higher doses.

Figure 6: Frequency Distribution of CIBIC-Plus Scores at Week 26

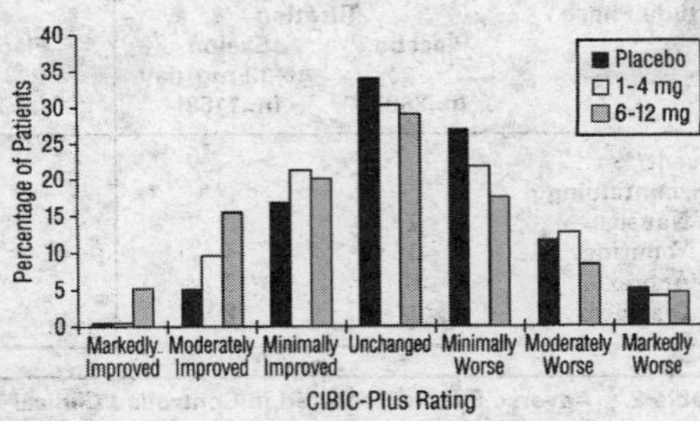

Age, Gender and Race: Patient's age, gender, or race did not predict clinical outcome to Exelon treatment.

Pharmacokinetics

Rivastigmine is well absorbed with absolute bioavailability of about 40% (3-mg dose). It shows linear pharmacokinetics up to 3 mg BID but is non-linear at higher doses. Doubling the dose from 3 to 6 mg BID results in a 3-fold increase in AUC. The elimination half-life is about 1.5 hours, with most elimination as metabolites via the urine.

Absorption: Rivastigmine is rapidly and completely absorbed. Peak plasma concentrations are reached in approximately 1 hour. Absolute bioavailability after a 3-mg dose is about 36%. Administration of Exelon with food delays absorption (t_{max}) by 90 min, lowers C_{max} by approximately 30% and increases AUC by approximately 30%.

Distribution: Rivastigmine is widely distributed throughout the body with a volume of distribution in the range of 1.8–2.7 L/kg. Rivastigmine penetrates the blood brain barrier, reaching CSF peak concentrations in 1.4-2.6 hours. Mean AUC_{1-12hr} ratio of CSF/plasma averaged 40 ± 0.5% following 1-6 mg BID doses.

Rivastigmine is about 40% bound to plasma proteins at concentrations of 1–400 ng/mL, which cover the therapeutic concentration range. Rivastigmine distributes equally between blood and plasma with a blood-to-plasma partition ratio of 0.9 at concentrations ranging from 1–400 ng/mL.

Metabolism: Rivastigmine is rapidly and extensively metabolized, primarily via cholinesterase-mediated hydrolysis to the decarbamylated metabolite. Based on evidence from *in vitro* and animal studies the major cytochrome P450 isozymes are minimally involved in rivastigmine metabolism. Consistent with these observations is the finding that no drug interactions related to cytochrome P450 have been observed in humans (see Drug-Drug Interactions).

Elimination: The major pathway of elimination is via the kidneys. Following administration of ^{14}C-rivastigmine to 6 healthy volunteers total recovery of radioactivity over 120 hours was 97% in urine and 0.4% in feces. No parent drug was detected in urine. The sulfate conjugate of the decarbamylated metabolite is the major component excreted in urine and represents 40% of the dose. Mean oral clearance of rivastigmine is 1.8 ± 0.6 L/min after 6 mg BID.

Special Populations

Hepatic Disease: Following a single 3-mg dose, mean oral clearance of rivastigmine was 60% lower in hepatically impaired patients (n=10, biopsy proven) than in healthy subjects (n=10). After multiple 6 mg BID oral dosing, the mean clearance of rivastigmine was 65% lower in mild (n=7, Child-Pugh score 5-6) and moderate (n=3, Child-Pugh score 7-9) hepatically impaired patients (biopsy proven, liver cirrhosis) than in healthy subjects (n=10). Dosage adjustment is not necessary in hepatically impaired patients as the dose of drug is individually titrated to tolerability.

Renal Disease: Following a single 3-mg dose, mean oral clearance of rivastigmine is 64% lower in moderately impaired renal patients (n=8, GFR=10-50 mL/min) than in healthy subjects (n=10, GFR≥60 mL/min); Cl/F=1.7 L/min (cv=45%) and 4.8 L/min (cv=80%), respectively. In severely impaired renal patients (n=8, GFR<10 mL/min), mean oral clearance of rivastigmine is 43% higher than in healthy subjects (n=10, GFR≥60 mL/min); Cl/F=6.9 L/min and 4.8 L/min, respectively. For unexplained reasons, the severely impaired renal patients had a higher clearance of rivastigmine than moderately impaired patients. However, dosage adjustment may not be necessary in renally impaired patients as the dose of the drug is individually titrated to tolerability.

Age: Following a single 2.5 mg oral dose to elderly volunteers (>60 years of age, n=24) and younger volunteers (n=24), mean oral clearance of rivastigmine was 30% lower in elderly (7 L/min) than in younger subjects (10 L/min).

Gender and Race: No specific pharmacokinetic study was conducted to investigate the effect of gender and race on the disposition of Exelon, but a population pharmacokinetic analysis indicates that gender (n=277 males and 348 females) and race (n=575 White, 34 Black, 4 Asian, and 12 Other) did not affect the clearance of Exelon.

Nicotine Use: Population PK analysis showed that nicotine use increases the oral clearance of rivastigmine by 23% (n=75 Smokers and 549 Nonsmokers).

Drug-Drug Interactions

Effect of Exelon on the Metabolism of Other Drugs: Rivastigmine is primarily metabolized through hydrolysis by esterases. Minimal metabolism occurs via the major cytochrome P450 isoenzymes. Based on *in vitro* studies, no pharmacokinetic drug interactions with drugs metabolized by the following isoenzyme systems are expected: CYP1A2, CYP2D6, CYP3A4/5, CYP2E1, CYP2C9, CYP2C8, or CYP2C19.

No pharmacokinetic interaction was observed between rivastigmine and digoxin, warfarin, diazepam, or fluoxetine in studies in healthy volunteers. The elevation of prothrombin time induced by warfarin is not affected by administration of Exelon.

Effect of Other Drugs on the Metabolism of Exelon: Drugs that induce or inhibit CYP450 metabolism are not expected to alter the metabolism of rivastigmine. Single dose pharmacokinetic studies demonstrated that the metabolism of rivastigmine is not significantly affected by concurrent administration of digoxin, warfarin, diazepam, or fluoxetine.

Population PK analysis with a database of 625 patients showed that the pharmacokinetics of rivastigmine were not influenced by commonly prescribed medications such as antacids (n=77), antihypertensives (n=72), β-blockers (n=42), calcium channel blockers (n=75), antidiabetics (n=21), nonsteroidal anti-inflammatory drugs (n=79), estrogens (n=70), salicylate analgesics (n=177), antianginals (n=35), and antihistamines (n=15). In addition, in clinical trials, no increased risk of clinically relevant untoward effects was observed in patients treated concomitantly with Exelon and these agents.

INDICATIONS AND USAGE

Exelon® (rivastigmine tartrate) is indicated for the treatment of mild to moderate dementia of the Alzheimer's type.

CONTRAINDICATIONS

Exelon® (rivastigmine tartrate) is contraindicated in patients with known hypersensitivity to rivastigmine, other carbamate derivatives or other components of the formulation (see DESCRIPTION).

WARNINGS

Gastrointestinal Adverse Reactions

Exelon® (rivastigmine tartrate) use is associated with significant gastrointestinal adverse reactions, including nausea and vomiting, anorexia, and weight loss.

Nausea and Vomiting: **In the controlled clinical trials, 47% of the patients treated with an Exelon dose in the therapeutic range of 6-12 mg/day (n=1189) developed nausea (compared with 12% in placebo). A total of 31% of Exelon-treated patients developed at least one episode of vomiting (compared with 6% for placebo). The rate of vomiting was higher during the titration phase (24% vs. 3% for placebo) than in the maintenance phase (14% vs. 3% for placebo). The rates were higher in women than men. Five percent of patients discontinued for vomiting, compared to less than 1% for patients on placebo. Vomiting was severe in 2% of Exelon-treated patients and was rated as mild or moderate each in 14% of patients. The rate of nausea was higher during the titration phase (43% vs. 9% for placebo) than in the maintenance phase (17% vs. 4% for placebo).**

Weight Loss: **In the controlled trials, approximately 26% of women on high doses of Exelon (greater than 9 mg/day) had weight loss of equal to or greater than 7% of their baseline weight compared to 6% in the placebo-treated patients. About 18% of the males in the high dose group experienced a similar degree of weight loss compared to 4% in placebo-treated patients. It is not clear how much of the weight loss was associated with anorexia, nausea, vomiting, and the diarrhea associated with the drug.**

Anorexia: In the controlled clinical trials, of the patients treated with an Exelon dose of 6–12 mg/day, 17% developed anorexia compared to 3% of the placebo patients. Neither the time course or the severity of the anorexia is known.

Peptic Ulcers/Gastrointestinal Bleeding: Because of their pharmacological action, cholinesterase inhibitors may be expected to increase gastric acid secretion due to increased cholinergic activity. Therefore, patients should be monitored closely for symptoms of active or occult gastrointestinal bleeding, especially those at increased risk for developing ulcers, e.g., those with a history of ulcer disease or those receiving concurrent nonsteroidal anti-inflammatory drugs (NSAIDS). Clinical studies of Exelon have shown no significant increase, relative to placebo, in the incidence of either peptic ulcer disease or gastrointestinal bleeding.

Anesthesia

Exelon as a cholinesterase inhibitor, is likely to exaggerate succinylcholine-type muscle relaxation during anesthesia.

Cardiovascular Conditions

Drugs that increase cholinergic activity may have vagotonic effects on heart rate (e.g., bradycardia). The potential for this action may be particularly important to patients with "sick sinus syndrome" or other supraventricular cardiac conduction conditions. In clinical trials, Exelon was not associated with any increased incidence of cardiovascular adverse events, heart rate or blood pressure changes, or ECG abnormalities. Syncopal episodes have been reported in 3% of patients receiving 6-12 mg/day of Exelon, compared to 2% of placebo patients.

Continued on next page

Exelon Oral Solution—Cont.

Genitourinary
Although this was not observed in clinical trials of Exelon, drugs that increase cholinergic activity may cause urinary obstruction.

Neurological Conditions
Seizures: Drugs that increase cholinergic activity are believed to have some potential for causing seizures. However, seizure activity also may be a manifestation of Alzheimer's Disease.

Pulmonary Conditions
Like other drugs that increase cholinergic activity, Exelon should be used with care in patients with a history of asthma or obstructive pulmonary disease.

PRECAUTIONS

Information for Patients and Caregivers
Caregivers should be advised of the high incidence of nausea and vomiting associated with the use of the drug along with the possibility of anorexia and weight loss. Caregivers should be encouraged to monitor for these adverse events and inform the physician if they occur.
Caregivers should be instructed in the correct procedure for administering Exelon® (rivastigmine tartrate) Oral Solution. In addition, they should be informed of the existence of an Instruction Sheet (included with the product) describing how the solution is to be administered. They should be urged to read this sheet prior to administering Exelon Oral Solution. Caregivers should direct questions about the administration of the solution to either their physician or pharmacist.

Drug-Drug Interactions
Effect of Exelon® on the Metabolism of Other Drugs: Rivastigmine is primarily metabolized through hydrolysis by esterases. Minimal metabolism occurs via the major cytochrome P450 isoenzymes. Based on *in vitro* studies, no pharmacokinetic drug interactions with drugs metabolized by the following isoenzyme systems are expected: CYP1A2, CYP2D6, CYP3A4/5, CYP2E1, CYP2C9, CYP2C8, or CYP2C19.
No pharmacokinetic interaction was observed between rivastigmine and digoxin, warfarin, diazepam, or fluoxetine in studies in healthy volunteers. The elevation of prothrombin time induced by warfarin is not affected by administration of Exelon.
Effect of Other Drugs on the Metabolism of Exelon: Drugs that induce or inhibit CYP450 metabolism are not expected to alter the metabolism of rivastigmine. Single dose pharmacokinetic studies demonstrated that the metabolism of rivastigmine is not significantly affected by concurrent administration of digoxin, warfarin, diazepam, or fluoxetine.
Population PK analysis with a database of 625 patients showed that the pharmacokinetics of rivastigmine were not influenced by commonly prescribed medications such as antacids (n=77), antihypertensives (n=72), β-blockers (n=42), calcium channel blockers (n=75), antidiabetics (n=21), nonsteroidal anti-inflammatory drugs (n=79), estrogens (n=70), salicylate analgesics (n=177), antianginals (n=35), and antihistamines (n=15).
Use with Anticholinergics: Because of their mechanism of action, cholinesterase inhibitors have the potential to interfere with the activity of anticholinergic medications.
Use with Cholinomimetics and Other Cholinesterase Inhibitors: A synergistic effect may be expected when cholinesterase inhibitors are given concurrently with succinylcholine, similar neuromuscular blocking agents or cholinergic agonists such as bethanechol.

Carcinogenesis, Mutagenesis, Impairment of Fertility
In carcinogenicity studies conducted at dose levels up to 1.1 mg-base/kg/day in rats and 1.6 mg-base/kg/day in mice, rivastigmine was not carcinogenic. These dose levels are approximately 0.9 times and 0.7 times the maximum recommended human daily dose of 12 mg per day on a mg/m^2 basis.
Rivastigmine was clastogenic in two *in vitro* assays in the presence, but not the absence, of metabolic activation. It caused structural chromosomal aberrations in V79 Chinese hamster lung cells and both structural and numerical (polyploidy) chromosomal aberrations in human peripheral blood lymphocytes. Rivastigmine was not genotoxic in three *in vitro* assays: the Ames test, the unscheduled DNA synthesis (UDS) test in rat hepatocytes (a test for induction of DNA repair synthesis), and the HGPRT test in V79 Chinese hamster cells. Rivastigmine was not clastogenic in the *in vivo* mouse micronucleus test.
Rivastigmine had no effect on fertility or reproductive performance in the rat at dose levels up to 1.1 mg-base/kg/day. This dose is approximately 0.9 times the maximum recommended human daily dose of 12 mg/day on a mg/m^2 basis.

Pregnancy
Pregnancy Category B: Reproduction studies conducted in pregnant rats at doses up to 2.3 mg-base/kg/day (approximately 2 times the maximum recommended human dose on a mg/m^2 basis) and in pregnant rabbits at doses up to 2.3 mg-base/kg/day (approximately 4 times the maximum recommended human dose on a mg/m^2 basis) revealed no evidence of teratogenicity. Studies in rats showed slightly decreased fetal/pup weights, usually at doses causing some maternal toxicity; decreased weights were seen at doses which were several fold lower than the maximum recommended human dose on a mg/m^2 basis. There are no adequate or well-controlled studies in pregnant women. Because animal reproduction studies are not always predictive of human response, Exelon should be used during pregnancy only if the potential benefit justifies the potential risk to the fetus.

Table 1. Most Frequent Adverse Events Leading to Withdrawal from Clinical Trials during Titration and Maintenance in Patients Receiving 6-12 mg/day Exelon® Using a Forced Dose Titration

Study Phase	Titration		Maintenance		Overall	
	Placebo (n=868)	Exelon ≥6-12 mg/day (n=1189)	Placebo (n=788)	Exelon ≥6-12 mg/day (n=987)	Placebo (n=868)	Exelon ≥6-12 mg/day (n=1189)
Event/% Discontinuing						
Nausea	<1	8	<1	1	1	8
Vomiting	<1	4	<1	1	<1	5
Anorexia	0	2	<1	1	<1	3
Dizziness	<1	2	<1	1	<1	2

Table 2. Adverse Events Reported in Controlled Clinical Trials in at Least 2% of Patients Receiving Exelon® (6–12 mg/day) and at a Higher Frequency than Placebo-treated Patients

Body System/Adverse Event	Placebo (n=868)	Exelon (6–12 mg/day) (n=1189)
Percent of Patients with any Adverse Event	79	92
Autonomic Nervous System		
Sweating increased	1	4
Syncope	2	3
Body as a Whole		
Accidental Trauma	9	10
Fatigue	5	9
Asthenia	2	6
Malaise	2	5
Influenza-like Symptoms	2	3
Weight Decrease	<1	3
Cardiovascular Disorders, General		
Hypertension	2	3
Central and Peripheral Nervous System		
Dizziness	11	21
Headache	12	17
Somnolence	3	5
Tremor	1	4
Gastrointestinal System		
Nausea	12	47
Vomiting	6	31
Diarrhea	11	19
Anorexia	3	17
Abdominal Pain	6	13
Dyspepsia	4	9
Constipation	4	5
Flatulence	2	4
Eructation	1	2
Psychiatric Disorders		
Insomnia	7	9
Confusion	7	8
Depression	4	6
Anxiety	3	5
Hallucination	3	4
Aggressive Reaction	2	3
Resistance Mechanism Disorders		
Urinary Tract Infection	6	7
Respiratory System		
Rhinitis	3	4

Nursing Mothers
It is not known whether rivastigmine is excreted in human breast milk. Exelon has no indication for use in nursing mothers.

Pediatric Use
There are no adequate and well-controlled trials documenting the safety and efficacy of Exelon in any illness occurring in children.

ADVERSE REACTIONS

Adverse Events Leading to Discontinuation
The rate of discontinuation due to adverse events in controlled clinical trials of Exelon® (rivastigmine tartrate) was 15% for patients receiving 6–12 mg/day compared to 5% for patients on placebo during forced weekly dose titration. While on a maintenance dose, the rates were 6% for patients on Exelon compared to 4% for those on placebo.
The most common adverse events leading to discontinuation, defined as those occurring in at least 2% of patients and at twice the incidence seen in placebo patients, are shown in Table 1.
[See table 1 above]

Most Frequent Adverse Clinical Events Seen in Association with the Use of Exelon
The most common adverse events, defined as those occurring at a frequency of at least 5% and twice the placebo rate, are largely predicted by Exelon's cholinergic effects. These include nausea, vomiting, anorexia, dyspepsia, and asthenia.
Gastrointestinal Adverse Reactions
Exelon use is associated with significant nausea, vomiting, and weight loss (see WARNINGS).

Adverse Events Reported in Controlled Trials
Table 2 lists treatment emergent signs and symptoms that were reported in at least 2% of patients in placebo-controlled trials and for which the rate of occurrence was greater for patients treated with Exelon doses of 6–12 mg/day than for those treated with placebo. The prescriber should be aware that these figures cannot be used to predict the frequency of adverse events in the course of usual medical practice when patient characteristics and other factors may differ from those prevailing during clinical studies. Similarly, the cited frequencies cannot be directly compared with figures obtained from other clinical investigations involving different treatments, uses, or investigators. An inspection of these frequencies, however, does provide the prescriber with one basis by which to estimate the relative contribution of drug and non-drug factors to the adverse event incidences in the population studied.
In general, adverse reactions were less frequent later in the course of treatment.
No systematic effect of race or age could be determined on the incidence of adverse events in the controlled studies. Nausea, vomiting and weight loss were more frequent in women than men.
[See table 2 above]
Other adverse events observed at a rate of 2% or more on Exelon 6–12 mg/day but at a greater or equal rate on placebo were chest pain, peripheral edema, vertigo, back pain, arthralgia, pain, bone fracture, agitation, nervousness, delusion, paranoid reaction, upper respiratory tract infections, infection (general), coughing, pharyngitis, bronchitis, rash (general), urinary incontinence.

Other Adverse Events Observed During Clinical Trials
Exelon has been administered to over 5297 individuals during clinical trials worldwide. Of these, 4326 patients have been treated for at least 3 months, 3407 patients have been treated for at least 6 months, 2150 patients have been treated for 1 year, 1250 have been treated for 2 years, and 168 have been treated for over 3 years. With regard to exposure to the highest dose, 2809 patients were exposed to doses of 10-12 mg, 2615 patients treated for 3 months, 2328 patients treated for 6 months, 1378 patients treated for 1 year, 917 patients treated for 2 years, and 129 treated for over 3 years.
Treatment emergent signs and symptoms that occurred during 8 controlled clinical trials and 9 open-label trials in North America, Western Europe, Australia, South Africa, and Japan were recorded as adverse events by the clinical

investigators using terminology of their own choosing. To provide an overall estimate of the proportion of individuals having similar types of events, the events were grouped into a smaller number of standardized categories using a modified WHO dictionary, and event frequencies were calculated across all studies. These categories are used in the listing below. The frequencies represent the proportion of 5297 patients from these trials who experienced that event while receiving Exelon. All adverse events occurring in at least 6 patients (approximately 0.1%) are included, except for those already listed elsewhere in labeling, WHO terms too general to be informative, relatively minor events, or events unlikely to be drug caused. Events are classified by body system and listed using the following definitions: frequent adverse events—those occurring in at least 1/100 patients; infrequent adverse events—those occurring in 1/100 to 1/1000 patients. These adverse events are not necessarily related to Exelon treatment and in most cases were observed at a similar frequency in placebo-treated patients in the controlled studies.

Autonomic Nervous System: *Infrequent:* Cold clammy skin, dry mouth, flushing, increased saliva.

Body as a Whole: *Frequent:* Accidental trauma, fever, edema, allergy, hot flushes, rigors. *Infrequent:* Edema periorbital or facial, hypothermia, edema, feeling cold, halitosis.

Cardiovascular System: *Frequent:* Hypotension, postural hypotension, cardiac failure.

Central and Peripheral Nervous System: *Frequent:* Abnormal gait, ataxia, paraesthesia, convulsions. *Infrequent:* Paresis, apraxia, aphasia, dysphonia, hyperkinesia, hyperreflexia, hypertonia, hypoesthesia, hypokinesia, migraine, neuralgia, nystagmus, peripheral neuropathy.

Endocrine System: *Infrequent:* Goitre, hypothyroidism.

Gastrointestinal System: *Frequent:* Fecal incontinence, gastritis. *Infrequent:* Dysphagia, esophagitis, gastric ulcer, gastritis, gastroesophagel reflux, GI hemorrhage, hernia, intestinal obstruction, melena, rectal hemorrhage, gastroenteritis, ulcerative stomatitis, duodenal ulcer, hematemesis, gingivitis, tenesmus, pancreatitis, colitis, glossitis.

Hearing and Vestibular Disorders: *Frequent:* Tinnitus.

Heart Rate and Rhythm Disorders: *Frequent:* Atrial fibrillation, bradycardia, palpitation. *Infrequent:* AV block, bundle branch block, sick sinus syndrome, cardiac arrest, supraventricular tachycardia, extrasystoles, tachycardia.

Liver and Biliary System Disorders: *Infrequent:* Abnormal hepatic function, cholecystitis.

Metabolic and Nutritional Disorders: *Frequent:* Dehydration, hypokalemia. *Infrequent:* Diabetes mellitus, gout, hypercholesterolemia, hyperlipernia, hypoglycemia, cachexia, thirst, hyperglycemia, hyponatremia.

Musculoskeletal Disorders: *Frequent:* Arthritis, leg cramps, myalgia. *Infrequent:* Cramps, hernia, muscle weakness.

Myo-, Endo-, Pericardial and Valve Disorders: *Frequent:* Angina pectoris, myocardial infarction.

Platelet, Bleeding, and Clotting Disorders: *Frequent:* Epistaxis. *Infrequent:* Hematoma, thrombocytopenia, purpura.

Psychiatric Disorders: *Frequent:* Paranoid reaction, confusion. *Infrequent:* Abnormal dreaming, amnesia, apathy, delirium, dementia, depersonalization, emotional lability, impaired concentration, decreased libido, personality disorder, suicide attempt, increased libido, neurosis, suicidal ideation, psychosis.

Red Blood Cell Disorders: *Frequent:* Anemia. *Infrequent:* Hypochromic anemia.

Reproductive Disorders (Female & Male): *Infrequent:* Breast pain, impotence, atrophic vaginitis.

Resistance Mechanism Disorders: *Infrequent:* Cellulitis, cystitis, herpes simplex, otitis media.

Respiratory System: *Infrequent:* Bronchospasm, laryngitis, apnea.

Skin and Appendages: *Frequent:* Rashes of various kinds (maculopapular, eczema, bullous, exfoliative, psoriaform, erythematous). *Infrequent:* Alopecia, skin ulceration, urticaria, dermatitis contact.

Special Senses: *Infrequent:* Perversion of taste, loss of taste.

Urinary System Disorders: *Frequent:* Hematuria. *Infrequent:* Albuminuria, oliguria, acute renal failure, dysuria, micturition urgency, nocturia, polyuria, renal calculus, urinary retention.

Vascular (extracardiac) Disorders: *Infrequent:* Hemorrhoids, peripheral ischemia, pulmonary embolism, thrombosis, thrombophlebitis deep, aneurysm, hemorrhage intracranial.

Vision Disorders: *Frequent:* Cataract. *Infrequent:* Conjunctival hemorrhage, blepharitis, diplopia, eye pain, glaucoma.

White Cell and Resistance Disorders: *Infrequent:* Lymphadenopathy, leukocytosis.

OVERDOSAGE

Because strategies for the management of overdose are continually evolving, it is advisable to contact a Poison Control Center to determine the latest recommendations for the management of an overdose of any drug.

As Exelon® (rivastigmine tartrate) has a short plasma half-life of about one hour and a moderate duration of acetylcholinesterase inhibition of 8–10 hours, it is recommended that in cases of asymptomatic overdoses, no further dose of Exelon should be administered for the next 24 hours.

As in any case of overdose, general supportive measures should be utilized. Overdosage with cholinesterase inhibitors can result in cholinergic crisis characterized by severe nausea, vomiting, salivation, sweating, bradycardia, hypotension, respiratory depression, collapse and convulsions. Increasing muscle weakness is a possibility and may result in death if respiratory muscles are involved. Atypical responses in blood pressure and heart rate have been reported with other drugs that increase cholinergic activity when coadministered with quaternary anticholinergics such as glycopyrrolate. Due to the short half-life of Exelon, dialysis (hemodialysis, peritoneal dialysis, or hemofiltration) would not be clinically indicated in the event of an overdose.

In overdoses accompanied by severe nausea and vomiting, the use of antiemetics should be considered. In a documented case of a 46 mg overdose with Exelon, the patient experienced vomiting, incontinence, hypertension, psychomotor retardation, and loss of consciousness. The patient fully recovered within 24 hours and conservative management was all that was required for treatment.

DOSAGE AND ADMINISTRATION

The dosage of Exelon® (rivastigmine tartrate) shown to be effective in controlled clinical trials is 6–12 mg/day, given as twice a day dosing (daily doses of 3 to 6 mg BID). There is evidence from the clinical trials that doses at the higher end of this range may be more beneficial.

The recommended starting dose of Exelon is 1.5 mg twice a day. If this dose is well tolerated, after a minimum of two weeks of treatment, the dose may be increased to 3 mg twice a day. Subsequent increases to 4.5 mg BID and 6 mg BID should be attempted after a minimum of 2 weeks at the previous dose. If adverse effects (e.g., nausea, vomiting, abdominal pain, loss of appetite) cause intolerance during treatment, the patient should be instructed to discontinue treatment for several doses and then restart at the same or next lower dose level. The maximum dose is 6 mg BID (12 mg/day).

Exelon should be taken with food in divided doses in the morning and evening.

Recommendations for Administration: Caregivers should be instructed in the correct procedure for administering Exelon Oral Solution. In addition, they should be directed to the Instruction Sheet (included with the product) describing how the solution is to be administered. Caregivers should direct questions about the administration of the solution to either their physician or pharmacist (see PRECAUTIONS: Information for Patients and Caregivers).

Patients should be instructed to remove the oral dosing syringe provided in its protective case, and using the provided syringe, withdraw the prescribed amount of Exelon Oral Solution from the container. Each dose of Exelon Oral Solution may be swallowed directly from the syringe or first mixed with a small glass of water, cold fruit juice or soda. Patients should be instructed to stir and drink the mixture.

Exelon Oral Solution and Exelon Capsules may be interchanged at equal doses.

HOW SUPPLIED

Exelon® (rivastigmine tartrate) Oral Solution is supplied as 120 mL of a clear, yellow solution (2.0 mg/mL base) in a 4 ounce USP Type III amber glass bottle with a child-resistant 28 mm cap, 0.5 mm foam liner, dip tube and self-aligning plug. The oral solution is packaged with a dispenser set which consists of an assembled oral dosing syringe that allows dipsensing a maximum volume of 3 mL corresponding to a 6 mg dose, with a plastic tube container.

Bottles of 120 mL .... NDC 0078-0339-31

Store below 77° F (25° C) in an upright position and protect from freezing.

When Exelon Oral Solution is combined with cold fruit juice or soda, the mixture is stable at room temperature for up to 4 hours.

Exelon® *(rivastigmine tartrate)* Oral Solution Instructions for Use

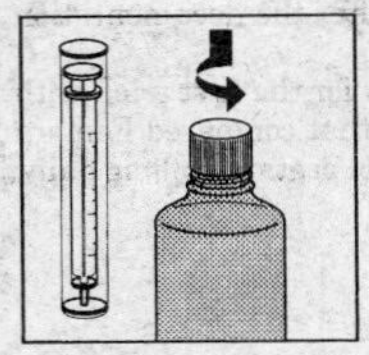

1. Remove oral dosing syringe from its protective case. Push down and twist child resistant closure to open bottle.

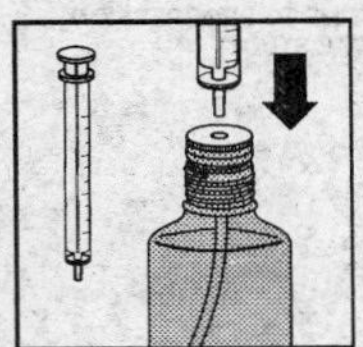

2. Insert tip of syringe into opening of white stopper.

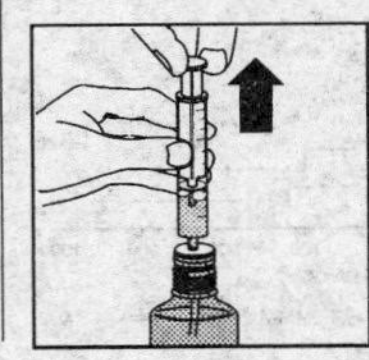

3. While holding the syringe, pull the plunger up to the level (see markings on side of syringe) that equals the dose prescribed by your doctor.

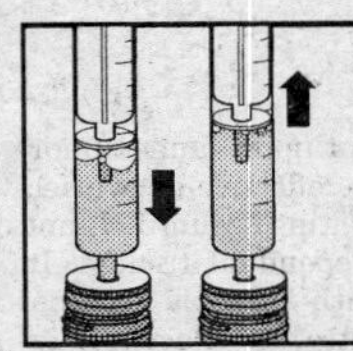

4. Before removing syringe containing prescribed dose from bottle, push out **large** bubbles by moving plunger up and down a few times. After the large bubbles are gone, pull the plunger again to the level that equals the dose prescribed by your doctor. Do not worry about a few tiny bubbles. This will not affect your dose in any way. Remove the syringe from the bottle.

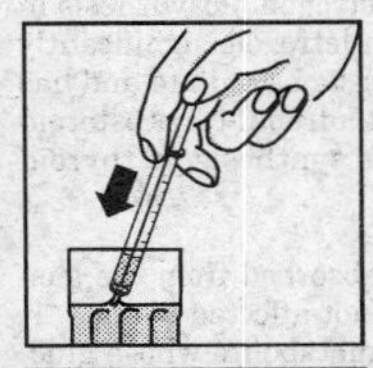

5. You may swallow Exelon Oral Solution directly from the syringe or mix with a small glass of water, cold fruit juice or soda. If mixing with water, juice or soda, be sure to stir completely and to drink the entire mixture. DO NOT MIX WITH OTHER LIQUIDS.

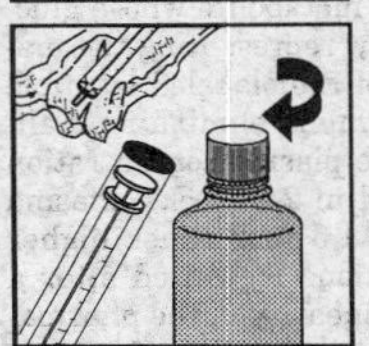

6. After use, wipe outside of syringe with a clean tissue and put it back into its case. Close bottle using child resistant closure.

Store Exelon Oral Solution at room temperature (below 77° F) in an upright position. Do not place in freezer.

(86000501 4/00)

 T2000–25

APRIL 2000 4048–2

Manufactured by
Novartis Consumer Health, Incorporated
Lincoln, Nebraska 68517
Manufactured for
Novartis Pharmaceuticals Corporation
East Hanover, New Jersey 07936

FEMARA® ℞

[fĕm-ara]
(letrozole tablets)
2.5 mg Tablets
Rx only

The following prescribing information is based on official labeling in effect July 2000.

DESCRIPTION

Femara (letrozole tablets) for oral administration contain 2.5 mg of letrozole, a nonsteroidal aromatase inhibitor (inhibitor of estrogen synthesis). It is chemically described as 4,4′-(1H-1,2,4-Triazol-1-ylmethylene)dibenzonitrile, and its structural formula is

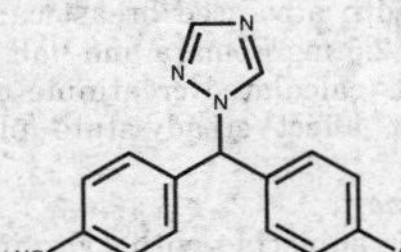

Letrozole is a white to yellowish crystalline powder, practically odorless, freely soluble in dichloromethane, slightly soluble in ethanol, and practically insoluble in water. It has a molecular weight of 285.31, empirical formula $C_{17}H_{11}N_5$, and a melting range of 184°C-185°C.

Femara (letrozole tablets) is available as 2.5 mg tablets for oral administration.

Inactive Ingredients. Colloidal silicon dioxide, ferric oxide, hydroxypropyl methylcellulose, lactose monohydrate, magnesium stearate, maize starch, microcrystalline cellulose, polyethylene glycol, sodium starch glycolate, talc, and titanium dioxide.

CLINICAL PHARMACOLOGY

Mechanism of Action

The growth of some cancers of the breast is stimulated or maintained by estrogens. Treatment of breast cancer thought to be hormonally responsive (i.e., estrogen and/or progesterone receptor positive or receptor unknown) has included a variety of efforts to decrease estrogen levels (ovariectomy, adrenalectomy, hypophysectomy) or inhibit estrogen effects (antiestrogens and progestational agents). These interventions lead to decreased tumor mass or delayed progression of tumor growth in some women.

In postmenopausal women, estrogens are mainly derived from the action of the aromatase enzyme, which converts adrenal androgens (primarily androstenedione and testosterone) to estrone and estradiol. The suppression of estrogen biosynthesis in peripheral tissues and in the cancer tissue itself can therefore be achieved by specifically inhibiting the aromatase enzyme.

Letrozole is a nonsteroidal competitive inhibitor of the aromatase enzyme system; it inhibits the conversion of an-

Continued on next page

Femara—Cont.

drogens to estrogens. In adult nontumor- and tumor-bearing female animals, letrozole is as effective as ovariectomy in reducing uterine weight, elevating serum LH, and causing the regression of estrogen-dependent tumors. In contrast to ovariectomy, treatment with letrozole does not lead to an increase in serum FSH. Letrozole selectively inhibits gonadal steroidogenesis but has no significant effect on adrenal mineralocorticoid or glucocorticoid synthesis.
Letrozole inhibits the aromatase enzyme by competitively binding to the heme of the cytochrome P450 subunit of the enzyme, resulting in a reduction of estrogen biosynthesis in all tissues. Treatment of women with letrozole significantly lowers serum estrone, estradiol and estrone sulfate and has not been shown to significantly affect adrenal corticosteroid synthesis, aldosterone synthesis, or synthesis of thyroid hormones.

Pharmacokinetics

Letrozole is rapidly and completely absorbed from the gastrointestinal tract and absorption is not affected by food. It is metabolized slowly to an inactive metabolite whose glucuronide conjugate is excreted renally, representing the major clearance pathway. About 90% of radiolabeled letrozole is recovered in urine. Letrozole's terminal elimination half-life is about 2 days and steady-state plasma concentration after daily 2.5 mg dosing is reached in 2-6 weeks. Plasma concentrations at steady-state are 1.5 to 2 times higher than predicted from the concentrations measured after a single dose, indicating a slight non-linearity in the pharmacokinetics of letrozole upon daily administration of 2.5 mg. These steady-state levels are maintained over extended periods, however, and continuous accumulation of letrozole does not occur. Letrozole is weakly protein bound and has a large volume of distribution (approximately 1.9 L/kg).

Metabolism and Excretion

Metabolism to a pharmacologically-inactive carbinol metabolite (4,4'-methanolbisbenzonitrile) and renal excretion of the glucuronide conjugate of this metabolite is the major pathway of letrozole clearance. Of the radiolabel recovered in urine, at least 75% was the glucuronide of the carbinol metabolite, about 9% was two unidentified metabolites, and 6% was unchanged letrozole.
In human microsomes with specific CYP isozyme activity, CYP 3A4 metabolized letrozole to the carbinol metabolite while CYP 2A6 formed both this metabolite and its ketone analog. In human liver microsomes, letrozole strongly inhibited CYP 2A6 and moderately inhibited CYP 2C19.

Special Populations

Pediatric, Geriatric and Race:

In the study populations (adults ranging in age from 35 to >80 years), no change in pharmacokinetic parameters was observed with increasing age. Differences in letrozole pharmacokinetics between adult and pediatric populations have not been studied. Differences in letrozole pharmacokinetics due to race have not been studied.

Renal Insufficiency:

In a study of volunteers with varying renal function (24-hour creatinine clearance: 9-116 mL/min), no effect of renal function on the pharmacokinetics of single doses of 2.5 mg of Femara (letrozole tablets) was found. In addition, in a study of 347 patients with advanced breast cancer, about half of whom received 2.5 mg Femara and half 0.5 mg Femara, renal impairment (calculated creatinine clearance: 20-50 mL/min) did not affect steady-state plasma letrozole concentration.

Hepatic Insufficiency:

In a study of subjects with varying degrees of non-metastatic hepatic dysfunction (e.g., cirrhosis, Child-Pugh classification A and B), the mean AUC values of the volunteers with moderate hepatic impairment were 37% higher than in normal subjects, but still within the range seen in subjects without impaired function. Patients with severe hepatic impairment (Child-Pugh classification C) have not been studied (see DOSAGE & ADMINISTRATION Hepatic Impairment).

Drug/Drug Interactions:

A pharmacokinetic interaction study with cimetidine showed no clinically significant effect on letrozole pharmacokinetics. An interaction study with warfarin showed no clinically significant effect of letrozole on warfarin pharmacokinetics.
There is no clinical experience to date on the use of Femara in combination with other anti-cancer agents.

Pharmacodynamics

In postmenopausal patients with advanced breast cancer, daily doses of 0.1 mg to 5 mg Femara suppress plasma concentrations of estradiol, estrone, and estrone sulfate by 75%-95% from baseline with maximal suppression achieved within two-three days. Suppression is dose-related, with doses of 0.5 mg and higher giving many values of estrone and estrone sulfate that were below the limit of detection in the assays. Estrogen suppression was maintained throughout treatment in all patients treated at 0.5 mg or higher.
Letrozole is highly specific in inhibiting aromatase activity. There is no impairment of adrenal steroidogenesis. No clinically-relevant changes were found in the plasma concentrations of cortisol, aldosterone, 11-deoxycortisol, 17-hydroxy-progesterone, ACTH or in plasma renin activity among postmenopausal patients treated with a daily dose of Femara 0.1 mg to 5 mg. The ACTH stimulation test performed after 6 and 12 weeks of treatment with daily doses of 0.1, 0.25, 0.5, 1, 2.5, and 5 mg did not indicate any attenuation of aldosterone or cortisol production. Glucocorticoid or mineralocorticoid supplementation is, therefore, not necessary.
No changes were noted in plasma concentrations of androgens (androstenedione and testosterone) among healthy postmenopausal women after 0.1, 0.5, and 2.5 mg single doses of Femara or in plasma concentrations of androstenedione among postmenopausal patients treated with daily doses of 0.1 mg to 5 mg. This indicates that the blockade of estrogen biosynthesis does not lead to accumulation of androgenic precursors. Plasma levels of LH and FSH were not affected by letrozole in patients, nor was thyroid function as evaluated by TSH levels, T3 uptake, and T4 levels.

Table I: Selected Study Population Demographics

Parameter	megestrol acetate study	aminoglutethimide study
No. of Participants	552	557
Receptor Status		
ER/PR Positive	57%	56%
ER/PR Unknown	43%	44%
Previous Therapy		
Adjuvant Only	33%	38%
Therapeutic +/- Adj.	66%	62%
Sites of Disease		
Visceral Metastases	40%	44%
Soft Tissue Metastases	56%	50%
Bony Metastases	50%	55%

Table 2: Megestrol Acetate Study Results

	Femara 0.5 mg N = 188	Femara 2.5 mg N = 174	Megestrol Acetate N = 190
Objective Response (CR + PR)	22 (11.7%)	41 (23.6%)	31 (16.3%)
Median Duration of Response	552 days	(Not reached)	561 days
Median Time to Progression	154 days	170 days	168 days
Median Survival	633 days	730 days	659 days
Odds Ratio for Response	Femara 2.5 : Femara 0.5 = 2.33 (95% CI: 1.32, 4.17); p=0.004*		Femara 2.5: Megestrol = 1.58 (95% CI: 0.94, 2.66); p = 0.08*
Relative Risk of Progression	Femara 2.5: Femara 0.5 = 0.81 (95% CI: 0.63, 1.03); p = 0.09*		Femara 2.5: Megestrol = 0.77 (95% CI: 0.60, 0.98), p = 0.03*

*two-sided p-value

Clinical Studies

Femara was initially studied at doses of 0.1 mg to 5.0 mg daily in six non-comparative phase I/II trials in 181 postmenopausal estrogen/progesterone receptor positive or unknown advanced breast cancer patients previously treated with at least antiestrogen therapy. Patients had received other hormonal therapies and also may have received cytotoxic therapy. Eight (20%) of forty patients treated with Femara 2.5 mg daily in phase I/II trials achieved an objective tumor response (complete or partial response).
Two large randomized controlled multinational (predominantly European) trials were conducted in patients with advanced breast cancer who had progressed despite antiestrogen therapy. Patients were randomized to Femara 0.5 mg daily, Femara 2.5 mg daily, or a comparator (megestrol acetate 160 mg daily in one study; and aminoglutethimide 250 mg bid with corticosteroid supplementation in the other study). In each study over 60% of the patients had received therapeutic antiestrogens, and about one-fifth of these patients had had an objective response. The megestrol acetate controlled study was double-blind; the other study was open label. Selected baseline characteristics for each study are shown in the following table:
[See table 1 above]
Confirmed objective tumor response (complete response plus partial response) was the primary endpoint of the trials. Responses were measured according to the Union Internationale Contre le Cancer (UICC) criteria and verified by independent, blinded review. All responses were confirmed by a second evaluation 4-12 weeks after the documentation of the initial response.
The following table shows the results for the first trial, with a minimum follow-up of 15 months, that compared Femara 0.5 mg, Femara 2.5 mg, and megestrol acetate 160 mg daily. (All analyses are unadjusted.)
[See table 2 above]

KAPLAN-MEIER ESTIMATES OF TIME TO PROGRESSION (MEGESTROL ACETATE STUDY)

TIME TO PROGRESSION (IN DAYS)

TREATMENT GROUP: —— FEMARA 0.5 MG ······ FEMARA 2.5 MG – – – MA

The Kaplan-Meier Curve for progression for the megestrol acetate study is shown below. The results for the study comparing Femara to aminoglutethimide, with a minimum follow-up of nine months, are shown in the following table. (Unadjusted analysis are used).
[See table 3 at top of next page]
The Kaplan-Meier Curve for progression for the aminoglutethimide study is shown below.

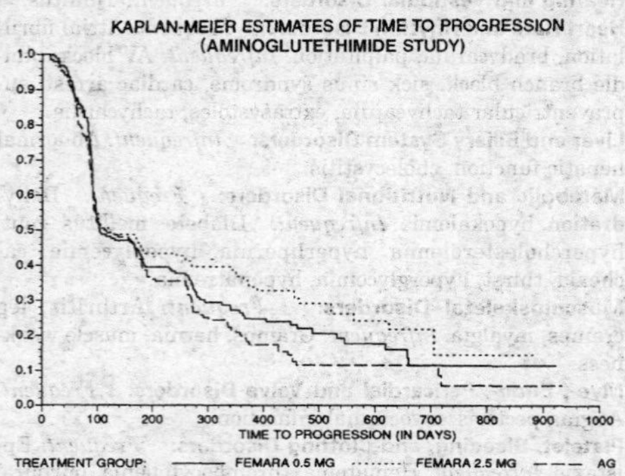

INDICATIONS AND USAGE

Femara (letrozole tablets) is indicated for the treatment of advanced breast cancer in postmenopausal women with disease progression following antiestrogen therapy.

CONTRAINDICATIONS

Femara is contraindicated in patients with known hypersensitivity to Femara or any of its excipients.

WARNINGS

Pregnancy

Letrozole may cause fetal harm when administered to pregnant women. Studies in rats at doses equal to or greater than 0.003 mg/kg (about 1/100 the daily maximum recommended human dose on a mg/m^2 basis) administered during the period of organogenesis, have shown that letrozole is embryotoxic and fetotoxic, as indicated by intrauterine mortality, increased resorption, increased postimplantation loss, decreased numbers of live fetuses and fetal anomalies including absence and shortening of renal papilla, dilation of ureter, edema and incomplete ossification of frontal skull and metatarsals. Letrozole was teratogenic in rats. A 0.03 mg/kg dose (about 1/10 the daily maximum recommended human dose on a mg/m^2 basis) caused fetal domed head and cervical/centrum vertebral fusion.
Letrozole is embryotoxic at doses equal to or greater than 0.002 mg/kg and fetotoxic when administered to rabbits at 0.02 mg/kg (about 1/100,000 and 1/10,000 the daily maximum recommended human dose on a mg/m^2 basis, respectively). Fetal anomalies included incomplete ossification of the skull, sternebrae, and fore- and hindlegs.
There are no studies in pregnant women. Femara is indicated for postmenopausal women. If there is exposure to letrozole during pregnancy, the patient should be apprised of the potential hazard to the fetus and potential risk for loss of the pregnancy.

PRECAUTIONS

Laboratory Tests

No dose-related effect of Femara on any hematologic or clinical chemistry parameter was evident. Moderate decreases in lymphocyte counts, of uncertain clinical significance, were observed in some patients receiving Femara (letrozole tablets) 2.5 mg. This depression was transient in about half

Table 3: Aminoglutethimide Study Results

	Femara 0.5 N = 193	Femara 2.5 N = 185	Aminoglutethimide N = 179
Objective Response (CR + PR)	34 (17.6%)	34 (18.4%)	22 (12.3%)
Median Duration of Response	619 days	706 days	450 days
Median Time to Progression	103 days	123 days	112 days
Median Survival	636 days	792 days	592 days
Odds Ratio for Response	Femara 2.5 : Femara 0.5 =1.05 (95% CI: 0.62, 1.79); p=0.85*		Femara 2.5: Aminoglutethimide =1.61 (95% CI: 0.90, 2.87); p = 0.11*
Relative Risk of Progression	Femara 2.5: Femara 0.5 =0.86 (95% CI: 0.68, 1.11); p = 0.25*		Femara 2.5: Aminoglutethimide =0.74 (95% CI: 0.57, 0.94), p = 0.02*

*two-sided p-value

Adverse Experience	Pooled Femara 2.5 mg (n=359) %	Pooled Femara 0.5 mg (n=380) %	Megestrol Acetate 160 mg (n=189) %	Aminoglutethimide 500 mg (n=178) %
	Percentage (%) of Patients with Adverse Events			
Body as a Whole				
Fatigue	8	6	11	3
Chest pain	6	3	7	3
Peripheral edema[1]	5	5	8	3
Asthenia	4	5	4	5
Weight increase	2	2	9	3
Cardiovascular				
Hypertension	5	7	5	6
Digestive System				
Nausea	13	15	9	14
Vomiting	7	7	5	9
Constipation	6	7	9	7
Diarrhea	6	5	3	4
Pain-abdominal	6	5	9	8
Anorexia	5	3	5	5
Dyspepsia	3	4	6	5
Infections/Infestations				
Viral infection	6	5	6	3
Lab Abnormality				
Hypercholesterolemia	3	3	0	6
Musculoskeletal System				
Musculoskeletal[2]	21	22	30	14
Arthralgia	8	8	8	3
Nervous System				
Headache	9	12	9	7
Somnolence	3	2	2	9
Dizziness	3	5	7	3
Respiratory System				
Dyspnea	7	9	16	5
Coughing	6	5	7	5
Skin and Appendages				
Hot flushes	6	5	4	3
Rash[3]	5	4	3	12
Pruritus	1	2	5	3

[1] Includes peripheral edema, leg edema, dependent edema, edema
[2] Includes musculoskeletal pain, skeletal pain, back pain, arm pain, leg pain
[3] Includes rash, erythematous rash, maculopapular rash, psoriaform rash, vesicular rash

of those affected. Two patients on Femara developed thrombocytopenia; relationship to the study drug was unclear. Patient withdrawal due to laboratory abnormalities, whether related to study treatment or not, was infrequent.

Increases in SGOT, SGPT, and gamma GT ≥5 times the upper limit of normal (ULN) and of bilirubin ≥1.5 times the ULN were most often associated with metastatic disease in the liver. About 3% of study participants receiving Femara had abnormalities in liver chemistries not associated with documented metastases; these abnormalities may have been related to study drug therapy. In the megestrol acetate comparative study about 8% of patients treated with megestrol acetate had abnormalities in liver chemistries that were not associated with documented liver metastases; in the aminoglutethimide study about 10% of aminoglutethimide-treated patients had abnormalities in liver chemistries not associated with hepatic metastases.

Drug Interactions

Clinical interaction studies with cimetidine and warfarin indicated that the coadministration of Femara with these drugs does not result in clinically-significant drug interactions. (See CLINICAL PHARMACOLOGY)

There is no clinical experience to date on the use of Femara in combination with other anti-cancer agents.

Drug/Laboratory Test-Interactions

None observed.

Carcinogenesis, Mutagenesis, Impairment of Fertility

A conventional carcinogenesis study in mice at doses of 0.6 to 60 mg/kg/day (about one to 100 times the daily maximum recommended human dose on a mg/m^2 basis) administered by oral gavage for up to 2 years revealed a dose-related increase in the incidence of benign ovarian stromal tumors. The incidence of combined hepatocellular adenoma and carcinoma showed a significant trend in females when the high dose group was excluded due to low survival. In a separate study, plasma $AUC_{0\text{-}12hr}$ levels in mice at 60 mg/kg/day were 55 times higher than the $AUC_{0\text{-}24hr}$ level in breast cancer patients at the recommended dose. The carcinogenicity study in rats at oral doses of 0.1 to 10 mg/kg/day (about 0.4 to 40 times the daily maximum recommended human dose on a mg/m^2 basis) for up to 2 years also produced an increase in the incidence of benign ovarian stromal tumors at 10 mg/kg/day. Ovarian hyperplasia was observed in females at doses equal to or greater than 0.1 mg/kg/day. At 10 mg/kg/day, plasma $AUC_{0\text{-}24hr}$ levels in rats were 80 times higher than the level in breast cancer patients at the recommended dose.

Letrozole was not mutagenic in *in vitro* tests (Ames and E.coli bacterial tests) but was observed to be a potential clastogen in *in vitro* assays (CHO K1 and CCL 61 Chinese hamster ovary cells). Letrozole was not clastogenic *in vivo* (micronucleus test in rats).

Studies to investigate the effect of letrozole on fertility have not been conducted; however, repeated dosing caused sexual inactivity in females and atrophy of the reproductive tract in males and females at doses of 0.6, 0.1 and 0.03 mg/kg in mice, rats and dogs, respectively (about one, 0.4 and 0.4 the daily maximum recommended human dose on a mg/m^2 basis, respectively).

Pregnancy: Pregnancy Category D (See WARNINGS).

Nursing Mothers

It is not known if letrozole is excreted in human milk. Because many drugs are excreted in human milk, caution should be exercised when letrozole is administered to a nursing woman (See WARNINGS AND PRECAUTIONS).

Pediatric Use

The safety and effectiveness in pediatric patients have not been established.

Geriatric Use

The mean age of patients in the two randomized trials, that compared Femara (0.5 mg and 2.5 mg) to megestrol acetate and to aminoglutethimide, was 64 years. Thirty percent of patients were ≥70 years old. The proportion of patients responding to each dose of Femara was similar for women ≥70 years old and <70 years old.

ADVERSE REACTIONS

Femara (letrozole tablets) was generally well tolerated in two controlled clinical trials.

Study discontinuations in the megestrol acetate comparison study for adverse events other than progression of tumor occurred in 5/188 (2.7%) of patients on Femara 0.5 mg, in 4/174 (2.3%) of the patients on Femara 2.5 mg, and in 15/190 (7.9%) of patients on megestrol acetate. There were fewer thromboembolic events at both Femara doses than on the megestrol acetate arm (2 of 362 patients or 0.6% vs. 9 of 190 patients or 4.7%). There was also less vaginal bleeding (1 of 362 patients or 0.3% vs. 6 of 190 patients or 3.2%) on letrozole than on megestrol acetate. In the aminoglutethimide comparison study, discontinuations for reasons other than progression occurred in 6/193 (3.1%) of patients on 0.5 mg Femara, 7/185 (3.8%) of patients on 2.5 mg Femara, and 7/178 (3.9%) of patients on aminoglutethimide.

Comparisons of the incidence of adverse events revealed no significant differences between the high and low dose Femara groups in either study. Most of the adverse events observed in all treatment groups were mild to moderate in severity and it was generally not possible to distinguish adverse reactions due to treatment from the consequences of the patient's metastatic breast cancer, the effects of estrogen deprivation, or intercurrent illness.

Adverse events, regardless of relationship to study drug, that were reported in at least 5% of the patients treated with Femara 0.5 mg, Femara 2.5 mg, megestrol acetate, or aminoglutethimide in the two controlled trials are shown in the following table:

[See second table above]

Other less frequent (<5%) adverse experiences considered consequential and reported in at least 3 patients treated with Femara, included hypercalcemia, fracture, depression, anxiety, pleural effusion, alopecia, increased sweating and vertigo.

OVERDOSAGE

No experience with Femara (letrozole tablets) overdose has been reported. In single dose studies the highest dose used was 30 mg, which was well tolerated; in multiple dose trials, the largest dose of 5 mg was well tolerated.

Lethality was observed in mice and rats following single oral doses that were equal to or greater than 2000 mg/kg (about 4000 to 8000 times the daily maximum recommended human dose on a mg/m^2 basis); death was associated with reduced motor activity, ataxia and dyspnea. Lethality was observed in cats following single IV doses that were equal to or greater than 10 mg/kg (about 50 times the daily maximum recommended human dose on a mg/m^2 basis); death was preceded by depressed blood pressure and arrhythmias.

There is no experience in humans with an overdose of Femara, so firm recommendations for treatment are not possible. Emesis could be induced if the patient is alert. In general, supportive care and frequent monitoring of vital signs is appropriate.

DOSAGE & ADMINISTRATION

Adult and Elderly Patients

The recommended dose of Femara (letrozole tablets) is one 2.5 mg tablet administered once a day, without regard to meals. Treatment with Femara should continue until tumor progression is evident. No dose adjustment is required for elderly patients. Patients treated with Femara do not require glucocorticoid or mineralocorticoid replacement therapy.

Renal Impairment

(See CLINICAL PHARMACOLOGY.) No dosage adjustment is required for patients with renal impairment if creatinine clearance is ≥10 mL/min.

Hepatic Impairment

(See CLINICAL PHARMACOLOGY.) Although letrozole blood concentrations were modestly increased in subjects with moderate hepatic impairment due to cirrhosis, no dosage adjustment is recommended for patients with mild-to-moderate hepatic impairment. Patients with severe impairment of liver function have not been studied. Because letrozole is eliminated almost exclusively by hepatic metabolism, patients with severe impairment of liver function should be dosed with caution.

HOW SUPPLIED

2.5 mg tablets - dark yellow, film-coated, round, slightly biconvex, with beveled edges (imprinted with the letters FV on one side and CG on the other side).

Packaged in HDPE bottles with a safety screw cap.

Bottles of 30 tablets .... NDC 0078-0249-15

Store at 25°C (77°F); excursions permitted to 15°C-30°C (59°F-86°F) [see USP Controlled Room Temperature].

REV: JUNE 2000 T2000-45

Shown in Product Identification Guide, page 325

LAMISIL® ℞

[la″mə′səl]

(terbinafine hydrochloride tablets)

Tablets

Rx only

The following prescribing information is based on official labeling in effect July 2000.

Continued on next page

Lamisil—Cont.

DESCRIPTION

Lamisil® (terbinafine hydrochloride tablets) Tablets contain the synthetic allylamine antifungal compound terbinafine hydrochloride.

Chemically, terbinafine hydrochloride is (E)-*N*-(6,6-dimethyl-2-hepten-4-ynyl)-*N*-methyl-1-naphthalenemethanamine hydrochloride. The empirical formula $C_{21}H_{26}ClN$ with a molecular weight of 327.90, and the following structural formula:

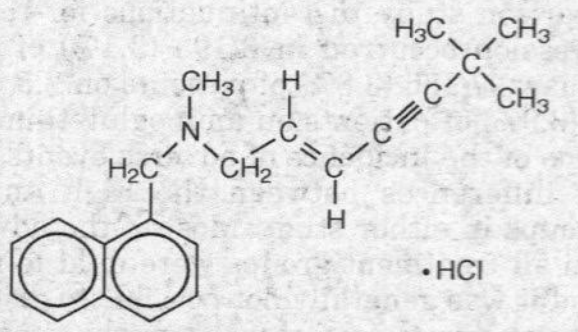

Terbinafine hydrochloride is a white to off-white fine crystalline powder. It is freely soluble in methanol and methylene chloride, soluble in ethanol, and slightly soluble in water.

Each tablet contains:

Active Ingredients: terbinafine hydrochloride (equivalent to 250 mg base)

Inactive Ingredients: colloidal silicon dioxide, NF; hydroxypropyl methylcellulose, USP; magnesium stearate, NF; microcrystalline cellulose, NF; sodium starch glycolate, NF

CLINICAL PHARMACOLOGY

Pharmacokinetics

Following oral administration, terbinafine is well absorbed (>70%) and the bioavailability of Lamisil® (terbinafine hydrochloride tablets) Tablets as a result of first-pass metabolism is approximately 40%. Peak plasma concentrations of 1 µg/mL appear within 2 h after a single 250 mg dose; the AUC (area under the curve) is approximately 4.56 µg•h/mL. An increase in the AUC of terbinafine of less than 20% is observed when Lamisil® is administered with food.

No clinically relevant age-dependent changes in steady-state plasma concentrations of terbinafine have been reported. In patients with renal impairment (creatinine clearance ≤50 mL/min) or hepatic cirrhosis, the clearance of terbinafine is decreased by approximately 50% compared to normal volunteers. No effect of gender on the blood levels of terbinafine was detected in clinical trials. In plasma, terbinafine is >99% bound to plasma proteins and there are no specific binding sites. At steady-state, in comparison to a single dose, the peak concentration of terbinafine is 25% higher and plasma AUC increases by a factor of 2.5; the increase in plasma AUC is consistent with an effective half-life of ~36 hours. Terbinafine is distributed to the sebum and skin. A terminal half-life of 200-400 h may represent the slow elimination of terbinafine from tissues such as skin and adipose. Prior to excretion, terbinafine is extensively metabolized. No metabolites have been identified that have antifungal activity similar to terbinafine. Approximately 70% of the administered dose is eliminated in the urine.

Microbiology

Terbinafine hydrochloride is a synthetic allylamine derivative. Terbinafine hydrochloride is hypothesized to act by inhibiting squalene epoxidase, thus blocking the biosynthesis of ergosterol, an essential component of fungal cell membranes. *In vitro*, mammalian squalene epoxidase is only inhibited at higher (4000 fold) concentrations than is needed for inhibition of the dermatophyte enzyme. Depending on the concentration of the drug and the fungal species test *in vitro*, terbinafine hydrochloride may be fungicidal. However, the clinical significance of *in vitro* data is unknown.

Terbinafine has been shown to be active against most strains of the following microorganisms both *in vitro* and in clinical infections as described in the *INDICATIONS AND USAGE* section:

Trichophyton mentagrophytes
Trichophyton rubrum

The following *in vitro* data are available, but their clinical significance is unknown. *In vitro*, terbinafine exhibits satisfactory MIC's against most strains of the following microorganisms; however, the safety and efficacy of terbinafine in treating clinical infections due to these microorganisms have not been established in adequate and well-controlled clinical trials:

Candida albicans
Epidermophyton floccosum
Scopulariopsis brevicaulis

CLINICAL STUDIES

The efficacy of Lamisil® (terbinafine hydrochloride tablets) Tablets in the treatment of onychomycosis is illustrated by the response of patients with toenail and/or fingernail infections who participated in three US/Canadian placebo-controlled clinical trials.

Results of the first toenail study, as assessed at week 48 (12 weeks of treatment with 36 weeks follow-up after completion of therapy), demonstrated mycological cure, defined as simultaneous occurrence of negative KOH plus negative culture, in 70% of patients. Fifty-nine percent (59%) of patients experienced effective treatment (mycological cure plus 0% nail involvement or >5mm of new unaffected nail growth); 38% of patients demonstrated mycological cure plus clinical cure (0% nail involvement).

In a second toenail study of dermatophytic onychomycosis, in which non-dermatophytes were also cultured, similar efficacy against the dermatophytes was demonstrated. The pathogenic role of the non-dermatophytes cultured in the presence of dermatophytic onychomycosis has not been established. The clinical significance of this association is unknown.

Results of the fingernail study, as assessed at week 24 (6 weeks of treatment with 18 weeks follow-up after completion of therapy), demonstrated mycological cure in 79% of patients, effective treatment in 75% of the patients, and mycological cure plus clinical cure in 59% of the patients.

The mean time to overall success was approximately 10 months for the first toenail study and 4 months for the fingernail study. In the first toenail study, for patients evaluated at least six months after achieving clinical cure and at least one year after completing Lamisil® therapy, the clinical relapse rate was approximately 15%.

INDICATIONS AND USAGE

Lamisil® (terbinafine hydrochloride tablets) Tablets are indicated for the treatment of onychomycosis of the toenail or fingernail due to dermatophytes (tinea unguium) *(see DOSAGE AND ADMINISTRATION and CLINICAL STUDIES).*

CONTRAINDICATIONS

Lamisil® (terbinafine hydrochloride tablets) Tablets are contraindicated in individuals with hypersensitivity to terbinafine or to any other ingredients of the formulation.

WARNINGS

Rare cases of symptomatic hepatobiliary dysfunction including cholestatic hepatitis have been reported. Treatment with Lamisil® (terbinafine hydrochloride tablets) Tablets should be discontinued if hepatobiliary dysfunction develops *(see PRECAUTIONS and ADVERSE REACTIONS).* There have been isolated reports of serious skin reactions (e.g., Stevens-Johnson Syndrome and toxic epidermal necrolysis). If progressive skin rash occurs, treatment with Lamisil® should be discontinued.

PRECAUTIONS

General

Changes in the ocular lens and retina have been reported following the use of Lamisil® (terbinafine hydrochloride tablets) Tablets in controlled trials. The clinical significance of these changes is unknown.

Hepatic function (hepatic enzyme) tests are recommended in patients administered Lamisil® (terbinafine hydrochloride tablets) Tablets for more than six weeks or in those who develop unexplained persistent nausea, anorexia, or fatigue or jaundice, dark urine, or pale stools *(see WARNINGS).*

In patients with either pre-existing liver disease or renal impairment (creatinine clearance ≤50 mL/min), the use of Lamisil® has not been adequately studied, and therefore, is not recommended *(see CLINICAL PHARMACOLOGY, Pharmacokinetics).*

Transient decreases in absolute lymphocyte counts (ALC) have been observed in controlled clinical trials. In placebo-controlled trials, 8/465 Lamisil®-treated patients (1.7%) and 3/137 placebo-treated patients (2.2%) had decreases in ALC to below 1000/mm^3 on two or more occasions. The clinical significance of this observation is unknown. However, in patients with known or suspected immunodeficiency, physicians should consider monitoring complete blood counts in individuals using Lamisil® therapy for greater than six weeks.

Isolated cases of severe neutropenia have been reported. These were reversible upon discontinuation of Lamisil®, with or without supportive therapy. If clinical signs and symptoms suggestive of secondary infection occur, a complete blood count should be obtained. If the neutrophil count is ≤1,000 cells/mm^3, Lamisil® should be discontinued and supportive management started.

Drug Interactions

In vitro studies with human liver microsomes showed that terbinafine does not inhibit the metabolism of tolbutamide, ethinylestradiol, ethoxycoumarin, and cyclosporine. *In vivo* drug-drug interaction studies conducted in normal volunteer subjects showed that terbinafine does not affect the clearance of antipyrine, digoxin, and the antihistamine terfenadine. Terbinafine decreases the clearance of intravenously administered caffeine by 19%. Terbinafine increases the clearance of cyclosporine by 15%.

Terbinafine clearance is increased 100% by rifampin, a CyP450 enzyme inducer, and decreased 33% by cimetidine, a CyP450 enzyme inhibitor. Terbinafine exposure (AUC) is increased 16% by terfenadine. Terbinafine clearance is unaffected by cyclosporine.

There is no information available from adequate drug-drug interaction studies with the following classes of drugs: oral contraceptives, hormone replacement therapies, hypoglycemics, theophyllines, phenytoins, thiazide diuretics, beta blockers, and calcium channel blockers.

Carcinogenesis, Mutagenesis, Impairment of Fertility

In a 28-month oral carcinogenicity study in rats, a marginal increase in the incidence of liver tumors was observed in males at the highest dose level, 69 mg/kg/day [3.6× the Maximum Recommended Human Dose (MRHD) based on body surface area (BSA)]. There was no dose-related trend and the mid-dose male rats (20 mg/kg/day; 1.0× the MRHD based on BSA) did not have any tumors. No increased incidence in liver tumors was noted in female rats at dose levels up to 97 mg/kg/day (4.5× the MRHD based on BSA) or in male or female mice treated orally for 23 months at doses up to 156 mg/kg/day (3.9× the MRHD based on BSA).

A wide range of *in vivo* studies in mice, rats, dogs, and monkeys, and *in vitro* studies using rat, monkey, and human hepatocytes suggest that the development of liver tumors in the high-dose male rats may be associated with peroxisome proliferation, and support the conclusion that this is a rat-specific finding. *In vivo* investigations included evaluations of the effects of Lamisil® on liver weight, morphology, and ultrastructure; hepatic cytochrome P450; and peroxisome proliferation assessed morphologically and biochemically (peroxisomal enzymes) in mice, rats, dogs, and monkeys. The effects of Lamisil® and two known metabolites on hepatic morphology and peroxisomal and P450 enzyme activities were also evaluated *in vivo* in male rats and *in vitro* in primary hepatocyte cultures from male rats and humans and from monkeys. The results of the *in vivo* investigations indicated that oral administration of Lamisil® (500 mg/kg/day) resulted in peroxisome proliferation in rats, and that these effects did not occur in mice, dogs, or monkeys. Further, *in vitro* studies indicated that peroxisome proliferation occurred in rat hepatocytes, but not in monkey or human hepatocytes.

Systemic exposure to Lamisil®, assessed by the steady-state plasma unbound fraction area under the curve (AUC) for terbinafine and metabolites, was 7.7 and 9.7 µg•h/mL for male and female rats, respectively, and 11.2 and 13.1 µg•h/mL for male and female mice, respectively, at doses comparable to the high doses in the carcinogenicity studies. In human subjects at the MRHD (a daily dose of 250 mg of Lamisil®), the unbound AUC was 0.466 µg•h/mL. The resulting safety margins for humans, based on relative systemic exposure (AUC unbound), in rats and mice were 17 to 21 and 24 to 28, respectively.

The results of a variety of *in vitro* (mutations in *E. coli* and *Salmonella*, DNA repair in rat hepatocytes, mutagenicity in Chinese hamster fibroblasts, chromosome aberration and sister chromatid exchanges in Chinese hamster lung cells), and *in vivo* (chromosome aberration in Chinese hamsters, micronucleus test in mice) genotoxicity tests gave no evidence of a mutagenic or clastogenic potential and demonstrated the absence of tumor-initiating or cell-proliferating activity.

Oral reproduction studies in rats at doses up to 300 mg/kg/day (approximately 12× the MRHD based on BSA) did not reveal any specific effects on fertility or other reproductive parameters. Intravaginal application of terbinafine hydrochloride at 150 mg/day in pregnant rabbits did not increase the incidence of abortions or premature deliveries nor affect fetal parameters.

Pregnancy

Pregnancy Category B: Oral reproduction studies have been performed in rabbits and rats at doses up to 300 mg/kg/day (9× to 12× the MRHD, in rabbits and rats, respectively, based on BSA) and have revealed no evidence of impaired fertility or harm to the fetus due to terbinafine. There are, however, no adequate and well-controlled studies in pregnant women. Because animal reproduction studies are not always predictive of human response, and because treatment of onychomycosis can be postponed until after pregnancy is completed, it is recommended that Lamisil® not be initiated during pregnancy.

Nursing Mothers

After oral administration, terbinafine is present in breast milk of nursing mothers. The ratio of terbinafine in milk to plasma is 7:1. Treatment with Lamisil® is not recommended in nursing mothers.

Pediatric Use

The safety and efficacy of Lamisil® have not been established in pediatric patients.

ADVERSE REACTIONS

The most frequently reported adverse events observed in the three US/Canadian placebo-controlled trials are listed in the table below. The adverse events reported encompass gastrointestinal symptoms (including diarrhea, dyspepsia, and abdominal pain), liver test abnormalities, rashes, urticaria, pruritus, and taste disturbances. In general, the adverse events were mild, transient, and did not lead to discontinuation from study participation.

	Adverse Event		Discontinuation	
	Lamisil® (%) n=465	Placebo (%) n=137	Lamisil® (%) n=465	Placebo (%) n=137
Headache	12.9	9.5	0.2	0.0
Gastrointestinal Symptoms:				
Diarrhea	5.6	2.9	0.6	0.0
Dyspepsia	4.3	2.9	0.4	0.0
Abdominal Pain	2.4	1.5	0.4	0.0
Nausea	2.6	2.9	0.2	0.0
Flatulence	2.2	2.2	0.0	0.0
Dermatological Symptoms:				
Rash	5.6	2.2	0.9	0.7
Pruritus	2.8	1.5	0.2	0.0
Urticaria	1.1	0.0	0.0	0.0

Liver Enzyme Abnormalities*	3.3	1.4	0.2	0.0
Taste Disturbance	2.8	0.7	0.2	0.0
Visual Disturbance	1.1	1.5	0.9	0.0

*Liver enzyme abnormalities ≥2× the upper limit of the normal range.

Rare adverse events, based on worldwide experience with Lamisil® (terbinafine hydrochloride tablets) Tablets use, include: symptomatic idiosyncratic hepatobiliary dysfunction (including cholestatic hepatitis and very rarely liver failure) *(see WARNINGS and PRECAUTIONS)*, serious skin reactions *(see WARNINGS)*, severe neutropenia *(see PRECAUTIONS)*, thrombocytopenia and allergic reactions (including anaphylaxis). Uncommonly, Lamisil® may cause taste disturbance (including taste loss) which usually recovers within several weeks after discontinuation of the drug. Other adverse reactions which have been reported include malaise, fatigue, vomiting, arthralgia, myalgia, and hair loss.

Clinical adverse effects reported spontaneously since the drug was marketed include altered prothrombin time (prolongation and reduction) in patients concomitantly treated with warfarin and Lamisil® (terbinafine hydrochloride tablets) Tablets and agranulocytosis (very rare).

OVERDOSAGE

Clinical experience regarding overdose with Lamisil® (terbinafine hydrochloride tablets) Tablets is limited. Doses up to 5 grams (20 times the therapeutic daily dose) have been taken without inducing serious adverse reactions. The symptoms of overdose included nausea, vomiting, abdominal pain, dizziness, rash, frequent urination, and headache.

DOSAGE AND ADMINISTRATION

Lamisil® (terbinafine hydrochloride tablets) Tablets, one 250 mg tablet, should be taken once daily for 6 weeks by patients with fingernail onychomycosis. Lamisil®, one 250 mg tablet, should be taken once daily for 12 weeks by patients with toenail onychomycosis. The optimal clinical effect is seen some months after mycological cure and cessation of treatment. This is related to the period required for outgrowth of healthy nail.

HOW SUPPLIED

Lamisil®
(terbinafine hydrochloride tablets)
Tablets

Supplied as white to yellow-tinged white circular, bi-convex, bevelled tablets containing 250 mg of terbinafine imprinted with "LAMISIL" in circular form on one side and code "250" on the other.

Bottles of 100 tablets
NDC 0078-0179-05
Bottles of 30 tablets
NDC 0078-0179-15

Store tablets below 25°C (77°F); in a tight container. Protect from light.

Manufactured by:
Novartis Pharmaceuticals Canada, Inc.
Dorval (Québec), Canada H9S 1A9
Distributed by:
Novartis Pharmaceuticals Corporation
East Hanover, New Jersey 07936
REV: NOVEMBER 1999 T1999-71

Shown in Product Identification Guide, page 325

LESCOL® ℞

[lěs-cōl]
(fluvastatin sodium)
Capsules
Rx only

The following prescribing information is based on official labeling in effect July 2000.

DESCRIPTION

Lescol® (fluvastatin sodium), is a water soluble cholesterol lowering agent which acts through the inhibition of 3-hydroxy-3-methylglutaryl-coenzyme A (HMG-CoA) reductase.

Fluvastatin sodium is [*R**,*S**-(*E*)]-(±)-7-[3-(4-fluorophenyl)-1-(1-methylethyl)-1*H*-indol-2-yl]-3,5-dihydroxy-6-heptenoic acid, monosodium salt. The structural formula is:

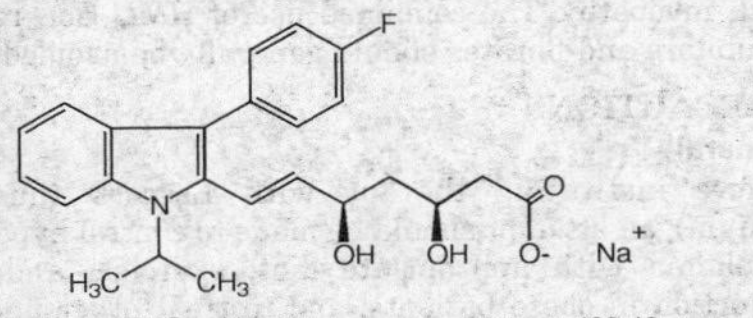

$C_{24}H_{25}FNO_4 \cdot Na$ Mol. wt. 433.46

This molecular entity is the first entirely synthetic HMG-CoA reductase inhibitor, and is in part structurally distinct from the fungal derivatives of this therapeutic class.

Fluvastatin sodium is a white to pale yellow, hygroscopic powder soluble in water, ethanol and methanol. Lescol®

	C_{max} (ng/mL) mean±SD (range)	AUC (ng·h/mL) mean±SD (range)	t_{max} (hr) mean±SD (range)	CL/F (L/hr) mean±SD (range)	$t_{1/2}$ (hr) mean±SD (range)
20 mg single dose (n=17)	166±106 (48.9-517)	207±65 (111-288)	0.9±0.4 (0.5-2.0)	107±38.1 (69.5-181)	2.5±1.7 (0.5-6.6)
20 mg b.i.d. (n=17)	200±86 (71.8-366)	275±111 (91.6-467)	1.2±0.9 (0.5-4.0)	87.8±45 (42.8-218)	2.8±1.7 (0.9-6.0)
40 mg single dose (n=16)	273±189 (72.8-812)	456±259 (207-1221)	1.2±0.7 (0.75-3.0)	108±44.7 (32.8-193)	2.7±1.3 (0.8-5.9)
40 mg b.i.d. (n=16)	432±236 (119-990)	697±275 (359-1559)	1.2±0.6 (0.5-2.5)	64.2±21.1 (25.7-111)	2.7±1.3 (0.7-5.0)

Median Percent Change in Lipid Parameters from Baseline to Week 24 Endpoint
All Placebo-Controlled Studies

	Total Chol.		TG		LDL		Apo B		HDL	
Dose	**N**	**%Δ**	**N**	**%Δ**	**N**	**%Δ**	**N**	**%Δ**	**N**	**%Δ**
All Patients										
Lescol 20 mg	747	-16.6	747	-11.9	747	-22.2	114	-19.3	747	+3.3
Lescol 40 mg	748	-18.6	748	-13.5	748	-25.0	125	-18.3	748	+4.4
Lescol 80 mg	257	-27.0	257	-17.8	257	-35.9	232	-28.4	257	+5.6
Baseline TG ≥200 mg/dL										
Lescol 20 mg	148	-16.4	148	-17.3	148	-21.6	23	-19.2	148	+5.8
Lescol 40 mg	179	-17.8	179	-19.6	179	-23.5	47	-18.3	179	+6.9
Lescol 80 mg	76	-26.8	76	-23.2	76	-34.6	69	-28.1	76	+9.0

(fluvastatin sodium) is supplied as capsules containing fluvastatin sodium, equivalent to 20 mg or 40 mg of fluvastatin, for oral administration.

Active Ingredient: fluvastatin sodium

Inactive Ingredients: gelatin, magnesium stearate, microcrystalline cellulose, pregelatinized starch, red iron oxide, sodium lauryl sulfate, talc, titanium dioxide, yellow iron oxide, and other ingredients.

May Also Include: benzyl alcohol, black iron oxide, butylparaben, carboxymethylcellulose sodium, edetate calcium disodium, methylparaben, propylparaben, silicon dioxide and sodium propionate.

CLINICAL PHARMACOLOGY

A variety of clinical studies have demonstrated that elevated levels of total cholesterol (Total-C), low density lipoprotein cholesterol (LDL-C), and apolipoprotein B (a membrane transport complex for LDL-C) promote human atherosclerosis. Similarly, decreased levels of HDL-cholesterol (HDL-C) and its transport complex, apolipoprotein A, are associated with the development of atherosclerosis. Epidemiologic investigations have established that cardiovascular morbidity and mortality vary directly with the level of Total-C and LDL-C and inversely with the level of HDL-C.

In patients with hypercholesterolemia, treatment with Lescol® (fluvastatin sodium) reduced Total-C, LDL-C, and apolipoprotein B. Lescol® (fluvastatin sodium) also moderately reduced triglycerides (TG) while producing an increase in HDL-C of variable magnitude. The agent had no consistent effect on either Lp(a) or fibrinogen. The effect of Lescol® (fluvastatin sodium)-induced changes in lipoprotein levels, including reduction of serum cholesterol, on cardiovascular morbidity or mortality has not been determined.

Mechanism of Action

Lescol® (fluvastatin sodium) is a competitive inhibitor of HMG-CoA reductase, which is responsible for the conversion of 3-hydroxy-3-methylglutaryl-coenzyme A (HMG-CoA) to mevalonate, a precursor of sterols, including cholesterol. The inhibition of cholesterol biosynthesis reduces the cholesterol in hepatic cells, which stimulates the synthesis of LDL receptors and thereby increases the uptake of LDL particles. The end result of these biochemical processes is a reduction of the plasma cholesterol concentration.

Pharmacokinetics/Metabolism

Oral Absorption

Fluvastatin is absorbed rapidly and completely following oral administration, with peak concentrations reached in less than 1 hour. Following administration of a 10 mg dose, the absolute bioavailability is 24% (range 9%-50%). Administration with food reduces the rate but not the extent of absorption. At steady-state, administration of fluvastatin with the evening meal results in a two-fold decrease in C_{max} and more than two-fold increase in t_{max} as compared to administration 4 hours after the evening meal. No significant difference in extent of absorption or in the lipid-lowering effects were observed between the two administrations. After single or multiple doses above 20 mg, fluvastatin exhibits saturable first-pass metabolism resulting in higher-than-expected plasma fluvastatin concentrations. The inactive enantiomer accounts for about 60% of the increase.

Distribution

Fluvastatin is 98% bound to plasma proteins. The mean volume of distribution (VD_{ss}) is estimated at 34.4 liters. The parent drug is targeted to the liver and no active metabolites are present systemically.

Metabolism

Fluvastatin is metabolized in the liver, primarily via hydroxylation of the indole ring at the 5- and 6-positions. N-dealkylation and beta-oxidation of the side-chain also occurs. The hydroxy metabolites have some pharmacologic activity, but do not circulate in the blood. Both enantiomers of fluvastatin are metabolized in a similar manner.

Elimination

Fluvastatin is primarily (about 90%) eliminated in the feces as metabolites, with less than 2% present as unchanged drug.

Special Populations

Renal Insufficiency: No significant (<6%) renal excretion of fluvastatin occurs in humans.

Hepatic Insufficiency: Fluvastatin is subject to saturable first-pass metabolism/sequestration by the liver and is eliminated primarily via the biliary route. Therefore, the potential exists for drug accumulation in patients with hepatic insufficiency. Caution should therefore be exercised when fluvastatin sodium is administered to patients with a history of liver disease or heavy alcohol ingestion *(see WARNINGS)*.

Age: Plasma levels of fluvastatin are not affected by age.

Gender: Women tend to have slightly higher (but statistically insignificant) fluvastatin concentrations than men. This is most likely due to body weight differences, as adjusting for body weight decreases the magnitude of the differences seen.

Pediatric: No data are available. Fluvastatin is not indicated for use in the pediatric population.

Steady-state plasma concentrations show no evidence of accumulation of fluvastatin following administration of up to 80 mg daily, as evidenced by a beta-elimination half-life of less than 3 hours. However, under conditions of maximum rate of absorption (i.e., fasting) systemic exposure to fluvastatin is increased 33% to 53% compared to a single 20 mg or 40 mg dose.

Single-dose and steady-state pharmacokinetic parameters in 33 subjects with hypercholesterolemia are summarized below:

[See first table above]

Clinical Studies

Hypercholesterolemia (heterozygous familial and non familial) and Mixed Dyslipidemia

In 12 placebo-controlled studies in patients with Type IIa and IIb hyperlipoproteinemia, Lescol® (fluvastatin sodium) alone was administered to 1621 patients in daily dose regimens of 20 mg, 40 mg, and 80 mg (40 mg b.i.d.) for at least 6 weeks duration. After 24 weeks of treatment, daily doses of 20 mg, 40 mg, and 80 mg (40 mg b.i.d.) resulted in median LDL-C reductions of 22% (N=747), 25% (N=748) and 36% (N=257), respectively. Lescol® (fluvastatin sodium) treatment produced dose-related reductions in Apo B and in triglycerides and variable increases in HDL-C. In the subgroup of patients with primary mixed dyslipidemia, defined as baseline TG levels ≥200 mg/dL, treatment with Lescol® (fluvastatin sodium) also produced significant decreases in Total-C, LDL-C, TG and Apo B and variable increases in HDL-C.

In a long term open label free titration study, after 96 weeks LDL-C decreases of 25% (20 mg, N=68), 31% (40 mg, N=298) and 34% (80 mg, N=209) were seen. No consistent effect on Lp(a) was observed.

[See second table above]

Although frequently found in association with low HDL-C, elevated plasma TG has not been established as an independent risk factor for coronary heart disease. The independent effect of raising HDL-C or lowering TG on the risk for coronary and cardiovascular morbidity and mortality has not been established.

Atherosclerosis

In the Lipoprotein and Coronary Atherosclerosis Study (LCAS), the effect of Lescol® (fluvastatin sodium) therapy on coronary atherosclerosis was assessed by quantitative coronary angiography (QCA) in patients with coronary artery disease and mild to moderate hypercholesterolemia (baseline LDL-C range 115-190 mg/dL). In this randomized

Continued on next page

Lescol—Cont.

double-blind, placebo controlled trial, 429 patients were treated with conventional measures (Step 1 AHA Diet) and either Lescol® (fluvastatin sodium) 40 mg/day or placebo. In order to provide treatment to patients receiving placebo with LDL-C levels ≥160 mg/dL at baseline, adjunctive therapy with cholestyramine was added after week 12 to all patients in the study with baseline LDL-C values of ≥160 mg/dL. These baseline levels were present in 25% of the study population. Quantitative coronary angiograms were evaluated at baseline and 2.5 years in 340 (79%) angiographic evaluable patients.

Lescol® (fluvastatin sodium) significantly slowed the progression of coronary atherosclerosis. Compared to placebo, Lescol® (fluvastatin sodium) significantly slowed the progression of lesions as measured by within-patient per-lesion change in minimum lumen diameter (MLD), the primary endpoint (see Figure 1 below), percent diameter stenosis (Figure 2), and the formation of new lesions (13% of all fluvastatin patients versus 22% of all placebo patients). Additionally, a significant difference in favor of Lescol® (fluvastatin sodium) was found between all fluvastatin and all placebo patients in the distribution among the three categories of definite progression, definite regression, and mixed or no change. Beneficial angiographic results (change in MLD) were independent of patients' gender and consistent across a range of baseline LDL-C levels.

Figure 1
Change in Minimum Lumen Diameter (mm)

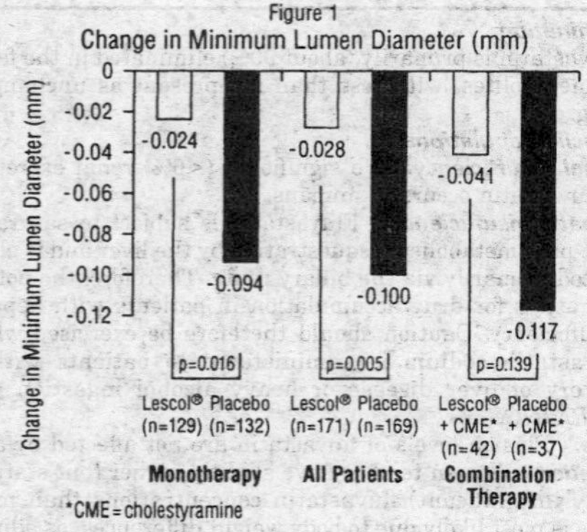

Figure 2
Change in % Diameter Stenosis

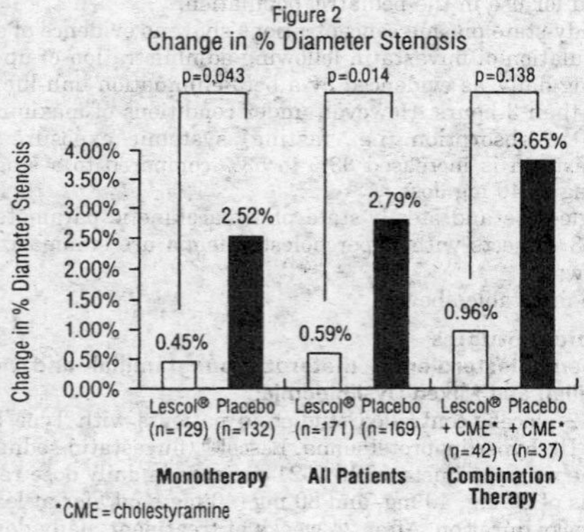

INDICATIONS AND USAGE

Therapy with lipid-altering agents should be a component of multiple risk factor intervention in those individuals at significantly increased risk for atherosclerosis vascular disease due to hypercholesterolemia.

Hypercholesterolemia (heterozygous familial and non familial) and Mixed Dyslipidemia

Lescol® (fluvastatin sodium) is indicated as an adjunct to diet in the treatment of elevated total cholesterol (Total-C), LDL-C, TG and Apo B levels in patients with primary hypercholesterolemia and mixed dyslipidemia (Frederickson Type IIa and IIb) whose response to dietary restriction of saturated fat and cholesterol and other nonpharmacological measures has not been adequate.

Atherosclerosis

Lescol® (fluvastatin sodium) is also indicated to slow the progression of coronary atherosclerosis in patients with coronary heart disease as part of a treatment strategy to lower total and LDL cholesterol to target levels.

Therapy with lipid-altering agents should be considered only after secondary causes for hyperlipidemia such as poorly controlled diabetes mellitus, hypothyroidism, nephrotic syndrome, dysproteinemias, obstructive liver disease, other medication, or alcoholism, have been excluded. Prior to initiation of fluvastatin sodium, a lipid profile should be performed to measure Total-C, HDL-C and TG. For patients with TG <400 mg/dL (<4.5 mmol/L), LDL-C can be estimated using the following equation:

LDL-C = Total-C − HDL-C − 1/5 TG

Definite Atherosclerotic Disease*	Two or More Other Risk Factors**	LDL-Cholesterol mg/dL (mmol/L) Initiation Level	Goal
NO	NO	≥190 (≥4.9)	<160 (<4.1)
NO	YES	≥160 (≥4.1)	<130 (<3.4)
YES	YES or NO	≥130 (≥3.4)	≤100 (≤2.6)

* Coronary heart disease or peripheral vascular disease (including symptomatic carotid artery disease).

** Other risk factors for coronary artery disease (CHD) include: age (males: ≥45 years; females: ≥55 years or premature menopause without estrogen replacement therapy); family history of premature CHD; current cigarette smoking; hypertension; confirmed HDL-C <35 mg/dL (<0.91 mmol/L); and diabetes mellitus. Subtract one risk factor if HDL-C is ≥60 mg/dL (≥1.6 mmol/L).

Classification of Hyperlipoproteinemias

Type	Lipoproteins Elevated	Lipid Elevations: Major	Lipid Elevations: Minor
I (rare)	Chylomicrons	TG	↑→C
IIa	LDL	C	–
IIb	LDL, VLDL	C	TG
III (rare)	IDL	C/TG	–
IV	VLDL	TG	↑→C
V (rare)	Chylomicrons, VLDL	TG	↑→C

C = cholesterol, TG = triglycerides, LDL = low density lipoprotein, VLDL = very low density lipoprotein, IDL = intermediate density lipoprotein

For TG levels >400 mg/dL (>4.5 mmol/L), this equation is less accurate and LDL-C concentrations should be determined by ultracentrifugation. In many hypertriglyceridemic patients LDL-C may be low or normal despite elevated Total-C. In such cases, Lescol® (fluvastatin sodium) is not indicated.

Lipid determinations should be performed at intervals of no less than 4 weeks and dosage adjusted according to the patient's response to therapy.

The National Cholesterol Education Program (NCEP) Treatment Guidelines are summarized below:

[See first table above]

Since the goal of treatment is to lower LDL-C, the NCEP recommends that the LDL-C levels be used to initiate and assess treatment response. Only if LDL-C levels are not available, should the Total-C be used to monitor therapy.

[See second table above]

Lescol® (fluvastatin sodium) has not been studied in conditions where the major abnormality is elevation of chylomicrons, VLDL, or IDL (i.e., hyperlipoproteinemia Types I, III, IV, or V).

CONTRAINDICATIONS

Hypersensitivity to any component of this medication. Lescol® (fluvastatin sodium) is contraindicated in patients with active liver disease or unexplained, persistent elevations in serum transaminases *(see WARNINGS)*.

Pregnancy and Lactation

Atherosclerosis is a chronic process and discontinuation of lipid-lowering drugs during pregnancy should have little impact on the out come of long-term therapy of primary hypercholesterolemia. Cholesterol and other products of cholesterol biosynthesis are essential components for fetal development (including synthesis of steroids and cell membranes). Since HMG-CoA reductase inhibitors decrease cholesterol synthesis and possibly the synthesis of other biologically active substances derived from cholesterol, they may cause fetal harm when administered to pregnant women. Therefore, HMG-CoA reductase inhibitors are contraindicated during pregnancy and in nursing mothers. **Fluvastatin sodium should be administered to women of childbearing age only when such patients are highly unlikely to conceive and have been informed of the potential hazards.** If the patient becomes pregnant while taking this class of drug, therapy should be discontinued and the patient apprised of the potential hazard to the fetus.

WARNINGS

Liver Enzymes

Biochemical abnormalities of liver function have been associated with HMG-CoA reductase inhibitors and other lipid-lowering agents. A small number of patients treated with Lescol® (fluvastatin sodium) in worldwide controlled trials (N=25, 1.1%) developed dose-related, persistent elevations of transaminase levels to more than 3 times the upper limit of normal. Fourteen of these patients (0.6%) were discontinued from therapy. In all clinical trials, a total of 33/2969 patients (1.1%) had persistent transaminase elevations with an average fluvastatin exposure of approximately 71.2 weeks; 19 of these patients (0.6%) were discontinued. The majority of patients with these abnormal biochemical findings were asymptomatic.

In a pooled analysis of all Lescol® (fluvastatin sodium) placebo-controlled studies persistent transaminase elevations (>3 times the upper limit of normal [ULN] on two consecutive weekly measurements) occurred in 0.2%, 1.5%, and 2.7% of patients treated with 20, 40, and 80 mg (40 mg b.i.d.) Lescol® (fluvastatin sodium), respectively. Ninety-one percent of the cases of persistent liver function test abnormalities (20 of 22 patients) occurred within 12 weeks of therapy and in all patients with persistent liver function test abnormalities there was an abnormal liver function test present at baseline or by week 8.

It is recommended that liver function tests be performed before initiation of therapy and at 12 weeks following initiation of treatment or elevation in dose. Patients who develop transaminase elevations or signs and symptoms of liver disease should be monitored to confirm the finding and should be followed thereafter with frequent liver function tests until the levels return to normal. Should an increase in AST or ALT of three times the upper limit of normal or greater persist (found on two consecutive occasions), withdrawal of fluvastatin sodium therapy is recommended.

Active liver disease or unexplained transaminase elevations are contraindications to the use of Lescol® (fluvastatin sodium) *(see CONTRAINDICATIONS)*. Caution should be exercised when fluvastatin sodium is administered to patients with a history of liver disease or heavy alcohol ingestion *(see CLINICAL PHARMACOLOGY: Pharmacokinetics/Metabolism)*. Such patients should be closely monitored.

Skeletal Muscle

Rhabdomyolysis with renal dysfunction secondary to myoglobinuria has been reported with fluvastatin and with other drugs in this class. Myopathy, defined as muscle aching or muscle weakness in conjunction with increases in creatine phosphokinase (CPK) values to greater than 10 times the upper limit of normal, has been reported rarely.

Myopathy should be considered in any patients with diffuse myalgias, muscle tenderness or weakness, and/or marked elevation of CPK. Patients should be advised to report promptly unexplained muscle pain, tenderness or weakness, particularly if accompanied by malaise or fever. Fluvastatin sodium therapy should be discontinued if markedly elevated CPK levels occur or myopathy is diagnosed or suspected. Fluvastatin sodium therapy should also be temporarily withheld in any patient experiencing an acute or serious condition predisposing to the development of renal failure secondary to rhabdomyolysis, e.g., sepsis; hypotension; major surgery; trauma; severe metabolic, endocrine, or electrolyte disorders; or uncontrolled epilepsy.

The risk of myopathy and or rhabdomyolysis during treatment with HMG-CoA reductase inhibitors has been reported to be increased if therapy with either cyclosporine, gemfibrozil, erythromycin, or niacin is administered concurrently. Myopathy was not observed in a clinical trial in 74 patients involving patients who were treated with fluvastatin sodium together with niacin.

Uncomplicated myalgia has been observed infrequently in patients treated with Lescol® (fluvastatin sodium) at rates indistinguishable from placebo.

The use of fibrates alone may occasionally be associated with myopathy. The combined use of HMG-CoA reductase inhibitors and fibrates should generally be avoided.

PRECAUTIONS

General

Before instituting therapy with Lescol® (fluvastatin sodium), an attempt should be made to control hypercholesterolemia with appropriate diet, exercise, and weight reduction in obese patients, and to treat other underlying medical problems *(see INDICATIONS AND USAGE)*.

The HMG-CoA reductase inhibitors may cause elevation of creatine phosphokinase and transaminase levels *(see WARNINGS and ADVERSE REACTIONS)*. This should be considered in the differential diagnosis of chest pain in a patient on therapy with fluvastatin sodium.

Homozygous Familial Hypercholesterolemia

HMG-CoA reductase inhibitors are reported to be less effective in patients with rare homozygous familial hypercholesterolemia, possibly because these patients have few functional LDL receptors.

Information for Patients

Patients should be advised to report promptly unexplained muscle pain, tenderness or weakness, particularly if accompanied by malaise or fever.

Women should be informed that if they become pregnant while receiving Lescol® (fluvastatin sodium) the drug should be discontinued immediately to avoid possible harmful effects on a developing fetus from a relative deficit of cholesterol and biological products derived from cholesterol. In addition, Lescol® (fluvastatin sodium) should not be taken during nursing. *(See CONTRAINDICATIONS).*

Drug Interactions

Immunosuppressive Drugs, Gemfibrozil, Niacin (Nicotinic Acid), Erythromycin: *See WARNINGS: Skeletal Muscle.*

Antipyrine: Administration of fluvastatin sodium does not influence the metabolism and excretion of antipyrine, either by induction or inhibition. Antipyrine is a model for drugs metabolized by the microsomal hepatic enzyme system; therefore, interactions with other drugs metabolized by this mechanism are not expected.

Niacin/Propranolol: Concomitant administration of fluvastatin sodium with niacin or propranolol has no effect on the bioavailability of fluvastatin sodium.

Cholestyramine: Administration of fluvastatin sodium concomitantly with, or up to 4 hours after cholestyramine, results in fluvastatin decreases of more than 50% for AUC and 50%-80% for C_{max}. However, administration of fluvastatin sodium 4 hours after cholestyramine resulted in a clinically significant additive effect compared with that achieved with either component drug.

Digoxin: In a crossover study involving 18 patients chronically receiving digoxin, a single 40 mg dose of fluvastatin had no effect on digoxin AUC, but had an 11% increase in digoxin C_{max} and small increase in digoxin urinary clearance. Patients taking digoxin should be monitored appropriately when fluvastatin therapy is initiated.

Cimetidine/Ranitidine/Omeprazole: Concomitant administration of fluvastatin sodium with cimetidine, ranitidine and omeprazole results in a significant increase in the fluvastatin C_{max} (43%, 70% and 50%, respectively) and AUC (24%-33%), with an 18%-23% decrease in plasma clearance.

Rifampicin: Administration of fluvastatin sodium to subjects pretreated with rifampicin results in significant reduction in C_{max} (59%) and AUC (51%), with a large increase (95%) in plasma clearance.

Warfarin: *In vitro* protein binding studies demonstrated no interaction at therapeutic concentrations. Concomitant administration of a single dose of warfarin (30 mg) in young healthy males receiving fluvastatin sodium (40 mg/day × 8 days) resulted in no elevation of racemic warfarin concentration. There was also no effect on prothrombin complex activity when compared to concomitant administration of placebo and warfarin. However, bleeding and/or increased prothrombin times have been reported in patients taking coumarin anticoagulants concomitantly with other HMG-CoA reductase inhibitors. Therefore, patients receiving warfarin-type anticoagulants should have their prothrombin times closely monitored when fluvastatin sodium is initiated or the dosage of fluvastatin sodium is changed.

Endocrine Function

HMG-CoA reductase inhibitors interfere with cholesterol synthesis and lower circulating cholesterol levels and, as such, might theoretically blunt adrenal or gonadal steroid hormone production.

Fluvastatin exhibited no effect upon non-stimulated cortisol levels and demonstrated no effect upon thyroid metabolism as assessed by TSH. Small declines in total testosterone have been noted in treated groups, but no commensurate elevation in LH occurred, suggesting that the observation was not due to a direct effect upon testosterone production. No effect upon FSH in males was noted. Due to the limited number of premenopausal females studied to date, no conclusions regarding the effect of fluvastatin upon female sex hormones may be made.

Two clinical studies in patients receiving fluvastatin at doses up to 80 mg daily for periods of 24 to 28 weeks demonstrated no effect of treatment upon the adrenal response to ACTH stimulation. A clinical study evaluated the effect of fluvastatin at doses up to 80 mg daily for 28 weeks upon the gonadal response to HCG stimulation. Although the mean total testosterone response was significantly reduced ($p<0.05$) relative to baseline in the 80 mg group, it was not significant in comparison to the changes noted in groups receiving either 40 mg of fluvastatin or placebo.

Patients treated with fluvastatin sodium who develop clinical evidence of endocrine dysfunction should be evaluated appropriately. Caution should be exercised if an HMG-CoA reductase inhibitor or other agent used to lower cholesterol levels is administered to patients receiving other drugs (e.g., ketoconazole, spironolactone, or cimetidine) that may decrease the levels of endogenous steroid hormones.

CNS Toxicity

CNS effects, as evidenced by decreased activity, ataxia, loss of righting reflex, and ptosis were seen in the following animal studies: the 18-month mouse carcinogenicity study at 50 mg/kg/day, the 6-month dog study at 36 mg/kg/day, the 6-month hamster study at 40 mg/kg/day, and in acute, high-dose studies in rats and hamsters (50 mg/kg), rabbits (300 mg/kg) and mice (1500 mg/kg). CNS toxicity in the acute high-dose studies was characterized (in mice) by conspicuous vacuolation in the ventral white columns of the spinal cord at a dose of 5000 mg/kg and (in rat) by edema with separation of myelinated fibers of the ventral spinal tracts and sciatic nerve at a dose of 1500 mg/kg. CNS toxicity, characterized by periaxonal vacuolation, was observed in the medulla of dogs that died after treatment for 5 weeks with 48 mg/kg/day; this finding was not observed in the remaining dogs when the dose level was lowered to 36 mg/kg/day. CNS vascular lesions, characterized by perivascular hemorrhages, edema, and mononuclear cell infiltration of perivascular spaces, have been observed in dogs treated with other members of this class. No CNS lesions have been observed after chronic treatment for up to 2 years with fluvastatin in the mouse (at doses up to 350 mg/kg/day), rat (up to 24 mg/kg/day), or dog (up to 16 mg/kg/day).

Prominent bilateral posterior Y suture lines in the ocular lens were seen in dogs after treatment with 1, 8, and 16 mg/kg/day for 2 years.

Carcinogenesis, Mutagenesis, Impairment of Fertility

A 2-year study was performed in rats at dose levels of 6, 9, and 18-24 (escalated after 1 year) mg/kg/day. These treatment levels represented plasma drug levels of approximately 9, 13, and 26-35 times the mean human plasma drug concentration after a 40 mg oral dose. A low incidence of forestomach squamous papillomas and 1 carcinoma of the forestomach at the 24 mg/kg/day dose level was considered to reflect the prolonged hyperplasia induced by direct contact exposure to fluvastatin sodium rather than to a systemic effect of the drug. In addition, an increased incidence of thyroid follicular cell adenomas and carcinomas was recorded for males treated with 18-24 mg/kg/day. The increased incidence of thyroid follicular cell neoplasm in male rats with fluvastatin sodium appears to be consistent with findings from other HMG-CoA reductase inhibitors. In contrast to other HMG-CoA reductase inhibitors, no hepatic adenomas or carcinomas were observed.

The carcinogenicity study conducted in mice at dose levels of 0.3, 15 and 30 mg/kg/day revealed, as in rats, a statistically significant increase in forestomach squamous cell papillomas in males and females at 30 mg/kg/day and in females at 15 mg/kg/day. These treatment levels represented plasma drug levels of approximately 0.05, 2, and 7 times the mean human plasma drug concentration after a 40 mg oral dose.

No evidence of mutagenicity was observed *in vitro*, with or without rat-liver metabolic activation, in the following studies: microbial mutagen tests using mutant strains of *Salmonella typhimurium* or *Escherichia coli;* malignant transformation assay in BALB/3T3 cells; unscheduled DNA synthesis in rat primary hepatocytes; chromosomal aberrations in V79 Chinese Hamster cells; HGPRT V79 Chinese Hamster cells. In addition, there was no evidence of mutagenicity *in vivo* in either a rat or mouse micronucleus test.

In a study in rats at dose levels for females of 0.6, 2 and 6 mg/kg/day and at dose levels for males of 2, 10 and 20 mg/kg/day, fluvastatin sodium had no adverse effects on the fertility or reproductive performance.

Seminal vesicles and testes were small in hamsters treated for 3 months at 20 mg/kg/day (approximately three times the 40 milligram human daily dose based on surface area, mg/m^2). There was tubular degeneration and aspermatogenesis in testes as well as vesiculitis of seminal vesicles. Vesiculitis of seminal vesicles and edema of the testes were also seen in rats treated for 2 years at 18 mg/kg/day (approximately 4 times the human C_{max} achieved with a 40 milligram daily dose).

Pregnancy

Pregnancy Category X

See CONTRAINDICATIONS.

Fluvastatin sodium produced delays in skeletal development in rats at doses of 12 mg/kg/day and in rabbits at doses of 10 mg/kg/day. Malaligned thoracic vertebrae were seen in rats at 36 mg/kg, a dose that produced maternal toxicity. These doses resulted in 2 times (rat at 12 mg/kg) or 5 times (rabbit at 10 mg/kg) the 40 mg human exposure based on mg/m^2 surface area. A study in which female rats were dosed during the third trimester at 12 and 24 mg/kg/day resulted in maternal mortality at or near term and postpartum. In addition, fetal and neonatal lethality were apparent. No effects on the dam or fetus occurred at 2 mg/kg/day. A second study at levels of 2, 6, 12 and 24 mg/kg/day confirmed the findings in the first study with neonatal mortality beginning at 6 mg/kg. A modified Segment III study was performed at dose levels of 12 or 24 mg/kg/day with or without the presence of concurrent supplementation with mevalonic acid, a product of HMG-CoA reductase which is essential for cholesterol biosynthesis. The concurrent administration of mevalonic acid completely prevented the maternal and neonatal mortality but did not prevent low body weights in pups at 24 mg/kg on days 0 and 7 postpartum. Therefore, the maternal and neonatal lethality observed with fluvastatin sodium reflect its exaggerated pharmacologic effect during pregnancy. There are no data with fluvastatin sodium in pregnant women. However, rare reports of congenital anomalies have been received following intrauterine exposure to other HMG-CoA reductase inhibitors. There has been one report of severe congenital bony deformity, tracheo-esophageal fistula, and anal atresia (VATER association) in a baby born to a woman who took another HMG-CoA reductase inhibitor with dextroamphetamine sulfate during the first trimester of pregnancy. **Lescol® (fluvastatin sodium) should be administered to women of child-bearing potential only when such patients are highly unlikely to conceive and have been informed of the potential hazards.** If a woman becomes pregnant while taking Lescol® (fluvastatin sodium), the drug should be discontinued and the patient advised again as to the potential hazards to the fetus.

Nursing Mothers

Based on preclinical data, drug is present in breast milk in a 2:1 ratio (milk:plasma). Because of the potential for serious adverse reactions in nursing infants, nursing women should not take Lescol® (fluvastatin sodium) *(see CONTRAINDICATIONS).*

Pediatric Use

Safety and effectiveness in individuals less than 18 years old have not been established. Treatment in patients less than 18 years of age is not recommended at this time.

Geriatric Use

The effect of age on the pharmacokinetics of fluvastatin sodium was evaluated. Results indicate that for the general patient population plasma concentrations of fluvastatin sodium do not vary either as a function of age or gender. *(See also CLINICAL PHARMACOLOGY: Pharmacokinetics/Metabolism.)* Elderly patients (≥65 years of age) demonstrated a greater treatment response in respect to LDL-C, Total-C and LDL/HDL ratio than patients <65 years of age.

ADVERSE REACTIONS

In all clinical studies, 1.0% (32/2969) of fluvastatin treated patients were discontinued due to adverse experiences attributed to study drug (mean exposure approximately 16 months ranging in duration from 1 to >36 months). This results in controlled studies in an exposure adjusted rate of 0.8% (32/4051) per patient year in fluvastatin patients compared to an incidence of 1.1% (4/355) in placebo patients. Adverse reactions have usually been of mild to moderate severity.

Adverse experiences occurring in controlled studies with a frequency >2% regardless of causality include the following:

Adverse Event	Lescol® (fluvastatin sodium) (%) (N=2326)	Placebo (%) (N=960)
Integumentary		
Rash	2.3	2.4
Musculoskeletal		
Back Pain	5.7	6.6
Myalgia	5.0	4.5
Arthralgia	4.0	4.1
Arthritis	2.1	2.0
Respiratory		
Upper Respiratory Tract Infection	16.2	16.5
Pharyngitis	3.8	3.8
Rhinitis	4.7	4.9
Sinusitis	2.6	1.9
Coughing	2.4	2.9
Gastrointestinal		
Dyspepsia	7.9	3.2
Diarrhea	4.9	4.2
Abdominal Pain	4.9	3.8
Nausea	3.2	2.0
Constipation	3.1	3.3
Flatulence	2.6	2.5
Misc. Tooth Disorder	2.1	1.7
Central Nervous System		
Dizziness	2.2	2.5
Psychiatric Disorders		
Insomnia	2.7	1.4
Miscellaneous		
Headache	8.9	7.8
Influenza-Like Symptoms	5.1	5.7
Accidental Trauma	5.1	4.8
Fatigue	2.7	2.3
Allergy	2.3	2.2

The following effects have been reported with drugs in this class. Not all the effects listed below have necessarily been associated with fluvastatin sodium therapy.

Skeletal: muscle cramps, myalgia, myopathy, rhabdomyolysis, arthralgias.

Neurological: dysfunction of certain cranial nerves (including alteration of taste, impairment of extra-ocular movement, facial paresis), tremor, dizziness, vertigo, memory loss, paresthesia, peripheral neuropathy, peripheral nerve palsy, psychic disturbances, anxiety, insomnia, depression.

Hypersensitivity Reactions: An apparent hypersensitivity syndrome has been reported rarely which has included one or more of the following features: anaphylaxis, angioedema, lupus erythematosus-like syndrome, polymyalgia rheumatica, vasculitis, purpura, thrombocytopenia, leukopenia, hemolytic anemia, positive ANA, ESR increase, eosinophilia, arthritis, arthralgia, urticaria, asthenia, photosensitivity, fever, chills, flushing, malaise, dyspnea, toxic epidermal necrolysis, erythema multiforme, including Stevens-Johnson syndrome.

Gastrointestinal: pancreatitis, hepatitis, including chronic active hepatitis, cholestatic jaundice, fatty change in liver,

Continued on next page

Lescol—Cont.

and, rarely, cirrhosis, fulminant hepatic necrosis, and hepatoma; anorexia, vomiting.
Skin: alopecia, pruritus. A variety of skin changes (e.g., nodules, discoloration, dryness of skin/mucous membranes, changes to hair/nails) have been reported.
Reproductive: gynecomastia, loss of libido, erectile dysfunction.
Eye: progression of cataracts (lens opacities), ophthalmoplegia.
Laboratory Abnormalities: elevated transaminases, alkaline phosphatase, γ-glutamyl transpeptidase, and bilirubin; thyroid function abnormalities.

Concomitant Therapy

Fluvastatin sodium has been administered concurrently with cholestyramine and nicotinic acid. No adverse reactions unique to the combination or in addition to those previously reported for this class of drugs alone have been reported. Myopathy and rhabdomyolysis (with or without acute renal failure) have been reported when another HMG-CoA reductase inhibitor was used in combination with immunosuppressive drugs, gemfibrozil, erythromycin, or lipid-lowering doses of nicotinic acid. Concomitant therapy with HMG-CoA reductase inhibitors and these agents is generally not recommended. *(See WARNINGS: Skeletal Muscle.)*

OVERDOSAGE

The approximate oral LD_{50} is greater than 2 g/kg in mice and greater than 0.7 g/kg in rats.
The maximum single oral dose received by healthy volunteers was 60 mg. No clinically significant adverse experiences were seen at this dose. There has been a single report of 2 children, one 2 years old and the other 3 years of age, either of whom may have possibly ingested fluvastatin sodium. The maximum amount of fluvastatin sodium that could have been ingested was 80 mg (4 × 20 mg capsules). Vomiting was induced by ipecac in both children and no capsules were noted in their emesis. Neither child experienced any adverse symptoms and both recovered from the incident without problems.
Should an accidental overdose occur, treat symptomatically and institute supportive measures as required. The dialyzability of fluvastatin sodium and of its metabolites in humans is not known at present.
Information about the treatment of overdose can often be obtained from a certified Regional Poison Control Center. Telephone numbers of certified Regional Poison Control Centers are listed in the Physicians' Desk Reference®.*

DOSAGE AND ADMINISTRATION

The patient should be placed on a standard cholesterol-lowering diet before receiving Lescol® (fluvastatin sodium) and should continue on this diet during treatment with Lescol® (fluvastatin sodium). (See NCEP Treatment Guidelines for details on dietary therapy.)
The recommended starting dose for the majority of patients is 20-40 mg once daily at bedtime. The recommended dosing range is 20-80 mg/day. The daily regimen of 80 mg should be administered in divided doses, i.e., 40 mg b.i.d., and should be reserved for those whose LDL-cholesterol response is inadequate at 40 mg/day. Lescol® (fluvastatin sodium) may be taken without regard to meals, since there are no apparent differences in the lipid-lowering effects of fluvastatin sodium administered with the evening meal or 4 hours after the evening meal. Since the maximal reductions in LDL-C of a given dose are seen within 4 weeks, periodic lipid determinations should be performed and dosage adjustment made according to the patient's response to therapy and established treatment guidelines. The therapeutic effect of Lescol® (fluvastatin sodium) is maintained with prolonged administration.

Concomitant Therapy

Lipid-lowering effects on total cholesterol and LDL cholesterol are additive when Lescol® (fluvastatin sodium) is combined with a bile-acid binding resin or niacin. When administering a bile-acid resin (e.g., cholestyramine) and fluvastatin sodium, Lescol® (fluvastatin sodium) should be administered at bedtime, at least 2 hours following the resin to avoid a significant interaction due to drug binding to resin. *(See also ADVERSE REACTIONS: Concomitant Therapy.)*

Dosage in Patients with Renal Insufficiency

Since fluvastatin sodium is cleared hepatically with less than 6% of the administered dose excreted into the urine, dose adjustments for mild to moderate renal impairment are not necessary. Caution should be exercised with severe impairment.

HOW SUPPLIED

Lescol® (fluvastatin sodium) Capsules

20 mg

Brown and light brown imprinted twice with "[logo]" and "20" on one half and "LESCOL" and the Lescol® (fluvastatin sodium) logo twice on the other half of the capsule.
Bottles of 30 capsules (NDC 0078-0176-15)
Bottles of 100 capsules (NDC 0078-0176-05)

40 mg

Brown and gold imprinted twice with "[logo]" and "40" on one half and "LESCOL" and the Lescol® (fluvastatin sodium) logo twice on the other half of the capsule.
Bottles of 30 capsules (NDC 0078-0234-15)
Bottles of 100 capsules (NDC 0078-0234-05)

Store and Dispense

Below 86° F (30° C) in a tight container. Protect from light.
*Trademark of Medical Economics Company, Inc.

REV: JANUARY 1999 T1999-08
Shown in Product Identification Guide, page 325

LOTENSIN® ℞

[lō' tĕnsĭn]
benazepril hydrochloride
Tablets
Rx only

The following prescribing information is based on official labeling in effect July 2000.

> **Use in Pregnancy**
> **When used in pregnancy during the second and third trimesters, ACE inhibitors can cause injury and even death to the developing fetus.** When pregnancy is detected, Lotensin should be discontinued as soon as possible. See **WARNINGS, Fetal/Neonatal Morbidity and Mortality.**

DESCRIPTION

Benazepril hydrochloride is a white to off-white crystalline powder, soluble (>100 mg/mL) in water, in ethanol, and in methanol. Benazepril's chemical name is 3-[[1-(ethoxy-carbonyl)-3-phenyl-(1S)-propyl]amino]-2,3,4,5-tetrahydro-2-oxo-1*H*-1-(3S)-benzazepine-1-acetic acid monohydrochloride; its structural formula is

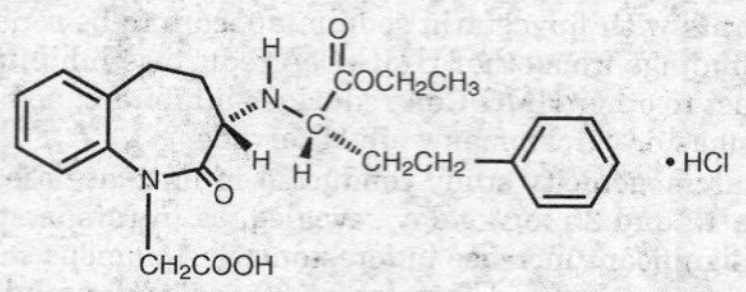

Its empirical formula is $C_{24}H_{28}N_2O_5 \bullet HCl$, and its molecular weight is 460.96.
Benazeprilat, the active metabolite of benazepril, is a non-sulfhydryl angiotensin-converting enzyme inhibitor. Benazepril is converted to benazeprilat by hepatic cleavage of the ester group.
Lotensin is supplied as tablets containing 5 mg, 10 mg, 20 mg, and 40 mg of benazepril for oral administration. The inactive ingredients are cellulose compounds, colloidal silicon dioxide, crospovidone, hydrogenated castor oil (5-mg, 10-mg, and 20-mg tablets), iron oxides, lactose, magnesium stearate (40-mg tablets), polysorbate 80, propylene glycol (5-mg and 40-mg tablets), starch, talc, and titanium dioxide.

CLINICAL PHARMACOLOGY

Mechanism of Action

Benazepril and benazeprilat inhibit angiotensin-converting enzyme (ACE) in human subjects and animals. ACE is a peptidyl dipeptidase that catalyzes the conversion of angiotensin I to the vasoconstrictor substance, angiotensin II. Angiotensin II also stimulates aldosterone secretion by the adrenal cortex.
Inhibition of ACE results in decreased plasma angiotensin II, which leads to decreased vasopressor activity and to decreased aldosterone secretion. The latter decrease may result in a small increase of serum potassium. Hypertensive patients treated with Lotensin alone for up to 52 weeks had elevations of serum potassium of up to 0.2 mEq/L. Similar patients treated with Lotensin and hydrochlorothiazide for up to 24 weeks had no consistent changes in their serum potassium (see PRECAUTIONS).
Removal of angiotensin II negative feedback on renin secretion leads to increased plasma renin activity. In animal studies, benazepril had no inhibitory effect on the vasopressor response to angiotensin II and did not interfere with the hemodynamic effects of the autonomic neurotransmitters acetylcholine, epinephrine, and norepinephrine.
ACE is identical to kininase, an enzyme that degrades bradykinin. Whether increased levels of bradykinin, a potent vasodepressor peptide, play a role in the therapeutic effects of Lotensin remains to be elucidated.
While the mechanism through which benazepril lowers blood pressure is believed to be primarily suppression of the renin-angiotensin-aldosterone system, benazepril has an antihypertensive effect even in patients with low-renin hypertension (see INDICATIONS AND USAGE).

Pharmacokinetics and Metabolism

Following oral administration of Lotensin, peak plasma concentrations of benazepril are reached within 0.5-1.0 hours. The extent of absorption is at least 37% as determined by urinary recovery and is not significantly influenced by the presence of food in the GI tract.
Cleavage of the ester group (primarily in the liver) converts benazepril to its active metabolite, benazeprilat. Peak plasma concentrations of benazeprilat are reached 1-2 hours after drug intake in the fasting state and 2-4 hours after drug intake in the nonfasting state. The serum protein binding of benazepril is about 96.7% and that of benazeprilat about 95.3%, as measured by equilibrium dialysis; on the basis of in vitro studies, the degree of protein binding should be unaffected by age, hepatic dysfunction, or concentration (over the concentration range of 0.24-23.6 μmol/L).
Benazepril is almost completely metabolized to benazeprilat, which has much greater ACE inhibitory activity than benazepril, and to the glucuronide conjugates of benazepril and benazeprilat. Only trace amounts of an administered dose of Lotensin can be recovered in the urine as unchanged benazepril, while about 20% of the dose is excreted as benazeprilat, 4% as benazepril glucuronide, and 8% as benazeprilat glucuronide.
The kinetics of benazepril are approximately dose-proportional within the dosage range of 10-80 mg.
The effective half-life of accumulation of benazeprilat following multiple dosing of benazepril hydrochloride is 10-11 hours. Thus, steady-state concentrations of benazeprilat should be reached after 2 or 3 doses of benazepril hydrochloride given once daily.
The kinetics did not change, and there was no significant accumulation during chronic administration (28 days) of once-daily doses between 5 mg and 20 mg. Accumulation ratios based on AUC and urinary recovery of benazeprilat were 1.19 and 1.27, respectively.
When dialysis was started two hours after ingestion of 10 mg of benazepril, approximately 6% of benazeprilat was removed in 4 hours of dialysis. The parent compound, benazepril, was not detected in the dialysate.
The disposition of benazepril and benazeprilat in patients with mild-to-moderate renal insufficiency (creatinine clearance > 30 mL/min) is similar to that in patients with normal renal function. In patients with creatinine clearance ≤ 30 mL/min, peak benazeprilat levels and the initial (alpha phase) half-life increase, and time to steady state may be delayed (see DOSAGE AND ADMINISTRATION).
Benazepril and benazeprilat are cleared predominantly by renal excretion in healthy subjects with normal renal function. Nonrenal (i.e., biliary) excretion accounts for approximately 11%-12% of benazeprilat excretion in healthy subjects. In patients with renal failure, biliary clearance may compensate to an extent for deficient renal clearance.
In patients with hepatic dysfunction due to cirrhosis, levels of benazeprilat are essentially unaltered. The pharmacokinetics of benazepril and benazeprilat do not appear to be influenced by age.
In studies in rats given ^{14}C-benazepril, benazepril and its metabolites crossed the blood-brain barrier only to an extremely low extent. Multiple doses of benazepril did not result in accumulation in any tissue except the lung, where, as with other ACE inhibitors in similar studies, there was a slight increase in concentration due to slow elimination in that organ.
Some placental passage occurred when the drug was administered to pregnant rats.

Pharmacodynamics

Single and multiple doses of 10 mg or more of Lotensin cause inhibition of plasma ACE activity by at least 80%-90% for at least 24 hours after dosing. Pressor responses to exogenous angiotensin I were inhibited by 60%-90% (up to 4 hours post-dose) at the 10-mg dose.
Administration of Lotensin to patients with mild-to-moderate hypertension results in a reduction of both supine and standing blood pressure to about the same extent with no compensatory tachycardia. Symptomatic postural hypotension is infrequent, although it can occur in patients who are salt- and/or volume-depleted (see WARNINGS).
In single-dose studies, Lotensin lowered blood pressure within 1 hour, with peak reductions achieved 2-4 hours after dosing. The antihypertensive effect of a single dose persisted for 24 hours. In multiple-dose studies, once-daily doses of 20-80 mg decreased seated pressure (systolic/diastolic) 24 hours after dosing by about 6-12 /4-7 mmHg. The trough values represent reductions of about 50% of that seen at peak.
Four dose-response studies using once-daily dosing were conducted in 470 mild-to-moderate hypertensive patients not using diuretics. The minimal effective once-daily dose of Lotensin was 10 mg; but further falls in blood pressure, especially at morning trough, were seen with higher doses in the studied dosing range (10-80 mg). In studies comparing the same daily dose of Lotensin given as a single morning dose or as a twice-daily dose, blood pressure reductions at the time of morning trough blood levels were greater with the divided regimen.
During chronic therapy, the maximum reduction in blood pressure with any dose is generally achieved after 1-2 weeks. The antihypertensive effects of Lotensin have continued during therapy for at least two years. Abrupt withdrawal of Lotensin has not been associated with a rapid increase in blood pressure.
In patients with mild-to-moderate hypertension, Lotensin 10-20 mg was similar in effectiveness to captopril, hydrochlorothiazide, nifedipine SR, and propranolol.
The antihypertensive effects of Lotensin were not appreciably different in patients receiving high- or low-sodium diets.
In hemodynamic studies in dogs, blood pressure reduction was accompanied by a reduction in peripheral arterial resistance, with an increase in cardiac output and renal blood flow and little or no change in heart rate. In normal human volunteers, single doses of benazepril caused an increase in renal blood flow but had no effect on glomerular filtration rate.
Use of Lotensin in combination with thiazide diuretics gives a blood-pressure-lowering effect greater than that seen with either agent alone. By blocking the renin-angiotensin-aldosterone axis, administration of Lotensin tends to reduce the potassium loss associated with the diuretic.

INDICATIONS AND USAGE

Lotensin is indicated for the treatment of hypertension. It may be used alone or in combination with thiazide diuretics.
In using Lotensin, consideration should be given to the fact that another angiotensin-converting enzyme inhibitor, captopril, has caused agranulocytosis, particularly in patients with renal impairment or collagen-vascular disease. Available data are insufficient to show that Lotensin does not have a similar risk (see WARNINGS).
Black patients receiving ACE-inhibitors have been reported to have a higher incidence of angioedema compared to nonblacks. It should also be noted that in controlled clinical trials ACE inhibitors have an effect on blood pressure that is less in black patients than in nonblacks.

CONTRAINDICATIONS

Lotensin is contraindicated in patients who are hypersensitive to this product or to any other ACE inhibitor.

WARNINGS

Anaphylactoid and Possibly Related Reactions

Presumably because angiotensin-converting enzyme inhibitors affect the metabolism of eicosanoids and polypeptides, including endogenous bradykinin, patients receiving ACE inhibitors (including Lotensin) may be subject to a variety of adverse reactions, some of them serious.

Angioedema: Angioedema of the face, extremities, lips, tongue, glottis, and larynx has been reported in patients treated with angiotensin-converting enzyme inhibitors. In U.S. clinical trials, symptoms consistent with angioedema were seen in none of the subjects who received placebo and in about 0.5% of the subjects who received Lotensin. Angioedema associated with laryngeal edema can be fatal. If laryngeal stridor or angioedema of the face, tongue, or glottis occurs, treatment with Lotensin should be discontinued and appropriate therapy instituted immediately. **Where there is involvement of the tongue, glottis, or larynx, likely to cause airway obstruction, appropriate therapy, e.g., subcutaneous epinephrine injection 1:1000 (0.3 mL to 0.5 mL) should be promptly administered (see ADVERSE REACTIONS).**

Anaphylactoid Reactions During Desensitization: Two patients undergoing desensitizing treatment with hymenoptera venom while receiving ACE inhibitors sustained life-threatening anaphylactoid reactions. In the same patients, these reactions were avoided when ACE inhibitors were temporarily withheld, but they reappeared upon inadvertent rechallenge.

Anaphylactoid Reactions During Membrane Exposure: Anaphylactoid reactions have been reported in patients dialyzed with high-flux membranes and treated concomitantly with an ACE inhibitor. Anaphylactoid reactions have also been reported in patients undergoing low-density lipoprotein apheresis with dextran sulfate absorption (a procedure dependent upon devices not approved in the United States).

Hypotension

Lotensin can cause symptomatic hypotension. Like other ACE inhibitors, benazepril has been only rarely associated with hypotension in uncomplicated hypertensive patients. Symptomatic hypotension is most likely to occur in patients who have been volume- and/or salt-depleted as a result of prolonged diuretic therapy, dietary salt restriction, dialysis, diarrhea, or vomiting. Volume- and/or salt-depletion should be corrected before initiating therapy with Lotensin.
In patients with congestive heart failure, with or without associated renal insufficiency, ACE inhibitor therapy may cause excessive hypotension, which may be associated with oliguria or azotemia and, rarely, with acute renal failure and death. In such patients, Lotensin therapy should be started under close medical supervision; they should be followed closely for the first 2 weeks of treatment and whenever the dose of benazepril or diuretic is increased.
If hypotension occurs, the patient should be placed in a supine position, and, if necessary, treated with intravenous infusion of physiological saline. Lotensin treatment usually can be continued following restoration of blood pressure and volume.

Neutropenia/Agranulocytosis

Another angiotensin-converting enzyme inhibitor, captopril, has been shown to cause agranulocytosis and bone marrow depression, rarely in uncomplicated patients, but more frequently in patients with renal impairment, especially if they also have a collagen-vascular disease such as systemic lupus erythematosus or scleroderma. Available data from clinical trials of benazepril are insufficient to show that benazepril does not cause agranulocytosis at similar rates. Monitoring of white blood cell counts should be considered in patients with collagen-vascular disease, especially if the disease is associated with impaired renal function.

Fetal/Neonatal Morbidity and Mortality

ACE inhibitors can cause fetal and neonatal morbidity and death when administered to pregnant women. Several dozen cases have been reported in the world literature. When pregnancy is detected, ACE inhibitors should be discontinued as soon as possible.
The use of ACE inhibitors during the second and third trimesters of pregnancy has been associated with fetal and neonatal injury, including hypotension, neonatal skull hypoplasia, anuria, reversible or irreversible renal failure, and death. Oligohydramnios has also been reported, presumably resulting from decreased fetal renal function; oligohydramnios in this setting has been associated with fetal limb contractures, craniofacial deformation, and hypoplastic lung development. Prematurity, intrauterine growth retardation, and patent ductus arteriosus have also been reported, although it is not clear whether these occurrences were due to the ACE inhibitor exposure.
These adverse effects do not appear to have resulted from intrauterine ACE inhibitor exposure that has been limited to the first trimester. Mothers whose embryos and fetuses are exposed to ACE inhibitors only during the first trimester should be so informed. Nonetheless, when patients become pregnant, physicians should make every effort to discontinue the use of benazepril as soon as possible.
Rarely (probably less often than once in every thousand pregnancies), no alternative to ACE inhibitors will be found. In these rare cases, the mothers should be apprised of the potential hazards to their fetuses, and serial ultrasound examinations should be performed to assess the intraamniotic environment.
If oligohydramnios is observed, benazepril should be discontinued unless it is considered life-saving for the mother. Contraction stress testing (CST), a nonstress test (NST), or biophysical profiling (BPP) may be appropriate, depending upon the week of pregnancy. Patients and physicians should be aware, however, that oligohydramnios may not appear until after the fetus has sustained irreversible injury.
Infants with histories of in utero exposure to ACE inhibitors should be closely observed for hypotension, oliguria, and hyperkalemia. If oliguria occurs, attention should be directed toward support of blood pressure and renal perfusion. Exchange transfusion or dialysis may be required as means of reversing hypotension and/or substituting for disordered renal function. Benazepril, which crosses the placenta, can theoretically be removed from the neonatal circulation by these means; there are occasional reports of benefit from these maneuvers with another ACE inhibitor, but experience is limited.
No teratogenic effects of Lotensin were seen in studies of pregnant rats, mice, and rabbits. On a mg/m^2 basis, the doses used in these studies were 60 times (in rats), 9 times (in mice), and more than 0.8 times (in rabbits) the maximum recommended human dose (assuming a 50-kg woman). On a mg/kg basis these multiples are 300 times (in rats), 90 times (in mice), and more than 3 times (in rabbits) the maximum recommended human dose.

Hepatic Failure

Rarely, ACE inhibitors have been associated with a syndrome that starts with cholestatic jaundice and progresses to fulminant hepatic necrosis and (sometimes) death. The mechanism of this syndrome is not understood. Patients receiving ACE inhibitors who develop jaundice or marked elevations of hepatic enzymes should discontinue the ACE inhibitor and receive appropriate medical follow-up.

PRECAUTIONS

General

Impaired Renal Function: As a consequence of inhibiting the renin-angiotensin-aldosterone system, changes in renal function may be anticipated in susceptible individuals. In patients with severe congestive heart failure whose renal function may depend on the activity of the renin-angiotensin-aldosterone system, treatment with angiotensin-converting enzyme inhibitors, including Lotensin, may be associated with oliguria and/or progressive azotemia and (rarely) with acute renal failure and/or death. In a small study of hypertensive patients with renal artery stenosis in a solitary kidney or bilateral renal artery stenosis, treatment with Lotensin was associated with increases in blood urea nitrogen and serum creatinine; these increases were reversible upon discontinuation of Lotensin or diuretic therapy, or both. When such patients are treated with ACE inhibitors, renal function should be monitored during the first few weeks of therapy. Some hypertensive patients with no apparent preexisting renal vascular disease have developed increases in blood urea nitrogen and serum creatinine, usually minor and transient, especially when Lotensin has been given concomitantly with a diuretic. This is more likely to occur in patients with preexisting renal impairment. Dosage reduction of Lotensin and/or discontinuation of the diuretic may be required. **Evaluation of the hypertensive patient should always include assessment of renal function (see DOSAGE AND ADMINISTRATION).**

Hyperkalemia: In clinical trials, hyperkalemia (serum potassium at least 0.5 mEq/L greater than the upper limit of normal) occurred in approximately 1% of hypertensive patients receiving Lotensin. In most cases, these were isolated values which resolved despite continued therapy. Risk factors for the development of hyperkalemia include renal insufficiency, diabetes mellitus, and the concomitant use of potassium-sparing diuretics, potassium supplements, and/or potassium-containing salt substitutes, which should be used cautiously, if at all, with Lotensin (see Drug Interactions).

Cough: Presumably due to the inhibition of the degradation of endogenous bradykinin, persistent nonproductive cough has been reported with all ACE inhibitors, always resolving after discontinuation of therapy. ACE inhibitor-induced cough should be considered in the differential diagnosis of cough.

Impaired Liver Function: In patients with hepatic dysfunction due to cirrhosis, levels of benazeprilat are essentially unaltered (see WARNINGS, Hepatic Failure).

Surgery/Anesthesia: In patients undergoing surgery or during anesthesia with agents that produce hypotension, benazepril will block the angiotensin II formation that could otherwise occur secondary to compensatory renin release. Hypotension that occurs as a result of this mechanism can be corrected by volume expansion.

Information for Patients

Pregnancy: Female patients of childbearing age should be told about the consequences of second- and third-trimester exposure to ACE inhibitors, and they should also be told that these consequences do not appear to have resulted from intrauterine ACE inhibitor exposure that has been limited to the first trimester. These patients should be asked to report pregnancies to their physicians as soon as possible.

Angioedema: Angioedema, including laryngeal edema, can occur at any time with treatment with ACE inhibitors. Patients should be so advised and told to report immediately any signs or symptoms suggesting angioedema (swelling of face, eyes, lips, or tongue, or difficulty in breathing) and to take no more drug until they have consulted with the prescribing physician.

Symptomatic Hypotension: Patients should be cautioned that lightheadedness can occur, especially during the first days of therapy, and it should be reported to the prescribing physician. Patients should be told that if syncope occurs, Lotensin should be discontinued until the prescribing physician has been consulted.
All patients should be cautioned that inadequate fluid intake or excessive perspiration, diarrhea, or vomiting can lead to an excessive fall in blood pressure, with the same consequences of lightheadedness and possible syncope.

Hyperkalemia: Patients should be told not to use potassium supplements or salt substitutes containing potassium without consulting the prescribing physician.

Neutropenia: Patients should be told to promptly report any indication of infection (e.g., sore throat, fever), which could be a sign of neutropenia.

Drug Interactions

Diuretics: Patients on diuretics, especially those in whom diuretic therapy was recently instituted, may occasionally experience an excessive reduction of blood pressure after initiation of therapy with Lotensin. The possibility of hypotensive effects with Lotensin can be minimized by either discontinuing the diuretic or increasing the salt intake prior to initiation of treatment with Lotensin. If this is not possible, the starting dose should be reduced (see DOSAGE AND ADMINISTRATION).

Potassium Supplements and Potassium-Sparing Diuretics: Lotensin can attenuate potassium loss caused by thiazide diuretics. Potassium-sparing diuretics (spironolactone, amiloride, triamterene, and others) or potassium supplements can increase the risk of hyperkalemia. Therefore, if concomitant use of such agents is indicated, they should be given with caution, and the patient's serum potassium should be monitored frequently.

Oral Anticoagulants: Interaction studies with warfarin and acenocoumarol failed to identify any clinically important effects on the serum concentrations or clinical effects of these anticoagulants.

Lithium: Increased serum lithium levels and symptoms of lithium toxicity have been reported in patients receiving ACE inhibitors during therapy with lithium. These drugs should be coadministered with caution, and frequent monitoring of serum lithium levels is recommended. If a diuretic is also used, the risk of lithium toxicity may be increased.

Other: No clinically important pharmacokinetic interactions occurred when Lotensin was administered concomitantly with hydrochlorothiazide, chlorthalidone, furosemide, digoxin, propranolol, atenolol, naproxen, or cimetidine.
Lotensin has been used concomitantly with beta-adrenergic-blocking agents, calcium-channel-blocking agents, diuretics, digoxin, and hydralazine, without evidence of clinically important adverse interactions. Benazepril, like other ACE inhibitors, has had less than additive effects with beta-adrenergic blockers, presumably because both drugs lower blood pressure by inhibiting parts of the renin-angiotensin system.

Carcinogenesis, Mutagenesis, Impairment of Fertility

No evidence of carcinogenicity was found when benazepril was administered to rats and mice for up to two years at doses of up to 150 mg/kg/day. When compared on the basis of body weights, this dose is 110 times the maximum recommended human dose. When compared on the basis of body surface areas, this dose is 18 and 9 times (rats and mice, respectively) the maximum recommended human dose (calculations assume a patient weight of 60 kg). No mutagenic activity was detected in the Ames test in bacteria (with or without metabolic activation), in an in vitro test for forward mutations in cultured mammalian cells, or in a nucleus anomaly test. In doses of 50-500 mg/kg/day (6-60 times the maximum recommended human dose based on mg/m^2 comparison and 37-375 times the maximum recommended human dose based on a mg/kg comparison), Lotensin had no adverse effect on the reproductive performance of male and female rats.

Pregnancy Categories C (first trimester) and D (second and third trimesters)

See WARNINGS, Fetal/Neonatal Morbidity and Mortality.

Nursing Mothers

Minimal amounts of unchanged benazepril and of benazeprilat are excreted into the breast milk of lactating women treated with benazepril. A newborn child ingesting entirely breast milk would receive less than 0.1% of the mg/kg maternal dose of benazepril and benazeprilat.

Continued on next page

Lotensin—Cont.

Geriatric Use

Of the total number of patients who received benazepril in U.S. clinical studies of Lotensin, 18% were 65 or older while 2% were 75 or older. No overall differences in effectiveness or safety were observed between these patients and younger patients, and other reported clinical experience has not identified differences in responses between the elderly and younger patients, but greater sensitivity of some older individuals cannot be ruled out.

Pediatric Use

Safety and effectiveness in pediatric patients have not been established.

ADVERSE REACTIONS

Lotensin has been evaluated for safety in over 6000 patients with hypertension; over 700 of these patients were treated for at least one year. The overall incidence of reported adverse events was comparable in Lotensin and placebo patients.

The reported side effects were generally mild and transient, and there was no relation between side effects and age, duration of therapy, or total dosage within the range of 2 to 80 mg. Discontinuation of therapy because of a side effect was required in approximately 5% of U.S. patients treated with Lotensin and in 3% of patients treated with placebo.

The most common reasons for discontinuation were headache (0.6%) and cough (0.5%) (see PRECAUTIONS, Cough).

The side effects considered possibly or probably related to study drug that occurred in U.S. placebo-controlled trials in more than 1% of patients treated with Lotensin are shown below.

PATIENTS IN U.S. PLACEBO-CONTROLLED STUDIES

	LOTENSIN (N=964)		PLACEBO (N=496)	
	N	%	N	%
Headache	60	6.2	21	4.2
Dizziness	35	3.6	12	2.4
Fatigue	23	2.4	11	2.2
Somnolence	15	1.6	2	0.4
Postural Dizziness	14	1.5	1	0.2
Nausea	13	1.3	5	1.0
Cough	12	1.2	5	1.0

Other adverse experiences reported in controlled clinical trials (in less than 1% of benazepril patients), and rarer events seen in postmarketing experience, include the following (in some, a causal relationship to drug use is uncertain):

Cardiovascular: Symptomatic hypotension was seen in 0.3% of patients, postural hypotension in 0.4%, and syncope in 0.1%; these reactions led to discontinuation of therapy in 4 patients who had received benazepril monotherapy and in 9 patients who had received benazepril with hydrochlorothiazide (see PRECAUTIONS and WARNINGS). Other reports included angina pectoris, palpitations, and peripheral edema.

Renal: Of hypertensive patients with no apparent preexisting renal disease, about 2% have sustained increases in serum creatinine to at least 150% of their baseline values while receiving Lotensin, but most of these increases have disappeared despite continuing treatment. A much smaller fraction of these patients (less than 0.1%) developed simultaneous (usually transient) increases in blood urea nitrogen and serum creatinine.

Fetal/Neonatal Morbidity and Mortality: See WARNINGS, Fetal/Neonatal Morbidity and Mortality.

Angioedema: Angioedema has been reported in patients receiving ACE inhibitors. During clinical trials in hypertensive patients with benazepril, 0.5% of patients experienced edema of the lips or face without other manifestations of angioedema. Angioedema associated with laryngeal edema and/or shock may be fatal. If angioedema of the face, extremities, lips, tongue, or glottis and/or larynx occurs, treatment with Lotensin should be discontinued and appropriate therapy instituted immediately (see WARNINGS).

Dermatologic: Stevens-Johnson syndrome, pemphigus, apparent hypersensitivity reactions (manifested by dermatitis, pruritus, or rash), photosensitivity, and flushing.

Gastrointestinal: Pancreatitis, constipation, gastritis, vomiting, and melena.

Hematologic: Thrombocytopenia and hemolytic anemia.

Neurologic and Psychiatric: Anxiety, decreased libido, hypertonia, insomnia, nervousness, and paresthesia.

Other: Asthma, bronchitis, dyspnea, sinusitus, urinary tract infection, infection, arthritis, impotence, alopecia, arthralgia, myalgia, asthenia, and sweating.

Another potentially important adverse experience, eosinophilic pneumonitis, has been attributed to other ACE inhibitors.

Clinical Laboratory Test Findings

Creatinine and Blood Urea Nitrogen: Of hypertensive patients with no apparent preexisting renal disease, about 2% have sustained increases in serum creatinine to at least 150% of their baseline values while receiving Lotensin, but most of these increases have disappeared despite continuing treatment. A much smaller fraction of these patients (less than 0.1%) developed simultaneous (usually transient) increases in blood urea nitrogen and serum creatinine. None of these increases required discontinuation of treatment. Increases in these laboratory values are more likely to occur in patients with renal insufficiency or those pretreated with a diuretic and, based on experience with other ACE inhibitors, would be expected to be especially likely in patients with renal artery stenosis (see PRECAUTIONS, General).

Potassium: Since benazepril decreases aldosterone secretion, elevation of serum potassium can occur. Potassium supplements and potassium-sparing diuretics should be given with caution, and the patient's serum potassium should be monitored frequently (see PRECAUTIONS).

Hemoglobin: Decreases in hemoglobin (a low value and a decrease of 5 g/dL) were rare, occurring in only 1 of 2014 patients receiving Lotensin alone and in 1 of 1357 patients receiving Lotensin plus a diuretic. No U.S. patients discontinued treatment because of decreases in hemoglobin.

Other (causal relationships unknown): Clinically important changes in standard laboratory tests were rarely associated with Lotensin administration.

Elevations of uric acid, blood glucose, serum bilirubin, and liver enzymes (see WARNINGS) have been reported, as have scattered incidents of hyponatremia, electrocardiographic changes, leukopenia, eosinophilia, and proteinuria. In U.S. trials, less than 0.5% of patients discontinued treatment because of laboratory abnormalities.

OVERDOSAGE

Single oral doses of 3 g/kg benazepril were associated with significant lethality in mice. Rats, however, tolerated single oral doses of up to 6 g/kg. Reduced activity was seen at 1 g/kg in mice and at 5 g/kg in rats. Human overdoses of benazepril have not been reported, but the most common manifestation of human benazepril overdosage is likely to be hypotension.

Laboratory determinations of serum levels of benazepril and its metabolites are not widely available, and such determinations have, in any event, no established role in the management of benazepril overdose.

No data are available to suggest physiological maneuvers (e.g., maneuvers to change the pH of the urine) that might accelerate elimination of benazepril and its metabolites. Benazepril is only slightly dialyzable, but dialysis might be considered in overdosed patients with severely impaired renal function (see WARNINGS).

Angiotensin II could presumably serve as a specific antagonist-antidote in the setting of benazepril overdose, but angiotensin II is essentially unavailable outside of scattered research facilities. Because the hypotensive effect of benazepril is achieved through vasodilation and effective hypovolemia, it is reasonable to treat benazepril overdose by infusion of normal saline solution.

DOSAGE AND ADMINISTRATION

The recommended initial dose for patients not receiving a diuretic is 10 mg once-a-day. The usual maintenance dosage range is 20-40 mg per day administered as a single dose or in two equally divided doses. A dose of 80 mg gives an increased response, but experience with this dose is limited. The divided regimen was more effective in controlling trough (pre-dosing) blood pressure than the same dose given as a once-daily regimen. Dosage adjustment should be based on measurement of peak (2-6 hours after dosing) and trough responses. If a once-daily regimen does not give adequate trough response, an increase in dosage or divided administration should be considered. If blood pressure is not controlled with Lotensin alone, a diuretic can be added. Total daily doses above 80 mg have not been evaluated.

Concomitant administration of Lotensin with potassium supplements, potassium salt substitutes, or potassium-sparing diuretics can lead to increases of serum potassium (see PRECAUTIONS).

In patients who are currently being treated with a diuretic, symptomatic hypotension occasionally can occur following the initial dose of Lotensin. To reduce the likelihood of hypotension, the diuretic should, if possible, be discontinued two to three days prior to beginning therapy with Lotensin (see WARNINGS). Then, if blood pressure is not controlled with Lotensin alone, diuretic therapy should be resumed.

If the diuretic cannot be discontinued, an initial dose of 5 mg Lotensin should be used to avoid excessive hypotension.

Dosage Adjustment in Renal Impairment

For patients with a creatinine clearance < 30 mL/min/1.73 m^2 (serum creatinine >3 mg/dL), the recommended initial dose is 5 mg Lotensin once daily. Dosage may be titrated upward until blood pressure is controlled or to a maximum total daily dose of 40 mg (see WARNINGS).

HOW SUPPLIED

Lotensin is available in tablets of 5 mg, 10 mg, 20 mg, and 40 mg, packaged with a desiccant in bottles of 90 and 100 tablets. Lotensin is also supplied in blister packages (1 tablet/blister), in Accu-Pak® Unit Dose boxes containing 10 strips of 10 blisters each.

Dose	Tablet Color	Bottle of 90	Bottle of 100	Accu-Pak® of 100
5 mg	light yellow	NDC 0083-0059-90	NDC 0083-0059-30	NDC 0083-0059-32
10 mg	dark yellow	NDC 0083-0063-90	NDC 0083-0063-30	NDC 0083-0063-32
20 mg	biege pink	NDC 0083-0079-90	NDC 0083-0079-30	NDC 0083-0079-32
40 mg	dark rose	NDC 0083-0094-90	NDC 0083-0094-30	NDC 0083-0094-32

Each tablet is imprinted with LOTENSIN on one side and the tablet strength ("5," "10," "20," or "40") on the other.

The National Drug Codes for the various packages are [See table below]

Storage: Do not store above 30°C (86°F). Protect from moisture.

Dispense in tight container (USP).

 T2000-15

REV: MAY 2000

Shown in Product Identification Guide, page 325

LOTENSIN HCT® ℞

[*lō tĕnsĭn*]

benazepril hydrochloride and hydrochlorothiazide USP Combination Tablets

5 mg/6.25 mg

10 mg/12.5 mg

20 mg/12.5 mg

20 mg/25 mg

Rx only

The following prescribing information is based on official labeling in effect July 2000.

USE IN PREGNANCY

When used in pregnancy during the second and third trimesters, ACE inhibitors can cause injury and even death to the developing fetus. When pregnancy is detected, Lotensin HCT should be discontinued as soon as possible. See **WARNINGS, Fetal/Neonatal Morbidity and Mortality**.

DESCRIPTION

Benazepril hydrochloride is a white to off-white crystalline powder, soluble (> 100 mg/mL) in water, in ethanol, and in methanol. Benazepril hydrochloride's chemical name is 3-[[1-(ethoxycarbonyl)-3-phenyl-(1S)-propyl]amino]-2,3,4,5-tetrahydro-2-oxo-1*H*-1-(3S)-benzazepine-1-acetic acid monohydrochloride; its structural formula is

Its empirical formula is $C_{24}H_{28}N_2O_5 \bullet HCl$, and its molecular weight is 460.96.

Benazeprilat, the active metabolite of benazepril, is a non-sulfhydryl angiotensin-converting enzyme inhibitor. Benazepril is converted to benazeprilat by hepatic cleavage of the ester group.

Hydrochlorothiazide USP is a white, or practically white, practically odorless, crystalline powder. It is slightly soluble in water; freely soluble in sodium hydroxide solution, in *n*-butylamine, and in dimethylformamide; sparingly soluble in methanol; and insoluble in ether, in chloroform, and in dilute mineral acids. Hydrochlorothiazide's chemical name is 6-chloro-3,4-dihydro-2*H*-1,2,4-benzothiadiazine-7-sulfonamide 1,1-dioxide; its structural formula is

Its empirical formula is $C_7H_8ClN_3O_4S_2$, and its molecular weight is 297.73. Hydrochlorothiazide is a thiazide diuretic. Lotensin HCT is a combination of benazepril hydrochloride and hydrochlorothiazide USP. The tablets are formulated for oral administration with a combination of 5, 10, or 20 mg of benazepril hydrochloride and 6.25, 12.5, or 25 mg of hydrochlorothiazide USP. The inactive ingredients of the tablets are cellulose compounds, crospovidone, hydrogenated castor oil, iron oxides (10/12.5-mg, 20/12.5-mg, and 20/25-mg tablets), lactose, polyethylene glycol, talc, and titanium dioxide.

CLINICAL PHARMACOLOGY

Mechanism of Action

Benazepril and benazeprilat inhibit angiotensin-converting enzyme (ACE) in human subjects and in animals. ACE is a peptidyl dipeptidase that catalyzes the conversion of angiotensin I to the vasoconstrictor substance, angiotensin II. Angiotensin II also stimulates aldosterone secretion by the adrenal cortex.

Inhibition of ACE results in decreased plasma angiotensin II, which leads to decreased vasopressor activity and to decreased aldosterone secretion. The latter decrease may result in a small increase of serum potassium. Hypertensive patients treated with benazepril alone for up to 52 weeks had elevations of serum potassium of up to 0.2 mEq/L. Similar patients treated with benazepril and hydrochlorothiazide for up to 24 weeks had no consistent changes in their serum potassium (see PRECAUTIONS).

Removal of angiotensin II negative feedback on renin secretion leads to increased plasma renin activity. In animal studies, benazepril had no inhibitory effect on the vasopressor response to angiotensin II and did not interfere with the hemodynamic effects of the autonomic neurotransmitters acetylcholine, epinephrine, and norepinephrine.

ACE is identical to kininase, an enzyme that degrades bradykinin. Whether increased levels of bradykinin, a potent vasodepressor peptide, play a role in the therapeutic effects of Lotensin HCT remains to be elucidated.

While the mechanism through which benazepril lowers blood pressure is believed to be primarily suppression of the renin-angiotensin-aldosterone system, benazepril has an antihypertensive effect even in patients with low-renin hypertension.

Hydrochlorothiazide is a thiazide diuretic. Thiazides affect the renal tubular mechanisms of electrolyte reabsorption, directly increasing excretion of sodium and chloride in approximately equivalent amounts. Indirectly, the diuretic action of hydrochlorothiazide reduces plasma volume, with consequent increases in plasma renin activity, increases in aldosterone secretion, increases in urinary potassium loss, and decreases in serum potassium. The renin-aldosterone link is mediated by angiotensin, so coadministration of an ACE inhibitor tends to reverse the potassium loss associated with these diuretics.

The mechanism of the antihypertensive effect of thiazides is unknown.

Pharmacokinetics and Metabolism

Following oral administration of Lotensin HCT, peak plasma concentrations of benazepril are reached within 0.5-1.0 hours. As determined by urinary recovery, the extent of absorption is at least 37%. The absorption of hydrochlorothiazide is somewhat slower (1-2.5 hours) and somewhat more complete (50%-80%). In fasting subjects, the rate and extent of absorption of benazepril and hydrochlorothiazide from Lotensin HCT are not different, respectively, from the rate and extent of absorption of benazepril and hydrochlorothiazide from immediate-release monotherapy formulations.

The absorption of benazepril from Lotensin® tablets is not influenced by the presence of food in the gastrointestinal tract, but possible effects of food upon absorption of either component from Lotensin HCT tablets have not been studied. The reported studies of food effects on hydrochlorothiazide absorption have been inconclusive. The absorption of hydrochlorothiazide is increased by agents that reduce gastrointestinal motility, but it is reported to be reduced by 50% in patients with congestive heart failure.

Cleavage of the ester group (primarily in the liver) converts benazepril to its active metabolite, benazeprilat. Peak plasma concentrations of benazeprilat are reached 1-2 hours after drug intake in the fasting state and 2-4 hours after drug intake in the nonfasting state. The serum protein binding of benazepril is about 96.7% and that of benazeprilat about 95.3%, as measured by equilibrium dialysis; on the basis of in vitro studies, the degree of protein binding should be unaffected by age, hepatic dysfunction, or — over the concentration range of 0.24-23.6 μmol/L — concentration.

Hydrochlorothiazide is not metabolized. Its apparent volume of distribution is 3.6-7.8 L/kg, and its measured plasma protein binding is 67.9%. The drug also accumulates in red blood cells, so that whole blood levels are 1.6-1.8 times those measured in plasma.

In studies of rats given ^{14}C-benazepril, benazepril and its metabolites crossed the blood-brain barrier only to an extremely low extent. Multiple doses of benazepril did not result in accumulation in any tissue except the lung, where, as with other ACE inhibitors in similar studies, there was a slight increase in concentration due to slow elimination in that organ.

Some placental passage occurred when benazepril was administered to pregnant rats. In humans, hydrochlorothiazide crosses the placenta freely, and levels in umbilical-cord blood are similar to those in the maternal circulation.

Benazepril is almost completely metabolized to benazeprilat, which has much greater ACE inhibitory activity than benazepril, and to the glucuronide conjugates of benazepril and benazeprilat. Only trace amounts of an administered dose of benazepril can be recovered unchanged in the urine; about 20% of the dose is excreted as benazeprilat, 4% as benazepril glucuronide, and 8% as benazeprilat glucuronide.

In patients with hepatic dysfunction due to cirrhosis, levels of benazeprilat are essentially unaltered. Similarly, the pharmacokinetics of benazepril and benazeprilat do not appear to be influenced by age.

The kinetics of benazepril are dose-proportional within the dosage range of 5-20 mg. Small deviations from dose proportionality were observed when the broader range of 2-80 mg was studied, possibly due to the saturable binding of the compound to ACE.

The effective half-life of accumulation of benazeprilat following multiple dosing of benazepril hydrochloride is 10-11 hours. Thus, steady-state concentrations of benazeprilat should be reached after 2 or 3 doses of benazepril hydrochloride given once daily.

During chronic administration (28 days) of once-daily doses of benazepril between 5 mg and 20 mg, the kinetics did not change, and there was no significant accumulation. Accumulation ratios based on AUC and urinary recovery of benazeprilat were 1.19 and 1.27, respectively.

When dialysis was started 2 hours after ingestion of 10 mg of benazepril, approximately 6% of benazeprilat was removed in 4 hours of dialysis. The parent compound, benazepril, was not detected in the dialysate.

Benazepril and benazeprilat are cleared predominantly by renal excretion in healthy subjects with normal renal function. Nonrenal (i.e., biliary) excretion accounts for approximately 11%-12% of benazeprilat excretion in healthy subjects. In patients with renal failure, biliary clearance may compensate to an extent for deficient renal clearance.

The disposition of benazepril and benazeprilat in patients with mild-to-moderate renal insufficiency (creatinine clearance > 30 mL/min) is similar to that in patients with normal renal function. In patients with creatinine clearance ≤ 30 mL/min, peak benazeprilat levels and the initial (alpha phase) half-life increase, and time to steady state may be delayed (see DOSAGE AND ADMINISTRATION).

Thiazide diuretics are eliminated by the kidney, with a terminal half-life of 5-15 hours. In a study of patients with impaired renal function (mean creatinine clearance of 19 mL/min), the half-life of hydrochlorothiazide elimination was lengthened to 21 hours.

Pharmacodynamics

Single and multiple doses of 10 mg or more of **benazepril** cause inhibition of plasma ACE activity by at least 80%-90% for at least 24 hours after dosing. For up to 4 hours after a 10-mg dose, pressor responses to exogenous angiotensin I were inhibited by 60%-90%.

Administration of benazepril to patients with mild-to-moderate hypertension results in a reduction of both supine and standing blood pressure to about the same extent, with no compensatory tachycardia.

Symptomatic postural hypotension is infrequent, although it can occur in patients who are salt and/or volume depleted (see WARNINGS, Hypotension).

In single-dose studies, benazepril lowered blood pressure within 1 hour, with peak reductions achieved 2-4 hours after dosing. The antihypertensive effect of a single dose persisted for 24 hours. In multiple-dose studies, once-daily doses of 20-80 mg decreased seated pressure (systolic/diastolic) 24 hours after dosing by about 6-12/4-7 mmHg. The reductions at trough are about 50% of those seen at peak.

Four dose-response studies of benazepril monotherapy using once-daily dosing were conducted in 470 mild-to-moderate hypertensive patients not using diuretics. The minimal effective once-daily dose of benazepril was 10 mg; further falls in blood pressure, especially at morning trough, were seen with higher doses in the studied dosing range (10-80 mg). In studies comparing the same daily dose of benazepril given as a single morning dose or as a twice-daily dose, blood pressure reductions at the time of morning trough blood levels were greater with the divided regimen.

During chronic therapy with benazepril, the maximum reduction in blood pressure with any given dose is generally achieved after 1-2 weeks. The antihypertensive effects of benazepril have continued during therapy for at least 2 years. Abrupt withdrawal of benazepril has not been associated with a rapid increase in blood pressure.

In patients with mild-to-moderate hypertension, total daily doses of Lotensin 20-40 mg were similar in effectiveness to total daily doses of captopril 50-100 mg, hydrochlorothiazide 25-50 mg, nifedipine SR 40-80 mg, and propranolol 80-160 mg.

The antihypertensive effects of benazepril were not appreciably different in patients receiving high- or low-sodium diets.

In hemodynamic studies in dogs, blood pressure reduction was accompanied by a reduction in peripheral arterial resistance, with an increase in cardiac output and renal blood flow and little or no change in heart rate. In normal human volunteers, single doses of benazepril caused an increase in renal blood flow but had no effect on glomerular filtration rate.

In clinical trials of **benazepril/hydrochlorothiazide** using benazepril doses of 5-20 mg and hydrochlorothiazide doses of 6.25-25 mg, the antihypertensive effects were sustained for at least 24 hours, and they increased with increasing dose of either component. Although benazepril monotherapy is somewhat less effective in blacks than in nonblacks, the efficacy of combination therapy appears to be independent of race.

By blocking the renin-angiotensin-aldosterone axis, administration of benazepril tends to reduce the potassium loss associated with the diuretic. In clinical trials of Lotensin HCT, the average change in serum potassium was near zero in subjects who received 5/6.25 mg or 20/12.5 mg, but the average subject who received 10/12.5 mg or 20/25 mg experienced a mild reduction in serum potassium, similar to that experienced by the average subject receiving the same dose of hydrochlorothiazide monotherapy.

INDICATIONS AND USAGE

Lotensin HCT is indicated for the treatment of hypertension.

This fixed combination drug is not indicated for the initial therapy of hypertension (see DOSAGE AND ADMINISTRATION).

In using Lotensin HCT, consideration should be given to the fact that another angiotensin-converting enzyme inhibitor, captopril, has caused agranulocytosis, particularly in patients with renal impairment or collagen-vascular disease. Available data are insufficient to show that benazepril does not have a similar risk (see WARNINGS, Neutropenia/Agranulocytosis).

Black patients receiving ACE inhibitors have been reported to have a higher incidence of angioedema compared to nonblacks.

CONTRAINDICATIONS

Lotensin HCT is contraindicated in patients who are anuric. Lotensin HCT is also contraindicated in patients who are hypersensitive to benazepril, to any other ACE inhibitor, to hydrochlorothiazide, or to other sulfonamide-derived drugs. Hypersensitivity reactions are more likely to occur in patients with a history of allergy or bronchial asthma.

WARNINGS

Anaphylactoid and Possibly Related Reactions

Presumably because angiotensin-converting enzyme inhibitors affect the metabolism of eicosanoids and polypeptides, including endogenous bradykinin, patients receiving ACE inhibitors (including Lotensin HCT) may be subject to a variety of adverse reactions, some of them serious.

Angioedema: Angioedema of the face, extremities, lips, tongue, glottis, and larynx has been reported in patients treated with angiotensin-converting enzyme inhibitors. In U.S. clinical trials, symptoms consistent with angioedema were seen in none of the subjects who received placebo and in about 0.5% of the subjects who received benazepril. Angioedema associated with laryngeal edema can be fatal. If laryngeal stridor or angioedema of the face, tongue, or glottis occurs, treatment with Lotensin HCT should be discontinued and appropriate therapy instituted immediately. *When involvement of the tongue, glottis, or larynx appears likely to cause airway obstruction, appropriate therapy, e.g., subcutaneous epinephrine injection 1:1000 (0.3-0.5 mL) should be promptly administered* (see PRECAUTIONS and ADVERSE REACTIONS).

Anaphylactoid Reactions During Desensitization: Two patients undergoing desensitizing treatment with hymenoptera venom while receiving ACE inhibitors sustained life-threatening anaphylactoid reactions. In the same patients, these reactions were avoided when ACE inhibitors were temporarily withheld, but they reappeared upon inadvertent rechallenge.

Anaphylactoid Reactions During Membrane Exposure: Anaphylactoid reactions have been reported in patients dialyzed with high-flux membranes and treated concomitantly with an ACE inhibitor. Anaphylactoid reactions have also been reported in patients undergoing low-density lipoprotein apheresis with dextran sulfate absorption.

Hypotension

Lotensin HCT can cause symptomatic hypotension. Like other ACE inhibitors, benazepril has been only rarely associated with hypotension in uncomplicated hypertensive patients. Symptomatic hypotension is most likely to occur in patients who have been volume and/or salt depleted as a result of prolonged diuretic therapy, dietary salt restriction, dialysis, diarrhea, or vomiting. Volume and/or salt depletion should be corrected before initiating therapy with Lotensin HCT.

Lotensin HCT should be used cautiously in patients receiving concomitant therapy with other antihypertensives. The thiazide component of Lotensin HCT may potentiate the action of other antihypertensive drugs, especially ganglionic or peripheral adrenergic-blocking drugs. The antihypertensive effects of the thiazide component may also be enhanced in the postsympathectomy patient.

In patients with congestive heart failure, with or without associated renal insufficiency, ACE inhibitor therapy may cause excessive hypotension, which may be associated with oliguria, azotemia, and (rarely) with acute renal failure and death. In such patients, Lotensin HCT therapy should be started under close medical supervision; they should be followed closely for the first 2 weeks of treatment and whenever the dose of benazepril or diuretic is increased.

If hypotension occurs, the patient should be placed in a supine position, and, if necessary, treated with intravenous infusion of physiological saline. Lotensin HCT treatment usually can be continued following restoration of blood pressure and volume.

Impaired Renal Function

Lotensin HCT should be used with caution in patients with severe renal disease. Thiazides may precipitate azotemia in such patients, and the effects of repeated dosing may be cumulative.

When the renin-angiotensin-aldosterone system is inhibited by benazepril, changes in renal function may be anticipated in susceptible individuals. In patients with **severe congestive heart failure,** whose renal function may depend on the activity of the renin-angiotensin-aldosterone system, treatment with angiotensin-converting enzyme inhibitors (including benazepril) may be associated with oliguria and/or progressive azotemia and (rarely) with acute renal failure and/or death.

In a small study of hypertensive patients with **unilateral or bilateral renal artery stenosis,** treatment with benazepril was associated with increases in blood urea nitrogen and serum creatinine; these increases were reversible upon discontinuation of benazepril therapy, concomitant diuretic therapy, or both. When such patients are treated with Lotensin HCT, renal function should be monitored during the first few weeks of therapy.

Some benazepril-treated hypertensive patients with **no apparent preexisting renal vascular disease** have developed increases in blood urea nitrogen and serum creatinine, usually minor and transient, especially when benazepril has been given concomitantly with a diuretic. Dosage reduction

Continued on next page

Lotensin HCT—Cont.

of Lotensin HCT may be required. **Evaluation of the hypertensive patient should always include assessment of renal function** (see DOSAGE AND ADMINISTRATION).

Neutropenia/Agranulocytosis

Another angiotensin-converting enzyme inhibitor, captopril, has been shown to cause agranulocytosis and bone marrow depression, rarely in uncomplicated patients (incidence probably less than once per 10,000 exposures) but more frequently (incidence possibly as great as once per 1000 exposures) in patients with renal impairment, especially those who also have collagen-vascular diseases such as systemic lupus erythematosus or scleroderma. Available data from clinical trials of benazepril are insufficient to show that benazepril does not cause agranulocytosis at similar rates. Monitoring of white blood cell counts should be considered in patients with collagen-vascular disease, especially if the disease is associated with impaired renal function.

Fetal/Neonatal Morbidity and Mortality

ACE inhibitors can cause fetal and neonatal morbidity and death when administered to pregnant women. Several dozen cases have been reported in the world literature. When pregnancy is detected, Lotensin HCT should be discontinued as soon as possible.

The use of ACE inhibitors during the second and third trimesters of pregnancy has been associated with fetal and neonatal injury, including hypotension, neonatal skull hypoplasia, anuria, reversible or irreversible renal failure, and death. Oligohydramnios has also been reported, presumably resulting from decreased fetal renal function; oligohydramnios in this setting has been associated with fetal limb contractures, craniofacial deformation, and hypoplastic lung development. Prematurity, intrauterine growth retardation, and patent ductus arteriosus have also been reported, although it is not clear whether these occurrences were due to the ACE-inhibitor exposure.

These adverse effects do not appear to have resulted from intrauterine ACE- inhibitor exposure that has been limited to the first trimester. Mothers whose embryos and fetuses are exposed to ACE inhibitors only during the first trimester should be so informed. Nonetheless, when patients become pregnant, physicians should make every effort to discontinue the use of benazepril as soon as possible.

Rarely (probably less often than once in every thousand pregnancies), no alternative to ACE inhibitors will be found. In these rare cases, the mothers should be apprised of the potential hazards to their fetuses, and serial ultrasound examinations should be performed to assess the intraamniotic environment.

If oligohydramnios is observed, benazepril should be discontinued unless it is considered life-saving for the mother. Contraction stress testing (CST), a nonstress test (NST), or biophysical profiling (BPP) may be appropriate, depending upon the week of pregnancy. Patients and physicians should be aware, however, that oligohydramnios may not appear until after the fetus has sustained irreversible injury.

Infants with histories of in utero exposure to ACE inhibitors should be closely observed for hypotension, oliguria, and hyperkalemia. If oliguria occurs, attention should be directed toward support of blood pressure and renal perfusion. Exchange transfusion or peritoneal dialysis may be required as means of reversing hypotension and/or substituting for disordered renal function. Benazepril, which crosses the placenta, can theoretically be removed from the neonatal circulation by these means; there are occasional reports of benefit from these maneuvers, but experience is limited.

Intrauterine exposure to thiazide diuretics is associated with fetal or neonatal jaundice, thrombocytopenia, and possibly other adverse reactions that have occurred in adults.

No teratogenic effects were seen when benazepril and hydrochlorothiazide were administered to pregnant rats at a dose ratio of 4:5. On a mg/kg basis, the doses used were up to 167 times the maximum recommended human dose. Similarly, no teratogenic effects were seen when benazepril and hydrochlorothiazide were administered to pregnant mice at total doses up to 160 mg/kg/day, with benazepril:hydrochlorothiazide ratios of 15:1. When hydrochlorothiazide was orally administered without benazepril to pregnant mice and rats during their respective periods of major organogenesis, at doses up to 3000 and 1000 mg/kg/day respectively, there was no evidence of harm to the fetus. Similarly, no teratogenic effects of benazepril were seen in studies of pregnant rats, mice, and rabbits; on a mg/kg basis, the doses used in these studies were 300 times (in rats), 90 times (in mice), and more than 3 times (in rabbits) the maximum recommended human dose.

Hepatic Failure

Rarely, ACE inhibitors have been associated with a syndrome that starts with cholestatic jaundice and progresses to fulminant hepatic necrosis and (sometimes) death. The mechanism of this syndrome is not understood. Patients receiving ACE inhibitors who develop jaundice or marked elevations of hepatic enzymes should discontinue the ACE inhibitor and receive appropriate medical follow-up.

Impaired Hepatic Function

Lotensin HCT should be used with caution in patients with impaired hepatic function or progressive liver disease, since minor alterations of fluid and electrolyte balance may precipitate hepatic coma (see Hepatic Failure, above). In patients with hepatic dysfunction due to cirrhosis, levels of benazeprilat are essentially unaltered. No formal pharmacokinetic studies have been carried out in hypertensive patients with impaired liver function.

Systemic Lupus Erythematosus

Thiazide diuretics have been reported to cause exacerbation or activation of systemic lupus erythematosus.

PRECAUTIONS

General

Derangements of Serum Electrolytes: In clinical trials of benazepril monotherapy, hyperkalemia (serum potassium at least 0.5 mEq/L greater than the upper limit of normal) occurred in approximately 1% of hypertensive patients receiving benazepril. In most cases, these were isolated values which resolved despite continued therapy. Risk factors for the development of hyperkalemia included renal insufficiency, diabetes mellitus, and the concomitant use of potassium-sparing diuretics, potassium supplements, and/or potassium-containing salt substitutes.

Conversely, treatment with thiazide diuretics has been associated with hypokalemia, hyponatremia, and hypochloremic alkalosis. These disturbances have sometimes been manifest as one or more of dryness of mouth, thirst, weakness, lethargy, drowsiness, restlessness, muscle pains or cramps, muscular fatigue, hypotension, oliguria, tachycardia, nausea, and vomiting. Hypokalemia can also sensitize or exaggerate the response of the heart to the toxic effects of digitalis. The risk of hypokalemia is greatest in patients with cirrhosis of the liver, in patients experiencing a brisk diuresis, in patients who are receiving inadequate oral intake of electrolytes, and in patients receiving concomitant therapy with corticosteroids or ACTH.

The opposite effects of benazepril and hydrochlorothiazide on serum potassium will approximately balance each other in many patients, so that no net effect upon serum potassium will be seen. In other patients, one or the other effect may be dominant. Initial and periodic determinations of serum electrolytes to detect possible electrolyte imbalance should be performed at appropriate intervals.

Chloride deficits are generally mild and require specific treatment only under extraordinary circumstances (e.g., in liver disease or renal disease). Dilutional hyponatremia may occur in edematous patients; appropriate therapy is water restriction rather than administration of salt, except in rare instances when the hyponatremia is life-threatening. In actual salt depletion, appropriate replacement is the therapy of choice.

Calcium excretion is decreased by thiazides. In a few patients on prolonged thiazide therapy, pathological changes in the parathyroid gland have been observed, with hypercalcemia and hypophosphatemia. More serious complications of hyperparathyroidism (renal lithiasis, bone resorption, and peptic ulceration) have not been seen.

Thiazides increase the urinary excretion of magnesium, and hypomagnesemia may result.

Other Metabolic Disturbances: Thiazide diuretics tend to reduce glucose tolerance and to raise serum levels of cholesterol, triglycerides, and uric acid. These effects are usually minor, but frank gout or overt diabetes may be precipitated in susceptible patients.

Cough: Presumably due to the inhibition of the degradation of endogenous bradykinin, persistent nonproductive cough has been reported with all ACE inhibitors, always resolving after discontinuation of therapy. ACE inhibitor-induced cough should be considered in the differential diagnosis of cough.

Surgery/Anesthesia: In patients undergoing surgery or during anesthesia with agents that produce hypotension, benazepril will block the angiotensin II formation that could otherwise occur secondary to compensatory renin release. Hypotension that occurs as a result of this mechanism can be corrected by volume expansion.

Information for Patients

Angioedema: Angioedema, including laryngeal edema, can occur at any time with treatment with ACE inhibitors. A patient receiving Lotensin HCT should be told to report immediately any signs or symptoms suggesting angioedema (swelling of face, eyes, lips, or tongue, or difficulty in breathing) and to take no more drug until after consulting with the prescribing physician.

Pregnancy: Female patients of childbearing age should be told about the consequences of second- and third-trimester exposure to ACE inhibitors, and they should also be told that these consequences do not appear to have resulted from intrauterine ACE-inhibitor exposure that has been limited to the first trimester. These patients should be asked to report pregnancies to their physicians as soon as possible.

Symptomatic Hypotension: A patient receiving Lotensin HCT should be cautioned that lightheadedness can occur, especially during the first days of therapy, and that it should be reported to the prescribing physician. The patient should be told that if syncope occurs, Lotensin HCT should be discontinued until the physician has been consulted.

All patients should be cautioned that inadequate fluid intake, excessive perspiration, diarrhea, or vomiting can lead to an excessive fall in blood pressure, with the same consequences of lightheadedness and possible syncope.

Hyperkalemia: A patient receiving Lotensin HCT should be told not to use potassium supplements or salt substitutes containing potassium without consulting the prescribing physician.

Neutropenia: Patients should be told to promptly report any indication of infection (e.g., sore throat, fever), which could be a sign of neutropenia.

Laboratory Tests

The hydrochlorothiazide component of Lotensin HCT may decrease serum PBI levels without signs of thyroid disturbance.

Therapy with Lotensin HCT should be interrupted for a few days before carrying out tests of parathyroid function.

Drug Interactions

Potassium Supplements and Potassium-Sparing Diuretics: As noted above (Derangements of Serum Electrolytes), the net effect of Lotensin HCT may be to elevate a patient's serum potassium, to reduce it, or to leave it unchanged. Potassium-sparing diuretics (spironolactone, amiloride, triamterene, and others) or potassium supplements can increase the risk of hyperkalemia. If concomitant use of such agents is indicated, they should be given with caution, and the patient's serum potassium should be monitored frequently.

Lithium: Increased serum lithium levels and symptoms of lithium toxicity have been reported in patients receiving ACE inhibitors during therapy with lithium. Because renal clearance of lithium is reduced by thiazides, the risk of lithium toxicity is presumably raised further when, as in therapy with Lotensin HCT, a thiazide diuretic is coadministered with the ACE inhibitor. Lotensin HCT and lithium should be coadministered with caution, and frequent monitoring of serum lithium levels is recommended.

Other: Benazepril has been used concomitantly with beta-adrenergic-blocking agents, calcium-blocking agents, cimetidine, diuretics, digoxin, hydralazine, and naproxen without evidence of clinically important adverse interactions. Other ACE inhibitors have had less than additive effects with beta-adrenergic blockers, presumably because drugs of both classes lower blood pressure by inhibiting parts of the renin-angiotensin system.

Interaction studies with warfarin and acenocoumarol have failed to identify any clinically important effects of benazepril on the serum concentrations or clinical effects of these anticoagulants.

Insulin requirements in diabetic patients may be increased, decreased, or unchanged.

Thiazides may decrease arterial responsiveness to norepinephrine, but not enough to preclude effectiveness of the pressor agent for therapeutic use.

Thiazides may increase the responsiveness to tubocurarine.

The diuretic, natriuretic, and antihypertensive effects of thiazide diuretics may be reduced by concurrent administration of nonsteroidal anti-inflammatory agents.

Cholestyramine and colestipol resins: Absorption of hydrochlorothiazide is impaired in the presence of anionic exchange resins. Single doses of either cholestyramine or colestipol resins bind the hydrochlorothiazide and reduce its absorption from the gastrointestinal tract by up to 85% and 43%, respectively.

Carcinogenesis, Mutagenesis, Impairment of Fertility

No evidence of carcinogenicity was found when **benazepril** was given to rats and mice for 104 weeks at doses up to 150 mg/kg/day. On a body-weight basis, this dose is over 100 times the maximum recommended human dose; on a body-surface-area basis, this dose is 18 times (rats) and 9 times (mice) the maximum recommended human dose. No mutagenic activity was detected in the Ames test in bacteria (with or without metabolic activation), in an in vitro test for forward mutations in cultured mammalian cells, or in a nucleus anomaly test. At doses of 50-500 mg/kg/day (38-375 times the maximum recommended human dose on a body-weight basis; 6-61 times the maximum recommended dose on a body-surface-area basis), benazepril had no adverse effect on the reproductive performance of male and female rats.

Under the auspices of the National Toxicology Program, rats and mice received **hydrochlorothiazide** in their feed for two years, at doses up to 600 mg/kg/day in mice and up to 100 mg/kg/day in rats. These studies uncovered no evidence of a carcinogenic potential of hydrochlorothiazide in rats or female mice, but there was equivocal evidence of hepatocarcinogenicity in male mice. Hydrochlorothiazide was not genotoxic in in vitro assays using strains TA 98, TA 100, TA 1535, TA 1537, and TA 1538 of *Salmonella typhimurium* (the Ames test); in the Chinese Hamster Ovary (CHO) test for chromosomal aberrations; or in in vivo assays using mouse germinal cell chromosomes, Chinese hamster bone marrow chromosomes, and the *Drosophila* sex-linked recessive lethal trait gene. Positive test results were obtained in the in vitro CHO Sister Chromatid Exchange (clastogenicity) test and in the Mouse Lymphoma Cell (mutagenicity) assays, using concentrations of hydrochlorothiazide of 43-1300 µg/mL. Positive test results were also obtained in the *Aspergillus nidulans* nondisjunction assay, using an unspecified concentration of hydrochlorothiazide.

Hydrochlorothiazide had no adverse effects on the fertility of mice and rats of either sex in studies wherein these species were exposed, via their diets, to doses up to 100 and 4 mg/kg/day, respectively, prior to mating and throughout gestation.

Pregnancy

Pregnancy Categories C (first trimester) and D (second and third trimesters): See WARNINGS, Fetal/Neonatal Morbidity and Mortality.

Nursing Mothers

Minimal amounts of unchanged benazepril and of benazeprilat are excreted into the breast milk of lactating women treated with benazepril, so that a newborn child ingesting nothing but breast milk would receive less than 0.1% of the maternal doses of benazepril and benazeprilat. Thiazides, on the other hand, are definitely excreted into breast milk. Because of the potential for serious adverse reactions in nursing infants from hydrochlorothiazide and the unknown effects of benazepril in infants, a decision should be made whether to discontinue nursing or to discontinue Lotensin HCT, taking into account the importance of the drug to the mother.

Geriatric Use

Of the total number of patients who received Lotensin HCT in U.S. clinical studies of Lotensin HCT, 19% were 65 or older while about 1.5% were 75 or older. Overall differences in effectiveness or safety were not observed between these patients and younger patients, and other reported clinical experience has not identified differences in responses between the elderly and younger patients, but greater sensitivity of some older individuals cannot be ruled out.

Pediatric Use

Safety and effectiveness in pediatric patients have not been established.

ADVERSE REACTIONS

Lotensin HCT has been evaluated for safety in over 2500 patients with hypertension; over 500 of these patients were treated for at least 6 months, and over 200 were treated for more than 1 year.

The reported side effects were generally mild and transient, and there was no relationship between side effects and age, sex, race, or duration of therapy. Discontinuation of therapy due to side effects was required in approximately 7% of U.S. patients treated with Lotensin HCT and in 4% of patients treated with placebo.

The most common reasons for discontinuation of therapy with Lotensin HCT in U.S. studies were cough (1.0%; see PRECAUTIONS), "dizziness" (1.0%), headache (0.6%), and fatigue (0.6%).

The side effects considered possibly or probably related to study drug that occurred in U.S. placebo-controlled trials in more than 1% of patients treated with Lotensin HCT are shown in the table below.

Reactions Possibly or Probably Drug Related
Patients in U.S. Placebo-Controlled Studies

	LOTENSIN HCT N=655		Placebo N=235	
	N	%	N	%
"Dizziness"	41	6.3	8	3.4
Fatigue	34	5.2	6	2.6
Postural Dizziness	23	3.5	1	0.4
Headache	20	3.1	10	4.3
Cough	14	2.1	3	1.3
Hypertonia	10	1.5	3	1.3
Vertigo	10	1.5	2	0.9
Nausea	9	1.4	2	0.9
Impotence	8	1.2	0	0.0
Somnolence	8	1.2	1	0.4

Other side effects considered possibly or probably related to study drug that occurred in U.S. placebo-controlled trials in 0.3% to 1.0% of patients treated with Lotensin HCT were the following:

Angioedema: Edema of the lips or face without other manifestations of angioedema (0.3%). See WARNINGS, Angioedema.

Cardiovascular: Hypotension (seen in 0.6% of patients), postural hypotension (0.3%), palpitations, and flushing.

Gastrointestinal: Vomiting, diarrhea, dyspepsia, anorexia, and constipation.

Neurologic and Psychiatric: Insomnia, nervousness, paresthesia, libido decrease, dry mouth, taste perversion, and tinnitus.

Dermatologic: Rash and sweating.

Other: Gout, urinary frequency, arthralgia, myalgia, asthenia, and pain (including chest pain and abdominal pain).

Other adverse experiences reported in 0.3% or more of Lotensin HCT patients in U.S. controlled clinical trials, and rarer events seen in postmarketing experience, were the following; asterisked entries occurred in more than 1% of patients (in some, a causal relationship to Lotensin HCT is uncertain):

Angioedema: Edema of the lips or face without other manifestations of angioedema. See WARNINGS, Angioedema.

Cardiovascular: Syncope, peripheral vascular disorder, and tachycardia.

Body as a Whole: Infection, back pain,* flu syndrome,* fever, chills, and neck pain.

Dermatologic: Photosensitivity and pruritus.

Gastrointestinal: Gastroenteritis, flatulence, and tooth disorder.

Neurologic and Psychiatric: Hypesthesia, abnormal vision, abnormal dreams, and retinal disorder.

Respiratory: Upper respiratory infection,* epistaxis, bronchitis, rhinitis,* sinusitis,* and voice alteration.

Other: Conjunctivitis, arthritis, urinary tract infection, alopecia, and urinary frequency.*

Fetal/Neonatal Morbidity and Mortality: See WARNINGS, Fetal/Neonatal Morbidity and Mortality.

Monotherapy with **benazepril** has been evaluated for safety in over 6000 patients. In clinical trials, the observed adverse reactions to benazepril were similar to those seen in trials of Lotensin HCT. In postmarketing experience with benazepril, there have been rare reports of Stevens-Johnson syndrome, pancreatitis, hemolytic anemia, pemphigus, and thrombocytopenia. Another potentially important adverse experience, eosinophilic pneumonitis, has been attributed to other ACE inhibitors.

Hydrochlorothiazide has been extensively prescribed for many years, but there has not been enough systematic collection of data to support an estimate of the frequency of the observed adverse reactions. Within organ-system groups, the reported reactions are listed here in decreasing order of severity, without regard to frequency.

Cardiovascular: Orthostatic hypotension (may be potentiated by alcohol, barbiturates, or narcotics).

Digestive: Pancreatitis, jaundice (intrahepatic cholestatic) (see WARNINGS), sialadenitis, vomiting, diarrhea, cramping, nausea, gastric irritation, constipation, and anorexia.

Neurologic: Vertigo, lightheadedness, transient blurred vision, headache, paresthesia, xanthopsia, weakness, and restlessness.

Musculoskeletal: Muscle spasm.

Hematologic: Aplastic anemia, agranulocytosis, leukopenia, and thrombocytopenia.

Metabolic: Hyperglycemia, glycosuria, and hyperuricemia.

Hypersensitivity: Necrotizing angiitis, Stevens-Johnson syndrome, respiratory distress (including pneumonitis and pulmonary edema), purpura, urticaria, rash, and photosensitivity.

Clinical Laboratory Test Findings

Serum Electrolytes: See PRECAUTIONS.

Creatinine: Minor reversible increases in serum creatinine were observed in patients with essential hypertension treated with Lotensin HCT. Such increases occurred most frequently in patients with renal artery stenosis (see PRECAUTIONS).

PBI and Tests of Parathyroid Function: See PRECAUTIONS.

Other (Causal Relationships Unknown): Other clinically important changes in standard laboratory tests were rarely associated with Lotensin HCT administration. Elevations in blood urea nitrogen, uric acid, glucose, SGOT, and SGPT (see WARNINGS) have been reported. In the somewhat larger patient population exposed to benazepril monotherapy in U.S. trials, the same abnormalities were reported, together with scattered accounts of hyponatremia, melena, electrocardiographic changes, leukopenia, eosinophilia, and proteinuria.

OVERDOSAGE

No specific information is available on the treatment of overdosage with Lotensin HCT; treatment should be symptomatic and supportive. Therapy with Lotensin HCT should be discontinued, and the patient should be observed. Dehydration, electrolyte imbalance, and hypotension should be treated by established procedures.

Single oral doses of 1 g/kg of benazepril caused reduced activity in mice, and doses of 3 g/kg were associated with significant lethality. Reduction of activity in rats was not seen until they had received doses of 5 g/kg, and doses of 6 g/kg were not lethal. In single-dose studies of hydrochlorothiazide, most rats survived doses up to 2.75 g/kg.

Data from human overdoses of benazepril are scanty, but the most common manifestation of human benazepril overdosage is likely to be hypotension. In human hydrochlorothiazide overdose, the most common signs and symptoms observed have been those of dehydration and electrolyte depletion (hypokalemia, hypochloremia, hyponatremia). If digitalis has also been administered, hypokalemia may accentuate cardiac arrhythmias.

Laboratory determinations of serum levels of benazepril and its metabolites are not widely available, and such determinations have, in any event, no established role in the management of benazepril overdose.

No data are available to suggest physiological maneuvers (e.g., maneuvers to change the pH of the urine) that might accelerate elimination of benazepril and its metabolites. Benazeprilat is only slightly dialyzable, but dialysis might be considered in overdosed patients with severely impaired renal function (see WARNINGS).

Angiotensin II could presumably serve as a specific antagonist-antidote in the setting of benazepril overdose, but angiotensin II is essentially unavailable outside of scattered research facilities. Because the hypotensive effect of benazepril is achieved through vasodilation and effective hypovolemia, it is reasonable to treat benazepril overdose by infusion of normal saline solution.

DOSAGE AND ADMINISTRATION

Benazepril is an effective treatment of hypertension in once-daily doses of 10-80 mg, while hydrochlorothiazide is effective in doses of 12.5-50 mg per day. In clinical trials of benazepril/hydrochlorothiazide combination therapy using benazepril doses of 5-20 mg and hydrochlorothiazide doses of 6.25-25 mg, the antihypertensive effects increased with increasing dose of either component.

The side effects (see WARNINGS) of benazepril are generally rare and apparently independent of dose; those of hydrochlorothiazide are a mixture of dose-dependent phenomena (primarily hypokalemia) and dose-independent phenomena (e.g., pancreatitis), the former much more common than the latter. Therapy with any combination of benazepril and hydrochlorothiazide will be associated with both sets of dose-independent side effects, but regimens in which benazepril is combined with low doses of hydrochlorothiazide produce minimal effects on serum potassium. In clinical trials of Lotensin HCT, the average change in serum potassium was near zero in subjects who received 5/6.25 mg or 20/12.5 mg, but the average subject who received 10/12.5 mg or 20/25 mg experienced a mild reduction in serum potassium, similar to that experienced by the average subject receiving the same dose of hydrochlorothiazide monotherapy.

To minimize dose-independent side effects, it is usually appropriate to begin combination therapy only after a patient has failed to achieve the desired effect with monotherapy.

Dose Titration Guided by Clinical Effect: A patient whose blood pressure is not adequately controlled with benazepril monotherapy may be switched to Lotensin HCT 10/12.5 or Lotensin HCT 20/12.5. Further increases of either or both components could depend on clinical response. The hydrochlorothiazide dose should generally not be increased until 2-3 weeks have elapsed. Patients whose blood pressures are adequately controlled with 25 mg of daily hydrochlorothiazide, but who experience significant potassium loss with this regimen, may achieve similar blood-pressure control without electrolyte disturbance if they are switched to Lotensin HCT 5/6.25.

Replacement Therapy: The combination may be substituted for the titrated individual components.

Use in Renal Impairment: Regimens of therapy with Lotensin HCT need not take account of renal function as long as the patient's creatinine clearance is $>$ 30 mL/min/1.73m^2 (serum creatinine roughly $\leq$ 3 mg/dL or 265 µmol/L). In patients with more severe renal impairment, loop diuretics are preferred to thiazides, so Lotensin HCT is not recommended (see WARNINGS).

HOW SUPPLIED

Lotensin HCT is available in tablets of four different strengths:

Benazepril	Hydrochlorothiazide	Tablet Color
5 mg	6.25 mg	white
10 mg	12.50 mg	light pink
20 mg	12.50 mg	grayish-violet
20 mg	25.00 mg	red

Tablets of each strength are supplied in bottles that contain a desiccant and 100 tablets.

The National Drug Codes for the various packages are

Dose	Bottle of 100
5/6.25	NDC 0083-0057-30
10/12.5	NDC 0083-0072-30
20/12.5	NDC 0083-0074-30
20/25	NDC 0083-0075-30

Tablets are oblong and scored, with "Lotensin HCT" on one side and a portion of the NDC code ("57," "72," "74," or "75") on the other.

Storage: Do not store above 30°C (86°F). Protect from moisture and light. *Dispense in tight, light-resistant container (USP).*

REV: FEBRUARY 1999 T1999-13

Shown in Product Identification Guide, page 326

LOTREL® ℞

[lō-trĕl]

amlodipine and benazepril hydrochloride
Combination Capsules
2.5 mg/10 mg
5 mg/10 mg
5 mg/20 mg
Rx only

The following prescribing information is based on official labeling in effect July 2000.

USE IN PREGNANCY
When used in pregnancy during the second and third trimesters, ACE inhibitors can cause injury and even death to the developing fetus. When pregnancy is detected, Lotrel should be discontinued as soon as possible. See **Warnings, Fetal/Neonatal Morbidity and Mortality.**

DESCRIPTION

Benazepril hydrochloride is a white to off-white crystalline powder, soluble (>100 mg/mL) in water, in ethanol, and in methanol. Benazepril hydrochloride's chemical name is 3-[[1-(ethoxycarbonyl)-3-phenyl-(1S)-propyl]amino]-2,3,4,5-tetrahydro-2-oxo-1*H*-1-(3S)-benzazepine-1-acetic acid monohydrochloride; its structural formula is

H O COOCH₂CH₃ N H CH₂CH₂ H O N CH₂COOH •HCl

Its empirical formula is $C_{24}H_{28}N_2O_5$•HCl, and its molecular weight is 460.96.

Continued on next page

Lotrel—Cont.

Benazeprilat, the active metabolite of benazepril, is a non-sulfhydryl angiotensin-converting enzyme (ACE) inhibitor. Benazepril is converted to benazeprilat by hepatic cleavage of the ester group.

Amlodipine besylate is a white to pale yellow crystalline powder, slightly soluble in water and sparingly soluble in ethanol. Its chemical name is (R,S)3-ethyl-5-methyl-2-(2-aminoethoxymethyl)-4-(2-chlorophenyl)-1,4-dihydro-6-methyl-3,5-pyridinedicarboxylate benzenesulfonate; its structural formula is

Its empirical formula is $C_{20}H_{25}ClN_2O_5 \cdot C_6H_6O_3S$, and its molecular weight is 567.1.

Amlodipine besylate is the besylate salt of amlodipine, a dihydropyridine calcium channel blocker.

Lotrel is a combination of amlodipine besylate and benazepril hydrochloride. The capsules are formulated for oral administration with a combination of amlodipine besylate equivalent to 2.5 mg or 5 mg of amlodipine and 10 mg or 20 mg of benazepril hydrochloride. The inactive ingredients of the capsules are calcium phosphate, cellulose compounds, colloidal silicon dioxide, crospovidone, gelatin, hydrogenated castor oil, iron oxides, lactose, magnesium stearate, polysorbate 80, silicon dioxide, sodium lauryl sulfate, sodium starch (potato) glycolate, starch (corn), talc, and titanium dioxide.

CLINICAL PHARMACOLOGY

Mechanism of Action

Benazepril and benazeprilat inhibit angiotensin-converting enzyme (ACE) in human subjects and in animals. ACE is a peptidyl dipeptidase that catalyzes the conversion of angiotensin I to the vasoconstrictor substance angiotensin II. Angiotensin II also stimulates aldosterone secretion by the adrenal cortex.

Inhibition of ACE results in decreased plasma angiotensin II, which leads to decreased vasopressor activity and to decreased aldosterone secretion. The latter decrease may result in a small increase of serum potassium. Hypertensive patients treated with benazepril and amlodipine for up to 56 weeks had elevations of serum potassium up to 0.2 mEq/L (see PRECAUTIONS).

Removal of angiotensin II negative feedback on renin secretion leads to increased plasma renin activity. In animal studies, benazepril had no inhibitory effect on the vasopressor response to angiotensin II and did not interfere with the hemodynamic effects of the autonomic neurotransmitters acetylcholine, epinephrine, and norepinephrine.

ACE is identical to kininase, an enzyme that degrades bradykinin. Whether increased levels of bradykinin, a potent vasodepressor peptide, play a role in the therapeutic effects of Lotrel remains to be elucidated.

While the mechanism through which benazepril lowers blood pressure is believed to be primarily suppression of the renin-angiotensin-aldosterone system, benazepril has an antihypertensive effect even in patients with low-renin hypertension.

Amlodipine is a dihydropyridine calcium antagonist (calcium ion antagonist or slow channel blocker) that inhibits the transmembrane influx of calcium ions into vascular smooth muscle and cardiac muscle. Experimental data suggest that amlodipine binds to both dihydropyridine and nondihydropyridine binding sites. The contractile processes of cardiac muscle and vascular smooth muscle are dependent upon the movement of extracellular calcium ions into these cells through specific ion channels. Amlodipine inhibits calcium ion influx across cell membranes selectively, with a greater effect on vascular smooth muscle cells than on cardiac muscle cells. Negative inotropic effects can be detected in vitro but such effects have not been seen in intact animals at therapeutic doses. Serum calcium concentration is not affected by amlodipine. Within the physiologic pH range, amlodipine is an ionized compound (pKa=8.6), and its kinetic interaction with the calcium channel receptor is characterized by a gradual rate of association and dissociation with the receptor binding site, resulting in a gradual onset of effect.

Amlodipine is a peripheral arterial vasodilator that acts directly on vascular smooth muscle to cause a reduction in peripheral vascular resistance and reduction in blood pressure.

Pharmacokinetics and Metabolism

The rate and extent of absorption of benazepril and amlodipine from Lotrel are not significantly different, respectively, from the rate and extent of absorption of benazepril and amlodipine from individual tablet formulations. Absorption from the individual tablets is not influenced by the presence of food in the gastrointestinal tract; food effects on absorption from Lotrel have not been studied. Following oral administration of Lotrel, peak plasma concentrations of benazepril are reached in 0.5-2 hours. Cleavage of the ester group (primarily in the liver) converts benazepril to its active metabolite, benazeprilat, which reaches peak plasma concentrations in 1.5-4 hours. The extent of absorption of benazepril is at least 37%.

Peak plasma concentrations of amlodipine are reached 6-12 hours after administration of Lotrel; the extent of absorption is 64%-90%.

The apparent volumes of **distribution** of amlodipine and benazeprilat are about 21 L/kg and 0.7 L/kg, respectively. Approximately 93% of circulating amlodipine is bound to plasma proteins, and the bound fraction of benazeprilat is slightly higher. On the basis of in vitro studies, benazeprilat's degree of protein binding should be unaffected by age, by hepatic dysfunction, or—over the therapeutic concentration range—by concentration.

Benazeprilat has much greater ACE-inhibitory activity than benazepril, and the **metabolism** of benazepril to benazeprilat is almost complete. Only trace amounts of an administered dose of benazepril can be recovered unchanged in the urine; about 20% of the dose is excreted as benazeprilat, 8% as benazeprilat glucuronide, and 4% as benazepril glucuronide.

Amlodipine is extensively metabolized in the liver, with 10% of the parent compound and 60% of the metabolites excreted in the urine. In patients with hepatic dysfunction, decreased clearance of amlodipine may increase the area-under-the-plasma-concentration curve by 40%-60%, and dosage reduction may be required (see DOSAGE AND ADMINISTRATION). In patients with renal impairment, the pharmacokinetics of amlodipine are essentially unaffected.

Benazeprilat's effective **elimination** half-life is 10-11 hours, while that of amlodipine is about 2 days, so steady-state levels of the two components are achieved after about a week of once-daily dosing. The clearance of benazeprilat from the plasma is primarily renal, but biliary excretion accounts for 11%-12% of benazepril elimination in normal subjects. In patients with severe renal insufficiency (creatinine clearance less than 30 mL/min), peak benazeprilat levels and the time to steady state may be increased (see DOSAGE AND ADMINISTRATION). In patients with hepatic impairment, on the other hand, the pharmacokinetics of benazeprilat are essentially unaffected.

Although the pharmacokinetics of benazepril and benazeprilat are unaffected by **age**, clearance of amlodipine is decreased in the elderly, with resulting increases of 35%-70% in peak plasma levels, elimination half-life, and area-under-the-plasma-concentration curve. Dose adjustment may be required.

Pharmacodynamics

Single and multiple doses of 10 mg or more of **benazepril** cause inhibition of plasma ACE activity by at least 80%-90% for at least 24 hours after dosing. For up to 4 hours after a 10-mg dose, pressor responses to exogenous angiotensin I were inhibited by 60%-90%.

Administration of benazepril to patients with mild-to-moderate hypertension results in a reduction of both supine and standing blood pressure to about the same extent, with no compensatory tachycardia. Symptomatic postural hypotension is infrequent, although it can occur in patients who are salt and/or volume depleted (see Warnings, Hypotension).

The antihypertensive effects of benazepril were not appreciably different in patients receiving high- or low-sodium diets.

In normal human volunteers, single doses of benazepril caused an increase in renal blood flow but had no effect on glomerular filtration rate.

Following administration of therapeutic doses to patients with hypertension, **amlodipine** produces vasodilation resulting in a reduction of supine and standing blood pressures. These decreases in blood pressure are not accompanied by a significant change in heart rate or plasma catecholamine levels with chronic dosing. Plasma concentrations correlate with effect in both young and elderly patients.

As with other calcium channel blockers, hemodynamic measurements of cardiac function at rest and during exercise (or pacing) in patients with normal ventricular function treated with amlodipine have generally demonstrated a small increase in cardiac index without significant influence on dP/dt or on left ventricular end diastolic pressure or volume. In hemodynamic studies, amlodipine has not been associated with a negative inotropic effect when administered in the therapeutic dose range to intact animals and humans, even when coadministered with beta blockers to humans.

Amlodipine does not change sinoatrial (SA) nodal function or atrioventricular (AV) conduction in intact animals or humans. In clinical studies in which amlodipine was administered in combination with beta blockers to patients with either hypertension or angina, no adverse effects on electrocardiographic parameters were observed.

Over 700 patients received Lotrel once daily in five double-blind, placebo-controlled studies. Lotrel lowered blood pressure within 1 hour, with peak reductions achieved 2-8 hours after dosing. The antihypertensive effect of a single dose persisted for 24 hours.

Once-daily doses of benazepril/amlodipine using benazepril doses of 10-20 mg and amlodipine doses of 2.5-5 mg decreased seated pressure (systolic/diastolic) 24 hours after dosing by about 10-25/6-13 mmHg.

Combination therapy was effective in blacks and nonblacks. Both components contributed to the antihypertensive efficacy in nonblacks, but virtually all of the antihypertensive effect in blacks could be attributed to the amlodipine component. Among nonblack patients in placebo-controlled trials comparing Lotrel to the individual components, the blood pressure lowering effects of the combination were shown to be additive and in some cases synergistic.

During chronic therapy with Lotrel, the maximum reduction in blood pressure with any given dose is generally achieved after 1-2 weeks. The antihypertensive effects of Lotrel have continued during therapy for at least 1 year. Abrupt withdrawal of Lotrel has not been associated with a rapid increase in blood pressure.

INDICATIONS AND USAGE

Lotrel is indicated for the treatment of hypertension.

This fixed combination drug is not indicated for the initial therapy of hypertension (see DOSAGE AND ADMINISTRATION).

In using Lotrel, consideration should be given to the fact that an ACE inhibitor, captopril, has caused agranulocytosis, particularly in patients with renal impairment or collagen-vascular disease. Available data are insufficient to show that benazepril does not have a similar risk (see Warnings, Neutropenia/Agranulocytosis).

Black patients receiving ACE inhibitors have been reported to have a higher incidence of angioedema compared to non-blacks.

CONTRAINDICATIONS

Lotrel is contraindicated in patients who are hypersensitive to benazepril, to any other ACE inhibitor, or to amlodipine.

WARNINGS

Anaphylactoid and Possibly Related Reactions

Presumably because angiotensin-converting enzyme inhibitors affect the metabolism of eicosanoids and polypeptides, including endogenous bradykinin, patients receiving ACE inhibitors (including Lotrel) may be subject to a variety of adverse reactions, some of them serious. These reactions usually occur after one of the first few doses of the ACE inhibitor, but they sometimes do not appear until after months of therapy.

Angioedema: Angioedema of the face, extremities, lips, tongue, glottis, and larynx has been reported in patients treated with ACE inhibitors. In U.S. clinical trials, symptoms consistent with angioedema were seen in none of the subjects who received placebo and in about 0.5% of the subjects who received benazepril. Angioedema associated with laryngeal edema can be fatal. If laryngeal stridor or angioedema of the face, tongue, or glottis occurs, treatment with Lotrel should be discontinued and appropriate therapy instituted immediately. *When involvement of the tongue, glottis, or larynx appears likely to cause airway obstruction, appropriate therapy, e.g., subcutaneous epinephrine injection 1:1000 (0.3-0.5 mL), should be promptly administered (see ADVERSE REACTIONS).*

Anaphylactoid Reactions During Desensitization: Two patients undergoing desensitizing treatment with hymenoptera venom while receiving ACE inhibitors sustained life-threatening anaphylactoid reactions. In the same patients, these reactions were avoided when ACE inhibitors were temporarily withheld, but they reappeared upon inadvertent rechallenge.

Anaphylactoid Reactions During Membrane Exposure: Anaphylactoid reactions have been reported in patients dialyzed with high-flux membranes and treated concomitantly with an ACE inhibitor. Anaphylactoid reactions have also been reported in patients undergoing low-density lipoprotein apheresis with dextran sulfate absorption.

Increased Angina and/or Myocardial Infarction: Rarely, patients, particularly those with severe obstructive coronary artery disease, have developed documented increased frequency, duration, and/or severity of angina or acute myocardial infarction on starting calcium channel blocker therapy or at the time of dosage increase. The mechanism of this effect has not been elucidated.

Hypotension

Lotrel can cause symptomatic hypotension. Like other ACE inhibitors, benazepril has been only rarely associated with hypotension in uncomplicated hypertensive patients. Symptomatic hypotension is most likely to occur in patients who have been volume and/or salt depleted as a result of prolonged diuretic therapy, dietary salt restriction, dialysis, diarrhea, or vomiting. Volume and/or salt depletion should be corrected before initiating therapy with Lotrel.

Since the vasodilation induced by amlodipine is gradual in onset, acute hypotension has rarely been reported after oral administration of amlodipine. Nonetheless, caution should be exercised when administering Lotrel as with any other peripheral vasodilator, particularly in patients with severe aortic stenosis.

In patients with congestive heart failure, with or without associated renal insufficiency, ACE inhibitor therapy may cause excessive hypotension, which may be associated with oliguria, azotemia, and (rarely) with acute renal failure and death. In such patients, Lotrel therapy should be started under close medical supervision; they should be followed closely for the first 2 weeks of treatment and whenever the dose of the benazepril component is increased or a diuretic is added or its dose increased.

If hypotension occurs, the patient should be placed in a supine position, and if necessary, treated with intravenous infusion of physiologic saline. Lotrel treatment usually can be continued following restoration of blood pressure and volume.

Neutropenia/Agranulocytosis

Another ACE inhibitor, captopril, has been shown to cause agranulocytosis and bone marrow depression, rarely in uncomplicated patients (incidence probably less than once per 10,000 exposures) but more frequently (incidence possibly as great as once per 1000 exposures) in patients with renal impairment, especially those who also have collagen-vascular diseases such as systemic lupus erythematosus or scleroderma. Available data from clinical trials of benazepril are insufficient to show that benazepril does not cause agranulocytosis at similar rates. Monitoring of white blood cell counts should be considered in patients with collagen-vascular disease, especially if the disease is associated with impaired renal function.

Fetal/Neonatal Morbidity and Mortality

ACE inhibitors can cause fetal and neonatal morbidity and death when administered to pregnant women. Several dozen cases have been reported in the world literature. When pregnancy is detected, Lotrel should be discontinued as soon as possible.

The use of ACE inhibitors during the second and third trimesters of pregnancy has been associated with fetal and neonatal injury, including hypotension, neonatal skull hypoplasia, anuria, reversible or irreversible renal failure, and death. Oligohydramnios has also been reported, presumably resulting from decreased fetal renal function; oligohydramnios in this setting has been associated with fetal limb contractures, craniofacial deformation, and hypoplastic lung development. Prematurity, intrauterine growth retardation, and patent ductus arteriosus have also been reported, although it is not clear whether these occurrences were due to the ACE inhibitor exposure.

These adverse effects do not appear to have resulted from intrauterine ACE inhibitor exposure that has been limited to the first trimester. Mothers whose embryos and fetuses are exposed to ACE inhibitors only during the first trimester should be so informed. Nonetheless, when patients become pregnant, physicians should make every effort to discontinue the use of benazepril as soon as possible.

Rarely (probably less often than once in every thousand pregnancies), no alternative to ACE inhibitors will be found. In these rare cases, the mothers should be apprised of the potential hazards to their fetuses, and serial ultrasound examinations should be performed to assess the intraamniotic environment.

If oligohydramnios is observed, benazepril should be discontinued unless it is considered life-saving for the mother. Contraction stress testing (CST), a nonstress test (NST), or biophysical profiling (BPP) may be appropriate, depending upon the week of pregnancy. Patients and physicians should be aware, however, that oligohydramnios may not appear until after the fetus has sustained irreversible injury.

Infants with histories of in utero exposure to ACE inhibitors should be closely observed for hypotension, oliguria, and hyperkalemia. If oliguria occurs, attention should be directed toward support of blood pressure and renal perfusion. Exchange transfusion or peritoneal dialysis may be required as means of reversing hypotension and/or substituting for disordered renal function. Benazepril, which crosses the placenta, can theoretically be removed from the neonatal circulation by these means; there are occasional reports of benefit from these maneuvers, but experience is limited.

Lotrel has not been adequately studied in pregnant women. When rats received benazepril:amlodipine at doses ranging from 5:2.5 to 50:25 mg/kg/day, dystocia was observed with increasing dose-related incidence at all doses tested. On a mg/m^2 basis, the 2.5 mg/kg/day dose of amlodipine is 3.6 times the amlodipine dose delivered when the maximum recommended dose of Lotrel is given to a 50-kg woman. Similarly, the 5 mg/kg/day dose of benazepril is approximately 2 times the benazepril dose delivered when the maximum recommended dose of Lotrel is given to a 50-kg woman.

No teratogenic effects were seen when benazepril and amlodipine were administered in combination to pregnant rats or rabbits. Rats received dose ratios up to 50:25 mg/kg/day (benazepril:amlodipine) (24 times the maximum recommended human dose on a mg/m^2 basis, assuming a 50-kg woman). Rabbits received doses of up to 1.5:0.75 (benazepril:amlodipine) mg/kg/day; on a mg/m^2 basis, this is 0.97 times the size of a maximum recommended dose of Lotrel given to a 50-kg woman.

Similar results were seen in animal studies involving benazepril alone and amlodipine alone.

Hepatic Failure

Rarely, ACE inhibitors have been associated with a syndrome that starts with cholestatic jaundice and progresses to fulminant hepatic necrosis and (sometimes) death. The mechanism of this syndrome is not understood. Patients receiving ACE inhibitors who develop jaundice or marked elevations of hepatic enzymes should discontinue the ACE inhibitor and receive appropriate medical follow-up.

PRECAUTIONS

General

Impaired Renal Function: Lotrel should be used with caution in patients with severe renal disease.

When the renin-angiotensin-aldosterone system is inhibited by benazepril, changes in renal function may be anticipated in susceptible individuals. In patients with **severe congestive heart failure**, whose renal function may depend on the activity of the renin-angiotensin-aldosterone system, treatment with ACE inhibitors (including benazepril) may be associated with oliguria and/or progressive azotemia and (rarely) with acute renal failure and/or death.

In a small study of hypertensive patients with **unilateral or bilateral renal artery stenosis**, treatment with benazepril was associated with increases in blood urea nitrogen and serum creatinine; these increases were reversible upon discontinuation of benazepril therapy, concomitant diuretic therapy, or both. When such patients are treated with Lotrel, renal function should be monitored during the first few weeks of therapy.

PERCENT INCIDENCE BY SEX OF CERTAIN ADVERSE EVENTS

	Benazepril/ Amlodipine		Benazepril		Amlodipine		Placebo	
	Male N=329	Female N=431	Male N=269	Female N=285	Male N=277	Female N=198	Male N=217	Female N=191
Edema	0.6	3.2	0.0	1.8	2.2	9.1	1.4	3.1
Flushing	0.3	0.0	0.0	0.7	0.4	2.0	0.5	0.0
Palpitations	0.3	0.5	0.4	1.4	0.4	2.0	0.5	0.5
Somnolence	0.3	0.0	0.4	0.4	0.4	0.5	0.0	0.0

Some benazepril-treated hypertensive patients with **no apparent preexisting renal vascular disease** have developed increases in blood urea nitrogen and serum creatinine, usually minor and transient, especially when benazepril has been given concomitantly with a diuretic. Dosage reduction of Lotrel may be required. **Evaluation of the hypertensive patient should always include assessment of renal function** (see Dosage and Administration).

Hyperkalemia: In U.S. placebo-controlled trials of Lotrel, hyperkalemia (serum potassium at least 0.5 mEq/L greater than the upper limit of normal) not present at baseline occurred in approximately 1.5% of hypertensive patients receiving Lotrel. Increases in serum potassium were generally reversible. Risk factors for the development of hyperkalemia include renal insufficiency, diabetes mellitus, and the concomitant use of potassium-sparing diuretics, potassium supplements, and/or potassium-containing salt substitutes.

Patients With Congestive Heart Failure: Although hemodynamic studies and a controlled trial in patients with NYHA Class II-III heart failure have shown that amlodipine did not lead to clinical deterioration as measured by exercise tolerance, left ventricular ejection fraction, and clinical symptomatology, studies have not been performed in patients with NYHA Class IV heart failure. In general, all calcium channel blockers should be used with caution in patients with heart failure.

Patients With Hepatic Failure: In patients with hepatic dysfunction due to cirrhosis, levels of benazeprilat are essentially unaltered. However, since amlodipine is extensively metabolized by the liver and the plasma elimination half-life (t 1/2) is 56 hours in patients with impaired hepatic function, caution should be exercised when administering Lotrel to patients with severe hepatic impairment (see also WARNINGS).

Cough: Presumably due to the inhibition of the degradation of endogenous bradykinin, persistent nonproductive cough has been reported with all ACE inhibitors, always resolving after discontinuation of therapy. ACE inhibitor-induced cough should be considered in the differential diagnosis of cough.

Surgery/Anesthesia: In patients undergoing surgery or during anesthesia with agents that produce hypotension, benazepril will block the angiotensin II formation that could otherwise occur secondary to compensatory renin release. Hypotension that occurs as a result of this mechanism can be corrected by volume expansion.

Drug Interactions

Diuretics: Patients on diuretics, especially those in whom diuretic therapy was recently instituted, may occasionally experience an excessive reduction of blood pressure after initiation of therapy with Lotrel. The possibility of hypotensive effects with Lotrel can be minimized by either discontinuing the diuretic or increasing the salt intake prior to initiation of treatment with Lotrel.

Potassium Supplements and Potassium-Sparing Diuretics: Benazepril can attenuate potassium loss caused by thiazide diuretics. Potassium-sparing diuretics (spironolactone, amiloride, triamterene, and others) or potassium supplements can increase the risk of hyperkalemia. If concomitant use of such agents is indicated, they should be given with caution, and the patient's serum potassium should be monitored frequently.

Lithium: Increased serum lithium levels and symptoms of lithium toxicity have been reported in patients receiving ACE inhibitors during therapy with lithium. Lotrel and lithium should be coadministered with caution, and frequent monitoring of serum lithium levels is recommended.

Other: Benazepril has been used concomitantly with oral anticoagulants, beta-adrenergic-blocking agents, calcium-blocking agents, cimetidine, diuretics, digoxin, hydralazine, and naproxen without evidence of clinically important adverse interactions.

In clinical trials, amlodipine has been safely administered with thiazide diuretics, beta blockers, ACE inhibitors, long-acting nitrates, sublingual nitroglycerin, digoxin, warfarin, nonsteroidal anti-inflammatory drugs, antibiotics, and oral hypoglycemic drugs.

In vitro data in human plasma indicate that amlodipine has no effect on the protein binding of drugs tested (digoxin, phenytoin, warfarin, and indomethacin). Special studies have indicated that the coadministration of amlodipine with digoxin did not change serum digoxin levels or digoxin renal clearance in normal volunteers; that coadministration with cimetidine did not alter the pharmacokinetics of amlodipine; and that coadministration with warfarin did not change the warfarin-induced prothrombin response time.

Carcinogenesis, Mutagenesis, Impairment of Fertility

No evidence of carcinogenicity was found when **benazepril** was given, via dietary administration, to rats and mice for 104 weeks at doses up to 150 mg/kg/day. On a body-weight basis, this dose is over 100 times the maximum recommended human dose; on a body-surface-area basis, this dose is 18 times (rats) and 9 times (mice) the maximum recommended human dose. No mutagenic activity was detected in the Ames test in bacteria, in an in vitro test for forward mutations in cultured mammalian cells, or in a nucleus anomaly test. At doses of 50-500 mg/kg/day (38-375 times the maximum recommended human dose on a body-weight basis; 6-61 times the maximum recommended dose on a body-surface-area basis), benazepril had no adverse effect on the reproductive performance of male and female rats.

Rats and mice treated with amlodipine in the diet for 2 years, at concentrations calculated to provide daily dosage levels of 0.5, 1.25, and 2.5 mg/kg/day, showed no evidence of carcinogenicity. For mice, but not for rats, the highest dose was close to the maximum tolerated dose. On a mg/m^2 basis, this dose given to mice was approximately equal to the maximum recommended clinical dose. On the same basis, the same dose given to rats was approximately twice the maximum recommended clinical dose.

Mutagenicity studies with amlodipine revealed no drug-related effects at either the gene or chromosome levels.

There was no effect on the fertility of rats treated with amlodipine (males for 64 days and females for 14 days prior to mating) at doses up to 10 mg/kg/day (8 times the maximum recommended human dose of 10 mg on a mg/m^2 basis, assuming a 50-kg person).

No adverse effects on fertility occurred when the benazepril:amlodipine combination was given orally to rats of either sex at dose ratios up to 15:7.5 mg/kg/day (benazepril:amlodipine), prior to mating and throughout gestation.

Pregnancy

Pregnancy Categories C (first trimester) and D (second and third trimesters): See Warnings, Fetal/Neonatal Morbidity and Mortality.

Nursing Mothers

Minimal amounts of unchanged benazepril and of benazeprilat are excreted into the breast milk of lactating women treated with benazepril, so that a newborn child ingesting nothing but breast milk would receive less than 0.1% of the maternal doses of benazepril and benazeprilat.

It is not known whether amlodipine is excreted in human milk. In the absence of this information, it is recommended that nursing be discontinued while Lotrel is administered.

Geriatric Use

Of the total number of patients who received Lotrel in U.S. clinical studies of Lotrel, 19% were 65 or older while about 2% were 75 or older. Overall differences in effectiveness or safety were not observed between these patients and younger patients. Clinical experience has not identified differences in responses between the elderly and younger patients, but greater sensitivity of some older individuals cannot be ruled out.

Pediatric Use

Safety and effectiveness in pediatric patients have not been established.

ADVERSE REACTIONS

Lotrel has been evaluated for safety in over 1600 patients with hypertension; over 500 of these patients were treated for at least 6 months, and over 400 were treated for more than 1 year.

The reported side effects were generally mild and transient, and there was no relationship between side effects and age, sex, race, or duration of therapy. Discontinuation of therapy due to side effects was required in approximately 4% of patients treated with Lotrel and in 3% of patients treated with placebo.

The most common reasons for discontinuation of therapy with Lotrel in U.S. studies were cough and edema.*

The side effects considered possibly or probably related to study drug that occurred in U.S. placebo-controlled trials in more than 1% of patients treated with Lotrel are shown in the table below.

PERCENT INCIDENCE IN U.S. PLACEBO-CONTROLLED TRIALS

	Benazepril/ Amlodipine N=760	Benazepril N=554	Amlodipine N=475	Placebo N=408
Cough	3.3	1.8	0.4	0.2
Headache	2.2	3.8	2.9	5.6
Dizziness	1.3	1.6	2.3	1.5
Edema*	2.1	0.9	5.1	2.2

*Edema refers to all edema, such as dependent edema, angioedema, facial edema.

The incidence of edema was statistically greater in patients treated with amlodipine monotherapy than in patients treated with the combination. Edema and certain other side effects are associated with amlodipine monotherapy in a

Continued on next page

Lotrel—Cont.

dose-dependent manner, and appear to affect women more than men. The addition of benazepril resulted in lower incidences as shown in the following table; the protective effect of benazepril was independent of race and (within the range of doses tested) of dose.

[See table at top of previous page]

Other side effects considered possibly or probably related to study drug that occurred in U.S. placebo-controlled trials of patients treated with Lotrel or in postmarketing experience were the following:

Angioedema: Includes edema of the lips or face without other manifestations of angioedema (see WARNINGS, Angioedema).

Body as a Whole: Asthenia and fatigue.

CNS: Insomnia, nervousness, anxiety, tremor, and decreased libido.

Dermatologic: Flushing, hot flashes, rash, skin nodule, and dermatitis.

Digestive: Dry mouth, nausea, abdominal pain, constipation, diarrhea, dyspepsia, and esophagitis.

Metabolic and Nutritional: Hypokalemia.

Musculoskeletal: Back pain, musculoskeletal pain, cramps, and muscle cramps.

Respiratory: Pharyngitis.

Urogenital: Sexual problems such as impotence, and polyuria.

Other infrequently reported events were seen in clinical trials (causal relationship unlikely) or in postmarketing experience. These included chest pain, ventricular extrasystole, gout, neuritis, tinnitus, and alopecia.

Fetal/Neonatal Morbidity and Mortality: See WARNINGS, Fetal/Neonatal Morbidity and Mortality.

Monotherapies of benazepril and amlodipine have been evaluated for safety in clinical trials in over 6000 and 11,000 patients, respectively. The observed adverse reactions to the monotherapies in these trials were similar to those seen in trials of Lotrel. In postmarketing experience with benazepril, there have been rare reports of Stevens-Johnson syndrome, pancreatitis, hemolytic anemia, pemphigus, and thrombocytopenia. Jaundice and hepatic enzyme elevations (mostly consistent with cholestasis) severe enough to require hospitalization have been reported in association with use of amlodipine. Other potentially important adverse experiences attributed to other ACE inhibitors and calcium channel blockers include: eosinophilic pneumonitis (ACE inhibitors) and gynecomastia (CCB's).

Clinical Laboratory Test Findings

Serum Electrolytes: See PRECAUTIONS.

Creatinine: Minor reversible increases in serum creatinine were observed in patients with essential hypertension treated with Lotrel. Increases in creatinine are more likely to occur in patients with renal insufficiency or those pretreated with a diuretic and, based on experience with other ACE inhibitors, would be expected to be especially likely in patients with renal artery stenosis (see PRECAUTIONS, General).

Other (causal relationships unknown): Clinically important changes in standard laboratory tests were rarely associated with Lotrel administration. Elevations of serum bilirubin and uric acid have been reported as have scattered incidents of elevations of liver enzymes.

OVERDOSAGE

Only a few cases of human overdose with amlodipine have been reported. One patient was asymptomatic after a 250-mg ingestion; another, who combined 70 mg of amlodipine with an unknown large quantity of a benzodiazepine, developed refractory shock and died.

Human overdoses with any combination of amlodipine and benazepril have not been reported. In scattered reports of human overdoses with benazepril and other ACE inhibitors, there are no reports of death.

When mice were given single oral doses of benazepril/amlodipine, mortality was 20% at 50:25 mg/kg, 10% at 100:50 mg/kg, and 100% at 500:250 mg/kg. In rats, mortality was 25% (pooling two studies) at 500:250 mg/kg and 100% at 900:450 mg/kg.

Treatment: To obtain up-to-date information about the treatment of overdose, a good resource is your certified Regional Poison-Control Center. Telephone numbers of certified poison-control centers are listed in the Physicians' Desk Reference (PDR). In managing overdose, consider the possibilities of multiple-drug overdoses, drug-drug interactions, and unusual drug kinetics in your patient.

The most likely effect of overdose with Lotrel is vasodilation, with consequent hypotension and tachycardia. Simple repletion of central fluid volume (Trendelenburg positioning, infusion of crystalloids) may be sufficient therapy, but pressor agents (norepinephrine or high-dose dopamine) may be required. Overdoses of other dihydropyridine calcium channel blockers are reported to have been treated with calcium chloride and glucagon, but evidence of a dose-response relation has not been seen, and these interventions must be regarded as unproven. With abrupt return of peripheral vascular tone, overdoses of other dihydropyridine calcium channel blockers have sometimes progressed to pulmonary edema, and patients must be monitored for this complication.

Analyses of bodily fluids for concentrations of amlodipine, benazepril, or their metabolites are not widely available. Such analyses are, in any event, not known to be of value in therapy or prognosis.

No data are available to suggest physiologic maneuvers (e.g., maneuvers to change the pH of the urine) that might accelerate elimination of amlodipine, benazepril, or their metabolites. Benazeprilat is only slightly dialyzable; attempted clearance of amlodipine by hemodialysis or hemoperfusion has not been reported, but amlodipine's high protein binding makes it unlikely that these interventions will be of value.

Angiotensin II could presumably serve as a specific antagonist-antidote to benazepril, but angiotensin II is essentially unavailable outside of scattered research laboratories.

DOSAGE AND ADMINISTRATION

Amlodipine is an effective treatment of hypertension in once-daily doses of 2.5-10 mg while benazepril is effective in doses of 10-80 mg. In clinical trials of amlodipine/benazepril combination therapy using amlodipine doses of 2.5-5 mg and benazepril doses of 10-20 mg, the antihypertensive effects increased with increasing dose of amlodipine in all patient groups, and the effects increased with increasing dose of benazepril in nonblack groups. All patient groups benefited from the reduction in amlodipine-induced edema (see below).

The hazards (see WARNINGS) of benazepril are generally independent of dose; those of amlodipine are a mixture of dose-dependent phenomena (primarily peripheral edema) and dose-independent phenomena, the former much more common than the latter. When benazepril is added to a regimen of amlodipine, the incidence of edema is substantially reduced. Therapy with any combination of amlodipine and benazepril will thus be associated with both sets of dose-independent hazards, but the incidence of edema will generally be less than that seen with similar (or higher) doses of amlodipine monotherapy.

Rarely, the dose-independent hazards of benazepril are serious. To minimize dose-independent hazards, it is usually appropriate to begin therapy with Lotrel only after a patient has either (a) failed to achieve the desired antihypertensive effect with one or the other monotherapy, or (b) demonstrated inability to achieve adequate antihypertensive effect with amlodipine therapy without developing edema.

Dose Titration Guided by Clinical Effect: A patient whose blood pressure is not adequately controlled with amlodipine (or another dihydropyridine) alone or with benazepril (or another ACE inhibitor) alone may be switched to combination therapy with Lotrel. The addition of benazepril to a regimen of amlodipine should not be expected to provide additional antihypertensive effect in African-Americans. However, all patient groups benefit from the reduction in amlodipine-induced edema. Dosage must be guided by clinical response; steady-state levels of benazepril and amlodipine will be reached after approximately 2 and 7 days of dosing, respectively.

In patients whose blood pressures are adequately controlled with amlodipine but who experience unacceptable edema, combination therapy may achieve similar (or better) blood-pressure control without edema. Especially in nonblacks, it may be prudent to minimize the risk of excessive response by reducing the dose of amlodipine as benazepril is added to the regimen.

Replacement Therapy: For convenience, patients receiving amlodipine and benazepril from separate tablets may instead wish to receive capsules of Lotrel containing the same component doses.

Use in Patients With Metabolic Impairments: Regimens of therapy with Lotrel need not take account of renal function as long as the patient's creatinine clearance is >30 mL/min/1.73m^2 (serum creatinine roughly ≤3 mg/dL or 265 µmol/L). In patients with more severe renal impairment, the recommended initial dose of benazepril is 5 mg. Lotrel is not recommended in these patients.

In small, elderly, frail, or hepatically impaired patients, the recommended initial dose of amlodipine, as monotherapy or as a component of combination therapy, is 2.5 mg.

HOW SUPPLIED

Lotrel is available as capsules containing amlodipine/benazepril HCl 2.5/10 mg, 5/10 mg, and 5/20 mg. All three strengths are packaged with a desiccant in bottles of 100 capsules.

Capsules are imprinted with "Lotrel" and a portion of the NDC code.

Dose	Capsule Color	NDC Code Bottle of 100
2.5/10 mg	white capsule with 2 gold bands	NDC 0083-2255-30
5/10 mg	light brown capsule with 2 white bands	NDC 0083-2260-30
5/20 mg	pink capsule with 2 white bands	NDC 0083-2265-30

Storage: Do not store above 30°C (86°F). Protect from moisture and light.

Dispense in tight, light-resistant container (USP).

REV: MAY 2000 T2000-14

Distributed by
Novartis Pharmaceuticals Corporation
East Hanover, New Jersey 07936

Shown in Product Identification Guide, page 326

MIACALCIN® ℞

[*mī "ă-kal 'sin*]
(calcitonin-salmon)
Injection, Synthetic

Rx only

The following prescribing information is based on official labeling in effect July 2000.

DESCRIPTION

Calcitonin is a polypeptide hormone secreted by the parafollicular cells of the thyroid gland in mammals and by the ultimobranchial gland of birds and fish.

Miacalcin® (calcitonin-salmon) Injection, Synthetic is a synthetic polypeptide of 32 amino acids in the same linear sequence that is found in calcitonin of salmon origin. This is shown by the following graphic formula:

H-Cys-Ser-Asn-Leu-Ser-Thr-Cys-Val-Leu-
1 2 3 4 5 6 7 8 9

Gly-Lys-Leu-Ser-Gln-Glu-Leu-His-Lys-Leu-
10 11 12 13 14 15 16 17 18 19

Gln-Thr-Tyr-Pro-Arg-Thr-Asn-Thr-Gly-Ser-
20 21 22 23 24 25 26 27 28 29

Gly-Thr-Pro-NH_2
30 31 32

It is provided in sterile solution for subcutaneous or intramuscular injection. Each milliliter contains: calcitonin-salmon 200 I.U., acetic acid, USP, 2.25 mg; phenol, USP, 5.0 mg; sodium acetate trihydrate, USP, 2.0 mg; sodium chloride, USP, 7.5 mg; water for injection, USP, qs to 1.0 mL. The activity of Miacalcin® (calcitonin-salmon) is stated in International Units based on bioassay in comparison with the International Reference Preparation of calcitonin-salmon for Bioassay, distributed by the National Institute for Biological Standards and Control, Holly Hill, London.

CLINICAL PHARMACOLOGY

Calcitonin acts primarily on bone, but direct renal effects and actions on the gastrointestinal tract are also recognized. Calcitonin-salmon appears to have actions essentially identical to calcitonins of mammalian origin, but its potency per mg is greater and it has a longer duration of action. The actions of calcitonin on bone and its role in normal human bone physiology are still incompletely understood.

Bone—Single injections of calcitonin cause a marked transient inhibition of the ongoing bone resorptive process. With prolonged use, there is a persistent, smaller decrease in the rate of bone resorption. Histologically, this is associated with a decreased number of osteoclasts and an apparent decrease in their resorptive activity. Decreased osteocytic resorption may also be involved. There is some evidence that initially bone formation may be augmented by calcitonin through increased osteoblastic activity. However, calcitonin will probably not induce a long-term increase in bone formation.

Animal studies indicate that endogenous calcitonin, primarily through its action on bone, participates with parathyroid hormone in the homeostatic regulation of blood calcium. Thus, high blood calcium levels cause increased secretion of calcitonin which, in turn, inhibits bone resorption. This reduces the transfer of calcium from bone to blood and tends to return blood calcium to the normal level. The importance of this process in humans has not been determined. In normal adults, who have a relatively low rate of bone resorption, the administration of exogenous calcitonin results in only a slight decrease in serum calcium. In normal children and in patients with generalized Paget's disease, bone resorption is more rapid and decreases in serum calcium are more pronounced in response to calcitonin.

Paget's Disease of Bone (osteitis deformans)—Paget's disease is a disorder of uncertain etiology characterized by abnormal and accelerated bone formation and resorption in one or more bones. In most patients only small areas of bone are involved and the disease is not symptomatic. In a small fraction of patients, however, the abnormal bone may lead to bone pain and bone deformity, cranial and spinal nerve entrapment, or spinal cord compression. The increased vascularity of the abnormal bone may lead to high output congestive heart failure.

Active Paget's disease involving a large mass of bone may increase the urinary hydroxyproline excretion (reflecting breakdown of collagen-containing bone matrix) and serum alkaline phosphatase (reflecting increased bone formation).

Calcitonin-salmon, presumably by an initial blocking effect on bone resorption, causes a decreased rate of bone turnover with a resultant fall in the serum alkaline phosphatase and urinary hydroxyproline excretion in approximately 2/3 of patients treated. These biochemical changes appear to correspond to changes toward more normal bone, as evidenced by a small number of documented examples of: 1) radiologic regression of Pagetic lesions, 2) improvement of impaired auditory nerve and other neurologic function, 3) decreases (measured) in abnormally elevated cardiac output. These improvements occur extremely rarely, if ever, spontaneously (elevated cardiac output may disappear over a period of years when the disease slowly enters a sclerotic phase; in the cases treated with calcitonin, however, the decreases were seen in less than one year.)

Some patients with Paget's disease who have good biochemical and/or symptomatic responses initially, later relapse.

Suggested explanations have included the formation of neutralizing antibodies and the development of secondary hyperparathyroidism, but neither suggestion appears to explain adequately the majority of relapses.
Although the parathyroid hormone levels do appear to rise transiently during each hypocalcemic response to calcitonin, most investigators have been unable to demonstrate persistent hypersecretion of parathyroid hormone in patients treated chronically with calcitonin-salmon.
Circulating antibodies to calcitonin after 2-18 months' treatment have been reported in about half of the patients with Paget's disease in whom antibody studies were done, but calcitonin treatment remained effective in many of these cases. Occasionally, patients with high antibody titers are found. These patients usually will have suffered a biochemical relapse of Paget's disease and are unresponsive to the acute hypocalcemic effects of calcitonin.
Hypercalcemia—In clinical trials, calcitonin-salmon has been shown to lower the elevated serum calcium of patients with carcinoma (with or without demonstrated metastases), multiple myeloma or primary hyperparathyroidism (lesser response). Patients with higher values for serum calcium tend to show greater reduction during calcitonin therapy. The decrease in calcium occurs about 2 hours after the first injection and lasts for about 6-8 hours. Calcitonin-salmon given every 12 hours maintained a calcium lowering effect for about 5-8 days, the time period evaluated for most patients during the clinical studies. The average reduction of 8-hour post-injection serum calcium during this period was about 9 percent.
Kidney—Calcitonin increases the excretion of filtered phosphate, calcium, and sodium by decreasing their tubular reabsorption. In some patients, the inhibition of bone resorption by calcitonin is of such magnitude that the consequent reduction of filtered calcium load more than compensates for the decrease in tubular reabsorption of calcium. The result in these patients is a decrease rather than an increase in urinary calcium.
Transient increases in sodium and water excretion may occur after the initial injection of calcitonin. In most patients, these changes return to pretreatment levels with continued therapy.
Gastrointestinal Tract—Increasing evidence indicates that calcitonin has significant actions on the gastrointestinal tract. Short-term administration results in marked transient decreases in the volume and acidity of gastric juice and in the volume and the trypsin and amylase content of pancreatic juice. Whether these effects continue to be elicited after each injection of calcitonin during chronic therapy has not been investigated.
Metabolism—The metabolism of calcitonin-salmon has not yet been studied clinically. Information from animal studies with calcitonin-salmon and from clinical studies with calcitonins of porcine and human origin suggest that calcitonin-salmon is rapidly metabolized by conversion to smaller inactive fragments, primarily in the kidneys, but also in the blood and peripheral tissues. A small amount of unchanged hormone and its inactive metabolites are excreted in the urine.
It appears that calcitonin-salmon cannot cross the placental barrier and its passage to the cerebrospinal fluid or to breast milk has not been determined.

INDICATIONS AND USAGE

Miacalcin® (calcitonin-salmon) Injection, Synthetic is indicated for the treatment of symptomatic Paget's disease of bone, for the treatment of hypercalcemia, and for the treatment of postmenopausal osteoporosis.
Paget's Disease—At the present time, effectiveness has been demonstrated principally in patients with moderate to severe disease characterized by polyostotic involvement with elevated serum alkaline phosphatase and urinary hydroxyproline excretion.
In these patients, the biochemical abnormalities were substantially improved (more than 30% reduction) in about 2/3 of patients studied, and bone pain was improved in a similar fraction. A small number of documented instances of reversal of neurologic deficits has occurred, including improvement in the basilar compression syndrome, and improvement of spinal cord and spinal nerve lesions. At present, there is too little experience to predict the likelihood of improvement of any given neurologic lesion. Hearing loss, the most common neurologic lesion of Paget's disease, is improved infrequently (4 of 29 patients studied audiometrically).
Patients with increased cardiac output due to extensive Paget's disease have had measured decreases in cardiac output while receiving calcitonin. The number of treated patients in this category is still too small to predict how likely such a result will be.
The large majority of patients with localized, especially monostotic disease do not develop symptoms and most patients with mild symptoms can be managed with analgesics. There is no evidence that the prophylactic use of calcitonin is beneficial in asymptomatic patients, although treatment may be considered in exceptional circumstances in which there is extensive involvement of the skull or spinal cord with the possibility of irreversible neurologic damage. In these instances, treatment would be based on the demonstrated effect of calcitonin on Pagetic bone, rather than on clinical studies in the patient population in question.
Hypercalcemia—Miacalcin® (calcitonin-salmon) Injection, Synthetic is indicated for early treatment of hypercalcemic emergencies, along with other appropriate agents, when a rapid decrease in serum calcium is required, until more specific treatment of the underlying disease can be accomplished. It may also be added to existing therapeutic regimens for hypercalcemia such as intravenous fluids and furosemide, oral phosphate or corticosteroids, or other agents.
Postmenopausal Osteoporosis—Miacalcin® (calcitonin-salmon) Injection, Synthetic is indicated for the treatment of postmenopausal osteoporosis in conjunction with adequate calcium and vitamin D intake to prevent the progressive loss of bone mass. No evidence currently exists to indicate whether or not Miacalcin® (calcitonin-salmon) decreases the risk of vertebral crush fractures or spinal deformity. A recent controlled study, which was discontinued prior to completion because of questions regarding its design and implementation, failed to demonstrate any benefit of salmon calcitonin on fracture rate. No adequate controlled trials have examined the effect of salmon calcitonin injection on vertebral bone mineral density beyond 1 year of treatment. Two placebo-controlled studies with salmon calcitonin have shown an increase in total body calcium at 1 year, followed by a trend to decreasing total body calcium (still above baseline) at 2 years. The minimum effective dose of Miacalcin® (calcitonin-salmon) for prevention of vertebral bone mineral density loss has not been established. It has been suggested that those postmenopausal patients having increased rates of bone turnover may be more likely to respond to anti-resorptive agents such as Miacalcin® (calcitonin-salmon).

CONTRAINDICATIONS

Clinical allergy to synthetic calcitonin-salmon.

WARNINGS

Allergic Reactions
Because calcitonin is protein in nature, the possibility of a systemic allergic reaction exists. **Administration of calcitonin-salmon has been reported in a few cases to cause serious allergic-type reactions (e.g. bronchospasm, swelling of the tongue or throat, and anaphylactic shock), and in one case, death attributed to anaphylaxis.** The usual provisions should be made for the emergency treatment of such a reaction should it occur. Allergic reactions should be differentiated from generalized flushing and hypotension.
For patients with suspected sensitivity to calcitonin, skin testing should be considered prior to treatment utilizing a dilute, sterile solution of Miacalcin® (calcitonin-salmon) Injection, Synthetic. Physicians may wish to refer patients who require skin testing to an allergist. A detailed skin testing protocol is available from the Medical Services Department of Novartis Pharmaceuticals Corporation.
The incidence of osteogenic sarcoma is known to be increased in Paget's disease. Pagetic lesions, with or without therapy, may appear by X-ray to progress markedly, possibly with some loss of definition of periosteal margins. Such lesions should be evaluated carefully to differentiate these from osteogenic sarcoma.

PRECAUTIONS

1. General
The administration of calcitonin possibly could lead to hypocalcemic tetany under special circumstances although no cases have yet been reported. Provisions for parenteral calcium administration should be available during the first several administrations of calcitonin.
2. Laboratory Tests
Periodic examinations of urine sediment of patients on chronic therapy are recommended.
Coarse granular casts and casts containing renal tubular epithelial cells were reported in young adult volunteers at bed rest who were given calcitonin-salmon to study the effect of immobilization on osteoporosis. There was no other evidence of renal abnormality and the urine sediment became normal after calcitonin was stopped. Urine sediment abnormalities have not been reported by other investigators.
3. Instructions for the Patient
Careful instruction in sterile injection technique should be given to the patient, and to other persons who may administer Miacalcin® (calcitonin-salmon) Injection, Synthetic.
4. Carcinogenesis, Mutagenesis, and Impairment of Fertility
An increased incidence of pituitary adenomas has been observed in one-year toxicity studies in Sprague-Dawley rats administered calcitonin-salmon at dosages of 20 and 80 I.U. kg/day and in Fisher 344 rats given 80 I.U./kg/day. The relevance of these findings to humans is unknown. Calcitonin-salmon was not mutagenic in tests using *Salmonella typhimurium, Escherichia coli,* and Chinese Hamster V79 cells.
5. Pregnancy: Teratogenic Effects
Category C
Calcitonin-salmon has been shown to cause a decrease in fetal birth weights in rabbits when given in doses 14-56 times the dose recommended for human use. Since calcitonin does not cross the placental barrier, this finding may be due to metabolic effects on the pregnant animal. There are no adequate and well-controlled studies in pregnant women. Miacalcin® (calcitonin-salmon) Injection, Synthetic should be used during pregnancy only if the potential benefit justifies the potential risk to the fetus.
6. Nursing Mothers
It is not known whether this drug is excreted in human milk. As a general rule, nursing should not be undertaken while a patient is on this drug since many drugs are excreted in human milk. Calcitonin has been shown to inhibit lactation in animals.
7. Pediatric Use
Disorders of bone in children referred to as juvenile Paget's disease have been reported rarely. The relationship of these disorders to adult Paget's disease has not been established and experience with the use of calcitonin in these disorders is very limited. There is no adequate data to support the use of Miacalcin® (calcitonin-salmon) Injection, Synthetic in children.

ADVERSE REACTIONS

Gastrointestinal System
Nausea with or without vomiting has been noted in about 10% of patients treated with calcitonin. It is most evident when treatment is first initiated and tends to decrease or disappear with continued administration.
Dermatologic/Hypersensitivity
Local inflammatory reactions at the site of subcutaneous or intramuscular injection have been reported in about 10% of patients. Flushing of face or hands occurred in about 2-5% of patients. Skin rashes, nocturia, pruritus of the ear lobes, feverish sensation, pain in the eyes, poor appetite, abdominal pain, edema of feet, and salty taste have been reported in patients treated with calcitonin-salmon. Administration of calcitonin-salmon has been reported in a few cases to cause serious allergic-type reactions (e.g. bronchospasm, swelling of the tongue or throat, and anaphylactic shock), and in one case, death attributed to anaphylaxis *(see WARNINGS).*

OVERDOSAGE

A dose of 1000 I.U. subcutaneously may produce nausea and vomiting as the only adverse effects. Doses of 32 units per kg per day for 1-2 days demonstrate no other adverse effects.
Data on chronic high dose administration are insufficient to judge toxicity.

DOSAGE AND ADMINISTRATION

Paget's Disease—The recommended starting dose of calcitonin-salmon in Paget's disease is 100 I.U. (0.5 mL) per day administered subcutaneously (preferred for outpatient self-administration) or intramuscularly. Drug effect should be monitored by periodic measurement of serum alkaline phosphatase and 24-hour urinary hydroxyproline (if available) and evaluations of symptoms. A decrease toward normal of the biochemical abnormalities is usually seen, if it is going to occur, within the first few months. Bone pain may also decrease during that time. Improvement of neurologic lesions, when it occurs, requires a longer period of treatment, often more than one year.
In many patients, doses of 50 I.U. (0.25 mL) per day or every other day are sufficient to maintain biochemical and clinical improvement. At the present time, however, there are insufficient data to determine whether this reduced dose will have the same effect as the higher dose on forming more normal bone structure. It appears preferable, therefore, to maintain the higher dose in any patient with serious deformity or neurological involvement.
In any patient with a good response initially who later relapses, either clinically or biochemically, the possibility of antibody formation should be explored. The patient may be tested for antibodies by an appropriate specialized test or evaluated for the possibility of antibody formation by critical clinical evaluation.
Patient compliance should also be assessed in the event of relapse.
In patients who relapse, whether because of antibodies or for unexplained reasons, a dosage increase beyond 100 I.U. per day does not usually appear to elicit an improved response.
Hypercalcemia—The recommended starting dose of Miacalcin® (calcitonin-salmon) Injection, Synthetic in hypercalcemia is 4 I.U./kg body weight every 12 hours by subcutaneous or intramuscular injection. If the response to this dose is not satisfactory after one or two days, the dose may be increased to 8 I.U./kg every 12 hours. If the response remains unsatisfactory after two more days, the dose may be further increased to a maximum of 8 I.U./kg every 6 hours.
Postmenopausal Osteoporosis—The minimum effective dose of salmon calcitonin for the prevention of vertebral bone mineral density loss has not been established. Data from a single one-year placebo-controlled study with salmon calcitonin injection suggested that 100 I.U. (subcutaneously or intramuscularly) every other day might be effective in preserving vertebral bone mineral density. Baseline and interval monitoring of biochemical markers of bone resorption/turnover (e.g., fasting AM, second-voided urine hydroxyproline to creatinine ratio) and of bone mineral density may be useful in achieving the minimum effective dose. Patients should also receive supplemental calcium such as calcium carbonate 1.5 g daily and an adequate vitamin D intake (400 units daily). An adequate diet is also essential.
If the volume of Miacalcin® (calcitonin-salmon) Injection, Synthetic to be injected exceeds 2 mL, intramuscular injection is preferable and multiple sites of injection should be used.
Parenteral drug products should be inspected visually for particulate matter and discoloration prior to administration whenever solution and container permit.

Continued on next page

Miacalcin Injection—Cont.

HOW SUPPLIED

Miacalcin® (calcitonin-salmon) Injection, Synthetic is available as a sterile solution in individual 2 mL vials containing 200 I.U. per mL (NDC 0078-0149-23).
Store in Refrigerator—Between 2°C-8°C (36°F-46°F).
Manufactured by
Novartis Pharma AG,
Basle, Switzerland for
Novartis Pharmaceuticals Corporation
East Hanover, NJ 07936
REV: MARCH 1999 30167404

MIACALCIN® ℞

[mī "ă-kal 'sin]
(calcitonin-salmon)
Nasal Spray

Rx only

The following prescribing information is based on official labeling in effect July 2000.

DESCRIPTION

Calcitonin is a polypeptide hormone secreted by the parafollicular cells of the thyroid gland in mammals and by the ultimobranchial gland of birds and fish.
Miacalcin® (calcitonin-salmon) Nasal Spray is a synthetic polypeptide of 32 amino acids in the same linear sequence that is found in calcitonin of salmon origin. This is shown by the following graphic formula:

```
H-Cys-Ser-Asn-Leu-Ser-Thr-Cys-Val-Leu-
  1   2   3   4   5   6   7   8   9
Gly-Lys-Leu-Ser-Gln-Glu-Leu-His-Lys-Leu-
10  11  12  13  14  15  16  17  18  19
Gln-Thr-Tyr-Pro-Arg-Thr-Asn-Thr-Gly-Ser-
20  21  22  23  24  25  26  27  28  29
Gly-Thr-Pro-NH2
30  31  32
```

It is provided in 2 mL fill glass bottles as a solution for nasal administration. This is sufficient medication for at least 14 doses.
Active Ingredient: calcitonin-salmon, 2200 I.U. per mL (corresponding to 200 I.U. per 0.09 mL actuation).
Inactive Ingredients: sodium chloride, benzalkonium chloride, nitrogen, hydrochloric acid (added as necessary to adjust pH) and purified water.
The activity of Miacalcin® (calcitonin-salmon) Nasal Spray is stated in International Units based on bioassay in comparison with the International Reference Preparation of calcitonin-salmon for Bioassay, distributed by the National Institute of Biologic Standards and Control, Holly Hill, London.

CLINICAL PHARMACOLOGY

Calcitonin acts primarily on bone, but direct renal effects and actions on the gastrointestinal tract are also recognized. Calcitonin-salmon appears to have actions essentially identical to calcitonins of mammalian origin, but its potency per mg is greater and it has a longer duration of action.
The information below, describing the clinical pharmacology of calcitonin, has been derived from studies with *injectable* calcitonin. The mean bioavailability of Miacalcin® (calcitonin-salmon) Nasal Spray is approximately 3% of that of injectable calcitonin in normal subjects and, therefore, the conclusions concerning the *CLINICAL PHARMACOLOGY* of this preparation may be different.
The actions of calcitonin on bone and its role in normal human bone physiology are still not completely elucidated, although calcitonin receptors have been discovered in osteoclasts and osteoblasts.
Single injections of calcitonin cause a marked transient inhibition of the ongoing bone resorptive process. With prolonged use, there is a persistent, smaller decrease in the rate of bone resorption. Histologically, this is associated with a decreased number of osteoclasts and an apparent decrease in their resorptive activity. *In vitro* studies have shown that calcitonin-salmon causes inhibition of osteoclast function with loss of the ruffled osteoclast border responsible for resorption of bone. This activity resumes following removal of calcitonin-salmon from the test system. There is some evidence from the *in vitro* studies that bone formation may be augmented by calcitonin through increased osteoblastic activity.
Animal studies indicate that endogenous calcitonin, primarily through its action on bone, participates with parathyroid hormone in the homeostatic regulation of blood calcium. Thus, high blood calcium levels cause increased secretion of calcitonin which, in turn, inhibits bone resorption. This reduces the transfer of calcium from bone to blood and tends to return blood calcium towards the normal level. The importance of this process in humans has not been determined. In normal adults, who have a relatively low rate of bone resorption, the administration of exogenous calcitonin results in only a slight decrease in serum calcium in the limits of the normal range. In normal children and in patients with Paget's disease in whom bone resorption is more rapid, decreases in serum calcium are more pronounced in response to calcitonin.
Bone biopsy and radial bone mass studies at baseline and after 26 months of daily injectable calcitonin indicate that calcitonin therapy results in formation of normal bone.
Postmenopausal Osteoporosis – Osteoporosis is a disease characterized by low bone mass and architectural deterioration of bone tissue leading to enhanced bone fragility and a consequent increase in fracture risk as patients approach or fall below a bone mineral density associated with increased frequency of fracture. The most common type of osteoporosis occurs in postmenopausal females. Osteoporosis is a result of a disproportionate rate of bone resorption compared to bone formation which disrupts the structural integrity of bone, rendering it more susceptible to fracture. The most common sites of these fractures are the vertebrae, hip, and distal forearm (Colles' fractures). Vertebral fractures occur with the highest frequency and are associated with back pain, spinal deformity and a loss of height.
Calcitonin, given by the intranasal route, has been shown to increase spinal bone mass in postmenopausal women with established osteoporosis but not in early postmenopausal women.
Calcium Homeostasis – In two clinical studies designed to evaluate the pharmacodynamic response to Miacalcin® (calcitonin-salmon) Nasal Spray, administration of 100-1600 I.U. to healthy volunteers resulted in rapid and sustained small decreases (but still within the normal range) in both total serum calcium and serum ionized calcium. Single doses greater than 400 I.U. did not produce any further biological response to the drug. The development of hypocalcemia has not been reported in studies in healthy volunteers or postmenopausal females.
Kidney – Studies with injectable calcitonin show increases in the excretion of filtered phosphate, calcium, and sodium by decreasing their tubular reabsorption. Comparable studies have not been carried out with Miacalcin® (calcitonin-salmon) Nasal Spray.
Gastrointestinal Tract – Some evidence from studies with injectable preparations suggest that calcitonin may have significant actions on the gastrointestinal tract. Short-term administration of injectable calcitonin results in marked transient decreases in the volume and acidity of gastric juice and in the volume and the trypsin and amylase content of pancreatic juice. Whether these effects continue to be elicited after each injection of calcitonin during chronic therapy has not been investigated. These studies have not been conducted with Miacalcin® (calcitonin-salmon) Nasal Spray.

Pharmacokinetics and Metabolism

The data on bioavailability of Miacalcin® (calcitonin-salmon) Nasal Spray obtained by various investigators using different methods show great variability. Miacalcin® (calcitonin-salmon) Nasal Spray is absorbed rapidly by the nasal mucosa. Peak plasma concentrations of drug appear 31-39 minutes after nasal administration compared to 16-25 minutes following parenteral dosing. In normal volunteers approximately 3% (range 0.3%-30.6%) of a nasally administered dose is bioavailable compared to the same dose administered by intramuscular injection. The half-life of elimination of calcitonin-salmon is calculated to be 43 minutes. There is no accumulation of the drug on repeated nasal administration at 10 hour intervals for up to 15 days. Absorption of nasally administered calcitonin has not been studied in postmenopausal women.

INDICATION AND USAGE

Postmenopausal Osteoporosis – Miacalcin® (calcitonin-salmon) Nasal Spray is indicated for the treatment of postmenopausal osteoporosis in females greater than 5 years postmenopause with low bone mass relative to healthy premenopausal females. Miacalcin® (calcitonin-salmon) Nasal Spray should be reserved for patients who refuse or cannot tolerate estrogens or in whom estrogens are contraindicated. Use of Miacalcin® (calcitonin-salmon) Nasal Spray is recommended in conjunction with an adequate calcium (at least 1000 mg elemental calcium per day) and vitamin D (400 I.U. per day) intake to retard the progressive loss of bone mass. The evidence of efficacy is based on increases in spinal bone mineral density observed in clinical trials.
Two randomized, placebo controlled trials were conducted in 325 postmenopausal females [227 Miacalcin® (calcitonin-salmon) Nasal Spray treated and 98 placebo treated] with spinal, forearm or femoral bone mineral density (BMD) at least one standard deviation below normal for healthy premenopausal females. These studies conducted over two years demonstrated that 200 I.U. daily of Miacalcin® (calcitonin-salmon) Nasal Spray increases lumbar vertebral BMD relative to baseline and relative to placebo in osteoporotic females who were greater than 5 years postmenopause. Miacalcin® (calcitonin-salmon) Nasal Spray produced statistically significant increases in lumbar vertebral BMD compared to placebo as early as six months after initiation of therapy with persistence of this level for up to 2 years of observation.
No effects of Miacalcin® (calcitonin-salmon) Nasal Spray on cortical bone of the forearm or hip were demonstrated. However, in one study, BMD of the hip showed a statistically significant increase compared with placebo in a region composed of predominantly trabecular bone after one year of treatment changing to a trend at 2 years that was no longer statistically significant.

CONTRAINDICATIONS

Clinical allergy to calcitonin-salmon.

WARNINGS

Allergic Reactions

Because calcitonin is a polypeptide, the possibility of a systemic allergic reaction exists. A few cases of allergic-type reactions have been reported in patients receiving Miacalcin® (calcitonin-salmon) Nasal Spray, including one case of anaphylactic shock, which appears to have been due to the preservative because the patient could tolerate injectable calcitonin-salmon without incident. With injectable calcitonin-salmon there have been a few reports of serious allergic-type reactions (e.g., bronchospasm, swelling of the tongue or throat, anaphylactic shock, and in one case death attributed to anaphylaxis). The usual provisions should be made for the emergency treatment of such a reaction should it occur. Allergic reactions should be differentiated from generalized flushing and hypotension.
For patients with suspected sensitivity to calcitonin, skin testing should be considered prior to treatment utilizing a dilute, sterile solution of Miacalcin® (calcitonin-salmon) Injection, Synthetic. Physicians may wish to refer patients who require skin testing to an allergist. A detailed skin testing protocol is available from the Medical Services Department of Novartis Pharmaceuticals Corporation.

PRECAUTIONS

1. Drug Interactions

Formal studies designed to evaluate drug interactions with calcitonin-salmon have not been done. No drug interaction studies have been performed with Miacalcin® (calcitonin-salmon) Nasal Spray ingredients.
Currently, no drug interactions with calcitonin-salmon have been observed. The effects of prior use of diphosphonates in postmenopausal osteoporosis patients have not been assessed; however, in patients with Paget's Disease prior diphosphonate use appears to reduce the anti-resorptive response to Miacalcin® (calcitonin-salmon) Nasal Spray.

2. Periodic Nasal Examinations

Periodic nasal examinations with visualization of the nasal mucosa, turbinates, septum and mucosal blood vessel status are recommended.
The development of mucosal alterations or transient nasal conditions occurred in up to 9% of patients who received Miacalcin® (calcitonin-salmon) Nasal Spray and in up to 12% of patients who received placebo nasal spray in studies in postmenopausal females. The majority of patients (approximately 90%) in whom nasal abnormalities were noted also reported nasally related complaints/symptoms as adverse events. Therefore, a nasal examination should be performed prior to start of treatment with nasal calcitonin and at any time nasal complaints occur.
In all postmenopausal patients treated with Miacalcin® (calcitonin-salmon) Nasal Spray, the most commonly reported nasal adverse events included rhinitis (12%), epistaxis (3.5%), and sinusitis (2.3%). Smoking was shown not to have any contributory effect on the occurrence of nasal adverse events. One patient (0.3%) treated with Miacalcin® (calcitonin-salmon) Nasal Spray who was receiving 400 I.U. daily developed a small nasal wound. In clinical trials in another disorder (Paget's Disease), 2.8% of patients developed nasal ulcerations.
If severe ulceration of the nasal mucosa occurs, as indicated by ulcers greater than 1.5 mm in diameter or penetrating below the mucosa, or those associated with heavy bleeding, Miacalcin® (calcitonin-salmon) Nasal Spray should be discontinued. Although smaller ulcers often heal without withdrawal of Miacalcin® (calcitonin-salmon) Nasal Spray, medication should be discontinued temporarily until healing occurs.

3. Information for Patients

Careful instructions on pump assembly, priming of the pump and nasal introduction of Miacalcin® (calcitonin-salmon) Nasal Spray should be given to the patient. Although instructions for patients are supplied with individual bottles, procedures for use should be demonstrated to each patient. Patients should notify their physician if they develop significant nasal irritation.
Patients should be advised of the following:

- Store new, unassembled bottles in the refrigerator between 36°-46°F (2°-8°C).
- Protect the product from freezing.
- Before priming the pump and using a new bottle, allow it to reach room temperature.
- Store bottle in use at room temperature in an upright position, for up to 30 days. Each bottle contains at least 14 doses.
- Store second bottle in refrigerator until ready to use. Protect from freezing.
- Discard all unrefrigerated bottles after 30 days.
- See *DOSAGE AND ADMINISTRATION, Priming (Activation) of Pump* for complete instructions on priming the pump and administering Miacalcin® (calcitonin-salmon) Nasal Spray.

4. Carcinogenicity, Mutagenicity, and Impairment of Fertility

An increased incidence of non-functioning pituitary adenomas has been observed in one-year toxicity studies in Sprague-Dawley and Fischer 344 Rats administered (subcutaneously) calcitonin-salmon at dosages of 80 I.U. per kilogram per day (16-19 times the recommended human parenteral dose and about 130-160 times the human intranasal dose based on body surface area). The findings suggest that calcitonin-salmon reduced the latency period for development of pituitary adenomas that do not produce hormones, probably through the perturbation of physiologic processes involved in the evolution of this commonly occurring endocrine lesion in the rat. Although administration of calcitonin-salmon reduces the latency period of the development of nonfunctional proliferative lesions in rats, it did not induce the hyperplastic/neoplastic process.

Calcitonin-salmon was tested for mutagenicity using *Salmonella typhimurium* (5 strains) and *Escherichia coli* (2 strains), with and without rat liver metabolic activation, and found to be non-mutagenic. The drug was also not mutagenic in a chromosome aberration test in mammalian V79 cells of the Chinese Hamster *in vitro*.

5. Laboratory Tests

Urine sediment abnormalities have not been reported in ambulatory volunteers treated with Miacalcin® (calcitonin-salmon) Nasal Spray. Coarse granular casts containing renal tubular epithelial cells were reported in young adult volunteers at bed rest who were given injectable calcitonin-salmon to study the effect of immobilization on osteoporosis. There was no evidence of renal abnormality and the urine sediment became normal after calcitonin was stopped. Periodic examinations of urine sediment should be considered.

6. Pregnancy

Teratogenic Effects

Category C

Calcitonin-salmon has been shown to cause a decrease in fetal birth weights in rabbits when given by injection in doses 8-33 times the parenteral dose and 70-278 times the intranasal dose recommended for human use based on body surface area.

Since calcitonin does not cross the placental barrier, this finding may be due to metabolic effects on the pregnant animal. There are no adequate and well controlled studies in pregnant women with calcitonin-salmon. Miacalcin® (calcitonin-salmon) Nasal Spray is *not* indicated for use in pregnancy.

7. Nursing Mothers

It is not known whether this drug is excreted in human milk. As a general rule, nursing should not be undertaken while a patient is on this drug since many drugs are excreted in human milk. Calcitonin has been shown to inhibit lactation in animals.

8. Geriatric Use

Clinical trials using Miacalcin® (calcitonin-salmon) Nasal Spray have included postmenopausal patients up to 77 years of age. No unusual adverse events or increased incidence of common adverse events have been noted in patients over 65 years of age.

9. Pediatric Use

There are no data to support the use of Miacalcin® (calcitonin-salmon) Nasal Spray in children. Disorders of bone in children referred to as idiopathic juvenile osteoporosis have been reported rarely. The relationship of these disorders to postmenopausal osteoporosis has not been established and experience with the use of calcitonin in these disorders is very limited.

ADVERSE REACTIONS

The incidence of adverse reactions reported in studies involving postmenopausal osteoporotic patients chronically exposed to Miacalcin® (calcitonin-salmon) Nasal Spray (N=341) and to placebo nasal spray (N=131) and reported in greater than 3% of Miacalcin® (calcitonin-salmon) Nasal Spray treated patients are presented below in the following table. Most adverse reactions were mild to moderate in severity. Nasal adverse events were most common with 70% mild, 25% moderate, and 5% severe in nature (placebo rates were 71% mild, 27% moderate, and 2% severe).

Adverse Reactions Occurring in at Least 3% of Postmenopausal Patients Treated Chronically

Adverse Reaction	Miacalcin® (calcitonin-salmon) Nasal Spray N=341 % of Patients	Placebo N=131 % of Patients
Rhinitis	12.0	6.9
Symptom of Nose†	10.6	16.0
Back Pain	5.0	2.3
Arthralgia	3.8	5.3
Epistaxis	3.5	4.6
Headache	3.2	4.6

†Symptom of nose includes: nasal crusts, dryness, redness or erythema, nasal sores, irritation, itching, thick feeling, soreness, pallor, infection, stenosis, runny/blocked, small wound, bleeding wound, tenderness, uncomfortable feeling and sore across bridge of of nose.

In addition, the following adverse events were reported in fewer than 3% of patients during chronic therapy with Miacalcin® (calcitonin-salmon) Nasal Spray. Adverse events reported in 1%-3% of patients are identified with an asterisk(*). The remainder occurred in less than 1% of patients. Other than flushing, nausea, possible allergic reactions, and possible local irritative effects in the respiratory tract, a relationship to Miacalcin® (calcitonin-salmon) Nasal Spray has not been established.

Body as a whole – General Disorders: influenza-like symptoms*, fatigue*, periorbital edema, fever
Integumentary: erythematous rash*, skin ulceration, eczema, alopecia, pruritus, increased sweating
Musculoskeletal/Collagen: arthrosis*, myalgia*, arthritis, polymyalgia rheumatica, stiffness
Respiratory/Special Senses: sinusitis*, upper respiratory tract infection*, bronchospasm*, pharyngitis, bronchitis, pneumonia, coughing, dyspnea, taste perversion, parosmia
Cardiovascular: hypertension*, angina pectoris*, tachycardia, palpitation, bundle branch block, myocardial infarction
Gastrointestinal: dyspepsia*, constipation*, abdominal pain*, nausea*, diarrhea*, vomiting, flatulence, increased appetite, gastritis, dry mouth
Liver/Metabolic: cholelithiasis, hepatitis, thirst, weight increase
Endocrine: goiter, hyperthyroidism
Urinary System: cystitis*, pyelonephritis, hematuria, renal calculus
Central and Peripheral Nervous System: dizziness*, paresthesia*, vertigo, migraine, neuralgia, agitation
Hearing/Vestibular: tinnitus, hearing loss, earache
Vision: abnormal lacrimation*, conjunctivitis*, blurred vision, vitreous floater
Vascular: flushing, cerebrovascular accident, thrombophlebitis
Hematologic/Resistance Mechanisms: lymphadenopathy*, infection*, anemia
Psychiatric: depression*, insomnia, anxiety, anorexia

Common adverse reactions associated with the use of injectable calcitonin-salmon occurred less frequently in patients treated with Miacalcin® (calcitonin-salmon) Nasal Spray than in those patients treated with injectable calcitonin. Nausea, with or without vomiting, which occurred in 1.8% of patients treated with the nasal spray (and 1.5% of those receiving placebo nasal spray) occurs in about 10% of patients who take injectable calcitonin-salmon. Flushing, which occurred in less than 1% of patients treated with the Nasal Spray, occurs in 2%-5% of patients treated with injectable calcitonin-salmon. Although the administered dosages of injectable and nasal spray calcitonin-salmon are comparable (50-100 units daily of injectable versus 200 units daily of nasal spray), the nasal dosage form has a mean bioavailability of about 3% (range 0.3%-30.6%) and therefore provides less drug to the systemic circulation, possibly accounting for the decrease in frequency of adverse reactions.

The collective foreign marketing experience with Miacalcin® (calcitonin-salmon) Nasal Spray does not show evidence of any notable difference in the incidence profile of reported adverse reactions when compared with that seen in the clinical trials.

OVERDOSAGE

No instances of overdose with Miacalcin® (calcitonin-salmon) Nasal Spray have been reported and no serious adverse reactions have been associated with high doses. There is no known potential for drug abuse for calcitonin-salmon.

Single doses of Miacalcin® (calcitonin-salmon) Nasal Spray up to 1600 I.U., doses up to 800 I.U. per day for three days and chronic administration of doses up to 600 I.U. per day have been studied without serious adverse effects. A dose of 1000 I.U. of Miacalcin® (calcitonin-salmon) injectable solution given subcutaneously may produce nausea and vomiting. A dose of Miacalcin® (calcitonin-salmon) injectable solution of 32 I.U. per kg per day for one or two days demonstrated no additional adverse effects.

There have been no reports of hypocalcemic tetany. However, the pharmacologic actions of Miacalcin® (calcitonin-salmon) Nasal Spray suggest that this could occur in overdose. Therefore, provisions for parenteral administration of calcium should be available for the treatment of overdose.

DOSAGE AND ADMINISTRATION

The recommended dose of Miacalcin® (calcitonin-salmon) Nasal Spray in postmenopausal osteoporotic females is one spray (200 I.U.) per day administered intranasally, alternating nostrils daily.

Drug effect may be monitored by periodic measurements of lumbar vertebral bone mass to document stabilization of bone loss or increases in bone density. Effects of Miacalcin® (calcitonin-salmon) Nasal Spray on biochemical markers of bone turnover have not been consistently demonstrated in studies in postmenopausal osteoporosis. Therefore, these parameters should not be solely utilized to determine clinical response to Miacalcin® (calcitonin-salmon) Nasal Spray therapy in these patients.

Priming (Activation) of Pump

Before the first dose and administration, Miacalcin® (calcitonin-salmon) Nasal Spray should be at room temperature. To prime the pump, the bottle should be held upright and the two white side arms of the pump depressed toward the bottle until a full spray is produced. The pump is primed once the first full spray is emitted. To administer, the nozzle should be carefully placed into the nostril with the head in the upright position, and the pump firmly depressed toward the bottle. The pump should not be primed before each daily dose.

HOW SUPPLIED

Miacalcin® (calcitonin-salmon) Nasal Spray

Available as a metered dose solution in 2 mL fill glass bottles. It is available in a dosage strength of 200 I.U. per activation (0.09 mL/spray). Screw-on pumps are provided. The pumps, following priming, will deliver 0.09 mL of solution. Miacalcin® (calcitonin-salmon) Nasal Spray contains 2200 I.U./mL calcitonin-salmon and is provided in individual boxes containing two glass bottles and two screw-on pumps (NDC 0078-0311-90).

Store and Dispense

Store unopened bottle(s) in refrigerator between 36°-46°F (2°-8°C). Protect from freezing.

Store bottle in use at room temperature in an upright position, for up to 30 days. Each bottle contains at least 14 doses.

Store second bottle in refrigerator until ready to use. Protect from freezing.

Discard all unrefrigerated bottles after 30 days.

666880

REV: DECEMBER 1998 30367905

Shown in Product Identification Guide, page 326

MIGRANAL® ℞

[*mĭ gră năl*]

(dihydroergotamine mesylate, USP)

Nasal Spray

The solution used in Migranal® (dihydroergotamine mesylate, USP) Nasal Spray (4 mg/mL) is intended for intranasal use and must not be injected.

Caution: Federal law prohibits dispensing without prescription.

The following prescribing information is based on official labeling in effect July 2000.

DESCRIPTION

Migranal® is ergotamine hydrogenated in the 9,10 position as the mesylate salt. Migranal® is known chemically as ergotaman-3′,6′,18-trione,9,10-dihydro-12′-hydroxy-2′-methyl-5′-(phenylmethyl)-,(5′α)-,monomethanesulfonate. Its molecular weight is 679.80 and its empirical formula is $C_{33}H_{37}N_5O_5 \bullet CH_4O_3S$. The chemical structure is:

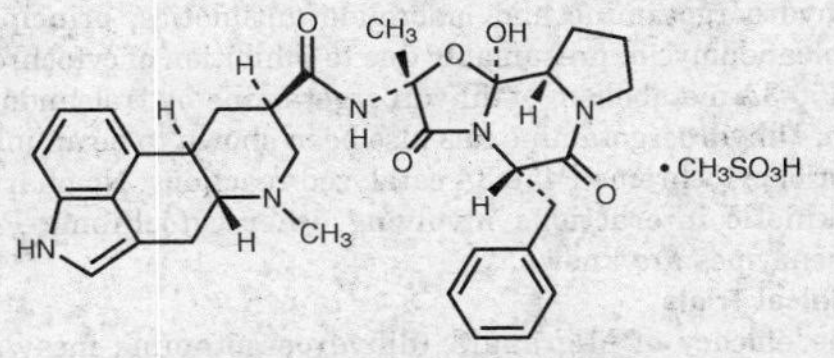

Dihydroergotamine mesylate

$C_{33}H_{37}N_5O_5 \bullet CH_4O_3S$ Mol. wt. 679.80

Migranal® (dihydroergotamine mesylate, USP) Nasal Spray is provided for intranasal administration as a clear, colorless to faintly yellow solution in an amber glass ampul containing:

dihydroergotamine mesylate, USP	4.0 mg
caffeine, anhydrous, USP	10.0 mg
dextrose, anhydrous, USP	50.0 mg
carbon dioxide	qs
water for injection, USP	qs 1.0 mL

CLINICAL PHARMACOLOGY

Mechanism of Action

Dihydroergotamine binds with high affinity to 5-$HT_{1D\alpha}$ and 5-$HT_{1D\beta}$ receptors. It also binds with high affinity to serotonin 5-HT_{1A}, 5-HT_{2A}, and 5-HT_{2C} receptors, noradrenaline α_{2A}, α_{2B} and α_1 receptors, and dopamine D_{2L} and D_3 receptors.

The therapeutic activity of dihydroergotamine in migraine is generally attributed to the agonist effect at 5-HT_{1D} receptors. Two current theories have been proposed to explain the efficacy of 5-HT_{1D} receptor agonists in migraine. One theory suggests that activation of 5-HT_{1D} receptors located on intracranial blood vessels, including those on arterio-venous anastomoses, leads to vasoconstriction, which correlates with the relief of migraine headache. The alternative hypothesis suggests that activation of 5-HT_{1D} receptors on sensory nerve endings of the trigeminal system results in the inhibition of pro-inflammatory neuropeptide release. In addition, dihydroergotamine possesses oxytocic properties. *(See CONTRAINDICATIONS)*

Pharmacokinetics

Absorption

Dihydroergotamine mesylate is poorly bioavailable following oral administration. Following intranasal administration, however, the mean bioavailability of dihydroergotamine mesylate is 32% relative to the injectable administration. Absorption is variable, probably reflecting both intersubject differences of absorption and the technique used for self-administration.

Distribution

Dihydroergotamine mesylate is 93% plasma protein bound. The apparent steady-state volume of distribution is approximately 800 liters.

Metabolism

Four dihydroergotamine mesylate metabolites have been identified in human plasma following oral administration. The major metabolite, 8′-β-hydroxydihydroergotamine, exhibits affinity equivalent to its parent for adrenergic and

Continued on next page

Migranal—Cont.

5-HT receptors and demonstrates equivalent potency in several venoconstrictor activity models, *in vivo* and *in vitro*. The other metabolites, i.e., dihydrolysergic acid, dihydrolysergic amide and a metabolite formed by oxidative opening of the proline ring are of minor importance. Following nasal administration, total metabolites represent only 20%-30% of plasma AUC. The systemic clearance of dihydroergotamine mesylate following I.V. and I.M. administration is 1.5 L/min. Quantitative pharmacokinetic characterization of the four metabolites has not been performed.

Excretion

The major excretory route of dihydroergotamine is via the bile in the feces. After intranasal administration the urinary recovery of parent drug amounts to about 2% of the administered dose compared to 6% after I.M. administration. The total body clearance is 1.5 L/min which reflects mainly hepatic clearance. The renal clearance (0.1 L/min) is unaffected by the route of dihydroergotamine administration. The decline of plasma dihydroergotamine is biphasic with a terminal half-life of about 10 hours.

Subpopulations

No studies have been conducted on the effect of renal or hepatic impairment, gender, race, or ethnicity on dihydroergotamine pharmacokinetics. Migranal® (dihydroergotamine mesylate, USP) Nasal Spray is contraindicated in patients with severely impaired hepatic or renal function. *(See CONTRAINDICATIONS)*

Interactions

The pharmacokinetics of dihydroergotamine did not appear to be significantly affected by the concomitant use of a local vasoconstrictor (e.g., fenoxazoline).

Multiple oral doses of the β-adrenoceptor antagonist propranolol, used for migraine prophylaxis, had no significant influence on the C_{max}, T_{max} or AUC of dihydroergotamine doses up to 4 mg.

Pharmacokinetic interactions (increased blood levels) have been reported in patients treated orally with dihydroergotamine and macrolide antibiotics, principally troleandomycin, presumably due to inhibition of cytochrome P450 3A metabolism of dihydroergotamine by troleandomycin. Dihydroergotamine has also been shown to be an inhibitor of cytochrome P450 3A catalyzed reactions. No pharmacokinetic interactions involving other cytochrome P450 isoenzymes are known.

Clinical Trials

The efficacy of Migranal® (dihydroergotamine mesylate, USP) Nasal Spray for the acute treatment of migraine headaches was evaluated in four randomized, double blind, placebo controlled studies in the U.S. The patient population for the trials was predominantly female (87%) and Caucasian (95%) with a mean age of 39 years (range 18 to 65 years). Patients treated a single moderate to severe migraine headache with a single dose of study medication and assessed pain severity over the 24 hours following treatment. Headache response was determined 0.5, 1, 2, 3 and 4 hours after dosing and was defined as a reduction in headache severity to mild or no pain. In studies 1 and 2, a four-point pain intensity scale was utilized; in studies 3 and 4, a five-point scale was used that included both pain response and restoration of function for "severe" or "incapacitating" pain, a less clear endpoint. Although rescue medication was allowed in all four studies, patients were instructed not to use them during the four hour observation period. In studies 3 and 4, a total dose of 2 mg was compared to placebo. In studies 1 and 2, doses of 2 and 3 mg were evaluated, and showed no advantage of the higher dose for a single treatment. In all studies, patients received a regimen consisting of 0.5 mg in each nostril, repeated in 15 minutes (and again in another 15 minutes for the 3 mg dose in studies 1 and 2). The percentage of patients achieving headache response 4 hours after treatment was significantly greater in patients receiving 2 mg doses of Migranal® (dihydroergotamine mesylate, USP) Nasal Spray compared to those receiving placebo in 3 of the 4 studies (see Tables 1 & 2 and Figures 1 & 2).

Table 1: Studies 1 and 2: Percentage of patients with headache response[a] 2 and 4 hours following a single treatment of study medication [Migranal® (dihydroergotamine mesylate, USP) Nasal Spray or Placebo]

		N	2 hours	4 hours
Study 1	Migranal®	105	61%**	70%**
	Placebo	98	23%	28%
Study 2	Migranal®	103	47%	56%*
	Placebo	102	33%	35%

[a] Headache response was defined as a reduction in headache severity to mild or no pain. Headache response was based on pain intensity as interpreted by the patient using a four-point pain intensity scale.

*p value < 0.01

**p value < 0.001

Table 2: Studies 3 and 4: Percentage of patients with headache response[a] 2 and 4 hours following a single treatment of study medication [Migranal® (dihydroergotamine mesylate, USP) Nasal Spray or Placebo]

		N	2 hours	4 hours
Study 3	Migranal®	50	32%	48%*
	Placebo	50	20%	22%
Study 4	Migranal®	47	30%	47%
	Placebo	50	20%	30%

[a] Headache response was defined as a reduction in headache severity to mild or no pain. Headache response was evaluated on a five-point scale that included both pain response and restoration of function for "severe" or "incapacitating" pain.

* p value < 0.01

Comparisons of drug performance based upon results obtained in different clinical trials are never reliable. Because studies are conducted at different times, with different samples of patients, by different investigators, employing different criteria and/or different interpretations of the same criteria, under different conditions (dose, dosing regimen, etc.), quantitative estimates of treatment response and the timing of response may be expected to vary considerably from study to study.

The Kaplan-Meier plots below (Figures 1 & 2) provides an estimate of the probability that a patient will have responded to a single 2 mg dose of Migranal® (dihydroergotamine mesylate, USP) Nasal Spray as a function of the time elapsed since initiation of treatment.

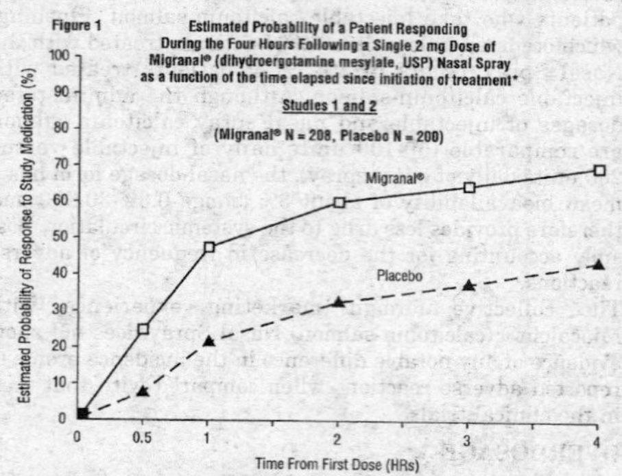

*The figure shows the probability over time of obtaining a response following treatment with Migranal® (dihydroergotamine mesylate, USP) Nasal Spray. Headache response was based on pain intensity as interpreted by the patient using a four-point pain intensity scale. Patients not achieving response within 4 hours were censored to 4 hours.

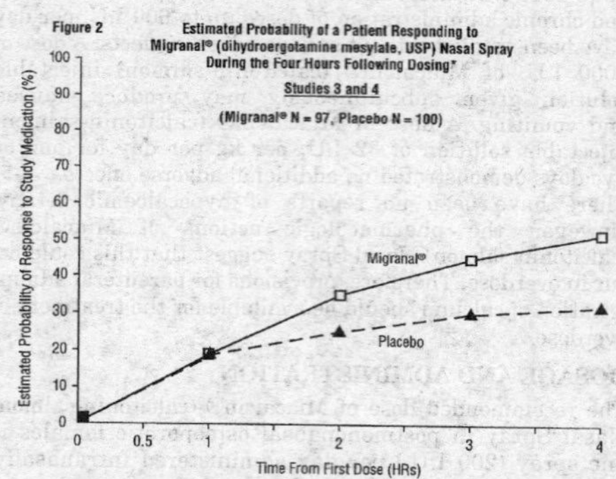

*The figure shows the probability over time of obtaining a response following treatment with Migranal® (dihydroergotamine mesylate, USP) Nasal Spray. Headache response was evaluated on a five-point scale that confounded pain response and restoration of function for "severe" or "incapacitating" pain. Patients not achieving response within 4 hours were censored to 4 hours.

For patients with migraine-associated nausea, photophobia, and phonophobia at baseline, there was a lower incidence of these symptoms at 2 and 4 hours following administration of Migranal® (dihydroergotamine mesylate, USP) Nasal Spray compared to placebo.

Patients were not allowed to use additional treatments for eight hours prior to study medication dosing and during the four hour observation period following study treatment. Following the 4 hour observation period, patients were allowed to use additional treatments. For all studies, the estimated probability of patients using additional treatments for their migraines over the 24 hours following the single 2 mg dose of study treatment is summarized in Figure 3 below.

[See figure at top of next column]

Neither age nor sex appear to effect the patient's response to Migranal® (dihydroergotamine mesylate, USP) Nasal Spray. While patients with menstrual migraine, migraine with aura, and migraine without aura by medical history were included in the clinical evaluation of Migranal® (dihydroergotamine mesylate, USP) Nasal Spray, patients

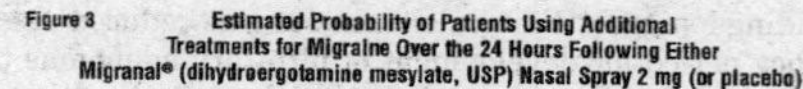

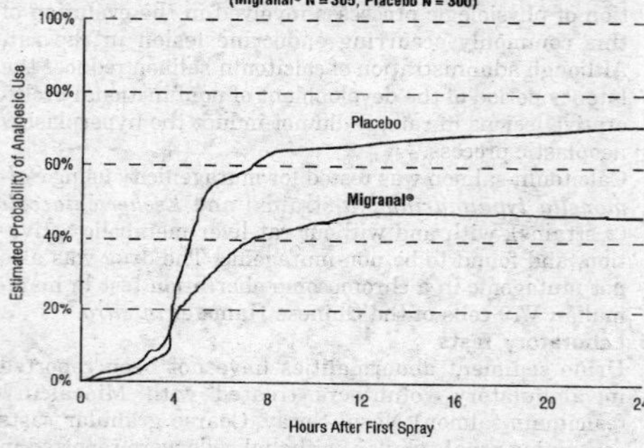

*Kaplan-Meier plot based on data obtained from all studies with patients not using additional treatments censored to 24 hours. All patients received a single treatment of study medication for their migraine attack. The plot also includes patients who had no response to the initial dose.

were not required to report the specific type of migraine treated with study medication. Thus, neither the effect of menses on migraine nor the presence or the absence of aura were assessed. The racial distribution of patients was insufficient to determine the effect of race on the efficacy of Migranal® (dihydroergotamine mesylate, USP) Nasal Spray.

INDICATIONS AND USAGE

Migranal® (dihydroergotamine mesylate, USP) Nasal Spray is indicated for the acute treatment of migraine headaches with or without aura.

Migranal® (dihydroergotamine mesylate, USP) Nasal Spray is not intended for the prophylactic therapy of migraine or for the management of hemiplegic or basilar migraine.

CONTRAINDICATIONS

Migranal® (dihydroergotamine mesylate, USP) Nasal Spray should not be given to patients with ischemic heart disease (angina pectoris, history of myocardial infarction, or documented silent ischemia) or to patients who have clinical symptoms or findings consistent with coronary artery vasospasm including Prinzmetal's variant angina. *(See WARNINGS)*

Because Migranal® (dihydroergotamine mesylate, USP) Nasal Spray may increase blood pressure, it should not be given to patients with uncontrolled hypertension.

Migranal® (dihydroergotamine mesylate, USP) Nasal Spray, 5-HT_1 agonists (e.g., sumatriptan), ergotamine-containing or ergot-type medications or methysergide should not be used within 24 hours of each other.

Migranal® (dihydroergotamine mesylate, USP) Nasal Spray should not be administered to patients with hemiplegic or basilar migraine.

In addition to those conditions mentioned above, Migranal® (dihydroergotamine mesylate, USP) Nasal Spray is also contraindicated in patients with known peripheral arterial disease, sepsis, following vascular surgery, and severely impaired hepatic or renal function.

Migranal® (dihydroergotamine mesylate, USP) Nasal Spray may cause fetal harm when administered to a pregnant woman. Dihydroergotamine possesses oxytocic properties and, therefore, should not be administered during pregnancy. If this drug is used during pregnancy, or if the patient becomes pregnant while taking this drug, the patient should be apprised of the potential hazard to the fetus.

There are no adequate studies of dihydroergotamine in human pregnancy, but developmental toxicity has been demonstrated in experimental animals. In embryofetal development studies of dihydroergotamine mesylate nasal spray, intranasal administration to pregnant rats throughout the period of organogenesis resulted in decreased fetal body weights and/or skeletal ossification at doses of 0.16 mg/day (associated with maternal plasma dihydroergotamine exposures [AUC] approximately 0.4-1.2 times the exposures in humans receiving the MRDD of 4 mg) or greater. A no effect level for embryo-fetal toxicity was not established in rats. Delayed skeletal ossification was also noted in rabbit fetuses following intranasal administration of 3.6 mg/day (maternal exposures approximately 7 times human exposures at the MRDD) during organogenesis. A no effect level was seen at 1.2 mg/day (maternal exposures approximately 2.5 times human exposures at the MRDD). When dihydroergotamine mesylate nasal spray was administered intranasally to female rats during pregnancy and lactation, decreased body weights and impaired reproductive function (decreased mating indices) were observed in the offspring at doses of 0.16 mg/day or greater. A no effect level was not established. Effects on development occurred at doses below those that produced evidence of significant maternal toxicity in these studies. Dihydroergotamine-induced intrauterine growth retardation has been attributed to reduced uteroplacental blood flow resulting from prolonged vasoconstriction of the uterine vessels and/or increased myometrial tone.

Migranal® (dihydroergotamine mesylate, USP) Nasal Spray is contraindicated in patients who have previously shown hypersensitivity to ergot alkaloids.

Dihydroergotamine mesylate should not be used by nursing mothers. *(See PRECAUTIONS)*

Dihydroergotamine mesylate should not be used with peripheral and central vasoconstrictors because the combination may result in additive or synergistic elevation of blood pressure.

WARNINGS

Migranal® (dihydroergotamine mesylate, USP) Nasal Spray should only be used where a clear diagnosis of migraine headache has been established.

Risk of Myocardial Ischemia and/or Infarction and Other Adverse Cardiac Events:

Migranal® (dihydroergotamine mesylate, USP) Nasal Spray should not be used by patients with documented ischemic or vasospastic coronary artery disease. *(See CONTRAINDICATIONS)* It is strongly recommended that Migranal® (dihydroergotamine mesylate, USP) Nasal Spray not be given to patients in whom unrecognized coronary artery disease (CAD) is predicted by the presence of risk factors (e.g., hypertension, hypercholesterolemia, smoker, obesity, diabetes, strong family history of CAD, females who are surgically or physiologically postmenopausal, or males who are over 40 years of age) unless a cardiovascular evaluation provides satisfactory clinical evidence that the patient is reasonably free of coronary artery and ischemic myocardial disease or other significant underlying cardiovascular disease. The sensitivity of cardiac diagnostic procedures to detect cardiovascular disease or predisposition to coronary artery vasospasm is modest, at best. If, during the cardiovascular evaluation, the patient's medical history or electrocardiographic investigations reveal findings indicative of or consistent with coronary artery vasospasm or myocardial ischemia, Migranal® (dihydroergotamine mesylate, USP) Nasal Spray should not be administered. *(See CONTRAINDICATIONS)*

For patients with risk factors predictive of CAD who are determined to have a satisfactory cardiovascular evaluation, it is strongly recommended that administration of the first dose of Migranal® (dihydroergotamine mesylate, USP) Nasal Spray take place in the setting of a physician's office or similar medically staffed and equipped facility unless the patient has previously received dihydroergotamine mesylate. Because cardiac ischemia can occur in the absence of clinical symptoms, consideration should be given to obtaining on the first occasion of use an electrocardiogram (ECG) during the interval immediately following Migranal® (dihydroergotamine mesylate, USP) Nasal Spray, in these patients with risk factors.

It is recommended that patients who are intermittent long-term users of Migranal® (dihydroergotamine mesylate, USP) Nasal Spray and who have or acquire risk factors predictive of CAD, as described above, undergo periodic interval cardiovascular evaluation as they continue to use Migranal® (dihydroergotamine mesylate, USP) Nasal Spray.

The systematic approach described above is currently recommended as a method to identify patients in whom Migranal® (dihydroergotamine mesylate, USP) Nasal Spray may be used to treat migraine headaches with an acceptable margin of cardiovascular safety.

Cardiac Events and Fatalities

No deaths have been reported in patients using Migranal® (dihydroergotamine mesylate, USP) Nasal Spray. However, the potential for adverse cardiac events exists. Serious adverse cardiac events, including acute myocardial infarction, life-threatening disturbances of cardiac rhythm, and death have been reported to have occurred following the administration of dihydroergotamine mesylate injection (e.g., D.H.E. 45® Injection). Considering the extent of use of dihydroergotamine mesylate in patients with migraine, the incidence of these events is extremely low.

Drug-Associated Cerebrovascular Events and Fatalities

Cerebral hemorrhage, subarachnoid hemorrhage, stroke, and other cerebrovascular events have been reported in patients treated with D.H.E. 45® Injection; and some have resulted in fatalities. In a number of cases, it appears possible that the cerebrovascular events were primary, the D.H.E. 45® Injection having been administered in the incorrect belief that the symptoms experienced were a consequence of migraine, when they were not. It should be noted that patients with migraine may be at increased risk of certain cerebrovascular events (e.g., stroke, hemorrhage, transient ischemic attack).

Other Vasospasm Related Events

Migranal® (dihydroergotamine mesylate, USP) Nasal Spray, like other ergot alkaloids, may cause vasospastic reactions other than coronary artery vasospasm. Myocardial and peripheral vascular ischemia have been reported with Migranal® (dihydroergotamine mesylate, USP) Nasal Spray.

Migranal® (dihydroergotamine mesylate, USP) Nasal Spray associated vasospastic phenomena may also cause muscle pains, numbness, coldness, pallor, and cyanosis of the digits. In patients with compromised circulation, persistent vasospasm may result in gangrene or death, Migranal® (dihydroergotamine mesylate, USP) Nasal Spray should be discontinued immediately if signs or symptoms of vasoconstriction develop.

Increase in Blood Pressure

Significant elevation in blood pressure has been reported on rare occasions in patients with and without a history of hypertension treated with Migranal® (dihydroergotamine mesylate, USP) Nasal Spray and dihydroergotamine mesylate injection. Migranal® (dihydroergotamine mesylate, USP) Nasal Spray is contraindicated in patients with uncontrolled hypertension. *(See CONTRAINDICATIONS)*

An 18% increase in mean pulmonary artery pressure was seen following dosing with another $5HT_1$ agonist in a study evaluating subjects undergoing cardiac catheterization.

Local Irritation

Approximately 30% of patients using Migranal® (dihydroergotamine mesylate, USP) Nasal Spray (compared to 9% of placebo patients) have reported irritation in the nose, throat, and/or disturbances in taste. Irritative symptoms include congestion, burning sensation, dryness, paraesthesia, discharge, epistaxis, pain, or soreness. The symptoms were predominantly mild to moderate in severity and transient. In approximately 70% of the above mentioned cases, the symptoms resolved within four hours after dosing with Migranal® (dihydroergotamine mesylate, USP) Nasal Spray. Examinations of the nose and throat in a small subset (N = 66) of study participants treated for up to 36 months (range 1-36 months) did not reveal any clinically noticeable injury. Other than this limited number of patients, the consequences of extended and repeated use of Migranal® (dihydroergotamine mesylate, USP) Nasal Spray on the nasal and/or respiratory mucosa have not been systematically evaluated in patients.

Nasal tissue in animals treated with dihydroergotamine mesylate daily at nasal cavity surface area exposures (in mg/mm^2) that were equal to or less than those achieved in humans receiving the maximum recommended daily dose of 0.08 mg/kg/day showed mild mucosal irritation characterized by mucous cell and transitional cell hyperplasia and squamous cell metaplasia. Changes in rat nasal mucosa at 64 weeks were less severe than at 13 weeks. Local effects on respiratory tissue after chronic intranasal dosing in animals have not been evaluated.

PRECAUTIONS

General

Migranal® (dihydroergotamine mesylate, USP) Nasal Spray may cause coronary artery vasospasm; patients who experience signs or symptoms suggestive of angina following its administration should, therefore, be evaluated for the presence of CAD or a predisposition to variant angina before receiving additional doses. Similarly, patients who experience other symptoms or signs suggestive of decreased arterial flow, such as ischemic bowel syndrome or Raynaud's syndrome following the use of any 5-HT agonist are candidates for further evaluation. *(See WARNINGS)*

Information for Patients

The text of a patient information sheet is printed at the end of this insert. To assure safe and effective use of Migranal® (dihydroergotamine mesylate, USP) Nasal Spray, the information and instructions provided in the patient information sheet should be discussed with patients.

Once the nasal spray applicator has been prepared, it should be discarded (with any remaining drug) after 8 hours.

Patients should be advised to report to the physician immediately any of the following: numbness or tingling in the fingers and toes, muscle pain in the arms and legs, weakness in the legs, pain in the chest, temporary speeding or slowing of the heart rate, swelling, or itching.

Prior to the initial use of the product by a patient, the prescriber should take steps to ensure that the patient understands how to use the product as provided. *(See Patient Information Sheet and product packaging)*

Drug Interactions

Vasoconstrictors

Migranal® (dihydroergotamine mesylate, USP) Nasal Spray should not be used with peripheral vasoconstrictors because the combination may cause synergistic elevation of blood pressure.

Sumatriptan

Sumatriptan has been reported to cause coronary artery vasospasm, and its effect could be additive with Migranal® (dihydroergotamine mesylate, USP) Nasal Spray. Sumatriptan and Migranal® (dihydroergotamine mesylate, USP) Nasal Spray should not be taken within 24 hours of each other. *(See CONTRAINDICATIONS)*

Beta Blockers

Although the results of a clinical study did not indicate a safety problem associated with the administration of Migranal® (dihydroergotamine mesylate, USP) Nasal Spray to subjects already receiving propranolol, there have been reports that propranolol may potentiate the vasoconstrictive action of ergotamine by blocking the vasodilating property of epinephrine.

Nicotine

Nicotine may provoke vasoconstriction in some patients, predisposing to a greater ischemic response to ergot therapy.

Macrolide Antibiotics

(e.g., erythromycin and troleandomycin)

Agents of the ergot alkaloid class, of which Migranal® (dihydroergotamine mesylate, USP) Nasal Spray is a member, have been shown to interact with antibiotics of the macrolide class, resulting in increased plasma levels of unchanged alkaloids and peripheral vasoconstriction. Vasospastic reactions have been reported with therapeutic doses of ergotamine-containing drugs when co-administered with these antibiotics.

SSRI's

Weakness, hyperreflexia, and incoordination have been reported rarely when $5HT_1$ agonists have been co-administered with SSRI's (e.g., fluoxetine, fluvoxamine, paroxetine, sertraline). There have been no reported cases from spontaneous reports of drug interaction between SSRI's and Migranal® (dihydroergotamine mesylate, USP) Nasal Spray or D.H.E. 45®.

Oral Contraceptives

The effect of oral contraceptives on the pharmacokinetics of Migranal® (dihydroergotamine mesylate, USP) Nasal Spray has not been studied.

Carcinogenesis, Mutagenesis, Impairment of Fertility

Carcinogenesis

Assessment of the carcinogenic potential of dihydroergotamine mesylate in mice and rats is ongoing.

Mutagenesis

Dihydroergotamine mesylate was clastogenic in two *in vitro* chromosomal aberration assays, the V79 Chinese hamster cell assay with metabolic activation and the cultured human peripheral blood lymphocyte assay. There was no evidence of mutagenic potential when dihydroergotamine mesylate was tested in the presence or absence of metabolic activation in two gene mutation assays (the Ames test and the *in vitro* mammalian Chinese hamster V79/HGPRT assay) and in an assay for DNA damage (the rat hepatocyte unscheduled DNA synthesis test). Dihydroergotamine was not clastogenic in the *in vivo* mouse and hamster micronucleus tests.

Impairment of Fertility

There was no evidence of impairment of fertility in rats given intranasal doses of Migranal® (dihydroergotamine mesylate, USP) Nasal Spray up to 1.6 mg/day (associated with mean plasma dihydroergotamine mesylate exposures [AUC] approximately 9 to 11 times those in humans receiving the MRDD of 4 mg).

Pregnancy

Pregnancy Category X. *See CONTRAINDICATIONS.*

Nursing Mothers

Ergot drugs are known to inhibit prolactin. It is likely that Migranal® (dihydroergotamine mesylate, USP) Nasal Spray is excreted in human milk, but there are no data on the concentration of dihydroergotamine in human milk. It is known that ergotamine is excreted in breast milk and may cause vomiting, diarrhea, weak pulse, and unstable blood pressure in nursing infants. Because of the potential for these serious adverse events in nursing infants exposed to Migranal® (dihydroergotamine mesylate, USP) Nasal Spray, nursing should not be undertaken with the use of Migranal® (dihydroergotamine mesylate, USP) Nasal Spray. *(See CONTRAINDICATIONS)*

Pediatric Use

Safety and effectiveness in pediatric patients have not been established.

Use in the Elderly

There is no information about the safety and effectiveness of Migranal® (dihydroergotamine mesylate, USP) Nasal Spray in this population because patients over age 65 were excluded from the controlled clinical trials.

ADVERSE REACTIONS

During clinical studies and the foreign postmarketing experience with Migranal® (dihydroergotamine mesylate, USP) Nasal Spray there have been no fatalities due to cardiac events.

Serious cardiac events, including some that have been fatal, have occurred following use of the parenteral form of dihydroergotamine mesylate (D.H.E. 45® Injection), but are extremely rare. Events reported have included coronary artery vasospasm, transient myocardial ischemia, myocardial infarction, ventricular tachycardia, and ventricular fibrillation. *(See CONTRAINDICATIONS, WARNINGS, and PRECAUTIONS)*

Incidence in Controlled Clinical Trials

Of the 1,796 patients and subjects treated with Migranal® (dihydroergotamine mesylate, USP) Nasal Spray doses 2 mg or less in U.S. and foreign clinical studies, 26 (1.4%) discontinued because of adverse events.

The adverse events associated with discontinuation were, in decreasing order of frequency: rhinitis 13, dizziness 2, facial edema 2, and one each due to cold sweats, accidental trauma, depression, elective surgery, somnolence, allergy, vomiting, hypotension, and paraesthesia.

The most commonly reported adverse events associated with the use of Migranal® (dihydroergotamine mesylate, USP) Nasal Spray during placebo-controlled, double-blind studies for the treatment of migraine headache and not reported at an equal incidence by placebo-treated patients were rhinitis, altered sense of taste, application site reactions, dizziness, nausea, and vomiting. The events cited reflect experience gained under closely monitored conditions of clinical trials in a highly selected patient population. In actual clinical practice or in other clinical trials, these frequency estimates may not apply, as the conditions of use, reporting behavior, and the kinds of patients treated may differ.

Migranal® (dihydroergotamine mesylate, USP) Nasal Spray was generally well tolerated. In most instances these events were transient and self-limited and did not result in patient discontinuation from a study. The following table summarizes the incidence rates of adverse events reported by at least 1% of patients who received Migranal®

Continued on next page

Migranal—Cont.

(dihydroergotamine mesylate, USP) Nasal Spray for the treatment of migraine headaches during placebo-controlled, double-blind clinical studies and were more frequent than in those patients receiving placebo.

Table 3: Adverse events reported by at least 1% of the Migranal® (dihydroergotamine mesylate, USP) Nasal Spray treated patients and occurred more frequently than in the placebo-group in the migraine placebo-controlled trials

	Migranal® N=597	Placebo N=631
Respiratory System		
Rhinitis	26%	7%
Pharyngitis	3%	1%
Sinusitis	1%	1%
Gastrointestinal System		
Nausea	10%	4%
Vomiting	4%	1%
Diarrhea	2%	<1%
Special Senses, Other		
Altered Sense of Taste	8%	1%
Application Site		
Application Site Reaction	6%	2%
Central and Peripheral Nervous System		
Dizziness	4%	2%
Somnolence	3%	2%
Paraesthesia	2%	2%
Body as a Whole, General		
Hot Flushes	1%	<1%
Fatigue	1%	1%
Asthenia	1%	0%
Autonomic Nervous System		
Mouth Dry	1%	1%
Musculoskeletal System		
Stiffness	1%	<1%

Other Adverse Events During Clinical Trials

In the paragraphs that follow, the frequencies of less commonly reported adverse clinical events are presented. Because the reports include events observed in open and uncontrolled studies, the role of Migranal® (dihydroergotamine mesylate, USP) Nasal Spray in their causation cannot be reliably determined. Furthermore, variability associated with adverse event reporting, the terminology used to describe adverse events, etc., limit the value of the quantitative frequency estimates provided. Event frequencies are calculated as the number of patients who used Migranal® (dihydroergotamine mesylate, USP) Nasal Spray in placebo-controlled trials and reported an event divided by the total number of patients (n=1796) exposed to Migranal® (dihydroergotamine mesylate, USP) Nasal Spray. All reported events are included except those already listed in the previous table, those too general to be informative, and those not reasonably associated with the use of the drug. Events are further classified within body system categories and enumerated in order of decreasing frequency using the following definitions: frequent adverse events are defined as those occurring in at least 1/100 patients; infrequent adverse events are those occurring in 1/100 to 1/1,000 patients; and rare adverse events are those occurring in fewer than 1/1,000 patients.

Skin and Appendages: *Infrequent:* petechia, pruritus, rash, cold clammy skin; *Rare:* papular rash, urticaria, herpes simplex.

Musculoskeletal: *Infrequent:* cramps, myalgia, muscular weakness, dystonia; *Rare:* arthralgia, involuntary muscle contractions, rigidity.

Central and Peripheral Nervous System: *Infrequent:* confusion, tremor, hypoesthesia, vertigo; *Rare:* speech disorder, hyperkinesia, stupor, abnormal gait, aggravated migraine.

Autonomic Nervous System: *Infrequent:* increased sweating.

Special Senses: *Infrequent:* sense of smell altered, photophobia, conjunctivitis, abnormal lacrimation, abnormal vision, tinnitus, earache; *Rare:* eye pain.

Psychiatric: *Infrequent:* nervousness, euphoria, insomnia, concentration impaired; *Rare:* anxiety, anorexia, depression.

Gastrointestinal: *Infrequent:* abdominal pain, dyspepsia, dysphagia, hiccup; *Rare:* increased salivation, esophagospasm.

Cardiovascular: *Infrequent:* edema, palpitation, tachycardia; *Rare:* hypotension, peripheral ischemia, angina.

Respiratory System: *Infrequent:* dyspnea, upper respiratory tract infections; *Rare:* bronchospasm, bronchitis, pleural pain, epistaxis.

Urinary System: *Infrequent:* increased frequency of micturition, cystitis.

Reproductive, Female: *Rare:* pelvic inflammation, vaginitis.

Body as a Whole - General: *Infrequent:* feeling cold, malaise, rigors, fever, periorbital edema; *Rare:* flu-like symptoms, shock, loss of voice, yawning.

Application Site: *Infrequent:* local anesthesia.

Post-introduction Reports

Voluntary reports of adverse events temporally associated with dihydroergotamine products used in the management of migraine that have been received since the introduction of the injectable formulation are included in this section save for those already listed above. Because of their source (open and uncontrolled clinical use), whether or not events reported in association with the use of dihydroergotamine are causally related to it cannot be determined.

There have been reports of pleural and retroperitoneal fibrosis in patients following prolonged daily use of injectable dihydroergotamine mesylate. Migranal® (dihydroergotamine mesylate, USP) Nasal Spray is not recommended for prolonged daily use. *(See DOSAGE AND ADMINISTRATION)*

DRUG ABUSE AND DEPENDENCE

Currently available data have not demonstrated drug abuse or psychological dependence with dihydroergotamine. However, cases of drug abuse and psychological dependence in patients on other forms of ergot therapy have been reported. Thus, due to the chronicity of vascular headaches, it is imperative that patients be advised not to exceed recommended dosages.

OVERDOSAGE

To date, there have been no reports of acute overdosage with this drug. Due to the risk of vascular spasm, exceeding the recommended dosages of Migranal® (dihydroergotamine mesylate, USP) Nasal Spray is to be avoided. Excessive doses of dihydroergotamine may result in peripheral signs and symptoms of ergotism. Treatment includes discontinuance of the drug, local application of warmth to the affected area, the administration of vasodilators, and nursing care to prevent tissue damage.

In general, the symptoms of an acute Migranal® (dihydroergotamine mesylate, USP) Nasal Spray overdose are similar to those of an ergotamine overdose, although there is less pronounced nausea and vomiting with Migranal® (dihydroergotamine mesylate, USP) Nasal Spray. The symptoms of an ergotamine overdose include the following: numbness, tingling, pain, and cyanosis of the extremities associated with diminished or absent peripheral pulses; respiratory depression; an increase and/or decrease in blood pressure, usually in that order; confusion, delirium, convulsions, and coma; and/or some degree of nausea, vomiting, and abdominal pain.

In laboratory animals, significant lethality occurs when dihydroergotamine is given at I.V. doses of 44 mg/kg in mice, 130 mg/kg in rats, and 37 mg/kg in rabbits.

Up-to-date information about the treatment of overdosage can often be obtained from a certified Regional Poison Control Center. Telephone numbers of certified Poison Control Centers are listed in the Physicians' Desk Reference® (PDR).*

DOSAGE AND ADMINISTRATION

The solution used in Migranal® (dihydroergotamine mesylate, USP) Nasal Spray (4 mg/mL) is intended for intranasal use and must not be injected.

In clinical trials, Migranal® (dihydroergotamine mesylate, USP) Nasal Spray has been effective for the acute treatment of migraine headaches with or without aura. One spray (0.5 mg) of Migranal® (dihydroergotamine mesylate, USP) Nasal Spray should be administered in each nostril. Fifteen minutes later, an additional one spray (0.5 mg) of Migranal® (dihydroergotamine mesylate, USP) Nasal Spray should be administered in each nostril, for a total dosage of four sprays (2.0 mg) of Migranal® (dihydroergotamine mesylate, USP) Nasal Spray. Studies have shown no additional benefit from acute doses greater than 2.0 mg for a single migraine administration. The safety of doses greater than 3.0 mg in a 24 hour period and 4.0 mg in a 7 day period has not been established.

Prior to administration, the pump must be primed (i.e., squeeze 4 times) before use. *(See Patient Information Sheet or Patient Instruction Booklet)*

Once the nasal spray applicator has been prepared, it should be discarded (with any remaining drug in opened ampul) after 8 hours.

HOW SUPPLIED

Migranal® (dihydroergotamine mesylate, USP) Nasal Spray is available (as a clear, colorless to faintly yellow solution) in 1 mL amber glass ampuls containing 4 mg of dihydroergotamine mesylate, USP (NDC 0078-0245-98).

Migranal® (dihydroergotamine mesylate, USP) Nasal Spray is provided in individual kits. The kits consist of four unit dose trays, a patient instruction booklet, one assembly case, and one patient information sheet packed in a carton. Each unit dose tray contains one ampul, a nasal spray applicator, and a breaker cap on the ampul.

Store below 77°F (25°C). Do not refrigerate or freeze.

Patient Information

Information for the Patient

Migranal® (dihydroergotamine mesylate, USP) Nasal Spray.

The solution used in Migranal® (dihydroergotamine mesylate, USP) Nasal Spray (4 mg/mL) is intended for intranasal use and must not be injected.

Please read this information carefully before using your Migranal® (dihydroergotamine mesylate, USP) Nasal Spray for the first time. Keep this information handy for future reference. This leaflet does not contain all of the information on Migranal® (dihydroergotamine mesylate, USP) Nasal Spray. Your pharmacist and/or health care provider can provide more detailed information.

Migranal® (dihydroergotamine mesylate, USP) Nasal Spray has been evaluated in a limited number of patients long term (e.g., 1 year or longer).

Purpose of your Medication

Migranal® (dihydroergotamine mesylate, USP) Nasal Spray is intended to treat an active migraine headache. Do not try to use it to prevent a headache if you have no symptoms. Do not use it to treat common tension headache or a headache that is not at all typical of your usual migraine headache.

Do not use Migranal® (dihydroergotamine mesylate, USP) Nasal Spray if you:

- are pregnant or nursing.
- have any disease affecting your heart, arteries, or circulation.

Important questions to consider before using Migranal® (dihydroergotamine mesylate, USP) Nasal Spray

Please answer the following questions before you use your Migranal® (dihydroergotamine mesylate, USP) Nasal Spray. If you answer YES to any of these questions or are unsure of the answer, you should talk to your doctor before using Migranal® (dihydroergotamine mesylate, USP) Nasal Spray.

- Do you have high blood pressure?
- Do you have chest pain, shortness of breath, heart disease, or have you had any surgery on your heart arteries?
- Do you have risk factors for heart disease (such as high blood pressure, high cholesterol, obesity, diabetes, smoking, strong family history of heart disease, or you are postmenopausal or a male over 40)?
- Do you have any problems with blood circulation in your arms or legs, fingers, or toes?
- Are you pregnant? Do you think you might be pregnant? Are you trying to become pregnant? Are you sexually active and not using birth control? Are you breast feeding?
- Have you ever had to stop taking this or any other medication because of an allergy or bad reaction?
- Are you taking any other migraine medications, erythromycin or other antibiotics, or medications for blood pressure prescribed by your doctor, or other medicines obtained from your drugstore without a doctor's prescription?
- Do you smoke?
- Have you had, or do you have, any disease of the liver or kidney?
- Is this headache different from your usual migraine attacks?

REMEMBER TO TELL YOUR DOCTOR IF YOU HAVE ANSWERED YES TO ANY OF THESE QUESTIONS BEFORE YOU USE MIGRANAL® (dihydroergotamine mesylate, USP) NASAL SPRAY.

Side Effects To Watch Out For

In clinical trials, most migraine patients have used Migranal® (dihydroergotamine mesylate, USP) Nasal Spray without serious side effects. You may experience some nasal congestion or irritation, altered sense of taste, sore throat, nausea, vomiting, dizziness, and fatigue after using Migranal® (dihydroergotamine mesylate, USP) Nasal Spray. These side effects are temporary and usually do not require you to stop using Migranal® (dihydroergotamine mesylate, USP) Nasal Spray. Although the following reactions rarely occur, they can be serious and should be reported to your physician immediately:

- Numbness or tingling in your fingers and toes
- Pain, tightness, or discomfort in your chest
- Muscle pain or cramps in your arms and legs
- Weakness in your legs
- Temporary speeding or slowing of your heart rate
- Swelling or itching

Dosing Information

- Each ampul contains one complete dose of Migranal® (dihydroergotamine mesylate, USP) Nasal Spray, which is 1 spray in each nostril followed in 15 minutes by an additional spray in each nostril, for a total of 4 sprays.
- Studies have shown no benefit from acute doses greater than 2.0 mg (4 sprays) for a single administration. The safety of doses greater than 3.0 mg in a 24 hour period has not been established.
- The safety of doses greater than 4.0 mg in a 7-day period has not been established.

Learn what to do in case of an Overdose

If you have used more medication than you have been instructed, contact your doctor, hospital emergency department, or nearest poison control center immediately.

How to use the Migranal® (dihydroergotamine mesylate, USP) Nasal Spray

1. Use available training materials.
   - Read and follow the instructions in the patient instruction booklet which is provided with the Migranal® (dihydroergotamine mesylate, USP) Nasal Spray package before attempting to use the product.
   - If there are any questions concerning the use of your Migranal® (dihydroergotamine mesylate, USP) Nasal Spray, ask your doctor or pharmacist, or call the Migranal® (dihydroergotamine mesylate, USP) Nasal Spray Information Line at 1-888-MY-RELIEF (1-888-697-3543) for training in the use of the spray.
2. Check the contents of the package.
   - Assembly Case
   - Well (which is part of the Assembly Case)
   - Unit Dose Tray

- Brown (amber) glass ampul with yellow breaker cap
- Nasal Sprayer with cover

3. Assemble the sprayer.

Assemble your Nasal Sprayer only when you are ready to use it.

- Tap top of ampul until all medication is in the bottom.
- Place ampul upright and straight in well of the Assembly Case with breaker cap pointing up.
- Push down the Assembly Case lid slowly but firmly, until you hear ampul snap open.
- Without removing ampul from well, push Nasal Sprayer onto ampul until it clicks. (To ensure that the ampul fits properly into the Nasal Sprayer, first look at the tube through the bottom of sprayer to make sure it is straight. If it is curved, straighten it with your finger.)

4. Using the sprayer:

- Remove cover from the Nasal Sprayer.
- Pump the Nasal Sprayer 4 times before using. (Point the Nasal Sprayer up and away from your face when pumping.) *Do not* prime the Nasal Sprayer more than 4 times. Although some medication will spray out, there is enough medication in each ampul to allow you to prepare your sprayer properly and still receive a full dose of Migranal® (dihydroergotamine mesylate, USP) Nasal Spray.
- Spray once in each nostril. You should not tilt head back or inhale through your nose while spraying.
- Wait 15 minutes, then spray once in each nostril again.

5. After completing these instructions:

- Carefully dispose of the Nasal Sprayer containing the ampul and the breaker cap containing the top of the ampul.
- Load a new Unit Dose Tray into your Assembly Case.
- Keep the Assembly Case for a maximum of 4 treatments, then discard it along with the Unit Dose Tray.

Important Notes:

- Once a Migranal® (dihydroergotamine mesylate, USP) Nasal Spray ampul has been opened, it must be thrown away after 8 hours.
- You should not sniff or tilt your head back when using Migranal® (dihydroergotamine mesylate, USP) Nasal Spray.

Storing Migranal® (dihydroergotamine mesylate, USP) Nasal Spray

- Keep medication in a safe place away from children.
- Keep Migranal® (dihydroergotamine mesylate, USP) Nasal Spray away from heat and light.
  - —Do not expose Migranal® (dihydroergotamine mesylate, USP) Nasal Spray to temperatures over 77°F.
  - —Never refrigerate or freeze Migranal® (dihydroergotamine mesylate, USP) Nasal Spray.
- Keep Migranal® (dihydroergotamine mesylate, USP) Nasal Spray components in the Unit Dose Tray.
- Keep the Unit Dose Tray loaded in the Assembly Case.
- Do not keep an opened Migranal® (dihydroergotamine mesylate, USP) Nasal Spray ampul for more than 8 hours.

Check the expiration date printed on the ampul containing medication. If the expiration date has passed, do not use it.

Answers to patients' questions about Migranal® (dihydroergotamine mesylate, USP) Nasal Spray

What if I need help in using my Migranal® (dihydroergotamine mesylate, USP) Nasal Spray?

If you have any questions or if you need help in opening, putting together, or using Migranal® (dihydroergotamine mesylate, USP) Nasal Spray, speak to your doctor or pharmacist, or call the Migranal® (dihydroergotamine mesylate, USP) Nasal Spray Information Line at 1-888-MY-RELIEF (1-888-697-3543).

How much medication should I use and how often?

Each ampul contains one complete dose of Migranal® (dihydroergotamine mesylate, USP) Nasal Spray, which is 1 spray in each nostril, followed by an additional spray in each nostril 15 minutes later for a total of 4 sprays. Do not use more than this amount unless instructed to do so by your doctor.

Why do I have to prime or pump the Nasal Sprayer 4 times before using? Am I wasting the medication?

You have to prime the Nasal Sprayer 4 times to make sure that you get the proper amount of medication when you use it. Although you will see some medication spray out, there is still enough medication in each ampul to allow you to prepare your sprayer properly and still receive a full dose of Migranal® (dihydroergotamine mesylate, USP) Nasal Spray.

Can I load the medication ampul into the Nasal Sprayer so it is ready before I need to use it?

No. The brown (amber) glass ampul containing your medication must remain unopened until you are ready to use it. It may not be fully effective if opened and not used within 8 hours. However, after each migraine attack, you should load a new plastic Unit Dose Tray containing an unopened Migranal® (dihydroergotamine mesylate, USP) Nasal Spray ampul and Nasal Sprayer into the Migranal® (dihydroergotamine mesylate, USP) Nasal Spray Assembly Case, so you will be prepared for your next migraine attack.

Can I reuse my Migranal® (dihydroergotamine mesylate, USP) Nasal Sprayer?

No. After completing the full dose, you must carefully dispose of your Migranal® (dihydroergotamine mesylate, USP) Nasal Sprayer containing the opened ampul. Each Unit Dose Tray contains a new Nasal Sprayer, an ampul of Migranal® (dihydroergotamine mesylate, USP) Nasal Spray medication, and a breaker cap on the ampul. But you should keep your Assembly Case and load it with a new Unit Dose Tray after each migraine so you are ready to treat your next migraine attack.

Can I use Migranal® (dihydroergotamine mesylate, USP) Nasal Spray if I have a stuffy nose, cold, or allergies?

Yes. Migranal® (dihydroergotamine mesylate, USP) Nasal Spray can be used if you have a stuffy nose, cold, or allergies. However, if you are taking any medications for your cold, or allergies, even those you can buy without a doctor's prescription, speak with your doctor before using Migranal® (dihydroergotamine mesylate, USP) Nasal Spray.

Do I need to sniff the medication when I spray it in my nostril?

No, you should not sniff because Migranal® (dihydroergotamine mesylate, USP) Nasal Spray should remain in the nose so that it can be absorbed into the bloodstream through the lining of the nose.

If you have any other unanswered question about Migranal® (dihydroergotamine mesylate, USP) Nasal Spray, consult your doctor or pharmacist.

*Trademark of Medical Economics Company, Inc.

DECEMBER 1997 30721901

Shown in Product Identification Guide, page 326

NEORAL® Soft Gelatin Capsules ℞

[nē ō 'ral]

(cyclosporine capsules, USP) MODIFIED

NEORAL® Oral Solution

(cyclosporine oral solution, USP) MODIFIED

Rx only

The following prescribing information is based on official labeling in effect July 2000.

WARNING

Only physicians experienced in management of systemic immunosuppressive therapy for the indicated disease should prescribe Neoral®. At doses used in solid organ transplantation, only physicians experienced in immunosuppressive therapy and management of organ transplant recipients should prescribe Neoral®. Patients receiving the drug should be managed in facilities equippped and staffed with adequate laboratory and supportive medical resources. The physician responsible for maintenance therapy should have complete information requisite for the follow-up of the patient.

Neoral®, a systemic immunosuppressant, may increase the susceptibility to infection and the development of neoplasia. In kidney, liver, and heart transplant patients Neoral® may be administered with other immunosuppressive agents. Increased susceptibility to infection and the possible development of lymphoma and other neoplasma may result from the increase in the degree of immunosuppression in transplant patients.

Neoral® Soft Gelatin Capsules (cyclosporine capsules, USP) MODIFIED and Neoral® Oral Solution (cyclosporine oral solution, USP) MODIFIED have increased bioavailability in comparison to Sandimmune® Soft Gelatin Capsules (cyclosporine capsules, USP) and Sandimmune® Oral Solution (cyclosporine oral solution, USP). Neoral® and Sandimmune® are not bioequivalent and cannot be used interchangeably without physician supervision. For a given trough concentration, cyclosporine exposure will be greater with Neoral® than with Sandimmune®. If a patient who is receiving exceptionally high doses of Sandimmune® is converted to Neoral®, particular caution should be exercised. Cyclosporine blood concentrations should be monitored in transplant and rheumatoid arthritis patients taking Neoral® to avoid toxicity due to high concentrations. Dose adjustments should be made in transplant patients to minimize possible organ rejection due to low concentrations. Comparison of blood concentrations in the published literature with blood concentrations obtained using current assays must be done with detailed knowledge of the assay methods employed.

For Psoriasis Patients *(See also Boxed* WARNINGS *above)*

Psoriasis patients previously treated with PUVA and to a lesser extent, methotrexate or other immunosuppressive agents, UVB, coal, tar, or radiation therapy, are at an increased risk of developing skin malignancies when taking Neoral®.

Cyclosporine, the active ingredient in Neoral®, in recommended dosages, can cause systemic hypertension and nephrotoxicity. The risk increases with increasing dose and duration of cyclosporine therapy. Renal dysfunction, including structural kidney damage, is a potential consequence of cyclosporine, and therefore, renal function must be monitored during therapy.

DESCRIPTION

Neoral® is an oral formulation of cyclosporine that immediately forms a microemulsion in an aqueous environment.

Cyclosporine, the active principle in Neoral®, is a cyclic polypeptide immunosuppressant agent consisting of 11 amino acids. It is produced as a metabolite by the fungus species *Beauveria nivea*.

Chemically, cyclosporine is designated as [*R*-[*R**,*R**-(*E*)]]-cyclic-(L-alanyl-D-alanyl-*N*-methyl-L-leucyl-*N*-methyl-L-leucyl-*N*-methyl-L-valyl-3-hydroxy-*N*,4-dimethyl-L-2-amino-6-octenoyl-L-α-amino-butyryl-*N*-methylglycyl-*N*-methyl-L-leucyl-L-valyl-*N*-methyl-L-leucyl).

Neoral® Soft Gelatin Capsules (cyclosporine capsules, USP) MODIFIED are available in 25 mg and 100 mg strengths.

Each 25 mg capsule contains:

cyclosporine .... 25 mg
alcohol, USP dehydrated .... 11.9% v/v (9.5% wt/vol.)

Each 100 mg capsule contains:

cyclosporine .... 100 mg
alcohol, USP dehydrated .... 11.9% v/v (9.5% wt/vol.)

Inactive Ingredients: Corn oil-mono-di-triglycerides, polyoxyl 40 hydrogenated castor oil NF, DL-α-tocopherol USP, gelatin NF, glycerol, iron oxide black, propylene glycol USP, titanium dioxide USP, carmine, and other ingredients.

Neoral® Oral Solution (cyclosporine oral solution, USP) MODIFIED is available in 50 mL bottles.

Each mL contains:

cyclosporine .... 100 mg/mL
alcohol, USP dehydrated .... 11.9% v/v (9.5% wt/vol.)

Inactive Ingredients: Corn oil-mono-di-triglycerides, polyoxyl 40 hydrogenated castor oil NF, DL-α-tocopherol USP, propylene glycol USP.

The chemical structure of cyclosporine (also known as cyclosporin A) is:

```
          H3C
             \
              CH
              ||
             HC
               \
                CH2
           H    |
       HO  |   CH-CH3
          \C/
           |
MeVal-N-CH-C-Abu-MeGly
   |  |    ||       |
MeLeu CH3  O      MeLeu
   |                |
MeLeu-D-Ala-Ala-MeLeu-Val
```

$C_{62}H_{111}N_{11}O_{12}$ Mol. Wt. 1202.63

CLINICAL PHARMACOLOGY: Cyclosporine is a potent immunosuppressive agent that in animals prolongs survival of allogeneic transplants involving skin, kidney, liver, heart, pancreas, bone marrow, small intestine, and lung. Cyclosporine has been demonstrated to suppress some humoral immunity and to a greater extent, cell-mediated immune reactions such as allograft rejection, delayed hypersensitivity, experimental allergic encephalomyelitis, Freund's adjuvant arthritis, and graft vs. host disease in many animal species for a variety of organs.

The effectiveness of cyclosporine results from specific and reversible inhibition of immunocompetent lymphocytes in the G_0- and G_1-phase of the cell cycle. T-lymphocytes are preferentially inhibited. The T-helper cell is the main target, although the T-suppressor cell may also be suppressed. Cyclosporine also inhibits lymphokine production and release including interleukin-2.

No effects on phagocytic function (changes in enzyme secretions, chemotactic migration of granulocytes, macrophage migration, carbon clearance *in vivo*) have been detected in animals. Cyclosporine does not cause bone marrow suppression in animal models or man.

Pharmacokinetics: The immunosuppressive activity of cyclosporine is primarily due to parent drug. Following oral administration, absorption of cyclosporine is incomplete. The extent of absorption of cyclosporine is dependent on the individual patient, the patient population, and the formulation. Elimination of cyclosporine is primarily biliary with only 6% of the dose (parent drug and metabolites) excreted in urine. The disposition of cyclosporine from blood is generally biphasic, with a terminal half-life of approximately 8.4 hours (range 5-18 hours). Following intravenous administration, the blood clearance of cyclosporine (assay: HPLC) is approximately 5-7 mL/min/kg in adult recipients of renal or liver allografts. Blood cyclosporine clearance appears to be slightly slower in cardiac transplant patients.

The Neoral® Soft Gelatin Capsules (cyclosporine capsules, USP) MODIFIED and Neoral® Oral Solution (cyclosporine oral solution, USP) MODIFIED are bioequivalent.

The relationship between administered dose and exposure (area under the concentration versus time curve, AUC) is linear within the therapeutic dose range. The intersubject variability (total, %CV) of cyclosporine exposure (AUC) when Neoral® or Sandimmune® is administered ranges from approximately 20% to 50% in renal transplant patients. This intersubject variability contributes to the need for individualization of the dosing regimen for optimal therapy (see *DOSAGE AND ADMINISTRATION*). Intrasubject variability of AUC in renal transplant recipients (%CV) was 9%-21% for Neoral® and 19%-26% for Sandimmune®. In the same studies, intrasubject variability of trough concentrations (%CV) was 17%-30% for Neoral® and 16%-38% for Sandimmune®.

Absorption: Neoral® has increased bioavailability compared to Sandimmune®. The absolute bioavailability of

Continued on next page

Neoral—Cont.

cyclosporine administered as Sandimmune® is dependent on the patient population, estimated to be less than 10% in liver transplant patients and as great as 89% in some renal transplant patients. The absolute bioavailability of cyclosporine administered as Neoral® has not been determined in adults. In studies of renal transplant, rheumatoid arthritis and psoriasis patients, the mean cyclosporine AUC was approximately 20% to 50% greater and the peak blood cyclosporine concentration (C_{max}) was approximately 40% to 106% greater following administration of Neoral® compared to following administration of Sandimmune®. The dose normalized AUC in *de novo* liver transplant patients administered Neoral® 28 days after transplantation was 50% greater and C_{max} was 90% greater than in those patients administered Sandimmune®. AUC and C_{max} are also increased (Neoral® relative to Sandimmune®) in heart transplant patients, but data are very limited. Although the AUC and C_{max} values are higher on Neoral® relative to Sandimmune®, the pre-dose trough concentrations (dose-normalized) are similar for the two formulations.

Following oral administration of Neoral®, the time to peak blood cyclosporine concentrations (T_{max}) ranged from 1.5-2.0 hours. The administration of food with Neoral® decreases the cyclosporine AUC and C_{max}. A high fat meal (669 kcal, 45 grams fat) consumed within one-half hour before Neoral® administration decreased the AUC by 13% and C_{max} by 33%. The effects of a low fat meal (667 kcal, 15 grams fat) were similar.

The effect of T-tube diversion of bile on the absorption of cyclosporine from Neoral® was investigated in eleven *de novo* liver transplant patients. When the patients were administered Neoral® with and without T-tube diversion of bile, very little difference in absorption was observed, as measured by the change in maximal cyclosporine blood concentrations from pre-dose values with the T-tube closed relative to when it was open: 6.9±41% (range -55% to 68%).

[See first table above]

Pharmacokinetic Parameters (mean ± SD)

Patient Population	Dose/day[1] (mg/d)	Dose/weight (mg/kg/d)	AUC[2] (ng•hr/mL)	C_{max} (ng/mL)	Trough[3] (ng/mL)	CL/F (mL/min)	CL/F (mL/min/kg)
De novo renal transplant[4] Week 4 (N=37)	597±174	7.95±2.81	8772±2089	1802±428	361±129	593±204	7.8±2.9
Stable renal transplant[4] (N=55)	344±122	4.10±1.58	6035±2194	1333±469	251±116	492±140	5.9±2.1
De novo liver transplant[5] Week 4 (N=18)	458±190	6.89±3.68	7187±2816	1555±740	268±101	577±309	8.6±5.7
De novo rheumatoid arthritis[6] (N=23)	182±55.6	2.37±0.36	2641±877	728±263	96.4±37.7	613±196	8.3±2.8
De novo psoriasis[6] Week 4 (N=18)	189±69.8	2.48±0.65	2324±1048	655±186	74.9±46.7	723±186	10.2±3.9

[1] Total daily dose was divided into two doses administered every 12 hours
[2] AUC was measured over one dosing interval
[3] Trough concentration was measured just prior to the morning Neoral® dose, approximately 12 hours after the previous dose
[4] Assay: TDx specific monoclonal fluorescence polarization immunoassay
[5] Assay: Cyclo-trac specific monoclonal radioimmunoassay
[6] Assay: INCSTAR specific monoclonal radioimmunoassay

Distribution: Cyclosporine is distributed largely outside the blood volume. The steady state volume of distribution during intravenous dosing has been reported as 3-5 L/kg in solid organ transplant recipients. In blood, the distribution is concentration dependent. Approximately 33%-47% is in plasma, 4%-9% in lymphocytes, 5%-12% in granulocytes, and 41%-58% in erythrocytes. At high concentrations, the binding capacity of leukocytes and erythrocytes becomes saturated. In plasma, approximately 90% is bound to proteins, primarily lipoproteins. Cyclosporine is excreted in human milk. (See *PRECAUTIONS, Nursing Mothers*)

Metabolism: Cyclosporine is extensively metabolized by the cytochrome P-450 III-A enzyme system in the liver, and to a lesser degree in the gastrointestinal tract, and the kidney. The metabolism of cyclosporine can be altered by the coadministration of a variety of agents. (See *PRECAUTIONS, Drug Interactions*) At least 25 metabolites have been identified from human bile, feces, blood, and urine. The biological activity of the metabolites and their contributions to toxicity are considerably less than those of the parent compound. The major metabolites (M1, M9, and M4N) result from oxidation at the 1-beta, 9-gamma, and 4-N-demethylated positions, respectively. At steady state following the oral administration of Sandimmune®, the mean AUCs for blood concentrations of M1, M9, and M4N are about 70%, 21%, and 7.5% of the AUC for blood cyclosporine concentrations, respectively. Based on blood concentration data from stable renal transplant patients (13 patients administered Neoral® and Sandimmune® in a crossover study), and bile concentration data from *de novo* liver transplant patients (4 administered Neoral®, 3 administered Sandimmune®), the percentage of dose present as M1, M9, and M4N metabolites is similar when either Neoral® or Sandimmune® is administered.

Excretion: Only 0.1% of a cyclosporine dose is excreted unchanged in the urine. Elimination is primarily biliary with only 6% of the dose (parent drug and metabolites) excreted in the urine. Neither dialysis nor renal failure alter cyclosporine clearance significantly.

Drug Interactions: (See *PRECAUTIONS, Drug Interactions*) When diclofenac or methotrexate was co-administered with cyclosporine in rheumatoid arthritis patients, the AUC of diclofenac and methotrexate, each was significantly increased. (See *PRECAUTIONS, Drug Interactions*) No clinically significant pharmacokinetic interactions occurred between cyclosporine and aspirin, ketoprofen, piroxicam, or indomethacin.

Special Populations: ***Pediatric Population:*** Pharmacokinetic data from pediatric patients administered Neoral® or Sandimmune® are very limited. In 15 renal transplant patients aged 3-16 years, cyclosporine whole blood clearance after IV administration of Sandimmune® was 10.6±3.7 mL/min/kg (assay: Cyclo-trac specific RIA). In a study of 7 renal transplant patients aged 2-16, the cyclosporine clearance ranged from 9.8-15.5 mL/min/kg. In 9 liver transplant patients aged 0.6-5.6 years, clearance was 9.3±5.4 mL/min/kg (assay: HPLC).

In the pediatric population, Neoral® also demonstrates an increased bioavailability as compared to Sandimmune®. In 7 liver *de novo* transplant patients aged 1.4-10 years, the absolute bioavailability of Neoral® was 43% (range 30%-68%) and for Sandimmune® in the same individuals absolute bioavailability was 28% (range 17%-42%).

[See second table above]

Pediatric Pharmacokinetic Parameters (mean ± SD)

Patient Population	Dose/day (mg/d)	Dose/weight (mg/kg/d)	AUC[1] (ng•hr/mL)	C_{max} (ng/mL)	CL/F (mL/min)	CL/F (mL/min/kg)
Stable renal transplant[2]						
Age 2-8, Dosed TID (N=9)	101±25	5.95±1.32	2163±801	629±219	285±94	16.6±4.3
Age 8-15, Dosed BID (N=8)	188±55	4.96±2.09	4272±1462	975±281	378±80	10.2±4.0
Stable liver transplant[3]						
Age 3, Dosed BID (N=1)	120	8.33	5832	1050	171	11.9
Age 8-15, Dosed BID (N=5)	158±55	5.51±1.91	4452±2475	1013±635	328±121	11.0±1.9
Stable liver transplant[3]						
Age 7-15, Dosed BID (N=5)	328±83	7.37±4.11	6922±1988	1827±487	418±143	8.7±2.9

[1] AUC was measured over one dosing interval
[2] Assay: Cyclo-trac specific monoclonal radioimmunoassay
[3] Assay: TDx specific monoclonal fluorescence polarization immunoassay

Geriatric Population: Comparison of single dose data from both normal elderly volunteers (N=18, mean age 69 years) and elderly rheumatoid arthritis patients (N=16, mean age 68 years) to single dose data in young adult volunteers (N=16, mean age 26 years) showed no significant difference in the pharmacokinetic parameters.

CLINICAL TRIALS: Rheumatoid Arthritis: The effectiveness of Sandimmune® and Neoral® in the treatment of severe rheumatoid arthritis was evaluated in 5 clinical studies involving a total of 728 cyclosporine treated patients and 273 placebo treated patients.

A summary of the results is presented for the "responder" rates per treatment group, with a responder being defined as a patient having *completed* the trial with a 20% improvement in the tender and the swollen joint count and a 20% improvement in 2 of 4 of investigator global, patient global, disability, and erythrocyte sedimentation rates (ESR) for the Studies 651 and 652 and 3 of 5 of investigator global, patient global, disability, visual analog pain, and ESR for Studies 2008, 654 and 302.

Study 651 enrolled 264 patients with active rheumatoid arthritis with at least 20 involved joints, who had failed at least one major RA drug, using a 3:3:2 randomization to one of the following three groups: (1) cyclosporine dosed at 2.5-5 mg/kg/day, (2) methotrexate at 7.5-15 mg/week, or (3) placebo. Treatment duration was 24 weeks. The mean cyclosporine dose at the last visit was 3.1 mg/kg/day. See Graph below.

Study 652 enrolled 250 patients with active RA with >6 active painful or tender joints who had failed at least one major RA drug. Patients were randomized using a 3:3:2 randomization to 1 of 3 treatment arms: (1) 1.5-5 mg/kg/day of cyclosporine, (2) 2.5-5 mg/kg/day of cyclosporine, and (3) placebo. Treatment duration was 16 weeks. The mean cyclosporine dose for group 2 at the last visit was 2.92 mg/kg/day. See Graph below.

Study 2008 enrolled 144 patients with active RA and >6 active joints who had unsuccessful treatment courses of aspirin and gold or Penicillamine. Patients were randomized to 1 of 2 treatment groups (1) cyclosporine 2.5-5 mg/kg/day with adjustments after the first month to achieve a target trough level and (2) placebo. Treatment duration was 24 weeks. The mean cyclosporine dose at the last visit was 3.63 mg/kg/day. See Graph below.

Study 654 enrolled 148 patients who remained with active joint counts of 6 or more despite treatment with maximally tolerated methotrexate doses for at least three months. Patients continued to take their current dose of methotrexate and were randomized to receive, in addition, one of the following medications: (1) cyclosporine 2.5 mg/kg/day with dose increases of 0.5 mg/kg/day at weeks 2 and 4 if there was no evidence of toxicity and further increases of 0.5 mg/kg/day at weeks 8 and 16 if a <30% decrease in active joint count occurred without any significant toxicity; dose decreases could be made at any time for toxicity or (2) placebo. Treatment duration was 24 weeks. The mean cyclosporine dose at the last visit was 2.8 mg/kg/day (range: 1.3-4.1). See Graph below.

Study 302 enrolled 299 patients with severe active RA, 99% of whom were unre sponsive or intolerant to at least one prior major RA drug. Patients were randomized to 1 of 2 treatment groups (1) Neoral® and (2) cyclosporine, both of which were started at 2.5 mg/kg/day and increased after 4 weeks for inefficacy in increments of 0.5 mg/kg/day to a maximum of 5 mg/kg/day and decreased at any time for toxicity. Treatment duration was 24 weeks. The mean cyclosporine dose at the last visit was 2.91 mg/kg/day (range: 0.72-5.17) for Neoral® and 3.27 mg/kg/day (range: 0.73-5.68) for cyclosporine. See Graph below.

[See graphic at top of next page]

INDICATIONS AND USAGE: Kidney, Liver, and Heart Transplantation: Neoral® is indicated for the prophylaxis of organ rejection in kidney, liver, and heart allogeneic transplants. Neoral® has been used in combination with azathioprine and corticosteroids.

Rheumatoid Arthritis: Neoral® is indicated for the treatment of patients with severe active, rheumatoid arthritis where the disease has not adequately responded to methotrexate. Neoral® can be used in combination with methotrexate in rheumatoid arthritis patients who do not respond adequately to methotrexate alone.

Psoriasis: Neoral® is indicated for the treatment of *adult, nonimmunocompromised* patients with severe (i.e., extensive and/or disabling), recalcitrant, plaque psoriasis who have failed to respond to at least one systemic therapy (eg., PUVA, retinoids, or methotrexate) or in patients for whom other systemic therapies are contraindicated, or cannot be tolerated.

While rebound rarely occurs, most patients will experience relapse with Neoral® as with other therapies upon cessation of treatment.

CONTRAINDICATIONS: General: Neoral® is contraindicated in patients with a hypersensitivity to cyclosporine or to any of the ingredients of the formulation.

Rheumatoid Arthritis: Rheumatoid arthritis patients with abnormal renal function, uncontrolled hypertension, or malignancies should not receive Neoral®.

Psoriasis: Psoriasis patients who are treated with Neoral® should not receive concomitant PUVA or UVB therapy, methotrexate or other immunosuppressive agents, coal tar or radiation therapy. Psoriasis patients with abnormal renal function, uncontrolled hypertension, or malignancies should not receive Neoral®.

WARNINGS: *(See also Boxed WARNING)* **All Patients:** Cyclosporine, the active ingredient of Neoral®, can cause nephrotoxicity and hepatotoxicity. The risk increases with increasing doses of cyclosporine. Renal dysfunction including structural kidney damage is a potential consequence of Neoral® and therefore renal function must be monitored during therapy. **Care should be taken in using cyclosporine with nephrotoxic drugs.** ***(See PRECAUTIONS)***

Patients receiving Neoral® require frequent monitoring of serum creatinine. *(See Special Monitoring under DOSAGE AND ADMINISTRATION)* Elderly patients should be monitored with particular care, since decreases in renal function also occur with age. If patients are not properly monitored and doses are not properly adjusted, cyclosporine therapy can be associated with the occurrence of structural kidney damage and persistent renal dysfunction.

An increase in serum creatinine and BUN may occur during Neoral® therapy and reflect a reduction in the glomerular filtration rate. Impaired renal function at any time requires close monitoring, and frequent dosage adjustment may be indicated. The frequency and severity of serum creatinine elevations increase with dose and duration of cyclosporine therapy. These elevations are likely to become more pronounced without dose reduction or discontinuation.

Because Neoral® is not bioequivalent to Sandimmune®, conversion from Neoral® to Sandimmune® using a 1:1 ratio (mg/kg/day) may result in lower cyclosporine blood concentrations. Conversion from Neoral® to Sandimmune® should be made with increased monitoring to avoid the potential of underdosing.

Kidney, Liver, and Heart Transplant: Cyclosporine, the active ingredient of Neoral®, can cause nephrotoxicity and hepatotoxicity when used in high doses. It is not unusual for serum creatinine and BUN levels to be elevated during cyclosporine therapy. These elevations in renal transplant patients do not necessarily indicate rejection, and each patient must be fully evaluated before dosage adjustment is initiated.

Based on the historical Sandimmune® experience with oral solution, nephrotoxicity associated with cyclosporine had been noted in 25% of cases of renal transplantation, 38% of cases of cardiac transplantation, and 37% of cases of liver transplantation. Mild nephrotoxicity was generally noted 2-3 months after renal transplant and consisted of an arrest in the fall of the pre-operative elevations of BUN and creatinine at a range of 35-45 mg/dl and 2.0-2.5 mg/dl respectively. These elevations were often responsive to cyclosporine dosage reduction.

More overt nephrotoxicity was seen early after transplantation and was characterized by a rapidly rising BUN and creatinine. Since these events are similar to renal rejection episodes, care must be taken to differentiate between them. This form of nephrotoxicity is usually responsive to cyclosporine dosage reduction.

Although specific diagnostic criteria which reliably differentiate renal graft rejection from drug toxicity have not been found, a number of parameters have been significantly associated with one or the other. It should be noted however, that up to 20% of patients may have simultaneous nephrotoxicity and rejection.

[See table above]

A form of a cyclosporine-associated nephropathy is characterized by serial deterioration in renal function and morphologic changes in the kidneys. From 5%-15% of transplant recipients who have received cyclosporine will fail to show a reduction in rising serum creatinine despite a decrease or discontinuation of cyclosporine therapy. Renal biopsies from these patients will demonstrate one or several of the following alterations: tubular vacuolization, tubular microcalcifications, peritubular capillary congestion, arteriolopathy, and a striped form of interstitial fibrosis with tubular atrophy. Though none of these morphologic changes is entirely specific, a diagnosis of cyclosporine-associated structural nephrotoxicity requires evidence of these findings.

When considering the development of cyclosporine-associated nephropathy, it is noteworthy that several authors have reported an association between the appearance of interstitial fibrosis and higher cumulative doses or persistently high circulating trough levels of cyclosporine. This is particularly true during the first 6 post-transplant months when the dosage tends to be highest and when, in kidney recipients, the organ appears to be most vulnerable to the toxic effects of cyclosporine. Among other contributing factors to the development of interstitial fibrosis in these patients are prolonged perfusion time, warm ischemia time, as well as episodes of acute toxicity, and acute and chronic rejection. The reversibility of interstitial fibrosis and its correlation to renal function have not yet been determined. Reversibility of arteriolopathy has been reported after stopping cyclosporine or lowering the dosage.

Impaired renal function at any time requires close monitoring, and frequent dosage adjustment may be indicated.

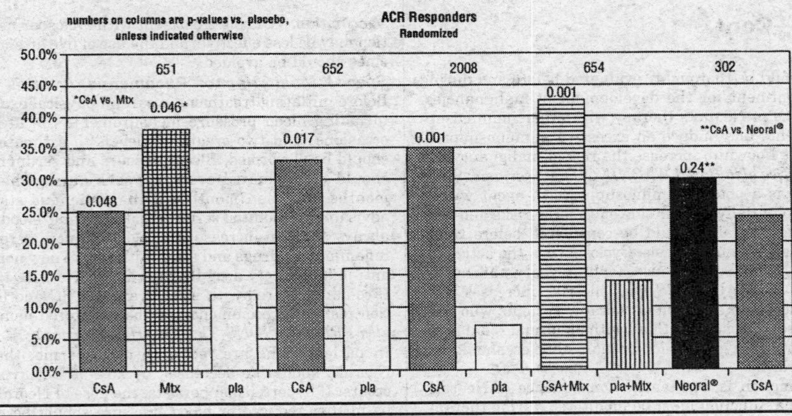

Nephrotoxicity vs. Rejection

Parameter	Nephrotoxicity	Rejection
History	Donor > 50 years old or hypotensive Prolonged kidney preservation Prolonged anastomosis time Concomitant nephrotoxic drugs	Anti-donor immune response Retransplant patient
Clinical	Often > 6 weeks postop[b] Prolonged initial nonfunction (acute tubular necrosis)	Often < 4 weeks postop[b] Fever > 37.5°C Weight gain > 0.5 kg Graft swelling and tenderness Decrease in daily urine volume > 500 mL (or 50%)
Laboratory	CyA serum trough level > 200 ng/mL Gradual rise in Cr (< 0.15 mg/dl/day)[a] Cr plateau < 25% above baseline BUN/Cr ≥ 20	CyA serum trough level < 150 ng/mL Rapid rise in Cr (> 0.3 mg/dl/day)[a] Cr > 25% above baseline BUN/Cr < 20
Biopsy	Arteriolopathy (medial hypertrophy[a], hyalinosis, nodular deposits, intimal thickening, endothelial vacuolization, progressive scarring) Tubular atrophy, isometric vacuolization, isolated calcifications Minimal edema Mild focal infiltrates[c] Diffuse interstitial fibrosis, often striped form	Endovasculitis[c] (proliferation[a], intimal arteritis[b], necrosis, sclerosis) Tubulitis with RBC[b] and WBC[b] casts, some irregular vacuolization Interstitial edema[c] and hemorrhage[b] Diffuse moderate to severe mononuclear infiltrates[d] Glomerulitis (mononuclear cells)[c]
Aspiration Cytology	CyA deposits in tubular and endothelial cells Fine isometric vacuolization of tubular cells	Inflammatory infiltrate with mononuclear phagocytes, macrophages, lymphoblastoid cells, and activated T-cells These strongly express HLA-DR antigens
Urine Cytology	Tubular cells with vacuolization and granularization	Degenerative tubular cells, plasma cells, and lymphocyturia > 20 % of sediment
Manometry	Intracapsular pressure < 40 mm Hg[b]	Intracapsular pressure > 40 mm Hg[b]
Ultrasonography	Unchanged graft cross sectional area	Increase in graft cross sectional area AP diameter ≥ Transverse diameter
Magnetic Resonance Imagery	Normal appearance	Loss of distinct corticomedullary junction, swelling image intensity of parachyma approaching that of psoas, loss of hilar fat
Radionuclide Scan	Normal or generally decreased perfusion Decrease in tubular function (^{131} I-hippuran) > decrease in perfusion (^{99m} Tc DTPA)	Patchy arterial flow Decrease in perfusion > decrease in tubular function Increased uptake of Indium 111 labeled platelets or Tc-99m in colloid
Therapy	Responds to decreased cyclosporine	Responds to increased steroids or antilymphocyte globulin

[a]$p < 0.05$, [b]$p < 0.01$, [c]$p < 0.001$, [d]$p < 0.0001$

In the event of severe and unremitting rejection, when rescue therapy with pulse steroids and monoclonal antibodies fail to reverse the rejection episode, it may be preferable to switch to alternative immunosuppressive therapy rather than increase the Neoral® dose to excessive levels.

Occasionally patients have developed a syndrome of thrombocytopenia and microangiopathic hemolytic anemia which may result in graft failure. The vasculopathy can occur in the absence of rejection and is accompanied by avid platelet consumption within the graft as demonstrated by Indium 111 labeled platelet studies. Neither the pathogenesis nor the management of this syndrome is clear. Though resolution has occurred after reduction or discontinuation of cyclosporine and 1) administration of streptokinase and heparin or 2) plasmapheresis, this appears to depend upon early detection with Indium 111 labeled platelet scans. *(See ADVERSE REACTIONS)*

Significant hyperkalemia (sometimes associated with hyperchloremic metabolic acidosis) and hyperuricemia have been seen occasionally in individual patients.

Hepatotoxicity associated with cyclosporine use had been noted in 4% of cases of renal transplantation, 7% of cases of cardiac transplantation, and 4% of cases of liver transplantation. This was usually noted during the first month of therapy when high doses of cyclosporine were used and consisted of elevations of hepatic enzymes and bilirubin. The chemistry elevations usually decreased with a reduction in dosage.

As in patients receiving other immunosuppressants, those patients receiving cyclosporine are at increased risk for development of lymphomas and other malignancies, particularly those of the skin. The increased risk appears related to the intensity and duration of immunosuppression rather than to the use of specific agents. Because of the danger of oversuppression of the immune system resulting in increased risk of infection or malignancy, a treatment regimen containing multiple immunosuppressants should be used with caution.

There have been reports of convulsions in adult and pediatric patients receiving cyclosporine, particularly in combination with high dose methylprednisolone.

Care should be taken in using cyclosporine with nephrotoxic drugs. *(See PRECAUTIONS)*

Rheumatoid Arthritis: Cyclosporine nephropathy was detected in renal biopsies of 6 out of 60 (10%) rheumatoid arthritis patients after the average treatment duration of 19 months. Only one patient, out of these 6 patients, was treated with a dose ≤4 mg/kg/day. Serum creatinine improved in all but one patient after discontinuation of cyclosporine. The "maximal creatinine increase" appears to be a factor in predicting cyclosporine nephropathy.

There is a potential, as with other immunosuppressive agents, for an increase in the occurrence of malignant lymphomas with cyclosporine. It is not clear whether the risk with cyclosporine is greater than that in Rheumatoid Arthritis patients or in Rheumatoid Arthritis patients on cytotoxic treatment for this indication. Five cases of lymphoma were detected: four in a survey of approximately 2,300 patients treated with cyclosporine for rheumatoid arthritis, and another case of lymphoma was reported in a clinical trial. Although other tumors (12 skin cancers, 24 solid tumors of diverse types, and 1 multiple myeloma) were also reported in this survey, epidemiologic analyses did not support a relationship to cyclosporine other than for malignant lymphomas.

Continued on next page

Neoral—Cont.

Patients should be thoroughly evaluated before and during Neoral® treatment for the development of malignancies. Moreover, use of Neoral® therapy with other immunosuppressive agents may induce an excessive immunosuppression which is known to increase the risk of malignancy.

Psoriasis: *(See also Boxed WARNINGS for Psoriasis)* Since cyclosporine is a potent immunosuppressive agent with a number of potentially serious side effects, the risks and benefits of using Neoral® should be considered before treatment of patients with psoriasis. Cyclosporine, the active ingredient in Neoral®, can cause nephrotoxicity and hypertension *(see PRECAUTIONS)* and the risk increases with increasing dose and duration of therapy. Patients who may be at increased risk such as those with abnormal renal function, uncontrolled hypertension or malignancies, should not receive Neoral®.

Renal dysfunction is a potential consequence of Neoral® therefore renal function must be monitored during therapy. Patients receiving Neoral® require frequent monitoring of serum creatinine. *(See Special Monitoring under DOSAGE AND ADMINISTRATION)* Elderly patients should be monitored with particular care, since decreases in renal function also occur with age. If patients are not properly monitored and doses are not properly adjusted, cyclosporine therapy can cause structural kidney damage and persistent renal dysfunction.

An increase in serum creatinine and BUN may occur during Neoral® therapy and reflects a reduction in the glomerular filtration rate.

Kidney biopsies from 86 psoriasis patients treated for a mean duration of 23 months with 1.2-7.6 mg/kg/day of cyclosporine showed evidence of cyclosporine nephropathy in 18/86 (21%) of the patients. The pathology consisted of renal tubular atrophy and interstitial fibrosis. On repeat biopsy of 13 of these patients maintained on various dosages of cyclosporine for a mean of 2 additional years, the number with cyclosporine induced nephropathy rose to 26/86 (30%). The majority of patients (19/26) were on a dose of ≥5.0 mg/kg/day (the highest recommended dose is 4 mg/kg/day). The patients were also on cyclosporine for greater than 15 months (18/26) and/or had a clinically significant increase in serum creatinine for greater than 1 month (21/26). Creatinine levels returned to normal range in 7 of 11 patients in whom cyclosporine therapy was discontinued.

There is an increased risk for the development of skin and lymphoproliferative malignancies in cyclosporine-treated psoriasis patients. The relative risk of malig nancies is comparable to that observed in psoriasis patients treated with other immunosuppressive agents.

Tumors were reported in 32 (2.2%) of 1439 psoriasis patients treated with cyclosporine worldwide from clinical trials. Additional tumors have been reported in 7 patients in cyclosporine postmarketing experience. Skin malignancies were reported in 16 (1.1%) of these patients; all but 2 of them had previously received PUVA therapy. Methotrexate was received by 7 patients. UVB and coal tar had been used by 2 and 3 patients, respectively. Seven patients had either a history of previous skin cancer or a potentially predisposing lesion was present prior to cyclosporine exposure. Of the 16 patients with skin cancer, 11 patients had 18 squamous cell carcinomas and 7 patients had 10 basal cell carcinomas. There were two lymphoproliferative malignancies; one case of non-Hodgkin's lymphoma which required chemo therapy, and one case of mycosis fungoides which regressed spontaneously upon discontinuation of cyclosporine. There were four cases of benign lymphocytic infiltration: 3 regressed spontaneously upon discon tinuation of cyclosporine, while the fourth regressed despite continuation of the drug. The remainder of the malignancies, 13 cases (0.9%), involved various organs.

Patients should not be treated concurrently with cyclosporine and PUVA or UVB, other radiation therapy, or other immunosuppressive agents, because of the possibility of excessive immunosuppression and the subsequent risk of malignancies. *(See CONTRAINDICATIONS)* Patients should also be warned to protect themselves appropriately when in the sun, and to avoid excessive sun exposure. Patients should be thoroughly evaluated before and during treatment for the presence of malignancies remembering that malignant lesions may be hidden by psoriatic plaques. Skin lesions not typical of psoriasis should be biopsied before starting treatment. Patients should be treated with Neoral® only after complete resolution of suspicious lesions, and only if there are no other treatment options. *(See Special Monitoring for Psoriasis Patients)*

PRECAUTIONS: General: ***Hypertension:*** Cyclosporine is the active ingredient of Neoral®. Hypertension is a common side effect of cyclosporine therapy which may persist. *(See ADVERSE REACTIONS and DOSAGE AND ADMINISTRATION for monitoring recommendations)* Mild or moderate hypertension is encountered more frequently than severe hypertension and the incidence decreases over time. In recipients of kidney, liver, and heart allografts treated with cyclosporine, antihypertensive therapy may be required. *(See Special Monitoring of Rheumatoid Arthritis and Psoriasis Patients)* However, since cyclosporine may cause hyperkalemia, potassium-sparing diuretics should not be used. While calcium antagonists can be effective agents in treating cyclosporine-associated hypertension, they can interfere with cyclosporine metabolism. *(See Drug Interactions)*

Vaccination: During treatment with cyclosporine, vaccination may be less effective; and the use of live attenuated vaccines should be avoided.

Special Monitoring of Rheumatoid Arthritis Patients: Before initiating treatment, a careful physical examination, including blood pressure measurements (on at least two occasions) and two creatinine levels to estimate baseline should be performed. Blood pressure and serum creatinine should be evaluated every 2 weeks during the initial 3 months and then monthly if the patient is stable. It is advisable to monitor serum creatinine and blood pressure always after an increase of the dose of non steroidal anti-inflammatory drugs and after initiation of new nonsteroidal anti-inflammatory drug therapy during Neoral® treatment. If co-administered with methotrexate, CBC and liver function tests are recommended to be monitored monthly. *(See also PRECAUTIONS, General, Hypertension)*

In patients who are receiving cyclosporine, the dose of Neoral® should be decreased by 25%-50% if hypertension occurs. If hypertension persists, the dose of Neoral® should be further reduced or blood pressure should be controlled with anti hyper tensive agents. In most cases, blood pressure has returned to baseline when cyclosporine was discontinued.

In placebo-controlled trials of rheumatoid arthritis patients, systolic hypertension (defined as an occurrence of two systolic blood pressure readings >140 mmHg) and diastolic hypertension (defined as two diastolic blood pressure readings >90 mmHg) occurred in 33% and 19% of patients treated with cyclosporine, respectively. The corresponding placebo rates were 22% and 8%.

Special Monitoring for Psoriasis Patients: Before initiating treatment, a careful dermatological and physical examination, including blood pressure measurements (on at least two occasions) should be performed. Since Neoral® is an immunosuppressive agent, patients should be evaluated for the presence of occult infection on their first physical examination and for the presence of tumors initially, and throughout treatment with Neoral®. Skin lesions not typical for psoriasis should be biopsied before starting Neoral®. Patients with malignant or premalignant changes of the skin should be treated with Neoral® only after appropriate treatment of such lesions and if no other treatment option exists.

Baseline laboratories should include serum creatinine (on two occasions), BUN, CBC, serum magnesium, potassium, uric acid, and lipids.

The risk of cyclosporine nephropathy is reduced when the starting dose is low (2.5 mg/kg/day), the maximum dose does not exceed 4.0 mg/kg/day, serum creatinine is monitored regularly while cyclosporine is administered, and the dose of Neoral® is decreased when the rise in creatinine is greater than or equal to 25% above the patients pretreatment level. The increase in creatinine is generally reversible upon timely decrease of the dose of Neoral® or its discontinuation.

Serum creatinine and BUN should be evaluated every 2 weeks during the initial 3 months of therapy and then monthly if the patient is stable. If the serum creatinine is greater than or equal to 25% above the patient's pretreatment level, serum creatinine should be repeated within two weeks. If the change in serum creatinine remains greater than or equal to 25% above baseline, Neoral® should be reduced by 25%-50%. If at **any time** the serum creatinine increases by greater than or equal to 50% above pretreatment level, Neoral® should be reduced by 25%-50%. Neoral® should be discontinued if reversibility (within 25% of baseline) of serum creatinine is not achievable after two dosage modifications. It is advisable to monitor serum creatinine after an increase of the dose of nonsteroidal anti-inflammatory drug and after initiation of new nonsteroidal anti-inflammatory therapy during Neoral® treatment.

Blood pressure should be evaluated every 2 weeks during the initial 3 months of therapy and then monthly if the patient is stable, or more frequently when dosage adjustments are made. Patients without a history of previous hypertension before initiation of treatment with Neoral®, should have the drug reduced by 25%-50% if found to have sustained hypertension. If the patient continues to be hypertensive despite multiple reductions of Neoral®, then Neoral® should be discontinued. For patients with treated hypertension, before the initiation of Neoral® therapy, their medication should be adjusted to control hypertension while on Neoral®. Neoral® should be discontinued if a change in hypertension management is not effective or tolerable.

CBC, uric acid, potassium, lipids, and magnesium should also be monitored every 2 weeks for the first 3 months of therapy, and then monthly if the patient is stable or more frequently when dosage adjustments are made. Neoral® dosage should be reduced by 25%-50% for any abnormality of clinical concern.

In controlled trials of cyclosporine in psoriasis patients, cyclosporine blood concentrations did not correlate well with either improvement or with side effects such as renal dysfunction.

Information for Patients: Patients should be advised that any change of cyclosporine formulation should be made cautiously and only under physician supervision because it may result in the need for a change in dosage.

Patients should be informed of the necessity of repeated laboratory tests while they are receiving cyclosporine. Patients should be advised of the potential risks during pregnancy and informed of the increased risk of neoplasia. Patients should also be informed of the risk of hypertension and renal dysfunction.

Patients should be advised that during treatment with cyclosporine, vaccination may be less effective and the use of live attenuated vaccines should be avoided.

Patients should be given careful dosage instructions. Neoral® Oral Solution (cyclosporine oral solution, USP) MODIFIED should be diluted, preferably with orange or apple juice that is at room temperature. The combination of Neoral® Oral Solution (cyclosporine oral solution, USP) MODIFIED with milk can be unpalatable.

Patients should be advised to take Neoral® on a consistent schedule with regard to time of day and relation to meals. Grapefruit and grapefruit juice affect metabolism, increasing blood concentration of cyclosporine, thus should be avoided.

Laboratory Tests: In all patients treated with cyclosporine, renal and liver functions should be assessed repeatedly by measurement of serum creatinine, BUN, serum bilirubin, and liver enzymes. Serum lipids, magnesium, and potassium should also be monitored. Cyclosporine blood concentrations should be routinely monitored in transplant patients *(see DOSAGE AND ADMINISTRATION, Blood Concentration Monitoring in Transplant Patients)*, and periodically monitored in rheumatoid arthritis patients.

Drug Interactions: All of the individual drugs cited below are well substantiated to interact with cyclosporine. In addition, concomitant non-steroidal anti- inflammatory drugs, particularly in the setting of dehydration, may potentiate renal dysfunction.

Drugs That May Potentiate Renal Dysfunction

Antibiotics	*Anti-inflammatory Drugs*
gentamicin	azapropazon
tobramycin	diclofenac
vancomycin	naproxen
trimethoprim with sulfamethoxazole	sulindac
	Gastrointestinal Agents
Antieoplastics	cimetidine
melphalan	ranitidine
Antifungals	*Immunosuppressives*
amphotericin B	tacrolimus
ketoconazole	

Drugs That Alter Cyclosporine Concentrations: Cyclosporine is extensively metabolized. Cyclosporine concentrations may be influenced by drugs that affect microsomal enzymes, particularly cytochrome P-450 III-A. Substances that inhibit this enzyme could decrease metabolism and increase cyclosporine concentrations. Substances that are inducers of cytochrome P-450 activity could increase metabolism and decrease cyclosporine concentrations. Monitoring of circulating cyclosporine concentrations and appropriate Neoral® dosage adjustment are essential when these drugs are used concomitantly. *(See Blood Concentration Monitoring)*

Drugs That Increase Cyclosporine Concentrations

Calcium Channel Blockers	*Glucocorticoids*
diltiazem	methylprednisolone
verapamil	*Other Drugs*
Antifungals	allopurinol
fluconazole	bromocriptine
itraconazole	danazol
ketoconazole	metoclopramide
Antibiotics	
clarithromycin	
erythromycin	

The HIV protease inhibitors (e.g., indinavir, nelfinavir, ritonavir, and saquinavir) are known to inhibit cytochrome P-450 III-A and increase the concentrations of drugs metabolized by the cytochrome P-450 system. The interaction between HIV protease inhibitors and cyclosporine has not been studied. Care should be exercised when these drugs are administered concomitantly.

Grapefruit and grapefruit juice affect metabolism, increasing blood concentrations of cyclosporine, thus should be avoided.

Drugs That Decrease Cyclosporine Concentrations

Antibiotics	*Other Drugs*
nafcillin	octreotide
rifampin	ticlopidine
Anticonvulsants	
carbamazepine	
phenobarbital	
phenytoin	

Rifabutin is known to increase the metabolism of other drugs metabolized by the cytochrome P-450 system. The interaction between rifabutin and cyclosporine has not been studied. Care should be exercised when these two drugs are administered concomitantly.

Nonsteroidal Anti-inflammatory Drug (NSAID) Interactions: Clinical status and serum creatinine should be closely monitored when cyclosporine is used with nonsteroidal anti-inflammatory agents in rheumatoid arthritis patients. *(See WARNINGS)*

Pharmacodynamic interactions have been reported to occur between cyclosporine and both naproxen and sulindac, in that concomitant use is associated with additive decreases in renal function, as determined by ^{99m}Tc-diethylenetriaminepentaacetic acid (DTPA) and (*p*-aminohippuric acid)

PAH clearances. Although concomitant administration of diclofenac does not affect blood levels of cyclosporine, it has been associated with approximate doubling of diclofenac blood levels and occasional reports of reversible decreases in renal function. Consequently, the dose of diclofenac should be in the lower end of the therapeutic range.

Methotrexate Interaction: Preliminary data indicate that when methotrexate and cyclosporine were co-administered to rheumatoid arthritis patients (N=20), methotrexate concentrations (AUCs) were increased approximately 30% and the concentrations (AUCs) of its metabolite, 7-hydroxy methotrexate, were decreased by approximately 80%. The clinical significance of this interaction is not known. Cyclosporine concentrations do not appear to have been altered (N=6).

Other Drug Interactions: Reduced clearance of prednisolone, digoxin, and lovastatin has been observed when these drugs are administered with cyclosporine. In addition, a decrease in the apparent volume of distribution of digoxin has been reported after cyclosporine administration. Severe digitalis toxicity has been seen within days of starting cyclosporine in several patients taking digoxin. Cyclosporine should not be used with potassium-sparing diuretics because hyperkalemia can occur.

During treatment with cyclosporine, vaccination may be less effective. The use of live vaccines should be avoided. Myositis has occurred with concomitant lovastatin, frequent gingival hyperplasia with nifedipine, and convulsions with high dose methylprednisolone.

Psoriasis patients receiving other immunosuppressive agents or radiation therapy (including PUVA and UVB) should not receive concurrent cyclosporine because of the possibility of excessive immunosuppression.

Carcinogenesis, Mutagenesis, and Impairment of Fertility: Carcinogenicity studies were carried out in male and female rats and mice. In the 78-week mouse study, evidence of a statistically significant trend was found for lymphocytic lymphomas in females, and the incidence of hepatocellular carcinomas in mid-dose males significantly exceeded the control value. In the 24-month rat study, pancreatic islet cell adenomas significantly exceeded the control rate in the low dose level. Doses used in the mouse and rat studies were 0.01 to 0.16 times the clinical maintenance dose (6 mg/kg). The hepatocellular carcinomas and pancreatic islet cell adenomas were not dose related. Published reports indicate that co-treatment of hairless mice with UV irradiation and cyclosporine or other immunosuppressive agents shorten the time to skin tumor formation compared to UV irradiation alone.

Cyclosporine was not mutagenic in appropriate test systems. Cyclosporine has not been found to be mutagenic/genotoxic in the Ames Test, the V79-HGPRT Test, the micronucleus test in mice and Chinese hamsters, the chromosome-aberration tests in Chinese hamster bone-marrow, the mouse dominant lethal assay, and the DNA-repair test in sperm from treated mice. A recent study analyzing sister chromatid exchange (SCE) induction by cyclosporine using human lymphocytes *in vitro* gave indication of a positive effect (i.e., induction of SCE), at high concentrations in this system.

No impairment in fertility was demonstrated in studies in male and female rats.

Widely distributed papillomatosis of the skin was observed after chronic treatment of dogs with cyclosporine at 9 times the human initial psoriasis treatment dose of 2.5 mg/kg, where doses are expressed on a body surface area basis. This papilloma tosis showed a spontaneous regression upon discontinuation of cyclosporine.

An increased incidence of malignancy is a recognized complication of immunosuppression in recipients of organ transplants and patients with rheumatoid arthritis and psoriasis. The most common forms of neoplasms are non-Hodgkin's lymphoma and carcinomas of the skin. The risk of malignancies in cyclosporine recipients is higher than in the normal, healthy population but similar to that in patients receiving other immunosuppressive therapies. Reduction or discontinuance of immunosuppression may cause the lesions to regress.

In psoriasis patients on cyclosporine, development of malignancies, especially those of the skin has been reported. *(See WARNINGS)* Skin lesions not typical for psoriasis should be biopsied before starting cyclosporine treatment. Patients with malignant or premalignant changes of the skin should be treated with cyclosporine only after appropriate treatment of such lesions and if no other treatment option exists.

Pregnancy: ***Pregnancy Category C.*** Cyclosporine was not teratogenic in appropriate test systems. Only at dose levels toxic to dams, were adverse effects seen in reproduction studies in rats. Cyclosporine has been shown to be embryo- and fetotoxic in rats and rabbits following oral administration at maternally toxic doses. Fetal toxicity was noted in rats at 0.8 and rabbits at 5.4 times the transplant doses in humans of 6.0 mg/kg, where dose corrections are based on body surface area. Cyclosporine was embryo- and fetotoxic as indicated by increased pre- and postnatal mortality and reduced fetal weight together with related skeletal retardation.

There are no adequate and well-controlled studies in pregnant women. Neoral® should be used during pregnancy only if the potential benefit justifies the potential risk to the fetus.

The following data represent the reported outcomes of 116 pregnancies in women receiving cyclosporine during pregnancy, 90% of whom were transplant patients, and most of whom received cyclosporine throughout the entire gestational period. The only consistent patterns of abnormality were premature birth (gestational period of 28 to 36 weeks) and low birth weight for gestational age. Sixteen fetal losses occurred. Most of the pregnancies (85 of 100) were complicated by disorders; including, pre-eclampsia, eclampsia, premature labor, abruptio placentae, oligohydramnios, Rh incompatibility, and fetoplacental dysfunction. Pre-term delivery occurred in 47%. Seven malformations were reported in 5 viable infants and in 2 cases of fetal loss. Twenty-eight percent of the infants were small for gestational age. Neonatal complications occurred in 27%. Therefore, the risks and benefits of using Neoral® during pregnancy should be carefully weighed.

Because of the possible disruption of maternal-fetal interaction, the risk/benefit ratio of using Neoral® in psoriasis patients during pregnancy should carefully be weighed with serious consideration for discontinuation of Neoral®.

Nursing Mothers: Since cyclosporine is excreted in human milk, breast-feeding should be avoided.

Pediatric Use: Although no adequate and well-controlled studies have been completed in children, transplant recipients as young as one year of age have received Neoral® with no unusual adverse effects. The safety and efficacy of Neoral® treatment in children with juvenile rheumatoid arthritis or psoriasis below the age of 18 have not been established.

Geriatric Use: In rheumatoid arthritis clinical trials with cyclosporine, 17.5% of patients were age 65 or older. These patients were more likely to develop systolic hypertension on therapy, and more likely to show serum creatinine rises ≥50% above the baseline after 3-4 months of therapy.

ADVERSE REACTIONS: Kidney, Liver, and Heart Transplantation: The principal adverse reactions of cyclosporine therapy are renal dysfunction, tremor, hirsutism, hypertension, and gum hyperplasia.

Hypertension, which is usually mild to moderate, may occur in approximately 50% of patients following renal transplantation and in most cardiac transplant patients.

Glomerular capillary thrombosis has been found in patients treated with cyclosporine and may progress to graft failure. The pathologic changes resembled those seen in the hemolytic-uremic syndrome and included thrombosis of the renal microvasculature, with platelet-fibrin thrombi occluding glomerular capillaries and afferent arterioles, microangiopathic hemolytic anemia, thrombocytopenia, and decreased renal function. Similar findings have been observed when other immunosuppressives have been employed post-transplantation.

Hypomagnesemia has been reported in some, but not all, patients exhibiting convulsions while on cyclosporine therapy. Although magnesium-depletion studies in normal subjects suggest that hypomagnesemia is associated with neurologic disorders, multiple factors, including hypertension, high dose methylprednisolone, hypocholesterolemia, and nephrotoxicity associated with high plasma concentrations of cyclosporine appear to be related to the neurological manifestations of cyclosporine toxicity.

In controlled studies, the nature, severity, and incidence of the adverse events that were observed in 493 transplanted patients treated with Neoral® were comparable with those observed in 208 transplanted patients who received Sandimmune® in these same studies when the dosage of the two drugs was adjusted to achieve the same cyclosporine blood trough concentrations.

Based on the historical experience with Sandimmune®, the following reactions occurred in 3% or greater of 892 patients involved in clinical trials of kidney, heart, and liver transplants.

Body System	Adverse Reactions	Randomized Kidney Patients: Sandimmune® (N=227) %	Randomized Kidney Patients: Azathioprine (N=228) %	Cyclosporine Patients (Sandimmune®): Kidney (N=705) %	Cyclosporine Patients (Sandimmune®): Heart (N=112) %	Cyclosporine Patients (Sandimmune®): Liver (N=75) %
Genitourinary	Renal Dysfunction	32	6	25	38	37
Cardiovascular	Hypertension	26	18	13	53	27
	Cramps	4	<1	2	<1	0
Skin	Hirsutism	21	<1	21	28	45
	Acne	6	8	2	2	1
Central Nervous System	Tremor	12	0	21	31	55
	Convulsions	3	1	1	4	5
	Headache	2	<1	2	15	4
Gastrointestinal	Gum Hyperplasia	4	0	9	5	16
	Diarrhea	3	<1	3	4	8
	Nausea/Vomiting	2	<1	4	10	4
	Hepatotoxicity	<1	<1	4	7	4
	Abdominal Discomfort	<1	0	<1	7	0
Antonomic Nervous System	Paresthesia	3	0	1	2	1
	Flushing	<1	0	4	0	4
Hematopoietic	Leukopenia	2	19	<1	6	0
	Lymphoma	<1	0	1	6	1
Respiratory	Sinusitis	<1	0	4	3	7
Miscellaneous	Gynecomastia	<1	0	<1	4	3

[See first table above]

Among 705 kidney transplant patients treated with cyclosporine oral solution (Sandimmune®) in clinical trials, the reason for treatment discontinuation was renal toxicity in 5.4%, infection in 0.9%, lack of efficacy in 1.4%, acute tubular necrosis in 1.0%, lymphoproliferative disorders in 0.3%, hypertension in 0.3%, and other reasons in 0.7% of the patients.

The following reactions occurred in 2% or less of Sandimmune®-treated patients: allergic reactions, anemia, anorexia, confusion, conjunctivitis, edema, fever, brittle fingernails, gastritis, hearing loss, hiccups, hyperglycemia, muscle pain, peptic ulcer, thrombocytopenia, tinnitus.

The following reactions occurred rarely: anxiety, chest pain, constipation, depression, hair breaking, hematuria, joint pain, lethargy, mouth sores, myocardial infarction, night sweats, pancreatitis, pruritus, swallowing difficulty, tingling, upper GI bleeding, visual disturbance, weakness, weight loss.

Infectious Complications in Historical Randomized Studies In Renal Transplant Patients Using Sandimmune®

Complication	Cyclosporine Treatment (N=227) % of Complications	Azathioprine with Steroids* (N=228) % of Complications
Septicemia	5.3	4.8
Abscesses	4.4	5.3
Systemic Fungal Infection	2.2	3.9
Local Fungal Infection	7.5	9.6
Cytomegalovirus	4.8	12.3
Other Viral Infections	15.9	18.4
Urinary Tract Infections	21.1	20.2
Wound and Skin Infections	7.0	10.1
Pneumonia	6.2	9.2

*Some patients also received ALG.

[See second table above]

There have been post-marketing reports of neurotoxicity associated with cyclosporine therapy. Signs of encephalopathy, convulsions, vision and movement disturbances and impaired consciousness have been described, especially in liver transplant patients. These alterations appear to be multifactorial in origin. Generally, reduction of dose has been observed to result in reversal of these changes.

Rheumatoid Arthritis: The principal adverse reactions associated with the use of cyclosporine in rheumatoid arthritis are renal dysfunction *(see WARNINGS)*, hypertension *(see PRECAUTIONS)*, headache, gastrointestinal disturbances, and hirsutism/hypertrichosis.

In rheumatoid arthritis patients treated in clinical trials within the recommended dose range, cyclosporine therapy was discontinued in 5.3% of the patients because of hypertension and in 7% of the patients because of increased creatinine. These changes are usually reversible with timely dose decrease or drug discontinuation. The frequency and severity of serum creatinine elevations increase with dose and duration of cyclosporine therapy. These elevations are

Continued on next page

Neoral—Cont.

likely to become more pronounced without dose reduction or discontinuation.

The following adverse events occurred in controlled clinical trials:

[See table below]

In addition, the following adverse events have been reported in 1% to <3% of the rheumatoid arthritis patients in the cyclosporine treatment group in controlled clinical trials.

Autonomic Nervous System: dry mouth, increased sweating;

Body as a Whole: allergy, asthenia, hot flushes, malaise, overdose, procedure NOS*, tumor NOS*, weight decrease, weight increase;

Cardiovascular: abnormal heart sounds, cardiac failure, myocardial infarction, peripheral ischemia;

Central and Peripheral Nervous System: hypoesthesia, neuropathy, vertigo;

Endocrine: goiter;

Gastrointestinal: constipation, dysphagia, enanthema, eructation, esophagitis, gastric ulcer, gastritis, gastroenteritis, gingival bleeding, glossitis, peptic ulcer, salivary gland enlargement, tongue disorder, tooth disorder;

Infection: abscess, bacterial infection, cellulitis, folliculitis, fungal infection, herpes simplex, herpes zoster, renal abscess, moniliasis, tonsillitis, viral infection;

Hematologic: anemia, epistaxis, leukopenia, lymphadenopathy;

Liver and Biliary System: bilirubinemia;

Metabolic and Nutritional: diabetes mellitus, hyperkalemia, hyperuricemia, hypoglycemia;

Musculoskeletal System: arthralgia, bone fracture, bursitis, joint dislocation, myalgia, stiffness, synovial cyst, tendon disorder;

Neoplasms: breast fibroadenosis, carcinoma;

Psychiatric: anxiety, confusion, decreased libido, emotional lability, impaired concentration, increased libido, nervousness, paroniria, somnolence;

Reproductive (Female): breast pain, uterine hemorrhage;

Respiratory System: abnormal chest sounds, bronchospasm;

Skin and Appendages: abnormal pigmentation, angioedema, dermatitis, dry skin, eczema, nail disorder, pruritus, skin disorder, urticaria;

Special Senses: abnormal vision, cataract, conjunctivitis, deafness, eye pain, taste perversion, tinnitus, vestibular disorder;

Urinary System: abnormal urine, hematuria, increased BUN, micturition urgency, nocturia, polyuria, pyelonephritis, urinary incontinence.

*NOS = Not Otherwise Specified.

Neoral®/Sandimmune® Rheumatoid Arthritis
Percentage of Patients with Adverse Events ≥3% in any Cyclosporine Treated Group

		Studies 651+652+2008	Study 302	Study 654	Study 654	Study 302	Studies 651+652+2008
Body System	**Preferred term**	**Sandimmune®† (N=269)**	**Sandimmune® (N=155)**	**Methotrexate & Sandimmune® (N=74)**	**Methotrtexate & Placebo (N=73)**	**Neoral® (N=143)**	**Placebo (N=201)**
Autonomic Nervous System Disorders							
	Flushing	2%	2%	3%	0%	5%	2%
Body As A Whole—General Disorders							
	Accidental Trauma	0%	1%	10%	4%	4%	0%
	Edema NOS*	5%	14%	12%	4%	10%	<1%
	Fatique	6%	3%	8%	12%	3%	7%
	Fever	2%	3%	0%	0%	2%	4%
	Influenza-like symptoms	<1%	6%	1%	0%	3%	2%
	Pain	6%	9%	10%	15%	13%	4%
	Rigors	1%	1%	4%	0%	3%	1%
Cardiovascular Disorders							
	Arrhythmia	2%	5%	5%	6%	2%	1%
	Chest Pain	4%	5%	1%	1%	6%	1%
	Hypertension	8%	26%	16%	12%	25%	2%
Central and Peripheral Nervous System Disorders							
	Dizziness	8%	6%	7%	3%	8%	3%
	Headache	17%	23%	22%	11%	25%	9%
	Migraine	2%	3%	0%	0%	3%	1%
	Paresthesia	8%	7%	8%	4%	11%	1%
	Tremor	8%	7%	7%	3%	13%	4%
Gastrointestinal System Disorders							
	Abdominal Pain	15%	15%	15%	7%	15%	10%
	Anorexia	3%	3%	1%	0%	3%	3%
	Diarrhea	12%	12%	18%	15%	13%	8%
	Dyspepsia	12%	12%	10%	8%	8%	4%
	Flatulence	5%	5%	5%	4%	4%	1%
	Gastrointestinal Disorders NOS*	0%	2%	1%	4%	4%	0%
	Gingivitis	4%	3%	0%	0%	0%	1%
	Gum Hyperplasia	2%	4%	1%	3%	4%	1%
	Nausea	23%	14%	24%	15%	18%	14%
	Rectal Hemorrhage	0%	3%	0%	0%	1%	1%
	Stomatitis	7%	5%	16%	12%	6%	8%
	Vomiting	9%	8%	14%	7%	6%	5%
Hearing and Vestibular Disorders							
	Ear Disorder NOS*	0%	5%	0%	0%	1%	0%
Metabolic and Nutritional Disorders							
	Hypomagnesemia	0%	4%	0%	0%	6%	0%
Musculoskeletal System Disorders							
	Arthropathy	0%	5%	0%	1%	4%	0%
	Leg Cramps/Involuntary Muscle Contractions	2%	11%	11%	3%	12%	1%
Psychiatric Disorders							
	Depression	3%	6%	3%	1%	1%	2%
	Insomnia	4%	1%	1%	0%	3%	2%
Renal							
	Creatinine elevations ≥30%	43%	39%	55%	19%	48%	13%
	Creatinine elevations ≥50%	24%	18%	26%	8%	18%	3%
Reproductive Disorders, Female							
	Leukorrhea	1%	0%	4%	0%	1%	0%
	Menstrual Disorder	3%	2%	1%	0%	1%	1%
Respiratory System Disorders							
	Bronchitis	1%	3%	1%	0%	1%	3%
	Coughing	5%	3%	5%	7%	4%	4%
	Dyspnea	5%	1%	3%	3%	1%	2%
	Infection NOS*	9%	5%	0%	7%	3%	10%
	Pharyngitis	3%	5%	5%	6%	4%	4%
	Pneumonia	1%	0%	4%	0%	1%	1%
	Rhinitis	0%	3%	11%	10%	1%	0%
	Sinusitis	4%	4%	8%	4%	3%	3%
	Upper Respiratory Tract	0%	14%	23%	15%	13%	0%
Skin and Appendages Disorders							
	Alopecia	3%	0%	1%	1%	4%	4%
	Bullous Eruption	1%	0%	4%	1%	1%	1%
	Hypertrichosis	19%	17%	12%	0%	15%	3%
	Rash	7%	12%	10%	7%	8%	10%
	Skin Ulceration	1%	1%	3%	4%	0%	2%
Urinary System Disorders							
	Dysuria	0%	0%	11%	3%	1%	2%
	Micturition Frequency	2%	4%	3%	1%	2%	2%
	NPN, Increased	0%	19%	12%	0%	18%	0%
	Urinary Tract Infection	0%	3%	5%	4%	3%	0%
Vascular (Extracardiac) Disorders							
	Purpura	3%	4%	1%	1%	2%	0%

†Includes patients in 2.5 mg/kg/day dose group only. *NOS = Not Otherwise Specified.

Psoriasis: The principal adverse reactions associated with the use of cyclosporine in patients with psoriasis are renal dysfunction, headache, hypertension, hypertriglyceridemia, hirsutism/hypertrichosis, paresthesia or hyperesthesia, influenza-like symptoms, nausea/vomiting, diarrhea, abdominal discomfort, lethargy, and musculoskeletal or joint pain.

In psoriasis patients treated in US controlled clinical studies within the recommended dose range, cyclosporine therapy was discontinued in 1.0% of the patients because of hypertension and in 5.4% of the patients because of increased creatinine. In the majority of cases, these changes were reversible after dose reduction or discontinuation of cyclosporine.

There has been one reported death associated with the use of cyclosporine in psoriasis. A 27 year old male developed renal deterioration and was continued on cyclosporine. He had progressive renal failure leading to death.

Frequency and severity of serum creatinine increases with dose and duration of cyclosporine therapy. These elevations are likely to become more pronounced and may result in irreversible renal damage without dose reduction or discontinuation.

[See table above]

Adverse Events Occurring in 3% or More of Psoriasis Patients in Controlled Clinical Trials

Body System*	Preferred Term	Neoral® (N=182)	Sandimmune® (N=185)
Infection or Potential Infection		24.7%	24.3%
	Influenza-like Symptoms	9.9%	8.1%
	Upper Respiratory Tract Infections	7.7%	11.3%
Cardiovascular System		28.0%	25.4%
	Hypertension**	27.5%	25.4%
Urinary System		24.2%	16.2%
	Increased Creatinine	19.8%	15.7%
Central and Peripheral Nervous System		26.4%	20.5%
	Headache	15.9%	14.0%
	Paresthesia	7.1%	4.8%
Musculoskeletal System		13.2%	8.7%
	Arthralgia	6.0%	1.1%
Body As a Whole—General		29.1%	22.2%
	Pain	4.4%	3.2%
Metabolic and Nutritional		9.3%	9.7%
Reproductive, female		8.5% (4 of 47 females)	11.5% (6 of 52 females)
Resistance Mechanism		18.7%	21.1%
Skin and Appendages		17.6%	15.1%
	Hypertrichosis	6.6%	5.4%
Respiratory System		5.0%	6.5%
	Bronchospasm, coughing, dyspnea, rhinitis	5.0%	4.9%
Psychiatric		5.0%	3.8%
Gastrointestinal System		19.8%	28.7%
	Abdominal pain	2.7%	6.0%
	Diarrhea	5.0%	5.9%
	Dyspepsia	2.2%	3.2%
	Gum hyperplasia	3.8%	6.0%
	Nausea	5.5%	5.9%
White cell and RES		4.4%	2.7%

*Total percentage of events within the system
**Newly occurring hypertension = SBP≥160 mm Hg and/or DBP≥90 mm Hg

The following events occurred in 1% to less than 3% of psoriasis patients treated with cyclosporine:

Body as a Whole: fever, flushes, hot flushes; ***Cardiovascular:*** chest pain; ***Central and Peripheral Nervous System:*** appetite increased, insomnia, dizziness, nervousness, vertigo; ***Gastrointestinal:*** abdominal distention, constipation, gingival bleeding; ***Liver and Biliary System:*** hyperbilirubinemia; ***Neoplasms:*** skin malignancies [squamous cell (0.9%) and basal cell (0.4%) carcinomas]; ***Reticuloendothelial:*** platelet, bleeding, and clotting disorders, red blood cell disorder; ***Respiratory:*** infection, viral and other infection; ***Skin and Appendages:*** acne, folliculitis, keratosis, pruritus, rash, dry skin; ***Urinary System:*** micturition frequency; ***Vision:*** abnormal vision.

Mild hypomagnesemia and hyperkalemia may occur but are asymptomatic. Increases in uric acid may occur and attacks of gout have been rarely reported. A minor and dose related hyperbilirubinemia has been observed in the absence of hepatocellular damage. Cyclosporine therapy may be associated with a modest increase of serum triglycerides or cholesterol. Elevations of triglycerides (>750 mg/dL) occur in about 15% of psoriasis patients; elevations of cholesterol (>300 mg/dL) are observed in less than 3% of psoriasis patients. Generally these laboratory abnormalities are reversible upon dose reduction or discontinuation of cyclosporine.

OVERDOSAGE: There is a minimal experience with cyclosporine overdosage. Forced emesis can be of value up to 2 hours after administration of Neoral®. Transient hepatotoxicity and nephrotoxicity may occur which should resolve following drug withdrawal. General supportive measures and symptomatic treatment should be followed in all cases of overdosage. Cyclosporine is not dialyzable to any great extent, nor is it cleared well by charcoal hemoperfusion. The oral dosage at which half of experimental animals are estimated to die is 31 times, 39 times, and >54 times the human maintenance dose for transplant patients (6mg/kg; corrections based on body surface area) in mice, rats, and rabbits.

DOSAGE AND ADMINISTRATION: Neoral® Soft Gelatin Capsules (cyclosporine capsules, USP) MODIFIED and Neoral® Oral Solution (cyclosporine oral solution, USP) MODIFIED

Neoral® has increased bioavailability in comparison to Sandimmune®. Neoral® and Sandimmune® are not bioequivalent and cannot be used interchangeably without physician supervision.

The daily dose of Neoral® should always be given in two divided doses (BID). It is recommended that Neoral® be administered on a consistent schedule with regard to time of day and relation to meals. Grapefruit and grapefruit juice affect metabolism, increasing blood concentration of cyclosporine, thus should be avoided.

Newly Transplanted Patients: The initial oral dose of Neoral® can be given 4-12 hours prior to transplantation or be given postoperatively. The initial dose of Neoral® varies depending on the transplanted organ and the other immunosuppressive agents included in the immunosuppressive protocol. In newly transplanted patients, the initial oral dose of Neoral® is the same as the initial oral dose of Sandimmune®. Suggested initial doses are available from the results of a 1994 survey of the use of Sandimmune® in US transplant centers. The mean ± SD initial doses were 9±3 mg/kg/day for renal transplant patients (75 centers), 8±4 mg/kg/day for liver transplant patients (30 centers), and 7±3 mg/kg/day for heart transplant patients (24 centers). Total daily doses were divided into two equal daily doses. The Neoral® dose is subsequently adjusted to achieve a pre-defined cyclosporine blood concentration. *(See Blood Concentration Monitoring in Transplant Patients, below)* If cyclosporine trough blood concentrations are used, the target range is the same for Neoral® as for Sandimmune®. Using the same trough concentration target range for Neoral® as for Sandimmune® results in greater cyclosporine exposure when Neoral® is administered. *(See Pharmacokinetics, Absorption)* Dosing should be titrated based on clinical assessments of rejection and tolerability. Lower Neoral® doses may be sufficient as maintenance therapy.

Adjunct therapy with adrenal corticosteroids is recommended initially. Different tapering dosage schedules of prednisone appear to achieve similar results. A representative dosage schedule based on the patient's weight started with 2.0 mg/kg/day for the first 4 days tapered to 1.0 mg/kg/day by 1 week, 0.6 mg/kg/day by 2 weeks, 0.3 mg/kg/day by 1 month, and 0.15 mg/kg/day by 2 months and thereafter as a maintenance dose. Steroid doses may be further tapered on an individualized basis depending on status of patient and function of graft. Adjustments in dosage of prednisone must be made according to the clinical situation.

Conversion from Sandimmune® to Neoral® in Transplant Patients: In transplanted patients who are considered for conversion to Neoral® from Sandimmune®, Neoral® should be started with the same daily dose as was previously used with Sandimmune® (1:1 dose conversion). The Neoral® dose should sub sequently be adjusted to attain the preconversion cyclosporine blood trough concentration. Using the same trough concentration target range for Neoral® as for Sandimmune® results in greater cyclosporine exposure when Neoral® is administered. *(See Pharmacokinetics, Absorption)* Patients with suspected poor absorption of Sandimmune® require different dosing strategies. *(See Transplant Patients with Poor Absorption of Sandimmune®, below)* In some patients, the increase in blood trough concentration is more pronounced and may be of clinical significance.

Until the blood trough concentration attains the pre-conversion value, it is strongly recommended that the cyclosporine blood trough concentration be monitored every 4 to 7 days after conversion to Neoral®. In addition, clinical safety parameters such as serum creatinine and blood pressure should be monitored every two weeks during the first two months after conversion. If the blood trough concentrations are outside the desired range and/or if the clinical safety parameters worsen, the dosage of Neoral® must be adjusted accordingly.

Transplant Patients with Poor Absorption of Sandimmune®: Patients with lower than expected cyclosporine blood trough concentrations in relation to the oral dose of Sandimmune® may have poor or inconsistent absorption of cyclosporine from Sandimmune®. After conversion to Neoral®, patients tend to have higher cyclosporine concentrations. **Due to the increase in bioavailability of cyclosporine following conversion to Neoral®, the cyclosporine blood trough concentration may exceed the target range. Particular caution should be exercised when converting patients to Neoral® at doses greater than 10 mg/kg/day.** The dose of Neoral® should be titrated individually based on cyclosporine trough concentrations, tolerability, and clinical response. In this population the cyclosporine blood trough concentration should be measured more frequently, at least twice a week (daily, if initial dose exceeds 10 mg/kg/day) until the concentration stabilizes within the desired range.

Rheumatoid Arthritis: The initial dose of Neoral® is 2.5 mg/kg/day, taken twice daily as a divided (BID) oral dose. Salicylates, nonsteroidal anti-inflammatory agents, and oral corticosteroids may be continued. *(See WARNINGS and PRECAUTIONS: Drug Interactions)* Onset of action generally occurs between 4 and 8 weeks. If insufficient clinical benefit is seen and tolerability is good (including serum creatinine less than 30% above baseline), the dose may be increased by 0.5-0.75 mg/kg/day after 8 weeks and again after 12 weeks to a maximum of 4 mg/kg/day. If no benefit is seen by 16 weeks of therapy, Neoral® therapy should be discontinued.

Dose decreases by 25%-50% should be made at any time to control adverse events, e.g., hypertension elevations in serum creatinine (30% above patient's pretreatment level) or clinically significant laboratory abnormalities. *(See WARNINGS and PRECAUTIONS)*

If dose reduction is not effective in controlling abnormalities or if the adverse event or abnormality is severe, Neoral® should be discontinued. The same initial dose and dosage range should be used if Neoral® is combined with the recommended dose of methotrexate. Most patients can be treated with Neoral® doses of 3 mg/kg/day or below when combined with methotrexate doses of up to 15 mg/week. *(See CLINICAL PHARMACOLOGY, Clinical Trials)*

There is limited long-term treatment data. Recurrence of rheumatoid arthritis disease activity is generally apparent within 4 weeks after stopping cyclosporine.

Psoriasis: The initial dose of Neoral® should be 2.5 mg/kg/day. Neoral® should be taken twice daily, as a divided (1.25 mg/kg BID) oral dose. Patients should be kept at that dose for at least 4 weeks, barring adverse events. If significant clinical improvement has not occurred in patients by that time, the patient's dosage should be increased at 2 week intervals. Based on patient response, dose increases of approximately 0.5 mg/kg/day should be made to a maximum of 4.0 mg/kg/day.

Dose decreases by 25%-50% should be made at any time to control adverse events, e.g., hypertension, elevations in serum creatinine (≥25% above the patient's pretreatment level), or clinically significant laboratory abnormalities. If dose reduction is not effective in controlling abnormalities, or if the adverse event or abnormality is severe, Neoral® should be discontinued. *(See Special Monitoring of Psoriasis Patients)*

Patients generally show some improvement in the clinical manifestations of psoriasis in 2 weeks. Satisfactory control and stabilization of the disease may take 12-16 weeks to achieve. Results of a dose-titration clinical trial with Neoral® indicate that an improvement of psoriasis by 75% or more (based on PASI) was achieved in 51% of the patients after 8 weeks and in 79% of the patients after 12 weeks. Treatment should be discontinued if satisfactory response cannot be achieved after 6 weeks at 4 mg/kg/day or the patient's maximum tolerated dose. Once a patient is adequately controlled and appears stable the dose of Neoral® should be lowered, and the patient treated with the lowest dose that maintains an adequate response (this should not necessarily be total clearing of the patient). In clinical trials, cyclosporine doses at the lower end of the recommended dosage range were effective in maintaining a satisfactory response in 60% of the patients. Doses below 2.5 mg/kg/day may also be equally effective.

Upon stopping treatment with cyclosporine, relapse will occur in approximately 6 weeks (50% of the patients) to 16 weeks (75% of the patients). In the majority of patients rebound does not occur after cessation of treatment with cyclosporine. Thirteen cases of transformation of chronic plaque psoriasis to more severe forms of psoriasis have been reported. There were 9 cases of pustular and 4 cases of erythrodermic psoriasis. Long term experience with Neoral® in psoriasis patients is limited and continuous treatment for extended periods greater than one year is not recommended. Alternation with other forms of treatment should be considered in the long term management of patients with this life long disease.

Neoral® Oral Solution (cyclosporine oral solution, USP) MODIFIED-Recommendations for Administration: To make Neoral® Oral Solution (cyclosporine oral solution,

Continued on next page

Neoral—Cont.

USP) MODIFIED more palatable, it should be diluted preferably with orange or apple juice that is at room temperature. Grapefruit juice affects metabolism of cyclosporine and should be avoided. The combination of Neoral® solution with milk can be unpalatable.
Take the prescribed amount of Neoral® Oral Solution (cyclosporine oral solution, USP) MODIFIED from the container using the dosing syringe supplied, after removal of the protective cover, and transfer the solution to a glass of orange or apple juice. Stir well and drink at once. Do not allow diluted oral solution to stand before drinking. Use a glass container (not plastic). Rinse the glass with more diluent to ensure that the total dose is consumed. After use, dry the outside of the dosing syringe with a clean towel and replace the protective cover. Do not rinse the dosing syringe with water or other cleaning agents. If the syringe requires cleaning, it must be completely dry before resuming use.
Blood Concentration Monitoring in Transplant Patients: Transplant centers have found blood concentration monitoring of cyclosporine to be an essential component of patient management. Of importance to blood concentration analysis are the type of assay used, the transplanted organ, and other immunosuppressant agents being administered. While no fixed relationship has been established, blood concentration monitoring may assist in the clinical evaluation of rejection and toxicity, dose adjustments, and the assessment of compliance.
Various assays have been used to measure blood concentrations of cyclosporine. Older studies using a nonspecific assay often cited concentrations that were roughly twice those of the specific assays. Therefore, comparison between concentrations in the published literature and an individual patient concentration using current assays must be made with detailed knowledge of the assay methods employed. Current assay results are also not interchangeable and their use should be guided by their approved labeling. A discussion of the different assay methods is contained in *Annals of Clinical Biochemistry* 1994;31:420-446. While several assays and assay matrices are available, there is a consensus that parent-compound-specific assays correlate best with clinical events. Of these, HPLC is the standard reference, but the monoclonal antibody RIAs and the monoclonal antibody FPIA offer sensitivity, reproducibility, and convenience. Most clinicians base their monitoring on trough cyclosporine concentrations. *Applied Pharmacokinetics, Principles of Therapeutic Drug Monitoring* (1992) contains a broad discussion of cyclosporine pharmacokinetics and drug monitoring techniques. Blood concentration monitoring is not a replacement for renal function monitoring or tissue biopsies.

HOW SUPPLIED

Neoral® Soft Gelatin Capsules (cyclosporine capsules, USP) MODIFIED
25 mg
Oval, blue-gray imprinted in red, "Neoral" over "25 mg." Packages of 30 unit-dose blisters (NDC 0078-0246-15).
100 mg
Oblong, blue-gray imprinted in red, "Neoral" over "100 mg." Packages of 30 unit-dose blisters (NDC 0078-0248-15).
Store and Dispense: In the original unit-dose container at controlled room temperature 68°-77°F (20°-25°C).
Neoral® Oral Solution (cyclosporine oral solution, USP) MODIFIED: A clear, yellow liquid supplied in 50 mL bottles containing 100 mg/mL (NDC 0078-0274-22).
Store and Dispense: In the original container at controlled room temperature 68°-77°F (20°-25°C). Do not store in the refrigerator. Once opened, the contents must be used within two months. At temperatures below 68°F (20°C) the solution may gel; light flocculation or the formation of a light sediment may also occur. There is no impact on product performance or dosing using the syringe provided. Allow to warm to room temperature 77°F (25°C) to reverse these changes.
Neoral® Soft Gelatin Capsules (cyclosporine capsules, USP) MODIFIED
Manufactured by R.P. Scherer GmbH, EBERBACH/BADEN, GERMANY
Manufactured for Novartis Pharmaceuticals Corporation, East Hanover, NJ 07936
Neoral® Oral Solution (cyclosporine oral solution, USP) MODIFIED
Manufactured by NOVARTIS PHARMA AG, Basle, Switzerland
Manufactured for Novartis Pharmaceuticals Corporation, East Hanover, NJ 07936

T1999-73
REV: NOVEMBER 1999 4061-42
Shown in Product Identification Guide, page 326

RITALIN® hydrochloride Ⓒ℞
[rit 'ah-lin]
methylphenidate hydrochloride tablets USP

RITALIN-SR® Ⓒ℞
methylphenidate hydrochloride USP sustained-release tablets
Rx only

The following prescribing information is based on official labeling in effect July 2000.

DESCRIPTION

Ritalin hydrochloride, methylphenidate hydrochloride USP, is a mild central nervous system (CNS) stimulant, available as tablets of 5, 10, and 20 mg for oral administration; Ritalin-SR is available as sustained-release tablets of 20 mg for oral administration. Methylphenidate hydrochloride is methyl α-phenyl-2-piperidineacetate hydrochloride, and its structural formula is

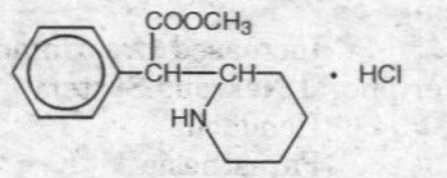

Methylphenidate hydrochloride USP is a white, odorless, fine crystalline powder. Its solutions are acid to litmus. It is freely soluble in water and in methanol, soluble in alcohol, and slightly soluble in chloroform and in acetone. Its molecular weight is 269.77.
Inactive Ingredients. Ritalin tablets: D&C Yellow No. 10 (5-mg and 20-mg tablets), FD&C Green No. 3 (10-mg tablets), lactose, magnesium stearate, polyethylene glycol, starch (5-mg and 10-mg tablets), sucrose, talc, and tragacanth (20-mg tablets).
Ritalin-SR tablets: Cellulose compounds, cetostearyl alcohol, lactose, magnesium stearate, mineral oil, povidone, titanium dioxide, and zein.

CLINICAL PHARMACOLOGY

Ritalin is a mild central nervous system stimulant.
The mode of action in man is not completely understood, but Ritalin presumably activates the brain stem arousal system and cortex to produce its stimulant effect.
There is neither specific evidence which clearly establishes the mechanism whereby Ritalin produces its mental and behavioral effects in children, nor conclusive evidence regarding how these effects relate to the condition of the central nervous system.
Ritalin in the SR tablets is more slowly but as extensively absorbed as in the regular tablets. Relative bioavailability of the SR tablet compared to the Ritalin tablet, measured by the urinary excretion of Ritalin major metabolite (α-phenyl-2-piperidine acetic acid) was 105% (49%-168%) in children and 101% (85%-152%) in adults. The time to peak rate in children was 4.7 hours (1.3-8.2 hours) for the SR tablets and 1.9 hours (0.3-4.4 hours) for the tablets. An average of 67% of SR tablet dose was excreted in children as compared to 86% in adults.
In a clinical study involving adult subjects who received SR tablets, plasma concentrations of Ritalin's major metabolite appeared to be greater in females than in males. No gender differences were observed for Ritalin plasma concentration in the same subjects.

INDICATIONS

Attention Deficit Disorders, Narcolepsy
Attention Deficit Disorders (previously known as Minimal Brain Dysfunction in Children). Other terms being used to describe the behavioral syndrome below include: Hyperkinetic Child Syndrome, Minimal Brain Damage, Minimal Cerebral Dysfunction, Minor Cerebral Dysfunction.
Ritalin is indicated as an integral part of a total treatment program which typically includes other remedial measures (psychological, educational, social) for a stabilizing effect in children with a behavioral syndrome characterized by the following group of developmentally inappropriate symptoms: moderate-to-severe distractibility, short attention span, hyperactivity, emotional lability, and impulsivity. The diagnosis of this syndrome should not be made with finality when these symptoms are only of comparatively recent origin. Nonlocalizing (soft) neurological signs, learning disability, and abnormal EEG may or may not be present, and a diagnosis of central nervous system dysfunction may or may not be warranted.
Special Diagnostic Considerations
Specific etiology of this syndrome is unknown, and there is no single diagnostic test. Adequate diagnosis requires the use not only of medical but of special psychological, educational, and social resources.
Characteristics commonly reported include: chronic history of short attention span, distractibility, emotional lability, impulsivity, and moderate-to-severe hyperactivity; minor neurological signs and abnormal EEG. Learning may or may not be impaired. The diagnosis must be based upon a complete history and evaluation of the child and not solely on the presence of one or more of these characteristics.
Drug treatment is not indicated for all children with this syndrome.
Stimulants are not intended for use in the child who exhibits symptoms secondary to environmental factors and/or primary psychiatric disorders, including psychosis. Appropriate educational placement is essential and psychosocial intervention is generally necessary. When remedial measures alone are insufficient, the decision to prescribe stimulant medication will depend upon the physician's assessment of the chronicity and severity of the child's symptoms.

CONTRAINDICATIONS

Marked anxiety, tension, and agitation are contraindications to Ritalin, since the drug may aggravate these symptoms. Ritalin is contraindicated also in patients known to be hypersensitive to the drug, in patients with glaucoma, and in patients with motor tics or with a family history or diagnosis of Tourette's syndrome.

WARNINGS

Ritalin should not be used in children under six years, since safety and efficacy in this age group have not been established.
Sufficient data on safety and efficacy of long-term use of Ritalin in children are not yet available. Although a causal relationship has not been established, suppression of growth (i.e., weight gain, and/or height) has been reported with the long-term use of stimulants in children. Therefore, patients requiring long-term therapy should be carefully monitored.
Ritalin should not be used for severe depression of either exogenous or endogenous origin. Clinical experience suggests that in psychotic children, administration of Ritalin may exacerbate symptoms of behavior disturbance and thought disorder.
Ritalin should not be used for the prevention or treatment of normal fatigue states.
There is some clinical evidence that Ritalin may lower the convulsive threshold in patients with prior history of seizures, with prior EEG abnormalities in absence of seizures, and, very rarely, in absence of history of seizures and no prior EEG evidence of seizures. Safe concomitant use of anticonvulsants and Ritalin has not been established. In the presence of seizures, the drug should be discontinued.
Use cautiously in patients with hypertension. Blood pressure should be monitored at appropriate intervals in all patients taking Ritalin, especially those with hypertension.
Symptoms of visual disturbances have been encountered in rare cases. Difficulties with accommodation and blurring of vision have been reported.

Drug Interactions
Ritalin may decrease the hypotensive effect of guanethidine. Use cautiously with pressor agents and MAO inhibitors.
Human pharmacologic studies have shown that Ritalin may inhibit the metabolism of coumarin anticoagulants, anticonvulsants (phenobarbital, diphenylhydantoin, primidone), phenylbutazone, and tricyclic drugs (imipramine, clomipramine, desipramine). Downward dosage adjustments of these drugs may be required when given concomitantly with Ritalin.

Usage in Pregnancy
Adequate animal reproduction studies to establish safe use of Ritalin during pregnancy have not been conducted. However, in a recently conducted study, methylphenidate has been shown to have teratogenic effects in rabbits when given in doses of 200 mg/kg/day, which is approximately 167 times and 78 times the maximum recommended human dose on a mg/kg and a mg/m^2 basis, respectively. In rats, teratogenic effects were not seen when the drug was given in doses of 75 mg/kg/day, which is approximately 62.5 and 13.5 times the maximum recommended human dose on a mg/kg and a mg/m^2 basis, respectively. Therefore, until more information is available, Ritalin should not be prescribed for women of childbearing age unless, in the opinion of the physician, the potential benefits outweigh the possible risks.

Drug Dependence
Ritalin should be given cautiously to emotionally unstable patients, such as those with a history of drug dependence or alcoholism, because such patients may increase dosage on their own initiative.
Chronically abusive use can lead to marked tolerance and psychic dependence with varying degrees of abnormal behavior. Frank psychotic episodes can occur, especially with parenteral abuse. Careful supervision is required during drug withdrawal, since severe depression as well as the effects of chronic overactivity can be unmasked. Long-term follow-up may be required because of the patient's basic personality disturbances.

PRECAUTIONS

Patients with an element of agitation may react adversely; discontinue therapy if necessary.
Periodic CBC, differential, and platelet counts are advised during prolonged therapy.
Drug treatment is not indicated in all cases of this behavioral syndrome and should be considered only in light of the complete history and evaluation of the child. The decision to prescribe Ritalin should depend on the physician's assessment of the chronicity and severity of the child's symptoms and their appropriateness for his/her age. Prescription should not depend solely on the presence of one or more of the behavioral characteristics.
When these symptoms are associated with acute stress reactions, treatment with Ritalin is usually not indicated.
Long-term effects of Ritalin in children have not been well established.

Carcinogenesis/Mutagenesis
In a lifetime carcinogenicity study carried out in B6C3F1 mice, methylphenidate caused an increase in hepatocellular adenomas and, in males only, an increase in hepatoblastomas, at a daily dose of approximately 60 mg/kg/day. This dose is approximately 30 times and 2.5 times the maximum recommended human dose on a mg/kg and mg/m^2 basis, respectively. Hepatoblastoma is a relatively rare rodent malignant tumor type. There was no increase in total malignant hepatic tumors. The mouse strain used is sensitive to the development of hepatic tumors, and the significance of these results to humans is unknown.

Methylphenidate did not cause any increases in tumors in a lifetime carcinogenicity study carried out in F344 rats; the highest dose used was approximately 45 mg/kg/day, which is approximately 22 times and 4 times the maximum recommended human dose on a mg/kg and mg/m^2 basis, respectively.
Methylphenidate was not mutagenic in the in vitro Ames reverse mutation assay or in the in vitro mouse lymphoma cell forward mutation assay. Sister chromatid exchanges and chromosome aberrations were increased, indicative of a weak clastogenic response, in an in vitro assay in cultured Chinese Hamster Ovary (CHO) cells. The genotoxic potential of methylphenidate has not been evaluated in an in vivo assay.

ADVERSE REACTIONS

Nervousness and insomnia are the most common adverse reactions but are usually controlled by reducing dosage and omitting the drug in the afternoon or evening. Other reactions include hypersensitivity (including skin rash, urticaria, fever, arthralgia, exfoliative dermatitis, erythema multiforme with histopathological findings of necrotizing vasculitis, and thrombocytopenic purpura); anorexia; nausea; dizziness; palpitations; headache; dyskinesia; drowsiness; blood pressure and pulse changes, both up and down; tachycardia; angina; cardiac arrhythmia; abdominal pain; weight loss during prolonged therapy. There have been rare reports of Tourette's syndrome. Toxic psychosis has been reported. Although a definite causal relationship has not been established, the following have been reported in patients taking this drug: instances of abnormal liver function, ranging from transaminase elevation to hepatic coma; isolated cases of cerebral arteritis and/or occlusion; leukopenia and/or anemia; transient depressed mood; a few instances of scalp hair loss. Very rare reports of neuroleptic malignant syndrome (NMS) have been received, and, in most of these, patients were concurrently receiving therapies associated with NMS. In a single report, a ten year old boy who had been taking methylphenidate for approximately 18 months experienced an NMS-like event within 45 minutes of ingesting his first dose of venlafaxine. It is uncertain whether this case represented a drug-drug interaction, a response to either drug alone, or some other cause.
In children, loss of appetite, abdominal pain, weight loss during prolonged therapy, insomnia, and tachycardia may occur more frequently; however, any of the other adverse reactions listed above may also occur.

DOSAGE AND ADMINISTRATION

Dosage should be individualized according to the needs and responses of the patient.

Adults

Tablets: Administer in divided doses 2 or 3 times daily, preferably 30 to 45 minutes before meals. Average dosage is 20 to 30 mg daily. Some patients may require 40 to 60 mg daily. In others, 10 to 15 mg daily will be adequate. Patients who are unable to sleep if medication is taken late in the day should take the last dose before 6 p.m.
SR Tablets: Ritalin-SR tablets have a duration of action of approximately 8 hours. Therefore, Ritalin-SR tablets may be used in place of Ritalin tablets when the 8-hour dosage of Ritalin-SR corresponds to the titrated 8-hour dosage of Ritalin. Ritalin-SR tablets must be swallowed whole and never crushed or chewed.

Children (6 years and over)

Ritalin should be initiated in small doses, with gradual weekly increments. Daily dosage above 60 mg is not recommended.
If improvement is not observed after appropriate dosage adjustment over a one-month period, the drug should be discontinued.
Tablets: Start with 5 mg twice daily (before breakfast and lunch) with gradual increments of 5 to 10 mg weekly.
SR Tablets: Ritalin-SR tablets have a duration of action of approximately 8 hours. Therefore, Ritalin-SR tablets may be used in place of Ritalin tablets when the 8-hour dosage of Ritalin-SR corresponds to the titrated 8-hour dosage of Ritalin. Ritalin-SR tablets must be swallowed whole and never crushed or chewed.
If paradoxical aggravation of symptoms or other adverse effects occur, reduce dosage, or, if necessary, discontinue the drug.
Ritalin should be periodically discontinued to assess the child's condition. Improvement may be sustained when the drug is either temporarily or permanently discontinued.
Drug treatment should not and need not be indefinite and usually may be discontinued after puberty.

OVERDOSAGE

Signs and symptoms of acute overdosage, resulting principally from overstimulation of the central nervous system and from excessive sympathomimetic effects, may include the following: vomiting, agitation, tremors, hyperreflexia, muscle twitching, convulsions (may be followed by coma), euphoria, confusion, hallucinations, delirium, sweating, flushing, headache, hyperpyrexia, tachycardia, palpitations, cardiac arrhythmias, hypertension, mydriasis, and dryness of mucous membranes.
Consult with a Certified Poison Control Center regarding treatment for up-to-date guidance and advice.
Treatment consists of appropriate supportive measures. The patient must be protected against self-injury and against external stimuli that would aggravate overstimulation already present. Gastric contents may be evacuated by gastric lavage. In the presence of severe intoxication, use a carefully titrated dosage of a *short-acting* barbiturate before performing gastric lavage. Other measures to detoxify the gut include administration of activated charcoal and a cathartic.
Intensive care must be provided to maintain adequate circulation and respiratory exchange; external cooling procedures may be required for hyperpyrexia.
Efficacy of peritoneal dialysis or extracorporeal hemodialysis for Ritalin overdosage has not been established.

HOW SUPPLIED

Tablets 5 mg — round, yellow (imprinted CIBA 7)
Bottles of 100 .... NDC 0083-0007-30
Tablets 10 mg — round, pale green, scored (imprinted CIBA 3)
Bottles of 100 .... NDC 0083-0003-30
Tablets 20 mg — round, pale yellow, scored (imprinted CIBA 34)
Bottles of 100 .... NDC 0083-0034-30
Do not store above 30°C (86°F). Protect from light.
Dispense in tight, light-resistant container (USP).
SR Tablets 20 mg — round, white, coated (imprinted CIBA 16)
Bottles of 100 .... NDC 0083-0016-30
Note: SR Tablets are color-additive free.
Do not store above 30°C (86°F). Protect from moisture.
Dispense in tight, light-resistant container (USP).

REV: NOVEMBER 1999 T1999-70
Shown in Product Identification Guide, page 326

SANDIMMUNE® Soft Gelatin Capsules ℞
(cyclosporine capsules, USP)

SANDIMMUNE® Oral Solution ℞
(cyclosporine oral solution, USP)

SANDIMMUNE® Injection ℞
(cyclosporine injection, USP)
FOR INFUSION ONLY
Rx only

The following prescribing information is based on official labeling in effect November 1999.

WARNING: Only physicians experienced in immunosuppressive therapy and management of organ transplant patients should prescribe Sandimmune® (cyclosporine). Patients receiving the drug should be managed in facilities equipped and staffed with adequate laboratory and supportive medical resources. The physician responsible for maintenance therapy should have complete information requisite for the follow-up of the patient.
Sandimmune® (cyclosporine) should be administered with adrenal corticosteroids but not with other immunosuppressive agents. Increased susceptibility to infection and the possible development of lymphoma may result from immunosuppression.

Sandimmune® soft gelatin capsules (cyclosporine capsules, USP) and Sandimmune® oral solution (cyclosporine oral solution, USP) have decreased bioavailability in comparison to Neoral® soft gelatin capsules (cyclsporine capsules, USP) MODIFIED and Neoral® oral solution (cyclosporine oral solution, USP) MODIFIED.
Sandimmune® and Neoral® are not bioequivalent and cannot be used interchangeably without physician supervision.
The absorption of cyclosporine during chronic administration of Sandimmune® soft gelatin capsules and oral solution was found to be erratic. It is recommended that patients taking the soft gelatin capsules or oral solution over a period of time be monitored at repeated intervals for cyclosporine blood levels and subsequent dose adjustments be made in order to avoid toxicity due to high levels and possible organ rejection due to low absorption of cyclosporine. This is of special importance in liver transplants. Numerous assays are being developed to measure blood levels of cyclosporine. Comparison of levels in published literature to patient levels using current assays must be done with detailed knowledge of the assay methods employed. *(See Blood Level Monitoring under DOSAGE AND ADMINISTRATION)*

DESCRIPTION

Cyclosporine, the active principle in Sandimmune® (cyclosporine) is a cyclic polypeptide immunosuppressant agent consisting of 11 amino acids. It is produced as a metabolite by the fungus species *Beauveria nivea*.
Chemically, cyclosporine is designated as [*R*-[*R**,*R**-(*E*)]]-cyclic(L-alanyl-D-alanyl-*N*-methyl-L-leucyl-*N*-methyl-L-leucyl-*N*-methyl-L-valyl-3-hydroxy-*N*,4-dimethyl-L-2-amino-6-octenoyl-L-α-amino-butyryl-*N*-methylglycyl-*N*-methyl-L-leucyl-L-valyl-*N*-methyl-L-leucyl).
Sandimmune® soft gelatin capsules (cyclosporine capsules, USP) are available in 25 mg, 50 mg, and 100 mg strengths.
Each 25 mg capsule contains:
cyclosporine, USP .... 25 mg
alcohol, USP dehydrated .... max 12.7% by volume
Each 50 mg capsule contains:
cyclosporine, USP .... 50 mg
alcohol, USP dehydrated .... max 12.7% by volume
Each 100 mg capsule contains:
cyclosporine, USP .... 100 mg
alcohol, USP dehydrated .... max 12.7% by volume
Inactive Ingredients: corn oil, gelatin, glycerol, Labrafil M 2125 CS (polyoxyethylated glycolysed glycerides), red iron oxide (25 mg and 100 mg capsule only), sorbitol, titanium dioxide, yellow iron oxide (50 mg capsule only), and other ingredients.
Sandimmune® oral solution (cyclosporine oral solution, USP) is available in 50 mL bottles.
Each mL contains:
cyclosporine, USP .... 100 mg
alcohol, Ph. Helv. .... 12.5% by volume
dissolved in an olive oil, Ph. Helv./Labrafil M 1944 CS (polyoxyethylated oleic glycerides) vehicle which must be further diluted with milk, chocolate milk, or orange juice before oral administration.
Sandimmune® injection (cyclosporine injection, USP) is available in a 5 mL sterile ampul for I.V. administration.
Each mL contains:
cyclosporine, USP .... 50 mg
*Cremophor® EL (polyoxyethylated castor oil) ...... 650 mg
alcohol, Ph. Helv. .... 32.9% by volume
nitrogen .... qs
which must be diluted further with 0.9% Sodium Chloride Injection or 5% Dextrose Injection before use.
The chemical structure of cyclosporine (also known as cyclosporin A) is:

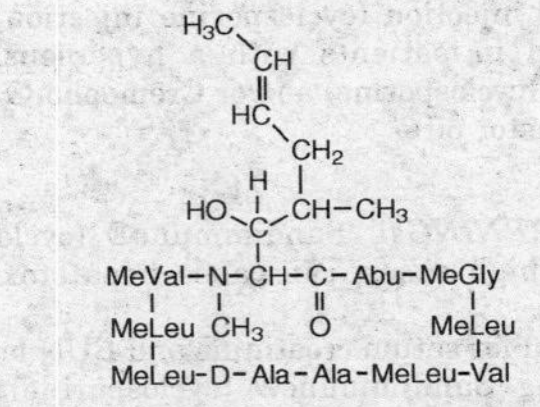

H3C–CH=CH–CH2–CH(CH3)–C(H)(OH)– (side chain)
MeVal–N–CH–C–Abu–MeGly
MeLeu CH3 O MeLeu
MeLeu–D–Ala–Ala–MeLeu–Val

$C_{62}H_{111}N_{11}O_{12}$ Mol. Wt. 1202.63

---

*Cremophor is the registered trademark of BASF Aktiengesellschaft.

CLINICAL PHARMACOLOGY

Sandimmune® (cyclosporine) is a potent immunosuppressive agent which in animals prolongs survival of allogeneic transplants involving skin, heart, kidney, pancreas, bone marrow, small intestine, and lung. Sandimmune® (cyclosporine) has been demonstrated to suppress some humoral immunity and to a greater extent, cell-mediated reactions such as allograft rejection, delayed hypersensitivity, experimental allergic encephalomyelitis, Freund's adjuvant arthritis, and graft vs. host disease in many animal species for a variety of organs.
Successful kidney, liver, and heart allogeneic transplants have been performed in man using Sandimmune® (cyclosporine).
The exact mechanism of action of Sandimmune® (cyclosporine) is not known. Experimental evidence suggests that the effectiveness of cyclosporine is due to specific and reversible inhibition of immunocompetent lymphocytes in the G_0- or G_1-phase of the cell cycle. T-lymphocytes are preferentially inhibited. The T-helper cell is the main target, although the T-suppressor cell may also be suppressed. Sandimmune® (cyclosporine) also inhibits lymphokine production and release including interleukin-2 or T-cell growth factor (TCGF).
No functional effects on phagocytic (changes in enzyme secretions not altered, chemotactic migration of granulocytes, macrophage migration, carbon clearance *in vivo*) or tumor cells (growth rate, metastasis) can be detected in animals. Sandimmune® (cyclosporine) does not cause bone marrow suppression in animal models or man.
The absorption of cyclosporine from the gastrointestinal tract is incomplete and variable. Peak concentrations (C_{max}) in blood and plasma are achieved at about 3.5 hours. C_{max} and area under the plasma or blood concentration/time curve (AUC) increase with the administered dose; for blood the relationship is curvilinear (parabolic) between 0 and 1400 mg. As determined by a specific assay, C_{max} is approximately 1.0 ng/mL/mg of dose for plasma and 2.7–1.4 ng/mL/mg of dose for blood (for low to high doses). Compared to an intravenous infusion, the absolute bioavailability of the oral solution is approximately 30% based upon the results in 2 patients. The bioavailability of Sandimmune® soft gelatin capsules (cyclosporine capsules, USP) is equivalent to Sandimmune® oral solution, (cyclosporine oral solution, USP).
Cyclosporine is distributed largely outside the blood volume. In the blood the distribution is concentration dependent. Approximately 33%–47% is in plasma, 4%–9% in lymphocytes, 5%–12% in granulocytes, and 41%–58% in erythrocytes. At high concentrations, the uptake by leukocytes and erythrocytes becomes saturated. In plasma, approximately 90% is bound to proteins, primarily lipoproteins.

Continued on next page

Sandimmune—Cont.

The disposition of cyclosporine from blood is biphasic with a terminal half-life of approximately 19 hours (range: 10–27 hours). Elimination is primarily biliary with only 6% of the dose excreted in the urine.

Cyclosporine is extensively metabolized but there is no major metabolic pathway. Only 0.1% of the dose is excreted in the urine as unchanged drug. Of 15 metabolites characterized in human urine, 9 have been assigned structures. The major pathways consist of hydroxylation of the Cγ-carbon of 2 of the leucine residues, Cη-carbon hydroxylation, and cyclic ether formation (with oxidation of the double bond) in the side chain of the amino acid 3-hydroxyl-*N*,4-dimethyl-L-2-amino-6-octenoic acid and *N*-demethylation of *N*-methyl leucine residues. Hydrolysis of the cyclic peptide chain or conjugation of the aforementioned metabolites do not appear to be important biotransformation pathways.

INDICATIONS AND USAGE

Sandimmune® (cyclosporine) is indicated for the prophylaxis of organ rejection in kidney, liver, and heart allogeneic transplants. It is always to be used with adrenal corticosteroids. The drug may also be used in the treatment of chronic rejection in patients previously treated with other immunosuppressive agents.

Because of the risk of anaphylaxis, Sandimmune® injection (cyclosporine injection, USP) should be reserved for patients who are unable to take the soft gelatin capsules or oral solution.

CONTRAINDICATIONS

Sandimmune® injection (cyclosporine injection, USP) is contraindicated in patients with a hypersensitivity to Sandimmune® (cyclosporine) and/or Cremophor® EL (polyoxyethylated castor oil).

WARNINGS

(See boxed WARNINGs): Sandimmune® (cyclosporine), when used in high doses, can cause hepatotoxicity and nephrotoxicity.

It is not unusual for serum creatinine and BUN levels to be elevated during Sandimmune® (cyclosporine) therapy. These elevations in renal transplant patients do not necessarily indicate rejection, and each patient must be fully evaluated before dosage adjustment is initiated.

Nephrotoxicity has been noted in 25% of cases of renal transplantation, 38% of cases of cardiac transplantation, and 37% of cases of liver transplantation. Mild nephrotoxicity was generally noted 2–3 months after transplant and consisted of an arrest in the fall of the preoperative elevations of BUN and creatinine at a range of 35–45 mg/dl and 2.0–2.5 mg/dl respectively. These elevations were often responsive to dosage reduction.

More overt nephrotoxicity was seen early after transplantation and was characterized by a rapidly rising BUN and creatinine. Since these events are similar to rejection episodes care must be taken to differentiate between them. This form of nephrotoxicity is usually responsive to Sandimmune® (cyclosporine) dosage reduction.

Although specific diagnostic criteria which reliably differentiate renal graft rejection from drug toxicity have not been found, a number of parameters have been significantly associated to one or the other. It should be noted however, that up to 20% of patients may have simultaneous nephrotoxicity and rejection.

[See table below]

A form of chronic progressive cyclosporine-associated nephrotoxicity is characterized by serial deterioration in renal function and morphologic changes in the kidneys. From 5%–15% of transplant recipients will fail to show a reduction in a rising serum creatinine despite a decrease or discontinuation of cyclosporine therapy. Renal biopsies from these patients will demonstrate an interstitial fibrosis with tubular atrophy. In addition, toxic tubulopathy, peritubular capillary congestion, arteriolopathy, and a striped form of interstitial fibrosis with tubular atrophy may be present. Though none of these morphologic changes is entirely specific, a histologic diagnosis of chronic progressive cyclosporine-associated nephrotoxicity requires evidence of these.

When considering the development of chronic nephrotoxicity it is noteworthy that several authors have reported an association between the appearance of interstitial fibrosis and higher cumulative doses or persistently high circulating trough levels of cyclosporine. This is particularly true during the first 6 posttransplant months when the dosage tends to be highest and when, in kidney recipients, the organ appears to be most vulnerable to the toxic effects of cyclosporine. Among other contributing factors to the development of interstitial fibrosis in these patients must be included, prolonged perfusion time, warm ischemia time, as well as episodes of acute toxicity, and acute and chronic rejection. The reversibility of interstitial fibrosis and its correlation to renal function have not yet been determined.

Impaired renal function at any time requires close monitoring, and frequent dosage adjustment may be indicated. In patients with persistent high elevations of BUN and creatinine who are unresponsive to dosage adjustments, consideration should be given to switching to other immunosuppressive therapy. In the event of severe and unremitting rejection, it is preferable to allow the kidney transplant to be rejected and removed rather than increase the Sandimmune® (cyclosporine) dosage to a very high level in an attempt to reverse the rejection.

Nephrotoxicity vs Rejection

Parameter	Nephrotoxicity	Rejection
History	Donor > 50 years old or hypotensive Prolonged kidney preservation Prolonged anastomosis time Concomitant nephrotoxic drugs	Antidonor immune response Retransplant patient
Clinical	Often > 6 weeks postop[b] Prolonged initial nonfunction (acute tubular necrosis)	Often < 4 weeks postop[b] Fever > 37.5°C Weight gain > 0.5 kg Graft swelling and tenderness Decrease in daily urine volume > 500 mL (or 50%)
Laboratory	CyA serum trough level > 200 ng/mL Gradual rise in Cr (< 0.15 mg/dl/day)[a] Cr plateau < 25% above baseline BUN/Cr ≥ 20	CyA serum trough level < 150 ng/mL Rapid rise in Cr (> 0.3 mg/dl/day)[a] Cr > 25% above baseline BUN/Cr < 20
Biopsy	Arteriolopathy (medial hypertrophy[a], hyalinosis, nodular deposits, intimal thickening, endothelial vacuolization, progressive scarring) Tubular atrophy, isometric vacuolization, isolated calcifications Minimal edema Mild focal infiltrates[c] Diffuse interstitial fibrosis, often striped form	Endovasculitis[c] (proliferation[a], intimal arteritis[b], necrosis, sclerosis) Tubulitis with RBC[b] and WBC[b] casts, some irregular vacuolization Interstitial edema[c] and hemorrhage[b] Diffuse moderate to severe mononuclear infiltrates[d] Glomerulitis (mononuclear cells)[c]
Aspiration Cytology	CyA deposits in tubular and endothelial cells Fine isometric vacuolization of tubular cells	Inflammatory infiltrate with mononuclear phagocytes, macrophages, lymphoblastoid cells, and activated T-cells These strongly express HLA-DR antigens
Urine Cytology	Tubular cells with vacuolization and granularization	Degenerative tubular cells, plasma cells, and lymphocyturia > 20% of sediment
Manometry	Intracapsular pressure < 40 mm Hg[b]	Intracapsular pressure > 40 mm Hg[b]
Ultrasonography	Unchanged graft cross sectional area	Increase in graft cross sectional area AP diameter ≥ Transverse diameter
Magnetic Resonance Imagery	Normal appearance	Loss of distinct corticomedullary junction, swelling, image intensity of parachyma approaching that of psoas, loss of hilar fat
Radionuclide Scan	Normal or generally decreased perfusion Decrease in tubular function (^{131} I-hippuran) > decrease in perfusion (^{99m} Tc DTPA)	Patchy arterial flow Decrease in perfusion > decrease in tubular function Increased uptake of Indium 111 labeled platelets or Tc-99m in colloid
Therapy	Responds to decreased Sandimmune® (cyclosporine)	Responds to increased steroids or antilymphocyte globulin

[a]$p < 0.05$, [b]$p < 0.01$, [c]$p < 0.001$, [d]$p < 0.0001$

Occasionally patients have developed a syndrome of thrombocytopenia and microangiopathic hemolytic anemia which may result in graft failure. The vasculopathy can occur in the absence of rejection and is accompanied by avid platelet consumption within the graft as demonstrated by Indium 111 labeled platelet studies. Neither the pathogenesis nor the management of this syndrome is clear. Though resolution has occurred after reduction or discontinuation of Sandimmune® (cyclosporine) and 1) administration of streptokinase and heparin or 2) plasmapheresis, this appears to depend upon early detection with Indium 111 labeled platelet scans. *(See ADVERSE REACTIONS)*

Significant hyperkalemia (sometimes associated with hyperchloremic metabolic acidosis) and hyperuricemia have been seen occasionally in individual patients.

Hepatotoxicity has been noted in 4% of cases of renal transplantation, 7% of cases of cardiac transplantation, and 4% of cases of liver transplantation. This was usually noted during the first month of therapy when high doses of Sandimmune® (cyclosporine) were used and consisted of elevations of hepatic enzymes and bilirubin. The chemistry elevations usually decreased with a reduction in dosage.

As in patients receiving other immunosuppressants, those patients receiving Sandimmune® (cyclosporine) are at increased risk for development of lymphomas and other malignancies, particularly those of the skin. The increased risk appears related to the intensity and duration of immunosuppression rather than to the use of specific agents. Because of the danger of oversuppression of the immune system, which can also increase susceptibility to infection, Sandimmune® (cyclosporine) should not be administered with other immunosuppressive agents except adrenal corticosteroids. The efficacy and safety of cyclosporine in combination with other immunosuppressive agents have not been determined.

There have been reports of convulsions in adult and pediatric patients receiving cyclosporine, particularly in combination with high dose methylprednisolone.

Rarely (approximately 1 in 1000), patients receiving Sandimmune® injection (cyclosporine injection, USP) have experienced anaphylactic reactions. Although the exact cause of these reactions is unknown, it is believed to be due to the Cremophor® EL (polyoxyethylated castor oil) used as the vehicle for the I.V. formulation. These reactions have consisted of flushing of the face and upper thorax, acute respiratory distress with dyspnea and wheezing, blood pressure changes, and tachycardia. One patient died after respiratory arrest and aspiration pneumonia. In some cases, the reaction subsided after the infusion was stopped.

Patients receiving Sandimmune® injection (cyclosporine injection, USP) should be under continuous observation for at least the first 30 minutes following the start of the infusion and at frequent intervals thereafter. If anaphylaxis occurs, the infusion should be stopped. An aqueous solution of epinephrine 1:1000 should be available at the bedside as well as a source of oxygen.

Anaphylactic reactions have not been reported with the soft gelatin capsules or oral solution which lack Cremophor® EL (polyoxyethylated castor oil). In fact, patients experiencing anaphylactic reactions have been treated subsequently with the soft gelatin capsules or oral solution without incident.

Care should be taken in using Sandimmune® (cyclosporine) with nephrotoxic drugs. *(See PRECAUTIONS)*

Because Sandimmune® is not bioequivalent to Neoral®, conversion from Neoral® to Sandimmune® using a 1:1 ratio (mg/kg/day) may result in a lower cyclosporine blood concentration. Conversion from Neoral® to Sandimmune® should be made with increased blood concentration monitoring to avoid the potential of underdosing.

PRECAUTIONS

General: Patients with malabsorption may have difficulty in achieving therapeutic levels with Sandimmune® soft gelatin capsules or oral solution.

Hypertension is a common side effect of Sandimmune® (cyclosporine) therapy. *(See ADVERSE REACTIONS)* Mild or moderate hypertension is more frequently encountered than severe hypertension and the incidence decreases over time. Antihypertensive therapy may be required. Control of blood pressure can be accomplished with any of the common anti hypertensive agents. However, since cyclosporine may cause hyperkalemia, potassium-sparing diuretics should not be used. While calcium antagonists can be effective agents in treating cyclosporine-associated hypertension, care should be taken since interference with cyclosporine metabolism may require a dosage adjustment. *(See Drug Interactions)*

During treatment with Sandimmune® (cyclosporine), vaccination may be less effective; and the use of live attenuated vaccines should be avoided.

Information for Patients: Patients should be advised that any change of cyclosporine formulation should be made cautiously and only under physician supervision because it may result in the need for a change in dosage.

Patients should be informed of the necessity of repeated laboratory tests while they are receiving the drug. They should be given careful dosage instructions, advised of the potential risks during pregnancy, and informed of the increased risk of neoplasia.

Patients using cyclosporine oral solution with its accompanying syringe for dosage measurement should be cautioned not to rinse the syringe either before or after use. Introduction of water into the product by any means will cause variation in dose.

Laboratory Tests: Renal and liver functions should be assessed repeatedly by measurement of BUN, serum creatinine, serum bilirubin, and liver enzymes.

Drug Interactions: All of the individual drugs cited below are well substantiated to interact with Sandimmune® (cyclosporine).

Drugs That Exhibit Nephrotoxic Synergy

gentamicin
tobramycin
vancomycin
amphotericin B
ketoconazole
melphalan
cimetidine
ranitidine
diclofenac
trimethoprim
 with sulfamethoxazole
azapropazon

Careful monitoring of renal function should be practiced when Sandimmune® (cyclosporine) is used with nephrotoxic drugs.

Drugs That Alter Cyclosporine Levels: Cyclosporine is extensively metabolized by the liver. Therefore, circulating cyclosporine levels may be influenced by drugs that affect hepatic microsomal enzymes, particularly the cytochrome P-450 system.

Substances known to inhibit these enzymes will decrease hepatic metabolism and increase cyclosporine levels. Substances that are inducers of cytochrome P-450 activity will increase hepatic metabolism and decrease cyclosporine levels. Monitoring of circulating cyclosporine levels and appropriate Sandimmune® (cyclosporine) dosage adjustment are essential when these drugs are used concomitantly. *(See Blood Level Monitoring)*

Drugs That Increase Cyclosporine Levels

diltiazem
nicardipine
verapamil
ketoconazole
fluconazole
itraconazole
danazol
bromocriptine
metoclopramide
erythromycin
methylprednisolone

Drugs That Decrease Cyclosporine Levels

rifampin
phenytoin
phenobarbital
carbamazepine

Other Drug Interactions: Reduced clearance of prednisolone, digoxin, and lovastatin has been observed when these drugs are administered with Sandimmune® (cyclosporine). In addition, a decrease in the apparent volume of distribution of digoxin has been reported after Sandimmune® (cyclosporine) administration. Severe digitalis toxicity has been seen within days of starting cyclosporine in several patients taking digoxin. Sandimmune® (cyclosporine) should not be used with potassium-sparing diuretics because hyperkalemia can occur. During treatment with Sandimmune® (cyclosporine), vaccination may be less effective; and the use of live vaccines should be avoided. Myositis has occurred with con comitant lovastatin, frequent gingival hyperplasia with nifedipine, and convulsions with high dose methylprednisolone. Further information on drugs that have been reported to interact with Sandimmune® (cyclosporine) is available from Novartis Pharmaceuticals Corporation.

Carcinogenesis, Mutagenesis, and Impairment of Fertility: Cyclosporine gave no evidence of mutagenic or teratogenic effects in appropriate test systems. Only at dose levels toxic to dams, were adverse effects seen in reproduction studies in rats. *(See Pregnancy)*

Carcinogenicity studies were carried out in male and female rats and mice. In the 78-week mouse study, at doses of 1, 4, and 16 mg/kg/day, evidence of a statistically significant trend was found for lymphocytic lymphomas in females, and the incidence of hepatocellular carcinomas in mid-dose males significantly exceeded the control value. In the 24-month rat study, conducted at 0.5, 2, and 8 mg/kg/day, pancreatic islet cell adenomas significantly exceeded the control rate in the low dose level. The hepatocellular carcinomas and pancreatic islet cell adenomas were not dose related.

No impairment in fertility was demonstrated in studies in male and female rats.

Cyclosporine has not been found mutagenic/genotoxic in the Ames Test, the V79-HGPRT Test, the micronucleus test in mice and Chinese hamsters, the chromosome-aberration tests in Chinese hamster bone-marrow, the mouse dominant lethal assay, and the DNA-repair test in sperm from treated mice. A recent study analyzing sister chromatid exchange (SCE) induction by cyclosporine using human lymphocytes *in vitro* gave indication of a positive effect (i.e., induction of SCE), at high concentrations in this system.

An increased incidence of malignancy is a recognized complication of immunosuppression in recipients of organ transplants. The most common forms of neoplasms are non-Hodgkin's lymphoma and carcinomas of the skin. The risk of malignancies in cyclosporine recipients is higher than in the normal, healthy population but similar to that in patients receiving other immunosuppressive therapies. It has been reported that reduction or discontinuance of immunosuppression may cause the lesions to regress.

Body System/ Adverse Reactions	Randomized Kidney Patients Sandimmune® (N=227) %	Randomized Kidney Patients Azathioprine (N=228) %	All Sandimmune® (cyclosporine) Patients Kidney (N=705) %	All Sandimmune® (cyclosporine) Patients Heart (N=112) %	All Sandimmune® (cyclosporine) Patients Liver (N=75) %
Genitourinary					
Renal Dysfunction	32	6	25	38	37
Cardiovascular					
Hypertension	26	18	13	53	27
Cramps	4	< 1	2	< 1	0
Skin					
Hirsutism	21	< 1	21	28	45
Acne	6	8	2	2	1
Central Nervous System					
Tremor	12	0	21	31	55
Convulsions	3	1	1	4	5
Headache	2	< 1	2	15	4
Gastrointestinal					
Gum Hyperplasia	4	0	9	5	16
Diarrhea	3	< 1	3	4	8
Nausea/Vomiting	2	< 1	4	10	4
Hepatotoxicity	< 1	< 1	4	7	4
Abdominal Discomfort	< 1	0	< 1	7	0
Autonomic Nervous System					
Paresthesia	3	0	1	2	1
Flushing	< 1	0	4	0	4
Hematopoietic					
Leukopenia	2	19	< 1	6	0
Lymphoma	< 1	0	1	6	1
Respiratory					
Sinusitis	< 1	0	4	3	7
Miscellaneous					
Gynecomastia	< 1	0	< 1	4	3

Renal Transplant Patients in Whom Therapy Was Discontinued

Reason for Discontinuation	Randomized Patients Sandimmune® (N=227) %	Randomized Patients Azathioprine (N=228) %	All Sandimmune® Patients (N=705) %
Renal Toxicity	5.7	0	5.4
Infection	0	0.4	0.9
Lack of Efficacy	2.6	0.9	1.4
Acute Tubular Necrosis	2.6	0	1.0
Lymphoma/Lymphoproliferative Disease	0.4	0	0.3
Hypertension	0	0	0.3
Hematological Abnormalities	0	0.4	0
Other	0	0	0.7

Pregnancy: *Pregnancy Category C.* Sandimmune® oral solution (cyclosporine oral solution, USP) has been shown to be embryo- and fetotoxic in rats and rabbits when given in doses 2–5 times the human dose. At toxic doses (rats at 30 mg/kg/day and rabbits at 100 mg/kg/day), Sandimmune® oral solution (cyclosporine oral solution, USP) was embryo- and fetotoxic as indicated by increased pre- and postnatal mortality and reduced fetal weight together with related skeletal retardations. In the well-tolerated dose range (rats at up to 17 mg/kg/day and rabbits at up to 30 mg/kg/day), Sandimmune® oral solution (cyclosporine oral solution, USP) proved to be without any embryolethal or teratogenic effects.

There are no adequate and well-controlled studies in pregnant women. Sandimmune® (cyclosporine) should be used during pregnancy only if the potential benefit justifies the potential risk to the fetus.

The following data represent the reported outcomes of 116 pregnancies in women receiving Sandimmune® (cyclosporine) during pregnancy, 90% of whom were transplant patients, and most of whom received Sandimmune® (cyclosporine) throughout the entire gestational period. Since most of the patients were not prospectively identified, the results are likely to be biased toward negative outcomes. The only consistent patterns of abnormality were premature birth (gestational period of 28 to 36 weeks) and low birth weight for gestational age. It is not possible to separate the effects of Sandimmune® (cyclosporine) on these pregnancies from the effects of the other immunosuppressants, the underlying maternal disorders, or other aspects of the transplantation milieu. Sixteen fetal losses occurred. Most of the pregnancies (85 of 100) were complicated by disorders; including, pre-eclampsia, eclampsia, premature labor, abruptio placentae, oligohydramnios, Rh incompatibility and fetoplacental dysfunction. Preterm delivery occurred in 47%. Seven malformations were reported in 5 viable infants and in 2 cases of fetal loss. Twenty-eight percent of the infants were small for gestational age. Neonatal complications occurred in 27%. In a report of 23 children followed up to 4 years, postnatal development was said to be normal. More information on cyclosporine use in pregnancy is available from Novartis Pharmaceuticals Corporation.

Nursing Mothers: Since Sandimmune® (cyclosporine) is excreted in human milk, nursing should be avoided.

Pediatric Use: Although no adequate and well controlled studies have been conducted in children, patients as young as 6 months of age have received the drug with no unusual adverse effects.

ADVERSE REACTIONS

The principal adverse reactions of Sandimmune® (cyclosporine) therapy are renal dysfunction, tremor, hirsutism, hypertension, and gum hyperplasia.

Hypertension, which is usually mild to moderate, may occur in approximately 50% of patients following renal transplantation and in most cardiac transplant patients.

Glomerular capillary thrombosis has been found in patients treated with cyclosporine and may progress to graft failure. The pathologic changes resemble those seen in the hemolytic-uremic syndrome and include throm bosis of the renal microvasculature, with platelet-fibrin thrombi occluding glomerular capillaries and afferent arterioles, microangiopathic hemolytic anemia, thrombocytopenia, and decreased renal function. Similar findings have been observed when other immunosuppressives have been employed posttransplantation.

Hypomagnesemia has been reported in some, but not all, patients exhibiting convulsions while on cyclosporine therapy. Although magnesium-depletion studies in normal subjects suggest that hypomagnesemia is associated with neurologic disorders, multiple factors, including hypertension, high dose methylprednisolone, hypocholesterolemia, and nephrotoxicity associated with high plasma concentrations of cyclosporine appear to be related to the neurological manifestations of cyclosporine toxicity.

The following reactions occurred in 3% or greater of 892 patients involved in clinical trials of kidney, heart, and liver transplants:

[See first table above]

Continued on next page

Sandimmune—Cont.

The following reactions occurred in 2% or less of patients: allergic reactions, anemia, anorexia, confusion, conjunctivitis, edema, fever, brittle fingernails, gastritis, hearing loss, hiccups, hyperglycemia, muscle pain, peptic ulcer, thrombocyto penia, tinnitus.

The following reactions occurred rarely: anxiety, chest pain, constipation, depression, hair breaking, hematuria, joint pain, lethargy, mouth sores, myocardial infarction, night sweats, pancreatitis, pruritus, swallowing difficulty, tingling, upper GI bleeding, visual disturbance, weakness, weight loss.

[See second table at top of previous page]

Sandimmune® (cyclosporine) was discontinued on a temporary basis and then restarted in 18 additional patients.

[See table below]

Cremophor® EL (polyoxyethylated castor oil) is known to cause hyperlipemia and electrophoretic abnormalities of lipoproteins. These effects are reversible upon discontinuation of treatment but are usually not a reason to stop treatment.

There have been post-marketing reports of neurotoxicity associated with cyclosporine therapy. Signs of encephalopathy, convulsions, vision and movement dis turbances and impaired consciousness have been described, especially in liver transplant patients. These alterations appear to be multifactorial in origin. Generally, reduction of dose has been observed to result in reversal of these changes.

OVERDOSAGE

There is a minimal experience with overdosage. Because of the slow absorption of Sandimmune® soft gelatin capsules or oral solution, forced emesis would be of value up to 2 hours after administration. Transient hepatotoxicity and nephrotoxicity may occur which should resolve following drug withdrawal. General supportive measures and symptomatic treatment should be followed in all cases of overdosage. Sandimmune® (cyclosporine) is not dialyzable to any great extent, nor is it cleared well by charcoal hemoperfusion. The oral LD_{50} is 2329 mg/kg in mice, 1480 mg/kg in rats, and > 1000 mg/kg in rabbits. The I.V. LD_{50} is 148 mg/kg in mice, 104 mg/kg in rats, and 46 mg/kg in rabbits.

DOSAGE AND ADMINISTRATION

Sandimmune® Soft Gelatin Capsules (cyclosporine capsules, USP) and Sandimmune® Oral Solution (cyclosporine oral solution, USP): Sandimmune® soft gelatin capsules (cyclosporine capsules, USP) and Sandimmune® oral solution (cyclosporine oral solution, USP) have decreased bioavailability in comparison to Neoral® soft gelatin capsules (cyclosporine capsules, USP) MODIFIED and Neoral® oral solution (cyclosporine oral solution, USP) MODIFIED. Sandimmune® and Neoral® are not bioequivalent and cannot be used interchangeably without physician supervision.

The initial oral dose of Sandimmune® (cyclosporine) should be given 4–12 hours prior to transplantation as a single dose of 15 mg/kg. Although a daily single dose of 14–18 mg/kg was used in most clinical trials, few centers continue to use the highest dose, most favoring the lower end of the scale. There is a trend towards use of even lower initial doses for renal transplantation in the ranges of 10–14 mg/kg/day. The initial single daily dose is continued postoperatively for 1–2 weeks and then tapered by 5% per week to a maintenance dose of 5–10 mg/kg/day. Some centers have successfully tapered the maintenance dose to as low as 3 mg/kg/day in selected renal transplant patients without an apparent rise in rejection rate.

(See Blood Level Monitoring below)

In pediatric usage, the same dose and dosing regimen may be used as in adults although in several studies children have required and tolerated higher doses than those used in adults.

Adjunct therapy with adrenal corticosteroids is recommended. Different tapering dosage schedules of prednisone appear to achieve similar results. A dosage schedule based on the patient's weight started with 2.0 mg/kg/day for the first 4 days tapered to 1.0 mg/kg/day by 1 week, 0.6 mg/kg/day by 2 weeks, 0.3 mg/kg/day by 1 month, and 0.15 mg/kg/day by 2 months and thereafter as a maintenance dose. Another center started with an initial dose of 200 mg tapered by 40 mg/day until reaching 20 mg/day. After 2 months at this dose, a further reduction to 10 mg/day was made. Adjustments in dosage of prednisone must be made according to the clinical situation.

To make Sandimmune® oral solution (cyclosporine oral solution, USP) more palatable, the oral solution may be diluted with milk, chocolate milk, or orange juice preferably at room temperature. Patients should avoid switching diluents frequently. Sandimmune® soft gelatin capsules and oral solution should be administered on a consistent schedule with regard to time of day and relation to meals.

Take the prescribed amount of Sandimmune® (cyclosporine) from the container using the dosage syringe supplied after removal of the protective cover, and transfer the solution to a glass of milk, chocolate milk, or orange juice. Stir well and drink at once. Do not allow to stand before drinking. It is best to use a glass container and rinse it with more diluent to ensure that the total dose is taken. After use, replace the dosage syringe in the protective cover. Do not rinse the dosage syringe with water or other cleaning agents either before or after use. If the dosage syringe requires cleaning, it must be completely dry before resuming use. Introduction of water into the product by any means will cause variation in dose.

Sandimmune® Injection (cyclosporine injection, USP)
FOR INFUSION ONLY

Note: Anaphylactic reactions have occurred with Sandimmune® injection (cyclosporine injection, USP). *(See WARNINGS)*

Patients unable to take Sandimmune® soft gelatin capsules or oral solution pre- or postoperatively may be treated with the I.V. concentrate. **Sandimmune® injection (cyclosporine injection, USP) is administered at 1/3 the oral dose.** The initial dose of Sandimmune® injection (cyclosporine injection, USP) should be given 4–12 hours prior to transplantation as a single I.V. dose of 5–6 mg/kg/day. This daily single dose is continued post operatively until the patient can tolerate the soft gelatin capsules or oral solution. Patients should be switched to Sandimmune® soft gelatin capsules or oral solution as soon as possible after surgery. In pediatric usage, the same dose and dosing regimen may be used, although higher doses may be required.

Adjunct steroid therapy is to be used. *(See aforementioned)*

Immediately before use, the I.V. concentrate should be diluted 1 mL Sandimmune® injection (cyclosporine injection, USP) in 20 mL-100 mL 0.9% Sodium Chloride Injection or 5% Dextrose Injection and given in a slow intravenous infusion over approximately 2–6 hours.

Diluted infusion solutions should be discarded after 24 hours.

The Cremophor® EL (polyoxyethylated castor oil) contained in the concentrate for intravenous infusion can cause phthalate stripping from PVC.

Parenteral drug products should be inspected visually for particulate matter and discoloration prior to administration, whenever solution and container permit.

Blood Level Monitoring: Several study centers have found blood level monitoring of cyclosporine useful in patient management. While no fixed relationships have yet been established, in one series of 375 consecutive cadaveric renal transplant recipients, dosage was adjusted to achieve specific whole blood 24-hour trough levels of 100–200 ng/mL as determined by high-pressure liquid chromatography (HPLC).

Of major importance to blood level analysis is the type of assay used. The above levels are specific to the parent cyclosporine molecule and correlate directly to the new monoclonal specific radioimmunoassays (mRIA-sp). Nonspecific assays are also available which detect the parent compound molecule and various of its metabolites. Older studies often cited levels using a nonspecific assay which were roughly twice those of specific assays. Assay results are not interchangeable and their use should be guided by their approved labeling. If plasma specimens are employed, levels will vary with the temperature at the time of separation from whole blood. Plasma levels may range from 1/2–1/5 of whole blood levels. Refer to individual assay labeling for complete instructions. In addition, *Transplantation Proceedings* (June 1990) contains position papers and a broad consensus generated at the Cyclosporine-Therapeutic Drug Monitoring conference that year. Blood level monitoring is not a replacement for renal function monitoring or tissue biopsies.

HOW SUPPLIED

Sandimmune® Soft Gelatin Capsules (cyclosporine capsules, USP)

25 mg: Oblong, pink, branded "Ⓢ 78/240". Unit dose packages of 30 capsules, 3 blister cards of 10 capsules (NDC 0078-0240-15).

50 mg: Oblong, corn-yellow, branded "Ⓢ 78/242". Unit dose packages of 30 capsules, 3 blister cards of 10 capsules (NDC 0078-0242-15).

100 mg: Oblong, dusty rose, branded "Ⓢ 78/241". Unit dose packages of 30 capsules, 3 blister cards of 10 capsules (NDC 0078-0241-15).

Store and Dispense: In the original unit dose container at temperatures below 86°F (30°C). An odor may be detected upon opening the unit dose container, which will dissipate shortly thereafter. This odor does not affect the quality of the product.

Sandimmune® Oral Solution (cyclosporine oral solution, USP): Supplied in 50 mL bottles containing 100 mg of cyclosporine per mL (NDC 0078-0110-22). A dosage syringe is provided for dispensing.

Store and Dispense: In the original container at temperatures below 86°F (30°C). Do not store in the refrigerator. Protect from freezing. Once opened, the contents must be used within 2 months.

Sandimmune® Injection (cyclosporine injection, USP)
FOR INTRAVENOUS INFUSION

Supplied as a 5 mL sterile ampul containing 50 mg of cyclosporine per mL, in boxes of 10 ampuls (NDC 0078-0109-01).

Store and Dispense: At temperatures below 86°F (30°C) and protected from light.

Sandimmune® Soft Gelatin Capsules (cyclosporine capsules, USP)

Manufactured by
R.P. Scherer GmbH, EBERBACH/BADEN, GERMANY
Manufactured for
Novartis Pharmaceuticals Corporation, East Hanover, NJ 07936

Sandimmune® Oral Solution (cyclosporine oral solution, USP) and Sandimmune® Injection (cyclosporine injection, USP)
FOR INFUSION ONLY

Manufactured by
NOVARTIS PHARMA AG, Basle, Switzerland
Manufactured for
Novartis Pharmaceuticals Corporation, East Hanover, NJ 07936

 T1999-55
REV: NOVEMBER 1999 4062-42

Shown in Product Identification Guide, page 326

IMMUNE GLOBULIN INTRAVENOUS (HUMAN) SANDOGLOBULIN® ℞

Lyophilized Preparation

Rx only

The following prescribing information is based on official labeling in effect July 2000.

DESCRIPTION

Immune Globulin Intravenous (Human), (IGIV) Sandoglobulin®, is a sterile, highly purified polyvalent antibody product containing in concentrated form all the IgG antibodies which regularly occur in the donor population (1). This immunoglobulin preparation is produced by cold alcohol fractionation from the plasma of volunteer US donors. Part of the fractionation may be performed by another US-licensed manufacturer. The fractionation process by which Sandoglobulin® is prepared from plasma includes several filtration steps which are carried out in the presence of filter aids; some of these filtration steps are used for the separation of a cold ethanol precipitate. Four of these steps were validated for virus *elimination*. The cumulative LRFs (log_{10} of reduction factors) were 15.5 for HIV (human immunodeficiency virus), 16.0 for PRV (pseudorabies virus), 9.3 for SFV (Semliki Forest virus), 12.4 for Sindbis virus, and 14.1 for BEV (bovine enterovirus). Sandoglobulin® is made suitable for intravenous use by treatment at acid pH in the presence of trace amounts of pepsin (2,3). Treatment with pepsin at pH4 rapidly *inactivates* enveloped viruses. LRFs were ≥6.1 for HIV, ≥5.3 for PRV, ≥4.4 for BVDV (bovine viral diarrhea virus), and ≥6.8 for SFV. PRV and the two model viruses for HCV (hepatitis C virus), BVDV and SFV, were all inactivated within 1/10, and HIV within 1/2 of the total incubation time used during production of Sandoglobulin®. *Overall viral clearance* by either *elimination* and/or *inactivation* during the manufacturing process has been documented to be ≥21 for HIV, ≥19 for PRV, ≥15 for SFV, and ≥14 for BEV (expressed as LRF). The preparation contains at least 96% of IgG and after reconstitution with a neutral unbuffered diluent has a pH of 6.6 ± 0.2. Most of the immunoglobulins are monomeric (7 S) IgG; the remainder consists of dimeric IgG and a small amount of polymeric IgG, traces of IgA and IgM and immunoglobulin fragments (4). The distribution of the IgG subclasses corresponds to that of normal serum (5,6,7,8). Final container lyophilized units are prepared so as to contain 1, 3, 6, or 12 g protein with 1.67 g sucrose and less than 20 mg NaCl per gram of protein. The lyophilized preparation is devoid of any preservatives and may be reconstituted with sterile water, 5% dextrose or 0.9% saline to a solution with protein concentrations ranging from 3%-12%. The patient's fluid, electrolyte, caloric requirements and renal function should be considered in selecting an appropriate diluent and concentration.

Infectious Complications in the Randomized Renal Transplant Patients

Complication	Sandimmune® Treatment (N=227) % of Complications	Standard Treatment* (N=228) % of Complications
Septicemia	5.3	4.8
Abscesses	4.4	5.3
Systemic Fungal Infection	2.2	3.9
Local Fungal Infection	7.5	9.6
Cytomegalovirus	4.8	12.3
Other Viral Infections	15.9	18.4
Urinary Tract Infections	21.1	20.2
Wound and Skin Infections	7.0	10.1
Pneumonia	6.2	9.2

* Some patients also received ALG.

Table 1
Calculated Sandoglobulin® Osmolality (mOsm/kg)

	Concentration			
Diluent	**3%**	**6%**	**9%**	**12%**
0.9% NaCl	498	690	882	1074
5% Dextrose	444	636	828	1020
Sterile Water	192	384	576	768

CLINICAL PHARMACOLOGY

This product contains a broad spectrum of antibody specificities against bacterial, viral, parasitic, and mycoplasma antigens, that are capable of both opsonization and neutralization of microbes and toxins. The 3 week half-life of Immune Globulin Intravenous (Human), Sandoglobulin®, corresponds to that of Immune Globulin (Human) for intramuscular use, although individual variations in half-life have been observed (9,10). Appropriate doses of Sandoglobulin® restore abnormally low immunoglobulin G levels to the normal range. One hundred percent of the infused dose is available in the recipient's circulation immediately after infusion. After approximately 6 days, an equilibrium is reached between the intra- and extravascular compartments, with immunoglobulin G being distributed approximately 50% intravascular and 50% extravascular. In comparison, after the intramuscular injection of immune globulin, the IgG requires 2-5 days to reach its maximum concentration in the intravascular compartment. This concentration corresponds to about 40% of the injected dose (10).

While Sandoglobulin® has been shown to be effective in some cases of Immune Thrombocytopenic Purpura (ITP) *(see INDICATIONS AND USAGE)*, the mechanism of action in ITP has not been fully elucidated.

Toxicity from overdose has not been observed on regimens of 0.4 g/kg body weight each day for 5 days (11,12,13). Sucrose is added to Sandoglobulin® for reasons of stability and solubility.

Since sucrose is excreted unchanged in the urine when given intravenously, Sandoglobulin® may be given to diabetics without compensatory changes in insulin dosage regimen. Please see *WARNINGS* section.

INDICATIONS AND USAGE

Immunodeficiency

Immune Globulin Intravenous (Human), Sandoglobulin®, is indicated for the maintenance treatment of patients with primary immunodeficiencies, e.g., in common variable immunodeficiency, severe combined immunodeficiency, and primary immunoglobulin deficiency syndromes such as X-linked agammaglobulinemia (12,14,15,16). Sandoglobulin® is preferable to intramuscular Immune Globulin (Human) preparations in treating patients who require an immediate and large increase in the intravascular immunoglobulin level (10), in patients with limited muscle mass, and in patients with bleeding tendencies for whom intramuscular injections are contraindicated. The infusions must be repeated at regular intervals. Please see *DOSAGE AND ADMINISTRATION* section.

Immune Thrombocytopenic Purpura (ITP)

Acute

A controlled study was performed in children in which Immune Globulin Intravenous (Human), Sandoglobulin®, was compared with steroids for the treatment of acute (defined as less than 6 months duration) ITP. In this study, sequential platelet levels of 30,000, 100,000, and 150,000/µl were all achieved faster with Sandoglobulin® than with steroids and without any of the side effects associated with steroids (11,17). However, it should be noted that many cases of acute ITP in childhood resolve spontaneously within weeks to months. Sandoglobulin® has been used with good results in the treatment of acute ITP in adult patients (18,19,20). In a study involving 10 adults with ITP of less than 16 weeks duration, Sandoglobulin® therapy raised the platelet count to the normal range after a 5 day course. This effect lasted a mean of over 173 days, ranging from 30-372 days (21).

Chronic

Children and adults with chronic (defined as greater than 6 months duration) ITP have also shown an increase (sometimes temporary) in platelet counts upon administration of Immune Globulin Intravenous (Human), Sandoglobulin®, (17,21,22,23,24,25). Therefore, in situations that require a rapid rise in platelet count, for example prior to surgery or to control excessive bleeding, use of Sandoglobulin® should be considered. In children with chronic ITP, Sandoglobulin® therapy resulted in a mean rise in platelet count of 312,000/µl with a duration of increase ranging from 2-6 months (22,25). Sandoglobulin® therapy may be considered as a means to defer or avoid splenectomy (24,25,26). In adults, Sandoglobulin® therapy has been shown to be effective in maintaining the platelet count in an acceptable range with or without periodic booster therapy. The mean rise in platelet count was 93,000/µl and the average duration of the increase was 20-24 days (21,22). However, it should be noted that not all patients will respond. Even in those patients who do respond, this treatment should not be considered to be curative.

CONTRAINDICATIONS

As with all blood products containing IgA, Immune Globulin Intravenous (Human), Sandoglobulin®, is contraindicated in patients with selective IgA deficiency, who possess antibody to IgA. It may also be contraindicated in patients who have had severe systemic reactions to the intravenous or intramuscular administration of human immune globulin.

WARNINGS

WARNING
Immune Globulin Intravenous (Human) (IGIV) products have been reported to be associated with renal dysfunction, acute renal failure, osmotic nephrosis, and death (27,28,29,30,31,32). Patients predisposed to acute renal failure include patients with any degree of pre-existing renal insufficiency, diabetes mellitus, age greater than 65, volume depletion, spesis, paraproteinemia, or patients receiving known nephrotoxic drugs. Especially in such patients, IGIV products should be administered at the minimum concentration available and the minimum rate of infusion practicable. While these reports of renal dysfunction and acute renal failure have been associated with the use of many of the licensed IGIV products, those containing sucrose as a stabilizer accounted for a disporportionate share of the total number.
See *PRECAUTIONS* and *DOSAGE AND ADMINISTRATION* sections for important information intended to reduce the risk of acute renal failure.

Immune Globulin Intravenous (Human), Sandoglobulin®, is made from human plasma. Products made from human plasma may contain infectious agents, such as viruses, that can cause disease. The risk that such products will transmit an infectious agent has been reduced by screening plasma donors for prior exposure to certain viruses, by testing for the presence of certain current virus infections, and by inactivating and/or removing certain viruses. The fractionation process by which Sandoglobulin® is prepared from plasma includes several filtration steps which are carried out in the presence of filter aids; some of these filtration steps are used for the separation of a cold ethanol precipitate. Four of these steps were validated for virus *elimination*. The cumulative LRFs (log_{10} of reduction factors) were 15.5 for HIV (human immunodeficiency virus), 16.0 for PRV (pseudorabies virus), 9.3 for SFV (Semliki Forest virus), 12.4 for Sindbis virus, and 14.1 for BEV (bovine enterovirus). Sandoglobulin® is made suitable for intravenous use by treatment at acid pH in the presence of trace amounts of pepsin (2,3). Treatment with pepsin at pH4 rapidly *inactivates* enveloped viruses. LRFs were ≥6.1 for HIV, ≥5.3 for PRV, ≥4.4 for BVDV (bovine viral diarrhea virus), and ≥6.8 for SFV. PRV and the two model viruses for HCV (hepatitis C virus), BVDV and SFV, were all inactivated within 1/10, and HIV within 1/2 of the total incubation time used during production of Sandoglobulin®. *Overall viral clearance* by either *elimination* and/or *inactivation* during the manufacturing process has been documented to be ≥21 for HIV, ≥19 for PRV, ≥15 for SFV, and ≥14 for BEV (expressed as LRF). Despite these measures, such products may carry a risk of transmitting infectious agents, e.g., viruses, and theoretically, the Creutzfeldt-Jakob disease (CJD) agent. There is also the possibility that unknown infectious agents may be present in such products. ALL infections thought by a physician possibly to have been transmitted by this product should be reported by the physician or other healthcare provider to Novartis Pharmaceuticals, 973-781-7500. The physician should discuss the risks and benefits of this product with the patient.

Patients with agamma- or extreme hypogammaglobulinemia who have never before received immunoglobulin substitution treatment or whose time from last treatment is greater than 8 weeks, may be at risk of developing inflammatory reactions on rapid infusion of Immune Globulin Intravenous (Human), Sandoglobulin®, (over 20 drops [1 mL] per minute). These reactions are manifested by a rise in temperature, chills, nausea, and vomiting. The patient's vital signs should be monitored continuously. The patient should be carefully observed throughout the infusion, since these reactions on rare occasions may lead to shock. Epinephrine should be available for treatment of an acute anaphylactic reaction.

PRECAUTIONS

Please see *DOSAGE AND ADMINISTRATION* below, for important information on Immune Globulin Intravenous (Human), Sandoglobulin®, compatibility with other medications or fluids. Assure that patients are not volume depleted prior to the initiation of the infusion of IGIV. Periodic monitoring of renal function tests and urine output is particularly important in patients judged to have a potential increased risk for developing acute renal failure. Renal function, including measurement of blood urea nitrogen (BUN)/serum creatinine, should be assessed prior to the initial infusion of Sandoglobulin® and again at appropriate intervals thereafter. If renal function deteriorates, discontinuation of the product should be considered. For patients judged to be at risk for developing renal dysfunction, it may be prudent to reduce the amount of product infused per unit time by infusing Sandoglobulin® at a rate less than 2 mg Ig/kg/min.

Information for Patients

Patients should be instructed to immediately report symptoms of decreased urine output, sudden weight gain, fluid retention/edema, and/or shortness of breath (which may suggest kidney damage) to their physicians.

Pregnancy

Pregnancy Category C: Animal reproduction studies have not been conducted with Immune Globulin Intravenous (Human), Sandoglobulin®. It is also not known whether Sandoglobulin® can cause fetal harm when administered to a pregnant woman or can affect reproduction capacity. Sandoglobulin® should be given to a pregnant woman only if clearly needed (20).

Intact immune globulins such as those contained in Sandoglobulin® cross the placenta from maternal circulation increasingly after 30 weeks gestation (33,34). In cases of maternal ITP where Sandoglobulin® was administered to the mother prior to delivery, the platelet response and clinical effect were similar in the mother and neonate (20,34-43).

Pediatric Use

High dose administration of Immune Globulin Intravenous (Human), Sandoglobulin®, in pediatric patients with acute or chronic Immune Thrombocytopenic Purpura did not reveal any pediatric-specific hazard (11).

Antibodies in Immune Globulin Intravenous (Human) may impair the efficacy of live attenuated viral vaccines such as measles, rubella, and mumps (44,45,46). Immunizing physicians should be informed of recent therapy with Immune Globulin Intravenous (Human) so that appropriate precautions may be taken.

Aseptic Meningitis Syndrome

An aseptic meningitis syndrome (AMS) has been reported to occur infrequently in association with Immune Globulin Intravenous (Human) (IGIV) treatment. The syndrome usually begins within several hours to two days following IGIV treatment. It is characterized by symptoms and signs including severe headache, nuchal rigidity, drowsiness, fever, photophobia, painful eye movements, and nausea and vomiting. Cerebrospinal fluid studies are frequently positive with pleocytosis up to several thousand cells per cu.mm., predominantly from the granulocytic series, and elevated protein levels up to several hundred mg/dl. Patients exhibiting such symptoms and signs should receive a thorough neurological examination, including CSF studies, to rule out other causes of meningitis. AMS may occur more frequently in association with high dose (2 g/kg) IGIV treatment. Discontinuation of IGIV treatment has resulted in remission of AMS within several days without sequelae.

ADVERSE REACTIONS

Increases in creatinine and blood urea nitrogen (BUN) have been observed as soon as one to two days following infusion. Progression to oliguria or anuria, requiring dialysis has been observed. Types of severe renal adverse events that have been seen following IGIV therapy include: acute renal failure, acute tubular necrosis, proximal tubular nephropathy and osmotic nephrosis (27,28,29,30,31,32,47,57-59).

Inflammatory adverse reactions have been described in agammaglobulinemic and hypogammaglobulinemic patients who have never received immunoglobulin substitution therapy before or in patients whose time from last treatment is greater than 8 weeks and whose initial infusion rate exceeds 20 drops (1 mL) per minute. This occurs in approximately 10% of such cases. Such reactions may also be observed in some patients during chronic substitution therapy.

These reactions, which generally become apparent only 30 minutes to 1 hour after the beginning of the infusion, are as follows: flushing of the face, feelings of tightness in the chest, chills, fever, dizziness, nausea, diaphoresis, and hypotension. In such cases the infusion should be temporarily stopped until the symptoms have subsided. Immediate anaphylactoid and hypersensitivity reactions due to previous sensitization of the recipient to certain antigens, most commonly IgA, may be observed in exceptional cases, described under *CONTRAINDICATIONS* (12,13,48).

In patients with ITP, who receive higher doses (0.4 g/kg/day or greater) 2.9% of infusions may result in adverse reactions (17). Headache, generally mild, is the most common symptom noted, occurring during or following 2% of infusions.

A few cases of usually mild hemolysis have been reported after infusion of intravenous immunoglobulin products (49,50). These were attributed to transferral of blood group (e.g., anti-D) antibodies (51,52).

DOSAGE AND ADMINISTRATION

It is generally advisable not to dilute plasma derivatives with other infusable drugs. Immune Globulin Intravenous (Human), Sandoglobulin®, should be given by a separate infusion line. No other medications or fluids should be mixed with the Sandoglobulin® preparation.

Sandoglobulin® should be used with caution in patients with pre-existing renal insufficiency and in patients judged to be at increased risk of developing renal insufficiency (including, but not limited to those with diabetes mellitus, age greater than 65, volume depletion, paraproteinemia, sepsis, and patients receiving known nephrotoxic drugs).

In these cases especially it is important to assure that patients are not volume depleted prior to Sandoglobulin® infusion. No prospective data are presently available to identify a maximum safe dose, concentration, and rate of infusion in patients determined to be at increased risk of acute renal failure. In the absence of prospective data, recommended doses should not be exceeded and the concentra-

Continued on next page

Sandoglobulin—Cont.

tion and infusion rate selected should be the minimum practicable. The product should be infused at a rate less than 2 mg Ig/kg/min.

Adult and Child Substitution Therapy

The usual dose of Immune Globulin Intravenous (Human), Sandoglobulin®, in immunodeficiency syndromes is 0.2 g/kg of body weight administered once a month by intravenous infusion. If the clinical response is inadequate, the dose may be increased to 0.3 g/kg of body weight or the infusion may be repeated more frequently than once a month (12,14,15,16).

The first infusion of Sandoglobulin® in previously untreated agammaglobulinemic or hypogammaglobulinemic patients must be given as a 3% immunoglobulin solution (use the total volume of fluid provided, or see *Table 2*, to reconstitute the lyophilized product). Start with a flow rate of 10-20 drops (0.5-1.0 mL) per minute. After 15-30 minutes the rate of infusion may be further increased to 30-50 drops (1.5-2.5 mL) per minute.

After the first bottle of 3% solution is infused and the patient shows good tolerance, subsequent in fusions may be administered at a higher rate or concentration. Such increases should be made gradually allowing 15-30 minutes before each increment.

The first infusion of Sandoglobulin® in previously untreated agammaglobulinemic and hypogammaglobulinemic patients may lead to systemic side effects. The nature of these effects has not been fully elucidated. Some of them may be due to the release of pro-inflammatory cytokines by activated macrophages in immunodeficient recipients (53,54). Subsequent administration of Sandoglobulin® to immunodeficient patients as well as to normal individuals usually does not cause further untoward side effects.

Therapy of Idiopathic Thrombocytopenic Purpura (ITP)

Induction

0.4 g/kg of body weight on 2-5 consecutive days.

Acute ITP-Childhood

In acute ITP of childhood, if an initial platelet count response to the first two doses is adequate (30-50,000/µl), therapy may be discontinued after the second day of the 5 day course (17).

Maintenance-Chronic ITP

In adults and children, if after induction therapy the platelet count falls to less than 30,000/µl and/or the patient manifests clinically significant bleeding, 0.4 g/kg of body weight may be given as a single infusion. If an adequate response does not result, the dose can be increased to 0.8-1.0 g/kg of body weight given as a single infusion (18,55,56).

Reconstitution

For a 3% solution using the transfer set

1. Tear off the protective caps from the bottle containing the solvent and the Immune Globulin Intravenous (Human), Sandoglobulin®. Disinfect both rubber stoppers with alcohol.
2. Remove the protective cover from one end of the transfer set and insert the needle through the rubber stopper into the bottle containing the solvent.
3. Remove the cover from the other needle and plunge the inverted Sandoglobulin® bottle onto it, as shown in picture #3.
4. Invert the two bottles so that the solvent flows into the Sandoglobulin® bottle until the required amount (see *Table 2*, above) has been transferred.
5. Discard any unused solvent and the transfer set.

For a 6% solution using the transfer set

1. Follow steps 1-3 aforementioned.
2. Invert the two bottles so that the solvent flows into the Sandoglobulin® bottle. Use the appropriate amount (see *Table 2*, above) of solvent by removing the solvent bottle with transfer needle as soon as the fluid reaches the 6% mark printed on the Sandoglobulin® label.
3. Discard any unused solvent and the transfer set.

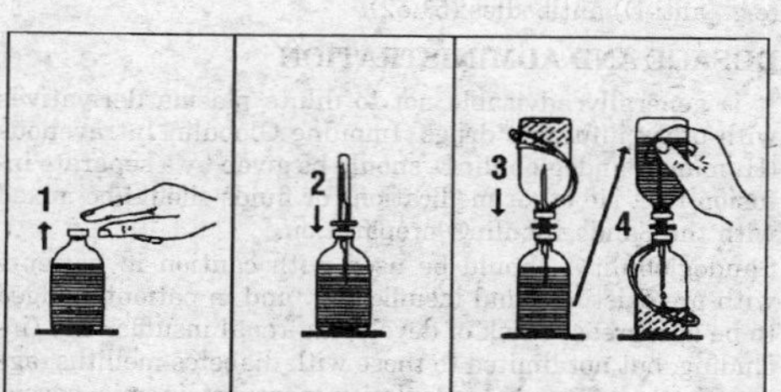

To reconstitute Sandoglobulin® from the individual vial package, or when using other diluents or higher concentrations, *Table 2* indicates the volume of sterile diluent required. Observing aseptic technique, this volume should be drawn into a sterile hypodermic syringe and needle. The diluent is then injected into the corresponding Sandoglobulin®, vial size.

Table 2
Required Diluent Volume*

Concentration	1 g Vial	3 g Vial	6 g Vial	12 g Vial
3%	33.0 cc	100 cc	200 cc	**
6%	16.5 cc	50 cc	100 cc	200 cc
9%	11.0 cc	33 cc	66 cc	132 cc
12%	8.3 cc	25 cc	50 cc	100 cc

* In patients judged to be at increased risk of developing renal insufficiency, the concentration and infusion rate of Sandoglobulin® should be the minimum practicable.

** Container not large enough to permit this concentration

If large doses of Sandoglobulin® are to be administered, several reconstituted vials of identical concentration and diluent may be pooled in an empty sterile glass or plastic i.v. infusion container using aseptic technique.

Sandoglobulin® normally dissolves within a few minutes, though in exceptional cases it may take up to 20 minutes.

DO NOT SHAKE! Excessive shaking will cause foaming.

Any undissolved particles should respond to careful rotation of the bottle. Avoid foaming. Parenteral drug products should be inspected visually for particulate matter and discoloration prior to administration, whenever solution and container permit.

Filtering of Sandoglobulin® is acceptable but not required. Pore sizes of 15 microns or larger will be less likely to slow infusion, especially with higher Sandoglobulin® concentrations. Antibacterial filters (0.2 microns) may be used.

When reconstitution of Sandoglobulin® occurs outside of sterile laminar air flow conditions, administration must begin promptly with partially used vials discarded. When reconstitution is carried out in a sterile laminar flow hood using aseptic technique, administration may begin within 24 hours provided the solution has been refrigerated during that time. Do not freeze Sandoglobulin® solution.

PROCEED WITH INFUSION ONLY IF SOLUTION IS CLEAR AND AT APPROXIMATELY ROOM TEMPERATURE!

HOW SUPPLIED

Immune Globulin Intravenous (Human), Sandoglobulin®, is available as a white lyophilized powder in 1, 3, 6 and 12 g size vials. The only diluents which may be used to reconstitute the product are sterile (0.9%) Sodium Chloride Injection USP, 5% Dextrose, or Sterile Water.

Sandoglobulin® is available in individual vial packages.

1 g

Individual vial package (NDC 0078-0120-94)

3 g

Individual vial package (NDC 0078-0122-95)

6 g

Individual vial package (NDC 0078-0124-96)

12 g

Individual vial package (NDC 0078-0244-93)

Please see *Table 1* for Calculated Sandoglobulin® Osmolality (mOsm/kg).

Store and Dispense

Immune Globulin Intravenous (Human), Sandoglobulin®, should be stored at room temperature not exceeding 30°C (86°F). The preparation should not be used after the expiration date printed on the label.

References

1. Gardi A: Quality control in the production of an immunoglobulin for intravenous use. *Blut* 1984; **48**:337-344.
2. Römer J, Morgenthaler JJ, Scherz R, et al: Characterization of various immunoglobulin-preparations for intravenous application. I. Protein composition and antibody content. *Vox Sang* 1982; **42**:62-73.
3. Römer J, Späth PJ, Skvaril F, et al: Characterization of various immunoglobulin preparations for intravenous application. II. Complement activation and binding to Staphylococcus protein A. *Vox Sang* 1982; **42**:74-80.
4. Römer J, Späth PJ: Molecular composition of immunoglobulin preparations and its relation to complement activation, in Nydegger UE (ed): *Immunohemotherapy: A Guide to Immunoglobulin Prophylaxis and Therapy*. London, Academic Press, 1981, pp 123-130.
5. Skvaril F, Roth-Wicky B, and Barandun S: IgG subclasses in human-γ-globulin preparations for intravenous use and their reactivity with Staphylococcus protein A. *Vox Sang* 1980; **38**:147.
6. Skvaril F: Qualitative and quantitative aspects of IgG subclasses in i.v. immunoglobulin preparations, in Nydegger UE (ed): *Immunohemotherapy: A Guide to Immunoglobulin Prophylaxis and Therapy*. London, Academic Press, 1981, pp 113-122.
7. Skvaril F, and Barandun S: In vitro characterization of immunoglobulins for intravenous use, in Alving BM, Finlayson JS (eds): *Immunoglobulins: Characteristics and Uses of Intravenous Preparations*, DHHS Publication No. (FDA)-80-9005. US Government Printing Office, 1980, pp 201-206.
8. Burckhardt JJ, Gardi A, Oxelius V, et al: Immunoglobulin G subclass distribution in three human intravenous immunoglobulin preparations. *Vox Sang* 1989; **57**:10-14.
9. Morell A, and Skvaril F: Struktur und biologische Eigenschaften von Immunoglobulinen und γ-Globulin-Präparaten. II. Eigenschaften von γ-Globulin-Präparaten. *Schweiz Med Wochenschr* 1980; **110**:80.
10. Morell A, Schürch B, Ryser D, et al: In vivo behavior of gamma globulin preparations. *Vox Sang* 1980; **38**:272.
11. Imbach P, Barandun S, d'Apuzzo V, et al: High-dose intravenous gamma globulin for idiopathic thrombocytopenic purpura in childhood. *Lancet* 1981; **1**:1228.
12. Barandun S, Morell A, Skvaril F: Clinical experiences with immunoglobulin for intravenous use, in Alving BM, Finlayson JS (eds): *Immunoglobulins: Characteristics and Uses of Intravenous Preparations*. DHHS Publication No. (FDA)-80-9005. US Government Printing Office, 1980, pp 31-35.
13. Schiff R, Sedlak D, Buckley R: Rapid infusion of Sandoglobulin® in patients with primary humoral immunodeficiency. *J Allergy Clin Immunol* 1991; **88**:61.
14. Joller PW, Barandun S, Hitzig WH: Neue Möglichkeiten der Immunoglobulin-Ersatztherapie bei Antikörpermangel. Syndrom. *Schweiz Med Wochenschr* 1980; **110**: 1451.
15. Barandun S, Imbach P, Morell A, et al: Clinical indications for immunoglobulin infusion, in Nydegger UE (ed): *Immunohemotherapy: A Guide to Immunoglobulin Prophylaxis and Therapy*. London, Academic Press, 1981, pp 275-282.
16. Cunningham-Rundles C, Smithwick EM, Siegal FP, et al: Treatment of primary humoral immunodeficiency disease with intravenous (pH 4.0 treated) gamma globulin, in Nydegger UE (ed): *Guide to Immunoglobulin Prophylaxis and Therapy*. London, Academic Press, 1981, pp 283-290.
17. Imbach P, Wagner HP, Berchtold W, et al: Intravenous immunoglobulin versus oral corticosteroids in acute immune thrombocytopenic purpura in childhood. *Lancet* 1985; **2**:464.
18. Fehr J, Hofmann V, Kappeler U: Transient reversal of thrombocytopenia in idiopathic thrombocytopenic purpura by high-dose intravenous gamma globulin. *N Engl J Med* 1982; **306**:1254.
19. Müeller-Eckhardt C, Küenzlen E, Thilo-Körner D, et al: High-dose intravenous immunoglobulin for posttransfusion purpura. *N Engl J Med* 1983; **308**:287.
20. Wenske G, Gaedicke G, Küenzlen E, et al: Treatment of idiopathic thrombocytopenic purpura in pregnancy by high-dose intravenous immunoglobulin. *Blut* 1983; **46**: 347-353.
21. Newland AC, Treleaven JG, Minchinton B, et al: High-dose intravenous IgG in adults with autoimmune thrombocytopenia. *Lancet* 1983; **1**:84-87.
22. Bussel JB, Kimberly RP, Inman RD, et al: Intravenous gammaglobulin for chronic idiopathic thrombocytopenic purpura. *Blood* 1983; **62**:480-486.
23. Abe T, Matsuda J, Kawasugi K, et al: Clinical effect of intravenous immunoglobulin in chronic idiopathic thrombocytopenic purpura. *Blut* 1983; **47**:69-75.
24. Bussel JB, Schulman I, Hilgartner MW, et al: Intravenous use of gamma globulin in the treatment of chronic immune thrombocytopenic purpura as a means to defer splenectomy. *J Pediatr* 1983; **103**:651-654.
25. Imholz B, et al: Intravenous immunoglobulin (i.v. IgG) for previously treated acute or for chronic idiopathic thrombocytopenic purpura (ITP) in childhood: A prospective multicenter study. *Blut* 1988; **56**:63-68.
26. Lusher JM, and Warrier I: Use of intravenous gamma globulin in children with idiopathic thrombocytopenic purpura and other immune thrombocytopenias. *Am J Med* 1987; **83(suppl 4A)**:10-16.
27. Winward DB, Brophy MT: Acute renal failure after administration of intravenous immunoglobulin: Review of the literature and case report. *Pharmacotherapy* 1995; **15**:765-772.
28. Cantú TG, Hoehn-Saric EW, Burgess KM, Racusen L, Scheel P: Acute renal failure associated with immunoglobulin therapy. *Am J Kidney Dis* 1995; **25**:228-234.
29. Cayco AV, Perazelly MA, Hayslett JP: Renal insufficiency after intravenous immune globulin therapy: A Report of Two Cases and an Analysis of the Literature. *J Amer Soc Nephrology* 1997; **8**:1788-1793.
30. Rault R, Pirano B, Johston J, Oral A: Pulmonary and renal toxicity of intravenous immunoglobulin. *Clin Nephrol* 1991; **36**:83-86.
31. Michail S, Nakopoulou L, Stravrianopoulos I, Stamatiadis D, Avdikou K, Vaiopoulos G, Stathakis C: Acute renal failure associated with immunoglobulin administration. *Nephrol Dial Transplant* 1997; **12**:1497-1499.
32. Ashan N, Wiegand LA, Abendroth CS, Manning EC: Acute renal failure following immunoglobulin therapy. *Am J Nephrol* 1996; **16**:532-536.
33. Hammarstrom L, and Smith CI: Placental transfer of intravenous immunoglobulin. *Lancet* 1986; **1**:681.
34. Sidiropoulos D, et al: Transplacental passage of intravenous immunoglobulin in the last trimester of pregnancy. *J Pediatr* 1986; **109**:505-508.
35. Wenske G, et al: Idiopathic thrombocytopenic purpura in pregnancy and neonatal period. *Blut* 1984; **48**:377-382.
36. Fabris P, et al: Successful treatment of a steroid-resistant form of idiopathic thrombocytopenic purpura in pregnancy with high doses of intravenous immunoglobulins. *Acta Haemat* 1987; **77**:107-110.
37. Coller BS, et al: Management of severe ITP during pregnancy with intravenous immunoglobulin (IVIgG). *Clin Res* 1985; **33**:545A.

38. Tchernia G, et al: Management of immune thrombocytopenia in pregnancy: Response to infusions of immunoglobulins. *Am J Obstet Gynecol* 1984; **148**:225-226.
39. Newland AC, et al: Intravenous IgG for autoimmune thrombocytopenia in pregnancy. *N Engl J Med* 1984; **310**:261-262.
40. Morgenstern GR, et al: Autoimmune thrombocytopenia in pregnancy: New approach to management. *Br Med J* 1983; **287**:584.
41. Ciccimarra F, et al: Treatment of neonatal passive immune thrombocytopenia. *J Pediat* 1984; **105**:677-678.
42. Rose VL, and Gordon LI: Idiopathic thrombocytopenic purpura in pregnancy. Successful management with immunoglobulin infusion. *JAMA* 1985; **254**:2626-2628.
43. Gounder MP, et al: Intravenous gammaglobulin therapy in the management of a patient with idiopathic thrombocytopenic purpura and a warm autoimmune erythrocyte panagglutinin during pregnancy. *Obstet Gynecol* 1986; **67**:741-746.
44. Siber GR, Werner BG, Halsey NA, et al: Interference of immune globulin with measles and rubella immunization. *J Pediatr* 1993; **122**:204-211.
45. American Academy of Pediatrics, Committee on Infectious Diseases. Recommended timing of routine measles immunization for children who have recently received immune globulin preparations. *Pediatrics* 1994; **93**:682-685.
46. Centers of Disease Control and Prevention. Measles, mumps, and rubella-vaccine use and strategies for elimination of measles, rubella, and congenital rubella syndrome and control of mumps: recommendations of the advisory committee on immunization practices (ACIP). *MMWR, Morbidity and Mortality Weekly Report* May 22, 1998; vol 47/No. RR-8, 1-57.
47. Phillips AO: Renal failure and intravenous immunoglobulin [letter;comment]. *Clin Nephrol* 1992; **36**:83-86.
48. Cunningham-Rundles C, Day NK, Wahn V, et al: Reactions to intravenous gamma globulin infusions and immune complex formation, in Nydegger UE (ed): *Immunohemotherapy: A Guide to Immunoglobulin Prophylaxis and Therapy*. London, Academic Press, 1981, pp 447-449.
49. Brox AG, Cournoyer D, et al: Hemolytic anemia following intravenous gamma globulin administration. *Am J Med* 1987; **82**:633-635.
50. Kim HC, Park CL, Cowan JH, et al: Massive intravascular hemolysis associated with intravenous immunoglobulin in bone marrow transplant recipients. *Am J Ped Hematol/Oncol* 1988; **10**:67-74.
51. Nicholls MD, Cummins JC, et al: Hemolysis induced by intravenously-administered immunoglobulin. *Med J of Australia* 1989; **150**:404-406.
52. Copelan EA, et al: Hemolysis following intravenous immune globulin therapy. *Transfusion* 1986; **26**:410-412.
53. Aukrust P, Froland SS, Liabakk N-B, Müller F, et al: Release of cytokines, soluble cytokine receptors, and interleukin-1 receptor antagonist after intravenous immunoglobulin administration in vivo. *Blood* 1994; **84**:2136-2143.
54. Bagdasarian A, Tonetta S, Harel W, Mamidi R, Uemura Y: IVIG adverse reactions: potential role of cytokines and vasoactive substances. *Vox Sang* 1998; **74**:74-82.
55. Bussel JB, Pham LC, Hilgartner MW, et al: Long-term maintenance of adults with ITP using intravenous gamma globulin. *Abstract, American Society of Hematology*. New Orleans, December, 1985.
56. Imbach PA, Kühne T, Holländer G: Immunologic aspects in the pathogenesis and treatment of immune thrombocytopenic purpura in children. Current opinion in *Pediatrics* 1997; **9**:35-40.
57. Anderson W, Bethea W: Renal lesions following administration of hypertonic solutions of sucrose. *JAMA*. 1940; **114**:1983-1987.
58. Lindberg H, Wald A: Renal lesions following the administration of hypertonic solutions: *Arch Intern Med*. 1939; **63**:907-918.
59. Rigdon RH, Cardwell ES: Renal lesions following the intravenous injection of hypertonic solution of sucrose: A clinical and experimental study. *Arch Intern Med*. 1942; **69**:670-690.

Manufactured by:
CENTRAL LABORATORY
BLOOD TRANSFUSION SERVICE
SWISS RED CROSS
Wankdorfstrasse 10, 3000 Berne 22
Switzerland
US License No. 647
Distributed by:
NOVARTIS PHARMACEUTICALS CORPORATION
East Hanover, NJ 07936
REV: FEBRUARY 2000 T2000-07
Shown in Product Identification Guide, page 326

SANDOSTATIN® ℞

[săn dō stăt ĭn]
octreotide acetate
Injection
Rx only

The following prescribing information is based on official labeling in effect May 1999.

DESCRIPTION

Sandostatin® (octreotide acetate) Injection, a cyclic octapeptide prepared as a clear sterile solution of octreotide, acetate salt, in a buffered lactic acid solution for administration by deep subcutaneous (intrafat) or intravenous injection. Octreotide acetate, known chemically as L-Cysteinamide, D-phenylalanyl-L-cysteinyl-L-phenylalanyl-D-tryptophyl-L-lysyl-L-threonyl-N-[2-hydroxy-1-(hydroxymethyl)propyl]-, cyclic (2→7)-disulfide; [R-(R*, R*)] acetate salt, is a long-acting octapeptide with pharmacologic actions mimicking those of the natural hormone somatostatin.

Sandostatin® (octreotide acetate) Injection is available as: sterile 1 mL ampuls in 3 strengths, containing 50, 100, or 500 mcg octreotide (as acetate), and sterile 5 mL multi-dose vials in 2 strengths, containing 200 and 1000 mcg/mL of octreotide (as acetate).

Each ampul also contains:

lactic acid, USP .... 3.4 mg
mannitol, USP .... 45 mg
sodium bicarbonate, USP .... qs to pH 4.2 ± 0.3
water for injection, USP .... qs to 1 mL

Each mL of the multi-dose vials also contains:

lactic acid, USP .... 3.4 mg
mannitol, USP .... 45 mg
phenol, USP .... 5.0 mg
sodium bicarbonate, USP .... qs to pH 4.2 ± 0.3
water for injection, USP .... qs to 1 mL

Lactic acid and sodium bicarbonate are added to provide a buffered solution, pH to 4.2 ± 0.3.

The molecular weight of octreotide acetate is 1019.3 (free peptide, $C_{49}H_{66}N_{10}O_{10}S_2$) and its amino acid sequence is:

H-D-Phe-Cys-Phe-D-Trp-Lys-Thr-Cys-Thr-ol,
x CH_3COOH where x = 1.4 to 2.5

CLINICAL PHARMACOLOGY

Sandostatin® (octreotide acetate) exerts pharmacologic actions similar to the natural hormone, somatostatin. It is an even more potent inhibitor of growth hormone, glucagon, and insulin than somatostatin. Like somatostatin, it also suppresses LH response to GnRH, decreases splanchnic blood flow, and inhibits release of serotonin, gastrin, vasoactive intestinal peptide, secretin, motilin, and pancreatic polypeptide.

By virtue of these pharmacological actions, Sandostatin® (octreotide acetate) has been used to treat the symptoms associated with metastatic carcinoid tumors (flushing and diarrhea), and Vasoactive Intestinal Peptide (VIP) secreting adenomas (watery diarrhea).

Sandostatin® (octreotide acetate) substantially reduces growth hormone and/or IGF-I (somatomedin C) levels in patients with acromegaly.

Single doses of Sandostatin® (octreotide acetate) have been shown to inhibit gallbladder contractility and to decrease bile secretion in normal volunteers. In controlled clinical trials the incidence of gallstone or biliary sludge formation was markedly increased *(See WARNINGS)*.

Sandostatin® (octreotide acetate) suppresses secretion of thyroid stimulating hormone (TSH).

Pharmacokinetics

After subcutaneous injection, octreotide is absorbed rapidly and completely from the injection site. Peak concentrations of 5.2 ng/mL (100 mcg dose) were reached 0.4 hours after dosing. Using a specific radioimmunoassay, intravenous and subcutaneous doses were found to be bioequivalent. Peak concentrations and area under the curve values were dose proportional both after subcutaneous or intravenous single doses up to 400 mcg and with multiple doses of 200 mcg t.i.d. (600 mcg/day). Clearance was reduced by about 66% suggesting non-linear kinetics of the drug at daily doses of 600 mcg/day as compared to 150 mcg/day. The relative decrease in clearance with doses above 600 mcg/day is not defined.

In healthy volunteers the distribution of octreotide from plasma was rapid (tα1/2 = 0.2 h), the volume of distribution (Vdss) was estimated to be 13.6 L, and the total body clearance was 10 L/hr.

In blood, the distribution into the erythrocytes was found to be negligible and about 65% was bound in the plasma in a concentration-independent manner. Binding was mainly to lipoprotein and, to a lesser extent, to albumin.

The elimination of octreotide from plasma had an apparent half-life of 1.7 hours compared with 1-3 minutes with the natural hormone. The duration of action of Sandostatin® (octreotide acetate) is variable but extends up to 12 hours depending upon the type of tumor. About 32% of the dose is excreted unchanged into the urine. In an elderly population, dose adjustments may be necessary due to a significant increase in the half-life (46%) and a significant decrease in the clearance (26%) of the drug.

In patients with acromegaly, the pharmacokinetics differ somewhat from those in healthy volunteers. A mean peak concentration of 2.8 ng/mL (100 mcg dose) was reached in 0.7 hours after subcutaneous dosing. The volume of distribution (Vdss) was estimated to be 21.6 ± 8.5 L and the total body clearance was increased to 18 L/h. The mean percent of the drug bound was 41.2%. The disposition and elimination half-lives were similar to normals.

In patients with severe renal failure requiring dialysis, clearance was reduced to about half that found in normal subjects (from approximately 10 L/h to 4.5 L/h). The effect of hepatic diseases on the disposition of octreotide is unknown.

INDICATIONS AND USAGE

Acromegaly

Sandostatin® (octreotide acetate) is indicated to reduce blood levels of growth hormone and IGF-I (somatomedin C) in acromegaly patients who have had inadequate response to or cannot be treated with surgical resection, pituitary irradiation, and bromocriptine mesylate at maximally tolerated doses. The goal is to achieve normalization of growth hormone and IGF-I (somatomedin C) levels *(See DOSAGE AND ADMINISTRATION)*. In patients with acromegaly, Sandostatin® (octreotide acetate) reduces growth hormone to within normal ranges in 50% of patients and reduces IGF-I (somatomedin C) to within normal ranges in 50%-60% of patients. Since the effects of pituitary irradiation may not become maximal for several years, adjunctive therapy with Sandostatin® (octreotide acetate) to reduce blood levels of growth hormone and IGF-I (somatomedin C) offers potential benefit before the effects of irradiation are manifested.

Improvement in clinical signs and symptoms or reduction in tumor size or rate of growth were not shown in clinical trials performed with Sandostatin® (octreotide acetate); these trials were not optimally designed to detect such effects.

Carcinoid Tumors

Sandostatin® (octreotide acetate) is indicated for the symptomatic treatment of patients with metastatic carcinoid tumors where it suppresses or inhibits the severe diarrhea and flushing episodes associated with the disease.

Sandostatin® (octreotide acetate) studies were not designed to show an effect on the size, rate of growth or development of metastases.

Vasoactive Intestinal Peptide Tumors (VIPomas)

Sandostatin® (octreotide acetate) is indicated for the treatment of the profuse watery diarrhea associated with VIP-secreting tumors. Sandostatin® (octreotide acetate) studies were not designed to show an effect on the size, rate of growth or development of metastases.

CONTRAINDICATIONS

Sensitivity to this drug or any of its components.

WARNINGS

Single doses of Sandostatin® (octreotide acetate) have been shown to inhibit gallbladder contractility and decrease bile secretion in normal volunteers. In clinical trials (primarily patients with acromegaly or psoriasis), the incidence of biliary tract abnormalities was 63% (27% gallstones, 24% sludge without stones, 12% biliary duct dilatation). The incidence of stones or sludge in patients who received Sandostatin® (octreotide acetate) for 12 months or longer was 52%. Less than 2% of patients treated with Sandostatin® (octreotide acetate) for 1 month or less developed gallstones. The incidence of gallstones did not appear related to age, sex or dose. Like patients without gallbladder abnormalities, the majority of patients developing gallbladder abnormalities on ultrasound had gastrointestinal symptoms. The symptoms were not specific for gallbladder disease. A few patients developed acute cholecystitis, ascending cholangitis, biliary obstruction, cholestatic hepatitis, or pancreatitis during Sandostatin® (octreotide acetate) therapy or following its withdrawal. One patient developed ascending cholangitis during Sandostatin® (octreotide acetate) therapy and died.

PRECAUTIONS

General

Sandostatin® (octreotide acetate) alters the balance between the counter-regulatory hormones, insulin, glucagon and growth hormone, which may result in hypoglycemia or hyperglycemia. Sandostatin® (octreotide acetate) also suppresses secretion of thyroid stimulating hormone, which may result in hypothyroidism. Cardiac conduction abnormalities have also occurred during treatment with Sandostatin® (octreotide acetate). However, the incidence of these adverse events during long-term therapy was determined vigorously only in acromegaly patients who, due to their underlying disease and/or the subsequent treatment they receive, are at an increased risk for the development of diabetes mellitus, hypothyroidism, and cardiovascular disease. Although the degree to which these abnormalities are related to Sandostatin® (octreotide acetate) therapy is not clear, new abnormalities of glycemic control, thyroid function and ECG developed during Sandostatin® (octreotide acetate) therapy as described below.

The hypoglycemia or hyperglycemia which occurs during Sandostatin® (octreotide acetate) therapy is usually mild, but may result in overt diabetes mellitus or necessitate dose changes in insulin or other hypoglycemic agents. Hypoglycemia and hyperglycemia occurred on Sandostatin® (octreotide acetate) in 3% and 16% of acromegalic patients, respectively. Severe hyperglycemia, subsequent pneumonia, and death following initiation of Sandostatin® (octreotide acetate) therapy was reported in one patient with no history of hyperglycemia.

In acromegalic patients, 12% developed biochemical hypothyroidism only, 8% developed goiter, and 4% required initiation of thyroid replacement therapy while receiving Sandostatin® (octreotide acetate). Baseline and periodic assessment of thyroid function (TSH, total and/or free T_4) is recommended during chronic therapy.

In acromegalics, bradycardia (<50 bpm) developed in 25%; conduction abnormalities occurred in 10% and arrhythmias occurred in 9% of patients during Sandostatin® (octreotide

Continued on next page

Sandostatin Injection—Cont.

acetate) therapy. Other EKG changes observed included QT prolongation, axis shifts, early repolarization, low voltage, R/S transition, and early R wave progression. These ECG changes are not uncommon in acromegalic patients. Dose adjustments in drugs such as beta-blockers that have bradycardia effects may be necessary. In one acromegalic patient with severe congestive heart failure, initiation of Sandostatin® (octreotide acetate) therapy resulted in worsening of CHF with improvement when drug was discontinued. Confirmation of a drug effect was obtained with a positive rechallenge.

Several cases of pancreatitis have been reported in patients receiving Sandostatin® (octreotide acetate) therapy.

Sandostatin® (octreotide acetate) may alter absorption of dietary fats in some patients.

In patients with severe renal failure requiring dialysis, the half-life of Sandostatin® (octreotide acetate) may be increased, necessitating adjustment of the maintenance dosage.

Depressed vitamin B_{12} levels and abnormal Schilling's tests have been observed in some patients receiving Sandostatin® (octreotide acetate) therapy, and monitoring of vitamin B_{12} levels is recommended during chronic Sandostatin® (octreotide acetate) therapy.

Information for Patients

Careful instruction in sterile subcutaneous injection technique should be given to the patients and to other persons who may administer Sandostatin® (octreotide acetate) Injection.

Laboratory Tests

Laboratory tests that may be helpful as biochemical markers in determining and following patient response depend on the specific tumor. Based on diagnosis, measurement of the following substances may be useful in monitoring the progress of therapy:

Acromegaly: Growth Hormone, IGF-I (somatomedin C) Responsiveness to Sandostatin® (octreotide acetate) may be evaluated by determining growth hormone levels at 1-4 hour intervals for 8-12 hours post dose. Alternatively, a single measurement of IGF-I (somatomedin C) level may be made two weeks after drug initiation or dosage change.

Carcinoid: 5-HIAA (urinary 5-hydroxyindole acetic acid), plasma serotonin, plasma Substance P

VIPoma: VIP (plasma vasoactive intestinal peptide)

Baseline and periodic total and/or free T_4 measurements should be performed during chronic therapy *(see PRECAUTIONS—General)*.

Drug Interactions

Sandostatin® (octreotide acetate) has been associated with alterations in nutrient absorption, so it may have an effect on absorption of orally administered drugs. Concomitant administration of Sandostatin® (octreotide acetate) with cyclosporine may decrease blood levels of cyclosporine and result in transplant rejection.

Patients receiving insulin, oral hypoglycemic agents, beta blockers, calcium channel blockers, or agents to control fluid and electrolyte balance, may require dose adjustments of these therapeutic agents.

Drug Laboratory Test Interactions

No known interference exists with clinical laboratory tests, including amine or peptide determinations.

Carcinogenesis/Mutagenesis/Impairment of Fertility

Studies in laboratory animals have demonstrated no mutagenic potential of Sandostatin® (octreotide acetate).

No carcinogenic potential was demonstrated in mice treated subcutaneously for 85-99 weeks at doses up to 2000 mcg/kg/day (8x the human exposure based on body surface area). In a 116-week subcutaneous study in rats, a 27% and 12% incidence of injection site sarcomas or squamous cell carcinomas was observed in males and females, respectively, at the highest dose level of 1250 mcg/kg/day (10x the human exposure based on body surface area) compared to an incidence of 8%-10% in the vehicle control groups. The increased incidence of injection site tumors was most probably caused by irritation and the high sensitivity of the rat to repeated subcutaneous injections at the same site. Rotating injection sites would prevent chronic irritation in humans. There have been no reports of injection site tumors in patients treated with Sandostatin® (octreotide acetate) for up to 5 years. There was also a 15% incidence of uterine adenocarcinomas in the 1250 mcg/kg/day females compared to 7% in the saline control females and 0% in the vehicle control females. The presence of endometritis coupled with the absence of corpora lutea, the reduction in mammary fibroadenomas, and the presence of uterine dilatation suggest that the uterine tumors were associated with estrogen dominance in the aged female rats which does not occur in humans.

Sandostatin® (octreotide acetate) did not impair fertility in rats at doses up to 1000 mcg/kg/day, which represents 7x the human exposure based on body surface area.

Pregnancy Category B

Reproduction studies have been performed in rats and rabbits at doses up to 16 times the highest human dose based on body surface area and have revealed no evidence of impaired fertility or harm to the fetus due to Sandostatin® (octreotide acetate). There are, however, no adequate and well-controlled studies in pregnant women. Because animal reproduction studies are not always predictive of human response, this drug should be used during pregnancy only if clearly needed.

Nursing Mothers

It is not known whether this drug is excreted in human milk. Because many drugs are excreted in milk, caution should be exercised when Sandostatin® (octreotide acetate) is administered to a nursing woman.

Pediatric Use

Experience with Sandostatin® (octreotide acetate) in the pediatric population is limited. The youngest patient to receive the drug was 1 month old. Doses of 1-10 mcg/kg body weight were well tolerated in the young patients. A single case of an infant (nesidioblastosis) was complicated by a seizure thought to be independent of Sandostatin® (octreotide acetate) therapy.

ADVERSE REACTIONS

Gallbladder Abnormalities

Gallbladder abnormalities, especially stones and/or biliary sludge, frequently develop in patients on chronic Sandostatin® (octreotide acetate) therapy *(See WARNINGS)*.

Cardiac

In acromegalics, sinus bradycardia (<50 bpm) developed in 25%; conduction abnormalities occurred in 10% and arrhythmias developed in 9% of patients during Sandostatin® (octreotide acetate) therapy *(see PRECAUTIONS — General)*.

Gastrointestinal

Diarrhea, loose stools, nausea and abdominal discomfort were each seen in 34%-61% of acromegalic patients in US studies although only 2.6% of the patients discontinued therapy due to these symptoms. These symptoms were seen in 5%-10% of patients with other disorders.

The frequency of these symptoms was not dose-related, but diarrhea and abdominal discomfort generally resolved more quickly in patients treated with 300 mcg/day than in those treated with 750 mcg/day. Vomiting, flatulence, abnormal stools, abdominal distention, and constipation were each seen in less than 10% of patients.

Hypo/Hyperglycemia

Hypoglycemia and hyperglycemia occurred in 3% and 16% of acromegalic patients, respectively, but only in about 1.5% of other patients. Symptoms of hypoglycemia were noted in approximately 2% of patients.

Hypothyroidism

In acromegalics, biochemical hypothyroidism alone occurred in 12% while goiter occurred in 6% during Sandostatin® (octreotide acetate) therapy *(See PRECAUTIONS — General)*. In patients without acromegaly, hypothyroidism has only been reported in several isolated patients and goiter has not been reported.

Other Adverse Events

Pain on injection was reported in 7.7%, headache in 6% and dizziness in 5%. Pancreatitis was also observed (See *WARNINGS* and *PRECAUTIONS*).

Other Adverse Events 1%-4%

Other events (relationship to drug not established), each observed in 1%-4% of patients, included fatigue, weakness, pruritus, joint pain, backache, urinary tract infection, cold symptoms, flu symptoms, injection site hematoma, bruise, edema, flushing, blurred vision, pollakiuria, fat malabsorption, hair loss, visual disturbance and depression.

Other Adverse Events <1%

Events reported in less than 1% of patients and for which relationship to drug is not established are listed: *Gastrointestinal:* hepatitis, jaundice, increase in liver enzymes, GI bleeding, hemorrhoids, appendicitis, gastric/peptic ulcer, gallbladder polyp; *Integumentary:* rash, cellulitis, petechiae, urticaria, basal cell carcinoma; *Musculoskeletal:* arthritis, joint effusion, muscle pain, Raynaud's phenomenon; *Cardiovascular:* chest pain, shortness of breath, thrombophlebitis, ischemia, congestive heart failure, hypertension, hypertensive reaction, palpitations, orthostatic BP decrease, tachycardia; *CNS:* anxiety, libido decrease, syncope, tremor, seizure, vertigo, Bell's Palsy, paranoia, pituitary apoplexy, increased intraocular pressure, amnesia, hearing loss, neuritis; *Respiratory:* pneumonia, pulmonary nodule, status asthmaticus; *Endocrine:* galactorrhea, hypoadrenalism, diabetes insipidus, gynecomastia, amenorrhea, polymenorrhea, oligomenorrhea, vaginitis; *Urogenital:* nephrolithiasis, hematuria; *Hematologic:* anemia, iron deficiency, epistaxis; *Miscellaneous:* otitis, allergic reaction, increased CK, weight loss.

Evaluation of 20 patients treated for at least 6 months has failed to demonstrate titers of antibodies exceeding background levels. However, antibody titers to Sandostatin® (octreotide acetate) were subsequently reported in three patients and resulted in prolonged duration of drug action in two patients. Anaphylactoid reactions, including anaphylactic shock, have been reported in several patients receiving Sandostatin® (octreotide acetate).

OVERDOSAGE

No frank overdose has occurred in any patient to date. Intravenous bolus doses of 1 mg (1000 mcg) given to healthy volunteers and of 30 mg (30,000 mcg) IV over 20 minutes and of 120 mg (120,000 mcg) IV over 8 hours to research patients have not resulted in serious ill effects.

Up-to-date information about the treatment of overdose can often be obtained from a certified Regional Poison Control Center. Telephone numbers of certified Regional Poison Control Centers are listed in the Physicians' Desk Reference®.*

Mortality occurred in mice and rats given 72 mg/kg and 18 mg/kg IV, respectively.

Drug Abuse and Dependence

There is no indication that Sandostatin® (octreotide acetate) has potential for drug abuse or dependence. Sandostatin® (octreotide acetate) levels in the central nervous system are negligible, even after doses up to 30,000 mcg.

DOSAGE AND ADMINISTRATION

Sandostatin® (octreotide acetate) may be administered subcutaneously or intravenously. Subcutaneous injection is the usual route of administration of Sandostatin® (octreotide acetate) for control of symptoms. Pain with subcutaneous administration may be reduced by using the smallest volume that will deliver the desired dose. Multiple subcutaneous injections at the same site within short periods of time should be avoided. Sites should be rotated in a systematic manner.

Parenteral drug products should be inspected visually for particulate matter and discoloration prior to administration. **Do not use if particulates and/or discoloration are observed.** Proper sterile technique should be used in the preparation of parenteral admixtures to minimize the possibility of microbial contamination. **Sandostatin® (octreotide acetate) is not compatible in Total Parenteral Nutrition (TPN) solutions because of the formation of a glycosyl octreotide conjugate which may decrease the efficacy of the product.**

Sandostatin® (octreotide acetate) is stable in sterile isotonic saline solutions or sterile solutions of dextrose 5% in water for 24 hours. It may be diluted in volumes of 50-200 mL and infused intravenously over 15-30 minutes or administered by IV push over 3 minutes. In emergency situations (e.g.: carcinoid crisis) it may be given by rapid bolus.

The initial dosage is usually 50 mcg administered twice or three times daily. Upward dose titration is frequently required. Dosage information for patients with specific tumors follows.

Acromegaly

Dosage may be initiated at 50 mcg t.i.d. Beginning with this low dose may permit adaptation to adverse gastrointestinal effects for patients who will require higher doses. IGF-I (somatomedin C) levels every 2 weeks can be used to guide titration. Alternatively, multiple growth hormone levels at 0-8 hours after Sandostatin® (octreotide acetate) administration permit more rapid titration of dose. The goal is to achieve growth hormone levels less than 5 ng/mL or IGF-I (somatomedin C) levels less than 1.9 U/mL in males and less than 2.2 U/mL in females. The dose most commonly found to be effective is 100 mcg t.i.d., but some patients require up to 500 mcg t.i.d. for maximum effectiveness. Doses greater than 300 mcg/day seldom result in additional biochemical benefit, and if an increase in dose fails to provide additional benefit, the dose should be reduced. IGF-I (somatomedin C) or growth hormone levels should be reevaluated at 6 month intervals.

Sandostatin® (octreotide acetate) should be withdrawn yearly for approximately 4 weeks from patients who have received irradiation to assess disease activity. If growth hormone or IGF-I (somatomedin C) levels increase and signs and symptoms recur, Sandostatin® (octreotide acetate) therapy may be resumed.

Carcinoid Tumors

The suggested daily dosage of Sandostatin® (octreotide acetate) during the first 2 weeks of therapy ranges from 100-600 mcg/day in 2-4 divided doses (mean daily dosage is 300 mcg). In the clinical studies, the **median** daily maintenance dosage was approximately 450 mcg, but clinical and biochemical benefits were obtained in some patients with as little as 50 mcg, while others required doses up to 1500 mcg/day. However, experience with doses above 750 mcg/day is limited.

VIPomas

Daily dosages of 200-300 mcg in 2-4 divided doses are recommended during the initial 2 weeks of therapy (range 150-750 mcg) to control symptoms of the disease. On an individual basis, dosage may be adjusted to achieve a therapeutic response, but usually doses above 450 mcg/day are not required.

HOW SUPPLIED

Sandostatin® (octreotide acetate) Injection is available in 1 mL ampuls and 5 mL multi-dose vials as follows:

Ampuls

50 mcg/mL octreotide (as acetate)
Package of 20 ampuls (NDC 0078-0180-03)
100 mcg/mL octreotide (as acetate)
Package of 20 ampuls (NDC 0078-0181-03)
500 mcg/mL octreotide (as acetate)
Package of 20 ampuls (NDC 0078-0182-03)

Multi-Dose Vials

200 mcg/mL octreotide (as acetate)
Box of one (NDC 0078-0183-25)
1000 mcg/mL octreotide (as acetate)
Box of one (NDC 0078-0184-25)

Storage

For prolonged storage, Sandostatin® (octreotide acetate) ampuls and multi-dose vials should be stored at refrigerated temperatures 2°-8°C (36°-46°F) and protected from light. At room temperature, (20°-30°C or 70°-86°F), Sandostatin® (octreotide acetate) is stable for 14 days if protected from light. The solution can be allowed to come to room temperature prior to administration. Do not warm artificially. After initial use, multiple dose vials should be discarded within 14 days. Ampuls should be opened just prior to administration and the unused portion discarded.

The ampuls and multi-dose vials are manufactured by:
NOVARTIS PHARMA AG, Basle, Switzerland
Distributed by:
Novartis Pharmaceuticals Corporation
East Hanover, New Jersey 07936
*Medical Economics Company, Inc.

REV: MAY 1999 T1999-40
Shown in Product Identification Guide, page 326

SANDOSTATIN LAR® DEPOT ℞

[săn dō stăt ĭn]
(octreotide acetate for injectable suspension)

Rx only
The following prescribing information is based on official labeling in effect July 2000.

DESCRIPTION

Octreotide is the acetate salt of a cyclic octapeptide. It is a long-acting octapeptide with pharmacologic properties mimicking those of the natural hormone somatostatin. Octreotide is known chemically as L-Cysteinamide, D-phenylalanyl-L-cysteinyl-L-phenylalanyl-D-tryptophyl-L-lysyl-L-threonyl-N-[2-hydroxy-1-(hydroxymethyl) propyl]-, cyclic (2→7)-disulfide; [R-(R*,R*)].

Sandostatin LAR® Depot (octreotide acetate for injectable suspension) is available in a vial containing the sterile drug product, which when mixed with diluent, becomes a suspension that is given as a monthly intragluteal injection. The octreotide is uniformly distributed within the microspheres which are made of a biodegradeable glucose star polymer, D,L-lactic and glycolic acids copolymer.

Sterile mannitol is added to the microspheres to improve suspendability.

Sandostatin LAR® Depot is available as: sterile 5 mL vials in 3 strengths delivering 10 mg, 20 mg or 30 mg octreotide free peptide. Each vial of Sandostatin LAR® Depot delivers:
[See first table above]

Each vial of diluent contains:

carboxymethylcellulose sodium	10.0 mg
mannitol	12.0 mg
water for injection	2.0 mL

The molecular weight of octreotide is 1019.3 (free peptide, $C_{49}H_{66}N_{10}O_{10}S_2$) and its amino acid sequence is:

H-D-Phe-Cys-Phe-D-Trp-Lys-Thr-Cys-Thr-ol•xCH_3COOH
where x = 1.4 to 2.5

CLINICAL PHARMACOLOGY

Sandostatin LAR® Depot (octreotide acetate for injectable suspension) is a long-acting dosage form consisting of microspheres of the biodegradable glucose star polymer, D,L-lactic and glycolic acids copolymer, containing octreotide. It maintains all of the clinical and pharmacological characteristics of the immediate-release dosage form Sandostatin® (octreotide acetate) Injection with the added feature of slow release of octreotide from the site of injection, reducing the need for frequent administration. This slow release occurs as the polymer biodegrades, primarily through hydrolysis. Sandostatin LAR® Depot is designed to be injected intramuscularly (intragluteally) once every four weeks.

Octreotide exerts pharmacologic actions similar to the natural hormone, somatostatin. It is an even more potent inhibitor of growth hormone, glucagon, and insulin than somatostatin. Like somatostatin, it also suppresses LH response to GnRH, decreases splanchnic blood flow, and inhibits release of serotonin, gastrin, vasoactive intestinal peptide, secretin, motilin, and pancreatic polypeptide.

By virtue of these pharmacological actions, octreotide has been used to treat the symptoms associated with metastatic carcinoid tumors (flushing and diarrhea), and Vasoactive Intestinal Peptide (VIP) secreting adenomas (watery diarrhea).

Octreotide substantially reduces and in many cases can normalize growth hormone and/or IGF-1 (somatomedin C) levels in patients with acromegaly.

Single doses of Sandostatin® Injection given subcutaneously have been shown to inhibit gallbladder contractility and to decrease bile secretion in normal volunteers. In controlled clinical trials the incidence of gallstone or biliary sludge formation was markedly increased *(See WARNINGS)*.

Octreotide may cause clinically significant suppression of thyroid stimulating hormone (TSH).

Pharmacokinetics

The magnitude and duration of octreotide serum concentrations after an intramuscular injection of the long-acting depot formulation Sandostatin LAR® Depot reflect the release of drug from the microsphere polymer matrix. Drug release is governed by the slow biodegradation of the microspheres in the muscle, but once present in the systemic circulation, octreotide distributes and is eliminated according to its known pharmacokinetic properties which are as follows:

1. Pharmacokinetics of Octreotide Acetate

According to data obtained with the immediate-release formulation, Sandostatin® Injection solution, after subcutaneous injection, octreotide is absorbed rapidly and completely from the injection site. Peak concentrations of 5.2 ng/mL (100 mcg dose) were reached 0.4 hours after dosing. Using a specific radioimmunoassay, intravenous and subcutaneous doses were found to be bioequivalent. Peak concentrations and area-under-the-curve values were dose proportional both after subcutaneous or intravenous single doses up to 400 mcg and with multiple doses of 200 mcg t.i.d. (600 mcg/day). Clearance was reduced by about 66% suggesting nonlinear kinetics of the drug at daily doses of 600 mcg/day as compared to 150 mcg/day. The relative decrease in clearance with doses above 600 mcg/day is not defined.

Name of Ingredient	10 mg	20 mg	30 mg
octreotide acetate	11.2 mg*	22.4 mg*	33.6 mg*
D, L-lactic and glycolic acids copolymer	188.8 mg	377.6 mg	566.4 mg
mannitol	41.0 mg	81.9 mg	122.9 mg

*Equivalent to 10/20/30 mg octreotide base.

Table 1
Hormonal Response in Acromegalic Patients Receiving 27-28 Injections During[1] Treatment with Sandostatin LAR® Depot

	Sandostatin® Injection S.C.		Sandostatin LAR® Depot	
Mean Hormone Level	N	%	N	%
GH <5.0 ng/mL	69/88	78	73/88	83
<2.5 ng/mL	44/88	50	41/88	47
<1.0 ng/mL	6/88	7	10/88	11
IGF-1 normalized	36/88	41	45/88	51
GH <5.0 ng/mL + IGF-1 normalized	36/88	41	45/88	51
<2.5 ng/mL + IGF-1 normalized	30/88	34	37/88	42
<1.0 ng/mL + IGF-1 normalized	5/88	6	10/88	11

[1]Average of monthly levels of GH and IGF-1 over the course of the trials

In healthy volunteers the distribution of octreotide from plasma was rapid ($t\alpha_{1/2}$ = 0.2 h), the volume of distribution (Vdss) was estimated to be 13.6 L and the total body clearance was 10 L/h.

In blood, the distribution of octreotide into the erythrocytes was found to be negligible and about 65% was bound in the plasma in a concentration-independent manner. Binding was mainly to lipoprotein and, to a lesser extent, to albumin.

The elimination of octreotide from plasma had an apparent half-life of 1.7 hours, compared with the 1-3 minutes with the natural hormone, somatostatin. The duration of action of subcutaneously administered Sandostatin® Injection solution is variable but extends up to 12 hours depending upon the type of tumor, necessitating multiple daily dosing with this immediate-release dosage form. About 32% of the dose is excreted unchanged into the urine. In an elderly population, dose adjustments may be necessary due to a significant increase in the half-life (46%) and a significant decrease in the clearance (26%) of the drug.

In patients with acromegaly, the pharmacokinetics differ somewhat from those in healthy volunteers. A mean peak concentration of 2.8 ng/mL (100 mcg dose) was reached in 0.7 hours after subcutaneous dosing. The volume of distribution (Vdss) was estimated to be 21.6 ± 8.5 L and the total body clearance was increased to 18 L/h. The mean percent of the drug bound was 41.2%. The disposition and elimination half-lives were similar to normals.

In patients with severe renal failure requiring dialysis, clearance was reduced to about half that found in healthy subjects (from approximately 10 L/h to 4.5 L/h).

The effect of hepatic diseases on the disposition of octreotide is unknown.

2. Pharmacokinetics of Sandostatin LAR® Depot

After a single IM injection of the long-acting depot dosage form Sandostatin LAR® Depot in healthy volunteer subjects, the serum octreotide concentration reached a transient initial peak of about 0.03 ng/mL/mg within 1 hour after administration progressively declining over the following 3 to 5 days to a nadir of <0.01 ng/mL/mg, then slowly increasing and reaching a plateau about two to three weeks post injection. Plateau concentrations were maintained over a period of nearly 2-3 weeks, showing dose proportional peak concentrations of about 0.07 ng/mL/mg. After about 6 weeks post injection, octreotide concentration slowly decreased, to <0.01 ng/mL/mg by weeks 12 to 13, concomitant with the terminal degradation phase of the polymer matrix of the dosage form. The relative bioavailability of the long-acting release Sandostatin LAR® Depot compared to immediate-release Sandostatin® Injection solution given subcutaneously was 60-63%.

In patients with acromegaly, the octreotide concentrations after single doses of 10 mg, 20 mg, and 30 mg Sandostatin LAR® Depot were dose proportional. The transient day 1 peak, amounting to 0.3 ng/mL, 0.8 ng/mL, and 1.3 ng/mL, respectively, was followed by plateau concentrations of 0.5 ng/mL, 1.3 ng/mL, and 2.0 ng/mL, respectively, achieved about 3 weeks post injection. These plateau concentrations were maintained for nearly two weeks.

Following multiple doses of Sandostatin LAR® Depot given every 4 weeks, steady-state octreotide serum concentrations were achieved after the third injection. Concentrations were dose proportional and higher by a factor of approximately 1.6 to 2.0 compared to the concentrations after a single dose. The steady-state octreotide concentrations were 1.2 ng/mL and 2.1 ng/mL, respectively, at trough and 1.6 ng/mL and 2.6 ng/mL, respectively, at peak with 20 mg and 30 mg Sandostatin LAR® Depot given every 4 weeks. No accumulation of octreotide beyond that expected from the overlapping release profiles occurred over a duration of up to 28 monthly injections of Sandostatin LAR® Depot. With the long-acting depot formulation Sandostatin LAR® Depot administered IM every 4 weeks the peak-to-trough variation in octreotide concentrations ranged from 44 to 68%, compared to the 163 to 209% variation encountered with the daily subcutaneous t.i.d. regimen of Sandostatin® Injection solution.

In patients with carcinoid tumors, the mean octreotide concentrations after 6 doses of 10 mg, 20 mg, and 30 mg Sandostatin LAR® Depot administered by IM injection every four weeks were 1.2 ng/mL, 2.5 ng/mL, and 4.2 ng/mL, respectively. Concentrations were dose proportional and steady-state concentrations were reached after two injections of 20 and 30 mg and after three injections of 10 mg.

Sandostatin LAR® Depot has not been studied in patients with renal impairment.

Sandostatin LAR® Depot has not been studied in patients with hepatic impairment.

CLINICAL TRIALS

The clinical trials of Sandostatin LAR® Depot (octreotide acetate for injectable suspension) were performed in patients who had been receiving Sandostatin® (octreotide acetate) Injection for a period of weeks to as long as 10 years. The acromegaly studies with Sandostatin LAR® Depot described below were performed in patients who achieved GH levels of <10 ng/mL (and, in most cases <5 ng/mL) while on subcutaneous Sandostatin® Injection. However, some patients enrolled were partial responders to subcutaneous Sandostatin® Injection, i.e., GH levels were reduced by >50% on subcutaneous Sandostatin® Injection compared to the untreated state, although not suppressed to <5 ng/mL.

Acromegaly

Sandostatin LAR® Depot was evaluated in three clinical trials in acromegalic patients.

In two of the clinical trials, a total of 101 patients were entered who had, in most cases, achieved a GH level <5 ng/mL on Sandostatin® Injection given in doses of 100 mcg or 200 mcg t.i.d. Most patients were switched to 20 mg or 30 mg doses of Sandostatin LAR® Depot given once every 4 weeks for up to 27 to 28 injections. A few patients received doses of 10 mg and a few required doses of 40 mg. Growth hormone and IGF-1 levels were at least as well-controlled with Sandostatin LAR® Depot as they had been on Sandostatin® Injection and this level of control remained for the entire duration of the trials.

A third trial was a 12-month study that enrolled 151 patients who had a GH level <10 ng/mL after treatment with Sandostatin® Injection (most had levels <5 ng/mL). The starting dose of Sandostatin LAR® Depot was 20 mg every 4 weeks for 3 doses. Thereafter, patients received 10, 20 or 30 mg every 4 weeks, depending upon the degree of GH suppression. (The recommended regimen for these dosage changes is described under *DOSAGE AND ADMINISTRATION*). Growth hormone and IGF-1 were at least as well-controlled on Sandostatin LAR® Depot as they had been on Sandostatin® Injection.

Table 1 summarizes the data on hormonal control (GH and IGF-1) for those patients in the first two clinical trials who received all 27-28 injections of Sandostatin LAR® Depot.

[See second table above]

For the 88 patients in Table 1, a mean GH level of <2.5 ng/mL was observed in 47% receiving Sandostatin LAR® Depot. Over the course of the trials 42% of patients maintained mean growth hormone levels of <2.5 ng/mL and mean normal IGF-1 levels.

Table 2 summarizes the data on hormonal control (GH and IGF-1) for those patients in the third clinical trial who received all 12 injections of Sandostatin LAR® Depot.

[See table 2 at top of next page]

Continued on next page

Sandostatin LAR—Cont.

For the 122 patients in Table 2, who received all 12 injections in the third trial, a mean GH level of <2.5 ng/mL was observed in 66% receiving Sandostatin LAR® Depot. Over the course of the trial 57% of patients maintained mean growth hormone levels of <2.5 ng/mL and mean normal IGF-1 levels. In comparing the hormonal response in these trials, note that a higher percentage of patients in the third trial suppressed their mean GH to <5 ng/mL on subcutaneous Sandostatin® Injection, 95%, compared to 78% across the two previous trials.

In all three trials, GH, IGF-1, and clinical symptoms were similarly controlled on Sandostatin LAR® Depot as they had been on Sandostatin® Injection.

Of the 25 patients who completed the trials and were partial responders to Sandostatin® Injection (GH >5.0 ng/mL but reduced by >50% relative to untreated levels), 1 patient (4%) responded to Sandostatin LAR® Depot with a reduction of GH to <2.5 ng/mL and 8 patients (32%) responded with a reduction of GH to <5.0 ng/mL.

Carcinoid Syndrome

A 6-month clinical trial of malignant carcinoid syndrome was performed in 93 patients who had previously been shown to be responsive to Sandostatin® Injection. Sixty-seven patients were randomized at baseline to receive, double-blind, doses of 10 mg, 20 mg, or 30 mg Sandostatin LAR® Depot every 28 days and 26 patients continued, unblinded, on their previous Sandostatin® Injection regimen (100 to 300 mcg t.i.d.).

In any given month after steady-state levels of octreotide were reached, approximately 35 to 40% of the patients who received Sandostatin LAR® Depot required supplemental subcutaneous Sandostatin® Injection therapy usually for a few days, to control exacerbation of carcinoid symptoms. In any given month the percentage of patients randomized to subcutaneous Sandostatin® Injection, who required supplemental treatment with an increased dose of Sandostatin® Injection, was similar to the percentage of patients randomized to Sandostatin LAR® Depot. Over the six-month treatment period approximately 50-70% of patients who completed the trial on Sandostatin LAR® Depot required subcutaneous Sandostatin® Injection supplemental therapy to control exacerbation of carcinoid symptoms although steady-state serum Sandostatin LAR® Depot levels had been reached.

Table 3 presents the average number of daily stools and flushing episodes in malignant carcinoid patients.

[See table 3 above]

Overall, mean daily stool frequency was as well-controlled on Sandostatin LAR® Depot as on Sandostatin® Injection (approximately 2 to 2.5 stools/day).

Mean daily flushing episodes were similar at all doses of Sandostatin LAR® Depot and on Sandostatin® Injection (approximately 0.5 to 1 episode/day).

In a subset of patients with variable severity of disease, median 24 hour urinary 5-HIAA (5-hydroxyindole acetic acid) levels were reduced by 38-50% in the groups randomized to Sandostatin LAR® Depot.

The reductions are within the range reported in the published literature for patients treated with octreotide (about 10-50%).

Seventy-eight patients with malignant carcinoid syndrome who had participated in this 6-month trial, subsequently participated in a 12-month extension study in which they received 12 injections of Sandostatin LAR® Depot at 4-week intervals. For those who remained in the extension trial, diarrhea and flushing were as well controlled as during the 6-month trial. Because malignant carcinoid disease is progressive, as expected, a number of deaths (8 patients: 10%) occurred due to disease progression or complications from the underlying disease. An additional 22% of patients prematurely discontinued Sandostatin LAR® Depot due to disease progression or worsening of carcinoid symptoms.

INDICATIONS AND USAGE

Acromegaly

Sandostatin LAR® Depot (octreotide acetate for injectable suspension) is indicated for long-term maintenance therapy in acromegalic patients for whom medical treatment is appropriate and who have been shown to respond to and can tolerate Sandostatin® (octreotide acetate) Injection. The goal of treatment in acromegaly is to reduce GH and IGF-1 levels to normal. Sandostatin LAR® Depot can be used in patients who have had an inadequate response to surgery or in those for whom surgical resection is not an option. It may also be used in patients who have received radiation and have had an inadequate therapeutic response *(See CLINICAL TRIALS and DOSAGE AND ADMINISTRATION)*.

Carcinoid Tumors

Sandostatin LAR® Depot is indicated for long-term treatment of the severe diarrhea and flushing episodes associated with metastatic carcinoid tumors in patients in whom initial treatment with Sandostatin® Injection has been shown to be effective and tolerated.

Vasoactive Intestinal Peptide Tumors (VIPomas)

Sandostatin LAR® Depot is indicated for long-term treatment of the profuse watery diarrhea associated with VIP-secreting tumors in patients in whom initial treatment with Sandostatin® Injection has been shown to be effective and tolerated.

Table 2
Hormonal Response in Acromegalic Patients Receiving 12 Injections During[1] Treatment with Sandostatin LAR® Depot

Mean Hormone Level	Sandostatin® Injection S.C. N	%	Sandostatin LAR® Depot N	%
GH <5.0 ng/mL	116/122	95	118/122	97
<2.5 ng/mL	84/122	69	80/122	66
<1.0 ng/mL	25/122	21	28/122	23
IGF-1 normalized	82/122	67	82/122	67
GH <5.0 ng/mL + IGF-1 normalized	80/122	66	82/122	67
<2.5 ng/mL + IGF-1 normalized	65/122	53	70/122	57
<1.0 ng/mL + IGF-1 normalized	23/122	19	27/122	22

[1]Average of monthly levels of GH and IGF-1 over the course of the trial

Table 3
Average No. of Daily Stools and Flushing Episodes in Patients with Malignant Carcinoid Syndrome

Treatment	N	Daily Stools (Average No.) Baseline	Last Visit	Daily Flushing Episodes (Average No.) Baseline	Last Visit
Sandostatin® Injection S.C.	26	3.7	2.6	3.0	0.5
Sandostatin LAR® Depot					
10 mg	22	4.6	2.8	3.0	0.9
20 mg	20	4.0	2.1	5.9	0.6
30 mg	24	4.9	2.8	6.1	1.0

In patients with acromegaly, carcinoid syndrome and VIPomas, the effect of Sandostatin® Injection and Sandostatin LAR® Depot on tumor size, rate of growth and development of metastases, has not been determined.

CONTRAINDICATIONS

Sensitivity to this drug or any of its components.

WARNINGS

Adverse events that have been reported in patients receiving Sandostatin® (octreotide acetate) Injection can also be expected in patients receiving Sandostatin LAR® Depot (octreotide acetate for injectable suspension). Incidence figures in the *WARNINGS* and *ADVERSE REACTIONS* sections, below, are those obtained in clinical trials of Sandostatin® Injection and Sandostatin LAR® Depot.

Gallbladder and Related Events

Single doses of Sandostatin® Injection have been shown to inhibit gallbladder contractility and decrease bile secretion in normal volunteers. In clinical trials with Sandostatin® Injection (primarily patients with acromegaly or psoriasis) in patients who had not previously received octreotide, the incidence of biliary tract abnormalities was 63% (27% gallstones, 24% sludge without stones, 12% biliary duct dilatation). The incidence of stones or sludge in patients who received Sandostatin® Injection for 12 months or longer was 52%. The incidence of gallbladder abnormalities did not appear to be related to age, sex or dose but was related to duration of exposure.

In clinical trials 52% of acromegalic patients, most of whom received Sandostatin LAR® Depot for 12 months or longer, developed new biliary abnormalities including gallstones, microlithiasis, sediment, sludge and dilatation. The incidence of new cholelithiasis was 22%, of which 7% were microstones.

In clinical trials 62% of malignant carcinoid patients who received Sandostatin LAR® Depot for up to 18 months developed new biliary abnormalities including gallstones, sludge and dilatation. New gallstones occurred in a total of 24% of patients.

Across all trials, a few patients developed acute cholecystitis, ascending cholangitis, biliary obstruction, cholestatic hepatitis, or pancreatitis during octreotide therapy or following its withdrawal. One patient developed ascending cholangitis during Sandostatin® Injection therapy and died. Despite the high incidence of new gallstones in patients receiving octreotide, 1% of patients developed acute symptoms requiring cholecystectomy.

PRECAUTIONS *(See ADVERSE REACTIONS)*

General

Growth hormone secreting tumors may sometimes expand and cause serious complications (e.g., visual field defects). Therefore, all patients with these tumors should be carefully monitored.

Octreotide alters the balance between the counter-regulatory hormones, insulin, glucagon and growth hormone, which may result in hypoglycemia or hyperglycemia. Octreotide also suppresses secretion of thyroid stimulating hormone, which may result in hypothyroidism. Cardiac conduction abnormalities have also occurred during treatment with octreotide.

Glucose Metabolism

The hypoglycemia or hyperglycemia which occurs during octreotide therapy is usually mild, but may result in overt diabetes mellitus or necessitate dose changes in insulin or other hypoglycemic agents. Severe hyperglycemia, subsequent pneumonia, and death following initiation of Sandostatin® (octreotide acetate) Injection therapy was reported in one patient with no history of hyperglycemia *(See ADVERSE REACTIONS)*.

Thyroid Function

Hypothyroidism has been reported in acromegaly and carcinoid patients receiving octreotide therapy. Baseline and periodic assessment of thyroid function (TSH, total and/or free T_4) is recommended during chronic octreotide therapy *(See ADVERSE REACTIONS)*.

Cardiac Function

In both acromegalic and carcinoid syndrome patients, bradycardia, arrhythmias and conduction abnormalities have been reported during octreotide therapy. Other EKG changes were observed such as QT prolongation, axis shifts, early repolarization, low voltage, R/S transition, early R wave progression, and non-specific ST-T wave changes. The relationship of these events to octreotide acetate is not established because many of these patients have underlying cardiac disease *(See PRECAUTIONS)*. Dose adjustments in drugs such as beta-blockers that have bradycardia effects may be necessary. In one acromegalic patient with severe congestive heart failure, initiation of Sandostatin® Injection therapy resulted in worsening of CHF with improvement when drug was discontinued. Confirmation of a drug effect was obtained with a positive rechallenge *(See ADVERSE REACTIONS)*.

Nutrition

Octreotide may alter absorption of dietary fats in some patients.

Depressed vitamin B_{12} levels and abnormal Schilling's tests have been observed in some patients receiving octreotide therapy, and monitoring of vitamin B_{12} levels is recommended during therapy with Sandostatin LAR® Depot (octreotide acetate for injectable suspension).

Octreotide has been investigated for the reduction of excessive fluid loss from the G.I. tract in patients with conditions producing such a loss. If such patients are receiving total parenteral nutrition (TPN), serum zinc may rise excessively when the fluid loss is reversed. Patients on TPN and octreotide should have periodic monitoring of zinc levels.

Information for Patients

Patients with carcinoid tumors and VIPomas should be advised to adhere closely to their scheduled return visits for reinjection in order to minimize exacerbation of symptoms.

Patients with acromegaly should also be urged to adhere to their return visit schedule to help assure steady control of GH and IGF-1 levels.

Laboratory Tests

Laboratory tests that may be helpful as biochemical markers in determining and following patient response depend on the specific tumor. Based on diagnosis, measurement of the following substances may be useful in monitoring the progress of therapy:

Acromegaly: Growth Hormone, IGF-1 (somatomedin C)

Responsiveness to octreotide may be evaluated by determining growth hormone levels at 1-4 hour intervals for 8-12 hours after subcutaneous injection of Sandostatin® Injection (not Sandostatin LAR® Depot). Alternatively, a single measurement of IGF-1 (somatomedin C) level may be made two weeks after initiation of Sandostatin® Injection or dosage change. After patients are switched from Sandostatin® Injection to Sandostatin LAR® Depot, GH and IGF-1 determinations may be made after 3 monthly injections of Sandostatin LAR® Depot. (Steady-state serum levels of octreotide are reached only after a period of 3 months of monthly injections.) Growth hormone can be determined using the mean of 4 assays taken at 1 hour intervals. Somatomedin C can be determined with a single assay. All GH and IGF-1 determinations should be made 4 weeks after the previous Sandostatin LAR® Depot.

Carcinoid: 5-HIAA (urinary 5-hydroxyindole acetic acid), plasma serotonin, plasma Substance P

VIPoma: VIP (plasma vasoactive intestinal peptide)
Baseline and periodic total and/or free T_4 measurements should be performed during chronic therapy *(See PRECAUTIONS - General)*.

Drug Interactions

Octreotide has been associated with alterations in nutrient absorption, so it may have an effect on absorption of orally administered drugs. Concomitant administration of octreotide injection with cyclosporine may decrease blood levels of cyclosporine and result in transplant rejection.

Patients receiving insulin, oral hypoglycemic agents, beta-blockers, calcium channel blockers, or agents to control fluid and electrolyte balance, may require dose adjustments of these therapeutic agents.

Drug Laboratory Test Interactions

No known interference exists with clinical laboratory tests, including amine or peptide determinations.

Carcinogenesis/Mutagenesis/Impairment of Fertility

Studies in laboratory animals have demonstrated no mutagenic potential of Sandostatin®. No mutagenic potential of the polymeric carrier in Sandostatin LAR® Depot, D,L-lactic and glycolic acids copolymer, was observed in the Ames mutagenicity test.

No carcinogenic potential was demonstrated in mice treated subcutaneously with octreotide for 85-99 weeks at doses up to 2000 mcg/kg/day (8× the human exposure based on body surface area). In a 116-week subcutaneous study in rats administered octreotide, a 27% and 12% incidence of injection site sarcomas or squamous cell carcinomas was observed in males and females, respectively, at the highest dose level of 1250 mcg/kg/day (10× the human exposure based on body surface area) compared to an incidence of 8-10% in the vehicle control groups. The increased incidence of injection site tumors was most probably caused by irritation and the high sensitivity of the rat to repeated subcutaneous injections at the same site. Rotating injection sites would prevent chronic irritation in humans. There have been no reports of injection site tumors in patients treated with Sandostatin® Injection for at least 5 years. There was also a 15% incidence of uterine adenocarcinomas in the 1250 mcg/kg/day females compared to 7% in the saline control females and 0% in the vehicle control females. The presence of endometritis coupled with the absence of corpora lutea, the reduction in mammary fibroadenomas, and the presence of uterine dilatation suggest that the uterine tumors were associated with estrogen dominance in the aged female rats which does not occur in humans.

Octreotide did not impair fertility in rats at doses up to 1000 mcg/kg/day, which represents 7× the human exposure based on body surface area.

Pregnancy Category B

Reproduction studies have been performed in rats and rabbits at doses up to 16 times the highest human dose based on body surface area and have revealed no evidence of impaired fertility or harm to the fetus due to octreotide. There are, however, no adequate and well-controlled studies in pregnant women. Because animal reproduction studies are not always predictive of human response, this drug should be used during pregnancy only if clearly needed.

Nursing Mothers

It is not known whether this drug is excreted in human milk. Because many drugs are excreted in milk, caution should be exercised when Sandostatin LAR® Depot is administered to a nursing woman.

Pediatric Use

Sandostatin LAR® Depot has not been studied in pediatric patients.

Experience with Sandostatin® Injection in the pediatric population is limited. Its use has been primarily in patients with congenital hyperinsulinism (also called nesidioblastosis). The youngest patient to receive the drug was 1 month old. At doses of 1 - 40 mcg/kg body weight/day, the majority of side effects observed were gastrointestinal - steatorrhea, diarrhea, vomiting and abdominal distension. Poor growth has been reported in several patients treated with Sandostatin® Injection for more than 1 year; catch-up growth occurred after Sandostatin® Injection was discontinued. A 16-month-old male with enterocutaneous fistula developed sudden abdominal pain and increased nasogastric drainage and died 8 hours after receiving a single 100 mcg subcutaneous dose of Sandostatin® Injection.

ADVERSE REACTIONS *(See WARNINGS and PRECAUTIONS)*

Gallbladder abnormalities, especially stones and/or biliary sludge, frequently develop in patients on chronic octreotide therapy *(See WARNINGS)*. Few patients, however, develop acute symptoms requiring cholecystectomy.

Cardiac

In acromegalics, sinus bradycardia (<50 bpm) developed in 25%; conduction abnormalities occurred in 10% and arrhythmias developed in 9% of patients during Sandostatin® (octreotide acetate) Injection therapy. Electrocardiograms were performed only in carcinoid patients receiving Sandostatin LAR® Depot (octreotide acetate for injectable suspension). In carcinoid syndrome patients sinus bradycardia developed in 19%; conduction abnormalities occurred in 9%, and arrhythmias developed in 3%. The relationship of these events to octreotide acetate is not established because many of these patients have underlying cardiac disease *(See PRECAUTIONS)*.

Gastrointestinal

The most common symptoms are gastrointestinal. The overall incidence of the most frequent of these symptoms in clinical trials of acromegalic patients treated for approximately 1 to 4 years is shown in Table 4.

[See table 4 above]

Table 4
Number (%) of Acromegalic Patients with Common G.I. Adverse Events

Adverse Event	Sandostatin® Injection S.C. t.i.d. n=114 N	%	Sandostatin LAR® Depot q. 28 days n=261 N	%
Diarrhea	66	(57.9)	95	(36.4)
Abdominal Pain or Discomfort	50	(43.9)	76	(29.1)
Flatulence	15	(13.2)	67	(25.7)
Constipation	10	(8.8)	49	(18.8)
Nausea	34	(29.8)	27	(10.3)
Vomiting	5	(4.4)	17	(6.5)

Only 2.6% of the patients on Sandostatin® (octreotide acetate) Injection in U.S. clinical trials discontinued therapy due to these symptoms. No acromegalic patient receiving Sandostatin LAR® Depot discontinued therapy for a G.I. event.

In patients receiving Sandostatin LAR® Depot the incidence of diarrhea was dose-related. Diarrhea, abdominal pain, and nausea developed primarily during the first month of treatment with Sandostatin LAR® Depot. Thereafter, new cases of these events were uncommon. The vast majority of these events were mild-to-moderate in severity.

In rare instances gastrointestinal adverse effects may resemble acute intestinal obstruction, with progressive abdominal distention, severe epigastric pain, abdominal tenderness, and guarding.

Dyspepsia, steatorrhea, discoloration of feces, and tenesmus were reported in 4% to 6% of patients.

In a clinical trial of carcinoid syndrome, nausea, abdominal pain, and flatulence were reported in 27% to 38% and constipation or vomiting in 15% to 21% of patients treated with Sandostatin LAR® Depot. Diarrhea was reported as an adverse event in 14% of patients but since most of the patients had diarrhea as a symptom of carcinoid syndrome, it is difficult to assess the actual incidence of drug-related diarrhea.

Hypo/Hyperglycemia

In acromegaly patients treated with either Sandostatin® Injection or Sandostatin LAR® Depot, hypoglycemia occurred in approximately 2% and hyperglycemia in approximately 15% of patients. In carcinoid patients, hypoglycemia occurred in 4% and hyperglycemia in 27% of patients treated with Sandostatin LAR® Depot *(See PRECAUTIONS)*.

Hypothyroidism

In acromegaly patients receiving Sandostatin® Injection, 12% developed biochemical hypothyroidism, 8% developed goiter, and 4% required initiation of thyroid replacement therapy while receiving Sandostatin® Injection. In acromegalics treated with Sandostatin LAR® Depot hypothyroidism was reported as an adverse event in 2% and goiter in 2%. Two patients receiving Sandostatin LAR® Depot, required initiation of thyroid hormone replacement therapy. In carcinoid patients, hypothyroidism has only been reported in isolated patients and goiter has not been reported *(See PRECAUTIONS)*.

Pain At the Injection Site

Pain on injection, which is generally mild-to-moderate, and short-lived (usually about 1 hour) is dose-related, being reported by 2%, 9%, and 11% of acromegalics receiving doses of 10 mg, 20 mg, and 30 mg, respectively, of Sandostatin LAR® Depot. In carcinoid patients, where a diary was kept, pain at the injection site was reported by about 20-25% at a 10-mg dose and about 30 to 50% at the 20-mg and 30-mg dose.

Other Adverse Events 16% - 20%

Other adverse events (relationship to drug not established) in acromegalic and/or carcinoid syndrome patients receiving Sandostatin LAR® Depot were upper respiratory infection, flu-like symptoms, fatigue, dizziness, headache, malaise, fever, dyspnea, back pain, chest pain, arthropathy.

Other Adverse Events 5% - 15%

Other adverse events (relationship to drug not established) occurring in an incidence of 5-15% in patients receiving Sandostatin LAR® Depot were:

Body As a Whole: asthenia, rigors, allergy
Cardiovascular: hypertension, peripheral edema
Central and Peripheral Nervous System: paresthesia, hypoesthesia
Gastrointestinal: dyspepsia, anorexia, hemorrhoids
Hearing and Vestibular: earache
Heart Rate and Rhythm: palpitations
Hematologic: anemia
Metabolic and Nutritional: dehydration, weight decrease
Musculoskeletal System: myalgia, leg cramps, arthralgia
Psychiatric: depression, anxiety, confusion, insomnia
Resistance Mechanism: viral infection, otitis media
Respiratory System: coughing, pharyngitis, rhinitis, sinusitis
Skin and Appendages: rash, pruritus, increased sweating
Urinary System: urinary tract infection, renal calculus

Other Adverse Events 1% - 4%

Other events (relationship to drug not established), each occurring in an incidence of 1-4% in patients receiving Sandostatin LAR® Depot and reported by at least 2 patients were:

Application Site: injection site inflammation
Body As a Whole: syncope, ascites, hot flushes
Cardiovascular: cardiac failure, angina pectoris, hypertension aggravated
Central and Peripheral Nervous System: vertigo, abnormal gait, neuropathy, neuralgia, tremor, dysphonia, hyperkinesia, hypertonia
Gastrointestinal: rectal bleeding, melena, gastritis, gastroenteritis, colitis, gingivitis, taste perversion, stomatitis, glossitis, dry mouth, dysphagia, steatorrhea, diverticulitis
Hearing and Vestibular: tinnitus
Heart Rate and Rhythm: tachycardia
Liver and Biliary: jaundice
Metabolic and Nutritional: hypokalemia, cachexia, gout, hypoproteinemia
Platelet, Bleeding, Clotting: pulmonary embolism, epistaxis
Psychiatric: amnesia, somnolence, nervousness, hallucinations
Reproductive, Female: menstrual irregularities, breast pain
Reproductive, Male: impotence
Resistance Mechanism: cellulitis, renal abcess, moniliasis, bacterial infection
Respiratory System: bronchitis, pneumonia, pleural effusion
Skin and Appendages: alopecia, urticaria, acne
Urinary System: incontinence, albuminuria
Vascular: cerebral vascular disorder, phlebitis, hematoma
Vision: abnormal vision

Rare Adverse Events

Other events (relationship to drug not established) of potential clinical significance occurring rarely (<1%) in clinical trials of octreotide either as Sandostatin® Injection or Sandostatin LAR® Depot, or reported post-marketing in patients with acromegaly, carcinoid syndrome, or other disorders include:

Body As a Whole: anaphylactoid reactions, including anaphylactic shock, facial edema, generalized edema, abdomen enlarged, malignant hyperpyrexia
Cardiovascular: aneurysm, myocardial infarction, angina pectoris, aggravated, pulmonary hypertension, cardiac arrest, orthostatic hypotension
Central and Peripheral Nervous System: hemiparesis, paresis, convulsions, paranoia, pituitary apoplexy, visual field defect, migraine, aphasia, scotoma, Bell's palsy
Endocrine Disorders: hypoadrenalism, diabetes insipidus, gynecomastia, galactorrhea
Gastrointestinal: G.I. hemorrhage, intestinal obstruction, hepatitis, increase in liver enzymes, fatty liver, peptic/gastric ulcer, gallbladder polyp, appendicitis, pancreatitis
Hearing and Vestibular: deafness
Heart Rate and Rhythm: atrial fibrillation
Hematologic: pancytopenia, thrombocytopenia
Metabolic and Nutritional: renal insufficiency, creatinine increased, CK increased, diabetes mellitus
Musculoskeletal: Raynaud's syndrome, arthritis, joint effusion
Neoplasms: breast carcinoma, basal cell carcinoma
Platelet, Bleeding, and Clotting: arterial thrombosis of the arm
Psychiatric: suicide attempt, libido decrease
Reproductive, Female: lactation, nonpuerperal
Respiratory: pulmonary nodule, status asthmaticus, pneumothorax
Skin and Appendages: cellulitis, petechiae, urticaria
Urinary System: renal failure, hematuria
Vascular: intracranial hemorrhage, retinal vein thrombosis
Vision: glaucoma

Antibodies to Octreotide

Studies to date have shown that antibodies to octreotide develop in up to 25% of patients treated with octreotide acetate. These antibodies do not influence the degree of efficacy response to octreotide; however, in two acromegalic patients who received Sandostatin® Injection, the duration of GH suppression following each injection was about twice as long as in patients without antibodies. It has not been determined whether octreotide antibodies will also prolong the duration of GH suppression in patients being treated with Sandostatin LAR® Depot.

OVERDOSAGE

No frank overdose has occurred in any patient to date. Sandostatin® (octreotide acetate) Injection given in intravenous bolus doses of 1 mg (1000 mcg) to healthy volunteers did not result in serious ill effects, nor did doses of 30 mg (30,000 mcg) given IV over 20 minutes and of 120 mg (120,000 mcg) given IV over 8 hours to research patients.

Continued on next page

Sandostatin LAR—Cont.

Doses of 2.5 mg (2500 mcg) of Sandostatin® Injection subcutaneously have, however, caused hypoglycemia, flushing, dizziness, and nausea.
Up-to-date information about the treatment of overdose can often be obtained from a certified Regional Poison Control Center. Telephone numbers of certified Regional Poison Control Centers are listed in the Physicians' Desk Reference®*.
Mortality occurred in mice and rats given 72 mg/kg and 18 mg/kg IV, respectively, of octreotide.

Drug Abuse and Dependence
There is no indication that octreotide has potential for drug abuse or dependence. Octreotide levels in the central nervous system are negligible, even after doses up to 30,000 mcg.

DOSAGE AND ADMINISTRATION

Sandostatin LAR® Depot (octreotide acetate for injectable suspension) must be administered under the supervision of a physician. It is important to closely follow the mixing instructions included in the packaging. Sandostatin LAR® Depot must be administered immediately after mixing.
Sandostatin LAR® Depot should be administered intragluteally at four-week intervals. Administration of Sandostatin LAR® Depot at intervals greater than 4 weeks is not recommended because there is no adequate information on whether such patients could be satisfactorily controlled.
Deltoid injections are to be avoided because of significant discomfort at the injection site when given in that area. **Sandostatin LAR® Depot should never be administered by the IV or S.C. routes.** The following dosage regimens are recommended.

Acromegaly
1. Patients Not Currently Receiving Octreotide Acetate
Patients not currently receiving octreotide acetate should begin therapy with Sandostatin® (octreotide acetate) Injection given subcutaneously in an initial dose of 50 mcg t.i.d. Beginning with this low dose may permit adaptation to adverse gastrointestinal effects for patients who require higher doses. Multiple growth hormone (GH) determinations at 0-8 hours after a subcutaneous Sandostatin® Injection will guide dosage titration. The goal is to attempt to normalize GH and IGF-1 (somatomedin C) levels. Most patients require doses of 100 mcg to 200 mcg t.i.d. for maximum effect but some patients require up to 500 mcg t.i.d. Injection sites should be rotated in a systematic manner to avoid irritation.
Although responsiveness of GH to octreotide acetate can be ascertained quickly, patients should be maintained on Sandostatin® Injection s.c. for at least 2 weeks to determine tolerance to octreotide.
The most common adverse events are gastrointestinal, which usually begin within the first few days of administration and usually subside within 2 to 8 weeks. In clinical trials, <3% of patients discontinued Sandostatin® Injection because of G.I. symptoms.
Patients who are considered to be "responders" to the drug, based on GH and IGF-1 levels, and who tolerate the drug, can then be switched to Sandostatin LAR® Depot in the dosage scheme described under 2, below [Patients Currently Receiving Sandostatin® Injection].

2. Patients Currently Receiving Sandostatin® (octreotide acetate) Injection
Patients currently receiving Sandostatin® Injection can be switched directly to Sandostatin LAR® Depot in a dose of 20 mg given IM intragluteally at 4 week intervals for 3 months. **(Deltoid injections are to be avoided because of significant discomfort at the injection site when given in that area.)** Gluteal injection sites should be alternated to avoid irritation.
At the end of 3 months Sandostatin LAR® Depot dosage may be continued at the same level or increased or decreased based on the following regimen:
GH ≤2.5 ng/mL, IGF-1 normal and clinical symptoms controlled: maintain Sandostatin LAR® Depot dosage at 20 mg every 4 weeks.
GH >2.5 ng/mL, IGF-1 elevated, and/or clinical symptoms uncontrolled, increase Sandostatin LAR® Depot dosage to 30 mg every 4 weeks.
GH ≤1 ng/mL, IGF-1 normal and clinical symptoms controlled, reduce Sandostatin LAR® Depot dosage to 10 mg every 4 weeks.
Patients whose GH, IGF-1, and symptoms are not adequately controlled at a dose of 30 mg may have the dose increased to 40 mg every 4 weeks. Doses higher than 40 mg are not recommended.
Administration of Sandostatin LAR® Depot at intervals greater than 4 weeks is not recommended because there is no adequate information on whether such patients could be satisfactorily controlled.
In patients who have received pituitary irradiation, Sandostatin LAR® Depot should be withdrawn yearly for approximately 8 weeks to assess disease activity. If GH or IGF-1 levels increase and signs and symptoms recur, Sandostatin LAR® Depot therapy may be resumed.

3. Special Populations: Renal Failure
In patients with renal failure requiring dialysis, the half-life of octreotide may be increased, necessitating adjustment of the maintenance dosage *(See CLINICAL PHARMACOLOGY and Pharmacokinetics of Octreotide)*.

Carcinoid Tumors and VIPomas
1. Patients Not Currently Receiving Octreotide Acetate
Patients not currently receiving octreotide acetate should begin therapy with Sandostatin® Injection given subcutaneously. The suggested daily dosage for carcinoid tumors during the first 2 weeks of therapy ranges from 100-600 mcg/day in 2-4 divided doses (mean daily dosage is 300 mcg). Some patients may require doses up to 1,500 mcg/day. The suggested daily dosage for VIPomas is 200-300 mcg in 2-4 divided doses (range 150-750 mcg); dosage may be adjusted on an individual basis to control symptoms but usually doses above 450 mcg/day are not required.
Sandostatin® Injection should be continued for at least 2 weeks. Thereafter, patients who are considered "responders" to octreotide acetate and who tolerate the drug may be switched to Sandostatin LAR® Depot in the dosage regimen described under 2, below [Patients Currently Receiving Sandostatin® Injection].

2. Patients Currently Receiving Sandostatin® (octreotide acetate) Injection
Patients currently receiving Sandostatin® Injection can be switched to Sandostatin LAR® Depot in a dosage of 20 mg given IM intragluteally at 4 week intervals for 2 months. **Deltoid injections are to be avoided because of significant discomfort at the injection site when given in that area.** Gluteal injection sites should be alternated to avoid irritation. Because of the need for serum octreotide to reach therapeutically effective levels following initial injection of Sandostatin LAR® Depot, carcinoid tumor and VIPoma patients should continue to receive Sandostatin® Injection s.c. for at least 2 weeks in the same dosage they were taking before the switch. Failure to continue subcutaneous injections for this period may result in exacerbation of symptoms. (Some patients may require 3 or 4 weeks of such therapy.)
After two months of a 20 mg dosage of Sandostatin LAR® Depot, dosage may be increased to 30 mg every 4 weeks if symptoms are not adequately controlled. Patients who achieve good control on a 20-mg dose may have their dose lowered to 10 mg for a trial period. If symptoms recur, dosage should then be increased to 20 mg every 4 weeks. Many patients can, however, be satisfactorily maintained at a 10 mg dosage every 4 weeks. A dose of 10 mg is not recommended as a starting dose, however, because therapeutically effective levels of octreotide are reached more rapidly with a 20-mg dose.
Dosages higher than 30 mg are not recommended because there is no information on their usefulness.
Despite good overall control of symptoms, patients with carcinoid tumors and VIPomas often experience periodic exacerbation of symptoms (regardless of whether they are being maintained on Sandostatin® Injection or Sandostatin LAR® Depot). During these periods they may be given Sandostatin® Injection s.c. for a few days at the dosage they were receiving prior to switch to Sandostatin LAR® Depot. When symptoms are again controlled, the Sandostatin® Injection s.c. can be discontinued.
Administration of Sandostatin LAR® Depot at intervals greater than 4 weeks is not recommended because there is no adequate information on whether such patients could be adequately controlled.

3. Special Populations: Renal Failure
In patients with renal failure requiring dialysis, the half-life of octreotide may be increased, necessitating adjustment of the maintenance dosage *(See CLINICAL PHARMACOLOGY and Pharmacokinetics of Octreotide)*.

HOW SUPPLIED

Sandostatin LAR® Depot (octreotide acetate for injectable suspension) is available in single use kits containing a 5 mL vial of 10 mg, 20 mg or 30 mg strength, a 2 mL vial of diluent, a 5 mL sterile plastic syringe, two sterile 1 1/2″ 20 gauge needles, and three alcohol wipes. An instruction booklet for the preparation of drug suspension for injection is also included with each kit.

Drug Product Kits

10 mg kit	NDC 0078-0340-84
20 mg kit	NDC 0078-0341-84
30 mg kit	NDC 0078-0342-84
Demonstration kit	NDC 0078-0340-97

Storage
For prolonged storage, Sandostatin LAR® Depot should be stored at refrigerated temperatures 2°C - 8°C (36°F - 46°F) and protected from light until the time of use. Sandostatin LAR® Depot drug product kit should remain at room temperature for 30-60 minutes prior to preparation of the drug suspension. However, after preparation the drug suspension must be administered immediately.

*Trademark of Medical Economics Company, Inc.

Sandostatin LAR® Depot vials are manufactured by:
Biochemie GmbH, Schaftenau, Austria
(Subsidiary of Novartis Pharma AG, Basle, Switzerland)
Distributed by:
Novartis Pharmaceuticals Corporation
East Hanover, New Jersey 07936
The diluent vials are manufactured by:
Novartis Pharma AG, Basle, Switzerland
Distributed by:
Novartis Pharmaceuticals Corporation
East Hanover, New Jersey 07936
667860
30774901 C98-53 (Rev. 11/98)

Shown in Product Identification Guide, page 326

SIMULECT® ℞

[sĭ mu lɘct]
(basiliximab)
For Injection
Rx only

The following prescribing information is based on official labeling in effect July 2000.

WARNING
Only physicians experienced in immunosuppression therapy and management of organ transplantation patients should prescribe Simulect® (basiliximab). The physician responsible for Simulect® administration should have complete information requisite for the follow-up of the patient. Patients receiving the drug should be managed in facilities equipped and staffed with adequate laboratory and supportive medical resources.

DESCRIPTION

Simulect® (basiliximab) is a chimeric (murine/human) monoclonal antibody (IgG_{1k}), produced by recombinant DNA technology, that functions as an immunosuppressive agent, specifically binding to and blocking the interleukin-2 receptor α-chain (IL-2Rα, also known as CD25 antigen) on the surface of activated T-lymphocytes. Based on the amino acid sequence, the calculated molecular weight of the protein is 144 kilodaltons. It is a glycoprotein obtained from fermentation of an established mouse myeloma cell line genetically engineered to express plasmids containing the human heavy and light chain constant region genes and mouse heavy and light chain variable region genes encoding the RFT5 antibody that binds selectively to the IL-2Rα.
The active ingredient, basiliximab, is water soluble. The drug product, Simulect®, is a sterile lyophilisate which is available in 6 mL colorless glass vials. Each vial contains 20 mg basiliximab, 7.21 mg monobasic potassium phosphate, 0.99 mg disodium hydrogen phosphate (anhydrous), 1.61 mg sodium chloride, 20 mg sucrose, 80 mg mannitol and 40 mg glycine, to be reconstituted in 5 mL of Sterile Water for Injection, USP. No preservatives are added.

CLINICAL PHARMACOLOGY

General
Mechanism of action: Basiliximab functions as an IL-2 receptor antagonist by binding with high affinity ($K_a = 1 \times 10^{10}\ M^{-1}$) to the alpha chain of the high affinity IL-2 receptor complex and inhibiting IL-2 binding. Basiliximab is specifically targeted against IL-2Rα, which is selectively expressed on the surface of activated T-lymphocytes. This specific high affinity binding of Simulect® (basiliximab) to IL-2Rα competitively inhibits IL-2-mediated activation of lymphocytes, a critical pathway in the cellular immune response involved in allograft rejection.
While in the circulation, Simulect® impairs the response of the immune system to antigenic challenges. Whether the ability to respond to repeated or ongoing challenges with those antigens returns to normal after Simulect® is cleared is unknown. *(See PRECAUTIONS)*

Pharmacokinetics
Adults: Single-dose and multiple-dose pharmacokinetic studies have been conducted in patients undergoing first kidney transplantation. Cumulative doses ranged from 15 mg up to 150 mg. Peak mean ± SD serum concentration following intravenous infusion of 20 mg over 30 minutes is 7.1 ± 5.1 mg/L. There is a dose-proportional increase in C_{max} and AUC up to the highest tested single dose of 60 mg. The volume of distribution at steady state is 8.6 ± 4.1 L. The extent and degree of distribution to various body compartments have not been fully studied. The terminal half-life is 7.2 ± 3.2 days. Total body clearance is 41 ± 19 mL/h. No clinically relevant influence of body weight or gender on distribution volume or clearance has been observed in adult patients. Elimination half-life was not influenced by age (20-69 years), gender or race. *(See DOSAGE AND ADMINISTRATION)*
Pediatric: The pharmacokinetics of Simulect® were assessed in 12 pediatric renal transplantation patients, children (2-11 years of age, n=8) and adolescents (12-15 years of age, n=4). These data indicate that in children, the volume of distribution at steady state was 5.2 ± 2.8 L, half-life was 11.5 ± 6.3 days and clearance was 17 ± 6 mL/h. Distribution volume and clearance are reduced by about 50% compared to adult renal transplantation patients. Disposition parameters were not influenced to a clinically relevant extent by age, body weight (9-37 kg) or body surface area (0.44-1.20 m^2) in this age group. In adolescents, the volume of distribution at steady state was 10.1 ± 7.6 L, half-life was 7.2 ± 3.6 days and clearance was 45 ± 25 mL/h. Disposition in adolescents was similar to that in adult renal transplantation patients. *(See DOSAGE AND ADMINISTRATION)*

Pharmacodynamics
Complete and consistent binding to IL-2Rα in adults is maintained as long as serum Simulect® levels exceed 0.2 μg/mL. As concentrations fall below this threshold, the IL-2Rα sites are no longer fully bound and the number of T-cells expressing unbound IL-2Rα returns to pretherapy values within 1-2 weeks. The relationship between serum concentration and receptor saturation was assessed in two pediatric patients (2 and 12 years of age) and was similar to that characterized in adult renal transplantation patients. *In vitro* studies using human tissues indicate that Simulect® binds only to lymphocytes.

At the recommended dosing regimen, the mean ± SD duration of basiliximab saturation of IL-2Rα was 36 ± 14 days (*See DOSAGE AND ADMINISTRATION*). The duration of clinically significant IL-2 receptor blockade after the recommended course of Simulect® is not known. No significant changes to circulating lymphocyte numbers or cell phenotypes were observed by flow cytometry.

Clinical Studies

The safety and efficacy of Simulect® for the prophylaxis of acute organ rejection in adults following first cadaveric- or living-donor renal transplantation were assessed in two randomized, double-blind, placebo-controlled, multicenter trials. These studies compared two 20 mg doses of Simulect® with placebo when each was administered intravenously as part of a standard immunosuppressive regimen comprised of cyclosporine oral solution USP (MODIFIED) and corticosteroids, administered starting on Day 0, to prevent acute renal allograft rejection. The first dose of Simulect® or placebo was administered within 2 hours prior to transplantation surgery (Day 0) and the second dose administered on Day 4 post-transplantation. The regimen of Simulect® was chosen to provide 30-45 days of IL-2Rα saturation. 729 patients were enrolled in the two studies, of which 363 Simulect®-treated patients and 358 placebo-treated patients underwent transplantation. One study was conducted at 21 sites in Europe and Canada (EU/CAN Study); the second was conducted at 21 sites in the USA (US Study). Patients 18-75 years of age undergoing first cadaveric (EU/CAN and US Studies) or living-donor (US only) renal transplantation, with ≥1 HLA mismatch, were enrolled. The primary efficacy endpoint in both studies was the incidence of death, graft loss or an episode of acute rejection during the first 6 months post-transplantation. Secondary efficacy endpoints included the primary efficacy variable measured during the first 12 months post-transplantation, the incidence of biopsy-confirmed acute rejection during the first 6 and 12 months post-transplantation, and patient survival and graft survival, each measured at 12 months post-transplantation. Table 1 summarizes the results of these studies. Figure 1 displays the Kaplan-Meier estimates of the percentage of patients by treatment group experiencing the primary efficacy endpoint during the first 12 months post-transplantation for the US study. Patients in both studies receiving Simulect® experienced a significantly lower incidence of biopsy-confirmed rejection episodes at both 6 and 12 months post-transplantation. There was no difference in the rate of delayed graft function, patient survival, or graft survival between Simulect®-treated patients and placebo-treated patients in either study.

There was no evidence that the clinical benefit of Simulect® was limited to specific subpopulations based on age, gender, race, donor type (cadaveric or living-donor allograft) or history of diabetes mellitus.

[See table 1 above]

Table 1
Efficacy Parameters (Percentage of Patients)

	EU/CAN Study			US Study		
	Placebo (N=185)	Simulect® (N=190)	p-value	Placebo (N=173)	Simulect® (N=173)	p-value
Primary endpoint						
Death, graft loss or acute rejection episode (0-6 months)	57%	42%	0.003	55%	38%	0.002
Secondary endpoints						
Death, graft loss or acute rejection episode (0-12 months)	60%	46%	0.007	58%	41%	0.001
Biopsy-confirmed rejection episode (0-6 months)	44%	30%	0.007	46%	33%	0.015
Biopsy-confirmed rejection episode (0-12 months)	46%	32%	0.005	49%	35%	0.009
Patient survival (12 months)	97%	95%	0.29	96%	97%	0.56
Patients with functioning graft (12 months)	87%	88%	0.70	93%	95%	0.50

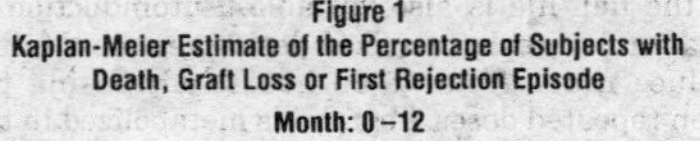
Figure 1
Kaplan-Meier Estimate of the Percentage of Subjects with Death, Graft Loss or First Rejection Episode
Month: 0–12

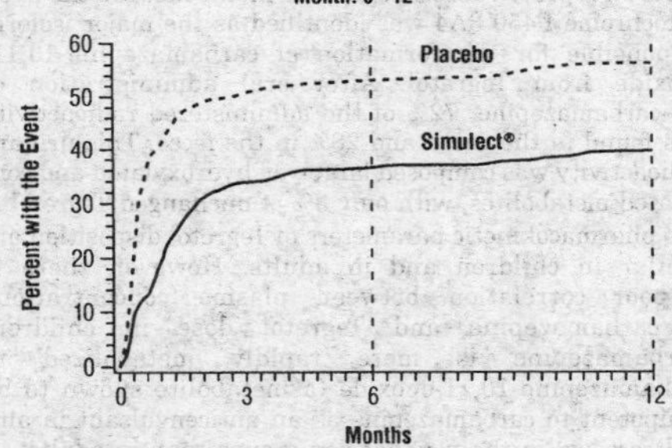

INDICATIONS AND USAGE

Simulect® (basiliximab) is indicated for the prophylaxis of acute organ rejection in patients receiving renal transplantation when used as part of an immunosuppressive regimen that includes cyclosporine and corticosteroids.

CONTRAINDICATIONS

Simulect® (basiliximab) is contraindicated in patients with known hypersensitivity to basiliximab or any other component of the formulation. See composition of Simulect® under *DESCRIPTION*.

WARNINGS: ***See Boxed WARNING.***

General

Simulect® (basiliximab) should be administered under qualified medical supervision. Patients should be informed of the potential benefits of therapy and the risks associated with administration of immunosuppressive therapy.

While neither the incidence of lymphoproliferative disorders nor opportunistic infections was higher in Simulect®-treated patients than in placebo-treated patients, patients on immunosuppressive therapy are at increased risk for developing these complications and should be monitored accordingly.

Hypersensitivity

Severe acute (onset within 24 hours) hypersensitivity reactions including anaphylaxis have been observed both on initial exposure to Simulect® and/or following re-exposure after several months. These reactions may include hypotension, tachycardia, cardiac failure, dyspnea, wheezing, bronchospasm, pulmonary edema, respiratory failure, urticaria, rash, pruritus, and/or sneezing. If a severe hypersensitivity reaction occurs, therapy with Simulect® should be permanently discontinued. Medications for the treatment of severe hypersensitivity reactions including anaphylaxis should be available for immediate use. Patients previously administered Simulect® should only be re-exposed to a subsequent course of therapy with extreme caution. The potential risks of such re-administration, specifically those associated with immunosuppression are not known.

PRECAUTIONS

General

It is not known whether Simulect® (basiliximab) use will have a long-term effect on the ability of the immune system to respond to antigens first encountered during Simulect®-induced immunosuppression.

Immunogenicity

Of renal transplantation patients treated with Simulect® (basiliximab) and tested for anti-idiotype antibodies, 1/246 developed an anti-idiotype antibody response, with no deleterious clinical effect upon the patient. In the US Study, the incidence of human anti-murine antibody (HAMA) in renal transplantation patients treated with Simulect® was 2/138 in patients not exposed to muromonab-CD3 and 4/34 in patients who subsequently received muromonab-CD3. The available clinical data on the use of muromonab-CD3 in patients previously treated with Simulect® suggest that subsequent use of muromonab-CD3 or other murine anti-lymphocytic antibody preparations is not precluded.

Drug Interactions

No formal drug-drug interaction studies have been conducted. The following medications have been administered in clinical trials with Simulect® (basiliximab) with no incremental increase in adverse reactions: ATG/ALG, azathioprine, corticosteroids, cyclosporine, mycophenolate mofetil, and muromonab-CD3.

Carcinogenesis, Mutagenesis and Impairment of Fertility

No mutagenic potential of Simulect® was observed in the *in vitro* assays with Salmonella (Ames) and V79 Chinese hamster cells. No long-term or fertility studies in laboratory animals have been performed to evaluate the potential of Simulect® to produce carcinogenicity or fertility impairment, respectively.

Pregnancy Category B

There are no adequate and well-controlled studies in pregnant women. No maternal toxicity, embryotoxicity, or teratogenicity was observed in cynomolgus monkeys 100 days post coitum following dosing with basiliximab during the organogenesis period; blood levels in pregnant monkeys were 13-fold higher than those seen in human patients. Immunotoxicology studies have not been performed in the offspring. Because IgG molecules are known to cross the placental barrier, because IL-2 receptor may play an important role in development of the immune system, and because animal reproduction studies are not always predictive of human response, Simulect® should only be used in pregnant women when the potential benefit justifies the potential risk to the fetus. Women of childbearing potential should use effective contraception before beginning Simulect® therapy, during therapy, and for 2 months after completion of Simulect® therapy.

Nursing Mothers

It is not known whether Simulect® is excreted in human milk. Because many drugs including human antibodies are excreted in human milk, and because of the potential for adverse reactions, a decision should be made to discontinue nursing or to discontinue the drug, taking into account the importance of the drug to the mother.

Pediatric Use

No adequate and well-controlled studies have been completed in pediatric patients. In an ongoing safety and pharmacokinetic study, pediatric patients [2-11 years of age (n=8), 12-15 years of age (n=4), median age 9.5 years] were treated with Simulect® via intravenous bolus injection in addition to standard immunosuppressive agents including cyclosporine, corticosteroids, azathioprine, and mycophenolate mofetil. Preliminary results indicate that 16.7% (2/12) of patients had experienced an acute rejection episode by 3 months post-transplantation. The most frequently reported adverse events were fever and urinary tract infections (41.7% each). Overall, the adverse event profile was consistent with general clinical experience in the pediatric renal transplantation population and with the profile in the controlled adult renal transplantation studies. The available pharmacokinetic data in children and adolescents are described in *CLINICAL PHARMACOLOGY and DOSAGE AND ADMINISTRATION.*

It is not known whether the immune response to vaccines, infection, and other antigenic stimuli administered or encountered during Simulect® therapy is impaired or whether such response will remain impaired after Simulect® therapy.

Geriatric Use

Controlled clinical studies of Simulect® have included a small number of patients 65 years and older (Simulect® 15; placebo 19). From the available data comparing Simulect®- and placebo-treated patients, the adverse event profile in patients ≥65 years of age is not different from patients <65 years of age and no age-related dosing adjustment is required. Caution must be used in giving immunosuppressive drugs to elderly patients.

ADVERSE REACTIONS

The incidence of adverse events for Simulect® (basiliximab) was determined in two randomized comparative double-blind trials for the prevention of renal allograft rejection. A total of 721 patients received renal allografts, of which 363 received Simulec® and 358 received placebo. All patients received concomitant cyclosporine oral solution USP (MODIFIED) and corticosteroids.

Simulect® did not appear to add to the background of adverse events seen in organ transplantation patients as a consequence of their underlying disease and the concurrent administration of immunosuppressants and other medications. Adverse events were reported by 99% of the patients in the placebo-treated group and 99% of the patients in the Simulect®-treated group. Simulect® did not increase the incidence of serious adverse events observed compared with placebo. The most frequently reported adverse events were gastrointestinal disorders, reported in 75% of Simulect®-treated patients and 73% of placebo-treated patients.

The incidence and types of adverse events were similar in Simulect®-treated and placebo-treated patients. The following adverse events occurred in ≥10% of Simulect®-treated patients: ***Gastrointestinal System:*** constipation, nausea, diarrhea, abdominal pain, vomiting, dyspepsia, moniliasis; ***Metabolic and Nutritional:*** hyperkalemia, hypokalemia, hyperglycemia, hyperuricemia, hypophosphatemia, hypocalcemia, weight increase, hypercholesterolemia, acidosis; ***Central and Peripheral Nervous System:*** headache, tremor, dizziness; ***Urinary System:*** dysuria, increased non-protein nitrogen, urinary tract infection; ***Body as a Whole-General:*** pain, peripheral edema, edema, fever, viral infection, leg edema, asthenia; ***Cardiovascular Disorders-General:*** hypertension; ***Respiratory System:*** dyspnea, upper respiratory tract infection, coughing, rhinitis, pharyngitis; ***Skin and Appendages:*** surgical wound complications, acne; ***Psychiatric:*** insomnia; ***Musculoskeletal System:*** leg pain, back pain; ***Red Blood Cell:*** anemia.

The following adverse events, not mentioned above, were reported with an incidence of ≥3% and <10% in patients treated with Simulect® in the two controlled clinical trials: ***Body as a Whole:*** accidental trauma, chest pain, increased drug level, face edema, fatigue, infection, malaise, generalized edema, rigors, sepsis; ***Cardiovascular:*** angina pectoris, cardiac failure, chest pain, abnormal heart sounds, aggravated hypertension, hypotension; ***Nervous System:*** hypoesthesia, neuropathy, paraesthesia; ***Endocrine:*** increased glucocorticoids; ***Gastrointestinal:*** enlarged abdomen, flatulence, gastrointestinal disorder, gastroenteritis, GI hemorrhage, gum hyperplasia, melena, esophagitis, ulcerative stomatitis; ***Heart Rate and Rhythm:*** arrhythmia, atrial fibrillation, tachycardia; ***Metabolic and Nutritional:*** dehydration, diabetes mellitus, fluid overload, hypercalcemia, hyperlipemia, hypoglycemia, hypoproteinemia, hypomagnesemia; ***Musculoskeletal:*** arthralgia, arthropathy, bone fracture, cramps, hernia, myalgia; ***Nervous Sys-***

Continued on next page

Simulect—Cont.

tem: paraesthesia, hypoesthesia; ***Platelet and Bleeding:*** hematoma, hemorrhage, purpura, thrombocytopenia, thrombosis; ***Psychiatric:*** agitation, anxiety, depression; ***Red Blood Cell:*** polycythemia; ***Reproductive Disorders, Male:*** impotence, genital edema; ***Respiratory:*** bronchitis, bronchospasm, abnormal chest sounds, pneumonia, pulmonary disorder, pulmonary edema, sinusitis; ***Skin and Appendages:*** cyst, herpes simplex, herpes zoster, hypertrichosis, pruritus, rash, skin disorder, skin ulceration; ***Urinary:*** albuminuria, bladder disorder, hematuria, frequent micturition, oliguria, abnormal renal function, renal tubular necrosis, surgery, ureteral disorder, urinary retention; ***Vascular Disorders:*** vascular disorder; ***Vision Disorders:*** cataract, conjunctivitis, abnormal vision.

Incidence of Malignancies: The overall incidence of malignancies among all patients in the two 12-month controlled trials was not significantly different between the Simulect® and placebo treatment groups. Overall, lymphoma/lymphoproliferative disease occurred in 1 patient (0.3%) in the Simulect® group compared with 2 patients (0.6%) in the placebo group. Other malignancies were reported among 5 patients (1.4%) in the Simulect® group compared with 7 patients (1.9%) in patients treated with placebo.

Incidence of Infectious Episodes: Cytomegalovirus infection was reported in 14% of Simulect®-treated patients and 18% of placebo-treated patients. The rates of infections, serious infections, and infectious organisms were similar in the Simulect® and placebo treatment groups.

Post-Marketing Experience

Severe acute hypersensitivity reactions including anaphylaxis characterized by hypotension, tachycardia, cardiac failure, dyspnea, wheezing, bronchospasm, pulmonary edema, respiratory failure, urticaria, rash, pruritus, and/or sneezing, as well as capillary leak syndrome and cytokine release syndrome, have been reported during post-marketing experience with Simulect®.

OVERDOSAGE

There have not been any reports of overdoses with Simulect® (basiliximab). A maximum tolerated dose has not been determined in patients. In clinical studies, Simulect® has been administered to renal transplantation patients in single doses of up to 60 mg without any associated serious adverse events.

DOSAGE AND ADMINISTRATION

Simulect® (basiliximab) is used as part of an immunosuppressive regimen that includes cyclosporine and corticosteroids. Simulect® is for central or peripheral intravenous administration only. Reconstituted Simulect® (20 mg in 5 mL) should be diluted to a volume of 50 mL with normal saline or dextrose 5% and administered as an intravenous infusion over 20 to 30 minutes.

Simulect® should only be administered once it has been determined that the patient will receive the graft and concomitant immunosuppression. Patients previously administered Simulect® should only be re-exposed to a subsequent course of therapy with extreme caution.

Adult: In adult patients, the recommended regimen is two doses of 20 mg each. The first 20 mg dose should be given within 2 hours prior to transplantation surgery. The recommended second 20 mg dose should be given 4 days after transplantation. The second dose should be withheld if complications such as severe hypersensitivity reactions to Simulect® or graft loss occur.

Pediatric: For children and adolescents from 2 up to 15 years of age, the recommended regimen is two doses of 12 mg/m^2 each, up to a maximum of 20 mg/dose. The first dose should be given within 2 hours prior to transplantation surgery. The recommended second dose should be given 4 days after transplantation. The second dose should be withheld if complications such as severe hypersensitivity reactions to Simulect® or graft loss occur.

RECONSTITUTION OF 20 mg Simulect® (basiliximab) VIAL

To prepare the infusion solution, add 5 mL of Sterile Water for Injection, USP, using aseptic technique, to the vial containing the Simulect® (basiliximab) powder. Shake the vial gently to dissolve the powder.

The reconstituted solution is isotonic and should be diluted to a volume of 50 mL with normal saline or dextrose 5% for infusion. When mixing the solution, gently invert the bag in order to avoid foaming; DO NOT SHAKE.

Parenteral drug products should be inspected visually for particulate matter and discoloration before administration. After reconstitution, Simulect® should be a clear to opalescent, colorless solution. If particulate matter is present or the solution is colored, do not use.

Care must be taken to assure sterility of the prepared solution because the drug product does not contain any antimicrobial preservatives or bacteriostatic agents.

It is recommended that after reconstitution the solution should be used immediately. If not used immediately, it can be stored at 2°C to 8°C for 24 hours or at room temperature for 4 hours. Discard the reconstituted solution if not used within 24 hours.

No incompatibility between Simulect® and polyvinyl chloride bags or infusion sets has been observed. No data are available on the compatibility of Simulect® with other intravenous substances. Other drug substances should not be added or infused simultaneously through the same intravenous line.

HOW SUPPLIED

Simulect® (basiliximab) is supplied in a single use glass vial containing 20 mg of basiliximab.

Each carton contains 1 Simulect® vial NDC 0078-0331-84

Store lyophilized Simulect® under refrigerated conditions (2°C to 8°C; 36°F to 46°F).

Do not use beyond the expiration date stamped on the vial.

T2000-02

REV: JUNE 2000

Distributed by: Novartis Pharmaceuticals Corporation
East Hanover, New Jersey 07936
©2000 Novartis
Manufactured by
Novartis Pharma AG
Basel, Switzerland

Shown in Product Identification Guide, page 326

TEGRETOL® ℞

[tē-grĕ-tōl]

carbamazepine USP
Chewable Tablets of 100 mg – red-speckled, pink
Tablets of 200 mg – pink
Suspension of 100 mg/5 mL

TEGRETOL®-XR ℞

(carbamazepine extended-release tablets)
100 mg, 200 mg, 400 mg
Rx only

The following prescribing information is based on official labeling in effect July 2000.

> WARNING
> APLASTIC ANEMIA AND AGRANULOCYTOSIS HAVE BEEN REPORTED IN ASSOCIATION WITH THE USE OF TEGRETOL. DATA FROM A POPULATION-BASED CASE CONTROL STUDY DEMONSTRATE THAT THE RISK OF DEVELOPING THESE REACTIONS IS 5-8 TIMES GREATER THAN IN THE GENERAL POPULATION. HOWEVER, THE OVERALL RISK OF THESE REACTIONS IN THE UNTREATED GENERAL POPULATION IS LOW, APPROXIMATELY SIX PATIENTS PER ONE MILLION POPULATION PER YEAR FOR AGRANULOCYTOSIS AND TWO PATIENTS PER ONE MILLION POPULATION PER YEAR FOR APLASTIC ANEMIA.
> ALTHOUGH REPORTS OF TRANSIENT OR PERSISTENT DECREASED PLATELET OR WHITE BLOOD CELL COUNTS ARE NOT UNCOMMON IN ASSOCIATION WITH THE USE OF TEGRETOL, DATA ARE NOT AVAILABLE TO ESTIMATE ACCURATELY THEIR INCIDENCE OR OUTCOME. HOWEVER, THE VAST MAJORITY OF THE CASES OF LEUKOPENIA HAVE NOT PROGRESSED TO THE MORE SERIOUS CONDITIONS OF APLASTIC ANEMIA OR AGRANULOCYTOSIS.
> BECAUSE OF THE VERY LOW INCIDENCE OF AGRANULOCYTOSIS AND APLASTIC ANEMIA, THE VAST MAJORITY OF MINOR HEMATOLOGIC CHANGES OBSERVED IN MONITORING OF PATIENTS ON TEGRETOL ARE UNLIKELY TO SIGNAL THE OCCURRENCE OF EITHER ABNORMALITY. NONETHELESS, COMPLETE PRETREATMENT HEMATOLOGICAL TESTING SHOULD BE OBTAINED AS A BASELINE. IF A PATIENT IN THE COURSE OF TREATMENT EXHIBITS LOW OR DECREASED WHITE BLOOD CELL OR PLATELET COUNTS, THE PATIENT SHOULD BE MONITORED CLOSELY. DISCONTINUATION OF THE DRUG SHOULD BE CONSIDERED IF ANY EVIDENCE OF SIGNIFICANT BONE MARROW DEPRESSION DEVELOPS.

Before prescribing Tegretol, the physician should be thoroughly familiar with the details of this prescribing information, particularly regarding use with other drugs, especially those which accentuate toxicity potential.

DESCRIPTION

Tegretol, carbamazepine USP, is an anticonvulsant and specific analgesic for trigeminal neuralgia, available for oral administration as chewable tablets of 100 mg, tablets of 200 mg, XR tablets of 100, 200, and 400 mg, and as a suspension of 100 mg/5 mL (teaspoon). Its chemical name is 5*H*-dibenz[*b,f*]azepine-5-carboxamide, and its structural formula is

CONH$_2$

Carbamazepine USP is a white to off-white powder, practically insoluble in water and soluble in alcohol and in acetone. Its molecular weight is 236.27.

Inactive Ingredients. Tablets: Colloidal silicon dioxide, D&C Red No. 30 Aluminum Lake (chewable tablets only), FD&C Red No. 40 (200-mg tablets only), flavoring (chewable tablets only), gelatin, glycerin, magnesium stearate, sodium starch glycolate (chewable tablets only), starch, stearic acid, and sucrose (chewable tablets only). Suspension: Citric acid, FD&C Yellow No. 6, flavoring, polymer, potassium sorbate, propylene glycol, purified water, sorbitol, sucrose, and xanthan gum. Tegretol-XR tablets: cellulose compounds, dextrates, iron oxides, magnesium stearate, mannitol, polyethylene glycol, sodium lauryl sulfate, titanium dioxide (200-mg tablets only).

CLINICAL PHARMACOLOGY

In controlled clinical trials, Tegretol has been shown to be effective in the treatment of psychomotor and grand mal seizures, as well as trigeminal neuralgia.

Mechanism of Action

Tegretol has demonstrated anticonvulsant properties in rats and mice with electrically and chemically induced seizures. It appears to act by reducing polysynaptic responses and blocking the post-tetanic potentiation. Tegretol greatly reduces or abolishes pain induced by stimulation of the infraorbital nerve in cats and rats. It depresses thalamic potential and bulbar and polysynaptic reflexes, including the linguomandibular reflex in cats. Tegretol is chemically unrelated to other anticonvulsants or other drugs used to control the pain of trigeminal neuralgia. The mechanism of action remains unknown.

The principal metabolite of Tegretol, carbamazepine-10,11-epoxide, has anticonvulsant activity as demonstrated in several in vivo animal models of seizures. Though clinical activity for the epoxide has been postulated, the significance of its activity with respect to the safety and efficacy of Tegretol has not been established.

Pharmacokinetics

In clinical studies, Tegretol suspension, conventional tablets, and XR tablets delivered equivalent amounts of drug to the systemic circulation. However, the suspension was absorbed somewhat faster, and the XR tablet slightly slower, than the conventional tablet. The bioavailability of the XR tablet was 89% compared to suspension. Following a b.i.d. dosage regimen, the suspension provides higher peak levels and lower trough levels than those obtained from the conventional tablet for the same dosage regimen. On the other hand, following a t.i.d. dosage regimen, Tegretol suspension affords steady-state plasma levels comparable to Tegretol tablets given b.i.d. when administered at the same total mg daily dose. Following a b.i.d. dosage regimen, Tegretol-XR tablets afford steady-state plasma levels comparable to conventional Tegretol tablets given q.i.d., when administered at the same total mg daily dose. Tegretol in blood is 76% bound to plasma proteins. Plasma levels of Tegretol are variable and may range from 0.5-25 µg/mL, with no apparent relationship to the daily intake of the drug. Usual adult therapeutic levels are between 4 and 12 µg/mL. In polytherapy, the concentration of Tegretol and concomitant drugs may be increased or decreased during therapy, and drug effects may be altered (see PRECAUTIONS, Drug Interactions). Following chronic oral administration of suspension, plasma levels peak at approximately 1.5 hours compared to 4-5 hours after administration of conventional Tegretol tablets, and 3-12 hours after administration of Tegretol-XR tablets. The CSF/serum ratio is 0.22, similar to the 24% unbound Tegretol in serum. Because Tegretol induces its own metabolism, the half-life is also variable. Autoinduction is completed after 3-5 weeks of a fixed dosing regimen. Initial half-life values range from 25-65 hours, decreasing to 12-17 hours on repeated doses. Tegretol is metabolized in the liver. Cytochrome P450 3A4 was identified as the major isoform responsible for the formation of carbamazepine-10,11-epoxide from Tegretol. After oral administration of ^{14}C-carbamazepine, 72% of the administered radioactivity was found in the urine and 28% in the feces. This urinary radioactivity was composed largely of hydroxylated and conjugated metabolites, with only 3% of unchanged Tegretol.

The pharmacokinetic parameters of Tegretol disposition are similar in children and in adults. However, there is a poor correlation between plasma concentrations of carbamazepine and Tegretol dose in children. Carbamazepine is more rapidly metabolized to carbamazepine-10,11-epoxide (a metabolite shown to be equipotent to carbamazepine as an anticonvulsant in animal screens) in the younger age groups than in adults. In children below the age of 15, there is an inverse relationship between CBZ-E/CBZ ratio and increasing age (in one report from 0.44 in children below the age of 1 year to 0.18 in children between 10-15 years of age).

The effects of race and gender on carbamazepine pharmacokinetics have not been systematically evaluated.

INDICATIONS AND USAGE

Epilepsy

Tegretol is indicated for use as an anticonvulsant drug. Evidence supporting efficacy of Tegretol as an anticonvulsant was derived from active drug-controlled studies that enrolled patients with the following seizure types:

1. Partial seizures with complex symptomatology (psychomotor, temporal lobe). Patients with these seizures appear to show greater improvement than those with other types.
2. Generalized tonic-clonic seizures (grand mal).
3. Mixed seizure patterns which include the above, or other partial or generalized seizures. Absence seizures (petit mal) do not appear to be controlled by Tegretol (see PRECAUTIONS, General).

Trigeminal Neuralgia

Tegretol is indicated in the treatment of the pain associated with true trigeminal neuralgia.

Beneficial results have also been reported in glossopharyngeal neuralgia.

This drug is not a simple analgesic and should not be used for the relief of trivial aches or pains.

CONTRAINDICATIONS

Tegretol should not be used in patients with a history of previous bone marrow depression, hypersensitivity to the drug, or known sensitivity to any of the tricyclic compounds, such as amitriptyline, desipramine, imipramine, protriptyline, nortriptyline, etc. Likewise, on theoretical grounds its use with monoamine oxidase inhibitors is not recommended. Before administration of Tegretol, MAO inhibitors should be discontinued for a minimum of 14 days, or longer if the clinical situation permits.

WARNINGS

Patients with a history of adverse hematologic reaction to any drug may be particularly at risk.

Severe dermatologic reactions, including toxic epidermal necrolysis (Lyell's syndrome) and Stevens-Johnson syndrome, have been reported with Tegretol. These reactions have been extremely rare. However, a few fatalities have been reported.

Tegretol has shown mild anticholinergic activity; therefore, patients with increased intraocular pressure should be closely observed during therapy.

Because of the relationship of the drug to other tricyclic compounds, the possibility of activation of a latent psychosis and, in elderly patients, of confusion or agitation should be borne in mind.

Usage in Pregnancy

Carbamazepine can cause fetal harm when administered to a pregnant woman.

Epidemiological data suggest that there may be an association between the use of carbamazepine during pregnancy and congenital malformations, including spina bifida. In treating or counseling women of childbearing potential, the prescribing physician will wish to weigh the benefits of therapy against the risks. If this drug is used during pregnancy, or if the patient becomes pregnant while taking this drug, the patient should be apprised of the potential hazard to the fetus.

Retrospective case reviews suggest that, compared with monotherapy, there may be a higher prevalence of teratogenic effects associated with the use of anticonvulsants in combination therapy. Therefore, if therapy is to be continued, monotherapy may be preferable for pregnant women.

In humans, transplacental passage of carbamazepine is rapid (30-60 minutes), and the drug is accumulated in the fetal tissues, with higher levels found in liver and kidney than in brain and lung.

Carbamazepine has been shown to have adverse effects in reproduction studies in rats when given orally in dosages 10-25 times the maximum human daily dosage (MHDD) of 1200 mg on a mg/kg basis or 1.5-4 times the MHDD on a mg/m^2 basis. In rat teratology studies, 2 of 135 offspring showed kinked ribs at 250 mg/kg and 4 of 119 offspring at 650 mg/kg showed other anomalies (cleft palate, 1; talipes, 1; anophthalmos, 2). In reproduction studies in rats, nursing offspring demonstrated a lack of weight gain and an unkempt appearance at a maternal dosage level of 200 mg/kg.

Antiepileptic drugs should not be discontinued abruptly in patients in whom the drug is administered to prevent major seizures because of the strong possibility of precipitating status epilepticus with attendant hypoxia and threat to life.

In individual cases where the severity and frequency of the seizure disorder are such that removal of medication does not pose a serious threat to the patient, discontinuation of the drug may be considered prior to and during pregnancy, although it cannot be said with any confidence that even minor seizures do not pose some hazard to the developing embryo or fetus.

Tests to detect defects using currently accepted procedures should be considered a part of routine prenatal care in childbearing women receiving carbamazepine.

There have been a few cases of neonatal seizures and/or respiratory depression associated with maternal Tegretol and other concomitant anticonvulsant drug use. A few cases of neonatal vomiting, diarrhea, and/or decreased feeding have also been reported in association with maternal Tegretol use. These symptoms may represent a neonatal withdrawal syndrome.

PRECAUTIONS

General

Before initiating therapy, a detailed history and physical examination should be made.

Tegretol should be used with caution in patients with a mixed seizure disorder that includes atypical absence seizures, since in these patients Tegretol has been associated with increased frequency of generalized convulsions (see INDICATIONS AND USAGE).

Therapy should be prescribed only after critical benefit-to-risk appraisal in patients with a history of cardiac, hepatic, or renal damage; adverse hematologic or hypersensitivity reaction to other drugs, including reactions to other anticonvulsants; or interrupted courses of therapy with Tegretol.

Hepatic effects, ranging from slight elevations in liver enzymes to rare cases of hepatic failure have been reported (see ADVERSE REACTIONS and PRECAUTIONS, Laboratory Tests). In some cases, hepatic effects may progress despite discontinuation of the drug.

Multi-organ hypersensitivity reactions occurring days to weeks or months after initiating treatment have been reported in rare cases (see ADVERSE REACTIONS, Other and PRECAUTIONS, Information for Patients).

Discontinuation of carbamazepine should be considered if any evidence of hypersensitivity develops.

Hypersensitivity reactions to carbamazepine have been reported in patients who previously experienced this reaction to anticonvulsants including phenytoin and phenobarbital. A history of hypersensitivity reactions should be obtained for a patient and the immediate family members. If positive, caution should be used in prescribing carbamazepine.

Since a given dose of Tegretol suspension will produce higher peak levels than the same dose given as the tablet, it is recommended that patients given the suspension be started on lower doses and increased slowly to avoid unwanted side effects (see DOSAGE AND ADMINISTRATION).

Information for Patients

Patients should be made aware of the early toxic signs and symptoms of a potential hematologic problem, as well as dermatologic, hypersensitivity or hepatic reactions. These symptoms may include, but are not limited to, fever, sore throat, rash, ulcers in the mouth, easy bruising, lymphadenopathy and petechial or purpuric hemorrhage, and in the case of liver reactions, anorexia, nausea/vomiting, or jaundice. The patient should be advised that, because these signs and symptoms may signal a serious reaction, that they must report any occurrence immediately to a physician. In addition, the patient should be advised that these signs and symptoms should be reported even if mild or when occurring after extended use.

Since dizziness and drowsiness may occur, patients should be cautioned about the hazards of operating machinery or automobiles or engaging in other potentially dangerous tasks.

Laboratory Tests

Complete pretreatment blood counts, including platelets and possibly reticulocytes and serum iron, should be obtained as a baseline. If a patient in the course of treatment exhibits low or decreased white blood cell or platelet counts, the patient should be monitored closely. Discontinuation of the drug should be considered if any evidence of significant bone marrow depression develops.

Baseline and periodic evaluations of liver function, particularly in patients with a history of liver disease, must be performed during treatment with this drug since liver damage may occur (see PRECAUTIONS, General and ADVERSE REACTIONS). Carbamazepine should be discontinued, based on clinical judgment, if indicated by newly occurring or worsening clinical or laboratory evidence of liver dysfunction or hepatic damage, or in the case of active liver disease.

Baseline and periodic eye examinations, including slit-lamp, funduscopy, and tonometry, are recommended since many phenothiazines and related drugs have been shown to cause eye changes.

Baseline and periodic complete urinalysis and BUN determinations are recommended for patients treated with this agent because of observed renal dysfunction.

Monitoring of blood levels (see CLINICAL PHARMACOLOGY) has increased the efficacy and safety of anticonvulsants. This monitoring may be particularly useful in cases of dramatic increase in seizure frequency and for verification of compliance. In addition, measurement of drug serum levels may aid in determining the cause of toxicity when more than one medication is being used.

Thyroid function tests have been reported to show decreased values with Tegretol administered alone.

Hyponatremia has been reported in association with Tegretol use, either alone or in combination with other drugs.

Interference with some pregnancy tests has been reported.

Drug Interactions

There has been a report of a patient who passed an orange rubbery precipitate in his stool the day after ingesting Tegretol suspension immediately followed by Thorazine® solution. Subsequent testing has shown that mixing Tegretol suspension and chlorpromazine solution (both generic and brand name) as well as Tegretol suspension and liquid Mellaril® resulted in the occurrence of this precipitate. Because the extent to which this occurs with other liquid medications is not known, Tegretol suspension should not be administered simultaneously with other liquid medicinal agents or diluents. (see DOSAGE AND ADMINISTRATION).

Clinically meaningful drug interactions have occurred with concomitant medications and include, but are not limited to, the following:

Agents That May Affect Tegretol Plasma Levels

CYP 3A4 inhibitors inhibit Tegretol metabolism and can thus increase plasma carbamazepine levels. Drugs that have been shown, or would be expected, to increase plasma carbamazepine levels include

cimetidine, danazol, diltiazem, macrolides, erythromycin, troleandomycin, clarithromycin, fluoxetine, loratadine, terfenadine, isoniazid, niacinamide, nicotinamide, propoxyphene, ketaconazole, itraconazole, verapamil, valproate.*

CYP 3A4 inducers can increase the rate of Tegretol metabolism. Drugs that have been shown, or that would be expected, to decrease plasma carbamazepine levels include

cisplatin, doxorubicin HCl, felbamate,† rifampin, phenobarbital, phenytoin, primidone, theophylline.

*increased levels of the active 10,11-epoxide

†decreased levels of carbamazepine and increased levels of the 10,11-epoxide

Effect of Tegretol on Plasma Levels of Concomitant Agents

Increased levels: clomipramine HCl, phenytoin, primidone

Tegretol induces hepatic CYP activity. Tegretol causes, or would be expected to cause, decreased levels of the following:

acetaminophen, alprazolam, clonazepam, clozapine, dicumarol, doxycycline, ethosuximide, haloperidol, lamotrigine, methsuximide, oral and other hormonal contraceptives, phensuximide, phenytoin, theophylline, tiagabine, topiramate, valproate, warfarin.

Concomitant administration of carbamazepine and lithium may increase the risk of neurotoxic side effects.

Alterations of thyroid function have been reported in combination therapy with other anticonvulsant medications.

Concomitant use of Tegretol with hormonal contraceptive products (e.g. oral, and levonorgestrel subdermal implant contraceptives) may render the contraceptives less effective because the plasma concentrations of the hormones may be decreased. Breakthrough bleeding and unintended pregnancies have been reported. Alternative or back-up methods of contraception should be considered.

Carcinogenesis, Mutagenesis, Impairment of Fertility

Carbamazepine, when administered to Sprague-Dawley rats for two years in the diet at doses of 25, 75, and 250 mg/kg/day, resulted in a dose-related increase in the incidence of hepatocellular tumors in females and of benign interstitial cell adenomas in the testes of males.

Carbamazepine must, therefore, be considered to be carcinogenic in Sprague-Dawley rats. Bacterial and mammalian mutagenicity studies using carbamazepine produced negative results. The significance of these findings relative to the use of carbamazepine in humans is, at present, unknown.

Usage in Pregnancy

Pregnancy Category D (see WARNINGS).

Labor and Delivery

The effect of Tegretol on human labor and delivery is unknown.

Nursing Mothers

Tegretol and its epoxide metabolite are transferred to breast milk. The ratio of the concentration in breast milk to that in maternal plasma is about 0.4 for Tegretol and about 0.5 for the epoxide. The estimated doses given to the newborn during breast feeding are in the range of 2-5 mg daily for Tegretol and 1-2 mg daily for the epoxide.

Because of the potential for serious adverse reactions in nursing infants from carbamazepine, a decision should be made whether to discontinue nursing or to discontinue the drug, taking into account the importance of the drug to the mother.

Pediatric Use

Substantial evidence of Tegretol's effectiveness for use in the management of children with epilepsy (see Indications for specific seizure types) is derived from clinical investigations performed in adults and from studies in several in vitro systems which support the conclusion that (1) the pathogenetic mechanisms underlying seizure propagation are essentially identical in adults and children, and (2) the mechanism of action of carbamazepine in treating seizures is essentially identical in adults and children.

Taken as a whole, this information supports a conclusion that the generally accepted therapeutic range of total carbamazepine in plasma (i.e., 4-12 mcg/mL) is the same in children and adults.

The evidence assembled was primarily obtained from short-term use of carbamazepine. The safety of carbamazepine in children has been systematically studied up to 6 months. No longer-term data from clinical trials is available.

Geriatric Use

No systematic studies in geriatric patients have been conducted.

ADVERSE REACTIONS

If adverse reactions are of such severity that the drug must be discontinued, the physician must be aware that abrupt discontinuation of any anticonvulsant drug in a responsive epileptic patient may lead to seizures or even status epilepticus with its life-threatening hazards.

The most severe adverse reactions have been observed in the hemopoietic system (see boxed WARNING), the skin, liver, and the cardiovascular system.

The most frequently observed adverse reactions, particularly during the initial phases of therapy, are dizziness, drowsiness, unsteadiness, nausea, and vomiting. To minimize the possibility of such reactions, therapy should be initiated at the low dosage recommended. The following additional adverse reactions have been reported:

Hemopoietic System: Aplastic anemia, agranulocytosis, pancytopenia, bone marrow depression, thrombocytopenia, leukopenia, leukocytosis, eosinophilia, acute intermittent porphyria.

Skin: Pruritic and erythematous rashes, urticaria, toxic epidermal necrolysis (Lyell's syndrome) (see WARNINGS), Stevens-Johnson syndrome (see WARNINGS), photosensitivity reactions, alterations in skin pigmentation, exfoliative dermatitis, erythema multiforme and nodosum, purpura, aggravation of disseminated lupus erythematosus, alopecia, and diaphoresis. In certain cases, discontinuation of therapy may be necessary. Isolated cases of hirsutism have been reported, but a causal relationship is not clear.

Cardiovascular System: Congestive heart failure, edema, aggravation of hypertension, hypotension, syncope and collapse, aggravation of coronary artery disease, arrhythmias and AV block, thrombophlebitis, thromboembolism, and adenopathy or lymphadenopathy.

Continued on next page

Tegretol—Cont.

Some of these cardiovascular complications have resulted in fatalities. Myocardial infarction has been associated with other tricyclic compounds.

Liver: Abnormalities in liver function tests, cholestatic and hepatocellular jaundice, hepatitis; very rare cases of hepatic failure.

Pancreatic: Pancreatitis.

Respiratory System: Pulmonary hypersensitivity characterized by fever, dyspnea, pneumonitis, or pneumonia.

Genitourinary System: Urinary frequency, acute urinary retention, oliguria with elevated blood pressure, azotemia, renal failure, and impotence. Albuminuria, glycosuria, elevated BUN, and microscopic deposits in the urine have also been reported.

Testicular atrophy occurred in rats receiving Tegretol orally from 4-52 weeks at dosage levels of 50-400 mg/kg/day. Additionally, rats receiving Tegretol in the diet for 2 years at dosage levels of 25, 75, and 250 mg/kg/day had a dose-related incidence of testicular atrophy and aspermatogenesis. In dogs, it produced a brownish discoloration, presumably a metabolite, in the urinary bladder at dosage levels of 50 mg/kg and higher. Relevance of these findings to humans is unknown.

Nervous System: Dizziness, drowsiness, disturbances of coordination, confusion, headache, fatigue, blurred vision, visual hallucinations, transient diplopia, oculomotor disturbances, nystagmus, speech disturbances, abnormal involuntary movements, peripheral neuritis and paresthesias, depression with agitation, talkativeness, tinnitus, and hyperacusis.

There have been reports of associated paralysis and other symptoms of cerebral arterial insufficiency, but the exact relationship of these reactions to the drug has not been established.

Isolated cases of neuroleptic malignant syndrome have been reported with concomitant use of psychotropic drugs.

Digestive System: Nausea, vomiting, gastric distress and abdominal pain, diarrhea, constipation, anorexia, and dryness of the mouth and pharynx, including glossitis and stomatitis.

Eyes: Scattered punctate cortical lens opacities, as well as conjunctivitis, have been reported. Although a direct causal relationship has not been established, many phenothiazines and related drugs have been shown to cause eye changes.

Musculoskeletal System: Aching joints and muscles, and leg cramps.

Metabolism: Fever and chills. Inappropriate antidiuretic hormone (ADH) secretion sydrome has been reported. Cases of frank water intoxication, with decreased serum sodium (hyponatremia) and confusion, have been reported in association with Tegretol use (see PRECAUTIONS, Laboratory Tests). Decreased levels of plasma calcium have been reported.

Other: Multi-organ hypersensitivity reactions occurring days to weeks or months after initiating treatment have been reported in rare cases. Signs or symptoms may include, but are not limited to fever, skin rashes, vasculitis, lymphadenopathy, disorders mimicking lymphoma, arthralgia, leukopenia, eosinophilia, hepato-splenomegaly and abnormal liver function tests. These signs and symptoms may occur in various combinations and not necessarily concurrently. Signs and symptoms may initially be mild. Various organs, including but not limited to, liver, skin, immune system, lungs, kidneys, pancreas, myocardium, and colon may be affected (see PRECAUTIONS, General and PRECAUTIONS, Information for Patients).

Isolated cases of a lupus erythematosus-like syndrome have been reported. There have been occasional reports of elevated levels of cholesterol, HDL cholesterol, and triglycerides in patients taking anticonvulsants.

A case of aseptic meningitis, accompanied by myoclonus and peripheral eosinophilia, has been reported in a patient taking carbamazepine in combination with other medications. The patient was successfully dechallenged, and the meningitis reappeared upon rechallenge with carbamazepine.

DRUG ABUSE AND DEPENDENCE

No evidence of abuse potential has been associated with Tegretol, nor is there evidence of psychological or physical dependence in humans.

OVERDOSAGE

Acute Toxicity

Lowest known lethal dose: adults, 3.2 g (a 24-year-old woman died of a cardiac arrest and a 24-year-old man died of pneumonia and hypoxic encephalopathy); children, 4 g (a 14-year-old girl died of a cardiac arrest), 1.6 g (a 3-year-old girl died of aspiration pneumonia).

Oral LD_{50} in animals (mg/kg): mice, 1100-3750; rats, 3850-4025; rabbits, 1500–2680; guinea pigs, 920.

Signs and Symptoms

The first signs and symptoms appear after 1-3 hours. Neuromuscular disturbances are the most prominent. Cardiovascular disorders are generally milder, and severe cardiac complications occur only when very high doses (> 60 g) have been ingested.

Respiration: Irregular breathing, respiratory depression.

Cardiovascular System: Tachycardia, hypotension or hypertension, shock, conduction disorders.

Nervous System and Muscles: Impairment of consciousness ranging in severity to deep coma. Convulsions, especially in small children. Motor restlessness, muscular twitching, tremor, athetoid movements, opisthotonos, ataxia, drowsiness, dizziness, mydriasis, nystagmus, adiadochokinesia, ballism, psychomotor disturbances, dysmetria. Initial hyperreflexia, followed by hyporeflexia.

Gastrointestinal Tract: Nausea, vomiting.

Kidneys and Bladder: Anuria or oliguria, urinary retention.

Laboratory Findings: Isolated instances of overdosage have included leukocytosis, reduced leukocyte count, glycosuria, and acetonuria. EEG may show dysrhythmias.

Combined Poisoning: When alcohol, tricyclic antidepressants, barbiturates, or hydantoins are taken at the same time, the signs and symptoms of acute poisoning with Tegretol may be aggravated or modified.

Treatment

The prognosis in cases of severe poisoning is critically dependent upon prompt elimination of the drug, which may be achieved by inducing vomiting, irrigating the stomach, and by taking appropriate steps to diminish absorption. If these measures cannot be implemented without risk on the spot, the patient should be transferred at once to a hospital, while ensuring that vital functions are safeguarded. There is no specific antidote.

Elimination of the Drug: Induction of vomiting.

Gastric lavage. Even when more than 4 hours have elapsed following ingestion of the drug, the stomach should be repeatedly irrigated, especially if the patient has also consumed alcohol.

Measures to Reduce Absorption: Activated charcoal, laxatives.

Measures to Accelerate Elimination: Forced diuresis. Dialysis is indicated only in severe poisoning associated with renal failure. Replacement transfusion is indicated in severe poisoning in small children.

Respiratory Depression: Keep the airways free; resort, if necessary, to endotracheal intubation, artificial respiration, and administration of oxygen.

Hypotension, Shock: Keep the patient's legs raised and administer a plasma expander. If blood pressure fails to rise despite measures taken to increase plasma volume, use of vasoactive substances should be considered.

Convulsions: Diazepam or barbiturates.

Warning: Diazepam or barbiturates may aggravate respiratory depression (especially in children), hypotension, and coma. However, barbiturates should not be used if drugs that inhibit monoamine oxidase have also been taken by the patient either in overdosage or in recent therapy (within 1 week).

Surveillance: Respiration, cardiac function (ECG monitoring), blood pressure, body temperature, pupillary reflexes, and kidney and bladder function should be monitored for several days.

Treatment of Blood Count Abnormalities: If evidence of significant bone marrow depression develops, the following recommendations are suggested: (1) stop the drug, (2) perform daily CBC, platelet, and reticulocyte counts, (3) do a bone marrow aspiration and trephine biopsy immediately and repeat with sufficient frequency to monitor recovery.

Special periodic studies might be helpful as follows: (1) white cell and platelet antibodies, (2) ^{59}Fe-ferrokinetic studies, (3) peripheral blood cell typing, (4) cytogenetic studies on marrow and peripheral blood, (5) bone marrow culture studies for colony-forming units, (6) hemoglobin electrophoresis for A_2 and F hemoglobin, and (7) serum folic acid and B_{12} levels.

A fully developed aplastic anemia will require appropriate, intensive monitoring and therapy, for which specialized consultation should be sought.

DOSAGE AND ADMINISTRATION

[See table below]

Tegretol suspension in combination with liquid chlorpromazine or thioridazine results in precipitate formation, and, in the case of chlorpromazine, there has been a report of a patient passing an orange rubbery precipitate in the stool following coadministration of the two drugs. (see Drug Interactions). Because the extent to which this occurs with other liquid medications is not known, Tegretol suspension should not be administered simultaneously with other liquid medications or diluents.

Monitoring of blood levels has increased the efficacy and safety of anticonvulsants (see PRECAUTIONS, Laboratory Tests). Dosage should be adjusted to the needs of the individual patient. A low initial daily dosage with a gradual increase is advised. As soon as adequate control is achieved, the dosage may be reduced very gradually to the minimum effective level. Medication should be taken with meals.

Since a given dose of Tegretol suspension will produce higher peak levels than the same dose given as the tablet, it is recommended to start with low doses (children 6-12 years: $^1/_2$ teaspoon q.i.d.) and to increase slowly to avoid unwanted side effects.

Conversion of patients from oral Tegretol tablets to Tegretol suspension: Patients should be converted by administering the same number of mg per day in smaller, more frequent doses (i.e., b.i.d. tablets to t.i.d. suspension).

Tegretol-XR is an extended-release formulation for twice-a-day administration. When converting patients from

Dosage Information

	Initial Dose			Subsequent Dose			Maximum Daily Dose		
Indication	Tablet*	XR†	Suspension	Tablet*	XR†	Suspension	Tablet*	XR†	Suspension
Epilepsy Under 6 yr	10-20 mg/kg/day b.i.d. or t.i.d.		10-20 mg/kg/day q.i.d.	Increase weekly to achieve optimal chemical response, t.i.d. or q.i.d.		Increase weekly to achieve optimal clinical response, t.i.d. or q.i.d.	35 mg/kg/24 hr (see Dosage and Administration section above)		35 mg/kg/24 hr (see Dosage and Administration section above)
6-12 yr	100 mg b.i.d. (200 mg/day)	100 mg b.i.d. (200 mg/day)	1/2 tsp q.i.d. (200 mg/day)	Add up to 100 mg/day at weekly intervals, t.i.d. or q.i.d.	Add 100 mg/day at weekly intervals, b.i.d.	Add up to 1 tsp (100 mg)/day at weekly intervals, t.i.d. or q.i.d.		1000 mg/24 hr	
Over 12 yr	200 mg b.i.d. (400 mg/day)	200 mg b.i.d. (400 mg/day)	1 tsp q.i.d. (400 mg/day)	Add up to 200 mg/day at weekly intervals. t.i.d. or q.i.d.	Add up to 200 mg/day at weekly intervals, b.i.d.	Add up to 2 tsp (200 mg)/day at weekly intervals, t.i.d. or q.i.d.		1000 mg/24 hr (12-15 yr) 1200 mg/24 hr (>15 yr) 1600 mg/24 hr (adults, in rare instances)	
Trigeminal Neuralgia	100 mg b.i.d. (200 mg/day)	100 mg b.i.d. (200 mg/day)	1/2 tsp q.i.d. (200 mg/day)	Add up to 200 mg/day in increments of 100 mg every 12 hr	Add up to 200 mg/day in increments of 100 mg every 12 hr	Add up to 2 tsp (200 mg)/day in increments of 50 mg (1/2 tsp) q.i.d.		1200 mg/24 hr	

*Tablet = Chewable or conventional tablets
†XR = Tegretol®-XR extended-release tablets

Tegretol conventional tablets to Tegretol-XR, the same total daily mg dose of Tegretol-XR should be administered. **Tegretol-XR tablets must be swallowed whole and never crushed or chewed.** Tegretol-XR tablets should be inspected for chips or cracks. Damaged tablets or tablets without a release portal should not be consumed. Tegretol-XR tablet coating is not absorbed and is excreted in the feces; these coatings may be noticeable in the stool.

Epilepsy (see INDICATIONS AND USAGE)

Adults and children over 12 years of age - Initial: Either 200 mg b.i.d. for tablets and XR tablets, or 1 teaspoon q.i.d. for suspension (400 mg/day). Increase at weekly intervals by adding up to 200 mg/day using a b.i.d. regimen of Tegretol-XR or a t.i.d. or q.i.d. regimen of the other formulations until the optimal response is obtained. Dosage generally should not exceed 1000 mg daily in children 12-15 years of age, and 1200 mg daily in patients above 15 years of age. Doses up to 1600 mg daily have been used in adults in rare instances.

Maintenance: Adjust dosage to the minimum effective level, usually 800-1200 mg daily.

Children 6-12 years of age - Initial: Either 100 mg b.i.d. for tablets or XR tablets, or 1/2 teaspoon q.i.d. for suspension (200 mg/day). Increase at weekly intervals by adding up to 100 mg/day using a b.i.d. regimen of Tegretol-XR or a t.i.d. or q.i.d. regimen of the other formulations until the optimal response is obtained. Dosage generally should not exceed 1000 mg daily. ***Maintenance:*** Adjust dosage to the minimum effective level, usually 400-800 mg daily.

Children under 6 years of age - Initial: 10-20 mg/kg/day b.i.d. or t.i.d. as tablets, or q.i.d. as suspension. Increase weekly to achieve optimal clinical response administered t.i.d. or q.i.d. ***Maintenance:*** Ordinarily, optimal clinical response is achieved at daily doses below 35 mg/kg. If satisfactory clinical response has not been achieved, plasma levels should be measured to determine whether or not they are in the therapeutic range. No recommendation regarding the safety of carbamazepine for use at doses above 35 mg/kg/24 hours can be made.

Combination Therapy: Tegretol may be used alone or with other anticonvulsants. When added to existing anticonvulsant therapy, the drug should be added gradually while the other anticonvulsants are maintained or gradually decreased, except phenytoin, which may have to be increased (see PRECAUTIONS, Drug Interactions, and Pregnancy Category D).

Trigeminal Neuralgia (see INDICATIONS AND USAGE)

Initial: On the first day, either 100 mg b.i.d. for tablets or XR tablets, or 1/2 teaspoon q.i.d. for suspension, for a total daily dose of 200 mg. This daily dose may be increased by up to 200 mg/day using increments of 100 mg every 12 hours for tablets or XR tablets, or 50 mg (1/2 teaspoon) q.i.d. for suspension, only as needed to achieve freedom from pain. Do not exceed 1200 mg daily. ***Maintenance:*** Control of pain can be maintained in most patients with 400-800 mg daily. However, some patients may be maintained on as little as 200 mg daily, while others may require as much as 1200 mg daily. At least once every 3 months throughout the treatment period, attempts should be made to reduce the dose to the minimum effective level or even to discontinue the drug.

HOW SUPPLIED

Chewable Tablets 100 mg - round, red-speckled, pink, single-scored (imprinted Tegretol on one side and 52 twice on the scored side)

Bottles of 100 .... NDC 0083-0052-30

Unit Dose (blister pack)

Box of 100 (strips of 10) .... NDC 0083-0052-32

Do not store above 30°C (86°F). *Protect from light and moisture.*

Dispense in tight, light-resistant container (USP).

Tablets 200 mg - capsule-shaped, pink, single-scored (imprinted Tegretol on one side and 27 twice on the partially scored side)

Bottles of 100 .... NDC 0083-0027-30

Bottles of 1000 .... NDC 0083-0027-40

Unit Dose (blister pack)

Box of 100 (strips of 10) .... NDC 0083-0027-32

Do not store above 30°C (86°F). *Protect from moisture. Dispense in tight container (USP).*

XR Tablets 100 mg - round, yellow, coated (imprinted T on one side and 100 mg on the other), release portal on one side

Bottles of 100 .... NDC 0083-0061-30

Unit Dose (blister pack)

Box of 100 (strips of 10) .... NDC 0083-0061-32

XR Tablets 200 mg - round, pink, coated (imprinted T on one side and 200 mg on the other), release portal on one side

Bottles of 100 .... NDC 0083-0062-30

Unit Dose (blister pack)

Box of 100 (strips of 10) .... NDC 0083-0062-32

XR Tablets 400 mg - round, brown, coated (imprinted T on one side and 400 mg on the other), release portal on one side

Bottles of 100 .... NDC 0083-0060-30

Unit Dose (blister pack)

Box of 100 (strips of 10) .... NDC 0083-0060-32

Store at controlled room temperature 15°C-30°C (59°F-86°F). *Protect from moisture. Dispense in tight container (USP).*

Suspension 100 mg/5 mL (teaspoon) - yellow-orange, citrus-vanilla flavored

Bottles of 450 mL .... NDC 0083-0019-76

Shake well before using.

Do not store above 30°C (86°F). *Dispense in tight, light-resistant container (USP).*

Tegretol Suspension Manufactured by:
Novartis Pharmaceuticals Canada Inc.
Dorval (Québec), Canada H9S 1A9

Novartis Pharmaceuticals Corporation
East Hanover, New Jersey 07936
REV: JUNE 2000 2257-25-00A
T2000-39

Shown in Product Identification Guide, page 326

TRILEPTAL® ℞

[trī lĕp-tăl]
(oxcarbazepine)
Tablets
Rx only

The following prescribing information is based on official labeling in effect July, 2000.

DESCRIPTION

Trileptal® (oxcarbazepine) is an antiepileptic drug available as 150 mg, 300 mg and 600 mg film-coated tablets for oral administration. Oxcarbazepine is 10,11-Dihydro-10-oxo-5*H*-dibenz[b,*f*]azepine-5-carboxamide, and its structural formula is

[structural formula: O, N, $CONH_2$]

Oxcarbazepine is a white to faintly orange crystalline powder. It is slightly soluble in chloroform, dichloromethane, acetone, and methanol and practically insoluble in ethanol, ether and water. Its molecular weight is 252.27.

Trileptal film-coated tablets contain the following inactive ingredients: colloidal silicon dioxide, crospovidone, hydroxypropyl methylcellulose, magnesium stearate, microcrystalline cellulose, polyethylene glycol, talc and titanium dioxide, yellow iron oxide.

CLINICAL PHARMACOLOGY

Mechanism of Action

The pharmacological activity of Trileptal® (oxcarbazepine) is primarily exerted through the 10-monohydroxy metabolite (MHD) of oxcarbazepine *(see Metabolism and Excretion subsection)*. The precise mechanism by which oxcarbazepine and MHD exert their antiseizure effect is unknown; however, *in vitro* electrophysiological studies indicate that they produce blockade of voltage-sensitive sodium channels, resulting in stabilization of hyperexcited neural membranes, inhibition of repetitive neuronal firing, and diminution of propagation of synaptic impulses. These actions are thought to be important in the prevention of seizure spread in the intact brain. In addition, increased potassium conductance and modulation of high-voltage activated calcium channels may contribute to the anticonvulsant effects of the drug. No significant interactions of oxcarbazepine or MHD with brain neurotransmitter or modulator receptor sites have been demonstrated.

Pharmacodynamics

Oxcarbazepine and its active metabolite (MHD) exhibit anticonvulsant properties in animal seizure models. They protected rodents against electrically induced tonic extension seizures and, to a lesser degree, chemically induced clonic seizures, and abolished or reduced the frequency of chronically recurring focal seizures in Rhesus monkeys with aluminum implants. No development of tolerance (i.e., attenuation of anticonvulsive activity) was observed in the maximal electroshock test when mice and rats were treated daily for 5 days and 4 weeks, respectively, with oxcarbazepine or MHD.

Pharmacokinetics

Following oral administration of Trileptal, oxcarbazepine is completely absorbed and extensively metabolized to its pharmacologically active 10-monohydroxy metabolite (MHD). The half-life of the parent is about 2 hours, while the half-life of MHD is about 9 hours, so that MHD is responsible for most antiepileptic activity.

After single dose administration of Trileptal to healthy male volunteers under fasted conditions, the median t_{max} was 4.5 (range 3 to 13 hours).

In a mass balance study in people, only 2% of total radioactivity in plasma was due to unchanged oxcarbazepine, with approximately 70% present as MHD, and the remainder attributable to minor metabolites. Food has no effect on the rate and extent of absorption of oxcarbazepine.

Steady-state plasma concentrations of MHD are reached within 2-3 days in patients when Trileptal is given twice a day. At steady-state the pharmacokinetics of MHD are linear and show dose proportionality over the dose range of 300 to 2400 mg/day.

Distribution

The apparent volume of distribution of MHD is 49L.

Approximately 40% of MHD is bound to serum proteins, predominantly to albumin. Binding is independent of the serum concentration within the therapeutically relevant range. Oxcarbazepine and MHD do not bind to alpha-1-acid glycoprotein.

Metabolism and Excretion

Oxcarbazepine is rapidly reduced by cytosolic enzymes in the liver to its 10-monohydroxy metabolite, MHD, which is primarily responsible for the pharmacological effect of Trileptal. MHD is metabolized further by conjugation with glucuronic acid. Minor amounts (4% of the dose) are oxidized to the pharmacologically inactive 10,11-dihydroxy metabolite (DHD).

Oxcarbazepine is cleared from the body mostly in the form of metabolites which are predominantly excreted by the kidneys. More than 95% of the dose appears in the urine, with less than 1% as unchanged oxcarbazepine. Fecal excretion accounts for less than 4% of the administered dose. Approximately 80% of the dose is excreted in the urine either as glucuronides of MHD (49%) or as unchanged MHD (27%); the inactive DHD accounts for approximately 3% and conjugates of MHD and oxcarbazepine account for 13% of the dose.

Special Populations

Hepatic Impairment

The pharmacokinetics and metabolism of oxcarbazepine and MHD were evaluated in healthy volunteers and hepatically-impaired subjects after a single 900 mg oral dose. Mild-to-moderate hepatic impairment did not affect the pharmacokinetics of oxcarbazepine and MHD. No dose adjustment for Trileptal is recommended in patients with mild-to-moderate hepatic impairment. The pharmacokinetics of oxcarbazepine and MHD have not been evaluated in severe hepatic impairment.

Renal Impairment

There is a linear correlation between creatinine clearance and the renal clearance of MHD. When Trileptal is administered as a single 300 mg dose in renally impaired patients (creatinine clearance <30 mL/min), the elimination half-life of MHD is prolonged to 19 hours, with a two fold increase in AUC. Dose adjustment for Trileptal is recommended in these patients *(see PRECAUTIONS and DOSAGE AND ADMINISTRATION sections)*.

Pediatric Use

After a single-dose administration of 5 or 15 mg/kg of Trileptal, the dose-adjusted AUC values of MHD were 30%-40% lower in children below the age of 8 years than in children above 8 years of age. The clearance in children greater than 8 years old approaches that of adults.

Geriatric Use

Following administration of single (300 mg) and multiple (600 mg/day) doses of Trileptal to elderly volunteers (60-82 years of age), the maximum plasma concentrations and AUC values of MHD were 30%-60% higher than in younger volunteers (18-32 years of age). Comparisons of creatinine clearance in young and elderly volunteers indicate that the difference was due to age-related reductions in creatinine clearance.

Gender

No gender related pharmacokinetic differences have been observed in children, adults, or the elderly.

Race

No specific studies have been conducted to assess what effect, if any, race may have on the disposition of oxcarbazepine.

CLINICAL STUDIES

The effectiveness of Trileptal® (oxcarbazepine) as adjunctive and monotherapy for partial seizures in adults, and as adjunctive therapy in children aged 4-16 was established in 6 multicenter randomized, double-blind controlled trials.

Trileptal Monotherapy Trials

Four randomized, double-blind, multicenter trials demonstrated the efficacy of Trileptal as monotherapy. Two trials compared Trileptal to placebo and two trials used a randomized withdrawal design to compare a high dose (2400 mg) with a low dose (300 mg) of Trileptal, after substituting Trileptal 2400 mg/day for one or more antiepileptic drugs (AEDs). All doses were administered on a BID schedule.

One placebo-controlled trial was conducted in 102 patients (11-62 years of age) with refractory partial seizures who had completed an inpatient evaluation for epilepsy surgery. Patients had been withdrawn from all AEDs and were required to have 2-10 partial seizures within 48 hours prior to randomization. Patients were randomized to receive either placebo or Trileptal given as 1500 mg/day on Day 1 and 2400 mg/day thereafter for an additional 9 days, or until one of the following three exit criteria occurred: 1) the occurrence of a fourth partial seizure, excluding Day 1, 2) two new-onset secondarily generalized seizures, where such seizures were not seen in the 1-year period prior to randomization, or 3) occurrence of serial seizures or status epilepticus. The primary measure of effectiveness was a between group comparison of the time to meet exit criteria. There was a statistically significant difference in favor of Trileptal *(see Figure 1)*, p=0.0001.

Figure 1: Kaplan-Meier estimates of exit rate by treatment group

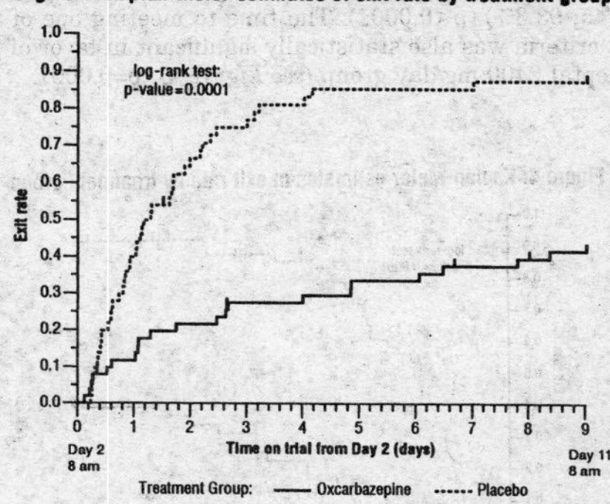

Continued on next page

Trileptal—Cont.

The second placebo-controlled trial was conducted in 67 untreated patients (8-69 years of age) with newly-diagnosed and recent-onset partial seizures. Patients were randomized to placebo or Trileptal, initiated at 300 mg BID and titrated to 1200 mg/day (given as 600 mg BID) in 6 days, followed by maintenance treatment for 84 days. The primary measure of effectiveness was a between group comparison of the time to first seizure. The difference between the two treatments was statistically significant in favor of Trileptal *(see Figure 2)*, p=0.046.

Figure 2: Kaplan-Meier estimates of first seizure event rate by treatment group

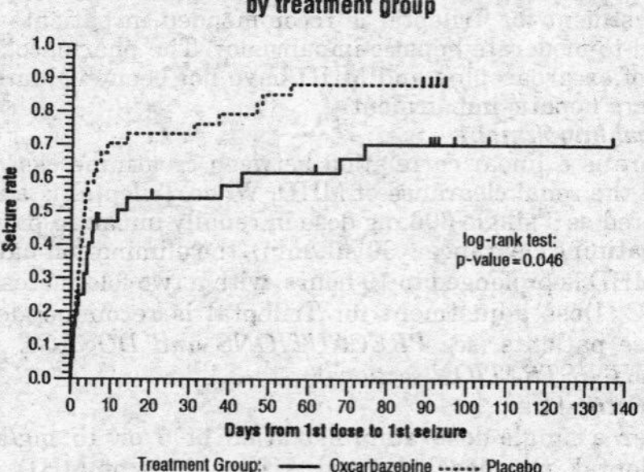

A third trial substituted Trileptal monotherapy at 2400 mg/day for carbamazepine in 143 patients (12-65 years of age) whose partial seizures were inadequately controlled on carbamazepine (CBZ) monotherapy at a stable dose of 800 to 1600 mg/day, and maintained this Trileptal dose for 56 days (baseline phase). Patients who were able to tolerate titration of Trileptal to 2400 mg/day during simultaneous carbamazepine withdrawal were randomly assigned to either 300 mg/day of Trileptal or 2400 mg/day Trileptal. Patients were observed for 126 days or until one of the following 4 exit criteria occurred: 1) a doubling of the 28-day seizure frequency compared to baseline, 2) a two fold increase in the highest consecutive 2-day seizure frequency during baseline, 3) a single generalized seizure if none had occurred during baseline, or 4) a prolonged generalized seizure. The primary measure of effectiveness was a between group comparison of the time to meet exit criteria. The difference between the curves was statistically significant in favor of the Trileptal 2400 mg/day group *(see Figure 3)*, p=0.0001.

Figure 3: Kaplan-Meier estimates of exit rate by treatment group

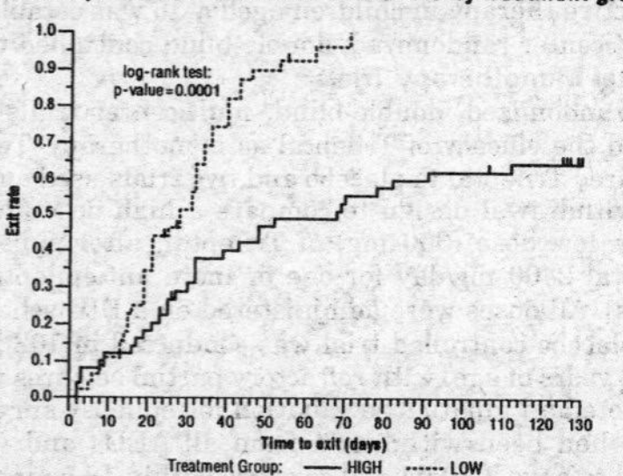

Another monotherapy substitution trial was conducted in 87 patients (11-66 years of age) whose seizures were inadequately controlled on 1 or 2 AEDs. Patients were randomized to either Trileptal 2400 mg/day or 300 mg/day and their standard AED regimen(s) were eliminated over the first 6 weeks of double-blind therapy. Double-blind treatment continued for another 84 days (total double-blind treatment of 126 days) or until one of the 4 exit criteria described for the previous study occurred. The primary measure of effectiveness was a between group comparison of the percentage of patients meeting exit criteria. The results were statistically significant in favor of the Trileptal 2400 mg/day group (14/34; 41.2%) compared to the Trileptal 300 mg/day group (42/45; 93.3%) (p<0.0001). The time to meeting one of the exit criteria was also statistically significant in favor of the Trileptal 2400 mg/day group *(see Figure 4)*, p=0.0001.

Figure 4: Kaplan-Meier estimates of exit rate by treatment group

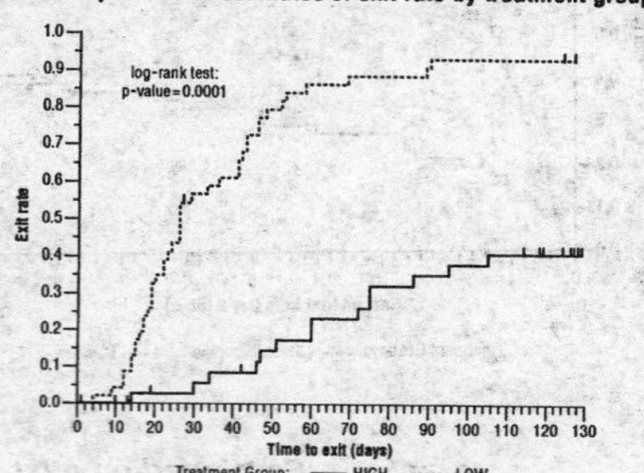

Table 1: Summary of percentage change in partial seizure frequency from baseline for placebo-controlled adjunctive therapy trials

Trial	Treatment Group	N	Baseline Median Seizure Rate*	Median % Reduction
1 (pediatrics)	Trileptal	136	12.5	34.8[1]
	Placebo	128	13.1	9.4
2 (adults)	Trileptal 2400 mg/day	174	10.0	49.9[1]
	Trileptal 1200 mg/day	177	9.8	40.2[1]
	Trileptal 600 mg/day	168	9.6	26.4[1]
	Placebo	173	8.6	7.6

[1]p=0.0001; *= # per 28 days

Trileptal Adjunctive Therapy Trials

The effectiveness of Trileptal as an adjunctive therapy for partial seizures was established in two multicenter, randomized, double-blind, placebo-controlled trials, one in 692 patients (15-66 years of age) and one in 264 pediatric patients (3-17 years of age). Patients in these trials were on 1-3 concomitant AEDs. In both of the trials, patients were stabilized on optimum dosages of their concomitant AEDs during an 8-week baseline phase. Patients who experienced at least 8 (minimum of 1-4 per month) partial seizures during the baseline phase were randomly assigned to placebo or to a specific dose of Trileptal in addition to their other AEDs. In these studies, the dose was increased over a 2-week period until either the assigned dose was reached, or intolerance prevented increases. Patients then entered a 14 (pediatrics) or 24 week (adults) maintenance period.

In the adult trial, patients received fixed doses of 600, 1200 or 2400 mg/day. In the pediatric trial, patients received maintenance doses in the range of 30-46 mg/kg/day, depending on baseline weight. The primary measure of effectiveness in both trials was a between group comparison of the percentage change in partial seizure frequency in the double-blind Treatment Phase relative to Baseline Phase. This comparison was statistically significant in favor of Trileptal at all doses tested in both trials (p=0.0001 for all doses for both trials). The number of patients randomized to each dose, the median baseline seizure rate, and the median percentage seizure rate reduction for each trial are shown in Table 1. It is important to note that in the high dose group in the study in adults, over 65% of patients discontinued treatment because of adverse events; only 46 (27%) of the patients in this group completed the 28-week study *(see ADVERSE REACTIONS section)*, an outcome not seen in the monotherapy studies.

[See table 1 above]

Subset analyses of the antiepileptic efficacy of Trileptal with regard to gender in these trials revealed no important differences in response between men and women. Because there were very few patients over the age of 65 in controlled trials, the effect of the drug in the elderly has not been adequately assessed.

INDICATIONS AND USAGE

Trileptal® (oxcarbazepine) is indicated for use as monotherapy or adjunctive therapy in the treatment of partial seizures in adults with epilepsy and as adjunctive therapy in the treatment of partial seizures in children ages 4-16 with epilepsy.

CONTRAINDICATIONS

Trileptal® (oxcarbazepine) should not be used in patients with a known hypersensitivity to oxcarbazepine or to any of its components.

WARNINGS

Hyponatremia

Clinically significant hyponatremia (sodium <125 mmol/L) can develop during Trileptal® (oxcarbazepine) use. In the 14 controlled epilepsy studies 2.5% of Trileptal treated patients (38/1524) had a sodium of less than 125 mmol/L at some point during treatment, compared to no such patients assigned placebo or active control (carbamazepine and phenobarbital for adjunctive and monotherapy substitution studies, and phenytoin and valproate for the monotherapy initiation studies). Clinically significant hyponatremia generally occurred during the first 3 months of treatment with Trileptal, although there were patients who first developed a serum sodium <125 mmol/L more than 1 year after initiation of therapy. Most patients who developed hyponatremia were asymptomatic but patients in the clinical trials were frequently monitored and some had their Trileptal dose reduced, discontinued, or had their fluid intake restricted for hyponatremia. Whether or not these maneuvers prevented the occurrence of more severe events is unknown. Cases of symptomatic hyponatremia have been reported during post-marketing use. In clinical trials, patients whose treatment with Trileptal was discontinued due to hyponatremia generally experienced normalization of serum sodium within a few days without additional treatment.

Measurement of serum sodium levels should be considered for patients during maintenance treatment with Trileptal, particularly if the patient is receiving other medications known to decrease serum sodium levels (for example, drugs associated with inappropriate ADH secretion) or if symptoms possibly indicating hyponatremia develop (e.g., nausea, malaise, headache, lethargy, confusion, or obtundation).

Patients with a Past History of Hypersensitivity Reaction to Carbamazepine

Patients who have had hypersensitivity reactions to carbamazepine should be informed that approximately 25%-30% of them will experience hypersensitivity reactions with Trileptal. For this reason patients should be specifically questioned about any prior experience with carbamazepine, and patients with a history of hypersensitivity reactions to carbamazepine should ordinarily be treated with Trileptal only if the potential benefit justifies the potential risk. If signs or symptoms of hypersensitivity develop, Trileptal should be discontinued immediately.

Withdrawal of AEDs

As with all antiepileptic drugs, Trileptal should be withdrawn gradually to minimize the potential of increased seizure frequency.

PRECAUTIONS

Cognitive/Neuropsychiatric Adverse Events

Use of Trileptal® (oxcarbazepine) has been associated with central nervous system related adverse events. The most significant of these can be classified into three general categories: 1) cognitive symptoms including psychomotor slowing, difficulty with concentration, and speech or language problems, 2) somnolence or fatigue, and 3) coordination abnormalities, including ataxia and gait disturbances.

In one, large, fixed dose study, Trileptal was added to existing AED therapy (up to three concomitant AEDs). By protocol, the dosage of the concomitant AEDs could not be reduced as Trileptal was added, reduction in Trileptal dosage was not allowed if intolerance developed, and patients were discontinued if unable to tolerate their highest target maintenance doses. In this trial, 65% of patients were discontinued because they could not tolerate the 2400 mg/day dose of Trileptal on top of existing AEDs. The adverse events seen in this study were primarily CNS related and the risk for discontinuation was dose related.

In this trial, 7.1% of oxcarbazepine-treated patients and 4% of placebo-treated patients experienced a cognitive adverse event. The risk of discontinuation for these events was about 6.5 times greater on oxcarbazepine than on placebo. In addition, 26% of oxcarbazepine-treated patients and 12% of placebo-treated patients experienced somnolence. The risk of discontinuation for somnolence was about 10 times greater on oxcarbazepine than on placebo. Finally, 28.7% of oxcarbazepine-treated patients and 6.4% of placebo-treated patients experienced ataxia or gait disturbances. The risk for discontinuation for these events was about 7 times greater on oxcarbazepine than on placebo.

In a single placebo-controlled monotherapy trial evaluating 2400 mg/day of Trileptal, no patients in either treatment group discontinued double-blind treatment because of cognitive adverse events, somnolence, ataxia, or gait disturbance.

In the two dose-controlled conversion to monotherapy trials comparing 2400 mg/day and 300 mg/day Trileptal, 1.1% of patients in the 2400 mg/day group discontinued double-blind treatment because of somnolence or cognitive adverse events compared to 0% in the 300 mg/day group. In these trials, no patients discontinued because of ataxia or gait disturbances in either treatment group.

Information for Patients

Patients who have exhibited hypersensitivity reactions to carbamazepine should be informed that approximately 25%-30% of these patients may experience hypersensitivity reactions with Trileptal. *(See WARNINGS section.)*

Female patients of childbearing age should be warned that the concurrent use of Trileptal with hormonal contraceptives may render this method of contraception less effective *(see Drug Interactions subsection)*. Additional non-hormonal forms of contraception are recommended when using Trileptal.

Caution should be exercised if alcohol is taken in combination with Trileptal therapy, due to a possible additive sedative effect.

Patients should be advised that Trileptal may cause dizziness and somnolence. Accordingly, patients should be advised not to drive or operate machinery until they have gained sufficient experience on Trileptal to gauge whether it adversely affects their ability to drive or operate machinery.

Laboratory Tests

Serum sodium levels below 125 mmol/L have been observed in patients treated with Trileptal *(see WARNINGS section)*. Experience from clinical trials indicates that serum sodium levels return toward normal when the Trileptal dosage is reduced or discontinued, or when the patient was treated conservatively (e.g., fluid restriction).

Laboratory data from clinical trials suggest that Trileptal use was associated with decreases in T_4, without changes in T_3 or TSH.

Drug Interactions

Oxcarbazepine can inhibit CYP2C19 and induce CYP3A4/5 with potentially important effects on plasma concentrations of other drugs. In addition, several AEDs that are cythochrome P450 inducers can decrease plasma concentrations of oxcarbazepine and MHD.

Oxcarbazepine was evaluated in human liver microsomes to determine its capacity to inhibit the major cytochrome P450 enzymes responsible for the metabolism of other drugs. Results demonstrate that oxcarbazepine and its pharmacologically active 10-monohydroxy metabolite (MHD) have little or no capacity to function as inhibitors for most of the human cytochrome P450 enzymes evaluated (CYP1A2, CYP2A6, CYP2C9, CYP2D6, CYP2E1, CYP4A9 and CYP4A11) with the exception of CYP2C19 and CYP3A4/5. Although inhibition of CYP3A4/5 by oxcarbazepine and MHD did occur at high concentrations, it is not likely to be of clinical significance. The inhibition of CYP2C19 by oxcarbazepine and MHD, however, is clinically relevant *(see below)*.

In vitro, the UDP-glucuronyl transferase level was increased, indicating induction of this enzyme. Increases of 22% with MHD and 47% with oxcarbazepine were observed. As MHD, the predominant plasma substrate, is only a weak inducer of UDP-glucuronyl transferase, it is unlikely to have an effect on drugs that are mainly eliminated by conjugation through UDP-glucuronyl transferase (e.g., valproic acid, lamotrigine).

In addition, oxcarbazepine and MHD induce a subgroup of the cytochrome P450 3A family (CYP3A4 and CYP3A5) responsible for the metabolism of dihydropyridine calcium antagonists and oral contraceptives, resulting in a lower plasma concentration of these drugs.

As binding of MHD to plasma proteins is low (40%), clinically significant interactions with other drugs through competition for protein binding sites are unlikely.

Antiepileptic Drugs

Potential interactions between Trileptal and other AEDs were assessed in clinical studies. The effect of these interactions on mean AUCs and C_{min} are summarized in Table 2: [See table 2 above]

In vivo, the plasma levels of phenytoin increased by up to 40% when Trileptal was given at doses above 1200 mg/day. Therefore, when using doses of Trileptal greater than 1200 mg/day during adjunctive therapy, a decrease in the dose of phenytoin may be required. The increase of phenobarbital level, however, is small (15%) when given with Trileptal.

Strong inducers of cytochrome P450 enzymes (i.e., carbamazepine, phenytoin and phenobarbital) have been shown to decrease the plasma levels of MHD (29%-40%).

No autoinduction has been observed with Trileptal.

Hormonal Contraceptives

Co-administration of Trileptal with an oral contraceptive has been shown to influence the plasma concentrations of the two hormonal components, ethinylestradiol (EE) and levonorgestrel (LNG). The mean AUC values of EE were decreased by 48% [90% CI: 22-65] in one study and 52% [90% CI: 38-52] in another study. The mean AUC values of LNG were decreased by 32% [90% CI: 20-45] in one study and 52% [90% CI: 42-52] in another study. Therefore, concurrent use of Trileptal with hormonal contraceptives may render these contraceptives less effective *(see Drug Interactions subsection)*. Studies with other oral or implant contraceptives have not been conducted.

Calcium Antagonists

After repeated co-administration of Trileptal, the AUC of felodipine was lowered by 28% [90% CI: 20-33].

Verapamil produced a decrease of 20% [90% CI: 18-27] of the plasma levels of MHD.

Other Drug Interactions

Cimetidine, erythromycin and dextropropoxyphene had no effect on the pharmacokinetics of MHD. Results with warfarin show no evidence of interaction with either single or repeated doses of Trileptal.

Drug/Laboratory Test Interactions

There are no known interactions of Trileptal with commonly used laboratory tests.

Carcinogenesis/Mutagenesis/Impairment of Fertility

In 2-year carcinogenicity studies, oxcarbazepine was administered in the diet at doses of up to 100 mg/kg/day to mice and by gavage at doses of up to 250 mg/kg to rats, and the pharmacologically active 10-hydroxy metabolite (MHD) was administered orally at doses of up to 600 mg/kg/day to rats. In mice, a dose-related increase in the incidence of hepatocellular adenomas was observed at oxcarbazepine doses ≥70 mg/kg/day or approximately 0.1 times the maximum recommended human dose [MRHD] on a mg/m^2 basis. In rats, the incidence of hepatocellular carcinomas was increased in females treated with oxcarbazepine at doses ≥25 mg/kg/day (0.1 times the MRHD on a mg/m^2 basis), and incidences of hepatocellular adenomas and/or carcinomas were increased in males and females treated with MHD at doses of 600 mg/kg/day (2.4 times the MRHD on a mg/m^2 basis) and ≥250 mg/kg/day (equivalent to the MRHD on a mg/m^2 basis), respectively. There was an increase in the incidence of benign testicular interstitial cell tumors in rats at 250 mg oxcarbazepine/kg/day and at ≥250 mg MHD/kg/day, and an increase in the incidence of granular cell tumors in the cervix and vagina in rats at 600 mg MHD/kg/day.

Oxcarbazepine increased mutation frequencies in the Ames test *in vitro* in the absence of metabolic activation in one of five bacterial strains. Both oxcarbazepine and MHD produced increases in chromosomal aberrations and polyploidy in the Chinese hamster ovary assay *in vitro* in the absence of metabolic activation. MHD was negative in the Ames test, and no mutagenic or clastogenic activity was found with either oxcarbazepine or MHD in V79 Chinese hamster cells *in vitro*. Oxcarbazepine and MHD were both negative for clastogenic or aneugenic effects (micronucleus formation) in an *in vivo* rat bone marrow assay.

In a fertility study in which rats were administered MHD (50, 150, or 450 mg/kg) orally prior to and during mating and early gestation, estrous cyclicity was disrupted and numbers of corpora lutea, implantations, and live embryos were reduced in females receiving the highest dose (approximately 2 times the MRHD on a mg/m^2 basis).

Table 2: Summary of AED Interactions with Trileptal

AED Co-administered	Dose of AED (mg/day)	Trileptal dose (mg/day)	Influence of Trileptal on AED Concentration (Mean change, 90% Confidence Interval)	Influence of AED on MHD Concentration (Mean change, 90% Confidence Interval)
Carbamazepine	400–2000	900	nc[1]	40% decrease [CI: 17% decrease, 57% decrease]
Phenobarbital	100-150	600-1800	14% increase [CI: 2% increase, 24% increase]	25% decrease [CI: 12% decrease, 51% decrease]
Phenytoin	250-500	600-1800 >1200-2400	nc[1,2] up to 40% increase[3] [CI: 12% increase, 60% increase]	30% decrease [CI: 3% decrease, 48% decrease]
Valproic acid	400-2800	600-1800	nc[1]	18% decrease [CI: 13% decrease, 40% decrease]

[1] nc denotes a mean change of less than 10%
[2] Pediatrics
[3] Mean increase in adults at high Trileptal doses

Table 3: Treatment-Emergent Adverse Event Incidence in a Controlled Clinical Study of Adjunctive Therapy in Adults (Events in at least 2% of patients treated with 2400 mg/day of Trileptal and numerically more frequent than in the placebo group)

	Oxcarbazepine Dosage (mg/day)			
Body System/ Adverse Event	OXC 600 N=163 %	OXC 1200 N=171 %	OXC 2400 N=126 %	Placebo N=166 %
Body as a Whole				
Fatigue	15	12	15	7
Asthenia	6	3	6	5
Edema Legs	2	1	2	1
Weight Increase	1	2	2	1
Feeling Abnormal	0	1	2	0
Cardiovascular System				
Hypotension	0	1	2	0
Digestive System				
Nausea	15	25	29	10
Vomiting	13	25	36	5
Pain Abnormal	10	13	11	5
Diarrhea	5	6	7	6
Dyspepsia	5	5	6	2
Constipation	2	1	6	4
Gastritis	2	1	2	1
Metabolic and Nutritional Disorders				
Hyponatremia	3	1	2	1
Musculoskeletal System				
Muscle Weakness	1	2	2	0
Sprains and Strains	0	2	2	1
Nervous System				
Headache	32	28	26	23
Dizziness	26	32	49	13
Somnolence	20	28	36	12
Ataxia	9	17	31	5
Nystagmus	7	20	26	5
Gait Abnormal	5	10	17	1
Insomnia	4	2	3	1
Tremor	3	8	16	5
Nervousness	2	4	2	1
Agitation	1	1	2	1
Coordination Abnormal	1	3	2	1
EEG Abnormal	0	0	2	0
Speech Disorder	1	1	3	0
Confusion	1	1	2	1
Cranial Injury NOS	1	0	2	1
Dysmetria	1	2	3	0
Thinking Abnormal	0	2	4	0
Respiratory System				
Rhinitis	2	4	5	4
Skin and Appendages				
Acne	1	2	2	0
Special Senses				
Diplopia	14	30	40	5
Vertigo	6	12	15	2
Vision Abnormal	6	14	13	4
Accommodation Abnormal	0	0	2	0

Pregnancy Category C

Increased incidences of fetal structural abnormalities and other manifestations of developmental toxicity (embryolethality, growth retardation) were observed in the offspring of animals treated with either oxcarbazepine or its active 10-hydroxy metabolite (MHD) during pregnancy at doses similar to the maximum recommended human dose.

When pregnant rats were given oxcarbazepine (30, 300, or 1000 mg/kg) orally throughout the period of organogenesis, increased incidences of fetal malformations (craniofacial, cardiovascular, and skeletal) and variations were observed at the intermediate and high doses (approximately 1.2 and 4 times, respectively, the maximum recommended human

Continued on next page

Trileptal—Cont.

dose [MRHD] on a mg/m² basis). Increased embryofetal death and decreased fetal body weights were seen at the high dose. Doses ≥300 mg/kg were also maternally toxic (decreased body weight gain, clinical signs), but there is no evidence to suggest that teratogenicity was secondary to the maternal effects.

In a study in which pregnant rabbits were orally administered MHD (20, 100, or 200 mg/kg) during organogenesis, embryofetal mortality was increased at the highest dose (1.5 times the MRHD on a mg/m² basis). This dose produced only minimal maternal toxicity.

In a study in which female rats were dosed orally with oxcarbazepine (25, 50, or 150 mg/kg) during the latter part of gestation and throughout the lactation period, a persistent reduction in body weights and altered behavior (decreased activity) were observed in offspring exposed to the highest dose (0.6 times the MRHD on a mg/m² basis). Oral administration of MHD (25, 75, or 250 mg/kg) to rats during gestation and lactation resulted in a persistent reduction in offspring weights at the highest dose (equivalent to the MRHD on a mg/m² basis).

There are no adequate and well-controlled clinical studies of Trileptal in pregnant women; however, Trileptal is closely related structurally to carbamazepine, which is considered to be teratogenic in humans. Given this fact, and the results of the animal studies described, it is likely that Trileptal is a human teratogen. Trileptal should be used during pregnancy only if the potential benefit justifies the potential risk to the fetus.

Labor and Delivery

The effect of Trileptal on labor and delivery in humans has not been evaluated.

Nursing Mothers

Oxcarbazepine and its active metabolite (MHD) are excreted in human breast milk. A milk-to-plasma concentration ratio of 0.5 was found for both. Because of the potential for serious adverse reactions to Trileptal in nursing infants, a decision should be made about whether to discontinue nursing or to discontinue the drug in nursing women, taking into account the importance of the drug to the mother.

Patients with Renal Impairment

In renally-impaired patients (creatinine clearance <30 mL/min), the elimination half-life of MHD is prolonged with a corresponding two fold increase in AUC *(see CLINICAL PHARMACOLOGY, Pharmacokinetics subsection).* Trileptal therapy should be initiated at one-half the usual starting dose and increased, if necessary, at a slower than usual rate until the desired clinical response is achieved.

Pediatric Use

Trileptal has been shown to be effective as adjunctive therapy for partial seizures in patients aged 4-16 years old. Trileptal has been given to about 623 patients between the ages of 3-17 in controlled clinical trials (185 treated as monotherapy) and about 615 patients between the ages of 3-17 in other trials. *(See ADVERSE REACTIONS for a description of the adverse events associated with Trileptal use in this population.)*

Geriatric Use

There were 52 patients over age 65 in controlled clinical trials and 565 patients over the age of 65 in other trials. Following administration of single (300 mg) and multiple (600 mg/day) doses of Trileptal in elderly volunteers (60-82 years of age), the maximum plasma concentrations and AUC values of MHD were 30%-60% higher than in younger volunteers (18-32 years of age). Comparisons of creatinine clearance in young and elderly volunteers indicate that the difference was due to age-related reductions in creatinine clearance.

Table 4: Treatment-Emergent Adverse Event Incidence in Controlled Clinical Studies of Monotherapy in Adults Previously Treated with Other AEDs (Events in at least 2% of patients treated with 2400 mg/day of Trileptal and numerically more frequent than in the low dose control group)

Body System/ Adverse Event	Oxcarbazepine Dosage (mg/day) 2400 N=86 %	300 N=86 %
Body as a Whole		
Fatigue	21	5
Fever	3	0
Allergy	2	0
Edema Generalized	2	1
Pain Chest	2	0
Digestive System		
Nausea	22	7
Vomiting	15	5
Diarrhea	7	5
Dyspepsia	6	1
Anorexia	5	3
Pain Abdominal	5	3
Mouth Dry	3	0
Hemorrhage Rectum	2	0
Toothache	2	1
Hemic and Lymphatic System		
Lymphadenopathy	2	0
Infections and Infestations		
Infection Viral	7	5
Infection	2	0
Metabolic and Nutritional Disorders		
Hyponatremia	5	0
Thirst	2	0
Nervous System		
Headache	31	15
Dizziness	28	8
Somnolence	19	5
Anxiety	7	5
Ataxia	7	1
Confusion	7	0
Nervousness	7	0
Insomnia	6	3
Tremor	6	3
Amnesia	5	1
Convulsions Aggravated	5	2
Emotional Lability	3	2
Hypoesthesia	3	1
Coordination Abnormal	2	1
Nystagmus	2	0
Speech Disorder	2	0
Respiratory System		
Upper Respiratory Tract Infection	10	5
Coughing	5	0
Bronchitis	3	0
Pharyngitis	3	0
Skin and Appendages		
Hot Flushes	2	1
Purpura	2	0
Special Senses		
Vision Abnormal	14	2
Diplopia	12	1
Taste Perversion	5	0
Vertigo	3	0
Ear Ache	2	1
Ear Infection NOS	2	0
Urogenital and Reproductive System		
Urinary Tract Infection	5	1
Micturition Frequency	2	1
Vaginitis	2	0

ADVERSE REACTIONS

Most Common Adverse Events in All Clinical Studies

Adjunctive Therapy/Monotherapy in Adults Previously Treated with other AEDs: The most commonly observed (≥5%) adverse experiences seen in association with Trileptal® (oxcarbazepine) and substantially more frequent than in placebo-treated patients were: Dizziness, somnolence, diplopia, fatigue, nausea, vomiting, ataxia, abnormal vision, abdominal pain, tremor, dyspepsia, abnormal gait.

Approximately 23% of these 1537 adult patients discontinued treatment because of an adverse experience. The adverse experiences most commonly associated with discontinuation were: Dizziness (6.4%), diplopia (5.9%), ataxia (5.2%), vomiting (5.1%), nausea (4.9%), somnolence (3.8%), headache (2.9%), fatigue (2.1%), abnormal vision (2.1%), tremor (1.8%), abnormal gait (1.7%), rash (1.4%), hyponatremia (1.0%).

Monotherapy in Adults not Previously Treated with other AEDs: The most commonly observed (≥5%) adverse experiences seen in association with Trileptal in these patients were similar to those in previously treated patients.

Approximately 9% of these 295 adult patients discontinued treatment because of an adverse experience. The adverse experiences most commonly associated with discontinuation were: Dizziness (1.7%), nausea (1.7%), rash (1.7%), headache (1.4%).

Adjunctive Therapy/Monotherapy in Pediatric Patients Previously Treated with other AEDs: The most commonly observed (≥5%) adverse experiences seen in association with Trileptal in these patients were similar to those seen in adults.

Approximately 11% of these 456 pediatric patients discontinued treatment because of an adverse experience. The adverse experiences most commonly associated with discontinuation were: Somnolence (2.4%), vomiting (2.0%), ataxia (1.8%), diplopia (1.3%), dizziness (1.3%), fatigue (1.1%), nystagmus (1.1%).

Incidence in Controlled Clinical Studies: The prescriber should be aware that the figures in Tables 3, 4, 5 and 6 cannot be used to predict the frequency of adverse experiences in the course of usual medical practice where patient characteristics and other factors may differ from those prevailing during clinical studies. Similarly, the cited frequencies cannot be directly compared with figures obtained from other clinical investigations involving different treatments, uses, or investigators. An inspection of these frequencies, however, does provide the prescriber with one basis to estimate the relative contribution of drug and nondrug factors to the adverse event incidences in the population studied.

Controlled Clinical Studies of Adjunctive Therapy/Monotherapy in Adults Previously Treated with other AEDs: Table 3 lists treatment-emergent signs and symptoms that occurred in at least 2% of adult patients with epilepsy treated with Trileptal or placebo as adjunctive treatment and were numerically more common in the patients treated with any dose of Trileptal. Table 4 lists treatment-emergent signs and symptoms in patients converted from other AEDs to either high dose Trileptal or low dose (300 mg) Trileptal. Note that in some of these monotherapy studies patients who dropped out during a preliminary tolerability phase are not included in the tables.

[See table 3 at top of previous page]

[See table 4 below]

Controlled Clinical Study of Monotherapy in Adults not Previously Treated with other AEDs: Table 5 lists treatment-emergent signs and symptoms in a controlled clinical study of monotherapy in adults not previously treated with other AEDs that occurred in at least 2% of adult patients with epilepsy treated with Trileptal or placebo and were numerically more common in the patients treated with Trileptal.

[See table 5 at bottom of next page]

Controlled Clinical Studies of Adjunctive Therapy/Monotherapy in Pediatric Patients Previously Treated with other AEDs: Table 6 lists treatment-emergent signs and symptoms that occurred in at least 2% of pediatric patients with epilepsy treated with Trileptal or placebo as adjunctive treatment and were numerically more common in the patients treated with Trileptal.

[See table 6 at bottom of next page]

Other Events Observed in Association with the Administration of Trileptal

In the paragraphs that follow, the adverse events other than those in the preceding tables or text, that occurred in a total of 565 children and 1574 adults exposed to Trileptal and that are reasonably likely to be related to drug use are presented. Events common in the population, events reflecting chronic illness and events likely to reflect concomitant illness are omitted particularly if minor. They are listed in order of decreasing frequency. Because the reports cite events observed in open label and uncontrolled trials, the role of Trileptal in their causation cannot be reliably determined.

Body as a Whole: Fever, malaise, pain chest precordial, rigors, weight decrease.

Cardiovascular System: Bradycardia, cardiac failure, cerebral hemorrhage, hypertension, hypotension postural, palpitation, syncope, tachycardia.

Digestive System: Appetite increased, blood in stool, cholelithiasis, colitis, duodenal ulcer, dysphagia, enteritis, eructation, esophagitis, flatulence, gastric ulcer, gingival bleeding, gum hyperplasia, hematemesis, hemorrhage rectum, hemorrhoids, hiccup, mouth dry, pain biliary, pain right hypochondrium, retching, sialoadenitis, stomatitis, stomatitis ulcerative.
Hemic and Lymphatic System: Leukopenia, thrombocytopenia.
Laboratory Abnormality: Gamma-GT increased, hyperglycemia, hypocalcemia, hypoglycemia, hypokalemia, liver enzymes elevated, serum transaminase increased.
Musculoskeletal System: Hypertonia muscle.
Nervous System: Aggressive reaction, amnesia, anguish, anxiety, apathy, aphasia, aura, convulsions aggravated, delirium, delusion, depressed level of consciousness, dysphonia, dystonia, emotional lability, euphoria, extrapyramidal disorder, feeling drunk, hemiplegia, hyperkinesia, hyperreflexia, hypoesthesia, hypokinesia, hyporeflexia, hypotonia, hysteria, libido decreased, libido increased, manic reaction, migraine, muscle contractions involuntary, nervousness, neuralgia, oculogyric crisis, panic disorder, paralysis, paroniria, personality disorder, psychosis, ptosis, stupor, tetany.
Respiratory System: Asthma, dyspnea, epistaxis, laryngismus, pleurisy.
Skin and Appendages: Acne, alopecia, angioedema, bruising, dermatitis contact, eczema, facial rash, flushing, folliculitis, heat rash, hot flushes, photosensitivity reaction, pruritus genital, psoriasis, purpura, rash erythematous, rash maculopapular, vitiligo.
Special Senses: Accommodation abnormal, cataract, conjunctival hemorrhage, edema eye, hemianopia, mydriasis, otitis externa, photophobia, scotoma, taste perversion, tinnitus, xerophthalmia.
Surgical and Medical Procedures: Procedure dental oral, procedure female reproductive, procedure musculoskeletal, procedure skin.
Urogenital and Reproductive System: Dysuria, hematuria, intermenstrual bleeding, leukorrhea, menorrhagia, micturition frequency, pain renal, pain urinary tract, polyuria, priapism, renal calculus.
Other: Systemic lupus erythematosus.

Post-Marketing and Other Experience

The following adverse events not seen in controlled clinical trials have been observed in named patient programs or post-marketing experience:
Body as a Whole: Multiorgan hypersensitivity disorders characterized by features such as rash, fever, lymphadenopathy, abnormal liver function tests, eosinophilia and arthralgia.
Skin and Appendages: Erythema multiforme, Stevens-Johnson syndrome, toxic epidermal necrolysis.

Table 5: Treatment-Emergent Adverse Event Incidence in a Controlled Clinical Study of Monotherapy in Adults not Previously Treated with Other AEDs (Events in at least 2% of patients treated with Trileptal and numerically more frequent than in the placebo group)

Body System/ Adverse Event	Oxcarbazepine N=55 %	Placebo N=49 %
Body as a Whole		
Falling Down NOS	4	0
Digestive System		
Nausea	16	12
Diarrhea	7	2
Vomiting	7	6
Constipation	5	0
Dyspepsia	5	4
Musculoskeletal System		
Pain Back	4	2
Nervous System		
Dizziness	22	6
Headache	13	10
Ataxia	5	0
Nervousness	5	2
Amnesia	4	2
Coordination Abnormal	4	2
Tremor	4	0
Respiratory System		
Upper Respiratory Tract Infection	7	0
Epistaxis	4	0
Infection Chest	4	0
Sinusitis	4	2
Skin and Appendages		
Rash	4	2
Special Senses		
Vision Abnormal	4	0

Table 6: Treatment-Emergent Adverse Event Incidence in Controlled Clinical Studies of Adjunctive Therapy/ Monotherapy in Pediatric Patients Previously Treated with Other AEDs (Events in at least 2% of patients treated with Trileptal and numerically more frequent than in the placebo group)

Body System/ Adverse Event	Oxcarbazepine N=171 %	Placebo N=139 %
Body as a Whole		
Fatigue	13	9
Allergy	2	0
Asthenia	2	1
Digestive System		
Vomiting	33	14
Nausea	19	5
Constipation	4	1
Dyspepsia	2	0
Nervous System		
Headache	31	19
Somnolence	31	13
Dizziness	28	8
Ataxia	13	4
Nystagmus	9	1
Emotional Lability	8	4
Gait Abnormal	8	3
Tremor	6	4
Speech Disorder	3	1
Concentration Impaired	2	1
Convulsions	2	1
Muscle Contractions Involuntary	2	1
Respiratory System		
Rhinitis	10	9
Pneumonia	2	1
Skin and Appendages		
Bruising	4	2
Sweating Increased	3	0
Special Senses		
Diplopia	17	1
Vision Abnormal	13	1
Vertigo	2	0

DRUG ABUSE AND DEPENDENCE

Abuse

The abuse potential of Trileptal® (oxcarbazepine) has not been evaluated in human studies.

Dependence

Intragastric injections of oxcarbazepine to four cynomolgus monkeys demonstrated no signs of physical dependence as measured by the desire to self administer oxcarbazepine by lever pressing activity.

OVERDOSAGE

Human Overdose Experience

Isolated cases of overdose with Trileptal® (oxcarbazepine) have been reported. The maximum dose taken was approximately 24,000 mg. All patients recovered with symptomatic treatment.

Treatment and Management

There is no specific antidote. Symptomatic and supportive treatment should be administered as appropriate. Removal of the drug by gastric lavage and/or inactivation by administering activated charcoal should be considered.

DOSAGE AND ADMINISTRATION

Trileptal® (oxcarbazepine) is recommended as adjunctive treatment and monotherapy in the treatment of partial seizures in adults and as adjunctive treatment for partial seizures in children ages 4-16. All dosing should be given in a twice a day (BID) regimen.
Trileptal can be taken with or without food.

Adults

Adjunctive Therapy

Treatment with Trileptal should be initiated with a dose of 600 mg/day, given in a BID regimen. If clinically indicated, the dose may be increased by a maximum of 600 mg/day at approximately weekly intervals; the recommended daily dose is 1200 mg/day. Daily doses above 1200 mg/day show somewhat greater effectiveness in controlled trials, but most patients were not able to tolerate the 2400 mg/day dose, primarily because of CNS effects. It is recommended that the patient be observed closely and plasma levels of the concomitant AEDs be monitored during the period of Trileptal titration, as these plasma levels may be altered, especially at Trileptal doses greater than 1200 mg/day *(see PRECAUTIONS, Drug Interactions subsection).*

Conversion to Monotherapy

Patients receiving concomitant AEDs may be converted to monotherapy by initiating treatment with Trileptal at 600 mg/day (given in a BID regimen) while simultaneously initiating the reduction of the dose of the concomitant AEDs. The concomitant AEDs should be completely withdrawn over 3-6 weeks, while the maximum dose of Trileptal should be reached in about 2-4 weeks. Trileptal may be increased as clinically indicated by a maximum increment of 600 mg/day at approximately weekly intervals to achieve the recommended daily dose of 2400 mg/day. A daily dose of 1200 mg/day has been shown in one study to be effective in patients in whom monotherapy has been initiated with Trileptal. Patients should be observed closely during this transition phase.

Initiation of Monotherapy

Patients not currently being treated with AEDs may have monotherapy initiated with Trileptal. In these patients, Trileptal should be initiated at a dose of 600 mg/day (given in a BID regimen); the dose should be increased by 300 mg/day every third day to a dose of 1200 mg/day. Controlled trials in these patients examined the effectiveness of a 1200 mg/day dose; a dose of 2400 mg/day has been shown to be effective in patients converted from other AEDs to Trileptal monotherapy *(see above).*

Pediatric Patients Age 4-16

Adjunctive Therapy

Treatment should be initiated at a daily dose of 8-10 mg/kg generally not to exceed 600 mg/day, given in a BID regimen. The target maintenance dose of Trileptal should be achieved over 2 weeks, and is dependent upon patient weight, according to the following chart:

20-29 kg - 900 mg/day
29.1-39 kg - 1200 mg/day
>39 kg - 1800 mg/day

In the clinical trial, in which the intention was to reach these target doses, the median daily dose was 31 mg/kg with a range of 6-51 mg/kg.
The pharmacokinetics of Trileptal are similar in older children (age >8 yrs) and adults. However, younger children (age <8 yrs) have an increased clearance (by about 30%-40%) compared with older children and adults. In the controlled trial, pediatric patients 8 years old and below received the highest maintenance doses.
Children below 2 years of age have not been studied in controlled clinical trials.

Patients with Hepatic Impairment

In general, dose adjustments are not required in patients with mild-to-moderate hepatic impairment *(see CLINICAL PHARMACOLOGY, Pharmacokinetics, Special Populations subsection).*

Patients with Renal Impairment

In patients with impaired renal function (creatine clearance <30 mL/min) Trileptal therapy should be initiated at one-half the usual starting dose (300 mg/day) and increased

Continued on next page

Trileptal—Cont.

slowly to achieve the desired clinical response *(see CLINICAL PHARMACOLOGY, Pharmacokinetics, Special Populations subsection).*

HOW SUPPLIED

150 mg Film-Coated Tablets: yellow, ovaloid, slightly biconvex, scored on both sides. Imprinted with T/D on one side and C/G on the other side.

Bottle of 100 .... NDC 0078-0336-05
Bottle of 1000 .... NDC 0078-0336-09
Unit Dose (blister pack)
Box of 100 (strips of 10) .... NDC 0078-0336-06

300 mg Film-Coated Tablets: yellow, ovaloid, slightly biconvex, scored on both sides. Imprinted with TE/TE on one side and CG/CG on the other side.

Bottle of 100 .... NDC 0078-0337-05
Bottle of 1000 .... NDC 0078-0337-09
Unit Dose (blister pack)
Box of 100 (strips of 10) .... NDC 0078-0337-06

600 mg Film-Coated Tablets: yellow, ovaloid, slightly biconvex, scored on both sides. Imprinted with TF/TF on one side and CG/CG on the other side.

Bottle of 100 .... NDC 0078-0338-05
Bottle of 1000 .... NDC 0078-0338-09
Unit Dose (blister pack)
Box of 100 (strips of 10) .... NDC 0078-0338-06

Store at 25°C (77°F); excursions permitted to 15°C-30°C (59°F-86°F) [see USP Controlled Room Temperature]. Dispense in tight container (USP).

REV: JANUARY 2000 T2000-01

Manufactured by:
Novartis Pharma Stein AG
Schaffhauserstrasse 48
CH-4332 Stein
Switzerland for
Novartis Pharmaceuticals Corporation
East Hanover, New Jersey 07936

Shown in Product Identification Guide, page 326

VIVELLE® ℞

estradiol transdermal system
Continuous delivery for twice-weekly application
Rx only
Prescribing Information

The following prescribing information is based on official labelling in effect November 2000.

ESTROGENS HAVE BEEN REPORTED TO INCREASE THE RISK OF ENDOMETRIAL CARCINOMA IN POSTMENOPAUSAL WOMEN.

Close clinical surveillance of all women taking estrogens is important. Adequate diagnostic measures, including endometrial sampling when indicated, should be undertaken to rule out malignancy in all cases of undiagnosed persistent or recurring abnormal vaginal bleeding. There is no evidence that "natural" estrogens are more or less hazardous than "synthetic" estrogens at equiestrogenic doses.

DESCRIPTION

The Vivelle estradiol transdermal system contains estradiol in a multipolymeric adhesive. The system is designed to release estradiol continuously upon application to intact skin. Five systems are available to provide nominal in vivo delivery of 0.025, 0.0375, 0.05, 0.075, or 0.1 mg of estradiol per day via skin of average permeability. Each corresponding system having an active surface area of 7.25, 11.0, 14.5, 22.0 or 29.0 cm^2 contains 2.17, 3.28, 4.33, 6.57, or 8.66 mg of estradiol USP, respectively. The composition of the systems per unit area is identical.

Estradiol USP is a white, crystalline powder, chemically described as estra-1,3,5 (10)-triene-3,17β-diol.

The structural formula is

The molecular formula of estradiol is $C_{18}H_{24}O_2$. The molecular weight is 272.39.

The Vivelle system comprises three layers. Proceeding from the visible surface toward the surface attached to the skin, these layers are (1) a translucent flexible film consisting of an ethylene vinyl alcohol copolymer film, a polyurethane film, urethane polymer and epoxy resin, (2) an adhesive formulation containing estradiol, acrylic adhesive, polyisobutylene, ethylene vinyl acetate copolymer, 1,3 butylene glycol, styrene-butadiene rubber, oleic acid, lecithin, propylene glycol, bentonite, mineral oil, and dipropylene glycol, and (3) a polyester release liner that is attached to the adhesive surface and must be removed before the system can be used. [See figure at top of next column]

The active component of the system is estradiol. The remaining components of the system are pharmacologically inactive.

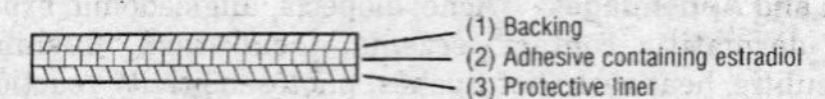

CLINICAL PHARMACOLOGY

Vivelle system provides systemic estrogen replacement therapy by releasing estradiol, the major estrogenic hormone secreted by the human ovary. Estrogens are largely responsible for the development and maintenance of the female reproductive system and secondary sexual characteristics. Although circulating estrogens exist in a dynamic equilibrium of metabolic interconversions, estradiol is the principal intracellular human estrogen and is substantially more potent than its metabolites, estrone and estriol at the receptor level. The primary source of estrogen in normally cycling adult women is the ovarian follicle, which secretes 70 to 500 µg of estradiol daily, depending on the phase of the menstrual cycle. After menopause, most endogenous estrogen is produced by conversion of androstenedione, secreted by the adrenal cortex, to estrone by peripheral tissues. Thus, estrone and the sulfate conjugated form, estrone sulfate, are the most abundant circulating estrogens in postmenopausal women.

Circulating estrogens modulate the pituitary secretion of the gonadotropins, luteinizing hormone (LH) and follicle stimulating hormone (FSH) through a negative feedback mechanism and estrogen replacement therapy acts to reduce the elevated levels of these hormones seen in postmenopausal women.

Pharmacokinetics

Absorption

In a multiple-dose study consisting of three consecutive patch applications of the Vivelle system, which was conducted in 17 healthy, postmenopausal women, blood levels of estradiol and estrone were compared following application of these units to sites on the abdomen and buttocks in a crossover fashion. Patches that deliver nominal estradiol doses of approximately 0.0375 mg/day and 0.1 mg/day were applied to abdominal application sites while the 0.1 mg/day doses were also applied to sites on the buttocks. These systems increased estradiol levels above baseline within 4 hours and maintained respective mean levels of 25 and 79 pg/mL above baseline following application to the abdomen; slightly higher mean levels of 88 pg/mL above baseline were observed following application to the buttocks. At the same time, increases in estrone plasma concentrations averaged about 12 and 50 pg/mL, respectively, following application to the abdomen and 61 pg/mL for the buttocks. While plasma concentrations of estradiol and estrone remained slightly above baseline at 12 hours following removal of the patches in this study, results from another study show these levels to return to baseline values within 24 hours following removal of the patches.

The figure (see Figure 1) illustrates the mean plasma concentrations of estradiol at steady-state during application of these patches at four different dosages.

Figure 1
Steady-State Estradiol Plasma Concentrations for Systems Applied to the Abdomen
Nonbaseline-corrected levels

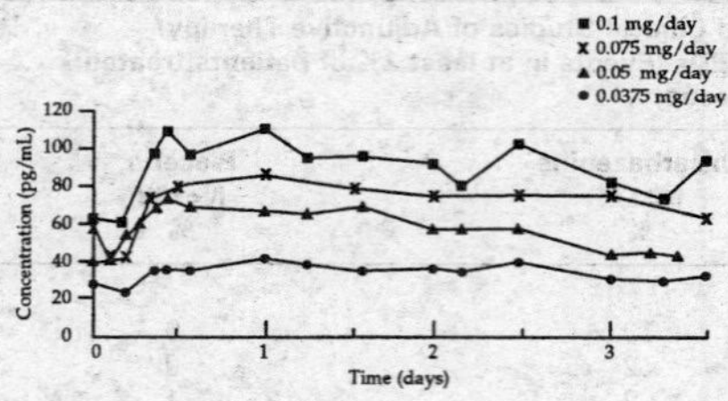

The corresponding pharmacokinetic parameters are summarized in the table below.

Steady-State Estradiol Pharmacokinetic Parameters for Systems Applied to the Abdomen (mean ± standard deviation)
Nonbaseline-corrected data*

Dosage (mg/day)	C_{max}† (pg/mL)	C_{avg}‡ (pg/mL)	C_{min} (84 hr)§ (pg/mL)
0.0375	46 ± 16	34 ± 10	30 ± 10
0.05	83 ± 41	57 ± 23#	41 ± 11#
0.075	99 ± 35	72 ± 24	60 ± 24
0.1	133 ± 51	89 ± 38	90 ± 44
0.1¶	145 ± 71	104 ± 52	85 ± 47

*Mean baseline estradiol concentration = 11.7 pg/mL
†Peak plasma concentration
‡Average plasma concentration
§Minimum plasma concentration at 84 hr
#Measured over 80 hr
¶Applied to the buttocks

Distribution

The distribution of exogenous estrogens is similar to that of endogenous estrogens. Estrogens are widely distributed in the body and are generally found in higher concentrations in the sex hormone target organs. Estradiol and other naturally occurring estrogens are bound mainly to sex hormone binding globulin (SHBG), and to a lesser degree to albumin.

Metabolism

Exogenous estrogens are metabolized in the same manner as endogenous estrogens. Circulating estrogens exist in a dynamic equilibrium of metabolic interconversions. These transformations take place mainly in the liver. Estradiol is converted reversibly to estrone, and both can be converted to estriol, which is the major urinary metabolite. Estrogens also undergo enterohepatic recirculation via sulfate and glucuronide conjugation in the liver, biliary secretion of conjugates into the intestine, and hydrolysis in the gut followed by reabsorption. In postmenopausal women, a significant portion of the circulating estrogens exist as sulfate conjugated, especially estrone sulfate, which serves as a circulating reservoir for the formation of more active estrogens.

Excretion

Estradiol, estrone, and estriol are excreted in the urine along with glucuronide and sulfate conjugates. Studies conducted with the Vivelle system show the drug has an apparent mean half-life of 4.4 ± 2.3 hours. After removal of the transdermal systems, serum concentrations of estradiol and estrone returned to baseline levels within 24 hours.

Special Populations

The Vivelle system has been studied only in healthy postmenopausal women (approximately 90% Caucasian). The Vivelle system has not been studied in patients with renal or hepatic impairment.

Drug Interactions

No drug interaction studies were conducted with the Vivelle system.

Adhesion

Data showing the number of systems in controlled studies that required replacement due to inadequate adhesion is not available.

Clinical Studies

In two controlled clinical trials of 356 subjects, the 0.075 and 0.1 mg doses were superior to placebo in relieving vasomotor symptoms at Week 4, and maintained efficacy through Weeks 8 and 12 of treatment. The 0.0375 and 0.05 mg doses, however, did not differ from placebo until approximately Week 6.

Therefore, an additional 12-week placebo-controlled study in 255 patients was performed to establish the efficacy of the lowest dose of 0.0375 mg. The baseline mean daily number of hot flushes in these 255 patients was 11.5. Results at Weeks 4, 8, and 12 of treatment are shown in the figure below. (See Figure 2)

Figure 2
Mean (SD) change from baseline in mean daily number of flushes for Vivelle 0.0375 mg versus Placebo in a 12-week trial.

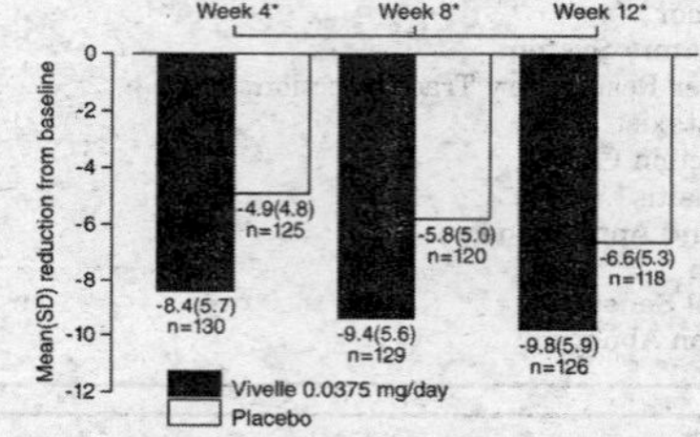

*Indicates statistically significant difference (p<0.05) between Vivelle and placebo

The 0.0375 mg dose was superior to placebo in reducing both the frequency and severity of vasomotor symptoms at Week 4 and maintained efficacy through Weeks 8 and 12 of treatment. All doses of Vivelle (0.0375 mg, 0.05 mg, 0.075 mg, and 0.1 mg) are effective for the control of vasomotor symptoms.

Efficacy and safety of the Vivelle system in the prevention of postmenopausal osteoporosis have been studied in a 2-year double-blind, randomized, placebo-controlled, parallel group study. A total of 261 hysterectomized (161) and non-hysterectomized (100), surgically or naturally menopausal women (within 5 years of menopause), with no evidence of osteoporosis (lumbar spine bone mineral density within 2 standard deviations of average peak bone mass, i.e., ≥ 0.827 g/cm^2) were enrolled in this study; 194 patients were randomized to one of the four doses of Vivelle (0.1, 0.05, 0.0375, or 0.025 mg/day) and 67 patients to placebo. Over 2 years, study systems were applied to the buttock or the abdomen twice a week. Non-hysterectomized women received oral medroxyprogesterone acetate (2.5 mg/day) throughout the study.

The study population comprised naturally (82%) or surgically (18%) menopausal, hysterectomized (61%) or non-hysterectomized (39%) women with a mean age of 52.0 years (range 27 to 62 years); the mean duration of menopause was 31.7 months (range 2 to 72 months). Two hundred thirty-two (89%) or randomized subjects (173 on active drug, 59 on placebo) contributed data to the analysis of percent change from baseline in bone mineral density (BMD) of the AP lumbar spine, the primary efficacy variable. Patients were given supplemental dietary calcium (1000 mg elemental calcium/day) but no supplemental vitamin D. There was an increase in BMD of the AP lumbar spine in all Vivelle dose groups; in contrast to this, a decrease in AP lumbar spine BMD was observed in placebo patients. All Vivelle doses were significantly superior to placebo (p<0.05) at all time points with the exception of Vivelle 0.05 mg/day at 6 months. The highest dose of Vivelle was superior to the three lower doses. There were no statistically significant differences in pairwise comparisons among the three lower doses. (See Figure 3.)

Figure 3
Bone mineral density - AP Lumbar spine
Least squares means of percentage change from baseline
All randomized patients with at least one post-baseline assessment available with last post-baseline observation carried forward

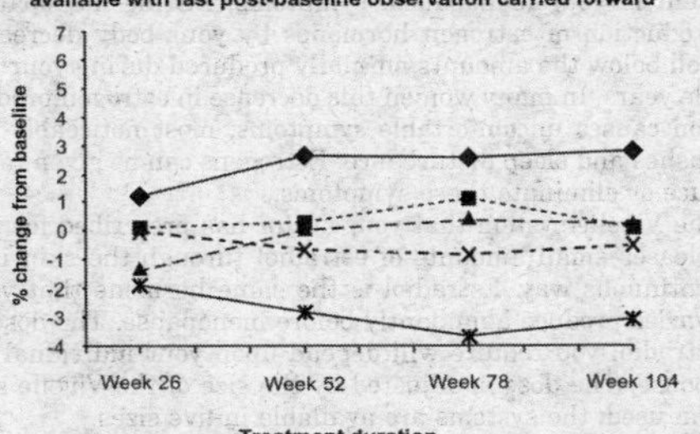

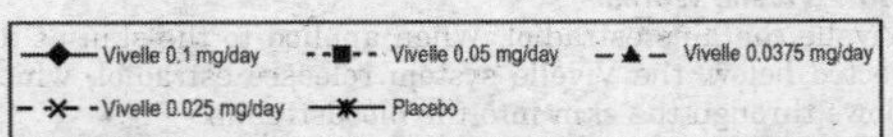

Analysis of percent change from baseline in femoral neck BMD, a secondary efficacy outcome variable, showed qualitatively similar results; all doses of Vivelle were significantly superior to placebo ($p<0.05$) at 24 months. The highest Vivelle dose was superior to placebo at all time points. A mixture of significant and non-significant results were obtained for the lower dose groups at earlier time points. The highest Vivelle dose was superior to the three lower doses, and there were no significant differenes among the three lower doses at this skeletal site. (See Figure 4.)

Figure 4
Bone mineral density - Femoral neck
Least squares means of percentage change from baseline
All randomized patients with at least one post-baseline assessment available with last post-baseline observation carried forward

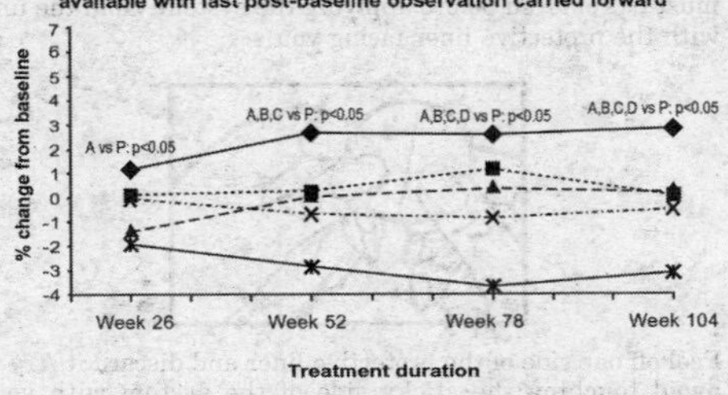

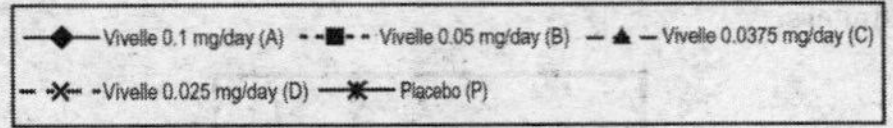

The mean serum osteocalcin (a marker of bone formation) and urinary excretion of cross-link N-telopeptides of type 1 collagen (a marker of bone resportion) decreased numerically in most of the active treatment groups relative to baseline. However, the decreases in both markers were inconsistent across treatment groups and the differences between active treatment groups and placebo were not statistically significant.

INDICATIONS AND USAGE

Vivelle® (estradiol transdermal system) is indicated in the following:

1. Treatment of moderate-to-severe vasomotor symptoms associated with the menopause.
2. Treatment of vulvar and vaginal atrophy.
3. Treatment of hypoestrogenism due to hypogonadism, castration, or primary ovarian failure.
4. Prevention of postmenopausal osteoporosis (in at-risk patients). Estrogen replacement therapy reduces bone resorption and retards postmenopausal bone loss. When estrogen therapy is discontinued, bone mass declines at a rate comparable to that of the immediate postmenopausal period.

   White and Asian women are at higher risk for osteoporosis than black women, and thin women are at a higher risk than heavier women, who generally have higher endogenous estrogen levels. Early menopause is one of the strongest predictors for the development of osteoporosis. Other factors associated with osteoporosis include genetic factors (small build, family history), lifestyle (cigarette smoking, alcohol abuse, sedentary exercise habits) and nutrition (below average body weight and dietary calcium intake).

   Essential to the prevention and management of osteoporosis are weight-bearing exercise and adequate calcium intake. Postmenopausal women absorb dietary calcium less efficiently than premenopausal women and require an average of 1500 mg/day of elemental calcium to remain in neutral calcium balance. The average calcium intake in the USA is 400–600 mg/day. Therefore, when not contraindicated, calcium supplementation may be helpful for women with suboptimal dietary intake.

CONTRAINDICATIONS

Patients with known hypersensitivity to any of the components of the therapeutic system should not use Vivelle.

Estrogens should not be used in individuals with any of the following conditions:

1. Known or suspected pregnancy (see PRECAUTIONS). Estrogen may cause fetal harm when administered to a pregnant woman.
2. Undiagnosed abnormal genital bleeding.
3. Known or suspected cancer of the breast.
4. Known or suspected estrogen-dependent neoplasia.
5. Active thrombophlebitis or thromboembolic disorders, or a documented history of these conditions.

WARNINGS

1. *Induction of Malignant Neoplasms.*

a. *Breast cancer.* While some epidemiologic studies suggest a very modest increase in breast cancer risk for estrogen alone users versus non-users, other studies have not shown any increased risk. The addition of progestin to estrogen may increase the risk for breast cancer over that noted in non-hormone users more significantly (by about 24–40%), although this is based solely on epidemiologic studies, and definitive conclusions await prospective, controlled clinical trials.

Women without a uterus who require hormone replacement should receive estrogen-alone therapy, and should not be exposed unnecessarily to progestins. Women with a uterus who are candidates for short-term combination estrogen/progestin therapy (for relief of vasomotor symptoms) are not felt to be at a substantially increased risk for breast cancer. Women with a uterus who are candidates for long-term use of estrogen/progestin therapy should be advised of potential benefits and risks (including the potential for an increased risk of breast cancer). All women should receive yearly breast exams by a health-care provider and perform monthly breast self-examinations. In addition, mammography examinations should be scheduled as suggested by providers based on patient age and risk factors.

b. *Endometrial cancer.* The reported endometrial cancer risk among unopposed estrogen users is about 2- to 12-fold greater than in nonusers and appears dependent on duration of treatment and on estrogen dose. Most studies show no significant increased risk associated with the use of estrogens for less than 1 year. The greatest risk appears associated with prolonged use with increased risks of 15- to 24-fold for five to 10 years or more. In three studies, persistence of risk was demonstrated for 8 to over 15 years after cessation of estrogen treatment. In one study, a significant decrease in the incidence of endometrial cancer occurred six months after estrogen withdrawal. Concurrent progestin therapy may offset this risk, but the overall health impact in postmenopausal women is not known (see PRECAUTIONS).

c. *Congenital reproductive tract disorders.* Estrogen therapy during pregnancy is associated with an increased risk of fetal congenital reproductive tract disorders. In female offspring, there is an increased risk of vaginal adenosis, squamous cell dysplasia of the cervix, and clear cell vaginal cancer later in life; in males, urogenital and possibly testicular abnormalities. Although some of these changes are benign, it is not known whether they are precursors of malignancy.

2. *Gallbladder Disease.* Two studies have reported a 2- to 4-fold increase in the risk of surgically confirmed gallbladder disease in postmenopausal women receiving oral estrogen replacement therapy, similar to the 2-fold increase previously noted in users of oral contraceptives.

3. *Cardiovascular Disease.* Large doses of estrogen (5 mg conjugated estrogens per day), comparable to those used to treat cancer of the prostate and breast, have been shown in a large prospective clinical trial in men to increase the risks of nonfatal myocardial infarction, pulmonary embolism, and thrombophlebitis. These risks cannot necessarily be extrapolated from men to women. However, to avoid the theoretical cardiovascular risk to women caused by high estrogen doses, the dose for estrogen replacement therapy should not exceed the lowest effective dose.

4. *Elevated Blood Pressure.* Occasional blood pressure increases during estrogen replacement therapy have been attributed to idiosyncratic reactions to estrogens. More often, blood pressure has remained the same or has dropped. Postmenopausal estrogen use does not increase the risk of stroke. Nonetheless, blood pressure should be monitored at regular intervals with estrogen use, especially if high doses are used. Ethinyl estradiol and conjugated estrogens have been shown to increase renin substrate. In contrast to these oral estrogens, transdermally administered estradiol does not affect renin substrate.

5. *Hypercalcemia.* Administration of estrogen may lead to severe hypercalcemia in patients with breast cancer and bone metastases. If this occurs, the drug should be stopped and appropriate measures taken to reduce the serum calcium level.

PRECAUTIONS

General

1. *Addition of a Progestin.* Studies of the addition of a progestin for 10 or more days of a cycle of estrogen administration or daily in an estrogen/progestin continuous regimen have reported a lower incidence of endometrial hyperplasia than would be induced by estrogen treatment alone. Morphologic and biochemical studies of endometria suggest that 10 to 14 days of progestin are needed to provide maximal maturation of the endometrium and to reduce the likelihood of hyperplastic changes.

There are, however, possible risks that may be associated with the use of progestins in estrogen replacement regimens. These include:

(1) adverse effects on lipoprotein metabolism (lowering HDL and raising LDL), which could diminish the purported cardioprotective effect of estrogen therapy (see PRECAUTIONS, below);
(2) impairment of glucose tolerance; and
(3) Possible enhancement of mitotic activity in breast epithelial tissue, although few epidemiologic data are available to address this point (see PRECAUTIONS, below).

The choice of progestin, its dose, and its regimen may be important in minimizing these adverse effects, but these issues will require further study before they are clarified.

2. *Cardiovascular Risk.* The effects of estrogen replacement on the risk of cardiovascular disease have not been adequately studied. However, data from the Heart and Estrogen/Progestin Replacement Study (HERS), a controlled clinical trial of secondary prevention of 2,763 postmenopausal women with documented heart disease, demonstrated no benefit. During an average follow-up of 4.1 years, treatment with oral conjugated estrogen plus medroxyprogesterone acetate did not reduce the overall rate of coronary heart disease (CHD) events in postmenopausal women with established coronary disease. There were more CHD events in the hormone treated group than in the placebo group in year 1, but fewer events in years 3 through 5.

3. *Physical Examination.* A complete medical and family history should be taken prior to the initiation of any estrogen therapy. The pretreatment and periodic physical examinations should include special reference to blood pressure, breasts, abdomen, and pelvic organs and should include a Papanicolaou smear. As a general rule, estrogen should not be prescribed for longer than one year without reexamining the patient.

4. *Hypercoagulability.* Some studies have shown that women taking estrogen replacement therapy have hypercoagulability, primarily related to decreased antithrombin activity. This effect appears dose- and duration-dependent and is less pronounced than that associated with oral contraceptive use. Also, postmenopausal women tend to have increased coagulation parameters at baseline compared to premenopausal women. Epidemiological studies, which employed primary orally administered estrogen products, have suggested that hormone replacement therapy (HRT) is associated with an increased relative risk of developing venous thromboembolism (VTE), e.g., deep venous thrombosis or pulmonary embolism. Risk/benefit should therefore be carefully weighed in consultation with the patient when prescribing any form of HRT to women with a risk factor for VTE.

5. *Familial Hyperlipoproteinemia.* Estrogen therapy may be associated with massive elevations of plasma triglycerides leading to pancreatitis and other complications in patients with familial defects of lipoprotein metabolism.

6. *Fluid Retention.* Because estrogens may cause some degree of fluid retention, conditions that might be exacerbated by this factor, such as asthma, epilepsy, migraine, and cardiac or renal dysfunction, require careful observation.

7. *Uterine Bleeding and Mastodynia.* Certain patients may develop undesirable manifestations of estrogenic stimulation, such as abnormal uterine bleeding and mastodynia.

8. *Impaired Liver Function.* Estrogens may be poorly metabolized in patients with impaired liver function and should be administered with caution.

Information for the Patient

See text of Patient Package Insert, which appears after the HOW SUPPLIED section.

Laboratory Tests

Estrogen administration should generally be guided by clinical response at the smallest dose, rather than laboratory monitoring, for relief of symptoms for those indications in which symptoms are observable.

Drug/Laboratory Test Interactions

Some of these drug/laboratory test interactions have been observed only with estrogen progestin combinations (oral contraceptives):

1. Accelerated prothrombin time, partial thromboplastin time, and platelet aggregation time; increased platelet count; increased factors II, VII antigen, VIII antigen, VIII coagulant activity, IX, X, XII, VII-X complex, II-VII-X complex; and beta-thromboglobulin; decreased levels of anti-factor Xa and antithrombin III; decreased antithrombin III activity; increased levels of fibrinogen and fibrinogen activity; increased plasminogen antigen and activity.
2. Increased thyroid-binding globulin (TBG) leading to increased circulating total thyroid hormone, as measured by protein-bound iodine (PBI), T_4 levels (by column or by radioimmunoassay) or T_3 levels by radioimmunoassay. T_3 resin uptake is decreased, reflecting the elevated TBG. Free T_4 and free T_3 concentrations are unaltered.
3. Other binding proteins may be elevated in serum, i.e., corticosteroid binding globulin (CBG), sex hormone-binding globulin (SHBG), leading to increased circulating corticosteroids and sex steroids, respectively. Free or biologically active hormone concentrations are unchanged. Other plasma proteins may be increased (angiotensinogen/renin substrate, alpha-1-antitrypsin, ceruloplasmin).
4. Increased plasma HDL and HDL_2 subfraction concentrations, reduced LDL cholesterol concentration, increased triglyceride levels.
5. Impaired glucose tolerance.
6. Reduced response to metyrapone test.
7. Reduced serum folate concentration.

Continued on next page

Vivelle—Cont.

Carcinogenesis, Mutagenesis, and Impairment of Fertility
Long-term, continuous administration of natural and synthetic estrogens in certain animal species increases the frequency of carcinomas of the breast, cervix, vagina, testis, and liver (see CONTRAINDICATIONS and WARNINGS).

Pregnancy Category X
Estrogens should not be used during pregnancy. There is no indication for estrogen therapy during pregnancy or during the immediate postpartum period. Estrogens are ineffective for the prevention or treatment of threatened or habitual abortion. Estrogens are not indicated for the prevention of postpartum breast engorgement.

Estrogen therapy during pregnancy is associated with an increased risk of congenital defects in the reproductive organs of the fetus, and possibly other birth defects. Studies of women who received diethylstilbestrol (DES) during pregnancy have shown that female offspring have an increased risk of vaginal adenosis, squamous cell dysplasia of the uterine cervix, and clear cell vaginal cancer later in life; male offspring have an increased risk of urogenital abnormalities and possibly testicular cancer later in life. The 1985 DES Task Force concluded that use of DES during pregnancy is associated with a subsequent increased risk of breast cancer in the mothers, although a causal relationship remains unproven and the observed level of excess risk is similar to that for a number of other breast cancer risk factors.

Nursing Mothers
Estrogen administration to nursing mothers has been shown to decrease the quantity and quality of the milk.

Pediatric Use
The safety and effectiveness in pediatric patients have not been established.

Geriatric Use
The safety and effectiveness in geriatric patients (over age 65) have not been established.

ADVERSE REACTIONS

See WARNINGS and Boxed Warning regarding the potential adverse effects on the fetus, the induction of malignant neoplasms, gallbladder disease, cardiovascular disease, elevated blood pressure, and hypercalcemia.

The most commonly reported systemic adverse event to the Vivelle system in controlled clinical trials was headache. This occurred in approximately 36% of patients treated with active systems and in 30% of patients treated with placebo. The most common topical adverse events in these trials were erythema and pruritus at the application site. Most cases were considered mild. Fewer than 5% of patients on active drug at the final visit of the study had reactions of greater than mild intensity. Rash was reported in approximately 5% of patients treated with active systems and in approximately 4% of patients treated with placebo in these trials. Two patients out of 356 were discontinued from the trials due to skin irritation/erythema.

In a 2-year controlled trial, back pain was reported in 13% of patients treated with the Vivelle system and 4.5% of patients treated with placebo. Local application site reactions (patch site erythema, itching, rash, burning, irritation) were reported in approximately 9% of patients treated with active systems and 10% of patients treated with placebo. In most cases, the local application site reactions were considered mild; none was considered severe. Two patients out of 259 were discontinued from the trial due to local application site reactions. Vaginal bleeding and breast tenderness were more common in the highest dose group (0.1 mg/day) than in the three other active treatment groups or in placebo-treated patients.

The following additional adverse reactions have been reported with estrogen therapy:

1. *Genitourinary system.* Changes in vaginal bleeding pattern and abnormal withdrawal bleeding or flow; breakthrough bleeding, spotting; increase in size of uterine leiomyomata; vaginal candidiasis; change in amount of cervical secretion.
2. *Breasts.* Tenderness, enlargement.
3. *Gastrointestinal.* Nausea, vomiting; abdominal cramps, bloating; cholestatic jaundice; gallbladder disease.
4. *Skin.* Chloasma or melasma that may persist when drug is discontinued; erythema multiforme; erythema nodosum; hemorrhagic eruption; loss of scalp hair; hirsutism.
5. *Eyes.* Steepening of corneal curvature; intolerance to contact lenses.
6. *Central Nervous System.* Headache, migraine, dizziness; mental depression; chorea.
7. *Miscellaneous.* Increase or decrease in weight; reduced carbohydrate tolerance; aggravation of porphyria; edema; changes in libido.

Post-Marketing Adverse Events
Although a causal relationship with Vivelle has not been established, adverse events reported from marketing experience include: isolated reports of anaphylaxis, rare elevated liver function tests, and reports of leg pain.

OVERDOSAGE

Serious ill effects have not been reported following acute ingestion of large doses of estrogen-containing oral contraceptives by young children. Overdosage of estrogen may cause nausea and vomiting, and withdrawal bleeding may occur in females.

DOSAGE AND ADMINISTRATION

The adhesive side of the Vivelle system should be placed on a clean, dry area of the trunk of the body (including the abdomen or buttocks). *The Vivelle system should not be applied to the breasts.* The Vivelle system should be replaced twice weekly. The sites of application must be rotated, with an interval of at least 1 week allowed between applications to a particular site. The area selected should not be oily, damaged, or irritated. The waistline should be avoided, since tight clothing may rub the system off. The system should be applied immediately after opening the pouch and removing the protective liner. The system should be pressed firmly in place with the palm of the hand for about 10 seconds, making sure there is good contact, especially around the edges. In the event that a system should fall off, the same system may be reapplied. If necessary, a new system may be applied. In either case, the original treatment schedule should be continued.

Initiation of Therapy
For treatment of moderate-to-severe vasomotor symptoms and vulvar and vaginal atrophy associated with the menopause, start therapy with Vivelle estradiol transdermal system 0.0375 mg/day applied to the skin twice weekly. In order to use the lowest dosage necessary for the control of symptoms, decisions to increase dosage should not be made until after the first month of therapy. Attempts to discontinue or taper medication should be made at 3-month to 6-month intervals.

In women not currently taking oral estrogens or in women switching from another estradiol transdermal therapy, treatment with the Vivelle estradiol transdermal system may be initiated at once. In women who are currently taking oral estrogens, treatment with the Vivelle estradiol transdermal system should be initiated 1 week after withdrawal of oral hormone replacement therapy, or sooner if menopausal symptoms reappear in less than 1 week.

For the prevention of postmenopausal osteoporosis, the minimum dose that has been shown to be effective is the 0.025 mg/day system. The dosage may be adjusted as necessary. Reproductive system-associated adverse events were encountered more frequently in the highest dose group (0.1 mg/day) than in other active treatment dose groups or in placebo-treated patients.

Therapeutic Regimen
Vivelle may be given continuously in patients who do not have an intact uterus. In those patients with an intact uterus, Vivelle may be given continuously or on a cyclic schedule (e.g., three weeks on drug followed by one week off drug) with a progestin.

HOW SUPPLIED

Vivelle estradiol transdermal system 0.025 mg/day—each 7.25 cm^2 system contains 2.17 mg of estradiol USP for nominal* delivery of 0.025 mg of estradiol per day.
Patient Calendar Pack of 8 systems ... NDC 0078-0348-42
Carton of 6 Patient Calendar Packs of 8 systems ..... NDC 0078-0348-44

Vivelle estradiol transdermal system 0.0375 mg/day—each 11.0 cm^2 system contains 3.28 mg of estradiol USP for nominal* delivery of 0.0375 mg of estradiol per day.
Patient Calendar Pack of 8 systems ... NDC 0083-2325-08
Carton of 6 Patient Calendar Packs of 8 systems ..... NDC 0083-2325-62
Carton of 24 systems .... NDC 0083-2325-25

Vivelle estradiol transdermal system 0.05 mg/day—each 14.5 cm^2 system contains 4.33 mg of estradiol USP for nominal* delivery of 0.05 mg of estradiol per day.
Patient Calendar Pack of 8 systems .. NDC 0083-2326-08
Carton of 6 Patient Calendar Packs of 8 systems ..... NDC 0083-2326-62
Carton of 24 systems .... NDC 0083-2326-25

Vivelle estradiol transdermal system 0.075 mg/day—each 22.0 cm^2 system contains 6.57 mg of estradiol USP for nominal* delivery of 0.075 mg of estradiol per day.
Patient Calendar Pack of 8 systems .. NDC 0083-2327-08
Carton of 6 Patient Calendar Packs of 8 systems ..... NDC 0083-2327-62
Carton of 24 systems .... NDC 0083-2327-25

Vivelle estradiol transdermal system 0.1 mg/day—each 29.0 cm^2 system contains 8.66 mg of estradiol USP for nominal* delivery of 0.1 mg of estradiol per day.
Patient Calendar Pack of 8 systems .. NDC 0083-2328-08
Carton of 6 Patient Calendar Packs of 8 systems ..... NDC 0083-2328-62
Carton of 24 systems .... NDC 0083-2328-25

*See DESCRIPTION

Do not store above 86°F (30°C). Do not store unpouched. Apply immediately upon removal from the protective pouch.

REV: AUGUST 2000 T2000-52

Information for the Patient

Vivelle®
estradiol transdermal system
Rx only

ESTROGENS INCREASE THE RISK OF CANCER OF THE UTERUS IN WOMEN WHO HAVE HAD THEIR MENOPAUSE ("CHANGE OF LIFE").
If you use any estrogen-containing drug, it is important to visit your doctor regularly and report any unusual vaginal bleeding right away. Vaginal bleeding after menopause may be a warning sign of uterine cancer. Your doctor should evaluate any unusual vaginal bleeding to find out the cause.

INTRODUCTION
Your doctor has prescribed the Vivelle system for the treatment of your menopausal symptoms. During menopause, production of estrogen hormones by your body decreases well below the amounts normally produced during your fertile years. In many women this decrease in estrogen production causes uncomfortable symptoms, most noticeably hot flushes and sleep disturbance. Estrogens can be given to reduce or eliminate these symptoms.

The Vivelle system that your doctor has prescribed for you releases small amounts of estradiol through the skin in a continuous way. Estradiol is the same hormone that your ovaries produce abundantly before menopause. The dose of estradiol you require will depend upon your individual response. The dose is adjusted by the size of the Vivelle system used; the systems are available in five sizes.

INFORMATION ABOUT VIVELLE

How Vivelle works
Vivelle contains estradiol. When applied to the skin as directed below, the Vivelle system releases estradiol, which flows through the skin into the bloodstream.

How and Where to Apply Vivelle
Each system is individually sealed in a protective pouch. Tear open this pouch at the indentation (do not use scissors) and remove the system.

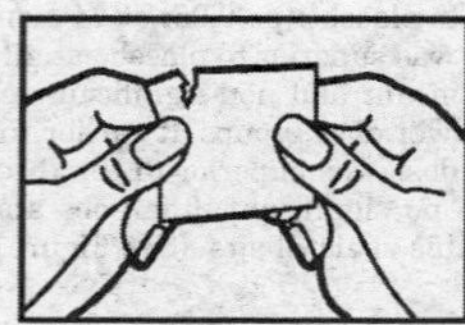

A stiff protective liner covers the adhesive side of the system – the side that will be placed against your skin. This liner must be removed before applying the system. Hold the unit with the protective liner facing you.

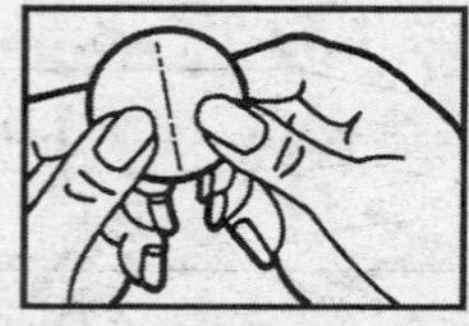

Peel off one side of the protective liner and discard it. Try to avoid touching the sticky side of the system with your fingers.

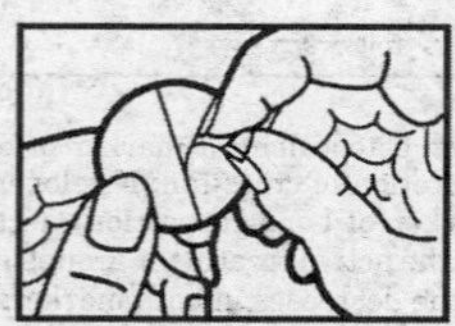

Using the other half of the liner as a handle, apply the sticky side of the system to a dry area of the skin on the trunk of the body (including the abdomen or buttocks). Press the sticky side on the skin and smooth down.

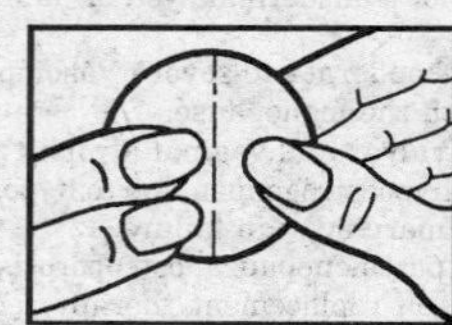

Fold back the remaining side of the system. Grasp the straight edge of the protective liner and pull it off the system.

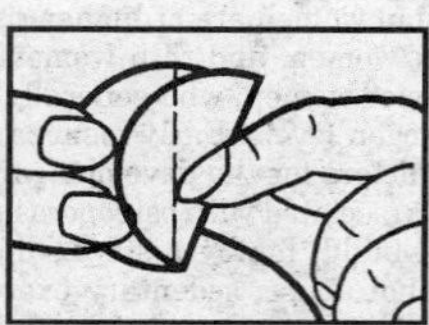

Press the system firmly in place.

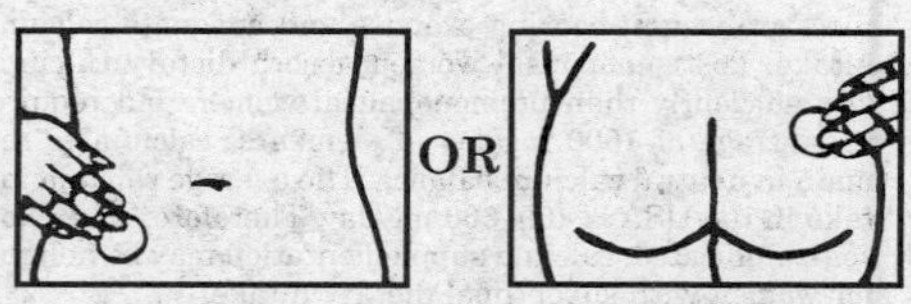

Some women may find that it is more comfortable to wear Vivelle on the buttocks. *Do not apply Vivelle to your breasts.* The sites of application must be rotated, with an interval of at least 1 week allowed between applications to a particular site. The area selected should not be oily, damaged, or irritated. Avoid the waistline, since tight clothing may rub the system off. Apply the system immediately after opening the pouch and removing the protective liner. Press the system firmly in place with the palm of your hand for about 10 seconds, making sure there is good contact, especially around the edges.

The Vivelle system should be worn continuously until it is time to replace it with a new system. You may wish to experiment with different locations when applying a new system, to find ones that are most comfortable for you and where clothing will not rub on the system.

When to Apply Vivelle

The Vivelle system should be replaced twice weekly. Your Vivelle package contains a calendar checklist on the back to help you remember a schedule. Mark the 2-day schedule you plan to follow. Always change the system on the 2 days of the week you have marked.

When changing the system, remove the used Vivelle system and discard it. Any adhesive that might remain on your skin can be easily rubbed off. Then place the new Vivelle system on a different skin site. (The same skin site should not be used again for at least 1 week after removal of the system.)

Please note: Contact with water when you are bathing, swimming, or showering will not affect the system. In the event that a system should fall off, put this same system back on and continue to follow your original treatment schedule. If necessary, you may apply a new system but continue to follow your original schedule.

Benefits of treatment with Vivelle

Regular use of the Vivelle twice weekly offers relief of moderate-to-severe symptoms of menopause.

Small quantities of the naturally occurring hormone estradiol are absorbed through the skin from the Vivelle system, ensuring a continuous supply of circulating hormone in the body.

USES OF ESTROGEN

To reduce moderate or severe menopausal symptoms. Estrogens are hormones produced by the ovaries. The decrease in the amount of estrogen that occurs in all women, usually between ages 45 and 55, causes the menopause. Sometimes the ovaries are removed by an operation, causing "surgical menopause." When the amount of estrogen begins to decrease, some women develop very uncomfortable symptoms, such as feelings of warmth in the face, neck, and chest, or sudden intense episodes of heat and sweating ("hot flashes"). The use of drugs containing estrogens can help the body adjust to lower estrogen levels.

Some women have only mild menopausal symptoms, or none at all, and do not need estrogen therapy for these particular symptoms. Other women may need estrogens for a few months while their bodies adjust to lower estrogen levels. For the treatment of menopausal symptoms only, most women need estrogen replacement therapy for no longer than 6 months.

To treat vulvar and vaginal atrophy (itching, burning, dryness in or around the vagina, difficulty or burning on urination) *associated with menopause.*

To treat certain conditions in which a young woman's ovaries do not produce enough estrogen naturally.

To help prevent osteoporosis (thinning of bones). Osteoporosis is a thinning of the bones that makes them weaker and allows them to break more easily. The bones of the spine, wrists, and hips break most often in osteporosis. Both men and women start to lose bone mass after about age 40, but women lose bone mass faster after the menopause. Women who are likely to develop osteoporosis often have one or more of the following characteristics: white or Asian race, slim, cigarette smokers, and a family history of osteoporosis in a mother, sister, or aunt. Women who have relatively early menopause, often because their ovaries were removed during an operation (surgical menopause), are more likely to develop osteoporosis than women whose menopause happens at the average age.

Using estrogens after the menopause slows down bone thinning and may prevent bones from breaking. Lifelong adequate calcium intake, either in the diet (such as dairy products) or by calcium supplements (to reach a total daily intake of 1000 milligrams per day before menopause of 1500 milligrams per day after menopause), may help to prevent osteoporosis. Regular weight-bearing exercise may also help to prevent osteoporosis. Before you change your calcium intake or exercise habits, it is important to discuss these lifestyle changes with your doctor to find out if they are safe for you.

WHEN ESTROGENS SHOULD NOT BE USED

During pregnancy. If you think you may be pregnant, do not use any form of estrogen-containing drug. Using estrogens while you are pregnant may cause your unborn child to have birth defects. Estrogens do not prevent miscarriage (spontaneous abortion) and are not needed in the days following childbirth. If you take estrogens during pregnancy, your unborn child has a greater than usual chance of having birth defects. The risk of developing these defects is small, but clearly larger than the risk in children whose mothers did not take estrogens during pregnancy. These birth defects may affect the baby's urinary system and sex organs. Daughters born to mothers who took DES (an estrogen drug) have a higher than usual chance of developing cancer of the vagina or cervix when they become teenagers or young adults. Sons may have a higher than usual chance of developing cancer of the testicles when they become teenagers or young adults.

If you have unusual vaginal bleeding which has not been evaluated by your doctor (see Boxed Warning). Unusual vaginal bleeding can be a warning sign of cancer of the uterus, especially if it happens after menopause. Your doctor must find out the cause of the bleeding so that he or she can recommend the proper treatment. Taking estrogens without visiting your doctor can cause you serious harm if your vaginal bleeding is caused by cancer of the uterus.

If you have had cancer. Since estrogens increase the risk of certain types of cancer, you should not use estrogens if you have or have ever had cancer of the breast or uterus.

If you have any circulation problems. Estrogen therapy should be used only after consultation with your doctor and only in recommended doses. Patients with current or past abnormal blood clotting should not use estrogens (see DANGERS OF ESTROGENS, below).

When they are ineffective. During menopause, some women develop nervous symptoms or depression. Estrogens do not relieve these symptoms. You may have heard that taking estrogens for years after menopause will keep your skin soft and supple and keep you feeling young. There is no evidence for these claims and such long-term estrogen use may have serious risks.

After childbirth or when breastfeeding a baby. Estrogens should not be used to try to stop the breasts from filling with milk after a baby is born. Such treatment may increase the risk of developing blood clots (see DANGERS OF ESTROGEN, below).

If you are breastfeeding, you should avoid using any drugs because many drugs pass through to the baby in the milk. While nursing a baby, you should take drugs only on the advice of your healthcare provider.

DANGERS OF ESTROGENS

Cancer of the uterus. The risk of developing cancer of the uterus gets higher the longer estrogens are used and when larger doses are taken. One study showed that when estrogens are discontinued, this increased risk of cancer seems to fall off quickly. Three other studies showed that the risk for uterine cancer stayed high for 8 to more than 15 years after stopping estrogen treatment. Because of this risk, *it is important to take the lowest dose that works and to take it only as long as you need it.* Using progestin therapy together with estrogen therapy may reduce the higher risk of uterine cancer related to estrogen use (see OTHER INFORMATION, below).

If you have had your uterus removed (total hysterectomy), there is no danger of developing cancer of the uterus.

Cancer of the breast. Studies examining the risk of breast cancer among women using estrogen alone and combined estrogen/progestin therapy have suggested that there may be a mildly increased risk of breast cancer in women taking the combined therapy.

If you do not have your uterus, there is no need for combined estrogen/progestin therapy since estrogen alone therapy is sufficient and may pose less risk for breast cancer.

If you do have your uterus, you should discuss the benefits and risks of combined estrogen/progestin therapy with your health care provider. Regular breast exams by a health professional and monthly self-exams are recommended for all women. Mammography may also be recommended depending on your age and risk factors.

Gallbladder disease. Women who use estrogens after menopause are more likely to develop gallbladder disease needing surgery than women who do not use estrogens.

Abnormal blood clotting. Taking estrogens may increase the risk of blood clots. These clots can cause a stroke, heart attack, or pulmonary embolus, any of which may cause death or long term serious disability.

SIDE EFFECTS

In addition to the risks listed above, the following side effects have been reported with estrogen use:

- Headache.
- Nausea and vomiting.
- Breast tenderness or enlargement.
- Enlargement of benign tumors ("fibroids") of the uterus.
- Retention of excess fluid. This may make some conditions worsen, such as asthma, epilepsy, migraine, heart disease, or kidney disease.
- A spotty darkening of the skin, particularly on the face. Skin irritation, redness, or rash may occur at the site of application.
- Back pain.
- Vaginal spotting or bleeding.

In Postmarketing experience, although a causal relationship with Vivelle has not been established, isolated reports of anaphylaxis as well as rare reports of elevated liver function tests have been received.

REDUCING RISK OF ESTROGEN USE

If you use estrogens, you can reduce your risks by doing these things:

See your doctor regularly. While you are using estrogens, it is important to visit your doctor at least once a year for a check-up. If you develop vaginal bleeding while taking estrogens, you may need further evaluation. If members of your family have had breast cancer or if you have ever had breast lumps or an abnormal mammogram (breast x-ray), you may need to have more frequent breast examinations.

Reassess your need for estrogens. You and your doctor should reevaluate whether or not you still need estrogens at least every six months.

Be alert for signs of trouble. Report these or any other unusual side effects to your doctor immediately:

- Abnormal bleeding from the vagina.
- Pains in the calves or chest, sudden shortness of breath, or coughing blood (indicating possible clots in the legs, heart, or lungs).
- Severe headache, dizziness, faintness, or changes in vision (indicating possible clots in the brain or eye).
- Breast lumps.
- Yellowing of the skin or eyes.
- Pain, swelling, or tenderness in the abdomen.
- Skin irritation, redness, or rash.

OTHER INFORMATION

If your uterus has not been removed, your doctor may choose to prescribe a progestin, a different hormonal drug to be used in association with estrogen treatment. Progestins lower the risk of developing endometrial hyperplasia, a possible precancerous condition of the uterine lining, which may occur while using estrogen. There are possible additional risks that may be associated with the inclusion of a progestin in estrogen treatment. The possible risks include unfavorable effects on blood fats and sugars, as well as a possible further increase in breast cancer risk that may be associated with long-term estrogen use.

Some research has suggested that estrogen taken *without progestins* may protect women against developing heart disease. However, this effect of estrogen is not certain.

You are cautioned to discuss very carefully with your doctor or healthcare provider all the possible risks and benefits of long-term estrogen and progestin treatment, as they affect you personally.

Your doctor has prescribed this drug for you and you alone. Do not give the drug to anyone else.

Keep this and all drugs out of the reach of children. In case of overdose, remove the system and call your doctor, hospital, or poison control center immediately.

This leaflet provides a summary of the most important information about estrogens. If you want more information, ask your doctor or pharmacist to show you the professional labeling.

 T2000-53
T2000-52/T2000-53
89008102

REV: AUGUST 2000
NOVARTIS
Distributed by
Novartis Pharmaceuticals Corporation
East Hanover, New Jersey 07936

Shown in Product Identification Guide, page 326

VIVELLE-DOT™ ℞

[*vī-vĕlle*]
(estradiol transdermal system)
0.0375, 0.05, 0.075 or 0.1 mg/day
Continuous delivery for twice-weekly application

Rx Only

The following prescribing information is based on official labeling in effect November 2000.

1. **ESTROGENS HAVE BEEN REPORTED TO INCREASE THE RISK OF ENDOMETRIAL CARCINOMA IN POSTMENOPAUSAL WOMEN.**
   Close clinical surveillance of all women taking estrogens is important. Adequate diagnostic measures, including endometrial sampling when indicated, should be undertaken to rule out malignancy in all cases of undiagnosed persistent or recurring abnormal vaginal bleeding. There is no evidence that "natural" estrogens are more or less hazardous than "synthetic" estrogens at equiestrogenic doses.
2. **ESTROGENS SHOULD NOT BE USED DURING PREGNANCY.**
   Estrogen therapy during pregnancy is associated with an increased risk of congenital defects in the reproductive organs of the fetus, and possibly other birth defects. Studies of women who received diethylstilbestrol (DES) during pregnancy have shown that female offspring have an increased risk of vaginal adenosis, squamous cell dysplasia of the uterine cervix, and clear cell vaginal cancer later in life; male offspring have an increased risk of urogenital abnormalities and possibly testicular cancer later in life. The 1985 DES Task Force concluded that use of DES during pregnancy is associated with a subsequent increased risk of breast cancer in the mothers, although a causal relationship remains unproven and the observed level of excess risk is similar to that for a number of other breast cancer risk factors.
   There is no indiction for estrogen therapy during pregnancy or during the immediate postpartum period. Estrogens are ineffective for the prevention or treatment of threatened or habitual abortion. Estrogens are not indicated for the prevention of postpartum breast engorgement.

DESCRIPTION

Vivelle-Dot™ (estradiol transdermal system) contains estradiol in a multipolymeric adhesive. The system is designed to release 17β-estradiol continuously upon application to intact skin.

Four systems are available to provide nominal in vivo delivery of 0.0375, 0.05, 0.075, or 0.1 mg of estradiol per day via

Continued on next page

Vivelle-Dot—Cont.

skin of average permeability. Each corresponding system having an active surface area of 3.75, 5.0, 7.5, or 10.0 cm^2 contains 0.585, 0.78, 1.17, or 1.56 mg of estradiol USP, respectively. The composition of the systems per unit area is identical.

Estradiol USP (17β-estradiol) is a white, crystalline powder, chemically described as estra-1,3,5 (10)-triene-3,17β-diol.

The structural formula is

The molecular formula of estradiol is $C_{18}H_{24}O_2$. The molecular weight is 272.39.

The Vivelle-Dot™ system comprises three layers. Proceeding from the visible surface toward the surface attached to the skin, these layers are (1) a translucent polyolefin film (2) an adhesive formulation containing estradiol, acrylic adhesive, silicone adhesive, oleyl alcohol, povidone and dipropylene glycol, and (3) a polyester release liner which is attached to the adhesive surface and must be removed before the system can be used.

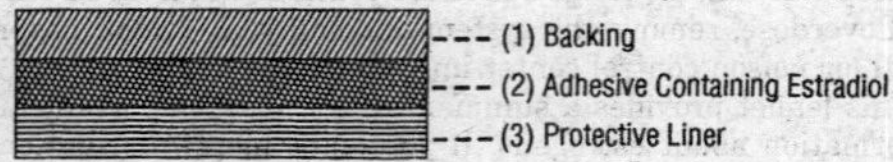

The active component of the system is estradiol. The remaining components of the system are pharmacologically inactive.

CLINICAL PHARMACOLOGY

Estrogens are largely responsible for the development and maintenance of the female reproductive system and secondary sexual characteristics. Although circulating estrogens exist in a dynamic equilibrium of metabolic interconversions, estradiol is the principal intracellular human estrogen and is substantially more potent than its metabolites, estrone and estriol, at the receptor level. The primary source of estrogen in normally cycling adult women is the ovarian follicle, which secretes 70 to 500 µg of estradiol daily, depending on the phase of the menstrual cycle. After menopause, most endogenous estrogen is produced by conversion of androstenedione, secreted by the adrenal cortex, to estrone by peripheral tissues. Thus, estrone and the sulfate conjugated form, estrone sulfate, are the most abundant circulating estrogens in postmenopausal women.

Circulating estrogens modulate the pituitary secretion of the gonadotropins, luteinizing hormone (LH) and follicle stimulating hormone (FSH) through a negative feedback mechanism and estrogen replacement therapy acts to reduce the elevated levels of these hormones seen in postmenopausal women.

The Vivelle-Dot™ system provides systemic estrogen replacement therapy. Estrogen receptors have been identified in tissues of the reproductive tract, breast, pituitary, hypothalamus, liver, and bone of women. Among numerous effects, estradiol is largely responsible for the development and maintenance of the female reproductive system and secondary sex characteristics. By a direct action, it causes growth and development of the vagina, uterus, and fallopian tubes. With other hormones, such as pituitary hormones and progesterone, it causes enlargement of the breasts through promotion of ductal growth, stromal development, and the accretion of fat. Estrogens contribute to the shaping of the skeleton, to the maintenance of tone and elasticity of urogenital structures, to changes in the epiphyses of the long bones that allow for the pubertal growth spurt and its termination, to the growth of axillary and pubic hair, and pigmentation of the nipples and genitals.

Estrogens are intricately involved with other hormones, especially progesterone, in the processes of the ovulatory menstrual cycle and pregnancy, and affect the release of pituitary gonadotropins.

Loss of ovarian estradiol secretion after menopause can result in instability of thermoregulation, causing hot flushes associated with sleep disturbance and excessive sweating, and urogenital atrophy, causing dyspareunia and urinary incontinence. Estradiol replacement therapy alleviates many of these symptoms of estradiol deficiency in the menopausal woman.

Pharmacokinetics

The skin metabolizes estradiol only to a small extent. In contrast, orally administered estradiol is rapidly metabolized by the liver to estrone and its conjugates, giving rise to higher circulating levels of estrone than estradiol. Therefore, transdermal administration produces therapeutic plasma levels of estradiol with lower circulating levels of estrone and estrone conjugates and requires smaller total doses than does oral therapy.

Absorption

In a multiple-dose study consisting of three consecutive patch applications of the original formulation (Vivelle® system) which was conducted in 17 healthy, postmenopausal women, blood levels of estradiol and estrone were compared following application of these units to sites on the abdomen and buttocks in a crossover fashion. Patches that deliver nominal estradiol doses of approximately 0.0375 mg/day and 0.1 mg/day were applied to abdominal application sites while the 0.1 mg/day doses were also applied to sites on the buttocks. These systems increased estradiol levels above baseline within 4 hours and maintained respective mean levels of 25 and 79 pg/mL above baseline following application to the abdomen; slightly higher mean levels of 88 pg/mL above baseline were observed following application to the buttocks. At the same time, increases in estrone plasma concentrations averaged about 12 and 50 pg/mL, respectively, following application to the abdomen and 61 pg/mL for the buttocks. While plasma concentrations of estradiol and estrone remained slightly above baseline at 12 hours following removal of the patches in this study, results from another study show these levels to return to baseline values within 24 hours following removal of the patches.

The graph illustrates the mean plasma concentrations of estradiol at steady-state during application of these patches at four different dosages.

Steady-State Estradiol Plasma Concentrations for Systems Applied to the Abdomen
Nonbaseline-corrected levels

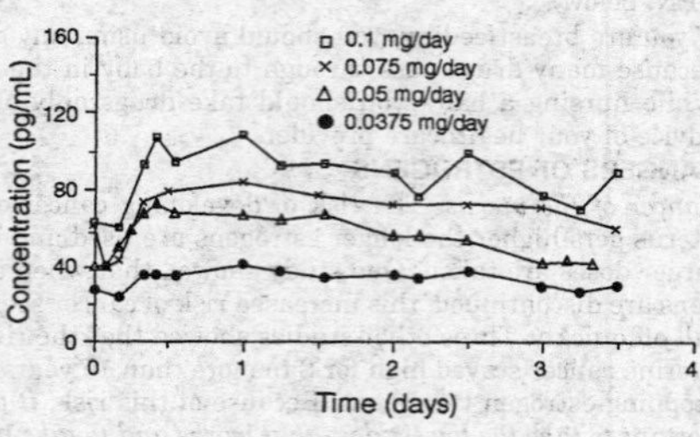

The corresponding pharmacokinetic parameters are summarized in the table below.

Steady-State Estradiol Pharmacokinetic Parameters for Systems Applied to the Abdomen (mean ± standard deviation)
Nonbaseline-corrected data*

Dosage (mg/day)	C_{max}† (pg/mL)	C_{avg}‡ (pg/mL)	C_{min}(84 hr)§ (pg/mL)
0.0375	46 ± 16	34 ± 10	30 ± 10
0.05	83 ± 41	57 ± 23#	41 ± 11#
0.075	99 ± 35	72 ± 24	60 ± 24
0.1	133 ± 51	89 ± 38	90 ± 44
0.1¶	145 ± 71	104 ± 52	85 ± 47

*Mean baseline estradiol concentration = 11.7 pg/mL
†Peak plasma concentration
‡Average plasma concentration
§Minimum plasma concentration at 84 hr
#Measured over 80 hr
¶Applied to the buttocks

The original formulation that was tested in clinical trials has been revised to reduce the patch sizes and the revised formulation was shown to be bioequivalent to the original formulation.

Distribution

The distribution of exogenous estrogens is similar to that of endogenous estrogens. Estrogens are widely distributed in the body and are generally found in higher concentrations in the sex hormone target organs.

Estradiol and other naturally occurring estrogens are bound mainly to sex hormone binding globulin (SHBG), and to lesser degree to albumin.

Metabolism

Exogenous estrogens are metabolized in the same manner as endogenous estrogens. Circulating estrogens exist in a dynamic equilibrium of metabolic interconversions. These transformations take place mainly in the liver. Estradiol is converted reversibly to estrone, and both can be converted to estriol, which is the major urinary metabolite. Estrogens also undergo enterohepatic recirculation via sulfate and glucuronide conjugation in the liver, biliary secretion of conjugates into the intestine, and hydrolysis in the gut followed by reabsorption. In postmenopausal women a significant portion of the circulating estrogens exist as sulfate conjugates, especially estrone sulfate, which serves as a circulating reservoir for the formation of more active estrogens.

Excretion

Estradiol, estrone and estriol are excreted in the urine along with glucuronide and sulfate conjugates. The half-life values calculated after dosing with the Vivelle-Dot™ systems ranged from 5.9 to 7.7 hours. After removal of the transdermal systems, serum concentrations of estradiol and estrone returned to baseline levels within 24 hours.

Special Populations

The Vivelle-Dot™ systems were investigated in postmenopausal women. No other special populations of volunteers were investigated.

Drug Interactions

No drug interaction studies were conducted with the Vivelle-Dot™ systems since estradiol is well characterized.

INDICATIONS AND USAGE

The Vivelle-Dot™ (estradiol transdermal system) is indicated in the following:

1. Treatment of moderate-to-severe vasomotor symptoms associated with the menopause. There is no adequate evidence that estrogens are effective for nervous symptoms or depression which might occur during menopause and they should not be used to treat these conditions.
2. Treatment of vulval and vaginal atrophy.
3. Treatment of hypoestrogenism due to hypogonadism, castration, or primary ovarian failure.

CONTRAINDICATIONS

Patients with known hypersensitivity to any of the components of the therapeutic system should not use the Vivelle-Dot™ system.

Estrogens should not be used in individuals with any of the following conditions:

1. Known or suspected pregnancy (see Boxed Warning). Estrogen may cause fetal harm when administered to a pregnant woman.
2. Undiagnosed abnormal genital bleeding.
3. Known or suspected cancer of the breast.
4. Known or suspected estrogen-dependent neoplasia.
5. Active thrombophlebitis or thromboembolic disorders, or a documented history of these conditions.

WARNINGS

1. **Induction of malignant neoplasms.**

   Breast Cancer.

   While some epidemiologic studies suggest a very modest increase in breast cancer risk for estrogen alone users versus non-users, other studies have not shown any increased risk. The addition of progestin to estrogen may increase the risk for breast cancer over that noted in non-hormone users more significantly (by about 24–40%), although this is based solely on epidemiologic studies, and definitive conclusions await prospective, controlled clinical trials.

   Women without a uterus who require hormone replacement should receive estrogen-alone therapy, and should not be exposed unnecessarily to progestins. Women with a uterus who are candidates for short-term combination estrogen/progestin therapy (for relief of vasomotor symptoms) are not felt to be at a substantially increased risk for breast cancer. Women with a uterus who are candidates for long-term use of estrogen/progestin therapy should be advised of potential benefits and risks (including the potential for an increased risk of breast cancer). All women should receive yearly breast exams by a health-care provider and perform monthly breast self-examinations. In addition, mammography examinations should be scheduled as suggested by providers based on patient age and risk factors. The reported endometrial cancer risk among unopposed estrogen users is about 2- to 12-fold greater than in nonusers and appears dependent on duration of treatment and on estrogen dose. Most studies show no significant increased risk associated with the use of estrogens for less than 1 year. The greatest risk appears associated with prolonged use with increased risks of 15- to 24-fold for five to 10 years or more. In three studies, persistence of risk was demonstrated for 8 to over 15 years after cessation of estrogen treatment. In one study, a significant decrease in the incidence of endometrial cancer occurred six months after estrogen withdrawal. Concurrent progestin therapy may offset this risk, but the overall health impact in postmenopausal women is not known (see PRECAUTIONS).

   Estrogen therapy during pregnancy is associated with an increased risk of fetal congenital reproductive tract disorders. In female offspring, there is an increased risk of vaginal adenosis, squamous cell dysplasia of the cervix, and clear cell vaginal cancer later in life; in males, urogenital and possibly testicular abnormalities. Although some of these changes are benign, it is not known whether they are precursors of malignancy.
2. **Gallbladder disease.** Two studies have reported a 2- to 4-fold increase in the risk of surgically confirmed gallbladder disease in postmenopausal women receiving oral estrogen replacement therapy, similar to the 2-fold increase previously noted in users of oral contraceptives.
3. **Cardiovascular disease.** Large doses of estrogen (5 mg conjugated estrogens per day), comparable to those used to treat cancer of the prostate and breast, have been shown in a large prospective clinical trial in men to increase the risks of nonfatal myocardial infarction, pulmonary embolism, and thrombophlebitis. These risks cannot necessarily be extrapolated from men to women. However, to avoid the theoretical cardiovascular risk to women caused by high estrogen doses, the dose for estrogen replacement therapy should not exceed the lowest effective dose.
4. **Elevated blood pressure.** Occasional blood pressure increases during estrogen replacement therapy have been attributed to idiosyncratic reactions to estrogens. More often, blood pressure has remained the same or has dropped.

   Postmenopausal estrogen use does not increase the risk of stroke. Nonetheless, blood pressure should be monitored at regular intervals with estrogen use, especially if high doses are used. Ethinyl estradiol and conjugated estrogens have been shown to increase renin substrate. In contrast to these oral estrogens, transdermally administered estradiol does not affect renin substrate.

5. **Hypercalcemia.** Administration of estrogen may lead to severe hypercalcemia in patients with breast cancer and bone metastases. If this occurs, the drug should be stopped and appropriate measures taken to reduce the serum calcium level.

PRECAUTIONS

A. General

1. **Addition of a progestin.** Studies of the addition of a progestin for 10 or more days of a cycle of estrogen administration have reported a lower incidence of endometrial hyperplasia than would be induced by estrogen treatment alone. Morphologic and biochemical studies of endometria suggest that 10 to 14 days of progestin are needed to provide maximal maturation of the endometrium and to reduce the likelihood of hyperplastic changes.
There are, however, possible risks that may be associated with the use of progestins in estrogen replacement regimens. These include:
(1) adverse effects on lipoprotein metabolism (lowering HDL and raising LDL) which could diminish the purported cardioprotective effect of estrogen therapy (see PRECAUTIONS, below);
(2) impairment of glucose tolerance; and
(3) possible enhancement of mitotic activity in breast epithelial tissue, although few epidemiologic data are available to address this point (see PRECAUTIONS, below).
The choice of progestin, its dose, and its regimen may be important in minimizing these adverse effects, but these issues will require further study before they are clarified.
2. **Cardiovascular risk.** The effects of estrogen replacement on the risk of cardiovascular disease have not been adequately studied. However, data from the Heart and Estrogen/Progestin Replacement Study (HERS), a controlled clinical trial of secondary prevention of 2,763 postmenopausal women with documented heart disease, demonstrated no benefit. During an average follow-up of 4.1 years, treatment with oral conjugated estrogen plus medroxyprogesterone acetate did not reduce the overall rate of coronary heart disease (CHD) events in post-menopausal women with established coronary disease. There were more CHD events in the hormone treated group than in the placebo group in year 1, but fewer events in years 3 through 5.
3. **Physical examination.** A complete medical and family history should be taken prior to the initiation of any estrogen therapy. The pretreatment and periodic physical examinations should include special reference to blood pressure, breasts, abdomen, and pelvic organs and should include a Papanicolaou smear. As a general rule, estrogen should not be prescribed for longer than one year without reexamining the patient.
4. **Hypercoagulability.** Some studies have shown that women taking estrogen replacement therapy have hypercoagulability, primarily related to decreased antithrombin activity. This effect appears dose- and duration-dependent and is less pronounced than that associated with oral contraceptive use. Also, postmenopausal women tend to have increased coagulation parameters at baseline compared to premenopausal women. Epidemiological studies, which employed primary orally administered estrogen products, have suggested that hormone replacement therapy (HRT) may be associated with an increased relative risk of developing venous thromboembolism (VTE), i.e., deep venous thrombosis or pulmonary embolism. Risk/benefit should therefore be carefully weighed in consultation with the patient when prescribing any form of HRT to women with a risk factor for VTE.
5. **Familial hyperlipoproteinemia.** Estrogen therapy may be associated with massive elevations of plasma triglycerides leading to pancreatitis and other complications in patients with familial defects of lipoprotein metabolism.
6. **Fluid retention.** Because estrogens may cause some degree of fluid retention, conditions that might be exacerbated by this factor, such as asthma, epilepsy, migraine, and cardiac or renal dysfunction, require careful observation.
7. **Uterine bleeding and mastodynia.** Certain patients may develop undesirable manifestations of estrogenic stimulation, such as abnormal uterine bleeding and mastodynia.
8. **Impaired liver function.** Estrogens may be poorly metabolized in patients with impaired liver function and should be administered with caution.

B. Information for the Patient. See text of Patient Package Insert, which appears after the HOW SUPPLIED section.

C. Laboratory Tests. Estrogen administration should generally be guided by clinical response at the smallest dose, rather than laboratory monitoring, for relief of symptoms for those indications in which symptoms are observable.

D. Drug/Laboratory Test Interactions. Some of these drug/laboratory test interactions have been observed only with estrogen progestin combinations (oral contraceptives):
1. Accelerated prothrombin time, partial thromboplastin time, and platelet aggregation time; increased platelet count; increased factors II, VII antigen, VIII antigen, VIII coagulant activity, IX, X, XII, VII-X complex, II-VII-X complex; and beta-thromboglobulin; decreased levels of anti-factor Xa and antithrombin III; decreased antithrombin III activity; increased levels of fibrinogen and fibrinogen activity; increased plasminogen antigen and activity.
2. Increased thyroid-binding globulin (TBG) leading to increased circulating total thyroid hormone, as measured by protein-bound iodine (PBI), T_4 levels (by column or by radioimmunoassay) or T_3 levels by radioimmunoassay. T_3 resin uptake is decreased, reflecting the elevated TBG. Free T_4 and free T_3 concentrations are unaltered.
3. Other binding proteins may be elevated in serum, i.e., corticosteroid binding globulin (CBG), sex hormone-binding globulin (SHBG), leading to increased circulating corticosteroids and sex steroids, respectively. Free or biologically active hormone concentrations are unchanged. Other plasma proteins may be increased (angiotensinogen/renin substrate, alpha-1-antitrypsin, ceruloplasmin).
4. Increased plasma HDL and HDL-2 subfraction concentrations, reduced LDL cholesterol concentration, increased triglycerides levels.
5. Impaired glucose tolerance.
6. Reduced response to metyrapone test.
7. Reduced serum folate concentration.

E. Carcinogenesis, Mutagenesis, and Impairment of Fertility. Long-term, continuous administration of natural and synthetic estrogens in certain animal species increases the frequency of carcinomas of the breast, cervix, vagina, testis, and liver (see CONTRAINDICATIONS and WARNINGS).

F. Pregnancy Category X. Estrogens should not be used during pregnancy (see CONTRAINDICATIONS and Boxed Warning).

G. Nursing Mothers. As a general principle, the administration of any drug to nursing mothers should be done only when clearly necessary since many drugs are excreted in human milk. In addition, estrogen administration to nursing mothers has been shown to decrease the quantity and quality of the milk.

H. Pediatric Use. The safety and effectiveness in pediatric patients have not been established.

ADVERSE REACTIONS

See WARNINGS and Boxed Warning regarding the potential adverse effects on the fetus, the induction of malignant neoplasms, gallbladder disease, cardiovascular disease, elevated blood pressure, and hypercalcemia.
The most commonly reported systemic adverse event with the Vivelle-Dot™ systems was mild headache. Topical irritancy evaluations showed that for the majority of the subjects, no erythema was observed at the application sites after removal of the systems. No occurrence of erythema was greater than mild in severity.
The following additional adverse reactions have been reported with estrogen therapy:
1. Genitourinary system. Changes in vaginal bleeding pattern and abnormal withdrawal bleeding or flow; breakthrough bleeding, spotting; increase in size of uterine leiomyomata; vaginal candidiasis; change in amount of cervical secretion.
2. Breasts. Tenderness, enlargement.
3. Gastrointestinal. Nausea, vomiting; abdominal cramps, bloating; cholestatic jaundice; gallbladder disease.
4. Skin. Chloasma or melasma that may persist when drug is discontinued; erythema multiforme; erythema nodosum; hemorrhagic eruption; loss of scalp hair; hirsutism.
5. Eyes. Steepening of corneal curvature; intolerance to contact lenses.
6. Central Nervous System. Headache, migraine, dizziness; mental depression; chorea.
7. Miscellaneous. Increase or decrease in weight; reduced carbohydrate tolerance; aggravation of porphyria; edema; changes in libido.

OVERDOSAGE

Serious ill effects have not been reported following acute ingestion of large doses of estrogen-containing oral contraceptives by young children. Overdosage of estrogen may cause nausea and vomiting, and withdrawal bleeding may occur in females.

DOSAGE AND ADMINISTRATION

The adhesive side of the Vivelle-Dot™ system should be placed on a clean, dry area of the abdomen. *The Vivelle-Dot™ system should not be applied to the breasts.* The Vivelle-Dot™ system should be replaced twice weekly. The sites of application must be rotated, with an interval of at least 1 week allowed between applications to a particular site. The area selected should not be oily, damaged, or irritated. The waistline should be avoided, since tight clothing may rub the system off. The system should be applied immediately after opening the pouch and removing the protective liner. The system should be pressed firmly in place with the palm of the hand for about 10 seconds, making sure there is good contact, especially around the edges. In the unlikely event that a system should fall off, the same system may be reapplied. If necessary, a new system may be applied. In either case, the original treatment schedule should be continued.

Initiation of Therapy

For treatment of moderate-to-severe vasomotor symptoms and vulval and vaginal atrophy associated with the menopause, start therapy with Vivelle-Dot™ (estradiol transdermal system) 0.05 mg/day applied to the skin twice weekly. In order to use the lowest dosage necessary for the control of symptoms, decisions to increase dosage should not be made until after the first month of therapy. Some women taking the 0.0375 mg/day dosage may experience a delayed onset of efficacy. Attempts to discontinue or taper medication should be made at 3-month to 6-month intervals.
In women not currently taking oral estrogens or in women switching from another estradiol transdermal therapy, treatment with the Vivelle-Dot™ system may be initiated at once. In women who are currently taking oral estrogens, treatment with the Vivelle-Dot™ system should be initiated 1 week after withdrawal of oral hormone replacement therapy, or sooner if menopausal symptoms reappear in less than 1 week.

Therapeutic Regimen

The Vivelle-Dot™ system may be given continuously in patients who do not have an intact uterus. In those patients with an intact uterus, the Vivelle-Dot™ system may be given on a cyclic schedule (e.g., three weeks on drug followed by one week off drug).

HOW SUPPLIED

Vivelle-Dot™ (estradiol transdermal system), 0.0375 mg/day - each 3.75 cm^2 system contains 0.585 mg of estradiol USP for nominal* delivery of 0.0375 mg of estradiol per day.
Patient Calendar Pack of 8 Systems
NDC 0078-0343-42
Carton of 3 Patient Calendar Packs of 8 Systems
NDC 0078-0343-45

Vivelle-Dot™ (estradiol transdermal system), 0.05 mg/day - each 5.0 cm^2 system contains 0.78 mg of estradiol USP for nominal* delivery of 0.05 mg of estradiol per day.
Patient Calendar Pack of 8 Systems
NDC 0078-0344-42
Carton of 3 Patient Calendar Packs of 8 Systems
NDC 0078-0344-45

Vivelle-Dot™ (estradiol transdermal system), 0.075 mg/day - each 7.5 cm^2 system contains 1.17 mg of estradiol USP for nominal* delivery of 0.075 mg of estradiol per day.
Patient Calendar Pack of 8 Systems
NDC 0078-0345-42
Carton of 3 Patient Calendar Packs of 8 Systems
NDC 0078-0345-45

Vivelle-Dot™ (estradiol transdermal system), 0.1 mg/day - each 10.0 cm^2 system contains 1.56 mg of estradiol USP for nominal* delivery of 0.1 mg of estradiol per day.
Patient Calendar Pack of 8 Systems
NDC 0078-0346-42
Carton of 3 Patient Calendar Packs of 8 Systems
NDC 0078-0346-45

*See DESCRIPTION.
Store at controlled room temperature at 25°C (77°F).
Do not store unpouched. Apply immediately upon removal from the protective pouch.
Rev. SEPTEMBER 2000 T2000-56

Information for the Patient

Vivelle-Dot™
(estradiol transdermal system)
Rx Only

1. ESTROGENS INCREASE THE RISK OF CANCER OF THE UTERUS IN WOMEN WHO HAVE HAD THEIR MENOPAUSE ("CHANGE OF LIFE").
If you use any estrogen-containing drug, it is important to visit your doctor regularly and report any unusual vaginal bleeding right away. Vaginal bleeding after menopause may be a warning sign of uterine cancer. Your doctor should evaluate any unusual vaginal bleeding to find out the cause.

2. ESTROGENS SHOULD NOT BE USED DURING PREGNANCY.
Estrogens do not prevent miscarriage (spontaneous abortion) and are not needed in the days following childbirth. If you take estrogens during pregnancy, your unborn child has a greater than usual chance of having birth defects. The risk of developing these defects is small, but clearly larger than the risk in children whose mothers did not take estrogens during pregnancy. These birth defects may affect the baby's urinary system and sex organs.
Daughters born to mothers who took DES (an estrogen drug) have a higher than usual chance of developing cancer of the vagina or cervix when they become teenagers or young adults. Sons may have a higher than usual chance of developing cancer of the testicles when they become teenagers or young adults.

INTRODUCTION

Your doctor has prescribed the Vivelle-Dot™ (estradiol transdermal system) for the treatment of your menopausal symptoms. During menopause, production of estrogen hormones by your body decreases well below the amounts normally produced during your fertile years. In many women this decrease in estrogen production causes uncomfortable symptoms, most noticeably hot flushes and sleep disturbance. Estrogens can be given to reduce or eliminate these symptoms.
The Vivelle-Dot™ system that your doctor has prescribed for you releases small amounts of estradiol through the skin in a continuous way. Estradiol is the same hormone that your ovaries produce abundantly before menopause. The dose of estradiol you require will depend upon your individual response. The dose is adjusted by the size of the Vivelle-Dot™ system used; the systems are available in four sizes.

Continued on next page

Vivelle-Dot—Cont.

INFORMATION ABOUT VIVELLE-DOT™
(estradiol transdermal system)
How the Vivelle-Dot™ system works
The Vivelle-Dot™ system contains estradiol. When applied to the skin as directed below, the Vivelle-Dot™ system releases estradiol, which flows through the skin into the bloodstream.
Application Instructions for Vivelle-Dot™
(estradiol transdermal system)

1. DETERMINE YOUR SCHEDULE FOR YOUR TWICE-A-WEEK APPLICATION

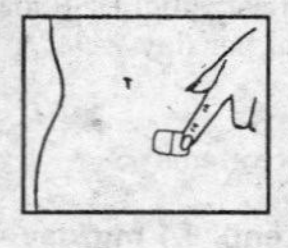

- Decide upon which two days you will change your patch.
- Your Vivelle-Dot™ individual carton contains a calendar card printed on its inner flap. Mark the two-day schedule you plan to follow on your carton's inner flap.
- **BE CONSISTENT.**
- If you forget to change your patch on the correct date, apply a new one as soon as you remember.
- No matter what day this happens, stick to the schedule you have marked on the inner flap of your carton (your calendar card).

2. WHERE TO APPLY THE VIVELLE-DOT™ SYSTEM

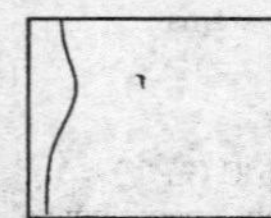

- Apply patch to lower abdomen, below the waistline. Avoid the waistline, since clothing may cause the patch to rub off.
- **DO NOT APPLY PATCH TO BREASTS.**
- When changing your patch, based on your twice-a-week schedule, apply your new patch to a different site. Do not apply a new patch to that same area for at least one week.

3. BEFORE YOU APPLY THE VIVELLE-DOT™ SYSTEM

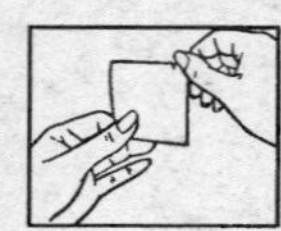

Make sure your skin is:
- Clean (freshly washed), dry and cool.
- Free of any powder, oil, moisturizer or lotion.
- Free of cuts and/or irritations (rashes or other skin problems).

4. HOW TO APPLY THE VIVELLE-DOT™ SYSTEM

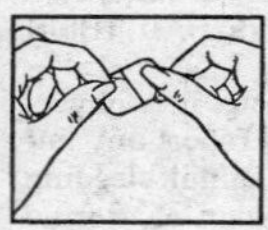

- Each patch is individually sealed in a protective pouch.
- Tear open the pouch at the tear notch (do not use scissors).
- Remove the patch.

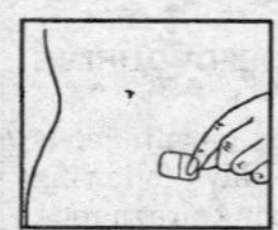

- **Apply the patch immediately after removing from pouch.**
- Holding the patch with the rigid protective liner facing you, remove **half** of the liner, which covers the sticky surface of the patch.

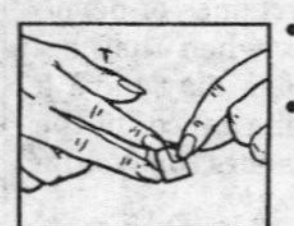

- **AVOID TOUCHING THE STICKY SIDE OF THE PATCH WITH YOUR FINGERS.**
- Using the other half of the rigid protective liner as a handle, apply the sticky side of the patch to the selected area of the abdomen.
- Press the sticky side of the patch firmly into place.
- Smooth it down.
- While still holding the sticky side down, fold back the other half of the patch.

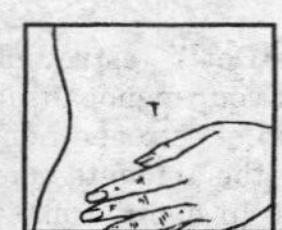

- Grasp an edge of the remaining protective liner and gently pull it off.
- **AVOID TOUCHING THE STICKY SIDE OF THE PATCH WITH YOUR FINGERS.**

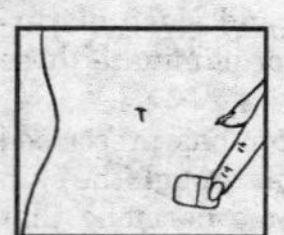

- Press the entire patch firmly into place with the palm of your hand.
- Continue to apply pressure, with the palm of your hand over the patch, for approximately 10 seconds.

- Make sure that the patch is properly adhered to your skin.
- Go over the edges with your finger to ensure good contact around the patch.

PLEASE NOTE:
- Contact with water while bathing, swimming or showering will not affect the patch.
- In the unlikely event that a patch should fall off, **AVOID TOUCHING THE STICKY SIDE WITH YOUR FINGERS.** Put the same patch back on a different site, making sure to press the patch firmly into place for at least 10 seconds.
- Continue to follow your original twice-a-week schedule you have marked on the inner flap of your individual carton (your calendar card).
- If necessary, you may apply a new system but continue to follow your original schedule.

5. HOW TO CHANGE AND DISCARD THE VIVELLE-DOT™ SYSTEM
- When changing the patch, peel off the used patch slowly.
- Fold the used patch in half (sticky sides together) and discard appropriately, in the trash.
- **PLEASE KEEP OUT OF REACH OF CHILDREN.**
- If any adhesive residue remains on your skin after removing the patch, allow the area to dry for 15 minutes. Then, gently rub the area with oil or lotion to remove the adhesive from your skin.
- Keep in mind, **the new patch must be applied to a different area of your abdomen.** This area must be clean, dry and cool; and free of powder, oil and/or lotion.

Benefits of treatment with Vivelle-Dot™
(estradiol transdermal system)
Regular use of the Vivelle-Dot™ system twice weekly offers relief of moderate-to-severe symptoms of menopause. Small quantities of the naturally occurring hormone estradiol are absorbed through the skin from the Vivelle-Dot™ system, ensuring a continuous supply of circulating hormone in the body.

USES OF ESTROGEN
- **To reduce moderate or severe menopausal symptoms.** Estrogens are hormones produced by the ovaries. The decrease in the amount of estrogen that occurs in all women, usually between ages 45 and 55, causes the menopause. Sometimes the ovaries are removed by an operation, causing "surgical menopause." When the amount of estrogen begins to decrease, some women develop very uncomfortable symptoms, such as feelings of warmth in the face, neck, and chest or sudden intense episodes of heat and sweating ("hot flashes"). The use of drugs containing estrogens can help the body adjust to lower estrogen levels. Some women have only mild menopausal symptoms, or none at all, and do not need estrogen therapy for these particular symptoms. Other women may need estrogens for a few months while their bodies adjust to lower estrogen levels. For the treatment of menopausal symptoms only, most women need estrogen replacement therapy for no longer than 6 months.
- **To treat vulval and vaginal atrophy** (itching, burning, dryness in or around the vagina, difficulty or burning on urination) associated with menopause.
- **To treat certain conditions in which a young woman's ovaries do not produce enough estrogen naturally.**

WHO SHOULD NOT USE ESTROGENS
Estrogens should not be used:
- **During pregnancy (see Boxed Warning).** If you think you may be pregnant, do not use any form of estrogen-containing drug. Using estrogens while you are pregnant may cause your unborn child to have birth defects. Estrogens do not prevent miscarriage.
- **If you have unusual vaginal bleeding which has not been evaluated by your doctor (see Boxed Warning).** Unusual vaginal bleeding can be a warning sign of cancer of the uterus, especially if it happens after menopause. Your doctor must find out the cause of the bleeding so that he or she can recommend the proper treatment. Taking estrogens without visiting your doctor can cause you serious harm if your vaginal bleeding is caused by cancer of the uterus.
- **If you have had cancer.** Since estrogens increase the risk of certain types of cancer, you should not use estrogens if you ever had cancer of the breast or uterus.
- **If you have any circulation problems.** Estrogen therapy should be used only after consultation with your doctor and only in recommended doses. Patients with a tendency for abnormal blood clotting should avoid estrogen use (see DANGERS OF ESTROGENS, below).
- **When they are ineffective.** During menopause, some women develop nervous symptoms or depression. Estrogens do not relieve these symptoms. You may have heard that taking estrogens for years after menopause will keep your skin soft and supple and keep you feeling young. There is no evidence for these claims and such long-term estrogen use may have serious risks.
- **After childbirth or when breastfeeding a baby.** Estrogens should not be used to try to stop the breasts from filling with milk after a baby is born. Such treatment may increase the risk of developing blood clots (see DANGERS OF ESTROGEN, below).
  If you are breastfeeding, you should avoid using any drugs because many drugs pass through to the baby in the milk. While nursing a baby, you should take drugs only on the advice of your healthcare provider.

DANGERS OF ESTROGENS
- **Cancer of the uterus.** The risk of developing cancer of the uterus gets higher the longer estrogens are used and when larger doses are taken. One study showed that when estrogens are discontinued, this increased risk of cancer seems to fall off quickly. Three other studies showed that the risk for uterine cancer stayed high for 8 to more than 15 years after stopping estrogen treatment. Because of this risk, **IT IS IMPORTANT TO TAKE THE LOWEST DOSE THAT WORKS AND TO TAKE IT ONLY AS LONG AS YOU NEED IT.**
  Using progestin therapy together with estrogen therapy may reduce the higher risk of uterine cancer related to estrogen use (see OTHER INFORMATION, below).
  If you have had your uterus removed (total hysterectomy), there is no danger of developing cancer of the uterus.
- **Cancer of the breast.** Studies examining the risk of breast cancer among women using estrogen alone and combined estrogen/progestin therapy have suggested that there may be a mildly increased risk of breast cancer in women taking the combined therapy.
  If you do not have your uterus, there is no need for combined estrogen/progestin therapy since estrogen alone therapy is sufficient and may pose less risk for breast cancer.
  If you do have your uterus, you should discuss the benefits and risks of combined estrogen/progestin therapy with your health care provider. Regular breast exams by a health professional and monthly self-exams are recommended for all women. Mammography may also be recommended depending on your age and risk factors.
- **Gallbladder disease.** Women who use estrogens after menopause are more likely to develop gallbladder disease needing surgery than women who do not use estrogens.
- **Abnormal blood clotting.** Taking estrogens may increase the risk of blood clots. These clots can cause a stroke, heart attack, or pulmonary embolus, any of which may be fatal.

SIDE EFFECTS
In addition to the risks listed above, the following side effects have been reported with estrogen use:
— Headache.
— Nausea and vomiting.
— Breast tenderness or enlargement.
— Enlargement of benign tumors ("fibroids") of the uterus.
— Retention of excess fluid. This may make some conditions worsen, such as asthma, epilepsy, migraine, heart disease, or kidney disease.
— A spotty darkening of the skin, particularly on the face.
Skin irritation, redness, or rash may occur at the site of application.

REDUCING RISK OF ESTROGEN USE
If you use estrogens, you can reduce your risks by doing these things:
- **See your doctor regularly.** While you are using estrogens, it is important to visit your doctor at least once a year for a check-up. If you develop vaginal bleeding while taking estrogens, you may need further evaluation. If members of your family have had breast cancer or if you have ever had breast lumps or an abnormal mammogram (breast x-ray), you may need to have more frequent breast examinations.
- **Reassess your need for estrogens.** You and your doctor should reevaluate whether or not you still need estrogens at least every six months.
- **Be alert for signs of trouble.** Report these or any other unusual side effects to your doctor immediately:
  — Abnormal bleeding from the vagina.
  — Pains in the calves or chest, sudden shortness of breath, or coughing blood (indicating possible clots in the legs, heart, or lungs).
  — Severe headache, dizziness, faintness, or changes in vision (indicating possible clots in the brain or eye).
  — Breast lumps.
  — Yellowing of the skin or eyes.
  — Pain, swelling, or tenderness in the abdomen.
  — Skin irritation, redness, or rash.

OTHER INFORMATION
If your uterus has not been removed, your doctor may choose to prescribe a progestin, a different hormonal drug to be used in association with estrogen treatment. Progestins lower the risk of developing endometrial hyperplasia, a possible precancerous condition of the uterine lining, which may occur while using estrogen. There are possible additional risks that may be associated with the inclusion of a progestin in estrogen treatment. The possible risks include unfavorable effects on blood fats and sugars, as well as a possible further increase in breast cancer risk that may be associated with long-term estrogen use.

Some research has suggested that estrogen taken without progestins may protect women against developing heart disease. However, this effect of estrogen is not certain.

You are cautioned to discuss very carefully with your doctor or healthcare provider all the possible risks and benefits of long-term estrogen and progestin treatment, as they affect you personally.

Your doctor has prescribed this drug for you and you alone. Do not give the drug to anyone else.

Keep this and all drugs out of the reach of children. In case of overdose, remove the system and call your doctor, hospital, or poison control center immediately.

This leaflet provides a summary of the most important information about estrogens. If you want more information, ask your doctor or pharmacist to show you the professional labeling.

T2000-56
Rev. SEPTEMBER 2000 T2000-56/T2000-57
Manufactured by Noven Pharmaceuticals Inc.
Miami, FL 33186
Distributed by Novartis Pharmaceuticals Corporation
East Hanover, NJ 07936
Shown in Product Identification Guide, page 326

Novo Nordisk Pharmaceuticals, Inc.

100 COLLEGE ROAD WEST
PRINCETON, NJ 08540

Direct Inquiries to:
Novo Nordisk Pharmaceuticals, Inc.
(800) 727-6500
In Emergencies after hours and weekends:
609-987-5800

NORDITROPIN® ℞

4 mg or 8 mg (approximately 12 or 24 IU) vials
Somatropin (rDNA origin) for subcutaneous injection

DESCRIPTION

Norditropin® is the Novo Nordisk Pharmaceuticals, Inc. registered trademark for somatropin, a polypeptide hormone of recombinant DNA origin. The hormone is synthesized by a special strain of *E.coli* bacteria that has been modified by the addition of a plasmid which carries the gene for human growth hormone. Norditropin® contains the identical sequence of 191 amino acids constituting the naturally occurring pituitary human growth hormone with a molecular weight of about 22,000 Daltons.
Norditropin® is a sterile, almost white, lyophilized powder. It is a highly purified preparation intended for subcutaneous injection in the thighs after reconstitution with 2 mL diluent.
Each vial of lyophilized drug contains the following:

4 mg (approximately 12 IU) Vial

Somatropin	4 mg
Glycine	8.8 mg
Disodium Phosphate Dihydrate (Na_2HPO_4,$2H_2O$)	1.3 mg
Sodium Dihydrogen Phosphate Dihydrate (NaH_2PO_4,$2H_2O$)	1.1 mg
Mannitol	44 mg

8 mg (approximately 24 IU) Vial

Somatropin	8 mg
Glycine	8.8 mg
Disodium Phosphate Dihydrate (Na_2HPO_4,$2H_2O$)	1.3 mg
Sodium Dihydrogen Phosphate Dihydrate (NaH_2PO_4,$2H_2O$)	1.1 mg
Mannitol	44 mg

Each vial of lyophilized drug is supplied in a combination package which also contains a vial of diluent. Each mL contains 1.5% benzyl alcohol as preservative.
The pH of the reconstituted solution is about 7.3.

CLINICAL PHARMACOLOGY

a. Tissue Growth
The primary and most intensively studied action of somatropin is the stimulation of linear growth. This effect is demonstrated in patients with somatropin deficiency.

1. Skeletal growth – the measurable increase in bone length after administration of somatropin results from its effect on the cartilaginous growth areas of long bones. Studies *in vitro* have shown that the incorporation of sulfate into proteoglycans is not due to a direct effect of somatropin, but rather is mediated by the somatomedins or insulin-like growth factors (IGF). The somatomedins, among them somatomedin C, are polypeptide hormones which are synthesized in the liver, kidney, and various other tissue. Somatomedin C is low in the serum of hypopituitary dwarfs and hypophysectomized humans or animals, but its presence can be demonstrated after treatment with somatropin.
2. Cell growth – it has been shown that the total number of skeletal muscle cells is markedly decreased in short stature children lacking endogenous somatropin compared with normal children, and that treatment with somatropin results in an increase in both the number and size of muscle cells.
3. Organ growth – somatropin influences the size of internal organs, and it also increases red cell mass.

b. Protein Metabolism
Linear growth is facilitated in part by increased cellular protein synthesis. This synthesis and growth are reflected by nitrogen retention which can be quantitated by observing the decline in urinary nitrogen excretion and blood urea nitrogen following the initiation of somatropin therapy.

c. Carbohydrate Metabolism
Hypopituitary children sometimes experience fasting hypoglycemia that may be improved by treatment with somatropin. In healthy subjects, large doses of somatropin may impair glucose tolerance. Although the precise mechanism of the diabetogenic effect of somatropin is not known, it is attributed to blocking the action of insulin rather than blocking insulin secretion. Insulin levels in serum actually increase as somatropin levels increase.

d. Fat Metabolism
Somatropin stimulates intracellular lipolysis, and administration of somatropin leads to an increase in plasma free fatty acids, cholesterol, and triglycerides. Untreated growth hormone deficiency is associated with increased body fat stores including increased subcutaneous adipose tissue. On somatropin replacement a general reduction of fat stores and of subcutaneous tissue in particular takes place.

e. Mineral Metabolism
Administration of somatropin results in the retention of total body potassium and phosphorus and to a lesser extent sodium. This retention is thought to be the result of cell growth. Serum levels of phosphate increase in patients with growth hormone deficiency after somatropin therapy due to metabolic activity associated with bone growth. Serum calcium levels are not altered. Although calcium excretion in the urine is increased, there is a simultaneous increase in calcium absorption from the intestine. Negative calcium balance, however, may occasionally occur during somatropin treatment.

f. Connective Tissue Metabolism
Somatropin stimulates the synthesis of chondroitin sulfate and collagen as well as the urinary excretion of hydroxyproline.

g. Pharmacokinetics
A 180-min IV infusion of Norditropin® (33 ng/kg/min) was given to 9 GHD patients. A mean (± SD) hGH steady-state serum level of approximately 23.1 (± 15.0) ng/mL was reached at 150 min and a mean clearance rate of approximately 2.3 (± 1.8) mL/min/kg or 139 (± 105) mL/min for hGH was obtained. Following infusion, serum hGH levels had a biexponential decay with a terminal elimination half-life ($T_{1/2}$) of approximately 21.1 (± 5.1) min.
In a study conducted in 18 GHD adult patients, where a SC dose of 0.024 mg/kg or 3 IU/m^2 was given in the thigh, the mean (± SD) C_{max} values of 13.8 (± 5.8) and 17.1 (± 10.0) ng/mL were obtained for the 4 and 8 mg Norditropin® vials, respectively, at approximately 4 to 5 hr. post dose. The mean apparent terminal $T_{1/2}$ values were estimated to be approximately 7 to 10 hr. However, the absolute bioavailability for Norditropin® after the SC route of administration is currently not known.

INDICATIONS AND USAGE

Norditropin® is indicated for the long-term treatment of children who have growth failure due to inadequate secretion of endogenous growth hormone.

CONTRAINDICATIONS

Norditropin® should not be used in subjects with closed epiphyses.
Norditropin® should not be used in hypopituitary children who have evidence of actively growing intracranial tumors. Therapy with somatropin should be discontinued if there is evidence of recurrent tumor growth.
Norditropin® should not be used in any subjects with known hypersensitivity to any of the constituents of the preparation.
Growth hormone should not be initiated to treat patients with acute critical illness due to complications following open heart or abdominal surgery, multiple accidental trauma or to patients having acute respiratory failure. Two placebo-controlled clinical trials in non-growth hormone deficient adult patients (n=522) with these conditions revealed a significant increase in morality (41.9% vs. 19.3%) among somatropin treated patients (doses 5.3-8 mg/day) compared to those receiving placebo (see WARNINGS).

WARNINGS

Benzyl alcohol as a preservative has been associated with toxicity in newborns. Norditropin® may be reconstituted in sterile water for injection. If Norditropin® is reconstituted in this manner, use only one dose per vial and discard the unused portion.
See CONTRAINDICATIONS for information on increased morality in patients with acute critical illnesses in intensive care units due to complications following open heart or abdominal surgery, multiple accidental trauma or with acute respiratory failure. The safety of continuing growth hormone treatment in patients receiving replacement doses for approved indications who concurrently develop these illnesses has not been established. Therefore, the potential benefit of treatment continuation with growth hormone in patients having acute critical illnesses should be weighed against the potential risk.

PRECAUTIONS

Norditropin® should be used only by physicians with experience in the diagnosis and management of patients with growth hormone deficiency.
Patients with growth hormone deficiency secondary to an intracranial lesion should be examined frequently for progression or recurrence of the underlying disease process.
Because growth hormone may induce a state of insulin resistance, patients should be observed for evidence of glucose intolerance.
Concomitant glucocorticoid therapy may inhibit the growth promoting effect of Norditropin®. Patients with coexisting ACTH deficiency should have their glucocorticoid replacement dose carefully adjusted to avoid an inhibitory effect on growth.
A state of hypothyroidism may develop during Norditropin® treatment. Since untreated hypothyroidism may interfere with the response to Norditropin®, patients should have a periodic thyroid function test and should be treated with thyroid hormone when indicated.
Patients with endocrine disorders, including growth hormone deficiency, may develop slipped capital epiphyses more frequently. Any child with the onset of a limp or complaints of hip or knee pain during growth hormone therapy should be evaluated.
Intracranial hypertension (IH) with papilledema, visual changes, headache, nausea and/or vomiting has been reported in a small number of patients treated with growth hormone products. Symptoms usually occurred within the first eight (8) weeks of the initiation of growth hormone therapy. In all reported cases, IH-associated signs and symptoms resolved after termination of therapy or a reduction of the growth hormone dose. Funduscopic examination of patients is recommended at the initiation and periodically during the course of growth hormone therapy.
Carcinogenesis, Mutagenesis, Impairment of Fertility: Long-term animal studies for carcinogenicity and impairment of fertility with Norditropin® have not been performed. There has been no evidence to date of Norditropin-induced mutagenicity.
Pregnancy: Pregnancy Category C. Reproduction studies have been performed in rats at doses up to 7 mg/m^2 or about 7 times the maximum recommended human dose on a body surface area basis (mg/m^2) and have revealed no evidence of impaired fertility or harm to the fetus due to Norditropin®. There are, however, no adequate and well-controlled studies in pregnant women. Because animal reproduction studies are not always predictive of human response, this drug should be used during pregnancy only if clearly needed.
Nursing Mothers: There have been no studies conducted with Norditropin® in nursing mothers. It is not known whether this drug is excreted in human milk. Because many drugs are excreted in human milk, caution should be exercised when Norditropin® is administered to a nursing woman.

ADVERSE REACTIONS

As with all protein drugs, a small percentage of patients may develop antibodies to the protein. Growth hormone antibody with binding capacity lower than 2 mg/L has not been associated with growth attenuation. In some cases, when binding capacity is greater than 2 mg/L, interference with growth response has been observed.
In clinical trials, patients receiving Norditropin® for up to 12 months have been tested for induction of antibodies and 0/358 patients developed antibodies with binding capacities above 2 mg/L. Among these patients, 165 had previously been treated with other preparations of growth hormone and 193 were previously untreated naive patients.
Since antibodies to somatropin have the potential to inhibit further linear growth, only patients failing to respond to treatment should be tested for antibodies.
The following adverse events have been reported from clinical studies: headache, localized muscle pain, weakness, mild hyperglycemia and glucosuria.
Leukemia has been reported in a small number of children who have been treated with growth hormone, including growth hormone of pituitary origin and recombinant somatrem and somatropin. On the basis of current evidence, experts cannot conclude that growth hormone therapy is responsible for these occurrences. If there is any risk to an individual patient, it is minimal.

OVERDOSAGE

The maximum dose generally recommended should not be exceeded due to the potential risk of side effects.

DOSAGE AND ADMINISTRATION

The Norditropin® dosage and schedule for administration must be individualized for each patient. Generally, subcutaneous administration in the evening, 6–7 times a week, is recommended. It is furthermore recommended to give the injections in the thighs and to vary the injection site on the thigh on a rotating basis. Dosage can be calculated according to body weight.

Generally recommended dosage:
Subcutaneous injection:
0.024–0.034 mg/kg body weight, 6–7 times a week.

Dissolution Procedure:
The Norditropin® solution for subcutaneous injection is prepared by adding the 2 mL diluent to the drug powder in the vial

1. Use a syringe and needle for injection. Before injection the rubber closures should be wiped with an antiseptic solution to prevent contamination of the contents after repeated needle insertions. Push the needle through the rubber closure on the top of the vial with the diluent. Draw up the diluent. It is easier to draw up the diluent if you have first injected air into the vial.
2. Pull out the needle. Take the vial with dry powder, push the needle through the rubber closure and inject the diluent into the vial aiming the stream of liquid against the glass wall.
3. Dissolve the dry powder completely by gently turning the vial upside down several times. DO NOT SHAKE the vial. The contents MUST NOT BE INJECTED if the solution is cloudy or contains particulate matter.

Continued on next page

Norditropin—Cont.

Measuring the Prescribed Dose:
4 mg (approximately 12 IU) Vial
After the dry powder has been dissolved, the solution contains 2 mg Norditropin® per mL. If the prescribed dose is e.g. 1 mg Norditropin®, draw up 0.5 mL of the solution into a syringe suitable for small volumes.
8 mg (approximately 24 IU) Vial
After the dry powder has been dissolved, the solution contains 4 mg Norditropin® per mL. If the prescribed dose is e.g. 1 mg Norditropin®, draw up 0.25 mL of the solution into a syringe suitable for small volumes.
Storage:
Before and after reconstitution with diluent Norditropin® must be stored at 2–8°C/36–46°F (refrigerator). Do not freeze. Avoid direct light.
Norditropin® retains its biological potency until the date of expiry indicated on the label. Reconstituted vials should be used within 14 days after dissolution.

HOW SUPPLIED

Norditropin® is supplied as 4 mg or 8 mg (approximately 12 or 24 IU) of lyophilized, sterile somatropin per vial.
Each 4 mg carton contains one vial of Norditropin® (4 mg per vial) and one vial of diluent (2 mL of Water for Injection USP with benzyl alcohol 1.5%).
NDC 0169-7774-11
Each 8 mg carton contains one vial of Norditropin® (8 mg per vial) and one vial of diluent (2 mL of Water for Injection USP with benzyl alcohol 1.5%).
NDC 0169-7778-12

Revised 3/99
Rx only

For information contact:
Novo Nordisk Pharmaceuticals, Inc.
100 College Road West
Princeton, NJ 08540

Manufactured by:
Novo Nordisk A/S
2880 Bagsvaerd, Denmark
Shown in Product Identification Guide, page 326

NORDITROPIN® CARTRIDGES ℞

[nŏrd" ĕ trōp' ĭn]
Somatropin (rDNA origin) injection
5 mg/1.5 mL, 10 mg/1.5 mL or 15 mg/1.5 mL

DESCRIPTION

Norditropin® is the Novo Nordisk Pharmaceuticals, Inc. registered trademark for somatropin, a polypeptide hormone of recombinant DNA origin. The hormone is synthesized by a special strain of *E. coli* bacteria that has been modified by the addition of a plasmid which carries the gene for human growth hormone. Norditropin® contains the identical sequence of 191 amino acids constituting the naturally occurring pituitary human growth hormone with a molecular weight of about 22,000 Daltons.
Norditropin® cartridges are supplied as solutions in ready-to-administer cartridges with a volume of 1.5 mL.
Each **Norditropin® cartridge** contains the following:

Component	5 mg/1.5 mL	10 mg/1.5 mL	15 mg/1.5 mL
Somatropin	5 mg	10 mg	15 mg
Histidine	1 mg	1 mg	1.7 mg
Poloxamer 188	4.5 mg	4.5 mg	4.5 mg
Phenol	4.5 mg	4.5 mg	4.5 mg
Mannitol	60 mg	60 mg	58 mg
HCl/NaOH	q.s.	q.s.	q.s.
Water for Injection	ad 1.5 mL	ad 1.5 mL	ad 1.5 mL

CLINICAL PHARMACOLOGY

a. Tissue Growth
The primary and most intensively studied action of somatropin is the stimulation of linear growth. This effect is demonstrated in patients with somatropin deficiency.

1. Skeletal growth – the measurable increase in bone length after administration of somatropin results from its effect on the cartilaginous growth areas of long bones. Studies *in vitro* have shown that the incorporation of sulfate into proteoglycans is not due to a direct effect of somatropin, but rather is mediated by the somatomedins or insulin-like growth factors (IGF). The somatomedins, among them somatomedin C, are polypeptide hormones which are synthesized in the liver, kidney, and various other tissue. Somatomedin C is low in the serum of hypopituitary dwarfs and hypophysectomized humans or animals, but its presence can be demonstrated after treatment with somatropin.
2. Cell growth – it has been shown that the total number of skeletal muscle cells is markedly decreased in short stature children lacking endogenous somatropin compared with normal children, and that treatment with somatropin results in an increase in both the number and size of muscle cells.
3. Organ growth – somatropin influences the size of internal organs, and it also increases red cell mass.

b. Protein Metabolism
Linear growth is facilitated in part by increased cellular protein synthesis. This synthesis and growth are reflected by nitrogen retention which can be quantitated by observing the decline in urinary nitrogen excretion and blood urea nitrogen following the initiation of somatropin therapy.
c. Carbohydrate Metabolism
Hypopituitary children sometimes experience fasting hypoglycemia that may be improved by treatment with somatropin. In healthy subjects, large doses of somatropin may impair glucose tolerance. Although the precise mechanism of the diabetogenic effect of somatropin is not known, it is attributed to blocking the action of insulin rather than blocking insulin secretion. Insulin levels in serum actually increase as somatropin levels increase.
d. Fat Metabolism
Somatropin stimulates intracellular lipolysis, and administration of somatropin leads to an increase in plasma free fatty acids, cholesterol, and triglycerides. Untreated growth hormone deficiency is associated with increased body fat stores including increased subcutaneous adipose tissue. On somatropin replacement a general reduction of fat stores and of subcutaneous tissue in particular takes place.
e. Mineral Metabolism
Administration of somatropin results in the retention of total body potassium and phosphorus and to a lesser extent sodium. This retention is thought to be the result of cell growth. Serum levels of phosphate increase in patients with growth hormone deficiency after somatropin therapy due to metabolic activity associated with bone growth. Serum calcium levels are not altered. Although calcium excretion in the urine is increased, there is a simultaneous increase in calcium absorption from the intestine. Negative calcium balance, however, may occasionally occur during somatropin treatment.
f. Connective Tissue Metabolism
Somatropin stimulates the synthesis of chrondroitin sulfate and collagen as well as the urinary excretion of hydroxyproline.
g. Pharmacokinetics
A 180-min IV infusion of Norditropin® (33 ng/kg/min) was given to 9 GHD patients. A mean (±SD) hGH steady-state serum level of approximately 23.1 (±15.0) ng/mL was reached at 150 min and a mean clearance rate of approximately 2.3 (±1.8) mL/min/kg or 139 (±105) mL/min for hGH was obtained. Following infusion, serum hGH levels had a biexponential decay with a terminal elimination half-life ($T_{1/2}$) of approximately 21.1 (±5.1) min.
In a study conducted in 18 GHD adult patients, where a SC dose of 0.024 mg/kg or 3 IU/m^2 was given in the thigh, the mean (±SD) C_{max} values of 13.8 (±5.8) and 17.1 (±10.0) ng/mL were obtained for the 4 and 8 mg Norditropin® vials, respectively, at approximately 4 to 5 hr. post dose. The mean apparent terminal $T_{1/2}$ values were estimated to be approximately 7 to 10 hr. However, the absolute bioavailability for Norditropin® after the SC route of administration is currently not known.
Norditropin® cartridge formulation is bioequivalent to Norditropin® vial formulation.

INDICATIONS AND USAGE

Norditropin® is indicated for the long-term treatment of children who have growth failure due to inadequate secretion of endogenous growth hormone.

CONTRAINDICATIONS

Norditropin® should not be used in subjects with closed epiphyses.
Norditropin® should not be used in hypopituitary children who have evidence of actively growing intracranial tumors. Therapy with somatropin should be discontinued if there is evidence of recurrent tumor growth.
Norditropin® should not be used or should be discontinued when there is any evidence of active malignancy. Anti-malignancy treatment must be complete with evidence of remission prior to the institution of growth hormone therapy.
Norditropin® should not be used in any subjects with known hypersensitivity to any of the constituents of the preparation.
Growth hormone should not be initiated to treat patients with acute critical illness due to complications following open heart or abdominal surgery, multiple accidental trauma or to patients having acute respiratory failure. Two placebo-controlled clinical trials in non-growth hormone deficient adult patients (n=522) with these conditions revealed a significant increase in mortality (41.9% vs. 19.3%) among somatropin treated patients (doses 5.3–8 mg/day) compared to those receiving placebo (see WARNINGS).

WARNINGS

Norditropin® (somatropin [rDNA origin] injection) cartridges must be used with their corresponding color-coded NordiPen™ delivery device. A Norditropin® cartridge must not be inserted into a pen with a different color code.
See CONTRAINDICATIONS for information on increased mortality in patients with acute critical illnesses in intensive care units due to complications following open heart or abdominal surgery, multiple accidental trauma or with acute respiratory failure. The safety of continuing growth hormone treatment in patients receiving replacement doses for approved indications who concurrently develop these illnesses has not been established. Therefore, the potential benefit of treatment continuation with growth hormone in patients having acute critical illnesses should be weighed against the potential risk.

PRECAUTIONS

Norditropin® should be used only by physicians with experience in the diagnosis and management of patients with growth hormone deficiency.
Patients with growth hormone deficiency secondary to an intracranial lesion should be examined frequently for progression or recurrence of the underlying disease process.
Because growth hormone may induce a state of insulin resistance, patients should be observed for evidence of glucose intolerance.
Concomitant glucocorticoid therapy may inhibit the growth promoting effect of Norditropin®. Patients with coexisting ACTH deficiency should have their glucocorticoid replacement dose carefully adjusted to avoid an inhibitory effect on growth.
A state of hypothyroidism may develop during Norditropin® treatment. Since untreated hypothyroidism may interfere with the response to Norditropin®, patients should have a periodic thyroid function test and should be treated with thyroid hormone when indicated.
Patients with endocrine disorders, including growth hormone deficiency, may develop slipped capital epiphyses more frequently. Any child with the onset of a limp or complaints of hip or knee pain during growth hormone therapy should be evaluated.
Intracranial hypertension (IH) with papilledema, visual changes, headache, nausea and/or vomiting has been reported in a small number of patients treated with growth hormone products. Symptoms usually occurred within the first eight (8) weeks of the initiation of growth hormone therapy. In all reported cases, IH-associated signs and symptoms resolved after termination of therapy or a reduction of the growth hormone dose. Funduscopic examination of patients is recommended at the initiation and periodically during the course of growth hormone therapy.
Progression of scoliosis can occur in children who experience rapid growth. Because growth hormone increases growth rate, patients with a history of scoliosis who are treated with growth hormone should be monitored for progression of scoliosis.
Carcinogenesis, Mutagenesis, Impairment of Fertility: Carcinogenicity, mutagenicity, and fertility studies have not been conducted with Norditropin® cartridges.
Pregnancy: Pregnancy Category C. Animal reproduction studies have not been conducted with Norditropin® cartridge formulation. It is also not known whether Norditropin® can cause fetal harm when administered to a pregnant woman or can affect reproduction capacity. Norditropin® should be given to a pregnant woman only if clearly needed.
Nursing Mothers: It is not known whether this drug is excreted in human milk. Because many drugs are excreted in human milk, caution should be exercised when Norditropin® is administered to a nursing woman.

ADVERSE REACTIONS

As with all protein drugs, a small percentage of patients may develop antibodies to the protein. Growth hormone antibody with binding capacity lower than 2 mg/L has not been associated with growth attenuation. In some cases, when binding capacity is greater than 2 mg/L, interference with growth response has been observed.
In clinical trials, patients receiving Norditropin® for up to 12 months have been tested for induction of antibodies and 0/358 patients developed antibodies with binding capacities above 2 mg/L. Among these patients, 165 had previously been treated with other preparations of growth hormone and 193 were previously untreated naive patients.
Since antibodies to somatropin have the potential to inhibit further linear growth, only patients failing to respond to treatment should be tested for antibodies.
The following adverse events have been reported from clinical studies: headache, localized muscle pain, weakness, mild hyperglycemia and glucosuria.
Leukemia has been reported in a small number of children who have been treated with growth hormone, including growth hormone of pituitary origin and recombinant somatrem and somatropin. On the basis of current evidence, experts cannot conclude that growth hormone therapy is responsible for these occurrences. If there is any risk to an individual patient, it is minimal.
Fluid retention and peripheral edema may occur.

OVERDOSAGE

The maximum dose generally recommended should not be exceeded due to the potential risk of side effects.

DOSAGE AND ADMINISTRATION

The Norditropin® dosage and schedule for administration must be individualized for each patient. Generally, subcutaneous administration in the evening, 6–7 times a week, is recommended. It is furthermore recommended to give the injections in the thighs and to vary the injection site on the thigh on a rotating basis. Dosage can be calculated according to body weight.
Generally recommended dosage:
Subcutaneous injection:
0.024–0.034 mg/kg body weight, 6–7 times a week.
Norditropin® cartridges must be administered using the NordiPen™ injection pen. Each cartridge size has a color-coded corresponding pen which is graduated to deliver the appropriate dose based on the concentration of Norditropin® in the cartridge.

Norditropin® MUST NOT BE INJECTED if the solution is cloudy or contains particulate matter. Use it only if it is clear and colorless.

Measuring the Prescribed Dose:

5 mg/1.5 mL, 10 mg/1.5 mL and 15 mg/1.5 mL Norditropin® cartridges

Each cartridge of Norditropin® must be inserted into its corresponding NordiPen™ injection pen. Instructions for delivering the dosage are provided in the NordiPen™ instruction booklet.

Storage:

Norditropin® cartridges must be stored at 2–8°C/36–46°F (refrigerator). Do not freeze. Avoid direct light.

Norditropin® cartridges retain their biological potency until the date of expiry indicated on the label. After a Norditropin® cartridge has been inserted into the NordiPen™ injector, it must be stored in the pen in the refrigerator and used within 4 weeks.

HOW SUPPLIED

Norditropin® (somatropin [rDNA origin] injection) 5 mg/1.5 mL, 10 mg/1.5 mL and 15 mg/1.5 mL cartridges:

Norditropin® is supplied in 5 mg/1.5 mL, 10 mg/1.5 mL or 15 mg/1.5 mL cartridges which must be administered using the corresponding color-coded NordiPen™ injection pen.

Norditropin® 5 mg/1.5 mL cartridge (orange) NDC 0169-7768-11

Norditropin® 10 mg/1.5 mL cartridge (blue) NDC 0169-7769-11

Norditropin® 15 mg/1.5 mL cartridge (green) NDC 0169-7770-11

Norditropin® and NordiPen™ are trademarks of Novo Nordisk A/S.

Revised 6/00

Rx Only

For information contact:

Novo Nordisk
Pharmaceuticals, Inc.
Princeton, New Jersey 08540
USA

Manufactured by:

Novo Nordisk A/S
2880 Bagsvaerd, Denmark

HUMAN INSULIN OTC

NOVOLIN® 70/30
70% NPH, Human Insulin Isophane Suspension and 30% Regular, Human Insulin Injection (recombinant DNA origin)
100 units/ml

WARNING

ANY CHANGE OF INSULIN SHOULD BE MADE CAUTIOUSLY AND ONLY UNDER MEDICAL SUPERVISION. CHANGES IN PURITY, STRENGTH, BRAND (MANUFACTURER), TYPE (REGULAR, NPH, LENTE®, ETC.), SPECIES (BEEF, PORK, BEEF-PORK, HUMAN) AND/OR METHOD OF MANUFACTURE (RECOMBINANT DNA VERSUS ANIMAL-SOURCE INSULIN) MAY RESULT IN THE NEED FOR A CHANGE IN DOSAGE.

SPECIAL CARE SHOULD BE TAKEN WHEN THE TRANSFER IS FROM A STANDARD BEEF OR MIXED SPECIES INSULIN TO A PURIFIED PORK OR HUMAN INSULIN. IF A DOSAGE ADJUSTMENT IS NEEDED, IT WILL USUALLY BECOME APPARENT EITHER IN THE FIRST FEW DAYS OR OVER A PERIOD OF SEVERAL WEEKS. ANY CHANGE IN TREATMENT SHOULD BE CAREFULLY MONITORED.

PLEASE READ THE SECTIONS "INSULIN REACTION AND SHOCK" AND "DIABETIC KETOACIDOSIS AND COMA" FOR SYMPTOMS OF HYPOGLYCEMIA (LOW BLOOD GLUCOSE) AND HYPERGLYCEMIA (HIGH BLOOD GLUCOSE).

INSULIN USE IN DIABETES

Your physician has explained that you have diabetes and that your treatment involves injections of insulin or insulin therapy combined with an oral antidiabetic medicine. Insulin is normally produced by the pancreas, a gland that lies behind the stomach. Without insulin, glucose (a simple sugar made from digested food) is trapped in the bloodstream and cannot enter the cells of the body. Some patients who don't make enough of their own insulin, or who cannot use the insulin they do make properly, must take insulin by injection in order to control their blood glucose levels.

Each case of diabetes is different and requires direct and continued medical supervision. Your physician has told you the type, strength and amount of insulin you should use and the time(s) at which you should inject it, and has also discussed with you a diet and exercise schedule. You should contact your physician if you experience any difficulties or if you have questions.

TYPES OF INSULINS

Standard and purified animal insulins as well as human insulins are available. Standard and purified insulins differ in their degree of purification and content of noninsulin material. Standard and purified insulins also vary in species source: they may be of beef, pork, or mixed beef and pork origin. Human insulin is identical in structure to the insulin produced by the human pancreas, and thus differs from animal insulins. Insulins vary in time of action and in strength; see PRODUCT DESCRIPTION and SYRINGES for additional information.

Your physician has prescribed the insulin that is right for you; be sure you have purchased the correct insulin and check it carefully before you use it.

PRODUCT DESCRIPTION

This vial contains **Novolin® 70/30** which is a mixture of 70% NPH, Human Insulin Isophane Suspension (recombinant DNA origin) and 30% Regular, Human Insulin Injection (recombinant DNA origin) USP. The concentration of this product is 100 units of insulin per milliliter. It is a cloudy or milky suspension of human insulin with protamine and zinc. The insulin substance (the cloudy material) settles at the bottom of the vial, therefore, the vial must be gently agitated or rotated so that the contents are uniformly mixed before a dose is withdrawn. **Novolin® 70/30** has an intermediate duration of action. The effect of **Novolin® 70/30** begins approximately $^1/_2$ hour after injection. The effect is maximal between 2 and approximately 12 hours. The full duration of action may last up to 24 hours after injection.

The time course of action of any insulin may vary considerably in different individuals, or at different times in the same individual. Because of this variation, the time periods listed here should be considered as general guidelines only. This human insulin (recombinant DNA origin) is structurally identical to the insulin produced by the human pancreas. This human insulin is produced by recombinant DNA technology utilziing Saccharomyces cerevisiae (bakers' yeast) as the production organism.

STORAGE

Insulin should be stored in a cold place, preferably in a refrigerator, but not in the freezing compartment. **Do not let it freeze.** Keep the insulin vial in its carton so that it will stay clean and protected from light. If refrigeration is not possible, the bottle of insulin which you are currently using can be kept unrefrigerated as long as it is kept as cool as possible and away from heat and sunlight.

Never use **Novolin® 70/30** if the precipitate (the white deposit at the bottom of the vial) has become lumpy or granular in appearance or has formed a deposit of solid particles on the wall of the vial. This insulin should not be used if the liquid in the vial remains clear after the vial has been gently agitated.

Never use insulin after the expiration date which is printed on the vial label and carton.

SYRINGES

Use the Correct Syringe

Doses of insulin are measured in units. Some insulins are available in two strengths: U-100 and U-40. One milliliter (ml) of U-100 contains 100 units of insulin. One milliliter (ml) of U-40 contains 40 units of insulin. Be sure to use the proper syringe for the strength of the insulin prescribed for you. Syringes are clearly marked **"For use with U-100 insulin"** or **"For use with U-40 insulin"**. Low dose U-100 syringes are also available. Failure to use the proper syringe can lead to mistakes in dosage.

Novo Nordisk insulin vials are intended for use with standard insulin syringes. Novo Nordisk has not evaluated the use of these vials with other devices for insulin delivery or with devices intended to aid in giving injections. Consult your doctor and the manufacturer of these devices before use with this product.

Disposable Syringes

Disposable syringes and needles require no sterilization provided the package is intact. They should be used only once and discarded.

Reusable Syringes

Reusable syringes and needles must be sterilized before each use.

1. Boil the syringe parts and needles in a pan of water for at least five minutes. Keep a special pan for this purpose. Heavily chlorinated water should not be used; distilled water is preferable.
   If boiling is not possible, the syringe parts and needles may be sterilized by immersion in 70% ethyl alcohol or 91% isopropyl alcohol for at least five minutes. **Do not use bathing, rubbing or medicated alcohol for sterilization.**
2. Assemble the syringe and fit the needle on the tip of the syringe being careful not to touch the surface of the plunger or needle.
3. Push the plunger in and out several times until the water (or alcohol) has been completely expelled. (The syringe should be thoroughly dried before its use.)

IMPORTANT

Failure to comply with the above and the following antiseptic measures may lead to infections at the injection site.

PREPARING THE INJECTION

1. Clean your hands and the injection site with soap and water or with alcohol. Wipe the rubber stopper with an alcohol swab. (Note: remove the tamper-resistant cap at first use. If the cap has already been removed, do not use this product, return it to your pharmacy.)
2. For insulin suspensions, roll the vial of insulin gently in your hands to mix it. Vigorous shaking immediately before the dose is drawn into the syringe may result in the formation of bubbles or froth which could cause dosage errors.
3. Pull back the plunger until the black tip reaches the marking for the number of units you will inject.
4. Push the needle through the rubber stopper into the vial.
5. Push the plunger all the way in. This inserts air into the bottle.
6. Turn the vial and syringe upside down and slowly pull the plunger back to a few units beyond the correct dose.
7. If there are air bubbles, flick the syringe firmly with your finger to raise the air bubbles to the needle, then slowly push the plunger to the correct unit marking.
8. Lift the vial off the syringe.

GIVING THE INJECTION

1. The following areas are suitable for subcutaneous insulin injection: thighs, upper arms, buttocks, abdomen. Do not change areas without consulting your physician. The actual point of injection should be changed each time; injection sites should be about an inch apart.
2. The injection site should be clean and dry. Pinch up skin area to be injected and hold it firmly.
3. Hold the syringe like a pencil and push the needle quickly and firmly into the pinched-up area.
4. Release the skin and push the plunger all the way in to inject insulin beneath the skin. To ensure that all the insulin is injected keep the needle in the skin for several seconds after injection with your finger on the plunger. Do not inject into a muscle unless your physician has advised it. You should never inject insulin into a vein.
5. Remove needle. If slight bleeding occurs, press lightly with a dry cotton swab for a few seconds—**do not rub.**

Note:

The dose should be injected over 2–4 seconds. Preparations of insulin suspensions which are injected slowly may clog the tip of the needle, resulting in an inability to complete the injection. Syringe plugging does not occur when the drug is injected more rapidly. Use the injection technique recommended by your physician.

MIXING INSULIN

Novolin® 70/30 is a premixed insulin containing 70% NPH, Human Insulin Isophane Suspension, recombinant DNA origin (**Novolin® N**) and 30% Regular, Human Insulin Injection, recombinant DNA origin (**Novolin® R**). You should not attempt to change the ratio of this product by adding additional NPH or Regular insulin to this vial. If your physician has prescribed insulin mixed in a proportion other than 70% NPH and 30% Regular, you should use the separate insulin formulations (**Novolin® N** and **Novolin® R**) in the amounts recommended by your physician.

USAGE IN PREGNANCY

It is particularly important to maintain good control of your diabetes during pregnancy and special attention must be paid to your diet, exercise and insulin regimens. If you are pregnant or nursing a baby, consult your physician or nurse educator.

INSULIN REACTION AND SHOCK

Insulin reaction ("hypoglycemia") occurs when the blood glucose falls very low. This can happen if you take too much insulin, miss or delay a meal, exercise more than usual or work too hard without eating, or become ill (especially with vomiting or fever). Hypoglycemia can also happen if you combine insulin therapy and other medications that lower blood glucose, such as an oral antidiabetic agents or other prescription and over-the-counter drugs. The first symptoms of an insulin reaction usually come on suddenly. They may include a cold sweat, fatigue, nervousness or shakiness, rapid heartbeat, or nausea. Personality change or confusion may also occur. If you drink or eat something right away (a glass of milk or orange juice, or several sugar candies), you can often stop the progression of symptoms. If symptoms persist, call your physician — an insulin reaction can lead to unconsciousness. If a reaction results in loss of consciousness, emergency medical care should be obtained immediately. If you have had repeated reactions or if an insulin reaction has led to a loss of consciousness, contact your physician. Severe hypoglycemia can result in temporary or permanent impairment of brain function and death. **In certain cases, the nature and intensity of the warning symptoms of hypoglycemia may change. A few patients have reported that after being transferred to human insulin, the early warning symptoms of hypoglycemia were less pronounced than they had been with animal-source insulin.**

DIABETIC KETOACIDOSIS AND COMA

Diabetic ketoacidosis may develop if your body has too little insulin. The most common causes are acute illness or infection or failure to take enough insulin by injection. If you are ill you should check your urine for ketones. The symptoms of diabetic ketoacidosis usually come on gradually, over a period of hours or days, and include a drowsy feeling, flushed face, thirst and loss of appetite. Notify your physician right away if the urine test is positive for ketones (acetone) or if you have any of these symptoms. Fast, heavy breathing and rapid pulse are more severe symptoms and you should have medical attention right away. Severe, sustained hyperglycemia may result in diabetic coma and death.

ADVERSE REACTIONS

A few people with diabetes develop red, swollen and itchy skin where the insulin has been injected. This is called a "local reaction" and it may occur if the injection is not properly made, if the skin is sensitive to the cleansing solution, or if you are allergic to the insulin being used. If you have a local reaction, tell your physician.

Generalized insulin allergy occurs rarely, but when it does it may cause a serious reaction, including skin rash over the

Continued on next page

Novolin 70/30—Cont.

body, shortness of breath, fast pulse, sweating, and a drop in blood pressure. If any of these symptoms develop, you should seek emergency medical care.
If severe allergic reactions to insulin have occurred (i.e., generalized rash, swelling or breathing difficulties) you should be skin-tested with **each** new insulin preparation before it is used.

IMPORTANT NOTES

1. A change in the type, strength, species or purity of insulin could require a dosage adjustment. Any change in insulin should be made under medical supervision.
2. You may have learned how to test your urine or your blood for glucose. It is important to do these tests regularly and to record the results for review with your physician or nurse educator.
3. If you have an acute illness, especially with vomiting or fever, continue taking your insulin. If possible, stay on your regular diet. If you have trouble eating, drink fruit juices, regular soft drinks, or clear soups; if you can, eat small amounts of bland foods. Test your urine for glucose and ketones and, if possible, test your blood glucose. Note the results and contact your physician for possible insulin dose adjustment. If you have severe and prolonged vomiting, seek emergency medical care.
4. You should always carry identification which states that you have diabetes.
5. Always ask your physician or pharmacist before taking any drug.

Always consult your physician if you have any questions about your condition or the use of insulin.

Helpful information for people with diabetes is published by American Diabetes Association, 1660 Duke Street, Alexandria, VA 22314.

For information contact: Novo Nordisk Pharmaceuticals, Inc., Princeton, NJ 08540

Manufactured by Novo Nordisk A/S, DK-2880 Bagsvaerd, Denmark and by Novo Nordisk Pharmaceutical Industries, Inc., 3612 Powhatan Road, Clayton, NC. 27520
Date of issue: December 1995

HOW SUPPLIED

Vials, U-100, 100 units/mL, 10 mL, (List No. 183711) (1's)
Novolin 70/30 Prefilled® Syringe, U-100, 100 units/mL, 1.5 mL, (List No. 001771) (5's)
Novolin® 70/30 PenFill® Cartridges, U-100, 100 units/mL, 1.5 mL, (List No. 183717) (5's)
Novolin® 70/30 PenFill® Cartridges, U-100, 100 units/mL, 3 mL, (List No. 347718) (5's)

HUMAN INSULIN NOVOLIN® L — OTC

Lente®, Human Insulin Zinc Suspension (recombinant DNA origin)
100 units/ml

PRODUCT DESCRIPTION

Novolin® L is commonly known as Lente® Human Insulin Zinc Suspension (recombinant DNA origin). The concentration of this product is 100 units of insulin per milliliter. It is a cloudy or milky suspension of 70% crystalline and 30% amorphous human insulin. The insulin substance (the cloudy material) settles at the bottom of the vial, therefore, the vial must be gently agitated or rotated so that the contents are uniformly mixed before a dose is withdrawn. **Novolin® L** has an intermediate duration of action. The effect of **Novolin® L** begins approximately $2^1/_2$ hours after injection. The effect is maximal between 7 and 15 hours and ends approximately 22 hours after injection. The time course of action of any insulin may vary considerably in different individuals or at different times in the same individual. Because of this variation, the periods listed here should be considered as general guidelines only.
This human insulin (recombinant DNA origin) is structurally identical to the insulin produced by the human pancreas. This human insulin is produced by recombinant DNA technology utilizing *Saccharomyces cerevisiae* (bakers' yeast) as the production organism.

STORAGE

Insulin should be stored in a cold place, preferably in a refrigerator, but not in the freezing compartment. **Do not let it freeze.** Keep the insulin vial in its carton so that it will stay clean and protected from light. If refrigeration is not possible, the bottle of insulin which you are currently using can be kept unrefrigerated as long as it is kept as cool as possible and away from heat and sunlight.
Never use **Novolin® L** if the precipitate (the white deposit at the bottom of the vial) has become lumpy or granular in appearance or has formed a deposit of solid particles on the wall of the vial. This insulin should not be used if the liquid in the vial remains clear after the vial has been gently agitated.

Never use insulin after the expiration date which is printed on the vial label and carton.

MIXING TWO TYPES OF INSULIN—SEE NOVOLIN® N

SEE NOVOLIN® 70/30 for complete package insert information on Warning: Insulin Use in Diabetes: Types of Insulins: Syringes: Needle-Free Injectors: Important Statement: Preparing the Injection: Giving the Injection: Usage in Pregnancy: Insulin Reaction and Shock: Diabetic Ketoacidosis and Coma: Adverse Reactions: Important Notes.

Date of Issue: February 1998

HOW SUPPLIED

Vials, U-100, 100 units/mL, 10 mL, (List No. 183511) (1's)

NOVOLIN® N — OTC

NPH, Human Insulin Isophane Suspension (recombinant DNA origin)
100 units/ml

PRODUCT DESCRIPTION

Novolin® N is commonly known as NPH, Human Insulin Isophane Suspension (recombinant DNA origin). The concentration of this product is 100 units of insulin per milliliter. It is a cloudy or milky suspension of human insulin with protamine and zinc. The insulin substance (the cloudy material) settles at the bottom of the vial, therefore, the vial must be gently agitated or rotated so that the contents are uniformly mixed before a dose is withdrawn. **Novolin® N** has an intermediate duration of action. The effect of **Novolin® N** begins approximately $1^1/_2$ hours after injection. The effect is maximal between 4 and 12 hours. The full duration of action may last up to 24 hours after injection. The time course of action of any insulin may vary considerably in different individuals, or at different times in the same individual. Because of this variation, the periods listed here should be considered as general guidelines only.
This human insulin (recombinant DNA origin) is structurally identical to the insulin produced by the human pancreas. This human insulin is produced by recombinant DNA technology utilizing *Saccharomyces cerevisiae* (bakers' yeast) as the production organism.

STORAGE

Insulin should be stored in a cold place, preferably in a refrigerator, but not in the freezing compartment. **Do not let it freeze.** Keep the insulin vial in its carton so that it will stay clean and protected from light. If refrigeration is not possible, the bottle of insulin which you are currently using can be kept unrefrigerated as long as it is kept as cool as possible and away from heat and sunlight.
Never use **Novolin® N** if the precipitate (the white deposit at the bottom of the vial) has become lumpy or granular in appearance or has formed a deposit of solid particles on the wall of the vial. This insulin should not be used if the liquid in the vial remains clear after the vial has been gently agitated.

Never use insulin after the expiration date which is printed on the vial label and carton.

MIXING TWO TYPES OF INSULIN

Different insulins should be mixed only under instruction from a physician. Hypodermic syringes may vary in the amount of space between the bottom line and the needle ("dead space"), so if you are mixing two types of insulin be sure to discuss any change in the model and brand of syringe you are using with your physician or pharmacist. When you are mixing two types of insulin, always draw the Regular (clear) insulin into the syringe first.
SEE NOVOLIN® 70/30 for complete package insert information on Warning: Insulin Use in Diabetes: Types of Insulin: Syringes: Needle-Free Injectors: Important Statement: Preparing the Injection: Giving the Injection: Usage in Pregnancy: Insulin Reaction and Shock; Diabetic Ketoacidosis and Coma: Adverse Reactions: Important Notes.

HOW SUPPLIED

Vials, U-100, 100 units/mL, 10 mL, (List No. 183411) (1's)
Novolin N Prefilled® Syringe, U-100, 100 units/mL, 1.5 mL, (List No. 004571) (5's)
Novolin® N PenFill® cartridges, U-100, 100 units/mL, 1.5 mL, (List No. 183417) (5's)
Novolin® N PenFill® cartridges, U-100, 100 units/mL, 3 mL (List No. 347418) (5's)
Manufactured by: Novo Nordisk A/S, DK-2880 Bagsvaerd, Denmark and by Novo Nordisk Pharmaceutical Industries, Inc., 3612 Powhatan Road, Clayton, NC. 27520
Date of Issue: February 1999

Shown in Product Identification Guide, page 327

NOVOLIN® R — OTC

Regular, Human Insulin Injection (recombinant DNA origin) USP
100 units/ml

PRODUCT DESCRIPTION

Novolin® R is commonly known as Regular, Human Insulin Injection (recombinant DNA origin) USP. The concentration of this product is 100 units of insulin per milliliter. It is a clear, colorless solution which has a short duration of action. The effect of **Novolin® R** begins approximately $^1/_2$ hour after injection. The effect is maximal between $2^1/_2$ and 5 hours and ends approximately 8 hours after injection. The time course of action of any insulin may vary considerably in different individuals or at different times in the same individual. Because of this variation, the time periods listed here should be considered as general guidelines only.
This human insulin (recombinant DNA origin) is structurally identical to the insulin produced by the human pancreas. This human insulin is produced by recombinant DNA technology utilizing *Saccharomyces cerevisiae* (bakers' yeast) as the production organism.

STORAGE

Insulin should be stored in a cold place, preferably in a refrigerator, but not in the freezing compartment. **Do not let it freeze.** Keep the insulin vial in its carton so that it will stay clean and protected from light. If refrigeration is not possible, the bottle of insulin which you are currently using can be kept unrefrigerated as long as it is kept as cool as possible and away from heat and sunlight.
Never use **Novolin® R** if it becomes viscous (thickened) or cloudy; use it only if it is clear and colorless.

Never use insulin after the expiration date which is printed on the vial label and carton.

MIXING TWO TYPES OF INSULIN—SEE NOVOLIN® N.

IMPORTANT NOTES

1. Due to risk of precipitation in some pump catheters, Novolin® R is not recommended for use in insulin pumps.
2. A change in the type, strength, species or purity of insulin could require a dosage adjustment. Any change in insulin should be made under medical supervision.
3. You may have learned how to test your urine or your blood for glucose. It is important to do these tests regularly and to record the results for review with your physician or nurse educator.
4. If you have an acute illness, especially with vomiting or fever, continue taking your insulin. If possible, stay on your regular diet. If you have trouble eating, drink fruit juices, regular soft drinks, or clear soups; if you can, eat small amounts of bland foods. Test your urine for glucose and ketones and, if possible, test your blood glucose. Note the results and contact your physician for possible insulin dose adjustment. If you have severe and prolonged vomiting, seek emergency medical care.
5. You should always carry identification which states that you have diabetes.
6. Always ask your physician or pharmacist before taking any drug.

Always consult your physician if you have any questions about your condition or the use of insulin.
See Novolin® 70/30 for complete package insert information on Warning: Insulin use in Diabetes: Types of Insulin: Syringes: Needle-Free Injectors: Important Statement: Preparing the Injection: Giving the Injection: Usage in Pregnancy: Insulin Reaction and Shock: Diabetic Ketoacidosis and Coma: Adverse Reactions.

HOW SUPPLIED

Vials, U-100, 100 units/mL, 10 mL, (List No. 183311) (1's)
Novolin R Prefilled® Syringe, U-100, 100 units/mL, 1.5 mL, (List No. 004471) (5's)
Novolin® R PenFill® cartridges, U-100, 100 units/mL, 1.5 mL, (List No. 183317) (5's)
Novolin® R Pen Fill® cartridges, U-100, 100 units/mL, 3 mL (List No. 347318) (5's)
Manufactured by: Novo Nordisk A/S, DK 2880 Bagsvaerd, Denmark and by Novo Nordisk Pharmaceutical Industries, Inc., 3612 Powhatan Road, Clayton, NC. 27520
Date of Issue: February 1999

Shown in Product Identification Guide, page 327

HUMAN INSULIN DELIVERY SYSTEMS

There are two types of Human Insulin Delivery Systems available from Novo Nordisk Pharmaceuticals, Inc.:

DURABLE INSULIN DELIVERY SYSTEM

For the durable insulin delivery system you will need the following items, which are sold separately:
1) **NovoPen® 3** Insulin Delivery Device
2) **NovoPen® 1.5** Insulin Delivery Device
3) **Novolin® PenFill®** Cartridges 1.5 mL and 3 mL
4) **NovoFine® 30** Disposable Needles
For information about obtaining NovoPen® Insulin Delivery Devices for patients, call 1-800-707-9856

DISPOSABLE INSULIN DELIVERY SYSTEM

For the disposable insulin delivery system you will need the following items, which are sold separately:
1) **Novolin Prefilled® Syringes**
2) **NovoFine® 30** Disposable Needles

HUMAN INSULIN NOVOLIN® 70/30 PenFill® — OTC

70% NPH, Human Insulin Isophane Suspension and 30% Regular, Human Insulin Injection (recombinant DNA origin)
100 units/ml

NOVOLIN® N PenFill® — OTC

NPH, Human Insulin Isophane Suspension (recombinant DNA origin)
100 units/ml

NOVOLIN® R PenFill® — OTC

Regular, Human Insulin Injection (recombinant DNA origin)
100 units/ml

Insulin Information for the Patient
Please read this leaflet carefully before using this product. Please note the special directions under "PREPARING THE INJECTION".
Novolin® PenFill® cartridges are designed for use with **NovoPen®** and **NovolinPen® Insulin Delivery Devices** and **NovoFine®** disposable needles or other products specifically recommended by Novo Nordisk.
PenFill® cartridge is for single person use only.
See Important Notes section.

WARNING

ANY CHANGE OF INSULIN SHOULD BE MADE CAUTIOUSLY AND ONLY UNDER MEDICAL SUPERVISION. CHANGES IN PURITY, STRENGTH, BRAND (MANUFACTURER), TYPE (REGULAR, NPH, LENTE®, ETC.), SPECIES (BEEF, PORK, BEEF-PORK, HUMAN), AND/OR METHOD OF MANUFACTURE (RECOMBINANT DNA VERSUS ANIMAL-SOURCE INSULIN) MAY RESULT IN THE NEED FOR A CHANGE IN DOSAGE.
SPECIAL CARE SHOULD BE TAKEN WHEN THE TRANSFER IS FROM A STANDARD BEEF OR MIXED SPECIES INSULIN TO A PURIFIED PORK OR HUMAN INSULIN. IF A DOSAGE ADJUSTMENT IS NEEDED, IT WILL USUALLY BECOME APPARENT EITHER IN THE FIRST FEW DAYS OR OVER A PERIOD OF SEVERAL WEEKS. ANY CHANGE IN TREATMENT SHOULD BE CAREFULLY MONITORED.
PLEASE READ THE SECTIONS "INSULIN REACTION AND SHOCK" AND "DIABETIC KETOACIDOSIS AND COMA" FOR SYMPTOMS OF HYPOGLYCEMIA (LOW BLOOD GLUCOSE) AND HYPERGLYCEMIA (HIGH BLOOD GLUCOSE).

INSULIN USE IN DIABETES

Your physician has explained that you have diabetes and that your treatment involves injections of insulin or insulin therapy combined with an oral antidiabetic medicine. Insulin is normally produced by the pancreas, a gland that lies behind the stomach. Without insulin, glucose (a simple sugar made from digested food) is trapped in the bloodstream and cannot enter the cells of the body. Some patients who don't make enough of their own insulin, or who cannot use properly the insulin they do make, must take insulin by injection in order to control their blood glucose levels. Each case of diabetes is different and requires direct and continued medical supervision. Your physician has told you the type, strength and amount of insulin you should use and the time(s) at which you should inject it, and has also discussed with you a diet and exercise schedule. You should contact your physician if you experience any difficulties or if you have questions.

TYPES OF INSULINS

Standard and purified animal insulins as well as human insulins are available. Standard and purified insulins differ in their degree of purification and content of noninsulin material. Standard and purified insulins also vary in species source: they may be of beef, pork, or mixed beef and pork origin. Human insulin is identical in structure to the insulin produced by the human pancreas, and thus differs from animal insulins. Insulins vary in time of action; see PRODUCT DESCRIPTION for additional information.
Your physician has prescribed the insulin that is right for you; be sure you have purchased the correct insulin and check it carefully before you use it.

PRODUCT DESCRIPTION

A package contains five (5) cartridges.
Novolin® 70/30 PenFill contain **Novolin® 70/30** which is a mixture of 70% NPH, Human Insulin Isophance Suspension (recombinant DNA origin) and 30% Regular, Human Insulin Injection (recombinant DNA origin) USP. The concentration of this product is 100 units of insulin per milliliter. It is a cloudy or milky suspension of human insulin with protamine and zinc. The insulin substance (the cloudy material) settles at the bottom of the cartridge, therefore, the cartridge must be rotated up and down as described under "PREPARING THE INJECTION" so that the contents are uniformly mixed before the dose is given.
Novolin® 70/30 has an intermediate duration of action. The effect of **Novolin® 70/30** begins approximately $^1/_2$ hour after injection. The effect is maximal between 2 and approximately 12 hours. The full duration of action may last up to 24 hours after injection.
The time course of action of any insulin may vary considerably in different individuals, or at different times in the same individual. Because of this variation, the time periods listed here should be considered as general guidelines only.
This human insulin (recombinant DNA origin) is structurally identical to the insulin produced by the human pancreas. This human insulin is produced by recombinant DNA technology utilizing *Saccharomyces cerevisiae* (bakers' yeast) as the production organism.
Novolin® N PenFill® cartridges contain **Novolin® N,** commonly known as NPH, Human Insulin Isophane Suspension (recombinant DNA origin). The concentration of this product is 100 units of insulin per milliliter. It is a cloudy or milky suspension of human insulin with protamine and zinc. The insulin substance (the cloudy material) settles at the bottom of the cartridge; therefore, the cartridge must be turned up and down at least 10 times or until the liquid appears uniformly white and cloudy (a glass ball inside the cartridge facilitates mixing).
Novolin® N has an intermediate duration of action. The effect of **Novolin® N** begins approximately 1½ hours after injection. The effect is maximal between 4 and 12 hours. The full duration of action may last up to 24 hours after injection. The time course of action of any insulin may vary considerably in different individuals, or at different times in the same individual. Because of this variation, the time periods listed here should be considered as general guidelines only.
This human insulin (recombinant DNA origin) is structurally identical to the insulin produced by the human pancreas. This human insulin is produced by recombinant DNA technology utilizing *Saccharomyces cerevisiae* (bakers' yeast) as the production organism.
Novolin® R PenFill® cartridges contain **Novolin® R,** commonly known as Regular, Human Insulin (recombinant DNA origin). The concentration of this product is 100 units of insulin per milliliter. It is a clear, colorless solution which has a short duration of action. The effect of **Novolin® R** begins approximately ½ hour after injection. The effect is maximal between 2½ and 5 hours and ends approximately 8 hours after injection. The time course of action of any insulin may vary considerably in different individuals, or at different times in the same individual. Because of this variation, the time periods listed here should be considered as general guidelines only.
This human insulin (recombinant DNA origin) is structurally identical to the insulin produced by the human pancreas. This human insulin is produced by recombinant DNA technology utilizing *Saccharomyces cerevisiae* (bakers' yeast) as the production organism.

STORAGE

Insulin should be stored in a cold place, preferably in a refrigerator, but not in the freezing compartment. **Do not let it freeze.** Keep **Novolin® 70/30 PenFill®, Novolin® N PenFill®** and **Novolin® R PenFill®** cartridges in the carton so that they will stay clean and protected from light. **Novolin® 70/30 PenFill®,** and **Novolin® N PenFill®** 1.5ml cartridges can be kept unrefrigerated for 7 days. **Novolin® N PenFill®** 3.0ml cartridges can be kept unrefrigerated for 14 days, and **Novolin® 70/30 PenFill®** 3.0ml cartridges can be kept unrefrigerated for 10 days. **Novolin® R PenFill®** 1.5ml and 3.0ml cartridges can be kept unrefrigerated for one (1) month. Unrefrigerated cartridges must be used within this time period or discarded. Be sure to protect cartridges from sunlight and extreme heat or cold.
Never use any **Novolin® 70/30 PenFill®** or **Novolin® N PenFill®** cartridge if the precipitate (the white deposit), has become lumpy or granular in appearance or has formed a deposit of solid particles on the wall of the cartridge. This insulin should not be used if the liquid in the cartridge remains clear after it has been mixed.
Never use any **Novolin® R PenFill®** if it becomes viscous (thickened) or cloudy; use it only if it is clear and colorless.
Never use insulin after the expiration date which is printed on the label and carton.

IMPORTANT

Failure to comply with the following antiseptic measures may lead to infections at the injection site.
— disposable needles are for single use; they should be used only once and destroyed.
— Clean your hands and the injection site with soap and water or with alcohol.
— Wipe the rubber stopper on the insulin cartridge with an alcohol swab.

PREPARING THE INJECTION

Novolin® R PenFill®
Place a single-use on the device. Be sure there is sufficient insulin in the cartridge to complete the injection. Refer to the instruction manual for your insulin delivery device for assistance in estimating the amount of insulin remaining in the cartridge.
Novolin® 70/30 PenFill® and **Novolin® N PenFill®**
Never place a single-use needle on your insulin delivery device until you are ready to give an injection, and remove it immediately after each injection. If the needle is not removed, some liquid may be expelled from the cartridge causing a change in the insulin concentration (strength).
The cloudy material in an insulin suspension will settle to the bottom of the cartridge, so the contents must be mixed before injection. These **Novolin® PenFill®** cartridges contain a glass ball to aid mixing.
When using a new cartridge, turn the cartridge up and down between positions A and B—See Figure 1. Do this at least 10 times until the liquid appears uniformly white and cloudy.

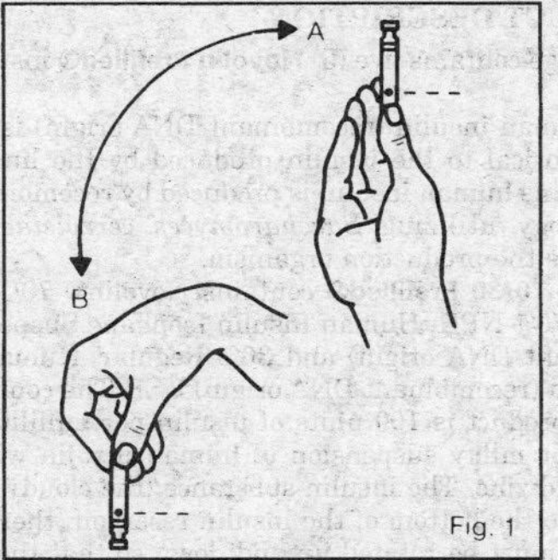

Fig. 1

Assemble your insulin delivery device following the directions in your instruction manual.
For subsequent injections when a cartridge is already in the device, turn the device up and down between positions A and B—See Figure 2. Do this at least 10 times until the liquid appears uniformly white and cloudy. Follow the directions in your insulin delivery device instruction manual.

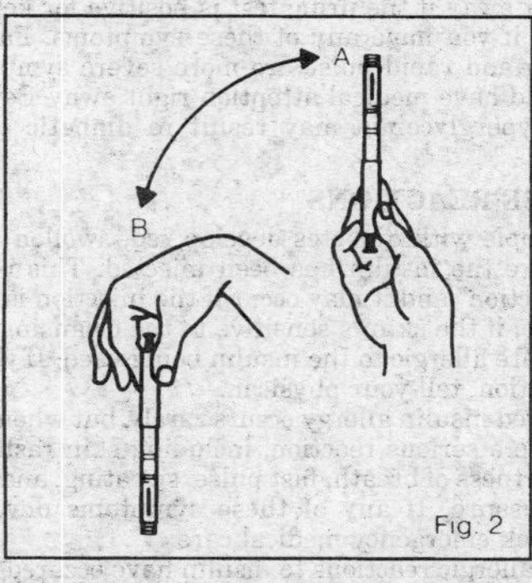

Fig. 2

Always be sure there is sufficient insulin in the cartridge to complete the injection. In order to help you estimate the amount of insulin in the cartridge, the width of the black band corresponds to 12 units of insulin.
Note: Never initiate a new injection unless there is sufficient insulin in the cartridge to ensure proper mixing (the glass ball needs adequate room for movement to mix the suspension). When using a **NovoPen®** device, never initiate a new injection once the leading edge of the plunger has passed the top edge of the black band.
Insulin PenFill® cartridges may contain a small amount of air. To prevent an injection of air and make certain insulin is delivered, an air shot must be done before each injection. Directions for performing an air shot are provided in your insulin delivery device instruction manual.

GIVING THE INJECTION

1. The following areas are suitable for subcutaneous insulin injection: thighs, upper arms, buttocks, abdomen. Do not change areas without consulting your physician. The actual point of injection should be changed each time; injection sites should be about an inch apart.
2. The injection site should be clean and dry. Pinch up skin area to be injected and hold it firmly.
3. Hold the device like a pencil and push the needle quickly and firmly into the pinched-up area.
4. Release the skin and push the push-button all the way in to inject insulin beneath the skin. To ensure that all the insulin is injected keep the needle in the skin for several seconds after injection with your thumb on the push-button. You should never inject insulin into a vein.
5. Remove needle. If slight bleeding occurs, press lightly with a dry cotton swab for a few seconds—**do not rub.**

Note: Use the injection Technique recommended by your physician.
For additional information see **GIVING THE INJECTION** on the reverse side of this insert.

USAGE IN PREGNANCY

It is particularly important to maintain good control of your diabetes during pregnancy and special attention must be paid to your diet, exercise and insulin regimens. If you are pregnant or nursing a baby, consult your physician or nurse educator.

INSULIN REACTION AND SHOCK

Insulin reaction (hypoglycemia) occurs when the blood glucose falls very low. This can happen if you take too much insulin, miss or delay a meal, exercise more than usual or work too hard without eating, or become ill (especially with vomiting or fever). Hypoglycemia can also happen if you combine insulin therapy and other medications that lower blood glucose, such as oral antidiabetic agents or other prescription and over-the-counter drugs. The first symptoms of an insulin reaction usually come on suddenly. They may include a cold sweat, fatigue, nervousness or shakiness, rapid heartbeat, or nausea. Personality change or confusion may also occur. If you drink or eat something right away (a glass of milk or orange juice, or several sugar candies), you can often stop the progression of symptoms. If symptoms persist, call your physician—an insulin reaction can lead to unconsciousness. If a reaction results in loss of consciousness, emergency medical care should be obtained immediately. If you have had repeated reactions or if an insulin reaction has led to a loss of consciousness, contact your physician. Severe hypoglycemia can result in temporary or permanent impairment of brain function and death.
In certain cases, the nature and intensity of the warning symptoms of hypoglycemia may change. A few patients have reported that after being transferred to human insulin, the early warning symptoms of hypoglycemia were less pronounced than they had been with animal-source insulin.

DIABETIC KETOACIDOSIS AND COMA

Diabetic ketoacidosis may develop if your body has too little insulin. The most common causes are acute illness or infec-

Continued on next page

Novolin 70/30 Penfill—Cont.

tion or failure to take enough insulin by injection. If you are ill you should check your urine for ketones. The symptoms of diabetic ketoacidosis usually come on gradually, over a period of hours or days, and include a drowsy feeling, flushed face, thirst and loss of appetite. Notify your physician right away if the urine test is positive for ketones (acetone) or if you have any of these symptoms. Fast, heavy breathing and rapid pulse are more severe symptoms and you should have medical attention right away. Severe, sustained hyperglycemia may result in diabetic coma and death.

ADVERSE REACTIONS

A few people with diabetes develop red, swollen and itchy skin where the insulin has been injected. This is called a "local reaction" and it may occur if the injection is not properly made, if the skin is sensitive to the cleansing solution, or if you are allergic to the insulin being used. If you have a local reaction, tell your physican.

Generalized insulin allergy occurs rarely, but when it does it may cause a serious reaction, including skin rash over the body, shortness of breath, fast pulse, sweating, and a drop in blood pressure. If any of these symptoms develop, you should seek emergency medical care.

If severe allergic reactions to insulin have occured (i.e., generalized rash, swelling or breathing difficulties) you should be skin-tested with **each** new insulin preparation before it is used.

IMPORTANT NOTES

1. A change in the type, strength, species or purity of insulin could require a dosage adjustment. Any change in insulin should be made under medical supervision.
2. To avoid possible transmission of disease, PenFill® cartridges is for single person use only.
3. Before use, check that the PenFill® cartridge is intact (e.g. no cracks). Do not use if any damage is seen, or if the rear rubber stopper is visible above the white bar code band when the PenFill® is pointing up.
4. You may have learned how to test your urine or your blood for glucose. It is important to do these tests regularly and to record the results for review with your physician or nurse educator.
5. If you have an acute illness, especially with vomiting or fever, continue taking your insulin. If possible, stay on your regular diet. If you have trouble eating, drink fruit juices, regular soft drinks, or clear soups; if you can, eat small amounts of bland foods. Test your urine for glucose and ketones and, if possible, test your blood glucose. Note the results and contact your physician for possible insulin dose adjustment. If you have severe and prolonged vomiting, seek emergency medical care.
6. You should always carry identification which states that you have diabetes.
7. Always ask your physician or pharmacist before taking any drug.
8. Do not try to refill a PenFill® cartridge.

Always consult your physician if you have any questions about your conditon or the use of insulin.

Helpful information for people with diabetes is published by American Diabetes Association, 1660 Duke Street, Alexandria, VA 22314

For information contact:
Novo Nordisk Pharmaceuticals, Inc.
100 College Road West
Princeton, NJ 08540
1-800-727-6500
Manufactured by
Novo Nordisk A/S
DK-2880 Bagsvaerd, Denmark
Novo Nordisk™, Novolin® PenFill®, NovoPen®, NovolinPen®, NovoFine® and Lente®
are trademarks owned by Novo Nordisk A/S
Date of issue: Feb. 2000
License under U.S. Patent No. 5,462,535 and Des. 347,894 restricted to use with Novo Nordisk insulin delivery devices and Novo Nordisk pen needles.

HOW SUPPLIED

Novolin® 70/30 PenFill® cartridges, U-100, 100 units/mL, 1.5 mL, (List No. 183717) (5's)
Novolin® 70/30 PenFill® cartridges, U100, 100 units/mL, 3mL, (List no. 347718) (5's)
Novolin® N PenFill® cartridges. U-100, 100 units/mL, 1.5 mL, (List No. 183417) (5's)
Novolin® N PenFill® cartridges, U100, 100 units/mL, 3 mL, (List no. 347418) (5's)
Novolin® R PenFill® cartridges, U-100, 100 units/mL, 1.5 mL, (List No. 183317) (5's)
Novolin® R PenFill® cartridges, U100, 100 units/mL, 3 mL, (List no. 347318) (5's)

Shown in Product Identification Guide, page 327

NovoFine® 30 ℞
Disposable Needle

DESCRIPTION

The self contained disposable needle consists of a protective plastic outer cap, a smooth plastic needle cap and a protective tab. (The needle should not be used if the protective tab is missing or damaged.)

Each **NovoFine® 30** is 30 gauge, one-third ($^1/_3$) inch (8mm) in length and is intended for single use only. Each **NovoFine® 30** is cut to a sharp, low-angle point and coated with silicone for easier penetration.

NovoFine® 30 is for use with all Novo Nordisk™ Insulin Delivery Systems.

List# 185250

NovoFine® trademark owned by Novo Nordisk A/S.

Shown in Product Identification Guide, page 327

HUMAN INSULIN
NOVOLIN 70/30 PREFILLED® OTC
70% NPH, Human Insulin Isophane Suspension and 30% Regular,
Human Insulin Injection
(recombinant DNA origin)
in a 1.5 ml Prefilled Syringe
100 units/ml

NOVOLIN N PREFILLED®
NPH, Human Insulin Isophane
Suspension (recombinant DNA origin)
in a 1.5 ml Prefilled Syringe
100 units/ml

NOVOLIN R PREFILLED®
Regular, Human Insulin Injection
(recombinant DNA origin)
in a 1.5 ml Prefilled Syringe
100 units/ml

Insulin Information For The Patient

Please read both sides of this leaflet carefully before using this product.

Novolin Prefilled® syringe is for single person use only. See Important Notes section.

WARNING

ANY CHANGE OF INSULIN SHOULD BE MADE CAUTIOUSLY AND ONLY UNDER MEDICAL SUPERVISION. CHANGES IN PURITY, STRENGTH, BRAND (MANUFACTURER), TYPE (REGULAR, NPH, LENTE® ETC.), SPECIES (BEEF, PORK, BEEF-PORK, HUMAN) AND/OR METHOD OF MANUFACTURE (RECOMBINANT DNA VERSUS ANIMAL-SOURCE INSULIN) MAY RESULT IN THE NEED FOR A CHANGE IN DOSAGE.

SPECIAL CARE SHOULD BE TAKEN WHEN THE TRANSFER IS FROM A STANDARD BEEF OR MIXED SPECIES INSULIN TO A PURIFIED PORK OR HUMAN INSULIN. IF A DOSAGE ADJUSTMENT IS NEEDED, IT WILL USUALLY BECOME APPARENT EITHER IN THE FIRST FEW DAYS OR OVER A PERIOD OF SEVERAL WEEKS, ANY CHANGE IN TREATMENT SHOULD BE CAREFULLY MONITORED.

PLEASE READ THE SECTIONS "INSULIN REACTION AND SHOCK" AND "DIABETIC KETOACIDOSIS AND COMA" FOR SYMPTOMS OF HYPOGLYCEMIA (LOW BLOOD GLUCOSE) AND HYPERGLYCEMIA (HIGH BLOOD GLUCOSE).

INSULIN USE IN DIABETES

Your physician has explained that you have diabetes and that your treatment involves injections of insulin or insulin therapy combined with an oral antidiabetic medicine. Insulin is normally produced by the pancreas, a gland that lies behind the stomach. Without insulin, glucose (a simple sugar made from digested food) is trapped in the bloodstream and cannot enter the cells of the body. Some patients who don't make enough of their own insulin, or who cannot properly use the insulin they do make, must take insulin by injection in order to control their blood glucose levels.

Each case of diabetes is different and requires direct and continued medical supervision. Your physician has told you the type, strength and amount of insulin you should use and the time(s) at which you should inject it, and has also discussed with you a diet and exercise schedule. You should contact your physician if you experience any difficulties or if you have questions.

TYPES OF INSULIN

Standard and purified animal insulin as well as human insulin are available. Standard and purified insulin differ in their degree of purification and content of noninsulin material. Standard and purified insulin also vary in species source: they may be of beef, pork, or mixed beef and pork origin. Human insulin is identical in structure to the insulin produced by the human pancreas, and thus differs from animals insulin. Insulin Products vary in time of action; see **PRODUCT DESCRIPTION** for additional information.

Your physician has prescribed the insulin that is right for you; be sure you have purchased the correct insulin and check it carefully before you use it.

PRODUCT DESCRIPTION

A package contains five (5) **Novolin Prefilled®** insulin syringes.

This human insulin (recombinant DNA origin) is structurally identical to the insulin produced by the human pancreas. This human insulin is produced by recombinant DNA technology utilizing *Saccharomyces cerevisiae* (bakers' yeast) as the production organism.

Novolin 70/30 Prefilled® contains Novolin® 70/30, a mixture of 70% NPH, Human Insulin Isophane Suspension (recombinant DNA origin) and 30% Regular, Human Insulin Injection (recombinant DNA origin) USP. The concentration of this product is 100 units of insulin per milliliter. It is a cloudy or milky suspension of human insulin with protamine and zinc. The insulin substance (the cloudy material) settles to the bottom of the insulin reservoir, therefore, the syringe must be rotated up and down so that the contents are uniformly mixed before a dose is given. Novolin® 70/30 has an intermediate duration of action. The effect of Novolin® 70/30 begins approximately $^1/_2$ hours after injection. The effect is maximal between 2 and approximately 12 hours. The full duration of action may last up to 24 hours after injection.

The time course of action of any insulin may vary considerably in different individuals, or at different times in the same individual. Because of the variation, the time periods listed here should be considered as general guidelines only.

Novolin N Prefilled® contains NPH, Human Insulin Isophane Suspension (recombinant DNA origin). The concentration of this product is 100 units of insulin per milliliter. It is a cloudy or milky suspension of human insulin with protamine and zinc. The insulin substance (the cloudy material) settles to the bottom of the insulin reservoir, therefore, the syringe must be rotated up and down so that the contents are uniformly mixed before a dose is given. Novolin® N has an intermediate duration of action. The effect of Novolin® N begins approximately $1^1/_2$ hours after injection. The effect is maximal between 4 and approximately 12 hours. The full duration of action may last up to 24 hours after injection.

Novolin R Prefilled® contains Regular, Human Insulin Injection (recombinant DNA origin) USP. The concentration of this product is 100 units of insulin per milliliter. It is a clear, colorless solution which has a short duration of action. The effect of Novolin® R begins approximately $^1/_2$ hour after injection. The effect is maximal between $2^1/_2$ and 5 hours and ends approximately 8 hours after injection.

STORAGE

Novolin Prefilled® insulin syringes should be stored in a cold place, preferably in a refrigerator, but not in the freezing compartment. **Do not let it freeze.** Keep **Novolin Prefilled®** in the carton so that they will stay clean and protected from light. **Novolin 70/30 Prefilled®** and **Novolin N Prefilled®** can be kept unrefrigerated for one (1) week.

Novolin R Prefilled® can be kept unrefrigerated for (1) month. Unrefrigerated syringes must be used within this time period or discarded. Be sure to protect syringes from sunlight and extreme heat or cold.

Never use any **Novolin R Prefilled®** if the insulin becomes viscous (thickend or cloudy); use it only if it is clear and colorless. Never use any **Novolin 70/30 Prefilled® or Novolin N Prefilled®** if the precipitate (the white deposit) has become lumpy or granular in appearance or has formed a deposit of solid particles on the wall of the insulin reservoir. This insulin should not be used if the liquid in the insulin reservoir remains clear after it has been mixed.

Never use insulin after the expiration date which is printed on the label and carton.

IMPORTANT

Failure to comply with the following antiseptic measures may lead to infections at the injection site.

— Disposable needles are for single use; they should be used only once and discarded properly.
— Clean your hands and the injection site with soap and water or with alcohol.
— Wipe the rubber stopper with an alcohol swab.

PREPARING THE INJECTION

Never place a single-use needle on your insulin delivery device until you are ready to give an injection, and remove it immediately after each injection. If the needle is not removed, some liquid may be expelled from the syringe causing a change in the insulin concentration (strength).

For **Novolin N Prefilled® & Novolin 70/30 Prefilled®**, the cloudy material in an insulin suspension will settle to the bottom of the insulin reservoir, so the contents must be mixed before injection. These syringes contain a glass ball to aid mixing.

Rotate the syringe up and down so that the contents are uniformly mixed before the dose is given.

Follow the directions for use of this syringe on the reverse side of this insert.

Insulin prefilled in cartridges may contain a small amount of air. To prevent an injection of air and make certain insulin is delivered an air shot must be done before each injection. Directions for performing an air shot are provided in your insulin delivery device instruction manual.

GIVING THE INJECTION

1. The following areas are suitable for subcutaneous insulin injection: thighs, upper arms, buttocks, abdomen. Do not change areas without consulting your physician. The actual point of injection should be changed each time; injection sites should be about an inch apart.
2. The injection site should be clean and dry. Pinch up skin area to be injected and hold it firmly.
3. Hold the syringe like a pencil and push the needle quickly and firmly into the pinched-up area. Release the skin and push the push-button all the way in to inject insulin beneath the skin. To ensure that all the insulin is injected keep the needle in the skin for several seconds after injection with your thumb on the push-button.
4. Do not inject into a muscle unless your physician has advised it. You should never inject insulin into a vein.
5. Remove needle. If slight bleeding occurs, press lightly with a dry cotton swab for a few seconds—**do not rub.**

For additional information see **GIVING THE INJECTION** on the reverse side of this insert.

USAGE IN PREGNANCY

It is particularly important to maintain good control of your diabetes during pregnancy and special attention must be paid to your diet, exercise and insulin regimens. If you are pregnant or nursing a baby, consult your physician or nurse educator.

INSULIN REACTION AND SHOCK

Insulin reaction (hypoglycemia) occurs when the blood glucose falls very low. This can happen if you take too much insulin, miss or delay a meal, exercise more than usual or work too hard without eating, or become ill (especially with vomiting or fever). Hypoglycemia can also happen if you combine insulin therapy and other medications that lower blood glucose, such as oral antidiabetic agents or other prescription and over-the-counter drugs. The first symptoms of an insulin reaction usually come on suddenly. They may include a cold sweat, fatigue, nervousness or shakiness, rapid heartbeat, or nausea. Personality change or confusion may also occur. If you drink or eat something right away (a glass of milk or orange juice, or several sugar candies), you can often stop the progression of symptoms. If symptoms persist, call your physician-an insulin reaction can lead to unconsciousness. If a reaction results in loss of consciousness, emergency medical care should be obtained immediately. If you have had repeated reactions or if an insulin reaction has led to a loss of consciousness, contact your physician. Severe hypoglycemia can result in temporary or permanent impairment of brain function and death.

In certain cases, the nature and intensity of the warning symptoms of hypoglycemia may change. A few patients have reported that after being transferred to human insulin, the early warning symptoms of hypoglycemia were less pronounced than they had been with animal-source insulin.

DIABETIC KETOACIDOSIS AND COMA

Diabetic ketoacidosis may develop if your body has too little insulin. The most common causes are acute illness or infection or failure to take enough insulin by injection. If you are ill you should check your urine for ketones. The symptoms of diabetic ketoacidosis usually come on gradually, over a period of hours or days, and include a drowsy feeling, flushed face, thirst and loss of appetite. Notify your physician right away if the urine test is positive for ketones (acetone) or if you have any of these symptoms. Fast, heavy breathing and rapid pulse are more severe symptoms and you should have medical attention right away. Severe sustained hyperglycemia may result in diabetic coma and death.

ADVERSE REACTIONS

A few people with diabetes develop red, swollen and itchy skin where the insulin has been injected. This is called a "local reaction" and it may occur if the injection is not properly made, if the skin is sensitive to the cleaning solution or if you are allergic to the insulin being used. If you have a local reaction, tell your physician.

Generalized insulin allergy occurs rarely, but when it does it may cause a serious reaction, including skin rash over the body, shortness of breath, fast pulse, sweating, and a drop in blood pressure. If any of these symptoms develop, you should seek emergency medical care.

If severe reactions to insulin have occurred (i.e. generalized rash, swelling or breathing difficulties) you should be skin-tested with each new insulin preparation before it is used.

IMPORTANT NOTES

1. A change in the type, strength, species or purity of insulin could require a dosage adjustment. Any change in insulin should be made under medical supervision.
2. To avoid possible transmission of disease, **Novolin Prefilled®** syringe is for single person use only.
3. You may have learned how to test your urine or your blood for glucose. It is important to do these tests regularly and to record the results for review with your physician or nurse educator.
4. If you have an acute illness, especially with vomiting or fever, continue taking your insulin. If possible, stay on your regular diet. If you have trouble eating, drink fruit juices, regular soft drinks, or clear soups; if you can, eat small amounts of bland foods. Test your urine for glucose and ketones and, if possible, test your blood glucose. Note the results and contact your physician for possible insulin dose adjustment. If you have severe and prolonged vomiting, seek emergency medical care.
5. You should always carry identification which states that you have diabetes.
6. Always ask your physician or pharmacist before taking any drug.

Always consult your physician if you have any questions about your condition or the use of insulin.

Helpful information for people with diabetes is published by American Diabetes Association, 1660 Duke Street, Alexandria, VA 22314.

For information contact:
Novo Nordisk Pharmaceuticals, Inc.
100 College Road West
Princeton, NJ 08540
1-800-727-6500
Manufactured by
Novo Nordisk A/S
DK-2880 Bagsvaerd, Denmark

License under U.S. Patent No. 5,462,535 and Des. 347,894 restricted to use with Novo Nordisk insulin delivery devices and Novo Nordisk pen needles.

Novo Nordisk®, Novolin®, PenFill®, NovoPen®, Novolin-Pen®, NovoFine® and Lente® are trademarks owned by Novo Nordisk A/S

Date of Issue: Dec 1998

HOW SUPPLIED

Novolin 70/30 Prefilled® Syringe, U-100, 100 units/ml, 1.5 ml, (List No. 001771) (5's)
Novolin N Prefilled® Syringe, U-100, 100 units/ml, 1.5 ml, (List No. 004571) (5's)
Novolin R Prefilled® Syringe, U-100, 100 units/ml, 1.5 ml, (List No. 004471) (5's)

Prefilled syringe directions for use

This is a disposable dial-a-dose insulin delivery system able to deliver 2–58 units in increments of 2 units. **Novolin Prefilled®** syringe is designed for use with **NovoFine®** single use needle or other products specifically recommended by Novo Nordisk. **Novolin Prefilled®** syringe is not recommended for the blind or visually impaired without the assistance of a sighted individual trained in the proper use of this product.

Please read these instructions completely before using this device.

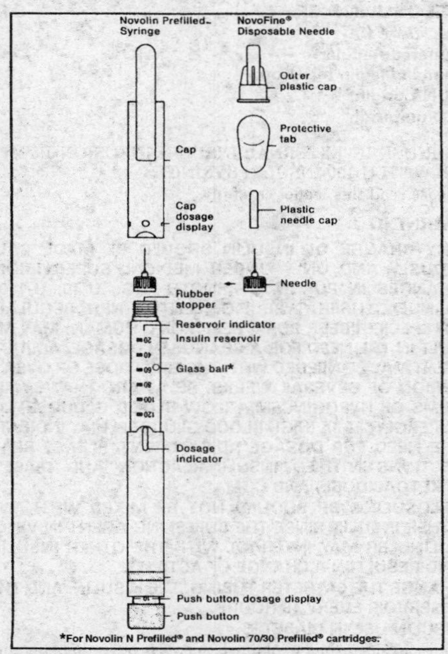

*For Novolin N Prefilled® and Novolin 70/30 Prefilled® cartridges.

1. Preparing the Syringe

Pull off the cap.

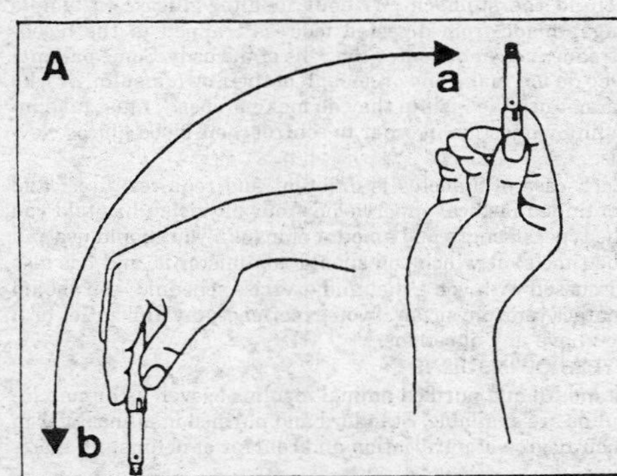

A. Turn the syringe up and down between **a** and **b** so the glass ball is moved from one end of the insulin reservoir to the other. Do this at least 10 times, until the liquid appears uniformly white and cloudy. Wipe rubber stopper with an alcohol swab. This step is not necessary with Novolin R Prefilled®.

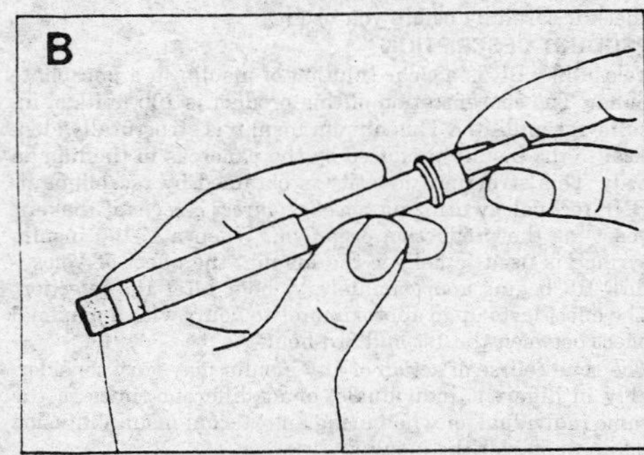

B. Remove the protective tab from disposable needle and screw the needle onto the syringe. Never place a disposable needle on your syringe until you are ready to give an injection. Remove the needle immediately after use. If the needle is not removed, some liquid may be expelled from the syringe causing a change in insulin concentration (strength).

Giving the air shot prior to each injection:

Small amounts of air may collect in the needle and insulin reservoir during normal use.

To avoid the injection of air and ensure proper dosing, hold the syringe with the needle upwards and tap the syringe gently with your finger so any air bubbles collect in the top of the reservoir. Remove both the plastic outer cap and the needle cap.

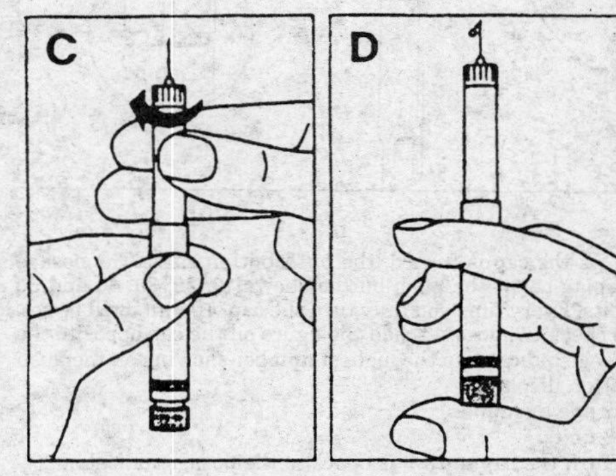

C. Holding the syringe with the needle pointing upwards, **slowly** turn the insulin reservoir clockwise (in the direction of the arrow, fig. C) to the first notch where resistance is felt ($^1/_5$ of a full rotation).

D. Still with the needle pointing upwards, press the push button as far as it will go and see if a drop of insulin appears at the needle tip (Fig. D).

Before the first use of Novolin Prefilled® you may need to perform up to 6 air shots to get a droplet of insulin at the needle tip. If you need to make more than 6 air shots do not use and return the product to Novo Nordisk.

If not, repeat the procedure until insulin appears. A small air bubble may remain but it will not be injected because the operating mechanism prevents the reservoir from being completely emptied.

2. Setting the dose

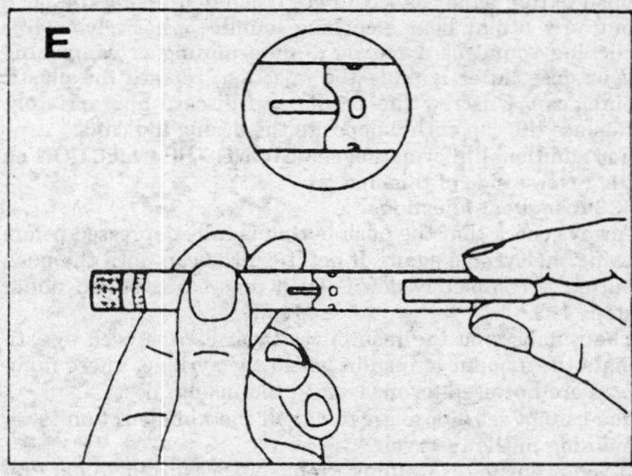

E. Replace the cap, so **0** is opposite the dosage indicator.

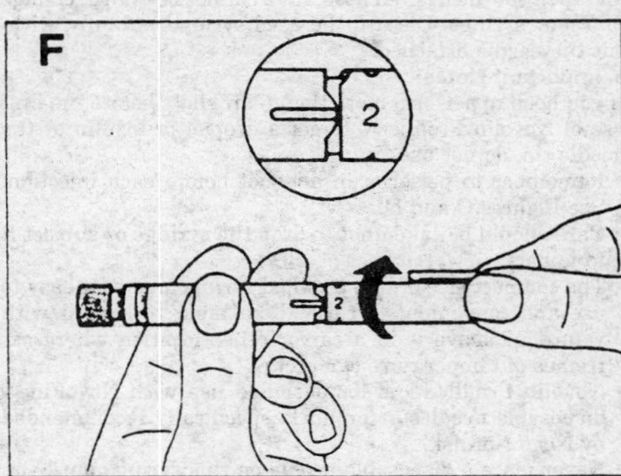

F. Hold the syringe horizontally and turn the cap in the direction of the arrow to set the required dose. Do not put your hand over the push button when dialing the dose. If the button is not allowed to rise freely, insulin will be pushed out of the needle. The dosage display on the cap shows **0, 2, 4, 6** and **8** units.

Continued on next page

Novolin Prefilled—Cont.

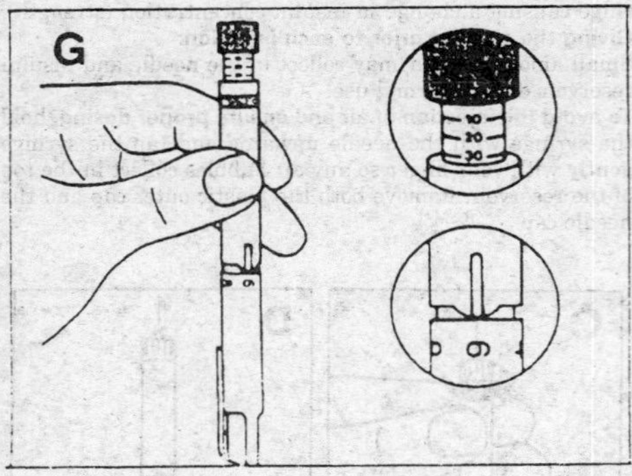

G. As the cap is turned, the push button rises. The dosage display below the push button shows **10, 20, 30, 40** and **50** units. Every time you fully turn the cap, 10 units will be set. To check the dose set, add the figure on the cap opposite the dosage indicator to the highest number showing on the push button display.

Dosage examples

- **8 units:**
  Turn the cap until **8** is opposite the dosage indicator.
- **36 units:**
  Turn the cap 3 full turns so **0** is opposite the dosage indicator. The 30-line will show on the push button display. Continue turning until **6** is opposite the dosage indicator (see **G**).

If you have set a wrong dose, simply turn the cap forwards or backwards until the right number of units has been set. **58 units is the maximum dose.** If you attempt to set a higher dose, insulin will be expelled from the needle and the dose will be wrong. If you set more than 58 units, turn the cap back as far as you can until resistance is felt and the push button is fully depressed. If the dosage indicator is not lined up with **0** when resistance is felt, remove the cap and replace it with **0** opposite the dosage indicator. Now start again, remembering that **58** units is the maximum dose. After the dose is set, remove the cap.

3. Giving the injection

Use the injection technique recommended by your doctor. Check that you have set the proper dose and depress the push button as far as it will go. When depressing the push button you may hear a clicking sound. Do not rely on this clicking sound as a means of determining or confirming your dose. After making the injection, replace the plastic outer cap. Unscrew the needle and discard appropriately. Replace the cap with **0** opposite the dosing indicator.

For additional information see **GIVING THE INJECTION** on the reverse side of this insert.

4. Subsequent Injections

Always check that the push button is fully depressed before using the syringe again. If not, turn the cap until the push button is completely down. Then proceed as stated under steps 1–3.

The numbers on the insulin reservoir can be used to estimate the amount of insulin left in the syringe. These numbers **are not** used for measuring the insulin dose.

You cannot set a dose greater then the number of units remaining in the reservoir.

If you are using Novolin N Prefilled® or Novolin 70/30 Prefilled® there must be at least 12 units left in the reservoir to give the glass ball space to move when mixing the insulin. If your dose is less than 12 units — and the reservoir is nearly empty — first dial up to 12 (to check that 12 units are left) and then set the desired dose. If 12 cannot be dialed, change to a new syringe. Discard the used syringe carefully, without the needle attached.

5. Important Notes

If you need to perform more than 6 air shots before the first use of Novolin Prefilled® to get a droplet of insulin at the needle tip, do not use.

- Remember to perform an air shot before each injection. See Figures C and D.
- Care should be taken not to drop the syringe or subject it to impact.
- The compact size of this prefilled syringe makes it easy to use and convenient to carry. Remember to keep it with you; don't leave it in a car or other location where extremes of temperature can occur.
- Novolin Prefilled® is for designed use with NovoFine® disposable needles or products specifically recommended by Novo Nordisk.
- Never place a disposable needle on this syringe until you are ready to use it. Remove the needle immediately after use. If the needle is not removed, some liquid may leak from the syringe causing a change in insulin concentration (strength).
- Always carry a spare Novolin Prefilled® syringe with you in case your prefilled syringe is damaged or lost.
- Novo Nordisk cannot be held responsible for adverse reactions occurring as a consequence of using this insulin delivery system with products that are not recommended by Novo Nordisk.
- Keep this syringe out of the reach of children.

For information contact:
Novo Nordisk Pharmaceuticals, Inc.
100 College Road West
Princeton, NJ 08540
1-800-727-6500
Manufactured by
Novo Nordisk A/S
DK-2880 Bagsvaerd, Denmark
License under U.S. Patent No. 5,462,535 and Des. 347,894 restricted to use with Novo Nordisk insulin delivery devices and Novo Nordisk pen needles.
Novo Nordisk®, Novolin®, PenFill®, NovoPen®, Novolin-Pen®, NovoFine® and Lente® are trademarks owned by Novo Nordisk A/S

Date of issue: December 1998

Shown in Product Identification Guide, page 327

VELOSULIN® BR OTC

[*vĕl" ŏs" ĕ lĭn*]

Buffered Regular
Human Insulin Injection
(rDNA origin)
100 units/mL

FOR USE IN EXTERNAL INSULIN INFUSION PUMPS OR WITH U-100 INSULIN SYRINGES

Please read this leaflet carefully.

WARNING

ANY CHANGE OF INSULIN SHOULD BE MADE CAUTIOUSLY AND ONLY UNDER MEDICAL SUPERVISION. CHANGES IN PURITY, STRENGTH (E.G., U-40, U-100), MANUFACTURER, TYPE (E.G., LENTE®, NPH, REGULAR) OR SPECIES (BEEF, PORK, BEEF/PORK, HUMAN) MAY RESULT IN THE NEED FOR A CHANGE IN DOSAGE. ADJUSTMENT MAY BE NEEDED WITH THE FIRST DOSE OR OVER A PERIOD OF SEVERAL WEEKS. BE AWARE THAT SYMPTOMS OF HYPOGLYCEMIA (LOW BLOOD GLUCOSE) OR HYPERGLYCEMIA (HIGH BLOOD GLUCOSE) MAY INDICATE THE NEED FOR DOSAGE ADJUSTMENT. PLEASE READ SECTIONS ENTITLED "INSULIN REACTION" AND "DIABETIC KETOACIDOSIS AND COMA".

VELOSULIN® BR SHOULD NOT BE MIXED WITH ANY OTHER INSULIN SINCE THE BUFFERING AGENT IN VELOSULIN® BR MAY INTERACT WITH THE OTHER INSULIN AND RESULT IN A CHANGE OF ACTIVITY.

CHANGE THE CATHETER TUBING, THE INSULIN, AND THE RESERVOIR EVERY 48 HOURS.

INSULIN USE IN DIABETES

Your physician has explained that you have diabetes and that your treatment involves the use of insulin or insulin therapy combined with an oral antidiabetic medicine. Insulin is normally produced by the pancreas, a gland that lies behind the stomach. Without insulin, glucose (a simple sugar made from digested food) is trapped in the bloodstream and cannot enter the cells of the body. Some patients who do not make any or enough of their own insulin, or who cannot use the insulin they do make properly, must take insulin by injection in order to control their blood glucose levels.

Each case of diabetes is different and requires direct and continued medical supervision. Your physician has told you the type, strength and amount of insulin you should use and the time(s) at which you should administer it, and has also discussed with you a diet and exercise schedule. You should contact your physician if you experience any difficulties or if you have any questions.

TYPES OF INSULINS

Standard and purified animal insulins as well as human insulins are available. Standard and purified insulins differ in their degree of purification and content of noninsulin material.

Standard and purified insulins also vary in species source: they may be of beef, pork, or mixed beef and pork origin. Human insulin is identical in structure to the insulin produced by the human pancreas, and thus differs from animal insulins. Insulins vary in time of action and in strength; see PRODUCT DESCRIPTION for additional information.

Your physician has prescribed the insulin that is right for you; be sure you have purchased the correct insulin and check it carefully before you use it.

PRODUCT DESCRIPTION

Velosulin® BR is a clear solution of insulin in a phosphate buffer. The concentration of this product is 100 units of insulin per milliliter. This human insulin is structurally identical to the insulin produced by the pancreas in the human body. This structural identity is obtained by recombinant-DNA technology utilizing *Saccharomyces cerevisiae* (bakers' yeast) as the production organism. When a U-100 insulin syringe is used to deliver the insulin, the effect of Velosulin® BR begins approximately $^1/_2$ hour after the injection. The effect lasts up to approximately 8 hours with a maximal effect between the 1st and 3rd hour.

The time course of action of any insulin may vary considerably in different individuals, or at different times in the same individual, or when using an external insulin infusion pump to deliver the insulin.

Because of this variation, the time periods listed here should be considered as general guidelines only when using U-100 insulin syringes to deliver the insulin.

STORAGE

Insulin should be stored in a cool place, preferably in a refrigerator, but not in the freezing compartment. **Do not use insulin if it has been frozen.** Keep the insulin in its carton so that it will stay clean and protected from light. If refrigeration is not possible, the bottle of insulin which you are currently using can be kept unrefrigerated as long as it is kept as cool as possible (below 86°F [30°C] and away from heat and sunlight. Never use Velosulin® BR if it becomes viscous (thickened) or cloudy. Use it only if it is clear and colorless. **Never use insulin after the expiration date which is printed on the vial label and carton.Once the vial has been opened, it should be used within four weeks (28 days).**

(Note: Remove the tamper-resistant cap at first use. If the cap has already been removed, do not use this product and return it to your pharmacy.)

EXTERNAL INSULIN INFUSION PUMPS

Velosulin® BR is indicated for use with external insulin infusion pumps. Novo Nordisk has demonstrated Velosulin® BR to be compatible with MiniMed® Model 506 external insulin infusion pump, using MiniMed® catheters of Polyfin™ and Sofset™ types without Quick Release. MiniMed® Models 506, 505, and 507 external insulin infusion pumps are equivalent with regard to insulin compatibility. If you have any questions on how to operate the pump, consult with your physician or diabetes educator. **It is important that you follow the instructions in your pump manual.** Failure to follow the instructions may result in an inaccurate insulin dose. The pump manual will also help you in the selection, use and sterilization of the appropriate accessories specific to your pump model. Use the correct reservoir and catheter for the pump that you are using to minimize catheter blockage. Follow your external insulin infusion pump instructions for filling a new reservoir making certain that there are no large air bubbles in the syringe or the catheter. Before inserting the needle, use soap and water to clean your hands and the skin of the infusion site to avoid infection. Choose a new site for each new needle.

Follow your instructions from your physician or diabetes educator regarding basal infusion rates and mealtime insulin bolus dosages. An insulin bolus should be followed by a meal within 30 minutes.

Velosulin® BR is for infusion under the skin. It should not be mixed with any other insulin. To get the most benefit from insulin, measure your blood sugar levels regularly. This will also help in detecting any possible malfunction of your insulin pump.

Change the catheter tubing, the insulin, and the reservoir every 48 hours.

NOTE: In case of pump interruption or failure, switch back to conventional insulin therapy using U-100 syringes and consult with your physician or diabetes educator. Please see the following information:

INSTRUCTIONS FOR INJECTION USING U-100 SYRINGES

A. PREPARING THE INJECTION

1. Clean your hands and the injection site with soap and water or with alcohol. Wipe the rubber stopper with an alcohol swab.
2. Pull back the plunger of the syringe until the rubber tip reaches the marking for the number of units you will inject.
3. Push the needle of the syringe through the rubber stopper into the vial.
4. Push the plunger all the way in. This inserts air into the vial.
5. Turn the vial and syringe upside down and slowly pull the plunger back to a few units beyond the correct dose.
6. If there are air bubbles, flick the syringe firmly with your finger to raise the air bubbles to the needle, then slowly push the plunger to the correct unit marking.
7. Remove the needle from the vial.

B. GIVING THE INJECTION

1. The following areas are suitable for subcutaneous insulin injection: thighs, upper arms, buttocks, or abdomen. Do not change areas without consulting your physician. The actual point of injection should be changed with each injection. Injection sites should be about an inch apart.
2. The injection site should be clean and dry. Pinch up skin area to be injected and hold it firmly.
3. Hold the syringe like a pencil and push the needle quickly and firmly into the pinched-up area.
4. Release the skin and push plunger all the way in to inject insulin beneath the skin. **To ensure that all the insulin is injected, keep the needle in the skin for several seconds after the injection with your finger on the plunger.** Do not inject into a muscle unless your physician has advised it. You should never inject insulin into a vein.
5. Remove the needle. If slight bleeding occurs, press lightly with a dry cotton swab for a few seconds—**do not rub.**

IMPORTANT

Failure to comply with the above instructions and the antiseptic measures may lead to infections at the injection site.

Note: you should use the injection technique recommended by your physician.

USAGE IN PREGNANCY

It is particularly important to maintain good control of your diabetes during pregnancy and special attention must be paid to your diet, exercise and insulin regimens. If you are pregnant or nursing a baby, consult your physician or diabetes educator.

INSULIN REACTION

Insulin reaction (too little sugar in the blood, also called hypoglycemia) can occur if the external infusion pump delivers too much insulin, if you take too large an insulin bolus, skip meals, exercise or work harder than normal. **Hypoglycemia can also happen if you combine insulin therapy and other medications that lower blood glucose, such as oral antidiabetic agents or other prescription and over-the-counter**

drugs. The symptoms, which usually come on suddenly, are hunger, dizziness, and sweating. Personality change or confusion may also occur. If you drink or eat something right away (a glass of milk or orange juice, or several sugar candies), you can often stop the progression of symptoms. If symptoms persist, call a physician; an insulin reaction can lead to unconsciousness. If a reaction results in loss of consciousness, emergency medical care should be obtained immediately. If you have had repeated reactions or if an insulin reaction has led to a loss of consciousness, contact your physician. Severe hypoglycemia can result in temporary or permanent impairment of brain function and death.

In certain cases, the nature and intensity of the warning symptoms of hypoglycemia may change. A few patients have reported that after being transferred to human insulin, the early warning symptoms of hypoglycemia were less pronounced than they had been with animal-source insulin.

DIABETIC KETOACIDOSIS AND COMA

Diabetic ketoacidosis may develop if your body has too little insulin. The most common causes are acute illness, infection, failure to take enough insulin by injection, or catheter clogging when used with an external insulin infusion pump. If you are ill, you should check your urine for ketones. The symptoms of diabetic ketoacidosis usually come on gradually, over a period of hours or days, and include a drowsy feeling, flushed face, thirst, and loss of appetite. Notify a physician immediately if the urine test is positive for ketones (acetone) or if you have any of these symptoms. More severe symptoms are fast, heavy breathing and rapid pulse; if these symptoms occur, you should seek medical attention right away. Severe, sustained hyperglycemia may result in diabetic coma and death.

ADVERSE REACTIONS

Insulin allergy occurs very rarely, but when it does, it may cause a serious reaction including a general skin rash over the body, shortness of breath, fast pulse, sweating and a drop in blood pressure. If any of these symptoms develop you should seek emergency medical care. The formation of fatty lumps at the infusion site or injection site is usually a sign of frequent needle insertion at the same site. Remember to choose new infusion sites or injection sites at which to insert each new needle and consult with your physician or diabetes educator if you develop these fatty lumps at the infusion site. The skin at the infusion site or injection site may also become red, swollen and itchy. This is a local reaction. It may occur if needle insertion is not properly made at the infusion site or injection site, or as a result of skin sensitivity to the cleansing solutions or if the patient is allergic to insulin. If you have a local reaction, consult with your physician or diabetes educator.

Patients with severe systemic allergic reactions to insulin (i.e. generalized urticaria, angioedema, anaphylaxis) should be skin tested with each new preparation to be used prior to initiation of therapy with that preparation.

IMPORTANT NOTES

1. A change in the type, strength, species or purity of insulin could require a dosage adjustment. Any change in insulin should be made under medical supervision.
2. You may have learned how to test your urine or your blood for glucose. It is important to do these tests regularly. Monitor your results and make appropriate dosage adjustments. Contact your physician or diabetes educator for assistance.
3. If you have an illness, especially with vomiting or fever, continue taking your insulin. If possible, stay on your regular diet. If you have trouble eating, drink fruit juices, regular soft drinks, or clear soups; if you can, eat small amounts of bland foods. Test your urine for glucose and ketones and, if possible, test your blood glucose. Note the results and adjust dosage accordingly or contact your physician or diabetes educator for assistance. If you have severe and prolonged vomiting, seek immediate emergency medical care.
4. You should always carry identification which states that you have diabetes.
5. Always consult with your physician or pharmacist before taking any new medication.

Contact your physician if you have any questions about your condition or the use of insulin.

Helpful information for people with diabetes is published by American Diabetes Association, 1160 Duke St., Alexandria, VA 22314.

Novo Nordisk™, Velosulin® and Lente® are trademarks of Novo Nordisk A/S

MiniMed®, Polyfin™, and Sofset™ are trademarks of MiniMed Inc.

For information contact: Novo Nordisk Pharmaceuticals, Inc., Princeton, NJ 08540

Manufactured by: Novo Nordisk A/S, DK-2880 Bagsvaerd, Denmark

Date of issue: July 1999

NOVOSEVEN® ℞

Coagulation Factor VIIa (Recombinant)
For Intravenous Use Only

DESCRIPTION

NovoSeven® is recombinant human coagulation Factor VIIa (rFVIIa), intended for promoting hemostasis by activating the extrinsic pathway of the coagulation cascade.[1] NovoSeven is a vitamin K-dependent glycoprotein consisting of 406 amino acid residues (MW 50 K Dalton). NovoSeven is structurally similar to human plasma-derived Factor VIIa.

The gene for human Factor VII is cloned and expressed in baby hamster kidney cells (BHK cells). Recombinant FVII is secreted into the culture media (containing newborn calf serum) in its single-chain form and then proteolytically converted by autocatalysis to the active two-chain form, rFVIIa, during a chromatographic purification process. The purification process has been demonstrated to remove exogenous viruses (MuLV, SV40, Pox virus, Reovirus, BEV, IBR virus). No human serum or other proteins are used in the production or formulation of NovoSeven.

NovoSeven is supplied as a sterile, white lyophilized powder of rFVIIa in single-use vials. Each vial of lyophilized drug contains the following:

Contents	1.2 mg (60 KIU) Vial	4.8 mg (240 KIU) Vial
rFVIIa	1200 µg	4800 µg
sodium chloride*	5.84 mg	23.36 mg
calcium chloride dihydrate*	2.94 mg	11.76 mg
glycylglycine	2.64 mg	10.56 mg
polysorbate 80	0.14 mg	0.56 mg
mannitol	60.0 mg	240.0 mg

*per mg of rFVIIa: 0.44 mEq sodium, 0.06 mEq calcium

After reconstitution with the appropriate volume of **Sterile Water for Injection, USP (not supplied)**, each vial contains approximately 0.6 mg/mL NovoSeven (corresponding to 600 µg/mL). The reconstituted vials have a pH of approximately 5.5 in sodium chloride (3 mg/mL), calcium chloride dihydrate (1.5 mg/mL), glycylglycine (1.3 mg/mL), polysorbate 80 (0.1 mg/mL), and mannitol (30 mg/mL).

The reconstituted product is a clear colorless solution which contains no preservatives. NovoSeven contains trace amounts of proteins derived from the manufacturing and purification processes such as mouse IgG (maximum of 1.2 ng/mg), bovine IgG (maximum of 30 ng/mg), and protein from BHK-cells and media (maximum of 19 ng/mg).

CLINICAL PHARMACOLOGY

Pharmacodynamics

NovoSeven is recombinant Factor VIIa and, when complexed with tissue factor can activate coagulation Factor X to Factor Xa, as well as coagulation Factor IX to Factor IXa. Factor Xa, in complex with other factors, then converts prothrombin to thrombin, which leads to the formation of a hemostatic plug by converting fibrinogen to fibrin and thereby inducing local hemostasis.

Pharmacokinetics

Single-dose pharmacokinetics of NovoSeven (17.5, 35, and 70 µg/kg) exhibited dose-porportional behavior in 15 subjects with hemophilia A or B.[2] Factor VII clotting activities were measured in plasma drawn prior to and during a 24-hour period after NovoSeven administration. The median apparent volume of distribution at steady state was 103 mL/kg (range 78–139). Median clearance was 33 mL/kg/hr (range 27–49). The median residence time was 3.0 hours (range 2.4–3.3), and the $t_{1/2}$ was 2.3 hours (range 1.7–2.7). The median *in vivo* plasma recovery was 44% (30–71%).

CLINICAL STUDIES

No direct comparisons to other coagulation products have been conducted, therefore no conclusions regarding the comparative safety or efficacy can be made.

Open Protocol Use

The largest number of patients who received NovoSeven during the investigational phase of product development were in an open protocol study[3,4,5] that began enrollment in 1988, shortly after the completion of the pharmacokinetic study. These patients included persons with hemophilia types A or B (with or without inhibitors), persons with acquired inhibitors to Factor VIII or Factor IX, and a few FVII deficient patients. The clinical situations were diverse and included muscle/joint bleeds, mucocutaneous bleeds, surgical prophylaxis, intracerebral bleeds, and other emergent situations. Dose schedules were suggested by Novo Nordisk, but they were subject to the option of the investigator. Clinical outcomes were not reported in a standardized manner. Therefore, the clinical data from the Open Protocol is problematic for the evaluation of the safety and efficacy of the product by statistical methods. The following two cases describe the extremes of the clinical outcomes that were observed under the Open Protocol:

Case #1: A one-year old hemophilia B patient had both an inhibitor to Factor IX and would experience severe anaphylactic reactions to any product containing Factor IX. His life threatening hypersensitivity reaction to Factor IX precluded the use of other coagulation products and NovoSeven was requested under the compassionate use program because it contained Factor VIIa and no other coagulation factors. Between the child's ages of one to three, he was successfully treated with NovoSeven for 23 spontaneous joint, muscle, and oral bleeds. NovoSeven was administered by intravenous bolus dosing at 90 µg/kg every two hours. Hemostasis was achieved each time within one to eight days therapy, without reported sequelae. Adverse events were infrequent, minor, and considered unrelated to NovoSeven treatment.

Case #2: A 36-year-old hemophilia A patient with long standing inhibitors experienced pain between his shoulder-blades (Day 0); he treated himself at home for three days with an activated Prothrombin Complex Concentrate (aPCC). From DAY 16-DAY 18, the patient treated himself at home with another aPCC. On DAY 18, he awoke with paraparesis of the lower extremities and was hospitalized. A large epidural hematoma (C6 to T12) was seen on MRI. The following day (DAY 19), the patient began treatment with NovoSeven, 90 µg/kg every 2 (and later every 3) hours (DAY 19–36). Neurologic and symptomatic improvement was observed. On DAY 29, the NovoSeven dose interval was increased to every four hours. On DAY 31, the patient experienced a massive upper gastrointestinal bleed secondary to stress ulcers (likely dexamethasone induced). He was hypotensive for over two hours, and by the next day, he was requiring large volumes of fluid support and developed abdominal pain. A laparotomy on DAY 32 revealed necrotic large bowel which required resection. Intraoperative and post operative hemostasis was satisfactory on NovoSeven and there was no evidence of thrombosis of the larger mesenteric vessels either at surgery or in the pathologic specimen. On the fourth day post-op (DAY 36), NovoSeven investigational supplies were depleted, and the patient began receiving an aPCC (72 U/kg every 6 hours) and four units of packed red cells per day. During aPCC therapy, bleeding increased; there was coffee ground emesis in the naso-gastric tube. After two days (DAY 38), additional NovoSeven was provided, but the patient was then experiencing severe adult respiratory distress syndrome (ARDS). Within 24 hours of resuming NovoSeven treatment (DAY 40), the patient's life support was voluntarily removed. An autopsy noted the history of bleeding ulcer, ischemic colon, thrombocytopenia, diffuse hemorrhage, lung changes consistent with ARDS, history of epidural hemorrhage, arthropathy, and generalized edema. His stomach had no signs of the ulcers seen the week before on endoscopy indicating healing. On gross neuropathologic exam, his epidural hematoma had resolved.

Dosing Study

A double-blind, randomized comparison trial[6] of two dose levels of NovoSeven in the treatment of joint, muscle and mucocutaneous hemorrhages was conducted in hemophilia A and B patients with and without inhibitors. Patients received NovoSeven as soon as they could be evaluated in the treatment centers (4 to 18 hours after experiencing a bleed). Thirty-five patients were treated at the 35 µg/kg dose (59 joint, 15 muscle and 5 mucocutaneous bleeding episodes) and 43 patients were treated at the 70 µg/kg dose (85 joint and 14 muscle bleeding episodes).

Dosing was to be repeated at 2.5 hour intervals but ranged up to four hours for some patients. Efficacy was assessed at 12±2 hours or at end of treatment, whichever occurred first. Based on a subjective evaluation by the investigator, the respective efficacy rates for the 35 and 70 µg/kg groups were: excellent 59% and 60%, effective 12% and 11%, and partially effective 17% and 20%. The average number of injections required to achieve hemostasis was 2.8 and 3.2 for the 35 and 70 µg/kg groups, respectively.

One patient in the 35 µg/kg group and three in the 70 µg/kg group experienced serious adverse events that were not considered related to NovoSeven. Two unrelated deaths occurred; one patient died of AIDS and the other of intracranial hemorrhage secondary to trauma.

INDICATIONS AND USAGE

NovoSeven is indicated for the treatment of bleeding episodes in hemophilia A or B patients with inhibitors to Factor VIII or Factor IX. NovoSeven should be administered to patients only under the direct supervision of a physician experienced in the treatment of hemophilia.

CONTRAINDICATIONS

NovoSeven Coagulation Factor VIIa (Recombinant) should not be administered to patients with known hypersensitivity to NovoSeven or any of the components of NovoSeven. NovoSeven is contraindicated in patients with known hypersensitivity to mouse, hamster, or bovine proteins.

WARNINGS

The extent of the risk of thrombotic adverse events after treatment with NovoSeven is not known, but is considered to be low. Patients with disseminated intravascular coagulation (DIC), advanced atherosclerotic disease, crush injury, or septicemia may have an increased risk of developing thrombotic events due to circulating TF or predisposing coagulopathy (See **ADVERSE REACTIONS**).

Additional data on the adverse event profile in general and regarding the frequency of thrombotic events in particular is being collected through a postmarket surveillance program. The NovoSeven Cooperative Registry surveillance program is designed to collect data on all uses of NovoSeven to expand the base of experience regarding the use of NovoSeven. All prescribers can obtain information regarding the contribution of patient data to this program by calling 1-877-362-7355.

PRECAUTIONS

General

Patients who receive NovoSeven should be monitored if they develop signs or symptoms of activation of the coagulation system or thrombosis. When there is laboratory confirmation of intravascular coagulation or presence of clinical

Continued on next page

NovoSeven—Cont.

thrombosis, the rFVIIa dosage should be reduced or the treatment stopped, depending on the patient's symptoms.
Due to limited clinical studies which clearly address the effect of post-hemostatic dosing, precautions should be exercised when NovoSeven is used for prolonged dosing (See DOSAGE AND ADMINISTRATION section).

Information for Patients
Patients receiving NovoSeven should be informed of the benefits and risks associated with treatment. Patients should be warned about the early signs of hypersensitivity reactions, including hives, urticaria, tightness of the chest, wheezing, hypotension, and anaphylaxis.

Laboratory Tests
Laboratory coagulation parameters may be used as an adjunct to the clinical evaluation of hemostasis in monitoring the effectiveness and treatment schedule of NovoSeven although these parameters have shown no direct correlation to achieving hemostasis. Assays of prothrombin time (PT), activated partial thromboplastin time (aPTT), and plasma FVII clotting activity (FVII:C), may give different results with different reagents. Treatment with NovoSeven has been shown to produce the following characteristics:

PT: As shown below, in patients with hemophilia A/B with inhibitors, the PT shortened to about a 7-second plateau at a FVII:C level of approximately 5 U/mL. For FVII:C levels > 5 U/mL, there is no further change in PT.

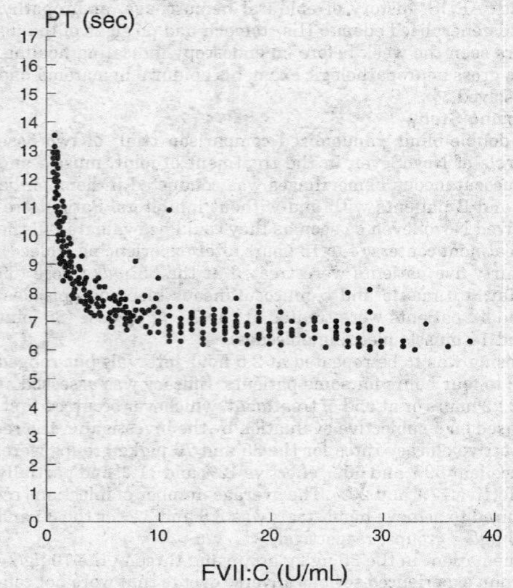

aPTT: While administration of NovoSeven shortens the prolonged aPTT in hemophilia A/B patients with inhibitors, normalization has usually not been observed in doses shown to induce clinical improvement. Data indicate that clinical improvement was associated with a shortening of aPTT of 15 to 20 seconds.

FVIIa:C: FVIIa:C levels were measured two hours after NovoSeven administration of 35 µg/kg and 90 µg/kg following two days of dosing at two hour intervals. Average steady state levels were 11 and 28 U/mL for the two dose levels, respectively.

Drug Interactions
The risk of a potential interactions between NovoSeven and coagulation factor concentrates has not been adequately evaluated in preclinical or clinical studies. Simultaneous use of activated prothrombin complex concentrates or prothrombin complex concentrates should be avoided.
Although the specific drug interaction was not studied in a clinical trial, there have been more than 50 episodes of concomitant use of antifibrinolytic therapies (*i.e.*, tranexamic acid, aminocaproic acid) and NovoSeven.
NovoSeven should not be mixed with infusion solutions until clinical data are available to direct this use.

Carcinogenesis, Mutagenesis, Impairment of Fertility
Two mutagenicity studies have given no indication of carcinogenic potential for NovoSeven. The clastogenic activity of NovoSeven was evaluated in both *in vitro* studies (*i.e.*, cultured human lymphocytes) and *in vivo* studies (*i.e.*, mouse micronucleus test). Neither of these studies indicated clastogenic activity of NovoSeven. Other gene mutation studies have not been performed with NovoSeven (*e.g.*, Ames test). No chronic carcinogenicity studies have been performed with NovoSeven.
A reproductive study in male and female rats at dose levels up to 3.0 mg/kg/day had no effect on mating performance, fertility, or litter characteristics.

Pregnancy
Pregnancy Category C. Treatment of rats and rabbits with NovoSeven in reproduction studies has been associated with mortality at doses up to 6 mg/kg and 5 mg/kg. At 6 mg/kg in rats, the abortion rate was 0 out of 25 litters; in rabbits at 5 mg/kg, the abortion rate was 2 out of 25 litters. Twenty-three out of 25 female rats given 6 mg/kg of NovoSeven gave birth successfully, however, two of the 23 litters died during the early period of lactation. No evidence of teratogenicity was observed after dosing with NovoSeven. There are no adequate and well-controlled studies in pregnant women. NovoSeven should be used during pregnancy only if the potential benefit justifies the potential risk to the fetus. The patients in whom NovoSeven is indicated are male.

Labor and Delivery
NovoSeven was administered to a FVII deficient patient (25 years of age, 66 kg) during a vaginal delivery (36 µg/kg) and during a tubal ligation (90 µg/kg). No adverse reactions were reported during labor, vaginal delivery, or the tubal ligation.

Nursing Mothers
It is not known whether NovoSeven is excreted in human milk. Because many drugs are excreted in human milk, and because of the potential for serious adverse reactions in nursing infants, a decision should be made whether to discontinue nursing or to discontinue the drug, taking into account the importance of the drug to the mother.

Pediatric Use
The safety and effectiveness of NovoSeven was not determined to be different in various age groups, from infants to adolescents (0 to 16 years of age). Clinical trials were conducted with dosing determined according to body weight and not according to age.

Geriatric Use
Clinical studies in hemophilia did not enroll geriatric patients.

ADVERSE REACTIONS

NovoSeven has been generally well tolerated in clinical studies in 298 patients with hemophilia A or B with inhibitors treated for 1,939 bleeding episodes. The table below lists adverse events that were reported in ≥2% of NovoSeven patients and were considered to be at least possibly related or of unknown relationship to NovoSeven administration.
[See table below]

Body System Event	# of episodes reported (n=1,939 treatments)	# of unique patients (n=298 patients)
Body as a whole		
Fever	16	13
Platelets, Bleeding, and Clotting		
Hemorrhage NOS	15	8
Fibrinogen plasma decreased	10	5
Skin and Musculoskeletal		
Hemarthrosis	14	8
Cardiovascular		
Hypertension	9	6

Events which were reported in 1% of patients and were considered to be at least possibly or of unknown relationship to NovoSeven administration were: allergic reaction, arhtrosis, bradycardia, coagulation disorder, DIC, edema, fibrinolysis increased, headache, hypotension, injection site reaction, pain, pneumonia, prothrombin decreased, pruritus, purpura, rash, renal function abnormal, therapeutic response decreased, and vomiting.
In the 298 hemophilia patients, thrombosis was reported in two patients.
Serious adverse events that were probably or possibly related, or where the relationship to NovoSeven was not specified occurred in 14 of the 298 patients (4.7%). Six of these 14 patients died of the following conditions: worsening of chronic renal failure, anesthesia complications during proctoscopy, renal failure complicating a retroperitoneal bleed, ruptured abscess leading to sepsis and DIC, pneumonia, and splenic hematoma and GI bleeding.

OVERDOSAGE

Dose limiting toxicities of NovoSeven Coagulation Factor VIIa (Recombinant) have not been investigated in clinical trials. Two cases of accidental overdose by bolus administration have occurred in the clinical program. One hemophilia B patient (16 years of age, 68 kg) received a single dose of 352 µg/kg and one hemophilia A patient (2 years of age, 14.6 kg) received doses ranging from 246 µg/kg to 986 µg/kg on five consecutive days. There were no reported complications in either case. The recommended dose schedule should not be intentionally increased, even in the case of lack of effect, due to the absence of information on the additional risk that may be incurred.

DOSAGE AND ADMINISTRATION

Dosage
NovoSeven is intended for intravenous bolus administration only. Evaluation of hemostasis should be used to determine the effectiveness of NovoSeven and to provide a basis for modification of the NovoSeven treatment schedule; coagulation parameters do not necessarily correlate with or predict the effectiveness of NovoSeven.
The recommended dose of NovoSeven for hemophilia A or B patients with inhibitors is 90 µg/kg given every two hours until hemostasis is achieved, or until the treatment has been judged to be inadequate. Doses between 35 and 120 µg/kg have been used successfully in clinical trials, and both the dose and administration interval may be adjusted based on the severity of the bleeding and degree of hemostasis achieved.[7] The minimal effective dose has not been established. For patients treated for joint or muscle bleeds, a decision on outcome was reached for a majority of patients within eight doses although more doses were required for severe bleeds. A majority of patients who reported adverse experiences received more than twelve doses.
Post-Hemostatic Dosing: The appropriate duration of post-hemostatic dosing has not been studied. For severe bleeds, dosing should continue at 3–6 hour intervals after hemostasis is achieved, to maintain the hemostatic plug. The biological and clinical effects of prolonged elevated levels of Factor VIIa have not been studied; therefore, the duration of post-hemostatic dosing should be minimized, and patients should be appropriately monitored by a physician experienced in the treatment of hemophilia during this time period.

Reconstitution
Reconstitution should be performed using the following procedures.

1. Always use aseptic technique.
2. Bring NovoSeven (white, lyophilized powder) and the specified volume of Sterile Water for Injection, USP, (diluent) to room temperature, but not above 37°C (98.6°F). The specified volume of diluent corresponding to the amount of NovoSeven is as follows.
   1.2 mg (1200 µg) vial + 2.2 mL **Sterile Water for Injection, USP**
   4.8 mg (4800 µg) vial + 8.5 mL **Sterile Water for Injection, USP**
   After reconstitution with the specified volume of diluent, each vial contains approximately 0.6 mg/mL NovoSeven (600 µg/mL).
3. Remove caps from the NovoSeven vials to expose the central portion of the rubber stopper. Cleanse the rubber stoppers with an alcohol swab and allow to dry prior to use.
4. Draw back the plunger of a sterile syringe (attached to sterile needle) and admit air into the syringe.
5. Insert the needle of the syringe into the sterile water for injection vial. Inject air into the vial and withdraw the quantity required for reconstitution.
6. Insert the syringe needle containing the diluent into the NovoSeven vial through the center of the rubber stopper, aiming the needle against the side so that the stream of liquid runs down the vial wall (the NovoSeven vial does not contain a vacuum). **Do not inject the diluent directly on the NovoSeven powder.**
7. Gently swirl the vial until all the material is dissolved. The reconstituted solution is a clear, colorless solution which may be used up to 3 hours after reconstitution.

Administration
Administration should take place within 3 hours after reconstitution. Any unused solution should be discarded. Do not store reconstituted NovoSeven in syringes. NovoSeven is intended for intravenous bolus injection only and should not be mixed with infusion solutions. As with all parenteral drug products, reconstituted NovoSeven should be inspected visually for particulate matter and discoloration prior to administration. Do not use if particulate matter or discoloration is observed. Administration should be performed using the following procedures.

1. Always use aseptic technique.
2. Draw back the plunger of a sterile syringe (attached to sterile needle) and admit air into the syringe.
3. Insert needle into the vial of reconstituted NovoSeven. Inject air into the vial and then withdraw the appropriate amount of reconstituted NovoSeven into the syringe.
4. Remove and discard the needle from the syringe; attach a suitable intravenous injection needle and administer as a slow bolus injection over 2 to 5 minutes, depending on the dose administered.
5. Discard any unused reconstituted NovoSeven after 3 hours.

HOW SUPPLIED

NovoSeven Coagulation Factor VIIa (Recombinant) is supplied as a white, lyophilized powder in single-use vials, one vial per carton. The vials are made of Class I, Type I, hydrolytic, neutral, white glass, closed with a latex-free, bromobutyl rubber stopper, and sealed with an aluminum cap. The vials are equipped with a snap-off polypropylene cap. The amount of rFVIIa in milligrams and in micrograms is stated on the label as follows.

1.2 mg per vial (1200 µg/vial) NDC 0169-7060-01
4.8 mg per vial (4800 µg/vial) NDC 0169-7062-01

Storage
Prior to reconstitution, keep refrigerated (2–8°C /36–46°F). Avoid exposure to direct sunlight. Do not use past the expiration date.
After reconstitution, NovoSeven may be stored either at room temperature or refrigerated for up to 3 hours. Do not freeze reconstituted NovoSeven or store it in syringes.

REFERENCES

1. Roberts, H.R.: Thoughts on the mechanism of action of FVIIa, 2nd Symposium on New Aspects of Hemophilia Treatment, Copenhagen, Denmark, 1991, pgs. 153–156.
2. Lindley, C.M., et al.: Pharmacokinetics and pharmacodynamics of recombinant Factor VIIa, Clinical Pharmacology & Therapeutics, Vol. 55, No. 6, June 1994, pgs. 638–648.
3. Lusher, J., et al.: Clinical experience with recombinant Factor VIIa, Blood Coagulation and Fibrinolysis 1998, 9:119–128.
4. Bech, M. R.: Recombinant Factor VIIa in Joint and Muscle Bleeding Episodes, Haemostasis 1996;26(suppl 1): 135–138.
5. Lusher, J.M.: Recombinant Factor VIIa (NovoSeven®) in the Treatment of Internal Bleeding in Patients with Factor VIII and IX Inhibitors, Haemostasis 1996; 26(suppl 1):124–130.
6. Macik, B.G., et al.: Safety and initial clinical efficacy of three dose levels of recombinant activated Factor VII (rFVIIa): results of a Phase 1 study, Blood Coagulation and Fibrinolysis 1993, 4:521–527.
7. Hedner, U.: Dosing and Monitoring NovoSeven® Treatment, Haemostasis 1996;26(suppl 1):102–108.

Rx only

U.S. Patent Nos. 4,382,083, 4,456,591, 4,479,938, and 5,180,583

License Number: 1261

NovoSeven® is a registered trademark of Novo Nordisk A/S.

For Information contact:
Novo Nordisk Pharmaceuticals, Inc.
100 College Road West
Princeton, NJ 08540
1-877-NOVO-777

Manufactured by: Revised: September, 1999
Novo Nordisk A/S
Novo Alle
DK-2880 Bagsvaerd
Denmark

PRANDIN® ℞
(repaglinide) Tablets
(0.5, 1, and 2 mg)

DESCRIPTION

PRANDIN® (repaglinide) is an oral blood glucose-lowering drug of the meglitinide class used in the management of type 2 diabetes mellitus (also known as non-insulin dependent diabetes mellitus or NIDDM). Repaglinide, S(+) 2-ethoxy-4(2((3-methyl-1-(2-(1-piperidinyl) phenyl)-butyl) amino)-2-oxoethyl) benzoic acid, is chemically unrelated to the oral sulfonylurea insulin secretagogues.

The structural formula is as shown below:

Repaglinide is a white to off-white powder with molecular formula $C_{27}H_{36}N_2O_4$ and a molecular weight of 452.6. PRANDIN® tablets contain 0.5 mg, 1 mg, or 2 mg of repaglinide. In addition each tablet contains the following inactive ingredients: calcium hydrogen phosphate (anhydrous), microcrystalline cellulose, maize starch, polacrilin potassium, povidone, glycerol (85%), magnesium stearate, meglumine, and poloxamer. The 1 mg and 2 mg tablets contain iron oxides (yellow and red, respectively) as coloring agents.

CLINICAL PHARMACOLOGY

Mechanism of Action

Repaglinide lowers blood glucose levels by stimulating the release of insulin from the pancreas. This action is dependent upon functioning beta (β) cells in the pancreatic islets. Insulin release is glucose-dependent and diminishes at low glucose concentrations.

Repaglinide closes ATP-dependent potassium channels in the β-cell membrane by binding at characterizable sites. This potassium channel blockade depolarizes the β-cell, which leads to an opening of calcium channels. The resulting increased calcium influx induces insulin secretion. The ion channel mechanism is highly tissue selective with low affinity for heart and skeletal muscle.

Pharmacokinetics

Absorption: After oral administration, repaglinide is rapidly and completely absorbed from the gastrointestinal tract. After single and multiple oral doses in healthy subjects or in patients, peak plasma drug levels (C_{max}) occur within 1 hour (T_{max}). Repaglinide is rapidly eliminated from the blood stream with a half-life of approximately 1 hour. The mean absolute bioavailability is 56%. When repaglinide was given with food, the mean T_{max} was not changed, but the mean C_{max} and AUC (area under the time/plasma concentration curve) were decreased 20% and 12.4%, respectively.

Distribution: After intravenous (IV) dosing in healthy subjects, the volume of distribution at steady state (V_{ss}) was 31 L, and the total body clearance (CL) was 38 L/h. Protein binding and binding to human serum albumin was greater than 98%.

PRANDIN® vs. Placebo Treatment: Mean FPG, PPG, and HbA_{1c} Changes from baseline after 3 months of treatment:

	FPG	(mg/dL)	PPG	(mg/dL)	HbA_{1c}	(%)
	PL	R	PL	R	PL	R
Baseline	215.3	220.2	245.2	261.7	8.1	8.5
Change from baseline (at last visit)	30.3	-31.0*	56.5	-47.6*	1.1	-0.6*

FPG = fasting plasma glucose
PPG = post-prandial glucose
PL = placebo (N=33)
R = repaglinide (N=66)
* $p<0.05$ for between group difference

Metabolism: Repaglinide is completely metabolized by oxidative biotransformation and direct conjugation with glucuronic acid after either an IV or oral dose. The major metabolites are an oxidized dicarboxylic acid (M2), the aromatic amine (M1), and the acyl glucuronide (M7). The cytochrome P-450 enzyme system, specifically 3A4, has been shown to be involved in the N-dealkylation of repaglinide to M2 and the further oxidation to M1. Metabolites do not contribute to the glucose-lowering effect of repaglinide.

Excretion: Within 96 hours after dosing with ^{14}C-repaglinide as a single, oral dose, approximately 90% of the radiolabel was recovered in the feces and approximately 8% in the urine. Only 0.1% of the dose is cleared in the urine as parent compound. The major metabolite (M2) accounted for 60% of the administered dose. Less than 2% of parent drug was recovered in feces.

Pharmacokinetic parameters: The pharmacokinetic parameters of repaglinide obtained from a single-dose, crossover study in healthy subjects and from a multiple-dose, parallel, dose-proportionality (0.5, 1, 2 and 4 mg) study in patients with type 2 diabetes are summarized in the following table:

Parameter	Patient with type 2 diabetes[a]
Dose 0.5 mg 1 mg 2 mg 4 mg	$AUC_{0-24\ hr}$ Mean ±SD (ng/mL*hr): 68.9 ± 154.4 125.8 ± 129.8 152.4 ± 89.6 447.4 ± 211.3
Dose 0.5 mg 1 mg 2 mg 4 mg	$C_{max\ 0-5\ hr}$ Mean ±SD (ng/mL): 9.8 ± 10.2 18.3 ± 9.1 26.0 ± 13.0 65.8 ± 30.1
Dose 0.5–4 mg	$T_{max\ 0-5\ hr}$ Means (SD) 1.0–1.4 (0.3–0.5) hr
Dose 0.5–4 mg	$T_{1/2}$ Means (Ind Range) 1.0–1.4 (0.4–8.0) hr
Parameter	Healthy Subjects
CL based on i.v.	38± 16 L/hr
V_{ss} based on i.v.	31± 12 L
AbsBio	56± 9%

a: dosed preprandially with three meals
CL = total body clearance
V_{ss} = volume of distribution at steady state
AbsBio = absolute bioavailability

These data indicate that repaglinide did not accumulate in serum. Clearance of oral repaglinide did not change over the 0.5–4 mg dose range, indicating a linear relationship between dose and plasma drug levels.

Variability of exposure: Repaglinide AUC after multiple doses of 0.25 to 4 mg with each meal varies over a wide range. The intra-individual and inter-individual coefficients of variation were 36% and 69%, respectively. AUC over the therapeutic dose range included 69 to 1005 ng/mL*hr, but AUC exposure up to 5417 ng/mL*hr was reached in dose escalation studies without apparent adverse consequences.

Special populations:

Geriatric. Healthy volunteers were treated with a regimen of 2 mg taken before each of 3 meals. There were no significant differences in repaglinide pharmacokinetics between the group of patients <65 years of age and a comparably sized group of patients ≥65 years of age. (See **PRECAUTIONS, Geriatric Use**)

Pediatric. No studies have been performed in pediatric patients.

Gender. A comparison of pharmacokinetics in males and females showed the AUC over the 0.5 mg to 4 mg dose range to be 15% to 70% higher in females with type 2 diabetes. This difference was not reflected in the frequency of hypoglycemic episodes (male: 16%; female: 17%) or other adverse events. With respect to gender, no change in general dosage recommendation is indicated since dosage for each patient should be individualized to achieve optimal clinical response.

Race. No pharmacokinetic studies to assess the effects of race have been performed, but in a U.S. 1-year study in patients with type 2 diabetes, the blood glucose-lowering effect was comparable between Caucasians (n=297) and African-Americans (n=33). In a U.S. dose-response study, there was no apparent difference in exposure (AUC) between Caucasians (n=74) and Hispanics (n=33).

Renal insufficiency. Single-dose and steady-state pharmacokinetics of repaglinide were evaluated in patients with various degrees of renal impairment. Measures of AUC and C_{max} after multiple dosing of 2 mg repaglinide were found to be higher in three groups of patients with reduced renal function ($AUC_{mild/moderate\ impairment}$: 90.8 ng/mL*hr to $AUC_{severe\ impairment}$: 137.7 ng/mL*hr versus $AUC_{healthy}$: 29.1 ng/mL*hr; $C_{max,\ mild/moderate\ impairment}$: 46.7 ng/mL to $C_{max,\ severe\ impairment}$: 44.0 ng/mL versus $C_{max,\ healthy}$: 20.6 ng/mL). Repaglinide AUC is only weakly correlated to creatinine clearance. Initial dosage adjustment does not appear to be necessary, but **subsequent increases in PRANDIN® should be made carefully in patients with type 2 diabetes who have renal function impairment or renal failure requiring hemodialysis.**

Hepatic insufficiency. A single-dose, open-label study was conducted in 12 healthy subjects and 12 patients with chronic liver disease (CLD) classified by caffeine clearance. Patients with moderate to severe impairment of liver function had higher and more prolonged serum concentrations of both total and unbound repaglinide than healthy subjects ($AUC_{healthy}$: 91.6 ng/mL*hr; $AUC_{CLD\ patients}$: 368.9 ng/mL*hr; $C_{max,\ healthy}$: 46.7 ng/mL; $C_{max,\ CLD\ patients}$: 105.4 ng/mL). AUC was statistically correlated with caffeine clearance. No difference in glucose profiles was observed across patient groups. Patients with impaired liver function may be exposed to higher concentrations of repaglinide and its associated metabolites than would patients with normal liver function receiving usual doses. Therefore, **PRANDIN® should be used cautiously in patients with impaired liver function. Longer intervals between dose adjustments should be utilized to allow full assessment of response.**

Clinical Trials

A four-week, double-blind, placebo-controlled dose-response trial was conducted in 138 patients with type 2 diabetes using doses ranging from 0.25 to 4 mg taken with each of three meals. PRANDIN® therapy resulted in dose-proportional glucose-lowering over the full dose range. Plasma insulin levels increased after meals and reverted toward baseline before the next meal. Most of the fasting blood glucose-lowering effect was demonstrated within 1–2 weeks.

In a double-blind, placebo-controlled, 3-month dose titration study, PRANDIN® or placebo doses for each patient were increased weekly from 0.25 mg through 0.5, 1, and 2 mg, to a maximum of 4 mg, until a fasting plasma glucose (FPG) level <160 mg/dL was achieved or the maximum dose reached. The dose that achieved the targeted control or the maximum dose was continued to end of study. FPG and 2-hour post-prandial glucose (PPG) increased in patients receiving placebo and decreased in patients treated with repaglinide. Differences between the repaglinide- and placebo-treated groups were -61 mg/dL (FPG) and -104 mg/dL (PPG). The between-group change in HbA_{1c}, which reflects long-term glycemic control, was 1.7% units.

[See table above]

Another double-blind, placebo-controlled trial was carried out in 362 patients treated for 24 weeks. The efficacy of 1 and 4 mg preprandial doses was demonstrated by lowering of fasting blood glucose and by HbA_{1c} at the end of the study. HbA_{1C} for the PRANDIN®-treated groups (1 and 4 mg groups combined) at the end of the study was decreased compared to the placebo-treated group in previously naive patients and in patients previously treated with oral hypoglycemic agents by 2.1% units and 1.7% units, respectively. In this fixed-dose trial, patients who were naive to oral hypoglycemic agent therapy and patients in relatively good glycemic control at baseline (HbA_{1c} below 8%) showed greater blood glucose-lowering including a higher frequency of hypoglycemia. Patients who were previously treated and who had baseline HbA_{1c} ≥8% reported hypoglycemia at the same rate as patients randomized to placebo. There was no average gain in body weight when patients previously treated with oral hypoglycemic agents were switched to PRANDIN®. The average weight gain in patients treated

Continued on next page

Prandin—Cont.

with PRANDIN® and not previously treated with sulfonylurea drugs was 3.3%.
The dosing of PRANDIN® relative to meal-related insulin release was studied in three trials including 58 patients. Glycemic control was maintained during a period in which the meal and dosing pattern was varied (2, 3, or 4 meals per day; before meals × 2, 3 or 4) compared with a period of 3 regular meals and 3 doses per day (before meals × 3). It was also shown that PRANDIN® can be administered at the start of a meal, 15 minutes before, or 30 minutes before the meal with the same blood glucose lowering effect.
PRANDIN® was compared to other insulin secretagogues in 1-year controlled trials to demonstrate comparability of efficacy and safety. Hypoglycemia was reported in 16% of 1228 PRANDIN® patients, 20% of 417 glyburide patients, and 19% of 81 glipizide patients. Of PRANDIN® treated patients with symptomatic hypoglycemia, none developed coma or required hospitalization.
PRANDIN® was studied in combination with metformin in 83 patients not satisfactorily controlled on exercise, diet, and metformin alone. Combination therapy with PRANDIN® and metformin resulted in synergistic improvement in glycemic control compared to repaglinide or metformin monotherapy. HbA_{1c} was improved by 1% unit and FPG decreased by an additional 35 mg/dL.

PRANDIN® and Metformin Therapy: Mean HbA_{1C} and FPG Changes from Baseline after 3 Months Treatment

	PRANDIN®	Combination	Metformin
N	28	27	27
HbA_{1c} (% units)	-0.38	-1.41*	-0.33
FPG (mg/dL)	8.8	-39.2*	-4.5

* $p<0.05$ for between group comparison

INDICATIONS AND USAGE

PRANDIN® is indicated as an adjunct to diet and exercise to lower the blood glucose in patients with type 2 diabetes mellitus (NIDDM) whose hyperglycemia cannot be controlled satisfactorily by diet and exercise alone.
PRANDIN® is also indicated for use in combination with metformin to lower blood glucose in patients whose hyperglycemia cannot be controlled by exercise, diet, and either repaglinide or metformin alone. If glucose control has not been achieved after a suitable trial of combination therapy, consideration should be given to discontinuing these drugs and using insulin. Judgments should be based on regular clinical and laboratory evaluations.
In initiating treatment for patients with type 2 diabetes, diet and exercise should be emphasized as the primary form of treatment. Caloric restriction, weight loss, and exercise are essential in the obese diabetic patient. Proper dietary management and exercise alone may be effective in controlling the blood glucose and symptoms of hyperglycemia. In addition to regular physical activity, cardiovascular risk factors should be identified and corrective measures taken where possible.
If this treatment program fails to reduce symptoms and/or blood glucose, the use of an oral blood glucose-lowering agent or insulin should be considered. Use of PRANDIN® must be viewed by both the physician and patient as a treatment in addition to diet, and not as a substitute for diet or as a convenient mechanism for avoiding dietary restraint. Furthermore, loss of blood glucose control on diet alone may be transient, thus requiring only short-term administration of PRANDIN®.
During maintenance programs, PRANDIN® should be discontinued if satisfactory lowering of blood glucose is no longer achieved. Judgments should be based on regular clinical and laboratory evaluations.
The Diabetes Control and Complications Trial (DCCT) demonstrated, in patients with type 1 diabetes, that improved glycemic control, as reflected by HbA_{1C} and fasting glucose levels, was associated with a reduction in the diabetic complications retinopathy, neuropathy, and nephropathy. In considering the use of PRANDIN® or other antidiabetic therapies, it should be recognized that controlling the blood glucose in type 2 diabetes has not been established to be effective in preventing the long-term cardiovascular and neural complications of diabetes. It has not been shown that the implications of the DCCT results also apply to patients with type 2 diabetes. Nonetheless, improved glycemic control appears to be an important goal in many patients with non-insulin-dependent disease because it is presumed that the mechanisms by which glucose causes complications is the same in both forms of diabetes.

CONTRAINDICATIONS

PRANDIN® is contraindicated in patients with:
1. Diabetic ketoacidosis, with or without coma. This condition should be treated with insulin.
2. Type 1 diabetes.
3. Known hypersensitivity to the drug or its inactive ingredients.

PRECAUTIONS

General: Hypoglycemia: All oral blood glucose-lowering drugs are capable of producing hypoglycemia. Proper patient selection, dosage, and instructions to the patients are important to avoid hypoglycemic episodes. Hepatic insufficiency may cause elevated repaglinide blood levels and may diminish gluconeogenic capacity, both of which increase the risk of serious hypoglycemia. Elderly, debilitated, or malnourished patients, and those with adrenal, pituitary, or hepatic insufficiency are particularly susceptible to the hypoglycemic action of glucose-lowering drugs.
Hypoglycemia may be difficult to recognize in the elderly and in people taking beta-adrenergic blocking drugs. Hypoglycemia is more likely to occur when caloric intake is deficient, after severe or prolonged exercise, when alcohol is ingested, or when more than one glucose-lowering drug is used.
The frequency of hypoglycemia is greater in patients with type 2 diabetes who have not been previously treated with oral blood glucose-lowering drugs (naive) or whose HbA_{1C} is less than 8%. PRANDIN® should be administered with meals to lessen the risk of hypoglycemia.
Loss of control of blood glucose: When a patient stabilized on any diabetic regimen is exposed to stress such as fever, trauma, infection, or surgery, a loss of glycemic control may occur. At such times, it may be necessary to discontinue PRANDIN® and administer insulin. The effectiveness of any hypoglycemic drug in lowering blood glucose to a desired level decreases in many patients over a period of time, which may be due to progression of the severity of diabetes or to diminished responsiveness to the drug. This phenomenon is known as secondary failure, to distinguish it from primary failure in which the drug is ineffective in an individual patient when the drug is first given. Adequate adjustment of dose and adherence to diet should be assessed before classifying a patient as a secondary failure.

Information for Patients

Patients should be informed of the potential risks and advantages of PRANDIN® and of alternative modes of therapy. They should also be informed about the importance of adherence to dietary instructions, of a regular exercise program, and of regular testing of blood glucose and HbA_{1C}. The risks of hypoglycemia, its symptoms and treatment, and conditions that predispose to its development and concomitant administration of other glucose-lowering drugs should be explained to patients and responsible family members. Primary and secondary failure should also be explained.
Patients should be instructed to take PRANDIN® before meals (2, 3, or 4 times a day preprandially). Doses are usually taken within 15 minutes of the meal but time may vary from immediately preceding the meal to as long as 30 minutes before the meal. **Patients who skip a meal (or add an extra meal) should be instructed to skip (or add) a dose for that meal.**

Laboratory Tests

Response to all diabetic therapies should be monitored by periodic measurements of fasting blood glucose and glycosylated hemoglobin levels with a goal of decreasing these levels towards the normal range. During dose adjustment, fasting glucose can be used to determine the therapeutic response. Thereafter, both glucose and glycosylated hemoglobin should be monitored. Glycosylated hemoglobin may be especially useful for evaluating long-term glycemic control.

Drug Interactions

In vitro data indicate that repaglinide metabolism may be inhibited by antifungal agents like ketoconazole and miconazole, and antibacterial agents like erythromycin. Drugs that induce the cytochrome P-450 enzyme system 3A4 may increase repaglinide metabolism; such drugs include troglitazone, rifampin, barbiturates, and carbamazepine. No systematically acquired data are available on increased or decreased plasma levels with 3A4 inhibitors or inducers.
Drug interaction studies performed in healthy volunteers show that PRANDIN® had no clinically relevant effect on the pharmacokinetic properties of digoxin, theophylline, or warfarin. Thus, no dosage adjustment is required for digoxin, theophylline, or warfarin on co-administration of PRANDIN®. Co-administration of cimetidine with PRANDIN® did not significantly alter the absorption and disposition of repaglinide.
The hypoglycemic action of oral blood glucose-lowering agents may be potentiated by certain drugs including nonsteroidal anti-inflammatory agents and other drugs that are highly protein bound, salicylates, sulfonamides, chloramphenicol, coumarins, probenecid, monoamine oxidase inhibitors, and beta adrenergic blocking agents. When such drugs are administered to a patient receiving oral blood glucose-lowering agents, the patient should be observed closely for hypoglycemia. When such drugs are withdrawn from a patient receiving oral blood glucose-lowering agents, the patient should be observed closely for loss of glycemic control.
Certain drugs tend to produce hyperglycemia and may lead to loss of glycemic control. These drugs include the thiazides and other diuretics, corticosteroids, phenothiazines, thyroid products, estrogens, oral contraceptives, phenytoin, nicotinic acid, sympathomimetics, calcium channel blocking drugs, and isoniazid. When these drugs are administered to a patient receiving oral blood glucose-lowering agents, the patient should be observed for loss of glycemic control. When these drugs are withdrawn from a patient receiving oral blood glucose-lowering agents, the patient should be observed closely for hypoglycemia.

Carcinogenesis, Mutagenesis, and Impairment of Fertility

Long-term carcinogenicity studies were performed for 104 weeks at doses up to and including 120 mg/kg body weight/day (rats) and 500 mg/kg body weight/day (mice) or approximately 60 and 125 times clinical exposure, respectively, on a mg/m^2 basis. No evidence of carcinogenicity was found in mice or female rats. In male rats, there was an increased incidence of benign adenomas of the thyroid and liver. The relevance of these findings to humans is unclear. The no-effect doses for these observations in male rats were 30 mg/kg body weight/day for thyroid tumors and 60 mg/kg body weight/day for liver tumors, which are over 15 and 30 times, respectively, clinical exposure on a mg/m^2 basis.
Repaglinide was non-genotoxic in a battery of *in vivo* and *in vitro* studies: Bacterial mutagenesis (Ames test), *in vitro* forward cell mutation assay in V79 cells (HGPRT), *in vitro* chromosomal aberration assay in human lymphocytes, unscheduled and replicating DNA synthesis in rat liver, and *in vivo* mouse and rat micronucleus tests.
Fertility of male and female rats was unaffected by repaglinide administration at doses up to 80 mg/kg body weight/day (females) and 300 mg/kg body weight/day (males); over 40 times clinical exposure on a mg/m^2 basis.

Pregnancy

Pregnancy category C
Teratogenic Effects: Safety in pregnant women has not been established. Repaglinide was not teratogenic in rats or rabbits at doses 40 times (rats) and approximately 0.8 times (rabbit) clinical exposure (on a mg/m^2 basis) throughout pregnancy. Because animal reproduction studies are not always predictive of human response, PRANDIN® should be used during pregnancy only if it is clearly needed.
Because recent information suggests that abnormal blood glucose levels during pregnancy are associated with a higher incidence of congenital abnormalities, many experts recommend that insulin be used during pregnancy to maintain blood glucose levels as close to normal as possible.
Nonteratogenic Effects: Offspring of rat dams exposed to repaglinide at 15 times clinical exposure on a mg/m^2 basis during days 17 to 22 of gestation and during lactation developed nonteratogenic skeletal deformities consisting of shortening, thickening, and bending of the humerus during the postnatal period. This effect was not seen at doses up to 2.5 times clinical exposure (on a mg/m^2 basis) on days 1 to 22 of pregnancy or at higher doses given during days 1 to 16 of pregnancy. Relevant human exposure has not occurred to date and therefore the safety of PRANDIN® administration throughout pregnancy or lactation cannot be established.

Nursing Mothers

In rat reproduction studies, measurable levels of repaglinide were detected in the breast milk of the dams and lowered blood glucose levels were observed in the pups. Cross fostering studies indicated that skeletal changes (see **Nonteratogenic Effects**) could be induced in control pups nursed by treated dams, although this occurred to a lesser degree than those pups treated *in utero*. Although it is not known whether repaglinide is excreted in human milk some oral agents are known to be excreted by this route. Because the potential for hypoglycemia in nursing infants may exist, and because of the effects on nursing animals, a decision should be made as to whether PRANDIN® should be discontinued in nursing mothers, or if mothers should discontinue nursing. If PRANDIN® is discontinued and if diet alone is inadequate for controlling blood glucose, insulin therapy should be considered.

Pediatric Use

No studies have been performed in pediatric patients.

Geriatric Use

In repaglinide clinical studies of 24 weeks or greater duration, 415 patients were over 65 years of age. In one-year, active-controlled trials, no differences were seen in effectiveness or adverse events between these subjects and those less than 65 other than the expected age-related increase in cardiovascular events observed for PRANDIN® and comparator drugs. There was no increase in frequency or severity of hypoglycemia in older subjects. Other reported clinical experience has not identified differences in responses between the elderly and younger patients, but greater sensitivity of some older individuals to PRANDIN® therapy cannot be ruled out.

ADVERSE REACTIONS

Hypoglycemia: See **Precautions** and **Overdosage** Sections.
PRANDIN® has been administered to 2931 individuals during clinical trials. Approximately 1500 of these individuals with type 2 diabetes have been treated for at least 3 months, 1000 for at least 6 months, and 800 for at least 1 year. The majority of these individuals (1228) received PRANDIN® in one of five 1-year, active-controlled trials. The comparator drugs in these 1-year trials were oral sulfonylurea drugs (SU) including glyburide and glipizide. Over one year, 13% of PRANDIN® patients were discontinued due to adverse events as were 14% of SU patients. The most common adverse events leading to withdrawal were hyperglycemia, hypoglycemia, and related symptoms (see **PRECAUTIONS**). Mild or moderate hypoglycemia occurred in 16% of PRANDIN® patients, 20% glyburide patients, and 19% of glipizide patients.
The following table lists common adverse events for PRANDIN® patients compared to both placebo (in trials 12 to 24 weeks duration) and to glyburide and glipizide in one year trials. The adverse event profile of PRANDIN® was generally comparable to that for sulfonylurea drugs (SU).
[See table at top of next page]

Commonly Reported Adverse Events (% of Patients)*

EVENT	PRANDIN N = 352	PLACEBO N = 108	PRANDIN N = 1228	SU N = 498
	Placebo controlled studies		Active controlled studies	
Metabolic				
Hypoglycemia	31**	7	16	20
Respiratory				
URI	16	8	10	10
Sinusitis	6	2	3	4
Rhinitis	3	3	7	8
Bronchitis	2	1	6	7
Gastrointestinal				
Nausea	5	5	3	2
Diarrhea	5	2	4	6
Constipation	3	2	2	3
Vomiting	3	3	2	1
Dyspepsia	2	2	4	2
Musculoskeletal				
Arthralgia	6	3	3	4
Back Pain	5	4	6	7
Other				
Headache	11	10	9	8
Paresthesia	3	3	2	1
Chest pain	3	1	2	1
Urinary tract infection	2	1	3	3
Tooth disorder	2	0	<1	<1
Allergy	2	0	1	<1

* Events ≥ 2% for the PRANDIN® group in the placebo-controlled studies and ≥ events in the placebo group
** See trial description in **CLINICAL PHARMACOLOGY, Clinical Trials**

Cardiovascular events also occur commonly in patients with type 2 diabetes. In one-year comparator trials, the incidence of individual events was not greater than 1% except for chest pain (1.8%) and angina (1.8%). The individual incidence of other cardiovascular events (hypertension, abnormal EKG, myocardial infarction, arrhythmias, and palpitations) was ≤ 1% and not different for PRANDIN® and the comparator drugs.
The incidence of serious cardiovascular adverse events added together, including ischemia, was slightly higher for repaglinide (4%) than for sulfonylurea drugs (3%) in controlled comparator clinical trials. In 1-year controlled trials, PRANDIN® treatment was not associated with excess mortality rates compared to rates observed with other oral hypoglycemic agent therapies.

Summary of Serious Cardiovascular Events (% of total patients with events)

	PRANDIN®	SU*
Total Exposed	1228	498
Serious CV Events	4%	3%
Cardiac Ischemic Events	2%	2%
Deaths due to CV Events	0.5%	0.4%

* glyburide and glipizide

Infrequent adverse events (<1% of patients)
Less common adverse clinical or laboratory events observed in clinical trials included elevated liver enzymes, thrombocytopenia, leukopenia, and anaphylactoid reactions (one patient).

OVERDOSAGE

In a clinical trial, patients received increasing doses of PRANDIN® up to 80 mg a day for 14 days. There were few adverse effects other than those associated with the intended effect of lowering blood glucose. Hypoglycemia did not occur when meals were given with these high doses. Hypoglycemic symptoms without loss of consciousness or neurologic findings should be treated aggressively with oral glucose and adjustments in drug dosage and/or meal patterns. Close monitoring may continue until the physician is assured that the patient is out of danger. Patients should be closely monitored for a minimum of 24 to 48 hours, since hypoglycemia may recur after apparent clinical recovery. There is no evidence that repaglinide is dialyzable using hemodialysis.
Severe hypoglycemic reactions with coma, seizure, or other neurological impairment occur infrequently, but constitute medical emergencies requiring immediate hospitalization. If hypoglycemic coma is diagnosed or suspected, the patient should be given a rapid intravenous injection of concentrated (50%) glucose solution. This should be followed by a continuous infusion of more dilute (10%) glucose solution at a rate that will maintain the blood glucose at a level above 100 mg/dL.

DOSAGE AND ADMINISTRATION

There is no fixed dosage regimen for the management of type 2 diabetes with PRANDIN®.
The patient's blood glucose should be monitored periodically to determine the minimum effective dose for the patient; to detect primary failure, i.e., inadequate lowering of blood glucose at the maximum recommended dose of medication; and to detect secondary failure, i.e., loss of an adequate blood glucose-lowering response after an initial period of effectiveness. Glycosylated hemoglobin levels are of value in monitoring the patient's longer term response to therapy.
Short-term administration of PRANDIN® may be sufficient during periods of transient blood loss of control in patients usually well controlled on diet.
PRANDIN® doses are usually taken within 15 minutes of the meal but time may vary from immediately preceding the meal to as long as 30 minutes before the meal.

Starting Dose
For patients not previously treated or whose HbA_{1C} is <8%, the starting dose should be 0.5 mg with each meal. For patients previously treated with blood glucose-lowering drugs and whose HbA_{1C} is ≥ 8%, the initial dose is 1 or 2 mg with each meal preprandially (see previous paragraph).

Dose Adjustment
Dosing adjustments should be determined by blood glucose response, usually fasting blood glucose. The preprandial dose should be doubled up to 4 mg with each meal until satisfactory blood glucose response is achieved. At least one week should elapse to assess response after each dose adjustment.
The recommended dose range is 0.5 mg to 4 mg taken with meals. PRANDIN® may be dosed preprandially 2, 3, or 4 times a day in response to changes in the patient's meal pattern. The maximum recommended daily dose is 16 mg.

Patient Management
Long-term efficacy should be monitored by measurement of HbA_{1c} levels approximately every 3 months. Failure to follow an appropriate dosage regimen may precipitate hypoglycemia or hyperglycemia. Patients who do not adhere to their prescribed dietary and drug regimen are more prone to exhibit unsatisfactory response to therapy including hypoglycemia.

Patients Receiving Other Oral Hypoglycemic Agents.
When PRANDIN® is used to replace therapy with other oral hypoglycemic agents, PRANDIN® may be started on the day after the final dose is given. Patients should then be observed carefully for hypoglycemia due to potential overlapping of drug effects. When transferred from longer half-life sulfonylurea agents (e.g., chloropropamide) to repaglinide, close monitoring may be indicated for up to one week or longer.

Combination Therapy
If PRANDIN® monotherapy does not result in adequate glycemic control, metformin may be added. Or, if metformin therapy does not provide adequate control, PRANDIN® may be added. The starting dose and dose adjustments for PRANDIN® combination therapy is the same as for PRANDIN® monotherapy. The dose of each drug should be carefully adjusted to determine the minimal dose required to achieve the desired pharmacologic effect. Failure to do so could result in an increase in the incidence of hypoglycemic episodes. Appropriate monitoring of FPG and HbA_{1c} measurements should be used to ensure that the patient is not subjected to excessive drug exposure or increased probability of secondary drug failure.

HOW SUPPLIED

PRANDIN® (repaglinide) tablets are supplied as unscored, biconvex tablets available in 0.5 mg (white), 1 mg (yellow) and 2 mg (peach) strengths. Tablets are embossed with the Novo Nordisk (Apis) bull symbol and colored to indicated strength.

0.5 mg tablets (white)	Bottles of 100	NDC 00169-0081-81
	Bottles of 500	NDC 00169-0081-82
	Bottles of 1000	NDC 00169-0081-83
1 mg tablets (yellow)	Bottles of 100	NDC 00169-0082-81
	Bottles of 500	NDC 00169-0082-82
	Bottles of 1000	NDC 00169-0082-83
2 mg tablets (peach)	Bottles of 100	NDC 00169-0084-81
	Bottles of 500	NDC 00169-0084-82
	Bottles of 1000	NDC 00169-0084-83

Do not store above 25°C (77°F). Protect from moisture. Keep bottles tightly closed.
Dispense in tight containers with safety closures.
Rx only

PRANDIN® is a trademark of Novo Nordisk A/S.

Manufactured in Germany for
Novo Nordisk Pharmaceuticals, Inc.
Princeton, NJ 08540.
1-800-727-6500

EDUCATIONAL MATERIAL

PATIENT EDUCATION MATERIALS
NOVO NORDISK DIABETES CARE®
SERVICE PROGRAMS THAT
EDUCATE AND SUPPORT
Novo Nordisk Diabetes Care® is a comprehensive service program encompassing patient education materials, professional education programs and a wide variety of services to support health care professionals and their patients with diabetes.
Some of the items available from Novo Nordisk Diabetes Care® are:

Professional Education
- CME, CNE & CPE Programs

Patient Education
- Self-management materials
- Materials for individualized treatment
  - — for children with diabetes and their parents
  - — for patients with type 2 diabetes
  - — for patients with complications
  - — for patients who read Spanish

For additional information call 1-800-727-6500.

Novogyne Pharmaceuticals

A joint venture between
Novartis Pharmaceuticals Corporation
EAST HANOVER, NEW JERSEY 07936
and
Noven Pharmaceuticals, Inc.
MIAMI, FLORIDA 33186

For Information Contact:
Customer Response Department
(888) NOW-NOVARTIS (888-669-6682)

Product information for **Vivelle®** (estradiol transdermal system) and **Vivelle-Dot™** (estradiol transdermal system) is referenced under the distributor, NOVARTIS PHARMACEUTICALS CORPORATION.

For information on over-the-counter drugs, consult **PDR For Nonprescription Drugs.**

Nutraceutics™ Corporation

4100 LACLEDE AVENUE
SUITE 112
ST. LOUIS, MO 63108

Direct Inquiries to:
1-800-391-0114

Q-BID™	OTC
(Coenzyme Q-10 in nanospheres)	100 mg
CARDIOTROPIN™	OTC
(Creatine Phosphate, L Carnitine)	
REDOX™	OTC
(Chewable Broad Spectrum Antioxidant)	
OSTEO I.P.™	OTC
(Slow Release Ipriflavone)	200 mg
PRO ENDORPHIN™	OTC
(Hypothalamic Protein, DL Phenylalanine)	
SAMe Plus	OTC
(S-adeno-sylmethionine, Betaine)	200 mg
SYMBIOTROPIN®	OTC
(Alpha-Glycerylphosphorylcholine, Hypothalamic protein)	

OSTEOMAX™ OTC

Effervescent Calcium Citrate Dietary Supplement

INGREDIENTS

Calcium Carbonate, Citric Acid, Magnesium Oxide, Vitamin D3, L Lysine, Sodium Bicarbonate, Sodium Carbonate, Polysorbate 80, Natural Orange Flavor.

One Effervescent Tablet Provides

500 mg of elemental Calcium, 200 mg of elemental Magnesium, 200 IU of Vitamin D3, and 100 mg of L Lysine.

DIRECTIONS

Dissolve one or two effervescent tablets in approximately 3 ounces of water, stir before drinking.

HOW SUPPLIED

OSTEOMAX effervescent tablets are supplied in a box of 28.

Oclassen Dermatologics

A Division of
Watson Pharma Inc.
CORONA, CA 92880

Direct Inquiries to:
Customer Service Department
(800) 272-5525
Fax (909) 735-2871

For Medical Information Contact:
Customer Service Department
(800) 272-5525
Fax (909) 737-8540

CONDYLOX® Gel 0.5% ℞

[*cŏn 'dy-lox*]
(podofilox gel)

DESCRIPTION

Podofilox is an antimitotic drug which can be chemically synthesized or purified from the plant families *Coniferae* and *Berberidaceae* (e.g. species of *Juniperus* and *Podophyllum*). Condylox® Gel 0.5% is formulated for topical administration. Each gram of gel contains 5mg of podofilox in a buffered alcoholic gel containing alcohol, glycerin, lactic acid, hydroxypropyl cellulose, sodium lactate, and butylated hydroxytoluene.

Podofilox has a molecular weight of 414.4 daltons, and is soluble in alcohol and sparingly soluble in water. Its chemical name is [5R-(5α,5aβ,8aα,9α)-5,8,8a,9-tetrahydro-9-hydroxy-5-(3,4,5-trimethoxyphenyl) furo[3′,4′:6,7]naphtho-[2,3,-d]-1,3-dioxol-6(5aH)-one.

Podofilox has the following structural formula:

OH
CH_3O OCH_3
OCH_3

CLINICAL PHARMACOLOGY

Mechanism of Action

Treatment of anogenital warts with podofilox results in necrosis of visible wart tissue. The exact mechanism of action is unknown.

Pharmacokinetics

In systemic absorption studies in 52 patients, topical application of 0.05mL of an ethanolic solution containing 0.5% podofilox to external genitalia did not result in detectable serum levels. Applications of 0.1 to 1.5mL resulted in peak serum levels of 1 to 17 ng/mL one to two hours after application. The elimination half-life ranged from 1.0 to 4.5 hours. The drug was not found to accumulate after multiple treatments.[1]

CLINICAL STUDIES

In the first multicenter clinical study in 326 patients with anogenital warts, Condylox® Gel 0.5% and its vehicle were applied in a double-blind fashion to comparable patient groups. Of the 260 patients with efficacy data, 176 were treated with Condylox® Gel 0.5%. Patients applied Condylox® Gel 0.5% twice daily for three consecutive days followed by a 4 day "rest" period.

At the end of 4 weeks, 38.4% of the patients had complete clearing of the wart tissue when treated with Condylox® Gel 0.5%.

In the second multicenter clinical trial in 108 evaluable patients with anogenital warts, Condylox® (podofilox) Topical Solution 0.5% was compared with Condylox® Gel 0.5% for efficacy. As in the first clinical trial, patients applied Condylox® Gel 0.5% twice daily for three consecutive days followed by a four day "rest" period.

Similar clearance rates were observed. At the end of 4 weeks, 25.6% of the patients had complete clearing of the wart tissue when treated with Condylox® Gel 0.5%.

INDICATIONS AND USAGE

Condylox® Gel 0.5% is indicated for the topical treatment of anogenital warts (external genital warts and perianal warts). This product is *not* indicated in the treatment of mucous membrane warts (see **PRECAUTIONS**).

Diagnosis

Although anogenital warts have a characteristic appearance, histopathologic confirmation should be obtained if there is any doubt of the diagnosis. Differentiating warts from squamous cell carcinoma and "Bowenoid papulosis" is of particular concern. Squamous cell carcinoma may also be associated with human papillomavirus which should not be treated with Condylox® Gel 0.5%.

CONTRAINDICATIONS

Condylox® Gel 0.5% is contraindicated for patients who develop hypersensitivity or intolerance to any components of the formulation.

WARNINGS

Correct diagnosis of the lesions to be treated is essential. See the **Diagnosis** subsection of the **INDICATIONS AND USAGE** section. Condylox® Gel 0.5% is intended for cutaneous use only. **Avoid contact with the eyes. If contact with the eyes occurs, patients should immediately flush the eyes with copious quantities of water and seek medical advice.**

Drug Product is Flammable. Keep Away From Open Flame.

PRECAUTIONS

General

Data are not available on the safe and effective use of this product for treatment of warts occurring on mucous membranes of the genital area (including the urethra, rectum and vagina). The recommended method of application, frequency of application, and duration of usage should not be exceeded (see **DOSAGE AND ADMINISTRATION**).

Information for Patients

Patients using Condylox® Gel 0.5% should receive the following information and instructions. This information is intended to aid in the safe and effective use of this medication. It is not intended to disclose all possible adverse or intended effects.

1) This medication should be used only as directed by the health care provider. Patients should be instructed to wash their hands thoroughly before and after each application. It is for external use only. Avoid contact with the eyes.
2) Patients should be advised not to use this medication for any disorder other than for which it was prescribed.
3) Patients should report any signs of adverse reactions to the health care provider.
4) If no improvement is observed after 4 weeks of treatment, discontinue the medication and consult the health care provider.

Carcinogenesis, Mutagenesis and Impairment of Fertility

An 80-week carcinogenicity study in the mouse was performed using a 0.5% podofilox solution applied dermally at 0.04, 0.2 and 1.0 mg/kg/day. There were no differences between the podofilox treated mice at any dose level and vehicle control in the incidence of neoplasia. Published animal studies, in general, have not shown the drug substance, podofilox, to be carcinogenic.[2,3,4,5,6] There are published reports that, in mouse studies, crude podophyllin resin (containing podofilox) applied topically to the cervix produced changes resembling carcinoma *in situ*.[7] These changes were reversible at five weeks after cessation of treatment. In one reported experiment, epidermal carcinoma of the vagina and cervix was found in 1 out of 18 mice after 120 applications of podophyllin[8] (the drug was applied twice weekly over a 15-month period).

Podofilox was not mutagenic in the Ames plate reverse mutation assay at concentrations up to 5mg/plate, with and without metabolic activation. No cell transformation related to potential oncogenicity was observed in BALB/3T3 cells after exposure to podofilox at concentration up to 0.008μg/mL, without metabolic activation and 12μg/mL podofilox with metabolic activation. Results from the mouse micronucleus *in vivo* assay using podofilox 0.5% solution at doses up to 25 mg/kg (75 mg/m^2), indicate that podofilox should be considered a potential clastogen (a chemical that induces disruption and breakage of chromosomes).

Daily topical application of 0.5% podofilox solution at doses up to the equivalent of 0.2mg/kg (1.18 mg/m^2, approximately equivalent to the human daily dose) to rats throughout gametogenesis, mating, gestation, parturition and lactation for two generation demonstrated no impairment of fertility.

Pregnancy

Pregnancy Category C: 0.5% podofilox solution was not teratogenic in the rabbit following topical application of up to 0.21 mg/kg (2.85 mg/m^2, approximately 2 times the maximum human dose) once daily for 13 days. The scientific literature contains references that podofilox is embryotoxic in rats when administered intaperitoneally at a dose of 5 mg/kg (29.5 mg/m^2, approximately 19 times the recommended maximum human dose).[9] Teratogenicity and embryotoxicity have not been studies with intravaginal application. Many antimitotic drug products are known to be embryotoxic. There are no adequate and well-controlled studies in pregnant women. Condylox® Gel 0.5% should be used during pregnancy only if the potential benefit justifies the potential risk to the fetus.

Nursing Mothers

It is not known whether this drug is excreted in human milk. Because of the potential for serious adverse reactions in nursing infants from podofilox, a decision should be made whether to discontinue nursing or to discontinue the drug, taking into account the importance of the drug to the mother.

Pediatric Use

Safety and effectiveness in pediatric patients have not been established.

ADVERSE REACTIONS

In clinical trials with Condylox® Gel 0.5%, the following local adverse reactions were reported during the treatment of anogenital warts. The severity of local adverse reactions were predominantly mild or moderate and did not increase during the treatment period. Severe reactions were most frequent within the first 2 weeks of treatment.

Adverse Reaction	Mild	Moderate	Severe
Inflammation	32.2%	30.4%	9.3%
Burning	37.1%	25.9%	11.5%
Erosion	27.0%	20.8%	8.9%
Pain	23.7%	20.4%	11.5%
Itching	32.2%	16.0%	7.8%
Bleeding	19.2%	3.0%	0.7%

Other local adverse reactions reported included stinging (7%), and erythema (5%); less commonly reported local adverse events included desquamation, scabbing, discoloration, tenderness, dryness, crusting, fissures, soreness, ulceration, swelling/edema, tingling, rash, and blisters.

The most common systemic adverse event reported during the clinical studies was headache (7%).

OVERDOSAGE

Topically applied podofilox may be absorbed systemically (see **CLINICAL PHARMACOLOGY** section). Toxicity reported following systemic administration of podofilox in investigational use for cancer treatment included: nausea, vomiting, fever, diarrhea, bone marrow depression, and oral ulcers. Following 5 to 10 daily intravenous doses of 0.5 to 1 mg/kg/day, significant hematological toxicity occurred but was reversible.[10] Other toxicities occurred at lower doses. Toxicity reported following systemic administration of podophyllum resin included: nausea, vomiting, fever, diarrhea, peripheral neuropathy, altered mental status, lethargy, coma, tachypnea, respiratory failure, leukocytosis, pancytosis, hematuria, renal failure and seizures.[11] Treatment of topical overdosage should include washing the skin free of any remaining drug and symptomatic and supportive therapy.

DOSAGE AND ADMINISTRATION

The prescriber should ensure that the patients is fully aware of the correct method of therapy and identify which specific warts should be treated.

Apply twice daily for 3 consecutive days, then discontinue for 4 consecutive days. This one week cycle of treatment may be repeated until there is no visible wart tissue or for a maximum of four cycles. **If there is incomplete response after four treatment cycles, discontinue treatment and consider alternative treatment. Safety and effectiveness of more than four treatment cycles has not been established.**

There is no evidence to suggest that more frequent application will increase efficacy, but additional applications would be expected to increase the rate of local adverse reactions and systemic absorptions.

Condylox® Gel 0.5% should be applied to the warts with the applicator tip or finger. Application on the surrounding normal tissue should be minimized. **Treatment should be limited to 10 cm^2 or less of wart tissue and to no more than 0.5g of the gel per day.**

Care should be taken to allow the gel to dry before allowing the return of opposing skin surfaces to their normal positions. Patients should be instructed to wash their hands thoroughly before and after each application.

HOW SUPPLIED

Condylox® Gel 0.5% is supplied as 3.5g of clear gel in aluminum tubes with an applicator tip. NDC 55515-102-01. Store at controlled room temperature between 15-30°C (59-86°F). **Avoid excessive heat. Do not freeze.**

Rx only

REFERENCES

1. von Krogh G. Podophyllotoxin in serum: Absorption subsequent to three day repeated applications of a 0.5% ethanolic preparation on condylomata acuminata. Sex Trans Disease 1982: 9: 26–33.
2. Berenblum I. The effect of podophyllotoxin on the skin of the mouse, with reference to carcinogenic, cocarcinogenic, and anticarcinogenic action. J Cancer Inst 11: 839–841, 1951.
3. Kaminetzky HA, Swerdlow M. Podophyllin and the mouse cervix: assessment of carcinogenic potential. Am J Obst Gyn 95:486–490, 1965.
4. McGrew EA, Kaminetzky HA. The genesis of experimental cervical epithelial dysplasia. Am J Clin Path 35: 538–545, 1961.
5. Roe FJC, Salaman MH. Further studies on incomplete carcinogenesis: triethylene melamine (T.E.M.) 1,2 benzanthracene and beta-propiolactone as initiators of skin tumor formation in the mouse. Brit J Cancer 9:177–203, 1955.
6. Taper HS. Induction of the deficient acid DNAase activity in mouse interfollicular epidermis by croton oil as a possible tumor promoting mechanism. Zeitschrift fur Krebsforschung und Klinisch Onkologie (Cancer Research and Clinical Oncology, Berlin) 90:197–210, 1977.
7. Kaminetzky HA, McGrew EA, Phillips RL. Experimental cervical epithelial dysplasia. J Obst Gyn 14:1–10, 1959.
8. Kaminetzky HA, McGrew EA: Podophyllin and mouse cervix: Effect of long term application. Arch Path 73: 481–485, 1962.
9. Thiersch JB. Effect of podophyllin (P) and podophyllotoxine (PT.) on the rat litter in utero. Soc Exptl Biol Med Proc 113:124–27, 1963.
10. Savel H.: Clinical experience with intravenous podophyllotoxin. Proc Amer Assoc Cancer Res, 1964; 5: 56.
11. Cassidy DE, Dewry J and Fanning JP: Podophyllum toxicity: A report of a fatal case and a review of the literature. J Toxicol Clinic Toxicol 1982: 19:35–44.

Mfd. for
OCLASSEN
DERMATOLOGICS
a division of Watson Pharma, Inc.
Corona CA 92880
by DPT Laboratories, Inc.
San Antonio, TX 78215

Revised March 10, 1998
127341-0398

Shown in Product Identification Guide, page 327

CONDYLOX® ℞

[*con 'de-lox*]
(podofilox)
Topical Solution 0.5%

DESCRIPTION

Condylox® is the brand name of podofilox, an antimitotic drug which can be chemically synthesized or purified from the plant families *Coniferae* and *Berberidaceae* (e.g. species of *Juniperus* and *Podophyllum*). Condylox® 0.5% Solution is formulated for topical administration. Each milliliter of solution contains 5 mg of podofilox, in a vehicle containing lactic acid and sodium lactate in alcohol 95%, USP.

Podofilox has a molecular weight of 414.4 daltons, and is soluble in alcohol and sparingly soluble in water. Its chemical name is 5,8,8a,9-Tetrahydro-9-hydroxy-5- (3,4,5-trimethoxylphenyl)furo [3′,4′:6,7] naphtho [2,3,d] -1,3-dioxol-6(5aH)-one. Podofilox has the following structural formula:

CLINICAL PHARMACOLOGY

Mechanism of Action

Treatment of genital warts with podofilox results in necrosis of visible wart tissue. The exact mechanism of action is unknown.

Pharmacokinetics

In systemic absorption studies in 52 patients, topical application of 0.05 mL of 0.5% podofilox solution to external genitalia did not result in detectable serum levels. Application of 0.1 to 1.5 mL resulted in peak serum levels of 1 to 17 ng/mL one to two hours after application. The elimination half-life ranged from 1.0 to 4.5 hours. The drug was not found to accumulate after multiple treatments.

CLINICAL STUDIES

In clinical studies with Condylox® Solution, the test product and its vehicle were applied in a double-blind fashion to comparable patient groups. Patients were treated for two to four weeks, and re-evaluated at a two-week follow-up examination. Although the number of patients and warts evaluated at each time period varied, the results among investigators were relatively consistent.

The following table represents the responses noted in terms of frequency of response by lesions treated and the overall response by patients. Data are presented for the 2-week follow-up only for those patients evaluated at that time point.

Responses in Treated Patients

	Initially Cleared*	Recurred after Clearing*	Cleared at 2-Week Follow-Up*
% Warts (n=524)	79% (412/524)	35% (146/412)	60% (269/449)
% Patients (n=70)	50% (35/70)	60% (21/35)	25% (14/57)

* Cleared and clearing mean no visible wart tissue remained at the treated sites

INDICATIONS AND USAGE

Condylox® 0.5% Solution is indicated for the topical treatment of external genital warts (Condyloma acuminatum). This product is *not* indicated in the treatment of perianal or mucous membrane warts (see **PRECAUTIONS**).

Diagnosis

Although genital warts have a characteristic appearance, histopathologic confirmation should be obtained if there is any doubt of the diagnosis. Differentiating warts from squamous cell carcinoma (so-called "Bowenoid papulosis") is of particular concern. Squamous cell carcinoma may also be associated with human papillomavirus but should not be treated with Condylox® 0.5% Solution.

CONTRAINDICATIONS

Condylox® 0.5% Solution is contraindicated for patients who develop hypersensitivity or intolerance to any component of the formulation.

WARNINGS

Correct diagnosis of the lesions to be treated is essential. See the "Diagnosis" subsection of the **INDICATIONS AND USAGE** statement.

Condylox® 0.5% Solution is intended for cutaneous use only. **Avoid contact with the eyes. If eye contact occurs, patients should immediately flush the eye with copious quantities of water and seek medical advice.**

PRECAUTIONS

General

Data are not available on the safe and effective use of this product for treatment of warts occurring in the perianal area or mucous membranes of the genital area (including the urethra, rectum and vagina). The recommended method of application, frequency of application, and duration of usage should not be exceeded (see **DOSAGE AND ADMINISTRATION**).

Information for Patients

The patient should be provided with a Patient Information leaflet when a Condylox® prescription is filled.

Carcinogenesis, Mutagenesis and Impairment of Fertility

Reports of lifetime carcinogenicity studies in mice are not available. Published animal studies, in general, have not shown the drug substance, podofilox, to be carcinogenic.[1,2,3,4,5] There are published reports that, in mouse studies, crude podophyllin resin (containing podofilox) applied topically to the cervix produced changes resembling carcinoma *in situ.*[6] These changes were reversible at five weeks after cessation of treatment. In one reported experiment, epidermal carcinoma of the vagina and cervix was found in 1 out of 18 mice after 120 applications of podophyllin[7] (the drug was applied twice weekly over a 15-month period).

Podofilox was not mutagenic in the Ames plate reverse mutation assay at concentrations up to 5 mg/plate, with and without metabolic activation. No cell transformation related to potential oncogenicity was observed in BALB/3T3 cells after exposure to podofilox at concentrations up to 0.008 μg/mL without metabolic activation and 12 μg/mL podofilox with metabolic activation. Results from the mouse micronucleus in vivo assay using podofilox 0.5% solution in concentrations up to 25 mg/kg, indicate that podofilox should be considered a potential clastogen (a chemical that induces disruption and breakage of chromosomes).

Daily topical applications of Condylox® 0.5% Solution at doses up to the equivalent of 0.2 mg/kg (5 times the recommended maximum human dose) to rats throughout gametogenesis, mating, gestation, parturition and lactation for two generations demonstrated no impairment of fertility.

Pregnancy

Pregnancy Category C: Podofilox was not teratogenic in the rabbit following topical application of up to 0.21 mg/kg (5 times the maximum human dose) once daily for 13 days. The scientific literature contains references that podofilox is embryotoxic in rats when administered systemically in a dose approximately 250 times the recommended maximum human dose.[8,9] Teratogenicity and embryotoxicity have not been studied with intravaginal application. Many antimitotic drug products are known to be embryotoxic. There are no adequate and well-controlled studies in pregnant women. Podofilox should be used in pregnancy only if the potential benefit justifies the potential risk to the fetus.

Nursing Mothers

It is not known whether this drug is excreted in human milk. Because of the potential for serious adverse reactions in nursing infants from podofilox, a decision should be made whether to discontinue nursing or to discontinue the drug, taking into account the importance of the drug to the mother.

Pediatric Use

Safety and effectiveness in pediatric patients have not been established.

ADVERSE REACTIONS

In clinical trials, the following local adverse reactions were reported at some point during treatment.

Adverse Experience	Males	Females
Burning	64%	78%
Pain	50%	72%
Inflammation	71%	63%
Erosion	67%	67%
Itching	50%	65%

Reports of burning and pain were more frequent and of greater severity in women than in men.

Adverse effects reported in less than 5% of the patients included pain with intercourse, insomnia, tingling, bleeding, tenderness, chafing, malodor, dizziness, scarring, vesicle formation, crusting, edema, dryness/peeling, foreskin irretraction, hematuria, vomiting and ulceration.

OVERDOSAGE

Topically applied podofilox may be absorbed systemically (see **CLINICAL PHARMACOLOGY** section). Toxicity reported following systemic administration of podofilox in investigational use for cancer treatment included: nausea, vomiting, fever, diarrhea, bone marrow depression, and oral ulcers. Following 5 to 10 daily intravenous doses of 0.5 to 1 mg/kg/day, significant hematological toxicity occurred but was reversible. Other toxicities occurred at lower doses. Toxicity reported following systemic administration of podophyllum resin included: nausea, vomiting, fever, diarrhea, peripheral neuropathy, altered mental status, lethargy, coma, tachypnea, respiratory failure, leukocytosis, pancytosis, hematuria, renal failure, and seizures. Treatment of topical overdosage should include washing the skin free of any remaining drug and symptomatic and supportive therapy.

DOSAGE AND ADMINISTRATION

In order to ensure that the patient is fully aware of the correct method of therapy and to identify which specific warts should be treated, the technique for initial application of the medication should be demonstrated by the prescriber.

Apply twice daily morning and evening (every 12 hours), for 3 consecutive days, then withhold use for 4 consecutive days. This one week cycle of treatment may be repeated up to four times until there is no visible wart tissue. **If there is incomplete response after four treatment weeks, alternative treatment should be considered. Safety and effectiveness of more than four treatment weeks have not been established.**

Condylox® 0.5% Solution is applied to the warts with a cotton-tipped applicator supplied with the drug. The drug-dampened applicator should be touched to the wart to be treated, applying the minimum amount of solution necessary to cover the lesion. **Treatment should be limited to less than 10 cm^2 of wart tissue and to no more than 0.5 mL of the solution per day.** There is no evidence to suggest that more frequent application will increase efficacy, but additional applications would be expected to increase the rate of local adverse reactions and systemic absorption.

Care should be taken to allow the solution to dry before allowing the return of opposing skin surfaces to their normal positions. After each treatment, the used applicator should be carefully disposed of and the patient should wash his or her hands.

HOW SUPPLIED

3.5 mL of Condylox® 0.5% Solution is supplied as a clear liquid in amber glass bottles with child-resistant screw caps. NDC #55515-101-01. Store at controlled room temperature between 15° and 30°C (59° and 86°F). **Avoid excessive heat. Do not freeze.**

Caution: Federal law prohibits dispensing without prescription.

REFERENCES

1. I. Berenblum, 1951. J. Natl. Cancer Inst. *11:* 839–841
2. H.A. Kaminetsky and M. Swerdlow, 1965. Am. J. Obst. Gyn. *95:* 486–490
3. E.A. McGrew and H.A. Kaminetsky. 1961. Am J. Clin. Pathol. *35:* 538–545
4. F.J.C. Roe and M.H. Salaman, 1955. Brit. J. Cancer. *9:* 177–203
5. H.S. Taper, 1977. Z. Kerbsforsch, *90:* 197–210
6. H.A. Kaminetsky and E.A. McGrew, and R.L. Phillips, 1959. Am. J. Obst. Gyn. *14:* 1–10
7. H.A. Kaminetsky and E.A. McGrew, 1962. Arch. Path. *73:* 481–485
8. K. Didcock, D. Jackson, and J.M. Robson, 1956. Brit. J. Pharmacol. *11:* 437–441
9. J. Thiersch, 1963. Soc. Exptl. Biol. Med. Proc. *113:* 124–127

Continued on next page

Condylox Topical Solution—Cont.

Revised: March, 1998
127339-0398
Mfd. for
OCLASSEN DERMATOLOGICS
A Division of Watson Pharma, Inc., Carona, CA 92880
by DPT Labs, Ltd., San Antonio, TX 78215
03-4709-R4
Shown in Product Identification Guide, page 327

CORDRAN® Lotion, 0.05% Flurandrenolide Lotion, USP ℞
[*kōr 'drăn*]

DESCRIPTION

Cordran® (Flurandrenolide, USP) is a potent corticosteroid intended for topical use. Flurandrenolide occurs as white to off-white, fluffy, crystalline powder and is odorless. Flurandrenolide is practically insoluble in water and in ether. One g dissolves in 72 mL of alcohol and in 10 mL of chloroform. The molecular weight of flurandrenolide is 436.52.
The chemical name of flurandrenolide is Pregn-4-ene-3,20-dione, 6-fluoro-11,21-dihydroxy-16,17-[(1-methylethylidene)bis (oxy)]-, (6α, 11β, 16α)-; its empirical formula is $C_{24}H_{33}FO_6$. The structure is as follows:

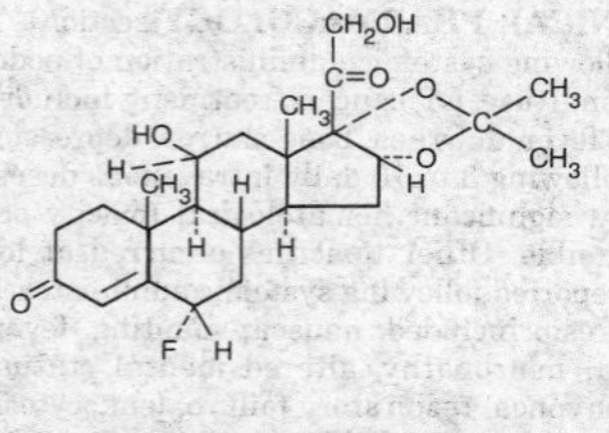

Each mL of Cordran Lotion contains 0.5 mg (1.145 µmol) (0.05%) flurandrenolide in an oil-in-water emulsion base composed of glycerin, cetyl alcohol, stearic acid, glyceryl monostearate, mineral oil, polyoxyl 40 stearate, menthol, benzyl alcohol, and purified water.

CLINICAL PHARMACOLOGY

Cordran is primarily effective because of its anti-inflammatory, antipruritic, and vasoconstrictive actions.
The mechanism of the anti-inflammatory effect of topical corticosteroids is not completely understood. Various laboratory methods, including vasoconstrictor assays, are used to compare and predict potencies and/or clinical efficacies of the topical corticosteroids. There is some evidence to suggest that a recognizable correlation exists between vasoconstrictor potency and therapeutic efficacy in man. Corticosteroids with anti-inflammatory activity may stabilize cellular and lysosomal membranes. There is also the suggestion that the effect on the membranes of lysosomes prevents the release of proteolytic enzymes and, thus, plays a part in reducing inflammation.
Evaporation of water from the lotion vehicle produces a cooling effect, which is often desirable in the treatment of acutely inflamed or weeping lesions.
Pharmacokinetics—The extent of percutaneous absorption of topical corticosteroids is determined by many factors, including the vehicle, the integrity of the epidermal barrier, and the use of occlusive dressings.
Topical corticosteroids can be absorbed from normal intact skin. Inflammation and/or other disease processes in the skin increase percutaneous absorption. Occlusive dressings substantially increase the percutaneous absorption of topical corticosteroids. Thus, occlusive dressings may be a valuable therapeutic adjunct for treatment of resistant dermatoses (*see* **DOSAGE AND ADMINISTRATION**).
Once absorbed through the skin, topical corticosteroids are handled through pharmacokinetic pathways similar to those of systematically administered corticosteroids. Corticosteroids are bound to plasma proteins in varying degrees. They are metabolized primarily in the liver and then excreted in the kidneys. Some of the topical corticosteroids and their metabolites are also excreted into the bile.

INDICATIONS AND USAGE

Cordran is indicated for the relief of the inflammatory and pruritic manifestations of corticosteroid-responsive dermatoses.

CONTRAINDICATIONS

Topical corticosteroids are contraindicated in patients with a history of hypersensitivity to any of the components of these preparations.

PRECAUTIONS

General—Systemic absorption of topical corticosteroids has produced reversible hypothalamic-pituitary-adrenal (HPA) axis suppression, manifestations of Cushing's syndrome, hyperglycemia, and glucosuria in some patients.
Conditions that augment systemic absorption include application of the more potent steroids, use over large surface areas, prolonged use, and the addition of occlusive dressings.
Therefore, patients receiving a large dose of a potent topical steroid applied to a large surface area or under an occlusive dressing should be evaluated periodically for evidence of HPA axis suppression using urinary-free cortisol and ACTH stimulation tests. If HPA axis suppression is noted, an attempt should be made to withdraw the drug, to reduce the frequency of application, or to substitute a less potent steroid.
Recovery of HPA axis function is generally prompt and complete on discontinuation of the drug. Infrequently, signs and symptoms of steroid withdrawal may occur, so that supplemental systemic corticosteroids are required.
Pediatric patients may absorb proportionately large amounts of topical corticosteroids and thus be more susceptible to systemic toxicity (*see Pediatric Use* under **PRECAUTIONS**).
If irritation develops, topical corticosteroids should be discontinued and appropriate therapy instituted.
In the presence of dermatologic infections, the use of an appropriate antifungal or antibacterial agent should be instituted. If a favorable response does not occur promptly, Cordran should be discontinued until the infection has been adequately controlled.
Information for the Patient—Patients using topical corticosteroids should receive the following information and instructions:

1. This medication is to be used as directed by the physician. It is for external use only. Avoid contact with the eyes.
2. Patients should be advised not to use this medication for any disorder other than that for which it was prescribed.
3. The treated skin area should not be bandaged or otherwise covered or wrapped in order to be occlusive unless the patient is directed to do so by the physician.
4. Patients should report any signs of local adverse reactions, especially under occlusive dressing.
5. Parents of pediatric patients should be advised not to use tight-fitting diapers or plastic pants on a patient being treated in the diaper area, because these garmets may constitute occlusive dressings.

Laboratory Tests—The following tests may be helpful in evaluating the HPA axis suppression:
Urinary-free cortisol test
ACTH stimulation test
Carcinogenesis, Mutagenesis, and Impairment of Fertility—Long-term animal studies have not been performed to evaluate the carcinogenic potential or the effect on fertility of topical corticosteroids.
Studies to determine mutagenicity with prednisolone and hydrocortisone have revealed negative results.
Usage in Pregnancy—Pregnancy Category C—Corticosteroids are generally teratogenic in laboratory animals when administered systemically at relatively low dosage levels. The more potent corticosteroids have been shown to be teratogenic after dermal application in laboratory animals. There are no adequate and well-controlled studies in pregnant women on teratogenic effects from topically applied corticosteroids. Therefore, topical corticosteroids should be used during pregnancy only if the potential benefit justifies the potential risk to the fetus. Drugs of this class should not be used extensively for pregnant patients or in large amounts or for prolonged periods of time.
Nursing Mothers—It is not known whether topical administration of corticosteroids could result in sufficient systemic absorption to produce detectable quantities in breast milk. Systemically administered corticosteroids are secreted into breast milk in quantities *not* likely to have a deleterious effect on the infant. Nevertheless, caution should be exercised when topical corticosteroids are administered to a nursing woman.
Pediatric Use—Pediatric patients may demonstrate greater susceptibility to topical corticosteroid-induced HPA axis suppression and Cushing's syndrome than do mature patients because of a larger skin surface area to body weight ratio.
Hypothalamic-pituitary-adrenal (HPA) axis suppression, Cushing's syndrome, and intracranial hypertension have been reported in pediatric patients receiving topical corticosteroids. Manifestations of adrenal suppression in pediatric patients include linear growth retardation, delayed weight gain, low plasma cortisol levels, and absence of response to ACTH stimulation. Manifestations of intracranial hypertension include bulging fontanelles, headaches, and bilateral papilledema.
Administration of topical corticosteroids to pediatric patients should be limited to the least amount compatible with an effective therapeutic regimen. Chronic corticosteroid therapy may interfere with the growth and development of pediatric patients.

ADVERSE REACTIONS

The following local adverse reactions are reported infrequently with topical corticosteroids but may occur more frequently with the use of occlusive dressings. These reactions are listed in an approximate decreasing order of occurrence:
Burning
Itching
Irritation
Dryness
Folliculitis
Hypertrichosis
Acneform eruptions
Hypopigmentation
Perioral dermatitis
Allergic contact dermatitis

The following may occur more frequently with occlusive dressings:
Maceration of the skin
Secondary infection
Skin atrophy
Striae
Miliaria

OVERDOSAGE

Topically applied corticosteroids can be absorbed in sufficient amounts to produce systemic effects (*see* **PRECAUTIONS**).

DOSAGE AND ADMINISTRATION

Topical corticosteroids are generally applied to the affected area as a thin film 1 to 4 times daily, depending on the severity of the condition.
A small quantity of Cordran Lotion should be rubbed gently into the affected area 2 or 3 times daily.
Occlusive dressings may be used for the management of psoriasis or recalcitrant conditions.
If an infection develops, the use of occlusive dressings should be discontinued and appropriate antimicrobial therapy instituted.

Use With Occlusive Dressings
The technique of occlusive dressings (for management of psoriasis and other persistant dermatoses) is as follows:

1. Remove as much as possible of the superficial scaling before applying Cordran Lotion. Soaking in a bath will help soften the scales and permit easier removal by brushing, picking, or rubbing.
2. Rub the lotion thoroughly into the affected areas.
3. Cover with an occlusive plastic film, such as polyethylene, Saran Wrap™, or Handi-Wrap®. (Added moisture may be provided by placing a slightly dampened cloth or gauze over the lesion before the plastic film is applied.)
4. Seal the edges to adjacent normal skin with tape or hold in place by a gauze wrapping.
5. For convenience, the patient may remove the dressing during the day. The dressing should then be reapplied each night.
6. For daytime therapy, the condition may be treated by rubbing Cordran Lotion sparingly into the affected areas.
7. In more resistant cases, leaving the dressing in place for 3 to 4 days at a time may result in a better response.
8. Thin polyethylene gloves are suitable for treatment of the hands and fingers; plastic garment bags may be utilized for treating lesions on the trunk or buttocks. A tight shower cap is useful in treating lesions on the scalp.

Occlusive Dressings Have the Following Advantages—

1. Percutaneous penetration of the corticosteroid is enhanced.
2. Medication is concentrated on the areas of skin where it is most needed.
3. This method of administration frequently is more effective in very resistant dermatoses than is the conventional application of Cordran.

Precautions to Be Observed in Therapy With Occlusive Dressings—Treatment should be continued for at least a few days after clearing of the lesions. If it is stopped too soon, a relapse may occur. Reinstitution of treatment frequently will cause remission.
Because of the increased hazard of secondary infection from resistant strains of staphylococci among hospitalized patients, it is suggested that the use of occlusive plastic films for corticosteroid therapy in such cases be restricted.
Generally, occlusive dressings should not be used on weeping, or exudative, lesions.
When large areas of the body are covered, thermal homeostasis may be impaired. If elevation of body temperature occurs, use of the occlusive dressing should be discontinued.
Rarely, a patient may develop miliaria, folliculitis, or a sensitivty to either the particular dressing material or a combination of Cordran and the occlusive dressing. If miliaria or folliculitis occurs, use of the occlusive dressing should be discontinued. Treatment by inunction with Codran Lotion may be continued. If the sensitivity is caused by the particular material of the dressing, substitution of a different material may be tried.
Warnings—Some plastic films are readily flammable. Patients should be cautioned against the use of any such material.
When plastic films are used on pediatric patients, the persons caring for the patients must be reminded of the danger of suffocation if the plastic material accidentally covers the face.

HOW SUPPLIED

Lotion (Plastic squeeze bottles):
0.05% (UC 5352)—(15 mL) NDC 55515-052-15; (60 mL) NDC 55515-052-60
Store at controlled room temperature, 59° to 86°F (15° to 30°C).
Rx only
Literature revised June 12, 1998
PV 2681 UCP
Mfd. for
OCLASSEN DERMATOLOGICS
a division of
Watson Pharma, Inc.
Corona CA 92880
by Eli Lily and Company
Indianapolis, IN 46285, U.S.A.
Shown in Product Identification Guide, page 327

CORDRAN® TAPE ℞

[*kōr 'drăn*]

Flurandrenolide Tape, USP

DESCRIPTION

Cordran® Tape (Flurandrenolide Tape, USP) is a transparent, inconspicuous, plastic surgical tape, impervious to moisture. It contains Cordran® (Flurandrenolide, USP), a potent corticosteroid for topical use. Flurandrenolide occurs as white to off-white, fluffy crystalline powder and is odorless. Flurandrenolide is practically insoluble in water and in ether. One g dissolves in 72 mL of alcohol and in 10 mL of chloroform. The molecular weight of flurandrenolide is 436.52.

The chemical name of flurandrenolide is Pregn-4-ene-3,20-dione, 6-fluoro-11,21-dihydroxy-16,17-[(1-methylethylidene)bis (oxy)]-, (6α, 11β, 16α)-; its empirical formula is $C_{24}H_{33}FO_6$. The structural formula is as follows:

Each square centimeter contains 4 µg (0.00916 µmol) flurandrenolide uniformly distributed in the adhesive layer. The tape is made of a thin, matte-finish polyethylene film that is slightly elastic and highly flexible.

The adhesive is a synthetic copolymer of acrylate ester and acrylic acid that is free from substances of plant origin. The pressure-sensitive adhesive surface is covered with a protective paper liner to permit handling and trimming before application.

CLINICAL PHARMACOLOGY

Cordran is primarily effective because of its anti-inflammatory, antipruritic, and vasoconstrictive actions.

The mechanism of the anti-inflammatory effect of topical corticosteroids is not completely understood. Various laboratory methods, including vasoconstrictor assays, are used to compare and predict potencies and/or clinical efficacies of the topical corticosteroids. There is some evidence to suggest that a recognizable correlation exists between vasoconstrictor potency and therapeutic efficacy in man. Corticosteroids with anti-inflammatory activity may stabilize cellular and lysosomal membranes. There is also the suggestion that the effect on the membranes of lysosomes prevents the release of proteolytic enzymes and, thus, plays a part in reducing inflammation.

The tape serves as both a vehicle and an occlusive dressing. Retention of insensible perspiration by the tape results in hydration of the stratum corneum and improved diffusion of the medication. The skin is protected from scratching, rubbing, desiccation, and chemical irritation. The tape acts as a mechanical splint to fissured skin. Since it prevents removal of the medication by washing or the rubbing action of clothing, the tape formulation provides a sustained action.

Pharmacokinetics—The extent of percutaneous absorption of topical corticosteroids is determined by many factors, including the vehicle, the integrity of the epidermal barrier, and the use of occlusive dressings.

Topical corticosteroids can be absorbed from normal intact skin. Inflammation and/or other disease processes in the skin increase percutaneous absorption. Occlusive dressings substantially increase the percutaneous absorption of topical corticosteroids. Thus, occlusive dressings may be a valuable therapeutic adjunct for treatment of resistant dermatoses (*see* **DOSAGE AND ADMINISTRATION**).

Once absorbed through the skin, topical corticosteroids are handled through pharmacokinetic pathways similar to those of systematically administered corticosteroids. Corticosteroids are bound to plasma proteins in varying degrees. They are metabolized primarily in the liver and then excreted in the kidneys. Some of the topical corticosteroids and their metabolites are also excreted into the bile.

INDICATIONS AND USAGE

For relief of the inflammatory and pruritic manifestations of corticosteroid-responsive dermatoses, particularly dry, scaling localized lesions.

CONTRAINDICATIONS

Topical corticosteroids are contraindicated in patients with a history of hypersensitivity to any of the components of these preparations.

Use of Cordran Tape is not recommended for lesions exuding serum or in intertriginous areas.

PRECAUTIONS

General—Systemic absorption of topical corticosteroids has produced reversible hypothalamic-pituitary-adrenal (HPA) axis suppression, manifestations of Cushing's syndrome, hyperglycemia, and glucosuria in some patients.

Conditions that augment systemic absorption include application of the more potent steroids, use over large surface areas, prolonged use, and the addition of occlusive dressings.

Therefore, patients receiving a large dose of a potent topical steroid applied to a large surface area or under an occlusive dressing shoul[illegible] valuated periodically for evidence of HPA axis suppres[illegible] using urinary-free cortisol and ACTH stimulation tests. I[illegible]PA axis suppression is noted, an attempt should be made to withdraw the drug, to reduce the frequency of application, or to substitute a less potent steroid.

Recovery of HPA axis function is generally prompt and complete on discontinuation of the drug. Infrequently, signs and symptoms of steroid withdrawal may occur, so that supplemental systemic corticosteroids are required.

Pediatric patients may absorb proportionately large amounts of topical corticosteroids and thus be more susceptible to systemic toxicity (*see* Pediatric Use under **PRECAUTIONS**).

If irritation develops, topical corticosteroids should be discontinued and appropriate therapy instituted.

In the presence of dermatologic infections, the use of an appropriate antifungal or antibacterial agent should be instituted. If a favorable response does not occur promptly, Cordran should be discontinued until the infection has been adequately controlled.

Information for the Patient—Patients using topical corticosteroids should receive the following information and instructions:

1. This medication is to be used as directed by the physician. It is for external use only. Avoid contact with the eyes.
2. Patients should be advised not to use this medication for any disorder other than that for which it was prescribed.
3. The treated skin area should not be bandaged or otherwise covered or wrapped in order to be occlusive unless the patient is directed to do so by the physician.
4. Patients should report any signs of local adverse reactions, especially under occlusive dressing.
5. Parents of pediatric patients should be advised not to use tight-fitting diapers or plastic pants on a patient being treated in the diaper area, because these garments may constitute occlusive dressings.

Laboratory Tests—The following tests may be helpful in evaluating the HPA axis suppression:

Urinary-free cortisol test
ACTH stimulation test

Carcinogenesis, Mutagenesis, and Impairment of Fertility—Long-term animal studies have not been performed to evaluate the carcinogenic potential or the effect on fertility of topical corticosteroids.

Studies to determine mutagenicity with prednisolone and hydrocortisone have revealed negative results.

Usage in Pregnancy—Pregnancy Category C—Corticosteroids are generally teratogenic in laboratory animals when administered systemically at relatively low dosage levels. The more potent corticosteroids have been shown to be teratogenic after dermal application in laboratory animals. There are no adequate and well-controlled studies in pregnant women on teratogenic effects from topically applied corticosteroids. Therefore, topical corticosteroids should be used during pregnancy only if the potential benefit justifies the potential risk to the fetus. Drugs of this class should not be used extensively for pregnant patients or in large amounts or for prolonged periods of time.

Nursing Mothers—It is not known whether topical administration of corticosteroids could result in sufficient systemic absorption to produce detectable quantities in breast milk. Systemically administered corticosteroids are secreted into breast milk in quantities *not* likely to have a deleterious effect on the infant. Nevertheless, caution should be exercised when topical corticosteroids are administered to a nursing woman.

Pediatric Use—Pediatric patients may demonstrate greater susceptibility to topical corticosteroid-induced HPA axis suppression and Cushing's syndrome than do mature patients because of a larger skin surface area to body weight ratio.

Hypothalamic-pituitary-adrenal (HPA) axis suppression, Cushing's syndrome, and intracranial hypertension have been reported in pediatric patients receiving topical corticosteroids. Manifestations of adrenal suppression in pediatric patients include linear growth retardation, delayed weight gain, low plasma-cortisol levels, and absence of response to ACTH stimulation. Manifestations of intracranial hypertension include bulging fontanelles, headaches, and bilateral papilledema.

Administration of topical corticosteroids to pediatric patients should be limited to the least amount compatible with an effective therapeutic regimen. Chronic corticosteroid therapy may interfere with the growth and development of pediatric patients.

ADVERSE REACTIONS

The following local adverse reactions are reported infrequently with topical corticosteroids but may occur more frequently with the use of occlusive dressings. These reactions are listed in an approximate decreasing order of occurrence:

Burning
Itching
Irritation
Dryness
Folliculitis
Hypertrichosis
Acneform eruptions
Hypopigmentation
Perioral dermatitis
Allergic contact dermatitis

The following may occur more frequently with occlusive dressings:

Maceration of the skin
Secondary infection
Skin atrophy
Striae
Miliaria

OVERDOSAGE

Topically applied corticosteroids can be absorbed in sufficient amounts to produce systemic effects (*see* **PRECAUTIONS**).

DOSAGE AND ADMINISTRATION

Occlusive dressings may be used for the management of psoriasis or recalcitrant conditions.

If an infection develops, the use of Cordran Tape and other occlusive dressings should be discontinued and appropriate antimicrobial therapy instituted.

Replacement of the tape every 12 hours produces the lowest incidence of adverse reactions, but it may be left in place for 24 hours if it is well tolerated and adheres satisfactorily. When necessary, the tape may be used at night only and removed during the day.

If ends of the tape loosen prematurely, they may be trimmed off and replaced with fresh tape.

The directions given below are included on a separate package insert for the patient to follow unless otherwise instructed by the physician.

APPLICATION OF CORDRAN TAPE

> IMPORTANT: Skin should be clean and *dry* before tape is applied. Tape should always be cut, never torn.

DIRECTIONS FOR USE:

1. Prepare skin as directed by your physician or as follows: Gently clean the area to be covered to remove scales, crusts, dried exudates, and any previously used ointments or creams. A germicidal soap or cleanser should be used to prevent the development of odor under the tape. Shave or clip the hair in the treatment area to allow good contact with the skin and comfortable removal. If shower or tub bath is to be taken, it should be completed before the tape is applied. The skin should be dry before application of the tape.
2. Remove tape from package and cut a piece slightly larger than area to be covered. Round off corners.
3. Pull white paper from transparent tape. Be careful that tape does not stick to itself.
4. Apply tape, keeping skin smooth; press tape into place.

REPLACEMENT OF TAPE.

Unless instructed otherwise by your physician, replace tape after 12 hours. Cleanse skin and allow it to dry for 1 hour before applying new tape.

IF IRRITATION OR INFECTION DEVELOPS, REMOVE TAPE AND CONSULT PHYSICIAN.

HOW SUPPLIED

Tape:

4 mcg/sq cm (UC 5350)—small roll, 24 in × 3 in (60 cm × 7.5 cm) NDC 55515-014-24

4 mcg/sq cm (UC 5350)—large roll, 80 in × 3 in (200 cm × 7.5 cm) NDC 55515-014-80

4 mcg/sq cm (UC 5350)—12 patches, each 2 in × 3 in (5.1 cm × 7.5 cm) NDC 55515-014-12

Directions for the patient are included in each package.

Store at controlled room temperature, 59° to 86°F (15° to 30°C).

Rx only

REFERENCES

Bard JW: Flurandrenolide tape in the treatment of lichen simplex chronicus. *J Ky Med Assoc* 1969;67:668.

Baxter DL, Stoughton RB: Mitotic index of psoriatic lesions treated with anthralin, glucocorticosteroid and occlusion only. *J Invest Dermatol* 1970;54:410.

Compilation of clinical reports on Cordran Tape received by Eli Lilly and Company.

Halprin KM, Fukui K, Ohkawara A: Flurandrenolone (Cordran) tape and carbohydrate metabolizing enzymes. *Arch Dermatol* 1969;100:336.

Labow TA, Eisert J, Sanders SL: Flurandrenolide tape in treatment of psoriasis. *NY State J Med* 1969;69:3138.

Ronchese F: Flurandrenolone tape therapy. *RI Med J* 1969;52:389.

Sellers FM: Investigative study of flurandrenolone tape in a series of ambulatory outpatients. *J Indiana State Med Assoc* 1970;63:34.

Weiner MA: Flurandrenolone tape, a new preparation for occlusive therapy, *J Invest Dermatol* 1966;47:63.

Literature revised February 22, 1999 PV 3052 UCP

Mfd. for

OCLASSEN DERMATOLOGICS

A Division of Watson Pharma, Inc.

Corona, CA 92880

Mfg. by Minnesota Mining and Manufacturing Company

St. Paul Minnesota 55101

Shown in Product Identification Guide, page 327

Continued on next page

CORMAX™ 0.05% CREAM ℞

(Clobetasol Propionate Cream, USP)
For Dermatologic Use Only—Not for Ophthalmic Use.

DESCRIPTION

Cormax™ Cream (Clobetasol Propionate Cream, USP) contains the active compound clobetasol propionate, a synthetic corticosteroid, for topical dermatologic use. Clobetasol, an analog of prednisolone, has a high degree of glucocorticoid activity and a slight degree of mineralocorticoid activity.
Chemically, clobetasol propionate is 21-chloro-9-fluoro-11β, 17-dihydroxy-16β-methylpregna-1,4-diene-3,20-dione, 17-propionate, and it has the following structural formula:

Clobetasol propionate has the molecular formula $C_{25}H_{32}ClFO_5$ and a molecular weight of 467. It is a white to cream-colored crystalline powder insoluble in water.
Each gram of Cormax™ Cream contains 0.5 mg clobetasol propionate in a base composed of white petrolatum, cetyl alcohol, stearyl alcohol, lanolin oil, PEG-8 stearate, polysorbate 60, glycol stearate, propylparaben, propylene glycol, methylparaben, sodium citrate, citric acid and purified water.

CLINICAL PHARMACOLOGY

The corticosteroids are a class of compounds comprising steroid hormones secreted by the adrenal cortex and their synthetic analogs. In pharmacologic doses, corticosteroids are used primarily for their anti-inflammatory and/or immunosuppressive effects. Topical corticosteroids such as clobetasol propionate are effective in the treatment of corticosteroid-responsive dermatoses primarily because of their anti-inflammatory, antipruritic, and vasoconstrictive actions. However, while the physiologic, pharmacologic, and clinical effects of the corticosteroids are well known, the exact mechanisms of their actions in each disease are uncertain. Clobetasol propionate, a corticosteroid, has been shown to have topical (dermatologic) and systemic pharmacologic and metabolic effects characteristic of this class of drugs.

Pharmacokinetics: The extent of percutaneous absorption of topical corticosteroids, including clobetasol propionate, is determined by many factors, including the vehicle, the integrity of the epidermal barrier, and the use of occlusive dressings (see **DOSAGE AND ADMINISTRATION**).
As with all topical corticosteroids, clobetasol propionate can be absorbed from normal intact skin. Inflammation and/or other disease processes in the skin may increase percutaneous absorption. Occlusive dressings substantially increase the percutaneous absorption of topical corticosteroids (see **DOSAGE AND ADMINISTRATION**).
Once absorbed through the skin, topical corticosteroids enter pharmacokinetic pathways similarly to systemically administered corticosteroids. Corticosteroids are bound to plasma proteins in varying degrees. Corticosteroids are metabolized primarily in the liver and are then excreted by the kidneys. Some of the topical corticosteroids, including clobetasol propionate and its metabolites, are also excreted into the bile.
Clobetasol propionate cream has been shown to depress the plasma levels of adrenal cortical hormones following repeated nonocclusive application to diseased skin in patients with psoriasis and eczematous dermatitis. These effects have been shown to be transient and reversible upon completion of a two-week course of treatment.

INDICATIONS AND USAGE

Cormax™ Cream (Clobetasol Propionate Cream, USP) is indicated for short-term treatment of inflammatory and pruritic manifestations of moderate to severe corticosteroid-responsive dermatoses. Treatment beyond two consecutive weeks is not recommended, and the total dosage should not exceed 50 g per week because of the potential for the drug to suppress the hypothalamic-pituitary-adrenal (HPA) axis.
This product is not recommended for use in children under 12 years of age.

CONTRAINDICATIONS

Cormax™ Cream (Clobetasol Propionate Cream, USP) is contraindicated in patients who are hypersensitive to clobetasol propionate, to other corticosteroids, or to any ingredient in this preparation.

PRECAUTIONS

General: Clobetasol propionate is a highly potent topical corticosteroid that has been shown to suppress the HPA axis at doses as low as 2 g per day. Systemic absorption of topical corticosteroids has resulted in reversible HPA axis suppression, manifestations of Cushing's syndrome, hyperglycemia, and glucosuria in some patients.
Conditions that augment systemic absorption include the application of the more potent corticosteroids, use over large surface areas, prolonged use, and the addition of occlusive dressings. Therefore, patients receiving a large dose of a potent topical steroid applied to a large surface area should be evaluated periodically for evidence of HPA axis suppression by using the urinary free cortisol and ACTH stimulation tests. If HPA axis suppression is noted, an attempt should be made to withdraw the drug, to reduce the frequency of application, or to substitute a less potent steroid.
Recovery of HPA axis function is generally prompt and complete upon discontinuation of the drug. Infrequently, signs and symptoms of steroid withdrawal may occur, requiring supplemental systemic corticosteroids.
Children may absorb proportionally larger amounts of topical corticosteroids and thus be more susceptible to systemic toxicity (see **PRECAUTIONS: Pediatric Use**).
If irritation develops, topical corticosteroids should be discontinued and appropriate therapy instituted.
In the presence of dermatologic infections, the use of an appropriate antifungal or antibacterial agent should be instituted. If a favorable response does not occur promptly, the corticosteroid should be discontinued until the infection has been adequately controlled.
Certain areas of the body, such as the face, groin, and axillae, are more prone to to atrophic changes than other areas of the body following treatment with corticosteroids. Frequent observation of the patient is important if these areas are to be treated.
As with other potent topical corticosteroids, Cormax™ Cream (Clobetasol Propionate Cream, USP) should not be used in the treatment of rosacea and perioral dermatitis. Topical corticosteroids in general should not be used in the treatment of acne or as sole therapy in widespread plaque psoriasis.

Information for Patients: Patients using Cormax™ Cream should receive the following information and instructions:
1. This medication is to be used as directed by the physician and should not be used longer than the prescribed time period. It is for external use only. Avoid contact with the eyes.
2. This medication should not be used for any disorder other than that for which it was prescribed.
3. The treated skin area should not be bandaged or otherwise covered or wrapped so as to be occlusive.
4. Patients should report any signs of local adverse reactions to the physician.

Laboratory Tests: The following tests may be helpful in evaluating HPA axis suppression:
Urinary free cortisol test
ACTH stimulation test

Carcinogenesis, Mutagenesis, Impairment of Fertility: Long-term animal studies have not been performed to evaluate the carcinogenic potential or the effect on fertility of topical corticosteroids.
Studies to determine mutagenicity with prednisolone have revealed negative results.

Pregnancy: Teratogenic Effects: Pregnancy Category C: The more potent corticosteroids have been shown to be teratogenic in animals after dermal application. Clobetasol propionate has not been tested for teratogenicity by this route; however, it is absorbed percutaneously, and when administered subcutaneously it was a significant teratogen in both the rabbit and the mouse. Clobetasol propionate has greater teratogenic potential than steroids that are less potent.
There are no adequate and well-controlled studies of the teratogenic effects of topically applied corticosteroids, including clobetasol, in pregnant women. Therefore, clobetasol and other topical corticosteroids should be used during pregnancy only if the potential benefit justifies the potential risk to the fetus, and they should not be used extensively on pregnant patients, in large amounts, or for prolonged periods of time.

Nursing Mothers: It is not known whether topical administration of corticosteroids could result in sufficient systemic absorption to produce detectable quantities in breast milk. Systemically administered corticosteroids are secreted into breast milk in quantities not likely to have a deleterious effect on the infant. Nevertheless, caution should be exercised when topical corticosteroids are prescribed for a nursing woman.

Pediatric Use: Use of Cormax™ Cream (Clobetasol Propionate Cream, USP) in children under 12 years of age is not recommended.
Pediatric patients may demonstrate greater susceptibility to topical corticosteroid-induced HPA axis suppression and Cushing's syndrome than mature patients because of a larger skin surface area to body weight ratio.
HPA axis suppression, Cushing's syndrome, and intracranial hypertension have been reported in children receiving topical corticosteroids. Manifestations of adrenal suppression in children include linear growth retardation, delayed weight gain, low plasma cortisol levels, and absence of response to ACTH stimulation. Manifestations of intracranial hypertension include bulging fontanelles, headaches, and bilateral papilledema.

ADVERSE REACTIONS

Cormax™ Cream (Clobetasol Propionate Cream, USP) is generally well tolerated when used for two-week treatment periods.
The most frequent adverse reactions reported to clobetasol propionate cream have been local and have included burning sensation and stinging sensation in approximately 1% of the patients. Less frequent adverse reactions were itching, skin atrophy, and cracking and fissuring of the skin.
The following local adverse reactions are reported infrequently when topical corticosteroids are used as recommended. These reactions are listed in an approximately decreasing order of occurrence: burning, itching, irritation, dryness, folliculitis, hypertrichosis, acneiform eruptions, popigmentation, perioral dermatitis, allergic contact dermatitis, maceration of the skin, secondary infection, skin atrophy, striae, and miliaria. Systemic absorption of topical corticosteroids has produced reversible HPA axis suppression, manifestations of Cushing's syndrome, hyperglycemia and glucosuria in some patients. In rare instances, treatment (or withdrawal of treatment) of psoriasis with corticosteroids is thought to have exacerbated the disease or provoked the pustular form of the disease, so careful patient supervision is recommended.

OVERDOSAGE

Topically applied Cormax™ Cream (Clobetasol Propionate Cream, USP) can be absorbed in sufficient amounts to produce systemic effects (see **PRECAUTIONS**).

DOSAGE AND ADMINISTRATION

A thin layer of Cormax™ Cream (Clobetasol Propionate Cream, USP) should be applied with gentle rubbing to the affected skin areas twice daily, once in the morning and once at night.
Cormax™ Cream is potent; therefore, **treatment must be limited to two consecutive weeks, and amounts greater than 50 g per week should not be used. Cormax™ Cream is not to be used with occlusive dressings.**

HOW SUPPLIED

Cormax™ Cream (Clobetasol Propionate Cream, USP) is supplied in 15 g (NDC 55515-420-15), 30 g (55515-420-30), and 45 g (NDC 55515-420-45) tubes.
Store at controlled room temperature 15°C to 30°C (59°F to 86°F).
Do not refrigerate.
Rx Only
Mfd. for
Oclassen
Dermatologics
A division of Watson Pharma, Inc., Corona, CA 92880
by DTP Labs, Ltd., San Antonio, TX 78215
Revised: July, 1998
127442-0798

Shown in Product Identification Guide, page 327

CORMAX™ OINTMENT 0.05% ℞

[kor ' māx]
(Clobetasol Propionate Ointment, USP)
For Dermatologic Use Only—
Not For Ophthalmic Use.

DESCRIPTION

Cormax™ Ointment (Clobetasol Propionate Ointment, USP) contains the active compound clobetasol propionate, a synthetic corticosteroid, for topical dermatologic use. Clobetasol, an analog of prednisolone, has a high degree of glucocorticoid activity and a slight degree of mineralocorticoid activity.
Chemically, clobetasol propionate is 21-chloro-9-fluoro-11β, 17-dihydroxy-16β-methylpregna-1, 4-diene-3,20-dione, 17-propionate, and it has the following structural formula:

Clobetasol propionate has the molecular formula $C_{25}H_{32}ClFO_5$ and a molecular weight of 467. It is a white to cream-colored crystalline powder insoluble in water.
Each gram of Cormax™ Ointment, contains 0.5 mg clobetasol propionate in a base composed of propylene glycol, sorbitan sesquioleate, and white petrolatum.

CLINICAL PHARMACOLOGY

The corticosteroids are a class of compounds comprising steroid hormones secreted by the adrenal cortex and their synthetic analogs. In pharmacologic doses, corticosteroids are used primarily for their anti-inflammatory and/or immunosuppressive effects. Topical corticosteroids such as clobetasol propionate are effective in the treatment of corticosteroid-responsive dermatoses primarily because of their anti-inflammatory, antipruritic, and vasoconstrictive actions. However, while the physiologic, pharmacologic, and clinical effects of the corticosteroids are well known, the exact mechanisms of their actions in each disease are uncertain. Clobetasol propionate, a corticosteroid, has been shown to have topical (dermatologic) and systemic pharmacologic and metabolic effects characteristic of this class of drugs.

Pharmacokinetics: The extent of percutaneous absorption of topical corticosteroids, including clobetasol propionate, is determined by many factors inclding the vehicle, the integrity of the epidermal barrier, and the use of occlusive dressings (see **DOSAGE AND ADMINISTRATION**).
As with all topical corticosteroids, clobetasol propionate can be absorbed from normal intact skin. Inflammation and/or other disease processes in the skin may increase percutaneous absorption. Occlusive dressings substantially increase the percutaneous absorption of topical corticosteroids (see **DOSAGE AND ADMINISTRATION**).

Once absorbed through the skin, topical corticosteroids enter pharmacokinetic pathways similarly to systemically administered corticosteroids.
Corticosteroids are bound to plasma proteins in varying degrees. Corticosteroids are metabolized primarily in the liver and are then excreted by the kidneys. Some of the topical corticosteroids, including clobetasol propionate and its metabolites, are also excreted into the bile.
Clobetasol propionate ointment has been shown to depress the plasma levels of adrenal cortical hormones following repeated nonocclusive application to diseased skin in patients with psoriasis and eczematous dermatitis. These effects have been shown to be transient and reversible upon completion of a two-week course of treatment.

INDICATIONS AND USAGE

Cormax™ Ointment (Clobetasol Propionate Ointment, USP) is indicated for short-term treatment of inflammatory and pruritic manifestations of moderate to severe corticosteroid-responsive dermatoses. Treatment beyond two consecutive weeks is not recommended, and the total dosage should not exceed 50 g per week because of the potential for the drug to suppress the hypothalamic-pituitary-adrenal (HPA) axis.
This product is not recommended for use in pediatric patients under 12 years of age.

CONTRAINDICATIONS

Cormax™ Ointment (Clobetasol Propionate Ointment, USP) is contraindicated in patients who are hypersensitive to clobetasol propionate, to other corticosteroids, or to any ingredient in this preparation.

PRECAUTIONS

General: Clobetasol propionate is a highly potent topical corticosteroid that has been shown to suppress the HPA axis at doses as low as 2 g per day. Systemic absorption of topical corticosteroids has resulted in reversible HPA axis supression, manifestations of Cushing's syndrome, hyperglycemia, and glucosuria in some patients.
Conditions that augment systemic absorption include the application of more potent corticosteroids, use over large surface areas, prolonged use, and the addition of occlusive dressings. Therefore, patients receiving a large dose of a potent topical steroid applied to a large surface area should be evaluated periodically for evidence of HPA axis' suppression by using the urinary free cortisol and ACTH stimulation tests. If HPA axis suppression is noted, an attempt should be made to withdraw the drug, to reduce the frequency of application, or to substitute a less potent steroid.
Recovery of HPA axis function is generally prompt and complete upon discontinuation of the drug. Infrequently, signs and symptoms of steroid withdrawal may occur, requiring supplemental systemic corticosteroids.
Pediatric patients may absorb proportionally larger amounts of topical corticosteroids and thus be more susceptible to systemic toxicity (see **PRECAUTIONS: Pediatric Use**).
If irritation develops, topical corticosteroids should be discontinued and appropriate therapy instituted.
In the presence of dermatologic infections, the use of an appropriate antifungal or antibacterial agent should be instituted. If a favorable response does not occur promptly, the corticosteroid should be discontinued until the infection has been adequately controlled.
Certain areas of the body, such as the face, groin, and axillae, are more prone to atrophic changes than other areas of the body following treatment with corticosteroids. Frequent observations of the patient is important if these areas are to be treated.
As with other potent topical corticosteroids, Cormax™ Ointment (Clobetasol Propionate Ointment, USP) should not be used in the treatment of rosacea and perioral dermatitis. Topical corticosteroids in general should not be used in the treatment of acne or as a sole therapy in widespread plaque psoriasis.
Information for patients: Patients using Cormax™ Ointment (Clobetasol Propionate Ointment, USP) should receive the following information and instructions:

1. This medication is to be used as directed by the physician and should not be used longer than the prescribed time period. It is for external use only. Avoid contact with the eyes.
2. This medication should not be used for any disorder other than that for which it is prescribed.
3. The treated skin area should not be bandaged or otherwise covered or wrapped so as to be occlusive.
4. Patients should report any signs of local adverse reactions to the physician.

Laboratory Tests: The following tests may be helpful in evaluating HPA axis suppression:

Urinary free cortisol test
ACTH stimulation test

Carcinogenesis, Mutagenesis, Impairment of Fertility: Long-term animal studies have not been performed to evaluate the carcinogenic potential or the effect on fertility of topical corticosteroids.
Studies to determine mutagenicity with prednisolone have revealed negative results.
Pregnancy: Teratogenic Effects: Pregnancy Category C: The more potent corticosteroids have been shown to be teratogenic in animals after dermal application. Clobetasol propionate has not been tested for teratogenicity by this route; however, it is absorbed percutaneously, and when administered subcutaneously it was a significant teratogen in both the rabbit and the mouse. Clobetasol propionate has greater teratogenic potential than steroids that are less potent.
There are no adequate and well-controlled studies of the teratogenic effects of topically applied corticosteroids, including clobetasol, in pregnant women. Therefore, clobetasol and other topical corticosteroids should be used during pregnancy only if the potential benefit justifies the potential risk to the fetus, and they should not be used extensively on pregnant patients, in large amounts, or for prolonged periods of time.
Nursing Mothers: It is not known whether topical administration of corticosteroids could result in sufficient systemic absorption to produce detectable quantities in breast milk. Systemically administered corticosteroids are secreted into breast milk in quantities **not** likely to have a deleterious effect on the infant. Nevertheless, caution should be exercised when topical corticosteroids are prescribed for a nursing woman.
Pediatric use: Use of Cormax™ Ointment, in pediatric patients is not recommended.
Pediatric patients may demonstrate greater susceptibility to topical corticosteroid-induced HPA axis suppression and Cushing's syndrome than mature patients because of a larger skin surface area to body weight ratio.
HPA axis suppression, Cushing's syndrome and intracranial hypertension have been reported in pediatric patients receiving topical corticosteroids. Manifestations of adrenal suppression in pediatric patients include linear growth retardation, delayed weight gain, low plasma cortisol levels, and absence of response to ACTH stimulation. Manifestations of intracranial hypertension include bulging fontanelles, headaches, and bilateral papilledema.

ADVERSE REACTIONS

Comax™ Ointment (Clobetasol Propionate Ointment, USP) is generally well tolerated when used for two-week treatment periods. The most frequent adverse reactions reported for clobetasol propionate ointment have been local and have included burning sensation, irritation, and itching. These occurred in approximately 0.5% of the patients. Less frequent adverse reactions wers stinging, cracking, erythema, folliculitis, numbness of fingers, skin atrophy, and telangiectasia, which occurred in approximately 0.3% of the patients.
The following local adverse reactions are reported infrequently when topical corticosteroids are used as recommended. These reactions are listed in an approximately decreasing order of occurrence: burning, itching, irritation, dryness, folliculitis, hypetrichosis, acneiform eruptions, hypopigmentation, perioral dermatitis, allergic contact dermatitis, maceration of the skin, secondary infection, skin atrophy, striae, miliaria. Systemic absorption of topical corticosteroids has produced reversible HPA axis suppression, manifestations of Cushing's syndrome, hyperglycemia, and glucosuria in some patients. In rare instances, treatment (or withdrawal of treatment) of psoriasis with corticosteroids is thought to have exacerbated the disease or provoked the pustular form of the disease, so careful patient supervision is recommended.

OVERDOSAGE

Topically applied Cormax™ Ointment (Clobetasol Propionate Ointment, USP) can be absorbed in sufficient amounts to produce systemic effects (see **PRECAUTIONS**).

DOSAGE AND ADMINISTRATION

A thin layer of Cormax™ Ointment (Clobetasol Propionate Ointment, USP) should be applied with gentle rubbing to the affected skin area twice daily, once in the morning and once at night.
Cormax™ Ointment is potent: therefore, **treatment must be limited to two consecutive weeks, and amounts greater than 50 g per week should not be used. Cormax™ Ointment is not to be used with occlusive dressings.**

HOW SUPPLIED

Cormax™ Ointment (Clobetasol Propionate Ointment, USP) 0.05% is supplied in 15 g (NDC 55515-410-15) and 45 g (NDC 55515-410-45) tubes.
Store at controlled room temperature 15°–30°C (59°–86°F).
Do not refrigerate.
Rx only
Mfd. for
OCLASSEN DERMATOLOGICS
a division of
Watson Pharma, Inc.
Corona CA 92880
by DPT Laboratories, Ltd.
San Antonio, TX 78215
Revised February 20, 1998.
127342-0298

Shown in Product Identification Guide, page 327

CORMAX™ ℞

[kor ' māx]
Scalp Application, 0.05% w/w
(Clobetasol Propionate Topical Solution, USP)
For Dermatologic Use Only
Not for Ophthalmic Use

DESCRIPTION

Cormax™ Scalp Application (Clobetasol Propionate Topical Solution, USP) contains the active compound clobetasol propionate, a synthetic corticosteroid, for topical dermatologic use. Clobetasol, an analog of prednisolone, has a high degree of glucocorticoid activity and a slight degree of mineralocorticoid activity.
Chemically, clobetasol propionate is 21-chloro-9-fluoro-11β, 17-dihydroxy-16β-methylpregna-1, 4-diene-3,20-dione 17-propionate, and it has the following structural formula:

Clobetasol propionate has the molecular formula $C_{25}H_{32}ClFO_5$ and a molecular weight of 467. It is a white to cream-colored crystalline powder insoluble in water.
Each gram of Cormax™ Scalp Application contains 0.5 mg clobetasol propionate in a base composed of purified water, isopropyl alcohol (40% w/w), carbomer 934P, and sodium hydroxide.

CLINICAL PHARMACOLOGY

The corticosteroids are a class of compounds comprising steroid hormones secreted by the adrenal cortex and their synthetic analogs. In pharmacologic doses, corticosteroids are used primarily for their anti-inflammatory and/or immunosuppressive effects. Topical corticosteroids such as clobetasol propionate are effective in the treatment of corticosteroid-responsive dermatoses primarily because of their anti-inflammatory, antipruritic, and vasconstrictive actions. However, while the physiologic, pharmacologic, and clinical effects of the corticosteroids are well known, the exact mechanisms of their actions in each disease are uncertain. Clobetasol propionate, a corticosteroid, has been shown to have topical (dermatologic) and systemic pharmacologic and metabolic effects characteristic of this class of drugs.
Pharmacokinetics
The extent of percutaneous absorption of topical corticosteroids, including clobetasol propionate, is determined by many factors, including the vehicle, the integrity of the epidermal barrier, and the use of occlusive dressings (see **DOSAGE AND ADMINISTRATION**).
As with all topical corticosteroids, clobetasol propionate can be absorbed from normal intact skin. Inflammation and/or other disease processes in the skin may increase percutaneous absorption. Occlusive dressings substantially increase the percutaneous absorption of topical corticosteroids (see **DOSAGE AND ADMINISTRATION**).
As with all topical corticosteroids, clobetasol propionate can be absorbed from normal intact skin. Inflammation and/or other disease processes in the skin may increase percutaneous absorption. Occlusive dressings substantially increase the percutanous absorption of topical corticosteroids (see **DOSAGE AND ADMINISTRATION**).
Once absorbed through the skin, topical corticosteroids enter pharmacokinetic pathways similarly to systemically administered corticosteroids. Corticosteroids are bound to plasma proteins in varying degrees. Corticosteroids are metabolized primarily in the liver and are then excreted by the kidneys. Some of the topical corticosteroids, including clobetasol propionate and its metabolites, are also excreted in the bile.
Following repeated nonocclusive application in the treatment of scalp psoriasis, there is some evidence that Cormax™ Scalp Application (Clobetasol Propionate Topical Solution, USP) has the potential to depress plasma cortisol levels in some patients. However, hypothalamic-pituitary-adrenal (HPA) axis effects produced by systemically absorbed clobetasol propionate have been shown to be transient and reversible upon completion of a two-week course of treatment.

INDICATIONS AND USAGE

Cormax™ Scalp Application (Clobetasol Propionate Topical Solution, USP) is indicated for short-term topical treatment of inflammatory and pruritic manifestations of moderate to severe corticosteroid-responsive dermatoses of the scalp. Treatment beyond two consecutive weeks is not recommended, and the total dosage should not exceed 50 mL per week because of the potential for the drug to suppress the HPA axis.
This product is not recommended for use in pediatric patients under 12 years of age.

CONTRAINDICATIONS

Cormax™ Scalp Application (Clobetasol Propionate Topical Solution, USP) is contraindicated in patients with primary infections of the scalp, or in patients who are hypersensitive to clobetasol propionate, to other corticosteroids, or to any ingredient in this preparation.

PRECAUTIONS

General
Clobetasol propionate is a highly potent topical corticosteroid that has been shown to suppress the HPA axis at doses as low as 2 g (of ointment) per day. Systemic absorption of

Continued on next page

Cormax Solution—Cont.

topical corticosteroids has resulted in reversible HPA axis suppression, manifestations of Cushing's syndrome, hyperglycemia, and glucosuria in some patients.
Conditions that augment systemic absorption include the application of the more potent corticosteroids, use over large surface areas, prolonged use and the addition of occlusive dressings. Therefore, patients receiving a large dose of potent topical steroid applied to a large surface area should be evaluated periodically for evidence of HPA axis suppression by using the urinary free cortisol and ACTH stimulation tests. If HPA axis suppression is noted, an attempt should be made to withdraw the drug, to reduce the frequency of application, or to substitute a less potent steroid.
Recovery of HPA axis function is generally prompt and complete upon discontinuation of the drug. Infrequently, signs and symptoms of steroid withdrawal may occur, requiring supplemental systemic corticosteroids.
Pediatric patients may absorb proportionally larger amounts of topical corticosteroids and thus be more susceptible to systemic toxicity (see **PRECAUTIONS: Pediatric Use**).
If irritation develops, topical corticosteroids should be discontinued and appropriate therapy instituted. Irritation is possible if Cormax™ Scalp Application (Clobetasol Propionate Topical Solution, USP) contacts the eye. If that should occur, immediate flushing of the eye with a large volume of water is recommended.
In the presence of dermatologic infections, the use of an appropriate antifungal or antibacterial agent should be instituted. If a favorable response does not occur promptly, the corticosteroid should be discontinued until the infection has been adequately controlled.
Although Cormax™ Scalp Application (Clobetasol Propionate Topical Solution, USP) is intended for the treatment of inflammatory conditions of the scalp, it should be noted that certain areas of the body, such as the face, groin, and axillae, are more prone to atrophic changes than other areas of the body following treatment with corticosteroids. Frequent observation of the patient is important if these areas are to be treated.
As with other potent topical corticosteroids, Cormax™ Scalp Application should not be used in the treatment of rosacea and perioral dermatitits. Topical corticosteroids in general should not be used in the treatment of acne or as sole therapy in widespread plaque psoriasis.

Information for Patients
Patients using Cormax™ Scalp Application should receive the following information and instructions:
1. This medication is to be used as directed by the physician and should not be used longer than the prescribed time period. It is for external use only. Avoid contact with the eyes.
2. This medication should not be used for any disorder other than that for which it is prescribed.
3. The treated skin area should not be bandaged or otherwise covered or wrapped so as to be occlusive.
4. Patients should report any signs of local adverse reactions to the physician.

Laboratory Tests
The following tests may be helpful in evaluating HPA axis suppression:
Urinary free cortisol test
ACTH stimulation test

Carcinogenesis, Mutagenesis, Impairment of Fertility
Long-term animal studies have not been performed to evaluate the carcinogenic potential or the effect on fertility of topical corticosteroids.
Studies to determine mutagenicity with prednisolone have revealed negative results.

Pregnancy: Teratogenic Effects: Pregnancy Category C
The more potent corticosteroids have been shown to be teratogenic in animals after dermal application. Clobetasol propionate has not been tested for teratogenicity by this route; however, it is absorbed percutaneously, and when administered subcutaneously it was a significant teratogen in both the rabbit and the mouse. Clobetasol propionate has greater teratogenic potential than steroids that are less potent.
There are no adequate and well-controlled studies of the teratogenic effects of topically applied corticosteroids, including clobetasol, in pregnant women. Therefore, clobetasol and other topical corticosteroids should be used during pregnancy only if the potential benefit justifies the potential risk to the fetus, and they should not be used extensively on pregnant patients, in large amounts, or for prolonged periods of time.

Nursing Mothers
It is not known whether topical administration of corticosteroids could result in sufficient systemic absorption to produce detectable quantities in breast milk. Systemically administered corticosteroids are secreted into breast milk in quantities not likely to have a deleterious effect on the infant. Nevertheless, caution should be exercised when topical corticosteroids are prescribed for a nursing woman.

Pediatric Use
Use of Cormax™ Scalp Application in pediatric patients under 12 years of age is not recommended.
Pediatric patients may demonstrate greater susceptibility to topical corticosteroids-induced HPA axis suppression and Cushing's syndrome than mature patients because of a larger skin surface area to body weight ratio.
HPA axis suppression, Cushing's syndrome and intracranial hypertension have been reported in pediatric patients receiving topical corticosteroids. Manifestations of adrenal suppression in pediatric patients include linear growth retardation, delayed weight gain, low plasma cortisol levels, and absence of response to ACTH stimulation. Manifestations of intercranial hypertension include bulging fontanelles, headaches, and bilateral papilledema.

ADVERSE REACTIONS
Cormax™ Scalp Application (Clobetasol Propionate Topical Solution, USP) is generally well tolerated when used for two-week treatment periods.
The most frequent adverse events reported have been local and have included burning and/or stinging sensation, which occurred in approximately 10% of the patients; scalp pustules, which occurred in approximately 1% of the patients; and tingling, and folliculitis, each of which occurred in approximately 0.6% of the patients. Less frequent adverse events were itching and tightness of the scalp, dermatitits, tenderness, headache, hair loss, and eye irritation, each of which occurred in approximately 0.3% of the patients.
The following local adverse reactions are reported infrequently when topical corticosteroids are used as recommended. These reactions are listed in an approximately decreasing order of occurrence: burning, itching, irritation, dryness, folliculitis, hypertrichosis, acneiform eruptions, hypopigmentation, perioral dermatitis, allergic contact dermatitis, maceration of the skin, secondary infection, skin atrophy, striae and miliaria. Systemic absorption of topical corticosteroids has produced reversible HPA axis suppression, manifestations of Cushing's syndrome, hyperglycemia, and glucosuria in some patients. In rare instances, treatment (or withdrawal of treatment) of psoriasis with corticosteroids is thought to have exacerbated the disease or provoked the pustular form of the disease, so careful patient supervision is recommended.

OVERDOSAGE
Topically applied Cormax™ Scalp Application (Clobetasol Propionate Topical Solution, USP) can be absorbed in sufficient amounts to produce systemic effects (see **PRECAUTIONS**).

DOSAGE AND ADMINISTRATION
Cormax™ Scalp Application (Clobetasol Propionate Topical Solution, USP) should be applied to the affected scalp areas twice daily, once in the morning and once at night. Cormax™ Scalp Application is potent; therefore, **treatment must be limited to two consecutive weeks and amounts greater than 50mL per week should not be used. Cormax™ Scalp Application is not be used with occlusive dressings.**

HOW SUPPLIED
Cormax™ Scalp Application (Clobetasol Propionate Topical Solution, USP), 0.05% w/w is supplied in plastic squeeze bottles of 25 mL (NDC 55515-430-25), and 50 mL (NDC 55515-430-50). Store at controlled room temperature 15°–30° C (59°–86°F). Do not refrigerate. Do not use near an open flame.
Rx only
Mfd for
OCLASSEN
DERMATOLOGICS
a division of Watson Pharma, Inc.,
Corona CA 92880
by DPT Laboratories, Ltd.
San Antonio, TX 78215
Revised: February 21, 1998.
127138-0298
Shown in Product Identification Guide, page 327

MONODOX® ℞
DOXYCYCLINE MONOHYDRATE CAPSULES
[mon 'o-dox]

DESCRIPTION
Doxycycline is a broad-spectrum antibiotic synthetically derived from oxytetracycline. Monodox® 100 mg and 50 mg capsules contain doxycycline monohydrate equivalent to 100 mg or 50 mg of doxycycline for oral administration. The chemical designation of the light-yellow crystalline powder is alpha-6-deoxy-5-oxytetracycline.
Structural formula:

OH O OH OH O CONH₂ • H₂O OH H H CH₃ H OH H N(CH₃)₂

$C_{22}H_{24}N_2O_8 \cdot H_2O$ M.W.=462.46

Doxycycline has a high degree of lipid solubility and a low affinity for calcium binding. It is highly stable in normal human serum. Doxycycline will not degrade into an epianhydro form.
Inert Ingredients: colloidal silicon dioxide; hard gelatin capsule; magnesium stearate; microcrystalline cellulose; and sodium starch glycolate.

CLINICAL PHARMACOLOGY
Tetracyclines are readily absorbed and are bound to plasma proteins in varying degrees. They are concentrated by the liver in the bile and excreted in the urine and feces at high concentrations in a biologically active form. Doxycycline is virtually completely absorbed after oral administration.

Following a 200 mg dose of doxycycline monohydrate, 24 normal adult volunteers averaged the following serum concentration values:
[See table at top of next page]

	Average Observed Values
Maximum Concentration	3.61 mcg/mL (± 0.9 sd)
Time of Maximum Concentration	2.60 hr (± 1.10 sd)
Elimination Rate Constant	0.049 per hr (± 0.030 sd)
Half-Life	16.33 hr (± 4.53 sd)

Excretion of doxycycline by the kidney is about 40%/72 hours in individuals with normal function (creatinine clearance about 75 mL/min). This percentage excretion may fall as low as 1-5%/72 hours in individuals with severe renal insufficiency (creatinine clearance below 10 mL/min). Studies have shown no significant difference in serum half-life of doxycycline (range 18-22 hours) in individuals with normal and severely impaired renal function.
Hemodialysis does not alter serum half-life.
Microbiology: The tetracyclines are primarily bacteriostatic and are thought to exert their antimicrobial effect by the inhibition of protein synthesis. The tetracyclines, including doxycycline, have a similar antimicrobial spectrum of activity against a wide range of gram-positive and gram-negative organisms. Cross-resistance of these organisms to tetracyclines is common.
While *in vitro* studies have demonstrated the susceptibility of most strains of the following microorganisms, clinical efficacy for infections other than those included in the INDICATIONS AND USAGE section has not been documented.

GRAM-NEGATIVE BACTERIA:
- *Neisseria gonorrhoeae*
- *Haemophilus ducreyi*
- *Haemophilus influenzae*
- *Yersinia pestis* (formerly *Pasteurella pestis*)
- *Francisella tularensis* (formerly *Pasteurella tularensis*)
- *Vibrio cholerae* (formerly *Vibrio comma*)
- *Bartonella bacilliformis*
- *Brucella species*

Because many strains of the following groups of gram-negative microorganisms have been shown to be resistant to tetracyclines, culture and susceptibility testing are recommended:
- *Escherichia coli*
- *Klebsiella species*
- *Enterobacter aerogenes*
- *Shigella species*
- *Acinetobacter species* (formerly *Mima* species and *Herellea* species)
- *Bacteroides* species

GRAM-POSITIVE BACTERIA:
Because many strains of the following groups of gram-positive microorganisms have been shown to be resistant to tetracyclines, culture and susceptibility testing are recommended. Up to 44 percent of strains of *Streptococcus pyogenes* and 74 percent of *Streptococcus faecalis* have been found to be resistant to tetracycline drugs. Therefore, tetracyclines should not be used to treat streptococcal infections unless the organism has been demonstrated to be susceptible.
- *Streptococcus pyogenes*
- *Streptococcus pneumoniae*
- *Enterococcus* group (*Streptococcus faecalis* and *Streptococcus faecium*)
- *Alpha-hemolytic streptococci (viridans* group)

OTHER MICROORGANISMS:
- *Chlamydia psittaci*
- *Chlamydia trachomatis*
- *Ureaplasma urealyticum*
- *Borrelia recurrentis*
- *Treponema pallidum*
- *Treponema pertenue*
- *Clostridium* species
- *Fusobacterium fusiforme*
- *Actinomyces* species
- *Bacillus anthracis*
- *Propionibacterium acnes*
- *Entamoeba* species
- *Balantidium coli*

Susceptibility tests: Diffusion Techniques: Quantitative methods that require measurement of zone diameters give the most precise estimate of the susceptibility of bacteria to antimicrobial agents.
One such standard procedure[1] which has been recommended for use with disks to test susceptibility of organisms to doxycycline uses the 30-mcg tetracycline-class disk or the 30-mcg doxycycline disk. Interpretation involves the correlation of the diameter obtained in the disk test with the minimum inhibitory concentration (MIC) for tetracycline or doxycycline, respectively.
Reports from the laboratory giving results of the standard single-disk susceptibility test with a 30-mcg tetracycline-class disk or the 30-mcg doxycycline disk should be interpreted according to the following criteria.

Zone Diameter (mm)		Interpretation
tetracycline	doxycycline	
≥19	≥16	Susceptible
15–18	13–15	Intermediate
≤14	≤12	Resistant

A report of "susceptible" indicates that the pathogen is likely to be inhibited by generally achievable blood levels. A report of "intermediate" suggests that the organism would be susceptible if a high dosage is used or if the infection is confined to tissues and fluids in which high antimicrobial levels are attained. A report of "resistant" indicates that achievable concentrations are unlikely to be inhibitory, and other therapy should be selected.
Standardized procedures require the use of laboratory control organisms. The 30-mcg tetracycline-class disk or the 30-mcg doxycycline disk should give the following zone diameters:

Organism	Zone Diameter	
	tetracycline	doxycycline
E. coli ATCC 25922	18–25	18–24
S. aureus ATCC 25923	19–28	23–29

Dilution Techniques:
Use a standardized dilution method[2] (broth, agar, microdilution) or equivalent with tetracycline powder. The MIC values obtained should be interpreted according to the following criteria:

MIC (mcg/mL)	Interpretation
≤4	Susceptible
8	Intermediate
≥16	Resistant

As with standard diffusion techniques, dilution methods require the use of laboratory control organisms. Standard tetracycline powder should provide the following MIC values:

Organism	MIC (mcg/mL)
S. aureus ATCC 29213	0.25–1
E. faecalis ATCC 29212	8–32
E. coli ATCC 25922	1–4
P. aeruginosa ATCC 27853	8–32

INDICATIONS AND USAGE

Doxycycline is indicated for the treatment of the following infections:
Rocky mountain spotted fever, typhus fever and the typhus group, Q fever, rickettsialpox, and tick fevers caused by Rickettsiae.
Respiratory tract infections caused by *Mycoplasma pneumoniae.*
Lymphogranuloma venereum caused by *Chlamydia trachomatis.*
Psittacosis (omithosis) caused by *Chlamydia psittaci.*
Trachoma caused by *Chlamydia trachomatis,* although the infectious agent is not always eliminated as judged by immunofluorescence.
Inclusion conjunctivitis caused by *Chlamydia trachomatis.*
Uncomplicated urethral, endocervical or rectal infections in adults caused by *Chlamydia trachomatis.*
Nongonococcal urethritis caused by *Ureaplasma urealyticum.*
Relapsing fever due to *Borrelia recurrentis.*
Doxycycline is also indicated for the treatment of infections caused by the following gram-negative microorganisms:
Chancroid caused by *Haemophilus ducreyi.*
Plague due to *Yersinia pestis* (formerly *Pasteurella pestis*).
Tularemia due to *Francisella tularensis* (formerly *Pasteurella tularensis*).
Cholera caused by *Vibrio cholerae* (formerly *Vibrio comma*).
Campylobacter fetus infections caused by *Campylobacter fetus* (formerly *Vibrio fetus*).
Brucellosis due to *Brucella* species (in conjunction with streptomycin).
Bartonellosis due to *Bartonella bacilliformis.*
Granuloma inguinale caused by *Calymmatobacterium granulomatis.*
Because many strains of the following groups of microorganisms have been shown to be resistant to doxycycline, culture and susceptibility testing are recommended.
Doxycycline is indicated for treatment of infections caused by the following gram-negative microorganisms, when bacteriologic testing indicates appropriate susceptibility to the drug:
Escherichia coli
Enterobacter aerogenes (formerly *Aerobacter aerogenes*)
Shigella species
Acinetobacter species (formerly *Mima* species and *Herellea* species)
Respiratory tract infections caused by *Haemophilus influenzae.*
Respiratory tract and urinary tract infections caused by *Klebsiella species.*
Doxycycline is indicated for treatment of infections caused by the following gram-positive microorganisms when bacteriologic testing indicates appropriate susceptibility to the drug:
Upper respiratory infections caused by *Streptococcus pneumoniae* (formerly *Diplococcus pneumoniae*).
Skin and skin structure infections caused by *Staphylococcus aureus.* Doxycycline is not the drug of choice in the treatment of any type of staphylococcal infections.
When penicillin is contraindicated, doxycycline is an alternative drug in the treatment of the following infections:
Uncomplicated gonorrhea caused by *Neisseria gonorrhoeae.*
Syphilis caused by *Treponema pallidum.*
Yaws caused by *Treponema pertenue.*
Listeriosis due to Listeria monocytogenes.

Time (hr):	0.5	1.0	1.5	2.0	3.0	4.0	8.0	12.0	24.0	48.0	72.0
Conc. (mcg/mL)	1.02	2.26	2.67	3.01	3.16	3.03	2.03	1.62	0.95	0.37	0.15

Anthrax due to *Bacillus anthracis.*
Vincent's infection caused by *Fusobacterium fusiforme.*
Actinomycosis caused by *Actinomyces israelii.*
Infections caused by *Clostridium* species.
In acute intestinal amebiasis, doxycycline may be a useful adjunct to amebicides.
In severe acne, doxycycline may be useful adjunctive therapy.

CONTRAINDICATIONS

This drug is contraindicated in persons who have shown hypersensitivity to any of the tetracyclines.

WARNINGS

THE USE OF DRUGS OF THE TETRACYCLINE CLASS DURING TOOTH DEVELOPMENT (LAST HALF OF PREGNANCY, INFANCY, AND CHILDHOOD TO THE AGE OF 8 YEARS) MAY CAUSE PERMANENT DISCOLORATION OF THE TEETH (YELLOW-GRAY-BROWN).
This adverse reaction is more common during long term use of the drugs but has been observed following repeated short-term courses. Enamel hypoplasia has also been reported.
TETRACYCLINE DRUGS, THEREFORE, SHOULD NOT BE USED IN THIS AGE GROUP UNLESS OTHER DRUGS ARE NOT LIKELY TO BE EFFECTIVE OR ARE CONTRAINDICATED.
All tetracyclines form a stable calcium complex in any bone-forming tissue. A decrease in the fibula growth rate has been observed in prematures given oral tetracycline in doses of 25 mg/kg every six hours. This reaction was shown to be reversible when the drug was discontinued.
Results of animal studies indicate that tetracyclines cross the placenta, are found in fetal tissues, and can have toxic effects on the developing fetus (often related to retardation of skeletal development). Evidence of embryo toxicity has been noted in animals treated early in pregnancy. If any tetracycline is used during pregnancy or if the patient becomes pregnant while taking these drugs, the patient should be apprised of the potential hazard to the fetus.
The antianabolic action of the tetracyclines may cause an increase in BUN. Studies to date indicate that this does not occur with the use of doxycycline in patients with impaired renal function.
Photosensitivity manifested by an exaggerated sunburn reaction has been observed in some individuals taking tetracyclines. Patients apt to be exposed to direct sunlight or ultraviolet light should be advised that this reaction can occur with tetracycline drugs, and treatment should be discontinued at the first evidence of skin erythema.

PRECAUTIONS

General:
As with other antibiotic preparations, use of this drug may result in overgrowth of non-susceptible organisms, including fungi. If superinfection occurs, the antibiotic should be discontinued and appropriate therapy instituted.
Bulging fontanels in infants and benign intracranial hypertension in adults have been reported in individuals receiving tetracyclines. These conditions disappeared when the drug was discontinued.
Incision and drainage or other surgical procedures should be performed in conjunction with antibiotic therapy when indicated.
Laboratory tests: In venereal disease when coexistent syphilis is suspected, a dark-field examination should be done before treatment is started and the blood serology repeated monthly for at least four months.
In long-term therapy, periodic laboratory evaluations of organ systems, including hematopoietic, renal, and hepatic studies should be performed.
Drug interactions: Because tetracyclines have been shown to depress plasma prothrombin activity, patients who are on anticoagulant therapy may require downward adjustment of their anticoagulant dosage.
Since bacteriostatic drugs may interfere with the bactericidal action of penicillin, it is advisable to avoid giving tetracyclines in conjunction with penicillin.
Absorption of tetracyclines is impaired by antacids containing aluminum, calcium, or magnesium, and iron-containing preparations.
Barbiturates, carbamazepine, and phenytoin decrease the half-life of doxycycline.
The concurrent use of tetracycline and methoxyflurane has been reported to result in fatal renal toxicity.
Concurrent use of tetracycline may render oral contraceptives less effective.
Drug/laboratory test interactions: False elevations of urinary catecholamine levels may occur due to interference with the fluorescence test.
Carcinogenesis, mutagenesis, impairment of fertility: Long-term studies in animals to evaluate the carcinogenic potential of doxycycline have not been conducted. However, there has been evidence of oncogenic activity in rats in studies with related antibiotics, oxytetracycline (adrenal and pituitary tumors) and minocycline (thyroid tumors). Likewise, although mutagenicity studies of doxycycline have not been conducted, positive results in *in vitro* mammalian cell assays have been reported for related antibiotics (tetracycline, oxytetracycline). Doxycycline administered orally at dosage levels as high as 250 mg/kg/day had no apparent effect on the fertility of female rats. Effect on male fertility has not been studied.
Pregnancy: Pregnancy Category D. (See **WARNINGS**).
Labor and Delivery: The effect of tetracyclines on labor and delivery is unknown.
Nursing mothers: Tetracyclines are present in the milk of lactating women who are taking a drug in this class. Because of the potential for serious adverse reactions in nursing infants from the tetracyclines, a decision should be made whether to discontinue nursing or discontinue the drug, taking into account the importance of the drug to the mother. (See **WARNINGS**).
Pediatric Use: See **WARNINGS** and **DOSAGE AND ADMINISTRATION** sections.

ADVERSE REACTIONS

Due to oral doxycycline's virtually complete absorption, side effects to the lower bowel, particularly diarrhea, have been infrequent. The following adverse reactions have been observed in patients receiving tetracyclines.
Gastrointestinal: Anorexia, nausea, vomiting, diarrhea, glossitis, dysphagia, enterocolitis, and inflammatory lesions (with monilial overgrowth) in the anogenital region. These reactions have been caused by both the oral and parenteral administration of tetracyclines. Rare instances of esophagitis and esophageal ulcerations have been reported in patients receiving capsule and tablet forms of drugs in the tetracycline class. Most of these patients took medications immediately before going to bed. (See **DOSAGE AND ADMINISTRATION**).
Skin: Maculopapular and erythematous rashes. Exfoliative dermatitis has been reported but is uncommon. Photosensitivity is discussed above. (See **WARNINGS.**)
Renal toxicity: Rise in BUN has been reported and is apparently dose related. (See **WARNINGS.**)
Hypersensitivity reactions: Urticaria, angioneurotic edema, anaphylaxis, anaphylactoid purpura, pericarditis, and exacerbation of systemic lupus erythematosus.
Blood: Hemolytic anemia, thrombocytopenia, neutropenia, and eosinophilia have been reported with tetracyclines.
Other: Bulging fontanels in infants and intracranial hypertension in adults. (See **PRECAUTIONS—General.**)
When given over prolonged periods, tetracyclines have been reported to produce brown-black microscopic discoloration of the thyroid gland. No abnormalities of thyroid function are known to occur.

OVERDOSAGE

In case of overdosage, discontinue medication, treat symptomatically and institute supportive measures. Dialysis does not alter serum half-life, and it would not be of benefit in treating cases of overdosage.

DOSAGE AND ADMINISTRATION

THE USUAL DOSAGE AND FREQUENCY OF ADMINISTRATION OF DOXYCYCLINE DIFFERS FROM THAT OF THE OTHER TETRACYCLINES. EXCEEDING THE RECOMMENDED DOSAGE MAY RESULT IN AN INCREASED INCIDENCE OF SIDE EFFECTS.
Adults: The usual dose of oral doxycycline is 200 mg on the first day of treatment (administered 100 mg every 12 hours or 50 mg every 6 hours) followed by a maintenance dose of 100 mg/day. The maintenance dose may be administered as a single dose or as 50 mg every 12 hours. In the management of more severe infections (particularly chronic infections of the urinary tract), 100 mg every 12 hours is recommended.
For pediatric patients above eight years of age: The recommended dosage schedule for pediatric patients weighing 100 pounds or less is 2 mg/lb of body weight divided into two doses on the first day of treatment, followed by 1 mg/lb of body weight given as a single daily dose or divided into two doses, on subsequent days. For more severe infections, up to 2 mg/lb of body weight may be used. For pediatric patients over 100 lbs the usual adult dose should be used.
Uncomplicated gonococcal infections in adults (except anorectal infections in men): 100 mg by mouth, twice a day for 7 days. As an alternate single visit dose, administer 300 mg stat followed in one hour by a second 300 mg dose.
Acute epididymo-orchitis caused by *N. gonorrhoeae* **:** 100 mg, by mouth, twice a day for at least 10 days.
Primary and secondary syphilis: 300 mg a day in divided doses for at least 10 days.
Uncomplicated urethral, endocervical, or rectal infection in adults caused by *Chlamydia trachomatis* : 100 mg, by mouth, twice a day for at least 7 days.
Nongonococcal urethritis caused by *C. trachomatis* and *U. urealyticum:* 100 mg, by mouth, twice a day for at least 7 days.
Acute epididymo-orchitis caused by *C. trachomatis:* 100 mg, by mouth, twice a day for at least 10 days.
When used in streptococcal infections, therapy should be continued for 10 days.
Administration of adequate amounts of fluid along with capsule and tablet forms of drugs in the tetracycline class is recommended to wash down the drugs and reduce the risk

Continued on next page

Monodox—Cont.

of esophageal irritation and ulceration. (See **ADVERSE REACTIONS**). If gastric irritation occurs, doxycycline may be given with food. Ingestion of a high fat meal has been shown to delay the time to peak plasma concentrations by an average of one hour and 20 minutes. However, in the same study, food enhanced the average peak concentration by 7.5% and the area under the curve by 5.7%.

HOW SUPPLIED

MONODOX® 50 mg Capsules have a white opaque body with a yellow opaque cap. The capsule bears the inscription "MONODOX 50" in brown and "M 260" in brown. Each capsule contains doxycycline monohydrate equivalent to 50 mg doxycycline.

MONODOX® 50 mg is available in: Bottles of 100 capsules, NDC 55515-260-06. MONODOX® 100 mg Capsules have a yellow opaque body with a brown opaque cap. The capsule bears the inscription "MONODOX 100" in white and "M 259" in brown. Each capsule contains doxycycline monohydrate equivalent to 100 mg of doxycycline. MONODOX® 100 mg is available in: Bottles of 50 capsules, NDC 55515-259-04 and in bottles of 250 capsules, NDC 55515-259-07.

STORE AT CONTROLLED ROOM TEMPERATURE 15°–30°C (59°–86°F). PROTECT FROM LIGHT.

ANIMAL PHARMACOLOGY AND ANIMAL TOXICOLOGY

Hyperpigmentation of the thyroid has been produced by members of the tetracycline class in the following species: in rats by oxytetracycline, doxycycline, tetracycline PO_4, and methacycline; in minipigs by doxycycline, minocycline, tetracycline PO_4, and methacycline; in dogs by doxycycline and minocycline; in monkeys by minocycline.

Minocycline, tetracycline PO_4, methacycline, doxycycline, tetracycline base, oxytetracycline HCl and tetracycline HCl were goitrogenic in rats fed a low iodine diet. This goitrogenic effect was accompanied by high radioactive iodine uptake. Administration of minocycline also produced a large goiter with high radioiodine uptake in rats fed a relatively high iodine diet.

Treatment of various animal species with this class of drugs has also resulted in the induction of thyroid hyperplasia in the following: in rats and dogs (minocycline), in chickens (chlortetracycline) and in rats and mice (oxytetracycline). Adrenal gland hyperplasia has been observed in goats and rats treated with oxytetracycline.

REFERENCES:

1. National Committee for Clinical Laboratory Standards, *Performance Standards for Antimicrobial Disk Susceptibility Tests,* Fourth Edition. Approved Standard NCCLS Document M2-A4, Vol. 10, No. 7 NCCLS, Villanova, PA, April 1990.
2. National Committee for Clinical Laboratory Standards, *Methods for Dilution Antimicrobial Susceptibility Tests for Bacteria That Grow Aerobically,* Second Edition. Approved Standard NCCLS Document M7-A2, Vol. 10, No. 8 NCCLS, Villanova, PA, April 1990.

Rx Only

Manufactured for
OCLASSEN
DERMATOLOGICS
A Division of Watson Pharma, Inc., Corona, CA 92880
by Vintage Pharmaceuticals, Inc., Charlotte, N.C.
Revised April 28, 1998 02-18391/R7

Shown in Product Identification Guide, page 327

Odyssey Pharmaceuticals, Inc.

72 DeFOREST AVE.
EAST HANOVER, NJ 07936

Direct Inquiries to:
(877) 427-9068

NYSTATIN VAGINAL TABLETS, USP

100,000 Units
15 Vaginal Tablets with Applicator

URECHOLINE® ℞

DESCRIPTION

Bethanechol chloride, a cholinergic agent, is a synthetic ester which is structurally and pharmacologically related to acetylcholine. It is designated chemically as 2-[(aminocarbonyl)oxy]-N, N, N-trimethyl-1-propanaminium chloride. Its molecular formula is $C_7H_{17}ClN_2O_2$ and its structural formula is:

$$\left[\begin{array}{c} CH_3CHCH_2N^{+4}(CH_3)_3 \\ OCONH_2 \end{array}\right] Cl^{-2}$$

It is a white, hygroscopic crystalline powder having a slight amine-like odor, freely soluble in water, and has a molecular weight of 196.68.

Each tablet for oral administration contains 25 mg bethanechol chloride, USP. Tablets also contain the following inactive ingredients: Anhydrous lactose, colloidal silicon dioxide, magnesium stearate, microcrystalline cellulose, sodium starch glycolate, D&C Yellow #10 and FD&C Yellow #6.

CLINICAL PHARMACOLOGY

Bethanechol chloride acts principally by producing the effects of stimulation of the parasympathetic nervous system. It increases the tone of the detrusor urinae muscle, usually producing a contraction sufficiently strong to initiate micturition and empty the bladder. It stimulates gastric motility, increases gastric tone and often restores impaired rhythmic peristalsis.

Stimulation of the parasympathetic nervous system releases acetylcholine at the nerve endings. When spontaneous stimulation is reduced and therapeutic intervention is required, acetylcholine can be given, but it is rapidly hydrolyzed by cholinesterase and its effects are transient. Bethanechol chloride is not destroyed by cholinesterase and its effects are more prolonged than those of acetylcholine.

Effects on the GI and urinary tracts sometimes appear within 30 minutes after oral administration of bethanechol chloride, but more often 60 to 90 minutes are required to reach maximum effectiveness. Following oral administration, the usual duration of action of bethanechol is one hour, although large doses (300 to 400 mg) have been reported to produce effects for up to six hours. Subcutaneous injection produces a more intense action on bladder muscle than does oral administration of the drug.

Because of the selective action of bethanechol, nicotinic symptoms of cholinergic stimulation are usually absent or minimal when orally or subcutaneously administered in therapeutic doses, while muscarinic effects are prominent. Muscarinic effects usually occur within 5 to 15 minutes after subcutaneous injection, reach a maximum in 15 to 30 minutes, and disappear within two hours. Doses that stimulate micturition and defecation and increase peristalsis do not ordinarily stimulate ganglia or voluntary muscles. Therapeutic test doses in normal human subjects have little effect on heart rate, blood pressure or peripheral circulation.

Bethanechol chloride does not cross the blood-brain barrier because of its charged quaternary amine moiety. The metabolic rate and mode of excretion of the drug have not been elucidated.

A clinical study (Diokno, A.C.; Lapides, J.; Urol 10: 23–24, July 1977) was conducted on the relative effectiveness of oral and subcutaneous doses of bethanechol chloride on the stretch response of bladder muscle in patients with urinary retention. Results showed that 5 mg of the drug given subcutaneously stimulated a response that was more rapid in onset and of larger magnitude than an oral dose of 50 mg, 100 mg, or 200 mg. All the oral doses, however, had a longer duration of effect than the subcutaneous dose. Although the 50 mg oral dose caused little change in intravesical pressure in this study, this dose has been found in other studies to be clinically effective in the rehabilitation of patients with decompensated bladders.

INDICATIONS AND USAGE

Bethanechol chloride is indicated for the treatment of acute postoperative and postpartum nonobstructive (functional) urinary retention and for neurogenic atony of the urinary bladder with retention.

CONTRAINDICATIONS

Hypersensitivity to bethanechol chloride tablets, hyperthyroidism, peptic ulcer, latent or active bronchial asthma, pronounced bradycardia or hypotension, vasomotor instability, coronary artery disease, epilepsy and parkinsonism.

Bethanechol chloride should not be employed when the strength or integrity of the gastrointestinal or bladder wall is in question, or in the presence of mechanical obstruction; when increased muscular activity of the gastrointestinal tract or urinary bladder might prove harmful, as following recent urinary bladder surgery, gastrointestinal resection and anastomosis, or when there is possible gastrointestinal obstruction; in bladder neck obstruction, spastic gastrointestinal disturbances, acute inflammatory lesions of the gastrointestinal tract, or peritonitis; or in marked vagotonia.

PRECAUTIONS

General: In urinary retention, if the sphincter fails to relax as bethanechol contracts the bladder, urine may be forced up the ureter into the kidney pelvis. If there is bacteriuria, this may cause reflux infection.

Information for Patients: Bethanechol chloride tablets should preferably be taken one hour before or two hours after meals to avoid nausea or vomiting. Dizziness, lightheadedness or fainting may occur, especially when getting up from a lying or sitting position.

Drug Interactions: Special care is required if this drug is given to patients receiving ganglion blocking compounds because a critical fall in blood pressure may occur. Usually, severe abdominal symptoms appear before there is such a fall in the blood pressure.

Carcinogenesis, Mutagenesis, Impairment of Fertility: Long-term studies in animals have not been performed to evaluate the effects upon fertility, mutagenic or carcinogenic potential of bethanechol chloride.

Pregnancy: ***Teratogenic Effects:*** Pregnancy Category C. Animal reproduction studies have not been conducted with bethanechol chloride. It is also not known whether bethanechol chloride can cause fetal harm when administered to a pregnant woman or can affect reproduction capacity. Bethanechol chloride should be given to a pregnant woman only if clearly needed.

Nursing Mothers: It is not known whether this drug is secreted in human milk. Because many drugs are secreted in human milk and because of the potential for serious adverse reactions from bethanechol chloride in nursing infants, a decision should be made whether to discontinue nursing or to discontinue the drug, taking into account the importance of the drug to the mother.

Pediatric Use: Safety and effectiveness in pediatric patients have not been established.

ADVERSE REACTIONS

Adverse reactions are rare following oral administration of bethanechol, but are more common following subcutaneous injection. Adverse reactions are more likely to occur when dosage is increased.

The following adverse reactions have been observed: *Body as a Whole*: malaise; *Digestive*: abdominal cramps or discomfort, colicky pain, nausea and belching, diarrhea, borborygmi, salivation; *Renal*: urinary urgency; *Nervous System*: headache; *Cardiovascular*: a fall in blood pressure with reflex tachycardia, vasomotor response; *Skin*: flushing producing a feeling of warmth, sensation of heat about the face, sweating; *Respiratory*: bronchial constriction, asthmatic attacks; *Special Senses*: lacrimation, miosis.

Causal Relationship Unknown: The following adverse reactions have been reported, and a causal relationship to therapy with bethanechol has not been established: *Body as a Whole*: malaise; *Nervous System*: seizures.

OVERDOSAGE

Early signs of overdosage are abdominal discomfort, salivation, flushing of the skin ("hot feeling"), sweating, nausea, and vomiting.

Atropine Sulfate is a specific antidote. The recommended dose for adults is 0.6 mg. Repeat doses can be given every two hours, according to clinical response. The recommended dosage in infants and children up to 12 years of age is 0.01 mg/kg (to a maximum single dose of 0.4 mg) repeated every two hours as needed until the desired effect is obtained or adverse effects of atropine preclude further usage. Subcutaneous injection of atropine is preferred except in emergencies when the intravenous route may be employed.

The oral LD_{50} of bethanechol chloride is 1510 mg/kg in the mouse.

DOSAGE AND ADMINISTRATION

Dosage must be individualized, depending on the type and severity of the condition to be treated.

Preferably give the drug when the stomach is empty. If taken soon after eating, nausea and vomiting may occur.

The usual adult oral dose ranges from 10 to 50 mg three or four times a day. The minimum effective dose is determined by giving 5 to 10 mg initially and repeating the same amount at hourly intervals until satisfactory response occurs, or until a maximum of 50 mg has been given. The effects of the drug sometimes appear within 30 minutes and are usually maximal within 60 to 90 minutes. The drug effects persist for about one hour.

If necessary, the effects of the drug can be abolished promptly by atropine (see **OVERDOSAGE**).

HOW SUPPLIED

Urecholine® Tablets 25 mg - Yellow, round, scored tablets in bottles of 100. Debossed OP 704

Dispense in a tight container as defined in the USP.

Store at controlled room temperature 15°–30°C (59°–86°F).

Distributed by Odyssey Pharmaceuticals, Inc., East Hanover, New Jersey 07936

Manufactured by Sidmak Laboratories, Inc., East Hanover, NJ 07936

Rev. 4/00

Organon Inc.

375 MT. PLEASANT AVE.
WEST ORANGE, NJ 07052

Direct Inquiries to:
(973) 325-4500

Currently available products are listed below. For complete product line information and price lists, direct inquiries to Organon Inc. Customer Service. For specific product information, contact Organon Inc. Medical Services Department.

FOLLISTIM®/ANTAGON™ KIT:

for FOLLISTIM® see page 2267

ANTAGON™ ℞
(ganirelix acetate) Injection
FOR SUBCUTANEOUS USE ONLY

DESCRIPTION
Antagon™ (ganirelix acetate) Injection is a synthetic decapeptide with high antagonistic activity against naturally occurring gonadotropin-releasing hormone (GnRH). Ganirelix acetate is derived from native GnRH with substitutions of amino acids at positions 1, 2, 3, 6, 8, and 10 to form the following molecular formula of the peptide: N-acetyl-3-(2-napthyl)-D-alanyl-4-chloro-D-phenylalanyl-3-(3-pyridyl)-D-alanyl-L-seryl-L-tyrosyl-N[9],N[10]-diethyl-D-homoarginyl-L-leucyl-N[9],N[10]-diethyl-L-homoarginyl-L-prolyl-D-alanylamide acetate. The molecular weight for ganirelix acetate is 1570.4 as an anhydrous free base. The structural formula is as follows:
Ganirelix acetate
[See graphic above]
Antagon™ is supplied as a colorless, sterile, ready-to-use, aqueous solution intended for SUBCUTANEOUS administration only. Each sterile, prefilled syringe contains 250 µg/0.5 mL of ganirelix acetate, 0.1 mg glacial acetic acid, 23.5 mg mannitol, and water for injection adjusted to pH 5.0 with acetic acid, NF and/or sodium hydroxide, NF.

CLINICAL PHARMACOLOGY
The pulsatile release of GnRH stimulates the synthesis and secretion of luteinizing hormone (LH) and follicle-stimulating hormone (FSH). The frequency of LH pulses in the mid and late follicular phase is approximately 1 pulse per hour. These pulses can be detected as transient rises in serum LH. At midcycle, a large increase in GnRH release results in an LH surge. The midcycle LH surge initiates several physiologic actions including: ovulation, resumption of meiosis in the oocyte, and luteinization. Luteinization results in a rise in serum progesterone with an accompanying decrease in estradiol levels.
Antagon™ (ganirelix acetate) Injection acts by competitively blocking the GnRH receptors on the pituitary gonadotroph and subsequent transduction pathway. It induces a rapid, reversible suppression of gonadotropin secretion. The suppression of pituitary LH secretion by Antagon™ is more pronounced than that of FSH. An initial release of endogenous gonadotropins has not been detected with Antagon™, which is consistent with an antagonist effect. Upon discontinuation of Antagon™, pituitary LH and FSH levels are fully recovered within 48 hours.

Pharmacokinetics
The pharmacokinetic parameters of single and multiple injections of Antagon™ (ganirelix acetate) Injection in healthy adult females are summarized in Table I. Steady state serum concentrations are reached after 3 days of treatment. The pharmacokinetics of ganirelix acetate are dose-proportional in the dose range of 125 to 500 µg.
[See table I above]

Absorption
Ganirelix acetate is rapidly absorbed following subcutaneous injection with maximum serum concentrations reached approximately one hour after dosing. The mean absolute bioavailability of Antagon™ following a single 250 µg subcutaneous injection to healthy female volunteers is 91.1%.

Distribution
The mean (SD) volume of distribution of Antagon™ in healthy females following intravenous administration of a single 250 µg dose is 43.7 (11.4) liters (L). *In vitro* protein binding to human plasma is 81.9%.

Metabolism
Following single dose intravenous administration of radiolabeled Antagon™ to healthy female volunteers, Antagon™ is the major compound present in the plasma (50–70% of total radioactivity in the plasma) up to 4 hours and urine (17.1–18.4% of administered dose) up to 24 hours. Antagon™ is not found in the feces. The 1–4 peptide and 1–6 peptide of Antagon™ are the primary metabolites observed in the feces.

Excretion
On average, 97.2% of the total radiolabeled Antagon™ dose is recovered in the feces and urine (75.1% and 22.1%, respectively) over 288 h following intravenous single dose administration of 1 mg [^{14}C]-ganirelix acetate. Urinary excretion is virtually complete in 24 h, whereas fecal excretion starts to plateau 192 h after dosing.

Special Populations
The pharmacokinetics of ganirelix acetate have not been determined in special populations such as geriatric, pediatric, renally impaired and hepatically impaired patients (see PRECAUTIONS).

Drug-Drug Interactions
Formal *in vivo* or *in vitro* drug-drug interaction studies have not been conducted (see PRECAUTIONS). Since Antagon™ can suppress the secretion of pituitary gonadotropins, dose adjustments of exogenous gonadotropins may be necessary when used during controlled ovarian hyperstimulation (COH).

Clinical Studies
The efficacy of Antagon™ (ganirelix acetate) Injection was established in two adequate and well-controlled clinical studies which included women with normal endocrine and pelvic ultra-sound parameters. The studies intended to exclude subjects with polycystic ovary syndrome (PCOS) and subjects with low or no ovarian reserve. One cycle of study medication was administered to each randomized subject. For both studies, the administration of exogenous recombinant FSH [Follistim® (follitropin beta for injection)] 150 IU daily was initiated on the morning of Day 2 or 3 of a natural menstrual cycle. Antagon™ was administered on the morning of Day 7 or 8 (Day 6 of recombinant FSH administration). The dose of recombinant FSH administered was adjusted according to individual responses starting on the day of initiation of Antagon™. Both recombinant FSH and Antagon™ were continued daily until at least three follicles were 17 mm or greater in diameter at which time hCG [Pregnyl® (chorionic gonadotropin for injection, USP)] was administered. Following hCG administration, Antagon™ and recombinant FSH administration were discontinued. Oocyte retrieval, followed by *in vitro* fertilization (IVF) or intracytoplasmatic sperm injection (ICSI), was subsequently performed.
In a multicenter, double-blind, randomized, dose-finding study, the safety and efficacy of Antagon™ were evaluated for the prevention of LH surges in women undergoing COH with recombinant FSH. Antagon™ doses ranging from 62.5 µg to 2000 µg and recombinant FSH were administered to 332 patients undergoing COH for IVF (see TABLE II). Median serum LH on the day of hCG administration decreased with increasing doses of Antagon™. Median serum E_2 (17β-estradiol) on the day of hCG administration was 1475, 1110, and 1160 pg/mL for the 62.5, 125, and 250 µg doses, respectively. Lower peak serum E_2 levels of 823, 703, and 441 pg/mL were seen at higher doses of Antagon™ 500, 1000, and 2000 µg, respectively. The highest pregnancy and implantation rates were achieved with the 250 µg dose of Antagon™ as summarized in Table II.
[See table II above]
Transient LH rises alone were not deleterious to achieving pregnancy with Antagon™ at doses of 125 µg (3/6 subjects) and 250 µg (1/1 subjects). In addition, none of the subjects with LH rises ≥ 10 mIU/mL had premature luteinization indicated by a serum progesterone above 2 ng/mL.
A multicenter, open-label, randomized study was conducted to assess the efficacy and safety of Antagon™ in women undergoing COH. Follicular phase treatment with Antagon™ 250 µg was studied using a luteal phase GnRH agonist as a reference treatment. A total of 463 subjects were treated with Antagon™ by subcutaneous injection once daily starting on Day 6 of recombinant FSH treatment. Recombinant FSH was maintained at 150 IU for the first 5 days of ovarian stimulation and was then adjusted by the investigator on the sixth day of gonadotropin use according to individual responses. The results for the Antagon™ arm are summarized in Table III.
[See table III at top of next page]
The mean number of days of Antagon™ treatment was 5.4 (2–14). There was no incidence of drug related allergic reactions within the adequate and well-controlled clinical studies.

LH Surges
The midcycle LH surge initiates several physiologic actions including: ovulation, resumption of meiosis in the oocyte, and luteinization. In 463 subjects administered Antagon™ 250 µg, a premature LH surge prior to hCG administration, (LH rise ≥ 10 mIU/mL with a significant rise in serum progesterone > 2 ng/mL, or a significant decline in serum estradiol) occurred in less than 1% of subjects.

INDICATIONS AND USAGE
Antagon™ (ganirelix acetate) Injection is indicated for the inhibition of premature LH surges in women undergoing controlled ovarian hyperstimulation.

CONTRAINDICATIONS
Antagon™ (ganirelix acetate) Injection is contraindicated under the following conditions:
- Known hypersensitivity to Antagon™ or to any of its components.
- Known hypersensitivity to GnRH or any other GnRH analog.
- Known or suspected pregnancy (see PRECAUTIONS).

WARNINGS
Antagon™ (ganirelix acetate) Injection should be prescribed by physicians who are experienced in infertility treatment.

Continued on next page

1 (D) 2 (D) 3 (D) 4 5 6 (D) 7 8 9 10 (D)
Ac-NH-CH-CO-pCl-Phe-NH-CH-CO-Ser-Tyr-NH-CH-CO-Leu-NH-CH-CO-Pro-Ala-NH_2
CH_2 CH_2 $(CH_2)_4$ $(CH_2)_4$
NH NH
HN C NH HN C NH $(CH_3COO^-)_2$
C_2H_5 C_2H_5 C_2H_5 C_2H_5
+ x $C_2H_4O_2$ + y H_2O

TABLE I: Mean (SD) pharmacokinetic parameters of 250 µg of Antagon™ following a single subcutaneous (SC) injection (n=15) and daily SC injections (n=15) for seven days.

	t_{max} h	$t_{1/2}$ h	C_{max} ng/mL	AUC ng•h/mL	CL/F L/h	V_d/F L
Antagon™ single dose	1.1 (0.3)	12.8 (4.3)	14.8 (3.2)	96 (12)	2.4 (0.2)†	43.7 (11.4)†
Antagon™ multiple dose	1.1 (0.2)	16.2 (1.6)	11.2 (2.4)	77.1 (9.8)	3.3 (0.4)	76.5 (10.3)

t_{max} Time to maximum concentration
$t_{1/2}$ Elimination half-life
C_{max} Maximum serum concentration
AUC Area under the curve; Single dose: $AUC_{0-\infty}$; multiple dose: AUC_{0-24}
V_d Volume of distribution
† Based on intravenous administration
CL Clearance = Dose/$AUC_{0-\infty}$
F Absolute bioavailability

TABLE II: Results from the multicenter, double-blind, randomized, dose-finding study to assess the efficacy of Antagon™ to prevent premature LH surges in women undergoing COH with recombinant FSH.

	Daily dose (µg) of Antagon™					
	62.5 µg	**125 µg**	**250 µg**	**500 µg**	**1000 µg**	**2000 µg**
No. subjects receiving Antagon™	31	66	70	69	66	30
No. subjects with ET†	27	61	62	54	61	27
No. of subjects with LH rise ≥ 10 mIU/mL*	4	6	1	0	0	0
Serum LH (mIU/mL) on day of hCG‡	3.6	2.5	1.7	1.0	0.6	0.3
5th–95th percentiles	0.6–19.9	0.6–11.4	<0.25–6.4	0.4–4.7	<0.25–2.2	<0.25–0.8
Serum E_2 (pg/mL) on day of hCG‡	1475	1110	1160	823	703	441
5th–95th percentiles	645–3720	424–3780	384–3910	279–2720	284–2360	166–1940
Vital pregnancy rate$^{\Omega}$						
per attempt, n (%)	7 (22.6)	17 (25.8)	25 (35.7)	8 (11.6)	9 (13.6)	2 (6.7)
per transfer, n (%)	7 (25.9)	17 (27.9)	25 (40.3)	8 (14.8)	9 (14.8)	2 (7.4)
Implantation rate (%)^{r}	14.2 (26.8)	16.3 (30.5)	21.9 (30.6)	9.0 (23.7)	8.5 (21.7)	4.9 (20.1)

(Protocol 38602)
* Following initiation of Antagon™ therapy. Includes subjects who have complied with daily injections
‡ Median values
^{r} Mean (standard deviation)
† ET: Embryo Transfer
$^{\Omega}$ As evidenced by ultrasound at 5–6 weeks following ET

Antagon—Cont.

Before starting treatment with Antagon™, pregnancy must be excluded. Safe use of Antagon™ during pregnancy has not been established (see CONTRAINDICATIONS and PRECAUTIONS).

PRECAUTIONS

General

Caution is advised in patients with hypersensitivity to GnRH. These patients should be carefully monitored after the first injection. Anaphylactic reactions or ganirelix antibody formation have not been reported in the clinical trials for Antagon™ (ganirelix acetate) Injection.

The packaging of this product contains natural rubber latex which may cause allergic reactions.

Information for Patients

Prior to therapy with Antagon™ (ganirelix acetate) Injection, patients should be informed of the duration of treatment and monitoring procedures that will be required. The risk of possible adverse reactions should be discussed (see ADVERSE REACTIONS).

Antagon™ should not be prescribed if the patient is pregnant.

Laboratory Tests

A neutrophil count ≥ 8.3 ($\times 10^9$/L) was noted in 11.9% (up to 16.8×10^9/L) of all subjects treated within the adequate and well-controlled clinical trials. In addition, downward shifts within the Antagon™ (ganirelix acetate) Injection group were observed for hematocrit and total bilirubin. The clinical significance of these findings was not determined.

Drug Interactions

No formal drug-drug interaction studies have been performed.

Carcinogenesis and Mutagenesis, Impairment of Fertility

Long-term toxicity studies in animals have not been performed with Antagon™ (ganirelix acetate) Injection to evaluate the carcinogenic potential of the drug. Antagon™ did not induce a mutagenic response in the Ames test *(S. typhimurium* and *E. coli)* or produce chromosomal aberrations in *in vitro* assay using Chinese Hamster Ovary cells.

Pregnancy

Pregnancy Category X

Antagon™ (ganirelix acetate) Injection is contraindicated in pregnant women. When administered from Day 7 to near term to pregnant rats and rabbits at doses up to 10 and 30 µg/day (approximately 0.4 to 3.2 times the human dose based on body surface area), Antagon™ increased the incidence of litter resorption. There was no increase in fetal abnormalities. No treatment related changes in fertility, physical, or behavioral characteristics were observed in the offspring of female rats treated with Antagon™ during pregnancy and lactation.

The effects on fetal resorption are logical consequences of the alteration in hormonal levels brought about by the antigonadotrophic properties of this drug and could result in fetal loss in humans. Therefore, this drug should not be used in pregnant women (see CONTRAINDICATIONS).

Nursing Mothers

Antagon™ (ganirelix acetate) Injection should not be used by lactating women. It is not known whether this drug is excreted in human milk.

Geriatric Use

Clinical studies with Antagon™ (ganirelix acetate) Injection did not include a sufficient number of subjects aged 65 and over.

ADVERSE REACTIONS

The safety of Antagon™ (ganirelix acetate) Injection was evaluated in two randomized, parallel-group, multicenter controlled clinical studies. Treatment duration for Antagon™ ranged from 1 to 14 days. Table IV represents adverse events (AEs) from first day of Antagon™ administration until confirmation of pregnancy by ultrasound at an incidence of ≥ 1% of Antagon™-treated subjects without regard to causality.

[See table IV above]

Congenital Anomalies

Ongoing clinical follow-up studies of 283 newborns of women administered Antagon™ were reviewed. There were three neonates with major congenital anomalies and 18 neonates with minor congenital anomalies. The major congenital anomalies were: hydrocephalus/meningocele, omphalocele, and Beckwith-Wiedemann Syndrome. The minor congenital anomalies were: nevus, skin tags, sacral sinus, hemangioma, torticollis/asymmetric skull, talipes, supernumerary digit finger, hip subluxation, torticollis/high palate, occiput/abnormal hand crease, hernia umbilicalis, hernia inguinalis, hydrocele, undescended testis, and hydronephrosis. The causal relationship between these congenital anomalies and Antagon™ is unknown. Multiple factors, genetic and others (including, but not limited to ICSI, IVF, gonadotropins, progesterone) may confound ART (Assisted Reproductive Technology) procedures.

OVERDOSAGE

There have been no reports of overdosage with Antagon™ (ganirelix acetate) Injection in humans.

DOSAGE AND ADMINISTRATION

After initiating FSH therapy on Day 2 or 3 of the cycle, Antagon™ (ganirelix acetate) Injection 250 µg may be administered subcutaneously once daily during the early to mid follicular phase. By taking advantage of endogenous pituitary FSH secretion, the requirement for exogenously administered FSH may be reduced. Treatment with Antagon™ should be continued daily until the day of hCG administration. When a sufficient number of follicles of adequate size are present, as assessed by ultrasound, final maturation of follicles is induced by administering hCG. The administration of hCG should be withheld in cases where the ovaries are abnormally enlarged on the last day of FSH therapy to reduce the chance of developing OHSS.

Directions for Using Antagon™ (ganirelix acetate) Injection

1. Antagon™ is supplied in a sterile, prefilled syringe and is intended for SUBCUTANEOUS administration only.
2. Wash hands thoroughly with soap and water.
3. The most convenient sites for SUBCUTANEOUS injection are in the abdomen around the navel or upper thigh.
4. The injection site should be swabbed with a disinfectant to remove any surface bacteria. Clean about two inches around the point where the needle will be inserted and let the disinfectant dry for at least one minute before proceeding.
5. Remove needle cover.
6. Pinch up a large area of skin between the finger and thumb. Vary the injection site a little with each injection.
7. The needle should be inserted at the base of the pinched-up skin at an angle of 45–90° to the skin surface.
8. When the needle is correctly positioned, it will be difficult to draw back on the plunger. If any blood is drawn into the syringe, the needle tip has penetrated a vein or artery. If this happens, withdraw the needle slightly and reposition the needle without removing it from the skin. Alternatively, remove the needle and use a new, sterile, prefilled syringe. Cover the injection site with a swab containing disinfectant and apply pressure; the site should stop bleeding within one or two minutes.
9. Once the needle is correctly placed, depress the plunger slowly and steadily, so the solution is correctly injected and the skin is not damaged.
10. Pull the syringe out quickly and apply pressure to the site with a swab containing disinfectant.
11. Use the sterile, prefilled syringe only once and dispose of it properly.

TABLE III: Results from the multicenter, open-label, randomized study to assess the efficacy and safety of Antagon™ in women undergoing COH.

	Antagon™ 250 µg
No. subjects treated	463
Duration of GnRH analog (days)§¥	5.4 (2.0)
Duration of recombinant FSH (days)§¥	9.6 (2.0)
Serum E_2 (pg/mL) on day of hCG‡ 5th–95th percentiles	1190 373–3105
Serum LH (mIU/mL) on day of hCG‡ 5th–95th percentiles	1.6 0.6–6.9
No. of subjects with LH rise ≥ 10 mIU/mL*	13
No. of follicles > 11 mm§¥	10.7 (5.3)
No. of subjects with oocyte retrieval	440
No. of occytes¥	8.7 (5.6)
Fertilization rate	62.1%
No. subjects with ET†	399
No. of embryos transferred¥	2.2 (0.6)
No. of embryos¥	6.0 (4.5)
Ongoing pregnancy rates^Ω§	
per attempt, n (%)^λ	94 (20.3)
per transfer, n (%)	93 (23.3)
Implantation rate (%)¥	15.7 (29)

(Protocol 38607)
* Following initiation of Antagon™ therapy
‡ Median values
§ Restricted to subjects with hCG injection
¥ Mean (standard deviation)
† ET: Embryo Transfer
Ω As evidenced by ultrasound at 12–16 weeks following ET
λ Includes one patient who achieved pregnancy with intrauterine induction.
Some centers were limited to the transfer of ≤ 2 embryos based on local practice standards

TABLE IV: Incidence of common adverse events (Incidence ≥1% in Antagon™-treated subjects). Completed controlled clinical studies (All-subjects-treated group).

Adverse Events Occurring in ≥ 1%	Antagon™ N=794 % (n)
Abdominal Pain (gynecological)	4.8 (38)
Death Fetal	3.7 (29)
Headache	3.0 (24)
Ovarian Hyperstimulation Syndrome	2.4 (19)
Vaginal Bleeding	1.8 (14)
Injection Site Reaction	1.1 (9)
Nausea	1.1 (9)
Abdominal Pain (gastrointestinal)	1.0 (8)

HOW SUPPLIED

Antagon™ (ganirelix acetate) Injection is supplied in:

Disposable, sterile, prefilled 1 mL glass syringes containing 250 µg/0.5 mL of ganirelix acetate. Each Antagon™ sterile, prefilled syringe is affixed with a 27 gauge × ½ inch needle and is blister-packed.

Single syringe	NDC 0052-0301-51
Box of 5	NDC 0052-0301-61
Box of 50	NDC 0052-0301-71

Storage

Store at 25°C (77°F); excursions permitted to 15–30°C (59–86°F) [see USP Controlled Room Temperature]. Protect from light.

Rx only

Manufactured for Organon Inc.
West Orange, NJ 07052
by Vetter Pharma-Fertigung GmbH & Co. KG
Ravensburg, Germany
and packaged by Organon (Ireland) Ltd, Swords Co.
Dublin, Ireland
5310194 6/99 08

TICE® BCG, BCG Live ℞
BCG VACCINE USP
(for Intravesical use)

Distributed by Organon Inc.
(See page 2293 complete product information.)

CALDEROL® ℞
[*kal-dah 'rol*]
(calcifediol capsules, USP)

HOW SUPPLIED

20 µg (white, soft elastic capsules) bottle of 60
50 µg (orange, soft elastic capsules) bottle of 60
Shown in Product Identification Guide, page 327

CORTROSYN® ℞
[*cōr-trō-sin*]
(cosyntropin) for injection
FOR DIAGNOSTIC USE ONLY

DESCRIPTION

Cortrosyn® (cosyntropin) for injection is a sterile lyophilized powder in vials containing 0.25 mg of Cortrosyn® and 10 mg of mannitol to be reconstituted with 1 mL sodium chloride for injection, USP as solvent. Administration is by intravenous or intramuscular injection. Cosyntropin is α 1-24 corticotropin, a synthetic subunit of ACTH. It is an open chain polypeptide containing, from the N terminus, the first 24 of the 39 amino acids of natural ACTH. The sequence of amino acids in the 1-24 compound is as follows:

Ser — Tyr — Ser — Met — Glu — His — Phe — Arg — Trp — Gly — Lys
1 2 3 4 5 6 7 8 9 10 11
Pro — Val — Gly — Lys — Lys — Arg — Arg — Pro — Val — Lys — Val
12 13 14 15 16 17 18 19 20 21 22
Tyr — Pro
23 24

CLINICAL PHARMACOLOGY

Cortrosyn® (cosyntropin) for injection exhibits the full corticosteroidogenic activity of natural ACTH. Various studies have shown that the biologic activity of ACTH resides in the N-terminal portion of the molecule and that the 1-20 amino acid residue is the minimal sequence retaining full activity. Partial or complete loss of activity is noted with progressive shortening of the chain beyond 20 amino acid residue. For example, the decrement from 20 to 19 results in a 70% loss of potency.

The pharmacologic profile of Cortrosyn® is similar to that of purified natural ACTH. It has been established that 0.25 mg of Cortrosyn® will stimulate the adrenal cortex maximally and to the same extent as 25 units of natural ACTH. This dose of Cortrosyn® will produce maximal secretion of 17-OH corticosteroids, 17-ketosteroids and/or 17-ketogenic steroids.

The extra-adrenal effects which natural ACTH and Cortrosyn® have in common include increased melanotropic activity, increased growth hormone secretion and an adipokinetic effect. These are considered to be without physiological or clinical significance.

Animal, human and synthetic ACTH (1-39) which all contain 39 amino acids exhibit similar immunologic activity. This activity resides in the C-terminal portion of the molecule and the 22-39 amino acid residues exhibit the greatest degree of antigenicity. In contrast, synthetic polypeptides containing 1-19 or fewer amino acids have no detectable immunologic activity. Those containing 1-26, 1-24 or 1-23 amino acids have very little immunologic although full biologic activity. This property of Cortrosyn® assumes added importance in view of the known antigenicity of natural ACTH.

INDICATIONS AND USAGE

Cortrosyn® (cosyntropin) for injection is intended for use as a diagnostic agent in the screening of patients presumed to have adrenocortical insufficiency. Because of its rapid effect on the adrenal cortex it may be utilized to perform a 30-minute test of adrenal function (plasma cortisol response) as an office or outpatient procedure, using only 2 venipunctures. (See DOSAGE AND ADMINISTRATION section for details.)

Severe hypofunction of the pituitary-adrenal axis is usually associated with subnormal plasma cortisol values but a low basal level is not per se evidence of adrenal insufficiency and does not suffice to make the diagnosis. Many patients with proven insufficiency will have normal basal levels and will develop signs of insufficiency only when stressed. For this reason a criterion which should be used in establishing the diagnosis is the failure to respond to adequate corticotropin stimulation. When presumptive adrenal insufficiency is diagnosed by a subnormal Cortrosyn® test, further studies are indicated to determine if it is primary or secondary.

Primary adrenal insufficiency (Addison's disease) is the result of an intrinsic disease process, such as tuberculosis within the gland. The production of adrenocortical hormones is deficient despite high ACTH levels (feedback mechanism). Secondary or relative insufficiency arises as the result of defective production of ACTH leading in turn to disuse atrophy of the adrenal cortex. It is commonly seen, for example, as a result of corticosteroid therapy, Sheehan's syndrome and pituitary tumors or ablation.

The differentiation of both types is based on the premise that a primarily defective gland cannot be stimulated by ACTH whereas a secondarily defective gland is potentially functional and will respond to adequate stimulation with ACTH. Patients selected for further study as the result of a subnormal Cortrosyn® test should be given a 3 or 4 day course of treatment with Repository Corticotropin Injection USP and then retested. Suggested doses are 40 USP units twice daily for 4 days or 60 USP units twice daily for 3 days. Under these conditions little or no increase in plasma cortisol levels will be seen in Addison's disease whereas higher or even normal levels will be seen in cases with secondary adrenal insufficiency.

CONTRAINDICATIONS

The only contraindication to Cortrosyn® (cosyntropin) for injection is a history of a previous adverse reaction to it.

PRECAUTIONS

General

Cortrosyn® (cosyntropin) for injection exhibits slight immunologic activity, does not contain animal protein and is therefore less risky to use than natural ACTH. Patients known to be sensitized to natural ACTH with markedly positive skin tests will, with few exceptions, react negatively when tested intradermally with Cortrosyn®. Most patients with a history of a previous hypersensitivity reaction to natural ACTH or a pre-existing allergic disease will tolerate Cortrosyn®. Despite this however, Cortrosyn® is not completely devoid of immunologic activity and hypersensitivity reactions including rare anaphylaxis are possible. Therefore, the physician should be prepared, prior to injection, to treat any possible acute hypersensitivity reaction.

Drug Interactions

Corticotropin may accentuate the electrolyte loss associated with diuretic therapy.

Carcinogenesis, Mutagenesis, Impairment of Fertility

Long term studies in animals have not been performed to evaluate carcinogenic or mutagenic potential or impairment of fertility. A study in rats noted inhibition of reproductive function like natural ACTH.

Pregnancy

Pregnancy Category C. Animal reproduction studies have not been conducted with Cortrosyn®. It is also not known whether Cortrosyn® can cause fetal harm when administered to a pregnant woman or can affect reproduction capacity. Cortrosyn® should be given to a pregnant woman only if clearly needed.

Nursing Mothers

It is not known whether this drug is excreted in human milk. Because many drugs are excreted in human milk, caution should be exercised when Cortrosyn® is administered to a nursing woman.

Pediatric Usage

(See DOSAGE AND ADMINISTRATION section for details.)

ADVERSE REACTIONS

Since Cortrosyn® (cosyntropin) for injection is intended for diagnostic and not therapeutic use, adverse reactions other than a rare hypersensitivity reaction are not anticipated. A rare hypersensitivity reaction usually associated with a pre-existing allergic disease and/or a previous reaction to natural ACTH is possible. Symptoms may include slight whealing with splotchy erythema at the injection site. There have been rare reports of anaphylactic reaction. The following adverse reactions have been reported in patients after the administration of Cortrosyn® and the association has been neither confirmed or refuted.

- bradycardia
- tachycardia
- hypertension
- peripheral edema
- rash

DOSAGE AND ADMINISTRATION

Cortrosyn® (cosyntropin) for injection may be administered intramuscularly or as a direct intravenous injection when used as a rapid screening test of adrenal function. It may also be given as an intravenous infusion over a 4 to 8 hour period to provide a greater stimulus to the adrenal glands. Doses of Cortrosyn® 0.25 to 0.75 mg have been used in clinical studies and a maximal response noted with the smallest dose.

A suggested method for a rapid screening test of adrenal function has been described by Wood and associates (1). A control blood sample of 6 to 7 mL is collected in a heparinized tube. Reconstitute 0.25 mg of Cortrosyn® in solvent (ampul of 1 mL sodium chloride injection USP — 0.9%) and inject intramuscularly. In the pediatric population, aged 2 years or less, a dose of 0.125 mg will often suffice. A second blood sample is collected exactly 30 minutes later. Both blood samples should be refrigerated until sent to the laboratory for determination of the plasma cortisol response by some appropriate method. If it is not possible to send them to the laboratory or perform the fluorimetric procedure within 12 hours, then the plasma should be separated and refrigerated or frozen according to need.

Two alternative methods of administration are intravenous injection and infusion. Cortrosyn® can be injected intravenously in 2 to 5 mL of saline over a 2-minute period. When given as an intravenous infusion: Cortrosyn®, 0.25 mg may be added to glucose or saline solutions and given at the rate of approximately 40 micrograms per hour over a 6-hour period. It should not be added to blood or plasma as it is apt to be inactivated by enzymes. Adrenal response may be measured in the usual manner by determining urinary steroid excretion before and after treatment or by measuring plasma cortisol levels before and at the end of the infusion. The latter is preferable because the urinary steroid excretion does not always accurately reflect the adrenal or plasma cortisol response to ACTH.

The usual normal response in most cases is an approximate doubling of the basal level, provided that the basal level does not exceed the normal range. Patients receiving cortisone, hydrocortisone or spironolactone should omit their pre-test doses on the day selected for testing. Patients taking inadvertent doses of cortisone or hydrocortisone on the test day and patients taking spironolactone or women taking drugs which contain estrogen may exhibit abnormally high basal plasma cortisol levels. A paradoxical response may be noted in the cortisone or hydrocortisone group as seen in a decrease in plasma cortisol values following a stimulating dose of Cortrosyn®. In the spironolactone or estrogen group only a normal incremental response is to be expected. Many patients with normal adrenal function, however, do not respond to the expected degree so that the following criteria have been established to denote a normal response:

1. The control plasma cortisol level should exceed 5 micrograms/100 mL.
2. The 30-minute level should show an increment of at least 7 micrograms/100 mL above the basal level.
3. The 30-minute level should exceed 18 micrograms/100 mL. Comparable figures have been reported by Greig and co-workers (2).

Plasma cortisol levels usually peak about 45 to 60 minutes after an injection of Cortrosyn® and some prefer the 60-minute interval for testing for this reason. While it is true that the 60-minute values are usually higher than the 30-minute values, the difference may not be significant enough in most cases to outweigh the disadvantage of a longer testing period. If the 60-minute test period is used, the criterion for a normal response is an approximate doubling of the basal plasma cortisol value.

In patients with a raised plasma bilirubin or in patients where the plasma contains free hemoglobin, falsely high fluorescence measurements will result. The test may be performed at any time during the day but because of the physiological diurnal variation of plasma cortisol the criteria listed by Wood cannot apply. It has been shown that basal plasma cortisol levels and the post Cortrosyn® increment exhibit diurnal changes. However, the 30-minute plasma cortisol level remains unchanged throughout the day so that only this single criterion should be used (3).

Parenteral drug products should be inspected visually for particulate matter and discoloration whenever solution and container permit. Reconstituted Cortrosyn® should not be retained.

HOW SUPPLIED

Box containing: 10 vials of Cortrosyn® (cosyntropin) for injection 0.25 mg
NDC # 0052-0731-10
10 ampuls of solvent (sodium chloride for injection, USP).
NDC # 0052-0318-01

Rx only

REFERENCES

1. Wood, J.B. et al. LANCET 1.243, 1965.
2. Greig, W.R. et al. J. ENDOCR 34.411, 1966.
3. McGill, P.E. et al. ANN RHEUM DIS 26.123, 1967.

Manufactured for ORGANON INC.
By BEN VENUE LABORATORIES, INC. • BEDFORD OHIO 44146
or by
ORGANON INC. • WEST ORANGE, NEW JERSEY 07052
PRINTED IN USA-731S 5310012 REVISED 3/99

COTAZYM® ℞
[*kōt 'a zīm*]
(pancrelipase capsules, USP)

DESCRIPTION

COTAZYM® (pancrelipase capsules, USP) contains pancrelipase obtained from the porcine pancreas. Pancrelipase is composed principally of lipase, amylase and protease and is used for oral digestive enzyme replacement. Each capsule contains not less than:

Lipase	8,000 USP Units
Protease	30,000 USP Units
Amylase	30,000 USP Units

At release, up to 25% more lipase may be present.

Each capsule also contains the inactive ingredients: cornstarch, precipitated calcium carbonate, gelatin, magnesium stearate, talc, titanium dioxide, FD&C Green #3 and D&C Yellow #10 as coloring.

Continued on next page

Cotazym—Cont.

CLINICAL PHARMACOLOGY

Pancrelipase, USP contains lipase, protease and amylase obtained from porcine pancreas. Normal pancreatic function includes secretion of proteolytic enzymes such as proteases (trypsin and chymotrypsin), nonproteolytic enzymes such as lipase and amylase, and electrolytes such as bicarbonate, chloride, sodium and potassium. Lipase, protease and amylase break down fat, protein, and starches, respectively, in the small intestine. Lipase hydrolyzes fats into glycerol and fatty acids. Protease converts proteins into proteoses and derived substances, while amylase converts starches into dextrins and sugars. Pancreatic enzymes are used to correct maldigestion, malabsorption and pain associated with pancreatic insufficiency. The major maldigestion/malabsorption problems arise from incomplete fat digestion. Exogenous pancrelipase reduces the amount of nitrogen and fat excreted in the stool. Activity of these products are dependent upon the amount of pancrelipase delivered to the small intestine. This delivery can be hampered by inactivation from low gastric pH, acidic precipitation of bile salts, and the proteolytic activity of the component protease. Pancreatic enzymes are more active at pH greater than 4, with lipase being the most sensitive of the pancreatic enzymes to inactivation by low pH. Malabsorption of fat is likely if an individual, ingesting 100 gm of fat per day, excretes more than 7 gm of fat (or 18 mmol) in a 24-hour period. Malabsorption of protein is likely if nitrogen excretion is greater than 2.5 gm per 24-hours (16% of protein by weight is nitrogen). In order for fat maldigestion to occur, a pancreas must secrete less than 10% of its normal output.

The enzymes contained in COTAZYM® (pancrelipase capsules, USP) are not absorbed systemically; therefore, pharmacokinetic studies of their absorption, distribution, metabolism, and excretion have not been conducted. The contents of COTAZYM® capsules are released in the stomach, whereupon some of the enzyme is inactivated by acid. The remaining enzymes traverse into the duodenum, where they facilitate digestion and subsequently are hydrolyzed to their constituent amino acids by proteases. Pancreatic extracts contain purines which are absorbed into the general circulation and are converted to uric acid. This uric acid could lead to hyperuricemia, hyperuricosuria, and possible kidney damage. Chymotrypsin activity in the stool is indicative of exocrine pancreatic function. Ingestion of pancrelipase enzymes result in an increase in chymotrypsin in the stool.

Clinical bioactivity and bioavailability studies in patients with exocrine pancreatic insufficiency from cystic fibrosis or chronic alcoholic pancreatitis have shown that the enzymes from COTAZYM® are released at the duodenojejunal junction.

A study was conducted in 6 patients (ages 43–58) with pancrelipase insufficiency secondary to chronic alcoholic pancreatitis. Four of the patients received 4 capsules of COTAZYM® with a standard test meal. The mean (±SEM) percent of ingested dose of lipase and trypsin delivered to the duodenum postprandially was 15.1% (±2.1) and 11.3% (±1.6), respectively. A randomized 3-way crossover study was also performed on this group of patients to further ascertain bioavailability. Each patient received 10 PANCREATIN® tablets per meal, 4 COTAZYM® capsules per meal, and 4 or 8 PANCREASE® capsules per meal in a randomized order. In patients who received COTAZYM®, PANCREASE®, or PANCREATIN® while on a 100 gm fat/day diet, the fat excretions were 15.0 gm, 13.0 gm, and 19.0 gm per 24 hours, respectively, while fat excretion was 31.0 gm/24 hours in the no enzyme treatment group.[1] An investigation was also conducted in 8 cystic fibrosis patients (ages 18–29) with steatorrhea who were already on some type of enzyme replacement therapy. Two patients were given a test meal together with 4 capsules of COTAZYM®. The mean delivery of lipase and trypsin to the duodenum postprandially was 7.6% (3.5–11.7%) and 14.5% (12–17%) of intake, respectively. A randomized 2-way crossover study was performed on 7 of these 8 patients. Each patient received 4 COTAZYM® capsules per meal or 8 PANCREASE® capsules per meal, while on a 100 gm fat/day diet. Steatorrhea was controlled with 19.2% of fat excreted (as % of fat intake) for COTAZYM® and 5.9% of fat excreted for PANCREASE®, reduced from 28% fat excreted with previous treatments.[2]

SPECIAL POPULATIONS

Pediatric and Geriatric Patients

There is no evidence to suggest that the bioactivity or bioavailability of COTAZYM® would differ markedly in pediatric or geriatric patients from other patient populations.

CLINICAL STUDIES

Cystic Fibrosis

In a single center, unblinded, non-randomized, active-controlled, one sequence, 2-period (with no washout period) crossover Canadian study of 15 patients, under the age of 4 years, with exocrine pancreatic insufficiency secondary to cystic fibrosis, COTAZYM® (pancrelipase capsules, USP) was compared to another pancreatic enzyme preparation for the treatment of fat malabsorption.[3]

COTAZYM® significantly reduced fecal fat as a percentage of intake when compared to baseline as follows:

	Baseline Mean ± SEM	COTAZYM® Mean ± SEM
Fecal Fat (as % of intake)	29.5 ± 5.2	14.7 ± 1.8 P value = 0.088

In a single center, randomized, double-blind, placebo controlled, 2-period crossover, 5-day treatment U.S. study in 10 male patients, ages 10–16 years, with exocrine pancreatic insufficiency secondary to cystic fibrosis, COTAZYM® and another pancreatic enzyme preparation were compared to placebo for treatment of fat malasbsorption.[4]

COTAZYM® significantly reduced fecal fat as compared to placebo as follows:

	Placebo Mean ± SEM	COTAZYM® Mean ± SEM
Fecal Fat Excretion (grams/day)	67.9 ± 13.1	29.9 ± 7.0 P value < 0.005

Chronic Pancreatitis

In a multicenter, randomized, unblinded, 3-period crossover, 6-day treatment U.S. study in 6 male patients, ages 43–58 years, with exocrine pancreatic insufficiency from chronic alcoholic pancreatitis, COTAZYM® (pancrelipase capsules, USP) and two other pancreatic enzyme preparations were compared to a no treatment control for the treatment of fat malabsorption.[1]

COTAZYM® significantly reduced fecal fat as compared to the no treatment control as follows:

	Control Mean ± SEM	COTAZYM® Mean ± SEM
Fecal Fat Excretion (grams/day)	31.0 ± 2.0	15.0 ± 2.0 P value < 0.005

INDICATIONS AND USAGE

COTAZYM® (pancrelipase capsules, USP) capsules are indicated for treatment of steatorrhea due to exocrine pancreatic enzyme deficiency in such conditions as cystic fibrosis and chronic pancreatitis.

CONTRAINDICATIONS

COTAZYM® (pancrelipase capsules, USP) is contraindicated in those individuals who are hypersensitive to antigens of porcine origin.

WARNINGS

(See PRECAUTIONS and DOSAGE AND ADMINISTRATION.)

PRECAUTIONS

General

Large doses of delayed release pancreatic enzyme preparations taken by patients with cystic fibrosis have been associated with fibrosing colonopathy (colonic stricture). While COTAZYM® (pancrelipase capsules, USP) is an immediate release product and such products have not generally been associated with the lesion, the doses recommended should not be exceeded unless justified by individual patient need and response (see DOSAGE AND ADMINISTRATION and ADVERSE REACTIONS). If capsules must be opened for any reason, care should be taken that the powder is not inhaled or spilled on hands; it may cause serious allergic reaction or be irritating to the skin or mucous membranes. A mask and gloves should be worn while handling opened capsules.

Folic acid supplementation during pregnancy is important. Daily oral supplementation with folic acid before conception and during pregnancy can substantially reduce the occurrence of neural tube defects (anencephaly and spina bifida). Women should take folic acid if they are pregnant, or are thinking of becoming pregnant during treatment with COTAZYM®.

Information for Patients

Physicians are advised to discuss the following issues with patients for whom they prescribe COTAZYM® (pancrelipase capsules, USP):

Taking the Capsules

Patients should be instructed not to increase their COTAZYM® (pancrelipase capsules, USP) dose without consulting their physician. If it becomes necessary to open the COTAZYM® capsules, inhalation of the powder or contact with the skin or mucous membranes should be avoided. It is suggested mask and gloves be worn when opening capsules. COTAZYM® should not be taken by patients with known hypersensitivity to antigens of porcine origin. Sensitive individuals may experience allergic reactions.

Folic acid supplementation during pregnancy is important. Daily oral supplementation with folic acid before conception and during pregnancy can substantially reduce the occurrence of neural tube defects (anencephaly and spina bifida). Women should take folic acid if they are pregnant, or are thinking of becoming pregnant during treatment with COTAZYM®.

Concomitant Medication

Patients should be advised not to take COTAZYM® (pancrelipase capsules, USP) together with a combination of calcium carbonate and magnesium hydroxide. Calcium carbonate and magnesium hydroxide may be found in certain antacids. Calcium carbonate can also be found in certain calcium or mineral supplements. COTAZYM® may interfere with the absorption of folic acid and iron. Patients should consult with their physician if taking folic acid or iron containing preparations.

Pregnancy

COTAZYM® (pancrelipase capsules, USP) may interfere with the absorption of folic acid. Folic acid supplementation during pregnancy is important. Daily oral supplementation with folic acid before conception and during pregnancy can substantially reduce the occurrence of neural tube defects (anencephaly and spina bifida). Patients should be advised to notify their physician if they are pregnant or are thinking of becoming pregnant during treatment with COTAZYM® (pancrelipase capsules, USP).

Nursing

Patients should be advised to notify their physician if they are breast-feeding an infant.

Drug Interactions

Antacids containing calcium carbonate and magnesium hydroxide should not be taken concurrently with pancrelipase. The combination of calcium carbonate and magnesium hydroxide with pancrelipase may precipitate glycine-conjugated bile acids and may form calcium and magnesium fatty acid soaps, causing a decrease in fat absorption and thus an increase in steatorrhea.

Carcinogenesis, Mutagenesis and Impairment of Fertility

Long-term animal studies for carcinogenesis and studies evaluating the potential for impairment of fertility or mutagenesis have not been performed with COTAZYM® (pancrelipase capsules, USP).

Pregnancy

Pregnancy Category C

Animal reproductive studies have not been conducted with COTAZYM® (pancrelipase capsules, USP). It is not known whether COTAZYM® can cause fetal harm when administered to a pregnant woman or can affect reproductive capacity. COTAZYM® should be given to a pregnant woman only if clearly needed.

Nursing Mothers

It is not known if COTAZYM® (pancrelipase capsules, USP) is excreted in human milk. Because many products are excreted in human milk, caution should be exercised when COTAZYM® is administered to nursing mothers.

ADVERSE REACTIONS

Adverse reactions to COTAZYM® (pancrelipase capsules, USP) have been reported uncommonly. The most frequent adverse reactions reported during clinical use are diarrhea and stool abnormalities, such as green stools. Other reactions reported include pharyngitis, vomiting, abdominal pain, gastric burning, syncope, mouth irritation, mouth ulcers, mild anemia, abnormal smell and taste, stomach trouble and belching. Hyperuricosuria and/or hyperuricemia have been reported in patients taking high doses of COTAZYM®; pancreatic extracts have high purine content. Renal damage has not been reported. Hypersensitivity reactions, such as anaphylaxis, allergy, nasal irritation, coughing spells and episodes of bronchospasm, can occur in people exposed to the enzyme powder from opened capsules. High doses of the powder may cause mouth or perianal excoriation. In addition, pancreatic enzyme preparations may interfere with folic acid and iron absorption.

There is a report of a child with cystic fibrosis who developed fibrosing colonopathy, and who has been treated with delayed-release pancreatic enzyme preparations as well as COTAZYM® prior to detection of the lesion.

OVERDOSAGE

No cases of acute overdose have been reported with COTAZYM® (pancrelipase capsules, USP). Hyperuricemia and/or hyperuricosuria have been reported in patients chronically taking high doses of COTAZYM® (pancrelipase capsules, USP). The minimum effective dose of COTAZYM® should be determined and adhered to for each patient. Large doses of delayed-release pancreatic enzyme preparations taken by patients with cystic fibrosis have been associated with fibrosing colonopathy (see PRECAUTIONS).

DOSAGE AND ADMINISTRATION

Cystic Fibrosis

The dosage of COTAZYM® (pancrelipase capsules, USP) must be individualized according to the patient's remaining exocrine pancreatic function, pH of the gut lumen (if such measurements are routinely taken) and intake of fat and protein. Dosage should depend on nutritional intake as well as body weight, and varies with age. A high caloric diet with unrestricted fat appropriate to age and clinical status should be consumed. While the dose may need to be adjusted for control of steatorrhea, a total daily dose should not exceed 2500 lipase units/kg per meal without careful evaluation of the patient. A dose higher than 6000 lipase units/kg per meal should not be administered[5] (see PRECAUTIONS).

Prior to treatment, the patient's stool should be evaluated microscopically for the presence of fat droplets. If visible, a 72-hour fat balance study should be performed while monitoring nutrient intake, to determine the extent of malabsorption. In patients with meconium ileus, a fat balance study is not required prior to establishing a dosage and beginning treatment with COTAZYM®. Do not exceed recommended dosage. Based on 2500 lipase units/kg per meal, the maximum recommended dosage for a 70 kg patient would be 20 capsules per meal (60 capsules/day for 3 meals). Dosages greater than 2500 lipase units/kg per meal should only be used with caution and only if safely tolerated by the patient and documented to be effective by 3 day fecal fat measures that indicate a significantly improved coefficient of absorption.[5] Infants should be given a total of 2000 to 4000 lipase units for each 120 mL (4 oz.) of formula or each breast feeding. For other children less than 4 years of age, dosing should begin with 1000 lipase units/kg for each meal. For children 4 years of age or older, 500 lipase units/kg for each meal should be initiated. For a snack, half the dose for a meal should be given.

Chronic Pancreatitis
One or two capsules should be administered for control of symptoms and adjusted as needed.

HOW SUPPLIED

COTAZYM® (pancrelipase capsules, USP) are opaque green capsules imprinted with "Organon" and "381". COTAZYM® is supplied in bottles of 100, NDC# 0052-0381-91, and bottles of 500, NDC# 0052-0381-95.

Storage: Not to exceed 25°C (77°F). Store in dry place when opened.

Dispense: In tight container as defined in the USP.

REFERENCES

1. Dutta SK, Rubin J, Harvey J. Comparative Evaluation of the Therapeutic Efficacy of a pH-Sensitive Enteric Coated Pancreatic Enzyme Preparation with Conventional Pancreatic Enzyme Therapy in the Treatment of Exocrine Pancreatic Insufficiency. *Gastroenterology* 1983;84:476–482.
2. Dutta SK, Hubbard VS, Appler M. Critical examination of therapeutic efficacy of a pH-sensitive enteric-coated pancreatic enzyme preparation in treatment of exocrine pancreatic insufficiency secondary to cystic fibrosis. *Dig Dis and Sci* 1988;33:1237–1244.
3. Data on File at Organon Inc., W. Orange, NJ, USA
4. Mischler EH, Parrell S, Farrell PM, Odell GB. Comparison of effectiveness of pancreatic enzyme preparations in cystic fibrosis. *Am J Dis Child* 1982;136:1060–1063.
5. Borowitz DS, Grand RJ, Durie PR, and the Consensus Committee. Use of pancreatic enzyme supplements for patients with cystic fibrosis in the context of fibrosing colonopathy. *J Ped* 1995;127:681–684.

Caution: Federal law prohibits dispensing without a prescription.

Organon Inc.
375 Mt. Pleasant Avenue
West Orange, NJ 07052

Shown in Product Identification Guide, page 327

Revision 8/97

COTAZYM®-S ℞

[*kōt 'a zīm-s*]
(pancrelipase, USP)
Enteric coated spheres

Each capsule contains not less than:

5,000	USP Units of Lipase
20,000	USP Units of Protease
20,000	USP Units of Amylase

HOW SUPPLIED

Bottles of 100 capsules
Bottles of 500 capsules

Shown in Product Identification Guide, page 327

DECA-DURABOLIN® Ⓒ℞

(nandrolone decanoate injection, USP)

HOW SUPPLIED

100 mg/mL—2 mL vials—NDC-0052-0697-02
200 mg/mL—1 mL vials—NDC-0052-0698-01

DESOGEN® ℞

(desogestrel and ethinyl estradiol) Tablets

PATIENTS SHOULD BE COUNSELED THAT THIS PRODUCT DOES NOT PROTECT AGAINST HIV INFECTION (AIDS) AND OTHER SEXUALLY TRANSMITTED DISEASES.
Rx only

DESCRIPTION

Desogen® 28 Tablets provide an oral contraceptive regimen of 21 white round tablets each containing 0.15 mg desogestrel (13-ethyl-11- methylene-18,19-dinor-17 alpha-pregn- 4-en- 20-yn-17-ol) and 0.03 mg ethinyl estradiol (19-nor-17 alpha-pregna-1,3,5 (10)-trien-20-yne-3,17-diol). Inactive ingredients include vitamin E, corn starch, povidone, stearic acid, colloidal silicon dioxide, lactose, hydroxypropyl methylcellulose, polyethylene glycol, titanium dioxide and talc. Desogen® 28 also contains 7 green round tablets containing the following inactive ingredients: lactose, corn starch, magnesium stearate, FD&C Blue No. 2 aluminum lake, ferric oxide, hydroxypropyl methylcellulose, polyethylene glycol, titanium dioxide and talc.

DESOGESTREL

ETHINYL ESTRADIOL

CLINICAL PHARMACOLOGY

Pharmacodynamics
Combination oral contraceptives act by suppression of gonadotropins. Although the primary mechanism of this action is inhibition of ovulation, other alterations include changes in the cervical mucus, which increase the difficulty of sperm entry into the uterus, and changes in the endometrium which reduce the likelihood of implantation.

Receptor binding studies, as well as studies in animals and humans, have shown that 3-keto-desogestrel, the biologically active metabolite of desogestrel, combines high progestational activity with minimal intrinsic androgenicity (91,92). Desogestrel, in combination with ethinyl estradiol, does not counteract the estrogen-induced increase in SHBG, resulting in lower serum levels of free testosterone (96–99).

Pharmacokinetics
Desogestrel is rapidly and almost completely absorbed and converted into 3-keto-desogestrel, its biologically active metabolite. Following oral administration, the relative bioavailability of desogestrel, as measured by serum levels of 3-keto-desogestrel, is approximately 84%.

In the third cycle of use after a single dose of Desogen®, maximum concentrations of 3-keto-desogestrel of 2,805±1,203 pg/mL (mean±SD) are reached at 1.4±0.8 hours. The area under the curve ($AUC_{0-\infty}$) is 33,858±11,043 pg/mL·hr after a single dose. At steady state, attained from at least day 19 onwards, maximum concentrations of 5,840±1,667 pg/mL are reached at 1.4±0.9 hours. The minimum plasma levels of 3-keto-desogestrel at steady state are 1,400±560 pg/mL. The AUC_{0-24} at steady state is 52,299±17,878 pg/mL·hr. The mean $AUC_{0-\infty}$ for 3-keto-desogestrel at single dose is significantly lower than the mean AUC_{0-24} at steady state. This indicates that the kinetics of 3-keto-desogestrel are non-linear due to an increase in binding of 3-keto-desogestrel to sex hormone-binding globulin in the cycle, attributed to increased sex hormone-binding globulin levels which are induced by the daily administration of ethinyl estradiol. Sex hormone-binding globulin levels increased significantly in the third treatment cycle from day 1 (150±64 nmol/L) to day 21 (230±59 nmol/L).

The elimination half-life of 3-keto-desogestrel is approximately 38±20 hours at steady state. In addition to 3-keto-desogestrel, other phase I metabolites are 3α-OH-desogestrel, 3β-OH-desogestrel, and 3α-OH-5α-H-desogestrel. These other metabolites are not known to have any pharmacologic effects, and are further converted in part by conjugation (phase II metabolism) into polar metabolites, mainly sulfates and glucuronides.

Ethinyl estradiol is rapidly and almost completely absorbed. In the third cycle of use after a single dose of Desogen®, the relative bioavailability is approximately 83%.

In the third cycle of use after a single dose of Desogen®, maximum concentrations of ethinyl estradiol of 95±34 pg/mL are reached at 1.5±0.8 hours. The $AUC_{0-\infty}$ is 1,471±268 pg/mL·hr after a single dose. At steady state, attained from at least day 19 onwards, maximum ethinyl estradiol concentrations of 141±48 pg/mL are reached at about 1.4±0.7 hours. The minimum serum levels of ethinyl estradiol at steady state are 24±8.3 pg/mL. The AUC_{0-24}, at steady state is 1,117±302 pg/mL·hr. The mean $AUC_{0-\infty}$ for ethinyl estradiol following a single dose during treatment cycle 3 does not significantly differ from the mean AUC_{0-24} at steady state. This finding indicates linear kinetics for ethinyl estradiol.

The elimination half-life is 26±6.8 hours at steady state. Ethinyl estradiol is subject to a significant degree of presystemic conjugation (phase II metabolism). Ethinyl estradiol escaping gut wall conjugation undergoes phase I metabolism and hepatic conjugation (phase II metabolism). Major phase I metabolites are 2-OH-ethinyl estradiol and 2-methoxy-ethinyl estradiol. Sulfate and glucuronide conjugates of both ethinyl estradiol and phase I metabolites, which are excreted in bile, can undergo enterohepatic circulation.

INDICATIONS AND USAGE

Desogen® Tablets are indicated for the prevention of pregnancy in women who elect to use oral contraceptives as a method of contraception.

Oral contraceptives are highly effective. Table I lists the typical accidental pregnancy rates for users of combination oral contraceptives and other methods of contraception. The efficacy of these contraceptive methods, except sterilization, depends upon the reliability with which they are used. Correct and consistent use of these methods can result in lower failure rates.

TABLE I: LOWEST EXPECTED AND TYPICAL FAILURE RATES (%) DURING THE FIRST YEAR OF USE OF A CONTRACEPTIVE METHOD

Method	Lowest Expected*	Typical**
Oral Contraceptives		3
combined	0.1	N/A
progestin only	0.5	N/A
Diaphragm with spermicidal cream or jelly	6	18
Spermicides alone (foam, creams, jellies and vaginal suppositories)	3	21
Vaginal Sponge		
nulliparous	6	18
parous	9	28
IUD (medicated)	2	3
Implant		
capsules	0.04	0.04
rods	0.03	0.03
Condom without spermicide	2	12
Cervical Cap	6	18
Periodic abstinence (all methods)	1–9	20
Female sterilization	0.2	0.4
Male sterilization	0.1	0.15
No contraception (planned pregnancy)	85	85

Adapted from J. Trussell, et al. Table 1, ref. #1.
N/A—Data not available.
* The author's best estimate of the percentage of women expected to experience an accidental pregnancy among couples who initiate a method (not necessarily for the first time) and who use it consistently and correctly during the first year, if they do not stop for any other reason.
** This term represents "typical" couples who initiate use of a method (not necessarily for the first time), who experience an accidental pregnancy during the first year, if they do not stop use for any other reason.

In clinical trials with Desogen®, 2,004 subjects completed 19,181 cycles and a total of 12 pregnancies were reported. This represents an overall user-efficacy pregnancy rate of 0.81 woman-years. This rate includes patients who did not take the drug correctly.

CONTRAINDICATIONS

Oral contraceptives should not be used in women who currently have the following conditions:
- Thrombophlebitis or thromboembolic disorders
- A past history of deep vein thrombophlebitis or thromboembolic disorders
- Cerebral vascular or coronary artery disease
- Known or suspected carcinoma of the breast
- Carcinoma of the endometrium or other known or suspected estrogen-dependent neoplasia
- Undiagnosed abnormal genital bleeding
- Cholestatic jaundice of pregnancy or jaundice with prior pill use
- Hepatic adenomas or carcinomas
- Known or suspected pregnancy

WARNINGS

Cigarette smoking increases the risk of serious cardiovascular side effects from oral contraceptive use. This risk increases with age and with heavy smoking (15 or more cigarettes per day) and is quite marked in women over 35 years of age. Women who use oral contraceptives should be strongly advised not to smoke.

The use of oral contraceptives is associated with increased risks of several serious conditions including myocardial infarction, thromboembolism, stroke, hepatic neoplasia, and gallbladder disease, although the risk of serious morbidity or mortality is very small in healthy women without underlying risk factors. The risk of morbidity and mortality increases significantly in the presence of other underlying risk factors such as hypertension, hyperlipidemias, obesity and diabetes.

Practitioners prescribing oral contraceptives should be familiar with the following information relating to these risks. The information contained in this package insert is principally based on studies carried out in patients who used oral contraceptives with formulations of higher doses of estrogens and progestogens than those in common use today. The effect of long-term use of the oral contraceptives with formulations of lower doses of both estrogens and progestogens remains to be determined.

Throughout this labeling, epidemiological studies reported are of two types: retrospective or case control studies and prospective or cohort studies. Case control studies provide a

Continued on next page

Desogen—Cont.

measure of the relative risk of a disease, namely, a *ratio* of the incidence of a disease among oral contraceptive users to that among non-users. The relative risk does not provide information on the actual clinical occurrence of a disease. Cohort studies provide a measure of attributable risk, which is the *difference* in the incidence of disease between oral contraceptive users and non-users. The attributable risk does provide information about the actual occurrence of a disease in the population (Adapted from refs. 2 and 3 with the author's permission). For further information, the reader is referred to a text on epidemiological methods.

1. THROMBOEMBOLIC DISORDERS AND OTHER VASCULAR PROBLEMS

a. Myocardial infarction

An increased risk of myocardial infarction has been attributed to oral contraceptive use. This risk is primarily in smokers or women with other underlying risk factors for coronary artery disease such as hypertension, hypercholesterolemia, morbid obesity, and diabetes. The relative risk of heart attack for current oral contraceptive users has been estimated to be two to six (4–10). The risk is very low in women under the age of 30.

Smoking in combination with oral contraceptive use has been shown to contribute substantially to the incidence of myocardial infarctions in women in their mid-thirties or older with smoking accounting for the majority of excess cases (11). Mortality rates associated with circulatory disease have been shown to increase substantially in smokers, especially in those 35 years of age and older among women who use oral contraceptives. (See Table II.)

TABLE II: CIRCULATORY DISEASE MORTALITY RATES PER 100,000 WOMAN-YEARS BY AGE, SMOKING STATUS AND ORAL CONTRACEPTIVE USE

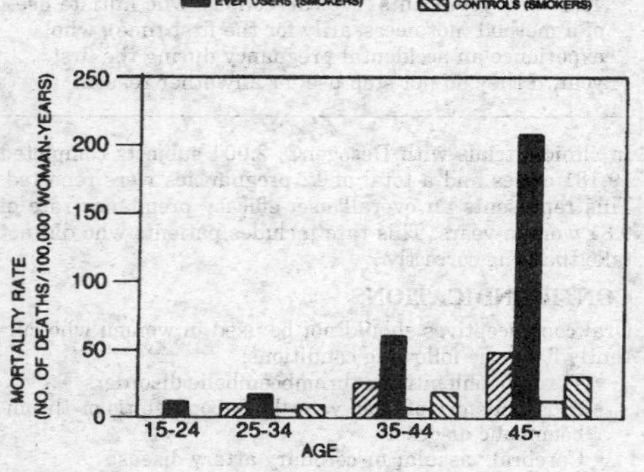

(Adapted from P.M. Layde and V. Beral, ref. #12.)

Oral contraceptives may compound the effects of well-known risk factors, such as hypertension, diabetes, hyperlipidemias, age and obesity (13). In particular, some progestogens are known to decrease HDL cholesterol and cause glucose intolerance, while estrogens may create a state of hyperinsulinism (14–18). Oral contraceptives have been shown to increase blood pressure among users (see section 9 in WARNINGS). Similar effects on risk factors have been associated with an increased risk of heart disease. Oral contraceptives must be used with caution in women with cardiovascular disease risk factors. Desogestrel has minimal androgenic activity (see CLINICAL PHARMACOLOGY) and there is some evidence that the risk of myocardial infarction associated with oral contraceptives is lower when the progestogen has minimal androgenic activity than when the activity is greater (100).

b. Thromboembolism

An increased risk of thromboembolic and thrombotic disease associated with the use of oral contraceptives is well established. Case control studies have found the relative risk of users compared to non-users to be 3 for the first episode of superficial venous thrombosis, 4 to 11 for deep vein thrombosis or pulmonary embolism, and 1.5 to 6 for women with predisposing conditions for venous thromboembolic disease (2,3,19–24). Cohort studies have shown the relative risk to be somewhat lower, about 3 for new cases and about 4.5 for new cases requiring hospitalization (25). The risk of thromboembolic disease associated with oral contraceptives is not related to length of use and disappears after pill use is stopped (2).

In two case-control studies and one cohort study of venous thromboembolism, third generation oral contraceptives, including those containing desogestrel, were reported to have a relative risk between 1.5 and 2.4 when compared to certain second generation oral contraceptives (101–103). These risks are within the above-mentioned range for deep vein thrombosis and pulmonary embolism. A relative risk of 2 would translate into an additional 1–2 cases of non-fatal venous thromboembolism per 10,000 women-years of use. The risk of venous thromboembolic disease associated with oral contraceptives does not increase with length of use and disappears after pill use is stopped.

A two- to four-fold increase in relative risk of post-operative thromboembolic complications has been reported with the use of oral contraceptives (9). The relative risk of venous thrombosis in women who have predisposing conditions is twice that of women without such medical conditions (26). If feasible, oral contraceptives should be discontinued at least four weeks prior to and for two weeks after elective surgery of a type associated with an increase in risk of thromboembolism and during and following prolonged immobilization. Since the immediate postpartum period is also associated with an increased risk of thromboembolism, oral contraceptives should be started no earlier than four weeks after delivery in women who elect not to breast feed.

TABLE III: ANNUAL NUMBER OF BIRTH-RELATED OR METHOD-RELATED DEATHS ASSOCIATED WITH CONTROL OF FERTILITY PER 100,000 NON-STERILE WOMEN, BY FERTILITY CONTROL METHOD ACCORDING TO AGE

Method of control and outcome	15–19	20–24	25–29	30–34	35–39	40–44
No fertility control methods*	7.0	7.4	9.1	14.8	25.7	28.2
Oral contraceptives non-smoker**	0.3	0.5	0.9	1.9	13.8	31.6
Oral contraceptives smoker**	2.2	3.4	6.6	13.5	51.1	117.2
IUD**	0.8	0.8	1.0	1.0	1.4	1.4
Condom*	1.1	1.6	0.7	0.2	0.3	0.4
Diaphragm/spermicide*	1.9	1.2	1.2	1.3	2.2	2.8
Periodic abstinence*	2.5	1.6	1.6	1.7	2.9	3.6

* Deaths are birth related
** Deaths are method related

Adapted from H.W. Ory, ref. #35.

c. Cerebrovascular diseases

Oral contraceptives have been shown to increase both the relative and attributable risks of cerebrovascular events (thrombotic and hemorrhagic strokes), although, in general, the risk is greatest among older (>35 years), hypertensive women who also smoke. Hypertension was found to be a risk factor for both users and non-users, for both types of strokes, and smoking interacted to increase the risk of stroke (27–29).

In a large study, the relative risk of thrombotic strokes has been shown to range from 3 for normotensive users to 14 for users with severe hypertension (30). The relative risk of hemorrhagic stroke is reported to be 1.2 for non-smokers who used oral contraceptives, 2.6 for smokers who did not use oral contraceptives, 7.6 for smokers who used oral contraceptives, 1.8 for normotensive users and 25.7 for users with severe hypertension (30). The attributable risk is also greater in older women (3).

d. Dose-related risk of vascular disease from oral contraceptives

A positive association has been observed between the amount of estrogen and progestogen in oral contraceptives and the risk of vascular disease (31–33). A decline in serum high-density lipoproteins (HDL) has been reported with many progestational agents (14–16). A decline in serum high-density lipoproteins has been associated with an increased incidence of ischemic heart disease. Because estrogens increase HDL cholesterol, the net effect of an oral contraceptive depends on a balance achieved between doses of estrogen and progestogen and the nature and absolute amount of progestogens used in the contraceptives. The amount of both hormones should be considered in the choice of an oral contraceptive.

Minimizing exposure to estrogen and progestogen is in keeping with good principles of therapeutics. For any particular estrogen/progestogen combination, the dosage regimen prescribed should be one which contains the least amount of estrogen and progestogen that is compatible with a low failure rate and the needs of the individual patient. New acceptors of oral contraceptive agents should be started on preparations containing 0.035 mg or less of estrogen.

e. Persistence of risk of vascular disease

There are two studies which have shown persistence of risk of vascular disease for ever-users of oral contraceptives. In a study in the United States, the risk of developing myocardial infarction after discontinuing oral contraceptives persists for at least 9 years for women 40–49 years old who had used oral contraceptives for five or more years, but this increased risk was not demonstrated in other age groups (8). In another study in Great Britain, the risk of developing cerebrovascular disease persisted for at least 6 years after discontinuation of oral contraceptives, although excess risk was very small (34). However, both studies were performed with oral contraceptive formulations containing 0.05 mg or higher of estrogens.

2. ESTIMATES OF MORTALITY FROM CONTRACEPTIVE USE

One study gathered data from a variety of sources which have estimated the mortality rate associated with different methods of contraception at different ages (Table III). These estimates include the combined risk of death associated with contraceptive methods plus the risk attributable to pregnancy in the event of method failure. Each method of contraception has its specific benefits and risks. The study concluded that with the exception of oral contraceptive users 35 and older who smoke and 40 and older who do not smoke, mortality associated with all methods of birth control is low and below that associated with childbirth.

The observation of an increase in risk of mortality with age for oral contraceptive users is based on data gathered in the 1970's (35). Current clinical recommendation involves the use of lower estrogen dose formulations and a careful consideration of risk factors. In 1989, the Fertility and Maternal Health Drugs Advisory Committee was asked to review the use of oral contraceptives in women 40 years of age and over. The Committee concluded that although cardiovascular disease risk may be increased with oral contraceptive use after age 40 in healthy non-smoking women (even with the newer low-dose formulations), there are also greater potential health risks associated with pregnancy in older women and with the alternative surgical and medical procedures which may be necessary if such women do not have access to effective and acceptable means of contraception. The Committee recommended that the benefits of low-dose oral contraceptive use by healthy non-smoking women over 40 may outweigh the possible risks.

Of course, older women, as all women who take oral contraceptives, should take an oral contraceptive which contains the least amount of estrogen and progestogen that is compatible with a low failure rate and individual patient needs.

[See table above]

3. CARCINOMA OF THE REPRODUCTIVE ORGANS AND BREASTS

Numerous epidemiological studies have been performed on the incidence of breast, endometrial, ovarian and cervical cancer in women using oral contraceptives. While there are conflicting reports, most studies suggest that the use of oral contraceptives is not associated with an overall increase in the risk of developing breast cancer. Some studies have reported an increased relative risk of developing breast cancer, particularly at a younger age. This increased relative risk appears to be related to duration of use (36–43, 79–89).

Some studies suggest that oral contraceptive use has been associated with an increase in the risk of cervical intra-epithelial neoplasia in some populations of women (45–48). However, there continues to be controversy about the extent to which such findings may be due to differences in sexual behavior and other factors.

4. HEPATIC NEOPLASIA

Benign hepatic adenomas are associated with oral contraceptive use, although the incidence of benign tumors is rare in the United States. Indirect calculations have estimated the attributable risk to be in the range of 3.3 cases/100,000 for users, a risk that increases after four or more years of use especially with oral contraceptives of higher dose (49). Rupture of rare, benign, hepatic adenomas may cause death through intra-abdominal hemorrhage (50,51).

Studies from Britain have shown an increased risk of developing hepatocellular carcinoma (52–54) in long-term (>8 years) oral contraceptive users. However, these cancers are rare in the U.S. and the attributable risk (the excess incidence) of liver cancers in oral contraceptive users approaches less than one per million users.

5. OCULAR LESIONS

There have been clinical case reports of retinal thrombosis associated with the use of oral contraceptives. Oral contraceptives should be discontinued if there is unexplained partial or complete loss of vision; onset of proptosis or diplopia; papilledema; or retinal vascular lesions. Appropriate diagnostic and therapeutic measures should be undertaken immediately.

6. ORAL CONTRACEPTIVE USE BEFORE OR DURING EARLY PREGNANCY

Extensive epidemiological studies have revealed no increased risk of birth defects in women who have used oral contraceptives prior to pregnancy (56–57). The majority of recent studies also do not indicate a teratogenic effect, particularly in so far as cardiac anomalies and limb reduction defects are concerned (55,56,58,59), when oral contraceptives are taken inadvertently during early pregnancy.

The administration of oral contraceptives to induce withdrawal bleeding should not be used as a test for pregnancy. Oral contraceptives should not be used during pregnancy to treat threatened or habitual abortion. It is recommended that for any patient who has missed two consecutive periods, pregnancy should be ruled out before continuing oral contraceptive use. If the patient has not adhered to the prescribed schedule, the possibility of pregnancy should be considered at the time of the first missed period. Oral contraceptive use should be discontinued until pregnancy is ruled out.

7. GALLBLADDER DISEASE
Earlier studies have reported an increased lifetime relative risk of gallbladder surgery in users of oral contraceptives and estrogens (60,61). More recent studies, however, have shown that the relative risk of developing gallbladder disease among oral contraceptive users may be minimal (62–64). The recent findings of minimal risk may be related to the use of oral contraceptive formulations containing lower hormonal doses of estrogens and progestogens.

8. CARBOHYDRATE AND LIPID METABOLIC EFFECTS
Oral contraceptives have been shown to cause a decrease in glucose tolerance in a significant percentage of users (17). This effect has been shown to be directly related to estrogen dose (65). In general, progestogens increase insulin secretion and create insulin resistance, this effect varying with different progestational agents (17,66). In the non-diabetic woman, oral contraceptives appear to have no effect on fasting blood glucose (67). Because of these demonstrated effects, prediabetic and diabetic women should be carefully monitored while taking oral contraceptives.
A small proportion of women will have persistent hypertriglyceridemia while on the pill. As discussed earlier (see WARNINGS 1.a. and 1.d.), changes in serum triglycerides and lipoprotein levels have been reported in oral contraceptive users.

9. ELEVATED BLOOD PRESSURE
An increase in blood pressure has been reported in women taking oral contraceptives (68) and this increase is more likely in older oral contraceptive users (69) and with extended duration of use (61).
Data from the Royal College of General Practitioners (12) and subsequent randomized trials have shown that the incidence of hypertension increases with increasing progestational activity.
Women with a history of hypertension or hypertension-related diseases, or renal disease (70) should be encouraged to use another method of contraception. If women elect to use oral contraceptives, they should be monitored closely and if significant elevation of blood pressure occurs, oral contraceptives should be discontinued. For most women, elevated blood pressure will return to normal after stopping oral contraceptives (69), and there is no difference in the occurrence of hypertension among former and never users (68,70,71).

10. HEADACHE
The onset or exacerbation of migraine or development of headache with a new pattern which is recurrent, persistent or severe requires discontinuation of oral contraceptives and evaluation of the cause.

11. BLEEDING IRREGULARITIES
Breakthrough bleeding and spotting are sometimes encountered in patients on oral contraceptives, especially during the first three months of use. Non-hormonal causes should be considered and adequate diagnostic measures taken to rule out malignancy or pregnancy in the event of breakthrough bleeding, as in the case of any abnormal vaginal bleeding. If pathology has been excluded, time or a change to another formulation may solve the problem. In the event of amenorrhea, pregnancy should be ruled out.
Some women may encounter post-pill amenorrhea or oligomenorrhea, especially when such a condition was pre-existent.

12. ECTOPIC PREGNANCY
Ectopic as well as intrauterine pregnancy may occur in contraceptive failures.

PRECAUTIONS

1. PHYSICAL EXAMINATION AND FOLLOW UP
It is good medical practice for all women to have annual history and physical examinations, including women using oral contraceptives. The physical examination, however, may be deferred until after initiation of oral contraceptives if requested by the woman and judged appropriate by the clinician. The physical examination should include special reference to blood pressure, breasts, abdomen and pelvic organs, including cervical cytology, and relevant laboratory tests. In case of undiagnosed, persistent or recurrent abnormal vaginal bleeding, appropriate measures should be conducted to rule out malignancy. Women with a strong family history of breast cancer or who have breast nodules should be monitored with particular care.

2. LIPID DISORDERS
Women who are being treated for hyperlipidemias should be followed closely if they elect to use oral contraceptives. Some progestogens may elevate LDL levels and may render the control of hyperlipidemias more difficult.

3. LIVER FUNCTION
If jaundice develops in any woman receiving such drugs, the medication should be discontinued. Steroid hormones may be poorly metabolized in patients with impaired liver function.

4. FLUID RETENTION
Oral contraceptives may cause some degree of fluid retention. They should be prescribed with caution, and only with careful monitoring, in patients with conditions which might be aggravated by fluid retention.

5. EMOTIONAL DISORDERS
Women with a history of depression should be carefully observed and the drug discontinued if depression recurs to a serious degree.

6. CONTACT LENSES
Contact lens wearers who develop visual changes or changes in lens tolerance should be assessed by an ophthalmologist.

7. DRUG INTERACTIONS
Reduced efficacy and increased incidence of breakthrough bleeding and menstrual irregularities have been associated with concomitant use of rifampin. A similar association, though less marked, has been suggested with barbiturates, phenylbutazone, phenytoin sodium, carbamazepine and possibly with griseofulvin, ampicillin and tetracyclines (72).

8. INTERACTIONS WITH LABORATORY TESTS
Certain endocrine and liver function tests and blood components may be affected by oral contraceptives:
a. Increased prothrombin and factors VII, VIII, IX and X; decreased antithrombin 3; increased norepinephrine-induced platelet aggregability.
b. Increased thyroid binding globulin (TBG) leading to increased circulating total thyroid hormone, as measured by protein-bound iodine (PBI), T4 by column or by radioimmunoassay. Free T3 resin uptake is decreased, reflecting the elevated TBG; free T4 concentration is unaltered.
c. Other binding proteins may be elevated in serum.
d. Sex hormone-binding globulins are increased and result in elevated levels of total circulating sex steroids; however, free or biologically active levels either decrease or remain unchanged.
e. High-density lipoprotein cholesterol (HDL-C) and triglycerides may be increased, while low-density lipoprotein cholesterol (LDL-C) and total cholesterol (Total-C) may be decreased or unchanged.
f. Glucose tolerance may be decreased.
g. Serum folate levels may be depressed by oral contraceptive therapy. This may be of clinical significance if a woman becomes pregnant shortly after discontinuing oral contraceptives.

9. CARCINOGENESIS
See WARNINGS section.

10. PREGNANCY
Pregnancy Category X. See CONTRAINDICATIONS and WARNINGS sections.

11. NURSING MOTHERS
Small amounts of oral contraceptive steroids have been identified in the milk of nursing mothers and a few adverse effects on the child have been reported, including jaundice and breast enlargement. In addition, oral contraceptives given in the postpartum period may interfere with lactation by decreasing the quantity and quality of breast milk. If possible, the nursing mother should be advised not to use oral contraceptives but to use other forms of contraception until she has completely weaned her child.

12. GENERAL
PATIENTS SHOULD BE COUNSELED THAT THIS PRODUCT DOES NOT PROTECT AGAINST HIV INFECTION (AIDS) AND OTHER SEXUALLY TRANSMITTED DISEASES.

INFORMATION FOR THE PATIENT

See Patient Labeling Printed Below

ADVERSE REACTIONS

An increased risk of the following serious adverse reactions has been associated with the use of oral contraceptives (see WARNINGS section):
- Thrombophlebitis and venous thrombosis with or without embolism
- Arterial thromboembolism
- Pulmonary embolism
- Myocardial infarction
- Cerebral hemorrhage
- Cerebral thrombosis
- Hypertension
- Gallbladder disease
- Hepatic adenomas or benign liver tumors

The following adverse reactions have been reported in patients receiving oral contraceptives and are believed to be drug-related:
- Nausea
- Vomiting
- Gastrointestinal symptoms (such as abdominal cramps and bloating)
- Breakthrough bleeding
- Spotting
- Change in menstrual flow
- Amenorrhea
- Temporary infertility after discontinuation of treatment
- Edema
- Melasma which may persist
- Breast changes: tenderness, enlargement, secretion
- Change in weight (increase or decrease)
- Change in cervical erosion and secretion
- Diminution in lactation when given immediately postpartum
- Cholestatic jaundice
- Migraine
- Rash (allergic)
- Mental depression
- Reduced tolerance to carbohydrates
- Vaginal candidiasis
- Change in corneal curvature (steepening)
- Intolerance to contact lenses

The following adverse reactions have been reported in users of oral contraceptives and the association has been neither confirmed nor refuted:
- Pre-menstrual syndrome
- Cataracts
- Changes in appetite
- Cystitis-like syndrome
- Headache
- Nervousness
- Dizziness
- Hirsutism
- Loss of scalp hair
- Erythema multiforme
- Erythema nodosum
- Hemorrhagic eruption
- Vaginitis
- Porphyria
- Impaired renal function
- Hemolytic uremic syndrome
- Acne
- Changes in libido
- Colitis
- Budd-Chiari Syndrome

OVERDOSAGE

Serious ill effects have not been reported following acute ingestion of large doses of oral contraceptives by young children. Overdosage may cause nausea, and withdrawal bleeding may occur in females.

NON-CONTRACEPTIVE HEALTH BENEFITS

The following non-contraceptive health benefits related to the use of oral contraceptives are supported by epidemiological studies which largely utilized oral contraceptive formulations containing estrogen doses exceeding 0.035 mg of ethinyl estradiol or 0.05 mg of mestranol (73–78).
Effects on menses:
- increased menstrual cycle regularity
- decreased blood loss and decreased incidence of iron deficiency anemia
- decreased incidence of dysmenorrhea

Effects related to inhibition of ovulation:
- decreased incidence of functional ovarian cysts
- decreased incidence of ectopic pregnancies

Effects from long-term use:
- decreased incidence of fibroadenomas and fibrocystic disease of the breast
- decreased incidence of acute pelvic inflammatory disease
- decreased incidence of endometrial cancer
- decreased incidence of ovarian cancer

DESOGEN®

DOSAGE AND ADMINISTRATION

To achieve maximum contraceptive effectiveness, Desogen® must be taken exactly as directed and at intervals not exceeding 24 hours. Desogen® may be initiated using either a Sunday start or a Day 1 start.
NOTE: Each cycle pack dispenser is preprinted with the days of the week, starting with Sunday, to facilitate a Sunday start regimen. Six different "day label strips" are provided with each cycle pack dispenser in order to accommodate a Day 1 start regimen. In this case, the patient should place the self-adhesive "day label strip" that corresponds to her starting day over the preprinted days.
IMPORTANT: The possibility of ovulation and conception prior to initiation of use of Desogen® should be considered. The use of Desogen® for contraception may be initiated 4 weeks postpartum in women who elect not to breast feed. When the tablets are administered during the postpartum period, the increased risk of thromboembolic disease associated with the postpartum period must be considered. (See CONTRAINDICATIONS and WARNINGS concerning thromboembolic disease. See also PRECAUTIONS for "Nursing Mothers".)
If the patient starts on Desogen® postpartum, and has not yet had a period, she should be instructed to use another method of contraception until a white tablet has been taken daily for 7 days.

SUNDAY START
When initiating a Sunday start regimen, another method of contraception should be used until after the first 7 consecutive days of administration.
Using a Sunday start, tablets are taken without interruption as follows: The first white tablet should be taken on the first Sunday after menstruation begins (if menstruation begins on Sunday, the first white tablet is taken on that day). One white tablet is taken daily for 21 days, followed by 1 green (inert) tablet daily for 7 days. For all subsequent cycles, the patient then begins a new 28-tablet regimen on the next day (Sunday) after taking the last green tablet. [If switching from a Sunday start oral contraceptive, the first

Continued on next page

Desogen—Cont.

Desogen® tablet should be taken on the second Sunday after the last tablet of a 21 day regimen or should be taken on the first Sunday after the last inactive tablet of a 28 day regimen.]

If a patient misses 1 white tablet, she should take the missed tablet as soon as she remembers. If the patient misses 2 consecutive white tablets in Week 1 or Week 2, the patient should take 2 tablets the day she remembers and 2 tablets the next day; thereafter, the patient should resume taking 1 tablet daily until she finishes the cycle pack. The patient should be instructed to use a back-up method of birth control if she has intercourse in the 7 days after missing pills. If the patient misses 2 consecutive white tablets in the third week or misses 3 or more white tablets in a row at any time during the cycle, the patient should keep taking 1 white tablet daily until the next Sunday. On Sunday the patient should throw out the rest of that cycle pack and start a new cycle pack that same day. The patient should be instructed to use a back-up method of birth control if she has intercourse in the 7 days after missing pills.

DAY 1 START

Counting the first day of menstruation as "Day 1", tablets are taken without interruption as follows: One white tablet daily for 21 days, then one green (inert) tablet daily for 7 days. For all subsequent cycles, the patient then begins a new 28-tablet regimen on the next day after taking the last green tablet. [If switching directly from another oral contraceptive, the first white tablet should be taken on the first day of menstruation which begins after the last ACTIVE tablet of the previous product.]

If a patient misses 1 white tablet, she should take the missed tablet as soon as she remembers. If the patient misses 2 consecutive white tablets in Week 1 or Week 2, the patient should take 2 tablets the day she remembers and 2 tablets the next day; thereafter, the patient should resume taking 1 tablet daily until she finishes the cycle pack. The patient should be instructed to use a back-up method of birth control if she has intercourse in the 7 days after missing pills. If the patient misses 2 consecutive white tablets in the third week or misses 3 or more white tablets in a row at any time during the cycle, the patient should throw out the rest of that cycle pack and start a new cycle pack that same day. The patient should be instructed to use a back-up method of birth control if she has intercourse in the 7 days after missing pills.

ALL ORAL CONTRACEPTIVES

Breakthrough bleeding, spotting, and amenorrhea are frequent reasons for patients discontinuing oral contraceptives. In breakthrough bleeding, as in all cases of irregular bleeding from the vagina, non-functional causes should be borne in mind. In undiagnosed persistent or recurrent abnormal bleeding from the vagina, adequate diagnostic measures are indicated to rule out pregnancy or malignancy. If both pregnancy and pathology have been excluded, time or a change to another preparation may solve the problem. Changing to an oral contraceptive with a higher estrogen content, while potentially useful in minimizing menstrual irregularity, should be done only if necessary since this may increase the risk of thromboembolic disease.

Use of oral contraceptives in the event of a missed menstrual period:

1. If the patient has not adhered to the prescribed schedule, the possibility of pregnancy should be considered at the time of the first missed period and oral contraceptive use should be discontinued until pregnancy is ruled out.
2. If the patient has adhered to the prescribed regimen and misses two consecutive periods, pregnancy should be ruled out before continuing oral contraceptive use.

HOW SUPPLIED

Desogen® 28 contains 21 round white tablets and 7 round green tablets in a blister card within a recyclable plastic dispenser. Each white tablet (debossed with "TR/5" on one side and "Organon" on the other side) contains 0.15 mg desogestrel and 0.03 mg ethinyl estradiol. Each green tablet (debossed with "KH/2" on one side and "Organon" on the other side) contains inert ingredients.

Boxes of 6 NDC# 0052-0261-06.

STORAGE: Store below 86°F (30°C)

CAUTION: Federal law prohibits dispensing without prescription.

REFERENCES

1. Reproduced with permission of the Population Council from J. Trussell and K. Kost: Contraceptive failure in the United States: A critical review of the literature. Studies in Family Planning, 18 (5), September–October 1987. **2.** Stadel BV. Oral contraceptives and cardiovascular disease. (Pt. 1). N Engl J Med 1981; 305:612–618. **3.** Stadel BV. Oral contraceptives and cardiovascular disease. (Pt. 2). N Engl J Med 1981; 305:672–677. **4.** Adam SA, Thorogood M. Oral contraception and myocardial infarction revisited: the effects of new preparations and prescribing patterns. Br J Obstet and Gynecol 1981; 88:838–845. **5.** Mann JI, Inman WH. Oral contraceptives and death from myocardial infarction. Br Med J 1975; 2(5965):245–248. **6.** Mann JI, Vessey MP, Thorogood M, Doll R. Myocardial infarction in young women with special reference to oral contraceptive practice. Br Med J 1975; 2(5956):241–245. **7.** Royal College of General Practitioners' Oral Contraception Study: Further analyses of mortality in oral contraceptive users. Lancet 1981; 1:541–546. **8.** Slone D, Shapiro S, Kaufman DW, Rosenberg L, Miettinen OS, Stolley PD. Risk of myocardial infarction in relation to current and discontinued use of oral contraceptives. N Engl J Med 1981; 305:420–424. **9.** Vessey MP. Female hormones and vascular disease—an epidemiological overview. Br J Fam Plann 1980; 6:1–12. **10.** Russell-Briefel RG, Ezzati TM, Fulwood R, Perlman JA, Murphy RS. Cardiovascular risk status and oral contraceptive use, United States, 1976–80. Prevent Med 1986; 15:352–362. **11.** Goldbaum GM, Kendrick JS, Hogelin GC, Gentry EM. The relative impact of smoking and oral contraceptive use on women in the United States. JAMA 1987; 258:1339–1342. **12.** Layde PM, Beral V. Further analyses of mortality in oral contraceptive users: Royal College General Practitioners' Oral Contraception Study. (Table 5) Lancet 1981; 1:541–546. **13.** Knopp RH. Arteriosclerosis risk: the roles of oral contraceptives and postmenopausal estrogens. J Reprod Med 1986; 31(9) (Supplement):913–921. **14.** Krauss RM, Roy S, Mishell DR, Casagrande J, Pike MC. Effects of two low-dose oral contraceptives on serum lipids and lipoproteins: Differential changes in high-density lipoproteins subclasses. Am J Obstet 1983; 145:446–452. **15.** Wahl P, Walden C, Knopp R, Hoover J, Wallace R, Heiss G, Rifkind B. Effect of estrogen/progestin potency on lipid/lipoprotein cholesterol. N Engl J Med 1983; 308: 862–867. **16.** Wynn V, Niththyananthan R. The effect of progestin in combined oral contraceptives on serum lipids with special reference to high-density lipoproteins. Am J Obstet Gynecol 1982; 142:766–771. **17.** Wynn V, Godsland I. Effects of oral contraceptives and carbohydrate metabolism. J Reprod Med 1986; 31 (9) (Supplement):892–897. **18.** LaRosa JC. Atherosclerotic risk factors in cardiovascular disease. J Reprod Med 1986; 31 (9) (Supplement): 906–912. **19.** Inman WH, Vessey MP. Investigation of death from pulmonary, coronary, and cerebral thrombosis and embolism in women of child-bearing age. Br Med J 1968; 2 (5599):193–199. **20.** Maguire MG, Tonascia J, Sartwell PE, Stolley PD, Tockman MS. Increased risk of thrombosis due to oral contraceptives: a further report. Am J Epidemiol 1979; 110 (2):188–195. **21.** Pettiti DB, Wingerd J, Pellegrin F, Ramacharan S. Risk of vascular disease in women: smoking, oral contraceptives, noncontraceptive estrogens, and other factors. JAMA 1979; 242:1150–1154. **22.** Vessey MP, Doll R. Investigation of relation between use of oral contraceptives and thromboembolic disease. Br Med J 1968; 2 (5599):199–205. **23.** Vessey MP, Doll R. Investigation of relation between use of oral contraceptives and thromboembolic disease. A further report. Br Med J 1969; 2 (5658):651–657. **24.** Porter JB, Hunter JR, Danielson DA, Jick H, Stergachis A. Oral contraceptives and non-fatal vascular disease—recent experience. Obstet Gynecol 1982; 59 (3): 299–302. **25.** Vessey M, Doll R, Peto R, Johnson B, Wiggins P. A long-term follow-up study of women using different methods of contraception: an interim report. Biosocial Sci 1976; 8: 375–427. **26.** Royal College of General Practitioners: Oral contraceptives, venous thrombosis, and varicose veins. J Royal Coll Gen Pract 1978; 28:393–399. **27.** Collaborative Group for the Study of Stroke in Young Women: Oral contraception and increased risk of cerebral ischemia or thrombosis. N Engl J Med 1973; 288:871–878. **28.** Petitti DB, Wingerd J. Use of oral contraceptives, cigarette smoking, and risk of subarachnoid hemorrhage. Lancet 1978; 2:234–236. **29.** Inman WH. Oral contraceptives and fatal subarachnoid hemorrhage. Br Med J 1979; 2 (6203):1468–70. **30.** Collaborative Group for the Study of Stroke in Young Women: Oral contraceptives and stroke in young women: associated risk factors. JAMA 1975; 231:718–722. **31.** Inman WH, Vessey MP, Westerholm B, Engelund A. Thromboembolic disease and the steroidal content of oral contraceptives. A report to the Committee on Safety of Drugs. Br Med J 1970; 2:203–209. **32.** Meade TW, Greenberg G, Thompson SG. Progestogens and cardiovascular reactions associated with oral contraceptives and a comparison of the safety of 50- and 35-mcg oestrogen preparations. Br Med J 1980; 280 (6224):1157–1161. **33.** Kay CR. Progestogens and arterial disease—evidence from the Royal College of General Practitioners' Study. Am J Obstet Gynecol 1982; 142:762–765. **34.** Royal College of General Practitioners: Incidence of arterial disease among oral contraceptive users. J Royal Coll Gen Pract 1983; 33:75–82. **35.** Ory HW. Mortality associated with fertility and fertility control: 1983. Family Planning Perspectives 1983; 15:50–56. **36.** The Cancer and Steroid Hormone Study of the Centers for Disease Control and the National Institute of Child Health and Human Development: Oral-contraceptive use and the risk of breast cancer. N Engl J Med 1986; 315:405–411. **37.** Pike MC, Henderson BE, Krailo MD, Duke A, Roy S. Breast cancer risk in young women and use of oral contraceptives: possible modifying effect of formulation and age at use. Lancet 1983; 2:926–929. **38.** Paul C, Skegg DG, Spears GFS, Kaldor JM. Oral contraceptives and breast cancer: A national study. Br Med J 1986; 293: 723–725. **39.** Miller DR, Rosenberg L, Kaufman DW, Schottenfeld D, Stolley PD, Shapiro S. Breast cancer risk in relation to early oral contraceptive use. Obstet Gynecol 1986; 68:863–868. **40.** Olson H, Olson KL, Moller TR, Ranstam J, Holm P. Oral contraceptive use and breast cancer in young women in Sweden (letter). Lancet 1985; 2:748–749. **41.** McPherson K, Vessey M, Neil A, Doll R, Jones L, Roberts M. Early contraceptive use and breast cancer: Results of another case-control study. Br J Cancer 1987; 56: 653–660. **42.** Huggins GR, Zucker PF. Oral contraceptives and neoplasia: 1987 update. Fertil Steril 1987; 47:733–761. **43.** McPherson K, Drife JO. The pill and breast cancer: why the uncertainty? Br Med J 1986; 293:709–710. **44.** Shapiro S. Oral contraceptives—time to take stock. N Engl J Med 1987; 315:450–451. **45.** Ory H, Naib Z, Conger SB, Hatcher RA, Tyler CW. Contraceptive choice and prevalence of cervical dysplasia and carcinoma in situ. Am J Obstet Gynecol 1976; 124:573–577. **46.** Vessey MP, Lawless M, McPherson K, Yeates D. Neoplasia of the cervix uteri and contraception: a possible adverse effect of the pill. Lancet 1983; 2:930. **47.** Brinton LA, Huggins GR, Lehman HF, Malli K, Savitz DA, Trapido E, Rosenthal J, Hoover R. Long-term use of oral contraceptives and risk of invasive cervical cancer. Int J Cancer 1986; 38:339–344. **48.** WHO Collaborative Study of Neoplasia and Steroid Contraceptives: Invasive cervical cancer and combined oral contraceptives. Br Med J 1985; 290:961–965. **49.** Rooks JB, Ory HW, Ishak KG, Strauss LT, Greenspan JR, Hill AP, Tyler CW. Epidemiology of hepatocellular adenoma: the role of oral contraceptive use. JAMA 1979; 242:644–648. **50.** Bein NN, Goldsmith HS. Recurrent massive hemorrhage from benign hepatic tumors secondary to oral contraceptives. Br J Surg 1977; 64:433–435. **51.** Klatskin G. Hepatic tumors: possible relationship to use of oral contraceptives. Gastroenterology 1977; 73:386–394. **52.** Henderson BE, Preston-Martin S, Edmondson HA, Peters RL, Pike MC. Hepatocellular carcinoma and oral contraceptives. Br J Cancer 1983; 48:437–440. **53.** Neuberger J, Forman D, Doll R, Williams R. Oral contraceptives and hepatocellular carcinoma. Br Med J 1986; 292:1355–1357. **54.** Forman D, Vincent TJ, Doll R. Cancer of the liver and oral contraceptives. Br Med J 1986; 292:1357–1361. **55.** Harlap S, Eldor J. Births following oral contraceptive failures. Obstet Gynecol 1980; 55:447–452. **56.** Savolainen E, Saksela E, Saxen L. Teratogenic hazards of oral contraceptives analyzed in a national malformation register. Am J Obstet Gynecol 1981; 140:521–524. **57.** Janerich DT, Piper JM, Glebatis DM. Oral contraceptives and birth defects. Am J Epidemiol 1980; 112:73–79. **58.** Ferencz C, Matanoski GM, Wilson PD, Rubin JD, Neill CA, Gutberlet R. Maternal hormone therapy and congenital heart disease. Teratology 1980; 21: 225–239. **59.** Rothman KJ, Fyler DC, Goldbatt A, Kreidberg MB. Exogenous hormones and other drug exposures of children with congenital heart disease. Am J Epidemiol 1979; 109:433–439. **60.** Boston Collaborative Drug Surveillance Program: Oral contraceptives and venous thromboembolic disease, surgically confirmed gallbladder disease, and breast tumors. Lancet 1973; 1:1399–1404. **61.** Royal College of General Practitioners: Oral contraceptives and health. New York, Pittman, 1974. **62.** Layde PM, Vessey MP, Yeates D. Risk of gallbladder disease: a cohort study of young women attending family planning clinics. J Epidemiol Community Health 1982; 36:274–278. **63.** Rome Group for the Epidemiology and Prevention of Cholelithiasis (GREPCO): Prevalence of gallstone disease in an Italian adult female population. Am J Epidemiol 1984; 119:796–805. **64.** Strom BL, Tamragouri RT, Morse ML, Lazar EL, West SL, Stolley PD, Jones JK. Oral contraceptives and other risk factors for gallbladder disease. Clin Pharmacol Ther 1986; 39:335–341. **65.** Wynn V, Adams PW, Godsland IF, Melrose J, Niththyananthan R, Oakley NW, Seedj A. Comparison of effects of different combined oral-contraceptive formulations on carbohydrate and lipid metabolism. Lancet 1979; 1:1045–1049. **66.** Wynn V. Effect of progesterone and progestins on carbohydrate metabolism. In Progesterone and Progestin. Edited by Bardin CW, Milgrom E, Mauvis-Jarvis P. New York, Raven Press, 1983 pp. 395–410. **67.** Perlman JA, Roussell-Briefel RG, Ezzati TM, Lieberknecht G. Oral glucose tolerance and the potency of oral contraceptive progestogens. J Chronic Dis 1985; 38:857–864. **68.** Royal College of General Practitioners' Oral Contraception Study: Effect on hypertension and benign breast disease of progestogen component in combined oral contraceptives. Lancet 1977; 1:624. **69.** Fisch IR, Frank J. Oral contraceptives and blood pressure. JAMA 1977; 237:2499–2503. **70.** Laragh AJ. Oral contraceptive induced hypertension—nine years later. Am J Obstet Gynecol 1976; 126:141–147. **71.** Ramcharan S, Peritz E, Pellegrin FA, Williams WT. Incidence of hypertension in the Walnut Creek Contraceptive Drug Study cohort. In Pharmacology of Steroid Contraceptive Drugs. Garattini S, Berendes HW. Eds. New York, Raven Press, 1977 pp. 277–288. (Monographs of the Mario Negri Institute for Pharmacological Research, Milan). **72.** Stockley I. Interactions with oral contraceptives. J Pharm 1976; 216:140–143. **73.** The Cancer and Steroid Hormone Study of the Centers for Disease Control and the National Institute of Child Health and Human Development: Oral contraceptive use and the risk of ovarian cancer. JAMA 1983; 249:1596–1599. **74.** The Cancer and Steroid Hormone Study of the Centers for Disease Control and the National Institute of Child Health and Human Development: Combination oral contraceptive use and the risk of endometrial cancer. JAMA 1987; 257:796–800. **75.** Ory HW. Functional ovarian cysts and oral contraceptives: negative association confirmed surgically. JAMA 1974; 228: 68–69. **76.** Ory HW, Cole P, Macmahon B, Hoover R. Oral contraceptives and reduced risk of benign breast disease. N Engl J Med 1976; 294:419–422. **77.** Ory HW. The noncontraceptive health benefits from oral contraceptive use. Fam Plann Perspect 1982; 14:182–184. **78.** Ory HW, Forrest JD, Lincoln R. Making Choices: Evaluating the health risks and benefits of birth control methods. New York, The Alan Guttmacher Institute, 1983; p. 1. **79.** Schlesselman J, Stadel BV, Murray P, Lai S. Breast Cancer in relation to early use of oral contraceptives 1988; 259:1828–1833. **80.** Hennekens CH, Speizer FE, Lipnick RJ, Rosner B, Bain C, Belanger C, Stampfer MJ, Willett W, Peto R. A case-controlled study of oral contraceptive use and breast cancer. JNCI 1984; 72:39–42. **81.** LaVecchia C, Decarli A, Fasoli M, Franceschi S, Gentile A, Negri E, Parazzini F, Tognoni G. Oral contraceptives and cancers of the breast and of the female genital tract. Interim results from a case-control study. Br. J. Cancer 1986; 54:311–317. **82.** Meirik O, Lund E, Adami H, Bergstrom R, Christoffersen T, Bergsjo P. Oral contraceptive use in breast cancer in young women. A Joint National Case-control study in Sweden and Norway. Lancet 1986; 11:650–654. **83.** Kay CR, Hannaford PC. Breast cancer and the pill—A further report from the Royal College of General Practitioners' oral contraception study. Br. J. Cancer 1988; 58:675–680. **84.** Stadel BV, Lai S, Schlesselman JJ, Murray P. Oral contraceptives and premenopausal breast cancer in nulliparous women. Contraception 1988; 38:287–299. **85.** Miller DR, Rosenberg L, Kaufman DW, Stolley P, Warshauer ME, Shapiro S. Breast cancer before age 45 and oral contraceptive use: New Findings. Am. J. Epidemiol 1989; 129:269–280. **86.** The UK National Case-Control Study Group, Oral contraceptive use and breast cancer risk in young women. Lancet 1989; 1:973–982. **87.** Schlesselman JJ. Cancer of the breast and reproductive tract in relation to use of oral contraceptives. Contraception 1989; 40:1–38. **88.** Vessey MP, McPherson K, Villard-Mackintosh L, Yeates D. Oral contraceptives and breast cancer: latest findings in a large cohert study. Br. J. Cancer 1989; 59:613–617. **89.** Jick SS, Walker AM, Stergachis A, Jick H. Oral contraceptives and breast cancer. Br. J. Cancer 1989; 59:618–621. **90.** Godsland, I et al. The effects of different formulations of oral contraceptive agents on lipid and carbohydrate metabolism. N Engl J Med 1990; 323:1375–81. **91.** Kloosterboer, HJ et al. Selectivity in progesterone and androgen receptor binding of progestogens used in oral contraception. Contraception, 1988; 38:325–32. **92.** Van der Vies, J and de Visser, J. Endocrinological studies with desogestrel. Arzneim. Forsch./Drug Res., 1983; 33(I),2:231–6. **93.** Data on file, Organon Inc. **94.** Fotherby, K. Oral contraceptives, lipids and cardiovascular diseases. Contraception, 1985; Vol. 31; 4:367–94. **95.** Lawrence, DM et al. Reduced sex hormone binding globulin and derived free testosterone levels in women with severe acne. Clinical Endocrinology, 1981; 15:87–91. **96.** Cullberg, G et al. Effects of a low-dose desogestrel-ethinyl estradiol combination on hirsutism, androgens and sex hormone binding globulin in women with a polycystic ovary syndrome. Acta Obstet Gynecol Scand, 1985; 64:195–202. **97.** Jung-Hoffmann, C and Kuhl, H. Divergent effects of two low-dose oral contraceptives on sex hormone-binding globulin and free testosterone. AJOG, 1987; 156:199–203. **98.** Hammond, G et al. Serum steroid binding protein concentrations, distribution of progestogens, and bioavailability of testosterone during treatment with contraceptives containing desogestrel or levonorgestrel. Fertil. Steril., 1984; 42:44–51. **99.** Palatsi, R et al. Serum total and unbound testosterone and sex hormone binding globulin (SHBG) in female acne patients treated with two different oral contraceptives. Acta Derm Venereol, 1984; 64:517–23. **100.** Lewis M, Spitzer WO, Heinemann LAJ, MacRae KD, Bruppacher R, Thorogood M on behalf of Transnational Research Group on Oral Contraceptives and Health of Young Women. Third generation oral contraceptives and risk of myocardial infarction: an international case-control study. Br Med J, 1996; 312:88–90. **101.** Jick H, Jick SS, Gurewich V, Myers MW, Vasilakis C. Risk of idiopathic cardiovascular death and non-fatal venous thromboembolism in women using oral contraceptives with differing progestagen components. Lancet, 1995; 346:1589–93. **102.** World Health Organization Collaborative Study of Cardiovascular Disease and Steroid Hormone Contraception. Effect of different progestagens in low oestrogen oral contraceptives on venous thromboembolic disease. Lancet, 1995; 346:1582–88. **103.** Spitzer WO, Lewis MA, Heinemann LAJ, Thorogood M, MacRae KD on behalf of Transnational Research Group on Oral Contraceptives and Health of Young Women. Third generation oral contraceptives and risk of venous thromboembolic disorders: an international case-control study. Br Med J 1996; 312:83–88.

BRIEF SUMMARY

PATIENT PACKAGE INSERT

THIS PRODUCT (LIKE ALL ORAL CONTRACEPTIVES) IS INTENDED TO PREVENT PREGNANCY. IT DOES NOT PROTECT AGAINST HIV INFECTION (AIDS) AND OTHER SEXUALLY TRANSMITTED DISEASES.

Oral contraceptives, also known as "birth control pills" or "the pill", are taken to prevent pregnancy, and when taken correctly, have a failure rate of about 1% per year when used without missing any pills. The typical failure rate of large numbers of pill users is less than 3% per year when women who miss pills are included. For most women, oral contraceptives are also free of serious or unpleasant side effects. However, forgetting to take pills considerably increases the chances of pregnancy.

For the majority of women, oral contraceptives can be taken safely. But there are some women who are at high risk of developing certain serious diseases that can be life-threatening or may cause temporary or permanent disability. The risks associated with taking oral contraceptives increase significantly if you:

- smoke
- have high blood pressure, diabetes, high cholesterol
- have or have had clotting disorders, heart attack, stroke, angina pectoris, cancer of the breast or sex organs, jaundice or malignant or benign liver tumors

Although cardiovascular disease risks may be increased with oral contraceptive use after age 40 in healthy, non-smoking women (even with the newer low-dose formulations), there are also greater potential health risks associated with pregnancy in older women.

You should not take the pill if you suspect you are pregnant or have unexplained vaginal bleeding.

Cigarette smoking increases the risk of serious cardiovascular side effects from oral contraceptive use. This risk increases with age and with heavy smoking (15 or more cigarettes per day) and is quite marked in women over 35 years of age. Women who use oral contraceptives are strongly advised not to smoke.

Most side effects of the pill are not serious. The most common such effects are nausea, vomiting, bleeding between menstrual periods, weight gain, breast tenderness, headache, and difficulty wearing contact lenses. These side effects, especially nausea and vomiting, may subside within the first three months of use.

The serious side effects of the pill occur very infrequently, especially if you are in good health and are young. However, you should know that the following medical conditions have been associated with or made worse by the pill:

1. Blood clots in the legs (thrombophlebitis) or lungs (pulmonary embolism), stoppage or rupture of a blood vessel in the brain (stroke), blockage of blood vessels in the heart (heart attack or angina pectoris) or other organs of the body. As mentioned above, smoking increases the risk of heart attacks and strokes, and subsequent serious medical consequences.
2. Liver tumors, which may rupture and cause severe bleeding. A possible but not definite association has been found with the pill and liver cancer. However, liver cancers are extremely rare. The chance of developing liver cancer from using the pill is thus even rarer.
3. High blood pressure, although blood pressure usually returns to normal when the pill is stopped.

The symptoms associated with these serious side effects are discussed in the detailed patient labeling given to you with your supply of pills. Notify your doctor or clinic if you notice any unusual physical disturbances while taking the pill. In addition, drugs such as rifampin, as well as some anticonvulsants and some antibiotics may decrease oral contraceptive effectiveness.

There is conflict among studies regarding breast cancer and oral contraceptive use. Some studies have reported an increase in the risk of developing breast cancer, particularly at a younger age. This increased risk appears to be related to duration of use. The majority of studies have found no overall increase in the risk of developing breast cancer. Some studies have found an increase in the incidence of cancer of the cervix in women who use oral contraceptives. However, this finding may be related to factors other than the use of oral contraceptives. There is insufficient evidence to rule out the possibility that pills may cause such cancers.

Taking the combination pill provides some important non-contraceptive benefits. These include less painful menstruation, less menstrual blood loss and anemia, fewer pelvic infections, and fewer cancers of the ovary and the lining of the uterus.

Be sure to discuss any medical condition you may have with your doctor or clinic. Your doctor or clinic will take a medical and family history before prescribing oral contraceptives and will examine you. The physical examination may be delayed to another time if you request it and your doctor or clinic believes that it is a good medical practice to postpone it. You should be reexamined at least once a year while taking oral contraceptives. The detailed patient information labeling gives you further information which you should read and discuss with your doctor or clinic.

DETAILED PATIENT LABELING

THIS PRODUCT (LIKE ALL ORAL CONTRACEPTIVES) IS INTENDED TO PREVENT PREGNANCY. IT DOES NOT PROTECT AGAINST HIV INFECTION (AIDS) AND OTHER SEXUALLY TRANSMITTED DISEASES.

PLEASE NOTE: This labeling is revised from time to time as important new medical information becomes available. Therefore, please review this labeling carefully.

The following oral contraceptive product contains a combination of a progestogen and estrogen, the two kinds of female hormones:

DESOGEN® 28 DAY REGIMEN

Each white tablet contains 0.15 mg desogestrel and 0.03 mg ethinyl estradiol. Each green tablet contains inert ingredients.

INTRODUCTION

Any woman who considers using oral contraceptives (the birth control pill or the pill) should understand the benefits and risks of using this form of birth control. This patient labeling will give you much of the information you will need to make this decision and will also help you determine if you are at risk of developing any of the serious side effects of the pill. It will tell you how to use the pill properly so that it will be as effective as possible. However, this labeling is not a replacement for a careful discussion between you and your doctor or clinic. You should discuss the information provided in this labeling with him or her, both when you first start taking the pill and during your revisits. You should also follow your doctor's or clinic's advice with regard to regular check-ups while you are on the pill.

EFFECTIVENESS OF ORAL CONTRACEPTIVES

Oral contraceptives or "birth control pills" or "the pill" are used to prevent pregnancy and are more effective than other non-surgical methods of birth control. When they are taken correctly, the chance of becoming pregnant is less than 1% (1 pregnancy per 100 women per year of use) when used perfectly, without missing any pills. Typical failure rates are actually 3% per year. The chance of becoming pregnant increases with each missed pill during a menstrual cycle.

In comparison, typical failure rates for other non-surgical methods of birth control during the first year of use are as follows:

IUD: 3%
Diaphragm with spermicides: 18%
Spermicides alone: 21%
Vaginal sponge: 18 to 28%
Implant: 0.03%
Condom alone: 12%
Periodic abstinence: 20%
No methods: 85%.

WHO SHOULD NOT TAKE ORAL CONTRACEPTIVES

Cigarette smoking increases the risk of serious cardiovascular side effects from oral contraceptive use. This risk increases with age and with heavy smoking (15 or more cigarettes per day) and is quite marked in women over 35 years of age. Women who use oral contraceptives are strongly advised not to smoke.

Some women should not use the pill. For example, you should not take the pill if you are pregnant or think you may be pregnant. You should also not use the pill if you have any of the following conditions:

- A history of heart attack or stroke
- Blood clots in the legs (thrombophlebitis), lungs (pulmonary embolism), or eyes
- A history of blood clots in the deep veins of your legs
- Chest pain (angina pectoris)
- Known or suspected breast cancer or cancer of the lining of the uterus, cervix or vagina
- Unexplained vaginal bleeding (until a diagnosis is reached by your doctor)
- Yellowing of the whites of the eyes or of the skin (jaundice) during pregnancy or during previous use of the pill
- Liver tumor (benign or cancerous)
- Known or suspected pregnancy.

Tell your doctor or clinic if you have ever had any of these conditions. Your doctor or clinic can recommend another method of birth control.

OTHER CONSIDERATIONS BEFORE TAKING ORAL CONTRACEPTIVES

Tell your doctor or clinic if you have or have had:

- Breast nodules, fibrocystic disease of the breast, an abnormal breast x-ray or mammogram
- Diabetes
- Elevated cholesterol or triglycerides
- High blood pressure
- Migraine or other headaches or epilepsy
- Mental depression
- Gallbladder, heart or kidney disease
- History of scanty or irregular menstrual periods.

Women with any of these conditions should be checked often by their doctor or clinic if they choose to use oral contraceptives.

Also, be sure to inform your doctor or clinic if you smoke or are on any medications.

RISKS OF TAKING ORAL CONTRACEPTIVES

1. Risk of developing blood clots

Blood clots and blockage of blood vessels are one of the most serious side effects of taking oral contraceptives and can cause death or serious disability. In particular, a clot in the legs can cause thrombophlebitis and a clot that travels to the lungs can cause a sudden blocking of the vessel carrying blood to the lungs. These risks may be greater with desogestrel-containing oral contraceptives such as Desogen® than with certain other low-dose pills. Rarely, clots occur in the blood vessels of the eye and may cause blindness, double vision, or impaired vision.

If you take oral contraceptives and need elective surgery, need to stay in bed for a prolonged illness or have recently delivered a baby, you may be at risk of developing blood clots. You should consult your doctor or clinic about stopping oral contraceptives three to four weeks before surgery and not taking oral contraceptives for two weeks after surgery or during bed rest. You should also not take oral contraceptives soon after delivery of a baby. It is advisable to wait for at least four weeks after delivery if you are not breast feeding or four weeks after a second trimester abortion. If you are breast feeding, you should wait until you have weaned your child before using the pill. (See also the section on Breast Feeding in General Precautions.)

The risk of circulatory disease in oral contraceptive users may be higher in users of high dose pills. The risk of venous thromboembolic disease associated with oral contraceptives does not increase with length of use and disappears after pill use is stopped. The risk of abnormal blood clotting increases with age in both users and non-users of oral contraceptives, but the increased risk from the oral contraceptive

Continued on next page

Desogen—Cont.

appears to be present at all ages. For women aged 20 to 44 it is estimated that about 1 in 2,000 using oral contraceptives will be hospitalized each year because of abnormal clotting. Among non-users in the same age group, about 1 in 20,000 would be hospitalized each year. For oral contraceptive users in general, it has been estimated that in women between the ages of 15 and 34 the risk of death due to a circulatory disorder is about 1 in 12,000 per year, whereas for non-users the rate is about 1 in 50,000 per year. In the age group 35 to 44, the risk is estimated to be about 1 in 2,500 per year for oral contraceptive users and about 1 in 10,000 per year for non-users.

2. Heart attacks and strokes

Oral contraceptives may increase the tendency to develop strokes (stoppage or rupture of blood vessels in the brain) and angina pectoris and heart attacks (blockage of blood vessels in the heart). Any of these conditions can cause death or serious disability.

Smoking greatly increases the possibility of suffering heart attacks and strokes. Furthermore, smoking and the use of oral contraceptives greatly increase the chances of developing and dying of heart disease.

3. Gallbladder disease

Oral contraceptive users probably have a greater risk than non-users of having gallbladder disease, although this risk may be related to pills containing high doses of estrogens.

4. Liver tumors

In rare cases, oral contraceptives can cause benign but dangerous liver tumors. These benign liver tumors can rupture and cause fatal internal bleeding. In addition, a possible but not definite association has been found with the pill and liver cancers in two studies, in which a few women who developed these very rare cancers were found to have used oral contraceptives for long periods. However, liver cancers are rare.

5. Cancer of the reproductive organs and breasts

There is conflict among studies regarding breast cancer and oral contraceptive use. Some studies have reported an increase in the risk of developing breast cancer, particularly at a younger age. This increased risk appears to be related to duration of use. The majority of studies have found no overall increase in the risk of developing breast cancer.

Some studies have found an increase in the incidence of cancer of the cervix in women who use oral contraceptives. However, this finding may be related to factors other than the use of oral contraceptives. There is insufficient evidence to rule out the possibility that pills may cause such cancers.

ESTIMATED RISK OF DEATH FROM A BIRTH CONTROL METHOD OR PREGNANCY

All methods of birth control and pregnancy are associated with a risk of developing certain diseases which may lead to disability or death. An estimate of the number of deaths associated with different methods of birth control and pregnancy has been calculated and is shown in the following table.

[See table below]

In the above table, the risk of death from any birth control method is less than the risk of childbirth, except for oral contraceptive users over the age of 35 who smoke and pill users over the age of 40 even if they do not smoke. It can be seen in the table that for women aged 15 to 39, the risk of death was highest with pregnancy (7–26 deaths per 100,000 women, depending on age). Among pill users who do not smoke, the risk of death is always lower than that associated with pregnancy for any age group, although over the age of 40, the risk increases to 32 deaths per 100,000 women, compared to 28 associated with pregnancy at that age. However, for pill users who smoke and are over the age of 35, the estimated number of deaths exceeds those for other methods of birth control. If a woman is over the age of 40 and smokes, her estimated risk of death is four times higher (117/100,000 women) than the estimated risk associated with pregnancy (28/100,000 women) in that age group.

The suggestion that women over 40 who do not smoke should not take oral contraceptives is based on information from older, higher-dose pills. An Advisory Committee of the FDA discussed this issue in 1989 and recommended that the benefits of low-dose oral contraceptive use by healthy, non-smoking women over 40 years of age may outweigh the possible risks.

WARNING SIGNALS

If any of these adverse effects occur while you are taking oral contraceptives, call your doctor or clinic immediately:

- Sharp chest pain, coughing of blood, or sudden shortness of breath (indicating a possible clot in the lung)
- Pain in the calf (indicating a possible clot in the leg)
- Crushing chest pain or heaviness in the chest (indicating a possible heart attack)
- Sudden severe headache or vomiting, dizziness or fainting, disturbances of vision or speech, weakness, or numbness in an arm or leg (indicating a possible stroke)
- Sudden partial or complete loss of vision (indicating a possible clot in the eye)
- Breast lumps (indicating possible breast cancer or fibrocystic disease of the breast; ask your doctor or clinic to show you how to examine your breasts)
- Severe pain or tenderness in the stomach area (indicating a possibly ruptured liver tumor)
- Difficulty in sleeping, weakness, lack of energy, fatigue, or change in mood (possibly indicating severe depression)
- Jaundice or a yellowing of the skin or eyeballs, accompanied frequently by fever, fatigue, loss of appetite, dark colored urine, or light colored bowel movements (indicating possible liver problems).

SIDE EFFECTS OF ORAL CONTRACEPTIVES

1. Vaginal bleeding

Irregular vaginal bleeding or spotting may occur while you are taking the pills. Irregular bleeding may vary from slight staining between menstrual periods to breakthrough bleeding which is a flow much like a regular period. Irregular bleeding occurs most often during the first few months of oral contraceptive use, but may also occur after you have been taking the pill for some time. Such bleeding may be temporary and usually does not indicate any serious problems. It is important to continue taking your pills on schedule. If the bleeding occurs in more than one cycle or lasts for more than a few days, talk to your doctor or clinic.

2. Contact lenses

If you wear contact lenses and notice a change in vision or an inability to wear your lenses, contact your doctor or clinic.

3. Fluid retention

Oral contraceptives may cause edema (fluid retention) with swelling of the fingers or ankles and may raise your blood pressure. If you experience fluid retention, contact your doctor or clinic.

4. Melasma

A spotty darkening of the skin is possible, particularly of the face, which may persist.

5. Other side effects

Other side effects may include nausea and vomiting, change in appetite, headache, nervousness, depression, dizziness, loss of scalp hair, rash, and vaginal infections.

If any of these side effects bother you, call your doctor or clinic.

GENERAL PRECAUTIONS

1. Missed periods and use of oral contraceptives before or during early pregnancy

There may be times when you may not menstruate regularly after you have completed taking a cycle of pills. If you have taken your pills regularly and miss one menstrual period, continue taking your pills for the next cycle but be sure to inform your doctor or clinic before doing so. If you have not taken the pills daily as instructed and missed a menstrual period, you may be pregnant. If you missed two consecutive menstrual periods, you may be pregnant. Check with your doctor or clinic immediately to determine whether you are pregnant. Do not continue to take oral contraceptives until you are sure you are not pregnant, but continue to use another method of contraception.

There is no conclusive evidence that oral contraceptive use is associated with an increase in birth defects, when taken inadvertently during early pregnancy. Previously, a few studies had reported that oral contraceptives might be associated with birth defects, but these findings have not been seen in more recent studies. Nevertheless, oral contraceptives or any other drugs should not be used during pregnancy unless clearly necessary and prescribed by your doctor or clinic. You should check with your doctor or clinic about risks to your unborn child of any medication taken during pregnancy.

2. While breast feeding

If you are breast feeding, consult your doctor or clinic before starting oral contraceptives. Some of the drug will be passed on to the child in the milk. A few adverse effects on the child have been reported, including yellowing of the skin (jaundice) and breast enlargement. In addition, oral contraceptives may decrease the amount and quality of your milk. If possible, do not use oral contraceptives while breast feeding. You should use another method of contraception since breast feeding provides only partial protection from becoming pregnant and this partial protection decreases significantly as you breast feed for longer periods of time. You should consider starting oral contraceptives only after you have weaned your child completely.

3. Laboratory tests

If you are scheduled for any laboratory tests, tell your doctor or clinic you are taking birth control pills. Certain blood tests may be affected by birth control pills.

4. Drug interactions

Certain drugs may interact with birth control pills to make them less effective in preventing pregnancy or cause an increase in breakthrough bleeding. Such drugs include rifampin, drugs used for epilepsy such as barbiturates (for example, phenobarbital), anticonvulsants such as carbamazepine (Tegretol is one brand of this drug), phenytoin (Dilantin is one brand of this drug), phenylbutazone (Butazolidin is one brand), and possibly certain antibiotics. You may need to use additional contraception when you take drugs which can make oral contraceptives less effective.

THIS PRODUCT (LIKE ALL ORAL CONTRACEPTIVES) IS INTENDED TO PREVENT PREGNANCY. IT DOES NOT PROTECT AGAINST TRANSMISSION OF HIV (AIDS) AND OTHER SEXUALLY TRANSMITTED DISEASES SUCH AS CHLAMYDIA, GENITAL HERPES, GENITAL WARTS, GONORRHEA, HEPATITIS B, AND SYPHILIS.

HOW TO TAKE THE PILL.

IMPORTANT POINTS TO REMEMBER.

BEFORE YOU START TAKING YOUR PILLS:

1. BE SURE TO READ THESE DIRECTIONS:
   Before you start taking your pills.
   Anytime you are not sure what to do.
2. THE RIGHT WAY TO TAKE THE PILL IS TO TAKE ONE PILL EVERY DAY AT THE SAME TIME.
   If you miss pills you could get pregnant. This includes starting the pack late. The more pills you miss, the more likely you are to get pregnant.
3. MANY WOMEN HAVE SPOTTING OR LIGHT BLEEDING, OR MAY FEEL SICK TO THEIR STOMACH DURING THE FIRST 1–3 PACKS OF PILLS.
   If you feel sick to your stomach, do not stop taking the pill. The problem will usually go away. If it doesn't go away, check with your doctor or clinic.
4. MISSING PILLS CAN ALSO CAUSE SPOTTING OR LIGHT BLEEDING, even when you make up these missed pills. On the days you take 2 pills to make up for missed pills, you could also feel a little sick to your stomach.
5. IF YOU HAVE VOMITING OR DIARRHEA, for any reason, or IF YOU TAKE SOME MEDICINES, including some antibiotics, your pills may not work as well.
   Use a back-up method (such as condoms, foam, or sponge) until you check with your doctor or clinic.
6. IF YOU HAVE TROUBLE REMEMBERING TO TAKE THE PILL, talk to your doctor or clinic about how to make pill-taking easier or about using another method of birth control.
7. IF YOU HAVE ANY QUESTIONS OR ARE UNSURE ABOUT THE INFORMATION IN THIS LEAFLET, call your doctor or clinic.

BEFORE YOU START TAKING YOUR PILLS:

1. DECIDE WHAT TIME OF DAY YOU WANT TO TAKE YOUR PILL. It is important to take it at about the same time every day.
2. LOOK AT YOUR PILL PACK TO SEE IF IT HAS 21 OR 28 PILLS:
   The **21-pill pack** has 21 "active" [white] pills (with hormones) to take for 3 weeks, followed by 1 week without pills.
   The **28-pill pack** has 21 "active" [white] pills (with hormones) to take for 3 weeks, followed by 1 week of reminder [green] pills (without hormones).
3. ALSO FIND:
   1) where on the pack to start taking the pills,
   2) in what order to take the pills (follow the arrows) and
   3) the week numbers printed on the pack.
4. BE SURE YOU HAVE READY AT ALL TIMES:
   ANOTHER KIND OF BIRTH CONTROL (such as condoms, foam or sponge) to use as a back-up in case you miss pills.
   AN EXTRA, FULL PILL PACK.

WHEN TO START THE FIRST PACK OF PILLS:

You have a choice of which day to start taking your first pack of pills. Decide with your doctor or clinic which is the best day for you. Pick a time of day which will be easy to remember.

DAY 1 START:

1. Pick the day label strip that starts with the first day of your period (this is the day you start bleeding or spotting, even if it is almost midnight when the bleeding begins).
2. Place this day label strip in the cycle tablet dispenser over the area that has the days of the week (starting with Sunday) imprinted in the plastic.
   Note: If the first day of your period is a Sunday, you can skip steps #1 and #2.
3. Take the first "active" [white] pill of the first pack during the first 24 hours of your period.
4. You will not need to use a back-up method of birth control, since you are starting the pill at the beginning of your period.

ANNUAL NUMBER OF BIRTH-RELATED OR METHOD-RELATED DEATHS ASSOCIATED WITH CONTROL OF FERTILITY PER 100,000 NON-STERILE WOMEN, BY FERTILITY CONTROL METHOD ACCORDING TO AGE

Method of control and outcome	15–19	20–24	25–29	30–34	35–39	40–44
No fertility control methods*	7.0	7.4	9.1	14.8	25.7	28.2
Oral contraceptives non-smoker**	0.3	0.5	0.9	1.9	13.8	31.6
Oral contraceptives smoker**	2.2	3.4	6.6	13.5	51.1	117.2
IUD**	0.8	0.8	1.0	1.0	1.4	1.4
Condom*	1.1	1.6	0.7	0.2	0.3	0.4
Diaphragm/spermicide*	1.9	1.2	1.2	1.3	2.2	2.8
Periodic abstinence*	2.5	1.6	1.6	1.7	2.9	3.6

* Deaths are birth related
** Deaths are method related

SUNDAY START:

1. Take the first "active" [white] pill of the first pack on the Sunday after your period starts, even if you are still bleeding. If your period begins on Sunday, start the pack that same day.
2. Use another method of birth control as a back-up method if you have sex anytime from the Sunday you start your first pack until the next Sunday (7 days). Condoms, foam or the sponge are good back-up methods of birth control.

WHAT TO DO DURING THE MONTH:

1. **TAKE ONE PILL AT THE SAME TIME EVERY DAY UNTIL THE PACK IS EMPTY.**
   Do not skip pills even if you are spotting or bleeding between monthly periods or feel sick to your stomach (nausea).
   Do not skip pills even if you do not have sex very often.
2. **WHEN YOU FINISH A PACK OR SWITCH YOUR BRAND OF PILLS:**
   21 pills: Wait 7 days to start the next pack. You will probably have your period during that week. Be sure that no more than 7 days pass between 21-day packs.
   28 pills: Start the next pack on the day after your last "reminder" pill. Do not wait any days between packs.

WHAT TO DO IF YOU MISS PILLS:

If you **MISS 1** [white] "active" pill:

1. Take it as soon as you remember. Take the next pill at your regular time. This means you take 2 pills in 1 day.
2. You do not need to use a back-up birth control method if you have sex.

If you **MISS 2** [white] "active" pills in a row in **WEEK 1 OR WEEK 2** of your pack:

1. Take 2 pills on the day you remember and 2 pills the next day.
2. Then take 1 pill a day until you finish the pack.
3. You MAY BECOME PREGNANT if you have sex in the 7 days after you miss pills.
   You MUST use another birth control method (such as condoms, foam, or sponge) as a back-up method for those 7 days.

If you **MISS 2** [white] "active" pills in a row in **THE 3RD WEEK:**

1. ***If you are a Day 1 Starter:***
   THROW OUT the rest of the pill pack and start a new pack that same day.
   If you are a Sunday Starter:
   Keep taking 1 pill every day until Sunday.
   On Sunday, THROW OUT the rest of the pack and start a new pack of pills that same day.
2. You may not have your period this month but this is expected. However, if you miss your period 2 months in a row, call your doctor or clinic because you might be pregnant.
3. You MAY BECOME PREGNANT if you have sex in the **7 days** after you miss pills. You MUST use another birth control method (such as condoms, foam, or sponge) as a back-up method for those 7 days.

If you **MISS 3 OR MORE** [white] "active" pills in a row (during the first 3 weeks):

1. ***If you are a Day 1 Starter:***
   THROW OUT the rest of the pill pack and start a new pack that same day.
   If you are a Sunday Starter:
   Keep taking 1 pill every day until Sunday.
   On Sunday, THROW OUT the rest of the pack and start a new pack of pills that same day.
2. You may not have your period this month but this is expected. However, if you miss your period 2 months in a row, call your doctor or clinic because you might be pregnant.
3. You MAY BECOME PREGNANT if you have sex in the **7 days** after you miss pills. You MUST use another birth control method (such as condoms, foam, or sponge) as a back-up method for those 7 days.

A REMINDER FOR THOSE ON 28-DAY PACKS:

If you forget any of the 7 [green] "reminder" pills in Week 4:
THROW AWAY the pills you missed.
Keep taking 1 pill each day until the pack is empty.
You do not need a back-up method.

FINALLY, IF YOU ARE STILL NOT SURE WHAT TO DO ABOUT THE PILLS YOU HAVE MISSED:

Use a BACK-UP METHOD anytime you have sex.
KEEP TAKING ONE [WHITE] "ACTIVE" PILL EACH DAY until you can reach your doctor or clinic.

PREGNANCY DUE TO PILL FAILURE

The incidence of pill failure resulting in pregnancy is approximately one percent (i.e., one pregnancy per 100 women per year) if taken every day as directed, but more typical failure rates are about 3%. If failure does occur, the risk to the fetus is minimal.

PREGNANCY AFTER STOPPING THE PILL

There may be some delay in becoming pregnant after you stop using oral contraceptives, especially if you had irregular menstrual cycles before you used oral contraceptives. It may be advisable to postpone conception until you begin menstruating regularly once you have stopped taking the pill and desire pregnancy.

There does not appear to be any increase in birth defects in newborn babies when pregnancy occurs soon after stopping the pill.

OVERDOSAGE

Serious ill effects have not been reported following ingestion of large doses of oral contraceptives by young children. Overdosage may cause nausea and withdrawal bleeding in females. In case of overdosage, contact your doctor, clinic or pharmacist.

OTHER INFORMATION

Your doctor or clinic will take a medical and family history before prescribing oral contraceptives and will examine you. The physical examination may be delayed to another time if you request it and your doctor or clinic believes that it is a good medical practice to postpone it. You should be reexamined at least once a year. Be sure to inform your doctor or clinic if there is a family history of any of the conditions listed previously in this leaflet. Be sure to keep all appointments with your doctor or clinic because this is a time to determine if there are early signs of side effects of oral contraceptive use.

Do not use the drug for any condition other than the one for which it was prescribed. This drug has been prescribed specifically for you; do not give it to others who may want birth control pills.

HEALTH BENEFITS FROM ORAL CONTRACEPTIVES

In addition to preventing pregnancy, use of combination oral contraceptives may provide certain benefits. They are:

- menstrual cycles may become more regular
- blood flow during menstruation may be lighter and less iron may be lost. Therefore, anemia due to iron deficiency is less likely to occur
- pain or other symptoms during menstruation may be encountered less frequently
- ectopic (tubal) pregnancy may occur less frequently
- non-cancerous cysts or lumps in the breast may occur less frequently
- acute pelvic inflammatory disease may occur less frequently
- oral contraceptive use may provide some protection against developing two forms of cancer: cancer of the ovaries and cancer of the lining of the uterus

If you want more information about birth control pills, ask your doctor, clinic or pharmacist. They have a more technical leaflet called the Professional Labeling, which you may wish to read. The Professional Labeling is also published in a book entitled *Physicians' Desk Reference,* available in many book stores and public libraries.

 1/00 23

Manufactured for Organon Inc.
West Orange, NJ 07052
by N.V. Organon, Oss, The Netherlands or
Organon (Ireland) Ltd, Swords, Co. Dublin, Ireland
Shown in Product Identification Guide, page 327

FOLLISTIM® ℞
(follitropin beta for injection)

FOR SUBCUTANEOUS OR INTRAMUSCULAR USE ONLY

DESCRIPTION

Follistim® (follitropin beta for injection) contains human follicle-stimulating hormone (hFSH), a glycoprotein hormone which is manufactured by recombinant DNA (rDNA) technology. Follitropin beta has a dimeric structure containing two glycoprotein subunits (alpha and beta). Both the 92 amino acid alpha-chain and the 111 amino acid beta-chain have complex heterogeneous structures arising from two N-linked oligosaccharide chains. Follitropin beta is synthesized in a Chinese hamster ovary (CHO) cell line that has been transfected with a plasmid containing the two subunit DNA sequences encoding for hFSH. The purification process results in a highly purified preparation with a consistent hFSH isoform profile and high specific activity[1]. The biological activity is determined by measuring the increase in ovary weight in female rats. The intrinsic luteinizing hormone (LH) activity in follitropin beta is less than 1 IU per 40,000 IU FSH. The compound is considered to contain no LH activity.

The amino acid sequence and tertiary structure of the product are indistinguishable from that of human follicle-stimulating hormone (hFSH) of urinary source. Also, based on available data derived from physio-chemical tests and bioassay, follitropin beta and follitropin alfa, another recombinant follicle-stimulating hormone product, are indistinguishable.

Follistim® is presented as a sterile, freeze-dried cake, intended for SUBCUTANEOUS or INTRAMUSCULAR administration after reconstitution with Sterile Water for Injection, USP. Each vial of Follistim® contains 75 IU of FSH activity plus 25.0 mg sucrose, NF; 7.35 mg sodium citrate dihydrate, USP; 0.10 mg polysorbate 20, NF, and hydrochloric acid, NF and/or sodium hydroxide, NF to adjust the pH in a sterile, lyophilized form. The pH of the reconstituted preparation is approximately 7.0. The recombinant protein in Follistim® has been standardized for FSH *in vivo* bioactivity in terms of the First International Reference Preparation for human menopausal gonadotropins (code 70/45), issued by the World Health Organization Expert Committee on Biological Standardization (1982). Under current storage conditions, Follistim® may contain up to 20% of oxidized follitropin beta.

In clinical trials with Follistim®, serum antibodies to FSH or anti-CHO cell derived proteins were not detected in any of the treated patients after exposure to Follistim® for up to three cycles.

Therapeutic Class: Infertility.

[1]As determined by the Ph. Eur. Test for FSH *in vivo* bioactivity and on the basis of the molar extinction coefficient at 277 nm (ϵ_s:$mg^{-1}cm^{-1}$) = 1.066.

CLINICAL PHARMACOLOGY

Follistim® (follitropin beta for injection) stimulates ovarian follicular growth in women who do not have primary ovarian failure. FSH, the active component of Follistim®, is required for normal follicular growth, maturation, and gonadal steroid production. In the female, the level of FSH is critical for the onset and duration of follicular development, and consequently for the timing and number of follicles reaching maturity. In order to effect the final phase of follicle maturation, resumption of meiosis and rupture of the follicle in the absence of an endogenous LH surge, human chorionic gonadotropin (hCG) must be given following the administration of Follistim® when patient monitoring indicates that appropriate follicular development parameters have been reached.

Pharmacokinetics

Absorption

The bioavailablity of Follistim® following subcutaneous and intramuscular administration was investigated in healthy, pituitary-suppressed, female subjects given a single 300 IU dose. After subcutaneous or intramuscular injection the apparent dose absorbed was 77.8% and 76.4%, respectively.

The subcutaneous (455.6 ± 141.4 IU*h/L) and intramuscular (445.7 ± 135.7 IU*h/L) routes of administration were equivalent with respect to area under the curve (AUC) in healthy, pituitary-suppressed, female subjects given a single 300 IU dose. However, equivalence could not be established for C_{max} between the subcutaneous (5.41 ± 0.72 IU/L) and intramuscular (6.86 ± 2.90 IU/L) routes of administration.

The pharmacokinetics and pharmacodynamics of a single, intramuscular dose (300 IU) of Follistim® were also investigated in a group of gonadotropin-deficient, but otherwise healthy women. Peak (C_{max}) serum FSH levels in these women were 4.3 ± 1.7 IU/L (mean ± SD) and it occurred approximately 27 hours after intramuscular administration.

A multiple, dose proportionality, pharmacokinetic study of Follistim® was completed in healthy, pituitary-suppressed, female subjects given intramuscular doses of 75 IU, 150 IU, or 225 IU for 7 days. Steady-state blood concentrations of FSH were reached with all doses after 4 days of treatment based on the minimum concentrations of FSH just prior to dosing (C_{min}). Peak blood concentrations with the 75 IU, 150 IU, and 225 IU dose were 4.65 ± 1.49 IU/L, 9.46 ± 2.57 IU/L and 11.30 ± 1.77 IU/L, respectively.

A multiple, dose proportionality, pharmacokinetic study of Follistim® was completed in healthy, pituitary-suppressed, female subjects given subcutaneous doses of 75 IU, 150 IU, or 225 IU for 7 days. Steady-state blood concentrations of FSH were reached with all doses after 5 days of treatment based on the minimum concentrations of FSH just prior to dosing (C_{min}). Peak blood concentrations with the 75 IU, 150 IU, and 225 IU dose were 4.30 ± 0.60 IU/L, 8.51 ± 1.16 IU/L and 13.92 ± 1.81 IU/L, respectively.

Distribution

The volume of distribution of Follistim® in healthy, pituitary-suppressed, female subjects following intravenous administration of a 300 IU dose was approximately 8 L.

Metabolism

The recombinant FSH in Follistim® is biochemically very similar to urinary FSH and it is therefore anticipated that it is metabolized in the same manner.

Elimination

The elimination half-life following a single intramuscular dose (300 IU) of Follistim® in female subjects was 43.9 ± 14.1 hours (mean ± SD). The elimination half-life following a 7-day intramuscular treatment with 75 IU, 150 IU, or 225 IU was 26.9 ± 7.8 hours (mean ± SD), 30.1 ± 6.2, and 28.9 ± 6.5, respectively.

Special Populations

The effect of body weight on the pharmacokinetics of Follistim® was evaluated in a group of European and Japanese women who were significantly different in terms of body weight. The European subjects had a body weight of (mean ± SD) 67.4 ± 13.5 kg and the Japanese subjects were 46.8 ± 11.6 kg. Following a single intramuscular dose of 300 IU of Follistim®, the AUC (IU*h/L) was significantly smaller in European subjects (339 ± 105) than in Japanese subjects (544 ± 201). However, clearance per kg of body weight was essentially the same for the respective groups (0.014 and 0.013 $1{*}h^{-1}kg^{-1}$).

Clinical Studies

The efficacy of Follistim® was established in four controlled, clinical studies [three studies for Assisted Reproductive Technologies (ART) and one study for Ovulation Induction], three of which are described below. In these comparative studies, there were no clinically significant differences between treatment groups in study outcomes.

Assisted Reproductive Technologies (ART)

Results from a randomized, assessor-blind, group comparative, multicenter safety and efficacy study of Follistim® (Protocol 37608) in 981 infertile women treated for one cycle with *in vitro* fertilization with Follistim® or Metrodin® after pituitary suppression with a GnRH agonist are summarized in Table I.

[See tables I & II at top of next page]

Continued on next page

Follistim—Cont.

Results from a randomized, assessor-blind, group comparative, single center safety and efficacy study of Follistim® (Protocol 37604) in 89 infertile women treated with *in vitro* fertilization with Follistim® or Humegon® without pituitary suppression with a GnRH agonist are summarized in Table III.

[See table III at right]

The outcomes of the 22 clinical pregnancies (14 in Follistim® and 8 in Humegon®) are shown in Table IV:

[See table IV at right]

Ovulation Induction

Results from a randomized, assessor-blind, group comparative, multicenter safety and efficacy study of Follistim® (Protocol 37609) in 172 chronic anovulatory women who failed to ovulate and/or conceive during clomiphene citrate treatment are summarized in Tables V, VI, and VII.

[See table V at right]
[See table VI at top of next page]

The outcomes of the 56 clinical pregnancies (35 in Follistim® and 21 in Metrodin®) are shown in Table VII:

[See table VII at top of next page]

INDICATIONS AND USAGE

Follistim® (follitropin beta for injection) is indicated for the development of multiple follicles in ovulatory patients participating in an Assisted Reproductive Technology (ART) program. Follistim® is also indicated for the induction of ovulation and pregnancy in anovulatory infertile patients in whom the cause of infertility is functional and not due to primary ovarian failure.

Selection of Patients

Before treatment with Follistim® is instituted:

1. A thorough gynecologic and endocrinologic evaluation of the patient must be performed. The evaluation should include a hysterosalpingogram (to rule out uterine and tubal pathology) and documentation of anovulation by means of reviewing a patient's history, performing a physical examination, determining serum hormonal levels as indicated, and optionally performing an endometrial biopsy. Patients with tubal pathology should receive Follistim® only if enrolled in an ART program.
2. Primary ovarian failure should be excluded by the determination of circulating gonadotropin levels.
3. Careful examination should be made to rule out early pregnancy.
4. Evaluation of the partner's fertility potential should be included in the workup procedure.

CONTRAINDICATIONS

Follistim® (follitropin beta for injection) is contraindicated in women who exhibit:

1. Prior hypersensitivity to recombinant hFSH products.
2. A high circulating FSH level indicating primary ovarian failure.
3. Uncontrolled thyroid or adrenal dysfunction.
4. Tumor of the ovary, breast, uterus, hypothalamus or pituitary gland.
5. Pregnancy.
6. Heavy or irregular vaginal bleeding of undetermined origin.
7. Ovarian cysts or enlargement not due to polycystic ovary syndrome (PCOS).

WARNINGS

Follistim® (follitropin beta for injection) should be used only by physicians who are experienced in infertility treatment. Follistim® is a potent gonadotropic substance capable of causing Ovarian Hyperstimulation Syndrome (OHSS) (see WARNINGS-Overstimulation of the Ovary During Follistim® Therapy) with or without pulmonary or vascular complications (see WARNINGS-Pulmonary and Vascular Complications) and multiple births (see WARNINGS-Multiple Births). Gonadotropin therapy requires the availability of appropriate monitoring facilities (see PRECAUTIONS-Laboratory Tests).

Overstimulation of the Ovary During Follistim® Therapy

In order to minimize the hazards associated with the occasional abnormal ovarian enlargement that may occur with Follistim® therapy, the lowest effective dose should be used (see DOSAGE AND ADMINISTRATION). Use of ultrasound monitoring of ovarian response and/or measurement of serum estradiol levels can further minimize the risk of overstimulation.

If the ovaries are abnormally enlarged on the last day of Follistim® therapy, hCG should not be administered in this course of treatment; this will reduce the chances of developing Ovarian Hyperstimulation Syndrome (OHSS).

The Ovarian Hyperstimulation Syndrome (OHSS): OHSS is a medical entity distinct from uncomplicated ovarian enlargement and may progress rapidly to become a serious medical event. OHSS is characterized by a dramatic increase in vascular permeability, which can result in a rapid accumulation of fluid in the peritoneal cavity, thorax, and potentially, the pericardium. The early warning signs of OHSS developing are severe pelvic pain, nausea, vomiting and weight gain. The following symptoms have been reported in cases of OHSS: abdominal pain, abdominal distension, gastrointestinal symptoms including nausea, vomiting and diarrhea, severe ovarian enlargement, weight gain, dyspnea, and oliguria. Clinical evaluation may reveal hypovolemia, hemoconcentration, electrolyte imbalances, ascites, hemoperitoneum, pleural effusions, hydrothorax, acute pulmonary distress, and thromboembolic events (see WARNINGS-Pulmonary and Vascular Complications).

During clinical trials with Follistim® therapy, OHSS occurred in 53 (5.2%) of the 1,029 women treated and of these 29 (2.8%) were hospitalized. Cases of OHSS are more common, more severe, and more protracted if pregnancy occurs; therefore, patients should be followed for at least two weeks after hCG administration. Most often, OHSS occurs after treatment has been discontinued and it can develop rapidly, reaching its maximum about seven to ten days following treatment. Usually, OHSS resolves spontaneously with the onset of menses. If there is evidence that OHSS may be developing prior to hCG administration (see PRECAUTIONS-Laboratory Tests), the hCG must be withheld.

TABLE I. Results From a Randomized, Assessor-blind, Group Comparative, Multicenter Safety and Efficacy Study of Follistim® (Protocol 37608) in Infertile Women Treated With *In Vitro* Fertilization With Follistim® or Metrodin® After Pituitary Suppression With a GnRH Agonist[1]

Parameter	Follistim® (n=585)	Metrodin® (n=396)
Total number of oocytes recovered	10.9	9.0
Number of mature oocytes recovered	9.1	7.3
Maximum serum estradiol before hCG (pmol/L)[2]	6637	5692
Treatment duration (days)	11.0 (range 1-29)	11.6 (range 1-21)
Ongoing[3] pregnancy rate/attempt	22.2%	18.2%
Ongoing[3] pregnancy rate/transfer[4]	26.0%	22.0%

[1] All values are means
[2] Conversion factor to pg/mL is 3.671
[3] A single vital or multiple vital pregnancy was termed ongoing when a pregnancy, at least 12 weeks after embryo transfer (ET), was confirmed by the investigator
[4] Transfers were limited to a maximum of three embryos
Metrodin® is a registered trademark of Serono Laboratories, Inc., Randolph, MA 02368.

The outcomes of the 286 clinical pregnancies (179 in Follistim® and 107 in Metrodin®) are shown in Table II:

TABLE II. Outcome for All Clinical* Pregnancies

	Follistim® (n=179)	Metrodin® (n=107)
Did not result in live birth	50 (28%)	35 (33%)
Single birth	87 (49%)	43 (40%)
Multiple birth	42 (23%)	29 (27%)

*Clinical pregnancies included ongoing pregnancies as well as miscarriages with or without proof of a vital fetus

TABLE III. Results From a Randomized, Assessor-blind, Group Comparative, Single Center Safety and Efficacy Study of Follistim® (Protocol 37604) in Infertile Women Treated With *In Vitro* Fertilization With Follistim® or Humegon® Without Pituitary Suppression With a GnRH Agonist[1]

Parameter	Follistim® (n=54)	Humegon® (n=35)
Total number of oocytes recovered	9.9	7.6
Number of mature oocytes recovered	9.4	6.9
Maximum serum estradiol before hCG (pmol/L)[2]	3791	3087
Treatment duration (days)	5.8 (range 1-9)	6.0 (range 2-10)
Ongoing[3] pregnancy rate/attempt	22.2%	17.1%
Ongoing[3] pregnancy rate/transfer[4]	30.8%	22.2%

[1] All values are means
[2] Conversion factor to pg/mL is 3.671
[3] A single vital or multiple vital pregnancy was termed ongoing when a pregnancy, at least 12 weeks after embryo transfer (ET), was confirmed by the investigator
[4] Transfers were limited to a maximum of three embryos

TABLE IV. Outcome for All Clinical* Pregnancies

	Follistim® (n=14)	Humegon® (n=8)
Did not result in live birth	2 (14%)	2 (25%)
Single birth	7 (50%)	4 (50%)
Multiple birth	5 (36%)	2 (25%)

*Clinical pregnancies included ongoing pregnancies as well as miscarriages with or without proof of a vital fetus

TABLE V. Cumulative Ovulation Rates From Protocol 37609

	Follistim® (n=105)	Metrodin® (n=67)
First treatment cycle	72%	63%
Second treatment cycle	82%	79%
Third treatment cycle	85%	82%

If serious OHSS occurs, treatment should be stopped and the patient should be hospitalized. Treatment is primarily symptomatic and should consist of bed rest, fluid and electrolyte management, and analgesics (if needed). Hemoconcentration associated with fluid loss into the peritoneal cavity, pleural cavity, and the pericardial cavity may occur and should be thoroughly assessed in the following manner: 1) fluid intake and output; 2) weight; 3) hematocrit; 4) serum and urinary electrolytes; 5) urine specific gravity; 6) BUN and creatinine; 7) total proteins with albumin: globulin ratio; 8) coagulation studies; 9) electrocardiogram to monitor for hyperkalemia and 10) abdominal girth. These determinations should be performed daily or more often based on clinical need.

OHSS increases the risk of injury to the ovary. The ascitic, pleural, and pericardial fluid should not be removed unless there is the necessity to relieve symptoms such as pulmonary distress or cardiac tamponade. Pelvic examination may cause rupture of an ovarian cyst, which may result in hemoperitoneum, and should therefore be avoided. If bleeding occurs and requires surgical intervention, the clinical objective should be to control the bleeding and retain as much ovarian tissue as possible. Intercourse should be prohibited in patients with significant ovarian enlargement after ovulation because of the danger of hemoperitoneum resulting from ruptured ovarian cysts.

The management of OHSS may be divided into three phases: an acute, a chronic, and a resolution phase. Because the use of diuretics can accentuate the diminished intravascular volume, diuretics should be avoided except in the late phase of resolution as described below.

Acute Phase: Management during the acute phase should be directed at preventing hemoconcentration due to loss of intravascular volume to the third space and minimizing the risk of thromboembolic phenomena and kidney damage. Treatment is intended to normalize electrolytes while maintaining an acceptable but somewhat reduced intravascular volume. Full correction of the intravascular volume deficit may lead to an unacceptable increase in the amount of third space fluid accumulation.

Management includes administration of limited intravenous fluids, electrolytes, human serum albumin and strict monitoring of fluid intake and output. Monitoring for the development of hyperkalemia is recommended.

Chronic Phase: After stabilizing the patient during the acute phase, excessive fluid accumulation in the third space should be limited by instituting severe potassium, sodium, and fluid restriction.

Resolution Phase: A fall in hematocrit and an increasing urinary output without an increased intake are observed due to the return of the third space fluid to the intravascular compartment. Peripheral and/or pulmonary edema may result if the kidneys are unable to excrete third space fluid as rapidly as it is mobilized. Diuretics may be indicated during the resolution phase, if necessary, to combat pulmonary edema.

Pulmonary and Vascular Complications

Serious pulmonary conditions (e.g., atelectasis, acute respiratory distress syndrome) have been reported in women treated with gonadotropins. In addition, thromboembolic events both in association with, and separate from, the Ovarian Hyperstimulation Syndrome have been reported following gonadotropin therapy. Intravascular thrombosis, which may originate in venous or arterial vessels, can result in reduced blood flow to vital organs or the extremities. Sequelae of such events have included venous thrombophlebitis, pulmonary embolism, pulmonary infarction, cerebral vascular occlusion (stroke), and arterial occlusion resulting in loss of limb. In rare cases, pulmonary complications and/or thromboembolic events have resulted in death.

Multiple Births

Reports of multiple births have been associated with Follistim® treatment. The patient and her partner should be advised of the potential risk of multiple births before starting treatment. In clinical trials with Follistim® and Metrodin®, multiple gestation rates in ART patients were 31% and 38%, respectively, and in ovulation induction patients, the rates were 8% in both groups.

PRECAUTIONS

General

Careful attention should be given to the diagnosis of infertility and in the selection of candidates for Follistim® (follitropin beta for injection) therapy (see INDICATIONS AND USAGE-Selection of Patients).

Information for Patients

Prior to therapy with Follistim®, patients should be informed of the duration of treatment and monitoring procedures that will be required. The risks of Ovarian Hyperstimulation Syndrome and multiple births (see WARNINGS), and other possible adverse reactions (see ADVERSE REACTIONS) should be discussed.

Laboratory Tests

In most instances, treatment with Follistim® will result only in follicular growth and maturation. In order to complete the final phase of follicular maturation and to induce ovulation, hCG must be given following the administration of Follistim® or when clinical assessment of the patient indicates that sufficient follicular maturation has occurred. This may be directly estimated by sonographic visualization of the ovaries and endometrial lining and/or measuring serum estradiol levels. The combination of both ultrasonography and measurement of estradiol levels is useful for monitoring the growth and development of follicles, timing hCG administration, as well as minimizing the risk of OHSS and multiple gestations.

The clinical evaluation of estrogenic activity (changes in vaginal cytology, changes in appearance and volume of cervical mucus, spinnbarkeit, and ferning of the cervical mucus) provides an indirect estimate of the estrogenic effect upon the target organs, and therefore it should only be used adjunctively with more direct estimates of follicular development (e.g., ultrasonography and serum estradiol determinations).

The clinical confirmation of ovulation is obtained by direct and indirect indices of progesterone production. The indices most generally used are as follows:

a) A rise in basal body temperature,
b) Increase in serum progesterone, and
c) Menstruation following the shift in basal body temperature.

When used in conjunction with indices of progesterone production, sonographic visualization of the ovaries will assist in determining if ovulation has occurred. Sonographic evidence of ovulation may include the following:

a) Fluid in the cul-de-sac,
b) Follicle showing marked decrease in size, and
c) Collapsed follicle.

Drug Interactions

No drug/drug interaction studies have been performed.

Carcinogenesis and Mutagenesis, Impairment of Fertility

Long-term toxicity studies in animals have not been performed with Follistim® to evaluate the carcinogenic potential of the drug. Follistim® was not mutagenic in the Ames test using *S. typhimurium* and *E. coli* tester strains and did not produce chromosomal aberrations in an *in vitro* assay using human lymphocytes.

Pregnancy

Pregnancy Category X: (See CONTRAINDICATIONS).

Nursing Mothers

It is not known whether this drug is excreted in human milk. Because many drugs are excreted in human milk and because of the potential for serious adverse reactions in the nursing infant from Follistim®, a decision should be made whether to discontinue nursing or to discontinue the drug, taking into account the importance of the drug to the mother.

Pediatric Use

Safety and effectiveness in pediatric patients have not been established.

Geriatric Use

Clinical studies of Follistim® did not include subjects aged 65 and over.

ADVERSE REACTIONS

Assisted Reproductive Technologies (ART)

Rates of adverse events from a randomized, assessor-blind, group comparative, multicenter safety and efficacy study of Follistim® (Protocol 37608) in 989 infertile women treated with *in vitro* fertilization with Follistim® or Metrodin® after pituitary suppression with a GnRH agonist are summarized in Table VIII.

[See table VIII above]

Ovulation Induction

Rates of adverse events from a randomized, assessor-blind, group comparative, multicenter safety and efficacy study of Follistim® (Protocol 37609) in 172 chronic anovulatory women who failed to ovulate and/or conceive during clomiphene citrate treatment are summarized in Table IX.

[See table IX above]

The following adverse events have been reported in women treated with gonadotropins: pulmonary and vascular complications (see WARNINGS), hemoperitoneum, adnexal torsion (as a complication of ovarian enlargement), dizziness, tachycardia, dyspnea, tachypnea, febrile reactions, flu-like symptoms including fever, chills, musculoskeletal aches, joint pains, nausea, headache and malaise, breast tenderness, and dermatological symptoms (dry skin, body rash, hair loss and hives).

There have been infrequent reports of ovarian neoplasms, both benign and malignant, in women who have undergone multiple drug regimens for ovulation induction; however, a causal relationship has not been established.

TABLE VI. Cumulative Ongoing[1] Pregnancy Rates From Protocol 37609

	Follistim® (n=105)	Metrodin® (n=67)
First treatment cycle	14%	10%
Second treatment cycle	19%	18%
Third treatment cycle	23%	19%

[1] All ongoing pregnancies were confirmed after at least 12 weeks after the hCG injection

TABLE VII. Outcome for All Clinical* Pregnancies

	Follistim® (n=35)	Metrodin® (n=21)
Did not result in live birth	11 (31%)	8 (38%)
Single birth	22 (63%)	12 (57%)
Multiple birth	2 (6%)	1 (5%)

*Clinical pregnancies included ongoing pregnancies as well as miscarriages with or without proof of a vital fetus

TABLE VIII. Incidence of Adverse Clinical Experiences (>1%) that Occurred in Protocol 37608

Adverse Event	Follistim® (n=591)	Metrodin® (n=398)
Miscarriage	11.0%	11.3%
Ovarian Hyperstimulation Syndrome	5.2%	4.3%
Ectopic pregnancy	3.0%	3.8%
Abdominal pain	2.5%	2.3%
Injection site pain	1.7%	0.5%
Vaginal hemorrhage	1.5%	0.8%

TABLE IX. Incidence of Adverse Clinical Experiences (>1%) that Occurred in Protocol 37609

Adverse Event	Follistim® (n=105)	Metrodin® (n=67)
Miscarriage	9.5%	9.0%
Ovarian Hyperstimulation Syndrome	7.6%	4.5%
Abdominal discomfort	2.9%	1.5%
Abdominal pain, lower	2.9%	1.5%
Abdominal pain	1.9%	3.0%
Ovarian cyst	2.9%	3.0%

Continued on next page

Follistim—Cont.

DRUG ABUSE AND DEPENDENCE

There have been no reports of abuse or dependence with Follistim® (follitropin beta for injection).

OVERDOSAGE

Aside from the possibility of Ovarian Hyperstimulation Syndrome (see WARNINGS-Overstimulation of the Ovary During Follistim® Therapy) and multiple gestations (see WARNINGS-Multiple Births), there is no additional information concerning the consequences of acute overdosage with Follistim® (follitropin beta for injection).

DOSAGE AND ADMINISTRATION

Assisted Reproductive Technologies (ART)

A starting dose of 150 to 225 IU of Follistim® (follitropin beta for injection) is recommended for at least the first four days of treatment. After this, the dose may be adjusted for the individual patient based upon their ovarian response. In clinical studies with patients who are responding, it was shown that daily maintenance dosages ranging from 75 to 300 IU for six to twelve days are sufficient, although longer treatment may be necessary. However, in patients that were low or poor responders, maintenance doses of 375 to 600 IU were administered according to individual response. This later category comprised approximately 10% of the women evaluated during clinical studies. The maximum, individualized, daily dose of Follistim® that has been used in clinical studies is 600 IU. When a sufficient number of follicles of adequate size are present, the final maturation of the follicles is induced by administering hCG at a dose of 5,000 IU to 10,000 IU. Oocyte (egg) retrieval is performed 34 to 36 hours later. The administration of hCG must be withheld in cases where the ovaries are abnormally enlarged on the last day of Follistim® therapy; this will reduce the chance of developing OHSS.

Ovulation Induction

There are a variety of treatment protocols available for ovulation induction. In studies using Follistim®, a stepwise gradually increasing dosing scheme was used. The starting dose was 75 IU of Follistim® for up to 14 days. The dose was then increased by 37.5 IU of Follistim® at weekly intervals until follicular growth and/or serum estradiol levels indicated an adequate response. The maximum, individualized, daily dose of Follistim® that has been safely used for ovulation induction patients during clinical trials is 300 IU. The patient should be treated until ultrasonic visualizations and/or serum estradiol determinations indicate pre-ovulatory conditions equivalent to or greater than those of the normal individual followed by hCG, 5,000 IU to 10,000 IU. If the ovaries are abnormally enlarged on the last day of Follistim® therapy, hCG must be withheld during this course of treatment; this will reduce the chances of developing OHSS.

During treatment with Follistim® and during a two week post-treatment period, patients should be examined at least every other day for signs of excessive ovarian stimulation. It is recommended that Follistim® administration be stopped if the ovaries become abnormally enlarged or abdominal pain occurs. Most OHSS occurs after treatment has been discontinued and reaches its maximum at about seven to ten days post-ovulation.

For ovulation induction, the couple should be encouraged to have intercourse daily, beginning on the day prior to the administration of hCG and until ovulation becomes apparent from the indices employed for the determination of progestational activity (see PRECAUTIONS-Laboratory Tests). Care should be taken to insure insemination. In the light of the foregoing indices and parameters mentioned, it should become obvious that, unless a physician is willing to devote considerable time to these patients and be familiar with and conduct these necessary laboratory studies, he/she should not use Follistim®.

Directions for using Follistim®

1. Wash hands thoroughly with soap and water.
2. Before injections, the septum tops of the vials should be wiped with an aseptic solution to prevent contamination of the contents.
3. To prepare the Follistim® solution, inject 1 mL of Sterile Water for Injection, USP into the vial of Follistim®. **DO NOT SHAKE**, but gently swirl until the solution is clear. Generally, the Follistim® dissolves immediately. Check the liquid in the container. If it is not clear or has particles in it, **DO NOT USE IT**.
4. For patients requiring a single injection from multiple vials of Follistim®, up to 4 vials can be reconstituted with 1 mL of Sterile Water for Injection, USP. This can be accomplished by reconstituting a single vial as described above (see step 3). Then draw the entire contents of the first vial into a syringe, and inject the contents into a second vial of lyophilized Follistim®. Gently swirl the second vial, as described above, once again checking to make sure the solution is clear and free of particles. This step can be repeated with 2 additional vials for a total of up to 4 vials of lyophilized Follistim® into 1 mL of diluent.
5. Immediately **ADMINISTER** the reconstituted Follistim® either **SUBCUTANEOUSLY** or **INTRAMUSCULARLY**. Any unused reconstituted material should be discarded.
6. Draw the reconstituted Follistim® into an empty, sterile syringe.
7. Hold the syringe pointing upwards and gently tap the side to force any air bubbles to the top; then squeeze the plunger gently until all the air has been expelled and only Follistim® solution is left in the syringe.
8. Follistim® only works if it is injected **SUBCUTANEOUSLY** or **INTRAMUSCULARLY**. The most convenient sites for **SUBCUTANEOUS** injection are either in the abdomen around the navel where there is a lot of loose skin and layers of fatty tissue or in the upper thigh. Pinch up a large are of skin between the finger and thumb. You should vary the injection site a little with each injection.
   The best site for **INTRAMUSCULAR** injection of Follistim® is the upper outer quadrant of the buttock muscle. This area contains a large volume of muscle with few blood vessels and major nerves. Stretching the skin helps the needle to go in more easily and pushes the tissue beneath the skin out of the way. This helps the solution disperse correctly.
9. The injection site should be swabbed with a disinfectant to remove any surface bacteria. Clean about two inches around the point where the needle will go in and let the disinfectant dry for at least one minute before proceeding.
10. For **SUBCUTANEOUS** injection the needle should be inserted at the base of the pinched-up skin at an angle of 45° to the skin surface.
    The needle for **INTRAMUSCULAR** injection should be inserted right up to the hilt at an angle of 90° to the skin surface. Pushing in with a quick thrust causes the least discomfort.
11. If the needle is correctly positioned it will be difficult to draw back on the plunger. Any blood drawn into the syringe means the needle tip has penetrated a vein or artery. If this happens, remove the syringe, cover the injection site with a swab containing disinfectant and apply pressure; the site should stop bleeding in a minute or two.
12. Once the needle is properly placed, depress the plunger **slowly** and steadily, so the solution is correctly injected and the skin or muscle tissue is not damaged.
13. Pull the syringe out quickly and apply pressure to the site with a swab containing disinfectant. A gentle massage of the site–while still maintaining pressure–helps disperse the Follistim® solution and relieve any discomfort.
14. Use the disposable syringe only once and dispose of it properly.

HOW SUPPLIED

Follistim® (follitropin beta for injection) is supplied in a sterile, freeze-dried form, as a white to off-white cake or powder in vials containing 75 IU of FSH activity. The following package combinations are available:

—1 vial 75 IU Follistim® and 1 vial 5 mL Sterile Water for Injection, USP.
NDC 0052-0306-18

—5 vials 75 IU Follistim® and 5 vials 5 mL Sterile Water for Injection, USP.
NDC 0052-0306-31

Storage

Lyophilized powder may be stored refrigerated or at room temperature (2°-25°C/36°-77°F). Protect from light. Use immediately after reconstitution.

Rx only

Manufactured by
Organon Inc.
West Orange, NJ 07052
Diluent manufactured by
Luitpold Pharmaceuticals, Inc.
Shirley, NY 11967

5310182 12/98

Shown in Product Identification Guide, page 327

HUMEGON® ℞

(menotropins for injection, USP)
FOR INTRAMUSCULAR INJECTION

DESCRIPTION

Humegon® (menotropins for injection, USP) is a purified preparation of gonadotropins. Menotropins are extracted from the urine of postmenopausal females and possess follicle-stimulating hormone (FSH) and luteinizing hormone (LH) activity. The ratio of FSH bioactivity and LH bioactivity in menotropins is adjusted to approximate unity by the addition of human chorionic gonadotropin purified from the urine of pregnant women. Each vial of Humegon® contains 75 IU of follicle-stimulating hormone activity and 75 IU of luteinizing hormone activity, plus 10.5 mg lactose, hydrous NF; 0.25 mg monosodium phosphate, monohydrate USP; 0.25 mg disodium phosphate, anhydrous USP; sodium hydroxide NF or phosphoric acid NF to adjust pH; in a sterile, lyophilized form. Humegon® is administered by intramuscular injection.

Humegon® is biologically standardized for FSH and LH gonadotropin activities and the potencies are based on the results of *in vivo* bioassays, which are in agreement with the recommendations of the World Health Organization Expert Committee on Biological Standardization (1982).

Both FSH and LH as well as hCG are glycoproteins that are acidic and water soluble.

Therapeutic class: Infertility.

CLINICAL PHARMACOLOGY

The geometric mean absolute bioavailability of FSH from the 150 IU intramuscular (IM) dose compared to the 150 IU intravenous (IV) dose was 76%. Following single dose IM injections of 75, 150, and 300 IU Humegon® (menotropins for injection, USP) to healthy male volunteers, FSH dose response was less than proportional between the 75 and 150 IU doses and between the 150 and 300 IU doses. The mean FSH elimination half-lives of 75, 150, and 300 IU IM were 37 hrs, 30 hrs, and 36 hrs, respectively, and 31 hrs following 150 IU IV administration.

Repeated daily IM administration of 150 IU Humegon® to seven women on 8 consecutive days led to a gradual accumulation of FSH levels which plateaued in 3–4 days. It took 4–5 days for the elevated FSH levels to return to pretreatment levels. These findings underline the importance of very careful and frequent monitoring of the patient in order to reduce the danger of ovarian hyperstimulation.

Women

Humegon® administered for seven to twelve days produces ovarian follicular growth in women who do not have primary ovarian failure. Treatment with Humegon® in most instances results only in follicular growth and maturation. In order to induce ovulation, human chorionic gonadotropin (hCG) must be given following the administration of Humegon® when clinical assessment of the patient indicates that sufficient follicular maturation has occurred.

Men

Humegon® administered concomitantly with human chorionic gonadotropin (hCG) for at least three months induces spermatogenesis in men with primary or secondary pituitary hypofunction who have achieved adequate masculinization with prior hCG therapy.

CLINICAL STUDIES

Women

The Induction of Ovulation

Results of clinical experience and effectiveness from the administration of Humegon® (menotropins for injection, USP) to 2,682 patients in 7,204 courses of therapy are summarized below:

Patients Ovulating	73.2%†
Clinical Pregnancies	26.2%
Patients Aborting	22%*
Multiple Pregnancies	19.5%

† Data reported for 2,409 out of 2,682 patients
* Data reported for 678 out of 704 clinical pregnancies

IVF, GIFT, ZIFT

Results of clinical experience and effectiveness from the administration of Humegon® in 1,081 cycles of therapy are summarized below:

% Cycles with Oocyte Retrieval	85†
% Cycles with Transfers	65.6*
# Clinical Pregnancies	182
% Clinical Pregnancy/Cycle	16.8
% Clincial Pregnancy/Retrieval	19.8
% Clinical Pregnancy/Transfer	25.6
% Abortion	32.7§

† Data reported for 773 cycles
* Data reported for 791 cycles
§ Data reported for 174 out of 182 clinical pregnancies

Men

Clinical results of treatment of men with hypogonadotropic hypogonadism and idiopathic infertility were summarized from the medical literature. Efficacy was evaluated in 246 patients, 22 with hypogonadotropic hypogonadism and 224 with idiopathic infertility. Treatment generally consisted of Humegon®, with or without concomitant administration of hCG 500–2,500 IU, two or three times per week for up to 48 months. Sperm count improved in 16 of 22 evaluable (73%) hypogonadotropic hypogonadism patients and in 86 of 224 evaluable (38%) idiopathic infertility patients. Overall, seven of 14 (50%) evaluable hypogonadotropic hypogonadism patients and 26 of 224 (12%) idiopathic infertility patients impregnated their partners following Humegon® treatment.

INDICATIONS AND USAGE

Women

Humegon® (menotropins for injection, USP) and hCG given in a sequential manner are indicated for the induction of ovulation and pregnancy in the anovulatory infertile patient, in whom the cause of anovulation is functional and is not due to primary ovarian failure.

Humegon® and hCG may also be used to stimulate the development of multiple follicles in ovulatory patients participating in an *in vitro* fertilization program.

Men

Humegon® with concomitant hCG is indicated for the stimulation of spermatogenesis in men who have primary or secondary hypogonadotropic hypogonadism, and idiopathic infertility.

Humegon® with concomitant hCG has proven effective in inducing spermatogenesis in men with primary hypogonadotropic hypogonadism due to a congenital factor or prepubertal hypophysectomy and in men with secondary hypogonadotropic hypogonadism due to hypophysectomy, craniopharyngioma, cerebral aneurysm, or chromophobe adenoma.

SELECTION OF PATIENTS

Women

1. Before treatment with Humegon® (menotropins for injection, USP) is instituted, a thorough gynecologic and endocrinologic evaluation must be performed. Except for

those patients enrolled in an *in vitro* fertilization program, this should include a hysterosalpingogram (to rule out uterine and tubal pathology) and documentation of anovulation by means of basal body temperature, serial vaginal smears, examination of cervical mucus, determination of serum (or urinary) progesterone, urinary pregnanediol, and endometrial biopsy. Patients with tubal pathology should receive Humegon® only if enrolled in an *in vitro* fertilization program.

2. Primary ovarian failure should be excluded by the determination of gonadotropin levels.
3. Careful examination should be made to rule out the presence of an early pregnancy.
4. Patients in late reproductive life have a greater predilection to endometrial carcinoma as well as a higher incidence of anovulatory disorders. Cervical dilation and curettage should always be done for diagnosis before starting Humegon® therapy in such patients who demonstrate abnormal uterine bleeding or other signs of endometrial abnormalities.
5. Evaluation of the partner's fertility potential should be included in the workup.

Men

Patient selection should be made based on a documented lack of pituitary function. Prior to hormonal therapy, these patients will have low testosterone levels and low or absent gonadotropin levels. Patients with primary hypogonadotropic hypogonadism will have a subnormal development of masculinization, and those with secondary hypogonadotropic hypogonadism will have decreased masculinization.

CONTRAINDICATIONS

Women

Humegon® (menotropins for injection, USP) is contraindicated in women who have:

1. A high FSH level indicating primary ovarian failure.
2. Uncontrolled thyroid and adrenal dysfunction.
3. An organic intracranial lesion such as a pituitary tumor.
4. The presence of any cause of infertility other than anovulation, unless they are candidates for *in vitro* fertilization.
5. Abnormal bleeding of undetermined origin.
6. Ovarian cysts or enlargement not due to polycystic ovary syndrome.
7. Prior hypersensitivity to menotropins.
8. Humegon® is contraindicated in women who are pregnant and may cause fetal harm. There are limited human data on the effects of Humegon® when administered during pregnancy.

Men

Humegon® is contraindicated in men who have:

1. Normal gonadotropin levels indicating normal pituitary function.
2. Elevated gonadotropin levels indicating primary testicular failure.
3. Infertility disorders other than hypogonadotropic hypogonadism.

WARNINGS

Humegon® (menotropins for injection, USP) is a drug that should only be used by physicians who are thoroughly familiar with infertility problems. It is a potent gonadotropic substance capable of causing mild to severe adverse reactions in women. Gonadotropin therapy requires a certain time commitment by physicians and supportive health professionals, and its use requires the availability of appropriate monitoring facilities (see PRECAUTIONS/Laboratory Tests). In female patients, it must be used with a great deal of care.

Overstimulation of the Ovary During Humegon® (menotropins for injection, USP) Therapy

Ovarian Enlargement: Mild to moderate uncomplicated ovarian enlargement which may be accompanied by abdominal distension and/or abdominal pain occurs in approximately 20% of those treated with Humegon® and hCG, and generally regresses without treatment within two or three weeks.

In order to minimize the hazard associated with the occasional abnormal ovarian enlargement which may occur with Humegon®-hCG therapy, the lowest dose consistent with expectation of good results should be used. Careful monitoring of ovarian response can further minimize the risk of overstimulation.

If the ovaries are abnormally enlarged on the last day of Humegon® therapy, hCG should not be administered in this course of therapy; this will reduce the chances of development of the Ovarian Hyperstimulation Syndrome.

The Ovarian Hyperstimulation Syndrome (OHSS): OHSS is a medical event distinct from uncomplicated ovarian enlargement. OHSS may progress rapidly to become a serious medical event. It is characterized by an apparent dramatic increase in vascular permeability which can result in a rapid accumulation of fluid in the peritoneal cavity, thorax, and potentially, the pericardium. The early warning signs of development of OHSS are severe pelvic pain, nausea, vomiting, and weight gain. The following symptomatology has been seen with cases of OHSS: abdominal pain, abdominal distension, gastrointestinal symptoms including nausea, vomiting and diarrhea, severe ovarian enlargement, weight gain, dyspnea, and oliguria. Clinical evaluation may reveal hypovolemia, hemoconcentration, electrolyte imbalances, ascites, hemoperitoneum, pleural effusions, hydrothorax, acute pulmonary distress, and thromboembolic events (see Pulmonary and Vascular Complications).

OHSS occurs in approximately 0.4% of patients when the recommended dose is administered and in 1.3% of patients when higher than recommended doses are administered. Cases of OHSS are more common, more severe, and more protracted if pregnancy occurs. OHSS develops rapidly; therefore, patients should be followed for at least two weeks after hCG administration. Most often, OHSS occurs after treatment has been discontinued and reaches its maximum at about seven to ten days following treatment. Usually, OHSS resolves spontaneously with the onset of menses. If there is evidence that OHSS may be developing prior to hCG administration (see PRECAUTIONS/Laboratory Tests), the hCG should be withheld.

If OHSS occurs, treatment should be stopped and the patient hospitalized. Treatment is primarily symptomatic, consisting of bed rest, fluid and electrolyte management, and analgesics, if needed. The phenomenon of hemoconcentration associated with fluid loss into the peritoneal cavity, pleural cavity, and the pericardial cavity has been seen to occur and should be thoroughly assessed in the following manner: 1) fluid intake and output, 2) weight, 3) hematocrit, 4) serum and urinary electrolytes, 5) urine specific gravity, 6) BUN and creatinine, and 7) abdominal girth. These determinations are to be performed daily or more often if the need arises.

With OHSS there is an increased risk of injury to the ovary. The ascitic, pleural, and pericardial fluid should not be removed unless absolutely necessary to relieve symptoms such as pulmonary distress or cardiac tamponade. Pelvic examination may cause rupture of an ovarian cyst, which may result in hemoperitoneum, and should therefore be avoided. If this does occur, and if bleeding becomes such that surgery is required, the surgical treatment should be designed to control bleeding and to retain as much ovarian tissue as possible. Intercourse should be prohibited in those patients in whom significant ovarian enlargement occurs after ovulation because of the danger of hemoperitoneum resulting from ruptured ovarian cysts.

The management of OHSS may be divided into three phases: an acute, a chronic, and a resolution phase. Because the use of diuretics can accentuate the diminished intravascular volume, diuretics should be avoided except in the late phase of resolution as described below.

Acute Phase: Management during the acute phase should be designed to prevent hemoconcentration due to loss of intravascular volume to the third space and to minimize the risk of thromboembolic phenomena and kidney damage. Treatment is designed to normalize electrolytes while maintaining an acceptable but somewhat reduced intravascular volume. Full correction of the intravascular volume deficit may lead to an unacceptable increase in the amount of third space fluid accumulation. Management includes administration of limited intravenous fluids, electrolytes, and human serum albumin. Monitoring for the development of hyperkalemia is recommended.

Chronic Phase: After stabilizing the patient during the acute phase, excessive fluid accumulation in the third space should be limited by instituting severe potassium, sodium, and fluid restriction.

Resolution Phase: A fall in hematocrit and an increasing urinary output without an increased intake are observed due to the return of third space fluid to the intravascular compartment. Peripheral and/or pulmonary edema may result if the kidneys are unable to excrete third space fluid as rapidly as it is mobilized. Diuretics may be indicated during the resolution phase if necessary to combat pulmonary edema.

Pulmonary and Vascular Complications

Serious pulmonary conditions (e.g., atelectasis, acute respiratory distress syndrome) have been reported. In addition, thromboembolic events both in association with, and separate from, the Ovarian Hyperstimulation Syndrome have been reported following Humegon® (menotropins for injection, USP) therapy. Intravascular thrombosis, which may originate in venous or arterial vessels, can result in reduced blood flow to vital organs or the extremities. Sequelae of such events have included venous thrombophlebitis, pulmonary embolism, pulmonary infarction, cerebral vascular occlusion (stroke), and arterial occlusion resulting in loss of limb. In rare cases, pulmonary complications and/or thromboembolic events have resulted in death.

Multiple Births

Data from a clinical trial revealed the following results regarding multiple births: Of the pregnancies following therapy with Humegon® (menotropins for injection, USP) and hCG, 80% resulted in single births. The patient and her partner should be advised of the frequency and potential hazards of multiple gestation before starting treatment.

PRECAUTIONS

General

Careful attention should be given to diagnosis in the selection of candidates for Humegon® (menotropins for injection, USP) therapy (see INDICATIONS AND USAGE/Selection of Patients).

Information for Patients

Prior to therapy with Humegon® (menotropins for injection, USP), patients should be informed of the duration of treatment and the monitoring of their condition that will be required. Possible adverse reactions (see ADVERSE REACTIONS) and the risk of multiple births should also be discussed.

Laboratory Tests

Women

Treatment for Induction of Ovulation

In most instances, treatment with Humegon® (menotropins for injection, USP) results only in follicular growth and maturation. In order to induce ovulation, hCG must be given following the administration of Humegon® when clinical assessment of the patient indicates that sufficient follicular maturation has occurred. This may be directly estimated by measuring serum (or urinary) estrogen levels and sonographic visualization of the ovaries. The combination of both estradiol levels and ultrasonography is useful for monitoring the growth and development of follicles, timing hCG administration, as well as minimizing the risk of the Ovarian Hyperstimulation Syndrome and multiple gestation.

Other clinical parameters which may have potential use for monitoring menotropins therapy include:

a) Changes in vaginal cytology;
b) Appearance and volume of cervical mucus;
c) Spinnbarkeit; and
d) Ferning of cervical mucus.

The above clinical indices provide an indirect estimate of the estrogenic effect upon the target organs, and therefore should only be used adjunctively with more direct estimates of follicular development, i.e., serum estradiol and ultrasonography.

The clinical confirmation of ovulation, with the exception of pregnancy, is obtained by direct and indirect indices of progesterone production. The indices most generally used are as follows:

a) A rise in basal body temperature;
b) Increase in serum progesterone; and
c) Menstruation following the shift in basal body temperature.

When used in conjunction with indices of progesterone production, sonographic visualization of the ovaries will assist in determining if ovulation has occurred. Sonographic evidence of ovulation may include the following:

a) Fluid in the cul-de-sac;
b) Ovarian stigmata; and
c) Collapsed follicle.

Because of the subjectivity of the various tests for the determination of follicular maturation and ovulation, it cannot be overemphasized that the physician should choose the test(s) with which he/she is thoroughly familiar.

Drug Interactions

No clinically significant drug/drug or drug/food adverse interactions have been reported during Humegon® (menotropins for injection, USP) therapy.

Carcinogenesis, Mutagenesis, Impairment of Fertility

Long-term toxicity studies in animals have not been performed to evaluate the carcinogenic potential of Humegon® (menotropins for injection, USP).

Pregnancy

Pregnancy Category X (see CONTRAINDICATIONS).

Males: No animal studies have been performed that examine the potential teratogenic effect associated with Humegon® (menotropins for injection, USP) therapy when prescribed for male infertility.

Nursing Mothers

It is not known whether this drug is excreted in human milk. Because many drugs are excreted in human milk, caution should be exercised if Humegon® (menotropins for injection, USP) is administered to a nursing woman.

ADVERSE REACTIONS

Women

The following adverse reactions, reported during Humegon® (menotropins for injection, USP) therapy, are listed in decreasing order of potential severity:

1. Pulmonary and vascular complications (see WARNINGS),
2. Ovarian Hyperstimulation Syndrome (see WARNINGS),
3. Hemoperitoneum,
4. Adnexal torsion (as a complication of ovarian enlargement),
5. Mild to moderate ovarian enlargement,
6. Ovarian cysts,
7. Abdominal pain,
8. Sensitivity to Humegon®,
   (Febrile reactions after the administration of Humegon® have occurred. It is not clear whether or not these were pyrogenic responses or possible allergic reactions. In addition, reports of "flu-like symptoms" including fever, chills, musculoskeletal aches, joint pains, nausea, headache and malaise have been received.)
9. Gastrointestinal symptoms (nausea, vomiting, diarrhea, abdominal cramps, bloating),
10. Pain, rash, swelling and/or irritation at the site of injection,
11. Body rashes,
12. Dizziness, tachycardia, dyspnea, tachypnea.

The following medical events have been reported subsequent to pregnancies resulting from Humegon® therapy:

1. Ectopic pregnancy
2. Congenital abnormalities
   From a large clinical trial comprising of 6,096 cycles (2,166 women) with 594 babies examined, the incidence of congenital malformation with Humegon®/hCG therapy was 1.7%. Of the major malformations (nine babies, 1.5%) there were two cases each of anencephaly and harelip, and one each of cleft palate, polydactyly, umbilical hernia, congenital dislocation of hip and equinovarus. There was one case (0.2%) of minor malformation (anomaly of auricle). The congenital anomaly rate after Humegon® therapy is then no higher than that expected for the general population.

Continued on next page

Humegon—Cont.

There have been infrequent reports of ovarian neoplasms, both benign and malignant, in women who have undergone multiple drug regimens for ovulation induction; however, a causal relationship has not been established.

Men

Gynecomastia, breast pain, mastitis, nausea, abnormal lipoprotein fraction, abnormal SGOT and SGPT may occur occasionally during Humegon®-hCG therapy.

DRUG ABUSE AND DEPENDENCE

There have been no reports of abuse or dependence with Humegon® (menotropins for injection, USP).

OVERDOSAGE

Aside from possible ovarian hyperstimulation (see WARNINGS), little is known concerning the consequences of acute overdosage with Humegon® (menotropins for injection, USP).

DOSAGE AND ADMINISTRATION

Women

The dose of Humegon® (menotropins for injection, USP) to produce maturation of the follicle must be individualized for each patient. It is recommended that the initial dose to any patient should be 75 IU of FSH/LH per day, **ADMINISTERED INTRAMUSCULARLY,** for seven to twelve days followed by hCG, 5,000 U to 10,000 U, one day after the last dose of Humegon®. Administration of Humegon® should not exceed 12 days in a single course of therapy. The patient should be treated until indices of estrogenic activity, as indicated under "Precautions" above, are equivalent to or greater than those of the normal individual. If serum or urinary estradiol determinations or ultrasonographic visualizations are available, they may be useful as a guide to therapy. If the ovaries are abnormally enlarged on the last day of Humegon® therapy, hCG should not be administered in this course of therapy; this will reduce the chances of development of the Ovarian Hyperstimulation Syndrome. If there is evidence of ovulation but no pregnancy, repeat this dosage regime for at least two more courses before increasing the dose of Humegon® to 150 IU of FSH/LH per day for seven to twelve days. As before, this dose should be followed by 5,000 U to 10,000 U of hCG one day after the last dose of Humegon®. A Humegon® dose of 150 IU of FSH/LH per day has proven to be the most effective dose especially for *in vitro* fertilization. If evidence of ovulation is present, but pregnancy does not ensue, repeat the same dose for two more courses. Doses larger than this are not routinely recommended.

During treatment with both Humegon® and hCG and during a two-week post-treatment period, patients should be examined at least every other day for signs of excessive ovarian stimulation. It is recommended that Humegon® administration be stopped if the ovaries become abnormally enlarged or abdominal pain occurs. Most of the Ovarian Hyperstimulation Syndrome occurs after treatment has been discontinued and reaches its maximum at about seven to ten days post-ovulation. Patients should be followed for at least two weeks after hCG administration.

For ovulation induction, the couple should be encouraged to have intercourse daily, beginning on the day prior to the administration of hCG until ovulation becomes apparent from the indices employed for the determination of progestational activity. Care should be taken to insure insemination. In the light of the foregoing indices and parameters mentioned, it should become obvious that, unless a physician is willing to devote considerable time to these patients and be familiar with and conduct the necessary laboratory studies, he/she should not use Humegon®.

Dissolve the contents of one vial of Humegon® in one to two mL of sterile saline and **ADMINISTER INTRAMUSCULARLY** immediately. Any unused reconstituted material should be discarded. Parenteral drug products should be inspected visually for particulate matter and discoloration prior to administration, whenever solution and container permit.

Men

Prior to concomitant therapy with Humegon® and hCG, pretreatment with hCG alone (5,000 U three times a week) is required. Treatment should continue for a period sufficient to achieve serum testosterone levels within the normal range and masculinization as judged by the appearance of secondary sex characteristics. Such pretreatment may require four to six months, then the recommended dose of Humegon® is 75 IU FSH/LH **ADMINISTERED INTRAMUSCULARLY, three times** a week and the recommended dose of hCG is 2,000 U **twice** a week. Therapy should be carried on for a minimum of four more months to insure detecting spermatozoa in the ejaculate, as it takes 74 ± 4 days in the human male for germ cells to reach the spermatozoa stage. If the patient has not responded with evidence of increased spermatogenesis at the end of four months of therapy, treatment may continue with 75 IU FSH/LH **three times** a week, or the dose can be increased to 150 IU FSH/LH **three times** a week, with the hCG dose unchanged.

Dissolve the contents of one vial of Humegon® in one to two mL of sterile saline and **ADMINISTER INTRAMUSCULARLY** immediately. Any unused reconstituted material should be discarded. Parenteral drug products should be inspected visually for particulate matter and discoloration prior to administration, whenever solution and container permit.

HOW SUPPLIED

Humegon® (menotropins for injection, USP) is supplied in sterile lyophilized form as a white to off-white powder in vials containing 75 IU FSH/LH activity. The following package combinations are available:

1 vial 75 IU Humegon® and 1 vial 2 mL Sodium Chloride Injection, USP.
NDC 0052-0300-17

5 vials 75 IU Humegon® and 5 vials 2 mL Sodium Chloride Injection, USP.
NDC 0052-0300-22

By biological assay, one IU of LH for the Second International Reference Preparation (2nd-IRP) for hMG is biologically equivalent to approximately 1/2 U of hCG.

Storage

Lyophilized powder may be stored refrigerated or at room temperature 2°–30°C (35°–86°F). Protect from light. Use immediately after reconstitution. Discard unused material.

Rx only

Organon Inc.
West Orange, New Jersey 07052
5310119 Iss. 9/98

MIRCETTE® ℞

(desogestrel/ethinyl estradiol and ethinyl estradiol) Tablets

Patients should be counseled that this product does not protect against HIV infection (AIDS) and other sexually transmitted diseases.

DESCRIPTION

Mircette® (desogestrel/ethinyl estradiol and ethinyl estradiol) Tablets provide an oral contraceptive regimen of 21 white round tablets each containing 0.15 mg desogestrel (13-ethyl-11- methylene-18,19-dinor-17 alpha-pregn- 4-en-20-yn-17-ol), 0.02 mg ethinyl estradiol (19-nor-17 alpha-pregna-1,3,5 (10)-trien-20-yne-3,17-diol), and inactive ingredients which include vitamin E, corn starch, povidone, stearic acid, colloidal silicon dioxide, lactose, hydroxypropyl methylcellulose, polyethylene glycol, titanium dioxide and talc, followed by 2 green round tablets with the following inactive ingredients: lactose, corn starch, magnesium stearate, FD&C Blue No. 2 aluminum lake, yellow ferric oxide, hydroxypropyl methylcellulose, polyethylene glycol, titanium dioxide and talc. Mircette® also contains 5 yellow round tablets containing 0.01 mg ethinyl estradiol (19-nor-17 alpha-pregna-1,3,5 (10)-trien-20-yne-3,17-diol) and inactive ingredients which include vitamin E, corn starch, povidone, stearic acid, colloidal silicon dioxide, lactose, hydroxypropyl methylcellulose, polyethylene glycol, titanium dioxide, talc, and yellow ferric oxide. The molecular weight for desogestrel and ethinyl estradiol are 310.48 and 296.41 respectively. The structural formulas are as follows:

DESOGESTREL

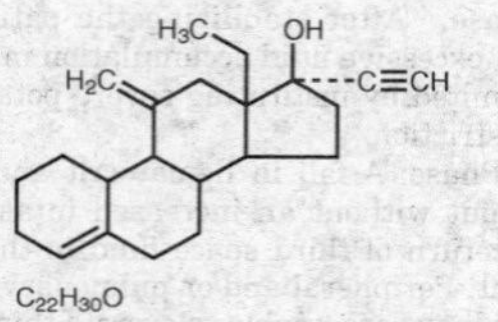

$C_{22}H_{30}O$

ETHINYL ESTRADIOL

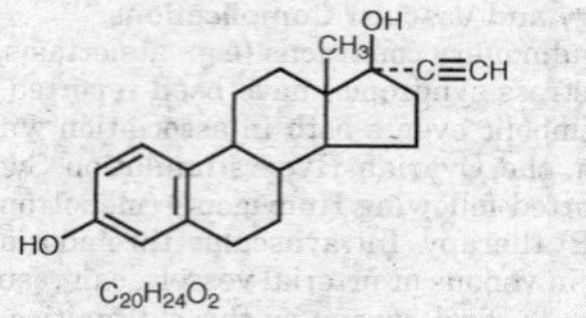

$C_{20}H_{24}O_2$

CLINICAL PHARMACOLOGY

Combination oral contraceptives act by suppression of gonadotropins. Although the primary mechanism of this action is inhibition of ovulation, other alterations include changes in the cervical mucus (which increase the difficulty of sperm entry into the uterus) and the endometrium (which reduce the likelihood of implantation).

Receptor binding studies, as well as studies in animals, have shown that etonogestrel, the biologically active metabolite of desogestrel, combines high progestational activity with minimal intrinsic androgenicity (91,92).

Pharmacokinetics

Absorption

Desogestrel is rapidly and almost completely absorbed and converted into etonogestrel, its biologically active metabolite. Following oral administration, the relative bioavailability of desogestrel compared to a solution, as measured by serum levels of etonogestrel, is approximately 100%. Mircette® (desogestrel/ethinyl estradiol and ethinyl estradiol) Tablets provide two different regimens of ethinyl estradiol; 0.02 mg in the combination tablet [white] as well as 0.01 mg in the yellow tablet. Ethinyl estradiol is rapidly and almost completely absorbed. After a single dose of Mircette® combination tablet [white], the relative bioavailability of ethinyl estradiol is approximately 93% while the relative bioavailability of the 0.01 mg tablet [yellow] is 99%. The effect of food on the bioavailability of Mircette® tablets following oral administration has not been evaluated.

The pharmacokinetics of etonogestrel and ethinyl estradiol following multiple dose administration of Mircette® tablets were determined during the third cycle in 17 subjects. Plasma concentrations of etonogestrel and ethinyl estradiol reached steady-state by Day 21. The $AUC_{(0-24)}$ for etonogestrel at steady-state on Day 21 was approximately 2.2 times higher than $AUC_{(0-24)}$ on Day 1 of the third cycle. The pharmacokinetic parameters of etonogestrel and ethinyl estradiol during the third cycle following multiple dose administration of Mircette® tablets are summarized in Table 1.

[See table below]

Distribution

Etonogestrel, the active metabolite of desogestrel, was found to be 99% protein bound, primarily to sex hormone-binding globulin (SHBG). Ethinyl estradiol is approximately 98.3% bound, mainly to plasma albumin. Ethinyl estradiol does not bind to SHBG, but induces SHBG synthesis. Desogestrel, in combination with ethinyl estradiol, does not counteract the estrogen-induced increase in SHBG, resulting in lower serum levels of free testosterone (96–99).

Metabolism

Desogestrel: Desogestrel is rapidly and completely metabolized by hydroxylation in the intestinal mucosa and on first pass through the liver to etonogestrel. Other metabolites (i.e., 3α-OH-desogestrel, 3β-OH-desogestrel, and 3α-OH-5α-H-desogestrel) with no pharmacologic actions also have been identified and these metabolites may undergo glucuronide and sulfate conjugation.

Ethinyl estradiol: Ethinyl estradiol is subject to a significant degree of presystemic conjugation (phase II metabolism). Ethinyl estradiol escaping gut wall conjugation undergoes phase I metabolism and hepatic conjugation (phase II metabolism). Major phase I metabolites are 2-OH-ethinyl estradiol and 2-methoxy-ethinyl estradiol. Sulfate and glucuronide conjugates of both ethinyl estradiol and phase I metabolites, which are excreted in bile, can undergo enterohepatic circulation.

Excretion

Etonogestrel and ethinyl estradiol are excreted in urine, bile and feces. At steady state, on Day 21, the elimination half-life of etonogestrel is 27.8±7.2 hours and the elimination half-life of ethinyl estradiol for the combination tablet is 23.9±25.5 hours. For the 0.01 mg ethinyl estradiol tablet [yellow], the elimination half-life at steady state, Day 28, is 18.9±8.3 hours.

Special Populations

Race

There is no information to determine the effect of race on the pharmacokinetics of Mircette® (desogestrel/ethinyl estradiol and ethinyl estradiol) Tablets.

TABLE I: MEAN (SD) PHARMACOKINETIC PARAMETERS OF Mircette® OVER A 28-DAY DOSING PERIOD IN THE THIRD CYCLE (n=17).

Etonogestrel

Day	Dose† mg	C_{max} pg/mL	T_{max} h	$t_{1/2}$ h	AUC_{0-24} pg/mL•hr	CL/F L/h
1	0.15	2503.6 (987.6)	2.4 (1.0)	29.8 (16.3)	17832 (5674)	5.4 (2.5)
21	0.15	4091.2 (1186.2)	1.6 (0.7)	27.8 (7.2)	39391(12134)	4.4 (1.4)

†Desogestrel

Ethinyl Estradiol

Day	Dose mg	C_{max} pg/mL	T_{max} h	$t_{1/2}$ h	AUC_{0-24} pg/mL•hr	CL/F L/h
1	0.02	51.9 (15.4)	2.9 (1.2)	16.5 (4.8)	566 (173)[a]	25.7 (9.1)
21	0.02	62.2 (25.9)	2.0 (0.8)	23.9 (25.5)	597 (127)[a]	35.1 (8.2)
24	0.01	24.6 (10.8)	2.4 (1.0)	18.8 (10.3)	246 (65)	43.6 (12.2)
28	0.01	35.3 (27.5)	2.1 (1.3)	18.9 (8.3)	312 (62)	33.2 (6.6)

[a]n=16

C_{max}—measured peak concentration

T_{max}—observed time of peak concentration

$t_{1/2}$—elimination half-life, calculated by $0.693/K_{elim}$

AUC_{0-24}—area under the concentration-time curve calculated by the linear trapezoidal rule (Time 0 to 24 hours)

CL/F—apparent clearance

Hepatic Insufficiency
No formal studies were conducted to evaluate the effect of hepatic disease on the disposition of Mircette®.
Renal Insufficiency
No formal studies were conducted to evaluate the effect of renal disease on the disposition of Mircette®.
Drug-Drug Interactions
Interactions between desogestrel/ethinyl estradiol and other drugs have been reported in the literature. No formal drug-drug interaction studies were conducted (see PRECAUTIONS section).

INDICATIONS AND USAGE

Mircette® (desogestrel/ethinyl estradiol and ethinyl estradiol) Tablets are indicated for the prevention of pregnancy in women who elect to use this product as a method of contraception.
Oral contraceptives are highly effective. Table II lists the typical accidental pregnancy rates for users of combination oral contraceptives and other methods of contraception. The efficacy of these contraceptive methods, except sterilization, depends upon the reliability with which they are used. Correct and consistent use of these methods can result in lower failure rates.
[See table above]

TABLE II: Percentage of women experiencing an unintended pregnancy during the first year of typical use and the first year of perfect use of contraception and the percentage continuing use at the end of the first year, United States.

Method (1)	% of Women Experiencing an Unintended Pregnancy within the First Year of Use: Typical Use[1] (2)	Perfect Use[2] (3)	% of Women Continuing Use at One Year[3] (4)
Chance[4]	85	85	
Spermicides[5]	26	6	40
Periodic abstinence	25		63
Calendar		9	
Ovulation Method		3	
Sympto-Thermal[6]		2	
Post-Ovulation		1	
Withdrawal	19	4	
Cap[7]			
Parous Women	40	26	42
Nulliparous Women	20	9	56
Sponge			
Parous Women	40	20	42
Nulliparous Women	20	9	56
Diaphragm[7]	20	6	56
Condom[8]			
Female (Reality)	21	5	56
Male	14	3	61
Pill	5		71
Progestin Only		0.5	
Combined		0.1	
IUD			
Progesterone T	2.0	1.5	81
Copper T 380A	0.8	0.6	78
LNg 20	0.1	0.1	81
Depo-Provera	0.3	0.3	70
Norplant and Norplant-2	0.05	0.05	88
Female sterilization	0.5	0.5	100
Male sterilization	0.15	0.10	100

Adapted from Hatcher et al., 1998, Ref#1.
[1] Among *typical* couples who initiate use of a method (not necessarily for the first time), the percentage who experience an accidental pregnancy during the first year if they do not stop use for any other reason.
[2] Among couples who initiate use of a method (not necessarily for the first time) and who use it *perfectly* (both consistently and correctly), the percentage who experience an accidental pregnancy during the first year if they do not stop use for any other reason.
[3] Among couples attempting to avoid pregnancy, the percentage who continue to use a method for one year.
[4] The percents becoming pregnant in columns (2) and (3) are based on data from populations where contraception is not used and from women who cease using contraception in order to become pregnant. Among such populations, about 89% become pregnant within one year. This estimate was lowered slightly (to 85%) to represent the percent who would become pregnant within one year among women now relying on reversible methods of contraception if they abandoned contraception altogether.
[5] Foams, creams, gels, vaginal suppositories, and vaginal film.
[6] Cervical mucus (ovulation) method supplemented by calendar in the pre-ovulatory and basal body temperature in the post-ovulatory phases.
[7] With spermicidal cream or jelly.
[8] Without spermicides.

CONTRAINDICATIONS

Oral contraceptives should not be used in women who currently have the following conditions:

- Thrombophlebitis or thromboembolic disorders
- A past history of deep vein thrombophlebitis or thromboembolic disorders
- Cerebral vascular or coronary artery disease
- Known or suspected carcinoma of the breast
- Carcinoma of the endometrium or other known or suspected estrogen-dependent neoplasia
- Undiagnosed abnormal genital bleeding
- Cholestatic jaundice of pregnancy or jaundice with prior pill use
- Hepatic adenomas of carcinomas
- Known or suspected pregnancy

WARNINGS

Cigarette smoking increases the risk of serious cardiovascular side effects from oral contraceptive use. This risk increases with age and with heavy smoking (15 or more cigarettes per day) and is quite marked in women over 35 years of age. Women who use oral contraceptives should be strongly advised not to smoke.

The use of oral contraceptives is associated with increased risks of several serious conditions including myocardial infarction, thromboembolism, stroke, hepatic neoplasia, and gallbladder disease, although the risk of serious morbidity or mortality is very small in healthy women without underlying risk factors. The risk of morbidity and mortality increases significantly in the presence of other underlying risk factors such as hypertension, hyperlipidemias, obesity and diabetes.
Practitioners prescribing oral contraceptives should be familiar with the following information relating to these risks.
The information contained in this package insert is principally based on studies carried out in patients who used oral contraceptives with formulations of higher doses of estrogens and progestogens than those in common use today. The effect of long-term use of the oral contraceptives with formulations of lower doses of both estrogens and progestogens remains to be determined.
Throughout this labeling, epidemiological studies reported are of two types: retrospective or case control studies and prospective or cohort studies. Case control studies provide a measure of the relative risk of a disease, namely, a *ratio* of the incidence of a disease among oral contraceptive users to that among non-users. The relative risk does not provide information on the actual clinical occurrence of a disease. Cohort studies provide a measure of attributable risk, which is the *difference* in the incidence of disease between oral contraceptive users and non-users. The attributable risk does provide information about the actual occurrence of a disease in the population (Adapted from refs. 2 and 3 with the author's permission). For further information, the reader is referred to a text on epidemiological methods.

1. THROMBOEMBOLIC DISORDERS AND OTHER VASCULAR PROBLEMS

a. Myocardial infarction
An increased risk of myocardial infarction has been attributed to oral contraceptive use. This risk is primarily in smokers or women with other underlying risk factors for coronary artery disease such as hypertension, hypercholesterolemia, morbid obesity, and diabetes. The relative risk of heart attack for current oral contraceptive users has been estimated to be two to six (4–10). The risk is very low in women under the age of 30.
Smoking in combination with oral contraceptive use has been shown to contribute substantially to the incidence of myocardial infarction in women in their mid-thirties or older with smoking accounting for the majority of excess cases (11). Mortality rates associated with circulatory disease have been shown to increase substantially in smokers, over the age of 35 and non-smokers over the age of 40 (Table III) among women who use oral contraceptives.
[See figure at top of next column]

TABLE III: CIRCULATORY DISEASE MORTALITY RATES PER 100,000 WOMAN-YEARS BY AGE, SMOKING STATUS AND ORAL CONTRACEPTIVE USE

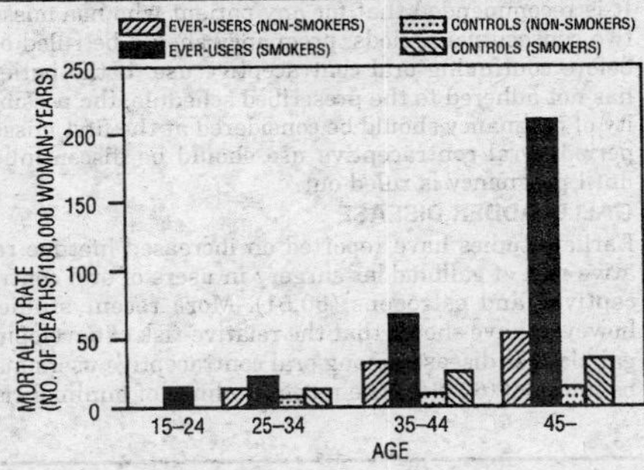

(Adapted from P.M. Layde and V. Beral, ref. #12.)

Oral contraceptives may compound the effects of well-known risk factors, such as hypertension, diabetes, hyperlipidemias, age and obesity (13). In particular, some progestogens are known to decrease HDL cholesterol and cause glucose intolerance, while estrogens may create a state of hyperinsulinism (14–18). Oral contraceptives have been shown to increase blood pressure among users (see section 9 in WARNINGS). Similar effects on risk factors have been associated with an increased risk of heart disease. Oral contraceptives must be used with caution in women with cardiovascular disease risk factors.

b. Thromboembolism
An increased risk of thromboembolic and thrombotic disease associated with the use of oral contraceptives is well established. Case control studies have found the relative risk of users compared to non-users to be 3 for the first episode of superficial venous thrombosis, 4 to 11 for deep vein thrombosis or pulmonary embolism, and 1.5 to 6 for women with predisposing conditions for venous thromboembolic disease (2,3,19–24). Cohort studies have shown the relative risk to be somewhat lower, about 3 for new cases and about 4.5 for new cases requiring hospitalization (25). The risk of thromboembolic disease associated with oral contraceptives is not related to length of use and disappears after pill use is stopped (2).
A two- to four-fold increase in relative risk of post-operative thromboembolic complications has been reported with the use of oral contraceptives (9,26). The relative risk of venous thrombosis in women who have predisposing conditions is twice that of women without such medical conditions (9,26). If feasible, oral contraceptives should be discontinued at least four weeks prior to and for two weeks after elective surgery of a type associated with an increase in risk of thromboembolism and during and following prolonged immobilization. Since the immediate postpartum period is also associated with an increased risk of thromboembolism, oral contraceptives should be started no earlier than four weeks after delivery in women who elect not to breast feed.

c. Cerebrovascular diseases
Oral contraceptives have been shown to increase both the relative and attributable risks of cerebrovascular events (thrombotic and hemorrhagic strokes), although, in general, the risk is greatest among older (>35 years), hypertensive women who also smoke. Hypertension was found to be a risk factor for both users and non-users, for both types of strokes, while smoking interacted to increase the risk for hemorrhagic strokes (27–29).
In a large study, the relative risk of thrombotic strokes has been shown to range from 3 for normotensive users to 14 for users with severe hypertension (30). The relative risk of hemorrhagic stroke is reported to be 1.2 for non-smokers who used oral contraceptives, 2.6 for smokers who did not use oral contraceptives, 7.6 for smokers who used oral contraceptives, 1.8 for normotensive users and 25.7 for users with severe hypertension (30). The attributable risk is also greater in older women (3).

d. Dose-related risk of vascular disease from oral contraceptives
A positive association has been observed between the amount of estrogen and progestogen in oral contraceptives and the risk of vascular disease (31–33). A decline in serum high-density lipoproteins (HDL) has been reported with many progestational agents (14–16). A decline in serum high-density lipoproteins has been associated with an increased incidence of ischemic heart

Continued on next page

Mircette—Cont.

disease. Because estrogens increase HDL cholesterol, the net effect of an oral contraceptive depends on a balance achieved between doses of estrogen and progestogen and the nature and absolute amount of progestogens used in the contraceptives. The amount of both hormones should be considered in the choice of an oral contraceptive.

Minimizing exposure to estrogen and progestogen is in keeping with good principles of therapeutics. For any particular estrogen/progestogen combination, the dosage regimen prescribed should be one which contains the least amount of estrogen and progestogen that is compatible with a low failure rate and the needs of the individual patient. New acceptors of oral contraceptive agents should be started on preparations containing the lowest estrogen content which produces satisfactory results in the individual.

e. Persistence of risk of vascular disease

There are two studies which have shown persistence of risk of vascular disease for ever-users of oral contraceptives. In a study in the United States, the risk of developing myocardial infarction after discontinuing oral contraceptives persists for at least 9 years for women 40–49 years old who had used oral contraceptives for five or more years, but this increased risk was not demonstrated in other age groups (8). In another study in Great Britain, the risk of developing cerebrovascular disease persisted for at least 6 years after discontinuation of oral contraceptives, although excess risk was very small (34). However, both studies were performed with oral contraceptive formulations containing 50 micrograms or more of estrogen.

2. ESTIMATES OF MORTALITY FROM CONTRACEPTIVE USE

One study gathered data from a variety of sources which have estimated the mortality rate associated with different methods of contraception at different ages (Table IV). These estimates include the combined risk of death associated with contraceptive methods plus the risk attributable to pregnancy in the event of method failure. Each method of contraception has its specific benefits and risks. The study concluded that with the exception of oral contraceptive users 35 and older who smoke and 40 and older who do not smoke, mortality associated with all methods of birth control is low and below that associated with childbirth.

The observation of a possible increase in risk of mortality with age for oral contraceptive users is based on data gathered in the 1970's - but not reported until 1983 (35). However, current clinical practice involves the use of lower estrogen formulations combined with careful consideration of risk factors.

Because of these changes in practice and, also, because of some limited new data which suggest that the risk of cardiovascular disease with the use of oral contraceptives may now be less than previously observed (100,101), the Fertility and Maternal Health Drugs Advisory Committee was asked to review the topic in 1989. The Committee concluded that although cardiovascular disease risks may be increased with oral contraceptive use after age 40 in healthy non-smoking women (even with the newer low-dose formulations), there are also greater potential health risks associated with pregnancy in older women and with the alternative surgical and medical procedures which may be necessary if such women do not have access to effective and acceptable means of contraception.

Therefore, the Committee recommended that the benefits of low-dose oral contraceptive use by healthy non-smoking women over 40 may outweigh the possible risks. Of course, older women, as all women who take oral contraceptives, should take the lowest possible dose formulation that is effective.

[See table below]

3. CARCINOMA OF THE REPRODUCTIVE ORGANS AND BREASTS

Numerous epidemiological studies have been performed on the incidence of breast, endometrial, ovarian and cervical cancer in women using oral contraceptives. While there are conflicting reports, most studies suggest that the use of oral contraceptives is not associated with an overall increase in the risk of developing breast cancer. Some studies have reported an increased relative risk of developing breast cancer, particularly at a younger age. This increased relative risk appears to be related to duration of use (36–43, 79–89).

Some studies suggest that oral contraceptive use has been associated with an increase in the risk of cervical intra-epithelial neoplasia in some populations of women (45–48). However, there continues to be controversy about the extent to which such findings may be due to differences in sexual behavior and other factors.

4. HEPATIC NEOPLASIA

Benign hepatic adenomas are associated with oral contraceptive use, although the incidence of benign tumors is rare in the United States. Indirect calculations have estimated the attributable risk to be in the range of 3.3 cases/100,000 for users, a risk that increases after four or more years of use especially with oral contraceptives of higher dose (49). Rupture of rare, benign, hepatic adenomas may cause death through intra-abdominal hemorrhage (50,51).

Studies from Britain have shown an increased risk of developing hepatocellular carcinoma (52–54) in long-term (>8 years) oral contraceptive users. However, these cancers are extremely rare in the U.S. and the attributable risk (the excess incidence) of liver cancers in oral contraceptive users approaches less than one per million users.

5. OCULAR LESIONS

There have been clinical case reports of retinal thrombosis associated with the use of oral contraceptives. Oral contraceptives should be discontinued if there is unexplained partial or complete loss of vision; onset of proptosis or diplopia; papilledema; or retinal vascular lesions. Appropriate diagnostic and therapeutic measures should be undertaken immediately.

6. ORAL CONTRACEPTIVE USE BEFORE OR DURING EARLY PREGNANCY

Extensive epidemiological studies have revealed no increased risk of birth defects in women who have used oral contraceptives prior to pregnancy (55–57). Studies also do not suggest a teratogenic effect, particularly in so far as cardiac anomalies and limb reduction defects are concerned (55,56,58,59), when oral contraceptives are taken inadvertently during early pregnancy.

The administration of oral contraceptives to induce withdrawal bleeding should not be used as a test for pregnancy. Oral contraceptives should not be used during pregnancy to treat threatened or habitual abortion. It is recommended that for any patient who has missed two consecutive periods, pregnancy should be ruled out before continuing oral contraceptive use. If the patient has not adhered to the prescribed schedule, the possibility of pregnancy should be considered at the first missed period. Oral contraceptive use should be discontinued until pregnancy is ruled out.

7. GALLBLADDER DISEASE

Earlier studies have reported an increased lifetime relative risk of gallbladder surgery in users of oral contraceptives and estrogens (60,61). More recent studies, however, have shown that the relative risk of developing gallbladder disease among oral contraceptive users may be minimal (62–64). The recent findings of minimal risk may be related to the use of oral contraceptive formulations containing lower hormonal doses of estrogens and progestogens.

8. CARBOHYDRATE AND LIPID METABOLIC EFFECTS

Oral contraceptives have been shown to cause a decrease in glucose tolerance in a significant percentage of users (17). Oral contraceptives containing greater than 75 micrograms of estrogens cause hyperinsulinism, while lower doses of estrogen cause less glucose intolerance (65). Progestogens increase insulin secretion and create insulin resistance, this effect varying with different progestational agents (17,66). However, in the non-diabetic woman, oral contraceptives appear to have no effect on fasting blood glucose (67). Because of these demonstrated effects, prediabetic and diabetic women should be carefully monitored while taking oral contraceptives.

A small proportion of women will have persistent hypertriglyceridemia while on the pill. As discussed earlier (see WARNINGS 1.a. and 1.d.), changes in serum triglycerides and lipoprotein levels have been reported in oral contraceptive users.

9. ELEVATED BLOOD PRESSURE

An increase in blood pressure has been reported in women taking oral contraceptives (68) and this increase is more likely in older oral contraceptive users (69) and with continued use (61). Data from the Royal College of General Practitioners (12) and subsequent randomized trials have shown that the incidence of hypertension increases with increasing quantities of progestogens.

Women with a history of hypertension or hypertension-related diseases, or renal disease (70) should be encouraged to use another method of contraception. If women elect to use oral contraceptives, they should be monitored closely and if significant elevation of blood pressure occurs, oral contraceptives should be discontinued. For most women, elevated blood pressure will return to normal after stopping oral contraceptives (69), and there is no difference in the occurrence of hypertension between ever- and never-users (68,70,71).

10. HEADACHE

The onset or exacerbation of migraine or development of headache with a new pattern which is recurrent, persistent, or severe requires discontinuation of oral contraceptives and evaluation of the cause.

11. BLEEDING IRREGULARITIES

Breakthrough bleeding and spotting are sometimes encountered in patients on oral contraceptives, especially during the first three months of use. Non-hormonal causes should be considered and adequate diagnostic measures taken to rule out malignancy or pregnancy in the event of breakthrough bleeding, as in the case of any abnormal vaginal bleeding. If pathology has been excluded, time or a change to another formulation may solve the problem. In the event of amenorrhea, pregnancy should be ruled out.

Some women may encounter post-pill amenorrhea or oligomenorrhea, especially when such a condition was preexistent.

12. ECTOPIC PREGNANCY

Ectopic as well as intrauterine pregnancy may occur in contraceptive failures.

PRECAUTIONS

1. GENERAL

Patients should be counseled that this product does not protect against HIV infection (AIDS) and other sexually transmitted diseases.

2. PHYSICAL EXAMINATION AND FOLLOW UP

It is good medical practice for all women to have annual history and physical examinations, including women using oral contraceptives. The physical examination, however, may be deferred until after initiation of oral contraceptives if requested by the woman and judged appropriate by the clinician. The physical examination should include special reference to blood pressure, breasts, abdomen and pelvic organs, including cervical cytology, and relevant laboratory tests. In case of undiagnosed, persistent or recurrent abnormal vaginal bleeding, appropriate measures should be conducted to rule out malignancy. Women with a strong family history of breast cancer or who have breast nodules should be monitored with particular care.

3. LIPID DISORDERS

Women who are being treated for hyperlipidemias should be followed closely if they elect to use oral contraceptives. Some progestogens may elevate LDL levels and may render the control of hyperlipidemias more difficult.

4. LIVER FUNCTION

If jaundice develops in any woman receiving such drugs, the medication should be discontinued. Steroid hormones may be poorly metabolized in patients with impaired liver function.

5. FLUID RETENTION

Oral contraceptives may cause some degree of fluid retention. They should be prescribed with caution, and only with careful monitoring, in patients with conditions which might be aggravated by fluid retention.

6. EMOTIONAL DISORDERS

Women with a history of depression should be carefully observed and the drug discontinued if depression recurs to a serious degree.

TABLE IV: ANNUAL NUMBER OF BIRTH-RELATED OR METHOD-RELATED DEATHS ASSOCIATED WITH CONTROL OF FERTILITY PER 100,000 NON-STERILE WOMEN, BY FERTILITY CONTROL METHOD ACCORDING TO AGE

Method of control and outcome	15–19	20–24	25–29	30–34	35–39	40–44
No fertility control methods*	7.0	7.4	9.1	14.8	25.7	28.2
Oral contraceptives non-smoker**	0.3	0.5	0.9	1.9	13.8	31.6
Oral contraceptives smoker**	2.2	3.4	6.6	13.5	51.1	117.2
IUD**	0.8	0.8	1.0	1.0	1.4	1.4
Condom*	1.1	1.6	0.7	0.2	0.3	0.4
Diaphragm/spermicide*	1.9	1.2	1.2	1.3	2.2	2.8
Periodic abstinence*	2.5	1.6	1.6	1.7	2.9	3.6

* Deaths are birth related
** Deaths are method related

Adapted from H.W. Ory, ref. #35.

7. CONTACT LENSES
Contact lens wearers who develop visual changes or changes in lens tolerance should be assessed by an ophthalmologist.

8. DRUG INTERACTIONS
Reduced efficacy and increased incidence of breakthrough bleeding and menstrual irregularities have been associated with concomitant use of rifampin. A similar association, though less marked, has been suggested with barbiturates, phenylbutazone, phenytoin sodium, carbamazepine and possibly with griseofulvin, ampicillin, and tetracyclines (72).

9. INTERACTIONS WITH LABORATORY TESTS
Certain endocrine and liver function tests and blood components may be affected by oral contraceptives:

a. Increased prothrombin and factors VII, VIII, IX and X; decreased antithrombin 3; increased norepinephrine-induced platelet aggregability.
b. Increased thyroid binding globulin (TBG) leading to increased circulating total thyroid hormone, as measured by protein-bound iodine (PBI), T4 by column or by radioimmunoassay. Free T3 resin uptake is decreased, reflecting the elevated TBG; free T4 concentration is unaltered.
c. Other binding proteins may be elevated in serum.
d. Sex hormone-binding globulins are increased and result in elevated levels of total circulating sex steroids; however, free or biologically active levels either decrease or remain unchanged.
e. High-density lipoprotein cholesterol (HDL-C) and triglycerides may be increased, while low-density lipoprotein cholesterol (LDL-C) and total cholesterol (Total-C) may be decreased or unchanged.
f. Glucose tolerance may be decreased.
g. Serum folate levels may be depressed by oral contraceptive therapy. This may be of clinical significance if a woman becomes pregnant shortly after discontinuing oral contraceptives.

10. CARCINOGENESIS
See WARNINGS section.

11. PREGNANCY
Pregnancy Category X (see CONTRAINDICATIONS and WARNINGS sections.)

12. NURSING MOTHERS
Small amounts of oral contraceptive steroids have been identified in the milk of nursing mothers and a few adverse effects on the child have been reported, including jaundice and breast enlargement. In addition, oral contraceptives given in the postpartum period may interfere with lactation by decreasing the quantity and quality of breast milk. If possible, the nursing mother should be advised not to use oral contraceptives but to use other forms of contraception until she has completely weaned her child.

13. PEDIATRIC USE
Safety and efficacy of Mircette® (desogestrel/ethinyl estradiol and ethinyl estradiol) Tablets have been established in women of reproductive age. Safety and efficacy are expected to be the same for postpubertal adolescents under the age of 16 and for users 16 years and older. Use of this product before menarche is not indicated.

INFORMATION FOR THE PATIENT
See Patient Labeling Printed Below

ADVERSE REACTIONS

An increased risk of the following serious adverse reactions has been associated with the use of oral contraceptives (see WARNINGS section):

- Thrombophlebitis and venous thrombosis with or without embolism
- Arterial thromboembolism
- Pulmonary embolism
- Myocardial infarction
- Cerebral hemorrhage
- Cerebral thrombosis
- Hypertension
- Gallbladder disease
- Hepatic adenomas or benign liver tumors

There is evidence of an association between the following conditions and the use of oral contraceptives:

- Mesenteric thrombosis
- Retinal thrombosis

The following adverse reactions have been reported in patients receiving oral contraceptives and are believed to be drug-related:

- Nausea
- Vomiting
- Gastrointestinal symptoms (such as abdominal cramps and bloating)
- Breakthrough bleeding
- Spotting
- Change in menstrual flow
- Amenorrhea
- Temporary infertility after discontinuation of treatment
- Edema
- Melasma which may persist
- Breast changes: tenderness, enlargement, secretion
- Change in weight (increase or decrease)
- Change in cervical erosion and secretion
- Diminution in lactation when given immediately postpartum
- Cholestatic jaundice
- Migraine
- Rash (allergic)
- Mental depression
- Reduced tolerance to carbohydrates
- Vaginal candidiasis
- Change in corneal curvature (steepening)
- Intolerance to contact lenses

The following adverse reactions have been reported in users of oral contraceptives and the association has been neither confirmed nor refuted:

- Pre-menstrual syndrome
- Cataracts
- Changes in appetite
- Cystitis-like syndrome
- Headache
- Nervousness
- Dizziness
- Hirsutism
- Loss of scalp hair
- Erythema multiforme
- Erythema nodosum
- Hemorrhagic eruption
- Vaginitis
- Porphyria
- Impaired renal function
- Hemolytic uremic syndrome
- Acne
- Changes in libido
- Colitis
- Budd-Chiari Syndrome

OVERDOSAGE

Serious ill effects have not been reported following acute ingestion of large doses of oral contraceptives by young children. Overdosage may cause nausea, and withdrawal bleeding may occur in females.

NON-CONTRACEPTIVE HEALTH BENEFITS
The following non-contraceptive health benefits related to the use of oral contraceptives are supported by epidemiological studies which largely utilized oral contraceptive formulations containing estrogen doses exceeding 0.035 mg of ethinyl estradiol or 0.05 mg of mestranol (73–78).

Effects on menses:
- increased menstrual cycle regularity
- decreased blood loss and decreased incidence of iron deficiency anemia
- decreased incidence of dysmenorrhea

Effects related to inhibition of ovulation:
- decreased incidence of functional ovarian cysts
- decreased incidence of ectopic pregnancies

Effects from long-term use:
- decreased incidence of fibroadenomas and fibrocystic disease of the breast
- decreased incidence of acute pelvic inflammatory disease
- decreased incidence of endometrial cancer
- decreased incidence of ovarian cancer

DOSAGE AND ADMINISTRATION

To achieve maximum contraceptive effectiveness, Mircette® (desogestrel/ethinyl estradiol and ethinyl estradiol) Tablets must be taken exactly as directed and at intervals not exceeding 24 hours. Mircette® may be initiated using either a Sunday start or a Day 1 start.

NOTE: Each cycle pack dispenser is preprinted with the days of the week, starting with Sunday, to facilitate a Sunday start regimen. Six different "day label strips" are provided with each cycle pack dispenser in order to accommodate a Day 1 start regimen. In this case, the patient should place the self-adhesive "day label strip" that corresponds to her starting day over the preprinted days.

IMPORTANT: The possibility of ovulation and conception prior to initiation of use of Mircette® should be considered. The use of Mircette® for contraception may be initiated 4 weeks postpartum in women who elect not to breast feed. When the tablets are administered during the postpartum period, the increased risk of thromboembolic disease associated with the postpartum period must be considered (see CONTRAINDICATIONS and WARNINGS concerning thromboembolic disease. See also PRECAUTIONS for "Nursing Mothers").

If the patient starts on Mircette® postpartum, and has not yet had a period, she should be instructed to use another method of contraception until a white tablet has been taken daily for 7 days.

SUNDAY START
When initiating a Sunday start regimen, another method of contraception should be used until after the first 7 consecutive days of administration.

Using a Sunday start, tablets are taken daily without interruption as follows: The first white tablet should be taken on the first Sunday after menstruation begins (if menstruation begins on Sunday, the first white tablet is taken on that day). One white tablet is taken daily for 21 days, followed by 1 green (inert) tablet daily for 2 days and 1 yellow (active) tablet daily for 5 days. For all subsequent cycles, the patient then begins a new 28-tablet regimen on the next day (Sunday) after taking the last yellow tablet. [If switching from a Sunday Start oral contraceptive, the first Mircette® (desogestrel/ethinyl estradiol and ethinyl estradiol) tablet should be taken on the second Sunday after the last tablet of a 21 day regimen or should be taken on the first Sunday after the last inactive tablet of a 28 day regimen.]

If a patient misses 1 white tablet, she should take the missed tablet as soon as she remembers. If the patient misses 2 consecutive white tablets in Week 1 or Week 2, the patient should take 2 tablets the day she remembers and 2 tablets the next day; thereafter, the patient should resume taking 1 tablet daily until she finishes the cycle pack. The patient should be instructed to use a back-up method of birth control if she has intercourse in the 7 days after missing pills. If the patient misses 2 consecutive white tablets in the third week or misses 3 or more white tablets in a row at any time during the cycle, the patient should keep taking 1 white tablet daily until the next Sunday. On Sunday the patient should throw out the rest of that cycle pack and start a new cycle pack that same day. The patient should be instructed to use a back-up method of birth control if she has intercourse in the 7 days after missing pills.

DAY 1 START
Counting the first day of menstruation as "Day 1", tablets are taken without interruption as follows: One white tablet daily for 21 days, one green (inert) tablet daily for 2 days followed by 1 yellow (ethinyl estradiol) tablet daily for 5 days. For all subsequent cycles, the patient then begins a new 28-tablet regimen on the next day after taking the last yellow tablet. [If switching directly from another oral contraceptive, the first white tablet should be taken on the first day of menstruation which begins after the last ACTIVE tablet of the previous product.]

If a patient misses 1 white tablet, she should take the missed tablet as soon as she remembers. If the patient misses 2 consecutive white tablets in Week 1 or Week 2, the patient should take 2 tablets the day she remembers and 2 tablets the next day; thereafter, the patient should resume taking 1 tablet daily until she finishes the cycle pack. The patient should be instructed to use a back-up method of birth control if she has intercourse in the 7 days after missing pills. If the patient misses 2 consecutive white tablets in the third week or if the patient misses 3 or more white tablets in a row at any time during the cycle, the patient should throw out the rest of that cycle pack and start a new cycle pack that same day. The patient should be instructed to use a back-up method of birth control if she has intercourse in the 7 days after missing pills.

ALL ORAL CONTRACEPTIVES
Breakthrough bleeding, spotting, and amenorrhea are frequent reasons for patients discontinuing oral contraceptives. In breakthrough bleeding, as in all cases of irregular bleeding from the vagina, non-functional causes should be borne in mind. In undiagnosed persistent or recurrent abnormal bleeding from the vagina, adequate diagnostic measures are indicated to rule out pregnancy or malignancy. If both pregnancy and pathology have been excluded, time or a change to another preparation may solve the problem. Changing to an oral contraceptive with a higher estrogen content, while potentially useful in minimizing menstrual irregularity, should be done only if necessary since this may increase the risk of thromboembolic disease.

Use of oral contraceptives in the event of a missed menstrual period:

1. If the patient has not adhered to the prescribed schedule, the possibility of pregnancy should be considered at the time of the first missed period and oral contraceptive use should be discontinued until pregnancy is ruled out.
2. If the patient has adhered to the prescribed regimen and misses two consecutive periods, pregnancy should be ruled out before continuing oral contraceptive use.

HOW SUPPLIED

Mircette® (desogestrel/ethinyl estradiol and ethinyl estradiol) Tablets contain 21 round white tablets, 2 round green tablets and 5 round yellow tablets in a blister card within a recyclable plastic dispenser. Each white tablet (debossed with "T_4R" on one side and "Organon" on the other side) contains 0.15 mg desogestrel and 0.02 mg ethinyl estradiol. Each green tablet (debossed with "K_2H" on one side and "Organon" on the other side) contains inert ingredients. Each yellow tablet (debossed with "K_2S" on one side and "Organon" on the other side) contains 0.01 mg ethinyl estradiol.

Boxes of 6 NDC 0052-0281-06

Storage
Store at controlled room temperature 20–25°C (68–77°F).

℞ only

REFERENCES

1. Hatcher RA, Trussell J, Stewart F et al. Contraceptive Technology: Seventeenth Revised Edition, New York: Irvington Publishers, 1998, in press. **2.** Stadel BV. Oral contraceptives and cardiovascular disease. (Pt. 1). N Engl J Med 1981; 305:612–618. **3.** Stadel BV. Oral contraceptives and cardiovascular disease. (Pt. 2). N Engl J Med 1981; 305: 672–677. **4.** Adam SA, Thorogood M. Oral contraception and myocardial infarction revisited: the effects of new preparations and prescribing patterns. Br J Obstet and Gynecol 1981; 88:838–845. **5.** Mann JI, Inman WH. Oral contraceptives and death from myocardial infarction. Br Med J 1975; 2(5965):245–248. **6.** Mann JI, Vessey MP, Thorogood M, Doll R. Myocardial infarction in young women with special reference to oral contraceptive practice. Br Med J 1975; 2(5956):241–245. **7.** Royal College of General Practitioners' Oral Contraception Study: Further analyses of mortality in oral contraceptive users. Lancet 1981; 1:541–546. **8.** Slone D, Shapiro S, Kaufman DW, Rosenberg L, Miettinen OS, Stolley PD. Risk of myocardial infarction in relation to current and discontinued use of oral contraceptives. N Engl J

Continued on next page

Mircette—Cont.

Med 1981; 305:420–424. **9.** Vessey MP. Female hormones and vascular disease—an epidemiological overview. Br J Fam Plann 1980; 6:1–12. **10.** Russell-Briefel RG, Ezzati TM, Fulwood R, Perlman JA, Murphy RS. Cardiovascular risk status and oral contraceptive use, United States, 1976–80. Prevent Med 1986; 15:352–362. **11.** Goldbaum GM, Kendrick JS, Hogelin GC, Gentry EM. The relative impact of smoking and oral contraceptive use on women in the United States. JAMA 1987; 258:1339–1342. **12.** Layde PM, Beral V. Further analyses of mortality in oral contraceptive users: Royal College General Practitioners' Oral Contraception Study. (Table 5) Lancet 1981; 1:541–546. **13.** Knopp RH. Arteriosclerosis risk: the roles of oral contraceptives and postmenopausal estrogens. J Reprod Med 1986; 31(9) (Supplement):913–921. **14.** Krauss RM, Roy S, Mishell DR, Casagrande J, Pike MC. Effects of two low-dose oral contraceptives on serum lipids and lipoproteins: Differential changes in high-density lipoproteins subclasses. Am J Obstet 1983; 145:446–452. **15.** Wahl P, Walden C, Knopp R, Hoover J, Wallace R, Heiss G, Rifkind B. Effect of estrogen/progestin potency on lipid/lipoprotein cholesterol. N Engl J Med 1983; 308:862–867. **16.** Wynn V, Niththyananthan R. The effect of progestin in combined oral contraceptives on serum lipids with special reference to high-density lipoproteins. Am J Obstet Gynecol 1982; 142:766–771. **17.** Wynn V, Godsland I. Effects of oral contraceptives and carbohydrate metabolism. J Reprod Med 1986; 31 (9) (Supplement):892–897. **18.** LaRosa JC. Atherosclerotic risk factors in cardiovascular disease. J Reprod Med 1986; 31 (9) (Supplement): 906–912. **19.** Inman WH, Vessey MP. Investigation of death from pulmonary, coronary, and cerebral thrombosis and embolism in women of child-bearing age. Br Med J 1968; 2 (5599):193–199. **20.** Maguire MG, Tonascia J, Sartwell PE, Stolley PD, Tockman MS. Increased risk of thrombosis due to oral contraceptives: a further report. Am J Epidemiol 1979; 110 (2):188–195. **21.** Pettiti DB, Wingerd J, Pellegrin F, Ramacharan S. Risk of vascular disease in women: smoking, oral contraceptives, noncontraceptive estrogens, and other factors. JAMA 1979; 242:1150–1154. **22.** Vessey MP, Doll R. Investigation of relation between use of oral contraceptives and thromboembolic disease. Br Med J 1968; 2 (5599):199–205. **23.** Vessey MP, Doll R. Investigation of relation between use of oral contraceptives and thromboembolic disease. A further report. Br Med J 1969; 2 (5658):651–657. **24.** Porter JB, Hunter JR, Danielson DA, Jick H, Stergachis A. Oral contraceptives and non-fatal vascular disease—recent experience. Obstet Gynecol 1982; 59 (3): 299–302. **25.** Vessey M, Doll R, Peto R, Johnson B, Wiggins P. A long-term follow-up study of women using different methods of contraception: an interim report. Biosocial Sci 1976; 8:375–427. **26.** Royal College of General Practitioners: Oral contraceptives, venous thrombosis, and varicose veins. J Royal Coll Gen Pract 1978; 28:393–399. **27.** Collaborative Group for the Study of Stroke in Young Women: Oral contraception and increased risk of cerebral ischemia or thrombosis. N Engl J Med 1973; 288:871–878. **28.** Pettiti DB, Wingerd J. Use of oral contraceptives, cigarette smoking, and risk of subarachnoid hemorrhage. Lancet 1978; 2:234–236. **29.** Inman WH. Oral contraceptives and fatal subarachnoid hemorrhage. Br Med J 1979; 2 (6203):1468–70. **30.** Collaborative Group for the Study of Stroke in Young Women: Oral contraceptives and stroke in young women: associated risk factors. JAMA 1975; 231:718–722. **31.** Inman WH, Vessey MP, Westerholm B, Engelund A. Thromboembolic disease and the steroidal content of oral contraceptives. A report to the Committee on Safety of Drugs. Br Med J 1970; 2:203–209. **32.** Meade TW, Greenberg G, Thompson SG. Progestogens and cardiovascular reactions associated with oral contraceptives and a comparison of the safety of 50- and 35-mcg oestrogen preparations. Br Med J 1980; 280 (6224):1157–1161. **33.** Kay CR. Progestogens and arterial disease—evidence from the Royal College of General Practitioners' Study. Am J Obstet Gynecol 1982; 142:762–765. **34.** Royal College of General Practitioners: Incidence of arterial disease among oral contraceptive users. J Royal Coll Gen Pract 1983; 33:75–82. **35.** Ory HW. Mortality associated with fertility and fertility control: 1983. Family Planning Perspectives 1983; 15:50–56. **36.** The Cancer and Steroid Hormone Study of the Centers for Disease Control and the National Institute of Child Health and Human Development: Oral-contraceptive use and the risk of breast cancer. N Engl J Med 1986; 315:405–411. **37.** Pike MC, Henderson BE, Krailo MD, Duke A, Roy S. Breast cancer risk in young women and use of oral contraceptives: possible modifying effect of formulation and age at use. Lancet 1983; 2:926–929. **38.** Paul C, Skegg DG, Spears GFS, Kaldor JM. Oral contraceptives and breast cancer: A national study. Br Med J 1986; 293:723–725. **39.** Miller DR, Rosenberg L, Kaufman DW, Schottenfeld D, Stolley PD, Shapiro S. Breast cancer risk in relation to early oral contraceptive use. Obstet Gynecol 1986; 68:863–868. **40.** Olson H, Olson KL, Moller TR, Ranstam J, Holm P. Oral contraceptive use and breast cancer in young women in Sweden (letter). Lancet 1985; 2:748–749. **41.** McPherson K, Vessey M, Neil A, Doll R, Jones L, Roberts M. Early contraceptive use and breast cancer: Results of another case-control study. Br J Cancer 1987; 56: 653–660. **42.** Huggins GR, Zucker PF. Oral contraceptives and neoplasia: 1987 update. Fertil Steril 1987; 47:733–761. **43.** McPherson K, Drife JO. The pill and breast cancer: why the uncertainty? Br Med J 1986; 293:709–710. **44.** Shapiro S. Oral contraceptives—time to take stock. N Engl J Med 1987; 315:450–451. **45.** Ory H, Naib Z, Conger SB, Hatcher RA, Tyler CW. Contraceptive choice and prevalence of cervical dysplasia and carcinoma in situ. Am J Obstet Gynecol 1976; 124:573–577. **46.** Vessey MP, Lawless M, McPherson K, Yeates D. Neoplasia of the cervix uteri and contraception: a possible adverse effect of the pill. Lancet 1983; 2:930. **47.** Brinton LA, Huggins GR, Lehman HF, Malli K, Savitz DA, Trapido E, Rosenthal J, Hoover R. Long-term use of oral contraceptives and risk of invasive cervical cancer. Int J Cancer 1986; 38:339–344. **48.** WHO Collaborative Study of Neoplasia and Steroid Contraceptives: Invasive cervical cancer and combined oral contraceptives. Br Med J 1985; 209:961–965. **49.** Rooks JB, Ory HW, Ishak KG, Strauss LT, Greenspan JR, Hill AP, Tyler CW. Epidemiology of hepatocellular adenoma: the role of oral contraceptive use. JAMA 1979; 242:644–648. **50.** Bein NN, Goldsmith HS. Recurrent massive hemorrhage from benign hepatic tumors secondary to oral contraceptives. Br J Surg 1977; 64:433–435. **51.** Klatskin G. Hepatic tumors: possible relationship to use of oral contraceptives. Gastroenterology 1977; 73:386–394. **52.** Henderson BE, Preston-Martin S, Edmondson HA, Peters RL, Pike MC. Hepatocellular carcinoma and oral contraceptives. Br J Cancer 1983; 48:437–440. **53.** Neuberger J, Forman D, Doll R, Williams R. Oral contraceptives and hepatocellular carcinoma. Br Med J 1986; 292:1355–1357. **54.** Forman D, Vincent TJ, Doll R. Cancer of the liver and oral contraceptives. Br Med J 1986; 292:1357–1361. **55.** Harlap S, Eldor J. Births following oral contraceptive failures. Obstet Gynecol 1980; 55:447–452. **56.** Savolainen E, Saksela E, Saxen L. Teratogenic hazards of oral contraceptives analyzed in a national malformation register. Am J Obstet Gynecol 1981; 140:521–524. **57.** Janerich DT, Piper JM, Glebatis DM. Oral contraceptives and birth defects. Am J Epidemiol 1980; 112:73–79. **58.** Ferencz C, Matanoski GM, Wilson PD, Rubin JD, Neill CA, Gutberlet R. Maternal hormone therapy and congenital heart disease. Teratology 1980; 21: 225–239. **59.** Rothman KJ, Fyler DC, Goldbatt A, Kreidberg MB. Exogenous hormones and other drug exposures of children with congenital heart disease. Am J Epidemiol 1979; 109:433–439. **60.** Boston Collaborative Drug Surveillance Program: Oral contraceptives and venous thromboembolic disease, surgically confirmed gallbladder disease, and breast tumors. Lancet 1973; 1:1399–1404. **61.** Royal College of General Practitioners: Oral contraceptives and health. New York, Pittman, 1974. **62.** Layde PM, Vessey MP, Yeates D. Risk of gallbladder disease: a cohort study of young women attending family planning clinics. J Epidemiol Community Health 1982; 36:274–278. **63.** Rome Group for the Epidemiology and Prevention of Cholelithiasis (GREPCO): Prevalence of gallstone disease in an Italian adult female population. Am J Epidemiol 1984; 119:796–805. **64.** Strom BL, Tamragouri RT, Morse ML, Lazar EL, West SL, Stolley PD, Jones JK. Oral contraceptives and other risk factors for gallbladder disease. Clin Pharmacol Ther 1986; 39:335–341. **65.** Wynn V, Adams PW, Godsland IF, Melrose J, Niththyananthan R, Oakley NW, Seedj A. Comparison of effects of different combined oral-contraceptive formulations on carbohydrate and lipid metabolism. Lancet 1979; 1:1045–1049. **66.** Wynn V. Effect of progesterone and progestins on carbohydrate metabolism. In Progesterone and Progestin. Edited by Bardin CW, Milgrom E, Mauvis-Jarvis P. New York, Raven Press, 1983 pp. 395–410. **67.** Perlman JA, Roussell-Briefel RG, Ezzati TM, Lieberknecht G. Oral glucose tolerance and the potency of oral contraceptive progestogens. J Chronic Dis 1985; 38:857–864. **68.** Royal College of General Practitioners' Oral Contraception Study: Effect on hypertension and benign breast disease of progestogen component in combined oral contraceptives. Lancet 1977; 1:624. **69.** Fisch IR, Frank J. Oral contraceptives and blood pressure. JAMA 1977; 237:2499–2503. **70.** Laragh AJ. Oral contraceptive induced hypertension—nine years later. Am J Obstet Gynecol 1976; 126:141–147. **71.** Ramcharan S, Peritz E, Pellegrin FA, Williams WT. Incidence of hypertension in the Walnut Creek Contraceptive Drug Study cohort. In Pharmacology of Steroid Contraceptive Drugs. Garattini S, Berendes HW. Eds. New York, Raven Press, 1977 pp. 277–288. (Monographs of the Mario Negri Institute for Pharmacological Research, Milan). **72.** Stockley I. Interactions with oral contraceptives. J Pharm 1976; 216:140–143. **73.** The Cancer and Steroid Hormone Study of the Centers for Disease Control and the National Institute of Child Health and Human Development: Oral contraceptive use and the risk of ovarian cancer. JAMA 1983; 249:1596–1599. **74.** The Cancer and Steroid Hormone Study of the Centers for Disease Control and the National Institute of Child Health and Human Development: Combination oral contraceptive use and the risk of endometrial cancer. JAMA 1987; 257:796–800. **75.** Ory HW. Functional ovarian cysts and oral contraceptives: negative association confirmed surgically. JAMA 1974; 228:68–69. **76.** Ory HW, Cole P, Macmahon B, Hoover R. Oral contraceptives and reduced risk of benign breast disease. N Engl J Med 1976; 294:419–422. **77.** Ory HW. The noncontraceptive health benefits from oral contraceptive use. Fam Plann Perspect 1982; 14:182–184. **78.** Ory HW, Forrest JD, Lincoln R. Making Choices: Evaluating the health risks and benefits of birth control methods. New York, The Alan Guttmacher Institute, 1983; p. 1. **79.** Schlesselman J, Stadel BV, Murray P, Lai S. Breast Cancer in relation to early use of oral contraceptives 1988; 259:1828–1833. **80.** Hennekens CH, Speizer FE, Lipnick RJ, Rosner B, Bain C, Belanger C, Stampfer MJ, Willett W, Peto R. A case-controlled study of oral contraceptive use and breast cancer. JNCI 1984; 72:39–42. **81.** LaVecchia C, Decarli A, Fasoli M, Franceschi S, Gentile A, Negri E, Parazzini F, Tognoni G. Oral contraceptives and cancers of the breast and of the female genital tract. Interim results from a case-control study. Br. J. Cancer 1986; 54:311–317. **82.** Meirik O, Lund E, Adami H, Bergstrom R, Christoffersen T, Bergsjo P. Oral contraceptive use in breast cancer in young women. A Joint National Case-control study in Sweden and Norway. Lancet 1986; 11:650–654. **83.** Kay CR, Hannaford PC. Breast cancer and the pill—A further report from the Royal College of General Practitioners' oral contraception study. Br. J. Cancer 1988; 58:675–680. **84.** Stadel BV, Lai S, Schlesselman JJ, Murray P. Oral contraceptives and premenopausal breast cancer in nulliparous women. Contraception 1988; 38:287–299. **85.** Miller DR, Rosenberg L, Kaufman DW, Stolley P, Warshauer ME, Shapiro S. Breast cancer before age 45 and oral contraceptive use: New Findings. Am. J. Epidemiol 1989; 129:269–280. **86.** The UK National Case-Control Study Group, Oral contraceptive use and breast cancer risk in young women. Lancet 1989; 1:973–982. **87.** Schlesselman JJ. Cancer of the breast and reproductive tract in relation to use of oral contraceptives. Contraception 1989; 40:1–38. **88.** Vessey MP, McPherson K, Villard-Mackintosh L, Yeates D. Oral contraceptives and breast cancer: latest findings in a large cohort study. Br. J. Cancer 1989; 59:613–617. **89.** Jick SS, Walker AM, Stergachis A, Jick H. Oral contraceptives and breast cancer. Br. J. Cancer 1989; 59:618–621. **90.** Godsland, I et al. The effects of different formulations of oral contraceptive agents on lipid and carbohydrate metabolism. N Engl J Med 1990; 323:1375–81. **91.** Kloosterboer, HJ et al. Selectivity in progesterone and androgen receptor binding of progestogens used in oral contraception. Contraception, 1988; 38:325–32. **92.** Van der Vies, J and de Visser, J. Endocrinological studies with desogestrel. Arzneim. Forsch./Drug Res., 1983; 33(I),2:231–6. **93.** Data on file, Organon Inc. **94.** Fotherby, K. Oral contraceptives, lipids and cardiovascular diseases. Contraception, 1985; Vol. 31; 4:367–94. **95.** Lawrence, DM et al. Reduced sex hormone binding globulin and derived free testosterone levels in women with severe acne. Clinical Endocrinology, 1981; 15:87–91. **96.** Cullberg, G et al. Effects of a low-dose desogestrel-ethinyl estradiol combination on hirsutism, androgens and sex hormone binding globulin in women with a polycystic ovary syndrome. Acta Obstet Gynecol Scand, 1985; 64:195–202. **97.** Jung-Hoffmann, C and Kuhl, H. Divergent effects of two low-dose oral contraceptives on sex hormone-binding globulin and free testosterone. AJOG, 1987; 156:199–203. **98.** Hammond, G et al. Serum steroid binding protein concentrations, distribution of progestogens, and bioavailability of testosterone during treatment with contraceptives containing desogestrel or levonorgestrel. Fertil. Steril., 1984; 42:44–51. **99.** Palatsi, R et al. Serum total and unbound testosterone and sex hormone binding globulin (SHBG) in female acne patients treated with two different oral contraceptives. Acta Derm Venereol, 1984; 64:517–23. **100.** Porter JB, Hunter J, Jick H et al. Oral contraceptives and nonfatal vascular disease. Obstet Gynecol 1985; 66:1–4. **101.** Porter JB, Jick H, Walker AM. Mortality among oral contraceptive users. Obstet Gynecol 1987; 7029–32.

PATIENT PACKAGE INSERT
BRIEF SUMMARY

Mircette® (desogestrel/ethinyl estradiol and ethinyl estradiol) Tablets

This product (like all oral contraceptives) is intended to prevent pregnancy. It does not protect against HIV infection (AIDS) and other sexually transmitted diseases.

Oral contraceptives, also known as "birth control pills" or "the pill", are taken to prevent pregnancy, and when taken correctly, have a failure rate of about 1% per year when used without missing any pills. The typical failure rate of large numbers of pill users is less than 5% per year when women who miss pills are included. For most women, oral contraceptives are also free of serious or unpleasant side effects. However, forgetting to take pills considerably increases the chances of pregnancy.

For the majority of women, oral contraceptives can be taken safely. But there are some women who are at high risk of developing certain serious diseases that can be life-threatening or may cause temporary or permanent disability. The risks associated with taking oral contraceptives increase significantly if you:

- smoke
- have high blood pressure, diabetes, high cholesterol
- have or have had clotting disorders, heart attack, stroke, angina pectoris, cancer of the breast or sex organs, jaundice, or malignant or benign liver tumors.

Although cardiovascular disease risks may be increased with oral contraceptive use after age 40 in healthy, non-smoking women (even with the newer low-dose formulations), there are also greater potential health risks associated with pregnancy in older women.

You should not take the pill if you suspect you are pregnant or have unexplained vaginal bleeding.

Cigarette smoking increases the risk of serious cardiovascular side effects from oral contraceptive use. This risk increases with age and with heavy smoking (15 or more cigarettes per day) and is quite marked in women over 35 years of age. Women who use oral contraceptives are strongly advised not to smoke.

Most side effects of the pill are not serious. The most common such effects are nausea, vomiting, bleeding between menstrual periods, weight gain, breast tenderness, headache, and difficulty wearing contact lenses. These side effects, especially nausea and vomiting, may subside within the first three months of use.

The serious side effects of the pill occur very infrequently, especially if you are in good health and are young. However, you should know that the following medical conditions have been associated with or made worse by the pill:

1. Blood clots in the legs (thrombophlebitis) or lungs (pulmonary embolism), stoppage or rupture of a blood vessel in the brain (stroke), blockage of blood vessels in the heart (heart attack or angina pectoris) or other organs of the body. As mentioned above, smoking increases the risk of heart attacks and strokes, and subsequent serious medical consequences.
2. Liver tumors, which may rupture and cause severe bleeding. A possible but not definite association has been found with the pill and liver cancer. However, liver cancers are extremely rare. The chance of developing liver cancer from using the pill is thus even rarer.
3. High blood pressure, although blood pressure usually returns to normal when the pill is stopped.

The symptoms associated with these serious side effects are discussed in the detailed leaflet given to you with your supply of pills. Notify your doctor or health care provider if you notice any unusual physical disturbances while taking the pill. In addition, drugs such as rifampin, as well as some anticonvulsants and some antibiotics may decrease oral contraceptive effectiveness.

There is conflict among studies regarding breast cancer and oral contraceptive use. Some studies have reported an increase in the risk of developing breast cancer, particularly at a younger age.

This increased risk appears to be related to duration of use. The majority of studies have found no overall increase in the risk of developing breast cancer. Some studies have found an increase in the incidence of cancer of the cervix in women who use oral contraceptives. However, this finding may be related to factors other than the use of oral contraceptives. There is insufficient evidence to rule out the possibility that pills may cause such cancers.

Taking the pill provides some important non-contraceptive benefits. These include less painful menstruation, less menstrual blood loss and anemia, fewer pelvic infections, and fewer cancers of the ovary and the lining of the uterus.

Be sure to discuss any medical condition you may have with your doctor or health care provider. Your doctor or health care provider will take a medical and family history before prescribing oral contraceptives and will examine you. The physical examination may be delayed to another time if you request it and your doctor or health care provider believes that it is a good medical practice to postpone it. You should be reexamined at least once a year while taking oral contraceptives. The detailed patient information leaflet gives you further information which you should read and discuss with your doctor or health care provider.

This product (like all oral contraceptives) is intended to prevent pregnancy. It does not protect against transmission of HIV (AIDS) and other sexually transmitted diseases such as chlamydia, genital herpes, genital warts, gonorrhea, hepatitis B, and syphilis.

INSTRUCTIONS TO PATIENTS
HOW TO TAKE THE PILL

IMPORTANT POINTS TO REMEMBER

BEFORE YOU START TAKING YOUR PILLS:

1. BE SURE TO READ THESE DIRECTIONS:
   Before you start taking your pills.
   Anytime you are not sure what to do.
2. THE RIGHT WAY TO TAKE THE PILL IS TO TAKE ONE PILL EVERY DAY AT THE SAME TIME.
   If you miss pills you could get pregnant. This includes starting the pack late.
   The more pills you miss, the more likely you are to get pregnant.
3. MANY WOMEN HAVE SPOTTING OR LIGHT BLEEDING, OR MAY FEEL SICK TO THEIR STOMACH DURING THE FIRST 1–3 PACKS OF PILLS.
   If you feel sick to your stomach, do not stop taking the pill. The problem will usually go away. If it doesn't go away, check with your doctor or health care provider.
4. MISSING PILLS CAN ALSO CAUSE SPOTTING OR LIGHT BLEEDING, even when you make up these missed pills.
   On the days you take 2 pills to make up for missed pills, you could also feel a little sick to your stomach.
5. IF YOU HAVE VOMITING OR DIARRHEA, for any reason, or IF YOU TAKE SOME MEDICINES, including some antibiotics, your pills may not work as well.
   Use a back-up method (such as condoms, foam, or sponge) until you check with your doctor or health care provider.
6. IF YOU HAVE TROUBLE REMEMBERING TO TAKE THE PILL, talk to your doctor or health care provider about how to make pill-taking easier or about using another method of birth control.
7. IF YOU HAVE ANY QUESTIONS OR ARE UNSURE ABOUT THE INFORMATION IN THIS LEAFLET, call your doctor or health care provider.

BEFORE YOU START TAKING YOUR PILLS

1. DECIDE WHAT TIME OF DAY YOU WANT TO TAKE YOUR PILL.
   It is important to take it at about the same time every day.
2. LOOK AT YOUR PILL PACK: IT WILL HAVE 28 PILLS:
   This **28-pill pack** has 26 "active" [white and yellow] pills (with hormones) and 2 "inactive" [green] pills (without hormones).
3. ALSO FIND:
   1) where on the pack to start taking the pills,
   2) in what order to take the pills (follow the arrows) and
   3) the week numbers as shown in the picture below.

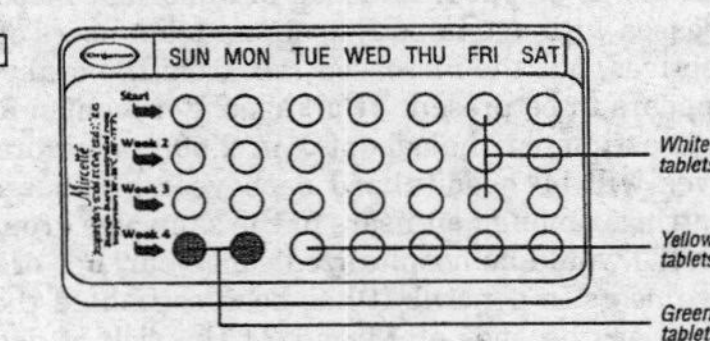

4. BE SURE YOU HAVE READY AT ALL TIMES:
   ANOTHER KIND OF BIRTH CONTROL (such as condoms, foam, or sponge) to use as a back-up in case you miss pills.
   AN EXTRA, FULL PILL PACK.

WHEN TO START THE FIRST PACK OF PILLS

You have a choice of which day to start taking your first pack of pills. Decide with your doctor or health care provider which is the best day for you. Pick a time of day which will be easy to remember.

DAY 1 START:

1. Pick the day label strip that starts with the first day of your period (this is the day you start bleeding or spotting, even if it is almost midnight when the bleeding begins).
2. Place this day label strip in the cycle tablet dispenser over the area that has the days of the week (starting with Sunday) imprinted in the plastic.

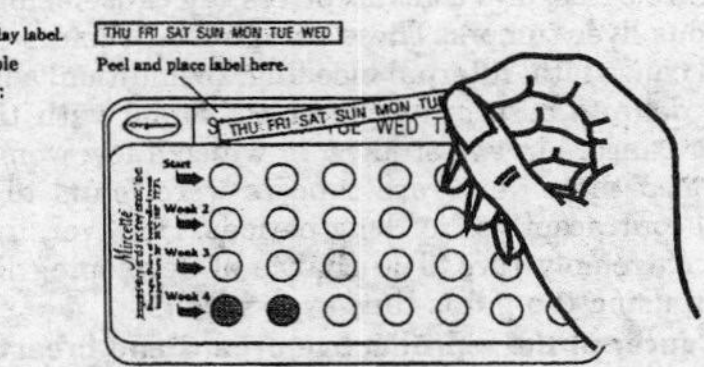

Note: If the first day of your period is a Sunday, you can skip steps #1 and #2.

3. Take the first "active" [white] pill of the first pack during the first 24 hours of your period.
4. You will not need to use a back-up method of birth control, since you are starting the pill at the beginning of your period.

SUNDAY START:

1. Take the first "active" [white] pill of the first pack on the Sunday after your period starts, even if you are still bleeding. If your period begins on Sunday, start the pack that same day.
2. Use another method of birth control as a back-up method if you have sex anytime from the Sunday you start your first pack until the next Sunday (7 days). Condoms, foam, or the sponge are good back-up methods of birth control.

WHAT TO DO DURING THE MONTH

1. **TAKE ONE PILL AT THE SAME TIME EVERY DAY UNTIL THE PACK IS EMPTY.**
   Do not skip pills even if you are spotting or bleeding between monthly periods or feel sick to your stomach (nausea).
   Do not skip pills even if you do not have sex very often.
2. **WHEN YOU FINISH A PACK OR SWITCH YOUR BRAND OF PILLS:**
   21 pills: Wait 7 days to start the next pack. You will probably have your period during that week. Be sure that no more than 7 days pass between 21-day packs.
   28 pills: Start the next pack on the day after your last pill. Do not wait any days between packs.

WHAT TO DO IF YOU MISS PILLS

If you **MISS 1** [white] "active" pill:

1. Take it as soon as you remember. Take the next pill at your regular time. This means you take 2 pills in 1 day.
2. You do not need to use a back-up birth control method if you have sex.

If you **MISS 2** [white] "active" pills in a row in **WEEK 1 OR WEEK 2** of your pack:

1. Take 2 pills on the day you remember and 2 pills the next day.
2. Then take 1 pill a day until you finish the pack.
3. You MAY BECOME PREGNANT if you have sex in the **7 days** after you miss pills.
   You MUST use another birth control method (such as condoms, foam, or sponge) as a back-up method for those 7 days.

If you **MISS 2** [white] "active" pills in a row in **THE 3RD WEEK:**

1. ***If you are a Day 1 Starter:***
   THROW OUT the rest of the pill pack and start a new pack that same day.
   If you are a Sunday Starter:
   Keep taking 1 pill every day until Sunday.
   On Sunday, THROW OUT the rest of the pack and start a new pack of pills that same day.
2. You may not have your period this month but this is expected. However, if you miss your period 2 months in a row, call your doctor or health care provider because you might be pregnant.
3. You MAY BECOME PREGNANT if you have sex in the **7 days** after you miss pills. You MUST use another birth control method (such as condoms, foam, or sponge) as a back-up method for those 7 days.

If you **MISS 3 OR MORE** [white] "active" pills in a row (during the first 3 weeks):

1. ***If you are a Day 1 Starter:***
   THROW OUT the rest of the pill pack and start a new pack that same day.
   If you are a Sunday Starter:
   Keep taking 1 pill every day until Sunday.
   On Sunday, THROW OUT the rest of the pack and start a new pack of pills that same day.
2. You may not have your period this month but this is expected. However, if you miss your period 2 months in a row, call your doctor or health care provider because you might be pregnant.
3. You MAY BECOME PREGNANT if you have sex in the **7 days** after you miss pills. You MUST use another birth control method (such as condoms, foam, or sponge) as a back-up method for those 7 days.

A REMINDER FOR THOSE ON 28-DAY PACKS:

If you forget any of the 2 [green] or 5 [yellow] pills in Week 4:
THROW AWAY the pills you missed.
Keep taking 1 pill each day until the pack is empty.
You do not need a back-up method.

FINALLY, IF YOU ARE STILL NOT SURE WHAT TO DO ABOUT THE PILLS YOU HAVE MISSED:

Use a BACK-UP METHOD anytime you have sex.
KEEP TAKING ONE [WHITE] "ACTIVE" PILL EACH DAY until you can reach your doctor or health care provider.

DETAILED PATIENT PACKAGE INSERT

Mircette® (desogestrel/ethinyl estradiol and ethinyl estradiol) Tablets

This product (like all oral contraceptives) is intended to prevent pregnancy. It does not protect against HIV infection (AIDS) and other sexually transmitted diseases.

℞ only

PLEASE NOTE: This labeling is revised from time to time as important new medical information becomes available. Therefore, please review this labeling carefully.

DESCRIPTION

The following oral contraceptive product contains a combination of a progestin and estrogen, the two kinds of female hormones:

Each white tablet contains 0.15 mg desogestrel and 0.02 mg ethinyl estradiol. Each green tablet contains inert ingredients and each yellow tablet contains 0.01 mg ethinyl estradiol.

INTRODUCTION

Any woman who considers using oral contraceptives (the birth control pill or the pill) should understand the benefits and risks of using this form of birth control. This leaflet will give you much of the information you will need to make this decision and will also help you determine if you are at risk of developing any of the serious side effects of the pill. It will tell you how to use the pill properly so that it will be as effective as possible. However, this leaflet is not a replacement for a careful discussion between you and your doctor or health care provider. You should discuss the information provided in this leaflet with him or her, both when you first start taking the pill and during your revisits. You should also follow your doctor's or health care provider's advice with regard to regular check-ups while you are on the pill.

EFFECTIVENESS OF ORAL CONTRACEPTIVES

Oral contraceptives or "birth control pills" or "the pill" are used to prevent pregnancy and are more effective than other non-surgical methods of birth control. When they are taken correctly, the chance of becoming pregnant is less than 1% (1 pregnancy per 100 women per year of use) when used perfectly, without missing any pills. Typical failure rates are actually 5% per year. The chance of becoming pregnant increases with each missed pill during a menstrual cycle.

In comparison, typical failure rates for other methods of birth control during the first year of use are as follows:

Implants (2 or 6 capsules): <1%
Injection: <1%
IUD: <1 to 2%
Diaphragm with spermicides: 20%
Spermicides alone: 26%
Vaginal sponge: 20 to 40%
Female sterilization: <1%

Continued on next page

Mircette—Cont.

Male sterilization: <1%
Cervical Cap with spermicides: 20 to 40%
Condom alone (male): 14%
Condom alone (female): 21%
Periodic abstinence: 25%
Withdrawal: 19%
No methods: 85%.

WHO SHOULD NOT TAKE ORAL CONTRACEPTIVES

Cigarette smoking increases the risk of serious cardiovascular side effects from oral contraceptive use. This risk increases with age and with heavy smoking (15 or more cigarettes per day) and is quite marked in women over 35 years of age. Women who use oral contraceptives are strongly advised not to smoke.

Some women should not use the pill. For example, you should not take the pill if you are pregnant or think you may be pregnant. You should also not use the pill if you have any of the following conditions:

- A history of heart attack or stroke
- Blood clots in the legs (thrombophlebitis), lungs (pulmonary embolism), or eyes
- A history of blood clots in the deep veins of your legs
- Chest pain (angina pectoris)
- Known or suspected breast cancer or cancer of the lining of the uterus, cervix or vagina
- Unexplained vaginal bleeding (until a diagnosis is reached by your doctor)
- Yellowing of the whites of the eyes or of the skin (jaundice) during pregnancy or during previous use of the pill
- Liver tumor (benign or cancerous)
- Known or suspected pregnancy.

Tell your doctor or health care provider if you have ever had any of these conditions. Your doctor or health care provider can recommend another method of birth control.

OTHER CONSIDERATIONS BEFORE TAKING ORAL CONTRACEPTIVES

Tell your doctor or health care provider if you have:

- Breast nodules, fibrocystic disease of the breast, an abnormal breast x-ray or mammogram
- Diabetes
- Elevated cholesterol or triglycerides
- High blood pressure
- Migraine or other headaches or epilepsy
- Mental depression
- Gallbladder, heart or kidney disease
- History of scanty or irregular menstrual periods.

Women with any of these conditions should be checked often by their doctor or health care provider if they choose to use oral contraceptives.

Also, be sure to inform your doctor or health care provider if you smoke or are on any medications.

RISKS OF TAKING ORAL CONTRACEPTIVES

1. Risk of developing blood clots

Blood clots and blockage of blood vessels are one of the most serious side effects of taking oral contraceptives. In particular, a clot in the legs can cause thrombophlebitis and a clot that travels to the lungs can cause a sudden blocking of the vessel carrying blood to the lungs. Rarely, clots occur in the blood vessels of the eye and may cause blindness, double vision, or impaired vision.

If you take oral contraceptives and need elective surgery, need to stay in bed for a prolonged illness or have recently delivered a baby, you may be at risk of developing blood clots. You should consult your doctor or health care provider about stopping oral contraceptives three to four weeks before surgery and not taking oral contraceptives for two weeks after surgery or during bed rest. You should also not take oral contraceptives soon after delivery of a baby. It is advisable to wait for at least four weeks after delivery if you are not breast feeding or four weeks after a second trimester abortion. If you are breast feeding, you should wait until you have weaned your child before using the pill (see Breast Feeding in GENERAL PRECAUTIONS).

The risk of circulatory disease in oral contraceptive users may be higher in users of high dose pills and may be greater with longer duration of oral contraceptive use. In addition, some of these increased risks may continue for a number of years after stopping oral contraceptives. The risk of venous thromboembolic disease associated with oral contraceptives does not increase with length of use and disappears after pill use is stopped. The risk of abnormal blood clotting increases with age in both users and non-users of oral contraceptives, but the increased risk from the oral contraceptive appears to be present at all ages. For women aged 20 to 44 it is estimated that about 1 in 2,000 using oral contraceptives will be hospitalized each year because of abnormal clotting. Among non-users in the same age group, about 1 in 20,000 would be hospitalized each year. For oral contraceptive users in general, it has been estimated that in women between the ages of 15 and 34 the risk of death due to a circulatory disorder is about 1 in 12,000 per year, whereas for non-users the rate is about 1 in 50,000 per year. In the age group 35 to 44, the risk is estimated to be about 1 in 2,500 per year for oral contraceptive users and about 1 in 10,000 per year for non-users.

2. Heart attacks and strokes

Oral contraceptives may increase the tendency to develop strokes (stoppage or rupture of blood vessels in the brain) and angina pectoris and heart attacks (blockage of blood vessels in the heart). Any of these conditions can cause death or serious disability.

Smoking greatly increases the possibility of suffering heart attacks and strokes. Furthermore, smoking and the use of oral contraceptives greatly increase the chances of developing and dying of heart disease.

3. Gallbladder disease

Oral contraceptive users probably have a greater risk than non-users of having gallbladder disease, although this risk may be related to pills containing high doses of estrogens.

4. Liver tumors

In rare cases, oral contraceptives can cause benign but dangerous liver tumors. These benign liver tumors can rupture and cause fatal internal bleeding. In addition, a possible but not definite association has been found with the pill and liver cancers in two studies, in which a few women who developed these very rare cancers were found to have used oral contraceptives for long periods. However, liver cancers are extremely rare. The chance of developing liver cancer from using the pill is thus even rarer.

5. Cancer of the reproductive organs and breasts

There is conflict among studies regarding breast cancer and oral contraceptive use. Some studies have reported an increase in the risk of developing breast cancer, particularly at a younger age. This increased risk appears to be related to duration of use. The majority of studies have found no overall increase in the risk of developing breast cancer.

Some studies have found an increase in the incidence of cancer of the cervix in women who use oral contraceptives. However, this finding may be related to factors other than the use of oral contraceptives. There is insufficient evidence to rule out the possibility that pills may cause such cancers.

ESTIMATED RISK OF DEATH FROM A BIRTH CONTROL METHOD OR PREGNANCY

All methods of birth control and pregnancy are associated with a risk of developing certain diseases which may lead to disability or death. An estimate of the number of deaths associated with different methods of birth control and pregnancy has been calculated and is shown in the following table.

[See table below]

In the above table, the risk of death from any birth control method is less than the risk of childbirth, except for oral contraceptive users over the age of 35 who smoke and pill users over the age of 40 even if they do not smoke. It can be seen in the table that for women aged 15 to 39, the risk of death was highest with pregnancy (7–26 deaths per 100,000 women, depending on age). Among pill users who do not smoke, the risk of death is always lower than that associated with pregnancy for any age group, although over the age of 40, the risk increases to 32 deaths per 100,000 women, compared to 28 associated with pregnancy at that age. However, for pill users who smoke and are over the age of 35, the estimated number of deaths exceeds those for other methods of birth control. If a woman is over the age of 40 and smokes, her estimated risk of death is four times higher (117/100,000 women) than the estimated risk associated with pregnancy (28/100,000 women) in that age group.

The suggestion that women over 40 who do not smoke should not take oral contraceptives is based on information from older, high-dose pills and on less selective use of pills than is practiced today. An Advisory Committee of the FDA discussed this issue in 1989 and recommended that the benefits of oral contraceptive use by healthy, non-smoking women over 40 years of age may outweigh the possible risks. However, all women, especially older women, are cautioned to use the lowest dose pill that is effective.

WARNING SIGNALS

If any of these adverse effects occur while your are taking oral contraceptives, call your doctor or health care provider immediately:

- Sharp chest pain, coughing of blood, or sudden shortness of breath (indicating a possible clot in the lung)
- Pain in the calf (indicating a possible clot in the leg)
- Crushing chest pain or heaviness in the chest (indicating a possible heart attack)
- Sudden severe headache or vomiting, dizziness or fainting, disturbances of vision or speech, weakness, or numbness in an arm or leg (indicating a possible stroke)
- Sudden partial or complete loss of vision (indicating a possible clot in the eye)
- Breast lumps (indicating possible breast cancer or fibrocystic disease of the breast; ask your doctor or health care provider to show you how to examine your breasts)
- Severe pain or tenderness in the stomach area (indicating a possibly ruptured liver tumor)
- Difficulty in sleeping, weakness, lack of energy, fatigue, or change in mood (possibly indicating severe depression)
- Jaundice or a yellowing of the skin or eyeballs, accompanied frequently by fever, fatigue, loss of appetite, dark colored urine, or light colored bowel movements (indicating possible liver problems).

SIDE EFFECTS OF ORAL CONTRACEPTIVES

1. Vaginal bleeding

Irregular vaginal bleeding or spotting may occur while you are taking the pills. Irregular bleeding may vary from slight staining between menstrual periods to breakthrough bleeding which is a flow much like a regular period. Irregular bleeding occurs most often during the first few months of oral contraceptive use, but may also occur after you have been taking the pill for some time. Such bleeding may be temporary and usually does not indicate any serious problems. It is important to continue taking your pills on schedule. If the bleeding occurs in more than one cycle or lasts for more than a few days, talk to your doctor or health care provider.

2. Contact lenses

If you wear contact lenses and notice a change in vision or an inability to wear your lenses, contact your doctor or health care provider.

3. Fluid retention

Oral contraceptives may cause edema (fluid retention) with swelling of the fingers or ankles and may raise your blood pressure. If you experience fluid retention, contact your doctor or health care provider.

4. Melasma

A spotty darkening of the skin is possible, particularly of the face.

5. Other side effects

Other side effects may include nausea and vomiting, change in appetite, headache, nervousness, depression, dizziness, loss of scalp hair, rash, and vaginal infections.

If any of these side effects bother you, call your doctor or health care provider.

GENERAL PRECAUTIONS

1. Missed periods and use of oral contraceptives before or during early pregnancy

There may be times when you may not menstruate regularly after you have completed taking a cycle of pills. If you have taken your pills regularly and miss one menstrual period, continue taking your pills for the next cycle but be sure to inform your doctor or health care provider before doing so. If you have not taken the pills daily as instructed and missed a menstrual period, or if you missed two consecutive menstrual periods, you may be pregnant. Check with your doctor or health care provider immediately to determine whether you are pregnant. Do not continue to take oral contraceptives until you are sure you are not pregnant, but continue to use another method of contraception.

There is no conclusive evidence that oral contraceptive use is associated with an increase in birth defects, when taken inadvertently during early pregnancy. Previously, a few studies had reported that oral contraceptives might be associated with birth defects, but these studies have not been confirmed. Nevertheless, oral contraceptives or any other drugs should not be used during pregnancy unless clearly necessary and prescribed by your doctor or health care pro-

ANNUAL NUMBER OF BIRTH-RELATED OR METHOD-RELATED DEATHS ASSOCIATED WITH CONTROL OF FERTILITY PER 100,000 NONSTERILE WOMEN, BY FERTILITY CONTROL METHOD ACCORDING TO AGE

Method of control and outcome	15–19	20–24	25–29	30–34	35–39	40–44
No fertility control methods*	7.0	7.4	9.1	14.8	25.7	28.2
Oral contraceptives non-smoker**	0.3	0.5	0.9	1.9	13.8	31.6
Oral contraceptives smoker**	2.2	3.4	6.6	13.5	51.1	117.2
IUD**	0.8	0.8	1.0	1.0	1.4	1.4
Condom*	1.1	1.6	0.7	0.2	0.3	0.4
Diaphragm/spermicide*	1.9	1.2	1.2	1.3	2.2	2.8
Periodic abstinence*	2.5	1.6	1.6	1.7	2.9	3.6

* Deaths are birth related
** Deaths are method related

vider. You should check with your doctor or health care provider about risks to your unborn child of any medication taken during pregnancy.

2. While breast feeding

If you are breast feeding, consult your doctor or health care provider before starting oral contraceptives. Some of the drug will be passed on to the child in the milk. A few adverse effects on the child have been reported, including yellowing of the skin (jaundice) and breast enlargement. In addition, oral contraceptives may decrease the amount and quality of your milk. If possible, do not use oral contraceptives while breast feeding. You should use another method of contraception since breast feeding provides only partial protection from becoming pregnant and this partial protection decreases significantly as you breast feed for longer periods of time. You should consider starting oral contraceptives only after you have weaned your child completely.

3. Laboratory tests

If you are scheduled for any laboratory tests, tell your doctor or health care provider you are taking birth control pills. Certain blood tests may be affected by birth control pills.

4. Drug interactions

Certain drugs may interact with birth control pills to make them less effective in preventing pregnancy or cause an increase in breakthrough bleeding. Such drugs include rifampin, drugs used for epilepsy such as barbiturates (for example, phenobarbital), phenytoin (Dilantin is one brand of this drug), phenylbutazone (Butazolidin is one brand), and possibly certain antibiotics. You may need to use additional contraception when you take drugs which can make oral contraceptives less effective.

5. Sexually transmitted diseases

This product (like all oral contraceptives) is intended to prevent pregnancy. It does not protect against transmission of HIV (AIDS) and other sexually transmitted diseases such as chlamydia, genital herpes, genital warts, gonorrhea, hepatitis B, and syphilis.

HOW TO TAKE THE PILL

IMPORTANT POINTS TO REMEMBER

BEFORE YOU START TAKING YOUR PILLS:

1. BE SURE TO READ THESE DIRECTIONS:
   Before you start taking your pills.
   Anytime you are not sure what to do.
2. THE RIGHT WAY TO TAKE THE PILL IS TO TAKE ONE PILL EVERY DAY AT THE SAME TIME.
   If you miss pills you could get pregnant. This includes starting the pack late.
   The more pills you miss, the more likely you are to get pregnant.
3. MANY WOMEN HAVE SPOTTING OR LIGHT BLEEDING, OR MAY FEEL SICK TO THEIR STOMACH DURING THE FIRST 1–3 PACKS OF PILLS.
   If you feel sick to your stomach, do not stop taking the pill. The problem will usually go away. If it doesn't go away, check with your doctor or health care provider.
4. MISSING PILLS CAN ALSO CAUSE SPOTTING OR LIGHT BLEEDING, even when you make up these missed pills.
   On the days you take 2 pills to make up for missed pills, you could also feel a little sick to your stomach.
5. IF YOU HAVE VOMITING OR DIARRHEA, for any reason, or IF YOU TAKE SOME MEDICINES, including some antibiotics, your pills may not work as well.
   Use a back-up method (such as condoms, foam, or sponge) until you check with your doctor or health care provider.
6. IF YOU HAVE TROUBLE REMEMBERING TO TAKE THE PILL, talk to your doctor or health care provider about how to make pill-taking easier or about using another method of birth control.
7. IF YOU HAVE ANY QUESTIONS OR ARE UNSURE ABOUT THE INFORMATION IN THIS LEAFLET, call your doctor or health care provider.

BEFORE YOU START TAKING YOUR PILLS

1. DECIDE WHAT TIME OF DAY YOU WANT TO TAKE YOUR PILL.
   It is important to take it at about the same time every day.
2. LOOK AT YOUR PILL PACK: IT WILL HAVE 28 PILLS:
   This **28-pill pack** has 26 "active" [white and yellow] pills (with hormones) and 2 "inactive" [green] pills (without hormones).
3. ALSO FIND:
   1) where on the pack to start taking the pills,
   2) in what order to take the pills (follow the arrows) and
   3) the week numbers as shown in the picture below.

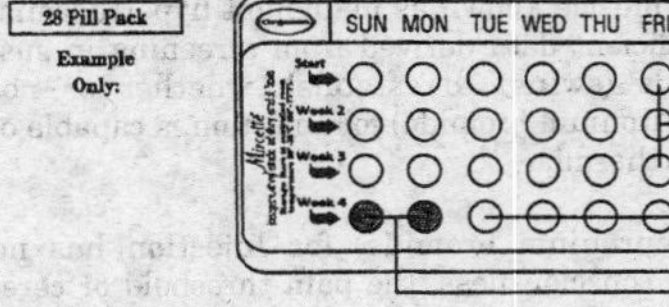

4. BE SURE YOU HAVE READY AT ALL TIMES:
   ANOTHER KIND OF BIRTH CONTROL (such as condoms, foam, or sponge) to use as a back-up in case you miss pills.
   AN EXTRA, FULL PILL PACK.

WHEN TO START THE FIRST PACK OF PILLS

You have a choice of which day to start taking your first pack of pills. Decide with your doctor or health care provider which is the best day for you. Pick a time of day which will be easy to remember.

DAY 1 START:

1. Pick the day label strip that starts with the first day of your period (this is the day you start bleeding or spotting, even if it is almost midnight when the bleeding begins).
2. Place this day label strip in the cycle tablet dispenser over the area that has the days of the week (starting with Sunday) imprinted in the plastic.

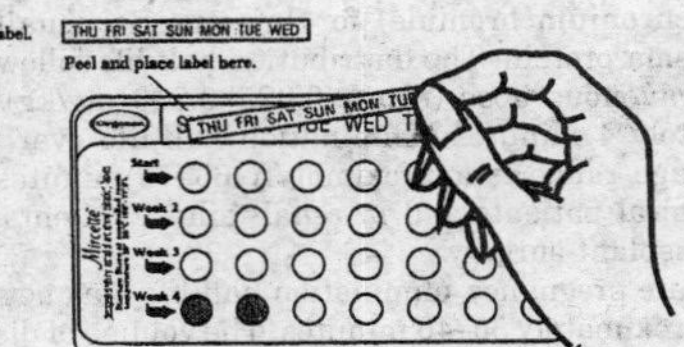

Note: If the first day of your period is a Sunday, you can skip steps #1 and #2.

3. Take the first "active" [white] pill of the first pack during the first 24 hours of your period.
4. You will not need to use a back-up method of birth control, since you are starting the pill at the beginning of your period.

SUNDAY START:

1. Take the first "active" [white] pill of the first pack on the Sunday after your period starts, even if you are still bleeding. If your period begins on Sunday, start the pack that same day.
2. Use another method of birth control as a back-up method if you have sex anytime from the Sunday you start your first pack until the next Sunday (7 days). Condoms, foam, or the sponge are good back-up methods of birth control.

WHAT TO DO DURING THE MONTH

1. **TAKE ONE PILL AT THE SAME TIME EVERY DAY UNTIL THE PACK IS EMPTY.**
   Do not skip pills even if you are spotting or bleeding between monthly periods or feel sick to your stomach (nausea).
   Do not skip pills even if you do not have sex very often.
2. **WHEN YOU FINISH A PACK OR SWITCH YOUR BRAND OF PILLS:**
   21 pills: Wait 7 days to start the next pack. You will probably have your period during that week. Be sure that no more than 7 days pass between 21-day packs.
   28 pills: Start the next pack on the day after your last pill. Do not wait any days between packs.

WHAT TO DO IF YOU MISS PILLS

If you **MISS 1** [white] "active" pill:

1. Take it as soon as you remember. Take the next pill at your regular time. This means you take 2 pills in 1 day.
2. You do not need to use a back-up birth control method if you have sex.

If you **MISS 2** [white] "active" pills in a row in **WEEK 1 OR WEEK 2** of your pack:

1. Take 2 pills on the day you remember and 2 pills the next day.
2. Then take 1 pill a day until you finish the pack.
3. You MAY BECOME PREGNANT if you have sex in the 7 days after you miss pills.
   You MUST use another birth control method (such as condoms, foam, or sponge) as a back-up method for those 7 days.

If you **MISS 2** [white] "active" pills in a row in **THE 3RD WEEK:**

1. ***If you are a Day 1 Starter:***
   THROW OUT the rest of the pill pack and start a new pack that same day.
   If you are a Sunday Starter:
   Keep taking 1 pill every day until Sunday.
   On Sunday, THROW OUT the rest of the pack and start a new pack of pills that same day.
2. You may not have your period this month but this is expected. However, if you miss your period 2 months in a row, call your doctor or health care provider because you might be pregnant.
3. You MAY BECOME PREGNANT if you have sex in the 7 days after you miss pills. You MUST use another birth control method (such as condoms, foam, or sponge) as a back-up method for those 7 days.

If you **MISS 3 OR MORE** [white] "active" pills in a row (during the first 3 weeks):

1. ***If you are a Day 1 Starter:***
   THROW OUT the rest of the pill pack and start a new pack that same day.
   If you are a Sunday Starter:
   Keep taking 1 pill every day until Sunday.
   On Sunday, THROW OUT the rest of the pack and start a new pack of pills that same day.
2. You may not have your period this month but this is expected. However, if you miss your period 2 months in a row, call your doctor or health care provider because you might be pregnant.
3. You MAY BECOME PREGNANT if you have sex in the 7 days after you miss pills. You MUST use another birth control method (such as condoms, foam, or sponge) as a back-up method for those 7 days.

A REMINDER FOR THOSE ON 28-DAY PACKS:

If you forget any of the 2 [green] or 5 [yellow] pills in Week 4:
THROW AWAY the pills you missed.
Keep taking 1 pill each day until the pack is empty.
You do not need a back-up method.

FINALLY, IF YOU ARE STILL NOT SURE WHAT TO DO ABOUT THE PILLS YOU HAVE MISSED:

Use a BACK-UP METHOD anytime you have sex.
KEEP TAKING ONE [WHITE] "ACTIVE" PILL EACH DAY until you can reach your doctor or health care provider.

PREGNANCY DUE TO PILL FAILURE

The incidence of pill failure resulting in pregnancy is approximately one percent (i.e., one pregnancy per 100 women per year) if taken every day as directed, but more typical failure rates are about 5%. If failure does occur, the risk to the fetus is minimal.

PREGNANCY AFTER STOPPING THE PILL

There may be some delay in becoming pregnant after you stop using oral contraceptives, especially if you had irregular menstrual cycles before you used oral contraceptives. It may be advisable to postpone conception until you begin menstruating regularly once you have stopped taking the pill and desire pregnancy.

There does not appear to be any increase in birth defects in newborn babies when pregnancy occurs soon after stopping the pill.

OVERDOSAGE

Serious ill effects have not been reported following ingestion of large doses of oral contraceptives by young children. Overdosage may cause nausea and withdrawal bleeding in females. In case of overdosage, contact your doctor, health care provider or pharmacist.

OTHER INFORMATION

Your doctor or health care provider will take a medical and family history before prescribing oral contraceptives and will examine you. The physical examination may be delayed to another time if you request it and your doctor or the health care provider believes that it is a good medical practice to postpone it. You should be reexamined at least once a year. Be sure to inform your doctor or health care provider if there is a family history of any of the conditions listed previously in this leaflet. Be sure to keep all appointments with your doctor or health care provider, because this is a time to determine if there are early signs of side effects of oral contraceptive use.

Do not use the drug for any condition other than the one for which it was prescribed. This drug has been prescribed specifically for you; do not give it to others who may want birth control pills.

HEALTH BENEFITS FROM ORAL CONTRACEPTIVES

In addition to preventing pregnancy, use of combination oral contraceptives may provide certain benefits. They are:

- menstrual cycles may become more regular.
- blood flow during menstruation may be lighter and less iron may be lost. Therefore, anemia due to iron deficiency is less likely to occur.
- pain or other symptoms during menstruation may be encountered less frequently.
- ectopic (tubal) pregnancy may occur less frequently.
- non-cancerous cysts or lumps in the breast may occur less frequently.
- acute pelvic inflammatory disease may occur less frequently.
- oral contraceptive use may provide some protection against developing two forms of cancer: cancer of the ovaries and cancer of the lining of the uterus.

If you want more information about birth control pills, ask your doctor, health care provider, or pharmacist. They have a more technical leaflet called the Prescribing Information which you may wish to read.

Manufactured for Organon Inc.
West Orange, NJ 07052 USA
by N.V. Organon, Oss, The Netherlands
and packaged by Organon (Ireland) Ltd.,
Swords, Co. Dublin, Ireland

Shown in Product Identification Guide, page 327

NORCURON® ℞
(vecuronium bromide) for Injection

THIS DRUG SHOULD BE ADMINISTERED BY ADEQUATELY TRAINED INDIVIDUALS FAMILIAR WITH ITS ACTIONS, CHARACTERISTICS, AND HAZARDS.

DESCRIPTION

NORCURON® (vecuronium bromide) for Injection is a nondepolarizing neuromuscular blocking agent of intermediate

Continued on next page

Norcuron—Cont.

duration, chemically designated as piperidinium, 1-[(2β, 3α, 5α, 16β, 17β)-3, 17-bis(acetyloxy)-2-(1-piperidinyl) androstan-16-yl]-1-methyl-, bromide. The structural formula is:

Its chemical formula is $C_{34}H_{57}BrN_2O_4$ with molecular weight 637.74.

Norcuron® is supplied as a sterile nonpyrogenic freeze-dried buffered cake of very fine microscopic crystalline particles for intravenous injection only. Each 10 mL vial contains 10 mg vecuronium bromide, 20.75 mg citric acid anhydrous, 16.25 mg sodium phosphate dibasic anhydrous, 97 mg mannitol (to adjust tonicity), sodium hydroxide and/or phosphoric acid to buffer and adjust to a pH of 4. Each 20 mL vial contains 20 mg of vecuronium bromide, 41.5 mg citric acid anhydrous, 32.5 mg sodium phosphate dibasic anhydrous, 194 mg mannitol (to adjust tonicity), sodium hydroxide and/or phosphoric acid to buffer and adjust to a pH of 4. Bacteriostatic water for injection, USP when supplied contains 0.9% w/v BENZYL ALCOHOL, WHICH IS NOT FOR USE IN NEWBORNS.

CLINICAL PHARMACOLOGY

Norcuron® (vecuronium bromide) for Injection is a nondepolarizing neuromuscular blocking agent possessing all of the characteristic pharmacological actions of this class of drugs (curariform). It acts by competing for cholinergic receptors at the motor end-plate. The antagonism to acetylcholine is inhibited and neuromuscular block is reversed by acetylcholinesterase inhibitors such as neostigmine, edrophonium, and pyridostigmine. Norcuron® is about $^1/_3$ more potent than pancuronium; the duration of neuromuscular blockade produced by Norcuron® is shorter than that of pancuronium at initially equipotent doses. The time to onset of paralysis decreases and the duration of maximum effect increases with increasing Norcuron® doses. The use of a peripheral nerve stimulator is recommended in assessing the degree of muscular relaxation with all neuromuscular blocking drugs. The ED_{90} (dose required to produce 90% suppression of the muscle twitch response with balanced anesthesia) has averaged 0.057 mg/kg (0.049 to 0.062 mg/kg in various studies). An initial Norcuron® dose of 0.08 to 0.10 mg/kg generally produces first depression of twitch in approximately 1 minute, good or excellent intubation conditions within 2.5 to 3 minutes, and maximum neuromuscular blockade within 3 to 5 minutes of injection in most patients.

Under balanced anesthesia, the time to recovery to 25% of control (clinical duration) is approximately 25 to 40 minutes after injection and recovery is usually 95% complete approximately 45–65 minutes after injection of intubating dose. The neuromuscular blocking action of Norcuron® is slightly enhanced in the presence of potent inhalation anesthetics. If Norcuron® is first administered more than 5 minutes after the start of the inhalation of enflurane, isoflurane, or halothane, or when steady-state has been achieved, the intubating dose of Norcuron® may be decreased by approximately 15% (see **DOSAGE AND ADMINISTRATION** section). Prior administration of succinylcholine may enhance the neuromuscular blocking effect of Norcuron® and its duration of action. With succinylcholine as the intubating agent, initial doses of 0.04–0.06 mg/kg of Norcuron® will produce complete neuromuscular block with clinical duration of action of 25–30 minutes. If succinylcholine is used prior to Norcuron®, the administration of Norcuron® should be delayed until the patient starts recovering from succinylcholine-induced neuromuscular blockade. The effect of prior use of other nondepolarizing neuromuscular blocking agents on the activity of Norcuron® has not been studied (see **Drug Interactions**).

Repeated administration of maintenance doses of Norcuron® has little or no cumulative effect on the duration of neuromuscular blockade. Therefore, repeat doses can be administered at relatively regular intervals with predictable results. After an initial dose of 0.08 to 0.10 mg/kg under balanced anesthesia, the first maintenance dose (suggested maintenance dose is 0.010 to 0.015 mg/kg) is generally required within 25 to 40 minutes; subsequent maintenance doses, if required, may be administered at approximately 12 to 15 minute intervals. Halothane anesthesia increases the clinical duration of the maintenance dose only slightly. Under enflurane a maintenance dose of 0.010 mg/kg is approximately equal to 0.015 mg/kg dose under balanced anesthesia.

The recovery index (time from 25% to 75% recovery) is approximately 15–25 minutes under balanced or halothane anesthesia. When recovery from Norcuron® neuromuscular blocking effect begins, it proceeds more rapidly than recovery from pancuronium. Once spontaneous recovery has started, the neuromuscular block produced by Norcuron® is readily reversed with various anticholinesterase agents, e.g., pyridostigmine, neostigmine, or edrophonium in conjunction with an anticholinergic agent such as atropine or glycopyrrolate. Rapid recovery is a finding consistent with Norcuron® short elimination half-life, although there have been occasional reports of prolonged neuromuscular blockade in patients in the intensive care unit (see **PRECAUTIONS**).

The administration of clinical doses of Norcuron® is not characterized by laboratory or clinical signs of chemically mediated histamine release. This does not preclude the possibility of rare hypersensitivity reactions (see **ADVERSE REACTIONS**).

Pharmacokinetics

At clinical doses of 0.04–0.10 mg/kg, 60–80% of Norcuron® (vecuronium bromide) for Injection is usually bound to plasma protein. The distribution half-life following a single intravenous dose (range 0.025–0.280 mg/kg) is approximately 4 minutes. Elimination half-life over this sample dosage range is approximately 65–75 minutes in healthy surgical patients and in renal failure patients undergoing transplant surgery.

In late pregnancy, elimination half-life may be shortened to approximately 35–40 minutes. The volume of distribution at steady-state is approximately 300–400 mL/kg; systemic rate of clearance is approximately 3–4.5 mL/minute/kg. In man, urine recovery of Norcuron® varies from 3–35% within 24 hours. Data derived from patients requiring insertion of a T-tube in the common bile duct suggests that 25–50% of a total intravenous dose of vecuronium may be excreted in bile within 42 hours. Only unchanged vecuronium has been detected in human plasma following use during surgery. In addition, one metabolite 3-desacetyl vecuronium has been rarely detected in human plasma following prolonged clinical use in the I.C.U. (see **PRECAUTIONS: Long-term Use in I.C.U.**). The 3-desacetyl vecuronium metabolite has been recovered in the urine of some patients in quantities that account for up to 10% of injected dose; 3-desacetyl vecuronium has also been recovered by T-tube in some patients accounting for up to 25% of the injected dose.

This metabolite has been judged by animal screening (dogs and cats) to have 50% or more of the potency of Norcuron®; equipotent doses are of approximately the same duration as Norcuron® in dogs and cats. Biliary excretion accounts for about half the dose of Norcuron® within 7 hours in the anesthetized rat. Circulatory bypass of the liver (cat preparation) prolongs recovery from Norcuron®. Limited data derived from patients with cirrhosis or cholestasis suggests that some measurements of recovery may be doubled in such patients. In patients with renal failure, measurements of recovery do not differ significantly from similar measurements in healthy patients.

Studies involving routine hemodynamic monitoring in good risk surgical patients reveal that the administration of Norcuron® in doses up to three times that needed to produce clinical relaxation (0.15 mg/kg) did not produce clinically significant changes in systolic, diastolic or mean arterial pressure. The heart rate, under similar monitoring, remained unchanged in some studies and was lowered by a mean of up to 8% in other studies. A large dose of 0.28 mg/kg administered during a period of no stimulation, while patients were being prepared for coronary artery bypass grafting was not associated with alterations in rate-pressure-product or pulmonary capillary wedge pressure. Systemic vascular resistance was lowered slightly and cardiac output was increased insignificantly. (The drug has not been studied in patients with hemodynamic dysfunction secondary to cardiac valvular disease.) Limited clinical experience with use of Norcuron® during surgery for pheochromocytoma has shown that administration of this drug is not associated with changes in blood pressure or heart rate.

Unlike other nondepolarizing skeletal muscle relaxants, Norcuron® has no clinically significant effects on hemodynamic parameters. Norcuron® will not counteract those hemodynamic changes or known side effects produced by or associated with anesthetic agents, other drugs or various other factors known to alter hemodynamics.

INDICATIONS AND USAGE

Norcuron® (vecuronium bromide) for Injection is indicated as an adjunct to general anesthesia, to facilitate endotracheal intubation and to provide skeletal muscle relaxation during surgery or mechanical ventilation.

CONTRAINDICATIONS

Norcuron® (vecuronium bromide) for Injection is contraindicated in patients known to have a hypersensitivity to it.

WARNINGS

NORCURON® (VECURONIUM BROMIDE) FOR INJECTION SHOULD BE ADMINISTERED IN CAREFULLY ADJUSTED DOSAGE BY OR UNDER THE SUPERVISION OF EXPERIENCED CLINICIANS WHO ARE FAMILIAR WITH ITS ACTIONS AND THE POSSIBLE COMPLICATIONS THAT MIGHT OCCUR FOLLOWING ITS USE. THE DRUG SHOULD NOT BE ADMINISTERED UNLESS FACILITIES FOR INTUBATION, ARTIFICIAL RESPIRATION, OXYGEN THERAPY, AND REVERSAL AGENTS ARE IMMEDIATELY AVAILABLE. THE CLINICIAN MUST BE PREPARED TO ASSIST OR CONTROL RESPIRATION, TO REDUCE THE POSSIBILITY OF PROLONGED NEUROMUSCULAR BLOCKADE AND OTHER POSSIBLE COMPLICATIONS THAT MIGHT OCCUR FOLLOWING LONG-TERM USE IN THE I.C.U., NORCURON® OR ANY OTHER NEUROMUSCULAR BLOCKING AGENT SHOULD BE ADMINISTERED IN CAREFULLY ADJUSTED DOSES BY OR UNDER THE SUPERVISION OF EXPERIENCED CLINICIANS WHO ARE FAMILIAR WITH ITS ACTIONS AND WHO ARE FAMILIAR WITH APPROPRIATE PERIPHERAL NERVE STIMULATOR MUSCLE MONITORING TECHNIQUES (see **PRECAUTIONS**).

In patients who are known to have myasthenia gravis or the myasthenic (Eaton-Lambert) syndrome, small doses of Norcuron® may have profound effects. In such patients, a peripheral nerve stimulator and use of a small test dose may be of value in monitoring the response to administration of muscle relaxants.

PRECAUTIONS

Renal Failure

Norcuron® (vecuronium bromide) for Injection is well tolerated without clinically significant prolongation of neuromuscular blocking effect in patients with renal failure who have been optimally prepared for surgery by dialysis. Under emergency conditions in anephric patients some prolongation of neuromuscular blockade may occur; therefore, if anephric patients cannot be prepared for non-elective surgery, a lower initial dose of Norcuron® should be considered.

Altered Circulation Time

Conditions associated with slower circulation time in cardiovascular disease, old age, edematous states resulting in increased volume of distribution may contribute to delay in onset time; therefore, dosage should not be increased.

Hepatic Disease

Experience in patients with cirrhosis or cholestasis has revealed prolonged recovery time in keeping with the role the liver plays in Norcuron® (vecuronium bromide) for Injection metabolism and excretion (see **Pharmacokinetics**). Data currently available do not permit dosage recommendations in patients with impaired liver function.

Long-term Use in I.C.U.

In the intensive care unit, long-term use of neuromuscular blocking drugs to facilitate mechanical ventilation may be associated with prolonged paralysis and/or skeletal muscle weakness, that may be first noted during attempts to wean such patients from the ventilator. Typically, such patients receive other drugs such as broad spectrum antibiotics, narcotics and/or steroids and may have electrolyte imbalance and diseases which lead to electrolyte imbalance, hypoxic episodes of varying duration, acid-base imbalance and extreme debilitation, any of which may enhance the actions of a neuromuscular blocking agent. Additionally, patients immobilized for extended periods frequently develop symptoms consistent with disuse muscle atrophy. The recovery picture may vary from regaining movement and strength in all muscles to initial recovery of movement of the facial and small muscles of the extremities then to the remaining muscles. In rare cases recovery may be over an extended period of time and may even, on occasion, involve rehabilitation. Therefore, when there is a need for long-term mechanical ventilation, the benefits-to-risk ratio of neuromuscular blockade must be considered.

Continuous infusion or intermittent bolus dosing to support mechanical ventilation, has not been studied sufficiently to support dosage recommendations. IN THE INTENSIVE CARE UNIT, APPROPRIATE MONITORING, WITH THE USE OF A PERIPHERAL NERVE STIMULATOR TO ASSESS THE DEGREE OF NEUROMUSCULAR BLOCKADE IS RECOMMENDED TO HELP PRECLUDE POSSIBLE PROLONGATION OF THE BLOCKADE. WHENEVER THE USE OF NORCURON® (VERCURONIUM BROMIDE) FOR INJECTION OR ANY NEUROMUSCULAR BLOCKING AGENT IS CONTEMPLATED IN THE I.C.U., IT IS RECOMMENDED THAT NEUROMUSCULAR TRANSMISSION BE MONITORED CONTINUOUSLY DURING ADMINISTRATION AND RECOVERY WITH THE HELP OF A NERVE STIMULATOR. ADDITIONAL DOSES OF NORCURON® OR ANY OTHER NEUROMUSCULAR BLOCKING AGENT SHOULD NOT BE GIVEN BEFORE THERE IS A DEFINITE RESPONSE TO T_1 OR TO THE FIRST TWITCH. IF NO RESPONSE IS ELICITED, INFUSION ADMINISTRATION SHOULD BE DISCONTINUED UNTIL A RESPONSE RETURNS.

Severe Obesity or Neuromuscular Disease

Patients with severe obesity or neuromuscular disease may pose airway and/or ventilatory problems requiring special care before, during and after the use of neuromuscular blocking agents such as Norcuron® (vecuronium bromide) for Injection.

Malignant Hyperthermia

Many drugs used in anesthetic practice are suspected of being capable of triggering a potentially fatal hypermetabolism of skeletal muscle known as malignant hyperthermia. There are insufficient data derived from screening in susceptible animals (swine) to establish whether or not Norcuron® (vecuronium bromide) for Injection is capable of triggering hyperthermia.

C.N.S.

Norcuron® (vecuronium bromide) for Injection has no known effect on consciousness, the pain threshold or cerebration. Administration must be accompanied by adequate anesthesia or sedation.

Drug Interactions

Prior administration of succinylcholine may enhance the neuromuscular blocking effect of Norcuron® (vecuronium bromide) for Injection and its duration of action. If succinyl-

choline is used before Norcuron® the administration of Norcuron® should be delayed until the succinylcholine effect shows signs of wearing off. With succinylcholine as the intubating agent, initial doses of 0.04–0.06 mg/kg of Norcuron® may be administered to produce complete neuromuscular block with clinical duration of action of 25–30 minutes (see **CLINICAL PHARMACOLOGY**).
The use of Norcuron® before succinylcholine, in order to attenuate some of the side effects of succinylcholine, has not been sufficiently studied.
Other nondepolarizing neuromuscular blocking agents (pancuronium, d-tubocurarine, metocurine, and gallamine) act in the same fashion as does Norcuron®; therefore, these drugs and Norcuron® may manifest an additive effect when used together. There are insufficient data to support concomitant use of Norcuron® and other competitive muscle relaxants in the same patient.

Inhalational Anesthetics

Use of volatile inhalational anesthetics such as enflurane, isoflurane, and halothane with Norcuron® (vecuronium bromide) for Injection will enhance neuromuscular blockade. Potentiation is most prominent with use of enflurane and isoflurane. With the above agents the initial dose of Norcuron® may be the same as the balanced anesthesia unless the inhalational anesthetic has been administered for a sufficient time at a sufficient dose to have reached clinical equilibrium (see **CLINICAL PHARMACOLOGY**).

Antibiotics

Parenteral/intraperitoneal administration of high doses of certain antibiotics may intensify or produce neuromuscular block on their own. The following antibiotics have been associated with various degrees of paralysis: aminoglycosides (such as neomycin, streptomycin, kanamycin, gentamicin, and dihydrostreptomycin); tetracyclines; bacitracin; polymyxin B; colistin; and sodium colistimethate. If these or other newly introduced antibiotics are used in conjunction with Norcuron® (vercuronium bromide) for Injection, unexpected prolongation of neuromuscular block should be considered a possibility.

Other

Experience concerning injection of quinidine during recovery from use of other muscle relaxants suggests that recurrent paralysis may occur. This possibility must also be considered for Norcuron® (vecuronium bromide) for Injection. Norcuron® induced neuromuscular blockade has been counteracted by alkalosis and enhanced by acidosis in experimental animals (cat). Electrolyte imbalance and diseases which lead to electrolyte imbalance, such as adrenal cortical insufficiency, have been shown to alter neuromuscular blockade. Depending on the nature of the imbalance, either enhancement or inhibition may be expected. Magnesium salts, administered for the management of toxemia of pregnancy may enhance the neuromuscular blockade.

Drug/Laboratory Test Interactions

None known.

Carcinogenesis, Mutagenesis, Impairment of Fertility

Long-term studies in animals have not been performed to evaluate carcinogenic or mutagenic potential or impairment of fertility.

Pregnancy

Pregnancy Category C: Animal reproduction studies have not been conducted with Norcuron® (vecuronium bromide) for Injection. It is also not known whether Norcuron® can cause fetal harm when administered to a pregnant woman or can affect reproduction capacity. Norcuron® should be given to a pregnant woman only if clearly needed.

Labor and Delivery

The use of Norcuron® (vecuronium bromide) for Injection in patients undergoing cesarean section has been reported in the literature. Following tracheal intubation with succinylcholine, Norcuron® dosages of 0.04 mg/kg (n=11) and 0.06 to 0.08 mg/kg (n=20) were administered.[1,2] The umbilical venous plasma concentrations were 11% of maternal concentrations at delivery and mean neonate APGAR scores at 5 minutes were $\geq$ 9 in both reports.[1,2] The action of neuromuscular blocking agents may be enhanced by magnesium salts administered for the management of toxemia of pregnancy.

Nursing Mothers

It is not known whether this drug is excreted in human milk. Because many drugs are excreted in human milk, caution should be exercised when Norcuron® (vecuronium bromide) for Injection is administered to a nursing woman.

Pediatric Use

Infants under 1 year of age but older than 7 weeks also tested under halothane anesthesia, are moderately more sensitive to Norcuron® (vecuronium bromide) for Injection on a mg/kg basis than adults and take about $1^1/_2$ times as long to recover. See **Use in Pediatrics** subsection of **DOSAGE AND ADMINISTRATION** for recommendations for use in pediatric patients 7 weeks to 16 years of age. The safety and effectiveness of Norcuron® in pediatric patients less than 7 weeks of age have not been established.

ADVERSE REACTIONS

The most frequent adverse reaction to nondepolarizing blocking agents as a class consists of an extension of the drug's pharmacological action beyond the time period needed. This may vary from skeletal muscle weakness to profound and prolonged skeletal muscle paralysis resulting in respiration insufficiency or apnea.
Inadequate reversal of the neuromuscular blockade is possible with Norcuron® (vecuronium bromide) for Injection as with all curariform drugs. These adverse reactions are managed by manual or mechanical ventilation until recovery is judged adequate. Little or no increase in intensity of blockade or duration of action with Norcuron® is noted from the use of thiobarbiturates, narcotic analgesics, nitrous oxide, or droperidol. See **OVERDOSAGE** for discussion of other drugs used in anesthetic practice which also cause respiratory depression.
Prolonged to profound extension of paralysis and/or muscle weakness as well as muscle atrophy have been reported after long-term use to support mechanical ventilation in the intensive care unit (see **PRECAUTIONS**). The administration of Norcuron® has been associated with rare instances of hypersensitivity reactions (bronchospasm, hypotension and/or tachycardia, sometimes associated with acute urticaria or erythema); (see also **CLINICAL PHARMACOLOGY**).

OVERDOSAGE

The possibility of iatrogenic overdosage can be minimized by carefully monitoring muscle twitch response to peripheral nerve stimulation.
Excessive doses of Norcuron® (vecuronium bromide) for Injection produce enhanced pharmacological effects. Residual neuromuscular blockade beyond the time period needed may occur with Norcuron® as with other neuromuscular blockers. This may be manifested by skeletal muscle weakness, decreased respiratory reserve, low tidal volume, or apnea. A peripheral nerve stimulator may be used to assess the degree of residual neuromuscular blockade from other causes of decreased respiratory reserve.
Respiratory depression may be due either wholly or in part to other drugs used during the conduct of general anesthesia such as narcotics, thiobarbiturates and other central nervous system depressants.
Under such circumstances the primary treatment is maintenance of a patent airway and manual or mechanical ventilation until complete recovery of normal respiration is assured. Regonol® (pyridostigmine bromide) Injection, neostigmine, or edrophonium, in conjunction with atropine or glycopyrrolate will usually antagonize the skeletal muscle relaxant action of Norcuron®. Satisfactory reversal can be judged by adequacy of skeletal muscle tone and by adequacy of respiration. A peripheral nerve stimulator may also be used to monitor restoration of twitch height. Failure of prompt reversal (within 30 minutes) may occur in the presence of extreme debilitation, carcinomatosis, and with concomitant use of certain broad spectrum antibiotics, or anesthetic agents and other drugs which enhance neuromuscular blockade or cause respiratory depression of their own. Under such circumstances the management is the same as that of prolonged neuromuscular blockade. Ventilation must be supported by artificial means until the patient has resumed control of his respiration. Prior to the use of reversal agents, reference should be made to the specific package insert of the reversal agent. The effects of hemodialysis and peritoneal dialysis on plasma levels of Norcuron® and its metabolite are unknown.

DOSAGE AND ADMINISTRATION

Norcuron® (vecuronium bromide) for Injection is for intravenous use only.
This drug should be administered by or under the supervision of experienced clinicians familiar with the use of neuromuscular blocking agents. Dosage must be individualized in each case. The dosage information which follows is derived from studies based upon units of drug per unit of body weight and is intended to serve as a guide only, especially regarding enhancement of neuromuscular blockade of Norcuron® by volatile anesthetics and by prior use of succinylcholine (see **PRECAUTIONS: Drug Interactions**). Parenteral drug products should be inspected visually for particulate matter and discoloration prior to administration whenever solution and container permit.
To obtain maximum clinical benefits of Norcuron® and to minimize the possibility of overdosage, the monitoring of muscle twitch response to peripheral nerve stimulation is advised.
The recommended initial dose of Norcuron® is 0.08 to 0.10 mg/kg (1.4 to 1.75 times the ED_{90}) given as an intravenous bolus injection. This dose can be expected to produce good or excellent non-emergency intubation conditions in 2.5 to 3 minutes after injection. Under balanced anesthesia, clinically required neuromuscular blockade lasts approximately 25 to 30 minutes, with recovery to 25% of control achieved approximately 25 to 40 minutes after injection and recovery to 95% of control achieved approximately 45–65 minutes after injection. In the presence of potent inhalation anesthetics, the neuromuscular blocking effect of Norcuron® is enhanced. If Norcuron® is first administered more than 5 minutes after the start of inhalation agent or when steady-state has been achieved, the initial Norcuron® dose may be reduced by approximately 15%, i.e., 0.060 to 0.085 mg/kg.
Prior administration of succinylcholine may enhance the neuromuscular blocking effect and duration of action of Norcuron®. If intubation is performed using succinylcholine, a reduction of initial dose of Norcuron® to 0.04–0.06 mg/kg with inhalation anesthesia and 0.05–0.06 mg/kg with balanced anesthesia may be required.
During prolonged surgical procedures, maintenance doses of 0.010 to 0.015 mg/kg of Norcuron® are recommended; after the initial Norcuron® injection, the first maintenance dose will generally be required within 25 to 40 minutes. However, clinical criteria should be used to determine the need for maintenance doses.
Since Norcuron® lacks clinically important cumulative effects, subsequent maintenance doses, if required, may be administered at relatively regular intervals for each patient, ranging approximately from 12 to 15 minutes under balanced anesthesia, slightly longer under inhalation agents. (If less frequent administration is desired, higher maintenance doses may be administered.)
Should there be reason for the selection of larger doses in individual patients, initial doses ranging from 0.15 mg/kg up to 0.28 mg/kg have been administered during surgery under halothane anesthesia without ill effects to the cardiovascular system being noted as long as ventilation is properly maintained (see **CLINICAL PHARMACOLOGY**).

Use by Continuous Infusion

After an intubating dose of 80–100 µg/kg, a continuous infusion of 1 µg/kg/min can be initiated approximately 20–40 min later. Infusion of Norcuron® (vecuronium bromide) for Injection should be initiated only after early evidence of spontaneous recovery from the bolus dose. Long-term intravenous infusion to support mechanical ventilation in the intensive care unit has not been studied sufficiently to support dosage recommendations (see **PRECAUTIONS**).
The infusion of Norcuron® (vecuronium bromide) for Injection should be individualized for each patient. The rate of administration should be adjusted according to the patient's twitch response as determined by peripheral nerve stimulation. An initial rate of 1 µg/kg/min is recommended, with the rate of the infusion adjusted thereafter to maintain a 90% suppression of twitch response. Average infusion rates may range from 0.8 to 1.2 µg/kg/min.
Inhalation anesthetics, particularly enflurane and isoflurane may enhance the neuromuscular blocking action of nondepolarizing muscle relaxants. In the presence of steady-state concentrations of enflurane or isoflurane, it may be necessary to reduce the rate of infusion 25–60 percent, 45–60 min after the intubating dose. Under halothane anesthesia it may not be necessary to reduce the rate of infusion.
Spontaneous recovery and reversal of neuromuscular blockade following discontinuation of Norcuron® infusion may be expected to proceed at rates comparable to that following a single bolus dose (see **CLINICAL PHARMACOLOGY**).
Infusion solutions of Norcuron® (vecuronium bromide) for Injection can be prepared by mixing Norcuron® with an appropriate infusion solution such as 5% glucose in water, 0.9% NaCl, 5% glucose in saline, or Lactated Ringers.
Unused portions of infusion solutions should be discarded.
Infusion rates of Norcuron® can be individualized for each patient using the following table:

Drug Delivery Rate (µg/kg/min)	Infusion Delivery Rate (mL/kg/min)	
	0.1 mg/mL*	0.2 mg/mL†
0.7	0.007	0.0035
0.8	0.008	0.0040
0.9	0.009	0.0045
1.0	0.010	0.0050
1.1	0.011	0.0055
1.2	0.012	0.0060
1.3	0.013	0.0065

* 10 mg of Norcuron® in 100 mL solution
† 20 mg of Norcuron® in 100 mL solution

The following table is a guideline for mL/min delivery for a solution of 0.1 mg/mL (10 mg in 100 mL) with an infusion pump.

NORCURON® INFUSION RATE — mL/MIN

Amount of Drug µg/kg/min	Patient Weight—kg 40	50	60	70	80	90	100
0.7	0.28	0.35	0.42	0.49	0.56	0.63	0.70
0.8	0.32	0.40	0.48	0.56	0.64	0.72	0.80
0.9	0.36	0.45	0.54	0.63	0.72	0.81	0.90
1.0	0.40	0.50	0.60	0.70	0.80	0.90	1.00
1.1	0.44	0.55	0.66	0.77	0.88	0.99	1.10
1.2	0.48	0.60	0.72	0.84	0.96	1.08	1.20
1.3	0.52	0.65	0.78	0.91	1.04	1.17	1.30

NOTE: If a concentration of 0.2 mg/mL is used (20 mg in 100 mL), the rate should be decreased by one-half.

Use in Pediatrics: Pediatric patients (10 to 16 years of age) have approximately the same dosage requirements (mg/kg) as adults and may be managed the same way. Younger pediatric patients (1 to 10 years of age) may require a slightly higher initial dose and may also require supplementation slightly more often than adults.
Infants under 1 year of age but older than 7 weeks are moderately more sensitive to Norcuron® (vecuronium bromide) for Injection on a mg/kg basis than adults and take about $1^1/_2$ times as long to recover. See also subsection of **PRECAUTIONS** titled **Pediatric Use**. Information presently available does not permit recommendation on usage in pediatric patients less than 7 weeks of age (see **PRECAUTIONS**). There are insufficient data concerning continuous infusion of vecuronium in pediatric patients, therefore, no dosing recommendations can be made.

Continued on next page

Norcuron—Cont.

COMPATIBILITY

Norcuron® (vecuronium bromide) for Injection is compatible in solution with:

- 0.9% NaCl solution
- 5% glucose in water
- Sterile water for injection
- 5% glucose in saline
- Lactated Ringers

Use within 24 hours of mixing with the above solutions.

Parenteral drug products should be inspected visually for particulate matter and discoloration prior to administration whenever solution and container permit.

HOW SUPPLIED

10 mL vials (10 mg vecuronium bromide) and 10 mL prefilled syringes of diluent (bacteriostatic water for injection, USP) 22 g $1^1/_4$" needle.

Boxes of 10 NDC No. 0052-0441-60

10 mL vials (10 mg vecuronium bromide) and 10 mL vials of diluent (bacteriostatic water for injection, USP).

Boxes of 10 NDC No. 0052-0441-17

10 mL vials (10 mg vecuronium bromide) only; DILUENT NOT SUPPLIED.

Boxes of 10 NDC No. 0052-0441-15

20 mL vials (20 mg vecuronium bromide) only; DILUENT NOT SUPPLIED.

Boxes of 10 NDC No. 0052-0442-46

Store at 15°–30°C (59°–86°F).

Protect from light.

AFTER RECONSTITUTION

- When reconstituted with supplied bacteriostatic water for injection: CONTAINS BENZYL ALCOHOL, WHICH IS NOT INTENDED FOR USE IN NEWBORNS. Use within 5 days. May be stored at room temperature or refrigerated.
- When reconstituted with sterile water for injection or other compatible I.V. solutions: Refrigerate vial. Use within 24 hours. Single use only. Discard unused portion.

Rx only

REFERENCES

1. Dailey PA, Fisher DM, Shnider SM et al. Pharmacokinetics, Placental Transfer, and Neonatal Effects of Vecuronium and Pancuronium Administered during Cesarean Section. *Anesthesiology* 1984;**60**:569–574.
2. Demetriou M, Depoix J-P, Diakite B, et al. Placental Transfer of ORG NC45 in Women Undergoing Caesarean Section. *Br J Anaesth* 1982;**54**:643–645.

ORGANON INC.
WEST ORANGE, NEW JERSEY 07052
PTD. IN USA-441, 442 5310125 REVISED 2/98

ORGARAN®

(danaparoid sodium) Injection ℞

SPINAL/EPIDURAL HEMATOMAS

When neuraxial anesthesia (epidural/spinal anesthesia) or spinal puncture is employed, patients anticoagulated or scheduled to be anticoagulated with low molecular weight heparins or heparinoids for prevention of thromboembolic complications are at risk of developing an epidural or spinal hematoma which can result in long-term or permanent paralysis.

The risk of these events is increased by the use of indwelling epidural catheters for administration of analgesia or by the concomitant use of drugs affecting hemostasis such as non steroidal anti-inflammatory drugs (NSAIDs), platelet inhibitors, or other anticoagulants. The risk also appears to be increased by traumatic or repeated epidural or spinal puncture.

Patient should be frequently monitored for signs and symptoms of neurological impairment. If neurologic compromise is noted, urgent treatment is necessary.

The physician should consider the potential benefit versus risk before intervention in patients anticoagulated or to be anticoagulated for thromboprophylaxis (see also WARNINGS, Hemorrhage and PRECAUTIONS, Drug Interactions).

DESCRIPTION

ORGARAN® (danaparoid sodium) Injection is a sterile, glycosaminoglycuronan antithrombotic agent. The active components of ORGARAN®, isolated from porcine intestinal mucosa, are heparan sulfate (~84%), dermatan sulfate (~12%) and a small amount of chondroitin sulfate (~4%). The average molecular weight is approximately 5500 Daltons.

ORGARAN® is intended for subcutaneous injection. Each prefilled syringe or ampule contains 750 anti-Xa units in 0.6 mL solution. ORGARAN® Injection is made isotonic with sodium chloride, adjusted to pH 7 with hydrochloric acid, or sodium hydroxide. ORGARAN® Injection contains 0.15% (w/v) sodium sulfite to prevent discoloration of the solution. The structural formula of the main repeating disaccharide units is as follows:

Structural Formula:
Main Repeating Disaccharide Units:

Heparan Sulfate: R_1 = H or SO^-_3

Heparan Sulfate: R_2 = $COCH_3$ or SO^-_3

Dermatan Sulfate
R = H or SO^-_3

Chondroitin Sulfate

CLINICAL PHARMACOLOGY

Pharmacodynamics: *Effect on Coagulation Factors:* ORGARAN® (danaparoid sodium) Injection is an antithrombotic agent. ORGARAN® prevents fibrin formation in the coagulation pathway via thrombin generation inhibition by anti-Xa and anti-IIa (thrombin) effects. The anti-Xa: anti-IIa activity ratio is greater than 22. Inactivation of factor Xa is mediated by antithrombin-III (AT-III) while factor IIa inactivation is mediated by both AT-III and heparin cofactor II (HC II). ORGARAN® has only minor effect on platelet function and platelet aggregability.

Measurements of Hemostasis: Because of its predominant anti-Xa activity, ORGARAN® (danaparoid sodium) Injection has little effect on clotting assays (*e.g.,* prothrombin time [PT], partial thromboplastin time [PTT]). ORGARAN® has minimal effect on fibrinolytic activity and bleeding time.

Pharmacokinetics: The pharmacokinetics of ORGARAN® (danaparoid sodium) Injection have been described by monitoring its biological activity (plasma anti-Xa activity) since no specific chemical assay methods are currently available for the components of ORGARAN®.

By subcutaneous route of administration, ORGARAN® was approximately 100% bioavailable, compared with the same dose administered intravenously. The maximum anti-Xa activity (T_{max}) occurred at approximately two to five hours. For single subcutaneous doses of 750, 1500, 2250, and 3250 anti-Xa units of ORGARAN® the mean peak plasma anti-Xa activities were 102.4, 206.1, 283.9, and 403.4 mU/mL, respectively. The mean value for the terminal half-life ($T^1/_2$) was about 24 hours and the clearance was 0.36 L/hour. Clearance was affected by body surface area in that the higher the body surface, the faster the clearance. ORGARAN® is mainly eliminated via the kidneys. In patients with severely impaired renal function, the half-life of elimination of plasma anti-Xa activity may be prolonged, therefore, monitoring such patients carefully is recommended.

Clinical Trials: In a European multicenter double-blind trial, ORGARAN® (danaparoid sodium) Injection was compared with placebo in 196 patients undergoing elective hip replacement surgery. The administration of ORGARAN® for 7 to 14 days post-operatively significantly reduced the overall incidence of DVT to 15% (15/98 patients) compared to the incidence of 57% (56/98 patients) observed with placebo.

Number (%) of Patients with DVT*
Intent-to-Treat

	ORGARAN® N=98	Placebo N=98	p-value[a]
Proximal; N (%)	8 (8)	26 (27)	0.001
Distal; N (%)	14 (14)	51 (52)	<0.001
Overall; N (%)	15 (15)	56 (57)	<0.001

* A patient may be counted more than once (proximal and/or distal)
[a] Using the Cochran Mantel-Haenszel test

In a United States multicenter trial, ORGARAN® was compared with warfarin in 396 patients undergoing elective hip replacement. A significant reduction in the overall incidence of DVT was observed with ORGARAN® (14.6%; 29/199 patients) compared with warfarin (26.9%; 53/197 patients), p=0.003.

Number (%) of Patients with DVT[a]
Intent-to-Treat

	ORGARAN® N=199	Warfarin N=197	p-value[b]
Proximal[c]; N (%)	3 (1.5)	8 (4.1)	0.13
Distal[d]; N (%)	28 (14.1)	49 (24.9)	0.007
Overall[e]; N (%)	29 (14.6)	53 (26.9)	0.003

[a] By positive venogram only
[b] Using the Cochran Mantel-Haenszel test
[c] Popliteal, iliac, and femoral
[d] Calf
[e] A patient may be counted more than once (proximal and distal)

Blood Loss and Transfusions
DVT and PE Prophylaxis for Orthopedic Hip Surgery
All Patients Treated

Blood Loss and Transfusions	Total N	ORGARAN®	Placebo	Warfarin	Other[a]
Total (728 Males: 1675 Females)		(N) Mean±SD	(N) Mean±SD	(N) Mean±SD	(N) Mean±SD
Intraoperative Blood Loss (mL)					
Males	596	(330) 694±555	(27) 586±737	(141) 689±499	(98) 754±661
Females	1259	(686) 486±430	(66) 416±252	(219) 471±306	(288) 530±456
Postoperative Blood Loss (mL)					
Males	580	(318) 954±879	(45) 908±812	(88) 817±585	(129) 1056±1055
Females	1256	(639) 700±778	(122) 715±520	(80) 619±352	(415) 798±779
Transfusions (units PRBCs)					
Males	462	(258) 2.6±1.8	(35) 2.7±1.4	(87) 2.5±1.4	(82) 2.9±2.1
Females	1152	(604) 2.6±1.7	(92) 2.8±1.4	(177) 2.1±1.1	(279) 2.8±2.0

[a] "Other" includes the following active reference agents: heparin, heparin/DHE, acetylsalicylic acid, dextran, and low-molecular weight heparins.
Total N = Total number of patients with available data across all treatment groups.
n = The number of patients with available data in each respective treatment group and by gender.

Incidence of Adverse Experiences (≥2%)
DVT and PE Prophylaxis for Elective Hip Surgery
All Patients Treated

Adverse Experience	ORGARAN® N=645 N(%)	Placebo N=135 N(%)	Warfarin N=243 N(%)	Other N=168 N(%)
Fever	143(22.2)	1(0.7)	138(56.8)	3(1.8)
Nausea	92(14.3)	3(2.2)	78(32.1)	8(4.8)
Constipation	73(11.3)	0(0.0)	70(28.8)	2(1.2)
Injection Site Pain	49(7.6)	4(3.0)	0(0.0)	34(20.2)
Rash	31(4.8)	0(0.0)	18(7.4)	2(1.2)
Pruritus	25(3.9)	1(0.7)	14(5.8)	0(0.0)
Peripheral Edema	21(3.3)	0(0.0)	19(7.8)	4(2.4)
Insomnia	20(3.1)	0(0.0)	32(13.2)	0(0.0)
Vomiting	19(2.9)	3(2.2)	20(8.2)	3(1.8)
Joint Disorder	17(2.6)	0(0.0)	15(6.2)	0(0.0)
Headache	17(2.6)	1(0.7)	13(5.3)	0(0.0)
Urinary Tract Infection	17(2.6)	1(0.7)	5(2.1)	5(3.0)
Edema	17(2.6)	0(0.0)	14(5.8)	2(1.2)
Asthenia	15(2.3)	0(0.0)	10(4.1)	1(0.6)
Dizziness	15(2.3)	0(0.0)	14(5.8)	0(0.0)
Anemia	14(2.2)	3(2.2)	5(2.1)	5(3.0)
Urinary Retention	13(2.0)	0(0.0)	14(5.8)	1(0.6)

Incidence of Adverse Experiences (≥2%)
DVT and PE Prophylaxis Indication
All Patients Treated

Adverse Experience	ORGARAN® N=2383 N(%)	Placebo N=276 N(%)	Warfarin N=421 N(%)	Other N=1163 N(%)
Injection Site Pain	327(13.7)	53(19.2)	0(0.0)	153(13.2)
Pain	207(8.7)	0(0.0)	202(48.0)	20(1.7)
Fever	173(7.3)	1(0.4)	150(35.6)	21(1.8)
Nausea	98(4.1)	3(1.1)	79(18.8)	13(1.1)
Urinary Tract Infection	96(4.0)	3(1.1)	27(6.4)	65(5.6)
Constipation	83(3.5)	0(0.0)	73(17.3)	3(0.3)
Rash	51(2.1)	0(0.0)	25(5.9)	5(0.4)
Infection	51(2.1)	3(1.1)	0(0.0)	47(4.0)

INDICATIONS AND USAGE

ORGARAN® (danaparoid sodium) Injection is indicated for the prophylaxis of post-operative deep venous thrombosis (DVT), which may lead to pulmonary embolism (PE), in patients undergoing elective hip replacement surgery.

CONTRAINDICATIONS

ORGARAN® (danaparoid sodium) Injection is contraindicated in the following conditions: severe hemorrhagic diathesis, e.g., hemophilia and idiopathic thrombocytopenic purpura; active major bleeding state, including hemorrhagic stroke in the acute phase; hypersensitivity to ORGARAN®; Type II thrombocytopenia associated with a positive *in vitro* test for antiplatelet antibody in the presence of ORGARAN® Injection. ORGARAN® is contraindicated in patients with known hypersensitivity to pork products.

WARNINGS

General: ORGARAN® (danaparoid sodium) Injection is not intended for intramuscular administration. Since a specific standard for the anti-Xa activity of ORGARAN® is used, the anti-Xa unit activity of ORGARAN® is not equivalent to that described for heparin or low-molecular weight heparin. Therefore, ORGARAN® cannot be dosed interchangeably (unit for unit) with either heparin or any low molecular weight heparin.

Miscellaneous: ORGARAN® (danaparoid sodium) Injection contains sodium sulfite which may cause allergic-type reactions, including anaphylactic symptoms and life-threatening or less severe asthmatic episodes in certain susceptible people. The overall prevalence of sulfite sensitivity in the general population is unknown and probably low. Sulfite sensitivity is seen more frequently in asthmatic than in non-asthmatic patients.

Hemorrhage: Hemorrhage can occur at virtually any site in patients receiving ORGARAN® (danaparoid sodium) Injection. An unexplained fall in hematocrit and/or fall in blood pressure should lead to serious consideration of a hemorrhagic event. ORGARAN®, like anticoagulants, should be used with extreme caution in disease states in which there is increased risk of hemorrhage, such as severe uncontrolled hypertension, acute bacterial endocarditis, congenital or acquired bleeding disorders, active ulcerative and angiodysplastic gastrointestinal disease, non-hemorrhagic stroke, shortly after brain, spinal or ophthalmological surgery and post-operative indwelling epidural catheter use.

Spinal or epidural hematomas can occur with the associated use of low molecular weight heparins or heparinoids and neuraxial (spinal/epidural) anesthesia or spinal puncture which can result in long-term or permanent paralysis. The risk of these events is higher with the use of post-operative indwelling epidural catheters or concomitant use of additional drugs affecting hemostasis such as NSAIDs (see boxed WARNING).

PRECAUTIONS

General: The risks and benefits of ORGARAN® (danaparoid sodium) Injection should be carefully considered before use in patients with severely impaired renal function or hemorrhagic disorders (see **DOSAGE AND ADMINISTRATION**).

Laboratory Tests: ORGARAN® (danaparoid sodium) Injection has only a small effect on factor IIa (thrombin) activity, therefore, when administered at recommended prophylaxis doses, routine coagulation tests (e.g. Prothrombin Time [PT], Activated Partial Thromboplastin Time [APTT], Kaolin Cephalin Clotting Time [KCCT], Whole Blood Clotting Time [WBCT], and Thrombin Time [TT]) are relatively insensitive measures of ORGARAN® activity and, therefore, unsuitable for monitoring.

Periodic complete blood counts, including platelet count, and stool occult blood tests are recommended during the course of treatment with ORGARAN®.

Thrombocytopenia: ORGARAN® (danaparoid sodium) Injection shows a low cross-reactivity with antiplatelet antibodies in individuals with Type II heparin-induced thrombocytopenia. No cases of white clot syndrome or cases of Type II thrombocytopenia have been reported in clinical studies for the prophylaxis of DVT in patients receiving multiple doses of ORGARAN® up to 14 days.

Drug Interactions: In clinical studies for the prophylaxis of DVT, no clinically significant drug interactions have been noted in the following drugs: digoxin, cloxacillin, ticarcillin, chlorthalidone, and pentobarbital.

ORGARAN® (danaparoid sodium) Injection should be used with caution in patients receiving oral anticoagulants and/or platelet inhibitors. Monitoring of anticoagulant activity of oral anticoagulants by Prothrombin Time and Thrombotest is unreliable within 5 hours after ORGARAN® Injection administration.

Carcinogenesis, Mutagenesis, Impairment of Fertility: No long term studies in animals have been performed to evaluate the carcinogenic potential of ORGARAN® (danaparoid sodium) Injection. ORGARAN® was not genotoxic in the Ames test, the *in vitro* CHL/HGPRT forward gene mutation assay, the *in vitro* CHO cell chromosome aberration test, the *in vitro* HeLa cell unscheduled DNA synthesis (UDS) test or the *in vivo* mouse micronucleus test. ORGARAN® at intravenous doses of up to 1090 anti-Xa units/kg/day was found to have no effect on fertility or reproductive performance of male and female rats. This dose is 5.9 times the recommended human subcutaneous dose based on body surface area (50 kg body weight and 1.46 m^2 body surface area assumed).

Pregnancy: Teratogenic effects. Pregnancy Category B. Teratology studies have been performed in pregnant rats at intravenous doses up to 1600 anti-Xa units/kg/day (8.7 times the recommended human dose based on body surface area) and pregnant rabbits at intravenous doses up to 780 anti-Xa units/kg/day (6 times the recommended human dose based on body surface area) and have not revealed evidence of impaired fertility or harm to the fetus due to ORGARAN® (danaparoid sodium) Injection. There are, however, no adequate and well-controlled studies in pregnant women. Because animal reproduction studies are not always predictive of human response, this drug should be used during pregnancy only if clearly needed.

Nursing Mothers: It is not known whether ORGARAN® (danaparoid sodium) Injection is excreted in breast milk. Because many drugs are excreted in human milk, caution should be exercised when ORGARAN® is administered to a nursing woman.

Pediatric Use: Safety and effectiveness of ORGARAN® (danaparoid sodium) Injection in pediatric patients have not been established.

ADVERSE REACTIONS

The following table summarizes adverse bleeding events that occurred in clinical trials which studied ORGARAN® (danaparoid sodium) Injection compared to placebo, warfarin, and others (heparin, heparin/DHE, acetylsalicylic acid, dextran, and low-molecular weight heparins).
[See table at bottom of previous page]

Other: The following table summarizes adverse events that occurred at a frequency greater than, or equal to, 2% of patients in clinical trials for the prophylaxis of DVT and PE following elective hip surgery which studied ORGARAN® (danaparoid sodium) Injection compared to placebo, warfarin, and others (dextran, heparin/DHE, aspirin).
[See first table above]

In addition, the following table summarizes adverse events that occurred at a frequency greater than, or equal to, 2% of patients in clinical trials for the prophylaxis of DVT and PE which studied ORGARAN® (danaparoid sodium) Injection compared to placebo, warfarin, and others (heparin, heparin sodium, heparin calcium, enoxaparin, dalteparin, dextran, heparin/DHE, aspirin).
[See second table above]

OVERDOSAGE

Symptoms/Treatment: Accidental overdosage following administration of ORGARAN® (danaparoid sodium) Injection may lead to bleeding complications. The effects of ORGARAN® on anti-Xa activity cannot be antagonized with any known agent at this time. Although protamine sulfate partially neutralizes the anti-Xa activity of ORGARAN® and can be safely co-administered, there is no evidence that protamine sulfate is capable of reducing severe non-surgical bleeding during treatment with ORGARAN®. In the event of serious bleeding, ORGARAN® should be stopped and blood or blood product transfusions should be administered as needed. Withdrawal of ORGARAN® may be expected to restore the coagulation balance without rebound phenomenon.

Single subcutaneous doses of ORGARAN® at 3800 anti-Xa units/kg (20.5 times the recommended human dose based on body surface area) and 15200 anti-Xa units/kg (82 times the recommended human dose based on body surface area) were lethal to female and male rats, respectively. Symptoms of acute toxicity after intravenous dosing were respiratory depression, prostration and twitching.

DOSAGE AND ADMINISTRATION

Usual Adult Dosage:

In patients undergoing hip replacement surgery, the recommended dose of ORGARAN® (danaparoid sodium) Injection is 750 anti-Xa units twice daily administered by subcutaneous injection beginning 1–4 hours pre-operatively, and then not sooner than two hours after surgery. Treatment should

Continued on next page

Organan—Cont.

be continued throughout the period of post-operative care until the risk of deep vein thrombosis has diminished. The average duration of administration in clinical trials was 7 to 10 days, up to 14 days. Patients with serum creatinine ≥ 2.0 mg/dL should be carefully monitored.

Administration:

ORGARAN® (danaparoid sodium) Injection is intended for subcutaneous administration and should not be administered by intramuscular injection. Subcutaneous injection technique: Patients should be lying down and ORGARAN® Injection administered by deep subcutaneous injection using a fine needle (25 to 26 gauge) to minimize tissue trauma. Administration should be alternated between the left and right anterolateral and left and right posterolateral abdominal wall. The whole length of the needle should be introduced into a skin fold held gently between the thumb and forefinger; the skin fold should be held throughout the injection and should neither be pinched nor rubbed afterwards.

Parenteral drug products should be inspected visually for particulate matter and discoloration prior to administration whenever solution and container permit.

HOW SUPPLIED

ORGARAN® (danaparoid sodium) Injection is supplied in:
—Ampules containing 0.6 mL (750 anti-Xa units) of danaparoid sodium:
boxes of 10, NDC 0052-0830-11.
—Disposable prefilled syringes containing 0.6 mL (750 anti-Xa) units of danaparoid sodium:
boxes of 10, NDC 0052-0830-61. Each ORGARAN® prefilled syringe is affixed with a 25 gauge × $^5/_8$ inch needle.

Storage:

—Ampules should be stored at temperatures of 2°–30°C (36°–86°F).
—Syringes should be stored at a refrigerated temperature of 2°–8°C (36°–46°F).
—Protect from light.

Rx only

Organon Inc.
West Orange, N.J. 07052

5310150 10/98 19

Shown in Product Identification Guide, page 327

PAVULON® ℞

[*pāv-u-lon*]
(pancuronium bromide) injection

HOW SUPPLIED

10 mL vials—1 mg/mL—boxes of 25—NDC-0052-0443-25

PREGNYL® ℞

(chorionic gonadotropin for injection, USP)

DESCRIPTION

Human chorionic gonadotropin (HCG), a polypeptide hormone produced by the human placenta, is composed of an alpha and a beta sub-unit. The alpha sub-unit is essentially identical to the alpha sub-units of the human pituitary gonadotropins, luteinizing hormone (LH) and follicle-stimulating hormone (FSH), as well as to the alpha sub-unit of human thyroid-stimulating hormone (TSH). The beta sub-units of these hormones differ in amino acid sequence.

PREGNYL® (chorionic gonadotropin for injection, USP) is a highly purified pyrogen-free preparation obtained from the urine of pregnant females. It is standardized by a biological assay procedure. It is available for intramuscular injection in multiple dose vials containing 10,000 USP Units of sterile dried powder with 5 mg monobasic sodium phosphate and 4.4 mg dibasic sodium phosphate. If required, pH is adjusted with sodium hydroxide and/or phosphoric acid. Each package also contains a 10 mL vial of solvent containing water for injection with 0.56% sodium chloride and 0.9% BENZYL ALCOHOL WHICH IS NOT FOR USE IN NEWBORNS. If required, pH is adjusted with sodium hydroxide and/or hydrochloric acid.

CLINICAL PHARMACOLOGY

The action of HCG is virtually identical to that of pituitary LH, although HCG appears to have a small degree of FSH activity as well. It stimulates production of gonadal steroid hormones by stimulating the interstitial cells (Leydig cells) of the testis to produce androgens and the corpus luteum of the ovary to produce progesterone.

Androgen stimulation in the male leads to the development of secondary sex characteristics and may stimulate testicular descent when no anatomical impediment to descent is present. This descent is usually reversible when HCG is discontinued. During the normal menstrual cycle, LH participates with FSH in the development and maturation of the normal ovarian follicle, and the mid-cycle LH surge triggers ovulation. HCG can substitute for LH in this function.

During a normal pregnancy, HCG secreted by the placenta maintains the corpus luteum after LH secretion decreases, supporting continued secretion of estrogen and progesterone and preventing menstruation. HCG HAS NO KNOWN EFFECT ON FAT MOBILIZATION, APPETITE OR SENSE OF HUNGER, OR BODY FAT DISTRIBUTION.

INDICATIONS AND USAGE

HCG HAS NOT BEEN DEMONSTRATED TO BE EFFECTIVE ADJUNCTIVE THERAPY IN THE TREATMENT OF OBESITY. THERE IS NO SUBSTANTIAL EVIDENCE THAT IT INCREASES WEIGHT LOSS BEYOND THAT RESULTING FROM CALORIC RESTRICTION, THAT IT CAUSES A MORE ATTRACTIVE OR "NORMAL" DISTRIBUTION OF FAT, OR THAT IT DECREASES THE HUNGER AND DISCOMFORT ASSOCIATED WITH CALORIE-RESTRICTED DIETS.

1. Prepubertal cryptorchidism not due to anatomical obstruction. In general, HCG is thought to induce testicular descent in situations when descent would have occurred at puberty. HCG thus may help predict whether or not orchiopexy will be needed in the future. Although, in some cases, descent following HCG administration is permanent, in most cases, the response is temporary. Therapy is usually instituted in children between the ages of 4 and 9.
2. Selected cases of hypogonadotropic hypogonadism (hypogonadism secondary to a pituitary deficiency) in males.
3. Induction of ovulation and pregnancy in the anovulatory, infertile woman in whom the cause of anovulation is secondary and not due to primary ovarian failure, and who has been appropriately pretreated with human menotropins.

CONTRAINDICATIONS

Precocious puberty, prostatic carcinoma or other androgen-dependent neoplasm, prior allergic reaction to HCG.

WARNINGS

HCG should be used in conjunction with human menopausal gonadotropins only by physicians experienced with infertility problems who are familiar with the criteria for patient selection, contraindications, warnings, precautions, and adverse reactions described in the package insert for menotropins.

The principal serious adverse reactions during this use are: (1) Ovarian hyperstimulation, a syndrome of sudden ovarian enlargement, ascites with or without pain, and/or pleural effusion, (2) Rupture of ovarian cysts with resultant hemoperitoneum, (3) Multiple births, and (4) Arterial thromboembolism.

PRECAUTIONS

General

Since androgens may cause fluid retention, HCG should be used with caution in patients with cardiac or renal disease, epilepsy, migraine, or asthma.

Pediatric Use

Induction of androgen secretion by HCG may induce precocious puberty in pediatric patients treated for cryptorchidism. Therapy should be discontinued if signs of precocious puberty occur.

Geriatric Use

Clinical studies of PREGNYL® (chorionic gonadotropin for injection, USP) did not include subjects aged 65 and over.

ADVERSE REACTIONS

Headache, irritability, restlessness, depression, fatigue, edema, precocious puberty, gynecomastia, pain at the site of injection.

DOSAGE AND ADMINISTRATION

For intramuscular use only. The dosage regimen employed in any particular case will depend upon the indication for the use, the age and weight of the patient, and the physician's preference. The following regimens have been advocated by various authorities:

Prepubertal cryptorchidism not due to anatomical obstruction. Therapy is usually instituted in children between the ages of 4 and 9.

1. 4,000 USP Units three times weekly for three weeks.
2. 5,000 USP Units every second day for four injections.
3. 15 injections for 500 to 1,000 USP Units over a period of six weeks.
4. 500 USP Units three times weekly for four to six weeks. If this course of treatment is not successful, another series is begun one month later, giving 1,000 USP Units per injection.

Selected cases of hypogonadotropic hypogonadism in males.

1. 500 to 1,000 USP Units three times a week for three weeks, followed by the same dose twice a week for three weeks.
2. 4,000 USP Units three times weekly for six to nine months, following which the dosage may be reduced to 2,000 USP Units three times weekly for an additional three months.

Induction of ovulation and pregnancy in the anovulatory, infertile woman in whom the cause of anovulation is secondary and not due to primary ovarian failure and who has been appropriately pretreated with human menotropins. (See prescribing information for menotropins for dosage and administration for that drug product.)

5,000 to 10,000 USP Units one day following the last dose of menotropins. (A dosage of 10,000 USP Units is recommended in the labeling for menotropins.)

Directions for Reconstitution

Two-vial package: Withdraw sterile air from lyophilized vial and inject into diluent vial. Remove 1–10 mL from diluent and add to lyophilized vial; agitate gently until powder is completely dissolved in solution.

Parenteral drug products should be inspected visually for particulate matter and discoloration prior to administration, whenever solution and container permit.

IMPORTANT: USE COMPLETELY AFTER RECONSTITUTION. RECONSTITUTED SOLUTION IS STABLE FOR 60 DAYS WHEN REFRIGERATED.

HOW SUPPLIED

Two-vial package containing:
1-10 mL lyophilized multiple dose vial containing:
10,000 USP Units chorionic gonadotropin per vial, NDC 0052-0315-10.
1-10 mL vial of solvent containing:
water for injection with sodium chloride 0.56% and benzyl alcohol 0.9%, NDC 0052-0325-10.
When reconstituted, each 10 mL vial contains:

Chorionic gonadotropin	10,000 USP Units
Monobasic sodium phosphate	5 mg
Dibasic sodium phosphate	4.4 mg
Sodium chloride	0.56%
Benzyl alcohol	0.9%

If required pH adjusted with sodium hydroxide and/or phosphoric acid.

Storage: Store at 15°–30°C (59°–86°F). Reconstituted solution is stable for 60 days when refrigerated.

Rx only

Manufactured by
Organon Inc.
West Orange, NJ 07052
5310122 Revised 8/98

RAPLON™ ℞

[*răp-lŏn*]
(rapacuronium bromide) for Injection

5310167 8/99 14

THIS DRUG SHOULD BE ADMINISTERED BY ADEQUATELY-TRAINED INDIVIDUALS FAMILIAR WITH ITS ACTIONS, CHARACTERISTICS AND HAZARDS.

DESCRIPTION

RAPLON™ (rapacuronium bromide) for Injection is a nondepolarizing neuromuscular blocking agent. Its chemical name is 1-[(2β,3α,5α,16β,17β)-3-(Acetyloxy)-17-(1-oxopropoxy)-2-(1-piperidinyl)androstan-16-yl]-1-(2-propenyl) piperidinium bromide. The chemical formula of the bromide salt is $C_{37}H_{61}BrN_2O_4$ with a molecular weight of 677.78. The structural formula is:

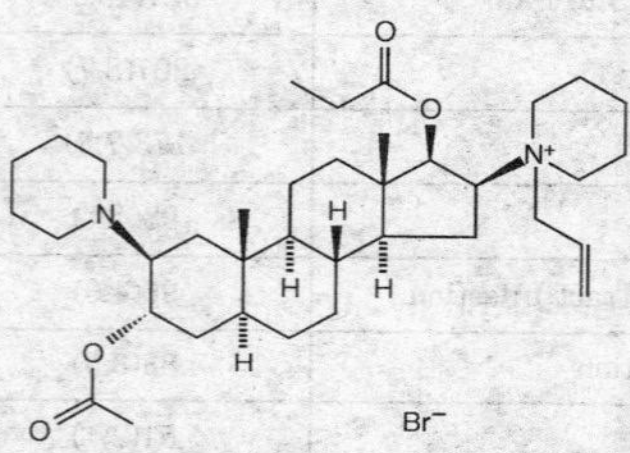

RAPLON™ is a synthetic steroid molecule with a monoquaternary structure in the form of a bromide salt. This chemical structure has a basic steroid framework similar to other neuromuscular blocking agents like vecuronium, pancuronium, rocuronium, and pipecuronium. Rapacuronium bromide is distinguished as being a propenyl bromide ammonium salt with a 17-hydroxy propionate carboxyester that has the same basic steroid backbone as the rest of the family of steroid neuromuscular blockers.

RAPLON™ is supplied as a sterile, nonpyrogenic lyophilized cake in 5 mL and 10 mL vials. Each 5 mL vial contains 100 mg of rapacuronium bromide base, 35.8 mg of citric acid anhydrous, 7.5 mg of sodium phosphate dibasic anhydrous, 137.5 mg of mannitol, and sodium hydroxide and/or phosphoric acid to buffer and adjust the pH. When the 5 mL vial is reconstituted to a volume of 5 mL with sterile water for injection or bacteriostatic water for injection, an isotonic preparation for intravenous injection is obtained at a pH of 4.0 with a concentration of 20 mg of rapacuronium bromide base per mL. Each 10 mL vial contains 200 mg of rapacuronium bromide base, 71.5 mg of citric acid anhydrous, 15.0 mg of sodium phosphate dibasic anhydrous, 275.0 mg of mannitol, and sodium hydroxide and/or phosphoric acid to buffer and adjust the pH. When the 10 mL vial is reconstituted to a volume of 10 mL with sterile water for injection or bacteriostatic water for injection, an isotonic preparation for intravenous injection is obtained at a pH of 4.0 with a concentration of 20 mg of rapacuronium bromide base per mL.

CLINICAL PHARMACOLOGY

RAPLON™ (rapacuronium bromide) for Injection is a nondepolarizing neuromuscular blocking agent with a rapid onset of action (mean onset approximately 90 seconds; range 35–219 seconds) and a dose-dependent duration of action. The recommended dose of 1.5 mg/kg in adults has a short clinical duration of action (mean duration approximately 15 minutes; range 6–30 minutes) (see CLINICAL PHARMACOLOGY—Clinical Studies). Rapacuronium acts by competing for cholinergic receptors at the motor end plate. Profound neuromuscular blockade induced by RAPLON™ can be reversed by neostigmine (see CLINICAL PHARMACOLOGY—Early Reversal).

Pharmacodynamics

The neuromuscular block seen after the intravenous administration of 1.5 mg/kg RAPLON™ (rapacuronium bromide) for Injection is primarily due to rapacuronium. Plasma levels of the major active metabolite of rapacuronium (the 3-hydroxy metabolite) are relatively low compared to the parent at a dose of 1.5 mg/kg of RAPLON™. Pharmacokinetic and pharmacodynamic modeling studies were conducted after the separate administration of rapacuronium bromide and the 3-hydroxy metabolite. These studies evaluated the effect of plasma drug concentrations on the neuromuscular block achieved as measured by mechanomyography [MMG] of the adductor pollicis muscle to indirect supramaximal train-of-four stimulation of the ulnar nerve. These results are shown in Tables 1 and 2. Comparison of κ_{eo} (rate constant for the equilibration between effect compartment and the outside effect compartment) and EC_{50} (concentration in the effect compartment at 50% drug effect) values of rapacuronium and the 3-hydroxy metabolite shows that the metabolite has slower onset and a higher potency than rapacuronium bromide. However, when comparing the ED_{90} (dose required to produce 90% suppression of the first $[T_1]$ mechanomyographic [MMG] response of the adductor pollicis muscle to indirect supramaximal train-of-four stimulation of the ulnar nerve) of rapacuronium bromide (1.03 mg/kg) and the 3-hydroxy metabolite (0.42 mg/kg) with the ED_{90} of rocuronium (0.3 mg/kg), vecuronium (0.05 mg/kg) and pancuronium (0.06 mg/kg), rapacuronium bromide and the 3-hydroxy metabolite may be viewed as low potency neuromuscular blocking drugs.

TABLE 1: Pharmacokinetic/pharmacodynamic Modeling Parameters of Rapacuronium Bromide After a Slow Intravenous Infusion of Rapacuronium Bromide in Ten Subjects at a Median Dose of 0.93 mg/kg Over a Median Time of Four Minutes and Forty Seconds [Mean (% CV)]

Parameter	
κ_{eo}, 1/minute	0.44 (41)
γ	2.97 (23)
EC_{50}, mcg/mL	4.44 (33)
ED_{90}, mg/kg	1.03 (33)

TABLE 2: Pharmacokinetic/pharmacodynamic Modeling Parameters of the 3-hydroxy Metabolite After a Slow Intravenous Infusion in Seven Subjects of a Median Dose of 0.68 mg/kg Over Three to Five Minutes [Mean (%CV)]

Parameter	
κ_{eo}, 1/minute	0.10 (40)
γ	4.83 (44)
EC_{50}, mcg/mL	2.06 (55)
ED_{90}, mg/kg	0.46 (33)

The ED_{50} for rapacuronium bromide (dose required to produce 50% suppression of the first $[T_1]$ mechanomyographic [MMG] response of the adductor pollicis muscle to indirect supramaximal train-of-four stimulation of the ulnar nerve) during opioid/nitrous oxide/oxygen anesthesia is approximately 0.3 mg/kg in adult (18 to 64 years) and geriatric (≥ 65 years) patients. The ED_{50} for rapacuronium bromide for pediatric patients (1 to 12 years) is 0.4 mg/kg and for infants (1 month to < 1 year) is 0.3 mg/kg (see PRECAUTIONS—Pediatric Use).

Tables 3 and 4 present the neuromuscular function parameters following an initial dose of RAPLON™ in adult patients (18 to 64 years) and geriatric patients (≥ 65 years).

[See table 3 above]

TABLE 3: Neuromuscular Function Parameters [Mean (SD)] Following an Initial Dose of RAPLON™ in Adults (18 to 64 years)

Dosage	Time to Maximum Block[a] (sec)	Maximum Block[b] (%)	Clinical Duration (min)[c]	25–75% T_1 Recovery Index (min)	Time to 70% T_4/T_1 Recovery[d] (min)
RAPLON™ 1.5 mg/kg	88 (47) (n=32)	99 (2) (n=49)	15 (5) (n=57)	9 (5) (n=38)	34 (15) (n=47)

a=Time from injection to maximum block (peak effect)
b=(100 − % T_1 control at peak effect)
c=Time from injection to return to 25% of control T_1
d=Time from injection to recovery of 70% T_4/T_1

In US clinical trials, in adult patients (18 to 64 years), the mean (SD) time to maximum block [time from injection to maximum block (peak effect)] following an initial 2.5 mg/kg dose of RAPLON™ was 72 (24) seconds (n=19). The mean (SD) clinical duration (time from injection to return to 25% of control T_1) in adult patients was 24 (8) minutes (n=45) with a mean (SD) 25–75% T_1 recovery index of 13 (7) minutes (n=23) and a mean (SD) time to 70% T_4/T_1 recovery (n=34) of 58 (15) minutes (time from injection to recovery of 70% T_4/T_1).

[See table 4 above]

TABLE 4: Neuromuscular Function Parameters [Mean (SD)] Following an Initial Dose of RAPLON™ in Geriatric Patients (≥ 65 years)

Dosage	Time to Maximum Block[a] (sec)	Maximum Block[b] (%)	Clinical Duration[c] (min)	25–75% T_1 Recovery Index (min)	Time to 70% T_4/T_1 Recovery[d] (min)
RAPLON™ 1.5 mg/kg	89 (6) (n=6)	98 (5) (n=17)	17 (5) (n=16)	11 (6) (n=4)	38 (5) (n=12)

a=Time from injection to maximum block (peak effect)
b=(100 − % T_1 control at peak effect)
c=Time from injection to return to 25% of control T_1
d=Time from injection to recovery of 70% T_4/T_1

In US clinical trials, in geriatric patients (≥ 65 years), the mean (SD) time to maximum block [time from injection to maximum block (peak effect)] following an initial 2.5 mg/kg dose of RAPLON™ was 51 (21) seconds (n=4). The mean (SD) clinical duration (time from injection to return to 25% of control T_1) was 43 (37) minutes (n=13) with a mean (SD) 25–75% T_1 recovery index of 17 (16) minutes (n=3) and a mean (SD) time to 70% T_4/T_1 recovery (n=9) of 76 (20) minutes (time from injection to recovery of 70% T_4/T_1).

Table 5 presents the neuromuscular function parameters following an initial dose of RAPLON™ in pediatric patients under halothane anesthesia.

[See table 5 above]

TABLE 5: Neuromuscular Function Parameters Following an Initial Dose of RAPLON™ in Pediatric Patients (1 month to ≤ 12 years)

Age Group	Dosage		Time to Maximum Block[a] (sec)	Maximum Block[b] (%)	Clinical Duration[c] (min)	25–75% T_1 Recovery Index (min)	Time to 70% T_4/T_1 Recovery[d] (min)
Infants (1 mo to < 2 yrs)	RAPLON™ (n=14)	1 mg/kg	88 (73)	96 (12)	9 (3) (n=13)	7 (4) (n=9)	20 (7) (n=12)
	RAPLON™ (n=16)	2 mg/kg	84 (66)	99 (3)	16 (7)	13 (11) (n=8)	34 (13)
Children (2 to 12 yrs)	RAPLON™ (n=23)	2 mg/kg	53 (16)	100 (1)	14 (7)	6 (4) (n=19)	26 (9) (n=21)
	RAPLON™ (n=21)	3 mg/kg	67 (44)	100 (2)	18 (3) (n=20)	11 (6) (n=12)	37 (9) (n=19)

a=Time from injection to maximum block (peak effect)
b=(100 − % T_1 control at peak effect)
c=Time from injection to return to 25% of control T_1
d=Time from injection to recovery of 70% T_4/T_1

Cardiac Patients

Hemodynamic parameters were assessed in patients with coronary artery and valvular disease receiving 1.5 mg/kg of RAPLON™ in one US (n=14) and one European (n=18) placebo controlled trial. Overall, there were mild to moderate changes in hemodynamic parameters (e.g., mean arterial pressure, heart rate, mean pulmonary artery pressure, pulmonary capillary wedge pressure, central venous pressure, cardiac index, and systemic vascular resistance index) measured invasively, in cardiac patients (valvular disease or coronary artery disease) receiving 1.5 mg/kg RAPLON™.

Obese Patients

Obese patients with a body mass index (BMI) ≥ 30 kg/m² were compared to normal weight subjects in a European study in which they received 1.5 mg/kg of RAPLON™ as part of a rapid sequence induction of anesthesia using either fentanyl/thiopental or alfentanil/propofol. Patients were dosed based on actual body weight. Acceptable (excellent or good) intubating conditions following 1.5 mg/kg of RAPLON™ were similar in obese (86% under fentanyl/thiopental, 92% under alfentanil/propofol) and normal weight subjects (87% under fentanyl/thiopental, 91% under alfentanil/propofol) at 60 seconds. The percent of excellent scores under fentanyl/thiopental or alfentanil/propofol were 48% and 65%, respectively in obese patients, and 44% and 52%, respectively, in normal weight patients.

Repeat Dosing in Adults

In three controlled clinical trials, after an initial intubating dose of RAPLON™ of 1.5 mg/kg, 3 additional doses of 0.5 to 0.55 mg/kg were administered at 25% recovery of T_1 or at the reappearance of T_3 (n=76). The duration of action of maintenance doses of 0.5 to 0.55 mg/kg ranged from 3 to 35 minutes. A statistically significant increase in the duration of action of RAPLON™ was noted with subsequent maintenance doses (see Table 6).

[See table 6 at top of next page]

Early Reversal

Administration of neostigmine (50 or 70 mcg/kg at 2 or 5 minutes) at profound neuromuscular block (≥ 90%) following administration of either 1.5 or 2.5 mg/kg of RAPLON™ in adults reduced the recovery time by approximately 50%. After early reversal with neostigmine, a decrease in neuromuscular function did not occur over the clinical trial period.

Table 7 presents the recovery parameters following reversal of profound block from a US study of adult patients. Anesthesia consisted of premedication with midazolam, induction with fentanyl and propofol, and maintenance with N_2O supplemented with fentanyl and propofol.

[See table 7 at top of next page]

Hemodynamics

After the administration of RAPLON™, dose-related increases in heart rate were observed, peaking within the first few minutes after RAPLON™ administration. These changes in heart rate were generally mild to moderate and were stable or near baseline levels within 5 to 10 minutes of RAPLON™ administration. After the administration of RAPLON™, dose-related decreases in mean arterial pressure (MAP) were observed. Decreases in MAP occurred after all doses of RAPLON™. These changes were observed to peak within 5 minutes after the administration of RAPLON™, returning toward baseline by 10 minutes.

Increases in heart rate and decreases in mean blood pressure were also observed in the pediatric population. In neonates, infants, and children treated with RAPLON™, the observed changes of increased heart rate and decreased mean blood pressure were generally small in magnitude (see CLINICAL PHARMACOLOGY—Clinical Studies).

Dose- and duration-related adverse ECG changes were observed in nonclinical studies in dogs. These changes included prolongation of the QT interval after dosing 2 times per week over 4 weeks, at a total dosage of 18 mg/kg/day given in 3 divided doses, and prolongation of QT interval, sinus arrhythmia, lengthened PR intervals, P wave widening, and AV dissociation following a bolus dose of 27 mg/kg given at 30 minutes after an uneventful first dose of 13.5 mg/kg. In the cat, right bundle branch block pattern and prolonged PR intervals were observed following a bolus dose of 26 mg/kg given at 30 minutes after an uneventful first dose of 13 mg/kg. Therefore, potential adverse ECG effects in humans should be considered when RAPLON™ is given in a high bolus dose or following prolonged infusion.

Electrocardiogram parameters (QT, QTc, and RR intervals) were assessed in patients during a 15 minute observation period after receiving 1.5 mg/kg RAPLON™ (n=18) and placebo (n=16) in a European study. Mean QT interval decreases up to 0.015 second from baseline were observed in the RAPLON™ group while small increases of up to 0.082 second were observed in the placebo group. Mean changes in the QTc interval during the 15-minute period ranged from a decrease of 0.025 second to an increase of 0.052 second from baseline in the RAPLON™ group compared to increases of up to 0.04 second in the placebo group. Mean changes in the RR interval ranged from 0.101 to 0.024 second in the RAPLON™ group and up to 0.113 second in the placebo group. The clinical significance of these changes is unknown.

Continued on next page

Raplon—Cont.

Histamine Release

Plasma histamine release were assessed following administration of RAPLON™ (1.0, 2.0, and 3.0 mg/kg) in a US study (n=46). Increases in plasma histamine levels peaked at 1 minute following 2.0 and 3.0 mg/kg of RAPLON™. The elevation in histamine levels was dose-related; 1/16, 2/15, and 6/15 subjects in the 1.0 mg/kg, 2.0 mg/kg, and 3.0 mg/kg groups, respectively, demonstrated clinically significant elevations of histamine levels (clinical significance defined as ≥ 1 ng/mL or 100% increase from baseline). Two of six patients in the 3.0 mg/kg group with clinically significant elevations of histamine levels had ≥ 30% increase in heart rate and ≥ 30% decrease in blood pressure after the administration of RAPLON™.

Events possibly related to histamine release (e.g., erythema, bronchospasm) occurred in 29 (5.1%) of 564 adult patients in US studies and in 43 (5.8%) of 736 adult patients in European studies.

Intraocular Pressure

In a clinical study, intraocular pressure following a single bolus dose of 1.5 mg/kg of RAPLON™ (n=8) decreased by a maximum of 15% at 3 minutes.

Pharmacokinetics

Data from the *in vivo* pharmacokinetic studies were used to develop population estimates of the parameters for the subpopulations represented (e.g., geriatric, pediatric, renal insufficiency, and hepatic insufficiency). These population-based estimates and a measure of the estimated variability are contained in the following sections.

Following intravenous administration of RAPLON™ (rapacuronium bromide) for Injection, plasma concentration data were best described by a three-compartment model. The pharmacokinetic model was parameterized in clearances and volumes. Estimates of these parameters were used subsequently to calculate volume of distribution at steady state and half-lives. Table 8 presents the results of a population pharmacokinetic analysis from 206 adult patients (18 to 83 years), including patients with end-state renal disease (n=7) and cirrhosis (n=8). The variability for these parameters is not available from this analysis. See Tables 11 and 12 for variability estimates for these parameters.

[See table 8 at right]

Distribution

The mean volume of distribution of RAPLON™ at steady state was 292 mL/kg in adult patients. The mean rapid distribution half-life was 4.56 minutes and the mean slow distribution half-life was 27.8 minutes.

Metabolism

Rapacuronium bromide undergoes hydrolysis of the acetyloxy-ester bond at the 3-position to form the 3-hydroxy metabolite, the major and active metabolite of rapacuronium. Relative to its parent, the 3-hydroxy metabolite has greater potency and a slower onset of action. This hydrolysis is nonspecific and can occur at physiological temperature and pH. This hydrolysis may also be catalyzed by esterases of unknown identity and at unknown sites. The cytochrome P450 enzyme system does not appear to be involved in the hydrolysis of rapacuronium bromide. A mass balance study suggests that there may be seven additional minor metabolites of unknown identity in addition to the 3-hydroxy metabolite.

Elimination

A mass balance study using 1.5 mg/kg of [^{14}C] rapacuronium bromide demonstrated that urine and feces are the main routes of elimination of [^{14}C] rapacuronium bromide (Table 9). The mean combined excretion in urine and feces at the end of the continuous 13.5-day collection period was approximately 56% (range: 50–64%), with approximately 28% excreted in urine samples and 28% in feces. Measurable concentrations of radiocarbon were also detected in urine samples collected once a week over four weeks after the end of the continuous 13.5-day collection period.

The estimated radioactivity excreted in expired CO_2 over 24 hours was approximately 0.6% of the administered dose. The apparent elimination half-life of radioactivity was estimated to be approximately 22 days, suggesting that complete excretion can take several weeks.

[See table 9 at right]

Rapacuronium bromide, in addition to undergoing hydrolysis to its 3-hydroxy metabolite, is also excreted unchanged in urine and feces. The 3-hydroxy metabolite is excreted unchanged in urine and feces without further biotransformation. Approximately 8% of the administered rapacuronium bromide dose was recovered from urine up to 48 hours after dosing as unchanged rapacuronium bromide and approximately 5% as the 3-hydroxy metabolite (Table 10).

[See table 10 at right]

The mean plasma clearance of rapacuronium bromide in adult patients was 6.56 mL/kg/min and the mean plasma elimination half-life ($t_{1/2}\beta$) was 141 minutes. However, this half-life may not represent the terminal elimination of rapacuronium bromide from the body as characterized in the mass balance study.

Protein Binding

Plasma protein binding of rapacuronium was studied *in vitro* for human plasma by equilibrium dialysis. The protein binding was variable and ranged between 50% and 88%, which was at least partly due to hydrolysis of rapacuronium bromide to its 3-hydroxy metabolite. The specific plasma protein to which rapacuronium binds is unknown. Plasma protein binding of the 3-hydroxy metabolite was not determined.

Special Populations

Geriatrics

In the pooled population pharmacokinetic analysis based on 206 adult patients ages 18 to 83 years, the analysis of covariates showed that total plasma clearance of rapacuronium bromide decreases with increasing age. However, as these changes were not clinically significant, no dosage adjustment is recommended for geriatric patients.

Pediatrics

Pharmacokinetic parameters in pediatric patients (n=49) ranging in age from 1 month to 12 years (median 3 years)

TABLE 6: Clinical Duration (25% Recovery of T_1) of Maintenance Doses of RAPLON™ (minutes) Following an Initial Intubating Dose of 1.5 mg/kg

	Study 1 RAPLON™ 0.55 mg/kg	Study 2 RAPLON™ 0.5 mg/kg	Study 3 RAPLON™ 0.5 mg/kg
Dose No. 1	(n=15)	(n=28)	(n=33)
Mean (SD)	7 (3)	12 (3)	13 (3)
Median	6	12	13
Range	3–12	6–19	7–20
Dose No. 2	(n=15)	(n=28)	(n=33)
Mean (SD)	8 (2)	14 (4)	15 (5)
Median	8	14	14
Range	5–12	6–22	8–29
Dose No. 3	(n=14)	(n=25)	Not measured
Mean (SD)	8 (2)	16 (6)	
Median	8	15	
Range	5–13	6–35	

TABLE 7: Recovery Profile Following Neostigmine Reversal at Profound RAPLON™-induced Block (> 90%) in Adults (18 to 64 years)

RAPLON™ Dose	Neostigmine Dose	Time of Neostigmine Administration	Clinical Duration (min)	25–75% T_1 Recovery Index (min)	Time to 70% T_4/T_1 Recovery (min)	Time to 80% T_4/T_1 Recovery (min)
1.5 mg/kg	None	N/A (n=11)	17 (5)[a]	12 (5)[a]	38 (10)[a]	43 (12)[a]
	50 mcg/kg	2 min (n=7)	8 (1)	5 (1)	17 (4)	20 (5)
		5 min (n=12)	9 (1)	5 (3)	17 (3)	19 (4)
	70 mcg/kg	2 min (n=10)	8 (1)	7 (4)	15 (3)	21 (7)
		5 min (n=9)	9 (1)	6 (2)	19 (8)	24 (8)
2.5 mg/kg	None	N/A (n=10)	24 (5)[a]	15 (6)[a]	56 (13)[a]	60 (11)[a]
	50 mcg/kg	2 min (n=12)	12 (2)	9 (4)	26 (7)	31 (8)
		5 min (n=8)	12 (3)	8 (3)	32 (13)	38 (18)
	70 mcg/kg	2 min (n=9)	12 (2)	12 (5)[b]	35 (8)	41 (10)
		5 min (n=9)	12 (2)	8 (3)	28 (9)	36 (12)

a=p ≤ 0.03 for comparisons with each early reversal with neostigmine
b=(p=NS)

TABLE 8: Population Pharmacokinetic Parameter Estimates for RAPLON™[a]

PK Parameter	Estimate	CV[b]
Plasma Clearance (mL/kg/min)	6.56	2.5%
Volume of Distribution at Steady State (mL/kg)	292	ND[c]

a=Based on basic three-compartment model without covariates
b=Coefficient of variation (%)
c=Not determined for derived parameters

TABLE 9: Recovery of Radioactivity[a] From Volunteers (n=8) Given [^{14}C] Rapacuronium

Source	Percentage Recovery Mean (SD)	Duration of Sampling
Urine	28.4 (4.3)	13.5 days
Stool	27.7 (4.2)	13.5 days
Exhaled Gas[b]	0.6 (0.07)	24 hours
Total[c]	56 (5) (range 50–64%)	13.5 days

a=Radioactivity recovery does not distinguish between rapacuronium and the 3-hydroxy metabolite
b=Sampling started 2 hours after anesthesia recovery and a total of 7 samples were collected
c=Excluding exhaled gas

TABLE 10: Recovery of Rapacuronium Bromide and the 3-hydroxy Metabolite From a 48-Hour Urine Collection of Volunteers (n=10) Given Unlabelled Rapacuronium Bromide

Compound Excreted in Urine Mean (SD)	Time After RAPLON™ 1.5 mg/kg Bolus 0–24 hours	0–48 hours
Rapacuronium Bromide (% excreted)	7.96 (2)	8.12 (2)
3-hydroxy Metabolite (% excreted)	3.43 (1)	4.96 (1.2)

were estimated using population pharmacokinetic (PK) analyses. The plasma concentration data were best described by a three-compartment model in which all PK parameters were proportional to body weight. The mean plasma clearance was 10.6 mL/kg/min. The mean volume of distribution at steady state was 495 mL/kg and the mean elimination half-life was 262 (see PRECAUTIONS—Pediatric Use).

Gender

In general, studies in normal adult subjects did not reveal any differences in the pharmacokinetics of RAPLON™ (rapacuronium bromide) for Injection due to gender.

Race

Race was not examined as a covariate in the pooled population pharmacokinetic analysis of RAPLON™.

Renal Insufficiency

Table 11 summarizes the results of conventional PK analyses from a US study of normal volunteers and patients with end-stage renal disease (ESRD) receiving a single bolus dose of 1.5 mg/kg of RAPLON™. Patients with renal insufficiency had a mean 30% reduction in clearance compared with normal adult patients. The volume of distribution was more variable in patients with renal insufficiency compared to normal volunteers.

Comparison of the concentration of the 3-hydroxy metabolite relative to that of rapacuronium bromide up to eight hours after rapacuronium bromide administration and the plasma concentration versus time profiles between the normal volunteer group and patients with ESRD showed that the pharmacokinetics of the 3-hydroxy metabolite were altered in patients with ESRD. In normal volunteers, the ratio of the 3-hydroxy metabolite to rapacuronium increased steadily through the 6-hour period but decreased by the 8-hour time point (from 0.03 at 3 minutes to 4.5 at 8 hours). In patients with ESRD, this ratio showed an increasing trend even at the 8-hour time point (from 0.02 at 3 minutes to 7.5 at 8 hours). The decrease in the plasma concentration of the 3-hydroxy metabolite in patients with ESRD was only 35% from peak levels (265 to 171 ng/mL) compared to an 87% decrease in the normal volunteer group (381 to 49 ng/mL). No clear elimination phase was observed at the end of 8 hours. Despite the persistence of the 3-hydroxy metabolite, neuromuscular function recovered completely with a mean time course to 70% T_4/T_1 only slightly longer in patients with ESRD, compared to that in healthy volunteers with normal renal function after a single 1.5 mg/kg bolus. However, it is likely that recovery from supplemental doses of RAPLON™ will be prolonged in patients with renal failure.

[See table 11 above]

Hepatic Insufficiency

The pharmacokinetic (PK) parameters for patients with mild to moderate hepatic insufficiency and patients with normal liver function are presented in Table 12. These estimates are based on conventional PK analyses. Plasma clearance and volume of distribution at steady-state are greater in patients with cirrhosis compared to patients with normal liver function. Pharmacokinetics of rapacuronium bromide in patients with severe hepatic impairment have not been evaluated.

[See table 12 above]

Drug-Drug Interactions

There were no specific pharmacokinetic studies conducted to examine the drug-drug interactions of RAPLON™ (see PRECAUTIONS).

Clinical Studies

In US studies, 929 patients received RAPLON™ (rapacuronium bromide) for Injection including 219 pediatric, 146 geriatric, and 20 obstetric patients. In European studies, 964 patients received RAPLON™ including 165 pediatric and 63 geriatric patients. The majority of patients, 91%, were ASA (American Society of Anesthesiologists) Class I or II, approximately 8% were ASA Class III, and approximately 1% were ASA Class IV.

Neuromuscular function parameters following administration of RAPLON™, succinylcholine, and mivacurium were compared in one clinical study. In direct comparision with succinylcholine and mivacurium, RAPLON™ at the recommended 1.5 mg/kg dose had a mean (SD) onset of action of 98 (46) seconds compared with 67 (27) seconds for succinylcholine and 127 (50) seconds for mivacurium. RAPLON™ had a mean (SD) clinical duration of 15 (6) minutes compared with 9 (3) minutes for succinylcholine and 21 (5) minutes for mivacurium. Table 13 presents these neuromuscular function parameters in patients 18 years of age and older.

[See table 13 above]

Intubating conditions following administration of RAPLON™ and succinylcholine were compared in three randomized, multicenter trials conducted in the US, France, and Germany. A blinded rater assessed intubating conditions on the Viby-Mogensen scale (see Table 14) 50 seconds after administration of the neuromuscular blocking agent. Several different anesthetic techniques were used. In the US study, fentanyl was given about 5 minutes before intubation followed by propofol one to two minutes before intubation. The French study was similar except that thiopental was used instead of propofol. The German study tested a rapid sequence, with initiation of administration of the neuromuscular blocking agent within a few seconds after the end of the injection of the hypnotic, either fentanyl and thio-

TABLE 11: Estimates of PK Parameters of RAPLON™ in Normal Volunteers and Patients With ESRD

PK Parameter	Normal Volunteers[a]	Patients with ESRD[a]
Elimination Half-Life[c] ($t_{1/2}\beta$, min)	240 (97)	198 (141)[b]
Volume of Distribution at Steady State (mL/kg)	431.7 (78)	440.3 (347)
Plasma Clearance (mL/kg/min)	9.4 (2.2)	6.1 (1.7)[b]

a=Normal volunteers n=10, patients with ESRD n=9, values are mean (SD)
b=p ≤ 0.05 for comparison with normal volunteers
c=May not represent the slow elimination kinetics of rapacuronium bromide

TABLE 12: Estimates of PK Parameters of RAPLON™ in Patients With Normal Liver Function and Patients With Hepatic Insufficiency

PK Parameter	Normal Liver Function[a]	Hepatic Insufficiency (cirrhotic)[a]
Elimination Half-Life[c] ($t_{1/2}\beta$, min)	84 (4)	88 (6)
Volume of Distribution at Steady State (mL/kg)	252 (77)	465 (82)[b]
Plasma Clearance (mL/kg/min)	6.6 (1.7)	9.0 (1.4)[b]

a=Normal liver function n=7, hepatic insufficiency n=6, values are mean (SD)
b=p ≤ 0.01 for comparison with normal patients
c=May not represent the slow elimination kinetics of rapacuronium bromide. Values are harmonic mean and standard error of harmonic mean. Harmonic mean is calculated based on 0.693/t≠beta.

TABLE 13: Neuromuscular Function Parameters Following an Initial Dose of RAPLON™, Succinylcholine, or Mivacurium in Adults (≥ 18 years)

Drug/ Dosage	Time to Maximum Block[a] (sec)	Maximum Block[b] (%)	Clinical Duration[c] (min)	25–75% T_1 Recovery Index (min)	Time to 70% T_4/T_1 Recovery[d] (min)
RAPLON™ 1.5 mg/kg					
n	28	28	25	22	16
Mean (SD)	98 (46)	99 (2)	15 (6)	8 (5)	38 (21)
Range	35–219	94–100	7–30	2–21	21–101
Succinylcholine 1 mg/kg					
n	30	30	29	29	N/A
Mean (SD)	67 (27)	99 (2)	9 (3)	2 (1)	
Range	31–138	90–100	5–15	1–4	
Mivacurium 0.25 mg/kg[e]					
n	25	25	21	24	18
Mean (SD)	127 (50)	100 (0.4)	21 (5)	9 (4)	32 (7)
Range	64–261	99–100	14–29	4–20	22–45

a=Time from injection to maximum block (peak effect)
b=(100− % T_1 control at peak effect)
c=Time from injection to return to 25% of control T_1
d=Time from injection to recovery of 70% T_4/T_1
e=Administered as a divided dose (0.15 mg/kg followed in 30 sec by 0.10 mg/kg), parameter measured from second dose

pental or alfentanil and propofol were used at random. Tables 15 and 16 show the intubation scores in adults (18 to 64 years) and in geriatric patients (≥ 65 years).

[See table 14 at top of next page]

Intubating dosages of 1.5 and 2.5 mg/kg of RAPLON™ were evaluated in 784 patients. A population of patients undergoing Cesarean section was also studied (see below).

[See table 15 at top of next page]
[See table 16 at top of next page]

Intubating conditions were also studied in pediatric patients (≥ 1 month to ≤ 12 years) in one non-comparative European study. Patients were premedicated with midazolam and induced with thiopental. Results are presented in Table 17.

[See table 17 at top of next page]

Cesarean Section

In a controlled clinical trial, patients undergoing rapid sequence induction of anesthesia for Cesarean section received thiopental 4–6 mg/kg followed by 2.5 mg/kg of RAPLON™ or 1.5 mg/kg of succinylcholine. Laryngoscopy was initiated 50 seconds after the muscle relaxant was administered and intubation completed by 60 seconds in all patients. Acceptable (excellent or good) intubating conditions were achieved in 14/15 (93%) patients receiving RAPLON™ and in 17/19 (89%) patients receiving succinylcholine. Excellent scores were recorded in 10/15 (67%) RAPLON™ patients and 13/19 (68%) succinylcholine patients.

No neonates born of mothers who received RAPLON™ during Cesarean section had APGAR scores below 6 at 5 minutes post-delivery or NAC (Neurological and Adaptive Capacity) scores < 30 at 24 hours post-delivery.

The venous umbilical/maternal concentrations of RAPLON™ (median 8.4%, range of 4.4 to 16.1%) and its 3-hydroxy metabolite (median 10.2%, range of 4.6 to 19.9%) demonstrated that there is some placental transfer of the drug from the maternal blood to the fetal blood at delivery.

Individualization of Dosage

DOSES OF RAPLON™ (rapacuronium bromide) FOR INJECTION SHOULD BE INDIVIDUALIZED AND A PERIPHERAL NERVE STIMULATOR SHOULD BE USED TO MEASURE NEUROMUSCULAR FUNCTION DURING RAPLON™ ADMINISTRATION IN ORDER TO MONITOR DRUG EFFECT, DETERMINE THE NEED FOR ADDITIONAL DOSES, AND CONFIRM RECOVERY FROM NEUROMUSCULAR BLOCK.

Based on the known actions of rapacuronium bromide and other neuromuscular blocking agents, the following factors should be considered when administering RAPLON™.

Renal or Hepatic Impairment

A slight delay in the onset of neuromuscular block and prolongation of duration of block were observed in patients with ESRD when compared to normal volunteers. A greater variability of onset and duration was also observed in patients with renal insufficiency. The mean time to 25–75% T_1 recovery was greater in patients with renal and hepatic impairment. Although dosage adjustments are not recommended in patients with renal or hepatic impairment, RAPLON™ should be used with caution in these patient populations.

The results of studies in patients with renal failure and hepatic dysfunction do not suggest any additional safety concerns in these patients when RAPLON™ is administered as a single dose.

Continued on next page

Raplon—Cont.

Reduced Plasma Cholinesterase Activity
RAPLON™ metabolism does not depend on plasma cholinesterase, therefore, no differences in clinical effect are expected in patients with reduced or normal plasma cholinesterase activity.

Drugs or Conditions Causing Potentiation of, or Resistance to, Neuromuscular Block
Use of inhalation anesthetics (enflurane, isoflurane, halothane, desflurane, sevoflurane) has been shown to enhance the activity of other neuromuscular blocking agents (see PRECAUTIONS—Drug Interactions—Inhalational Anesthetics).
Magnesium salts, lithium, local anesthetics, procainamide, quinidine, and certain antibiotics have been shown to increase the duration of neuromuscular block and decrease infusion requirements of other neuromuscular blocking agents. In patients in whom potentiation of neuromuscular block may be anticipated, a decrease from the recommended initial dose of RAPLON™ should be considered (see PRECAUTIONS—Drug Interactions—Other).
Severe acid-base and/or electrolyte abnormalities may potentiate or cause resistance to the neuromuscular blocking action of RAPLON™.
Resistance to non-depolarizing agents, consistent with up-regulation of skeletal muscle acetylcholine receptors, is associated with burns, disuse atrophy, denervation, and direct muscle trauma. Receptor up-regulation may also contribute to the resistance to nondepolarizing muscle relaxants that sometimes develops in patients with cerebral palsy and in patients with chronic exposure to anticonvulsant or nondepolarizing agents (see PRECAUTIONS—Drug Interactions).
Other nondepolarizing neuromuscular blocking agents have been found to exhibit profound effects in cachectic or debilitated patients, patients with neuromuscular diseases, and patients with carcinomatosis. In these or other patients in whom potentiation of neuromuscular block or difficulty with reversal may be anticipated, a decrease from the recommended initial dose of RAPLON™ should be considered.

Obesity
In obese patients, the initial dose of RAPLON™ should be based upon the patient's actual body weight (see CLINICAL PHARMACOLOGY—Obese Patients).
The neuromuscular blocking effect of 1.5 mg/kg RAPLON™ was determined in a group of obese patients (body mass index ≥ 30) and a group of non-obese patients (body mass index 20–28). When dosed by actual body weight, the obese group had approximately the same percentage of patients with acceptable (excellent or good) intubating conditions as the non-obese group.
Although RAPLON™ has not been formally studied in morbidly obese patients (body mass index ≥ 40), clinicians should consider dosing this patient population based on ideal body weight. As with other neuromuscular blocking drugs, RAPLON™ may exhibit prolonged duration and delayed spontaneous recovery when the morbidly obese are dosed based on actual body weight.

Burns
Patients with burns are known to develop resistance to non-depolarizing neuromuscular blocking agents, probably due to up-regulation of post-synaptic skeletal muscle cholinergic receptors.

INDICATIONS AND USAGE

RAPLON™ (rapacuronium bromide) for Injection is indicated as an adjunct to general anesthesia to facilitate tracheal intubation, and to provide skeletal muscle relaxation during surgical procedures.

CONTRAINDICATIONS

RAPLON™ (rapacuronium bromide) for Injection is contraindicated in patients known to have hypersensitivity to rapacuronium bromide.

WARNINGS

RAPLON™ (rapacuronium bromide) FOR INJECTION SHOULD BE ADMINISTERED IN CAREFULLY ADJUSTED DOSAGE BY OR UNDER THE SUPERVISION OF EXPERIENCED CLINICIANS WHO ARE FAMILIAR WITH THE DRUG'S ACTIONS AND THE POSSIBLE COMPLICATIONS OF ITS USE. THE DRUG SHOULD NOT BE ADMINISTERED UNLESS PERSONNEL AND FACILITIES FOR RESUSCITATION AND LIFE SUPPORT (TRACHEAL INTUBATION, ARTIFICIAL VENTILATION, OXYGEN THERAPY), AND AN ANTAGONIST OF RAPLON™ ARE IMMEDIATELY AVAILABLE. IT IS RECOMMENDED THAT ADEQUATE NEUROMUSCULAR MONITORING EQUIPMENT, SUCH AS A PERIPHERAL NERVE STIMULATOR, BE USED TO MEASURE NEUROMUSCULAR FUNCTION DURING THE ADMINISTRATION OF RAPLON™ IN ORDER TO MONITOR DRUG EFFECT, DETERMINE THE NEED FOR ADDITIONAL DOSES, AND CONFIRM RECOVERY FROM NEUROMUSCULAR BLOCK.
RAPLON™ HAS NO KNOWN EFFECT ON CONSCIOUSNESS, PAIN THRESHOLD, OR CEREBRATION. TO AVOID DISTRESS TO THE PATIENT, NEUROMUSCULAR BLOCK SHOULD NOT BE INDUCED BEFORE UNCONSCIOUSNESS. THEREFORE, ADMINISTRATION OF RAPLON™ MUST BE ACCOMPANIED BY ADEQUATE ANESTHESIA OR SEDATING AGENTS.

TABLE 14: Viby-Mogensen Scale

	CLINICALLY ACCEPTABLE		
	Excellent†	Good†	Poor†
Vocal Cord Position	Abducted	Intermediate	Closed
Vocal Cord Movement	None	Moving	Closing
Easiness of Laryngoscopy*	Easy	Fair	Difficult
Airway Reaction	None	Diaphragm	Sustained > 10 sec
Movement of Limbs	None	Slight	Vigorous

*Easy: Jaw relaxed; no resistance
Fair: Jaw relaxed; slight resistance
†Excellent: All items excellent
Good: All items excellent or good
Poor: Any item poor

TABLE 15: Intubation Scores in Adults (18 to 64 years) With Laryngoscopy Initiated at 50 Seconds Following Administration of RAPLON™ or Succinylcholine

Study	US		France		Germany	
Drug/Dosage	RAPLON™ 1.5 mg/kg n=124	Succinylcholine 1.0 mg/kg n=112	RAPLON™ 1.5 mg/kg n=128	Succinylcholine 1.0 mg/kg n=128	RAPLON™ 1.5 mg/kg n=160	Succinylcholine 1.0 mg/kg n=166
Excellent	43%	67%	30%	48%	51%	73%
Good	44%	29%	55%	41%	39%	24%
Poor	13%	4%	9%	9%	11%	3%
Impossible	0%	2%	5%	2%	0%	0%

TABLE 16: Intubation Scores in Geriatric Patients (≥ 65 years) With Laryngoscopy Initiated at 50 Seconds After Administration of RAPLON™ or Succinylcholine

Study	US		France	
Drug/Dosage	RAPLON™ 1.5 mg/kg n=26	Succinylcholine 1.0 mg/kg n=28	RAPLON™ 1.5 mg/kg n=25	Succinylcholine 1.0 mg/kg n=26
Excellent	50%	79%	32%	62%
Good	46%	21%	48%	35%
Poor	4%	0%	4%	0%
Impossible	0%	0%	16%	4%

TABLE 17: Intubation Scores in Pediatric Patients With Laryngoscopy Initiated at 50 Seconds After Administration of RAPLON™

	Infants (1 mo to 1 yr) 2.0 mg/kg n=9	Children (1 to 12 yrs) 2.0 mg/kg n=17
Excellent	100%	59%
Good	0%	41%
Poor	0%	0%
Impossible	0%	0%

Long-Term Use
RAPLON™ (rapacuronium bromide) FOR INJECTION SHOULD NOT BE ADMINISTERED BY INFUSION, PARTICULARLY IN THE INTENSIVE CARE UNIT (ICU) OR DURING LONG SURGICAL PROCEDURES. In an infusion study (n=90) with RAPLON™, one patient displayed a deterioration of neuromuscular function after attaining evidence of adequate spontaneous recovery. Six minutes after spontaneously recovering to a T_4/T_1 of 70%, the T_4/T_1 decreased to 64%. Thirteen minutes later T_4/T_1 recovered to 80%. This patient did not receive neostigmine and had no respiratory problems that required reintubation or mask assisted breathing.
Radioisotope studies have demonstrated that only 56% of the original RAPLON™ dose had been excreted two weeks following a single IV bolus. Excretion of ^{14}C-labeled rapacuronium continued for at least six weeks. Accumulation of rapacuronium bromide following repeat dosing is likely to occur but has not been studied.
ECG abnormalities have been observed in animals following repeat doses and large single doses of rapacuronium bromide (see CLINICAL PHARMACOLOGY—Hemodynamics).
During pregnancy there is passage of low levels of rapacuronium across the placenta and slow elimination following a single maternal dose (see CLINICAL PHARMACOLOGY—Pharmacokinetics). The risk to the developing fetus from extended low-dose intrauterine exposure to a neuromuscular blocking agent is unknown. Because of these concerns and because animal reproduction studies are not always predictive of human response, this drug should not be used during pregnancy unless the potential benefit to the patient outweighs the potential risk to the fetus. This warning does not extend to use of RAPLON™ during Cesarean section, but appropriate monitoring of the infant is recommended after delivery (see CLINICAL PHARMACOLOGY—Clinical Studies).
In patients with myasthenia gravis or myasthenic (Eaton-Lambert) syndrome, small doses of nondepolarizing neuromuscular blocking agents may have profound effects. In such patients, a peripheral nerve stimulator and use of a small test dose may be of value in monitoring the response to administration of muscle relaxants.
Reconstituted RAPLON™, which has an acid pH of 4.0, should not be mixed with alkaline solutions (e.g., barbiturate solutions) in the same syringe or administered simultaneously during intravenous infusion through the same needle.

PRECAUTIONS

Repeat Dosing
It is strongly recommended that during administration of RAPLON™ (rapacuronium bromide) for Injection, neuromuscular transmission and recovery be monitored continuously using a nerve stimulator. Additional doses of RAPLON™ should not be given until there is a definite response (one twitch of the train-of-four) to nerve stimulation. Repeat dosing in adults after intubating doses greater than 1.5 mg/kg, and repeat dosing in pediatric patients have not been studied, and are, therefore, not recommended.
The experience with a limited number of patients indicates that repeat bolus dosing of RAPLON™ may have a potential for prolonged block. Theoretically, increased histamine effects may result from slow elimination of the drug from the body; however, no studies to date have been conducted to substantiate this possibility (see CLINICAL PHARMACOLOGY—Pharmacokinetics).
In three European studies, adult patients were given an intubating dose of 1.5 mg/kg of RAPLON™ followed by three maintenance doses of RAPLON™ 0.5 mg/kg (n=61) or 0.55 mg/kg (n=19). In one study, median (range) clinical durations of the three doses of 0.55 mg/kg were 6 (3–12), 8 (5–12), and 8 (5–13) minutes. In the second study, the three maintenance doses of 0.5 mg/kg had median (range) clinical durations of 12 (6–19), 14 (6–22), and 15 (6–35) minutes. Neostigmine was administered to half the patients in this study after the third dose when T_1 returned to 25%, and the median (range) time to recover to 70% T_4/T_1 was 6 (2–9)

minutes (n=14). The remaining half of the patients had spontaneous recovery after the third dose. The median spontaneous recovery from 25% T_1 to 70% T_4/T_1 was 57 minutes and ranged from 44 to 80 minutes (n=11). In the third study, the median (range) clinical durations of the first and second maintenance doses of 0.5 mg/kg were 13 (7–20) and 14 (8–29) minutes. Neostigmine (n=12) or edrophonium (n=13) were administered two minutes after the third dose of RAPLON™. Median (range) recovery time to 70% T_4/T_1 was 14 (7–24) minutes after neostigmine and 33 (19–49) minutes after edrophonium (see CLINICAL PHARMACOLOGY—Repeat Dosing in Adults).

In the 80 patients who received three maintenance doses following a bolus dose of 1.5 mg/kg or RAPLON™, adverse events reported in separate patients during or following the maintenance doses consisted of hypotension, tachycardia, respiratory depression, and bronchospasm.

Drug Interactions

Inhalation Anesthetics

Use of inhalation anesthetics (enflurane, isoflurane, halothane, desflurane, sevoflurane) have been shown to enhance the activity of other neuromuscular blocking agents and may enhance the activity of RAPLON™ (rapacuronium bromide) for Injection.

Intravenous Anesthetics

In clinical studies, the use of propofol for induction and maintenance of anesthesia did not alter the clinical duration or recovery characteristics of recommended doses of RAPLON™.

Anticonvulsants

As with other nondepolarizing neuromuscular blocking drugs, if RAPLON™ is administered to patients chronically receiving anticonvulsant agents such as carbamazepine or phenytoin, shorter durations of neuromuscular block may occur and infusion rates may be higher due to the development of resistance to nondepolarizing muscle relaxants. While the mechanism for development of this resistance is not known, receptor up-regulation may be a contributing factor.

Antibiotics

Certain antibiotics (e.g., aminoglycosides, vancomycin, tetracyclines, bacitracin, polymyxin, and colistin) may enhance the neuromuscular blocking action of nondepolarizing agents such as RAPLON™. If these antibiotics are used in conjunction with RAPLON™, prolongation of neuromuscular block should be considered a possibility.

Other

Magnesium salts, administered for the management of toxemia of pregnancy, may enhance neuromuscular blockade. Experience concerning injection of quinidine during recovery from use of other muscle relaxants suggests that recurrent paralysis may occur. This possibility must also be considered for RAPLON™.

Other drugs that may possibly enhance the neuromuscular blocking action of nondepolarizing muscle relaxants, such as RAPLON™, include lithium, local anesthetics, procainamide, and quinidine.

Acid-base and/or serum electrolyte abnormalities may potentiate or antagonize the action of neuromuscular blocking agents.

Carcinogenesis, Mutagenesis, Impairment of Fertility

Studies in animals to evaluate carcinogenic potential or impairment of fertility with rapacuronium bromide have not been performed. Mutagenicity studies conducted with rapacuronium using the Ames test and the Mouse Lymphoma L5178Y cell assay were negative. An *in vivo* rat bone marrow micronucleus assay for clastogenic activity was also negative for rapacuronium. Two *in vitro* human lymphocyte chromosomal aberration assays for clastogenic potential were conducted with rapacuronium. Both assays were negative in the presence of metabolic activation, while in the absence of metabolic activation the first assay was inconclusive and the second assay was positive.

Pregnancy

Pregnancy Category C

Reproduction studies have been performed in pregnant nonventilated New Zealand White rabbits and nonventilated Sprague Dawley rats. Throughout gestation days 6–18, rabbits received 0.75, 1.5, or 3 mg/kg/day of rapacuronium bromide by continuous infusion. Rats, during gestation days 6–17, received intravenous doses of 0.75, 1.5, or 2.25 mg/kg/day of rapacuronium bromide in 3 divided doses at 30 minute intervals on each treatment day. No teratogenic effects were observed in rabbits or rats at the highest doses tested. The high doses of 3 and 2.25 mg/kg are approximately 0.3 and 0.1 times the maximum recommended human intravenous dose for adults on a mg/m^2 basis, respectively. Post-implantation losses, as evidenced by increased resorption, were observed in rabbits at and above the lowest dose of 0.75 mg/kg, which is approximately 0.1 times the maximum recommended human intravenous dose for adults on a mg/m^2 basis.

Fetotoxicity, as evidenced by increased fetal deaths and subsequent resorption, was observed in rats at the high dose of 2.25 mg/kg, which is approximately 0.1 times the maximum recommended human intravenous dose for adults on a mg/m^2 basis. There are no adequate and well-controlled studies in pregnant women.

During pregnancy there is passage of low levels of rapacuronium across the placenta and slow elimination following a single maternal dose (see CLINICAL PHARMACOLOGY—Clinical Studies—Cesarean Section). The risk to the developing fetus from extended low-dose intrauterine exposure to a neuromuscular blocking agent is unknown. Because of these concerns and because animal reproduction studies are not always predictive of human response, this drug should not be used during pregnancy unless the potential benefit to the patient outweighs the potential risk to the fetus.

Labor and Delivery

The use of RAPLON™ (rapacuronium bromide) for Injection in Cesarean section has been studied in a limited number of patients (see CLINICAL PHARMACOLOGY—Clinical Studies).

Nursing Mothers

It is not known whether this drug is excreted in human milk or what effects it may have after oral administration. Since many drugs are excreted in human milk, caution should be exercised when RAPLON™ (rapacuronium bromide) for Injection is administered to nursing mothers.

Pediatric Use

RAPLON™ (rapacuronium bromide) for Injection single bolus dose administration has been studied in 397 pediatric patients, the majority of whom were ASA Class I and II.

The use of RAPLON™ has not been studied in pediatric and adolescent patients aged 13 to 17 years.

There are insufficient data to recommend the use of RAPLON™ in infants < 1 month of age until more is known about the safety of RAPLON™ in this population.

The intravenous administration of RAPLON™ has been studied in pediatric patients from 1 month up to 12 years of age (see CLINICAL PHARMACOLOGY—Clinical Studies and DOSAGE AND ADMINISTRATION). Initial doses of 2 mg/kg intravenously in pediatric patients (ages 1 month to 12 years) under halothane anesthesia produce acceptable intubating conditions within 60 seconds. Mean maximum block occurred within 90 seconds in most pediatric patients and had a mean clinical duration of 15 minutes. Intubating doses of 3.0 mg/kg in children (2 to 12 years) provided maximum block within 90 seconds and a mean clinical duration of 18 minutes. Sufficient numbers of pediatric patients 1 month of age and older have received RAPLON™ to establish the safety of single-dose administration in this age group.

No long-term follow-up data are available in pediatric patients exposed to RAPLON™. Studies have demonstrated small quantities of residual drug remaining in tissues of animals administered a single bolus injection of rapacuronium one week after injection. This small residual was primarily observed in kidney, heart, lung, and pituitary. Elimination kinetics in pediatric patients have not been studied, although elimination in adult humans is known to be slower than in animal species tested. Measurable concentrations of radiolabeled rapacuronium in human urine samples following single-dose administration in adults were detected over a period of 6 weeks. The effect of sequestered drug in tissues theoretically may affect development; however, no studies to date have been conducted to substantiate this possibility.

Geriatric Use

RAPLON™ (rapacuronium bromide) for Injection has been studied in 209 patients ≥ 65 years of age. Advanced age or other conditions associated with slower circulation time, e.g., cardiovascular disease, may be associated with a delay in onset time. Nevertheless, the recommended dosage of 1.5 mg/kg should not be increased in these patients to reduce onset time, as higher doses produce a longer duration of action (see CLINICAL PHARMACOLOGY—Pharmacodynamics—Special Populations).

RAPLON™ is known to be substantially excreted by the kidney, and the risk of prolonged effect or other toxic reactions to this drug may be greater in patients with impaired renal function. While elderly patients are more likely to have altered renal function, no dosage adjustments are recommended in geriatric patients.

Hepatic Disease

Resistance to neuromuscular blocking agents in patients with hepatic insufficiency has been ascribed to an increase in volume of distribution. RAPLON™ (rapacuronium bromide) for Injection at a dose of 1.5 mg/kg has been studied in a limited number of patients with cirrhosis (n=6) under isoflurane anesthesia. Following 1.5 mg/kg of RAPLON™, the median (range) of clinical duration and recovery rate in patients with cirrhosis were 14 (8–18) minutes and 14 (9–18) minutes, respectively. These times were similar to the median times of 16 minutes clinical duration and recovery rate of 14 minutes in patients with normal hepatic function. The plasma clearance of rapacuronium was faster and the volume of distribution was greater in patients with cirrhosis compared to normal controls.

Renal Failure

RAPLON™ (rapacuronium bromide) for Injection has been studied at a dose of 1.5 mg/kg in one US study, in patients with end-stage renal disease (n=9) under isoflurane anesthesia. The median (range) onset time in patients with ESRD [83 (38–180) seconds] was slow compared to normal volunteers (median onset time 66 seconds). The median clinical duration of 12 minutes (range 6 to 39 minutes) in patients with ESRD was similar to the median time of 13 minutes in normal volunteers. The recovery time from 25–75% T_1 ranged from 6 to 68 minutes in patients with ESRD.

Malignant Hyperthermia (MH)

RAPLON™ (rapacuronium bromide) for Injection has not been studied in MH-susceptible patients. No subjects exposed to RAPLON™ developed MH or any other syndrome suggestive of MH during premarketing clinical studies. In a study with MH-susceptible swine, the administration of RAPLON™ did not trigger malignant hyperthermia. Since RAPLON™ is always used with other agents, and the occurrence of malignant hyperthermia during anesthesia is possible even in the absence of known triggering agents, clinicians should be prepared to diagnose and treat malignant hyperthermia during the administration of any anesthetic.

Use in Patients With Elevated Intracranial Pressure

In a clinical trial enrolling patients with head injury in which intracranial pressure was monitored, the effects of RAPLON™ (rapacuronium bromide) for Injection and vecuronium were compared. One patient in the RAPLON™-treated group developed an increase in intracranial pressure from 17 to 34 mm Hg two minutes after receiving 1.5 mg/kg of RAPLON™. In the same study, a patient in the vecuronium-treated group developed a rise in intracranial pressure from 26 to 45 mm Hg six minutes after receiving vecuronium 0.1 mg/kg. The results of this study were not conclusive.

ADVERSE REACTIONS

Premarketing Clinical Trial Experience

The safety of RAPLON™ (rapacuronium bromide) for Injection was evaluated in 2036 subjects in prospective clinical trials. The majority of use in clinical trials was single bolus intravenous exposure.

Incidence of Adverse Events in Controlled Clinical Trials

The most common adverse event with an incidence of > 5% seen with RAPLON™ in controlled clinical trials was hypotension (5.2%). Table 18 lists treatment-emergent signs and symptoms that occurred in at least 1% of patients receiving RAPLON™ in controlled clinical trials that were numerically more frequent than in the active control.

[See table 18 above]

TABLE 18: Most Frequent Adverse Events Seen With RAPLON™ in Controlled Clinical Trials

Body System Adverse Clinical Experience	RAPLON™ n=1956	Succinylcholine n=572	Other Active Controls[a] n=141
Cardiovascular			
Hypotension	5.2%	6.5%	4.3%
Tachycardia	3.2%	0.52%	1.4%
Bradycardia	1.5%	1%	2.1%
Respiratory			
Bronchospasm	3.2%	2.1%	0.71%

a=Active controls include rocuronium bromide, vecuronium bromide, and mivacurium

Incidence of Other Adverse Events During Premarketing Evaluation of RAPLON™—in All Treated Patients

In the following tabulation, the frequencies represent the proportion of the 1956 patients exposed to at least one dose of RAPLON™ who experienced an event of the type cited on at least one occasion while receiving RAPLON™. All events reported are included except those already listed in the previous table. Although events reported occurred during treatment with RAPLON™, a causal relationship has not necessarily been established.

Events are further classified within body system categories and enumerated in order of decreasing frequency using the following definitions: frequent adverse events are defined as those occurring in at least 1/100 patients; infrequent adverse events are those occurring in 1/100 to 1/1000 patients; rare events are those occurring in fewer than 1/1000 patients.

Body as a Whole: *Infrequent*: fever, rigors, back pain, hypothermia, chest pain, peripheral edema, pain; *Rare*: asthenia, fatigue, non-inflammatory swelling, therapeutic response decrease.

Cardiovascular: *Infrequent*: hypertension, extrasystoles, abnormal ECG, arrhythmia, cerebrovascular disorder, ventricular fibrillation, atrial fibrillation, ventricular tachycardia; *Rare*: atria arrhythmia, cardiac failure, right cardiac failure, cardio-respiratory arrest, cardiac arrest, thrombophlebitis, supraventricular extrasystoles, supraventricular tachycardia, myocardial infarction, left bundle branch block.

Digestive: *Frequent*: vomiting, nausea; *Infrequent*: ileus, saliva increased; *Rare*: abdominal pain, cholelithiasis, nonspecific gastrointestinal disorder, rectal hemorrhage, esophagospasm, oral hemorrhage, tooth disorder.

Continued on next page

Raplon—Cont.

Hemic and Lymphatic: *Infrequent*: thrombosis, post-operative bleeding; *Rare*: epistaxis, coagulation factor decrease, purpura, anemia, hemoperitoneum.
Metabolic and Nutritional: *Rare*: acidosis.
Musculoskeletal: *Infrequent*: myalgia; *Rare*: muscle weakness, neonatal hypotonia.
Nervous: *Infrequent*: hypoesthesia, hemiparesis, hypertonia, prolonged neuromuscular block, prolonged anesthesia emergence; *Rare*: headache, cerebral hemorrhage, intracranial pressure increased, migraine, ptosis, tetany, breath holding, confusion, anxiety.
Respiratory: *Infrequent*: hypoxia, increased airway pressure, hypoventilation, laryngismus, coughing, apnea, respiratory depression, upper airway obstruction, neonatal respiratory distress syndrome, pneumothorax, pulmonary edema, respiratory insufficiency, stridor; *Rare*: pharyngitis, larynx edema, dyspnea, neonatal respiratory depression, hyperventilation, rhinitis, sputum increase.
Skin: *Frequent*: erythematous rash; *Infrequent*: injection site reaction, injection site pain, rash, urticaria, pruritus, sweating increased; *Rare*: paravenous injection.
Special Senses: *Rare*: corneal ulceration, meiosis, decreased hearing.
Urogenital: *Infrequent*: urinary retention, oliguria; *Rare*: abnormal renal function, urinary tract infection, pelvic inflammation, vaginal bleeding.

OVERDOSAGE

In premarketing clinical studies, one case of accidental overdose with RAPLON™ (rapacuronium bromide) for Injection was reported. A 22-year-old obstetric patient received 5 mg/kg of RAPLON™ during rapid sequence induction for Cesarean section. The patient did not meet extubating criteria until more than two hours after administration of RAPLON™. Complete recovery was reached 19 minutes after the sixth dose of 1.0 mg of neostigmine. There was no evidence of recurarization or respiratory distress in the recovery room. The premature newborn did not demonstrate evidence of neuromuscular weakness.
Overdosage with neuromuscular blocking agents may result in neuromuscular block extending beyond the time needed for surgery and anesthesia. The primary treatment is maintenance of a patent airway and controlled ventilation until recovery of neuromuscular function is assured.

ANTAGONISM OF NEUROMUSCULAR BLOCKADE

THE USE OF A NERVE STIMULATOR TO DOCUMENT RECOVERY AND ANTAGONISM OF NEUROMUSCULAR BLOCKADE IS RECOMMENDED. Patients should be evaluated for adequate clinical evidence of antagonism, e.g., 5 second head lift, ventilation, and upper airway maintenance. Ventilation must be supported until recovery of normal respiration is assured. A 1.5 mg/kg or 2.5 mg/kg dose of RAPLON™ (rapacuronium bromide) for Injection may be reversed 2 minutes after administration with neostigmine 50 mcg/kg in order to reduce the duration by approximately 50%.
Antagonism may be delayed in the presence of debilitation, carcinomatosis, and concomitant use of certain broad-spectrum antibiotics, anesthetic agents, and other drugs that enhance neuromuscular blockade or separately cause respiratory depression. Under such circumstances, clinical management is the same as that for prolonged neuromuscular blockade.

DOSAGE AND ADMINISTRATION

RAPLON™ (rapacuronium bromide) FOR INJECTION IS INTENDED FOR INTRAVENOUS USE ONLY. THIS DRUG SHOULD BE ADMINISTERED BY OR UNDER THE SUPERVISION OF EXPERIENCED CLINICIANS FAMILIAR WITH THE USE OF NEUROMUSCULAR BLOCKING AGENTS. THE DOSAGE INFORMATION PROVIDED BELOW IS INTENDED AS A GUIDE ONLY (see CLINICAL PHARMACOLOGY). THE USE OF ADEQUATE NEUROMUSCULAR MONITORING EQUIPMENT, SUCH AS A PERIPHERAL NERVE STIMULATOR, WILL PERMIT THE MOST ADVANTAGEOUS USE OF RAPLON™, MINIMIZE THE POSSIBILITY OF OVERDOSAGE OR UNDERDOSAGE, AND ASSIST IN THE EVALUATION OF RECOVERY.

Dose for Tracheal Intubation

The recommended initial dose of RAPLON™ (rapacuronium bromide) for Injection in adult and geriatric patients is 1.5 mg/kg for short surgical procedures. In US and European studies, acceptable intubation scores were present in at least 85% of patients within 60 seconds after administration of 1.5 mg/kg of RAPLON™. Maximum block was achieved in most patients by 90 seconds. This dose had a mean clinical duration of approximately 15 minutes. In patients undergoing Cesarean section, the recommended RAPLON™ intubating dose, with thiopental induction, is 2.5 mg/kg.

Repeat Dosing in Adults (Bolus)

Following an intubating dose of 1.5 mg/kg, up to three maintenance doses of 0.50 mg/kg of RAPLON™ (rapacuronium bromide) for Injection, administered at 25% recovery of control T_1 provided a mean clinical duration of 12 to 16 minutes under opioid/nitrous oxide/oxygen anesthesia. The duration of neuromuscular blockade was noted to increase with each additional dose. Repeat dosing should always be guided based on the clinical duration of the previous dose and should not be administered until recovery of neuromuscular function is evident (see PRECAUTIONS—Repeat Dosing).

Use in Pediatrics

Initial doses of RAPLON™ (rapacuronium bromide) for Injection of 2.0 mg/kg intravenously in pediatric patients (ages 1 month to 12 years) under halothane anesthesia produced acceptable intubating conditions within 60 seconds. Mean maximum block occurred within 90 seconds in most pediatric patients and had a mean clinical duration of approximately 15 minutes. When administration is being considered for patients 13 to 17 years of age, clinicians should consider the physical maturity, height, and weight of the patient in determining the dose of RAPLON™. The adult (1.5 mg/kg), pediatric (2.0 mg/kg), and Cesarean section (2.5 mg/kg) dosing recommendations may serve as a general guideline in determining an intubating dose in this age group.

Use in Geriatrics

The clinical duration of RAPLON™ (rapacuronium bromide) for Injection is not prolonged in geriatric patients at a dose of 1.5 mg/kg, and the median spontaneous recovery time is not different from that in other adults. No dosage adjustment is recommended in elderly patients.

Compatibility

RAPLON™ (rapacuronium bromide) for Injection is compatible in solution with:

0.9% NaCl solution	sterile water for injection
5% dextrose in water	lactated Ringers
5% dextrose in saline	bacteriostatic water for injection

Use within 24 hours of mixing with the above solutions. Prepared solutions may be stored at room temperature.
Studies have shown that RAPLON™ is physically compatible when mixed with the following drugs:
alfentanil
aminophylline (compatible if used within 4 hours)
atropine sulfate
ceftazidime (compatible if used within 4 hours)
droperidol
epinephrine
fentanyl
gentamicin
glycopyrrolate
heparin sulfate
ketamine
labetalol
lidocaine
methohexital
metoclopramide
midazolam
morphine
potassium chloride
propranolol
ranitidine
remifentanil
sufentanil
verapamil
RAPLON™ is physically incompatible when mixed with the following drugs:
cefuroxime
danaparoid sodium
diazepam
nitroglycerin
thiopental
Parenteral drug products should be inspected visually for particulate matter and clarity prior to administration, whenever solution and container permit. Do not use solution if particulate matter is present.

Safety and Handling

There is no specific work-exposure limit for RAPLON™ (rapacuronium bromide) for Injection. In case of eye contact, flush with water for at least 10 minutes.

HOW SUPPLIED

RAPLON™ (rapacuronium bromide) for Injection is available in the following:
5 mL vials containing 100 mg of rapacuronium bromide base and when reconstituted to 5 mL with sterile water for injection or bacteriostatic water for injection provides 20 mg of rapacuronium bromide base per milliliter (20 mg/mL) at pH of 4.0
Box of 10 NDC 0052-0490-15
10 mL vials containing 200 mg of rapacuronium bromide base and when reconstituted to 10 mL with sterile water for injection or bacteriostatic water for injection provides 20 mg of rapacuronium bromide base per milliliter (20 mg/mL) at a pH of 4.0
Box of 10 NDC 0052-0495-16
The packaging of this product contains **no** natural rubber (latex).

Storage

Store at 2–25°C (36–77°F).

After Reconstitution

When reconstituted with sterile water for injection or other compatible I.V. solutions, keep vial at room temperature or refrigerated 2–25°C (36–77°F) and use within 24 hours. Discard unused portion. Single use only.
When reconstituted with bacteriostatic water for injection, keep vial at room temperature or refrigerated 2–25°C (36–77°F) and use within 24 hours. Bacteriostatic water for injection CONTAINS BENZYL ALCOHOL, WHICH IS NOT INTENDED FOR USE IN NEWBORNS.

Rx only
Organon Inc.
West Orange, NJ 07052
5310167 8/99 14

Shown in Product Identification Guide, page 327

REGONOL® ℞

[re-gō-nol]
(pyridostigmine bromide) injection, USP

HOW SUPPLIED

5 mg/mL: 2 mL ampuls—boxes of 25—NDC-0052-0460-02
5 mg/mL: 5 mL vials— boxes of 25—NDC-0052-0460-05

REMERON® ℞

(mirtazapine) Tablets

DESCRIPTION

REMERON® (mirtazapine) Tablets are an antidepressant for oral administration. Mirtazapine has a tetracyclic chemical structure unrelated to selective serotonin reuptake inhibitors, tricyclics or monoamine oxidase inhibitors (MAOI). Mirtazapine belongs to the piperazino-azepine group of compounds. It is designated 1,2,3,4,10,14b-hexahydro-2-methylpyrazino [2,1-a] pyrido [2,3-c] benzazepine and has the empirical formula of $C_{17}H_{19}N_3$. Its molecular weight is 265.36. The structural formula is the following and it is the racemic mixture:

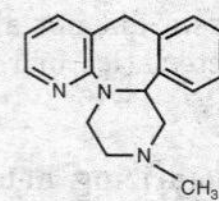

Mirtazapine is a white to creamy white crystalline powder which is slightly soluble in water.
REMERON® is supplied for oral administration as scored film-coated tablets containing 15 or 30 mg of mirtazapine, and unscored film-coated tablets containing 45 mg of mirtazapine. Each tablet also contains corn starch, hydroxypropyl cellulose, magnesium stearate, colloidal silicon dioxide, lactose, and other inactive ingredients.

CLINICAL PHARMACOLOGY

Pharmacodynamics

The mechanism of action of REMERON® (mirtazapine) Tablets, as with other antidepressants, is unknown.
Evidence gathered in preclinical studies suggests that mirtazapine enhances central noradrenergic and serotonergic activity. These studies have shown that mirtazapine acts as an antagonist at central presynaptic α_2 adrenergic inhibitory autoreceptors and heteroreceptors, an action that is postulated to result in an increase in central noradrenergic and serotonergic activity.
Mirtazapine is a potent antagonist of 5-HT_2 and 5-HT_3 receptors. Mirtazapine has no significant affinity for the 5-HT_{1A} and 5-HT_{1B} receptors.
Mirtazapine is a potent antagonist of histamine (H_1) receptors, a property that may explain its prominent sedative effects.
Mirtazapine is a moderate peripheral α_1 adrenergic antagonist, a property that may explain the occasional orthostatic hypotension reported in association with its use.
Mirtazapine is a moderate antagonist at muscarinic receptors, a property that may explain the relatively low incidence of anticholinergic side effects associated with its use.

Pharmacokinetics

REMERON® (mirtazapine) Tablets are rapidly and completely absorbed following oral administration and have a half-life of about 20–40 hours. Peak plasma concentrations are reached within about 2 hours following an oral dose. The presence of food in the stomach has a minimal effect on both the rate and extent of absorption and does not require a dosage adjustment.
Mirtazapine is extensively metabolized after oral administration. Major pathways of biotransformation are demethylation and hydroxylation followed by glucuronide conjugation. In vitro data from human liver microsomes indicate that cytochrome 2D6 and 1A2 are involved in the formation of the 8-hydroxy metabolite of mirtazapine, whereas cytochrome 3A is considered to be responsible for the formation of the N-desmethyl and N-oxide metabolite. Mirtazapine has an absolute bioavailability of about 50%. It is eliminated predominantly via urine (75%) with 15% in feces. Several unconjugated metabolites possess pharmacological activity but are present in the plasma at very low levels. The (−) enantiomer has an elimination half-life that is approximately twice as long as the (+) enantiomer and therefore achieves plasma levels that are about three times as high as that of the (+) enantiomer.
Plasma levels are linearly related to dose over a dose range of 15 to 80 mg. The mean elimination half-life of mirtazapine after oral administration ranges from approximately 20–40 hours across age and gender subgroups, with females of all ages exhibiting significantly longer elimination half-lives than males (mean half-life of 37 hours for females vs. 26 hours for males). Steady state plasma levels of mirtazapine are attained within 5 days, with about 50% accumulation (accumulation ratio = 1.5).
Mirtazapine is approximately 85% bound to plasma proteins over a concentration range of 0.01 to 10 μg/mL.

Special Populations

Geriatric
Following oral administration of REMERON® (mirtazapine) Tablets 20 mg/day for 7 days to subjects of varying ages (range, 25–74), oral clearance of mirtazapine was reduced in

the elderly compared to the younger subjects. The differences were most striking in males, with a 40% lower clearance in elderly males compared to younger males, with the clearance in elderly females was only 10% lower compared to younger females. Caution is indicated in administering REMERON® to elderly patients (see PRECAUTIONS and DOSAGE AND ADMINISTRATION).

Pediatrics

Safety and effectiveness of mirtazapine in the pediatric population have not been established (see PRECAUTIONS).

Gender

The mean elimination half-life of mirtazapine after oral administration ranges from approximately 20–40 hours across age and gender subgroups, with females of all ages exhibiting significantly longer elimination half-lives than males (mean half-life of 37 hours for females vs 26 hours for males) (see Pharmacokinetics).

Race

There have been no clinical studies to evaluate the effect of race on the pharmacokinetics of REMERON®

Renal Insufficiency

The disposition of mirtazapine was studied in patients with varying degrees of renal function. Elimination of mirtazapine is correlated with creatinine clearance. Total body clearance of mirtazapine was reduced approximately 30% in patients with moderate (Clcr = 11–39 mL/min/1.73 m^2) and approximately 50% in patients with severe (Clcr = < 10 mL/min/1.73 m^2) renal impairment when compared to normal subjects. Caution is indicated in administering REMERON® to patients with compromised renal function (see PRECAUTIONS and DOSAGE AND ADMINISTRATION).

Hepatic Insufficiency

Following a single 15 mg oral dose of REMERON®, the oral clearance of mirtazapine was decreased by approximately 30% in hepatically impaired patients compared to subjects with normal hepatic function. Caution is indicated in administering REMERON® to patients with compromised hepatic function (see PRECAUTIONS and DOSAGE AND ADMINISTRATION).

Clinical Trials Showing Effectiveness

The efficacy of REMERON® (mirtazapine) Tablets as a treatment for depression was established in four placebo-controlled, 6-week trials in adult outpatients meeting DSM-III criteria for major depression. Patients were titrated with mirtazapine from a dose range of 5 mg up to 35 mg/day. Overall, these studies demonstrated mirtazapine to be superior to placebo on at least three of the following four measures: 21-Item Hamilton Depression Rating Scale (HDRS) total score; HDRS Depressed Mood Item; CGI Severity score; and Montgomery and Asberg Depression Rating Scale (MADRS). Superiority of mirtazapine over placebo was also found for certain factors of the HDRS, including anxiety/somatization factor and sleep disturbance factor. The mean mirtazapine dose for patients who completed these four studies ranged from 21 to 32 mg/day. A fifth study of similar design utilized a higher dose (up to 50 mg) per day and also showed effectiveness.

Examination of age and gender subsets of the population did not reveal any differential responsiveness on the basis of these subgroupings.

INDICATIONS AND USAGE

REMERON® (mirtazapine) Tablets are indicated for the treatment of depression.

The efficacy of REMERON® in the treatment of depression was established in six week controlled trials of outpatients whose diagnoses corresponded most closely to the Diagnostic and Statistical Manual of Mental Disorders – 3rd edition (DSM-III) category of major depressive disorder (see CLINICAL PHARMACOLOGY).

A major depressive episode (DSM-IV) implies a prominent and relatively persistent (nearly every day for at least 2 weeks) depressed or dysphoric mood that usually interferes with daily functioning, and includes at least five of the following nine symptoms: depressed mood, loss of interest in usual activities, significant change in weight and/or appetite, insomnia or hypersomnia, psychomotor agitation or retardation, increased fatigue, feelings of guilt or worthlessness, slowed thinking or impaired concentration, a suicide attempt or suicidal ideation.

The antidepressant effectiveness of REMERON® in hospitalized depressed patients has not been adequately studied. The effectiveness of REMERON® in long-term use, that is, for more than 6 weeks, has not been systematically evaluated in controlled trials. Therefore, the physician who elects to use REMERON® for extended periods should periodically evaluate the long-term usefulness of the drug for the individual patient.

CONTRAINDICATIONS

REMERON® (mirtazapine) Tablets are contraindicated in patients with a known hypersensitivity to mirtazapine.

WARNINGS

Agranulocytosis

In premarketing clinical trials, two (one with Sjögren's Syndrome) out of 2,796 patients treated with REMERON® (mirtazapine) Tablets developed agranulocytosis (absolute neutrophil count (ANC) < 500/mm^3 with associated signs and symptoms, e.g., fever, infection, etc.) and a third patient developed severe neutropenia (ANC < 500/mm^3 without any associated symptoms). For these three patients, onset of severe neutropenia was detected on days 61, 9, and 14 of treatment, respectively. All three patients recovered after REMERON® was stopped. These three cases yield a crude incidence of severe neutropenia (with or without associated infection) of approximately 1.1 per thousand patients exposed, with a very wide 95% confidence interval, i.e., 2.2 cases per 10,000 to 3.1 cases per 1000. If a patient develops a sore throat, fever, stomatitis or other signs of infection, along with a low WBC count, treatment with REMERON® should be discontinued and the patient should be closely monitored.

MAO Inhibitors

In patients receiving other antidepressants in combination with a monoamine oxidase inhibitor (MAOI) and in patients who have recently discontinued an antidepressant drug and then are started on an MAOI, there have been reports of serious, and sometimes fatal, reactions, e.g., including nausea, vomiting, flushing, dizziness, tremor, myoclonus, rigidity, diaphoresis, hyperthermia, autonomic instability with rapid fluctuations of vital signs, seizures, and mental status changes ranging from agitation to coma. Although there are no human data pertinent to such an interaction with REMERON® (mirtazapine) Tablets, it is recommended that REMERON® not be used in combination with an MAOI, or within 14 days of initiating or discontinuing therapy with an MAOI.

PRECAUTIONS

General

Somnolence

In U.S. controlled studies, somnolence was reported in 54% of patients treated with REMERON® (mirtazapine) Tablets, compared to 18% for placebo and 60% for amitriptyline. In these studies, somnolence resulted in discontinuation for 10.4% of REMERON® treated patients, compared to 2.2% for placebo. It is unclear whether or not tolerance develops to the somnolent effects of REMERON®. Because of REMERON®'s potentially significant effects on impairment of performance, patients should be cautioned about engaging in activities requiring alertness until they have been able to assess the drug's effect on their own psychomotor performance (see Information for Patients).

Dizziness

In U.S. controlled studies, dizziness was reported in 7% of patients treated with REMERON®, compared to 3% for placebo and 14% for amitriptyline. It is unclear whether or not tolerance develops to the dizziness observed in association with the use of REMERON®.

Increased Appetite/Weight Gain

In U.S. controlled studies, appetite increase was reported in 17% of patients treated with REMERON®, compared to 2% for placebo and 6% for amitriptyline. In these same trials, weight gain of ≥ 7% of body weight was reported in 7.5% of patients treated with mirtazapine, compared to 0% for placebo and 5.9% for amitriptyline. In a pool of premarketing U.S. studies, including many patients for long-term, open label treatment, 8% of patients receiving REMERON® discontinued for weight gain.

Cholesterol/Triglycerides

In U.S. controlled studies, nonfasting cholesterol increases to ≥ 20% above the upper limits of normal were observed in 15% of patients treated with REMERON®, compared to 7% for placebo and 8% for amitriptyline. In these same studies, nonfasting triglyceride increases to ≥ 500 mg/dL were observed in 6% of patients treated with mirtazapine, compared to 3% for placebo and 3% for amitriptyline.

Transaminase Elevations

Clinically significant ALT (SGPT) elevations (≥ 3 times the upper limit of the normal range) were observed in 2.0% (8/424) of patients exposed to REMERON® in a pool of short-term U.S. controlled trials, compared to 0.3% (1/328) of placebo patients and 2.0% (3/181) of amitriptyline patients. Most of these patients with ALT increases did not develop signs or symptoms associated with compromised liver function. While some patients were discontinued for the ALT increases, in other cases, the enzyme levels returned to normal despite continued REMERON® treatment. REMERON® should be used with caution in patients with impaired hepatic function (see CLINICAL PHARMACOLOGY and DOSAGE AND ADMINISTRATION).

Activation of Mania/Hypomania

Mania/hypomania occurred in approximately 0.2% (3/1,299 patients) of REMERON® treated patients in U.S. studies. Although the incidence of mania/hypomania was very low during treatment with mirtazapine, it should be used carefully in patients with a history of mania/hypomania.

Seizure

In premarketing clinical trials only one seizure was reported among the 2,796 U.S. and non-U.S. patients treated with REMERON®. However, no controlled studies have been carried out in patients with a history of seizures. Therefore, care should be exercised when mirtazapine is used in these patients.

Suicide

Suicidal ideation is inherent in depression and may persist until significant remission occurs. As with any patient receiving antidepressants, high-risk patients should be closely supervised during initial drug therapy. Prescriptions of REMERON® should be written for the smallest quantity consistent with good patient management, in order to reduce the risk of overdose.

Use in Patients with Concomitant Illness

Clinical experience with REMERON® in patients with concomitant systemic illness is limited. Accordingly, care is advisable in prescribing mirtazapine for patients with diseases or conditions that affect metabolism or hemodynamic responses.

REMERON® has not been systematically evaluated or used to any appreciable extent in patients with a recent history of myocardial infarction or other significant heart disease. REMERON® was not associated with clinically significant ECG abnormalities in U.S. and non-U.S. placebo controlled trials. REMERON® was associated with significant orthostatic hypotension in early clinical pharmacology trials with normal volunteers. Orthostatic hypotension was infrequently observed in clinical trials with depressed patients. REMERON® should be used with caution in patients with known cardiovascular or cerebrovascular disease that could be exacerbated by hypotension (history of myocardial infarction, angina, or ischemic stroke) and conditions that would predispose patients to hypotension (dehydration, hypovolemia, and treatment with antihypertensive medication).

Mirtazapine clearance is decreased in patients with moderate [glomerular filtration rate (GFR) = 11–39 mL/min/1.73 m^2] and severe [GFR < 10 mL/min/1.73 m^2] renal impairment, and also in patients with hepatic impairment. Caution is indicated in administering REMERON® to such patients (see CLINICAL PHARMACOLOGY and DOSAGE ADMINISTRATION).

Information for Patients

Physicians are advised to discuss the following issues with patients for whom they prescribe REMERON® (mirtazapine) Tablets:

Agranulocytosis

Patients who are to receive REMERON® should be warned about the risk of developing agranulocytosis. Patients should be advised to contact their physician if they experience any indication of infection such as fever, chills, sore throat, mucous membrane ulceration or other possible signs of infection. Particular attention should be paid to any flu-like complaints or other symptoms that might suggest infection.

Interference with Cognitive and Motor Performance

REMERON® may impair judgement, thinking, and particularly, motor skills, because of its prominent sedative effect. The drowsiness associated with mirtazapine use may impair a patient's ability to drive, use machines or perform tasks that require alertness. Thus, patients should be cautioned about engaging in hazardous activities until they are reasonably certain that REMERON® therapy does not adversely affect their ability to engage in such activities.

Completing Course of Therapy

While patients may notice improvement with REMERON® therapy in 1 to 4 weeks, they should be advised to continue therapy as directed.

Concomitant Medication

Patients should be advised to inform their physician if they are taking, or intend to take, any prescription or over-the-counter drugs since there is a potential for REMERON® to interact with other drugs.

Alcohol

The impairment of cognitive and motor skills produced by REMERON® has been shown to be additive with those produced by alcohol. Accordingly, patients should be advised to avoid alcohol while taking mirtazapine.

Pregnancy

Patients should be advised to notify their physician if they become pregnant or intend to become pregnant during REMERON® therapy.

Nursing

Patients should be advised to notify their physician if they are breast-feeding an infant.

Laboratory Tests

There are no routine laboratory tests recommended.

Drug Interactions

As with other drugs, the potential for interaction by a variety of mechanisms (e.g., pharmacodynamic, pharmacokinetic inhibition or enhancement, etc.) is a possibility (see CLINICAL PHARMACOLOGY).

Drugs Affecting Hepatic Metabolism

The metabolism and pharmacokinetics of REMERON® (mirtazapine) Tablets may be affected by the induction or inhibition of drug-metabolizing enzymes.

Drugs that are Metabolized by and/or Inhibit Cytochrome P450 Enzymes

Many drugs are metabolized by and/or inhibit various cytochrome P450 enzymes, e.g., 2D6, 1A2, 3A4, etc. In vitro studies have shown that mirtazapine is a substrate for several of these enzymes, including 2D6, 1A2, and 3A4. While in vitro studies have shown that mirtazapine is not a potent inhibitor of any of these enzymes, an indication that mirtazapine is not likely to have a clinically significant inhibitory effect on the metabolism of other drugs that are substrates for these cytochrome P450 enzymes, the concomitant use of REMERON® with most other drugs metabolized by these enzymes has not been formally studied. Consequently, it is not possible to make any definitive statements about the risks of coadministration of REMERON® with such drugs.

Alcohol

Concomitant administration of alcohol (equivalent to 60 g) had a minimal effect on plasma levels of mirtazapine (15 mg) in 6 healthy male subjects. However, the impairment of cognitive and motor skills produced by REMERON® were

Continued on next page

Remeron—Cont.

shown to be additive with those produced by alcohol. Accordingly, patients should be advised to avoid alcohol while taking REMERON®.

Diazepam

Concomitant administration of diazepam (15 mg) had a minimal effect on plasma levels of mirtazapine (15 mg) in 12 healthy subjects. However, the impairment of motor skills produced by REMERON® has been shown to be additive with those caused by diazepam. Accordingly, patients should be advised to avoid diazepam and other similar drugs while taking REMERON®.

Carcinogenesis, Mutagenesis, Impairment of Fertility

Carcinogenesis

Carcinogenicity studies were conducted with mirtazapine given in the diet at doses of 2, 20, and 200 mg/kg/day to mice and 2, 20, and 60 mg/kg/day to rats. The highest doses used are approximately 20 and 12 times the maximum recommended human dose (MRHD) of 45 mg/day on a mg/m^2 basis in mice and rats, respectively. There was an increased incidence of hepatocellular adenoma and carcinoma in male mice at the high dose. In rats, there was an increase in hepatocellular adenoma in females at the mid and high doses and in hepatocellular tumors and thyroid follicular adenoma/cystadenoma and carcinoma in males at the high dose. The data suggest that the above effects could possibly be mediated by non-genotoxic mechanisms, the relevance of which to humans is not known.

The doses used in the mouse study may not have been high enough to fully characterize the carcinogenic potential of REMERON® (mirtazapine) Tablets.

Mutagenesis

Mirtazapine was not mutagenic or clastogenic and did not induce general DNA damage as determined in several genotoxicity tests: Ames test, in vitro gene mutation assay in Chinese hamster V 79 cells, in vitro sister chromatid exchange assay in cultured rabbit lymphocytes, in vivo bone marrow micronucleus test in rats, and unscheduled DNA synthesis assay in HeLa cells.

Impairment of Fertility

In a fertility study in rats, mirtazapine was given at doses up to 100 mg/kg (20 times the maximum recommended human dose (MRHD) on a mg/m^2 basis). Mating and conception were not affected by the drug, but estrous cycling was disrupted at doses that were 3 or more times the MRHD and pre-implantation losses occurred at 20 times the MRHD.

Pregnancy

Teratogenic Effects – Pregnancy Category C

Reproduction studies in pregnant rats and rabbits at doses up to 100 mg/kg and 40 mg/kg, respectively (20 and 17 times the maximum recommended human dose (MRHD) on a mg/m^2 basis, respectively), have revealed no evidence of teratogenic effects. However, in rats, there was an increase in post-implantation losses in dams treated with mirtazapine. There was an increase in pup deaths during the first 3 days of lactation and a decrease in pup birth weights. The cause of these deaths is not known. These effects occurred at doses that were 20 times the MRHD, but not at 3 times the MRHD, on a mg/m^2 basis. There are no adequate and well controlled studies in pregnant women. Because animal reproduction studies are not always predictive of human response, this drug should be used during pregnancy only if clearly needed.

Nursing Mothers

It is not known whether mirtazapine is excreted in human milk. Because many drugs are excreted in human milk, caution should be exercised when REMERON® (mirtazapine) Tablets are administered to nursing women.

Pediatric Use

Safety and effectiveness in pediatric patients have not been established.

Geriatric Use

Approximately 190 elderly individuals (≥ 65 years of age) participated in clinical studies with REMERON® (mirtazapine) Tablets. This drug is known to be substantially excreted by the kidney (75%), and the risk of decreased clearance of this drug is greater in patients with impaired renal function. Because elderly patients are more likely to have decreased renal function, care should be taken in dose selection. Sedating drugs may cause confusion and over-sedation in the elderly. No unusual adverse age-related phenomena were identified in this group. Pharmacokinetic studies revealed a decreased clearance in the elderly. Caution is indicated in administering REMERON® to elderly patients (see CLINICAL PHARMACOLOGY and DOSAGE AND ADMINISTRATION).

ADVERSE REACTIONS

Associated with Discontinuation of Treatment

Approximately 16 percent of the 453 patients who received REMERON® (mirtazapine) Tablets in U.S. 6-week controlled clinical trials discontinued treatment due to an adverse experience, compared to 7 percent of the 361 placebo-treated patients in those studies. The most common events (≥ 1%) associated with discontinuation and considered to be drug related (i.e., those events associated with dropout at a rate at least twice that of placebo) included:

Common Adverse Events Associated with Discontinuation of Treatment in 6-Week U.S. REMERON® Trials

Adverse Event	Percentage of Patients Discontinuing with Adverse Event	
	REMERON® (n=453)	Placebo (n=361)
Somnolence	10.4%	2.2%
Nausea	1.5%	0%

Commonly Observed Adverse Events in U.S. Controlled Clinical Trials

The most commonly observed adverse events associated with the use of REMERON® (mirtazapine) Tablets (incidence of 5% or greater) and not observed at an equivalent incidence among placebo-treated patients (REMERON® incidence at least twice that for placebo) were:

Common Treatment-Emergent Adverse Events Associated with the Use of REMERON® in 6-Week U.S. Trials

Adverse Event	Percentage of Patients Reporting Adverse Event	
	REMERON® (n=453)	Placebo (n=361)
Somnolence	54%	18%
Increased Appetite	17%	2%
Weight Gain	12%	2%
Dizziness	7%	3%

Adverse Events Occurring at an Incidence of 1% or More Among REMERON®-Treated Patients

The table that follows enumerates adverse events that occurred at an incidence of 1% or more, and were more frequent than in the placebo group, among REMERON® (mirtazapine) Tablets-treated patients who participated in short-term U.S. placebo-controlled trials in which patients were dosed in a range of 5 to 60 mg/day. This table shows the percentage of patients in each group who had at least one episode of an event at some time during their treatment. Reported adverse events were classified using a standard COSTART-based dictionary terminology.

The prescriber should be aware that these figures cannot be used to predict the incidence of side effects in the course of usual medical practice where patient characteristics and other factors differ from those which prevailed in the clinical trials. Similarly, the cited frequencies cannot be compared with figures obtained from other investigations involving different treatments, uses and investigators. The cited figures, however, do provide the prescribing physician with some basis for estimating the relative contribution of drug and non-drug factors to the side effect incidence rate in the population studied.

INCIDENCE OF ADVERSE CLINICAL EXPERIENCES[1] (≥ 1%) IN SHORT-TERM U.S. CONTROLLED STUDIES

Body System Adverse Clinical Experience	REMERON® (n=453)	Placebo (n=361)
Body as a Whole		
Asthenia	8%	5%
Flu Syndrome	5%	3%
Back Pain	2%	1%
Digestive System		
Dry Mouth	25%	15%
Increased Appetite	17%	2%
Constipation	13%	7%
Metabolic and Nutritional Disorders		
Weight Gain	12%	2%
Peripheral Edema	2%	1%
Edema	1%	0%
Musculoskeletal System		
Myalgia	2%	1%
Nervous System		
Somnolence	54%	18%
Dizziness	7%	3%
Abnormal Dreams	4%	1%
Thinking Abnormal	3%	1%
Tremor	2%	1%
Confusion	2%	0%
Respiratory System		
Dyspnea	1%	0%
Urogenital System		
Urinary Frequency	2%	1%

[1] Events reported by at least 1% of patients treated with REMERON® are included, except the following events which had an incidence on placebo ≥ REMERON®: headache, infection, pain, chest pain, palpitation, tachycardia, postural hypotension, nausea, dyspepsia, diarrhea, flatulence, insomnia, nervousness, libido decreased, hypertonia, pharyngitis, rhinitis, sweating, amblyopia, tinnitus, taste perversion.

ECG Changes

In an analysis of ECGs obtained in U.S. placebo-controlled clinical trials, REMERON® (mirtazapine) Tablets and placebo-treated patients had a similar incidence of abnormal changes from baseline at 6–8 weeks of approximately 3%. The abnormalities were generally not considered clinically significant.

Other Adverse Events Observed During the Premarketing Evaluation of REMERON®

During its premarketing assessment, multiple doses of REMERON® (mirtazapine) Tablets were administered to 2,796 patients in clinical studies. The conditions and duration of exposure to mirtazapine varied greatly, and included (in overlapping categories) open and double-blind studies, uncontrolled and controlled studies, inpatient and outpatient studies, fixed dose and titration studies. Untoward events associated with this exposure were recorded by clinical investigators using terminology of their own choosing. Consequently, it is not possible to provide a meaningful estimate of the proportion of individuals experiencing adverse events without first grouping similar types of untoward events into a smaller number of standardized event categories.

In the tabulations that follow, reported adverse events were classified using a standard COSTART-based dictionary terminology. The frequencies presented, therefore, represent the proportion of the 2,796 patients exposed to multiple doses of REMERON® who experienced an event of the type cited on at least one occasion while receiving REMERON®. All reported events are included except those already listed in the previous table, those adverse experiences subsumed under COSTART terms that are either overly general or excessively specific so as to be uninformative, and those events for which a drug cause was very remote.

It is important to emphasize that, although the events reported occurred during treatment with REMERON®, they were not necessarily caused by it.

Events are further categorized by body system and listed in order of decreasing frequency according to the following definitions: frequent adverse events are those occurring on one or more occasions in at least 1/100 patients; infrequent adverse events are those occurring in 1/100 to 1/1000 patients; rare events are those occurring in fewer than 1/1000 patients. Only those events not already listed in the previous table appear in this listing. Events of major clinical importance are also described in the WARNINGS and PRECAUTIONS sections.

Body as a Whole: *frequent:* malaise, abdominal pain, abdominal syndrome acute; *infrequent:* chills, fever, face edema, ulcer, photosensitivity reaction, neck rigidity, neck pain, abdomen enlarged; *rare:* cellulitis, chest pain substernal.

Cardiovascular System: *frequent:* hypertension, vasodilatation; *infrequent:* angina pectoris, myocardial infarction, bradycardia, ventricular extrasystoles, syncope, migraine, hypotension; *rare:* atrial arrhythmia, bigeminy, vascular headache, pulmonary embolus, cerebral ischemia, cardiomegaly, phlebitis, left heart failure.

Digestive System: *frequent:* vomiting, anorexia; *infrequent:* eructation, glossitis, cholecystitis, nausea and vomiting, gum hemorrhage, stomatitis, colitis, liver function tests abnormal; *rare:* tongue discoloration, ulcerative stomatitis, salivary gland enlargement, increased salivation, intestinal obstruction, pancreatitis, aphthous stomatitis, cirrhosis of liver, gastritis, gastroenteritis, oral moniliasis, tongue edema.

Endocrine System: *rare:* goiter, hypothyroidism.

Hemic and Lymphatic System: *rare:* lymphadenopathy, leukopenia, petechia, anemia, thrombocytopenia, lymphocytosis, pancytopenia.

Metabolic and Nutritional Disorders: *frequent:* thirst; *infrequent:* dehydration, weight loss; *rare:* gout, SGOT increased, healing abnormal, acid phosphatase increased, SGPT increased, diabetes mellitus.

Musculoskeletal System: *frequent:* myasthenia, arthralgia; *infrequent:* arthritis, tenosynovitis; *rare:* pathologic fracture, osteoporosis fracture, bone pain, myositis, tendon rupture, arthrosis, bursitis.
Nervous System: *frequent:* hypesthesia, apathy, depression, hypokinesia, vertigo, twitching, agitation, anxiety, amnesia, hyperkinesia, paresthesia; *infrequent:* ataxia, delirium, delusions, depersonalization, dyskinesia, extrapyramidal syndrome, libido increased, coordination abnormal, dysarthria, hallucinations, manic reaction, neurosis, dystonia, hostility, reflexes increased, emotional lability, euphoria, paranoid reaction; *rare:* aphasia, nystagmus, akathisia, stupor, dementia, diplopia, drug dependence, paralysis, grand mal convulsion, hypotonia, myoclonus, psychotic depression, withdrawal syndrome.
Respiratory System: *frequent:* cough increased, sinusitis; *infrequent:* epistaxis, bronchitis, asthma, pneumonia; *rare:* asphyxia, laryngitis, pneumothorax, hiccup.
Skin and Appendages: *frequent:* pruritus, rash; *infrequent:* acne, exfoliative dermatitis, dry skin, herpes simplex, alopecia; *rare:* urticaria, herpes zoster, skin hypertrophy, seborrhea, skin ulcer.
Special Senses: *infrequent:* eye pain, abnormality of accommodation, conjunctivitis, deafness, keratoconjunctivitis, lacrimation disorder, glaucoma, hyperacusis, ear pain; *rare:* blepharitis, partial transitory deafness, otitis media, taste loss, parosmia.
Urogenital System: *frequent:* urinary tract infection; *infrequent:* kidney calculus, cystitis, dysuria, urinary incontinence, urinary retention, vaginitis, hematuria, breast pain, amenorrhea, dysmenorrhea, leukorrhea, impotence; *rare:* polyuria, urethritis, metrorrhagia, menorrhagia, abnormal ejaculation, breast engorgement, breast enlargement, urinary urgency.

DRUG ABUSE AND DEPENDENCE

Controlled Substance Class
REMERON® (mirtazapine) Tablets are not a controlled substance.

Physical and Psychological Dependence
REMERON® (mirtazapine) Tablets has not been systematically studied in animals or humans for its potential for abuse, tolerance or physical dependence. While clinical trials did not reveal any tendency for any drug-seeking behavior, these observations were not systematic and it is not possible to predict on the basis of this limited experience the extent to which a CNS-active drug will be misused, diverted and/or abused once marketed. Consequently, patients should be evaluated carefully for history of drug abuse, and such patients should be observed closely for signs of REMERON® misuse or abuse (e.g., development of tolerance, incrementations of dose, drug-seeking behavior).

OVERDOSAGE

Human Experience
There is very limited experience with REMERON® (mirtazapine) Tablets overdose. In premarketing clinical studies, there were eight reports of REMERON® overdose alone or in combination with other pharmacological agents. The only drug overdose death reported while taking REMERON® was in combination with amitriptyline and chlorprothixene in a non-U.S. clinical study. Based on plasma levels, the REMERON® dose taken was 30–45 mg, while plasma levels of amitriptyline and chlorprothixene were found to be at toxic levels. All other premarketing overdose cases resulted in full recovery. Signs and symptoms reported in association with overdose included disorientation, drowsiness, impaired memory, and tachycardia. There were no reports of ECG abnormalities, coma or convulsions following overdose with REMERON® alone.

Overdose Management
Treatment should consist of those general measures employed in the management of overdose with any antidepressant. Ensure an adequate airway, oxygenation, and ventilation. Monitor cardiac rhythm and vital signs. General supportive and symptomatic measures are also recommended. Indication of emesis is not recommended. Gastric lavage with a large-bore orogastric tube with appropriate airway protection, if needed, may be indicated if performed soon after ingestion, or in symptomatic patients.
Activated charcoal should be administered. There is no experience with the use of forced diuresis, dialysis, hemoperfusion or exchange transfusion in the treatment of mirtazapine overdosage. No specific antidotes for mirtazapine are known.
In managing overdosage, consider the possibility of multiple-drug involvement. The physician should consider contacting a poison control center for additional information on the treatment of any overdose. Telephone numbers for certified poison control centers are listed in the *Physicians' Desk Reference* (PDR).

DOSAGE AND ADMINISTRATION

Initial Treatment
The recommended starting dose for REMERON® (mirtazapine) Tablets is 15 mg/day, administered in a single dose, preferably in the evening prior to sleep. In the controlled clinical trials establishing the antidepressant efficacy of REMERON®, the effective dose range was generally 15–45 mg/day. While the relationship between dose and antidepressant response for REMERON® has not been adequately explored, patients not responding to the initial 15 mg dose may benefit from dose increases up to a maximum of 45 mg/day. REMERON® has an elimination half-life of approximately 20–40 hours; therefore, dose changes should not be made at intervals of less than one to two weeks in order to allow sufficient time for evaluation of the therapeutic response to a given dose.

Elderly and Patients with Renal or Hepatic Impairment
The clearance of mirtazapine is reduced in elderly patients and in patients with moderate to severe renal or hepatic impairment. Consequently, the prescriber should be aware that plasma mirtazapine levels may be increased in these patient groups, compared to levels observed in younger adults without renal or hepatic impairment (see PRECAUTIONS and CLINICAL PHARMACOLOGY).

Maintenance/Extended Treatment
There is no body of evidence available from controlled trials to indicate how long the depressed patient should be treated with REMERON® (mirtazapine) Tablets. It is generally agreed, however, that pharmacological treatment for acute episodes of depression should continue for up to six months or longer. Whether the dose of antidepressant needed to induce remission is identical to the dose needed to maintain euthymia is unknown.

Switching Patients To or From a Monoamine Oxidase Inhibitor
At least 14 days should elapse between discontinuation of an MAOI and initiation of therapy with REMERON® (mirtazapine) Tablets. In addition, at least 14 days should be allowed after stopping REMERON® before starting an MAOI.

HOW SUPPLIED

REMERON® (mirtazapine) Tablets are supplied as:
15 mg Tablets — oval, scored, yellow, coated, with "Organon" debossed on one side and "TZ/3" on the other side.

Bottles of 30	NDC 0052-0105-30
Bottles of 100	NDC 0052-0105-91
Unit Dose, Box of 100	NDC 0052-0105-90*

30 mg Tablets — oval, scored, red-brown, coated, with "Organon" debossed on one side and "TZ/5" on the other side.

Bottles of 30	NDC 0052-0107-30
Bottles of 100	NDC 0052-0107-91
Unit Dose, Box of 100	NDC 0052-0107-90*

45 mg Tablets — oval, white, coated, with "Organon" debossed on one side and "TZ/7" on the other side.

Bottles of 30	NDC 0052-0109-30

*Unit dose packs are provided as a blisterpack with 10 strips, each of which contains 10 tablets.

Storage
Store at 25°C (77°F); excursions permitted to 15–30°C (59–86°F) [see USP Controlled Room Temperature]. Protect from light and moisture.

Rx only

Organon
Manufactured for Organon Inc.
West Orange, NJ 07052
by N.V. Organon, OSS, The Netherlands
5310179 3/99 07

Shown in Product Identification Guide, page 327

REVERSOL® ℞
(edrophonium chloride) injection, USP

HOW SUPPLIED

10 mg/mL: 10 mL Multiple Dose Vials-boxes of 25-NDC-0052-0466-34

SUCCINYLCHOLINE CHLORIDE INJECTION, USP ℞

HOW SUPPLIED

20 mg/mL: 10 mL vials-boxes of 25-NDC-0052-0445-10

BCG LIVE
(FOR INTRAVESICAL USE)
TICE® BCG ℞

WARNING
TICE® BCG contains live, attenuated mycobacteria. Because of the potential risk for transmission, it should be prepared, handled, and disposed of as a biohazard material (see PRECAUTIONS and DOSAGE AND ADMINISTRATION).
BCG infections have been reported in health care workers, primarily from exposures resulting from accidental needle sticks or skin lacerations during the preparation of BCG for administration. Nosocomial infections have been reported in patients receiving parenteral drugs that were prepared in areas in which BCG was reconstituted. BCG is capable of dissemination when administered by the intravesical route, and serious infections, including fatal infections, have been reported in patients receiving intravesical BCG (see WARNINGS, PRECAUTIONS, and ADVERSE REACTIONS).

DESCRIPTION

TICE® BCG for intravesical use, is an attenuated, live culture preparation of the Bacillus of Calmette and Guerin (BCG) strain of *Mycobacterium bovis.*[1] The TICE® strain was developed at the University of Illinois from a strain originated at the Pasteur Institute.
The medium in which the BCG organism is grown for preparation of the freeze-dried cake is composed of the following ingredients: glycerin, asparagine, citric acid, potassium phosphate, magnesium sulfate, and iron ammonium citrate. The final preparation prior to freeze drying also contains lactose. The freeze-dried BCG preparation is delivered in glass vials, each containing 1 to 8×10^8 colony forming units (CFU) of TICE® BCG which is equivalent to approximately 50 mg wet weight. Determination of *in-vitro* potency is achieved through colony counts derived from a serial dilution assay. A single dose consists of 1 reconstituted vial (See DOSAGE AND ADMINISTRATION).
For intravesical use the entire vial is reconstituted with sterile saline. TICE® BCG is viable upon reconstitution. No preservatives have been added.

CLINICAL PHARMACOLOGY

TICE® BCG induces a granulomatous reaction at the local site of administration. Intravesical TICE® BCG has been used as a therapy for, and prophylaxis against, recurrent tumors in patients with carcinoma *in situ* (CIS) of the urinary bladder, and to prevent recurrence of Stage TaT1 papillary tumors of the bladder at high risk of recurrence. The precise mechanism of action is unknown.

CLINICAL STUDIES

To evaluate the efficacy of intravesical administration of TICE® BCG in the treatment of carcinoma *in situ*, patients were identified who had been treated with TICE® BCG under six different Investigational New Drug (IND) applications in which the most important shared aspect was the use of an induction plus maintenance schedule. Patients received TICE® BCG (50 mg; 1 - 8×10^8 CFU) intravesically, once weekly for at least 6 weeks and once monthly thereafter for up to 12 months. A longer maintenance was given in some cases. The study population consisted of 153 patients, 132 males, 19 females, and 2 unidentified as to gender. Thirty patients lacking baseline documentation of CIS and four patients lost to follow-up were not evaluable for treatment response. Therefore, 119 patients were available for efficacy evaluation. The mean age was 69 years (range: 38–97 years). There were two categories of clinical response: (1) Complete Histological Response (CR), defined as complete resolution of carcinoma *in situ* documented by cystoscopy and cytology, with or without biopsy; and (2) Complete Clinical Response Without Cytology (CRNC), defined as an apparent complete disappearance of tumor upon cystoscopy. The results of a 1987 analysis of the evaluable patients are shown in Table I.
[See table I at top of next page]
A 1989 update of these data is presented in Table II. The median duration of follow-up was 47 months.
[See table II at top of next page]
There was no significant difference in response rates between patients with or without prior intravesical chemotherapy. The median duration of response, calculated from the Kaplan-Meier curve as median time to recurrence, is estimated at 4 years or greater. The incidence of cystectomy for 90 patients who achieved a complete response (CR or CRNC) was 11%. The median time to cystectomy in patients who achieved a complete response (CR or CRNC) exceeded 74 months.
The efficacy of intravesical TICE® BCG in preventing the recurrence of a TaT1 bladder cancer after complete transurethral resection of all papillary tumors was evaluated in two open-label randomized phase III clinical trials. Initial diagnosis of patients included in the studies was determined by cystoscopic biopsies. One was conducted by the Southwestern Oncology Group (SWOG) in patients at high risk of recurrence. High risk was defined as two occurrences of tumor within 56 weeks, any stage T1 tumor, or three or more tumors presenting simultaneously. The second study was conducted at the Nijmegen University Hospital; Nijmegen, The Netherlands. In this study patients were not selected for high risk of recurrence. In both studies treatment was initiated between 1 and 2 weeks after TUR.
In the SWOG trial (study 8795) patients were randomized to TICE® BCG or mitomycin C (MMC). Both drugs were given intravesically weekly for 6 weeks, at 8 and 12 weeks, and then monthly for a total treatment duration of 1 year. Cystoscopy and urinary cytology were performed every 3 months for 2 years. Patients with progressive disease or residual or recurrent disease at or after the 6 month follow-up were removed from the study and were classified as treatment failures.
A total of 469 patients was entered into the study: 237 to the TICE® BCG arm and 232 to the MMC arm. Twenty-two patients were subsequently found to be ineligible, and 66 patients had concurrent CIS, and were analyzed separately. Four patients were lost to follow-up, leaving 191 evaluable patients in the TICE® BCG arm and 186 in the MMC arm. Of the patients, 84% were male and 16% were female. The average age of these patients was 65 years old.
The Kaplan-Meier estimates of 2 year disease-free survival are shown in Table III. The difference in disease-free survival time between the two groups was statistically significant by the log rank test (p=0.03). The 95% confidence interval of the difference in 2 year disease-free survival was 12% ± 10%. No statistically significant differences between the groups were noted in time to tumor progression, tumor invasion, or overall survival.
[See table III at top of next page]

Continued on next page

Tice BCG—Cont.

In the Nijmegen study, the efficacy of three treatments was compared: TICE substrain BCG, *Rijksinstituut voor Volksgezondheid en Milieuhygiene* substrain BCG (BCG-RIVM), and MMC.

TICE® BCG and BCG-RIVM were given intravesically weekly for 6 weeks. In contrast to the SWOG study, maintenance BCG was not given. Mitomycin C was given intravesically weekly for 4 weeks and then monthly for a total duration of treatment of 6 months. Cystoscopy and urinary cytology were performed every 3 months until recurrence.

A total of 469 patients was enrolled and randomized. Thirty-two patients were not evaluable, 17 were ineligible, 15 were withdrawn before treatment, and 50 had concurrent CIS and were analyzed separately, leaving 387 evaluable patients: 117 in the TICE® BCG arm, 134 in the BCG-RIVM arm, and 136 in the MMC arm. Twenty-eight patients (24%) in the TICE® BCG arm, 32 patients (24%) in the BCG-RIVM arm and 24 patients (18%) in the MMC arm had TaG1 tumors. The median duration of follow-up was 22 months (range 3–54 months).

The Kaplan-Meier estimates of 2 year disease-free survival are shown in Table IV. The differences in disease-free survival among the three arms were not statistically significant by the log-rank test (p=0.08).

[See table IV above]

In both the SWOG 8795 study and the Nijmegen study, acute toxicity was more common, and usually more severe, with TICE® BCG than with MMC (see ADVERSE REACTIONS).

TABLE I: THE RESPONSE OF PATIENTS WITH CIS BLADDER CANCER IN SIX IND STUDIES

	Entered	Evaluable	CR	CRNC	Overall Response
No. (%)Of Patients	153	119 (78%)	54 (46%)	36 (30%)	90 (76%)

TABLE II: FOLLOW-UP RESPONSE OF PATIENTS WITH CIS BLADDER CANCER IN SIX IND STUDIES

	1989 Status of 90 Responders (CR or CRNC)			
Response	1987/CR n = 54	1987/CRNC n = 36	1987 Response n = 90	Percent
CR	30	15	45	50
CRNC	0	0	0	0
Unrelated Deaths	6	6	12	13
Failure	18	15	33	37

TABLE III: RESULTS OF SWOG STUDY 8795

	TICE® BCG Arm N = 191	MMC Arm N = 186
Estimated Disease-Free Survival at 2 years	57%	45%
95% Confidence Interval (CI)	(50%, 65%)	(38%, 53%)

TABLE IV: RESULTS OF NIJMEGEN STUDY

	TICE® BCG Arm N = 117	BCG-RIVM Arm N = 134	MMC Arm N = 136
Estimated Disease-Free Survival at 2 years	53%	62%	64%
95% Confidence Interval (CI)	(44%, 64%)	(53%, 72%)	(55%, 74%)

INDICATIONS AND USAGE

TICE® BCG is indicated for the treatment and prophylaxis of carcinoma *in situ* (CIS) of the urinary bladder, and for the prophylaxis of primary or recurrent stage Ta and/or T1 papillary tumors following transurethral resection (TUR). TICE® BCG is not recommended for stage TaG1 papillary tumors, unless they are judged to be at high risk of tumor recurrence.

TICE® BCG is not indicated for papillary tumors of stages higher than T1.

CONTRAINDICATIONS

TICE® BCG should not be used in immunosuppressed patients or persons with congenital or acquired immune deficiencies, whether due to concurrent disease (e.g., AIDS, leukemia, lymphoma) cancer therapy (e.g., cytotoxic drugs, radiation) or immunosuppressive therapy (e.g. corticosteroids).

Treatment should be postponed until resolution of a concurrent febrile illness, urinary tract infection, or gross hematuria. Seven to 14 days should elapse before BCG is administered following biopsy, TUR, or traumatic catheterization.

TICE® BCG should not be administered to persons with active tuberculosis. Active tuberculosis should be ruled out in individuals who are PPD positive before starting treatment with TICE® BCG.

WARNINGS

BCG LIVE (TICE® BCG) is not a vaccine for the prevention of cancer. BCG Vaccine, U.S.P., not BCG LIVE (TICE® BCG), should be used for the prevention of tuberculosis. For vaccination use, refer to BCG Vaccine, U.S.P. prescribing information.

TICE® BCG is an infectious agent. Physicians using this product should be familiar with the literature on the prevention and treatment of BCG-related complications, and should be prepared in such emergencies to contact an infectious disease specialist with experience in treating the infectious complications of intravesical BCG. The treatment of the infectious complications of BCG requires long-term, multiple-drug antibiotic therapy. Special culture media are required for mycobacteria, and physicians administering intravesical BCG or those caring for these patients should have these media readily available.

Instillation of TICE® BCG with an actively bleeding mucosa may promote systemic BCG infection. Treatment should be postponed for at least one week following transurethral resection, biopsy, traumatic catheterization, or gross hematuria.

Deaths have been reported as a result of systemic BCG infection and sepsis.[2,3] Patients should be monitored for the presence of symptoms and signs of toxicity after each intravesical treatment. Febrile episodes with flu-like symptoms lasting more than 72 hours, fever ≥ 103°F, systemic manifestations increasing in intensity with repeated instillations, or persistent abnormalities of liver function tests suggest systemic BCG infection and may require antituberculous therapy. Local symptoms (prostatitis, epididymitis, orchitis) lasting more than 2–3 days may also suggest active infection (See ***Management of Serious BCG Complications*** subsection of WARNINGS).

The use of TICE® BCG may cause tuberculin sensitivity. Since this is a valuable aid in the diagnosis of tuberculosis, it is advisable to determine the tuberculin reactivity by PPD skin testing before treatment.

Intravesical instillations of BCG should be postponed during treatment with antibiotics, since antimicrobial therapy may interfere with the effectiveness of TICE® BCG (see PRECAUTIONS). TICE® BCG should not be used in individuals with concurrent infections.

Small bladder capacity has been associated with increased risk of severe local reactions and should be considered in deciding to use TICE® BCG therapy.

Management of Serious BCG Complications.

Acute, localized irritative toxicities of TICE® BCG may be accompanied by systemic manifestations, consistent with a "flu-like" syndrome. Systemic adverse effects of 1–2 days' duration such as malaise, fever, and chills often reflect hypersensitivity reactions. However, **symptoms such as fever of ≥ 38.5°C (101.3°F), or acute localized inflammation such as epididymitis, prostatitis, or orchitis persisting longer than 2–3 days suggest active infection, and evaluation for serious infectious complication should be considered.**

In patients who develop persistent fever or experience an acute febrile illness consistent with BCG infection, two or more antimycobacterial agents should be administered while diagnostic evaluation, including cultures, is conducted. **BCG treatment should be discontinued.** Negative cultures do not necessarily rule out infection. Physicians using this product should be familiar with the literature on prevention, diagnosis, and treatment of BCG-related complications and, when appropriate, should consult an infectious disease specialist or other physician with experience in the diagnosis and treatment of mycobacterial infections.

TICE® BCG is sensitive to the most commonly used antituberculous agents (isoniazid, rifampin and ethambutol). **TICE® BCG is not sensitive to pyrazinamide.**

PRECAUTIONS

General

TICE® BCG contains live mycobacteria and should be prepared and handled using aseptic technique (See **Preparation of Agent** subsection of DOSAGE AND ADMINISTRATION). BCG infections have been reported in health care workers preparing BCG for administration. Needle stick injuries should be avoided during the handling and mixing of TICE® BCG. Nosocomial infections have been reported in patients receiving parenteral drugs which were prepared in areas in which BCG was prepared.[4]

BCG is capable of dissemination when administered by intravesical route and serious reactions, including fatal infections, have been reported in patients receiving intravesical BCG.[3] Care should be taken not to traumatize the urinary tract or to introduce contaminants into the urinary system. Seven to 14 days should elapse before TICE® BCG is administered following TUR, biopsy, or traumatic catheterization.

TICE® BCG should be administered with caution to persons in groups at high risk for HIV infection.

Laboratory Tests

The use of TICE® BCG may cause tuberculin sensitivity. It is advisable to determine the tuberculin reactivity of patients receiving TICE® BCG by PPD skin testing before treatment is initiated.

Information for Patients

TICE® BCG is retained in the bladder for 2 hours and then voided. Patients should void while seated in order to avoid splashing of urine. For the 6 hours after treatment, urine voided should be disinfected for 15 minutes with an equal volume of household bleach before flushing. Patients should be instructed to increase fluid intake in order to "flush" the bladder in the hours following BCG treatment. Patients may experience burning with the first void after treatment. Patients should be attentive to side effects, such as fever, chills, malaise, flu-like symptoms, or increased fatigue. If the patient experiences severe urinary side effects, such as burning or pain on urination, urgency, frequency of urination, blood in urine, or other symptoms such as joint pain, cough, or skin rash, the physician should be notified.

Drug Interaction

Drug combinations containing immunosuppressants and/or bone marrow depressants and/or radiation interfere with the development of the immune response and should not be used in combination with TICE® BCG. Antimicrobial therapy for other infections may interfere with the effectiveness of TICE® BCG. There are no data to suggest that the acute, local urinary tract toxicity common with BCG is due to mycobacterial infection and **antituberculosis drugs (e.g. isoniazid) should not be used to prevent or treat the local, irritative toxicities of TICE® BCG.**

Carcinogenesis, Mutagenesis, Impairment of Fertility

TICE® BCG has not been evaluated for its carcinogenic, mutagenic potentials or impairment of fertility.

Pregnancy

Teratogenic Effects – Pregnancy Category C

Animal reproduction studies have not been conducted with TICE® BCG. It is also not known whether TICE® BCG can cause fetal harm when administered to a pregnant woman or can affect reproductive capacity. TICE® BCG should not be given to a pregnant woman except when clearly needed. Women should be advised not to become pregnant while on therapy.

Nursing Mothers

It is not known whether TICE® BCG is excreted in human milk. Because many drugs are excreted in human milk and because of the potential for serious adverse reactions from TICE® BCG in nursing infants, it is advisable to discontinue nursing or to discontinue the drug, taking into account the importance of the drug to the mother.

Pediatric Use

Safety and effectiveness of TICE® BCG for the treatment of superficial bladder cancer in pediatric patients have not been established.

Geriatric Use

Of the total number of subjects in clinical studies of TICE® BCG, the average age was 66 years old. No overall difference in safety or effectiveness was observed between older and younger subjects. Other reported clinical experience has not identified differences in response between elderly and younger patients, but greater sensitivity of some older individual to BCG cannot be ruled out.

ADVERSE REACTIONS

Symptoms of bladder irritability, related to the inflammatory response induced, are reported in approximately 60% of patients receiving TICE® BCG. The symptoms typically begin 4–6 hours after instillation and last 24–72 hours. The irritative side effects are usually seen following the third instillation, and tend to increase in severity after each administration.

The irritative bladder adverse effects can usually be managed symptomatically with products such as pyridium, propantheline bromide, oxybutynin chloride and acetaminophen. The mechanism of action of the irritative side effects has not been firmly established, but is most consistent with an immunological mechanism.[3] There is no evidence that dose reduction or antituberculous drug therapy can prevent or lessen the irritative toxicity of TICE® BCG.

"Flu-like" symptoms (malaise, fever, and chills) which may accompany the localized, irritative toxicities often reflect hypersensitivity reactions which can be treated symptomatically. Antihistamines have also been used.[5]

Adverse reactions to TICE® BCG tend to be progressive in frequency and severity with subsequent instillation. Delay or postponement of subsequent treatment may or may not reduce the severity of a reaction during subsequent instillation.

Although uncommon, serious infectious complications of intravesical BCG have been reported.[2,3,6] The most serious infectious complication of BCG is disseminated sepsis with associated mortality. In addition, *M. bovis* infections have been reported in lung, liver, bone, bone marrow, kidney, regional lymph nodes, and prostate in patients who have received intravesical BCG. Some male genitourinary tract in-

TABLE V: SUMMARY OF ADVERSE EFFECTS SEEN IN 674 PATIENTS WITH SUPERFICIAL BLADDER CANCER, INCLUDING 153 WITH CARCINOMA *IN SITU*

Adverse Event	N	Overall (Grade ≥3)	Adverse Event	N	Overall (Grade ≥3)
	Percent of Patients			Percent of Patients	
Dysuria	401	60% (11%)	Arthritis/Myalgia	18	3% (<1%)
Urinary Frequency	272	40% (7%)	Headache/Dizziness	16	2% (0)
Flu-Like Syndrome	224	33% (9%)	Urinary Incontinence	16	2% (0)
Hematuria	175	26% (7%)	Anorexia/Weight Loss	15	2% (<1%)
Fever	134	20% (8%)	Urinary Debris	15	2% (<1%)
Malaise/Fatigue	50	7% (0)	Allergy	14	2% (<1%)
Cystitis	40	6% (2%)	Cardiac (Unclassified)	13	2% (1%)
Urgency	39	6% (1%)	Genital Inflammation/ Abscess	12	2% (<1%)
Nocturia	30	5% (1%)	Respiratory (Unclassified)	11	2% (<1%)
Cramps/Pain	27	4% (1%)	Urinary Tract Infection	10	2% (1%)
Rigors	22	3% (1%)	Abdominal Pain	10	2% (1%)
Nausea/Vomiting	20	3% (<1%)			

TABLE VI: MOST COMMON ADVERSE REACTIONS IN SWOG STUDY 8795*

	Study Arm			
	TICE® BCG (N = 222)		MMC (N = 220)	
Adverse Event	All Grades	Grade ≥3	All Grades	Grade ≥3
Dysuria	115 (52%)	6 (3%)	77 (35%)	5 (2%)
Urgency/Frequency	112 (50%)	5 (2%)	63 (29%)	7 (3%)
Hematuria	85 (38%)	6 (3%)	56 (25%)	5 (2%)
Flu-Like Symptoms	54 (24%)	1 (<1%)	29 (13%)	0
Fever	37 (17%)	1 (<1%)	7 (3%)	0
Pain (Not Specified)	37 (17%)	4 (2%)	22 (10%)	1 (<1%)
Hemorrhagic Cystitis	19 (9%)	3 (1%)	10 (5%)	0
Chills	19 (9%)	0	2 (1%)	0
Bladder Cramps	18 (8%)	0	9 (4%)	0
Nausea	16 (7%)	0	12 (5%)	0
Incontinence	8 (4%)	0	3 (1%)	0
Myalgia/Arthralgia	7 (3%)	0	0	0
Diaphoresis	7 (3%)	0	1 (<1%)	0
Rash	6 (3%)	1 (<1%)	16 (7%)	2 (1%)

*The adverse reaction profile of TICE® BCG was similar in the Nijmegen study.[8]

fections (orchitis/epididymitis) have been resistant to multiple drug antituberculous therapy and required orchiectomy.

If a patient develops persistent fever or experiences an acute febrile illness consistent with BCG infection, BCG treatment should be discontinued and the patient immediately evaluated and treated for systemic infection (See Warnings).

The local and systemic adverse reactions reported in a review of 674 patients with superficial bladder cancer, including 153 patient with carcinoma *in situ*, are summarized in Table V.

[See table V above]

The following adverse events were reported in ≤1% of patients: anemia, BCG sepsis, coagulopathy, contracted bladder, diarrhea, epididymitis/prostatitis, hepatic granuloma, hepatitis, leukopenia, neurologic (unclassified), orchitis, pneumonitis, pyuria, rash, thrombocytopenia, urethritis, and urinary obstruction.

In SWOG study 8795, toxicity evaluations were available on a total of 222 TICE® BCG-treated patients and 220 MMC-treated patients. Direct bladder toxicity (cramps, dysuria, frequency, urgency, hematuria, hemorrhagic cystitis, or incontinence) was seen more often with TICE® BCG, with 356 events compared to 234 events for MMC. Grade ≤ 2 toxicity was seen significantly more frequently following TICE® BCG treatment (p=0.003). No life-threatening toxicity was seen in either arm. Systemic toxicity with TICE® BCG was markedly increased compared to that of MMC, with 181 events for TICE® BCG compared to 80 for MMC. The frequency of toxicity was increased in all grades, particularly for grades 2 and 3. The most common complaints were malaise, fatigue and lethargy, fever, and abdominal pain. Thirty-two TICE® BCG patients were reported to have been treated with isoniazid. Five TICE® BCG patients had liver enzyme elevation, including two with grade 3 elevations. Eighteen of the 222 (8.1%) TICE® BCG patients failed to complete the prescribed protocol compared to 6.2% in the MMC group. Table VI summarizes the most common adverse reactions reported in this trial.[7]

[See table VI above]

OVERDOSAGE

Overdosage occurs if more than one vial of TICE® BCG is administered per instillation. If overdosage occurs, the patient should be closely monitored for signs of active local or systemic BCG infection. For acute local or systemic reactions suggesting active infection, an infectious disease specialist experienced in BCG complications should be consulted.

DOSAGE AND ADMINISTRATION

The dose for the intravesical treatment of carcinoma *in situ* and for the prophylaxis of recurrent papillary tumors consists of one vial of TICE® BCG suspended in 50 ml preservative-free saline.

Do not inject subcutaneously or intravenously.

Preparation of Agent

The preparation of the TICE® BCG suspension should be done using aseptic technique. To avoid cross-contamination, parenteral drugs should not be prepared in areas where BCG has been prepared. A separate area for the preparation of the TICE® BCG suspension is recommended. All equipment, supplies and receptacles in contact with TICE® BCG should be handled and disposed of as biohazardous. The pharmacist or individual responsible for mixing the agent should wear gloves and take precautions to avoid contact of BCG with broken skin. If preparation cannot be performed in a biocontainment hood, then a mask and gown should be worn to avoid inhalation of BCG organisms and inadvertent exposure to broken skin.

Draw 1 ml of sterile, preservative-free saline (0.9% Sodium Chloride Injection U.S.P.) at 4–25°C, into a small syringe (e.g., 3 ml) and add to one vial of TICE® BCG to resuspend. Gently swirl the vial until a homogenous suspension is obtained. Avoid forceful agitation which may cause clumping of the mycobacteria.

Dispense the cloudy TICE® BCG suspension into the top end of a catheter-tip syringe which contains 49 ml of saline diluent, bringing the total volume to 50 ml. To mix, gently rotate the syringe. The suspended TICE® BCG should be used immediately after preparation. Discard after two hours.

Note: DO NOT filter the contents of the TICE® BCG vial. Precautions should be taken to avoid exposing the TICE® BCG to direct sunlight. Bacteriostatic solutions must be avoided. In addition, use only sterile preservative-free saline, 0.9% Sodium Chloride Injection U.S.P. as diluent.

Treatment and Schedule

Allow 7–14 days to elapse after bladder biopsy before TICE® BCG is administered. Patients should not drink fluids for 4 hours before treatment and should empty their bladder prior to TICE® BCG administration. The reconstituted TICE® BCG is instilled into the bladder by gravity flow via the catheter. **DO NOT** depress plunger and force the flow of the TICE® BCG. The TICE® BCG is retained in the bladder 2 hours and then voided. Patients unable to retain the suspension for 2 hours should be allowed to void sooner, if necessary.

While the BCG is retained in the bladder, the patient ideally should be repositioned from left side to right side and also should lie upon the back and the abdomen, changing these positions every 15 minutes to maximize bladder surface exposure to the agent.

A standard treatment schedule consists of one intravesical instillation per week for 6 weeks. This schedule may be repeated once if tumor remission has not been achieved and if the clinical circumstances warrant. Thereafter, intravesical TICE® BCG administration should continue at approximately monthly intervals for at least 6–12 months. There are no data to support the interchangeability of BCG LIVE products.

HOW SUPPLIED

TICE® BCG is supplied in a box of one vial of TICE® BCG. Each vial contains 1 to 8 × 10^8 CFU, which is equivalent to approximately 50 mg (wet weight), as lyophilized (freeze-dried) powder, NDC 0052-0602-02.

STORAGE

The intact vials of TICE® BCG should be stored refrigerated, at 2–8°C (36–46°F).

This agent contains live bacteria and should be protected from **direct** sunlight. The product should not be used after the expiration date printed on the label.

Rx Only

REFERENCES

1. DeJager R, Guinan P, Lamm D, Khanna O, Brosman S, DeKernion J, et al. Long-Term Complete Remission in Bladder Carcinoma in Situ with Intravesical TICE Bacillus Calmette Guerin. *Urology* 1991;38:507–513.
2. Rawls WH, Lamm DL, Lowe BA, Crawford ED, Sarosdy MF, Montie JE, Grossman HB, Scardino PT. Fatal Sepsis Following Intravesical Bacillus Calmette-Guerin Administration For Bladder Cancer. *J Urol* 1990;144: 1328–1330.
3. Lamm DL, van der Meijden APM, Morales A, Brosman SA, Catalona WJ, Herr HW, et al. Incidence and Treatment of Complications of Bacillus Calmette-Guerin Intravesical Therapy in Superficial Bladder Cancer. *J. Urol* 1992; 147: 596–600.
4. Stone MM, Vannier AM, Storch SK, Nitta AT, Zhang Y. Brief Report: Meningitis Due to Iatrogenic BCG Infection in Two Immunocompromised Children. *NEJM* 1995: 333: 561–563.
5. Steg A, Leleu C, Debre B, Gibod-Boccon L, Sicard D. Systemic Bacillus Calmette-Guerin Infection in Patients Treated by Intravesical BCG Therapy for Superficial Bladder Cancer. *EORTC Genitourinary Group Monograph 6: BCG in Superficial Bladder Cancer*. Edited by F.M. J. Debruyne, L. Denis and A.P.M. van der Meijden. New York: Alan R. Liss Inc., pp. 325–334.
6. van der Meijden, APM. Practical Approaches to the Prevention and Treatment of Adverse Reactions to BCG. *Eur Urol* 1995;27(suppl 1):23–28.
7. Lamm DL, Blumenstein BA, Crawford ED, Crissman JD, Lowe BA, Smith JA, Sarosdy MF, Schellhammer PF, Sagalowsky AI, Messing EM, et al. Randomized Intergroup Comparison of Bacillus Calmette-Guerin Immunotherapy and Mitomycin C Chemotherapy Prophylaxis in Superficial Transitional Cell Carcinoma of the Bladder. *Urol Oncol* 1995; 1:119–126.
8. Witjes JA, van der Meijden APM, Witjes WPJ, et al. A Randomized Prospective Study Comparing Intravesical Instillations of Mitomycin-C, BCG-Tice, and BCG-RIVM in pTa-pT1 Tumours and Primary Carcinoma *In Situ* of the Urinary Bladder. *Eur J Cancer* 1993;29A(12):1672–1676.

Manufactured for: Organon, Inc.
West Orange, NJ 07052
Manufactured by: Organon Teknika Corporation
100 Akzo Avenue
Durham, NC 27712
U.S. License No. 956

TICE® is a registered trademark owned by the University of Illinois and licensed to Organon Teknika Corporation.

RM129 November 1998

Shown in Product Identification Guide, page 327

WIGRAINE® ℞

(ergotamine tartrate and caffeine tablets, USP)

DESCRIPTION

Wigraine® Tablets: Each tablet contains the following:
Ergotamine Tartrate, USP .... 1 mg
Caffeine, USP .... 100 mg

Each tablet also contains: Lactose, Magnesium Stearate, Microcrystalline Cellulose, Corn Starch, Glycerin, Acacia Powder, Colloidal Silicon Dioxide, and Purified Water as inactive ingredients.

Wigraine® tablets are uncoated and prepared to insure rapid disintegration (by an exclusive manufacturing process) and facilitate quick absorption. Rapid onset of effect is important for the satisfactory treatment of acute attacks of vascular headaches.

CLINICAL PHARMACOLOGY

Ergotamine is an alpha adrenergic blocking agent with a direct stimulating effect on the smooth muscle of peripheral and cranial blood vessels and produces depression of central vasomotor centers. The compound also has the properties of serotonin antagonism. In comparison to hydrogenated ergotamine, the adrenergic blocking actions are less pronounced and vasoconstrictive actions are greater. Caffeine, also a cranial vasoconstrictor is added to further enhance the vasoconstrictive effect without the necessity of increasing ergotamine dosage.

INDICATIONS AND USAGE

Wigraine® (ergotamine tartrate and caffeine tablets, USP) is indicated as therapy to abort or prevent vascular headaches such as migraine, migraine variants, or so-called histamine cephalalgia.

CONTRAINDICATIONS

Wigraine® can cause fetal harm when administered to a pregnant women. It can produce prolonged uterine contractions which can result in abortion. Wigraine® is contraindicated in women who are or may become pregnant. If this is used during pregnancy, or if the patient becomes pregnant while taking this drug, the patient should be advised of the potential hazard to the fetus.

Peripheral vascular disease, coronary heart disease, hypertension, impaired hepatic or renal function, sepsis and hypersensitivity to any of the components.

Continued on next page

Wigraine—Cont.

PRECAUTIONS

Although signs and symptoms of ergotism rarely develop even after long term intermittent use of the orally administered drug, care should be exercised to remain within the limits of recommended dosage.

Pregnancy Category X. See Contraindications section.

Nursing Mothers. It is not known whether the ergotamine tartrate in Wigraine® is excreted in human milk. Because some ergot alkaloids have been found in the milk of nursing mothers resulting in symptoms of ergotism in their children, a decision should be made whether to discontinue nursing or to discontinue the drug, taking into account the importance of the drug to the mother.

Pediatric Usage. Safety and effectiveness in children have not been established.

ADVERSE REACTIONS

In order of decreasing severity; precordial distress and pain, muscle pains in the extremities, numbness and tingling in fingers and toes, transient tachycardia or bradycardia, vomiting, nausea, weakness in the legs, diarrhea, localized edema and itching.

DOSAGE AND ADMINISTRATION

Best results are obtained if the tablets are administered at the first sign of an attack.

The average adult dose is 2 tablets at the start of a vascular headache (migraine) attack; followed by 1 additional tablet every $^1/_2$ hour if needed, up to 6 tablets per attack. Total weekly dosage should not exceed 10 tablets.

OVERDOSAGE

The toxic effects of an acute overdosage of Wigraine® are due primarily to the ergotamine component. The amount of caffeine is such that its toxic effects will be overshadowed by those of ergotamine. Symptoms include vomiting, numbness, tingling, pain and cyanosis of the extremities associated with diminished or absent peripheral pulses, hypertension or hypotension, drowsiness, stupor, coma, convulsions and shock. Treatment consists of removal of the offending drug by induction of emesis, gastric lavage and catharsis. Maintenance of adequate pulmonary ventilation, correction of hypotension, and control of convulsions are important considerations. Treatment of peripheral vasospasm should consist of warmth, but not heat, and protection of the ischemic limbs. Vasodilators may be used with benefit but caution must be exercised to avoid aggravating an already existing hypotension. The LD50 limits of the various components as outlined in NIOSH 1978 Registry of Toxic Effects of Chemical Substances, published by U.S. Department of Health, Education and Welfare are as follows: Ergotamine Tartrate IV LD50 in rats = 80mg/Kg, Caffeine IV LD50 in rats = 105mg/Kg.

HOW SUPPLIED

Wigraine® tablets are white tablets embossed with "ORGANON 542" on one side. They are individually foil stripped and packaged in boxes of 20's NDC #0052-0542-20 and 100's NDC #0052-0542-91.

STORAGE

Wigraine® tablets should be stored at a maximum of 30°C (86°F).

CAUTION

℞ only

5310108 Revised 3/98

Organon Inc.
West Orange, NJ 07052

Shown in Product Identification Guide, page 327

ZEMURON® ℞

(rocuronium bromide) Injection

THIS DRUG SHOULD BE ADMINISTERED BY ADEQUATELY-TRAINED INDIVIDUALS FAMILIAR WITH ITS ACTIONS, CHARACTERISTICS, AND HAZARDS.

DESCRIPTION

ZEMURON® (rocuronium bromide) Injection is a nondepolarizing neuromuscular blocking agent with a rapid to intermediate onset depending on dose and intermediate duration. Rocuronium bromide is chemically designated as 1-[17β-(acetyloxy)-3α-hydroxy-2β-(4-morpholinyl)-5α-androstan-16β-yl]-1-(2-propenyl)pyrrolidinium bromide.

The structural formula is:

The chemical formula is $C_{32}H_{53}BrN_2O_4$ with a molecular weight of 609.70. The partition coefficient of rocuronium bromide in n-octanol/water is 0.5 at 20°C.

Table 1. Intubating Conditions in Patients with Intubation Initiated at 60 to 70 seconds. Percent, Median (Range)

ZEMURON® Dose (mg/kg) Administered over 5 sec	Percent of patients with excellent or good intubating conditions	Time to completion of intubation (min)
Adults* 18–64 yr		
0.45 (n=43)	86%	1.6 (1.0–7.0)
0.6 (n=51)	96%	1.6 (1.0–3.2)
Infants 3 mo–1 yr		
0.6 (n=18)	100%	1.0 (1.0–1.5)
Pediatric 1–12 yr		
0.6 (n=12)	100%	1.0 (0.5–2.3)

* Excludes patients undergoing cesarean section

Excellent intubating conditions = jaw relaxed, vocal cords apart and immobile, no diaphragmatic movement.

Good intubating conditions = same as excellent but with some diaphragmatic movement.

Table 2. Time to Onset and Clinical Duration following Initial (intubating) Dose during Opioid/Nitrous Oxide/Oxygen Anesthesia (Adults) and Halothane Anesthesia (Pediatric Patients), Median (Range)

ZEMURON® Dose (mg/kg) Administered over 5 sec	Time to ≥ 80% Block (min)	Time to Maximum Block (min)	Clinical Duration (min)
Adults 18–64 yr			
0.45 (n=50)	1.3 (0.8–6.2)	3.0 (1.3–8.2)	22 (12–31)
0.6 (n=142)	1.0 (0.4–6.0)	1.8 (0.6–13.0)	31 (15–85)
0.9 (n=20)	1.1 (0.3–3.8)	1.4 (0.8–6.2)	58 (27–111)
1.2 (n=18)	0.7 (0.4–1.7)	1.0 (0.6–4.7)	67 (38–160)
Geriatric ≥ 65 yr			
0.6 (n=31)	2.3 (1.0–8.3)	3.7 (1.3–11.3)	46 (22–73)
0.9 (n=5)	2.0 (1.0–3.0)	2.5 (1.2–5.0)	62 (49–75)
1.2 (n=7)	1.0 (0.8–3.5)	1.3 (1.2–4.7)	94 (64–138)
Infants 3 mo–1 yr			
0.6 (n=17)	—	0.8 (0.3–3.0)	41 (24–68)
0.8 (n=9)	—	0.7 (0.5–0.8)	40 (27–70)
Pediatric 1–12 yr			
0.6 (n=27)	0.8 (0.4–2.0)	1.0 (0.5–3.3)	26 (17–39)
0.8 (n=18)	—	0.5 (0.3–1.0)	30 (17–56)

n = the number of patients who had Time to Maximum Block recorded.

Clinical duration = time until return to 25% of control T_1. Patients receiving doses of 0.45 mg/kg who achieved less than 90% block (16% of these patients) had about 12 to 15 minutes to 25% recovery.

ZEMURON® (rocuronium bromide) Injection is supplied as a sterile, nonpyrogenic, isotonic solution for intravenous injection only. Each mL contains 10 mg rocuronium bromide and 2 mg sodium acetate. The aqueous solution is adjusted to isotonicity with sodium chloride and to a pH of 4 with acetic acid and/or sodium hydroxide.

CLINICAL PHARMACOLOGY

ZEMURON® (rocuronium bromide) Injection is a nondepolarizing neuromuscular blocking agent with a rapid to intermediate onset depending on dose and intermediate duration. It acts by competing for cholinergic receptors at the motor end-plate. This action is antagonized by acetylcholinesterase inhibitors, such as neostigmine and edrophonium.

Pharmacodynamics: The ED_{95} (dose required to produce 95% suppression of the first [T_1] mechanomyographic [MMG] response of the adductor pollicis muscle [thumb] to indirect supramaximal train-of-four stimulation of the ulnar nerve) during opioid/nitrous oxide/oxygen anesthesia is approximately 0.3 mg/kg. Patient variability around the ED_{95} dose suggests that 50% of patients will exhibit T_1 depression of 91–97%.

Table 1 presents intubating conditions in patients with intubation initiated at 60 to 70 seconds.

[See table 1 above]

Table 2 presents the time to onset and clinical duration for the initial dose of ZEMURON® (rocuronium bromide) under opioid/nitrous oxide/oxygen anesthesia in adults and geriatric patients, and under halothane anesthesia in pediatric patients.

[See table 2 above]

The time to ≥ 80% block and clinical duration as a function of dose are presented in Figures 1 and 2.

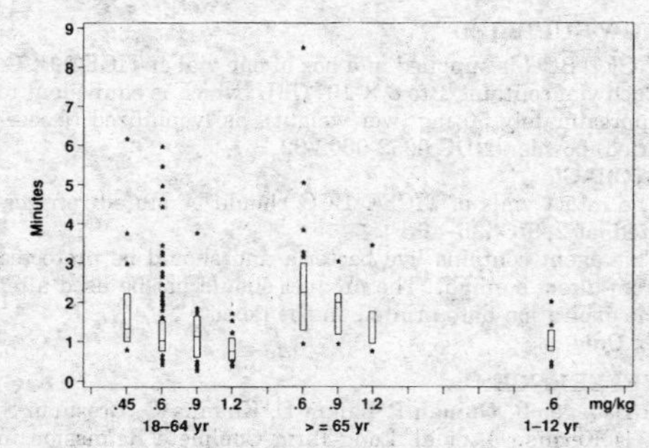

Figure 1. Time to ≥ 80% Block *vs.* Initial Dose of ZEMURON® By Age Group (Median, 25th and 75th percentile, and individual values).

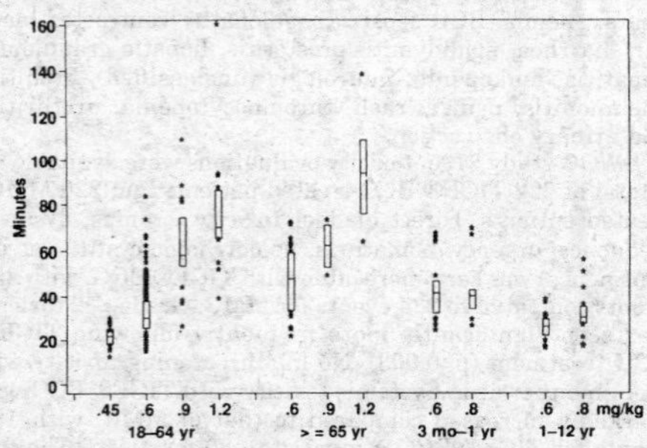

Figure 2. Duration of Clinical Effect *vs.* Initial Dose of ZEMURON® By Age Group (Median, 25th and 75th percentile, and individual values).

The clinical durations for the first five maintenance doses, in patients receiving five or more maintenance doses are represented in Figure 3 (see also Maintenance Dosing subsection of DOSAGE AND ADMINISTRATION).

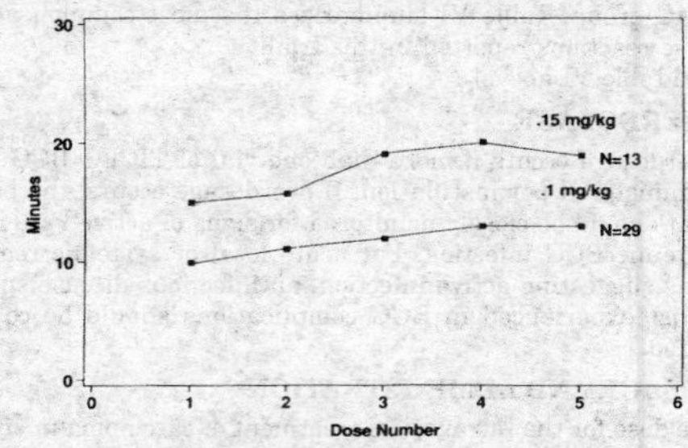

Figure 3. Duration of Clinical Effect *vs.* Number of ZEMURON® Maintenance Doses, by Dose.

Once spontaneous recovery has reached 25% of control T_1, the neuromuscular block produced by ZEMURON® is readily reversed with anticholinesterase agents, e.g., edrophonium or neostigmine.

The median spontaneous recovery from 25 to 75% T_1 was 13 minutes in adult patients. When neuromuscular block was reversed in 36 adults at a T_1 of 22–27%, recovery to a T_1 of 89 (50–132)% and T_4/T_1 of 69 (38–92)% was achieved within

5 minutes. Only five of 320 adults reversed received an additional dose of reversal agent. The median (range) dose of neostigmine was 0.04 (0.01 to 0.09) mg/kg and the median (range) dose of edrophonium was 0.5 (0.3 to 1.0) mg/kg.

In geriatric patients (n=51) reversed with neostigmine, the median T_4/T_1 increased from 40 to 88% in 5 minutes.

Pediatric patients (n=27) who received 0.5 mg/kg edrophonium had increases in the median T_4/T_1 from 37% at reversal to 93% after 2 minutes. Pediatric patients (n=58) who received 1 mg/kg edrophonium had increases in the median T_4/T_1 from 72% at reversal to 100% after 2 minutes. Infants (n=10) who were reversed with 0.03 mg/kg neostigmine recovered from 25 to 75% T_1 within 4 minutes.

There were no reports of less than satisfactory clinical recovery of neuromuscular function.

The neuromuscular blocking action of ZEMURON® may be enhanced in the presence of potent inhalation anesthetics (see Inhalation Anesthetics subsection of PRECAUTIONS).

Hemodynamics: There were no dose-related effects on the incidence of changes from baseline (≥ 30%) in mean arterial blood pressure (MAP) or heart rate associated with ZEMURON® (rocuronium bromide) Injection administration over the dose range of 0.12 to 1.2 mg/kg (4 × ED_{95}) within 5 minutes after ZEMURON® administration and prior to intubation. Increases or decreases in MAP were observed in 2–5% of geriatric and other adult patients, and in about 1% of pediatric patients. Heart rate changes (≥ 30%) occurred in 0–2% of geriatric and other adult patients. Tachycardia (≥ 30%) occurred in 12 of 127 pediatric patients. Most of the pediatric patients developing tachycardia were from a single study where the patients were anesthetized with halothane and who did not receive atropine for induction (see Pediatric subsection of Clinical Trials). In U.S. studies, laryngoscopy and tracheal intubation following ZEMURON® administration were accompanied by transient tachycardia (≥ 30% increases) in about one-third of adult patients under opioid/nitrous oxide/oxygen anesthesia. Animal studies have indicated that the ratio of vagal:neuromuscular block following ZEMURON® administration is less than vecuronium but greater than pancuronium. The tachycardia observed in some patients may result from this vagal blocking activity.

Histamine Release: In studies of histamine release, clinically significant concentrations of plasma histamine occurred in 1 of 88 patients. Clinical signs of histamine release (flushing, rash, or bronchospasm) associated with the administration of ZEMURON® (rocuronium bromide) Injection were assessed in clinical trials and reported in 9 of 1137 (0.8%) patients.

Pharmocokinetics: *In an effort to maximize the information gathered in the in vivo pharmacokinetic studies the data from the studies was used to develop population estimates of the parameters for the subpopulations represented (e.g., geriatric, pediatric, renal, and hepatic insufficiency). These population based estimates and a measure of the estimate variability are contained in the following section.*

Following IV administration of ZEMURON® (rocuronium bromide) Injection, plasma levels of rocuronium follow a three compartment open model. The rapid distribution half-life is 1–2 minutes and the slower distribution half-life is 14–18 minutes. Rocuronium is approximately 30% bound to human plasma proteins. In geriatric and other adult surgical patients undergoing either opioid/nitrous oxide/oxygen or inhalational anesthesia the observed pharmacokinetic profile was essentially unchanged.

Table 3. Pharmacokinetic Parameters in Adults (n=22; ages 27–58 yr) and Geriatric (n=20; ≥ 65 yr) During Opioid/Nitrous Oxide/Oxygen Anesthesia (Mean ± SD)

PK Parameters	Adults (Ages 27–58 yr)	Geriatrics (≥ 65 yr)
Clearance (L/kg/hr)	0.25 ± 0.08	0.21 ± 0.06
Volume of Distribution at Steady State (L/kg)	0.25 ± 0.04	0.22 ± 0.03
$T_{1/2}$ β Elimination (hr)	1.4 ± 0.4	1.5 ± 0.4

[See table 3 above]

In general, studies with normal adult subjects did not reveal any differences in the pharmacokinetics of rocuronium due to gender.

Studies of distribution, metabolism, and excretion in cats and dogs indicate that rocuronium is eliminated primarily by the liver. The rocuronium analog 17-desacetyl-rocuronium, a metabolite, has been rarely observed in the plasma or urine of humans administered single doses of 0.5–1 mg/kg with or without a subsequent infusion (for up to 12 hr) of rocuronium. In the cat, 17-desacetyl-rocuronium has approximately one-twentieth the neuromuscular blocking potency of rocuronium. The effects of renal failure and hepatic disease on the pharmacokinetics and pharmacodynamics of rocuronium in humans are consistent with these findings.

In general, patients undergoing cadaver kidney transplant have a small reduction in clearance which is offset pharmacokinetically by a corresponding increase in volume, such that the net effect is an unchanged plasma half-life. Patients with demonstrated liver cirrhosis have a marked increase in their volume of distribution resulting in a plasma half-life approximately twice that of patients with normal hepatic function. Table 4 shows the pharmacokinetic parameters in subjects with either impaired renal or hepatic function.

Table 4. Pharmacokinetic Parameters in Adults with Normal Renal and Hepatic Function (n=10, ages 23–65), Renal Transplant Patients (n=10, ages 21–45) and Hepatic Dysfunction Patients (n=9, ages 31–67) During Isoflurane Anesthesia (Mean ± SD)

PK Parameters	Normal Renal and Hepatic Function	Renal Transplant Patients	Hepatic Dysfunction Patients
Clearance (L/kg/hr)	0.16 ± 0.05*	0.13 ± 0.04	0.13 ± 0.06
Volume of Distribution at Steady State (L/kg)	0.26 ± 0.03	0.34 ± 0.11	0.53 ± 0.14
$T_{1/2}$ β Elimination (hr)	2.4 ± 0.8*	2.4 ± 1.1	4.3 ± 2.6

* Differences in the calculated $T_{1/2}$ β and Cl between this study and the study in young adults *vs.* geriatrics (≥ 65 years) is related to the different sample populations and anesthetic techniques.

[See table 4 above]

The net result of these findings is that subjects with renal failure have clinical durations that are similar to but somewhat more variable than the duration that one would expect in subjects with normal renal function. Hepatically impaired patients, due to the large increase in volume, may demonstrate clinical durations approaching 1.5 times that of subjects with normal hepatic function. In both populations the clinician should individualize the dose to the needs of the patient (see INDIVIDUALIZATION OF DOSAGE).

Tissue redistribution accounts for most (about 80%) of the initial amount of rocuronium administered. As tissue compartments fill with continued dosing (4–8 hours), less drug is redistributed away from the site of action and, for an infusion-only dose, the rate to maintain neuromuscular blockade falls to about 20% of the initial infusion rate. The use of a loading dose and a smaller infusion rate reduces the need for adjustment of dose.

Special Populations—Pediatrics: The clinical duration of effects of ZEMURON® (rocuronium bromide) Injection did not vary with age in patients 4 months to 8 years of age. The terminal half-life and other pharmacokinetic parameters of rocuronium in these pediatric patients are presented in Table 5.

Table 5. Pharmacokinetic Parameters of Rocuronium in Pediatric Patients (ages 3- < 12 mo, n=6; 1- < 3 yr, n=5; 3- < 8 yr, n=7) During Halothane Anesthesia (Mean ± SD)

PK Parameters	Patient Age Range: 3- < 12 mo	1- < 3yr	3- < 8 yr
Clearance (L/kg/hr)	0.35 ± 0.08	0.32 ± 0.07	0.44 ± 0.16
Volume of Distribution at Steady State (L/kg)	0.30 ± 0.04	0.26 ± 0.06	0.21 ± 0.03
$T_{1/2}$ β Elimination (hr)	1.3 ± 0.5	1.1 ± 0.7	0.8 ± 0.3

[See table 5 above]

Clinical Trials

In U.S. clinical trials a total of 1,137 patients received ZEMURON® (rocuronium bromide) Injection including 176 pediatric, 140 geriatric, 55 obstetric, and 766 other adults. Most patients (90%) were ASA physical status I or II, about 9% were ASA III, and 10 patients (undergoing coronary artery bypass grafting or valvular surgery) were ASA IV. In European clinical trials, a total of 1,394 patients received ZEMURON® including 52 pediatric, 128 geriatric (≥ 65 years) and 1,214 other adults.

Adult Patients: Intubation using doses of ZEMURON® (rocuronium bromide) Injection 0.6 to 0.85 mg/kg was evaluated in 203 adults in 11 clinical trials. Excellent to good intubating conditions were generally achieved within 2 minutes and maximum block occurred within 3 minutes in most patients. Doses within this range provide clinical relaxation for a median (range) time of 33 (14–85) minutes under opioid/nitrous oxide/oxygen anesthesia. Larger doses (0.9 and 1.2 mg/kg) were evaluated in two trials with 19 and 16 patients under opioid/nitrous oxide/oxygen anesthesia and provided 58 (27–111) and 67 (38–160) minutes of clinical relaxation, respectively.

Cardiovascular Disease: In one clinical trial, 10 patients with clinically significant cardiovascular disease undergoing coronary artery bypass graft received an initial dose of 0.6 mg/kg ZEMURON® (rocuronium bromide) Injection. Neuromuscular block was maintained during surgery with bolus maintenance doses of 0.3 mg/kg. Following induction, continuous 0.008 mg/kg/min infusion of ZEMURON® produced relaxation sufficient to support mechanical ventilation for 6 to 12 hours in the surgical intensive care unit (SICU) while the patients were recovering from surgery. Hypertension and tachycardia were reported in some patients but these occurrences were less frequent in patients receiving beta or calcium channel blocking drugs. In 7 of these 10 patients ZEMURON® was associated with transient increases (≥ 30%) in pulmonary vascular resistance. In another clinical trial of 17 patients undergoing abdominal aortic surgery, transient increases (≥ 30%) in pulmonary vascular resistance were observed in 4 of 17 patients receiving ZEMURON® 0.6 or 0.9 mg/kg.

Rapid Sequence Intubation: Intubating conditions were assessed in 230 patients in six clinical trials where anesthesia was induced with either thiopental (3 to 6 mg/kg) or propofol (1.5 to 2.5 mg/kg) in combination with either fentanyl (2 to 5 mcg/kg) or alfentanil (1 mg). Most of the patients also received a premedication such as midazolam or temazepam. Most patients had intubation attempted within 60 to 90 seconds of administration of ZEMURON® (rocuronium bromide) Injection 0.6 mg/kg or succinylcholine 1 to 1.5 mg/kg. Excellent or good intubating conditions were achieved in 119/120 (99% [95% confidence interval 95–99.9%]) patients receiving ZEMURON® and in 108/110 (98% [94–99.8%]) patients receiving succinylcholine. The duration of action of ZEMURON® 0.6 mg/kg is longer than succinylcholine and at this dose is approximately equivalent to the duration of other intermediate acting neuromuscular blocking drugs.

Geriatric Patients: ZEMURON® (rocuronium bromide) Injection was evaluated in 55 geriatric patients (ages 65–80 years) in six clinical trials. Doses of 0.6 mg/kg provided excellent to good intubating conditions in a median (range) time of 2.3 (1–8) minutes. Recovery times from 25% to 75% after these doses were not prolonged in geriatric patients compared to other adult patients.

Pediatric Patients: ZEMURON® (rocuronium bromide) Injection 0.6 or 0.8 mg/kg was evaluated for intubation in 75 pediatric patients (n=28; age 3–12 months, n=47; age 1–12 years) in three trials using halothane (1–5%) nitrous oxide (60–70%) in oxygen. Of the pediatric patients anesthetized with halothane who did not receive atropine for induction, about 80% experienced a transient increase (≥ 30%) in heart rate after intubation. One of the 19 infants anesthetized with halothane and fentanyl who received atropine for induction experienced this magnitude of change.

Obese Patients: ZEMURON® (rocuronium bromide) Injection was dosed according to actual body weight (ABW) in most clinical trials. The administration of ZEMURON® in the 47 of 330 (14%) patients who were at least 30% or more above their ideal body weight (IBW) was not associated with clinically significant differences in the onset, duration, recovery, or reversal of ZEMURON®-induced neuromuscular block.

In one clinical trial in obese patients, ZEMURON® 0.6 mg/kg was dosed according to ABW (n=12) or IBW (n=11). Obese patients dosed according to IBW had a longer time to maximum block, a shorter clinical duration of 25 (14–29) minutes, and did not achieve intubating conditions comparable to those dosed based on ABW. These results support the recommendation that obese patients be dosed based on actual body weight.

Obstetric Patients: ZEMURON® (rocuronium bromide) Injection 0.6 mg/kg was administered with thiopental, 3–4 mg/kg (n=13) or 4–6 mg/kg (n=42), for rapid sequence induction of anesthesia for cesarean section. No neonate had APGAR scores < 7 at 5 minutes. The umbilical venous plasma concentrations were 18% of maternal concentrations at delivery. Intubating conditions were poor or inadequate in 5 of 13 women receiving 3–4 mg/kg thiopental when intubation was attempted 60 seconds after drug injection. Therefore, ZEMURON® is not recommended for rapid sequence induction in cesarean section patients.

INDIVIDUALIZATION OF DOSAGE

DOSES OF ZEMURON® (rocuronium bromide) INJECTION SHOULD BE INDIVIDUALIZED AND A PERIPH-

Continued on next page

Zemuron—Cont.

ERAL NERVE STIMULATOR SHOULD BE USED TO MEASURE NEUROMUSCULAR FUNCTION DURING ZEMURON® ADMINISTRATION IN ORDER TO MONITOR DRUG EFFECT, DETERMINE THE NEED FOR ADDITIONAL DOSES, AND CONFIRM RECOVERY FROM NEUROMUSCULAR BLOCK.

Based on the known actions of ZEMURON®, the following factors should be considered when administering ZEMURON®:

Renal or Hepatic Impairment: No differences from patients with normal hepatic and kidney function were observed for onset time at a dose of 0.6 mg/kg ZEMURON® (rocuronium bromide) Injection. When compared to patients with normal renal and hepatic function, the mean clinical duration is similar in patients with end-stage renal disease undergoing renal transplant, and is about 1.5 times longer in patients with hepatic disease. Patients with renal failure may have a greater variation in duration of effect (see Pharmacokinetics subsection of CLINICAL PHARMACOLOGY and Renal Failure and Hepatic Disease subsections of PRECAUTIONS).

Reduced Plasma Cholinesterase Activity: No differences from patients with normal plasma cholinesterase activity is expected since rocuronium metabolism does not depend on plasma cholinesterase.

Drugs or Conditions Causing Potentiation of or Resistance to Neuromuscular Block: The neuromuscular blocking action of ZEMURON® (rocuronium bromide) Injection is potentiated by isoflurane and enflurane anesthesia. Potentiation is minimal when administration of the recommended dose of ZEMURON® occurs prior to the administration of these potent inhalation agents. The median clinical duration of a dose of 0.57–0.85 mg/kg was 34, 38, and 42 minutes under opioid/nitrous oxide/oxygen, enflurane and isoflurane maintenance anesthesia, respectively. During 1–2 hr of infusion, the infusion rate of ZEMURON® required to maintain about 95% block was decreased by as much as 40% under enflurane and isoflurane anesthesia (see Inhalation Anesthetics subsection of PRECAUTIONS).

When ZEMURON® is administered to patients chronically receiving anticonvulsant agents such as carbamazepine or phenytoin, shorter durations of neuromuscular block may occur and infusion rates may be higher due to the development of resistance to nondepolarizing muscle relaxants (see Anticonvulsants subsection of PRECAUTIONS).

Pulmonary Hypertension: ZEMURON® (rocuronium bromide) Injection may be associated with increased pulmonary vascular resistance so caution is appropriate in patients with pulmonary hypertension or valvular heart disease (see Clinical Trials subsection of CLINICAL PHARMACOLOGY).

Obesity: In obese patients, the initial dose of ZEMURON® (rocuronium bromide) Injection 0.6 mg/kg should be based upon the patient's actual body weight (see Obese Patients subsection of Clinical Trials).

Based on the known actions of other nondepolarizing neuromuscular blocking agents the following additional factors should be considered when administering ZEMURON®:

Drugs or Conditions Causing Potentiation of or Resistance to Neuromuscular Block: Resistance to nondepolarizing agents, consistent with up-regulation of skeletal muscle acetylcholine receptors, is associated with burns, disuse atrophy, denervation, and direct muscle trauma. Receptor up-regulation may also contribute to the resistance to nondepolarizing muscle relaxants which sometimes develops in patients with cerebral palsy, patients chronically receiving anticonvulsant agents such as carbamazepine or phenytoin or with chronic exposure to nondepolarizing agents (see PRECAUTIONS).

Other nondepolarizing neuromuscular blocking agents have been found to exhibit profound neuromuscular blocking effects in cachectic or debilitated patients, patients with neuromuscular diseases, and patients with carcinomatosis. In these or other patients in whom potentiation of neuromuscular block or difficulty with reversal may be anticipated, a decrease from the recommended initial dose should be considered.

Certain antibiotics, magnesium salts, lithium, local anesthetics, procainamide, and quinidine have been shown to increase the duration of neuromuscular block and decrease infusion requirements of other neuromuscular blocking agents. In patients in whom potentiation of neuromuscular block may be anticipated, a decrease from the recommended initial dose should be considered (see Antibiotics and Other subsections of PRECAUTIONS).

Severe acid-base and/or electrolyte abnormalities may potentiate or cause resistance to the neuromuscular blocking action of ZEMURON® (rocuronium bromide) Injection (see Other subsection of PRECAUTIONS). No data are available in such patients and no dosing recommendations can be made.

Burns: Patients with burns are known to develop resistance to nondepolarizing neuromuscular blocking agents, probably due to up-regulation of post-synaptic skeletal muscle cholinergic receptors (see INDIVIDUALIZATION OF DOSAGE).

INDICATIONS AND USAGE

ZEMURON® (rocuronium bromide) Injection is a nondepolarizing neuromuscular blocking agent with a rapid to intermediate onset depending on dose and intermediate duration and is indicated for inpatients and outpatients as an adjunct to general anesthesia to facilitate both rapid sequence and routine tracheal intubation, and to provide skeletal muscle relaxation during surgery or mechanical ventilation.

CONTRAINDICATIONS

ZEMURON® (rocuronium bromide) Injection is contraindicated in patients known to have hypersensitivity to rocuronium bromide.

WARNINGS

ZEMURON® (rocuronium bromide) INJECTION SHOULD BE ADMINISTERED IN CAREFULLY ADJUSTED DOSAGES BY OR UNDER THE SUPERVISION OF EXPERIENCED CLINICIANS WHO ARE FAMILIAR WITH THE DRUG'S ACTIONS AND THE POSSIBLE COMPLICATIONS OF ITS USE. THE DRUG SHOULD NOT BE ADMINISTERED UNLESS FACILITIES FOR INTUBATION, ARTIFICIAL RESPIRATION, OXYGEN THERAPY, AND AN ANTAGONIST ARE IMMEDIATELY AVAILABLE. IT IS RECOMMENDED THAT CLINICIANS ADMINISTERING NEUROMUSCULAR BLOCKING AGENTS SUCH AS ZEMURON® EMPLOY A PERIPHERAL NERVE STIMULATOR TO MONITOR DRUG RESPONSE, NEED FOR ADDITIONAL RELAXANT, AND ADEQUACY OF SPONTANEOUS RECOVERY OR ANTAGONISM.

ZEMURON® HAS NO KNOWN EFFECT ON CONSCIOUSNESS, PAIN THRESHOLD, OR CEREBRATION. THEREFORE, ITS ADMINISTRATION MUST BE ACCOMPANIED BY ADEQUATE ANESTHESIA OR SEDATION.

In patients with myasthenia gravis or myasthenic (Eaton-Lambert) syndrome, small doses of nondepolarizing neuromuscular blocking agents may have profound effects. In such patients, a peripheral nerve stimulator and use of a small test dose may be of value in monitoring the response to administration of muscle relaxants.

ZEMURON®, which has an acid pH, should not be mixed with alkaline solutions (e.g., barbiturate solutions) in the same syringe or administered simultaneously during intravenous infusion through the same needle.

PRECAUTIONS

Long-term Use in I.C.U.: ZEMURON® (rocuronium bromide) Injection has not been studied for long-term use in the I.C.U. As with other nondepolarizing neuromuscular blocking drugs, apparent tolerance to ZEMURON® may develop rarely during chronic administration in the I.C.U. While the mechanism for development of this resistance is not known, receptor up-regulation may be a contributing factor. It is STRONGLY RECOMMENDED THAT NEUROMUSCULAR TRANSMISSION BE MONITORED CONTINUOUSLY DURING ADMINISTRATION AND RECOVERY WITH THE HELP OF A NERVE STIMULATOR. ADDITIONAL DOSES OF ZEMURON® OR ANY OTHER NEUROMUSCULAR BLOCKING AGENT SHOULD NOT BE GIVEN UNTIL THERE IS A DEFINITE RESPONSE (ONE TWITCH OF THE TRAIN-OF-FOUR) TO NERVE STIMULATION. Prolonged paralysis and/or skeletal muscle weakness may be noted during initial attempts to wean from the ventilator patients who have chronically received neuromuscular blocking drugs in the I.C.U. Therefore, ZEMURON® should only be used in this setting if, in the opinion of the prescribing physician, the specific advantages of the drug outweigh the risk.

Labor and Delivery: The use of ZEMURON® (rocuronium bromide) Injection in cesarean section has been studied in a limited number of patients. ZEMURON® is not recommended for rapid sequence induction in cesarean section patients (see Clinical Trials subsection of CLINICAL PHARMACOLOGY).

Hepatic Disease: Since ZEMURON® (rocuronium bromide) Injection is primarily excreted by the liver it should be used with caution in patients with clinically significant hepatic disease. ZEMURON® 0.6 mg/kg has been studied in a limited number of patients (n=9) with clinically significant hepatic disease under steady-state isoflurane anesthesia. After ZEMURON® 0.6 mg/kg, the median (range) clinical duration of 60 (35–166) minutes was moderately prolonged compared to 42 minutes in patients with normal hepatic function. The median recovery time of 53 minutes was also prolonged in patients with cirrhosis compared to 20 minutes in patients with normal hepatic function. Four of eight patients with cirrhosis, who received ZEMURON® 0.6 mg/kg under opioid/nitrous oxide/oxygen anesthesia, did not achieve complete block. These findings are consistent with the increase in volume of distribution at steady state observed in patients with significant hepatic disease (see Pharmacokinetics subsection of CLINICAL PHARMACOLOGY). If used for rapid sequence induction in patients with ascites, an increased initial dosage may be necessary to assure complete block. Duration will be prolonged in these cases. The use of doses higher than 0.6 mg/kg has not been studied.

Renal Failure: Due to the limited role of the kidney in the excretion of ZEMURON® (rocuronium bromide) Injection, usual dosing guidelines should be adequate. ZEMURON® 0.6 mg/kg has been evaluated in three single center trials (n=30, ages 19–61 years) in patients undergoing renal transplant surgery, or shunt procedures in preparation for dialysis. After ZEMURON® 0.6 mg/kg, the time to maximum block was about 1–2 minutes and was not different from patients without renal dysfunction. The mean ± SD clinical duration of 54 ± 22 minutes was not considered prolonged compared to 46 ± 12 minutes in normal patients; however, there was substantial variation (range, 22–90 minutes). The spontaneous recovery rate from 25 to 75% of control in renal dysfunction patients of 27 ± 11 minutes was similar to 28 ± 20 minutes in normal patients (see Pharmacokinetics subsection of CLINICAL PHARMACOLOGY).

Malignant Hyperthermia (MH): In an animal study in MH-susceptible swine, the administration of ZEMURON® (rocuronium bromide) Injection did not appear to trigger malignant hyperthermia. ZEMURON® has not been studied in MH-susceptible patients. Because ZEMURON® is always used with other agents, and the occurrence of malignant hyperthermia during anesthesia is possible even in the absence of known triggering agents, clinicians should be familiar with early signs, confirmatory diagnosis and treatment of malignant hyperthermia prior to the start of any anesthetic.

Altered Circulation Time: Conditions associated with slower circulation time, e.g., cardiovascular disease or advanced age, may be associated with a delay in onset time. Because higher doses of ZEMURON® (rocuronium bromide) Injection produce a longer duration of action, the initial dosage should usually not be increased in these patients to reduce onset time; instead, when feasible, more time should be allowed for the drug to achieve onset of effect.

Drug Interactions: The use of ZEMURON® (rocuronium bromide) Injection before succinylcholine, for the purpose of attenuating some of the side effects of succinylcholine, has not been studied.

If ZEMURON® is administered following administration of succinylcholine, it should not be given until recovery from succinylcholine has been observed. The median duration of action of ZEMURON® 0.6 mg/kg administered after a 1 mg/kg dose of succinylcholine when T_1 returned to 75% of control was 36 minutes (range 14–57, n=12) *vs.* 28 minutes (17–51, n=12) without succinylcholine.

There are no controlled studies documenting the use of ZEMURON® before or after other nondepolarizing muscle relaxants. Interactions have been observed when other nondepolarizing muscle relaxants have been administered in succession.

Inhalation Anesthetics: Use of inhalation anesthetics has been shown to enhance the activity of other neuromuscular blocking agents, enflurane > isoflurane > halothane.

Isoflurane and enflurane may also prolong the duration of action of initial and maintenance doses of ZEMURON® (rocuronium bromide) Injection and decrease the average infusion requirement of ZEMURON® by 40% compared to opioid/nitrous oxide/oxygen anesthesia. No definite interaction between ZEMURON® and halothane has been demonstrated. In one study, use of enflurane in 10 patients resulted in a 20% increase in mean clinical duration of the initial intubating dose, and a 37% increase in the duration of subsequent maintenance doses, when compared in the same study to 10 patients under opioid/nitrous oxide/oxygen anesthesia. The clinical duration of initial doses of ZEMURON® of 0.57–0.85 mg/kg under enflurane or isoflurane anesthesia, as used clinically, was increased by 11% and 23%, respectively. The duration of maintenance doses was affected to a greater extent, increasing by 30 to 50% under either enflurane or isoflurane anesthesia. Potentiation by these agents is also observed with respect to the infusion rates of ZEMURON® required to maintain approximately 95% neuromuscular block. Under isoflurane and enflurane anesthesia, the infusion rates are decreased by approximately 40% compared to opioid/nitrous oxide/oxygen anesthesia. The median spontaneous recovery time (from 25 to 75% of control T_1) is not affected by halothane, but is prolonged by enflurane (15% longer) and isoflurane (62% longer). Reversal-induced recovery of ZEMURON® neuromuscular block is minimally affected by anesthetic technique.

Intravenous Anesthetics: The use of propofol for induction and maintenance of anesthesia does not alter the clinical duration or recovery characteristics following recommended doses of ZEMURON® (rocuronium bromide) Injection.

Anticonvulsants: In 2 of 4 patients receiving chronic anticonvulsant therapy apparent resistance to the effects of ZEMURON® (rocuronium bromide) Injection was observed in the form of diminished magnitude of neuromuscular block, or shortened clinical duration. As with other nondepolarizing neuromuscular blocking drugs, if ZEMURON® is administered to patients chronically receiving anticonvulsant agents such as carbamazepine or phenytoin, shorter durations of neuromuscular block may occur and infusion rates may be higher due to the development of resistance to nondepolarizing muscle relaxants. While the mechanism for development of this resistance is not known, receptor up-regulation may be a contributing factor (see INDIVIDUALIZATION OF DOSAGE).

Antibiotics: Drugs which may enhance the neuromuscular blocking action of nondepolarizing agents such as ZEMURON® (rocuronium bromide) Injection include certain antibiotics (e.g., aminoglycosides; vancomycin; tetracyclines; bacitracin; polymyxins; colistin; and sodium colistimethate). If these antibiotics are used in conjunction with ZEMURON®, prolongation of neuromuscular block should be considered a possibility.

Other: Experience concerning injection of quinidine during recovery from use of other muscle relaxants suggests that recurrent paralysis may occur. This possibility must also be considered for ZEMURON® (rocuronium bromide) Injection.

ZEMURON®-induced neuromuscular blockade was modified by alkalosis and acidosis in experimental pigs. Both respiratory and metabolic acidosis prolonged the recovery time. The potency of ZEMURON® was significantly enhanced in metabolic acidosis and alkalosis, but was reduced in respiratory alkalosis. In addition, experience with other drugs has suggested that acute (e.g., diarrhea) or chronic (e.g., adrenocortical insufficiency) electrolyte imbalance may alter neuromuscular blockade. Since electrolyte imbalance and acid-base imbalance are usually mixed, either enhancement or inhibition may occur. Magnesium salts, administered for the management of toxemia of pregnancy, may enhance neuromuscular blockade.

A local tolerance study in rabbits demonstrated that ZEMURON® was well tolerated following intravenous, intra-arterial and perivenous administration with only a slight irritation of surrounding tissues observed after perivenous administration. In humans, if extravasation occurs it may be associated with signs or symptoms of local irritation; the injection or infusion should be terminated immediately and restarted in another vein (see DOSAGE AND ADMINISTRATION).

Drug/Laboratory Test Interactions: None known.

Carcinogenesis, Mutagenesis, Impairment of Fertility: Studies in animals have not been performed to evaluate carcinogenic potential or impairment of fertility. Mutagenicity studies (Ames test, analysis of chromosomal aberrations in mammalian cells, and micronucleus test) conducted with ZEMURON® (rocuronium bromide) Injection did not suggest mutagenic potential.

Pregnancy Category B: A teratogenicity study has been conducted in rats using intravenously administered doses of ZEMURON® (rocuronium bromide) Injection approximating the clinical dose in humans (0.3 mg/kg). No teratogenic effects were observed in this study. There are no adequate and well-controlled studies in pregnant women. ZEMURON® should be used during pregnancy only if the potential benefit justifies the potential risk to the fetus.

Pediatric Use: The use of ZEMURON® (rocuronium bromide) Injection in pediatric patients less than 3 months of age and greater than 14 years of age has not been studied. See Pharmacodynamics subsection of CLINICAL PHARMACOLOGY and Use in Pediatrics subsection of DOSAGE AND ADMINISTRATION for clinical experience and recommendations for use in pediatric patients 3 months to 14 years of age.

ADVERSE REACTIONS

Clinical studies in the U.S. (n=1,137) and Europe (n=1,394) totaled 2,531 patients. Prolonged neuromuscular block is associated with neuromuscular blockers as a class. Prolonged neuromuscular block (166 minutes) occurred after 0.6 mg/kg ZEMURON® (rocuronium bromide) Injection in an obese 67 year-old female with hepatic dysfunction who had received gentamicin before surgery. The patients exposed in the U.S. clinical studies provide the basis for calculation of adverse reaction rates. The following adverse experiences were reported in patients administered ZEMURON® Injection (all events judged by investigators during the clinical trials to have a possible causal relationship):

Adverse experiences in greater than 1% patients:—NONE

Adverse experiences in less than 1% of patients Probably Related or Relationship Unknown:

Cardiovascular:	arrhythmia, abnormal electrocardiogram, tachycardia
Digestive:	nausea, vomiting
Respiratory:	asthma (bronchospasm, wheezing, or rhonchi), hiccup
Skin and Appendages:	rash, injection site edema, pruritus

In the European studies, the most commonly reported adverse experiences were transient hypotension (2%) and hypertension (2%); it is in greater frequency than the U.S. studies (0.1% and 0.1%). Changes in heart rate and blood pressure were defined differently from the U.S. studies in which changes in cardiovascular parameters were not considered as adverse events unless judged by the investigator as unexpected, clinically significant, or thought to be histamine related.

In clinical practice, there have been rare reports of allergic reactions (anaphylactic and anaphylactoid) with ZEMURON® (rocuronium bromide) Injection.

OVERDOSAGE

No cases of significant accidental or intentional overdose with ZEMURON® (rocuronium bromide) Injection have been reported. Overdosage with neuromuscular blocking agents may result in neuromuscular block beyond the time needed for surgery and anesthesia. The primary treatment is maintenance of a patent airway and controlled ventilation until recovery of normal neuromuscular function is assured. Once evidence of recovery from neuromuscular block is observed, further recovery may be facilitated by administration of an anticholinesterase agent (e.g., neostigmine, edrophonium) in conjunction with an appropriate anticholinergic agent (see Antagonism of Neuromuscular Blockade).

Antagonism of Neuromuscular Blockade

ANTAGONISTS (SUCH AS NEOSTIGMINE) SHOULD NOT BE ADMINISTERED PRIOR TO THE DEMONSTRATION OF SOME SPONTANEOUS RECOVERY FROM NEUROMUSCULAR BLOCKADE. THE USE OF A NERVE STIMULATOR TO DOCUMENT RECOVERY AND ANTAGONISM OF NEUROMUSCULAR BLOCKADE IS RECOMMENDED.

Patients should be evaluated for adequate clinical evidence of antagonism, e.g., 5 sec head lift, adequate phonation, ventilation, and upper airway maintenance. Ventilation must be supported until no longer required.

Antagonism may be delayed in the presence of debilitation, carcinomatosis, and concomitant use of certain broad spectrum antibiotics, or anesthetic agents and other drugs which enhance neuromuscular blockade or separately cause respiratory depression. Under such circumstances the management is the same as that of prolonged neuromuscular blockade.

Table 6. Infusion Rates Using ZEMURON® Injection (0.5 mg/mL)*

Patient Weight (kg)	(Lbs)	Drug Delivery Rate (μg/kg/min) 4	5	6	7	8	9	10	12	14	16
		Infusion Delivery Rate (mL/hr)									
10	22	4.8	6.0	7.2	8.4	9.6	10.8	12.0	14.4	16.8	19.2
15	33	7.2	9.0	10.8	12.6	14.4	16.2	18.0	21.6	25.2	28.8
20	44	9.6	12.0	14.4	16.8	19.2	21.6	24.0	28.8	33.6	38.4
25	55	12.0	15.0	18.0	21.0	24.0	27.0	30.0	36.0	42.0	48.0
35	77	16.8	21.0	25.2	29.4	33.6	37.8	42.0	50.4	58.8	67.2
50	110	24.0	30.0	36.0	42.0	48.0	54.0	60.0	72.0	84.0	96.0
60	132	28.8	36.0	43.2	50.4	57.6	64.8	72.0	86.4	100.8	115.2
70	154	33.6	42.0	50.4	58.8	67.2	75.6	84.0	100.8	117.6	134.4
80	176	38.4	48.0	57.6	67.2	76.8	86.4	96.0	115.2	134.4	153.6
90	198	43.2	54.0	64.8	75.6	86.4	97.2	108.0	129.6	151.2	172.8
100	220	48.0	60.0	72.0	84.0	96.0	108.0	120.0	144.0	168.0	192.0

Table 7. Infusion Rates Using ZEMURON® Injection (1 mg/mL)**

Patient Weight (kg)	(Lbs)	Drug Delivery Rate (μg/kg/min) 4	5	6	7	8	9	10	12	14	16
		Infusion Delivery Rate (mL/hr)									
10	22	2.4	3.0	3.6	4.2	4.8	5.4	6.0	7.2	8.4	9.6
15	33	3.6	4.5	5.4	6.3	7.2	8.1	9.0	10.8	12.6	14.4
20	44	4.8	6.0	7.2	8.4	9.6	10.8	12.0	14.4	16.8	19.2
25	55	6.0	7.5	9.0	10.5	12.0	13.5	15.0	18.0	21.0	24.0
35	77	8.4	10.5	12.6	14.7	16.8	18.9	21.0	25.2	29.4	33.6
50	110	12.0	15.0	18.0	21.0	24.0	27.0	30.0	36.0	42.0	48.0
60	132	14.4	18.0	21.6	25.2	28.8	32.4	36.0	43.2	50.4	57.6
70	154	16.8	21.0	25.2	29.4	33.6	37.8	42.0	50.4	58.8	67.2
80	176	19.2	24.0	28.8	33.6	38.4	43.2	48.0	57.6	67.2	76.8
90	198	21.6	27.0	32.4	37.8	43.2	48.6	54.0	64.8	75.6	86.4
100	220	24.0	30.0	36.0	42.0	48.0	54.0	60.0	72.0	84.0	96.0

* 50 mg ZEMURON® in 100 mL solution
** 100 mg ZEMURON® in 100 mL solution

DOSAGE AND ADMINISTRATION

ZEMURON® (rocuronium bromide) INJECTION IS FOR INTRAVENOUS USE ONLY. THIS DRUG SHOULD BE ADMINISTERED BY OR UNDER THE SUPERVISION OF EXPERIENCED CLINICIANS FAMILIAR WITH THE USE OF NEUROMUSCULAR BLOCKING AGENTS. INDIVIDUALIZATION OF DOSAGE SHOULD BE CONSIDERED IN EACH CASE (see INDIVIDUALIZATION OF DOSAGE).

The dosage information which follows is derived from studies based upon units of drug per unit of body weight. It is expressed in this section in units of mg/kg to assist the clinician in calculating individual patient dosage requirements relative to the product as supplied for clinical use. It is intended to serve as an initial guide to clinicians familiar with other neuromuscular blocking agents to acquire experience with ZEMURON®. The monitoring of twitch response is recommended to evaluate recovery from ZEMURON® and decrease the hazards of overdosage if additional doses are administered (see Pharmacodynamics subsection of CLINICAL PHARMACOLOGY and Maintenance Dosing subsection).

It is recommended that clinicians administering neuromuscular blocking agents such as ZEMURON® employ a peripheral nerve stimulator to monitor drug response, determine the need for additional relaxant and adequacy of spontaneous recovery or antagonism.

Rapid Sequence Intubation: In appropriately premedicated and adequately anesthetized patients, ZEMURON® (rocuronium bromide) Injection 0.6–1.2 mg/kg will provide excellent or good intubating conditions in most patients in less than 2 minutes (see Clinical Trials subsection of CLINICAL PHARMACOLOGY).

Dose for Tracheal Intubation: The recommended initial dose regardless of anesthetic technique is 0.6 mg/kg. Neuromuscular block sufficient for intubation (≥ 80% block) is attained in a median (range) time of 1 (0.4–6) minute(s) and most patients have intubation completed within 2 minutes. Maximum blockade is achieved in most patients in less than 3 minutes. This dose may be expected to provide 31 (15–85) minutes of clinical relaxation under opioid/nitrous oxide/oxygen anesthesia. Under halothane, isoflurane, and enflurane anesthesia, some extension of the period of clinical relaxation should be expected (see Inhalation Anesthetics subsection of PRECAUTIONS).

A lower dose of ZEMURON® (rocuronium bromide) Injection (0.45 mg/kg) may be used. Neuromuscular block sufficient for intubation (≥ 80% block) is attained in a median (range) time of 1.3 (0.8–6.2) minute(s) and most patients have intubation completed within 2 minutes. Maximum blockade is achieved in most patients in less than 4 minutes. This dose may be expected to provide 22 (12–31) minutes of clinical relaxation under opioid/nitrous oxide/oxygen anesthesia. Patients receiving this low dose of 0.45 mg/kg who achieve less than 90% block (about 16% of these patients) may have a more rapid time to 25% recovery, 12–15 minutes.

Should there be reason for the selection of a larger bolus dose in individual patients, initial doses of 0.9 or 1.2 mg/kg can be administered during surgery under opioid/nitrous oxide/oxygen anesthesia without adverse effects to the cardiovascular system. These doses will provide ≥ 80% block in most patients in less than 2 minutes, with maximum blockade occurring in most patients in less than 3 minutes. Doses of 0.9 and 1.2 mg/kg may be expected to provide 58 (27–111) and 67 (38–160) minutes, respectively, of clinical relaxation under opioid/nitrous oxide/oxygen anesthesia.

Maintenance Dosing: Maintenance doses of 0.1, 0.15, and 0.2 mg/kg ZEMURON® (rocuronium bromide) Injection, administered at 25% recovery of control T_1 (defined as 3 twiches of train-of-four), provide a median (range) of 12 (2–31), 17 (6–50) and 24 (7–69) minutes of clinical duration under opioid/nitrous oxide/oxygen anesthesia (see Pharmacodynamics subsection of CLINICAL PHARMACOLOGY). In all cases, dosing should be guided based on the clinical duration following initial dose or prior maintenance dose and not administered until recovery of neuromuscular function is evident. A clinically insignificant cumulation of effect with repetitive maintenance dosing has been observed (see Pharmacodynamics subsection of CLINICAL PHARMACOLOGY).

Use by Continuous Infusion: Infusion at an initial rate of 0.01 to 0.012 mg/kg/min of ZEMURON® (rocuronium bromide) Injection should be initiated only after early evidence of spontaneous recovery from an intubating dose. Due to rapid redistribution (see Pharmacokinetics subsection of CLINICAL PHARMACOLOGY) and the associated rapid spontaneous recovery, initiation of the infusion after substantial return of neuromuscular function (more than 10% of control T_1), may necessitate additional bolus doses to maintain adequate block for surgery.

Upon reaching the desired level of neuromuscular block, the infusion of ZEMURON® must be individualized for each patient. The rate of administration should be adjusted according to the patient's twitch response as monitored with the use of a peripheral nerve stimulator. In clinical trials, infusion rates have ranged from 0.004 to 0.016 mg/kg/min.

Continued on next page

Zemuron—Cont.

Inhalation anesthetics, particularly enflurane and isoflurane may enhance the neuromuscular blocking action of nondepolarizing muscle relaxants. In the presence of steady-state concentrations of enflurane or isoflurane, it may be necessary to reduce the rate of infusion by 30 to 50%, at 45–60 minutes after the intubating dose.

Spontaneous recovery and reversal of neuromuscular blockade following discontinuation of ZEMURON® infusion may be expected to proceed at rates comparable to that following comparable total doses administered by repetitive bolus injections (see Pharmacodynamics subsection of CLINICAL PHARMACOLOGY).

Infusion solutions of ZEMURON® can be prepared by mixing ZEMURON® with an appropriate infusion solution such as 5% glucose in water or Lactated Ringers (see Compatibility). Unused portions of infusion solutions should be discarded.

Infusion rates of ZEMURON® can be individualized for each patient using the following tables as guidelines:

[See table 6 at top of previous page]

[See table 7 at top of previous page]

Use in Pediatrics: Initial doses of 0.6 mg/kg in pediatric patients under halothane anesthesia produce excellent to good intubating conditions within 1 minute. The median (range) time to maximum block was 1 (0.5–3.3) minute(s). This dose will provide a median (range) time of clinical relaxation of 41 (24–68) minutes in 3 months–1 year infants and 27 (17–41) minutes in 1–12 year-old pediatric patients. Maintenance doses of 0.075–0.125 mg/kg, administered upon return of T_1 to 25% of control, provide clinical relaxation for 7–10 minutes.

Spontaneous recovery proceeds at approximately the same rate in infants (3 months–1 year) as in adults, but is more rapid in pediatric patients (1–12 years) than adults (see Tables 2 and 4 in Pharmacodynamics subsection of CLINICAL PHARMACOLOGY). A continuous infusion of ZEMURON® (rocuronium bromide) Injection initiated at a rate of 0.012 mg/kg/min upon return of T_1 to 10% of control (one twitch present in the train-of-four), may also be used to maintain neuromuscular blockade in pediatric patients. The infusion of ZEMURON® must be individualized for each patient. The rate of administration should be adjusted according to the patient's twitch response as monitored with the use of a peripheral nerve stimulator. Spontaneous recovery and reversal of neuromuscular blockade following discontinuation of ZEMURON® infusion may be expected to proceed at rates comparable to that following similar total exposure to single bolus doses (see Pharmacodynamics subsection of CLINICAL PHARMACOLOGY).

Use in Obese Patients: An analysis across all U.S. controlled clinical studies indicates that the pharmacodynamics of ZEMURON® (rocuronium bromide) Injection are not different between obese and non-obese patients when dosed based upon their actual body weight.

Use in Geriatrics: Geriatric patients (≥ 65 years) exhibited a slightly prolonged median (range) clinical duration of 46 (22–73), 62 (49–75), and 94 (64–138) minutes under opioid/nitrous oxide/oxygen anesthesia following doses of 0.6, 0.9 and 1.2 mg/kg, respectively. Maintenance doses of 0.1 and 0.15 mg/kg ZEMURON® (rocuronium bromide) Injection, administered at 25% recovery of T_1, provide approximately 13 and 33 minutes of clinical duration under opioid/nitrous oxide/oxygen anesthesia. The median (range) rate of spontaneous recovery of T_1 from 25 to 75% in geriatric patients is 17 (7–56) minutes which is not different from that in other adults (see Pharmacokinetics and Pharmacodynamics subsections of CLINICAL PHARMACOLOGY).

Compatibility: ZEMURON® (rocuronium bromide) Injection is compatible in solution with:

0.9% NaCl solution	Sterile water for injection
5% glucose in water	Lactated Ringers
5% glucose in saline	

Use within 24 hours of mixing with the above solutions.

Parenteral drug products should be inspected visually for particulate matter and clarity prior to administration whenever solution and container permit. Do not use solution if particulate matter is present.

Safety and Handling: There is no specific work exposure limit for ZEMURON® (rocuronium bromide) Injection. In case of eye contact, flush with water for at least 10 minutes.

HOW SUPPLIED

ZEMURON® (rocuronium bromide) Injection is available in the following forms:

ZEMURON® 5 mL multiple dose vials containing 50 mg rocuronium bromide injection (10 mg/mL)

Boxes of 10 NDC No. 0052-0450-15

ZEMURON® 10 mL multiple dose vials containing 100 mg rocuronium bromide injection (10 mg/mL)

Boxes of 10 NDC No. 0052-0450-16

Storage: ZEMURON® (rocuronium bromide) Injection should be stored under refrigeration, 2° to 8°C (36° to 46°F). DO NOT FREEZE. Upon removal from refrigeration to room temperature storage conditions (25°C/77°F), use ZEMURON® within 60 days. Use opened vials of ZEMURON® within 30 days.

Caution: Federal law prohibits dispensing without prescription.

ORGANON INC. WEST ORANGE, NEW JERSEY 07052

5310153 7/97

Shown in Product Identification Guide, page 327

ZYMASE® ℞

(pancrelipase, USP)
enteric coated spheres

DESCRIPTION

Zymase® capsules contain enteric coated spheres of pancrelipase, a substance containing enzymes, principally lipase, with amylase and protease obtained from the pancreas of the hog. Each capsule contains not less than:

Lipase—12,000 USP Units
Protease—24,000 USP Units
Amylase—24,000 USP Units

Each capsule also contains: Gelatin, purified water, starch, talc, titanium dioxide, FD&C Green #3, FD&C Yellow #10, and other inactive ingredients.

CLINICAL PHARMACOLOGY

Zymase® is protected against inactivation by gastric acidity, and active enzymes are released in the duodenum. The enzymes promote hydrolysis of fats into glycerol and fatty acids, protein into proteases and derived substances, and starch into dextrans and sugars.

INDICATIONS AND USAGE

Zymase® is indicated in conditions where pancreatic enzymes are either absent or deficient with resultant inadequate fat digestion. Such conditions include but are not limited to chronic pancreatitis, pancreatectomy, cystic fibrosis and steatorrhea of diverse etiologies.

CONTRAINDICATIONS

Known hypersensitivity to pork protein.

PRECAUTIONS

To maintain enteric coating integrity, do not chew or crush spheres.

ADVERSE REACTIONS

No adverse reactions have been reported. It should be noted, however, that extremely high doses of exogenous pancreatic enzymes have been associated with hyperuricosuria and hyperuricemia.

DOSAGE AND ADMINISTRATION

One to two capsules with each meal or snack. Individual cases may require higher dosage and dietary adjustment. Where swallowing of capsules is difficult, capsules may be opened and the spheres taken with liquids or soft foods which do not require chewing.

STORAGE

Not to exceed 25°C (77°F). Store in dry place when opened.

DISPENSE

In tight container as defined in the USP.

HOW SUPPLIED

Bottles of 100, NDC 0052-0393-91

5308530 393 91 5/99 04

Revised 4/93

Shown in Product Identification Guide, page 327

Ortho Biotech Products, L.P.

RARITAN, NJ 08869-0602

Direct Inquiries to:
(800) 325-7504
Prompt #1, Customer Service
Prompt #2, Medical Information
FAX: (908) 526-9230
(908) 526-6457

LEUSTATIN® ℞

(cladribine) Injection
For Intravenous Infusion Only

WARNING

LEUSTATIN (cladribine) Injection should be administered under the supervision of a qualified physician experienced in the use of antineoplastic therapy. Suppression of bone marrow function should be anticipated. This is usually reversible and appears to be dose dependent. Serious neurological toxicity (including irreversible paraparesis and quadraparesis) has been reported in patients who received LEUSTATIN Injection by continuous infusion at high doses (4 to 9 times the recommended dose for Hairy Cell Leukemia). Neurologic toxicity appears to demonstrate a dose relationship; however, severe neurological toxicity has been reported rarely following treatment with standard cladribine dosing regimens.

Acute nephrotoxicity has been observed with high doses of LEUSTATIN (4 to 9 times the recommended dose for Hairy Cell Leukemia), especially when given concomitantly with other nephrotoxic agents/therapies.

DESCRIPTION

LEUSTATIN (cladribine) Injection (also commonly known as 2-chloro-2′-deoxy-β-D-adenosine) is a synthetic antineoplastic agent for continuous intravenous infusion. It is a clear, colorless, sterile, preservative-free, isotonic solution. LEUSTATIN Injection is available in single-use vials containing 10 mg (1 mg/mL) of cladribine, a chlorinated purine nucleoside analog. Each milliliter of LEUSTATIN Injection contains 1 mg of the active ingredient and 9 mg (0.15 mEq) of sodium chloride as an inactive ingredient. The solution has a pH range of 5.5 to 8.0. Phosphoric acid and/or dibasic sodium phosphate may have been added to adjust the pH to 6.3±0.3.

The chemical name for cladribine is 2-chloro-6-amino-9-(2-deoxy-β-D-erythropento-furanosyl) purine and the structure is represented below:

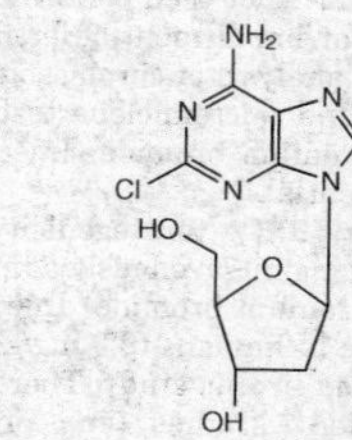

cladribine

MW 285.7

CLINICAL PHARMACOLOGY

Cellular Resistance and Sensitivity:

The selective toxicity of 2-chloro-2′-deoxy-β-D-adenosine towards certain normal and malignant lymphocyte and monocyte populations is based on the relative activities of deoxycytidine kinase and deoxynucleotidase. Cladribine passively crosses the cell membrane. In cells with a high ratio of deoxycytidine kinase to deoxynucleotidase, it is phosphorylated by deoxycytidine kinase to 2-chloro-2′-deoxy-β-D-adenosine monophosphate (2-CdAMP). Since 2-chloro-2′-deoxy-β-D-adenosine is resistant to deamination by adenosine deaminase and there is little deoxynucleotide deaminase in lymphocytes and monocytes, 2-CdAMP accumulates intracellularly and is subsequently converted into the active triphosphate deoxynucleotide, 2-chloro-2′-deoxy-β-D-adenosine triphosphate (2-CdATP). It is postulated that cells with high deoxycytidine kinase and low deoxynucleotidase activities will be selectively killed by 2-chloro-2′-deoxy-β-D-adenosine as toxic deoxynucleotides accumulate intracellularly.

Cells containing high concentrations of deoxynucleotides are unable to properly repair single-strand DNA breaks. The broken ends of DNA activate the enzyme poly (ADP-ribose) polymerase resulting in NAD and ATP depletion and disruption of cellular metabolism. There is evidence, also, that 2-CdATP is incorporated into the DNA of dividing cells, resulting in impairment of DNA synthesis. Thus, 2-chloro-2′-deoxy-β-D-adenosine can be distinguished from other chemotherapeutic agents affecting purine metabolism in that it is cytotoxic to both actively dividing and quiescent lymphocytes and monocytes, inhibiting both DNA synthesis and repair.

HUMAN PHARMACOLOGY

In a clinical investigation, 17 patients with Hairy Cell Leukemia and normal renal function were treated for 7 days with the recommended treatment regimen of LEUSTATIN Injection (0.09 mg/kg/day) by continuous intravenous infusion. The mean steady-state serum concentration was estimated to be 5.7 ng/mL with an estimated systemic clearance of 663.5 mL/h/kg when LEUSTATIN was given by continuous infusion over 7 days. In Hairy Cell Leukemia patients, there does not appear to be a relationship between serum concentrations and ultimate clinical outcome.

In another study, 8 patients with hematologic malignancies received a two (2) hour infusion of LEUSTATIN Injection (0.12 mg/kg). The mean end-of-infusion plasma LEUSTATIN concentration was 48±19 ng/mL. For 5 of these patients, the disappearance of LEUSTATIN could be described by either a biphasic or triphasic decline. For these patients with normal renal function, the mean terminal half-life was 5.4 hours. Mean values for clearance and steady-state volume of distribution were 978±422 mL/h/kg and 4.5±2.8 L/kg, respectively.

Plasma concentrations are reported to decline multi-exponentially after intravenous infusions with terminal half-lives ranging from approximately 3-22 hours. In general, the apparent volume of distribution of cladribine is very large (mean approximately 9 L/kg), indicating an extensive distribution of cladribine in body tissues. The mean half-life of cladribine in leukemic cells has been reported to be 23 hours.

Cladribine penetrates into cerebrospinal fluid. One report indicates that concentrations are approximately 25% of those in plasma.

LEUSTATIN is bound approximately 20% to plasma proteins.

Except for some understanding of the mechanism of cellular toxicity, no other information is available on the metabolism of LEUSTATIN in humans. An average of 18% of the administered dose has been reported to be excreted in urine of patients with solid tumors during a 5-day continuous intravenous infusion of 3.5-8.1 mg/m^2/day of LEUSTATIN. The effect of renal and hepatic impairment on the elimination of cladribine has not been investigated in humans.

Two single-center open label studies of LEUSTATIN (cladribine) have been conducted in patients with Hairy Cell Leukemia with evidence of active disease requiring therapy. In the study conducted at the Scripps Clinic and Research Foundation (Study A), 89 patients were treated with a single course of LEUSTATIN Injection given by continuous intravenous infusion for 7 days at a dose of 0.09 mg/kg/day. In the study conducted at the M.D. Anderson Cancer Center (Study B), 35 patients were treated with a 7-day continuous intravenous infusion of LEUSTATIN Injection at a comparable dose of 3.6 mg/m^2/day. A complete response (CR) required clearing of the peripheral blood and bone marrow of hairy cells and recovery of the hemoglobin to 12 g/dL, platelet count to 100 × 10^9/L, and absolute neutrophil count to 1500 × 10^6/L. A good partial response (GPR) required the same hematologic parameters as a complete response, and that fewer than 5% hairy cells remain in the bone marrow. A partial response (PR) required that hairy cells in the bone marrow be decreased by at least 50% from baseline and the same response for hematologic parameters as for complete response. A pathologic relapse was defined as an increase in bone marrow hairy cells to 25% of pretreatment levels. A clinical relapse was defined as the recurrence of cytopenias, specifically, decreases in hemoglobin ≥2 g/dL, ANC ≥25% or platelet counts ≥50,000. Patients who met the criteria for a complete response but subsequently were found to have evidence of bone marrow hairy cells (<25% of pretreatment levels) were reclassified as partial responses and were not considered to be complete responses with relapse.

Among patients evaluable for efficacy (N=106), using the hematologic and bone marrow response criteria described above, the complete response rates in patients treated with LEUSTATIN Injection were 65% and 68% for Study A and Study B, respectively, yielding a combined complete response rate of 66%. Overall response rates (i.e., Complete plus Good Partial plus Partial Responses) were 89% and 86% in Study A and Study B, respectively, for a combined overall response rate of 88% in evaluable patients treated with LEUSTATIN Injection.

Using an intent-to-treat analysis (N=123) and further requiring no evidence of splenomegaly as a criterion for CR (i.e., no palpable spleen on physical examination and ≤13 cm on CT scan), the complete response rates for Study A and Study B were 54% and 53%, respectively, giving a combined CR rate of 54%. The overall response rates (CR + GPR + PR) were 90% and 85%, for Studies A and B, respectively, yielding a combined overall response rate of 89%.

RESPONSE RATES TO LEUSTATIN TREATMENT IN PATIENTS WITH HAIRY CELL LEUKEMIA

	CR	Overall
Evaluable Patients N=106	66%	88%
Intent-to-treat Population N=123	54%	89%

In these studies, 60% of the patients had not received prior chemotherapy for Hairy Cell Leukemia or had undergone splenectomy as the only prior treatment and were receiving LEUSTATIN as a first-line treatment. The remaining 40% of the patients received LEUSTATIN as a second-line treatment, having been treated previously with other agents, including α-interferon and/or deoxycoformycin. The overall response rate for patients without prior chemotherapy was 92%, compared with 84% for previously treated patients. LEUSTATIN is active in previously treated patients; however, retrospective analysis suggests that the overall response rate is decreased in patients previously treated with splenectomy or deoxycoformycin and in patients refractory to α-interferon.

OVERALL RESPONSE RATES (CR + GPR + PR) TO LEUSTATIN TREATMENT IN PATIENTS WITH HAIRY CELL LEUKEMIA

	OVERALL RESPONSE (N=123)	NR + RELAPSE
No Prior Chemotherapy	68/74 92%	6 + 4 14%
Any Prior Chemotherapy	41/49 84%	8 + 3 22%
Previous Splenectomy	32/41* 78%	9 + 1 24%
Previous Interferon	40/48 83%	8 + 3 23%
Interferon Refractory	6/11* 55%	5 + 2 64%
Previous Deoxycoformycin	3/6* 50%	3 + 1 66%

NR = No Response
* $P < 0.05$

After a reversible decline, normalization of peripheral blood counts (Hemoglobin >12.0 g/dL, Platelets >100 × 10^9/L, Absolute Neutrophil Count (ANC) >1500 × 10^6/L) was achieved by 92% of evaluable patients. The median time to normalization of peripheral counts was 9 weeks from the start of treatment (Range: 2 to 72). The median time to normalization of Platelet Count was 2 weeks, the median time to normalization of ANC was 5 weeks and the median time to normalization of Hemoglobin was 8 weeks. With normalization of Platelet Count and Hemoglobin, requirements for platelet and RBC transfusions were abolished after Months 1 and 2, respectively, in those patients with complete response. Platelet recovery may be delayed in a minority of patients with severe baseline thrombocytopenia. Corresponding to normalization of ANC, a trend toward a reduced incidence of infection was seen after the third month, when compared to the months immediately preceding LEUSTATIN therapy. (see also WARNINGS, PRECAUTIONS and ADVERSE REACTIONS)

LEUSTATIN TREATMENT IN PATIENTS WITH HAIRY CELL LEUKEMIA TIME TO NORMALIZATION OF PERIPHERAL BLOOD COUNTS

Parameter	Median Time to Normalization of Count*
Platelet Count	2 weeks
Absolute Neutrophil Count	5 weeks
Hemoglobin	8 weeks
ANC, Hemoglobin and Platelet Count	9 weeks

*Day 1 = First day of infusion

For patients achieving a complete response, the median time to response (i.e., absence of hairy cells in bone marrow and peripheral blood together with normalization of peripheral blood parameters), measured from treatment start, was approximately 4 months. Since bone marrow aspiration and biopsy were frequently not performed at the time of peripheral blood normalization, the median time to complete response may actually be shorter than that which was recorded. At the time of data cut-off, the median duration of complete response was greater than 8 months and ranged to 25+ months. Among 93 responding patients, seven had shown evidence of disease progression at the time of the data cut-off. In four of these patients, disease was limited to the bone marrow without peripheral blood abnormalities (pathologic progression), while in three patients there were also peripheral blood abnormalities (clinical progression). Seven patients who did not respond to a first course of LEUSTATIN received a second course of therapy. In the five patients who had adequate follow-up, additional courses did not appear to improve their overall response.

INDICATIONS FOR USE

LEUSTATIN Injection is indicated for the treatment of active Hairy Cell Leukemia as defined by clinically significant anemia, neutropenia, thrombocytopenia or disease-related symptoms.

CONTRAINDICATIONS

LEUSTATIN is contraindicated in those patients who are hypersensitive to this drug or any of its components.

WARNINGS

Severe bone marrow suppression, including neutropenia, anemia and thrombocytopenia, has been commonly observed in patients treated with LEUSTATIN, especially at high doses. At initiation of treatment, most patients in the clinical studies had hematologic impairment as a manifestation of active Hairy Cell Leukemia. Following treatment with LEUSTATIN, further hematologic impairment occurred before recovery of peripheral blood counts began. During the first two weeks after treatment initiation, mean Platelet Count, ANC, and Hemoglobin concentration declined and subsequently increased with normalization of mean counts by Day 12, Week 5 and Week 8, respectively. The myelosuppressive effects of LEUSTATIN were most notable during the first month following treatment. Forty-four percent (44%) of patients received transfusions with RBCs and 14% received transfusions with platelets during Month 1. Careful hematologic monitoring, especially during the first 4 to 8 weeks after treatment with LEUSTATIN Injection, is recommended. (see PRECAUTIONS)

Fever (T≥100°F) was associated with the use of LEUSTATIN in approximately two-thirds of patients (131/196) in the first month of therapy. Virtually all of these patients were treated empirically with parenteral antibiotics. Overall, 47% (93/196) of all patients had fever in the setting of neutropenia (ANC ≤1000), including 62 patients (32%) with severe neutropenia (i.e., ANC ≤500).

In a Phase I investigational study using LEUSTATIN in high doses (4 to 9 times the recommended dose for Hairy Cell Leukemia) as part of a bone marrow transplant conditioning regimen, which also included high dose cyclophosphamide and total body irradiation, acute nephrotoxicity and delayed onset neurotoxicity were observed. Thirty-one (31) poor-risk patients with drug-resistant acute leukemia in relapse (29 cases) or non-Hodgkins Lymphoma (2 cases) received LEUSTATIN for 7 to 14 days prior to bone marrow transplantation. During infusion, 8 patients experienced gastrointestinal symptoms. While the bone marrow was initially cleared of all hematopoietic elements, including tumor cells, leukemia eventually recurred in all treated patients. Within 7 to 13 days after starting treatment with LEUSTATIN, 6 patients (19%) developed manifestations of renal dysfunction (e.g., acidosis, anuria, elevated serum creatinine, etc.) and 5 required dialysis. Several of these patients were also being treated with other medications having known nephrotoxic potential. Renal dysfunction was reversible in 2 of these patients. In the 4 patients whose renal function had not recovered at the time of death, autopsies were performed; in 2 of these, evidence of tubular damage was noted. Eleven (11) patients (35%) experienced delayed onset neurologic toxicity. In the majority, this was characterized by progressive irreversible motor weakness (paraparesis/quadriparesis), of the upper and/or lower extremities, first noted 35 to 84 days after starting high dose therapy with LEUSTATIN. Non-invasive testing (electromyography and nerve conduction studies) was consistent with demyelinating disease. Severe neurologic toxicity has also been noted with high doses of another drug in this class.

Axonal peripheral polyneuropathy was observed in a dose escalation study at the highest dose levels (approximately 4 times the recommended dose for Hairy Cell Leukemia) in patients not receiving cyclophosphamide or total body irradiation. Severe neurological toxicity has been reported rarely following treatment with standard cladribine dosing regimens.

In patients with Hairy Cell Leukemia treated with the recommended treatment regimen (0.09 mg/kg/day for 7 consecutive days), there have been no reports of nephrologic toxicities.

Of the 196 Hairy Cell Leukemia patients entered in the two trials, there were 8 deaths following treatment. Of these, 6 were of infectious etiology, including 3 pneumonias, and 2 occurred in the first month following LEUSTATIN therapy. Of the 8 deaths, 6 occurred in previously treated patients who were Refractory to α-interferon.

Benzyl alcohol is a constituent of the recommended diluent for the 7-day infusion solution. Benzyl alcohol has been reported to be associated with a fatal "Gasping Syndrome" in premature infants. (see DOSAGE AND ADMINISTRATION)

Pregnancy Category D: LEUSTATIN Injection should not be given during pregnancy.

Cladribine is teratogenic in mice and rabbits and consequently has the potential to cause fetal harm when administered to a pregnant woman. A significant increase in fetal variations was observed in mice receiving 1.5 mg/kg/day (4.5 mg/m^2) and increased resorptions, reduced litter size and increased fetal malformations were observed when mice received 3.0 mg/kg/day (9 mg/m^2). Fetal death and malformations were observed in rabbits that received 3.0 mg/kg/day (33.0 mg/m^2). No fetal effects were seen in mice at 0.5 mg/kg/day (1.5 mg/m^2) or in rabbits at 1.0 mg/kg/day (11.0 mg/m^2).

Although there is no evidence of teratogenicity in humans due to LEUSTATIN, other drugs which inhibit DNA synthesis (e.g., methotrexate and aminopterin) have been reported to be teratogenic in humans. LEUSTATIN has been shown to be embryotoxic in mice when given at doses equivalent to the recommended dose.

There are no adequate and well controlled studies in pregnant women. If LEUSTATIN is used during pregnancy, or if the patient becomes pregnant while taking this drug, the patient should be apprised of the potential hazard to the fetus. Women of childbearing age should be advised to avoid becoming pregnant.

PRECAUTIONS

General: LEUSTATIN Injection is a potent antineoplastic agent with potentially significant toxic side effects. It should be administered only under the supervision of a physician experienced with the use of cancer chemotherapeutic agents. Patients undergoing therapy should be closely observed for signs of hematologic and non-hematologic toxicity. Periodic assessment of peripheral blood counts, particu

Continued on next page

Leustatin—Cont.

larly during the first 4 to 8 weeks post-treatment, is recommended to detect the development of anemia, neutropenia and thrombocytopenia and for early detection of any potential sequelae (e.g., infection or bleeding). As with other potent chemotherapeutic agents, monitoring of renal and hepatic function is also recommended, especially in patients with underlying kidney or liver dysfunction. (see WARNINGS and ADVERSE REACTIONS)

Fever was a frequently observed side effect during the first month on study. Since the majority of fevers occurred in neutropenic patients, patients should be closely monitored during the first month of treatment and empiric antibiotics should be initiated as clinically indicated. Although 69% of patients developed fevers, less than 1/3 of febrile events were associated with documented infection. Given the known myelosuppressive effects of LEUSTATIN, practitioners should carefully evaluate the risks and benefits of administering this drug to patients with active infections. (see WARNINGS and ADVERSE REACTIONS)

There are inadequate data on dosing of patients with renal or hepatic insufficiency. Development of acute renal insufficiency in some patients receiving high doses of LEUSTATIN has been described. Until more information is available, caution is advised when administering the drug to patients with known or suspected renal or hepatic insufficiency. (see WARNINGS)

Rare cases of tumor lysis syndrome have been reported in patients treated with cladribine with other hematologic malignancies having a high tumor burden.

LEUSTATIN Injection must be diluted in designated intravenous solutions prior to administration. (see DOSAGE AND ADMINISTRATION)

Laboratory Tests: During and following treatment, the patient's hematologic profile should be monitored regularly to determine the degree of hematopoietic suppression. In the clinical studies, following reversible declines in all cell counts, the mean Platelet Count reached 100 × 10^9/L by Day 12, the mean Absolute Neutrophil Count reached 1500 × 10^6/L by Week 5 and the mean Hemoglobin reached 12 g/dL by Week 8. After peripheral counts have normalized, bone marrow aspiration and biopsy should be performed to confirm response to treatment with LEUSTATIN. Febrile events should be investigated with appropriate laboratory and radiologic studies. Periodic assessment of renal function and hepatic function should be performed as clinically indicated.

Drug Interactions: There are no known drug interactions with LEUSTATIN Injection. Caution should be exercised if LEUSTATIN Injection is administered before, after, or in conjunction with other drugs known to cause immunosuppression or myelosuppression. (See WARNINGS)

Carcinogenesis: No animal carcinogenicity studies have been conducted with cladribine. However, its carcinogenic potential cannot be excluded based on demonstrated genotoxicity of cladribine.

Mutagenesis: As expected for compounds in this class, the actions of cladribine yield DNA damage. In mammalian cells in culture, cladribine caused the accumulation of DNA strand breaks. Cladribine was also incorporated into DNA of human lymphoblastic leukemia cells. Cladribine was not mutagenic *in vitro* (Ames and Chinese hamster ovary cell gene mutation tests) and did not induce unscheduled DNA synthesis in primary rat hepatocyte cultures. However, cladribine was clastogenic both *in vitro* (chromosome aberrations in Chinese hamster ovary cells) and *in vivo* (mouse bone marrow micronucleus test).

Impairment of Fertility: When administered intravenously to Cynomolgus monkeys, cladribine has been shown to cause suppression of rapidly generating cells, including testicular cells. The effect on human fertility is unknown.

Pregnancy: Pregnancy Category D: (see WARNINGS)

Nursing Mothers: It is not known whether this drug is excreted in human milk. Because many drugs are excreted in human milk and because of the potential for serious adverse reactions in nursing infants from cladribine, a decision should be made whether to discontinue nursing or discontinue the drug, taking into account the importance of the drug for the mother.

Pediatric Use: Safety and effectiveness in pediatric patients have not been established. In a Phase I study involving patients 1–21 years old with relapsed acute leukemia; LEUSTATIN was given by continuous intravenous infusion in doses ranging from 3 to 10.7 mg/m^2/day for 5 days (one-half to twice the dose recommended in Hairy Cell Leukemia). In this study, the dose-limiting toxicity was severe myelosuppression with profound neutropenia and thrombocytopenia. At the highest dose (10.7 mg/m^2/day), 3 of 7 patients developed irreversible myelosuppression and fatal systemic bacterial or fungal infections. No unique toxicities were noted in this study.(1) (see WARNINGS and ADVERSE REACTIONS)

ADVERSE REACTIONS

Safety data are based on 196 patients with Hairy Cell Leukemia: the original cohort of 124 patients plus an additional 72 patients enrolled at the same two centers after the original enrollment cutoff. In Month 1 of the Hairy Cell Leukemia clinical trials, severe neutropenia was noted in 70% of patients, fever in 69%, and infection was documented in 28%. Other adverse experiences reported frequently during the first 14 days after initiating treatment included: fatigue (45%), nausea (28%), rash (27%), headache (22%) and injection site reactions (19%). Most non-hematologic adverse experiences were mild to moderate in severity.

Myelosuppression was frequently observed during the first month after starting treatment. Neutropenia (ANC <500 × 10^6/L) was noted in 70% of patients, compared with 26% in whom it was present initially. Severe anemia (Hemoglobin <8.5 g/dL) developed in 37% of patients, compared with 10% initially and thrombocytopenia (Platelets <20 × 10^9/L) developed in 12% of patients, compared to 4% in whom it was noted initially.

During the first month, 54 of 196 patients (28%) exhibited documented evidence of infection. Serious infections (e.g., septicemia, pneumonia) were reported in 6% of all patients; the remainder were mild or moderate. Several deaths were attributable to infection and/or complications related to the underlying disease. During the second month, the overall rate of documented infection was 6%; these infections were mild to moderate and no severe systemic infections were seen. After the third month, the monthly incidence of infection was either less than or equal to that of the months immediately preceding LEUSTATIN therapy.

During the first month, 11% of patients experienced severe fever (i.e., ≥104°F). Documented infections were noted in fewer than one-third of febrile episodes. Of the 196 patients studied, 19 were noted to have a documented infection in the month prior to treatment. In the month following treatment, there were 54 episodes of documented infection: 23 (42%) were bacterial, 11 (20%) were viral and 11 (20%) were fungal. Seven (7) of 8 documented episodes of herpes zoster occurred during the month following treatment. Fourteen (14) of 16 episodes of documented fungal infections occurred in the first two months following treatment. Virtually all of these patients were treated empirically with antibiotics. (see WARNINGS and PRECAUTIONS)

Analysis of lymphocyte subsets indicates that treatment with cladribine is associated with prolonged depression of the CD4 counts. Prior to treatment, the mean CD4 count was 766/μL. The mean CD4 count nadir, which occurred 4 to 6 months following treatment, was 272/μL. Fifteen (15) months after treatment, mean CD4 counts remained below 500/μL. CD8 counts behaved similarly, though increasing counts were observed after 9 months. The clinical significance of the prolonged CD4 lymphopenia is unclear.

Another event of unknown clinical significance includes the observation of prolonged bone marrow hypocellularity. Bone marrow cellularity of <35% was noted after 4 months in 42 of 124 patients (34%) treated in the two pivotal trials. This hypocellularity was noted as late as day 1010. It is not known whether the hypocellularity is the result of disease related marrow fibrosis or if it is the result of cladribine toxicity. There was no apparent clinical effect on the peripheral blood counts.

The vast majority of rashes were mild and occurred in patients who were receiving or had recently been treated with other medications (e.g., allopurinol or antibiotics) known to cause rash.

Most episodes of nausea were mild, not accompanied by vomiting, and did not require treatment with antiemetics. In patients requiring antiemetics, nausea was easily controlled, most frequently with chlorpromazine.

Adverse reactions reported during the first 2 weeks following treatment initiation (regardless of relationship to drug) by >5% of patients included:

Body as a Whole: fever (69%), fatigue (45%), chills (9%), asthenia (9%), diaphoresis (9%), malaise (7%), trunk pain (6%)

Gastrointestinal: nausea (28%), decreased appetite (17%), vomiting (13%), diarrhea (10%), constipation (9%), abdominal pain (6%)

Hemic/Lymphatic: purpura (10%), petechiae (8%), epistaxis (5%)

Nervous System: headache (22%), dizziness (9%), insomnia (7%)

Cardiovascular System: edema (6%), tachycardia (6%)

Respiratory System: abnormal breath sounds (11%), cough (10%), abnormal chest sounds (9%), shortness of breath (7%)

Skin/Subcutaneous Tissue: rash (27%), injection site reactions (19%), pruritis (6%), erythema (6%)

Musculoskeletal System: myalgia (7%), arthralgia (5%)

Adverse experiences related to intravenous administration included: injection site reactions (9%) (i.e., redness, swelling, pain), thrombosis (2%), phlebitis (2%) and a broken catheter (1%). These appear to be related to the infusion procedure and/or indwelling catheter, rather than the medication or the vehicle.

From Day 15 to the last follow-up visit, the only events reported by >5% of patients were: fatigue (11%), rash (10%), headache (7%), cough (7%), and malaise (5%).

For a description of adverse reactions associated with use of high doses in non-Hairy Cell Leukemia patients, see WARNINGS.

The following additional adverse events have been reported since the drug became commercially available. These adverse events have been reported primarily in patients who received multiple courses of LEUSTATIN Injection:

Hematologic: bone marrow suppression with prolonged pancytopenia, including some reports of aplastic anemia; hemolytic anemia, which was reported in patients with lymphoid malignancies, occurring within the first few weeks following treatment.

Hepatic: reversible, generally mild increases in bilirubin and transaminases.

Nervous System: Neurological toxicity; however, severe neurotoxicity has been reported rarely following treatment with standard cladribine dosing regimens.

Respiratory System: pulmonary interstitial infiltrates; in most cases, an infectious etiology was identified.

Skin/Subcutaneous: urticaria, hypereosinophilia. In isolated cases Stevens-Johnson and toxic epidermal necrolysis have been reported in patients who were receiving or had recently been treated with other medications (e.g., allopurinol or antibiotics) known to cause these syndromes.

Opportunistic infections have occurred in the acute phase of treatment due to the immunosuppression mediated by LEUSTATIN Injection.

OVERDOSAGE

High doses of LEUSTATIN have been associated with: irreversible neurologic toxicity (paraparesis/quadriparesis), acute nephrotoxicity, and severe bone marrow suppression resulting in neutropenia, anemia and thrombocytopenia. (see WARNINGS) There is no known specific antidote to overdosage. Treatment of overdosage consists of discontinuation of LEUSTATIN, careful observation and appropriate supportive measures. It is not known whether the drug can be removed from the circulation by dialysis or hemofiltration.

DOSAGE AND ADMINISTRATION

Usual Dose:

The recommended dose and schedule of LEUSTATIN Injection for active Hairy Cell Leukemia is as a single course given by continuous infusion for 7 consecutive days at a dose of 0.09 mg/kg/day. Deviations from this dosage regimen are not advised. If the patient does not respond to the initial course of LEUSTATIN Injection for Hairy Cell Leukemia, it is unlikely that they will benefit from additional courses. Physicians should consider delaying or discontinuing the drug if neurotoxicity or renal toxicity occurs. (see WARNINGS)

Specific risk factors predisposing to increased toxicity from LEUSTATIN have not been defined. In view of the known toxicities of agents of this class, it would be prudent to proceed carefully in patients with known or suspected renal insufficiency or severe bone marrow impairment of any etiology. Patients should be monitored closely for hematologic and non-hematologic toxicity. (see WARNINGS and PRECAUTIONS).

Preparation and Administration of Intravenous Solutions: LEUSTATIN Injection must be diluted with the designated diluent prior to administration. Since the drug product does not contain any anti-microbial preservative or bacteriostatic agent, **aseptic technique and proper environmental precautions must be observed in preparation of LEUSTATIN Injection solutions.**

To prepare a single daily dose: Add the calculated dose (0.09 mg/kg or 0.09 mL/kg) of LEUSTATIN Injection to an infusion bag containing 500 mL of 0.9% Sodium Chloride Injection, USP. Infuse continuously over 24 hours. Repeat daily for a total of 7 consecutive days. **The use of 5% dextrose as a diluent is not recommended because of increased degradation of cladribine.** Admixtures of LEUSTATIN Injection are chemically and physically stable for at least 24 hours at room temperature under normal room fluorescent light in Baxter Viaflex®† PVC infusion containers. **Since limited compatability data are available, adherence to the recommended diluents and infusion systems is advised.**

	Dose of LEUSTATIN Injection	Recommended Diluent	Quantity of Diluent
24-hour infusion method	1 (day) × 0.09 mg/kg	0.9% Sodium Chloride Injection, USP	500 mL

To prepare a 7-day infusion: The 7-day infusion solution should only be prepared with Bacteriostatic 0.9% Sodium Chloride Injection, USP (0.9% benzyl alcohol preserved). In order to minimize the risk of microbial contamination, both LEUSTATIN Injection and the diluent should be passed through a sterile 0.22μ disposable hydrophilic syringe filter as each solution is being introduced into the infusion reservoir. First add the calculated dose of LEUSTATIN Injection (7 days × 0.09 mg/kg or mL/kg) to the infusion reservoir through the sterile filter. Then add a calculated amount of Bacteriostatic 0.9% Sodium Chloride Injection, USP (0.9% benzyl alcohol preserved) also through the filter to bring the total volume of the solution to 100 mL. After completing solution preparation, clamp off the line, disconnect and discard the filter. Aseptically aspirate air bubbles from the reservoir as necessary using the syringe and a dry second sterile filter or a sterile vent filter assembly. Reclamp the line and discard the syringe and filter assembly. Infuse continuously over 7 days. Solutions prepared with Bacteriostatic Sodium Chloride Injection for individuals weighing more than 85 kg may have reduced preservative effectiveness due to greater dilution of the benzyl alcohol preservative. Admixtures for the 7-day infusion have demonstrated acceptable chemical and physical stability for at least 7 days in the SIMS Deltec MEDICATION CASSETTE™ Reservoir‡.

	Dose of LEUSTATIN Injection	Recommended Diluent	Quantity of Diluent
7-day infusion method (use sterile 0.22μ filter when preparing infusion solution)	7 (days) × 0.09 mg/kg	Bacteriostatic 0.9% Sodium Chloride Injection, USP (0.9% benzyl alcohol)	q.s. to 100 mL

Since limited compatibility data are available, adherence to the recommended diluents and infusion systems is advised. Solutions containing LEUSTATIN Injection should not be mixed with other intravenous drugs or additives or infused simultaneously via a common intravenous line, since compatibility testing has not been performed. Preparations containing benzyl alcohol should not be used in neonates. (see WARNINGS)

Care must be taken to assure the sterility of prepared solutions. Once diluted, solutions of LEUSTATIN Injection should be administered promptly or stored in the refrigerator (2° to 8°C) for no more than 8 hours prior to start of administration. Vials of LEUSTATIN Injection are for single-use only. Any unused portion should be discarded in an appropriate manner. (see Handling and Disposal)

Parenteral drug products should be inspected visually for particulate matter and discoloration prior to administration, whenever solution and container permit. A precipitate may occur during the exposure of LEUSTATIN Injection to low temperatures; it may be resolubilized by allowing the solution to warm naturally to room temperature and by shaking vigorously. **DO NOT HEAT OR MICROWAVE.**

Chemical Stability of Vials:

When stored in refrigerated conditions between 2° to 8°C (36° to 46°F) protected from light, unopened vials of LEUSTATIN Injection are stable until the expiration date indicated on the package. Freezing does not adversely affect the solution. If freezing occurs, thaw naturally to room temperature. DO NOT heat or microwave. Once thawed, the vial of LEUSTATIN Injection is stable until expiry if refrigerated. DO NOT refreeze. Once diluted, solutions containing LEUSTATIN Injection should be administered promptly or stored in the refrigerator (2° to 8°C) for no more than 8 hours prior to administration.

Handling and Disposal:

The potential hazards associated with cytotoxic agents are well established and proper precautions should be taken when handling, preparing, and administering LEUSTATIN Injection. The use of disposable gloves and protective garments is recommended. If LEUSTATIN Injection contacts the skin or mucous membranes, wash the involved surface immediately with copious amounts of water. Several guidelines on this subject have been published.[2–8] There is no general agreement that all of the procedures recommended in the guidelines are necessary or appropriate. Refer to your Institution's guidelines and all applicable state/local regulations for disposal of cytotoxic waste.

HOW SUPPLIED

LEUSTATIN Injection is supplied as a sterile, preservative-free, isotonic solution containing 10 mg (1 mg/mL) of cladribine as 10 mL filled into a single-use clear flint glass 20 mL vial. LEUSTATIN Injection is supplied in 10 mL (1 mg/mL) single-use vials (NDC 59676-201-01) available in a treatment set (case) of seven vials.

Store refrigerated 2° to 8°C (36° to 46°F). Protect from light during storage.

References:

1. Santana VM, Mirro J, Harwood FC, *et al:* A phase I clinical trial of 2-Chloro-deoxyadenosine in pediatric patients with acute leukemia. J. Clin. Onc., **9:** 416 (1991).
2. Recommendations for the Safe Handling of Parenteral Antineoplastic Drugs. NIH Publication No. 83-2621. For sale by the Superintendent of Documents, U. S. Government Printing Office, Washington, D.C. 20402.
3. AMA Council Report. Guidelines for Handling Parenteral Antineoplastics, JAMA, March 15 (1985).
4. National Study Commission on Cytotoxic Exposure—Recommendations for Handling Cytotoxic Agents. Available from Louis P. Jeffrey, Sc.D., Chairman, National Study Commission of Cytotoxic Exposure, Massachusetts College of Pharmacy and Allied Health Sciences, 179 Longwood Avenue, Boston, Massachusetts 02115.
5. Clinical Oncological Society of Australia: Guidelines and Recommendations for Safe Handling of Antineoplastic Agents, Med. J. Australia **1**:425 (1983).
6. Jones RB, *et al.* Safe Handling of Chemotherapeutic Agents: A Report from the Mount Sinai Medical Center. Ca—A Cancer Journal for Clinicians, Sept/Oct. 258–263 (1983).
7. American Society of Hospital Pharmacists Technical Assistance Bulletin on Handling Cytotoxic Drugs in Hospitals. Am. J. Hosp. Pharm., **42**:131 (1985).
8. OSHA Work-Practice Guidelines for Personnel Dealing with Cytotoxic (antineoplastic) Drugs. Am. J. Hosp. Pharm., **43**:1193 (1986).

CAUTION: Federal law prohibits dispensing without prescription.

† Viaflex® containers, manufactured by Baxter Healthcare Corporation - Code No. 2B8013 (testing in 1991)

‡ MEDICATION CASSETTE™ Reservoir, manufactured by SIMS Deltec, Inc. - Reorder No. 602100A (tested in 1991)

ORTHO BIOTECH PRODUCTS, L.P.
Raritan, New Jersey 08869 ORTHO BIOTECH
©OBI 1996 638-10-940-5
Revised December 1996 LEU-533

Shown in Product Identification Guide, page 327

ORTHOCLONE OKT®3 Sterile Solution ℞

(muromonab-CD3)
For Intravenous Use Only

WARNING:
Only physicians experienced in immunosuppressive therapy and management of solid organ transplant patients should use ORTHOCLONE OKT3 (muromonab-CD3). Patients treated with ORTHOCLONE OKT3 must be managed in a facility equipped and staffed for cardiopulmonary resuscitation and where the patient can be closely monitored for an appropriate period based on his or her health status.
Anaphylactic and anaphylactoid reactions may occur following administration of any dose or course of ORTHOCLONE OKT3. In addition, serious, occasionally life-threatening or lethal, systemic, cardiovascular, and central nervous system reactions have been reported following administration of ORTHOCLONE OKT3. These have included: pulmonary edema, especially in patients with volume overload; shock, cardiovascular collapse, cardiac or respiratory arrest, seizures, coma, cerebral edema, cerebral herniation, blindness, and paralysis. Fluid status should be carefully monitored prior to and during ORTHOCLONE OKT3 administration. Pretreatment with methylprednisolone is recommended to minimize symptoms of Cytokine Release Syndrome. (See: WARNINGS: Cytokine Release Syndrome, Central Nervous System Events, Anaphylactic Reactions; DOSAGE AND ADMINISTRATION)

DESCRIPTION

ORTHOCLONE OKT3 (muromonab-CD3) Sterile Solution is a murine monoclonal antibody to the CD3 antigen of human T cells which functions as an immunosuppressant. It is for intravenous use only. The antibody is a biochemically purified IgG_{2a} immunoglobulin with a heavy chain of approximately 50,000 daltons and a light chain of approximately 25,000 daltons. It is directed to a glycoprotein with a molecular weight of 20,000 in the human T cell surface which is essential for T cell functions. Because it is a monoclonal antibody preparation, ORTHOCLONE OKT3 Sterile Solution is a homogeneous, reproducible antibody product with consistent, measurable reactivity to human T cells.

Each 5 mL ampule of ORTHOCLONE OKT3 Sterile Solution contains 5 mg (1 mg/mL) of muromonab-CD3 in a clear colorless solution which may contain a few fine translucent protein particles. Each ampule contains a buffered solution (pH 7.0 ± 0.5) of monobasic sodium phosphate (2.25 mg), dibasic sodium phosphate (9.0 mg), sodium chloride (43 mg), and polysorbate 80 (1.0 mg) in water for injection.

The proper name, muromonab-CD3, is derived from the descriptive term murine monoclonal antibody. The CD3 designation identifies the specificity of the antibody as the Cell Differentiation (CD) cluster 3 defined by the First International Workshop on Human Leukocyte Differentiation Antigens.

CLINICAL PHARMACOLOGY

ORTHOCLONE OKT3 reverses graft rejection, probably by blocking the function of T cells which play a major role in acute allograft rejection. ORTHOCLONE OKT3 reacts with and blocks the function of a 20,000 dalton molecule (CD3) in the membrane of human T cells that has been associated *in vitro* with the antigen recognition structure of T cells and is essential for signal transduction. In *in vitro* cytolytic assays, ORTHOCLONE OKT3 blocks both the generation and function of effector cells. Binding of ORTHOCLONE OKT3 to T lymphocytes results in early activation of T cells, which leads to cytokine release, followed by blocking T cell functions. After termination of ORTHOCLONE OKT3 therapy, T cell function usually returns to normal within one week.

In vivo, ORTHOCLONE OKT3 reacts with most peripheral blood T cells and T cells in body tissues, but has not been found to react with other hematopoietic elements or other tissues of the body.

A rapid and concomitant decrease in the number of circulating CD3 positive cells, including those that are CD2, CD4, or CD8 positive has been observed in patients studied within minutes after the administration of ORTHOCLONE OKT3. This decrease in the number of CD3 positive T cells results from the specific interaction between ORTHOCLONE OKT3 and the CD3 antigen on the surface of all T lymphocytes. T cell activation results in the release of numerous cytokines/lymphokines, which are felt to be responsible for many of the acute clinical manifestations seen following ORTHOCLONE OKT3 administration. (See: WARNINGS: Cytokine Release Syndrome, Central Nervous System Events)

While CD3 positive cells are not detectable between days two and seven, increasing numbers of circulating CD2, CD4, and CD8 positive cells have been observed. The presence of these CD2, CD4, and CD8 positive cells has not been shown to affect reversal of rejection. After termination of ORTHOCLONE OKT3 therapy, CD3 positive cells reappear rapidly and reach pre-treatment levels within a week. In some patients however, increasing numbers of CD3 positive cells have been observed prior to termination of ORTHOCLONE OKT3 therapy. This reappearance of CD3 positive cells has been attributed to the development of neutralizing antibodies to ORTHOCLONE OKT3, which in turn block its ability to bind to the CD3 antigen on T lymphocytes. (See: PRECAUTIONS: Sensitization)

Pediatric patients are known to have higher CD3 lymphocyte counts than adults. Pediatric patients receiving ORTHOCLONE OKT®3 therapy often require progressively higher doses of ORTHOCLONE OKT3 to achieve depletion of CD3 positive cells (<25 cells/mm^3) and ensure therapeutic ORTHOCLONE OKT3 serum concentrations (>800 ng/mL). (See: DOSAGE AND ADMINISTRATION; PRECAUTIONS: Laboratory Tests)

Serum levels of ORTHOCLONE OKT3 are measurable using an enzyme-linked immunosorbent assay (ELISA). During the initial clinical trials in renal allograft rejection, in patients treated with 5 mg per day for 14 days, mean serum trough levels of the drug rose over the first three days and then averaged 900 ng/mL on days 3 to 14. Serum concentrations measured daily during treatment with ORTHOCLONE OKT3 in renal, hepatic, and cardiac allograft recipients revealed that pediatric patients less than 10 years of age have higher levels than patients 10–50 years of age. Subsequent clinical experience has demonstrated that serum levels greater than or equal to 800 ng/mL of ORTHOCLONE OKT3 blocks the function of cytotoxic T cells *in vitro* and *in vivo*. Reduced T cell clearance or low plasma ORTHOCLONE OKT3 levels provide a basis for adjusting ORTHOCLONE OKT3 dosage or for discontinuing therapy. (See: WARNINGS: Anaphylactic Reactions; PRECAUTIONS: Laboratory Tests; ADVERSE EVENTS: Hypersensitivity Reactions; DOSAGE AND ADMINISTRATION)

Following administration of ORTHOCLONE OKT3 *in vivo*, leukocytes have been observed in cerebrospinal and peritoneal fluids. The mechanism for this effect is not completely understood, but probably is related to cytokines altering membrane permeability, rather than an active inflammatory process. (See: WARNINGS: Cytokine Release Syndrome, Central Nervous System Events)

CLINICAL STUDIES

Acute Renal Rejection:

In a controlled randomized clinical trial, ORTHOCLONE OKT3 was compared with conventional high-dose steroid therapy in reversing acute renal allograft rejection. In this trial, 122 evaluable patients undergoing acute rejection of cadaveric renal transplants were treated either with ORTHOCLONE OKT3 daily for a mean of 14 days, with concomitant lowering of the dosage of azathioprine and maintenance steroids (62 patients), or with conventional high-dose steroids (60 patients). ORTHOCLONE OKT3 reversed 94% of the rejections compared to a 75% reversal rate obtained with conventional high-dose steroid treatment (p=0.006). The one year Kaplan-Meier (actuarial) estimates of graft survival rates for these patients who had acute rejection were 62% and 45% for ORTHOCLONE OKT3 and steroid-treated patients, respectively (p=0.04). At two years the rates were 56% and 42%, respectively (p=0.06).

One- and two-year patient survivals were not significantly different between the two groups, being 85% and 75% for ORTHOCLONE OKT3 treated patients and 90% and 85% for steroid-treated patients.

In additional open clinical trials, the observed rate of reversal of acute renal allograft rejection was 92% (n=126) for ORTHOCLONE OKT3 therapy. ORTHOCLONE OKT3 was also effective in reversing acute renal allograft rejections in 65% (n=225) of cases where steroids and lymphocyte immune globulin preparations were contraindicated or were not successful.

The effectiveness of ORTHOCLONE OKT3 for prophylaxis of renal allograft rejection has not been established.

Acute Cardiac or Hepatic Allograft Rejection:

ORTHOCLONE OKT3 was studied for use in reversing acute cardiac and hepatic allograft rejection in patients who are unresponsive to high-doses of steroids. The rate of reversal in acute cardiac allograft rejection was 90% (n = 61) and was 83% for hepatic allograft rejection (n = 124) in patients unresponsive to treatment with steroids.

Controlled randomized trials have not been conducted to evaluate the effectiveness of ORTHOCLONE OKT3 compared to conventional therapy as first line treatment for acute cardiac and hepatic allograft rejection.

INDICATIONS AND USAGE

ORTHOCLONE OKT3 is indicated for the treatment of acute allograft rejection in renal transplant patients.

ORTHOCLONE OKT3 is indicated for the treatment of steroid-resistant acute allograft rejection in cardiac and hepatic transplant patients.

Continued on next page

Orthoclone—Cont.

The dosage of other immunosuppressive agents used in conjunction with ORTHOCLONE OKT3 should be reduced to the lowest level compatible with an effective therapeutic response. (See: WARNINGS and ADVERSE EVENTS: Infections, Neoplasia; DOSAGE AND ADMINISTRATION)

CONTRAINDICATIONS

ORTHOCLONE OKT3 should not be given to patients who:

- are hypersensitive to this or any other product of murine origin;
- have anti-mouse antibody titers ≥1:1000;
- are in (uncompensated) heart failure or in fluid overload, as evidenced by chest X-ray or a greater than 3 percent weight gain within the week prior to planned ORTHOCLONE OKT3 administration;
- have uncontrolled hypertension;
- have a history of seizures, or are predisposed to seizures;
- are determined or suspected to be pregnant, or who are breast-feeding. (See: PRECAUTIONS: Pregnancy, Nursing Mothers)

WARNINGS

SEE BOXED WARNING

Cytokine Release Syndrome

Most patients develop an acute clinical syndrome [i.e., Cytokine Release Syndrome (CRS)] that has been attributed to the release of cytokines by activated lymphocytes or monocytes and is temporally associated with the administration of the first few doses of ORTHOCLONE OKT®3 (particularly, the first two to three doses). This clinical syndrome has ranged from a more frequently reported mild, self-limited, "flu-like" illness to a less frequently reported severe, life-threatening shock-like reaction, which may include serious cardiovascular and central nervous system manifestations. The syndrome typically begins approximately 30 to 60 minutes after administration of a dose of ORTHOCLONE OKT3 (but may occur later) and may persist for several hours. The frequency and severity of this symptom complex is usually greatest with the first dose. With each successive dose of ORTHOCLONE OKT3, both the frequency and severity of the Cytokine Release Syndrome tends to diminish. Increasing the amount of ORTHOCLONE OKT3 or resuming treatment after a hiatus may result in a reappearance of the CRS.

Common clinical manifestations of CRS may include: high fever (often spiking, up to 107°F), chills/rigors, headache, tremor, nausea/vomiting, diarrhea, abdominal pain, malaise, muscle/joint aches and pains, and generalized weakness. Less frequently reported adverse experiences include: minor dermatologic reactions (e.g., rash, pruritus, etc.) and a spectrum of often serious, occasionally fatal, cardiorespiratory and central nervous system adverse experiences.

Cardiorespiratory findings may include: dyspnea, shortness of breath, bronchospasm/wheezing, tachypnea, respiratory arrest/failure/distress, cardiovascular collapse, cardiac arrest, angina/myocardial infarction, chest pain/tightness, tachycardia (including ventricular), hypertension, hemodynamic instability, hypotension including profound shock, heart failure, pulmonary edema (cardiogenic and non-cardiogenic), adult respiratory distress syndrome, hypoxemia, apnea, and arrhythmias. (See: BOXED WARNING; PRECAUTIONS; ADVERSE EVENTS)

In the initial studies of renal allograft rejection, potentially fatal, severe pulmonary edema occurred in 5% of the initial 107 patients. Fluid overload was present before treatment in all of these cases. It occurred in none of the subsequent 311 patients treated with first-dose volume/weight restrictions. In subsequent trials and in post-marketing experience, severe pulmonary edema has occurred in patients who appeared to be euvolemic. The pathogenesis of pulmonary edema may involve all or some of the following: volume overload; increased pulmonary vascular permeability; and/or reduced left ventricular compliance/contractility.

During the first 1 to 3 days of ORTHOCLONE OKT3 therapy, some patients have experienced an acute and transient decline in the glomerular filtration rate (GFR) and diminished urine output with a resulting increase in the level of serum creatinine. Massive release of cytokines appears to lead to reversible renal functional impairment and/or delayed renal allograft function. Similarly, transient elevations in hepatic transaminases have been reported following administration of the first few doses of ORTHOCLONE OKT3.

Patients at risk for more serious complications of CRS may include those with the following conditions: unstable angina; recent myocardial infarction or symptomatic ischemic heart disease; heart failure of any etiology; pulmonary edema of any etiology; any form of chronic obstructive pulmonary disease; intravascular volume overload or depletion of any etiology (e.g., excessive dialysis, recent intensive diuresis, blood loss, etc.); cerebrovascular disease; patients with advanced symptomatic vascular disease or neuropathy; a history of seizures; and septic shock. Efforts should be made to correct or stabilize background conditions prior to the initiation of therapy. (See: PRECAUTIONS)

Prior to administration of ORTHOCLONE OKT3, the patient's volume (fluid) status and a chest x-ray should be assessed to rule out volume overload, uncontrolled hypertension, or uncompensated heart failure. Patients should not weigh >3% above their minimum weight during the week prior to injection.

The Cytokine Release Syndrome is associated with increased serum levels of cytokines (e.g., TNF-α, IL-2, IL-6, IFN-γ) that peak between 1 and 4 hours following administration of ORTHOCLONE OKT3. The serum levels of cytokines and the manifestations of CRS may be reduced by pretreatment with 8 mg/kg of methylprednisolone (i.e., high-dose steroids), given 1 to 4 hours prior to administration of the first dose of ORTHOCLONE OKT3, and by closely following recommendations for dosage and treatment duration. (See: DOSAGE AND ADMINISTRATION) It is not known if corticosteroid pretreatment decreases organ damage and sequelae associated with CRS. For example, increased intracranial pressure and cerebral herniation have occurred despite pretreatment with currently recommended doses and schedules of methylprednisolone.

If any of the more serious presentations of the Cytokine Release Syndrome occur, intensive treatment including oxygen, intravenous fluids, corticosteroids, pressor amines, antihistamines, intubation, etc., may be required.

Central Nervous System Events

Seizures, encephalopathy, cerebral edema, aseptic meningitis, and headache have been reported, even following the first dose, during therapy with ORTHOCLONE OKT®3. Seizures, some accompanied by loss of consciousness or cardiorespiratory arrest, or death, have occurred independently or in conjunction with any of the neurologic syndromes described below.

A few cases of fatal cerebral herniations subsequent to cerebral edema have been reported. All patients, particularly pediatric patients, must be carefully evaluated for fluid retention and hypertension before the initiation of ORTHOCLONE OKT3 therapy. Close monitoring for neurologic symptoms must be performed during the first twenty-four (24) hours following each of the first few doses of ORTHOCLONE OKT3 injection.

Patients should be closely monitored for convulsions and manifestations of encephalopathy, including: impaired cognition, confusion, obtundation, altered mental status, disorientation, auditory/visual hallucinations, psychosis (delirium, paranoia), mood changes (e.g., mania, agitation, combativeness, etc.), diffuse hypotonus, hyperreflexia, myoclonus, tremor, asterixis, involuntary movements, major motor seizures, lethargy/stupor/coma, and diffuse weakness. Approximately one-third of patients with a diagnosis of encephalopathy may have had coexisting aseptic meningitis syndrome.

Signs and symptoms of the aseptic meningitis syndrome described in association with the use of ORTHOCLONE OKT3 have included: fever, headache, meningismus (stiff neck), and photophobia. Diagnosis is confirmed by cerebrospinal fluid (CSF) analysis demonstrating leukocytosis with pleocytosis, elevated protein and normal or decreased glucose, with negative viral, bacterial, and fungal cultures. The possibility of infection should be evaluated in any immunosuppressed transplant patient with clinical findings suggesting meningitis. Approximately one-third of the patients with a diagnosis of aseptic meningitis had coexisting signs and symptoms of encephalopathy. Most patients with the aseptic meningitis syndrome had a benign course and recovered without any permanent sequelae during therapy or subsequent to its completion or discontinuation. However, because meningitis is a frequent infection encountered in pediatric allograft recipients, and the immunosuppression associated with transplantation increases the risk of opportunistic infection, pediatric patients with signs or symptoms suggestive of meningeal irritation while receiving ORTHOCLONE OKT3 should have lumbar punctures performed to rule out an infectious etiology. (See: PRECAUTIONS: Pediatric Use)

Signs or symptoms of encephalopathy, meningitis, seizures, and cerebral edema, with or without headache, typically have been reversible. Headache, aseptic meningitis, seizures, and less severe forms of encephalopathy resolved in most patients despite continued treatment with ORTHOCLONE OKT3. However, some events resulted in permanent neurologic impairment.

The following additional central nervous system events have each been reported: irreversible blindness, impaired vision, quadri- or paraparesis/plegia, cerebrovascular accident (hemiparesis/plegia), aphasia, transient ischemic attack, subarachnoid hemorrhage, palsy of the VI cranial nerve, hearing decrease, and deafness.

Patients who may be at greater risk for CNS adverse experiences include those: with known or suspected CNS disorders (e.g., history of seizure disorder, etc.); with cerebrovascular disease (small or large vessel); with conditions having associated neurologic problems (e.g., head trauma, uremia, infection, fluid and electrolyte disturbance, etc.); with underlying vascular diseases; or who are receiving a medication concomitantly that may, by itself, affect the central nervous system. (See: WARNINGS, PRECAUTIONS and ADVERSE EVENTS: Cytokine Release Syndrome)

Anaphylactic Reactions

Serious and occasionally fatal, immediate (usually within 10 minutes) hypersensitivity (anaphylactic) reactions have been reported in patients treated with ORTHOCLONE OKT3. **Manifestations of anaphylaxis may appear similar to manifestations of the Cytokine Release Syndrome (described above). It may be impossible to determine the mechanism responsible for any systemic reaction(s).** Reactions attributed to hypersensitivity have been reported less frequently than those attributed to cytokine release. Acute hypersensitivity reactions may be characterized by: cardiovascular collapse, cardiorespiratory arrest, loss of consciousness, hypotension/shock, tachycardia, tingling, angioedema (including laryngeal, pharyngeal, or facial edema), airway obstruction, bronchospasm, dyspnea, urticaria, and pruritus.

Serious allergic events, including anaphylactic or anaphylactoid reactions, have been reported in patients re-exposed to ORTHOCLONE OKT3 subsequent to their initial course of therapy. Pretreatment with antihistamines and/or steroids may not reliably prevent anaphylaxis in this setting. Possible allergic hazards of retreatment should be weighed against expected therapeutic benefits and alternatives. If a patient is retreated with ORTHOCLONE OKT3, it is particularly important that epinephrine and other emergency life-support equipment should be immediately available.

If hypersensitivity is suspected, discontinue the drug immediately; do not resume therapy or re-expose the patient to ORTHOCLONE OKT3. Serious acute hypersensitivity reactions may require emergency treatment with 0.3 mL to 0.5 mL aqueous epinephrine (1:1000 dilution) subcutaneously and other resuscitative measures including oxygen, intravenous fluids, antihistamines, corticosteroids, pressor amines, and airway management, as clinically indicated. (See: PRECAUTIONS: Cytokine Release Syndrome vs. Anaphylactic Reactions; ADVERSE EVENTS: Hypersensitivity Reactions)

Consequences of Immunosuppression

Serious and sometimes fatal infections and neoplasias have been reported in association with all immunosuppressive therapies, including those regimens containing ORTHOCLONE OKT®3.

Infections: ORTHOCLONE OKT3 is usually added to immunosuppressive therapeutic regimens, thereby augmenting the degree of immunosuppression. This increase in the total amount of immunosuppression may alter the spectrum of infections observed and increase the risk, the severity, and the morbidity of infectious complications. During the first month post-transplant, patients are at greatest risk for the following infections: (1) those present prior to transplant, perhaps exacerbated by post-transplant immunosuppression; (2) infection conveyed by the donor organ; and (3) the usual post-operative urinary tract, intravenous line related, wound, or pulmonary infections due to bacterial pathogens. (See: ADVERSE EVENTS: Infections)

Approximately one to six months post-transplant, patients are at risk for viral infections [e.g., cytomegalovirus (CMV), Epstein-Barr virus (EBV), herpes simplex virus (HSV), etc.] which produce serious systemic disease and which also increase the overall state of immunosuppression.

Reactivation (1 to 4 months post-transplant) of EBV and CMV has been reported. When administration of an anti-lymphocyte antibody, including ORTHOCLONE OKT3, is followed by an immunosuppressive regimen including cyclosporine, there is an increased risk of reactivating CMV and impaired ability to limit its proliferation, resulting in symptomatic and disseminated disease. EBV infection, either primary or reactivated, may play an important role in the development of post-transplant lymphoproliferative disorders. (See: WARNINGS and ADVERSE EVENTS: Neoplasia)

In the pediatric transplant population, viral infections often include pathogens uncommon in adults, such as varicella zoster virus (VZV), adenovirus, and respiratory syncytial virus (RSV). A large proportion of pediatric patients have not been infected with the herpes viruses prior to transplantation and, therefore, are susceptible to developing primary infections from the grafted organ and/or blood products.

Anti-infective prophylaxis may reduce the morbidity associated with certain potential pathogens and should be considered for pediatric and other high-risk patients. Judicious use of immunosuppressive drugs, including type, dosage, and duration, may limit the risk and seriousness of some opportunistic infections. It is also possible to reduce the risk of serious CMV or EBV infection by avoiding transplantation of a CMV-seropositive (donor) and/or EBV-seropositive (donor) organ into a seronegative patient.

Neoplasia: As a result of depressed cell-mediated immunity from immunosuppressive agents, organ transplant patients have an increased risk of developing malignancies. This risk is evidenced almost exclusively by the occurrence of lymphoproliferative disorders, squamous cell carcinomas of the skin and lip, and sarcomas. In immunosuppressed patients, T cell cytotoxicity is impaired allowing for transformation and proliferation of EBV-infected B lymphocytes. Transformed B lymphocytes are thought to initiate oncogenesis, which ultimately culminates in the development of most post-transplant lymphoproliferative disorders. Patients, especially pediatric patients, with primary EBV infection may be at a higher risk for the development of EBV-associated lymphoproliferative disorders. Data support an association between the development of lymphoproliferative disorders at the time of active EBV infection and ORTHOCLONE OKT3 administration in pediatric liver allograft recipients. (See: ADVERSE EVENTS, Infections, Neoplasia)

Following the initiation of ORTHOCLONE OKT3 therapy, patients should be continuously monitored for evidence of lymphoproliferative disorders through physical examination and histological evaluation of any suspect lymphoid tissue. Close surveillance is advised, since early detection with subsequent reduction of total immunosuppression may result in regression of some of these lymphoproliferative disorders. Since the potential for the development of lymphoproliferative disorders is related to the duration and extent (intensity) of total immunosuppression, physicians are advised: to adhere to the recommended dosage and duration of ORTHOCLONE OKT3 therapy; to limit the number of courses of ORTHOCLONE OKT3 and other anti- T lymphocyte antibody preparations administered within a short period of time; and, if appropriate, to reduce the dosage(s) of immunosuppressive drugs used concomitantly to the lowest level compatible with an effective therapeutic response. (See: DOSAGE AND ADMINISTRATION)

A recent study examined the incidence of non-Hodgkin's lymphoma (NHL) among 45,000 kidney transplant recipients and over 7,500 heart transplant recipients. This study suggested that all transplant patients, regardless of the immunosuppressive regimen employed, are at increased risk of NHL over the general population. The relative risk was highest among those receiving the most aggressive regimens.

The long-term risk of neoplastic events in patients being treated with ORTHOCLONE OKT3 has not been determined.

PRECAUTIONS

General

When using combinations of immunosuppressive agents, the dose of each agent, including ORTHOCLONE OKT®3, should be reduced to the lowest level compatible with an effective therapeutic response so as to reduce the potential for and severity of infections and malignant transformations.

Fever: If the temperature of the patient exceeds 37.8°C (100°F), it should be lowered by antipyretics before administration of each dose of ORTHOCLONE OKT3. The possibility of infection should be evaluated.

Severe Cytokine Release Syndrome Versus Anaphylactic Reactions: **It may not be possible to distinguish between an acute hypersensitivity reaction (e.g., anaphylaxis, angioedema, etc.) and the Cytokine Release Syndrome. Potentially serious signs and symptoms having an immediate onset (usually within 10 minutes) following administration of ORTHOCLONE OKT3 are probably due to acute hypersensitivity. If hypersensitivity is suspected, discontinue the drug immediately; do not resume therapy or re-expose the patient to ORTHOCLONE OKT3.** Clinical manifestations beginning approximately 30 to 60 minutes (or later) following administration of ORTHOCLONE OKT3 are more likely cytokine-mediated. (See: WARNINGS: Cytokine Release Syndrome, Anaphylactic Reactions)

Central Nervous System Events: Since some seizures (and other serious central nervous system events) following ORTHOCLONE OKT3 administration have been life-threatening, anti-seizure precautions (e.g., an airway ready for use, if needed) should be taken. (See: WARNINGS and ADVERSE EVENTS: Central Nervous System Events)

Infection / Viral-Induced Lymphoproliferative Disorders: If infection or a viral induced lymphoproliferative disorder occurs, culture or biopsy as soon as possible, promptly institute appropriate anti-infective therapy, and (if possible) reduce/discontinue immunosuppressive therapy. (See: WARNINGS, ADVERSE EVENTS)

Low Protein-Binding Filter: Use a low protein-binding 0.2 or 0.22 micrometer (μm) filter to prepare the injections. (See: ADMINISTRATION INSTRUCTIONS)

Sensitization: ORTHOCLONE OKT3 is a mouse (immunoglobulin) protein that can induce human anti-mouse antibody production (i.e., sensitization) in some patients following exposure; a titer ≥1:1000 is a contraindication for use. (See: WARNINGS, ADVERSE EVENTS)

In the initial clinical trials using low doses of prednisone and azathioprine during ORTHOCLONE OKT3 therapy for renal allograft rejection, antibodies to ORTHOCLONE OKT3 were observed with an incidence of 21% (n=43) for IgM, 86% (n=43) for IgG and 29% (n=35) for IgE. The mean time of appearance of IgG antibodies was 20 ± 2 days (mean ± SD). Early IgG antibodies appeared towards the end of the second week of treatment in 3% (n=86) of the patients. Subsequent clinical experience has shown that the dose, duration, and type of immunosuppressive medications used in combination with ORTHOCLONE OKT3 may affect both the incidence and magnitude of the host antibody response. Furthermore, immunosuppressive agents used concomitantly with ORTHOCLONE OKT3 (i.e., steroids, azathioprine, prednisone, or cyclosporine) have altered the time course of anti-mouse antibody development and the specificity of the antibodies formed (i.e., idiotypic, isotypic, allotypic).

Thrombosis: As with other immunosuppressive therapies, arterial, venous, and capillary thromboses of allografts and other vascular beds (e.g., heart, lungs, brain, bowel, etc.) have been reported in patients treated with ORTHOCLONE OKT3. In addition, microangiopathic changes (e.g., platelet microthrombi) in the renal allograft associated in some patients with microangiopathic hemolytic anemia have been reported. This was observed in 5 of 93 (5%) patients receiving doses above the recommended dose. The relationship to dose remains uncertain; however, the relative risk appears to be greater with doses above the recommended dose. Patients with a history of thrombosis or underlying vascular disease should be given ORTHOCLONE OKT3 only when the potential benefits clearly outweigh the increased risks of therapy.

Information for Patients:

Patients should be advised:

- of the signs and symptoms associated with the Cytokine Release Syndrome and the potentially serious nature of this syndrome (e.g., systemic, cardiovascular, central nervous system events).
- to seek medical attention for skin rash, urticaria, rapid heart beat, respiratory distress, dysphagia, or any swelling suggesting an allergic reaction or angioedema.
- that ORTHOCLONE OKT3 may impair mental alertness and coordination and may effect the ability to operate an automobile or machinery.
- of other risks associated with the use of ORTHOCLONE OKT3. (See: BOXED WARNING; WARNINGS; PRECAUTIONS; ADVERSE EVENTS)

Laboratory Tests: The following tests should be monitored prior to and during ORTHOCLONE OKT®3 therapy:

- Renal: BUN, serum creatinine, etc.;
- Hepatic: transaminases, alkaline phosphatase, bilirubin;
- Hematopoietic: WBCs and differential, platelet count, etc.;
- Chest X-ray within 24 hours before initiating ORTHOCLONE OKT3 treatment to rule out heart failure or fluid overload.
- Blood Tests: Periodic assessment of organ system functions (renal, hepatic, and hematopoietic) should be performed.

During therapy with ORTHOCLONE OKT3: In adults, periodic monitoring to ensure plasma ORTHOCLONE OKT3 levels (≥800 ng/mL) or T cell clearance (CD3 positive T cells <25 cells/mm^3) is recommended. In pediatric patients, both plasma ORTHOCLONE OKT3 levels (≥800 ng/mL) and T cell clearance (CD3 positive T cells <25 cells/mm^3) should be monitored daily. (See: CLINICAL PHARMACOLOGY)

Carcinogenesis: Long-term studies have not been performed in laboratory animals to evaluate the carcinogenic potential of ORTHOCLONE OKT3; however, neoplasia has been reported in patients receiving this product. (See: WARNINGS and ADVERSE EVENTS: Neoplasia)

Pregnancy Category C: Animal reproductive studies have not been conducted with ORTHOCLONE OKT3. It is also not known whether ORTHOCLONE OKT3 can cause fetal harm when administered to a pregnant woman or can affect reproduction capacity. However, ORTHOCLONE OKT3 is an IgG antibody and may cross the human placenta. The effect on the fetus of the release of cytokines and/or immunosuppression after treatment with ORTHOCLONE OKT3 is not known. ORTHOCLONE OKT3 should be given to a pregnant woman only if clearly needed. If this drug is used during pregnancy, or the patient becomes pregnant while taking this drug, the patient should be apprised of the potential hazard to the fetus. (See: CONTRAINDICATIONS, WARNINGS, and ADVERSE EVENTS)

Nursing Mothers: It is not known whether ORTHOCLONE OKT3 is excreted in human milk. Because many drugs are excreted in human milk and because of the potential for serious adverse events/oncogenesis shown for ORTHOCLONE OKT3 in human studies, a decision should be made to discontinue nursing or to discontinue the drug, taking into account the importance of the drug to the mother. (See: CONTRAINDICATIONS)

Pediatric Use: Safety and effectiveness have been established in infants (1 mo. up to 2 yr.); children (2 yr. up to 12 yr.); and adolescents (12 yr. up to 16 yr.). Use of ORTHOCLONE OKT3 in these age groups is supported by clinical studies that included adults and pediatric patients. In those studies, the safety and efficacy of ORTHOCLONE OKT3 in pediatric patients receiving renal or hepatic transplants was similar to that in the overall cohort. There were insufficient data to compare the safety and efficacy of ORTHOCLONE OKT3 in pediatric patients in a study of patients receiving cardiac transplants. Additional pharmacokinetic, pharmacodynamic, and clinical studies in infants, children, and adolescents have been reported in published literature. Pediatric patients are known to have higher CD3 lymphocyte counts than adults; therefore, progressively higher doses of ORTHOCLONE OKT3 are often required to achieve therapeutic levels of lymphocyte clearance. (See: DOSAGE AND ADMINISTRATION)

<u>Specific Safety Concerns in Pediatric Patients</u>

Deaths due to Cerebral Herniation:

The postmarketing data base indicates that pediatric patients may be at increased risk of developing cerebral edema with or without herniation compared to adults. In the period between 1986 and 1996, twenty-five cases (6 in pediatric patients) of cerebral edema were identified with subsequent cerebral herniation and death in five cases (4 in pediatric patients). Herniation in the pediatric patients and one 19 year old subject occurred within a few hours to one day after the first dose (2.5 or 5 mg) of ORTHOCLONE OKT3 administered in the investigational setting for prophylaxis of renal allograft rejection. All pediatric patients and especially those receiving a renal allograft must be carefully evaluated for fluid retention and hypertension before the initiation of ORTHOCLONE OKT3 therapy (See: WARNINGS: Cytokine Release Syndrome; DOSAGE AND ADMINISTRATION: General). Patients should be closely monitored for neurologic symptoms during the first twenty four (24) hours following each of the first few doses of ORTHOCLONE OKT3 injection.

Other Serious Central Nervous System Adverse Events:

Other significant neurologic complications reported in pediatric transplant recipients receiving ORTHOCLONE OKT3 include status epilepticus, cerebral edema, diffuse encephalopathy, cerebritis, seizures, cortical dysfunction, and intracranial hemorrhage. Permanent neurologic impairments(e.g., blindness, deafness, paralysis) have been reported rarely. Because meningitis is a frequent infection encountered in pediatric allograft recipients, and the immunosuppression associated with transplantation increases the risk of opportunistic infection, patients with meningeal irritation following treatment with ORTHOCLONE OKT3 therapy should be evaluated with lumbar puncture as early as possible to rule out an infectious etiology.

Viral Infection:

The overall incidence of infections appeared to be similar in pediatric patients compared to the overall population studied. In the pediatric population, viral infections often include pathogens uncommon in adults, such as varicella zoster virus (VZV), adenovirus, enterovirus, parainfluenza virus, and respiratory syncytial virus (RSV). In addition, many viral diseases often manifest differently in pediatric patients than they do in adults. Because a large proportion of pediatric patients have not been infected by herpes viruses (e.g., EBV, HSV, CMV) prior to transplantation they may be more susceptible to acquiring primary infections from the grafted organ and/or blood products when immunosuppressed. Antiviral prophylactic therapy may be particularly useful in these high risk pediatric patients. (See: ADVERSE EVENTS: Infections)

Neoplasia:

Patients with primary EBV infection may be at higher risk for the development of EBV-associated lymphoproliferative disorders. There are data to support an association between the development of lymphoproliferative disorders at the time of active EBV infection and ORTHOCLONE OKT®3 administration in pediatric liver allograft recipients. Antiviral prophylactic therapy may be particularly useful in these high risk pediatric patients.

Gastrointestinal Fluid Losses:

Parenteral hydration may be required for gastrointestinal fluid loss secondary to diarrhea and/or vomiting resulting from the "Cytokine Release Syndrome".

Thrombosis:

Pediatric patients may be at an increased risk of thrombosis. Pediatric patients weighing less than 15 kg are at high-risk for hepatic artery thrombosis. Thrombosis has been reported in pediatric transplant recipients treated with ORTHOCLONE OKT3. A number of factors, including surgical technique, the presence of a hypercoagulable state, and the absence of prior dialysis experience may be relevant to the pathophysiology of the increased risk of thrombosis. (See: BOXED WARNING; WARNINGS; PRECAUTIONS; ADVERSE EVENTS; DOSAGE AND ADMINISTRATION)

ADVERSE EVENTS

Cytokine Release Syndrome

In controlled clinical trials for treatment of acute renal allograft rejection, patients treated with ORTHOCLONE OKT3 plus concomitant low-dose immunosuppressive therapy (primarily azathioprine and corticosteroids) were observed to have an increased incidence of adverse experiences during the first two days of treatment, as compared with the group of patients receiving azathioprine and high-dose steroid therapy. During this period the majority of patients experienced pyrexia (90%), of which 19% were 40.0°C (104°F) or above, and chills (59%). In addition, other adverse experiences occurring in 8% or more of the patients during the first two days of ORTHOCLONE OKT3 therapy included: dyspnea (21%), nausea (19%), vomiting (19%), chest pain (14%), diarrhea (14%), tremor (13%), wheezing (13%), headache (11%), tachycardia (10%), rigor (8%), and hypertension (8%). A similar spectrum of clinical manifestations has been observed in open clinical studies and in post-marketing experience involving patients treated with ORTHOCLONE OKT3 for rejection following renal, cardiac, and hepatic transplantation.

Additional serious and occasionally fatal cardiorespiratory manifestations have been reported following any of the first few doses. (See: WARNINGS: Cytokine Release Syndrome; ADVERSE EVENTS: Cardiovascular, Respiratory)

In the acute renal allograft rejection trials, potentially fatal pulmonary edema had been reported following the first two doses in less than 2% of the patients treated with ORTHOCLONE OKT3. Pulmonary edema was usually associated with fluid overload. However, post-marketing experience revealed that pulmonary edema has occurred in patients who appeared to be euvolemic, presumably as a consequence of cytokine-mediated increased vascular permeability ("leaky capillaries") and/or reduced myocardial contractility/compliance (i.e., left ventricular dysfunction). (See: WARNINGS: Cytokine Release Syndrome; DOSAGE AND ADMINISTRATION)

Infections

In the controlled randomized renal allograft rejection trial conducted before cyclosporine was marketed, the most common infections during the first 45 days of ORTHOCLONE OKT3 therapy were due to herpes simplex virus (27%) and cytomegalovirus (19%). Other severe and life-threatening infections were *Staphylococcus epidermidis* (5%), *Pneumocystis carinii* (3%), *Legionella* (2%), *Cryptococcus* (2%), *Serratia* (2%) and gram-negative bacteria (2%). The incidence of infections was similar in patients treated with ORTHOCLONE OKT3 and in patients treated with high-dose steroids.

In a clinical trial of acute hepatic allograft rejection, refractory to conventional treatment, the most common infections reported in patients treated with ORTHOCLONE OKT3 during the first 45 days of the study were cytomegalovirus (16% of patients, of which 43% of infections were severe), fungal infections (15% of patients, of which 30% were severe), and herpes simplex virus (8% of patients, of which

Continued on next page

Orthoclone—Cont.

10% were severe). Other severe and life-threatening infections were gram-positive infections (9% of patients), gram-negative infections (8% of patients), viral infections (2% of patients), and *Legionella* (1% of patients). In another trial studying the use of ORTHOCLONE OKT®3 in patients with hepatic allografts, the incidence of fungal infections was 34% and infections with the herpes simplex virus was 31%.

In a clinical trial studying the use of ORTHOCLONE OKT3 in patients with acute cardiac rejection refractory to conventional treatment, the most common infections in the ORTHOCLONE OKT3 group reported during the first 45 days of the study were herpes simplex virus (5% of patients, of which 20% were severe), fungal infections (4% of patients, of which 75% were severe), and cytomegalovirus (3% of patients, of which 33% were severe). No other severe or life-threatening infections were reported during this period.

In a retrospective analysis of pediatric patients treated for acute hepatic rejection, the most common infections reported in patients treated with ORTHOCLONE OKT3 therapy were due to bacterial infections (47%), fungal infections (21%), cytomegalovirus (19%), herpes simplex virus (15%), adenovirus (8%), and Epstein-Barr virus (8%). The overall rates of viral, fungal, and bacterial infections were similar in patients treated with ORTHOCLONE OKT3 (n = 53) and in patients whose rejection was treated with steroids alone (n = 27). In another study of 149 pediatric liver allograft patients where 59 episodes of steroid-resistant rejection were treated with ORTHOCLONE OKT3, the incidence of invasive cytomegalovirus infection was higher in patients receiving ORTHOCLONE OKT3 than in those receiving steroids alone.

Clinically significant infections (e.g., pneumonia, sepsis, etc.) due to the following pathogens have been reported:

Bacterial: *Clostridium* species (including *perfringens*), *Corynebacterium*, Enterococcus, *Enterobacter aerogenes*, *Escherichia coli*, *Klebsiella* species, *Lactobacillus*, *Legionella*, *Listeria monocytogenes*, *Mycobacteria* species, *Nocardia asteroides*, *Proteus* species, *Providencia* species, *Pseudomonas aeruginosa*, *Serratia* species, *Staphylococcus* species, *Streptococcus* species, *Yersinia enterocolitica*, and other gram-negative bacteria.

*Fungal:** *Aspergillus, Candida, Cryptococcus, Dermatophytes.*

Protozoa: *Pneumocystis carinii, Toxoplasma gondii.*

Viral: cytomegalovirus* (CMV), Epstein-Barr virus* (EBV), herpes simplex virus* (HSV), hepatitis viruses, varicella zoster virus (VZV), adenovirus, enterovirus, respiratory syncytial virus (RSV), parainfluenza virus.

As a consequence of being a potent immunosuppressive, the incidence and severity of infections with designated(*) pathogens, especially the herpes family of viruses, may be increased. (See: WARNINGS: Infections)

Neoplasia

In patients treated with ORTHOCLONE OKT3, post-transplant lymphoproliferative disorders have ranged from lymphadenopathy or benign polyclonal B cell hyperplasias to malignant and often fatal monoclonal B cell lymphomas. In post-marketing experience, approximately one-third of the lymphoproliferations reported were benign and two-thirds were malignant. Lymphoma types included: B cell, large cell, polyclonal, non-Hodgkin's, lymphocytic, T cell, Burkitt's. The majority were not histologically classified. Malignant lymphomas appear to develop early after transplantation, the majority within the first four months post-treatment. Many of these have been rapidly progressive. Some were fulminant, involving the allografted organ and were widely disseminated at the time of diagnosis. Carcinomas of the skin included: basal cell, squamous cell, sarcoma, melanoma, and keratoacanthoma. Other neoplasms infrequently reported include: multiple myeloma, leukemia, carcinoma of the breast, adenocarcinoma, cholangiocarcinoma, and recurrences of pre-existing hepatoma and renal cell carcinoma. (See: WARNINGS: Neoplasia)

Hypersensitivity Reactions

Reported adverse reactions resulting from the formation of antibodies to ORTHOCLONE OKT3 have included antigen-antibody (immune complex) mediated syndromes and IgE-mediated reactions. Hypersensitivity reactions have ranged from a mild, self-limited rash or pruritus to severe, life-threatening anaphylactic reactions/shock or angioedema (including: swelling of lips, eyelids, laryngeal spasm and airway obstruction with hypoxia). (See: WARNINGS: Anaphylactic Reactions)

Other hypersensitivity reactions have included: ineffectiveness of treatment, serum sickness, arthritis, allergic interstitial nephritis, immune complex deposition resulting in glomerulonephritis, vasculitis (including temporal and retinal), and eosinophilia.

Adverse Reactions by Body System

Adverse events reported in greater than or equal to 1% of clinical trial patients treated with ORTHOCLONE OKT3 (n=393) are shown in Table 1:

Table 1: Adverse Events Reported in Clinical Trials (≥1% incidence, n=393)

Body System	Incidence (%)
Autonomic Nervous System Disorders	
Diaphoresis	7
Vasodilation	7
Body as a Whole, General Disorders	
Anorexia	4
Asthenia	10
Chills	43
Fatigue	9
Lethargy	6
Malaise	5
Pain, trunk	6
Pyrexia	77
Cardiovascular Disorders, General	
Arrhythmia	4
Bradycardia	4
Hypertension	19
Hypotension	25
Pain, chest	9
Tachycardia	26
Vascular Occlusion	2
Central & Peripheral Nervous System Disorders	
Convulsions	1
Dizziness	6
Headache	28
Meningitis	1
Tremor	14
Gastrointestinal System Disorders	
Diarrhea	37
Nausea	32
Pain, abdominal	6
Pain, GI	7
Vomiting	25
Hematopoietic Disorders	
Anemia	2
Leukocytosis	1
Thrombocytopenia	2
Metabolic and Nutritional Disorders	
Edema	12
Musculoskeletal System Disorders	
Arthralgia	7
Myalgia	1
Psychiatric Disorders	
Confusion	6
Depression	3
Nervousness	5
Somnolence	2
Renal Disorders	
Renal Dysfunction	3
Respiratory System Disorders	
Abnormal Chest Sound	10
Dyspnea	16
Hyperventilation	7
Hypoxia	1
Pneumonia	1
Pulmonary Edema	2
Respiratory Congestion	4
Wheezing	6
Skin and Appendages Disorders	
Pruritus	7
Rash	14
Rash Erythematous	2
Special Senses	
Photophobia	1
Tinnitus	1
White Cell & Reticuloendothelial System Disorders	
Leukopenia	7

Selected Adverse Events Reported In Clinical Trials (< 1% incidence, n=393):

Cardiovascular Disorders, General: Angina, Cardiac Arrest, Fluctuation in Blood Pressure, Heart Failure, Myocardial Infarction, Shock, Thrombosis.

Central & Peripheral Nervous System Disorders: Coma, Encephalopathy, Epilepsy, Hypotonia.

Gastrointestinal Disorders: Gastrointestinal Hemorrhage.

Hemapoietic Disorders: Coagulation Disorder, Lymphadenopathy, Lymphopenia.

Hepatobiliary: Hepatitis, SGOT Increased, SGPT Increased.

Psychiatric Disorders: Hallucinations, Mood Changes, Paranoia, Psychosis.

Renal Disorders: Anuria, Oliguria.

Respiratory System Disorders: Apnea, Pneumonitis.

Special Senses: Conjunctivitis, Hearing Decrease.

Worldwide Postmarketing Experience - Body Systems/Events Listed Alphabetically:

Body As A Whole, General Disorders: Fever (including spiking temperatures as high as 107°F), Flu-like Syndrome.

Cardiovascular Disorders: Cardiovascular Collapse, Hemodynamic Instability, Left Ventricular Dysfunction.

Central & Peripheral Nervous System Disorders: Agitation, Aphasia, Asterixis, Cerebritis, Cerebral Edema, Cerebral Herniation, Cerebrovascular Accident, CNS Infection, CNS Malignancy, Cranial Nerve VI Palsy, Encephalitis, Hyperreflexia, Involuntary Movements, Intracranial Hemorrhage, Impaired Cognition, Myoclonus, Obnubilation, Paresis/plegia including quadriparesis/plegia, Status Epilepticus, Stupor, Transient Ischemic Attack, Vertigo.

In a post-marketing survey involving 214 renal transplant patients, the incidence of aseptic meningitis syndrome was 6%. Fever (89%), headache (44%), neck stiffness (14%), and photophobia (10%) were the most commonly reported symptoms; a combination of these four symptoms occurred in 5% of patients.

Between 1987 and 1992, 75 post-marketing reports have described seizures, averaging about 12 per year, and including 23 fatalities. More than two-thirds of these reports (53) were of domestic spontaneous origin, and their age and sex distributions were broad. Post-licensure reports generally provide insufficient data to allow accurate estimation of risk or of incidence.

Gastrointestinal Disorders: Bowel Infarction.

Hematopoietic Disorders: Aplastic anemia, Arterial, Venous and Capillary Thrombosis of allografts and other vascular beds e.g., heart, lung, brain and bowel etc., Disseminated Intravascular Coagulation, Microangiopathic Changes (e.g., platelet microthrombi), Microangiopathic Hemolytic Anemia, Neutropenia, Pancytopenia.

Hepatobiliary: Hepatitis or Hepato/splenomegaly, usually secondary to viral infection or lymphoma.

Musculoskeletal Disorders: Arthritis, Stiffness/Aches/Pains.

Renal Disorders: Azotemia, Abnormal Urinary Cytology including exfoliation of damaged lymphocytes, collecting duct cells and cellular casts, Delayed Graft Function, Renal Insufficiency/Renal Failure, usually transient and reversible and occasionally in association with Cytokine Release Syndrome.

Respiratory System Disorders: Adult Respiratory Distress Syndrome, Respiratory Arrest, Respiratory Failure.

Skin and Appendages: Erythema, Flushing, Stevens-Johnson Syndrome, Urticaria.

Special Senses: Blindness, Blurred Vision, Deafness, Diplopia, Otitis Media, Nasal and Ear Stuffiness, Papilledema.

OVERDOSAGE

Symptoms of overdosage with ORTHOCLONE OKT®3 may include hyperthermia, severe chills, myalgia, vomiting, diarrhea, edema, oliguria, pulmonary edema, and acute renal failure. A high incidence (5%) of microangiopathic hemolytic anemia/HUS syndrome in patients receiving 10 mg per day of ORTHOCLONE OKT3 was also reported. In the event of acute overdosage with ORTHOCLONE OKT3, the patient should be carefully observed and given symptomatic and supportive treatment.

DOSAGE AND ADMINISTRATION

Adults

The recommended dose of ORTHOCLONE OKT3 for the treatment of acute renal, steroid-resistant cardiac, or steroid-resistant hepatic allograft rejection is 5 mg per day in a single (bolus) intravenous injection in less than one minute for 10 to 14 days. For acute renal rejection, treatment should begin upon diagnosis. For steroid-resistant cardiac or hepatic allograft rejection, treatment should begin when the treating physician deems a rejection has not been reversed by an adequate course of corticosteroid therapy. (See: CLINICAL PHARMACOLOGY; PRECAUTIONS: Sensitization, Laboratory Tests)

Pediatric Patients

The initial recommended dose is 2.5 mg per day in pediatric patients weighing less than or equal to 30 kg and 5 mg per day in pediatric patients weighing greater than 30 kg in a single (bolus) intravenous injection in less than one minute for 10 to 14 days. Daily increases in ORTHOCLONE OKT3 doses (i.e., 2.5 mg increments) may be required to achieve depletion of CD3 positive cells (<25 cells/mm^3) and ensure therapeutic ORTHOCLONE OKT3 serum concentrations (> 800 ng/mL). Pediatric patients may require augmentation of the ORTHOCLONE OKT3 dose. For acute renal rejection, treatment should begin upon diagnosis. For steroid-resistant cardiac or hepatic allograft rejection, treatment should begin when the treating physician deems a rejection has not been reversed by an adequate course of corticosteroid therapy. (See: CLINICAL PHARMACOLOGY; PRECAUTIONS: Laboratory Tests; Pediatric Use)

General

For the first few doses, patients should be monitored in a facility equipped and staffed for cardiopulmonary resuscitation (CPR). Patients receiving subsequent doses of ORTHOCLONE OKT3, should also be monitored in a facility equipped and staffed for CPR. Vital signs should be monitored frequently. Patients receiving ORTHOCLONE OKT3 should also be carefully monitored for signs and symptoms of Cytokine Release Syndrome, particularly after the first few doses but also after a treatment hiatus with resumption of therapy. The patient's temperature should be lowered to <37.8°C (100°F) before the administration of any dose of ORTHOCLONE OKT3.

Prior to administration of ORTHOCLONE OKT3, the patient's volume status should be assessed carefully. It is imperative, especially prior to the first few doses, that there be no clinical evidence of volume overload, uncontrolled hypertension, or uncompensated heart failure. Patients should have a clear chest X-ray and should not weigh more than 3% above their minimum weight during the week prior to injection.

To decrease the incidence and severity of Cytokine Release Syndrome, associated with the first dose of ORTHOCLONE OKT3, it is strongly recommended that methylprednisolone sodium succinate 8.0 mg/kg be administered intravenously

1 to 4 hours prior to the initial dose of ORTHOCLONE OKT3. Acetaminophen and antihistamines given concomitantly with ORTHOCLONE OKT3 may also help to reduce some early reactions. (See: WARNINGS and ADVERSE EVENTS: Cytokine Release Syndrome)

When using concomitant immunosuppressive drugs, the dose of each should be reduced to the lowest level compatible with an effective therapeutic response in order to reduce the potential for malignancy and infections. Maintenance immunosuppression should be resumed approximately three days prior to the cessation of ORTHOCLONE OKT®3 therapy. (See: WARNINGS and ADVERSE EVENTS: Infection, Neoplasia)

Reduced T cell clearance or low plasma ORTHOCLONE OKT3 levels provide a basis for adjusting ORTHOCLONE OKT3 dosage or for discontinuing therapy. (See: WARNINGS: Anaphylactic Reactions; PRECAUTIONS: Laboratory Tests; ADVERSE EVENTS: Hypersensitivity Reactions)

ADMINISTRATION INSTRUCTIONS

1. Before administration, ORTHOCLONE OKT3 should be inspected for particulate matter and discoloration. Because ORTHOCLONE OKT3 is a protein solution, it may develop fine translucent particles (shown not to affect potency).
2. No bacteriostatic agent is present in this product. Adherence to aseptic technique is advised. Once the ampule is opened, use immediately and discard the unused portion.
3. Prepare ORTHOCLONE OKT3 for injection by drawing solution into a syringe through a low protein-binding 0.2 or 0.22 micrometer (μm) filter. Detach filter and attach a new needle for a single intravenous (bolus) injection.
4. Because no data is available on compatibility of ORTHOCLONE OKT3 with other intravenous substances or additives, other medications/substances should not be added or infused simultaneously through the same intravenous line. If the same intravenous line is used for sequential infusion of several different drugs, the line should be flushed with saline before and after injection of ORTHOCLONE OKT3.
5. Administer ORTHOCLONE OKT3 as a single intravenous (bolus) injection in less than one minute. Do **not** administer by intravenous infusion or in conjunction with other drug solutions.

HOW SUPPLIED

ORTHOCLONE OKT3 is supplied as a sterile solution in packages of 5 ampules (NDC 59676-101-01). Each 5 mL ampule contains 5 mg of muromonab-CD3.

Storage: Store in a refrigerator at 2° to 8°C (36° to 46°F). DO NOT FREEZE OR SHAKE.

REFERENCES

1. Adair JC, Woodley SL, O'Connell JB, et al. Aseptic Meningitis following Cardiac Transplantation: Clinical Characteristics and Relationship to Immunosuppressive Regimen. Neurology 41:249–252, 1991.
2. Chatenoud L, Legendre C, Ferran C, *et al.* Corticosteroid Inhibition of the OKT3 - Induced Cytokine-Related Syndrome - Dosage and Kinetics Prerequisites. Transplantation 51:334–338, 1991.
3. Cockfield SM, Preiksaitis J, Harvey E, Jones C, Herbert D, Keown P, and Halloran PF, *et al.* Is Sequential Use of ALG and OKT3 in Renal Transplants Associated with an Increased Incidence of Fulminant Post Transplant Lymphoproliferative Disorders? Transplant. Proc. 23: 1106–1107, 1991.
4. Ettenger RB, Marik J, Rosenthal JT, *et al.* OKT3 for Rejection Reversal in Pediatric Renal Transplantation. Clin. Transplantation 2:180–184, 1988.
5. Gaston RS, Deierhoi MH, Patterson T, *et al.* OKT3 First-Dose Reaction: Association with T Cell Subsets and Cytokine Release. Kid. International 39:141–148, 1991.
6. Goldman M, Abramowicz D, DePauw L, *et al.* OKT3-Induced Cytokine Released Attenuation by High-Dose Methylprednisolone. Lancet 2:802–803, 1989.
7. Ortho Multicenter Transplant Study Group. A Randomized Clinical Trial of OKT3 Monoclonal Antibody for Acute Rejection of Cadaveric Renal Transplants. N. Engl. J. Med. 313:337–342, 1985.
8. Penn I. The Changing Patterns of Posttransplant Malignancies. Transplant. Proc. 23:1101–1103,1991.
9. Rubin RH and Tolkoff-Rubin NE. The Impact of Infection on the Outcome of Transplantation. Transplant. Proc. 23:2068–2074, 1991.
10. Schroeder TJ, Ryckman FC, Hurtubise PE, *et al.* Immunological Monitoring During and Following OKT3 Therapy in Children. Clin. Transplantation 5:191–196, 1991.
11. Goldstein G, Fuccello AJ, Norman DJ, *et al.* OKT3 Monoclonal Antibody Plasma Levels During Therapy and the Subsequent Development of Host Antibodies to OKT3. Transplantation 42:507–511, 1986.
12. Schroeder TJ, Michael AT, First MR, *et al.* Variations in Serum OKT3 Concentration Based Upon Age, Sex, Transplanted Organ, Treatment Regimen, and Anti-OKT3 Status. Therapeutic Drug Monitoring 16:361–367, 1994.
13. First MR, Schroeder TJ, Hurtubise PE, *et al.* Immune Monitoring During Retreatment with OKT3. Transplan. Proc. 21:1753–1754, 1989.

ORTHO BIOTECH PRODUCTS, L.P.
Raritan, New Jersey 08869
U.S.A.
631-10-191-2
Revised February 1999

PROCRIT® ℞

EPOETIN ALFA

PROCRIT registered trademark of distributor
FOR INJECTION

DESCRIPTION

Erythropoietin is a glycoprotein which stimulates red blood cell production. It is produced in the kidney and stimulates the division and differentiation of committed erythroid progenitors in the bone marrow. PROCRIT (Epoetin alfa), a 165 amino acid glycoprotein manufactured by recombinant DNA technology, has the same biological effects as endogenous erythropoietin.[1] It has a molecular weight of 30,400 daltons and is produced by mammalian cells into which the human erythropoietin gene has been introduced. The product contains the identical amino acid sequence of isolated natural erythropoietin.

PROCRIT is formulated as a sterile, colorless, liquid in an isotonic sodium chloride/sodium citrate or a sodium chloride/sodium phosphate buffered solution for intravenous (IV) or subcutaneous (SC) administration.

Single-Dose, Preservative-Free Vial: 1 mL (2,000, 3,000, 4,000 or 10,000 Units/mL). Each 1 mL of solution contains 2,000, 3,000, 4,000 or 10,000 Units of Epoetin alfa, 2.5 mg Albumin (Human), 5.8 mg sodium citrate, 5.8 mg sodium chloride, and 0.06 mg citric acid in Water for Injection, USP (pH 6.9±0.3). This formulation contains no preservative.

Single-Dose, Preservative-Free Vial: 1 mL (40,000 Units/mL). Each 1 mL of solution contains 40,000 Units of Epoetin alfa, 2.5 mg Albumin (Human), 1.164 mg sodium phosphate monobasic monohydrate, 1.766 mg sodium phosphate dibasic anhydrate, 0.696 mg sodium citrate, 5.78 mg sodium chloride, and 6.8 mcg citric acid in Water for Injection, USP (pH 6.9±0.3). This formulation contains no preservative.

Multidose, Preserved Vial: 2 mL (20,000 Units, 10,000 Units/mL). Each 1 mL of solution contains 10,000 Units of Epoetin alfa, 2.5 mg Albumin (Human), 1.3 mg sodium citrate, 8.2 mg sodium chloride, 0.11 mg citric acid, and 1% benzyl alcohol as preservative in Water for Injection, USP (pH 6.1±0.3).

Multidose, Preserved Vial: 1 mL (20,000 Units/mL). Each 1 mL of solution contains 20,000 Units of Epoetin alfa, 2.5 mg Albumin (Human), 1.3 mg sodium citrate, 8.2 mg sodium chloride, 0.11 mg citric acid, and 1% benzyl alcohol as preservative in Water for Injection, USP (pH 6.1±0.3).

CLINICAL PHARMACOLOGY

Chronic Renal Failure Patients

Endogenous production of erythropoietin is normally regulated by the level of tissue oxygenation. Hypoxia and anemia generally increase the production of erythropoietin, which in turn stimulates erythropoiesis.[2] In normal subjects, plasma erythropoietin levels range from 0.01 to 0.03 Units/mL, and increase up to 100- to 1000-fold during hypoxia or anemia.[2] In contrast, in patients with chronic renal failure (CRF), production of erythropoietin is impaired, and this erythropoietin deficiency is the primary cause of their anemia.[3,4]

Chronic renal failure is the clinical situation in which there is a progressive and usually irreversible decline in kidney function. Such patients may manifest the sequelae of renal dysfunction, including anemia, but do not necessarily require regular dialysis. Patients with end-stage renal disease (ESRD) are those patients with CRF who require regular dialysis or kidney transplantation for survival.

PROCRIT has been shown to stimulate erythropoiesis in anemic patients with CRF, including both patients on dialysis and those who do not require regular dialysis.[4–13] The first evidence of a response to the three times weekly (T.I.W.) administration of PROCRIT is an increase in the reticulocyte count within 10 days, followed by increases in the red cell count, hemoglobin, and hematocrit, usually within 2–6 weeks.[4,5] Because of the length of time required for erythropoiesis—several days for erythroid progenitors to mature and be released into the circulation—a clinically significant increase in hematocrit is usually not observed in less than 2 weeks and may require up to 6 weeks in some patients. Once the hematocrit reaches the suggested target range (30–36%), that level can be sustained by PROCRIT therapy in the absence of iron deficiency and concurrent illnesses.

The rate of hematocrit increase varies between patients and is dependent upon the dose of PROCRIT, within a therapeutic range of approximately 50–300 Units/kg (T.I.W.).[4] A greater biologic response is not observed at doses exceeding 300 Units/kg (T.I.W.).[6] Other factors affecting the rate and extent of response include availability of iron stores, the baseline hematocrit, and the presence of concurrent medical problems.

Zidovudine-treated HIV-infected Patients

Responsiveness to PROCRIT in HIV-infected patients is dependent upon the endogenous serum erythropoietin level prior to treatment. Patients with endogenous serum erythropoietin levels ≤ 500 mUnits/mL, and who are receiving a dose of zidovudine ≤ 4,200 mg/week, may respond to PROCRIT therapy. Patients with endogenous serum erythropoietin levels > 500 mUnits/mL do not appear to respond to PROCRIT therapy. In a series of four clinical trials involving 255 patients, 60% to 80% of HIV-infected patients treated with zidovudine had endogenous serum erythropoietin levels ≤ 500 mUnits/mL.

Response to PROCRIT in zidovudine-treated, HIV-infected patients is manifested by reduced transfusion requirements and increased hematocrit.

Cancer Patients on Chemotherapy

Anemia in cancer patients may be related to the disease itself or the effect of concomitantly administered chemotherapeutic agents. PROCRIT has been shown to increase hematocrit and decrease transfusion requirements after the first month of therapy (months 2 and 3), in anemic cancer patients undergoing chemotherapy.

A series of clinical trials enrolled 131 anemic cancer patients who were receiving cyclic cisplatin- or non cisplatin-containing chemotherapy. Endogenous baseline serum erythropoietin levels varied among patients in these trials with approximately 75% (N=83/110) having endogenous serum erythropoietin levels ≤ 132 mUnits/mL, and approximately 4% (N=4/110) of patients having endogenous serum erythropoietin levels > 500 mUnits/mL. In general, patients with lower baseline serum erythropoietin levels responded more vigorously to PROCRIT than patients with higher baseline erythropoietin levels. Although no specific serum erythropoietin level can be stipulated above which patients would be unlikely to respond to PROCRIT therapy, treatment of patients with grossly elevated serum erythropoietin levels (e.g., > 200 mUnits/mL) is not recommended.

Pharmacokinetics

Intravenously administered PROCRIT is eliminated at a rate consistent with first order kinetics with a circulating half-life ranging from approximately 4 to 13 hours in adult and pediatric patients with CRF.[14–16] Within the therapeutic dose range, detectable levels of plasma erythropoietin are maintained for at least 24 hours. After subcutaneous administration of PROCRIT to patients with CRF, peak serum levels are achieved within 5–24 hours after administration and decline slowly thereafter. There is no apparent difference in half-life between adult patients not on dialysis whose serum creatinine levels were greater than 3, and adult patients maintained on dialysis.

In normal volunteers, the half-life of intravenously administered PROCRIT is approximately 20% shorter than the half-life in CRF patients. The pharmacokinetics of PROCRIT have not been studied in HIV-infected patients. The pharmacokinetic profile of Epoetin alfa in children and adolescents appears to be similar to that of adults. Limited data are available in neonates.[17]

It has been demonstrated in normal volunteers that the 10,000 U/mL citrate-buffered Epoetin alfa formulation and the 40,000 U/mL phosphate-buffered Epoetin alfa formulation are bioequivalent after subcutaneous administration of single 750 Units/kg doses. The C_{max} and $t_{1/2}$ after administration of the phosphate buffered Epoetin alfa formulation were 1.80 ± 0.7 U/mL and 19.0 ± 5.9 hours (mean ± SD), respectively. The corresponding mean ± SD values for the citrate-buffered Epoetin alfa formulation were 2 ± 0.9 U/mL and 16.3 ± 3.0 hours. There was minimal accumulation in serum after two weekly 750 Units/kg subcutaneous doses of Epoetin alfa.

INDICATIONS AND USAGE

Treatment of Anemia of Chronic Renal Failure Patients

PROCRIT is indicated in the treatment of anemia associated with chronic renal failure, including patients on dialysis (end-stage renal disease) and patients not on dialysis. PROCRIT is indicated to elevate or maintain the red blood cell level (as manifested by the hematocrit or hemoglobin determinations) and to decrease the need for transfusions in these patients.

Non-dialysis patients with symptomatic anemia considered for therapy should have a hematocrit less than 30%.

PROCRIT is not intended for patients who require immediate correction of severe anemia. PROCRIT may obviate the need for maintenance transfusions but is not a substitute for emergency transfusion.

Prior to initiation of therapy, the patient's iron stores should be evaluated. Transferrin saturation should be at least 20% and ferritin at least 100 ng/mL. Blood pressure should be adequately controlled prior to initiation of PROCRIT therapy, and must be closely monitored and controlled during therapy.

PROCRIT should be administered under the guidance of a qualified physician (see "DOSAGE AND ADMINISTRATION").

Treatment of Anemia in Zidovudine-treated HIV-infected Patients

PROCRIT is indicated for the treatment of anemia related to therapy with zidovudine in HIV-infected patients. PROCRIT is indicated to elevate or maintain the red blood cell level (as manifested by the hematocrit or hemoglobin determinations) and to decrease the need for transfusions in these patients. PROCRIT is not indicated for the treatment of anemia in HIV-infected patients due to other factors such as iron or folate deficiencies, hemolysis or gastrointestinal bleeding, which should be managed appropriately.

PROCRIT, at a dose of 100 Units/kg three times per week, is effective in decreasing the transfusion requirement and increasing the red blood cell level of anemic, HIV-infected patients treated with zidovudine, when the endogenous serum erythropoietin level is ≤ 500 mUnits/mL and when patients are receiving a dose of zidovudine ≤ 4,200 mg/week.

Treatment of Anemia in Cancer Patients on Chemotherapy

PROCRIT is indicated for the treatment of anemia in patients with non-myeloid malignancies where anemia is due to the effect of concomitantly administered chemotherapy. PROCRIT is indicated to decrease the need for transfusions in patients who will be receiving concomitant chemotherapy

Continued on next page

Procrit—Cont.

for a minimum of 2 months. PROCRIT is not indicated for the treatment of anemia in cancer patients due to other factors such as iron or folate deficiencies, hemolysis or gastrointestinal bleeding which should be managed appropriately.

Reduction of Allogeneic Blood Transfusion in Surgery Patients

PROCRIT is indicated for the treatment of anemic patients (hemoglobin >10 to ≤13 g/dL) scheduled to undergo elective, noncardiac, nonvascular surgery to reduce the need for allogeneic blood transfusions.[18-20] PROCRIT is indicated for patients at high risk for perioperative transfusions with significant, anticipated blood loss. PROCRIT is not indicated for anemic patients who are willing to donate autologous blood. The safety of the perioperative use of PROCRIT has been studied only in patients who are receiving anticoagulant prophylaxis.

Clinical Experience: Response to PROCRIT

Chronic Renal Failure Patients

Response to PROCRIT was consistent across all studies. In the presence of adequate iron stores (see "Iron Evaluation"), the time to reach the target hematocrit is a function of the baseline hematocrit and the rate of hematocrit rise.

The rate of increase in hematocrit is dependent upon the dose of PROCRIT administered and individual patient variation. In clinical trials at starting doses of 50–150 Units/kg (T.I.W.), adult patients responded with an average rate of hematocrit rise of:

HEMATOCRIT INCREASE

STARTING DOSE (T.I.W. IV)	POINTS/DAY	POINTS/ 2 WEEKS
50 Units/kg	0.11	1.5
100 Units/kg	0.18	2.5
150 Units/kg	0.25	3.5

Over this dose range, approximately 95% of all patients responded with a clinically significant increase in hematocrit, and by the end of approximately 2 months of therapy virtually all patients were transfusion-independent. Changes in the quality of life of adult patients treated with PROCRIT were assessed as part of a Phase III clinical trial.[5,8] Once the target hematocrit (32–38%) was achieved, statistically significant improvements were demonstrated for most quality of life parameters measured, including energy and activity level, functional ability, sleep and eating behavior, health status, satisfaction with health, sex life, well-being, psychological effect, life satisfaction, and happiness. Patients also reported improvement in their disease symptoms. They showed a statistically significant increase in exercise capacity (VO_2 max), energy, and strength with a significant reduction in aching, dizziness, anxiety, shortness of breath, muscle weakness, and leg cramps.[8,21]

Adult Patients On Dialysis: Thirteen clinical studies were conducted, involving intravenous administration to a total of 1,010 anemic patients on dialysis for 986 patient-years of PROCRIT therapy. In the three largest of these clinical trials, the median maintenance dose necessary to maintain the hematocrit between 30–36% was approximately 75 Units/kg (T.I.W.). In the U.S. multicenter Phase III study, approximately 65% of the patients required doses of 100 Units/kg (T.I.W.), or less, to maintain their hematocrit at approximately 35%. Almost 10% of patients required a dose of 25 Units/kg, or less, and approximately 10% required a dose of more than 200 Units/kg (T.I.W.) to maintain their hematocrit at this level.

A multicenter unit dose study was also conducted in 119 patients receiving peritoneal dialysis who self-administered PROCRIT subcutaneously for approximately 109 patient-years of experience. Patients responded to PROCRIT administered subcutaneously in a manner similar to patients receiving intravenous administration.[22]

Pediatric Patients On Dialysis: One hundred twenty-eight children from 2 months to 19 years of age with CRF requiring dialysis were enrolled in 4 clinical studies of PROCRIT. The largest study was a placebo-controlled, randomized trial in 113 children with anemia (hematocrit ≤ 27%) undergoing peritoneal dialysis or hemodialysis. The initial dose of PROCRIT was 50 Units/kg IV or SC (T.I.W.). The dose of study drug was titrated to achieve either a hematocrit of 30% to 36% or an absolute increase in hematocrit of 6 percentage points over baseline.

At the end of the initial 12 weeks, a statistically significant rise in mean hematocrit (9.4% vs 0.9%) was observed only in the PROCRIT arm. The proportion of children achieving a hematocrit of 30%, or an increase in hematocrit of 6 percentage points over baseline, at any time during the first 12 weeks was higher in the PROCRIT arm (96% vs 58%). Within 12 weeks of initiating PROCRIT therapy, 92.3% of the pediatric patients were transfusion-independent as compared to 65.4% who received placebo. Among patients who received 36 weeks of PROCRIT, hemodialysis patients required a higher median maintenance dose (167 Units/kg/week [n=28] vs 76 Units/kg/week [n=36]) and took longer to achieve a hematocrit of 30% to 36% (median time to response 69 days vs 32 days) than patients undergoing peritoneal dialysis.

Patients With CRF Not Requiring Dialysis: Four clinical trials were conducted in patients with CRF not on dialysis involving 181 patients treated with PROCRIT for approximately 67 patient-years of experience. These patients responded to PROCRIT therapy in a manner similar to that observed in patients on dialysis. Patients with CRF not on dialysis demonstrated a dose-dependent and sustained increase in hematocrit when PROCRIT was administered by either an intravenous (IV) or subcutaneous (SC) route, with similar rates of rise of hematocrit when PROCRIT was administered by either route. Moreover, PROCRIT doses of 75–150 Units/kg per week have been shown to maintain hematocrits of 36–38% for up to six months. Correcting the anemia of progressive renal failure will allow patients to remain active even though their renal function continues to decrease.[23-24]

Zidovudine-treated HIV-infected Patients

PROCRIT has been studied in four placebo-controlled trials enrolling 297 anemic (hematocrit < 30%) HIV-infected (AIDS) patients receiving concomitant therapy with zidovudine, (all patients were treated with Epoetin alfa manufactured by Amgen Inc.). In the subgroup of patients (89/125 PROCRIT, and 88/130 placebo) with prestudy endogenous serum erythropoietin levels ≤ 500 mUnits/mL PROCRIT reduced the mean cumulative number of units of blood transfused per patient by approximately 40%, as compared to the placebo group.[25] Among those patients who required transfusions at baseline, 43% of patients treated with PROCRIT versus 18% of placebo-treated patients were transfusion-independent during the second and third months of therapy. PROCRIT therapy also resulted in significant increases in hematocrit in comparison to placebo. When examining the results according to the weekly dose of zidovudine received during Month 3 of therapy, there was a statistically significant ($p < 0.003$) reduction in transfusion requirements in patients treated with PROCRIT (N=51) compared to placebo-treated patients (N=54) whose mean weekly zidovudine dose was ≤ 4,200 mg/week.[25]

Approximately 17% of the patients with endogenous serum erythropoietin levels ≤ 500 mUnits/mL receiving PROCRIT in doses from 100–200 Units/kg three times weekly (T.I.W.) achieved a hematocrit of 38% without administration of transfusions or a significant reduction in zidovudine dose. In the subgroup of patients whose prestudy endogenous serum erythropoietin levels were > 500 mUnits/mL, PROCRIT therapy did not reduce transfusion requirements or increase hematocrit, compared to the corresponding responses in placebo-treated patients.

In a six month open-label PROCRIT study, patients responded with decreased transfusion requirements and sustained increases in hematocrit and hemoglobin with doses of PROCRIT up to 300 Units/kg (T.I.W.).[25-27]

Responsiveness to PROCRIT therapy may be blunted by intercurrent infectious/inflammatory episodes and by an increase in zidovudine dosage. Consequently, the dose of PROCRIT must be titrated based on these factors to maintain the desired erythropoietic response.

Cancer Patients on Chemotherapy

PROCRIT has been studied in a series of placebo-controlled, double-blind trials in a total of 131 anemic cancer patients. Within this group, 72 patients were treated with concomitant noncisplatin-containing chemotherapy regimens and 59 patients were treated with concomitant cisplatin-containing chemotherapy regimens. Patients were randomized to PROCRIT 150 Units/kg or placebo subcutaneously (T.I.W.) for 12 weeks.

PROCRIT therapy was associated with a significantly ($p<0.008$) greater hematocrit response than in the corresponding placebo-treated patients (see TABLE).[25]

HEMATOCRIT (%): MEAN CHANGE FROM BASELINE TO FINAL VALUE[a]

STUDY	PROCRIT	PLACEBO
Chemotherapy	7.6	1.3
Cisplatin	6.9	0.6

[a]Significantly higher in PROCRIT patients than in placebo patients ($p <0.008$)

In the two types of chemotherapy studies [utilizing a PROCRIT dose of 150 Units/kg (T.I.W.)] the mean number of units of blood transfused per patient after the first month of therapy was significantly ($p < 0.02$) lower in patients treated with PROCRIT (0.71 units in Months 2, 3) than in corresponding placebo-treated patients (1.84 units in Months 2, 3). Moreover, the proportion of patients transfused during Months 2 and 3 of therapy combined was significantly ($p < 0.03$) lower in the patients treated with PROCRIT than in the corresponding placebo-treated patients (22% versus 43%).[25]

Comparable intensity of chemotherapy in the PROCRIT and placebo groups in the chemotherapy trials was suggested by a similar area under the neutrophil time curve in patients treated with PROCRIT and placebo-treated patients as well as by a similar proportion of patients in groups treated with PROCRIT and placebo-treated groups whose absolute neutrophil counts fell below 1,000 cells/μL. Available evidence suggests that patients with lymphoid and solid cancers respond equivalently to PROCRIT therapy, and that patients with or without tumor infiltration of the bone marrow respond equivalently to PROCRIT therapy.

Surgery Patients

PROCRIT has been studied in a placebo-controlled, double-blind trial enrolling 316 patients scheduled for major, elective orthopedic hip or knee surgery who were expected to require ≥2 units of blood and who were not able or willing to participate in an autologous blood donation program. Based on previous studies which demonstrated that pretreatment hemoglobin is a predictor of risk of receiving transfusion[20,28], patients were stratified into one of three groups based on their pretreatment hemoglobin [≤10 (n=2), >10 to ≤13 (n=96), and >13 to ≤15 g/dL (n=218)] and then randomly assigned to receive 300 U/kg PROCRIT, 100 U/kg PROCRIT or placebo by subcutaneous injection for 10 days before surgery, on the day of surgery, and for four days after surgery[18]. All patients received oral iron and a low dose postoperative warfarin regimen.[18]

Treatment with PROCRIT 300 U/kg significantly (p=0.024) reduced the risk of allogeneic transfusion in patients with a pretreatment hemoglobin of >10 to ≤13 g/dL; 5/31 (16%) of PROCRIT 300 U/kg, 6/26 (23%) of PROCRIT 100 U/kg and 13/29 (45%) of placebo-treated patients were transfused.[18]

There was no significant difference in the number of patients transfused between PROCRIT (9% 300 U/kg, 6% 100 U/kg) and placebo (13%) in the >13 to ≤15 g/dL hemoglobin stratum. There were too few patients in the ≤10 g/dL group to determine if PROCRIT is useful in this hemoglobin strata.

In the >10 to ≤13 g/dL pretreatment stratum, the mean number of units transfused per PROCRIT-treated patient (0.45 units blood for 300 U/kg, 0.42 units blood for 100 U/kg) was less than the mean transfused per placebo-treated patient (1.14 units) (overall p=0.028). In addition, mean hemoglobin, hematocrit and reticulocyte counts increased significantly during the presurgery period in PROCRIT-treated patients.[18]

PROCRIT was also studied in an open-label, parallel-group trial enrolling 145 subjects with a pretreatment hemoglobin level of ≥10 to ≤13 g/dL who were scheduled for major orthopedic hip or knee surgery and who were not participating in an autologous program.[19] Subjects were randomly assigned to receive one of two subcutaneous dosing regimens of PROCRIT (600 U/kg once weekly for three weeks prior to surgery and on the day of surgery or 300 U/kg once daily for 10 days prior to surgery, on the day of surgery and for four days after surgery). All subjects received oral iron and appropriate pharmacologic anticoagulation therapy.

From pretreatment to presurgery, the mean increase in hemoglobin in 600 U/kg weekly group (1.44 g/dL) was greater than observed in the 300 U/kg daily group.[19] The mean increase in absolute reticulocyte count was smaller in the weekly group (0.11 x $10^6/mm^3$) compared to the daily group (0.17 x $10^6/mm^3$). Mean hemoglobin levels were similar for the two treatment groups throughout the postsurgical period.

The erythropoietic response observed in both treatment groups resulted in similar transfusion rates [11/69 (16%) in the 600 U/kg weekly group and 14/71 (20%) in the 300 U/kg daily group].[19] The mean number of units transfused per subject was approximately 0.3 units in both treatment groups.

CONTRAINDICATIONS

PROCRIT is contraindicated in patients with:

1) Uncontrolled hypertension.
2) Known hypersensitivity to mammalian cell-derived products.
3) Known hypersensitivity to Albumin (Human).

WARNINGS

Pediatric Use

The multidose preserved formulation contains benzyl alcohol. Benzyl alcohol has been reported to be associated with an increased incidence of neurological and other complications in premature infants which are sometimes fatal.

Thrombotic Events and Increased Mortality

A randomized, prospective trial of 1265 hemodialysis patients with clinically evident cardiac disease (ischemic heart disease or congestive heart failure) was conducted in which patients were assigned to PROCRIT treatment targeted to a maintenance hematocrit of either 42 ± 3% or 30 ± 3%. Increased mortality was observed in 634 patients randomized to a target hematocrit of 42% [221 deaths (35% mortality)] compared to 631 patients targeted to remain at a hematocrit of 30% [185 deaths (29% mortality)]. The reason for increased mortality observed in these studies is unknown, however the incidence of non-fatal myocardial infarctions (3.1% vs. 2.3%), vascular access thrombosis (39% vs. 29%) and all other thrombotic events (22% vs. 18%) were also higher in the group randomized to achieve a hematocrit of 42%.

Increased mortality was observed in a randomized placebo-controlled study of PROCRIT in adult patients who did not have chronic renal failure who were undergoing coronary artery bypass surgery (7 deaths in 126 patients randomized to PROCRIT vs. no deaths among 56 patients receiving placebo). Four of these deaths occurred during the period of study drug administration and all 4 deaths were associated with thrombotic events. While the extent of the population affected is unknown, in patients at risk for thrombosis, the anticipated benefits of PROCRIT treatment should be weighed against the potential for increased risks associated with therapy.

Chronic Renal Failure Patients

Hypertension: Patients with uncontrolled hypertension should not be treated with PROCRIT; blood pressure should be controlled adequately before initiation of therapy. Up to 80% of patients with CRF have a history of hypertension.[29] Although there does not appear to be any direct pressor effects of PROCRIT, blood pressure may rise during

PROCRIT therapy. During the early phase of treatment when the hematocrit is increasing, approximately 25% of patients on dialysis may require initiation of, or increases in, antihypertensive therapy. Hypertensive encephalopathy and seizures have been observed in patients with CRF treated with PROCRIT.

Special care should be taken to closely monitor and aggressively control blood pressure in patients treated with PROCRIT. Patients should be advised as to the importance of compliance with antihypertensive therapy and dietary restrictions. If blood pressure is difficult to control by initiation of appropriate measures, the hematocrit may be reduced by decreasing or withholding the dose of PROCRIT. A clinically significant decrease in hematocrit may not be observed for several weeks.

It is recommended that the dose of PROCRIT be decreased if the hematocrit increase exceeds 4 points in any two-week period, because of the possible association of excessive rate of rise of hematocrit with an exacerbation of hypertension. In chronic renal failure patients on hemodialysis with clinically evident ischemic heart disease or congestive heart failure, the hematocrit should be managed carefully, not to exceed 36%. (see "Thrombotic Events")

Seizures: Seizures have occurred in patients with CRF participating in PROCRIT clinical trials.

In adult patients on dialysis, there was a higher incidence of seizures during the first 90 days of therapy (occurring in approximately 2.5% of patients) as compared with later timepoints.

Given the potential for an increased risk of seizures during the first 90 days of therapy, blood pressure and the presence of premonitory neurologic symptoms should be monitored closely. Patients should be cautioned to avoid potentially hazardous activities such as driving or operating heavy machinery during this period.

While the relationship between seizures and the rate of rise of hematocrit is uncertain, it is recommended that the dose of PROCRIT be decreased if the hematocrit increase exceeds 4 points in any two-week period.

Thrombotic Events: During hemodialysis, patients treated with PROCRIT may require increased anticoagulation with heparin to prevent clotting of the artificial kidney. (See "ADVERSE REACTIONS" for more information about thrombotic events.)

Other thrombotic events (e.g., myocardial infarction, cerebrovascular accident, transient ischemic attack) have occurred in clinical trials at an annualized rate of less than 0.04 events per patient-year of PROCRIT therapy. These trials were conducted in patients with CRF (whether on dialysis or not) in whom the target hematocrit was 32–40%. However, the risk of thrombotic events, including vascular access thromboses, was significantly increased in adult patients with ischemic heart disease or congestive heart failure receiving PROCRIT therapy with the goal of reaching a normal hematocrit (42%) as compared to a target hematocrit of 30%. Patients with pre-existing cardiovascular disease should be monitored closely.

Zidovudine-treated HIV-infected Patients

In contrast to CRF patients, PROCRIT therapy has not been linked to exacerbation of hypertension, seizures, and thrombotic events in HIV-infected patients.

PRECAUTIONS

The parenteral administration of any biologic product should be attended by appropriate precautions in case allergic or other untoward reactions occur (see "CONTRAINDICATIONS"). In clinical trials, while transient rashes were occasionally observed concurrently with PROCRIT therapy, no serious allergic or anaphylactic reactions were reported. (See "ADVERSE REACTIONS" for more information regarding allergic reactions.)

The safety and efficacy of PROCRIT therapy have not been established in patients with a known history of a seizure disorder or underlying hematologic disease (e.g., sickle cell anemia, myelodysplastic syndromes, or hypercoagulable disorders).

In some female patients, menses have resumed following PROCRIT therapy; the possibility of pregnancy should be discussed and the need for contraception evaluated.

Hematology: Exacerbation of porphyria has been observed rarely in patients with CRF treated with PROCRIT. However, PROCRIT has not caused increased urinary excretion of porphyrin metabolites in normal volunteers, even in the presence of a rapid erythropoietic response. Nevertheless, PROCRIT should be used with caution in patients with known porphyria.

In preclinical studies in dogs and rats, but not in monkeys, PROCRIT therapy was associated with subclinical bone marrow fibrosis. Bone marrow fibrosis is a known complication of CRF in humans and may be related to secondary hyperparathyroidism or unknown factors. The incidence of bone marrow fibrosis was not increased in a study of adult patients on dialysis who were treated with PROCRIT for 12–19 months, compared to the incidence of bone marrow fibrosis in a matched group of patients who had not been treated with PROCRIT.

Hematocrit in CRF patients should be measured twice a week; zidovudine-treated HIV-infected and cancer patients should have hematocrit measured once a week until hematocrit has been stabilized, and measured periodically thereafter.

Delayed or Diminished Response: If the patient fails to respond or to maintain a response to doses within the recommended dosing range, the following etiologies should be considered and evaluated:

1) Iron deficiency: Virtually all patients will eventually require supplemental iron therapy. (See "Iron Evaluation").
2) Underlying infectious, inflammatory, or malignant processes.
3) Occult blood loss.
4) Underlying hematologic diseases (i.e., thalassemia, refractory anemia, or other myelodysplastic disorders).
5) Vitamin deficiencies: folic acid or vitamin B12.
6) Hemolysis.
7) Aluminum intoxication.
8) Osteitis fibrosa cystica.

Iron Evaluation: During PROCRIT therapy, absolute or functional iron deficiency may develop. Functional iron deficiency, with normal ferritin levels but low transferrin saturation, is presumably due to the inability to mobilize iron stores rapidly enough to support increased erythropoiesis. Transferrin saturation should be at least 20% and ferritin should be at least 100 ng/mL.

Prior to and during PROCRIT therapy, the patient's iron status, including transferrin saturation (serum iron divided by iron binding capacity) and serum ferritin, should be evaluated. Virtually all patients will eventually require supplemental iron to increase or maintain transferrin saturation to levels which will adequately support erythropoiesis stimulated by PROCRIT. All surgery patients being treated with PROCRIT should receive adequate iron supplementation throughout the course of therapy in order to support erythropoiesis and avoid depletion of iron stores.

Drug Interactions: No evidence of interaction of PROCRIT with other drugs was observed in the course of clinical trials.

Carcinogenesis, Mutagenesis, and Impairment of Fertility: Carcinogenic potential of PROCRIT has not been evaluated. PROCRIT does not induce bacterial gene mutation (Ames Test), chromosomal aberrations in mammalian cells, micronuclei in mice, or gene mutation at the HGPRT locus. In female rats treated intravenously with PROCRIT, there was a trend for slightly increased fetal wastage at doses of 100 and 500 Units/kg.

Pregnancy Category C: PROCRIT has been shown to have adverse effects in rats when given in doses five times the human dose. There are no adequate and well-controlled studies in pregnant women. PROCRIT should be used during pregnancy only if potential benefit justifies the potential risk to the fetus.

In studies in female rats, there were decreases in body weight gain, delays in appearance of abdominal hair, delayed eyelid opening, delayed ossification, and decreases in the number of caudal vertebrae in the F1 fetuses of the 500 Units/kg group. In female rats treated intravenously, there was a trend for slightly increased fetal wastage at doses of 100 and 500 Units/kg. PROCRIT has not shown any adverse effect at doses as high as 500 Units/kg in pregnant rabbits (from day 6 to 18 of gestation).

Nursing Mothers: Postnatal observations of the live offspring (F1 generation) of female rats treated with PROCRIT during gestation and lactation revealed no effect of PROCRIT at doses of up to 500 Units/kg. There were, however, decreases in body weight gain, delays in appearance of abdominal hair, eyelid opening, and decreases in the number of caudal vertebrae in the F1 fetuses of the 500 Units/kg group. There were no PROCRIT related effects on the F2 generation fetuses.

It is not known whether PROCRIT is excreted in human milk. Because many drugs are excreted in human milk, caution should be exercised when PROCRIT is administered to a nursing woman.

Pediatric Use:

See WARNINGS, Pediatric Use.

Pediatric Patients on Dialysis: PROCRIT is indicated in infants (1 month to 2 years), children (2 years to 12 years), and adolescents (12 years to 16 years) for the treatment of anemia associated with CRF requiring dialysis. Safety and effectiveness in pediatric patients less than 1 month old have not been established (see CLINICAL EXPERIENCE, Chronic Renal Failure, *Pediatric Patients on Dialysis*). The safety data from these studies show that there is no increased risk to pediatric CRF patients on dialysis when compared to the safety profile of PROCRIT in adult CRF patients (see ADVERSE REACTIONS and WARNINGS). Published literature[30–33] provides supportive evidence of the safety and effectiveness of PROCRIT in pediatric CRF patients on dialysis.

Pediatric Patients Not Requiring Dialysis: Published literature[33,34] has reported the use of PROCRIT in 133 pediatric patients with anemia associated with CRF not requiring dialysis, ages 3 months to 20 years, treated with 50 to 250 Units/kg SC or IV, Q.W. to T.I.W. Dose-dependent increases in hemoglobin and hematocrit were observed with reductions in transfusion requirements.

Pediatric HIV-infected Patients: Published literature[35,36] has reported the use of PROCRIT in 20 zidovudine-treated anemic HIV-infected pediatric patients ages 8 months to 17 years, treated with 50 to 400 Units/kg SC or IV, 2 to 3 times per week (T.I.W.). Increases in hemoglobin levels and in reticulocyte counts, and decreases in or elimination of blood transfusions were observed.

Pediatric Cancer Patients on Chemotherapy: Published literature[37,38] has reported the use of PROCRIT in approximately 64 anemic pediatric cancer patients ages 6 months to 18 years, treated with 25 to 300 Units/kg SC or IV, 3 to 7 times per week (T.I.W.). Increases in hemoglobin and decreases in transfusion requirements were noted.

Chronic Renal Failure Patients

Patients with CRF Not Requiring Dialysis: Blood pressure and hematocrit should be monitored no less frequently than for patients maintained on dialysis. Renal function and fluid and electrolyte balance should be closely monitored, as an improved sense of well-being may obscure the need to initiate dialysis in some patients.

Hematology: Sufficient time should be allowed to determine a patient's responsiveness to a dosage of PROCRIT before adjusting the dose. Because of the time required for erythropoiesis and the red cell half-life, an interval of 2–6 weeks may occur between the time of a dose adjustment (initiation, increase, decrease, or discontinuation) and a significant change in hematocrit.

In order to avoid reaching the suggested target hematocrit too rapidly, or exceeding the suggested target range (hematocrit of 30–36%), the guidelines for dose and frequency of dose adjustments (see "DOSAGE AND ADMINISTRATION") should be followed.

For patients who respond to PROCRIT with a rapid increase in hematocrit (e.g., more than 4 points in any two-week period), the dose of PROCRIT should be reduced because of the possible association of excessive rate of rise of hematocrit with an exacerbation of hypertension.

The elevated bleeding time characteristic of CRF decreases toward normal after correction of anemia in patients treated with PROCRIT. Reduction of bleeding time also occurs after correction of anemia by transfusion.

Laboratory Monitoring: The hematocrit should be determined twice a week until it has stabilized in the suggested target range and the maintenance dose has been established. After any dose adjustment, the hematocrit should also be determined twice weekly for at least 2–6 weeks until it has been determined that the hematocrit has stabilized in response to the dose change. The hematocrit should then be monitored at regular intervals.

A complete blood count with differential and platelet count should be performed regularly. During clinical trials, modest increases were seen in platelets and white blood cell counts. While these changes were statistically significant, they were not clinically significant and the values remained within normal ranges.

In patients with CRF, serum chemistry values [including blood urea nitrogen (BUN), uric acid, creatinine, phosphorus, and potassium] should be monitored regularly. During clinical trials in patients on dialysis, modest increases were seen in BUN, creatinine, phosphorus, and potassium. In some patients with CRF not on dialysis, treated with PROCRIT, modest increases in serum uric acid and phosphorus were observed. While changes were statistically significant, the values remained within the ranges normally seen in patients with CRF.

Diet: As the hematocrit increases and patients experience an improved sense of well-being and quality of life, the importance of compliance with dietary and dialysis prescriptions should be reinforced. In particular, hyperkalemia is not uncommon in patients with CRF. In U.S. studies in patients on dialysis, hyperkalemia has occurred at an annualized rate of approximately 0.11 episodes per patient-year of PROCRIT therapy, often in association with poor compliance to medication, diet and/or dialysis.

Dialysis Management: Therapy with PROCRIT results in an increase in hematocrit and a decrease in plasma volume which could affect dialysis efficiency. In studies to date, the resulting increase in hematocrit did not appear to adversely affect dialyzer function[9,10] or the efficiency of high flux hemodialysis.[11] During hemodialysis, patients treated with PROCRIT may require increased anticoagulation with heparin to prevent clotting of the artificial kidney.

Patients who are marginally dialyzed may require adjustments in their dialysis prescription. As with all patients on dialysis, the serum chemistry values (including BUN, creatinine, phosphorus, and potassium) in patients treated with PROCRIT should be monitored regularly to assure the adequacy of the dialysis prescription.

Information for Patients: In those situations in which the physician determines that a home dialysis patient can safely and effectively self-administer PROCRIT, the patient should be instructed as to the proper dosage and administration. Home dialysis patients should be referred to the full "INFORMATION FOR HOME DIALYSIS PATIENTS" section attached; it is not a disclosure of all possible effects. Patients should be informed of the signs and symptoms of allergic drug reaction and advised of appropriate actions. If home use is prescribed for a home dialysis patient, the patient should be thoroughly instructed in the importance of proper disposal and cautioned against the reuse of needles, syringes, or drug product. A puncture-resistant container for the disposal of used syringes and needles should be available to the patient. The full container should be disposed of according to the directions provided by the physician.

Renal Function: In adult patients with CRF not on dialysis, renal function and fluid and electrolyte balance should be closely monitored, as an improved sense of well-being may obscure the need to initiate dialysis in some patients. In patients with CRF not on dialysis, placebo-controlled studies of progression of renal dysfunction over periods of greater than one year have not been completed. In shorter-

Continued on next page

Procrit—Cont.

term trials in adult patients with CRF not on dialysis, changes in creatinine and creatinine clearance were not significantly different in patients treated with PROCRIT, compared with placebo-treated patients. Analysis of the slope of 1/serum creatinine vs. time plots in these patients indicates no significant change in the slope after the initiation of PROCRIT therapy.

Zidovudine-treated HIV-infected Patients

Hypertension: Exacerbation of hypertension has not been observed in zidovudine-treated HIV-infected patients treated with PROCRIT. However, PROCRIT should be withheld in these patients if pre-existing hypertension is uncontrolled, and should not be started until blood pressure is controlled. In double-blind studies, a single seizure has been experienced by a patient treated with PROCRIT.[25]

Cancer Patients on Chemotherapy

Hypertension: Hypertension, associated with a significant increase in hematocrit, has been noted rarely in cancer patients treated with PROCRIT. Nevertheless, blood pressure in patients treated with PROCRIT should be monitored carefully, particularly in patients with an underlying history of hypertension or cardiovascular disease.

Seizures: In double-blind, placebo-controlled trials, 3.2% (N=2/63) of patients treated with PROCRIT and 2.9% (N=2/68) of placebo-treated patients had seizures. Seizures in 1.6% (N=1/63) of patients treated with PROCRIT occurred in the context of a significant increase in blood pressure and hematocrit from baseline values. However, both patients treated with PROCRIT also had underlying CNS pathology which may have been related to seizure activity.

Thrombotic Events: In double-blind, placebo-controlled trials, 3.2% (N=2/63) of patients treated with PROCRIT and 11.8% (N=8/68) of placebo-treated patients had thrombotic events (e.g., pulmonary embolism, cerebrovascular accident).

Growth Factor Potential: PROCRIT is a growth factor that primarily stimulates red cell production. However, the possibility that PROCRIT can act as a growth factor for any tumor type, particularly myeloid malignancies, cannot be excluded.

Surgery Patients

Thrombotic/Vascular Events: In perioperative clinical trials with orthopedic patients, the overall incidence of thrombotic/vascular events was similar in Epoetin alfa and placebo-treated patients who had a pretreatment hemoglobin of >10 to ≤13 g/dL. In patients with a hemoglobin of >13 g/dL treated with 300 U/kg of Epoetin alfa, the possibility that PROCRIT treatment may be associated with an increased risk of postoperative thrombotic/vascular events cannot be excluded.[18–20,28]

In one study in which Epoetin alfa was administered in the perioperative period to patients undergoing coronary artery bypass graft surgery, there were seven deaths in the Epoetin alfa-treated groups (N=126) and no deaths in the placebo-treated group (N=56). Among the seven deaths in the Epoetin alfa-treated patients, four were at the time of therapy (between study day 2 and 8). The four deaths at the time of therapy (3%) were associated with thrombotic/vascular events. A causative role of Epoetin alfa cannot be excluded. (See "WARNINGS")

Hypertension: Blood pressure may rise in the perioperative period in patients being treated with PROCRIT. Therefore, blood pressure should be monitored carefully.

ADVERSE REACTIONS

Chronic Renal Failure Patients

PROCRIT is generally well-tolerated. The adverse events reported are frequent sequelae of CRF and are not necessarily attributable to PROCRIT therapy. In double-blind, placebo-controlled studies involving over 300 patients with CRF, the events reported in greater than 5% of patients treated with PROCRIT during the blinded phase were:

PERCENT OF PATIENTS REPORTING EVENT

Event	Patients Treated with Epoetin alfa (N=200)	PLACEBO-Treated Patients (N=135)
Hypertension	24%	19%
Headache	16%	12%
Arthralgias	11%	6%
Nausea	11%	9%
Edema	9%	10%
Fatigue	9%	14%
Diarrhea	9%	6%
Vomiting	8%	5%
Chest Pain	7%	9%
Skin Reaction (Administration Site)	7%	12%
Asthenia	7%	12%
Dizziness	7%	13%
Clotted Access	7%	2%

Significant adverse events of concern in patients with CRF treated in double-blind, placebo-controlled trials occurred in the following percent of patients during the blinded phase of the studies:

Seizure	1.1%	1.1%
CVA/TIA	0.4%	0.6%
MI	0.4%	1.1%
Death	0	1.7%

In the U.S. PROCRIT studies in adult patients on dialysis (over 567 patients), the incidence (number of events per patient-year) of the most frequently reported adverse events were: hypertension (0.75), headache (0.40), tachycardia (0.31), nausea/vomiting (0.26), clotted vascular access (0.25), shortness of breath (0.14), hyperkalemia (0.11), and diarrhea (0.11). Other reported events occurred at a rate of less than 0.10 events per patient per year.

Events reported to have occurred within several hours of administration of PROCRIT were rare, mild, and transient, and included injection site stinging in dialysis patients and flu-like symptoms such as arthralgias and myalgias.

In all studies analyzed to date, PROCRIT administration was generally well-tolerated, irrespective of the route of administration.

Pediatric CRF Patients: In pediatric patients with CRF on dialysis, the pattern of most adverse events was similar to that found in adults. Additional adverse events reported during the double-blind phase in > 10% of pediatric patients in either treatment group were: abdominal pain, dialysis access complications including access infections and peritonitis in those receiving peritoneal dialysis, fever, upper respiratory infection, cough, pharyngitis, and constipation. The rates are similar between the treatment groups for each event.

Hypertension: Increases in blood pressure have been reported in clinical trials, often during the first 90 days of therapy. On occasion, hypertensive encephalopathy and seizures have been observed in patients with CRF treated with PROCRIT. When data from all patients in the U.S. Phase III multicenter trial were analyzed, there was an apparent trend of more reports of hypertensive adverse events in patients on dialysis with a faster rate of rise of hematocrit (greater than 4 hematocrit points in any two-week period). However, in a double-blind, placebo-controlled trial, hypertensive adverse events were not reported at an increased rate in the group treated with PROCRIT (150 Units/kg T.I.W.) relative to the placebo group.

Seizures: There have been 47 seizures in 1,010 patients on dialysis treated with PROCRIT in clinical trials, with an exposure of 986 patient-years for a rate of approximately 0.048 events per patient-year. However, there appeared to be a higher rate of seizures during the first 90 days of therapy (occurring in approximately 2.5% of patients) when compared to subsequent 90-day periods. The baseline incidence of seizures in the untreated dialysis population is difficult to determine; it appears to be in the range of 5–10% per patient-year.[39–41]

Thrombotic Events: In clinical trials where the maintenance hematocrit was 35 ± 3% on PROCRIT, clotting of the vascular access (A-V shunt) has occurred at an annualized rate of about 0.25 events per patient-year, and other thrombotic events (e.g. myocardial infarction, cerebrovascular accident, transient ischemic attack, and pulmonary embolism) occurred at a rate of 0.04 events per patient-year. In a separate study of 1,111 untreated dialysis patients, clotting of the vascular access occurred at a rate of 0.5 events per patient-year. However, in chronic renal failure patients on hemodialysis who also had clinically evident ischemic heart disease or congestive heart failure, the risk of A-V shunt thrombosis was higher (39% vs 29%, p<0.001), and myocardial infarction, vascular ischemic events, and venous thrombosis were increased in patients targeted to a hematocrit of 42 ± 3% compared to those maintained at 30 ± 3%. (see "WARNINGS")

In patients treated with commercial PROCRIT, there have been rare reports of serious or unusual thrombo-embolic events including migratory thrombophlebitis, microvascular thrombosis, pulmonary embolus, and thrombosis of the retinal artery, and temporal and renal veins. A causal relationship has not been established.

Allergic Reactions: There have been no reports of serious allergic reactions or anaphylaxis associated with PROCRIT administration during clinical trials. Skin rashes and urticaria have been observed rarely and when reported have generally been mild and transient in nature.

In over 125,000 patients treated with commercial PROCRIT, there have been rare reports of potentially serious allergic reactions including urticaria with associated respiratory symptoms or circumoral edema (<0.0001 events per patient-year), or urticaria alone (<0.0001 events per patient-year). Most reactions occurred in situations where a causal relationship could not be established. Many of these patients resumed PROCRIT therapy without recurrence of symptoms, some in conjunction with antihistamine pretreatment. However, symptoms recurred with rechallenge in a few instances, suggesting that allergic reactivity, although rare, may occasionally be associated with PROCRIT therapy.

There has been no evidence for development of antibodies to erythropoietin in patients tested to date, including those receiving PROCRIT for over 4 years. Nevertheless, if an anaphylactoid reaction occurs, PROCRIT should be immediately discontinued and appropriate therapy initiated.

Zidovudine-treated HIV-infected Patients

Adverse events reported in clinical trials with PROCRIT in zidovudine-treated HIV-infected patients were consistent with the progression of HIV infection. In double-blind, placebo-controlled studies of three-months duration involving approximately 300 zidovudine-treated HIV-infected patients, adverse events with an incidence of ≥10% in either patients treated with PROCRIT or placebo-treated patients were:

Percent of Patients Reporting Event

Event	Patients Treated with PROCRIT (N=144)	PLACEBO-Treated Patients (N=153)
Pyrexia	38%	29%
Fatigue	25%	31%
Headache	19%	14%
Cough	18%	14%
Diarrhea	16%	18%
Rash	16%	8%
Congestion, Respiratory	15%	10%
Nausea	15%	12%
Shortness of Breath	14%	13%
Asthenia	11%	14%
Skin Reaction, (Administration Site)	10%	7%
Dizziness	9%	10%

There were no statistically significant differences between treatment groups in the incidence of the above events.

In the 297 patients studied, PROCRIT was not associated with significant increases in opportunistic infections or mortality.[25] In 71 patients from this group treated with PROCRIT at 150 Units/kg (T.I.W.), serum p24 antigen levels did not appear to increase.[27] Preliminary data showed no enhancement of HIV replication in infected cell lines *in vitro*.[25]

Peripheral white blood cell and platelet counts are unchanged following PROCRIT therapy.

Allergic Reactions: Two zidovudine-treated HIV-infected patients had urticarial reactions within 48 hours of their first exposure to study medication. One patient was treated with PROCRIT and one was treated with placebo (PROCRIT vehicle alone). Both patients had positive immediate skin tests against their study medication with a negative saline control. The basis for this apparent pre-existing hypersensitivity to components of the PROCRIT formulation is unknown, but may be related to HIV-induced immunosuppression or prior exposure to blood products.

Seizures: In double-blind and open-label trials of PROCRIT in zidovudine-treated HIV-infected patients, ten patients have experienced seizures.[25] In general, these seizures appear to be related to underlying pathology such as meningitis or cerebral neoplasms, not PROCRIT therapy.

Cancer Patients on Chemotherapy

Adverse experiences reported in clinical trials with PROCRIT in cancer patients were consistent with the underlying disease state. In double-blind, placebo-controlled studies of up to 3-months duration involving 131 cancer patients, adverse events with an incidence > 10% in either patients treated with PROCRIT or placebo-treated patients were as indicated below.

Percent of Patients Reporting Event

Event	Patients Treated with PROCRIT (N=63)	PLACEBO-Treated Patients (N=68)
Pyrexia	29%	19%
Diarrhea	21%[a]	7%
Nausea	17%[b]	32%
Vomiting	17%	15%
Edema	17%[c]	1%
Asthenia	13%	16%
Fatigue	13%	15%
Shortness of Breath	13%	9%
Paresthesia	11%	6%
Upper Respiratory Infection	11%	4%
Dizziness	5%	12%
Trunk Pain	3%[d]	16%

[a] p = 0.041 [c] p = 0.0016
[b] p = 0.069 [d] p = 0.017

Although some statistically significant differences between patients treated with PROCRIT and placebo-treated patients were noted, the overall safety profile of PROCRIT appeared to be consistent with the disease process of advanced cancer. During double-blind and subsequent open-label therapy in which patients (N=72 for total exposure to PROCRIT) were treated for up to 32 weeks with doses as high as 927 Units/kg, the adverse experience profile of PROCRIT was consistent with the progression of advanced cancer.

Based on comparable survival data and on the percentage of patients treated with PROCRIT and placebo-treated patients who discontinued therapy due to death, disease progression or adverse experiences (22% and 13%, respectively; p = 0.25), the clinical outcome in patients treated with

PROCRIT and placebo-treated patients appeared to be similar. Available data from animal tumor models and measurement of proliferation of solid tumor cells from clinical biopsy specimens in response to PROCRIT suggest that PROCRIT does not potentiate tumor growth. Nevertheless, as a growth factor, the possibility that PROCRIT may potentiate growth of some tumors, particularly myeloid tumors, cannot be excluded. A randomized controlled Phase IV study is currently ongoing to further evaluate this issue.

The mean peripheral white blood cell count was unchanged following PROCRIT therapy compared to the corresponding value in the placebo-treated group.

Surgery Patients

Adverse events with an incidence of $\geq$10% are shown in the following table:

[See first table above]

Thrombotic/vascular events: In three double-blind, placebo-controlled orthopedic surgery studies, the rate of deep venous thrombosis (DVT) was similar among Epoetin alfa and placebo-treated patients in the recommended population of patients with a pretreatment hemoglobin of >10 to $\leq$13 g/dL.[18,19,28] However, in 2 of 3 orthopedic surgery studies the overall rate (all pretreatment hemoglobin groups combined) of DVTs detected by postoperative ultrasonography and/or surveillance venography was higher in the group treated with Epoetin alfa than in the placebo-treated group (11% vs. 6%). This finding was attributable to the difference in DVT rates observed in the subgroup of patients with pretreatment hemoglobin >13 g/dL. However, the incidence of DVTs was within the range of that reported in the literature for orthopedic surgery patients.

In the orthopedic surgery study of patients with pretreatment hemoglobin of >10 to $\leq$13 g/dL which compared two dosing regimens (600 U/kg weekly × 4 and 300 U/kg daily × 15), four subjects in the 600 U/kg weekly PROCRIT group (5%) and no subjects in the 300 U/kg daily group had a thrombotic vascular event during the study period.[19]

In a study examining the use of Epoetin alfa in 182 patients scheduled for coronary artery bypass graft surgery, 23% of patients treated with Epoetin alfa and 29% treated with placebo experienced thrombotic/vascular events. There were 4 deaths among the Epoetin alfa-treated patients that were associated with a thrombotic/vascular event. A causative role of Epoetin alfa cannot be excluded. (See "WARNINGS")

OVERDOSAGE

The maximum amount of PROCRIT that can be safely administered in single or multiple doses has not been determined. Doses of up to 1,500 Units/kg (T.I.W.) for three to four weeks have been administered to adults without any direct toxic effects of PROCRIT itself.[6] Therapy with PROCRIT can result in polycythemia if the hematocrit is not carefully monitored and the dose appropriately adjusted. If the suggested target range is exceeded, PROCRIT may be temporarily withheld until the hematocrit returns to the suggested target range; PROCRIT therapy may then be resumed using a lower dose (see "DOSAGE AND ADMINISTRATION"). If polycythemia is of concern, phlebotomy may be indicated to decrease the hematocrit.

DOSAGE AND ADMINISTRATION

Chronic Renal Failure Patients

Starting doses of PROCRIT over the range of 50–100 Units/kg three times weekly (T.I.W.) for adult patients. The recommended starting dose for pediatric CRF patients on dialysis is 50 Units/kg three times weekly (T.I.W.). The dose of PROCRIT should be reduced as the hematocrit approaches 36% or increases by more than 4 points in any 2-week period. The dosage of PROCRIT must be individualized to maintain the hematocrit within the suggested target range. At the physician's discretion, the suggested target hematocrit range may be expanded to achieve maximal patient benefit.

PROCRIT may be given either as an intravenous (IV) or subcutaneous (SC) injection. In patients on hemodialysis, PROCRIT usually has been administered as an IV bolus (T.I.W.). While the administration of PROCRIT is independent of the dialysis procedure, PROCRIT may be administered into the venous line at the end of the dialysis procedure to obviate the need for additional venous access. In adult patients with CRF not on dialysis, PROCRIT may be given either as an IV or SC injection.

Patients who have been judged competent by their physicians to self-administer PROCRIT without medical or other supervision may give themselves either an IV or SC injection. The table below provides general therapeutic guidelines for patients with CRF:

[See second table above]

During therapy, hematological parameters should be monitored regularly (see "Laboratory Monitoring").

Pre-Therapy Iron Evaluation: Prior to and during PROCRIT therapy, the patient's iron stores, including transferrin saturation (serum iron divided by iron binding capacity) and serum ferritin, should be evaluated. Transferrin saturation should be at least 20%, and ferritin should be at least 100 ng/mL. Virtually all patients will eventually require supplemental iron to increase or maintain transferrin saturation to levels that will adequately support erythropoiesis stimulated by PROCRIT.

Dose Adjustment: Following PROCRIT therapy, a period of time is required for erythroid progenitors to mature and be released into circulation resulting in an eventual increase in hematocrit. Additionally, red blood cell survival time affects hematocrit and may vary due to uremia. As a result, the time required to elicit a clinically significant

	Percent of Patients Reporting Event				
Event	Patients Treated with PROCRIT 300 U/kg (N=112)[a]	Patients Treated with PROCRIT 100 U/kg (N=101)[a]	PLACEBO-Treated Patients (N=103)[a]	PROCRIT 600 U/kg (N=73)[b]	PROCRIT 300 U/kg (N=72)[b]
Pyrexia	51%	50%	60%	47%	42%
Nausea	48%	43%	45%	45%	58%
Constipation	43%	42%	43%	51%	53%
Skin Reaction, (Administration Site)	25%	19%	22%	26%	29%
Vomiting	22%	12%	14%	21%	29%
Skin Pain	18%	18%	17%	5%	4%
Pruritus	16%	16%	14%	14%	22%
Insomnia	13%	16%	13%	21%	18%
Headache	13%	11%	9%	10%	19%
Dizziness	12%	9%	12%	11%	21%
Urinary Tract Infection	12%	3%	11%	11%	8%
Hypertension	10%	11%	10%	5%	10%
Diarrhea	10%	7%	12%	10%	6%
Deep Venous Thrombosis	10%	3%	5%	0%[c]	0%[c]
Dyspepsia	9%	11%	6%	7%	8%
Anxiety	7%	2%	11%	11%	4%
Edema	6%	11%	8%	11%	7%

[a]Study including patients undergoing orthopedic surgery treated with PROCRIT or placebo for 15 days

[b] Study including patients undergoing orthopedic surgery treated with PROCRIT 600 U/kg weekly × 4 or 300 U/kg daily ×15

[c]Determined by clinical symptoms

Starting Dose	Reduce Dose If	Increase Dose When	Maintenance Dose	Suggested Hct. Range
Adults 50-100 Units/kg T.I.W.; IV or SC	1) Hct. approaches 36%, or	Hct. does not increase by 5-6 points after 8 weeks of therapy, and hct. is below suggested target range	Individually titrate	30-36%
Pediatric Patients 50 Units/kg T.I.W.; IV or SC	2) Hct. increases > 4 points in any 2-week period			

change in hematocrit (increase or decrease) following any dose adjustment may be 2–6 weeks.

Dose adjustment should not be made more frequently than once a month, unless clinically indicated. After any dose adjustment, the hematocrit should be determined twice weekly for at least 2–6 weeks (see "Laboratory Monitoring").

- If the hematocrit is increasing and approaching 36%, the dose should be reduced to maintain the suggested target hematocrit range. If the reduced dose does not stop the rise in hematocrit, and it exceeds 36%, doses should be temporarily withheld until the hematocrit begins to decrease, at which point therapy should be reinitiated at a lower dose.
- At any time, if the hematocrit increases by more than 4 points in a 2-week period, the dose should be immediately decreased. After the dose reduction, the hematocrit should be monitored twice weekly for 2–6 weeks, and further dose adjustments should be made as outlined in "Maintenance Dose".
- If a hematocrit increase of 5–6 points is not achieved after an 8-week period and iron stores are adequate (see "Delayed or Diminished Response"), the dose of PROCRIT may be incrementally increased. Further increases may be made at 4–6 week intervals until the desired response is attained.

Maintenance Dose: The maintenance dose must be individualized for each patient on dialysis. In the U.S. Phase III multicenter trial in patients on hemodialysis, the median maintenance dose was 75 Units/kg (T.I.W.), with a range from 12.5 to 525 Units/kg (T.I.W.). Almost 10% of the patients required a dose of 25 Units/kg, or less, and approximately 10% of the patients required more than 200 Units/kg (T.I.W.) to maintain their hematocrit in the suggested target range. In pediatric hemodialysis and peritoneal dialysis patients, the median maintenance dose was 167 Units/kg/week (49 to 447 Units/kg per week) and 76 Units/kg per week (24 to 323 Units/kg/week) administered in divided doses (T.I.W. or B.I.W.), respectively to achieve the target range of 30% to 36%.

If the hematocrit remains below, or falls below, the suggested target range, iron stores should be re-evaluated. If the transferrin saturation is less than 20%, supplemental iron should be administered. If the transferrin saturation is greater than 20%, the dose of PROCRIT may be increased. Such dose increases should not be made more frequently than once a month, unless clinically indicated, as the response time of the hematocrit to a dose increase can be 2–6 weeks. Hematocrit should be measured twice weekly for 2–6 weeks following dose increases. In adult patients with CRF not on dialysis, the maintenance dose must also be individualized. PROCRIT doses of 75–150 Units/kg per week have been shown to maintain hematocrits of 36–38% for up to 6 months.

Delayed or Diminished Response: Over 95% of patients with CRF responded with clinically significant increases in hematocrit, and virtually all patients were transfusion-independent within approximately two months of initiation of PROCRIT therapy.

If a patient fails to respond or maintain a response, other etiologies should be considered and evaluated as clinically indicated. (See "PRECAUTIONS" section for discussion of delayed or diminished response.)

Zidovudine-treated HIV-infected Patients

Prior to beginning PROCRIT, it is recommended that the endogenous serum erythropoietin level be determined (prior to transfusion). Available evidence suggests that patients receiving zidovudine with endogenous serum erythropoietin levels > 500 mUnits/mL are unlikely to respond to therapy with PROCRIT.

Starting Dose: For adult patients with serum erythropoietin levels $\leq$ 500 mUnits/mL who are receiving a dose of zidovudine $\leq$ 4,200 mg/week, the recommended starting dose of PROCRIT is 100 Units/kg as an intravenous or subcutaneous injection three times weekly (T.I.W.) for 8 weeks. For pediatric patients, see "PRECAUTIONS, Pediatric Use."

Increase Dose: During the dose adjustment phase of therapy, the hematocrit should be monitored weekly. If the response is not satisfactory in terms of reducing transfusion requirements or increasing hematocrit after 8 weeks of therapy, the dose of PROCRIT can be increased by 50–100 Units/kg (T.I.W.). Response should be evaluated every 4–8 weeks thereafter and the dose adjusted accordingly by 50–100 Units/kg increments (T.I.W.). If patients have not responded satisfactorily to a PROCRIT dose of 300 Units/kg (T.I.W.), it is unlikely that they will respond to higher doses of PROCRIT.

Maintenance Dose: After attainment of the desired response (i.e., reduced transfusion requirements or increased hematocrit), the dose of PROCRIT should be titrated to maintain the response based on factors such as variations in zidovudine dose and the presence of intercurrent infectious or inflammatory episodes. If the hematocrit exceeds 40%, the dose should be discontinued until the hematocrit drops to 36%. The dose should be reduced by 25% when treatment is resumed and then titrated to maintain the desired hematocrit.

Cancer Patients on Chemotherapy

Baseline endogenous serum erythropoietin levels varied among patients in these trials with approximately 75% (N=83/110) having endogenous serum erythropoietin levels < 132 mUnits/mL, and approximately 4% (N=4/110) of patients having endogenous serum erythropoietin levels > 500 mUnits/mL. In general, patients with lower baseline serum erythropoietin levels responded more vigorously to PROCRIT than patients with higher erythropoietin levels. Although no specific serum erythropoietin level can be stip-

Continued on next page

Procrit—Cont.

ulated above which patients would be unlikely to respond to PROCRIT therapy, treatment of patients with grossly elevated serum erythropoietin levels (e.g., > 200 mUnits/mL) is not recommended. The hematocrit should be monitored on a weekly basis in patients receiving PROCRIT therapy until hematocrit becomes stable.

Starting Dose: The recommended starting dose of PROCRIT for adults is 150 Units/kg subcutaneously (T.I.W.). For pediatric patients, see "PRECAUTIONS, Pediatric Use."

Dose Adjustment: If the response is not satisfactory in terms of reducing transfusion requirements or increasing hematocrit after 8 weeks of therapy, the dose of PROCRIT can be increased up to 300 Units/kg (T.I.W.). If patients have not responded satisfactorily to a PROCRIT dose of 300 Units/kg (T.I.W.), it is unlikely that they will respond to higher doses of PROCRIT. If the hematocrit exceeds 40%, the dose of PROCRIT should be withheld until the hematocrit falls to 36%. The dose of PROCRIT should be reduced by 25% when treatment is resumed and titrated to maintain the desired hematocrit. If the initial dose of PROCRIT includes a very rapid hematocrit response (e.g., an increase of more than 4 percentage points in any 2-week period), the dose of PROCRIT should be reduced.

Surgery Patients

Prior to initiating treatment with PROCRIT a hemoglobin should be obtained to establish that it is >10 to ≤13 g/dL.[18] The recommended dose of PROCRIT is 300 U/kg/day subcutaneously for 10 days before surgery, on the day of surgery, and for 4 days after surgery.

An alternate dose schedule is 600 U/kg PROCRIT subcutaneously in once weekly doses (21, 14 and 7 days before surgery) plus a fourth dose on day of surgery.[19]

All patients should receive adequate iron supplementation. Iron supplementation should be initiated no later than the beginning of treatment with PROCRIT and should continue throughout the course of therapy.

PREPARATION AND ADMINISTRATION OF PROCRIT

1. DO NOT SHAKE. It is not necessary to shake PROCRIT. Prolonged vigorous shaking may denature any glycoprotein, rendering it biologically inactive.
2. Parenteral drug products should be inspected visually for particulate matter and discoloration prior to administration. Do not use any vials exhibiting particulate matter or discoloration.
3. Using aseptic techniques, attach a sterile needle to a sterile syringe. Remove the flip top from the vial containing PROCRIT, and wipe the septum with a disinfectant. Insert the needle into the vial, and withdraw into the syringe an appropriate volume of solution.
4. **Single-dose** 1 mL vial contains no preservative. Use one dose per vial; do not re-enter vial. Discard unused portions. **Multidose** 1 mL and 2 mL vials contain preservative. Store at 2 to 8°C after initial entry and between doses. Discard 21 days after initial entry.
5. Do not dilute or administer in conjunction with other drug solutions. However, at the time of subcutaneous administration, preservative-free PROCRIT from single-use vials may be admixed in a syringe with bacteriostatic 0.9% sodium chloride injection, USP, with benzyl alcohol 0.9% (bacteriostatic saline) at a 1:1 ratio using aseptic technique. The benzyl alcohol in the bacteriostatic saline acts as a local anesthetic which may ameliorate subcutaneous injection site discomfort. Admixing is not necessary when using the multidose vials of PROCRIT containing benzyl alcohol.

HOW SUPPLIED

PROCRIT, containing Epoetin alfa, is available in vials containing color coded labels.

1 mL **Single-Dose, Preservative-Free** Solution

Each dosage form is supplied in the following packages:

Cartons containing six (6) **single-dose** vials:
- 2,000 Units/mL (NDC 59676-302-01) (Purple)
- 3,000 Units/mL (NDC 59676-303-01) (Magenta)
- 4,000 Units/mL (NDC 59676-304-01) (Green)
- 10,000 Units/mL (NDC 59676-310-01) (Red)

Cartons containing four (4) **single-dose** vials:
- 40,000 Units/mL (NDC 59676-340-01) (Orange)

Trays containing twenty-five (25) **single-dose** vials:
- 2,000 Units/mL (NDC 59676-302-02) (Purple)
- 3,000 Units/mL (NDC 59676-303-02) (Magenta)
- 4,000 Units/mL (NDC 59676-304-02) (Green)
- 10,000 Units/mL (NDC 59676-310-02) (Red)

2 mL **Multidose, Preserved** Solution

Cartons containing six (6) **multidose** vials:
- 10,000 Units/mL (NDC 59676-312-01) (Blue)

1 mL **Multidose, Preserved** Solution

Cartons containing six (6) **multidose** vials:
- 20,000 Units/mL (NDC 59676-320-01) (Lime)

STORAGE

Store at 2° to 8° C (36° to 46° F). Do not freeze or shake.

REFERENCES:

1. Egrie JC, Strickland TW, Lane J, *et al.*, (1986). "Characterization and Biological Effects of Recombinant Human Erythropoietin." *Immunobiol.* 72:213–224.
2. Graber SE and Krantz SB, (1978). "Erythropoietin and the Control of Red Cell Production." *Ann. Rev. Med.* 29:51–66.
3. Eschbach JW and Adamson JW, (1985). "Anemia of End-Stage Renal Disease (ESRD)." *Kidney Intl.* 28:1–5.
4. Eschbach JW, Egrie JC, Downing MR, Browne JK, and Adamson JW, (1987). "Correction of the Anemia of End-Stage Renal Disease with Recombinant Human Erythropoietin." *NEJM* 316:73–78.
5. Eschbach JW, Abdulhadi MH, Browne JK, *et al.*, (1989). "Recombinant Human Erythropoietin in Anemic Patients with End-Stage Renal Disease." *Ann. Intern. Med.* 111:992–1000.
6. Eschbach JW, Egrie JC, Downing MR, Browne JK, Adamson JW, (1989). "The Use of Recombinant Human Erythropoietin (r-HuEPO): Effect in End-Stage Renal Disease (ESRD)," *Prevention Of Chronic Uremia*, (Friedman, Beyer, DeSanto, Giordano, eds.), Field and Wood Inc., Philadelphia, PA, pp 148–155.
7. Egrie JC, Eschbach JW, McGuire T, and Adamson JW, (1988). "Pharmacokinetics of Recombinant Human Erythropoietin (r-HuEPO) Administered to Hemodialysis (HD) Patients." *Kidney Intl.* 33:262.
8. Evans RW, Rader B, Manninen DL, *et al.*, (1990). "The Quality of Life of Hemodialysis Recipients Treated with Recombinant Human Erythropoietin." *JAMA* 263:825–830.
9. Paganini E, Garcia J, Ellis P, Bodnar D, and Magnussen M, (1988). "Clinical Sequelae of Correction of Anemia with Recombinant Human Erythropoietin (r-HuEPO); Urea Kinetics, Dialyzer Function and Reuse." *Am. J. Kid. Dis.* 11: 16.
10. Delano BG, Lundin AP, Golansky R, Quinn RM, Rao TKS, and Friedman EA, (1988). "Dialyzer Urea and Creatinine Clearances Not Significantly Changed in r-HuEPO Treated Maintenance Hemodialysis (MD) Patients." *Kidney Intl.* 33:219.
11. Stivelman J, Van Wyck D, and Ogden D, (1988). "Use of Recombinant Erythropoietin (r-HuEPO) with High Flux Dialysis (HFD) Does Not Worsen Azotemia or Shorten Access Survival." *Kidney Intl.* 33:239.
12. Lim VS, DeGowin RL, Zavala D, Kirchner PT, Abels R, Perry P, and Fangman J, (1989). "Recombinant Human Erythropoietin Treatment in Pre-Dialysis Patients: A Double-Blind Placebo-Controlled Trial." *Ann. Int. Med.* 110:108–114.
13. Stone WJ, Graber SE, Krantz SB, *et al.*, (1988). "Treatment of the Anemia of Pre-Dialysis Patients with Recombinant Human Erythropoietin: A Randomized, Placebo-Controlled Trial." *Am. J. Med. Sci.* 296:171–179.
14. Braun A, Ding R, Seidel C, *et al.*, (1993). "Pharmacokinetics of recombinant human erythropoietin applied subcutaneously to children with chronic renal failure." *Pediatr Nephrol.* 7:61–64.
15. Geva P and Sherwood JB, (1991). "Pharmacokinetics of recombinant human erythropoietin (rHuEPO) in pediatric patients on chronic cycling peritoneal dialysis (CCPD)." *Blood.* 78 (Suppl 1):91a.
16. Jabs K, Grant JR, Harmon W, *et al.*, (1991). "Pharmacokinetics of Epoetin alfa (rHuEPO) in pediatric hemodialysis (HD) patients." *J Am Soc Nephrol.* 2:380.
17. Kling PJ, Widness JA, Guillery EN, *et al.*, (1992). "Pharmacokinetics and pharmacodynamics of erythropoietin during therapy in an infant with renal failure." *J Pediatr.* 121: 822–825.
18. de Andrade JR and Jove M, (1996). "Baseline Hemoglobin as a Predictor of Risk of Transfusion and Response to Epoetin alfa in Orthopedic Surgery Patients." *Am. J. of Orthoped.* 25(8): 533–542.
19. Goldberg MA and McCutchen JW, (1996). "A Safety and Efficacy Comparison Study of Two Dosing Regimens of Epoetin alfa in Patients Undergoing Major Orthopedic Surgery." *Am. J. of Orthoped.* 25(8): 544–552.
20. Faris PM and Ritter MA, (1996). "The Effects of Recombinant Human Erythropoietin on Perioperative Transfusion Requirements in Patients Having a Major Orthopaedic Operation." *J. Bone and Joint Surg.* 78-A:62–72.
21. Lundin AP, Akerman MJH, Chesler RM, Delano BG, Goldberg N, Stein RA, and Friedman EA, (1991). "Exercise in Hemodialysis Patients after Treatment with Recombinant Human Erythropoietin" *Nephron.* 58:315–319.
22. Data on file, Amgen Inc.
23. Eschbach JW, Kelly MR, Galey NR, Abels RI and Adamson JU (1989). "Treatment of the Anemia of Progressive Renal Failure with Recombinant Human Erythropoietin," *NEJM* 321:158–163.
24. The US Recombinant Human Erythropoietin Predialysis Study Group (1991). "Double-Blind, Placebo-Controlled Study of the Therapeutic Use of Recombinant Human Erythropoietin for Anemia Associated with Chronic Renal Failure in Predialysis Patients," *Am. J. Kid. Dis.* 18(1):50–59.
25. Data on file, Ortho Biologics, Inc.
26. Danna RP, Rudnick SA, and Abels RI, (1990). "Erythropoietin Therapy for the Anemia Associated with AIDS and AIDS Therapy and Cancer." *Erythropoietin in Clinical Applications—An International Perspective*, (MB Garnick, ed.), Marcel Dekker, New York, NY, pp. 301–324.
27. Fischl M, Galpin JE, Levine JD, *et al.*, (1990). "Recombinant Human Erythropoietin for Patients with AIDS Treated with Zidovudine." *NEJM* 322:1488–1493.
28. Laupacis A, (1993). "Effectiveness of Perioperative Recombinant Human Erythropoietin in Elective Hip Replacement." *Lancet* 341:1228–1232.
29. Kerr DN, (1979). "Chronic Renal Failure," *Cecil Textbook of Medicine*, (Beeson PB, McDermott W, Wyngaarden JB, eds.), W.B. Saunders, Philadelphia, PA, pp 1351–1367.
30. Campos A and Garin EH. (1992). "Therapy of renal anemia in children and adolescents with recombinant human erythropoietin (rHuEPO)." *Clin Pediatr* (Phila). 31:94–99.
31. Montini G, Zacchello G, Baraldi E, et al., (1990). "Benefits and risks of anemia correction with recombinant human erythropoietin in children maintained by hemodialysis." *J Pediatr.* 117:556–560.
32. Offner G, Hoyer PF, Latta K, et al., (1990). "One year's experience with recombinant erythropoietin in children undergoing continuous ambulatory or cycling peritoneal dialysis." *Pediatr Nephrol.* 4:498–500.
33. Muller-Wiefel DE and Scigalla P, (1988). "Specific problems of renal anemia in childhood." *Contrib Nephrol.* 66:71–84.
34. Scharer K, Klare B, Dressel P, and Gretz N, (1993) "Treatment of renal anemia by subcutaneous erythropoietin in children with preterminal chronic renal failure." *Acta Paediatr.* 82:953–958.
35. Mueller BU, Jacobsen RN, Jarosinski P, et al. (1994). "Erythropoietin for zidovudine-associated anemia in children with HIV infection." *Pediatr AIDS and HIV Infect: Fetus to Adolesc.* 5:169–173.
36. Zuccotti GV, Plebani A, Biasucci G, et al. (1996). "Granulocyte-colony stimulating factor and erythropoietin therapy in children with human immunodeficiency virus infection." *J Int Med Res.* 24:115–121.
37. Beck MN and Beck D, (1995). "Recombinant erythropoietin in acute chemotherapy-induced anemia of children with cancer." *Med Pediatr Oncol.* 25:17–21.
38. Bennetts G, Bertolone S, Bray G, et al., (1995). "Erythropoietin reduces volumes of red cell transfusions required in some subsets of children with acute lymphocytic leukemia." *Blood.* 86:853a.
39. Raskin NH and Fishman RA, (1976). "Neurologic Disorders in Renal Failure (First of Two Parts)." *NEJM* 294:143–148.
40. Raskin NH and Fishman RA, (1976). "Neurologic Disorders in Renal Failure (Second of Two Parts)." *NEJM* 294: 204–210.
41. Messing RO and Simon RP,(1986). "Seizures as a Manifestation of Systemic Disease." *Neurologic Clinics* 4:563–584.

Manufactured by:
Amgen, Inc.
U.S. Lic. # 1080
Thousand Oaks, California 91320–1789

Distributed by:
Ortho Biotech Products, L.P.
Raritan, New Jersey 08869-0670

 638-29-979-8
6300G020
Revised March 2000 3193602

PROCRIT®
EPOETIN ALFA

INFORMATION FOR HOME DIALYSIS PATIENTS

What is PROCRIT and how does it work?

PROCRIT is a copy of human erythropoietin, a hormone produced primarily by healthy kidneys. PROCRIT replaces the erythropoietin that the failed kidneys can no longer produce, and signals the bone marrow to make the oxygen-carrying red blood cells once again. PROCRIT is produced in mammalian cells that have been genetically altered by the addition of a gene of the natural substance erythropoietin.

How should I take PROCRIT?

In those situations where your doctor has determined that you, as a home dialysis patient, can self-administer PROCRIT, you will receive instruction on how much PROCRIT to use, how to inject it, how often you should inject it, and how you should dispose of the unused portions of each vial.

You will be instructed to monitor your blood pressure carefully everyday and to report any changes outside of the guidelines that your doctor has given you. When the number of red blood cells increases, your blood pressure can also increase, so your doctor may prescribe some new or additional blood pressure medication. Be sure to follow your doctor's orders. You may also be instructed to have certain laboratory tests, such as additional hematocrit or iron level measurements, done more frequently. You may be asked to report these tests to your doctor or dialysis center. Also, your doctor may prescribe additional iron for you to take. Be sure to comply with your doctor's orders.

Continue to check your access, as your doctor or nurse has shown you, to make sure it is working. Be sure to let your health care professional know right away if there is a problem.

Allergy to PROCRIT

Patients occasionally experience redness, swelling, or itching at the site of injection of PROCRIT. This may indicate an allergy to the components of PROCRIT, or it may indicate a local reaction. If you have a local reaction, consult your doctor. A potentially more serious reaction would be a generalized allergy to PROCRIT, which could cause a rash over the whole body, shortness of breath, wheezing, reduction in blood pressure, fast pulse, or sweating. Severe cases of generalized allergy may be life-threatening. If you think you are having a generalized allergic reaction, stop taking PROCRIT and notify a doctor or emergency medical personnel immediately.

How will I know if PROCRIT is working?

The effectiveness of PROCRIT is measured by the increase in hematocrit (the amount of red blood cells in the blood) that results from PROCRIT therapy. The rise in hematocrit is not immediate. It usually takes about 2–6 weeks before the hematocrit starts to rise. The amount of time it takes, and the dose of PROCRIT that is needed to make the hematocrit increase, varies from patient to patient.

What is the most important information I should know about PROCRIT and CHRONIC RENAL FAILURE?

PROCRIT has been prescribed for you by your doctor because you:

1. Have anemia due to your kidney disease.
2. Are able to dialyze at home.
3. Have been determined to be able to administer PROCRIT without direct medical or other supervision.

A lack of energy or feeling of tiredness is the major symptom of anemia. Additional symptoms include shortness of breath, chest pain, and feeling cold all the time. The reason for these symptoms is that there is a lack of red blood cells. Red blood cells carry oxygen, which is important for all of the body's functions. When there are fewer red blood cells, the body does not get all the oxygen it needs.

Kidneys remove toxins from the blood; they also measure the amount of oxygen in the blood. If there is not enough oxygen, the kidneys will produce a hormone called erythropoietin. Erythropoietin is released into the bloodstream and travels to the bone marrow where red blood cells are made. Erythropoietin signals the bone marrow to make more oxygen-carrying red blood cells.

As the kidneys fail, they stop cleansing toxins from your blood. They also make less erythropoietin than they should. Therefore, the bone marrow does not receive a strong-enough signal to make the oxygen-carrying red blood cells. Fewer red blood cells are produced so the muscles, brain, and other parts of the body do not get the oxygen they need to function properly.

Most patients treated with PROCRIT no longer need blood transfusions. However, certain medical conditions, or unexpected blood loss, may result in the need for a transfusion.

What do I need to know if I am giving myself PROCRIT injections?

When you receive your PROCRIT from the dialysis center, doctor's office or home dialysis supplier, always check to see that:

1. The name PROCRIT appears on the carton and vial label.
2. You will be able to use PROCRIT before the expiration date stamped on the package.

The PROCRIT solution in the vial should always be clear and colorless. Do not use PROCRIT if the contents of the vial appear discolored or cloudy, or if the vial appears to contain lumps, flakes, or particles. In addition, if the vial has been shaken vigorously, the solution may appear to be frothy and should not be used. Therefore, care should be taken not to shake the PROCRIT vial vigorously before use. Unless you have been prescribed Multidose PROCRIT (1 mL or 2 mL vials with a big "M" on the label, each containing a total of 20,000 Units of PROCRIT), vials of PROCRIT are for single use. Any unused portion of a vial should not be used. However, Multidose PROCRIT may be stored in the refrigerator between doses for up to 21 days, and can be used for multiple doses. Follow your dialysis center's instructions on what to do with the used vials.

How should I store PROCRIT?

PROCRIT should be stored in the refrigerator, but not in the freezing compartment. Do not let the vial freeze and do not leave it in direct sunlight. Do not use a vial of PROCRIT that has been frozen or after the expiration date that is stamped on the label. If you have any questions about the safety of a vial of PROCRIT that has been subjected to temperature extremes, be sure to check with your dialysis unit staff.

Always use the correct syringe.

Your doctor has instructed you on how to give yourself the correct dosage of PROCRIT. This dosage will usually be measured in Units per milliliter or cc's. It is important to use a syringe that is marked in tenths of milliliters (for example, 0.2 mL or cc). Failure to use the proper syringe can lead to a mistake in dosage, and you may receive too much or too little PROCRIT. Too little PROCRIT may not be effective in increasing your hematocrit, and too much PROCRIT may lead to a hematocrit that is too high. Only use disposable syringes and needles as they do not require sterilization; they should be used once and disposed of as instructed by your doctor.

IMPORTANT: TO HELP AVOID CONTAMINATION AND POSSIBLE INFECTION, FOLLOW THESE INSTRUCTIONS EXACTLY.

PREPARING THE DOSE

1. Wash your hands thoroughly with soap and water before preparing the medication.
2. Check the date on the PROCRIT vial to be sure that the drug has not expired.

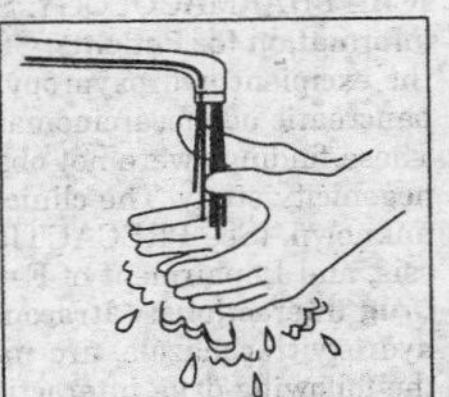

3. Remove the vial of PROCRIT from the refrigerator and allow it to reach room temperature. Each PROCRIT vial is designed to be used only once; do not reenter the vial. It is not necessary to shake PROCRIT. Prolonged vigorous shaking may damage the product. Assemble the other supplies you will need for your injection.

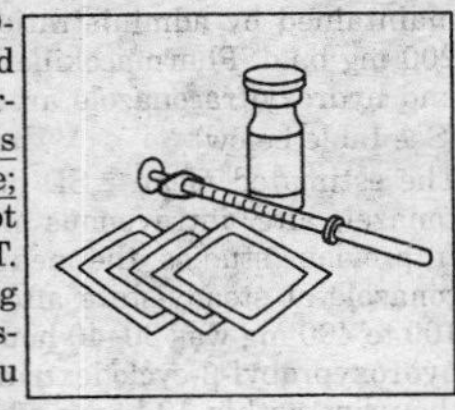

4. Hemodialysis patients should wipe off the venous port of the hemodialysis tubing with an antiseptic swab. Peritoneal dialysis patients should cleanse the skin with an antiseptic swab where the injection is to be made.

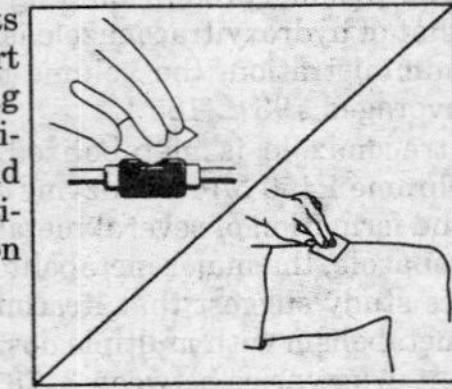

5. Flip off the red protective cap but do not remove the gray rubber stopper. Wipe the top of the gray rubber stopper with an antiseptic swab.

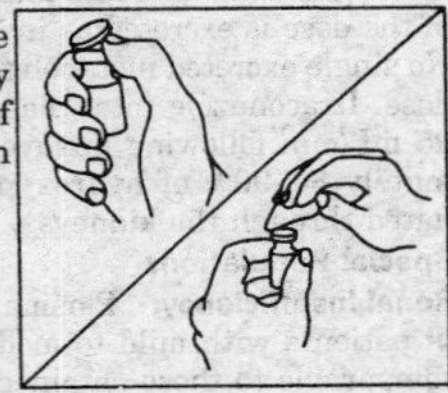

6. Using a syringe and needle designed for subcutaneous injection, draw air into the syringe by pulling back on the plunger. The amount of air should be equal to your PROCRIT dose.

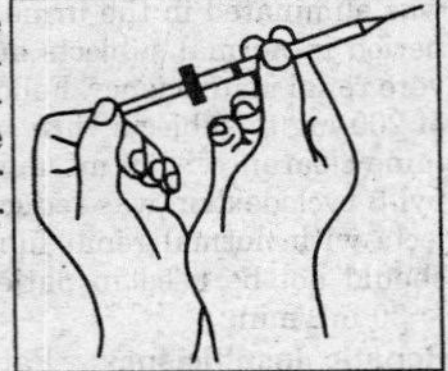

7. Carefully remove the needle cover. Put the needle through the gray rubber stopper of the PROCRIT vial.
8. Push the plunger in to discharge air into the vial. The air injected into the vial will allow PROCRIT to be easily withdrawn into the syringe.

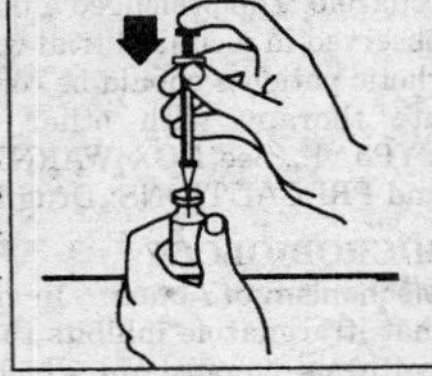

9. Turn the vial and syringe upside down in one hand. Be sure the tip of the needle is in the PROCRIT solution. Your other hand will be free to move the plunger. Draw back on the plunger slowly to draw the correct dose of PROCRIT into the syringe.
10. Check for air bubbles. The air is harmless, but too large an air bubble will reduce the PROCRIT dose. To remove air bubbles, gently tap the syringe to move the air bubbles to the top of the syringe, then use the plunger to push the solution and the air back into the vial. Then re-measure your correct dose of PROCRIT.
11. Double check your dose. Remove the needle from the vial. Do not lay the syringe down or allow the needle to touch anything.

INJECTING THE DOSE

Patients on home hemodialysis using the intravenous injection route:

1. Insert the needle of the syringe into the previously cleansed venous port and inject the PROCRIT.
2. Remove the syringe and dispose of the whole unit. Use the disposable syringe only once. Dispose of syringes and needles as directed by your doctor, by following these simple steps:

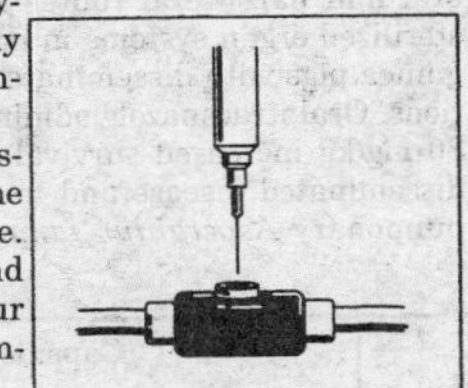

— Place all used needles and syringes in a hard plastic container with a screw-on-cap, or a metal container with a plastic lid, such as a coffee can properly labeled as to content. If a metal container is used, cut a small hole in the plastic lid and tape the lid to the metal container. If a hard-plastic container is used, always screw the cap on tightly after each use. When the container is full, tape around the cap or lid, and dispose of according to your doctor's instructions.
— Do not use glass or clear plastic containers, or any container that will be recycled or returned to a store.
— Always store the container out of the reach of children.
— Please check with your doctor, nurse, or pharmacist for other suggestions. There may be special state and local laws that they will discuss with you.

Patients on home peritoneal dialysis or home hemodialysis using the subcutaneous route:

1. With one hand, stabilize the previously cleansed skin by spreading it or by pinching up a large area with your free hand.
2. Hold the syringe with the other hand, as you would a pencil. Double check that the correct amount of PROCRIT is in the syringe. Insert the needle straight into the skin (90 degree angle). Pull the plunger back slightly. If blood comes into the syringe, do not inject PROCRIT, as the needle has entered a blood vessel; withdraw the syringe and inject at a different site. Inject the PROCRIT by pushing the plunger all the way down.

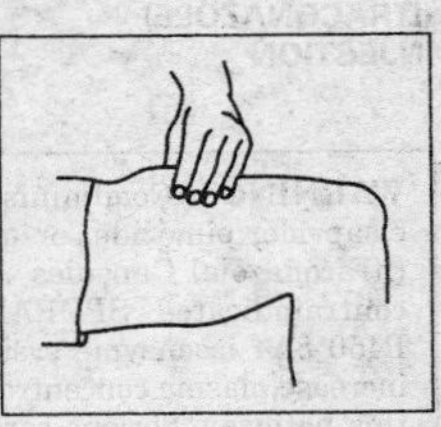

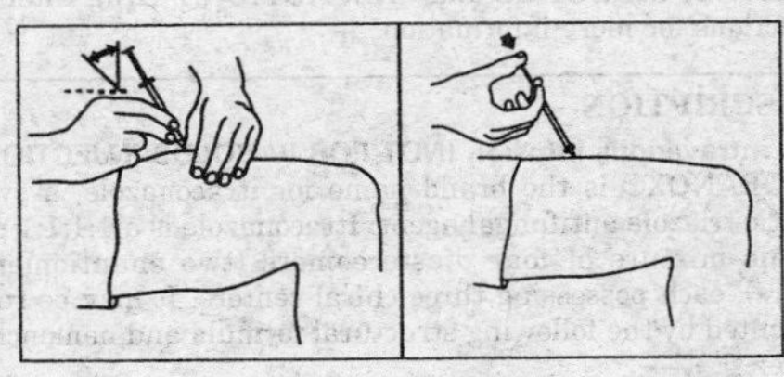

3. Hold an antiseptic swab near the needle and pull the needle straight out of the skin. Press the antiseptic swab over the injection site for several seconds.
4. **Use the disposable syringe only once.** Dispose of syringes and needles as directed by your doctor, by following these simple steps:

— Place all used needles and syringes in a hard plastic container with a screw-on-cap, or a metal container with a plastic lid, such as a coffee can properly labeled as to content. If a metal container is used, cut a small hole in the plastic lid and tape the lid to the metal container. If a hard-plastic container is used, always screw the cap on tightly after each use. When the container is full, tape around the cap or lid, and dispose of according to your doctor's instructions.
— Do not use glass or clear plastic containers, or any container that will be recycled or returned to a store.
— Always store the container out of the reach of children.
— Please check with your doctor, nurse, or pharmacist for other suggestions. There may be special state and local laws that they will discuss with you.

5. Always change the site for each injection as directed. Occasionally a problem may develop at the injection site. If you notice a lump, swelling, or bruising that doesn't go away, contact your doctor. You may wish to record the site just used so that you can keep track.

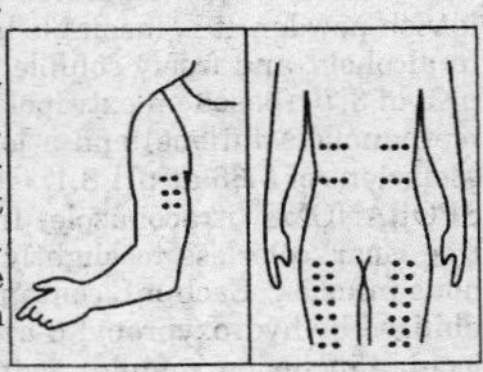

USAGE IN PREGNANCY

If you are pregnant or nursing a baby, consult your doctor before using PROCRIT.

IMPORTANT NOTES

Since you are a home dialysis patient and your doctor allows you to self-administer PROCRIT, please note the following:

1. Always follow the instructions of your doctor concerning the dosage and administration of PROCRIT. Do not change the dose or instructions for administration of PROCRIT without consulting your doctor.
2. Your doctor will tell you what to do if you miss a dose of PROCRIT. Always keep a spare syringe and needle on hand.
3. Always consult your doctor if you notice anything unusual about your condition or your use of PROCRIT.

Manufactured by:
Amgen Inc.
U.S. Lic. # 1080
Thousand Oaks, California 91320-1789
Distributed by:
Ortho Biotech Products, L.P.
Raritan, New Jersey 08869-0670
© OBI 1994

638-29-979-8
6300G020
Revised March 2000 3193602

Shown in Product Identification Guide, page 327 and 328

SPORANOX ℞
[*spə 'ah-näks"*]
(itraconazole)
100 mg capsules

(For full prescribing information, see listing under JANSSEN PHARMACEUTICA PRODUCTS, L.P.)
Shown in Product Identification Guide, page 328

Continued on next page

SPORANOX® ℞

[spŏr-a-nŏx]
(ITRACONAZOLE) INJECTION

WARNING: Coadministration of astemizole, cisapride, pimozide, or quinidine with SPORANOX® (itraconazole) Capsules, Injection or Oral Solution is contraindicated. SPORANOX®, a potent cytochrome P450 3A4 isoenzyme system (CYP3A4) inhibitor, may increase plasma concentrations of drugs metabolized by this pathway. Serious cardiovascular events, including QT prolongation, torsades de pointes, ventricular tachycardia, cardiac arrest, and/or sudden death have occurred in patients using astemizole, cisapride, pimozide, or quinidine, concomitantly with SPORANOX® and/or other CYP3A4 inhibitors. See CONTRAINDICATIONS, WARNINGS and PRECAUTIONS: Drug Interactions for more information.

DESCRIPTION

For intravenous infusion (NOT FOR IV BOLUS INJECTION)
SPORANOX® is the brand name for itraconazole, a synthetic triazole antifungal agent. Itraconazole is a 1:1:1:1 racemic mixture of four diastereomers (two enantiomeric pairs), each possessing three chiral centers. It may be represented by the following structural formula and nomenclature:

(±)-1-[(R*)-sec-butyl-4-[p-[4-[p-[[(2R*,4S*)-2-(2,4-dichlorophenyl)-2-(1H-1,2,4-triazol-1-ylmethyl)-1,3-dioxolan-4-yl]methoxy]phenyl]-1-piperazinyl]phenyl]-Δ^2-1,2,4-triazolin-5-one mixture with (±)-1-[(R*)-sec-butyl]-4-[p-[4-[p-[[2S*, 4R*)-2-(2,4-dichlorophenyl)-2-(1H-1,2,4-triazol-1-ylmethyl)-1,3-dioxolan-4-yl]methoxy] phenyl]-1-piperazinyl]phenyl]-Δ^2-1,2,4-triazolin-5-one

or

(±)-1-[(RS)-sec-butyl]-4-[p-4-[p-[[(2R,4S)-2-(2,4-dichlorophenyl)-2-(1H-1,2,4-triazol-1-ylmethyl)-1,3-dioxolan-4-yl]methoxy]phenyl-1-piperazinyl]phenyl]-Δ^2-1,2,4-triazolin-5-one

Itraconazole has a molecular formula of $C_{35}H_{38}Cl_2N_8O_4$ and a molecular weight of 705.64. It is a white to slightly yellowish powder. It is insoluble in water, very slightly soluble in alcohols, and freely soluble in dichloromethane. It has a pKa of 3.70 (based on extrapolation of values obtained from methanolic solutions) and a log (n-octanol/water) partition coefficient of 5.66 at pH 8.1.

SPORANOX® (itraconazole) Injection is a sterile pyrogen-free clear, colorless to slightly yellow solution for intravenous infusion. Each mL contains 10 mg of itraconazole, solubilized by hydroxypropyl-β-cyclodextrin (400 mg) as a molecular inclusion complex, with 3.8 µL hydrochloric acid, 25 µL propylene glycol, and sodium hydroxide for pH adjustment to 4.5, in water for injection. SPORANOX® Injection is packaged in 25 mL colorless glass ampules, containing 250 mg of itraconazole, contents of which are diluted in 50 mL 0.9% Sodium Chloride Injection, USP (Normal Saline) prior to infusion. When properly administered, contents of one ampule will supply 200 mg of itraconazole.

CLINICAL PHARMACOLOGY

Pharmacokinetics and Metabolism: NOTE: The plasma concentrations reported below were measured by high-performance liquid chromatography (HPLC) specific for itraconazole. When itraconazole in plasma is measured by a bioassay, values reported may be higher than those obtained by HPLC due to the presence of the bioactive metabolite, hydroxyitraconazole. (See MICROBIOLOGY.)

The pharmacokinetics of SPORANOX® (itraconazole) Injection (200 mg b.i.d. for two days, then 200 mg q.d. for five days) followed by oral dosing of SPORANOX® Capsules were studied in patients with advanced HIV infection. Steady-state plasma concentrations were reached after the fourth dose for itraconazole and by the seventh dose for hydroxyitraconazole. Steady-state plasma concentrations were maintained by administration of SPORANOX® Capsules, 200 mg b.i.d. Pharmacokinetic parameters for itraconazole and hydroxyitraconazole are presented in the table below: [See table below]

Parameter	Injection Day 7 n=29		Capsules, 200 mg b.i.d. Day 36 n=12	
	itraconazole	hydroxyitraconazole	itraconazole	hydroxyitraconazole
C_{max} (ng/mL)	2856 ± 866*	1906 ± 612	2010 ± 1420	2614 ± 1703
t_{max} (hr)	1.08 ± 0.14	8.53 ± 6.36	3.92 ± 1.83	5.92 ± 6.14
$AUC_{0\text{-}12h}$ (ng•h/mL)	—	—	18768 ± 13933	28516 ± 19149
$AUC_{0\text{-}24h}$ (ng•h/mL)	30605 ± 8961	42445 ± 13282	—	—

*mean ± standard deviation

The estimated mean ±SD half-life at steady-state of itraconazole after intravenous infusion was 35.4 ± 29.4 hours. In previous studies, the mean elimination half-life for itraconazole at steady-state after daily oral administration of 100 to 400 mg was 30–40 hours. Approximately 93–101% of hydroxypropyl-β-cyclodextrin was excreted unchanged in the urine within 12 hours after dosing.

The plasma protein binding of itraconazole is 99.8% and that of hydroxyitraconazole is 99.5%. Following intravenous administration, the volume of distribution of itraconazole averaged 796 ± 185 L.

Itraconazole is metabolized predominately by the cytochrome P450 3A4 isoenzyme system (CYP3A4), resulting in the formation of several metabolites, including hydroxyitraconazole, the major metabolite. Results of a pharmacokinetics study suggest that itraconazole may undergo saturable metabolism with multiple dosing. Fecal excretion of the parent drug varies between 3–18% of the dose. Renal excretion of the parent drug is less than 0.03% of the dose. About 40% of the dose is excreted as inactive metabolites in the urine. No single excreted metabolite represents more than 5% of a dose. Itraconazole total plasma clearance averaged 381 ± 95 mL/min following intravenous administration. Approximately 80–90% of hydroxypropyl-β-cyclodextrin is eliminated through the kidneys.

Special Populations

Renal Insufficiency: Plasma concentrations of itraconazole in patients with mild to moderate renal insufficiency were comparable to those obtained in healthy subjects. The majority of the 8-gram dose of hydroxypropyl-β-cyclodextrin was eliminated in the urine during the 120-hour collection period in normal subjects and in patients with mild to severe renal insufficiency. Following a single intravenous dose of 200 mg to subjects with severe renal impairment (creatinine clearance ≤ 19 mL/minute), clearance of hydroxypropyl-β-cyclodextrin was reduced six-fold compared with subjects with normal renal function. SPORANOX® Injection should not be used in patients with creatinine clearance < 30 mL/min.

Hepatic Insufficiency: Patients with impaired hepatic function should be carefully monitored when taking itraconazole. The prolonged elimination half-life of itraconazole observed in a clinical trial with itraconazole capsules in cirrhotic patients should be considered when deciding to initiate therapy with other medications metabolized by CYP3A4. (See BOX WARNING, CONTRAINDICATIONS, and PRECAUTIONS: Drug Interactions.)

MICROBIOLOGY

Mechanism of Action: In vitro studies have demonstrated that itraconazole inhibits the cytochrome P-450-dependent synthesis of ergosterol, which is a vital component of fungal cell membranes.

Activity In Vitro and In Vivo: Itraconazole exhibits in vitro activity against *Blastomyces dermatitidis, Histoplasma capsulatum, Histoplasma duboisii, Aspergillus flavus, Aspergillus fumigatus, Candida albicans,* and *Cryptococcus neoformans.* Itraconazole also exhibits varying in vitro activity against *Sporothrix schenckii, Trichophyton* species, *Candida krusei,* and other *Candida* species. The bioactive metabolite, hydroxyitraconazole, has not been evaluated against *Histoplasma capsulatum* and *Blastomyces dermatitidis.* Correlation between minimum inhibitory concentration (MIC) results in vitro and clinical outcome has yet to be established for azole antifungal agents.

Itraconazole administered orally was active in a variety of animal models of fungal infection using standard laboratory strains of fungi. Fungistatic activity has been demonstrated against disseminated fungal infections caused by *Blastomyces dermatitidis, Histoplasma duboisii, Aspergillus fumigatus, Coccidioides immitis, Cryptococcus neoformans, Paracoccidioides brasiliensis, Sporothix schenckii, Trichophyton rubrum,* and *Trichophyton mentagrophytes.*

Itraconazole administered at 2.5 mg/kg and 5 mg/kg via the oral and parenteral routes increased survival rates and sterilized organ systems in normal and immunosuppressed guinea pigs with disseminated *Aspergillus fumigatus* infections. Oral itraconazole administered daily at 40 mg/kg and 80 mg/kg increased survival rates in normal rabbits with disseminated disease and in immunosuppressed rats with pulmonary *Aspergillus fumigatus* infection, respectively.

Itraconazole has demonstrated antifungal activity in a variety of animal models infected with *Candida albicans* and other *Candida* species.

Resistance: Isolates from several fungal species with decreased susceptibility to itraconazole have been isolated in vitro and from patients receiving prolonged therapy.

Several in vitro studies reported that some fungal clinical isolates, including *Candida* species, with reduced susceptibility to one azole antifungal agent may also be less susceptible to other azole derivatives. The finding of cross-resistance is dependent on a number of factors, including the species evaluated, its clinical history, the particular azole compounds compared, and the type of susceptibility test that is performed. The relevance of these in vitro susceptibility data to clinical outcome remains to be elucidated.

Studies (both in vitro and in vivo) suggest that the activity of amphotericin B may be suppressed by prior azole antifungal therapy. As with other azoles, itraconazole inhibits the ^{14}C-demethylation step in the synthesis of ergosterol, a cell wall component of fungi. Ergosterol is the active site for amphotericin B. In one study the antifungal activity of amphotericin B against *Aspergillus fumigatus* infections in mice was inhibited by ketoconazole therapy. The clinical significance of test results obtained in this study is unknown.

INDICATIONS AND USAGE

SPORANOX® (itraconazole) Injection is indicated for the treatment of the following fungal infections in immunocompromised and non-immunocompromised patients:

1. Blastomycosis, pulmonary and extrapulmonary;
2. Histoplasmosis, including chronic cavitary pulmonary disease and disseminated, non-meningeal histoplasmosis; and
3. Aspergillosis, pulmonary and extrapulmonary, in patients who are intolerant of or who are refractory to amphotericin B therapy.

Specimens for fungal cultures and other relevant laboratory studies (wet mount, histopathology, serology) should be obtained prior to therapy to isolate and identify causative organisms. Therapy may be instituted before the results of the cultures and other laboratory studies are known; however, once these results become available, anti-infective therapy should be adjusted accordingly.

CONTRAINDICATIONS

Concomitant administration of SPORANOX® (itraconazole) Capsules, Injection, or Oral Solution and certain drugs metabolized by the cytochrome P450 3A4 isoenzyme system (CYP3A4) may result in increased plasma concentrations of those drugs, leading to potentially serious and/or life-threatening adverse events. Astemizole, cisapride, oral midazolam, pimozide, quinidine, and triazolam are contraindicated with SPORANOX®, HMG CoA-reductase inhibitors metabolized by CYP3A4, such as lovastatin and simvastatin, are also contraindicated with SPORANOX®. (See BOX WARNING, and PRECAUTIONS: Drug Interactions.)

SPORANOX® is contraindicated in patients who have shown hypersensitivity to itraconazole or its excipients. There is no information regarding cross-hypersensitivity between itraconazole and other azole antifungal agents. Caution should be used when prescribing SPORANOX® to patients with hypersensitivity to other azoles.

WARNINGS

SPORANOX® (itraconazole) Injection contains the excipient hydroxypropyl-β-cyclodextrin which produced pancreatic adenocarcinomas in a rat carcinogenicity study. These findings were not observed in a similar mouse carcinogenicity study. The clinical relevance of these findings is unknown. (See PRECAUTIONS: Carcinogenesis, Mutagenesis, and Impairment of Fertility.)

Hepatitis: There have been rare cases of reversible idiosyncratic hepatitis reported among patients taking SPORANOX® Capsules. SPORANOX® has been associated with rare cases of serious hepatotoxicity, including fatalities, primarily in patients with serious underlying medical conditions taking multiple medications. The causal association with SPORANOX® is uncertain. If clinical signs and symptoms develop that are consistent with liver disease and may be attributable to itraconazole, SPORANOX® should be discontinued.

Cardiac Dysrhythmias: Life-threatening cardiac dysrhythmias and/or sudden death have occurred in patients using astemizole, cisapride, pimozide or quinidine concomitantly with SPORANOX® and/or other CYP3A4 inhibitors. Concomitant administration of these drugs with SPORANOX® is contraindicated. (See BOX WARNING, CONTRAINDICATIONS, and PRECAUTIONS: Drug Interactions.)

PRECAUTIONS

General: Hepatic enzyme test values should be monitored in patients with pre-existing hepatic function abnormalities or those who have experienced liver toxicity with other medications. Hepatic enzyme test values should be monitored periodically in all patients receiving continuous treatment for more than 1 month, or at any time a patient develops signs or symptoms suggestive of liver dysfunction.

As severe renal impairment prolongs the elimination rate of hydroxypropyl-β-cyclodextrin, SPORANOX® (itraconazole) Injection should not be used in patients with severe renal dysfunction (creatinine clearance < 30 mL/min). (See CLINICAL PHARMACOLOGY: Special populations.)

Information for Patients: SPORANOX® Injection contains the excipient hydroxypropyl-β-cyclodextrin which produced pancreatic adenocarcinomas in a rat carcinogenicity study. These findings were not observed in a similar mouse carcinogenicity study. The clinical relevance of these findings is unknown. (See PRECAUTIONS: Carcinogenesis, Mutagenesis, and Impairment of Fertility.)

Drug Interactions: Itraconazole and its major metabolite, hydroxyitraconazole, are inhibitors of CYP3A4. Therefore, the following drug interactions may occur.

(See Table 1 below and the following drug class subheadings that follow):

1. SPORANOX® may decrease the elimination of drugs metabolized by CYP3A4, resulting in increased plasma concentrations of these drugs when they are administered with SPORANOX®. These elevated plasma concentrations may increase or prolong both therapeutic and adverse effects of these drugs. Whenever possible, plasma concentrations of these drugs should be monitored, and dosage adjustments made after concomitant SPORANOX® therapy is initiated. When appropriate, clinical monitoring for signs or symptoms of increased or prolonged pharmacologic effects is advised. Upon discontinuation, depending on the dose and duration of treatment, itraconazole plasma concentrations decline gradually (especially in patients with hepatic cirrhosis or in those receiving CYP3A4 inhibitors). This is particularly important when initiating therapy with drugs whose metabolism is affected by itraconazole.
2. Inducers of CYP3A4 may decrease the plasma concentrations of itraconazole. SPORANOX® may not be effective in patients concomitantly taking SPORANOX® and one of these drugs. Therefore, administration of these drugs with SPORANOX® is not recommended.
3. Other inhibitors of CYP3A4 may increase the plasma concentrations of itraconazole. Patients who must take SPORANOX® concomitantly with one of these drugs should be monitored closely for signs or symptoms of increased or prolonged pharmacologic effects of SPORANOX®.

[See table above]

Table 1. Selected Drugs that are predicted to alter the plasma concentration of itraconazole or have their plasma concentration altered by SPORANOX®[1]

Drug plasma concentration increased by itraconazole	
Antiarrhythmics	digoxin, quinidine[2]
Anticonvulsants	carbamazepine
Antihistamines	astemizole[2]
Antimycobacterials	rifabutin
Antineoplastics	busulfan, docetaxel, vinca alkaloids
Antipsychotics	pimozide[2]
Benzodiazepines	alprazolam, diazepam, midazolam,[2,3] triazolam[2]
Calcium Channel Blockers	dihydropyridines, verapamil
Gastrointestinal Motility Agents	cisapride[2]
HMG CoA-Reductase Inhibitors	atorvastatin, cerivastatin, lovastatin,[2] simvastatin[2]
Immunosuppressants	cyclosporine, tacrolimus, sirolimus
Oral Hypoglycemics	oral hypoglycemics
Protease Inhibitors	indinavir, ritonavir, saquinavir
Other	alfentanil, buspirone, methylprednisolone, trimetrexate, warfarin
Decrease plasma concentration of itraconazole	
Anticonvulsants	carbamazepine, phenobarbital, phenytoin
Antimycobacterials	isoniazid, rifabutin, rifampin
Reverse Transcriptase Inhibitors	nevirapine
Increase plasma concentration of itraconazole	
Macrolide Antibiotics	clarithromycin
Protease Inhibitors	indinavir, ritonavir

[1] This list is not all-inclusive.
[2] Contraindicated with SPORANOX® based on clinical and/or pharmacokinetics studies. (See WARNINGS and below.)
[3] For information on parenterally administered midazolam, see the benzodiazepine paragraph below.

Antiarrhythmics: The class IA antiarrhythmic quinidine is known to prolong the QT interval. Coadministration of quinidine with SPORANOX® increases plasma concentrations of quinidine which could result in serious cardiovascular events. Therefore, concomitant administration of SPORANOX® and quinidine is contraindicated. (See BOX WARNING, CONTRAINDICATIONS, and WARNINGS.)
Concomitant administration of digoxin and SPORANOX® has led to increased plasma concentrations of digoxin.

Anticonvulsants: Reduced plasma concentrations of itraconazole were reported when SPORANOX® was administered concomitantly with phenytoin. Carbamazepine, phenobarbital, and phenytoin are all inducers of CYP3A4. Although interactions with carbamazepine and phenobarbital have not been studied, concomitant administration of SPORANOX® and these drugs would be expected to result in decreased plasma concentrations of itraconazole. In addition, in vivo studies have demonstrated an increase in plasma carbamazepine concentrations in subjects concomitantly receiving ketoconazole. Although there are no data regarding the effect of itraconazole on carbamazepine metabolism, because of the similarities between ketoconazole and itraconazole, concomitant administration of SPORANOX® and carbamazepine may inhibit the metabolism of carbamazepine.

Antihistamines: Coadministration of astemizole with SPORANOX® has led to elevated plasma concentrations of astemizole and desmethylastemizole which could result in serious cardiovascular events. Therefore, concomitant administration of SPORANOX® with astemizole is contraindicated. (See BOX WARNING, CONTRAINDICATIONS, and WARNINGS.)

Antimycobacterials: Drug interaction studies have demonstrated that plasma concentrations of azole antifungal agents and their metabolites, including itraconazole and hydroxyitraconazole, were significantly decreased when these agents were given concomitantly with rifabutin or rifampin. In vivo data suggest that rifabutin is metabolized in part by CYP3A4. SPORANOX® may inhibit the metabolism of rifabutin. Although no formal study data are available for isoniazid, similar effects should be anticipated. Therefore, the efficacy of SPORANOX® could be substantially reduced if given concomitantly with one of these agents. Coadministration is not recommended.

Antineoplastics: SPORANOX® may inhibit the metabolism of busulfan, docetaxel, and vinca alkaloids.

Antipsychotics: Pimozide is known to prolong the QT interval and is partially metabolized by CYP3A4. Coadministration of pimozide with SPORANOX® could result in serious cardiovascular events. Therefore, concomitant administration of SPORANOX® and pimozide is contraindicated. (See BOX WARNING, CONTRAINDICATIONS, and WARNINGS.)

Benzodiazepines: Concomitant administration of SPORANOX® and alprazolam, diazepam, oral midazolam, or triazolam could lead to increased plasma concentrations of these benzodiazepines. Increased plasma concentrations could potentiate and prolong hypnotic and sedative effects. Concomitant administration of SPORANOX® and oral midazolam or triazolam is contraindicated. (See CONTRAINDICATIONS and WARNINGS.) If midazolam is administered parenterally, special precaution and patient monitoring is required since the sedative effect may be prolonged.

Calcium Channel Blockers: SPORANOX® may inhibit the metabolism of the dihydropyridines and verapamil.

Gastrointestinal Motility Agents: Coadministration of SPORANOX® with cisapride can elevate plasma cisapride concentrations which could result in serious cardiovascular events. Therefore, concomitant administration of SPORANOX® with cisapride is contraindicated. (See BOX WARNING, CONTRAINDICATIONS, and WARNINGS.)

HMG CoA-Reductase Inhibitors: Human pharmacokinetic data suggest that SPORANOX® inhibits the metabolism of atorvastatin, cerivastatin, lovastatin, and simvastatin, which may increase the risk of skeletal muscle toxicity, including rhabdomyolysis. Concomitant adminstration of SPORANOX® and lovastatin or simvastatin is contraindicated. (See CONTRAINDICATIONS and WARNINGS.)

Immunosuppressants: Concomitant administration of SPORANOX® and cyclosporine or tacrolimus has led to increased plasma concentrations of these immunosuppressants. Concomitant administration of SPORANOX® and sirolimus could increase plasma concentrations of sirolimus.

Macrolide Antibiotics: Clarithromycin is a known inhibitor of CYP3A4 and may increase plasma concentrations of itraconazole. There is no data regarding the pharmacokinetic effects of other macrolides on itraconazole.

Oral Hypoglycemic Agents: Severe hypoglycemia has been reported in patients concomitantly receiving azole antifungal agents and oral hypoglycemic agents. Blood glucose concentrations should be carefully monitored when SPORANOX® and oral hypoglycemic agents are coadministered.

Polyenes: Prior treatment with itraconazole, like other azoles, may reduce or inhibit the activity of polyenes such as amphoterecin B. However, the clinical significance of this drug effect has not been clearly defined.

Protease Inhibitors: Concomitant administration of SPORANOX® and protease inhibitors metabolized by CYP3A4, such as indinavir, ritonavir, and saquinavir, may increase plasma concentrations of these protease inhibitors. In addition, concomitant administration of SPORANOX® and indinavir and ritonavir (but not saquinavir) may increase plasma concentrations of itraconazole. Caution is advised when SPORANOX® and protease inhibitors must be given concomitantly.

Reverse Transcriptase Inhibitors: Nevirapine is an inducer of CYP3A4. In vivo studies have shown that nevirapine induces the metabolism of ketoconazole, significantly reducing the bioavailability of ketoconazole. Studies involving nevirapine and itraconazole have not been conducted. However, because of the similarities between ketoconazole and itraconazole, concomitant administration of SPORANOX® and nevirapine is not recommended. In a clinical study, when 8 HIV-infected subjects were treated concomitantly with SPORANOX® Capsules 100 mg twice daily and the nucleoside reverse transcriptase inhibitor zidovudine 8 ± 0.4 mg/kg/day, the pharmacokinetics of zidovudine were not affected. Other nucleoside reverse transcriptase inhibitors have not been studied.

Other:

- In vitro data suggest that alfentanil is metabolized by CYP3A4. Administration with SPORANOX® may increase plasma concentrations of alfentanil.
- Human pharmacokinetic data suggest that concomitant administration of SPORANOX® and buspirone results in significant increases in plasma concentrations of buspirone.
- SPORANOX® may inhibit the metabolism of methylprednisolone.
- In vitro data suggest that trimetrexate is extensively metabolized by CYP3A4. In vitro animal models have demonstrated that ketoconazaole potently inhibits the metabolism of trimetrexate. Although there are no data regarding the effect of itraconazole on trimetrexate metabolism, because of the similarities between ketoconazole and itraconazole, concomitant administration of SPORANOX® and trimetrexate may inhibit the metabolism of trimetrexate.
- SPORANOX® enhances the anticoagulant effect of coumarin-like drugs, such as warfarin.

Carcinogenesis, Mutagenesis and Impairment of Fertility: Itraconazole showed no evidence of carcinogenicity potential in mice treated orally for 23 months at dosage levels up to 80 mg/kg/day (approximately 10× the maximum recommended human dose [MRHD]). Male rats treated with 25 mg/kg/day (3.1× MRHD) had a slightly increased incidence of soft tissue sarcoma. These sarcomas may have been a consequence of hypercholesterolemia, which is a response of rats, but not dogs or humans, to chronic itraconazole administration. Female rats treated with 50 mg/kg/day (6.25× MRHD) had an increased incidence of squamous cell carcinoma of the lung (2/50) as compared to the untreated group. Although the occurrence of squamous cell carcinoma in the lung is extremely uncommon in untreated rats, the increase in this study was not statistically significant.
Hydroxypropyl-β-cyclodextrin (HP-β-CD), the solubilizing excipient used in SPORANOX® Injection and Oral Solution, was found to produce pancreatic exocrine hyperplasia and neoplasia when administered orally to rats at doses of 500, 2000 or 5000 mg/kg/day for 25 months. Adenocarcinomas of

Continued on next page

Sporanox Injection—Cont.

the exocrine pancreas produced in the treated animals were not seen in the untreated group and are not reported in the historical controls. Development of these tumors may be related to a mitogenic action of cholecystokinin. This finding was not observed in the mouse carcinogenicity study at doses of 500, 2000 or 5000 mg/kg/day for 22–23 months; however, the clinical relevance of these findings is unknown. Based on body surface area comparisons, the exposure to humans of HP-β-CD at the recommended clinical dose of SPORANOX® Oral Solution, is approximately equivalent to 1.7 times the exposure at the lowest dose in the rat study. The relevance of the findings with orally administered HP-β-CD to potential carcinogenic effects for SPORANOX® Injection is uncertain.

Itraconazole produced no mutagenic effects when assayed in DNA repair test (unscheduled DNA synthesis) in primary rat hepatocytes, in Ames tests with *Salmonella typhimurium* (6 strains) and *Escherichia coli*, in the mouse lymphoma gene mutation tests, in a sex-linked recessive lethal mutation (*Drosphila melanogaster*) test, in chromosome aberration tests in human lymphocytes, in a cell transformation test with C3H/10T$^{1}/_{2}$ C18 mouse embryo fibroblasts cells, in a dominant lethal mutation test in male and female mice, and in micronucleus tests in mice and rats.

Itraconazole did not affect the fertility of male or female rats treated orally with dosage levels of up to 40 mg/kg/day (5× MRHD), even though parental toxicity was present at this dosage level. More severe signs of parental toxicity, including death, were present in the next higher dosage level, 160 mg/kg/day (20× MRHD).

Pregnancy: Teratogenic Effects. Pregnancy Category C: Itraconazole was found to cause a dose-related increase in maternal toxicity, embryotoxicity, and teratogenicity in rats at dosage levels of approximately 40–160 mg/kg/day (5–20× MRHD), and in mice at dosage levels of approximately 80 mg/kg/day (10× MRHD). In rats, the teratogenicity consisted of major skeletal defects; in mice, it consisted of encephaloceles and/or macroglossia.

There are no studies in pregnant women. SPORANOX® should be used for the treatment of systemic fungal infections in pregnancy only if the benefit outweighs the potential risk.

Nursing Mothers: Itraconazole is excreted in human milk; therefore, the expected benefits of SPORANOX® therapy for the mother should be weighed against the potential risk from exposure of itraconazole to the infant. The U.S. Public Health Service Centers for Disease Control and Prevention advises HIV-infected women not to breast-feed to avoid potential transmission of HIV to uninfected infants.

Pediatric Use: The safety and efficacy of SPORANOX® have not been established in pediatric patients. No pharmacokinetic data on SPORANOX® Capsules or Injection are available in children. A small number of patients ages 3 to 16 years have been treated with 100 mg/day of itraconazole capsules for systemic fungal infections, and no serious unexpected adverse effects have been reported. SPORANOX® Oral Solution (5 mg/kg/day) has been administered to pediatric patients (N=26; ages 6 months to 12 years) for 2 weeks and no serious unexpected adverse events were reported.

The long-term effects of itraconazole on bone growth in children are unknown. In three toxicology studies using rats, itraconazole induced bone defects at dosage levels as low as 20 mg/kg/day (2.5× MRHD). The induced defects included reduced bone plate activity, thinning of the zona compacta of the large bones, and increased bone fragility. At a dosage level of 80 mg/kg/day (10× MRHD) over 1 year or 160 mg/kg/day (20× MRHD) for 6 months, itraconazole induced small tooth pulp with hypocellular appearance in some rats. No such bone toxicity has been reported in adult patients.

Summary of possibly or definitely drug-related adverse events reported by ≥1% of SPORANOX® Injection patients (TOTAL)

Adverse Event	Total SPORANOX® Injection (N=360) %	Comparative Studies		
		SPORANOX® Injection (N=234) %	Intravenous Fluconazole (N=32) %	Intravenous Amphotericin B (N=202) %
Gastrointestinal system disorders				
Nausea	8	9	0	15
Diarrhea	6	6	3	9
Vomiting	4	6	0	10
Abdominal pain	2	2	0	3
Metabolic and nutritional disorders				
Hypokalemia	5	8	0	29
Alkaline phosphatase increased	1	2	3	2
Serum creatinine increased	2	2	3	26
Hypo-magnesemia	1	1	0	5
Liver and biliary system disorders				
Bilirubinemia	4	6	9	3
SGPT/ALT increased	2	3	3	1
Hepatic function abnormal	1	2	0	2
Jaundice	1	2	0	1
SGOT/AST increased	1	2	0	1
Body as a whole – General disorders				
Pain	1	2	0	1
Edema	1	1	0	1
Skin and appendages disorders				
Rash	3	3	3	3
Sweating increased	1	2	0	1
Central and peripheral nervous system disorders				
Dizziness	1	2	0	1
Headache	2	2	0	3
Urinary system disorders				
Renal function abnormal	1	1	0	11
Albuminuria	1	0	0	0
Application site disorder				
Application site reaction	4	0	0	0
Vascular (extracardiac) disorders				
Vein disorder	3	0	0	0

Geriatric Use: Clinical studies of SPORANOX® Injection did not include sufficient numbers of subjects aged 65 and over to determine whether they respond differently from younger subjects. Other reported clinical experience has not identified differences in responses between the elderly and younger patients. In general, dose selection for an elderly patient should be cautious reflecting the greater frequency of decreased hepatic, renal, or cardiac function, and of concomitant disease or other drug therapy.

ADVERSE REACTIONS

Rare cases of reversible idiosyncratic hepatitis have been reported among patients taking SPORANOX® (itraconazole) Capsules. SPORANOX® has been associated with rare cases of serious hepatotoxicity, including fatalities, primarily in patients with serious underlying medical conditions who are taking multiple medications. The causal association with SPORANOX® is uncertain. If clinical signs and symptoms consistent with liver disease develop and could be attributed to itraconazole, SPORANOX® should be discontinued. (See WARNINGS.)

Adverse events considered at least possibly drug related are listed below and are based on the experience of 360 patients treated with SPORANOX® Injection in four pharmacokinetic, one uncontrolled and four active controlled studies where the control was amphotericin B or fluconazole. Nearly all patients were neutropenic or were otherwise immunocompromised and were treated empirically for febrile episodes, for documented systemic fungal infections, or in trials to determine pharmacokinetics. The dose of SPORANOX® Injection was 200 mg twice daily for the first two days followed by a single daily dose of 200 mg for the remainder of the intravenous treatment period. The majority of patients received between 7 and 14 days of SPORANOX® Injection.

[See table below]

The following adverse events occurred in less than 1% of patients in clinical trials of SPORANOX® Injection: constipation, hyperglycemia, hepatitis, fever, rigors, dyspnea, and hypotension.

Post-marketing Experience

In worldwide post-marketing experience with SPORANOX® Capsules, allergic reactions, including rash, pruritus, urticaria, angioedema, and, in rare instances, anaphylaxis and Stevens-Johnson syndrome, have been reported. Post-marketing experiences have also included reports of elevated liver enzymes and rarely, hepatitis. Although the causal association with SPORANOX® is uncertain, rare cases of alopecia, hypertriglyceridemia, menstrual disorders, and neutropenia, and isolated cases of neuropathy have also been reported.

OVERDOSAGE

Itraconazole is not removed by dialysis.

There are limited data on the outcomes of patients ingesting high doses of itraconazole. In patients taking either 100 mg of SPORANOX® (itraconazole) Oral Solution or up to 3000 mg of SPORANOX® Capsules, the adverse event profile was similar to that observed at recommended doses.

DOSAGE AND ADMINISTRATION

Use only the components [SPORANOX® (itraconazole) Injection ampule, 0.9% Sodium Chloride Injection, USP (Normal Saline) bag and filtered infusion set] provided in the kit: **DO NOT SUBSTITUTE.**

SPORANOX® Injection should not be diluted with 5% Dextrose Injection, USP, or with Lactated Ringer's Injection, USP, alone or in combination with any other diluent. The compatibility of SPORANOX® Injection with diluents other than 0.9% Sodium Chloride Injection, USP (Normal Saline) is not known. **NOT FOR IV BOLUS INJECTION.**

NOTE: After reconstitution, the diluted SPORANOX® Injection may be stored refrigerated (2–8°C) or at room temperature (15–25°C) for up to 48 hours, when protected from direct light. During administration, exposure to normal room light is acceptable.

NOTE: Use only a dedicated infusion line for administration of SPORANOX® Injection. Do not introduce concomitant medication in the same bag nor through the same line as SPORANOX® Injection. Other medications may be administered after flushing the line/catheter with 0.9% Sodium Chloride Injection, USP, as described below, and removing and replacing the entire infusion line. Alternatively, utilize another lumen, in the case of a multi-lumen catheter.

Add the full contents (25 mL) of the SPORANOX® Injection ampule into the infusion bag provided, which contains 50 mL of 0.9% Sodium Chloride Injection, USP (Normal Saline). Mix gently after the solution is completely transferred. Using a flow control device, infuse 60 mL of the dilute solution (3.33 mg/mL = 200 mg itraconazole, pH apx. 48) intravenously over 60 minutes, using an extension line and the infusion set provided. After administration, flush the infusion set with 15–20 mL of 0.9% Sodium Chloride Injection, USP, over 30 seconds-15 minutes, via the two-way stopcock. Discard the entire infusion line.

Parenteral drug products should be inspected visually for particulate matter and discoloration prior to administration, whenever solution and container permit.

Treatment of Blastomycosis, Histoplasmosis and Aspergillosis: The recommended intravenous dose is 200 mg b.i.d. for four doses, followed by 200 mg q.d. Each intravenous dose should be infused over 1 hour.

For the treatment of blastomycosis, histoplasmosis and aspergillosis, SPORANOX® can be given as oral capsules or intravenously. The safety and efficacy of SPORANOX® Injection administered for greater than 14 days is not known. Total itraconazole therapy (SPORANOX® Injection followed by SPORANOX® Capsules) should be continued for a minimum of 3 months and until clinical parameters and laboratory tests indicate that the active fungal infection has subsided. An inadequate period of treatment may lead to recurrence of active infection.

SPORANOX® Injection should not be used in patients with creatinine clearance < 30 mL/min.

HOW SUPPLIED

SPORANOX® (itraconazole) Injection for intravenous infusion is supplied as a kit (NDC 50458-298-01), containing one 25 mL colorless glass ampule of itraconazole 10 mg/mL sterile, pyrogen-free solution (NDC 50458-297-10), one 50 mL bag (100 mL capacity) of 0.9% Sodium Chloride Injection, USP (Normal Saline) and one filtered infusion set. Store at or below 25°C (77°F). Protect from light and freezing.

Distributed by:
Ortho Biotech Products, L.P.
Raritan, NJ 08869 631-10-938-2
Manufactured by: U.S. Patents 4,267,179; 4,791,111
Abbott Laboratories, Inc. 58-6011-R2
March 2000
North Chicago, IL 60064 ©JPPLP 2000

Shown in Product Identification Guide, page 328

SPORANOX® ℞

[*spŏr-a-nŏx*]
(ITRACONAZOLE)
ORAL SOLUTION

WARNING: Coadministration of astemizole, cisapride, pimozide, or quinidine with SPORANOX® (itraconazole) Capsules, Injection or Oral Solution is contraindicated. SPORANOX®, a potent cytochrome P450 3A4 isoenzyme system (CYP3A4) inhibitor, may increase plasma concentrations of drugs metabolized by this pathway. Serious cardiovascular events, including QT prolongation, torsades de pointes, ventricular tachycardia, cardiac arrest, and/or sudden death have occurred in patients using astemizole, cisapride, pimozide, or quinidine, concomitantly with SPORANOX® and/or other CYP3A4 inhibitors. See CONTRAINDICATIONS, WARNINGS, and PRECAUTIONS: Drug Interactions for more information.

DESCRIPTION

SPORANOX® is the brand name for itraconazole, a synthetic antifungal agent. Itraconazole is a 1:1:1:1 racemic mixture of four diastereomers (two enantiomeric pairs), each possessing three chiral centers. It may be represented by the following nomenclature:

(±)-1-[(R*)-sec-butyl]-4-[p-[4-[p-[[(2R*,4S*)-2-(2,4-dichlorophenyl)-2-(1H-1,2,4-triazol-1-ylmethyl)-1,3-dioxolan-4-yl-]methoxy]phenyl]-1-piperazinyl]phenyl]-Δ^2-1,2,4-triazolin-5-one mixture with (±)-1-[(R*)-sec-butyl]-4-[p-[4-[p-[[(2S*,4R*)-2-(2,4-dichlorophenyl)-2-(1H-1,2,4-triazol-1-ylmethyl)-1,3-dioxolan-4-yl]methoxy]phenyl]-1-piperazinyl]phenyl]-Δ^2-1,2,4-triazolin-5-one

or

(±)-1-[(RS)-sec-butyl]-4-[p-[4-[p-[[(2R,4S)-2-(2,4-dichlorophenyl)-2-(1H-1,2,4-triazol-1-ylmethyl)-1,3-dioxolan-4-yl-]methoxy]phenyl]-1-piperazinyl]phenyl]-Δ^2-1,2,4-triazolin-5-one.

Itraconazole has a molecular formula of $C_{35}H_{38}Cl_2N_8O_4$ and a molecular weight of 705.64. It is a white to slightly yellowish powder. It is insoluble in water, very slightly soluble in alcohols, and freely soluble in dichloromethane. It has a pKa of 3.70 (based on extrapolation of values obtained from methanolic solutions) and a log (n-octanol/water) partition coefficient of 5.66 at pH 8.1.

SPORANOX® (itraconazole) Oral Solution contains 10 mg of itraconazole per mL, solubilized by hydroxypropyl-β-cyclodextrin (400 mg/mL) as a molecular inclusion complex. SPORANOX® Oral Solution is clear and yellowish in color with a target pH of 2. Other ingredients are hydrochloric acid, propylene glycol, purified water, sodium hydroxide, sodium saccharin, sorbitol, cherry flavor 1, cherry flavor 2 and caramel flavor.

CLINICAL PHARMACOLOGY

Pharmacokinetics and Metabolism: NOTE: The plasma concentrations reported below were measured by high-performance liquid chromatography (HPLC) specific for itraconazole. When itraconazole in plasma is measured by a bioassay, values reported may be higher than those obtained by HPLC due to the presence of the bioactive metabolite, hydroxyitraconazole. (See MICROBIOLOGY.) The absolute bioavailability of itraconazole administered as a non-marketed solution formulation under fed conditions was 55% in 6 healthy male volunteers. However, the bioavailability of SPORANOX® (itraconazole) Oral Solution is increased under fasted conditions reaching higher maximum plasma concentrations (C_{max}) in a shorter period of time. In 27 healthy male volunteers, the steady-state area under the plasma concentration versus time curve (AUC_{0-24h}) of itraconazole (SPORANOX® Oral Solution, 200 mg daily for 15 days) under fasted conditions was 131 ± 30% of that obtained under fed conditions. Therefore, unlike SPORANOX® Capsules, it is recommended that SPORANOX® Oral Solution be administered without food. Presented in the table below are the steady-state (Day 15) pharmacokinetic parameters for itraconazole and hydroxyitraconazole (SPORANOX® Oral Solution) under fasted and fed conditions:

[See first table above]

	Itraconazole		Hydroxyitraconazole	
	Fasted	Fed	Fasted	Fed
C_{max} (ng/mL)	1963 ± 601*	1435 ± 477	2055 ± 487	1781 ± 397
T_{max} (hours)	2.5 ± 0.8	4.4 ± 0.7	5.3 ± 4.3	4.3 ± 1.2
AUC_{0-24h} (ng·h/mL)	29271 ± 10285	22815 ± 7098	45184 ± 10981	38823 ± 8907
$t_{1/2}$ (hours)	39.7 ± 13	37.4 ± 13	27.3 ± 13	26.1 ± 10

*mean ± standard deviation

The bioavailability of SPORANOX® Oral Solution relative to SPORANOX® Capsules was studied in 30 healthy male volunteers who received 200 mg of itraconazole as the oral solution and capsules under fed conditions. The $AUC_{0-\infty}$ from SPORANOX® Oral Solution was 149 ± 68% of that obtained from SPORANOX® Capsules; a similar increase was observed for hydroxyitraconazole. In addition, a cross study comparison of itraconazole and hydroxyitraconazole pharmacokinetics following the administration of single 200 mg doses of SPORANOX® Oral Solution (under fasted conditions) or SPORANOX® Capsules (under fed conditions) indicates that when these two formulations are administered under conditions which optimize their systemic absorption, the bioavailability of the solution relative to capsules is expected to be increased further. Therefore, it is recommended that SPORANOX® Oral Solution and SPORANOX® Capsules not be used interchangeably. The following table contains pharmacokinetic parameters for itraconazole and hydroxyitraconazole following single 200 mg doses of SPORANOX® Oral Solution (n=27) or SPORANOX® Capsules (n=30) administered to healthy male volunteers under fasted and fed conditions, respectively:

[See second table above]

	Itraconazole		Hydroxyitraconazole	
	Oral Solution fasted	Capsules fed	Oral Solution fasted	Capsules fed
C_{max} (ng/mL)	544 ± 213*	302 ± 119	622 ± 116	504 ± 132
T_{max} (hours)	2.2 ± 0.8	5 ± 0.8	3.5 ± 1.2	5 ± 1
AUC_{0-24h} (ng·h/mL)	4505 ± 1670	2682 ± 1084	9552 ± 1835	7293 ± 2144

*mean ± standard deviation

The plasma protein binding of itraconazole is 99.8% and that of hydroxyitraconazole is 99.5%. Following intravenous administration, the volume of distribution of itraconazole averaged 796 ± 185 L.

Itraconazole is metabolized predominately by the cytochrome P450 3A4 isoenzyme system (CYP3A4), resulting in the formation of several metabolites, including hydroxyitraconazole, the major metabolite. Results of a pharmacokinetics study suggest that itraconazole may undergo saturable metabolism with multiple dosing. Fecal excretion of the parent drug varies between 3–18% of the dose. Renal excretion of the parent drug is less than 0.03% of the dose. About 40% of the dose is excreted as inactive metabolites in the urine. No single excreted metabolite represents more than 5% of a dose. Itraconazole total plasma clearance averaged 381 ± 95 mL/minute following intravenous administration.

Special Populations:

Pediatrics: The pharmacokinetics of SPORANOX® Oral Solution were studied in 26 pediatric patients requiring systemic antifungal therapy. Patients were stratified by age: 6 months to 2 years (n=8), 2 to 5 years (n=7) and 5 to 12 years (n=11), and received itraconazole oral solution 5 mg/kg once daily for 14 days. Pharmacokinetic parameters at steady-state (Day 14) were not significantly different among the age strata and are summarized in the table below for all 26 patients:

	Itraconazole	Hydroxyitraconazole
C_{max} (ng/mL)	582.5 ± 382.4*	692.4 ± 355.0
C_{min} (ng/mL)	187.5 ± 161.4	403.8 ± 336.1
AUC_{0-24h} (ng·h/mL)	7706.7 ± 5245.2	13356.4 ± 8942.4
$t_{1/2}$ (hours)	35.8 ± 35.6	17.7 ± 13.0

*mean ± standard deviation

Renal Insufficiency: A pharmacokinetic study using a single 200-mg dose of itraconazole (four 50-mg capsules) was conducted in three groups of patients with renal impairment (uremia: n=7; hemodialysis: n=7; and continuous ambulatory peritoneal dialysis: n=5). In uremic subjects with a mean creatinine clearance of 13 mL/min. × 1.73 m², the bioavailability was slightly reduced compared with normal population parameters. This study did not demonstrate any significant effect of hemodialysis or continuous ambulatory peritoneal dialysis on the pharmacokinetics of itraconazole (T_{max}, C_{max}, and AUC_{0-8}). Plasma concentration-versus-time profiles showed wide intersubject variation in all three groups.

Hepatic Insufficiency: Patients with impaired hepatic function should be carefully monitored when taking itraconazole. The prolonged elimination half-life of itraconazole observed in cirrhotic patients should be considered when deciding to initiate therapy with other medications metabolized by CYP3A4. (See BOX WARNING, CONTRAINDICATIONS, and PRECAUTIONS: Drug Interactions.)

MICROBIOLOGY

Mechanism of Action: In vitro studies have demonstrated that itraconazole inhibits the cytochrome P-450-dependent synthesis of ergosterol, which is a vital component of fungal cell membranes.

Activity in Vitro and in Vivo: Itraconazole exhibits in vitro activity against *Blastomyces dermatitidis, Histoplasma capsulatum, Histoplasma duboisii, Aspergillus flavus, Aspergillus fumigatus, Candida albicans,* and *Cryptococcus neoformans.* Intraconazole also exhibits varying in vitro activity against *Sporothrix schenckii, Trichophyton* species, *Candida krusei,* and other *Candida* species. The bioactive metabolite, hydroxyitraconazole, has not been evaluated against *Histoplasma capsulatum* and *Blastomyces dermatitidis.* Correlation between minimum inhibitory concentration (MIC) results in vitro and clinical outcome has yet to be established for azole antifungal agents.

Itraconazole administered orally was active in a variety of animal models of fungal infection using standard laboratory strains of fungi. Fungistatic activity has been demonstrated against disseminated fungal infections caused by *Blastomyces dermatitidis, Histoplasma duboisii, Aspergillus fumigatus, Coccidioides immitis, Cryptococcus neoformans, Paracoccidioides brasiliensis, Sporothrix schenckii, Trichophyton rubrum,* and *Trichophyton mentagrophytes.*

Itraconazole administered at 2.5 mg/kg and 5 mg/kg via the oral and parenteral routes increased survival rates and sterilized organ systems in normal and immunosuppressed guinea pigs with disseminated *Aspergillus fumigatus* infections. Oral itraconazole administered daily at 40 mg/kg and 80 mg/kg increased survival rates in normal rabbits with disseminated disease and in immunosuppressed rats with pulmonary *Aspergillus fumigatus* infection, respectively. Itraconazole has demonstrated antifungal activity in a variety of animal models infected with *Candida albicans* and other *Candida* species.

Resistence: Isolates from several fungal species with decreased susceptibility to itraconazole have been isolated in vitro and from patients receiving prolonged therapy.

Several in vitro studies have reported that some fungal clinical isolates, including *Candida* species, with reduced susceptibility to one azole antifungal agent may also be less susceptible to other azole derivatives. The finding of cross-resistance is dependent on a number of factors, including the species evaluated, its clinical history, the particular azole compounds compared, and the type of susceptibility test that is performed. The relevance of these in vitro susceptibility data to clinical outcome remains to be elucidated.

Studies (both in vitro and in vivo) suggest that the activity of amphotericin B may be suppressed by prior azole antifungal therapy. As with other azoles, itraconazole inhibits the ^{14}C-demethylation step in the synthesis of ergosterol, a cell wall component of fungi. Ergosterol is the active site for amphotericin B. In one study the antifungal activity of amphotericin B against *Aspergillus fumigatus* infections in mice was inhibited by ketoconazole therapy. The clinical significance of test results obtained in this study is unknown.

INDICATIONS AND USAGE

SPORANOX® (itraconazole) Oral Solution is indicated for the treatment of oropharyngeal and esophageal candidiasis.

Description of Clinical Studies:

Oropharyngeal Candidiasis: Two randomized, controlled studies for the treatment of oropharyngeal candidiasis have

Continued on next page

Sporanox Oral Solution—Cont.

been conducted (total n=344). In one trial, clinical response to either 7 or 14 days of itraconazole oral solution, 200 mg/day, was similar to fluconazole tablets and averaged 84% across all arms. Clinical response in this study was defined as cured or improved (only minimal signs and symptoms with no visible lesions). Approximately 5% of subjects were lost to follow-up before any evaluations could be performed. Response to 14 days therapy of itraconazole oral solution was associated with a lower relapse rate than 7 days of itraconazole therapy. In another trial, the clinical response rate (defined as cured or improved) for itraconazole oral solution was similar to clotrimazole troches and averaged approximately 71% across both arms, with approximately 3% of subjects lost to follow-up before any evaluations could be performed. Ninety-two percent of the patients in these studies were HIV seropositive.

In an uncontrolled, open-label study of selected patients clinically unresponsive to fluconazole tablets (n=74, all patients HIV seropositive), patients were treated with itraconazole oral solution 100 mg b.i.d. (Clinically unresponsive to fluconazole in this study was defined as having received a dose of fluconazole tablets at least 200 mg/day for a minimum of 14 days.) Treatment duration was 14–28 days based on response. Approximately 55% of patients had complete resolution of oral lesions. Of patients who responded and then entered a follow-up phase (n=22), all relapsed within 1 month (median 14 days) when treatment was discontinued. Although baseline endoscopies had not been performed, several patients in this study developed symptoms of esophageal candidiasis while receiving therapy with itraconazole oral solution. Itraconazole oral solution has not been directly compared to other agents in a controlled trial of similar patients.

Esophageal Candidiasis: A double-blind randomized study (n=119, 111 of whom were HIV seropositive) compared itraconazole oral solution (100 mg/day) to fluconazole tablets (100 mg/day). The dose of each was increased to 200 mg/day for patients not responding initially. Treatment continued for 2 weeks following resolution of symptoms, for a total duration of treatment of 3–8 weeks. Clinical response (a global assessment of cured or improved) was not significantly different between the two study arms, and averaged approximately 86% with 8% lost to follow-up. Six of 53 (11%) itraconazole-treated patients and 12/57 (21%) fluconazole-treated patients were escalated to the 200 mg dose in this trial. Of the subgroup of patients who responded and entered a follow-up phase (n=88), approximately 23% relapsed across both arms within 4 weeks.

Table 1. Selected Drugs that are predicted to alter the plasma concentration of itraconazole or have their plasma concentration altered by SPORANOX®[1]

Drug plasma concentration increased by itraconazole	
Antiarrhythmics	digoxin, quinidine[2]
Anticoagulants	warfarin
Anticonvulsants	carbamazepine
Antihistamines	astemizole[2]
Antimycobacterials	rifabutin
Antineoplastics	busulfan, docetaxel, vinca alkaloids
Antipsychotics	pimozide[2]
Benzodiazepines	alprazolam, diazepam, midazolam,[2,3] triazolam[2]
Calcium Channel Blockers	dihydropyridines, verapamil
Gastrointestinal Motility Agents	cisapride[2]
HMG CoA-Reductase Inhibitors	atorvastatin, cerivastatin, lovastatin,[2] simvastatin[2]
Immunosuppressants	cyclosporine, tacrolimus, sirolimus
Oral Hypoglycemics	oral hypoglycemics
Protease Inhibitors	indinavir, ritonavir, saquinavir
Other	alfentanil, buspirone, methylprednisolone, trimetrexate
Decrease plasma concentration of itraconazole	
Anticonvulsants	carbamazepine, phenobarbital, phenytoin
Antimycobacterials	isoniazid, rifabutin, rifampin
Gastric Acid Suppressors/Neutralizers	antacids, H_2-receptor antagonists, proton pump inhibitors
Reverse Transcriptase Inhibitors	nevirapine
Increase plasma concentration of itraconazole	
Macrolide Antibiotics	clarithromycin
Protease Inhibitors	indinavir, ritonavir

[1] This list is not all-inclusive.
[2] Contraindicated with SPORANOX® based on clinical and/or pharmacokinetics studies. (See WARNINGS and below.)
[3] For information on parenterally administered midazolam, see the Benzodiazepine paragraph below.

CONTRAINDICATIONS

Concomitant administration of SPORANOX® (itraconazole) Capsules, Injection, or Oral Solution and certain drugs metabolized by the cytochrome P450 3A4 isoenzyme system (CYP3A4) may result in increased plasma concentrations of those drugs, leading to potentially serious and/or life-threatening adverse events. Astemizole, cisapride, oral midazolam, pimozide, quinidine, and triazolam are contraindicated with SPORANOX®. HMG CoA-reductase inhibitors metabolized by CYP3A4, such as lovastatin and simvastatin, are also contraindicated with SPORANOX®. (See BOX WARNING, and PRECAUTIONS: Drug Interactions.)

SPORANOX® is contraindicated for patients who have shown hypersensitivity to itraconazole or its excipients. There is no information regarding cross-hypersensitivity between itraconazole and other azole antifungal agents. Caution should be used when prescribing SPORANOX® to patients with hypersensitivity to other azoles.

WARNINGS

SPORANOX® (itraconazole) Oral Solution and SPORANOX® Capsules should not be used interchangeably. Only SPORANOX® Oral Solution has been demonstrated effective for oral and/or esophageal candidiasis. SPORANOX® Oral Solution contains the excipient hydroxypropyl-β-cyclodextrin which produced pancreatic adenocarcinomas in a rat carcinogenicity study. These findings were not observed in a similar mouse carcinogenicity study. The clinical relevance of these findings is unknown. (See Carcinogenesis, Mutagenesis, and Impairment of Fertility.)

Hepatitis: Rare cases of reversible idiosyncratic hepatitis have been reported among patients taking SPORANOX® Capsules. SPORANOX® has been associated with rare cases of serious hepatotoxicity, including death, primarily in patients with serious underlying medical conditions who are taking multiple medications. The causal association with SPORANOX® is uncertain. If clinical signs and symptoms develop that are consistent with liver disease and may be attributable to itraconazole, SPORANOX® should be discontinued.

Cardiac Dysrhythmias: Life-threatening cardiac dysrhythmias and/or sudden death have occurred in patients using astemizole, cisapride, pimozide or quinidine concomitantly with SPORANOX® and/or other CYP3A4 inhibitors. Concomitant administration of these drugs with SPORANOX® is contraindicated. (See BOX WARNING, CONTRAINDICATIONS, and PRECAUTIONS: Drug Interactions.)

PRECAUTIONS

General: Hepatic enzyme test values should be monitored in patients with pre-existing hepatic function abnormalities or those who have experienced liver toxicity with other medications. Hepatic enzyme test values should be monitored periodically in all patients receiving continuous treatment for more than 1 month, or at any time a patient develops signs or symptoms suggestive of liver dysfunction.

Information for Patients: Only SPORANOX® Oral Solution has been demonstrated effective for oral and/or esophageal candidiasis. SPORANOX® Oral Solution contains the excipient hydroxypropyl-β-cyclodextrin which produced pancreatic adenocarcinomas in a rat carcinogenicity study. These findings were not observed in a similar mouse carcinogenicity study. The clinical relevence of these findings is unknown. (See Carcinogenesis, Mutagenesis, and Impairment of Fertility.)

Taking SPORANOX® Oral Solution under fasted conditions improves the systemic availability of itraconazole. Instruct patients to take SPORANOX® Oral Solution without food, if possible.

Instruct patients to report any signs and symptoms that may suggest liver dysfunction so that the appropriate laboratory testing can be done. Such signs and symptoms may include unusual fatigue, anorexia, nausea and/or vomiting, jaundice, dark urine or pale stools.

Instruct patients to contact their physician before taking any concomitant medications with itraconazole to ensure there are no potential drug interactions.

Drug Interactions: Itraconazole and its major metabolite, hydroxyitraconazole, are inhibitors of CYP3A4. Therefore, the following drug interactions may occur (See Table 1 below and the following drug class subheadings that follow):

1. SPORANOX® may decrease the elimination of drugs metabolized by CYP3A4, resulting in increased plasma concentrations of these drugs when they are administered with SPORANOX®. These elevated plasma concentrations may increase or prolong both therapeutic and adverse effects of these drugs. Whenever possible, plasma concentrations of these drugs should be monitored, and dosage adjustments made after concomitant SPORANOX® therapy is initiated. When appropriate, clinical monitoring for signs or symptoms of increased or prolonged pharmacologic effects is advised. Upon discontinuation, depending on the dose and duration of treatment, itraconazole plasma concentrations decline gradually (especially in patients with hepatic cirrhosis or in those receiving CYP3A4 inhibitors). This is particularly important when initiating therapy with drugs whose metabolism is affected by intraconazole.
2. Inducers of CYP3A4 may decrease the plasma concentrations of itraconazole. SPORANOX® may not be effective in patients concomitantly taking SPORANOX® and one of these drugs. Therefore, administration of these drugs with SPORANOX® is not recommended.
3. Other inhibitors of CYP3A4 may increase the plasma concentrations of itraconazole. Patients who must take SPORANOX® concomitantly with one of these drugs should be monitored closely for signs or symptoms of increased or prolonged pharmacologic effects of SPORANOX®.

[See table above]

Antiarrhythmics: The class IA antiarrhythmic quinidine is known to prolong the QT interval. Coadministration of quinidine with SPORANOX® increases plasma concentrations of quinidine which could result in serious cardiovascular events. Therefore, concomitant administration of SPORANOX® and quinidine is contraindicated. (See BOX WARNING, CONTRAINDICATIONS, and WARNINGS.)

Concomitant administration of digoxin and SPORANOX® has led to increased plasma concentrations of digoxin.

Anticoagulants: SPORANOX® enhances the anticoagulant effect of coumarin-like drugs, such as warfarin.

Anticonvulsants: Reduced plasma concentrations of itraconazole were reported when SPORANOX® was administered concomitantly with phenytoin. Carbamazepine, phenobarbital, and phenytoin are all inducers of CYP3A4. Although interactions with carbamazepine and phenobarbital have not been studied, concomitant administration of SPORANOX® and these drugs would be expected to result in decreased plasma concentrations of itraconazole. In addition, in vivo studies have demonstrated an increase in plasma carbamazepine concentrations in subjects concomitantly receiving ketoconazole. Although there are no data regarding the effect of itraconazole on carbamazepine metabolism, because of the similarities between ketoconazole and itraconazole, concomitant administration of SPORANOX® and carbamazepine may inhibit the metabolism of carbamazepine.

Antihistamines: Coadministration of astemizole with SPORANOX® has led to elevated plasma concentrations of astemizole and desmethyl-astemizole which could result in serious cardiovascular events. Therefore, concomitant administration of SPORANOX® with astemizole is contraindicated. (See BOX WARNING, CONTRAINDICATIONS, and WARNINGS.)

Antimycobacterials: Drug interaction studies have demonstrated that plasma concentrations of azole antifungal agents and their metabolites, including itraconazole and hydroxyitraconazole, were significantly decreased when these agents were given concomitantly with rifabutin or rifampin. In vivo data suggest that rifabutin is metabolized in part by CYP3A4. SPORANOX® may inhibit the metabolism of rifabutin. Although no formal study data are available for isoniazid, similar effects should be anticipated. Therefore, the efficacy of SPORANOX® could be substantially reduced if given concomitantly with one of these agents. Coadministration is not recommended.

Body System/Adverse Event	Itraconazole Total n=350*	Itraconazole All controlled studies n=272	Fluconazole n=125**	Clotrimazole n=81***
Gastrointestinal disorders				
Nausea	11.1%	10.3%	11.2%	4.9%
Diarrhea	10.9%	10.3%	10.4%	3.7%
Vomiting	7.1%	5.5%	8.0%	1.2%
Abdominal Pain	5.7%	4.0%	7.2%	7.4%
Constipation	2.0%	2.2%	0.8%	0%
Body as a whole				
Fever	6.6%	6.3%	8.0%	4.9%
Chest pain	2.6%	2.9%	2.4%	0%
Pain	2.3%	1.8%	4.0%	0%
Fatigue	2.0%	1.1%	1.6%	0%
Respiratory disorders				
Coughing	4.0%	4.4%	9.6%	0%
Dyspnea	2.3%	2.6%	4.8%	1.2%
Pneumonia	2.0%	1.5%	0%	0%
Sinusitis	2.0%	1.8%	4.0%	0%
Sputum increased	2.0%	2.6%	3.2%	1.2%
Skin and appendages disorders				
Rash	4.0%	4.8%	4.0%	6.2%
Increased sweating	3.4%	3.7%	6.4%	1.2%
Skin disorder, unspecified	2.3%	2.2%	2.4%	1.2%
Central/peripheral nervous system				
Headache	4.3%	4.4%	5.6%	6.2%
Dizziness	2.0%	1.5%	4.0%	1.2%
Resistance mechanism disorders				
Pneumocystis carinii infection	2.3%	1.5%	1.6%	0%
Psychiatric disorders				
Depression	2.0%	1.1%	0%	1.2%

* Of the 350 patients, 209 were treated for oropharyngeal candidiasis in controlled studies, 63 were treated for esophageal candidiasis in controlled studies and 78 were treated for oropharyngeal candidiasis in an open study.

** Of the 125 patients, 62 were treated for oropharyngeal candidiasis and 63 were treated for esophageal candidiasis.

*** All 81 patients were treated for oropharyngeal candidiasis.

Antineoplastics: SPORANOX® may inhibit the metabolism of busulfan, docetaxel, and vinca alkaloids.

Antipsychotics: Pimozide is known to prolong the QT interval and is partially metabolized by CYP3A4. Coadministration of pimozide with SPORANOX® could result in serious cardiovascular events. Therefore, concomitant administration of SPORANOX® and pimozide is contraindicated. (See BOX WARNING, CONTRAINDICATIONS, and WARNINGS.)

Benzodiazepines: Concomitant administration of SPORANOX® and alprazolam, diazepam, oral midazolam, or triazolam could lead to increased plasma concentrations of these benzodiazepines. Increased plasma concentrations could potentiate and prolong hypnotic and sedative effects. Concomitant administration of SPORANOX® and oral midazolam or triazolam is contraindicated. (See CONTRAINDICATIONS and WARNINGS.) If midazolam is administered parenterally, special precaution and patient monitoring is required since the sedative effect may be prolonged.

Calcium Channel Blockers: SPORANOX® may inhibit the metabolism of the dihydropyridines and verapamil.

Gastric Acid Suppressors/Neutralizers: Reduced plasma concentrations of itraconazole were reported when SPORANOX® Capsules were administered concomitantly with H_2-receptor antagonists. Studies have shown that absorption of itraconazole is impaired when gastric acid production is decreased. Therefore, SPORANOX® should be administered with a cola beverage if the patient has achlorhydria or is taking H_2-receptor antagonists or other gastric acid suppressors. Antacids should be administered at least 1 hour before or 2 hours after administration of SPORANOX® Capsules. In a clinical study, when SPORANOX® Capsules were administered with omeprazole (a proton pump inhibitor), the bioavailability of itraconazole was significantly reduced. However, as itraconazole is already dissolved in SPORANOX® Oral Solution, the effect of H_2 antagonists is expected to be substantially less than with the capsules. Nevertheless, caution is advised when the two drugs are coadministered.

Gastrointestinal Motility Agents: Coadministration of SPORANOX® with cisapride can elevate plasma cisapride concentrations which could result in serious cardiovascular events. Therefore, concomitant administration of SPORANOX® with cisapride is contraindicated. (See BOX WARNING, CONTRAINDICATIONS, and WARNINGS.)

HMG CoA-Reductase Inhibitors: Human pharmacokinetic data suggest that SPORANOX® inhibits the metabolism of atorvastatin, cerivastatin, lovastatin, and simvastatin, which may increase the risk of skeletal muscle toxicity, including rhabdomyolysis. Concomitant administration of SPORANOX® and lovastatin or simvastatin is contraindicated. (See CONTRAINDICATIONS, and WARNINGS.)

Immunosuppressants: Concomitant administration of SPORANOX® and cyclosporine or tacrolimus has led to increased plasma concentrations of these immunosuppressants. Concomitant administration of SPORANOX® and sirolimus could increase plasma concentrations of sirolimus.

Macrolide Antibiotics: Clarithromycin is a known inhibitor of CYP3A4 and may increase plasma concentrations of itraconazole.

Oral Hypoglycemic Agents: Severe hypoglycemia has been reported in patients concomitantly receiving azole antifungal agents and oral hypoglycemic agents. Blood glucose concentrations should be carefully monitored when SPORANOX® and oral hypoglycemic agents are coadministered.

Polyenes: Prior treatment with itraconazole, like other azoles, may reduce or inhibit the activity of polyenes such as amphotericin B. However, the clinical significance of this drug effect has not been clearly defined.

Protease Inhibitors: Concomitant administration of SPORANOX® and protease inhibitors metabolized by CYP3A4, such as indinavir, ritonavir, and saquinavir, may increase plasma concentrations of these protease inhibitors. In addition, concomitant administration of SPORANOX® and indinavir and ritonavir (but not saquinavir) may increase plasma concentrations of itraconazole. Caution is advised when SPORANOX® and protease inhibitors must be given concomitantly.

Reverse Transcriptase Inhibitors: Nevirapine is an inducer of CYP3A4. In vivo studies have shown that nevirapine induces the metabolism of ketoconazole, significantly reducing the bioavailability of ketoconazole. Studies involving nevirapine and itraconazole have not been conducted. However, because of the similarities between ketoconazole and itraconazole, concomitant administration of SPORANOX® and nevirapine is not recommended. In a clinical study, when 8 HIV-infected subjects were treated concomitantly with SPORANOX® Capsules 100mg twice daily and the nucleoside reverse transcriptase inhibitor zidovudine 8 ± 0.4 mg/kg/day, the pharmacokinetics of zidovudine were not affected. Other nucleoside reverse transcriptase inhibitors have not been studied.

Other:

- In vitro data suggest that alfentanil is metabolized by CYP3A4. Administration with SPORANOX® may increase plasma concentrations of alfentanil.
- Human pharmacokinetic data suggest that concomitant administration of SPORANOX® and buspirone results in significant increases in plasma concentrations of buspirone.
- SPORANOX® may inhibit the metabolism of methylprednisolone.
- In vitro data suggest that trimetrexate is extensively metabolized by CYP3A4. In vitro animal models have demonstrated that ketoconazole potently inhibits the metabolism of trimetrexate. Although there are no data regarding the effect of itraconazole on trimetrexate metabolism, because of the similarities between ketoconazole and itraconazole, concomitant administration of SPORANOX® and trimetrexate may inhibit the metabolism of trimetrexate.

Carcinogenesis, Mutagenesis, and Impairment of Fertility: Itraconazole showed no evidence of carcinogenicity potential in mice treated orally for 23 months at dosage levels up to 80 mg/kg/day (approximately 10× the maximum recommended human dose [MRHD]). Male rats treated with 25 mg/kg/day (3.1× MRHD) had a slightly increased incidence of soft tissue sarcoma. These sarcomas may have been a consequence of hypercholesterolemia, which is a response of rats, but not dogs or humans, to chronic itraconazole administration. Female rats treated with 50 mg/kg/day (6.25× MRHD) had an increased incidence of squamous cell carcinoma of the lung (2/50) as compared to the untreated group. Although the occurrence of squamous cell carcinoma in the lung is extremely uncommon in untreated rats, the increase in this study was not statistically significant.

Hydroxypropyl-β-cyclodextrin (HP-β-CD), the solubilizing excipient used in SPORANOX® Oral Solution, was found to produce pancreatic exocrine hyperplasia and neoplasia when administered orally to rats at doses of 500, 2000 or 5000 mg/kg/day for 25 months. Adenocarcinomas of the exocrine pancreas produced in the treated animals were not seen in the untreated group and are not reported in the historical controls. Development of these tumors may be related to a mitogenic action of cholecystokinin. This finding was not observed in the mouse carcinogenicity study at doses of 500, 2000 or 5000 mg/kg/day for 22–23 months; however, the clinical relevance of these findings is unknown. Based on body surface area comparisons, the exposure to humans of HP-β-CD at the recommended clinical dose of SPORANOX® Oral Solution, is approximately equivalent to 1.7 times the exposure at the lowest dose in the rat study.

Itraconazole produced no mutagenic effects when assayed in a DNA repair test (unscheduled DNA synthesis) in primary rat hepatocytes, in Ames tests with *Salmonella typhimurium* (6 strains) and *Escherichia coli*, in the mouse lymphoma gene mutation tests, in a sex-linked recessive lethal mutation (*Drosophila melanogaster*) test, in chromosome aberration tests in human lymphocytes, in a cell transformation test with C3H/10T$^1/_2$ C18 mouse embryo fibroblasts cells, in a dominant lethal mutation test in male and female mice, and in micronucleus tests in mice and rats.

Itraconazole did not affect the fertility of male or female rats treated orally with dosage levels of up to 40 mg/kg/day (5× MRHD), even though parental toxicity was present at this dosage level. More severe signs of parental toxicity, including death, were present in the next higher dosage level, 160 mg/kg/day (20× MRHD).

Pregnancy: Teratogenic Effects. Pregnancy Category C: Itraconazole was found to cause a dose-related increase in maternal toxicity, embryotoxicity, and teratogenicity in rats at dosage levels of approximately 40–160 mg/kg/day (5–20× MRHD), and in mice at dosage levels of approximately 80 mg/kg/day (10× MRHD). In rats, the teratogenicity consisted of major skeletal defects; in mice, it consisted of encephaloceles and/or macroglossia.

There are no studies in pregnant women. SPORANOX® should be used in pregnancy only if the benefit outweighs the potential risk.

Nursing Mothers: Itraconazole is excreted in human milk; therefore, the expected benefits of SPORANOX® therapy for the mother should be weighed against the potential risk from exposure of itraconazole to the infant. The U.S. Public Health Service Centers for Disease Control and Prevention advises HIV-infected women not to breast-feed to avoid potential transmission of HIV to uninfected infants.

Pediatric Use: The efficacy and safety of SPORANOX® have not been established in pediatric patients. A pharmacokinetic study was conducted with SPORANOX® Oral Solution in 26 pediatric patients, ages 6 months to 12 years, requiring systemic antifungal treatment. Itraconazole was dosed at 5 mg/kg once daily for two weeks and no serious unexpected adverse events were reported. (See CLINICAL PHARMACOLOGY.)

The long-term effects of itraconazole on bone growth in children are unknown. In three toxicology studies using rats, itraconazole induced bone defects at dosage levels as low as 20 mg/kg/day (2.5× MRHD). The induced defects included reduced bone plate activity, thinning of the zona compacta of the large bones, and increased bone fragility. At a dosage level of 80 mg/kg/day (10× MRHD) over 1 year or 160 mg/kg/day (20× MRHD) for 6 months, itraconazole induced small tooth pulp with hypocellular appearance in some rats. No such bone toxicity has been reported in adult patients.

ADVERSE REACTIONS

Rare cases of reversible idiosyncratic hepatitis have been reported among patients taking SPORANOX® (itraconazole) Capsules. SPORANOX® has been associated with rare cases of serious hepatotoxicity, including fatalities, primarily in patients with serious underlying medical conditions who are taking multiple medications. The causal association with SPORANOX® is uncertain. If clinical signs and symptoms consistent with liver disease develop and could be attributed to itraconazole. SPORANOX® should be discontinued. (See WARNINGS.)

U.S. adverse experience data are derived from 350 immunocompromised patients (332 HIV seropositive/AIDS) treated for oropharyngeal or esophageal candidiasis. The table below lists adverse events reported by at least 2% of patients treated with SPORANOX® Oral Solution in U.S. clinical trials. Data on patients receiving comparator agents in these trials are included for comparison.

[See table above]

Adverse events reported by less than 2% of patients in U.S. clinical trials with SPORANOX® included: adrenal insuffi-

Continued on next page

Sporanox Oral Solution—Cont.

ciency, asthenia, back pain, dehydration, dyspepsia, dysphagia, flatulence, gynecomastia, hematuria, hemorrhoids, hot flushes, implantation complication, infection unspecified, injury, insomnia, male breast pain, myalgia, pharyngitis, pruritus, rhinitis, rigors, stomatitis ulcerative, taste perversion, tinnitus, upper respiratory tract infection, vision abnormal, and weight decrease. Edema, hypokalemia and menstrual disorders have been reported in clinical trials with itraconazole capsules.

Post-marketing Experience

In worldwide post-marketing experience with SPORANOX® Capsules, allergic reactions, including rash, pruritus, urticaria, angioedema, and, in rare instances, anaphylaxis and Stevens-Johnson syndrome, have been reported. Post-marketing experiences have also included reports of elevated liver enzymes and rarely, hepatitis. Although the causal association with SPORANOX® is uncertain, rare cases of alopecia, hypertriglyceridemia, menstrual disorders, neutropenia, and isolated cases of neuropathy have also been reported.

OVERDOSAGE

Itraconazole is not removed by dialysis. In the event of accidental overdosage, supportive measures, including gastric lavage with sodium bicarbonate, should be employed.

There are limited data on the outcomes of patients ingesting high doses of itraconazole. In patients taking either 1000 mg of SPORANOX® (itraconazole) Oral Solution or up to 3000 mg of SPORANOX® Capsules, the adverse event profile was similar to that observed at recommended doses.

DOSAGE AND ADMINISTRATION

The solution should be vigorously swished in the mouth (10 mL at a time) for several seconds and swallowed.

The recommended dosage of SPORANOX® (itraconazole) Oral Solution for oropharyngeal candidiasis is 200 mg (20 mL) daily for 1 to 2 weeks. Clinical signs and symptoms of oropharyngeal candidiasis generally resolve within several days.

For patients with oropharyngeal candidiasis unresponsive/refractory to treatment with fluconazole tablets, the recommended dose is 100 mg (10 mL) b.i.d. For patients responding to therapy, clinical response will be seen in 2 to 4 weeks. Patients may be expected to relapse shortly after discontinuing therapy. Limited data on the safety of long-term use (>6 months) of SPORANOX® Oral Solution are available at this time.

The recommended dosage of SPORANOX® Oral Solution for esophageal candidiasis is 100 mg (10 mL) daily for a minimum treatment of three weeks. Treatment should continue for 2 weeks following resolution of symptoms. Doses up to 200 mg (20 mL) per day may be used based on medical judgement of the patient's response to therapy.

SPORANOX® Oral Solution and SPORANOX® Capsules should not be used interchangeably. Patients should be instructed to take SPORANOX® Oral Solution without food, if possible. Only SPORANOX® Oral Solution has been demonstrated effective for oral and/or esophageal candidiasis.

HOW SUPPLIED

SPORANOX® (itraconazole) Oral Solution is available in 150 mL amber glass bottles (NDC 50458-295-15) containing 10 mg of itraconazole per mL.

Store at or below 25°C (77°F). Do not freeze.

631-10-939-2

U.S. Patent Nos. 4,267,179; 4,791,111; 5,707,975; 4,727,064

February 1997, February 2000

© JPPLP 2000

Manufactured by:
Janssen Pharmaceutica N.V.
Beerse, Belgium
Distributed by:
Ortho Biotech Products, L.P.
Raritan, NJ 08869

Shown in Product Identification Guide, page 328

Ortho Dermatological

199 GRANDVIEW ROAD
SKILLMAN, NJ 08558

For Medical Information Contact:
Dermatological Medical Information
(800) 426-7762

DERMATOP® EMOLLIENT CREAM ℞

[dur' mə-täp]

(prednicarbate emollient cream)* 0.1%
FOR DERMATOLOGIC USE ONLY.
NOT FOR USE IN EYES.

Prescribing Information

DESCRIPTION

DERMATOP® Emollient Cream (prednicarbate emollient cream) 0.1% contains prednicarbate, a synthetic corticosteroid for topical dermatologic use. The chemical name of prednicarbate is 11β, 17, 21-trihydroxypregna-1,4-diene-3,20-dione 17-(ethyl carbonate) 21-propionate. Prednicarbate has the empirical formula $C_{27}H_{36}O_8$ and a molecular weight of 488.58. Topical corticosteroids constitute a class of primarily synthetic steroids used topically as anti-inflammatory and antipruritic agents.

The CAS Registry Number is 73771-04-7. The chemical structure is:

Prednicarbate is a practically odorless white to yellow-white powder insoluble to practically insoluble in water and freely soluble in ethanol.

Each gram of DERMATOP Emollient Cream 0.1% contains 1.0 mg of prednicarbate in a base consisting of white petrolatum USP, purified water USP, isopropyl myristate NF, lanolin alcohols NF, mineral oil USP, cetostearyl alcohol NF, aluminum stearate, edetate disodium USP, lactic acid USP, and magnesium stearate DAB 9.

CLINICAL PHARMACOLOGY

In common with other topical corticosteroids, prednicarbate has anti-inflammatory, antipruritic, and vasoconstrictive properties. In general, the mechanism of the anti-inflammatory activity of topical steroids is unclear. However, corticosteroids are thought to act by the induction of phospholipase A_2 inhibitory proteins, collectively called lipocortins. It is postulated that these proteins control the biosynthesis of potent mediators of inflammation such as prostaglandins and leukotrienes by inhibiting the release of their common precursor arachidonic acid. Arachidonic acid is released from membrane phospholipids by phospholipase A_2.

Pharmacokinetics

The extent of percutaneous absorption of topical corticosteroids is determined by many factors, including the vehicle and the integrity of the epidermal barrier. Use of occlusive dressings with hydrocortisone for up to 24 hours have not been shown to increase penetration; however, occlusion of hydrocortisone for 96 hours does markedly enhance penetration. Topical corticosteroids can be absorbed from normal intact skin. Inflammation and/or other disease processes in the skin increase percutaneous absorption.

Studies performed with DERMATOP Emollient Cream (prednicarbate emollient cream) 0.1% indicate that the drug product is in the medium range of potency compared with other topical corticosteroids.

INDICATIONS AND USAGE

DERMATOP Emollient Cream 0.1% is a medium-potency corticosteroid indicated for the relief of the inflammatory and pruritic manifestations of corticosteroid-responsive dermatoses. DERMATOP Emollient Cream 0.1% may be used with caution in pediatric patients 1 year of age or older. The safety and efficacy of drug use for longer than 3 weeks in this population have not been established. Since safety and efficacy of DERMATOP Emollient Cream 0.1% have not been established in pediatric patients below 1 year of age, its use in this age group is not recommended.

CONTRAINDICATIONS

DERMATOP Emollient Cream 0.1% is contraindicated in those patients with a history of hypersensitivity to any of the components in the preparations.

PRECAUTIONS

General

Systemic absorption of topical corticosteroids can produce reversible hypothalamic-pituitary-adrenal (HPA) axis suppression with the potential for glucocorticosteroid insufficiency after withdrawal of treatment. Manifestations of Cushing's syndrome, hyperglycemia, and glucosuria can also be produced in some patients by systemic absorption of topical corticosteroids while on treatment.

Patients applying a topical steroid to a large surface area or under occlusion should be evaluated periodically for evidence of HPA-axis suppression. This may be done by using the ACTH stimulation, AM plasma cortisol, and urinary free cortisol tests.

DERMATOP Emollient Cream 0.1% did not produce significant HPA-axis suppression when used at a dose of 30 g/day for a week in 10 adult patients with extensive psoriasis or atopic dermatitis. DERMATOP Emollient Cream 0.1% did not produce HPA-axis suppression in any of 59 pediatric patients with extensive atopic dermatitis when applied BID for 3 weeks to >20% of the body surface **(See PRECAUTIONS, Pediatric Use.)**

If HPA-axis suppression is noted, an attempt should be made to withdraw the drug, to reduce the frequency of application, or to substitute a less potent corticosteroid. Recovery of HPA-axis function is generally prompt upon discontinuation of topical corticosteroids. Infrequently, signs and symptoms of glucocorticosteroid insufficiency may occur, requiring supplemental systemic corticosteroids. For information on systemic supplementation, see prescribing information for those products.

Pediatric patients may be more susceptible to systemic toxicity from equivalent doses due to their larger skin surface to body mass ratios. **(See PRECAUTIONS, Pediatric Use.)**

If irritation develops, DERMATOP Emollient Cream 0.1% should be discontinued and appropriate therapy instituted. Allergic contact dermatitis with corticosteroids is usually diagnosed by observing a *failure to heal* rather than noting a clinical exacerbation, as observed with most topical products not containing corticosteroids. Such an observation should be corroborated with appropriate diagnostic patch testing.

If concomitant skin infections are present or develop, an appropriate antifungal or antibacterial agent should be used. If a favorable response does not occur promptly, use of DERMATOP Emollient Cream 0.1% should be discontinued until the infection has been adequately controlled.

Information for Patients

Patients using topical corticosteroids should receive the following information and instructions:

1. This medication is to be used as directed by the physician. It is for external use only. Avoid contact with the eyes.
2. This medication should not be used for any disorder other than that for which it was prescribed.
3. The treated skin area should not be bandaged, otherwise covered or wrapped so as to be occlusive, unless directed by the physician.
4. Patients should report to their physician any signs of local adverse reactions.
5. Parents of pediatric patients should be advised not to use this medication in the treatment of diaper dermatitis. This medication should not be applied in the diaper area as diapers or plastic pants may constitute occlusive dressing. **(See DOSAGE AND ADMINISTRATION.)**
6. This medication should not be used on the face, underarms, or groin areas.
7. As with other corticosteroids, therapy should be discontinued when control is achieved. If no improvement is seen within two weeks, contact the physician.

Laboratory Tests

The following tests may be helpful in evaluating patients for HPA-axis suppression:

ACTH stimulation test
AM plasma cortisol test
Urinary free cortisol test

Carcinogenesis, Mutagenesis, and Impairment of Fertility

In a study of the effect of prednicarbate on fertility, pregnancy, and postnatal development in rats, no effect was noted on the fertility or pregnancy of the parent animals or postnatal development of the offspring after administration of up to 0.80 mg/kg of prednicarbate subcutaneously.

Prednicarbate has been evaluated in the Salmonella reversion test (Ames test) over a wide range of concentrations in the presence and absence of an S-9 liver microsomal fraction, and did not demonstrate mutagenic activity. Similarly, prednicarbate did not produce any significant changes in the numbers of micronuclei seen in erythrocytes when mice were given doses ranging from 1 to 160 mg/kg of the drug.

Pregnancy: Teratogenic Effects: Pregnancy Category C.

Corticosteroids have been shown to be teratogenic in laboratory animals when administered systemically at relatively low dosage levels. Some corticosteroids have been shown to be teratogenic after dermal application in laboratory animals.

Prednicarbate has been shown to be teratogenic and embryotoxic in Wistar rats and Himalayan rabbits when given subcutaneously during gestation at doses 1900 times and 45 times the recommended topical human dose, assuming a percutaneous absorption of approximately 3%.

In the rats, slightly retarded fetal development and an incidence of thickened and wavy ribs higher than the spontaneous rate were noted.

In rabbits, increased liver weights and slight increase in the fetal intrauterine death rate were observed. The fetuses that were delivered exhibited reduced placental weight, increased frequency of cleft palate, ossification disorders in the sternum, omphalocele, and anomalous posture of the forelimbs.

There are no adequate and well-controlled studies in pregnant women on teratogenic effects of prednicarbate. DERMATOP Emollient Cream (prednicarbate emollient cream) 0.1% should be used during pregnancy only if the potential benefit justifies the potential risk to the fetus.

Nursing Mothers

Systemically administered corticosteroids appear in human milk and could suppress growth, interfere with endogenous corticosteroid production, or cause other untoward effects. It is not known whether topical administration of corticosteroids could result in sufficient systemic absorption to produce detectable quantities in human milk. Because many drugs are excreted in human milk, caution should be exercised when DERMATOP Emollient Cream 0.1% is administered to a nursing woman.

Pediatric Use

DERMATOP Emollient Cream 0.1% may be used with caution in pediatric patients 1 year of age or older, although the safety and efficacy of drug use longer than 3 weeks have not been established. The use of DERMATOP Emollient Cream (prednicarbate emollient cream) 0.1% is supported by results of a three-week, uncontrolled study in 59 pediatric patients between the ages of 4 months and 12 years of age with atopic dermatitis. None of the 59 pediatric patients showed evidence of HPA-axis suppression. Safety and efficacy of DERMATOP Emollient Cream 0.1% in pediatric patients below 1 year of age have not been established, therefore use in this age group is not recommended. Because of a higher ratio of skin surface area to body mass, pediatric patients are at a greater risk than adults of HPA-axis suppression and Cushing's syndrome when they are treated with topical corticosteroids. They are therefore also at greater risk of adrenal insufficiency during and/or after withdrawal of treatment. In an uncontrolled study in pediatric patients with atopic dermatitis, the incidence of adverse reactions possibly or probably associated with the use of DERMATOP Emollient Cream 0.1% was limited. Mild signs of atrophy developed in 5 patients (5/59, 8%) during the clinical trial, with 2 patients exhibiting more than one sign. Two patients (2/59, 3%) developed shininess, and 2 patients (2/59, 3%) developed thinness. Three patients (3/59, 5%) were observed with mild telangectasia. It is unknown whether prior use of topical corticosteroids was a contributing factor in the development of telangectasia in 2 of the patients. Adverse effects including striae have also been reported with inappropriate use of topical corticosteroids in infants and children. Pediatric patients applying topical corticosteroids to greater than 20% of body surface are at higher risk for HPA-axis suppression.

HPA axis suppression, Cushing's syndrome, linear growth retardation, delayed weight gain and intracranial hypertension have been reported in children receiving topical corticosteroids. Manifestations of adrenal suppression in children include low plasma cortisol levels, and absence of response to ACTH stimulation. Manifestations of intracranial hypertension include bulging fontanelles, headaches, and bilateral papilledema.

DERMATOP Emollient Cream 0.1% should not be used in the treatment of diaper dermatitis.

ADVERSE REACTIONS

In controlled adult clinical studies, the incidence of adverse reactions probably or possibly associated with the use of DERMATOP Emollient Cream 0.1% was approximately 4%. Reported reactions included mild signs of skin atrophy in 1% of treated patients, as well as the following reactions which were reported in less than 1% of patients: pruritis, edema, paresthesia, urticaria, burning, allergic contact dermatitis and rash.

In an uncontrolled study in pediatric patients with atopic dermatitis, the incidence of adverse reactions possibly or probably associated with the use of DERMATOP Emollient Cream 0.1% was limited. Mild signs of atrophy developed in 5 patients (5/59, 8%) during the clinical trial, with 2 patients exhibiting more than one sign. Two patients (2/59, 3%) developed shininess, and 2 patients (2/59, 3%) developed thinness. Three patients (3/59, 5%) were observed with mild telangectasia. It is unknown whether prior use of topical corticosteroids was a contributing factor in the development of telangectasia in 2 of the patients (See PRECAUTIONS, Pediatric Use.)

The following additional local adverse reactions have been reported infrequently with topical corticosteroids, but may occur more frequently with the use of occlusive dressings. These reactions are listed in an approximate decreasing order of occurrence: folliculitis, acneiform eruptions, hypopigmentation, perioral dermatitis, secondary infection, striae and miliaria.

OVERDOSAGE

Topically applied corticosteroids can be absorbed in sufficient amounts to produce systemic effects. (See PRECAUTIONS.)

DOSAGE AND ADMINISTRATION

Apply a thin film of DERMATOP Emollient Cream (prednicarbate emollient cream) 0.1% to the affected skin areas twice daily. Rub in gently.

DERMATOP Emollient Cream (prednicarbate emollient cream) 0.1% may be used in pediatric patients 1 year of age or older. Safety and efficacy of DERMATOP Emollient cream 0.1% in pediatric patients for more than 3 weeks of use have not been established. Use in pediatric patients under 1 year of age is not recommended.

As with other corticosteroids, therapy should be discontinued when control is achieved. If no improvement is seen within 2 weeks, reassessment of the diagnosis may be necessary.

DERMATOP Emollient Cream 0.1% should not be used with occlusive dressings unless directed by the physician. DERMATOP Emollient Cream 0.1% should not be applied in the diaper area if the child still requires diapers or plastic pants as these garments may constitute occlusive dressing.

HOW SUPPLIED

DERMATOP Emollient Cream (prednicarbate emollient cream) 0.1% is supplied in 15 g (NDC 0062-0351-15) and 60 g (NDC 0062-0351-60) tubes.

Store between 41° and 77°F (5 and 25°C).

Prescribing Information as of December 1998

Dermatop REG TM HOECHST AG

U.S. Patent 4,242,334

Manufactured by:
Hoechst Marion Roussel
Deutschland GmbH and
Distributed by:
Ortho Dermatological
Division of Ortho-McNeil Pharmaceutical, Inc.
Raritan, NJ
651-44-590-2

Shown in Product Identification Guide, page 328

GRIFULVIN V ® ℞

[*gri 'fulvən*]

(griseofulvin tablets) microsize and (griseofulvin oral suspension) microsize Suspension and Tablets

DESCRIPTION

Griseofulvin is an antibiotic derived from a species of *Penicillium.* Each GRIFULVIN V Tablet contains either 250 mg or 500 mg of griseofulvin microsize, and also contains calcium stearate, colloidal silicon dioxide, starch, and wheat gluten. Additionally, the 250 mg tablet also contains dibasic calcium phosphate. Each 5 mL of GRIFULVIN V Suspension contains 125 mg of griseofulvin microsize and also contains alcohol 0.2%, docusate sodium, FD&C Red No. 40, FD&C Yellow No. 6, flavors, magnesium aluminium silicate, menthol, methylparaben, propylene glycol, propylparaben, saccharin sodium, simethicone emulsion, sodium alginate, sucrose, and purified water.

CLINICAL PHARMACOLOGY

GRIFULVIN V (griseofulvin microsize) acts systemically to inhibit the growth of *Trichophyton, Microsporum* and *Epidermophyton* genera of fungi. Fungistatic amounts are deposited in the keratin, which is gradually exfoliated and replaced by noninfected tissue.

Griseofulvin absorption from the gastrointestinal tract varies considerably among individuals, mainly because of insolubility of the drug in aqueous media of the upper G.I. tract. The peak serum level found in fasting adults given 0.5 g occurs at about four hours and ranges between 0.5 and 2.0 mcg/mL.

It should be noted that some individuals are consistently "poor absorbers" and tend to attain lower blood levels at all times. This may explain unsatisfactory therapeutic results in some patients. Better blood levels can probably be attained in most patients if the tablets are administered after a meal with a high fat content.

INDICATIONS AND USAGE

Major indications for GRIFULVIN V are:
- Tinea capitis (ringworm of the scalp)
- Tinea corporis (ringworm of the body)
- Tinea pedis (athlete's foot)
- Tinea unguium (onychomycosis; ringworm of the nails)
- Tinea cruris (ringworm of the thigh)
- Tinea barbae (barber's itch)

GRIFULVIN V inhibits the growth of those genera of fungi that commonly cause ringworm infections of the hair, skin, and nails, such as:
- *Trichophyton rubrum*
- *Trichophyton tonsurans*
- *Trichophyton mentagrophytes*
- *Trichophyton interdigitalis*
- *Trichophyton verrucosum*
- *Trichophyton sulphureum*
- *Trichophyton schoenleini*
- *Microsporum audouini*
- *Microsporum canis*
- *Microsporum gypseum*
- *Epidermophyton floccosum*
- *Trichophyton megnini*
- *Trichophyton gallinae*
- *Trichophyton crateriform*

Note: Prior to therapy, the type of fungi responsible for the infection should be identified. The use of the drug is not justified in minor or trivial infections which will respond to topical antifungal agents alone.

It is *not* effective in:
- Bacterial infections
- Candidiasis (Moniliasis)
- Histoplasmosis
- Actinomycosis
- Sporotrichosis
- Chromoblastomycosis
- Coccidioidomycosis
- North American Blastomycosis
- Cryptococcosis (Torulosis)
- Tinea versicolor
- Nocardiosis

CONTRAINDICATIONS

This drug is contraindicated in patients with porphyria, hepatocellular failure, and in individuals with a history of hypersensitivity to griseofulvin.

Two cases of conjoined twins have been reported in patients taking griseofulvin during the first trimester of pregnancy. Griseofulvin should not be prescribed to pregnant patients.

WARNINGS

Prophylactic Usage: Safety and efficacy of prophylactic use of this drug have not been established.

Chronic feeding of griseofulvin, at levels ranging from 0.5-2.5% of the diet, resulted in the development of liver tumors in several strains of mice, particularly in males. Smaller particle sizes result in an enhanced effect. Lower oral dosage levels have not been tested. Subcutaneous administration of relatively small doses of griseofulvin once a week during the first three weeks of life has also been reported to induce hepatomata in mice. Although studies in other animal species have not yielded evidence of tumorigenicity, these studies were not of adequate design to form a basis for conclusions in this regard.

In subacute toxicity studies, orally administered griseofulvin produced hepatocellar necrosis in mice, but this has not been seen in other species. Disturbances in porphyrin metabolism have been reported in griseofulvin-treated laboratory animals. Griseofulvin has been reported to have a colchicine-like effect on mitosis and cocarcinogenicity with methylcholanthrene in cutaneous tumor induction in laboratory animals.

Reports of animal studies in the Soviet literature state that a griseofulvin preparation was found to be embryotoxic and teratogenic on oral administration to pregnant Wistar rats. Rat reproduction studies done in the United States and Great Britain were inconclusive in this regard. Pups with abnormalities have been reported in the litters of a few bitches treated with griseofulvin. Because the potential for adverse effects on the human fetus cannot be ruled out, additional contraceptive precautions should be taken during treatment with griseofulvin and for a month after termination of treatment. GRIFULVIN V should not be prescribed to women intending to become pregnant within one month following cessation of therapy.

Suppression of spermatogenesis has been reported to occur in rats but investigation in man failed to confirm this. Griseofulvin interferes with chromosomal distribution during cell division, causing aneuploidy in plant and mammalian cells. These effects have been demonstrated *in vitro* at concentrations that may be achieved in the serum with the recommended therapeutic dosage.

Since griseofulvin has demonstrated harmful effects *in vitro* on the genotype in bacteria, plants, and fungi, males should wait at least six months after completing griseofulvin therapy before fathering a child.

PRECAUTIONS

Patients on prolonged therapy with any potent medication should be under close observation. Periodic monitoring of organ system function, including renal, hepatic and hemopoietic, should be done.

Since griseofulvin is derived from species of penicillin, the possibility of cross sensitivity with penicillin exists; however, known penicillin-sensitive patients have been treated without difficulty.

Since a photosensitivity reaction is occasionally associated with griseofulvin therapy, patients should be warned to avoid exposure to intense natural or artificial sunlight. Should a photosensitivity reaction occur, lupus erythematosus may be aggravated.

Drug Interactions: Patients on warfarin-type anticoagulant therapy may require dosage adjustment of the anticoagulant during and after griseofulvin therapy. Concomitant use of barbiturates usually depresses griseofulvin activity and may necessitate raising the dosage.

The concomitant administration of griseofulvin has been reported to reduce the efficacy of oral contraceptives and to increase the incidence of breakthrough bleeding.

ADVERSE REACTIONS

When adverse reactions occur, they are most commonly of the hypersensitivity type such as skin rashes, urticaria and rarely, angioneurotic edema or erythema multiforme-like drug reaction, and may necessitate withdrawal of therapy and appropriate countermeasures. Paresthesias of the hands and feet have been reported rarely after extended therapy. Other side effects reported occasionally are oral thrush, nausea, vomiting, epigastric distress, diarrhea, headache, fatigue, dizziness, insomnia, mental confusion and impairment of performance of routine activities.

Proteinuria and leukopenia have been reported rarely. Administration of the drug should be discontinued if granulocytopenia occurs.

When rare, serious reactions occur with griseofulvin, they are usually associated with high dosages, long periods of therapy, or both.

DOSAGE AND ADMINISTRATION

Accurate diagnosis of the infecting organism is essential. Identification should be made either by direct microscopic examination of a mounting of infected tissue in a solution of potassium hydroxide or by culture on an appropriate medium.

Medication must be continued until the infecting organism is completely eradicated as indicated by appropriate clinical or laboratory examination. Representative treatment periods are tinea capitis, 4 to 6 weeks; tinea corporis, 2 to 4 weeks; tinea pedis, 4 to 8 weeks; tinea unguium—depending on rate of growth—fingernails, at least 4 months; toenails, at least 6 months.

General measures in regard to hygiene should be observed to control sources of infection or reinfection. Concomitant use of appropriate topical agents is usually required, particularly in treatment of tinea pedis since in some forms of athlete's foot, yeasts and bacteria may be involved. Griseofulvin will not eradicate the bacterial or monilial infection.

Adults: A daily dose of 500 mg. will give a satisfactory response in most patients with tinea corporis, tinea cruris, and tinea capitis.

For those fungus infections more difficult to eradicate such as tinea pedis and tinea unguium, a daily dose of 1.0 g is recommended.

Children: Approximately 5 mg per pound of body weight per day is an effective dose for most children. On this basis the following dosage schedule for children is suggested:

Children weighing 30 to 50 pounds—125 mg to 250 mg daily.

Continued on next page

Grifulvin V—Cont.

Children weighing over 50 pounds—250 mg to 500 mg daily.

HOW SUPPLIED

GRIFULVIN V 250 mg Tablets in bottles of 100 (NDC 0062-0211-60) (white, scored, imprinted "ORTHO 211").
GRIFULVIN V 500 mg Tablets in bottles of 100 (NDC 0062-0214-60) and 500 (NDC 0062-0214-70) (white, scored, imprinted "ORTHO 214").
Dispense GRIFULVIN V Tablets in a tight container as defined in the USP.
GRIFULVIN V Suspension 125 mg per 5 mL in bottles of 4 fl oz (120mL) (NDC 0062-0206-04).
Dispense GRIFULVIN V Suspension in tight, light-resistant container as defined in the USP.
STORE AT ROOM TEMPERATURE
Revised January 1997
631-10-560-2
Shown in Product Identification Guide, page 328

RENOVA® ℞

[*rē' novă*]
(TRETINOIN EMOLLIENT CREAM) 0.05%
FOR TOPICAL USE ON THE FACE ONLY

Prescribing Information

DESCRIPTION

RENOVA (tretinoin emollient cream) 0.05% contains the active ingredient tretinoin (a retinoid) in an emollient cream base. Tretinoin is a yellow to light orange crystalline powder having a characteristic floral odor. Tretinoin is soluble in dimethylsulfoxide, slightly soluble in polyethylene glycol 400, octanol, and 100% ethanol. It is practically insoluble in water and mineral oil, and it is insoluble in glycerin. The chemical name for tretinoin is (all-E)-3,7-dimethyl-9-(2,6,6-trimethyl-1-cyclonexen-1-yl)-2,4,6,8-nonatetraenoic acid. Tretinoin is also referred to as all-*trans*-retinoic acid and has a molecular weight of 300.44. The structural formula is represented below.

H_3C CH_3 CH_3 CH_3 COOH CH_3
TRETINOIN

Tretinoin is available as RENOVA at a concentration of 0.05% w/w in a water in oil emulsion formulation consisting of light mineral oil, NF; sorbitol solution, USP; hydroxyoctacosanyl hydroxystearate; methoxy PEG-22/dodecyl glycol copolymer; PEG-45/dodecyl glycol copolymer; stearoxytrimethylsilane and stearyl alcohol; dimethicone 50 cs; methylparaben, NF; edetate disodium, USP; quaternium-15; butylated hydroxytoluene, NF; citric acid monohydrate, USP; fragrance; and purified water, USP.

CLINICAL PHARMACOLOGY

The exact mechanism of action of tretinoin is unknown although retinoids are believed to exert an effect on the growth and differentiation of various epithelial cells. When applied topically, however, there was no noted increase in desmosine, hydroxyproline, or elastin mRNA in human skin. In addition, the role of the irritative nature of this product in effecting the positive effects attributed to this product for its indication has not yet been fully determined.
The transdermal absorption of tretinoin from various topical formulations ranged from 1% to 31% of applied dose, depending on whether it was applied to healthy skin or dermatitic skin. When percutaneous absorption of RENOVA was assessed in healthy male subjects (n=14) after a single application, as well as after repeated daily applications for 28 days, the absorption of tretinoin was less than 2% and endogenous concentrations of tretinoin and its major metabolites were unaltered.

INDICATIONS AND USAGE

(To understand fully the indication for this product, please read the entire INDICATIONS AND USAGE section of the labeling.)
RENOVA (tretinoin emollient cream) 0.05% is indicated as an adjunctive agent (see second bullet point below) for use in the mitigation (palliation) of fine wrinkles, mottled hyperpigmentation, and tactile roughness of facial skin in patients who do not achieve such palliation using comprehensive skin care and sun avoidance programs alone (see bullet point 3 for populations in which effectiveness has not been established). **RENOVA DOES NOT ELIMINATE WRINKLES, REPAIR SUN DAMAGED SKIN, REVERSE PHOTO-AGING, or RESTORE A MORE YOUTHFUL or YOUNGER DERMAL HISTOLOGIC PATTERN.** Many patients achieve desired palliative effects on fine wrinkling, mottled hyperpigmentation, and tactile roughness of facial skin with the use of comprehensive skin care and sun avoidance programs including sunscreens, protective clothing, and emollient creams NOT containing tretinoin.

- RENOVA has demonstrated NO MITIGATING EFFECT on significant signs of chronic sun exposure such as coarse or deep wrinkling, skin yellowing, lentigines, telangiectasia, skin laxity, keratinocytic atypia, melanocytic atypia, or dermal elastosis.

FINE WRINKLING	NO IMPROVEMENT	MINIMAL IMPROVEMENT	MODERATE IMPROVEMENT
RENOVA +CSP*	36%	40%	24%
Vehicle + CSP	62%	30%	8%

MOTTLED HYPERPIGMENTATION	NO IMPROVEMENT	MINIMAL IMPROVEMENT	MODERATE IMPROVEMENT
RENOVA +CSP	35%	27%	38%
Vehicle + CSP	53%	21%	27%

TACTILE SKIN ROUGHNESS	NO IMPROVEMENT	MINIMAL IMPROVEMENT	MODERATE IMPROVEMENT
RENOVA +CSP	49%	35%	16%
Vehicle + CSP	67%	23%	10%

* CSP = Comprehensive skin protection and sun avoidance programs including use of sunscreens, protective clothing, and emollient cream.

- RENOVA should only be used under medical supervision as an adjunct to a comprehensive skin care and sun avoidance program that includes the use of effective sunscreens (minimum SPF of 15) and protective clothing when desired results on fine wrinkles, mottled hyperpigmentation, and roughness of facial skin have not been achieved with a comprehensive skin care and sun avoidance program alone.
- The effectiveness of RENOVA in the mitigation of fine wrinkles, mottled hyperpigmentation, and tactile roughness of facial skin has not been established in people greater than 50 years of age OR in people with moderately to heavily pigmented skin. In addition, patients with visible actinic keratoses and patients with a history of skin cancer were excluded from clinical trials of RENOVA. Thus the effectiveness and safety of RENOVA in these populations are not known at this time.
- Neither the safety nor the effectiveness of RENOVA for the prevention or treatment of actinic keratoses or skin neoplasms has been established.
- Neither the safety nor the efficacy of using RENOVA daily for greater than 48 weeks has been established, and daily use beyond 48 weeks has not been systematically and histologically investigated in adequate and well-controlled trials. (See **WARNINGS** section.)

CLINICAL TRIALS DATA:

Two adequate and well-controlled trials were conducted involving a total of 161 evaluable patients (under 50 years of age) treated with RENOVA and 154 evaluable patients treated with the vehicle emollient cream on the face for 24 weeks as an adjunct to a comprehensive skin care and sun avoidance program, to assess the effects on fine wrinkling, mottled hyperpigmentation, and tactile skin roughness. Patients were evaluated at baseline on a 10 point scale and changes from that baseline rating were categorized as follows:

No Improvement	No change or an increase of 1 unit or more.
Minimal Improvement	Reduction of 1 unit.
Moderate Improvement	Reduction of 2 units or more.

In these trials, the fine wrinkles, mottled hyperpigmentation, and tactile roughness of the facial skin were thought to be caused by multiple factors which included intrinsic aging or environmental factors, such as chronic sun exposure.
The results of these assessments are as follows:
[See table above]
Most of the improvement in these signs was noted during the first 24 weeks of therapy. Thereafter, therapy primarily maintained the improvement realized during the first 24 weeks.
A majority of patients will lose most mitigating effects of RENOVA on fine wrinkles, mottled hyperpigmentation, and tactile roughness of facial skin with discontinuation of a comprehensive skin care and sun avoidance program including RENOVA; however, the safety and effectiveness of using RENOVA daily for greater than 48 weeks have not been established.

CONTRAINDICATIONS

This drug is contraindicated in individuals with a history of sensitivity reactions to any of its components. It should be discontinued if hypersensitivity to any of its ingredients is noted.

WARNINGS

- RENOVA is a dermal irritant, and the results of continued irritation of the skin for greater than 48 weeks in chronic, long term use are not known. There is evidence of atypical changes in melanocytes and keratinocytes, and of increased dermal elastosis in some patients treated with RENOVA for longer than 48 weeks. The significance of these findings is unknown.
- Safety and effectiveness of RENOVA in individuals with moderately or heavily pigmented skin have not been established.
- RENOVA should not be administered if the patient is also taking drugs known to be photosensitizers (e.g., thiazides, tetracyclines, fluoroquinolones, phenothiazines, sulfonamides) because of the possibility of augmented phototoxicity.

Because of heightened burning susceptibility, exposure to sunlight (including sunlamps) should be avoided or minimized during use of RENOVA. Patients must be warned to use sunscreens (minimum of SPF of 15) and protective clothing when using RENOVA. Patients with sunburn should be advised not to use RENOVA until fully recovered. Patients who may have considerable sun exposure due to their occupation and those patients with inherent sensitivity to sunlight should exercise particular caution when using RENOVA and assure that the precautions outlined in the Patient Package Insert are observed.
RENOVA should be kept out of the eyes, mouth, angles of the nose, and mucous membranes. Topical use may cause severe local erythema, pruritus, burning, stinging, and peeling at the site of application. If the degree of local irritation warrants, patients should be directed to use less medication, decrease the frequency of application, discontinue use temporarily or discontinue use altogether.
Tretinoin has been reported to cause severe irritation on eczematous skin and should be used only with utmost caution in patients with this condition.
Application of larger amounts of medication than recommended will not lead to more rapid or better results, and marked redness, peeling, or discomfort may occur.

PRECAUTIONS

General: RENOVA should only be used as an adjunct to a comprehensive skin care and sun avoidance program. (See **INDICATIONS AND USAGE** section.)
If a drug sensitivity, chemical irritation, or a systemic adverse reaction develops, use of RENOVA should be discontinued.
Weather extremes, such as wind or cold, may be more irritating to patients using RENOVA.
Information for Patients: See Patient Package Insert.
Drug Interactions: Concomitant topical medication, medicated or abrasive soaps, shampoos, cleansers, cosmetics with a strong drying effect, products with high concentration of alcohol, astringents, spices or lime, permanent wave solutions, electrolysis, hair depilatories or waxes, and products that may irritate the skin should be used with caution in patients being treated with RENOVA because they may increase irritation with RENOVA.
RENOVA should not be administered if the patient is also taking drugs known to be photosensitizers (e.g., thiazides, tetracyclines, fluoroquinolones, phenothiazines, sulfonamides) because of the possibility of augmented phototoxicity.
Carcinogenesis, Mutagenesis, Impairment of Fertility: In a life-time dermal study in CD-1 mice, at 100 and 200 times the average recommended human topical clinical dose, a few skin tumors in the female mice and liver tumors in male mice were observed. The biological significance of these findings is not clear because they occurred at doses that exceeded the dermal maximally tolerated dose (MTD) of tretinoin and because they were within the background natural occurrence rate for these tumors in this strain of mice. There was no evidence of carcinogenic potential when tretinoin was administered topically at a dose 5 times the average recommended human topical clinical dose. For purposes of comparisons of the animal exposure to human exposure,

the "recommended human topical clinical dose" is defined as 500 mg of 0.05% RENOVA applied daily to a 50 kg person. In a chronic, two-year bioassay of Vitamin A acid in mice performed by Tsubura and Yamamoto, generalized amyloid deposition was reported in all groups in the basal layer of the Vitamin A treated skin. In CD-1 mice, a similar study reported hyalinization at the treated skin sites and the incidence of this finding was 0/50, 3/50, 3/50, and 2/50 in male mice and 1/50, 0/50, 4/50, and 2/50 in female mice from the vehicle control, 0.25 mg/kg, 0.5 mg/kg, and 1 mg/kg groups, respectively.

Studies in hairless albino mice suggest that tretinoin may enhance the tumorigenic potential of carcinogenic doses of UVB and UVA light from a solar simulator. In other studies, when lightly pigmented hairless mice treated with tretinoin were exposed to carcinogenic doses of UVB light, the incidence and rate of development of skin tumors were either reduced or no effect was seen. Due to significantly different experimental conditions, no strict comparison of these disparate data is possible at this time. Although the significance of these studies to humans is not clear, patients should minimize exposure to sun.

The mutagenic potential of tretinoin was evaluated in the Ames assay and in the in vivo mouse micronucleus assay, both of which were negative.

Dermal Segment I and III studies with RENOVA have not been performed in any species. In oral Segment I and Segment III studies in rats with tretinoin, decreased survival of neonates and growth retardation were observed at doses in excess of 2 mg/kg/day (>400 times the average recommended human topical clinical dose).

Pregnancy:

Teratogenic effects: Pregnancy Category C.

ORAL tretinoin has been shown to be teratogenic in rats, mice, rabbits, hamsters, and subhuman primates. It was teratogenic and fetotoxic in rats when given orally in doses of 1000 times the average recommended human topical clinical dose. However, variations in teratogenic doses among various strains of rats have been reported. In the cynomolgus monkey, which, metabolically, is closer to humans for tretinoin than the other species examined, fetal malformations were reported at doses of 10 mg/kg/day or greater, but none were observed at 5 mg/kg/day (1000 times the average recommended human topical clinical dose), although increased skeletal variations were observed at all doses. A dose-related increased embryolethality and abortion was reported. Similar results have also been reported in pigtail macaques.

TOPICAL tretinoin in animal teratogenicity tests has generated equivocal results. There is evidence for teratogenicity (shortened or kinked tail) of topical tretinoin in Wistar rats at doses greater than 1 mg/kg/day (200 times the recommended human topical clinical dose). Anomalies (humerus: short 13%, bent 6%, os parietal incompletely ossified 14%) have also been reported when 10 mg/kg/day was dermally applied.

There are other reports in New Zealand White rabbits with doses of approximately 80 times the recommended human topical clinical dose of an increased incidence of domed head and hydrocephaly, typical of retinoid-induced fetal malformations in this species.

In contrast, several well-controlled animal studies have shown that dermally applied tretinoin was not teratogenic at doses of 100 and 200 times the recommended human topical clinical dose, in rats and rabbits, respectively.

With widespread use of any drug, a small number of birth defect reports associated temporally with the administration of the drug would be expected by chance alone. Thirty cases of temporally-associated congenital malformations have been reported during two decades of clinical use of another formulation of topical tretinoin (Retin-A). Although no definite pattern of teratogenicity and no causal association has been established from these cases, 5 of the reports describe the rare birth defect category holoprosencephaly (defects associated with incomplete midline development of the forebrain). The significance of these spontaneous reports in terms of risk to the fetus is not known.

Non-teratogenic effects:

Dermal tretinoin has been shown to be fetotoxic in rabbits when administered in doses 100 times the recommended topical human clinical dose. Oral tretinoin has been shown to be fetotoxic in rats when administered in doses 500 times the recommended topical human clinical dose.

There are, however, no adequate and well-controlled studies in pregnant women. RENOVA should not be used during pregnancy.

Nursing Mothers: It is not known whether this drug is excreted in human milk. Because many drugs are excreted in human milk, caution should be exercised when RENOVA is administered to a nursing women.

Pediatric Use: Safety and effectiveness in patients less than 18 years of age have not been established.

Geriatric Use: Safety and effectiveness in individuals older than 50 years of age have not been established.

ADVERSE REACTIONS

(See **WARNINGS** and **PRECAUTIONS** sections.)

In double-blind, vehicle-controlled studies involving 179 patients who applied RENOVA to their face, adverse reactions associated with the use of RENOVA were limited primarily to the skin. During these trials, 4% of patients had to discontinue use of RENOVA because of adverse reactions. These discontinuations were due to skin irritation or related cutaneous adverse reactions.

Local reactions such as peeling, dry skin, burning, stinging, erythema, and pruritus were reported by almost all subjects during therapy with RENOVA. These signs and symptoms were usually of mild to moderate severity and generally occurred early in therapy. In most patients the dryness, peeling, and redness recurred after an initial (24 week) decline.

OVERDOSAGE

Application of larger amounts of medication than recommended will not lead to more rapid or better results, and marked redness, peeling, or discomfort may occur. Oral ingestion of the drug may lead to the same side effects as those associated with excessive oral intake of Vitamin A.

DOSAGE AND ADMINISTRATION

- Do NOT use RENOVA if the patient is pregnant or is attempting to become pregnant or is at high risk of pregnancy,
- Do NOT use RENOVA if the patient is sunburned or if the patient has eczema or other chronic skin condition(s),
- Do NOT use RENOVA if the patient is inherently sensitive to sunlight,
- Do NOT use RENOVA if the patient is also taking drugs known to be photosensitizers (e.g., thiazides, tetracyclines, fluoroquinolones, phenothiazines, sulfonamides) because of the possibility of augmented phototoxicity.

Patients require detailed instruction to obtain maximal benefits and to understand all the precautions necessary to use this product with greatest safety. The physician should review the Patient Package Insert.

RENOVA should be applied to the face once a day before retiring using only enough to cover the entire affected area lightly. Patients should gently wash their face with a mild soap, pat the skin dry, and wait 20 to 30 minutes before applying RENOVA. The patient should apply a pea-sized amount of cream to cover the entire face lightly. Special caution should be taken when applying the cream to avoid the eyes, ears, nostrils, and mouth.

Application of RENOVA may cause a transitory feeling of warmth or slight stinging.

Mitigation (palliation) of facial fine wrinkling, mottled hyperpigmentation and tactile roughness may occur gradually over the course of therapy. Up to six months of therapy may be required before the effects are seen. Most of the improvement noted with RENOVA is seen during the first 24 weeks of therapy. Thereafter, therapy primarily maintains the improvement realized during the first 24 weeks.

With discontinuation of RENOVA therapy, a majority of patients will lose most mitigating effects of RENOVA on fine wrinkles, mottled hyperpigmentation, and tactile roughness of facial skin; **however, the safety and effectiveness of using RENOVA daily for greater than 48 weeks have not been established.**

Application of larger amounts of medication than recommended will not lead to more rapid or better results, and marked redness, peeling, or discomfort may occur.

Patients treated with RENOVA may use cosmetics but the areas to be treated should be cleansed thoroughly before the medication is applied. (See **PRECAUTIONS** section.)

HOW SUPPLIED

RENOVA is available in these sizes:

NDC 0062-0185-00	20 gram tube
NDC 0062-0185-05	40 gram tube
NDC 0062-0185-03	60 gram tube

Storage: Store between 15° and 25°C (59° and 77°F). DO NOT FREEZE.

QUESTIONS: Physicians and Pharmacists can call 1-800-426-7762, from 8:30 a.m. to 4:30 p.m. Eastern Time, Monday through Friday.

Rx only.

DERMATOLOGICAL DIVISION
ORTHO PHARMACEUTICAL CORPORATION
Raritan, New Jersey 08869

©OPC 1991 Revised February 1998

U.S. Patents 4,603,146, 4,423,041 and 4,877,805

653-10-870-5

Shown in Product Identification Guide, page 328

RETIN-A® MICRO® ℞

(tretinoin gel) microsphere, 0.1%

For Topical Use Only

DESCRIPTION

Retin-A Micro (tretinoin gel) microsphere, 0.1%, is a formulation containing 0.1% by weight tretinoin for the topical treatment of acne vulgaris. This formulation uses patented methy methacrylate/glycol dimethacrylate crosspolymer porous microspheres (MICROSPONGE® System) to enable inclusion of the active ingredient, tretinoin, in an aqueous gel. Other components of this formulation are purified water, carbomer 934P, glycerin, disodium EDTA, propylene glycol, sorbic acid, PPG-20 methyl glucose ether distearate, cyclomethicone and dimethicone copolyol, benzyl alcohol, trolamine, and butylated hydroxytoluene.

Chemically, tretinoin is all-*trans*-retinoic acid, also known as (all-E) 3,7-dimethyl-9-(2,6,6-trimethyl-1-cyclohexen-1-yl)-2,4,6,8-nonatetraenoic acid. It is a member of the retinoid family of compounds, and an endogenous metabolite of naturally occurring Vitamin A. Tretinoin has the following structure:

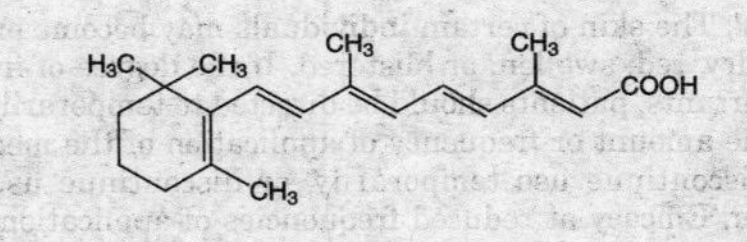

CLINICAL PHARMACOLOGY

Mode of Action: Although the exact mode of action of tretinoin is unknown, current evidence suggests that the effectiveness of tretinoin in acne is due primarily to its ability to modify abnormal follicular keratinization. Comedones form in follicles with an excess of keratinized epithelial cells. Tretinoin promotes detachment of cornified cells and the enhanced shedding of corneocytes from the follicle. By increasing the mitotic activity of follicular epithelia, tretinoin also increases the turnover rate of thin, loosely-adherent corneocytes. Through these actions, the comedo contents are extruded and the formation of the microcomedo, the precursor lesion of acne vulgaris, is reduced.

Additionally, tretinoin acts by modulating the proliferation and differentiation of epidermal cells. These effects are mediated by tretinoin's interaction with a family of nuclear retinoic acid receptors. Activation of these nuclear receptors causes changes in gene expression. The exact mechanisms whereby tretinoin-induced changes in gene expression regulate skin function are not understood.

Irritation Potential:

Acne clinical trial results

In clinical trials with acne patients treated with Retin-A Micro (tretinoin gel) microsphere, 0.1%, analysis over the twelve week treatment period showed that cutaneous irritation scores for erytherna, peeling, burning/stinging, or itching peaked during the initial 2 weeks of therapy, decreasing thereafter. Throughout, no more than 3% of patients had scores indicative of a severe irritation rating; although, 6% (14/224) of patients treated with Retin-A Micro (tretinoin gel) microsphere, 0.1%, discontinued treatment due to irritation. Of these 14 patients, four had severe irritation after 3 to 5 days of treatment, with blistering in one patient.

Results in studies of subjects without acne

In a half-face comparison trial conducted for up to 14 days in women with sensitive skin, but without acne, Retin-A Micro (tretinoin gel) microsphere, 0.1% was statistically less irritating than tretinoin cream, 0.1%. In addition, a cumulative 21 day irritation evaluation in subjects with normal skin showed that Retin-A Micro (tretinoin gel) microsphere, 0.1%, had a lower irritation profile than tretinoin cream, 0.1%. The clinical significance of these irritation studies for patients with acne is not established. Comparable effectiveness of Retin-A Micro (tretinoin gel) microsphere, 0.1%, and tretinoin cream, 0.1% has not been established. The lower irritancy of Retin-A Micro (tretinoin gel) microsphere, 0.1%, in subjects without acne may be attributable to the properties of its vehicle. The contribution to decreased irritancy by the MICROSPONGE® System has not been established.

Pharmacokinetics: Tretinoin is an endogenous metabolite of Vitamin A metabolism in man. Percutaneous absorption, as determined by the cumulative excretion of radiolabeled drug into urine and feces, was assessed in 44 healthy men and women. Estimates of in vivo bioavailability, mean (SD) %, following both single and multiple daily applications, for a period of 28 days, were 0.82 (0.11)% and 1.41 (0.54)%, respectively. The plasma concentrations of tretinoin and its metabolites, 13-*cis*-retinoic acid, all-*trans*-4-oxo-retinoic acid, and 13-*cis*-4-oxo-retinoic acid, generally ranged from 1 to 3 ng/ml and were essentially unaltered after either single or multiple daily applications relative to baseline levels.

INDICATIONS AND USAGE

Retin-A Micro (tretinoin gel) microsphere, 0.1%, is indicated for topical application in the treatment of acne vulgaris. The safety and efficacy of the use of this product in the treatment of other disorders have not been established.

CLINICAL STUDIES

In two vehicle-controlled clinical studies, Retin-A Micro (tretinoin gel) microsphere, 0.1%, applied once daily was significantly more effective than vehicle in reducing the severity of acne lesion counts. The mean reductions in lesion counts from baseline after treatment for 12 weeks are shown in the following table:

[See table at top of next page]

Retin-A Micro (tretinoin gel) microsphere, 0.1%, was also significantly superior to the vehicle in the investigator's global evaluation of the clinical response. In study #1, thirty-five percent (35%) of patients using Retin-A Micro (tretinoin gel) microsphere, 0.1%, achieved an excellent result compared to eleven percent (11%) of patients on vehicle control. In study #2, twenty-eight percent (28%) of patients using Retin-A Micro (tretinoin gel) microsphere, 0.1%, achieved an excellent result compared to nine percent (9%) of patients on vehicle control.

CONTRAINDICATIONS

This drug is contraindicated in individuals with a history of sensitivity reactions to any of its components. It should be discontinued if hypersensitivity to any of its ingredients is noted.

Continued on next page

Retin-A Micro—Cont.

Mean Percent Reduction In Lesion Counts

	Retin-A Micro (tretinoin gel) microsphere, 0.1%		Vehicle gel	
	Study #1 72 pts	Study #2 71 pts	Study #1 72 pts	Study #2 67 pts
Non-inflammatory lesion counts	49%	32%	22%	3%
Inflammatory lesion counts	37%	29%	18%	24%
Total lesion counts	45%	32%	23%	16%

PRECAUTIONS

General: The skin of certain individuals may become excessively dry, red, swollen, or blistered. If the degree of irritation warrants, patients should be directed to temporarily reduce the amount or frequency of application of the medication, discontinue use temporarily, or discontinue use all together. Efficacy at reduced frequencies of application has not been established. If a reaction suggesting sensitivity occurs, use of the medication should be discontinued. Excessive skin dryness may also be experienced; if so, use of an appropriate emollient during the day may be helpful. Unprotected exposure to sunlight, including sunlamps, should be minimized during the use of Retin-A Micro (tretinoin gel) microsphere, 0.1%, and patients with sunburn should be advised not to use the product until fully recovered because of heightened susceptibility to sunlight as a result of the use of tretinoin. Patients who may be required to have considerable sun exposure due to their occupation and those with inherent sensitivity to the sun should exercise particular caution. Use of sunscreen products (SPF 15) and protective clothing over treated areas are recommended when exposure cannot be avoided. Weather extremes, such as wind or cold, also may be irritating to patients being treated with tretinoin. Retin-A Micro (tretinoin gel) microsphere, 0.1%, should be kept away from the eyes, the mouth, paranasal creases of the nose, and mucous membranes. Tretinoin has been reported to cause severe irritation on eczematous skin and should be used with utmost caution in patients with this condition.

Information for Patients: See Patient Information leaflet.

Drug Interactions: Concomitant topical medication, medicated or abrasive soaps and cleansers, products that have a strong drying effect, products with high concentrations of alcohol, astringents, or spices should be used with caution because of possible interaction with tretinoin. Avoid contact with the peel of limes. Particular caution should be exercised with the concomitant use of topical over-the-counter acne preparations containing benzoyl peroxide, sulfur, resorcinol, or salicylic acid with Retin-A Micro (tretinoin gel) microsphere, 0.1%. It also is advisable to allow the effects of such preparations to subside before use of Retin-A Micro (tretinoin gel) microsphere, 0.1%, is begun.

Carcinogenesis, Mutagenesis, Impairment of Fertility: In a life-time dermal study in CD-1 mice, there was no evidence of carcinogenic potential when tretinoin was administered topically at a dose of 1.25 times the recommended clinical dose. For purposes of comparisons of animal exposure to human exposure, the "recommended human clinical dose" is defined as 1.0 g of 0.1% Retin-A Micro (tretinoin gel) microsphere applied to a 50 kg person. In the same study, at 25 and 50 times the recommended human clinical dose, the dermal maximum tolerated dose (MTD) of tretinoin was exceeded, yet there were no biologically significant findings.

Dermal carcinogenicity testing has not been performed with the microspheres or Retin-A Micro (tretinoin gel) microsphere, 0.1%. The components of the microspheres have not demonstrated carcinogenic potential when evaluated individually. The components of the microspheres have shown mutagenic and teratogenic potential with chronic exposure at doses several orders of magnitude higher than the human clinical dose. The very low levels of these components in microsponge polymer (< 25 ppm), used in the drug formulation, indicate an insignificant human risk under usage conditions.

Studies in hairless albino mice suggest that tretinoin may enhance the tumorigenic potential of ultraviolet (UV) light from a solar simulator. In other studies, when lightly pigmented hairless mice treated with tretinoin were exposed to carcinogenic doses of UVA/UVB light, the incidence and rate of development of skin tumors were either reduced or no effect was seen. Due to significantly different experimental conditions, no strict comparison of these disparate data is possible. Although the significance of these studies to humans is not clear, patients should avoid or minimize exposure to sun.

Tretinoin had no mutagenic potential when evaluated in the Ames assay and the in vivo mouse micronucleus assay.

The microspheres had no mutagenic potential when evaluated in the Ames assay.

Dermal fertility and perinatal development studies with Retin-A Micro (tretinoin gel) microsphere, 0.1%, have not been performed in any species. In oral fertility and perinatal development studies in rats with tretinoin, decreased survival of neonates and growth retardation were observed at doses in excess of 2 mg/kg/day (> 100 times the recommended human clinical dose which is 1.0 g/50kg adult).

Pregnancy: Teratogenic effects. Pregnancy Category C. No teratogenic effects were seen in pregnant rats with topical application of Retin-A Micro (tretinoin gel) microsphere, 0.1%, at doses up to 50 times the recommended daily human topical dose. In one study in New Zealand white rabbits treated with Retin-A Micro (tretinoin gel) microsphere, 0.1%, where doses of 0.2, 0.5 and 1.0 mg/kg/day of tretinoin were administered topically for 24 hours a day to pregnant rabbits, there appeared to be an association of the dosages with increased incidences of domed head and hydrocephaly in some of the fetuses, typical of retinoid-induced fetal malformations in this species. No abnormalities were observed at 0.2 mg/kg/day, 10 times the normal human topical dose of tretinoin. In a repeat study of the highest topical dose (1.0 mg/kg/day) in pregnant rabbits, these effects were not seen. Other pregnant rabbits exposed to six hours of 0.5 or 1.0 mg/kg/day tretinoin with proper controls to prevent oral ingestion, did not show any teratogenic effects up to 50 times (1.0 mg/kg/day) the human topical dose. In addition, topical tretinoin in non Retin-A Micro (tretinoin gel) microsphere, 0.1%, formulations was not teratogenic in rats and rabbits when given in doses of 250 and 80 times the recommended human clinical topical dose, respectively, (assuming a 50 kg adult applied a daily dose of 1.0 g of 0.1% gel topically). At these topical doses, however, delayed ossification of several bones occurred in rabbits. In rats, a dose-dependent increase of supernumerary ribs was observed.

Oral tretinoin has been shown to be teratogenic in rats, mice, rabbits, hamsters, and subhuman primates. Tretinoin is teratogenic in rats when given orally in doses 500 times the human clinical topical dose. However, variations in teratogenic doses among various strains of rats have been reported. In the cynomolgus monkey, which metabolically is more similar to humans than other species in its handling of tretinoin, no malformations were reported at 5 mg/kg/day (250 times the recommended human clinical topical dose), although increased skeletal variations were observed. A dose-related increased embryolethality was also reported. Similar results have also been reported in pigtail macaques.

There have been isolated reports of birth defects among babies born to women exposed to topical tretinoin during pregnancy. To date, there have been no adequate and well-controlled studies performed in pregnant women, and the teratogenic blood level of tretinoin is not known. However, a well-conducted retrospective cohort study of babies born to women exposed to topical tretinoin during the first trimester of pregnancy found no excess birth defects among these babies when compared to babies born to women in the same cohort who were not similarly exposed. Nevertheless, topical tretinoin should be used during pregnancy only if the potential benefit justifies the potential risk to the fetus.

Pregnancy: Non-teratogenic Effects: Oral tretinoin has been shown to be fetotoxic in rats when administered in doses 125 times the recommended human clincal topical dose.

Preclinical toxicity studies: In male mice treated topically with Retin-A Micro (tretinoin gel) microsphere, 0.1%, at 0.5, 2.0 or 5.0 mg/kg/day tretinoin (25, 100 or 250 times the recommended human dose) for 90 days, a reduction in testicular weight, but with no pathological changes, was observed at 100 and 250 times the human topical dose. Similarly, in female mice, there was a reduction in ovarian weights, but without any underlying pathological changes, at 5.0 mg/kg/day (250 times the recommended human dose). In this study there was a dose-related increase in the plasma concentration of tretinoin 4 hours after the first dose. A separate toxicokinetic study in mice indicates that systemic exposure is greater after topical application to unrestrained animals than to restrained animals, suggesting that the systemic toxicity observed is probably related to oral ingestion. Male and female dogs treated with Retin-A Micro (tretinoin gel) microsphere, 0.1%, at 0.2, 0.5 or 1.0 mg/kg/day tretinoin (10, 25 or 50 times the human dose, respectively) for 90 days showed no evidence of reduced testicular or ovarian weights or pathological changes.

Nursing Mothers: It is not known whether this drug is excreted in human milk. Because many drugs are excreted in human milk, caution should be exercised when Retin-A Micro (tretinoin gel) microsphere, 0.1%, is administered to a nursing woman.

Pediatric Use: Safety and effectiveness in children below the age of 12 have not been established.

Geriatric Use: Safety and effectiveness in a geriatric population have not been established.

ADVERSE REACTIONS

The skin of certain sensitive individuals may become excessively red, edematous, blistered, or crusted. If these effects occur, the medication should be either discontinued until the integrity of the skin is restored, or the medication should be adjusted temporarily to a level the patient can tolerate. However, efficacy has not been established for lower dosing frequencies. True contact allergy to topical tretinoin is rarely encountered. Temporary hyper- or hypopigmentation has been reported with repeated application of tretinoin. Some individuals have been reported to have heightened susceptibility to sunlight while under treatment with tretinoin. To date, all adverse effects of tretinoin have been reversible upon discontinuance of therapy (see Dosage and Administration Section).

OVERDOSAGE

Retin-A Micro (tretinoin gel) microsphere, 0.1%, is intended for topical use only. If medication is applied excessively, no more rapid or better results will be obtained, and marked redness, peeling, or discomfort may occur. Oral ingestion of large amounts of the drug may lead to the same side effects as those associated with excessive oral intake of Vitamin A.

DOSAGE AND ADMINISTRATION

Retin-A Micro (tretinoin gel) microsphere, 0.1%, should be applied once a day, before retiring, to the skin areas where acne lesions appear, using enough to cover the entire affected area lightly. Application of excessive amounts of gel may result in "caking" of the gel, and will not provide incremental efficacy.

A transitory feeling of warmth or slight stinging may be noted on application. In cases where it has been necessary to temporarily discontinue therapy or to reduce the frequency of application, therapy may be resumed or the frequency of application increased as the patient becomes able to tolerate the treatment. Frequency of application should be closely monitored by careful observation of the clinical therapeutic response and skin tolerance. Efficacy has not been established for less than once daily dosing frequencies.

During the early weeks of therapy, an apparent exacerbation of inflammatory lesions may occur. If tolerated, this should not be considered a reason to discontinue therapy.

Therapeutic results may be noticed after two weeks, but more than seven weeks of therapy are required before consistent beneficial effects are observed.

Patients treated with Retin-A Micro (tretinoin gel) microsphere, 0.1%, may use cosmetics, but the areas to be treated should be cleansed thoroughly before the medication is applied.

HOW SUPPLIED

Retin-A Micro (tretinoin gel) microsphere, 0.1%, is supplied as:

20g (NDC 0062-0190-02) and 45g (NDC 0062-0190-03) tubes.

Storage Conditions: Store at 15°–25°C (59°–77°F).

Rx only.

Ortho Dermatological
Division of Ortho-McNeil Pharmaceutical, Inc.
Skillman, New Jersey 08558

 Revised November 1999 643-11-477-4

Shown in Product Identification Guide, page 328

SPECTAZOLE® ℞

['spek-ti-zōl]

(econazole nitrate 1%)
Cream
For Topical Use Only

DESCRIPTION

SPECTAZOLE Cream contains the antifungal agent, econazole nitrate 1%, in a water-miscible base consisting of pegoxol 7 stearate, peglicol 5 oleate, mineral oil, benzoic acid, butylated hydroxyanisole and purified water. The white to off-white soft cream is for topical use only.

Chemically, econazole nitrate is 1-[2-[(4-chlorophenyl) methoxy]-2-(2,4-dichlorophenyl)ethyl]-1H-imidazole mononitrate. Its structure is as follows:

CLINICAL PHARMACOLOGY

After topical application to the skin of normal subjects, systemic absorption of econazole nitrate is extremely low. Although most of the applied drug remains on the skin surface, drug concentrations were found in the stratum corneum which, by far, exceeded the minimum inhibitory concentration for dermatophytes. Inhibitory concentrations were achieved in the epidermis and as deep as the middle region of the dermis. Less than 1% of the applied dose was recovered in the urine and feces.

Microbiology: Econazole nitrate has been shown to be active against most strains of the following microorganisms, both *in vitro* and in clinical infections as described in the INDICATIONS AND USAGE section.

Dermatophytes	Yeasts
Epidermophyton floccosum	*Candida albicans*
Microsporum audouini	*Malassezia furfur*
Microsporum canis	
Microsporum gypseum	
Trichophyton mentagrophytes	
Trichophyton rubrum	
Trichophyton tonsurans	

Econazole nitrate exhibits broad-spectrum antifungal activity against the following organisms *in vitro*, but the clinical significance of these data is unknown.

Dermatophytes	Yeasts
Trichophyton verrucosum	*Candida guillermondii*
	Candida parapsilosis
	Candida tropicalis

INDICATIONS AND USAGE

SPECTAZOLE Cream is indicated for topical application in the treatment of tinea pedis, tinea cruris, and tinea corporis caused by *Trichophyton rubrum, Trichophyton mentagrophytes, Trichophyton tonsurans, Microsporum canis, Microsporum audouini, Microsporum gypseum,* and *Epidermophyton floccosum,* in the treatment of cutaneous candidiasis, and in the treatment of tinea versicolor.

CONTRAINDICATIONS

SPECTAZOLE Cream is contraindicated in individuals who have shown hypersensitivity to any of its ingredients.

WARNINGS

SPECTAZOLE is not for ophthalmic use.

PRECAUTIONS

General: If a reaction suggesting sensitivity or chemical irritation should occur, use of the medication should be discontinued.

For external use only. Avoid introduction of SPECTAZOLE Cream into the eyes.

Carcinogenicity Studies: Long-term animal studies to determine carcinogenic potential have not been performed.

Fertility (Reproduction): Oral administration of econazole nitrate in rats has been reported to produce prolonged gestation. Intravaginal administration in humans has not shown prolonged gestation or other adverse reproductive effects attributable to econazole nitrate therapy.

Pregnancy: Pregnancy Category C. Econazole nitrate has not been shown to be teratogenic when administered orally to mice, rabbits or rats. Fetotoxic or embryotoxic effects were observed in Segment I oral studies with rats receiving 10 to 40 times the human dermal dose. Similar effects were observed in Segment II or Segment III studies with mice, rabbits and/or rats receiving oral doses 80 or 40 times the human dermal dose.

Econazole nitrate should be used in the first trimester of pregnancy only when the physician considers it essential to the welfare of the patient. The drug should be used during the second and third trimesters of pregnancy only if clearly needed.

Nursing Mothers: It is not known whether econazole nitrate is excreted in human milk. Following oral administration of econazole nitrate to lactating rats, econazole and/or metabolites were excreted in milk and were found in nursing pups. Also, in lactating rats receiving large oral doses (40 or 80 times the human dermal dose), there was a reduction in postpartum viability of pups and survival to weaning; however, at these high doses, maternal toxicity was present and may have been a contributing factor. Caution should be exercised when econazole nitrate is administered to a nursing woman.

ADVERSE REACTIONS

During clinical trials, approximately 3% of patients treated with econazole nitrate 1% cream reported side effects thought possibly to be due to the drug, consisting mainly of burning, itching, stinging and erythema. One case of pruritic rash has also been reported.

OVERDOSE

Overdosage of econazole nitrate in humans has not been reported to date. In mice, rats, guinea pigs and dogs, the oral LD 50 values were found to be 462, 668, 272, and > 160 mg/kg, respectively.

DOSAGE AND ADMINISTRATION

Sufficient SPECTAZOLE Cream should be applied to cover affected areas once daily in patients with tinea pedis, tinea cruris, tinea corporis, and tinea versicolor, and twice daily (morning and evening) in patients with cutaneous candidiasis.

Early relief of symptoms is experienced by the majority of patients and clinical improvement may be seen fairly soon after treatment is begun; however, candidal infections and tinea cruris and corporis should be treated for two weeks and tinea pedis for one month in order to reduce the possibility of recurrence. If a patient shows no clinical improvement after the treatment period, the diagnosis should be redetermined. Patients with tinea versicolor usually exhibit clinical and mycological clearing after two weeks of treatment.

HOW SUPPLIED

SPECTAZOLE (econazole nitrate 1%) Cream is supplied in tubes of 15 grams (NDC 0062-5460-02), 30 grams (NDC 0062-5460-01), and 85 grams (NDC 0062-5460-03).

Store SPECTAZOLE Cream below 86°F.

Revised June 1996 631-10-331-9

Shown in Product Identification Guide, page 328

Ortho-Clinical Diagnostics, Inc.

A Johnson & Johnson Company
1001 U.S. HWY 202
RARITAN, NEW JERSEY 08869-0606

Direct Inquiries to:
Customer Service
(800) 828-6316

MICRhoGAM® ℞

[mīcrō gam]
Rh_o(D) Immune Globulin (Human)
Ultra-Filtered

Micro-dose for use *only* after spontaneous or induced abortion or termination of ectopic pregnancy up to and including 12 weeks' gestation.

Rx Only

For Intramuscular Injection Only

DESCRIPTION

MICRhoGAM Rh_o(D) Immune Globulin (Human) is a sterile solution containing IgG anti-D(RH1) for use in preventing Rh immunization. A single dose of MICRhoGAM contains sufficient anti-D(RH1) (approximately 50 µg)† to suppress the immune response to 2.5 mL (or less) of Rh positive red blood cells.

All donors are carefully screened to reduce the risk of transmitting disease from individuals in high-risk groups. Fractionation of the plasma is performed by a modification of the cold alcohol procedure. Following fractionation, a viral-clearance filtration step is incorporated into the manufacturing process. This filtration step removes viruses via a size-exclusion mechanism utilizing a patented Viresolve* 180 ultrafiltration membrane with defined pore-size distribution. The filter is inert to the product. This virus removal process has been shown in laboratory spiking studies to reduce the levels of some viruses ranging from 18 to 200 nm in size, including enveloped viruses as well as non-enveloped viruses. Non-enveloped viruses are known to be resistant to chemical and physical inactivation.

The final product contains approximately 5±1% gamma globulin, 2.9 mg/mL sodium chloride, 0.01% polysorbate 80 and 0.003% thimerosal (mercury derivative), with glycine (15 mg/mL) as a stabilizer.

This product is for intramuscular injection only.

† A full dose of Rh_o(D) Immune Globulin (Human) has traditionally been referred to as a "300 µg" dose and this usage is employed here for convenience in terminology. *It should not be construed as the actual anti-D content.* Each full dose of Rh_o(D) Immune Globulin (Human) must contain at least as much anti-D as 1 milliliter of the U.S. Reference Rh_o(D) Immune Globulin (Human). Studies performed at the Food and Drug Administration have shown that the U.S. Reference contains 820 international units (IU) of anti-D per milliliter. When the conversion factor determined for the International (WHO) Reference Preparation is used, 820 IU per milliliter is equivalent to 164 µg per milliliter of anti-D. MICRhoGAM contains approximately one-sixth the amount of anti-D contained in the full dose.

*Viresolve is a trademark of Millipore Corporation.

CLINICAL PHARMACOLOGY

Intramuscular Rh_o(D) human immune globulins prepared by cold alcohol fractionation have not been reported to transmit hepatitis or other infectious diseases.

MICRhoGAM acts by suppressing the immune response of Rh negative individuals to Rh positive red blood cells. The risk of immunization is related to the number of D positive red blood cells received. The risk was found to be 3% when 0.1 mL of fetal red blood cells is present in the mother and 65% when 5 mL is present. In the first 12 weeks of gestation, the total volume of red blood cells in the fetus is estimated at less than 2.5 mL.

Clinical studies demonstrated that administration of MICRhoGAM within three (3) hours following abortion was 100% effective in preventing Rh immunization. Studies showed MICRhoGAM to be effective when given as long as 72 hours after the infusion of Rh positive red cells. A lesser degree of protection is afforded if the antibody is administered beyond this time period.

INDICATIONS AND USAGE

MICRhoGAM is indicated for an Rh negative woman following spontaneous or induced abortion or termination of ectopic pregnancy up to and including 12 weeks' gestation, unless the father can be shown conclusively to be Rh negative.

CONTRAINDICATIONS

MICRhoGAM must not be used for any indication with continuation of pregnancy. RhoGAM® Rh_o(D) Immune Globulin (Human) is recommended for any indication beyond 12 weeks' gestation.

Individuals known to have had an anaphylactic or severe systemic reaction to human globulin should not receive MICRhoGAM or any other Rh_o(D) Immune Globulin (Human).

WARNINGS

Do not inject intravenously.

MICRhoGAM is made from human plasma. Products made from human plasma may contain infectious agents, such as viruses, and theoretically the Creutzfeldt-Jakob disease (CJD) agent, that can cause disease. The risk that such products will transmit an infectious agent has been reduced by screening plasma donors for prior exposure to certain viruses, by testing for the presence of certain current viral infections and by removing certain viruses during the manufacturing process. Following fractionation, a viral-clearance filtration step is incorporated into the manufacturing process. This filtration step removes viruses via a size-exclusion mechanism utilizing a patented Viresolve 180 ultrafiltration membrane with defined pore-size distribution. The filter is inert to the product. This virus removal process has been shown in laboratory spiking studies to reduce the levels of some viruses ranging from 18 to 200 nm in size, including enveloped viruses as well as non-enveloped viruses. Despite these measures, such products can still potentially transmit disease. There is also the possibility that unknown infectious agents may be present in such products. ALL infections thought by a physician possibly to have been transmitted by this product should be reported by the physician or other healthcare provider in the U.S. to Ortho-Clinical Diagnostics, Inc. at 1-800-322-6374. Outside of the U.S., the company distributing this product should be contacted. The physician should discuss the risks and benefits of this product with the patient.

PRECAUTIONS

Pregnancy Category C

Animal reproduction studies have not been conducted with MICRhoGAM. It is also not known whether Rh_o(D) Immune Globulin (Human) can cause fetal harm when administered to a pregnant woman or can affect reproduction capacity. Rh_o(D) Immune Globulin (Human) should be given to a pregnant woman only if clearly needed.

ADVERSE REACTIONS

Systemic reactions associated with administration of MICRhoGAM are extremely rare. Discomfort at the site of injection has been reported and a small number of women have noted a slight elevation in temperature.

DOSAGE AND ADMINISTRATION

Parenteral drug products should be inspected visually for particulate matter and discoloration prior to administration, whenever solution and container permit.

A single dose (approximately 50 µg)† is contained in each prefilled syringe of MICRhoGAM. This will completely suppress the immune response to 2.5 mL of Rh positive red blood cells (packed cells, not whole blood).

Administer MICRhoGAM intramuscularly as soon as possible after termination of a pregnancy up to and including 12 weeks' gestation. At or beyond 13 weeks' gestation, it is recommended that a single dose of RhoGAM be given instead of MICRhoGAM. Do not inject intravenously.

†See footnote under Description

HOW SUPPLIED

MICRhoGAM is available in packages containing:

5 prefilled single-dose syringes of MICRhoGAM (Product Code 780805) NDC 0562-7808-05
5 package inserts
5 control forms
5 patient identification cards
and
25 prefilled single-dose syringes of MICRhoGAM (Product Code 780825) NDC 0562-7808-25
25 package inserts
25 control forms
25 patient identification cards

STORAGE

Store at 2 to 8°C. Do not store frozen.

RhoGAM® ℞

[rō gam]
Rh_o(D) Immune Globulin (Human)
Ultra-Filtered

Rx Only

For Intramuscular Injection Only

DESCRIPTION

RhoGAM Rh_o(D) Immune Globulin (Human) is a sterile solution containing IgG anti-D(RH1) for use in preventing Rh immunization. A single dose of RhoGAM contains sufficient anti-D(RH1) (approximately 300 µg)† to suppress the immune response to 15 mL (or less) of Rh positive red blood cells.

Continued on next page

RhoGAM—Cont.

All donors are carefully screened to reduce the risk of transmitting disease from individuals in high-risk groups. Fractionation of the plasma is performed by a modification of the cold alcohol procedure. Following fractionation, a viral-clearance filtration step is incorporated into the manufacturing process. This filtration step removes viruses via a size-exclusion mechanism utilizing a patented Viresolve* 180 ultrafiltration membrane with defined pore-size distribution. The filter is inert to the product. This virus removal process has been shown in laboratory spiking studies to reduce the levels of some viruses ranging from 18 to 200 nm in size, including enveloped viruses as well as non-enveloped viruses. Non-enveloped viruses are known to be resistant to chemical and physical inactivation.

The final product contains approximately 5±1% gamma globulin, 2.9 mg/mL sodium chloride, 0.01% polysorbate 80 and 0.003% thimerosal (mercury derivative), with glycine (15 mg/mL) as a stabilizer.

This product is for intramuscular injection only.

†A full dose of Rh_o(D) Immune Globulin (Human) has traditionally been referred to as a "300 µg" dose and this usage is employed here for convenience in terminology. *It should not be construed as the actual anti-D content.* Each full dose of Rh_o(D) Immune Globulin (Human) must contain at least as much anti-D as 1 milliliter of the U.S. Reference Rh_o(D) Immune Globulin (Human). Studies performed at the Food and Drug Administration have shown that the U.S. Reference contains 820 international units (IU) of anti-D per milliliter. When the conversion factor determined for the International (WHO) Reference Preparation is used, 820 IU per milliliter is equivalent to 164 µg per milliliter of anti-D.

*Viresolve is a trademark of Millipore Corporation.

CLINICAL PHARMACOLOGY

Intramuscular Rh_o(D) human immune globulins prepared by cold alcohol fractionation have not been reported to transmit hepatitis or other infectious diseases.

RhoGAM acts by suppressing the immune response of Rh negative individuals to Rh positive red blood cells.

The obstetrical patient may be exposed to red blood cells from her Rh positive fetus during the normal course of pregnancy. Clinical studies have proven that the incidence of Rh immunization as a result of pregnancy was reduced to 1–2% from 12–13% when RhoGAM was given within 72 hours following delivery. Further studies in which patients received Rh immune globulin, antepartum at 28 to 32 weeks and postpartum, reduced the risk of immunization to less than 0.1%.

An Rh negative individual transfused with one unit of Rh positive red blood cells has about an 80% likelihood of producing anti-D. Protection from Rh immunization is accomplished by administering the appropriate dose of RhoGAM.

INDICATIONS AND USAGE

Pregnancy and Other Obstetric Conditions

RhoGAM is indicated whenever it is known or suspected that fetal red blood cells have entered the circulation of an Rh negative mother unless the fetus or the father can be shown conclusively to be Rh negative.

Transfusion

RhoGAM is indicated for any Rh negative female of child-bearing age who receives any Rh positive red blood cells or component such as platelets or granulocytes prepared from Rh positive blood.

CONTRAINDICATIONS

Individuals known to have had an anaphylactic or severe systemic reaction to human globulin should not receive RhoGAM or any other Rh_o(D) Immune Globulin (Human).

WARNINGS

Do not inject intravenously.

Do not inject infant.

RhoGAM is made from human plasma. Products made from human plasma may contain infectious agents, such as viruses, and theoretically the Creutzfeldt-Jakob disease (CJD) agent, that can cause disease. The risk that such products will transmit an infectious agent has been reduced by screening plasma donors for prior exposure to certain viruses, by testing for the presence of certain current viral infections and by removing certain viruses during the manufacturing process. Following fractionation, a viral-clearance filtration step is incorporated into the manufacturing process. This filtration step removes viruses via a size-exclusion mechanism utilizing a patented Viresolve 180 ultrafiltration membrane with defined pore-size distribution. The filter is inert to the product. This virus removal process has been shown in laboratory spiking studies to reduce the levels of some viruses ranging from 18 to 200 nm in size, including enveloped viruses as well as non-enveloped viruses. Despite these measures, such products can still potentially transmit disease. There is also the possibility that unknown infectious agents may be present in such products. ALL infections thought by a physician possibly to have been transmitted by this product should be reported by the physician or other healthcare provider in the U.S. to Ortho-Clinical Diagnostics, Inc. at 1-800-322-6374. Outside of the U.S., the company distributing this product should be contacted. The physician should discuss the risks and benefits of this product with the patient.

PRECAUTIONS

The presence of passively acquired anti-D in the maternal serum may cause a positive antibody screening test. This does not preclude further antepartum or postpartum prophylaxis.

Some babies born of women given Rh_o(D) Immune Globulin (Human) antepartum have weakly positive direct antiglobulin tests at birth.

Late in pregnancy or following delivery there may be sufficient fetal red blood cells in the maternal circulation to cause a positive antiglobulin test for weak D(D^u). When there is any doubt as to the patient's Rh type, RhoGAM should be administered.

Pregnancy Category C

Animal reproduction studies have not been conducted with RhoGAM. It is also not known whether Rh_o(D) Immune Globulin (Human) can cause fetal harm when administered to a pregnant woman or can affect reproduction capacity. Rh_o(D) Immune Globulin (Human) should be given to a pregnant woman only if clearly needed. However, use of Rh antibody during the third trimester in full doses of antibody has been reported to produce no evidence of hemolysis in the infant.

ADVERSE REACTIONS

Systemic reactions associated with administration of RhoGAM are extremely rare. Discomfort at the site of injection has been reported and a small number of women have noted a slight elevation in temperature. About one-quarter of a group of 22 individuals who were given multiple doses of RhoGAM to treat mismatched transfusions noted fever, myalgia and lethargy. Bilirubin levels of 0.4 to 6.8 mg/dL were observed in some of the treated individuals and one had splenomegaly.

DOSAGE AND ADMINISTRATION

Parenteral drug products should be inspected visually for particulate matter and discoloration prior to administration, whenever solution and container permit.

A single dose (approximately 300 µg)† is contained in each prefilled syringe of RhoGAM. This is the usual dose for the indications associated with pregnancy unless there is clinical or laboratory evidence of a fetal-maternal hemorrhage in excess of 15 mL of Rh positive red blood cells. The indications and recommended dosage for RhoGAM are summarized in the following table.

Indications and Recommended Dosage

Indication	Dose (approximately)
Threatened abortion at any stage of gestation with continuation of pregnancy	300 µg†
Abortion or termination of pregnancy at or beyond 13 weeks' gestation**	300 µg
Genetic amniocentesis, chorionic villus sampling (CVS) and percutaneous umbilical blood sampling (PUBS)	300 µg
Abdominal trauma	300 µg
Antepartum prophylaxis at 26 to 28 weeks' gestation††	300 µg
Postpartum (if newborn Rh positive)	300 µg

†See footnote under Description

**If abortion or termination of pregnancy occurs up to and including 12 weeks' gestation, a single dose of MICRhoGAM® Rh_o(D) Immune Globulin (Human) (approximately 50 µg)† may be used instead of RhoGAM.

††If antepartum prophylaxis is indicated, it is essential that the mother receive a postpartum dose if the infant is Rh positive.

If an adverse event requires the administration of RhoGAM early in the pregnancy, there is an obligation to maintain a level of passively acquired anti-D by administration of RhoGAM at 12-week intervals. RhoGAM should be given within 72 hours after delivery if the baby is Rh positive. If delivery occurs within three weeks after the last antepartum dose, the postpartum dose may be withheld, but a test for fetal-maternal hemorrhage (FMH) should still be performed to determine a bleed greater than 15 mL of packed red blood cells.

Whenever there is a fetal-maternal hemorrhage in excess of 15 mL of Rh positive red blood cells, multiple doses of RhoGAM are required. A fetal-maternal hemorrhage of this magnitude is unlikely prior to the last trimester of pregnancy. Patients who may need multiple doses of RhoGAM can be identified by a fetal-maternal hemorrhage screening test. If the test is positive, the volume of the fetal-maternal bleed should be determined by a quantitative method. A single dose of RhoGAM should be administered for every 15 mL of fetal red blood cells. If the dose calculation results in a fraction, administer the next number of whole syringes of RhoGAM.

Multiple doses of RhoGAM are usual for indications associated with transfusion. For every 15 mL of Rh positive red blood cells transfused, the patient should receive a single dose of RhoGAM. If multiple doses are required, consult your pharmacy for pooling directions.

Administer RhoGAM intramuscularly. Do not inject intravenously. Multiple doses may be administered at the same time or at spaced intervals, as long as the total dose is administered within three days of exposure.

HOW SUPPLIED

RhoGAM is available in packages containing:

5 prefilled single-dose syringes of RhoGAM (Product Code 780705) NDC 0562-7807-05
5 package inserts
5 control forms
5 patient identification cards
and
25 prefilled single-dose syringes of RhoGAM (Product Code 780725) NDC 0562-7807-25
25 package inserts
25 control forms
25 patient identification cards
and
100 prefilled single-dose syringes of RhoGAM (Product Code 780795) NDC 0562-7807-10
100 package inserts
100 control forms
100 patient identification cards

STORAGE

Store at 2 to 8°C. Do not store frozen.

Ortho-McNeil Pharmaceutical

RARITAN, NJ 08869-0602

www.ortho-mcneil.com

For Medical Information/Emergencies Contact:

Generally:
(800) 682-6532

In Emergencies:
(908) 218-7325

ACI–JEL® Therapeutic Vaginal Jelly ℞

DESCRIPTION

ACI-JEL Vaginal Jelly is a bland, non-irritating, water-dispersible, buffered acid jelly for intravaginal use. ACI-JEL is classified as a Vaginal Therapeutic Jelly. ACI-JEL contains 0.921% glacial acetic acid ($C_2H_4O_2$), 0.025% oxyquinoline sulfate ($C_{18}H_{16}N_2O_6S$), 0.7% ricinoleic acid ($C_{18}H_{34}O_3$), and 5% glycerin ($C_3H_8O_3$) compounded with tragacanth, acacia, propylparaben, potassium hydroxide, stannous chloride, egg albumen, potassium bitartrate, perfume and purified water. ACI-JEL is formulated to pH 3.9–4.1.

CLINICAL PHARMACOLOGY

ACI-JEL acts to restore and maintain normal vaginal acidity through its buffer action.

INDICATIONS AND USAGE

ACI-JEL is indicated as adjunctive therapy in those cases where restoration and maintenance of vaginal acidity is desirable.

CONTRAINDICATIONS

None known.

WARNINGS

No serious adverse reactions or potential safety hazards have been reported with the use of ACI-JEL.

PRECAUTIONS

General: No special care is required for the safe and effective use of ACI-JEL. *Drug Interactions:* No incidence of drug interactions have been reported with concomitant use of ACI-JEL and any other medications. *Laboratory Tests:* The monitoring of vaginal acidity (pH) may be helpful in following the patient's response. (The normal vaginal pH has been shown to be in the range of 4.0 to 5.0.) *Carcinogenesis:* No long-term studies in animals have been performed to evaluate carcinogenic potential. *Pregnancy:* Pregnancy Category C. Animal reproduction studies have not been conducted with ACI-JEL. It is also not known whether ACI-JEL can cause fetal harm when administered to a pregnant woman or can affect reproduction capacity. ACI-JEL should be given to a pregnant woman only if clearly needed. *Nursing Mothers:* It is not known whether this drug is excreted in human milk. Because many drugs are excreted in human milk, caution should be exercised when ACI-JEL is administered to a nursing woman.

ADVERSE REACTIONS

Occasional cases of local stinging and burning have been reported.

DOSAGE AND ADMINISTRATION

The usual dose is one applicatorful, administered intravaginally, morning and evening. Duration of treatment may be determined by the patient's response to therapy.

HOW SUPPLIED

85g Tube (NDC 0062-5421-01) with ORTHO® Measured-Dose Applicator.

Revised June 1998 643-10-310-3

DIENESTROL Cream ℞

(See ORTHO® Dienestrol Cream.)

FLOXIN® I.V. ℞
(ofloxacin injection)
FOR INTRAVENOUS INFUSION

DESCRIPTION
FLOXIN® (ofloxacin injection) I.V. is a synthetic, broad-spectrum antimicrobial agent for intravenous administration. Chemically, ofloxacin, a fluorinated carboxyquinolone, is the racemate, (±)-9-fluoro-2,3-dihydro-3-methyl-10-(4-methyl-1-piperazinyl)-7-oxo-7H-pyrido[1,2,3-de]-1,4-benzoxazine-6-carboxylic acid. The chemical structure is:

Its empirical formula is $C_{18}H_{20}FN_3O_4$, and its molecular weight is 361.4. Ofloxacin is an off-white to pale yellow crystalline powder. The relative solubility characteristics of ofloxacin at room temperature, as defined by USP nomenclature, indicate that ofloxacin is considered to be *soluble* in aqueous solutions with pH between 2 and 5. It is *sparingly* to *slightly soluble* in aqueous solutions with pH 7 (solubility falls to 4 mg/mL) and *freely soluble* in aqueous solutions with pH above 9. Ofloxacin has the potential to form stable coordination compounds with many metal ions. This *in vitro* chelation potential has the following formation order: $Fe^{+3} > Al^{+3} > Cu^{+2} > Ni^{+2} > Pb^{+2} > Zn^{+2} > Mg^{+2} > Ca^{+2} > Ba^{+2}$.

FLOXIN I.V. IN SINGLE-USE VIALS is a sterile, preservative-free aqueous solution of ofloxacin with pH ranging from 3.5 to 5.5. FLOXIN I.V. IN PRE-MIXED BOTTLES and IN PRE-MIXED FLEXIBLE CONTAINERS are sterile, preservative-free aqueous solutions of ofloxacin with pH ranging from 3.8 to 5.8. The color of FLOXIN I.V. may range from light yellow to amber. This does not adversely affect product potency. FLOXIN I.V. IN SINGLE-USE VIALS contains ofloxacin in Water for Injection. FLOXIN I.V. IN PRE-MIXED BOTTLES and IN PRE-MIXED FLEXIBLE CONTAINERS are dilute, non-pyrogenic, nearly isotonic pre-mixed solutions that contain ofloxacin in 5% Dextrose (D_5W). Hydrochloric acid and sodium hydroxide may have been added to adjust the pH.

The flexible container is fabricated from a specially formulated non-plasticized, thermoplastic copolyester (CR3). The amount of water that can permeate from the container into the overwrap is insufficient to affect the solution significantly. Solutions in contact with the flexible container can leach out certain of the container's chemical components in very small amounts within the expiration period. The suitability of the container material has been confirmed by tests in animals according to USP biological tests for plastic containers.

CLINICAL PHARMACOLOGY
Following a single 60-minute intravenous infusion of 200 mg or 400 mg of ofloxacin to normal volunteers, the mean maximum plasma concentrations attained were 2.7 and 4.0 µg/mL, respectively; the concentrations at 12 hours (h) after dosing were 0.3 and 0.7 µg/mL, respectively.

Steady-state concentrations were attained after four doses, and the area under the curve (AUC) was approximately 40% higher than the AUC after a single dose. The mean peak and trough plasma steady-state levels attained following intravenous administration of 200 mg of ofloxacin q 12 h for seven days were 2.9 and 0.5 µg/mL, respectively. Following intravenous doses of 400 mg of ofloxacin q 12 h, the mean peak and trough plasma steady-state levels ranged, in two different studies, from 5.5 to 7.2 µg/mL and 1.2 to 1.9 µg/mL, respectively.

Following 7 days of intravenous administration, the elimination half-life of ofloxacin was 6 h (range 5 to 10 h). The total clearance and the volume of distribution were approximately 15 L/h and 120 L, respectively.

Elimination of ofloxacin is primarily by renal excretion. Approximately 65% of a dose is excreted renally within 48 h. Studies indicate that <5% of an administered dose is recovered in the urine as the desmethyl or N-oxide metabolites. Four to eight percent of an ofloxacin dose is excreted in the feces. This indicates a small degree of biliary excretion of ofloxacin.

In vitro, approximately 32% of the drug in plasma is protein bound.

The single dose and steady-state plasma profiles of ofloxacin injection were comparable in extent of exposure (AUC) to those of ofloxacin tablets when the injectable and tablet formulations of ofloxacin were administered in equal doses (mg/mg). The mean $AUC_{(0-12)}$ attained after the intravenous administration of 400 mg over 60 min was 43.5 µg·h/mL; the mean $AUC_{(0-12)}$ attained after the oral administration of 400 mg was 41.2 µg•h/mL (two one-sided t-test, 90% confidence interval was 103–109). [See following chart.]

[See figure at top of next column]

Between 0 and 6 h following the administration of a single 200 mg oral dose of ofloxacin to 12 healthy volunteers, the average urine ofloxacin concentration was approximately 220 µg/mL. Between 12 and 24 h after administration, the average urine ofloxacin level was approximately 34 µg/mL.

Following oral administration of recommended therapeutic doses, ofloxacin has been detected in blister fluid, cervix,

Gram-positive aerobes		
Staphylococcus epidermidis (excluding methicillin-resistant strains)	*Staphylococcus haemolyticus*	
	Staphylococcus saprophyticus	
Gram-negative aerobes		
Acinetobacter calcoaceticus	*Enterobacter cloacae*	*Proteus vulgaris*
Aeromonas caviae	*Haemophilus ducreyi*	*Providencia rettgeri*
Aeromonas hydrophila	*Klebsiella oxytoca*	*Providencia stuartii*
Bordetella parapertussis	*Moraxella catarrhalis*	*Serratia marcescens*
Bordetella pertussis	*Morganella morganii*	*Vibrio parahaemolyticus*
Citrobacter freundii		
Anaerobes		
Clostridium perfringens	*Gardnerella vaginalis*	
Other organisms		
Chlamydia pneumoniae	*Mycobacterium tuberculosis* (including multiple drug-resistant strains)	*Mycoplasma hominis*
Legionella pneumophila		*Mycoplasma pneumoniae*
		Ureaplasma urealyticum

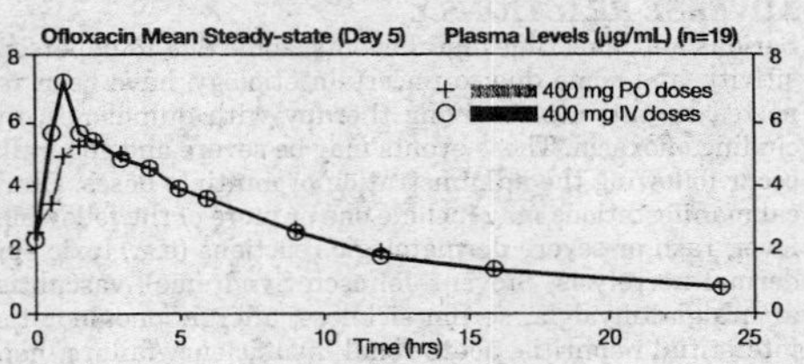

lung tissue, ovary, prostatic fluid, prostatic tissue, skin, and sputum. The mean concentration of ofloxacin in each of these various body fluids and tissues after one or more doses was 0.8 to 1.5 times the concurrent plasma level. Inadequate data are presently available on the distribution or levels of ofloxacin in the cerebrospinal fluid or brain tissue.

Following the administration of oral doses of ofloxacin to healthy elderly volunteers (64–74 years of age) with normal renal function, the apparent half-life of ofloxacin was 7 to 8 h, as compared to approximately 6 h in younger adults.

Clearance of ofloxacin is reduced in patients with impaired renal function (creatinine clearance ≤ 50 mL/min), and dosage adjustment is necessary. (See ***PRECAUTIONS: General*** and ***DOSAGE AND ADMINISTRATION***.)

Microbiology

Ofloxacin has *in vitro* activity against a broad-spectrum of gram-positive and gram-negative aerobic and anaerobic bacteria. Ofloxacin is often bactericidal at concentrations equal to or slightly greater than inhibitory concentrations. Ofloxacin is thought to exert a bactericidal effect on susceptible microorganisms by inhibiting DNA gyrase, an essential enzyme that is a critical catalyst in the duplication, transcription, and repair of bacterial DNA.

Ofloxacin has been shown to be active against most strains of the following microorganisms, both in vitro and in clinical infections as described in the ***INDICATIONS AND USAGE*** section:

Gram-positive aerobes

Staphylococcus aureus	*Streptococcus pyogenes*
Streptococcus pneumoniae	

Gram-negative aerobes

Citrobacter diversus	*Klebsiella pneumoniae*
Enterobacter aerogenes	*Neisseria gonorrhoeae*
Escherichia coli	*Proteus mirabilis*
Haemophilus influenzae	*Pseudomonas aeruginosa*

Other microorganisms

Chlamydia trachomatis

The following *in vitro* data are available, **but their clinical significance is unknown.**

Ofloxacin exhibits *in vitro* minimum inhibitory concentrations (MIC's) of 2 µg/mL or less against most (≥90%) strains of the following microorganisms; however, the safety and effectiveness of ofloxacin in treating clinical infections due to these microorganisms have not been established in adequate and well-controlled clinical trials:

[See table above]

Ofloxacin is not active against *Treponema pallidum*. (See ***WARNINGS***.)

Many strains of other streptococcal species, *Enterococcus* species, and anaerobes are resistant to ofloxacin.

Resistance to ofloxacin due to spontaneous mutation *in vitro* is a rare occurrence (range: 10^{-9} to 10^{-11}). To date, emergence of resistance has been relatively uncommon in clinical practice. With the exception of *Pseudomonas aeruginosa* (10%), less than a 4% rate of resistance emergence has been reported for most other species. Although cross-resistance has been observed between ofloxacin and other fluoroquinolones, some organisms resistant to other quinolones may be susceptible to ofloxacin.

Susceptibility Tests

Dilution techniques:

Quantitative methods are used to determine antimicrobial minimal inhibitory concentrations (MIC's). These MIC's provide estimates of the susceptibility of bacteria to antimicrobial compounds. The MICs should be determined using a standardized procedure. Standardized procedures are based on a dilution method[1] (broth or agar) or equivalent with standardized inoculum concentrations and standardized concentrations of ofloxacin powder. The MIC values should be interpreted according to the following criteria:

MIC (µg/mL)	Interpretation
≤2	Susceptible (S)
4	Intermediate (I)
≥8	Resistant (R)

A report of "Susceptible" indicates that the pathogen is likely to be inhibited if the antimicrobial compound in the blood reaches the concentrations usually achievable. A report of "Intermediate" indicates that the result should be considered equivocal, and, if the microorganism is not fully susceptible to alternative, clinically feasible drugs, the test should be repeated. This category implies possible clinical applicability in body sites where the drug is physiologically concentrated or in situations where high dosage of drug can be used. This category also provides a buffer zone which prevents small uncontrolled technical factors from causing major discrepancies in interpretation. A report of "Resistant" indicates that the pathogen is not likely to be inhibited if the antimicrobial compound in the blood reaches the concentrations usually achievable; other therapy should be selected.

Standardized susceptibility test procedures require the use of laboratory control microorganisms to control the technical aspects of the laboratory procedures. Standard ofloxacin powder should provide the following MIC values:

Microorganism		MIC (µg/mL)
Escherichia coli	ATCC 25922	0.015–0.12
Staphylococcus aureus	ATCC 29213	0.12–1.0
Pseudomonas aeruginosa	ATCC 27853	1.0–8.0
Haemophilus influenzae	ATCC 49247	0.016–0.06
Neisseria gonorrhoeae	ATCC 49226	0.004–0.016

Diffusion techniques:

Quantitative methods that require measurement of zone diameters also provide reproducible estimates of the susceptibility of bacteria to antimicrobial compounds. One such standardized procedure[2] requires the use of standardized inoculum concentrations. This procedure uses paper disks impregnated with 5-µg ofloxacin to test the susceptibility of microorganisms to ofloxacin.

Reports from the laboratory providing results of the standard single-disk susceptibility test with a 5-µg ofloxacin disk should be interpreted according to the following criteria:

Zone Diameter (mm)	Interpretation
≥16	Susceptible (S)
13–15	Intermediate (I)
≤12	Resistant (R)

Interpretation should be as stated above for results using dilution techniques. Interpretation involves correlation of the diameter obtained in the disk test with the MIC for ofloxacin.

As with standardized dilution techniques, diffusion methods require the use of laboratory control microorganisms that are used to control the technical aspects of the laboratory procedures. For the diffusion technique, the 5-µg ofloxacin disk should provide the following zone diameters in these laboratory test quality control strains:

Microorganism		Zone Diameter (mm)
Escherichia coli	ATCC 25922	29–33
Pseudomonas aeruginosa	ATCC 27853	17–21
Haemophilus influenzae	ATCC 49247	31–40
Neisseria gonorrhoeae	ATCC 49226	43–51
Staphylococcus aureus	ATCC 25923	24–28

INDICATIONS AND USAGE
FLOXIN (ofloxacin injection) I.V. is indicated for the treatment of adults with mild to moderate infections (unless otherwise indicated) caused by susceptible strains of the designated microorganisms in the infections listed below – when intravenous administration offers a route of administration

Continued on next page

Floxin I.V.—Cont.

advantageous to the patient, (e.g., patient cannot tolerate an oral dosage form). Please see ***DOSAGE AND ADMINISTRATION*** for specific recommendations.

The safety and effectiveness of the intravenous formulation in treating patients with severe infections have not been established.

NOTE: IN THE ABSENCE OF VOMITING OR OTHER FACTORS INTERFERING WITH THE ABSORPTION OF ORALLY ADMINISTERED DRUG, PATIENTS RECEIVE ESSENTIALLY THE SAME SYSTEMIC ANTIMICROBIAL THERAPY AFTER EQUIVALENT DOSES OF OFLOXACIN ADMINISTERED BY EITHER THE ORAL OR THE INTRAVENOUS ROUTE. THEREFORE, THE INTRAVENOUS FORMULATION DOES NOT PROVIDE A HIGHER DEGREE OF EFFICACY OR MORE POTENT ANTIMICROBIAL ACTIVITY THAN AN EQUIVALENT DOSE OF THE ORAL FORMULATION OF OFLOXACIN.

Acute bacterial exacerbation of chronic bronchitis due to *Haemophilus influenzae* or *Streptococcus pneumoniae*.

Community-acquired Pneumonia due to *Haemophilus influenzae* or *Streptococcus pneumoniae*.

Uncomplicated skin and skin structure infections due to *Staphylococcus aureus, Streptococcus pyogenes*, or *Proteus mirabilis*.

Acute, uncomplicated urethral and cervical gonorrhea due to *Neisseria gonorrhoeae*. (See ***WARNINGS***.)

Nongonococcal urethritis and cervicitis due to *Chlamydia trachomatis*. (See ***WARNINGS***.)

Mixed infections of the urethra and cervix due to *Chlamydia trachomatis* and *Neisseria gonorrhoeae*. (See ***WARNINGS***.)

Acute pelvic inflammatory disease (including severe infection) due to *Chlamydia trachomatis* and/or *Neisseria gonorrhoeae*. (See ***WARNINGS***.)

NOTE: If anaerobic microorganisms are suspected of contributing to the infection, appropriate therapy for anaerobic pathogens should be administered.

Uncomplicated cystitis due to *Citrobacter diversus, Enterobacter aerogenes, Escherichia coli, Klebsiella pneumoniae, Proteus mirabilis*, or *Pseudomonas aeruginosa*.

Complicated urinary tract infections due to *Escherichia coli, Klebsiella pneumoniae, Proteus mirabilis, Citrobacter diversus**, or *Pseudomonas aeruginosa**.

Prostatitis due to *Escherichia coli*.

*= Although treatment of infections due to this organism in this organ system demonstrated a clinically significant outcome, efficacy was studied in fewer than 10 patients.

Appropriate culture and susceptibility tests should be performed before treatment in order to isolate and identify organisms causing the infection and to determine their susceptibility to ofloxacin. Therapy with ofloxacin may be initiated before results of these tests are known; once results become available, appropriate therapy should be continued.

As with other drugs in this class, some strains of *Pseudomonas aeruginosa* may develop resistance fairly rapidly during treatment with ofloxacin. Culture and susceptibility testing performed periodically during therapy will provide information not only on the therapeutic effect of the antimicrobial agent but also on the possible emergence of bacterial resistance.

CONTRAINDICATIONS

FLOXIN (ofloxacin) is contraindicated in persons with a history of hypersensitivity associated with the use of ofloxacin or any member of the quinolone group of antimicrobial agents.

WARNINGS

THE SAFETY AND EFFICACY OF OFLOXACIN IN CHILDREN, ADOLESCENTS (UNDER THE AGE OF 18 YEARS), PREGNANT WOMEN, AND LACTATING WOMEN HAVE NOT BEEN ESTABLISHED. (SEE PEDIATRIC USE, USE IN PREGNANCY, AND NURSING MOTHERS SUBSECTIONS IN THE PRECAUTIONS SECTION.)

In the immature rat, the oral administration of ofloxacin at 5 to 16 times the recommended maximum human dose based on mg/kg or 1–3 times based on mg/m^2 increased the incidence and severity of osteochondrosis. The lesions did not regress after 13 weeks of drug withdrawal. Other quinolones also produce similar erosions in the weight-bearing joints and other signs of arthropathy in immature animals of various species. (See ***ANIMAL PHARMACOLOGY***.)

Convulsions, increased intracranial pressure, and toxic psychosis have been reported in patients receiving quinolones, including ofloxacin. Quinolones, including ofloxacin, may also cause central nervous system stimulation which may lead to: tremors, restlessness/agitation, nervousness/anxiety, lightheadedness, confusion, hallucinations, paranoia and depression, nightmares, insomnia, and rarely suicidal thoughts or acts. These reactions may occur following the first dose. If these reactions occur in patients receiving ofloxacin, the drug should be discontinued and appropriate measures instituted. As with all quinolones, ofloxacin should be used with caution in patients with a known or suspected CNS disorder that may predispose to seizures or lower the seizure threshold (e.g., severe cerebral arteriosclerosis, epilepsy) or in the presence of other risk factors that may predispose to seizures or lower the seizure threshold (e.g., certain drug therapy, renal dysfunction). (See ***PRECAUTIONS: General, Information for Patients, Drug Interactions*** and ***ADVERSE REACTIONS***.)

Serious and occasionally fatal hypersensitivity (anaphylactic/anaphylactoid) reactions have been reported in patients receiving therapy with quinolones, including ofloxacin. These reactions often occur following the first dose. Some reactions were accompanied by cardiovascular collapse, hypotension/shock, seizure, loss of consciousness, tingling, angioedema (including tongue, laryngeal, throat or facial edema/swelling), airway obstruction (including bronchospasm, shortness of breath and acute respiratory distress), dyspnea, urticaria/hives, itching, and other serious skin reactions. A few patients had a history of hypersensitivity reactions. The drug should be discontinued immediately at the first appearance of a skin rash or any other sign of hypersensitivity. Serious acute hypersensitivity reactions may require treatment with epinephrine and other resuscitative measures, including oxygen, intravenous fluids, antihistamines, corticosteroids, pressor amines, and airway management, as clinically indicated. (See ***PRECAUTIONS*** and ***ADVERSE REACTIONS***.)

Serious and sometimes fatal events, some due to hypersensitivity, and some due to uncertain etiology, have been reported in patients receiving therapy with quinolones, including ofloxacin. These events may be severe and generally occur following the administration of multiple doses. Clinical manifestations may include one or more of the following: fever, rash or severe dermatologic reactions (e.g., toxic epidermal necrolysis, Stevens-Johnson Syndrome); vasculitis; arthralgia; myalgia; serum sickness; allergic pneumonitis; interstitial nephritis; acute renal insufficiency/failure; hepatitis; jaundice; acute hepatic necrosis/failure; anemia, including hemolytic and aplastic; thrombocytopenia, including thrombotic thrombocytopenic purpura; leukopenia; agranulocytosis; pancytopenia; and/or other hematologic abnormalities. The drug should be discontinued immediately at the first appearance of a skin rash or any other sign of hypersensitivity and supportive measures instituted. (See ***PRECAUTIONS: Information for Patients*** and ***ADVERSE REACTIONS***.)

Pseudomembranous colitis has been reported with nearly all antibacterial agents, including ofloxacin, and may range in severity from mild to life-threatening. Therefore, it is important to consider this diagnosis in patients who present with diarrhea subsequent to the administration of any antibacterial agent.

Treatment with antibacterial agents alters the normal flora of the colon and may permit overgrowth of clostridia. Studies indicate a toxin produced by *Clostridium difficile* is one primary cause of "antibiotic-associated colitis".

After the diagnosis of pseudomembranous colitis has been established, therapeutic measures should be initiated. Mild cases of pseudomembranous colitis usually respond to drug discontinuation alone. In moderate to severe cases, consideration should be given to management with fluids and electrolytes, protein supplementation, and treatment with an oral antibacterial drug clinically effective against *C. difficile* colitis. (See ***ADVERSE REACTIONS***.)

Ruptures of the shoulder, hand, and Achilles tendons that required surgical repair or resulted in prolonged disability have been reported with ofloxacin and other quinolones. Ofloxacin should be discontinued if the patient experiences pain, inflammation, or rupture of a tendon. Patients should rest and refrain from exercise until the diagnosis of tendinitis or tendon rupture has been confidently excluded. Tendon rupture can occur at any time during or after therapy with ofloxacin.

Ofloxacin has not been shown to be effective in the treatment of syphilis. Antimicrobial agents used in high doses for short periods of time to treat gonorrhea may mask or delay the symptoms of incubating syphilis. All patients with gonorrhea should have a serologic test for syphilis at the time of diagnosis. Patients treated with ofloxacin for gonorrhea should have a follow-up serologic test for syphilis after three months and, if positive, treatment with an appropriate antimicrobial should be instituted.

PRECAUTIONS

General:

Because a rapid or bolus intravenous injection may result in hypotension, **OFLOXACIN INJECTION SHOULD ONLY BE ADMINISTERED BY SLOW INTRAVENOUS INFUSION OVER A PERIOD OF 60 MINUTES.** (See ***DOSAGE AND ADMINISTRATION***.)

Adequate hydration of patients receiving ofloxacin should be maintained to prevent the formation of a highly concentrated urine.

Administer ofloxacin with caution in the presence of renal or hepatic insufficiency/impairment. In patients with known or suspected renal or hepatic insufficiency/impairment, careful clinical observation and appropriate laboratory studies should be performed prior to and during therapy since elimination of ofloxacin may be reduced. In patients with impaired renal function (creatinine clearance $\leq$ 50 mg/mL), alteration of the dosage regimen is necessary. (See ***CLINICAL PHARMACOLOGY*** and ***DOSAGE AND ADMINISTRATION***.)

Moderate to severe phototoxicity reactions have been observed in patients exposed to direct sunlight while receiving some drugs in this class, including ofloxacin. Excessive sunlight should be avoided. Therapy should be discontinued if phototoxicity (e.g., a skin eruption) occurs.

As with other quinolones, ofloxacin should be used with caution in any patient with a known or suspected CNS disorder that may predispose to seizures or lower the seizure threshold (e.g., severe cerebral arteriosclerosis, epilepsy) or in the presence of other risk factors that may predispose to seizures or lower the seizure threshold (e.g., certain drug therapy, renal dysfunction). (See ***WARNINGS*** and ***Drug Interactions***.)

A possible interaction between oral hypoglycemic drugs (e.g., glyburide/glibenclamide) or with insulin and fluoroquinolone antimicrobial agents have been reported resulting in a potentiation of the hypoglycemic action of these drugs. The mechanism for this interaction is not known. If a hypoglycemic reaction occurs in a patient being treated with ofloxacin, discontinue ofloxacin immediately and consult a physician. (See ***Drug Interactions*** and ***ADVERSE REACTIONS***.)

As with any potent drug, periodic assessment of organ system functions, including renal, hepatic, and hematopoietic, is advisable during prolonged therapy. (See ***WARNINGS*** and ***ADVERSE REACTIONS***.)

Information for Patients:

Patients should be advised:

— to drink fluids liberally if able to take fluids by the oral route;

— that ofloxacin may cause neurologic adverse effects (e.g., dizziness, lightheadedness) and that patients should know how they react to ofloxacin before they operate an automobile or machinery or engage in activities requiring mental alertness and coordination (See ***WARNINGS*** and ***ADVERSE REACTIONS***);

— that ofloxacin may be associated with hypersensitivity reactions, even following the first dose, to discontinue the drug at the first sign of a skin rash, hives or other skin reactions, a rapid heartbeat, difficulty in swallowing or breathing, any swelling suggesting angioedema (e.g., swelling of the lips, tongue, face; tightness of the throat, hoarseness), or any other symptom of an allergic reaction (See ***WARNINGS*** and ***ADVERSE REACTIONS***);

— to avoid excessive sunlight or artificial ultraviolet light while receiving ofloxacin and to discontinue therapy if phototoxicity (e.g., skin eruption) occurs;

— to discontinue treatment and inform their physician if they experience pain, inflammation, or rupture of a tendon, and to rest and refrain from exercise until the diagnosis of tendinitis or tendon rupture has been confidently excluded;

— that if they are diabetic and are being treated with insulin or an oral hypoglycemic agent, to discontinue ofloxacin immediately if a hypoglycemic reaction occurs and consult a physician (See ***PRECAUTIONS: General*** and ***Drug Interactions***);

— that convulsions have been reported in patients taking quinolones, including ofloxacin, and to notify their physician before taking this drug if there is a history of this condition.

Drug Interactions:

Antacids, Sucralfate, Metal Cations, Multi-Vitamins: There are no data concerning an interaction of **intravenous** quinolones with **oral** antacids, sucralfate, multi-vitamins, or metal cations. However, no quinolone should be co-administered with any solution containing multivalent cations, e.g., magnesium, through the same intravenous line. (See ***DOSAGE AND ADMINISTRATION***.)

Caffeine: Interactions between ofloxacin and caffeine have not been detected.

Cimetidine: Cimetidine has demonstrated interference with the elimination of some quinolones. This interference has resulted in significant increases in half-life and AUC of some quinolones. The potential for interaction between ofloxacin and cimetidine has not been studied.

Cyclosporine: Elevated serum levels of cyclosporine have been reported with concomitant use of cyclosporine with some other quinolones. The potential for interaction between ofloxacin and cyclosporine has not been studied.

Drugs metabolized by Cytochrome P450 enzymes: Most quinolone antimicrobial drugs inhibit cytochrome P450 enzyme activity. This may result in a prolonged half-life for some drugs that are also metabolized by this system (e.g., cyclosporine, theophylline/methylxanthines, warfarin) when co-administered with quinolones. The extent of this inhibition varies among different quinolones. (See other ***Drug Interactions***.)

Non-steroidal anti-inflammatory drugs: The concomitant administration of a non-steroidal anti-inflammatory drug with a quinolone, including ofloxacin, may increase the risk of CNS stimulation and convulsive seizures. (See ***WARNINGS*** and ***PRECAUTIONS: General***.)

Probenecid: The concomitant use of probenecid with certain other quinolones has been reported to affect renal tubular secretion. The effect of probenecid on the elimination of ofloxacin has not been studied.

Theophylline: Steady-state theophylline levels may increase when ofloxacin and theophylline are administered concurrently. As with other quinolones, concomitant administration of ofloxacin may prolong the half-life of theophylline, elevate serum theophylline levels, and increase the risk of theophylline-related adverse reactions. Theophylline levels should be closely monitored and theophylline dosage adjustments made, if appropriate, when ofloxacin is co-administered. Adverse reactions (including seizures) may occur with or without an elevation in the serum theophylline level. (See ***WARNINGS*** and ***PRECAUTIONS: General***.)

Warfarin: Some quinolones have been reported to enhance the effects of the oral anticoagulant warfarin or its derivatives. Therefore, if a quinolone antimicrobial is administered concomitantly with warfarin or its derivatives, the prothrombin time or other suitable coagulation test should be closely monitored.

Antidiabetic agents (e.g., insulin, glyburide/glibenclamide): Since disturbances of blood glucose, including hyperglycemia and hypoglycemia, have been reported in patients treated concurrently with quinolones and an antidiabetic agent, careful monitoring of blood glucose is recommended when these agents are used concomitantly (See ***PRECAUTIONS: General*** and ***Information for Patients.***)

Carcinogenesis, Mutagenesis, Impairment of Fertility:
Long-term studies to determine the carcinogenic potential of ofloxacin have not been conducted.
Ofloxacin was not mutagenic in the Ames bacterial test, *in vitro* and *in vivo* cytogenetic assay, sister chromatid exchange (Chinese Hamster and Human Cell Lines), unscheduled DNA Repair (UDS) using human fibroblasts, dominant lethal assays, or mouse micronucleus assay. Ofloxacin was positive in the UDS test using rat hepatocytes and Mouse Lymphoma Assay.

Pregnancy: Teratogenic Effects. Pregnancy Category C.
Ofloxacin has not been shown to have any teratogenic effects at oral doses as high as 810 mg/kg/day (11 times the recommended maximum human dose based on mg/m^2 or 50 times based on mg/kg) and 160 mg/kg/day (4 times the recommended maximum human dose based on mg/m^2 or 10 times based on mg/kg) when administered to pregnant rats and rabbits, respectively. Additional studies in rats with oral doses up to 360 mg/kg/day (5 times the recommended maximum human dose based on mg/m^2 or 23 times based on mg/kg) demonstrated no adverse effect on late fetal development, labor, delivery, lactation, neonatal viability, or growth of the newborn. Doses equivalent to 50 and 10 times the recommended maximum human dose of ofloxacin (based on mg/kg) were fetotoxic (i.e., decreased fetal body weight and increased fetal mortality) in rats and rabbits, respectively. Minor skeletal variations were reported in rats receiving doses of 810 mg/kg/day, which is more than 10 times higher than the recommended maximum human dose based on mg/m^2.
There are, however, no adequate and well-controlled studies in pregnant women. Ofloxacin should be used during pregnancy only if the potential benefit justifies the potential risk to the fetus. (See ***WARNINGS.***)

Nursing Mothers:
In lactating females, a single oral 200-mg dose of ofloxacin resulted in concentrations of ofloxacin in milk that were similar to those found in plasma. Because of the potential for serious adverse reactions from ofloxacin in nursing infants, a decision should be made whether to discontinue nursing or to discontinue the drug, taking into account the importance of the drug to the mother. (See ***WARNINGS*** and ***ADVERSE REACTIONS.***)

Pediatric Use:
Safety and effectiveness in children and adolescents below the age of 18 years have not been established. Ofloxacin causes arthropathy (arthrosis) and osteochondrosis in juvenile animals of several species. (See ***WARNINGS.***)

ADVERSE REACTIONS

The following is a compilation of the data for ofloxacin based on clinical experience with both the oral and intravenous formulations. The incidence of drug-related adverse reactions in patients during Phase 2 and 3 clinical trials was 11%. Among patients receiving multiple-dose therapy, 4% discontinued ofloxacin due to adverse experiences.
In clinical trials, the following events were considered likely to be drug-related in patients receiving multiple doses of ofloxacin:

nausea 3%, insomnia 3%, headache 1%, dizziness 1%, diarrhea 1%, vomiting 1%, rash 1%, pruritus 1%, external genital pruritus in women 1%, vaginitis 1%, dysgeusia 1%.

Local injection site reactions (phlebitis, swelling, erythema) were reported in approximately 2% of patients treated with the 3.63 mg/mL final infusion concentration of intravenous ofloxacin used in the clinical safety trials. The final infusion concentration of intravenous ofloxacin in the commercially available intravenous preparations is 4.0 mg/mL. To date, individuals administered the 4.0 mg/mL concentration of the intravenous ofloxacin have demonstrated clinically acceptable rates of local injection site reactions. Due to the small difference in concentration, significant differences in local site reactions are unexpected with the 4.0 mg/mL concentration.

In clinical trials, the most frequently reported adverse events, regardless of relationship to drug, were:

nausea 10%, headache 9%, insomnia 7%, external genital pruritus in women 6%, dizziness 5%, vaginitis 5%, diarrhea 4%, vomiting 4%.

In clinical trials, the following events, regardless of relationship to drug occurred in 1 to 3% of patients:

Abdominal pain and cramps, chest pain, decreased appetite, dry mouth, dysgeusia, fatigue, flatulence, gastrointestinal distress, nervousness, pharyngitis, pruritus, fever, rash, sleep disorders, somnolence, trunk pain, vaginal discharge, visual disturbances, and constipation.

Additional events, occurring in clinical trials at a rate of less than 1%, regardless of relationship to drug, were:

Body as a whole:	asthenia, chills, malaise, extremity pain, pain, epistaxis
Cardiovascular System:	cardiac arrest, edema, hypertension, hypotension, palpitations, vasodilation
Gastrointestinal System:	dyspepsia
Genital/Reproductive System:	burning, irritation, pain and rash of the female genitalia; dysmenorrhea; menorrhagia; metrorrhagia
Musculoskeletal System:	arthralgia, myalgia
Nervous System:	seizures, anxiety, cognitive change, depression, dream abnormality, euphoria, hallucinations, paresthesia, syncope, vertigo, tremor, confusion
Nutritional/Metabolic:	thirst, weight loss
Respiratory System:	respiratory arrest, cough, rhinorrhea
Skin/Hypersensitivity:	angioedema, diaphoresis, urticaria, vasculitis
Special Senses:	decreased hearing acuity, tinnitus, photophobia
Urinary System:	dysuria, urinary frequency, urinary retention

The following laboratory abnormalities appeared in ≥ 1.0% of patients receiving multiple doses of ofloxacin. It is not known whether these abnormalities were caused by the drug or the underlying conditions being treated.

Hematopoietic:	anemia, leukopenia, leukocytosis, neutropenia, neutrophilia, increased band forms, lymphocytopenia, eosinophilia, lymphocytosis, thrombocytopenia, thrombocytosis, elevated ESR
Hepatic:	elevated: alkaline phosphatase, AST (SGOT), ALT (SGPT)
Serum chemistry:	hyperglycemia, hypoglycemia, elevated creatinine, elevated BUN
Urinary:	glucosuria, proteinuria, alkalinuria, hyposthenuria, hematuria, pyuria

Post-Marketing Adverse Events:
Additional adverse events, regardless of relationship to drug, reported from worldwide marketing experience with quinolones, including ofloxacin:

Clinical:

Cardiovascular System:	cerebral thrombosis, pulmonary edema, tachycardia, hypotension/shock, syncope
Endocrine/Metabolic:	hyper- or hypoglycemia, especially in diabetic patients on insulin or oral hypoglycemic agents (See ***PRECAUTIONS: General*** and ***Drug Interactions.***)
Gastrointestinal System:	hepatic dysfunction including: hepatic necrosis, jaundice (cholestatic or hepatocellular), hepatitis; intestinal perforation; pseudomembranous colitis (the onset of pseudomembranous colitis symptoms may occur during or after antimicrobial treatment), GI hemorrhage; hiccough, painful oral mucosa, pyrosis (See ***WARNINGS.***)
Genitourinary System:	vaginal candidiasis
Hematopoietic:	anemia, including hemolytic and aplastic; hemorrhage, pancytopenia, agranulocytosis, leukopenia, reversible bone marrow depression, thrombocytopenia, thrombotic thrombocytopenic purpura, petechiae, ecchymosis/bruising (See ***WARNINGS.***)
Musculoskeletal:	tendinitis/rupture; weakness; rhabdomyolysis
Nervous System:	nightmares; suicidal thoughts or acts, disorientation, psychotic reactions, paranoia; phobia, agitation, restlessness, aggressiveness/hostility, manic reaction, emotional lability; peripheral neuropathy, ataxia, incoordination; possible exacerbation of: myasthenia gravis and extrapyramidal disorders; dysphasia, lightheadedness (See ***WARNINGS*** and ***PRECAUTIONS.***)
Respiratory System:	dyspnea, bronchospasm, allergic pneumonitis, stridor (See ***WARNINGS.***)
Skin/Hypersensitivity:	anaphylactic (-toid) reactions/shock; purpura, serum sickness, erythema multiforme/Stevens-Johnson Syndrome, erythema nodosum, exfoliative dermatitis, hyperpigmentation, toxic epidermal necrolysis, conjunctivitis, photosensitivity, vesiculobullous eruption (See ***WARNINGS*** and ***PRECAUTIONS.***)
Special Senses:	diplopia, nystagmus, blurred vision, disturbances of: taste, smell, hearing and equilibrium, usually reversible following discontinuation
Urinary System:	anuria, polyuria, renal calculi, renal failure, interstitial nephritis, hematuria (See ***WARNINGS*** and ***PRECAUTIONS.***)

Laboratory:

Hematopoietic:	prolongation of prothrombin time
Serum chemistry:	acidosis, elevation of: serum triglycerides, serum cholesterol, serum potassium, liver function tests including: GGTP, LDH, bilirubin
Urinary:	albuminuria, candiduria

In clinical trials using multiple-dose therapy, ophthalmologic abnormalities, including cataracts and multiple punctate lenticular opacities, have been noted in patients undergoing treatment with other quinolones. The relationship of the drugs to these events is not presently established.
CRYSTALLURIA and CYLINDRURIA HAVE BEEN REPORTED with other quinolones.

OVERDOSAGE

Information on overdosage with ofloxacin is limited. One incident of accidental overdosage has been reported. In this case, an adult female received 3 grams of ofloxacin intravenously over 45 minutes. A blood sample obtained 15 minutes after the completion of the infusion revealed an ofloxacin level of 39.3 µg/mL. In 7 h, the level had fallen to 16.2 µg/mL, and by 24 h to 2.7 µg/mL. During the infusion, the patient developed drowsiness, nausea, dizziness, hot and cold flushes, subjective facial swelling and numbness, slurring of speech, and mild to moderate disorientation. All complaints except the dizziness subsided within 1 h after discontinuation of the infusion. The dizziness, most bothersome while standing, resolved in approximately 9 h. Laboratory testing reportedly revealed no clinically significant changes in routine parameters in this patient.
In the event of acute overdose, the patient should be observed and appropriate hydration maintained. Ofloxacin is not efficiently removed by hemodialysis or peritoneal dialysis.

DOSAGE AND ADMINISTRATION

FLOXIN I.V. should only be administered by **intravenous** infusion. It is not for intramuscular, intrathecal, intraperitoneal, or subcutaneous administration.
CAUTION: RAPID OR BOLUS INTRAVENOUS INFUSION MUST BE AVOIDED. Ofloxacin injection should be infused intravenously slowly over a period of not less than 60 minutes. (See ***PRECAUTIONS.***)
Single-use vials require dilution prior to administration. (See ***PREPARATION FOR ADMINISTRATION.***)
The usual dose of FLOXIN (ofloxacin injection) I.V. is 200 mg to 400 mg administered by slow infusion over 60 minutes every 12 h as described in the following dosing chart. These recommendations apply to patients with mild to moderate infection and normal renal function (i.e., creatinine clearance >50 mL/min). For patients with altered renal function (i.e., creatinine clearance ≤50 mL/min), see the ***Patients with Impaired Renal Function*** subsection.

Patients with Normal Renal Function:
[See table at top of next page]

Patients with Impaired Renal Function:
Dosage should be adjusted for patients with a creatinine clearance ≤ 50 mL/min. **After a normal initial dose,** dosage should be adjusted as follows:

Creatinine Clearance	Maintenance Dose	Frequency
20-50 mL/min	the usual recommended unit dose	q24h
<20 mL/min	1/2 the usual recommended unit dose	q24h

When only the serum creatinine is known, the following formula may be used to estimate creatinine clearance.

Men: Creatinine clearance (mL/min) =

$$\frac{\text{Weight (kg)} \times (140\text{-age})}{72 \times \text{serum creatinine (mg/dL)}}$$

Women: 0.85 × the value calculated for men.

The serum creatinine should represent a steady-state of renal function.

Patients with Cirrhosis:
The excretion of ofloxacin may be reduced in patients with severe liver function disorders (e.g., cirrhosis with or without ascites). A maximum dose of 400 mg of ofloxacin per day should therefore not be exceeded.

PREPARATION OF OFLOXACIN INJECTION FOR ADMINISTRATION

FLOXIN I.V. IN SINGLE-USE VIALS:
FLOXIN I.V. is supplied in single-use vials containing a concentrated ofloxacin solution with the equivalent of 400 mg of

Continued on next page

Floxin I.V.—Cont.

ofloxacin in Water for Injection. The 10 mL vials contain 40 mg of ofloxacin/mL. **THESE FLOXIN I.V. SINGLE-USE VIALS MUST BE FURTHER DILUTED WITH AN APPROPRIATE SOLUTION PRIOR TO INTRAVENOUS ADMINISTRATION. (See COMPATIBLE INTRAVENOUS SOLUTIONS.)** The concentration of the resulting diluted solution should be 4 mg/mL prior to administration.

This parenteral drug product should be inspected visually for discoloration and particulate matter prior to administration.

Since no preservative or bacteriostatic agent is present in this product, aseptic technique must be used in preparation of the final parenteral solution. **Since the vials are for single-use only, any unused portion should be discarded.**

Since only limited data are available on the compatibility of ofloxacin intravenous injection with other intravenous substances, **additives or other medications should not be added to FLOXIN I.V. in single-use vials or infused simultaneously through the same intravenous line.** If the same intravenous line is used for sequential infusion of several different drugs, the line should be flushed before and after infusion of FLOXIN I.V. with an infusion solution compatible with FLOXIN I.V. and with any other drug(s) administered via this common line.

Prepare the desired dosage of ofloxacin according to the following chart:

Desired Dosage Strength	From 10 mL Vial, Withdraw Volume	Volume of Diluent	Infusion Time
200 mg	5 mL	qs 50 mL	60 min
300 mg	7.5 mL	qs 75 mL	60 min
400 mg	10 mL	qs 100 mL	60 min

For example, to prepare a 200-mg dose using the 10 mL vial (40 mg/mL), withdraw 5 mL and dilute with a compatible intravenous solution to a total volume of 50 mL.

Compatible Intravenous Solutions:

Any of the following intravenous solutions may be used to prepare a 4 mg/mL ofloxacin solution with the approximate pH values:

Intravenous Fluids	pH of 4 mg/mL FLOXIN I.V. Solution
0.9% Sodium Chloride Injection, USP	4.69
5% Dextrose Injection, USP	4.57
5% Dextrose/0.9% NaCl Injection	4.56
5% Dextrose in Lactated Ringers	4.94
5% Sodium Bicarbonate Injection	7.95
Plasma-Lyte® 56/5% Dextrose Injection	5.02
5% Dextrose, 0.45% Sodium Chloride, and 0.15% Potassium Chloride Injection	4.64
Sodium Lactate Injection (M/6)	5.64
Water for Injection	4.66

FLOXIN I.V. PRE-MIXED IN SINGLE-USE FLEXIBLE CONTAINERS:

FLOXIN I.V. is also supplied in 50 mL and 100 mL flexible containers containing a pre-mixed, ready-to-use ofloxacin solution in D_5W for single-use. **NO FURTHER DILUTION OF THIS PREPARATION IS NECESSARY. Each 50 mL pre-mixed flexible container already contains a dilute solution with the equivalent of 200 mg of ofloxacin (4 mg/mL) in 5% Dextrose (D_5W). Each 100 mL pre-mixed flexible container already contains a dilute solution with the equivalent of 400 mg of ofloxacin (4 mg/mL) in 5% Dextrose (D_5W).**

This parenteral drug product should be inspected visually for discoloration and particulate matter prior to administration.

Since no preservative or bacteriostatic agent is present in this product, aseptic technique must be used in preparation of the final parenteral solution. **Since the pre-mixed flexible containers are for single-use only, any unused portion should be discarded.**

Since only limited data are available on the compatibility of ofloxacin intravenous injection with other intravenous substances, **additives or other medications should not be added to FLOXIN I.V. in flexible containers or infused simultaneously through the same intravenous line.** If the same intravenous line is used for sequential infusion of several different drugs, the line should be flushed before and after infusion of FLOXIN I.V. with an infusion solution compatible with FLOXIN I.V. and with any other drug(s) administered via this common line.

Instructions for the Use of FLOXIN I.V. PRE-MIXED IN FLEXIBLE CONTAINERS:

To open:

1. Tear outer wrap at the notch and remove solution container.
2. Check the container for minute leaks by squeezing the inner bag firmly. If leaks are found, or if the seal is not intact, discard the solution, as the sterility may be compromised.
3. Do not use if the solution is cloudy or a precipitate is present.
4. Use sterile equipment.
5. **WARNING: Do not use flexible containers in series connections.** Such use could result in air embolism due to residual air being drawn from the primary container before administration of the fluid from the secondary container is complete.

Patients with Normal Renal Function:

Infection†	Unit Dose	Frequency	Duration	Daily Dose
Acute Bacterial Exacerbation of Chronic Bronchitis	400 mg	q12h	10 days	800 mg
Comm. Acquired Pneumonia	400 mg	q12h	10 days	800 mg
Uncomplicated Skin and Skin Structure Infections	400 mg	q12h	10 days	800 mg
Acute, Uncomplicated Urethral and Cerivcal Gonorrhea	400 mg	single dose	1 day	400 mg
Nongonococcal Cervicitis/ Urethritis due toC. *trachomatis*	300 mg	q12h	7 days	600 mg
Mixed infection of the urethra and cervix due to *C. trachomatis* and *N. gonorrhoeae*	300 mg	q12h	7 days	600 mg
Acute Pelvic Inflammatory Disease	400 mg	q12h	10-14 days	800 mg
Uncomplicated Cystitis due to *E. coli* or *K. pneumoniae*	200 mg	q12h	3 days	400 mg
Uncomplicated Cystitis due to other approved pathogens	200 mg	q12h	7 days	400 mg
Complicated UTI's	200 mg	q12h	10 days	400 mg
Prostatitis due to *E. coli*	300 mg	q12h	6 wks‡	600 mg

†DUE TO THE DESIGNATED PATHOGENS (See ***INDICATIONS AND USAGE***.)

‡BECAUSE THERE ARE NO SAFETY DATA PRESENTLY AVAILABLE TO SUPPORT THE USE OF THE INTRAVENOUS FORMULATION OF OFLOXACIN FOR MORE THAN 10 DAYS, THERAPY AFTER 10 DAYS SHOULD BE SWITCHED TO THE ORAL TABLET FORMULATION OR OTHER APPROPRIATE THERAPY.

Preparation for administration:

1. Close flow control clamp of administration set.
2. Remove cover from port at bottom of container.
3. Insert piercing pin of administration set into port with a twisting motion until the pin is firmly seated. **NOTE: See full directions on administration set carton.**
4. Suspend container from hanger.
5. Squeeze and release drip chamber to establish proper fluid level in chamber during infusion of FLOXIN I.V. IN PRE-MIXED FLEXIBLE CONTAINERS.
6. Open flow control clamp to expel air from set. Close clamp.
7. Regulate rate of administration with flow control clamp.

Stability of FLOXIN I.V. as Supplied:

When stored under recommended conditions, FLOXIN I.V., as supplied in 10 mL vials, and 50 mL and 100 mL flexible containers, is stable through the expiration date printed on the label.

Stability of FLOXIN I.V. Following Dilution:

FLOXIN I.V., when diluted in a compatible intravenous fluid to a concentration between 0.4 mg/mL and 4 mg/mL, is stable for 72 h when stored at or below 75°F or 24°C and for 14 days when stored under refrigeration at 41°F or 5°C in glass bottles or plastic intravenous containers. Solutions that are diluted in a compatible intravenous solution and frozen in glass bottles or plastic intravenous containers are stable for 6 months when stored at -4°F or -20°C. Once thawed, the solution is stable for up to 14 days, if refrigerated at 36°F to 46°F (2°C to 8°C). **THAW FROZEN SOLUTIONS AT ROOM TEMPERATURE (77°F OR 25°C) OR IN A REFRIGERATOR (46°F OR 8°C). DO NOT FORCE THAW BY MICROWAVE IRRADIATION OR WATER BATH IMMERSION. DO NOT REFREEZE AFTER INITIAL THAWING.**

HOW SUPPLIED

SINGLE-USE VIALS:

FLOXIN (ofloxacin injection) I.V. is supplied in single-use vials. Each vial contains a concentrated solution with the equivalent of 400 mg of ofloxacin.

40 mg/mL, 10 mL vials (NDC 0062-1550-01)

FLOXIN I.V. SINGLE-USE VIALS are manufactured for ORTHO-McNEIL PHARMACEUTICAL, INC. by Schering-Plough Products, Inc., Manati, PR 00674.

PRE-MIXED IN FLEXIBLE CONTAINERS:

FLOXIN (ofloxacin injection) I.V. PRE-MIXED IN FLEXIBLE CONTAINERS is supplied as a single-use, pre-mixed solution in 50 mL and 100 mL flexible containers. Each contains a dilute solution with the equivalent of 200 mg or 400 mg of ofloxacin, respectively, in 5% Dextrose (D_5W).

4 mg/mL (200 mg), 50 mL flexible container (NDC 0062-1553-01)

4 mg/mL (400 mg), 100 mL flexible container (NDC 0062-1552-02)

FLOXIN I.V. PRE-MIXED IN FLEXIBLE CONTAINERS is manufactured for ORTHO-McNEIL, PHARMACEUTICAL, INC. by Abbott Laboratories, North Chicago, IL 60064.

FLOXIN (ofloxacin injection) I.V. in SINGLE-USE VIALS should be stored at controlled room temperature 59°F to 86°F (15°C to 30°C) and protected from light. FLOXIN I.V. PRE-MIXED IN FLEXIBLE CONTAINERS should be stored at or below 77°F or 25°C; however, brief exposure up to 104°F or 40°C does not adversely affect the product. Avoid excessive heat and protect from freezing and light.

Also Available:

TABLETS

Ofloxacin is also available as FLOXIN TABLETS (ofloxacin tablets) 200, 300 and 400 mg.

ANIMAL PHARMACOLOGY

Ofloxacin, as well as other drugs of the quinolone class, has been shown to cause arthropathies (arthrosis) in immature dogs and rats. In addition, these drugs are associated with an increased incidence of osteochondrosis in rats as compared to the incidence observed in vehicle-treated rats. (See ***WARNINGS***.) There is no evidence of arthropathies in fully mature dogs at intravenous doses up to 3 times the recommended maximum human dose (on a mg/m^2 basis or 5 times based on a mg/kg basis) for a one-week exposure period.

Long-term, high-dose systemic use of other quinolones in experimental animals has caused lenticular opacities; however, this finding was not observed in any animal studies with ofloxacin.

Reduced serum globulin and protein levels were observed in animals treated with other quinolones. In one ofloxacin study, minor decreases in serum globulin and protein levels were noted in female cynomolgus monkeys dosed orally with 40 mg/kg ofloxacin daily for one year. These changes, however, were considered to be within normal limits for monkeys.

Crystalluria and ocular toxicity were not observed in any animals treated with ofloxacin.

Rx only.

FLOXIN® is a trademark of ORTHO-McNEIL PHARMACEUTICAL, INC. U.S. Patent No. 4,382,892

REFERENCES

1. National Committee for Clinical Laboratory Standards. Methods for Dilution Antimicrobial Susceptibility Tests for Bacteria That Grow Aerobically — Third Edition. Approved Standard NCCLS Document M7-A3, Vol. 13, No. 25, NCCLS, Villanova, PA, December, 1993.
2. National Committee for Clinical Laboratory Standards. Performance Standards for Antimicrobial Disk Susceptibility Tests — Fifth Edition. Approved Standard NCCLS Document M2-A5, Vol. 13, No. 24, NCCLS, Villanova, PA, December, 1993.

ORTHO-McNEIL PHARMACEUTICAL, INC.
Raritan, NJ USA 08869

 Revised March 1998 635-10-267-4

Shown in Product Identification Guide, page 328

FLOXIN® Tablets ℞
(ofloxacin tablets)

DESCRIPTION

FLOXIN® (ofloxacin tablets) Tablets is a synthetic broad-spectrum antimicrobial agent for oral administration. Chemically, ofloxacin, a fluorinated carboxyquinolone, is the racemate, (±)-9-fluoro-2,3-dihydro-3-methyl-10-(4-methyl-1-piperazinyl)-7-oxo-7H-pyrido[1,2,3-de]-1,4-benzoxazine-6-carboxylic acid. The chemical structure is:

[See chemical structure at top of next column]

Its empirical formula is $C_{18}H_{20}FN_3O_4$, and its molecular weight is 361.4. Ofloxacin is an off-white to pale yellow crystalline powder. The molecule exists as a zwitterion at the pH conditions in the small intestine. The relative solubility characteristics of ofloxacin at room temperature, as defined by USP nomenclature, indicate that ofloxacin is considered to be *soluble* in aqueous solutions with pH between 2 and 5. It is *sparingly* to *slightly soluble* in aqueous solutions with pH 7 (solubility falls to 4 mg/mL) and *freely soluble* in aqueous solutions with pH above 9. Ofloxacin has the potential to form stable coordination compounds with many metal ions. This *in vitro* chelation potential has the following formation order: $Fe^{+3} > Al^{+3} > Cu^{+2} > Ni^{+2} > Pb^{+2} > Zn^{+2} > Mg^{+2} > Ca^{+2} > Ba^{+2}$.

FLOXIN Tablets contain the following inactive ingredients: anhydrous lactose, corn starch, hydroxypropyl cellulose, hydroxypropyl methylcellulose, magnesium stearate, polyethylene glycol, polysorbate 80, sodium starch glycolate, titanium dioxide and may also contain synthetic yellow iron oxide.

CLINICAL PHARMACOLOGY

Following oral administration, the bioavailability of ofloxacin in the tablet formulation is approximately 98%. Maximum serum concentrations are achieved one to two hours after an oral dose. Absorption of ofloxacin after single or multiple doses of 200 to 400 mg is predictable, and the amount of drug absorbed increases proportionately with the dose. Ofloxacin has biphasic elimination. Following multiple oral doses at steady-state administration, the half-lives are approximately 4–5 hours and 20–25 hours. However, the longer half-life represents less than 5% of the total AUC. Accumulation at steady-state can be estimated using a half-life of 9 hours. The total clearance and volume of distribution are approximately similar after single or multiple doses. Elimination is mainly by renal excretion. The following are mean peak serum concentrations in healthy 70–80 kg male volunteers after single oral doses of 200, 300, or 400 mg of ofloxacin or after multiple oral doses of 400 mg.

[See table above]

Oral Dose	Serum Concentration 2 hours after admin. (μg/mL)	Area Under the Curve ($AUC_{(0-\infty)}$) (μg•h/mL)
200 mg single dose	1.5	14.1
300 mg single dose	2.4	21.2
400 mg single dose	2.9	31.4
400 mg steady-state	4.6	61.0

Steady-state concentrations were attained after four oral doses, and the area under the curve (AUC) was approximately 40% higher than the AUC after single doses. Therefore, after multiple-dose administration of 200 mg and 300 mg doses, peak serum levels of 2.2 μg/mL and 3.6 μg/mL, respectively, are predicted at steady-state.

In vitro, approximately 32% of the drug in plasma is protein bound.

The single dose and steady-state plasma profiles of ofloxacin injection were comparable in extent of exposure (AUC) to those of ofloxacin tablets when the injectable and tablet formulations of ofloxacin were administered in equal doses (mg/mg) to the same group of subjects. The mean steady-state $AUC_{(0\text{-}12)}$ attained after the intravenous administration of 400 mg over 60 min was 43.5 μg•h/mL; the mean steady-state $AUC_{(0\text{-}12)}$ attained after the oral administration of 400 mg was 41.2 μg•h/mL (two one-sided t-test, 90% confidence interval was 103–109).

(See following chart.)

Ofloxacin Mean Steady-state (Day 5) Plasma Levels (μg/mL) (n=19)

+ 400 mg PO doses
○ 400 mg IV doses

Time (hrs)

Between 0 and 6 h following the administration of a single 200 mg oral dose of ofloxacin to 12 healthy volunteers, the average urine ofloxacin concentration was approximately 220 μg/mL. Between 12 and 24 hours after administration, the average urine ofloxacin level was approximately 34 μg/mL.

Following oral administration of recommended therapeutic doses, ofloxacin has been detected in blister fluid, cervix, lung tissue, ovary, prostatic fluid, prostatic tissue, skin, and sputum. The mean concentration of ofloxacin in each of these various body fluids and tissues after one or more doses was 0.8 to 1.5 times the concurrent plasma level. Inadequate data are presently available on the distribution or levels of ofloxacin in the cerebrospinal fluid or brain tissue.

Ofloxacin has a pyridobenzoxazine ring that appears to decrease the extent of parent compound metabolism. Between 65% and 80% of an administered oral dose of ofloxacin is excreted unchanged via the kidneys within 48 hours of dosing. Studies indicate that less than 5% of an administered dose is recovered in the urine as the desmethyl or N-oxide metabolites. Four to eight percent of an ofloxacin dose is excreted in the feces. This indicates a small degree of biliary excretion of ofloxacin.

The administration of FLOXIN with food does not affect the C_{max} and AUC_{∞} of the drug, but T_{max} is prolonged.

Clearance of ofloxacin is reduced in patients with impaired renal function (creatinine clearance rate ≤ 50 mL/min), and dosage adjustment is necessary. (See ***PRECAUTIONS: General*** and ***DOSAGE AND ADMINISTRATION.***)

Following oral administration to healthy elderly subjects (65–81 years of age), maximum plasma concentrations are usually achieved one to two hours after single and multiple twice-daily doses, indicating that the rate of oral absorption is unaffected by age or gender. Mean peak plasma concentrations in elderly subjects were 9–21% higher than those observed in younger subjects. Gender differences in the pharmacokinetic properties of elderly subjects have been observed. Peak plasma concentrations were 114% and 54% higher in elderly females compared to elderly males following single and multiple twice-daily doses. [This interpretation was based on study results collected from two separate studies.] Plasma concentrations increase dose-dependently with the increase in doses after single oral dose and at steady state. No differences were observed in the volume of distribution values between elderly and younger subjects. As in younger subjects, elimination is mainly by renal excretion as unchanged drug in elderly subjects, although less drug is recovered from renal excretion in elderly subjects. Consistent with younger subjects, less than 5% of an administered dose was recovered in the urine as the desmethyl and N-oxide metabolites in the elderly. A longer plasma half-life of approximately 6.4 to 7.4 hours was observed in elderly subjects, compared with 4 to 5 hours for young subjects. Slower elimination of ofloxacin is observed in elderly subjects as compared with younger subjects which may be attributable to the reduced renal function and renal clearance observed in the elderly subjects. Because ofloxacin is known to be substantially excreted by the kidney, and elderly patients are more likely to have decreased renal function, dosage adjustment is necessary for elderly patients with impaired renal function as recommended for all patients. (See ***PRECAUTIONS: General*** and ***DOSAGE AND ADMINISTRATION.***)

Microbiology

Ofloxacin is a quinolone antimicrobial agent. The mechanism of action of ofloxacin and other fluoroquinolone antimicrobials involves inhibition of bacterial topoisomerase IV and DNA gyrase (both of which are type II topoisomerases), enzymes required for DNA replication, transcription, repair and recombination.

Ofloxacin has *in vitro* activity against a wide range of gram-negative and gram-positive microorganisms. Ofloxacin is often bactericidal at concentrations equal to or slightly greater than inhibitory concentrations.

Fluoroquinolones, including ofloxacin, differ in chemical structure and mode of action from aminoglycosides, macrolides and β-lactam antibiotics, including penicillins. Fluoroquinolones may, therefore, be active against bacteria resistant to these antimicrobials.

Resistance to ofloxacin due to spontaneous mutation *in vitro* is a rare occurrence (range: 10^{-9} to 10^{-11}). Although cross-resistance has been observed between ofloxacin and some other fluoroquinolones, some microorganisms resistant to other fluoroquinolones may be susceptible to ofloxacin.

Ofloxacin has been shown to be active against most strains of the following microorganisms both *in vitro* and in clinical infections as described in the ***INDICATIONS AND USAGE*** section:

Aerobic gram-positive microorganisms
Staphylococcus aureus (methicillin-susceptible strains)
Streptococcus pneumoniae (penicillin-susceptible strains)
Streptococcus pyogenes

Aerobic gram-negative microorganisms
Citrobacter (diversus) koseri
Enterobacter aerogenes
Escherichia coli
Haemophilus influenzae
Klebsiella pneumoniae
Neisseria gonorrhoeae
Proteus mirabilis
Pseudomonas aeruginosa

As with other drugs in this class, some strains of *Pseudomonas aeruginosa* may develop resistance fairly rapidly during treatment with ofloxacin.

Other microorganisms
Chlamydia trachomatis

The following *in vitro* data are available, **but their clinical significance is unknown.**

Ofloxacin exhibits *in vitro* minimum inhibitory concentrations (MIC values) of 2 μg/mL or less against most (≥ 90%) strains of the following microorganisms; however, the safety and effectiveness of ofloxacin in treating clinical infections due to these microorganisms have not been established in adequate and well-controlled trials:

Aerobic gram-positive microorganisms
Staphylococcus epidermidis (methicillin-susceptible strains)
Staphylococcus saprophyticus
Streptococcus pneumoniae (penicillin-resistant strains)

Aerobic gram-negative microorganisms
Acinetobacter calcoaceticus
Bordetella pertussis
Citrobacter freundii
Enterobacter cloacae
Haemophilus ducreyi
Klebsiella oxytoca
Moraxella catarrhalis
Morganella morganii
Proteus vulgaris
Providencia rettgeri
Providencia stuartii
Serratia marcescens

Anaerobic microorganisms
Clostridium perfringes

Other microorganisms
Chlamydia pneumoniae
Gardnerella vaginalis
Legionella pneumophila
Mycoplasma hominis
Mycoplasma pneumoniae
Ureaplasma urealyticum

Ofloxacin is not active against Treponema pallidum. (See ***WARNINGS.***)

Many strains of other streptococcal species, *Enterococcus* species, and anaerobes are resistant to ofloxacin.

Susceptibility Tests

Dilution techniques: Quantitative methods are used to determine antimicrobial minimum inhibitory concentrations (MIC values). These MIC values provide estimates of the susceptibility of bacteria to antimicrobial compounds. The MIC values should be determined using a standardized procedure. Standardized procedures are based on a dilution method[1] (broth or agar) or equivalent with standardized inoculum concentrations and standardized concentrations of ofloxacin powder. The MIC values should be interpreted according to the following criteria:

For testing aerobic microorganisms other than *Haemophilus influenzae*, *Neisseria gonorrhoeae*, and *Streptococcus pneumoniae*:

MIC (μg/mL)	Interpretation
≤2	Susceptible (S)
4	Intermediate (I)
≥8	Resistant (R)

For testing *Haemophilus influenzae*:[a]

MIC (μg/mL)	Interpretation
≤2.0	Susceptible (S)

[a] This interpretive standard is applicable only to broth microdilution susceptibility tests with *Haemophilus influenzae* using *Haemophilus* Test Medium[1].

The current absence of data on resistant strains precludes defining any results other than "Susceptible." Strains yielding MIC results suggestive of a "nonsusceptible" category should be submitted to a reference laboratory for further testing.

For testing *Neisseria gonorrhoeae*:[b]

MIC (μg/mL)	Interpretation
≤0.25	Susceptible (S)
0.5–1	Intermediate (I)
≥2	Resistant (R)

[b] These interpretive standards are applicable only to agar dilution tests using GC agar base and 1% defined growth supplement incubated in 5% CO_2.

For testing *Streptococcus* species including *Streptococcus pneumoniae*:[c]

MIC (μg/mL)	Interpretation
≤2	Susceptible (S)
4	Intermediate (I)
≥8	Resistant (R)

[c] These interpretive standards are applicable only to broth microdilution susceptibility tests using cation-adjusted Mueller-Hinton broth with 2–5% lysed horse blood.

A report of "Susceptible" indicates that the pathogen is likely to be inhibited if the antimicrobial compound in the blood reaches the concentrations usually achievable. A report of "Intermediate" indicates that the result should be considered equivocal, and, if the microorganism is not fully susceptible to alternative, clinically feasible drugs, the test should be repeated. This category implies possible clinical applicability in body sites where the drug is physiologically concentrated or in situations where high dosage of drug can be used. This category also provides a buffer zone which prevents small uncontrolled technical factors from causing major discrepancies in interpretation. A report of "Resistant" indicates that the pathogen is not likely to be inhibited if

Continued on next page

Floxin Tablets—Cont.

the antimicrobial compound in the blood reaches the concentrations usually achievable; other therapy should be selected.
Standardized susceptibility test procedures require the use of laboratory control microorganisms to control the technical aspects of the laboratory procedures. Standard ofloxacin powder should provide the following MIC values:
[See first table above]
Diffusion techniques: Quantitative methods that require measurement of zone diameters also provide reproducible estimates of the susceptibility of bacteria to antimicrobial compounds. One such standardized procedure[2] requires the use of standardized inoculum concentrations. This procedure uses paper disks impregnated with 5-μg ofloxacin to test the susceptibility of microorganisms to ofloxacin.
Reports from the laboratory providing results of the standard single-disk susceptibility test with a 5-μg ofloxacin disk should be interpreted according to the following criteria:

For testing aerobic microorganisms other than *Haemophilus influenzae*, *Neisseria gonorrhoeae*, and *Streptococcus pneumoniae*:

Zone Diameter (mm)	Interpretation
≥16	Susceptible (S)
13–16	Intermediate (I)
≤12	Resistant (R)

For testing *Haemophilus influenzae*:[g]

Zone Diameter (mm)	Interpretation
≥16	Susceptible (S)

[g] This zone diameter standard is applicable only to disk diffusion tests with *Haemophilus influenzae* using *Haemophilus* Test Medium (HTM)[2] incubated in 5% CO_2.

The current absence of data on resistant strains precludes defining any results other than "Susceptible." Strains yielding zone diameter results suggestive of a "nonsusceptible" category should be submitted to a reference laboratory for further testing.

For testing *Neisseria gonorrhoea*:[h]

Zone Diameter (mm)	Interpretation
≥31	Susceptible (S)
25–30	Intermediate (I)
≤24	Resistant (R)

[h] These zone diameter standards are applicable only to disk diffusion tests using GC agar base and 1% defined growth supplement incubated in 5% CO_2.

For testing *Streptococcus* species including *Streptococcus pneumoniae*:[i]

Zone Diameter (mm)	Interpretation
≥16	Susceptible (S)
13–15	Intermediate (I)
≤12	Resistant (R)

[i] These zone diameter standards are applicable only to disk diffusion tests performed using Mueller-Hinton agar supplemented with 5% defibrinated sheep blood and incubated in 5% CO_2.

Interpretation should be as stated above for results using dilution techniques. Interpretation involves correlation of the diameter obtained in the disk test with the MIC for ofloxacin.
As with standardized dilution techniques, diffusion methods require the use of laboratory control microorganisms that are used to control the technical aspects of the laboratory procedures. For the diffusion technique, the 5-μg ofloxacin disk should provide the following zone diameters in these laboratory quality control strains:
[See second table above]

Microorganism		MIC (μg/mL)
Escherichia coli	ATCC 25922	0.015–0.12
Haemophilus influenzae	ATCC 49247[d]	0.016–0.06
Neisseria gonorrhoeae	ATCC 49226[e]	0.004–0.016
Pseudomonas aeruginosa	ATCC 27853	1–8
Staphylococcus aureus	ATCC 29213	0.12–1
Streptococcus pneumoniae	ATCC 49619[f]	1–4

[d] This quality control range is applicable only to *H. influenzae* ATCC 49247 tested by a microdilution procedure using *Haemophilus* Test Medium (HTM)[1].
[e] This quality control range is applicable only to *N. gonorrhoeae* ATCC 49226 tested by an agar dilution procedure using GC agar base with 1% defined growth supplement incubated in 5% CO_2.
[f] This quality control range is applicable only to *S. pneumoniae* ATCC 49619 tested by a microdilution procedure using cation-adjusted Mueller-Hinton broth with 2–5% lysed horse blood.

Microorganism		Zone Diameter (mm)
Escherichia coli	ATCC 25922	29–33
Haemophilus influenzae	ATCC 49247[j]	31–40
Neisseria gonorrhoeae	ATCC 49226[k]	43–51
Pseudomonas aeruginosa	ATCC 27853	17–21
Staphylococcus aureus	ATCC 25923	24–28
Streptococcus pneumoniae	ATCC 49619[l]	16–21

[j] This quality control range is applicable only to *H. influenzae* ATCC 49247 tested by a disk diffusion procedure using *Haemophilus* Test Medium (HTM)[2] incubated in 5% CO_2.
[k] This quality control range is applicable only to *N. gonorrhoeae* ATCC 49226 tested by a disk diffusion procedure using GC agar base with 1% defined growth supplement incubated in 5% CO_2.
[l] This quality control range is applicable only to *S. pneumoniae* ATCC 49619 tested by a disk diffusion procedure using Mueller-Hinton agar supplemented with 5% defibrinated sheep blood and incubated in 5% CO_2.

INDICATIONS AND USAGE

FLOXIN (ofloxacin tablets) Tablets are indicated for the treatment of adults with mild to moderate infections (unless otherwise indicated) caused by susceptible strains of the designated microorganisms in the infections listed below. Please see ***DOSAGE AND ADMINISTRATION*** for specific recommendations.

Acute bacterial exacerbations of chronic bronchitis due to *Haemophilus influenzae* or *Streptococcus pneumoniae*.
Community-acquired Pneumonia due to *Haemophilus influenzae* or *Streptococcus pneumoniae*.
Uncomplicated skin and skin structure infections due to *Staphylococcus aureus, Streptococcus pyogenes*, or *Proteus mirabilis*.
Acute, uncomplicated urethral and cervical gonorrhea due to *Neisseria gonorrhoeae*. (See ***WARNINGS.***)
Nongonococcal urethritis and cervicitis due to *Chlamydia trachomatis*. (See ***WARNINGS.***)
Mixed infections of the urethra and cervix due to *Chlamydia trachomatis* and *Neisseria gonorrhoeae*. (See ***WARNINGS.***)
Acute pelvic inflammatory disease (including severe infection) due to *Chlamydia trachomatis* and/or *Neisseria gonorrhoeae*. (See ***WARNINGS.***)
NOTE: If anaerobic microorganisms are suspected of contributing to the infection, appropriate therapy for anaerobic pathogens should be administered.
Uncomplicated cystitis due to *Citrobacter diversus, Enterobacter aerogenes, Escherichia coli, Klebsiella pneumoniae, Proteus mirabilis*, or *Pseudomonas aeruginosa*.
Complicated urinary tract infections due to *Escherichia coli, Klebsiella pneumoniae, Proteus mirabilis, Citrobacter diversus**, or *Pseudomonas aeruginosa**.
Prostatitis due to *Escherichia coli*.

* = Although treatment of infections due to this organism in this organ system demonstrated a clinically significant outcome, efficacy was studied in fewer than 10 patients.

Appropriate culture and susceptibility tests should be performed before treatment in order to isolate and identify organisms causing the infection and to determine their susceptibility to ofloxacin. Therapy with ofloxacin may be initiated before results of these tests are known; once results become available, appropriate therapy should be continued. As with other drugs in this class, some strains of *Pseudomonas aeruginosa* may develop resistance fairly rapidly during treatment with ofloxacin. Culture and susceptibility testing performed periodically during therapy will provide information not only on the therapeutic effect of the antimicrobial agent but also on the possible emergence of bacterial resistance.

CONTRAINDICATIONS

FLOXIN (ofloxacin) is contraindicated in persons with a history of hypersensitivity associated with the use of ofloxacin or any member of the quinolone group of antimicrobial agents.

WARNINGS

THE SAFETY AND EFFICACY OF OFLOXACIN IN PEDIATRIC PATIENTS AND ADOLESCENTS (UNDER THE AGE OF 18 YEARS), PREGNANT WOMEN, AND LACTATING WOMEN HAVE NOT BEEN ESTABLISHED. (See **PRECAUTIONS: Pediatric Use, Pregnancy, and Nursing Mothers** subsections.)
In the immature rat, the oral administration of ofloxacin at 5 to 16 times the recommended maximum human dose based on mg/kg or 1–3 times based on mg/m^2 increased the incidence and severity of osteochondrosis. The lesions did not regress after 13 weeks of drug withdrawal. Other quinolones also produce similar erosions in the weight-bearing joints and other signs of arthropathy in immature animals of various species. (See ***ANIMAL PHARMACOLOGY.***)
Convulsions, increased intracranial pressure, and toxic psychosis have been reported in patients receiving quinolones, including ofloxacin. Quinolones, including ofloxacin, may also cause central nervous system stimulation which may lead to: tremors, restlessness/agitation, nervousness/anxiety, lightheadedness, confusion, hallucinations, paranoia and depression, nightmares, insomnia, and rarely suicidal thoughts or acts. These reactions may occur following the first dose. If these reactions occur in patients receiving ofloxacin, the drug should be discontinued and appropriate measures instituted. Insomnia may be more common with ofloxacin than some other products in the quinolone class. As with all quinolones, ofloxacin should be used with caution in patients with a known or suspected CNS disorder that may predispose to seizures or lower the seizure threshold (e.g., severe cerebral arteriosclerosis, epilepsy) or in the presence of other risk factors that may predispose to seizures or lower the seizure threshold (e.g., certain drug therapy, renal dysfunction). (See ***PRECAUTIONS: General, Information for Patients, Drug Interactions*** and ***ADVERSE REACTIONS.***)
Serious and occasionally fatal hypersensitivity (anaphylactic/anaphylactoid) reactions have been reported in patients receiving therapy with quinolones, including ofloxacin. These reactions often occur following the first dose. Some reactions were accompanied by cardiovascular collapse, hypotension/shock, seizure, loss of consciousness, tingling, angioedema (including tongue, laryngeal, throat or facial edema/swelling), airway obstruction (including bronchospasm, shortness of breath and acute respiratory distress), dyspnea, urticaria/hives, itching, and other serious skin reactions. A few patients had a history of hypersensitivity reactions. The drug should be discontinued immediately at the first appearance of a skin rash or any other sign of hypersensitivity. Serious acute hypersensitivity reactions may require treatment with epinephrine and other resuscitative measures, including oxygen, intravenous fluids, antihistamines, corticosteroids, pressor amines, and airway management, as clinically indicated. (See ***PRECAUTIONS*** and ***ADVERSE REACTIONS.***)
Serious and sometimes fatal events, some due to hypersensitivity, and some due to uncertain etiology, have been reported in patients receiving therapy with quinolones, including ofloxacin. These events may be severe and generally occur following the administration of multiple doses. Clinical manifestations may include one or more of the following: fever, rash or severe dermatologic reactions (e.g., toxic epidermal necrolysis, Stevens-Johnson Syndrome); vasculitis; arthralgia; myalgia; serum sickness; allergic pneumonitis; interstitial nephritis; acute renal insufficiency/failure; hepatitis; jaundice; acute hepatic necrosis/failure; anemia, including hemolytic and aplastic; thrombocytopenia, including thrombotic thrombocytopenic purpura; leukopenia; agranulocytosis; pancytopenia; and/or other hematologic abnormalities. The drug should be discontinued immediately at the first appearance of a skin rash or any other sign of hypersensitivity and supportive measures instituted. (See ***PRECAUTIONS: Information for Patients*** and ***ADVERSE REACTIONS.***)
Pseudomembranous colitis has been reported with nearly all antibacterial agents, including ofloxacin, and may range in severity from mild to life-threatening. Therefore, it is important to consider this diagnosis in patients who present with diarrhea subsequent to the administration of any antibacterial agents.
Treatment with antibacterial agents alters the normal flora of the colon and may permit overgrowth of clostridia. Studies indicate a toxin produced by *Clostridium difficile* is one primary cause of "antibiotic-associated colitis".
After the diagnosis of pseudomembranous colitis has been established, therapeutic measures should be initiated. Mild cases of pseudomembranous colitis usually respond to drug discontinuation alone. In moderate to severe cases, consideration should be given to management with fluids and electrolytes, protein supplementation, and treatment with an antibacterial drug clinically effective against *C. difficile* colitis. (See ***ADVERSE REACTIONS.***)
Ruptures of the shoulder, hand, and Achilles tendons that required surgical repair or resulted in prolonged disability have been reported with ofloxacin and other quinolones. Ofloxacin should be discontinued if the patient experiences pain, inflammation, or rupture of a tendon. Patients should rest and refrain from exercise until the diagnosis of tendinitis or tendon rupture has been confidently excluded. Tendon rupture can occur at any time during or after therapy with ofloxacin.
Ofloxacin has not been shown to be effective in the treatment of syphilis. Antimicrobial agents used in high doses for short periods of time to treat gonorrhea may mask or delay the symptoms of incubating syphilis. All patients with

gonorrhea should have a serologic test for syphilis at the time of diagnosis. Patients treated with ofloxacin for gonorrhea should have a follow-up serologic test for syphilis after three months and, if positive, treatment with an appropriate antimicrobial should be instituted.

PRECAUTIONS

General:

Adequate hydration of patients receiving ofloxacin should be maintained to prevent the formation of a highly concentrated urine.

Administer ofloxacin with caution in the presence of renal or hepatic insufficiency/impairment. In patients with known or suspected renal or hepatic insufficiency/impairment, careful clinical observation and appropriate laboratory studies should be performed prior to and during therapy since elimination of ofloxacin may be reduced. In patients with impaired renal function (creatinine clearance ≤ 50 mg/mL), alteration of the dosage regimen is necessary. (See ***CLINICAL PHARMACOLOGY*** and ***DOSAGE AND ADMINISTRATION.***)

Moderate to severe phototoxicity reactions have been observed in patients exposed to direct sunlight while receiving some drugs in this class, including ofloxacin. Excessive sunlight should be avoided. Therapy should be discontinued if phototoxicity (e.g., a skin eruption) occurs.

As with other quinolones, ofloxacin should be used with caution in any patient with a known or suspected CNS disorder that may predispose to seizures or lower the seizure threshold (e.g., severe cerebral arteriosclerosis, epilepsy) or in the presence of other risk factors that may predispose to seizures or lower the seizure threshold (e.g., certain drug therapy, renal dysfunction). (See ***WARNINGS*** and ***Drug Interactions.***)

A possible interaction between oral hypoglycemic drugs (e.g., glyburide/glibenclamide) or with insulin and fluoroquinolone antimicrobial agents have been reported resulting in a potentiation of the hypoglycemic action of these drugs. The mechanism for this interaction is not known. If a hypoglycemic reaction occurs in a patient being treated with ofloxacin, discontinue ofloxacin immediately and consult a physician. (See ***Drug Interactions*** and ***ADVERSE REACTIONS.***)

As with any potent drug, periodic assessment of organ system functions, including renal, hepatic, and hematopoietic, is advisable during prolonged therapy. (See ***WARNINGS*** and ***ADVERSE REACTIONS.***)

Information for Patients:

Patients should be advised:

— to drink fluids liberally;

— that mineral supplements, vitamins with iron or minerals, calcium-, aluminum-, or magnesium-based antacids, sucralfate or Videx®, (Didanosine), chewable/buffered tablets or the pediatric powder for oral solution should not be taken within the two-hour period before or within the two-hour period after taking ofloxacin (See ***Drug Interactions***);

— that ofloxacin can be taken without regard to meals;

— that ofloxacin may cause neurologic adverse effects (e.g., dizziness, lightheadedness) and that patients should know how they react to ofloxacin before they operate an automobile or machinery or engage in activities requiring mental alertness and coordination (See ***WARNINGS*** and ***ADVERSE REACTIONS***);

— to discontinue treatment and inform their physician if they experience pain, inflammation, or rupture of a tendon, and to rest and refrain from exercise until the diagnosis of tendinitis or tendon rupture has been confidently excluded;

— that ofloxacin may be associated with hypersensitivity reactions, even following the first dose, to discontinue the drug at the first sign of a skin rash, hives or other skin reactions, a rapid heartbeat, difficulty in swallowing or breathing, any swelling suggesting angioedema (e.g., swelling of the lips, tongue, face; tightness of the throat, hoarseness), or any other symptom of an allergic reaction (See ***WARNINGS*** and ***ADVERSE REACTIONS***);

— to avoid excessive sunlight or artificial ultraviolet light while receiving ofloxacin and to discontinue therapy if phototoxicity (e.g., skin eruption) occurs;

— that if they are diabetic and are being treated with insulin or an oral hypoglycemic drug, to discontinue ofloxacin immediately if a hypoglycemic reaction occurs and consult a physician (See ***PRECAUTIONS*: *General*** and ***Drug Interactions***);

— that convulsions have been reported in patients taking quinolones, including ofloxacin, and to notify their physician before taking this drug if there is a history of this condition.

Drug Interactions:

Antacids, Sucralfate, Metal Cations, Multivitamins: Quinolones form chelates with alkaline earth and transition metal cations. Administration of quinolones with antacids containing calcium, magnesium, or aluminum, with sucralfate, with divalent or trivalent cations such as iron, or with multivitamins containing zinc or with Videx®, (Didanosine), chewable/buffered tablets or the pediatric powder for oral solution may substantially interfere with the absorption of quinolones resulting in systemic levels considerably lower than desired. These agents should not be taken within the two-hour period before or within the two-hour period after ofloxacin administration. (See ***DOSAGE AND ADMINISTRATION.***)

Caffeine: Interactions between ofloxacin and caffeine have not been detected.

Cimetidine: Cimetidine has demonstrated interference with the elimination of some quinolones. This interference has resulted in significant increases in half-life and AUC of some quinolones. The potential for interaction between ofloxacin and cimetidine has not been studied.

Cyclosporine: Elevated serum levels of cyclosporine have been reported with concomitant use of cyclosporine with some other quinolones. The potential for interaction between ofloxacin and cyclosporine has not been studied.

Drugs metabolized by Cytochrome P450 enzymes: Most quinolone antimicrobial drugs inhibit cytochrome P450 enzyme activity. This may result in a prolonged half-life for some drugs that are also metabolized by this system (e.g., cyclosporine, theophylline/methylxanthines, warfarin) when co-administered with quinolones. The extent of this inhibition varies among different quinolones. (See other ***Drug Interactions.***)

Non-steroidal anti-inflammatory drugs: The concomitant administration of a non-steroidal anti-inflammatory drug with a quinolone, including ofloxacin, may increase the risk of CNS stimulation and convulsive seizures. (See ***WARNINGS*** and ***PRECAUTIONS*: *General.***)

Probenecid: The concomitant use of probenecid with certain other quinolones has been reported to affect renal tubular secretion. The effect of probenecid on the elimination of ofloxacin has not been studied.

Theophylline: Steady-state theophylline levels may increase when ofloxacin and theophylline are administered concurrently. As with other quinolones, concomitant administration of ofloxacin may prolong the half-life of theophylline, elevate serum theophylline levels, and increase the risk of theophylline-related adverse reactions. Theophylline levels should be closely monitored and theophylline dosage adjustments made, if appropriate, when ofloxacin is co-administered. Adverse reactions (including seizures) may occur with or without an elevation in the serum theophylline level. (See ***WARNINGS*** and ***PRECAUTIONS*: *General.***)

Warfarin: Some quinolones have been reported to enhance the effects of the oral anticoagulant warfarin or its derivatives. Therefore, if a quinolone antimicrobial is administered concomitantly with warfarin or its derivatives, the prothrombin time or other suitable coagulation test should be closely monitored.

Antidiabetic agents (e.g., insulin, glyburide/glibenclamide): Since disturbances of blood glucose, including hyperglycemia and hypoglycemia, have been reported in patients treated concurrently with quinolones and an antidiabetic agent, careful monitoring of blood glucose is recommended when these agents are used concomitantly. (See ***PRECAUTIONS*: *General*** and ***Information for Patients.***)

Carcinogenesis, Mutagenesis, Impairment of Fertility:

Long-term studies to determine the carcinogenic potential of ofloxacin have not been conducted.

Ofloxacin was not mutagenic in the Ames bacterial test, *in vitro* and *in vivo* cytogenetic assay, sister chromatid exchange (Chinese Hamster and Human Cell Lines), unscheduled DNA Repair (UDS) using human fibroblasts, dominant lethal assays, or mouse micronucleus assay. Ofloxacin was positive in the UDS test using rat hepatocytes and Mouse Lymphoma Assay.

Pregnancy: Teratogenic Effects. Pregnancy Category C.

Ofloxacin has not been shown to have any teratogenic effects at oral doses as high as 810 mg/kg/day (11 times the recommended maximum human dose based on mg/m^2 or 50 times based on mg/kg) and 160 mg/kg/day (4 times the recommended maximum human dose based on mg/m^2 or 10 times based on mg/kg) when administered to pregnant rats and rabbits, respectively. Additional studies in rats with oral doses up to 360 mg/kg/day (5 times the recommended maximum human dose based on mg/m^2 or 23 times based on mg/kg) demonstrated no adverse effect on late fetal development, labor, delivery, lactation, neonatal viability, or growth of the newborn. Doses equivalent to 50 and 10 times the recommended maximum human dose of ofloxacin (based on mg/kg) were fetotoxic (i.e., decreased fetal body weight and increased fetal mortality) in rats and rabbits, respectively. Minor skeletal variations were reported in rats receiving doses of 810 mg/kg/ day, which is more than 10 times higher than the recommended maximum human dose based on mg/m^2.

There are, however, no adequate and well-controlled studies in pregnant women. Ofloxacin should be used during pregnancy only if the potential benefit justifies the potential risk to the fetus. (See ***WARNINGS.***)

Nursing Mothers:

In lactating females, a single oral 200-mg dose of ofloxacin resulted in concentrations of ofloxacin in milk that were similar to those found in plasma. Because of the potential for serious adverse reactions from ofloxacin in nursing infants, a decision should be made whether to discontinue nursing or to discontinue the drug, taking into account the importance of the drug to the mother. (See ***WARNINGS*** and ***ADVERSE REACTIONS.***)

Pediatric Use:

Safety and effectiveness in pediatric patients and adolescents below the age of 18 years have not been established. Ofloxacin causes arthropathy (arthrosis) and osteochondrosis in juvenile animals of several species. (See ***WARNINGS.***)

Geriatric Use:

In phase 2/3 clinical trials with ofloxacin, 688 patients (14.2%) were ≥ 65 years of age. Of these, 436 patients (9.0%) were between the ages of 65 and 74 and 252 patients (5.2%) were 75 years or older. There was no apparent difference in the frequency or severity of adverse reactions in elderly adults compared with younger adults. The pharmacokinetic properties of ofloxacin in elderly subjects are similar to those in younger subjects. Drug absorption appears to be unaffected by age. Dosage adjustment is necessary for elderly patients with impaired renal function (creatinine clearance rate ≤ 50 mL/min) due to reduced clearance of ofloxacin. In comparative studies, the frequency and severity of most drug-related nervous system events in patients ≥ 65 years of age were comparable for ofloxacin and control drugs. The only differences identified were an increase in reports of insomnia (3.9% vs 1.5%) and headache (4.7% vs 1.8%) with ofloxacin. It is important to note that these geriatric safety data are extracted from 44 comparative studies where the adverse reaction information from 20 different controls (other antibiotics or placebo) were pooled for comparison with ofloxacin. The clinical significance of such a comparison is not clear. (See ***CLINICAL PHARMACOLOGY*** and ***DOSAGE AND ADMINISTRATION.***)

ADVERSE REACTIONS

The following is a compilation of the data for ofloxacin based on clinical experience with both the oral and intravenous formulations. The incidence of drug-related adverse reactions in patients during Phase 2 and 3 clinical trials was 11%. Among patients receiving multiple-dose therapy, 4% discontinued ofloxacin due to adverse experiences.

In clinical trials, the following events were considered likely to be drug-related in patients receiving multiple doses of ofloxacin:

nausea 3%, insomnia 3%, headache 1%, dizziness 1%, diarrhea 1%, vomiting 1%, rash 1%, pruritus 1%, external genital pruritus in women 1%, vaginitis 1%, dysgeusia 1%.

In clinical trials, the most frequently reported adverse events, regardless of relationship to drug, were:

nausea 10%, headache 9%, insomnia 7%, external genital pruritus in women 6%, dizziness 5%, vaginitis 5%, diarrhea 4%, vomiting 4%.

In clinical trials, the following events, regardless of relationship to drug, occurred in 1 to 3% of patients:

Abdominal pain and cramps, chest pain, decreased appetite, dry mouth, dysgeusia, fatigue, flatulence, gastrointestinal distress, nervousness, pharyngitis, pruritus, fever, rash, sleep disorders, somnolence, trunk pain, vaginal discharge, visual disturbances, and constipation.

Additional events, occurring in clinical trials at a rate of less than 1%, regardless of relationship to drug, were:

Body as a whole:	asthenia, chills, malaise, extremity pain, pain, epistaxis
Cardiovascular System:	cardiac arrest, edema, hypertension, hypotension, palpitations, vasodilation
Gastrointestinal System:	dyspepsia
Genital/Reproductive System:	burning, irritation, pain and rash of the female genitalia; dysmenorrhea; menorrhagia; metrorrhagia
Musculoskeletal System:	arthralgia, myalgia
Nervous System:	seizures, anxiety, cognitive change, depression, dream abnormality, euphoria, hallucinations, paresthesia, syncope, vertigo, tremor, confusion
Nutritional/Metabolic:	thirst, weight loss
Respiratory System:	respiratory arrest, cough, rhinorrhea
Skin/Hypersensitivity:	angioedema, diaphoresis, urticaria, vasculitis
Special Senses:	decreased hearing acuity, tinnitus, photophobia
Urinary System:	dysuria, urinary frequency, urinary retention

The following laboratory abnormalities appeared in ≥ 1.0% of patients receiving multiple doses of ofloxacin. It is not known whether these abnormalities were caused by the drug or the underlying conditions being treated.

Hematopoietic:	anemia, leukopenia, leukocytosis, neutropenia, neutrophilia, increased band forms, lymphocytopenia, eosinophilia, lymphocytosis, thrombocytopenia, thrombocytosis, elevated ESR
Hepatic:	elevated: alkaline phosphatase, AST (SGOT), ALT (SGPT)
Serum chemistry:	hyperglycemia, hypoglycemia, elevated creatinine, elevated BUN
Urinary:	glucosuria, proteinuria, alkalinuria, hyposthenuria, hematuria, pyuria

Post-Marketing Adverse Events:

Additional adverse events, regardless of relationship to drug, reported from worldwide marketing experience with quinolones, including ofloxacin:

Clinical:

Cardiovascular System:	cerebral thrombosis, pulmonary edema, tachycardia, hypotension/shock, syncope

Continued on next page

Floxin Tablets—Cont.

Endocrine/Metabolic:	hyper- or hypoglycemia, especially in diabetic patients on insulin or oral hypoglycemic agents (See ***PRECAUTIONS**: **General** and **Drug Interactions**.*)
Gastrointestinal System:	hepatic dysfunction including: hepatic necrosis, jaundice (cholestatic or hepatocellular), hepatitis; intestinal perforation; pseudomembranous colitis (the onset of pseudomembranous colitis symptoms may occur during or after antimicrobial treatment), GI hemorrhage; hiccough, painful oral mucosa, pyrosis (See ***WARNINGS.***)
Genital/Reproductive System:	vaginal candidiasis
Hematopoietic:	anemia, including hemolytic and aplastic; hemorrhage, pancytopenia, agranulocytosis, leukopenia, reversible bone marrow depression, thrombocytopenia, thrombotic thrombocytopenic purpura, petechiae, ecchymosis/bruising (See ***WARNINGS.***)
Musculoskeletal:	tendinitis/rupture; weakness; rhabdomyolysis
Nervous System:	nightmares; suicidal thoughts or acts, disorientation, psychotic reactions, paranoia; phobia, agitation, restlessness, aggressiveness/hostility, manic reaction, emotional lability; peripheral neuropathy, ataxia, incoordination; possible exacerbation of: myasthenia gravis and extrapyramidal disorders; dysphasia, lightheadedness (See ***WARNINGS*** and ***PRECAUTIONS.***)
Respiratory System:	dyspnea, bronchospasm, allergic pneumonitis, stridor (See ***WARNINGS.***)
Skin/Hypersensitivity:	anaphylactic (-toid) reactions/shock; purpura, serum sickness, erythema multiforme/Stevens-Johnson Syndrome, erythema nodosum, exfoliative dermatitis, hyperpigmentation, toxic epidermal necrolysis, conjunctivitis, photosensitivity, vesiculobullous eruption (See ***WARNINGS*** and ***PRECAUTIONS.***)
Special Senses:	diplopia, nystagmus, blurred vision, disturbances of: taste, smell, hearing and equilibrium, usually reversible following discontinuation
Urinary System:	anuria, polyuria, renal calculi, renal failure, interstitial nephritis, hematuria (See ***WARNINGS*** and ***PRECAUTIONS.***)
Laboratory:	
Hematopoietic:	prolongation of prothrombin time
Serum chemistry:	acidosis, elevation of: serum triglycerides, serum cholesterol, serum potassium, liver function tests including: GGTP, LDH, bilirubin
Urinary:	albuminuria, candiduria

In clinical trials using multiple-dose therapy, ophthalmologic abnormalities, including cataracts and multiple punctate lenticular opacities, have been noted in patients undergoing treatment with other quinolones. The relationship of the drugs to these events is not presently established.

CRYSTALLURIA and CYLINDRURIA HAVE BEEN REPORTED with other quinolones.

OVERDOSAGE

Information on overdosage with ofloxacin is limited. One incident of accidental overdosage has been reported. In this case, an adult female received 3 grams of ofloxacin intravenously over 45 minutes. A blood sample obtained 15 minutes after the completion of the infusion revealed an ofloxacin level of 39.3 μg/mL. In 7 h, the level had fallen to 16.2 μg/mL, and by 24 h to 2.7 μg/mL. During the infusion, the patient developed drowsiness, nausea, dizziness, hot and cold flushes, subjective facial swelling and numbness, slurring of speech, and mild to moderate disorientation. All complaints except the dizziness subsided within 1 h after discontinuation of the infusion. The dizziness, most bothersome while standing, resolved in approximately 9 h. Laboratory testing reportedly revealed no clinically significant changes in routine parameters in this patient.

Patients with Normal Renal Function:

Infection†	Unit Dose	Frequency	Duration	Daily Dose
Acute Bacterial Exacerbation of Chronic Bronchitis	400 mg	q12h	10 days	800 mg
Comm. Acquired Pneumonia	400 mg	q12h	10 days	800 mg
Uncomplicated Skin and Skin Structure Infections	400 mg	q12h	10 days	800 mg
Acute, Uncomplicated Urethral and Cervical Gonorrhea	400 mg	single dose	1 day	400 mg
Nongonococcal Cervicitis/Urethritis due to *C. trachomatis*	300 mg	q12h	7 days	600 mg
Mixed Infection of the urethra and cervix due to *C. trachomatis* and *N. gonorrhoeae*	300 mg	q12h	7 days	600 mg
Acute Pelvic Inflammatory Disease	400 mg	q12h	10–14 days	800 mg
Uncomplicated Cystitis due to *E. coli* or *K. pneumoniae*	200 mg	q12h	3 days	400 mg
Uncomplicated Cystitis due to other approved pathogens	200 mg	q12h	7 days	400 mg
Complicated UTI's	200 mg	q12h	10 days	400 mg
Prostatitis due to *E. coli*	300 mg	q12h	6 weeks	600 mg

† DUE TO THE DESIGNATED PATHOGENS (See ***INDICATIONS AND USAGE.***)

Creatinine Clearance	Maintenance Dose	Frequency
20–50 mL/min	the usual recommended unit dose	q24h
< 20 mL/min	½ the usual recommended unit dose	q24h

$$\text{Men: Creatinine clearance (mL/min)} = \frac{\text{Weight (kg)} \times (140-\text{age})}{72 \times \text{serum creatinine (mg/dL)}}$$

Women: 0.85 × the value calculated for men.

In the event of an acute overdose, the stomach should be emptied. The patient should be observed and appropriate hydration maintained. Ofloxacin is not efficiently removed by hemodialysis or peritoneal dialysis.

DOSAGE AND ADMINISTRATION

The usual dose of FLOXIN (ofloxacin tablets) Tablets is 200 mg to 400 mg orally every 12 h as described in the following dosing chart. These recommendations apply to patients with normal renal function (i.e., creatinine clearance > 50 mL/min). For patients with altered renal function (i.e., creatinine clearance ≤ 50 mL/min), see the ***Patients with Impaired Renal Function*** subsection.

Patients with Normal Renal Function:

[See first table above]

Antacids containing calcium, magnesium, or aluminum; sucralfate; divalent or trivalent cations such as iron; or multivitamins containing zinc; or Videx®, (Didanosine), chewable/buffered tablets or the pediatric powder for oral solution should not be taken within the two-hour period before or within the two-hour period after taking ofloxacin. (See ***PRECAUTIONS.***)

Patients with Impaired Renal Function:

Dosage should be adjusted for patients with a creatinine clearance ≤ 50 mL/min.

After a normal initial dose, dosage should be adjusted as follows:

[See second table above]

When only the serum creatinine is known, the following formula may be used to estimate creatinine clearance.

[See third table above]

The serum creatinine should represent a steady-state of renal function.

Patients with Cirrhosis:

The excretion of ofloxacin may be reduced in patients with severe liver function disorders (e.g., cirrhosis with or without ascites). A maximum dose of 400 mg of ofloxacin per day should therefore not be exceeded.

HOW SUPPLIED

FLOXIN (ofloxacin tablets) Tablets are supplied as 200 mg light yellow, 300 mg white, and 400 mg pale gold film-coated tablets. Each tablet is distinguished by "FLOXIN" and the appropriate strength. FLOXIN Tablets are packaged in bottles and in unit-dose blister strips in the following configurations:

200 mg tablets—UROPAK unit-dose/6 tablets (NDC 0062-1540-09)
200 mg tablets—bottles of 50 (NDC 0062-1540-02)
200 mg tablets—unit-dose/100 tablets (NDC 0062-1540-05)
300 mg tablets—bottles of 50 (NDC 0062-1541-02)
300 mg tablets—unit-dose/100 tablets (NDC 0062-1541-05)
400 mg tablets—bottles of 100 (NDC 0062-1542-01)
400 mg tablets—unit-dose/100 tablets (NDC 0062-1542-05)

FLOXIN Tablets should be stored in well-closed containers. Store below 86°F (30°C).

Also Available:

Ofloxacin is also available for intravenous administration in the following configurations:

FLOXIN (ofloxacin injection) I.V. IN SINGLE-USE VIALS (10 mL) containing a concentrated solution with the equivalent of 400 mg of ofloxacin.

FLOXIN (ofloxacin injection) I.V. PRE-MIXED IN FLEXIBLE CONTAINERS (50 mL and 100 mL) containing a dilute solution with the equivalent of 200 mg or 400 mg of ofloxacin, respectively, in 5% Dextrose (D_5W).

ANIMAL PHARMACOLOGY

Ofloxacin, as well as other drugs of the quinolone class, has been shown to cause arthropathies (arthrosis) in immature dogs and rats. In addition, these drugs are associated with an increased incidence of osteochondrosis in rats as compared to the incidence observed in vehicle-treated rats. (See ***WARNINGS.***) There is no evidence of arthropathies in fully mature dogs at intravenous doses up to 3 times the recommended maximum human dose (on a mg/m^2 basis or 5 times based on mg/kg basis), for a one-week exposure period.

Long-term, high-dose systemic use of other quinolones in experimental animals has caused lenticular opacities; however, this finding was not observed in any animal studies with ofloxacin.

Reduced serum globulin and protein levels were observed in animals treated with other quinolones. In one ofloxacin study, minor decreases in serum globulin and protein levels were noted in female cynomolgus monkeys dosed orally with 40 mg/kg ofloxacin daily for one year. These changes, however, were considered to be within normal limits for monkeys.

Crystalluria and ocular toxicity were not observed in any animals treated with ofloxacin.

FLOXIN® is a trademark of ORTHO-McNEIL PHARMACEUTICAL, INC.

U.S. Patent No. 4,382,892

REFERENCES

1. National Committee for Clinical Laboratory Standards. Methods for Dilution Antimicrobial Susceptibility Tests for Bacteria That Grow Aerobically—Fourth Edition. Approved Standard NCCLS Document M7-A4, Vol. 17, No. 2, NCCLS, Wayne, PA, January, 1997.
2. National Committee for Clinical Laboratory Standards. Performance Standards for Antimicrobial Disk Susceptibility Tests—Sixth Edition. Approved Standard NCCLS Document M2-A6, Vol. 17, No. 1, NCCLS, Wayne, PA, January, 1997.

ORTHO-McNEIL
PHARMACEUTICAL, INC.
Raritan, New Jersey 08869

 Revised February 2000 7516001

Shown in Product Identification Guide, page 328

HALDOL® ℞

brand of
haloperidol
[hal 'dawl]
Tablets/Concentrate/Injection
(For Immediate Release)

DESCRIPTION

Haloperidol is the first of the butyrophenone series of major tranquilizers. The chemical designation is 4-[4-(p-chlorophenyl)-4-hydroxypiperidino]-4′-fluorobutyrophenone and it has the following structural formula:

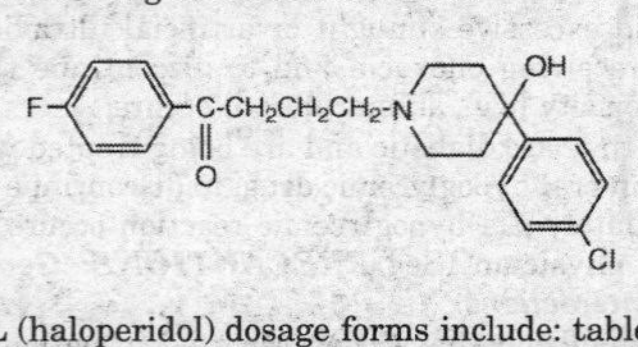

HALDOL (haloperidol) dosage forms include: tablets ($^1/_2$, 1, 2, 5, 10 and 20 mg); a concentrate with 2 mg per mL haloperidol (as the lactate); and a sterile parenteral form for intramuscular injection. The injection provides 5 mg haloperidol (as the lactate) with 1.8 mg methylparaben and 0.2 mg propylparaben per mL, and lactic acid for pH adjustment between 3.0–3.6.

Inactive ingredients: tablets—calcium phosphate, calcium stearate, corn starch and flavor—1 mg contains D&C Yellow No. 10 and FD&C Red No. 40; 2 mg contains D&C Red No. 33 and FD&C Blue No. 2; 5 mg contains FD&C Blue No. 1, D&C Yellow No. 10 and D&C Red No. 30; 10 mg contains FD&C Blue No. 1, D&C Yellow No. 10 and D&C Red No. 30; and 20 mg contains FD&C Red No. 40; concentrate - lactic acid and methylparaben.

ACTIONS

The precise mechanism of action has not been clearly established.

INDICATIONS

HALDOL (haloperidol) is indicated for use in the management of manifestations of psychotic disorders.
HALDOL is indicated for the control of tics and vocal utterances of Tourette's Disorder in children and adults.
HALDOL is effective for the treatment of severe behavior problems in children of combative, explosive hyperexcitability (which cannot be accounted for by immediate provocation). HALDOL is also effective in the short-term treatment of hyperactive children who show excessive motor activity with accompanying conduct disorders consisting of some or all of the following symptoms: impulsivity, difficulty sustaining attention, aggressivity, mood lability and poor frustration tolerance. HALDOL should be reserved for these two groups of children only after failure to respond to psychotherapy or medications other than antipsychotics.

CONTRAINDICATIONS

HALDOL haloperidol is contraindicated in severe toxic central nervous system depression or comatose states from any cause and in individuals who are hypersensitive to this drug or have Parkinson's disease.

WARNINGS

Tardive Dyskinesia

A syndrome consisting of potentially irreversible, involuntary, dyskinetic movements may develop in patients treated with antipsychotic drugs. Although the prevalence of the syndrome appears to be highest among the elderly, especially elderly women, it is impossible to rely upon prevalence estimates to predict, at the inception of antipsychotic treatment, which patients are likely to develop the syndrome. Whether antipsychotic drug products differ in their potential to cause tardive dyskinesia is unknown.
Both the risk of developing tardive dyskinesia and the likelihood that it will become irreversible are believed to increase as the duration of treatment and the total cumulative dose of antipsychotic drugs administered to the patient increase. However, the syndrome can develop, although much less commonly, after relatively brief treatment periods at low doses.
There is no known treatment for established cases of tardive dyskinesia, although the syndrome may remit, partially or completely, if antipsychotic treatment is withdrawn. Antipsychotic treatment, itself, however, may suppress (or partially suppress) the signs and symptoms of the syndrome and thereby may possibly mask the underlying process. The effect that symptomatic suppression has upon the long-term course of the syndrome is unknown.
Given these considerations, antipsychotic drugs should be prescribed in a manner that is most likely to minimize the occurrence of tardive dyskinesia. Chronic antipsychotic treatment should generally be reserved for patients who suffer from a chronic illness that, 1) is known to respond to antipsychotic drugs, and 2) for whom alternative, equally effective, but potentially less harmful treatments are **not** available or appropriate. In patients who do require chronic treatment, the smallest dose and the shortest duration of treatment producing a satisfactory clinical response should be sought. The need for continued treatment should be reassessed periodically.
If signs and symptoms of tardive dyskinesia appear in a patient on antipsychotics, drug discontinuation should be considered. However, some patients may require treatment despite the presence of the syndrome.
(For further information about the description of tardive dyskinesia and its clinical detection, please refer to ADVERSE REACTIONS.)

Neuroleptic Malignant Syndrome (NMS)

A potentially fatal symptom complex sometimes referred to as Neuroleptic Malignant Syndrome (NMS) has been reported in association with antipsychotic drugs. Clinical manifestations of NMS are hyperpyrexia, muscle rigidity, altered mental status (including catatonic signs) and evidence of autonomic instability (irregular pulse or blood pressure, tachycardia, diaphoresis, and cardiac dysrhythmias). Additional signs may include elevated creatine phosphokinase, myoglobinuria (rhabdomyolysis) and acute renal failure.
The diagnostic evaluation of patients with this syndrome is complicated. In arriving at a diagnosis, it is important to identify cases where the clinical presentation includes both serious medical illness (e.g., pneumonia, systemic infection, etc.) and untreated or inadequately treated extrapyramidal signs and symptoms (EPS). Other important considerations in the differential diagnosis include central anticholinergic toxicity, heat stroke, drug fever and primary central nervous system (CNS) pathology.
The management of NMS should include 1) immediate discontinuation of antipsychotic drugs and other drugs not essential to concurrent therapy, 2) intensive symptomatic treatment and medical monitoring, and 3) treatment of any concomitant serious medical problems for which specific treatments are available. There is no general agreement about specific pharmacological treatment regimens for uncomplicated NMS.
If a patient requires antipsychotic drug treatment after recovery from NMS, the potential reintroduction of drug therapy should be carefully considered. The patient should be carefully monitored, since recurrences of NMS have been reported.
Hyperpyrexia and heat stroke, not associated with the above symptom complex, have also been reported with HALDOL.

Usage in Pregnancy

Rodents given 2 to 20 times the usual maximum human dose of haloperidol by oral or parenteral routes showed an increase in incidence of resorption, reduced fertility, delayed delivery and pup mortality. No teratogenic effect has been reported in rats, rabbits or dogs at dosages within this range, but cleft palate has been observed in mice given 15 times the usual maximum human dose. Cleft palate in mice appears to be a nonspecific response to stress or nutritional imbalance as well as to a variety of drugs, and there is no evidence to relate this phenomenon to predictable human risk for most of these agents.
There are no well controlled studies with HALDOL (haloperidol) in pregnant women. There are reports, however, of cases of limb malformations observed following maternal use of HALDOL along with other drugs which have suspected teratogenic potential during the first trimester of pregnancy. Causal relationships were not established in these cases. Since such experience does not exclude the possibility of fetal damage due to HALDOL, this drug should be used during pregnancy or in women likely to become pregnant only if the benefit clearly justifies a potential risk to the fetus. Infants should not be nursed during drug treatment.

Combined Use of HALDOL and Lithium

An encephalopathic syndrome (characterized by weakness, lethargy, fever, tremulousness and confusion, extrapyramidal symptoms, leukocytosis, elevated serum enzymes, BUN, and FBS) followed by irreversible brain damage has occurred in a few patients treated with lithium plus HALDOL. A causal relationship between these events and the concomitant administration of lithium and HALDOL has not been established; however, patients receiving such combined therapy should be monitored closely for early evidence of neurological toxicity and treatment discontinued promptly if such signs appear.

General

A number of cases of bronchopneumonia, some fatal, have followed the use of antipsychotic drugs, including HALDOL. It has been postulated that lethargy and decreased sensation of thirst due to central inhibition may lead to dehydration, hemoconcentration and reduced pulmonary ventilation. Therefore, if the above signs and symptoms appear, especially in the elderly, the physician should institute remedial therapy promptly.
Although not reported with HALDOL, decreased serum cholesterol and/or cutaneous and ocular changes have been reported in patients receiving chemically-related drugs.
HALDOL may impair the mental and/or physical abilities required for the performance of hazardous tasks such as operating machinery or driving a motor vehicle. The ambulatory patient should be warned accordingly.
The use of alcohol with this drug should be avoided due to possible additive effects and hypotension.

PRECAUTIONS

HALDOL (haloperidol) should be administered cautiously to patients:

- with severe cardiovascular disorders, because of the possibility of transient hypotension and/or precipitation of anginal pain. Should hypotension occur and a vasopressor be required, epinephrine should not be used since HALDOL may block its vasopressor activity and paradoxical further lowering of the blood pressure may occur. Instead, metaraminol, phenylephrine or norepinephrine should be used.
- receiving anticonvulsant medications, with a history of seizures, or with EEG abnormalities, because HALDOL may lower the convulsive threshold. If indicated, adequate anticonvulsant therapy should be concomitantly maintained.
- with known allergies, or with a history of allergic reactions to drugs.
- receiving anticoagulants, since an isolated instance of interference occurred with the effects of one anticoagulant (phenindione).

If concomitant antiparkinson medication is required, it may have to be continued after HALDOL is discontinued because of the difference in excretion rates. If both are discontinued simultaneously, extrapyramidal symptoms may occur. The physician should keep in mind the possible increase in intraocular pressure when anticholinergic drugs, including antiparkinson agents, are administered concomitantly with HALDOL.
As with other antipsychotic agents, it should be noted that HALDOL may be capable of potentiating CNS depressants such as anesthetics, opiates, and alcohol.
In a study of 12 schizophrenic patients coadministered haloperidol and rifampin, plasma haloperidol levels were decreased by a mean of 70% and mean scores on the Brief Psychiatric Rating Scale were increased from baseline. In 5 other schizophrenic patients treated with haloperidol and rifampin, discontinuation of rifampin produced a mean 3.3-fold increase in haloperidol concentrations. Thus, careful monitoring of clinical status is warranted when rifampin is administered or discontinued in haloperidol-treated patients.
When HALDOL is used to control mania in cyclic disorders, there may be a rapid mood swing to depression.
Severe neurotoxicity (rigidity, inability to walk or talk) may occur in patients with thyrotoxicosis who are also receiving antipsychotic medication, including HALDOL.
No mutagenic potential of haloperidol was found in the Ames Salmonella microsomal activation assay. Negative or inconsistent positive findings have been obtained in *in vitro* and *in vivo* studies of effects of haloperidol on chromosome structure and number. The available cytogenetic evidence is considered too inconsistent to be conclusive at this time.
Carcinogenicity studies using oral haloperidol were conducted in Wistar rats (dosed at up to 5 mg/kg daily for 24 months) and in Albino Swiss mice (dosed at up to 5 mg/kg daily for 18 months). In the rat study survival was less than optimal in all dose groups, reducing the number of rats at risk for developing tumors. However, although a relatively greater number of rats survived to the end of the study in high dose male and female groups, these animals did not have a greater incidence of tumors than control animals. Therefore, although not optimal, this study does suggest the absence of a haloperidol related increase in the incidence of neoplasia in rats at doses up to 20 times the usual daily human dose for chronic or resistant patients.
In female mice at 5 and 20 times the highest initial daily dose for chronic or resistant patients, there was a statistically significant increase in mammary gland neoplasia and total tumor incidence; at 20 times the same daily dose there was a statistically significant increase in pituitary gland neoplasia. In male mice, no statistically significant differences in incidences of total tumors or specific tumor types were noted.

Antipsychotic drugs elevate prolactin levels; the elevation persists during chronic administration. Tissue culture experiments indicate that approximately one-third of human breast cancers are prolactin dependent *in vitro*, a factor of potential importance if the prescription of these drugs is contemplated in a patient with a previously detected breast cancer. Although disturbances such as galactorrhea, amenorrhea, gynecomastia, and impotence have been reported, the clinical significance of elevated serum prolactin levels is unknown for most patients. An increase in mammary neoplasms has been found in rodents after chronic administration of antipsychotic drugs. Neither clinical studies nor epidemiologic studies conducted to date, however, have shown an association between chronic administration of these drugs and mammary tumorigenesis; the available evidence is considered too limited to be conclusive at this time.
Geriatric Use—Clinical studies of haloperidol did not include sufficient numbers of subjects aged 65 and over to determine whether they respond differently from younger subjects. Other reported clinical experience has not consistently identified differences in responses between the elderly and younger patients. However, the prevalence of tardive dyskinesia appears to be highest among the elderly, especially elderly women (see WARNINGS, Tardive dyskinesia). Also, the pharmacokinetics of haloperidol in geriatric patients generally warrants the use of lower doses (see DOSAGE AND ADMINISTRATION).

ADVERSE REACTIONS

CNS Effects:

Extrapyramidal Symptoms (EPS)—EPS during the administration of HALDOL (haloperidol) have been reported frequently, often during the first few days of treatment. EPS can be categorized generally as Parkinson-like symptoms, akathisia, or dystonia (including opisthotonos and oculogyric crisis). While all can occur at relatively low doses, they occur more frequently and with greater severity at higher doses. The symptoms may be controlled with dose reductions or administration of antiparkinson drugs such as benztropine mesylate USP or trihexyphenidyl hydrochloride USP. It should be noted that persistent EPS have been reported; the drug may have to be discontinued in such cases.
Withdrawal Emergent Neurological Signs—Generally, patients receiving short-term therapy experience no problems with abrupt discontinuation of antipsychotic drugs. However, some patients on maintenance treatment experience transient dyskinetic signs after abrupt withdrawal. In certain of these cases the dyskinetic movements are indistinguishable from the syndrome described below under "Tardive Dyskinesia" except for duration. It is not known whether gradual withdrawal of antipsychotic drugs will reduce the rate of occurrence of withdrawal emergent neurological signs but until further evidence becomes available, it seems reasonable to gradually withdraw use of HALDOL.
Tardive Dyskinesia—As with all antipsychotic agents HALDOL has been associated with persistent dyskinesias. Tardive dyskinesia, a syndrome consisting of potentially irreversible, involuntary, dyskinetic movements, may appear in some patients on long-term therapy or may occur after drug therapy has been discontinued. The risk appears to be greater in elderly patients on high-dose therapy, especially females. The symptoms are persistent and in some patients appear irreversible. The syndrome is characterized by rhythmical involuntary movements of tongue, face, mouth or jaw (e.g., protrusion of tongue, puffing of cheeks, puckering of mouth, chewing movements). Sometimes these may be accompanied by involuntary movements of extremities and the trunk.
There is no known effective treatment for tardive dyskinesia; antiparkinson agents usually do not alleviate the symptoms of this syndrome. It is suggested that all antipsychotic agents be discontinued if these symptoms appear. Should it

Continued on next page

Haldol—Cont.

be necessary to reinstitute treatment, or increase the dosage of the agent, or switch to a different antipsychotic agent, this syndrome may be masked.

It has been reported that fine vermicular movement of the tongue may be an early sign of tardive dyskinesia and if the medication is stopped at that time the full syndrome may not develop.

Tardive Dystonia—Tardive dystonia, not associated with the above syndrome, has also been reported. Tardive dystonia is characterized by delayed onset of choreic or dystonic movements, is often persistent, and has the potential of becoming irreversible.

Other CNS Effects—Insomnia, restlessness, anxiety, euphoria, agitation, drowsiness, depression, lethargy, headache, confusion, vertigo, grand mal seizures, exacerbation of psychotic symptoms including hallucinations, and catatonic-like behavioral states which may be responsive to drug withdrawal and/or treatment with anticholinergic drugs.

Body as a Whole: Neuroleptic malignant syndrome (NMS), hyperpyrexia and heat stroke have been reported with HALDOL. (See WARNINGS for further information concerning NMS.)

Cardiovascular Effects: Tachycardia, hypotension, hypertension and ECG changes including prolongation of the Q-T interval and ECG pattern changes compatible with the polymorphous configuration of torsade de pointes.

Hematologic Effects: Reports have appeared citing the occurrence of mild and usually transient leukopenia and leukocytosis, minimal decreases in red blood cell counts, anemia, or a tendency toward lymphomonocytosis. Agranulocytosis has rarely been reported to have occurred with the use of HALDOL, and then only in association with other medication.

Liver Effects: Impaired liver function and/or jaundice have been reported.

Dermatologic Reactions: Maculopapular and acneiform skin reactions and isolated cases of photosensitivity and loss of hair.

Endocrine Disorders: Lactation, breast engorgement, mastalgia, menstrual irregularities, gynecomastia, impotence, increased libido, hyperglycemia, hypoglycemia and hyponatremia.

Gastrointestinal Effects: Anorexia, constipation, diarrhea, hypersalivation, dyspepsia, nausea and vomiting.

Autonomic Reactions: Dry mouth, blurred vision, urinary retention, diaphoresis and priapism.

Respiratory Effects: Laryngospasm, bronchospasm and increased depth of respiration.

Special Senses: Cataracts, retinopathy and visual disturbances.

Other: Cases of sudden and unexpected death have been reported in association with the administration of HALDOL. The nature of the evidence makes it impossible to determine definitively what role, if any, HALDOL played in the outcome of the reported cases. The possibility that HALDOL caused death cannot, of course, be excluded, but it is to be kept in mind that sudden and unexpected death may occur in psychotic patients when they go untreated or when they are treated with other antipsychotic drugs.

Postmarketing Events: Hyperammonemia has been reported in a $5^1/_2$ year old child with citrullinemia, an inherited disorder of ammonia excretion, following treatment with HALDOL.

OVERDOSAGE

Manifestations

In general, the symptoms of overdosage would be an exaggeration of known pharmacologic effects and adverse reactions, the most prominent of which would be: 1) severe extrapyramidal reactions, 2) hypotension, or 3) sedation. The patient would appear comatose with respiratory depression and hypotension which could be severe enough to produce a shock-like state. The extrapyramidal reaction would be manifest by muscular weakness or rigidity and a generalized or localized tremor as demonstrated by the akinetic or agitans types respectively. With accidental overdosage, hypertension rather than hypotension occurred in a two-year old child. The risk of ECG changes associated with torsades de pointes should be considered. (For further information regarding torsades de pointes, please refer to ADVERSE REACTIONS.)

Treatment

Gastric lavage or induction of emesis should be carried out immediately followed by administration of activated charcoal. Since there is no specific antidote, treatment is primarily supportive. A patent airway must be established by use of an oropharyngeal airway or endotracheal tube or, in prolonged cases of coma, by tracheostomy. Respiratory depression may be counteracted by artificial respiration and mechanical respirators. Hypotension and circulatory collapse may be counteracted by use of intravenous fluids, plasma, or concentrated albumin, and vasopressor agents such as metaraminol, phenylephrine and norepinephrine. Epinephrine should not be used. In case of severe extrapyramidal reactions, antiparkinson medication should be administered. ECG and vital signs should be monitored especially for signs of Q-T prolongation or dysrhythmias and monitoring should continue until the ECG is normal. Severe arrhythmias should be treated with appropriate anti-arrhythmic measures.

DOSAGE AND ADMINISTRATION

There is considerable variation from patient to patient in the amount of medication required for treatment. As with all antipsychotic drugs, dosage should be individualized according to the needs and response of each patient. Dosage adjustments, either upward or downward, should be carried out as rapidly as practicable to achieve optimum therapeutic control.

To determine the initial dosage, consideration should be given to the patient's age, severity of illness, previous response to other antipsychotic drugs, and any concomitant medication or disease state. Children, debilitated or geriatric patients, as well as those with a history of adverse reactions to antipsychotic drugs, may require less HALDOL haloperidol. The optimal response in such patients is usually obtained with more gradual dosage adjustments and at lower dosage levels, as recommended below.

Clinical experience suggests the following recommendations:

Oral Administration

Initial Dosage Range

Adults

Moderate Symptomatology	0.5 mg to 2.0 mg b.i.d. or t.i.d.
Severe Symptomatology	3.0 mg to 5.0 mg b.i.d. or t.i.d.

To achieve prompt control, higher doses may be required in some cases.

Geriatric or Debilitated Patients	0.5 mg to 2.0 mg b.i.d. or t.i.d.
Chronic or Resistant Patients	3.0 mg to 5.0 mg b.i.d. or t.i.d.

Patients who remain severly disturbed or inadequately controlled may require dosage adjustment. Daily dosages up to 100 mg may be necessary in some cases to achieve an optimal response. Infrequently, HALDOL has been used in doses above 100 mg for severely resistant patients; however, the limited clinical usage has not demonstrated the safety of prolonged administration of such doses.

Children

The following recommendations apply to children between the ages of 3 and 12 years (weight range 15 to 40 kg). HALDOL is not intended for children under 3 years old. Therapy should begin at the lowest dose possible (0.5 mg per day). If required, the dose should be increased by an increment of 0.5 mg at 5 to 7 day intervals until the desired therapeutic effect is obtained. (See chart below).

The total dose may be divided, to be given b.i.d. or t.i.d.

Psychotic Disorders	0.05 mg/kg/day to 0.15 mg/kg/day
Non-Psychotic Behavior Disorders and Tourette's Disorder	0.05 mg/kg/day to 0.075 mg/kg/day

Severely disturbed psychotic children may require higher doses. In severely disturbed, non-psychotic children or in hyperactive children with accompanying conduct disorders, who have failed to respond to psychotherapy or medications other than antipsychotics, it should be noted that since these behaviors may be short-lived, short-term administration of HALDOL may suffice. There is no evidence establishing a maximum effective dosage. There is little evidence that behavior improvement is further enhanced in dosages beyond 6 mg per day.

Maintenance Dosage

Upon achieving a satisfactory therapeutic response, dosage should then be gradually reduced to the lowest effective maintenance level.

Intramuscular Administration

Adults

Parenteral medication, administered intramuscularly in doses of 2 to 5 mg, is utilized for prompt control of the acutely agitated patient with moderately severe to very severe symptoms. Depending on the response of the patient, subsequent doses may be given, administered as often as every hour, although 4 to 8 hour intervals may be satisfactory.

Controlled trials to establish the safety and effectiveness of intramuscular administration in children have not been conducted.

Parenteral drug products should be inspected visually for particulate matter and discoloration prior to administration, whenever solution and container permit.

Switchover Procedure

The oral form should supplant the injectable as soon as practicable. In the absence of bioavailability studies establishing bioequivalence between these two dosage forms the following guidelines for dosage are suggested. For an initial approximation of the total daily dose required, the parenteral dose administered in the preceding 24 hours may be used. Since this dose is only an initial estimate, it is recommended that careful monitoring of clinical signs and symptoms, including clinical efficacy, sedation, and adverse effects, be carried out periodically for the first several days following the initiation of switchover. In this way, dosage adjustments, either upward or downward, can be quickly accomplished. Depending on the patient's clinical status, the first oral dose should be given within 12–24 hours following the last parenteral dose.

HOW SUPPLIED

HALDOL® brand of haloperidol Tablets with a cut-out "H" design, Scored, Imprinted "McNeil" and "HALDOL" with the mg strength of the tablet:

		Bottles Containing 100
1/2 mg, white	NDC 0045-0240-60	x
1 mg, yellow	NDC 0045-0241-60	x
2 mg, pink	NDC 0045-0242-60	x
5 mg, green	NDC 0045-0245-60	x
10 mg, aqua	NDC 0045-0246-60	x
20 mg, salmon	NDC 0045-0248-60	x

HALDOL® brand of haloperidol Concentrate 2 mg per mL (as the lactate) Colorless, Odorless, and Tasteless Solution—NDC 0045-0250-15, bottles of 15 mL and NDC 0045-0250-04, bottles of 120 mL.

HALDOL® brand of haloperidol Injection (For Immediate Release) 5 mg per mL (as the lactate)—NDC 0045-0255-01, units of 10 × 1 mL ampuls and NDC 0045-0255-49, 10 mL multiple-dose vial.

Store HALDOL® haloperidol Tablets at controlled room temperature (15°-30°C, 59°-86°F). Protect from light.

Store HALDOL® haloperidol Concentrate at controlled room temperature (15°-30°C, 59°-86°F). Protect from light. Do not freeze.

Store HALDOL® haloperidol Injection at controlled room temperature (15°-30°C, 59°-86°F). Protect from light. Do not freeze.

Dispense the HALDOL haloperidol tablets and concentrate in a tight, light-resistent container as defined in the official compendium.

McNEIL PHARMACEUTICAL
McNEILAB, INC.
SPRING HOUSE, PA 19477

643-94-066-4 Revised October 1998

Shown in Product Identification Guide, page 328

HALDOL® Decanoate 50 (haloperidol) ℞
HALDOL® Decanoate 100 (haloperidol) ℞

[*hal 'dawl dek "ah-nō 'ōt*]

For IM Injection Only

DESCRIPTION

Haloperidol decanoate is the decanoate ester of the butyrophenone, HALDOL (haloperidol). It has a markedly extended duration of effect. It is available in sesame oil in sterile form for intramuscular (IM) injection. The structural formula of haloperidol decanoate, 4-(4-chlorophenyl)-1-[4-(4-fluorophenyl)-4-oxobutyl]-4 piperidinyl decanoate, is:

Haloperidol decanoate is almost insoluble in water (0.01 mg/mL), but is soluble in most organic solvents.

Each mL of HALDOL Decanoate 50 for IM injection contains 50 mg haloperidol (present as haloperidol decanoate 70.52 mg) in a sesame oil vehicle, with 1.2% (w/v) benzyl alcohol as a preservative.

Each mL of HALDOL Decanoate 100 for IM injection contains 100 mg haloperidol (present as haloperidol decanoate 141.04 mg) in a sesame oil vehicle, with 1.2% (w/v) benzyl alcohol as a preservative.

CLINICAL PHARMACOLOGY

HALDOL Decanoate 50 and HALDOL Decanoate 100 are the long-acting forms of HALDOL (haloperidol). The basic effects of haloperidol decanoate are no different from those of HALDOL with the exception of duration of action. Haloperidol blocks the effects of dopamine and increases its turnover rate; however, the precise mechanism of action is unknown.

Administration of haloperidol decanoate in sesame oil results in slow and sustained release of haloperidol. The plasma concentrations of haloperidol gradually rise, reaching a peak at about 6 days after the injection, and falling thereafter, with an apparent half-life of about 3 weeks. Steady state plasma concentrations are achieved after the third or fourth dose. The relationship between dose of haloperidol decanoate and plasma haloperidol concentration is roughly linear for doses below 450 mg. It should be noted, however, that the pharmacokinetics of haloperidol decanoate following intramuscular injections can be quite variable between subjects.

INDICATIONS AND USAGE

HALDOL Decanoate 50 and HALDOL Decanoate 100 are long-acting parenteral antipsychotic drugs intended for use in the management of patients requiring prolonged parenteral antipsychotic therapy (e.g., patients with chronic schizophrenia).

CONTRAINDICATIONS

Since the pharmacologic and clinical actions of HALDOL Decanoate 50 and HALDOL Decanoate 100 are attributed to HALDOL (haloperidol) as the active medication, Contraindications, Warnings, and additional information are those of HALDOL, modified only to reflect the prolonged action.
HALDOL is contraindicated in severe toxic central nervous system depression or comatose states from any cause and in individuals who are hypersensitive to this drug or have Parkinson's disease.

WARNINGS

Tardive Dyskinesia

A syndrome consisting of potentially irreversible, involuntary, dyskinetic movements may develop in patients treated with antipsychotic drugs. Although the prevalence of the syndrome appears to be highest among the elderly, especially elderly women, it is impossible to rely upon prevalence estimates to predict, at the inception of antipsychotic treatment, which patients are likely to develop the syndrome. Whether antipsychotic drug products differ in their potential to cause tardive dyskinesia is unknown.
Both the risk of developing tardive dyskinesia and the likelihood that it will become irreversible are believed to increase as the duration of treatment and the total cumulative dose of antipsychotic drugs administered to the patient increase. However, the syndrome can develop, although much less commonly, after relatively brief treatment periods at low doses.
There is no known treatment for established cases of tardive dyskinesia, although the syndrome may remit, partially or completely, if antipsychotic treatment is withdrawn. Antipsychotic treatment, itself, however, may suppress (or partially suppress) the signs and symptoms of the syndrome and thereby may possibly mask the underlying process. The effect that symptomatic suppression has upon the long-term course of the syndrome is unknown.
Given these considerations, antipsychotic drugs should be prescribed in a manner that is most likely to minimize the occurrence of tardive dyskinesia. Chronic antipsychotic treatment should generally be reserved for patients who suffer from a chronic illness that 1) is known to respond to antipsychotic drugs, and 2) for whom alternative, equally effective, but potentially less harmful treatments are **not** available or appropriate. In patients who do require chronic treatment, the smallest dose and the shortest duration of treatment producing a satisfactory clinical response should be sought. The need for continued treatment should be reassessed periodically.
If signs and symptoms of tardive dyskinesia appear in a patient on antipsychotics, drug discontinuation should be considered. However, some patients may require treatment despite the presence of the syndrome. (For further information about the description of tardive dyskinesia and its clinical detection, please refer to ADVERSE REACTIONS.)

Neuroleptic Malignant Syndrome (NMS)

A potentially fatal symptom complex sometimes referred to as Neuroleptic Malignant Syndrome (NMS) has been reported in association with antipsychotic drugs. Clinical manifestations of NMS are hyperpyrexia, muscle rigidity, altered mental status (including catatonic signs) and evidence of autonomic instability (irregular pulse or blood pressure, tachycardia, diaphoresis, and cardiac dysrhythmias). Additional signs may include elevated creatine phosphokinase, myoglobinuria (rhabdomyolysis) and acute renal failure.
The diagnostic evaluation of patients with this syndrome is complicated. In arriving at a diagnosis, it is important to identify cases where the clinical presentation includes both serious medical illness (e.g., pneumonia, systemic infection, etc.) and untreated or inadequately treated extrapyramidal signs and symptoms (EPS). Other important considerations in the differential diagnosis include central anticholinergic toxicity, heat stroke, drug fever and primary central nervous system (CNS) pathology.
The management of NMS should include 1) immediate discontinuation of antipsychotic drugs and other drugs not essential to concurrent therapy, 2) intensive symptomatic treatment and medical monitoring, and 3) treatment of any concomitant serious medical problems for which specific treatments are available. There is no general agreement about specific pharmacological treatment regimens for uncomplicated NMS.
If a patient requires antipsychotic drug treatment after recovery from NMS, the potential reintroduction of drug therapy should be carefully considered. The patient should be carefully monitored, since recurrences of NMS have been reported.
Hyperpyrexia and heat stroke, not associated with the above symptom complex, have also been reported with HALDOL.

General

A number of cases of bronchopneumonia, some fatal, have followed the use of antipsychotic drugs, including HALDOL (haloperidol). It has been postulated that lethargy and decreased sensation of thirst due to central inhibition may lead to dehydration, hemoconcentration and reduced pulmonary ventilation. Therefore, if the above signs and symptoms appear, especially in the elderly, the physician should institute remedial therapy promptly.
Although not reported with HALDOL, decreased serum cholesterol and/or cutaneous and ocular changes have been reported in patients receiving chemically-related drugs.

PRECAUTIONS

HALDOL Decanoate 50 and HALDOL Decanoate 100 should be administered cautiously to patients:
— with severe cardiovascular disorders, because of the possibility of transient hypotension and/or precipitation of anginal pain. Should hypotension occur and a vasopressor be required, epinephrine should not be used since HALDOL (haloperidol) may block its vasopressor activity, and paradoxical further lowering of the blood pressure may occur. Instead, metaraminol, phenylephrine or norepinephrine should be used.
— receiving anticonvulsant medications, with a history of seizures, or with EEG abnormalities, because HALDOL may lower the convulsive threshold. If indicated, adequate anticonvulsant therapy should be concomitantly maintained.
— with known allergies, or with a history of allergic reactions to drugs.
— receiving anticoagulants, since an isolated instance of interference occurred with the effects of one anticoagulant (phenindione).

If concomitant antiparkinson medication is required, it may have to be continued after HALDOL Decanoate 50 or HALDOL Decanoate 100 is discontinued because of the prolonged action of haloperidol decanoate. If both drugs are discontinued simultaneously, extrapyramidal symptoms may occur. The physician should keep in mind the possible increase in intraocular pressure when anticholinergic drugs, including antiparkinson agents, are administered concomitantly with haloperidol decanoate.
In patients with thyrotoxicosis who are also receiving antipsychotic medication, including haloperidol decanoate, severe neurotoxicity (rigidity, inability to walk or talk) may occur.
When HALDOL is used to control mania in bipolar disorders, there may be a rapid mood swing to depression.

Information for Patients

Haloperidol decanoate may impair the mental and/or physical abilities required for the performance of hazardous tasks such as operating machinery or driving a motor vehicle. The ambulatory patient should be warned accordingly.
The use of alcohol with this drug should be avoided due to possible additive effects and hypotension.

Drug Interactions

An encephalopathic syndrome (characterized by weakness, lethargy, fever, tremulousness and confusion, extrapyramidal symptoms, leukocytosis, elevated serum enzymes, BUN, and FBS) followed by irreversible brain damage has occurred in a few patients treated with lithium plus HALDOL. A causal relationship between these events and the concomitant administration of lithium and HALDOL has not been established; however, patients receiving such combined therapy should be monitored closely for early evidence of neurological toxicity and treatment discontinued promptly if such signs appear.
As with other antipsychotic agents, it should be noted that HALDOL may be capable of potentiating CNS depressants such as anesthetics, opiates, and alcohol.
In a study of 12 schizophrenic patients coadministered oral haloperidol and rifampin, plasma haloperidol levels were decreased by a mean of 70% and mean scores on the Brief Psychiatric Rating Scale were increased from baseline. In 5 other schizophrenic patients treated with oral haloperidol and rifampin, discontinuation of rifampin produced a mean 3.3-fold increase in haloperidol concentrations. Thus, careful monitoring of clinical status is warranted when rifampin is administered or discontinued in haloperidol-treated patients.

Carcinogenesis, Mutagenesis, and Impairment of Fertility

No mutagenic potential of haloperidol decanoate was found in the Ames Salmonella microsomal activation assay. Negative or inconsistent positive findings have been obtained in *in vitro* and *in vivo* studies of effects of short-acting haloperidol on chromosome structure and number. The available cytogenetic evidence is considered too inconsistent to be conclusive at this time.
Carcinogenicity studies using oral haloperidol were conducted in Wistar rats (dosed at up to 5 mg/kg daily for 24 months) and in Albino Swiss mice (dosed at up to 5 mg/kg daily for 18 months). In the rat study survival was less than optimal in all dose groups, reducing the number of rats at risk for developing tumors. However, although a relatively greater number of rats survived to the end of the study in high dose male and female groups, these animals did not have a greater incidence of tumors than control animals. Therefore, although not optimal, this study does suggest the absence of a haloperidol related increase in the incidence of neoplasia in rats at doses up to 20 times the usual daily human dose for chronic or resistant patients.
In female mice at 5 and 20 times the highest initial daily dose for chronic or resistant patients, there was a statistically significant increase in mammary gland neoplasia and total tumor incidence; at 20 times the same daily dose there was a statistically significant increase in pituitary gland neoplasia. In male mice, no statistically significant differences in incidences of total tumors or specific tumor types were noted.
Antipsychotic drugs elevate prolactin levels; the elevation persists during chronic administration. Tissue culture experiments indicate that approximately one-third of human breast cancers are prolactin dependent *in vitro*, a factor of potential importance if the prescription of these drugs is contemplated in a patient with a previously detected breast cancer. Although disturbances such as galactorrhea, amenorrhea, gynecomastia, and impotence have been reported, the clinical significance of elevated serum prolactin levels is unknown for most patients.
An increase in mammary neoplasms has been found in rodents after chronic administration of antipsychotic drugs. Neither clinical studies nor epidemiologic studies conducted to date, however, have shown an association between chronic administration of these drugs and mammary tumorigenesis; the available evidence is considered too limited to be conclusive at this time.

Usage in Pregnancy

Pregnancy Category C. Rodents given up to 3 times the usual maximum human dose of haloperidol decanoate showed an increase in incidence of resorption, fetal mortality, and pup mortality. No fetal abnormalities were observed.
Cleft palate has been observed in mice given oral haloperidol at 15 times the usual maximum human dose. Cleft palate in mice appears to be a non-specific response to stress or nutritional imbalance as well as to a variety of drugs, and there is no evidence to relate this phenomenon to predictable human risk for most of these agents.
There are no adequate and well-controlled studies in pregnant women. There are reports, however, of cases of limb malformations observed following maternal use of HALDOL along with other drugs which have suspected teratogenic potential during the first trimester of pregnancy. Causal relationships were not established with these cases. Since such experience does not exclude the possibility of fetal damage due to HALDOL, haloperidol decanoate should be used during pregnancy or in women likely to become pregnant only if the benefit clearly justifies a potential risk to the fetus.

Nursing Mothers

Since haloperidol is excreted in human breast milk, infants should not be nursed during drug treatment with haloperidol decanoate.

Pediatric Use

Safety and effectiveness of haloperidol decanoate in children have not been established.

Geriatric Use

Clinical studies of haloperidol did not include sufficient numbers of subjects aged 65 and over to determine whether they respond differently from younger subjects. Other reported clinical experience has not consistently identified differences in responses between the elderly and younger patients. However, the prevalence of tardive dyskinesia appears to be highest among the elderly, especially elderly women (see WARNINGS, Tardive Dyskinesia). Also, the pharmacokinetics of haloperidol in geriatric patients generally warrants the use of lower doses (see DOSAGE AND ADMINISTRATION).

ADVERSE REACTIONS

Adverse reactions following the administration of HALDOL Decanoate 50 or HALDOL Decanoate 100 are those of HALDOL (haloperidol). Since vast experience has accumulated with HALDOL, the adverse reactions are reported for that compound as well as for haloperidol decanoate. As with all injectable medications, local tissue reactions have been reported with haloperidol decanoate.

CNS Effects:

Extrapyramidal Symptoms (EPS) —EPS during the administration of HALDOL (haloperidol) have been reported frequently, often during the first few days of treatment. EPS can be categorized generally as Parkinson-like symptoms, akathisia, or dystonia (including opisthotonos and oculogyric crisis). While all can occur at relatively low doses, they occur more frequently and with greater severity at higher doses. The symptoms may be controlled with dose reductions or administration of antiparkinson drugs such as benztropine mesylate USP or trihexyphenidyl hydrochloride USP. It should be noted that persistent EPS have been reported; the drug may have to be discontinued in such cases.
Withdrawal Emergent Neurological Signs —Generally, patients receiving short term therapy experience no problems with abrupt discontinuation of antipsychotic drugs. However, some patients on maintenance treatment experience transient dyskinetic signs after abrupt withdrawal. In certain of these cases the dyskinetic movements are indistinguishable from the syndrome described below under "Tardive Dyskinesia" except for duration. Although the long acting properties of haloperidol decanoate provide gradual withdrawal, it is not known whether gradual withdrawal of antipsychotic drugs will reduce the rate of occurrence of withdrawal emergent neurological signs.
Tardive Dyskinesia —As with all antipsychotic agents HALDOL has been associated with persistent dyskinesias. Tardive dyskinesia, a syndrome consisting of potentially ir-

Continued on next page

Haldol Decanoate—Cont.

reversible, involuntary, dyskinetic movements, may appear in some patients on long-term therapy with haloperidol decanoate or may occur after drug therapy has been discontinued. The risk appears to be greater in elderly patients on high-dose therapy, especially females. The symptoms are persistent and in some patients appear irreversible. The syndrome is characterized by rhythmical involuntary movements of tongue, face, mouth, or jaw (e.g., protrusion of tongue, puffing of cheeks, puckering of mouth, chewing movements). Sometimes these may be accompanied by involuntary movements of extremities and the trunk.
There is no known effective treatment for tardive dyskinesia; antiparkinson agents usually do not alleviate the symptoms of this syndrome. It is suggested that all antipsychotic agents be discontinued if these symptoms appear. Should it be necessary to reinstitute treatment, or increase the dosage of the agent, or switch to a different antipsychotic agent, this syndrome may be masked.
It has been reported that fine vermicular movement of the tongue may be an early sign of tardive dyskinesia and if the medication is stopped at that time the full syndrome may not develop.
Tardive Dystonia —Tardive dystonia, not associated with the above syndrome, has also been reported. Tardive dystonia is characterized by delayed onset of choreic or dystonic movements, is often persistent, and has the potential of becoming irreversible.
Other CNS effects —Insomnia, restlessness, anxiety, euphoria, agitation, drowsiness, depression, lethargy, headache, confusion, vertigo, grand mal seizures, exacerbation of psychotic symptoms including hallucinations, and catatonic-like behavioral states which may be responsive to drug withdrawal and/or treatment with anticholinergic drugs.
Body as a Whole: Neuroleptic malignant syndrome (NMS); hyperpyrexia and heat stroke have been reported with HALDOL. (See WARNINGS for further information concerning NMS.)
Cardiovascular Effects: Tachycardia, hypotension, hypertension and ECG changes including prolongation of the Q-T interval and ECG pattern changes compatible with the polymorphous configuration of torsades de pointes.
Hematologic Effects: Reports have appeared citing the occurrence of mild and usually transient leukopenia and leukocytosis, minimal decreases in red blood cell counts, anemia, or a tendency toward lymphomonocytosis. Agranulocytosis has rarely been reported to have occurred with the use of HALDOL, and then only in association with other medication.
Liver Effects: Impaired liver function and/or jaundice have been reported.
Dermatologic Reactions: Maculopapular and acneiform skin reactions and isolated cases of photosensitivity and loss of hair.
Endocrine Disorders: Lactation, breast engorgement, mastalgia, menstrual irregularities, gynecomastia, impotence, increased libido, hyperglycemia, hypoglycemia and hyponatremia.
Gastrointestinal Effects: Anorexia, constipation, diarrhea, hypersalivation, dyspepsia, nausea and vomiting.
Autonomic Reactions: Dry mouth, blurred vision, urinary retention, diaphoresis and priapism.
Respiratory Effects: Laryngospasm, bronchospasm and increased depth of respiration.
Special Senses: Cataracts, retinopathy and visual disturbances.
Other: Cases of sudden and unexpected death have been reported in association with the administration of HALDOL. The nature of the evidence makes it impossible to determine definitively what role, if any, HALDOL played in the outcome of the reported cases. The possibility that HALDOL caused death cannot, of course, be excluded, but it is to be kept in mind that sudden and unexpected death may occur in psychotic patients when they go untreated or when they are treated with other antipsychotic drugs.
Postmarketing Events: Hyperammonemia has been reported in a $5^1/_2$ year old child with citrullinemia, an inherited disorder of ammonia excretion, following treatment with HALDOL.

OVERDOSAGE

While overdosage is less likely to occur with a parenteral than with an oral medication, information pertaining to HALDOL (haloperidol) is presented, modified only to reflect the extended duration of action of haloperidol decanoate.
Manifestations —In general, the symptoms of overdosage would be an exaggeration of known pharmacologic effects and adverse reactions, the most prominent of which would be: 1) severe extrapyramidal reactions, 2) hypotension, or 3) sedation. The patient would appear comatose with respiratory depression and hypotension which could be severe enough to produce a shock-like state. The extrapyramidal reactions would be manifested by muscular weakness or rigidity and a generalized or localized tremor, as demonstrated by the akinetic or agitans types, respectively. With accidental overdosage, hypertension rather than hypotension occurred in a two-year old child. The risk of ECG changes associated with torsades de pointes should be considered. (For further information regarding torsades de pointes, please refer to ADVERSE REACTIONS.)
Treatment —Since there is no specific antidote, treatment is primarily supportive. A patent airway must be established by use of an oropharyngeal airway or endotracheal tube or, in prolonged cases of coma, by tracheostomy. Respiratory depression may be counteracted by artificial respiration and mechanical respirators. Hypotension and circulatory collapse may be counteracted by use of intravenous fluids, plasma, or concentrated albumin, and vasopressor agents such as metaraminol, phenylephrine and norepinephrine. Epinephrine should not be used. In case of severe extrapyramidal reactions, antiparkinson medication should be administered, and should be continued for several weeks, and then withdrawn gradually as extrapyramidal symptoms may emerge. ECG and vital signs should be monitored especially for signs of Q-T prolongation or dysrhythmias and monitoring should continue until the ECG is normal. Severe arrhythmias should be treated with appropriate anti-arrhythmic measures.

DOSAGE AND ADMINISTRATION

HALDOL Decanoate 50 and HALDOL Decanoate 100 should be administered by deep intramuscular injection. A 21 gauge needle is recommended. The maximum volume per injection site should not exceed 3 mL. DO NOT ADMINISTER INTRAVENOUSLY.
Parenteral drug products should be inspected visually for particulate matter and discoloration prior to administration, whenever solution and container permit.
HALDOL Decanoate 50 and HALDOL Decanoate 100 are intended for use in chronic psychotic patients who require prolonged parenteral antipsychotic therapy. These patients should be previously stabilized on antipsychotic medication before considering a conversion to haloperidol decanoate. Furthermore, it is recommended that patients being considered for haloperidol decanoate therapy have been treated with, and tolerate well, short-acting HALDOL (haloperidol) in order to reduce the possibility of an unexpected adverse sensitivity to haloperidol. Close clinical supervision is required during the initial period of dose adjustment in order to minimize the risk of overdosage or reappearance of psychotic symptoms before the next injection. During dose adjustment or episodes of exacerbation of psychotic symptoms, haloperidol decanoate therapy can be supplemented with short-acting forms of haloperidol.
The dose of HALDOL Decanoate 50 or HALDOL Decanoate 100 should be expressed in terms of its haloperidol content. The starting dose of haloperidol decanoate should be based on the patient's age, clinical history, physical condition, and response to previous antipsychotic therapy. The preferred approach to determining the minimum effective dose is to begin with lower initial doses and to adjust the dose upward as needed. For patients previously maintained on low doses of antipsychotics (e.g. up to the equivalent of 10 mg/day oral haloperidol), it is recommended that the initial dose of haloperidol decanoate be 10–15 times the previous daily dose in oral haloperidol equivalents; limited clinical experience suggests that lower initial doses may be adequate.

Initial Therapy

Conversion from oral haloperidol to haloperidol decanoate can be achieved by using an initial dose of haloperidol decanoate that is 10 to 20 times the previous daily dose in oral haloperidol equivalents.
In patients who are elderly, debilitated, or stable on low doses of oral haloperidol (e.g. up to the equivalent of 10 mg/day oral haloperidol), a range of 10 to 15 times the previous daily dose in oral haloperidol equivalents is appropriate for initial conversion.
In patients previously maintained on higher doses of antipsychotics for whom a low dose approach risks recurrence of psychiatric decompensation and in patients whose long-term use of haloperidol has resulted in a tolerance to the drug, 20 times the previous daily dose in oral haloperidol equivalents should be considered for initial conversion, with downward titration on succeeding injections.
The initial dose of haloperidol decanoate should not exceed 100 mg regardless of previous antipsychotic dose requirements. If, therefore, conversion requires more than 100 mg of haloperidol decanoate as an initial dose, that dose should be administered in two injections, i.e. a maximum of 100 mg initially followed by the balance in 3 to 7 days.

Maintenance Therapy

The maintenance dosage of haloperidol decanoate must be individualized with titration upward or downward based on therapeutic response. The usual maintenance range is 10 to 15 times the previous daily dose in oral haloperidol equivalents dependent on the clinical response of the patient. [See table below]
Close clinical supervision is required during initiation and stabilization of haloperidol decanoate therapy.
Haloperidol decanoate is usually administered monthly or every 4 weeks. However, variation in patient response may dictate a need for adjustment of the dosing interval as well as the dose (See CLINICAL PHARMACOLOGY).
Clinical experience with haloperidol decanoate at doses greater than 450 mg per month has been limited.

HALDOL DECANOATE DOSING RECOMMENDATIONS

Patients	Monthly 1st Month	Maintenance
Stabilized on low daily oral doses (up to 10 mg/day) Debilitated or Elderly	10–15 x Daily Oral Dose	10—15 x Previous Daily Oral Dose
High Dose Risk of relapse Tolerant to oral HALDOL®	20 x Daily Oral Dose	10–15 x Previous Daily Oral Dose

HOW SUPPLIED

HALDOL® (haloperidol) Decanoate 50 for IM injection, 50 mg haloperidol as 70.5 mg per mL haloperidol decanoate—NDC 0045-0253, 10 × 1 mL ampuls, 3 × 1 mL ampuls and 5 mL multiple dose vials.
HALDOL® (haloperidol) Decanoate 100 for IM injection, 100 mg haloperidol as 141.04 mg per mL haloperidol decanoate—NDC 0045-0254, 5 × 1 mL ampuls and 5 mL multiple dose vials.
Store at controlled room temperature (15°–30°C, 59°–86°F). Do not refrigerate or freeze.
Protect from light.
McNeil Pharmaceutical, McNEILAB, INC., Spring House, PA 19477
643-94-253-3 Revised October 1998
Shown in Product Identification Guide, page 328

LEVAQUIN® Tablets/Injection ℞

(levofloxacin tablets/injection)
Prescribing Information

DESCRIPTION

LEVAQUIN® (levofloxacin tablets/injection) Tablets/Injection are synthetic broad spectrum antibacterial agents for oral and intravenous administration. Chemically, levofloxacin, a chiral fluorinated carboxyquinolone, is the pure (-)-(S)-enantiomer of the racemic drug substance ofloxacin. The chemical name is (-)-(S)-9-fluoro-2,3-dihydro-3-methyl-10-(4-methyl-1-piperazinyl)-7-oxo-7H-pyrido[1,2,3-de]-1,4-benzoxazine-6-carboxylic acid hemihydrate.
The chemical structure is:

Its empirical formula is $C_{18}H_{20}FN_3O_4 \cdot {}^1/_2\ H_2O$ and its molecular weight is 370.38. Levofloxacin is a light yellowish-white to yellow-white crystal or crystalline powder. The molecule exists as a zwitterion at the pH conditions in the small intestine.
The data demonstrate that from pH 0.6 to 5.8, the solubility of levofloxacin is essentially constant (approximately 100 mg/mL). Levofloxacin is considered *soluble to freely soluble* in this pH range, as defined by USP nomenclature. Above pH 5.8, the solubility increases rapidly to its maximum at pH 6.7 (272 mg/mL) and is considered *freely soluble* in this range. Above pH 6.7, the solubility decreases and reaches a minimum value (about 50 mg/mL) at a pH of approximately 6.9.
Levofloxacin has the potential to form stable coordination compounds with many metal ions. This *in vitro* chelation potential has the following formation order: $Al^{+3}>Cu^{+2}>Zn^{+2}>Mg^{+2}>Ca^{+2}$.
LEVAQUIN Tablets are available as film-coated tablets and contain the following inactive ingredients: 250-mg (as expressed in the anhydrous form): hydroxypropyl methylcellulose, crospovidone, microcrystalline cellulose, magnesium stearate, polyethylene glycol, titanium dioxide, polysorbate 80 and synthetic red iron oxide.
500-mg (as expressed in the anhydrous form): hydroxypropyl methylcellulose, crospovidone, microcrystalline cellulose, magnesium stearate, polyethylene glycol, titanium dioxide, polysorbate 80 and synthetic red and yellow iron oxides.
LEVAQUIN Injection in Single-Use Vials is a sterile, preservative-free aqueous solution of levofloxacin with pH ranging from 3.8 to 5.8. LEVAQUIN Injection in Premix Flexible Containers is a sterile, preservative-free aqueous solution of levofloxacin with pH ranging from 3.8 to 5.8. The appearance of LEVAQUIN Injection may range from a clear yellow to a greenish-yellow solution. This does not adversely affect product potency.
LEVAQUIN Injection in Single-Use Vials contains levofloxacin in Water for Injection. LEVAQUIN Injection in Premix Flexible Containers is a dilute, non-pyrogenic, nearly isotonic premixed solution that contains levofloxacin in 5% Dextrose (D_5W). Solutions of hydrochloric acid and sodium hydroxide may have been added to adjust the pH.
The flexible container is fabricated from a specially formulated non-plasticized, thermoplastic copolyester (CR3). The

amount of water that can permeate from the container into the overwrap is insufficient to affect the solution significantly. Solutions in contact with the flexible container can leach out certain of the container's chemical components in very small amounts within the expiration period. The suitability of the container material has been confirmed by tests in animals according to USP biological tests for plastic containers.

CLINICAL PHARMACOLOGY

Absorption

Levofloxacin is rapidly and essentially completely absorbed after oral administration. Peak plasma concentrations are usually attained one to two hours after oral dosing. Following a single 60-minute intravenous infusion of 500-mg of levofloxacin to healthy volunteers, the mean peak plasma concentration attained was 6.2 μg/mL. The absolute bioavailability of a 500-mg oral dose of levofloxacin is approximately 99%.

Levofloxacin pharmacokinetics are linear and predictable after single and multiple oral and i.v. dosing regimens. Steady-state is reached within 48 hours following a 500-mg once-daily regimen. The peak and trough plasma concentrations attained following multiple once-daily oral 500-mg regimens were approximately 5.7 and 0.5 μg/mL, respectively. The peak and trough plasma concentrations attained following multiple once-daily i.v. 500-mg regimens were approximately 6.4 and 0.6 μg/mL, respectively.

Oral administration with food slightly prolongs the time to peak concentration by approximately 1 hour and slightly decreases the peak concentration by approximately 14%. Therefore, levofloxacin can be administered without regard to food.

The plasma concentration profile of levofloxacin after i.v. administration is similar and comparable in extent of exposure (AUC) to that observed for levofloxacin tablets when equal doses (mg/mg) are administered. Therefore, the oral and i.v. routes of administration can be considered interchangeable. (See following chart.)

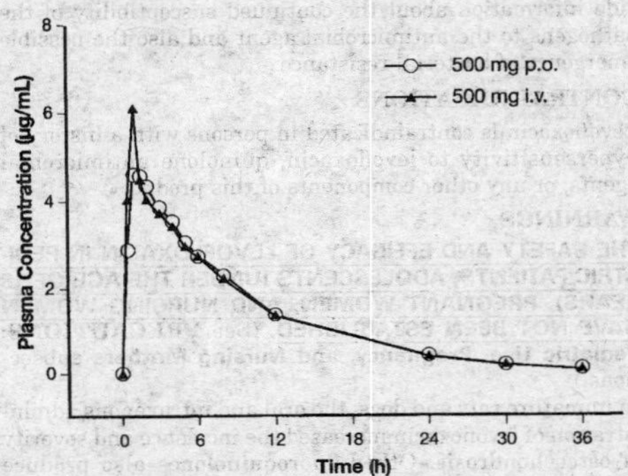

Distribution

The mean volume of distribution of levofloxacin generally ranges from 89 to 112 L after single and multiple 500-mg doses, indicating widespread distribution into body tissues. Penetration of levofloxacin into blister fluid is rapid and extensive. The blister fluid to plasma AUC ratio is approximately 1. Levofloxacin also penetrates well into lung tissues. Lung tissue concentrations were generally 2- to 5- fold higher than plasma concentrations and ranged from approximately 2.4 to 11.3 μg/g over a 24-hour period after a single 500-mg oral dose.

In vitro, over a clinically relevant range (1 to 10 μg/mL) of serum/plasma levofloxacin concentrations, levofloxacin is approximately 24 to 38% bound to serum proteins across all species studied, as determined by the equilibrium dialysis method. Levofloxacin is mainly bound to serum albumin in humans. Levofloxacin binding to serum proteins is independent of the drug concentration.

Metabolism

Levofloxacin is stereochemically stable in plasma and urine and does not invert metabolically to its enantiomer, D-ofloxacin. Levofloxacin undergoes limited metabolism in humans and is primarily excreted as unchanged drug in the urine. Following oral administration, approximately 87% of an administered dose was recovered as unchanged drug in urine within 48 hours, whereas less than 4% of the dose was recovered in feces in 72 hours. Less than 5% of an administered dose was recovered in the urine as the desmethyl and N-oxide metabolites, the only metabolites identified in humans. These metabolites have little relevant pharmacological activity.

Excretion

Levofloxacin is excreted largely as unchanged drug in the urine. The mean terminal plasma elimination half-life of levofloxacin ranges from approximately 6 to 8 hours following single or multiple doses of levofloxacin given orally or intravenously. The mean apparent total body clearance and renal clearance range from approximately 144 to 226 mL/min and 96 to 142 mL/min, respectively. Renal clearance in excess of the glomerular filtration rate suggests that tubular secretion of levofloxacin occurs in addition to its glomerular filtration. Concomitant administration of either cimetidine or probenecid results in approximately 24% and 35% reduction in the levofloxacin renal clearance, respectively, indicating that secretion of levofloxacin occurs in the renal proximal tubule. No levofloxacin crystals were found in any of the urine samples freshly collected from subjects receiving levofloxacin.

Special Populations

Geriatric: There are no significant differences in levofloxacin pharmacokinetics between young and elderly subjects when the subjects' differences in creatinine clearance are taken into consideration. Following a 500-mg oral dose of levofloxacin to healthy elderly subjects (66–80 years of age), the mean terminal plasma elimination half-life of levofloxacin was about 7.6 hours, as compared to approximately 6 hours in younger adults. The difference was attributable to the variation in renal function status of the subjects and was not believed to be clinically significant. Drug absorption appears to be unaffected by age. Levofloxacin dose adjustment based on age alone is not necessary.

Pediatric: The pharmacokinetics of levofloxacin in pediatric subjects have not been studied.

Gender: There are no significant differences in levofloxacin pharmacokinetics between male and female subjects when subjects' differences in creatinine clearance are taken into consideration. Following a 500-mg oral dose of levofloxacin to healthy male subjects, the mean terminal plasma elimination half-life of levofloxacin was about 7.5 hours, as compared to approximately 6.1 hours in female subjects. This difference was attributable to the variation in renal function status of the male and female subjects and was not believed to be clinically significant. Drug absorption appears to be unaffected by the gender of the subjects. Dose adjustment based on gender alone is not necessary.

Race: The effect of race on levofloxacin pharmacokinetics was examined through a covariate analysis performed on data from 72 subjects: 48 white and 24 nonwhite. The apparent total body clearance and apparent volume of distribution were not affected by the race of the subjects.

Renal insufficiency: Clearance of levofloxacin is reduced and plasma elimination half-life is prolonged in patients with impaired renal function (creatinine clearance ≤80 mL/min), requiring dosage adjustment in such patients to avoid accumulation. Neither hemodialysis nor continuous ambulatory peritoneal dialysis (CAPD) is effective in removal of levofloxacin from the body, indicating that supplemental doses of levofloxacin are not required following hemodialysis or CAPD. (See **PRECAUTIONS: General** and **DOSAGE AND ADMINISTRATION**.)

Hepatic insufficiency: Pharmacokinetic studies in hepatically impaired patients have not been conducted. Due to the limited extent of levofloxacin metabolism, the pharmacokinetics of levofloxacin are not expected to be affected by hepatic impairment.

Bacterial infection: The pharmacokinetics of levofloxacin in patients with serious community-acquired bacterial infections are comparable to those observed in healthy subjects.

Drug-drug interactions: The potential for pharmacokinetic drug interactions between levofloxacin and theophylline, warfarin, cyclosporine, digoxin, probenecid, cimetidine, sucralfate, and antacids has been evaluated. (See **PRECAUTIONS: Drug Interactions.**)

The mean (± SD) pharmacokinetic parameters of levofloxacin determined under single and steady state conditions following oral (p.o.) or intravenous (i.v.) doses of levofloxacin are summarized as follows:

[See table above]

Regimen	C_{max} (μg/mL)	T_{max} (h)	AUC (μg·h/mL)	CL/F[1] (mL/min)	Vd/F[2] (L)	$t_{1/2}$ (h)	CLR (mL/min)
Single dose							
250 mg p.o.[3]	2.8 ± 0.4	1.6 ± 1.0	27.2 ± 3.9	156 ± 20	ND	7.3 ± 0.9	142 ± 21
500 mg p.o.[3]*	5.1 ± 0.8	1.3 ± 0.6	47.9 ± 6.8	178 ± 28	ND	6.3 ± 0.6	103 ± 30
500 mg i.v.[3]	6.2 ± 1.0	1.0 ± 0.1	48.3 ± 5.4	175 ± 20	90 ± 11	6.4 ± 0.7	112 ± 25
Multiple dose							
500 mg q24h p.o.[3]	5.7 ± 1.4	1.1 ± 0.4	47.5 ± 6.7	175 ± 25	102 ± 22	7.6 ± 1.6	116 ± 31
500 mg q24h i.v.[3]	6.4 ± 0.8	ND	54.6 ± 11.1	158 ± 29	91 ± 12	7.0 ± 0.8	99 ± 28
500 mg or 250 mg q24h i.v., patients with bacterial infection[4]	8.7 ± 4.0[5]	ND	72.5 ± 51.2[5]	154 ± 72	111 ± 58	ND	ND
500 mg p.o. single dose, effects of gender and age:							
male[6]	5.5 ± 1.1	1.2 ± 0.4	54.4 ± 18.9	166 ± 44	89 ± 13	7.5 ± 2.1	126 ± 38
female[7]	7.0 ± 1.6	1.7 ± 0.5	67.7 ± 24.2	136 ± 44	62 ± 16	6.1 ± 0.8	106 ± 40
young[8]	5.5 ± 1.0	1.5 ± 0.6	47.5 ± 9.8	182 ± 35	83 ± 18	6.0 ± 0.9	140 ± 33
elderly[9]	7.0 ± 1.6	1.4 ± 0.5	74.7 ± 23.3	121 ± 33	67 ± 19	7.6 ± 2.0	91 ± 29
500 mg p.o. single dose, patients with renal insufficiency:							
CL_{CR} 50-80 mL/min	7.5 ± 1.8	1.5 ± 0.5	95.6 ± 11.8	88 ± 10	ND	9.1 ± 0.9	57 ± 8
CL_{CR} 20-49 mL/min	7.1 ± 3.1	2.1 ± 1.3	182.1 ± 62.6	51 ± 19	ND	27 ± 10	26 ± 13
CL_{CR} <20 mL/min	8.2 ± 2.6	1.1 ± 1.0	263.5 ± 72.5	33 ± 8	ND	35 ± 5	13 ± 3
hemodialysis	5.7 ± 1.0	2.8 ± 2.2	ND	ND	ND	76 ± 42	ND
CAPD	6.9 ± 2.3	1.4 ± 1.1	ND	ND	ND	51 ± 24	ND

[1] clearance/bioavailability
[2] volume of distribution/bioavailability
[3] healthy males 18-53 years of age
[4] 500 mg q48h for patients with moderate renal impairment (CL_{CR} 20-50 mL/min) and infections of the respiratory tract or skin
[5] dose-normalized values (to 500 mg dose), estimated by population pharmacokinetic modeling
[6] healthy males 22-75 years of age
[7] healthy females 18-80 years of age
[8] young healthy male and female subjects 18-36 years of age
[9] healthy elderly male and female subjects 66-80 years of age
* Absolute bioavailability; F = 0.99 ± 0.08; ND = not determined.

MICROBIOLOGY

Levofloxacin is the L-isomer of the racemate, ofloxacin, a quinolone antimicrobial agent. The antibacterial activity of ofloxacin resides primarily in the L-isomer. The mechanism of action of levofloxacin and other fluoroquinolone antimicrobials involves inhibition of bacterial topoisomerase IV and DNA gyrase (both of which are type II topoisomerases), enzymes required for DNA replication, transcription, repair and recombination.

Levofloxacin has *in vitro* activity against a wide range of gram-negative and gram-positive microorganisms. Levofloxacin is often bactericidal at concentrations equal to or slightly greater than inhibitory concentrations.

Fluoroquinolones, including levofloxacin, differ in chemical structure and mode of action from aminoglycosides, macrolides and β-lactam antibiotics, including penicillins. Fluoroquinolones may, therefore, be active against bacteria resistant to these antimicrobials.

Resistance to levofloxacin due to spontaneous mutation *in vitro* is a rare occurrence (range: 10^{-9} to 10^{-10}). Although cross-resistance has been observed between levofloxacin and some other fluoroquinolones, some microorganisms resistant to other fluoroquinolones may be susceptible to levofloxacin.

Levofloxacin has been shown to be active against most strains of the following microorganisms both *in vitro* and in clinical infections as described in the **INDICATIONS AND USAGE** section:

Aerobic gram-positive microorganisms

Enterococcus faecalis (many strains are only moderately susceptible)
Staphylococcus aureus (methicillin-susceptible strains)
Staphylococcus saprophyticus
Streptococcus pneumoniae (including penicillin-resistant strains*)
Streptococcus pyogenes

*Note: penicillin-resistant *S. pneumoniae* are those strains with a penicillin MIC value of ≥2 μg/mL

Aerobic gram-negative microorganisms

Enterobacter cloacae
Escherichia coli
Haemophilus influenzae
Haemophilus parainfluenzae
Klebsiella pneumoniae
Legionella pneumophila
Moraxella catarrhalis
Proteus mirabilis
Pseudomonas aeruginosa

As with other drugs in this class, some strains of *Pseudomonas aeruginosa* may develop resistance fairly rapidly during treatment with levofloxacin.

Other microorganisms

Chlamydia pneumoniae
Mycoplasma pneumoniae

The following *in vitro* data are available, **but their clinical significance is unknown.**

Levofloxacin exhibits *in vitro* minimum inhibitory concentrations (MIC values) of 2 μg/mL or less against most (≥ 90%) strains of the following microorganisms; however, the safety and effectiveness of levofloxacin in treating clinical infections due to these microorganisms have not been established in adequate and well-controlled trials.

Aerobic gram-positive microorganisms

Staphylococcus epidermidis
(methicillin-susceptible strains)

Continued on next page

Levaquin—Cont.

Streptococcus (Group C/F)
Streptococcus (Group G)
Streptococcus agalactiae
Viridans group streptococci
Aerobic gram-negative microorganisms
Acinetobacter baumannii
Acinetobacter calcoaceticus
Acinetobacter lwoffii
Bordetella pertussis
Citrobacter (diversus) koseri
Citrobacter freundii
Enterobacter aerogenes
Enterobacter sakazakii
Klebsiella oxytoca
Morganella morganii
Pantoea (Enterobacter) agglomerans
Proteus vulgaris
Providencia rettgeri
Providencia stuartii
Pseudomonas fluorescens
Serratia marcescens
Anaerobic gram-positive microorganisms
Clostridium perfringens

Susceptibility Tests

Susceptibility testing for levofloxacin should be performed, as it is the optimal predictor of activity.

Dilution techniques: Quantitative methods are used to determine antimicrobial minimal inhibitory concentrations (MIC values). These MIC values provide estimates of the susceptibility of bacteria to antimicrobial compounds. The MIC values should be determined using a standardized procedure. Standardized procedures are based on a dilution method[1] (broth or agar) or equivalent with standardized inoculum concentrations and standardized concentrations of levofloxacin powder. The MIC values should be interpreted according to the following criteria:

For testing aerobic microorganisms other than *Haemophilus influenzae, Haemophilus parainfluenzae,* and *Streptococcus* spp. including *S. pneumoniae:*

MIC (µg/mL)	Interpretation
≤2	Susceptible (S)
4	Intermediate (I)
≥8	Resistant (R)

For testing *Haemophilus influenzae* and *Haemophilus parainfluenzae.*[a]

MIC (µg/mL)	Interpretation
≤2	Susceptible (S)

[a]These interpretive standards are applicable only to broth microdilution susceptibility testing with *Haemophilus influenzae* and *Haemophilus parainfluenzae* using Haemophilus Test Medium.[1]

The current absence of data on resistant strains precludes defining any categories other than "Susceptible". Strains yielding MIC results suggestive of a "nonsusceptible" category should be submitted to a reference laboratory for further testing.

For testing *Streptococcus* spp. including *S. pneumoniae.*[b]

MIC (µg/mL)	Interpretation
≤2	Susceptible (S)
4	Intermediate (I)
≥8	Resistant (R)

[b]These interpretive standards are applicable only to broth microdilution susceptibility tests using cation-adjusted Mueller-Hinton broth with 2-5% lysed horse blood.

A report of "Susceptible" indicates that the pathogen is likely to be inhibited if the antimicrobial compound in the blood reaches the concentrations usually achievable. A report of "Intermediate" indicates that the result should be considered equivocal, and, if the microorganism is not fully susceptible to alternative, clinically feasible drugs, the test should be repeated. This category implies possible clinical applicability in body sites where the drug is physiologically concentrated or in situations where a high dosage of drug can be used. This category also provides a buffer zone which prevents small uncontrolled technical factors from causing major discrepancies in interpretation. A report of "Resistant" indicates that the pathogen is not likely to be inhibited if the antimicrobial compound in the blood reaches the concentrations usually achievable; other therapy should be selected.

Standardized susceptibility test procedures require the use of laboratory control microorganisms to control the technical aspects of the laboratory procedures. Standard levofloxacin powder should give the following MIC values:

Microorganism		MIC (µg/mL)
Enterococcus faecalis	ATCC 29212	0.25 – 2
Escherichia coli	ATCC 25922	0.008 – 0.06
Escherichia coli	ATCC 35218	0.015 – 0.06
Pseudomonas aeruginosa	ATCC 27853	0.5 – 4
Staphylococcus aureus	ATCC 29213	0.06 – 0.5
Haemophilus influenzae	ATCC 49247[c]	0.008 – 0.03
Streptococcus pneumoniae	ATCC 49619[d]	0.5 – 2

[c]This quality control range is applicable to only *H. influenzae* ATCC 49247 tested by a broth microdilution procedure using Haemophilus Test Medium (HTM).[1]

[d]This quality control range is applicable to only *S. pneumoniae* ATCC 49619 tested by a broth microdilution procedure using cation-adjusted Mueller-Hinton broth with 2-5% lysed horse blood.

Diffusion techniques: Quantitative methods that require measurement of zone diameters also provide reproducible estimates of the susceptibility of bacteria to antimicrobial compounds. One such standardized procedure[2] requires the use of standardized inoculum concentrations. This procedure uses paper disks impregnated with 5-µg levofloxacin to test the susceptibility of microorganisms to levofloxacin.

Reports from the laboratory providing results of the standard single-disk susceptibility test with a 5-µg levofloxacin disk should be interpreted according to the following criteria:

For aerobic microorganisms other than *Haemophilus influenzae, Haemophilus parainfluenzae,* and *Streptococcus* spp. including *S. pneumoniae:*

Zone diameter (mm)	Interpretation
≥17	Susceptible (S)
14–16	Intermediate (I)
≤13	Resistant (R)

For *Haemophilus influenzae* and *Haemophilus parainfluenzae.*[e]

Zone diameter (mm)	Interpretation
≥17	Susceptible (S)

[e]These interpretive standards are applicable only to disk diffusion susceptibility testing with *Haemophilus influenzae* and *Haemophilus parainfluenzae* using Haemophilus Test Medium.[2]

The current absence of data on resistant strains precludes defining any categories other than "Susceptible". Strains yielding zone diameter results suggestive of a "nonsusceptible" category should be submitted to a reference laboratory for further testing.

For *Streptococcus* spp. including *S. pneumoniae.*[f]

Zone diameter (mm)	Interpretation
≥17	Susceptible (S)
14–16	Intermediate (I)
≤13	Resistant (R)

[f]These zone diameter standards for *Streptococcus* spp. including *S. pneumoniae* apply only to tests performed using Mueller-Hinton agar supplemented with 5% sheep blood and incubated in 5% CO_2.

Interpretation should be as stated above for results using dilution techniques. Interpretation involves correlation of the diameter obtained in the disk test with the MIC for levofloxacin.

As with standardized dilution techniques, diffusion methods require the use of laboratory control microorganisms to control the technical aspects of the laboratory procedures. For the diffusion technique, the 5-µg levofloxacin disk should provide the following zone diameters in these laboratory test quality control strains:

Microorganism		Zone Diameter (mm)
Escherichia coli	ATCC 25922	29 – 37
Pseudomonas aeruginosa	ATCC 27853	19 – 26
Staphylococcus aureus	ATCC 25923	25 – 30
Haemophilus influenzae	ATCC 49247[g]	32 – 40
Streptococcus pneumoniae	ATCC 49619[h]	20 – 25

[g] This quality control range is applicable to only *H. influenzae* ATCC 49247 tested by a disk diffusion procedure using Haemophilus Test Medium (HTM).[2]

[h] This quality control range is applicable to only *S. pneumoniae* ATCC 49619 tested by a disk diffusion procedure using Mueller-Hinton agar supplemented with 5% sheep blood and incubated in 5% CO_2.

INDICATIONS AND USAGE

LEVAQUIN Tablets/Injection are indicated for the treatment of adults (≥ 18 years of age) with mild, moderate, and severe infections caused by susceptible strains of the designated microorganisms in the conditions listed below. LEVAQUIN Injection is indicated when intravenous administration offers a route of administration advantageous to the patient (e.g., patient cannot tolerate an oral dosage form). Please see **DOSAGE AND ADMINISTRATION** for specific recommendations.

Acute maxillary sinusitis due to *Streptococcus pneumoniae, Haemophilus influenzae,* or *Moraxella catarrhalis.*

Acute bacterial exacerbation of chronic bronchitis due to *Staphylococcus aureus, Streptococcus pneumoniae, Haemophilus influenzae, Haemophilus parainfluenzae,* or *Moraxella catarrhalis.*

Community-acquired pneumonia due to *Staphylococcus aureus, Streptococcus pneumoniae* (including penicillin-resistant strains, MIC value for penicillin ≥2 µg/mL), *Haemophilus influenzae, Haemophilus parainfluenzae, Klebsiella pneumoniae, Moraxella catarrhalis, Chlamydia pneumoniae, Legionella pneumophila,* or *Mycoplasma pneumoniae.* (See **CLINICAL STUDIES.**)

Uncomplicated skin and skin structure infections (mild to moderate) including abscesses, cellulitis, furuncles, impetigo, pyoderma, wound infections, due to *Staphylococcus aureus,* or *Streptococcus pyogenes.*

Complicated urinary tract infections (mild to moderate) due to *Enterococcus faecalis, Enterobacter cloacae, Escherichia coli, Klebsiella pneumoniae, Proteus mirabilis,* or *Pseudomonas aeruginosa.*

Acute pyelonephritis (mild to moderate) caused by *Escherichia coli.*

Uncomplicated urinary tract infections (mild to moderate) due to *Escherichia coli, Klebsiella pneumoniae,* or *Staphylococcus saprophyticus.*

Appropriate culture and susceptibility tests should be performed before treatment in order to isolate and identify organisms causing the infection and to determine their susceptibility to levofloxacin. Therapy with levofloxacin may be initiated before results of these tests are known; once results become available, appropriate therapy should be selected.

As with other drugs in this class, some strains of *Pseudomonas aeruginosa* may develop resistance fairly rapidly during treatment with levofloxacin. Culture and susceptibility testing performed periodically during therapy will provide information about the continued susceptibility of the pathogens to the antimicrobial agent and also the possible emergence of bacterial resistance.

CONTRAINDICATIONS

Levofloxacin is contraindicated in persons with a history of hypersensitivity to levofloxacin, quinolone antimicrobial agents, or any other components of this product.

WARNINGS

THE SAFETY AND EFFICACY OF LEVOFLOXACIN IN PEDIATRIC PATIENTS, ADOLESCENTS (UNDER THE AGE OF 18 YEARS), PREGNANT WOMEN, AND NURSING WOMEN HAVE NOT BEEN ESTABLISHED. (See **PRECAUTIONS: Pediatric Use, Pregnancy,** and **Nursing Mothers** subsections.)

In immature rats and dogs, the oral and intravenous administration of levofloxacin increased the incidence and severity of osteochondrosis. Other fluoroquinolones also produce similar erosions in the weight bearing joints and other signs of arthropathy in immature animals of various species. (See **ANIMAL PHARMACOLOGY.**)

Convulsions and toxic psychoses have been reported in patients receiving quinolones, including levofloxacin. Quinolones may also cause increased intracranial pressure and central nervous system stimulation which may lead to tremors, restlessness, anxiety, lightheadedness, confusion, hallucinations, paranoia, depression, nightmares, insomnia, and, rarely, suicidal thoughts or acts. These reactions may occur following the first dose. If these reactions occur in patients receiving levofloxacin, the drug should be discontinued and appropriate measures instituted. As with other quinolones, levofloxacin should be used with caution in patients with a known or suspected CNS disorder that may predispose to seizures or lower the seizure threshold (e.g., severe cerebral arteriosclerosis, epilepsy) or in the presence of other risk factors that may predispose to seizures or lower the seizure threshold (e.g., certain drug therapy, renal dysfunction.) (See **PRECAUTIONS: General, Information for Patients, Drug Interactions** and **ADVERSE REACTIONS.**)

Serious and occasionally fatal hypersensitivity and/or anaphylactic reactions have been reported in patients receiving therapy with quinolones, including levofloxacin. These reactions often occur following the first dose. Some reactions have been accompanied by cardiovascular collapse, hypotension/shock, seizure, loss of consciousness, tingling, angioedema (including tongue, laryngeal, throat, or facial edema/swelling), airway obstruction (including bronchospasm, shortness of breath, and acute respiratory distress), dyspnea, urticaria, itching, and other serious skin reactions. Levofloxacin should be discontinued immediately at the first appearance of a skin rash or any other sign of hypersensitivity. Serious acute hypersensitivity reactions may require treatment with epinephrine and other resuscitative measures, including oxygen, intravenous fluids, antihistamines, corticosteroids, pressor amines, and airway management, as clinically indicated. (See **PRECAUTIONS** and **ADVERSE REACTIONS.**)

Serious and sometimes fatal events, some due to hypersensitivity, and some due to uncertain etiology, have been reported rarely in patients receiving therapy with quinolones, including levofloxacin. These events may be severe and generally occur following the administration of multiple doses.

Clinical manifestations may include one or more of the following: fever, rash or severe dermatologic reactions (e.g., toxic epidermal necrolysis, Stevens-Johnson Syndrome); vasculitis; arthralgia; myalgia; serum sickness; allergic pneumonitis; interstitial nephritis; acute renal insufficiency or failure; hepatitis; jaundice; acute hepatic necrosis or failure; anemia, including hemolytic and aplastic; thrombocytopenia, including thrombotic thrombocytopenic purpura; leukopenia; agranulocytosis; pancytopenia; and/or other hematologic abnormalities. The drug should be discontinued immediately at the first appearance of a skin rash or any other sign of hypersensitivity and supportive measures instituted. (See **PRECAUTIONS: Information for Patients** and **ADVERSE REACTIONS**.)

Pseudomembranous colitis has been reported with nearly all antibacterial agents, including levofloxacin, and may range in severity from mild to life-threatening. Therefore, it is important to consider this diagnosis in patients who present with diarrhea subsequent to the administration of any antibacterial agent.

Treatment with antibacterial agents alters the normal flora of the colon and may permit overgrowth of clostridia. Studies indicate that a toxin produced by *Clostridium difficile* is one primary cause of "antibiotic-associated colitis."

After the diagnosis of pseudomembranous colitis has been established, therapeutic measures should be initiated. Mild cases of pseudomembranous colitis usually respond to drug discontinuation alone. In moderate to severe cases, consideration should be given to management with fluids and electrolytes, protein supplementation, and treatment with an antibacterial drug clinically effective against *C. difficile* colitis. (See **ADVERSE REACTIONS**.)

Ruptures of the shoulder, hand, or Achilles tendons that required surgical repair or resulted in prolonged disability have been reported in patients receiving quinolones, including levofloxacin. Levofloxacin should be discontinued if the patient experiences pain, inflammation, or rupture of a tendon. Patients should rest and refrain from exercise until the diagnosis of tendinitis or tendon rupture has been confidently excluded. Tendon rupture can occur during or after therapy with quinolones, including levofloxacin.

PRECAUTIONS

General

Because a rapid or bolus intravenous injection may result in hypotension, LEVOFLOXACIN INJECTION SHOULD ONLY BE ADMINISTERED BY SLOW INTRAVENOUS INFUSION OVER A PERIOD OF 60 MINUTES. (See **DOSAGE AND ADMINISTRATION**.)

Although levofloxacin is more soluble than other quinolones, adequate hydration of patients receiving levofloxacin should be maintained to prevent the formation of a highly concentrated urine.

Administer levofloxacin with caution in the presence of renal insufficiency. Careful clinical observation and appropriate laboratory studies should be performed prior to and during therapy since elimination of levofloxacin may be reduced. In patients with impaired renal function (creatinine clearance ≤80 mL/min), adjustment of the dosage regimen is necessary to avoid the accumulation of levofloxacin due to decreased clearance. (See **CLINICAL PHARMACOLOGY** and **DOSAGE AND ADMINISTRATION**.)

Moderate to severe phototoxicity reactions have been observed in patients exposed to direct sunlight while receiving drugs in this class. Excessive exposure to sunlight should be avoided. However, in clinical trials with levofloxacin, phototoxicity has been observed in less than 0.1% of patients. Therapy should be discontinued if phototoxicity (e.g., a skin eruption) occurs.

As with other quinolones, levofloxacin should be used with caution in any patient with a known or suspected CNS disorder that may predispose to seizures or lower the seizure threshold (e.g., severe cerebral arteriosclerosis, epilepsy) or in the presence of other risk factors that may predispose to seizures or lower the seizure threshold (e.g., certain drug therapy, renal dysfunction). (See **WARNINGS** and **Drug Interactions**.)

As with other quinolones, disturbances of blood glucose, including symptomatic hyper- and hypoglycemia, have been reported, usually in diabetic patients receiving concomitant treatment with an oral hypoglycemic agent (e.g., glyburide/glibenclamide) or with insulin. In these patients, careful monitoring of blood glucose is recommended. If a hypoglycemic reaction occurs in a patient being treated with levofloxacin, levofloxacin should be discontinued immediately and appropriate therapy should be initiated immediately. (See **Drug Interactions** and **ADVERSE REACTIONS**.)

Some quinolones have been associated with prolongation of the QT interval on the electrocardiogram and infrequent cases of arrhythmia. During post-marketing surveillance, extremely rare cases of torsades de pointes, have been reported in patients taking levofloxacin. These reports generally involve patients who had other concurrent medical conditions and the relationship to levofloxacin has not been established. Among drugs known to cause prolongation of the QT interval, the risk of arrhythmias may be reduced by avoiding use in the presence of hypokalemia, significant bradycardia, or concurrent treatment with class Ia or class III antiarrhythmic agents.

As with any potent antimicrobial drug, periodic assessment of organ system functions, including renal, hepatic, and hematopoietic, is advisable during therapy. (See **WARNINGS** and **ADVERSE REACTIONS**.)

Information for Patients

Patients should be advised:

- to drink fluids liberally;
- that antacids containing magnesium, or aluminum, as well as sucralfate, metal cations such as iron, and multivitamin preparations with zinc or Videx®, (Didanosine), chewable/buffered tablets or the pediatric powder for oral solution should be taken at least two hours before or two hours after oral levofloxacin administration. (See **Drug Interactions**);
- that oral levofloxacin can be taken without regard to meals;
- that levofloxacin may cause neurologic adverse effects (e.g., dizziness, lightheadedness) and that patients should know how they react to levofloxacin before they operate an automobile or machinery or engage in other activities requiring mental alertness and coordination. (See **WARNINGS** and **ADVERSE REACTIONS**);
- to discontinue treatment and inform their physician if they experience pain, inflammation, or rupture of a tendon, and to rest and refrain from exercise until the diagnosis of tendinitis or tendon rupture has been confidently excluded;
- that levofloxacin may be associated with hypersensitivity reactions, even following the first dose, and to discontinue the drug at the first sign of a skin rash, hives or other skin reactions, a rapid heartbeat, difficulty in swallowing or breathing, any swelling suggesting angioedema (e.g., swelling of the lips, tongue, face, tightness of the throat, hoarseness), or other symptoms of an allergic reaction. (See **WARNINGS** and **ADVERSE REACTIONS**);
- to avoid excessive sunlight or artificial ultraviolet light while receiving levofloxacin and to discontinue therapy if phototoxicity (i.e., skin eruption) occurs;
- that if they are diabetic and are being treated with insulin or an oral hypoglycemic agent and a hypoglycemic reaction occurs, they should discontinue levofloxacin and consult a physician. (See **PRECAUTIONS: General** and **Drug Interactions**.);
- that concurrent administration of warfarin and levofloxacin has been associated with increases of the International Normalized Ratio (INR) or prothrombin time and clinical episodes of bleeding. Patients should notify their physician if they are taking warfarin.
- that convulsions have been reported in patients taking quinolones, including levofloxacin, and to notify their physician before taking this drug if there is a history of this condition.

Drug Interactions

Antacids, Sucralfate, Metal Cations, Multivitamins

LEVAQUIN Tablets: While the chelation by divalent cations is less marked than with other quinolones, concurrent administration of LEVAQUIN Tablets with antacids containing magnesium, or aluminum, as well as sucralfate, metal cations such as iron, and multivitamin preparations with zinc may interfere with the gastrointestinal absorption of levofloxacin, resulting in systemic levels considerably lower than desired. Tablets with antacids containing magnesium, aluminum, as well as sucralfate, metal cations such as iron, and multivitamins preparations with zinc or Videx®, (Didanosine), chewable/buffered tablets or the pediatric powder for oral solution may substantially interfere with the gastrointestinal absorption of levofloxacin, resulting in systemic levels considerably lower than desired. These agents should be taken at least two hours before or two hours after levofloxacin administration.

LEVAQUIN Injection: There are no data concerning an interaction of **intravenous** quinolones with **oral** antacids, sucralfate, multivitamins, Videx®, (Didanosine), or metal cations. However, no quinolone should be co-administered with any solution containing multivalent cations, e.g., magnesium, through the same intravenous line. (See **DOSAGE AND ADMINISTRATION**.)

Theophylline: No significant effect of levofloxacin on the plasma concentrations, AUC, and other disposition parameters for theophylline was detected in a clinical study involving 14 healthy volunteers. Similarly, no apparent effect of theophylline on levofloxacin absorption and disposition was observed. However, concomitant administration of other quinolones with theophylline has resulted in prolonged elimination half-life, elevated serum theophylline levels, and a subsequent increase in the risk of theophylline-related adverse reactions in the patient population. Therefore, theophylline levels should be closely monitored and appropriate dosage adjustments made when levofloxacin is co-administered. Adverse reactions, including seizures, may occur with or without an elevation in serum theophylline levels. (See **WARNINGS** and **PRECAUTIONS: General**.)

Warfarin: No significant effect of levofloxacin on the peak plasma concentrations, AUC, and other disposition parameters for R- and S- warfarin was detected in a clinical study involving healthy volunteers. Similarly, no apparent effect of warfarin on levofloxacin absorption and disposition was observed. There have been reports during the post-marketing experience in patients that levofloxacin enhances the effects of warfarin. Elevations of the prothrombin time in the setting of concurrent warfarin and levofloxacin use have been associated with episodes of bleeding. Prothrombin time, International Normalized Ratio (INR), or other suitable anticoagulation tests should be closely monitored if levofloxacin is administered concomitantly with warfarin. Patients should also be monitored for evidence of bleeding.

Cyclosporine: No significant effect of levofloxacin on the peak plasma concentrations, AUC, and other disposition parameters for cyclosporine was detected in a clinical study involving healthy volunteers. However, elevated serum levels of cyclosporine have been reported in the patient population when co-administered with some other quinolones. Levofloxacin C_{max} and k_e were slightly lower while T_{max} and $t_{1/2}$ were slightly longer in the presence of cyclosporine than those observed in other studies without concomitant medication. The differences, however, are not considered to be clinically significant. Therefore, no dosage adjustment is required for levofloxacin or cyclosporine when administered concomitantly.

Digoxin: No significant effect of levofloxacin on the peak plasma concentrations, AUC, and other disposition parameters for digoxin was detected in a clinical study involving healthy volunteers. Levofloxacin absorption and disposition kinetics were similar in the presence or absence of digoxin. Therefore, no dosage adjustment for levofloxacin or digoxin is required when administered concomitantly.

Probenecid and Cimetidine: No significant effect of probenecid or cimetidine on the rate and extent of levofloxacin absorption was observed in a clinical study involving healthy volunteers. The AUC and $t_{1/2}$ of levofloxacin were 27–38% and 30% higher, respectively, while CL/F and CL_R were 21–35% lower during concomitant treatment with probenecid or cimetidine compared to levofloxacin alone. Although these differences were statistically significant, the changes were not high enough to warrant dosage adjustment for levofloxacin when probenecid or cimetidine is co-administered.

Non-steroidal anti-inflammatory drugs: The concomitant administration of a non-steroidal anti-inflammatory drug with a quinolone, including levofloxacin, may increase the risk of CNS stimulation and convulsive seizures. (See **WARNINGS** and **PRECAUTIONS: General**.)

Antidiabetic agents: Disturbances of blood glucose, including hyperglycemia and hypoglycemia, have been reported in patients treated concomitantly with quinolones and an antidiabetic agent. Therefore, careful monitoring of blood glucose is recommended when these agents are co-administered.

Carcinogenesis, Mutagenesis, Impairment of Fertility

In a long term carcinogenicity study in rats, levofloxacin exhibited no carcinogenic or tumorigenic potential following daily dietary administration for 2 years; the highest dose was 2 or 10 times the recommended human dose based on surface area or body weight, respectively.

Levofloxacin was not mutagenic in the following assays; Ames bacterial mutation assay (*S. typhimurium* and *E. coli*), CHO/HGPRT forward mutation assay, mouse micronucleus test, mouse dominant lethal test, rat unscheduled DNA synthesis assay, and the mouse sister chromatid exchange assay. It was positive in the *in vitro* chromosomal aberration (CHL cell line) and sister chromatid exchange (CHL/IU cell line) assays.

Levofloxacin caused no impairment of fertility or reproductive performance in rats at oral doses as high as 360 mg/kg/day (2124 mg/m^2), corresponding to 3.0 or 18 times the recommended maximum human dose based on surface area or body weight, respectively, and intravenous doses as high as 100 mg/kg/day (590 mg/m^2), corresponding to 1.0 or 5 times the recommended maximum human dose based on surface area or body weight, respectively.

Pregnancy: Teratogenic Effects. Pregnancy Category C.

Levofloxacin was not teratogenic in rats at oral doses as high as 810 mg/kg/day (4779 mg/m^2), which corresponds to 14 or 82 times the recommended maximum human dose based on surface area or body weight, respectively, or at intravenous doses as high as 160 mg/kg/day (944 mg/m^2) corresponding to 2.7 or 16 times the recommended maximum human dose based on surface area or body weight, respectively. Doses equivalent to 26 or 81 times the recommended maximum human dose of levofloxacin (based on surface area or body weight, respectively) caused decreased fetal body weight and increased fetal mortality in rats when administered orally at 810 mg/kg/day (8910 mg/m^2). No teratogenicity was observed when rabbits were dosed orally as high as 50 mg/kg/day (550 mg/m^2) which corresponds to 1.6 or 5.0 times the recommended maximum human dose based on surface area or body weight, respectively, or when dosed intravenously as high as 25 mg/kg/day (275 mg/m^2), corresponding to 0.8 or 2.5 times the maximum recommended human dose based on surface area or body weight, respectively.

There are, however, no adequate and well-controlled studies in pregnant women. Levofloxacin should be used during pregnancy only if the potential benefit justifies the potential risk to the fetus. (See **WARNINGS**.)

Nursing Mothers

Levofloxacin has not been measured in human milk. Based upon data from ofloxacin, it can be presumed that levofloxacin will be excreted in human milk. Because of the potential for serious adverse reactions from levofloxacin in nursing infants, a decision should be made whether to discontinue nursing or to discontinue the drug, taking into account the importance of the drug to the mother.

Pediatric Use

Safety and effectiveness in pediatric patients and adolescents below the age of 18 years have not been established.

Continued on next page

Levaquin—Cont.

Quinolones, including levofloxacin, cause arthropathy and osteochondrosis in juvenile animals of several species. (See **WARNINGS.**)

Geriatric Use

In phase 3 clinical trials, 898 levofloxacin-treated patients (26%) were ≥65 years of age. Of these, 514 patients (15%) were between the ages of 65 and 74 and 384 patients (11%) were 75 years or older. No overall differences in safety or effectiveness were observed between these subjects and younger subjects, and other reported clinical experience has not identified differences in responses between the elderly and younger patients, but greater sensitivity of some older individuals cannot be ruled out.

The pharmacokinetic properties of levofloxacin in younger adults and elderly adults do not differ significantly when creatinine clearance is taken into consideration. However since the drug is known to be substantially excreted by the kidney, the risk of toxic reactions to this drug may be greater in patients with impaired renal function. Because elderly patients are more likely to have decreased renal function, care should be taken in dose selection, and it may be useful to monitor renal function.

ADVERSE REACTIONS

The incidence of drug-related adverse reactions in patients during Phase 3 clinical trials conducted in North America was 6.2%. Among patients receiving levofloxacin therapy, 3.4% discontinued levofloxacin therapy due to adverse experiences.

In clinical trials, the following events were considered likely to be drug-related in patients receiving levofloxacin: nausea 1.3%, diarrhea 1.1%, vaginitis 0.7%, pruritus 0.5%, abdominal pain 0.4%, dizziness 0.4%, flatulence 0.4%, rash 0.4%, dyspepsia 0.3%, genital moniliasis 0.3%, insomnia 0.3%, taste perversion 0.2%, vomiting 0.2%, anorexia 0.1%, anxiety 0.1%, constipation 0.1%, edema 0.1%, fatigue 0.1%, fungal infection 0.1%, headache 0.1%, increased sweating 0.1%, leukorrhea 0.1%, malaise 0.1%, nervousness 0.1%, sleep disorders 0.1%, tremor 0.1%, urticaria 0.1%.

In clinical trials, the following events occurred in >3% of patients, regardless of drug relationship: nausea 7.1%, headache 6.4%, diarrhea 5.6%, injection site reaction 5.6%, insomnia 4.0%.

In clinical trials, the following events occurred in 1 to 3% of patients, regardless of drug relationship: constipation 2.9%, dizziness 2.9%, injection site pain 2.7%, abdominal pain 2.6%, dyspepsia 2.5%, vomiting 2.2%, rash 1.7%, flatulence 1.6%, vaginitis 1.6%, injection site inflammation 1.5%, pruritus 1.5%, fatigue 1.3%, back pain 1.2%, pain 1.2%, chest pain 1.1%, pharyngitis 1.1%, rhinitis 1.1%, taste perversion 1.0%.

In clinical trials, the following events occurred in 0.5 to less than 1% of patients, regardless of drug relationship: anorexia, anxiety, arthralgia, coughing, dry mouth, dyspnea, ear disorder (not otherwise specified), edema, fever, fungal infection, genital pruritus, increased sweating, skin disorder, somnolence.

In clinical trials, the following events, of potential medical importance, occurred at a rate of less than 0.5% regardless of drug relationship: abnormal coordination, abnormal dreaming, abnormal hepatic function, abnormal platelets, abnormal renal function, abnormal vision, acute renal failure, aggravated diabetes mellitus, aggressive reaction, agitation, anemia, angina pectoris, ARDS, arrhythmia, arthritis, arthrosis, asthenia, asthma, atrial fibrillation, bradycardia, cardiac arrest, cardiac failure, carcinoma, cerebrovascular disorder, cholelithiasis, circulatory failure, coma, confusion, conjunctivitis, convulsions (seizures), coronary thrombosis, dehydration, delirium, depression, diplopia, dysphagia, ejaculation failure, embolism (blood clot), emotional lability, epistaxis, erythema nodosum, face edema, gastroenteritis, genital moniliasis, G.I. hemorrhage, granulocytopenia, haematuria, haemoptysis, hallucination, heart block, hepatic coma, hyperglycemia, hyperkalemia, hyperkinesia, hypertension, hypertonia, hypoaesthesia, hypoglycemia, hypokalemia, hypotension, hypoxia, impaired concentration, impotence, increased LDH, involuntary muscle contractions, jaundice, leukocytosis, leukopenia, lymphadenopathy, malaise, manic reaction, mental deficiency, muscle weakness, myalgia, myocardial infarction, nervousness, palpitation, pancreatitis, paraesthesia, paralysis, paranoia, parosmia, phlebitis, pleural effusion, postural hypotension, pseudomembranous colitis, purpura, respiratory insufficiency, rhabdomyolysis, rigors, skin exfoliation, skin ulceration, sleep disorders, speech disorder, stupor, substernal chest pain, supraventricular tachycardia, syncope, synovitis, tachycardia, tendinitis, thrombocytopenia, tinnitus, tongue edema, tremor, urticaria, ventricular fibrillation, vertigo, weight decrease, WBC abnormal (not otherwise specified), withdrawal syndrome.

In clinical trials using multiple-dose therapy, ophthalmologic abnormalities, including cataracts and multiple punctate lenticular opacities, have been noted in patients undergoing treatment with other quinolones. The relationship of the drugs to these events is not presently established.

Crystalluria and cylindruria have been reported with other quinolones.

The following laboratory abnormalities appeared in 2.1 to 2.3% of patients receiving levofloxacin. It is not known whether these abnormalities were caused by the drug or the underlying condition being treated.

Patients with Normal Renal Function

Infection*	Unit Dose	Freq.	Duration**	Daily Dose
Acute Bacterial Exacerbation of Chronic Bronchitis	500 mg	q24h	7 days	500 mg
Comm. Acquired Pneumonia	500 mg	q24h	7–14 days	500 mg
Acute Maxillary Sinusitis	500 mg	q24h	10–14 days	500 mg
Uncomplicated SSSI	500 mg	q24h	7–10 days	500 mg
Complicated UTI	250 mg	q24h	10 days	250 mg
Acute pyelonephritis	250 mg	q24h	10 days	250 mg
Uncomplicated UTI	250 mg	q24h	3 days	250 mg

*DUE TO THE DESIGNATED PATHOGENS (See **INDICATIONS AND USAGE.**)
**Sequential therapy (intravenous to oral) may be instituted at the discretion of the physician.

Patients with Impaired Renal Function

Renal Status	Initial Dose	Subsequent Dose
Acute Bacterial Exacerbation of Chronic Bronchitis / Comm. Acquired Pneumonia / Acute Maxillary Sinusitis / Uncomplicated SSSI		
CL_{CR} from 50 to 80 mL/min	No dosage adjustment required	
CL_{CR} from 20 to 49 mL/min	500 mg	250 mg q24h
CL_{CR} from 10 to 19 mL/min	500 mg	250 mg q48h
Hemodialysis	500 mg	250 mg q48h
CAPD	500 mg	250 mg q48h
Complicated UTI / Acute Pyelonephritis		
CL_{CR} ≥20 mL/min	No dosage adjustment required	
CL_{CR} from 10 to 19 mL/min	250 mg	250 mg q48h
Uncomplicated UTI	No dosage adjustment required	

CL_{CR}=creatinine clearances
CAPD=chronic ambulatory peritoneal dialysis

Desired Dosage Strength	From 20 mL Vial, Withdraw Volume	Volume of Diluent	Infusion Time
250 mg	10 mL	40 mL	60 min
500 mg	20 mL	80 mL	60 min

Blood Chemistry: decreased glucose
Hematology: decreased lymphocytes

Post-Marketing Adverse Reactions

Additional adverse events reported from worldwide post-marketing experience with levofloxacin include: allergic pneumonitis, anaphylactic shock, anaphylactoid reaction, dysphonia, abnormal EEG, encephalopathy, eosinophilia, erythema multiforme, hemolytic anemia, multi-system organ failure, increased International Normalized Ratio (INR)/prothrombin time, Stevens-Johnson Syndrome, tendon rupture, torsades de pointes, vasodilation.

OVERDOSAGE

Levofloxacin exhibits a low potential for acute toxicity. Mice, rats, dogs and monkeys exhibited the following clinical signs after receiving a single high dose of levofloxacin: ataxia, ptosis, decreased locomotor activity, dyspnea, prostration, tremors, and convulsions. Doses in excess of 1500 mg/kg orally and 250 mg/kg i.v. produced significant mortality in rodents. In the event of an acute overdosage, the stomach should be emptied. The patient should be observed and appropriate hydration maintained. Levofloxacin is not efficiently removed by hemodialysis or peritoneal dialysis.

DOSAGE AND ADMINISTRATION

LEVAQUIN Injection should only be administered by intravenous infusion. It is not for intramuscular, intrathecal, intraperitoneal, or subcutaneous administration.

CAUTION: RAPID OR BOLUS INTRAVENOUS INFUSION MUST BE AVOIDED. Levofloxacin Injection should be infused intravenously slowly over a period of not less than 60 minutes. (See **PRECAUTIONS.**)

Single-use vials require dilution prior to administration. (See **PREPARATION FOR ADMINISTRATION.**)

The usual dose of LEVAQUIN Tablets/Injection is 500 mg administered orally or by slow infusion over 60 minutes every 24 hours as described in the following dosing chart. These recommendations apply to patients with normal renal function (i.e., creatinine clearance > 80 mL/min). For patients with altered renal function (i.e., creatinine clearance ≤ 80 mL/min), see the **Patients with Impaired Renal Function** subsection. Oral doses should be administered at least two hours before or two hours after antacids containing magnesium, aluminum, as well as sucralfate, metal cations such as iron, and multivitamin preparations with zinc or Videx®, (Didanosine), chewable/buffered tablets or the pediatric powder for oral solution.

Patients with Normal Renal Function

[See first table above]

Patients with Impaired Renal Function

[See second table above]

When only the serum creatinine is known, the following formula may be used to estimate creatinine clearance.

Men: Creatinine Clearance (mL/min) =

$$\frac{\text{Weight (kg)} \times (140 - \text{age})}{72 \times \text{serum creatinine (mg/dL)}}$$

Women: 0.85 × the value calculated for men.

The serum creatinine should represent a steady state of renal function.

Preparation of Levofloxacin Injection for Administration

LEVAQUIN Injection in Single-Use Vials: LEVAQUIN Injection is supplied in single-use vials containing a concentrated levofloxacin solution with the equivalent of 500 mg of levofloxacin in Water for Injection. The 20 mL vials contain 25 mg of levofloxacin/mL. **THESE LEVAQUIN INJECTION SINGLE-USE VIALS MUST BE FURTHER DILUTED WITH AN APPROPRIATE SOLUTION PRIOR TO INTRAVENOUS ADMINISTRATION.** (See **COMPATIBLE INTRAVENOUS SOLUTIONS.**) The concentration of the resulting diluted solution should be 5 mg/mL prior to administration.

This intravenous drug product should be inspected visually for particulate matter prior to administration. Samples containing visible particles should be discarded.

Since no preservative or bacteriostatic agent is present in this product, aseptic technique must be used in preparation of the final intravenous solution. **Since the vials are for single-use only, any unused portion remaining in the vial should be discarded. When used to prepare two 250 mg doses, the full content of the vial should be withdrawn at once using a single-entry procedure, and a second dose should be prepared and stored for subsequent use.** (See **Stability of LEVAQUIN Injection Following Dilution.**)

Since only limited data are available on the compatibility of levofloxacin intravenous injection with other intravenous substances, **additives or other medications should not be added to LEVAQUIN Injection in single-use vials or infused simultaneously through the same intravenous line.** If the same intravenous line is used for sequential infusion of several different drugs, the line should be flushed before and after infusion of LEVAQUIN Injection with an infusion solution compatible with LEVAQUIN Injection and with any other drug(s) administered via this common line.

Prepare the desired dosage of levofloxacin according to the following chart:

[See third table above]

For example, to prepare a 500-mg dose using the 20 mL vial (25 mg/mL), withdraw 20 mL and dilute with a compatible intravenous solution to a total volume of 100 mL.

Compatible Intravenous Solutions: Any of the following intravenous solutions may be used to prepare a 5 mg/mL levofloxacin solution with the approximate pH values:

Intravenous Fluids	Final pH of LEVAQUIN Solution
0.9% Sodium Chloride Injection, USP	4.71
5% Dextrose Injection, USP	4.58
5% Dextrose/0.9% NaCl Injection	4.62
5% Dextrose in Lactated Ringers	4.92
Plasma-Lyte® 56/5% Dextrose Injection	5.03
5% Dextrose, 0.45% Sodium Chloride, and 0.15% Potassium Chloride Injection	4.61
Sodium Lactate Injection (M/6)	5.54

LEVAQUIN Injection Premix in Single-Use Flexible Containers: LEVAQUIN Injection is also supplied in 100 mL flexible containers containing a premixed, ready-to-use levofloxacin solution in D_5W for single-use. The fill volume is either 50 or 100 mL. **NO FURTHER DILUTION OF THIS PREPARATION IS NECESSARY. Consequently each 50 mL and 100 mL premix flexible container already contains a dilute solution with the equivalent of 250 mg and 500 mg of levofloxacin, respectively (5 mg/mL) in 5% Dextrose (D_5W).** This parenteral drug product should be inspected visually for particulate matter prior to administration. Samples containing visible particles should be discarded.

Pathogen	No. Pathogens	Microbiologic Eradiction Rate (%)
H. influenzae	55	98
S. pneumoniae	83	95
S. aureus	17	88
M. catarrhalis	18	94
H. parainfluenzae	19	95
K. pneumoniae	10	100.0

Since the premix flexible containers are for single-use only, any unused portion should be discarded.

Since only limited data are available on the compatibility of levofloxacin intravenous injection with other intravenous substances, **additives or other medications should not be added to LEVAQUIN Injection in flexible containers or infused simultaneously through the same intravenous line.** If the same intravenous line is used for sequential infusion of several different drugs, the line should be flushed before and after infusion of LEVAQUIN Injection with an infusion solution compatible with LEVAQUIN Injection and with any other drug(s) administered via this common line.

Instructions for the Use of LEVAQUIN Injection Premix in Flexible Containers

To open:

1. Tear outer wrap at the notch and remove solution container.
2. Check the container for minute leaks by squeezing the inner bag firmly. If leaks are found, or if the seal is not intact, discard the solution, as the sterility may be compromised.
3. Do not use if the solution is cloudy or a precipitate is present.
4. Use sterile equipment.
5. **WARNING: Do not use flexible containers in series connections.** Such use could result in air embolism due to residual air being drawn from the primary container before administration of the fluid from the secondary container is complete.

Preparation for administration:

1. Close flow control clamp of administration set.
2. Remove cover from port at bottom of container.
3. Insert piercing pin of administration set into port with a twisting motion until the pin is firmly seated. **NOTE: See full directions on administration set carton.**
4. Suspend container from hanger.
5. Squeeze and release drip chamber to establish proper fluid level in chamber during infusion of LEVAQUIN Injection in Premix Flexible Containers.
6. Open flow control clamp to expel air from set. Close clamp.
7. Regulate rate of administration with flow control clamp.

Stability of LEVAQUIN Injection as Supplied

When stored under recommended conditions, LEVAQUIN Injection, as supplied in 20 mL vials and 100 mL flexible containers, is stable through the expiration date printed on the label.

Stability of LEVAQUIN Injection Following Dilution

LEVAQUIN Injection, when diluted in a compatible intravenous fluid to a concentration of 5 mg/mL, is stable for 72 h when stored at or below 25°C (77°F) and for 14 days when stored under refrigeration at 5°C (41°F) in plastic intravenous containers. Solutions that are diluted in a compatible intravenous solution and frozen in glass bottles or plastic intravenous containers are stable for 6 months when stored at –20°C (–4°F). **THAW FROZEN SOLUTIONS AT ROOM TEMPERATURE 25°C (77°F) OR IN A REFRIGERATOR 8°C (46°F). DO NOT FORCE THAW BY MICROWAVE IRRADIATION OR WATER BATH IMMERSION. DO NOT REFREEZE AFTER INITIAL THAWING.**

HOW SUPPLIED

LEVAQUIN Tablets

LEVAQUIN (levofloxacin tablets) Tablets are supplied as 250- and 500-mg modified rectangular, film-coated tablets. LEVAQUIN Tablets are packaged in bottles and in unit-dose blister strips in the following configurations:

250-mg tablets: color: terra cotta pink
debossing: "LEVAQUIN" on side 1 and "250" on side 2
bottles of 50 (NDC 0045-1520-50)
unit-dose/100 tablets (NDC 0045-1520-10)

500-mg tablets: color: peach
debossing: "LEVAQUIN" on side 1 and "500" on side 2
bottles of 50 (NDC 0045-1525-50)
unit-dose/100 tablets (NDC 0045-1525-10)

LEVAQUIN Tablets should be stored at 15° to 30°C (59° to 86°F) in well-closed containers.

LEVAQUIN Tablets are manufactured for ORTHO-McNEIL PHARMACEUTICAL, INC. by Johnson & Johnson Pharmaceutical Partners, Gurabo, Puerto Rico 00778.

LEVAQUIN Injection

Single-Use Vials: LEVAQUIN (levofloxacin injection) Injection is supplied in single-use vials. Each vial contains a concentrated solution with the equivalent of 500 mg of levofloxacin.

25 mg/mL, 20 mL vials (NDC 0045-0069-51)

LEVAQUIN Injection in Single-Use Vials should be stored at controlled room temperature and protected from light.

LEVAQUIN Injection in Single-Use Vials is manufactured for ORTHO-McNEIL PHARMACEUTICAL, INC. by OMJ Pharmaceuticals, Inc., San German, Puerto Rico, 00683.

Premix in Flexible Containers: LEVAQUIN (levofloxacin injection) Injection is supplied as a single-use, premixed solution in flexible containers. Each bag contains a dilute solution with the equivalent of 250 mg or 500 mg of levofloxacin, respectively, in 5% Dextrose (D_5W).

5 mg/mL (250 mg), 50 mL flexible container (NDC 0045-0067-01)

5 mg/mL (500 mg), 100 mL flexible container (NDC 0045-0068-01)

LEVAQUIN Injection Premix in Flexible Containers should be stored at or below 25°C (77°F); however, brief exposure up to 40°C (104°F) does not adversely affect the product. Avoid excessive heat and protect from freezing and light.

LEVAQUIN Injection Premix in Flexible Containers is manufactured for ORTHO-McNEIL PHARMACEUTICAL, INC. by ABBOTT Laboratories, North Chicago, IL 60064.

CLINICAL STUDIES

Community-Acquired Bacterial Pneumonia

Adult inpatients and outpatients with a diagnosis of community-acquired bacterial pneumonia were evaluated in two pivotal clinical studies. In the first study, 590 patients were enrolled in a prospective, multi-center, unblinded randomized trial comparing levofloxacin 500 mg once daily orally or intravenously for 7 to 14 days to ceftriaxone 1 to 2 grams intravenously once or in equally divided doses twice daily followed by cefuroxime axetil 500 mg orally twice daily for a total of 7 to 14 days. Patients assigned to treatment with the control regimen were allowed to receive erythromycin (or doxycycline if intolerant of erythromycin) if an infection due to atypical pathogens was suspected or proven. Clinical and microbiologic evaluations were performed during treatment, 5 to 7 days posttherapy, and 3 to 4 weeks posttherapy. Clinical success (cure plus improvement) with levofloxacin at 5 to 7 days posttherapy, the primary efficacy variable in this study, was superior (95%) to the control group (83%) [95% CI of –19,–6]. In the second study, 264 patients were enrolled in a prospective, multi-center, non-comparative trial of 500 mg levofloxacin administered orally or intravenously once daily for 7 to 14 days. Clinical success for clinically evaluable patients was 93%. For both studies, the clinical success rate in patients with atypical pneumonia due to *Chlamydia pneumoniae, Mycoplasma pneumoniae,* and *Legionella pneumophila* were 96%, 96%, and 70%, respectively. Microbiologic eradication rates across both studies were as follows:

[See table above]

Additional studies were initiated to evaluate the utility of LEVAQUIN in community-acquired pneumonia due to *S. pneumoniae*, with particular interest in penicillin-resistant strains (MIC value for penicillin ≥ 2 μg/mL). In addition to the studies previously discussed, inpatients and outpatients with mild to severe community-acquired pneumonia were evaluated in six additional clinical studies; one double-blind study, two open label randomized studies, and three open label non-comparative studies. The total number of clinically evaluable patients with *S. pneumoniae* across all 8 studies was 250 for levofloxacin and 41 for comparators. The clinical success rate (cured or improved) among the 250 levofloxacin-treated patients with *S. pneumoniae* was 245/250 (98%). The clinical success rate among the 41 comparator-treated patients with *S. pneumoniae* was 39/41 (95%).

Across these 8 studies, 18 levofloxacin-treated and 4 non-quinolone comparator-treated patients with community-acquired pneumonia due to penicillin-resistant *S. pneumoniae* (MIC value for penicillin ≥ 2 μg/mL) were identified. Of the 18 levofloxacin-treated patients, 15 were evaluable following the completion of therapy. Fifteen out of the 15 evaluable levofloxacin-treated patients with community-acquired pneumonia due to penicillin-resistant *S. pneumoniae* achieved clinical success (cure or improvement). Of these 15 patients, 6 were bacteremic and 5 were classified as having severe disease. Of the 4 comparator-treated patients with community-acquired pneumonia due to penicillin-resistant *S. pneumoniae*, 3 were evaluable for clinical efficacy. Three out of the 3 evaluable comparator-treated patients achieved clinical success. All three of the comparator-treated patients were bacteremic and had disease classified as severe.

ANIMAL PHARMACOLOGY

Levofloxacin and other quinolones have been shown to cause arthropathy in immature animals of most species tested. (See **WARNINGS.**) In immature dogs (4–5 months old), oral doses of 10 mg/kg/day for 7 days and intravenous doses of 4 mg/kg/day for 14 days of levofloxacin resulted in arthropathic lesions. Administration at oral doses of 300 mg/kg/day for 7 days and intravenous doses of 60 mg/kg/day for 4 weeks produced arthropathy in juvenile rats.

When tested in a mouse ear swelling bioassay, levofloxacin exhibited phototoxicity similar in magnitude to ofloxacin, but less phototoxicity than other quinolones.

While crystalluria has been observed in some intravenous rat studies, urinary crystals are not formed in the bladder, being present only after micturition and are not associated with nephrotoxicity.

In mice, the CNS stimulatory effect of quinolones is enhanced by concomitant administration of nonsteroidal anti-inflammatory drugs.

In dogs, levofloxacin administered at 6 mg/kg or higher by rapid intravenous injection produced hypotensive effects. These effects were considered to be related to histamine release.

In vitro and *in vivo* studies in animals indicate that levofloxacin is neither an enzyme inducer or inhibitor in the human therapeutic plasma concentration range; therefore, no drug metabolizing enzyme-related interactions with other drugs or agents are anticipated.

REFERENCES

1. National Committee for Clinical Laboratory Standards. Methods for Dilution Antimicrobial Susceptibility Tests for Bacteria That Grow Aerobically Fourth Edition. Approved Standard NCCLS Document M7-A4, Vol. 17, No. 2, NCCLS, Wayne, PA, January, 1997.
2. National Committee for Clinical Laboratory Standards. Performance Standards for Antimicrobial Disk Susceptibility Tests Sixth Edition. Approved Standard NCCLS Document M2-A6, Vol. 17, No. 1, NCCLS, Wayne, PA, January, 1997.

Patient Information About:

LEVAQUIN®
(levofloxacin tablets)
250 mg Tablets and 500 mg Tablets

This leaflet contains important information about LEVAQUIN® (levofloxacin), and should be read completely before you begin treatment. This leaflet does not take the place of discussions with your doctor or health care professional about your medical condition or your treatment. This leaflet does not list all benefits and risks of LEVAQUIN®. The medicine described here can be prescribed only by a licensed health care professional. If you have any questions about LEVAQUIN® talk to your health care professional. Only your health care professional can determine if LEVAQUIN® is right for you.

What is LEVAQUIN®?

LEVAQUIN® is a quinolone antibiotic used to treat lung, sinus, skin, and urinary tract infections caused by certain germs called bacteria. LEVAQUIN® kills many of the types of bacteria that can infect the lungs, sinuses, skin, and urinary tract and has been shown in a large number of clinical trials to be safe and effective for the treatment of bacterial infections.

Sometimes viruses rather than bacteria may infect the lungs and sinuses (for example the common cold). LEVAQUIN®, like other antibiotics, does not kill viruses.

You should contact your health care professional if you think that your condition is not improving while taking LEVAQUIN®. LEVAQUIN® Tablets are either terra cotta pink for the 250 mg tablet or peach colored for the 500 mg tablet.

How and when should I take LEVAQUIN®?

LEVAQUIN® should be taken once a day for 3, 7, 10, or 14 days depending on your prescription. It should be swallowed and may be taken with or without food. Try to take the tablet at the same time each day and drink fluids liberally.

You may begin to feel better quickly; however, in order to make sure that all bacteria are killed, you should complete the full course of medication. Do not take more than the prescribed dose of LEVAQUIN® even if you missed a dose by mistake. You should not take a double dose.

Who should not take LEVAQUIN®?

You should not take LEVAQUIN® if you have ever had a severe allergic reaction to any of the group of antibiotics known as "quinolones" such as ciprofloxacin. Serious and occasionally fatal allergic reactions have been reported in patients receiving therapy with quinolones, including LEVAQUIN®.

If you are pregnant or are planning to become pregnant while taking LEVAQUIN®, talk to your health care professional before taking this medication. LEVAQUIN® is not recommended for use during pregnancy or nursing, as the effects on the unborn child or nursing infant are unknown. LEVAQUIN® is not recommended for children.

What are possible side effects of LEVAQUIN®?

LEVAQUIN® is generally well tolerated. The most common side effects caused by LEVAQUIN®, which are usually mild, include nausea, diarrhea, itching, abdominal pain, dizziness, flatulence, rash and vaginitis in women.

You should be careful about driving or operating machinery until you are sure LEVAQUIN® is not causing dizziness.

Allergic reactions have been reported in patients receiving quinolones including LEVAQUIN®, even after just one dose. If you develop hives, skin rash or other symptoms of an allergic reaction, you should stop taking this medication and call your health care professional.

Ruptures of shoulder, hand, or Achilles tendons have been reported in patients receiving quinolones, including LEVAQUIN®. If you develop pain, swelling, or rupture of a tendon you should stop taking LEVAQUIN® and contact your health care professional.

Some quinolone antibiotics have been associated with the development of phototoxicity ("sunburns" and "blistering sunburns") following exposure to sunlight or other sources of ultraviolet light such as artificial ultraviolet light used in tanning salons. LEVAQUIN® has been infrequently associated with phototoxicity. You should avoid excessive exposure to sunlight or artificial ultraviolet light while you are taking LEVAQUIN®.

If you have diabetes and you develop a hypoglycemic reaction while on LEVAQUIN®, you should stop taking LEVAQUIN® and call your health care professional.

Continued on next page

Levaquin—Cont.

Convulsions have been reported in patients receiving quinolone antibiotics including LEVAQUIN®. If you have experienced convulsions in the past, be sure to let your physician know that you have a history of convulsions.

Quinolones, including LEVAQUIN®, may also cause central nervous system stimulation which may lead to tremors, restlessness, anxiety, lightheadedness, confusion, hallucinations, paranoia, depression, nightmares, insomnia, and, rarely, suicidal thoughts or acts.

If you notice any side-effects not mentioned in this leaflet or you have concerns about the side effects you are experiencing, please inform your health care professional.

For more complete information regarding levofloxacin, please refer to the full prescribing information, which may be obtained from your health care professional, pharmacist, or the Physicians Desk Reference (PDR).

What about other medicines I am taking?

Taking warfarin (Coumadin®) and LEVAQUIN® together can further predispose you to the development of bleeding problems. If you take warfarin, be sure to tell your health care professional.

Many antacids and multivitamins may interfere with the absorption of LEVAQUIN® and may prevent it from working properly. You should take LEVAQUIN® either 2 hours before or 2 hours after taking these products.

It is important to let your health care professional know all of the medicines you are using.

Other Information

Take your dose of LEVAQUIN® once a day.

Complete the course of medication even if you are feeling better.

Keep this medication out of the reach of children.

This information does not take the place of discussions with your doctor or health care professional about your medical condition on your treatment.

ORTHO-McNEIL
OMP DIVISION
ORTHO-McNEIL PHARMACEUTICAL, INC.
Raritan, New Jersey 08869
U.S. Patent No. 4,382,892 and U.S. Patent No. 5,053,407

Shown in Product Identification Guide, page 328

MICRONOR® Tablets ℞
(norethindrone) 0.35 mg

Patients should be counseled that this product does not protect against HIV infection (AIDS) and other sexually transmitted diseases.

DESCRIPTION

MICRONOR® 28 Day Regimen

Each tablet contains 0.35 mg norethindrone. Inactive ingredients include D&C Green No. 5, D&C Yellow No. 10, lactose, magnesium stearate, povidone and starch.

norethindrone

CLINICAL PHARMACOLOGY

1. MODE OF ACTION

MICRONOR progestin-only oral contraceptives prevent conception by suppressing ovulation in approximately half of users, thickening the cervical mucus to inhibit sperm penetration, lowering the midcycle LH and FSH peaks, slowing the movement of the ovum through the fallopian tubes, and altering the endometrium.

2. PHARMACOKINETICS

Serum progestin levels peak about two hours after oral administration, followed by rapid distribution and elimination. By 24 hours after drug ingestion, serum levels are near baseline, making efficacy dependent upon rigid adherence to the dosing schedule. There are large variations in serum levels among individual users. Progestin-only administration results in lower steady-state serum progestin levels and a shorter elimination half-life than concomitant administration with estrogens.

INDICATIONS AND USAGE

1. Indications

Progestin-only oral contraceptives are indicated for the prevention of pregnancy.

2. Efficacy

If used perfectly, the first-year failure rate for progestin-only oral contraceptives is 0.5%. However, the typical failure rate is estimated to be closer to 5%, due to late or omitted pills. Table 1 lists the pregnancy rates for users of all major methods of contraception

[See table I above]

CONTRAINDICATIONS

Progestin-only oral contraceptives (POPs) should not be used by women who currently have the following conditions:

- Known or suspected pregnancy
- Known or suspected carcinoma of the breast
- Undiagnosed abnormal genital bleeding
- Hypersensitivity to any component of this product

TABLE I: PERCENTAGE OF WOMEN EXPERIENCING AN UNINTENDED PREGNANCY DURING THE FIRST YEAR OF TYPICAL USE AND THE FIRST YEAR OF PERFECT USE OF CONTRACEPTION AND THE PERCENTAGE CONTINUING USE AT THE END OF THE FIRST YEAR. UNITED STATES.

	% of Women Experiencing an Unintended Pregnancy within the First Year of Use		% of Women Continuing Use at One Year[3]
Method (1)	Typical Use[1] (2)	Perfect Use[2] (3)	(4)
Chance[4]	85	85	
Spermicides[5]	26	6	40
Periodic abstinence	25		63
Calendar		9	
Ovulation method		3	
Sympto-Thermal[6]		2	
Post-Ovulation		1	
Withdrawal	19	4	
Cap[7]			
Parous Women	40	26	42
Nulliparous Women	20	9	56
Sponge			
Parous Women	40	20	42
Nulliparous Women	20	9	56
Diaphragm[7]	20	6	56
Condom[8]			
Female (Reality)	21	5	56
Male	14	3	61
Pill	5		71
Progestin Only		0.5	
Combined		0.1	
IUD			
Progesterone T	2.0	1.5	81
Copper T380A	0.8	0.6	78
LNg 20	0.1	0.1	81
Depo-Provera	0.3	0.3	70
Norplant and Norplant-2	0.05	0.05	88
Female Sterilization	0.5	0.5	100
Male Sterilization	0.15	0.10	100

Adapted from Trussel J. Contraceptive efficacy. In Hatcher RA, Trussel J, Stewart F, Cates W, Stewart GK, Kowal D, Guest F, Contraceptive Technology: Seventeenth Revised Edition. New York NY: Irvington Publishers, 1998, in press.

1. Among *typical* couples who initiate use of a method (not necessarily for the first time), the percentage who experience an accidental pregnancy during the first year if they do not stop use for any other reason.
2. Among couples who initiate use of a method (not necessarily for the first time) and who use it *perfectly* (both consistently and correctly), the percentage who experience an accidental pregnancy during the first year if they do not stop use for any other reason.
3. Among couples attempting to avoid pregnancy, the percentage who continue to use a method for one year.
4. The percents becoming pregnant in columns (2) and (3) are based on data from populations where contraception is not used and from women who cease using contraception in order to become pregnant. Among such populations, about 89% become pregnant within one year. This estimate was lowered slightly (to 85%) to represent the percent who would become pregnant within one year among women now relying on reversible methods of contraception if they abandoned contraception altogether.
5. Foams, creams, gels, vaginal suppositories, and vaginal film.
6. Cervical mucus (ovulation) method supplemented by calendar in the pre-ovulatory and basal body temperature in the post-ovulatory phases.
7. With spermicidal cream or jelly.
8. Without spermicides.

- Benign or malignant liver tumors
- Acute liver disease

WARNINGS

Cigarette smoking increases the risk of serious cardiovascular disease. Women who use oral contraceptives should be strongly advised not to smoke.

MICRONOR does not contain estrogen and, therefore, this insert does not discuss the serious health risks that have been associated with the estrogen component of combined oral contraceptives (COCs). The health care provider is referred to the prescribing information of combined oral contraceptives for a discussion of those risks. The relationship between progestin-only oral contraceptives and these risks is not fully defined. The physician should remain alert to the earliest manifestation of symptoms of any serious disease and discontinue oral contraceptive therapy when appropriate.

1. Ectopic Pregnancy

The incidence of ectopic pregnancies for progestin-only oral contraceptive users is 5 per 1000 woman-years. Up to 10% of pregnancies reported in clinical studies of progestin-only oral contraceptive users are extrauterine. Although symptoms of ectopic pregnancy should be watched for, a history of ectopic pregnancy need not be considered a contraindication to use of this contraceptive method. Health providers should be alert to the possibility of an ectopic pregnancy in women who become pregnant or complain of lower abdominal pain while on progestin-only oral contraceptives.

2. Delayed Follicular Atresia/Ovarian Cysts

If follicular development occurs, atresia of the follicle is sometimes delayed and the follicle may continue to grow beyond the size it would attain in a normal cycle. Generally these enlarged follicles disappear spontaneously. Often they are asymptomatic; in some cases they are associated with mild abdominal pain. Rarely they may twist or rupture, requiring surgical intervention.

3. Irregular Genital Bleeding

Irregular menstrual patterns are common among women using progestin-only oral contraceptives. If genital bleeding is suggestive of infection, malignancy or other abnormal conditions, such nonpharmacologic causes should be ruled out. If prolonged amenorrhea occurs, the possibility of pregnancy should be evaluated.

4. Carcinoma of the Breast and Reproductive Organs

Some epidemiological studies of oral contraceptive users have reported an increased relative risk of developing breast cancer, particularly at a younger age and apparently related to duration of use. These studies have predominantly involved combined oral contraceptives and there is insufficient data to determine whether the use of POPs similarly increases the risk.

A meta-analysis of 54 studies found a small increase in the frequency of having breast cancer diagnosed for women who were currently using combined oral contraceptives or had used them within the past ten years. This increase in the frequency of breast cancer diagnosis, within ten years of stopping use, was generally accounted for by cancers localized to the breast. There was no increase in the frequency of having breast cancer diagnosed ten or more years after cessation of use.

Women with breast cancer should not use oral contraceptives because the role of female hormones in breast cancer has not been fully determined.

Some studies suggest that oral contraceptive use has been associated with an increase in the risk of cervical intraepithealial neoplasia in some populations of women. However, there continues to be controversy about the extent to which such findings may be due to differences in sexual behavior and other factors. There is insufficient data to determine whether the use of POPs increases the risk of developing cervical intraepithelial neoplasia.

5. Hepatic Neoplasia

Benign hepatic adenomas are associated with combined oral contraceptive use, although the incidence of benign tumors is rare in the United States. Rupture of benign, hepatic adenomas may cause death through intraabdominal hemorrhage.

Studies have shown an increased risk of developing hepatocellular carcinoma in combined oral contraceptive users. However, these cancers are rare in the U.S. There is insufficient data to determine whether POPs increase the risk of developing hepatic neoplasia.

PRECAUTIONS

1. General
Patients should be counseled that this product does not protect against HIV infection (AIDS) and other sexually transmitted diseases.

2. Physical Examination and Follow up
It is considered good medical practice for sexually active women using oral contraceptives to have annual history and physical examinations. The physical examination may be deferred until after initiation of oral contraceptives if requested by the woman and judged appropriate by the clinician.

3. Carbohydrate and Lipid Metabolism
Some users may experience slight deterioration in glucose tolerance, with increases in plasma insulin but women with diabetes mellitus who use progestin-only oral contraceptives do not generally experience changes in their insulin requirements. Nonetheless, prediabetic and diabetic women in particular should be carefully monitored while taking POPs.
Lipid metabolism is occasionally affected in that HDL, HDL2, and apolipoprotein A-I and A-II may be decreased; hepatic lipase may be increased. There is usually no effect on total cholesterol, HDL_3, LDL, or VLDL.

4. Drug Interactions
The effectiveness of progestin-only pills is reduced by hepatic enzyme-inducing drugs such as the anticonvulsants phenytoin, carbamazepine, and barbiturates, and the antituberculosis drug rifampin. No significant interaction has been found with broad-spectrum antibiotics.

5. Interactions with Laboratory Tests
The following endocrine tests may be affected by progestin-only oral contraceptive use:

- Sex hormone-binding globulin (SHBG) concentrations may be decreased.
- Thyroxine concentrations may be decreased, due to a decrease in thyroid binding globulin (TBG).

6. Carcinogenesis
See WARNINGS section.

7. Pregnancy
Many studies have found no effects on fetal development associated with long-term use of contraceptive doses of oral progestins. The few studies of infant growth and development that have been conducted have not demonstrated significant adverse effects. It is nonetheless prudent to rule out suspected pregnancy before initiating any hormonal contraceptive use.

8. Nursing Mothers
No adverse effects have been found on breastfeeding performance or on the health, growth or development of the infant. Small amounts of progestin pass into the breast milk, resulting in steroid levels in infant plasma of 1-6% of the levels of maternal plasma.

9. Pediatric Use
Safety and efficacy of MICRONOR Tablets have been established in women of reproductive age. Safety and efficacy are expected to be the same for postpubertal adolescents under the age of 16 and for users 16 years and older. Use of this product before menarche is not indicated.

10. Fertility Following Discontinuation
The limited available data indicate a rapid return of normal ovulation and fertility following discontinuation of progestin-only oral contraceptives.

11. Headache
The onset or exacerbation of migraine or development of severe headache with focal neurological symptoms which is recurrent or persistent requires discontinuation of progestin-only contraceptives and evaluation of the cause.

INFORMATION FOR THE PATIENT

1. See Detailed Patient Labeling for detailed information.
2. Counseling issues
The following points should be discussed with prospective users before prescribing progestin-only oral contraceptives:

- The necessity of taking pills at the same time every day, including throughout all bleeding episodes.
- The need to use a backup method such as condoms and spermicides for the next 48 hours whenever a progestin-only oral contraceptive is taken 3 or more hours late.
- The potential side effects of progestin-only oral contraceptives, particularly menstrual irregularities.
- The need to inform the clinician of prolonged episodes of bleeding, amenorrhea or severe abdominal pain.
- The importance of using a barrier method in addition to progestin-only oral contraceptives if a woman is at risk of contracting or transmitting STDs/HIV.

ADVERSE REACTIONS

Adverse reactions reported with the use of POPs include:

- Menstrual irregularity is the most frequently reported side effect.
- Frequent and irregular bleeding are common, while long duration of bleeding episodes and amenorrhea are less likely.
- Headache, breast tenderness, nausea, and dizziness are increased among progestin-only oral contraceptive users in some studies.
- Androgenic side effects such as acne, hirsutism, and weight gain occur rarely.

TABLE II: PERCENTAGE OF WOMEN EXPERIENCING AN UNINTENDED PREGNANCY DURING THE FIRST YEAR OF TYPICAL USE AND THE FIRST YEAR OF PERFECT USE OF CONTRACEPTION AND THE PERCENTAGE CONTINUING USE AT THE END OF THE FIRST YEAR. UNITED STATES.

	% of Women Experiencing an Unintended Pregnancy within the First Year of Use		% of Women Continuing Use at One Year[3]
Method (1)	Typical Use[1] (2)	Perfect Use[2] (3)	(4)
Chance[4]	85	85	
Spermicides[5]	26	6	40
Periodic abstinence	25		63
Calendar		9	
Ovulation method		3	
Sympto-Thermal[6]		2	
Post-Ovulation		1	
Withdrawal	19	4	
Cap[7]			
Parous Women	40	26	42
Nulliparous Women	20	9	56
Sponge			
Parous Women	40	20	42
Nulliparous Women	20	9	56
Diaphragm[7]	20	6	56
Condom[8]			
Female (Reality)	21	5	56
Male	14	3	61
Pill	5		71
Progestin Only		0.5	
Combined		0.1	
IUD			
Progesterone T	2.0	1.5	81
Copper T380A	0.8	0.6	78
LNg 20	0.1	0.1	81
Depo-Provera	0.3	0.3	70
Norplant and Norplant-2	0.05	0.05	88
Female Sterilization	0.5	0.5	100
Male Sterilization	0.15	0.10	100

Adapted from Trussel J. Contraceptive efficacy. In Hatcher RA, Trussel J, Stewart F, Cates W, Stewart GK, Kowal D, Guest F, Contraceptive Technology: Seventeenth Revised Edition. New York NY: Irvington Publishers, 1998, in press.

1. Among *typical* couples who initiate use of a method (not necessarily for the first time), the percentage who experience an accidental pregnancy during the first year if they do not stop use for any other reason.
2. Among couples who initiate use of a method (not necessarily for the first time) and who use it *perfectly* (both consistently and correctly), the percentage who experience an accidental pregnancy during the first year if they do not stop use for any other reason.
3. Among couples attempting to avoid pregnancy, the percentage who continue to use a method for one year.
4. The percents becoming pregnant in columns (2) and (3) are based on data from populations where contraception is not used and from women who cease using contraception in order to become pregnant. Among such populations, about 89% become pregnant within one year. This estimate was lowered slightly (to 85%) to represent the percent who would become pregnant within one year among women now relying on reversible methods of contraception if they abandoned contraception altogether.
5. Foams, creams, gels, vaginal suppositories, and vaginal film.
6. Cervical mucous (ovulation) method supplemented by calendar in the pre-ovulatory and basal body temperature in the post-ovulatory phases.
7. With spermicidal cream or jelly.
8. Without spermicides.

OVERDOSAGE

There have been no reports of serious ill effects from overdosage, including ingestion by children.

DOSAGE AND ADMINISTRATION

To achieve maximum contraceptive effectiveness, MICRONOR must be taken exactly as directed. One tablet is taken every day, at the same time. Administration is continuous, with no interruption between pill packs. See Detailed Patient Labeling for detailed instruction.

HOW SUPPLIED

MICRONOR Tablets are available in a DIALPAK® Tablet Dispenser (NDC 0062-1411-01) containing 28 green tablets (0.35 mg norethindrone).
STORAGE: Store at controlled room temperature (15-30°C; 59-86°F).

REFERENCE

McCann M, and Potter L. Progestin-Only Oral Contraceptives: A Comprehensive Review. Contraception, 50:60 (Suppl. 1), December 1994.

DETAILED PATIENT LABELING

MICRONOR® (norethindrone) Tablets

This product (like all oral contraceptives) is used to prevent pregnancy. It does not protect against HIV infection (AIDS) or other sexually transmitted diseases.

DESCRIPTION

MICRONOR® 28 Day Regimen
Each tablet contains 0.35 mg norethindrone. Inactive ingredients include D&C Green No. 5, D&C Yellow No. 10, lactose, magnesium stearate, povidone and starch.

INTRODUCTION

This leaflet is about birth control pills that contain one hormone, a progestin. Please read this leaflet before you begin to take your pills. It is meant to be used along with talking with your doctor or clinic.
Progestin-only pills are often called "POPs" or "the mini-pill". POPs have less progestin than the combined birth control pill (or "the pill") which contains both an estrogen and a progestin.

HOW EFFECTIVE ARE POPs?

About 1 in 200 POP users will get pregnant in the first year if they all take POPs perfectly (that is, on time, every day). About 1 in 20 "typical" POP users (including women who are late taking pills or miss pills) gets pregnant in the first year of use. Table 2 will help you compare the efficacy of different methods.
[See table II above]

HOW DO POPs WORK?

POPs can prevent pregnancy in different ways including:

- They make the cervical mucus at the entrance to the womb (the uterus) too thick for the sperm to get through to the egg.
- They prevent ovulation (release of the egg from the ovary) in about half of the cycles.
- They also affect other hormones, the fallopian tubes and the lining of the uterus.

YOU SHOULD NOT TAKE POPs

- If there is any chance you may be pregnant.
- If you have breast cancer.
- If you have bleeding between your periods that has not been diagnosed.
- If you are taking certain drugs for epilepsy (seizures) or for TB. (See "Using POPs with Other Medicines" below.)
- If you are hypersensitive, or allergic, to any component of this product.
- If you have liver tumors, either benign or cancerous.
- If you have acute liver disease.

RISKS OF TAKING POPs

Cigarette smoking greatly increases the possibility of suffering heart attacks and strokes. Women who use oral contraceptives are strongly advised not to smoke.

WARNING: If you have sudden or severe pain in your lower abdomen or stomach area, you may have an ectopic pregnancy or an ovarian cyst. If this happens, you should contact your doctor or clinic immediately.

Continued on next page

Micronor—Cont.

Ectopic Pregnancy
An ectopic pregnancy is a pregnancy outside the womb. Because POPs protect against pregnancy, the chance of having a pregnancy outside the womb is very low. If you do get pregnant while taking POPs, you have a slightly higher chance that the pregnancy will be ectopic than do users of some other birth control methods.

Ovarian Cysts
These cysts are small sacs of fluid in the ovary. They are more common among POP users than among users of most other birth control methods. They usually disappear without treatment and rarely cause problems.

Cancer of the Reproductive Organs and Breasts
Some studies in women who use combined oral contraceptives that contain both estrogen and a progestin have reported an increase in the risk of developing breast cancer, particularly at a younger age and apparently related to duration of use. There is insufficient data to determine whether the use of POPs similarly increases this risk.
A meta-analysis of 54 studies found a small increase in the frequency of having breast cancer diagnosed for women who were currently using combined oral contraceptives or had used them within the past ten years. This increase in the frequency of breast cancer diagnosis, within ten years of stopping use, was generally accounted for by cancers localized to the breast. There was no increase in the frequency of having breast cancer diagnosed ten or more years after cessation of use.
Some studies have found an increase in the incidence of cancer of the cervix in women who use oral contraceptives. However, this finding may be related to factors other than the use of oral contraceptives and there is insufficient data to determine whether the use of POPs increases the risk of developing cancer of the cervix.

Liver Tumors
In rare cases, combined oral contraceptives can cause benign but dangerous liver tumors. These benign liver tumors can rupture and cause fatal internal bleeding. In addition, some studies report an increased risk of developing liver cancer among women who use combined oral contraceptives. However, liver cancers are rare. There is insufficient data to determine whether POPs increase the risk of liver tumors.

Diabetic Women
Diabetic women taking POPs do not generally require changes in the amount of insulin they are taking. However, your physician may monitor you more closely under these conditions.

SEXUALLY TRANSMITTED DISEASES (STDs)
WARNING: POPs do not protect against getting or giving someone HIV (AIDS) or any other STD, such as chlamydia, gonorrhea, genital warts or herpes.

SIDE EFFECTS
Irregular Bleeding:
The most common side effect of POPs is a change in menstrual bleeding. Your periods may be either early or late, and you may have some spotting between periods. Taking pills late or missing pills can result in some spotting or bleeding.

Other Side Effects:
Less common side effects include headaches, tender breasts, nausea and dizziness. Weight gain, acne and extra hair on your face and body have been reported, but are rare.
If you are concerned about any of these side effects, check with your doctor or clinic.

USING POPs WITH OTHER MEDICINES
Before taking a POP, inform your health care provider of any other medication, including over-the-counter medicine, that you may be taking.
These medicines can make POPs less effective:
Medicines for seizures such as:
- Phenytoin (Dilantin)
- Carbamazepine (Tegretol)
- Phenobarbital

Medicine for TB:
- Rifampin (Rifampicin)

Before you begin taking any new medicines be sure your doctor or clinic knows you are taking a progestin-only birth control pill.

HOW TO TAKE POPs

IMPORTANT POINTS TO REMEMBER

- POPs must be taken at the same time every day, so choose a time and then take the pill at that same time every day. Every time you take a pill late, and especially if you miss a pill, you are more likely to get pregnant.
- Start the next pack the day after the last pack is finished. There is no break between packs. Always have your next pack of pills ready.
- You may have some menstrual spotting between periods. Do not stop taking your pills if this happens.
- If you vomit soon after taking a pill, use a backup method (such as a condom and/or a spermicide) for 48 hours.
- If you want to stop taking POPs, you can do so at any time, but, if you remain sexually active and don't wish to become pregnant, be certain to use another birth control method.
- If you are not sure about how to take POPs, ask your doctor or clinic.

STARTING POPs

- It's best to take your first POP on the first day of your menstrual period.
- If you decide to take your first POP on another day, use a backup method (such as a condom and/or a spermicide) every time you have sex during the next 48 hours.
- If you have had a miscarriage or an abortion, you can start POPs the next day.

IF YOU ARE LATE OR MISS TAKING YOUR POPs

- If you are more than 3 hours late or you miss one or more POPs:

(1) **TAKE** a missed pill as soon as you remember that you missed it,
(2) **THEN** go back to taking POPs at your regular time,
(3) **BUT** be sure to use a backup method (such as a condom and/or a spermcide) every time you have sex for the next 48 hours.

- If you are not sure what to do about the pills you have missed, keep taking POPs and use a backup method until you can talk to your doctor or clinic.

IF YOU ARE BREASTFEEDING

- If you are fully breastfeeding (not giving your baby any food or formula), you may start your pills 6 weeks after delivery.
- If you are partially breastfeeding (giving your baby some food or formula), you should start taking pills by 3 weeks after delivery.

IF YOU ARE SWITCHING PILLS

- If you are switching from the combined pills to POPs, take the first POP the day after you finish the last active combined pill. Do not take any of the 7 inactive pills from the combined pill pack. You should know that many women have irregular periods after switching to POPs, but this is normal and to be expected.
- If you are switching from POPs to the combined pills, take the first active combined pill on the first day of your period, even if your POPs pack is not finished.
- If you switch to another brand of POPs, start the new brand anytime.
- If you are breastfeeding, you can switch to another method of birth control at any time, except do not switch to the combined pills until you stop breastfeeding or at least until 6 months after delivery.

PREGNANCY WHILE ON THE PILL
If you think you are pregnant, contact your physician. Even though research has shown that POPs do not cause harm to the unborn baby, it is always best not to take any drugs or medicines that you don't need when you are pregnant.
You should get a pregnancy test:
- If your period is late and you took one or more pills late or missed taking them and had sex without a backup method.
- Anytime it has been more than 45 days since the beginning of your last period.

WILL POPs AFFECT YOUR ABILITY TO GET PREGNANT LATER?
If you want to become pregnant, simply stop taking POPs. POPs will not delay your ability to get pregnant.

BREASTFEEDING
If you are breastfeeding, POPs will not affect the quality or amount of your breastmilk or the health of your nursing baby.

OVERDOSE
No serious problems have been reported when many pills were taken by accident, even by a small child, so there is usually no reason to treat an overdose.

OTHER QUESTIONS OR CONCERNS
If you have any questions or concerns, check with your doctor or clinic. You can also ask for the more detailed "Professional Labeling" written for doctors and other health care providers.

HOW TO STORE YOUR POPs
Store your POPs at room temperature (between 59° and 86°F).

ORTHO-McNEIL
PHARMACEUTICAL, INC.
Raritan, New Jersey 08869

REVISED JUNE 1998 635-10-895-5
Shown in Product Identification Guide, page 328

ORTHO-CEPT® ℞
(desogestrel and ethinyl estradiol) Tablets

Patients should be counseled that this product does not protect against HIV infection (AIDS) and other sexually transmitted diseases.

DESCRIPTION
ORTHO-CEPT 21 and ORTHO-CEPT 28 Tablets provide an oral contraceptive regimen of 21 orange round tablets each containing 0.15 mg desogestrel (13-ethyl-11-methylene-18,19-dinor-17 alpha-pregn-4-en-20-yn-17-ol) and 0.03 mg ethinyl estradiol (19-nor-17 alpha-pregna-1,3,5 (10)-trien-20-yne-3,17,diol). Inactive ingredients include vitamin E, pregelatinized starch, stearic acid, lactose, hydroxypropyl methylcellulose, polyethylene glycol, titanium dioxide, talc and ferric oxide. ORTHO-CEPT 28 also contains 7 green tablets containing the following inactive ingredients: lactose, pregelatinized starch, magnesium stearate, FD&C Blue No. 1 Aluminum Lake, ferric oxide, hydroxypropyl methylcellulose, polyethylene glycol, titanium dioxide and talc.

desogestrel

H_3C OH
H_2C —C≡CH

ethinyl estradiol

CH_3 OH
—C≡CH
HO

CLINICAL PHARMACOLOGY
Pharmacodynamics
Combination oral contraceptives act by suppression of gonadotropins. Although the primary mechanism of this action is inhibition of ovulation, other alterations include changes in the cervical mucus, which increase the difficulty of sperm entry into the uterus, and changes in the endometrium which reduce the likelihood of implantation.
Receptor binding studies, as well as studies in animals and humans, have shown that 3-keto-desogestrel, the biologically active metabolite of desogestrel, combines high progestational activity with minimal intrinsic androgenicity[91,92]. Desogestrel, in combination with ethinyl estradiol, does not counteract the estrogen-induced increases in SHBG, resulting in lower serum levels of free testosterone[96–99].
Pharmacokinetics
Desogestrel is rapidly and almost completely absorbed and converted into 3-keto-desogestrel, its biologically active metabolite. Following oral administration, the relative bioavailability of desogestrel, as measured by serum levels of 3-keto-desogestrel, is approximately 84%.
In the third cycle of use after a single dose of ORTHO-CEPT, maximum concentrations of 3-keto-desogestrel of 2,805±1,203 pg/mL (mean±SD) are reached at 1.4±0.8 hours. The area under the curve ($AUC_{0-\infty}$) is 33,858±11,043 pg/mL·hr after a single dose. At steady state, attained from at least day 19 onwards, maximum concentrations of 5,840±1,667 pg/mL are reached at 1.4±0.9 hours. The minimum plasma levels of 3-keto-desogestrel at steady state are 1,400±560 pg/mL. The AUC_{0-24} at steady state is 52,299±17,878 pg/mL·hr. The mean $AUC_{0-\infty}$ for 3-keto-desogestrel at single dose is significantly lower than the mean AUC_{0-24} at steady state. This indicates that the kinetics of 3-keto-desogestrel are non-linear due to an increase in binding of 3-keto-desogestrel to sex hormone-binding globulin in the cycle, attributed to increased sex hormone-binding globulin levels which are induced by the daily administration of ethinyl estradiol. Sex hormone-binding globulin levels increased significantly in the third treatment cycle from day 1 (150±64 nmol/L) to day 21 (230±59 nmol/L).
The elimination half-life for 3-keto-desogestrel is approximately 38±20 hours at steady state. In addition to 3-keto-desogestrel, other phase I metabolites are 3α-OH-desogestrel, 3β-OH-desogestrel, and 3α-OH-5α-H-desogestrel. These other metabolites are not known to have any pharmacologic effects, and are further converted in part by conjugation (phase II metabolism) into polar metabolites, mainly sulfates and glucuronides.
Ethinyl estradiol is rapidly and almost completely absorbed. In the third cycle of use after a single dose of ORTHO-CEPT, the relative bioavailability is approximately 83%.
In the third cycle of use after a single dose of ORTHO-CEPT, maximum concentrations of ethinyl estradiol of 95±34 pg/mL are reached at 1.5±0.8 hours. The $AUC_{0-\infty}$ is 1,471±268 pg/mL·hr after a single dose. At steady state, attained from at least day 19 onwards, maximum ethinyl estradiol concentrations of 141±48 pg/mL are reached at about 1.4±0.7 hours. The minimum serum levels of ethinyl estradiol at steady state are 24±8.3 pg/mL. The AUC_{0-24}, at steady state is 1,117±302 pg/mL·hr. The mean $AUC_{0-\infty}$ for ethinyl estradiol following a single dose during treatment cycle 3 does not significantly differ from the mean AUC_{0-24} at steady state. This finding indicates linear kinetics for ethinyl estradiol.
The elimination half-life is 26±6.8 hours at steady state. Ethinyl estradiol is subject to a significant degree of presystemic conjugation (phase II metabolism). Ethinyl estradiol

escaping gut wall conjugation undergoes phase I metabolism and hepatic conjugation (phase II metabolism). Major phase I metabolites are 2-OH-ethinyl estradiol and 2-methoxy-ethinyl estradiol. Sulfate and glucuronide conjugates of both ethinyl estradiol and phase I metabolites, which are excreted in bile, can undergo enterohepatic circulation.

INDICATIONS AND USAGE

ORTHO-CEPT Tablets are indicated for the prevention of pregnancy in women who elect to use oral contraceptives as a method of contraception.

Oral contraceptives are highly effective. Table I lists the typical accidental pregnancy rates for users of combination oral contraceptives and other methods of contraception. The efficacy of these contraceptive methods, except sterilization, depends upon the reliability with which they are used. Correct and consistent use of these methods can result in lower failure rates.

[See table above]

In a clinical trial with ORTHO-CEPT, 1,195 subjects completed 11,656 cycles and a total of 10 pregnancies were reported. This represents an overall user-efficacy (typical user-efficacy) pregnancy rate of 1.12 per 100 women-years. This rate includes patients who did not take the drug correctly.

CONTRAINDICATIONS

Oral contraceptives should not be used in women who currently have the following conditions:

- Thrombophlebitis or thromboembolic disorders
- A past history of deep vein thrombophlebitis or thromboembolic disorders
- Cerebral vascular or coronary artery disease
- Known or suspected carcinoma of the breast
- Carcinoma of the endometrium or other known or suspected estrogen-dependent neoplasia
- Undiagnosed abnormal genital bleeding
- Cholestatic jaundice of pregnancy or jaundice with prior pill use
- Hepatic adenomas or carcinomas
- Known or suspected pregnancy

WARNINGS

Cigarette smoking increases the risk of serious cardiovascular side effects from oral contraceptive use. This risk increases with age and with heavy smoking (15 or more cigarettes per day) and is quite marked in women over 35 years of age. Women who use oral contraceptives should be strongly advised not to smoke.

The use of oral contraceptives is associated with increased risks of several serious conditions including myocardial infarction, thromboembolism, stroke, hepatic neoplasia, and gallbladder disease, although the risk of serious morbidity or mortality is very small in healthy women without underlying risk factors. The risk of morbidity and mortality increases significantly in the presence of other underlying risk factors such as hypertension, hyperlipidemias, obesity and diabetes.

Practitioners prescribing oral contraceptives should be familiar with the following information relating to these risks.

The information contained in this package insert is principally based on studies carried out in patients who used oral contraceptives with formulations of higher doses of estrogens and progestogens than those in common use today. The effect of long term use of the oral contraceptives with formulations of lower doses of both estrogens and progestogens remains to be determined.

Throughout this labeling, epidemiological studies reported are of two types: retrospective or case control studies and prospective or cohort studies. Case control studies provide a measure of the relative risk of a disease, namely, a *ratio* of the incidence of a disease among oral contraceptive users to that among nonusers. The relative risk does not provide information on the actual clinical occurrence of a disease. Cohort studies provide a measure of attributable risk, which is the *difference* in the incidence of disease between oral contraceptive users and nonusers. The attributable risk does provide information about the actual occurrence of a disease in the population (Adapted from refs. 2 and 3 with the author's permission). For further information, the reader is referred to a text on epidemiological methods.

1. THROMBOEMBOLIC DISORDERS AND OTHER VASCULAR PROBLEMS

a. Myocardial infarction

An increased risk of myocardial infarction has been attributed to oral contraceptive use. This risk is primarily in smokers or women with other underlying risk factors for coronary artery disease such as hypertension, hypercholesterolemia, morbid obesity, and diabetes. The relative risk of heart attack for current oral contraceptive users has been estimated to be two to six[4–10]. The risk is very low in women under the age of 30.

Smoking in combination with oral contraceptive use has been shown to contribute substantially to the incidence of myocardial infarctions in women in their mid-thirties or older with smoking accounting for the majority of excess cases[11]. Mortality rates associated with circulatory disease have been shown to increase substantially in smokers, especially in those 35 years of age and older among women who use oral contraceptives. (See Table II)

[See figure at top of next column]

TABLE I: PERCENTAGE OF WOMEN EXPERIENCING AN UNINTENDED PREGNANCY DURING THE FIRST YEAR OF TYPICAL USE AND THE FIRST YEAR OF PERFECT USE OF CONTRACEPTION AND THE PERCENTAGE CONTINUING USE AT THE END OF THE FIRST YEAR. UNITED STATES

	% of Women Experiencing an Unintended Pregnancy within the First Year of Use		% of Women Continuing Use at One Year[3]
Method (1)	Typical Use[1] (2)	Perfect Use[2] (3)	(4)
Chance[4]	85	85	
Spermicides[5]	26	6	40
Periodic abstinence	25		63
Calendar		9	
Ovulation Method		3	
Sympto-Thermal[6]		2	
Post-Ovulation		1	
Withdrawal	19	4	
Cap[7]			
Parous Women	40	26	42
Nulliparous Women	20	9	56
Sponge			
Parous Women	40	20	42
Nulliparous Women	20	9	56
Diaphragm[7]	20	6	56
Condom[8]			
Female (Reality)	21	5	56
Male	14	3	61
Pill	5		71
Progestin Only		0.5	
Combined		0.1	
IUD			
Progesterone T	2.0	1.5	81
Copper T380A	0.8	0.6	78
LNg 20	0.1	0.1	81
Depo-Provera	0.3	0.3	70
Norplant and Norplant-2	0.05	0.05	88
Female Sterilization	0.5	0.5	100
Male Sterilization	0.15	0.10	100

Adapted from Hatcher et al., 1998 Ref. #1.

[1]Among *typical* couples who initiate use of a method (not necessarily for the first time), the percentage who experience an accidental pregnancy during the first year if they do not stop use for any other reason.

[2]Among couples who initiate use of a method (not necessarily for the first time) and who use it *perfectly* (both consistently and correctly), the percentage who experience an accidental pregnancy during the first year if they do not stop use for any other reason.

[3]Among couples attempting to avoid pregnancy, the percentage who continue to use a method for one year.

[4]The percents becoming pregnant in columns (2) and (3) are based on data from populations where contraception is not used and from women who cease using contraception in order to become pregnant. Among such populations, about 89% become pregnant within one year. This estimate was lowered slightly (to 85%) to represent the percent who would become pregnant within one year among women now relying on reversible methods of contraception if they abandoned contraception altogether.

[5]Foam, creams, gels, vaginal suppositories, and vaginal film.

[6]Cervical mucus (ovulation) method supplementary by calendar in the pre-ovulatory and basal body temperature in the post-ovulatory phases.

[7]With spermicidal cream or jelly.

[8]Without spermicides.

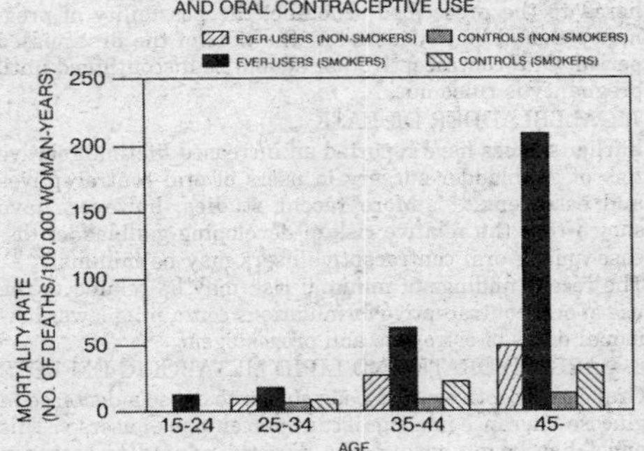

TABLE II. (Adapted from P.M. Layde and V. Beral, ref. #12.)

Oral contraceptives may compound the effects of well-known risk factors, such as hypertension, diabetes, hyperlipidemias, age and obesity.[13] In particular, some progestogens are known to decrease HDL cholesterol and cause glucose intolerance, while estrogens may create a state of hyperinsulinism[14–18]. Oral contraceptives have been shown to increase blood pressure among users (see section 9 in WARNINGS). Similar effects on risk factors have been associated with an increased risk of heart disease. Oral contraceptives must be used with caution in women with cardiovascular disease risk factors.

Desogestrel has minimum androgenic activity (See CLINICAL PHARMACOLOGY), and there is some evidence that the risk of myocardial infarction associated with oral contraceptives is lower when the progestogen has minimal androgenic activity than when the activity is greater.[100]

b. Thromboembolism

An increased risk of thromboembolic and thrombotic disease associated with the use of oral contraceptives is well established. Data from case-control and cohort studies report that oral contraceptives containing desogestral (ORTHO-CEPT contains desogestrel) are associated with a two-fold increase in the risk of venous thromboembolic disease as compared to other low-dose (containing less than 50 mcg of estrogen) pills containing other progestins. According to these studies, this two-fold risk increases the yearly occurrence of venous thromboembolic disease by about 10-15 cases per 100,000 women.

Earlier case control studies on older formulations have found the relative risk of users compared to nonusers to be 3 for the first episode of superficial venous thrombosis, 4 to 11 for deep vein thrombosis or pulmonary embolism, and 1.5 to 6 for women with predisposing conditions for venous thromboembolic disease[2,3,19-24]. Cohort studies have shown the relative risk to be somewhat lower, about 3 for new cases and about 4.5 for new cases requiring hospitalization[25]. The risk of thromboembolic disease associated with oral contraceptives is not related to length of use and disappears after pill use is stopped[2].

A two- to four-fold increase in relative risk of post-operative thromboembolic complications has been reported with the use of oral contraceptives[9]. The relative risk of venous thrombosis in women who have predisposing conditions is twice that of women without such medical conditions[26]. If feasible, oral contraceptives should be discontinued at least four weeks prior to and for two weeks after elective surgery of a type associated with an increase in risk of thromboembolism and during and following prolonged immobilization. Since the immediate postpartum period is also associated with an increased risk of thromboembolism, oral contraceptives should be started no earlier than four weeks after delivery in women who elect not to breast feed.

c. Cerebrovascular diseases

Oral contraceptives have been shown to increase both the relative and attributable risks of cerebrovascular events (thrombotic and hemorrhagic strokes), although, in general, the risk is greatest among older (>35 years), hypertensive women who also smoke. Hypertension was found to be a risk factor for both users and nonusers, for both types of strokes, and smoking interacted to increase the risk of stroke[27–29].

In a large study, the relative risk of thrombotic strokes has been shown to range from 3 for normotensive users to 14 for users with severe hypertension[30]. The relative risk of hemorrhagic stroke is reported to be 1.2 for non-smokers who

Continued on next page

Ortho-Cept—Cont.

used oral contraceptives, 2.6 for smokers who did not use oral contraceptives, 7.6 for smokers who used oral contraceptives, 1.8 for normotensive users and 25.7 for users with severe hypertension[30]. The attributable risk is also greater in older women[3].

d. Dose-related risk of vascular disease from oral contraceptives

A positive association has been observed between the amount of estrogen and progestogen in oral contraceptives and the risk of vascular disease[31–33]. A decline in serum high density lipoproteins (HDL) has been reported with many progestational agents[14–16]. A decline in serum high density lipoproteins has been associated with an increased incidence of ischemic heart disease. Because estrogens increase HDL cholesterol, the net effect of an oral contraceptive depends on a balance achieved between doses of estrogen and progestogen and the nature and absolute amount of progestogens used in the contraceptives. The amount of both hormones should be considered in the choice of an oral contraceptive.

Minimizing exposure to estrogen and progestogen is in keeping with good principles of therapeutics. For any particular estrogen/progestogen combination, the dosage regimen prescribed should be one which contains the least amount of estrogen and progestogen that is compatible with a low failure rate and the needs of the individual patient. New acceptors of oral contraceptive agents should be started on preparations containing 0.035 mg or less of estrogen.

e. Persistence of risk of vascular disease

There are two studies which have shown persistence of risk of vascular disease for ever-users of oral contraceptives. In a study in the United States, the risk of developing myocardial infarction after discontinuing oral contraceptives persists for at least 9 years for women 40–49 years old who had used oral contraceptives for five or more years, but this increased risk was not demonstrated in other age groups[8]. In another study in Great Britain, the risk of developing cerebrovascular disease persisted for at least 6 years after discontinuation of oral contraceptives, although excess risk was very small[34]. However, both studies were performed with oral contraceptive formulations containing 0.050 mg or higher of estrogens.

2. ESTIMATES OF MORTALITY FROM CONTRACEPTIVE USE

One study gathered data from a variety of sources which have estimated the mortality rate associated with different methods of contraception at different ages (Table III). These estimates include the combined risk of death associated with contraceptive methods plus the risk attributable to pregnancy in the event of method failure. Each method of contraception has its specific benefits and risks. The study concluded that with the exception of oral contraceptive users 35 and older who smoke and 40 and older who do not smoke, mortality associated with all methods of birth control is low and below that associated with childbirth.

The observation of an increase in risk of mortality with age for oral contraceptive users is based on data gathered in the 1970's[35]. Current clinical recommendation involves the use of lower estrogen dose formulations and a careful consideration of risk factors. In 1989, the Fertility and Maternal Health Drugs Advisory Committee was asked to review the use of oral contraceptives in women 40 years of age and over. The Committee concluded that although cardiovascular disease risk may be increased with oral contraceptive use after age 40 in healthy non-smoking women (even with the newer low-dose formulations), there are also greater potential health risks associated with pregnancy in older women and with the alternative surgical and medical procedures which may be necessary if such women do not have access to effective and acceptable means of contraception. The Committee recommended that the benefits of low-dose oral contraceptive use by healthy non-smoking women over 40 may outweigh the possible risks.

Of course, older women, as all women who take oral contraceptives, should take an oral contraceptive which contains the least amount of estrogen and progestogen that is compatible with a low failure rate and individual patient needs. [See table below]

3. CARCINOMA OF THE REPRODUCTIVE ORGANS AND BREASTS

Numerous epidemiological studies have been performed on the incidence of breast, endometrial, ovarian and cervical cancer in women using oral contraceptives. While there are conflicting reports, most studies suggest that use of oral contraceptives is not associated with an overall increase in the risk of developing breast cancer. Some studies have reported an increased relative risk of developing breast cancer particularly at a younger age. This increased relative risk has been reported to be related to duration of use[36–44,79–89].

A meta-analysis of 54 studies found a small increase in the frequency of having breast cancer diagnosed for women who were currently using combined oral contraceptives or had used them within the past ten years. This increase in the frequency of breast cancer diagnosis, within ten years of stopping use, was generally accounted for by cancers localized to the breast. There was no increase in the frequency of having breast cancer diagnosed ten or more years after cessation of use.[101]

Some studies suggest that oral contraceptive use has been associated with an increase in the risk of cervical intraepithelial neoplasia in some populations of women[45–48]. However, there continues to be controversy about the extent to which such findings may be due to differences in sexual behavior and other factors.

4. HEPATIC NEOPLASIA

Benign hepatic adenomas are associated with oral contraceptive use, although the incidence of benign tumors is rare in the United States. Indirect calculations have estimated the attributable risk to be in the range of 3.3 cases/100,000 for users, a risk that increases after four or more years of use especially with oral contraceptives of higher dose[49].

Rupture of benign, hepatic adenomas may cause death through intra-abdominal hemorrhage[50,51].

Studies have shown an increased risk of developing hepatocellular carcinoma[52–54,102] in oral contraceptive users. However, these cancers are rare in the U.S.

5. OCULAR LESIONS

There have been clinical case reports of retinal thrombosis associated with the use of oral contraceptives. Oral contraceptives should be discontinued if there is unexplained partial or complete loss of vision; onset of proptosis or diplopia; papilledema; or retinal vascular lesions. Appropriate diagnostic and therapeutic measures should be undertaken immediately.

6. ORAL CONTRACEPTIVE USE BEFORE OR DURING EARLY PREGNANCY

Extensive epidemiological studies have revealed no increased risk of birth defects in women who have used oral contraceptives prior to pregnancy[56–57]. The majority of recent studies also do not indicate a teratogenic effect, particularly in so far as cardiac anomalies and limb reduction defects are concerned[55,56,58,59], when oral contraceptives are taken inadvertently during early pregnancy.

The administration of oral contraceptives to induce withdrawal bleeding should not be used as a test for pregnancy. Oral contraceptives should not be used during pregnancy to treat threatened or habitual abortion.

It is recommended that for any patient who has missed two consecutive periods, pregnancy should be ruled out before continuing oral contraceptive use. If the patient has not adhered to the prescribed schedule, the possibility of pregnancy should be considered at the time of the first missed period. Oral contraceptive use should be discontinued until pregnancy is ruled out.

7. GALLBLADDER DISEASE

Earlier studies have reported an increased lifetime relative risk of gallbladder surgery in users of oral contraceptives and estrogens[60,61]. More recent studies, however, have shown that the relative risk of developing gallbladder disease among oral contraceptive users may be minimal[62–64]. The recent findings of minimal risk may be related to the use of oral contraceptive formulations containing lower hormonal doses of estrogens and progestogens.

8. CARBOHYDRATE AND LIPID METABOLIC EFFECTS

Oral contraceptives have been shown to cause a decrease in glucose tolerance in a significant percentage of users[17]. This effect has been shown to be directly related to estrogen dose[65]. In general, progestogens increase insulin secretion and create insulin resistance, this effect varying with different progestational agents[17,66]. In the nondiabetic woman, oral contraceptives appear to have no effect on fasting blood glucose[67]. Because of these demonstrated effects, prediabetic and diabetic women should be carefully monitored while taking oral contraceptives.

A small proportion of women will have persistent hypertriglyceridemia while on the pill. As discussed earlier (see WARNINGS 1.a. and 1.d.), changes in serum triglycerides and lipoprotein levels have been reported in oral contraceptive users.

9. ELEVATED BLOOD PRESSURE

An increase in blood pressure has been reported in women taking oral contraceptives[68] and this increase is more likely in older oral contraceptive users[69] and with extended duration of use[61]. Data from the Royal College of General Practitioners[12] and subsequent randomized trials have shown that the incidence of hypertension increases with increasing progestational activity.

Women with a history of hypertension or hypertension-related diseases, or renal disease[70] should be encouraged to use another method of contraception. If women elect to use oral contraceptives, they should be monitored closely and if significant elevation of blood pressure occurs, oral contraceptives should be discontinued. For most women, elevated blood pressure will return to normal after stopping oral contraceptives[69], and there is no difference in the occurrence of hypertension among former and never users[68,70,71].

10. HEADACHE

The onset or exacerbation of migraine or development of headache with a new pattern which is recurrent, persistent or severe requires discontinuation of oral contraceptives and evaluation of the cause.

11. BLEEDING IRREGULARITIES

Breakthrough bleeding and spotting are sometimes encountered in patients on oral contraceptives, especially during the first three months of use. Nonhormonal causes should be considered and adequate diagnostic measures taken to rule out malignancy or pregnancy in the event of breakthrough bleeding, as in the case of any abnormal vaginal bleeding. If pathology has been excluded, time or a change to another formulation may solve the problem. In the event of amenorrhea, pregnancy should be ruled out.

Some women may encounter post-pill amenorrhea or oligomenorrhea, especially when such a condition was pre-existent.

12. ECTOPIC PREGNANCY

Ectopic as well as intrauterine pregnancy may occur in contraceptive failures.

PRECAUTIONS

1. PHYSICAL EXAMINATION AND FOLLOW UP

It is good medical practice for all women to have annual history and physical examinations, including women using oral contraceptives. The physical examination, however, may be deferred until after initiation of oral contraceptives if requested by the woman and judged appropriate by the clinician. The physical examination should include special reference to blood pressure, breasts, abdomen and pelvic organs, including cervical cytology, and relevant laboratory tests. In case of undiagnosed, persistent or recurrent abnormal vaginal bleeding, appropriate measures should be conducted to rule out malignancy. Women with a strong family history of breast cancer or who have breast nodules should be monitored with particular care.

2. LIPID DISORDERS

Women who are being treated for hyperlipidemias should be followed closely if they elect to use oral contraceptives. Some progestogens may elevate LDL levels and may render the control of hyperlipidemias more difficult.

3. LIVER FUNCTION

If jaundice develops in any woman receiving such drugs, the medication should be discontinued. Steroid hormones may be poorly metabolized in patients with impaired liver function.

4. FLUID RETENTION

Oral contraceptives may cause some degree of fluid retention. They should be prescribed with caution, and only with careful monitoring, in patients with conditions which might be aggravated by fluid retention.

5. EMOTIONAL DISORDERS

Women with a history of depression should be carefully observed and the drug discontinued if depression recurs to a serious degree.

6. CONTACT LENSES

Contact lens wearers who develop visual changes or changes in lens tolerance should be assessed by an ophthalmologist.

7. DRUG INTERACTIONS

Reduced efficacy and increased incidence of breakthrough bleeding and menstrual irregularities have been associated with concomitant use of rifampin. A similar association, though less marked, has been suggested with barbiturates, phenylbutazone, phenytoin sodium, carbamazepine and possibly with griseofulvin, ampicillin and tetracyclines[72].

8. INTERACTIONS WITH LABORATORY TESTS

Certain endocrine and liver function tests and blood components may be affected by oral contraceptives:

a. Increased prothrombin and factors VII, VIII, IX and X; decreased antithrombin 3; increased norepinephrine-induced platelet aggregability.

b. Increased thyroid binding globulin (TBG) leading to increased circulating total thyroid hormone, as measured by protein-bound iodine (PBI), T4 by column or by radioimmunoassay. Free T3 resin uptake is decreased, reflecting the elevated TBG; free T4 concentration is unaltered.

TABLE III—ANNUAL NUMBER OF BIRTH-RELATED OR METHOD-RELATED DEATHS ASSOCIATED WITH CONTROL OF FERTILITY PER 100,000 NON-STERILE WOMEN, BY FERTILITY CONTROL METHOD ACCORDING TO AGE

Method of control and outcome	15–19	20–24	25–29	30–34	35–39	40–44
No fertility control methods*	7.0	7.4	9.1	14.8	25.7	28.2
Oral contraceptives non-smoker**	0.3	0.5	0.9	1.9	13.8	31.6
Oral contraceptives smoker**	2.2	3.4	6.6	13.5	51.1	117.2
IUD**	0.8	0.8	1.0	1.0	1.4	1.4
Condom*	1.1	1.6	0.7	0.2	0.3	0.4
Diaphragm/spermicide*	1.9	1.2	1.2	1.3	2.2	2.8
Periodic abstinence*	2.5	1.6	1.6	1.7	2.9	3.6

* Deaths are birth-related
** Deaths are method-related

Adapted from H.W. Ory, ref. #35.

c. Other binding proteins may be elevated in serum.
d. Sex hormone binding globulins are increased and result in elevated levels of total circulating sex steroids however, free or biologically active levels either decrease or remain unchanged.
e. High-density lipoprotein (HDL-C) and triglycerides may be increased, while low-density lipoprotein cholesterol (LDL-C) and total cholesterol (Total-C) may be decreased or unchanged.
f. Glucose tolerance may be decreased.
g. Serum folate levels may be depressed by oral contraceptive therapy. This may be of clinical significance if a woman becomes pregnant shortly after discontinuing oral contraceptives.

9. CARCINOGENESIS
See WARNINGS section.

10. PREGNANCY
Pregnancy Category X. See CONTRAINDICATIONS and WARNINGS sections.

11. NURSING MOTHERS
Small amounts of oral contraceptive steroids have been identified in the milk of nursing mothers and a few adverse effects on the child have been reported, including jaundice and breast enlargement. In addition, oral contraceptives given in the postpartum period may interfere with lactation by decreasing the quantity and quality of breast milk. If possible, the nursing mother should be advised not to use oral contraceptives but to use other forms of contraception until she has completely weaned her child.

12. PEDIATRIC USE
Safety and efficacy of ORTHO-CEPT Tablets have been established in women of reproductive age. Safety and efficacy are expected to be the same for postpubertal adolescents under the age of 16 and for users 16 years and older. Use of this product before menarche is not indicated.

13. SEXUALLY TRANSMITTED DISEASES
Patients should be counseled that this product does not provide against HIV infection (AIDS) and other sexually transmitted diseases.

INFORMATION FOR THE PATIENT

See Patient Labeling Printed Below

ADVERSE REACTIONS

An increased risk of the following serious adverse reactions has been associated with the use of oral contraceptives (see WARNINGS section).

- Thrombophlebitis and venous thrombosis with or without embolism
- Arterial thromboembolism
- Pulmonary embolism
- Myocardial infarction
- Cerebral hemorrhage
- Cerebral thrombosis
- Hypertension
- Gallbladder disease
- Hepatic adenomas or benign liver tumors

The following adverse reactions have been reported in patients receiving oral contraceptives and are believed to be drug-related:

- Nausea
- Vomiting
- Gastrointestinal symptoms (such as abdominal cramps and bloating)
- Breakthrough bleeding
- Spotting
- Change in menstrual flow
- Amenorrhea
- Temporary infertility after discontinuation of treatment
- Edema
- Melasma which may persist
- Breast changes: tenderness, enlargement, secretion
- Change in weight (increase or decrease)
- Change in cervical erosion and secretion
- Diminution in lactation when given immediately postpartum
- Cholestatic jaundice
- Migraine
- Rash (allergic)
- Mental depression
- Reduced tolerance to carbohydrates
- Vaginal candidiasis
- Change in corneal curvature (steepening)
- Intolerance to contact lenses

The following adverse reactions have been reported in users of oral contraceptives and the association has been neither confirmed nor refuted:

- Pre-menstrual syndrome
- Cataracts
- Changes in appetite
- Cystitis-like syndrome
- Headache
- Nervousness
- Dizziness
- Hirsutism
- Loss of scalp hair
- Erythema multiforme
- Erythema nodosum
- Hemorrhagic eruption
- Vaginitis
- Porphyria
- Impaired renal function
- Hemolytic uremic syndrome
- Acne
- Changes in libido
- Colitis
- Budd-Chiari Syndrome

OVERDOSAGE

Serious ill effects have not been reported following acute ingestion of large doses of oral contraceptives by young children. Overdosage may cause nausea, and withdrawal bleeding may occur in females.

NON-CONTRACEPTIVE HEALTH BENEFITS

The following non-contraceptive health benefits related to the use of oral contraceptives are supported by epidemiological studies which largely utilized oral contraceptive formulations containing estrogen doses exceeding 0.035 mg of ethinyl estradiol or 0.05 mg of mestranol[73–78].

Effects on menses:

- increased menstrual cycle regularity
- decreased blood loss and decreased incidence of iron deficiency anemia
- decreased incidence of dysmenorrhea

Effects related to inhibition of ovulation:

- decreased incidence of functional ovarian cysts
- decreased incidence of ectopic pregnancies

Effects from long-term use:

- decreased incidence of fibroadenomas and fibrocystic disease of the breast
- decreased incidence of acute pelvic inflammatory disease
- decreased incidence of endometrial cancer
- decreased incidence of ovarian cancer

DOSAGE AND ADMINISTRATION

To achieve maximum contraceptive effectiveness, ORTHO-CEPT must be taken exactly as directed and at intervals not exceeding 24 hours. ORTHO-CEPT is available in the DIALPAK® Tablet Dispenser which is preset for a Sunday Start. Day 1 Start is also provided.

21-Day Regimen (Day 1 Start)

The dosage of ORTHO-CEPT 21 for the initial cycle of therapy is one tablet administered daily from the 1st day through the 21st day of the menstrual cycle, counting the first day of menstrual flow as "Day 1". For subsequent cycles, no tablets are taken for 7 days, then a new course is started of one tablet a day for 21 days. The dosage regimen then continues with 7 days of no medication, followed by 21 days of medication, instituting a three-weeks-on, one-week-off dosage regimen.

The use of ORTHO-CEPT 21 for contraception may be initiated 4 weeks postpartum in women who elect not to breast feed. When the tablets are administered during the postpartum period, the increased risk of thromboembolic disease associated with the postpartum period must be considered. (See CONTRAINDICATIONS and WARNINGS concerning thromboembolic disease. See also PRECAUTIONS for "Nursing Mothers".) If the patient starts on ORTHO-CEPT postpartum, and has not yet had a period, she should be instructed to use another method of contraception until an orange tablet has been taken daily for 7 days. The possibility of ovulation and conception prior to initiation of medication should be considered. If the patient misses one (1) active tablet in Weeks 1, 2, or 3, the tablet should be taken as soon as she remembers. If the patient misses two (2) active tablets in Week 1 or Week 2, the patient should take two (2) tablets the day she remembers and two (2) tablets the next day; and then continue taking one (1) tablet a day until she finishes the pack. The patient should be instructed to use a back-up method of birth control if she has sex in the seven (7) days after missing pills. If the patient misses two (2) active tablets in the third week or misses three (3) or more active tablets in a row, the patient should throw out the rest of the pack and start a new pack that same day. The patient should be instructed to use a back-up method of birth control if she has sex in the seven (7) days after missing pills.

21-Day Regimen (Sunday Start)

When taking ORTHO-CEPT 21, the first orange tablet should be taken on the first Sunday after menstruation begins. If period begins on Sunday, the first orange tablet is taken on that day. If switching directly from another oral contraceptive, the first orange tablet should be taken on the first Sunday after the last ACTIVE tablet of the previous product. One orange tablet is taken daily for 21 days. For subsequent cycles, no tablets are taken for seven days, then a new course is started of one tablet a day for 21 days instituting a 3-weeks-on, one-week-off dosage regimen. When initiating a Sunday start regimen, another method of contraception should be used until after the first 7 consecutive days of administration.

The use of ORTHO-CEPT 21 for contraception may be initiated 4 weeks postpartum in women who elect not to breast feed. When the tablets are administered during the postpartum period, the increased risk of thromboembolic disease associated with the postpartum period must be considered. (See CONTRAINDICATIONS and WARNINGS concerning thromboembolic disease. See also PRECAUTIONS for "Nursing Mothers".) If the patient starts on ORTHO-CEPT postpartum, and has not yet had a period, she should be instructed to use another method of contraception until an orange tablet has been taken daily for 7 days. The possibility of ovulation and conception prior to initiation of medication should be considered. If the patient misses one (1) active tablet in Weeks 1, 2, or 3, the tablet should be taken as soon as she remembers. If the patient misses two (2) active tablets in Week 1 or Week 2, the patient should take two (2) tablets the day she remembers and two (2) tablets the next day; and then continue taking one (1) tablet a day until she finishes the pack. The patient should be instructed to use a back-up method of birth control if she has sex in the seven (7) days after missing pills. If the patient misses two (2) active tablets in the third week or misses three (3) or more tablets in a row, the patient should continue taking one tablet every day until Sunday. On Sunday the patient should throw out the rest of the pack and start a new pack that same day. The patient should be instructed to use a back-up method of birth control if she has sex in the seven (7) days after missing pills.

28-Day Regimen (Day 1 Start)

The dosage of ORTHO-CEPT 28 for the initial cycle of therapy is one tablet administered daily from the 1st day through 21st day of the menstrual cycle, counting the first day of menstrual flow as "Day 1". Tablets are taken without interruption as follows: One orange tablet daily for 21 days, then one green tablet daily for 7 days. After 28 tablets have been taken, a new course is started and an orange tablet is taken the next day.

The use of ORTHO-CEPT 28 for contraception may be initiated 4 weeks postpartum in women who elect not to breast feed. When the tablets are administered during the postpartum period, the increased risk of thromboembolic disease associated with the postpartum period must be considered. (See CONTRAINDICATIONS and WARNINGS concerning thromboembolic disease. See also PRECAUTIONS for "Nursing Mothers".) If the patient starts on ORTHO-CEPT postpartum, and has not yet had a period, she should be instructed to use another method of contraception until an orange tablet has been taken daily for 7 days. The possibility of ovulation and conception prior to initiation of medication should be considered. If the patient misses one (1) active tablet in Weeks 1, 2, or 3, the tablet should be taken as soon as she remembers. If the patient misses two (2) active tablets in Week 1 or Week 2, the patient should take two (2) tablets the day she remembers and two (2) tablets the next day; and then continue taking one (1) tablet a day until she finishes the pack. The patient should be instructed to use a back-up method of birth control if she has sex in the seven (7) days after missing pills. If the patient misses two (2) active tablets in the third week or misses three (3) or more active tablets in a row, the patient should throw out the rest of the pack and start a new pack that same day. The patient should be instructed to use a back-up method of birth control if she has sex in the seven (7) days after missing pills.

28-Day Regimen (Sunday Start)

When taking ORTHO-CEPT 28, the first orange tablet should be taken on the first Sunday after menstruation begins. If period begins on Sunday, the first orange tablet is taken on that day. If switching directly from another oral contraceptive, the first orange tablet should be taken on the first Sunday after the last ACTIVE tablet of the previous product. Tablets are taken without interruption as follows: One orange tablet daily for 21 days, then one green tablet daily for 7 days. After 28 tablets have been taken, a new course is started and an orange tablet is taken the next day (Sunday). When initiating a Sunday start regimen, another method of contraception should be used until after the first 7 consecutive days of administration.

The use of ORTHO-CEPT 28 for contraception may be initiated 4 weeks postpartum. When the tablets are administered during the postpartum period, the increased risk of thromboembolic disease associated with the postpartum period must be considered. (See CONTRAINDICATIONS and WARNINGS concerning thromboembolic disease. See also PRECAUTIONS for "Nursing Mothers".) If the patient starts on ORTHO-CEPT postpartum, and has not yet had a period, she should be instructed to use another method of contraception until an orange tablet has been taken daily for 7 days. The possibility of ovulation and conception prior to initiation of medication should be considered. If the patient misses one (1) active tablet in Weeks 1, 2, or 3, the tablet should be taken as soon as she remembers. If the patient misses two (2) active tablets in Week 1 or Week 2, the patient should take two (2) tablets the day she remembers and two (2) tablets the next day; and then continue taking one (1) tablet a day until she finishes the pack. The patient should be instructed to use a back-up method of birth control if she has sex in the seven (7) days after missing pills. If the patient misses two (2) active tablets in the third week or misses three (3) or more tablets in a row, the patient should continue taking one tablet every day until Sunday. On Sunday the patient should throw out the rest of the pack and start a new pack that same day. The patient should be instructed to use a back-up method of birth control if she has sex in the seven (7) days after missing pills.

ALL ORAL CONTRACEPTIVES

Breakthrough bleeding, spotting, and amenorrhea are frequent reasons for patients discontinuing oral contraceptives. In breakthrough bleeding, as in all cases of irregular bleeding from the vagina, nonfunctional causes should be borne in mind. In undiagnosed persistent or recurrent abnormal bleeding from the vagina, adequate diagnostic measures are indicated to rule out pregnancy or malignancy. If pathology has been excluded, time or a change to another formulation may solve the problem. Changing to an oral contraceptive with a higher estrogen content, while potentially useful in minimizing menstrual irregularity, should be done only if necessary since this may increase the risk of thromboembolic disease.

Use of oral contraceptives in the event of a missed menstrual period:

Continued on next page

Ortho-Cept—Cont.

1. If the patient has not adhered to the prescribed schedule, the possibility of pregnancy should be considered at the time of the first missed period and oral contraceptive use should be discontinued until pregnancy is ruled out.
2. If the patient has adhered to the prescribed regimen and misses two consecutive periods, pregnancy should be ruled out before continuing oral contraceptive use.

HOW SUPPLIED

ORTHO-CEPT® 21 Tablets are available in a DIALPAK® Tablet Dispenser (NDC 0062-1795-15) containing 21 orange tablets (0.15 mg desogestrel and 0.03 mg ethinyl estradiol) which are unscored with "ORTHO" on one side and "D 150" on the opposite side.

ORTHO-CEPT 28 Tablets are available in a DIALPAK Tablet Dispenser (NDC 0062-1796-15) containing 28 tablets, as follows: 21 orange tablets as described under ORTHO-CEPT 21, and 7 green tablets containing inert ingredients. ORTHO-CEPT 28 is available for clinic usage in a VERIDATE Tablet Dispenser (unfilled) and VERIDATE Refills (NDC 0062-1796-20).

STORAGE: Store below 86° F (30° C).

REFERENCES

1. Trussel J. Contraceptive efficacy. In Hatcher RA, Trussel J, Stewart F, Cates W, Stewart GK, Kowal D, Guest F, Contraceptive Technology: Seventeenth Revised Edition. New York NY: Irvington Publishers, 1998, in press.**2.** Stadel BV. Oral contraceptives and cardiovascular disease. (Pt. 1). N Engl J Med 1981; 305:612–618. **3.** Stadel BV. Oral contraceptives and cardiovascular disease. (Pt. 2). N Engl J Med 1981; 305:672–677. **4.** Adam SA, Thorogood M. Oral contraception and myocardial infarction revisited: the effects of new preparations and prescribing patterns. Br J Obstet and Gynecol 1981; 88:838–845. **5.** Mann JI, Inman WH. Oral contraceptives and death from myocardial infarction. Br Med J 1975; 2(5965):245–248. **6.** Mann JI, Vessey MP, Thorogood M. Doll R. Myocardial infarction in young women with special reference to oral contraceptive practice. Br Med J 1975; 2(5956):241–245. **7.** Royal College of General Practitioners' Oral Contraception Study: Further analyses of mortality in oral contraceptive users. Lancet 1981;1:541–546. **8.** Slone D, Shapiro S, Kaufman DW, Rosenberg L, Miettinen OS, Stolley PD. Risk of myocardial infarction in relation to current and discontinued use of oral contraceptives. N Engl J Med 1981; 305:420–424. **9.** Vessey MP. Female hormones and vascular disease—an epidemiological overview. Br J Fam Plann 1980; 6:1–12. **10.** Russell-Briefel RG, Ezzati TM. Fulwood R, Perlman JA, Murphy RS. Cardiovascular risk status and oral contraceptive use, United States, 1976–80. Prevent Med 1986; 15:352–362. **11.** Goldbaum GM, Kendrick JS, Hogelin GC, Gentry EM. The relative impact of smoking and oral contraceptive use on women in the United States. JAMA 1987; 258:1339–1342. **12.** Layde PM, Beral V. Further analyses of mortality in oral contraceptive users: Royal College General Practitioners' Oral Contraception Study. (Table 5) Lancet 1981; 1:541–546. **13.** Knopp RH. Arteriosclerosis risk: the roles of oral contraceptives and postmenopausal estrogens. J Reprod Med 1986; 31(9) (Supplement):913–921. **14.** Krauss RM, Roy S, Mishell DR, Casagrande J, Pike MC. Effects of two low-dose oral contraceptives on serum lipids and lipoproteins: Differential changes in high-density lipoproteins subclasses. Am J Obstet 1983; 145:446–452. **15.** Wahl P, Walden C, Knopp R, Hoover J, Wallace R, Heiss G, Rifkind B. Effect of estrogen/progestin potency on lipid/lipoprotein cholesterol. N Engl J Med 1983; 308:862–867. **16.** Wynn V, Niththyananthan R. The effect of progestin in combined oral contraceptives on serum lipids with special reference to high-density lipoproteins. Am J Obstet Gynecol 1982; 142:766–771. **17.** Wynn V, Godsland I. Effects of oral contraceptives and carbohydrate metabolism. J Reprod Med 1986; 31 (9) (Supplement):892–897. **18.** LaRosa JC, Atherosclerotic risk factors in cardiovascular disease. J Reprod Med 1986;31 (9) (Supplement): 906–912. **19.** Inman WH, Vessey MP. Investigation of death from pulmonary, coronary, and cerebral thrombosis and embolism in women of childbearing age. Br Med J 1968; 2 (5599):193–199. **20.** Maguire MG, Tonascia J, Sartwell PE, Stolley PD, Tockman MS. Increased risk of thrombosis due to oral contraceptives: a further report. Am J Epidemiol 1979; 110(2):188–195. **21.** Pettiti DB, Wingerd J, Pellegrin F, Ramacharan S. Risk of vascular disease in women: smoking, oral contraceptives, noncontraceptive estrogens, and other factors. JAMA 1979; 242:1150–1154. **22.** Vessey MP, Doll R. Investigation of relation between use of oral contraceptives and thromboembolic disease. Br Med J 1968; 2(5599):199–205. **23.** Vessey MP, Doll R. Investigation of relation between use of oral contraceptives and thromboembolic disease. A further report. Br Med J 1969; 2 (5658):651–657. **24.** Porter JB, Hunter JR, Danielson DA, Jick H, Stergachis A. Oral contraceptives and non-fatal vascular disease—recent experience. Obstet Gynecol 1982; 59 (3): 299–302. **25.** Vessey M, Doll R, Peto R. Johnson B, Wiggins P. A long-term follow-up study of women using different methods of contraception: an interim report. J Biosocial Sci 1976; 8:375–427. **26.** Royal College of General Practitioners: Oral contraceptives, venous thrombosis, and varicose veins. J Royal Coll Gen Pract 1978; 28:393–399. **27.** Collaborative Group for the Study of Stroke in Young Women: Oral contraception and increased risk of cerebral ischemia or thrombosis. N Engl J Med 1973; 288:871–878. **28.** Petitti DB, Wingerd J. Use of oral contraceptives, cigarette smoking, and risk of subarachnoid hemorrhage. Lancet 1978; 2:234–236. **29.** Inman WH. Oral contraceptives and fatal subarachnoid hemorrhage. Br Med J 1979; 2 (6203):1468–70. **30.** Collaborative Group for the study of Stroke in Young Women: Oral contraceptives and stroke in young women: associated risk factors. JAMA 1975; 231:718–722. **31.** Inman WH, Vessey MP, Westerholm B, Engelund A. Thromboembolic disease and the steroidal content of oral contraceptives. A report to the Committee on Safety of Drugs. Br Med J 1970; 2:203–209. **32.** Meade TW, Greenberg G, Thompson SG. Progestogens and cardiovascular reactions associated with oral contraceptives and a comparison of the safety of 50- and 35-mcg oestrogen preparations. Br Med J 1980; 280 (6224):1157–1161. **33.** Kay, CR. Progestogens and arterial disease—evidence from the Royal College of General Practitioners' Study. Am J Obstet Gynecol 1982; 142:762–765. **34.** Royal College of General Practitioners: Incidence of arterial disease among oral contraceptive users. J Royal Coll Gen Pract 1983; 33:75–82. **35.** Ory HW. Mortality associated with fertility and fertility control: 1983. Family Planning Perspectives 1983; 15:50–56. **36.** The Cancer and Steroid Hormone Study of the Centers for Disease Control and the National Institute of Child Health and Human Development: Oral contraceptive use and the risk of breast cancer. N Engl J Med 1986; 315:405–411. **37.** Pike MC, Henderson BE, Krailo MD, Duke A, Roy S. Breast cancer risk in young women and use of oral contraceptives: possible modifying effect of formulation and age at use. Lancet 1983; 2:926–929. **38.** Paul C, Skegg DG, Spears GFS, Kaldor JM. Oral contraceptives and breast cancer: A national study. Br Med J 1986; 293:723–725. **39.** Miller DR, Rosenberg L, Kaufman DW, Schottenfeld D, Stolley PD, Shapiro S. Breast cancer risk in relation to early oral contraceptive use. Obstet Gynecol 1986; 68:863–868. **40.** Olson H, Olson KL, Moller TR, Ranstam J, Holm P. Oral contraceptive use and breast cancer in young women in Sweden (letter). Lancet 1985; 2:748–749. **41.** McPherson K, Vessey M, Neil A, Doll R, Jones L, Roberts M. Early contraceptive use and breast cancer: Results of another case-control study. Br J Cancer 1987; 56: 653–660. **42.** Huggins GR, Zucker PF. Oral contraceptives and neoplasia: 1987 update. Fertil Steril 1987; 47:733–761. **43.** McPherson K, Drife JO. The pill and breast cancer: why the uncertainty? Br Med J 1986; 293:709–710. **44.** Shapiro S. Oral contraceptives—time to take stock. N Engl J Med 1987; 315:450–451. **45.** Ory H, Naib Z, Conger SB, Hatcher RA, Tyler CW. Contraceptive choice and prevalence of cervical dysplasia and carcinoma in situ. Am J Obstet Gynecol 1976;124:573–577. **46.** Vessey MP, Lawless M, McPherson K, Yeates D. Neoplasia of the cervix uteri and contraception: a possible adverse effect of the pill. Lancet 1983; 2:930. **47.** Brinton LA, Huggins GR, Lehman HF, Malli K, Savitz DA, Trapido E, Rosenthal J, Hoover R. Long term use of oral contraceptives and risk of invasive cervical cancer. Int J Cancer 1986; 38:339–344. **48.** WHO Collaborative Study of Neoplasia and Steroid Contraceptives: Invasive cervical cancer and combined oral contraceptives. Br Med J 1985; 290:961–965. **49.** Rooks JB, Ory HW, Ishak KG, Strauss LT, Greenspan JR, Hill AP, Tyler CW. Epidemiology of hepatocellular adenoma: the role of oral contraceptive use. JAMA 1979; 242:644–648. **50.** Bein NN, Goldsmith HS. Recurrent massive hemorrhage from benign hepatic tumors secondary to oral contraceptives. Br J Surg 1977; 64:433–435. **51.** Klatskin G. Hepatic tumors: possible relationship to use of oral contraceptives. Gastroenterology 1977; 73:386–394. **52.** Henderson BE, Preston-Martin S, Edmondson HA, Peters RL, Pike MC. Hepatocellular carcinoma and oral contraceptives. Br J Cancer 1983; 48:437–440. **53.** Neuberger J, Forman D, Doll R, Williams R. Oral contraceptives and hepatocellular carcinoma. Br Med J 1986; 292:1355–1357. **54.** Forman D, Vincent TJ, Doll R. Cancer of the liver and oral contraceptives. Br Med J 1986; 292:1357–1361. **55.** Harlap S, Eldor J. Births following oral contraceptive failures. Obstet Gynecol 1980; 55:447–452. **56.** Savolainen E, Saksela E, Saxen L. Teratogenic hazards of oral contraceptives analyzed in a national malformation register. Am J Obstet Gynecol 1981; 140:521–524. **57.** Janerich DT, Piper JM, Glebatis DM. Oral contraceptives and birth defects. Am J Epidemiol 1980; 112:73–79. **58.** Ferencz C, Matanoski GM, Wilson PD, Rubin JD, Neill CA, Gutberlet R. Maternal hormone therapy and congenital heart disease. Teratology 1980; 21: 225–239. **59.** Rothman KJ, Fyler DC, Goldbatt A, Kreidberg MB. Exogenous hormones and other drug exposures of children with congenital heart disease. Am J Epidemiol 1979; 109:433–439. **60.** Boston Collaborative Drug Surveillance Program: Oral contraceptives and venous thromboembolic disease, surgically confirmed gall-bladder disease, and breast tumors. Lancet 1973; 1:1399–1404. **61.** Royal College of General Practitioners: Oral contraceptives and health. New York, Pittman, 1974. **62.** Layde PM, Vessey MP, Yeates D. Risk of gall bladder disease: a cohort study of young women attending family planning clinics. J Epidemiol Community Health 1982; 36:274–278. **63.** Rome Group for the Epidemiology and Prevention of Cholelithiasis (GREPCO): Prevalence of gallstone disease in an Italian adult female population. Am J Epidemiol 1984; 119:796–805. **64.** Strom BL, Tamragouri RT, Morse ML, Lazar EL, West SL, Stolley PD, Jones JK. Oral contraceptives and other risk factors for gall bladder disease. Clin Pharmacol Ther 1986; 39:335–341. **65.** Wynn V, Adams PW, Godsland IF, Melrose J, Niththyananthan R, Oakley NW, Seedj A. Comparison of effects of different combined oral-contraceptive formulations on carbohydrate and lipid metabolism. Lancet 1979; 1:1045–1049. **66.** Wynn V. Effect of progesterone and progestins on carbohydrate metabolism. In Progesterone and Progestin. Edited by Bardin CW, Milgrom E, Mauvis-Jarvis P. New York, Raven Press, 1983 pp. 395–410. **67.** Perlman JA, Roussell-Briefel RG, Ezzati TM, Lieberknecht G. Oral glucose tolerance and the potency of oral contraceptive progestogens. J Chronic Dis 1985; 38:857–864. **68.** Royal College of General Practitioners' Oral Contraception Study: Effect on hypertension and benign breast disease of progestogen component in combined oral contraceptives. Lancet 1977; 1:624. **69.** Fisch IR, Frank J. Oral contraceptives and blood pressure. JAMA 1977; 237:2499–2503. **70.** Laragh AJ. Oral contraceptive induced hypertension—nine years later. Am J Obstet Gynecol 1976; 126:141–147. **71.** Ramcharan S, Peritz E, Pellegrin FA, Williams WT. Incidence of hypertension in the Walnut Creek Contraceptive Drug Study cohort. In Pharmacology of Steroid Contraceptive Drugs. Garattini S, Berendes HW. Eds. New York, Raven Press, 1977 pp. 277–278. (Monographs of the Mario Negri Institute for Pharmacological Research, Milan). **72.** Stockley I. Interactions with oral contraceptives. J Pharm 1976; 216:140–143. **73.** The Cancer and Steroid Hormone Study of the Centers for Disease Control and the National Institute of Child Health and Human Development: Oral contraceptive use and the risk of ovarian cancer. JAMA 1983; 249:1596–1599. **74.** The Cancer and Steroid Hormone Study of the Centers for Disease Control and the National Institute of Child Health and Human Development: Combination oral contraceptive use and the risk of endometrial cancer. JAMA 1987; 257:796–800. **75.** Ory HW. Functional ovarian cysts and oral contraceptives: negative association confirmed surgically. JAMA 1974; 228:68–69. **76.** Ory HW. Cole P. Macmahon B, Hoover R. Oral contraceptives and reduced risk of benign breast disease. N Engl J Med 1976; 294:419–422. **77.** Ory HW. The noncontraceptive health benefits from oral contraceptive use. Fam Plann Perspect 1982; 14:182–184. **78.** Ory HW, Forrest JD, Lincoln R. Making Choices: Evaluating the health risks and benefits of birth control methods. New York, The Alan Guttmacher Institute, 1983; p. 1. **79.** Schlesselman J, Stadel BV, Murray P, Lai S. Breast Cancer in relation to early use of oral contraceptives 1988; 259: 1828–1833. **80.** Hennekens CH, Speizer FE, Lipnick RJ, Rosner B, Bain C, Belanger C, Stampfer MJ, Willett W, Peto R. A case-controlled study of oral contraceptive use and breast cancer. JNCI 1984;72:39–42. **81.** LaVecchia C, Decarli A, Fasoli M, Franceschi S, Gentile A, Negri E, Parazzini F, Tognoni G. Oral contraceptives and cancers of the breast and of the female genital tract. Interim results from a case-control study. Br J Cancer 1986; 54:311–317. **82.** Meirik O, Lund E, Adami H, Bergstrom R, Christoffersen T, Bergsjo P. Oral contraceptive use in breast cancer in young women. A Joint National Case-control study in Sweden and Norway. Lancet 1986; 11:650–654. **83.** Kay CR, Hannaford PC. Breast cancer and the pill—A further report from the Royal College of General Practitioners' oral contraception study. Br J Cancer 1988; 58:675–680. **84.** Stadel BV, Lai S, Schlesselman JJ, Murray P. Oral contraceptives and premenopausal breast cancer in nulliparous women. Contraception 1988; 38:287–299. **85.** Miller DR, Rosenberg L, Kaufman DW, Stolley P, Warshauer ME, Shapiro S. Breast cancer before age 45 and oral contraceptive use: New Findings. Am J Epidemiol 1989; 129:269–280. **86.** The UK National Case-Control Study Group, Oral contraceptive use and breast cancer risk in young women. Lancet 1989; 1:973–982. **87.** Schlesselman JJ. Cancer of the breast and reproductive tract in relation to use of oral contraceptives. Contraception 1989; 40:1–38. **88.** Vessey MP, McPherson K, Villard-Mackintosh L, Yeates D. Oral contraceptives and breast cancer: latest findings in a large cohort study. Br J Cancer 1989; 59:613–617. **89.** Jick SS, Walker AM, Stergachis A, Jick H. Oral contraceptives and breast cancer. Br J Cancer 1989; 59:618–621. **90.** Godsland, I et al. The effects of different formulations of oral contraceptive agents on lipid and carbohydrate metabolism. N Engl J Med 1990;323: 1375–81. **91.** Kloosterboer, HJ et al. Selectivity in progesterone and androgen receptor binding of progestogens used in oral contraception. Contraception, 1988;38:325–32. **92.** Van der Vies, J and de Visser, J. Endocrinological studies with desogestrel. Arzneim. Forsch./Drug Res., 1983;33(l),2: 231–6. **93.** Data on file, Organon Inc. **94.** Fotherby, K. Oral contraceptives, lipids and cardiovascular diseases. Contraception, 1985; Vol. 31; 4:367–94. **95.** Lawrence, DM et al. Reduced sex hormone binding globulin and derived free testosterone levels in women with severe acne. Clinical Endocrinology, 1981; 15:87–91. **96.** Cullberg, G et al. Effects of a low-dose desogestrel-ethinyl estradiol combination on hirsutism, androgens and sex hormone binding globulin in women with a polycystic ovary syndrome. Acta Obstet Gynecol Scand, 1985;64:195–202. **97.** Jung-Hoffmann, C and Kuhl, H. Divergent effects of two low-dose oral contraceptives on sex hormone-binding globulin and free testosterone. AJOG, 1987; 156:199–203. **98.** Hammond, G et al. Serum steroid binding protein concentrations, distribution of progestogens, and bioavailability of testosterone during treatment with contraceptives containing desogestrel or levonorgestrel. Fertil Steril, 1984;42:44–51. **99.** Palatsi, R et al. Serum total and unbound testosterone and sex hormone binding globulin (SHBG) in female acne patients treated with two different oral contraceptives. Acta Derm Venereol, 1984; 64:517–23. **100.** Lewis M, Spitzer WO, Heinemann LAJ, MacRae KD, Bruppacher R, Thorogood M on behalf of Transnational Research Group on Oral Contraceptives and Health of Young Women. Third generation oral contraceptives and risk of myocardial infarction: an international case-control study. Br Med J 1996; 312:88–90. **101.** Collaborative Group on Hormonal Factors in Breast Cancer. Breast Cancer and hormonal contraceptives: collaborative reanalysis of individual data on 53 297 women with breast cancer and 100 239 women without breast cancer from 54 epidemiological studies. Lancet 1996; 347:1713–1727. **102.** Palmer JR, Rosenberg L, Kaufman DW, Warshauer ME, Stolley P, Shapiro S. Oral Contraceptive Use and Liver Cancer. Am J Epidemiol 1989; 130:878–882.

BRIEF SUMMARY PATIENT PACKAGE INSERT

This product (like all oral contraceptives) is intended to prevent pregnancy. It does not protect against HIV infection (AIDS) and other sexually transmitted diseases.

Oral contraceptives, also known as "birth control pills" or "the pill", are taken to prevent pregnancy, and when taken correctly, have a failure rate of about 1% per year when used without missing any pills. The typical failure rate of large numbers of pill users is less than 3% per year when women who miss pills are included. For most women, oral contraceptives are also free of serious or unpleasant side effects. However, forgetting to take pills considerably increases the chances of pregnancy.

For the majority of women, oral contraceptives can be taken safely. But there are some women who are at high risk of developing certain serious diseases that can be life-threatening or may cause temporary or permanent disability. The risks associated with taking oral contraceptives increase significantly if you:

- smoke
- have high blood pressure, diabetes, high cholesterol
- have or have had clotting disorders, heart attack, stroke, angina pectoris, cancer of the breast or sex organs, jaundice or malignant or benign liver tumors

Although cardiovascular disease risks may be increased with oral contraceptive use after age 40 in healthy, nonsmoking women (even with the newer low-dose formulations), there are also greater potential health risks associated with pregnancy in older women.

You should not take the pill if you suspect you are pregnant or have unexplained vaginal bleeding.

Cigarette smoking increases the risk of serious cardiovascular side effects from oral contraceptive use. This risk increases with age and with heavy smoking (15 or more cigarettes per day) and is quite marked in women over 35 years of age. Women who use oral contraceptives are strongly advised not to smoke.

Most side effects of the pill are not serious. The most common such effects are nausea, vomiting, bleeding between menstrual periods, weight gain, breast tenderness, headache, and difficulty wearing contact lenses. These side effects, especially nausea and vomiting, may subside within the first three months of use.

The serious side effects of the pill occur very infrequently, especially if you are in good health and are young. However, you should know that the following medical conditions have been associated with or made worse by the pill:

1. Blood clots in the legs (thrombophlebitis) or lungs (pulmonary embolism), stoppage or rupture of a blood vessel in the brain (stroke), blockage of blood vessels in the heart (heart attack or angina pectoris) or other organs of the body. As mentioned above, smoking increases the risk of heart attacks and strokes, and subsequent serious medical consequences.
2. In rare cases, oral contraceptives can cause benign but dangerous liver tumors. The benign liver tumors can rupture and cause fatal internal bleeding. In addition, some studies report an increased risk of developing liver cancer. However, liver cancers are rare.
3. High blood pressure, although blood pressure usually returns to normal when the pill is stopped.

The symptoms associated with these serious side effects are discussed in the detailed patient labeling given to you with your supply of pills. Notify your doctor or clinic if you notice any unusual physical disturbances while taking the pill. In addition, drugs such as rifampin, as well as some anticonvulsants and some antibiotics may decrease oral contraceptive effectiveness.

There is conflict among studies regarding breast cancer and oral contraceptive use. Some studies have reported an increase in the risk of developing breast cancer, particularly at a younger age. This increased risk appears to be related to duration of use. The majority of studies have found no overall increase in the risk of developing breast cancer.

Some studies have found an increase in the incidence of cancer of the cervix in women who use oral contraceptives. However, this finding may be related to factors other than the use of oral contraceptives. There is insufficient evidence to rule out the possibility that pills may cause such cancers.

Taking the pill provides some important non-contraceptive benefits. These include less painful menstruation, less menstrual blood loss and anemia, few pelvic infections, and fewer cancers of the ovary and the lining of the uterus.

Be sure to discuss any medical condition you may have with your doctor or clinic. Your doctor or clinic will take a medical and family history before prescribing oral contraceptives and will examine you. The physical examination may be delayed to another time if you request it and the health care provider believes that it is good medical practice to postpone it. You should be reexamined at least once a year while taking oral contraceptives. The detailed patient information labeling gives you further information which you should read and discuss with your doctor or clinic.

This product (like all oral contraceptives) is intended to prevent pregnancy. It does not protect against transmission of HIV (AIDS) and other sexually transmitted diseases such as chlamydia, genital herpes, genital warts, gonorrhea, hepatitis B, and syphilis.

DETAILED PATIENT LABELING

This product (like all oral contraceptives) is intended to prevent pregnancy. It does not protect against HIV infection (AIDS) and other sexually transmitted diseases.

PLEASE NOTE: This labeling is revised from time to time as important new medical information becomes available. Therefore, please review this labeling carefully.

The following oral contraceptive products contain a combination of a progestogen and estrogen, the two kinds of female hormones:

ORTHO-CEPT® □ 21 Day Regimen

ORTHO-CEPT® □ 28 Day Regimen

Each orange tablet contains 0.15 mg desogestrel and 0.03 mg ethinyl estradiol. Each green tablet in the ORTHO-CEPT 28 day regimen contains inert ingredients.

INTRODUCTION

Any woman who considers using oral contraceptives (the birth control pill or the pill) should understand the benefits and risks of using this form of birth control. This patient labeling will give you much of the information you will need to make this decision and will also help you determine if you are at risk of developing any of the serious side effects of the pill. It will tell you how to use the pill properly so that it will be as effective as possible. However, this labeling is not a replacement for a careful discussion between you and your doctor or clinic. You should discuss the information provided in this labeling with him or her, both when you first start taking the pill and during your revisits. You should also follow your doctor's or clinic's advice with regard to regular check-ups while you are on the pill.

EFFECTIVENESS OF ORAL CONTRACEPTIVES

Oral contraceptives or "birth control pills" or "the pill" are used to prevent pregnancy and are more effective than other non-surgical methods of birth control. When they are taken correctly, the chance of becoming pregnant is less than 1% (1 pregnancy per 100 women per year of use) when used perfectly, without missing any pills. Typical failure rates are actually 3% per year. The chance of becoming pregnant increases with each missed pill during a menstrual cycle.

In comparison, typical failure rates for other non-surgical methods of birth control during the first year of use are as follows:

Implant: <1%
Injection: <1%
IUD: 1 to 2%
Diaphragm with spermicides: 20%
Spermicides alone: 26%
Vaginal sponge: 20 to 40%
Female sterilization: <1%
Male sterilization: <1%
Cervical Cap with spermicides: 20 to 40%
Condom alone (male): 14%
Condom alone (female): 21%
Periodic abstinence: 25%
Withdrawal: 19%
No methods: 85%

WHO SHOULD NOT TAKE ORAL CONTRACEPTIVES

Cigarette smoking increases the risk of serious cardiovascular side effects from oral contraceptive use. This risk increases with age and with heavy smoking (15 or more cigarettes per day) and is quite marked in women over 35 years of age. Women who use oral contraceptives are strongly advised not to smoke.

Some women should not use the pill. For example, you should not take the pill if you are pregnant or think you may be pregnant. You should also not use the pill if you have any of the following conditions:

- A history of heart attack or stroke
- Blood clots in the legs (thrombophlebitis), lungs (pulmonary embolism), or eyes
- A history of blood clots in the deep veins of your legs
- Chest pain (angina pectoris)
- Known or suspected breast cancer or cancer of the lining of the uterus, cervix or vagina
- Unexplained vaginal bleeding (until a diagnosis is reached by your doctor)
- Yellowing of the whites of the eyes or of the skin (jaundice) during pregnancy or during previous use of the pill
- Liver tumor (benign or cancerous)
- Known or suspected pregnancy

Tell your doctor or clinic if you have ever had any of these conditions. Your doctor or clinic can recommend another method of birth control.

OTHER CONSIDERATIONS BEFORE TAKING ORAL CONTRACEPTIVES

Tell your doctor or clinic if you have or have had:

- Breast nodules, fibrocystic disease of the breast, an abnormal breast x-ray or mammogram
- Diabetes
- Elevated cholesterol or triglycerides
- High blood pressure
- Migraine or other headaches or epilepsy
- Mental depression
- Gallbladder, heart or kidney disease
- History of scanty or irregular menstrual periods

Women with any of these conditions should be checked often by their doctor or clinic if they choose to use oral contraceptives.

Also, be sure to inform your doctor or clinic if you smoke or are on any medications.

RISKS OF TAKING ORAL CONTRACEPTIVES

1. Risk of developing blood clots

Blood clots and blockage of blood vessels are one of the most serious side effects of taking oral contraceptives and can cause death or serious disability. In particular, a clot in the legs can cause thrombophlebitis and a clot that travels to the lungs can cause a sudden blocking of the vessel carrying blood to the lungs. These risks are greater with desogestrel–containing oral contraceptives, such as ORTHO-CEPT, than with other low-dose pills. Rarely, clots occur in the blood vessels of the eye and may cause blindness, double vision, or impaired vision.

If you take oral contraceptives and need elective surgery, need to stay in bed for a prolonged illness or have recently delivered a baby, you may be at risk of developing blood clots. You should consult your doctor or clinic about stopping oral contraceptives three to four weeks before surgery and not taking oral contraceptives for two weeks after surgery or during bed rest. You should also not take oral contraceptives soon after delivery of a baby. It is advisable to wait for at least four weeks after delivery if you are not breast feeding or four weeks after a second trimester abortion. If you are breast feeding, you should wait until you have weaned your child before using the pill. (See also the section on Breast Feeding in General Precautions.)

The risk of circulatory disease in oral contraceptive users may be higher in users of high dose pills. The risk of venous thromboembolic disease associated with oral contraceptives does not increase with length of use and disappears after pill use is stopped. The risk of abnormal blood clotting increases with age in both users and nonusers of oral contraceptives, but the increased risk from the oral contraceptive appears to be present at all ages. For women aged 20 to 44 it is estimated that about 1 in 2,000 using oral contraceptives will be hospitalized each year because of abnormal clotting. Among nonusers in the same age group, about 1 in 20,000 would be hospitalized each year. For oral contraceptive users in general, it has been estimated that in women between the ages of 15 and 34 the risk of death due to a circulatory disorder is about 1 in 12,000 per year, whereas for nonusers the rate is about 1 in 50,000 per year. In the age group 35 to 44, the risk is estimated to be about 1 in 2,500 per year for oral contraceptive users and about 1 in 10,000 per year for nonusers.

2. Heart attacks and strokes

Oral contraceptives may increase the tendency to develop strokes (stoppage or rupture of blood vessels in the brain) and angina pectoris and heart attacks (blockage of blood vessels in the heart). Any of these conditions can cause death or serious disability.

Smoking greatly increases the possibility of suffering heart attacks and strokes. Furthermore, smoking and the use of oral contraceptives greatly increase the chances of developing and dying of heart disease.

3. Gallbladder disease

Oral contraceptive users probably have a greater risk than nonusers of having gallbladder disease, although this risk may be related to pills containing high doses of estrogens.

4. Liver tumors

In rare cases, oral contraceptives can cause benign but dangerous liver tumors. These benign liver tumors can rupture and cause fatal internal bleeding. In addition, some studies report an increased risk of developing liver cancer. However, liver cancers are rare.

5. Cancer of the reproductive organs and breasts

There is conflict among studies regarding breast cancer and oral contraceptive use. Some studies have reported an increase in the risk of developing breast cancer, particularly at a younger age. This increased risk appears to be related to duration of use. The majority of studies have found no overall increase in the risk of developing breast cancer.

A meta-analysis of 54 studies found a small increase in the frequency of having breast cancer diagnosed for women who are currently using combined oral contraceptives or had used them within the past ten years. This increase in the frequency of breast cancer diagnosis, within ten years of stopping use, was generally accounted for by cancers localized to the breast. There was no increase in the frequency of having breast cancer diagnosed ten or more years after cessation of use.

Some studies have found an increase in the incidence of cancer of the cervix in women who use oral contraceptives. However, this finding may be related to factors other than the use of oral contraceptives. There is insufficient evidence to rule out the possibility that pills may cause such cancers.

ESTIMATED RISK OF DEATH FROM A BIRTH CONTROL METHOD OR PREGNANCY

All methods of birth control and pregnancy are associated with a risk of developing certain diseases which may lead to disability or death. An estimate of the number of deaths as-

Continued on next page

Ortho-Cept—Cont.

sociated with different methods of birth control and pregnancy has been calculated and is shown in the following table.
[See table below]
In the above table, the risk of death from any birth control method is less than the risk of childbirth, except for oral contraceptive users over the age of 35 who smoke and pill users over the age of 40 even if they do not smoke. It can be seen in the table that for women aged 15 to 39, the risk of death was highest with pregnancy (7–26 deaths per 100,000 women, depending on age). Among pill users who do not smoke, the risk of death is always lower than that associated with pregnancy for any age group, although over the age of 40, the risk increases to 32 deaths per 100,000 women, compared to 28 associated with pregnancy at that age. However, for pill users who smoke and are over the age of 35, the estimated number of deaths exceeds those for other methods of birth control. If a woman is over the age of 40 and smokes, her estimated risk of death is four times higher (117/100,000 women) than the estimated risk associated with pregnancy (28/100,000 women) in that age group. The suggestion that women over 40 who do not smoke should not take oral contraceptives is based on information from older, higher-dose pills. An Advisory Committee of the FDA discussed this issue in 1989 and recommended that the benefits of low-dose oral contraceptive use by healthy, non-smoking women over 40 years of age may outweigh the possible risks.

WARNING SIGNALS

If any of these adverse effects occur while you are taking oral contraceptives, call your doctor or clinic immediately:

- Sharp chest pain, coughing of blood, or sudden shortness of breath (indicating a possible clot in the lung)
- Pain in the calf (indicating a possible clot in the leg)
- Crushing chest pain or heaviness in the chest (indicating a possible heart attack)
- Sudden severe headache or vomiting, dizziness or fainting, disturbances of vision or speech, weakness, or numbness in an arm or leg (indicating a possible stroke)
- Sudden partial or complete loss of vision (indicating a possible clot in the eye)
- Breast lumps (indicating possible breast cancer or fibrocystic disease of the breast; ask your doctor or clinic to show you how to examine your breasts)
- Severe pain or tenderness in the stomach area (indicating a possibly ruptured liver tumor)
- Difficulty in sleeping, weakness, lack of energy, fatigue, or change in mood (possibly indicating severe depression)
- Jaundice or a yellowing of the skin or eyeballs, accompanied frequently by fever, fatigue, loss of appetite, dark colored urine, or light colored bowel movements (indicating possible liver problems)

SIDE EFFECTS OF ORAL CONTRACEPTIVES

1. Vaginal bleeding
Irregular vaginal bleeding or spotting may occur while you are taking the pills. Irregular bleeding may vary from slight staining between menstrual periods to breakthrough bleeding which is a flow much like a regular period. Irregular bleeding occurs most often during the first few months of oral contraceptive use, but may also occur after you have been taking the pill for some time. Such bleeding may be temporary and usually does not indicate any serious problems. It is important to continue taking your pills on schedule. If the bleeding occurs in more than one cycle or lasts for more than a few days, talk to your doctor or clinic.
2. Contact lenses
If you wear contact lenses and notice a change in vision or an inability to wear your lenses, contact your doctor or clinic.
3. Fluid retention
Oral contraceptives may cause edema (fluid retention) with swelling of the fingers or ankles and may raise your blood pressure. If you experience fluid retention, contact your doctor or clinic.
4. Melasma
A spotty darkening of the skin is possible, particularly of the face, which may persist.
5. Other side effects
Other side effects may include nausea and vomiting, change in appetite, headache, nervousness, depression, dizziness, loss of scalp hair, rash, and vaginal infections.
If any of these side effects bother you, call your doctor or clinic.

GENERAL PRECAUTIONS

1. Missed periods and use of oral contraceptives before or during early pregnancy
There may be times when you may not menstruate regularly after you have completed taking a cycle of pills. If you have taken your pills regularly and miss one menstrual period, continue taking your pills for the next cycle but be sure to inform your doctor or clinic before doing so. If you have not taken the pills daily as instructed and missed a menstrual period, you may be pregnant. If you missed two consecutive menstrual periods, you may be pregnant. Check with your doctor or clinic immediately to determine whether you are pregnant. Do not continue to take oral contraceptives until you are sure you are not pregnant, but continue to use another method of contraception.
There is no conclusive evidence that oral contraceptive use is associated with an increase in birth defects, when taken inadvertently during early pregnancy. Previously, a few studies had reported that oral contraceptives might be associated with birth defects, but these findings have not been seen in more recent studies. Nevertheless, oral contraceptives or any other drugs should not be used during pregnancy unless clearly necessary and prescribed by your doctor or clinic. You should check with your doctor or clinic about risks to your unborn child of any medication taken during pregnancy.
2. While breast feeding
If you are breast feeding, consult your doctor or clinic before starting oral contraceptives. Some of the drug will be passed on to the child in the milk. A few adverse effects on the child have been reported, including yellowing of the skin (jaundice) and breast enlargement. In addition, oral contraceptives may decrease the amount and quality of your milk. If possible, do not use oral contraceptives while breast feeding. You should use another method of contraception since breast feeding provides only partial protection from becoming pregnant and this partial protection decreases significantly as you breast feed for longer periods of time. You should consider starting oral contraceptives only after you have weaned your child completely.
3. Laboratory tests
If you are scheduled for any laboratory tests, tell your doctor or clinic you are taking birth control pills. Certain blood tests may be affected by birth control pills.
4. Drug interactions
Certain drugs may interact with birth control pills to make them less effective in preventing pregnancy or cause an increase in breakthrough bleeding. Such drugs include rifampin, drugs used for epilepsy such as barbiturates (for example, phenobarbital), anticonvulsants such as carbamazepine (Tegretol is one brand of this drug), phenytoin (Dilantin is one brand of this drug), phenylbutazone (Butazolidin is one brand), and possibly certain antibiotics. You may need to use additional contraception when you take drugs which can make oral contraceptives less effective.
5. Sexually transmitted diseases
This product (like all oral contraceptives) is intended to prevent pregnancy. It does not protect against transmission of HIV (AIDS) and other sexually transmitted diseases such as chlamydia, genital herpes, genital warts, gonorrhea, hepatitis B, and syphilis.

HOW TO TAKE THE PILL

IMPORTANT POINTS TO REMEMBER

BEFORE YOU START TAKING YOUR PILLS:
1. BE SURE TO READ THESE DIRECTIONS:
Before you start taking your pills.
Anytime you are not sure what to do.
2. THE RIGHT WAY TO TAKE THE PILL IS TO TAKE ONE PILL EVERY DAY AT THE SAME TIME.
If you miss pills you could get pregnant. This includes starting the pack late. The more pills you miss, the more likely you are to get pregnant.
3. MANY WOMEN HAVE SPOTTING OR LIGHT BLEEDING, OR MAY FEEL SICK TO THEIR STOMACH DURING THE FIRST 1–3 PACKS OF PILLS. If you feel sick to your stomach, do not stop taking the pill. The problem will usually go away. If it doesn't go away, check with your doctor or clinic.
4. MISSING PILLS CAN ALSO CAUSE SPOTTING OR LIGHT BLEEDING, even when you make up these missed pills.
On the days you take 2 pills to make up for missed pills, you could also feel a little sick to your stomach.
5. IF YOU HAVE VOMITING OR DIARRHEA, for any reason, or IF YOU TAKE SOME MEDICINES, including some antibiotics, your pills may not work as well.
Use a back-up method (such as condoms, foam, or sponge) until you check with your doctor or clinic.
6. IF YOU HAVE TROUBLE REMEMBERING TO TAKE THE PILL, talk to your doctor or clinic about how to make pill-taking easier or about using another method of birth control.
7. IF YOU HAVE ANY QUESTIONS OR ARE UNSURE ABOUT THE INFORMATION IN THIS LEAFLET, call your doctor or clinic.

BEFORE YOU START TAKING YOUR PILLS

1. DECIDE WHAT TIME OF DAY YOU WANT TO TAKE YOUR PILL.
It is important to take it at about the same time every day.
2. LOOK AT YOUR PILL PACK TO SEE IF IT HAS 21 OR 28 PILLS:
The 21-pill pack has 21 "active" orange pills (with hormones) to take for 3 weeks, followed by 1 week without pills.
The 28-pill pack has 21 "active" orange pills (with hormones) to take for 3 weeks, followed by 1 week of "reminder" green pills (without hormones).
3. ALSO FIND:
1) where on the pack to start taking pills,
2) in what order to take the pills.
CHECK PICTURE OF PILL PACK AND ADDITIONAL INSTRUCTIONS FOR USING THIS PACKAGE IN THE BRIEF SUMMARY PATIENT PACKAGE INSERT.
4. BE SURE YOU HAVE READY AT ALL TIMES:
ANOTHER KIND OF BIRTH CONTROL (such as condoms, foam, or sponge) to use as a back-up method in case you miss pills.
AN EXTRA, FULL PILL PACK

WHEN TO START THE FIRST PACK OF PILLS

You have a choice of which day to start taking your first pack of pills. ORTHO-CEPT is available in the DIALPAK® Tablet Dispenser which is preset for a Sunday Start. Day 1 start is also provided. Decide with your doctor or clinic which is the best day for you. Pick a time of day which will be easy to remember.
DAY 1 START:
1. Take the first "active" orange pill of the first pack during the first 24 hours of your period.
2. You will not need to use a back-up method of birth control, since you are starting the pill at the beginning of your period.
SUNDAY START:
1. Take the first "active" orange pill of the first pack on the Sunday after your period starts, even if you are still bleeding. If your period begins on Sunday, start the pack that same day.
2. Use another method of birth control as a back-up method if you have sex anytime from the Sunday you start your first pack until the next Sunday (7 days). Condoms, foam, or the sponge are good back-up methods of birth control.

WHAT TO DO DURING THE MONTH

1. TAKE ONE PILL AT THE SAME TIME EVERY DAY UNTIL THE PACK IS EMPTY.
Do not skip pills even if you are spotting or bleeding between monthly periods or feel sick to your stomach (nausea).
Do not skip pills even if you do not have sex very often.
2. WHEN YOU FINISH A PACK OR SWITCH YOUR BRAND OF PILLS:
21 pills: Wait 7 days to start the next pack. You will probably have your period during that week. Be sure that no more than 7 days pass between 21-day packs.
28 pills: Start the next pack on the day after your last "reminder" pill. Do not wait any days between packs.

WHAT TO DO IF YOU MISS PILLS

If you **MISS 1** orange "active" pill:
1. Take it as soon as you remember. Take the next pill at your regular time. This means you may take 2 pills in 1 day.
2. You do not need to use a back-up birth control method if you have sex.
If you **MISS 2** orange "active" pills in a row in **WEEK 1 OR WEEK 2** of your pack:
1. Take 2 pills on the day you remember and 2 pills the next day.
2. Then take 1 pill a day until you finish the pack.
3. You MAY BECOME PREGNANT if you have sex in the 7 days after you miss pills. You MUST use another birth control method (such as condoms, foam, or sponge) as a back-up method for those 7 days.
If you **MISS 2** orange "active" pills in a row in **THE 3RD WEEK:**
1. If you are a Day 1 Starter:
THROW OUT the rest of the pill pack and start a new pack that same day.
If you are a Sunday Starter:
Keep taking 1 pill every day until Sunday. On Sunday, THROW OUT the rest of the pack and start a new pack of pills that same day.

ANNUAL NUMBER OF BIRTH-RELATED OR METHOD-RELATED DEATHS ASSOCIATED WITH CONTROL OF FERTILITY PER 100,000 NONSTERILE WOMEN, BY FERTILITY CONTROL METHOD ACCORDING TO AGE

Method of control and outcome	15–19	20–24	25–29	30–34	35–39	40–44
No fertility control methods*	7.0	7.4	9.1	14.8	25.7	28.2
Oral contraceptives non-smoker**	0.3	0.5	0.9	1.9	13.8	31.6
Oral contraceptives smoker**	2.2	3.4	6.6	13.5	51.1	117.2
IUD**	0.8	0.8	1.0	1.0	1.4	1.4
Condom*	1.1	1.6	0.7	0.2	0.3	0.4
Diaphragm/spermicide*	1.9	1.2	1.2	1.3	2.2	2.8
Periodic abstinence*	2.5	1.6	1.6	1.7	2.9	3.6

* Deaths are birth-related
** Deaths are method-related

2. You may not have your period this month but this is expected. However, if you miss your period 2 months in a row, call your doctor or clinic because you might be pregnant.
3. You MAY BECOME PREGNANT if you have sex in the 7 days after you miss pills. You MUST use another birth control method (such as condoms, foam, or sponge) as a back-up method for those 7 days.
If you **MISS 3 OR MORE** orange "active" pills in a row (during the first 3 weeks).
1. **If you are a Day 1 Starter:**
THROW OUT the rest of the pill pack and start a new pack that same day.
If you are a Sunday Starter:
Keep taking 1 pill every day until Sunday. On Sunday, THROW OUT the rest of the pack and start a new pack of pills that same day.
2. You may not have your period this month but this is expected. However, if you miss your period 2 months in a row, call your doctor or clinic because you might be pregnant.
3. You MAY BECOME PREGNANT if you have sex in the 7 days after you miss pills. You MUST use another birth control method (such as condoms, foam, or sponge) as a back-up method for those 7 days.

A REMINDER FOR THOSE ON 28-DAY PACKS:
If you forget any of the 7 green "reminder" pills in Week 4:
THROW AWAY the pills you missed.
Keep taking 1 pill each day until the pack is empty.
You do not need a back-up method.

FINALLY, IF YOU ARE STILL NOT SURE WHAT TO DO ABOUT THE PILLS YOU HAVE MISSED:
Use a BACK-UP METHOD anytime you have sex.
KEEP TAKING ONE "ACTIVE" PILL EACH DAY until you can reach your doctor or clinic.

PREGNANCY DUE TO PILL FAILURE

The incidence of pill failure resulting in pregnancy is approximately one percent (i.e., one pregnancy per 100 women per year) if taken every day as directed, but more typical failure rates are about 3%. If failure does occur, the risk to the fetus is minimal.

PREGNANCY AFTER STOPPING THE PILL

There may be some delay in becoming pregnant after you stop using oral contraceptives, especially if you had irregular menstrual cycles before you used oral contraceptives. It may be advisable to postpone conception until you begin menstruating regularly once you have stopped taking the pill and desire pregnancy.
There does not appear to be any increase in birth defects in newborn babies when pregnancy occurs soon after stopping the pill.

OVERDOSAGE

Serious ill effects have not been reported following ingestion of large doses of oral contraceptives by young children. Overdosage may cause nausea and withdrawal bleeding in females. In cases of overdosage, contact your doctor, clinic or pharmacist.

OTHER INFORMATION

Your doctor or clinic will take a medical and family history before prescribing oral contraceptives and will examine you. The physical examination may be delayed to another time if you request it and the health care provider believes that it is a good medical practice to postpone it.You should be reexamined at least once a year. Be sure to inform your doctor or clinic if there is a family history of any of the conditions listed previously in this leaflet. Be sure to keep all appointments with your doctor or clinic because this is a time to determine if there are early signs of side effects of oral contraceptive use.
Do not use the drug for any condition other than the one for which it was prescribed. This drug has been prescribed specifically for you; do not give it to others who may want birth control pills.

HEALTH BENEFITS FROM ORAL CONTRACEPTIVES

In addition to preventing pregnancy, use of combination oral contraceptives may provide certain benefits. They are:
- menstrual cycles may become more regular
- blood flow during menstruation may be lighter and less iron may be lost. Therefore, anemia due to iron deficiency is less likely to occur.
- pain or other symptoms during menstruation may be encountered less frequently
- ectopic (tubal) pregnancy may occur less frequently
- noncancerous cysts or lumps in the breast may occur less frequently
- acute pelvic inflammatory disease may occur less frequently
- oral contraceptive use may provide some protection against developing two forms of cancer: cancer of the ovaries and cancer of the lining of the uterus.

If you want more information about birth control pills, ask your doctor, clinic or pharmacist. They have a more technical leaflet called the Professional Labeling, which you may wish to read. The professional labeling is also published in a book entitled *Physicians' Desk Reference*, available in many book stores and public libraries.

Packaged and Distributed by
ORTHO-McNEIL PHARMACEUTICAL, INC.
Raritan, New Jersey 08869
Jointly Manufactured by
ORTHO-McNEIL PHARMACEUTICAL, INC.
Raritan, New Jersey 08869 and
DIOSYNTH bv Oss, The Netherlands
©OPC 1998 Revised February 1999 PO7-220
631-10-840-6
Shown in Product Identification Guide, page 328

ORTHO® DIAPHRAGM KITS ℞

This product contains dry natural rubber.

DESCRIPTION

ORTHO Diaphragm Kits include two different types in a variety of sizes.
1. The ALL-FLEX® Arcing Spring Diaphragm is a molded, buff-colored, dry natural rubber vaginal diaphragm containing a distortion-free, dual spring-within-a-spring which provides unique arcing action no matter where the rim is compressed. It is appropriate not only where ordinary diaphragms are indicated, but also in patients with mild cystocele, rectocele or retroversion.
2. The ORTHO® Coil Spring Diaphragm is a molded dry natural rubber vaginal diaphragm. The rim encases a tension-adjusted spring which allows for compressibility in one plane only, thus allowing insertion with the ORTHO UNIVERSAL INTRODUCER.

ACTION

These Diaphragms when properly fitted serve two purposes:
a. To stop the sperm from entering the cervical canal;
b. To hold the spermicide.

INDICATIONS

ORTHO Diaphragms, in conjunction with an appropriate spermicide, are indicated for the prevention of pregnancy in women who elect to use diaphragms as a method of contraception.
The diaphragm should always be used in combination with a spermicidal jelly (or cream) [e.g., ORTHO OPTIONS™ GYNOL II® Original Formula Contraceptive Jelly, ORTHO OPTIONS™ ORTHO-GYNOL Contraceptive Jelly.

CONTRAINDICATIONS

Known hypersensitivity to dry natural rubber and/or prior history of Toxic Shock Syndrome (TSS).

WARNINGS

An association has been reported between diaphragm use and toxic shock syndrome (TSS), a serious condition which can be fatal.
For contraceptive effectiveness, the diaphragm should remain in place for six hours after intercourse and *should be removed as soon as possible thereafter*.
Continuous wearing of a contraceptive diaphragm for more than twenty-four hours is not recommended. Removal of the diaphragm before six hours may increase the risk of becoming pregnant. Retention of the diaphragm for any period of time may encourage the growth of certain bacteria in the vaginal tract. It has been suggested that under certain as yet unestablished conditions, overgrowth of these bacteria may lead to symptoms of toxic shock syndrome.
Primary symptoms of TSS are sudden high fever (usually 102° or more), and vomiting, diarrhea, fainting or near fainting when standing up, dizziness or a rash that looks like sunburn. There may also be other signs of TSS such as aching of muscles and joints, redness of the eyes, sore throat and weakness. Patients should be instructed that if they experience sudden high fever and one or more of the other symptoms, they should remove the diaphragm and consult their physician or health care provider immediately.

Latex or Natural Rubber Sensitivity
The ORTHO Diaphragm contains dry natural rubber proteins. Persons sensitive to latex or natural rubber may have an allergic reaction to the diaphragm. If this occurs, discontinue use and consult your doctor or health care provider.

PRECAUTIONS

Diaphragm users should be instructed to consult their physician or health care provider:
1. If they are not sure about the insertion and placement of the diaphragm.
2. If they or their partner feel or are made uncomfortable by the presence of the diaphragm.
3. If you experience any discomfort or pain while the diaphragm is in place. This may be due to incorrect diaphragm insertion, an abnormal pelvic condition, constipation or incorrect diaphragm size.
4. If the diaphragm slips out of place when walking, coughing, or straining.
5. If the diaphragm no longer fits snugly above the pubic bone.
6. If at times other than menstruation there is blood on the diaphragm when it is removed.
7. If there are any holes, tears or other deterioration of the diaphragm.
8. If unable to remove the diaphragm.
9. **IMPORTANT**—For contraceptive effectiveness, the diaphragm should remain in place for six hours after intercourse and *should be removed as soon as possible thereafter*. Continuous wearing of a contraceptive diaphragm for more than twenty-four hours is not recommended. Removal of the diaphragm before six hours may increase the risk of becoming pregnant. Retention of the diaphragm for any period of time may encourage the growth of certain bacteria in the vaginal tract. It has been suggested that under certain as yet unestablished conditions, overgrowth of these bacteria may lead to symptoms of toxic shock syndrome. Primary symptoms of TSS are sudden high fever (usually 102° or more), and vomiting, diarrhea, fainting or near fainting when standing up, dizziness or a rash that looks like a sunburn. There may also be other signs of TSS such as aching of muscles and joints, redness of the eyes, sore throat and weakness. If the patient has a sudden high fever and one or more of the other symptoms, the diaphragm should be removed immediately and TSS should be considered.
10. Diaphragm users should have another diaphragm fitting if they have lost or gained more than ten pounds, have had the diaphragm for more than a year, or have had a baby or an abortion. As a matter of routine, each time a pelvic examination is performed, refitting should be done. The size and shape of the vagina changes and this may require a new size diaphragm. Even if the diaphragm size does not change, it is advisable to replace the diaphragm every two years or sooner.
11. Diaphragms may increase the risk of urinary tract infections especially if not properly fitted. Patients should be instructed to consult their physician if they experience any of the signs or symptoms of this type of infection which include pain on urination, blood in the urine, elevated temperature, frequent urination, or a sensation of obstruction while urinating.
12. Persons sensitive to dry natural rubber may have an allergic reaction to diaphragm use.
13. Persons sensitive to spermicides used with the diaphragm should discontinue use.
14. Petroleum jelly, mineral oil, vegetable oil and cold cream lubricants should **NOT** be used concurrently with the diaphragm.

INSTRUCTIONS

1. Proper placement of the diaphragm is vital for effectiveness.
2. To be fully effective the diaphragm should never be used without contraceptive cream or jelly. The contraceptive cream or jelly must be spread around the inner surface of the diaphragm as well as around the rim.
3. To avoid pregnancy the diaphragm must be used every time there is intercourse.
4. The diaphragm may be inserted up to six hours before intercourse. If more than six hours has elapsed between insertion of the diaphragm and intercourse, additional contraceptive jelly or cream must be inserted. The diaphragm should not be removed to insert this additional cream or jelly.

The following Patient Instructions for insertion and removal are contained in the leaflet "After your doctor or health care provider Prescribes your Ortho Diaphragm" which is included in each Ortho Diaphragm Kit.

Preparing for insertion
Cleanse the diaphragm before initial use by washing it with mild, non-perfumed soap and warm water, rinsing and dry it carefully.
Empty your bladder (urinate) and wash your hands thoroughly before insertion.
Examine the diaphragm carefully before use by holding it in front of a light to make sure it has no cracks or tiny holes. Take care not to stretch or puncture the diaphragm with sharp fingernails. Do not use if you observe any visible cracks or holes.
The diaphragm should always be inserted before intercourse. To prepare your diaphragm for insertion, you should put the spermicide into the cup of the diaphragm. This ensures that the spermicide is placed between the cervix and the diaphragm. Use the amount of spermicide recommended by the manufacturer of the spermicide you use.
Using your finger tip, spread some of the spermicidal jelly (or cream) around the rim of the diaphragm that will be in contact with the cervix (entrance to the womb). If the amount applied to the rim is excessive, it will be difficult to control the diaphragm during insertion.

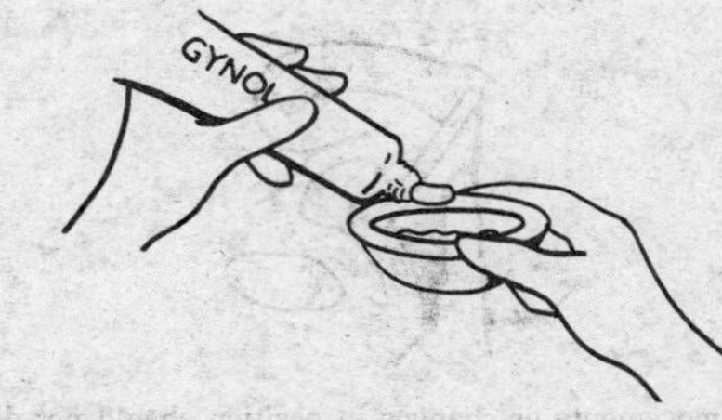

You can insert the diaphragm while you are standing with one leg up, squatting, or lying down. The position of the cervix and the walls of the vagina will be different depending on your position. If you are used to one position and then

Continued on next page

Ortho Diaphragm—Cont.

change to another, take extra care in positioning the diaphragm to be sure the cervix is covered.

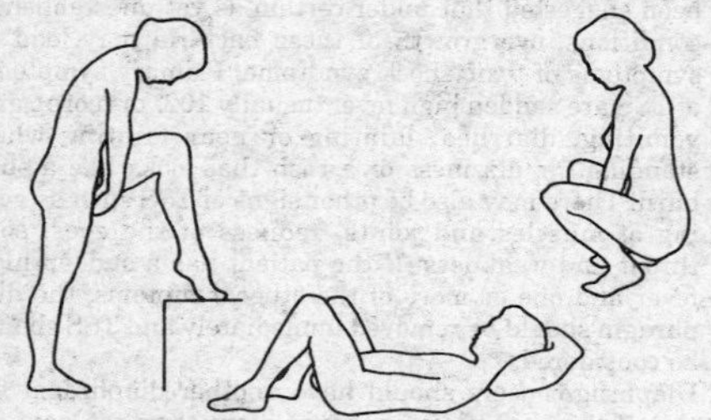

Inserting the diaphragm
Hold the diaphragm with the dome down (spermicide up) and press the opposite sides of the rim together between your thumb and third finger. The diaphragm can be held from above or below.

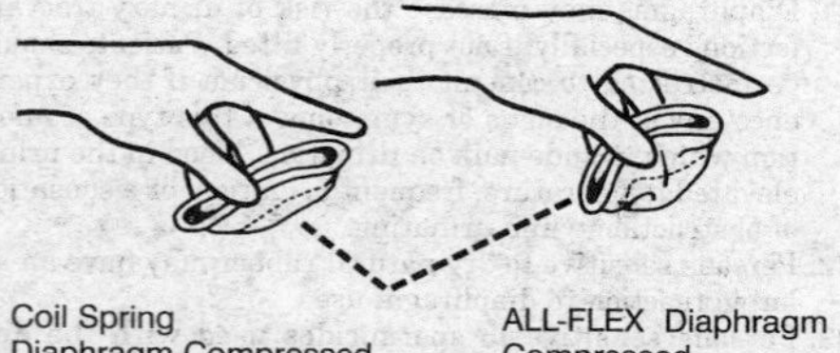

Coil Spring Diaphragm Compressed ALL-FLEX Diaphragm Compressed

Separate the lips of your vagina with your free hand. Hold the compressed diaphragm with the dome down (spermicide up) and push it gently inward, along the rear wall of the vaginal canal, directing it backwards as far as it can go. Your index finger, kept on the outer rim of the diaphragm, helps to guide the diaphragm into place.

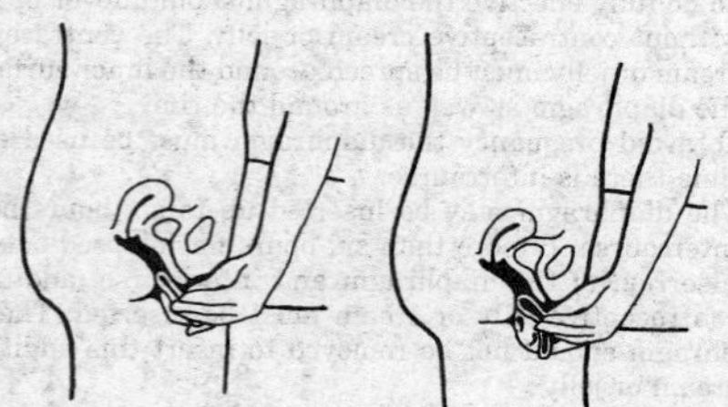

Coil Spring Diaphragm being introduced ALL-FLEX Diaphragm being introduced

Always insert the diaphragm as far back as it will go behind the mouth of the cervix. Then push the front rim of the diaphragm up until it is locked in place just behind the pubic bone.

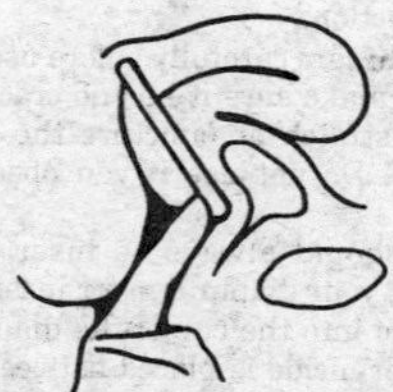

It is important that the cervix be covered by the spermicide and the diaphragm and that the diaphragm be locked in place between the upper edge of the pubic bone and the rear wall of the vagina. Test for correct position by running the index or middle finger over the diaphragm's dome to be sure it covers the cervix.
The cervix will feel like the end of your nose. It is normal to feel folds in the diaphragm when it is in place.

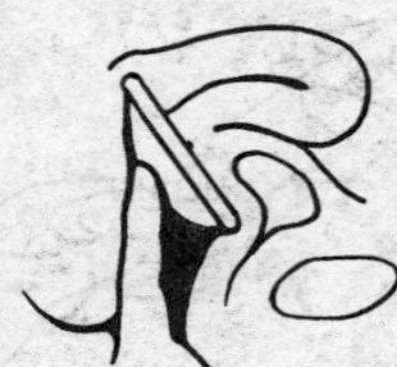

Bodily movements or changes in position should not dislodge a correctly-inserted diaphragm. A properly-fitted diaphragm should stay in place during urination or bowel movement.

Preparing the diaphragm when using an introducer
The introducer has been designed to insert diaphragms from size 60mm through 90mm. The introducer is slightly indented and used to hold one side of the diaphragm rim for insertion. The ORTHO Diaphragm has the size molded into the side of the rubber dome so that it is easy to read throughout the life of the diaphragm.
Hold the introducer in either hand with the notched-side down. Hold the diaphragm in your other hand with the dome up. Squeeze the opposite sides of the diaphragm together and place one end of the diaphragm's rim into the notched end of the introducer, then fit the other end of the diaphragm over the notch corresponding to your diaphragm size (sizes are shown next to each notch on the introducer.) Turn the introducer over and insert the amount of spermicidal jelly (or cream) recommended by the manufacturer of the spermicide you use into the folds formed on the top of the diaphragm (the cup side.) This ensures that the spermicide is placed between the cervix and the diaphragm. Using your fingertip, spread some of the spermicidal jelly (or cream) around the rim of the diaphragm to make insertion easier and to help seal the diaphragm in place.

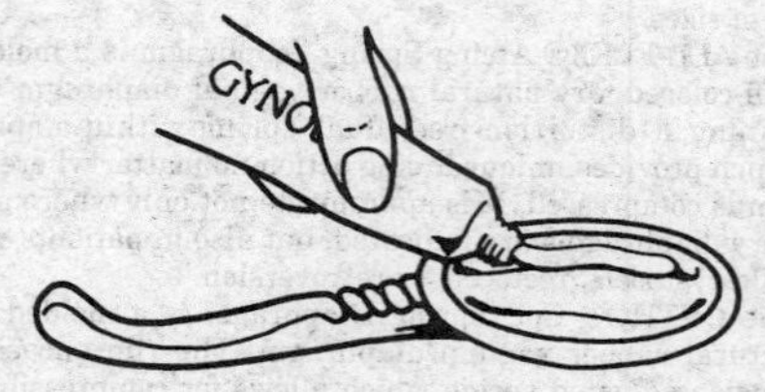

Inserting the diaphragm when using an introducer
With the spermicide up, insert the introducer into the vagina. Press gently inward along the rear wall of the vagina until the diaphragm has been inserted as far as possible.

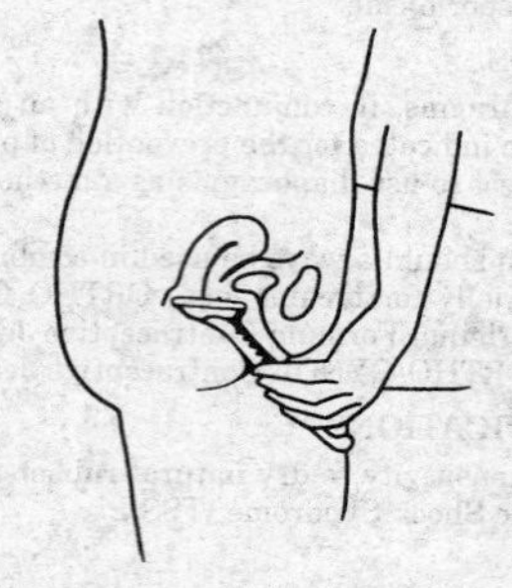

Once the diaphragm is in place, twist the introducer slightly to the left or right to release the diaphragm. Then, gently withdraw the introducer. Using your index finger, check to ensure the near rim of the diaphragm is pushed up behind the pubic bone.

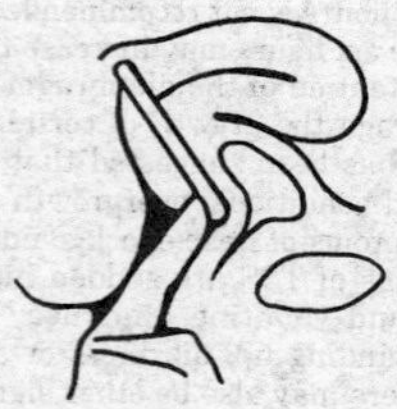

Test for correct position by running the index or middle finger over the diaphragm's dome to be sure it covers the cervix. The cervix will feel like the end of your nose. It is normal to feel folds in the diaphragm when it is in place.

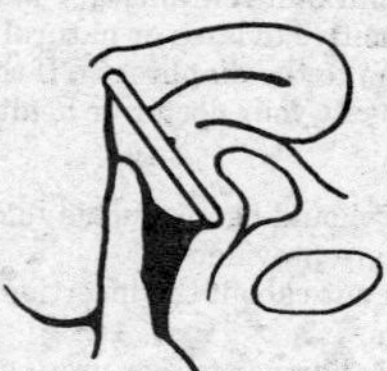

To cleanse the introducer, wash with soap and warm water, rinse and dry.

Removing the Diaphragm
To reduce the risk of TSS the diaphragm should be removed six (to eight) hours after intercourse (depending upon which brand of spermicide you use.) Continuous wearing of a diaphragm for more than 24 hours is not recommended. (See WARNINGS AND PRECAUTIONS FOR USE.)
Removal of the diaphragm before six (to eight) hours after intercourse (depending on which brand of spermicide you use), may increase your risk of becoming pregnant.
Do not douche until the diaphragm is removed. To remove the diaphragm, put your index finger behind the from rim and pull the diaphragm down and out. Avoid puncturing the diaphragm with your fingernails.
[See figure at top of next column]

To facilitate removal, straining down as with a bowel movement may help to push the rim down so that the index finger can reach the rim more easily. If suction is holding the diaphragm, the suction may be broken by placing a finger between the vaginal wall and the rim.
If your menstrual period begins while the diaphragm is in place and blood is found in the cup of the diaphragm when it is removed, do not be concerned as this is not harmful.

CARE OF THE DIAPHRAGM
After removal of the diaphragm, it should be cleansed thoroughly with mild, non-perfumed soap and water, rinsed and dried carefully. Powders should not be used with the diaphragm. Never boil the diaphragm or use antiseptic solutions in cleaning it.
Store the diaphragm, unrolled, in its original container. Do not allow the diaphragm to dry in the open. Prolonged exposure to light or heat will deteriorate the rubber.
Never stretch or puncture the diaphragm with sharp fingernails. With regular use, and in the absence of evident deterioration, the diaphragm should be replaced every 1–2 years.
Some vaginal medications and lubricating agents may contain ingredients that can damage a contraceptive diaphragm. You should discuss the use of any such vaginal preparation with your doctor, health care provider, pharmacist or the manufacturer or distributor. Petroleum jelly, mineral oil, vegetable oil and cold cream lubricants should NOT be used concurrently with the diaphragm.

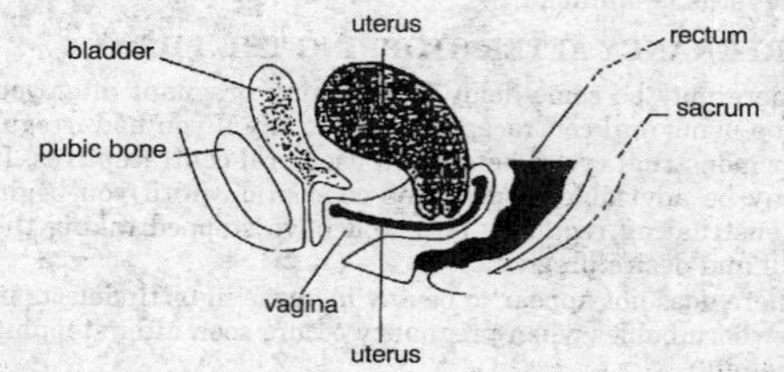

Where to purchase Ortho Contraceptive Products
The ORTHO® Universal Introducer is available by prescription through pharmacies.
These Ortho contraceptive jelly brands for use with diaphragms are available without a prescription at most pharmacies and some grocery stores.
ORTHO OPTIONS™ GYNOL II® Original Formula large tube only—3.8 oz.
ORTHO OPTIONS™ GYNOL II® Extra Strength includes applicator w/small tube
ORTHO OPTIONS™ ORTHO-GYNOL® large tube only—3.8 oz.
If added vaginal lubrication is necessary, you may want to consider K-Y® BRAND Jelly Personal Lubricant which is available without a prescription in a .4 oz., 2 oz. and a 4 oz. tube. K-Y® Liquid and K-Y® Long Lasting™ vaginal moisturizer. K-Y® BRAND Jelly Personal Lubricant is not a contraceptive.

HOW SUPPLIED
All ORTHO Diaphragm Kits are available individually and contain a tube of ORTHO OPTIONS™ GYNOL II Original Formula Contraceptive Jelly.
1. The ALL-FLEX Arcing Spring Diaphragm is available in sizes 55mm through 95mm in 5mm increments.
2. The ORTHO Coil Spring Diaphragm is available in sizes 55mm through 95mm in 5mm increments.

HOW TO FIT ORTHO DIAPHRAGMS
1. To measure for diaphragm size:
Hold index and middle fingers together and insert into vagina up to the posterior fornix. Raise hand to bring surface of index finger to contact with pubic arch.
Use tip of thumb to mark the point directly beneath the inferior margin of the pubic bone and withdraw finger in this position.
2. To determine diaphragm size:
Place one end of rim of fitting diaphragm or ring on tip of middle finger. The opposite end should lie just in front of the thumb tip. This is the approximate diameter of the diaphragm needed.
Insert a fitting diaphragm or ring of the appropriate size into the vagina.
Try both a larger and a smaller size before making a decision.
3. The proper size will fit snugly in the posterior fornix and behind the pubic arch without undue pressure.

Revised May 2000

Shown in Product Identification Guide, page 328

ORTHO® Dienestrol Cream ℞

1. ESTROGENS HAVE BEEN REPORTED TO INCREASE THE RISK OF ENDOMETRIAL CARCINOMA.

Three independent case control studies have shown an increased risk of endometrial cancer in postmenopausal women exposed to exogenous estrogens for prolonged periods.[1–3] This risk was independent of the other known risk factors for endometrial cancer. These studies are further supported by the finding that incidence rates of endometrial cancer have increased sharply since 1969 in eight different areas of the United States with population-based cancer reporting systems, an increase which may be related to the rapidly expanding use of estrogens during the last decade.[4]

The three case control studies reported that the risk of endometrial cancer in estrogen users was about 4.5 to 13.9 times greater than in nonusers. The risk appears to depend on both duration of treatment[1] and on estrogen dose.[3] In view of these findings, when estrogens are used for the treatment of menopausal symptoms, the lowest dose that will control symptoms should be utilized and medication should be discontinued as soon as possible. When prolonged treatment is medically indicated, the patient should be reassessed on at least a semiannual basis to determine the need for continued therapy. Although the evidence must be considered preliminary, one study suggests that cyclic administration of low doses of estrogen may carry less risk than continuous administration;[3] it therefore appears prudent to utilize such a regimen.

Close clinical surveillance of all women taking estrogens is important. In all cases of undiagnosed persistent or recurring abnormal vaginal bleeding, adequate diagnostic measures should be undertaken to rule out malignancy.

There is no evidence at present that "natural" estrogens are more or less hazardous than "synthetic" estrogens at equiestrogenic doses.

2. ESTROGENS SHOULD NOT BE USED DURING PREGNANCY

The use of female sex hormones, both estrogens and progestogens, during early pregnancy may seriously damage the offspring. It has been shown that females exposed *in utero* to diethylstilbestrol, a non-steroidal estrogen, have an increased risk of developing in later life a form of vaginal or cervical cancer that ordinarily is extremely rare.[5,6] This risk has been estimated as not greater than 4 per 1000 exposures.[7] Furthermore, a high percentage of such exposed women (from 30 to 90 percent) have been found to have vaginal adenosis,[8,13] epithelial changes of the vagina and cervix. Although these changes are histologically benign, it is not known whether they are precursors of malignancy. Although similar data are not available with the use of other estrogens, it cannot be presumed they would not induce similar changes.

Several reports suggest an association between intrauterine exposure to female sex hormones and congenital anomalies, including congenital heart defects and limb reduction defects.[13–16] One case control study[16] estimated a 4.7 fold increased risk of limb reduction defects in infants exposed *in utero* to sex hormones (oral contraceptives, hormone withdrawal tests for pregnancy, or attempted treatment for threatened abortion). Some of these exposures were very short and involved only a few days of treatment. The data suggest that the risk of limb reduction defects in exposed fetuses is somewhat less than 1 per 1000.

In the past, female sex hormones have been used during pregnancy in an attempt to treat threatened or habitual abortion. There is considerable evidence that estrogens are ineffective for these indications, and there is no evidence from well controlled studies that progestogens are effective for these uses.

If ORTHO Dienestrol Cream is used during pregnancy, or if the patient becomes pregnant while using this drug, she should be apprised of the potential risks to the fetus, and the advisability of pregnancy continuation.

DESCRIPTION

ORTHO Dienestrol Cream
Cream for Intravaginal use only

Active ingredient: Dienestrol 0.01%.

Dienestrol is a synthetic, non-steroidal estrogen. It is compounded in a cream base suitable for intravaginal use only. The cream base is composed of glyceryl monostearate, peanut oil, glycerin, benzoic acid, glutamic acid, butylated hydroxyanisole, citric acid, sodium hydroxide and water. The pH is approximately 4.3.

HO—C₆H₄—C(=CH—CH₃)—C(=CH—CH₃)—C₆H₄—OH

4,4'-(Diethylideneethylene)diphenol

CLINICAL PHARMACOLOGY

Systemic absorption and mode of action of dienestrol are undetermined.

INDICATIONS AND USAGE

ORTHO Dienestrol Cream is indicated in the treatment of atrophic vaginitis and kraurosis vulvae.

ORTHO DIENESTROL CREAM HAS NOT BEEN SHOWN TO BE EFFECTIVE FOR ANY PURPOSE DURING PREGNANCY AND ITS USE MAY CAUSE SEVERE HARM TO THE FETUS (*SEE* BOXED WARNING).

CONTRAINDICATIONS

Estrogens may cause fetal harm when administered to a pregnant woman (*see* Boxed Warning). Estrogens are contraindicated in women who are or may become pregnant. If this drug is used during pregnancy, or if the patient becomes pregnant while using this drug, the patient should be apprised of the potential hazard to the fetus.

Estrogens should also not be used in women with any of the following conditions:

1. Known or suspected cancer of the breast.
2. Known or suspected estrogen-dependent neoplasia.
3. Undiagnosed abnormal genital bleeding.
4. Active thrombophlebitis or thromboembolic disorders.
5. A past history of thrombophlebitis, thrombosis, or thromboembolic disorders associated with previous estrogen use.

WARNINGS

1. *Induction of malignant neoplasms.* Long-term continuous administration of natural and synthetic estrogens in certain animal species increases the frequency of carcinomas of the breast, cervix, vagina, and liver. There is now evidence that estrogens increase the risk of carcinoma of the endometrium in humans. (*See* Boxed Warning.)

At the present time there is no satisfactory evidence that estrogens given to postmenopausal women increase the risk of cancer of the breast,[18] although a recent long-term followup of a single physician's practice has raised this possibility.[18a] Because of the animal data, there is a need for caution in prescribing estrogens for women with a strong family history of breast cancer or who have breast nodules, fibrocystic disease, or abnormal mammograms.

2. *Gallbladder disease.* A recent study has reported a 2- to 3-fold increase in the risk of surgically confirmed gall bladder disease in women receiving postmenopausal estrogens,[18] similar to the 2-fold increase previously noted in users of oral contraceptives.[19,24] In the case of oral contraceptives the increased risk appeared after two years of use.[24]

3. *Effects similar to those caused by estrogen-progestogen oral contraceptives.* There are several serious adverse effects of oral contraceptives, most of which have not, up to now, been documented as consequences of postmenopausal estrogen therapy. This may reflect the comparatively low doses of estrogen used in postmenopausal women. It would be expected that the larger doses of estrogen used to treat prostatic or breast cancer or postpartum breast engorgement are more likely to result in these adverse effects, and, in fact, it has been shown that there is an increased risk of thrombosis in men receiving estrogens for prostatic cancer and women for postpartum breast engorgement.[20–23]

a. *Thromboembolic disease.* It is now well established that users of oral contraceptives have an increased risk of various thromboembolic and thrombotic vascular diseases, such as thrombophlebitis, pulmonary embolism, stroke, and myocardial infarction.[24–31] Cases of retinal thrombosis, mesenteric thrombosis, and optic neuritis have been reported in oral contraceptive users. There is evidence that the risk of several of these adverse reactions is related to the dose of the drug.[32,33] An increased risk of postsurgery thromboembolic complications has also been reported in users of oral contraceptives.[34,35] If feasible, estrogen should be discontinued at least 4 weeks before surgery of the type associated with an increased risk of thromboembolism, or during periods of prolonged immobilization.

While an increased rate of thromboembolic and thrombotic disease in postmenopausal users of estrogens has not been found,[18,36] this does not rule out the possibility that such an increase may be present or that subgroups of women who have underlying risk factors or who are receiving large doses of estrogens may have increased risk. Therefore estrogens should not be used in persons with active thrombophlebitis or thromboembolic disorders, and they should not be used (except in treatment of malignancy) in persons with a history of such disorders in association with estrogen use. They should be used with caution in patients with cerebral vascular or coronary artery disease and only for those in whom estrogens are clearly needed.

Large doses of estrogen (5 mg conjugated estrogens per day), comparable to those used to treat cancer of the prostate and breast, have been shown in a large prospective clinical trial in men to increase the risk of nonfatal myocardial infarction, pulmonary embolism and thrombophlebitis. When estrogen doses of this size are used, any of the thromboembolic and thrombotic adverse effects associated with oral contraceptive use should be considered a clear risk.

b. *Hepatic adenoma.* Benign hepatic adenomas appear to be associated with the use of oral contraceptives.[38–40] Although benign, and rare, these may rupture and may cause death through intra-abdominal hemorrhage. Such lesions have not yet been reported in association with other estrogen or progestogen preparations but should be considered in estrogen users having abdominal pain and tenderness, abdominal mass, or hypovolemic shock. Hepatocellular carcinoma has also been reported in women taking estrogen-containing oral contraceptives.[39] The relationship of this malignancy to these drugs is not known at this time.

c. *Elevated blood pressure.* Increased blood pressure is not uncommon in women using oral contraceptives. There is now a report that this may occur with the use of estrogens during menopause.[41] Blood pressure should be monitored with estrogen use, especially if high doses are used.

d. *Glucose tolerance.* A worsening of glucose tolerance has been observed in a significant percentage of patients on estrogen-containing oral contraceptives. For this reason, diabetic patients should be carefully observed while receiving estrogen.

4. *Hypercalcemia.* Administration of estrogens may lead to severe hypercalcemia in patients with breast cancer and bone metastases. If this occurs, the drug should be stopped and appropriate measures taken to reduce the serum calcium level.

PRECAUTIONS

A. General

1. A complete medical and family history should be taken prior to the initiation of any estrogen therapy. The pretreatment and periodic physical examinations should include special reference to blood pressure, breasts, abdomen, and pelvic organs, and should include a Papanicolaou smear. As a general rule, estrogen should not be prescribed for longer than one year without another physical examination being performed.
2. Fluid retention—Because estrogens may cause some degree of fluid retention, conditions which might be influenced by this factor such as epilepsy, migraine, and cardiac or renal dysfunction, require careful observation.
3. Certain patients may develop undesirable manifestations of excessive estrogenic stimulation, such as abnormal or excessive uterine bleeding, mastodynia, etc.
4. Oral contraceptives appear to be associated with an increased incidence of mental depression.[24] Although it is not clear whether this is due to the estrogenic or progestogenic component of the contraceptive, patients with a history of depression should be carefully observed.
5. Preexisting uterine leiomyomata may increase in size during estrogen use.
6. The pathologist should be advised of estrogen therapy when relevant specimens are submitted.
7. Patients with a past history of jaundice during pregnancy have an increased risk of recurrence of jaundice while receiving estrogen-containing oral contraceptive therapy. If jaundice develops in any patient receiving estrogen, the medication should be discontinued while the cause is investigated.
8. Estrogens may be poorly metabolized in patients with impaired liver function and they should be administered with caution in such patients.
9. Because estrogens influence the metabolism of calcium and phosphorus, they should be used with caution in patients with metabolic bone diseases that are associated with hypercalcemia or in patients with renal insufficiency.
10. Because of the effects of estrogens on epiphyseal closure, they should be used judiciously in young patients in whom bone growth is not complete.
11. The lowest effective dose appropriate for the specific indication should be utilized. Studies of the addition of a progestin for seven or more days of a cycle of estrogen administration have reported a lowered incidence of endometrial hyperplasia. Morphological and biochemical studies of endometrium suggest that 10 to 13 days of progestin are needed to provide maximal maturation of the endometrium and to eliminate any hyperplastic changes. Whether this will provide protection from endometrial carcinoma has not been clearly established. There are possible additional risks which may be associated with the inclusion of progestin in estrogen replacement regimens.The potential risks include adverse effects on carbohydrate and lipid metabolism. The choice of progestin and dosage may be important in minimizing these adverse effects.

B. Information for Patients: See text of Patient Package Information which is reproduced below.

C. Drug/Laboratory Test Interactions

Certain endocrine and liver function tests may be affected by estrogen-containing oral contraceptives. The following similar changes may be expected with larger doses of estrogen:

1. Increased sulfobromophthalein retention.
2. Increased prothrombin and factors VII, VIII, IX and X; decreased antithrombin 3; increased norepinephrine-induced platelet aggregability.
3. Increased thyroid-binding globulin (TBG) leading to increased circulating total thyroid hormone, as measured by PBI, T4 by column, or T4 by radioimmunoassay. Free T3 resin uptake is decreased, reflecting the elevated TBG; free T4 concentration is unaltered.
4. Impaired glucose tolerance.
5. Decreased pregnanediol excretion.
6. Reduced response to metyrapone test.
7. Reduced serum folate concentration.
8. Increased serum triglyceride and phospholipid concentration.

D. Carcinogenesis, Mutagenesis, Impairment of Fertility: See "Warnings" section for information on carcinogenesis, mutagenesis and impairment of fertility.

E. Pregnancy:

Teratogenic Effects.

Pregnancy Category X.

See "Contraindications" section.

Continued on next page

Ortho Dienestrol—Cont.

F. Nursing Mothers: It is not known whether this drug is excreted in human milk. Because many drugs are excreted in human milk, caution should be exercised when estrogens are administered to a nursing woman.

ADVERSE REACTIONS

(*See* Warnings regarding induction of neoplasia, adverse effects on the fetus, increased incidence of gall bladder disease, and adverse effects similar to those of oral contraceptives, including thromboembolism.) The following additional adverse reactions have been reported with estrogenic therapy, including oral contraceptives:

1. *Genitourinary system.*
Increase in size of uterine fibromyomata.
Vaginal candidiasis.
Breakthrough bleeding, spotting, change in menstrual flow.
Dysmenorrhea.
Premenstrual-like syndrome.
Amenorrhea during and after treatment.
Change in cervical eversion and in degree of cervical secretion.
Cystitis-like syndrome.
2. *Breasts.*
Tenderness, enlargement, secretion.
3. *Gastrointestinal.*
Cholestatic jaundice.
Nausea, vomiting.
Abdominal cramps, bloating.
4. *Skin.*
Erythema multiforme.
Erythema nodosum.
Hemorrhagic eruption.
Loss of scalp hair.
Hirsutism.
Chloasma or melasma which may persist when drug is discontinued.
5. *Eyes.*
Steepening of corneal curvature.
Intolerance to contact lenses.
6. *CNS.*
Mental depression.
Headache, migraine, dizziness.
Chorea.
7. *Miscellaneous.*
Reduced carbohydrate tolerance.
Aggravation of porphyria.
Edema.
Changes in libido.
Increase or decrease in weight.

OVERDOSAGE

Numerous reports of ingestion of large doses of estrogen-containing oral contraceptives by young children indicate that serious ill effects do not occur. Overdosage of estrogen may cause nausea, and withdrawal bleeding may occur in females.

DOSAGE AND ADMINISTRATION

Given cyclically for short term use only:
For treatment of atrophic vaginitis, or kraurosis vulvae associated with the menopause.
The lowest dose that will control symptoms should be chosen and medication should be discontinued as promptly as possible.
Attempts to discontinue or taper medication should be made at 3 to 6 month intervals.
The usual dosage range is one or two applicatorsful per day for one or two weeks, then gradually reduced to one half initial dosage for a similar period. A maintenance dosage of one applicatorful, one to three times a week, may be used after restoration of the vaginal mucosa has been achieved.
Treated patients with an intact uterus should be monitored closely for signs of endometrial cancer and appropriate diagnostic measures should be taken to rule out malignancy in the event of persistent or recurring abnormal vaginal bleeding.

HOW SUPPLIED

Available in 2.75 oz. (78g) tubes with or without ORTHO® Measured Dose Applicator.
With applicator: NDC 0062-5450-77
Without applicator: NDC 0062-5450-00
Store at controlled room temperature.

REFERENCES

1. Ziel, H.K. and W.D. Finkle, "Increased Risk of Endometrial Carcinoma Among Users of Conjugated Estrogens," *New England Journal of Medicine,* 293:1167–1170, 1975.
2. Smith, D.C., R. Prentice, D.J. Thompson, and W.L. Hermann, "Association of Exogenous Estrogen and Endometrial Carcinoma," *New England Journal of Medicine,* 293:1164–1167, 1975.
3. Mack, T.M., M.C. Pike, B.E. Henderson, R.I. Pfeffer, V.R. Gerkins, M. Arthur, and S.E. Brown, "Estrogens and Endometrial Cancer in a Retirement Community," *New England Journal of Medicine,* 294:1267–1287, 1976.
4. Weiss, N.S., D.R. Szekely and D.F. Austin, "Increasing Incidence of Endometrial Cancer in the United States," *New England Journal of Medicine,* 294:1259–1262, 1976.
5. Herbst, A.L., H. Ulfelder and D.C. Poskanzer, "Adenocarcinoma of Vagina," *New England Journal of Medicine,* 284: 878–881, 1971.
6. Greenwald, P., J. Barlow, P. Nasca, and W. Burnett, "Vaginal Cancer after Maternal Treatment with Synthetic Estrogens," *New England Journal of Medicine,* 285:390–392, 1971.
7. Lanier, A., K. Noller, D. Decker, L. Elveback, and L. Kurland, "Cancer and Stilbestrol. A Follow-up of 1719 Persons Exposed to Estrogens in Utero and Born 1943–1959," *Mayo Clinic Proceedings,* 48:793–799, 1973.
8. Herbst, A., R. Kurman, and R. Scully, "Vaginal and Cervical Abnormalities After Exposure to Stilbestrol In Utero," *Obstetrics and Gynecology,* 40:287–298, 1972.
9. Herbst, A., S. Robboy, G. Macdonald, and R. Scully, "The Effects of Local Progesterone on Stilbestrol-Associated Vaginal Adenosis," *American Journal of Obstetrics and Gynecology* 118:607–615, 1974.
10. Herbst, A., D. Poskanzer, S. Robboy, L. Friedlander, and R. Scully, "Prenatal Exposure to Stilbestrol, A Prospective Comparison of Exposed Female Offspring with Unexposed Controls," *New England Journal of Medicine,* 292:334–339, 1975.
11. Staffi, A., R. Mattingly, D. Foley, and W. Fetherston, "Clinical Diagnosis of Vaginal Adenosis," *Obstetrics and Gynecology,* 43:118–128, 1974.
12. Sherman, A.I., M. Goldrath, A. Berlin, V. Vakhariya, F. Banooni, W. Michaels, P. Goodman, S. Brown, "Cervical-Vaginal Adenosis After *In Utero* Exposure to Synthetic Estrogens," *Obstetrics and Gynecology,* 44:531–545, 1974.
13. Gal, I., B. Kirman, and J. Stern, "Hormone Pregnancy Tests and Congenital Malformation," *Nature,* 216:83, 1967.
14. Levy, E.P., A. Cohen, and F.C. Fraser, "Hormone Treatment During Pregnancy and Congenital Heart Defects," *Lancet,* 1:611, 1973.
15. Nora, J. and A. Nora, "Birth Defects and Oral Contraceptives," *Lancet,* 1:941–942, 1973.
16. Janerich, D.T., J.M. Piper, and D.M. Glebatis, "Oral Contraceptives and Congenital Limb-Reduction Defects," *New England Journal of Medicine,* 291:697–700, 1974.
17. "Estrogens for Oral or Parenteral Use," *Federal Register,* 40:8212, 1975.
18. Boston Collaborative Drug Surveillance Program, "Surgically Confirmed Gall Bladder Disease, Venous Thromboembolism and Breast Tumors in Relation to Post-Menopausal Estrogen Therapy," *New England Journal of Medicine,* 290:15–19, 1974.
18a. Hoover, R., L.A. Gray, Sr., P. Cole, and B. MacMahon, "Menopausal Estrogens and Breast Cancer," *New England Journal of Medicine,* 295:401–405, 1976.
19. Boston Collaborative Drug Surveillance Program, "Oral Contraceptives and Venous Thromboembolic Disease, Surgically Confirmed Gall Bladder Disease, and Breast Tumors," *Lancet* 1:1399–1404, 1973.
20. Daniel, D.G., H. Campbell, and A.C. Turnbull, "Puerperal Thromboembolism and Suppression of Lactation," *Lancet,* 2:287–289, 1967.
21. The Veterans Administration Cooperative Urological Research Group, "Carcinoma of the Prostate: Treatment Comparisons," *Journal of Urology,* 98:516–522, 1967.
22. Bailar, J.C., "Thromboembolism and Oestrogen Therapy," *Lancet,* 2:560, 1967.
23. Blackard, C., R. Doe, G. Mellinger, and D. Byar, "Incidence of Cardiovascular Disease and Death In Patients Receiving Diethylstilbestrol for Carcinoma of the Prostate," *Cancer,* 26:249–256, 1970.
24. Royal College of General Practitioners, "Oral Contraception and Thromboembolic Disease," *Journal of the Royal College of General Practitioners,* 13:267–279, 1967.
25. Inman, W.H.W. and M.P. Vessey, "Investigation of Deaths from Pulmonary, Coronary, and Cerebral Thrombosis and Embolism in Women of Child-Bearing Age," *British Medical Journal,* 2:193–199, 1968.
26. Vessey, M.P. and R. Doll, "Investigation of Relation Between Use of Oral Contraceptives and Thromboembolic Disease, A Further Report," *British Medical Journal,* 2:651–657, 1969.
27. Sartwell, P.E., A.T. Masi, F.G. Arthes, G.R. Greene, and H.E. Smith, "Thromboembolism and Oral Contraceptives: An Epidemiological Case Control Study," *American Journal of Epidemiology,* 90:365–380, 1969.
28. Collaborative Group for the Study of Stroke In Young Women, "Oral Contraception and Increased Risk of Cerebral Ischemia or Thrombosis," *New England Journal of Medicine,* 288:871–878, 1973.
29. Collaborative Group for the Study of Stroke in Young Women, "Oral Contraceptives and Stroke in Young Women: Associated Risk Factors," *Journal of the American Medical Association,* 231:718–722, 1975.
30. Mann, J.I. and W.H.W. Inman, "Oral Contraceptives and Death from Myocardial Infarction," *British Medical Journal,* 2:245–248, 1975.
31. Mann, J.I., M.P. Vessey, M. Thorogood, and R. Doll., "Myocardial Infarction in Young Women with Special Reference to Oral Contraceptive Practice," *British Medical Journal,* 2:241–245, 1975.
32. Inman, W.H.W., V.P. Vessey, B. Westerholm, and A. Engelund, "Thromboembolic Disease and the Steroidal Content of Oral Contraceptives," *British Medical Journal,* 2:203–209, 1970.
33. Stolley, P.D., J.A. Tonascia, M.S. Tockman, P.E. Sartwell, A.H. Rutledge, and M.P. Jacobs, "Thrombosis with Low-Estrogen Oral Contraceptives," *American Journal of Epidemiology,* 102:197–208, 1975.
34. Vessey, M.P., R. Doll, A.S. Fairbairn, and G. Glober, "Post-Operative Thromboembolism and the Use of the Oral Contraceptives," *British Medical Journal,* 3:123–126, 1970.
35. Greene, G.R. and P.E. Sartwell, "Oral Contraceptive Use in Patients with Thromboembolism Following Surgery, Trauma or Infection," *American Journal of Public Health,* 62:680–685, 1972.
36. Rosenberg, L., M.B. Armstrong and H. Jick, "Myocardial Infarction and Estrogen Therapy in Postmenopausal Women," *New England Journal of Medicine,* 294:1256–1259, 1976.
37. Coronary Drug Project Research Group, "The Coronary Drug Project: Initial Findings Leading to Modifications of Its Research Protocol," *Journal of the American Medical Association,* 214:1303–1313, 1970.
38. Baum, J., F. Holtz, J.J. Bookstein, and E.W. Klein, "Possible Association between Benign Hepatomas and Oral Contraceptives," *Lancet,* 2:926–928, 1973.
39. Mays, E.T., W.M. Christopherson, M.M. Mahr, and H.C. Williams, "Hepatic Changes in Young Women Ingesting Contraceptive Steroids, Hepatic Hemorrhage and Primary Hepatic Tumors." *Journal of the American Medical Association,* 235:730–782, 1976.
40. Edmondson, H.A., B. Henderson, and B. Benton, "Liver Cell Adenomas Associated with the Use of Oral Contraceptives," *New England Journal of Medicine,* 294:470–472, 1976.
41. Pfeffer, R.I. and S. Van Den Noore, "Estrogen Use and Stroke Risk in Postmenopausal Women," *American Journal of Epidemiology,* 103:445–456, 1976.

PATIENT INFORMATION ABOUT ESTROGENS

Estrogens are female hormones produced by the ovaries. The ovaries make several different kinds of estrogens. In addition, scientists have been able to make a variety of synthetic estrogens. As far as we know, all these synthetic estrogens have similar properties and therefore much the same usefulness, side effects, and risks. This leaflet is intended to help you understand what estrogens are used for, some of the risks involved in their use, and to help minimize these risks.
This leaflet includes important information about estrogens, but not all the information. If you want to know more, you can ask your doctor or pharmacist to let you read the package insert prepared for the doctor.

USES OF ESTROGEN

THERE IS NO PROPER USE OF ESTROGENS IN A PREGNANT WOMAN
Estrogens are prescribed by doctors for a number of purposes, including:

1. To provide estrogen during a period of adjustment when a woman's ovaries no longer produce it, in order to prevent certain uncomfortable symptoms of estrogen deficiency. (All women normally decrease the production of estrogens, generally between the ages of 45 and 55; this is called the menopause.)
2. To prevent symptoms of estrogen deficiency when a woman's ovaries have been removed surgically before the natural menopause.
3. To prevent pregnancy. (Estrogens are given along with a progestogen, another female hormone; these combinations are called oral contraceptives or birth control pills. Patient labeling is available to women taking oral contraceptives and they will not be discussed in this leaflet.)
4. To treat certain cancers in women and men.
5. To prevent painful swelling of the breasts after pregnancy in women who choose not to nurse their babies.

ESTROGENS IN THE MENOPAUSE

In the natural course of their lives, all women eventually experience a decrease in estrogen production. This usually occurs between ages 45 and 55 but may occur earlier or later. Sometimes the ovaries may need to be removed by an operation before natural menopause, producing a "surgical menopause."
When the amount of estrogen in the blood begins to decrease, many women may develop typical symptoms: Feelings of warmth in the face, neck, and chest or sudden intense episodes of heat and sweating throughout the body (called "hot flashes" or "hot flushes"). These symptoms are sometimes very uncomfortable. A few women eventually develop changes in the vagina (called "atrophic vaginitis") which cause discomfort, especially during and after intercourse.
Estrogens can be prescribed to treat these symptoms of the menopause. It is estimated that considerably more than half of all women undergoing the menopause have only mild symptoms or no symptoms at all and therefore do not need estrogens. Other women may need estrogens for a few months, while their bodies adjust to lower estrogen levels. Sometimes the need will be for periods longer than six months. In an attempt to avoid over-stimulation of the uterus (womb), estrogens are usually given cyclically during each month of use, that is three weeks of pills followed by one week without pills.
Sometimes women experience nervous symptoms or depression during menopause. There is no evidence that estrogens are effective for such symptoms and they should not be used to treat them, although other treatment may be needed.
You may have heard that taking estrogens for long periods (years) after the menopause will keep your skin soft and supple and keep you feeling young. There is no evidence that this is so, however, and such long-term treatment carries important risks.

ESTROGENS TO PREVENT SWELLING OF THE BREASTS AFTER PREGNANCY

If you do not breast-feed your baby after delivery, your breasts may fill up with milk and become painful and engorged. This usually begins about three to four days after delivery and may last for a few days to up to a week or more. Sometimes the discomfort is severe, but usually it is not and can be controlled by pain-relieving drugs such as aspirin and by binding the breasts up tightly. Estrogens can be used to try to prevent the breasts from filling up. While this treatment is sometimes successful, in many cases the breasts fill up to some degree in spite of treatment. The dose of estrogens needed to prevent pain and swelling of the breasts is much larger than the dose needed to treat symptoms of the menopause and this may increase your chances of developing blood clots in the legs or lungs (see below). Therefore, it is important that you discuss the benefits and the risks of estrogen use with your doctor if you have decided not to breast-feed your baby.

SOME OF THE DANGERS OF ESTROGEN

1. *Cancer of the uterus.* If estrogens are used in the post-menopausal period for more than a year, there is an increased risk of *endometrial cancer* (cancer of the uterus). Women taking estrogens have roughly five to ten times as great a chance of getting this cancer as women who take no estrogens. To put this another way, while a postmenopausal woman not taking estrogens has one chance in 1,000 each year of getting cancer of the uterus, a woman taking estrogens has five to ten chances in 1,000 each year. For this reason *it is important to take estrogens only when you really need them.*

The risk of this cancer is greater the longer estrogens are used and also seems to be greater when larger doses are taken. For this reason *it is important to take the lowest dose of estrogen that will control symptoms and to take it only as long as it is needed.* If estrogens are needed for longer periods of time, your doctor will want to reevaluate your need for estrogens at least every six months.

Women using estrogens should report any irregular vaginal bleeding to their doctors; such bleeding may be of no importance, but it can be an early warning of cancer of the uterus. If you have undiagnosed vaginal bleeding, you should not use estrogens until a diagnosis is made and you are certain there is no cancer of the uterus.

If you have had your uterus completely removed (total hysterectomy), there is no danger of developing cancer of the uterus.

2. *Other possible cancers.* Estrogens can cause development of other tumors in animals, such as tumors of the breast, cervix, vagina, or liver, when given for a long time. At present there is no good evidence that women using estrogen in the menopause have an increased risk of such tumors, but there is no way yet to be sure they do not; and one study raises the possibility that use of estrogens in the menopause may increase the risk of breast cancer many years later. This is a further reason to use estrogens only when clearly needed. While you are taking estrogens, it is important that you go to your doctor at least once a year for a physical examination. Also, if members of your family have had breast cancer or if you have breast nodules or abnormal mammograms (breast x-rays), your doctor may wish to carry out more frequent examinations of your breasts.

3. *Gall bladder disease.* Women who use estrogens after menopause are more likely to develop gall bladder disease needing surgery than women who do not use estrogens. Birth control pills have a similar effect.

4. *Abnormal blood clotting.* Oral contraceptives, some of which contain estrogens, increase the risk of blood clotting in various parts of the body. This can result in a stroke (if the clot is in the brain), a heart attack (clot in a blood vessel of the heart), or a pulmonary embolus (a clot which forms in the legs or pelvis, then breaks off and travels to the lungs). Any of these can be fatal. Blood clots may result in the loss of a limb, paralysis or loss of sight, depending on where the blood clot is formed or lodges if it breaks loose.

The larger doses of estrogen used to prevent swelling of the breasts after pregnancy have been reported to cause clotting in the legs and lungs.

It is recommended that if you have had any blood clotting disorders including clotting in the legs or lungs, or a heart attack or stroke, you should not use estrogens.

SPECIAL WARNING ABOUT PREGNANCY

You should not receive estrogen if you are pregnant. If this should occur, there is a greater than usual chance that the developing child will be born with a birth defect, although the possibility remains fairly small. A female child may have an increased risk of developing cancer of the vagina or cervix later in life (in the teens or twenties). Every possible effort should be made to avoid exposure to estrogens during pregnancy. If exposure occurs, see your doctor.

SOME OTHER EFFECTS OF ESTROGENS

In addition to the serious known risks of estrogens described above, estrogens have the following side effects and potential risks:

1. *Nausea and vomiting.* The most common side effect of estrogen therapy is nausea. Vomiting is less common.

2. *Effects on breasts.* Estrogens may cause breast tenderness or enlargement and may cause the breasts to secrete a liquid.

3. *Effects on the uterus.* Estrogens may cause benign fibroid tumors of the uterus to get larger. Some women will have menstrual bleeding when estrogens are stopped. But if the bleeding occurs on days you are still taking estrogens you should report this to your doctor.

4. *Effects on liver.* Women taking estrogens develop on rare occasions a tumor of the liver which can rupture and bleed into the abdomen. You should report any swelling or unusual pain or tenderness in the abdomen to your doctor immediately.

Women with a past history of jaundice (yellowing of the skin and white parts of the eyes) may get jaundice again during estrogen use.

5. *Other effects.* Estrogens may cause excess fluid to be retained in the body. This may make some conditions worse, such as epilepsy, migraine, heart disease, or kidney disease. If any of the above occur, stop taking estrogens and call your doctor.

SUMMARY

Estrogens have important uses, but they have serious risks as well. You must decide, with your doctor, whether the risks are acceptable to you in view of the benefits of treatment. Except where your doctor has prescribed estrogens for use in special cases of cancer of the breast or prostate, you should not use estrogens if you have cancer of the breast or uterus, are pregnant, have undiagnosed abnormal vaginal bleeding, blood clotting disorders including clotting in the legs or lungs, or have had a stroke, heart attack or angina.

You must understand that your doctor will require regular physical examinations while you are taking them and will try to discontinue the drug as soon as possible and use the smallest dose possible. You can help minimize the risk by being alert for signs of trouble including:

1. Abnormal bleeding from the vagina.
2. Pains in the calves or chest or sudden shortness of breath, or coughing blood (indicating possible clots in the legs, heart or lungs).
3. Severe headache, dizziness, faintness, or changes in vision (indicating possible developing clots in the brain or eye).
4. Breast lumps (you should ask your doctor how to examine your own breasts).
5. Jaundice (yellowing of the skin).
6. Mental depression.
7. *Any* other unusual condition or problem.

Based on his or her assessment of your medical needs, your doctor has prescribed this drug for you. Do not give the drug to anyone else.

HOW SUPPLIED

Available in 2.75 oz. (78g) tubes with or without ORTHO® Measured-Dose Applicator.
With applicator: NDC 0062-5450-77
Without applicator: NDC 0062-5450-00
Store at controlled room temperature.

ORTHO-NOVUM® 1/50 tablets ℞
(norethindrone/mestranol)

Patients should be counseled that this product does not protect against HIV infection (AIDS) and other sexually transmitted diseases.

DESCRIPTION

Each of the following products is a combination oral contraceptive containing the progestational compound norethindrone and the estrogenic compound mestranol:

ORTHO-NOVUM 1/50 □ 28 Tablets: Each yellow tablet contains 1 mg norethindrone and 0.05 mg of mestranol. Inactive ingredients include D&C Yellow No. 10, lactose, magnesium stearate and pregelatinized starch. Each green tablet in the ORTHO-NOVUM 1/50 □ 28 package contains only inert ingredients, as follows: D&C Yellow No. 10 Aluminum Lake, FD&C Blue No. 2 Aluminum Lake, lactose, magnesium stearate, microcrystalline cellulose and pregelatinized starch.

The chemical name for norethindrone is 17-hydroxy-19-nor-17α-pregn-4-en-20-yn-3-one, and for mestranol is 3-methoxy-19-nor-17α-pregna-1,3,5(10)-trien-20-yn-17-ol. Their structural formulas are as follows:

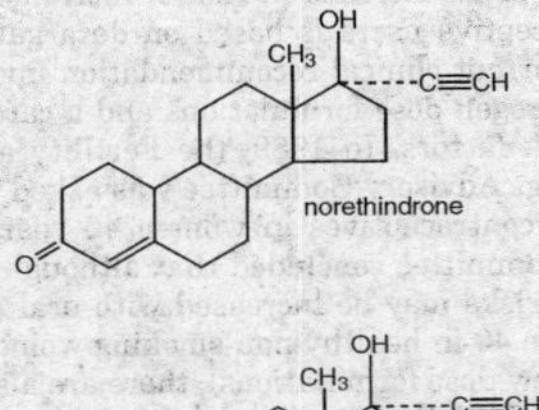

norethindrone

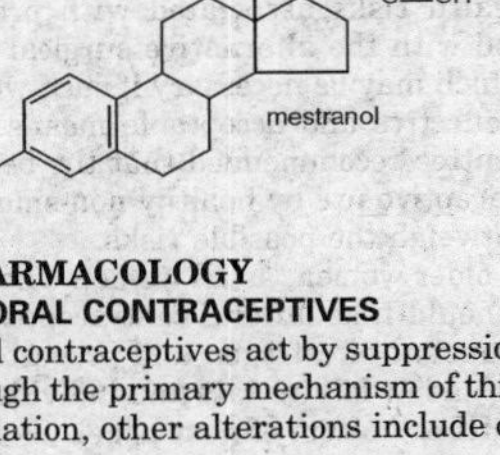

mestranol

CLINICAL PHARMACOLOGY

COMBINATION ORAL CONTRACEPTIVES

Combination oral contraceptives act by suppression of gonadotropins. Although the primary mechanism of this action is inhibition of ovulation, other alterations include changes in the cervical mucus (which increase the difficulty of sperm entry into the uterus) and the endometrium (which reduce the likelihood of implantation).

INDICATIONS AND USAGE

Oral contraceptives are indicated for the prevention of pregnancy in women who elect to use this product as a method of contraception. Oral contraceptive products such as ORTHO-NOVUM 1/50 □ 28-Day, which contains 50 mcg of estrogen, should not be used unless medically indicated.

Oral contraceptives are highly effective. Table I lists the typical accidental pregnancy rates for users of combination oral contraceptives and other methods of contraception. The efficacy of these contraceptive methods, except sterilization, depends upon the reliability with which they are used. Correct and consistent use of methods can result in lower failure rates.

[See table I at top of next page]

CONTRAINDICATIONS

Oral contraceptives should not be used in women who currently have the following conditions:

- Thrombophlebitis or thromboembolic disorders
- A past history of deep vein thrombophlebitis or thromboembolic disorders
- Cerebral vascular or coronary artery disease.
- Known or suspected carcinoma of the breast
- Carcinoma of the endometrium or other known or suspected estrogen-dependent neoplasia
- Undiagnosed abnormal genital bleeding
- Cholestatic jaundice of pregnancy or jaundice with prior pill use.
- Hepatic adenomas or carcinomas
- Known or suspected pregnancy

WARNINGS

Cigarette smoking increases the risk of serious cardiovascular side effects from oral contraceptive use. This risk increases with age and with heavy smoking (15 or more cigarettes per day) and is quite marked in women over 35 years of age. Women who use oral contraceptives should be strongly advised not to smoke.

The use of oral contraceptives is associated with increased risks of several serious conditions including myocardial infarction, thromboembolism, stroke, hepatic neoplasia, and gallbladder disease, although the risk of serious morbidity or mortality is very small in healthy women without underlying risk factors. The risk of morbidity and mortality increases significantly in the presence of other underlying risk factors such as hypertension, hyperlipidemias, obesity and diabetes.

Practitioners prescribing oral contraceptives should be familiar with the following information relating to these risks.

The information contained in this package insert is principally based on studies carried out in patients who used oral contraceptives with higher formulations of estrogens and progestogens than those in common use today. The effect of long-term use of the oral contraceptives with lower formulations of both estrogens and progestogens remains to be determined.

Throughout this labeling, epidemiological studies reported are of two types: retrospective or case control studies and prospective or cohort studies. Case control studies provide a measure of the relative risk of a disease, namely, a *ratio* of the incidence of a disease among oral contraceptive users to that among nonusers. The relative risk does not provide information on the actual clinical occurrence of a disease. Cohort studies provide a measure of attributable risk, which is the *difference* in the incidence of disease between oral contraceptive users and nonusers. The attributable risk does provide information about the actual occurrence of a disease in the population (adapted from refs. 2 and 3 with the author's permission). For further information, the reader is referred to a text on epidemiological methods.

1. THROMBOEMBOLIC DISORDERS AND OTHER VASCULAR PROBLEMS

a. Myocardial Infarction

An increased risk of myocardial infarction has been attributed to oral contraceptive use. This risk is primarily in smokers or women with other underlying risk factors for coronary artery disease such as hypertension, hypercholesterolemia, morbid obesity, and diabetes. The relative risk of heart attack for current oral contraceptive users has been estimated to be two to six.[4–10]. The risk is very low under the age of 30.

Smoking in combination with other oral contraceptive use has been shown to contribute substantially to the incidence of myocardial infarctions in women in their mid-thirties or older with smoking accounting for the majority of excess cases.[11] Mortality rates associated with circulatory disease have been shown to increase substantially in smokers, especially in those 35 years of age and older among women who use oral contraceptives.

[See figure at top of next column]

Oral contraceptives may compound the effects of well-known risk factors, such as hypertension, diabetes, hyperlipidemias, age and obesity.[13] In particular, some progestogens are known to decrease HDL cholesterol and cause glucose intolerance, while estrogens may create a state of hyperinsulinism.[14–18] Oral contraceptives have been shown

Continued on next page

Ortho-Novum 1/50—Cont.

TABLE II: CIRCULATORY DISEASE MORTALITY RATES PER 100,000 WOMAN-YEARS BY AGE, SMOKING STATUS AND ORAL CONTRACEPTIVE USE

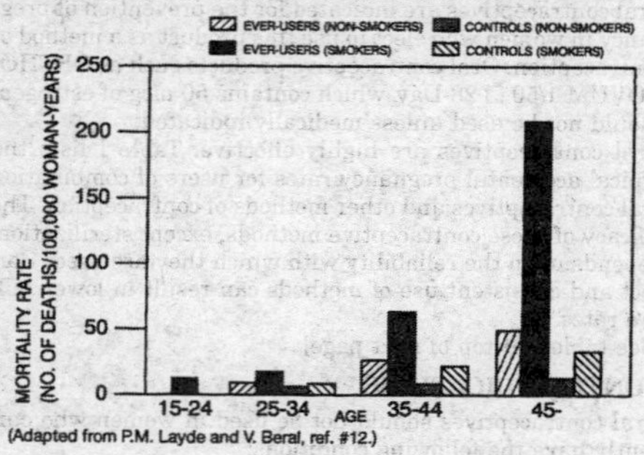

(Adapted from P.M. Layde and V. Beral, ref. #12.)

to increase blood pressure among users (see Section 9 in WARNINGS). Similar effects on risk factors have been associated with an increased risk of heart disease. Oral contraceptives must be used with caution in women with cardiovascular disease risk factors.

b. Thromboembolism

An increased risk of thromboembolic and thrombotic disease associated with the use of oral contraceptives is well established. Case control studies have found the relative risk of users compared to nonusers to be 3 for the first episode of superficial venous thrombosis, 4 to 11 for deep vein thrombosis or pulmonary embolism, and 1.5 to 6 for women with predisposing conditions for venous thromboembolic disease.[2,3,19–24]

Cohort studies have shown the relative risk to be somewhat lower, about 3 for new cases and about 4.5 for new cases requiring hospitalization.[25] The risk of thromboembolic disease associated with oral contraceptives is not related to length of use and disappears after pill use is stopped.[2]

A two- to four-fold increase in relative risk of post-operative thromboembolic complications has been reported with the use of oral contraceptives.[9] The relative risk of venous thrombosis in women who have predisposing conditions is twice that of women without such medical conditions.[26] If feasible, oral contraceptives should be discontinued at least four weeks prior to and for two weeks after elective surgery of a type associated with an increase in risk of thromboembolism and during and following prolonged immobilization. Since the immediate postpartum period is also associated with an increased risk of thromboembolism, oral contraceptives should be started no earlier than four weeks after delivery in women who elect not to breast feed or four weeks after a second trimester abortion.

c. Cerebrovascular diseases

Oral contraceptives have been shown to increase both the relative and attributable risks of cerebrovascular events (thrombotic and hemorrhagic strokes), although, in general, the risk is greatest among older (>35 years), hypertensive women who also smoke. Hypertension was found to be a risk factor for both users and nonusers, for both types of strokes, and smoking interacted to increase the risk of stroke.[27–29]

In a large study, the relative risk of thrombotic strokes has been shown to range from 3 for normotensive users to 14 for users with severe hypertension.[30] The relative risk of hemorrhagic stroke is reported to be 1.2 for non-smokers who used oral contraceptives, 2.6 for smokers who did not use oral contraceptives, 7.6 for smokers who used oral contraceptives, 1.8 for normotensive users and 25.7 for users with severe hypertension.[30] The attributable risk is also greater in older women.[3]

d. Dose-related risk of vascular disease from oral contraceptives

A positive association has been observed between the amount of estrogen and progestogen in oral contraceptives and the risk of vascular disease.[31–33] A decline in serum high density lipoproteins (HDL) has been reported with many progestational agents.[14–16] A decline in serum high density lipoproteins has been associated with an increased incidence of ischemic heart disease. Because estrogens increase HDL cholesterol, the net effect of an oral contraceptive depends on a balance achieved between doses of estrogen and progestogen and the activity of the progestogen used in the contraceptives. The activity and amount of both hormones should be considered in the choice of an oral contraceptive.

Minimizing exposure to estrogen and progestogen is in keeping with good principles of therapeutics. For any particular estrogen/progestogen combination, the dosage regimen prescribed should be one which contains the least amount of estrogen and progestogen that is compatible with a low failure rate and the needs of the individual patient. New acceptors of oral contraceptive agents should be started on preparations containing 0.035 mg or less of estrogen. Products containing 50 mcg estrogen should be used only when medically indicated.

e. Persistence of risk of vascular disease

There are two studies which have shown persistence of risk of vascular disease for ever-users of oral contraceptives. In a study in the United States, the risk of developing myocardial infarction after discontinuing oral contraceptives persists for at least 9 years for women 40–49 years who had used oral contraceptives for five or more years, but this increased risk was not demonstrated in other age groups.[8] In another study in Great Britain, the risk of developing cerebrovascular disease persisted for at least 6 years after discontinuation of oral contraceptives, although excess risk was very small.[34] However, both studies were performed with oral contraceptive formulations containing 50 micrograms or higher of estrogens.

TABLE I: PERCENTAGE OF WOMEN EXPERIENCING AN UNINTENDED PREGNANCY DURING THE FIRST YEAR OF TYPICAL USE AND THE FIRST YEAR OF PERFECT USE OF CONTRACEPTION AND THE PERCENTAGE CONTINUING USE AT THE END OF THE FIRST YEAR. UNITED STATES.

Method (1)	% of Women Experiencing an Unintended Pregnancy within the First Year of Use: Typical Use[1] (2)	Perfect Use[2] (3)	% of Women Continuing Use at One Year[3] (4)
Chance[4]	85	85	
Spermicides[5]	26	6	40
Periodic abstinence	25		63
Calendar		9	
Ovulation method		3	
Sympto-Thermal[6]		2	
Post-Ovulation		1	
Withdrawal	19	4	
Cap[7]			
Parous Women	40	26	42
Nulliparous Women	20	9	56
Sponge			
Parous Women	40	20	42
Nulliparous Women	20	9	56
Diaphragm[7]	20	6	56
Condom[8]			
Female (Reality)	21	5	56
Male	14	3	61
Pill	5		71
Progestin Only		0.5	
Combined		0.1	
IUD			
Progesterone T	2.0	1.5	81
Copper T380A	0.8	0.6	78
LNg 20	0.1	0.1	81
Depo-Provera	0.3	0.3	70
Norplant and Norplant-2	0.05	0.05	88
Female Sterilization	0.5	0.5	100
Male Sterilization	0.15	0.10	100

Adapted from Hatcher et al., 1998 Ref. #1.

1. Among *typical* couples who initiate use of a method (not necessarily for the first time), the percentage who experience an accidental pregnancy during the first year if they do not stop use for any other reason.
2. Among couples who initiate use of a method (not necessarily for the first time) and who use it *perfectly* (both consistently and correctly), the percentage who experience an accidental pregnancy during the first year if they do not stop use for any other reason.
3. Among couples attempting to avoid pregnancy, the percentage who continue to use a method for one year.
4. The percents becoming pregnant in columns (2) and (3) are based on data from population where contraception is not used and from women who cease using contraception in order to become pregnant. Among such populations, about 89% become pregnant within one year. This estimate was lowered slightly (to 85%) to represent the percent who would become pregnant within one year among women now relying on reversible methods of contraception if they abandoned contraception altogether.
5. Foams, creams, gels, vaginal suppositories, and vaginal film.
6. Cervical musus (ovulation) method supplemented by calendar in the pre-ovulatory and basal body temperature in the post-ovulatory phases.
7. With spermicidal cream or jelly.
8. Without spermicides.

2. ESTIMATES OF MORTALITY FROM CONTRACEPTIVE USE

One study gathered data from a variety of sources which have estimated the mortality rate associated with different methods of contraception at different ages (Table III). These estimates include the combined risk of death associated with contraceptive methods plus the risk attributable to pregnancy in the event of method failure. Each method of contraception has its specific benefits and risks. The study concluded that with the exception of oral contraceptive users 35 and older who smoke, and 40 and older who do not smoke, mortality associated with all methods of birth control is low and below that associated with childbirth. The observation of an increase in risk of morality with age for oral contraceptive users is based on data gathered in the 1970's.[35] Current clinical recommendation involves the use of lower estrogen dose formulations and a careful consideration of risk factors. In 1989, the Fertility and Maternal Health Drugs Advisory Committee was asked to review the use of oral contraceptives in women 40 years of age and over. The Committee concluded that although cardiovascular disease risks may be increased with oral contraceptive use after age 40 in healthy non-smoking women (even with the newer low-dose formulations), there are also greater potential health risks associated with pregnancy in older women and with the alternative surgical and medical procedures which may be necessary if such women do not have access to effective and acceptable means of contraception. The Committee recommended that the benefits of low-dose oral contraceptive use by healthy non-smoking women over 40 may outweigh the possible risks.

Of course, older women, as all women who take oral contraceptives, should take an oral contraceptive which contains the least amount of estrogen and progestogen that is compatible with a low failure rate and individual patient needs.

[See table III at bottom of next page]

3. CARCINOMA OF THE REPRODUCTIVE ORGANS AND BREASTS

Numerous epidemiological studies have been performed on the incidence of breast, endometrial, ovarian and cervical cancer in women using oral contraceptives. While there are conflicting reports, most studies suggest that use of oral contraceptives is not associated with an overall increase in the risk of developing breast cancer. Some studies have reported an increased relative risk of developing breast cancer particularly at a younger age. This increased relative risk has been reported to be related to duration of use.[36–44,79–89]

A meta-analysis of 54 studies found a small increase in the frequency of having breast cancer diagnosed for women who were currently using combined oral contraceptives or had used them within the past ten years. This increase in the frequency of breast cancer diagnosis, within ten years of stopping use, was generally accounted for by cancers localized to the breast. There was no increase in the frequency of having breast cancer diagnosed ten or more years after cessation of use.[90]

Some studies suggest that oral contraceptive use has been associated with an increase in the risk of cervical neoplasia in some populations of women.[45–48] However, there continues to be controversy about the extent to which such findings may be due to differences in sexual behavior and other factors.

4. HEPATIC NEOPLASIA

Benign hepatic adenomas are associated with oral contraceptive use, although the incidence of benign tumors is rare in the United States. Indirect calculations have estimated the attributable risk to be in the range of 3.3 cases/100,000 for users, a risk that increases after four or more years of use especially with oral contraceptives of higher dose.[49] Rupture of benign, hepatic adenomas may cause death through intra-abdominal hemorrhage.[50,51]

Studies have shown an increased risk of developing hepatocellular carcinoma[52–54,91] in oral contraceptive users. However, these cancers are rare in the U.S.

5. OCULAR LESIONS

There have been clinical case reports of retinal thrombosis associated with the use of oral contraceptives. Oral contraceptives should be discontinued if there is unexplained partial or complete loss of vision; onset of proptosis or diplopia; papilledema; or retinal vascular lesions. Appropriate diagnostic and therapeutic measures should be undertaken immediately.

6. ORAL CONTRACEPTIVE USE BEFORE OR DURING EARLY PREGNANCY

Extensive epidemiological studies have revealed no increased risk of birth defects in women who have used oral contraceptives prior to pregnancy.[56,57] The majority of recent studies also do not indicate a teratogenic effect, particularly in so far as cardiac anomalies and limb reduction defects are concerned,[55,56,58,59] when taken inadvertently during early pregnancy.

The administration of oral contraceptives to induce withdrawal bleeding should not be used as a test for pregnancy. Oral contraceptives should not be used during pregnancy to treat threatened or habitual abortion.

It is recommended that for any patient who has missed two consecutive periods, pregnancy should be ruled out before continuing oral contraceptive use. If the patient has not adhered to the prescribed schedule, the possibility of pregnancy should be considered at the time of the first missed period. Oral contraceptive use should be discontinued until pregnancy is ruled out.

7. GALLBLADDER DISEASE

Earlier studies have reported an increased lifetime relative risk of gallbladder surgery in users of oral contraceptives and estrogens.[60,61] More recent studies, however, have shown that the relative risk of developing gallbladder disease among oral contraceptive users may be minimal.[62–64] The recent findings of minimal risk may be related to the use of oral contraceptive formulations containing lower hormonal doses of estrogens and progestogens.

8. CARBOHYDRATE AND LIPID METABOLIC EFFECTS

Oral contraceptives have been shown to cause a decrease in glucose tolerance in a significant percentage of users.[17] This effect has been shown to be directly related to estrogen dose.[65] Progestogens increase insulin secretion and create insulin resistance, this effect varying with different progestational agents.[17,66] However, in the non-diabetic woman, oral contraceptives appear to have no effect on fasting blood glucose.[67] Because of these demonstrated effects, prediabetic and diabetic women in particular should be carefully monitored while taking oral contraceptives.

A small proportion of women will have persistent hypertriglyceridemia while on the pill. As discussed earlier (see WARNINGS 1a and 1d), changes in serum triglycerides and lipoprotein levels have been reported in oral contraceptive users.

9. ELEVATED BLOOD PRESSURE

An increase in blood pressure has been reported in women taking oral contraceptives[68] and this increase is more likely in older oral contraceptive users[69] and with extended duration of use.[61] Data from the Royal College of General Practitioners[12] and subsequent randomized trials have shown that the incidence of hypertension increases with increasing progestational activity.

Women with a history of hypertension or hypertension-related diseases, or renal disease[70] should be encouraged to use another method of contraception. If women elect to use oral contraceptives, they should be monitored closely and if significant elevation of blood pressure occurs, oral contraceptives should be discontinued. For most women, elevated blood pressure will return to normal after stopping oral contraceptives, and there is no difference in the occurrence of hypertension between former and never users.[68–71]

10. HEADACHE

The onset or exacerbation of migraine or development of headache with a new pattern which is recurrent, persistent or severe requires discontinuation of oral contraceptives and evaluation of the cause.

11. BLEEDING IRREGULARITIES

Breakthrough bleeding and spotting are sometimes encountered in patients on oral contraceptives, especially during the first three months of use. Nonhormonal causes should be considered and adequate diagnostic measures taken to rule out malignancy or pregnancy in the event of breakthrough bleeding, as in the case of any abnormal vaginal bleeding. If pathology has been excluded, time or a change to another formulation may solve the problem. In the event of amenorrhea, pregnancy should be ruled out.

Some women may encounter post-pill amenorrhea or oligomennorrhea, especially when such a condition was preexistent.

12. ECTOPIC PREGNANCY

Ectopic as well as intrauterine pregnancy may occur in contraceptive failures.

PRECAUTIONS

1. PHYSICAL EXAMINATION AND FOLLOW UP

It is good medical practice for all women to have annual history and physical examinations, including women using oral contraceptives. The physical examination, however, may be deferred until after initiation of oral contraceptives if requested by the woman and judged appropriate by the clinician. The physical examination should include special reference to blood pressure, breasts, abdomen and pelvic organs, including cervical cytology, and relevant laboratory tests. In case of undiagnosed, persistent or recurrent abnormal vaginal bleeding, appropriate measures should be conducted to rule out malignancy. Women with a strong family history of breast cancer or who have breast nodules should be monitored with particular care.

2. LIPID DISORDERS

Women who are being treated for hyperlipidemias should be followed closely if they elect to use oral contraceptives. Some progestogens may elevate LDL levels and may render the control of hyperlipidemias more difficult.

3. LIVER FUNCTION

If jaundice develops in any woman receiving such drugs, the medication should be discontinued. Steroid hormones may be poorly metabolized in patients with impaired liver function.

4. FLUID RETENTION

Oral contraceptives may cause some degree of fluid retention. They should be prescribed with caution, and only with careful monitoring, in patients with conditions which might be aggravated by fluid retention.

5. EMOTIONAL DISORDERS

Women with a history of depression should be carefully observed and the drug discontinued if depression recurs to a serious degree.

6. CONTACT LENSES

Contact lens wearers who develop visual changes or changes in lens tolerance should be assessed by an ophthalmologist.

7. DRUG INTERACTIONS

Reduced efficacy and increased incidence of breakthrough bleeding and menstrual irregularities have been associated with concomitant use of rifampin. A similar association, though less marked, has been suggested with barbiturates, phenylbutazone, phenytoin sodium, carbamazepine, and possibly with griseofulvin, ampicillin and tetracyclines.[72]

8. INTERACTIONS WITH LABORATORY TESTS

Certain endocrine and liver function tests and blood components may be affected by oral contraceptives:

a. Increased prothrombin and factors, VII, VIII, IX, and X; decreased antithrombin 3; increased norepinephrine-induced platelet aggregability.
b. Increased thyroid binding globulin (TBG) leading to increased circulating total thyroid hormone, as measured by protein-bound iodine (PBI), T4 by column or by radioimmunoassay. Free T3 resin uptake is decreased, reflecting the elevated TBG, free T4 concentration is unaltered.
c. Other binding proteins may be elevated in serum.
d. Sex-binding globulins are increased and result in elevated levels of total circulating sex steroids and corticoids; however, free or biologically active levels remain unchanged.
e. Triglycerides may be increased.
f. Glucose tolerance may be decreased.
g. Serum folate levels may be depressed by oral contraceptive therapy. This may be of clinical significance if a woman becomes pregnant shortly after discontinuing oral contraceptives.

9. CARCINOGENESIS

See WARNINGS Section.

10. PREGNANCY

Pregnancy Category X. See CONTRAINDICATIONS and WARNINGS Sections.

11. NURSING MOTHERS

Small amounts of oral contraceptive steroids have been identified in the milk of nursing mothers and a few adverse effects on the child have been reported, including jaundice and breast enlargement. In addition, oral contraceptives given in the postpartum period may interfere with lactation by decreasing the quantity and quality of breast milk. If possible, the nursing mother should be advised not to use combination oral contraceptives but to use other forms of contraception until she has completely weaned her child.

12. PEDIATRIC USE

Safety and efficacy of ORTHO-NOVUM 1/50 Tablets have been established in women of reproductive age. Safety and efficacy are expected to be the same for postpubertal adolescents under the age of 16 and for users 16 years and older. Use of this product before menarche is not indicated.

13. SEXUALLY TRANSMITTED DISEASES

Patients should be counseled that this product does not protect against HIV infection (AIDS) and other sexually transmitted diseases.

INFORMATION FOR THE PATIENT

See Patient Labeling printed below.

ADVERSE REACTIONS

An increased risk of the following serious adverse reactions has been associated with the use of oral contraceptives (See WARNINGS Section).

- Thrombophlebitis and venous thrombosis with or without embolism
- Arterial thromboembolism
- Pulmonary embolism
- Myocardial infarction
- Cerebral hemorrhage
- Cerebral thrombosis
- Hypertension
- Gallbladder disease
- Hepatic ademonas or benign liver tumors

The following adverse reactions have been reported in patients receiving oral contraceptives and are believed to be drug-related:

- Nausea
- Vomiting
- Gastrointestinal symptoms (such as abdominal cramps and bloating)
- Breakthrough bleeding
- Spotting
- Change in menstrual flow
- Amenorrhea
- Temporary infertility after discontinuation of treatment
- Edema
- Melasma which may persist
- Breast changes: tenderness, enlargement, secretion
- Change in weight (increase or decrease)
- Change in cervical erosion and secretion
- Diminution in lactation when given immediately postpartum
- Cholestatic jaundice
- Migraine
- Rash (allergic)
- Mental depression
- Reduced tolerance to carbohydrates
- Vaginal candidiasis
- Change in corneal curvature (steepening)
- Intolerance to contact lenses

The following adverse reactions have been reported in users of oral contraceptives and the association has been neither confirmed nor refuted:

- Pre-menstrual syndrome
- Cataracts
- Changes in appetite
- Cystitis-like syndrome
- Headache
- Nervousness
- Dizziness
- Hirsutism
- Loss of scalp hair
- Erythema multiforme
- Erythema nodosum
- Hemorrhagic eruption
- Vaginitis
- Porphyria

Continued on next page

TABLE III: ANNUAL NUMBER OF BIRTH-RELATED OR METHOD-RELATED DEATHS ASSOCIATED WITH CONTROL OF FERTILITY PER 100,000 NONSTERILE WOMEN, BY FERTILITY CONTROL METHOD ACCORDING TO AGE

Method of control and outcome	15–19	20–24	25–29	30–34	35–39	40–44
No fertility control methods*	7.0	7.4	9.1	14.8	25.7	28.2
Oral contraceptives non-smoker**	0.3	0.5	0.9	1.9	13.8	31.6
Oral contraceptives smoker**	2.2	3.4	6.6	13.5	51.1	117.2
IUD**	0.8	0.8	1.0	1.0	1.4	1.4
Condom*	1.1	1.6	0.7	0.2	0.3	0.4
Diaphragm/ spermicide*	1.9	1.2	1.2	1.3	2.2	2.8
Periodic abstinence*	2.5	1.6	1.6	1.7	2.9	3.6

*Deaths are birth-related
** Deaths are method-related

Adapted from H.W. Ory, ref. #35.

Ortho-Novum 1/50—Cont.

- Impaired renal function
- Hemolytic uremic syndrome
- Acne
- Changes in libido
- Colitis
- Budd-Chiari Syndrome

OVERDOSAGE

Serious ill effects have not been reported following acute ingestion of large doses of oral contraceptives by young children. Overdosage may cause nausea, and withdrawal bleeding may occur in females.

NON-CONTRACEPTIVE HEALTH BENEFITS

The following non-contraceptive health benefits related to the use of combination oral contraceptives are supported by epidemiological studies which largely utilized oral contraceptive formulations containing estrogen doses exceeding 0.035 mg of ethinyl estradiol or 0.05 mg mestranol.[73-78]

Effects on menses:
- increased menstrual cycle regularity
- decreased blood loss and decreased incidence of iron deficiency anemia
- decreased incidence of dysmenorrhea

Effects related to inhibition of ovulation:
- decreased incidence of functional ovarian cysts
- decreased incidence of ectopic pregnancies

Other effects:
- decreased incidence of fibroademonas and fibrocystic disease of the breast
- decreased incidence of acute pelvic inflammatory disease
- decreased incidence of endometrial cancer
- decreased incidence of ovarian cancer

DOSAGE AND ADMINISTRATION

To achieve maximum contraceptive effectiveness, ORTHO-NOVUM 1/50 Tablets must be taken exactly as directed and at intervals not exceeding 24 hours. ORTHO-NOVUM 1/50 Tablets are available in the DIALPAK® Tablet Dispenser which is preset for a Sunday Start. Day 1 Start is also available.

28-Day Regimen (Sunday Start)

When taking ORTHO-NOVUM 1/50 □ 28, the first tablet should be taken on the first Sunday after menstruation begins. If period begins on Sunday, the first tablet should be taken that day. Take one active tablet daily for 21 days followed by one green placebo tablet daily for 7 days. After 28 tablets have been taken, a new course is started the next day (Sunday). For the first cycle of a Sunday Start regimen, another method of contraception should be used until after the first 7 consecutive days of administration.

If the patient misses one (1) active tablet in Weeks 1, 2, or 3, the tablet should be taken as soon as she remembers. If the patient misses two (2) active tablets in Week 1 or Week 2, the patient should take two (2) tablets the day she remembers and two (2) tablets the next day; and then continue taking one (1) tablet a day until she finishes the pack. The patient should be instructed to use a back-up method of birth control if she has sex in the seven (7) days after missing pills. If the patient misses two (2) active tablets in the third week or misses three (3) or more active tablets in a row, the patient should continue taking one tablet every day until Sunday. On Sunday the patient should throw out the rest of the pack and start a new pack that same day. The patient should be instructed to use a back-up method of birth control if she has sex in the seven (7) days after missing pills.

Complete instructions to facilitate patient counseling on proper pill usage may be found in the Detailed Patient Labeling ("How to Take the Pill" section).

28-Day Regimen (Day 1 Start)

The dosage of ORTHO-NOVUM 1/50 □ 28, for the initial cycle of therapy is one active tablet administered daily from the 1st through the 21st day of the menstrual cycle, counting the first day of menstrual flow as "Day 1" followed by one green tablet daily for 7 days. Tablets are taken without interruption for 28 days. After 28 tablets have been taken, a new course is started the next day.

If the patient misses one (1) active tablet in Weeks 1, 2, or 3, the tablet shoud be taken as soon as she remembers. If the patient misses two (2) active tablets in Week 1 or Week 2, the patient should take two (2) tablets the day she remembers and two (2) tablets the next day; and then continue taking one (1) tablet a day until she finishes the pack. The patient should be instructed to use a back-up method of birth control if she has sex in the seven (7) days after missing pills. If the patient misses two (2) active tablets in the third week or misses three (3) or more active tablets in a row, the patient should throw out the rest of the pack and start a new pack that same day. The patient should be instructed to use a back-up method of birth control if she has sex in the seven (7) days after missing pills.

Complete instructions to facilitate patient counseling on proper pill usage may be found in the Detailed Patient Labeling ("How to Take the Pill" section).

The use of ORTHO-NOVUM 1/50 for contraception may be initiated 4 weeks postpartum in women who elect not to breast feed. When the tablets are administered during the postpartum period, the increased risk of thromboembolic disease associated with the postpartum period must be considered. (See CONTRAINDICATIONS and WARNINGS concerning thromboembolic disease. See also PRECAUTIONS for "Nursing Mothers.") The possibility of ovulation and conception prior to initiation of medication should be considered.

(See Discussion of Dose-Related Risk of Vascular Disease from Oral Contraceptives.)

ADDITIONAL INSTRUCTIONS FOR ALL DOSING REGIMENS

Breakthrough bleeding, spotting, and amenorrhea are frequent reasons for patients discontinuing oral contraceptives. In breakthrough bleeding, as in all cases of irregular bleeding from the vagina, nonfunctional causes should be borne in mind. In undiagnosed persistent or recurrent abnormal bleeding from the vagina, adequate diagnostic measures are indicated to rule out pregnancy or malignancy. If pathology has been excluded, time or a change to another formulation may solve the problem. Changing to an oral contraceptive with a higher estrogen content, while potentially useful in minimizing menstrual irregularity, should be done only if necessary since this may increase the risk of thromboembolic disease.

Use of oral contraceptives in the event of a missed menstrual period:

1. If the patient has not adhered to the prescribed schedule, the possibility of pregnancy should be considered at the time of the first missed period and oral contraceptive use should be discontinued until pregnancy is ruled out.
2. If the patient has adhered to the prescribed regimen and misses two consecutive periods, pregnancy should be ruled out before continuing oral contraceptive use.

HOW SUPPLIED

ORTHO-NOVUM 1/50 □ 28 Tablets are available in a DIALPAK Tablet Dispenser (NDC 0062-1332-15) containing 28 tablets, as follows: 21 yellow tablets (1 mg norethindrone and 0.05 mg mestranol) which are unscored with "Ortho" and "150" debossed on each side, and 7 green tablets containing inert ingredients.

REFERENCES

1. Trussel J. Contraceptive efficacy. In Hatcher RA, Trussel J, Stewart F, Cates W, Stewart GK, Kowal D, Guest F, Contraceptive Technology: Seventeenth Revised Edition. New York NY: Irvington Publishers, 1998, in press. **2.** Stadel BV, Oral contraceptives and cardiovascular disease. (Pt. 1). N Engl J Med 1981; 305:612-618. **3.** Stadel BV, Oral contraceptives and cardiovascular disease. (Pt. 2). N Engl J Med 1981; 305:672-677. **4.** Adam SA, Thorogood M. Oral contraception and myocardial infarction revisited: the effects of new preparations and prescribing patterns. Br J Obstet Gynaecol 1981; 88:838-845. **5.** Mann JI, Inman WH. Oral contraceptives and death from myocardial infarction. Br Med J 1975; 2(5965):245-248. **6.** Mann JI, Vessey MP, Thorogood M, Doll R. Myocardial infarction in young women with special reference to oral contraceptive practice. Br Med J 1975; 2(5956):241-245. **7.** Royal College of General Practitioners' Oral Contraception Study: further analyses of mortality in oral contraceptive users. Lancet 1981; 1:541-546. **8.** Slone D, Shapiro S, Kaufman DW, Rosenberg L, Miettinen OS, Stolley PD. Risk of myocardial infarction in relation to current and discounted use of oral contraceptives. N Engl J Med 1981; 305:420-424. **9.** Vessey MP. Female hormones and vascular disease – an epidemiological overview. Br J Fam Plann 1980; 6 (Supplement): 1-12. **10.** Russell-Briefel RG, Ezzati TM, Fulwood R, Perlman JA, Murphy RS. Cardiovascular risk status and oral contraceptive use, United States, 1976-80. Prevent Med 1986; 15:352-362. **11.** Goldbaum GM, Kendrick JS, Hogelin GC, Gentry EM. The relative impact of smoking and oral contraceptive use on women in the United States. JAMA 1987; 258:1339-1342. **12.** Layde PM, Beral V. Further analyses of mortality in oral contraceptive users; Royal College of General Practitioners' Oral Contraception Study. (Table 5) Lancet 1981; 1:541-546. **13.** Knopp RH. Arteriosclerosis risk: the roles of oral contraceptives and postmenopausal estrogens. J Reprod Med 1986; 31(9) (Supplement): 913-921. **14.** Krauss RM, Roy S, Mishell DR, Casagrande J, Pike MC. Effects of two low-dose oral contraceptives on serum lipids and lipoproteins: Differential changes in high-density lipoproteins subclasses. Am J Obstet 1983; 145:446-452. **15.** Wahl P, Walden C, Knopp R, Hoover J, Wallace R, Heiss G, Rifkind B. Effect of estrogen/progestin potency on lipid/lipoprotein cholesterol. N Engl J Med 1983; 308:862-867. **16.** Wynn V, Niththyananthan R. The effect of progestin in combined oral contraceptives on serum lipids with special reference to high density lipoproteins. Am J Obstet Gynecol 1982; 142:766-771. **17.** Wynn V, Godsland I. Effects of oral contraceptives on carbohydrate metabolism. J Reprod Med 1986; 31(9)(Supplement):892-897. **18.** LaRosa JC. Atherosclerotic risk factors in cardiovascular disease. J Reprod Med 1986; 31(9)(Supplement): 906-912. **19.** Inman WH, Vessey MP. Investigation of death from pulmonary, coronary, and cerebral thrombosis and embolism in women of child-bearing age. Br Med J 1968; 2(5599):193-199. **20.** Maguire MG, Tonascia J, Sartwell PE, Stolley PD, Tockman MS. Increased risk of thrombosis due to oral contraceptives: a further report. Am J Epidemiol 1979; 110(2):188-195. **21.** Petitti DB, Wingerd J, Pellegrin F, Ramacharan S. Risk of vascular disease in women: smoking, oral contraceptives, noncontraceptive estrogens, and other factors. JAMA 1979; 242:1150-1154. **22.** Vessey MP, Doll R. Investigation of relation between use of oral contraceptives and thromboembolic disease. Br Med J 1968; 2(5599):199-205. **23.** Vessey MP, Doll R. Investigation of relation between use of oral contraceptives and thromboembolic disease. A further report. Br Med J 1969; 2(5658):651-657. **24.** Porter JB, Hunter JR, Danielson DA, Jick H, Stergachis A. Oral contraceptives and non-fatal vascular disease – recent experience. Obstet Gynecol 1982; 59(3):299-302. **25.** Vessey M, Doll R, Peto R, Johnson B, Wiggins P. A long-term follow-up study of women using different methods of contraception: an interim report. J Biosocial Sci 1976; 8:375-427. **26.** Royal College of General Practitioners: Oral Contraceptives, venous thrombosis, and varicose veins. J Royal Coll Gen Pract 1978; 28:393-399. **27.** Collaborative Group for the Study of Stroke in Young Women: Oral contraception and increased risk of cerebral ischemia or thrombosis. N Engl J Med 1973; 288:871-878. **28.** Petitti DB, Wingerd J. Use of oral contraceptives, cigarette smoking, and risk of subarachnoid hemorrhage. Lancet 1978; 2:234-236. **29.** Inman WH. Oral contraceptives and fatal subarachnoid hemorrhage. Br Med J 1979; 2(6203):1468-1470. **30.** Collaborative Group for the Study of Stroke in Young Women: Oral Contraceptives and stroke in young women: associated risk factors. JAMA 1975; 231:718-722. **31.** Inman WH, Vessey MP, Westerholm B, Engelund A. Thromboembolic disease and the steroidal content of oral contraceptives. A report to the Committee on Safety of Drugs. Br Med J 1970; 2:203-209. **32.** Meade TW, Greenberg G, Thompson SG. Progestogens and cardiovascular reactions associated with oral contraceptives and a comparison of the safety of 50- and 35-mcg oestrogen preparations. Br Med J 1980; 280(6224):1157-1161. **33.** Kay CR. Progestogens and arterial disease – evidence from the Royal College of General Practitioners' Study Am J Obstet Gynecol 1982; 142:762-765. **34.** Royal College of General Practitioners: incidence of arterial disease among oral contraceptive users. J Royal Coll Gen Pract 1983; 33:75-82. **35.** Ory HW. Mortality associated with fertility and fertility control: 1983. Family Planning Perspectives 1983; 15:50-56. **36.** The Cancer and Steroid Hormone Study of the Centers for Disease Control and the National Institute of Child Health and Human Development: Oral contraceptive use and the risk of breast cancer. N Engl J Med 1986; 315:405-411. **37.** Pike MC, Henderson BE, Krailo BE, Krailo MD, Duke A. Roy S. Breast cancer in young women and use of oral contraceptives: possible modifying effect of formulation and age at use. Lancet 1983; 2:926-929. **38.** Paul C, Skegg DG, Spears GFS, Kaldor JM. Oral contraceptives and breast cancer: A national study. Br Med J 1986; 293:723-725. **39.** Miller DR, Rosenberg L, Kaufman DW, Schottenfeld D, Stolley PD, Shapiro S. Breast cancer risk in relation to early oral contraceptive use. Obstet Gynecol 1986; 68:863-868. **40.** Olson H, Olson KL, Moller TR, Ranstam J, Holm P. Oral contraceptive use and breast cancer in young women in Sweden (letter). Lancet 1985; 2:748-749. **41.** McPherson K, Vessey M, Neil A, Doll R, Jones L, Roberts M. Early contraceptive use and breast cancer: Results of another case-control study. Br J Cancer 1987; 56:653-660. **42.** Huggins GR, Zucker PF. Oral contraceptives and neoplasia: 1987 update. Fertil Steril 1987; 47:733-761. **43.** McPherson K, Drife JO. The pill and breast cancer: why the uncertainty? Br Med J 1986; 293:709-710. **44.** Shapiro S. Oral contraceptives – time to take stock. N Engl J Med 1987; 315: 450-451. **45.** Ory H, Naib Z, Conger SB, Hatcher RA, Tyler CW. Contraceptive choice and prevalence of cervical dysplasia and carcinoma in situ. Am J Obstet Gynecol 1976; 124: 573-577. **46.** Vessey MP, Lawless M, McPherson K, Yeates D. Neoplasia of the cervix uteri and contraception: a possible adverse effect of the pill. Lancet 1983; 2:930. **47.** Brinton LA, Huggins GR, Lehman HF, Malli K, Savitz DA, Trapido E, Rosenthal J, Hoover R. Long term use of oral contraceptives and risk of invasive cervical cancer. Int J Cancer 1986; 38:339-344. **48.** WHO Collaborative Study of Neoplasia and Steroid Contraceptives: Invasive cervical cancer and combined oral contraceptives. Br Med J 1985; 290:961-965. **49.** Rooks JB, Ory HW, Ishak KG, Strauss LT, Greenspan JR, Hill AP, Tyler CW. Epidemiology of hepatocellular adenoma: the role of oral contraceptive use. JAMA 1979; 242:644-648. **50.** Bein NN, Goldsmith HS. Recurrent massive hemorrhage from benign hepatic tumors secondary to oral contraceptives. Br J Surg 1977; 64:433-435. **51.** Klatskin G. Hepatic tumors: possible relationship to use of oral contraceptives. Gastroenterology 1977; 73:386-394. **52.** Henderson BE, Preston-Martin S, Edmondson HA, Peters RL, Pike MC. Hepatocellular carcinoma and oral contraceptives. Br J Cancer 1983; 48:437-440. **53.** Neuberger J, Forman D, Doll R, Williams R. Oral contraceptives and hepatocellular carcinoma. Br Med J 1986; 292:1355-1357. **54.** Forman D, Vincent TJ, Doll R. Cancer of the liver and oral contraceptives. Br Med J 1986; 292:1357-1361. **55.** Harlap S, Eldor J. Births following oral contraceptive failures. Obstet Gynecol 1980; 55:447-452. **56.** Savolainen E, Saksela L, Saxen, L. Teratogenic hazards of oral contraceptives analyzed in a national malformation register. Am J Obstet Gynecol 1981; 140:521-524. **57.** Janerich DT, Piper JM, Glebatis DM. Oral contraceptives and birth defects. Am J Epidemiol 1980; 112:73-79. **58.** Ferencz C, Matanoski GM, Wilson PD, Rubin JD, Neill CA, Gutberlet R. Maternal hormone therapy and congenital heart disease. Teratology 1980; 21:225-239. **59.** Rothman KJ, Fyler DC, Goldblatt A, Kreidberg MB. Exogenous hormones and other drug exposures of children with congenital heart disease. Am J Epidemiol 1979; 109:433-439. **60.** Boston Collaborative Drug Surveillance Program: Oral contraceptives and venous thromboembolic disease, surgically comfirmed gallbladder disease, and breast tumors. Lancet 1973; 1:1399-1404. **61.** Royal College of General Practitioners: Oral contraceptives and health. New York, Pittman 1974. **62.** Layde PM, Vessey MP, Yeates D. Risk of gallbladder disease: a cohort study of young women attending family planning clinics. J Epidemiol Community Health 1982;

36:274-278. **63.** Rome Group for Epidemiology and Prevention of Cholelithiasis (GREPCO): Prevalence of gallstone disease in an Italian adult female population. Am J Epidemiol 1984; 119:796-805. **64.** Storm BL, Tamragouri RT, Morse ML, Lazar EL, West SL, Stolley PD, Jones JK. Oral contraceptives and other risk factors for gallbladder disease. Clin Pharmacol Ther 1986; 39:335-341. **65.** Wynn V, Adams PW, Godsland IF, Melrose J, Niththyananthan R, Oakley NW, Seedj A. Comparison of effects of different combined oral contraceptive formulations on carbohydrate and lipid metabolism. Lancet 1979; 1:1045-1049. **66.** Wynn V. Effect of progesterone and progestins on carbohydrate metabolism. In: Progesterone and Progestin. Bardin CW, Milgrom E, Mauvis-Jarvis P. eds. New York, Raven Press, 1983; pp. 395-410. **67.** Perlman JA, Roussell-Briefel RG, Ezzati TM, Lieberknecht G. Oral glucose tolerance and the potency of oral contraceptive progestogens. J Chronic Dis 1985; 38: 857-864. **68.** Royal College of General Practitioners' Oral Contraception Study: Effect on hypertension and benign breast disease of progestogen component in combined oral contraceptives. Lancet 1977; 1:624. **69.** Fisch IR, Frank J. Oral contraceptives and blood pressure. JAMA 1977; 237: 2499-2503. **70.** Laragh AJ. Oral contraceptive induced hypertension – nine years later. Am J Obstet Gynecol 1976; 126:141-147. **71.** Ramcharan S, Peritz E, Pellegrin FA, Williams WT. Incidence of hypertension in the Walnut Creek Contraceptive Drug Study cohort: In: Pharmacology of steroid contraceptive drugs. Garattini S, Berendes HW. Eds. New York, Raven Press, 1977; pp. 277-288, (Monographs of the Mario Negri Institute for Pharmacological Research Milan.) **72.** Stockley I. Interactions with oral contraceptives. J Pharm 1976; 216:140-143. **73.** The Cancer and Steroid Hormone Study of the Centers for Disease Control and the National Institute of Child Health and Human Development: Oral contraceptive use and the risk of ovarian cancer. JAMA 1983; 249:1596-1599. **74.** The Cancer and Steroid Hormone Study of the Centers for Disease Control and the National Institute of Child Health and Human Development: Combination oral contraceptive use and the risk of endometrial cancer. JAMA 1987; 257:796-800. **75.** Ory HW. Functional ovarian cysts and oral contraceptives: negative association confirmed surgically. JAMA 1974; 228:68-69. **76.** Ory HW, Cole P, MacMahon B, Hoover R. Oral contraceptives and reduced risk of benign breast disease. N Engl J Med 1976; 294:419-422. **77.** Ory HW. The noncontraceptive health benefits from oral contraceptive use. Fam Plann Perspect 1982; 14:182-184. **78.** Ory HW, Forrest JD, Lincoln R. Making choices: Evaluating the health risks and benefits of birth control methods. New York, The Alan Guttmacher Institute, 1983; p. 1. **79.** Schlesselman J, Stadel BV, Murray P, Lai S. Breast cancer in relation to early use of oral contraceptives. JAMA 1988; 259:1828-1833. **80.** Hennekens CH, Speizer FE, Lipnick RJ, Rosner B, Bain C, Belanger C, Stampfer MJ, Willett W, Peto R. A case-control study of oral contraceptive use and breast cancer. JNCI 1984; 72:39-42. **81.** LaVecchia C, Decarli A, Fasoli M, Franceschi S, Gentile A, Negri E, Parazzini R, Tognoni G. Oral contraceptives and cancers of the breast and of the female genital tract. Interim results from a case-control study. Br J Cancer 1986; 54:311-317. **82.** Meirik O, Lund E, Adami H, Bergstrom R, Christoffersen T, Bergsjo P. Oral contraceptive use and breast cancer in young women. A Joint National Case-control study in Sweden and Norway. Lancet 1986; 11:650-654. **83.** Kay CR, Hannaford PC. Breast cancer and the pill – A further report from the Royal College of General Practitioners' oral contraception study. Br J Cancer 1988; 58:675-680. **84.** Stadel BV, Lai S, Schlesselman JJ, Murray P. Oral contraceptives and premenopausal breast cancer in nulliparous women. Contraception 1988; 38:287-299. **85.** Miller DR, Rosenberg L, Kaufman DW, Stolley P. Warshauer ME, Shapiro S. Breast cancer before age 45 and oral contraceptive use: New Findings. Am J Epidemiol 1989; 129:269-280. **86.** The UK National Case-Control Study Group, Oral contraceptive use and breast cancer in young women. Lancet 1989; 1:973-982. **87.** Schlesselman JJ. Cancer of the breast and reproductive tract in relation to the use of oral contraceptives. Contraception 1989; 40:1-38. **88.** Vessey MP, McPherson K, Villard-Mackintosh L, Yeates D. Oral contraceptives and breast cancer: latest findings in a large cohort study. Br J Cancer 1989; 59:613-617. **89.** Jick SS, Walker AM, Stergachis A, Jick H. Oral contraceptives and breast cancer. Br J Cancer 1989; 59:618-621. **90.** Collaborative Group on Hormonal Factors in Breast Cancer. Breast cancer and hormonal contraceptives: collaborative reanalysis of individual data on 53 297 women with breast cancer and 100 239 women without breast cancer from 54 epidemiological studies. Lancet 1996; 347:1713-1727. **91.** Palmer JR, Rosenberg L, Kaufman DW, Warshauer ME, Stolley P, Shapiro S. Oral Contraceptive Use and Liver Cancer. Am J Epidemiol 1989; 130:878-882.

BRIEF SUMMARY PATIENT PACKAGE INSERT

Oral contraceptives, also known as "birth control pills" or "the pill," are taken to prevent pregnancy and when taken correctly, have a failure rate of less than 1% per year when used without missing any pills. The typical failure rate of large numbers of pill users is less than 3% per year when women who miss pills are included. For most women oral contraceptives are also free of serious or unpleasant side effects. However, forgetting to take pills considerably increases the chances of pregnancy.

For the majority of women, oral contraceptives can be taken safely. But there are some women who are at high risk of developing certain serious diseases that can be fatal or may cause temporary or permanent disability. The risks associated with taking oral contraceptives increases significantly if you:

- smoke
- have high blood pressure, diabetes, high cholesterol
- have or have had clotting disorders, heart attack, stroke, angina pectoris, cancer of the breast or sex organs, jaundice or malignant or benign liver tumors.

Although cardiovascular disease risks may be increased with oral contraceptive use after age 40 in healthy, nonsmoking women (even with the newer low-dose formulations), there are also greater potential health risks associated with pregnancy in older women.

You should not take the pill if you suspect you are pregnant or have unexplained vaginal bleeding.

Cigarette smoking increases the risk of serious cardiovascular side effects from oral contraceptive use. This risk increases with age and with heavy smoking (15 or more cigarettes per day) and is quite marked in women over 35 years of age. Women who use oral contraceptives are strongly advised not to smoke.

Most side effects of the pill are not serious. The most common side effects are nausea, vomiting, bleeding between menstrual periods, weight gain, breast tenderness, and difficulty wearing contact lenses. These side effects, especially nausea and vomiting, may subside within the first three months of use.

The serious side effects of the pill may occur very infrequently, especially if you are in good health and are young. However, you should know that the following medical conditions have been associated with or made worse by the pill:

1. Blood clots in the legs (thrombophlebitis), lungs (pulmonary embolism), stoppage or rupture of a blood vessel in the brain (stroke), blockage of blood vessels in the heart (heart attack or angina pectoris) or other organs of the body. As mentioned above, smoking increases the risk of heart attacks and strokes and subsequent serious medical consequences.
2. In rare cases, oral contraceptives can cause benign but dangerous liver tumors. These benign liver tumors can rupture and cause fatal internal bleeding. In addition, some studies report an increased risk of developing liver cancer. However, liver cancers are rare.
3. High blood pressure, although blood pressure usually returns to normal when the pill is stopped.

The symptoms associated with these serious side effects are discussed in the detailed leaflet given to you with your supply of pills. Notify your doctor or health care provider if you notice any unusual physical disturbances while taking the pill. In addition, drugs such as rifampin, as well as some anticonvulsants and some antibiotics may decrease oral contraceptive effectiveness.

There is conflict among studies regarding breast cancer and oral contraceptive use. Some studies have reported an increase in the risk of developing breast cancer, particularly at a younger age. This increased risk appears to be related to duration of use. The majority of studies have found no overall increase in the risk of developing breast cancer. Some studies have found an increase in the incidence of cancer of the cervix in women who use oral contraceptives. However, this finding may be related to factors other than the use of oral contraceptives. There is insufficient evidence to rule out the possibility that pills may cause such cancers.

Taking the combination pill provides some important noncontraceptive benefits. These include less painful menstruation, less menstrual blood loss and anemia, fewer pelvic infections, and fewer cancers of the ovary and the lining of the uterus.

Be sure to discuss any medical condition you may have with your health care provider. Your health care provider will take a medical and family history before prescribing oral contraceptives and will examine you. The physical examination may be delayed to another time if you request it and the health care provider believes that it is a good medical practice to postpone it. You should be reexamined at least once a year while taking oral contraceptives. Your pharmacist should have given you the detailed patient information labeling which gives you further information which you should read and discuss with your health care provider.

This product (like all oral contraceptives) is intended to prevent pregnancy. It does not protect against transmission of HIV (AIDS) and other sexually transmitted diseases such as chlamydia, genital herpes, genital warts, gonorrhea, hepatitis B, and syphilis.

DETAILED PATIENT LABELING

PLEASE NOTE: This labeling is revised from time to time as important new medical information becomes available. Therefore, please review this labeling carefully.

The following oral contraceptive product contains a combination of estrogen and progestogen, the two kinds of female hormones:

Each yellow tablet contains 1 mg norethindrone and 0.05 mg mestranol. Each green tablet in ORTHO-NOVUM 1/50 □ 28 Day Regimen contains inert ingredients.

INTRODUCTION

You should not use ORTHO-NOVUM 1/50 □ 28 Day, which contains higher doses of estrogen than other oral contraceptives, unless specifically recommended by your health care provider. Any woman who considers using oral contraceptives (the birth control pill or the pill) should understand the benefits and risks of using this form of birth control. This patient labeling will give you much of the information you will need to make this decision and will also help you determine if you are at risk of developing any of the serious side effects of the pill. It will tell you how to use the pill properly so that it will be as effective as possible. However, this labeling is not a replacement for a careful discussion between you and your health care provider. You should discuss the information provided in this labeling with him or her, both when you first start taking the pill and during your revisits. You should also follow your health care provider's advice with regard to regular check-ups while you are on the pill.

EFFECTIVENESS OF ORAL CONTRACEPTIVES

Oral contraceptives or "birth control pills" or "the pill" are used to prevent pregnancy and are more effective than other non-surgical methods of birth control. When they are taken correctly, the chance of becoming pregnant is less than 1% (1 pregnancy per 100 women per year of use) when used perfectly, without missing any pills. Typical failure rates are actually 3% per year. The chance of becoming pregnant increases with each missed pill during a menstrual cycle.

In comparison, typical failure rates for other non-surgical methods of birth control during the first year of use are as follows:

Implant: <1%	Cervical Cap 18 to 36%
Injection: <1%	Condom alone (male): 12%
IUD: 1 to 2%	Condom alone (female): 21%
Diaphragm with spermicides: 18%	Periodic abstinence: 20%
Spermicides alone: 21%	No methods: 85%
Vaginal sponge: 18 to 36%	

WHO SHOULD NOT TAKE ORAL CONTRACEPTIVES

Cigarette smoking increases the risk of serious cardiovascular side effects from oral contraceptive use. This risk increases with age and with heavy smoking (15 or more cigarettes per day) and is quite marked in women over 35 years of age. Women who use oral contraceptives are strongly advised not to smoke.

Some women should not use the pill. For example, you should not take the pill if you are pregnant or think you may be pregnant. You should also not use the pill if you have any of the following conditions:

- A history of heart attack or stroke
- Blood clots in the legs (thrombophlebitis), lungs (pulmonary embolism), or eyes
- A history of blood clots in the deep veins of your legs
- Chest pain (angina pectoris)
- Known or suspected breast cancer or cancer of the lining of the uterus, cervix or vagina
- Unexplained vaginal bleeding (until a diagnosis is reached by your doctor)
- Yellowing of the whites of the eyes or of the skin (jaundice) during pregnancy or during previous use of the pill
- Liver tumor (benign or cancerous)
- Known or suspected pregnancy

Tell your health care provider if you have ever had any of these conditions. Your health care provider can recommend a safer method of birth control.

OTHER CONSIDERATIONS BEFORE TAKING ORAL CONTRACEPTIVES

Tell your health care provider if you have or have had:

- Breast nodules, fibrocystic disease of the breast, an abnormal breast x-ray or mammogram
- Diabetes
- Elevated cholesterol or triglycerides
- High blood pressure
- Migraine or other headaches or epilepsy
- Mental depression
- Gallbladder, heart or kidney disease
- History of scanty or irregular menstrual periods

Women with any of these conditions should be checked often by their health care provider if they choose to use oral contraceptives.

Also, be sure to inform your doctor or health care provider if you smoke or are on any medications.

RISKS OF TAKING ORAL CONTRACEPTIVES

1. Risk of developing blood clots

Blood clots and blockage of blood vessels are one of the most serious side effects of taking oral contraceptives and can cause death or serious disability. In particular, a clot in the legs can cause thrombophlebitis and a clot that travels to the lungs can cause a sudden blocking of the vessel carrying blood to the lungs. Rarely, clots occur in the blood vessels of the eye and may cause blindness, double vision, or impaired vision.

If you take oral contraceptives and need elective surgery, need to stay in bed for a prolonged illness or have recently delivered a baby, you may be at risk of developing blood clots. You should consult your doctor about stopping oral contraceptives three to four weeks before surgery and not taking oral contraceptives for two weeks after surgery or during bed rest. You should also not take oral contraceptives soon after delivery of a baby. It is advisable to wait for at least four weeks after delivery if you are not breast feeding

Continued on next page

Ortho-Novum 1/50—Cont.

or four weeks after a second trimester abortion. If you are breast feeding, you should wait until you have weaned your child before using the pill. (See also in the section on Breast Feeding in General Precautions.)

The risk of circulatory disease in oral contraceptive users may be higher in users of high dose pills and may be greater with longer duration of oral contraceptive use. In addition, some of these increased risks may continue for a number of years after stopping oral contraceptives. The risk of abnormal blood clotting increases with age in both users and nonusers of oral contraceptives, but the increased risk from the oral contraceptive appears to be present at all ages. For women aged 20 to 44, it is estimated that about 1 in 2,000 using oral contraceptives will be hospitalized each year because of abnormal clotting. Among nonusers in the same age group, about 1 in 20,000 would be hospitalized each year. For oral contraceptive users in general, it has been estimated that in women between the ages of 15 and 34 the risk of death due to a circulatory disorder is about 1 in 12,000 per year, whereas for nonusers the rate is about 1 in 50,000 per year. In the age group 35 to 44, the risk is estimated to be about 1 in 2,500 per year for oral contraceptive users and about 1 in 10,000 per year for nonusers.

2. Heart attacks and strokes

Oral contraceptives may increase the tendency to develop strokes (stoppage or rupture of blood vessels in the brain) and angina pectoris and heart attacks (blockage of blood vessels in the heart). Any of these conditions can cause death or serious disability.

Smoking greatly increases the possibility of suffering heart attacks and strokes. Furthermore, smoking and the use of oral contraceptives greatly increase the chances of developing and dying of heart disease

3. Gallbladder disease

Oral contraceptive users probably have a greater risk than nonusers of having gallbladder disease, although this risk may be related to pills containing high doses of estrogens.

4. Liver tumors

In rare cases, oral contraceptives can cause benign but dangerous liver tumors. These benign liver tumors can rupture and cause fatal internal bleeding. In addition, some studies report an increased risk of developing liver cancer. However, liver cancers are rare.

5. Cancer of the reproductive organs and breast

There is conflict among studies regarding breast cancer and oral contraceptive use. Some studies have reported an increase in the risk of developing breast cancer, particularly at a younger age. This increased risk appears to be related to duration of use. The majority of studies have found no overall increase in the risk of developing breast cancer.

A meta-analyses of 54 studies found a small increase in the frequency of having breast cancer diagnosed for women who were currently using combined oral contraceptives or had used them within the past ten years. This increase in the frequency of breast cancer diagnosis, within ten years of stopping use, was generally accounted for by cancers localized to the breast. There was no increase in the frequency of having breast cancer diagnosed ten or more years after cessation of use.

Some studies have found an increase in the incidence of cancer of the cervix in women who use oral contraceptives. However, this finding may be related to factors other than the use of oral contraceptives. There is insufficient evidence to rule out the possibility that pills may cause such cancers.

ESTIMATED RISK OF DEATH FROM A BIRTH CONTROL METHOD OR PREGNANCY

All methods of birth control and pregnancy are associated with a risk of developing certain diseases which may lead to disability or death. An estimate of the number of deaths associated with different methods of birth control and pregnancy has been calculated and is shown in the following table.

[See table below]

In the above table, the risk of death from any birth control method is less than the risk of childbirth, except for oral contraceptive users over the age of 35 who smoke and pill users over the age of 40 even if they do not smoke. It can be seen in the table that for women aged 15 to 39, the risk of death was highest with pregnancy (7–26 deaths per 100,000 women, depending on age). Among pill users who do not smoke, the risk of death was always lower than that associated with pregnancy for any age group, although over the age of 40, the risk increases to 32 deaths per 100,000 women, compared to 28 associated with pregnancy at that age. However, for pill users who smoke and are over the age of 35, the estimated number of deaths exceed those for other methods of birth control. If a woman is over the age of 40 and smokes, her estimated risk of death is four times higher (117/100,000 women) than the estimated risk associated with pregnancy (28/100,000 women) in that age group.

The suggestion that women over 40 who do not smoke should not take oral contraceptives is based on information from older, higher-dose pills. An Advisory Committee of the FDA discussed this issue in 1989 and recommended that the benefits of low-dose oral contraceptive use by healthy, nonsmoking women over 40 years of age may outweigh the possible risks.

WARNINGS SIGNALS

If any of these adverse effects occur while you are taking oral contraceptives, call your doctor immediately:

- Sharp chest pain, coughing of blood, or sudden shortness of breath (indicating a possible clot in the lung)
- Pain in the calf (indicating a possible clot in the leg)
- Crushing chest pain or heaviness in the chest (indicating a possible heart attack)
- Sudden severe headache or vomiting, dizziness, or fainting, disturbances of vision or speech, weakness, or numbness in an arm or leg (indicating a possible stroke)
- Sudden partial or complete loss of vision (indicating a possible clot in the eye)
- Breast lumps (indicating possible breast cancer or fibrocystic disease of the breast; ask your doctor or health care provider to show you how to examine your breasts)
- Severe pain or tenderness in the stomach area (indicating a possibly ruptured liver tumor)
- Difficulty in sleeping, weakness, lack of energy, fatigue, or change in mood (possibly indicating severe depression)
- Jaundice or yellowing of the skin or eyeballs, accompanied frequently by fever, fatigue, loss of appetite, dark colored urine, or light colored bowel movements (indicating possible liver problems)

SIDE EFFECTS OF ORAL CONTRACEPTIVES

1. Vaginal bleeding

Irregular vaginal bleeding or spotting may occur while you are taking the pills. Irregular bleeding may vary from slight staining between menstrual periods to breakthrough bleeding which is a flow much like a regular period. Irregular bleeding occurs most often during the first few months of oral contraceptive use, but may also occur after you have been taking the pill for some time. Such bleeding may be temporary and usually does not indicate any serious problems. It is important to continue taking your pills on schedule. If the bleeding occurs in more than one cycle or last for more than a few days, talk to your doctor or health care provider.

ANNUAL NUMBER OF BIRTH-RELATED OR METHOD-RELATED DEATHS ASSOCIATED WITH CONTROL OF FERTILITY PER 100,000 NONSTERILE WOMEN, BY FERTILITY CONTROL METHOD ACCORDING TO AGE

Method of control and outcome	15–19	20–24	25–29	30–34	35–39	40–44
No fertility control methods*	7.0	7.4	9.1	14.8	25.7	28.2
Oral contraceptives non-smoker**	0.3	0.5	0.9	1.9	13.8	31.6
Oral contraceptives smoker**	2.2	3.4	6.6	13.5	51.1	117.2
IUD**	0.8	0.8	1.0	1.0	1.4	1.4
Condom*	1.1	1.6	0.7	0.2	0.3	0.4
Diaphragm/ spermicide*	1.9	1.2	1.2	1.3	2.2	2.8
Periodic abstinence*	2.5	1.6	1.6	1.7	2.9	3.6

*Deaths are birth-related
**Deaths are method-related

2. Contact lenses

If you wear contact lenses and notice a change in vision or an inability to wear your lenses, contact your doctor or health care provider.

3. Fluid retention

Oral contraceptives may cause edema (fluid retention) with swelling of the fingers or ankles and may raise your blood pressure. If you experience fluid retention, contact your doctor or health care provider.

4. Melasma

A spotty darkening of the skin is possible, particularly of the face, which may persist.

5. Other side effects

Other side effects may include nausea and vomiting, change in appetite, headache, nervousness, depression, dizziness, loss of scalp hair, rash, and vaginal infections.

If any of these side effects bother you, call your doctor or health care provider.

GENERAL PRECAUTIONS

1. Missed periods and use of oral contraceptives before or during early pregnancy

There may be times when you may not menstruate regularly after you have completed taking a cycle of pills. If you have taken your pills regularly and miss one menstrual period, continue taking your pills for the next cycle but be sure to inform your health care provider before doing so. If you have not taken the pills daily as instructed and missed a menstrual period, you may be pregnant. If you missed two consecutive menstrual periods, you may be pregnant. Check with your health care provider immediately to determine whether you are pregnant. Do not continue to take oral contraceptives until you are sure you are not pregnant, but continue to use another method of contraception.

There is no conclusive evidence that oral contraceptive use is associated with an increase in birth defects, when taken inadvertently during early pregnancy. Previously, a few studies had reported that oral contraceptives might be associated with birth defects, but these findings have not been seen in more recent studies. Nevertheless, oral contraceptives or any other drugs should not be used during pregnancy unless clearly necessary and prescribed by your doctor. You should check with your doctor about risks to your unborn child of any medication taken during pregnancy.

2. While breast feeding

If you are beast feeding, consult your doctor before starting oral contraceptives. Some of the drug will be passed on to the child in the milk. A few adverse effects on the child have been reported, including yellowing of the skin (jaundice) and breast enlargement. In addition, combination oral contraceptives may decrease the amount and quality of your milk. If possible, do not use oral contraceptives while breast feeding. You should use another method of contraception since breast feeding provides only partial protection from becoming pregnant and this partial protection decreases significantly as you breast feed for longer periods of time. You should consider starting oral contraceptives only after you have weaned your child completely.

3. Laboratory tests

If you are scheduled for any laboratory tests, tell your doctor you are taking birth control pills. Certain blood tests may be affected by birth control pills.

4. Drug interactions

Certain drugs may interact with birth control pills to make them less effective in preventing pregnancy or cause an increase in breakthrough bleeding. Such drugs include rifampin, drugs used for epilepsy such as barbiturates (for example, phenobarbital), anticonvulsants such as carbamazepine (Tegretol is one brand of this drug), phenytoin (Dilantin is one brand of this drug), phenylbutazone (Butazolidin is one brand), and possibly certain antibiotics. You may need to use additional contraception when you take drugs which can make oral contraceptives less effective.

5. Sexually transmitted diseases

This product (like all oral contraceptives) is intended to prevent pregnancy. It does not protect against transmission of HIV (AIDS) and other sexually transmitted diseases such as chlamydia, genital herpes, genital warts, gonorrhea, hepatitis B, and syphilis.

HOW TO TAKE THE PILL

IMPORTANT POINTS TO REMEMBER

BEFORE YOU START TAKING YOUR PILLS:

1. BE SURE TO READ THESE DIRECTIONS:
Before you start taking your pills.
Anytime you are not sure what to do.

2. THE RIGHT WAY TO TAKE THE PILL IS TO TAKE ONE PILL EVERY DAY AT THE SAME TIME
If you miss pills you could get pregnant. This includes starting the pack late.
The more pills you miss, the more likely you are to get pregnant.

3. MANY WOMEN HAVE SPOTTING OR LIGHT BLEEDING, OR MAY FEEL SICK TO THEIR STOMACH DURING THE FIRST 1–3 PACKS OF PILLS. If you feel sick to your stomach, do not stop taking the pill. The problem will usually go away. If it doesn't go away, check with your doctor or clinic.

4. MISSING PILLS CAN ALSO CAUSE SPOTTING OR LIGHT BLEEDING, even when you make up these missed pills.
On the days you take 2 pill to make up for missed pills, you could also feel a little sick to your stomach.

5. IF YOU HAVE VOMITING OR DIARRHEA, for any reason, or IF YOU TAKE SOME MEDICINES, including some antibiotics, your pills may not work as well. Use a back-up method (such as condoms, foam, or sponge) until you check with your doctor or clinic.
6. IF YOU HAVE TROUBLE REMEMBERING TO TAKE THE PILL, talk to your doctor or clinic about how to make pill-taking easier or about using another method of birth control.
7. IF YOU HAVE ANY QUESTIONS OR ARE UNSURE ABOUT THE INFORMATION IN THIS LEAFLET, call your doctor or clinic.

BEFORE YOU START TAKING YOUR PILLS

1. DECIDE WHAT TIME OF DAY YOU WANT TO TAKE YOUR PILL.
It is important to take it at about the same time every day.
2. LOOK AT YOUR PILL PACK TO SEE IF IT HAS 28 PILLS:
The 28-pill pack has 21 yellow "active" pills (with hormones) to take for 3 weeks. This is followed by 1 week of "reminder" green pills (without hormones).
3. ALSO FIND:
1) where on the pack to start taking the pills,
2) in what order to take the pills.
CHECK PICTURE OF PILL PACK AND ADDITIONAL INSTRUCTIONS FOR USING THIS PACKAGE IN THE BRIEF SUMMARY PATIENT PACKAGE INSERT.
4. BE SURE YOU HAVE READY AT ALL TIMES:
ANOTHER KIND OF BIRTH CONTROL (such as condoms, foam, or sponge) to use as a back-up method in case you miss pills.
AN EXTRA, FULL PILL PACK.

WHEN TO START THE FIRST PACK OF PILLS

You have a choice of which day to start taking your first pack of pills. ORTHO-NOVUM 1/50 is available in the DIALPAK® Tablet Dispenser which is preset for a Sunday Start. Day 1 Start is also provided. Decide with your doctor or clinic which is the best day for you. Pick a time of day which will be easy to remember.

SUNDAY START:
Take the first "active" yellow pill of the first pack on the Sunday after your period starts, even if you are still bleeding If your period begins on Sunday, start the pack the same day.
Use another method of birth control as a back-up method if you have sex anytime from the Sunday you start your first pack of until the next Sunday (7 days). Condoms, foam, or the sponge are good back-up methods of birth control.

DAY 1 START:
Take the first "active" yellow pill of the first pack during the first 24 hours of your period.
You will not need to use a back-up method of birth control, since you are starting the pill at the beginning of your period.

WHAT TO DO DURING THE MONTH

1. TAKE ONE PILL AT THE SAME TIME EVERY DAY UNTIL THE PACK IS EMPTY.
Do not skip pills even if you are spotting or bleeding between monthly periods or feel sick to your stomach (nausea).
Do not skip pills even if you do not have sex very often.
2. WHEN YOU FINISH A PACK OR SWITCH YOUR BRAND OF PILLS:
Start the next pack on the day after your last "reminder" pill. Do not wait any days between packs.

WHAT TO DO IF YOU MISS PILLS

If you **MISS 1** yellow "active" pill.
1. Take it as soon as you remember. Take the next pill at your regular time. This means you may take 2 pills in 1 day.
2. You do not need to use a back-up birth control method if you have sex.
If you **MISS 2** yellow "active" pills in a row in **WEEK 1 OR WEEK 2** of your pack:
1. Take 2 pills on the day you remember and 2 pills the next day.
2. Then take 1 pill a day until you finish the pack.
3. You MAY BECOME PREGNANT if you have sex in the 7 days after you miss pills. You MUST use another birth control method (such as condoms, foam or sponge) as a back-up method for those 7 days.
If you **MISS 2** yellow "active" pills in a row in **THE 3RD WEEK:**
1. **If you are a Sunday Starter:**
Keep taking 1 pill every day until Sunday. On Sunday, THROW OUT the rest of the pack and start a new pack of pills that same day.
If you are a Day 1 Starter:
THROW OUT the rest of the pill pack and start a new pack that same day.
2. You may not have our period this month but this is expected. However, if you miss your period 2 months in a row, call your doctor or clinic because you might be pregnant.
3. You MAY BECOME PREGNANT if you have sex in the 7 days after you miss pills. You MUST use another birth control method (such as condoms, foam, or sponge) as a back-up method for those 7 days.

If you **MISS 3 OR MORE** yellow "active" pills in a row (during the first 3 weeks):
1. **If you are a Sunday Starter:**
Keep taking 1 pill every day until Sunday. On Sunday, THROW OUT the rest of the pack and start a new pack of pills that same day.
If you are a Day 1 Starter:
THROW OUT the rest of the pill pack and start a new pack that same day.
2. You may not have your period this month but this is expected. However, if you miss your period 2 months in a row, call your doctor or clinic because you might be pregnant.
3. You MAY BECOME PREGNANT if you have sex in the 7 days after you miss pills. You MUST use another birth control method (such as condoms, foam, or sponge) as a back-up method for those 7 days.

A REMINDER FOR ON 28-DAY PACKS:
If you forget any of the 7 green "reminder" pills in Week 4:
THROW AWAY the pills you missed.
Keep taking 1 pill each day until the pack is empty.
You do not need a back-up method.

FINALLY, IF YOU ARE STILL NOT SURE WHAT TO DO ABOUT THE PILLS YOU HAVE MISSED:
Use a BACK-UP METHOD anytime you have sex.
KEEP TAKING ONE "ACTIVE" PILL EACH DAY until you can reach your doctor or clinic.

PREGNANCY DUE TO PILL FAILURE

Combination Oral Contraceptives
The incidence of pill failure resulting in pregnancy is approximately one percent (i.e., one pregnancy per 100 women per year) if taken every day as directed, but more typical failure rates are about 3%. If failure does occur, the risk to the fetus is minimal.

PREGNANCY AFTER STOPPING THE PILL

There may be some delay in becoming pregnant after you stop using oral contraceptives, especially if you had irregular menstrual cycles before you used oral contraceptives. It may be advisable to postpone conception until you begin menstruating regularly once you have stopped taking the pill and desire pregnancy.
There does not appear to be any increase in birth defects in newborn babies when pregnancy occurs soon after stopping the pill.

OVERDOSAGE

Serious ill effects have not been reported following ingestion of large doses of oral contraceptives by young children. Overdosage may cause nausea and withdrawal bleeding in females. In case of overdosage, contact your health care provider or pharmacist.

OTHER INFORMATION

Your health care provider will take a medical and family history before prescribing oral contraceptives and will examine you. The physical examination may be delayed to another time if you request it and the health care provider believes that it is a good medical practice to postpone it. You should be reexamined at least once a year. Be sure to inform your health provider if there is a family history of any of the conditions listed previously in this leaflet. Be sure to keep all appointments with your health care provider, because this is a time to determine if there are early signs of side effects of oral contraceptive use.
Do not use the drug for any condition other than the one for which it was prescribed. This drug has been prescribed specifically for you; do not give it to others who may want birth control pills.

HEALTH BENEFITS FROM ORAL CONTRACEPTIVES

In addition to preventing pregnancy, use of combination oral contraceptives may provide certain benefits. They are:

- menstrual cycles may become more regular
- blood flow during menstruation may be lighter and less iron may be lost. Therefore, anemia due to iron deficiency is less likely to occur.
- pain or other symptoms during menstruation may be encountered less frequently
- ectopic (tubal) pregnancy may occur less frequently
- noncancerous cysts or lumps in the breast may occur less frequently
- acute pelvic inflammatory disease may occur less frequently
- oral contraceptive use may provide some protection against developing two forms of cancer: cancer of the ovaries and cancer of the lining of the uterus.

If you want more information about birth control pills, ask your doctor or pharmacist. They have a more technical leaflet called the Professional Labeling, which you may wish to read. The professional labeling is also published in a book called *Physicians' Desk Reference*, available in many book stores and public libraries.
ORTHO-McNEIL PHARMACEUTICAL, INC.
Raritan, New Jersey 08869
© OPC 1998 Revised July 1998 635-50-800-3
Shown in Product Identification Guide, page 328

ORTHO–NOVUM® Tablets ℞
(norethindrone/ethinyl estradiol)
and MODICON® Tablets ℞
(norethindrone/ethinyl estradiol)

Patients should be counseled that this product does not protect against HIV infection (AIDS) and other sexually transmitted diseases.

COMBINATION ORAL CONTRACEPTIVES
Each of the following products is a combination oral contraceptive containing the progestational compound norethindrone and the estrogenic compound ethinyl estradiol.
ORTHO-NOVUM 7/7/7 □ 21 Tablets and ORTHO-NOVUM 7/7/7 □ 28 Tablets: Each white tablet contains 0.5 mg of norethindrone and 0.035 mg of ethinyl estradiol. Inactive ingredients include lactose, magnesium stearate and pregelatinized starch. Each light peach tablet contains 0.75 of norethindrone and 0.035 mg of ethinyl estradiol. Inactive ingredients include FD&C Yellow No. 6, lactose, magnesium stearate and pregelatinized starch. Each peach tablet contains 1 mg of norethindrone and 0.035 mg of ethinyl estradiol. Inactive ingredients include FD&C Yellow No. 6, lactose, magnesium stearate and pregelatinized starch. Each green tablet in the ORTHO-NOVUM 7/7/7 □ 28 package contains only inert ingredients, as follows: D&C Yellow No. 10 Aluminum Lake, FD&C Blue No. 2 Aluminum Lake, lactose, magnesium stearate, microcrystalline cellulose and pregelatinized starch.
ORTHO-NOVUM 10/11 □ 21 Tablets and ORTHO-NOVUM 10/11 □ 28 Tablets: Each white tablet contains 0.5 mg of norethindrone and 0.035 mg of ethinyl estradiol. Inactive ingredients include lactose, magnesium stearate and pregelatinized starch. Each peach tablet contains 1 mg norethindrone and 0.035 mg ethinyl estradiol. Inactive ingredients include FD&C Yellow No. 6, lactose, magnesium stearate and pregelatinized starch. Each green tablet in the ORTHO-NOVUM 10/11 □ 28 package contains only inert ingredients, as listed under green tablets in ORTHO-NOVUM 7/7/7 □ 28.
ORTHO-NOVUM 1/35 □ 21 Tablets and ORTHO-NOVUM 1/35 □ 28 Tablets: Each peach tablet contains 1 mg of norethindrone and 0.035 mg of ethinyl estradiol. Inactive ingredients include FD&C Yellow No. 6, lactose, magnesium stearate and pregelatinized starch. Each green tablet in the ORTHO-NOVUM 1/35 □ 28 package contains only inert ingredients, as listed under green tablets in ORTHO-NOVUM 7/7/7 □ 28.
MODICON 21 Tablets and MODICON 28 Tablets: Each white tablet contains 0.5 mg of norethindrone and 0.035 mg of ethinyl estradiol. Inactive ingredients include lactose, magnesium stearate and pregelatinized starch. Each green tablet in the MODICON 28 package contains only inert ingredients, as listed under green tablets in ORTHO-NOVUM 7/7/7 □ 28.
The chemical name for norethindrone is 17-hydroxy-19-nor-17α-pregn-4-en-20-yn-3-one, for ethinyl estradiol is 19-nor-17α-pregna-1,3,5(10)-trien-20-yne-3, 17-diol. Their structural formulas are as follows:

norethindrone

ethinyl estradiol

CLINICAL PHARMACOLOGY
COMBINATION ORAL CONTRACEPTIVES
Combination oral contraceptives act by suppression of gonadotropins. Although the primary mechanism of this action is inhibition of ovulation, other alterations include changes in the cervical mucus (which increase the difficulty of sperm entry into the uterus) and the endometrium (which reduce the likelihood of implantation).

INDICATIONS AND USAGE
ORTHO-NOVUM 7/7/7 □ 21, ORTHO-NOVUM 7/7/7 □ 28, ORTHO-NOVUM 10/11 □ 21, ORTHO-NOVUM 10/11 □ 28, ORTHO-NOVUM 1/35 □ 21, ORTHO-NOVUM 1/35 □ 28, MODICON 21, and **MODICON 28** are indicated for the prevention of pregnancy in women who elect to use this product as a method of contraception.
Oral contraceptives are highly effective. Table I lists the typical accidental pregnancy rates for users of combination oral contraceptives and other methods of contraception. The efficacy of these contraceptive methods, except sterilization, depends upon the reliability with which they are used. Correct and consistent use of methods can result in lower failure rates.
[See table at top of next page]

CONTRAINDICATIONS
Oral contraceptives should not be used in women who currently have the following conditions:

Continued on next page

Ortho-Novum Tablets—Cont.

- Thrombophlebitis or thromboembolic disorders
- A past history of deep vein thrombophlebitis or thromboembolic disorders
- Cerebral vascular or coronary artery disease
- Known or suspected carcinoma of the breast
- Carcinoma of the endometrium or other known or suspected estrogen-dependent neoplasia
- Undiagnosed abnormal genital bleeding
- Cholestatic jaundice of pregnancy or jaundice with prior pill use
- Hepatic adnenomas or carcinomas
- Known or suspected pregnancy

WARNINGS

Cigarette smoking increase the risk of serious cardiovascular side effects from oral contraceptive use. This risk increases with age and with heavy smoking (15 or more cigarettes per day) and is quite marked in women over 35 years of age. Women who use oral contraceptives should be strongly advised not to smoke.

The use of oral contraceptives is associated with increased risks of several serious conditions including myocardial infarction, thromboembolism, stroke, hepatic neoplasia, and gallbladder disease, although the risk of serious morbidity or mortality is very small in healthy women without underlying risk factors. The risk of morbidity and mortality increases significantly in the presence of other underlying risk factors such as hypertension, hyperlipidemias, obesity and diabetes.

Practitioners prescribing oral contraceptives should be familiar with the following information relating to these risks.

The information contained in this package insert is principally based on studies carried out in patients who used oral contraceptives with higher formulations of estrogens and progestogens than those in common use today. The effect of long-term use of the oral contraceptives with lower formulations of both estrogens and progestogens remains to be determined.

Throughout this labeling, epidemiological studies reported are of two types: retrospective or case control studies and prospective or cohort studies. Case control studies provide a measure of the relative risk of disease, namely, a *ratio* of the incidence of a disease among oral contraceptive users to that among nonusers. The relative risk does not provide information on the actual clinical occurrence of a disease. Cohort studies provide a measure of attributable risk, which is the *difference* in the incidence of disease between oral contraceptive users and nonusers. The attributable risk does provide information about the actual occurrence of a disease in the population (adapted from refs. 2 and 3 with the author's permission). For further information, the reader is referred to a text on epidemiological methods.

1. THROMBOEMBOLIC DISORDERS AND OTHER VASCULAR PROBLEMS

a. Myocardial Infarction

An increased risk of myocardial infarction has been attributed to oral contraceptive use. This risk is primarily in smokers or women with other underlying risk factors for coronary artery disease such as hypertension, hypercholesterolemias, morbid obesity, and diabetes. The relative risk of heart attack for current oral contraceptive users has been estimated to be two to six.[4–10] The risk is very low under the age of 30.

Smoking in combination with oral contraceptive use has been shown to contribute substantially to the incidence of myocardial infarctions in women in their mid-thirties or older with smoking accounting for the majority of excess cases.[11] Mortality rates associated with circulatory disease have been shown to increase substantially in smokers, especially in those 35 years of age and older among women who use oral contraceptives.

TABLE II: CIRCULATORY DISEASE MORTALITY RATES PER 100,000 WOMAN-YEARS BY AGE, SMOKING STATUS AND ORAL CONTRACEPTIVE USE

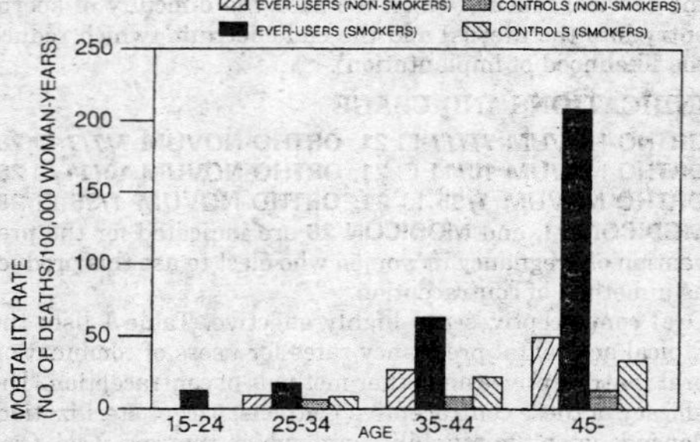

(Adapted from P.M. Layde and V. Beral, ref. #12.)

Oral contraceptives may compound the effects of well-known risk factors, such as hypertension, diabetes, hyperlipidemias, age and obesity.[13] In particular, some progestogens are known to decrease HDL cholesterol and cause glucose intolerance, while estrogens may create a state of hyperinsulinism.[14–18] Oral contraceptives have been shown to increase blood pressure among users (see Section 9 in WARNINGS). Similar effects on risk factors have been associated with an increased risk of heart disease. Oral contraceptives must be used with caution in women with cardiovascular disease risk factors.

b. Thromboembolism

An increased risk of thromboembolic and thrombotic disease associated with the use of oral contraceptives is well established. Case control studies have found the relative risk of users compared to nonusers to be 3 for the first episode of superficial venous thrombosis, 4 to 11 for deep vein thrombosis or pulmonary embolism, and 1.5 to 6 for women with predisposing conditions for venous thromboembolic disease.[2,3,19–24] Cohort studies have shown the relative risk to be somewhat lower, about 3 for new cases and about 4.5 for new cases requiring hospitalization.[25] The risk of thromboembolic disease associated with oral contraceptives is not related to length of use and disappears after pill use is stopped.[2]

A two- to four-fold increase in relative risk of post-operative thromboembolic complications has been reported with the use of oral contraceptives.[9] The relative risk of venous thrombosis in women who have predisposing conditions is twice that of women without such medical conditions.[26] If feasible, oral contraceptives should be discontinued at least four weeks prior to and for two weeks after elective surgery of a type associated with an increase in risk of thromboembolism and during and following prolonged immobilization. Since the immediate postpartum period is also associated with an increased risk of thromboembolism, oral contraceptives should be started no earlier than four weeks after delivery in women who elect not to breast feed or four weeks after a second trimester abortion.

c. Cerebrovascular diseases

Oral contraceptives have been shown to increase both the relative and attributable risks of cerebrovascular events (thrombotic and hemorrhagic strokes), although, in general, the risk is greatest among older (>35 years), hypertensive women who also smoke. Hypertension was found to be a risk factor for both users and nonusers, for both types of strokes, and smoking interacted to increase the risk of stroke.[27–29]

In a large study, the relative risk of thrombotic strokes has been shown to range from 3 for normotensive users to 14 for users with severe hypertension.[30] The relative risk of hemorrhagic stroke is reported to be 1.2 for non-smokers who used oral contraceptives, 2.6 for smokers who did not use oral contraceptives, 7.6 for smokers who used oral contraceptives, 1.8 for normotensive users and 25.7 for users with severe hypertension.[30] The attributable risk is also greater in older women.[3]

d. Dose-related risk of vascular disease from oral contraceptives

A positive association has been observed between the amount of estrogen and progestogen in oral contraceptives and the risk of vascular disease.[31–33] A decline in serum high density lipoproteins (HDL) has been reported with many progestational agents.[14–16] A decline in serum high density lipoproteins has been associated with an increased incidence of ischemic heart disease. Because estrogens increase HDL cholesterol, the net effect of an oral contraceptive depends on a balance achieved between doses of estrogen and progestogen and the activity of the progestogen used in the contraceptives. The activity and amount of both hormones should be considered in the choice of an oral contraceptive.

Minimizing exposure to estrogen and progestogen is in keeping with good principles of therapeutics. For any particular estrogen/progestogen combination, the dosage regimen prescribed should be one which contains the least amount of estrogen and progestogen that is compatible with a low failure rate and the needs of the individual patient. New acceptors of oral contraceptive agents should be started on preparations containing 0.035 mg or less of estrogen.

e. Persistence of risk of vascular disease

There are two studies which have shown persistence of risk of vascular disease for ever-users of oral contraceptives. In a study in the United States, the risk of developing myocardial infarction after discontinuing oral contraceptives persists for at least 9 years for women 40–49 years who had used oral contraceptives for five or more years, but this increased risk was not demonstrated in other age groups.[8] In another study in Great Britain, the risk of developing cerebrovascular disease persisted for at least 6 years after discontinuation of oral contraceptives, although excess risk was very small.[34] However, both studies were performed with oral contraceptive formulations containing 50 micrograms or higher of estrogens.

TABLE I: PERCENTAGE OF WOMEN EXPERIENCING AN UNINTENDED PREGNANCY DURING THE FIRST YEAR OF TYPICAL USE AND THE FIRST YEAR OF PERFECT USE OF CONTRACEPTION AND THE PERCENTAGE CONTINUING USE AT THE END OF THE FIRST YEAR. UNITED STATES.

	% of Women Experiencing an Unintended Pregnancy within the First Year of Use		% of Women Continuing Use at One Year[3]
Method (1)	Typical Use[1] (2)	Perfect Use[2] (3)	(4)
Chance[4]	85	85	
Spermicides[5]	26	6	40
Periodic abstinence	25		63
Calender		9	
Ovulation Method		3	
Sympto-Thermal[6]		2	
Post-Ovulation		1	
Withdrawal	19	4	
Cap[7]			
Parous Women	40	26	42
Nulliparous Women	20	9	56
Sponge			
Parous Women	40	20	42
Nulliparous Women	20	9	56
Diaphragm[7]	20	6	56
Condom[8]			
Female (Reality)	21	5	56
Male	14	3	61
Pill	5		71
Progestin Only		0.5	
Combined		0.1	
IUD			
Progesterone T	2.0	1.5	81
Copper T380A	0.8	0.6	78
LNg 20	0.1	0.1	81
Depo-Provera	0.3	0.3	70
Norplant and Norplant-2	0.05	0.05	88
Female Sterilization	0.5	0.5	100
Male Sterilization	0.15	0.10	100

Adapted from Hatcher et al., 1998 Ref. #1.

[1]Among *typical* couples who initiate use of a method (not necessarily for the first time), the percentage who experience an accidental pregnancy during the first year if they do not stop use for any other reason.

[2]Among couples who initiate use of a method (not necessarily for the first time) and who use it *perfectly* (both consistently and correctly), the percentage who experience an accidental pregnancy during the first year if they do not stop use for any other reason.

[3]Among couples attempting to avoid pregnancy, the percentage who continue to use a method for one year.

[4]The percents becoming pregnant in columns (2) and (3) are based on data from populations where contraception is not used and from women who cease using contraception in order to become pregnant. Among such populations, about 89% become pregnant within one year. This estimate was lowered slightly (to 85%) to represent the percent who would become pregnant within one year among women now relying on reversible methods of contraception if they abandoned contraception altogether.

[5]Foams, creams gels, vaginal suppositories, and vaginal film.

[6]Cervical mucus (ovulation) method supplemented by calendar in the pre-ovulatory and basal body temperature in the post-ovulatory phases.

[7]With spermicidal cream or jelly.

[8]Without spermicides.

2. ESTIMATES OF MORTALITY FROM CONTRACEPTIVE USE

One study gathered data from a variety of sources which have estimated the mortality rate associated with different methods of contraception at different ages (Table III). These estimates include the combined risk of death associated with contraceptive methods plus the risk attributable to pregnancy in the event of method failure. Each method of contraception has its specific benefits and risks. The study concluded that with the exception of oral contraceptive users 35 and older who smoke, and 40 and older who do not smoke, mortality associated with all methods of birth control is low and below that associated with childbirth. The observation of an increase in risk of mortality with age for oral contraceptive users is based on data gathered in the 1970's.[35] Current clinical recommendation involves the use of lower estrogen dose formulations and a careful consideration of risk factors. In 1989, the Fertility and Maternal Health Drugs Advisory Committee was asked to review the use of oral contraceptive in women 40 years of age and over. The committee concluded that although cardiovascular disease risks may be increased with oral contraceptive use after age 40 in healthy non-smoking women (even with the newer low-dose formulations), there are also greater potential health risks associated with pregnancy in older women and with the alternative surgical and medical procedures which may be necessary if such women do not have access to effective and acceptable means of contraception. The Committee recommended that the benefits of low-dose oral contraceptive use by healthy non-smoking women over 40 may outweigh the possible risks.

Of course, older women, as all women who take oral contraceptives, should take an oral contraceptive which contains the least amount of estrogen and progestogen that is compatible with a low failure rate and individual patient needs.

[See table III above]

3. CARCINOMA OF THE REPRODUCTIVE ORGANS AND BREASTS

Numerous epidemiological studies have been performed on the incidence of breast, endometrial, ovarian and cervical cancer in women using oral contraceptives. While there are conflicting reports, most studies suggest that use of oral contraceptives is not associated with an overall increase in the risk of developing breast cancer. Some studies have reported an increased relative risk of developing breast cancer particularly at a younger age. This increased relative risk has been reported to be related to duration of use.[36–44,79–89]

A meta-analysis of 54 studies found a small increase in the frequency of having breast cancer diagnosed for women who were currently using combined oral contraceptives or had used them within the past ten years. This increase in the frequency of breast cancer diagnosis, within ten years of stopping use, was generally accounted for by cancers localized to the breast. There was no increase in the frequency of having breast cancer diagnosed ten or more years after cessation of use.[90]

Some studies suggest that oral contraceptive use has been associated with an increase in the risk of cervical intraepithelial neoplasia in some populations of women.[45–48] However, there continues to be controversy about the extent to which such findings may be due to differences in sexual behavior and other factors.

4. HEPATIC NEOPLASIA

Benign hepatic adenomas are associated with oral contraceptive use, although the incidence of benign tumors is rare in the United States. Indirect calculations have estimated the attributable risk to be in the range of 3.3 cases/100,000 for users, a risk that increases after four or more years of use especially with oral contraceptives of higher dose.[49] Rupture of benign, hepatic adenomas may cause death through intra-abdominal hemorrhage.[50,51]

Studies have shown an increased risk of developing hepatocellular carcinoma[52–54,91] in oral contraceptive users. However, these cancers are rare in the U.S.

5. OCULAR LESIONS

There have been clinical case reports of retinal thrombosis associated with the use of oral contraceptives. Oral contraceptives should be discontinued if there is unexplained partial or complete loss of vision; onset of proptosis or diplopia; papilledema; or retinal vascular lesions. Appropriate diagnostic and therapeutic measures should be undertaken immediately.

6. ORAL CONTRACEPTIVE USE BEFORE OR DURING EARLY PREGNANCY

Extensive epidemiological studies have revealed no increased risk of birth defects in women who have used oral contraceptives prior to pregnancy.[56,57] The majority of recent studies also do not indicate a teratogenic effect, particularly in so far as cardiac anomalies and limb reduction defects are concerned,[55,56,58,59] when taken inadvertently during early pregnancy.

The administration of oral contraceptives to induce withdrawal bleeding should not be used as a test for pregnancy. Oral contraceptives should not be used during pregnancy to treat threatened or habitual abortion.

It is recommended that for any patient who has missed two consecutive periods, pregnancy should be ruled out before continuing oral contraceptive use. If the patient has not adhered to the prescribed schedule, the possibility of pregnancy should be considered at the time of the first missed period. Oral contraceptive use should be discontinued until pregnancy is ruled out.

TABLE III: ANNUAL NUMBER OF BIRTH-RELATED OR METHOD-RELATED DEATHS ASSOCIATED WITH CONTROL OF FERTILITY PER 100,000 NONSTERILE WOMEN, BY FERTILITY CONTROL METHOD ACCORDING TO AGE

Method of control and outcome	15-19	20-24	25-29	30-34	35-39	40-44
No fertility control methods*	7.0	7.4	9.1	14.8	25.7	28.2
Oral contraceptives non-smoker**	0.3	0.5	0.9	1.9	13.8	31.6
Oral contraceptives smoker**	2.2	3.4	6.6	13.5	51.1	117.2
IUD**	0.8	0.8	1.0	1.0	1.4	1.4
Condom*	1.1	1.6	0.7	0.2	0.3	0.4
Diaphragm/ spermicide*	1.9	1.2	1.2	1.3	2.2	2.8
Periodic abstinence*	2.5	1.6	1.6	1.7	2.9	3.6

*Deaths are birth-related
**Deaths are method-related

Adapted from H.W. Ory, ref. #35.

7. GALLBLADDER DISEASE

Earlier studies have reported an increased lifetime relative risk of gallbladder surgery in users of oral contraceptives and estrogens.[60,61] More recent studies, however, have shown that the relative risk of developing gallbladder disease among oral contraceptive users may be minimal.[62–64] The recent findings of minimal risk may be related to the use of oral contraceptive formulations containing lower hormonal doses of estrogens and progestogens.

8. CARBOHYDRATE AND LIPID METABOLIC EFFECTS

Oral contraceptives have been shown to cause a decrease in glucose tolerance in a significant percentage of users.[17] This effect has been shown to be directly related to estrogen dose.[65] Progestogens increase insulin secretion and create insulin resistance, this effect varying with different progestational agents.[17,66] However, in the non-diabetic woman, oral contraceptives appear to have no effect on fasting blood glucose.[67] Because of these demonstrated effects, prediabetic and diabetic women in particular should be carefully monitored while taking oral contraceptives.

A small proportion of women will have persistent hypertriglyceridemia while on the pill. As discussed earlier (see WARNINGS 1a and 1d), changes in serum triglycerides and lipoprotein levels have been reported in oral contraceptive users.

9. ELEVATED BLOOD PRESSURE

An increase in blood pressure has been reported in women taking oral contraceptives[68] and this increase is more likely in older oral contraceptive users[69] and with extended duration of use.[61] Data from the Royal College of General Practitioners[12] and subsequent randomized trials have shown that the incidence of hypertension increases with increasing progestational activity.

Women with a history of hypertension or hypertension-related diseases, or renal disease[70] should be encouraged to use another method of contraception. If women elect to use oral contraceptives, they should be monitored closely and if significant elevation of blood pressure occurs, oral contraceptives should be discontinued. For most women, elevated blood pressure will return to normal after stopping oral contraceptives, and there is no difference in the occurrence of hypertension between former and never users.[68–71]

10. HEADACHE

The onset or exacerbation of migraine or development of headache with a new pattern which is recurrent, persistent or severe requires discontinuation of oral contraceptives and evaluation of the cause.

11. BLEEDING IRREGULARITIES

Breakthrough bleeding and spotting are sometimes encountered in patients on oral contraceptives, especially during the first three months of use. Nonhormonal causes should be considered and adequate diagnostic measures taken to rule out malignancy or pregnancy in the event of breakthrough bleeding, as in the case of any abnormal vaginal bleeding. If pathology has been excluded, time or a change to another formulation may solve the problem. In the event of amenorrhea, pregnancy should be ruled out.

Some women may encounter post-pill amenorrhea or oligomenorrhea, especially when such a condition was preexistent.

12. ECTOPIC PREGNANCY

Ectopic as well as intrauterine pregnancy may occur in contraceptive failures.

PRECAUTIONS

1. PHYSICAL EXAMINATION AND FOLLOW UP

It is good medical practice for all women to have annual history and physical examinations, including women using oral contraceptives. The physical examination, however, may be deferred until after initiation of oral contraceptives if requested by the woman and judged appropriate by the clinician. The physical examination should include special reference to blood pressure, breasts, abdomen and pelvic organs, including cervical cytology, and relevant laboratory tests. In case of undiagnosed, persistent or recurrent abnormal vaginal bleeding, appropriate measures should be conducted to rule out malignancy. Women with a strong family history of breast cancer or who have breast nodules should be monitored with particular care.

2. LIPID DISORDERS

Women who are being treated for hyperlipidemias should be followed closely if they elect to use oral contraceptives. Some progestogens may elevate LDL levels and may render the control of hyperlipidemias more difficult.

3. LIVER FUNCTION

If jaundice develops in any woman receiving such drugs, the medication should be discontinued. Steroid hormones may be poorly metabolized in patients with impaired liver function.

4. FLUID RETENTION

Oral contraceptives may cause some degree of fluid retention. They should be prescribed with caution, and only with careful monitoring, in patients with conditions which might be aggravated by fluid retention.

5. EMOTIONAL DISORDERS

Women with a history of depression should be carefully observed and the drug discontinued if depression recurs to a serious degree.

6. CONTACT LENSES

Contact lens wearers who develop visual changes or changes in lens tolerance should be assessed by an ophthalmologist.

7. DRUG INTERACTIONS

Reduced efficacy and increased incidence of breakthrough bleeding and menstrual irregularities have been associated with concomitant use of rifampin. A similar association, though less marked, has been suggested with barbiturates, phenylbutazone, phenytoin sodium, carbamazepine, and possibly with griseofulvin, ampicillin and tetracyclines.[72]

8. INTERACTIONS WITH LABORATORY TESTS

Certain endocrine and liver function tests and blood components may be affected by oral contraceptives:

a. Increased prothrombin and factors VII, VIII, IX, and X; decreased antithrombin 3; increased norepinephrine-induced platelet aggregability.
b. Increased thyroid binding globulin (TBG) leading to increased circulating total thyroid hormone, as measured by protein-bound iodine (PBI), T4 by column or by radioimmunoassay. Free T3 resin uptake is decreased, reflecting the elevated TBG, free T4 concentration is unaltered.
c. Other binding proteins may be elevated in serum.
d. Sex-binding globulins are increased and result in elevated levels of total circulating sex steroids and corticoids; however, free or biologically active levels remain unchanged.
e. Triglycerides may be increased.
f. Glucose tolerance may be decreased.
g. Serum folate levels may be depressed by oral contraceptive therapy. This may be of clinical significance if a woman becomes pregnant shortly after discontinuing oral contraceptives.

9. CARCINOGENESIS

See WARNINGS Section.

10. PREGNANCY

Pregnancy Category X. See CONTRAINDICATIONS and WARNINGS Sections.

11. NURSING MOTHERS

Small amounts of oral contraceptive steroids have been identified in the milk of nursing mothers and a few adverse effects on the child have been reported, including jaundice and breast enlargement. In addition, combination oral contraceptives given in the postpartum period may interfere with lactation by decreasing the quantity of breast milk. If possible, the nursing mother should be advised not to use combination oral contraceptives but to use other forms of contraception until she has completely weaned her child.

12. PEDIATRIC USE

Safety and efficacy of ORTHO-NOVUM Tablets and MODICON Tablets has been established in women of reproductive age. Safety and efficacy are expected to be the same for post-

Continued on next page

Ortho-Novum Tablets—Cont.

pubertal adolescents under the age of 16 and for users 16 years and older. Use of this product before menarche is not indicated.

13. SEXUALLY TRANSMITTED DISEASES

Patients should be counseled that this product does not protect against HIV infection (AIDS) and other sexually transmitted diseases.

INFORMATION FOR THE PATIENT

See Patient Labeling printed below.

ADVERSE REACTIONS

An increased risk of the following serious adverse reactions has been associated with the use of oral contraceptives (See WARNINGS Section).

- Thrombophlebitis and venous thrombosis with or without embolism.
- Arterial thromboembolism
- Pulmonary embolism
- Myocardial infarction
- Cerebral hemorrhage
- Cerebral thrombosis
- Hypertension
- Gallbladder disease
- Hepatic adenomas or benign liver tumors

The following adverse reactions have been reported in patients receiving oral contraceptives and are believed to be drug-related:

- Nausea
- Vomiting
- Gastrointestinal symptoms (such as abdominal cramps and bloating)
- Breakthrough bleeding
- Spotting
- Change in menstrual flow
- Amenorrhea
- Temporary infertility after discontinuation of treatment
- Edema
- Melasma which may persist
- Breast changes: tenderness, enlargement, secretion
- Change in weight (increase or decrease)
- Change in cervical erosion and secretion
- Diminution in lactation when given immediately postpartum
- Cholestatic jaundice
- Migraine
- Rash (allergic)
- Mental depression
- Reduced tolerance to carbohydrates
- Vaginal candidiasis
- Change in corneal curvature (steepening)
- Intolerance to contact lenses

The following adverse reactions have been reported in users of oral contraceptives and the association has been neither confirmed nor refuted:

- Pre-menstrual syndrome
- Cataracts
- Changes in appetite
- Cystitis-like syndrome
- Headache
- Nervousness
- Dizziness
- Hirsutism
- Loss of scalp hair
- Erythema multiforme
- Erythema nodosum
- Hemorrhagic eruption
- Vaginitis
- Porphyria
- Impaired renal function
- Hemolytic uremic syndrome
- Acne
- Changes in libido
- Colitis
- Budd-Chiari Syndrome

OVERDOSAGE

Serious ill effects have not been reported following acute ingestion of large doses of oral contraceptives by young children. Overdosage may cause nausea, and withdrawal bleeding may occur in females.

NON-CONTRACEPTIVE HEALTH BENEFITS

The following non-contraceptive health benefits related to the use of combination oral contraceptives are supported by epidemiological studies which largely utilized oral contraceptive formulations containing estrogen doses exceeding 0.035 mg of ethinyl estradiol or 0.05 mg mestranol.[73–78]

Effect on menses:

- increased menstrual cycle regularity
- decreased blood loss and decreased incidence of iron deficiency anemia
- decreased incidence of dysmenorrhea

Effects related to inhibition of ovulation:

- decreased incidence of functional ovarian cysts
- decreased incidence of ectopic pregnancies

Other effects:

- decreased incidence of fibroadenomas and fibrocystic disease of the breast
- decreased incidence of acute pelvic inflammatory disease
- decreased incidence of endometrial cancer
- decreased incidence of ovarian cancer

DOSAGE AND ADMINISTRATION

To achieve maximum contraceptive effectiveness, ORTHO-NOVUM Tablets and MODICON Tablets must be taken exactly as directed and in intervals not exceeding 24 hours. ORTHO-NOVUM Tablets and MODICON Tablets are available in the DIALPAK® Tablet Dispenser which is preset for a Sunday Start. Day 1 Start is also available.

21-Day Regimen (Sunday Start)

When taking ORTHO-NOVUM 7/7/7 □ 21, ORTHO-NOVUM 10/11 □ 21, ORTHO-NOVUM 1/35 □ 21, and MODICON 21, the first tablet should be taken on the first Sunday after menstruation begins. If period begins on Sunday, the first tablet is taken on that day. One tablet is taken daily for 21 days. For subsequent cycles, no tablets are taken for 7 days, then a tablet is taken the next day (Sunday). For the first cycle of a Sunday Start regimen, another method of contraception should be used until after the first 7 consecutive days of administration.

If the patient misses one (1) active tablet in Weeks 1, 2, or 3, the tablet should be taken as soon as she remembers. If the patient misses two (2) active tablets in Week 1 or Week 2, the patient should take two (2) tablets the day she remembers and two (2) tablets the next day; and then continue taking one (1) tablet a day until she finishes the pack. The patient should be instructed to use a back-up method of birth control if she has sex in the seven (7) days after missing pills. If the patient misses two (2) active tablets in the third week or misses three (3) or more active tablets in a row, the patient should continue taking one tablet every day until Sunday. On Sunday the patient should throw out the rest of the pack and start a new pack that same day. The patient should be instructed to use a back-up method of birth control if she has sex in the seven (7) days after missing pills.

Complete instructions to facilitate patient counseling on proper pill usage may be found in the Detailed Patient Labeling ("How to Take the Pill" section).

21-Day Regimen (Day 1 Start)

The dosage of ORTHO-NOVUM 7/7/7 □ 21, ORTHO-NOVUM 10/11 □ 21, ORTHO-NOVUM 1/35 □ 21, and MODICON 21, for the initial cycle of therapy is one tablet administered daily from the 1st day through the 21st day of the menstrual cycle, counting the first day of menstrual flow as "Day 1." For subsequent cycles, no tablets are taken for 7 days, then a new course is started of one tablet a day for 21 days. The dosage regimen then continues with 7 days of no medication, followed by 21 days of medication, instituting a three-weeks-on, one-week-off dosage regimen.

If the patient misses one (1) active tablet in Weeks 1, 2, or 3, the tablet should be taken as soon as she remembers. If the patient misses two (2) active tablets in Week 1 or Week 2, the patient should take two (2) tablets the day she remembers and two (2) tablets the next day; and then continue taking one (1) tablet a day until she finishes the pack. The patient should be instructed to use a back-up method of birth control if she has sex in the seven (7) days after missing pills. If the patient misses two (2) active tablets in the third week or misses three (3) or more active tablets in a row, the patient should throw out the rest of the pack and start a new pack that same day. The patient should be instructed to use a back-up method of birth control if she has sex in the seven (7) days after missing pills.

Complete instructions to facilitate patient counseling on proper pill usage may be found in the Detailed Patient Labeling ("How to Take the Pill" section).

28-Day Regimen (Sunday Start)

When taking ORTHO-NOVUM 7/7/7 □ 28, ORTHO-NOVUM 10/11 □ 28, ORTHO-NOVUM 1/35 □ 28, and MODICON 28, the first tablet should be taken on the first Sunday after menstruation begins. If period begins on Sunday, the first tablet should be taken that day. Take one active tablet daily for 21 days followed by one green placebo tablet daily for 7 days. After 28 tablets have been taken, a new course is started the next day (Sunday). For the first cycle of a Sunday Start regimen, another method of contraception should be used until after the first 7 consecutive days of administration.

If the patient misses one (1) active tablet in Weeks 1, 2, or 3, the tablet should be taken as soon as she remembers. If the patient misses two (2) active tablets in Week 1 or Week 2, the patient should take two (2) tablets the day she remembers and two (2) tablets the next day; and then continue taking one (1) tablet a day until she finishes the pack. The patient should be instructed to use a back-up method of birth control if she has sex in the seven (7) days after missing pills. If the patient misses two (2) active tablets in the third week or misses three (3) or more active tablets in a row, the patient should continue taking one tablet every day until Sunday. On Sunday the patient should throw out the rest of the pack and start a new pack that same day. The patient should be instructed to use a back-up method of birth control if she has sex in the seven (7) days after missing pills.

Complete instructions to facilitate patient counseling on proper pill usage may be found in the Detailed Patient Labeling ("How to Take the Pill" section).

28-Day Regimen (Day 1 Start)

The dosage of ORTHO-NOVUM 7/7/7 □ 28, ORTHO-NOVUM 10/11 □ 28, ORTHO-NOVUM 1/35 □ 28, and MODICON 28, for the first initial cycle of therapy is one active tablet administered daily from the 1st through the 21st day of the menstrual cycle, counting the first day of menstrual flow as "Day 1" followed by one green tablet daily for 7 days. Tablets are taken without interruption for 28 days. After 28 tablets have been taken, a new course is started the next day.

If the patient misses one (1) active tablet in Weeks 1, 2, or 3, the tablet should be taken as soon as she remembers. If the patient misses two (2) active tablets in Week 1 or Week 2, the patient should take two (2) tablets the day she remembers and two (2) tablets the next day; and then continue taking one (1) tablet a day until she finishes the pack. The patient should be instructed to use a back-up method of birth control if she has sex in the seven (7) days after missing pills. If the patient misses two (2) active tablets in the third week or misses three (3) or more active tablets in a row, the patient should throw out the rest of the pack and start a new pack that same day. The patient should be instructed to use a back-up method of birth control if she has sex in the seven (7) days after missing pills.

Complete instructions to facilitate patient counseling on proper pill usage may be found in the Detailed Patient Labeling ("How to Take the Pill" section).

The use of ORTHO-NOVUM 7/7/7, ORTHO-NOVUM 10/11, ORTHO-NOVUM 1/35, and MODICON for contraception may be initiated 4 weeks postpartum in women who elect not to breast feed. When the tablets are administered during the postpartum period, the increased risk of thromboembolic disease associated with the postpartum period must be considered. (See CONTRAINDICATIONS and WARNINGS concerning thromboembolic disease. See also PRECAUTIONS for "Nursing Mothers.") The possibility of ovulation and conception prior to initiation of medication should be considered.

(See Discussion of Dose-Related Risk of Vascular Disease from Oral Contraceptives.)

ADDITIONAL INSTRUCTIONS FOR ALL DOSING REGIMENS

Breakthrough bleeding, spotting, and amenorrhea are frequent reasons for patients discontinuing oral contraceptives. In breakthrough bleeding, as in all cases of irregular bleeding from the vagina, nonfunctional causes should be borne in mind. In undiagnosed persistent or recurrent abnormal bleeding from the vagina, adequate diagnostic measures are indicated to rule out pregnancy or malignancy. If pathology has been excluded, time or a change to another formulation may solve the problem. Changing to an oral contraceptive with a higher estrogen content, while potentially useful in minimizing menstrual irregularity, should be done only if necessary since this may increase the risk of thromboembolic disease.

Use of oral contraceptives in the event of a missed menstrual period:

1. If the patient has not adhered to the prescribed schedule, the possibility of pregnancy should be cosidered at the time of the first missed period and oral contraceptive use should be discontinued until pregnancy is ruled out.
2. If the patient has adhered to the prescribed regimen and misses two consecutive periods, pregnancy should be ruled out before continuing oral contraceptive use.

HOW SUPPLIED

ORTHO-NOVUM 7/7/7 □ 21 Tablets are available in a DIALPAK® Tablet Dispenser (NDC 0062-1780-15) containing 21 tablets, as follows: 7 white tablets (0.5 mg norethindrone and 0.035 mg ethinyl estradiol), 7 light peach tablets (0.75 mg norethindrone and 0.035 mg ethinyl estradiol) and 7 peach tablets (1 mg norethindrone and 0.035 mg ethinyl estradiol). The white tablets are unscored with "Ortho" and "535" debossed on each side; the light peach tablets are unscored with "Ortho" and "75" debossed on each side; the peach tablets are unscored with "Ortho" and "135" debossed on each side.

ORTHO-NOVUM 7/7/7 □ 21 is available for clinic usage in a VERIDATE® Tablet Dispenser (unfilled) and VERIDATE Refills (NDC 0062-1780-20).

ORTHO-NOVUM 7/7/7 □ 28 Tablets are available in a DIALPAK Tablet Dispenser (NDC 0062-1781-15) containing 28 tablets, as follows: 7 white, 7 light peach and 7 peach tablets as described under ORTHO-NOVUM 7/7/7 □ 21, and 7 green tablets containing inert ingredients.

ORTHO-NOVUM 7/7/7 □ 28 is available for clinic usage in a VERIDATE Tablet Dispenser (unfilled) and VERIDATE Refills (NDC 0062-1781-20).

ORTHO-NOVUM 10/11 □ 21 Tablets are available in a DIALPAK Tablet Dispenser (NDC 0062-1770-15) containing 21 tablets, as follows: 10 white tablets (0.5 mg norethindrone and 0.035 mg ethinyl estradiol) and 11 peach tablets (1 mg norethindrone and 0.035 mg ethinyl estradiol). The white tablets are unscored with "Ortho" and "535" debossed on each side; the peach tablets are unscored with "Ortho" and "135" debossed on each side.

ORTHO-NOVUM 10/11 □ 28 Tablets are available in a DIALPAK Tablet Dispenser (NDC 0062-1771-15) containing 28 tablets, as follows: 10 white and 11 peach tablets as described under ORTHO-NOVUM 10/11 □ 21, and 7 green tablets containing inert ingredients.

ORTHO-NOVUM 10/11 □ 28 is avalable for clinic usage in a VERIDATE Tablet Dispenser (unfilled) and VERIDATE Refills (NDC 0062-1771-20)

ORTHO-NOVUM 1/35 □ 21 Tablets are available in a DIALPAK Tablet Dispenser (NDC 0062-1760-15) containing 21 peach tablets (1 mg norethindrone and 0.035 mg ethinyl estradiol) which are unscored with "Ortho" and "135" debossed on each side.

ORTHO-NOVUM 1/35 □ 21 is available for clinic usage in a VERIDATE Tablet Dispenser (unfilled) and VERIDATE Refills (NDC 0062-1760-20).

ORTHO-NOVUM 1/35 □ 28 Tablets are available in a DIALPAK Tablet Dispenser (NDC 0062-1761-15) containing 28 tablets, as follows: 21 peach tablets as described under ORTHO-NOVUM 1/35 ☐ 21, and 7 green tablets containing inert ingredients.

ORTHO-NOVUM 1/35 ☐ 28 is available for clinic usage in a VERIDATE Tablet Dispenser (unfilled) and VERIDATE Refills (NDC 0062-1761-20).

MODICON 21 Tablets are available in a DIALPAK Tablet Dispenser (NDC 0062-1712-15) containing 21 white tablets (0.5 mg norethindrone and 0.035 mg ethinyl estradiol) which are unscored with "Ortho" and "535" debossed on each side.

MODICON 28 Tablets are available in a DIALPAK Tablet Dispenser (NDC 0062-1714-15) containing 28 tablets, as follows: 21 white tablets as described under MODICON 21, and 7 green tablets containing inert ingredients.

MODICON 28 is available for clinic usage in a VERIDATE Tablet Dispenser (unfilled) and VERIDATE Refills (NDC 0062-1714-20).

Rx only

REFERENCES

1. Trussel J. Contraceptive efficacy. In Hatcher RA, Trussel J, Stewart F, Cates W, Stewart GK, Kowal D, Guest F, Contraceptive Technology: Seventeenth Revised Edition. New York NY: Irvington Publishers, 1998, in press **2.** Stadel BV, Oral contraceptives and cardiovascular disease. (Pt. 1). N Engl J Med 1981; 305:612–618. **3.** Stadel BV, Oral contraceptives and cardiovascular disease. (Pt. 2). N Engl J Med 1981; 305:672–677. **4.** Adam SA, Thorogood M. Oral contraception and myocardial infarction revisited: the effects of new preparations and prescribing patterns. Br J Obstet Gynaecol 1981; 88:838–845. **5.** Mann JI, Inman WH. Oral contraceptives and death from myocardial infarction. Br Med J 1975; 2(5965):245–248. **6.** Mann JI, Vessey MP, Thorogood M, Doll R. Myocardial infarction in young women with special reference to oral contraceptive practice. Br Med J 1975; 2(5956):241–245. **7.** Royal College of General Practitioners' Oral Contraception Study: further analyses of mortality in oral contraceptive users. Lancet 1981; 1:541–546. **8.** Slone D, Shapiro S, Kaufman DW, Rosenberg L, Miettinen OS, Stolley PD. Risk of myocardial infarction in relation to current and discontinued use of oral contraceptives. N Engl J Med 1981; 305:420–424. **9.** Vessey MP. Female hormones and vascular disease—an epidemiological overview. Br J Fam Plann 1980; 6 (Supplement): 1–12. **10.** Russel-Briefel RG, Ezzati TM, Fulwood R, Perlman JA, Murphy RS. Cardiovascular risk satus and oral contraceptive use, United States, 1976–80. Prevent Med 1986; 15:352–362. **11.** Goldbaum GM, Kendrick JS, Hogelin GC, Gentry EM. The relative impact of smoking and oral contraceptive use on women in the United States. JAMA 1987; 258:1339–1342. **12.** Layde PM, Beral V. Further analyses of mortality in oral contraceptive users; Royal College of General Practitioners' Oral Contraception Study. (Table 5) Lancet 1981; 1:541–546. **13.** Knopp RH. Arteriosclerosis risk: the roles of oral contraceptives and postmenopausal estrogens. J Reprod Med 1986; 31(9) (Supplement): 913–921. **14.** Krauss RM, Roy S, Mishell DR, Casagrande J, Pike MC. Effects of two low-dose oral contraceptives on serum lipids and lipoproteins: Differential changes in high-density lipoproteins subclasses. Am J Obstet 1983; 145:446–452. **15.** Wahl P, Walden C, Knopp R, Hoover J, Wallace R, Heiss G, Rifkind B. Effect of estrogen/progestin potency on lipid/lipoprotein cholesterol. N Engl J Med 1983; 308:862–867. **16.** Wynn V. Niththyananthan R. The effect of progestin in combined oral contraceptives on serum lipids with special reference to high density lipoproteins. Am J Obstet Gynecol 1982; 142:766–771. **17.** Wynn V, Godsland I. Effects of oral contraceptives on carbohydrate metabolism. J Reprod Med 1986; 31(9)(Supplement):892–897. **18.** LaRosa JC. Atherosclerotic risk factors in cardiovascular disease. J Reprod Med 1986; 31(9)(Supplement): 906–912. **19.** Inman WH, Vessey MP. Investigation of death from pulmonary, coronary, and cerebral thrombosis and embolism in women of child-bearing age. Br Med J 1968; 2(5599):193–199. **20.** Maguire MG, Tonascia J, Sartwell PE, Stolley PD, Tockman MS. Increased risk of thrombosis due to oral contraceptives: a further report. Am J Epidemiol 1979; 110(2):188–195. **21.** Petitti DB, Wingerd J, Pellegrin F, Ramacharan S. Risk of vascular disease in women: smoking, oral contraceptives, noncontraceptive estrogens, and other factors, JAMA 1979; 242:1150–1154. **22.** Vessey MP, Doll R. Investigation of relation between use of oral contraceptives and thromboembolic disease. Br Med J 1968; 2(5599):199–205. **23.** Vessey MP, Doll R. Investigation of relation between use of oral contraceptives and thromboembolic disease. A further report. Br Med J 1969; 2(5658):651–657. **24.** Porter JB, Hunter JR, Danielson DA, Jick H, Stergachis A. Oral contraceptives and non-fatal vascular disease—recent experience. Obstet Gynecol 1982; 59(3): 299–302. **25.** Vessey M, Doll R, Peto R, Johnson B, Wiggins P. A long-term follow-up study of women using different methods of contraception: an interim report. J Biosocial Sci 1976; 8:375–427. **26.** Royal College of General Practitioners: Oral Contraceptives, venous thrombosis, and varicose veins. J Royal Coll Gen Pract 1978; 28:393–399. **27.** Collaborative Group for the Study of Stroke in Young Women: Oral contraception and increased risk of cerebral ischemia or thrombosis. N Engl J Med 1973; 288:871–878. **28.** Petitti DB, Wingerd J. Use of oral contraceptives, cigarette smoking, and risk of subarachnoid hemorrhage. Lancet 1978; 2:234–236. **29.** Inman WH. Oral contraceptives and fatal subarachnoid hemorrhage. Br Med J 1979; 2(6203):1468–1470. **30.** Collaborative Group for the Study of Stroke in Young Women: Oral Contraceptives and stroke in young women: associated risk factors. JAMA 1975; 231:718–722. **31.** Inman WH, Vessey MP, Westerholm B, Engelund A. Thromboembolic disease and the steroidal content of oral contraceptives. A report to the Committee on Safety of Drugs. Br Med J 1970; 2:203–209. **32.** Meade TW, Greenberg G, Thompson SG. Progestogens and cardiovascular reactions associated with oral contraceptives and a comparison of the safety of 50- and 35-mcg oestrogen preparations. Br Med J 1980; 280(6224):1157–1161. **33.** Kay CR. Progestogens and arterial disease—evidence from the Royal College of General Practitioners' Study. Am J Obstet Gynecol 1982; 142:762–765. **34.** Royal College of General Practitioners: Incidence of arterial disease among oral contraceptive users. J Royal Coll Gen Pract 1983; 33:75–82. **35.** Ory HW. Mortality associated with fertility and fertility control: 1983. Family Planning Perspectives 1983; 15:50–56. **36.** The Cancer and Steroid Hormone Study of the Centers for Disease Control and the National Institute of Child Health and Human Development: Oral contraceptive use and the risk of breast cancer. N Engl J Med 1986; 315:405–411. **37.** Pike MC, Henderson BE, Krailo MD, Duke A, Roy S. Breast cancer in young women and use of oral contraceptives: possible modifying effect of formulation and age at use. Lancet 1983; 2:926–929. **38.** Paul C, Skegg DG, Spears GFS, Kaldor JM. Oral contraceptives and breast cancer: A national study. Br Med J 1986; 293:723–725. **39.** Miller DR, Rosenberg L, Kaufman DW, Shottenfeld D, Stolley PD, Shapiro S. Breast cancer risk in relation to early oral contraceptive use. Obstet Gynecol 1986; 68:863–868. **40.** Olson H, Olson KL, Moller TR, Ranstam J, Holm P. Oral contraceptive use and breast cancer in young women in Sweden (letter). Lancet 1985; 2:748–749. **41.** McPherson K, Vessey M, Neil A, Doll R, Jones L, Roberts M. Early contraceptive use and breast cancer: Results of another case-control study. Br J Cancer 1987; 56: 653–660. **42.** Huggins GR, Zucker PF. Oral contraceptives and neoplasia: 1987 update. Fertil Steril 1987; 47:733–761. **43.** McPherson K, Drife JO. The pill and breast cancer: why the uncertainty? Br J Med 1986; 293:709–710. **44.** Shapiro S. Oral contraceptives—time to take stock. N Engl J Med 1987; 315:450–451. **45.** Ory H, Naib Z, Conger SB, Hatcher RA, Tyler CW. Contraceptive choice and prevalence of cervical dysplasia and carcinoma in situ. Am J Obstet Gynecol 1976; 124:573–577. **46.** Vessey MP, Lawless M, McPherson K, Yeates D. Neoplasia of the cervix uteri and contraception: a possible adverse effect of the pill. Lancet 1983; 2:930. **47.** Brinton LA, Huggins GR, Lehman HF, Malli K, Savitz DA, Trapido E, Rosenthal J, Hoover R. Long term use of oral contraceptives and risk of invasive cervical cancer. Int J Cancer 1986; 38:339–344. **48.** WHO Collaborative Study of Neoplasia and Steroid Contraceptives: Invasive cervical cancer and combined oral contraceptives. Br Med J 1985; 290:961–965. **49.** Rooks JB, Ory HW, Ishak KG, Strauss LT, Greenspan JR, Hill AP, Tyler CW. Epidemiology of hepatocellular adenoma: the role of oral contraceptive use. JAMA 1979; 242:644–648. **50.** Bein NN, Goldsmith HS. Recurrent massive hemorrhage from benign hepatic tumors secondary to oral contraceptives. Br J Surg 1977; 64:433–435. **51.** Klatskin G. Hepatic tumors: possible relationship to use of oral contraceptives. Gastroenterology 1977; 73:386–394. **52.** Henderson BE, Preston-Martin S, Edmondson HA, Peters RL, Pike MC. Hepatocellular carcinoma and oral contraceptives. Br J Cancer 1983; 48:437–440. **53.** Neuberger J, Forman D, Doll R, Williams R. Oral contraceptives and hepatocellular carcinoma. Br Med J 1986; 292:1355–1357. **54.** Forman D, Vincent TJ, Doll R. Cancer of the liver and oral contraceptives. Br Med J 1986; 292:1357–1361. **55.** Harlap S, Eldor J. Births following oral contraceptive failures. Obstet Gynecol 1980; 55:447–452. **56.** Savolainen E, Saksela E, Saxen L. Teratogenic hazards of oral contraceptives analyzed in a national malformation register. Am J Obstet Gynecol 1981; 140:521–524. **57.** Janerick DT, Piper JM, Glebatis DM. Oral contraceptives and birth defects. Am J Epidemiol 1980; 112:73–79. **58.** Ferencz C, Matanoski GM, Wilson PD, Rubin JD, Neill CA, Gutberlet R. Maternal hormone therapy and congenital heart disease. Teratology 1980; 21: 225–239. **59.** Rothman KJ, Fyler DC, Goldblatt A, Kreidberg MB. Exogenous hormones and other drug exposures of children with congenital heart disease. Am J Epidemiol 1979; 109:433–439. **60.** Boston Collaborative Drug Surveillance Program: Oral contraceptives and venous thromboembolic disease, surgicaly confirmed gallbladder disease, and breast tumors. Lancet 1973; 1:1399–1404. **61.** Royal College of General Practitioners: Oral contraceptives and health. New York, Pittman 1974. **62.** Layde PM, Vessey MP, Yeates D. Risk of gallbladder disease: a cohort study of young women attending family planning clinics. J Epidemiol Community Health 1982; 36:274–278. **63.** Rome Group for Epidemiology and Prevention of Cholelithiasis (GREPCO): Prevalence of gallstone disease in an Italian adult female population. Am J Epidemiol 1984; 119:796–805. **64.** Storm BL, Tamragouri RT, Morse ML, Lazar EL, West SL, Stolley PD, Jones JK. Oral contraceptives and other risk factors for gallbladder disease. Clin Pharmacol Ther 1986; 39:335–341. **65.** Wynn V, Adams PW, Godsland IF, Melrose J. Niththyananthan R, Oakley NW, Seedj A. Comparison of effects of different combined oral contraceptive formulations on carbohydrate and lipid metabolism. Lancet 1979; 1:1045–1049. **66.** Wynn V. Effect of progesterone and progestins on carbohydrate metabolism. In: Progesterone and Progestin. Bardin CW, Milgrom E, Mauvis-Jarvis P. eds. New York, Raven Press, 1983; pp. 395–410. **67.** Perlman JA, Roussell-Briefel RG, Ezzati TM, Lieberknecht G. Oral glucose tolerance and the potency of oral contraceptive progestogens. J Chronic Dis 1985; 38: 857–864. **68.** Royal College of General Practitioners' Oral Contraception Study: Effect on hypertension and benign breast disease of progestogen component in combined oral contraceptives. Lancet 1977; 1:624. **69.** Fisch IR, Frank J. Oral contraceptives and blood pressure. JAMA 1977; 237: 2499–2503. **70.** Laragh AJ. Oral contraceptive induced hypertension—nine years later. Am J Obstet Gynecol 1976; 126:141–147. **71.** Ramcharan S, Peritz E, Pellegrin FA, Williams WT. Incidence of hypertension in the Walnut Creek Contraceptive Drug Study cohort: In: Pharmacology of steroid contraceptive drugs. Garattini S, Berendes HW. Eds. New York, Raven Press, 1977; pp. 277–288, (Monographs of the Mario Negri Institute for Pharmacological Research Milan.) **72.** Stockley I. Interactions with oral contraceptives. J Pharm 1976; 216:140–143. **73.** The Cancer and Steroid Hormone Study of the Centers for Disease Control and the National Institute of Child Health and Human Development: Oral contraceptive use and the risk of ovarian cancer. JAMA 1983; 249:1596–1599. **74.** The Cancer and Steroid Hormone Study of the Centers for Disease Control and the National Institute of Child Health and Human Development: Combination oral contraceptive use and the risk of endometrial cancer. JAMA 1987; 257:796–800. **75.** Ory HW. Functional ovarian cysts and oral contraceptives: negative association confirmed surgically. JAMA 1974; 228:68–69. **76.** Ory HW, Cole P, MacMahon B, Hoover R. Oral contraceptives and reduced risk of benign breast disease. N Engl J Med 1976; 294:419–422. **77.** Ory HW. The noncontraceptive health benefits from oral contraceptive use. Fam Plann Perspect 1982; 14:182–184. **78.** Ory HW, Forrest JD, Lincoln R. Making choices: Evaluating the health risks and benefits of birth control methods. New York, The Alan Guttmacher Institute, 1983; p. 1. **79.** Schlesselman J, Stadel BV, Murray P, Lai S. Breast cancer in relation to early use of oral contraceptives. JAMA 1988; 259:1828–1833. **80.** Hennekens CH, Speizer FE, Lipnick RJ, Rosner B, Bain C, Belanger C, Stampfer MJ, Willett W, Peto R. A case-control study of oral contraceptive use and breast cancer. JNCI 1984; 72:39–42. **81.** LaVecchia C, Decarli A, Fasoli M, Franceschi S, Gentile A, Negri E, Parazzini F, Tognoni G. Oral contraceptives and cancers of the breast and of the female genital tract. Interim results from a case-control study. Br J Cancer 1986; 54:311–317. **82.** Meirik O, Lund E, Adami H, Bergstrom R, Christoffersen T, Bergsjo P. Oral contraceptive use and breast cancer in young women. A Joint National Case-control study in Sweden and Norway. Lancet 1986; 11:650–654. **83.** Kay CR, Hannaford PC. Breast cancer and the pill—A further report from the Royal College of General Practitioners' oral contraception study. Br J Cancer 1988; 58:675–680. **84.** Stadel BV, Lai S, Schlesselman JJ, Murray P. Oral contraceptives and premenopausal breast cancer in nulliparous women. Contraception 1988; 38:287–299. **85.** Miller DR, Rosenberg L, Kaufman DW, Stolley P, Warshauer ME, Shapiro S. Breast cancer before age 45 and oral contraceptive use: New Findings. Am J Epidemiol 1989; 129:269–280. **86.** The UK National Case-Control Study Group, Oral contraceptive use and breast cancer risk in young women. Lancet 1989; 1:973–982. **87.** Schlesselman JJ. Cancer of the breast and reproductive tract in relation to use of oral contraceptives. Contraception 1989; 40:1–38. **88.** Vessey MP, McPherson K, Villard-Mackintosh L, Yeates D. Oral contraceptives and breast cancer: latest findings in large cohort study. Br J Cancer 1989; 59:613–617. **89.** Jick SS, Walker AM, Stergachis A, Jick H. Oral contraceptives and breast cancer. Br J Cancer 1989; 59:618–621. **90.** Collaborative Group on Hormonal Factors in Breast Cancer. Breast cancer and hormonal contraceptives: collaborative reanalysis of individual data on 53 297 women with breast cancer and 100 239 women without breast cancer from 54 epidemiological studies. Lancet 1996; 347:1713–1727. **91.** Palmer JR, Rosenberg L, Kaufman DW, Warshauer ME, Stolley P, Shapiro S. Oral Contraceptive Use and Liver Cancer. Am J Epidemiol 1989; 130:878–882.

BRIEF SUMMARY PATIENT PACKAGE INSERT

Oral contraceptives, also known as "birth control pills" or "the pill," are taken to prevent pregnancy and when taken correctly, have a failure rate of less than 1% per year when used without missing any pills. The typical failure rate of large numbers of pill users is less than 3% per year when women who miss pills are included. For most women oral contraceptives are also free of serious or unpleasant side effects. However, forgetting to take pills considerably increases the chances of pregnancy.

For the majority of women, oral contraceptives can be taken safely. But there are some women who are at high risk of developing certain serious diseases that can be fatal or may cause temporary or permanent disability. The risks associated with taking oral contraceptives increase significantly if you:

- smoke
- have high blood pressure, diabetes, high cholesterol
- have or have had clotting disorders, heart attack, stroke, angina pectoris, cancer of the breast or sex organs, jaundice or malignant or benign liver tumors.

Although cardiovascular disease risks may be increased with oral contraceptive use after age 40 in healthy, nonsmoking women (even with the newer low-dose formulations), there are also greater potential health risks associated with pregnancy in older women.

You should not take the pill if you suspect you are pregnant or have unexplained vaginal bleeding.

Continued on next page

Ortho-Novum Tablets—Cont.

Cigarette smoking increases the risk of serious cardiovascular side effects from oral contraceptive use. This risk increases with age and with heavy smoking (15 or more cigarettes per day) and is quite marked in women over 35 years of age. Women who use oral contraceptives are strongly advised not to smoke.

Most side effects of the pill are not serious. The most common such effects are nausea, vomiting, bleeding between menstrual periods, weight gain, breast tenderness, and difficulty wearing contact lenses. These side effects, especially nausea and vomiting, may subside within the first three months of use.

The serious side effects of the pill occur very infrequently, especially if you are in good health and are young. However, you should know that the follwing medical conditions have been associated with or made worse by the pill:

1. Blood clots in the legs (thrombophlebitis), lungs (pulmonary embolism), stoppage or rupture of a blood vessel in the brain (stroke), blockage of blood vessels in the heart (heart attack or angina pectoris) or other organs of the body. As mentioned above, smoking increases the risk of heart attacks and strokes and subsequent serious medical consequences.

2. In rare cases, oral contraceptives can cause benign but dangerous liver tumors. These benign liver tumors can rupture and cause fatal internal bleeding. In addition, some studies report an increased risk of developing liver cancer. However, liver cancers are rare.

3. High blood pressure, although blood pressure usually returns to normal when the pill is stopped.

The symptoms associated with these serious side effects are discussed in the detailed leaflet given to you with your supply of pills. Notify your doctor or health care provider if you notice any unusual physical disturbances while taking the pill. In addition, drugs such as rifampin, as well as some anticonvulsants and some antibiotics may decrease oral contraceptive effectiveness.

There is conflict among studies regarding breast cancer and oral contraceptive use. Some studies have reported an increase in the risk of developing breast cancer, particularly at a younger age. This increased risk appears to be related to duration of use. The majority of studies have found no overall increase in the risk of developing breast cancer. Some studies have found an increase in the incidence of cancer of the cervix in women who use oral contraceptives. However, this finding may be related to factors other than the use of oral contraceptives. There is insufficient evidence to rule out the possibility that pills may cause such cancers.

Taking the combination pill provides some important noncontraceptive benefits. These include less painful menstruation, less menstrual blood loss and anemia, fewer pelvic infections, and fewer cancers of the ovary and the lining of the uterus.

Be sure to discuss any medical condition you may have with your health care provider. Your health care provider will take a medical and family history before prescribing oral contraceptives and will examine you. The physical examination may be delayed to another time if you request it and the health care provider believes that it is a good medical practice to postpone it. You should be reexamined at least once a year while taking oral contraceptives. Your pharmacist should have given you the detailed patient information labeling which gives you further information which you should read and discuss with your health care provider.

This product (like all oral contraceptives) is intended to prevent pregnancy. It does not protect against transmission of HIV (AIDS) and other sexually transmitted diseases such as chlamydia, genital herpes, genital warts, gonorrhea, hepatitis B, and syphilis.

DETAILED PATIENT LABELING

PLEASE NOTE: This labeling is revised from time to time as important new medical information becomes available. Therefore, please review this labeling carefully.

The following oral contraceptive products contain a combination of an estrogen and progestogen, the two kinds of female hormones:

ORTHO-NOVUM 7/7/7 □ 21 Day Regimen and ORTHO-NOVUM 7/7/7 □ 28 Day Regimen

Each white tablet contains 0.5 mg norethindrone and 0.035 mg ethinyl estradiol. Each light peach tablet contains 0.75 mg norethindrone and 0.035 mg ethinyl estradiol. Each peach tablet contains 1 mg norethindrone and 0.035 mg ethinyl estradiol. Each green tablet in ORTHO-NOVUM 7/7/7 □ 28 Day Regimen contains inert ingredients.

ORTHO-NOVUM 10/11 □ 21 Day Regimen and ORTHO-NOVUM 10/11 □ 28 Day Regimen

Each white tablet contains 0.5 mg norethindrone and 0.035 mg ethinyl estradiol. Each peach tablet contains 1 mg norethindrone and 0.035 mg ethinyl estradiol. Each green tablet in ORTHO-NOVUM 10/11 □ 28 Day Regimen contains inert ingredients.

ORTHO-NOVUM 1/35 □ 21 Day Regimen and ORTHO-NOVUM 1/35 □ 28 Day Regimen

Each peach tablet contains 1 mg norethindrone and 0.035 mg ethinyl estradiol. Each green tablet in ORTHO-NOVUM 1/35 □ 28 Day Regimen contains inert ingredients.

MODICON 21 Day Regimen and MODICON 28 Day Regimen

Each white tablet contains 0.5 mg norethindrone and 0.035 mg ethinyl estradiol. Each green tablet in MODICON 28 Day Regimen contains inert ingredients.

INTRODUCTION

Any woman who considers using oral contraceptives (the birth control pill or the pill) should understand the benefits and the risks of using this form of birth control. This patient labeling will give you much of the information you will need to make this decision and will also help you determine if you are at risk of developing any of the serious side effects of the pill. It will tell you how to use the pill properly so that it will be as effective as possible. However, this labeling is not a replacement for a careful discussion between you and your health care provider. You should discuss the information provided in this labeling with him or her, both when you first start taking the pill and during your revisits. You should also follow your health care provider's advice with regard to regular check-ups while you are on the pill.

EFFECTIVENESS OF ORAL CONTRACEPTIVES

Oral contraceptives or "birth control pills" or "the pill" are used to prevent pregnancy and are more effective than other non-surgical methods of birth control. When they are taken correctly, the chance of becoming pregnant is less than 1% (1 pregnancy per 100 women per year of use) when used perfectly, without missing any pills. Typical failure rates are actually 3% per year. The chance of becoming pregnant increases with each missed pill during a menstrual cycle.

In comparison, typical failure rates for other non-surgical methods of birth control during the first year of use are as follows:

Implant: <1%
Injection: <1%
IUD: 1 to 2%
Diaphragm with spermicides: 18%
Spermicides alone: 21%
Vaginal sponge: 18 to 36%
Cervical Cap: 18 to 36%
Condom alone (male): 12%
Condom alone (female): 21%
Periodic abstinence: 20%
No methods: 85%

WHO SHOULD NOT TAKE ORAL CONTRACEPTIVES

Cigarette smoking increases the risk of serious cardiovascular side effects from oral contraceptive use. This risk increases with age and with heavy smoking (15 or more cigarettes per day) and is quite marked in women over 35 years of age. Women who use oral contraceptives are strongly advised not to smoke.

Some women should not use the pill. For example, you should not take the pill if you are pregnant or think you may be pregnant. You should also not use the pill if you have any of the following conditions:

- A history of heart attack or stroke
- Blood clots in the legs (thrombophlebitis), lungs (pulmonary embolism), or eyes
- A history of blood clots in the deep veins of your legs
- Chest pain (angina pectoris)
- Known or suspected breast cancer or cancer of the lining of the uterus, cervix or vagina
- Unexplained vaginal bleeding (until a diagnosis is reached by your doctor)
- Yellowing of the whites of the eyes or of the skin (jaundice) during pregnancy or during previous use of the pill
- Liver tumor (benign or cancerous)
- Known or suspected pregnancy

Tell your health care provider if you have ever had any of these conditions. Your health care provider can recommend a safer method of brith control.

OTHER CONSIDERATIONS BEFORE TAKING ORAL CONTRACEPTIVES

Tell your health care provider if you have or have had:

- Breast nodules, fibrocystic disease of the breast, an abnormal breast x-ray or mammogram
- Diabetes
- Elevated cholesterol or triglycerides
- High blood pressure
- Migraine or other headaches or epilepsy
- Mental depression
- Gallbladder, heart or kidney disease
- History of scanty or irregular menstrual periods

Women with any of these conditions should be checked often by their health care provider if they choose to use oral contraceptives.

Also, be sure to inform your doctor or health care provider if you smoke or are on any medications.

RISKS OF TAKING ORAL CONTRACEPTIVES

1. Risk of developing blood clots

Blood clots and blockage of blood vessels are one of the most serious side effects of taking oral contraceptives and can cause death or serious disability. In particular, a clot in the legs can cause thrombophlebitis and a clot that travels to the lungs can cause a sudden blocking of the vessel carrying blood to the lungs. Rarely, clots occur in the blood vessels of the eye and may cause blindness, double vision, or impaired vision.

If you take oral contraceptives and need elective surgery, need to stay in bed for a prolonged illness or have recently delivered a baby, you may be at risk of develping blood clots. You should consult your doctor about stopping oral contraceptives three to four weeks before surgery and not taking oral contraceptives for two weeks after surgery or during bed rest. You should also not take oral contraceptives soon after delivery of a baby. It is advisable to wait for at least four weeks after delivery if you are not breast feeding or four weeks after a second trimester abortion. If you are breast feeding, you should wait until you have weaned your child before using the pill. (See also the section on Breast Feeding in General Precautions.)

The risk of circulatory disease in oral contraceptive users may be higher in users of high dose pills and may be greater with longer duration of oral contraceptive use. In addition, some of these increased risks may continue for a number of years after stopping oral contraceptives. The risk of abnormal blood clotting increases with age in both users and nonusers of oral contraceptives, but the increased risk from the oral contraceptive appears to be present at all ages. For women aged 20 to 44, it is estimated that about 1 in 2,000 using oral contraceptives will be hospitalized each year because of abnormal clotting. Among nonusers in the same age group, about 1 in 20,000 would be hospitalized each year. For oral contraceptive users in general, it has been estimated that in women between the ages of 15 and 34 the risk of death due to a circulatory disorder is about 1 in 12,000 per year, whereas for nonusers the rate is about 1 in 50,000 per year. In the age group 35 to 44, the risk is estimated to be about 1 in 2,500 per year for oral contraceptive users and about 1 in 10,000 per year for nonusers.

2. Heart attacks and strokes

Oral contraceptives may increase the tendency to develop strokes (stoppage or rupture of blood vessels in the brain) and angina pectoris and heart attacks (blockage of blood vessels in the heart). Any of these conditions can cause death or serious disability.

Smoking greatly increases the possibility of suffering heart attacks and strokes. Furthermore, smoking and the use of oral contraceptives greatly increase the chances of developing and dying of heart disease.

3. Gallbladder disease

Oral contraceptive users probably have a greater risk than nonusers of having gallbladder disease, although this risk may be related to pills containing high doses of estrogens.

4. Liver tumors

In rare cases, oral contraceptives can cause benign but dangerous liver tumors. These benign liver tumors can rupture and cause fatal internal bleeding. In addition, some studies report an increased risk of developing liver cancer. However, liver cancers are rare.

5. Cancer of the reproductive organs and breasts

There is conflict among studies regarding breast cancer and oral contraceptive use. Some studies have reported an increase in the risk of developing breast cancer, particularly at a younger age. This increased risk appears to be related to duration of use. The majority of studies have found no overall increase in the risk of developing breast cancer.

A meta-analysis of 54 studies found a small increase in the frequency of having breast cancer diagnosed for women who were currently using combined oral contraceptives or had used them within the past ten years. This increase in the frequency of breast cancer diagnosis, within ten years of stopping use, was generally accounted for by cancers localized to the breast. There was no increase in the frequency of having breast cancer diagnosed ten or more years after cessation of use.

Some studies have found an increase in the incidence of cancer of the cervix in women who use oral contraceptives. However, this finding may be related to factors other than the use of oral contraceptives. There is insufficient evidence to rule out the possibility that pills may cause such cancers.

ESTIMATED RISK OF DEATH FROM A BIRTH CONTROL METHOD OR PREGNANCY

All methods of birth control and pregnancy are associated with a risk of developing certain diseases which may lead to disability or death. An estimate of the number of deaths associated with different methods of birth control and pregnancy has been calculated and is shown in the following table.

[See table at bottom of next page]

In the above table, the risk of death from any birth control method is less than the risk of childbirth, except for oral contraceptive users over the age of 35 who smoke and pill users over the age of 40 even if they do not smoke. It can be seen in the table that for women aged 15 to 39, the risk of death was highest with pregnancy (7–26 deaths per 100,000 women, depending on age). Among pill users who do not smoke, the risk of death was always lower than that associated with pregnancy for any age group, although over the age of 40, the risk increases to 32 deaths per 100,000 women, compared to 28 associated with pregnancy at that age. However, for pill users who smoke and are over the age of 35, the estimated number of deaths exceed those for other methods of birth control. If a woman is over the age of 40 and smokes, her estimated risk of death is four times higher (117/100,000 women) than the estimated risk associated with pregnancy (28/100,000 women) in that age group.

The suggestion that women over 40 who do not smoke should not take oral contraceptives is based on information from older, higher-dose pills. An Advisory Committee of the FDA discussed this issue in 1989 and recommended that the benefits of low-dose oral contraceptive use by healthy, non-smoking women over 40 years of age may outweigh the possible risks.

WARNING SIGNALS

If any of these adverse effects occur while you are taking oral contraceptives, call your doctor immediately:

- Sharp chest pain, coughing of blood, or sudden shortness of breath (indicating a possible clot in the lung)
- Pain in the calf (indicating a possible clot in the leg)
- Crushing chest pain or heaviness in the chest (indicating a possible heart attack)
- Sudden severe headache or vomiting, dizziness or fainting, disturbances of vision or speech, weakness, or numbness in an arm or leg (indicating a possible stroke)
- Sudden partial or complete loss of vision (indicating a possible clot in the eye)
- Breast lumps (indicating possible breast cancer or fibrocystic disease of the breast; ask your doctor or health care provider to show you how to examine your breasts)
- Severe pain or tenderness in the stomach area (indicating a possibly ruptured liver tumor)
- Difficulty in sleeping, weakness, lack of energy, fatigue, or change in mood (possibly indicating severe depression)
- Jaundice or a yellowing of the skin or eyeballs, accompanied frequently by fever, fatigue, loss of appetite, dark colored urine, or light colored bowel movements (indicating possible liver problems)

SIDE EFFECTS OF ORAL CONTRACEPTIVES

1. Vaginal bleeding

Irregular vaginal bleeding or spotting may occur while you are taking the pills. Irregular bleeding may vary from slight staining between menstrual periods to breakthrough bleeding which is a flow much like regular period. Irregular bleeding occurs most often during the first few months of oral contraceptive use, but may also occur after you have been taking the pill for some time. Such bleeding may be temporary and usually does not indicate any serious problems. It is important to continue taking your pills on schedule. If the bleeding occurs in more than one cycle or lasts for more than a few days, talk to your doctor or health care provider.

2. Contact lenses

If you wear contact lenses and notice a change in vision or an inability to wear your lenses, contact your doctor or health care provider.

3. Fluid retention

Oral contraceptives may cause edema (fluid retention) with swelling of the fingers or ankles and may raise your blood pressure. If you experience fluid retention, contact your doctor or health care provider.

4. Melasma

A spotty darkening of the skin is possible, particularly of the face, which may persist.

5. Other side effects

Other side effects may include nausea and vomiting, change in appetite, headache, nervousness, depression, dizziness, loss of scalp hair, rash, and vaginal infections.

If any of these side effects bother you, call your doctor or health care provider.

GENERAL PRECAUTIONS

1. Missed periods and use of oral contraceptives before or during early pregnancy

There may be times when you may not menstruate regularly after you have completed taking a cycle of pills. If you have taken your pills regularly and miss one menstrual period, continue taking your pills for the next cycle but be sure to inform your health care provider before doing so. If you have not taken the pills daily as instructed and missed a menstrual period, you may be pregnant. If you missed two consecutive menstrual periods, you may be pregnant. Check with your health care provider immediately to determine whether you are pregnant. Do not continue to take oral contraceptives until you are sure you are not pregnant, but continue to use another method of contraception.

There is no conclusive evidence that oral contraceptive use is associated with an increase in birth defects, when taken inadvertently during early pregnancy. Previously, a few studies had reported that oral contraceptives might be associated with birth defects, but these findings have not been seen in more recent studies. Nevertheless, oral contraceptives or any other drugs should not be used during pregnancy unless clearly necessary and prescribed by your doctor. You should check with your doctor about risks to your unborn child of any medication taken during pregnancy.

2. While breast feeding

If you are breast feeding, consult your doctor before starting oral contraceptives. Some of the drug will be passed on to the child in the milk. A few adverse effects on the child have been reported, including yellowing of the skin (jaundice) and breast enlargement. In addition, combination oral contraceptives may decrease the amount and quality of your milk. If possible, do not use combination oral contraceptives while breast feeding. You should use another method of contraception since breast feeding provides only partial protection from becoming pregnant and this partial protection decreases significantly as you breast feed for longer periods of time. You should consider starting combination oral contraceptives only after you have weaned your child completely.

3. Laboratory tests

If you are scheduled for any laboratory tests, tell your doctor you are taking birth control pills. Certain blood tests may be affected by birth control pills.

4. Drug interactions

Certain drugs may interact with birth control pills to make them less effective in preventing pregnancy or cause an increase in breakthrough bleeding. Such drugs include rifampin, drugs used for epilepsy such as barbiturates (for example, phenobarbital), anticonvulsants such as carbamazepine (Tegretol is one brand of this drug), phenytoin (Dilantin is one brand of this drug), phenylbutazone (Butazolidin is one brand), and possibly certain antibiotics. You may need to use addtional contraception when you take drugs which can make oral contraceptives less effective.

5. Sexually transmitted diseases

This product (like all oral contraceptives) is intended to prevent pregnancy. It does not protect against transmission of HIV (AIDS) and other sexually transmitted diseases such as chlamydia, genital herpes, genital warts, gonorrhea, hepatitis B, and syphilis.

HOW TO TAKE THE PILL

IMPORTANT POINTS TO REMEMBER

BEFORE YOU START TAKING YOUR PILLS:

1. BE SURE TO READ THESE DIRECTIONS:
Before you start taking your pills.
Anytime you are not sure what to do.

2. THE RIGHT WAY TO TAKE THE PILL IS TO TAKE ONE PILL EVERY DAY AT THE SAME TIME.
If you miss pills you could get pregnant. This includes starting the pack late.
The more pills you miss, the more likely you are to get pregnant.

3. MANY WOMEN HAVE SPOTTING OR LIGHT BLEEDING, OR MAY FEEL SICK TO THEIR STOMACH DURING THE FIRST 1–3 PACKS OF PILLS: If you feel sick to your stomach, do not stop taking the pill. The problem will usually go away. If it doesn't go away, check with your doctor or clinic.

4. MISSING PILLS CAN ALSO CAUSE SPOTTING OR LIGHT BLEEDING, even when you make up these missed pills.
On the days you take 2 pills to make up for missed pills, you could also feel a little sick to your stomach.

5. IF YOU HAVE VOMITING OR DIARRHEA, for any reason, or IF YOU TAKE SOME MEDICINES, including some antibiotics, your pills may not work as well. Use a back-up method (such as condoms, foam, or sponge) until you check with your doctor or clinic.

6. IF YOU HAVE TROUBLE REMEMBERING TO TAKE THE PILL, talk to your doctor or clinic about how to make pill-taking easier or about using another method of birth control.

7. IF YOU HAVE ANY QUESTIONS OR ARE UNSURE ABOUT THE INFORMATION IN THIS LEAFLET, call your doctor or clinic.

ANNUAL NUMBER OF BIRTH-RELATED OR METHOD-RELATED DEATHS ASSOCIATED WITH CONTROL OF FERTILITY PER 100,000 NONSTERILE WOMEN, BY FERTILITY CONTROL METHOD ACCORDING TO AGE

Method of control and outcome	15-19	20-24	25-29	30-34	35-39	40-44
No fertility control methods*	7.0	7.4	9.1	14.8	25.7	28.2
Oral contraceptives non-smoker**	0.3	0.5	0.9	1.9	13.8	31.6
Oral contraceptives smoker**	2.2	3.4	6.6	13.5	51.1	117.2
IUD**	0.8	0.8	1.0	1.0	1.4	1.4
Condom*	1.1	1.6	0.7	0.2	0.3	0.4
Diaphragm/spermicide*	1.9	1.2	1.2	1.3	2.2	2.8
Periodic abstinence*	2.5	1.6	1.6	1.7	2.9	3.6

*Deaths are birth-related
**Deaths are method-related

BEFORE YOU START TAKING YOUR PILLS

1. DECIDE WHAT TIME OF DAY YOU WANT TO TAKE YOUR PILL.
It is important to take it at about the same time every day.

2. LOOK AT YOUR PILL PACK TO SEE IF IT HAS 21 OR 28 PILLS:
The 21-pill pack has 21 "active" pills (with hormones) to take for 3 weeks. This is followed by 1 week without pills.
The 28-pill pack has 21 "active" pills (with hormones) to take for 3 weeks. This is followed by 1 week of "reminder" green pills (without hormones).
ORTHO-NOVUM 7/7/7: There are 7 white "active" pills, 7 light peach "active" pills, and 7 peach "active" pills.
ORTHO–NOVUM 10/11: There are 10 white "active" pills and 11 peach "active" pills.
ORTHO-NOVUM 1/35: There are 21 peach "active" pills.
MODICON: There are 21 white "active" pills.

3. ALSO FIND:
1) where on the pack to start taking pills,
2) in what order to take the pills.
CHECK PICTURE OF PILL PACK AND ADDITIONAL INSTRUCTIONS FOR USING THIS PACKAGE IN THE BRIEF SUMMARY PATIENT PACKAGE INSERT.

4. BE SURE YOU HAVE READY AT ALL TIMES:
ANOTHER KIND OF BIRTH CONTROL (such as condoms, foam, or sponge) to use as a back-up method in case you miss pills.
AN EXTRA, FULL PILL PACK.

WHEN TO START THE FIRST PACK OF PILLS

You have a choice of which day to start taking your first pack of pills. ORTHO-NOVUM 7/7/7, ORTHO-NOVUM 10/11, ORTHO-NOVUM 1/35, and MODICON are available in the DIALPAK® Tablet Dispenser which is preset for a Sunday Start. Day 1 Start is also provided. Decide with your doctor or clinic which is the best day for you. Pick a time of day which will be easy to remember.

SUNDAY START:

ORTHO-NOVUM 7/7/7: Take the first "active" white pill of the first pack on the Sunday after your period starts, even if you are still bleeding. If your period begins on Sunday, start the pack the same day.

ORTHO-NOVUM 10/11: Take the first "active" white pill of the first pack on the Sunday after your period starts, even if you are still bleeding. If your period begins on Sunday, start the pack the same day.

ORTHO-NOVUM 1/35: Take the first "active" peach pill of the first pack on the Sunday after your period starts, even if you are still bleeding. If your period begins on Sunday, start the pack the same day.

MODICON: Take the first "active" white pill of the first pack on the Sunday after your period starts, even if you are still bleeding. If your period begins on Sunday, start the pack the same day.

Use another method of birth control as a back-up method if you have sex anytime from the Sunday you start your first pack until the next Sunday (7 days). Condoms, foam, or the sponge are good back-up methods of birth control.

DAY 1 START:

ORTHO-NOVUM 7/7/7: Take the first "active" white pill of the first pack during the first 24 hours of your period.

ORTHO-NOVUM 10/11: Take the first "active" white pill of the first pack during the first 24 hours of your period.

ORTHO-NOVUM 1/35: Take the first "active" peach pill of the first pack during the first 24 hours of your period.

MODICON: Take the first "active" white pill of the first pack during the first 24 hours of your period.

You will not need to use a back-up method of birth control, since you are starting the pill at the beginning of your period.

WHAT TO DO DURING THE MONTH

1. TAKE ONE PILL AT THE SAME TIME EVERY DAY UNTIL THE PACK IS EMPTY.

Do not skip pills even if you are spotting or bleeding between monthly periods or feel sick to your stomach (nausea).

Do not skip pills even if you do not have sex very often.

2. WHEN YOU FINISH A PACK OR SWITCH YOUR BRAND OF PILLS:

21 pills: Wait 7 days to start the next pack. You will probably have your period during that week. Be sure that no more than 7 days pass between 21-day packs.

28 pills: Start the next pack on the day after your last "reminder" pill. Do not wait any days between packs.

WHAT TO DO IF YOU MISS PILLS

ORTHO-NOVUM 7/7/7:

If you **MISS 1** white, light peach, or peach "active" pill:

1. Take it as soon as you remember. Take the next pill at your regular time. This means you may take 2 pills in 1 day.
2. You do not need to use a back-up birth control method if you have sex.

If you **MISS 2** white or light peach "active" pills in a row in **WEEK 1 OR WEEK 2** of your pack:

Continued on next page

Ortho-Novum Tablets—Cont.

1. Take 2 pills on the day you remember and 2 pills the next day.
2. Then take 1 pill a day until you finish the pack.
3. You MAY BECOME PREGNANT if you have sex in the 7 days after you miss pills. You MUST use another birth control method (such as condoms, foam, or sponge) as a back-up method for those 7 days.

If you **MISS 2** peach "active" pills in a row in **THE 3RD WEEK:**

1. **If you are a Sunday Starter:**
Keep taking 1 pill every day until Sunday. On Sunday, THROW OUT the rest of the pack and start a new pack of pills that same day.
If you are a Day 1 Starter:
THROW OUT the rest of the pill pack and start a new pack that same day.
2. You may not have your period this month but this is expected. However, if you miss your period 2 months in a row, call your doctor or clinic because you might be pregnant.
3. You MAY BECOME PREGNANT if you have sex in the 7 days after you miss pills. You MUST use another birth control method (such as condoms, foam, or sponge) as a back-up method for those 7 days.

If you **MISS 3 OR MORE** white, light peach, or peach "active" pills in a row (during the first 3 weeks):

1. **If you are a Sunday Starter:**
Keep taking 1 pill every day until Sunday. On Sunday, THROW OUT the rest of the pack and start a new pack of pills that same day.
If you are a Day 1 Starter:
THROW OUT the rest of the pill pack and start a new pack that same day.
2. You may not have your period this month but this is expected. However, if you miss your period 2 months in a row, call your doctor or clinic because you might be pregnant.
3. You MAY BECOME PREGNANT if you have sex in the 7 days after you miss pills. You MUST use another birth control method (such as condoms, foam, or sponge) as a back-up method for those 7 days.

ORTHO-NOVUM 10/11:

If you **MISS 1** white or peach "active" pill:

1. Take it as soon as you remember. Take the next pill at your regular time. This means you may take 2 pills in 1 day.
2. You do not need to use a back-up birth control method if you have sex.

If you **MISS 2** white or peach "active" pills in a row in **WEEK 1 OR WEEK 2** of your pack:

1. Take 2 pills on the day you remember and 2 pills the next day.
2. Then take 1 pill a day until you finish the pack.
3. You MAY BECOME PREGNANT if you have sex in the 7 days after you miss pills. You MUST use another birth control method (such as condoms, foam, or sponge) as a back-up method for those 7 days.

If you **MISS 2** peach "active" pills in a row in **THE 3RD WEEK:**

1. **If you are a Sunday Starter:**
Keep taking 1 pill every day until Sunday. On Sunday, THROW OUT the rest of the pack and start a new pack of pills that same day.
If you are a Day 1 Starter:
THROW OUT the rest of the pill pack and start a new pack that same day.
2. You may not have your period this month but this is expected. However, if you miss your period 2 months in a row, call your doctor or clinic because you might be pregnant.
3. You MAY BECOME PREGNANT if you have sex in the 7 days after you miss pills. You MUST use another birth control method (such as condoms, foam, or sponge) as a back-up method for those 7 days.

If you **MISS 3 OR MORE** white or peach "active" pills in a row (during the first 3 weeks):

1. **If you are a Sunday Starter:**
Keep taking 1 pill every day until Sunday. On Sunday, THROW OUT the rest of the pack and start a new pack of pills that same day.
If you are a Day 1 Starter:
THROW OUT the rest of the pill pack and start a new pack that same day.
2. You may not have your period this month but this is expected. However, if you miss your period 2 months in a row, call your doctor or clinic because you might be pregnant.
3. You MAY BECOME PREGNANT if you have sex in the 7 days after you miss pills. You MUST use another birth control method (such as condoms, foam, or sponge) as a back-up method for those 7 days.

ORTHO-NOVUM 1/35:

If you **MISS 1** peach "active" pill:

1. Take it as soon as you remember. Take the next pill at your regular time. This means you may take 2 pills in 1 day.
2. You do not need to use a back-up birth control method if you have sex.

If you **MISS 2** peach "active" pills in a row in **WEEK 1 OR WEEK 2** of your pack:

1. Take 2 pills on the day you remember and 2 pills the next day.
2. Then take 1 pill a day until you finish the pack.
3. You MAY BECOME PREGNANT if you have sex in the 7 days after you miss pills. You MUST use another birth control method (such as condoms, foam, or sponge) as a back-up method for those 7 days.

If you **MISS 2** peach "active" pills in a row in **THE 3RD WEEK:**

1. **If you are a Sunday Starter:**
Keep taking 1 pill every day until Sunday. On Sunday, THROW OUT the rest of the pack and start a new pack of pills that same day.
If you are a Day 1 Starter:
THROW OUT the rest of the pill pack and start a new pack that same day.
2. You may not have your period this month but this is expected. However, if you miss your period 2 months in a row, call your doctor or clinic because you might be pregnant.
3. You MAY BECOME PREGNANT if you have sex in the 7 days after you miss pills. You MUST use another birth control method (such as condoms, foam, or sponge) as a back-up method for those 7 days.

If you **MISS 3 OR MORE** peach "active" pills in a row (during the first 3 weeks):

1. **If you are a Sunday Starter:**
Keep taking 1 pill every day until Sunday. On Sunday, THROW OUT the rest of the pack and start a new pack of pills that same day.
If you are a Day 1 Starter:
THROW OUT the rest of the pill pack and start a new pack that same day.
2. You may not have your period this month but this is expected. However, if you miss your period 2 months in a row, call your doctor or clinic because you might be pregnant.
3. You MAY BECOME PREGNANT if you have sex in the 7 days after you miss pills. You MUST use another birth control method (such as condoms, foam, or sponge) as a back-up method for those 7 days.

MODICON:

If you **MISS 1** white "active" pill:

1. Take it as soon as you remember. Take the next pill at your regular time. This means you may take 2 pills in 1 day.
2. You do not need to use a back-up birth control method if you have sex.

If you **MISS 2** white "active" pills in a row in **WEEK 1 OR WEEK 2** of your pack:

1. Take 2 pills on the day you remember and 2 pills the next day.
2. Then take 1 pill a day until you finish the pack.
3. You MAY BECOME PREGNANT if you have sex in the 7 days after you miss pills. You MUST use another birth control method (such as condoms, foam, or sponge) as a back-up method for those 7 days.

If you **MISS 2** white "active" pills in a row in **THE 3RD WEEK:**

1. **If you are a Sunday Starter:**
Keep taking 1 pill every day until Sunday. On Sunday, THROW OUT the rest of the pack and start a new pack of pills that same day.
If you are a Day 1 Starter:
THROW OUT the rest of the pill pack and start a new pack that same day.
2. You may not have your period this month but this is expected. However, if you miss your period 2 months in a row, call your doctor or clinic because you might be pregnant.
3. You MAY BECOME PREGNANT if you have sex in the 7 days after you miss pills. You MUST use another birth control method (such as condoms, foam, or sponge) as a back-up method for those 7 days.

If you **MISS 3 OR MORE** white "active" pills in a row (during the first 3 weeks):

1. **If you are a Sunday Starter:**
Keep taking 1 pill every day until Sunday. On Sunday, THROW OUT the rest of the pack and start a new pack of pills that same day.
If you are a Day 1 Starter:
THROW OUT the rest of the pill pack and start a new pack that same day.
2. You may not have your period this month but this is expected. However, if you miss your period 2 months in a row, call your doctor or clinic because you might be pregnant.
3. You MAY BECOME PREGNANT if you have sex in the 7 days after you miss pills. You MUST use another birth control method (such as condoms, foam, or sponge) as a back-up method for those 7 days.

A REMINDER FOR THOSE ON 28-DAY PACKS:
If you forget any of the 7 green "reminder" pills in Week 4:
THROW AWAY the pills you missed.
Keep taking 1 pill each day until the pack is empty.
You do not need a back-up method.

FINALLY, IF YOU ARE STILL NOT SURE WHAT TO DO ABOUT THE PILLS YOU HAVE MISSED:
Use a BACK-UP METHOD anytime you have sex.
KEEP TAKING ONE "ACTIVE" PILL EACH DAY until you can reach your doctor or clinic.

PREGNANCY DUE TO PILL FAILURE

Combination Oral Contraceptives
The incidence of pill failure resulting in pregnancy is approximately one percent (i.e., one pregnancy per 100 women per year) if taken every day as directed, but more typical failure rates are about 3%. If failure does occur, the risk to the fetus is minimal.

PREGNANCY AFTER STOPPING THE PILL

There may be some delay in becoming pregnant after you stop using oral contraceptives, especially if you had irregular menstrual cycles before you used oral contraceptives. It may be advisable to postpone conception until you begin menstruating regularly once you have stopped taking the pill and desire pregnancy.
There does not appear to be any increase in birth defects in newborn babies when pregnancy occurs soon after stopping the pill.

OVERDOSAGE

Serious ill effects have not been reported following ingestion of large doses of oral contraceptives by young children. Overdosage may cause nausea and withdrawal bleeding in females. In case of overdosage, contact your health care provider or pharmacist.

OTHER INFORMATION

Your health care provider will take a medical and family history before prescribing oral contraceptives and will examine you. The physical examination may be delayed to another time if you request it and the health care provider believes that it is a good medical practice to postpone it. You should be reexamined at least once a year. Be sure to inform your health care provider if there is a family history of any of the conditions listed previously in this leaflet. Be sure to keep all appointments with your health care provider, because this is a time to determine if there are early signs of side effects of oral contraceptive use.
Do not use the drug for any condition other than the one for which it was prescribed. This drug has been prescribed specifically for you; do not give it to others who may want birth control pills.

HEALTH BENEFITS FROM ORAL CONTRACEPTIVES

In addition to preventing pregnancy, use of combination oral contraceptives may provide certain benefits. They are:

- menstrual cycles may become more regular
- blood flow during menstruation may be lighter and less iron may be lost. Therefore, anemia due to iron deficiency is less likely to occur.
- pain or other symptoms during menstruation may be encountered less frequently
- ectopic (tubal) pregnancy may occur less frequently
- noncancerous cysts or lumps in the breast may occur less frequently
- acute pelvic inflammatory disease may occur less frequently
- oral contraceptive use may provide some protection against developing two forms of cancer: cancer of the ovaries and cancer of the lining of the uterus.

If you want more information about birth control pills, ask your doctor or pharmacist. They have a more technical leaflet called the Professional Labeling, which you may wish to read. The professional labeling is also published in a book entitled *Physicians' Desk Reference*, available in many book stores and public libraries.
ORTHO-McNEIL PHARMACEUTICAL, INC.
Raritan, New Jersey 08869
© OMP 1998 REVISED MAY 1998 635-50-700-3
Shown in Product Identification Guide, page 328

ORTHO-PREFEST™ ℞

[*orthō-prē-fĕst*]
(17β-estradiol/norgestimate)
tablets

Prescribing Information

DESCRIPTION

The ORTHO-PREFEST™ regimen provides for a single oral tablet to be taken once daily. The pink tablet containing 1.0 mg estradiol is taken on days one through three of therapy; the white tablet containing 1.0 mg estradiol and 0.09 mg norgestimate is taken on days four through six of therapy. This pattern is then repeated continuously to produce the constant estrogen/intermittent progestogen regimen of ORTHO-PREFEST™.
The estrogenic component of ORTHO-PREFEST™ is 17β-estradiol. It is a white, crystalline solid, chemically described as estra-1,3,5(10)-triene-3,17β-diol. It has an empirical formula of $C_{18}H_{24}O_2$ and molecular weight of 272.39. The structural formula is:

The progestational component of ORTHO-PREFEST™ is micronized norgestimate, a white powder which is chemically described as (17α)-17-(Acetyloxyl)-13-ethyl-18,19-dinorpregn-4-en-20-yn-3-one3-oxime. It has an empirical formula of $C_{23}H_{31}NO_3$ and a molecular weight of 369.50. The structural formula is:
[See chemical structure at top of next column]
Each tablet for oral administration contains 1.0 mg estradiol alone or 1.0 mg estradiol and 0.09 mg of norgestimate, and the following inactive ingredients: croscarmellose sodium, microcrystalline cellulose, magnesium stearate, ferric oxide red, and lactose monohydrate.

CLINICAL PHARMACOLOGY

Estrogens are important in the development and maintenance of the female reproductive system and secondary sex characteristics. By a direct action, they cause growth and development of the uterus, fallopian tubes, and vagina. With other hormones, such as pituitary hormones and progesterone, they cause enlargement of the breasts through promotion of ductal growth, stromal development, and the accretion of fat. Estrogens are intricately involved with other hormones, especially progesterone, in the processes of the ovulatory menstrual cycle and pregnancy and affect the release of pituitary gonadotropins. They also contribute to the shaping of the skeleton, maintenance of tone and elasticity of urogenital structures, changes in the epiphyses of the long bones that allow for the pubertal growth spurt and its termination, and pigmentation of the nipples and genitals.

Although circulating estrogens exist in a dynamic equilibrium of metabolic interconversions, estradiol is the principal intracellular human estrogen and is substantially more potent than its metabolites, estrone and estriol at the receptor level. The primary source of estrogen in adult women with normal menstrual cycles is the ovarian follicle, which secretes 70 to 500 micrograms of estradiol daily, depending on the phase of the menstrual cycle. After menopause, most endogenous estrogens are produced by conversion of androstenedione, secreted by the adrenal cortex, to estrone by the peripheral tissues. Thus, estrone and the sulfate conjugated form, estrone sulfate, are the most abundant circulating estrogens in postmenopausal women.

Circulating estrogens modulate the pituitary secretion of the gonadotropins, luteinizing hormone (LH) and follicle stimulating hormone (FSH) through a negative feedback mechanism and estrogen replacement therapy acts to reduce the elevated levels of these hormones seen in postmenopausal women.

Norgestimate is a derivative of 19-nortestosterone and binds to androgen and progestogen receptors, similar to that of the natural hormone progesterone; it does not bind to estrogen receptors. Progestins counter the estrogenic effects by decreasing the number of nuclear estradiol receptors and suppressing epithelial DNA synthesis in endometrial tissue.

Pharmacokinetics

Absorption:
Estradiol reaches its peak serum concentration (C_{max}) at approximately 7 hours in postmenopausal women receiving ORTHO-PREFEST™ (Table 1). Norgestimate is completely metabolized; its primary active metabolite, 17-deacetylnorgestimate, reaches C_{max} at approximately 2 hours after dose (Table 1). Upon co-administration of ORTHO-PREFEST™ with a high fat meal, the C_{max} values for estrone and estrone sulfate were increased by 14% and 24% respectively, and the C_{max} for 17-deacetylnorgestimate was decreased by 16%. The AUC values for these analytes were not significantly affected by food.

Distribution:
The distribution of exogenous estrogens is similar to that of endogenous estrogens. Estrogens are widely distributed in the body and are generally found in higher concentrations in the sex hormone target organs. Estradiol is bound mainly to sex hormone binding globulin (SHBG), and to albumin. 17-deacetylnorgestimate, the primary active metabolite of norgestimate, does not bind to SHBG but to other serum proteins. The percent protein binding of 17-deacetylnorgestimate is approximately 99%.

Metabolism:
Exogenous estrogens are metabolized in the same manner as endogenous estrogens. Circulating estrogens exist in a dynamic equilibrium of metabolic interconversions. These transformations take place mainly in the liver. Estradiol is converted reversibly to estrone, and both can be converted to estriol, which is the major urinary metabolite. Estrogens also undergo enterohepatic recirculation via sulfate and glucuronide conjugation in the liver, biliary secretion of conjugates into the intestine, and hydrolysis in the gut followed by reabsorption. In postmenopausal women a significant portion of the circulating estrogens exist as sulfate conjugates, especially estrone sulfate, which serves as a circulating reservoir for the formation of more active estrogens. Norgestimate is extensively metabolized by first-pass mechanisms in gastrointestinal tract and/or liver. Norgestimate's primary active metabolite is 17-deacetylnorgestimate.

Excretion:
Estradiol, estrone, and estriol are excreted in the urine along with glucuronide and sulfate conjugates. Norgestimate metabolites are eliminated in the urine and feces. The half-life ($t_{1/2}$) of estradiol and 17-deacetylnorgestimate in postmenopausal women receiving ORTHO-PREFEST™ is approximately 16 and 37 hours, respectively.

Special Populations

Pediatric: ORTHO-PREFEST™ is not indicated in children.

Table 1: Mean Pharmacokinetic Parameters of E_2, E_1, E_1S, and 17d-NGM[1] Following Single and Multiple Dosing of ORTHO-PREFEST™

Analyte	Parameter[2]	Units	First Dose E_2	First Dose E_2/NGM	Mutiple Dose E_2	Multiple Dose E_2/NGM
E_2	C_{max}	pg/mL	27.4	39.3	49.7	46.2
	t_{max}	h	7	7	7	7
	AUC(0–24 h)	pg. h/mL	424	681	864	779
E_1	C_{max}	pg/mL	210	285	341	325
	t_{max}	h	6	6	7	6
	AUC(0–24 h)	pg. h/mL	2774	4153	5429	4957
E_1S	C_{max}	ng/mL	11.1	13.9	14.9	14.5
	t_{max}	h	5	4	6	5
	AUC(0–24 h)	ng.h/mL	135	180	198	198
17d-NGM	C_{max}	pg/mL	NA[3]	515	NA	643
	t_{max}	h	NA	2	NA	2
	AUC(0–24 h)	pg. h/mL	NA	2146	NA	5322
	t½	h	NA	37	NA	NA

[1] E_2 = 17β-Estradiol, E_1 = Estrone, E_1S = Estrone Sulfate, 17d-NGM = 17-deacetylnorgestimate. Baseline uncorrected data are reported for E_2, E_1 and E_1S.
[2] C_{max} = peak serum concentration, t_{max} = time to reach peak serum concentration, AUC(0–24 h) = area under serum concentration vs. time curve from 0 to 24 hours after dose, $t_{1/2}$ = half-life.
[3] NA= Not available or not applicable.

Geriatric: ORTHO-PREFEST™ has not been studied in geriatric patients

Gender: ORTHO-PREFEST™ is indicated in women only.

Effects of Race, Age, and Body Weight: The effects of race, age, and body weight on the pharmacokinetics of 17β-estradiol, norgestimate, and their metabolites were evaluated in 164 healthy postmenopausal women (100 Caucasians, 61 Hispanics, 2 Blacks, and 1 Asian). No significant pharmacokinetic difference was observed between the Caucasian and the Hispanic postmenopausal women. No significant difference due to age (40–66 years) was observed. No significant difference due to body weight was observed in women in the 60 to 80 kg weight range. Women with body weight higher than 80 kg, however, had approximately 40% lower peak serum levels of 17-deacetylnorgestimate, 30% lower AUC values for 17-deacetylnorgestimate and 30% lower C_{max} values for norgestrel. The clinical relevance of these observations is unknown.

Renal Insufficiency: It has been reported in the literature that at both baseline and after estradiol ingestion, postmenopausal women with end stage renal disease (ESRD) had higher free serum estradiol levels than the control subjects. No pharmacokinetic study with norgestimate or a hormone combination with norgestimate has been conducted in postmenopausal women with ESRD.

Hepatic Insufficiency: No pharmacokinetic study for ORTHO-PREFEST™ has been conducted in postmenopausal women with hepatic impairment.

[See table 1 above]

Drug-Drug Interactions

Estradiol, norgestimate, and their metabolites inhibit a variety of P450 enzymes in human liver microsomes. However, the clinical and toxicological consequences of such interaction are likely to be insignificant because, under the recommended dosing regimen, the in vivo concentrations of these steroids, even at the peak serum levels, are relatively low compared to the inhibitory constant (Ki). Results of a subset population (n=24) from a clinical study conducted in 36 healthy postmenopausal women indicated that the steady state serum estradiol levels during the estradiol plus norgestimate phase of the regimen may be lower by 12-18% as compared with estradiol administered alone. The serum estrone levels may decrease by 4% and the serum estrone sulfate levels may increase by 17% during the estradiol plus norgestimate phase as compared with estradiol administered alone. The clinical relevance of these observations is unknown.

CLINICAL STUDIES

Efficacy on Postmenopausal Symptoms

The effect of the estrogen component of ORTHO-PREFEST™ on vasomotor symptoms was confirmed in a 12-week placebo-controlled trial of healthy postmenopausal women with moderate-to-severe vasomotor symptoms (MSVS). The addition of norgestimate to estrogen (i.e., the ORTHO-PREFEST™ regimen) was studied in two 12-month trials in healthy postmenopausal women (n=1212) for endometrial protection. Results from a subset population (n=119) of these 12-month trials (women with MSVS) are shown in Table 2.

Table 2: Change in the Mean Number of Moderate-to-Severe Vasomotor Symptoms (Subset of Subjects with ≥ 7 Moderate-to-Severe Hot Flushes per Day)

	1 mg E_2		ORTHO-PREFEST™	
	N	Mean	N	Mean
Baseline	29	11.0	26	10.9
Week 4	29	3.3	26	2.6
Week 8	29	1.1	23	0.9
Week 12	29	1.1	23	0.7

The effects of the addition of norgestimate on steady state estrogen levels and the clinical relevance thereof have been discussed in **CLINICAL PHARMACOLOGY** (see **Drug-Drug Interactions**).

Efficacy on Vulvar and Vaginal Atrophy

The effect of the estrogen component of ORTHO-PREFEST™ on vulvovaginal atrophy was confirmed in a 12-week placebo-controlled trial of healthy postmenopausal women with moderate-to-severe vasomotor symptoms (MSVS). The addition of norgestimate to estrogen (i.e., the ORTHO-PREFEST™ regimen) was studied in a 12-month trial in healthy postmenopausal women for endometrial protection. Results from a subset population (n=69) with paired tests for maturation index of the vaginal mucosa are shown in Table 3.

[See table 3 at top of next page]

Effects on the Endometrium

The effect of ORTHO-PREFEST™ on the endometrium was evaluated in two 12-month trials. The combined results are shown in (Table 4).

[See table 4 at top of next page]

In another 12-month controlled clinical trial for endometrial protection an additional 190 postmenopausal women were treated with ORTHO-PREFEST™. No subject had a diagnosis of endometrial hyperplasia after treatment.

Control of Uterine Bleeding

The effect of ORTHO-PROFEST™ on uterine bleeding was evaluated in two 12-month trials.
Combined results are shown in Figure 1.

Figure 1: Subjects with Cumulative Amenorrhea Over Time (Intent To Treat Population)

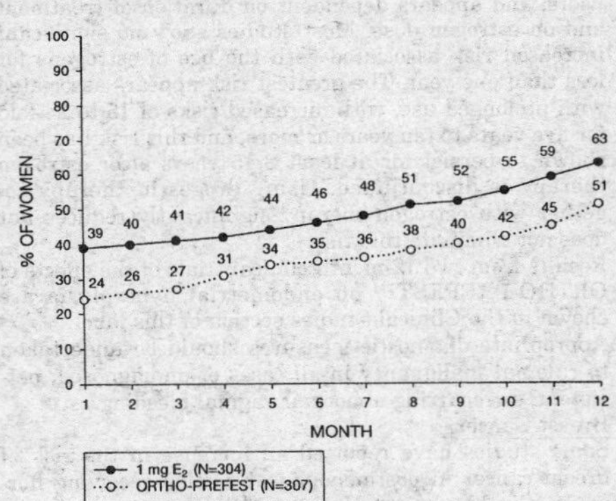

Note: At each month, the percentage of women who were amenorrheic in that month and through month 12 is shown.

Metabolic Parameters

Effects on Lipids:
The effect of ORTHO-PREFEST™ on lipids was evaluated in a 12-month metabolic trial of healthy postmenopausal women.
Results are shown in Table 5.

Table 5: Effects on Blood Lipoproteins at Month 12

	1 mg E_2		ORTHO-PREFEST™	
	N	Mean % Change	N	Mean % Change
Total Cholesterol	36	1.2	31	−1.9
HDL	36	12.0	31	9.7
LDL	31	1.7	30	1.2
Triglycerides	36	29.0	31	9.4

INDICATIONS AND USAGE

ORTHO-PREFEST™ therapy is indicated in women with an intact uterus for the:

1. Treatment of moderate to severe vasomotor symptoms associated with the menopause.

Continued on next page

Ortho-Prefest—Cont.

2. Treatment of vulvar and vaginal atrophy.
3. Prevention of osteoporosis.

Most prospective studies of efficacy for this indication have been carried out in white postmenopausal women, without stratification by other risk factors, and tend to show a universally beneficial effect on bone. Since estrogen administration is associated with risk, patient selection must be individualized based on the balance of risk and benefits.

Case-control studies have shown an approximately 60-percent reduction in hip and wrist fractures in women whose estrogen replacement was begun within a few years after menopause. Studies also suggest that estrogen reduces the rate of vertebral fractures. When estrogen therapy is discontinued, bone mass declines at a rate comparable to the immediate postmenopausal period.

White and Asian women are at higher risk for osteoporosis than Black women, and thin women are at higher risk than heavier women, who generally have higher endogenous estrogen levels. Early menopause is one of the strongest predictors for the development of osteoporosis. Other factors associated with osteoporosis include genetic factors (small build, family history), lifestyle (cigarette smoking, alcohol abuse, sedentary exercise habits) and nutrition (below average body weight and dietary calcium intake).

The mainstays of prevention and management of osteoporosis are weight-bearing exercise, adequate lifetime calcium intake, and, when indicated, estrogen. Postmenopausal women absorb dietary calcium less efficiently than premenopausal women and require an average of 1500 mg/day of elemental calcium to remain in neutral calcium balance. The average calcium intake in the USA is 400–600 mg/day. Therefore, when not contraindicated, calcium supplementation may be helpful for women with suboptimal dietary intake.

CONTRAINDICATIONS

Estrogens/progestins should not be used in individuals with any of the following conditions:

1. Known or suspected pregnancy.
2. Undiagnosed abnormal genital bleeding.
3. Known or suspected cancer of the breast.
4. Known or suspected estrogen-dependent neoplasia.
5. Active or past history of thrombophlebitis or thromboembolic disorders.
6. Hypersensitivity to any components of this product.

WARNINGS

Based on experience with estrogens and/or progestins:

1. Induction of Malignant Neoplasms

Endometrial Cancer:

The reported endometrial cancer risk among unopposed estrogen users is about 2 to 12-fold greater than in non-users, and appears dependent on duration of treatment and on estrogen dose. Most studies show no significant increased risk associated with the use of estrogens for less than one year. The greatest risk appears associated with prolonged use, with increased risks of 15 to 24-fold for five years to ten years or more, and this risk has been shown to persist for at least 8-15 years after estrogen therapy is discontinued. Using progestin therapy together with estrogen therapy significantly reduces but does not eliminate this risk.

Results from two 12-month clinical trials of the effects of ORTHO-PREFEST™ on endometrial hyperplasia are shown in the Clinical Studies section of this label.

Appropriate diagnostic measures should be undertaken to rule out malignancy in all cases of undiagnosed, persistent, or recurring abnormal vaginal bleeding.

Breast Cancer:

Some studies have reported an increase in the risk of breast cancer in postmenopausal women receiving hormone replacement therapy. A meta-analysis of 51 clinical studies suggests that this increased risk is comparable to that observed in women with every year of delay of natural menopause. This increased risk decreases after cessation of use of hormone replacement therapy and is not apparent five years following cessation of treatment. Breast cancers found in current or recent users of hormone replacement therapy are more likely to be localized to the breast than those in non-users. Concurrent progestin use does not appear to protect against this risk. Therefore, a careful appraisal of the risk/benefit ratio should be undertaken before the initiation of long-term treatment.

Women on hormone replacement therapy should have regular examinations and should be instructed in breast self-examination, and women over the age of 50 should have regular mammograms.

2. Venous Thromboembolism

Epidemiologic studies have reported an increased risk of venous thromboembolism (VTE) in users of estrogen replacement therapy (ERT) who did not have predisposing conditions for VTE, such as past history of cardiovascular disease or a recent history of pregnancy, surgery, trauma, or serious illness. The increased risk was found only in current ERT users; it did not persist in former users. The findings were similar for ERT alone or with added progestin and pertain to commonly used ERT types and doses, including 0.625 mg or more per day orally of conjugated estrogens, 1 mg or more per day orally of estradiol, and 50 micrograms or more per day or transdermal estradiol. The studies found the VTE risk to be about one case per 10,000 women per year among women not using ERT and without predisposing conditions. The risk in current ERT users was increased to 2–3 cases per 10,000 women per year.

Table 3: Summary of Maturation Index Results in Subjects with Paired Tests Following 7 Months Treatment with ORTHO-PREFEST™ or Estradiol

	Pretreatment Mean	Month 7 Mean	Mean Change
		1 mg Estradiol (N=37)	
Parabasal Cells (%)	25.1	2.7	−22.4
Intermediate Cells (%)	69.2	76.4	7.2
Superficial Cells (%)	5.7	20.9	15.3
		ORTHO-PREFEST™ (N=32)	
Parabasal Cells (%)	31.9	0.0	−31.9
Intermediate Cells (%)	64.2	80.9	16.7
Superficial Cells (%)	3.9	19.1	15.2

Table 4: Incidence of Endometrial Hyperplasia After 12 Months of Treatment (Intent To Treat Population)

	Continuous 1 mg estradiol	ORTHO-PREFEST™
Total No. Subjects	265	242
Total No. Evaluable Biopsies	256 (97%)	227 (94%)
Normal endometrium	182 (71%)	227 (100%)
Simple hyperplasia	64 (25%)	0 (0%)
Complex hyperplasia	2 (0.8%)	0 (0%)
Hyperplasia with cytological atypia	8 (3%)	0 (0%)

3. Cardiovascular Disease

Large doses of estrogens (5 mg conjugated estrogens per day), comparable to those used to treat cancer of the prostate and breast, have been shown to increase the risks of nonfatal myocardial infarction, pulmonary embolism, and thrombophlebitis in a large prospective clinical trial in men.

4. Hypercalcemia

Administration of estrogens may lead to severe hypercalcemia in patients with breast cancer and bone metastases. If this occurs, the drugs should be stopped and appropriate measures taken to reduce the serum calcium level.

5. Gallbladder Disease

A 2 to 4-fold increase in the risk of gallbladder disease requiring surgery in women receiving postmenopausal estrogens has been reported.

PRECAUTIONS

General

Based on experience with estrogens and/or progestins:

1. Addition of a progestin when a women has not had a hysterectomy

Studies of the addition of a progestin for 10 or more days of a cycle of estrogen administration, or daily with estrogen in a continuous regimen, have reported a lowered incidence of endometrial hyperplasia than would be induced by estrogen treatment alone.

There are, however, possible risks that may be associated with the use of progestins in estrogen replacement regimens. These include:

a. adverse effects on lipoprotein metabolism (lowering HDL and raising LDL).
b. impairment of glucose tolerance;
and;
c. possible enhancement of mitotic activity in breast epithelial tissue. There is minimal epidemiological data available to address this point.

The choice of progestin, its dose, and its regimen may be important in minimizing these adverse effects.

2. Endometrial hyperplasia

In pharmacokinetic studies with ORTHO-PREFEST™, women with body weight greater than 80 kg, had approximately 40% lower peak serum levels of 17-deacetylnorgestimate, 30% lower AUC values for 17-deacetylnorgestimate and 30% lower C_{max} values for norgestrel. 17-deacetylnorgestimate and norgestrel are metabolites of the progestin norgestimate.

Although the clinical relevance of these observations is unknown, the underlying risk of endometrial hyperplasia is known to be higher in overweight women. Therefore, clinical surveillance is important. Appropriate diagnostic measures, including endometrial sampling when indicated, should be undertaken to rule out malignancy in all cases of undiagnosed persistent or recurring abnormal vaginal bleeding or in women with other risk factors for endometrial hyperplasia.

3. Elevated blood pressure

Occasional increases in blood pressure during estrogen replacement therapy have been attributed to idiosyncratic reactions to estrogens in a small number of case reports. A generalized effect of estrogen therapy on blood pressure was not found in the one randomized, placebo-controlled study that has been reported. This effect was also not observed in clinical studies with ORTHO-PREFEST™.

4. Familial hyperlipoproteinemia

Estrogen therapy may be associated with elevations of plasma triglycerides leading to pancreatitis and other complications in patients with familial defects of lipoprotein metabolism.

5. Impaired liver function

Estrogens may be poorly metabolized in patients with impaired liver function.

Information For The Patient

See text of PATIENT LABELING, below.

Drug/Laboratory Test Interactions

1. Accelerated prothrombin time, partial thromboplastin time, and platelet aggregation time; increased platelet count; increased factors II, VII antigen, VIII antigen, VIII coagulant activity, IX, X, XII, VII-X complex, II-VII-X complex, and beta-thromboglobulin; decreased levels of anti-factor Xa and antithrombin III, decreased antithrombin III activity; increased levels of fibrinogen and fibrinogen activity; increased plasminogen antigen and activity.
2. Increased thyroid-binding globulin (TBG) leading to increased circulating total thyroid hormone, as measured by protein-bound iodine (PBI), T4 levels (by column or by radioimmunoassay) or T3 levels by radioimmunoassay. T3 resin uptake is decreased, reflecting the elevated TBG. Free T4 and free T3 concentrations are unaltered.
3. Other binding proteins may be elevated in serum, i.e., corticosteroid binding globulin (CBG), sex hormone-binding globulin (SHBG), leading to increased circulating corticosteroids and sex steroids respectively. Free or biologically active hormone concentrations are unchanged. Other plasma proteins may be increased (angiotensinogen/renin substrate, alpha-1-antitrypsin, ceruloplasmin).
4. Increased plasma HDL and HDL-2 subfraction concentrations, reduced LDL cholesterol concentration, increased triglycerides levels.
5. Impaired glucose tolerance. For this reason, diabetic patients should be carefully observed while receiving estrogen/progestin therapy.
6. Reduced response to metyrapone test.
7. Reduced serum folate concentration.

Carcinogenesis, Mutagenesis, and Impairment of Fertility

Long-term continuous administration of natural and synthetic estrogens in certain animal species increases the frequency of carcinomas of the breasts, uterus, cervix, vagina, testis, and liver (See **CONTRAINDICATIONS** and **WARNINGS**.)

Pregnancy Category X

ORTHO-PREFEST™ should not be used during pregnancy. (See **CONTRAINDICATIONS**.)

Nursing Mothers

As a general principle, the administration of any drug to nursing mothers should be done only when clearly necessary since many drugs are excreted in human milk. Estrogen administration to nursing mothers has been shown to decrease the quantity and quality of the milk. Estrogens are not indicated for the prevention of postpartum breast engorgement.

ADVERSE REACTIONS

In four 12-month trials that included 579 healthy postmenopausal women treated with ORTHO-PREFEST™ the following treatment-emergent adverse events occurred at a rate ≥5% (Table 6):

Table 6: All Treatment-Emergent Adverse Events Regardless Of Drug Relationship Reported at a Frequency of ≥ 5% with ORTHO-PREFEST™

Four 12-Month Clinical Trials	
	ORTHO-PREFEST™ (estradiol and NGM) (N = 579) n (%)
Body as a Whole	
Back pain	69 (12%)
Fatigue	32 (6%)
Influenza-like symptoms	64 (11%)
Pain	37 (6%)

Digestive System	
Abdominal pain	70 (12%)
Flatulence	29 (5%)
Nausea	34 (6%)
Tooth disorder	27 (5%)
Musculoskeletal System	
Arthralgia	51 (9%)
Myalgia	30 (5%)
Nervous System	
Dizziness	27 (5%)
Headache	132 (23%)
Psychiatric Disorders	
Depression	27 (5%)
Reproductive System	
Breast pain	92 (16%)
Dysmenorrhea	48 (8%)
Vaginal bleeding (all)	52 (9%)
Vaginitis	42 (7%)
Resistance Mechanism Disorders	
Viral infection	35 (6%)
Respiratory System	
Coughing	28 (5%)
Pharyngitis	38 (7%)
Sinusitis	44 (8%)
Upper respiratory-tract infection	121 (21%)

Endometrial Hyperplasia
See Table 4 for incidence of endometrial hyperplasia in clinical trials for efficacy.
In all clinical studies, endometrial biopsy specimens initially were read for safety by a single pathologist. All biopsies were subsequently evaluated by at least 2 blinded expert pathologists as per study protocol. Those biopsy specimens initially read as hyperplasia were reported in the safety database, were evaluated by the expert pathologist panel, and were determined not to be cases of hyperplasia.
The following additional adverse reactions have been reported with estrogen therapy (see **WARNINGS** and **PRECAUTIONS** regarding induction of neoplasia, increased incidence of gallbladder disease, cardiovascular disease, elevated blood pressure, and hypercalcemia).
1. **Genitourinary System.** Changes in vaginal bleeding pattern and abnormal withdrawal bleeding or flow; breakthrough bleeding, spotting; increase in size of uterine leiomyomata; vaginal candidiasis; change in amount of cervical secretion.
2. **Breasts.** Tenderness, enlargement, galactorrhea.
3. **Gastrointestinal.** Cholestatic jaundice, nausea, vomiting; abdominal cramps, bloating, increased incidence of gallbladder disease.
4. **Skin.** Chloasma or melasma; which may persist when drug is discontinued; erythema multiforme; erythema nodosum; hemorrhagic eruption; loss of scalp hair; hirsutism.
5. **Central Nervous System.** Headache, migraine, dizziness; mental depression; chorea.
6. **Eyes.** Steepening of corneal curvature; intolerance to contact lenses.
7. **Miscellaneous.** Increase or decrease in weight; reduced carbohydrate tolerance; aggravation of porphyria; edema; changes in libido.

OVERDOSAGE

No serious ill effects have been reported following acute ingestion of large doses of estrogen/progestin-containing oral contraceptives by young children. Overdosage may cause nausea and vomiting, and withdrawal bleeding may occur in females.

DOSAGE AND ADMINISTRATION

ORTHO-PREFEST™ regimen consists of the daily administration of a single tablet containing 1 mg estradiol (pink color) for three days followed by a single tablet of 1 mg estradiol combined with 0.09 mg norgestimate (white color) for three days. This regimen is repeated continuously without interruption.

1. For treatment of moderate to severe vasomotor symptoms and vulvar and vaginal atrophy associated with menopause, the patient should start with the first tablet in the first row, and place the weekday schedule sticker which starts with the weekday of first tablet intake in the appropriate space. After all tablets from the blister card have been used, the first tablet from a new blister card should be taken on the following day.
   This dose may not be the lowest effective dose for treatment of vulvar and vaginal atrophy.
   Patients should be re-evaluated at three-month to six-month intervals to determine if treatment for symptoms is still necessary.
2. For prevention of osteoporosis, the patient should start with the first tablet in the first row, and place the weekday schedule sticker which starts with the weekday of first tablet intake in the appropriate space. After all tablets from the blister card have been used, the first tablet from a new blister card should be taken on the following day.
   This dose may not be the lowest effective dose for the prevention of osteoporosis.

Missed Tablets
If a tablet is missed for one or more days, therapy should be resumed with the next available tablet. The patient should continue to take only one tablet each day in sequence.

HOW SUPPLIED

ORTHO-PREFEST™ is available as two separate, round-shaped tablets for oral administration supplied in a blister card with the following configuration: 3 pink tablets, followed by 3 white tablets for a total of 30 tablets per blister card.
Each blister card contains 15 tablets of each of the following components:
1 mg estradiol: pink tablets embossed with "1" and "J-C" on one side and "E2" and "O-M" on the other side.
1 mg estradiol/0.09mg norgestimate: white tablets embossed with "1/90" and "J-C" on one side and "E2/N" and "O-M" on the other side.
NDC: 0062-1840-01 ORTHO-PREFEST™, 30 Tablets/Blister
This product is stable for 18 months. Store at 25°C (77°F); excursions permitted to 15–30°C (59–86°F).

PATIENT INSTRUCTIONS

INFORMATION FOR THE PATIENT

INTRODUCTION

This leaflet describes when and how to use estrogens/progestins, and the risks and benefits of estrogen/progestin treatment.
Estrogens/progestins have important benefits but also some risks. You must decide, with your doctor, whether the risks are acceptable in comparison to the benefits. If you use estrogens, make sure you are using the lowest possible dose that works, and that you don't use them longer than necessary. How long you need to use estrogens will depend on the reason for use.

ESTROGENS INCREASE THE RISK OF CANCER OF THE UTERUS

THIS FINDING REFERS TO ESTROGENS GIVEN WITHOUT PROGESTIN

Progestin drugs taken with estrogen-containing drugs significantly reduce, but do not eliminate, this risk.
If you use any drug containing estrogen, it is important to visit your doctor regularly and report any unusual vaginal bleeding right away. Vaginal bleeding after menopause may be a warning sign of uterine cancer. Your doctor should evaluate any unusual vaginal bleeding to find out the cause.
If you take ORTHO-PREFEST™ and later find you were pregnant when you took it, be sure to discuss this with your doctor as soon as possible.

USES OF ESTROGEN

Not every estrogen drug is approved for every use listed in this section. If you want to know which of these uses are approved for the medicine prescribed for you, ask your doctor or pharmacist to show you the professional labeling.
To reduce moderate or severe menopausal symptoms. Estrogens are hormones made by the ovaries of normal women. Between ages 45 and 55, the ovaries normally stop making estrogens. This leads to a drop in body estrogen levels, which causes the "change of life" or menopause (the end of monthly menstrual periods). If both ovaries are removed during an operation before natural menopause takes place, the sudden drop in estrogen levels causes "surgical menopause."
When the estrogen levels begin dropping some women develop very uncomfortable symptoms such as feelings of warmth in the face, neck, and chest, or sudden intense episodes of heat and sweating ("hot flashes" or "hot flushes"). Using estrogen drugs can help the body adjust to lower estrogen levels and reduce these symptoms. Most women have only mild menopausal symptoms or none at all and do not need to use estrogen drugs for these symptoms. Others may need to take estrogens for a few months while their bodies adjust to lower estrogen levels. The majority of women do not need estrogen replacement for longer than six months for these symptoms.
To treat vulvar and vaginal atrophy (itching, burning, dryness in or around the vagina, difficulty or burning on urination) associated with menopause.
To prevent thinning of bones (osteoporosis). Osteoporosis is a thinning of the bones that makes them weaker and allows them to break more easily. The bones of the spine, wrists and hips break most often in osteoporosis. Both men and women start to lose bone mass after about age 40, but women lose bone mass faster after the menopause. Using estrogens after the menopause slows down bone thinning and may prevent bones from breaking. Lifelong adequate calcium intake, either in the diet (such as dairy products) or by calcium supplements (to reach a total daily intake of 1000 milligrams per day before menopause or 1500 milligrams per day after menopause), may help to prevent osteoporosis. Regular weight-bearing exercise may also help to prevent osteoporosis. Before you change your calcium intake or exercise habits, it is important to discuss these lifestyle changes with your doctor to find out if they are safe for you.
Since estrogen use has some risks, women who are likely to develop osteoporosis should use estrogens for prevention. Women who are likely to develop osteoporosis often have one or more of the following characteristics: White or Asian race, slim, cigarette smokers, and a family history of osteoporosis in a mother, sister, or aunt. Women who have relatively early menopause, often because their ovaries were removed during an operation (surgical menopause), are also more likely to develop osteoporosis than women whose menopause happens at the average age.

WHO SHOULD NOT USE ESTROGENS

Estrogens should not be used:
During pregnancy
If you think you may be pregnant, do not use any form of estrogen-containing drug. Using some types of estrogens while you are pregnant may cause your unborn child to have birth defects. Estrogens do not prevent miscarriage.
If you have unusual vaginal bleeding which has not been evaluated by your doctor
Unusual vaginal bleeding can be a warning sign of cancer of the uterus, especially if it happens after menopause. Your doctor must find out the cause of the bleeding so that he or she can recommend the proper treatment.
If you have had cancer
Since estrogens may increase the risk of certain types of breast and uterine cancer, you should not use estrogens unless your doctor recommends that you take it. (For certain patients with breast or prostate cancer, estrogens may help.)
If you have any circulation problems
Women with abnormal blood clotting conditions should avoid estrogen use (see **RISKS OF ESTROGENS AND/OR PROGESTINS**, below).
After childbirth or when breast-feeding a baby
Estrogens should not be used to try to stop the breasts from filling with milk after a baby is born. Such treatment may increase the risk of developing blood clots (see **RISKS OF ESTROGENS AND/OR PROGESTINS**, below).

RISKS OF ESTROGENS AND/OR PROGESTINS

Cancer of the uterus
Your risk of developing cancer of the uterus gets higher the longer you use estrogens and the larger the dose you use. Because of this risk, it is important to take the lowest dose that works and to take it only as long as you need it.
Using progestin therapy together with estrogen therapy reduces, but does not eliminate, the higher risk of uterine cancer related to estrogen use (see also **OTHER INFORMATION**, below).
If you have had your uterus removed (total hysterectomy), there is no danger of developing cancer of the uterus.
Cancer of the breast
Studies suggest a higher risk of breast cancer in women who have used estrogens for long periods of time (especially more than 10 years), or who use higher doses for shorter time periods. The effects of added progestin on the risks of breast cancer are unknown.
Regular breast examinations by a health professional and monthly self-examination are recommended for all women. Yearly mammography is recommended for women beginning at age 50.
Abnormal blood clotting
Taking estrogens may cause changes in your blood clotting system. These changes allow the blood to clot more easily, possibly allowing clots to form in your bloodstream. If blood clots do form in your bloodstream, they can cut off the blood supply to vital organs, causing serious problems. These problems may include a stroke (by cutting off blood to the brain), heart attack (by cutting off blood to the heart), a pulmonary clot (by cutting off blood to the lungs), or other problems. Any of these conditions may cause death or serious long-term disability.
Gallbladder disease
Women who use estrogens after menopause are more likely to develop gallbladder disease needing surgery than women who do not use estrogens.

SIDE EFFECTS

In addition to the risks listed above, the following side effects have been reported with estrogen and/or progestin use:
- Nausea and vomiting
- Breast tenderness or enlargement
- Enlargement of benign tumors of the uterus ("fibroids")
- Retention of excess fluid
- A spotty darkening of the skin, particularly on the face
- Irregular vaginal bleeding or spotting
- Headache, migraine, dizziness, faintness or change in vision including intolerance to contact lenses
- Mental depression
- Vaginal yeast infections

USE IN CHILDREN

Estrogen treatment has not been shown either effective or safe for use by infants, children or adolescent boys or girls.

REDUCING THE RISKS OF ESTROGEN USE

While you are using ORTHO-PREFEST™:
See your doctor regularly
Visit your doctor regularly for a check-up. If you develop vaginal bleeding, you may need further evaluation.
Reassess your need for treatment
You and your doctor should reevaluate whether or not you still need ORTHO-PREFEST™ every six months.
Be alert for signs of trouble
If any of these warning signals (or any other unusual symptoms) happen while you are using ORTHO-PREFEST™, call your doctor immediately:
- Abnormal bleeding from the vagina (possible uterine cancer).
- Pains in the calves or chest, a sudden shortness of breath or coughing blood (indicating possible clots in the legs, heart, or lungs).

Continued on next page

Ortho-Prefest—Cont.

- Severe headache or vomiting, dizziness, faintness, or changes in vision or speech, weakness or numbness of an arm or leg (indicating possible clots in the brain or eye).
- Breast lumps (possible breast cancer; ask your doctor or health professional to show you how to examine your breasts monthly).
- Yellowing of the skin and/or whites of the eyes (possible liver problems).
- Pain, swelling, or tenderness in the abdomen (possible gallbladder problem).

OTHER INFORMATION

Estrogens increase the risk of developing a condition (endometrial hyperplasia) that may lead to cancer of the lining of the uterus. Taking progestins, another hormonal drug, with estrogens lowers the risk of developing this condition. Since you still have your uterus, your doctor has prescribed ORTHO-PREFEST™ which has both an estrogen and progestin.

Your doctor has prescribed this drug for you and you alone. Do not give the drug to anyone else.

Keep this and all drugs out of the reach of children. In case of overdose, call your doctor, hospital, or poison control center immediately.

HOW SUPPLIED

ORTHO-PREFEST™ therapy consists of the daily administration of a single tablet containing 1 mg estradiol (pink color) for three days followed by a single tablet of 1 mg estradiol combined with 0.09 mg norgestimate (white color) for three days. The three days of pink tablets followed by 3-days of white tablets are repeated continuously during treatment.

ORTHO-PREFEST™ is available as two separate, round-shaped tablets for oral administration and is supplied in a blister card with the following configuration: 4 rows of 7 tablets each and one row with 2 tablets, with space on the blister to place one of 7 weekday schedules.

ORTHO-McNEIL PHARMACEUTICAL, INC.
Raritan, NJ 08869

 Issued December 1999 638-10-785-1

Shown in Product Identification Guide, page 328

ORTHO TRI-CYCLEN® Tablets ℞
ORTHO-CYCLEN® Tablets
(norgestimate/ethinyl estradiol)

Prescribing Information

Patients should be counseled that this product does not protect against HIV infection (AIDS) and other sexually transmitted diseases.

DESCRIPTION

Each of the following products is a combination oral contraceptive containing the progestational compound norgestimate and the estrogenic compound ethinyl estradiol.

ORTHO TRI-CYCLEN □ 21 Tablets and ORTHO TRI-CYCLEN □ 28 Tablets.

Each white tablet contains 0.180 mg of the progestational compound, norgestimate (18,19-Dinor-17-pregn-4-en-20-yn-3-one,17-(acetyloxy)-13-ethyl-,oxime,(17α)-(+)-) and 0.035 mg of the estrogenic compound, ethinyl estradiol (19-nor-17α-pregna,1,3,5(10)-trien-20-yne-3,17-diol). Inactive ingredients include lactose, magnesium stearate, and pregelatinized starch.

Each light blue tablet contains 0.215 mg of the progestational compound norgestimate (18,19-Dinor-17-pregn-4-en-20-yn-3-one,17-(acetyloxy)-13-ethyl-,oxime,(17α)-(+)-) and 0.035 mg of the estrogenic compound, ethinyl estradiol (19-nor-17α-pregna,1,3,5(10)-trien-20-yne-3,17-diol). Inactive ingredients include FD&C Blue No. 2 Aluminum Lake, lactose, magnesium stearate, and pregelatinized starch.

Each blue tablet contains 0.250 mg of the progestational compound norgestimate (18,19-Dinor-17-pregn-4-en-20-yn-3-one,17-(acetyloxy)-13-ethyl-,oxime,(17α)-(+)-) and 0.035 mg of the estrogenic compound, ethinyl estradiol (19-nor-17α-pregna,1,3,5(10)-trien-20-yne-3,17-diol). Inactive ingredients include FD&C Blue No. 2 Aluminum Lake, lactose, magnesium stearate, and pregelatinized starch.

Each green tablet in the ORTHO TRI-CYCLEN □ 28 package contains only inert ingredients, as follows: D&C Yellow No. 10 Aluminum Lake, FD&C Blue No. 2 Aluminum Lake, lactose, magnesium stearate, microcrystalline cellulose and pregelatinized starch.

ORTHO-CYCLEN □ 21 Tablets and ORTHO-CYCLEN □ 28 Tablets.

Each blue tablet contains 0.250 mg of the progestational compound norgestimate (18,19-Dinor-17-pregn-4-en-20-yn-3-one,17-(acetyloxy)-13-ethyl-,oxime,(17α)-(+)-) and 0.035 mg of the estrogenic compound, ethinyl estradiol (19-nor-17α-pregna,1,3,5(10)-trien-20-yne-3,17-diol). Inactive ingredients include FD&C Blue No. 2 Aluminum Lake, lactose, magnesium stearate, and pregelatinized starch.

Each green tablet in the ORTHO-CYCLEN □ 28 package contains only inert ingredients, as follows: D&C Yellow No. 10 Aluminum Lake, FD&C Blue No. 2 Aluminum Lake, lactose, magnesium stearate, microcrystalline cellulose and pregelatinized starch.

[See chemical structures at top of next column]

Norgestimate

Ethinyl Estradiol

CLINICAL PHARMACOLOGY

ORAL CONTRACEPTION

Combination oral contraceptives act by suppression of gonadotropins. Although the primary mechanism of this action is inhibition of ovulation, other alterations include changes in the cervical mucus (which increase the difficulty of sperm entry into the uterus) and the endometrium (which reduce the likelihood of implantation).

Receptor binding studies, as well as studies in animals and humans, have shown that norgestimate and 17-deacetyl norgestimate, the major serum metabolite, combine high progestational activity with minimal intrinsic androgenicity.[90–93] Norgestimate, in combination with ethinyl estradiol, does not counteract the estrogen-induced increases in sex hormone binding globulin (SHBG), resulting in lower serum testosterone.[90,91,94]

ACNE

Acne is a skin condition with a multifactorial etiology. The combination of ethinyl estradiol and norgestimate may increase sex hormone binding globulin (SHBG) and decrease free testosterone resulting in a decrease in the severity of facial acne in otherwise healthy women with this skin condition.

Norgestimate and ethinyl estradiol are well absorbed following oral administration of ORTHO-CYCLEN and ORTHO TRI-CYCLEN. On the average, peak serum concentrations of norgestimate and ethinyl estradiol are observed within two hours (0.5–2.0 hr for norgestimate and 0.75–3.0 hr for ethinyl estradiol) after administration followed by a rapid decline due to distribution and elimination. Although norgestimate serum concentrations following single or multiple dosing were generally below assay detection within 5 hours, a major norgestimate serum metabolite, 17-deacetyl norgestimate, (which exhibits a serum half-life ranging from 12 to 30 hours) appears rapidly in serum with concentrations greatly exceeding that of norgestimate. The 17-deacetylated metabolite is pharmacologically active and the pharmacologic profile is similar to that of norgestimate. The elimination half-life of ethinyl estradiol ranged from approximately 6 to 14 hours.

Both norgestimate and ethinyl estradiol are extensively metabolized and eliminated by renal and fecal pathways. Following administration of ^{14}C-norgestimate, 47% (45–49%) and 37% (16–49%) of the administered radioactivity was eliminated in the urine and feces, respectively. Unchanged norgestimate was not detected in the urine. In addition to 17-deacetyl norgestimate, a number of metabolites of norgestimate have been identified in human urine following administration of radiolabeled norgestimate. These include 18,19-Dinor-17-pregn-4-en-20-yn-3-one,17-hydroxy-13-ethyl,(17α)-(-);18,19-Dinor-5β-17-pregnan-20-yn,3α,17β-dihydroxy-13-ethyl,(17α), various hydroxylated metabolites and conjugates of these metabolites. Ethinyl estradiol is metabolized to various hydroxylated products and their glucuronide and sulfate conjugates.

INDICATIONS AND USAGE

ORTHO-CYCLEN and ORTHO TRI-CYCLEN Tablets are indicated for the prevention of pregnancy in women who elect to use oral contraceptives as a method of contraception.

ORTHO TRI-CYCLEN is indicated for the treatment of moderate acne vulgaris in females, ≥ 15 years of age, who have no known contraindications to oral contraceptive therapy, desire contraception, have achieved menarche and are unresponsive to topical anti-acne medications.

Oral contraceptives are highly effective. Table I lists the typical accidental pregnancy rates for users of combination oral contraceptives and other methods of contraception. The efficacy of these contraceptive methods, except sterilization, depends upon the reliability with which they are used. Correct and consistent use of methods can result in lower failure rates.

[See table I at bottom of next page]

In clinical trials with ORTHO-CYCLEN, 1,651 subjects completed 24,272 cycles and a total of 18 pregnancies were reported. This represents an overall use-efficacy (typical user efficacy) pregnancy rate of 0.96 per 100 women-years. This rate includes patients who did not take the drug correctly.

In four clinical trials with ORTHO TRI-CYCLEN, the use-efficacy pregnancy rate ranged from 0.68 to 1.47 per 100 women-years. In total, 4,756 subjects completed 45,244 cycles and a total of 42 pregnancies were reported. This represents an overall use-efficacy rate of 1.21 per 100 women-years. One of these 4 studies was a randomized comparative clinical trial in which 4,633 subjects completed 22,312 cycles. Of the 2,312 patients on ORTHO TRI-CYCLEN, 8 pregnancies were reported. This represents an overall use-efficacy pregnancy rate of 0.94 per 100 women-years.

In two double-blind, placebo-controlled, six month, multicenter clinical trials, ORTHO TRI-CYCLEN showed a statistically significant decrease in inflammatory lesion count and total lesion count (Table II). The adverse reaction profile of ORTHO TRI-CYCLEN from these two controlled clinical trials is consistent with what has been noted from previous studies involving ORTHO TRI-CYCLEN and are the known risks associated with oral contraceptives.

TABLE II: Acne Vulgaris Indication
Combined Results: Two Multicenter,
Placebo-Controlled Trials Primary Efficacy Variables:
Evaluable-for-Efficacy Population

	ORTHO TRI-CYCLEN®	Placebo
	N = 163	N = 161
Mean Age at Enrollment	27.3 years	28.0
Inflammatory Lesions– Mean Percent Reduction	56.6	36.6
Total Lesions– Mean Percent Reduction	49.6	30.3

CONTRAINDICATIONS

Oral contraceptives should not be used in women who currently have the following conditions:

- Thrombophlebitis or thromboembolic disorders
- A past history of deep vein thrombophlebitis or thromboembolic disorders
- Cerebral vascular or coronary artery disease
- Known or suspected carcinoma of the breast
- Carcinoma of the endometrium or other known or suspected estrogen-dependent neoplasia
- Undiagnosed abnormal genital bleeding
- Cholestatic jaundice of pregnancy or jaundice with prior pill use
- Hepatic adenomas or carcinomas
- Known or suspected pregnancy

WARNINGS

Cigarette smoking increases the risk of serious cardiovascular side effects from oral contraceptive use. This risk increases with age and with heavy smoking (15 or more cigarettes per day) and is quite marked in women over 35 years of age. Women who use oral contraceptives should be strongly advised not to smoke.

The use of oral contraceptives is associated with increased risks of several serious conditions including myocardial infarction, thromboembolism, stroke, hepatic neoplasia, and gallbladder disease, although the risk of serious morbidity or mortality is very small in healthy women without underlying risk factors. The risk of morbidity and mortality increases significantly in the presence of other underlying risk factors such as hypertension, hyperlipidemias, obesity and diabetes.

Practitioners prescribing oral contraceptives should be familiar with the following information relating to these risks.

The information contained in this package insert is principally based on studies carried out in patients who used oral contraceptives with higher formulations of estrogens and progestogens than those in common use today. The effect of long-term use of the oral contraceptives with lower formulations of both estrogens and progestogens remains to be determined.

Throughout this labeling, epidemiological studies reported are of two types: retrospective or case control studies and prospective or cohort studies. Case control studies provide a measure of the relative risk of a disease, namely, a *ratio* of the incidence of a disease among oral contraceptive users to that among nonusers. The relative risk does not provide information on the actual clinical occurrence of a disease. Cohort studies provide a measure of attributable risk, which is the *difference* in the incidence of disease between oral contraceptive users and nonusers. The attributable risk does provide information about the actual occurrence of a disease in the population (adapted from refs. 2 and 3 with the author's permission). For further information, the reader is referred to a text on epidemiological methods.

1. THROMBOEMBOLIC DISORDERS AND OTHER VASCULAR PROBLEMS

a. Myocardial Infarction

An increased risk of myocardial infarction has been attributed to oral contraceptive use. This risk is primarily in smokers or women with other underlying risk factors for coronary artery disease such as hypertension, hypercholesterolemia, morbid obesity, and diabetes. The relative risk of heart attack for current oral contraceptive users has been estimated to be two to six.[4–10] The risk is very low under the age of 30.

Smoking in combination with oral contraceptive use has been shown to contribute substantially to the incidence of myocardial infarctions in women in their mid-thirties or older with smoking accounting for the majority of excess cases.[11] Mortality rates associated with circulatory disease have been shown to increase substantially in smokers, especially in those 35 years of age and older among women who use oral contraceptives.

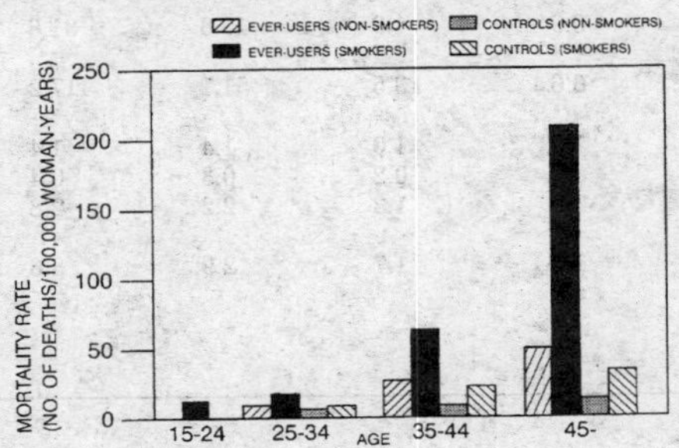

TABLE III. (Adapted from P.M. Layde and V. Beral, ref. #12.)

Oral contraceptives may compound the effects of well-known risk factors, such as hypertension, diabetes, hyperlipidemias, age and obesity.[13] In particular, some progestogens are known to decrease HDL cholesterol and cause glucose intolerance, while estrogens may create a state of hyper insulinism.[14–18] Oral contraceptives have been shown to increase blood pressure among users (see Section 9 in WARNINGS). Similar effects on risk factors have been associated with an increased risk of heart disease. Oral contraceptives must be used with caution in women with cardiovascular disease risk factors.

Norgestimate has minimal androgenic activity (see CLINICAL PHARMACOLOGY), and there is some evidence that the risk of myocardial infarction associated with oral contraceptives is lower when the progestogen has minimal androgenic activity than when the activity is greater[97].

b. Thromboembolism

An increased risk of thromboembolic and thrombotic disease associated with the use of oral contraceptives is well established. Case control studies have found the relative risk of users compared to nonusers to be 3 for the first episode of superficial venous thrombosis, 4 to 11 for deep vein thrombosis or pulmonary embolism, and 1.5 to 6 for women with predisposing conditions for venous thromboembolic disease.[2,3,19–24] Cohort studies have shown the relative risk to be somewhat lower, about 3 for new cases and about 4.5 for new cases requiring hospitalization.[25] The risk of thromboembolic disease associated with oral contraceptives is not related to length of use and disappears after pill use is stopped.[2]

A two- to four-fold increase in relative risk of post-operative thromboembolic complications has been reported with the use of oral contraceptives.[9] The relative risk of venous thrombosis in women who have predisposing conditions is twice that of women without such medical conditions.[26] If feasible, oral contraceptives should be discontinued at least four weeks prior to and for two weeks after elective surgery of a type associated with an increase in risk of thromboembolism and during and following prolonged immobilization. Since the immediate postpartum period is also associated with an increased risk of thromboembolism, oral contraceptives should be started no earlier than four weeks after delivery in women who elect not to breast feed or four weeks after a second trimester abortion.

c. Cerebrovascular diseases

Oral contraceptives have been shown to increase both the relative and attributable risks of cerebrovascular events (thrombotic and hemorrhagic strokes), although, in general, the risk is greatest among older (>35 years), hypertensive women who also smoke. Hypertension was found to be a risk factor for both users and nonusers, for both types of strokes, and smoking interacted to increase the risk of stroke.[27–29]

In a large study, the relative risk of thrombotic strokes has been shown to range from 3 for normotensive users to 14 for users with severe hypertension.[30] The relative risk of hemorrhagic stroke is reported to be 1.2 for non-smokers who used oral contraceptives, 2.6 for smokers who did not use oral contraceptives, 7.6 for smokers who used oral contraceptives, 1.8 for normotensive users and 25.7 for users with severe hypertension.[30] The attributable risk is also greater in older women.[3]

TABLE I: PERCENTAGE OF WOMEN EXPERIENCING AN UNINTENDED PREGNANCY DURING THE FIRST YEAR OF TYPICAL USE AND THE FIRST YEAR OF PERFECT USE OF CONTRACEPTION AND THE PERCENTAGE CONTINUING USE AT THE END OF THE FIRST YEAR. UNITED STATES.

Method (1)	% of Women Experiencing an Unintended Pregnancy within the First Year of Use: Typical Use[1] (2)	Perfect Use[2] (3)	% of Women Continuing Use at One Year[3] (4)
Chance [4]	85	85	
Spermicides[5]	26	6	40
Periodic abstinence	25		63
Calendar		9	
Ovulation Method		3	
Sympto-Thermal[6]		2	
Post-Ovulation		1	
Withdrawal	19	4	
Cap[7]			
Parous Women	40	26	42
Nulliparous Women	20	9	56
Sponge			
Parous Women	40	20	42
Nulliparous Women	20	9	56
Diaphragm[7]	20	6	56
Condom[8]			
Female (Reality)	21	5	56
Male	14	3	61
Pill	5		71
Progestin Only		0.5	
Combined		0.1	
IUD			
Progesterone T	2.0	1.5	81
Copper T380A	0.8	0.6	78
LNg 20	0.1	0.1	81
Depo-Provera	0.3	0.3	70
Norplant and Norplant-2	0.05	0.05	88
Female Sterilization	0.5	0.5	100
Male Sterilization	0.15	0.10	100

Adapted from Hatcher et al., 1998 Ref. #1.

[1] Among typical couples who initiate use of a method (not necessarily for the first time), the percentage who experience an accidental pregnancy during the first year if they do not stop use for any other reason.

[2] Among couples who initiate use of a method (not necessarily for the first time) and who use it perfectly (both consistently and correctly), the percentage who experience an accidental pregnancy during the first year if they do not stop use for any other reason.

[3] Among couples attempting to avoid pregnancy, the percentage who continue to use a method for one year.

[4] The percents becoming pregnant in columns (2) and (3) are based on data from populations where contraception is not used and from women who cease using contraception in order to become pregnant. Among such populations, about 89% become pregnant within one year. This estimate was lowered slightly (to 85%) to represent the percent who would become pregnant within one year among women now relying on reversible methods of contraception if they abandoned contraception altogether.

[5] Foams, creams, gels, vaginal suppositories, and vaginal film.

[6] Cervical mucus (ovulation) method supplemented by calendar in the pre-ovulatory and basal body temperature in the post-ovulatory phases.

[7] With spermicidal cream or jelly.

[8] Without spermicides.

d. Dose-related risk of vascular disease from oral contraceptives

A positive association has been observed between the amount of estrogen and progestogen in oral contraceptives and the risk of vascular disease.[31–33] A decline in serum high density lipoproteins (HDL) has been reported with many progestational agents.[14–16] A decline in serum high density lipoproteins has been associated with an increased incidence of ischemic heart disease. Because estrogens increase HDL cholesterol, the net effect of an oral contraceptive depends on a balance achieved between doses of estrogen and progestogen and the activity of the progestogen used in the contraceptives. The activity and amount of both hormones should be considered in the choice of an oral contraceptive.

Minimizing exposure to estrogen and progestogen is in keeping with good principles of therapeutics. For any particular estrogen/progestogen combination, the dosage regimen prescribed should be one which contains the least amount of estrogen and progestogen that is compatible with a low failure rate and the needs of the individual patient. New acceptors of oral contraceptive agents should be started on preparations containing 0.035 mg or less of estrogen.

e. Persistence of risk of vascular disease

There are two studies which have shown persistence of risk of vascular disease for ever-users of oral contraceptives. In a study in the United States, the risk of developing myocardial infarction after discontinuing oral contraceptives persists for at least 9 years for women 40-49 years who had used oral contraceptives for five or more years, but this increased risk was not demonstrated in other age groups.[8] In another study in Great Britain, the risk of developing cerebrovascular disease persisted for at least 6 years after discontinuation of oral contraceptives, although excess risk was very small.[34] However, both studies were performed with oral contraceptive formulations containing 50 micrograms or higher of estrogens.

2. ESTIMATES OF MORTALITY FROM CONTRACEPTIVE USE

One study gathered data from a variety of sources which have estimated the mortality rate associated with different methods of contraception at different ages (Table IV). These estimates include the combined risk of death associated with contraceptive methods plus the risk attributable to pregnancy in the event of method failure. Each method of contraception has its specific benefits and risks. The study concluded that with the exception of oral contraceptive users 35 and older who smoke, and 40 and older who do not smoke, mortality associated with all methods of birth control is low and below that associated with childbirth. The observation of an increase in risk of mortality with age for oral contraceptive users is based on data gathered in the 1970's.[35] Current clinical recommendation involves the use of lower estrogen dose formulations and a careful consideration of risk factors. In 1989, the Fertility and Maternal Health Drugs Advisory Committee was asked to review the use of oral contraceptives in women 40 years of age and over. The Committee concluded that although cardiovascular disease risks may be increased with oral contraceptive use after age 40 in healthy non-smoking women (even with the newer low-dose formulations), there are also greater potential health risks associated with pregnancy in older women and with the alternative surgical and medical procedures which may be necessary if such women do not have access to effective and acceptable means of contraception. The Committee recommended that the benefits of low-dose oral contraceptive use by healthy non-smoking women over 40 may outweigh the possible risks.

Of course, older women, as all women, who take oral contraceptives, should take an oral contraceptive which contains the least amount of estrogen and progestogen that is compatible with a low failure rate and individual patient needs.

[See table IV at top of next page]

3. CARCINOMA OF THE REPRODUCTIVE ORGANS AND BREASTS

Numerous epidemiological studies have been performed on the incidence of breast, endometrial, ovarian, and cervical cancer in women using oral contraceptives. While there are conflicting reports, most studies suggest that use of oral contraceptives is not associated with an overall increase in the risk of developing breast cancer. Some studies have reported an increased relative risk of developing breast cancer, particularly at a younger age. This increased relative risk has been reported to be related to duration of use.[36–44,79–89]

A meta-analysis of 54 studies found a small increase in the frequency of having breast cancer diagnosed for women who were currently using combined oral contraceptives or had used them within the past ten years. This increase in the frequency of breast cancer diagnosis, within ten years of stopping use, was generally accounted for by cancers localized to the breast. There was no increase in the frequency of having breast cancer diagnosed ten or more years after cessation of use.[95]

Some studies suggest that oral contraceptive use has been associated with an increase in the risk of cervical intraepithelial neoplasia in some populations of women.[45–48] However, there continues to be controversy about the extent to which such findings may be due to differences in sexual behavior and other factors.

Continued on next page

Ortho Tri-Cyclen—Cont.

4. HEPATIC NEOPLASIA
Benign hepatic adenomas are associated with oral contraceptive use, although the incidence of benign tumors is rare in the United States. Indirect calculations have estimated the attributable risk to be in the range of 3.3 cases/100,000 for users, a risk that increases after four or more years of use especially with oral contraceptives of higher dose.[49] Rupture of benign, hepatic adenomas may cause death through intra-abdominal hemorrhage.[50,51]
Studies have shown an increased risk of developing hepatocellular carcinoma[52–54, 96] in oral contraceptive users. However, these cancers are rare in the U.S.
5. OCULAR LESIONS
There have been clinical case reports of retinal thrombosis associated with the use of oral contraceptives. Oral contraceptives should be discontinued if there is unexplained partial or complete loss of vision; onset of proptosis or diplopia; papilledema; or retinal vascular lesions. Appropriate diagnostic and therapeutic measures should be undertaken immediately.
6. ORAL CONTRACEPTIVE USE BEFORE OR DURING EARLY PREGNANCY
Extensive epidemiological studies have revealed no increased risk of birth defects in women who have used oral contraceptives prior to pregnancy.[56,57] The majority of recent studies also do not indicate a teratogenic effect, particularly in so far as cardiac anomalies and limb reduction defects are concerned,[55,56,58,59] when taken inadvertently during early pregnancy.
The administration of oral contraceptives to induce withdrawal bleeding should not be used as a test for pregnancy. Oral contraceptives should not be used during pregnancy to treat threatened or habitual abortion.
It is recommended that for any patient who has missed two consecutive periods, pregnancy should be ruled out before continuing oral contraceptive use. If the patient has not adhered to the prescribed schedule, the possibility of pregnancy should be considered at the time of the first missed period. Oral contraceptive use should be discontinued until pregnancy is ruled out.
7. GALLBLADDER DISEASE
Earlier studies have reported an increased lifetime relative risk of gallbladder surgery in users of oral contraceptives and estrogens.[60,61] More recent studies, however, have shown that the relative risk of developing gallbladder disease among oral contraceptive users may be minimal.[62–64] The recent findings of minimal risk may be related to the use of oral contraceptive formulations containing lower hormonal doses of estrogens and progestogens.
8. CARBOHYDRATE AND LIPID METABOLIC EFFECTS
Oral contraceptives have been shown to cause a decrease in glucose tolerance in a significant percentage of users.[17] This effect has been shown to be directly related to estrogen dose.[65] Progestogens increase insulin secretion and create insulin resistance, this effect varying with different progestational agents.[17,66] However, in the non-diabetic woman, oral contraceptives appear to have no effect on fasting blood glucose.[67] Because of these demonstrated effects, prediabetic and diabetic women in particular should be carefully monitored while taking oral contraceptives.
A small proportion of women will have persistent hypertriglyceridemia while on the pill. As discussed earlier (see WARNINGS 1a and 1d), changes in serum triglycerides and lipoprotein levels have been reported in oral contraceptive users.
In clinical studies with ORTHO-CYCLEN there were no clinically significant changes in fasting blood glucose levels. No statistically significant changes in mean fasting blood glucose levels were observed over 24 cycles of use. Glucose tolerance tests showed minimal, clinically insignificant changes from baseline to cycles 3, 12, and 24.
In clinical studies with ORTHO TRI-CYCLEN there were no clinically significant changes in fasting blood glucose levels. Minimal statistically significant changes were noted in glucose levels over 24 cycles of use. Glucose tolerance tests showed no clinically significant changes from baseline to cycles 3, 12, and 24.
9. ELEVATED BLOOD PRESSURE
An increase in blood pressure has been reported in women taking oral contraceptives[68] and this increase is more likely in older oral contraceptive users[69] and with extended duration of use.[61] Data from the Royal College of General Practitioners[12] and subsequent randomized trials have shown that the incidence of hypertension increases with increasing progestational activity.
Women with a history of hypertension or hypertension-related diseases, or renal disease[70] should be encouraged to use another method of contraception. If women elect to use oral contraceptives, they should be monitored closely and if significant elevation of blood pressure occurs, oral contraceptives should be discontinued. For most women, elevated blood pressure will return to normal after stopping oral contraceptives, and there is no difference in the occurrence of hypertension between former and never users.[68–71]
It should be noted that in two separate large clinical trials (N = 633 and N = 911), no statistically significant changes in mean blood pressure were observed with ORTHO-CYCLEN.

TABLE IV: ANNUAL NUMBER OF BIRTH-RELATED OR METHOD-RELATED DEATHS ASSOCIATED WITH CONTROL OF FERTILITY PER 100,000 NON-STERILE WOMEN, BY FERTILITY CONTROL METHOD ACCORDING TO AGE

Method of control and outcome	15–19	20–24	25–29	30–34	35–39	40–44
No fertility control methods*	7.0	7.4	9.1	14.8	25.7	28.2
Oral contraceptives non-smoker**	0.3	0.5	0.9	1.9	13.8	31.6
Oral contraceptives smoker**	2.2	3.4	6.6	13.5	51.1	117.2
IUD**	0.8	0.8	1.0	1.0	1.4	1.4
Condom*	1.1	1.6	0.7	0.2	0.3	0.4
Diaphragm/ spermicide*	1.9	1.2	1.2	1.3	2.2	2.8
Periodic abstinence*	2.5	1.6	1.6	1.7	2.9	3.6

*Deaths are birth-related
**Deaths are method-related

Adapted from H.W. Ory, ref. #35.

10. HEADACHE
The onset or exacerbation of migraine or development of headache with a new pattern which is recurrent, persistent or severe requires discontinuation of oral contraceptives and evaluation of the cause.
11. BLEEDING IRREGULARITIES
Breakthrough bleeding and spotting are sometimes encountered in patients on oral contraceptives, especially during the first three months of use. Non-hormonal causes should be considered and adequate diagnostic measures taken to rule out malignancy or pregnancy in the event of breakthrough bleeding, as in the case of any abnormal vaginal bleeding. If pathology has been excluded, time or a change to another formulation may solve the problem. In the event of amenorrhea, pregnancy should be ruled out.
Some women may encounter post-pill amenorrhea or oligomenorrhea, especially when such a condition was preexistent.
12. ECTOPIC PREGNANCY
Ectopic as well as intrauterine pregnancy may occur in contraceptive failures.

PRECAUTIONS

1. PHYSICAL EXAMINATION AND FOLLOW UP
It is good medical practice for all women to have annual history and physical examinations, including women using oral contraceptives. The physical examination, however, may be deferred until after initiation of oral contraceptives if requested by the woman and judged appropriate by the clinician. The physical examination should include special reference to blood pressure, breasts, abdomen and pelvic organs, including cervical cytology, and relevant laboratory tests. In case of undiagnosed, persistent or recurrent abnormal vaginal bleeding, appropriate measures should be conducted to rule out malignancy. Women with a strong family history of breast cancer or who have breast nodules should be monitored with particular care.
2. LIPID DISORDERS
Women who are being treated for hyperlipidemias should be followed closely if they elect to use oral contraceptives. Some progestogens may elevate LDL levels and may render the control of hyperlipidemias more difficult.
3. LIVER FUNCTION
If jaundice develops in any woman receiving such drugs, the medication should be discontinued. Steroid hormones may be poorly metabolized in patients with impaired liver function.
4. FLUID RETENTION
Oral contraceptives may cause some degree of fluid retention. They should be prescribed with caution, and only with careful monitoring, in patients with conditions which might be aggravated by fluid retention.
5. EMOTIONAL DISORDERS
Women with a history of depression should be carefully observed and the drug discontinued if depression recurs to a serious degree.
6. CONTACT LENSES
Contact lens wearers who develop visual changes or changes in lens tolerance should be assessed by an ophthalmologist.
7. DRUG INTERACTIONS
Reduced efficacy and increased incidence of breakthrough bleeding and menstrual irregularities have been associated with concomitant use of rifampin. A similar association, though less marked, has been suggested with barbiturates, phenylbutazone, phenytoin sodium, carbamazepine, and possibly with griseofulvin, ampicillin and tetracyclines.[72]
8. INTERACTIONS WITH LABORATORY TESTS
Certain endocrine and liver function tests and blood components may be affected by oral contraceptives:
a. Increased prothrombin and factors VII, VIII, IX, and X; decreased antithrombin 3; increased norepinephrine-induced platelet aggregability.
b. Increased thyroid binding globulin (TBG) leading to increased circulating total thyroid hormone, as measured by protein-bound iodine (PBI), T4 by column or by radioimmunoassay. Free T3 resin uptake is decreased, reflecting the elevated TBG, free T4 concentration is unaltered.
c. Other binding proteins may be elevated in serum.
d. Sex hormone binding globulins are increased and result in elevated levels of total circulating sex steroids; however, free or biologically active levels either decrease or remain unchanged.
e. High-density lipoprotein (HDL-C) and total cholesterol (Total-C) may be increased, low-density lipoprotein (LDL-C) may be increased or decreased, while LDL-C/HDL-C ratio may be decreased and triglycerides may be unchanged.
f. Glucose tolerance may be decreased.
g. Serum folate levels may be depressed by oral contraceptive therapy. This may be of clinical significance if a woman becomes pregnant shortly after discontinuing oral contraceptives.
9. CARCINOGENESIS
See WARNINGS Section.
10. PREGNANCY
Pregnancy Category X. See CONTRAINDICATIONS and WARNINGS Sections.
11. NURSING MOTHERS
Small amounts of oral contraceptive steroids have been identified in the milk of nursing mothers and a few adverse effects on the child have been reported, including jaundice and breast enlargement. In addition, combination oral contraceptives given in the postpartum period may interfere with lactation by decreasing the quantity and quality of breast milk. If possible, the nursing mother should be advised not to use combination oral contraceptives but to use other forms of contraception until she has completely weaned her child.
12. PEDIATRIC USE
Safety and efficacy of ORTHO-CYCLEN Tablets and ORTHO TRI-CYCLEN Tablets has been established in women of reproductive age. Safety and efficacy are expected to be the same for postpubertal adolescents under the age of 16 and for users 16 years and older. Use of this product before menarche is not indicated.
13. SEXUALLY TRANSMITTED DISEASES
Patients should be counseled that this product does not protect against HIV infection (AIDS) and other sexually transmitted diseases.

INFORMATION FOR THE PATIENT
See Patient Labeling printed below.

ADVERSE REACTIONS

An increased risk of the following serious adverse reactions has been associated with the use of oral contraceptives (See WARNINGS Section).

- Thrombophlebitis and venous thrombosis with or without embolism
- Arterial thromboembolism
- Pulmonary embolism
- Myocardial infarction
- Cerebral hemorrhage
- Cerebral thrombosis
- Hypertension
- Gallbladder disease
- Hepatic adenomas or benign liver tumors

The following adverse reactions have been reported in patients receiving oral contraceptives and are believed to be drug-related:

- Nausea
- Vomiting
- Gastrointestinal symptoms (such as abdominal cramps and bloating)
- Breakthrough bleeding
- Spotting
- Change in menstrual flow
- Amenorrhea
- Temporary infertility after discontinuation of treatment
- Edema
- Melasma which may persist
- Breast changes: tenderness, enlargement, secretion
- Change in weight (increase or decrease)
- Change in cervical erosion and secretion
- Diminution in lactation when given immediately postpartum
- Cholestatic jaundice
- Migraine
- Rash (allergic)

- Mental depression
- Reduced tolerance to carbohydrates
- Vaginal candidiasis
- Change in corneal curvature (steepening)
- Intolerance to contact lenses

The following adverse reactions have been reported in users of oral contraceptives and the association has been neither confirmed nor refuted:

- Pre-menstrual syndrome
- Cataracts
- Changes in appetite
- Cystitis-like syndrome
- Headache
- Nervousness
- Dizziness
- Hirsutism
- Loss of scalp hair
- Erythema multiforme
- Erythema nodosum
- Hemorrhagic eruption
- Vaginitis
- Porphyria
- Impaired renal function
- Hemolytic uremic syndrome
- Acne
- Changes in libido
- Colitis
- Budd-Chiari Syndrome

OVERDOSAGE

Serious ill effects have not been reported following acute ingestion of large doses of oral contraceptives by young children. Overdosage may cause nausea and withdrawal bleeding may occur in females.

NON-CONTRACEPTIVE HEALTH BENEFITS

The following non-contraceptive health benefits related to the use of combination oral contraceptives are supported by epidemiological studies which largely utilized oral contraceptive formulations containing estrogen doses exceeding 0.035 mg of ethinyl estradiol or 0.05 mg mestranol.[73–78]

Effects on menses:

- increased menstrual cycle regularity
- decreased blood loss and decreased incidence of iron deficiency anemia
- decreased incidence of dysmenorrhea

Effects related to inhibition of ovulation:

- decreased incidence of functional ovarian cysts
- decreased incidence of ectopic pregnancies

Other effects:

- decreased incidence of fibroadenomas and fibrocystic disease of the breast
- decreased incidence of acute pelvic inflammatory disease
- decreased incidence of endometrial cancer
- decreased incidence of ovarian cancer

DOSAGE AND ADMINISTRATION

ORAL CONTRACEPTION

To achieve maximum contraceptive effectiveness, ORTHO TRI-CYCLEN Tablets and ORTHO-CYCLEN Tablets must be taken exactly as directed and at intervals not exceeding 24 hours. ORTHO TRI-CYCLEN and ORTHO-CYCLEN are available in the DIALPAK® Tablet Dispenser which is preset for a Sunday Start. Day 1 Start is also provided.

21-Day Regimen (Sunday Start)

When taking ORTHO TRI-CYCLEN □ 21 and ORTHO-CYCLEN □ 21, the first tablet should be taken on the first Sunday after menstruation begins. If period begins on Sunday, the first tablet is taken on that day. One tablet is taken daily for 21 days. For subsequent cycles, no tablets are taken for 7 days, then a tablet is taken the next day (Sunday). For the first cycle of a Sunday Start regimen, another method of contraception should be used until after the first 7 consecutive days of administration.

If the patient misses one (1) active tablet in Weeks 1, 2, or 3, the tablet should be taken as soon as she remembers. If the patient misses two (2) active tablets in Week 1 or Week 2, the patient should take two (2) tablets the day she remembers and two (2) tablets the next day; and then continue taking one (1) tablet a day until she finishes the pack. The patient should be instructed to use a back-up method of birth control if she has sex in the seven (7) days after missing pills. If the patient misses two (2) active tablets in the third week or misses three (3) or more active tablets in a row, the patient should continue taking one tablet every day until Sunday. On Sunday the patient should throw out the rest of the pack and start a new pack that same day. The patient should be instructed to use a back-up method of birth control if she has sex in the seven (7) days after missing pills.

Complete instructions to facilitate patient counseling on proper pill usage may be found in the Detailed Patient Labeling ("How to Take the Pill" section).

21-Day Regimen (Day 1 Start)

The dosage of ORTHO TRI-CYCLEN □ 21 and ORTHO-CYCLEN □ 21, for the initial cycle of therapy is one tablet administered daily from the 1st day through the 21st day of the menstrual cycle, counting the first day of menstrual flow as "Day 1." For subsequent cycles, no tablets are taken for 7 days, then a new course is started of one tablet a day for 21 days. The dosage regimen then continues with 7 days of no medication, followed by 21 days of medication, instituting a three-weeks-on, one-week-off dosage regimen.

If the patient misses one (1) active tablet in Weeks 1, 2, or 3, the tablet should be taken as soon as she remembers. If the patient misses two (2) active tablets in Week 1 or Week 2, the patient should take two (2) tablets the day she remembers and two (2) tablets the next day; and then continue taking one (1) tablet a day until she finishes the pack. The patient should be instructed to use a back-up method of birth control if she has sex in the seven (7) days after missing pills. If the patient misses two (2) active tablets in the third week or misses three (3) or more active tablets in a row, the patient should throw out the rest of the pack and start a new pack that same day. The patient should be instructed to use a back-up method of birth control if she has sex in the seven (7) days after missing pills.

Complete instructions to facilitate patient counseling on proper pill usage may be found in the Detailed Patient Labeling ("How to Take the Pill" section).

28-Day Regimen (Sunday Start)

When taking ORTHO TRI-CYCLEN □ 28 and ORTHO-CYCLEN □ 28 the first tablet should be taken on the first Sunday after menstruation begins. If period begins on Sunday, the first tablet should be taken that day. Take one active tablet daily for 21 days followed by one green tablet daily for 7 days. After 28 tablets have been taken, a new course is started the next day (Sunday). For the first cycle of a Sunday Start regimen, another method of contraception should be used until after the first 7 consecutive days of administration.

If the patient misses one (1) active tablet in Weeks 1, 2, or 3, the tablet should be taken as soon as she remembers. If the patient misses two (2) active tablets in Week 1 or Week 2, the patient should take two (2) tablets the day she remembers and two (2) tablets the next day; and then continue taking one (1) tablet a day until she finishes the pack. The patient should be instructed to use a back-up method of birth control if she has sex in the seven (7) days after missing pills. If the patient misses two (2) active tablets in the third week or misses three (3) or more active tablets in a row, the patient should continue taking one tablet every day until Sunday. On Sunday the patient should throw out the rest of the pack and start a new pack that same day. The patient should be instructed to use a back-up method of birth control if she has sex in the seven (7) days after missing pills.

Complete instructions to facilitate patient counseling on proper pill usage may be found in the Detailed Patient Labeling ("How to Take the Pill" section).

28-Day Regimen (Day 1 Start)

The dosage of ORTHO TRI-CYCLEN □ 28 and ORTHO-CYCLEN □ 28, for the initial cycle of therapy is one active tablet administered daily from the 1st day through the 21st day of the menstrual cycle, counting the first day of menstrual flow as "Day 1" followed by one green tablet daily for 7 days. Tablets are taken without interruption for 28 days. After 28 tablets have been taken, a new course is started the next day.

If the patient misses one (1) active tablet in Weeks 1, 2, or 3, the tablet should be taken as soon as she remembers. If the patient misses two (2) active tablets in Week 1 or Week 2, the patient should take two (2) tablets the day she remembers and two (2) tablets the next day; and then continue taking one (1) tablet a day until she finishes the pack. The patient should be instructed to use a back-up method of birth control if she has sex in the seven (7) days after missing pills. If the patient misses two (2) active tablets in the third week or misses three (3) or more active tablets in a row, the patient should throw out the rest of the pack and start a new pack that same day. The patient should be instructed to use a back-up method of birth control if she has sex in the seven (7) days after missing pills.

Complete instructions to facilitate patient counseling on proper pill usage may be found in the Detailed Patient Labeling ("How to Take the Pill" section).

The use of ORTHO TRI-CYCLEN and ORTHO-CYCLEN for contraception may be initiated 4 weeks postpartum in women who elect not to breast feed. When the tablets are administered during the postpartum period, the increased risk of thromboembolic disease associated with the postpartum period must be considered. (See CONTRAINDICATIONS and WARNINGS concerning thromboembolic disease. See also PRECAUTIONS for "Nursing Mothers.") The possibility of ovulation and conception prior to initiation of medication should be considered.

(See Discussion of Dose-Related Risk of Vascular Disease from Oral Contraceptives.)

ADDITIONAL INSTRUCTIONS FOR ALL DOSING REGIMENS

Breakthrough bleeding, spotting, and amenorrhea are frequent reasons for patients discontinuing oral contraceptives. In breakthrough bleeding, as in all cases of irregular bleeding from the vagina, nonfunctional causes should be borne in mind. In undiagnosed persistent or recurrent abnormal bleeding from the vagina, adequate diagnostic measures are indicated to rule out pregnancy or malignancy. If pathology has been excluded, time or a change to another formulation may solve the problem. Changing to an oral contraceptive with a higher estrogen content, while potentially useful in minimizing menstrual irregularity, should be done only if necessary since this may increase the risk of thromboembolic disease.

Use of oral contraceptives in the event of a missed menstrual period:

1. If the patient has not adhered to the prescribed schedule, the possibility of pregnancy should be considered at the time of the first missed period and oral contraceptive use should be discontinued until pregnancy is ruled out.
2. If the patient has adhered to the prescribed regimen and misses two consecutive periods, pregnancy should be ruled out before continuing oral contraceptive use.

ACNE

The timing of initiation of dosing with ORTHO TRI-CYCLEN for acne should follow the guidelines for use of ORTHO TRI-CYCLEN as an oral contraceptive. **Consult the DOSAGE AND ADMINISTRATION section for oral contraceptives.** The dosage regimen for ORTHO TRI-CYCLEN for treatment of facial acne, as available in a DIALPAK® Tablet Dispenser, utilizes a 21-day active and a 7-day placebo schedule. Take one active tablet daily for 21 days followed by one green tablet for 7 days. After 28 tablets have been taken, a new course is started the next day.

HOW SUPPLIED

ORTHO TRI-CYCLEN □ 21 Tablets are available in a DIALPAK® Tablet Dispenser (NDC 0062-1902-15) containing 21 tablets. Each white tablet contains 0.180 mg of the progestational compound, norgestimate, together with 0.035 mg of the estrogenic compound, ethinyl estradiol. Each light blue tablet contains 0.215 mg of the progestational compound, norgestimate, together with 0.035 mg of the estrogenic compound, ethinyl estradiol. Each blue tablet contains 0.250 mg of the progestational compound, norgestimate, together with 0.035 mg of the estrogenic compound, ethinyl estradiol.

The white tablets are unscored, with "Ortho" and "180" debossed on each side; the light blue tablets are unscored with "Ortho" and "215" debossed on each side; the blue tablets are unscored with "Ortho" and "250" debossed on each side.

ORTHO TRI-CYCLEN □ 28 Tablets are available in a DIALPAK® Tablet Dispenser (NDC 0062-1903-15) containing 28 tablets. Each white tablet contains 0.180 mg of the progestational compound, norgestimate, together with 0.035 mg of the estrogenic compound, ethinyl estradiol. Each light blue tablet contains 0.215 mg of the progestational compound, norgestimate, together with 0.035 mg of the estrogenic compound, ethinyl estradiol. Each blue tablet contains 0.250 mg of the progestational compound, norgestimate, together with 0.035 mg of the estrogenic compound, ethinyl estradiol. Each green tablet contains inert ingredients.

The white tablets are unscored, with "Ortho" and "180" debossed on each side; the light blue tablets are unscored with "Ortho" and "215" debossed on each side; the blue tablets are unscored with "Ortho" and "250" debossed on each side.

ORTHO TRI-CYCLEN □ 28 Tablets are available for clinic usage in a VERIDATE® Tablet Dispenser (unfilled) and VERIDATE Refills (NDC 0062-1903-20).

ORTHO-CYCLEN □ 21 Tablets are available in a DIALPAK® Tablet Dispenser (NDC 0062-1900-15) containing 21 tablets. Each blue tablet contains 0.250 mg of the progestational compound, norgestimate, together with 0.035 mg of the estrogenic compound, ethinyl estradiol which are unscored with "Ortho" and "250" debossed on each side.

ORTHO-CYCLEN □ 28 Tablets are available in a DIALPAK® Tablet Dispenser (NDC 0062-1901-15) containing 28 tablets as follows: 21 blue tablets as described under ORTHO-CYCLEN □ 21 Tablets, and 7 green tablets containing inert ingredients.

ORTHO-CYCLEN □ 28 Tablets are available for clinic usage in a VERIDATE® Tablet Dispenser (unfilled) and VERIDATE Refills (NDC 0062-1901-20).

Rx only.

REFERENCES

1. Trussel J. Contraceptive efficacy. In Hatcher RA, Trussel J, Stewart F, Cates W, Stewart GK, Kowal D, Guest F, Contraceptive Technology: Seventeenth Revised Edition. New York NY: Irvington Publishers, 1998, in press. **2.** Stadel BV, Oral contraceptives and cardiovascular disease. (Pt. 1). N Engl J Med 1981; 305:612-618. **3.** Stadel BV, Oral contraceptives and cardiovascular disease. (Pt. 2). N Engl J Med 1981; 305:672-677. **4.** Adam SA, Thorogood M. Oral contraception and myocardial infarction revisited: the effects of new preparations and prescribing patterns. Br J Obstet Gynaecol 1981; 88:838-845. **5.** Mann JI, Inman WH. Oral contraceptives and death from myocardial infarction. Br Med J 1975; 2(5965):245-248. **6.** Mann JI, Vessey MP, Thorogood M, Doll R. Myocardial infarction in young women with special reference to oral contraceptive practice. Br Med J 1975; 2(5956):241-245. **7.** Royal College of General Practitioners' Oral Contraception Study: further analyses of mortality in oral contraceptive users. Lancet 1981; 1:541-546. **8.** Slone D, Shapiro S, Kaufman DW, Rosenberg L, Miettinen OS, Stolley PD. Risk of myocardial infarction in relation to current and discontinued use of oral contraceptives. N Engl J Med 1981; 305:420-424. **9.** Vessey MP. Female hormones and vascular disease – an epidemiological overview. Br J Fam Plann 1980; 6 (Supplement): 1–12. **10.** Russell-Briefel RG, Ezzati TM, Fulwood R, Perlman JA, Murphy RS. Cardiovascular risk status and oral contraceptive use, United States, 1976-80. Prevent Med 1986; 15:352-362. **11.** Goldbaum GM, Kendrick JS, Hogelin GC, Gentry EM. The relative impact of smoking and oral contraceptive use on women

Continued on next page

Ortho Tri-Cyclen—Cont.

in the United States. JAMA 1987; 258:1339-1342. **12.** Layde PM, Beral V. Further analyses of mortality in oral contraceptive users: Royal College of General Practitioners' Oral Contraception Study. (Table 5) Lancet 1981; 1:541-546. **13.** Knopp RH. Arteriosclerosis risk: the roles of oral contraceptives and postmenopausal estrogens. J Reprod Med 1986; 31(9)(Supplement): 913-921. **14.** Krauss RM, Roy S, Mishell DR, Casagrande J, Pike MC. Effects of two low-dose oral contraceptives on serum lipids and lipoproteins: Differential changes in high-density lipoproteins subclasses. Am J Obstet 1983; 145:446-452. **15.** Wahl P, Walden C, Knopp R, Hoover J, Wallace R, Heiss G, Rifkind B. Effect of estrogen/progestin potency on lipid/lipoprotein cholesterol. N Engl J Med 1983; 308:862-867. **16.** Wynn V, Niththyananthan R. The effect of progestin in combined oral contraceptives on serum lipids with special reference to high density lipoproteins. Am J Obstet Gynecol 1982; 142: 766-771. **17.** Wynn V, Godsland I. Effects of oral contraceptives on carbohydrate metabolism. J Reprod Med 1986; 31(9)(Supplement):892-897. **18.** LaRosa JC. Atherosclerotic risk factors in cardiovascular disease. J Reprod Med 1986; 31(9)(Supplement): 906-912. **19.** Inman WH, Vessey MP. Investigation of death from pulmonary, coronary, and cerebral thrombosis and embolism in women of child-bearing age. Br Med J 1968; 2(5599):193-199. **20.** Maguire MG, Tonascia J, Sartwell PE, Stolley PD, Tockman MS. Increased risk of thrombosis due to oral contraceptives: a further report. Am J Epidemiol 1979; 110(2):188-195. **21.** Petitti DB, Wingerd J, Pellegrin F, Ramacharan S. Risk of vascular disease in women: smoking, oral contraceptives, noncontraceptive estrogens, and other factors. JAMA 1979; 242:1150-1154. **22.** Vessey MP, Doll R. Investigation of relation between use of oral contraceptives and thromboembolic disease. Br Med J 1968; 2(5599):199-205. **23.** Vessey MP, Doll R. Investigation of relation between use of oral contraceptives and thromboembolic disease. A further report. Br Med J 1969; 2(5658): 651-657. **24.** Porter JB, Hunter JR, Danielson DA, Jick H, Stergachis A. Oral contraceptives and non-fatal vascular disease – recent experience. Obstet Gynecol 1982; 59(3):299-302. **25.** Vessey M, Doll R, Peto R, Johnson B, Wiggins P. A long-term follow-up study of women using different methods of contraception: an interim report. J Biosocial Sci 1976; 8:375-427. **26.** Royal College of General Practitioners: Oral Contraceptives, venous thrombosis, and varicose veins. J Royal Coll Gen Pract 1978; 28:393-399. **27.** Collaborative Group for the Study of Stroke in Young Women: Oral contraception and increased risk of cerebral ischemia or thrombosis. N Engl J Med 1973; 288:871-878. **28.** Petitti DB, Wingerd J. Use of oral contraceptives, cigarette smoking, and risk of subarachnoid hemorrhage. Lancet 1978; 2:234-236. **29.** Inman WH. Oral contraceptives and fatal subarachnoid hemorrhage. Br Med J 1979; 2(6203):1468-1470. **30.** Collaborative Group for the Study of Stroke in Young Women: Oral Contraceptives and stroke in young women: associated risk factors. JAMA 1975; 231:718-722. **31.** Inman WH, Vessey MP, Westerholm B, Engelund A. Thromboembolic disease and the steroidal content of oral contraceptives. A report to the Committee on Safety of Drugs. Br Med J 1970; 2:203-209. **32.** Meade TW, Greenberg G, Thompson SG. Progestogens and cardiovascular reactions associated with oral contraceptives and a comparison of the safety of 50- and 35-mcg oestrogen preparations. Br Med J 1980; 280(6224):1157-1161. **33.** Kay CR. Progestogens and arterial disease – evidence from the Royal College of General Practitioners' Study. Am J Obstet Gynecol 1982; 142:762-765. **34.** Royal College of General Practitioners: Incidence of arterial disease among oral contraceptive users. J Royal Coll Gen Pract 1983; 33:75-82. **35.** Ory HW. Mortality associated with fertility and fertility control: 1983. Family Planning Perspectives 1983; 15:50-56. **36.** The Cancer and Steroid Hormone Study of the Centers for Disease Control and the National Institute of Child Health and Human Development: Oral contraceptive use and the risk of breast cancer. N Engl J Med 1986; 315:405-411. **37.** Pike MC, Henderson BE, Krailo MD, Duke A, Roy S. Breast cancer in young women and use of oral contraceptives: possible modifying effect of formulation and age at use. Lancet 1983; 2:926-929. **38.** Paul C, Skegg DG, Spears GFS, Kaldor JM. Oral contraceptives and breast cancer: A national study. Br Med J 1986; 293:723-725. **39.** Miller DR, Rosenberg L, Kaufman DW, Schottenfeld D, Stolley PD, Shapiro S. Breast cancer risk in relation to early oral contraceptive use. Obstet Gynecol 1986; 68:863-868. **40.** Olson H, Olson KL, Moller TR, Ranstam J, Holm P. Oral contraceptive use and breast cancer in young women in Sweden (letter). Lancet 1985; 2:748-749. **41.** McPherson K, Vessey M, Neil A, Doll R, Jones L, Roberts M. Early contraceptive use and breast cancer: Results of another case-control study. Br J Cancer 1987; 56: 653-660. **42.** Huggins GR, Zucker PF. Oral contraceptives and neoplasia: 1987 update. Fertil Steril 1987; 47:733-761. **43.** McPherson K, Drife JO. The pill and breast cancer: why the uncertainty? Br Med J 1986; 293:709-710. **44.** Shapiro S. Oral contraceptives – time to take stock. N Engl J Med 1987; 315:450-451. **45.** Ory H, Naib Z, Conger SB, Hatcher RA, Tyler CW. Contraceptive choice and prevalence of cervical dysplasia and carcinoma in situ. Am J Obstet Gynecol 1976; 124:573-577. **46.** Vessey MP, Lawless M, McPherson K, Yeates D. Neoplasia of the cervix uteri and contraception: a possible adverse effect of the pill. Lancet 1983; 2:930. **47.** Brinton LA, Huggins GR, Lehman HF, Malli K, Savitz DA, Trapido E, Rosenthal J, Hoover R. Long term use of oral contraceptives and risk of invasive cervical cancer. Int J Cancer 1986; 38:339-344. **48.** WHO Collaborative Study of Neoplasia and Steroid Contraceptives: Invasive cervical cancer and combined oral contraceptives. Br Med J 1985; 290:961-965. **49.** Rooks JB, Ory HW, Ishak KG, Strauss LT, Greenspan JR, Hill AP, Tyler CW. Epidemiology of hepatocellular adenoma: the role of oral contraceptive use. JAMA 1979; 242:644-648. **50.** Bein NN, Goldsmith HS. Recurrent massive hemorrhage from benign hepatic tumors secondary to oral contraceptives. Br J Surg 1977; 64:433-435. **51.** Klatskin G. Hepatic tumors: possible relationship to use of oral contraceptives. Gastroenterology 1977; 73:386-394. **52.** Henderson BE, Preston-Martin S, Edmondson HA, Peters RL, Pike MC. Hepatocellular carcinoma and oral contraceptives. Br J Cancer 1983; 48:437-440. **53.** Neuberger J, Forman D, Doll R, Williams R. Oral contraceptives and hepatocellular carcinoma. Br Med J 1986; 292:1355-1357. **54.** Forman D, Vincent TJ, Doll R. Cancer of the liver and oral contraceptives. Br Med J 1986; 292:1357-1361. **55.** Harlap S, Eldor J. Births following oral contraceptive failures. Obstet Gynecol 1980; 55:447-452. **56.** Savolainen E, Saksela E, Saxen L. Teratogenic hazards of oral contraceptives analyzed in a national malformation register. Am J Obstet Gynecol 1981; 140:521-524. **57.** Janerich DT, Piper JM, Glebatis DM. Oral contraceptives and birth defects. Am J Epidemiol 1980; 112:73-79. **58.** Ferencz C, Matanoski GM, Wilson PD, Rubin JD, Neill CA, Gutberlet R. Maternal hormone therapy and congenital heart disease. Teratology 1980; 21: 225-239. **59.** Rothman KJ, Fyler DC, Goldblatt A, Kreidberg MB. Exogenous hormones and other drug exposures of children with congenital heart disease. Am J Epidemiol 1979; 109:433-439. **60.** Boston Collaborative Drug Surveillance Program: Oral contraceptives and venous thromboembolic disease, surgically confirmed gallbladder disease, and breast tumors. Lancet 1973; 1:1399-1404. **61.** Royal College of General Practitioners: Oral contraceptives and health. New York, Pittman 1974. **62.** Layde PM, Vessey MP, Yeates D. Risk of gallbladder disease: a cohort study of young women attending family planning clinics. J Epidemiol Community Health 1982; 36:274-278. **63.** Rome Group for Epidemiology and Prevention of Cholelithiasis (GREPCO): Prevalence of gallstone disease in an Italian adult female population. Am J Epidemiol 1984; 119:796-805. **64.** Storm BL, Tamragouri RT, Morse ML, Lazar EL, West SL, Stolley PD, Jones JK. Oral contraceptives and other risk factors for gallbladder disease. Clin Pharmacol Ther 1986; 39:335-341. **65.** Wynn V, Adams PW, Godsland IF, Melrose J, Niththyananthan R, Oakley NW, Seedj A. Comparison of effects of different combined oral contraceptive formulations on carbohydrate and lipid metabolism. Lancet 1979; 1:1045-1049. **66.** Wynn V. Effect of progesterone and progestins on carbohydrate metabolism. In: Progesterone and Progestin. Bardin CW, Milgrom E, Mauvis-Jarvis P. eds. New York, Raven Press 1983; pp. 395-410. **67.** Perlman JA, Roussell-Briefel RG, Ezzati TM, Lieberknecht G. Oral glucose tolerance and the potency of oral contraceptive progestogens. J Chronic Dis 1985; 38:857-864. **68.** Royal College of General Practitioners' Oral Contraception Study: Effect on hypertension and benign breast disease of progestogen component in combined oral contraceptives. Lancet 1977; 1:624. **69.** Fisch IR, Frank J. Oral contraceptives and blood pressure. JAMA 1977; 237:2499-2503. **70.** Laragh AJ. Oral contraceptive induced hypertension – nine years later. Am J Obstet Gynecol 1976; 126:141-147. **71.** Ramcharan S, Peritz E, Pellegrin FA, Williams WT. Incidence of hypertension in the Walnut Creek Contraceptive Drug Study cohort: In: Pharmacology of steroid contraceptive drugs. Garattini S, Berendes HW. eds. New York, Raven Press, 1977; pp. 277-288, (Monographs of the Mario Negri Institute for Pharmacological Research Milan.) **72.** Stockley I. Interactions with oral contraceptives. J Pharm 1976; 216:140-143. **73.** The Cancer and Steroid Hormone Study of the Centers for Disease Control and the National Institute of Child Health and Human Development: Oral contraceptive use and the risk of ovarian cancer. JAMA 1983; 249:1596-1599. **74.** The Cancer and Steroid Hormone Study of the Centers for Disease Control and the National Institute of Child Health and Human Development: Combination oral contraceptive use and the risk of endometrial cancer. JAMA 1987; 257:796-800. **75.** Ory HW. Functional ovarian cysts and oral contraceptives: negative association confirmed surgically. JAMA 1974; 228:68-69. **76.** Ory HW, Cole P, MacMahon B, Hoover R. Oral contraceptives and reduced risk of benign breast disease. N Engl J Med 1976; 294:419-422. **77.** Ory HW. The noncontraceptive health benefits from oral contraceptive use. Fam Plann Perspect 1982; 14:182-184. **78.** Ory HW, Forrest JD, Lincoln R. Making choices: evaluating the health risks and benefits of birth control methods. New York, The Alan Guttmacher Institute, 1983; p. 1. **79.** Schlesselman J, Stadel BV, Murray P, Lai S. Breast cancer in relation to early use of oral contraceptives. JAMA 1988; 259:1828-1833. **80.** Hennekens CH, Speizer FE, Lipnick RJ, Rosner B, Bain C, Belanger C, Stampfer MJ, Willett W, Peto R. A case-control study of oral contraceptive use and breast cancer. JNCI 1984; 72:39-42. **81.** LaVecchia C, Decarli A, Fasoli M, Franceschi S, Gentile A, Negri E, Parazzini F, Tognoni G. Oral contraceptives and cancers of the breast and of the female genital tract. Interim results from a case-control study. Br J Cancer 1986; 54:311-317. **82.** Meirik O, Lund E, Adami H, Bergstrom R, Christoffersen T, Bergsjo P. Oral contraceptive use and breast cancer in young women. A Joint National Case-control study in Sweden and Norway. Lancet 1986; 11:650-654. **83.** Kay CR, Hannaford PC. Breast cancer and the pill – A further report from the Royal College of General Practitioners' oral contraception study. Br J Cancer 1988; 58:675-680. **84.** Stadel BV, Lai S, Schlesselman JJ, Murray P. Oral contraceptives and premenopausal breast cancer in nulliparous women. Contraception 1988; 38:287-299. **85.** Miller DR, Rosenberg L, Kaufman DW, Stolley P, Warshauer ME, Shapiro S. Breast cancer before age 45 and oral contraceptive use: New findings. Am J Epidemiol 1989; 129:269-280. **86.** The UK National Case-Control Study Group, Oral contraceptive use and breast cancer risk in young women. Lancet 1989; 1:973-982. **87.** Schlesselman JJ. Cancer of the breast and reproductive tract in relation to use of oral contraceptives. Contraception 1989; 40:1-38. **88.** Vessey MP, McPherson K, Villard-Mackintosh L, Yeates D. Oral contraceptives and breast cancer: latest findings in a large cohort study. Br J Cancer 1989; 59:613-617. **89.** Jick SS, Walker AM, Stergachis A, Jick H. Oral contraceptives and breast cancer. Br J Cancer 1989; 59:618-621. **90.** Anderson FD. Selectivity and minimal androgenicity of norgestimate in monophasic and triphasic oral contraceptives. Acta Obstet Gynecol Scand 1992; 156 (Supplement):15-21. **91.** Chapdelaine A, Desmaris J-L, Derman RJ. Clinical evidence of minimal androgenic activity of norgestimate. Int J Fertil 1989; 34(51):347-352. **92.** Phillips A, Demarest K, Hahn DW, Wong F, McGuire JL. Progestational and androgenic receptor binding affinities and in vivo activities of norgestimate and other progestins. Contraception 1989; 41(4):399-409. **93.** Phillips A, Hahn DW, Klimek S, McGuire JL. A comparison of the potencies and activities of progestogens used in contraceptives. Contraception 1987; 36(2):181-192. **94.** Janaud A, Rouffy J, Upmalis D, Dain M-P. A comparison study of lipid and androgen metabolism with triphasic oral contraceptive formulations containing norgestimate or levonorgestrel. Acta Obstet Gynecol Scand 1992; 156 (Supplement):34-38. **95.** Collaborative Group on Hormonal Factors in Breast Cancer. Breast cancer and hormonal contraceptives: collaborative reanalysis of individual data on 53 297 women with breast cancer and 100 239 women without breast cancer from 54 epidemiological studies. Lancet 1996; 347:1713-1727. **96.** Palmer JR, Rosenberg L, Kaufman DW, Warshauer ME, Stolley P, Shapiro S. Oral Contraceptive Use and Liver Cancer. Am J Epidemiol 1989; 130:878-882. **97.** Lewis M, Spitzer WO, Heinemann LAJ, MacRae KD, Bruppacher R, Thorogood M, on behalf of Transnational Research Group on Oral Contraceptives and Health of Young Women. Third generation oral contraceptives and risk of myocardial infarction: an international case-control study. Br Med J 1996;312:88-90.

BRIEF SUMMARY PATIENT PACKAGE INSERT

Oral contraceptives, also known as "birth control pills" or "the pill," are taken to prevent pregnancy. ORTHO TRI-CYCLEN may also be taken to treat moderate acne in females who are able to use the pill. When taken correctly to prevent pregnancy, oral contraceptives have a failure rate of less than 1% per year when used without missing any pills. The typical failure rate of large numbers of pill users is less than 3% per year when women who miss pills are included. For most women oral contraceptives are also free of serious or unpleasant side effects. However, forgetting to take pills considerably increases the chances of pregnancy.

For the majority of women, oral contraceptives can be taken safely. But there are some women who are at high risk of developing certain serious diseases that can be fatal or may cause temporary or permanent disability. The risks associated with taking oral contraceptives increase significantly if you:

- smoke
- have high blood pressure, diabetes, high cholesterol
- have or have had clotting disorders, heart attack, stroke, angina pectoris, cancer of the breast or sex organs, jaundice or malignant or benign liver tumors.

Although cardiovascular disease risks may be increased with oral contraceptive use after age 40 in healthy, non-smoking women (even with the newer low-dose formulations), there are also greater potential health risks associated with pregnancy in older women.

You should not take the pill if you suspect you are pregnant or have unexplained vaginal bleeding.

Cigarette smoking increases the risk of serious cardiovascular side effects from oral contraceptive use. This risk increases with age and with heavy smoking (15 or more cigarettes per day) and is quite marked in women over 35 years of age. Women who use oral contraceptives and strongly advised not to smoke.

Most side effects of the pill are not serious. The most common such effects are nausea, vomiting, bleeding between menstrual periods, weight gain, breast tenderness, and difficulty wearing contact lenses. These side effects, especially nausea and vomiting, may subside within the first three months of use.

The serious side effects of the pill occur very infrequently, especially if you are in good health and are young. However, you should know that the following medical conditions have been associated with or made worse by the pill:

1. Blood clots in the legs (thrombophlebitis), lungs (pulmonary embolism), stoppage or rupture of a blood vessel in the brain (stroke), blockage of blood vessels in the heart (heart attack or angina pectoris) or other organs of the body. As mentioned above, smoking increases the risk of heart attacks and strokes and subsequent serious medical consequences.

2. In rare cases, oral contraceptives can cause benign but dangerous liver tumors. These benign liver tumors can rupture and cause fatal internal bleeding. In addition, some studies report an increased risk of developing liver cancer. However, liver cancers are rare.

3. High blood pressure, although blood pressure usually returns to normal when the pill is stopped.

The symptoms associated with these serious side effects are discussed in the detailed leaflet given to you with your supply of pills. Notify your doctor or health care provider if you notice any unusual physical disturbances while taking the pill. In addition, drugs such as rifampin, as well as some anticonvulsants and some antibiotics may decrease oral contraceptive effectiveness.

There is conflict among studies regarding breast cancer and oral contraceptive use. Some studies have reported an increase in the risk of developing breast cancer, particularly at a younger age. This increased risk appears to be related to duration of use. The majority of studies have found no overall increase in the risk of developing breast cancer. Some studies have found an increase in the incidence of cancer of the cervix in women who use oral contraceptives. However, this finding may be related to factors other than the use of oral contraceptives. There is insufficient evidence to rule out the possibility pills may cause such cancers.

Taking the combination pill provides some important noncontraceptive benefits. These include less painful menstruation, less menstrual blood loss and anemia, fewer pelvic infections, and fewer cancers of the ovary and the lining of the uterus.

Be sure to discuss any medical condition you may have with your health care provider. Your health care provider will take a medical and family history before prescribing oral contraceptives and will examine you. The physical examination may be delayed to another time if you request it and the health care provider believes that it is a good medical practice to postpone it. You should be reexamined at least once a year while taking oral contraceptives. Your pharmacist should have given you the detailed patient information labeling which gives you further information which you should read and discuss with your health care provider.

ORTHO-CYCLEN and ORTHO TRI-CYCLEN (like all oral contraceptives) are intended to prevent pregnancy. ORTHO TRI-CYCLEN is also used to treat moderate acne in females who are able to take oral contraceptives. Oral contraceptives do not protect against transmission of HIV (AIDS) and other sexually transmitted diseases such as chlamydia, genital herpes, genital warts, gonorrhea, hepatitis B, and syphilis.

DETAILED PATIENT LABELING

PLEASE NOTE: This labeling is revised from time to time as important new medical information becomes available. Therefore, please review this labeling carefully.

ORTHO TRI-CYCLEN ☐ 21 Day Regimen and
ORTHO TRI-CYCLEN ☐ 28 Day Regimen

Each white tablet contains 0.180 mg norgestimate and 0.035 mg ethinyl estradiol. Each light blue tablet contains 0.215 mg norgestimate and 0.035 mg ethinyl estradiol. Each blue tablet contains 0.250 mg norgestimate and 0.035 mg ethinyl estradiol. Each green tablet in ORTHO TRI-CYCLEN ☐ 28 Day Regimen contains inert ingredients.

ORTHO-CYCLEN ☐ 21 Day Regimen and
ORTHO-CYCLEN ☐ 28 Day Regimen

Each blue tablet contains 0.250 mg norgestimate and 0.035 mg ethinyl estradiol. Each green tablet in ORTHO-CYCLEN ☐ 28 Day Regimen contains inert ingredients.

INTRODUCTION

Any woman who considers using oral contraceptives (the birth control pill or the pill) should understand the benefits and risks of using this form of birth control. This patient labeling will give you much of the information you will need to make this decision and will also help you determine if you are at risk of developing any of the serious side effects of the pill. It will tell you how to use the pill properly so that it will be as effective as possible. However, this labeling is not a replacement for a careful discussion between you and your health care provider. You should discuss the information provided in this labeling with him or her, both when you first start taking the pill and during your revisits. You should also follow your health care provider's advice with regard to regular check-ups while you are on the pill.

EFFECTIVENESS OF ORAL CONTRACEPTIVES FOR CONTRACEPTION

Oral contraceptives or "birth control pills" or "the pill" are used to prevent pregnancy and are more effective than other non-surgical methods of birth control. When they are taken correctly, the chance of becoming pregnant is less than 1% (1 pregnancy per 100 women per year of use) when used perfectly, without missing any pills. Typical failure rates are actually 3% per year. The chance of becoming pregnant increases with each missed pill during a menstrual cycle.

In comparison, typical failure rates for other non-surgical methods of birth control during the first year of use are as follows:

Implant: <1%
Injection: <1%
IUD: 1 to 2%
Diaphragm with spermicides: 20%
Spermicides alone: 26%
Vaginal sponge: 20 to 40%
Female sterilization: <1%
Male sterilization: <1%
Cervical Cap with spermicides: 20 to 40%
Condom alone (male): 14%
Condom alone (female): 21%
Periodic abstinence: 25%
Withdrawal: 19%
No methods: 85%

ANNUAL NUMBER OF BIRTH-RELATED OR METHOD-RELATED DEATHS ASSOCIATED WITH CONTROL OF FERTILITY PER 100,000 NON-STERILE WOMEN, BY FERTILITY CONTROL METHOD ACCORDING TO AGE

Method of control and outcome	15–19	20–24	25–29	30–34	35–39	40–44
No fertility control methods*	7.0	7.4	9.1	14.8	25.7	28.2
Oral contraceptives non-smoker**	0.3	0.5	0.9	1.9	13.8	31.6
Oral contraceptives smoker**	2.2	3.4	6.6	13.5	51.1	117.2
IUD**	0.8	0.8	1.0	1.0	1.4	1.4
Condom*	1.1	1.6	0.7	0.2	0.3	0.4
Diaphragm/ spermicide*	1.9	1.2	1.2	1.3	2.2	2.8
Periodic abstinence*	2.5	1.6	1.6	1.7	2.9	3.6

*Deaths are birth-related
**Deaths are method-related

Adapted from H.W. Ory, ref. #35.

WHO SHOULD NOT TAKE ORAL CONTRACEPTIVES

Cigarette smoking increases the risk of serious cardiovascular side effects from oral contraceptive use. This risk increases with age and with heavy smoking (15 to more cigarettes per day) and is quite marked in women over 35 years of age. Women who use oral contraceptives are strongly advised not to smoke.

Some women should not use the pill. For example, you should not take the pill if you are pregnant or think you may be pregnant. You should also not use the pill if you have any of the following conditions:

- A history of heart attack or stroke
- Blood clots in the legs (thrombophlebitis), lungs (pulmonary embolism), or eyes
- A history of blood clots in the deep veins of your legs
- Chest pain (angina pectoris)
- Known or suspected breast cancer or cancer of the lining of the uterus, cervix or vagina
- Unexplained vaginal bleeding (until a diagnosis is reached by your doctor)
- Yellowing of the whites of the eyes or of the skin (jaundice) during pregnancy or during previous use of the pill
- Liver tumor (benign or cancerous)
- Known or suspected pregnancy

Tell your health care provider if you have ever had any of these conditions. Your health care provider can recommend a safer method of birth control.

OTHER CONSIDERATIONS BEFORE TAKING ORAL CONTRACEPTIVES

Tell your health care provider if you have or have had:

- Breast nodules, fibrocystic disease of the breast, an abnormal breast x-ray or mammogram
- Diabetes
- Elevated cholesterol or triglycerides
- High blood pressure
- Migraine or other headaches or epilepsy
- Mental depression
- Gallbladder, heart or kidney disease
- History of scanty or irregular menstrual periods

Women with any of these conditions should be checked often by their health care provider if they choose to use oral contraceptives.

Also, be sure to inform your doctor or health care provider if you smoke or are on any medications.

RISKS OF TAKING ORAL CONTRACEPTIVES

1. Risk of developing blood clots

Blood clots and blockage of blood vessels are one of the most serious side effects of taking oral contraceptives and can cause death or serious disability. In particular, a clot in the legs can cause thrombophlebitis and a clot that travels to the lungs can cause a sudden blocking of the vessel carrying blood to the lungs. Rarely, clots occur in the blood vessels of the eye and may cause blindness, double vision, or impaired vision.

If you take oral contraceptives and need elective surgery, need to stay in bed for a prolonged illness or have recently delivered a baby, you may be at risk of developing blood clots. You should consult your doctor about stopping oral contraceptives four weeks before surgery and not taking oral contraceptives for two weeks after surgery or during bed rest. You should also not take oral contraceptives soon after delivery of a baby. It is advisable to wait for at least four weeks after delivery if you are not breast feeding or four weeks after a second trimester abortion. If you are breast feeding, you should wait until you have weaned your child before using the pill. (See also the section on Breast Feeding in General Precautions.)

The risk of circulatory disease in oral contraceptive users may be higher in users of high-dose pills and may be greater with longer duration of oral contraceptive use. In addition, some of these increased risks may continue for a number of years after stopping oral contraceptives. The risk of abnormal blood clotting increases with age in both users and nonusers of oral contraceptives, but the increased risk from the oral contraceptive appears to be present at all ages. For women aged 20 to 44 it is estimated that about 1 in 2,000 using oral contraceptives will be hospitalized each year because of abnormal clotting. Among nonusers in the same age group, about 1 in 20,000 would be hospitalized each year. For oral contraceptive users in general, it has been estimated that in women between the ages of 15 and 34 the risk of death due to a circulatory disorder is about 1 in 12,000 per year, whereas for nonusers the rate is about 1 in 50,000 per year. In the age group 35 to 44, the risk is estimated to be about 1 in 2,500 per year for oral contraceptive users and about 1 in 10,000 per year for nonusers.

2. Heart attacks and strokes

Oral contraceptives may increase the tendency to develop strokes (stoppage or rupture of blood vessels in the brain) and angina pectoris and heart attacks (blockage of blood vessels in the heart). Any of these conditions can cause death or serious disability.

Smoking greatly increases the possibility of suffering heart attacks and strokes. Furthermore, smoking and the use of oral contraceptives greatly increase the chances of developing and dying of heart disease.

3. Gallbladder disease

Oral contraceptive users probably have a greater risk than nonusers of having gallbladder disease, although this risk may be related to pills containing high doses of estrogens.

4. Liver tumors

In rare cases, oral contraceptives can cause benign but dangerous liver tumors. These benign liver tumors can rupture and cause fatal internal bleeding. In addition, some studies report an increased risk of developing liver cancer. However, liver cancers are rare.

5. Cancer of the reproductive organs and breasts

There is conflict among studies regarding breast cancer and oral contraceptive use. Some studies have reported an increase in the risk of developing breast cancer, particularly at a younger age. This increased risk appears to be related to duration of use. The majority of studies have found no overall increase in the risk of developing breast cancer.

A meta-analysis of 54 studies found a small increase in the frequency of having breast cancer diagnosed for women who were currently using combined oral contraceptives or had used them within the past ten years. This increase in the frequency of breast cancer diagnosis, within ten years of stopping use, was generally accounted for by cancers localized to the breast. There was no increase in the frequency of having breast cancer diagnosed ten or more years after cessation of use.

Some studies have found an increase in the incidence of cancer of the cervix in women who use oral contraceptives. However, this finding may be related to factors other than the use of oral contraceptives. There is insufficient evidence to rule out the possibility that pills may cause such cancers.

ESTIMATED RISK OF DEATH FROM A BIRTH CONTROL METHOD OR PREGNANCY

All methods of birth control and pregnancy are associated with a risk of developing certain diseases which may lead to disability or death. An estimate of the number of deaths as-

Continued on next page

Ortho Tri-Cyclen—Cont.

sociated with different methods of birth control and pregnancy has been calculated and is shown in the following table.

[See table at top of previous page]

In the above table, the risk of death from any birth control method is less than the risk of childbirth, except for oral contraceptive users over the age of 35 who smoke and pill users over the age of 40 even if they do not smoke. It can be seen in the table that for women aged 15 to 39, the risk of death was highest with pregnancy (7–26 deaths per 100,000 women, depending on age). Among pill users who do not smoke, the risk of death was always lower than that associated with pregnancy for any age group, although over the age of 40, the risk increases to 32 deaths per 100,000 women, compared to 28 associated with pregnancy at that age. However, for pill users who smoke and are over the age of 35, the estimated number of deaths exceed those for other methods of birth control. If a woman is over the age of 40 and smokes, her estimated risk of death is four times higher (117/100,000 women) than the estimated risk associated with pregnancy (28/100,000 women) in that age group.

The suggestion that women over 40 who do not smoke should not take oral contraceptives is based on information from older, higher-dose pills. An Advisory Committee of the FDA discussed this issue in 1989 and recommended that the benefits of low-dose oral contraceptive use by healthy, non-smoking women over 40 years of age may outweigh the possible risks.

WARNING SIGNALS

If any of these adverse effects occur while you are taking oral contraceptives, call your doctor immediately:

- Sharp chest pain, coughing of blood, or sudden shortness of breath (indicating a possible clot in the lung)
- Pain in the calf (indicating a possible clot in the leg)
- Crushing chest pain or heaviness in the chest (indicating a possible heart attack)
- Sudden severe headache or vomiting, dizziness or fainting, disturbances of vision or speech, weakness, or numbness in an arm or leg (indicating a possible stroke)
- Sudden partial or complete loss of vision (indicating a possible clot in the eye)
- Breast lumps (indicating possible breast cancer or fibrocystic disease of the breast; ask your doctor or health care provider to show you how to examine your breasts)
- Severe pain or tenderness in the stomach area (indicating a possibly ruptured liver tumor)
- Difficulty in sleeping, weakness, lack of energy, fatigue, or change in mood (possibly indicating severe depression)
- Jaundice or a yellowing of the skin or eyeballs, accompanied frequently by fever, fatigue, loss of appetite, dark colored urine, or light colored bowel movements (indicating possible liver problems)

SIDE EFFECTS OF ORAL CONTRACEPTIVES

1. Vaginal bleeding

Irregular vaginal bleeding or spotting may occur while you are taking the pills. Irregular bleeding may vary from slight staining between menstrual periods to breakthrough bleeding which is a flow much like a regular period. Irregular bleeding occurs most often during the first few months of oral contraceptive use, but may also occur after you have been taking the pill for some time. Such bleeding may be temporary and usually does not indicate any serious problems. It is important to continue taking your pills on schedule. If the bleeding occurs in more than one cycle or lasts for more than a few days, talk to your doctor or health care provider.

2. Contact lenses

If you wear contact lenses and notice a change in vision or an inability to wear your lenses, contact your doctor or health care provider.

3. Fluid retention

Oral contraceptives may cause edema (fluid retention) with swelling of the fingers or ankles and may raise your blood pressure. If you experience fluid retention, contact your doctor or health care provider.

4. Melasma

A spotty darkening of the skin is possible, particularly of the face, which may persist.

5. Other side effects

Other side effects may include nausea and vomiting, change in appetite, headache, nervousness, depression, dizziness, loss of scalp hair, rash, and vaginal infections.

If any of these side effects bother you, call your doctor or health care provider.

GENERAL PRECAUTIONS

1. Missed periods and use of oral contraceptives before or during early pregnancy

There may be times when you may not menstruate regularly after you have completed taking a cycle of pills. If you have taken your pills regularly and miss one menstrual period, continue taking your pills for the next cycle but be sure to inform your health care provider before doing so. If you have not taken the pills daily as instructed and missed a menstrual period, you may be pregnant. If you missed two consecutive menstrual periods, you may be pregnant. Check with your health care provider immediately to determine whether you are pregnant. Do not continue to take oral contraceptives until you are sure you are not pregnant, but continue to use another method of contraception.

There is no conclusive evidence that oral contraceptive use is associated with an increase in birth defects, when taken inadvertently during early pregnancy. Previously, a few studies had reported that oral contraceptives might be associated with birth defects, but these findings have not been seen in more recent studies. Nevertheless, oral contraceptives or any other drugs should not be used during pregnancy unless clearly necessary and prescribed by your doctor. You should check with your doctor about risks to your unborn child of any medication taken during pregnancy.

2. While breast feeding

If you are breast feeding, consult your doctor before starting oral contraceptives. Some of the drug will be passed on to the child in the milk. A few adverse effects on the child have been reported, including yellowing of the skin (jaundice) and breast enlargement. In addition, combination oral contraceptives may decrease the amount and quality of your milk. If possible, do not use combination oral contraceptives while breast feeding. You should use another method of contraception since breast feeding provides only partial protection from becoming pregnant and this partial protection decreases significantly as you breast feed for longer periods of time. You should consider starting combination oral contraceptives only after you have weaned your child completely.

3. Laboratory tests

If you are scheduled for any laboratory tests, tell your doctor you are taking birth control pills. Certain blood tests may be affected by birth control pills.

4. Drug interactions

Certain drugs may interact with birth control pills to make them less effective in preventing pregnancy or cause an increase in breakthrough bleeding. Such drugs include rifampin, drugs used for epilepsy such as barbiturates (for example, phenobarbital), anticonvulsants such as carbamazepine (Tegretol is one brand of this drug), phenytoin (Dilantin is one brand of this drug), phenylbutazone (Butazolidin is one brand) and possibly certain antibiotics. You may need to use additional contraception when you take drugs which can make oral contraceptives less effective.

5. Sexually transmitted diseases

ORTHO-CYCLEN and ORTHO TRI-CYCLEN (like all oral contraceptives) are intended to prevent pregnancy. ORTHO TRI-CYCLEN is also used to treat moderate acne in females who are able to take oral contraceptives. Oral contraceptives do not protect against transmission of HIV (AIDS) and other sexually transmitted diseases such as chlamydia, genital herpes, genital warts, gonorrhea, hepatitis B, and syphilis.

HOW TO TAKE THE PILL

IMPORTANT POINTS TO REMEMBER

BEFORE YOU START TAKING YOUR PILLS:

1. BE SURE TO READ THESE DIRECTIONS:
Before you start taking your pills.
Anytime you are not sure what to do.

2. THE RIGHT WAY TO TAKE THE PILL IS TO TAKE ONE PILL EVERY DAY AT THE SAME TIME.
If you miss pills you could get pregnant. This includes starting the pack late. The more pills you miss, the more likely you are to get pregnant.

3. MANY WOMEN HAVE SPOTTING OR LIGHT BLEEDING, OR MAY FEEL SICK TO THEIR STOMACH DURING THE FIRST 1-3 PACKS OF PILLS. If you feel sick to your stomach, do not stop taking the pill. The problem will usually go away. If it doesn't go away, check with your doctor or clinic.

4. MISSING PILLS CAN ALSO CAUSE SPOTTING OR LIGHT BLEEDING, even when you make up these missed pills.
On the days you take 2 pills to make up for missed pills, you could also feel a little sick to your stomach.

5. IF YOU HAVE VOMITING OR DIARRHEA, for any reason, or IF YOU TAKE SOME MEDICINES, including some antibiotics, your pills may not work as well. Use a back-up method (such as condoms, foam, or sponge) until you check with your doctor or clinic.

6. IF YOU HAVE TROUBLE REMEMBERING TO TAKE THE PILL, talk to your doctor or clinic about how to make pill-taking easier or about using another method of birth control.

7. IF YOU HAVE ANY QUESTIONS OR ARE UNSURE ABOUT THE INFORMATION IN THIS LEAFLET, call your doctor or clinic.

BEFORE YOU START TAKING YOUR PILLS

1. DECIDE WHAT TIME OF DAY YOU WANT TO TAKE YOUR PILL.
It is important to take it at about the same time every day.

2. LOOK AT YOUR PILL PACK TO SEE IF IT HAS 21 OR 28 PILLS:
The 21-pill pack has 21 "active" pills (with hormones) to take for 3 weeks. This is followed by 1 week without pills.
The 28-pill pack has 21 "active" pills (with hormones) to take for 3 weeks. This is followed by 1 week of "reminder" green pills (without hormones).
ORTHO TRI-CYCLEN: There are 7 white "active" pills, 7 light blue "active" pills, and 7 blue "active" pills.
ORTHO-CYCLEN: There are 21 blue "active" pills.

3. ALSO FIND:
1) where on the pack to start taking pills,
2) in what order to take the pills.
CHECK PICTURE OF PILL PACK AND ADDITIONAL INSTRUCTIONS FOR USING THIS PACKAGE IN THE BRIEF SUMMARY PATIENT PACKAGE INSERT.

4. BE SURE YOU HAVE READY AT ALL TIMES:
ANOTHER KIND OF BIRTH CONTROL (such as condoms, foam, or sponge) to use as a back-up method in case you miss pills.
AN EXTRA, FULL PILL PACK.

WHEN TO START THE FIRST PACK OF PILLS

You have a choice of which day to start taking your first pack of pills. ORTHO TRI-CYCLEN and ORTHO-CYCLEN are available in the DIALPAK® Tablet Dispenser which is preset for a Sunday Start. Day 1 Start is also provided. Decide with your doctor or clinic which is the best day for you. Pick a time of day which will be easy to remember.

SUNDAY START:

ORTHO TRI-CYCLEN: Take the first "active" white pill of the first pack on the Sunday after your period starts, even if you are still bleeding. If your period begins on Sunday, start the pack that same day.

ORTHO-CYCLEN: Take the first "active" blue pill of the first pack on the Sunday after your period starts, even if you are still bleeding. If your period begins on Sunday, start the pack that same day.

Use another method of birth control as a back-up method if you have sex anytime from the Sunday you start your first pack until the next Sunday (7 days). Condoms, foam, or the sponge are good back-up methods of birth control.

DAY 1 START:

ORTHO TRI-CYCLEN: Take the first "active" white pill of the first pack during the first 24 hours of your period.

ORTHO-CYCLEN: Take the first "active" blue pill of the first pack during the first 24 hours of your period.

You will not need to use a back-up method of birth control, since you are starting the pill at the beginning of your period.

WHAT TO DO DURING THE MONTH

1. TAKE ONE PILL AT THE SAME TIME EVERY DAY UNTIL THE PACK IS EMPTY.

Do not skip pills even if you are spotting or bleeding between monthly periods or feel sick to your stomach (nausea).

Do not skip pills even if you do not have sex very often.

2. WHEN YOU FINISH A PACK OR SWITCH YOUR BRAND OF PILLS:

21 pills: Wait 7 days to start the next pack. You will probably have your period during that week. Be sure that no more than 7 days pass between 21-day packs.

28 pills: Start the next pack on the day after your last "reminder" pill. Do not wait any days between packs.

WHAT TO DO IF YOU MISS PILLS

ORTHO TRI-CYCLEN:

If you **MISS 1** white, light blue, or blue "active" pill:

1. Take it as soon as you remember. Take the next pill at your regular time. This means you may take 2 pills in 1 day.
2. You do not need to use a back-up birth control method if you have sex.

If you **MISS 2** white or light blue "active" pills in a row in **WEEK 1 OR WEEK 2** of your pack:

1. Take 2 pills on the day you remember and 2 pills the next day.
2. Then take 1 pill a day until you finish the pack.
3. You MAY BECOME PREGNANT if you have sex in the 7 days after you miss pills. You MUST use another birth control method (such as condoms, foam, or sponge) as a back-up method for those 7 days.

If you **MISS 2** blue "active" pills in a row in **THE 3RD WEEK:**

1. **If you are a Sunday Starter:**
Keep taking 1 pill every day until Sunday. On Sunday, THROW OUT the rest of the pack and start a new pack of pills that same day.
If you are a Day 1 Starter:
THROW OUT the rest of the pill pack and start a new pack that same day.
2. You may not have your period this month but this is expected. However, if you miss your period 2 months in a row, call your doctor or clinic because you might be pregnant.
3. You MAY BECOME PREGNANT if you have sex in the 7 days after you miss pills. You MUST use another birth control method (such as condoms, foam, or sponge) as a back-up method for those 7 days.

If you **MISS 3 OR MORE** white, light blue, or blue "active" pills in a row (during the first 3 weeks):

1. **If you are a Sunday Starter:**
Keep taking 1 pill every day until Sunday. On Sunday, THROW OUT the rest of the pack and start a new pack of pills that same day.
If you are a Day 1 Starter:
THROW OUT the rest of the pill pack and start a new pack that same day.
2. You may not have your period this month but this is expected. However, if you miss your period 2 months in a row, call your doctor or clinic because you might be pregnant.

3. You MAY BECOME PREGNANT if you have sex in the 7 days after you miss pills. You MUST use another birth control method (such as condoms, foam, or sponge) as a back-up method for those 7 days.

ORTHO-CYCLEN:

If you **MISS 1** blue "active" pill:

1. Take it as soon as you remember. Take the next pill at your regular time. This means you may take 2 pills in 1 day.
2. You do not need to use a back-up birth control method if you have sex.

If you **MISS 2** blue "active" pills in a row in **WEEK 1 OR WEEK 2** of your pack:

1. Take 2 pills on the day you remember and 2 pills the next day.
2. Then take 1 pill a day until you finish the pack.
3. You MAY BECOME PREGNANT if you have sex in the 7 days after you miss pills. You MUST use another birth control method (such as condoms, foam, or sponge) as a back-up method for those 7 days.

If you **MISS 2** blue "active" pills in a row in **THE 3RD WEEK:**

1. **If you are a Sunday Starter:**
Keep taking 1 pill every day until Sunday. On Sunday, THROW OUT the rest of the pack and start a new pack of pills that same day.
If you are a Day 1 Starter:
THROW OUT the rest of the pill pack and start a new pack that same day.
2. You may not have your period this month but this is expected. However, if you miss your period 2 months in a row, call your doctor or clinic because you might be pregnant.
3. You MAY BECOME PREGNANT if you have sex in the 7 days after you miss pills. You MUST use another birth control method (such as condoms, foam, or sponge) as a back-up method for those 7 days.

If you **MISS 3 OR MORE** blue "active" pills in a row (during the first 3 weeks):

1. **If you are a Sunday Starter:**
Keep taking 1 pill every day until Sunday. On Sunday, THROW OUT the rest of the pack and start a new pack of pills that same day.
If you are a Day 1 Starter:
THROW OUT the rest of the pill pack and start a new pack that same day.
2. You may not have your period this month but this is expected. However, if you miss your period 2 months in a row, call your doctor or clinic because you might be pregnant.
3. You MAY BECOME PREGNANT if you have sex in the 7 days after you miss pills. You MUST use another birth control method (such as condoms, foam, or sponge) as a back-up method for those 7 days.

A REMINDER FOR THOSE ON 28-DAY PACKS:

If you forget any of the 7 green "reminder" pills in Week 4:
THROW AWAY the pills you missed.
Keep taking 1 pill each day until the pack is empty.
You do not need a back-up method.

FINALLY, IF YOU ARE STILL NOT SURE WHAT TO DO ABOUT THE PILLS YOU HAVE MISSED:

Use a BACK-UP METHOD anytime you have sex.
KEEP TAKING ONE "ACTIVE" PILL EACH DAY until you can reach your doctor or clinic.

PREGNANCY DUE TO PILL FAILURE

The incidence of pill failure resulting in pregnancy is approximately one percent (i.e., one pregnancy per 100 women per year) if taken every day as directed, but more typical failure rates are about 3%. If failure does occur, the risk to the fetus is minimal.

PREGNANCY AFTER STOPPING THE PILL

There may be some delay in becoming pregnant after you stop using oral contraceptives, especially if you had irregular menstrual cycles before you used oral contraceptives. It may be advisable to postpone conception until you begin menstruating regularly once you have stopped taking the pill and desire pregnancy.

There does not appear to be any increase in birth defects in newborn babies when pregnancy occurs soon after stopping the pill.

OVERDOSAGE

Serious ill effects have not been reported following ingestion of large doses of oral contraceptives by young children. Overdosage may cause nausea and withdrawal bleeding in females. In case of overdosage, contact your health care provider or pharmacist.

OTHER INFORMATION

Your health care provider will take a medical and family history before prescribing oral contraceptives and will examine you. The physical examination may be delayed to another time if you request it and the health care provider believes that it is a good medical practice to postpone it. You should be reexamined at least once a year. Be sure to inform your health care provider if there is a family history of any of the conditions listed previously in this leaflet. Be sure to keep all appointments with your health care provider, because this is a time to determine if there are early signs of side effects of oral contraceptive use.

Do not use the drug for any condition other than the one for which it was prescribed. This drug has been prescribed specifically for you; do not give it to others who may want birth control pills.

HEALTH BENEFITS FROM ORAL CONTRACEPTIVES

In addition to preventing pregnancy, use of combination oral contraceptives may provide certain benefits. They are:

- menstrual cycles may become more regular
- blood flow during menstruation may be lighter and less iron may be lost. Therefore, anemia due to iron deficiency is less likely to occur.
- pain or other symptoms during menstruation may be encountered less frequently
- ectopic (tubal) pregnancy may occur less frequently
- noncancerous cysts or lumps in the breast may occur less frequently
- acute pelvic inflammatory disease may occur less frequently
- oral contraceptive use may provide some protection against developing two forms of cancer: cancer of the ovaries and cancer of the lining of the uterus.

If you want more information about birth control pills, ask your doctor/health care provider or pharmacist. They have a more technical leaflet called the Professional Labeling, which you may wish to read. The professional labeling is also published in a book entitled *Physicians' Desk Reference*, available in many book stores and public libraries.

ORTHO-McNEIL
ORTHO-McNEIL PHARMACEUTICAL, INC.
Raritan, New Jersey 08869
 REVISED JANUARY 2000 635-50-900-5
Shown in Product Identification Guide, page 328

PANCREASE® ℞

[*pan 'kre-āce*]
brand of PANCRELIPASE
ENTERIC COATED MICROSPHERES
Capsules

DESCRIPTION

PANCREASE® (pancrelipase) Capsules are a pancreatic enzyme supplement for oral administration. Pancrelipase, the active ingredient in PANCREASE Capsules, is a natural product harvested by extraction from the pancreas of the hog. Pancrelipase powder is a slightly brown amorphous powder with a faint characteristic odor. It is partly soluble in water and practically insoluble in alcohol or ether.

PANCREASE Capsules contain enteric-coated microspheres of porcine pancreatic enzyme concentrate in the following theoretical quantities:

Lipase	4,500 U.S.P. Units
Amylase	20,000 U.S.P. Units
Protease	25,000 U.S.P. Units

Inactive ingredients are povidone, sodium starch glycolate, sugar (sucrose) spheres, cellulose acetate phthalate, diethyl phthalate, talc, corn starch, titanium dioxide, gelatin, and other trace ingredients.

PRECLINICAL

Studies in a small number of rats administered indomethacin or ibuprofen and pancrelipase enzymes concomitantly revealed intestinal and liver lesions. The clinical significance of these findings is not known.

CLINICAL PHARMACOLOGY

The enteric-coated microspheres contained in PANCREASE Capsules resist gastric inactivation and deliver enzymes into the duodenum. The enzymes in PANCREASE act locally in the gastrointestinal tract. The enzymes are present in the form of pH-sensitive enteric-coated microspheres of less than 3 mm in diameter which are filled into gelatin capsules. The microspheres, which are released from the capsule into the stomach, are enteric coated to resist inactivation at low pH. Once released the microspheres are distributed into the stomach and pass into the duodenum where, when the pH reaches approximately 5.5, the enteric coating begins to dissolve and the release of the enzymes is initiated. The enzymes catalyze the hydrolysis of fats into glycerol and fatty acids, protein into proteoses and derived substances, and starch into dextrins and sugars. Duodenal availability studies in adults indicate that following oral administration of PANCREASE to adults, measurable levels of enzymes are present in the duodenum. Once thay have accomplished their digestive function the enzymes may be digested in the intestine. The constituents may be partially absorbed and subsequently excreted in the urine. Any undigested enzymes are excreted in the feces.

INDICATIONS AND USAGE

PANCREASE is indicated for the treatment of steatorrhea secondary to pancreatic insufficiency such as cystic fibrosis or chronic alcoholic pancreatitis.

CONTRAINDICATIONS

PANCREASE Capsules are contraindicated in patients known to be hypersensitive to pork protein or any other component of this product.

WARNINGS

Cases of fibrotic strictures in the colon have been reportedly primarily in cystic fibrosis patients with the use of enzyme supplements, generally at dosages above the recommended range. Some cases required surgery including resection of the bowel. If symptoms suggestive of gastrointestinal obstruction occur, the possibility of bowel strictures should be considered.

Any change in pancreatic enzyme replacement therapy (e.g., dose or brand of medication) should be made cautiously and only under medical supervision. It is recommended that therapy be initiated at a low dose, followed by titration to an effective dose. The titration schedule should be guided by measured changes in 3-day fecal fat excretion. (See **DOSAGE AND ADMINISTRATION.**)

PRECAUTIONS

General

TO PROTECT THE ENTERIC COATING, MICROSPHERES SHOULD NOT BE CRUSHED OR CHEWED. Intact capsules should be swallowed with liquids at mealtime. If an intact capsule can not be swallowed, it may be opened and the contents taken with small amounts of food that do not require chewing. (See **DOSAGE AND ADMINISTRATION.**)

Information for Patients

Patients should be advised that:

- PANCREASE Capsules must not be crushed or chewed;
- intact capsules should be swallowed with liquid at mealtimes;
- the microspheres from opened capsules should be swallowed immediately and not be retained in the mouth;
- doses should only be taken with meals or snacks;
- fluids should be consumed liberally while dosing with PANCREASE;
- any change in pancreatic enzyme replacement therapy (e.g., dose or brand of medication) should be made only under medical supervision.

Pregnancy: Teratogenic Effects

Pregnancy Category B

Reproduction studies have been conducted in rats and rabbits at doses 0.44 times and 0.35 times the maximum daily human dose, respectively, and have revealed no evidence of impaired fertility or harm to the fetus due to PANCREASE. No fertility or peri-/postnatal studies have been performed in animals. There are, however, no adequate and well-controlled studies in pregnant women. Because animal reproduction studies are not always predictive of human response, this drug should be used during pregnancy only if clearly needed.

Nursing Mothers

Pancreatic enzymes act locally in the gastrointestinal tract and are not likely to be systematically absorbed. Some of the constituent amino and nucleic acids are likely to be absorbed along with dietary proteins. The possibility of the protein constituents appearing in the breast milk can not be excluded.

Pediatric Use

Colonic strictures, particularly in children with cystic fibrosis, have been associated with doses generally above the recommended dosing range (See **WARNINGS.**) Patients currently receiving doses >2,500 lipase units/kg/meal or 4,000 lipase units/gm fat/day should be re-evaluated and the dosage either immediately decreased or titrated downward to the lowest effective clinical dose as assessed by 3-day fecal fat excretion.

Geriatric Use

Studies on the relationship of age to the effects of pancrelipase have not been conducted. However, geriatric-specific problems that would limit the usefulness of this medication in the elderly are not expected.

ADVERSE REACTIONS

Clinical evidence indicates that PANCREASE Capsules are well-tolerated.

The most frequently reported adverse events resulting from the post-marketing experience with PANCREASE were gastrointestinal and include diarrhea, abdominal pain, intestinal obstruction, vomiting, flatulence, nausea, constipation, melena, and perianal irritation. Frequently reported adverse events in other body systems included weight decrease and pain. Hyperuricemia and hyperuricosuria have been reported with the use of pancrelipase products, primarily with non-enteric coaated formulations. Cases of fibrosing colonopathy have been reported primarily in cystic fibrosis. (See **WARNINGS**)

OVERDOSAGE

There have been no reports of acute overdosage.

DOSAGE AND ADMINISTRATION

General

Patients with pancreatic insufficiency should consume a high-calorie diet with unrestricted fat which is appropriate for age and clinical status. A nutritional assessment should be performed regularly as a component of routine care and additionally, when dosing of pancreatic enzyme replacement is altered.

Dosage should be individualized and determined by the degree of steatorrhea and the fat content of the diet. Therapy should be initiated at the lowest possible dose and gradually incresed until the desired control of steatorrhea is obtained. Dosage should be adjusted based on 3-day fecal fat studies. PANCREASE Capsules should only be taken with meals or snacks.

It is important to ensure that patients ingest a liberal amount of liquids to maintain adequate hydration while dosing with PANCREASE.

Continued on next page

Pancrease—Cont.

Whenever possible, PANCREASE Capsules should be swallowed intact with generous amounts of liquid. However, if swallowing of capsules is difficult, they may be opened and the microspheres sprinkled onto a small quantity of soft food on a teaspoon or tablespoon and ingested immediately. Foods which do not require chewing and have a pH lower than 7.3 are recommended. Examples of such foods are apricot, banana and sweet potato baby foods, applesauce, instant pudding and gelatin snacks. Contact of the microspheres with foods having a pH greater than 7.3 (e.g., milk, custard, ice cream, and many other dairy products) can dissolve the protective enteric coating and destroy enzyme activity.
To avoid irritation of the mouth, lips, and tongue, opened PANCREASE Capsules should be swallowed immediately before regular feedings or meals to minimize the likelihood that the microspheres are retained in the mouth. Proteolytic enzymes present in pancrelipase, when retained in the mouth, may begin to digest the mucous membranes and cause ulcerations.
There is considerable variation among individuals in response to enzymes with respect to control of steatorrhea; therefore, a range of doses is suggested.

Infants: (up to 12 months)
Fat-consumption scheme
2,000–4000 U.S.P. lipase units per 120 mL of formula or per breast feeding. This provides approximately 450–900 lipase units per gram of fat ingested (based on 4.5 grams of fat per 120 mL standard cow's milk-based infant formula).
Higher doses are used in infants because on average, infants ingest 5 grams of fat per kilogram of body weight per day, whereas adults tend to ingest about 2 grams of fat per kilogram per day.

Children and Older
Weight-based scheme
< 4 yrs: Begin with 1,000 U.S.P. lipase units/kg/meal to a maximum of 2,500 lipase units/kg/meal.
> 4 yrs: Begin with 400 U.S.P. lipase units/kg/meal to a maximum of 2,500 units/kg/meal.
Enzyme doses, expressed as lipase units/kg/meal, should be decreased in older patients since they weigh more but tend to ingest less fat per kilogram. Usually, half the mealtime dose is given with a snack. The total daily dose reflects approximately three meals and two to three snacks per day.
If doses greater than 2,500 lipase units/kg/meal (4,000 lipase units/gm fat/day) are required to control malabsorption, further investigation is warranted to rule out other causes of malabsorption. Doses greater than 2,500 lipase units/kg/meal should be used with caution and only if they are documented to be effective by 3-day fecal fat measures. It is unknown whether doses above 2,500 lipase units/kg/meal are safe.
Colonic strictures, particularly in children with cystic fibrosis, have been associated with doses generally above the recommended dosing range (See **WARNINGS**.) Patients currently receiving doses >2,500 lipase units/kg/meal or 4,000 lipase units/gm/fat/day should be re-evaluated and the dosage either immediately decreased or titrated downward to the lowest effective clinical dose as assessed by 3-day fecal fat excretion.

HOW SUPPLIED

PANCREASE (pancrelipase) Capsules are supplied as white body, clear cap, dye-free capsules. PANCREASE Capsules are imprinted with "McNEIL" and "Pancrease" and are packaged in bottles of:
100–(NDC 0045-0095-60)
250–(NDC 0045-0095-69)

Storage
PANCREASE Capsules should be stored in a dry place below 25° C (77° F) in well-closed containers. Do not refrigerate.
Rx only.
PANCREASE is manufactured and distributed by:
McNEIL PHARMACEUTICAL
McNEILAB, INC.
SPRING HOUSE, PA 19477
©McNEILAB, Inc. — 1992
Patent No. 4,079,125
Revised 6/98 643-10-106-4
Shown in Product Identification Guide, page 328

PANCREASE® MT ℞
[pan 'kre-āce MT]
brand of PANCRELIPASE
ENTERIC COATED MICROTABLETS
Capsules

DESCRIPTION

PACREASE® MT (pancrelipase) Capsules are a pancreatic enzyme supplement for oral administration. Pancrelipase, the active ingredient in PANCREASE MT Capsules, is a natural product harvested by extraction from the pancreas of the hog. Pancrelipase powder is a slightly brown amorphous powder with a faint characteristic odor. It is partly soluble in water and practically insoluble in alcohol or ether. PANCREASE MT Capsules contain enteric-coated microtablets of porcine pancreatic enzyme concentrate in the following theoretical quantities:

PANCREASE MT 4 Capsules:	
Lipase	4,000 U.S.P. Units
Amylase	12,000 U.S.P. Units
Protease	12,000 U.S.P. Units
PANCREASE MT 10 Capsules:	
Lipase	10,000 U.S.P. Units
Amylase	30,000 U.S.P. Units
Protease	30,000 U.S.P. Units
PANCREASE MT 16 Capsules:	
Lipase	16,000 U.S.P. Units
Amylase	48,000 U.S.P. Units
Protease	48,000 U.S.P. Units
PANCREASE MT 20 Capsules:	
Lipase	20,000 U.S.P. Units
Amylase	56,000 U.S.P. Units
Protease	44,000 U.S.P. Units

Inactive ingredients are cellulose, crospovidone, magnesium stearate, colloidal silicon dioxide, methacrylic acid copolymer, triethyl citrate, talc, polydimethylsiloxane, wax, gelatin, iron oxide, polysorbate 80, sodium lauryl sulfate, titanium dioxide, and other trace ingredients.

PRECLINICAL

Studies in small number of rats administered indomethacin or ibuprofen and pancrelipase enzymes concomitantly revealed intestinal and liver lesions. The clinical significance of these findings is not known.

CLINICAL PHARMACOLOGY

The enteric-coated microtablets contained in PANCREASE MT Capsules resist gastric inactivation and deliver enzymes into the duodenum. The enzymes in PANCREASE MT act locally in the gastrointestinal tract. The enzymes are present in the form of pH-sensitive enteric-coated microtablets of less than 3 mm in diameter which are filled into gelatin capsules. The microtablets, which are released from the capsule into the stomach, are enteric coated to resist inactivation at low pH. Once released, the microtablets are distributed into the stomach and pass into the duodenum where, when the pH reaches approximately 5.5, the enteric coating begins to dissolve and release of the enzymes is initiated. The enzymes catalyze the hydrolysis of fats into glycerol and fatty acids, protein into proteoses and derived substances, and starch into dextrins and sugars. Duodenal availability studies in adults indicate that following oral administration of PANCREASE MT to adults, measurable levels of enzymes are present in the duodenum. Once they have accomplished their digestive function the enzymes may be digested in the intestine. The constituents may be partially absorbed and subsequently excreted in the urine. Any undigested enzymes are excreted in the feces.

INDICATIONS AND USAGE

PANCREASE MT is indicated for the treatment of steatorrhea secondary to pancreatic insufficiency such as cystic fibrosis or chronic alcoholic pancreatitis.

CONTRAINDICATIONS

PANCREASE MT Capsules are contraindicated in patients known to be hypersensitive to pork protein or any other component of this product.

WARNINGS

Cases of fibrotic strictures in the colon have been reported primarily in cystic fibrosis patients with the use of enzyme supplements, generally at dosages above the recommended range. Some cases required surgery including resection of the bowel. If symptoms suggestive of gastrointestinal obstruction occur, the possibility of bowel strictures should be considered.
Any change in pancreatic enzyme replacement therapy (e.g., dose or brand of medication) should be made cautiously and only under medical supervision. It is recommended that therapy be initiated at a low dose, followed by titration to an effective dose. The titration schedule should be guided by measured changes in 3-day fecal fat excretion. (See **DOSAGE AND ADMINISTRATION**.)

PRECAUTIONS
General
TO PROTECT THE ENTERIC COATING, MICROTABLETS SHOULD NOT BE CRUSHED OR CHEWED. Intact capsules should be swallowed with liquids at mealtime. If an intact capsule can not be swallowed, it may be opened and the contents taken with small amounts of food that do not require chewing. (See **DOSAGE AND ADMINISTRATION**.)

Information for Patients
Patients should be advised that:
- PANCREASE MT Capsules must not be crushed or chewed;
- intact capsules should be swallowed with liquid at mealtimes;
- the microtablets from opened capsules should be swallowed immediately and not be retained in the mouth;
- doses should only be taken with meals or snacks;
- fluids should be consumed liberally while dosing with PANCREASE MT;
- any change in pancreatic enzyme replacement therapy (e.g., dose or brand of medication) should be made only under medical supervision.

Pregnancy: Teratogenic Effects
Pregnancy Category B
Reproduction studies have been conducted in rats and rabbits at doses 0.44 times and 0.35 times the maximum daily human dose, respectively, and have revealed no evidence of impaired fertility or harm to the fetus due to PANCREASE MT. No fertility or peri-/postnatal studies have been performed in animals. There are, however, no adequate and well-controlled studies in pregnant women. Because animal reproduction studies are not always predictive of human response, this drug should be used during pregnancy only if clearly needed.

Nursing Mothers
Pancreatic enzymes act locally in the gastrointestinal tract and are not likely to be systemically absorbed. Some of the constituent amino and nucleic acids are likely to be absorbed along with dietary proteins. The possibility of the protein constituents appearing in the breast milk can not be excluded.

Pediatric Use
Colonic strictures, particularly in children with cystic fibrosis, have been associated with doses generally above the recommended dosing range. (See **WARNINGS**.) Patients currently receiving doses >2,500 lipase units/kg/meal or 4,000 lipase units/gm fat/day should be re-evaluated and the dosage either immediately decreased or titrated downward to the lowest effective clinical dose as assessed by 3-day fecal fat excretion.

Geriatric Use
Studies on the relationship of age to the effects of pancrelipase have not been conducted. However, geriatric-specific problems that would limit the usefulness of this medication in the elderly are not expected.

ADVERSE REACTIONS

Clinical evidence indicates that PANCREASE MT Capsules are well-tolerated.
The most frequently reported adverse events resulting from the post-marketing experience with PANCREASE MT were gastrointestinal in nature and include diarrhea, abdominal pain, intestinal obstruction, vomiting, intestinal stenosis, and constipation. Frequently reported adverse events in other body systems include dermatitis. Hyperuricemia and hyperuricosuria have been reported with the use of pancrelipase products, primarily with non-enteric coated formulations. Cases of fibrosing colonopathy have been reported primarily in cystic fibrosis patients. (See **WARNINGS**.)

OVERDOSAGE

There have been no reports of acute overdosage.

DOSAGE AND ADMINISTRATION
General
Patients with pancreatic insufficiency should consume a high-calorie diet with unrestricted fat which is appropriate for age and clinical status. A nutritional assessment should be performed regularly as a component of routine care and additionally, when dosing of pancreatic enzyme replacement is altered.
Dosage should be individualized and determined by the degree of steatorrhea and the fat content of the diet. Therapy should be initiated at the lowest possible dose and gradually increased until the desired control of steatorrhea is obtained. Dosage should be adjusted based on 3-day fecal fat studies.
PANCREASE MT Capsules should only be taken with meals or snacks.
It is important to ensure that patients ingest a liberal amount of liquids to maintain adequate hydration while dosing with PANCREASE MT.
Whenever possible, PANCREASE MT Capsules should be swallowed intact with generous amounts of liquid. However, if swallowing of capsules is difficult, they may be opened and the microtablets sprinkled onto a small quantity of soft food on a teaspoon or tablespoon and ingested immediately. Foods which do not require chewing and have a pH lower than 7.3 are recommended. Examples of such foods are apricot, banana and sweet potato baby foods, applesauce, instant pudding and gelatin snacks. Contact of the microtablets with foods having a pH greater than 7.3 (e.g., milk, custard, ice cream, and many other dairy products) can dissolve the protective enteric coating and destroy the enzyme activity.
To avoid irritation of the mouth, lips, and tongue, opened PANCREASE MT Capsules should be swallowed immediately before regular feedings or meals to minimize the likelihood that the microtablets are retained in the mouth. Proteolytic enzymes present in pancrealipase, when retained in the mouth, may begin to digest the mucous membranes and cause ulcerations.
There is considerable variation among individuals in response to enzymes with respect to control of steatorrhea; therefore, a range of doses is suggested.

Infants: (up to 12 months)
Fat-consumption scheme
2,000–4,000 U.S.P. lipase units per 120 mL of formula or per breast feeding. This provides approximately 450–900 lipase units per gram of fat ingested (based on 4.5 grams of fat per 120 mL standard cow's milk-based infant formula).
Higher doses are used in infants because on average, infants ingest 5 grams of fat per kilogram of body weight per day, whereas adults tend to ingest about 2 grams of fat per kilogram per day.

Children and Older
Weight-based scheme
<4 yrs: Begin with 1,000 U.S.P. lipase units/kg/meal to a maximum of 2,500 lipase units/kg/meal.
>4 yrs: Begin with 400 U.S.P. lipase units/kg/meal to a maximum of 2,500 lipase units/kg/meal.

Enzyme doses, expressed as lipase units/kg/meal, should be decreased in older patients since they weigh more but tend to ingest less fat per kilogram. Usually, half the mealtime dose is given with a snack. The total daily dose reflects approximately three meals and two to three snacks per day.

If doses greater than 2,500 lipase units/kg/meal (4,000 lipase units/gm fat/day) are required to control malabsorption, further investigation is warranted to rule out other causes of malabsorption. Doses greater than 2,500 lipase units/kg/meal should be used with caution and only if they are documented to be effective by 3-day fecal fat measures. It is unknown whether doses above 2,500 lipase units/kg/meal are safe.

Colonic strictures, particularly in children with cystic fibrosis, have been associated with doses generally above the recommended dosing range. (See **WARNINGS**.) Patients currently receiving doses >2,500 lipase units/kg/meal or 4,000 lipase units/gm fat/day should be re-evaluated and the dosage either immediately decreased or titrated downward to the lowest effective clinical dose as assessed by 3-day fecal fat excretion.

HOW SUPPLIED

PANCREASE MT 4 (pancrelipase) Capsules are supplied as yellow opaque body, clear cap capsules imprinted with "McNEIL" and "PANCREASE MT 4" and packaged in bottles of 100–(NDC 0045-0341-60).

PANCREASE MT 10 (pancrelipase) Capsules are supplied as pink opaque body, clear cap capsules imprinted with "McNEIL" and "PANCREASE MT 10" and packaged in bottles of 100–(NDC 0045-0342-60).

PANCREASE MT 16 (pancrelipase) Capsules are supplied as salmon opaque body, clear cap capsules imprinted with "McNEIL" and "PANCREASE MT 16" and packaged in bottles of 100–(NDC 0045-0343-60).

PANCREASE MT 20 (pancrelipase) Capsules are supplied as white opaque body, cap with yellow band capsules imprinted with "McNEIL" and "PANCREASE MT 20" and packaged in bottles of 100–(NDC 0045-0346-60).

Storage

PANCREASE MT Capsules should be stored in a dry place below 25° C (77° F) in well-closed containers. Do not refrigerate.

Rx only.

Microtablets manufactured by Knoll AG Uetersen, Germany.

McNEIL PHARMACEUTICAL
McNEILAB, INC.
SPRING HOUSE, PA 19477
©McNEILAB, Inc.—1994

Revised 6/98 643-10-104-4

Shown in Product Identification Guide, page 329

PARAFON FORTE® DSC ℞

[par 'a-fahn for 'ta]

(chlorzoxazone) Caplets 500 mg
For Painful Musculoskeletal Conditions
NSN 6505-01-264-4453—100's
NSN 6505-01-288-0524—100's (10x10)

DESCRIPTION

Each caplet (capsule shaped tablet) contains:
Chlorzoxazone* .... 500 mg

Inactive ingredients: FD&C Blue No. 1, microcrystalline cellulose, docusate sodium, lactose (hydrous), magnesium stearate, sodium benzoate, sodium starch glycolate, pregelatinized corn starch, D&C Yellow No. 10.

*5-chlorobenzoxazolinone

ACTIONS

Chlorzoxazone is a centrally-acting agent for painful musculoskeletal conditions. Data available from animal experiments as well as human study indicate that chlorzoxazone acts primarily at the level of the spinal cord and subcortical areas of the brain where it inhibits multisynaptic reflex arcs involved in producing and maintaining skeletal muscle spasm of varied etiology. The clinical result is a reduction of the skeletal muscle spasm with relief of pain and increased mobility of the involved muscles. Blood levels of chlorzoxazone can be detected in people during the first 30 minutes and peak levels may be reached, in the majority of the subjects, in about 1 to 2 hours after oral administration of chlorzoxazone. Chlorzoxazone is rapidly metabolized and is excreted in the urine, primarily in a conjugated form as the glucuronide. Less than one percent of a dose of chlorzoxazone is excreted unchanged in the urine in 24 hours.

INDICATIONS

PARAFON FORTE DSC chlorzoxazone is indicated as an adjunct to rest, physical therapy, and other measures for the relief of discomfort associated with acute, painful musculoskeletal conditions. The mode of action of this drug has not been clearly identified, but may be related to its sedative properties. Chlorzoxazone does not directly relax tense skeletal muscles in man.

CONTRAINDICATIONS

PARAFON FORTE DSC chlorzoxazone is contraindicated in patients with known intolerance to the drug.

WARNINGS

Serious (including fatal) hepatocellular toxicity has been reported rarely in patients receiving chlorzoxazone. The mechanism is unknown but appears to be idiosyncratic and unpredictable. Factors predisposing patients to this rare event are not known. Patients should be instructed to report early signs and/or symptoms of hepatotoxicity such as fever, rash, anorexia, nausea, vomiting, fatigue, right upper quandrant pain, dark urine, or jaundice. Chlorzoxazone should be discontinued immediately and a physician consulted if any of these signs or symptoms develop. Chlorzoxazone use should also be discontinued if a patient develops abnormal liver enzymes (eg. AST, ALT, alkaline phosphatase and bilirubin).

The concomitant use of alcohol or other central nervous system depressants may have an additive effect.

Usage in Pregnancy: The safe use of PARAFON FORTE DSC chlorzoxazone has not been established with respect to the possible adverse effects upon fetal development. Therefore, it should be used in women of childbearing potential only when, in the judgment of the physician, the potential benefits outweigh the possible risks.

PRECAUTIONS

PARAFON FORTE DSC chlorzoxazone should be used with caution in patients with known allergies or with a history of allergic reactions to drugs. If a sensitivity reaction occurs such as urticaria, redness, or itching of the skin, the drug should be stopped.

If any signs or symptoms suggestive of liver dysfunction are observed, the drug should be discontinued.

ADVERSE REACTIONS

Chlorzoxazone containing products are usually well tolerated. It is possible in rare instances that chlorzoxazone may have been associated with gastrointestinal bleeding. Drowsiness, dizziness, light-headedness, malaise, or overstimulation may be noted by an occasional patient. Rarely, allergic-type skin rashes, petechiae, or ecchymoses may develop during treatment. Angioneurotic edema or anaphylactic reactions are extremely rare. There is no evidence that the drug will cause renal damage. Rarely, a patient may note discoloration of the urine resulting from a phenolic metabolite of chlorzoxazone. This finding is of no known clinical significance.

DOSAGE AND ADMINISTRATION

Usual Adult Dosage: One caplet three or four times daily. If adequate reponse is not obtained with this dose, it may be increased to $1^1/_2$ caplets (750 mg) three or four times daily. As improvement occurs dosage can usually be reduced.

OVERDOSAGE

Symptoms: Initially, gastrointestinal disturbances such as nausea, vomiting, or diarrhea together with drowsiness, dizziness, lightheadedness or headache may occur. Early in the course there may be malaise or sluggishness followed by marked loss of muscle tone, making voluntary movement impossible. The deep tendon reflexes may be decreased or absent. The sensorium remains intact, and there is no peripheral loss of sensation. Respiratory depression may occur with rapid, irregular respiration and intercostal and substernal retraction. The blood pressure is lowered, but shock has not been observed.

Treatment: Gastric lavage or induction of emesis should be carried out, followed by administration of activated charcoal. Thereafter, treatment is entirely supportive. If respirations are depressed, oxygen and artificial respiration should be employed and a patent airway assured by use of an oropharyngeal airway or endotracheal tube. Hypotension may be counteracted by use of dextran, plasma, concentrated albumin or a vasopressor agent such as norepinephrine. Cholinergic drugs or analeptic drugs are of no value and should not be used.

HOW SUPPLIED

PARAFON FORTE® DSC (chlorzoxazone) 500 mg caplets, (capsule shaped tablet, colored light green, imprinted "PARAFON FORTE DSC" and "McNEIL", scored).

NDC 0045-0325, bottles of 100, 500 and unit dose 100's.

Dispense in a tight container as defined in the official compendium.

Store at controlled room temperature (15°–30°C, 59°–86°F).

Revised 3/01/95 643-10-098-2

McNeil Pharmaceutical, McNEILAB, Inc.
Spring House, PA 19477

Shown in Product Identification Guide, page 329

PARAGARD® T 380A ℞

Intrauterine Copper Contraceptive

Patients should be counseled that this product does not protect against HIV Infection (AIDS) and other sexually transmitted diseases.

NOTICE

You have received a Patient Package Insert that Federal Regulations (21 CFR 310.502) require you to furnish to each patient who is considering the use of the ParaGard® T 380A.

The Patient Package Insert contains information on the safety and efficacy of the ParaGard® T 380A. Before inserting the ParaGard® T 380A:

- You should read the physician prescription labeling and be familiar with all the information it contains.
- You should counsel the patient and answer her questions about contraception, the ParaGard® T 380A, and the information in the Patient Package Insert.
- You and the patient should read each section of the Patient Package Insert, and if the patient agrees, she may sign a consent form provided for your convenience.

The Patient Package Insert is also available in Spanish and other foreign languages. Address requests to Ortho-McNeil Pharmaceutical, Inc. telephone 1-800-322-4966.

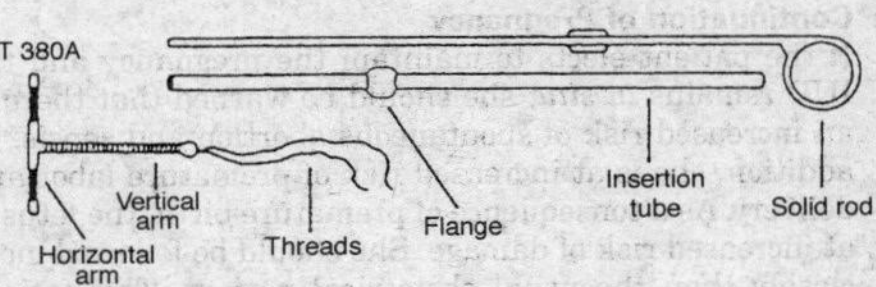

DESCRIPTION

The polyethylene body of the ParaGard® T 380A is wound with approximately 176 mg of copper wire and carries a copper collar of approximately 68.7 mg of copper on each of its transverse arms. The exposed surface areas of copper are 380 ± 23 mm^2. The dimensions of the ParaGard® T 380A are 36 mm in the vertical direction and 32 mm in the horizontal direction. The tip of the vertical arm of the ParaGard® T 380A is enlarged to form a bulb having a diameter of 3 mm. The ParaGard® T 380A is equipped with a monofilament polyethylene thread which is tied through the bulb, resulting in two threads at the tip to aid in removal of the IUD. The ParaGard® T 380A contains barium sulfate to render it radiopaque.

The ParaGard® T 380A is packaged together with an insertion tube and solid rod in a Tyvek®-polyethylene pouch and then sterilized. The insertion tube is equipped with a movable flange to aid in gauging the depth to which the insertion tube is inserted through the cervical canal and into the uterine cavity.

CLINICAL PHARMACOLOGY

Available data indicate that the contraceptive effectiveness of the ParaGard® T 380A is enhanced by copper being released continuously from the copper coil and sleeves into the uterine cavity. The exact mechanism by which metallic copper enhances the contraceptive effect of an IUD has not been conclusively demonstrated. Various hypotheses have been advanced, including interference with sperm transport, fertilization, and implantation. Clinical studies with copper-bearing IUDs also suggest that fertilization is prevented either due to an altered number or lack of viability of spermatozoa.[1]

INDICATIONS AND USAGE

The ParaGard® T 380A is indicated for intrauterine contraception. ParaGard® T 380A is highly effective. Table II and Table III list an expected pregnancy rate for one year between 0.7 and 0.5, respectively. ParaGard® T 380A should not be kept in place longer than 10 years.

RECOMMENDED PATIENT PROFILE

The ParaGard® T 380A is recommended for women who have had at least one child, are in a stable, mutually monogamous relationship, and have no history of pelvic inflammatory disease.

CONTRAINDICATIONS

The ParaGard® T 380A should not be inserted when one or more of the following conditions exist:

1. Pregnancy or suspicion of pregnancy.
2. Abnormalities of the uterus resulting in distortion of the uterine cavity.
3. Acute pelvic inflammatory disease or a history of pelvic inflammatory disease.
4. Postpartum endometritis or infected abortion in the past 3 months.
5. Known or suspected uterine or cervical malignancy, including unresolved, abnormal "Pap" smear.
6. Genital bleeding of unknown etiology.
7. Untreated acute cervicitis or vaginitis, including bacterial vaginosis, until infection is controlled.
8. Copper-containing IUDs should not be inserted in the presence of diagnosed Wilson's disease.
9. Known allergy to copper.
10. Patient or her partner has multiple sexual partners.
11. Conditions associated with increased susceptibility to infections with microorganisms. Such conditions include, but are not limited to, leukemia, acquired immune deficiency syndrome (AIDS), and I.V. drug abuse.
12. Genital actinomycosis.
13. A previously inserted IUD that has not been removed.

WARNINGS

1. PREGNANCY

Effects on the offspring when pregnancy occurs with the ParaGard® T 380A in place are unknown.

a. Septic Abortion

Reports indicate an increased incidence of septic abortion with septicemia, septic shock, and death in patients becoming pregnant with an IUD in place. Most of these reports have been associated with, but are not limited to, the mid-trimester of pregnancy. In some cases, the initial symptoms have been insidious and not easily recognized. If pregnancy should occur with an IUD *in situ*, the IUD

Continued on next page

Paragard T—Cont.

should be removed if the string is visible and removal is easily accomplished. Of course, manipulation may result in spontaneous abortion. If removal proves to be difficult, or if threads are not visible, interruption of the pregnancy should be considered and offered as an option. Rates of mortality with and without contraception are shown in Table 1.

b. Continuation of Pregnancy
If the patient elects to maintain the pregnancy and the IUD remains *in situ*, she should be warned that there is an increased risk of spontaneous abortion and sepsis. In addition, she is at increased risk of premature labor and delivery. As a consequence of premature birth, the fetus is at increased risk of damage. She should be followed more closely than the usual obstetrical patient. The patient must be advised to report immediately all abnormal symptoms, such as flu-like syndrome, fever, abdominal cramping or pain, bleeding or vaginal discharge, because generalized symptoms of septicemia may be insidious.

2. ECTOPIC PREGNANCY

a. Patients with a history of ectopic pregnancy are at an increased risk of subsequent pregnancies being ectopic. Although current data indicate that there is no increased risk of ectopic pregnancy in patients using the ParaGard® T 380A and some data suggest there may be a lower risk than the general population using no method of contraception, a pregnancy which occurs with the ParaGard® T 380A in place is more likely to be ectopic than a pregnancy occurring without the ParaGard® T 380A[2–4]. Therefore, patients who become pregnant while using the ParaGard® T 380A should be carefully evaluated for the possibility of an ectopic pregnancy.
b. Special attention should be directed to patients with delayed menses, slight metrorrhagia and/or unilateral pelvic pain, and to those patients who wish to terminate a pregnancy because of IUD failure, to determine whether ectopic pregnancy has occurred.

3. PELVIC INFECTION (PELVIC INFLAMMATORY DISEASE, PID)

The ParaGard® T 380A is contraindicated in the presence of PID or in women with a history of PID. Use of all IUDs, including the ParaGard® T 380A, has been associated with an increased incidence of PID. Therefore, a decision to use the ParaGard® T 380A must include consideration of the risks of PID. The highest rate of PID has been reported to occur after insertion and up to four months thereafter. A study suggests that the highest incidence occurs within 20 days postinsertion, then falls, remaining constant thereafter.[5] Administration of prophylactic antibiotics has been reported, although studies do not confirm the utility of this prophylactic measure in reducing PID. PID can necessitate hysterectomy and can also lead to tubo-ovarian abscesses, tubal occlusion and infertility, and tubal damage that can predispose to ectopic pregnancy. PID can result in peritonitis and, infrequently, in death. The effect of PID on fertility is especially important for women who may wish to have children at a later date.

a. Women at special risk of PID
The risk of PID appears to be greater for women who have multiple sexual partners and also for those women whose sexual partners have multiple sexual partners, as PID is most frequently caused by sexually transmitted diseases.

b. PID warning to ParaGard® T 380A users
All women who choose the ParaGard® T 380A must be informed prior to insertion that IUD use has been associated with an increased incidence of PID and that PID can necessitate hysterectomy, can cause tubal damage leading to ectopic pregnancy or infertility or, in infrequent cases, can cause death. Patients must be taught to recognize and report to their physician promptly any symptoms of pelvic inflammatory disease. These symptoms include development of menstrual disorders (prolonged or heavy bleeding), unusual vaginal discharge, abdominal or pelvic pain or tenderness, dyspareunia, chills, and fever.

c. Asymptomatic PID
PID may be asymptomatic but still result in tubal damage and its sequelae.[6,7]

d. Treatment of PID
Following diagnosis of PID, or suspected PID, bacteriologic specimens should be obtained and antibiotic therapy should be initiated promptly. Removal of the ParaGard® T 380A after initiation of antibiotic therapy is usually appropriate. Time should be allowed for therapeutic blood levels to be reached prior to removal. Guidelines for PID treatment are available from the Center for Disease Control (CDC), Atlanta, Georgia. A copy of the printed guidelines has been provided to you by Ortho-McNeil Pharmaceutical, Inc. The guidelines were established after deliberation by a group of experts and staff of the CDC, but they should not be construed as rules suitable for use in all patients. Adequate PID treatment requires the application of current standards of therapy prevailing at the time of occurrence of the infection with reference to the prescription labeling of the antibiotic selected.

Genital actinomycosis has been associated primarily with long-term IUD use. If actinomycosis occurs, promptly institute appropriate antibiotic therapy and remove the ParaGard® T 380A.

4. EMBEDMENT

Partial penetration or embedment of the ParaGard® T 380A in the endometrium or myometrium can result in difficult removal. In some cases this can result in breakage of the IUD, necessitating surgical removal.

5. PERFORATION

Partial or total perforation of the uterine wall or cervix may occur with use of the ParaGard® T 380A. The rate of perforation in randomized trials of the ParaGard® T 380A has been 1 in 1,360. Insertions immediately after the expulsion of the placenta are not known to be associated with increased risks of perforation, but insertion later in the first postpartum month, particularly during lactation, has been associated with an increased risk of perforation.[8,9] Thus, unless performed immediately postpartum, insertion should be delayed to the second postpartum month. IUD insertion immediately postabortion in the first trimester is not known to be associated with increased risks of perforation, but insertion after second trimester abortion should be delayed until the second postabortion month.

The possibility of perforation must be kept in mind during insertion and at the time of any subsequent examination. If perforation occurs, the ParaGard® T 380A should be removed as soon as possible. A surgical procedure may be required. Abdominal adhesions, intestinal penetration, intestinal obstruction, and local inflammatory reaction with abscess formation and erosion of adjacent viscera may result if the ParaGard® T 380A is left in the peritoneal cavity. There are reports of migration after insertion.

6. MEDICAL DIATHERMY

The use of medical diathermy (short-wave and microwave) in a patient with a metal-containing IUD may cause heat injury to the surrounding tissue. Therefore, medical diathermy to the abdominal and sacral areas should not be used on patients with a ParaGard® T 380A in place.

7. EFFECTS OF COPPER

Additional amounts of copper available to the body from the ParaGard® T 380A may precipitate symptoms in women with Wilson's disease. The incidence of Wilson's disease is approximately 1 in 200,000. The long-term effects of intrauterine copper to a child conceived in the presence of an IUD are unknown.

8. RISKS OF MORTALITY

The available data from a variety of sources have been analyzed to estimate the risk of death associated with various methods of contraception. The estimates of risk of death include the combined risk of the contraceptive method plus the risk of pregnancy or abortion in the event of method failure. The findings of the analysis are shown in Table I.[10]
[See table below]

PRECAUTIONS

Patients should be counseled that this product does not protect against HIV Infection (AIDS) and other sexually transmitted diseases.

1. Patient Counseling

Prior to insertion, the physician, nurse, or other trained health professional must provide the patient with the Patient Package Insert. The patient should be given the opportunity to read the information and discuss fully any questions she may have concerning the ParaGard® T 380A as well as other methods of contraception.

2. Patient Evaluation and Clinical Considerations

a. A complete medical and social history, including that of the partner, should be obtained to determine conditions that might influence the selection of an IUD. A physical examination should include a pelvic examination, a "Pap" smear, and appropriate tests for any other forms of genital disease, such as gonorrhea and chlamydia laboratory evaluations, if indicated. If actinomyces-like organisms are detected on the Pap smear, they should be cultured to determine whether genital actinomyces is present. The physician should determine that the patient is not pregnant.
b. The uterus should be carefully sounded prior to the insertion to determine the degree of patency of the endocervical canal and the internal os, and the direction and depth of the uterine cavity. In occasional cases, severe cervical stenosis may be encountered. Do not use excessive force to overcome this resistance.
c. The uterus should sound to a depth of 6 to 9 centimeters (cm). Insertion of an IUD into a uterine cavity measuring less than 6.0 cm by sounding may increase the incidence of expulsion, bleeding, pain, perforation, and possibly, pregnancy.
d. Clinicians are cautioned that it is imperative for them to become thoroughly familiar with the instructions for use before attempting placement of the ParaGard® T 380A. To reduce the possibility of insertion in the presence of an existing undetermined pregnancy, the optimal time for insertion is the latter part of the menstrual period, or one or two days thereafter. The ParaGard® T 380A should not be inserted postpartum or postabortion until involution of the uterus is complete. The incidence of perforation and expulsion is greater if involution is not complete. Data also suggest that there may be an increased risk of perforation and expulsion if the woman is lactating.[8,9] Other recent studies report no increased incidence of perforation or expulsion in lactating women.[11,12]
The ParaGard® T 380A should be placed at the fundus of the uterine cavity. Proper placement enhances contraceptive effectiveness and helps avoid perforation and partial or complete expulsion that could result in pregnancy.
e. Patients experiencing menorrhagia and/or metrorrhagia following IUD insertion may be at risk for the development of hypochromic microcytic anemia. Careful consideration of this risk must be given before insertion in patients with anemia or a history of menorrhagia or hypermenorrhea. Patients receiving anticoagulants or having a coagulopathy may have a greater risk of menorrhagia or hypermenorrhea.
f. Syncope, bradycardia, or other neurovascular episodes may occur during insertion or removal of IUDs, especially in patients with a previous disposition to these conditions or cervical stenosis.
g. Use of an IUD in patients with cervicitis should be postponed until treatment has eradicated the infection.
h. Patients with valvular or congenital heart disease are more prone to develop subacute bacterial endocarditis than patients who do not have valvular or congenital heart disease. Use of an IUD in these patients may represent a potential source of septic emboli. Patients with known congenital heart disease who may be at increased risk should be treated with appropriate antibiotics at the time of insertion.
i. Patients requiring chronic corticosteroid therapy or insulin for diabetes should be monitored with special care for infection.
j. Since the ParaGard® T 380A may be partially or completely expelled, patients should be reexamined and evaluated shortly after the first postinsertion menses, but no later than 3 months afterwards. Thereafter, annual examination with appropriate evaluation, including a "Pap" smear, should be carried out. The ParaGard® T 380A should be kept in place no longer than 10 years.
k. The patient should be told that some bleeding or cramps may occur during the first few weeks after insertion. If these symptoms continue or are severe she should report them to her physician. She should be instructed on how to check to make certain that the threads still protrude from the cervix and cautioned that there is no contraceptive protection if the ParaGard® T 380A has been expelled. She should check frequently, at least after each menstrual period. She should be cautioned not to dislodge the ParaGard® T 380A by pulling on the thread. If a partial expulsion occurs, removal is indicated.
l. Rarely, a copper-induced urticarial allergic skin reaction may develop in women using a copper-containing IUD. If the symptoms of such an allergic response occur, the patient should be instructed to tell the consulting physician that a copper-containing device is being used.
m. The effect of magnetic resonance imaging of the pelvis was investigated in one study[13] in women with the CU-7® (Intrauterine Copper Contraceptive) and the LIPPES LOOP™ IUD. The CU-7® has a different configuration and contains less copper than the ParaGard® T 380A. The results of the study indicate that neither the CU-7® nor the LIPPES LOOP™ were moved under the influence of the magnetic field nor did they heat during the spin-echo sequences usually employed for pelvic imaging.

TABLE I—Annual Number of Birth-Related or Method-Related Deaths Associated with Control of Fertility per 100,000 Non-sterile Women by Fertility Control Method, by Age.

Methods	Age Group 15–19	20–24	25–29	30–34	35–39	40–44
No Birth Control Method/Term	4.7	5.4	4.8	6.3	11.7	20.6
No Birth Control Method/AB	2.1	2.0	1.6	1.9	2.8	5.3
IUD	0.2	0.3	0.2	0.1	0.3	0.6
Periodic Abstinence	1.4	1.3	0.7	1.0	1.0	1.9
Withdrawal	0.9	1.7	0.9	1.3	0.8	1.5
Condom	0.6	1.2	0.6	0.9	0.5	1.0
Diaphragm/Cap	0.6	1.1	0.6	0.9	1.6	3.1
Sponge	0.8	1.5	0.8	1.1	2.2	4.1
Spermicides	1.6	1.9	1.4	1.9	1.5	2.7
Oral Contraceptives	0.8	1.3	1.1	1.8	1.0	1.9
Implants/Injectables	0.2	0.6	0.5	0.8	0.5	0.6
Tubal Sterilization	1.3	1.2	1.1	1.1	1.2	1.3
Vasectomy	0.1	0.1	0.1	0.1	0.1	0.2

TABLE II

ParaGard® T 380A(Intrauterine Copper Contraceptive)
GROSS ANNUAL TERMINATION AND CONTINUATION RATES PER 100* USERS
All Copper T 380A IUD Acceptors
Combined Population Council and WHO Studies

	YEAR									
RATE OF ITEM	**1**	**2**	**3**	**4**	**5**	**6**	**7**	**8**	**9**	**10**
Pregnancy	0.7	0.3	0.6	0.2	0.3	0.2	0.0	0.4	0.0	0.0
Expulsion	5.7	2.5	1.6	1.2	0.3	0.0	0.6	1.7	0.2	0.4
Bleeding/Pain	11.9	9.8	7.0	3.5	3.7	2.7	3.0	2.5	2.2	3.7
Other Medical	2.5	2.1	1.6	1.7	0.1	0.3	1.0	0.4	0.7	0.3
Continuation	76.8	78.3	81.2	86.2	89.0	91.9	87.9	88.1	92.0	91.8
No. of Women:										
At Start of Year	4932	3149	2018	1121	872	621	563	483	423	325
At End of Year	3149	2018	1121	872	621	563	483	423	325	230

* Rates were calculated by weighing the annual rates by the number of subjects starting each year for each of the Population Council (3536 acceptors) and the World Health Organization (1396 acceptors) trials.

TABLE IV—Percentage of women experiencing a contraceptive failure during the first year of typical use and the first year of perfect use and the percentage continuing use at the end of the first year, United States.[16]

	% of Women Experiencing an Accidental Pregnancy Within the First Year of Use		% of Women Continuing Use at One Year[3]
Method	**Typical Use[1]**	**Perfect Use[2]**	
Chance[4]	85	85	
Spermicides[5]	21	6	43
Periodic Abstinence	20		67
Calendar		9	
Ovulation Method		3	
Sympto-Thermal[6]		2	
Post-Ovulation		1	
Withdrawal	19	4	
Cap[7]			
Parous Women	36	26	45
Nulliparous Women	18	9	58
Sponge			
Parous Women	36	20	45
Nulliparous Women	18	9	58
Diaphragm[7]	18	6	58
Condom[8]			
Female (Reality)	21	5	56
Male	12	3	63
Pill	3		72
Progestin Only		0.5	
Combined		0.1	
IUD			
Progesterone T	2.0	1.5	81
Copper T 380A (ParaGard® T 380A)	0.8	0.6	78
Depo-Provera®	0.3	0.3	70
Norplant® (6 Capsules)	0.09	0.09	85
Female Sterilization	0.4	0.4	100
Male Sterilization	0.15	0.10	100

Emergency Contraceptive Pills: Treatment initiated within 72 hours after unprotected intercourse reduces the risk of pregnancy by at least 75%[9].
Lactational Amenorrhea Method: LAM is a highly effective temporary method of contraception.[10]

Footnotes to **Table IV**

1. Among *typical* couples who initiate use of a method (not necessarily for the first time), the percentage who experience an accidental pregnancy during the first year if they do not stop use for any other reason.
2. Among couples who initiate use of a method (not necessarily for the first time) and who use it *perfectly* (both consistently and correctly), the percentage who experience an accidental pregnancy during the first year if they do not stop use for any other reason.
3. Among couples attempting to avoid pregnancy, the percentage who continue to use a method for one year.
4. The percentages failing in columns (2) and (3) are based on data from populations where contraception is not used and from women who cease using contraception in order to become pregnant. Among such populations, about 89% become pregnant within one year. This estimate was lowered slightly (to 85%) to represent the percentage who would become pregnant within 1 year among women now relying on reversible methods of contraception if they abandoned contraception altogether.
5. Foams, creams, gels, vaginal suppositories, and vaginal film.
6. Cervical mucus (ovulation) method supplemented by calendar in the pre-ovulatory and basal body temperature in the post-ovulatory phases.
7. With spermicidal cream or jelly.
8. Without spermicides.
9. The treatment schedule is one dose as soon as possible (but no more than 72 hours) after unprotected intercourse, and a second dose 12 hours after the first dose. The hormones that have been studied in the clinical trials of postcoital hormonal contraception are found in Nordette, Levlen, Lo/Orval (1 dose is 4 pills), Triphasil, Tri-Levlin (1 dose is 4 yellow pills), and Ovral (1 dose is 2 pills).
10. However, to maintain effective protection against pregnancy, another method of contraception must be used as soon as menstruation resumes, the frequency or duration of breastfeeds is reduced, bottle feeds are introduced, or the baby reaches 6 months of age.

3. Insertion Prophylaxis

Observe strict asepsis at insertion; clean the endocervix with an antiseptic solution, because the presence of organisms capable of establishing PID cannot be determined by appearance, and because IUD insertion may be associated with introduction of vaginal bacteria into the uterus. Data do not confirm the utility of prophylactic administration of antibiotics in reducing the incidence of PID, and their use in nursing women is not recommended.

4. Requirements for Continuation and Removal

a. The ParaGard® T 380A must be replaced before the end of the tenth year of use. There is no evidence of decreasing contraceptive efficacy with time before ten years, but the contraceptive effectiveness at longer times has not been established; therefore, the patient should be informed of the known duration of contraceptive efficacy and be advised to return in 10 years for removal and possible insertion of a new ParaGard® T 380A.

b. The ParaGard® T 380A should be removed for the following medical reasons: menorrhagia- and/or metrorrhagia-producing anemia; pelvic infection; genital actinomycosis; intractable pelvic pain; dyspareunia; pregnancy; endometrial or cervical malignancy; uterine or cervical perforation; increase in length of the threads extending from the cervix, or any other indication of partial expulsion. Insertions immediately following placental delivery or first trimester abortion may result in threads becoming slightly longer as the uterus involutes and may not represent expulsion or partial expulsion.

c. If the retrieval threads cannot be visualized, they may have retracted into the uterus or have been broken, or the ParaGard® T 380A may have been broken, or the ParaGard® T 380A may have been expelled. Localization may be made by feeling with a probe, X-ray, or sonography. When the physician elects to recover a ParaGard® T 380A with the threads not visible, the removal instructions should be reviewed.

d. Should the patient's relationship cease to be mutually monogamous, or should her partner become HIV positive, or acquire a sexually transmitted disease, she should be instructed to report this change to her clinician immediately. It may be advisable to recommend the use of a barrier method as a partial protection against acquiring sexually transmitted diseases until the ParaGard® T 380A can be removed.

5. Continuing Care of Patients Using ParaGard® T 380A

a. Any inquiries regarding pain, odorous discharge, bleeding, fever, genital lesions or sores, or a missed period should be promptly responded to and prompt examination is recommended.

b. If examination during visits subsequent to insertion reveals that the length of the threads has visibly or palpably changed from their length at time of insertion, the ParaGard® T 380A should be considered displaced and should be removed. A new ParaGard® T 380A may be inserted at that time or during the next menses if it is certain that conception has not occurred. Under no circumstances should reinsertion with an expelled ParaGard® T 380A be attempted. A new ParaGard® T 380A should be inserted.

c. Since the ParaGard® T 380A may be partially or completely expelled, patients should be reexamined and evaluated shortly after the first postinsertion menses, but no later than 3 months afterwards. Thereafter, at least annual examination with appropriate evaluation, including a "Pap" smear, and if indicated, gonococcal and chlamydial laboratory evaluations, should be carried out. The ParaGard® T 380A should be kept in place no longer than 10 years.

d. In the event a pregnancy is confirmed during ParaGard® T 380A use, the following steps should be taken:

- Determine whether pregnancy is ectopic and take appropriate measures if it is.
- Inform patient of the risks of leaving an IUD *in situ* or removing it during pregnancy, and of the lack of data on the long term effects of the ParaGard® T 380A on the offspring of women who have had it *in utero* during conception or gestation (see WARNINGS). This information should include the risk of septic spontaneous abortion with the IUD *in situ*.
- If possible, the ParaGard® T 380A should be removed after the patient has been warned of the risks of removal. If removal is difficult, the patient should be counseled about and offered pregnancy termination.
- If the ParaGard® T 380A is left in place, the patient's course should be followed closely.

ADVERSE REACTIONS

These adverse reactions are not listed in any order of frequency or severity.

Reported adverse reactions with intrauterine contraceptives include: endometritis; spontaneous abortion; septic abortion; septicemia; perforation of the uterus and cervix; embedment; fragmentation of the IUD; pelvic infection; tubo-ovarian abscess; tubal damage; vaginitis; leukorrhea; cervical erosion; pregnancy; ectopic pregnancy; fetal damage; difficult removal; complete or partial expulsion of the IUD, particularly in those patients with uteri measuring less than 6.0 cm by sounding; menstrual spotting; prolongation of menstrual flow; anemia; amenorrhea or delayed menses; pain and cramping; dysmenorrhea; backaches; dyspareunia; neurovascular episodes, including bradycardia and syncope secondary to insertion. Uterine perforation and IUD displacement into the abdomen have been followed by peritonitis, abdominal adhesions, intestinal penetration, intestinal obstruction, and cystic masses in the pelvis. (Certain of these adverse reactions can lead to loss of fertility, partial or total removal of reproductive organs, hormonal imbalance, or death). Urticarial allergic skin reaction may occur.

CLINICAL STUDIES

Different event rates have been reported with the use of different intrauterine contraceptives. Inasmuch as these rates are usually derived from separate studies conducted by different investigators in several populations, they cannot be compared with precision. Considerably different rates are likely to be obtained because event rates per unit of time tend to decrease as studies are extended, since more susceptible subjects discontinue due to expulsions, adverse reactions, or pregnancy, leaving the study population richer in less susceptible subjects. In clinical trials conducted by The Population Council[14,15] and WHO, use-effectiveness of the ParaGard® T 380A as calculated by the life table method was determined through ten (10) years of use.

Data suggest a higher pregnancy rate in women under 20.[14,15,17]

[See table II above]

Continued on next page

Paragard T—Cont.

TABLE III
GROSS ANNUAL EVENT RATES PER 100 CONTINUING USERS BY YEAR AND PARITY

	1 Year Parous
Pregnancy	0.5
Expulsion	2.3
Bleeding/Pain	3.4
Infection	0.3
Other Medical	0.5
Planning Pregnancy	0.6
Other Personal	0.7
Continuation	92.1
No. Completed	1842.0

Rates were calculated by combining the experience on a weighted basis from both an international study by the World Health Organization (2110 women) and a U.S. study by GynoPharma Inc. (230 women).

The lowest expected and typical failure rates during the first year of continuous use of all contraceptive methods are listed in Table IV (Adapted from Reference 16).

[See table IV at top of previous page]

HOW SUPPLIED

Available in cartons of one (NDC 54765-380-01) or five (NDC 54765-380-05) sterile units. Each ParaGard® T 380A is packaged in a Tyvek®-polyethylene pouch, together with an insertion tube and solid rod.

INSTRUCTIONS FOR USE
Paragard®T 380A
(Intrauterine Copper Contraceptive)
CLINICIANS SHOULD HAVE DEMONSTRATED CLINICAL COMPETENCE IN PARAGARD® T 380A INSERTIONS RECEIVED UNDER SUPERVISION. PREVIOUS EDUCATION RE: SURGICAL PROCEDURES WILL REQUIRE VARYING LEVELS OF EXPERIENCE.
The ParaGard® T 380A (Intrauterine Copper Contraceptive) represents a different design in intrauterine contraceptives. Physicians are, therefore, cautioned that they should become thoroughly familiar with instructions for insertion before attempting placement of the ParaGard® T 380A. The insertion technique is different in several respects from that employed with other intrauterine contraceptives and the physician should pay particular attention to the drawings and commentary accompanying these instructions.
A single ParaGard® T 380A is placed at the fundus of the uterine cavity.
The ParaGard® T 380A may be inserted at any time during the cycle. However, it is essential that pregnancy be ruled out before insertion.
The ParaGard® T 380A is indicated for use up to 10 years. Therefore, the ParaGard® T 380A must be removed and a new one inserted on or before 10 years from the date of insertion.

PRELIMINARY PREPARATION AND INSERTION

1. Before insertion, you and the patient will want to review the Patient Package Insert. If the patient agrees, she may sign the Consent Form provided for your records.
2. Take a medical and social history.
3. Refer to CONTRAINDICATIONS, WARNINGS, and PRECAUTIONS.
4. Pelvic examination is to be performed prior to insertion of the ParaGard® T 380A, including a cervical "Pap" smear, and gonococcal and chlamydial evaluations, if indicated, and any other necessary specific tests.
5. If appropriate, commence antibiotic prophylaxis one hour before insertion.
6. Use of aseptic technique during insertion is essential.
7. The endocervix should be cleansed with an antiseptic solution and a tenaculum applied to the cervix with downward traction for correction of the angulation as well as stabilization of the cervix.
8. With a speculum in place, gently insert a sterile sound to determine the depth and direction of the uterine canal. Be sure to determine the position of the uterus before insertion.

CAUTION

Any intrauterine procedure can result in severe pain, bradycardia, and syncope.
It is generally believed that perforations, if they occur, are encountered at the time of insertion, although the perforation may not be detected until some time later. The position of the uterus should be determined during the preinsertion examination. Great care must be exercised during the preinsertion sounding and subsequent insertion. No attempt should be made to force the insertion.

HOW TO LOAD AND INSERT ParaGard® T 380A
STEP 1
To minimize the chance of introducing contamination, do not remove the ParaGard® T 380A from the insertion tube prior to placement in the uterus. Do not bend the arms of the ParaGard® T 380A earlier than 5 minutes before it is to be introduced into the uterus.
In the absence of sterile gloves, this can be accomplished without destroying sterility by folding the arms in the partially opened package. Place the partially opened package on a flat surface and pull the solid rod partially from the package so it will not interfere with assembly. Place thumb and index finger on top of package on ends of the horizontal arms. Push insertion tube against arms of ParaGard® T 380A as indicated by arrow in Fig. 1A to start arms folding.
[See figure at top of next column]

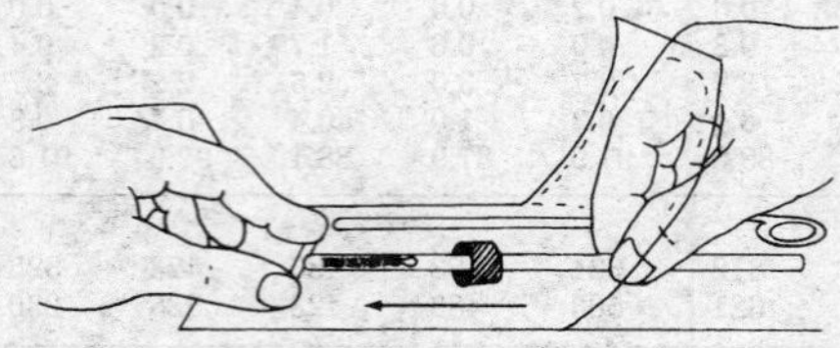

Fig. 1A

Complete the bending by bringing the thumb and index finger together using the other hand to maneuver the insertion tube to pick up the arms of the ParaGard® T 380A (Fig. 1B). Insert no further than necessary to insure retention of the arms. Introduce the solid rod into the insertion tube from the bottom alongside the threads until it touches the bottom of the ParaGard® T 380A.

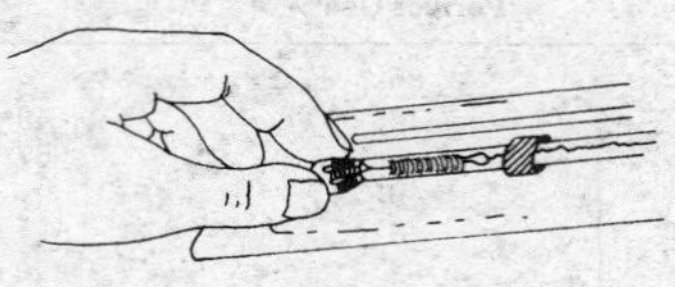

Fig. 1B

STEP 2
Adjust the movable flange so that it indicates the depth to which the ParaGard® T 380A should be inserted and the direction in which the arms of the ParaGard® T 380A will open. At this point, make certain that the horizontal arms of the ParaGard® T 380A and the long axis of the flange lie in the same horizontal plane. Introduce the loaded insertion tube through the cervical canal and upwards until the ParaGard® T 380A lies in contact with the fundus. The movable flange should be at the cervix (Fig. 2).
DO NOT FORCE THE INSERTION.

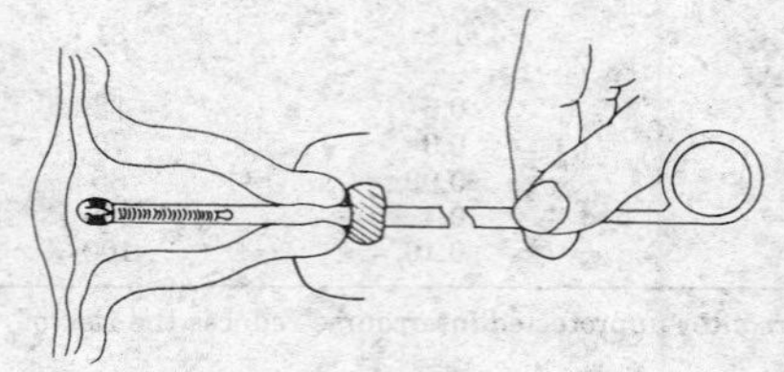

Fig. 2

STEP 3
To release the arms of the ParaGard® T 380A, withdraw the insertion tube not more than $^1/_2$ inch while the solid rod is not permitted to move. This releases the arms of the ParaGard® T 380A (Fig. 3).

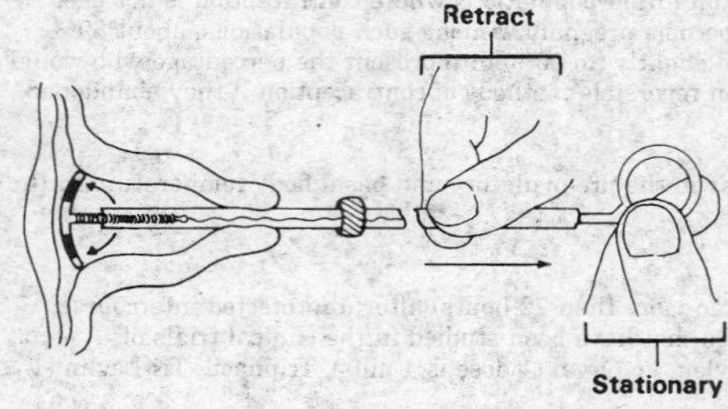

Fig. 3

STEP 4
After the arms are released, the insertion tube should be moved upward gently until the resistance of the fundus is felt. This will assure placement of the T at the highest possible position within the endometrial cavity (Fig. 4).
[See figure 4 at top of next column]
STEP 5
Withdraw the solid rod while holding the insertion tube stationary (Fig. 5).
[See figure 5 at top of next column]
STEP 6
Withdraw the insertion tube from the cervix. Be sure sufficient length of the threads are visible (approximately 1 in. or 2.5 cm.) to facilitate checking for the presence of the

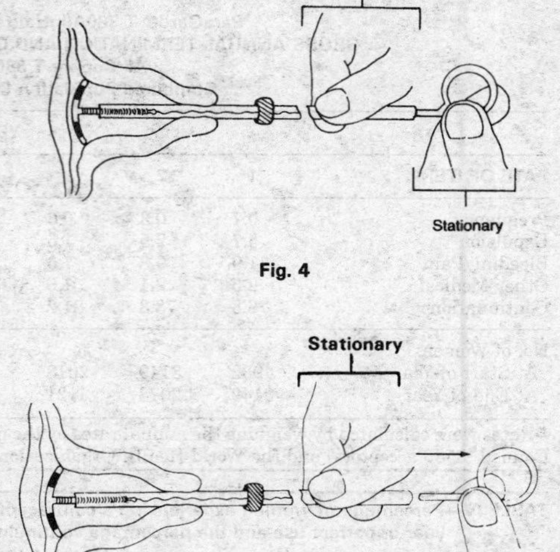

Fig. 4

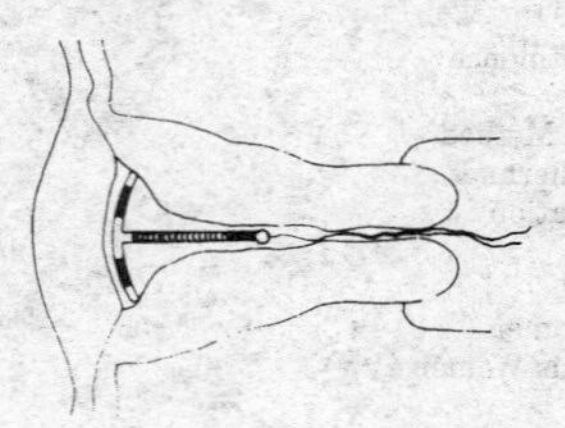

Fig. 5

ParaGard® T 380A (Fig. 6). Notation of length of the threads should be made in patient record.

Fig. 6

HOW TO REMOVE ParaGard® T 380A

To remove the ParaGard® T 380A, pull gently on the exposed threads. The arms of the ParaGard® T 380A will fold upwards as it is withdrawn from the uterus. Even if removal proves difficult, the ParaGard® T 380A should not remain in the uterus after 10 years.

REFERENCES

1. Alvarez F et al: New insights on the mode of action on intrauterine contraceptives in women. *Fertil Steril* 1988; 49:768–773.
2. World Health Organization's Special Programme of Research, Development and Research Training in Human Reproduction: A multinational case-control study of ectopic pregnancy. *Clin Reprod Fertil* 1985; 3:131–143.
3. Ory HW, Women's Health Study: Ectopic pregnancy and intrauterine contraceptive devices: New perspectives. *Obstet Gynecol* 1981; 57:137–144.
4. Marchbanks PA et al: Risk factors for ectopic pregnancy: A population-based study. *JAMA* 1988; 259:1823–1827.
5. Farley TMM et al: Intrauterine devices and pelvic inflammatory disease: An international perspective. *Lancet* 1992; 339:785–788.
6. Cramer DW et al: Tubal infertility and the intrauterine device. *N Engl J Med* 1985; 312:941–947.
7. Daling JR et al: Primary tubal infertility in relation to the use of an intrauterine device. *N Engl J Med* 1985; 312:937–941.
8. Heartwell SF, Schlesselman S: Risk of uterine perforation among users of intrauterine devices. *Obstet Gynecol* 1983; 61:31–36.
9. Chi I-C, Kelly E: Is lactation a risk factor of IUD and sterilization-related uterine perforations? A hypothesis. *Int J Gynaecol Obstet* 1984; 22:315–317.
10. Harlap S, Kost K, Forrest JD: Preventing pregnancy, protecting health: a new look at birth control choices in the United States. The Alan Guttmacher Institute 1991: 1–129.
11. Chi I-C et al: Performance of the Copper T 380A Intrauterine device in breast feeding women. *Contraception* 1989; 39:603–618.
12. Farr G. Rivera R: Interactions between intrauterine contraceptive device use and breast-feeding status at time of intrauterine contraceptive device insertion. Analysis of TCu-380A acceptors in developing countries. *Am J Obstet Gynecol* 1992; 167:144–151.
13. Mark AS, Hricak H: Intrauterine contraceptive devices: MR imaging. *Radiology* 1987; 311–314.
14. Sivin, I, Stern J: Long-acting, more effective Copper T IUDs: A summary of US experience, 1970–1975, *Stud Fam Plann* 1979; 10:263–281.
15. Sivin I, Schmidt F: Effectiveness of IUDs: A review. *Contraception* 1987; 36:55–84.
16. Trussell J: The Essentials of Contraception, in R.A. Hatcher, et al: *Contraceptive Technology,* 16th Revised Ed., New York, Irvington, 1994, 113–114.
17. World Health Organization (WHO): Mechanism of action, safety, and efficacy of intrauterine devices. Report of a WHO Scientific Group. Technical Report Series 753. Geneva; World Health Organization, 1987, p. 22.

Manufactured for
ORTHO-McNEIL PHARMACEUTICAL, INC.
Raritan, New Jersey 08869
by FEI Products, Inc.
N. Tonawanda, New York 14120
© OPC 1998
Revised April 1999
631-40-410-4

Shown in Product Identification Guide, page 329

REGRANEX® Gel 0.01% ℞
[*rĕ grən 'x*]
(becaplermin)

DESCRIPTION

REGRANEX® Gel contains becaplermin, a recombinant human platelet-derived growth factor (rhPDGF-BB) for topical administration. Becaplermin is produced by recombinant DNA technology by insertion of the gene for the B chain of platelet-derived growth factor (PDGF) into the yeast, *Saccharomyces cerevisiae*. Becaplermin has a molecular weight of approximately 25 KD and is a homodimer composed of two identical polypeptide chains that are bound together by disulfide bonds. Becaplermin Concentrate is produced by Chiron Corp. and supplied to OMJ Pharmaceuticals under a shared manufacturing arrangement. REGRANEX Gel is a non-sterile, low bioburden, preserved, sodium carboxymethylcellulose-based (CMC) topical gel, containing the active ingredient becaplermin and the following inactive ingredients: sodium chloride, sodium acetate trihydrate, glacial acetic acid, water for injection, and methylparaben, propylparaben, and m-cresol as preservatives and l-lysine hydrochloride as a stabilizer. Each gram of REGRANEX Gel contains 100 µg of becaplermin.

CLINICAL PHARMACOLOGY

REGRANEX has biological activity similar to that of endogenous platelet-derived growth factor, which includes promoting the chemotactic recruitment and proliferation of cells involved in wound repair and enhancing the formation of granulation tissue.

Pharmacokinetics

Ten patients with Stage III or IV (as defined in the International Association of Enterostomal Therapy (IAET) guide to chronic wound staging, *J. Enterostomal Ther* 15:4, 1988 and *Decubitis* 2:24, 1989) lower extremity diabetic ulcers received topical applications of becaplermin gel 0.01% at a dose range of 0.32–2.95 µg/kg (7µg/cm^2) daily for 14 days. Six patients had non-quantifiable PDGF levels at baseline and throughout the study, two patients had PDGF levels at baseline which did not increase substantially, and two patients had PDGF levels that increased sporadically above their baseline values during the 14 day study period.

Systemic bioavailability of becaplermin was less than 3% in rats with full thickness wounds receiving single or multiple (5 days) topical applications of 127 µg/kg (20.1 µg/cm^2 of wound area) of becaplermin gel.

Clinical Studies

The effects of REGRANEX Gel on the incidence of and time to complete healing in lower extremity diabetic ulcers were assessed in four randomized controlled studies. Of 922 patients studied, 478 received either REGRANEX Gel 0.003% or 0.01%. All study participants had lower extremity diabetic neuropathic ulcers that extended into the subcutaneous tissue or beyond (Stages III and IV of the IAET guide to chronic wound staging). Ninety-three percent of the patients enrolled in these four trials had foot ulcers. The remaining 7% of the patients had ankle or leg ulcers. The diabetic ulcers were of at least 8 weeks duration and had an adequate blood supply (defined as $T_cpO_2 > 30$ mm Hg). In the four trials, ninety-five percent of the ulcers measured in area up to 10 cm^2, and the median ulcer size at baseline ranged from 1.4 cm^2 to 3.5 cm^2. All treatment groups received a program of good ulcer care consisting of initial complete sharp debridement, a non-weight-bearing regimen, systemic treatment for wound-related infection if present, moist saline dressings changed twice a day, and additional debridement as necessary. REGRANEX Gel 0.003% or 0.01% or placebo gel was applied once a day and covered with a saline moistened dressing. After approximately 12 hours, the gel was gently rinsed off and a saline moistened dressing was then applied for the remainder of the day. Patients were treated until complete healing, or for a period of up to 20 weeks. Patients were considered a treatment failure if their ulcer did not show an approximately 30% reduction in initial ulcer area after eight to ten weeks of REGRANEX Gel therapy.

The primary endpoint, incidence of complete ulcer closure within 20 weeks, for all treatment arms is shown in Figure 1. In each study, REGRANEX Gel in conjunction with good ulcer care was compared to placebo gel plus good ulcer care or good ulcer care alone.

In Study 1, a multicenter, double-blind, placebo controlled trial of 118 patients, the incidence of complete ulcer closure for REGRANEX Gel 0.003% (n=61) was 48% versus 25% for placebo gel (n=57; p=0.02, logistic regression analysis).

In Study 2, a multicenter, double-blind, placebo controlled trial of 382 patients, the incidence of complete ulcer closure for REGRANEX Gel 0.01% (n=123), was 50% versus 36% for REGRANEX Gel 0.003% (n=132), and 35% for placebo gel (n=127). Only REGRANEX Gel 0.01% was significantly different from placebo gel (p=0.01, logistic regression analysis).

The primary goal of Study 3, a multicenter controlled trial of 172 patients, was to assess the safety of vehicle gel (placebo; n=70) compared to good ulcer care alone (n=68). The study included a small (n=34) REGRANEX Gel 0.01% arm. Incidences of complete ulcer closure were 44% for REGRANEX Gel, 36% for placebo gel and 22% for good ulcer care alone.

In Study 4, a multicenter, evaluator-blind, controlled trial of 250 patients, the incidences of complete ulcer closure in the REGRANEX Gel 0.01% arm (n=128) (36%) and good ulcer care alone (n=122) (32%) were not statistically different.

Figure 1: Incidence of Complete Healing

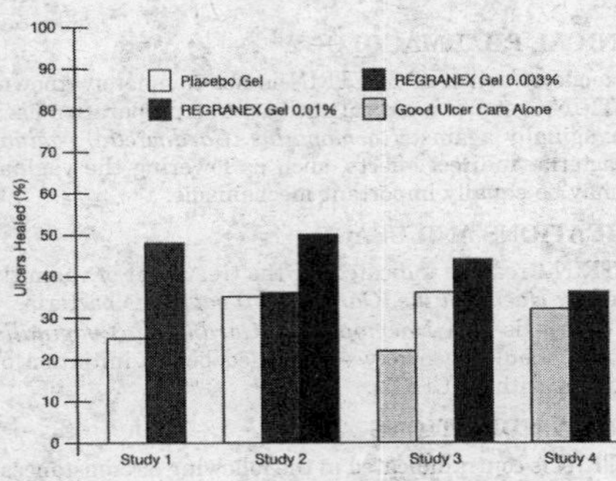

In general, where REGRANEX Gel was associated with higher incidences of complete ulcer closure, differences in the incidence first became apparent after approximately 10 weeks and increased with continued treatment (Table 1).

Table 1: Life Table Estimates of the Incidence (%) of Complete Healing Over Time for Study 2

	REGRANEX Gel 0.01% (%)	Placebo Gel (%)
Week 2	1	0
Week 4	6	2
Week 6	9	6
Week 8	16	14
Week 10	23	18
Week 12	34	25
Week 14	37	28
Week 16	43	33
Week 18	46	34
Week 20	50	37

In a 3-month follow-up period where no standardized regimen of preventative care was utilized, the incidence of ulcer recurrence was approximately 30% in all treatment groups, demonstrating that the durability of ulcer closure was comparable in all treatment groups.

The efficacy of REGRANEX Gel for the treatment of non-diabetic ulcers is under evaluation.

INDICATIONS AND USAGE

REGRANEX Gel is indicated for the treatment of lower extremity diabetic neuropathic ulcers that extend into the subcutaneous tissue or beyond and have an adequate blood supply. When used as an adjunct to, and not a substitute for, good ulcer care practices including initial sharp debridement, pressure relief and infection control, REGRANEX Gel increases the incidence of complete healing of diabetic ulcers.

The efficacy of REGRANEX Gel for the treatment of diabetic neuropathic ulcers that do not extend through the dermis into subcutaneous tissue (Stage I or II, IAET staging classification) or ischemic diabetic ulcers has not been evaluated.

CONTRAINDICATIONS

REGRANEX Gel is contraindicated in patients with:
— known hypersensitivity to any component of this product (e.g., parabens);
— known neoplasm(s) at the site(s) of application.

WARNINGS

REGRANEX (becaplermin) Gel is a non-sterile, low bioburden preserved product. Therefore, it should not be used in wounds that close by primary intention.

PRECAUTIONS

For external use only.

If application site reactions occur, the possibility of sensitization or irritation caused by parabens or m-cresol should be considered.

The effects of becaplermin on exposed joints, tendons, ligaments, and bone have not been established in humans. In pre-clinical studies, rats injected at the metatarsals with 3 or 10 µg/site (approximately 60 or 200 µg/kg) of becaplermin every other day for 13 days displayed histological changes indicative of accelerated bone remodeling consisting of periosteal hyperplasia and subperiosteal bone resorption and exostosis. The soft tissue adjacent to the injection site had fibroplasia with accompanying mononuclear cell infiltration reflective of the ability of PDGF to stimulate connective tissue growth.

Information for Patients

Patients should be advised that:
— hands should be washed thoroughly before applying REGRANEX Gel;
— the tip of the tube should not come into contact with the ulcer or any other surface; the tube should be recapped tightly after each use;
— a cotton swab, tongue depressor, or other application aid should be used to apply REGRANEX Gel;
— REGRANEX Gel should only be applied once a day in a carefully measured quantity (see Dosage and Administration section). The measured quantity of gel should be spread evenly over the ulcerated area to yield a thin continuous layer of approximately $^1/_{16}$ of an inch thickness. The measured length of the gel to be squeezed from the tube should be adjusted according to the size of the ulcer. The amount of REGRANEX Gel to be applied daily should be recalculated at weekly or biweekly intervals by the physician or wound care giver;

Step-by-step instructions for application of REGRANEX Gel are as follows:
- Squeeze the calculated length of gel on to a clean, firm, non-absorbable surface, e.g., wax paper.
- With a clean cotton swab, tongue depressor, or similar application aid, spread the measured REGRANEX Gel over the ulcer surface to obtain an even layer.
- Cover with a saline moistened gauze dressing.

— after approximately 12 hours, the ulcer should be gently rinsed with saline or water to remove residual gel and covered with a saline-moistened gauze dressing (without REGRANEX Gel);
— it is important to use REGRANEX Gel together with a good ulcer care program, including a strict non-weight-bearing program;
— excess application of REGRANEX Gel has not been shown to be beneficial;
— REGRANEX Gel should be stored in the refrigerator. Do not freeze REGRANEX Gel;
— REGRANEX Gel should not be used after the expiration date on the bottom, crimped end of the tube.

Drug Interactions

It is not known if REGRANEX Gel interacts with other topical medications applied to the ulcer site. The use of REGRANEX Gel with other topical drugs has not been studied.

Carcinogenesis, Mutagenesis, Impairment of Fertility

Becaplermin was not genotoxic in a battery of *in vitro* assays, (including those for bacterial and mammalian cell point mutation, chromosomal aberration, and DNA damage/repair). Becaplermin was also not mutagenic in an *in vivo* assay for the induction of micronuclei in mouse bone marrow cells.

Carcinogenesis and reproductive toxicity studies have not been conducted with REGRANEX Gel.

Pregnancy: Category C

Animal reproduction studies have not been conducted with REGRANEX Gel. It is also not known whether REGRANEX Gel can cause fetal harm when administered to a pregnant woman or can affect reproductive capacity. REGRANEX Gel should be given to pregnant women only if clearly needed.

Nursing Mothers

It is not known whether becaplermin is excreted in human milk. Because many drugs are secreted in human milk, caution should be exercised when REGRANEX Gel is administered to nursing women.

Pediatric Use

Safety and effectiveness of REGRANEX Gel in pediatric patients below the age of 16 years have not been established.

ADVERSE REACTIONS

Patients receiving REGRANEX Gel, placebo gel, and good ulcer care alone had a similar incidence of ulcer-related adverse events such as infection, cellulitis, or osteomyelitis. However, erythematous rashes occurred in 2% of patients treated with REGRANEX Gel and placebo, and none in patients receiving good ulcer care alone. The incidence of cardiovascular, respiratory, musculoskeletal and central and peripheral nervous system disorders was not different across all treatment groups. Mortality rates were also similar across all treatment groups. Patients treated with REGRANEX Gel did not develop neutralizing antibodies against becaplermin.

DOSAGE AND ADMINISTRATION

The amount of REGRANEX Gel to be applied will vary depending upon the size of the ulcer area. To calculate the length of gel to apply to the ulcer, measure the greatest length of the ulcer by the greatest width of the ulcer in either inches or centimeters. To calculate the length of gel in inches, use the formula shown below in Table 2, and to calculate the length of gel in centimeters, use the formula shown below in Table 3.

Table 2: Formula to Calculate Length of Gel in Inches to be Applied Daily

	INCHES
Tube Size	Formula
15 or 7.5 g tube	length × width × 0.6
2 g tube	length × width × 1.3

Using the calculation, each square inch of ulcer surface will require approximately $^2/_3$ inch length of gel squeezed from a

Continued on next page

Regranex—Cont.

15g or 7.5g tube, or approximately 1⅓ inch length of the gel from a 2g tube. For example, if the ulcer measures 1 inch by 2 inches, then a 1¼ inch length of gel should be used for 15g or 7.5g tubes (1 × 2 × 0.6 = 1¼) and 2¾ inch gel length should be used for 2g tube (1 × 2 × 1.3 = 2¾).

Table 3: Formula to Calculate Length of Gel in Centimeters to be Applied Daily

	CENTIMETERS
Tube Size	Formula
15 or 7.5 g tube	length × width ÷ 4
2 g tube	length × width ÷ 2

Using the calculations for ulcer size in centimeters, each square centimeter of ulcer surface will require approximately a 0.25 centimeter length of gel squeezed from a 15g or 7.5g tube, or approximately a 0.5 centimeter length of gel from a 2g tube. For example, if the ulcer measures 4 cm by 2 cm, then a 2 centimeter length of gel should be used for 15g or 7.5g tube [(4 × 2) ÷ 4 = 2] and a 4 centimeter length of gel should be used for 2g tube [(4 × 2) ÷ 2 = 4].

The amount of REGRANEX Gel to be applied should be recalculated by the physician or wound care giver at weekly or biweekly intervals depending on the rate of change in ulcer area. The weight of REGRANEX Gel from 7.5g and 15g tubes is 0.65g per inch length and 0.25g per centimeter length.

To apply REGRANEX Gel, the calculated length of gel should be squeezed on to a clean measuring surface, e.g., wax paper. The measured REGRANEX Gel is transferred from the clean measuring surface using an application aid and then spread over the entire ulcer area to yield a thin continuous layer of approximately 1/16 of an inch thickness. The site(s) of application should then be covered by a saline moistened dressing and left in place for approximately 12 hours. The dressing should then be removed and the ulcer rinsed with saline or water to remove residual gel and covered again with a second moist dressing (without REGRANEX Gel) for the remainder of the day. REGRANEX Gel should be applied once daily to the ulcer until complete healing has occurred. If the ulcer does not decrease in size by approximately 30% after 10 weeks of treatment or complete healing has not occurred in 20 weeks, continued treatment with REGRANEX Gel should be reassessed. The step-by-step instructions for applying REGRANEX Gel for home administration are described under "Information for Patients".

HOW SUPPLIED

REGRANEX (becaplermin) Gel, supplied as a clear, colorless to straw-colored preserved gel containing 100µg of becaplermin per gram of gel, is available in multi-use tubes in the following sizes:

2g tubes	NDC 0045-0810-02
7.5g tubes	NDC 0045-0810-07
15g tubes	NDC 0045-0810-15

REGRANEX Gel is for external use only.

Storage

Store refrigerated, 2–8° C (36–46° F). DO NOT FREEZE. DO NOT USE THE GEL AFTER THE EXPIRATION DATE AT THE BOTTOM OF THE TUBE.

U.S. Patent #5,457,093

Distributed by:
OMP DIVISION
ORTHO-McNEIL
PHARMACEUTICAL, INC.
Raritan, New Jersey 08869

Manufactured by:
OMJ Pharmaceuticals, Inc.
U.S. License No. 1196
San German, Puerto Rico 00683

Becaplermin Concentrate provided by: Chiron Corp.,
U.S. License No. 1106, Emeryville, CA 94608

©OMP 1998 Revised March 1999 635-10-240-3

Shown in Product Identification Guide, page 329

SULTRIN® Triple Sulfa Cream ℞
(sulfathiazole/sulfacetamide/sulfabenzamide)

DESCRIPTION

SULTRIN Cream contains sulfathiazole (Benzenesulfonamide,4-amino-N-2-thiazolyl-N[1]-2-thiazolylsulfanilamide) 3.42%, sulfacetamide (Acetamide,N-[(4-aminophenyl) sulfonyl]-N-Sulfanilylacetamide) 2.86%, and sulfabenzamide (Benzamide,N-[(4-aminophenyl) sulfonyl]-N-Sulfanilylbenzamide) 3.7%, compounded with cetyl alcohol 2%, cholesterol, diethylaminoethyl stearamide, glyceryl monostearate, lanolin, lecithin, methylparaben, peanut oil, phosphoric acid, propylene glycol, propylparaben, purified water, stearic acid and urea.

SULTRIN Cream is a topical antibacterial preparation available for intravaginal administration.

H_2N–C₆H₄–$SO_2NHC(=O)$–C₆H₅

Sulfabenzamide

NH_2–C₆H₄–$SO_2NHCOCH_3$

Sulfacetamide

H_2N–C₆H₄–SO_2NH–(thiazolyl)

Sulfathiazole

CLINICAL PHARMACOLOGY

The mode of action of SULTRIN is not completely known. SULTRIN Cream is a topical antibacterial preparation used intravaginally against *Haemophilus (Gardnerella) vaginalis* bacteria. Indirect effects, such as lowering the vaginal pH, may be equally important mechanisms.

INDICATIONS AND USAGE

SULTRIN Cream is indicated for the treatment of vaginitis caused by *Haemophilus (Gardnerella) vaginalis* bacteria. The diagnosis of a *Haemophilus (Gardnerella) vaginalis* vaginitis should be firmly established before initiation of treatment with SULTRIN.

CONTRAINDICATIONS

SULTRIN is contraindicated in the following circumstances: kidney disease; hypersensitivity to sulfonamides; in pregnancy at term and during the nursing period because sulfonamides cross the placenta, are excreted in breast milk and may cause Kernicterus.

WARNINGS

Deaths associated with the administration of sulfonamides have been reported from hypersensitivity reactions, agranulocytosis, aplastic anemia and other blood dyscrasias.

The presence of clinical signs such as sore throat, fever, pallor, purpura or jaundice may be early indications of serious blood disorders.

PRECAUTIONS

Because sulfonamides may be absorbed from the vaginal mucosa, the usual precautions for oral sulfonamides apply. Patients should be observed for skin rash or evidence of systemic toxicity, and if these develop, the medications should be discontinued.

Laboratory tests: Standard office diagnostic procedures for vaginitis are usually sufficient to establish the diagnosis of *Haemophilus (Gardnerella) vaginalis* and to rule out a trichomonal or monilial infection. These include noting a fish-like odor upon addition of 10% KOH to vaginal discharge and microscopic identification of "clue cells" in a wet mount preparation. If cultures are obtained, care must be taken to use appropriate media and methods for *Haemophilus (Gardnerella) vaginalis.*

Carcinogenesis, mutagenesis, impairment of fertility: The sulfonamides bear certain chemical similarities to some goitrogens. Rats appear to be especially susceptible to the goitrogenic effects of sulfonamides, and long-term administration has produced thyroid malignancies in this species.

Pregnancy:

Teratogenic Effects: Pregnancy Category C: The safe use of sulfonamides in pregnancy has not been established. The teratogenicity potential of most sulfonamides has not been thoroughly investigated in either animals or humans. However, a significant increase in the incidence of cleft palate and other bony abnormalities of offspring has been observed when certain sulfonamides of the short, intermediate and long-acting types were given to pregnant rats and mice at high oral doses (7 to 25 times the human therapeutic dose).

Nursing Mothers: Because of the potential for serious adverse reactions in nursing infants from SULTRIN, a decision should be made whether to discontinue nursing or to discontinue the drug, taking into account the importance of the drug to the mother. See CONTRAINDICATIONS.

Pediatric use: Safety and effectiveness in children have not been established.

ADVERSE REACTIONS

There has been one reported case of Agranulocytosis in a patient receiving SULTRIN Cream. The most frequent adverse reactions to SULTRIN are localized irritation and/or allergy including rare reports of Stevens-Johnson syndrome which may be fatal.

DOSAGE AND ADMINISTRATION

SULTRIN Cream. One full applicator intravaginally twice daily for four to six days. This course of therapy may be repeated if necessary; the dosage may be reduced one-half to one-quarter.

HOW SUPPLIED

Cream—78 g tubes with the ORTHO* Measured-Dose Applicator.

NDC 0062-5440-77

REVISED October 1998 643-10-370-7

TERAZOL® 3 ℞
VAGINAL CREAM 0.8%
(terconazole)

DESCRIPTION

TERAZOL® 3 (terconazole) Vaginal Cream 0.8% is a white to off-white, water washable cream for intravaginal administration containing 0.8% of the antifungal agent terconazole, *cis* -1-[*p*-[[2-(2,4-Dichlorophenyl)-2-(1H-1,2,4-triazol-1-ylmethyl)-1,3-dioxolan-4-yl] methoxy] phenyl]-4-isopropylpiperazine, compounded in a cream base consisting of butylated hydroxyanisole, cetyl alcohol, isopropyl myristate, polysorbate 60, polysorbate 80, propylene glycol, stearyl alcohol, and purified water.

The structural formula of terconazole is as follows:

$C_{26}H_{31}Cl_2N_5O_3$

Terconazole, a triazole derivative, is a white to almost white powder with a molecular weight of 532.47. It is insoluble in water; sparingly soluble in ethanol; and soluble in butanol.

CLINICAL PHARMACOLOGY

Following daily intravaginal administration of 0.8% terconazole 40 mg (0.8% cream × 5 g) for seven days to normal humans, plasma concentrations were low and gradually rose to a daily peak (mean of 5.9 ng/mL or 0.006 mcg/mL) at 6.6 hours. Results from similar studies in patients with vulvovaginal candidiasis indicate that the slow rate of absorption, the lack of accumulation, and the mean peak plasma concentration of terconazole was not different from that observed in healthy women. The absorption characteristics of terconazole 0.8% in pregnant or nonpregnant patients with vulvovaginal candidiasis were also similar to those found in normal volunteers.

Following oral (30 mg) administration of ^{14}C-labelled terconazole, the harmonic half-life of elimination from the blood for the parent terconazole was 6.9 hours (range 4.0–11.3). Terconazole is extensively metabolized; the plasma AUC for terconazole compared to the AUC for total radioactivity was 0.6%. Total radioactivity was eliminated from the blood with a harmonic half-life of 52.2 hours (range 44–60). Excretion of radioactivity was both by renal (32–56%) and fecal (47–52%) routes.

In vitro, terconazole is highly protein bound (94.9%) and the degree of binding is independent of the drug concentration.

Photosensitivity reactions were observed in some normal volunteers following repeated dermal application of terconazole 2.0% and 0.8% creams under conditions of filtered artificial ultraviolet light. Photosensitivity reactions have not been observed in U.S. and foreign clinical trials in patients who were treated with terconazole 0.8% vaginal cream.

Microbiology: Terconazole exhibits fungicidal activity *in vitro* against *Candida albicans.* Antifungal activity also has been demonstrated against other fungi. The MIC values for terconazole against most species of lactic acid bacteria typically found in the human vagina were ≥128 mcg/mL. The exact pharmacologic mode of action of terconazole is uncertain; however, it may exert its antifungal activity by the disruption of normal fungal cell membrane permeability. No resistance to terconazole has developed during successive passages of *C. albicans.*

INDICATIONS AND USAGE

TERAZOL 3 Vaginal Cream is indicated for the local treatment of vulvovaginal candidiasis (moniliasis). As TERAZOL 3 Vaginal Cream is effective only for vulvovaginitis caused by the genus *Candida,* the diagnosis should be confirmed by KOH smears and/or cultures.

CONTRAINDICATIONS

Patients known to be hypersensitive to terconazole or to any of the components of the cream.

WARNINGS

None.

PRECAUTIONS

General: Discontinue use and do not retreat with terconazole if sensitization, irritation, fever, chills or flu-like symptoms are reported during use.

Laboratory Tests: If there is lack of response to TERAZOL 3 Vaginal Cream, appropriate microbiologic studies (standard KOH smear and/or cultures) should be repeated to confirm the diagnosis and rule out other pathogens.

Drug Interactions: The levels of estradiol (E2) and progesterone did not differ significantly when 0.8% terconazole vaginal cream was administered to healthy female volunteers established on a low dose oral contraceptive.

Carcinogenesis, Mutagenesis, Impairment of Fertility:

Carcinogenesis: Studies to determine the carcinogenic potential of terconazole have not been performed.

Mutagenicity: Terconazole was not mutagenic when tested *in vitro* for induction of microbial point mutations (Ames test) or for inducing cellular transformation, or *in vivo* for chromosome breaks (micronucleus test) or dominant lethal mutations in mouse germ cells.

Impairment of Fertility: No impairment of fertility occurred when female rats were administered terconazole orally up to 40 mg/kg/day for a three month period.

PREGNANCY: Teratogenic Effects.
Pregnancy Category C.
There was no evidence of teratogenicity when terconazole was administered orally up to 40 mg/kg/day or subcutaneously up to 20 mg/kg/day in rats. Dosages at or below 10 mg/kg/day produced no embryotoxicity; however, there was a delay in fetal ossification at 10 mg/kg/day in rats. There was some evidence of embryotoxicity in rabbits and rats at 20–40 mg/kg. In rats, this was reflected as a decrease in litter size and number of viable young and reduced fetal weight. There was also delay in ossification and an increased incidence of skeletal variants. The no-effect oral dose of 10/mg/kg/day resulted in a mean peak plasma level of terconazole in pregnant rats of 0.176 mcg/mL which exceeds by 30 times the mean peak plasma level (0.006 mcg/mL) seen in normal subjects after intravaginal administration of terconazole 0.8% vaginal cream. This safety assessment does not account for possible exposure of the fetus through direct transfer of terconazole from the irritated vagina by diffusion across amniotic membranes. Since terconazole is absorbed from the human vagina, it should not be used in the first trimester of pregnancy unless the physician considers it essential to the welfare of the patient.
Nursing Mothers: It is not known whether this drug is excreted in human milk. Animal studies have shown that rat offspring exposed via the milk of treated (40 mg/kg/orally) dams showed decreased survival during the first few postpartum days, but overall pup weight and weight gain were comparable to or greater than controls throughout lactation. Because many drugs are excreted in human milk, and because of the potential for adverse reaction in nursing infants from terconazole, a decision should be made whether to discontinue nursing or to discontinue the drug, taking into account the importance of the drug to the mother.
Pediatric Use: Safety and efficacy in children have not been established.

ADVERSE REACTIONS

During controlled clinical studies conducted in the United States, patients with vulvovaginal candidiasis were treated with terconazole 0.8% vaginal cream for three days. Based on comparative analyses with placebo and a standard agent, the adverse experiences considered most likely related to terconazole 0.8% vaginal cream were headache (21% vs. 16% with placebo) and dysmenorrhea (6% vs. 2% with placebo). Genital complaints in general, and burning and itching in particular, occurred less frequently in the terconazole 0.8% vaginal cream 3 day regimen (5% vs. 6%–9% with placebo). Other adverse experiences reported with terconazole 0.8% vaginal cream were abdominal pain (3.4% vs. 1% with placebo) and fever (1% vs. 0.3% with placebo). The therapy related dropout rate was 2.0% for the terconazole 0.8% vaginal cream. The adverse drug experience most frequently causing discontinuation of therapy was vulvovaginal itching, 0.7% with the terconazole 0.8% vaginal cream group and 0.3% with the placebo group.

OVERDOSAGE

Overdose of terconazole in humans has not been reported to date. In the rat, the oral LD 50 values were found to be 1741 and 849 mg/kg for the male and female, respectively. The oral LD 50 values for the male and female dog were ≅1280 and ≥640 mg/kg, respectively.

DOSAGE AND ADMINISTRATION

One full applicator (5 g) of TERAZOL 3 Vaginal Cream (40 mg terconazole) should be administered intravaginally once daily at bedtime for three consecutive days. Before prescribing another course of therapy, the diagnosis should be reconfirmed by smears and/or cultures and other pathogens commonly associated with vulvovaginitis ruled out. The therapeutic effect of TERAZOL 3 Vaginal Cream is not affected by menstruation.

HOW SUPPLIED

TERAZOL 3 (terconazole) Vaginal Cream 0.8% is available in 20 g (NDC 0062-5356-01) tubes with an ORTHO® Measured-Dose Applicator. Store at controlled room temperature 15–30°C (59–86°F).
Caution: Federal (U.S.A.) law prohibits dispensing without prescription.
631-11-314-4 Revised March 1995
Shown in Product Identification Guide, page 329

TERAZOL® 3 ℞
Vaginal Suppositories 80 mg
(terconazole)

DESCRIPTION

TERAZOL 3 Vaginal Suppositories are white to off-white suppositories for intravaginal administration containing 80 mg of the antifungal agent terconazole, *cis* -1-[*p*-[[2-(2,4-Dichlorophenyl)-2-(1H-1,2,4-triazol-1-ylmethyl)-1,3-dioxolan-4-yl]methoxy]phenyl]-4-isopropylpiperazine, in triglycerides derived from coconut and/or palm kernel oil (a base of hydrogenated vegetable oils) and butylated hydroxyanisole.
[See chemical structure at top of next column]
Terconazole, a triazole derivative, is a white to almost white powder with a molecular weight of 532.47. It is insoluble in water; sparingly soluble in ethanol; and soluble in butanol.

TERCONAZOLE

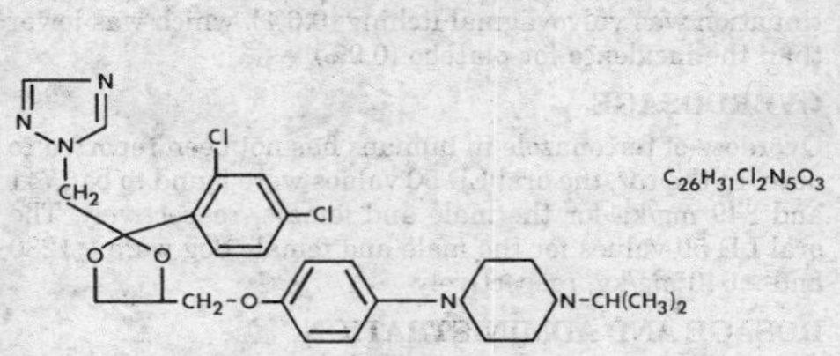

$C_{26}H_{31}Cl_2N_5O_3$

CLINICAL PHARMACOLOGY

Microbiology: Terconazole exhibits fungicidal activity *in vitro* against *Candida albicans.* The MIC values for terconazole against most species of lactic acid bacteria typically found in the human vagina were ≥128 mcg/mL, therefore, these beneficial bacteria are not affected by drug treatment. The exact pharmacologic mode of action of terconazole is uncertain; however, it may exert its antifungal activity by the disruption of normal fungal cell membrane permeability. No resistance to terconazole has developed during successive passages of *C. albicans.*
Human Pharmacology: Following intravaginal administration of terconazole in humans, absorption ranged from 5–8% in three hysterectomized subjects and 12–16% in two non-hysterectomized subjects with tubal ligations. Following oral (30 mg) administration of ^{14}C-labelled terconazole, the half-life of elimination from the blood for the parent terconazole was 6.9 hours (range 4.0–11.3). Terconazole is extensively metabolized; the plasma AUC for terconazole compared to the AUC for total radioactivity was 0.6%. Total radioactivity was eliminated from the blood with a half-life of 52.2 hours (range 44–60). Excretion of radioactivity was both by renal (32–56%) and fecal (47–52%) routes.
Photosensitivity reactions were observed in some normal volunteers following repeated dermal application of terconazole 2.0% and 0.8% creams under conditions of filtered artificial ultraviolet light.
Photosensitivity reactions have not been observed in U.S. and foreign clinical trials in patients who were treated vaginally with terconazole suppositories or cream.

INDICATIONS AND USAGE

TERAZOL 3 Vaginal Suppositories are indicated for the local treatment of vulvovaginal candidiasis (moniliasis). As TERAZOL 3 Vaginal Suppositories are effective only for vulvovaginitis caused by the genus *Candida*, the diagnosis should be confirmed by KOH smears and/or cultures.

CONTRAINDICATIONS

Patients known to be hypersensitive to terconazole or to any components of the suppository.

WARNINGS

None.

PRECAUTIONS

General: Discontinue use and do not retreat with terconazole if sensitization, irritation, fever, chills or flu-like symptoms are reported during use. The base contained in the suppository formulation may interact with certain rubber or latex products, such as those used in vaginal contraceptive diaphragms, therefore concurrent use is not recommended. If there is lack of response to TERAZOL 3 Vaginal Suppositories, appropriate microbiological studies (standard KOH smear and/or cultures) should be repeated to confirm the diagnosis and rule out other pathogens.
Drug Interactions: The therapeutic effect of TERAZOL 3 Vaginal Suppositories is not affected by oral contraceptive usage.
Carcinogenesis, Mutagenesis, Impairment of Fertility
Carcinogenesis: Studies to determine the carcinogenic potential of terconazole have not been performed.
Mutagenicity: Terconazole was not mutagenic when tested *in vitro* for induction of microbial point mutations (Ames test), or for inducing cellular transformation, or *in vivo* for chromosome breaks (micronucleus test) or dominant lethal mutations in mouse germ cells.
Impairment of Fertility: No impairment of fertility occurred when female rats were administered terconazole orally up to 40 mg/kg/day.
Pregnancy: Pregnancy Category C
There was no evidence of teratogenicity when terconazole was administered orally up to 40 mg/kg/day (25 × the recommended intravaginal human dose) in rats, or 20 mg/ kg/ day in rabbits, or subcutaneously in rats up to 20 mg/kg/ day. Dosages at or below 10 mg/kg/day produced no embryotoxicity; however, there was a delay in fetal ossification at 10 mg/kg/day in rats. There was some evidence of embryotoxicity in rabbits and rats at 20–40 mg/kg. In rats this was reflected as a decrease in litter size and number of viable young and reduced fetal weight. There was also delay in ossification and an increased incidence of skeletal variants.
The no-effect oral dose of 10 mg/kg/day resulted in a mean peak plasma level of terconazole in pregnant rats of 0.176 mcg/mL which exceeds by 44 times the mean peak plasma level (0.004 mcg/mL) seen in normal subjects after intravaginal administration of terconazole. This assessment does not account for possible exposure of the fetus through direct transfer of terconazole from the irritated vagina to the fetus by diffusion across amniotic membranes.
Since terconazole is absorbed from the human vagina, it should not be used in the first trimester of pregnancy unless the physician considers it essential to the welfare of the patient.
Nursing Mothers: It is not known whether terconazole is excreted in human milk. Animal studies have shown that rat off-spring exposed via the milk of treated (40 mg/kg/ orally) dams showed decreased survival during the first few post-partum days. Because many drugs are excreted in human milk, and because of the potential for adverse reaction in nursing infants from terconazole, a decision should be made whether to discontinue nursing or to discontinue the drug, taking into account the importance of the drug to the mother.
Pediatric Use: Safety and efficacy in children have not been established.

ADVERSE REACTIONS

During controlled clinical studies conducted in the United States, 284 patients with vulvovaginal candidiasis were treated with terconazole 80 mg vaginal suppositories. Based on comparative analyses with placebo (295 patients) the adverse experiences considered adverse reactions most likely related to terconazole 80 mg vaginal suppositories were headache (30.3% vs 20.7% with placebo) and pain of the female genitalia (4.2% vs 0.7% with placebo). Adverse reactions that were reported but were not statistically significantly different from placebo were burning (15.2% vs 11.2% with placebo) and body pain (3.9% vs 1.7% with placebo). Fever (2.8% vs 1.4% with placebo) and chills (1.8% vs 0.7% with placebo) have also been reported. The therapy-related dropout rate was 3.5% and the placebo therapy-related dropout rate was 2.7%. The adverse drug experience on terconazole most frequently causing discontinuation was burning (2.5% vs 1.4% with placebo) and pruritus (1.8% vs 1.4% with placebo).

DOSAGE AND ADMINISTRATION

One TERAZOL 3 Vaginal Suppository (80 mg terconazole) is administered intravaginally once daily at bedtime for three consecutive days. Before prescribing another course of therapy, the diagnosis should be reconfirmed by smears and/or cultures and other pathogens commonly associated with vulvovaginitis ruled out. The therapeutic effect of TERAZOL 3 Vaginal Suppositories is not affected by menstruation.

HOW SUPPLIED

TERAZOL 3 (terconazole) Vaginal Suppositories 80 mg are available as 2.5 g, elliptically shaped white to off-white suppositories in packages of three (NDC 0062-5351-01) with a vaginal applicator. Store at Controlled Room Temperature 15°–30°C (59°–86°F)
Caution: Federal (USA) law prohibits dispensing without a prescription.
631-11-303-7 REVISED March 1995
Shown in Product Identification Guide, page 329

TERAZOL® 7 ℞
Vaginal Cream 0.4%
(terconazole)

DESCRIPTION

TERAZOL 7 Vaginal Cream is a white to off-white, water washable cream for intravaginal administration containing 0.4% of the antifungal agent terconazole, *cis* -1-[*p*-[[2-(2,4-Dichlorophenyl)-2-(1H-1, 2, 4-triazol-1-ylmethyl)-1,3-dioxolan-4-yl]methoxy]phenyl]-4-isopropylpiperazine, compounded in a cream base consisting of butylated hydroxyanisole, cetyl alcohol, isopropyl myristate, polysorbate 60, polysorbate 80, propylene glycol, stearyl alcohol, and purified water.

TERCONAZOLE

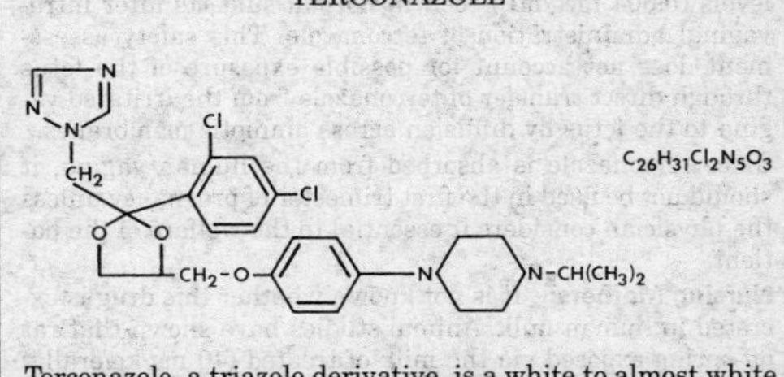

$C_{26}H_{31}Cl_2N_5O_3$

Terconazole, a triazole derivative, is a white to almost white powder with a molecular weight of 532.47. It is insoluble in water; sparingly soluble in ethanol; and soluble in butanol.

CLINICAL PHARMACOLOGY

Microbiology: Terconazole exhibits fungicidal activity *in vitro* against *Candida albicans.* Antifungal activity also has been demonstrated against other fungi. The MIC values for terconazole against most species of lactic acid bacteria typically found in the human vagina were ≥128 mcg/mL, therefore these beneficial bacteria are not affected by drug treatment.
The exact pharmacologic mode of action of terconazole is uncertain; however, it may exert its antifungal activity by the disruption of normal fungal cell membrane permeability. No resistance to terconazole has developed during successive passages of *C. albicans.*
Human Pharmacology: Following intravaginal administration of terconazole in humans, absorption ranged from 5–8% in three hysterectomized subjects and 12–16% in two non-hysterectomized subjects with tubal ligations.
Following oral (30 mg) administration of ^{14}C-labelled terconazole, the half-life of elimination from the blood for the

Continued on next page

Terazol 7 Cream—Cont.

parent terconazole was 6.9 hours (range 4.0–11.3). Terconazole is extensively metabolized; the plasma AUC for terconazole compared to the AUC for total radioactivity was 0.6%. Total radioactivity was eliminated from the blood with a half-life of 52.2 hours (range 44–60). Excretion of radioactivity was both by renal (32–56%) and fecal (47–52%) routes.

Photosensitivity reactions were observed in some normal volunteers following repeated dermal application of terconazole 2.0% and 0.8% creams under conditions of filtered artificial ultraviolet light. Photosensitivity reactions have not been observed in U.S. and foreign clinical trials in patients who were treated with terconazole 0.4% vaginal cream.

INDICATIONS AND USAGE

TERAZOL 7 Vaginal Cream is indicated for the local treatment of vulvovaginal candidiasis (moniliasis). As TERAZOL 7 Vaginal Cream is effective only for vulvovaginitis caused by the genus *Candida*, the diagnosis should be confirmed by KOH smears and/or cultures.

CONTRAINDICATIONS

Patients known to be hypersensitive to terconazole or to any of the components of the cream.

WARNINGS

None.

PRECAUTIONS

General: Discontinue use and do not retreat with terconazole if sensitization, irritation, fever, chills or flu-like symptoms are reported during use. If there is lack of response to TERAZOL 7 Vaginal Cream, appropriate microbiological studies (standard KOH smear and/or cultures) should be repeated to confirm the diagnosis and rule out other pathogens.

Drug Interactions: The therapeutic effect of TERAZOL 7 Vaginal Cream is not affected by oral contraceptive usage.

Carcinogenesis, Mutagenesis, Impairment of Fertility:

Carcinogenesis: Studies to determine the carcinogenic potential of terconazole have not been performed.

Mutagenicity: Terconazole was not mutagenic when tested *in vitro* for induction of microbial point mutations (Ames test) or for inducing cellular transformation, or *in vivo* for chromosome breaks (micronucleus test) or dominant lethal mutations in mouse germ cells.

Impairment of Fertility: No impairment of fertility occurred when female rats were administered terconazole orally up to 40 mg/kg/day.

Pregnancy: Pregnancy Category C.

There was no evidence of teratogenicity when terconazole was administered orally up to 40 mg/kg/day (100 × the recommended intravaginal human dose) in rats, or 20 mg/kg/day in rabbits, or subcutaneously in rats up to 20 mg/kg/day.

Dosages at or below 10 mg/kg/day produced no embryotoxicity; however, there was a delay in fetal ossification at 10 mg/kg/day in rats. There was some evidence of embryotoxicity in rabbits and rats at 20–40 mg/kg. In rats this was reflected as a decrease in litter size and number of viable young and reduced fetal weight. There was also delay in ossification and an increased incidence of skeletal variants.

The no-effect oral dose of 10 mg/kg/day resulted in a mean peak plasma level of terconazole in pregnant rats of 0.176 mcg/mL which exceeds by 44 times the mean peak plasma levels (0.004 mcg/mL) seen in normal subjects after intravaginal administration of terconazole. This safety assessment does not account for possible exposure of the fetus through direct transfer of terconazole from the irritated vagina to the fetus by diffusion across amniotic membranes.

Since terconazole is absorbed from the human vagina, it should not be used in the first trimester of pregnancy unless the physician considers it essential to the welfare of the patient.

Nursing Mothers: It is not known whether this drug is excreted in human milk. Animal studies have shown that rat off-spring exposed via the milk of treated (40 mg/kg/orally) dams showed decreased survival during the first few postpartum days, but overall pup weight and weight gain were comparable to or greater than controls throughout lactation. Because many drugs are excreted in human milk, and because of the potential for adverse reaction in nursing infants from terconazole, a decision should be made whether to discontinue nursing or to discontinue the drug, taking into account the importance of the drug to the mother.

Pediatric Use: Safety and efficacy in children have not been established.

ADVERSE REACTIONS

During controlled clinical studies conducted in the United States, 521 patients with vulvovaginal candidiasis were treated with terconazole 0.4% vaginal cream. Based on comparative analyses with placebo, the adverse experiences considered most likely related to terconazole 0.4% vaginal cream were headaches (26% *vs* 17% with placebo) and body pain (2.1% *vs* 0% with placebo). Vulvovaginal burning (5.2%), itching (2.3%) or irritation (3.1%) occurred less frequently with terconazole 0.4% vaginal cream than with the vehicle placebo. Fever (1.7% *vs* 0.5% with placebo) and chills (0.4% *vs* 0.0% with placebo) have also been reported. The therapy-related dropout rate was 1.9%. The adverse drug experience on terconazole most frequently causing discontinuation was vulvovaginal itching (0.6%), which was lower than the incidence for placebo (0.9%).

OVERDOSAGE

Overdose of terconazole in humans has not been reported to date. In the rat, the oral LD 50 values were found to be 1741 and 849 mg/kg for the male and female, respectively. The oral LD 50 values for the male and female dog were ≅1280 and ≥640 mg/kg, respectively.

DOSAGE AND ADMINISTRATION

One full applicator (5 g) of TERAZOL 7 Vaginal Cream (20 mg terconazole) is administered intravaginally once daily at bedtime for seven consecutive days. Before prescribing another course of therapy, the diagnosis should be reconfirmed by smears and/or cultures and other pathogens commonly associated with vulvovaginitis ruled out. The therapeutic effect of TERAZOL 7 Vaginal Cream is not affected by menstruation.

HOW SUPPLIED

TERAZOL® 7 (terconazole) Vaginal Cream 0.4% is available in 45 g (NDC 0062-5350-01) tubes with an ORTHO® Measured-Dose Applicator. Store at controlled room temperature 15°–30°C (59°–86°F).

Caution: Federal (USA) law prohibits dispensing without a prescription.

631-11-301-6 Revised September 1996

Shown in Product Identification Guide, page 329

TOLECTIN® 200 (tolmetin sodium) ℞
[*to-lek 'tin*]
200 mg Tablets
NSN 6505-01-038-7460—100's
TOLECTIN® DS (tolmetin sodium) ℞
400 mg Capsules
NSN 6505-01-091-9624—100's
NSN 6505-01-039-4469—U/D 100's
TOLECTIN® 600 (tolmetin sodium) ℞
600 mg Tablets
NSN 6505-01-322-8539—100's
For Oral Administration

DESCRIPTION

TOLECTIN 200 (tolmetin sodium) tablets for oral administration contain tolmetin sodium as the dihydrate in an amount equivalent to 200 mg of tolmetin (scored for 100 mg). Each tablet contains 18 mg (0.784 mEq) of sodium and the following inactive ingredients: cellulose, magnesium stearate, silicon dioxide, corn starch and talc.

TOLECTIN DS (tolmetin sodium) capsules for oral administration contain tolmetin sodium as the dihydrate in an amount equivalent to 400 mg of tolmetin. Each capsule contains 36 mg (1.568 mEq) of sodium and the following inactive ingredients: gelatin, magnesium stearate, corn starch, talc, FD&C Red No. 3, FD&C Yellow No. 6 and titanium dioxide.

TOLECTIN 600 (tolmetin sodium) tablets for oral administration contain tolmetin sodium as the dihydrate in an amount equivalent to 600 mg of tolmetin. Each tablet contains 54 mg (2.35 mEq) of sodium and the following inactive ingredients: cellulose, silicon dioxide, crospovidone, hydroxypropyl methyl cellulose, magnesium stearate, polyethylene glycol, corn starch, titanium dioxide, FD&C Yellow No. 6 and D&C Yellow No. 10.

The pKa of tolmetin is 3.5 and tolmetin sodium is freely soluble in water.

Tolmetin sodium is a nonsteroidal anti-inflammatory agent. The structural formula is:

H_3C–(C₆H₄)–C(=O)–(pyrrole, N–CH_3)–CH_2–$COO^-Na^+ \cdot 2H_2O$

Sodium 1-methyl-5-(4-methylbenzoyl)-1*H* -pyrrole-2-acetate dihydrate.

CLINICAL PHARMACOLOGY

Studies in animals have shown TOLECTIN (tolmetin sodium) to possess anti-inflammatory, analgesic and antipyretic activity. In the rat, TOLECTIN prevents the development of experimentally induced polyarthritis and also decreases established inflammation.

The mode of action of TOLECTIN is not known. However, studies in laboratory animals and man have demonstrated that the anti-inflammatory action of TOLECTIN is *not* due to pituitary-adrenal stimulation. TOLECTIN inhibits prostaglandin synthetase *in vitro* and lowers the plasma level of prostaglandin E in man. This reduction in prostaglandin synthesis may be responsible for the anti-inflammatory action. TOLECTIN does not appear to alter the course of the underlying disease in man.

In patients with rheumatoid arthritis and in normal volunteers, tolmetin sodium is rapidly and almost completely absorbed with peak plasma levels being reached within 30–60 minutes after an oral therapeutic dose. In controlled studies, the time to reach peak tolmetin plasma concentration is approximately 20 minutes longer following administration of a 600 mg tablet, compared to an equivalent dose given as 200 mg tablets. The clinical meaningfulness of this finding, if any, is unknown. Tolmetin displays a biphasic elimination from the plasma consisting of a rapid phase with a half-life of one to 2 hours followed by a slower phase with a half-life of about 5 hours. Peak plasma levels of approximately 40 µg/mL are obtained with a 400 mg oral dose. Essentially all of the administered dose is recovered in the urine in 24 hours either as an inactive oxidative metabolite or as conjugates of tolmetin. An 18-day multiple dose study demonstrated no accumulation of tolmetin when compared with a single dose.

In two fecal blood loss studies of 4 to 6 days duration involving 15 subjects each, TOLECTIN did not induce an increase in blood loss over that observed during a 4-day drug-free control period. In the same studies, aspirin produced a greater blood loss than occurred during the drug-free control period, and a greater blood loss than occurred during the TOLECTIN treatment period. In one of the two studies, indomethacin produced a greater fecal blood loss than occurred during the drug-free control period; in the second study, indomethacin did not induce a significant increase in blood loss.

TOLECTIN is effective in treating both the acute flares and in the long-term management of the symptoms of rheumatoid arthritis, osteoarthritis and juvenile rheumatoid arthritis.

In patients with either rheumatoid arthritis or osteaoarthritis, TOLECTIN is as effective as aspirin and indomethacin in controlling disease activity, but the frequency of the milder gastrointestinal adverse effects and tinnitus was less than in aspirin-treated patients, and the incidence of central nervous system adverse effects was less than in indomethacin-treated patients.

In patients with juvenile rheumatoid arthritis, TOLECTIN is as effective as aspirin in controlling disease activity, with a similar incidence of adverse reactions. Mean SGOT values, initially elevated in patients on previous aspirin therapy, remained elevated in the aspirin group and decreased in the TOLECTIN group.

TOLECTIN has produced additional therapeutic benefit when added to a regimen of gold salts and, to a lesser extent, with corticosteroids. TOLECTIN should not be used in conjunction with salicylates since greater benefit from the combination is not likely, but the potential for adverse reactions is increased.

INDICATIONS AND USAGE

TOLECTIN (tolmetin sodium) is indicated for the relief of signs and symptoms of rheumatoid arthritis and osteoarthritis. TOLECTIN is indicated in the treatment of acute flares and the long-term management of the chronic disease.

TOLECTIN is also indicated for treatment of juvenile rheumatoid arthritis. The safety and effectiveness of TOLECTIN have not been established in children under 2 years of age (see PRECAUTIONS—Pediatric Use and DOSAGE AND ADMINISTRATION).

CONTRAINDICATIONS

Anaphylactoid reactions have been reported with TOLECTIN as with other nonsteroidal anti-inflammatory drugs. Because of the possibility of cross-sensitivity to other nonsteroidal anti-inflammatory drugs, particularly zomepirac sodium, anaphylactoid reactions may be more likely to occur in patients who have exhibited allergic reactions to these compounds. For this reason, TOLECTIN should not be given to patients in whom aspirin and other nonsteroidal anti-inflammatory drugs induce symptoms of asthma, rhinitis, urticaria and other symptoms of allergic or anaphylactoid reactions. Patients experiencing anaphylactoid reactions on TOLECTIN should be treated with conventional therapy, such as epinephrine, antihistamines and/or steroids.

WARNINGS

Risk of GI Ulceration, Bleeding and Perforation with NSAID Therapy:

Serious gastrointestinal toxicity such as bleeding, ulceration, and perforation, can occur at any time, with or without symptoms, in patients treated chronically with NSAID (Nonsteroidal Anti-Inflammatory Drug) therapy. Although minor upper gastrointestinal problems, such as dyspepsia, are common, usually developng early in therapy, physicians should remain alert for ulceration and bleeding in patients treated chronically with NSAID's even in the absence of previous GI tract symptoms. In patients observed in clinical trials of several months to two years duration, symptomatic upper GI ulcers, gross bleeding or perforation appear to occur in approximately 1% of patients treated for 3–6 months, and in about 2–4% of patients treated for one year. Physicians should inform patients about the signs and/or symptoms of serious GI toxicity and what steps to take if they occur.

Studies to date have not identified any subset of patients not at risk of developing peptic ulceration and bleeding. Except for a prior history of serious GI events and other risk factors known to be associated with peptic ulcer disease, such as alcoholism, smoking, etc., no risk factors (e.g., age, sex) have been associated with increased risk. Elderly or debilitated patients seem to tolerate ulceration or bleeding less well than other individuals and most spontaneous reports of fatal GI events are in this population. Studies to date are inconclusive concerning the relative risk of various NSAID's in causing such reactions. High doses of any NSAID probably carry a greater risk of these reactions, although controlled clinical trials showing this do not exist in most cases. In considering the use of relatively large doses (within the recommended dosage range), sufficient benefit should be anticipated to offset the potential increased risk of GI toxicity.

PRECAUTIONS

General

Because of ocular changes observed in animals and reports of adverse eye findings with nonsteroidal anti-inflammatory agents, it is recommended that patients who develop visual disturbances during treatment with TOLECTIN have ophthalmologic evaluations.

As with other nonsteroidal anti-inflammatory drugs, long-term administration of tolmetin to animals has resulted in renal papillary necrosis and other abnormal renal pathology. In humans, there have been reports of acute interstitial nephritis with hematuria, proteinuria, and occasionally nephrotic syndrome.

A second form of renal toxicity has been seen in patients with prerenal conditions leading to a reduction in renal blood flow or blood volume, where the renal prostaglandins have a supportive role in the maintenance of renal perfusion. In these patients administration of an NSAID may cause a dose dependent reduction in prostaglandin formation and may precipitate overt renal decompensation. Patients at greatest risk of this reaction are those with heart failure, liver dysfunction, those taking diuretics, and the elderly. Discontinuation of NSAID therapy is typically followed by recovery to the pretreatment state.

Since TOLECTIN and its metabolites are eliminated primarily by the kidneys, patients with impaired renal function should be closely monitored, and it should be anticipated that they will require lower doses.

TOLECTIN prolongs bleeding time. Patients who may be adversely affected by prolongation of bleeding time should be carefully observed when TOLECTIN is administered.

In patients receiving concomitant TOLECTIN-steroid therapy, any reduction in steroid dosage should be gradual to avoid the possible complications of sudden steroid withdrawal.

Peripheral edema has been reported in some patients receiving TOLECTIN therapy. Therefore, as with other nonsteroidal anti-inflammatory drugs, TOLECTIN should be used with caution in patients with compromised cardiac function, hypertension, or other conditions predisposing to fluid retention.

The antipyretic and anti-inflammatory activities of the drug may reduce fever and inflammation, thus diminishing their utility as diagnostic signs in detecting complications of presumed non-infectious, non-inflammatory painful conditions.

As with other nonsteroidal anti-inflammatory drugs, borderline elevations of one or more liver tests may occur in up to 15% of patients. These abnormalities may progress, may remain essentially unchanged, or may be transient with continued therapy. The SGPT (ALT) test is probably the most sensitive indicator of liver dysfunction. Meaningful (3 times the upper limit of normal) elevations of SGPT or SGOT (AST) occurred in controlled clinical trials in less than 1% of patients. A patient with symptoms and/or signs suggesting liver dysfunction, or in whom an abnormal liver test has occurred, should be evaluated for evidence of the development of more severe hepatic reaction while on therapy with TOLECTIN. Severe hepatic reactions, including jaundice and fatal hepatitis, have been reported with TOLECTIN as with other nonsteroidal anti-inflammatory drugs. Although such reactions are rare, if abnormal liver tests persist or worsen, if clinical signs and symptoms consistent with liver disease develop, or if systemic manifestations occur (e.g. eosinophilia, rash, etc.), TOLECTIN should be discontinued.

Carcinogenesis, Mutagenesis, Impairment of Fertility

Tolmetin sodium did not possess any carcinogenic liability in the following long-term studies: a 24-month study in rats at doses as high as 75 mg/kg/day, and an 18-month study in mice at doses as high as 50 mg/kg/day.

No mutagenic potential of tolmetin sodium was found in the Ames Salmonella-Microsomal Activation Test.

Reproductive studies revealed no impairment of fertility in animals. Effects on parturition have been shown, however, as with other prostaglandin inhibitors. This information is detailed in the Pregnancy section below.

Pregnancy

Pregnancy Category C. Reproduction studies in rats and rabbits at doses up to 50 mg/kg (1.5 times the maximum clinical dose based on a body weight of 60 kg) revealed no evidence of teratogenesis or impaired fertility due to TOLECTIN. However, TOLECTIN is an inhibitor of prostaglandin synthetase. Drugs in this class have known effects on the fetal cardiovascular system which may cause constriction of the ductus arteriosus *in utero* during the third trimester of pregnancy, which may result in persistent pulmonary hypertension of the newborn.

There are no adequate and well-controlled studies in pregnant women. TOLECTIN should be used during pregnancy only if the potential benefit justifies the potential risk to the fetus.

Non-Teratogenic Effects

Prostaglandin inhibitors have also been shown to increase the incidence of dystocia and delayed parturition in animals.

Nursing Mothers

TOLECTIN has been shown to be secreted in human milk. Because of the possible adverse effects of prostaglandin inhibiting drugs on neonates, use in nursing mothers should be avoided.

Pediatric Use

The safety and effectiveness of TOLECTIN in children under 2 years of age have not been established.

Drug Interactions

The *in vitro* binding of warfarin to human plasma proteins is unaffected by tolmetin, and tolmetin does not alter the prothrombin time of normal volunteers. However, increased prothrombin time and bleeding have been reported in patients on concomitant TOLECTIN and warfarin therapy. Therefore, caution should be exercised when administering TOLECTIN to patients on anticoagulants.

In adult diabetic patients under treatment with either sulfonylureas or insulin there is no change in the clinical effects of either TOLECTIN or the hypoglycemic agents.

Caution should be used if TOLECTIN is administered concomitantly with methotrexate. TOLECTIN and other nonsteroidal anti-inflammatory drugs have been reported to reduce the tubular secretion of methotrexate in an animal model, possibly enhancing the toxicity of methotrexate.

Laboratory Tests

Because serious GI tract ulceration and bleeding can occur without warning symptoms, physicians should follow chronically treated patients for the signs and symptoms of ulceration and bleeding and should inform them of the importance of this follow-up (see WARNINGS—Risk of GI Ulceration, Bleeding and Perforation with NSAID Therapy).

Drug/Laboratory Test Interaction

The metabolites of tolmetin sodium in urine have been found to give positive tests for proteinuria using tests which rely on acid precipitation as their endpoint (e.g. sulfosalicylic acid). No interference is seen in the tests for proteinuria using dye-impregnated commercially available reagent strips (e.g., Albustix®, Uristix®, etc.).

Drug-Food Interaction

In a controlled single dose study, administration of TOLECTIN with milk had no effect on peak plasma tolmetin concentrations, but decreased total tolmetin bioavailability by 16%. When TOLECTIN was taken immediately after a meal, peak plasma tolmetin concentrations were reduced by 50% while total bioavailability was again decreased by 16%.

Information for Patients

TOLECTIN, like other drugs of its class, is not free of side effects. The side effects of these drugs can cause discomfort and, rarely, there are more serious side effects, such as gastrointestinal bleeding, which may result in hospitalization and even fatal outcomes.

NSAID's (Nonsteroidal Anti-Inflammatory Drugs) are often essential agents in the management of arthritis, but they also may be commonly employed for conditions which are less serious.

Physicians may wish to discuss with their patients the potential risks (see WARNINGS, PRECAUTIONS, and ADVERSE REACTIONS sections) and likely benefits of NSAID treatment, particularly when the drugs are used for less serious conditions where treatment without NSAID's may represent an acceptable alternative to both the patient and physician.

ADVERSE REACTIONS

The adverse reactions which have been observed in clinical trials encompass observations in about 4370 patients treated with TOLECTIN (tolmetin sodium), over 800 of whom have undergone at least one year of therapy. These adverse reactions, reported below by body system, are among those typical of nonsteroidal anti-inflammatory drugs and, as expected, gastrointestinal complaints were most frequent. In clinical trials with TOLECTIN, about 10% of patients dropped out because of adverse reactions, mostly gastrointestinal in nature.

Incidence Greater Than 1%

The following adverse reactions which occurred more frequently than 1 in 100 were reported in controlled clinical trials.

Gastrointestinal: Nausea (11%), dyspepsia,* gastrointestinal distress,* abdominal pain,* diarrhea,* flatulence,* vomiting,* constipation, gastritis, and peptic ulcer. Forty percent of the ulcer patients had a prior history of peptic ulcer disease and/or were receiving concomitant anti-inflammatory drugs including corticosteroids, which are known to produce peptic ulceration.

Body as a Whole: Headache,* asthenia,* chest pain

Cardiovascular: Elevated blood pressure,* edema*

Central Nervous System: Dizziness,* drowsiness, depression

Metabolic/Nutritional: Weight gain,* weight loss*

Dermatologic: Skin irritation

Special Senses: Tinnitus, visual disturbance

Hematologic: Small and transient decreases in hemoglobin and hematocrit not associated with gastrointestinal bleeding have occurred. These are similar to changes reported with other nonsteroidal anti-inflammatory drugs.

Urogenital: Elevated BUN, urinary tract infection

*Reactions occurring in 3% to 9% of patients treated with TOLECTIN. Reactions occurring in fewer than 3% of the patients are unmarked.

Incidence Less Than 1%
(Causal Relationship Probable)

The following adverse reactions were reported less frequently than 1 in 100 in controlled clinical trials or were reported since marketing. The probability exists that there is a causal relationship between TOLECTIN and these adverse reactions.

Gastrointestinal: Gastrointestinal bleeding with or without evidence of peptic ulcer, perforation, glossitis, stomatitis, hepatitis, liver function abnormalities

Body as a Whole: Anaphylactoid reactions, fever, lymphadenopathy, serum sickness

Hematologic: Hemolytic anemia, thrombocytopenia, granulocytopenia, agranulocytosis

Cardiovascular: Congestive heart failure in patients with marginal cardiac function

Dermatologic: Urticaria, purpura, erythema multiforme, toxic epidermal necrolysis

Urogenital: Hematuria, proteinuria, dysuria, renal failure

Incidence Less Than 1%
(Causal Relationship Unknown)

Other adverse reactions were reported less frequently than 1 in 100 in controlled clinical trials or were reported since marketing, but a causal relationship between TOLECTIN and the reaction could not be determined. These rarely reported reactions are being listed as alerting information for the physician since the possibility of a causal relationship cannot be excluded.

Body as Whole: Epistaxis

Special Senses: Optic neuropathy, retinal and macular changes

MANAGEMENT OF OVERDOSAGE

In the event of overdosage, the stomach should be emptied by inducing vomiting or by gastric lavage followed by the administration of activated charcoal.

DOSAGE AND ADMINISTRATION

In adults with rheumatoid arthritis or osteoarthritis, the recommended starting dose is 400 mg three times daily (1200 mg daily), preferably including a dose on arising and a dose at bedtime. To achieve optimal therapeutic effect the dose should be adjusted according to the patient's response after one to two weeks. Control is usually achieved at doses of 600–1800 mg daily in divided doses (generally t.i.d.). Doses larger than 1800 mg/day have not been studied and are not recommended.

The recommended starting dose for children (2 years and older) is 20 mg/kg/day in divided doses (t.i.d. or q.i.d.). When control has been achieved, the usual dose ranges from 15 to 30 mg/kg/day. Doses higher than 30 mg/kg/day have not been studied and, therefore, are not recommended.

A therapeutic response to TOLECTIN (tolmetin sodium) can be expected in a few days to a week. Progressive improvement can be anticipated during succeeding weeks of therapy. If gastrointestinal symptoms occur, TOLECTIN can be administered with antacids other than sodium bicarbonate. TOLECTIN bioavailability and pharmacokinetics are not significantly affected by acute or chronic administration of magnesium and aluminum hydroxides; however, bioavailability is affected by food or milk (see PRECAUTIONS—Drug-Food Interaction).

HOW SUPPLIED

TOLECTIN® 200 (tolmetin sodium) tablets 200 mg (white, scored, imprinted "TOLECTIN," "200" and "McNEIL"), NDC 0045-0412, bottles of 100.

TOLECTIN® DS (tolmetin sodium) capsules 400 mg (colored orange opaque, with contrasting parallel bands, imprinted "TOLECTIN DS" and "McNEIL"), NDC 0045-0414, bottles of 100, 500.

TOLECTIN® 600 (tolmetin sodium) tablets 600 mg (colored orange, film coated, imprinted "TOLECTIN 600" and "McNEIL"), NDC 0045-0416, bottles of 100 and 500.

Dispense in tight, light-resistant container as defined in the official compendium.

Store at controlled room temperature (15°–30°C, 59°–86°F). Protect from light.

McNeil Pharmaceutical, McNEILAB, Inc.
Spring House, PA 19477
Revised June 1997 643-10-089-2

Shown in Product Identification Guide, page 329

TOPAMAX® ℞
[*tō ′-p-ă-măx*]
(topiramate)
Tablets
TOPAMAX® ℞
(topiramate capsules)
Sprinkle Capsules
Prescribing Information

DESCRIPTION

Topiramate is a sulfamate-substituted monosaccharide that is intended for use as an antiepileptic drug. TOPAMAX® (topiramate) Tablets are available as 25 mg, 100 mg, and 200 mg round tablets for oral administration. TOPAMAX® (topiramate capsules) Sprinkle Capsules are available as 15 mg and 25 mg sprinkle capsules for oral administration as whole capsules or opened and sprinkled onto soft food.

Topiramate is a white crystalline powder with a bitter taste. Topiramate is most soluble in alkaline solutions containing sodium hydroxide or sodium phosphate and having a pH of 9 to 10. It is freely soluble in acetone, chloroform, dimethylsulfoxide, and ethanol. The solubility in water is 9.8 mg/mL. Its saturated solution has a pH of 6.3. Topiramate has the molecular formula $C_{12}H_{21}NO_8S$ and a molecular weight of 339.37. Topiramate is designated chemically as 2,3:4,5-

Continued on next page

Topamax—Cont.

Di-*O*-isopropylidene-β-D-fructopyranose sulfamate and has the following structural formula:

TOPAMAX® (topiramate) Tablets contain the following inactive ingredients: lactose monohydrate, pregelatinized starch, microcrystalline cellulose, sodium starch glycolate, magnesium stearate, purified water, carnauba wax, hydroxypropyl methylcellulose, titanium dioxide, polyethylene glycol, synthetic iron oxide (100 and 200 mg tablets) and polysorbate 80.

TOPAMAX® (topiramate capsules) Sprinkle Capsules contain topiramate coated beads in a hard gelatin capsule. The inactive ingredients are: sugar spheres (sucrose and starch), povidone, cellulose acetate, gelatin, silicone dioxide, sodium lauryl sulfate, titanium dioxide, and black pharmaceutical ink.

CLINICAL PHARMACOLOGY

Mechanism of Action:

The precise mechanism by which topiramate exerts its antiseizure effect is unknown; however, electrophysiological and biochemical studies of the effects of topiramate on cultured neurons have revealed three properties that may contribute to topiramate's antiepileptic efficacy. First, action potentials elicited repetitively by a sustained depolarization of the neurons are blocked by topiramate in a time-dependent manner, suggestive of a state-dependent sodium channel blocking action. Second, topiramate increases the frequency at which γ-aminobutyrate (GABA) activates $GABA_A$ receptors, and enhances the ability of GABA to induce a flux of chloride ions into neurons, suggesting that topiramate potentiates the activity of this inhibitory neurotransmitter. This effect was not blocked by flumazenil, a benzodiazepine antagonist, nor did topiramate increase the duration of the channel open time, differentiating topiramate from barbiturates that modulate $GABA_A$ receptors. Third, topiramate antagonizes the ability of kainate to activate the kainate/AMPA (α-amino-3-hydroxy-5-methylisoxazole-4-propionic acid; non-NMDA) subtype of excitatory amino acid (glutamate) receptor, but has no apparent effect on the activity of N-methyl-D-aspartate (NMDA) at the NMDA receptor subtype. These effects of topiramate are concentration-dependent within the range of 1 µM to 200 µM.

Topiramate also inhibits some isoenzymes of carbonic anhydrase (CA-II and CA-IV). This pharmacologic effect is generally weaker than that of acetazolamide, a known carbonic anhydrase inhibitor, and is not thought to be a major contributing factor to topiramate's antiepileptic activity.

Pharmacodynamics:

Topiramate has anticonvulsant activity in rat and mouse maximal electroshock seizure (MES) tests. Topiramate is only weakly effective in blocking clonic seizures induced by the $GABA_A$ receptor antagonist, pentylenetetrazole. Topiramate is also effective in rodent models of epilepsy, which include tonic and absence-like seizures in the spontaneous epileptic rat (SER) and tonic and clonic seizures induced in rats by kindling of the amygdala or by global ischemia.

Pharmacokinetics:

The sprinkle formulation is bioequivalent to the immediate release tablet formulation and, therefore, may be substituted as a therapeutic equivalent.

Absorption of topiramate is rapid, with peak plasma concentrations occurring at approximately 2 hours following a 400 mg oral dose. The relative bioavailability of topiramate from the tablet formulation is about 80% compared to a solution. The bioavailability of topiramate is not affected by food.

The pharmacokinetics of topiramate are linear with dose proportional increases in plasma concentration over the dose range studied (200 to 800 mg/day). The mean plasma elimination half-life is 21 hours after single or multiple doses. Steady state is thus reached in about 4 days in patients with normal renal function. Topiramate is 13–17% bound to human plasma proteins over the concentration range of 1–250 µg/mL.

Metabolism and Excretion:

Topiramate is not extensively metabolized and is primarily eliminated unchanged in the urine (approximately 70% of an administered dose). Six metabolites have been identified in humans, none of which constitutes more than 5% of an administered dose. The metabolites are formed via hydroxylation, hydrolysis, and glucuronidation. There is evidence of renal tubular reabsorption of topiramate. In rats, given probenecid to inhibit tubular reabsorption, along with topiramate, a significant increase in renal clearance of topiramate was observed. This interaction has not been evaluated in humans. Overall, oral plasma clearance (CL/F) is approximately 20 to 30 mL/min in humans following oral administration.

Pharmacokinetic Interactions (see also Drug Interactions):

Antiepileptic Drugs

Potential interactions between topiramate and standard AEDs were assessed in controlled clinical pharmacokinetic studies in patients with epilepsy. The effect of these interactions on mean plasma AUCs are summarized under **PRECAUTIONS (Table 3).**

Table 1: Topiramate Dose Summary During the Stabilization Periods of Each of Five Double-Blind, Placebo-Controlled, Add-On Trials in Adults with Partial Onset Seizures[b]

			Target Topiramate Dosage (mg/day)				
Protocol	Stabilization Dose	Placebo[a]	200	400	600	800	1,000
YD	N	42	42	40	41	—	—
	Mean Dose	5.9	200	390	556	—	—
	Median Dose	6.0	200	400	600	—	—
YE	N	44	—	—	40	45	40
	Mean Dose	9.7	—	—	544	739	796
	Median Dose	10.0	—	—	600	800	1,000
Y1	N	23	—	19	—	—	—
	Mean Dose	3.8	—	395	—	—	—
	Median Dose	4.0	—	400	—	—	—
Y2	N	30	—	—	28	—	—
	Mean Dose	5.7	—	—	522	—	—
	Median Dose	6.0	—	—	600	—	—
Y3	N	28	—	—	—	25	—
	Mean Dose	7.9	—	—	—	568	—
	Median Dose	8.0	—	—	—	600	—

[a] Placebo dosages are given as the number of tablets. Placebo target dosages were as follows: Protocol Y1, 4 tablets/day; Protocol YD and Y2, 6 tablets/day; Protocol Y3, 8 tablets/day; Protocol YE, 10 tablets/day.

[b] Dose ranging studies were not conducted for other indications or pediatric partial onset seizures.

Table 2: Key Efficacy Results in Double-Blind, Placebo-Controlled, Add-On Trials

			Target Topiramate Dosage (mg/day)					
Protocol	Efficacy Results	Placebo	200	400	600	800	1,000	≈6 mg/kg/day*
Partial Onset Seizures Studies in Adults								
YD	N	45	45	45	46	—	—	—
	Median % Reduction	11.6	27.2[a]	47.5[b]	44.7[c]	—	—	—
	% Responders	18	24	44[d]	46[d]	—	—	—
YE	N	47	—	—	48	48	47	—
	Median % Reduction	1.7	—	—	40.8[c]	41.0[c]	36.0[c]	—
	% Responders	9	—	—	40[c]	41[c]	36[d]	—
Y1	N	24	—	23	—	—	—	—
	Median % Reduction	1.1	—	40.7[e]	—	—	—	—
	% Responders	8	—	35[d]	—	—	—	—
Y2	N	30	—	—	30	—	—	—
	Median % Reduction	−12.2	—	—	46.4[f]	—	—	—
	% Responders	10	—	—	47[c]	—	—	—
Y3	N	28	—	—	—	28	—	—
	Median % Reduction	−20.6	—	—	—	24.3[c]	—	—
	% Responders	0	—	—	—	43[c]	—	—
Studies in Pediatric Patients								
YP	N	45	—	—	—	—	—	41
	Median % Reduction	10.5	—	—	—	—	—	33.1[d]
	% Responders	20	—	—	—	—	—	39
Primary Generalized Tonic-Clonic[g]								
YTC	N	40	—	—	—	—	—	39
	Median % Reduction	9.0	—	—	—	—	—	56.7[d]
	% Responders	20	—	—	—	—	—	56[c]

Comparisons with placebo: [a]p=0.080; [b]p≤0.010; [c]p≤0.001; [d]p≤0.050; [e]p=0.065; [f]p≤0.005; [g] Median % reduction and % responders are reported for PGTC Seizures

*For Protocols YP and YTC, protocol-specified target dosages (<9.3 mg/kg/day) were assigned based on subject's weight to approximate a dosage of 6 mg/kg per day; these dosages corresponded to mg/day dosages of 125, 175, 225, and 400 mg/day.

Table 3: Summary of AED Interactions with TOPAMAX®

AED Co-administered	AED Concentration	Topiramate Concentration
Phenytoin	NC or 25% increase[a]	48% decrease
Carbamazepine (CBZ)	NC	40% decrease
CBZ epoxide[b]	NC	NE
Valproic acid	11% decrease	14% decrease
Phenobarbital	NC	NE
Primidone	NC	NE

a = Plasma concentration increased 25% in some patients, generally those on a b.i.d. dosing regimen of phenytoin.
b = is not administered but is an active metabolite of carbamazepine.
NC = Less than 10% change in plasma concentration.
AED = Antiepileptic drug.
NE = Not Evaluated.

Special Populations:

Renal Impairment:

The clearance of topiramate was reduced by 42% in moderately renally impaired (creatinine clearance 30–69 mL/min/1.73m²) and by 54% in severely renally impaired subjects (creatinine clearance <30 mL/min/1.73m²) compared to normal renal function subjects (creatinine clearance >70 mL/min/1.73m²). Since topiramate is presumed to undergo significant tubular reabsorption, it is uncertain whether this experience can be generalized to all situations of renal impairment. It is conceivable that some forms of renal disease could differentially affect glomerular filtration rate and tubular reabsorption resulting in a clearance of topiramate not predicted by creatinine clearance. In general, however, use of one-half the usual dose is recommended in patients with moderate or severe renal impairment.

Hemodialysis:

Topiramate is cleared by hemodialysis. Using a high efficiency, counterflow, single pass-dialysate hemodialysis procedure, topiramate dialysis clearance was 120 mL/min with blood flow through the dialyzer at 400 mL/min. This high clearance (compared to 20–30 mL/min total oral clearance in healthy adults) will remove a clinically significant amount of topiramate from the patient over the hemodialysis treatment period. Therefore, a supplemental dose may be required (see **DOSAGE AND ADMINISTRATION**).

Hepatic Impairment:

In hepatically impaired subjects, the clearance of topiramate may be decreased; the mechanism underlying the decrease is not well understood.

Age, Gender, and Race:

Clearance of topiramate in adults was not affected by age (18–67 years), gender, or race.

Pediatric Pharmacokinetics:

Pharmacokinetics of topiramate were evaluated in patients ages 4 to 17 years receiving one or two other antiepileptic drugs. Pharmacokinetic profiles were obtained after one week at doses of 1, 3, and 9 mg/kg/day. Clearance was independent of dose.

Pediatric patients have a 50% higher clearance and consequently shorter elimination half-life than adults. Consequently, the plasma concentration for the same mg/kg dose may be lower in pediatric patients compared to adults. As in adults, hepatic enzyme-inducing antiepileptic drugs decrease the steady state plasma concentrations of topiramate.

CLINICAL STUDIES

The results of controlled clinical trials established the efficacy of TOPAMAX® (topiramate) as adjunctive therapy in adults and pediatric patients ages 2–16 years with partial onset seizures or primary generalized tonic-clonic seizures.

Controlled Trials in Patients With Partial Onset Seizures

Adults With Partial Onset Seizures

The studies described in the following section were conducted using TOPAMAX® (topiramate) Tablets.

The effectiveness of topiramate as an adjunctive treatment for adults with partial onset seizures was established in five multicenter, randomized, double-blind, placebo-controlled trials, two comparing several dosages of topiramate and placebo and three comparing a single dosage with placebo, in patients with a history of partial onset seizures, with or without secondarily generalized seizures.

Patients in these studies were permitted a maximum of two antiepileptic drugs (AEDs) in addition to TOPAMAX® Tablets or placebo. In each study, patients were stabilized on optimum dosages of their concomitant AEDs during an 8–12 week baseline phase. Patients who experienced at least 12 (or 8, for 8-week baseline studies) partial onset seizures, with or without secondary generalization, during the baseline phase were randomly assigned to placebo or a specified dose of TOPAMAX® Tablets in addition to their other AEDs.

Following randomization, patients began the double-blind phase of treatment. Patients received active drug beginning at 100 mg per day; the dose was then increased by 100 mg or 200 mg/day increments weekly or every other week until the assigned dose was reached, unless intolerance prevented increases. After titration, patients entered an 8 or 12-week stabilization period. The numbers of patients randomized to each dose, and the actual mean, and median doses in the stabilization period are shown in Table 1.

Pediatric Patients Ages 2–16 Years With Partial Onset Seizures

The effectiveness of topiramate as an adjunctive treatment for pediatric patients with partial onset seizures was established in a multicenter, randomized, double-blind, placebo-controlled trial, comparing topiramate and placebo in patients with a history of partial onset seizures, with or without secondarily generalized seizures.

Patients in this study were permitted a maximum of two antiepileptic drugs (AEDs) in addition to TOPAMAX® Tablets or placebo. In this study, patients were stabilized on optimum dosages of their concomitant AEDs during an 8 week baseline phase. Patients who experienced at least six partial onset seizures, with or without secondarily generalized seizures, during the baseline phase were randomly assigned to placebo or TOPAMAX® Tablets in addition to their other AEDs.

Following randomization, patients began the double-blind phase of treatment. Patients received active drug beginning at 25 or 50 mg per day; the dose was then increased by 25 mg to 150 mg/day increments every other week until the assigned dosage of 125, 175, 225, or 400 mg/day based on patients' weight to approximate a dosage of 6 mg/kg per day was reached, unless intolerance prevented increases. After titration, patients entered an 8-week stabilization period.

Controlled Trials in Patients With Primary Generalized Tonic-Clonic Seizures

The effectiveness of topiramate as an adjunctive treatment for primary generalized tonic-clonic seizures was established in a multicenter randomized, double-blind, placebo-controlled trial, comparing a single dosage of topiramate and placebo.

Patients in this study were permitted a maximum of two antiepileptic drugs (AEDs) in addition to TOPAMAX® or placebo. Patients were stabilized on optimum dosages of their concomitant AEDs during an 8 week baseline phase. Patients who experienced at least three primary generalized tonic-clonic seizures during the baseline phase were randomly assigned to placebo or TOPAMAX® in addition to their other AEDs.

Following randomization, patients began the double-blind phase of treatment. Patients received active drug beginning at 50 mg per day for four weeks; the dose was then increased by 50 mg to 150 mg/day increments every other week until the assigned dose of 175, 225, or 400 mg/day based on patients' body weight to approximate a dosage of 6 mg/kg per day was reached, unless intolerance prevented increases. After titration, patients entered a 12-week stabilization period.

[See table 1 at top of previous page]

In all add-on trials, the reduction in seizure rate from baseline during the entire double-blind phase was measured. The median percent reductions in seizure rates and the responder rates (fraction of patients with at least a 50% reduction) by treatment group for each study are shown below in Table 2.

[See table 2 at top of previous page]

Subset analyses of the antiepileptic efficacy of TOPAMAX® Tablets in these studies showed no differences as a function of gender, race, age, baseline seizure rate, or concomitant AED.

Table 4: Incidence (1%) of Treatment-Emergent Adverse Events in Placebo-Controlled, Add-On Trials in Adults[a,b]

Body System/ Adverse Event[c]	Placebo (N=291)	TOPAMAX® Dosage (mg/day) 200–400 (N=183)	600–1,000 (N=414)
Body as a Whole—General Disorders			
Fatigue	13	15	30
Asthenia	1	6	3
Back Pain	4	5	3
Chest Pain	3	4	2
Influenza-Like Symptoms	2	3	4
Leg Pain	2	2	4
Hot Flushes	1	2	1
Allergy	1	2	3
Edema	1	2	1
Body Odor	0	1	0
Rigors	0	1	<1
Central & Peripheral Nervous System Disorders			
Dizziness	15	25	32
Ataxia	7	16	14
Speech Disorders/Related Speech Problems	2	13	11
Paresthesia	4	11	19
Nystagmus	7	10	11
Tremor	6	9	9
Language Problems	1	6	10
Coordination Abnormal	2	4	4
Hypoaesthesia	1	2	1
Gait Abnormal	1	3	2
Muscle Contractions Involuntary	1	2	2
Stupor	0	2	1
Vertigo	1	1	2
Gastro-Intestinal System Disorders			
Nausea	8	10	12
Dyspepsia	6	7	6
Abdominal Pain	4	6	7
Constipation	2	4	3
Gastroenteritis	1	2	1
Dry Mouth	1	2	4
Gingivitis	<1	1	1
GI Disorder	<1	1	0
Hearing and Vestibular Disorders			
Hearing Decreased	1	2	1
Metabolic and Nutritional Disorders			
Weight Decrease	3	9	13
Muscle-Skeletal System Disorders			
Myalgia	1	2	2
Skeletal Pain	0	1	0
Platelet, Bleeding, & Clotting Disorders			
Epistaxis	1	2	1
Psychiatric Disorders			
Somnolence	12	29	28
Nervousness	6	16	19
Psychomotor Slowing	2	13	21
Difficulty with Memory	3	12	14
Anorexia	4	10	12
Confusion	5	11	14
Depression	5	5	13
Difficulty with Concentration/Attention	2	6	14
Mood Problems	2	4	9
Agitation	2	3	3
Aggressive Reaction	2	3	3
Emotional Lability	1	3	3
Cognitive Problems	1	3	3
Libido Decreased	1	2	<1
Apathy	1	1	3
Depersonalization	1	1	2

(continued on next page)

INDICATIONS AND USAGE

TOPAMAX® (topiramate) Tablets and TOPAMAX® (topiramate capsules) Sprinkle Capsules are indicated as adjunctive therapy for adults and pediatric patients ages 2–16 years with partial onset seizures, or primary generalized tonic-clonic seizures.

CONTRAINDICATIONS

TOPAMAX® is contraindicated in patients with a history of hypersensitivity to any component of this product.

WARNINGS

Withdrawal of AEDs

Antiepileptic drugs, including TOPAMAX®, should be withdrawn gradually to minimize the potential of increased seizure frequency.

Cognitive/Neuropsychiatric Adverse Events

Adults

Adverse events most often associated with the use of TOPAMAX® were central nervous system-related. In adults, the most significant of these can be classified into two general categories: 1) psychomotor slowing, difficulty with concentration, and speech or language problems, in particular, word-finding difficulties and 2) somnolence or fatigue. Additional nonspecific CNS effects occasionally observed with topiramate as add-on therapy include dizziness or imbalance, confusion, memory problems, and exacerbation of mood disturbances (e.g., irritability and depression).

Reports of psychomotor slowing, speech and language problems, and difficulty with concentration and attention were common in adults. Although in some cases these events were mild to moderate, they at times led to withdrawal from treatment. The incidence of psychomotor slowing is only marginally dose-related, but both language problems and difficulty with concentration or attention clearly increased in frequency with increasing dosage in the five double-blind trials [see **ADVERSE REACTIONS, Table 5**].

Somnolence and fatigue were the most frequently reported adverse events during clinical trials with TOPAMAX®. These events were generally mild to moderate and occurred early in therapy. While the incidence of somnolence does not appear to be dose-related, that of fatigue increases at dosages above 400 mg/day.

Pediatric Patients

In double-blind clinical studies, the incidences of cognitive/neuropsychiatric adverse events in pediatric patients were generally lower than previously observed in adults. These events included psychomotor slowing, difficulty with concentration/attention, speech disorders/related speech problems and language problems. The most frequently reported neuropsychiatric events in this population were somnolence and fatigue. No patients discontinued treatment due to adverse events in double-blind trials.

Sudden Unexplained Death in Epilepsy (SUDEP)

During the course of premarketing development of TOPAMAX® (topiramate) Tablets, 10 sudden and unexplained deaths were recorded among a cohort of treated patients (2,796 subject years of exposure). This represents an incidence of 0.0035 deaths per patient year. Although this rate exceeds that expected in a healthy population matched for age and sex, it is within the range of estimates for the incidence of sudden unexplained deaths in patients with epilepsy not receiving TOPAMAX® (ranging from 0.0005 for the general population of patients with epilepsy, to 0.003 for a clinical trial population similar to that in the TOPAMAX® program, to 0.005 for patients with refractory epilepsy).

PRECAUTIONS

General:

Kidney Stones

A total of 32/2,086 (1.5%) of adults exposed to topiramate during its development reported the occurrence of kidney

Continued on next page

Topamax—Cont.

Table 4: Incidence (1%) of Treatment-Emergent Adverse Events in Placebo-Controlled, Add-On Trials in Adults[a,b]

Body System/ Adverse Event[c]	Placebo (N=291)	TOPAMAX® Dosage (mg/day) 200–400 (N=183)	600–1,000 (N=414)
Reproductive Disorders, Female			
Breast Pain	2	4	0
Amenorrhea	1	2	2
Menorrhagia	0	2	1
Menstrual Disorder	1	2	1
Reproductive Disorders, Male			
Prostatic Disorder	<1	2	0
Resistance Mechanism Disorders			
Infection	1	2	1
Infection Viral	1	2	<1
Moniliasis	<1	1	0
Respiratory System Disorders			
Pharyngitis	2	6	3
Rhinitis	6	7	6
Sinusitis	4	5	6
Dyspnea	1	1	2
Skin and Appendages Disorders			
Skin Disorder	<1	2	1
Sweating Increased	<1	1	<1
Rash Erythematous	<1	1	<1
Special Sense Other, Disorders			
Taste Perversion	0	2	4
Urinary System Disorders			
Hematuria	1	2	<1
Urinary Tract Infection	1	2	3
Micturition Frequency	1	1	2
Urinary Incontinence	<1	2	1
Urine Abnormal	0	1	<1
Vision Disorders			
Vision Abnormal	2	13	10
Diplopia	5	10	10
White Cell and RES Disorders			
Leukopenia	1	2	1

[a] Patients in these add-on trials were receiving 1 to 2 concomitant antiepileptic drugs in addition to TOPAMAX® or placebo.
[b] Values represent the percentage of patients reporting a given adverse event. Patients may have reported more than one adverse event during the study and can be included in more than one adverse event category.
[c] Adverse events reported by at least 1% of patients in the TOPAMAX® 200–400 mg/day group and more common than in the placebo group are listed in this table.

Table 5: Incidence (%) of Dose-Related Adverse Events From Placebo-Controlled, Add-On Trials in Adults with Partial Onset Seizures[a]

		TOPAMAX® Dosage (mg/day)		
Adverse Event	Placebo (N = 216)	200 (N = 45)	400 (N = 68)	600–1,000 (N = 414)
Fatigue	13	11	12	30
Nervousness	7	13	18	19
Difficulty with Concentration/Attention	1	7	9	14
Confusion	4	9	10	14
Depression	6	9	7	13
Anorexia	4	4	6	12
Language problems	<1	2	9	10
Anxiety	6	2	3	10
Mood problems	2	0	6	9
Weight decrease	3	4	9	13

[a] Dose-ranging studies were not conducted for other indications or for pediatric population.

stones, an incidence about 2–4 times that expected in a similar, untreated population. As in the general population, the incidence of stone formation among topiramate treated patients was higher in men. Kidney stones have also been reported in pediatric patients.

An explanation for the association of TOPAMAX® and kidney stones may lie in the fact that topiramate is a weak carbonic anhydrase inhibitor. Carbonic anhydrase inhibitors, e.g., acetazolamide or dichlorphenamide, promote stone formation by reducing urinary citrate excretion and by increasing urinary pH. The concomitant use of TOPAMAX® with other carbonic anhydrase inhibitors or potentially in patients on a ketogenic diet may create a physiological environment that increases the risk of kidney stone formation, and should therefore be avoided.

Increased fluid intake increases the urinary output, lowering the concentration of substances involved in stone formation. Hydration is recommended to reduce new stone formation.

Paresthesia

Paresthesia, an effect associated with the use of other carbonic anhydrase inhibitors, appears to be a common effect of TOPAMAX.®

Adjustment of Dose in Renal Failure

The major route of elimination of unchanged topiramate and its metabolites is via the kidney. Dosage adjustment may be required (see **DOSAGE AND ADMINISTRATION**).

Decreased Hepatic Function

In hepatically impaired patients, topiramate should be administered with caution as the clearance of topiramate may be decreased.

Information for Patients

Patients, particularly those with predisposing factors, should be instructed to maintain an adequate fluid intake in order to minimize the risk of renal stone formation [See **PRECAUTIONS: General,** for support regarding hydration as a preventative measure].

Patients should be warned about the potential for somnolence, dizziness, confusion, and difficulty concentrating and advised not to drive or operate machinery until they have gained sufficient experience on topiramate to gauge whether it adversely affects their mental and/or motor performance.

Additional food intake may be considered if the patient is losing weight while on this medication.

Please refer to the end of the product labeling for important information on how to take TOPAMAX® (topiramate capsules) Sprinkle Capsules.

Drug Interactions:

Antiepileptic Drugs

Potential interactions between topiramate and standard AEDs were assessed in controlled clinical pharmacokinetic studies in patients with epilepsy. The effects of these interactions on mean plasma AUCs are summarized in the following table:

In Table 3, the second column (AED concentration) describes what happens to the concentration of the AED listed in the first column when topiramate is added.

The third column (topiramate concentration) describes how the coadministration of a drug listed in the first column modifies the concentration of topiramate in experimental settings when TOPAMAX® was given alone.

[See table at top of page 2392]

Other Drug Interactions

Digoxin: In a single-dose study, serum digoxin AUC was decreased by 12% with concomitant TOPAMAX® administration. The clinical relevance of this observation has not been established.

CNS Depressants: Concomitant administration of TOPAMAX® and alcohol or other CNS depressant drugs has not been evaluated in clinical studies. Because of the potential of topiramate to cause CNS depression, as well as other cognitive and/or neuropsychiatric adverse events, topiramate should be used with extreme caution if used in combination with alcohol and other CNS depressants.

Oral Contraceptives: In a pharmacokinetic interaction study with oral contraceptives using a combination product containing norethindrone and ethinyl estradiol, TOPAMAX® did not significantly affect the clearance of norethindrone. The mean oral clearance of ethinyl estradiol at 800 mg/day dose was increased by 47% (range: 13–107%). The mean total exposure to the estrogenic component decreased by 18%, 21%, and 30% at daily doses of 200, 400, and 800 mg/day, respectively. Therefore, efficacy of oral contraceptives may be compromised by topiramate. Patients taking oral contraceptives should be asked to report any change in their bleeding patterns. The effect of oral contraceptives on the pharmacokinetics of topiramate is not known.

Others: Concomitant use of TOPAMAX®, a weak carbonic anhydrase inhibitor, with other carbonic anhydrase inhibitors, e.g., acetazolamide or dichlorphenamide, may create a physiological environment that increases the risk of renal stone formation, and should therefore be avoided.

Laboratory Tests: There are no known interactions of topiramate with commonly used laboratory tests.

Carcinogenesis, Mutagenesis, Impairment of Fertility:

An increase in urinary bladder tumors was observed in mice given topiramate (20, 75, and 300 mg/kg) in the diet for 21 months. The elevated bladder tumor incidence, which was statistically significant in males and females receiving 300 mg/kg, was primarily due to the increased occurrence of a smooth muscle tumor considered histomorphologically unique to mice. Plasma exposures in mice receiving 300 mg/kg were approximately 0.5 to 1 times steady state exposures measured in patients receiving topiramate monotherapy at the recommended human dose (RHD) of 400 mg, and 1.5 to 2 times steady state topiramate exposures in patients receiving 400 mg of topiramate plus phenytoin. The relevance of this finding to human carcinogenic risk is uncertain. No evidence of carcinogenicity was seen in rats following oral administration of topiramate for 2 years at doses up to 120 mg/kg (approximately 3 times the RHD on a mg/m^2 basis).

Topiramate did not demonstrate genotoxic potential when tested in a battery of *in vitro* and *in vivo* assays. Topiramate was not mutagenic in the Ames test or the *in vitro* mouse lymphoma assay; it did not increase unscheduled DNA synthesis in rat hepatocytes *in vitro*; and it did not increase chromosomal aberrations in human lymphocytes *in vitro* or in rat bone marrow *in vivo*.

No adverse effects on male or female fertility were observed in rats at doses up to 100 mg/kg (2.5 times the RHD on a mg/m^2 basis).

Pregnancy: Pregnancy Category C.

Topiramate has demonstrated selective developmental toxicity, including teratogenicity, in experimental animal studies. When oral doses of 20, 100, or 500 mg/kg were administered to pregnant mice during the period of organogenesis, the incidence of fetal malformations (primarily craniofacial defects) was increased at all doses. The low dose is approximately 0.2 times the recommended human dose (RHD=400 mg/day) on a mg/m^2 basis. Fetal body weights and skeletal ossification were reduced at 500 mg/kg in conjunction with decreased maternal body weight gain.

In rat studies (oral doses of 20, 100, and 500 mg/kg or 0.2, 2.5, 30 and 400 mg/kg), the frequency of limb malformations (ectrodactyly, micromelia, and amelia) was increased among the offspring of dams treated with 400 mg/kg (10 times the RHD on a mg/m^2 basis) or greater during the organogenesis period of pregnancy. Embryotoxicity (reduced fetal body weights, increased incidence of structural variations) was observed at doses as low as 20 mg/kg (0.5 times the RHD on a mg/m^2 basis). Clinical signs of maternal toxicity were seen at 400 mg/kg and above, and maternal body weight gain was reduced during treatment with 100 mg/kg or greater.

In rabbit studies (20, 60, and 180 mg/kg or 10, 35, and 120 mg/kg orally during organogenesis), embryo/fetal mortality was increased at 35 mg/kg (2 times the RHD on a mg/m^2 basis) or greater, and teratogenic effects (primarily rib and vertebral malformations) were observed at 120 mg/kg (6 times the RHD on a mg/m^2 basis). Evidence of maternal toxicity (decreased body weight gain, clinical signs, and/or mortality) was seen at 35 mg/kg and above.

When female rats were treated during the latter part of gestation and throughout lactation (0.2, 4, 20, and 100 mg/kg or 2, 20, and 200 mg/kg), offspring exhibited decreased viability and delayed physical development at 200 mg/kg (5 times the RHD on a mg/m^2 basis) and reductions in pre- and/or postweaning body weight gain at 2 mg/kg (0.05 times the RHD on a mg/m^2 basis) and above. Maternal toxicity (decreased body weight gain, clinical signs) was evident at 100 mg/kg or greater.

In a rat embryo/fetal development study with a postnatal component (0.2, 2.5, 30 or 400 mg/kg during organogenesis; noted above), pups exhibited delayed physical development at 400 mg/kg (10 times the RHD on a mg/m^2 basis) and persistent reductions in body weight gain at 30 mg/kg (1 times the RHD on a mg/m^2 basis) and higher.

There are no studies using TOPAMAX® in pregnant women. TOPAMAX® should be used during pregnancy only if the potential benefit outweighs the potential risk to the fetus.

In post-marketing experience, cases of hypospadias have been reported in male infants exposed in utero to topiramate, with or without other anticonvulsants; however, a causal relationship with topiramate has not been established.

Labor and Delivery:

In studies of rats where dams were allowed to deliver pups naturally, no drug-related effects on gestation length or parturition were observed at dosage levels up to 200 mg/kg/day. The effect of TOPAMAX® on labor and delivery in humans is unknown.

Nursing Mothers:

Topiramate is excreted in the milk of lactating rats. It is not known if topiramate is excreted in human milk. Since many drugs are excreted in human milk, and because the potential for serious adverse reactions in nursing infants to TOPAMAX® is unknown, the potential benefit to the mother should be weighed against the potential risk to the infant when considering recommendations regarding nursing.

Pediatric Use:

Safety and effectiveness in patients below the age of 2 years have not been established.

Geriatric Use:

In clinical trials, 2% of patients were over 60. No age related difference in effectiveness or adverse effects were seen. There were no pharmacokinetic differences related to age alone, although the possibility of age-associated renal functional abnormalities should be considered.

Race and Gender Effects:

Evaluation of effectiveness and safety in clinical trials has shown no race or gender related effects.

ADVERSE REACTIONS

The data described in the following section were obtained using TOPAMAX® (topiramate) Tablets.

The most commonly observed adverse events associated with the use of topiramate at dosages of 200 to 400 mg/day in controlled trials in adults with partial onset seizures, primary generalized tonic-clonic seizures, or Lennox-Gastaut syndrome, that were seen at greater frequency in topiramate-treated patients and did not appear to be dose-related were: somnolence, dizziness, ataxia, speech disorders and related speech problems, psychomotor slowing, abnormal vision, difficulty with memory, paresthesia and diplopia [see Table 4]. The most common dose-related adverse events at dosages of 200 to 1,000 mg/day were: fatigue, nervousness, difficulty with concentration or attention, confusion, depression, anorexia, language problems, anxiety, mood problems, and weight decrease [see Table 5].

Adverse events associated with the use of topiramate at dosages of 5 to 9 mg/kg/day in controlled trials in pediatric patients with partial onset seizures, primary generalized tonic-clonic seizures, or Lennox-Gastaut syndrome, that were seen at greater frequency in topiramate-treated patients were: fatigue, somnolence, anorexia, nervousness, difficulty with concentration/attention, difficulty with memory, aggressive reaction, and weight decrease [see Table 6].

In controlled clinical trials in adults, 11% of patients receiving topiramate 200 to 400 mg/day as adjunctive therapy discontinued due to adverse events. This rate appeared to increase at dosages above 400 mg/day. Adverse events associated with discontinuing therapy included somnolence, dizziness, anxiety, difficulty with concentration or attention, fatigue, and paresthesia and increased at dosages above 400 mg/day. None of the pediatric patients who received topiramate adjunctive therapy at 5 to 9 mg/kg/day in controlled clinical trials discontinued due to adverse events.

Approximately 28% of the 1,757 adults with epilepsy who received topiramate at dosages of 200 to 1,600 mg/day in clinical studies discontinued treatment because of adverse events; an individual patient could have reported more than one adverse event. These adverse events were: psychomotor slowing (4.0%), difficulty with memory (3.2%), fatigue (3.2%), confusion (3.1%), somnolence (3.2%), difficulty with concentration/attention (2.9%), anorexia (2.7%), depression (2.6%), dizziness (2.5%), weight decrease (2.5%), nervousness (2.3%), ataxia (2.1%), and paresthesia (2.0%). Approximately 11% of the 310 pediatric patients who received topiramate at dosages up to 30 mg/kg/day discontinued due to adverse events. Adverse events associated with discontinuing therapy included aggravated convulsions (2.3%), difficulty with concentration attention (1.6%), language problems (1.3%), personality disorder (1.3%), and somnolence (1.3%).

Incidence in Controlled Clinical Trials - Add-On Therapy

Table 4 lists treatment-emergent adverse events that occurred in at least 1% of adults treated with 200 to 400 mg/day topiramate in controlled trials that were numerically more common at this dose than in the patients treated with placebo. In general, most patients who experienced adverse events during the first eight weeks of these trials no longer experienced them by their last visit. Table 6 lists treatment-emergent adverse events that occurred in at least 1% of pediatric patients treated with 5 to 9 mg/kg topiramate in controlled trials that were numerically more common than in patients treated with placebo.

The prescriber should be aware that these data were obtained when TOPAMAX® was added to concurrent antiepileptic drug therapy and cannot be used to predict the frequency of adverse events in the course of usual medical practice where patient characteristics and other factors may differ from those prevailing during clinical studies. Similarly, the cited frequencies cannot be directly compared with data obtained from other clinical investigations involving different treatments, uses, or investigators. Inspection of these frequencies, however, does provide the prescribing physician with a basis to estimate the relative contribution of drug and non-drug factors to the adverse event incidences in the population studied.

[See table 4 at top of pages 2393 and 2394]

[See table 5 at top of previous page]

[See table 6 above]

Table 6: Incidence (%) of Treatment-Emergent Adverse Events in Placebo-Controlled, Add-On Trials in Pediatric Patients Ages 2–16 Years[a,b]
(Events that Occurred in at Least 1% of Topiramate-Treated Patients and Occurred More Frequently in Topiramate-Treated Than Placebo-Treated Patients)

Body System/ Adverse Event	Placebo (N=101)	Topiramate (N=98)
Body as a Whole—General Disorders		
Fatigue	5	16
Injury	13	14
Allergic Reaction	1	2
Back Pain	0	1
Pallor	0	1
Cardiovascular Disorders, General		
Hypertension	0	1
Central & Peripheral Nervous System Disorders		
Gait Abnormal	5	8
Ataxia	2	6
Hyperkinesia	4	5
Dizziness	2	4
Speech Disorders/Related Speech Problems	2	4
Hyporeflexia	0	2
Convulsions Grand Mal	0	1
Fecal Incontinence	0	1
Paresthesia	0	1
Gastro-Intestinal System Disorders		
Nausea	5	6
Saliva Increased	4	6
Constipation	4	5
Gastroenteritis	2	3
Dysphagia	0	1
Flatulence	0	1
Gastroesophageal Reflux	0	1
Glossitis	0	1
Gum Hyperplasia	0	1
Heart Rate and Rhythm Disorders		
Bradycardia	0	1
Metabolic and Nutritional Disorders		
Weight Decrease	1	9
Thirst	1	2
Hypoglycemia	0	1
Weight Increase	0	1
Platelet, Bleeding, & Clotting Disorders		
Purpura	4	8
Epistaxis	1	4
Hematoma	0	1
Prothrombin Increased	0	1
Thrombocytopenia	0	1
Psychiatric Disorders		
Somnolence	16	26
Anorexia	15	24
Nervousness	7	14
Personality Disorder (Behavior Problems)	9	11
Difficulty with Concentration/Attention	2	10
Aggressive Reaction	4	9
Insomnia	7	8
Difficulty with Memory NOS	0	5
Confusion	3	4
Psychomotor Slowing	2	3
Appetite Increased	0	1
Neurosis	0	1
Reproductive Disorders, Female		
Leukorrhoea	0	2
Resistance Mechanism Disorders		
Infection Viral	3	7
Respiratory System Disorders		
Pneumonia	1	5
Respiratory Disorder	0	1
Skin and Appendages Disorders		
Skin Disorder	2	3
Alopecia	1	2
Dermatitis	0	2
Hypertrichosis	1	2
Rash Erythematous	0	2
Eczema	0	1
Seborrhoea	0	1
Skin Discoloration	0	1
Urinary System Disorders		
Urinary Incontinence	2	4
Nocturia	0	1
Vision Disorders		
Eye Abnormality	1	2
Vision Abnormal	1	2
Diplopia	0	1
Lacrimation Abnormal	0	1
Myopia	0	1
White Cell and RES Disorders		
Leukopenia	0	2

[a] Patients in these add-on trials were receiving 1 to 2 concomitant antiepileptic drugs in addition to TOPAMAX® or placebo.
[b] Values represent the percentage of patients reporting a given adverse event. Patients may have reported more than one adverse event during the study and can be included in more than one adverse event category.

Other Adverse Events Observed

Other events that occurred in more than 1% of adults treated with 200 to 400 mg of topiramate in placebo-controlled trials but with equal or greater frequency in the placebo group were: headache, injury, anxiety, rash, pain, convulsions aggravated, coughing, fever, diarrhea, vomiting, muscle weakness, insomnia, personality disorder, dysmenorrhea, upper respiratory tract infection, and eye pain.

Other Adverse Events Observed During All Clinical Trials

Topiramate, initiated as adjunctive therapy, has been administered to 1,757 adults and 310 pediatric patients with

Continued on next page

Topamax—Cont.

epilepsy during all clinical studies. During these studies, all adverse events were recorded by the clinical investigators using terminology of their own choosing. To provide a meaningful estimate of the proportion of individuals having adverse events, similar types of events were grouped into a smaller number of standardized categories using modified WHOART dictionary terminology. The frequencies presented represent the proportion of patients who experienced an event of the type cited on at least one occasion while receiving topiramate. Reported events are included except those already listed in the previous table or text, those too general to be informative, and those not reasonably associated with the use of the drug.

Events are classified within body system categories and enumerated in order of decreasing frequency using the following definitions: *frequent* occurring in at least 1/100 patients; *infrequent* occurring in 1/100 to 1/1000 patients; *rare* occurring in fewer than 1/1000 patients.

Autonomic Nervous System Disorders: *Infrequent:* vasodilation.

Body as a Whole: *Frequent:* fever, malaise. *Infrequent:* syncope, halitosis, abdomen enlarged. *Rare:* alcohol intolerance, substernal chest pain.

Cardiovascular Disorders, General: *Infrequent:* hypotension, postural hypotension.

Central & Peripheral Nervous System Disorders: *Frequent:* hypertonia. *Infrequent:* leg cramps, neuropathy, migraine, apraxia, hyperaesthesia, dyskinesia, dysphonia, scotoma, ptosis, dystonia, visual field defect, coma, encephalopathy, upper motor neuron lesion, EEG abnormal. *Rare:* cerebellar syndrome, tongue paralysis.

Endocrine Disorders: *Infrequent:* goiter. *Rare:* thyroid disorder.

Gastrointestinal System Disorders: *Frequent:* diarrhea, vomiting, hemorrhoids. *Infrequent:* tooth caries, stomatitis, melena, gastritis, hiccough, tongue edema, esophagitis. *Rare:* eructation.

Hearing and Vestibular Disorders: *Frequent:* tinnitus. *Infrequent:* earache, hyperacusis.

Heart Rate and Rhythm Disorders: *Frequent:* palpitation. *Infrequent:* AV block, bradycardia, bundle branch block. *Rare:* arrhythmia, arrhythmia atrial, fibrillation atrial.

Liver and Biliary System Disorders: *Infrequent:* SGPT increased, SGOT increased, gall bladder disorders including cholelithiasis, gamma-GT increased.

Metabolic and Nutritional Disorders: *Frequent:* dehydration. *Infrequent:* hypokalemia, alkaline phosphatase increased, hypocalcemia, hyperlipemia, acidosis, hyperglycemia, hyperchloremia, xerophthalmia. *Rare:* diabetes mellitus, hypernatremia, abnormal serum folate, hyponatremia, hypocholesterolemia, hypophosphatemia, creatinine increased.

Musculoskeletal System Disorders: *Frequent:* arthralgia, muscle weakness. *Infrequent:* arthrosis, osteoporosis.

Myo-, Endo-, Pericardial & Valve Disorders: *Infrequent:* angina pectoris.

Neoplasms: *Infrequent:* basal cell carcinoma, thrombocythemia. *Rare:* polycythemia.

Platelet, Bleeding, and Clotting Disorders: *Infrequent:* gingival bleeding, pulmonary embolism.

Psychiatric Disorders: *Frequent:* impotence, hallucination, euphoria, psychosis. *Infrequent:* paranoid reaction, delusion, paranoia, delirium, abnormal dreaming, neurosis, libido increased, manic reaction, suicide attempt.

Red Blood Cell Disorders: *Frequent:* anemia. *Rare:* marrow depression, pancytopenia.

Reproductive Disorders, Female: *Frequent:* intermenstrual bleeding, vaginitis.

Reproductive Disorders, Male: *Infrequent:* ejaculation disorder, breast discharge.

Respiratory System Disorders: *Frequent:* coughing, bronchitis. *Infrequent:* asthma, bronchospasm, laryngismus.

Skin and Appendages Disorders: *Frequent:* acne, nail disorder, folliculitis, dry skin, urticaria. *Infrequent:* photosensitivity reaction, sweating decreased, abnormal hair texture. *Rare:* chloasma.

Special Senses Other, Disorders: *Infrequent:* taste loss, parosmia.

Urinary System Disorders: *Frequent:* dysuria, renal calculus. *Infrequent:* urinary retention, face edema, renal pain, albuminuria, polyuria, oliguria.

Vascular (Extracardiac) Disorders: *Infrequent:* flushing, deep vein thrombosis, phlebitis. *Rare:* vasospasm.

Vision Disorders: *Frequent:* conjunctivitis. *Infrequent:* abnormal accommodation, photophobia, strabismus, color blindness, mydriasis, cataract. *Rare:* corneal opacity, iritis.

White Cell and Reticuloendothelial System Disorders: *Infrequent:* lymphadenopathy, eosinophilia, lymphopenia, granulocytopenia, lymphocytosis.

Postmarketing and Other Experience

In addition to the adverse experiences reported during clinical testing of TOPAMAX®, the following adverse experiences have been reported in patients receiving marketed TOPAMAX® from worldwide use since approval. These adverse experiences have not been listed above and data are insufficient to support an estimate of their incidence or to establish causation. The listing is alphabetized: hepatic failure, hepatitis, pancreatitis, and renal tubular acidosis.

DRUG ABUSE AND DEPENDENCE

The abuse and dependence potential of TOPAMAX® has not been evaluated in human studies.

OVERDOSAGE

In acute TOPAMAX® overdose, if the ingestion is recent, the stomach should be emptied immediately by lavage or by induction of emesis. Activated charcoal has not been shown to adsorb topiramate *in vitro*. Therefore, its use in overdosage is not recommended. Treatment should be appropriately supportive. Hemodialysis is an effective means of removing topiramate from the body. However, in the few cases of acute overdosage reported, hemodialysis has not been necessary.

DOSAGE AND ADMINISTRATION

TOPAMAX® has been shown to be effective in adults and pediatric patients with partial onset seizures or primary generalized tonic-clonic seizures. In the controlled add-on trials, no correlation has been demonstrated between trough plasma concentrations of topiramate and clinical efficacy. No evidence of tolerance has been demonstrated in humans. Doses above 400 mg/day (600, 800, or 1000 mg/day) have not been shown to improve responses in dose-ranging studies in adults with partial onset seizures.

It is not necessary to monitor topiramate plasma concentrations to optimize TOPAMAX® therapy. On occasion, the addition of TOPAMAX® to phenytoin may require an adjustment of the dose of phenytoin to achieve optimal clinical outcome. Addition or withdrawal of phenytoin and/or carbamazepine during adjunctive therapy with TOPAMAX® may require adjustment of the dose of TOPAMAX®. Because of the bitter taste, tablets should not be broken. TOPAMAX® can be taken without regard to meals.

Adults (17 Years of Age and Over)

The recommended total daily dose of TOPAMAX® as adjunctive therapy is 400 mg/day in two divided doses. In studies of adults with partial onset seizures, a daily dose of 200 mg/day has inconsistent effects and is less effective than 400 mg/day. It is recommended that therapy be initiated at 25–50 mg/day followed by titration to an effective dose in increments of 25–50 mg/week. Titrating in increments of 25 mg/week may delay the time to reach an effective dose. Daily doses above 1,600 mg have not been studied.

In the study of primary generalized tonic-clonic seizures the initial titration rate was slower than in previous studies; the assigned dose was reached at the end of 8 weeks (see **CLINICAL STUDIES, Controlled Trials in Patients With Primary Generalized Tonic-Clonic Seizures**).

Pediatric Patients Ages 2–16 Years

The recommended total daily dose of TOPAMAX® (topiramate) as adjunctive therapy is approximately 5 to 9 mg/kg/day in two divided doses. Titration should begin at 25 mg (or less, based on a range of 1 to 3 mg/kg/day) nightly for the first week. The dosage should then be increased at 1- or 2-week intervals by increments of 1 to 3 mg/kg/day (administered in two divided doses), to achieve optimal clinical response. Dose titration should be guided by clinical outcome.

In the study of primary generalized tonic-clonic seizures the initial titration rate was slower than in previous studies; the assigned dose of 6 mg/kg/day was reached at the end of 8 weeks (see **CLINICAL STUDIES, Controlled Trials in Patients With Primary Generalized Tonic-Clonic Seizures**).

Administration of TOPAMAX® Sprinkle Capsules

TOPAMAX® (topiramate capsules) Sprinkle Capsules may be swallowed whole or may be administered by carefully opening the capsule and sprinkling the entire contents on a small amount (teaspoon) of soft food. This drug/food mixture should be swallowed immediately and not chewed. It should not be stored for future use.

Patients with Renal Impairment:

In renally impaired subjects (creatinine clearance less than 70 mL/min/1.73m^2), one half of the usual adult dose is recommended. Such patients will require a longer time to reach steady-state at each dose.

Patients Undergoing Hemodialysis:

Topiramate is cleared by hemodialysis at a rate that is 4 to 6 times greater than a normal individual. Accordingly, a prolonged period of dialysis may cause topiramate concentration to fall below that required to maintain an anti-seizure effect. To avoid rapid drops in topiramate plasma concentration during hemodialysis, a supplemental dose of topiramate may be required. The actual adjustment should take into account 1) the duration of dialysis period, 2) the clearance rate of the dialysis system being used, and 3) the effective renal clearance of topiramate in the patient being dialyzed.

Patients with Hepatic Disease:

In hepatically impaired patients topiramate plasma concentrations may be increased. The mechanism is not well understood.

HOW SUPPLIED

TOPAMAX® (topiramate) Tablets is available as debossed, coated, round tablets in the following strengths and colors:

25 mg white (coded "TOP" on one side; "25" on the other)

100 mg yellow (coded "TOPAMAX" on one side; "100" on the other)

200 mg salmon (coded "TOPAMAX" on one side; "200" on the other)

They are supplied as follows:

25 mg tablets—bottles of 60 count with desiccant (NDC 0045-0639-65)

100 mg tablets—bottles of 60 count with desiccant (NDC 0045-0641-65)

200 mg tablets—bottles of 60 count with desiccant (NDC 0045-0642-65)

TOPAMAX® (topiramate capsules) Sprinkle Capsules contain small, white to off white spheres. The gelatin capsules are white and clear.

They are marked as follows:

15 mg capsule with "TOP" and "15 mg" on the side

25 mg capsule with "TOP" and "25 mg" on the side

The capsules are supplied as follows:

15 mg capsules—bottles of 60 (NDC 0045-0647-65)

25 mg capsules—bottles of 60 (NDC 0045-0645-65)

TOPAMAX® (topiramate) Tablets should be stored in tightly-closed containers at controlled room temperature, (59 to 86°F, 15 to 30°C). Protect from moisture.

TOPAMAX® (topiramate capsules) Sprinkle Capsules should be stored in tightly-closed containers at or below 25°C (77°F). Protect from moisture.

TOPAMAX® (topiramate) and TOPAMAX® (topiramate capsules) are trademarks of Ortho-McNeil Pharmaceutical.

HOW TO TAKE

TOPAMAX® (topiramate capsules) SPRINKLE CAPSULES

A Guide for Patients and Their Caregivers

Your doctor has given you a prescription for TOPAMAX® (topiramate capsules) Sprinkle Capsules. Here are your instructions for taking this medication. Please read these instructions prior to use.

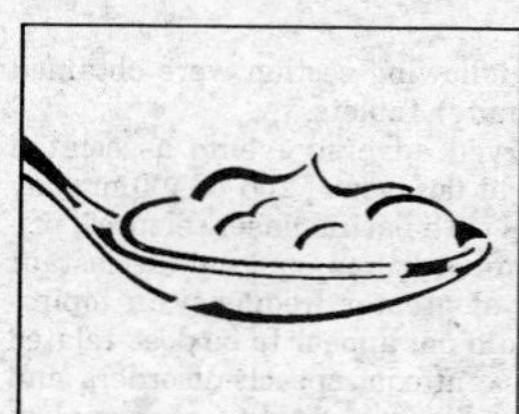

To Take With Food

You may sprinkle the contents of TOPAMAX® Sprinkle Capsules on a small amount (teaspoon) of soft food, such as applesauce, custard, ice cream, oatmeal, pudding, or yogurt.

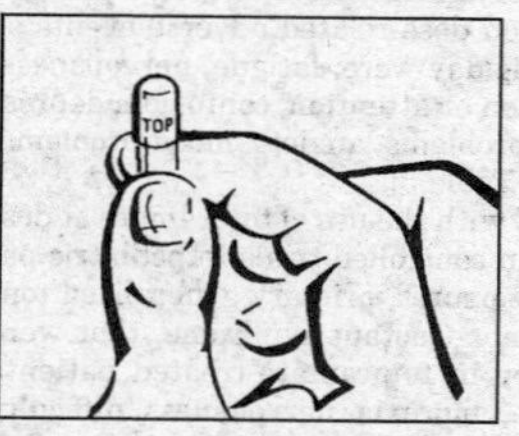

Hold the capsule upright so that you can read the word "TOP".

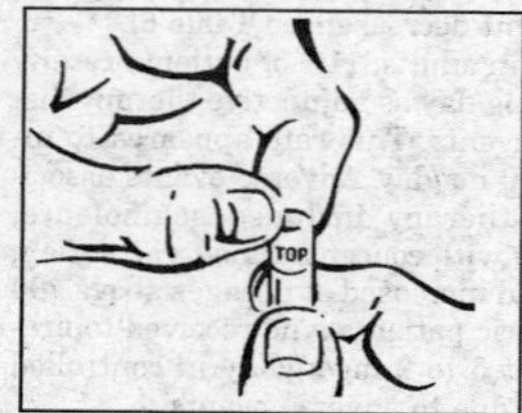

Carefully twist off the clear portion of the capsule. You may find it best to do this over the small portion of the food onto which you will be pouring the sprinkles.

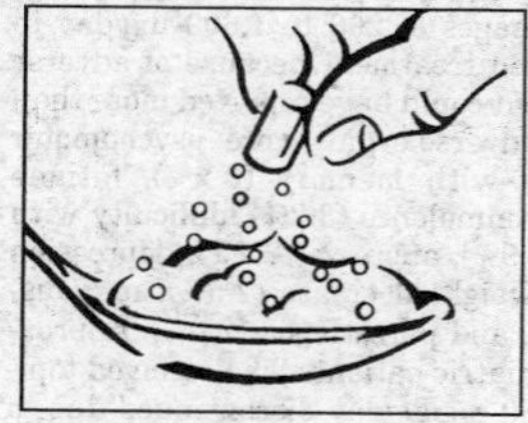

Sprinkle all of the capsule's contents onto a spoonful of soft food, taking care to see that the entire prescribed dosage is sprinkled onto the food.

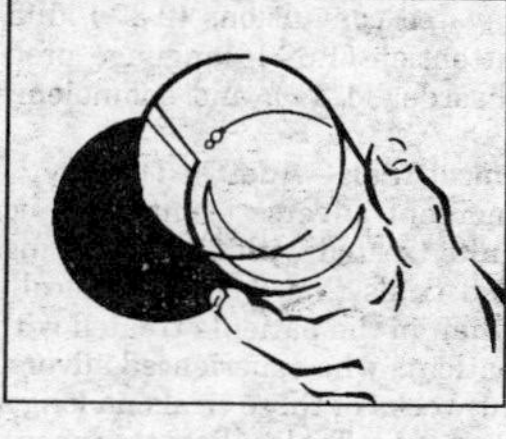

Be sure the patient swallows the entire spoonful of the sprinkle/food mixture immediately. Chewing should be avoided. It may be helpful to have the patient drink fluids immediately in order to make sure all of the mixture is swallowed.

IMPORTANT: Never store any sprinkle/food mixture for use at a later time.

To Take Without Food

TOPAMAX® Sprinkle Capsules may also be swallowed as whole capsules.

For more information about TOPAMAX® Sprinkle Capsules, ask your doctor or pharmacist.

ORTHO-McNEIL
OMP DIVISION
ORTHO-McNEIL PHARMACEUTICAL, INC.
Raritan, NJ 08869

 Revised May 2000 643-10-445-3

Shown in Product Identification Guide, page 329

TYLENOL® with Codeine ℞

[ti 'len-awl co' dēn]

tablets Ⓒ III

(acetaminophen and codeine phosphate tablets)

elixir Ⓒ V

(acetaminophen and codeine phosphate oral solution USP)

Analgesic For Oral Use

DESCRIPTION

Each tablet contains:

No. 3 Codeine Phosphate	30 mg
Acetaminophen	300 mg
No. 4 Codeine Phosphate	60 mg
Acetaminophen	300 mg
Each 5 mL of elixir contains:	
Codeine Phosphate	12 mg
Acetaminophen	120 mg
Alcohol 7%	

Inactive ingredients: tablets—powdered cellulose, magnesium stearate, sodium metabisulfite†, pregelatinized starch, starch (corn); elixir—alcohol, citric acid, propylene glycol, sodium benzoate, saccharin sodium, sucrose, natural and artificial flavors, FD&C Yellow No. 6.

Acetaminophen, 4′-hydroxyacetanilide, is a non-opiate, non-salicylate analgesic and antipyretic which occurs as a white, odorless, crystalline powder, possessing a slightly bitter taste. Its structure is as follows:

$C_8H_9NO_2$ M.W. 151.16

Codeine is an alkaloid, obtained from opium or prepared from morphine by methylation. Codeine phosphate occurs as fine, white, needle-shaped crystals, or white, crystalline powder. It is affected by light. Its chemical name is: 7,8-didehydro- 4,5α-epoxy-3-methoxy-17-methylmorphinan-6α-ol phosphate (1:1) (salt) hemihydrate. Its structure is as follows:

$C_{18}H_{21}NO_3.H_3PO_4.\ {}^1/_2H_2O$ M.W. 406.37

†See WARNINGS

CLINICAL PHARMACOLOGY

TYLENOL with Codeine (acetaminophen and codeine phosphate tablets and oral solution USP) combine the analgesic effects of a centrally acting analgesic, codeine, with a peripherally acting analgesic, acetaminophen. Both ingredients are well absorbed orally. The plasma elimination half-life ranges from 1 to 4 hours for acetaminophen, and from 2.5 to 3 hours for codeine.

Codeine retains at least one-half of its analgesic activity when administered orally. A reduced first-pass metabolism of codeine by the liver accounts for the greater oral efficacy of codeine when compared to most other morphine-like narcotics. Following absorption, codeine is metabolized by the liver and metabolic products are excreted in the urine. Approximately 10 percent of the administered codeine is demethylated to morphine, which may account for its analgesic activity.

Acetaminophen is distributed throughout most fluids of the body, and is metabolized primarily in the liver. Little unchanged drug is excreted in the urine, but most metabolic products appear in the urine within 24 hours.

INDICATIONS AND USAGE

TYLENOL with Codeine tablets (acetaminophen and codeine phosphate tablets) are indicated for the relief of mild to moderately severe pain.

TYLENOL with Codeine elixir (acetaminophen and codeine phosphate oral solution USP) is indicated for the relief of mild to moderate pain.

CONTRAINDICATIONS

TYLENOL with Codeine tablets or elixir (acetaminophen and codeine phosphate tablets and oral solution USP) should not be administered to patients who have previously exhibited hypersensitivity to any component.

WARNINGS

TYLENOL with Codeine tablets (acetaminophen and codeine phosphate tablets) contain sodium metabisulfite, a sulfite that may cause allergic-type reactions including anaphylactic symptoms and life-threatening or less severe asthmatic episodes in certain susceptible people. The overall prevalence of sulfite sensitivity in the general population is unknown and probably low. Sulfite sensitivity is seen more frequently in asthmatic than in nonasthmatic people.

PRECAUTIONS

General

Head Injury and Increased Intracranial Pressure: The respiratory depressant effects of narcotics and their capacity to elevate cerebrospinal fluid pressure may be markedly exaggerated in the presence of head injury, other intracranial lesions or a pre-existing increase in intracranial pressure. Furthermore, narcotics produce adverse reactions which may obscure the clinical course of patients with head injuries.

Acute Abdominal Conditions: The administration of this product or other narcotics may obscure the diagnosis or clinical course of patients with acute abdominal conditions.

Special Risk Patients: This drug should be given with caution to certain patients such as the elderly or debilitated, and those with severe impairment of hepatic or renal function, hypothyroidism, Addison's disease, and prostatic hypertrophy or urethral stricture.

Information for Patients

Codeine may impair the mental and/or physical abilities required for the performance of potentially hazardous tasks such as driving a car or operating machinery. The patient using this drug should be cautioned accordingly.

The patient should understand the single-dose and 24 hour dose limits, and the time interval between doses.

Drug Interactions

Patients receiving other narcotic analgesics, antipsychotics, antianxiety agents, or other CNS depressants (including alcohol) concomitantly with this drug may exhibit an additive CNS depression. When such combined therapy is contemplated, the dose of one or both agents should be reduced.

The concurrent use of anticholinergics with codeine may produce paralytic ileus.

Carcinogenesis, Mutagenesis, Impairment of Fertility

No long-term studies in animals have been performed with acetaminophen or codeine to determine carcinogenic potential or effects on fertility.

Acetaminophen and codeine have been found to have no mutagenic potential using the Ames Salmonella-Microsomal Activation test, the Basc test on Drosophila germ cells, and the Micronucleus test on mouse bone marrow.

Pregnancy

Teratogenic Effects: Pregnancy Category C.

Codeine: A study in rats and rabbits reported no teratogenic effect of codeine administered during the period of organogenesis in doses ranging from 5 to 120 mg/kg. In the rat, doses at the 120 mg/kg level, in the toxic range for the adult animal, were associated with an increase in embryo resorption at the time of implantation. In another study a single 100 mg/kg dose of codeine administered to pregnant mice reportedly resulted in delayed ossification in the offspring. There are no studies in humans, and the significance of these findings to humans, if any, is not known.

TYLENOL with Codeine (acetaminophen and codeine phosphate tablets and oral solution USP) should be used during pregnancy only if the potential benefit justifies the potential risk to the fetus.

Nonteratogenic Effects:

Dependence has been reported in newborns whose mothers took opiates regularly during pregnancy. Withdrawal signs include irritability, excessive crying, tremors, hyperreflexia, fever, vomiting, and diarrhea. These signs usually appear during the first few days of life.

Labor and Delivery

Narcotic analgesics cross the placental barrier. The closer to delivery and the larger the dose used, the greater the possibility of respiratory depression in the newborn. Narcotic analgesics should be avoided during labor if delivery of a premature infant is anticipated. If the mother has received narcotic analgesics during labor, newborn infants should be observed closely for signs of respiratory depression. Resuscitation may be required (see OVERDOSAGE). The effect of codeine, if any, on the later growth, development, and functional maturation of the child is unknown.

Nursing Mothers

Some studies, but not others, have reported detectable amounts of codeine in breast milk. The levels are probably not clinically significant after usual therapeutic dosage. The possibility of clinically important amounts being excreted in breast milk in individuals abusing codeine should be considered.

Pediatric Use

Safe dosage of TYLENOL with Codeine elixir (acetaminophen and codeine phosphate oral solution USP) has not been established in children below the age of three years.

ADVERSE REACTIONS

The most frequently observed adverse reactions include lightheadedness, dizziness, sedation, shortness of breath, nausea and vomiting. These effects seem to be more prominent in ambulatory than in non-ambulatory patients, and some of these adverse reactions may be alleviated if the patient lies down. Other adverse reactions include allergic reactions, euphoria, dysphoria, constipation, abdominal pain and pruritus.

At higher doses, codeine has most of the disadvantages of morphine including respiratory depression.

DRUG ABUSE AND DEPENDENCE

TYLENOL with Codeine tablets (acetaminophen and codeine phosphate tablets) are a Schedule III controlled substance.

TYLENOL with Codeine elixir (acetaminophen and codeine phosphate oral solution USP) is a Schedule V controlled substance.

Codeine can produce drug dependence of the morphine type and, therefore, has the potential for being abused. Psychic dependence, physical dependence and tolerance may develop upon repeated administration of this drug, and it should be prescribed and administered with the same degree of caution appropriate to the use of other oral narcotic-containing medications.

OVERDOSAGE

Acetaminophen

Signs and Symptoms: In acute acetaminophen overdosage, dose-dependent, potentially fatal hepatic necrosis is the most serious adverse effect. Renal tubular necrosis, hypoglycemic coma and thrombocytopenia may also occur.

In adults, hepatic toxicity has rarely been reported with acute overdoses of less than 10 grams and fatalities with less than 15 grams. Importantly, young children seem to be more resistant than adults to the hepatotoxic effect of an acetaminophen overdose. Despite this, the measures outlined below should be initiated in any adult or child suspected of having ingested an acetaminophen overdose.

Early symptoms following a potentially hepatotoxic overdose may include: nausea, vomiting, diaphoresis and general malaise. Clinical and laboratory evidence of hepatic toxicity may not be apparent until 48 to 72 hours post-ingestion.

Treatment: The stomach should be emptied promptly by lavage or by induction of emesis with syrup of ipecac. Patients' estimates of the quantity of a drug ingested are notoriously unreliable. Therefore, if an acetaminophen overdose is suspected, a serum acetaminophen assay should be obtained as early as possible, but no sooner than four hours following ingestion. Liver function studies should be obtained initially and repeated at 24-hour intervals.

The antidote, N-acetylcysteine, should be administered as early as possible, preferably within 16 hours of the overdose ingestion for optimal results, but in any case, within 24 hours. Following recovery, there are no residual, structural or functional hepatic abnormalities.

Codeine

Signs and Symptoms: Serious overdose with codeine is characterized by respiratory depression (a decrease in respiratory rate and/or tidal volume, Cheyne-Stokes respiration, cyanosis), extreme somnolence progressing to stupor or coma, skeletal muscle flaccidity, cold and clammy skin, and sometimes bradycardia and hypotension. In severe overdosage, apnea, circulatory collapse, cardiac arrest and death may occur.

Treatment: Primary attention should be given to the reestablishment of adequate respiratory exchange through provision of a patent airway and the institution of assisted or controlled ventilation. The narcotic antagonist naloxone is a specific antidote against respiratory depression which may result from overdosage or unusual sensitivity to narcotics, including codeine. Therefore, an appropriate dose of naloxone hydrochloride (see package insert) should be administered, preferably by the intravenous route, and simultaneously with efforts at respiratory resuscitation. Since the duration of action of codeine may exceed that of the antagonist, the patient should be kept under continued surveillance and repeated doses of the antagonist should be administered as needed to maintain adequate respiration.

An antagonist should not be administered in the absence of clinically significant respiratory or cardiovascular depression. Oxygen, intravenous fluids, vasopressors and other supportive measures should be employed as indicated.

Gastric emptying may be useful in removing unabsorbed drug.

DOSAGE AND ADMINISTRATION

Dosage should be adjusted according to severity of pain and response of the patient.

It should be kept in mind, however, that tolerance to codeine can develop with continued use and that the incidence of untoward effects is dose related. Adult doses of codeine higher than 60 mg fail to give commensurate relief of pain but merely prolong analgesia and are associated with an appreciably increased incidence of undesirable side effects. Equivalently high doses in children would have similar effects.

The usual adult dosage for tablets is:

	Single Doses (Range)	Maximum 24 Hour Dose
Codeine Phosphate	15mg–60mg	360mg
Acetaminophen	300mg–1000mg	4000mg

Doses may be repeated up to every 4 hours.

The prescriber must determine the number of tablets per dose, and the maximum number of tablets per 24 hours, based upon the above dosage guidance. This information should be conveyed in the prescription.

For children, the dose of codeine phosphate is 0.5 mg/kg.

TYLENOL with Codeine elixir (acetaminophen and codeine phosphate oral solution USP) contains 120 mg of acetaminophen and 12 mg of codeine phosphate/5 mL and is given orally.

Continued on next page

Tylenol w/Codeine—Cont.

The usual doses are:

Children:	*(7 to 12 years):* 10 mL (2 teaspoonfuls) 3 or 4 times daily.
	(3 to 6 years): 5 mL (1 teaspoonful) 3 or 4 times daily.
	(under 3 years): safe dosage has not been established.
Adults:	15 mL (1 tablespoonful) every 4 hours as needed.

HOW SUPPLIED

TYLENOL with Codeine tablets (acetaminophen and codeine phosphate tablets): (round, white, imprinted "McNEIL," "TYLENOL CODEINE" and either "3" or "4"): No. 3—NDC 0045-0513-60 bottles of 100, NDC 0045-0513-70 bottles of 500, NDC 0045-0513-80 bottles of 1000, NDC 0045-0513-72 unit dose (20 × 25); No. 4—NDC 0045-0515-60 bottles of 100, NDC 0045-0515-70 bottles of 500.

TYLENOL with Codeine elixir (acetaminophen and codeine phosphate oral solution USP) contains 120 mg acetaminophen and 12 mg codeine phosphate/5 mL (colored amber, cherry flavored) — NDC 0045-0508-16, bottles of 1 pint.

Store TYLENOL with Codeine tablets at controlled room temperature (15–30°C, 59–86°F).

Store TYLENOL with Codeine elixir at controlled room temperature (15–30°C, 59–86°F). Protect from light. Do not refrigerate. Do not freeze.

Dispense in tight, light-resistant container as defined in the official compendium.

OMP DIVISION
ORTHO-MCNEIL
PHARMACEUTICAL, INC.
RARITAN, NEW JERSEY 08869

633-10-057-3 Revised July 2000

Shown in Product Identification Guide, page 329

TYLOX® Capsules Ⓒ℞

[ti 'lox]

(oxycodone and acetaminophen capsules USP)
NSN 6505-01-210-4450-100's
NSN 6505-01-211-6803-Unit Dose (100's)

DESCRIPTION

Each capsule of TYLOX (oxycodone and acetaminophen capsules USP) contains:

Oxycodone Hydrochloride USP	5 mg*
Warning —May be habit forming.	
Acetaminophen USP	500 mg

Inactive ingredients: docusate sodium, gelatin, magnesium stearate, sodium benzoate, sodium metabisulfite†, corn starch, FD&C Blue No. 1, FD&C Red No. 3, FD&C Red No. 40, and titanium dioxide.

Acetaminophen occurs as a white, odorless crystalline powder, possessing a slightly bitter taste.

The oxycodone component is 14-hydroxydihydrocodeinone, a white, odorless crystalline powder having a saline, bitter taste. It is derived from the opium alkaloid thebaine, and may be represented by the following structural formula:

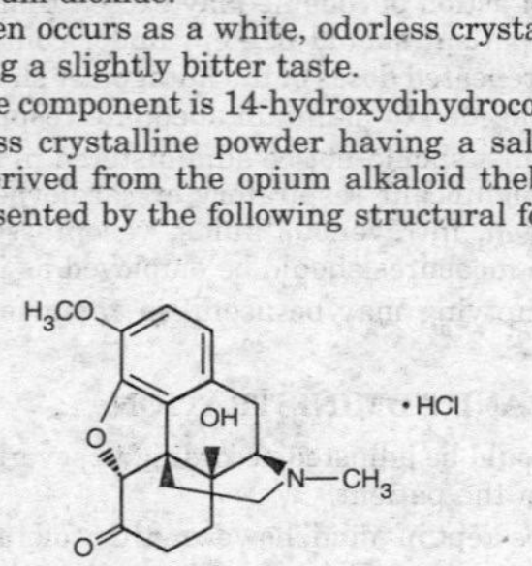

*5 mg oxycodone hydrochloride is equivalent to 4.4815 mg oxycodone

†See WARNINGS

CLINICAL PHARMACOLOGY

The principal ingredient, oxycodone, is a semisynthetic narcotic analgesic with multiple actions qualitatively similar to those of morphine; the most prominent of these involve the central nervous system and organs composed of smooth muscle. The principal actions of therapeutic value of the oxycodone in TYLOX (oxycodone and acetaminophen capsules) are analgesia and sedation.

Oxycodone is similar to codeine and methadone in that it retains at least one-half of its analgesic activity when administered orally.

Acetaminophen is a non-opiate, non-salicylate analgesic and antipyretic.

INDICATIONS AND USAGE

TYLOX (oxycodone and acetaminophen capsules) are indicated for the relief of moderate to moderately severe pain.

CONTRAINDICATIONS

TYLOX (oxycodone and acetaminophen capsules) should not be administered to patients who are hypersensitive to any component.

WARNINGS

Contains sodium metabisulfite, a sulfite that may cause allergic-type reactions including anaphylactic symptoms and life-threatening or less severe asthmatic episodes in certain susceptible people. The overall prevalence of sulfite sensitivity in the general population is unknown and probably low. Sulfite sensitivity is seen more frequently in asthmatic than in nonasthmatic people.

Drug Dependence

Oxycodone can produce drug dependence of the morphine type and, therefore, has the potential for being abused. Psychic dependence, physical dependence and tolerance may develop upon repeated administration of TYLOX (oxycodone and acetaminophen capsules), and it should be prescribed and administered with the same degree of caution appropriate to the use of other oral narcotic-containing medications. Like other narcotic-containing medications, TYLOX is subject to the Federal Control Substances Act (Schedule II).

PRECAUTIONS

General

Head Injury and Increased Intracranial Pressure: The respiratory depressant effects of narcotics and their capacity to elevate cerebrospinal fluid pressure may be markedly exaggerated in the presence of head injury, other intracranial lesions or a pre-existing increase in intracranial pressure. Furthermore, narcotics produce adverse reactions which may obscure the clinical course of patients with head injuries.

Acute Abdominal Conditions: The administration of TYLOX (oxycodone and acetaminophen capsules) or other narcotics may obscure the diagnosis or clinical course in patients with acute abdominal conditions.

Special Risk Patients: TYLOX should be given with caution to certain patients such as the elderly or debilitated, and those with severe impairment of hepatic or renal function, hypothyroidism, Addison's disease, and prostatic hypertrophy or urethral stricture.

Information for Patients

Oxycodone may impair the mental and/or physical abilities required for the performance of potentially hazardous tasks such as driving a car or operating machinery. The patient using TYLOX should be cautioned accordingly.

Drug Interactions

Patients receiving other narcotic analgesics, general anesthetics, phenothiazines, other tranquilizers, sedative-hypnotics or other CNS depressants (including alcohol) concomitantly with TYLOX may exhibit an additive CNS depression. When such combined therapy is contemplated, the dose of one or both agents should be reduced.

The concurrent use of anticholinergics with narcotics may produce paralytic ileus.

Usage in Pregnancy

Pregnancy Category C. Animal reproductive studies have not been conducted with TYLOX. It is also not known whether TYLOX can cause fetal harm when administered to a pregnant woman or can affect reproductive capacity. TYLOX should not be given to a pregnant woman unless in the judgment of the physician, the potential benefits outweigh the possible hazards.

Nonteratogenic Effects: Use of narcotics during pregnancy may produce physical dependence in the neonate.

Labor and Delivery

As with all narcotics, administration of TYLOX to the mother shortly before delivery may result in some degree of respiratory depression in the newborn and the mother, especially if higher doses are used.

Nursing Mothers

It is not known whether the components of TYLOX are excreted in human milk. Because many drugs are excreted in human milk, caution should be exercised when TYLOX is administered to a nursing woman.

Pediatric Use

Safety and effectiveness in children have not been established.

ADVERSE REACTIONS

The most frequently observed adverse reactions include lightheadedness, dizziness, sedation, nausea and vomiting. These effects seem to be more prominent in ambulatory than in non-ambulatory patients, and some of these adverse reactions may be alleviated if the patient lies down.

Other adverse reactions include allergic reactions, euphoria, dysphoria, constipation, skin rash and pruritus. At higher doses, oxycodone has most of the disadvantages of morphine including respiratory depression.

DRUG ABUSE AND DEPENDENCE

TYLOX capsules are a Schedule II controlled substance. Oxycodone can produce drug dependence and has the potential for being abused. (See WARNINGS)

OVERDOSAGE

Acetaminophen

Signs and Symptoms: In acute acetaminophen overdosage, dose-dependent potentially fatal hepatic necrosis is the most serious adverse effect. Renal tubular necrosis, hypoglycemic coma and thrombocytopenia may also occur.

In adults, hepatic toxicity has rarely been reported with acute overdoses of less than 10 grams and fatalities with less than 15 grams. Importantly, young children seem to be more resistant than adults to the hepatotoxic effect of an acetaminophen overdose. Despite this, the measures outlined below should be initiated in any adult or child suspected of having ingested an acetaminophen overdose.

Early symptoms following a potentially hepatotoxic overdose may include: nausea, vomiting, diaphoresis, and general malaise. Clinical and laboratory evidence of hepatic toxicity may not be apparent until 48 to 72 hours post-ingestion.

Treatment: The stomach should be emptied promptly by lavage or by induction of emesis with syrup of ipecac. Patients' estimates of the quantity of a drug ingested are notoriously unreliable. Therefore, if an acetaminophen overdose is suspected, a serum acetaminophen assay should be obtained as early as possible, but no sooner than four hours following ingestion. Liver function studies should be obtained initially and repeated at 24-hour intervals.

The antidote, N-acetylcysteine, should be administered as early as possible, and within 16 hours of the overdose ingestion for optimal results. Following recovery, there are no residual, structural, or functional hepatic abnormalities.

Oxycodone

Signs and symptoms: Serious overdosage with oxycodone is characterized by respiratory depression (a decrease in respiratory rate and/or tidal volume, Cheyne-Stokes respiration, cyanosis), extreme somnolence progressing to stupor or coma, skeletal muscle flaccidity, cold and clammy skin, and sometimes bradycardia and hypotension. In severe overdosage, apnea, circulatory collapse, cardiac arrest, and death may occur.

Treatment: Primary attention should be given to the reestablishment of adequate respiratory exchange through provision of a patent airway and the institution of assisted or controlled ventilation. The narcotic antagonist naloxone hydrochloride is a specific antidote against respiratory depression which may result from overdosage or unusual sensitivity to narcotics, including oxycodone. Therefore, an appropriate dose of naloxone hydrochloride (usual initial adult dose 0.4 mg to 2 mg) should be administered preferably by the intravenous route and simultaneously with efforts at respiratory resuscitation (see package insert). Since the duration of action of oxycodone may exceed that of the antagonist, the patient should be kept under continued surveillance and repeated doses of the antagonist should be administered as needed to maintain adequate respiration.

An antagonist should not be administered in the absence of clinically significant respiratory or cardiovascular depression. Oxygen, intravenous fluids, vasopressors and other supportive measures should be employed as indicated.

Gastric emptying may be useful in removing unabsorbed drug.

DOSAGE AND ADMINISTRATION

Dosage should be adjusted according to the severity of the pain and the response of the patient. However, it should be kept in mind that tolerance to oxycodone can develop with continued use and that the incidence of untoward effects is dose related. This product is inappropriate even in high doses for severe or intractable pain.

TYLOX (oxycodone and acetaminophen capsules) are given orally. The usual adult dosage is one TYLOX capsule every 6 hours as needed for pain.

HOW SUPPLIED

TYLOX (oxycodone and acetaminophen capsules USP): (colored red, imprinted "TYLOX" "McNEIL") NDC 0045-0526—bottles of 100 and unit dose 100's.

Dispense in tight, light-resistant container as defined in the official compendium.

Store at controlled room temperature (15°–30°C, 59°–86°F). Protect from moisture.

McNeil Pharmaceutical, McNEILAB, Inc.
Spring House, PA 19477

Revised June 1997 643-10-561-3

Shown in Product Identification Guide, page 329

ULTRAM® ℞

(tramadol hydrochloride tablets)

DESCRIPTION

ULTRAM® (tramadol hydrochloride tablets) is a centrally acting analgesic. The chemical name for tramadol hydrochloride is (±)*cis*-2-[(dimethylamino)methyl]-1-(3-methoxyphenyl) cyclohexanol hydrochloride. Its structural formula is:

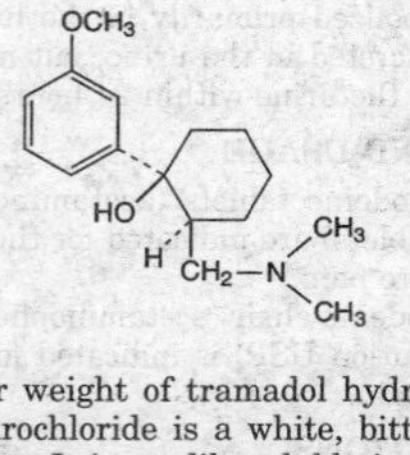

The molecular weight of tramadol hydrochloride is 299.8. Tramadol hydrochloride is a white, bitter, crystalline and odorless powder. It is readily soluble in water and ethanol and has a pKa of 9.41. The water/n-octanol partition coefficient is 1.35 at pH 7. ULTRAM tablets contain 50 mg of tramadol hydrochloride and are white in color. Inactive ingredients in the tablet are corn starch, hydroxypropyl methylcellulose, lactose, magnesium stearate, microcrystalline cellulose, polyethylene glycol, polysorbate 80, sodium starch glycolate, titanium dioxide and wax.

CLINICAL PHARMACOLOGY

Pharmacodynamics

ULTRAM is a centrally acting synthetic analgesic compound. Although its mode of action is not completely under-

chronic nonmalignant pain. Of these patients, 375 were 65 years old or older. Table 2 reports the cumulative incidence rate of adverse reactions by 7, 30 and 90 days for the most frequent reactions (5% or more by 7 days). The most frequently reported events were in the central nervous system and gastrointestinal system. Although the reactions listed in the table are felt to be probably related to ULTRAM administration, the reported rates also include some events that may have been due to underlying disease or concomitant medication. The overall incidence rates of adverse experiences in these trials were similar for ULTRAM and the active control groups, TYLENOL® with Codeine #3 (acetaminophen 300 mg with codeine phosphate 30 mg), and aspirin 325 mg with codeine phosphate 30 mg.

[See table 2 at top of previous page]

Incidence 1% to less than 5%, possibly causally related: the following lists adverse reactions that occurred with an incidence of 1% to less than 5% in clinical trials, and for which the possibility of a causal relationship with ULTRAM exists.

Body as a Whole: Malaise.
Cardiovascular: Vasodilation.
Central Nervous System: Anxiety, Confusion, Coordination disturbance, Euphoria, Nervousness, Sleep disorder.
Gastrointestinal: Abdominal pain, Anorexia, Flatulence.
Musculoskeletal: Hypertonia.
Skin: Rash.
Special Senses: Visual disturbance.
Urogenital: Menopausal symptoms, Urinary frequency, Urinary retention.

Incidence less than 1%, possibly causally related: the following lists adverse reactions that occurred with an incidence of less than 1% in clinical trials and/or reported in post-marketing experience.

Body as a Whole: Accidental injury, Allergic reaction, Anaphylaxis, Suicidal tendency, Weight loss.
Cardiovascular: Orthostatic hypotension, Syncope, Tachycardia.
Central Nervous System: Abnormal gait, Amnesia, Cognitive dysfunction, Depression, Difficulty in concentration, Hallucinations, Paresthesia, Seizure (see WARNINGS), Tremor.
Respiratory: Dyspnea.
Skin: Stevens-Johnson syndrome/Toxic epidermal necrolysis, Urticaria, Vesicles.
Special Senses: Dysgeusia.
Urogenital: Dysuria, Menstrual disorder.

Other adverse experiences, causal relationship unknown: A variety of other adverse events were reported infrequently in patients taking ULTRAM during clinical trials and/or reported in post-marketing experience. A causal relationship between ULTRAM and these events has not been determined. However, the most significant events are listed below as alerting information to the physician.

Cardiovascular: Abnormal ECG, Hypertension, Hypotension, Myocardial ischemia, Palpitations.
Central Nervous System: Migraine, Speech disorders.
Gastrointestinal: Gastrointestinal bleeding, Hepatitis, Stomatitis.
Laboratory Abnormalities: Creatinine increase, Elevated liver enzymes, Hemoglobin decrease, Proteinuria.
Sensory: Cataracts, Deafness, Tinnitus.

DRUG ABUSE AND DEPENDENCE

ULTRAM has a potential to cause psychic and physical dependence of the morphine-type (μ-opioid). The drug has been associated with craving, drug-seeking behavior and tolerance development. Cases of abuse and dependence on ULTRAM have been reported. ULTRAM should not be used in opioid-dependent patients. ULTRAM can reinitiate physical dependence in patients that have been previously dependent or chronically using other opioids. In patients with a tendency to drug abuse, a history of drug dependence, or are chronically using opioids, treatment with ULTRAM is not recommended.

OVERDOSAGE

Cases of overdose with tramadol have been reported. Estimates of ingested dose in foreign fatalities have been in the range of 3 to 5 g. A 3 g intentional overdose by a patient in the clinical studies produced emesis and no sequelae. The lowest dose reported to be associated with fatality was possibly between 500 and 1000 mg in a 40 kg woman, but details of the case are not completely known.

Serious potential consequences of overdosage are respiratory depression and seizure. In treating an overdose, primary attention should be given to maintaining adequate ventilation along with general supportive treatment. While naloxone will reverse some, but not all, symptoms caused by overdosage with ULTRAM the risk of seizures is also increased with naloxone administration. In animals convulsions following the administration of toxic doses of tramadol could be suppressed with barbiturates or benzodiazepines but were increased with naloxone. Naloxone administration did not change the lethality of an overdose in mice. Hemodialysis is not expected to be helpful in an overdose because it removes less than 7% of the administered dose in a 4-hour dialysis period.

DOSAGE AND ADMINISTRATION

For patients with moderate to moderately severe chronic pain not requiring rapid onset of analgesic effect, the tolerability of ULTRAM can be improved by initiating therapy with the following titration regimen: ULTRAM should be started at 25 mg/day qAM and titrated in 25 mg increments as separate doses every 3 days to reach 100 mg/day (25 mg q.i.d.). Thereafter the total daily dose may be increased by 50 mg as tolerated every 3 days to reach 200 mg/day (50 mg q.i.d.). After titration, ULTRAM 50 to 100 mg can be administered as needed for pain relief every 4 to 6 hours **not to exceed 400 mg/day.**

For the subset of patients for whom rapid onset of analgesic effect is required and for whom the benefits outweigh the risk of discontinuation due to adverse events associated with higher initial doses, ULTRAM 50 mg to 100 mg can be administered as needed for pain relief every four to six hours, **not to exceed 400 mg per day.**

Individualization of Dose

Available data do not suggest that a dosage adjustment is necessary in elderly patients 65 to 75 years of age unless they also have renal or hepatic impairment. For elderly patients **over 75 years old,** not more than 300 mg/day in divided doses as above is recommended. In all patients with **creatinine clearance less than 30 mL/min,** it is recommended that the dosing interval of ULTRAM be increased to 12 hours, with a maximum daily dose of 200 mg. Since only 7% of an administered dose is removed by hemodialysis, **dialysis patients** can receive their regular dose on the day of dialysis. The recommended dose for patients with **cirrhosis** is 50 mg every 12 hours. Patients receiving chronic **carbamazepine** doses up to 800 mg daily may require up to twice the recommended dose of ULTRAM.

HOW SUPPLIED

ULTRAM (tramadol hydrochloride tablets) Tablets - 50 mg (white, scored, film-coated capsule-shaped tablet) debossed "ULTRAM" on one side and "06 59" on the other side.
100's—NDC 0045-0659-60 bottles of 100 tablets
500's—NDC 0045-0659-70 bottles of 500 tablets
packages of 100 unit doses in blister packs—NDC 0045-0659-10 (10 cards of 10 tablets each).
Dispense in a tight container. Store at controlled room temperature (up to 25°C, 77°F).

OMP DIVISION
ORTHO-McNEIL
PHARMACEUTICAL, INC.
Raritan, New Jersey 08869
U.S. Patents 3,652,589 and 3,830,934
© OMP 1998 Issued December 1999 635-79-227-1

[See figure at top of next column]
Shown in Product Identification Guide, page 329

VASCOR® ℞
(bepridil hydrochloride)
Tablets
For Oral Administration

DESCRIPTION

VASCOR (bepridil hydrochloride) is a calcium channel blocker that has well characterized anti-anginal properties and known but poorly characterized type 1 anti-arrhythmic and anti-hypertensive properties. It has inhibitory effects on both the slow calcium and fast sodium inward currents in myocardial and vascular smooth muscle, interferes with calcium binding to calmodulin, and blocks both voltage and receptor operated calcium channels. It is not related chemically to other calcium channel blockers such as diltiazem hydrochloride, nifedipine and verapamil hydrochloride.

Bepridil hydrochloride monohydrate is a white to off-white, crystalline powder with a bitter taste. It is slightly soluble in water, very soluble in ethanol, methanol and chloroform, and freely soluble in acetone. The molecular weight of bepridil hydrochloride monohydrate is 421.02. Its molecular formula is $C_{24}H_{34}N_2O \cdot HCl \cdot H_2O$. The structural formula is:

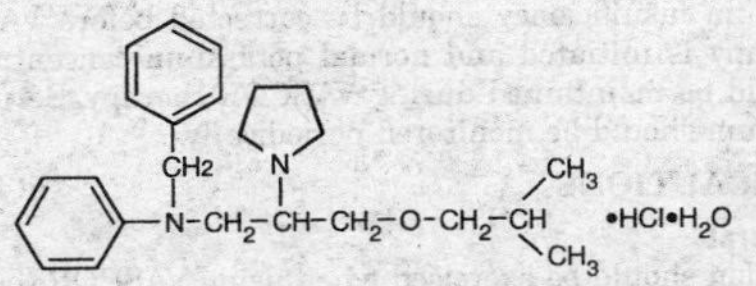

(±)-β-[(2-Methylpropoxy)methyl]-N-phenyl-*N*-(phenylmethyl)-1-pyrrolidineethanamine monohydrochloride monohydrate

VASCOR is available as film-coated tablets for oral use containing 200, 300, or 400 mg of bepridil hydrochloride monohydrate. Inactive ingredients: hydroxypropyl methylcellulose, lactose, magnesium stearate, microcrystalline cellulose, polyethylene glycol, silicon dioxide, pregelatinized corn starch, corn starch, titanium dioxide, FD&C Blue #1.

CLINICAL PHARMACOLOGY

VASCOR (bepridil hydrochloride) inhibits the transmembrane influx of calcium ions into cardiac and vascular smooth muscle. This has been demonstrated in isolated myocardial and vascular smooth muscle preparations in which both the slope of the calcium dose response curve and the maximum calcium-induced inotropic response were significantly reduced by bepridil hydrochloride. In cardiac myocytes *in vitro,* bepridil hydrochloride was shown to be tightly bound to actin. A negative inotropic effect can be seen in the isolated guinea pig atria.

In *in vitro* studies, bepridil hydrochloride has also been demonstrated to inhibit the sodium inward current. Reductions in the maximal upstroke velocity and the amplitude of the action potential, as well as increases in the duration of the normal action potential, have been observed. Additionally, bepridil hydrochloride has been shown to possess local anesthetic activity in isolated myocardial preparations. It effects electrophysiological changes that are observed with several classes of anti-arrhythmic agents.

Clinical Studies

In controlled clinical studies with 200–400 mg of VASCOR, given as a once daily dose, exercise tolerance was improved and angina frequency and daily nitroglycerin use was reduced compared to placebo. Improvement in exercise performance was dose related. In one controlled clinical study, VASCOR was added to propranolol in daily doses of up to 240 mg. The 200–400 mg dose of VASCOR was well tolerated [patients entered were not allowed to be in NYHA Class III or IV heart failure] and there was an added effect of VASCOR on exercise tolerance.

In another controlled clinical study, VASCOR in doses of up to 400 mg/day, significantly improved exercise tolerance compared to diltiazem hydrochloride in patients refractory to diltiazem hydrochloride therapy.

Mechanism of Action: The precise mechanism of action for VASCOR as an anti-anginal agent remains to be fully determined, but is believed to include the following mechanisms: VASCOR regularly reduces heart rate and arterial pressure at rest and at a given level of exercise by dilating peripheral arterioles and reducing total peripheral resistance (afterload) against which the heart works. In exercise tolerance tests in patients with stable angina the heart rate/blood pressure product was reduced with VASCOR for a given work load.

Hemodynamic Effects: VASCOR produces dose dependent slowing of the heart, and reflex tachycardia is not seen. The mean decrease in heart rate in US clinical trials was 3 b.p.m. Orally administered VASCOR also produces modest decreases (less than 5 mm Hg) in systolic and diastolic blood pressure in normotensive patients and somewhat larger decreases in hypertensive patients.

Intravenous administration of VASCOR is associated with a modest reduction in left ventricular contractility (dP/dt), and increased filling pressure, but radionuclide cineangiography studies in angina patients demonstrated improvement in ejection fraction at rest and during exercise following oral VASCOR therapy. Patients with impaired cardiac function [overt heart failure] were not included in these studies.

Electrophysiological Effects: Intravenous administration of VASCOR in man prolongs the effective refractory periods of the atria and ventricles, and the functional refractory period of the AV node. There was a tendency for the AV node effective refractory period and A-H interval to be increased as well. Intravenous and oral administration of VASCOR slow heart rate, prolong the QT and QTc intervals, and alter the morphology of the T-wave (indentation). In clinical trials with angina patients, the mean percent prolongation of the QTc interval was approximately 8%, and of QT about 10%. The prolongation of QT is dose related, varying from about 0.030 sec at doses of 200 mg once a day to 0.055 sec at 400 mg once a day. Upon cessation of therapy, the ECG gradually normalizes. No instances of greater than first-degree heart block have been observed in US controlled or open clinical studies with VASCOR, and first-degree heart block occurred in 0.2% of patients in these studies.

Pulmonary Function: In healthy subjects and asthmatic patients, intravenous VASCOR did not cause bronchoconstriction. VASCOR has been safely used in asthmatic patients and in patients with chronic obstructive lung disease.

Pharmacokinetics and Metabolism: In studies with healthy volunteers, VASCOR is rapidly and completely absorbed after oral administration. The time to peak bepridil plasma concentration is about 2 to 3 hours. Over a ten day period, approximately 70% of a single dose of VASCOR is excreted in the urine and 22% in the feces, as metabolites of bepridil. Excretion of unmetabolized drug is negligible. In healthy male volunteers, the relationship between dose and steady-state blood levels of bepridil was linear over the range of 200 to 400 mg/day. Elimination of bepridil is biphasic, with a distribution half-life of about 2 hours. The terminal elimination half-life following the cessation of multiple dosing averaged 42 hours (range 26–64 hours). However, during a given dosing interval, decay from the peak concentration occurs relatively rapidly indicating a dosing interval half-life shorter than 24 hours. Following once-daily dosing with therapeutic doses, steady-state was reached in about 8 days in healthy volunteers. The clearance of bepridil decreases after multiple dosing.

Clearance of bepridil in angina patients was lower than that in healthy volunteers, resulting in higher average plasma bepridil concentrations. At steady state, maximum bepridil concentrations averaged 2332 ng/ml (range 1451 to 3609) and mean minimum concentrations were 1174 ng/ml (range 226 to 2639) in angina patients following 300 mg/day doses of VASCOR.

Bepridil is more than 99% bound to plasma proteins. Administration of VASCOR after a meal resulted in a clinically

Continued on next page

Vascor—Cont.

insignificant delay in time to peak concentration, but neither peak bepridil plasma levels nor the extent of absorption was changed.

Bepridil is known to be substantially excreted by the kidney, and the risk of toxic reactions to this drug is greater in patients with impaired renal function. Peak plasma concentration of bepridil was increased 3-fold and $t_{1/2}$ was increased more than 2-fold in elderly (>74 years) receiving oral bepridil 100 mg twice daily for 3 weeks compared to younger volunteers (see **PRECAUTIONS—Geriatric Use**). Bepridil passes through the placental barrier. Bepridil may cause uterine hypotonia.

INDICATIONS AND USAGE

Chronic Stable Angina (Classic Effort-Associated Angina)

VASCOR (bepridil hydrochloride) is indicated for the treatment of chronic stable angina (classic effort-associated angina). Because VASCOR has caused serious ventricular arrhythmias, including torsades de pointes type ventricular tachycardia, and the occurrence of cases of agranulocytosis associated with its use (see **WARNINGS**), it should be reserved for patients who have failed to respond optimally to, or are intolerant of, other anti-anginal medication.

VASCOR may be used alone or in combination with beta blockers and/or nitrates. Controlled clinical studies have shown an added effect when VASCOR is administered to patients already receiving propranolol.

CONTRAINDICATIONS

VASCOR (bepridil hydrochloride) is contraindicated in patients with a known sensitivity to bepridil hydrochloride.

VASCOR is contraindicated in (1) patients with a history of serious ventricular arrhythmias (see **WARNINGS**—Induction of New Serious Arrhythmias), (2) patients with sick sinus syndrome or patients with second- or third-degree AV block, except in the presence of a functioning ventricular pacemaker, (3) patients with hypotension (less than 90 mm Hg systolic), (4) patients with uncompensated cardiac insufficiency, (5) patients with congenital QT interval prolongation (see **WARNINGS**), and (6) patients taking other drugs that prolong QT interval (see **PRECAUTIONS**-Drug Interactions).

WARNINGS

Induction of New Serious Arrhythmias

VASCOR (bepridil hydrochloride) has Class 1 anti-arrhythmic properties and, like other such drugs, can induce new arrhythmias, including VT/VF. In addition, because of its ability to prolong the QT interval, VASCOR can cause torsades de pointes type ventricular tachycardia. Because of these properties VASCOR should be reserved for patients in whom other anti-anginal agents do not offer a satisfactory effect.

In US clinical trials, the QT and QTc intervals were commonly prolonged by VASCOR in a dose-related fashion. While the mean prolongation of QTc was 8% and of QT was 10%. Increases of 25% or more were not uncommon, occurring in 5% of the studied population for QTc and 8.7% of the studied population for QT. Increased QT and QTc may be associated with torsades de pointes type VT, which was seen at least briefly, in about 1.0% of patients in US trials; in many cases, however, patients with marked prolongation of QTc were taken off VASCOR therapy. All of the US patients with torsades de pointes had a prolonged QT interval and relatively low serum potassium. French marketing experience has reported over one hundred verified cases of torsades de pointes. While this number, based on total use, represents a rate of only 0.01%, the true rate is undoubtedly much higher, as spontaneous reporting systems all suffer from substantial under reporting.

Torsades de pointes is a polymorphic ventricular tachycardia often but not always associated with a prolonged QT interval, and often drug induced. The relation between the degree of QT prolongation and the development of torsades de pointes is not linear and the likelihood of torsades appears to be increased by hypokalemia, use of potassium wasting diuretics, and the presence of antecedent bradycardia. While the safe upper limit of QT is not defined, it is suggested that the interval not be permitted to exceed 0.52 seconds during treatment. If dose reduction does not eliminate the excessive prolongation, VASCOR should be stopped.

Because most domestic and foreign cases of torsades have developed in patients with hypokalemia, usually related to diuretic use or significant liver disease, if concomitant diuretics are needed, low doses and addition or primary use of a potassium sparing diuretic should be considered and serum potassium should be monitored.

VASCOR has been associated with the usual range of pro-arrhythmic effects characteristic of Class 1 anti-arrhythmics (increased premature ventricular contraction rates, new sustained VT, and VT/VF that is more resistant to sinus rhythm conversion). Use in patients with severe arrhythmias (who are most susceptible to certain pro-arrhythmic effects) has been limited, so that risk in these patients is not defined.

In the National Heart, Lung and Blood Institute's Cardiac Arrhythmia Suppression Trial (CAST), a long-term, multi-centered, randomized, double-blind study in patients with asymptomatic non-life-threatening ventricular arrhythmias who had myocardial infarctions more than six days but less than two years previously, an excess mortality/non-fatal cardiac arrest rate was seen in patients treated with encainide or flecainide (56/730) compared with that seen in patients assigned to matched placebo-treated groups (22/725). The applicability of these results to other populations (e.g., those without recent myocardial infarction) or to other anti-arrhythmic drugs is uncertain, but at present it is prudent to consider any drug documented to provoke new serious arrhythmias or worsening of pre-existing arrhythmias as having a similar risk and to avoid their use in the post-infarction period.

Adverse Experiences by Body System and Treatment in Greater Than 2% of Bepridil Patients in Controlled Trials

Adverse Reaction	Bepridil HCl (N = 529)	Nifedipine (N = 50)	Propranolol (N = 88)	Diltiazem (N = 41)	Placebo (N = 190)
Body as a Whole					
Asthenia	9.83	22.00	22.73	12.20	7.37
Headache	11.34	22.00	13.64	7.32	14.21
Flu Syndrome	2.08	8.00	2.27	—[α]	1.05
Cardiovascular/Respiratory					
Palpitations	2.27	6.00	2.27	0.00	1.58
Dyspnea	3.59	4.00	5.68	4.88	2.11
Respiratory Infection	2.84	4.00	3.41	4.88	3.68
Gastrointestinal					
Dyspepsia	6.81	4.00	5.68	4.88	1.58
G.I. Distress	4.35	10.00	6.82	—[α]	2.11
Nausea	12.29	14.00	11.36	2.44	3.68
Dry Mouth	3.40	0.00	0.00	2.44	2.63
Anorexia	3.02	0.00	2.27	0.00	1.58
Diarrhea	7.75	2.00	9.09	2.44	2.63
Abdominal Pain	3.02	4.00	1.14	—[α]	3.16
Constipation	2.84	6.00	1.14	4.88	2.11
Central Nervous System					
Drowsy	3.78	4.00	4.55	—[α]	3.68
Insomnia	2.65	6.00	3.41	—[α]	1.05
Dizziness	14.74	30.00	10.23	4.88	9.47
Tremor	4.91	4.00	0.00	—[α]	1.05
Tremor of Hand	3.02	4.00	0.00	—[α]	0.53
Paresthesia	2.46	2.00	1.14	4.88	3.16
Psychiatric					
Nervous	7.37	16.00	1.14	2.44	3.68

[α] No data available.

Agranulocytosis: In US clinical trials of over 800 patients treated with VASCOR for up to five years, two cases of marked leukopenia and neutropenia were reported. Both patients were diabetic and elderly. One died with overwhelming gram-negative sepsis, itself a possible cause of marked leukopenia. The other patient recovered rapidly when VASCOR was stopped.

Congestive Heart Failure: Congestive heart failure has been observed infrequently (about 1%) during US controlled clinical trials, but experience with the use of VASCOR in patients with significantly impaired ventricular function is limited. There is little information on the effect of concomitant administration of VASCOR and digoxin; therefore, caution should be exercised in treating patients with congestive heart failure.

Hepatic Enzyme Elevation: In US clinical studies with VASCOR in about 1000 patients and subjects, clinically significant (at least 2 times the upper limit of normal) transaminase elevations were observed in approximately 1% of the patients. None of these patients became clinically symptomatic or jaundiced and values returned to normal when the drug was stopped.

Hypokalemia: In clinical trials VASCOR has not been reported to reduce serum potassium levels. Because hypokalemia has been associated with ventricular arrhythmias, potassium insufficiency should be corrected before VASCOR therapy is initiated and normal potassium concentrations should be maintained during VASCOR therapy. Serum potassium should be monitored periodically.

PRECAUTIONS

General

Caution should be exercised when using VASCOR (bepridil hydrochloride) in patients with left bundle branch block or sinus bradycardia (less than 50 b.p.m.). Care should also be exercised in patients with serious hepatic or renal disorders because such patients have not been studied and bepridil is highly metabolized, with metabolites excreted primarily in the urine.

Recent Myocardial Infarction

In US clinical trials with VASCOR, patients with myocardial infarctions within three months prior to initiation of drug treatment were excluded. The initiation of VASCOR therapy in such patients, therefore, cannot be recommended.

Pulmonary Infiltration

There have been cases of noninfective, noncardiogenic pulmonary interstitial infiltrates (with or without the presence of eosinophilia), including cases of pulmonary fibrosis in patients taking VASCOR. These cases may present as dyspnea or cough within a few weeks of commencing VASCOR; infiltrates may be seen on chest x-ray.

Although the relationship of pulmonary infiltration to VASCOR is unclear, any patient who develops dyspnea or cough of unspecified etiology should be adequately evaluated. If other causes cannot be identified, discontinuation of VASCOR therapy should be considered.

Information for Patients

Since QT prolongation is not associated with defined symptomatology, patients should be instructed on the importance of maintaining any potassium supplementation or potassium sparing diuretic, and the need for routine electrocardiograms and periodic monitoring of serum potassium.

The following Patient Information is printed on the carton label of each unit of use bottle of 30 tablets:

> As with any medication that you take, you should notify your physician of any changes in your overall condition. Be sure to follow your physician's instructions regarding follow-up visits. Please notify any physician who treats you for a medical condition that you are taking VASCOR® (bepridil hydrochloride), as well as any other medications.

Drug Interactions

Nitrates: The concomitant use of VASCOR with long- and short-acting nitrates has been safely tolerated in patients with stable angina pectoris. Sublingual nitroglycerin may be taken if necessary for the control of acute angina attacks during VASCOR therapy.

Beta-blocking Agents: The concomitant use of VASCOR and beta-blocking agents has been well tolerated in patients with stable angina. Available data are not sufficient, however, to predict the effects of concomitant medication on patients with impaired ventricular function or cardiac conduction abnormalities (see **CLINICAL PHARMACOLOGY** and **DOSAGE AND ADMINISTRATION**).

Digoxin: In controlled studies in healthy volunteers, bepridil hydrochloride either had no effect (one study) or was associated with modest increases, about 30% (two studies) in steady-state serum digoxin concentrations. Limited clinical data in angina patients receiving concomitant bepridil hydrochloride and digoxin therapy indicate no discernible changes in serum digoxin levels. Available data are neither sufficient to rule out possible increases in serum digoxin with concomitant treatment in some patients, nor other possible interactions, particularly in patients with cardiac conduction abnormalities (Also see **WARNINGS**-Congestive Heart Failure).

Oral Hypoglycemics: VASCOR has been safely used in diabetic patients without significantly lowering their blood glucose levels or altering their need for insulin or oral hypoglycemic agents.

General Interactions: Certain drugs could increase the likelihood of potentially serious adverse effects with bepridil hydrochloride. In general, these are drugs that have one or more pharmacologic activities similar to bepridil hydrochloride, including anti-arrhythmic agents such as quinidine and procainamide, cardiac glycosides and tricyclic anti-depressants. Anti-arrhythmics and tricyclic anti-depressants could exaggerate the prolongation of the QT interval observed with bepridil hydrochloride. Cardiac glycosides could exaggerate the depression of AV nodal conduction observed with bepridil hydrochloride.

Carcinogenesis, Mutagenesis, Impairment of Fertility

No evidence of carcinogenicity was revealed in one lifetime study in mice at dosages up to 60 times (for a 60 kg subject) the maximum recommended dosage in man. Unilateral follicular adenomas of the thyroid were observed in a study in rats following lifetime administration of high doses of bepridil hydrochloride, i.e., ≥ 100 mg/kg/day (20 times the usual recommended dose in man). No mutagenic or other genotoxic potential of bepridil hydrochloride was found in the following standard laboratory tests: the Micronucleus Test for Chromosomal Effects, the Liver Microsome Activated Bacterial Assay for Mutagenicity, the Chinese Hamster Ovary Cell Assay for Mutagenicity, and the Sister Chromatid Exchange Assay. No intrinsic effect on fertility by bepridil hydrochloride was demonstrated in rats.

Adverse Experiences by Body System and Treatment In Greater Than 5% of Bepridil Patients in Controlled Trials

Adverse Reaction	Bepridil HCl 200 mg (N = 43)	Bepridil HCl 300 mg (N = 46)	Bepridil HCl 400 mg (N = 44)	Placebo (N = 44)
Body as a Whole				
Asthenia	13.95	6.52	11.36	2.27
Headache	6.98	8.70	13.64	15.91
Cardiovascular/ Respiratory				
Palpitations	0.00	6.52	4.55	0.00
Dyspnea	2.33	8.70	0.00	2.27
Gastrointestinal				
G.I. Distress	6.98	0.00	4.55	4.55
Nausea	6.98	26.09	18.18	2.27
Anorexia	0.00	2.17	6.82	2.27
Diarrhea	0.00	10.87	6.82	0.00
Central Nervous System				
Drowsy	6.98	6.52	0.00	4.55
Dizziness	11.63	15.22	27.27	6.82
Tremor	6.98	0.00	4.55	0.00
Tremor of Hand	9.30	0.00	4.55	0.00
Psychiatric				
Nervous	11.63	8.70	11.36	0.00
Special Senses				
Tinnitus	0.00	6.52	2.27	2.27

Most Common Events Resulting in Discontinuation

Adverse Reaction	Bepridil (N = 515) n (%)	Placebo (N = 288) n (%)	Positive Control (N = 119) n (%)
Dizziness	5 (0.97)	0 (0.0)	2 (1.68)
Gastrointestinal Symptoms	5 (0.97)	0 (0.0)	5 (4.20)
Ventricular Arrhythmia	5 (0.97)	0 (0.0)	0 (0.0)
Syncope	3 (0.58)	0 (0.0)	0 (0.0)

In monkeys, at 200 mg/kg/day, there was a decrease in testicular weight and spermatogenesis. There were no systematic studies in man related to this point. In rats, at doses up to 300 mg/kg/day, there was no observed alteration of mating behavior nor of reproductive performance.

Usage in Pregnancy

Pregnancy Category C. Reproductive studies (fertility and peri-postnatal) have been conducted in rats. Reduced litter size at birth and decreased pup survival during lactation was observed at maternal dosages 37 times (on a mg/kg basis) the maximum daily recommended therapeutic dosage.

In teratology studies, no effects were observed in rats or rabbits at these same dosages.

There are no well-controlled studies in pregnant women. Use VASCOR in pregnant or nursing women only if the potential benefit justifies the potential risk.

Nursing Mothers

Bepridil is excreted in human milk. Bepridil concentration in human milk is estimated to reach about one third the concentration in serum. Because of the potential for serious adverse reactions in nursing infants from VASCOR a decision should be made whether to discontinue nursing or to discontinue the drug, taking into account the importance of the drug to the mother.

Pediatric Use

The safety and effectiveness of VASCOR in children have not been established.

Geriatric Use

Clinical studies of bepridil did not include sufficient numbers of subjects aged 65 and over to determine whether they respond differently from younger subjects. Other reported clinical experience has not identified differences in responses between the elderly and younger patients. In general, dose selection for an elderly patient should be cautious, usually starting at the low end of the dosing range, reflecting the greater frequency of decreased hepatic, renal, or cardiac function, and of concomitant disease or other drug therapy.

Bepridil is known to be substantially excreted by the kidney, and the risk of toxic reactions to this drug is greater in patients with impaired renal function (see **CLINICAL PHARMACOLOGY—Pharmacokinetics and Metabolism**).

ADVERSE REACTIONS

Adverse reactions were assessed in placebo and active-drug controlled trials of 4–12 weeks duration and longer-term uncontrolled studies. The most common side effects occurring more frequently than in control groups were upper gastrointestinal complaints (nausea, dyspepsia or GI distress) in about 22%, diarrhea in about 8%, dizziness in about 15%, asthenia in about 10% and nervousness in about 7%. The adverse reactions seen in at least 2% of bepridil patients in controlled trials are shown in the following table.

[See table at top of previous page]

In one twelve week controlled study, daily doses of 200, 300, and 400 mg were compared to placebo. The following table shows the rates of more common reactions (at least 5% in at least one bepridil group).

[See first table above]

Adverse experiences in long-term open studies were generally similar to those seen in controlled trials.

Although adverse experiences were frequent (at least one being reported in 71% of patients participating in controlled clinical trials), most were well-tolerated. About 15% of patients however, discontinued bepridil treatment because of adverse experiences. In controlled clinical trials, these were principally gastrointestinal (1.0%), dizziness (1.0%) ventricular arrhythmias (1.0%) and syncope (0.6%). The major reasons for discontinuation, with comparison to control agents, are shown below.

[See second table above]

Across all controlled and uncontrolled trials, VASCOR was evaluated in over 800 patients with chronic angina. In addition to the adverse reactions noted above, the following were observed in 0.5 to 2.0% of the VASCOR patients or are rarer, but potentially important events seen in clinical studies or reported in post marketing experience. In most cases it is not possible to determine whether there is a causal relationship to bepridil treatment.

Body as a Whole: Fever, pain, myalgic asthenia, superinfection, flu syndrome.

Cardiovascular/Respiratory: Sinus tachycardia, sinus bradycardia, hypertension, vasodilation, edema, ventricular premature contractions, ventricular tachycardia, prolonged QT interval, rhinitis, cough, pharyngitis.

Gastrointestinal: Flatulence, gastritis, appetite increase, dry mouth, constipation.

Musculoskeletal: Arthritis.

Central Nervous System: Fainting, vertigo, akathisia, drowsiness, insomnia, tremor.

Psychiatric: Depression, anxiousness, adverse behavior effect.

Skin: Rash, sweating, skin irritation.

Special Senses: Blurred vision, tinnitus, taste change.

Urogenital: Loss of libido, impotence.

Abnormal Lab Values: Abnormal liver function test, SGPT increase.

In postmarketing experience with other calcium blockers, gynecomastia has been rarely observed.

Certain cardiovascular events, such as acute myocardial infarction (about 3% of patients) worsened heart failure (1.9%), worsened angina (4.5%), severe arrhythmia (about 2.4% VT/VF) and sudden death (1.6%) have occurred in patients receiving bepridil, but have not been included as adverse events because they appear to be, and cannot be distinguished from, manifestations of the patient's underlying cardiac disease. Such events as torsades de pointes arrhythmias, prolonged QT/QTc, bradycardia, first degree heart block, which are probably related to bepridil, are included in the tables.

OVERDOSAGE

In the event of overdosage, we recommend close observation in a cardiac care facility for a minimum of 48 hours and use of appropriate supportive measures in addition to gastric lavage. Beta-adrenergic stimulation or parenteral administration of calcium solutions may increase transmembrane calcium ion influx. Clinically significant hypotensive reactions or high-degree AV block should be treated with vasopressor agents or cardiac pacing, respectively. Ventricular tachycardia should be handled by cardioversion and, if persistent, by overdrive pacing.

In a few reported cases, overdose with calcium channel blockers has been associated with hypotension and bradycardia, initially refractory to atropin but becoming more responsive to this treatment when the patients received large doses (close to 1 gram/hour for more than 24 hours) of calcium chloride.

There has been one experience with overdosage in which a patient inadvertently took a single dose of 1600 mg of VASCOR (bepridil hydrochloride). The patient was observed for 72 hours in intensive care, but no significant adverse experiences were noted.

DOSAGE AND ADMINISTRATION

Therapy with VASCOR (bepridil hydrochloride) should be individualized according to each patient's response and the physician's clinical judgement. The usual starting dose of VASCOR is 200 mg once daily. After 10 days, dosage may be adjusted upward depending upon the patient's response (e.g., ability to perform activities of daily living, QT interval, heart rate, and frequency and severity of angina). This long interval for dosage adjustment is needed because steady-state blood levels are not achieved until 8 days of therapy. In clinical trials, most patients were maintained at a dose of VASCOR of 300 mg once daily. The maximum daily dose of VASCOR is 400 mg and the established minimum effective dose is 200 mg daily.

The starting dose for elderly patients does not differ from that for young patients. After therapeutic response is demonstrated, however, elderly patients may require more frequent monitoring.

Food does not interfere with the absorption of VASCOR. (see **CLINICAL PHARMACOLOGY—**Pharmacokinetics and Metabolism). If nausea is experienced with VASCOR, the drug may be given at meals or at bedtime.

VASCOR has not been studied adequately in patients with impaired hepatic or renal function. It is therefore possible that dosage adjustments may be necessary in these patients.

Concomitant Use with Other Agents

The concomitant use of VASCOR and beta-blocking agents in patients without heart failure is safely tolerated. Physicians wishing to switch patients from beta-blocker therapy to VASCOR therapy may initiate VASCOR before terminating the beta blocker in the usual gradual fashion (see **CLINICAL PHARMACOLOGY** and **PRECAUTIONS).**

HOW SUPPLIED

VASCOR® (bepridil hydrochloride) tablets 200 mg (film coated light blue, scored, printed VASCOR and 200), 90 tablets (3 bottles of 30) (NDC 0045-0682-33)

VASCOR® (bepridil hydrochloride) tablets 300 mg (film coated blue, printed VASCOR and 300), 90 tablets (3 bottles of 30) (NDC 0045-0683-33).

Store at 15°–25° C (59°–77° F). Protect from light.

Revised March 2000 633–10–692–4

OMP Division
ORTHO-MCNEIL PHARMACEUTICAL, INC.
RARITAN, NEW JERSEY 08869

Shown in Product Identification Guide, page 329

EDUCATIONAL MATERIAL

LEVAQUIN® Tablets/Injection (levofloxacin tablets/injection)

"Patient Information on Acute Bacterial Exacerbation of Chronic Bronchitis"

"Patient Information on Acute Sinusitis"

"Patient Information on Community-Acquired Pneumonia"

Available at no charge to patients, physicians and pharmacists through representatives or directly from Ortho-McNeil Pharmaceutical (908) 218-6000.

AUA Video Library

Male/Female Urogenital System Diagram Pads

Available at no charge to physicians through representatives or directly from Ortho-McNeil Pharmaceutical (908) 218-6000.

PANCREASE® (pancrelipase) and PANCREASE® MT (pancrelipase) capsules

Educational materials are available at no charge to people with CF and their families and caregivers, physicians, nurses, and pharmacists by calling 1-800-356-3475 or through the Internet at www.cfcare.com or www.pancrease.com.

TOPAMAX® (topiramate) tablets and TOPAMAX® (topiramate capsules) sprinkle capsules

Daily Seizure Diary

"A Guide to Understanding and Living with Epilepsy" by Orrin Devinsky, MD

"Managing Seizures in Children" Video

All are available at no charge to patients, physicians and pharmacists through representatives or directly from Ortho-McNeil Pharmaceutical (908) 218-6000.

ULTRAM® (tramadol hydrochloride tablets)

"Exercises for Low Back Pain"

"Exercises for the Painful Neck and Shoulder"

"Information for You About ULTRAM"

"Helping Your Doctor Treat Your Chronic Pain"

All are available at no charge to patients, physicians and pharmacists through representatives or directly from Ortho-McNeil Pharmaceutical (908) 218-6000.

Otsuka America Pharma, Inc.

2440 RESEARCH BLVD
ROCKVILLE, MD 20850

For Direct Inquiries Contact:
Medical Affairs
Otsuka America Pharma, Inc.
1-800-441-6763
fax 301-212-8577
To request routine or emergency Medical Information, or to report an adverse experience, please call: 1-800-441-6771

PLETAL® ℞

[*PLAY-tal*]
(cilostazol) (sil-OS-tah-zol)
Tablets

CONTRAINDICATION
Cilostazol and several of its metabolites are inhibitors of phosphodiesterase III. Several drugs with this pharmacologic effect have caused decreased survival compared to placebo in patients with class III-IV congestive heart failure. PLETAL is contraindicated in patients with congestive heart failure of any severity.

DESCRIPTION

PLETAL (cilostazol) is a quinolinone derivative that inhibits cellular phosphodiesterase (more specific for phosphodiesterase III). The empirical formula of cilostazol is $C_{20}H_{27}N_5O_2$, and its molecular weight is 369.47. Cilostazol is 6-[4-(1-cyclohexyl-1*H*-tetrazol-5-yl)butoxy]-3,4-dihydro-2(1*H*)-quinolinone, CAS-73963-72-1.
The structural formula is:

CILOSTAZOL

Cilostazol occurs as white to off-white crystals or as a crystalline powder that is slightly soluble in methanol and ethanol, and is practically insoluble in water, 0.1 N HCl, and 0.1 N NaOH.
PLETAL (cilostazol) tablets for oral administration are available in 50 mg triangular and 100 mg round, white debossed tablets. Each tablet, in addition to the active ingredient, contains the following inactive ingredients: carboxymethylcellulose calcium, corn starch, hydroxypropyl methylcellulose 2910, magnesium stearate, and microcrystalline cellulose.

CLINICAL PHARMACOLOGY

Mechanism of Action:
The mechanism of the effects of PLETAL on the symptoms of intermittent claudication is not fully understood. PLETAL and several of its metabolites are cyclic AMP (cAMP) phosphodiesterase III inhibitors (PDE III inhibitors), inhibiting phosphodiesterase activity and suppressing cAMP degradation with a resultant increase in cAMP in platelets and blood vessels, leading to inhibition of platelet aggregation and vasodilation, respectively.
PLETAL reversibly inhibits platelet aggregation induced by a variety of stimuli, including thrombin, ADP, collagen, arachidonic acid, epinephrine, and shear stress. Effects on circulating plasma lipids have been examined in patients taking PLETAL. After 12 weeks, as compared to placebo, PLETAL 100 mg b.i.d. produced a reduction in triglycerides of 29.3 mg/dL (15%) and an increase in HDL-cholesterol of 4.0 mg/dL (≅10%).
Cardiovascular Effects:
Cilostazol affects both vascular beds and cardiovascular function. It produces non-homogenous dilation of vascular beds, with greater dilation in femoral beds than in vertebral, carotid, or superior mesenteric arteries. Renal arteries were not responsive to the effects of cilostazol.
In dogs or cynomolgous monkeys, cilostazol increased heart rate, myocardial contractile force, and coronary blood flow as well as ventricular automaticity, as would be expected for a PDE III inhibitor. Left ventricular contractility was increased at doses required to inhibit platelet aggregation. A-V conduction was accelerated. In humans, heart rate increased in a dose-proportional manner by a mean of 5.1 and 7.4 beats per minute in patients treated with 50 and 100 mg b.i.d., respectively. In 264 patients evaluated with Holter monitors, numerically more cilostazol-treated patients had increases in ventricular premature beats and non-sustained ventricular tachycardia events than did placebo-treated patients; the increases were not dose-related.
Pharmacokinetics:
PLETAL is absorbed after oral administration. A high fat meal increases absorption, with an approximately 90% increase in C_{max} and a 25% increase in AUC. Absolute bioavailability is not known. Cilostazol is extensively metabolized by hepatic cytochrome P-450 enzymes, mainly 3A4, with metabolites largely excreted in urine. Two metabolites are active, with one metabolite appearing to account for at least 50% of the pharmacologic (PDE III inhibition) activity after administration of PLETAL. Pharmacokinetics are approximately dose proportional. Cilostazol and its active metabolites have apparent elimination half-lives of about 11–13 hours. Cilostazol and its active metabolites accumulate about 2-fold with chronic administration and reach steady state blood levels within a few days. The pharmacokinetics of cilostazol and its two major active metabolites were similar in healthy normal subjects and patients with intermittent claudication due to peripheral arterial disease (PAD).
The mean ± SEM plasma concentration-time profile at steady state after multiple dosing of PLETAL 100 mg b.i.d. is shown below:

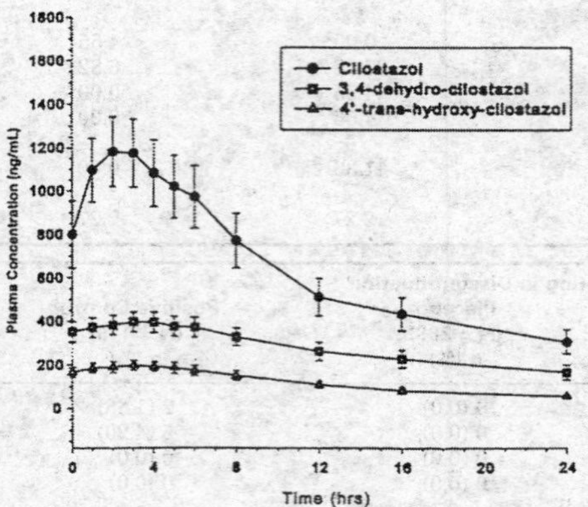

Distribution:
Plasma Protein and Erythrocyte Binding:
Cilostazol is 95%–98% protein bound, predominantly to albumin. The mean percent binding for 3,4-dehydro-cilostazol is 97.4% and for 4'-trans-hydroxy-cilostazol is 66%. Mild hepatic impairment did not affect protein binding. The free fraction of cilostazol was 27% higher in subjects with renal impairment than in normal volunteers. The displacement of cilostazol from plasma proteins by erythromycin, quinidine, warfarin, and omeprazole was not clinically significant.
Metabolism and Excretion:
Cilostazol is eliminated predominately by metabolism and subsequent urinary excretion of metabolites. Based on *in vitro* studies, the primary isoenzymes involved in cilostazol's metabolism are CYP3A4 and, to a lesser extent, CYP2C19. The enzyme responsible for metabolism of 3,4-dehydro-cilostazol, the most active of the metabolites, is unknown.
Following oral administration of 100 mg radiolabeled cilostazol, 56% of the total analytes in plasma was cilostazol, 15% was 3,4-dehydro-cilostazol (4–7 times as active as cilostazol), and 4% was 4'-trans-hydroxy-cilostazol (one fifth as active as cilostazol). The primary route of elimination was via the urine (74%), with the remainder excreted in the feces (20%). No measurable amount of unchanged cilostazol was excreted in the urine, and less than 2% of the dose was excreted as 3,4-dehydro-cilostazol. About 30% of the dose was excreted in the urine as 4'-trans-hydroxy-cilostazol. The remainder was excreted as other metabolites, none of which exceeded 5%. There was no evidence of induction of hepatic microenzymes.
Special Populations:
Age and Gender:
The total and unbound oral clearances, adjusted for body weight, of cilostazol and its metabolites were not significantly different with respect to age and/or gender across a 50-to-80-year-old age range.
Smokers:
Population pharmacokinetic analysis suggests that smoking decreased cilostazol exposure by about 20%.
Hepatic Impairment:
The pharmacokinetics of cilostazol and its metabolites were similar in subjects with mild hepatic disease as compared to healthy subjects.
Patients with moderate or severe hepatic impairment have not been studied.
Renal Impairment:
The total pharmacologic activity of cilostazol and its metabolites was similar in subjects with mild to moderate renal impairment and in normal subjects. Severe renal impairment increases metabolite levels and alters protein binding of the parent and metabolites. The expected pharmacologic activity, however, based on plasma concentrations and relative PDE III inhibiting potency of parent drug and metabolites, appeared little changed. Patients on dialysis have not been studied, but, it is unlikely that cilostazol can be removed efficiently by dialysis because of its high protein binding (95%–98%).
Pharmacokinetic and Pharmacodynamic Drug-Drug Interactions:
Cilostazol could have pharmacodynamic interactions with other inhibitors of platelet function and pharmacokinetic interactions because of effects of other drugs on its metabolism by CYP3A4 or CYP2C19. Cilostazol does not appear to inhibit CYP3A4 (see *Pharmacokinetic and Pharmacodynamic Drug-Drug Interactions,* Lovastatin).
Aspirin:
Short-term (≤4 days) coadministration of aspirin with PLETAL showed a 23%–35% increase in inhibition of ADP-induced *ex vivo* platelet aggregation compared to aspirin alone; there was no clinically significant impact on PT, aPTT, or bleeding time compared to aspirin alone. There was no additive or synergistic effect on arachidonic acid-induced platelet aggregation. Effects of long-term coadministration in the general population are unknown. In eight randomized, placebo-controlled, double-blind clinical trials, aspirin was coadministered with cilostazol to 201 patients. The most frequent doses and mean durations of aspirin therapy were 75–81 mg daily for 137 days (107 patients) and 325 mg daily for 54 days (85 patients). There was no apparent greater incidence of hemorrhagic adverse effects in patients taking cilostazol and aspirin compared to patients taking placebo and equivalent doses of aspirin.
Warfarin:
The cytochrome P-450 isoenzymes involved in the metabolism of R-warfarin are CYP3A4, CYP1A2, and CYP2C19, and in the metabolism of S-warfarin, CYP2C9. Cilostazol did not inhibit either the metabolism or the pharmacologic effects (PT, aPTT, bleeding time, or platelet aggregation) of R- and S-warfarin after a single 25 mg dose of warfarin. The effect of concomitant multiple dosing of warfarin and PLETAL on the pharmacokinetics and pharmacodynamics of both drugs is unknown.
Omeprazole:
Coadministration of omeprazole did not significantly affect the metabolism of cilostazol, but the systemic exposure to 3,4-dehydro-cilostazol was increased by 69%, probably the result of omeprazole's potent inhibition of CYP2C19 (see DOSAGE AND ADMINISTRATION).
Erythromycin and other macrolide antibiotics:
Erythromycin is a moderately strong inhibitor of CYP3A4. Coadministration of erythromycin 500 mg q 8h with a single dose of cilostazol 100 mg increased cilostazol C_{max} by 47% and AUC by 73%. Inhibition of cilostazol metabolism by erythromycin increased the AUC of 4'-trans-hydroxy-cilostazol by 141%. Other macrolide antibiotics would be expected to have a similar effect (see DOSAGE AND ADMINISTRATION).
Diltiazem:
Diltiazem, a moderate inhibitor of CYP3A4, has been shown to increase cilostazol plasma concentrations by approximately 53% (see DOSAGE AND ADMINISTRATION).
This information was obtained from population pharmacokinetic analysis.
Quinidine:
Concomitant administration of quinidine with a single dose of cilostazol 100 mg did not alter cilostazol pharmacokinetics.
Strong Inhibitors of CYP3A4:
Strong inhibitors of CYP3A4, such as ketoconazole, itraconazole, fluconazole, miconazole, fluvoxamine, fluoxetine, nefazodone, and sertraline, have not been studied in combination with cilostazol but would be expected to cause a greater increase in plasma levels of cilostazol and its metabolites than erythromycin.
Lovastatin:
Coadministration of a single dose of lovastatin 80 mg with cilostazol at steady state did not result in clinically significant increases in lovastatin and its hydroxyacid metabolite plasma concentrations.
Clinical Efficacy:
The ability of PLETAL to improve walking distance in patients with stable intermittent claudication was studied in eight large, randomized, placebo-controlled, double-blind trials of 12 to 24 weeks' duration using dosages of 50 mg b.i.d. (n=303), 100 mg b.i.d. (n=998), and placebo (n=973). Efficacy was determined primarily by the change in maximal walking distance from baseline (compared to change on placebo) on one of several standardized exercise treadmill tests.
Compared to patients treated with placebo, patients treated with PLETAL 50 or 100 mg b.i.d. experienced statistically significant improvements in walking distances both for the distance before the onset of claudication pain and the distance before exercise-limiting symptoms supervened (maximal walking distance). The effect of PLETAL on walking distance was seen as early as the first on-therapy observation point of two or four weeks.
The following figure depicts the mean percentage improvement in maximal walking distance, respectively, at study end for each of the eight studies.

Mean Percentage Improvement in Maximal Walking Distance at Study End for the Eight Randomized, Double-Blind, Placebo-Controlled Clinical Trials

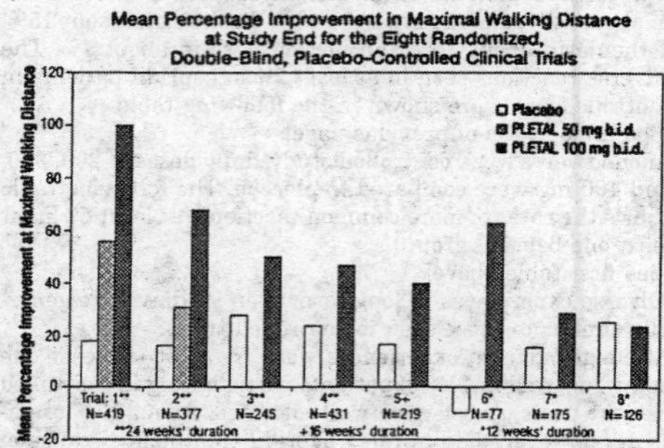

Across the eight clinical trials, the range of improvement in maximal walking distance in patients treated with PLETAL 100 mg b.i.d., expressed as the percent mean change from baseline, was 28% to 100%.
The corresponding changes in the placebo group were −10% to 30%.
The Walking Impairment Questionnaire, which was administered in six of the eight clinical trials, assesses the impact of a therapeutic intervention on walking ability. In a pooled analysis of the six trials, patients treated with either PLETAL 100 mg b.i.d. or 50 mg b.i.d. reported improvements in their walking speed and walking distance as compared to placebo. Improvements in walking performance were seen in the various subpopulations evaluated, including those defined by gender, smoking status, diabetes mellitus, duration of peripheral artery disease, age, and concomitant use of beta blockers or calcium channel blockers. PLETAL has not been studied in patients with rapidly progressing claudication or in patients with leg pain at rest, ischemic leg ulcers, or gangrene. Its long-term effects on limb preservation and hospitalization have not been evaluated. No reliable estimate of its effect on survival is available (see PRECAUTIONS).

INDICATIONS AND USAGE

PLETAL is indicated for the reduction of symptoms of intermittent claudication, as indicated by an increased walking distance.

CONTRAINDICATIONS

Cilostazol and several of its metabolites are inhibitors of phosphodiesterase III. Several drugs with this pharmacologic effect have caused decreased survival compared to placebo in patients with class III-IV congestive heart failure. PLETAL is contraindicated in patients with congestive heart failure of any severity.
PLETAL is contraindicated in patients with known or suspected hypersensitivity to any of its components.

PRECAUTIONS

PLETAL is contraindicated in patients with congestive heart failure. In patients without congestive heart failure, the long-term effects of PDE III inhibitors (including PLETAL) are unknown. Patients in the 3–6 month placebo-controlled trials of PLETAL were relatively stable (no recent myocardial infarction or strokes, no rest pain or other signs of rapidly progressing disease) and only 19 patients died (0.7% in the placebo group and 0.8% in the PLETAL group). The calculated relative risk of death of 1.2 has a wide 95% confidence limit (0.5–3.1). There are no data as to longer-term risk or risk in patients with more severe underlying heart disease.
Use with Clopidogrel.
There is no information with respect to the efficacy or safety of the concurrent use of cilostazol and clopidogrel, a platelet-aggregation inhibiting drug indicated for use in patients with peripheral arterial disease. Studies of concomitant use of cilostazol and clopidogrel are planned.
Information for Patients:
Please refer to the patient package insert.
Patients should be advised:

- to read the patient package insert for PLETAL carefully before starting therapy and to reread it each time therapy is renewed in case the information has changed.
- to take PLETAL at least one-half hour before or two hours after food.
- that the beneficial effects of PLETAL on the symptoms of intermittent claudication may not be immediate. Although the patient may experience benefit in 2 to 4 weeks after initiation of therapy, treatment for up to 12 weeks may be required before a beneficial effect is experienced.
- about the uncertainty concerning cardiovascular risk in long-term use or in patients with severe underlying heart disease, as described under PRECAUTIONS.

Hepatic Impairment:
Patients with moderate or severe hepatic impairment have not been studied in clinical trials.
Drug Interactions:
Since PLETAL is extensively metabolized by cytochrome P-450 isoenzymes, caution should be exercised when PLETAL is coadministered with inhibitors of CYP3A4 such as ketoconazole and erythromycin or inhibitors of CYP2C19 such as omeprazole. Pharmacokinetic studies have demonstrated that omeprazole and erythromycin significantly increased the systemic exposure of cilostazol and/or its major metabolites. Population pharmacokinetic studies showed higher concentrations of cilostazol among patients concurrently treated with diltiazem, an inhibitor of CYP3A4 (see CLINICAL PHARMACOLOGY, *Pharmacokinetic and Pharmacodynamic Drug-Drug Interactions*). PLETAL does not, however, appear to cause increased blood levels of drugs metabolized by CYP3A4, as it had no effect on lovastatin, a drug with metabolism very sensitive to CYP3A4 inhibition.
Cardiovascular Toxicity:
Repeated oral administration of cilostazol to dogs (30 or more mg/kg/day for 52 weeks, 150 or more mg/kg/day for 13 weeks, and 450 mg/kg/day for 2 weeks), produced cardiovascular lesions that included endocardial hemorrhage, hemosiderin deposition and fibrosis in the left ventricle, hemorrhage in the right atrial wall, hemorrhage and necrosis of the smooth muscle in the wall of the coronary artery, intimal thickening of the coronary artery, and coronary arteritis and periarteritis. At the lowest dose associated with cardiovascular lesions in the 52-week study, systemic exposure (AUC) to unbound cilostazol was less than that seen in humans at the maximum recommended human dose (MRHD) of 100 mg b.i.d. Similar lesions have been reported in dogs following the administration of other positive inotropic agents (including PDE III inhibitors) and/or vasodilating agents. No cardiovascular lesions were seen in rats following 5 or 13 weeks of administration of cilostazol at doses up to 1500 mg/kg/day. At this dose, systemic exposures (AUCs) to unbound cilostazol were only about 1.5 and 5 times (male and female rats, respectively) the exposure seen in humans at the MRHD. Cardiovascular lesions were also not seen in rats following 52 weeks of administration of cilostazol at doses up to 150 mg/kg/day. At this dose, systemic exposures (AUCs) to unbound cilostazol were about 0.5 and 5 times (male and female rats, respectively) the exposure in humans at the MRHD. In female rats, cilostazol AUCs were similar at 150 and 1500 mg/kg/day.
Cardiovascular lesions were also not observed in monkeys after oral administration of cilostazol for 13 weeks at doses up to 1800 mg/kg/day. While this dose of cilostazol produced pharmacologic effects in monkeys, plasma cilostazol levels were less than those seen in humans given the MRHD, and those seen in dogs given doses associated with cardiovascular lesions.
Carcinogenesis, Mutagenesis, Impairment of Fertility:
Dietary administration of cilostazol to male and female rats and mice for up to 104 weeks, at doses up to 500 mg/kg/day in rats and 1000 mg/kg/day in mice, revealed no evidence of carcinogenic potential. The maximum doses administered in both rat and mouse studies were, on a systemic exposure basis, less than the human exposure at the MRHD of the drug. Cilostazol tested negative in bacterial gene mutation, bacterial DNA repair, mammalian cell gene mutation, and mouse *in vivo* bone marrow chromosomal aberration assays. It was, however, associated with a significant increase in chromosomal aberrations in the *in vitro* Chinese Hamster Ovary Cell assay.
Cilostazol did not affect fertility or mating performance of male and female rats at doses as high as 1000 mg/kg/day. At this dose, systemic exposures (AUCs) to unbound cilostazol were less than 1.5 times in males, and about 5 times in females, the exposure in humans at the MRHD.
Pregnancy:
Pregnancy Category C: In a rat developmental toxicity study, oral administration of 1000 mg cilostazol/kg/day was associated with decreased fetal weights, and increased incidences of cardiovascular, renal, and skeletal anomalies (ventricular septal, aortic arch and subclavian artery abnormalities; renal pelvic dilation; 14th rib; and retarded ossification). At this dose, systemic exposure to unbound cilostazol in nonpregnant rats was about 5 times the exposure in humans given the MRHD. Increased incidences of ventricular septal defect and retarded ossification were also noted at 150 mg/kg/day (5 times the MRHD on a systemic exposure basis). In a rabbit developmental toxicity study, an increased incidence of retardation of ossification of the sternum was seen at doses as low as 150 mg/kg/day. In nonpregnant rabbits given 150 mg/kg/day, exposure to unbound cilostazol was considerably lower than that seen in humans given the MRHD, and exposure to 3,4-dehydro-cilostazol was barely detectable.
When cilostazol was administered to rats during late pregnancy and lactation, an increased incidence of stillborn and decreased birth weights of offspring was seen at doses of 150 mg/kg/day (5 times the MRHD on a systemic exposure basis). There are no adequate and well-controlled studies in pregnant women.
Nursing Mothers:
Transfer of cilostazol into milk has been reported in experimental animals (rats). Because of the potential risk to nursing infants, a decision should be made to discontinue nursing or to discontinue PLETAL.
Pediatric Use:
The safety and effectiveness of PLETAL in pediatric patients have not been established.
Geriatric Use:
Of the total number of subjects (n = 2274) in clinical studies of PLETAL, 56 percent were 65-years-old and over, while 16 percent were 75-years-old and over. No overall differences in safety or effectiveness were observed between these subjects and younger subjects, and other reported clinical experience has not identified differences in responses between the elderly and younger patients, but greater sensitivity of some older individuals cannot be ruled out. Pharmacokinetic studies have not disclosed any age-related effects on the absorption, distribution, metabolism, and elimination of cilostazol and its metabolites.

ADVERSE REACTIONS

Adverse events were assessed in eight placebo-controlled clinical trials involving 2274 patients exposed to either 50 or 100 mg b.i.d. PLETAL (n=1301) or placebo (n=973), with a median treatment duration of 127 days for patients on PLETAL and 134 days for patients on placebo.
The only adverse event resulting in discontinuation of therapy in ≥3% of patients treated with PLETAL 50 or 100 mg b.i.d. was headache, which occurred with an incidence of 1.3%, 3.5%, and 0.3% in patients treated with PLETAL 50 mg b.i.d., 100 mg b.i.d., or placebo, respectively. Other frequent causes of discontinuation included palpitation and diarrhea, both 1.1% for cilostazol (all doses) versus 0.1% for placebo.
The most commonly reported adverse events, occurring in ≥2% of patients treated with PLETAL 50 or 100 mg b.i.d., are shown in the table (to the right).
Other events seen with an incidence of ≥2%, but occurring in the placebo group at least as frequently as in the 100 mg b.i.d. group, were: asthenia, hypertension, vomiting, leg cramps, hyperesthesia, paresthesia, dyspnea, rash, hematuria, urinary tract infection, flu syndrome, angina pectoris, arthritis, and bronchitis.
[See table above]

Most Commonly Reported AEs (Incidence ≥2%) in Patients on PLETAL (PLT) 50 mg b.i.d. or 100 mg b.i.d. and Occurring at a Rate in the 100 mg b.i.d. Group Higher Than in Patients on Placebo

Adverse Events (AEs) by Body System	PLT 50 mg b.i.d. (N=303) %	PLT 100 mg b.i.d. (N=998) %	Placebo (N=973) %
BODY AS A WHOLE			
Abdominal pain	4	5	3
Back pain	6	7	6
Headache	27	34	14
Infection	14	10	8
CARDIOVASCULAR			
Palpitation	5	10	1
Tachycardia	4	4	1
DIGESTIVE			
Abnormal stools	12	15	4
Diarrhea	12	19	7
Dyspepsia	6	6	4
Flatulence	2	3	2
Nausea	6	7	6
METABOLIC & NUTRITIONAL			
Peripheral edema	9	7	4
MUSCULO-SKELETAL			
Myalgia	2	3	2
NERVOUS			
Dizziness	9	10	6
Vertigo	3	1	1
RESPIRATORY			
Cough increased	3	4	3
Pharyngitis	7	10	7
Rhinitis	12	7	5

Less frequent adverse events (<2%) that were experienced by patients exposed to PLETAL 50 mg b.i.d. or 100 mg b.i.d. in the eight controlled clinical trials and that occurred at a frequency in the 100 mg b.i.d. group greater than in the placebo group, regardless of suspected drug relationship, are listed below.

Continued on next page

Pletal—Cont.

Body as a whole: Chills, face edema, fever, generalized edema, malaise, neck rigidity, pelvic pain, retroperitoneal hemorrhage.
Cardiovascular: Atrial fibrillation, atrial flutter, cerebral infarct, cerebral ischemia, congestive heart failure, heart arrest, hemorrhage, hypotension, myocardial infarction, myocardial ischemia, nodal arrhythmia, postural hypotension, supraventricular tachycardia, syncope, varicose vein, vasodilation, ventricular extrasystoles, ventricular tachycardia.
Digestive: Anorexia, cholelithiasis, colitis, duodenal ulcer, duodenitis, esophageal hemorrhage, esophagitis, increased GGT, gastritis, gastroenteritis, gum hemorrhage, hematemesis, melena, peptic ulcer, periodontal abscess, rectal hemorrhage, stomach ulcer, tongue edema.
Endocrine: Diabetes mellitus.
Hemic and Lymphatic: Anemia, ecchymosis, iron deficiency anemia, polycythemia, purpura.
Metabolic and Nutritional: Increased creatinine, gout, hyperlipemia, hyperuricemia.
Musculo-skeletal: Arthralgia, bone pain, bursitis.
Nervous: Anxiety, insomnia, neuralgia.
Respiratory: Asthma, epistaxis, hemoptysis, pneumonia, sinusitis.
Skin and Appendages: Dry skin, furunculosis, skin hypertrophy, urticaria.
Special Senses: Amblyopia, blindness, conjunctivitis, diplopia, ear pain, eye hemorrhage, retinal hemorrhage, tinnitus.
Urogenital: Albuminuria, cystitis, urinary frequency, vaginal hemorrhage, vaginitis.

OVERDOSAGE

Information on acute overdosage with PLETAL in humans is limited. The signs and symptoms of an acute overdose can be anticipated to be those of excessive pharmacologic effect: severe headache, diarrhea, hypotension, tachycardia, and possibly cardiac arrhythmias. The patient should be carefully observed and given supportive treatment. Since cilostazol is highly protein-bound, it is unlikely that it can be efficiently removed by hemodialysis or peritoneal dialysis. The oral LD_{50} of cilostazol is >5.0 g/kg in mice and rats and >2.0 g/kg in dogs.

DOSAGE AND ADMINISTRATION

The recommended dosage of PLETAL is 100 mg b.i.d. taken at least half an hour before or two hours after breakfast and dinner. A dose of 50 mg b.i.d. should be considered during coadministration of such inhibitors of CYP3A4 as ketoconazole, itraconazole, erythromycin and diltiazem, and during coadministration of such inhibitors of CYP2C19 as omeprazole. CPY3A4 is also inhibited by grapefruit juice. Because the magnitude and timing of this interaction have not yet been investigated, patients receiving PLETAL should avoid consuming grapefruit juice.
Patients may respond as early as 2 to 4 weeks after the initiation of therapy, but treatment for up to 12 weeks may be needed before a beneficial effect is experienced.
Discontinuation of Therapy: The available data suggest that the dosage of PLETAL can be reduced or discontinued without rebound (i.e., platelet hyperaggregability).

HOW SUPPLIED

PLETAL is supplied as 50 mg and 100 mg tablets. The 50 mg tablets are white, triangular, debossed with PLETAL 50, and provided in bottles of 60 tablets (NDC #59148-003-16), and hospital unit dose packs of 100 tablets (NDC #59148-003-35). The 100 mg tablets are white, round, debossed with PLETAL 100, and provided in bottles of 60 tablets (NDC #59148-002-16), and hospital unit dose packs of 100 tablets (NDC #59148-002-35).
Rx ONLY.
STORAGE
Store PLETAL tablets at 25°C (77°F); excursions permitted to 15–30°C (59–86°F) [See USP Controlled Room Temperature].
Manufactured for
OTSUKA AMERICA PHARMACEUTICAL, INC.
Rockville, MD 20850
Copromoted with
PHARMACIA & UPJOHN
Kalamazoo, MI 49001
Manufactured by
OTSUKA PHARMACEUTICAL CO., LTD
Tokushima 771-0192, Japan
1073/01-99
U.S. Patent No. 4,277,479
Shown in Product Identification Guide, page 329

For information on over-the-counter drugs, consult **PDR For Nonprescription Drugs.**

Paddock Laboratories, Inc.

3940 QUEBEC AVENUE NORTH
MINNEAPOLIS, MN 55427

Direct Inquiries to:
(800) 328-5113

For Medical Information Contact:
Regulatory Affairs Department
(800) 328-5113

ACTIDOSE® with SORBITOL OTC

[act 'ĭ –dose]
(Activated Charcoal with Sorbitol Suspension)

DESCRIPTION

Actidose with Sorbitol is supplied in bottles and tubes. Each 120 mL package contains 25 grams of activated charcoal in suspension and 48 grams of sorbitol. Each 240 mL package contains 50 grams of activated charcoal in suspension and 96 grams of sorbitol. Each milliliter contains 208 mg (0.208 gram) activated in charcoal and 400 mg (0.4 gram) sorbitol.

HOW SUPPLIED

25 g unit-of-use bottle NDC 0574-0120-04
50 g unit-of-use bottle NDC 0574-0120-08
25 g unit-of-use tube NDC 0574-0120-74
50 g unit-of-use tube NDC 0574-0120-76

ACTIDOSE®–AQUA OTC

[act 'ĭ 'dose a–qua]
(Activated Charcoal Suspension)

DESCRIPTION

Actidose-Aqua is supplied in bottles and tubes. Each 72 mL package contains 15 grams of activated charcoal in suspension, each 120 mL package contains 25 grams of activated charcoal in suspension and each 240 mL package contains 50 grams of activated charcoal in suspension. Each milliliter contains 208 mg (0.208 gram) activated charcoal.

HOW SUPPLIED

25 g unit-of-use bottle NDC 0574-0121-04
50 g unit-of-use bottle NDC 0574-0121-08
15 g unit-of-use tube NDC 0574-0121-25
25 g unit-of-use tube NDC 0574-0121-74
50 g unit-of-use tube NDC 0574-0121-76

COLOCORT™ ℞

[cō-lō-cŏrt]
Hydrocortisone Enema, USP
(Retention)
100 mg/60 mL
Disposable Unit for Rectal Use Only

DESCRIPTION

Hydrocortisone is a white to practically white, odorless, crystalline powder, very slightly soluble in water. The empirical formula for hydrocortisone is $C_{21}H_{30}O_5$. Its molecular weight is 362.47. The chemical name for hydrocortisone is Pregn-4-ene-3,20-dione, 11,17,21-trihydroxy-,(11β)-. Hydrocortisone enema is a convenient disposable single-dose enema designed for ease of self-administration.
Each disposable unit (60 mL) for rectal administration contains: Hydrocortisone, 100 mg in an aqueous solution containing carbomer 934P, polysorbate 80, purified water, sodium hydroxide and methylparaben, 0.18% as a preservative.

CLINICAL PHARMACOLOGY

Hydrocortisone is a naturally occurring glucocorticoid (adrenal corticosteroid) which, similar to its acetate and sodium hemisuccinate derivatives, is partially absorbed following rectal administration. Absorption studies in ulcerative colitis patients have shown up to 50% absorption of hydrocortisone administered as hydrocortisone retention enema and up to 30% of hydrocortisone acetate administered in an identical vehicle.
Colocort™ provides the potent anti-inflammatory effect of hydrocortisone. Because this drug is absorbed from the colon, it acts both topically and systemically. Although rectal hydrocortisone, used as recommended for hydrocortisone retention enema, has a low incidence of reported adverse reactions, prolonged use presumably may cause systemic reactions associated with oral dosage forms.

INDICATIONS AND USAGE

Colocort™ is indicated as adjunctive therapy in the treatment of ulcerative colitis, especially distal forms, including ulcerative proctitis, ulcerative proctosigmoiditis, and left-sided ulcerative colitis. It has proved useful also in some cases involving the transverse and ascending colons.

CONTRAINDICATIONS

Systemic fungal infections; and ileocolostomy during the immediate or early postoperative period.

WARNINGS

In severe ulcerative colitis, it is hazardous to delay needed surgery while awaiting response to medical treatment.
Damage to the rectal wall can result from careless or improper insertion of an enema tip.
In patients on corticosteroid therapy subjected to unusual stress, increased dosage of rapidly acting corticosteroids before, during, and after the stressful situation is indicated.
Corticosteroids may mask some signs of infection, and new infections may appear during their use. There may be decreased resistance and inability to localize infection when corticosteroids are used.
Prolonged use of corticosteroids may produce posterior subcapsular cataracts, glaucoma with possible damage to the optic nerves, and may enhance the establishment of secondary ocular infections due to fungi or viruses.
Usage in pregnancy: Since adequate human reproduction studies have not been done with corticosteroids, the use of these drugs in pregnancy, nursing mothers or women of childbearing potential requires that the possible benefits of the drug be weighed against the potential hazards to the mother and embryo or fetus. Infants born of mothers who have received substantial doses of corticosteroid during pregnancy should be carefully observed for signs of hypoadrenalism.
Average and large doses of hydrocortisone or cortisone can cause elevation of blood pressure, salt and water retention, and increased excretion of potassium. These effects are less likely to occur with the synthetic derivatives except when used in large doses. Dietary salt restriction and potassium supplementation may be necessary. All corticosteroids increase calcium excretion.
While on corticosteroid therapy, patients should not be vaccinated against smallpox. Other immunization procedures should not be undertaken in patients who are on corticosteroids, especially on high dose, because of possible hazards of neurological complications and a lack of antibody response.
Persons who are on drugs which suppress the immune system are more susceptible to infections than healthy individuals. Chicken pox and measles, for example, can have a more serious or even fatal course in nonimmune children or adults on corticosteroids. In such children or adults who have not had these diseases, particular care should be taken to avoid exposure. How the dose, route and duration of corticosteroid administration affects the risk of developing a disseminated infection is not known. The contribution of the underlying disease and/or prior corticosteroid treatment to the risk is also not known. If exposed to chicken pox, prophylaxis with varicella zoster immune globulin (VZIG) may be indicated. If exposed to measles, prophylaxis with pooled intramuscular immunoglobulin (IG) may be indicated. (See the respective package inserts for complete VZIG and IG prescribing information.) If chicken pox develops, treatment with antiviral agents may be considered.
If corticosteroids are indicated in patients with latent tuberculosis or tuberculin reactivity, close observation is necessary as reactivation of the disease may occur. During prolonged corticosteroid therapy, these patients should receive chemoprophylaxis.

PRECAUTIONS

Colocort™ hydrocortisone retention enema should be used with caution where there is a probability of impending perforation, abscess or other pyogenic infection; fresh intestinal anastomoses; obstruction; or extensive fistulas and sinus tracts. Use with caution in presence of active or latent peptic ulcer; diverticulitis; renal insufficiency; hypertension; osteoporosis; and myasthenia gravis.
Steroid therapy might impair prognosis in surgery by increasing the hazard of infection. If infection is suspected, appropriate antibiotic therapy must be administered, usually in larger than ordinary doses.
Drug-induced secondary adrenocortical insufficiency may occur with prolonged Colocort™ therapy. This is minimized by gradual reduction of dosage. This type of relative insufficiency may persist for months after discontinuation of therapy; therefore, in any situation of stress occurring during that period, hormone therapy should be reinstituted. Since mineralocorticoid secretion may be impaired, salt and/or a mineralocorticoid should be administered concurrently. There is an enhanced effect of corticosteroids on patients with hypothyroidism and in those with cirrhosis.
Corticosteroid should be used cautiously in patients with ocular herpes simplex because of possible corneal perforation.
The lowest possible dose of corticosteroid should be used to control the conditions under treatment, and when reduction in dosage is possible, the reduction should be gradual.
Psychic derangement may appear when corticosteroids are used, ranging from euphoria, insomnia, mood swings, personality changes, and severe depression, to frank psychotic manifestations. Also, existing emotional instability or psychotic tendencies may be aggravated by corticosteroids.
Aspirin should be used cautiously in conjunction with corticosteroids in hypoprothrombinemia.
Growth and development of pediatric patients on prolonged corticosteroid therapy should carefully observed.
Information for Patients: Persons who are on immunosuppressant doses of corticosteroids should be warned to avoid exposure to chicken pox or measles. Patients should also be advised that if they are exposed, medical advice should be sought without delay.

ADVERSE REACTIONS

Local pain or burning and rectal bleeding attributed to hydrocortisone retention enema have been reported rarely. Apparent exacerbations or sensitivity reactions also occur rarely. The following adverse reactions should be kept in mind whenever corticosteroids are given by rectal administration.

Fluid and Electrolyte Disturbances: Sodium retention; fluid retention; congestive heart failure in susceptible patients; potassium loss; hypokalemic alkalosis; hypertension. **Musculoskeletal:** Muscle weakness; steroid myopathy; loss of muscle mass; osteoporosis; vertebral compression fractures; asceptic necrosis of femoral and humeral heads; pathologic fracture of long bones. **Gastrointestinal:** Peptic ulcer with possible perforation and hemorrhage; pancreatitis; abdominal distention; ulcerative esophagitis. **Dermatologic:** Impaired wound healing; thin fragile skin; petechiae and ecchymoses; facial erythema; increased sweating; may suppress reactions to skin tests. **Neurological:** Convulsions; increased intracranial pressure with papilledema (pseudotumor cerebri) usually after treatment; vertigo; headache. **Endocrine:** Menstrual irregularities; development of Cushingoid state; suppression of growth in children; secondary adrenocortical and pituitary unresponsiveness, particularly in times of stress, as in trauma, surgery or illness, decreased carbohydrate tolerance; manifestations of latent diabetes mellitus; increased requirements for insulin or oral hypoglycemic agents in diabetics. **Ophthalmic:** Posterior subcapsular cataracts; increased intraocular pressure; glaucoma; exophthalmos. **Metabolic:** Negative nitrogen balance due to protein catabolism.

DOSAGE AND ADMINISTRATION

The use of Colocort™ hydrocortisone retention enema is predicated upon the concomitant use of modern supportive measures such as rational dietary control, sedatives, antidiarrheal agents, antibacterial therapy, blood replacement if necessary, etc.

The usual course of therapy is one Colocort™ nightly for 21 days, or until the patient comes into remission both clinically and proctologically. Clinical symptoms usually subside promptly within 3 to 5 days. Improvement in the appearance of the mucosa, as seen by sigmoidoscopic examination, may lag somewhat behind clinical improvement. Difficult cases may require as long as 2 to 3 months of Colocort™ treatment. Where the course of therapy extends beyond 21 days, Colocort™ should be discontinued gradually by reducing administration to every other night for 2 or 3 weeks.

If clinical or proctologic improvement fails to occur within 2 or 3 weeks after starting Colocort™, discontinue its use.

Symptomatic improvement, evidenced by decreased diarrhea and bleeding; weight gain; improved appetite; lessened fever; and decrease in leukocytosis, may be misleading and should not be used as the sole criterion in judging efficacy. Sigmoidoscopic examination and X-ray visualization are essential for adequate monitoring of ulcerative colitis. Biopsy is useful for differential diagnosis.

Patient instructions for administering Colocort™ are enclosed in each box. We recommend the patient lie on his/her left side during administration and for 30 minutes thereafter, so that the fluid will distribute throughout the left colon. Every effort should be made to retain the enema for at least an hour and preferably, all night. This may be facilitated by prior sedation and/or antidiarrheal medication, especially early in therapy, when the urge to evacuate is great.

HOW SUPPLIED

Colocort™, Hydrocortisone Enema, USP, (Retention) 100 mg/60 mL, is supplied as disposable single-dose bottles with lubricated rectal applicator tips, in boxes of seven × 60 mL (NDC 0574-2020-07) and boxes of one × 60 mL (NDC 0574-2020-01).

Store at controlled room temperature, 15°–30°C (59°–86°F).

Rx only

124148(03-99)

COMPRO™ ℞

[*cŏm-prō*]

PROCHLORPERAZINE
SUPPOSITORIES USP, 25mg
Rx only
ANTIEMETIC - TRANQUILIZER

DESCRIPTION

Prochlorperazine is a clear, pale yellow, viscous liquid. It is sensitive to light, very slightly soluble in water, freely soluble in alcohol, in chloroform, and in ether.

Each suppository, for rectal administration, contains 25mg of prochlorperazine; with glycerin, glyceryl monopalmitate, glyceryl monostearate, hydrogenated coconut oil fatty acids and hydrogenated palm kernel oil fatty acids.

Prochlorperazine has the molecular formula $C_{20}H_{24}ClN_3S$. Its molecular weight is 373.95. The chemical name for prochlorperazine is 2-Chloro-10-[3-(4-methyl-1-piperazinyl) propyl] phenothiazine.

CLINICAL PHARMACOLOGY

Prochlorperazine is a propylpiperazine derivative of phenothiazine. Like other phenothiazines, it exerts an antiemetic effect through a depressant action on the chemoreceptor trigger zone.

INDICATIONS AND USAGE

Prochlorperazine 25mg suppositories are indicated in the control of severe nausea and vomiting in adults.

CONTRAINDICATIONS

Do not use in comatose states or in the presence of large amounts of central nervous system depressants (alcohol, barbiturates, narcotics, etc.).

Do not use in pediatric surgery.

Do not use in children under 2 years of age or under 20 lbs.

Do not use in children for conditions for which dosage has not been established.

WARNINGS

The extrapyramidal symptoms which can occur secondary to prochlorperazine may be confused with the central nervous system signs of an undiagnosed primary disease responsible for the vomiting, e.g., Reye's Syndrome or other encephalopathy. The use of prochlorperazine and other potential hepatotoxins should be avoided in children and adolescents whose signs and symptoms suggest Reye's Syndrome.

Tardive Dyskinesia: Tardive dyskinesia, a syndrome consisting of potentially irreversible, involuntary, dyskinetic movements, may develop in patients treated with neuroleptic (antipsychotic) drugs. Although the prevalence of the syndrome appears to be highest among the elderly, especially elderly women, it is impossible to rely upon prevalence estimates to predict, at the inception of neuroleptic treatment, which patients are likely to develop the syndrome. Whether neuroleptic drug products differ in their potential to cause tardive dyskinesia is unknown.

Both the risk of developing the syndrome and the likelihood that it will become irreversible are believed to increase as the duration of treatment and the total cumulative dose of neuroleptic drugs administered to the patient increase. However, the syndrome can develop, although much less commonly, after relatively brief treatment periods at low doses.

There is no known treatment for established cases of tardive dyskinesia, although the syndrome may remit, partially or completely, if neuroleptic treatment is withdrawn. Neuroleptic treatment itself, however, may suppress (or partially suppress) the signs and symptoms of the syndrome and thereby may possibly mask the underlying disease process.

The effect that symptomatic suppression has upon the long-term course of the syndrome is unknown.

Given these considerations, neuroleptics should be prescribed in a manner that is most likely to minimize the occurrence of tardive dyskinesia. Chronic neuroleptic treatment should generally be reserved for patients who suffer from a chronic illness that, 1) is known to respond to neuroleptic drugs, and 2) for whom alternative, equally effective, but potentially less harmful treatments are *not* available or appropriate. In patients who do require chronic treatment, the smallest dose and the shortest duration of treatment producing a satisfactory clinical response should be sought. The need for continued treatment should be reassessed periodically.

If signs and symptoms of tardive dyskinesia appear in a patient on neuroleptics, drug discontinuation should be considered. However, some patients may require treatment despite the presence of the syndrome.

For further information about the description of tardive dyskinesia and its clinical detection, please refer to the sections on PRECAUTIONS and ADVERSE REACTIONS.

Neuroleptic Malignant Syndrome (NMS): A potentially fatal symptom complex sometimes referred to as Neuroleptic Malignant Syndrome (NMS) has been reported in association with antipsychotic drugs. Clinical manifestations of NMS are hyperpyrexia, muscle rigidity, altered mental status and evidence of autonomic instability (irregular pulse or blood pressure, tachycardia, diaphoresis and cardiac dysrhythmias).

The diagnostic evaluation of patients with this syndrome is complicated. In arriving at a diagnosis, it is important to identify cases where the clinical presentation includes both serious medical illness (e.g., pneumonia, systemic infection, etc.) and untreated or inadequately treated extrapyramidal signs and symptoms (EPS). Other important considerations in the differential diagnosis include central anticholinergic toxicity, heat stroke, drug fever and primary central nervous system (CNS) pathology.

The management of NMS should include 1) immediate discontinuation of antipsychotic drugs and other drugs not essential to concurrent therapy, 2) intensive symptomatic treatment and medical monitoring, and 3) treatment of any concomitant serious medical problems for which specific treatments are available. There is no general agreement about specific pharmacological treatment regimens for uncomplicated NMS.

If a patient requires antipsychotic drug treatment after recovery from NMS, the potential reintroduction of drug therapy should be carefully considered. The patient should be carefully monitored, since recurrences of NMS have been reported.

General: Patients with bone marrow depression or who have previously demonstrated a hypersensitivity reaction (e.g., blood dyscrasias, jaundice) with a phenothiazine should not receive any phenothiazine, including prochlorperazine, unless in the judgement of the physician the potential benefits of treatment outweigh the possible hazards.

Prochlorperazine may impair mental and/or physical abilities, especially during the first few days of therapy. Therefore, caution patients about activities requiring alertness (e.g., operating vehicles or machinery).

Phenothiazines may intensify or prolong the action of central nervous system depressants (e.g., alcohol, anesthetics, narcotics).

Usage in Pregnancy: Safety for the use of prochlorperazine during pregnancy has not been established. Therefore, prochlorperazine is not recommended for use in pregnant patients except in cases of severe nausea and vomiting that are so serious and intractable that, in the judgment of the physician, drug intervention is required and potential benefits outweigh possible hazards.

There have been reported instances of prolonged jaundice, extrapyramidal signs, hyperreflexia or hyporeflexia in newborn infants whose mothers received phenothiazines.

Nursing Mothers: There is evidence that phenothiazines are excreted in the breast milk of nursing mothers.

PRECAUTIONS

The antiemetic action of prochlorperazine may mask the signs and symptoms of overdosage of other drugs and may obscure the diagnosis and treatment of other conditions such as intestinal obstruction, brain tumor and Reye's Syndrome (see WARNINGS).

When prochlorperazine is used with cancer chemotherapeutic drugs, vomiting as a sign of the toxicity of these agents may be obscured by the antiemetic effect of prochlorperazine.

Because hypotension may occur, large doses and parenteral administration should be used cautiously in patients with impaired cardiovascular systems. If hypotension occurs after parenteral or oral dosing, place patient in head-low position with legs raised. If a vasoconstrictor is required, norepinephrine bitartrate and phenylephrine hydrochloride are suitable. Other pressor agents, including epinephrine, should not be used because they may cause a paradoxical further lowering of blood pressure.

Aspiration of vomitus has occurred in a few post-surgical patients who have received prochlorperazine as an antiemetic. Although no causal relationship has been established, this possibility should be borne in mind during surgical aftercare.

Deep sleep, from which patients can be aroused, and coma have been reported, usually with overdosage.

Neuroleptic drugs elevate prolactin levels; the elevation persists during chronic administration. Tissue culture experiments indicate that approximately one third of human breast cancers are prolactin-dependent *in vitro*, a factor of potential importance if the prescribing of these drugs is contemplated in a patient with a previously detected breast cancer. Although disturbances such as galactorrhea, amenorrhea, gynecomastia and impotence have been reported, the clinical signficance of elevated serum prolactin levels is unknown for most patients. An increase in mammary neoplasms has been found in rodents after chronic administration of neuroleptic drugs. Neither clinical nor epidemiologic studies conducted to date, however, have shown an association between chronic administration of these drugs and mammary tumorigenesis; the available evidence is considered too limited to be conclusive at this time.

Chromosomal aberrations in spermatocytes and abnormal sperm have been demonstrated in rodents treated with certain neuroleptics.

As with all drugs which exert an anticholinergic effect, and/or cause mydriasis, prochlorperazine should be used with caution in patients with glaucoma.

Because phenothiazines may interfere with thermoregulatory mechanisms, use with caution in persons who will be exposed to extreme heat.

Phenothiazines can diminish the effect of oral anticoagulants.

Phenothiazines can produce alpha-adrenergic blockade.

Thiazide diuretics may accentuate the orthostatic hypotension that may occur with phenothiazines.

Antihypertensive effects of guanethidine and related compounds may be counteracted when phenothiazines are used concomitantly.

Concomitant administration of propranolol with phenothiazines results in increased plasma levels of both drugs.

Phenothiazines may lower the convulsive threshold; dosage adjustments of anticonvulsants may be necessary. Potentiation of anticonvulsant effects does not occur. However, it has been reported that phenothiazines may interfere with the metabolism of phenytoin and thus precipitate phenytoin toxicity.

The presence of phenothiazines may produce false-positive phenylketonuria (PKU) test results.

Long-Term Therapy: Given the likelihood that some patients exposed chronically to neuroleptics will develop tardive dyskinesia, it is advised that all patients in whom chronic use is contemplated be given, if possible, full information about this risk. The decision to inform patients and/or their guardians must obviously take into account the clinical circumstances and the competency of the patient to understand the information provided.

To lessen the likelihood of adverse reactions related to cumulative drug effect, patients with a history of long-term therapy with prochlorperazine and/or other neuroleptics

Continued on next page

Compro—Cont.

should be evaluated periodically to decide whether the maintenance dosage could be lowered or drug therapy discontinued.

Children with acute illnesses (e.g., chicken pox, CNS infections, measles, gastroenteritis) or dehydration seem to be much more susceptible to neuromuscular reactions, particularly dystonias, than are adults. In such patients, the drug should be used only under close supervision.

Drugs which lower the seizure threshold, including phenothiazine derivatives, should not be used with metrizamide. As with other phenothiazine derivatives, prochlorperazine should be discontinued at least 48 hours before myelography, should not be resumed for at least 24 hours postprocedure, and should not be used for the control of nausea and vomiting occurring either prior to myelography with metrizamide, or postprocedure.

ADVERSE REACTIONS

Drowsiness, dizziness, amenorrhea, blurred vision, skin reactions and hypotension may occur.

Cholestatic jaundice has occurred. If fever with grippe-like symptoms occurs, appropriate liver studies should be conducted. If tests indicate an abnormality, stop treatment. There have been a few observations of fatty changes in the livers of patients who have died while receiving the drug. No causal relationship has been established.

Leukopenia and agranulocytosis have occurred. Warn patients to report the sudden appearance of sore thoat or other signs of infection. If white blood cell and differential counts indicate leukocyte depression, stop treatment and start antibiotic and other suitable therapy.

Neuromuscular (Extrapyramidal) Reactions

These symptoms are seen in a significant number of hospitalized mental patients. They may be characterized by motor restlessness, be of the dystonic type, or they may resemble parkinsonism.

Depending on the severity of symptoms, dosage should be reduced or discontinued. If therapy is reinstituted, it should be at a lower dosage. Should these symptoms occur in children or pregnant patients, the drug should be stopped and not reinstituted. In most cases barbiturates by suitable route of administration will suffice. (Or, injectable diphenhydramine may be useful.) In more severe cases, the administration of an anti-parkinsonism agent, except levodopa (see *PDR*), usually produces rapid reversal of symptoms. Suitable supportive measures such as maintaining a clear airway and adequate hydration should be employed.

Motor Restlessness: Symptoms may include agitation or jitteriness and sometimes insomnia. These symptoms often disappear spontaneously. At times these symptoms may be similar to the original neurotic or psychotic symptoms. Dosage should not be increased until these side effects have subsided.

If these symptoms become too troublesome, they can usually be controlled by a reduction of dosage or change of drug. Treatment with anti-parkinsonian agents, benzodiazepines or propranolol may be helpful.

Dystonias: Symptoms may include: spasm of the neck muscles, sometimes progressing to torticollis; extensor rigidity of back muscles, sometimes progressing to opisthotonos; carpopedal spasm, trismus, swallowing difficulty, oculogyric crisis and protrusion of the tongue.

These usually subside within a few hours, and almost always within 24 to 48 hours, after the drug has been discontinued.

In mild cases, reassurance or a barbiturate is often sufficient. *In moderate cases,* barbiturates will usually bring rapid relief. *In more severe adult cases,* the administration of an anti-parkinsonism agent, except levodopa (see *PDR*), usually produces rapid reversal of symptoms. *In children,* reassurance and barbiturates will usually control symptoms. (Or, injectable diphenhydramine may be useful. Note: See diphenhydramine prescribing information for appropriate *children's* dosage.) If appropriate treatment with anti-parkinsonism agents or diphenhydramine fails to reverse the signs and symptoms, the diagnosis should be reevaluated.

Pseudo-parkinsonism: Symptoms may include: mask-like facies; drooling; tremors; pillrolling motion; cogwheel rigidity; and shuffling gait. Reassurance and sedation are important. In most cases these symptoms are readily controlled when an anti-parkinsonism agent is administered concomitantly. Anti-parkinsonism agents should be used only when required. Generally, therapy of a few weeks to 2 or 3 months will suffice. After this time patients should be evaluated to determine their need for continued treatment. (Note: Levodopa has not been found effective in pseudo-parkinsonism.) Occasionally it is necessary to lower the dosage of prochlorperazine or to discontinue the drug.

Tardive Dyskinesia: As with all antipsychotic agents, tardive dyskinesia may appear in some patients on long-term therapy or may appear after drug therapy has been discontinued. The syndrome can also develop, although much less frequently, after relatively brief treatment periods at low doses. This syndrome appears in all age groups. Although its prevalence appears to be highest among elderly patients, especially elderly women, it is impossible to rely upon prevalence estimates to predict at the inception of neuroleptic treatment which patients are likely to develop the syndrome. The symptoms are persistent and in some patients appear to be irreversible. The syndrome is characterized by rhythmical involuntary movements of the tongue, face, mouth or jaw (e.g., protrusion of tongue, puffing of cheeks, puckering of mouth, chewing movements). Sometimes these may be accompanied by involuntary movements of extremities. In rare instances, these involuntary movements of the extremities are the only manifestations of tardive dyskinesia. A variant of tardive dyskinesia, tardive dystonia, has also been described.

There is no known effective treatment for tardive dyskinesia; anti-parkinsonism agents do not alleviate the symptoms of this syndrome. It is suggested that all antipsychotic agents be discontinued if these symptoms appear.

Should it be necessary to reinstitute treatment, or increase the dosage of the agent, or switch to a different antipsychotic agent, the syndrome may be masked.

It has been reported that fine vermicular movements of the tongue may be an early sign of the syndrome and if the medication is stopped at that time the syndrome may not develop.

Adverse Reactions Reported with Prochlorperazine or Other Phenothiazine Derivatives: Adverse reactions with different phenothiazines vary in type, frequency and mechanism of occurrence, i.e., some are dose-related, while others involve individual patient sensitivity. Some adverse reactions may be more likely to occur, or occur with greater intensity, in patients with special medical problems, e.g., patients with mitral insufficiency or pheochromocytoma have experienced severe hypotension following recommended doses of certain phenothiazines.

Not all of the following adverse reactions have been observed with every phenothiazine derivative, but they have been reported with 1 or more and should be borne in mind when drugs of this class are administered: extrapyramidal symptoms (opisthotonos, oculogyric crisis, hyperreflexia, dystonia, akathisia, dyskinesia, parkinsonism) some of which have lasted months and even years—particularly in elderly patients with previous brain damage; grand mal and petit mal convulsions, particularly in patients with EEG abnormalities or history of such disorders; altered cerebrospinal fluid proteins; cerebral edema; intensification and prolongation of the action of central nervous system depressants (opiates, analgesics, antihistamines, barbiturates, alcohol), atropine, heat, organophosphorus insecticides; autonomic reactions (dryness of the mouth, nasal congestion, headache, nausea, constipation, obstipation, adynamic ileus, ejaculatory disorders/impotence, priapism, atonic colon, urinary retention, miosis and mydriasis); reactivation of psychotic processes, catatonic-like states; hypotension (sometimes fatal); cardiac arrest; blood dyscrasias (pancytopenia, thrombocytopenic purpura, leukopenia, agranulocytosis, eosinophilia, hemolytic anemia, aplastic anemia); liver damage (jaundice, biliary stasis); endocrine disturbances (hyperglycemia, hypoglycemia, glycosuria, lactation, galactorrhea, gynecomastia, menstrual irregularities, false-positive pregnancy tests); skin disorders (photosensitivity, itching, erythema, urticaria, eczema up to exfoliative dermatitis); other allergic reactions (asthma, laryngeal edema, angioneurotic edema, anaphylactoid reactions); peripheral edema; reversed epinephrine effect; hyperpyrexia; mild fever after large I.M. doses; increased appetite; increased weight; a systemic lupus erythematosus-like syndrome; pigmentary retinopathy; with prolonged administration of substantial doses, skin pigmentation, epithelial keratopathy, and lenticular and corneal deposits.

EKG changes—particularly nonspecific, usually reversible Q and T wave distortions—have been observed in some patients receiving phenothiazine tranquilizers.

Although phenothiazines cause neither psychic nor physical dependence, sudden discontinuance in long-term psychiatric patients may cause temporary symptoms, e.g., nausea and vomiting, dizziness, tremulousness.

Note: There have been occasional reports of sudden death in patients receiving phenothiazines. In some cases, the cause appeared to be cardiac arrest or asphyxia due to failure of the cough reflex.

OVERDOSAGE

(See also ADVERSE REACTIONS).

SYMPTOMS—Primarily involvement of the extrapyramidal mechanism producing some of the dystonic reactions described above.

Symptoms of central nervous system depression to the point of somnolence or coma. Agitation and restlessness may also occur. Other possible manifestations include convulsions, EKG changes and cardiac arrhythmias, fever and autonomic reactions such as hypotension, dry mouth and ileus.

TREATMENT—It is important to determine other medications taken by the patient since multiple-dose therapy is common in overdosage situations. Treatment is essentially symptomatic and supportive. Early gastric lavage is helpful. Keep patient under observation and maintain an open airway, since involvement of the extrapyramidal mechanism may produce dysphagia and respiratory difficulty in severe overdosage. **Do not attempt to induce emesis because a dystonic reaction of the head or neck may develop that could result in aspiration of vomitus.** Extrapyramidal symptoms may be treated with anti-parkinsonism drugs, barbiturates or diphenhydramine. See prescribing information for these products. Care should be taken to avoid increasing respiratory depression.

If administration of a stimulant is desirable, amphetamine, dextroamphetamine or caffeine with sodium benzoate is recommended.

Stimulants that may cause convulsions (e.g., picrotoxin or pentylenetetrazol) should be avoided.

If hypotension occurs, the standard measures for managing circulatory shock should be initiated. If it is desirable to administer a vasoconstrictor, norepinephrine bitartrate and phenylephrine hydrochloride are most suitable. Other pressor agents, including epinephrine, are not recommended because phenothiazine derivatives may reverse the usual elevating action of these agents and cause a further lowering of blood pressure.

Limited experience indicates that phenothiazines are *not* dialyzable.

DOSAGE AND ADMINISTRATION

Adults: Dosage should be increased more gradually in debilitated or emaciated patients.

Elderly Patients: In general, dosages in the lower range are sufficient for most elderly patients. Since they appear to be more susceptible to hypotension and neuromuscular reactions, such patients should be observed closely. Dosage should be tailored to the individual, response carefully monitored and dosage adjusted accordingly. Dosage should be increased more gradually in elderly patients.

To Control Severe Nausea and Vomiting: Adjust dosage to the response of the individual. Begin with the lowest recommended dosage.

Rectal Dosage: 25mg twice daily.

HOW SUPPLIED

Compro™ Prochlorperazine Suppositories USP, 25mg (for adults) are easy to open, and available in boxes of 12.

12's—NDC 0574-7226-12

Store between 15° and 30°C (59° and 86°F).

Do not remove from wrapper until ready to use.

124140 (06-99)

GLUTOSE 15™ GLUTOSE 45™ OTC
(Oral Glucose Gel)

DESCRIPTION

Glutose gel is a lemon-flavored, dye-free oral glucose gel for treatment of insulin reaction or hypoglycemia. Glutose gel contains Dextrose (d-glucose) USP 40%.

HOW SUPPLIED

Glutose 15: 3 x 15g unit-of-use tubes per package NDC 0574-0069-30

Glutose 45: 1 x 45g multi-use tube per package NDC 0574-0069-45

KIONEX™ ℞
[*ky-oněx*]
Sodium Polystyrene Sulfonate, USP

Cation-Exchange Resin

DESCRIPTION

Kionex™ brand of sodium polystyrene sulfonate is a benzene, diethenyl-, polymer with ethenylbenzene, sulfonated, sodium salt.

The drug is a light brown to brown finely ground, powdered form of sodium polystyrene sulfonate, a cation-exchange resin prepared in the sodium phase with an *in vitro* exchange capacity of approximately 3.1 mEq (*in vivo* approximately 1 mEq) of potassium per gram. The sodium content is approximately 100 mg (4.1 mEq) per gram of the drug. It can be administered orally or in an enema.

CLINICAL PHARMACOLOGY

As the resin passes along the intestine or is retained in the colon after administration by enema, the sodium ions from the resin are partially released and are replaced by potassium ions. For the most part, this action occurs in the large intestine, which excretes potassium ions to a greater degree than does the small intestine. The efficiency of this process is limited and unpredictably variable. It commonly approximates the order of 33 percent but the range is so large that definitive indices of electrolyte balance must be clearly monitored. Metabolic data are unavailable.

INDICATIONS AND USAGE

Kionex is indicated for the treatment of hyperkalemia.

CONTRAINDICATIONS

Kionex is contraindicated in patients with hypokalemia or those patients who are hypersensitive to it.

WARNINGS

Alternative Therapy in Severe Hyperkalemia: Since effective lowering of serum potassium with this product may take hours to days, treatment with this drug alone may be insufficient to rapidly correct severe hyperkalemia associated with states of rapid tissue breakdown (e.g., burns and renal failure) or hyperkalemia so marked as to constitute a medical emergency. Therefore, other definitive measures, including dialysis, should always be considered and may be imperative.

Hypokalemia: Serious potassium deficiency can occur from therapy with Kionex. The effect must be carefully controlled by frequent serum potassium determinations within each 24 hour period. Since intracellular potassium deficiency is not always reflected by serum potassium levels, the level at which treatment with Kionex should be discontinued must be determined individually for each patient. Important aids in making this determination are the patient's clinical condition and electrocardiogram. Early clinical signs of severe hypokalemia include a pattern of irritable confusion and delayed thought processes. Electrocardiographically, severe hypokalemia is often associated with a lengthened Q-T interval, widening, flattening, or inversion of the T wave, and prominent U waves. Also, cardiac arrhythmias may occur, such as premature atrial, nodal, and ventricular contractions, and supraventricular and ventricular tachycardias. The toxic effects of digitalis are likely to be exaggerated. Marked hypokalemia can also be manifested by severe muscle weakness, at times extending into frank paralysis.

Electrolyte Disturbances: Like all cation-exchange resins, Kionex is not totally selective (for potassium) in its actions, and small amounts of other cations such as calcium and magnesium can also be lost during treatment. Accordingly patients receiving Kionex should be monitored for all applicable electrolyte disturbances.

Systemic Alkalosis: Systemic alkalosis has been reported after cation-exchange resins were administered orally in combination with nonabsorbable cation-donating antacids and laxatives such as magnesium hydroxide and aluminum carbonate. Magnesium hydroxide should not be administered with Kionex. One case of grand mal seizure has been reported in a patient with chronic hypocalcemia of renal failure who was given sodium polystyrene sulfonate with magnesium hydroxide as a laxative. (See PRECAUTIONS, Drug Interactions.)

PRECAUTIONS

Caution is advised when Kionex is administered to patients who cannot tolerate even a small increase in sodium loads (i.e., severe congestive heart failure, severe hypertension, or marked edema). In such instances, compensatory restriction of sodium intake from other sources may be indicated.

If constipation occurs, patients should be treated with sorbitol (from 10 to 20 mL of 70 percent syrup every two hours or as needed to produce 1 or 2 watery stools daily), a measure which also reduces any tendency to fecal impaction.

Drug Interactions

Antacids: The simultaneous oral administration of Kionex with nonabsorbable cation-donating antacids and laxatives may reduce the resin's potassium exchange capability.

Systemic alkalosis has been reported after cation-exchange resins were administered orally in combination with nonabsorbable cation-donating antacids and laxatives such as magnesium hydroxide and aluminum carbonate. Magnesium hydroxide should not be administered with Kionex. One case of grand mal seizure has been reported in a patient with chronic hypocalcemia of renal failure who was given sodium polystyrene sulfonate with magnesium hydroxide as a laxative.

Intestinal obstruction due to concretions of aluminum hydroxide when used in combination with sodium polystyrene sulfonate has been reported.

Digitalis: The toxic effects of digitalis on the heart, especially various ventricular arrhythmias and A-V nodal dissociation, are likely to be exaggerated by hypokalemia, even in the face of serum digoxin concentrations in the "normal range". (See WARNINGS.)

Carcinogenesis, Mutagenesis, Impairment of Fertility

Studies have not been performed.

Pregnancy Category C

Animal reproduction studies have not been conducted with Kionex. It is also not known whether Kionex can cause fetal harm when administered to a pregnant woman or can affect reproduction capacity. Kionex should be given to a pregnant woman only if clearly needed.

Nursing Mothers

It is not known whether this drug is excreted in human milk. Because many drugs are excreted in human milk, caution should be exercised when Kionex is administered to a nursing woman.

ADVERSE REACTIONS

Kionex may cause some degree of gastric irritation. Anorexia, nausea, vomiting, and constipation may occur especially if high doses are given. Also, hypokalemia, hypocalcemia, and significant sodium retention may occur. Occasionally diarrhea develops. Large doses in elderly individuals may cause fecal impaction (see PRECAUTIONS). This effect may be obviated through usage of the resin in enemas as described under DOSAGE AND ADMINISTRATION. Rare instances of colonic necrosis have been reported. Intestinal obstruction due to concretions of aluminum hydroxide, when used in combination with sodium polystyrene sulfonate, has been reported.

DOSAGE AND ADMINISTRATION

Suspension of this drug should be freshly prepared and not stored beyond 24 hours.

The average daily adult dose of the resin is 15 g to 60 g. This is best provided by administering 15 grams (approximately 4 *level teaspoons*) of Kionex one to four times daily. One gram of Kionex contains 4.1 mEq of sodium; one level teaspoon contains approximately 3.5 grams of Kionex and 15 mEq of sodium. (A heaping teaspoon may contain as much as 10 to 12 grams of Kionex.) Since the *in vivo* efficiency of sodium-potassium exchange resins is approximately 33 percent, about one third of the resin's actual sodium content is being delivered to the body.

In smaller children and infants, lower doses should be employed by using as a guide a rate of 1 mEq of potassium per gram of resin as the basis for calculation.

Each dose should be given as a suspension in a small quantity of water or, for greater palatability, in syrup. The amount of fluid usually ranges from 20 to 100 mL, depending on the dose, or may be simply determined by allowing 3 to 4 mL per gram resin. Sorbitol may be administered in order to combat constipation.

The resin may be introduced into the stomach through a plastic tube and, if desired, mixed with a diet appropriate for a patient in renal failure.

The resin may also be given, although with less effective results, in an enema consisting (for adults) of 30 g to 50 g every six hours. Each dose is administered as a warm emulsion (at body temperature) in 100 mL of aqueous vehicle, such as sorbitol. The emulsion should be agitated gently during administration. The enema should be retained as long as possible and followed by a cleansing enema.

After an initial cleansing enema, a soft, large size (French 28) rubber tube is inserted into the rectum for a distance of about 20 cm, with the tip well into the sigmoid colon, and taped in place. The resin is then suspended in the appropriate amount of aqueous vehicle at body temperature and introduced by gravity, while the particles are kept in suspension by stirring. The suspension is flushed with 50 mL or 100 mL of fluid, following which the tube is clamped and left in place. If back leakage occurs, the hips are elevated on pillows or a knee-chest position is taken temporarily. A somewhat thicker suspension may be used, but care should be taken that no paste is formed, because the latter has a greatly reduced exchange surface and will be particularly ineffective if deposited in the rectal ampulla. The suspension is kept in the sigmoid colon for several hours, if possible. Then the colon is irrigated with nonsodium containing solution at body temperature in order to remove the resin. Two quarts of flushing solution may be necessary. The returns are drained constantly through a Y tube connection. Particular attention should be paid to this cleansing enema when sorbitol has been used.

The intensity and duration of therapy depend upon the severity and resistance of hyperkalemia.

HOW SUPPLIED

Store at controlled room temperature 15–30°C (59–86°F). Kionex should not be heated for to do so may alter the exchange properties of the resin.

Dispense in a tight, light-resistant container as defined in the USP.

Rx only

Kionex™ (Sodium Polystyrene Sulfonate, USP) is available as a powder in containers of:

1 Pound (454 grams) NDC 0574-2004-16

Packaged by:

PADDOCK LABORATORIES, INC.
Minneapolis, Minnesota 55427

Revised April 1993 124142 (04.93)

NYSTOP® ℞

Nystatin Topical Powder USP
Rx only
For topical use only.
Not for ophthalmic use.

DESCRIPTION

Nystatin is a polyene antifungal antibiotic obtained from *Streptomyces nursei*.

Nystatin Topical Powder USP is for dermatologic use.

Nystatin Topical Powder USP contains 100,000 USP nystatin units per gram dispersed in talc.

CLINICAL PHARMACOLOGY

Pharmacokinetics

Nystatin is not absorbed from intact skin or mucous membrane.

Microbiology

Nystatin is an antibiotic which is both fungistatic and fungicidal *in vitro* against a wide variety of yeasts and yeast-like fungi, including *Candida albicans, C. parapsilosis, C. tropicalis, C. guilliermondi, C. pseudotropicalis, C. krusei, Torulopsis glabrata, Tricophyton rubrum, T. mentagrophytes.*

Nystatin acts by binding to sterols in the cell membrane of susceptible species resulting in a change in membrane permeability and the subsequent leakage of intracellular components. On repeated subculturing with increasing levels of nystatin, *Candida albicans* does not develop resistance to nystatin. Generally, resistance to nystatin does not develop during therapy. However, other species of *Candida (C. tropicalis, C. guilliermondi, C. krusei, and C. stellatoides)* become quite resistant on treatment with nystatin and simultaneously become cross resistant to amphotericin as well. This resistance is lost when the antibiotic is removed. Nystatin exhibits no appreciable activity against bacteria, protozoa, or viruses.

INDICATIONS AND USAGE

Nystatin Topical Powder is indicated in the treatment of cutaneous or mucocutaneous mycotic infections caused by *Candida albicans* and other susceptible *Candida* species.

This preparation is not indicated for systemic, oral, intravaginal or ophthalmic use.

CONTRAINDICATIONS

Nystatin Topical Powder is contraindicated in patients with a history of hypersensitivity to any of its components.

PRECAUTIONS

General

Nystatin Topical Powder should not be used for the treatment of systemic, oral, intravaginal or ophthalmic infections.

If irritation or sensitization develops, treatment should be discontinued and appropriate measures taken as indicated. It is recommended that KOH smears, cultures, or other diagnostic methods be used to confirm the diagnosis of cutaneous or mucocutaneous candidiasis and to rule out infection caused by other pathogens.

ADVERSE REACTIONS

The frequency of adverse events reported in patients using nystatin topical preparations is less than 0.1%. The more common events that were reported include allergic reactions, burning, itching, rash, eczema, and pain on application. (See **PRECAUTIONS**: **General.**)

DOSAGE AND ADMINISTRATION

Very moist lesions are best treated with the topical dusting powder.

Adults and Pediatric Patients (Neonates and Older):

Apply to candidal lesions two or three times daily until healing is complete. For fungal infection of the feet caused by *Candida* species, the powder should be dusted on the feet, as well as, in all foot wear.

HOW SUPPLIED

Nystop® Nystatin Topical Powder USP is supplied as 100,000 units nystatin per gram in 15 g plastic squeeze bottles.

(NDC 0574-2008-15)

STORAGE

Store at controlled room temperature 15°–30°C (59°—86°F); avoid excessive heat (40°C; 104°F).

(12-99)

PADDOCK™ NYSTATIN
NYSTATIN, USP ℞

For Extemporaneous Preparation of Oral Suspension

DESCRIPTION

Nystatin USP is an antifungal antibiotic obtained from *Streptomyces noursei*. It is known to be a mixture, but the composition has not been completely elucidated. Nystatin A is closely related to amphotericin B. Each is a macrocyclic lactone containing a ketal ring, an all-*trans* polyene system, and a mycosamine (3-amino-3-deoxy-rhamnose) moiety. Nystatin A has a molecular formula of $C_{47}H_{75}NO_{17}$ and a molecular weight of 926.11.

Nystatin USP is a ready-to-use, non-sterile powder for oral administration which contains no excipients or preservatives. It is available in containers of 50 million, 150 million, 500 million, 2 billion, and 5 billion units. Each mg contains a minimum of 5,000 units.

HOW SUPPLIED

Product Code (NDC)	Size (units)	Approx. Weight (grams)
0574-0404-05	50 million	8.3 – 10
0574-0404-15	150 million	25 – 30
0574-0404-50	500 million	83 – 100
0574-0404-02	2 billion	333 – 400
0574-0404-00	5 billion	833 – 1,000

Storage: Store in a refrigerator. 2°–8°C (36°–46°F). Protect from light.

PODOCON-25® ℞

(25% podophyllin in benzoin tincture)

DESCRIPTION

Podocon-25® is composed of Podophyllin (Podophyllum Resin, American) 25% in Benzoin Tincture. Podophyllum Resin is the powdered mixture of resins removed from the May apple or Mandrake (*Podophyllum peltatum Linne'*), a perennial plant of northern and middle United States[1]. The podophyllum resin used in this product is exclusively the American podophyllin (rather than the Indian resin). American podophyllin typically has a reduced level of podophyllotoxin (see below).

CLINICAL PHARMACOLOGY

Podophyllin is a cytotoxic agent that has been used topically in the treatment of genital warts. It arrests mitosis in metaphase, an effect it shares with other cytotoxic agents such as

Continued on next page

Podocon-25—Cont.

the vinca alkaloids[2]. The active agent is podophyllotoxin, whose concentration varies with the type of podophyllin used; the American source normally containing one-fourth the amount of podophyllotoxin as the Indian source[3].

NOTE: PODOCON-25 IS TO BE APPLIED ONLY BY A PHYSICIAN. IT IS NOT TO BE DISPENSED TO THE PATIENT.

INDICATIONS

Podocon-25 (25% podophyllin in benzoin tincture) is indicated for the removal of soft genital (venereal) warts (condylomata acuminata)[4].

CONTRAINDICATIONS

Podocon-25 is contraindicated in diabetics, patients using steroids or with poor blood circulation. **Podocon-25** should not be used on bleeding warts, moles, birthmarks or unusual warts with hair growing from them. It is recommended that **Podocon-25** not be used during pregnancy (see Pregnancy warning below).

WARNINGS

Podophyllin is a powerful caustic and severe irritant. Keep away from the eyes; if eye contact occurs, flush with copious amounts of warm water and consult physician or poison control center immediately for advice.

PRECAUTIONS

Do not use **Podocon-25** if wart or surrounding tissue is inflamed or irritated. Do not use on bleeding warts, moles, birthmarks or unusual warts with hair growing from them.

ADVERSE REACTIONS

The use of topical podophyllin has been known to result in paresthesia, polyneuritis, paralytic ileus, pyrexia, leukopenia, thrombocytopenia, coma and death[5].

Pregnancy: There have been reports of complications associated with the topical use of podophyllin on condylomata of pregnant patients including birth defects, fetal death and stillbirth[6]. In the absence of controlled safety studies, podophyllin remains contraindicated for use on pregnant patients.

Nursing Mothers: It is not known whether podophyllin is excreted in human milk following topical application. In the absence of controlled safety studies, podophyllin remains contraindicated for use on nursing patients.

DOSAGE AND ADMINISTRATION

PODOCON-25 IS TO BE APPLIED ONLY BY A PHYSICIAN. IT IS NOT TO BE DISPENSED TO THE PATIENT. Thoroughly cleanse affected area. Use supplied applicator to apply **Podocon-25 sparingly** to lesion. Avoid contact with healthy tissue. Allow to dry thoroughly. Only intact (no bleeding) lesions should be treated. As podophyllin is a powerful caustic and severe irritant, it is recommended the first application of **Podocon-25** be left in contact for only a short time (30 to 40 minutes) to determine patient's sensitivity. To avoid systemic absorption, time of contact should be minimum time necessary to produce the desired result (1 to 4 hours, depending on condititon of lesion and of patient), the physician developing his/her own experience and technique. Large areas or numerous warts should not be treated at once.

After treatment time has elapsed, remove dried **Podocon-25 thoroughly** with alcohol or soap and water.

HOW SUPPLIED

Podocon-25 is available in 15-mL bottles with tapered tip applicator attached inside cap. **NDC 0574-0601-15**

Store at room temperature 15°–30° C (59°–86° F) in tight, light-resistant containers.

Rx only

1) Blumgarten, A.F.: Text Book of Materia Medica, Pharmacology and Therapeutics; Ed. 7, New York, The Macmillan Company, 1937, pp. 220 and 223.
2) Green, L.K., Klima, M., Burns, T.; Arch Dermatol. Vol 124, Nov 1988, p. 1718.
3) Martindale, 28th Ed. London, 1982, pp. 1366, 1367.
4) Medical Letter; Vol 26, New Rochelle, N.Y., 1984, p10.
5) Fisher: Severe Systemic and Local Reactions to Topical Podophyllum Resins; Cutis, Volume 28, 1981.
6) Zackheim: Hazards of Topical Mitotic-Blocking Agents; Arch. Dermat. Volume 113, 1977.

IDENTIFICATION PROBLEM?
Turn to the **Product Identification Guide,**
where you'll find more than
1600 products pictured in actual
size and full color.

Par Pharmaceutical, Inc.

**ONE RAM RIDGE ROAD
SPRING VALLEY, NY 10977**

Direct Inquiries to:
Customer Service
(800) 828-9393
(845) 425-7100

The following is a listing of products currently available from Par Pharmaceutical, Inc.

NDC # 49884-	Product
587	Acebutolol Capsules 200 mg
588	Acebutolol Capsules 400 mg
565	Acyclovir Capsules 200 mg
566	Acyclovir Capsules 400 mg
567	Acyclovir Capsules 800 mg
602	Allopurinol Tablets 100 mg
603	Allopurinol Tablets 300 mg
448	Alprazolam Tablets 0.25 mg
449	Alprazolam Tablets 0.5 mg
450	Alprazolam Tablets 1 mg
400	Alprazolam Tablets 2 mg
117	Amiloride HCl Tablets 5 mg
458	Amiodarone HCl Tablets 200 mg
568	Amoxicillin Capsules 250 mg
569	Amoxicillin Capsules 500 mg
570	Amoxicillin Oral Suspension 125 mg
571	Amoxicillin Oral Suspension 250 mg
574	Ampicillin Capsules 250 mg
575	Ampicillin Capsules 500 mg
576	Ampicillin Oral Suspension 125 mg
577	Ampicillin Oral Suspension 250 mg
164	Benztropine Mesylate Tablets 0.5 mg
165	Benztropine Mesylate Tablets 1 mg
166	Benztropine Mesylate Tablets 2 mg
619	Captopril Tablets 12.5 mg
620	Captopril Tablets 25 mg
621	Captopril Tablets 50 mg
622	Captopril Tablets 100 mg
246	Carisoprodol and Aspirin Tablets 200 mg/325 mg
701	Clomiphene Tablets 50 mg
495	Clonazepam Tablets 0.5 mg
496	Clonazepam Tablets 1 mg
497	Clonazepam Tablets 2 mg
043	Cyproheptadine Tablets 4 mg
083	Dexamethasone Tablets 0.25 mg
084	Dexamethasone Tablets 0.5 mg
085	Dexamethasone Tablets 0.75 mg
086	Dexamethasone Tablets 1.5 mg
087	Dexamethasone Tablets 4 mg
129	Dexamethasone Tablets 6 mg
771	Diphenoxylate w/Atropine Sulfate Tablet 2.5 mg/.025 mg
217	Doxepin HCl Capsules 10 mg
218	Doxepin HCl Capsules 25 mg
219	Doxepin HCl Capsules 50 mg
220	Doxepin HCl Capsules 75 mg
221	Doxepin HCl Capsules 100 mg
222	Doxepin HCl Capsules 150 mg
596	Etodolac Tablets 500 mg
061	Fluphenazine HCl Tablets 1 mg
062	Fluphenazine HCl Tablets 2.5 mg
076	Fluphenazine HCl Tablets 5 mg
064	Fluphenazine HCl Tablets 10 mg
193	Flurazepam HCl Capsules 15 mg
194	Flurazepam HCl Capsules 30 mg
572	Guanfacine Tablets 1 mg
573	Guanfacine Tablets 2 mg
029	Hydralazine HCl Tablets 10 mg
027	Hydralazine HCl Tablets 25 mg
028	Hydralazine HCl Tablets 50 mg
121	Hydralazine HCl Tablets 100 mg
143	Hydra-Zide (Hydralazine HCl and Hydrochloro-thiazide) Capsules 25 mg/25 mg
144	Hydra-Zide (Hydralazine HCl and Hydrochloro-thiazide) Capsules 50 mg/50 mg
145	Hydra-Zide (Hydralazine HCl and Hydrochloro-thiazide) Capsules 100 mg/50 mg
724	Hydroxyurea Capsules 500 mg
200	Ibuprofen Tablets 200 mg
200	Ibuprofen Capsules 200 mg
162	Ibuprofen Tablets 400 mg
467	IBU (Ibuprofen Tablets) 400 mg
163	Ibuprofen Tablets 600 mg
468	IBU (Ibuprofen Tablets) 600 mg
216	Ibuprofen Tablets 800 mg
469	IBU (Ibuprofen Tablets) 800 mg
494	Ibuprofen Suspension 100 mg/5 ml
054	Imipramine HCl Tablets 10 mg
055	Imipramine HCl Tablets 25 mg
056	Imipramine HCl Tablets 50 mg
589	Indapamide Tablets 1.25 mg
590	Indapamide Tablets 2.5 mg
009	Isosorbide Dinitrate Tablets 30 mg
034	Meclizine HCl Tablets 12.5 mg
035	Meclizine HCl Tablets 25 mg
289	Megestrol Acetate Tablets 20 mg
290	Megestrol Acetate Tablets 40 mg
640	Methimazole Tablets 5 mg
641	Methimmazole Tablets 10 mg
643	Minocycline Capsules 50 mg
644	Minocycline Capsules 100 mg
249	Methocarbamol and Aspirin Tablets 400 mg/325 mg
490	Methylprednisolone Tablets 4 mg
256	Minoxidil Tablets 2.5 mg
257	Minoxidil Tablets 10 mg
542	Naproxen Sodium 220 mg
498	Nicardipine Capsules 20 mg
499	Nicardipine Capsules 30 mg
472	Orphengesic (Orphenadrine Citrate/Asa/Caff) Tablets 25 mg/385 mg/30 mg
473	Orphengesic Forte (Orphenadrine Citrate/Asa/Caff) Tablets 50 mg/770 mg/60 mg
578	Penicillin V Potassium Tablets 250 mg
579	Penicillin V Potassium Tablets 500 mg
580	Penicillin V Potassium Susp 125 mg
581	Penicillin V Potassium Susp 250 mg
549	Prochlorperazine Tablets 5 mg
550	Prochlorperazine Tablets 10 mg
544	Ranitidine Tablets 150 mg
545	Ranitidine Tablets 300 mg
610	Selegiline Tablets 5 mg
582	Sotolol Tablets 80 mg
583	Sotolol Tablets 120 mg
584	Sotolol Tablets 160 mg
585	Sotolol Tablets 240 mg
600	SSD (1% Silver Sulfadiazine) Cream
601	SSD AF (1% Silver Sulfadiazine) Cream
240	Temazepam Capsules 15 mg
241	Temazepam Capsules 30 mg
599	Ticlopidine HCl Tablets 250 mg
453	Triazolam Tablets 0.125 mg
454	Triazolam Tablets 0.25 mg
057	Zorprin Tablets 800 mg

Parkedale Pharmaceuticals

**870 PARKDALE ROAD
ROCHESTER, MI 48307**

Direct Inquiries to:
888-401-2879
FAX: 423-989-6279
Medical Emergency Contact:
Kathy Montgomery
800-546-4906
248-650-6407

APLISOL® ℞

[ăp' lĭsōl]

(Tuberculin Purified Protein Derivative, Diluted [Stabilized Solution])
Diagnostic Antigen
For Intradermal Injection Only

DESCRIPTION

Aplisol (tuberculin PPD, diluted) is a sterile aqueous solution of purified protein fraction for intradermal administration as an aid in the diagnosis of tuberculosis. The solution is stabilized with polysorbate (Tween)80, buffered with potassium and sodium phosphates and contains approximately 0.35% phenol as a preservative. This product is ready for immediate use without further dilution.

The purified protein fraction is isolated from culture media filtrates of a human strain of *Mycobacterium tuberculosis* by the method of F.B. Seibert.[1,2] Tuberculin PPD, diluted, is prepared from Tuberculin PPD Powder Master Lot 154616 which is clinically bioequivalent in potency to the standard PPD-S* (5 TU** per 0.1mL) of the U.S. Public Health Service, National Centers for Disease Control. This product is made from a single master lot (No. 154616) to eliminate lot to lot variation inherent in manufacturing.

The potency of each lot of tuberculin PPD, diluted is determined in sensitized guinea pigs.

CLINICAL PHARMACOLOGY

In the United States, the prevalence of *Mycobacterium tuberculosis* infection and active disease varies for different segments of the population; however, the risk for *M. tuberculosis* infection in the overall population is low. Tuberculosis (TB) case rates declined steadily for decades in the United States. However, in 1985 the TB case rate stabilized and subsequently increased through 1992, accompanied by a 14% increase in the TB mortality rate in 1988. This has been attributed to several complex social and medical factors, including the human immunodeficiency virus (HIV) epidemic, the occurrence of TB in foreign-born persons from countries that have a high prevalence of TB, the emergence of drug-resistant strains of TB, and the transmission of *M. tuberculosis* in congregate settings. (e.g., health-care facilities, correctional facilities, drug-treatment centers, and homeless shelters). Because the overall risk of acquiring M. tuberculosis is low for the total U.S. population, the primary strategy for preventing and controlling TB in the United States is to minimize the risk transmission by the early identification and treatment of patients who have active infectious TB, finding screening persons who have been in contact with active infectious TB patients and screening high-risk populations.

Tuberculin PPD is recommended by the American Lung Association as an aid in the detection of infection with *Mycobacterium tuberculosis*.[3,4] After a person becomes infected with mycobacteria, T lymphocytes proliferate and become sensitized. These sensitized T cells enter the bloodstream and circulate for months or years. This sensitization process occurs principally in the regional lymph nodes and may take 2–10 weeks to develop following infection. Once acquired, tuberculin sensitivity tends to persist, although it often wanes with time and advancing age. The injection of tuberculin into the skin stimulates the lymphocytes and activates a series of events leading to a delayed-type hypersensitivity (DTH) response. This response is called "delayed" because the reaction becomes evident hours after injection. Dermal reactivity involves vasodilation, edema, and the infiltration of lymphocytes, basophils, monocytes, and neutrophils into the site of antigen injection. Antigen-specific T lymphocytes proliferate and release lymphokines, which mediate the accumulation of other cells at the site. The area of induration reflects DTH activity.[5] In most tuberculin-sensitive individuals, the delayed hypersensitivity reaction is evident 5–6 hours after administration of a tuberculin skin test and is maximal 48–72 hours. In geriatric patients or in patients receiving a tuberculin skin test for the first time, the reaction may develop more slowly and may not be maximal until after 72 hours.[6] Because their immune systems are immature, many neonates and infants < 6 weeks of age, who are infected with *M. tuberculosis*, do not react at all to tuberculin tests.[5]

Immediate erythematous or other hypersensitivity reactions to tuberculin or the constituents of the diluent may occur at the injection site. A possible decrease in responsiveness to skin testing may occur in the presence of tuberculous infections including viral infections, live virus vaccination, overwhelming tuberculosis, other bacterial infections, drugs and malignancy.

Tuberculin skin-test results are also less reliable as CD4 counts decline in HIV infected individuals.[3]

The 5TU dose of Tuberculin PPD intradermally (Mantoux) is recommended as the standard tuberculin test, and Tuberculin PPD is recommended by the American Lung Association as an aid in the detection of infection with *Mycobacterium tuberculosis*. Reactions to the Mantoux test are interpreted on the basis of a quantitative measurement of the response to a specific dose (5 TU PPD-S or equivalent) of Tuberculin PPD[7].

To determine that Tuberculin PPD Master Lot 154616 is clinically bioequivalent in potency to standard 5TU PPD-S*, 3 dose-response studies were conducted in the following populations (1) persons with a history of bacteriologically confirmed TB; (2) healthy volunteers in a geographical region of low endemicity of atypical mycobacterial infection; and (3) healthy volunteers in a geographical location of high endemicity of atypical mycobacterial infection.

*PPD-S (No. 49608) World Health Organization International PPD-Tuberculin Standard (PPD-S is a dried powder from which WHO and U.S. Standard tuberculin solutions are made.)

**U.S. Tuberculin Unit

INDICATIONS AND USAGE

Tuberculin PPD is recommended by the American Lung Association as an aid in the detection of infection with *Mycobacterium tuberculosis*. The standard tuberculin test recommended employs the intradermal (Mantoux) test using a 5TU dose of tuberculin PPD.[7] The 0.1-mL test dose of Aplisol (tuberculin PPD, diluted) is equivalent to the 5 TU dose recommended as clinically established and standardized with PPD-S. Tuberculin skin testing is not contraindicated for persons who have been vaccinated with BCG and the skin-test results of such persons are used to support or exclude the diagnosis of *M. tuberculosis* infections.[4]

HIV infection is a strong risk factor for the development of TB disease in persons having TB infection. All HIV-infected persons should receive a PPD-tuberculin skin test.[3]

CONTRAINDICATIONS

Aplisol is contraindicated in patients with known hypersensitivity or allergy to Aplisol or any of its components. Aplisol should not be administered to persons who have previously experienced a severe reaction (e.g., vesiculation, ulceration, or necrosis) because of the severity of reactions that may occur at the test site.

WARNINGS

Tuberculin should be administered with caution to known tuberculin-positive reactors because of the severity of reactions (e.g., vesiculation, ulceration, or necrosis) that may occur at the test site in very sensitive individuals.

Not all infected persons will have a delayed hypersensitivity reaction to a tuberculin test. A number of factors have been reported to cause a decreased ability to respond to the tuberculin test, such as the presence of tuberculous infection or viral infections (measles, mumps chickenpox, and HIV), live virus vaccination (measles, mumps, rubella, oral polio and yellow fever), overwhelming tuberculosis, other bacterial infections, drugs (corticosteroids and other immunosuppressive agents) and malignancy.[8,9]

Any condition that impairs or attenuates cell mediated immunity potentially can cause a false negative reaction.

Tuberculin skin test results are less reliable in HIV-infected individuals as CD4 counts decline (see CLINICAL PHARMACOLOGY).[3]

Aplisol should not be administered to persons who previously experienced a severe reaction (e.g., vesiculation, ulceration, or necrosis) because of the severity of reactions that may occur at the test site (see CONTRAINDICATIONS).

Avoid injecting tuberculin subcutaneously. If this occurs, no local reaction develops, but a general febrile reaction and/or acute inflammation around old tuberculous lesions may occur in highly sensitive individuals.

PRECAUTIONS

General

The predictive value of the tuberculin skin test depends on the prevalence of infection with *M. tuberculosis* and the relative prevalence of cross-reactions with nontuberculous mycobacteria.[9,10]

A separate, sterile, single-use disposable syringes and needles should be used for each individual patient to prevent possible transmission of serum hepatitis virus and other infectious agents from one person to another.

Special care should be taken to ensure that the product is injected intradermally and not into a blood vessel.

Before administration of Aplisol, a review of the patient's history with respect to possible immediate-type hypersensitivity to the product, determination of previous use of Aplisol and the presence of any contraindication to the test should be made (see CONTRAINDICATIONS). As with any biological product, epinephrine should be immediately available in case an anaphylactoid or acute hypersensitivity reaction occurs.

Failure to store and handle Aplisol as recommended may result in a loss of potency and inaccurate test results.[11,8]

Reactivity to the test may be depressed or suppressed for as long as 5–6 weeks in individuals following immunization with certain live viral vaccines, viral infections or discontinuation of corticosteroids or immunosuppressive agents.[8,9]

Information to Patients

Patients should be instructed to report adverse events such as vesiculation, ulceration or necrosis which may occur at the test site in highly sensitive individuals. Patients should be informed that pain, pruritus and discomfort may occur at injection site.

Patient should be informed of the need to return to their physician or health care provider for the reading of the test and of the need to keep and maintain a personal immunization record.

Drug Interactions

In patients who are receiving corticosteroids or immunosuppressive agents, reactivity to the test may be depressed or suppressed. This reduced reactivity may present for as long as 5–6 weeks after discontinuation of therapy (see PRECAUTIONS-General).[9]

The reactivity to PPD may be temporarily depressed by certain live virus vaccines. Therefore, if a tuberculin test is to be performed, it should be administered either before or simultaneously with the use of oral polio and/or injection of measles, mumps and rubella vaccines in combined form or as separate antigens, or testing should be postponed for 4–6 weeks.[10]

Carcinogenesis, Mutagenesis, Impairment of Fertility

No long term studies have been conducted in animals or in humans to evaluate carcinogenic or mutagenic potential or effects on fertility with Aplisol.

Pregnancy

Teratogenic effects: Pregnancy Category C. Animal reproduction studies have not been conducted with Aplisol. It is also not known whether Aplisol can cause fetal harm when administered to a pregnant woman or can affect the reproduction capacity. Aplisol should be given to a pregnant woman only if clearly needed.

However, the risk of unrecognized tuberculosis and the postpartum contact between a mother with active disease and an infant leaves the infant in grave danger of tuberculosis and complications such as tuberculous meningitis. Although there have not been any reported adverse effects upon the fetus recognized as being due to tuberculosis skin testing, the prescribing physician will want to consider if the potential benefits outweigh the possible risks for performing the tuberculin test on a pregnant woman or a woman of childbearing age, particularly in certain high risk populations.

ADVERSE REACTIONS

In highly sensitive individuals, strongly positive reactions including vesiculation, ulceration or necrosis may occur at the test site. Cold packs or topical steroid preparations may be employed for symptomatic relief of the associated pain, pruritus and discomfort.

Strongly positive test reactions may result in scarring at the test site. Immediate erythematous or other reactions may occur at the injection site.

DOSAGE AND ADMINISTRATION

Aplisol vials should be inspected visually for both particulate matter and discoloration prior to administration and discarded of either is seen. Vials in use for more than 30 days should be discarded.

Standard Method (Mantoux Test)

The Mantoux test is performed by **intradermally** injecting with a syringe and needle exactly 0.1mL of Aplisol. The result is read 48 to 72 hours later and **induration only is considered in interpreting the test.**

Induration is a hard, raised area with clearly defined margins at and around the injection site. Erythema may develop at the injection site but has no diagnostic value. The standard test is performed as follows:

1. The site of the test is usually the flexor or dorsal surface of the forearm about 4" below the elbow. Other skin sites may be used, but the flexor surface of the forearm is preferred. The use of a skin area free of lesions and away from any veins is recommended.[7]
2. The skin at the injection site is cleansed with 70% alcohol and allowed to dry.
3. The test material is administered with a tuberculin syringe (0.5 or 1.0mL) fitted with a short (1/2") 26 or 27 gauge needle.
4. A separate, sterile, single-use disposable syringe and needles should be used for each individual patient.
5. The diaphragm of the vial-stopper should be wiped with 70% alcohol.
6. The needle is inserted through the stopper diaphragm of the inverted vial. Exactly 0.1 mL is filled into the syringe with care being taken to exclude air bubbles and to maintain the lumen of the needle filled.
7. The point of the needle is inserted into the most superficial layers of the skin with the needle bevel pointed upward. **As the tuberculin solution is injection, a pale bleb 6 to 10mm in size (1/3) will rise over the point of the needle.** This is quickly absorbed and no dressing is required.

In the event the injection is delivered subcutaneously (i.e., no bleb will form), or if a significant part of the dose leaks from the injection site, the test should be repeated immediately at another site at least 5cm (2") removed.

The Mantoux test is the standard of comparison for all other tuberculin tests.

Interpretation of tuberculin Reaction

Readings of Mantoux reactions should be made during the period from 48 to 72 hours after the injection. **Induration only should be considered in interpreting the test.** The diameter of induration should be measured transversely to the long axis of the forearm and recorded in millimeters. Erythema has no diagnostic value and should be disregarded. The presence and size of necrosis and edema if present should be recorded although not used in the interpretation of the test. In the absence of induration, an area of erythema greater than 10 mm is diameter may indicate the injection was made too deeply and retesting is indicated.

Reactions should be interpreted as follows:

Positive—A positive reaction to the tuberculin skin test may not be seen until 2–10 weeks after the infection.[7] Based in current guidelines,[3,12] interpretation of positive reactions (depending on the age, immune status or risk factors of the persons tested) is:

1. An induration of ≥5mm is classified as positive in the following:
   - Person who have had recent close contact with persons who have active TB;
   - Persons who have human immunodeficiency virus (HIV) infection or risk factors for HIV infection but unknown HIV status;
   - Persons who have fibrotic chest radiographs consistent with healed TB.
2. An induration of ≥10mm is classified as positive in all persons who do not meet any of the above criteria, but who belong to one or more of the following groups at high risk for TB:
   - Injecting-drug users known to be HIV seronegative;
   - Persons who have other medical conditions that have been reported to increase the risk for progressing from latent TB infection to active TB infection. These medical conditions include diabetes mellitus, conditions requiring prolonged high-dose corticosteroid therapy and other immunosuppressive therapy (including bone marrow and organ transplantation), chronic renal failure, some hematologic disorders (e.g., leukemias and lymphomas), other specific malignancies (e.g., carcinoma of the head or neck), weight loss of ≥10% below ideal body weight, silicosis, gastrectomy, jejunileal bypass;
   - Residents and employees of high-risk congregate settings; prisons and jails, nursing homes and other long-term facilities for the elderly, health-care facilities (including some residential mental health facilities), and homeless shelters;
   - Foreign-born persons recently arrived (i.e., within the last 5 years) from countries having a high prevalence or incidence of TB;
   - Some medically underserved, low-income populations, including migrant farm workers and homeless persons;
   - High-risk racial or ethnic minority populations, as defined locally;
   - Children <4 years of age or infants, children and adolescents exposed to adults in high-risk categories.
3. An induration of ≥ 15mm is classified as positive in persons who do not meet any of the above criteria.

Negative—Induration of less than 5 mm. This indicates a lack of hypersensitivity to tuberculoprotein and tuberculous infection is highly unlikely.

Continued on next page

Aplisol—Cont.

Booster Effect—Infection of an individual with tubercle bacilli or other mycobacteria or BCG vaccination results in a delayed hypersensitivity response to tuberculin which is demonstrated by the skin test. The delayed hypersensitivity response may gradually wane over a period of years. If a person receives a tuberculin test at this time, a significant reaction may not be detected. However, the stimulus of the test may boost or increase the size of the reaction to a second test, sometimes causing an apparent conversion or development of sensitivity. This booster effect can be seen on a second test done one week after the initial stimulating test and can persist for a year, and perhaps longer. When routine periodic tuberculin testing of adults is done, initially two-stage testing should be considered to minimize the likelihood of interpreting a boosted reaction as a conversion.[13,14]

It should be noted that reactivity to tuberculin may be depressed or suppressed for as long as 5–6 weeks by viral infections, live virus vaccines (i.e., measles, smallpox, polio, rubella and mumps), or after discontinuation of therapy with corticosteroids or immunosuppressive agents.

Malnutrition may also have a similar effect. When of diagnostic importance, a negative test should be accepted as proof that hypersensitivity is absent only after normal reactivity to non-specific irritants has been demonstrated. A primary injection of tuberculin may possibly have a boosting effect on subsequent tuberculin reactions.

A pediatric patient who is known to have been exposed to a person with tuberculosis must not be adjudged free of infection until that patient has a negative tuberculin reaction at least ten weeks after contact with tuberculous person has ceased.[15] Annual testing is generally recommended for pediatric patients in high risk populations, such as persons from countries with a high prevalence of tuberculosis and low-income groups.[16]

A positive tuberculin reaction does not necessarily signify the presence of active disease. Further diagnostic procedures (e.g., chest radiograph, sputum smear and/or culture examination) should be carried out before a diagnosis of tuberculosis is made. A small percentage of responders may not have been infected with *M. tuberculosis* but by some other mycobacterium. The negative tuberculin skin test should never be used to exclude the possibility of active tuberculosis among persons for whom the diagnosis is being considered (symptoms compatible with tuberculosis).

HOW SUPPLIED

Tuberculin PPD-Aplisol bioequivalent to 5US units (TU) PPD-S per test dose (0.1mL) is available in the following presentations:

NDC 64029-4525-3 (Bio. 1525)

1 mL (10 tests) - rubber-diaphragm-capped vial

NDC 64029-4525-4 (Bio. 1607)

5 mL (50 tests) - rubber-diaphragm-capped vial

This product is ready for use without further dilution.

Storage

DO NOT FREEZE

This product should be stored at 2°–8°C (36°–46°F) and protected from light.

Vials in use more than 30 days should be discarded due to possible oxidation and degradation which may affect potency.

REFERENCES

1. Seibert, F.B.: Am Rev Tuberc, 30:713, 1934
2. Seibert, F.B., and Glenn, J.T.: Am Rev Tuberc, 44:9, 1941
3. MMWR, 1995:44 RR-11
4. MMWR, 1996:45 RR-4
5. Huebner RE, Shein MF, Bass JB, The Tuberculin Skin Test, *Clin Infect Dis*, 1993;17:968-75
6. AHFS Drug Information, 1997, 36:84 pp 1962-1968
7. American Thoracic Society: Diagnostic Standards and classification of tuberculosis, 1990 Am Rev Respir Dis, 142:725-735
8. Am Rev Respir Dis, 1985;886
9. Brickman HF et.Al., The Timing of Tuberculin Tests in Relation to Immunization with Live Viral Vaccines, *Pediatrics*; 1975;55:392
10. Red Book Report of the Committee on Infectious Disease, (1994)
11. Landi S, Held HR, Stability of a dilute solution of tuberculin purified derivative at extreme temperatures, *J Biol Stand*, 1981; 9:195
12. Diagnosis of TB Infection and TB Disease, Centers For Disease Control and Prevention(CDC), March 21, 1996, Doc#2250102
13. Sewell, E.M., O'Hare, D., and Kendig, E.L., Jr.: The Tuberculin Test, Pediatrics, Vol.54, No. 5, Nov.1974.
14. Advisory Committee of Elimination of Tuberculosis (ACET/CDC: Prevention and control of tuberculosis in facilities providing long-term care to the elderly, 1990. MMWR 39(10): 7–13,15.
15. ACET(CDC): The use of preventative therapy therapy for tuberculosis infection in the United States, 1990. MMWR 39(8):9–12.
16. ACET(CDC): Screening for tuberculosis and tuberculosis infection in high risk populations. Recommendations of the ACET, 1990. MMWR 39(8):1–7.

Rx only.

Rev. 7/98

0932906

Manufactured by: Parkedale Pharmaceuticals, Inc.
Rochester, MI 48307

Shown in Product Identification Guide, page 329

INFLUENZA VIRUS VACCINE, TRIVALENT, TYPES A AND B FLUOGEN® ℞

2000–2001 Formula

Subvirion Vaccine/Immunizing Antigen, Ether Extracted

DESCRIPTION

Fluogen (Influenza Virus Vaccine, Trivalent, Types A and B) is a sterile product for intramuscular injection composed of the antigens of the strains of influenza virus recommended for vaccine use during the 2000–2001 season by the US Public Health Service. It is formulated to contain no less than 45 micrograms of hemagglutinin antigen (HA) content per 0.5 mL dose in the recommended ratio of 15µg of HA of the A influenza virus component representative of A/New Caledonia/20/99 (H1N1), 15 µg of HA of the A influenza virus component representative of A/Panama/2007/99 (A/Moscow/10/99-like) (H3N2), and 15 µg of HA of the B influenza virus component representative of B/Yamanashi/166/98 (B/Beijing/184/93-like).

Influenza virus is propagated in embryonated chicken eggs using an inoculum containing approximately 1 mg/mL streptomycin sulfate. The allantoic fluids containing the virus are harvested, clarified by filtration, and concentrated and refined by ultracentrifugation and zonal centrifugation. Polysorbate 80, USP, is added to the refined concentrate, which is subsequently extracted with ethyl ether to disrupt the virus and allow removal of a high proportion of pyrogenic substances. The extracted concentrate is inactivated with formaldehyde. The vaccine is diluted to its final volume with phosphate-buffered-saline solution. Thimerosal (mercury derivative) 0.01% is added as a preservative. Streptomycin sulfate is undetectable (less than the limit of detection of the assay) in the final product.

Treatment of the influenza virus with ethyl ether results in disruption or "splitting" of the virus. The active immunizing antigens, hemagglutinin and neuraminidase, are retained while a high proportion of egg protein and pyrogenic substances are removed. The resultant split-virus vaccine has been shown to be less reactogenic than whole-virus vaccines in younger age groups.

CLINICAL PHARMACOLOGY

The inoculation of antigen prepared from inactivated influenza virus stimulates the production of specific antibodies. Protection is afforded only against those strains of virus from which the vaccine is prepared or closely related strains.

The effectiveness of influenza vaccine in preventing or attenuating illness varies, depending primarily on the age and immunocompetence of the vaccine recipient and the degree of similarity between the virus strains included in the vaccine and those that circulate during the influenza season. When a good match exists between vaccine and circulating viruses, influenza vaccine has been shown to prevent illness in approximately 70%–90% of healthy persons ages less than 65 years. Under these circumstances, studies also have indicated that the effectiveness of influenza vaccine in preventing hospitalization for pneumonia and influenza among elderly persons living in settings other than nursing homes or similar chronic-care facilities ranges from 30%–70%. Among elderly persons residing in nursing homes, influenza vaccine is most effective in preventing severe illness, secondary complications, and death. Studies in this population have indicated that the vaccine can be 50%–60% effective in preventing hospitalization and pneumonia and 80% effective in preventing death, even though efficacy in preventing influenza illness may often be in the range of 30%–40% among the frail elderly. Achieving a high rate of vaccination among nursing home residents can reduce the spread of infection in a facility, thus preventing disease through herd immunity. Vaccination of health care workers in nursing homes has also been demonstrated to reduce the impact of influenza among residents.

Based on the most recent epidemiological and laboratory data, the US Public Health Service anticipates that the strains prevalent in 2000–2001 will be closely related to A/New Caledonia/20/99 (H1N1), A/Panama/2007/99 (A/Moscow/10/99-like) (H3N2), and B/Yamanashi/166/98 (B/Beijing/184/93-like). Therefore, these strains will be included in the influenza virus vaccine for use during the 2000–2001 season.

INDICATIONS AND USAGE

Fluogen is indicated for the production of immunity to influenza virus containing antigens related to those in the vaccine.

Influenza vaccine is strongly recommended for any person 6 months of age or older who, because of age or underlying medical condition, is at increased risk for complications of influenza. Health-care workers and others (including household members) in close contact with persons in high-risk groups should also be vaccinated. In addition, influenza vaccine may be administered to any person aged ≥ 6 months who wishes to reduce the chance of becoming infected with influenza. Guidelines for the use of vaccine among certain patient populations follow.[1]

TARGET GROUPS FOR SPECIAL VACCINATION PROGRAMS

To maximize protection of high-risk persons, they and their close contacts should be targeted for organized vaccination programs.

Groups at increased risk for influenza-related complications:

1. Persons 50 years of age or older.
2. Residents of nursing homes and other chronic-care facilities that house persons of any age who have chronic medical conditions.
3. Adults and pediatric patients with chronic disorders of the pulmonary or cardiovascular systems, including asthma.
4. Adults and pediatric patients who have required regular medical follow-up or hospitalization during the preceding year because of chronic metabolic diseases (including diabetes mellitus), renal dysfunction, hemoglobinopathies, or immunosuppression (including immunosuppression caused by medications or by human immunodeficiency virus).
5. Pediatric patients and young adults (6 months to 18 years of age) who are receiving long-term aspirin therapy and, therefore, may be at risk for developing Reye syndrome after influenza.

Groups that can transmit influenza to persons at high risk: Persons who are clinically or subclinically infected and who care for or live with members of high-risk groups can transmit influenza virus to them. Some persons at high risk (eg, the elderly, transplant recipients, and persons with acquired immunodeficiency syndrome [AIDS]) can have a low antibody response to influenza vaccine. Efforts to protect these members of high-risk groups against influenza might be improved by reducing the likelihood of influenza exposure from their caregivers.

Therefore, the following groups should be vaccinated:

1. Physicians, nurses, and other personnel in both hospital and outpatient-care settings.
2. Employees of nursing homes and chronic-care facilities who have contact with patients or residents.
3. Employees of assisted living and other residences for persons in high-risk groups.
4. Providers of home care to persons at high risk (eg, visiting nurses, volunteer workers).
5. Household-members (including the pediatric population 6 months of age or older) of persons in high-risk groups.

VACCINATION OF OTHER GROUPS

General population: Physicians should administer influenza vaccine to any person greater than or equal to age 6 months who wishes to reduce the likelihood of becoming ill with influenza. Persons who provide essential community services should be considered for vaccination to minimize disruption of essential activities during influenza outbreaks. Students or other persons in institutional settings, such as those who reside in dormitories, should be encouraged to receive vaccine to minimize the disruption of routine activities during epidemics.

Pregnant women: Influenza-associated excess mortality among pregnant women has not been documented except during the pandemics of 1918–19 and 1957–58. However, because death-certificate data often do not indicate whether a woman was pregnant at the time of death, studies conducted during interpandemic periods may underestimate the impact of influenza in this population. Case reports and limited studies suggest that pregnancy may increase the risk for serious medical complications of influenza as a result of increases in heart rate, stroke volume and oxygen consumption, decreases in lung capacity, and changes in immunologic function. A recent study of the impact of influenza during 17 interpandemic influenza seasons documented that the relative risk of hospitalization for selected cardiorespiratory conditions among pregnant women increased from 1.4 during weeks 14–20 of gestation to 4.7 during weeks 37–42 compared with rates among women who were 1–6 months postpartum. Women in their third trimester of pregnancy were hospitalized at a rate comparable to that of nonpregnant women who have high-risk medical conditions for whom influenza vaccine was traditionally recommended. Physicians generally avoid prescribing unnecessary drugs and biologics for pregnant women especially in the first trimester; however, there are no data specifically to contraindicate vaccination with the available killed virus vaccine in pregnant women who have underlying high-risk conditions. (See also PRECAUTIONS.)

Persons infected with human immunodeficiency virus (HIV): Limited information exists regarding the frequency and severity of influenza illness or the benefits of influenza vaccination among persons with human immunodeficiency virus (HIV) infection. However, a recent retrospective study of young and middle-aged women enrolled in Tennessee's Medicaid program found that the attributable risk for cardiopulmonary hospitalizations among women with HIV infection was higher during influenza seasons than in the peri-influenza periods. The risk of hospitalization for HIV-infected women was higher than the risk for women with other well-recognized high-risk conditions for influenza complications, including chronic heart and lung diseases. Other reports suggest that influenza symptoms might be prolonged and the risk for complications from influenza increased for some HIV-infected persons.

Influenza vaccine has produced substantial antibody titers against influenza in vaccinated HIV-infected persons who have minimal acquired immunodeficiency syndrome-related symptoms and high $CD4_+$ T-lymphocyte cell counts. However, in patients who have advanced HIV disease and low $CD4_+$ T-lymphocyte cell counts, influenza vaccine might not induce protective antibody titers; a second dose of vaccine does not improve the immune response in these persons. Because influenza can result in serious illness and complications and because influenza vaccination can result in the production of protective antibody titers vaccination will benefit many HIV-infected patients, including HIV-infected pregnant women.

Foreign travelers: The risk for exposure to influenza during foreign travel varies, depending on season and destination. In the tropics, influenza can occur throughout the year; in the Southern Hemisphere, most activity occurs from April through September. Because of the short incubation period for influenza, exposure to the virus during travel can result in clinical illness that begins while travelling, an inconvenience or potential danger, especially for persons at increased risk for complications. Persons preparing to travel to the tropics at any time of year, travel with large organized tourist groups at any time of year, or to travel to the Southern Hemisphere from April through September should review their influenza vaccination histories. If they were not vaccinated the previous fall/winter, they should consider influenza vaccination before travel. Persons in the high-risk categories should be especially encouraged to receive the most current vaccine. Persons at high risk who received the previous season's vaccine before travel should be revaccinated in the fall/winter with the current vaccine.

TIMING OF INFLUENZA VACCINATION ACTIVITIES

Beginning each September, when vaccine for the upcoming influenza season becomes available, persons at high risk who are seen by health-care providers for routine care or as a result of hospitalization should be offered influenza vaccine. Opportunities to vaccinate persons at high risk for complications of influenza should not be missed.

The optimal time for organized vaccination campaigns for persons in high-risk groups is usually the period from the beginning of October through mid-November. In the United States, influenza activity generally peaks between late December and early March. High levels of influenza activity infrequently occur in the contiguous 48 states before December. Although vaccine generally becomes available in August or September, in some years, vaccine for the upcoming influenza season might not be available in some locations until later in the fall. To minimize the possibility that large organized vaccination campaigns will need to be canceled because vaccine is unavailable, persons planning large organized vaccination campaigns may consider scheduling these events after mid-October because the availability of vaccine in any location cannot be assured consistently in the early fall. Administering vaccine too far in advance of the influenza season should be avoided in facilities such as nursing homes because antibody levels might begin to decline within a few months of vaccination. Vaccination programs can be undertaken as soon as current vaccine is available if regional influenza activity is expected to begin earlier than December.

Pediatric patients under 9 years of age who have not been vaccinated previously should receive two doses of vaccine at least one month apart to maximize the likelihood of a satisfactory antibody response to all three vaccine antigens. The second dose should be administered before December, if possible. Vaccine should be offered to both the pediatric and adult populations up to and even after influenza virus activity is documented in a community.

The degree of protection afforded by immunization with any vaccine may not be sufficient to prevent the disease if the exposure to the influenza virus strains is overwhelming or if the virus strains are not closely related antigenically to those used in the production of vaccine.

CONTRAINDICATIONS

INFLUENZA VIRUS VACCINE SHOULD NOT BE ADMINISTERED TO INDIVIDUALS WITH A HISTORY OF HYPERSENSITIVITY (ALLERGY) TO CHICKEN EGGS OR TO OTHER COMPONENTS OF INFLUENZA VIRUS VACCINE, INCLUDING THIMEROSAL (see ADVERSE REACTIONS).

In persons suspected of having an allergic condition, immunization procedures should be preceded by testing and/or desensitization procedures conducted under the supervision of a physician. A positive skin reaction contraindicates immunization with the vaccine. See PRECAUTIONS.

Immunization should be deferred in the presence of any acute respiratory disease or other active infection.

WARNING

Persons being given immunosuppressive therapy or other immunosuppressed individuals may experience a lower than expected antigenic response.

The packaging of this product contains natural rubber latex which may cause allergic reactions.

PRECAUTIONS

General

A separate sterile syringe and needle should be used for each patient to prevent transmission of hepatitis B virus or other infectious agents from one person to another.

Although current influenza vaccines contain only a minute quantity of egg protein, they do, on rare occasions, provoke anaphylactic hypersensitivity reactions. Epinephrine 1 mg/mL (1:1000) should be available and ready for immediate use should such reactions occur.

Because of the possibility of a febrile reaction following immunization with influenza virus vaccine, the wisdom of attempting to immunize patients with a history of febrile convulsion should be given careful consideration. Persons with acute febrile illnesses usually should not be vaccinated until their temporary symptoms have abated.

Proper precautions should be taken for persons with known sensitivity to latex, which is present in packaging components of this product.

Drug Interactions

Although influenza vaccination can inhibit the clearance of warfarin and theophylline, studies have failed to show any adverse clinical effects attributable to these drugs in patients receiving influenza vaccine.

Concomitant influenza vaccination and immunosuppressive therapy (eg, corticosteroids, chemotherapy) may be associated with impaired immune response to the vaccine.

Pregnancy

Pregnancy Category C:

Animal reproduction studies have not been conducted with influenza vaccine. It is also not known whether influenza vaccine can cause fetal harm when administered to a pregnant woman or can affect reproduction capacity. Influenza vaccine should be given to a pregnant woman only if clearly needed. (See also INDICATIONS AND USAGE.)

Nursing Mothers

Influenza vaccine does not affect the safety of breastfeeding for mothers or infants. Breastfeeding does not adversely affect immune response and is not a contraindication for vaccination.

Pediatric Use

The safety and effectiveness of Fluogen in infants below the age of 6 months have not been established.

ADVERSE REACTIONS

Side effects of influenza vaccine administration are generally inconsequential in adults and occur at low frequency. The most frequent side effect of vaccination is soreness at the vaccination site that lasts for up to two days. Severe reactions are uncommon in adults, and truly disabling effects appear to be exceedingly rare.

The following types of systemic reactions to influenza vaccine have occurred:

Fever, malaise, myalgia, and other systemic symptoms of toxicity occurring 6 to 12 hours after vaccination and persisting one or two days. These responses to influenza vaccine are usually attributed to characteristics of the influenza virus antigens (even though the virus is inactivated) and represent the bulk of the side effects of influenza vaccination. Such effects occur most frequently in persons who have had no exposure to the influenza virus antigen in the vaccine (eg, young children).

Immediate, presumably allergic, responses, such as hives, angioedema, allergic asthma, and systemic anaphylaxis, are expressions of hypersensitivity. These reactions occur rarely after influenza vaccination. They probably derive from exquisite sensitivity to some vaccine component, most likely to residual egg protein.

Neurologic disorders, including such central nervous system conditions as encephalopathy, have a temporal association with influenza vaccination.

Rare occurrences of optic neuritis and vasiculitis following administration of influenza vaccine have been recently reported in the literature.

The 1976 swine influenza vaccine was associated with an increased frequency of Guillain-Barré syndrome(GBS). Among persons who received the swine influenza vaccine in 1976, the rate of GBS that exceeded the background rate was slightly less than 10 cases per million persons vaccinated. Evidence for a casual relationship of GBS with subsequent vaccines prepared from other virus strains is less clear. Obtaining strong epidemiologic evidence for a possible small increase in risk is difficult for a rare condition such as GBS, which has an annual incidence of only 10–20 cases per million adults, and stretches the limits of epidemiologic investigation. More definitive data probably will require the use of other methodologies such as laboratory studies of the pathophysiology of GBS.

During three of four influenza seasons studied from 1977–1991, the overall relative risk estimates for GBS after influenza vaccination were slightly elevated but were not statistically significant in any of these studies. However, in a study of the 1992–1993 and 1993–1994 seasons, the overall relative risk for GBS was 1.7 (95% confidence interval = 1.0–2.8; p = 0.04) during the 6 weeks following vaccination, representing an excess of slightly more than one additional case of GBS per million persons vaccinated; the combined number of GBS cases peaked 2 weeks after vaccination. Thus, investigations to date suggest no large increase in GBS associated with influenza vaccines (other than the swine influenza vaccine in 1976) and that if influenza vaccine does pose a risk, it is probably quite small—slightly more than one additional case per million persons vaccinated. Cases of GBS following influenza infection have been reported, but no epidemiologic studies have documented such an association. Good evidence exists that several infectious illnesses, most notably *Campylobacter jejuni* as well as upper respiratory tract infections in general, are associated with GBS.

Even if GBS were a true side effect of vaccination in the years after 1976, the estimated risk for GBS of slightly more than one additional case per million persons vaccinated is substantially less than the risk for severe influenza, which could be prevented by vaccination in all age groups, especially persons aged >65 years and those who have medical indications for influenza vaccination. During different epidemics occurring from 1972 through 1981, estimated rates of influenza-associated hospitalization have ranged from approximately 200 to 300 hospitalizations per million population for previously healthy persons aged 5–44 years and from 2,000 to > 10,000 hospitalizations per million population for persons aged >65 years. During epidemics from 1972–1973 through 1994–1995, estimated rates of influenza-associated death have ranged from approximately 300 to > 1,500 per million persons aged >65 years, who account for more than 90% of all influenza-associated deaths. The potential benefits of influenza vaccination in preventing serious illness, hospitalization, and death greatly outweigh the possible risks for developing vaccine-associated GBS.

The average case-fatality ratio for GBS is 6% and increases with age. However, no evidence indicates that the case-fatality ratio for GBS differs among vaccinated persons and those not vaccinated.

The incidence of GBS in the general population is very low, but persons with a history of GBS have a substantially greater likelihood of subsequently developing GBS than persons without such a history. Thus, the likelihood of coincidentally developing GBS after influenza vaccination is expected to be greater among persons with a history of GBS than among persons with no history of this syndrome. Whether influenza vaccination specifically might increase the risk for recurrence of GBS is not known. Therefore, it would seem prudent to avoid influenza vaccination of persons who are not at high risk for severe influenza complications and who are known to have developed GBS within 6 weeks of a previous influenza vaccination. However, many experts believe that for most persons who have a history of GBS and who are at high risk for severe complications from influenza, the established benefits of influenza vaccination justify yearly vaccination.

DOSAGE AND ADMINISTRATION

Although the current influenza vaccine can contain one or more of the antigens administered in previous years, annual vaccination with the current vaccine is necessary because immunity declines in the year following vaccination.

Because the 2000–2001 vaccine differs from the 1999–2000 vaccine, supplies of 1999–2000 vaccine should not be administered to provide protection for the 2000–2001 influenza season.[1]

Two doses administered at least one month apart may be required for satisfactory antibody responses among pediatric patients under 9 years of age who are receiving influenza vaccine for the first time. (See timing for vaccination under INDICATIONS AND USAGE.) To minimize febrile reactions, only subvirion or purified-surface-antigen preparations should be used for pediatric patients 6 months to 12 years of age.[1] Studies of vaccines similar to those being used currently have indicated little or no improvement in antibody response when a second dose is administered to adults during the same season.[1]

The intramuscular route is recommended for influenza vaccine. Adults and older children should be vaccinated in the deltoid muscle. Infants and young children should be vaccinated in the anterolateral aspect of the thigh.[1] *Do Not Inject Intravenously.*

Parenteral drug products should be inspected visually for particulate matter and discoloration prior to administration whenever solution and containers permit.

The dosage may be administered by the intramuscular route as follows:

1. Persons 9 years and older, a single injection of 0.5 mL.
2. Persons 3 years through 8 years, one or two injections of 0.5 mL.*
3. Persons 6 months through 35 months, one or two injections of 0.25 mL.*†

*Two doses administered at least one month apart are recommended for children under 9 years of age who are receiving influenza virus vaccine for the first time.

† Note: based on limited data. Because the likelihood of febrile convulsions is greater in this age group, special care should be taken in weighing risks and benefits.

HOW SUPPLIED

NDC 64029-2000-2—5 mL multiple-dose vials.

NDC 64029-2000-1—0.5 mL disposable syringes. Supplied in packages of 10.

Storage—Store at temperature between 2° and 8°C (36° and 46°).

Freezing destroys potency.

Shake before use.

REFERENCES

1. Centers for Disease Control and Prevention. Recommendations of the Public Health Service Advisory Committee on Immunization Practices—Prevention and Control of Influenza. *MMWR*, Vol. 49, No. RR-3(April 14, 2000).
2. Centers for Disease Control. Recommendation of the Public Health Service Immunization Practices Advisory Committee—Influenza Vaccines, 1983–1984. *MMWR*, Vol. 32, No. 26 (July 8, 1983).

IMPORTANT INFORMATION for Group Immunization Programs

If any portion of this product is to be used in an immunization program sponsored by any organization WHERE A TRADITIONAL PHYSICIAN/PATIENT RELATIONSHIP DOES NOT EXIST, each recipient (or legal guardian) should be made aware of the benefits and risks, including a

Continued on next page

Fluogen—Cont.

possible risk of a form of paralysis sometimes known as Guillain-Barré syndrome. These are summarized in the current labeling, and informed consent should be obtained from the recipient (or legal guardian) before immunization.
PLEASE CONTACT YOUR LOCAL MONARCH REPRESENTATIVE for copies of the following group immunization forms:
1. Group immunization acknowledgment form
2. Group immunization patient informed consent form (sample)
3. Posters announcing the group immunization program

Rx only

Manufactured by: Parkdale Pharmaceuticals, Inc.
Rochester, MI 48307
Rev. 5/00
2000G120
273

Parke-Davis

A Warner-Lambert Division
A Pfizer Company
201 TABOR ROAD
MORRIS PLAINS, NEW JERSEY 07950

For Medical Information Contact:
During working hours:
Customer Service
Product/Medical Information
(800) 223-0432
FAX: (973) 385-2248
After Hours and Weekend Emergencies:
(973) 385-6089
Distribution:
1855 Shelby Oaks Drive North
Memphis, TN 38134
(901) 387-5200
Customer Service:
(800) 533-4535

EXPORT INQUIRIES:
Pfizer International Inc.
(212) 573-2323

PARCODE®
(Parke-Davis Accurate Recognition Code)

Code Number	Product Name
001-006	*Unassigned*
007	**Dilantin® Infatabs®** Each tablet contains 50 mg phenytoin, USP.
008-143	*Unassigned*
144	**femhrt® Tablets** Each white D-shaped tablet contains 1 mg norethindrone acetate and 5 mcg ethinyl estradiol.
145-154	*Unassigned*
155	**Lipitor® Tablets** Each tablet contains atorvastatin calcium equivalent to 10 mg atorvastatin.
156	**Lipitor® Tablets** Each tablet contains atorvastatin calcium equivalent to 20 mg atorvastatin.
157	**Lipitor® Tablets** Each tablet contains atorvastatin calcium equivalent to 40 mg atorvastatin.
158-219	*Unassigned*
220	**Accuretic™ Tablets** Each tablet contains 20 mg quinapril and 12.5 mg hydrochlorothiazide.
221	*Unassigned*
222	**Accuretic™ Tablets** Each tablet contains 10 mg quinapril and 12.5 mg hydrochlorothiazide.
223	**Accuretic™ Tablets** Each tablet contains 20 mg quinapril and 25 mg hydrochlorothiazide.
224-236	*Unassigned*
237	**Zarontin® Capsules** Each capsule contains 250 mg ethosuximide, USP.
238-269	*Unassigned*
270	**Nardil® Tablets** Each tablet contains 15 mg phenelzine sulfate, USP.
271-361	*Unassigned*
362	**Dilantin® Kapseals®** Each Kapseal contains 100 mg extended phenytoin sodium, USP. The Kapseal is a No. 3 capsule with Orange band. (The Orange band on White capsule is a trademark registered in the US Patent Office.)
363-364	*Unassigned*
365	**Dilantin® Kapseals®** Each Kapseal contains 30 mg extended phenytoin sodium, USP. The Kapseal is a No. 4 capsule with Pink opaque band.
366-424	Unassigned
425	**Estrostep® Tablets** Each tablet contains 1 mg norethindrone acetate and 30 mcg ethinyl estradiol.
426	*Unassigned*
427	**Estrostep® Tablets** Each tablet contains 1 mg norethindrone acetate and 20 mcg ethinyl estradiol.
428-524	*Unassigned*
525	**Celontin® Kapseals®** Each Kapseal contains 300 mg methsuximide, USP. The Kapseal is a Yellow Tint No. 2 capsule with Orange band.
526	*Unassigned*
527	**Accupril® Tablets** Each tablet contains quinapril hydrochloride equivalent to 5 mg quinapril.
528-529	*Unassigned*
530	**Accupril® Tablets** Each tablet contains quinapril hydrochloride equivalent to 10 mg quinapril.
531	*Unassigned*
532	**Accupril® Tablets** Each tablet contains quinapril hydrochloride equivalent to 20 mg quinapril.
533-534	*Unassigned*
535	**Accupril® Tablets** Each tablet contains quinapril hydrochloride equivalent to 40 mg quinapril.
536	*Unassigned*
537	**Celontin® Kapseals®** Each Kapseal contains 150 mg methsuximide, USP.
538-554	*Unassigned*
555	**Estrostep® Tablets** Each tablet contains 1 mg norethindrone acetate and 35 mcg ethinyl estradiol.
556-621	*Unassigned*
622	**Ferrous Fumarate Tablets** Each tablet contains 75 mg ferrous fumarate.
623-736	*Unassigned*
737	**Lopid® Tablets** Each tablet contains 600 mg gemfibrozil.
738-914	*Unassigned*
915	**Loestrin® 1/20 Tablets** Each tablet contains norethindrone acetate, 1 mg; ethinyl estradiol, 20 mcg.
916	**Loestrin® 1.5/30 Tablets** Each tablet contains norethindrone acetate, 1.5 mg; ethinyl estradiol, 30 mcg.
917-999	*Unassigned*

ACCUPRIL® ℞
(Quinapril Hydrochloride Tablets)

> **USE IN PREGNANCY**
> **When used in pregnancy during the second and third trimesters, ACE inhibitors can cause injury and even death to the developing fetus.** When pregnancy is detected, ACCUPRIL should be discontinued as soon as possible. See WARNINGS, Fetal/Neonatal Morbidity and Mortality.

DESCRIPTION

ACCUPRIL® (quinapril hydrochloride) is the hydrochloride salt of quinapril, the ethyl ester of a nonsulfhydryl, angiotensin-converting enzyme (ACE) inhibitor, quinaprilat.
Quinapril hydrochloride is chemically described as [3S-[2[R*(R*)], 3R*]]-2-[2-[[1-(ethoxycarbonyl)-3-phenylpropyl]amino] -1- oxopropyl]-1,2,3,4- tetrahydro -3- isoquinolinecarboxylic acid, monohydrochloride. Its empirical formula is $C_{25}H_{30}N_2O_5$·HCl and its structural formula is:
[See chemical structure at top of next column]
Quinapril hydrochloride is a white to off-white amorphous powder that is freely soluble in aqueous solvents.
ACCUPRIL tablets contain 5 mg, 10 mg, 20 mg, or 40 mg of quinapril for oral administration. Each tablet also contains

• HCl

M.W.=474.98

candelilla wax, crospovidone, gelatin, lactose, magnesium carbonate, magnesium stearate, synthetic red iron oxide, and titanium dioxide.

CLINICAL PHARMACOLOGY

Mechanism of Action: Quinapril is deesterified to the principal metabolite, quinaprilat, which is an inhibitor of ACE activity in human subjects and animals. ACE is a peptidyl dipeptidase that catalyzes the conversion of angiotensin I to the vasoconstrictor, angiotensin II. The effect of quinapril in hypertension and in congestive heart failure (CHF) appears to result primarily from the inhibition of circulating and tissue ACE activity, thereby reducing angiotensin II formation. Quinapril inhibits the elevation in blood pressure caused by intravenously administered angiotensin I, but has no effect on the pressor response to angiotensin II, norepinephrine or epinephrine. Angiotensin II also stimulates the secretion of aldosterone from the adrenal cortex, thereby facilitating renal sodium and fluid reabsorption. Reduced aldosterone secretion by quinapril may result in a small increase in serum potassium. In controlled hypertension trials, treatment with ACCUPRIL alone resulted in mean increases in potassium of 0.07 mmol/L (see PRECAUTIONS). Removal of angiotensin II negative feedback on renin secretion leads to increased plasma renin activity (PRA).
While the principal mechanism of antihypertensive effect is thought to be through the renin-angiotensin-aldosterone system, quinapril exerts antihypertensive actions even in patients with low renin hypertension. ACCUPRIL was an effective antihypertensive in all races studied, although it was somewhat less effective in blacks (usually a predominantly low renin group) than in nonblacks. ACE is identical to kininase II, an enzyme that degrades bradykinin, a potent peptide vasodilator; whether increased levels of bradykinin play a role in the therapeutic effect of quinapril remains to be elucidated.
Pharmacokinetics and Metabolism: Following oral administration, peak plasma quinapril concentrations are observed within one hour. Based on recovery of quinapril and its metabolites in urine, the extent of absorption is at least 60%. The rate and extent of quinapril absorption are diminished moderately (approximately 25–30%) when ACCUPRIL tablets are administered during a high-fat meal. Following absorption, quinapril is deesterified to its major active metabolite, quinaprilat (about 38% of oral dose), and to other minor inactive metabolites. Following multiple oral dosing of ACCUPRIL, there is an effective accumulation half-life of quinaprilat of approximately 3 hours, and peak plasma quinaprilat concentrations are observed approximately 2 hours post-dose. Quinaprilat is eliminated primarily by renal excretion, up to 96% of an IV dose, and has an elimination half-life in plasma of approximately 2 hours and a prolonged terminal phase with a half-life of 25 hours. The pharmacokinetics of quinapril and quinaprilat are linear over a single-dose range of 5–80 mg doses and 40–160 mg in multiple daily doses. Approximately 97% of either quinapril or quinaprilat circulating in plasma is bound to proteins.
In patients with renal insufficiency, the elimination half-life of quinaprilat increases as creatinine clearance decreases. There is a linear correlation between plasma quinaprilat clearance and creatinine clearance. In patients with end-stage renal disease, chronic hemodialysis or continuous ambulatory peritoneal dialysis has little effect on the elimination of quinapril and quinaprilat. Elimination of quinaprilat may be reduced in elderly patients (≥65 years) and in those with heart failure; this reduction is attributable to decrease in renal function (see DOSAGE AND ADMINISTRATION). Quinaprilat concentrations are reduced in patients with alcoholic cirrhosis due to impaired deesterification of quinapril. Studies in rats indicate that quinapril and its metabolites do not cross the blood-brain barrier.

Pharmacodynamics and Clinical Effects

Hypertension: Single doses of 20 mg of ACCUPRIL provide over 80% inhibition of plasma ACE for 24 hours. Inhibition of the pressor response to angiotensin I is shorter-lived, with a 20 mg dose giving 75% inhibition for about 4 hours, 50% inhibition for about 8 hours, and 20% inhibition at 24 hours. With chronic dosing, however, there is substantial inhibition of angiotensin II levels at 24 hours by doses of 20–80 mg.
Administration of 10 to 80 mg of ACCUPRIL to patients with mild to severe hypertension results in a reduction of sitting and standing blood pressure to about the same extent with minimal effect on heart rate. Symptomatic postural hypotension is infrequent although it can occur in patients who are salt- and/or volume-depleted (see WARNINGS). Antihypertensive activity commences within 1 hour with peak effects usually achieved by 2 to 4 hours after dosing. During chronic therapy, most of the blood pressure lowering effect of a given dose is obtained in 1–2 weeks. In multiple-dose studies, 10–80 mg per day in single or divided doses lowered systolic and diastolic blood pressure throughout the dosing interval, with a trough effect of about 5–11/3–7 mm Hg. The trough effect represents about 50% of the peak effect. While the dose-response relationship is rela-

tively flat, doses of 40–80 mg were somewhat more effective at trough than 10–20 mg, and twice daily dosing tended to give a somewhat lower trough blood pressure than once daily dosing with the same total dose. The antihypertensive effect of ACCUPRIL continues during long-term therapy, with no evidence of loss of effectiveness.

Hemodynamic assessments in patients with hypertension indicate that blood pressure reduction produced by quinapril is accompanied by a reduction in total peripheral resistance and renal vascular resistance with little or no change in heart rate, cardiac index, renal blood flow, glomerular filtration rate, or filtration fraction.

Use of ACCUPRIL with a thiazide diuretic gives a blood-pressure lowering effect greater than that seen with either agent alone.

In patients with hypertension, ACCUPRIL 10–40 mg was similar in effectiveness to captopril, enalapril, propranolol, and thiazide diuretics.

Therapeutic effects appear to be the same for elderly (≥65 years of age) and younger adult patients given the same daily dosages, with no increase in adverse events in elderly patients.

Heart Failure: In a placebo-controlled trial involving patients with congestive heart failure treated with digitalis and diuretics, parenteral quinaprilat, the active metabolite of quinapril, reduced pulmonary capillary wedge pressure and systemic vascular resistance and increased cardiac output/index. Similar favorable hemodynamic effects were seen with oral quinapril in baseline-controlled trials, and such effects appeared to be maintained during chronic oral quinapril therapy. Quinapril reduced renal hepatic vascular resistance and increased renal and hepatic blood flow with glomerular filtration rate remaining unchanged.

A significant dose response relationship for improvement in maximal exercise tolerance has been observed with ACCUPRIL therapy. Beneficial effects on the severity of heart failure as measured by New York Heart Association (NYHA) classification and Quality of Life and on symptoms of dyspnea, fatigue, and edema were evident after 6 months in a double blind, placebo controlled study. Favorable effects were maintained for up to two years of open label therapy. The effects of quinapril on long-term mortality in heart failure have not been evaluated.

INDICATIONS AND USAGE

Hypertension

ACCUPRIL is indicated for the treatment of hypertension. It may be used alone or in combination with thiazide diuretics.

Heart Failure

ACCUPRIL is indicated in the management of heart failure as adjunctive therapy when added to conventional therapy including diuretics and/or digitalis.

In using ACCUPRIL, consideration should be given to the fact that another angiotensin converting enzyme inhibitor, captopril, has caused agranulocytosis, particularly in patients with renal impairment or collagen vascular disease. Available data are insufficient to show that ACCUPRIL does not have a similar risk (see WARNINGS).

Angioedema in black patients:

Black patients receiving ACE inhibitor monotherapy have been reported to have a higher incidence of angioedema compared to non-blacks. It should also be noted that in controlled clinical trials ACE inhibitors have an effect on blood pressure that is less in black patients than in non-blacks.

CONTRAINDICATIONS

ACCUPRIL is contraindicated in patients who are hypersensitive to this product and in patients with a history of angioedema related to previous treatment with an ACE inhibitor.

WARNINGS

Anaphylactoid and Possibly Related Reactions

Presumably because angiotensin-converting inhibitors affect the metabolism of eicosanoids and polypeptides, including endogenous bradykinin, patients receiving ACE inhibitors (including Accupril) may be subject to a variety of adverse reactions, some of them serious.

Angioedema: Angioedema of the face, extremities, lips, tongue, glottis, and larynx has been reported in patients treated with ACE inhibitors and has been seen in 0.1% of patients receiving ACCUPRIL.

In two similarly sized U.S. postmarketing trials that, combined, enrolled over 3,000 black patients and over 19,000 non-blacks, angioedema was reported in 0.30% and 0.55% of blacks (in study 1 and 2 respectively) and 0.39% and 0.17% of non-blacks.

Angioedema associated with laryngeal edema can be fatal. If laryngeal stridor or angioedema of the face, tongue, or glottis occurs, treatment with ACCUPRIL should be discontinued immediately, the patient treated in accordance with accepted medical care, and carefully observed until the swelling disappears. In instances where swelling is confined to the face and lips, the condition generally resolves without treatment; antihistamines may be useful in relieving symptoms. **Where there is involvement of the tongue, glottis, or larynx likely to cause airway obstruction, emergency therapy including, but not limited to, subcutaneous epinephrine solution 1:1000 (0.3 to 0.5 mL) should be promptly administered** (see ADVERSE REACTIONS).

Patients with a history of angioedema: Patients with a history of angioedema unrelated to ACE inhibitor therapy may be at increased risk of angioedema while receiving an ACE inhibitor (see also CONTRAINDICATIONS).

Anaphylactoid reactions during desensitization: Two patients undergoing desensitizing treatment with hymenoptera venom while receiving ACE inhibitors sustained life-threatening anaphylactoid reactions. In the same patients, these reactions were avoided when ACE inhibitors were temporarily withheld, but they reappeared upon inadvertent rechallenge.

Anaphylactoid reactions during membrane exposure: Anaphylactoid reactions have been reported in patients dialyzed with high-flux membranes and treated concomitantly with an ACE inhibitor. Anaphylactoid reactions have also been reported in patients undergoing low-density lipoprotein apheresis with dextran sulfate absorption.

Hepatic Failure: Rarely, ACE inhibitors have been associated with a syndrome that starts with cholestatic jaundice and progresses to fulminant hepatic necrosis and (sometimes) death. The mechanism of this syndrome is not understood. Patients receiving ACE inhibitors who develop jaundice or marked elevations of hepatic enzymes should discontinue the ACE inhibitor and receive appropriate medical follow-up.

Hypotension: Excessive hypotension is rare in patients with uncomplicated hypertension treated with ACCUPRIL alone. Patients with heart failure given ACCUPRIL commonly have some reduction in blood pressure, but discontinuation of therapy because of continuing symptomatic hypotension usually is not necessary when dosing instructions are followed. Caution should be observed when initiating therapy in patients with heart failure (see DOSAGE AND ADMINISTRATION). In controlled studies, syncope was observed in 0.4% of patients (N=3203); this incidence was similar to that observed for captopril (1%) and enalapril (0.8%).

Patients at risk of excessive hypotension, sometimes associated with oliguria and/or progressive azotemia, and rarely with acute renal failure and/or death, include patients with the following conditions or characteristics: heart failure, hyponatremia, high dose diuretic therapy, recent intensive diuresis or increase in diuretic dose, renal dialysis, or severe volume and/or salt depletion of any etiology. It may be advisable to eliminate the diuretic (except in patients with heart failure), reduce the diuretic dose or cautiously increase salt intake (except in patients with heart failure) before initiating therapy with ACCUPRIL in patients at risk for excessive hypotension who are able to tolerate such adjustments.

In patients at risk of excessive hypotension, therapy with ACCUPRIL should be started under close medical supervision. Such patients should be followed closely for the first two weeks of treatment and whenever the dose of ACCUPRIL and/or diuretic is increased. Similar considerations may apply to patients with ischemic heart or cerebrovascular disease in whom an excessive fall in blood pressure could result in a myocardial infarction or a cerebrovascular accident.

If excessive hypotension occurs, the patient should be placed in the supine position and, if necessary, receive an intravenous infusion of normal saline. A transient hypotensive response is not a contraindication to further doses of ACCUPRIL, which usually can be given without difficulty once the blood pressure has stabilized. If symptomatic hypotension develops, a dose reduction or discontinuation of ACCUPRIL or concomitant diuretic may be necessary.

Neutropenia/Agranulocytosis: Another ACE inhibitor, captopril, has been shown to cause agranulocytosis and bone marrow depression rarely in patients with uncomplicated hypertension, but more frequently in patients with renal impairment, especially if they also have a collagen vascular disease, such as systemic lupus erythematosus or scleroderma. Agranulocytosis did occur during ACCUPRIL treatment in one patient with a history of neutropenia during previous captopril therapy. Available data from clinical trials of ACCUPRIL are insufficient to show that, in patients without prior reactions to other ACE inhibitors, ACCUPRIL does not cause agranulocytosis at similar rates. As with other ACE inhibitors, periodic monitoring of white blood cell counts in patients with collagen vascular disease and/or renal disease should be considered.

Fetal/Neonatal Morbidity and Mortality: ACE inhibitors can cause fetal and neonatal morbidity and death when administered to pregnant women. Several dozen cases have been reported in the world literature. When pregnancy is detected, ACE inhibitors should be discontinued as soon as possible.

The use of ACE inhibitors during the second and third trimesters of pregnancy has been associated with fetal and neonatal injury, including hypotension, neonatal skull hypoplasia, anuria, reversible or irreversible renal failure, and death. Oligohydramnios has also been reported, presumably resulting from decreased fetal renal function; oligohydramnios in this setting has been associated with fetal limb contractures, craniofacial deformation, and hypoplastic lung development. Prematurity, intrauterine growth retardation, and patent ductus arteriosus have also been reported, although it is not clear whether these occurrences were due to the ACE inhibitor exposure.

These adverse effects do not appear to have resulted from intrauterine ACE inhibitor exposure that has been limited to the first trimester. Mothers whose embryos and fetuses are exposed to ACE inhibitors only during the first trimester should be so informed. Nonetheless, when patients become pregnant, physicians should make every effort to discontinue the use of ACCUPRIL as soon as possible.

Rarely (probably less often than once in every thousand pregnancies), no alternative to ACE inhibitors will be found. In these rare cases, the mothers should be apprised of the potential hazards to their fetuses, and serial ultrasound examinations should be performed to assess the intraamniotic environment.

If oligohydramnios is observed, ACCUPRIL should be discontinued unless it is considered life-saving for the mother. Contraction stress testing (CST), a non-stress test (NST), or biophysical profiling (BPP) may be appropriate, depending upon the week of pregnancy. Patients and physicians should be aware, however, that oligohydramnios may not appear until after the fetus has sustained irreversible injury.

Infants with histories of *in utero* exposure to ACE inhibitors should be closely observed for hypotension, oliguria, and hyperkalemia. If oliguria occurs, attention should be directed toward support of blood pressure and renal perfusion. Exchange transfusion or dialysis may be required as a means of reversing hypotension and/or substituting for disordered renal function. Removal of ACCUPRIL, which crosses the placenta, from the neonatal circulation is not significantly accelerated by these means.

No teratogenic effects of ACCUPRIL were seen in studies of pregnant rats and rabbits. On a mg/kg basis, the doses used were up to 180 times (in rats) and one time (in rabbits) the maximum recommended human dose.

PRECAUTIONS

General

Impaired renal function: As a consequence of inhibiting the renin-angiotensin-aldosterone system, changes in renal function may be anticipated in susceptible individuals. In patients with severe heart failure whose renal function may depend on the activity of the renin-angiotensin-aldosterone system, treatment with ACE inhibitors, including ACCUPRIL, may be associated with oliguria and/or progressive azotemia and rarely acute renal failure and/or death.

In clinical studies in hypertensive patients with unilateral or bilateral renal artery stenosis, increases in blood urea nitrogen and serum creatinine have been observed in some patients following ACE inhibitor therapy. These increases were almost always reversible upon discontinuation of the ACE inhibitor and/or diuretic therapy. In such patients, renal function should be monitored during the first few weeks of therapy.

Some patients with hypertension or heart failure with no apparent preexisting renal vascular disease have developed increases in blood urea and serum creatinine, usually minor and transient, especially when ACCUPRIL has been given concomitantly with a diuretic. This is more likely to occur in patients with preexisting renal impairment. Dosage reduction and/or discontinuation of any diuretic and/or ACCUPRIL may be required.

Evaluation of patients with hypertension or heart failure should always include assessment of renal function (see DOSAGE AND ADMINISTRATION).

Hyperkalemia and potassium-sparing diuretics: In clinical trials, hyperkalemia (serum potassium ≥5.8 mmol/L) occurred in approximately 2% of patients receiving ACCUPRIL. In most cases, elevated serum potassium levels were isolated values which resolved despite continued therapy. Less than 0.1% of patients discontinued therapy due to hyperkalemia. Risk factors for the development of hyperkalemia include renal insufficiency, diabetes mellitus, and the concomitant use of potassium-sparing diuretics, potassium supplements, and/or potassium-containing salt substitutes, which should be used cautiously, if at all, with ACCUPRIL (see PRECAUTIONS, Drug Interactions).

Cough: Presumably due to the inhibition of the degradation of endogenous bradykinin, persistent nonproductive cough has been reported with all ACE inhibitors, always resolving after discontinuation of therapy. ACE inhibitor-induced cough should be considered in the differential diagnosis of cough.

Surgery/anesthesia: In patients undergoing major surgery or during anesthesia with agents that produce hypotension, ACCUPRIL will block angiotensin II formation secondary to compensatory renin release. If hypotension occurs and is considered to be due to this mechanism, it can be corrected by volume expansion.

Information for Patients

Pregnancy: Female patients of childbearing age should be told about the consequences of second- and third-trimester exposure to ACE inhibitors, and they should also be told that these consequences do not appear to have resulted from intrauterine ACE-inhibitor exposure that has been limited to the first trimester. These patients should be asked to report pregnancies to their physicians as soon as possible.

Angioedema: Angioedema, including laryngeal edema, can occur with treatment with ACE inhibitors, especially following the first dose. Patients should be so advised and told to report immediately any signs or symptoms suggesting angioedema (swelling of face, extremities, eyes, lips, tongue, difficulty in swallowing or breathing) and to stop taking the drug until they have consulted with their physician (see WARNINGS).

Continued on next page

This product information was prepared in June 2000. On these and other Parke-Davis Products, information may be obtained by addressing PARKE-DAVIS, a Warner-Lambert Division, Morris Plains, New Jersey 07950.

Accupril—Cont.

Symptomatic hypotension: Patients should be cautioned that lightheadedness can occur, especially during the first few days of ACCUPRIL therapy, and that it should be reported to a physician. If actual syncope occurs, patients should be told to not take the drug until they have consulted with their physician (see WARNINGS).
All patients should be cautioned that inadequate fluid intake or excessive perspiration, diarrhea, or vomiting can lead to an excessive fall in blood pressure because of reduction in fluid volume, with the same consequences of lightheadedness and possible syncope.
Patients planning to undergo any surgery and/or anesthesia should be told to inform their physician that they are taking an ACE inhibitor.
Hyperkalemia: Patients should be told not to use potassium supplements or salt substitutes containing potassium without consulting their physician (see PRECAUTIONS).
Neutropenia: Patients should be told to report promptly any indication of infection (eg, sore throat, fever) which could be a sign of neutropenia.
NOTE: As with many other drugs, certain advice to patients being treated with ACCUPRIL is warranted. This information is intended to aid in the safe and effective use of this medication. It is not a disclosure of all possible adverse or intended effects.

Drug Interactions

Concomitant diuretic therapy: As with other ACE inhibitors, patients on diuretics, especially those on recently instituted diuretic therapy, may occasionally experience an excessive reduction of blood pressure after initiation of therapy with ACCUPRIL. The possibility of hypotensive effects with ACCUPRIL may be minimized by either discontinuing the diuretic or cautiously increasing salt intake prior to initiation of treatment with ACCUPRIL. If it is not possible to discontinue the diuretic, the starting dose of quinapril should be reduced (see DOSAGE AND ADMINISTRATION).
Agents increasing serum potassium: Quinapril can attenuate potassium loss caused by thiazide diuretics and increase serum potassium when used alone. If concomitant therapy of ACCUPRIL with potassium-sparing diuretics (eg, spironolactone, triamterene, or amiloride), potassium supplements, or potassium-containing salt substitutes is indicated, they should be used with caution along with appropriate monitoring of serum potassium (see PRECAUTIONS).
Tetracycline and other drugs that interact with magnesium: Simultaneous administration of tetracycline with ACCUPRIL reduced the absorption of tetracycline by approximately 28% to 37%, possibly due to the high magnesium content in ACCUPRIL tablets. This interaction should be considered if coprescribing ACCUPRIL and tetracycline or other drugs that interact with magnesium.
Lithium: Increased serum lithium levels and symptoms of lithium toxicity have been reported in patients receiving concomitant lithium and ACE inhibitor therapy. These drugs should be coadministered with caution and frequent monitoring of serum lithium levels is recommended. If a diuretic is also used, it may increase the risk of lithium toxicity.
Other agents: Drug interaction studies of ACCUPRIL with other agents showed:

- Multiple dose therapy with propranolol or cimetidine has no effect on the pharmacokinetics of single doses of ACCUPRIL.
- The anticoagulant effect of a single dose of warfarin (measured by prothrombin time) was not significantly changed by quinapril coadministration twice-daily.
- ACCUPRIL treatment did not affect the pharmacokinetics of digoxin.
- No pharmacokinetic interaction was observed when single doses of ACCUPRIL and hydrochlorothiazide were administered concomitantly.

Carcinogenesis, Mutagenesis, Impairment of Fertility
Quinapril hydrochloride was not carcinogenic in mice or rats when given in doses up to 75 or 100 mg/kg/day (50 to 60 times the maximum human daily dose, respectively, on an mg/kg basis and 3.8 to 10 times the maximum human daily dose when based on an mg/m^2 basis) for 104 weeks. Female rats given the highest dose level had an increased incidence of mesenteric lymph node hemangiomas and skin/subcutaneous lipomas. Neither quinapril nor quinaprilat were mutagenic in the Ames bacterial assay with or without metabolic activation. Quinapril was also negative in the following genetic toxicology studies: *in vitro* mammalian cell point mutation, sister chromatid exchange in cultured mammalian cells, micronucleus test with mice, *in vitro* chromosome aberration with V79 cultured lung cells, and in an *in vivo* cytogenetic study with rat bone marrow. There were no adverse effects on fertility or reproduction in rats at doses up to 100 mg/kg/day (60 and 10 times the maximum daily human dose when based on mg/kg and mg/m^2, respectively).

Pregnancy

Pregnancy Categories C (first trimester) and D (second and third trimesters): See WARNINGS, Fetal/Neonatal Morbidity and Mortality.

Nursing Mothers
Because ACCUPRIL is secreted in human milk, caution should be exercised when this drug is administered to a nursing woman.

Geriatric Use
Of the total number of subjects in clinical studies of ACCUPRIL, 21% were 65 and over. (There was no distinction between patients over 65 or over 75 years.) No overall differences in safety or effectiveness were observed between these subjects and younger subjects, and other reported clinical experience has not identified differences in responses between the elderly and younger patients, but greater sensitivity of some older individuals cannot be ruled out.
This drug is known to be substantially excreted by the kidney, and the risk of toxic reactions to this drug may be greater in patients with impaired renal function. Because elderly patients are more likely to have decreased renal function, care should be taken in dose selection, and it may be useful to monitor renal function.
Elderly patients exhibited increased area under the plasma concentration time curve and peak levels for quinaprilat compared to values observed in younger patients; this appeared to relate to decreased renal function rather than to age itself.

Pediatric Use
The safety and effectiveness of ACCUPRIL in pediatric patients have not been established.

ADVERSE REACTIONS

Hypertension
ACCUPRIL has been evaluated for safety in 4960 subjects and patients. Of these, 3203 patients, including 655 elderly patients, participated in controlled clinical trials. ACCUPRIL has been evaluated for long-term safety in over 1400 patients treated for 1 year or more.
Adverse experiences were usually mild and transient.
In placebo-controlled trials, discontinuation of therapy because of adverse events was required in 4.7% of patients with hypertension.
Adverse experiences probably or possibly related to therapy or of unknown relationship to therapy occurring in 1% or more of the 1563 patients in placebo-controlled hypertension trials who were treated with ACCUPRIL are shown below.

Adverse Events in Placebo-Controlled Trials

	Accupril (N=1563) Incidence (Discontinuance)	Placebo (N=579) Incidence (Discontinuance)
Headache	5.6 (0.7)	10.9 (0.7)
Dizziness	3.9 (0.8)	2.6 (0.2)
Fatigue	2.6 (0.3)	1.0
Coughing	2.0 (0.5)	0.0
Nausea and/or Vomiting	1.4 (0.3)	1.9 (0.2)
Abdominal Pain	1.0 (0.2)	0.7

Heart Failure
Accupril has been evaluated for safety in 1222 ACCUPRIL treated patients. Of these, 632 patients participated in controlled clinical trials. In placebo-controlled trials, discontinuation of therapy because of adverse events was required in 6.8% of patients with congestive heart failure.
Adverse experiences probably or possibly related or of unknown relationship to therapy occurring in 1% or more of the 585 patients in placebo-controlled congestive heart failure trials who were treated with ACCUPRIL are shown below.

	Accupril (N=585) Incidence (Discontinuance)	Placebo (N=295) Incidence (Discontinuance)
Dizziness	7.7 (0.7)	5.1 (1.0)
Coughing	4.3 (0.3)	1.4
Fatigue	2.6 (0.2)	1.4
Nausea and/or Vomiting	2.4 (0.2)	0.7
Chest Pain	2.4	1.0
Hypotension	2.9 (0.5)	1.0
Dyspnea	1.9 (0.2)	2.0
Diarrhea	1.7	1.0
Headache	1.7	1.0 (0.3)
Myalgia	1.5	2.0
Rash	1.4 (0.2)	1.0
Back Pain	1.2	0.3

See PRECAUTIONS. Cough.

Hypertension and/or Heart Failure
Clinical adverse experiences probably, possibly, or definitely related, or of uncertain relationship to therapy occurring in 0.5% to 1.0% (except as noted) of the patients with CHF or hypertension treated with ACCUPRIL (with or without concomitant diuretic) in controlled or uncontrolled trials (N=4847) and less frequent, clinically significant events seen in clinical trials or post-marketing experience (the rarer events are in italics) include (listed by body system):
General: back pain, malaise, viral infections
Cardiovascular: palpitation, vasodilation, tachycardia, *heart failure, hyperkalemia, myocardial infarction, cerebrovascular accident, hypertensive crisis, angina pectoris, orthostatic hypotension, cardiac rhythm disturbances, cardiogenic shock*
Hematology: *hemolytic anemia*
Gastrointestinal: dry mouth or throat, constipation, *gastrointestinal hemorrhage, pancreatitis, abnormal liver function tests*
Nervous/Psychiatric: somnolence, vertigo, syncope, nervousness, depression, insomnia, paresthesia
Integumentary: alopecia, increased sweating, pemphigus, pruritus, *exfoliative dermatitis, photosensitivity reaction, dermatopolymyositis*
Urogenital: impotence, *acute renal failure, worsening renal failure*
Respiratory: *eosinophilic pneumonitis*
Other: amblyopia, pharyngitis, *agranulocytosis, hepatitis, thrombocytopenia*

Fetal/Neonatal Morbidity and Mortality
See WARNINGS, Fetal/Neonatal Morbidity and Mortality.

Angioedema
Angioedema has been reported in patients receiving ACCUPRIL (0.1%). Angioedema associated with laryngeal edema may be fatal. If angioedema of the face, extremities, lips, tongue, glottis, and/or larynx occurs, treatment with ACCUPRIL should be discontinued and appropriate therapy instituted immediately. (See WARNINGS.)

Clinical Laboratory Test Findings
Hematology: (See WARNINGS)
Hyperkalemia: (See PRECAUTIONS)
Creatinine and Blood Urea Nitrogen: Increases (>1.25 times the upper limit of normal) in serum creatinine and blood urea nitrogen were observed in 2% and 2%, respectively, of all patients treated with ACCUPRIL alone. Increases are more likely to occur in patients receiving concomitant diuretic therapy than in those on ACCUPRIL alone. These increases often remit on continued therapy. In controlled studies of heart failure, increases in blood urea nitrogen and serum creatinine were observed in 11% and 8%, respectively, of patients treated with ACCUPRIL; most often these patients were receiving diuretics with or without digitalis.

OVERDOSAGE

No data are available with respect to overdosage in humans. Doses of 1440 to 4280 mg/kg of quinapril cause significant lethality in mice and rats.
The most likely clinical manifestation would be symptoms attributable to severe hypotension.
Laboratory determinations of serum levels of quinapril and its metabolites are not widely available, and such determinations have, in any event, no established role in the management of quinapril overdose.
No data are available to suggest physiological maneuvers (eg, maneuvers to change pH of the urine) that might accelerate elimination of quinapril and its metabolites.
Hemodialysis and peritoneal dialysis have little effect on the elimination of quinapril and quinaprilat. Angiotensin II could presumably serve as a specific antagonist-antidote in the setting of quinapril overdose, but angiotensin II is essentially unavailable outside of scattered research facilities. Because the hypotensive effect of quinapril is achieved through vasodilation and effective hypovolemia, it is reasonable to treat quinapril overdose by infusion of normal saline solution.

DOSAGE AND ADMINISTRATION

Hypertension
Monotherapy: The recommended initial dose of ACCUPRIL in patients not on diuretics is 10 or 20 mg once daily. Dosage should be adjusted according to blood pressure response measured at peak (2–6 hours after dosing) and trough (predosing). Generally, dosage adjustments should be made at intervals of at least 2 weeks. Most patients have required dosages of 20, 40, or 80 mg/day, given as a single dose or in two equally divided doses. In some patients treated once daily, the antihypertensive effect may diminish toward the end of the dosing interval. In such patients an increase in dosage or twice daily administration may be warranted. In general, doses of 40–80 mg and divided doses give a somewhat greater effect at the end of the dosing interval.
Concomitant Diuretics: If blood pressure is not adequately controlled with ACCUPRIL monotherapy, a diuretic may be added. In patients who are currently being treated with a diuretic, symptomatic hypotension occasionally can occur following the initial dose of ACCUPRIL. To reduce the likelihood of hypotension, the diuretic should, if possible, be discontinued 2 to 3 days prior to beginning therapy with ACCUPRIL (see WARNINGS). Then, if blood pressure is not controlled with ACCUPRIL alone, diuretic therapy should be resumed.
If the diuretic cannot be discontinued, an initial dose of 5 mg ACCUPRIL should be used with careful medical supervision for several hours and until blood pressure has stabilized.
The dosage should subsequently be titrated (as described above) to the optimal response (see WARNINGS, PRECAUTIONS, and Drug Interactions).
Renal Impairment: Kinetic data indicate that the apparent elimination half-life of quinaprilat increases as creatinine clearance decreases. Recommended starting doses, based on clinical and pharmacokinetic data from patients with renal impairment, are as follows:

Creatinine Clearance	Maximum Recommend Initial Dose
>60 mL/min	10 mg
30–60 mL/min	5 mg
10–30 mL/min	2.5 mg
<10 mL/min	Insufficient data for dosage recommendation

Patients should subsequently have their dosage titrated (as described above) to the optimal response.

Elderly (≥65 years): The recommended initial dosage of ACCUPRIL in elderly patients is 10 mg given once daily followed by titration (as described above) to the optimal response.

Heart Failure

ACCUPRIL is indicated as adjunctive therapy when added to conventional therapy including diuretics and/or digitalis. The recommended starting dose is 5 mg twice daily. This dose may improve symptoms of heart failure, but increases in exercise duration have generally required higher doses. Therefore, if the initial dosage of ACCUPRIL is well tolerated, patients should then be titrated at weekly intervals until an effective dose, usually 20 to 40 mg daily given in two equally divided doses, is reached or undesirable hypotension, orthostasis, or azotemia (see WARNINGS) prohibit reaching this dose.

Following the initial dose of ACCUPRIL, the patient should be observed under medical supervision for at least two hours for the presence of hypotension or orthostasis and, if present, until blood pressure stabilizes. The appearance of hypotension, orthostasis, or azotemia early in dose titration should not preclude further careful dose titration. Consideration should be given to reducing the dose of concomitant diuretics.

DOSE ADJUSTMENTS IN PATIENTS WITH HEART FAILURE AND RENAL IMPAIRMENT OR HYPONATREMIA

Pharmacokinetic data indicate that quinapril elimination is dependent on level of renal function. In patients with heart failure and renal impairment, the recommended initial dose of ACCUPRIL is 5 mg in patients with a creatinine clearance above 30 mL/min and 2.5 mg in patients with a creatinine clearance of 10 to 30 mL/min. There is insufficient data for dosage recommendation in patients with a creatinine clearance less than 10 mL/min. (See DOSAGE AND ADMINISTRATION, Heart Failure, WARNINGS, and PRECAUTIONS, Drug Interactions.)

If the initial dose is well tolerated, ACCUPRIL may be administered the following day as a twice daily regimen. In the absence of excessive hypotension or significant deterioration of renal function, the dose may be increased at weekly intervals based on clinical and hemodynamic response.

HOW SUPPLIED

ACCUPRIL tablets are supplied as follows:

5-mg tablets: brown, film-coated, elliptical, scored tablets, coded "PD 527" on one side and "5" on the other.
N0071-0527-23 bottles of 90 tablets
N0071-0527-40 10 × 10 unit dose blisters

10-mg tablets: brown, film-coated, triangular tablets, coded "PD 530" on one side and "10" on the other.
N0071-0530-23 bottles of 90 tablets
N0071-0530-40 10 × 10 unit dose blisters

20-mg tablets: brown, film-coated, round tablets, coded "PD 532" on one side and "20" on the other.
N0071-0532-23 bottles of 90 tablets
N0071-0532-40 10 × 10 unit dose blisters

40-mg tablets: brown, film-coated, elliptical tablets, coded "PD 535" on one side and "40" on the other.
N0071-0535-23 bottles of 90 tablets

Dispense in well-closed containers as defined in the USP.

Storage: Store at controlled room temperature 15°–30°C (59°–86°F). Protect from light.

Rx only

Revised July 1999

Manufactured by:
Parke Davis Pharmaceuticals, Ltd.
Vega Baja, PR 00694
Distributed by:
PARKE-DAVIS
Div of Warner-Lambert Co.
Morris Plains, NJ 07950 USA

0527G077

Shown in Product Identification Guide, page 329

ACCURETIC™ ℞
(quinapril HCl/hydrochlorothiazide) Tablets

USE IN PREGNANCY

When used in pregnancy during the second and third trimesters, ACE inhibitors can cause injury and even death to the developing fetus. When pregnancy is detected, ACCURETIC should be discontinued as soon as possible. See **WARNINGS: Fetal/Neonatal Morbidity and Mortality.**

DESCRIPTION

ACCURETIC is a fixed-combination tablet that combines an angiotensin-converting enzyme (ACE) inhibitor, quinapril hydrochloride, and a thiazide diuretic, hydrochlorothiazide.

Quinapril hydrochloride is chemically described as [3S-[2[R*(R*)], 3R*]]-2-[2-[[1-(ethoxycarbonyl)-3-phenylpropyl]amino]-1-oxopropyl]-1,2,3,4-tetrahydro-3-isoquinolinecarboxylic acid, monohydrochloride. Its empirical formula is $C_{25}H_{30}N_2O_5$ HCl and its structural formula is:

• HCl
M.W. = 474.98

Quinapril hydrochloride is a white to off-white amorphous powder that is freely soluble in aqueous solvents.

Hydrochlorothiazide is chemically described as: 6-Chloro-3,4-dihydro-2H-1,2,4-benzothiadiazine-7-sulfonamide 1,1-dioxide. Its empirical formula is $C_7H_8ClN_3O_4S_2$ and its structural formula is:

M.W. = 297.72

Hydrochlorothiazide is a white to off-white, crystalline powder which is slightly soluble in water but freely soluble in sodium hydroxide solution.

ACCURETIC is available for oral use as fixed combination tablets in three strengths of quinapril with hydrochlorothiazide: 10 mg with 12.5 mg (ACCURETIC 10/12.5), 20 mg with 12.5 mg (ACCURETIC 20/12.5), and 20 mg with 25 mg (ACCURETIC 20/25). Inactive ingredients: candelilla wax, crospovidone, hydroxypropyl cellulose, hydroxypropylmethyl cellulose, iron oxide red, iron oxide yellow, lactose, magnesium carbonate, magnesium stearate, polyethylene glycol, povidone, and titanium dioxide.

CLINICAL PHARMACOLOGY

Mechanism of Action: The principal metabolite of quinapril, quinaprilat, is an inhibitor of ACE activity in human subjects and animals. ACE is peptidyl dipeptidase that catalyzes the conversion of angiotensin I to the vasoconstrictor, angiotensin II. The effect of quinapril in hypertension appears to result primarily from the inhibition of circulating and tissue ACE activity, thereby reducing angiotensin II formation. Quinapril inhibits the elevation in blood pressure caused by intravenously administered angiotensin I, but has no effect on the pressor response to angiotensin II, norepinephrine, or epinephrine. Angiotensin II also stimulates the secretion of aldosterone from the adrenal cortex, thereby factilitating renal sodium and fluid reabsorption. Reduced aldosterone secretion by quinapril may result in a small increase in serum potassium. In controlled hypertension trials, treatment with quinapril alone resulted in mean increases in potassium of 0.07 mmol/L (see **PRECAUTIONS**). Removal of angiotensin II negative feedback on renin secretion leads to increased plasma renin activity (PRA).

While the principal mechanism of antihypertensive effect is thought to be through the renin-angiotensin-aldosterone system, quinapril exerts antihypertensive actions even in patients with low renin hypertension. Quinapril was an effective antihypertensive in all races studied, although it was somewhat less effective in blacks (usually a predominantly low renin group) than in non-blacks. ACE is identical to kininase II, an enzyme that degrades bradykinin, a potent peptide vasodilator; whether increased levels of bradykinin play a role in the therapeutic effect of quinapril remains to be elucidated.

Hydrochlorothiazide is a thiazide diuretic. Thiazides affect the renal tubular mechanisms of electrolyte reabsorption, directly increasing excretion of sodium and chloride in approximately equivalent amounts. Indirectly, the diuretic action of hydrochlorothiazide reduces plasma volume, with consequent increases in plasma renin activity, increases in aldosterone secretion, increases in urinary potassium loss, and decreases in serum potassium. The renin-aldolsterone link is mediated by angiotensin, so coadministration of an ACE inhibitor tends to reverse the potassium loss associated with these diuretics.

The mechanism of the antihypertensive effect of thiazides is unknown.

Pharmacokinetics and Metabolism: The rate and extent of absorption of quinapril and hydrochlorothiazide from ACCURETIC tablets are not different, respectively, from the rate and extent of absorption of quinapril and hydrochlorothiazide from immediate-release monotherapy formulations, either administered concurrently or separately. Following oral administration of Accupril (quinapril monotherapy) tablets, peak plasma quinapril concentrations are observed within 1 hour. Based on recovery of quinapril and its metabolites in urine, the extent of absorption is at least 60%. The absorption of hydrochlorothiazide is somewhat slower (1 to 2.5 hours) and more complete (50% to 80%).

The rate of quinapril absorption was reduced by 14% when ACCURETIC tablets were administered with a high-fat meal as compared to fasting, while the extent of absorption was not affected. The rate of hydrochlorothiazide absorption was reduced by 12% when ACCURETIC tablets were administered with a high-fat meal, while the extent of absorption was not significantly affected. Therefore, ACCURETIC may be administered without regard to food.

Following absorption, quinapril is deesterified to its major active metabolite, quinaprilat (about 38% of oral dose), and to other minor inactive metabolites. Following multiple oral dosing of quinapril, there is an effective accumulation half-life of quinaprilat of approximately 3 hours, and peak plasma quinaprilat concentrations are observed approximately 2 hours postdose. Approximately 97% of either quinapril or quinaprilat circulating in plasma is bound to proteins. Hydrochlorothiazide is not metabolized. Its apparent volume of distribution is 3.6 to 7.8 L/kg, consistent with measured plasma protein binding of 67.9%. The drug also accumulates in red blood cells, so that whole blood levels are 1.6 to 1.8 times those measured in plasma.

Some placental passage occurred when quinapril was administered to pregnant rats. Studies in rats indicate that quinapril and its metabolites do not cross the blood-brain barrier. Hydrochlorothiazide crosses the placenta freely but not the blood-brain barrier. Quinaprilat is eliminated primarily by renal excretion, up to 96% of an IV dose, an has an elimination half-life in plasma of approximately 2 hours and a prolonged terminal phase with a half-life of 25 hours. Hydrochlorothiazide is excreted unchanged by the kidney. When plasma levels have been followed for at least 24 hours, the plasma half-life has been observed to vary between 4 to 15 hours. At least 61% of the oral dose is eliminated unchanged within 24 hours.

In patients with renal insufficiency, the elimination half-life of quinaprilat increases as creatinine clearance decreases. There is a linear correlation between plasma quinaprilat clearance and creatinine clearance. In patients with end-stage renal disease, chronic hemodialysis or continuous ambulatory peritoneal dialysis have little effect on the elimination of quinapril and quinaprilat. Elimination of quinaprilat is reduced in elderly patients (≥65 years) and in those with heart failure; this reduction is attributable to decrease in renal function (see **DOSAGE AND ADMINISTRATION**). Quinaprilat concentrations are reduced in patients with alcoholic cirrhosis due to impaired deesterification of quinapril. In a study of patients with impaired renal function (mean creatinine clearance of 19 mL/min), the half-life of hydrochlorothiazide elimination was lengthened to 21 hours.

The pharmacokinetics of quinapril and quinaprilat are linear over a single-dose range of 5- to 80-mg doses and 40- to 160-mg in multiple daily doses.

Pharmacodynamics and Clinical Effects: Single doses of 20 mg of quinapril provide over 80% inhibition of plasma ACE for 24 hours. Inhibition of the pressor response to angiotensin I is shorter-lived, with a 20-mg dose giving 75% inhibition for about 4 hours, 50% inhibition for about 8 hours, and 20% inhibition at 24 hours. With chronic dosing, however, there is substantial inhibition of angiotensin II levels at 24 hours by doses of 20 to 80 mg.

Administration of 10 to 80 mg of quinapril to patients with mild to severe hypertension results in a reduction of sitting and standing blood pressure to about the same extent with minimal effect on heart rate. Symptomatic postural hypotension is infrequent, although it can occur in patients who are salt- and/or volume-depleted (see **WARNINGS**).

Antihypertensive activity commences within 1 hour with peak effects usually achieved by 2 to 4 hours after dosing. During chronic therapy, most of the blood pressure lowering effect of a given dose is obtained in 1 to 2 weeks. In multiple-dose studies, 10 to 80 mg per day in single or divided doses lowered systolic and diastolic blood pressure throughout the dosing interval, with a trough effect of about 5 to 11/3 to 7 mm Hg. The trough effect represents about 50% of the peak effect.

While the dose-response relationship is relatively flat, doses of 40 to 80 mg were somewhat more effective at trough than 10 to 20 mg, and twice-daily dosing tended to give a somewhat lower trough blood pressure than once-daily dosing with the same total dose. The antihypertensive effect of quinapril continues during long-term therapy, with no evidence of loss of effectiveness.

Hemodynamic assessments in patients with hypertension indicate that blood pressure reduction produced by quinapril is accompanied by a reduction in total peripheral resistance and renal vascular resistance with little or no change in heart rate, cardiac index, renal blood flow, glomerular filtration rate, or filtration fraction.

Therapeutic effects of quinapril appear to be the same for elderly (≥65 years of age) and younger adult patients given the same daily dosages, with no increase in adverse events in elderly patients. In patients with hypertension, quinapril 10 to 40 mg was similar in effectiveness to captopril, enalapril, propranolol, and thiazide diuretics.

After oral administration of hydrochlorothiazide, diuresis begins within 2 hours, peaks in about 4 hours, and lasts about 6 to 12 hours. Use of quinapril with a thiazide diuretic gives blood pressure lowering effect greater than that

Continued on next page

This product information was prepared in June 2000. On these and other Parke-Davis Products, information may be obtained by addressing PARKE-DAVIS, a Warner-Lambert Division, Morris Plains, New Jersey 07950.

Accuretic—Cont.

seen with either agent alone. In clinical trials of quinapril/hydrochlorothiazide using quinapril doses of 2.5 to 40 mg and hydrochlorothiazide doses at 6.25 to 25 mg, the antihypertensive effects were sustained for at least 24 hours, and increased with increasing dose of either component. Although quinapril monotherapy is somewhat less effective in blacks than in non-blacks, the efficacy of combination therapy appears to be independent of race. By blocking the renin-angiotensin-aldosterone axis, administration of quinapril tends to reduce the potassium loss associated with the diuretic. In clinical trials of ACCURETIC, the average change in serum potassium was near zero when 2.5 to 40 mg of quinapril was combined with hydrochlorothiazide 6.25 mg, and the average subject who received 10 to 20/12.5 to 25 mg experienced a milder reduction in serum potassium than that experienced by the average subject receiving the same dose of hydrochlorothiazide monotherapy.

INDICATIONS AND USAGE

ACCURETIC is indicated for the treatment of hypertension. This fixed combination is not indicated for the initial therapy of hypertension (see **DOSAGE AND ADMINISTRATION**).

In using ACCURETIC, consideration should be given to the fact that another angiotensin-converting enzyme inhibitor, captopril, has caused agranulocytosis, particularly in patients with renal impairment or collagen-vascular disease. Available data are insufficient to show that quinapril does not have a similar risk (see **WARNINGS: Neutropenia/Agranulocytosis**).

Angioedema in Black Patients: Black patients receiving ACE inhibitor monotherapy have been reported to have a higher incidence of angioedema compared to non-blacks. It should also be noted that in controlled clinical trials, ACE inhibitors have an effect on blood pressure that is less in black patients than in non-blacks.

CONTRAINDICATIONS

ACCURETIC is contraindicated in patients who are hypersensitive to quinapril or hydrochlorothiazide and in patients with a history of angioedema related to previous treatment with an ACE inhibitor.

Because of the hydrochlorothiazide components, this product is contraindicated in patients with anuria or hypersensitivity to other sulfonamide-derived drugs.

WARNINGS

Anaphylactoid and Possibly Related Reactions: Presumably because angiotensin converting inhibitors affect the metabolism of eicosanoids and polypeptides, including endogenous bradykinin, patients receiving ACE inhibitors (including quinapril) may be subject to a variety of adverse reactions, some of them serious.

Angioedema: Angioedema of the face, extremities, lips, tongue, glottis, and larynx has been reported in patients treated with ACE inhibitors and has been seen in 0.1% of patients receiving quinapril. In two similarly sized US postmarketing quinapril trials that, combined, enrolled over 3,000 black patients and over 19,000 non-blacks, angioedema was reported in 0.30% and 0.55% of blacks (in Study 1 and 2, respectively) and 0.39% and 0.17% of non-blacks. Angioedema associated with laryngeal edema can be fatal. If laryngeal stridor or angioedema of the face, tongue, or glottis occurs, treatment with ACCURETIC should be discontinued immediately, the patient treated in accordance with accepted medical care, and carefully observed until the swelling disappears. In instances where swelling is confined to the face and lips, the condition generally resolves without treatment; antihistamines may be useful in relieving symptoms. **Where there is involvement of the tongue, glottis, or larynx likely to cause airway obstruction, emergency therapy including, but not limited to, subcutaneous epinephrine solution 1:1000 (0.3 to 0.5 mL) should be promptly administered** (see **PRECAUTIONS** and **ADVERSE REACTIONS**).

Patients With a History of Angioedema: Patients with a history of angioedema unrelated to ACE inhibitor therapy may be at increased risk of angioedema while receiving an ACE inhibitor (see also **CONTRAINDICATIONS**).

Anaphylactoid Reactions During Desensitization: Two patients undergoing desensitizing treatment with Hymenoptera venom while receiving ACE inhibitors sustained life-threatening anaphylactoid resections. In the same patients, these reactions were avoided when ACE inhibitors were temporarily withheld, but they reappeared upon inadvertent challenge.

Anaphylactoid Reactions During Membrane Exposure: Anaphylactoid reactions have been reported in patients dialyzed with high-flux membranes an treated concomitantly with an ACE inhibitor. Anaphylactoid reactions have also been reported in patients undergoing low-density lipoprotein apheresis with dextran sulfate absorption.

Hepatic Failure: Rarely, ACE inhibitors have been associated with a syndrome that starts with cholestatic jaundice and progresses to fulminant hepatic necrosis and (sometimes) death. The mechanism of this syndrome is not understood. Patients receiving ACE inhibitors who develop jaundice or marked elevations of hepatic enzymes should discontinue the ACE inhibitor and receive appropriate medical follow-up.

Hypotension: ACCURETIC can cause symptomatic hypotension, probably not more frequently than either monotherapy. It was reported in 1.2% of 1,571 patients receiving ACCURETIC during clinical trials. Like other ACE inhibitors, quinapril has been only rarely associated with hypotension in uncomplicated hypertensive patients.

Symptomatic hypotension sometimes associated with oliguria and/or progressive azotemia, and rarely acute renal failure and/or death, include patients with the following conditions or characteristics: heart failure, hyponatremia, high dose diuretic therapy, recent intensive diuresis or increase in diuretic dose, renal dialysis or severe volume and/or salt depletion of any etiology. Volume and/or salt depletion should be corrected before initiating therapy with ACCURETIC.

ACCURETIC should be used cautiously in patients receiving concomitant therapy with other antihypertensives. The thiazide component of ACCURETIC may potentiate the action of other antihypertensive drugs, especially ganglionic or peripheral adrenergic-blocking agents. The antihypertensive effects of the thiazide component may also be enhanced in the postsympathectomy patients.

In patients at risk of excessive hypotension, therapy with ACCURETIC should be started under close medical supervision. Such patients should be followed closely for the first 2 weeks of treatment and whenever the dosage of quinapril or diuretic is increased. Similar considerations may apply to patients with ischemic heart or cerebrovascular disease in whom an excessive fall in blood pressure could result in myocardial infarction or cerebrovascular accident.

If excessive hypotension occurs, the patient should be placed in a supine position and, if necessary, treated with intravenous infusion of normal saline. ACCURETIC treatment usually can be continued following restoration of blood pressure and volume. If symptomatic hypotension develops, a dose reduction or discontinuation of ACCURETIC may be necessary.

Impaired Renal Function: ACCURETIC should be used with caution in patients with severe renal disease. Thiazides may precipitate azotemia in such patients, and the effects of repeated dosing may be cumulative.

When the renin-angiotensin-aldosterone system is inhibited by quinapril, changes in renal function may be anticipated in susceptible individuals. In patients with severe congestive heart failure, whose renal function may depend on the activity of the renin-angiotensin-aldosterone system, treatment with angiotensin-converting enzyme inhibitors (including quinapril) may be associated with oliguria and/or progressive azotemia and (rarely) with acute renal failure and/or death.

In clinical studies in hypertensive patients with unilateral renal artery stenosis, treatment with ACE inhibitors was associated with increases in blood urea nitrogen and serum creatinine; these increases were reversible upon discontinuation of ACE inhibitor, concomitant diuretic, or both. When such patients are treated with ACCURETIC, renal function should be monitored during the first few weeks of therapy.

Some quinapril-treated hypertensive patients with no apparent preexisting renal vascular diseases have developed increases in blood urea nitrogen and serum creatinine, usually minor and transient, especially when quinapril has been given concomitantly with a diuretic. This is more likely to occur in patients with pre-existing renal impairment. Dosage reduction of ACCURETIC may be required. **Evaluation of the hypertensive patients should also include assessment of the renal function.** (see **DOSAGE AND ADMINISTRATION**).

Neutropenia/Agranulocytosis: Another ACE inhibitor, captopril, has been shown to cause agranulocytosis and bone marrow depression rarely in patients with uncomplicated hypertension, but more frequently in patients with renal impairment, especially if they also have a collagen vascular disease, such as systemic lupus erythematosus or scleroderma. Agranulocytosis did occur during quinapril treatment in one patient with a history of neutropenia during previous captopril therapy. Available data from clinical trials of quinapril are insufficient to show that, in patients without prior reactions to other ACE inhibitors, quinapril does not cause agranulocytosis at similar rates. As with other ACE inhibitors, periodic monitoring of white blood cell counts in patients with collagen vascular disease and/or renal disease should be considered.

Fetal/Neonatal Morbidity and Mortality: ACE inhibitors can cause fetal and neonatal morbidity and death when administered to pregnant women. Several dozen cases have been reported in the world literature. When pregnancy is detected, ACCURETIC should be discontinued as soon as possible.

The use of ACE inhibitors during the second and third trimesters of pregnancy has been associated with fetal and neonatal injury, including hypotension, neonatal skull hypoplasia, anuria, reversible or irreversible renal failure, and death. Oligohydramnios has also been reported, presumably resulting from decreased fetal renal function; oligohydramnios in this setting has been associated with fetal limb contractures, craniofacial deformation, and hypoplastic lung development. Prematurity, intrauterine growth retardation, and patent ductus arteriosus have also been reported, although it is not clear whether these occurences were due to the ACE inhibitor exposure.

These adverse effects do not appear to have resulted from intrauterine ACE inhibitor exposure that has been limited to the first trimester. Mothers whose embryos and fetuses are exposed to ACE inhibitors only during the first trimester should be so informed. Nonetheless, when patients become pregnant, physicians should make every effort to discontinue the use of quinapril as soon as possible.

Rarely (probably less often than once in every thousand pregnancies), no alternative to ACE inhibitors will be found. In these rare cases, the mothers should be apprised of the potential hazards to their fetuses, and serial ultrasound examinations should be performed to assess the intraamniotic environment.

If oligohydramnios is observed, quinapril should be discontinued unless it is considered life-saving for the mother. Contraction stress testing (CST), a nonstress test (NST), or biophysical profiling (BPP) may be appropriate, depending upon the week of pregnancy. Patients and physicians should be aware, however, that oligohydramnios may not appear until after the fetus has sustained irreversible injury.

Infants with histories of *in utero* exposure to ACE inhibitors should be closely observed for hypotension, oliguria, and hyperkalemia. If oliguria occurs, attention should be directed toward support of blood pressure and renal perfusion. Exchange transfusion or peritoneal dialysis may be required as a means of reversing hypotension and/or substituting for disordered renal function. Removal of quinapril, which crosses the placenta, from the neonatal circulation is not significantly accelerated by these means.

Intrauterine exposure to thiazide diuretics is associated with fetal or neonatal jaundice, thrombocytopenia, and possibly other adverse reactions that occurred in adults.

No teratogenic effects of quinapril were seen in studies of pregnant rats and rabbits. On a mg/kg basis, the doses used were up to 180 times (in rats) and one time (in rabbits) the maximum recommended human dose. No teratogenic effects of ACCURETIC were seen in studies of pregnant rats and rabbits. On a mg/kg (quinapril/hydrochlorothiazide) basis, the doses used were up to 188/94 times (in rats) and 0.6/0.3 times (in rabbits) the maximum recommended human dose.

Impaired Hepatic Function: ACCURETIC should be used with caution in patients with impaired hepatic function or progressive liver disease, since minor alterations of fluid and electrolyte balance may precipitate hepatic coma. Also, since the metabolism of quinapril to quinaprilat is normally dependent upon hepatic esterases, patients with impaired liver function could develop markedly elevated plasma levels of quinapril. No normal pharmacokinetic studies have been carried out in hypertensive patients with impaired liver function.

Systemic Lupus Erythematosus: Thiazide diuretics have been reported to cause exacerbation or activation of systemic lupus erythematosus.

PRECAUTIONS

General

Derangements of Serum Electrolytes: In clinical trials, hyperkalemia (serum potassium ≥5.8 mmol/L) occurred in approximately 2% of patients receiving quinapril. In most cases, elevated serum potassium levels were isolated values which resolved despite continued therapy. Less than 0.1% of patients discontinued therapy due to hyperkalemia. Risk factors for the development of hyperkalemia include renal insufficiency, diabetes mellitus, and the concomitant use of potassium-sparing diuretics, potassium supplements, and/or potassium-containing salt substitutes.

Treatment with thiazide diuretics has been associated with hypokalemia, hyponatremia, and hypochloremic alkalosis. These disturbances have sometimes been manifest as one or more of dryness of mouth, thirst, weakness, lethargy, drowsiness, restlessness, muscle pains or cramps, muscular fatigue, hypotension, oliguria, tachycardia, nausea, and vomiting. Hypokalemia can also sensitize or exaggerate the response of the heart to the toxic effects of digitalis. The risk of hypokalemia is greatest in patients with cirrhosis of the liver, in patients experiencing a brisk diuresis, in patients who are receiving inadequate oral intake of electrolytes, and in patients receiving concomitant therapy with corticosteroids or ACTH.

The opposite effects of quinapril and hydrochlorothiazide on serum potassium will approximately balance each other in many patients, so that no net effect upon serum potassium will be seen. In other patients, one or the other effect may be dominant. Initial and periodic determinations of serum electrolytes to detect possible electrolyte imbalance should be performed at appropriate intervals.

Chloride deficits secondary to thiazide therapy are generally mild and require specific treatment only under extraordinary circumstances (eg, in liver disease or renal disease).

Dilutional hyponatremia may occur in edematous patients in hot weather; appropriate therapy is water restriction rather than administration of salt, except in rare instances when the hyponatremia is life threatening. In actual salt depletion, appropriate replacement is the therapy of choice.

Calcium excretion is decreased by thiazides. In a few patients on prolonged thiazide therapy, pathological changes in the parathyroid gland have been observed, with hypercalcemia and hypophosphatemia. More serious complications of hyperparathyroidism (renal lithiasis, bone resorption, and peptic ulceration) have not been seen.

Thiazides increase the urinary excretion of magnesium, and hypomegnesemia may result.

Other Metabolic Disturbances: Thiazide diuretics tend to reduce glucose tolerance and to raise serum levels of cholesterol, triglycerides, and uric acid. These effects are usually minor, but frank gout or overt diabetes may be precipitated in susceptible patients.

Cough: Presumably due to the inhibition of the degradation of endogenous bradykinin, persistent nonproductive cough has been reported with all ACE inhibitors, resolving after discontinuation of therapy. ACE inhibitor-induced cough should be considered in the differential diagnosis of cough.

Surgery/Anesthesia: In patients undergoing surgery or during anesthesia with agents that produce hypotension, quinapril will block the angiotensin II formation that could otherwise secure secondary to compensatory renin release. Hypotension that occurs as a result of this mechanism can be corrected by volume expansion.

Information for Patients

Angioedema: Angioedema, including laryngeal edema, can occur with treatment of ACE inhibitors, especially following the first dose. Patients receiving ACCURETIC should be told to report immediately any signs or symptoms suggesting angioedema (swelling of face, eyes, lips, or tongue, or difficulty in breathing) and to take no more drug until after consulting with the prescribing physician.

Pregnancy: Female patients of childbearing age should be told about the consequences of second- and third-trimester exposure to ACE inhibitors, and they should also be told that these consequences do not appear to have resulted from intrauterine ACE-inhibitor exposure that has been limited to the first trimester. These patients should be asked to report pregnancies to their physicians as soon as possible.

Symptomatic Hypotension: A patient receiving ACCURETIC should be cautioned that lightheadedness can occur, especially during the first days of therapy, and that it should be reported to the prescribing physician. The patient should be told that if syncope occurs, ACCURETIC should be discontinued until the physician has been consulted.

All patients should be cautioned that inadequate fluid intake, excessive perspiration, diarrhea, or vomiting can lead to an excessive fall in blood pressure because of reduction in fluid volume, with the same consequences of lightheadedness and possible syncope.

Patients planning to undergo major surgery and/or general or spinal anesthesia should be told to inform their physicians that they are taking an ACE inhibitor.

Hyperkalemia: A patient receiving ACCURETIC should be told not to use potassium supplements or salt substitutes containing potassium without consulting the prescribing physician.

Neutropenia: Patients should be told to promptly report any indication of infection (eg, sore throat, fever) which could be a sign of neutropenia.

NOTE: As with many other drugs, certain advice to patients being treated with quinapril is warranted. This information is intended to aid in the safe and effective use of this medication. It is not a disclosure of all possible adverse or intended effects.

Laboratory Tests

The hydrochlorothiazide component of ACCURETIC may decrease serum PBI levels without signs of thyroid disturbance.

Therapy with ACCURETIC should be interrupted for a few days before carrying out tests of parathyroid function.

Drug Interactions

Potassium Supplements and Potassium-Sparing Diuretics: As noted above ("Derangements of Serum Electrolytes"), the net effect of ACCURETIC may be to elevate a patient's serum potassium, to reduce it, or to leave it unchanged. Potassium-sparing diuretics (spironolactone, amiloride, triamterene, and others) or potassium supplements can increase the risk of hyperkalemia. If concomitant use of such agents is indicated, they should be given with caution, and the patient's serum potassium should be monitored frequently.

Lithium: Increased serum lithium levels and symptoms of lithium toxicity have been reported in patients receiving ACE inhibitors during therapy with lithium. Because renal clearance of lithium is reduced by thiazides, the risk of lithium toxicity is presumably raised further when, as in therapy with ACCURETIC, a thiazide diuretic is coadministered with the ACE inhibitor. ACCURETIC and lithium should be coadministered with caution, and frequent monitoring of serum lithium levels is recommended.

Tetracycline and Other Drugs That Interact with Magnesium: Simultaneous administration of tetracycline with quinapril reduced the absorption of tetracycline by approximately 28% to 37%, possibly due to the high magnesium content in quinapril tablets. This interaction should be considered if coprescribing quinapril and tetracycline or other drugs that interact with magnesium.

Other Agents:

Drug interaction studies of quinapril and other agents showed:

- Multiple dose therapy with propranolol or cimetidine has no effect on the pharmacokinetics of single doses of quinapril.
- The anticoagulant effect of a single dose of warfarin (measured by prothrombin time) was not significantly changed by quinapril coadministration twice daily.
- Quinapril treatment did not affect the pharmacokinetics of digoxin.
- No pharmacokinetic interaction was observed when single doses of quinapril and hydrochlorothiazide were administered concomitantly.

When administered concurrently, the following drugs may interact with thiazide diuretics:

- Alcohol, Barbiturates, or Narcotics—potentiation of orthostatic hypotension may occur.
- Antidiabetic Drugs (oral hypoglycemic agents and insulin)—dosage adjustments of the antidiabetic drug may be required.
- Cholestyramine and Colestipol Resin—absorption of hydrochlorothiazide is impaired in the presence of anionic exchange resins. Single doses of either cholestyramine or colestipol resins bind the hydrochlorothiazide and reduce its absorption from the gastrointestinal tract by up to 85% and 43%, respectively.
- Corticosteroids, ACTH—intensified electrolyte depletion, particularly hypokalemia.
- Pressor Amines (eg, norepinephrine)—possible decreased response to pressor amines, but not sufficient to preclude their therapeutic use.
- Skeletal Muscle Relaxants, Nondepolarizing (eg, tubocurarine)—possible increased responsiveness to the muscle relaxant.
- Nonsteroidal Antiinflammatory Drugs—the diuretic, natriuretic, and antihypertensive effects of thiazide diuretics may be reduced by concurrent administration of nonsteroidal antiinflammatory agents.

Carcinogenesis, Mutagenesis, Impairment of Fertility

Carcinogenicity, mutagenicity, and fertility studies have not been conducted in animals with ACCURETIC.

Quinapril hydrochloride was not carcinogenic in mice or rats when given in doses up to 75 or 100 mg/kg/day (50 or 60 times the maximum human daily dose, respectively, on a mg/kg basis and 3.8 or 10 times the maximum human daily dose on a mg/m^2 basis) for 104 weeks. Female rats given the highest dose level had an increased incidence of mesenteric lymph node hemangiomas and skin/subcutaneous lipomas. Neither quinapril nor quinaprilat were mutagenic in the Ames bacterial assay with or without metabolic activation. Quinapril was also negative in the following genetic toxicology studies: *in vitro* mammalian cell point mutation, sister chromatid exchange in cultured mammalian cells, micronucleus test with mice, *in vitro* chromosome aberration with V79 cultured lung cells, and in an *in vivo* cytogenetic study with rat bone marrow. There were no adverse effects on fertility or reproduction in rats at doses up to 100 mg/kg/day (60 and 10 times the maximum daily human dose when based on mg/kg and mg/m^2, respectively).

Under the auspices of the National Toxicology Program, rats and mice received hydrochlorothiazide in their feed for 2 years, at doses up to 600 mg/kg/day in mice and up to 100 mg/kg/day in rats. These studies uncovered no evidence of a carcinogenic potential of hydrochlorothiazide in rats or female mice, but there was "equivocal" evidence of hepatocarcinogenicity in male mice. Hydrochlorothiazide was not genotoxic in *in vitro* assays using strains TA 98, TA 100, TA 1535, TA 1537, and TA 1538 of *Salmonella typhimurium* (the Ames test); in the Chinese hamster ovary (CHO) test for chormosomal aberrations; or *in vivo* assays using mouse germinal cell chromosomes, Chinese hamster bone marrow chromosomes, and the *Drosophila* sex-liked recessive lethal trait gene. Positive test results were obtained in the *in vitro* CHO sister chromatid exchange (clastogenicity) test and in the mouse lymphoma cell (mutagenicity) assays, using concentrations of hydrochlorothiazide of 43 to 1300 μg/mL. Positive test results were also obtained in the *Aspergillus nidulans* nondisjunction assay, using an unspecified concentration of hydrochlorothiazide.

Hydrochlorothiazide had no adverse effects on the fertility of mice and rats of either sex in studies wherein these species were exposed, via their diets, to doses of up to 100 and 4 mg/kg/day, respectively, prior to mating and throughout gestation.

Pregnancy

Pregnancy Categories C (first trimester) and D (second and third trimesters): See WARNINGS: Fetal/Neonatal Morbidity and Mortality.

Nursing Mothers

Because quinapril and hydrochlorothiazide are secreted in human milk, caution should be exercised when ACCURETIC is administered to a nursing woman.

Because of the potential for serious adverse reactions in nursing infants from hydrochlorothiazide and the unknown effects of quinapril in infants, a decision should be made whether to discontinue nursing or to discontinue ACCURETIC, taking into account the importance of the drug to the mother.

Geriatric Use

Clinical studies of quinapril HCl/hydrochlorothiazide did not include sufficient numbers of subjects aged 65 and over to determine whether they respond differently from younger subjects. Other reported clinical experience has not identified differences in responses between the elderly and younger patients. In general, dose selection for an elderly patient should be cautious, usually starting at the low end of the dosing range, reflecting the greater frequency of decreased hepatic, renal, or cardiac function, and of concomitant disease or other drug therapy.

Pediatric Use

Safety and effectiveness of ACCURETIC in children have not been established.

ADVERSE REACTIONS

ACCURETIC has been evaluated for safety in 1571 patients in controlled and uncontrolled studies. Of these, 498 were given quinapril plus hydrochlorothiazide for at least 1 year, with 153 patients extending combination therapy for over 2 years. In clinical trials with ACCURETIC, no adverse experience specific to the combination has been observed. Adverse experiences that have occurred have been limited to those that have been previously reported with quinapril or hydrochlorothiazide.

Adverse experiences were usually mild and transient, and there was no relationship between side effects and age, sex, race, or duration of therapy. Discontinuation of therapy because of adverse effects was required in 2.1% of patients in controlled studies. The most common reasons for discontinuation of therapy with ACCURETIC were cough (1.0%; see **PRECAUTIONS**) and headache (0.7%).

	Percent of Patients in Controlled Trials	
	Quinapril/HCTZ N = 943	Placebo N = 100
Headache	6.7	30.0
Dizziness	4.8	4.0
Coughing	3.2	2.0
Fatigue	2.9	3.0
Myalgia	2.4	5.0
Viral Infection	1.9	4.0
Rhinitis	2.0	3.0
Nausea and/or Vomiting	1.8	6.0
Abdominal Pain	1.7	4.0
Back Pain	1.5	2.0
Diarrhea	1.4	1.0
Upper Respiratory Infection	1.3	4.0
Insomnia	1.2	2.0
Somnolence	1.2	0.0
Bronchitis	1.2	1.0
Dyspepsia	1.2	2.0
Asthenia	1.1	1.0
Pharyngitis	1.1	2.0
Vasodilatation	1.0	1.0
Vertigo	1.0	2.0
Chest Pain	1.0	2.0

BODY AS A WHOLE:	Asthenia, Malaise
CARDIOVASCULAR:	Palpitation, Tachycardia, *Heart Failure, Hyperkalemia, Myocardial Infarction, Cerebrovascular Accident, Hypertensive Crisis, Angina Pectoris, Orthostatic Hypotension, Cardiac Rhythm Disturbance*
GASTROINTESTINAL:	Mouth or Throat Dry, *Gastrointestinal Hemorrhage, Pancreatitis, Abnormal Liver Function Tests*
NERVOUS/PSYCHIATRIC:	Nervousness, Vertigo, *Paresthesia*
RESPIRATORY:	Sinusitis, Dyspnea
INTEGUMENTARY:	Pruritus, Sweating Increased, *Erythema Multiforme, Exfoliative Dermatitis, Photosensitivity Reaction, Alopecia, Pemphigus*
UROGENITAL SYSTEM:	*Acute Renal Failure, Impotence*
OTHER:	*Agranulocytosis, Thrombocytopenia, Arthralgia*
Angioedema:	Angioedema has been reported in 0.1% of patients receiving quinapril (0.1%) (see **WARNINGS**).
Fetal/Neonatal Morbidity and Mortality:	See **WARNINGS:** Fetal/Neonatal Morbidity and Mortality

Continued on next page

This product information was prepared in June 2000. On these and other Parke-Davis Products, information may be obtained by addressing PARKE-DAVIS, a Warner-Lambert Division, Morris Plains, New Jersey 07950.

Accuretic—Cont.

Adverse experiences probably or possibly related to therapy or of unknown relationship to therapy occurring in 1% or more of the 943 patients treated with quinapril plus hydrochlorothiazide in controlled trials are shown below.
[See first table at top of previous page]
Clinical adverse experiences probably, possibly, or definitely related or of uncertain relationship to therapy occurring in ≥0.5% to <1.0% (except as noted) of the patients treated with quinapril/HCTZ in controlled and uncontrolled trials (N=1571) and less frequent, clinically significant events seen in clinical trials or postmarketing experience (the rarer events are in italics) include (listed by body system):
[See second table at top of previous page]

Postmarketing Experience
The following serious nonfatal adverse events, regardless of their relationship to quinapril and HCTZ combination tablets, have been reported during extensive postmarketing experience:
BODY AS A WHOLE: Shock, accidental injury, neoplasm, cellulitis, ascites, generalized edema, and hernia.
CARDIOVASCULAR SYSTEM: Bradycardia, cor pulmonale, vasculitis, and deep thrombosis.
DIGESTIVE SYSTEM: Gastrointestinal carcinoma, cholestatic jaundice, hepatitis, esophagitis, vomiting, and diarrhea.
HEMIC SYSTEM: Anemia.
METABOLIC AND NUTRITIONAL DISORDERS: Weight loss.
MUSCULOSKELETAL SYSTEM: Myopathy, myositis, and arthritis.
NERVOUS SYSTEM: Paralysis, hemiplegia, speech disorder, abnormal gait, meningism, and amnesia.
RESPIRATORY SYSTEM: Pneumonia, asthma, respiratory infiltration, and lung disorder.
SKIN AND APPENDAGES: Urticaria, macropapular rash, and petechiases.
SPECIAL SENSES: Abnormal vision.
UROGENITAL SYSTEM: Kidney function abnormal, albuminuria, pyuria, hematuria, and nephrosis.
Quinapril monotherapy has been evaluated for safety in 4960 patient. In clinical trials adverse events which occurred with quinapril were also seen with ACCURETIC. In addition, the following were reported for quinapril at an incidence >0.5%: depression, back pain, constipation, syncope, and amblyopia.
Hydrochlorothiazide has been extensively prescribed for many years, but there has not been enough systematic collection of data to support an estimate of the frequency of the observed adverse reactions. Within organ-system groups, the reported reactions are listed here in decreasing order of severity, without regard to frequency.
[See table below]

Clinical Laboratory Test Findings
Serum Electrolytes: See **PRECAUTIONS**.
Creatinine, Blood Urea Nitrogen: Increases (>1.25 times the upper limit of normal) in serum creatinine and blood urea nitrogen were observed in 3% and 4%, respectively, of patients treated with ACCURETIC. Most increases were minor and reversible, which can occur in patients with essential hypertension but most frequently in patients with renal artery stenosis (see **PRECAUTIONS**).
PBI and Tests of Parathyroid Function: See **PRECAUTIONS**.
Hematology: See **WARNINGS**.
Other (causal relationships unknown): Other clinically important changes in standard laboratory tests were rarely associated with ACCURETIC administration. Elevations in uric acid, glucose, magnesium, cholesterol, triglyceride, and calcium (see **PRECAUTIONS**) have been reported.

OVERDOSAGE

No specific information is available on the treatment of overdosage with ACCURETIC or quinapril monotherapy; treatment should be symptomatic and supportive. Therapy with ACCURETIC should be discontinued, and the patient should be observed.
Dehydration, electrolyte imbalance, and hypotension should be treated by established procedures.
The oral median lethal dose of quinapril/hydrochlorothiazide in combination ranges from 1063/664 to 4640/2896 mg/kg in mice and rats. Doses of 1440 to 4280 mg/kg of quinapril cause significant lethality in mice and rats. In single-dose studies of hydrochlorothiazide, most rats survived doses up to 2.75 g/kg.
Data from human overdoses of ACE inhibitors are scanty; the most likely manifestation of human quinapril overdosage is hypotension. In human hydrochlorothiazide overdose, the most common signs and symptoms observed have been those of dehydration and electrolyte depletion (hypokalemia, hypochloremia, hyponatremia). If digitalis has also been administered, hypokalemia may accentuate cardiac arrhythmias.
Laboratory determinations of serum levels of quinapril and its metabolites are not widely available, and such determinations have, in any event, no established role in the management of quinapril overdose.
No data are available to suggest physiological maneuvers (eg, maneuvers to change the pH of the urine) that might accelerate elimination of quinapril and its metabolites. Hemodialysis and peritoneal dialysis have little effect on the elimination of quinapril and quinaprilat.
Angiotensin II could presumably serve as a specific antagonist-antidote in the setting of quinapril overdose, but angiotensin II is essentially unavailable outside of scattered research facilities. Because the hypotensive effect of quinapril is achieved through vasodilation and effective hypovolemia, it is reasonable to treat quinapril overdose by infusion of normal saline solution.

DOSAGE AND ADMINISTRATION

As individual monotherapy, quinapril is an effective treatment of hypertension in once-daily doses of 10 to 80 mg and hydrochlorothiazide is effective in doses of 12.5 to 50 mg. In clinical trials of quinapril/hydrochlorothiazide combination therapy using quinapril doses of 2.5 to 40 mg and hydrochlorothiazide doses of 6.25 to 25 mg, the antihypertensive effects increased with increasing dose of either component.
The side effects (see **WARNINGS**) of quinapril are generally rare and apparently independent of dose; those of hydrochlorothiazide are a mixture of dose-dependent phenomena (primarily hypokalemia) and dose-independent phenomena (eg, pancreatitis), the former much more common than the latter. Therapy with any combination of quinapril and hydrochlorothiazide will be associated with both sets of dose-independent side effects, but regimens that combine low doses of hydrochlorothiazide with quinapril produce minimal effects on serum potassium. In clinical trials of ACCURETIC, the average change in serum potassium was near zero in subjects who received HCTZ 6.25 mg in the combination, and the average subject who received 10 to 40/12.5 to 25 mg experienced a milder reduction in serum potassium than that experienced by the average subject receiving the same dose of hydrochlorothiazide monotherapy.
To minimize dose-independent side effects, it is usually appropriate to begin combination therapy only after a patient has failed to achieve the desired effect with monotherapy.

Therapy Guided by Clinical Effect
Patients whose blood pressures are not adequately controlled with quinapril monotherapy may instead be given ACCURETIC 10/12.5 or 20/12.5. Further increases of either or both components could depend on clinical response. The hydrochlorothiazide dose should generally not be increased until 2 to 3 weeks have elapsed. Patients whose blood pressures are adequately controlled with 25 mg of daily hydrochlorothiazide, but who experience significant potassium loss with this regimen, may achieve blood pressure control with less electrolyte disturbance if they are switched to ACCURETIC 10/12.5 or 20/12.5.

Replacement Therapy
For convenience, patients who are adequately treated with 20 mg of quinapril and 25 mg of hydrochlorothiazide and experience no significant electrolyte disturbances may instead wish to receive ACCURETIC 20/25.

Use in Renal Impairment
Regimens of therapy with ACCURETIC need not take account of renal function as long as the patient's creatinine clearance is >30 mL/min/1.73 m^2 (serum creatinine roughly ≤3 mg/dL or 265 μmol/L). In patients with more severe renal impairment, loop diuretics are preferred to thiazides. Therefore, ACCURETIC is not recommended for use in these patients.

HOW SUPPLIED

ACCURETIC is available in tablets of three different strengths:
10/12.5 tablets: pink, scored elliptical, biconvex, film-coated tablets. Each tablet contains 10 mg of quinapril and 12.5 mg of hydrochlorothiazide.
N0071-0222-06: 30 tablets (3 blisters - 10 tablets each)
20/12.5 tablets: pink, scored triangular, film-coated tablets. Each tablet contains 20 mg of quinapril and 12.5 mg of hydrochlorothiazide.
N0071-0220-06: 30 tablets (3 blisters - 10 tablets each)
20/25 tablets: pink, scored round, biconvex, film-coated tablets. Each tablet contains 20 mg of quinapril and 25 mg of hydrochlorothiazide.
N0071-0223-06: 30 tablets (3 blisters - 10 tablets each)
Dispense in well-closed containers as defined in the USP.
Store at Controlled Room Temperature 20°–25°C (68°–77°F) [see USP].
℞ only.
Manufactured by:
Parke Davis Pharmaceuticals, Ltd.
Vega Baja, PR 00694
MADE IN GERMANY
Distributed by:
PARKE-DAVIS
Div of Warner-Lambert Co
Morris Plains, NJ 07950 USA
©1999–00, PDPL
January 2000 0222G021
Shown in Product Identification Guide, page 329

BENADRYL® ℞

[*bĕ 'nă-dril*]
(Diphenhydramine Hydrochloride Injection, USP)

DESCRIPTION

Benadryl (diphenhydramine hydrochloride) is an antihistamine drug having the chemical name 2-(Diphenylmethoxy)-N, N-dimethylethylamine hydrochloride. It occurs as a white, crystalline powder, is freely soluble in water and alcohol and has a molecular weight of 291.82. The molecular formula is $C_{17}H_{21}NO \cdot HCl$.

H H+
C—O—$CH_2CH_2N(CH_3)_2$ Cl^-

Benadryl in the parenteral form is a sterile, pyrogen-free solution available in a concentration of 50 mg of diphenhydramine hydrochloride per mL. The solutions for parenteral use have been adjusted to a pH between 5.0 and 6.0 with either sodium hydroxide or hydrochloric acid. The multidose Steri-Vials® contain 0.1 mg/mL benzethonium chloride as a germicidal agent.

CLINICAL PHARMACOLOGY

Diphenhydramine hydrochloride is an antihistamine with anticholinergic (drying) and sedative side effects. Antihistamines appear to compete with histamine for cell receptor sites on effector cells.
Benadryl in the injectable form has a rapid onset of action. Diphenhydramine hydrochloride is widely distributed throughout the body, including the CNS. A portion of the drug is excreted unchanged in the urine, while the rest is metabolized via the liver. Detailed information on the pharmacokinetics of Diphenhydramine Hydrochloride Injection is not available.

INDICATIONS AND USAGE

Benadryl in the injectable form is effective in adults and pediatric patients, other than premature infants and neonates, for the following conditions when Benadryl in the oral form is impractical.
Antihistaminic: For amelioration of allergic reactions to blood or plasma, in anaphylaxis as an adjunct to epinephrine and other standard measures after the acute symptoms have been controlled, and for other uncomplicated allergic conditions of the immediate type when oral therapy is impossible or contraindicated.
Motion Sickness: For active treatment of motion sickness.
Antiparkinsonism: For use in parkinsonism, when oral therapy is impossible or contraindicated, as follows: parkinsonism in the elderly who are unable to tolerate more potent agents, mild cases of parkinsonism in other age groups, and in other cases of parkinsonism in combination with centrally acting anticholinergic agents.

CONTRAINDICATIONS

Use in Neonates or Premature Infants
This drug should *not* be used in neonates or premature infants.
Use in Nursing Mothers
Because of the higher risk of antihistamines for infants generally, and for neonates and prematures in particular, antihistamine therapy is contraindicated in nursing mothers.
Use as a Local Anesthetic
Because of the risk of local necrosis, this drug should not be used as a local anesthetic.
Antihistamines are also contraindicated in the following conditions:
Hypersensitivity to diphenhydramine hydrochloride and other antihistamines of similar chemical structure.

WARNINGS

Antihistamines should be used with considerable caution in patients with narrow-angle glaucoma, stenosing peptic ulcer, pyloroduodenal obstruction, symptomatic prostatic hypertrophy, or bladder-neck obstruction.
Local necrosis has been associated with the use of subcutaneous or intradermal use of intravenous Benadryl.
Use in Pediatric Patients
In pediatric patients, especially, antihistamines in *overdosage* may cause hallucinations, convulsions, or death.
As in adults, antihistamines may diminish mental alertness in pediatric patients. In the young pediatric patient, particularly, they may produce excitation.

BODY AS A WHOLE:	Weakness.
CARDIOVASCULAR:	Orthostatic hypotension (may be potentiated by alcohol, barbiturates, or narcotics).
DIGESTIVE:	Pancreatitis, jaundice (intrahepatic cholestatic), sialadenitis, vomiting, diarrhea, cramping, nausea, gastric irritation, constipation, and anorexia.
NEUROLOGIC:	Vertigo, lightheadedness, transient blurred vision, headache, paresthesia, xanthopsia, weakness, and restlessness.
MUSCULOSKELETAL:	Muscle spasm.
HEMATOLOGIC:	Aplastic anemia, agranulocytosis, leukopenia, thrombocytopenia, and hemolytic anemia.
RENAL:	Renal failure, renal dysfunction, interstitial nephritis See **WARNINGS**).
METABOLIC:	Hyperglycemia, glycosuria, and hyperuricemia.
HYPERSENSITIVITY:	Necrotizing angiitis, Stevens-Johnson syndrome, respiratory distress (including pneumonitis and pulmonary edema), purpura, urticaria, rash, and photosensitivity.

Use in the Elderly (approximately 60 years or older)
Antihistamines are more likely to cause dizziness, sedation, and hypotension in elderly patients.

PRECAUTIONS

General
Diphenhydramine hydrochloride has an atropine-like action and, therefore, should be used with caution in patients with a history of bronchial asthma, increased intraocular pressure, hyperthyroidism, cardiovascular disease or hypertension. Use with caution in patients with lower respiratory disease including asthma.

Information for Patients
Patients taking diphenhydramine hydrochloride should be advised that this drug may cause drowsiness and has an additive effect with alcohol.
Patients should be warned about engaging in activities requiring mental alertness such as driving a car or operating appliances, machinery, etc.

Drug Interactions
Diphenhydramine hydrochloride has additive effects with alcohol and other CNS depressants (hypnotics, sedatives, tranquilizers, etc).
MAO inhibitors prolong and intensify the anticholinergic (drying) effects of antihistamines.

Carcinogenesis, Mutagenesis, Impairment of Fertility
Long-term studies in animals to determine mutagenic and carcinogenic potential have not been performed.

Pregnancy
Pregnancy Category B. Reproduction studies have been performed in rats and rabbits at doses up to 5 times the human dose and have revealed no evidence of impaired fertility or harm to the fetus due to diphenhydramine hydrochloride. There are, however, no adequate and well-controlled studies in pregnant women. Because animal reproduction studies are not always predictive of human response, this drug should be used during pregnancy only if clearly needed.

Pediatric Use
Benadryl should not be used in neonates and premature infants (see CONTRAINDICATIONS).
Benadryl may diminish mental alertness, or, in the young pediatric patient, cause excitation. Overdosage may cause hallucinations, convulsions, or death (see WARNINGS, and OVERDOSAGE).
See also DOSAGE AND ADMINISTRATION Section.

ADVERSE REACTIONS

The most frequent adverse reactions are underscored.

1. *General:* Urticaria, drug rash, anaphylactic shock, photosensitivity, excessive perspiration, chills, dryness of mouth, nose, and throat
2. *Cardiovascular System:* Hypotension, headache, palpitations, ta chycardia, extrasystoles
3. *Hematologic System:* Hemolytic anemia, thrombocytopenia, agranulocytosis
4. *Nervous System:* Sedation, sleepiness, dizziness, disturbed coordination, fatigue, confusion, restlessness, excitation, nervousness, tremor, irritability, insomnia, euphoria, paresthesia, blurred vision, diplopia, vertigo, tinnitus, acute labyrinthitis, neuritis, convulsions
5. *GI System:* Epigastric distress, anorexia, nausea, vomiting, diarrhea, constipation
6. *GU System:* Urinary frequency, difficult urination, urinary retention, early menses
7. *Respiratory System:* Thickening of bronchial secretions, tightness of chest or throat and wheezing, nasal stuffiness

OVERDOSAGE

Antihistamine overdosage reactions may vary from central nervous system depression to stimulation. Stimulation is particularly likely in pediatric patients. Atropine-like signs and symptoms, dry mouth; fixed, dilated pupils; flushing, and gastrointestinal symptoms may also occur.
Stimulants should not be used.
Vasopressors may be used to treat hypotension.

DOSAGE AND ADMINISTRATION

THIS PRODUCT IS FOR INTRAVENOUS OR INTRAMUSCULAR ADMINISTRATION ONLY.
Benadryl in the injectable form is indicated when the oral form is impractical.
Parenteral drug products should be inspected visually for particulate matter and discoloration prior to administration, whenever solution and container permit.
DOSAGE SHOULD BE INDIVIDUALIZED ACCORDING TO THE NEEDS AND THE RESPONSE OF THE PATIENT.
Pediatric Patients, other than premature infants and neonates: 5 mg/kg/24 hr or 150 mg/m^2/24 hr. Maximum daily dosage is 300 mg. Divide into four doses, administered intravenously at a rate generally not exceeding 25 mg/min, or deep intramuscularly.
Adults: 10 to 50 mg intravenously at a rate generally not exceeding 25 mg/min, or deep intramuscularly, 100 mg if required; maximum daily dosage is 400 mg.

HOW SUPPLIED

Benadryl in parenteral form is supplied as:
Benadryl Steri-Vials®—Sterile, pyrogen-free solution containing 50 mg diphenhydramine hydrochloride in each milliliter of solution with 0.1 mg/mL benzethonium chloride as a germicidal agent. Available in 10-mL (N-0071-4402-10) Steri-Vials.
—sterile, pyrogen-free solution containing 50 mg diphenhydramine hydrochloride in each milliliter of solution. Available in packages of twenty-five 1-mL (N 0071-4259-13) Steri-Vials.
Benadryl Steri-Dose®—sterile, pyrogen-free solution containing 50 mg diphenhydramine hydrochloride in a 1-mL disposable syringe (Steri-Dose). Available in packages of ten syringes (N 0071-4259-45).
Benadryl Ampoule—sterile, pyrogen-free solution containing 50 mg diphenhydramine hydrochloride in a 1-mL ampoule. Available in packages of ten (N 0071-4259-03).

STORAGE CONDITIONS

Store at controlled room temperature 15°–30°C (59°–86°F).
Protect from freezing and light.
Rx only

Manufactured by:
Parkedale Pharmaceuticals, Inc.
Rochester, MI 48307
For:
PARKE-DAVIS
Div of Warner-Lambert Co.
Morris Plains, NJ 07950 USA
Revised April 1998 4259G444

CELONTIN® ℞

[cĕ 'lŏn 'tĭn]
(methsuximide capsules, USP)

DESCRIPTION

Celontin (methsuximide) is an anticonvulsant succinimide, chemically designated as N,2-Dimethyl-2-phenylsuccinimide.

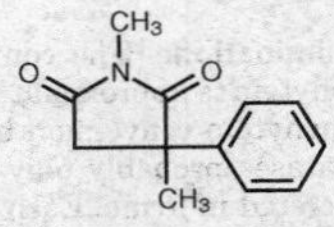

Each Celontin capsule contains 150 mg or 300 mg methsuximide, USP. Also contains starch, NF. The capsule contains colloidal silicon dioxide, NF; D&C yellow No. 10; FD&C yellow No. 6; gelatin, NF; and sodium lauryl sulfate, NF.

CLINICAL PHARMACOLOGY

Methsuximide suppresses the paroxysmal three cycle per second spike and wave activity associated with lapses of consciousness which is common in absence (petit mal) seizures. The frequency of epileptiform attacks is reduced, apparently by depression of the motor cortex and elevation of the threshold of the central nervous system to convulsive stimuli.

INDICATIONS AND USAGE

Celontin is indicated for the control of absence (petit mal) seizures that are refractory to other drugs.

CONTRAINDICATIONS

Methsuximide should not be used in patients with a history of hypersensitivity to succinimides.

WARNINGS

Blood dyscrasias, including some with fatal outcome, have been reported to be associated with the use of succinimides; therefore, periodic blood counts should be performed. Should signs and/or symptoms of infection (eg sore throat, fever) develop, blood counts should be considered at that point.
It has been reported that succinimides have produced morphological and functional changes in animal liver. For this reason, methsuximide should be administered with extreme caution to patients with known liver or renal disease. Periodic urinalysis and liver function studies are advised for all patients receiving the drug.
Cases of systemic lupus erythematosus have been reported with the use of succinimides. The physician should be alert to this possibility.

Usage in Pregnancy:

Reports suggest an association between the use of anticonvulsant drugs by women with epilepsy and an elevated incidence of birth defects in children born to these women. Data are more extensive with respect to phenytoin and phenobarbital, but these are also the most commonly prescribed anticonvulsants; less systematic or anecdotal reports suggest a possible similar association with the use of all known anticonvulsant drugs.
The reports suggesting an elevated incidence of birth defects in children of drug-treated epileptic women cannot be regarded as adequate to prove a definite cause and effect relationship. There are intrinsic methodologic problems in obtaining adequate data on drug teratogenicity in humans; the possibility also exists that other factors, eg, genetic factors or the epileptic condition itself, may be more important than drug therapy in leading to birth defects. The great majority of mothers on anticonvulsant medication deliver normal infants. It is important to note that anticonvulsant drugs should not be discontinued in patients in whom the drug is administered to prevent major seizures because of the strong possibility of precipitating status epilepticus with attendant hypoxia and threat to life. In individual cases where the severity and frequency of the seizure disorder are such that the removal of medication does not pose a serious threat to the patient, discontinuation of the drug may be considered prior to and during pregnancy, although it cannot be said with any confidence that even minor seizures do not pose some hazard to the developing embryo or fetus.
The prescribing physician will wish to weigh these considerations in treating or counseling epileptic women of childbearing potential.

PRECAUTIONS

General:
It is recommended that the physician withdraw the drug slowly on the appearance of unusual depression, aggressiveness, or other behavioral alterations.
As with other anticonvulsants, it is important to proceed slowly when increasing or decreasing dosage, as well as when adding or eliminating other medication. Abrupt withdrawal of anticonvulsant medication may precipitate absence (petit mal) status.
Methsuximide, when used alone in mixed types of epilepsy, may increase the frequency of grand mal seizures in some patients.

Information for Patients:
Methsuximide may impair the mental and/or physical abilities required for the performance of potentially hazardous tasks, such as driving a motor vehicle or other such activity requiring alertness, therefore, the patient should be cautioned accordingly.
Patients taking methsuximide should be advised of the importance of adhering strictly to the prescribed dosage regimen.
Patients should be instructed to promptly contact their physician if they develop signs and/or symptoms suggesting an infection (eg sore throat, fever).
ADVICE TO THE PHARMACIST AND PATIENT: Since methsuximide has a relatively low melting temperature (124°F), storage conditions which may promote high temperatures (closed cars, delivery vans, or storage near steam pipes) should be avoided. Do not dispense or use capsules that are not full or in which contents have melted. Effectiveness may be reduced. Protect from excessive heat (104°F).

Drug Interactions:
Since Celontin (methsuximide) may interact with concurrently administered antiepileptic drugs, periodic serum level determinations of these drugs may be necessary (eg methsuximide may increase the plasma concentrations of phenytoin and phenobarbital).

Pregnancy:
See WARNINGS.

Pediatric Use:
See DOSAGE AND ADMINISTRATION.

ADVERSE REACTIONS

Gastrointestinal System: Gastrointestinal symptoms occur frequently and have included nausea or vomiting, anorexia, diarrhea, weight loss, epigastric and abdominal pain, and constipation.
Hemopoietic System: Hemopoietic complications associated with the administration of methsuximide have included eosinophilia, leukopenia, monocytosis, and pancytopenia with or without bone marrow suppression.
Nervous System: Neurologic and sensory reactions reported during therapy with methsuximide have included drowsiness, ataxia or dizziness, irritability and nervousness, headache, blurred vision, photophobia, hiccups, and insomnia. Drowsiness, ataxia, and dizziness have been the most frequent side effects noted. Psychologic abnormalities have included confusion, instability, mental slowness, depression, hypochondriacal behavior, and aggressiveness. There have been rare reports of psychosis, suicidal behavior, and auditory hallucinations.
Integumentary System: Dermatologic manifestations which have occurred with the administration of methsuximide have included urticaria, Stevens-Johnson syndrome, and pruritic erythematous rashes.
Cardiovascular: Hyperemia.
Genitourinary system: Proteinuria, microscopic hematuria
Body as a Whole: Periorbital edema.

OVERDOSAGE

Acute overdoses may produce nausea, vomiting, and CNS depression including coma with respiratory depression. Methsuximide poisoning may follow a biphasic course. Following an initial comatose state, patients have awakened and then relapsed into a coma within 24 hours. It is believed that an active metabolite of methsuximide, N-desmethylmethsuximide, is responsible for this biphasic profile. It is important to follow plasma levels of N-desmethylmethsuximide in methsuximide poisonings. Levels greater than 40 µg/mL have caused toxicity and coma has been seen at levels of 150 µg/mL.

Treatment:
Treatment should include emesis (unless the patient is or could rapidly become obtunded, comatose, or convulsing) or

Continued on next page

This product information was prepared in June 2000. On these and other Parke-Davis Products, information may be obtained by addressing PARKE-DAVIS, a Warner-Lambert Division, Morris Plains, New Jersey 07950.

Celontin—Cont.

gastric lavage, activated charcoal, cathartics, and general supportive measures. Charcoal hemoperfusion may be useful in removing the N-desmethyl metabolite of methsuximide. Forced diuresis and exchange transfusions are ineffective.

DOSAGE AND ADMINISTRATION

Optimum dosage of Celontin must be determined by trial. A suggested dosage schedule is 300 mg per day for the first week. If required, dosage may be increased thereafter at weekly intervals by 300 mg per day for the three weeks following to a daily dosage of 1.2 g. Because therapeutic effect and tolerance vary among patients, therapy with Celontin must be individualized according to the response of each patient. Optimal dosage is that amount of Celontin which is barely sufficient to control seizures so that side effects may be kept to a minimum. The smaller capsule (150 mg) facilitates administration to small children.

Celontin may be administered in combination with other anticonvulsants when other forms of epilepsy coexist with absence (petit mal).

HOW SUPPLIED

N 0071-0525-24 (P-D 525)—Celontin capsules, #1 capsule each containing 300 mg methsuximide; bottles of 100.

N 0071-0537-24 (P-D 537)—Celontin capsules, Half Strength, #3 capsule each containing 150 mg methsuximide, bottles of 100.

Store at 25°C (77°F); excursions permitted to 15–30°C (59–86°F) [see USP Controlled Room Temperature].

Protect from light and moisture.

Protect from excessive heat 40°C (104°F).

Rx only

Revised April 2000 0537G150

PARKE-DAVIS

Div. of Warner-Lambert Co

Morris Plains, NJ 07950 USA

MADE IN FRANCE

Shown in Product Identification Guide, page 329

CEREBYX® ℞

(Fosphenytoin Sodium Injection)

DESCRIPTION

Cerebyx® (fosphenytoin sodium injection) is a prodrug intended for parenteral administration; its active metabolite is phenytoin. Each Cerebyx vial contains 75 mg/mL fosphenytoin sodium (hereafter referred to as fosphenytoin) **equivalent to 50 mg/mL phenytoin sodium** after administration. Cerebyx is supplied in vials as a ready-mixed solution in Water for Injection, USP, and Tromethamine, USP (TRIS), buffer adjusted to pH 8.6 to 9.0 with either Hydrochloric Acid, NF, or Sodium Hydroxide, NF. Cerebyx is a clear, colorless to pale yellow, sterile solution.

The chemical name of fosphenytoin is 5,5-diphenyl-3-[(phosphonooxy)methyl]-2,4-imidazolidinedione disodium salt. The molecular structure of fosphenytoin is:

The molecular weight of fosphenytoin is 406.24.

IMPORTANT NOTE: Throughout all Cerebyx® product labeling, the amount and concentration of fosphenytoin is expressed in terms of phenytoin sodium equivalents (PE). Fosphenytoin's weight is expressed as phenytoin sodium equivalents to avoid the need to perform molecular weight-based adjustments when converting between fosphenytoin and phenytoin sodium doses. Cerebyx should always be prescribed and dispensed in phenytoin sodium equivalent units (PE) (see DOSAGE AND ADMINISTRATION).

CLINICAL PHARMACOLOGY

Introduction

Following parenteral administration of Cerebyx, fosphenytoin is converted to the anticonvulsant phenytoin. For every mmol of fosphenytoin administered, one mmol of phenytoin is produced. The pharmacological and toxicological effects of fosphenytoin include those of phenytoin. However, the hydrolysis of fosphenytoin to phenytoin yields two metabolites, phosphate and formaldehyde. Formaldehyde is subsequently converted to formate, which is in turn metabolized via a folate dependent mechanism. Although phosphate and formaldehyde (formate) have potentially important biological effects, these effects typically occur at concentrations considerably in excess of those obtained when Cerebyx is administered under conditions of use recommended in this labeling.

Mechanism of Action

Fosphenytoin is a prodrug of phenytoin and accordingly, its anticonvulsant effects are attributable to phenytoin.

After IV administration to mice, fosphenytoin blocked the tonic phase of maximal electroshock seizures at doses equivalent to those effective for phenytoin. In addition to its ability to suppress maximal electroshock seizures in mice and rats, phenytoin exhibits anticonvulsant activity against kindled seizures in rats, audiogenic seizures in mice, and seizures produced by electrical stimulation of the brainstem in rats. The cellular mechanisms of phenytoin thought to be responsible for its anticonvulsant actions include modulation of voltage-dependent sodium channels of neurons, inhibition of calcium flux across neuronal membranes, modulation of voltage-dependent calcium channels of neurons, and enhancement of the sodium-potassium ATPase activity of neurons and glial cells. The modulation of sodium channels may be a primary anticonvulsant mechanism because this property is shared with several other anticonvulsants in addition to phenytoin.

Pharmacokinetics and Drug Metabolism

Fosphenytoin

Absorption/Bioavailability: *Intravenous:* When Cerebyx is administered by IV infusion, maximum plasma fosphenytoin concentrations are achieved at the end of the infusion. Fosphenytoin has a half-life of approximately 15 minutes.

Intramuscular: Fosphenytoin is completely bioavailable following IM administration of Cerebyx. Peak concentrations occur at approximately 30 minutes postdose. Plasma fosphenytoin concentrations following IM administration are lower but more sustained than those following IV administration due to the time required for absorption of fosphenytoin from the injection site.

Distribution: Fosphenytoin is extensively bound (95% to 99%) to human plasma proteins, primarily albumin. Binding to plasma proteins is saturable with the result that the percent bound decreases as total fosphenytoin concentrations increase. Fosphenytoin displaces phenytoin from protein binding sites. The volume of distribution of fosphenytoin increases with Cerebyx dose and rate. and ranges from 4.3 to 10.8 liters.

Metabolism and Elimination: The conversion half-life of fosphenytoin to phenytoin is approximately 15 minutes. The mechanism of fosphenytoin conversion has not been determined, but phosphatases probably play a major role. Fosphenytoin is not excreted in urine. Each mmol of fosphenytoin is metabolized to 1 mmol of phenytoin, phosphate, and formate (see CLINICAL PHARMACOLOGY, Introduction and PRECAUTIONS, Phosphate Load for Renally Impaired Patients).

Phenytoin (after Cerebyx administration)

In general, IM administration of Cerebyx generates systemic phenytoin concentrations that are similar enough to oral phenytoin sodium to allow essentially interchangeable use.

The pharmacokinetics of fosphenytoin following IV administration of Cerebyx, however, are complex, and when used in an emergency setting (eg, status epilepticus), differences in rate of availability of phenytoin could be critical. Studies have therefore empirically determined an infusion rate for Cerebyx that gives a rate and extent of phenytoin systemic availability similar to that of a 50 mg/min phenytoin sodium infusion.

A dose of 15 to 20 mg PE/kg of Cerebyx infused at 100 to 150 mg PE/min yields plasma free phenytoin concentrations over time that approximate those achieved when an equivalent dose of phenytoin sodium (eg, parenteral Dilantin®) is administered at 50 mg/min (see DOSAGE AND ADMINISTRATION, WARNINGS).

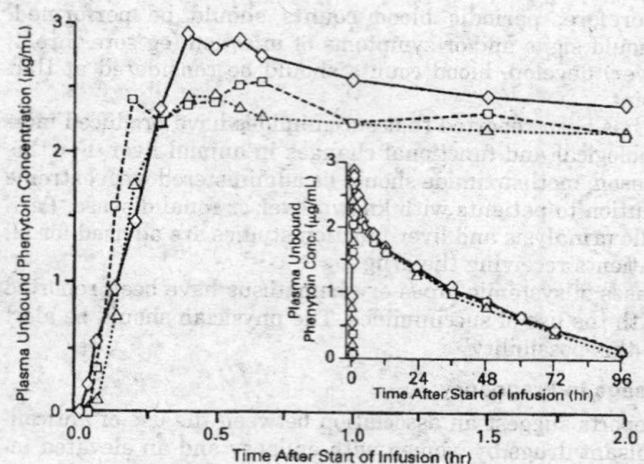

FIGURE 1. Mean plasma unbound phenytoin concentrations following IV administration of 1200 mg PE Cerebyx infused at 100 mg PE/min (triangles) or 150 mg PE/min (squares) and 1200 mg Dilantin infused at 50 mg/min (diamonds) to healthy subjects (N = 12). Inset shows time course for the entire 96-hour sampling period.

Following administration of single IV Cerebyx doses of 400 to 1200 mg PE, mean maximum total phenytoin concentrations increase in proportion to dose, but do not change appreciably with changes in infusion rate. In contrast, mean maximum unbound phenytoin concentrations increase with both dose and rate.

Absorption/Bioavailability: Fosphenytoin is completely converted to phenytoin following IV administration, with a half-life of approximately 15 minutes. Fosphenytoin is also completely converted to phenytoin following IM administration and plasma total phenytoin concentrations peak in approximately 3 hours.

Distribution: Phenytoin is highly bound to plasma proteins, primarily albumin, although to a lesser extent than fosphenytoin. In the absence of fosphenytoin, approximately 12% of total plasma phenytoin is unbound over the clinically relevant concentration range. However, fosphenytoin displaces phenytoin from plasma protein binding sites. This increases the fraction of phenytoin unbound (up to 30% unbound) during the period required for conversion of fosphenytoin to phenytoin (approximately 0.5 to 1 hour postinfusion).

Metabolism and Elimination: Phenytoin derived from administration of Cerebyx is extensively metabolized in the liver and excreted in urine primarily as 5-(p-hydroxyphenyl)-5-phenythydantoin and its glucuronide; little unchanged phenytoin (1%-5% of the Cerebyx dose) is recovered in urine. Phenytoin hepatic metabolism is saturable, and following administration of single IV Cerebyx doses of 400 to 1200 mg PE, total and unbound phenytoin AUC values increase disproportionately with dose. Mean total phenytoin half-life values (12.0 to 28.9 hr) following Cerebyx administration at these doses are similar to those after equal doses of parenteral Dilantin and tend to be greater at higher plasma phenytoin concentrations.

Special Populations

Patients with Renal or Hepatic Disease: Due to an increased fraction of unbound phenytoin in patients with renal or hepatic disease, or in those with hypoalbuminemia, the interpretation of total phenytoin plasma concentrations should be made with caution (see DOSAGE AND ADMINISTRATION). Unbound phenytoin concentrations may be more useful in these patient populations. After IV administration of Cerebyx to patients with renal and/or hepatic disease, or in those with hypoalbuminemia, fosphenytoin clearance to phenytoin may be increased without similar increase in phenytoin clearance. This has the potential to increase the frequency and severity of adverse events (see PRECAUTIONS).

Age: The effect of age was evaluated in patients 5 to 98 years of age. Patient age had no significant impact on fosphenytoin pharmacokinetics. Phenytoin clearance tends to decrease with increasing age (20% less in patients over 70 years of age relative to that in patients 20–30 years of age). Phenytoin dosing requirements are highly variable and must be individualized (see DOSAGE AND ADMINISTRATION).

Gender and Race: Gender and race have no significant impact on fosphenytoin or phenytoin pharmacokinetics.

Pediatrics: Only limited pharmacokinetic data are available in children (N=8; age 5 to 10 years). In these patients with status epilepticus who received loading doses of Cerebyx, the plasma fosphenytoin, total phenytoin, and unbound phenytoin concentration-time profiles did not signal any major differences from those in adult patients with status epilepticus receiving comparable doses.

Clinical Studies

Infusion tolerance was evaluated in clinical studies. One double-blind study assessed infusion-site tolerance of equivalent loading doses (15–20 mg PE/kg) of Cerebyx infused at 150 mg PE/min or phenytoin infused at 50 mg/min. The study demonstrated better local tolerance (pain and burning at the infusion site), fewer disruptions of the infusion, and a shorter infusion period for Cerebyx-treated patients (Table 1).

TABLE 1. Infusion Tolerance of Equivalent Loading Doses of IV Cerebyx and IV Phenytoin

	IV Cerebyx N=90	IV Phenytoin N=22
Local Intolerance	9%[a]	90%
Infusion Disrupted	21%	67%
Average Infusion Time	13 min	44 min

[a] Percent of patients.

Cerebyx-treated patients, however, experienced more systemic sensory disturbances (see PRECAUTIONS, Sensory Disturbances).

Infusion disruptions in Cerebyx-treated patients were primarily due to systemic burning, pruritus, and/or paresthesia while those in phenytoin-treated patients were primarily due to pain and burning at the infusion site (see Table 1).

In a double-blind study investigating temporary substitution of Cerebyx for oral phenytoin, IM Cerebyx was as well-tolerated as IM placebo. IM Cerebyx resulted in a slight increase in transient, mild to moderate local itching (23% of patients vs 11% of IM placebo-treated patients at any time during the study). This study also demonstrated that equimolar doses of IM Cerebyx may be substituted for oral phenytoin sodium with no dosage adjustments needed when initiating IM or returning to oral therapy. In contrast, switching between IM and oral phenytoin requires dosage adjustments because of slow and erratic phenytoin absorption from muscle.

INDICATIONS AND USAGE

Cerebyx is indicated for short-term parenteral administration when other means of phenytoin administration are unavailable, inappropriate, or deemed less advantageous. The safety and effectiveness of Cerebyx in this use has not been systematically evaluated for more than 5 days.

Cerebyx can be used for the control of generalized convulsive status epilepticus and prevention and treatment of seizures occurring during neurosurgery. It can also be substituted, short-term, for oral phenytoin.

CONTRAINDICATIONS

Cerebyx is contraindicated in patients who have demonstrated hypersensitivity to Cerebyx or its ingredients, or to phenytoin or other hydantoins.

Because of the effect of parenteral phenytoin on ventricular automaticity, Cerebyx is contraindicated in patients with sinus bradycardia, sino-atrial block, second and third degree A-V block, and Adams-Strokes syndrome.

WARNINGS

DOSES OF CEREBYX ARE EXPRESSED AS THEIR PHENYTOIN SODIUM EQUIVALENTS IN THIS LABELING (PE=phenytoin sodium equivalent).

DO NOT, THEREFORE, MAKE ANY ADJUSTMENT IN THE RECOMMENDED DOSES WHEN SUBSTITUTING CEREBYX FOR PHENYTOIN SODIUM OR VICE VERSA.

The following warnings are based on experience with Cerebyx or phenytoin.

Status Epilepticus Dosing Regimen

• Do not administer Cerebyx at a rate greater than 150 mg PE/min.

The dose of IV Cerebyx (15 to 20 mg PE/kg) that is used to treat status epilepticus is administered at a maximum rate of 150 mg PE/min. The typical Cerebyx infusion administered to a 50 kg patient would take between 5 and 7 minutes. Note that the delivery of an identical molar dose of phenytoin using parenteral Dilantin or generic phenytoin sodium injection cannot be accomplished in less than 15 to 20 minutes because of the untoward cardiovascular effects that accompany the direct intravenous administration of phenytoin at rates greater than 50 mg/min.

If rapid phenytoin loading is a primary goal, IV administration of Cerebyx is preferred because the time to achieve therapeutic plasma phenytoin concentrations is greater following IM than that following IV administration (see DOSAGE AND ADMINISTRATION).

Withdrawal Precipitated Seizure, Status Epilepticus

Antiepileptic drugs should not be abruptly discontinued because of the possibility of increased seizure frequency, including status epilepticus. When, in the judgement of the clinician, the need for dosage reduction, discontinuation, or substitution of alternative medication arises, this should be done gradually. However, in the event of an allergic or hypersensitivity reaction, rapid substitution of alternative therapy may be necessary. In this case, alternative therapy should be an antiepileptic drug not belonging to the hydantoin chemical class.

Cardiovascular Depression

Hypotension may occur, especially after IV administration at high doses and high rates of administration. Following administration of phenytoin, severe cardiovascular reactions and fatalities have been reported with atrial and ventricular conduction depression and ventricular fibrillation. Severe complications are most commonly encountered in elderly or gravely ill patients. Therefore, careful cardiac monitoring is needed when administering IV loading doses of Cerebyx. Reduction in rate of administration or discontinuation of dosing may be needed.

Cerebyx should be used with caution in patients with hypotension and severe myocardial insufficiency.

Rash

Cerebyx should be discontinued if a skin rash appears. If the rash is exfoliative, purpuric, or bullous, or if lupus erythematosus, Stevens-Johnson syndrome, or toxic epidermal necrolysis is suspected, use of this drug should not be resumed and alternative therapy should be considered. If the rash is of a milder type (measles-like scarlatiniform), therapy may be resumed after the rash has completely disappeared. If the rash recurs upon reinstitution, further Cerebyx or phenytoin administration is contraindicated.

Hepatic Injury

Cases of acute hepatotoxicity, including infrequent cases of acute hepatic failure, have been reported with phenytoin. These incidents have been associated with a hypersensitivity syndrome characterized by fever, skin eruptions, and lymphadenopathy, and usually occur within the first 2 months of treatment. Other common manifestations include jaundice, hepatomegaly, elevated serum transaminase levels, leukocytosis, and eosinophilia. The clinical course of acute phenytoin hepatotoxicity ranges from prompt recovery to fatal outcomes. In these patients with acute hepatotoxicity, Cerebyx should be immediately discontinued and not readministered.

Hemopoietic System

Hemopoietic complications, some fatal, have occasionally been reported in association with administration of phenytoin. These have included thrombocytopenia, leukopenia, granulocytopenia, agranulocytosis, and pancytopenia with or without bone marrow suppression.

There have been a number of reports that have suggested a relationship between phenytoin and the development of lymphadenopathy (local or generalized), including benign lymph node hyperplasia, pseudolymphoma, lymphoma, and Hodgkin's disease. Although a cause and effect relationship has not been established, the occurrence of lymphadenopathy indicates the need to differentiate such a condition from other types of lymph node pathology. Lymph node involvement may occur with or without symptoms and signs resembling serum sickness, eg, fever, rash, and liver involvement. In all cases of lymphadenopathy, follow-up observation for an extended period is indicated and every effort should be made to achieve seizure control using alternative antiepileptic drugs.

Alcohol Use

Acute alcohol intake may increase plasma phenytoin concentrations while chronic alcohol use may decrease plasma concentrations.

Usage in Pregnancy

Clinical:

A. Risks to Mother. An increase in seizure frequency may occur during pregnancy because of altered phenytoin pharmacokinetics. Periodic measurements of plasma phenytoin concentrations may be valuable in the management of pregnant women as a guide to appropriate adjustment of dosage (see PRECAUTIONS, Laboratory Tests). However, postpartum restoration of the original dosage will probably be indicated.

B. Risks to the Fetus. If this drug is used during pregnancy, or if the patient becomes pregnant while taking the drug, the patient should be apprised of the potential harm to the fetus.

Prenatal exposure to phenytoin may increase the risks for congenital malformations and other adverse developmental outcomes. Increased frequencies of major malformations (such as orofacial clefts and cardiac defects), minor anomalies (dysmorphic facial features, nail and digit hypoplasia), growth abnormalities (including microcephaly), and mental deficiency have been reported among children born to epileptic women who took phenytoin alone or in combination with other antiepileptic drugs during pregnancy. There have also been several reported cases of malignancies, including neuroblastoma, in children whose mothers received phenytoin during pregnancy. The overall incidence of malformations for children of epileptic women treated with antiepileptic drugs (phenytoin and/or others) during pregnancy is about 10%, or two-to three-fold that in the general population. However, the relative contributions of antiepileptic drugs and other factors associated with epilepsy to this increased risk are uncertain and in most cases it has not been possible to attribute specific developmental abnormalities to particular antiepileptic drugs.

Patients should consult with their physicians to weigh the risks and benefits of phenytoin during pregnancy.

C. Postpartum Period. A potentially life-threatening bleeding disorder related to decreased levels of vitamin K-dependent clotting factors may occur in newborns exposed to phenytoin *in utero* . This drug-induced condition can be prevented with vitamin K administration to the mother before delivery and to the neonate after birth.

Preclinical: Increased frequencies of malformations (brain, cardiovascular, digit, and skeletal anomalies), death, growth retardation, and functional impairment (chromodacryorrhea, hyperactivity, circling) were observed among the offspring of rats receiving fosphenytoin during pregnancy. Most of the adverse effects of embryo-fetal development occurred at doses of 33 mg PE/kg or higher (approximately 30% of the maximum human loading dose or higher on a mg/m^2 basis), which produced peak maternal plasma phenytoin concentrations of approximately 20 μg/mL or greater. Maternal toxicity was often associated with these doses and plasma concentrations, however, there is no evidence to suggest that the developmental effects were secondary to the maternal effects. The single occurrence of a rare brain malformation at a non-maternotoxic dose of 17 mg PE/kg (approximately 10% of the maximum human loading dose on a mg/m^2 basis) was also considered drug-induced. The developmental effects of fosphenytoin in rats were similar to those which have been reported following administration of phenytoin to pregnant rats.

No effects on embryo-fetal development were observed when rabbits were given up to 33 mg PE/kg of fosphenytoin (approximately 50% of the maximum human loading dose on a mg/m^2 basis) during pregnancy. Increased resorption and malformation rates have been reported following administration of phenytoin doses of 75 mg/kg or higher (approximately 120% of the maximum human loading dose or higher on a mg/m^2 basis) to pregnant rabbits.

PRECAUTIONS

General: (Cerebyx specific)

Sensory Disturbances

Severe burning, itching, and/or paresthesia were reported by 7 of 16 normal volunteers administered IV Cerebyx at a dose of 1200 mg PE at the maximum rate of administration (150 mg PE/min). The severe sensory disturbance lasted from 3 to 50 minutes in 6 of these subjects and for 14 hours in the seventh subject. In some cases, milder sensory disturbances persisted for as long as 24 hours. The location of the discomfort varied among subjects with the groin mentioned most frequently as an area of discomfort. In a separate cohort of 16 normal volunteers (taken from 2 other studies) who were administered IV Cerebyx at a dose of 1200 mg PE at the maximum rate of administration (150 mg PE/min), none experienced severe disturbances, but most experienced mild to moderate itching or tingling.

Patients administered Cerebyx at doses of 20 mg PE/kg at 150 mg PE/min are expected to experience discomfort of some degree. The occurrence and intensity of the discomfort can be lessened by slowing or temporarily stopping the infusion.

The effect of continuing infusion unaltered in the presence of these sensations is unknown. No permanent sequelae have been reported thus far. The pharmacologic basis for these positive sensory phenomena is unknown, but other phosphate ester drugs, which deliver smaller phosphate loads, have been associated with burning, itching, and/or tingling predominantly in the groin area.

Phosphate Load

The phosphate load provided by Cerebyx (0.0037 mmol phosphate/mg PE Cerebyx) should be considered when treating patients who require phosphate restriction, such as those with severe renal impairment.

IV Loading in Renal and/or Hepatic Disease or in Those With Hypoalbuminemia

After IV administration to patients with renal and/or hepatic disease, or in those with hypoalbuminemia, fosphenytoin clearance to phenytoin may be increased without a similar increase in phenytoin clearance. This has the potential to increase the frequency and severity of adverse events (see CLINICAL PHARMACOLOGY: Special Populations, and DOSAGE AND ADMINISTRATION: Dosing in Special Populations).

General: (phenytoin associated)

Cerebyx is *not* indicated for the treatment of *absence seizures.*

A small percentage of individuals who have been treated with phenytoin have been shown to metabolize the drug slowly. *Slow metabolism* may be due to limited enzyme availability and lack of induction; it appears to be genetically determined.

Phenytoin and other hydantoins are contraindicated in patients who have experienced phenytoin hypersensitivity. Additionally, caution should be exercised if using structurally similar (eg, barbiturates, succinimides, oxazolidinediones, and other related compounds) in these same patients.

Phenytoin has been infrequently associated with the exacerbation of *porphyria.* Caution should be exercised when Cerebyx is used in patients with this disease.

Hyperglycemia, resulting from phenytoin's inhibitory effect on insulin release, has been reported. Phenytoin may also raise the serum glucose concentrations in diabetic patients.

Plasma concentrations of phenytoin sustained above the optimal range may produce confusional states referred to as "delirium," "psychosis," or "encephalopathy," or rarely, irreversible cerebellar dysfunction. Accordingly, at the first sign of *acute toxicity,* determination of plasma phenytoin concentrations is recommended (see PRECAUTIONS: Laboratory Tests). Cerebyx dose reduction is indicated if phenytoin concentrations are excessive, if symptoms persist, administration of Cerebyx should be discontinued.

The liver is the primary site of biotransformation of phenytoin; patients with impaired liver function, elderly patients, or those who are gravely ill may show early signs of toxicity.

Phenytoin and other hydantoins are not indicated for seizures due to hypoglycemic or other metabolic causes. Appropriate diagnostic procedures should be performed as indicated.

Phenytoin has the potential to lower serum folate levels.

Laboratory Tests

Phenytoin doses are usually selected to attain therapeutic plasma total phenytoin concentrations of 10 to 20 μg/mL, (unbound phenytoin concentrations of 1 to 2 μg/mL). Following Cerebyx administration, it is recommended that phenytoin concentrations not be monitored until conversion to phenytoin is essentially complete. This occurs within approximately 2 hours after the end of IV infusion and 4 hours after IM injection.

Prior to complete conversion, commonly used immunoanalytical techniques, such as TDx®/TDxFLx™ (fluorescence polarization) and Emit® 2000 (enzyme multiplied), may significantly overestimate plasma phenytoin concentrations because of cross-reactivity with fosphenytoin. The error is dependent on plasma phenytoin and fosphenytoin concentration (influenced by Cerebyx dose, route and rate of administration, and time of sampling relative to dosing), and analytical method. Chromatographic assay methods accurately quantitate phenytoin concentrations in biological fluids in the presence of fosphenytoin. Prior to complete conversion, blood samples for phenytoin monitoring should be collected in tubes containing EDTA as an anticoagulant to minimize *ex vivo* conversion of fosphenytoin to phenytoin. However, even with specific assay methods, phenytoin concentrations measured before conversion of fosphenytoin is complete will not reflect phenytoin concentrations ultimately achieved.

Drug Interactions

No drugs are known to interfere with the conversion of fosphenytoin to phenytoin. Conversion could be affected by alterations in the level of phosphatase activity, but given the abundance and wide distribution of phosphatases in the body it is unlikely that drugs would affect this activity enough to affect conversion of fosphenytoin to phenytoin. Drugs highly bound to albumin could increase the unbound fraction of fosphenytoin. Although, it is unknown whether this could result in clinically significant effects, caution is advised when administering Cerebyx with other drugs that significantly bind to serum albumin.

The pharmacokinetics and protein binding of fosphenytoin, phenytoin, and diazepam were not altered when diazepam and Cerebyx were concurrently administered in single submaximal doses.

Continued on next page

This product information was prepared in June 2000. On these and other Parke-Davis Products, information may be obtained by addressing PARKE-DAVIS, a Warner-Lambert Division, Morris Plains, New Jersey 07950.

Cerebyx—Cont.

The most significant drug interactions following administration of Cerebyx are expected to occur with drugs that interact with phenytoin. Phenytoin is extensively bound to serum plasma proteins and is prone to competitive displacement. Phenytoin is metabolized by hepatic cytochrome P450 enzymes and is particularly susceptible to inhibitory drug interactions because it is subject to saturable metabolism. Inhibition of metabolism may produce significant increases in circulating phenytoin concentrations and enhance the risk of drug toxicity. Phenytoin is a potent inducer of hepatic drug-metabolizing enzymes.

The most commonly occurring drug interactions are listed below:

- Drugs that may increase plasma phenytoin concentrations include: acute alcohol intake, amiodarone, chloramphenicol, chlordiazepoxide, cimetidine, diazepam, dicumarol, disulfiram, estrogens, ethosuximide, fluoxetine, H_2-antagonists, halothane, isoniazid, methylphenidate, phenothiazines, phenylbutazone, salicylates, succinimides, sulfonamides, tolbutamide, trazodone.
- Drugs that may decrease plasma phenytoin concentrations include: carbamazepine, chronic alcohol abuse, reserpine.
- Drugs that may either increase or decrease plasma phenytoin concentrations include: phenobarbital, valproic acid, and sodium valproate. Similarly, the effects of phenytoin on phenobarbital, valproic acid and sodium plasma valproate concentrations are unpredictable.
- Although not a true drug interaction, tricyclic antidepressants may precipitate seizures in susceptible patients and Cerebyx dosage may need to be adjusted.
- Drugs whose efficacy is impaired by phenytoin include: anticoagulants, corticosteroids, coumarin, digitoxin, doxycycline, estrogens, furosemide, oral contraceptives, rifampin, quinidine, theophylline, vitamin D.

Monitoring of plasma phenytoin concentrations may be helpful when possible drug interactions are suspected (see Laboratory Tests).

Drug/Laboratory Test Interactions

Phenytoin may decrease serum concentrations of T_4. It may also produce artifactually low results in dexamethasone or metyrapone tests. Phenytoin may also cause increased serum concentrations of glucose, alkaline phosphatase, and gamma glutamyl transpeptidase (GGT).

Care should be taken when using immunoanalytical methods to measure plasma phenytoin concentrations following Cerebyx administration (see Laboratory Tests).

Carcinogenesis, Mutagenesis, Impairment of Fertility

The carcinogenic potential of fosphenytoin has not been studied. Assessment of the carcinogenic potential of phenytoin in mice and rats is ongoing.

Structural chromosome aberration frequency in cultured V79 Chinese hamster lung cells was increased by exposure to fosphenytoin in the presence of metabolic activation. No evidence of mutagenicity was observed in bacteria (Ames test) or Chinese hamster lung cells *in vitro,* and no evidence for clastogenic activity was observed in an *in vivo* mouse bone marrow micronucleus test.

No effects on fertility were noted in rats of either sex given fosphenytoin. Maternal toxicity and altered estrous cycles, delayed mating, prolonged gestation length, and developmental toxicity were observed following administration of fosphenytoin during mating, gestation, and lactation at doses of 50 mg PE/kg or higher (approximately 40% of the maximum human loading dose or higher on a mg/m^2 basis).

Pregnancy-Category D: (see WARNINGS)

Use in Nursing Mothers

It is not known whether fosphenytoin is excreted in human milk.

Following administration of Dilantin, phenytoin appears to be excreted in low concentrations in human milk. Therefore, breast-feeding is not recommended for women receiving Cerebyx.

Pediatric Use

The safety of Cerebyx in pediatric patients has not been established.

Geriatric Use

No systematic studies in geriatric patients have been conducted. Phenytoin clearance tends to decrease with increasing age (see CLINICAL PHARMACOLOGY: Special Populations).

ADVERSE REACTIONS

The more important adverse clinical events caused by the IV use of Cerebyx or phenytoin are cardiovascular collapse and/or central nervous system depression. Hypotension can occur when either drug is administered rapidly by the IV route. The rate of administration is very important; for Cerebyx, it should not exceed 150 mg PE/min.

The adverse clinical events most commonly observed with the use of Cerebyx in clinical trials were nystagmus, dizziness, pruritus, paresthesia, headache, somnolence, and ataxia. With two exceptions, these events are commonly associated with the administration of IV phenytoin. Paresthesia and pruritus, however, were seen much more often following Cerebyx administration and occurred more often with IV Cerebyx administration than with IM Cerebyx administration. These events were dose and rate related; most alert patients (41 of 64; 64%) administered doses of ≥15 mg PE/kg at 150 mg PE/min experienced discomfort of some degree. These sensations, generally described as itching, burning, or tingling, were usually not at the infusion site. The location of the discomfort varied with the groin mentioned most frequently as a site of involvement. The paresthesia and pruritus were transient events that occurred within several minutes of the start of infusion and generally resolved within 10 minutes after completion of Cerebyx infusion. Some patients experienced symptoms for hours. These events did not increase in severity with repeated administration.

Concurrent adverse events or clinical laboratory change suggesting an allergic process were not seen (see PRECAUTIONS, Sensory Disturbances).

Approximately 2% of the 859 individuals who received Cerebyx in premarketing clinical trials discontinued treatment because of an adverse event. The adverse events most commonly associated with withdrawal were pruritus (0.5%), hypotension (0.3%), and bradycardia (0.2%).

Dose and Rate Dependency of Adverse Events Following IV Cerebyx: The incidence of adverse events tended to increase as both dose and infusion rate increased. In particular, at doses of ≥15 mg PE/kg and rates ≥150 mg PE/min, transient pruritus, tinnitus, nystagmus, somnolence, and ataxia occurred 2 to 3 times more often than at lower doses or rates.

Incidence in Controlled Clinical Trials

All adverse events were recorded during the trials by the clinical investigators using terminology of their own choosing. Similar types of events were grouped into standardized categories using modified COSTART dictionary terminology. These categories are used in the tables and listings below with the frequencies representing the proportion of individuals exposed to Cerebyx or comparative therapy.

The prescriber should be aware that these figures cannot be used to predict the frequency of adverse events in the course of usual medical practice where patient characteristics and other factors may differ from those prevailing during clinical studies. Similarly, the cited frequencies cannot be directly compared with figures obtained from other clinical investigations involving different treatments, uses or investigators. An inspection of these frequencies, however, does provide the prescribing physician with one basis to estimate the relative contribution of drug and nondrug factors to the adverse event incidences in the population studied.

Incidence in Controlled Clinical Trials-IV Administration To Patients With Epilepsy or Neurosurgical Patients: Table 2 lists treatment-emergent adverse events that occurred in at least 2% of patients treated with IV Cerebyx at the maximum dose and rate in a randomized, double-blind, controlled clinical trial where the rates for phenytoin and Cerebyx administration would have resulted in equivalent systemic exposure to phenytoin.

TABLE 2. Treatment-Emergent Adverse Event Incidence Following IV Administration at the Maximum Dose and Rate to Patients With Epilepsy or Neurosurgical Patients

(Events in at Least 2% of Cerebyx-Treated Patients)

BODY SYSTEM Adverse Event	IV Cerebyx N=90	IV Phenytoin N=22
BODY AS A WHOLE		
Pelvic Pain	4.4	0.0
Asthenia	2.2	0.0
Back Pain	2.2	0.0
Headache	2.2	4.5
CARDIOVASCULAR		
Hypotension	7.7	9.1
Vasodilatation	5.6	4.5
Tachycardia	2.2	0.0
DIGESTIVE		
Nausea	8.9	13.6
Tongue Disorder	4.4	0.0
Dry Mouth	4.4	4.5
Vomiting	2.2	9.1
NERVOUS		
Nystagmus	44.4	59.1
Dizziness	31.1	27.3
Somnolence	20.0	27.3
Ataxia	11.1	18.2
Stupor	7.7	4.5
Incoordination	4.4	4.5
Paresthesia	4.4	0.0
Extrapyramidal Syndrome	4.4	0.0
Tremor	3.3	9.1
Agitation	3.3	0.0
Hypesthesia	2.2	9.1
Dysarthria	2.2	0.0
Vertigo	2.2	0.0
Brain Edema	2.2	4.5
SKIN AND APPENDAGES		
Pruritus	48.9	4.5
SPECIAL SENSES		
Tinnitus	8.9	9.1
Diplopia	3.3	0.0
Taste Perversion	3.3	0.0
Amblyopia	2.2	9.1
Deafness	2.2	0.0

Incidence in Controlled Trials-IM Administration to Patients With Epilepsy. Table 3 lists treatment-emergent adverse events that occurred in at least 2% of Cerebyx-treated patients in a double-bind, randomized controlled clinical trial of adult epilepsy patients receiving either IM Cerebyx substituted for oral Dilantin or continuing oral Dilantin. Both treatments were administered for 5 days.

TABLE 3. Treatment-Emergent Adverse Event Incidence Following Substitution of IM Cerebyx for Oral Dilantin in Patients With Epilepsy

(Events in at Least 2% of Cerebyx-Treated Patients)

BODY SYSTEM Adverse Event	IM Cerebyx N=179	Oral Dilantin N=61
BODY AS A WHOLE		
Headache	8.9	4.9
Asthenia	3.9	3.3
Accidental Injury	3.4	6.6
DIGESTIVE		
Nausea	4.5	0.0
Vomiting	2.8	0.0
HEMATOLOGIC AND LYMPHATIC		
Ecchymosis	7.3	4.9
NERVOUS		
Nystagmus	15.1	8.2
Tremor	9.5	13.1
Ataxia	8.4	8.2
Incoordination	7.8	4.9
Somnolence	6.7	9.8
Dizziness	5.0	3.3
Paresthesia	3.9	3.3
Reflexes Decreased	2.8	4.9
SKIN AND APPENDAGES		
Pruritus	2.8	0.0

Adverse Events During All Clinical Trials

Cerebyx has been administered to 859 individuals during all clinical trials. All adverse events seen at least twice are listed in the following, except those already included in previous tables and listings. Events are further classified within body system categories and enumerated in order of decreasing frequency using the following definitions: frequent adverse events are defined as those occurring in greater than 1/100 individuals; infrequent adverse events are those occurring in 1/100 to 1/1000 individuals.

Body As a Whole: *Frequent:* fever, injection-site reaction, infection, chills, face edema, injection-site pain; *Infrequent:* sepsis, injection-site inflammation, injection-site edema, injection-site hemorrhage, flu syndrome, malaise, generalized edema, shock, photosensitivity reaction, cachexia, cryptococcosis.

Cardiovascular: *Frequent:* hypertension; *Infrequent:* cardiac arrest, migraine, syncope, cerebral hemorrhage, palpitation, sinus bradycardia, atrial flutter, bundle branch block, cardiomegaly, cerebral infarct, postural hypotension, pulmonary embolus. QT interval prolongation, thrombophlebitis, ventricular extrasystoles, congestive heart failure.

Digestive: *Frequent:* constipation; *Infrequent:* dyspepsia, diarrhea, anorexia, gastrointestinal hemorrhage, increased salivation, liver function tests abnormal, tenesmus, tongue edema, dysphagia, flatulence, gastritis, ileus.

Endocrine: *Infrequent:* diabetes insipidus.

Hematologic and Lymphatic: *Infrequent:* thrombocytopenia, anemia, leukocytosis, cyanosis, hypochromic anemia, leukopenia, lymphadenopathy, petachia.

Metabolic and Nutritional: *Frequent:* hypokalemia; *Infrequent:* hyperglycemia, hypophosphatemia, alkalosis, acidosis, dehydration, hyperkalemia, ketosis.

Musculoskeletal: *Frequent:* myasthenia; *Infrequent:* myopathy, leg cramps, arthralgia, myalgia.

Nervous: *Frequent:* reflexes increased, speech disorder, dysarthria, intracranial hypertension, thinking abnormal, nervousness, hypesthesia; *Infrequent:* confusion, twitching, Babinski sign positive, circumoral paresthesia, hemiplegia, hypotonia, convulsion, extrapyramidal syndrome, insomnia, meningitis, depersonalization, CNS depression, depression, hypokinesia, hyperkinesia, brain edema, paralysis, psychosis, aphasia, emotional lability, coma, hyperesthesia, myoclonus, personality disorder, acute brain syndrome, encephalitis, subdural hematoma, encephalopathy, hostility, akathisia, amnesia, neurosis.

Respiratory: *Frequent:* pneumonia; *Infrequent:* pharyngitis, sinusitis, hyperventilation, rhinitis, apnea, aspiration pneumonia, asthma, dyspnea, atelectasis, cough increased, sputum increased, epistaxis, hypoxia, pneumothorax, hemoptysis, bronchitis.

Skin and Appendages: *Frequent:* rash; *Infrequent:* maculopapular rash, urticaria, sweating, skin discoloration, contact dermatitis, pustular rash, skin nodule.

Special Senses: *Frequent:* taste perversion; *Infrequent:* deafness, visual field defect, eye pain, conjunctivitis, photophobia, hyperacusis, mydriasis, parosmia, ear pain, taste loss.

Urogenital: *Infrequent:* urinary retention, oliguria, dysuria, vaginitis, albuminuria, genital edema, kidney failure, polyuria, urethral pain, urinary incontinence, vaginal moniliasis.

OVERDOSAGE

There is no experience with Cerebyx overdosage in humans. The median lethal dose of fosphenytoin given intravenously in mice and rats was 156 mg PE/kg and approximately 250 mg PE/kg, or about 0.6 and 2 times, respectively, the maximum human loading dose on a mg/m^2 basis. Signs of acute toxicity in animals included ataxia, labored breathing, ptosis, and hypoactivity.

Because Cerebyx is a prodrug of phenytoin, the following information may be helpful. Initial symptoms of acute phenytoin toxicity are nystagmus, ataxia, and dysarthria. Other signs include tremor, hyperreflexia, lethargy, slurred speech, nausea, vomiting, coma, and hypotension. Depression of respiratory and circulatory systems leads to death. There are marked variations among individuals with respect to plasma phenytoin concentrations where toxicity occurs. Lateral gaze nystagmus usually appears at 20 μg/mL, ataxia at 30 μg/mL, and dysarthria and lethargy appear when the plasma concentration is over 40 μg/mL. However, phenytoin concentrations as high as 50 μg/mL have been reported without evidence of toxicity. As much as 25 times the therapeutic phenytoin dose has been taken, resulting in plasma phenytoin concentrations over 100 μg/mL, with complete recovery.

Treatment is nonspecific since there is no known antidote to Cerebyx or phenytoin overdosage. The adequacy of the respiratory and circulatory systems should be carefully observed, and appropriate supportive measures employed. Hemodialysis can be considered since phenytoin is not completely bound to plasma proteins. Total exchange transfusion has been used in the treatment of severe intoxication in children. In acute overdosage the possibility of other CNS depressants, including alcohol, should be borne in mind.

Formate and phosphate are metabolites of fosphenytoin and therefore may contribute to signs of toxicity following overdosage. Signs of formate toxicity are similar to those of methanol toxicity and are associated with severe anion-gap metabolic acidosis. Large amounts of phosphate, delivered rapidly, could potentially cause hypocalcemia with paresthesia, muscle spasms, and seizures. Ionized free calcium levels can be measured and, if low, used to guide treatment.

DOSAGE AND ADMINISTRATION

The dose, concentration in dosing solutions, and infusion rate of IV Cerebyx is expressed as phenytoin sodium equivalents (PE) to avoid the need to perform molecular weight-based adjustments when converting between fosphenytoin and phenytoin sodium doses. Cerebyx should always be prescribed and dispensed in phenytoin sodium equivalent units (PE). Cerebyx has important differences in administration from those for parenteral phenytoin sodium (see below).

Products with particulate matter or discoloration should not be used. Prior to IV infusion, dilute Cerebyx in 5% dextrose or 0.9% saline solution for injection to a concentration ranging from 1.5 to 25 mg PE/mL.

Status Epilepticus

- The loading dose of Cerebyx is 15 to 20 mg PE/kg administered at 100 to 150 mg PE/min.
- Because of the risk of hypotension, fosphenytoin should be administered no faster than 150 mg PE/min. Continuous monitoring of the electrocardiogram, blood pressure, and respiratory function is essential and the patient should be observed throughout the period where maximal serum phenytoin concentrations occur, approximately 10 to 20 minutes after the end of Cerebyx infusions.
- Because the full antiepileptic effect of phenytoin, whether given as Cerebyx or parenteral phenytoin is not immediate, other measures, including concomitant administration of an IV benzodiazepine, will usually be necessary for the control of status epilepticus.
- The loading dose should be followed by maintenance doses of Cerebyx, or phenytoin either orally or parenterally.

If administration of Cerebyx does not terminate seizures, the use of other anticonvulsants and other appropriate measures should be considered.

IM Cerebyx should not be used in the treatment of status epilepticus because therapeutic phenytoin concentrations may not be reached as quickly as with IV administration. If IV access is impossible, loading doses of Cerebyx have been given by the IM route for other indications.

Nonemergent Loading and Maintenance Dosing

The loading dose of Cerebyx is 10-20 mg PE/kg given IV or IM. The rate of administration for IV Cerebyx should be no greater than 150 mg PE/min. Continuous monitoring of the electrocardiogram, blood pressure, and respiratory function is essential and the patient should be observed throughout the period where maximal serum phenytoin concentrations occur, approximately 10 to 20 minutes after the end of Cerebyx infusions.

The initial daily maintenance dose of Cerebyx is 4-6 mg PE/kg/day.

IM or IV Substitution For Oral Phenytoin Therapy

Cerebyx can be substituted for oral phenytoin sodium therapy at the same total daily dose.

Dilantin capsules are approximately 90% bioavailable by the oral route. Phenytoin, supplied as Cerebyx, is 100% bioavailable by both the IM and IV routes. For this reason, plasma phenytoin concentrations may increase modestly when IM or IV Cerebyx is substituted for oral phenytoin sodium therapy.

The rate of administration for IV Cerebyx should be no greater than 150 mg PE/min.

In controlled trials, IM Cerebyx was administered as a single daily dose utilizing either 1 or 2 injection sites. Some patients may require more frequent dosing.

Dosing in Special Populations

Patients with Renal or Hepatic Disease: Due to an increased fraction of unbound phenytoin in patients with renal or hepatic disease, or in those with hypoalbuminemia, the interpretation of total phenytoin plasma concentrations should be made with caution (see CLINICAL PHARMACOLOGY: Special Populations). Unbound phenytoin concentrations may be more useful in these patient populations. After IV Cerebyx administration to patients with renal and/or hepatic disease, or in those with hypoalbuminemia, fosphenytoin clearance to phenytoin may be increased without a similar increase in phenytoin clearance. This has the potential to increase the frequency and severity of adverse events (see PRECAUTIONS).

Elderly Patients: Age does not have a significant impact on the pharmacokinetics of fosphenytoin following Cerebyx administration. Phenytoin clearance is decreased slightly in elderly patients and lower or less frequent dosing may be required.

Pediatric: The safety of Cerebyx in pediatric patients has not been established.

HOW SUPPLIED

Cerebyx Injection is supplied as follows:

10 mL per vial—Each vial contains fosphenytoin sodium 750 mg equivalent to 500 mg of phenytoin sodium:
N 0071-4008-10 Packages of 10.

2 mL per vial—Each vial contains fosphenytoin sodium 150 mg equivalent to 100 mg of phenytoin sodium:
N 0071-4007-05. Packages of 25.

Both sizes of vials contain Tromethamine, USP (TRIS), Hydrochloric Acid, NF, or Sodium Hydroxide, NF, and Water for Injection, USP.

Cerebyx should always be prescribed in phenytoin sodium equivalent units (PE) (see DOSAGE AND ADMINISTRATION).

Storage

Store under refrigeration at 2°C to 8°C (36°F to 46°F). The product should not be stored at room temperature for more than 48 hours. Vials that develop particulate matter should not be used.

Rx only

Revised September 1998

PARKE-DAVIS

Div of Warner-Lambert Co.
Morris Plains, NJ 07950 USA 4007G210

MADE IN IRELAND

KAPSEALS®
DILANTIN® ℞
[*dī-lăn 'tĭn"*]
(Extended Phenytoin Sodium Capsules, USP)

DESCRIPTION

Phenytoin Sodium is an antiepileptic drug. Phenytoin sodium is related to the barbiturates in chemical structure, but has a five-membered ring. The chemical name is sodium 5,5-diphenyl-2,4-imidazolidinedione having the following structural formula:

H N ONa N O

Each Dilantin—*Extended Phenytoin Sodium Capsule* USP contains 30 mg or 100 mg phenytoin sodium USP. Also contains lactose, NF; confectioner's sugar, NF; talc, USP; and magnesium stearate, NF. The capsule shell and band contain colloidal silicon dioxide, NF; FD&C red No. 3; gelatin, NF; glyceryl monooleate; sodium lauryl sulfate, NF. The Dilantin 30-mg capsule shell and band also contain citric acid, USP; FD&C blue No. 1; sodium benzoate, NF; titanium dioxide, USP. The Dilantin 100-mg capsule shell and band also contain FD&C yellow no. 6; purified water, USP; polyethylene glycol 200. Product *in vivo* performance is characterized by a slow and extended rate of absorption with peak blood concentrations expected in 4 to 12 hours as contrasted to *Prompt Phenytoin Sodium Capsules* USP with a rapid rate of absorption with peak blood concentration expected in $1^1/_2$ to 3 hours.

CLINICAL PHARMACOLOGY

Phenytoin is an antiepileptic drug which can be useful in the treatment of epilepsy. The primary site of action appears to be *the motor cortex* where spread of seizure activity is inhibited. Possibly by promoting sodium efflux from neurons, phenytoin tends to *stabilize* the threshold against hyperexcitability caused by excessive stimulation or environmental changes capable of reducing membrane sodium gradient. This includes the reduction of posttetanic potentiation at synapses. Loss of posttetanic potentiation prevents cortical seizure foci from detonating adjacent cortical areas. Phenytoin reduces the maximal activity of brain stem centers responsible for the tonic phase of tonic-clonic (grand mal) seizures.

The plasma half-life in man after oral administration of phenytoin averages 22 hours, with a range of 7 to 42 hours. Steady-state therapeutic levels are achieved 7 to 10 days after initiation of therapy with recommended doses of 300 mg/day.

When serum level determinations are necessary, they should be obtained at least 5-7 half-lives after treatment initiation, dosage change, or addition or subtraction of another drug to the regimen so that equilibrium or steady-state will have been achieved. Trough levels provide information about clinically effective serum level range and confirm patient compliance and are obtained just prior to the patient's next scheduled dose. Peak levels indicate an individual's threshold for emergence of dose-related side effects and are obtained at the time of expected peak concentration. For Dilantin Kapseals peak serum levels occur 4-12 hours after administration.

Optimum control without clinical signs of toxicity occurs more often with serum levels between 10 and 20 mcg/ml, although some mild cases of tonic-clonic (grand mal) epilepsy may be controlled with lower serum levels of phenytoin.

In most patients maintained at a steady dosage, stable phenytoin serum levels are achieved. There may be wide interpatient variability in phenytoin serum levels with equivalent dosages. Patients with unusually low levels may be noncompliant or hypermetabolizers of phenytoin. Unusually high levels result from liver disease, congenital enzyme deficiency or drug interactions which result in metabolic interference. The patient with large variations in phenytoin plasma levels, despite standard doses, presents a difficult clinical problem. Serum level determinations in such patients may be particularly helpful. As phenytoin is highly protein bound, free phenytoin levels may be altered in patients whose protein binding characteristics differ from normal.

Most of the drug is excreted in the bile as inactive metabolites which are then reabsorbed from the intestinal tract and excreted in the urine. Urinary excretion of phenytoin and its metabolites occurs partly with glomerular filtration but more importantly, by tubular secretion. Because phenytoin is hydroxylated in the liver by an enzyme system which is saturable at high plasma levels, small incremental doses may increase the half-life and produce very substantial increases in serum levels, when these are in the upper range. The steady-state level may be disproportionately increased, with resultant intoxication, from an increase in dosage of 10% or more.

INDICATIONS AND USAGE

Dilantin is indicated for the control of generalized tonic-clonic (grand mal) and complex partial (psychomotor, temporal lobe) seizures and prevention and treatment of seizures occurring during or following neurosurgery.

Phenytoin serum level determinations may be necessary for optimal dosage adjustments (see Dosage and Administration and Clinical Pharmacology sections).

CONTRAINDICATIONS

Phenytoin is contraindicated in those patients who are hypersensitive to phenytoin or other hydantoins.

WARNINGS

Abrupt withdrawal of phenytoin in epileptic patients may precipitate status epilepticus. When, in the judgment of the clinician, the need for dosage reduction, discontinuation, or substitution of alternative antiepileptic medication arises, this should be done gradually. However, in the event of an allergic or hypersensitivity reaction, rapid substitution of alternative therapy may be necessary. In this case, alternative therapy should be an antiepileptic drug not belonging to the hydantoin chemical class.

There have been a number of reports suggesting a relationship between phenytoin and the development of lymphadenopathy (local or generalized) including benign lymph node hyperplasia, pseudolymphoma, lymphoma, and Hodgkin's Disease. Although a cause and effect relationship has not been established, the occurrence of lymphadenopathy indicates the need to differentiate such a condition from other types of lymph node pathology. Lymph node involvement may occur with or without symptoms and signs resembling serum sickness, eg, fever, rash and liver involvement.

In all cases of lymphadenopathy, follow-up observation for an extended period is indicated and every effort should be made to achieve seizure control using alternative antiepileptic drugs.

Acute alcoholic intake may increase phenytoin serum levels while chronic alcoholic use may decrease serum levels.

In view of isolated reports associating phenytoin with exacerbation of porphyria, caution should be exercised in using this medication in patients suffering from this disease.

Continued on next page

This product information was prepared in June 2000. On these and other Parke-Davis Products, information may be obtained by addressing PARKE-DAVIS, a Warner-Lambert Division, Morris Plains, New Jersey 07950.

Dilantin Kapseals—Cont.

Usage in Pregnancy:
A number of reports suggests an association between the use of antiepileptic drugs by women with epilepsy and a higher incidence of birth defects in children born to these women. Data are more extensive with respect to phenytoin and phenobarbital, but these are also the most commonly prescribed antiepileptic drugs; less systematic or anecdotal reports suggest a possible similar association with the use of all known antiepileptic drugs.
The reports suggesting a higher incidence of birth defects in children of drug-treated epileptic women cannot be regarded as adequate to prove a definite cause and effect relationship. There are intrinsic methodologic problems in obtaining adequate data on drug teratogenicity in humans; genetic factors or the epileptic condition itself may be more important than drug therapy in leading to birth defects. The great majority of mothers on antiepileptic medication deliver normal infants. It is important to note that antiepileptic drugs should not be discontinued in patients in whom the drug is administered to prevent major seizures, because of the strong possibility of precipitating status epilepticus with attendant hypoxia and threat to life. In individual cases where the severity and frequency of the seizure disorder are such that the removal of medication does not pose a serious threat to the patient, discontinuation of the drug may be considered prior to and during pregnancy, although it cannot be said with any confidence that even minor seizures do not pose some hazard to the developing embryo or fetus. The prescribing physician will wish to weigh these considerations in treating or counseling epileptic women of childbearing potential.
In addition to the reports of increased incidence of congenital malformation, such as cleft lip/palate and heart malformations in children of women receiving phenytoin and other antiepileptic drugs, there have more recently been reports of a fetal hydantoin syndrome. This consists of prenatal growth deficiency, microcephaly and mental deficiency in children born to mothers who have received phenytoin, barbiturates, alcohol, or trimethadione. However, these features are all interrelated and are frequently associated with intrauterine growth retardation from other causes.
There have been isolated reports of malignancies, including neuroblastoma, in children whose mothers received phenytoin during pregnancy.
An increase in seizure frequency during pregnancy occurs in a high proportion of patients, because of altered phenytoin absorption or metabolism. Periodic measurement of serum phenytoin levels is particularly valuable in the management of a pregnant epileptic patient as a guide to an appropriate adjustment of dosage. However, postpartum restoration of the original dosage will probably be indicated.
Neonatal coagulation defects have been reported within the first 24 hours in babies born to epileptic mothers receiving phenobarbital and/or phenytoin. Vitamin K has been shown to prevent or correct this defect and has been recommended to be given to the mother before delivery and to the neonate after birth.

PRECAUTIONS

General:
The liver is the chief site of biotransformation of phenytoin; patients with impaired liver function, elderly patients, or those who are gravely ill may show early signs of toxicity.
A small percentage of individuals who have been treated with phenytoin have been shown to metabolize the drug slowly. Slow metabolism may be due to limited enzyme availability and lack of induction; it appears to be genetically determined.
Phenytoin should be discontinued if a skin rash appears (see "Warnings" section regarding drug discontinuation). If the rash is exfoliative, purpuric, or bullous or if lupus erythematosus, Stevens-Johnson syndrome, or toxic epidermal necrolysis is suspected, use of the drug should not be resumed and alternative therapy should be considered. (See ADVERSE REACTIONS section.) If the rash is of a milder type (measles-like or scarlatiniform), therapy may be resumed after the rash has completely disappeared. If the rash recurs upon reinstitution of therapy, further phenytoin medication is contraindicated.
Phenytoin and other hydantoins are contraindicated in patients who have experienced phenytoin hypersensitivity. Additionally, caution should be exercised if using structurally similar compounds (eg, barbiturates, succinimides, oxazolidinediones and other related compounds) in these same patients.
Hyperglycemia, resulting from the drug's inhibitory effects on insulin release, has been reported. Phenytoin may also raise the serum glucose level in diabetic patients.
Osteomalacia has been associated with phenytoin therapy and is considered to be due to phenytoin's interference with Vitamin D metabolism.
Phenytoin is not indicated for seizures due to hypoglycemic or other causes. Appropriate diagnostic procedures should be performed as indicated.
Phenytoin is not effective for absence (petit mal) seizures. If tonic-clonic (grand-mal) and absence (petit mal) seizures are present, combined drug therapy is needed.
Serum levels of phenytoin sustained above the optimal range may produce confusional states referred to as "delirium," "psychosis," or "encephalopathy," or rarely irreversible cerebellar dysfunction. Accordingly, at the first sign of acute toxicity, plasma levels are recommended. Dose reduction of phenytoin therapy is indicated if plasma levels are excessive; if symptoms persist, termination is recommended. (See Warnings section.)

Information for Patients:
Patients taking phenytoin should be advised of the importance of adhering strictly to the prescribed dosage regimen, and of informing the physician of any clinical condition in which it is not possible to take the drug orally as prescribed, eg, surgery, etc.
Patients should also be cautioned on the use of other drugs or alcoholic beverages without first seeking the physician's advice.
Patients should be instructed to call their physician if skin rash develops.
The importance of good dental hygiene should be stressed in order to minimize the development of gingival hyperplasia and its complications.

Laboratory Tests:
Phenytoin serum level determinations may be necessary to achieve optimal dosage adjustments.

Drug Interactions:
There are many drugs which may increase or decrease phenytoin levels or which phenytoin may affect. Serum level determinations for phenytoin are especially helpful when possible drug interactions are suspected. The most commonly occurring drug interactions are listed below.

1. Drugs which may increase phenytoin serum levels include: acute alcohol intake, amiodarone, chloramphenicol, chlordiazepoxide, diazepam, dicumarol, disulfiram, estrogens, H_2-antagonists, halothane, isoniazid, methylphenidate, phenothiazines, phenylbutazone, salicylates, succinimides, sulfonamides, tolbutamide, trazodone.
2. Drugs which may decrease phenytoin levels include: carbamazepine, chronic alcohol abuse, reserpine, and sucralfate. Moban® brand of molindone hydrochloride contains calcium ions which interfere with the absorption of phenytoin. Ingestion times of phenytoin and antacid preparations containing calcium should be staggered in patients with low serum phenytoin levels to prevent absorption problems.
3. Drugs which may either increase or decrease phenytoin serum levels include: phenobarbital, sodium valproate, and valproic acid. Similarly, the effect of phenytoin on phenobarbital, valproic acid and sodium valproate serum levels is unpredictable.
4. Although not a true drug interaction, tricyclic antidepressants may precipitate seizures in susceptible patients and phenytoin dosage may need to be adjusted.
5. Drugs whose efficacy is impaired by phenytoin include: corticosteroids, coumarin anticoagulants, digitoxin, doxycycline, estrogens, furosemide, oral contraceptives, quinidine, rifampin, theophylline, vitamin D.

Drug/Laboratory Test Interactions:
Phenytoin may cause decreased serum levels of protein-bound iodine (PBI). It may also produce lower than normal values for dexamethasone or metyrapone tests. Phenytoin may cause increased serum levels of glucose, alkaline phosphatase, and gamma glutamyl transpeptidase (GGT).

Carcinogenesis:
See 'Warnings' section for information on carcinogenesis.

Pregnancy:
See WARNINGS section.

Nursing Mothers:
Infant breast feeding is not recommended for women taking this drug because phenytoin appears to be secreted in low concentrations in human milk.

ADVERSE REACTIONS

Central Nervous System: The most common manifestations encountered with phenytoin therapy are referable to this system and are usually dose-related. These include nystagmus, ataxia, slurred speech, decreased coordination, and mental confusion. Dizziness, insomnia, transient nervousness, motor twitchings, and headaches have also been observed. There have also been rare reports of phenytoin induced dyskinesias, including chorea, dystonia, tremor and asterixis, similar to those induced by phenothiazine and other neuroleptic drugs.
A predominantly sensory peripheral polyneuropathy has been observed in patients receiving long-term phenytoin therapy.
Gastrointestinal System: Nausea, vomiting, constipation, toxic hepatitis and liver damage.
Integumentary System: Dermatological manifestations sometimes accompanied by fever have included scarlatiniform or morbilliform rashes. A morbilliform rash (measles-like) is the most common; other types of dermatitis are seen more rarely. Other more serious forms which may be fatal have included bullous, exfoliative or purpuric dermatitis, lupus erythematosus, Stevens-Johnson syndrome, and toxic epidermal necrolysis (see Precautions section).
Hemopoietic System: Hemopoietic complications, some fatal, have occasionally been reported in association with administration of phenytoin. These have included thrombocytopenia, leukopenia, granulocytopenia, agranulocytosis, and pancytopenia with or without bone marrow suppression. While macrocytosis and megaloblastic anemia have occurred, these conditions usually respond to folic acid therapy. Lymphadenopathy including benign lymph node hyperplasia, pseudolymphoma, lymphoma, and Hodgkin's Disease have been reported (see WARNINGS section).
Connective Tissue System: Coarsening of the facial features, enlargement of the lips, gingival hyperplasia, hypertrichosis, and Peyronie's Disease.
Cardiovascular: Periarteritis nodosa.
Immunologic: Hypersensitivity syndrome (which may include, but is not limited to, symptoms such as arthralgias, eosinophilia, fever, liver dysfunction, lymphadenopathy or rash), systemic lupus erythematosus, immunoglobulin abnormalities.

OVERDOSAGE

The lethal dose in pediatric patients is not known. The lethal dose in adults is estimated to be 2 to 5 grams. The initial symptoms are nystagmus, ataxia, and dysarthria. Other signs are tremor, hyperflexia, lethargy, slurred speech, nausea, vomiting. The patient may become comatose and hypotensive. Death is due to respiratory and circulatory depression.
There are marked variations among individuals with respect to phenytoin plasma levels where toxicity may occur. Nystagmus, on lateral gaze, usually appears at 20 mcg/ml, ataxia at 30 mcg/ml, dysarthria and lethargy appear when the plasma concentration is over 40 mcg/ml, but as high a concentration as 50 mcg/ml has been reported without evidence of toxicity. As much as 25 times the therapeutic dose has been taken to result in a serum concentration over 100 mcg/ml with complete recovery.

Treatment:
Treatment is nonspecific since there is no known antidote. The adequacy of the respiratory and circulatory systems should be carefully observed and appropriate supportive measures employed. Hemodialysis can be considered since phenytoin is not completely bound to plasma proteins. Total exchange transfusion has been used in the treatment of severe intoxication in pediatric patients.
In acute overdosage, the possibility of other CNS depressants, including alcohol, should be borne in mind.

DOSAGE AND ADMINISTRATION

Serum concentrations should be monitored in changing from extended Phenytoin Sodium Capsules USP (Dilantin) to Prompt Phenytoin Sodium Capsules USP, and from the sodium salt to the free acid form.
Dilantin® Kapseals® and Dilantin Parenteral are formulated with the sodium salt of phenytoin. The free acid form of phenytoin is used in Dilantin-125 Suspension and Dilantin Infatabs. Because there is approximately an 8% increase in drug content with the free acid form over that of the sodium salt, dosage adjustments and serum level monitoring may be necessary when switching from a product formulated with the free acid to a product formulated with the sodium salt and vice versa.

General:
Dosage should be individualized to provide maximum benefit. In some cases, serum blood level determinations may be necessary for optimal dosage adjustments—the clinically effective serum level is usually 10-20 mcg/ml. With recommended dosage, a period of seven to ten days may be required to achieve steady-state blood levels with phenytoin and changes in dosage (increase or decrease) should not be carried out at intervals shorter than seven to ten days.

Adult Dosage:

Divided Daily Dosage
Patients who have received no previous treatment may be started on one 100-mg Dilantin (Extended Phenytoin Sodium Capsule) three times daily and the dosage then adjusted to suit individual requirements. For most adults, the satisfactory maintenance dosage will be one capsule three to four times a day. An increase up to two capsules three times a day may be made, if necessary.

Once-a-Day Dosage:
In adults, if seizure control is established with divided doses of three 100 mg Dilantin capsules daily, once-a-day dosage with 300 mg of extended phenytoin sodium capsules may be considered. Studies comparing divided doses of 300 mg with a single daily dose of this quantity indicated absorption, peak plasma levels, biologic half-life, difference between peak and minimum values, and urinary recovery were equivalent. Once-a-day dosage offers a convenience to the individual patient or to nursing personnel for institutionalized patients and is intended to be used only for patients requiring this amount of drug daily. A major problem in motivating noncompliant patients may also be lessened when the patient can take this drug once a day. However, patients should be cautioned not to miss a dose, inadvertently.
Only extended phenytoin sodium capsules are recommended for once-a-day dosing. Inherent differences in dissolution characteristics and resultant absorption rates of phenytoin due to different manufacturing procedures and/or dosage forms preclude such recommendation for other phenytoin products. When a change in the dosage form or brand is prescribed, careful monitoring of phenytoin serum levels should be carried out.

Loading Dose:
Some authorities have advocated use of an oral loading dose of phenytoin in adults who require rapid steady-state serum levels and where intravenous administration is not desirable. This dosing regimen should be reserved for patients in a clinic or hospital setting where phenytoin serum levels can be closely monitored. Patients with a history of renal or liver disease should not receive the oral loading regimen.
Initially, one gram of phenytoin capsules is divided into 3 doses (400 mg, 300 mg, 300 mg) and administered at two-

hourly intervals. Normal maintenance dosage is then instituted 24 hours after the loading dose, with frequent serum level determinations.

Pediatric Dosage:

Initially, 5 mg/kg/day in two or three equally divided doses, with subsequent dosage individualized to a maximum of 300 mg daily. A recommended daily maintenance dosage is usually 4 to 8 mg/kg. Children over 6 years old and adolescents may require the minimum adult dose (300 mg/day).

HOW SUPPLIED

N 0071-0362 (Kapseal 362, transparent #3 capsule with an orange band)—Dilantin 100 mg; in 100's, 1,000's, and unit dose 100's.

N 0071-0365 (Kapseal 365, transparent #4 capsule with a pink band)—Dilantin 30 mg; in 100's.

Store below 30°C (86°F). Protect from light and moisture.

Also available as:

N 0071-2214—Dilantin-125® Suspension 125 mg phenytoin/5 ml with a maximum alcohol content not greater than 0.6 percent, available in 8-oz bottles. The minimum sales unit is 100 pouches.

N 0071-0007 (Tablet 7)—Dilantin Infatabs® each contain 50 mg phenytoin, 100's and unit dose 100's.

For Parenteral Use:

N 0071-4488-47 (Steri-Dose® 4488)-Dilantin ready-mixed solution containing 50 mg phenytoin sodium per milliliter is supplied in a 2-mL sterile disposable syringe (22 gauge × $1^1/_4$ inch needle). Packages of ten syringes.

N 0071-4488-45 Dilantin ready-mixed solution containing 50 mg phenytoin sodium per milliliter is supplied in 2-mL Steri-Vials.® Packages of twenty-five.

N 0071-4475-45 Dilantin ready-mixed solution containing 50 mg phenytoin sodium per milliliter is supplied in 5-mL Steri-Vials.® Packages of twenty-five.

Store below 30°C (86°F). Protect from light and moisture.

Rx only

Revised May 1999

 0362G550

Shown in Product Identification Guide, page 329

INFATABS®
DILANTIN® ℞

[*dī-lăn 'tĭn " ĭn 'fă-tăbs "*]

(Phenytoin Tablets, USP)

NOT FOR ONCE A DAY DOSING

DESCRIPTION

Dilantin is an antiepileptic drug.

Dilantin (phenytoin) is related to the barbiturates in chemical structure, but has a five-membered ring. The chemical name is 5,5-diphenyl-2,4-imidazolidinedione having the following structural formula:

[structural formula: H, N, O, NH, O]

Each Dilantin Infatab, for oral administration, contains 50 mg phenytoin, USP. Also contains: D&C yellow No. 10, Al lake; FD&C yellow No. 6, Al lake flavor; saccharin sodium, USP; sucrose, NF; talc, USP; and other ingredients.

CLINICAL PHARMACOLOGY

Phenytoin is an antiepileptic drug which can be useful in the treatment of epilepsy. The primary site of action appears to be the motor cortex where spread of seizure activity is inhibited. Possibly by promoting sodium efflux from neurons, phenytoin tends to stabilize the threshold against hyperexcitability caused by excessive stimulation or environmental changes capable of reducing membrane sodium gradient. This includes the reduction of posttetanic potentiation at synapses. Loss of posttetanic potentiation prevents cortical seizure foci from detonating adjacent cortical areas. Phenytoin reduces the maximal activity of brain stem centers responsible for the tonic phase of tonic-clonic (grand mal) seizures.

Clinical studies using Dilantin Infatabs have shown an average plasma half-life of 14 hours with a range of 7 to 29 hours. Steady-state therapeutic levels are achieved at least 7 to 10 days (5-7 half-lives) after initiation of therapy with recommended doses of 300 mg/day.

When serum level determinations are necessary, they should be obtained at least 5-7 half-lives after treatment initiation, dosage change, or addition or subtraction of another drug to the regimen so that equilibrium or steady-state will have been achieved. Trough levels provide information about clinically effective serum level range and confirm patient compliance and are obtained just prior to the patient's next scheduled dose. Peak levels indicate an individual's threshold for emergence of dose-related side effects and are obtained at the time of expected peak concentration. For Dilantin Infatabs peak levels occur $1^1/_2$-3 hours after administration.

Optimum control without clinical signs of toxicity occurs more often with serum levels between 10 and 20 mcg/ml, although some mild cases of tonic-clonic (grand mal) epilepsy may be controlled with lower serum levels of phenytoin.

In most patients maintained at a steady dosage, stable phenytoin serum levels are achieved. There may be wide interpatient variability in phenytoin serum levels with equivalent dosages. Patients with unusually low levels may be noncompliant or hypermetabolizers of phenytoin. Unusually high levels result from liver disease, congenital enzyme deficiency or drug interactions which result in metabolic interference. The patient with large variations in phenytoin plasma levels, despite standard doses, presents a difficult clinical problem. Serum level determinations in such patients may be particularly helpful. As phenytoin is highly protein bound, free phenytoin levels may be altered in patients whose protein binding characteristics differ from normal.

Most of the drug is excreted in the bile as inactive metabolites which are then reabsorbed from the intestinal tract and excreted in the urine. Urinary excretion of phenytoin and its metabolites occurs partly with glomerular filtration but more importantly, by tubular secretion. Because phenytoin is hydroxylated in the liver by an enzyme system which is saturable at high plasma levels small incremental doses may increase the half-life and produce very substantial increases in serum levels, when these are in the upper range. The steady-state level may be disproportionately increased, with resultant intoxication, from an increase in dosage of 10% or more.

Clinical studies show that chewed and unchewed Dilantin Infatabs are bioequivalent, yield approximately equivalent plasma levels, and are more rapidly absorbed than 100-mg Dilantin Kapseals.®

INDICATIONS AND USAGE

Dilantin Infatabs (Phenytoin Tablets, USP) are indicated for the control of generalized tonic-clonic (grand mal) and complex partial (psychomotor, temporal lobe) seizures and prevention and treatment of seizures occurring during or following neurosurgery. Phenytoin serum level determinations may be necessary for optimal dosage adjustments (see Dosage and Administration and Clinical Pharmacology sections).

CONTRAINDICATIONS

Phenytoin is contraindicated in those patients who are hypersensitive to phenytoin or other hydantoins.

WARNINGS

Abrupt withdrawal of phenytoin in epileptic patients may precipitate status epilepticus. When, in the judgment of the clinician, the need for dosage reduction, discontinuation, or substitution of alternative antiepileptic medication arises, this should be done gradually. However, in the event of an allergic or hypersensitivity reaction, rapid substitution of alternative therapy may be necessary. In this case, alternative therapy should be an antiepileptic drug not belonging to the hydantoin chemical class.

There have been a number of reports suggesting a relationship between phenytoin and the development of lymphadenopathy (local or generalized) including benign lymph node hyperplasia, pseudolymphoma, lymphoma, and Hodgkin's Disease. Although a cause and effect relationship has not been established, the occurrence of lymphadenopathy indicates the need to differentiate such a condition from other types of lymph node pathology. Lymph node involvement may occur with or without symptoms and signs resembling serum sickness eg, fever, rash and liver involvement. In all cases of lymphadenopathy, follow-up observation for an extended period is indicated and every effort should be made to achieve seizure control using alternative antiepileptic drugs.

Acute alcoholic intake may increase phenytoin serum levels while chronic alcoholic use may decrease serum levels.

In view of isolated reports associating phenytoin with exacerbation of porphyria, caution should be exercised in using this medication in patients suffering from this disease.

Usage in Pregnancy

A number of reports suggest an association between the use of antiepileptic drugs by women with epilepsy and a higher incidence of birth defects in children born to these women. Data are more extensive with respect to phenytoin and phenobarbital, but these are also the most commonly prescribed antiepileptic drugs; less systematic or anecdotal reports suggest a possible similar association with the use of all known antiepileptic drugs.

The reports suggesting a higher incidence of birth defects in children of drug-treated epileptic women cannot be regarded as adequate to prove a definite cause and effect relationship. There are intrinsic methodologic problems in obtaining adequate data on drug teratogenicity in humans: genetic factors or the epileptic condition itself, may be more important than drug therapy in leading to birth defects. The great majority of mothers on antiepileptic medication deliver normal infants. It is important to note that antiepileptic drugs should not be discontinued in patients in whom the drug is administered to prevent major seizures, because of the strong possibility of precipitating status epilepticus with attendant hypoxia and threat to life. In individual cases where the severity and frequency of the seizure disorder are such that the removal of medication does not pose a serious threat to the patient, discontinuation of the drug may be considered prior to and during pregnancy, although it cannot be said with any confidence that even minor seizures do not pose some hazard to the developing embryo or fetus. The prescribing physician will wish to weigh these considerations in treating or counseling epileptic women of childbearing potential.

In addition to the reports of increased incidence of congenital malformations, such as cleft lip/palate and heart malformations in children of women receiving phenytoin and other antiepileptic drugs, there have more recently been reports of a fetal hydantoin syndrome. This consists of prenatal growth deficiency, microcephaly and mental deficiency in children born to mothers who have received phenytoin, barbiturates, alcohol, or trimethadione. However, these features are all interrelated and are frequently associated with intrauterine growth retardation from other causes.

There have been isolated reports of malignancies, including neuroblastoma, in children whose mothers received phenytoin during pregnancy.

An increase in seizure frequency during pregnancy occurs in a high proportion of patients, because of altered phenytoin absorption or metabolism. Periodic measurement of serum phenytoin levels is particularly valuable in the management of a pregnant epileptic patient as a guide to an appropriate adjustment of dosage. However, postpartum restoration of the original dosage will probably be indicated.

Neonatal coagulation defects have been reported within the first 24 hours in babies born to epileptic mothers receiving phenobarbital and/or phenytoin. Vitamin K has been shown to prevent or correct this defect and has been recommended to be given to the mother before delivery and to the neonate after birth.

PRECAUTIONS

General

The liver is the chief site of biotransformation of phenytoin; patients with impaired liver function, elderly patients, or those who are gravely ill may show early signs of toxicity.

A small percentage of individuals who have been treated with phenytoin have been shown to metabolize the drug slowly. Slow metabolism may be due to limited enzyme availability and lack of induction; it appears to be genetically determined.

Phenytoin should be discontinued if a skin rash appears (see "Warnings" section regarding drug discontinuation). If the rash is exfoliative, purpuric, or bullous or if lupus erythematosus, Stevens-Johnson syndrome, or toxic epidermal necrolysis is suspected, use of this drug should not be resumed, and alternative therapy should be considered (see Adverse Reactions). If the rash is of a milder type (measles-like or scarlatiniform), therapy may be resumed after the rash has completely disappeared. If the rash recurs upon reinstitution of therapy, further phenytoin medication is contraindicated.

Phenytoin and other hydantoins are contraindicated in patients who have experienced phenytoin hypersensitivity. Additionally, caution should be exercised if using structurally similar (eg barbiturates, succinimides, oxazolidinediones and other related compounds) in these same patients.

Hyperglycemia, resulting from the drug's inhibitory effects on insulin release, has been reported. Phenytoin may also raise the serum glucose level in diabetic patients.

Osteomalacia has been associated with phenytoin therapy and is considered to be due to phenytoin's interference with Vitamin D metabolism.

Phenytoin is not indicated for seizures due to hypoglycemic or other metabolic causes. Appropriate diagnostic procedures should be performed as indicated.

Phenytoin is not effective for absence (petit mal) seizures. If tonic-clonic (grand-mal) and absence (petit mal) seizures are present, combined drug therapy is needed.

Serum levels of phenytoin sustained above the optimal range may produce confusional states referred to as "delirium," "psychosis," or "encephalopathy," or rarely irreversible cerebellar dysfunction. Accordingly, at the first sign of acute toxicity, plasma levels are recommended. Dose reduction of phenytoin therapy is indicated if plasma levels are excessive; if symptoms persist, termination is recommended. (See Warnings).

Information for Patients

Patients taking phenytoin should be advised of the importance of adhering strictly to the prescribed dosage regimen, and of informing the physician of any clinical condition in which it is not possible to take the drug orally as prescribed, eg, surgery, etc.

Patients should also be cautioned on the use of other drugs or alcoholic beverages without first seeking the physician's advice.

Patients should be instructed to call their physician if skin rash develops.

The importance of good dental hygiene should be stressed in order to minimize the development of gingival hyperplasia and its complications.

Laboratory Tests

Phenytoin serum level determinations may be necessary to achieve optimal dosage adjustments.

Drug Interactions

There are many drugs which may increase or decrease phenytoin levels or which phenytoin may affect. Serum level

Continued on next page

This product information was prepared in June 2000. On these and other Parke-Davis Products, information may be obtained by addressing PARKE-DAVIS, a Warner-Lambert Division, Morris Plains, New Jersey 07950.

Dilantin Infatabs—Cont.

determinations for phenytoin are especially helpful when possible drug interactions are suspected. The most commonly occurring drug interactions are listed below:
1. Drugs which may increase phenytoin serum levels include: acute alcohol intake, amiodarone, chloramphenicol, chlordiazepoxide, diazepam, dicumarol, disulfiram, estrogens, H_2-antagonists, halothane, isoniazid, methylphenidate, phenothiazines, phenylbutazone, salicylates, succinimides, sulfonamides, tolbutamide, trazodone.
2. Drugs which may decrease phenytoin serum levels include: carbamazepine, chronic alcohol abuse, reserpine, and sucralfate. Moban® brand of Molindone Hydrochloride contains calcium ions which interfere with the absorption of phenytoin. Ingestion times of phenytoin and antacid preparations containing calcium should be staggered in patients with low serum phenytoin levels to prevent absorption problems.
3. Drugs which may either increase or decrease phenytoin serum levels include: phenobarbital, sodium valproate, and valproic acid. Similarly, the effect of phenytoin on phenobarbital, valproic acid and sodium valproate serum levels is unpredictable.
4. Although not a true drug interaction, tricyclic antidepressants may precipitate seizures in susceptible patients and phenytoin dosage may need to be adjusted.
5. Drugs whose efficacy is impaired by phenytoin include: corticosteroids, coumarin anticoagulants, digitoxin, doxycycline, estrogens, furosemide, oral contraceptives, quinidine, rifampin, theophylline, vitamin D.

Drug/Laboratory Test Interactions
Phenytoin may cause decreased serum levels of protein-bound iodine (PBI). It may also produce lower than normal values for dexamethasone or metyrapone tests. Phenytoin may cause increased serum levels of glucose, alkaline phosphatase, and gamma glutamyl transpeptidase (GGT).

Carcinogenesis
See 'Warnings' section for information on carcinogenesis.

Pregnancy
See Warnings Section.

Nursing Mothers
Infant breast-feeding is not recommended for women taking this drug because phenytoin appears to be secreted in low concentrations in human milk.

ADVERSE REACTIONS

Central Nervous System: The most common manifestations encountered with phenytoin therapy are referable to this system and are usually dose-related. These include nystagmus, ataxia, slurred speech, decreased coordination and mental confusion. Dizziness, insomnia, transient nervousness, motor twitchings, and headache have also been observed.
There have also been rare reports of phenytoin induced dyskinesias, including chorea, dystonia, tremor and asterixis, similar to those induced by phenothiazine and other neuroleptic drugs.
A predominantly sensory peripheral polyneuropathy has been observed in patients receiving long-term phenytoin therapy.
Gastrointestinal System: Nausea, vomiting, constipation, toxic hepatitis and liver damage.
Integumentary System: Dermatological manifestations sometimes accompanied by fever have included scarlatiniform or morbilliform rashes. A morbilliform rash (measles-like) is the most common; other types of dermatitis are seen more rarely. Other more serious forms which may be fatal have included bullous, exfoliative or purpuric dermatitis, lupus erythematosus, Stevens-Johnson syndrome, and toxic epidermal necrolysis (see Precautions section).
Hemopoietic System: Hemopoietic complications, some fatal, have occasionally been reported in association with administration of phenytoin. These have included thrombocytopenia, leukopenia, granulocytopenia, agranulocytosis, and pancytopenia with or without bone marrow suppression. While macrocytosis and megaloblastic anemia have occurred, these conditions usually respond to folic acid therapy. Lymphadenopathy including benign lymph node hyperplasia, pseudolymphoma, lymphoma, and Hodgkin's Disease have been reported (see Warnings section).
Connective Tissue System: Coarsening of the facial features, enlargement of the lips, gingival hyperplasia, hypertrichosis, and Peyronie's Disease.
Cardiovascular: Periarteritis nodosa.
Immunologic: Hypersensitivity syndrome (which may include, but is not limited to, symptoms such as arthralgias, eosinophilia, fever, liver dysfunction, lymphadenopathy or rash), systemic lupus erythematosus, and immunoglobulin abnormalities.

OVERDOSAGE

The lethal dose in pediatric patients is not known. The lethal dose in adults is estimated to be 2 to 5 grams. The initial symptoms are nystagmus, ataxia, and dysarthria. Other signs are tremor, hyperflexia, lethargy, slurred speech, nausea, vomiting. The patient may become comatose and hypotensive. Death is due to respiratory and circulatory depression.
There are marked variations among individuals with respect to phenytoin plasma levels where toxicity may occur. Nystagmus on lateral gaze usually appears at 20 mcg/ml, ataxia at 30 mcg/ml, dysarthria and lethargy appear when the plasma concentration is over 40 mcg/ml, but as high a concentration as 50 mcg/ml has been reported without evidence of toxicity. As much as 25 times the therapeutic dose has been taken to result in a serum concentration over 100 mcg/ml with complete recovery.

Treatment
Treatment is nonspecific since there is no known antidote. The adequacy of the respiratory and circulatory systems should be carefully observed and appropriate supportive measures employed. Hemodialysis can be considered since phenytoin is not completely bound to plasma proteins. Total exchange transfusion has been used in the treatment of severe intoxication in pediatric patients.
In acute overdosage the possibility of other CNS depressants, including alcohol, should be borne in mind.

DOSAGE AND ADMINISTRATION

When given in equal doses, Dilantin Infatabs yield higher plasma levels than Dilantin Kapseals.® For this reason serum concentrations should be monitored and care should be taken when switching a patient from the sodium salt to the free acid form.
Dilantin® Kapseals,® Dilantin Parenteral, and Dilantin with Phenobarbital are formulated with the sodium salt of phenytoin. The free acid form of phenytoin is used in Dilantin-30 Pediatric and Dilantin-125 Suspensions and Dilantin Infatabs. Because there is approximately an 8% increase in drug content with the free acid form over that of the sodium salt, dosage adjustments and serum level monitoring may be necessary when switching from a product formulated with the free acid to a product formulated with the sodium salt and vice versa.

General
Not for once a day dosing.
Dosage should be individualized to provide maximum benefit. In some cases, serum blood level determinations may be necessary for optimal dosage adjustments—the clinically effective serum level is usually 10–20 mcg/ml. With recommended dosage, a period of seven to ten days may be required to achieve steady-state blood levels with phenytoin and changes in dosage (increase or decrease) should not be carried out at intervals shorter than seven to ten days.
Dilantin Infatabs can be either chewed thoroughly before being swallowed or swallowed whole.

Adult Dosage
Patients who have received no previous treatment may be started on two Infatabs three times daily, and the dose is then adjusted to suit individual requirements. For most adults, the satisfactory maintenance dosage will be six to eight Infatabs daily; an increase to twelve Infatabs daily may be made, if necessary.

Pediatric Dosage
Initially, 5 mg/kg/day in two or three equally divided doses, with subsequent dosage individualized to a maximum of 300 mg daily. A recommended daily maintenance dosage is usually 4 to 8 mg/kg. Children over 6 years old and adolescents may require the minimum adult dose (300 mg/day). If the daily dosage cannot be divided equally, the larger dose should be given before retiring.

HOW SUPPLIED

Dilantin Infatabs are supplied as:
N 0071-0007-24—Bottle of 100.
Store at a room temperature below 30°C (86°F).
N 0071-0007-40—Unit dose (10/10's).
Store at controlled room temperature 15°–30°C (59°–86°F). Protect from moisture.
Each tablet contains 50 mg phenytoin in a yellow triangular scored chewable tablet.
Dilantin is also supplied in the following forms:
N 0071-0362-24—Bottle of 100.
N 0071-0362-32—Bottle of 1000.
N 0071-0362-40—Unit dose (10/10's).
Each Kapseal® contains 100 mg phenytoin sodium.
N 0071-0365-24—Bottle of 100.
Each Kapseal® contains 30 mg phenytoin sodium.
N 0071-2214-20—8 oz bottle.
Each 5 ml of suspension contains 125 mg phenytoin with a maximum alcohol content not greater than 0.6 percent.
N 0071-4488-47—2-ml prefilled Steri-Dose® syringes.
A sterile solution for parenteral use containing 50 mg phenytoin sodium per mL in a disposable syringe (22 gauge × $1^1/_4$ inch needle). Supplied in packages of ten.
N 0071-4488-45 Dilantin ready-mixed solution containing 50 mg phenytoin sodium per milliliter is supplied in 2-mL Steri-Vials.® Packages of twenty-five.
N 0071-4475-45 Dilantin ready-mixed solution containing 50 mg phenytoin sodium per milliliter is supplied in 5 mL Steri-Vials.® Packages of twenty-five.
Rx only
Manufactured by:
Parke Davis Pharmaceuticals, Ltd.
Vega Baja, PR 00694
Distributed by:
PARKE-DAVIS
Div of Warner-Lambert Co.
Morris Plains, NJ 07950 USA

Revised May 1998 0007G166

Shown in Product Identification Guide, page 329

DILANTIN-125® ℞

[dī-lăn 'tĭn]
(Phenytoin Oral Suspension, USP)

DESCRIPTION

Dilantin (phenytoin) is related to the barbiturates in chemical structure, but has a five-membered ring. The chemical name is 5,5-diphenyl-2,4 imidazolidinedione having the following structural formula:

Each teaspoonful of suspension contains 125 mg of phenytoin, USP with a maximum alcohol content not greater than 0.6 percent. Also contains carboxymethylcellulose sodium, USP; citric acid, anhydrous, USP; flavors; glycerin, USP; magnesium aluminum silicate, NF; polysorbate 40, NF; purified water, USP; sodium benzoate, NF; sucrose, NF; vanillin, NF; and FD&C yellow No. 6.

CLINICAL PHARMACOLOGY

Phenytoin is an antiepileptic drug which can be useful in the treatment of epilepsy. The primary site of action appears to be *the motor cortex* where spread of seizure activity is inhibited. Possibly by promoting sodium efflux from neurons, phenytoin tends to *stabilize* the threshold against hyperexcitability caused by excessive stimulation or environmental changes capable of reducing membrane sodium gradient. This includes the reduction of posttetanic potentiation at synapses. Loss of posttetanic potentiation prevents cortical seizure foci from detonating adjacent cortical areas. Phenytoin reduces the maximal activity of brain stem centers responsible for the tonic phase of tonic-clonic (grand mal) seizures.
The plasma half-life in man after oral administration of phenytoin averages 22 hours, with a range of 7 to 42 hours. Steady-state therapeutic levels are achieved at least 7 to 10 days (5–7 half-lives) after initiation of therapy with recommended doses of 300 mg/day.
When serum level determinations are necessary, they should be obtained at least 5–7 half-lives after treatment initiation, dosage change, or addition or subtraction of another drug to the regimen so that equilibrium or steady-state will have been achieved. Trough levels provide information about clinically effective serum level range and confirm patient compliance and are obtained just prior to the patient's next scheduled dose. Peak levels indicate an individual's threshold for emergence of dose-related side effects and are obtained at the time of expected peak concentration. For Dilantin-125 Suspension peak levels occur $1^1/_2$–3 hours after administration.
Optimum control without clinical signs of toxicity occurs more often with serum levels between 10 and 20 mcg/mL, although some mild cases of tonic-clonic (grand mal) epilepsy may be controlled with lower serum levels of phenytoin.
In most patients maintained at a steady dosage, stable phenytoin serum levels are achieved. There may be wide interpatient variability in phenytoin serum levels with equivalent dosages. Patients with unusually low levels may be noncompliant or hypermetabolizers of phenytoin. Unusually high levels result from liver disease, congenital enzyme deficiency or drug interactions which result in metabolic interference. The patient with large variations in phenytoin plasma levels, despite standard doses, presents a difficult clinical problem. Serum level determinations in such patients may be particularly helpful. As phenytoin is highly protein bound, free phenytoin levels may be altered in patients whose protein binding characteristics differ from normal.
Most of the drug is excreted in the bile as inactive metabolites which are then reabsorbed from the intestinal tract and excreted in the urine. Urinary excretion of phenytoin and its metabolites occurs partly with glomerular filtration but more importantly, by tubular secretion. Because phenytoin is hydroxylated in the liver by an enzyme system which is saturable at high plasma levels small incremental doses may increase the half-life and produce very substantial increases in serum levels, when these are in the upper range. The steady-state level may be disproportionately increased, with resultant intoxication, from an increase in dosage of 10% or more.

INDICATIONS AND USAGE

Dilantin (phenytoin) is indicated for the control of tonic-clonic (grand mal) and psychomotor (temporal lobe) seizures.
Phenytoin serum level determinations may be necessary for optimal dosage adjustments (see Dosage and Administration and Clinical Pharmacology sections).

CONTRAINDICATIONS

Dilantin is contraindicated in those patients with a history of hypersensitivity to phenytoin or other hydantoins.

WARNINGS

Abrupt withdrawal of phenytoin in epileptic patients may precipitate status epilepticus. When in the judgment of the clinician the need for dosage reduction, discontinuation, or substitution of alternative anticonvulsant medication arises, this should be done gradually. In the event of an allergic or hypersensitivity reaction, more rapid substitution of alternative therapy may be necessary. In this case, alternative therapy should be an anticonvulsant not belonging to the hydantion chemical class.

There have been a number of reports suggesting a relationship between phenytoin and the development of lymphadenopathy (local or generalized) including benign lymph node hyperplasia, pseudolymphoma, lymphoma, and Hodgkin's Disease. Although a cause and effect relationship has not been established, the occurrence of lymphadenopathy indicates the need to differentiate such a condition from other types of lymph node pathology. Lymph node involvement may occur with or without symptoms and signs resembling serum sickness eg, fever, rash and liver involvement.

In all cases of lymphadenopathy, follow-up observation for an extended period is indicated and every effort should be made to achieve seizure control using alternative antiepileptic drugs.

Acute alcoholic intake may increase phenytoin serum levels while chronic alcoholic use may decrease serum levels.

In view of isolated reports associating phenytoin with exacerbation of porphyria, caution should be exercised in using this medication in patients suffering from this disease.

Usage in Pregnancy: A number of reports suggests an association between the use of antiepileptic drugs by women with epilepsy and a higher incidence of birth defects in children born to these women. Data are more extensive with respect to phenytoin and phenobarbital, but these are also the most commonly prescribed antiepileptic drugs; less systematic or anecdotal reports suggest a possible similar association with the use of all known antiepileptic drugs.

The reports suggesting a higher incidence of birth defects in children of drug-treated epileptic women cannot be regarded as adequate to prove a definite cause and effect relationship. There are intrinsic methodologic problems in obtaining adequate data on drug teratogenicity in humans; genetic factors or the epileptic condition itself may be more important than drug therapy in leading to birth defects. The great majority of mothers on antiepileptic medication deliver normal infants. It is important to note that antiepileptic drugs should not be discontinued in patients in whom the drug is administered to prevent major seizures, because of the strong possibility of precipitating status epilepticus with attendant hypoxia and threat to life. In individual cases where the severity and frequency of the seizure disorder are such that the removal of medication does not pose a serious threat to the patient, discontinuation of the drug may be considered prior to and during pregnancy, although it cannot be said with any confidence that even minor seizures do not pose some hazards to the developing embryo or fetus. The prescribing physician will wish to weigh these considerations in treating and counseling epileptic women of childbearing potential.

In addition to the reports of increased incidence of congenital malformation, such as cleft lip/palate and heart malformations in children of women receiving phenytoin and other antiepileptic drugs, there have more recently been reports of a fetal hydantoin syndrome. This consists of prenatal growth deficiency, microcephaly and mental deficiency in children born to mothers who have received phenytoin, barbiturates, alcohol, or trimethadione. However, these features are all interrelated and are frequently associated with intrauterine growth retardation from other causes.

There have been isolated reports of malignancies, including neuroblastoma, in children whose mothers received phenytoin during pregnancy.

An increase in seizure frequency during pregnancy occurs in a high proportion of patients, because of altered phenytoin absorption or metabolism. Periodic measurement of serum phenytoin levels is particularly valuable in the management of a pregnant epileptic patient as a guide to an appropriate adjustment of dosage. However, postpartum restoration of the original dosage will probably be indicated.

Neonatal coagulation defects have been reported within the first 24 hours in babies born to epileptic mothers receiving phenobarbital and/or phenytoin. Vitamin K has been shown to prevent or correct this defect and has been recommended to be given to the mother before delivery and the neonate after birth.

PRECAUTIONS

General: The liver is the chief site of biotransformation of phenytoin; patients with impaired liver function, elderly patients, or those who are gravely ill may show early signs of toxicity.

A small percentage of individuals who have been treated with phenytoin have been shown to metabolize the drug slowly. Slow metabolism may be due to limited enzyme availability and lack of induction; it appears to be genetically determined.

Phenytoin should be discontinued if a skin rash appears (see "Warnings" section regarding drug discontinuation). If the rash is exfoliative, purpuric, or bullous or if lupus erythematosus, Stevens-Johnson syndrome, or toxic epidermal necrolysis is suspected, use of this drug should not be resumed and alternative therapy should be considered. (See Adverse Reactions section). If the rash is of a milder type (measles-like or scarlatiniform), therapy may be resumed after the rash has completely disappeared. If the rash recurs upon reinstitution of therapy, further phenytoin medication is contraindicated. Phenytoin and other hydantoins are contraindicated in patients who have experienced phenytoin hypersensitivity. Additionally, caution should be exercised if using structurally similar (eg, barbiturates, succinamides, oxazolidinediones and other related compounds) in these same patients. Hyperglycemia, resulting from the drug's inhibitory effects on insulin release, has been reported. Phenytoin may also raise the serum glucose level in diabetic patients.

Osteomalacia has been associated with phenytoin therapy and is considered to be due to phenytoin's interference with Vitamin D metabolism.

Phenytoin is not indicated for seizures due to hypoglycemic or other metabolic causes. Appropriate diagnostic procedures should be performed as indicated.

Phenytoin is not effective for absence (petit mal) seizures. If tonic-clonic (grand mal) and absence (petit mal) seizures are present, combined drug therapy is needed.

Serum levels of phenytoin sustained above the optimal range may produce confusional states referred to as "delirium," "psychosis" or "encephalopathy," or rarely irreversible cerebellar dysfunction. Accordingly, at the first sign of acute toxicity, plasma levels are recommended. Dose reduction of phenytoin therapy is indicated if plasma levels are excessive; if symptoms persist, termination is recommended. (See Warnings section).

Information for Patients: Patients taking phenytoin should be advised of the importance of adhering strictly to the prescribed dosage regimen, and of informing the physician of any clinical condition in which it is not possible to take the drug orally as prescribed, eg, surgery, etc. Patients should be instructed to use an accurately calibrated measuring device when using this medication to ensure accurate dosing.

Patients should also be cautioned on the use of other drugs or alcoholic beverages without first seeking the physician's advice.

Patients should be instructed to call their physician if skin rash develops.

The importance of good dental hygiene should be stressed in order to minimize the development of gingival hyperplasia and its complications.

Laboratory Tests: Phenytoin serum level determinations may be necessary to achieve optimal dosage adjustments.

Drug Interactions: There are many drugs which may increase or decrease phenytoin levels or which phenytoin may affect. Serum level determinations for phenytoin are especially helpful when possible drug interactions are suspected. The most commonly occurring drug interactions are:

1. Drugs which may increase phenytoin serum levels include: acute alcohol intake, amiodarone, chloramphenicol, chlordiazepoxide, diazepam, dicumarol, disulfiram, estrogens, ethosuximide, fluoxetine, H_2-antagonists, halothane, isoniazid, methylphenidate, phenothiazines, phenylbutazone, salicylates, succinimides, sulfonamides, tolbutamide, trazodone.
2. Drugs which may decrease phenytoin levels include: carbamazepine, chronic alcohol abuse, reserpine and sucralfate. Moban® brand of molindone hydrochloride contains calcium ions which interfere with the absorption of phenytoin. Ingestion times of phenytoin and antacid preparations containing calcium should be staggered in patients with low serum phenytoin levels to prevent absorption problems.
3. Drugs which may either increase or decrease phenytoin serum levels include: phenobarbital, sodium valproate, and valproic acid. Similarly, the effect of phenytoin on phenobarbital, valproic acid and sodium valproate serum levels is unpredictable.
4. Although not a true drug interaction, tricyclic antidepressants may precipitate seizures in susceptible patients and phenytoin dosage may need to be adjusted.
5. Drugs whose efficacy is impaired by phenytoin include: corticosteroids, coumarin anticoagulants, digitoxin, doxycycline, estrogens, furosemide, oral contraceptives, quinidine, rifampin, theophylline, vitamin D.

Drug/Laboratory Test Interactions: Phenytoin may cause decreased serum levels of protein-bound iodine (PBI). It may also produce lower than normal values for dexamethasone or metyrapone tests. Phenytoin may cause increased serum levels of glucose, alkaline phosphatase, and gamma glutamyl transpeptidase (GGT).

Carcinogenesis: See 'Warnings' section for information on carcinogenesis.

Pregnancy: See Warnings section.

Nursing Mothers: Infant breast feeding is not recommended for women taking this drug because phenytoin appears to be secreted in low concentrations in human milk.

Pediatric Use: See DOSAGE AND ADMINISTRATION section.

ADVERSE REACTIONS

Central Nervous System: The most common manifestations encountered with phenytoin therapy are referable to this system and are usually dose-related. These include nystagmus, ataxia, slurred speech, decreased coordination, and mental confusion. Dizziness, insomnia, transient nervousness, motor twitchings, and headaches have also been observed. There have also been rare reports of phenytoin induced dyskinesias, including chorea, dystonia, tremor and asterixis, similar to those induced by phenothiazine and other neuroleptic drugs.

A predominantly sensory peripheral polyneuropathy has been observed in patients receiving long-term phenytoin therapy.

Gastrointestinal System: Nausea, vomiting, constipation, toxic hepatitis and liver damage.

Integumentary System: Dermatological manifestations sometimes accompanied by fever have included scarlatiniform or morbilliform rashes. A morbilliform rash (measles-like) is the most common; other types of dermatitis are seen more rarely. Other more serious forms which may be fatal have included bullous, exfoliative or purpuric dermatitis, lupus erythematosus, Stevens-Johnson syndrome, and toxic epidermal necrolysis (see Precautions section).

Hemopoietic System: Hemopoietic complications, some fatal, have occasionally been reported in association with administration of phenytoin. These have included thrombocytopenia, leukopenia, granulocytopenia, agranulocytosis, and pancytopenia with or without bone marrow suppression. While macrocytosis and megaloblastic anemia have occurred, these conditions usually respond to folic acid therapy. Lymphadenopathy including benign lymph node hyperplasia, pseudolymphoma, lymphoma, and Hodgkin's Disease have been reported (see Warnings section).

Connective Tissue System: Coarsening of the facial features, enlargement of the lips, gingival hyperplasia, hypertrichosis, and Peyronie's Disease.

Cardiovascular: Periarteritis nodosa.

Immunologic: Hypersensitivity syndrome (which may include, but is not limited to, symptoms such as arthralgias, eosinophilia, fever, liver dysfunction, lymphadenopathy or rash), systemic lupus erythematosus, and immunoglobulin abnormalities.

OVERDOSAGE

The lethal dose in pediatric patients is not known. The lethal dose in adults is estimated to be 2 to 5 grams. The initial symptoms are nystagmus, ataxia, and dysarthria. Other signs are tremor, hyperflexia, lethargy, slurred speech, nausea, vomiting. The patient may become comatose and hypotensive. Death is due to respiratory and circulatory depression.

There are marked variations among individuals with respect to phenytoin plasma levels where toxicity may occur. Nystagmus, on lateral gaze, usually appears at 20 mcg/mL, ataxia at 30 mcg/mL, dysarthria and lethargy appear when the plasma concentration is over 40 mcg/mL, but as high a concentration as 50 mcg/mL has been reported without evidence of toxicity. As much as 25 times the therapeutic dose has been taken to result in a serum concentration over 100 mcg/mL with complete recovery.

Treatment: Treatment is nonspecific since there is no known antidote.

The adequacy of the respiratory and circulatory systems should be carefully observed and appropriate supportive measures employed. Hemodialysis can be considered since phenytoin is not completely bound to plasma proteins. Total exchange transfusion has been used in the treatment of severe intoxication in pediatric patients.

In acute overdosage the possibility of other CNS depressants, including alcohol, should be borne in mind.

DOSAGE AND ADMINISTRATION

Serum concentrations should be monitored and care should be taken when switching a patient from the sodium salt to the free acid form.

Dilantin® Kapseals®, Dilantin Parenteral, and Dilantin with Phenobarbital are formulated with the sodium salt of phenytoin. The free acid form of phenytoin is used in Dilantin-125 Suspension and Dilantin Infatabs. Because there is approximately an 8% increase in drug content with the free acid form over that of the sodium salt, dosage adjustments and serum level monitoring may be necessary when switching from a product formulated with the free acid to a product formulated with the sodium salt and vice versa.

General: Dosage should be individualized to provide maximum benefit. In some cases serum blood level determinations may be necessary for optimal dosage adjustments—the clinically effective serum level is usually 10–20 mcg/mL. With recommended dosage, a period of seven to ten days may be required to achieve steady-state blood levels with phenytoin and changes in dosage (increase or decrease) should not be carried out at intervals shorter than seven to ten days.

Adult Dose: Patients who have received no previous treatment may be started on one teaspoonful (5 mL) of Dilantin-125 Suspension three times daily, and the dose is then adjusted to suit individual requirements. An increase to five teaspoonfuls daily may be made, if necessary.

Pediatric Dose: Initially, 5 mg/kg/day in two or three equally divided doses, with subsequent dosage individualized to a maximum of 300 mg daily. A recommended daily maintenance dosage is usually 4 to 8 mg/kg. Children over 6 years and adolescents may require the minimum adult dose (300 mg/day).

HOW SUPPLIED

N 0071-2214—Dilantin-125® Suspension (phenytoin oral suspension, USP), 125 mg phenytoin/5 mL with a maximum

Continued on next page

This product information was prepared in June 2000. On these and other Parke-Davis Products, information may be obtained by addressing PARKE-DAVIS, a Warner-Lambert Division, Morris Plains, New Jersey 07950.

Dilantin-125—Cont.

alcohol content not greater than 0.6 percent, an orange suspension with an orange-vanilla flavor; available in 8-oz bottles.

Store at controlled Room Temperature 20°–25°C (68°–77°F) [See USP]

Also available as:

N 0071-0362 (Kapseal® 362)—Dilantin (extended phenytoin sodium capsules, USP) 100 mg; in 100's, 1000's, unit dose 100's.

N 0071-0365 (Kapseal 365)—Dilantin (extended phenytoin sodium capsules, USP) 30 mg, in 100's.

N 0071-0007 (Tablet 7)—Dilantin Infatabs® (phenytoin tablets, USP) each contain 50 mg phenytoin; 100's and unit dose 100's.

For Parenteral Use:

N 0071-4488-47 (Steri-Dose® 4488)-Dilantin ready-mixed solution containing 50 mg phenytoin sodium per milliliter is supplied in a 2-mL sterile disposable syringe (22 gauge × $1^1/_4$ inch needle). Packages of ten syringes.

N 0071-4488-45 Dilantin ready-mixed solution containing 50 mg phenytoin sodium per milliliter is supplied in 2 mL Steri-Vials.® Packages of twenty-five.

N 0071-4475-45 Dilantin ready-mixed solution containing 50 mg phenytoin sodium per milliliter is supplied in 5 mL Steri-Vials.® Packages of twenty-five.

Storage: Store at Controlled Room Temperature 20°–25°C (68°–77°F) [See USP]

Rx only

Revised May 1999 2214G132

ESTROSTEP® ℞

(Norethindrone Acetate and Ethinyl Estradiol Tablets, USP)

ESTROSTEP® 21 ℞

(Each white triangular tablet contains 1 mg norethindrone acetate and 20 mcg ethinyl estradiol; each white square tablet contains 1 mg norethindrone acetate and 30 mcg ethinyl estradiol; each white round tablet contains 1 mg norethindrone acetate and 35 mcg ethinyl estradiol.)

ESTROSTEP® Fe ℞

(Each white triangular tablet contains 1 mg norethindrone acetate and 20 mcg ethinyl estradiol; each white square tablet contains 1 mg norethindrone acetate and 30 mcg ethinyl estradiol; each white round tablet contains 1 mg norethindrone and 35 mcg ethinyl estradiol; each brown tablet contains 75 mg ferrous fumarate.)

Patients should be counseled that this product does not protect against HIV infection (AIDS) and other sexually transmitted diseases.

DESCRIPTION

Estrostep is a graduated estrophasic providing estrogen in a graduated sequence over a 21-day period with a constant dose of progestogen.

Estrostep **21** provides for a 21-day dosage regimen of oral contraceptive tablets.

Estrostep **Fe** provides for a continuous dosage regimen consisting of 21 oral contraceptive tablets and seven ferrous fumarate tablets. The ferrous fumarate tablets are present to facilitate ease of drug administration via a 28-day regimen, are non-hormonal, and do not serve any therapeutic purpose.

Each white triangle-shaped tablet contains 1 mg norethindrone acetate [(17 alpha)-17-(acetyloxy)-19-nonpregna-4-en-20-yn-3-one] and 20 mcg ethinyl estradiol [(17 alpha)-19-norpregna-1,3,5(10)-trien-20-yne-3,17-diol]; each white square-shaped tablet contains 1 mg norethindrone acetate and 30 mcg ethinyl estradiol; and each white round tablet contains 1 mg norethindrone acetate, 35 mcg ethinyl estradiol. Each tablet also contains calcium stearate; lactose; microcrystalline cellulose; and starch.

The structural formulas are as follows:

Ethinyl Estradiol

Norethindrone Acetate

Each brown tablet contains microcrystalline cellulose; ferrous fumarate; magnesium stearate; povidone; sodium starch glycolate; sucrose with modified dextrins.

Each Estrostep **21** tablet dispenser contains five white triangular tablets, seven white square tablets, and nine white round tablets. These tablets are to be taken in the following order: one triangular tablet each day for five days, followed by one square tablet each day for seven days, and then one round tablet each day for nine days.

Each Estrostep **Fe** tablet dispenser contains five white triangular tablets, seven white square tablets, nine white round tablets, and seven brown tablets. These tablets are to be taken in the following order: one triangular tablet each day for five days, then one square tablet each day for seven days, followed by one round tablet each day for nine days, and then one brown tablet each day for seven days.

CLINICAL PHARMACOLOGY

Combination oral contraceptives act by suppression of gonadotropins. Although the primary mechanism of this action is inhibition of ovulation, other alterations include changes in the cervical mucus (which increase the difficulty of sperm entry into the uterus) and the endometrium (which reduce the likelihood of implantation).

In vitro and animal studies have shown that norethindrone combines high progestational activity with low intrinsic androgenicity. In humans, norethindrone acetate in combination with ethinyl estradiol does not counteract estrogen-induced increases in sex hormone binding globulin (SHBG). Following multiple-dose administration of Estrostep, serum SHBG concentrations increase two- to three-fold and free testosterone concentrations decrease by 47% to 64%, indicating minimal androgenic activity.

Pharmacokinetics

Absorption

Norethindrone acetate appears to be completely and rapidly deacetylated to norethindrone after oral administration, since the disposition of norethindrone acetate is indistinguishable from that of orally administered norethindrone (1). Norethindrone acetate and ethinyl estradiol are rapidly absorbed, with maximum plasma concentrations of norethindrone and ethinyl estradiol occurring 1 to 2 hours postdose. Both are subject to first-pass metabolism after oral dosing, resulting in an absolute bioavailability of approximately 64% for norethindrone and 43% for ethinyl estradiol (1–3).

Administration of norethindrone acetate/ethinyl estradiol with a high fat meal decreases rate, but not extent, of ethinyl estradiol absorption. The extent of norethindrone absorption is increased by 27% following administration with food.

Plasma concentrations of norethindrone and ethinyl estradiol following chronic administration of Estrostep to 17 women are shown below (Figure 1). Mean steady-state concentrations of norethindrone for the 1/20, 1/30, and 1/35 tablet strengths increased as ethinyl estradiol dose increased over the 21-day dose regimen, due to dose-dependent effects of ethinyl estradiol on serum SHBG concentrations (Table 1). Mean steady-state plasma concentrations of ethinyl estradiol for the 1/20, 1/30, and 1/35 tablet strengths were proportional to ethinyl estradiol dose (Table 1).

[See figure at top of page]

[See table I above]

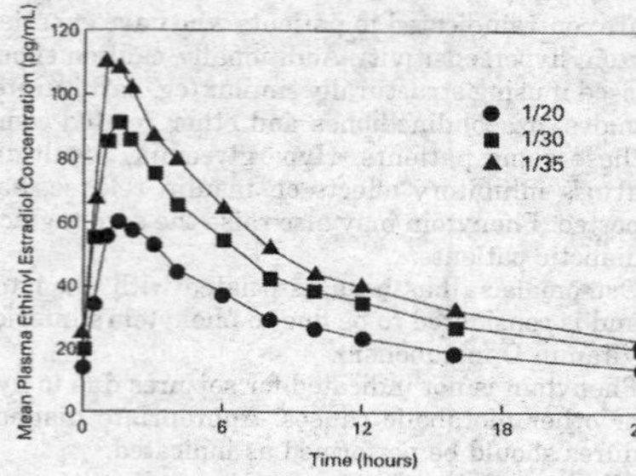

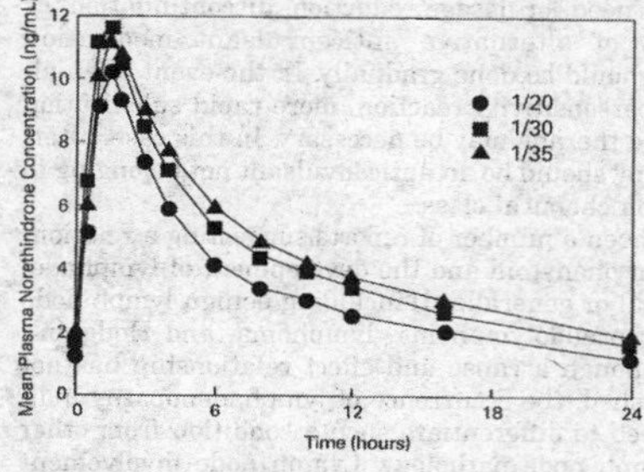

FIGURE 1. Mean Steady-State Plasma Ethinyl Estradiol and Norethindrone Concentrations Following Chronic Administration of Estrostep

TABLE I. Mean(SD) Steady-State Pharmacokinetic Parameters[a] Following Chronic Administration of Estrostep

Norethindrone Acetate/Ethinyl Estradiol Dose	Cycle Day	Cmax	AUC	CL/F	SHBG[b]
	Norethindrone				
mg/μg		ng/mL	ng·hr/mL	mL/min	nmol/L
1/20	5	10.8 (3.9)	81.1 (28.5)	220 (137)	120 (33)
1/30	12	12.7 (4.1)	102 (32)	166 (85)	139 (42)
1/35	21	12.7 (4.1)	109 (32)	152 (73)	163 (40)
	Ethinyl Estradiol				
mg/μg		pg/mL	pg·hr/mL	mL/min	nmol/L
1/20	5	61.0 (16.8)	661 (190)	549 (171)	
1/30	12	92.4 (26.9)	973 (293)	546 (199)	
1/35	21	113 (44)	1149 (372)	568 (219)	

[a] Cmax = Maximum plasma concentration; AUC (0–24)=Area under the plasma concentration-time curve over the dosing interval; CL/F=Apparent oral clearance

[b] Mean (SD) baseline value=55 (29) nmol/L

Distribution

Volume of distribution of norethindrone and ethinyl estradiol ranges from 2 to 4 L/kg (1–3). Plasma protein binding of both steroids is extensive (>95%); norethindrone binds to both albumin and sex hormone binding globulin, whereas ethinyl estradiol binds only to albumin (4). Although ethinyl estradiol does not bind to SHBG, it induces SHBG synthesis. Estrostep increases serum SHBG concentrations two- to three-fold (Table 1).

Metabolism

Norethindrone undergoes extensive biotransformation, primarily via reduction, followed by sulfate and glucuronide conjugation. The majority of metabolites in the circulation are sulfates, with glucuronides accounting for most of the urinary metabolites (5). A small amount of norethindrone acetate is metabolically converted to ethinyl estradiol. Ethinyl estradiol is also extensively metabolized, both by oxidation and by conjugation with sulfate and glucuronide. Sulfates are the major circulating conjugates of ethinyl estradiol and glucuronides predominate in urine. The primary oxidative metabolite is 2-hydroxy ethinyl estradiol, formed by the CYP3A4 isoform of cytochrome P450. Part of the first-pass metabolism of ethinyl estradiol is believed to occur in gastrointestinal mucosa. Ethinyl estradiol may undergo enterohepatic circulation (6).

Excretion

Norethindrone and ethinyl estradiol are excreted in both urine and feces, primarily as metabolites (5,6). Plasma clearance values for norethindrone and ethinyl estradiol are similar (approximately 0.4 L/hr/kg) (1–3). Steady-state elimination half-lives of norethindrone and ethinyl estradiol following administration of Estrostep are approximately 13 hours and 19 hours, respectively.

Special Population

Race:

The effect of race on the disposition of Estrostep has not been evaluated.

Renal Insufficiency

The effect of renal disease on the disposition of Estrostep has not been evaluated. In premenopausal women with chronic renal failure undergoing peritoneal dialysis who received multiple doses of an oral contraceptive containing ethinyl estradiol and norethindrone, plasma ethinyl estradiol concentrations were higher and norethindrone concentrations were unchanged compared to concentrations in premenopausal women with normal renal function.

Hepatic Insufficiency

The effect of hepatic disease on the disposition of Estrostep has not been evaluated. However, ethinyl estradiol and norethindrone may be poorly metabolized in patients with impaired liver function.

TABLE II
LOWEST EXPECTED AND TYPICAL FAILURE RATES DURING THE FIRST YEAR OF CONTINUOUS USE OF A METHOD
% of Women Experiencing an Unintended Pregnancy in the First Year of Continuous Use

Method	Lowest Expected*	Typical**
(No contraception)	(85)	(85)
Oral contraceptives		3
combined	0.1	N/A***
progestin only	0.5	N/A***
Diaphragm with spermicidal cream or jelly	6	20
Spermicides alone (foam, creams, gels, vaginal suppositories, and vaginal film)	6	26
Vaginal Sponge		
nulliparous	9	20
parous	20	40
Implant	0.05	0.05
Injection: depot medroxyprogesterone acetate	0.3	0.3
IUD		
progesterone T	1.5	2.0
copper T 380A	0.6	0.8
LNg 20	0.1	0.1
Condom without spermicides		
female	5	21
male	3	14
Cervical Cap with spermicidal cream or jelly		
nulliparous	9	20
parous	26	40
Periodic abstinence (all methods)	1–9	25
Withdrawal	4	19
Female sterilization	0.5	0.5
Male sterilization	0.10	0.15

Adapted from RA Hatcher et al, Reference 7.
*The authors' best guess of the percentage of women expected to experience an accidental pregnancy among couples who initiate a method (not necessarily for the first time) and who use it consistently and correctly during the first year if they do not stop for any other reason.
**This term represents "typical" couples who initiate use of a method (not necessarily for the first time), who experience an accidental pregnancy during the first year if they do not stop use for any other reason.
***N/A—Data not available.

Drug-Drug Interactions
Numerous drug-drug interactions have been reported for oral contraceptives. A summary of these is found under PRECAUTIONS, Drug Interactions.

INDICATIONS AND USAGE

Estrostep is indicated for the prevention of pregnancy in women who elect to use oral contraceptives as a method of contraception.

Oral contraceptives are highly effective. Table II lists the typical accidental pregnancy rates for users of combination oral contraceptives and other methods of contraception. The efficacy of these contraceptive methods, except sterilization, depends upon the reliability with which they are used. Correct and consistent use of methods can result in lower failure rates.

[See table II above]

CONTRAINDICATIONS

Oral contraceptives should not be used in women who currently have the following conditions:

- Thrombophlebitis or thromboembolic disorders
- A past history of deep vein thrombophlebitis or thromboembolic disorders
- Cerebral vascular or coronary artery disease
- Known or suspected carcinoma of the breast
- Carcinoma of the endometrium or other known or suspected estrogen-dependent neoplasia
- Undiagnosed abnormal genital bleeding
- Cholestatic jaundice of pregnancy or jaundice with prior pill use
- Hepatic adenomas or carcinomas
- Known or suspected pregnancy

WARNINGS

Cigarette smoking increases the risk of serious cardiovascular side effects from oral contraceptive use. This risk increases with age and with heavy smoking (15 or more cigarettes per day) and is quite marked in women over 35 years of age. Women who use oral contraceptives should be strongly advised not to smoke.

The use of oral contraceptives is associated with increased risks of several serious conditions including myocardial infarction, thromboembolism, stroke, hepatic neoplasia, and gallbladder disease, although the risk of serious morbidity or mortality is very small in healthy women without underlying risk factors. The risk of morbidity and mortality increases significantly in the presence of other underlying risk factors such as hypertension, hyperlipidemias, obesity, and diabetes.

Practitioners prescribing oral contraceptives should be familiar with the following information relating to these risks.

The information contained in this package insert is principally based on studies carried out in patients who used oral contraceptives with higher formulations of estrogens and progestogens than those in common use today. The effect of long-term use of the oral contraceptives with lower formulations of both estrogens and progestogens remains to be determined.

Throughout this labeling, epidemiological studies reported are of two types: retrospective or case control studies and prospective or cohort studies. Case control studies provide a measure of the relative risk of a disease, namely, a *ratio* of the incidence of a disease among oral contraceptive users to that among nonusers. The relative risk does not provide information on the actual clinical occurrence of a disease. Cohort studies provide a measure of attributable risk, which is the *difference* in the incidence of disease between oral contraceptive users and nonusers. The attributable risk does provide information about the actual occurrence of a disease in the population (adapted from References 8 and 9 with the author's permission). For further information, the reader is referred to a text on epidemiological methods.

1. Thromboembolic Disorders and Other Vascular Problems

a. Myocardial infarction

An increased risk of myocardial infarction has been attributed to oral contraceptive use. This risk is primarily in smokers or women with other underlying risk factors for coronary artery disease such as hypertension, hypercholesterolemia, morbid obesity, and diabetes. The relative risk of heart attack for current oral contraceptive users has been estimated to be two to six (10–16). The risk is very low under the age of 30.

Smoking in combination with oral contraceptive use has been shown to contribute substantially to the incidence of myocardial infarctions in women in their mid-thirties or older with smoking accounting for the majority of excess cases (17). Mortality rates associated with circulatory disease have been shown to increase substantially in smokers over the age of 35 and non-smokers over the age of 40 (Table III) among women who use oral contraceptives.

[See figure at top of next column]

Oral contraceptives may compound the effects of well-known risk factors, such as hypertension, diabetes, hyperlipidemias, age and obesity (19). In particular, some progestogens are known to decrease HDL cholesterol and cause glucose intolerance, while estrogens may create a state of hyperinsulinism (20–24). Oral contraceptives have been shown to increase blood pressure among users (see Section 9 in WARNINGS). Similar effects on risk factors have been associated with an increased risk of heart disease. Oral contraceptives must be used with caution in women with cardiovascular disease risk factors.

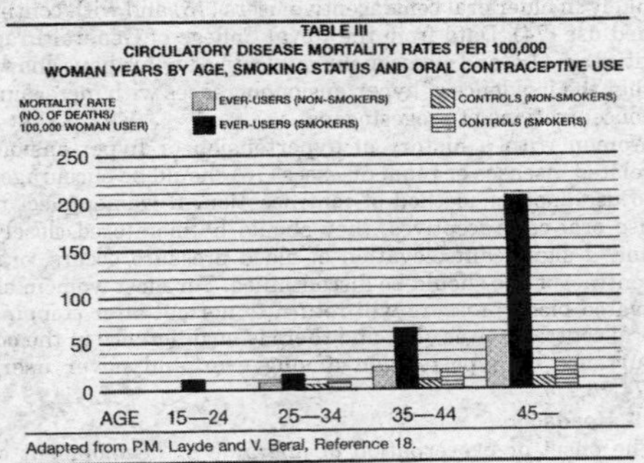

Adapted from P.M. Layde and V. Beral, Reference 18.

b. Thromboembolism

An increased risk of thromboembolic and thrombotic disease associated with the use of oral contraceptives is well established. Case control studies have found the relative risk of users compared to nonusers to be 3 for the first episode of superficial venous thrombosis, 4 to 11 for deep vein thrombosis or pulmonary embolism, and 1.5 to 6 for women with predisposing conditions for venous thromboembolic diseas (9,10,25–30). Cohort studies have shown the relative risk to be somewhat lower, about 3 for new cases and about 4.5 for new cases requiring hospitalization (31). The risk of thromboembolic disease due to oral contraceptives is not related to length of use and disappears after pill use is stopped (8).

A two- to four-fold increase in relative risk of postoperative thromboembolic complications has been reported with the use of oral contraceptives (15,32). The relative risk of venous thrombosis in women who have predisposing conditions is twice that of women without such medical conditions (15,32). If feasible, oral contraceptives should be discontinued at least 4 weeks prior to and for 2 weeks after elective surgery of a type associated with an increase in risk of thromboembolism and during and following prolonged immobilization. Since the immediate postpartum period is also associated with an increased risk of thromboembolism, oral contraceptives should be started no earlier than 4 to 6 weeks after delivery in women who elect not to breast feed.

c. Cerebrovascular disease

Oral contraceptives have been shown to increase both the relative and attributable risks of cerebrovascular events (thrombotic and hemorrhagic strokes), although, in general, the risk is greatest among older (>35 years), hypertensive women who also smoke. Hypertension was found to be a risk factor for both users and nonusers, for both types of strokes, while smoking interacted to increase the risk for hemorrhagic strokes (33–35).

In a large study, the relative risk of thrombotic strokes has been shown to range from 3 for normotensive users to 14 for users with severe hypertension (36). The relative risk of hemorrhagic stroke is reported to be 1.2 for non-smokers who used oral contraceptives, 2.6 for smokers who did not use oral contraceptives, 7.6 for smokers who used oral contraceptives, 1.8 for normotensive users, and 25.7 for users with severe hypertension (36). The attributable risk is also greater in older women (9).

d. Dose-related risk of vascular disease from oral contraceptives

A positive association has been observed between the amount of estrogen and progestogen in oral contraceptives and the risk of vascular disease (37–39). A decline in serum high-density lipoproteins (HDL) has been reported with many progestational agents (20–22). A decline in serum high-density lipoproteins has been associated with an increased incidence of ischemic heart disease. Because estrogens increase HDL cholesterol, the net effect of an oral contraceptive depends on a balance achieved between doses of estrogen and progestin and the nature of the progestin used in the contraceptives. The amount and activity of both hormones should be considered in the choice of an oral contraceptive.

Minimizing exposure to estrogen and progestogen is in keeping with good principles of therapeutics. For any particular oral contraceptive, the dosage regimen prescribed should be one which contains the least amount of estrogen and progestogen that is compatible with the needs of the individual patient. New acceptors of oral contraceptive agents should be started on preparations containing the lowest dose of estrogen which produces satisfactory results for the patient.

e. Persistence of risk of vascular disease

There are two studies which have shown persistence of risk of vascular disease for ever-users of oral contraceptives. In a study in the United States, the risk of developing myocardial infarction after discontinuing oral contraceptives persists for at least 9 years for women 40–49 years who had used oral contraceptives for 5 or more years, but this increased risk was not demonstrated in other age groups (14). In another study in Great Britain, the risk of developing cerebrovascular disease persisted for at least 6 years after discontinuation of oral contraceptives, although excess risk was very small (40). However, both studies were performed with oral contraceptive formulations containing 50 mcg or higher of estrogens.

2. Estimates of Mortality from Contraceptive Use

One study gathered data from a variety of sources which have estimated the mortality rate associated with different methods of contraception at different ages (Table IV). These estimates include the combined risk of death associated with contraceptive methods plus the risk attributable to pregnancy in the event of method failure. Each method of contraception has its specific benefits and risks. The study concluded that with the exception of oral contraceptive users 35 and older who smoke and 40 and older who do not smoke, mortality associated with all methods of birth con-

Continued on next page

This product information was prepared in June 2000. On these and other Parke-Davis Products, information may be obtained by addressing PARKE-DAVIS, a Warner-Lambert Division, Morris Plains, New Jersey 07950.

Estrostep—Cont.

trol is low and below that associated with childbirth. The observation of a possible increase in risk of mortality with age for oral contraceptive users is based on data gathered in the 1970's but not reported until 1983 (41). However, current clinical practice involves the use of lower estrogen dose formulations combined with careful restriction of oral contraceptive use to women who do not have the various risk factors listed in this labeling.

Because of these changes in practice and, also, because of some limited new data which suggest that the risk of cardiovascular disease with the use of oral contraceptives may now be less than previously observed (Porter JB, Hunter J, Jick H, et al. Oral contraceptives and nonfatal vascular disease. Obstet Gynecol 1985;66:1–4; and Porter JB, Hershel J, Walker AM. Mortality among oral contraceptive users. Obstet Gynecol 1987;70:29–32), the Fertility and Maternal Health Drugs Advisory Committee was asked to review the topic in 1989. The Committee concluded that although cardiovascular disease risks may be increased with oral contraceptive use after age 40 in healthy non-smoking women (even with the newer low-dose formulations), there are greater potential health risks associated with pregnancy in older women and with the alternative surgical and medical procedures which may be necessary if such women do not have access to effective and acceptable means of contraception.

Therefore, the Committee recommended that the benefits of oral contraceptive use by healthy non-smoking women over 40 may outweigh the possible risks. Of course, older women, as all women who take oral contraceptives, should take the lowest possible dose formulation that is effective.

[See table below]

3. Carcinoma of the Reproductive Organs

Numerous epidemiological studies have been performed on the incidence of breast, endometrial, ovarian, and cervical cancer in women using oral contraceptives. Most of the studies on breast cancer and oral contraceptive use report that the use of oral contraceptives is not associated with an increase in the risk of developing breast cancer (42, 44, 89). Some studies have reported an increased risk of developing breast cancer in certain subgroups of oral contraceptive users, but the findings reported in these studies are not consistent (43, 45–49, 85–88).

Some studies suggest that oral contraceptive use has been associated with an increase in the risk of cervical intraepithelial neoplasia in some populations of women (51–54). However, there continues to be controversy about the extent to which such findings may be due to differences in sexual behavior and other factors.

In spite of many studies of the relationship between oral contraceptive use and breast and cervical cancers, a cause and effect relationship has not been established.

4. Hepatic Neoplasia

Benign hepatic adenomas are associated with oral contraceptive use, although the incidence of benign tumors is rare in the United States. Indirect calculations have estimated the attributable risk to be in the range of 3.3 cases/100,000 for users, a risk that increases after 4 or more years of use (55). Rupture of rare, benign, hepatic adenomas may cause death through intra-abdominal hemorrhage (56,57).

Studies from Britain have shown an increased risk of developing hepatocellular carcinoma (58–60) in long-term (>8 years) oral contraceptive users. However, these cancers are extremely rare in the U.S. and the attributable risk (the excess incidence) of liver cancers in oral contraceptive users approaches less than one per million users.

5. Ocular Lesions

There have been clinical case reports of retinal thrombosis associated with the use of oral contraceptives. Oral contraceptives should be discontinued if there is unexplained partial or complete loss of vision; onset of proptosis or diplopia; papilledema; or retinal vascular lesions. Appropriate diagnostic and therapeutic measures should be undertaken immediately.

6. Oral Contraceptive Use Before and During Early Pregnancy

Extensive epidemiological studies have revealed no increased risk of birth defects in women who have used oral contraceptives prior to pregnancy (61–63). Studies also do not suggest a teratogenic effect, particularly insofar as cardiac anomalies and limb reduction defects are concerned (61,62,64,65), when taken inadvertently during early pregnancy.

The administration of oral contraceptives to induce withdrawal bleeding should not be used as a test for pregnancy. Oral contraceptives should not be used during pregnancy to treat threatened or habitual abortion.

It is recommended that for any patient who has missed two consecutive periods, pregnancy should be ruled out before continuing oral contraceptive use. If the patient has not adhered to the prescribed schedule, the possibility of pregnancy should be considered at the time of the first missed period. Oral contraceptive use should be discontinued if pregnancy is confirmed.

7. Gallbladder Disease

Earlier studies have reported an increased lifetime relative risk of gallbladder surgery in users of oral contraceptives and estrogens (66,67). More recent studies, however, have shown that the relative risk of developing gallbladder disease among oral contraceptive users may be minimal (68–70). The recent findings of minimal risk may be related to the use of oral contraceptive formulations containing lower hormonal doses of estrogens and progestogens.

8. Carbohydrate and Lipid Metabolic Effects

Oral contraceptives have been shown to cause glucose intolerance in a significant percentage of users (23). Oral contraceptives containing greater than 75 mcg of estrogens cause hyperinsulinism, while lower doses of estrogen cause less glucose intolerance (71). Progestogens increase insulin secretion and create insulin resistance, this effect varying with different progestational agents (23,72). However, in the non-diabetic woman, oral contraceptives appear to have no effect on fasting blood glucose (73). Because of these demonstrated effects, prediabetic women should be carefully observed while taking oral contraceptives.

A small proportion of women will have persistent hypertriglyceridemia while on the pill. As discussed earlier (see WARNINGS 1a. and 1d.), changes in serum triglycerides and lipoprotein levels have been reported in oral contraceptive users.

9. Elevated Blood Pressure

An increase in blood pressure has been reported in women taking oral contraceptives (74) and this increase is more likely in older oral contraceptive users (75) and with continued use (74). Data from the Royal College of General Practitioners (18) and subsequent randomized trials have shown that the incidence of hypertension increases with increasing concentrations of progestogens.

Women with a history of hypertension or hypertension-related diseases or renal diseases (76) should be encouraged to use another method of contraception. If women elect to use oral contraceptives, they should be monitored closely, and if significant elevation of blood pressure occurs, oral contraceptives should be discontinued. For most women, elevated blood pressure will return to normal after stopping oral contraceptives (75), and there is no difference in the occurrence of hypertension among ever and never users (74,76,77).

10. Headache

The onset or exacerbation of migraine or development of headache with a new pattern which is recurrent, persistent, or severe requires discontinuation of oral contraceptives and evaluation of the cause.

11. Bleeding Irregularities

Breakthrough bleeding and spotting are sometimes encountered in patients on oral contraceptives, especially during the first three months of use. Non-hormonal causes should be considered, and adequate diagnostic measures taken to rule out malignancy or pregnancy in the event of prolonged breakthrough bleeding, as in the case of any abnormal vaginal bleeding. If pathology has been excluded, time or a change to another formulation may solve the problem. In the event of amenorrhea, pregnancy should be ruled out.

Some women may encounter post-pill amenorrhea or oligomenorrhea, especially when such a condition was preexistent.

PRECAUTIONS

1. Patients should be counseled that this product does not protect against HIV infection (AIDS) and other sexually transmitted diseases.

2. Physical Examination and Follow-Up

It is good medical practice for all women to have annual history and physical examinations, including women using oral contraceptives. The physical examination, however, may be deferred until after initiation of oral contraceptives if requested by the woman and judged appropriate by the clinician. The physical examination should include special reference to blood pressure, breasts, abdomen and pelvic organs, including cervical cytology, and relevant laboratory tests. In case of undiagnosed, persistent or recurrent abnormal vaginal bleeding, appropriate measures should be conducted to rule out malignancy. Women with a strong family history of breast cancer or who have breast nodules should be monitored with particular care.

3. Lipid Disorders

Women who are being treated for hyperlipidemia should be followed closely if they elect to use oral contraceptives. Some progestogens may elevate LDL levels and may render the control of hyperlipidemias more difficult.

4. Liver Function

If jaundice develops in any woman receiving such drugs, the medication should be discontinued. Steroid hormones may be poorly metabolized in patients with impaired liver function.

5. Fluid Retention

Oral contraceptives may cause some degree of fluid retention. They should be prescribed with caution, and only with careful monitoring, in patients with conditions which might be aggravated by fluid retention.

6. Emotional Disorders

Women with a history of depression should be carefully observed and the drug discontinued if depression recurs to a serious degree.

7. Contact Lenses

Contact lens wearers who develop visual changes or changes in lens tolerance should be assessed by an ophthalmologist.

8. Drug Interactions

Effects of Other Drugs on Oral Contraceptives (78)

Rifampin: Metabolism of both norethindrone and ethinyl estradiol is increased by rifampin. A reduction in contraceptive effectiveness and increased incidence of breakthrough bleeding and menstrual irregularities have been associated with concomitant use of rifampin.

Anticonvulsants: Anticonvulsants such as phenobarbital, phenytoin, and carbamazepine, have been shown to increase the metabolism of ethinyl estradiol and/or norethindrone, which could result in a reduction in contraceptive effectiveness.

Troglitazone: Administration of troglitazone with an oral contraceptive containing ethinyl estradiol and norethindrone reduced the plasma concentrations of both by approximately 30%, which could result in a reduction in contraceptive effectiveness.

Antibiotics: Pregnancy while taking oral contraceptives has been reported when the oral contraceptives were administered with antimicrobials such as ampicillin, tetracycline, and griseofulvin. However, clinical pharmacokinetic studies have not demonstrated any consistent effect of antibiotics (other than rifampin) on plasma concentrations of synthetic steroids.

Atorvastatin: Coadministration of atorvastatin and an oral contraceptive increased AUC values for norethindrone and ethinyl estradiol by approximately 30% and 20%, respectively.

Other: Ascorbic acid and acetaminophen may increase plasma ethinyl estradiol concentrations, possibly by inhibition of conjugation. A reduction in contraceptive effectiveness and increased incidence of breakthrough bleeding has been suggested with phenylbutazone.

Effects of Oral Contraceptives on Other Drugs

Oral contraceptive combinations containing ethinyl estradiol may inhibit the metabolism of other compounds. Increased plasma concentrations of cyclosporine, prednisolone, and theophylline have been reported with concomitant administration of oral contraceptives. In addition, oral contraceptives may induce the conjugation of other compounds. Decreased plasma concentrations of acetaminophen and increased clearance of temazepam, salicylic acid, morphine, and clofibric acid have been noted when these drugs were administered with oral contraceptives.

9. Interactions with Laboratory Tests

Certain endocrine and liver function tests and blood components may be affected by oral contraceptives:

a. Increased prothrombin and factors VII, VIII, IX, and X; decreased antithrombin 3; increased noepinephrine-induced platelet aggregability.

b. Increased thyroid binding globulin (TBG) leading to increased circulating total thyroid hormone, as measured by protein-bound iodine (PBI), T_4 by column or by radioimmunoassay. Free T_3 resin uptake is decreased, reflecting the elevated TBG; free T_4 concentration is unaltered.

c. Other binding proteins may be elevated in serum.

d. Sex-binding globulins are increased and result in elevated levels of total circulating sex steroids and corticoids; however, free or biologically active levels remain unchanged.

e. Triglycerides may be increased.

f. Glucose tolerance may be decreased.

g. Serum folate levels may be depressed by oral contraceptive therapy. This may be of clinical significance if a woman becomes pregnant shortly after discontinuing oral contraceptives.

10. Carcinogenesis

See **WARNINGS** section.

11. Pregnancy

Pregnancy Category X. See **CONTRAINDICATIONS** and **WARNINGS** sections.

TABLE IV
ANNUAL NUMBER OF BIRTH-RELATED OR METHOD-RELATED DEATHS ASSOCIATED WITH CONTROL OF FERTILITY PER 100,000 NONSTERILE WOMEN BY FERTILITY CONTROL METHOD ACCORDING TO AGE

Method of control and outcome	15–19	20–24	25–29	30–34	35–39	40–44
No fertility control methods*	7.0	7.4	9.1	14.8	25.7	28.2
Oral contraceptives non-smoker**	0.3	0.5	0.9	1.9	13.8	31.6
Oral contraceptives smoker**	2.2	3.4	6.6	13.5	51.1	117.2
IUD**	0.8	0.8	1.0	1.0	1.4	1.4
Condom*	1.1	1.6	0.7	0.2	0.3	0.4
Diaphragm/spermicide*	1.9	1.2	1.2	1.3	2.2	2.8
Periodic abstinence*	2.5	1.6	1.6	1.7	2.9	3.6

*Deaths are birth related.
**Deaths are method related.

Adapted from H.W. Ory, Reference 41.

12. Nursing Mothers
Small amounts of oral contraceptive steroids have been identified in the milk of nursing mothers, and a few adverse effects on the child have been reported, including jaundice and breast enlargement. In addition, oral contraceptives given in the postpartum period may interfere with lactation by decreasing the quantity and quality of breast milk. If possible, the nursing mother should be advised not to use oral contraceptives but to use other forms of contraception until she has completely weaned her child.

13. Pediatric Use
Safety and efficacy of Estrostep have been established in women of reproductive age. Safety and efficacy are expected to be the same for postpubertal adolescents under the age of 16 and for users 16 years and older. Use of this product before menarche is not indicated.

INFORMATION FOR THE PATIENT
See patient labeling printed below.

ADVERSE REACTIONS

An increased risk of the following serious adverse reactions has been associated with the use of oral contraceptives (see WARNINGS section):
- Thrombophlebitis
- Arterial thromboembolism
- Pulmonary embolism
- Myocardial infarction
- Cerebral hemorrhage
- Cerebral thrombosis
- Hypertension
- Gallbladder disease
- Hepatic adenomas or benign liver tumors

There is evidence of an association between the following conditions and the use of oral contraceptives, although additional confirmatory studies are needed:
- Mesenteric thrombosis
- Retinal thrombosis

The following adverse reactions have been reported in patients receiving oral contraceptives and are believed to be drug-related:
- Nausea
- Vomiting
- Gastrointestinal symptoms (such as abdominal cramps and bloating)
- Breakthrough bleeding
- Spotting
- Change in menstrual flow
- Amenorrhea
- Temporary infertility after discontinuation of treatment
- Edema
- Melasma which may persist
- Breast changes: tenderness, enlargement, secretion
- Change in weight (increase or decrease)
- Change in cervical erosion and secretion
- Diminution in lactation when given immediately postpartum
- Cholestatic jaundice
- Migraine
- Rash (allergic)
- Mental depression
- Reduced tolerance to carbohydrates
- Vaginal candidiasis
- Change in corneal curvature (steepening)
- Intolerance to contact lenses

The following adverse reactions have been reported in users of oral contraceptives and the association has been neither confirmed nor refuted:
- Pre-menstrual syndrome
- Cataracts
- Changes in appetite
- Cystitis-like syndrome
- Headache
- Nervousness
- Dizziness
- Hirsutism
- Loss of scalp hair
- Erythema multiforme
- Erythema nodosum
- Hemorrhagic eruption
- Vaginitis
- Porphyria
- Impaired renal function
- Hemolytic uremic syndrome
- Budd-Chiari syndrome
- Acne
- Changes in libido
- Colitis

OVERDOSAGE

Serious ill effects have not been reported following acute ingestion of large doses of oral contraceptives by young children. Overdosage may cause nausea, and withdrawal bleeding may occur in females.

NON-CONTRACEPTIVE HEALTH BENEFITS
The following non-contraceptive health benefits related to the use of oral contraceptives are supported by epidemiological studies which largely utilized oral contraceptive formulations containing estrogen doses exceeding 0.035 mg of ethinyl estradiol or 0.05 mg of mestranol (79–84).

Effects on menses:
- Increased menstrual cycle regularity
- Decreased blood loss and decreased incidence of iron deficiency anemia
- Decreased incidence of dysmenorrhea

Effects related to inhibition of ovulation:
- Decreased incidence of functional ovarian cysts
- Decreased incidence of ectopic pregnancies

Effects from long-term use:
- Decreased incidence of fibroadenomas and fibrocystic disease of the breast
- Decreased incidence of acute pelvic inflammatory disease
- Decreased incidence of endometrial cancer
- Decreased incidence of ovarian cancer

DOSAGE AND ADMINISTRATION

The tablet dispenser has been designed to make oral contraceptive dosing as easy and as convenient as possible. The tablets are arranged in either three or four rows of seven tablets each, with the days of the week appearing on the tablet dispenser above the first row of tablets.

Note: Each tablet dispenser has been preprinted with the days of the week, starting with Sunday, to facilitate a Sunday-Start regimen. Six different day label strips have been provided with the Detailed Patient & Brief Summary Patient Package Insert in order to accomodate a Day-1 Start Regimen. If the patient is using the Day-1 Start regimen, she should place the self-adhesive day label strip that corresponds to her starting day over the preprinted days.

Important: The patient should be instructed to use an additional method of protection until after the first week of administration in the initial cycle when utilizing the Sunday-Start regimen.

The possibility of ovulation and conception prior to initiation of use should be considered.

Dosage and Administration for 21-Day Dosage Regimen
To achieve maximum contraceptive effectiveness, Estrostep **21** must be taken exactly as directed and at intervals not exceeding 24 hours. Estrostep **21** provides the patient with a convenient tablet schedule of "3 weeks on–1 week off." Two dosage regimens are described, one of which may be more convenient or suitable than the other for an individual patient. For the initial cycle of therapy, the patient begins her tablets according to the Day-1 Start or Sunday-Start regimen. With either regimen, the patient takes one tablet daily for 21 consecutive days followed by one week of no tablets.

A. Sunday-Start Regimen: The patient begins taking tablets from the top row on the first Sunday after menstrual flow begins. When menstrual flow begins on Sunday, the first tablet is taken on the same day. The last tablet in the dispenser will then be taken on a Saturday, followed by no tablets for a week (7 days). For all subsequent cycles, the patient then begins a new 21-tablet regimen on the eighth day, Sunday, after taking her last tablet. Following this regimen, of 21 days on–7 days off, the patient will start all subsequent cycles on a Sunday.

B. Day-1 Start Regimen: The first day of menstrual flow is Day 1. The patient places the self-adhesive day label strip that corresponds to her starting day over the preprinted days on the tablet dispenser. She starts taking one tablet daily, beginning with the first tablet in the top row. The patient completes her 21-tablet regimen when she has taken the last tablet in the tablet dispenser. She will then take no tablets for a week (7 days). For all subsequent cycles, the patient begins a new 21-tablet regimen on the eighth day after taking her last tablet, again starting with the first tablet in the top row after placing the appropriate day label strip over the preprinted days on the tablet dispenser. Following this regimen of 21 days on–7 days off, the patient will start all subsequent cycles on the same day of the week as the first course. Likewise, the interval of no tablets will always start on the same day of the week.

Tablets should be taken regularly at the same time each day and can be taken without regard to meals. It should be stressed that efficacy of medication depends on strict adherence to the dosage schedule.

Special Notes on Administration
Menstruation usually begins two or three days, but may begin as late as the fourth or fifth day, after discontinuing medication. If spotting occurs while on the usual regimen of one tablet daily, the patient should continue medication without interruption.

If a patient forgets to take one or more *white* tablets, the following is suggested:

One tablet is missed
- take tablet as soon as remembered
- take next tablet at the regular time

Two consecutive tablets are missed (week *1* or week *2*)
- take *two* tablets as soon as remembered
- take *two* tablets the next day
- use another birth control method for seven days following the missed tablets

Two consecutive tablets are missed (week *3*)

Sunday-Start Regimen:
- take *one* tablet daily until Sunday
- discard remaining tablets
- start new pick of tablets immediately (Sunday)
- use another birth control method for seven days following the missed tablets

Day-1 Start Regimen:
- discard remaining tablets
- start new pack of tablets that same day
- use another birth control method for seven days following the missed tablets

Three (or more) consecutive tablets are missed

Sunday-Start Regimen:
- take *one* tablet daily until Sunday
- discard remaining tablets
- start new pack of tablets immediately (Sunday)
- use another birth control method for seven days following the missed tablets

Day-1 Start Regimen:
- discard remaining tablets
- start new pack of tablets that same day
- use another birth control method for seven days following the missed tablets

The possibility of ovulation occurring increases with each successive day that scheduled tablets are missed. While there is little likelihood of ovulation occurring if only one tablet is missed, the possibility of spotting or bleeding is increased. This is particularly likely to occur if two or more consecutive tablets are missed.

In the rare case of bleeding which resembles menstruation, the patient should be advised to discontinue medication and then begin taking tablets from a new tablet dispenser on the next Sunday or the first day (Day 1), depending on her regime. Persistent bleeding which is not controlled by this method indicates the need for reexamination of the patient, at which time nonfunctional causes should be considered.

Dosage and Administration for 28-Day Dosage Regimen
To achieve maximum contraceptive effectiveness, Estrostep **Fe** should be taken exactly as directed and at intervals not exceeding 24 hours.

Estrostep **Fe** provides a continuous administration regimen consisting of 21 white tablets of Estrostep and seven brown non-hormone containing tablets of ferrous fumarate. The ferrous fumarate tablets are present to facilitate ease of drug administration via a 28-day regimen and do not serve any therapeutic purpose. There is no need for the patient to count days between cycles because there are no "off-tablet days."

A. Sunday-Start Regimen: The patient begins taking the first white tablet from the top row of the dispenser (labeled Sunday) on the first Sunday after menstrual flow begins. When the menstrual flow begins on Sunday, the first white tablet is taken on the same day. The patient takes one white tablet daily for 21 days. The last white tablet in the dispenser will be taken on a Saturday. Upon completion of all 21 white tablets, and without interruption, the patient takes one brown tablet daily for 7 days. Upon completion of this first course of tablets, the patient begins a second course of 28-day tablets, without interruption, the next day (Sunday), starting with the Sunday white tablet in the top row. Adhering to this regimen of one white tablet daily for 21 days, followed without interruption by one brown tablet daily for 7 days, the patient will start all subsequent cycles on a Sunday.

B. Day-1 Start Regimen: The first day of menstrual flow is Day 1. The patient places the self-adhesive day label strip that corresponds to her starting day over the preprinted days on the tablet dispenser. She starts taking one white tablet daily, beginning with the first white tablet in the top row. After the last white tablet (at the end of the third row) has been taken, the patient will then take the brown tablets for a week (7 days). For all subsequent cycles, the patient begins a new 28 tablet regimen on the eighth day after taking her last white tablet, again starting with the first tablet in the top row after placing the appropriate day label strip over the preprinted days on the tablet dispenser. Following this regimen of 21 white tablets and 7 brown tablets, the patient will start all subsequent cycles on the same day of the week as the first course.

Tablets should be taken regularly at the same time each day and can be taken without regard to meals. It should be stressed that efficacy of medication depends on strict adherence to the dosage schedule.

Special Notes on Administration
Menstruation usually begins two or three days, but may begin as late as the fourth or fifth day, after the brown tablets have been started. In any event, the next course of tablets should be started without interruption. If spotting occurs while the patient is taking white tablets, continue medication without interruption.

If the patient forgets to take one or more *white* tablets, the following is suggested:

One tablet is missed
- take tablet as soon as remembered
- take next tablet at the regular time

Two consecutive tablets are missed (week *1* or week *2*)
- take *two* tablets as soon as remembered
- take *two* tablets the next day
- use another birth control method for seven days following the missed tablets

Two consecutive tablets are missed (week *3*)

Sunday-Start Regimen:
- take *one* tablet daily until Sunday
- discard remaining tablets
- start new pack of tablets immediately (Sunday)
- use another birth control method for seven days following the missed tablets

Day-1 Start Regimen:
- discard remaining tablets
- start new pack of tablets that same day

Continued on next page

This product information was prepared in June 2000. On these and other Parke-Davis Products, information may be obtained by addressing PARKE-DAVIS, a Warner-Lambert Division, Morris Plains, New Jersey 07950.

Estrostep—Cont.

- use another birth control method for seven days following the missed tablets

Three (or more) consecutive tablets are missed

Sunday-Start Regimen:

- take *one* tablet daily until Sunday
- discard remaining tablets
- start new pack of tablets immediately (Sunday)
- use another birth control method for seven days following the missed tablets

Day-1 Start Regimen:

- discard remaining tablets
- start new pack of tablets that same day
- use another birth control method for seven days following the missed tablets

The possibility of ovulation occurring increases with each successive day that scheduled white tablets are missed. While there is little likelihood of ovulation occurring if only one white tablet is missed, the possibility of spotting or bleeding is increased. This is particularly likely to occur if two or more consecutive white tablets are missed.

If the patient forgets to take any of the seven brown tablets in week four, those brown tablets that were missed are discarded and one brown tablet is taken each day until the pack is empty. A back-up birth control method is not required during this time. A new pack of tablets should be started no later than the eighth day after the last white tablet was taken.

In the rare case of bleeding which resembles menstruation, the patient should be advised to discontinue medication and then begin taking tablets from a new tablet dispenser on the next Sunday or the first day (Day 1), depending on her regimen. Persistent bleeding which is not controlled by this method indicates the need for reexamination of the patient, at which time nonfunctional causes should be considered.

Use of Oral Contraceptives in the Event of a Missed Menstrual Period

1. If the patient has not adhered to the prescribed dosage regimen, the possibility of pregnancy should be considered after the first missed period and oral contraceptives should be withheld until pregnancy has been ruled out.

2. If the patient has adhered to the prescribed regimen and misses two consecutive periods, pregnancy should be ruled out before continuing the contraceptive regimen.

After several months on treatment, bleeding may be reduced to a point of virtual absence. This reduced flow may occur as a result of medication, in which event it is not indicative of pregnancy.

HOW SUPPLIED

Estrostep **21** is available in dispensers each containing 21 white tablets. The first five triangle tablets each contain 1 mg of norethindrone acetate and 20 mcg of ethinyl estradiol; the next seven square tablets each contain 1 mg of norethindrone acetate and 30 mcg of ethinyl estradiol; the last nine round tablets each contain 1 mg of norethindrone acetate and 35 mcg of ethinyl estradiol. Available in packages of five dispensers.

Estrostep **Fe** is available in dispensers each containing 21 white tablets. The first five triangle tablets each contain 1 mg of norethindrone acetate and 20 mcg of ethinyl estradiol; the next seven square tablets each contain 1 mg of norethindrone acetate and 30 mcg of ethinyl estradiol; the next nine round tablets each contain 1 mg of norethindrone acetate and 35 mcg of ethinyl estradiol; and the last seven (brown) tablets each contain 75 mg ferrous fumarate. Available in packages of five dispensers.

Storage—Do not store above 25° C (77° F). Protect from light.

Store tablets inside pouch when not in use.

REFERENCES

1. Back DJ, Breckenridge AM, Crawford FE, McIver M, Orme ML'E, Rowe PH and Smith E: Kinetics of norethindrone in women II. Single-dose kinetics. Clin Pharmacol Ther 1978;24:448–453.

2. Hümpel M, Nieuweboer B, Wendt H and Speck U: Investigations of pharmacokinetics of ethinyloestradiol to specific consideration of a possible first-pass effect in women. Contraception 1979;19:421–432.

3. Back DJ, Breckenridge AM, Crawford FE, MacIver M, Orme ML'E, Rowe PH and Watts MJ. An investigation of the pharmacokinetics of ethynylestradiol in women using radioimmunoassay. Contraception 1979;20:263–273.

4. Hammond GL, Lähteenmäki PLA, Lähteenmäki P and Luukkainen T. Distribution and percentages of non-protein bound contraceptive steroids in human serum. J Steriod Biochem 1982;17:375–380.

5. Fotherby K. Pharmacokinetics and metabolism of progestins in humans, in Pharmacology of the contraceptive steroids, Goldzieher JW, Fotherby K (eds), Raven Press, Ltd.., New York, 1994, 99–126.

6. Goldzieher JW. Pharmacokinetics and metabolism of ethynyl estrogens, in Pharmacology of the contraceptive steroids, Goldzieher JW, Foterhby K (eds), Raven Press Ltd., New York, 1994, 127–151.

7. Hatcher RA, et al. 1998. Contraceptive Technology, Seventeenth Edition. New York: Irvington Publishers.

8. Stadel B.V.: Oral contraceptives and cardiovascular disease. (Pt. 1). *New England Journal of Medicine,* 305: 612–618, 1981.

9. Stadel, B.V.: Oral contraceptives and cardiovascular disease. (Pt. 2). *New England Journal of Medicine,* 305: 672–677, 1981.

10. Adam, S.A., and M. Thorogood: Oral contraception and myocardial infarction revisited: The effects of new preparations and prescribing patterns. *Brit. J. Obstet. and Gynec.,* 88:838–845, 1981.

11. Mann, J.I., and W.H. Inman: Oral contraceptives and death from myocardial infarction. *Brit. Med. J.,* 2(5965): 245–248, 1975.

12. Mann, J.I., M.P. Vessey, M. Thorogood, and R. Doll: Myocardial infarction in young women with special reference to oral contraceptive practice. *Brit. Med. J.,* 2(5956): 241–245, 1975.

13. Royal College of General Practitioners' Oral Contraception Study: Further analyses of mortality in oral contraceptive users. *Lancet,* 1:541–546, 1981.

14. Slone, D., S. Shapiro, D.W. Kaufman, L. Rosenberg, O.S. Miettinen, and P.D. Stolley: Risk of myocardial infarction in relation to current and discontinued use of oral contraceptives. *N.E.J.M.,* 305:420–424, 1981.

15. Vessey, M.P.; Female hormone and vascular disease: An epidemiological overview. *Brit. J. Fam. Plann.,* 6:1–12, 1980.

16. Russell-Briefel, R.G., T.M. Ezzati, R. Fulwood, J.A. Perlman, and R.S. Murphy: Cardiovascular risk status and oral contraceptive use, United States, 1976–80. *Preventive Medicine,* 15:352–362, 1986.

17. Goldbaum, G.M., J.S. Kendrick, G.C. Hogelin, and E.M. Gentry: The relative impact of smoking and oral contraceptive use on women in the United States. *J.A.M.A.,* 258:1339–1342, 1987.

18. Layde, P.M., and V. Beral; Further analyses of mortality in oral contraceptive users: Royal College General Practitioners' Oral Contraception Study. (Table 5) *Lancet,* 1:541–546, 1981.

19. Knopp, R.H.: Arteriosclerosis risk: The roles of oral contraceptives and postmenopausal estrogens. *J. of Reprod. Med.,* 31(9)(Supplement): 913–921, 1986.

20. Krauss, R.M., S. Roy, D.R. Mishell, J. Casagrande, and M.C. Pike: Effects of two low-dose oral contraceptives on serum lipids and lipoproteins: Differential changes in high-density lipoproteins subclasses. Am. *J. Obstet. Gyn.,* 145:446–452, 1983.

21. Wahl, P., C. Walden, R. Knopp, J. Hoover, R. Wallace, G. Heiss, and B. Rifkind: Effect of estrogen/progestin potency on lipid/lipoprotein cholesterol. *N.E.J.M.,* 308:862–867, 1983.

22. Wynn, V., and R. Niththyananthan: The effect of progestin in combined oral contraceptives on serum lipids with special reference to high-density lipoproteins. *Am. J. Obstet. and Gyn.,* 142:766–771, 1982.

23. Wynn, V., and I. Godsland: Effects of oral contraceptives on carbohydrate metabolism. *J. Reprod. Medicine,* 31 (9)(Supplement): 892–897, 1986.

24. LaRosa, J.C.: Atherosclerotic risk factors in cardiovascular disease. *J. Reprod. Med.,* 31(9)(Supplement): 906–912, 1986.

25. Inman, W.H., and M.P. Vessey: Investigations of death from pulmonary, coronary, and cerebral thrombosis and embolism in women of child-bearing age. *Brit. Med. J.,* 2(5599): 193–199, 1968.

26. Maguire, M.G., J. Tonascia, P.E. Sartwell, P.D. Stolley, and M.S. Tockman: Increased risk of thrombosis due to oral contraceptives: A further report. *Am. J. Epidemiology,* 110(2): 188–195, 1979.

27. Pettiti, D.B., J. Wingerd, F. Pellegrin, and S. Ramacharan: Risk of vascular disease in women: Smoking, oral contraceptives, noncontraceptive estrogens, and other factors. *J.A.M.A.,* 242:1150–1154, 1979.

28. Vessey, M.P. and R. Doll: Investigation of relation between use of oral contraceptives and thromboembolic disease. *Brit. Med. J.,* 2(5599): 199–205, 1968.

29. Vessey, M.P., and R. Doll: Investigation of relation between use of oral contraceptives and thromboembolic disease; A further report. *Brit. Med. J.,* 2(5658): 651–657, 1969.

30. Porter, J.B., J.R. Hunter, D.A. Danielson, H. Jick, and A. Stergachis: Oral contraceptives and non-fatal vascular disease: Recent experience. *Obstet. and Gyn.,* 59(3):299–302, 1982.

31. Vessey, M., R. Doll, R. Peto, B. Johnson, and P. Wiggins: A long-term follow-up study of women using different methods of contraception: An interim report. *J. Biosocial. Sci.,* 8:375–427, 1976.

32. Royal College of General Practitioners: Oral contraceptives, venous thrombosis, and varicose veins. *J. of Royal College of General Practitioners,* 28:393–399, 1978.

33. Collaborative Group for the study of stroke in young women: Oral contraception and increased risk of cerebral ischemia or thrombosis. *N.E.J.M.,* 288:871–878, 1973.

34. Petitti, D.B., and J. Wingerd: Use of oral contraceptives, cigarette smoking, and risk of subarachnoid hemorrhage. *Lancet,* 2:234–236, 1978.

35. Inman, W.H.: Oral contraceptives and fatal subarachnoid hemorrhage. *Brit. Med. J.,* 2(6203): 1468–70, 1979.

36. Collaborative Group for the study of stroke in young women: Oral contraceptives and stroke in young women: Associated risk factors. *J.A.M.A.,* 231:718–722, 1975.

37. Inman, W.H., M.P. Vessey, B. Westerholm, and A. Engelund: Thromboembolic disease and the steroidal content of oral contraceptives. A report to the Committee on Safety of Drugs. *Brit. Med. J.,* 2:203–209, 1970.

38. Meade, T.W., G. Greenberg, and S.G. Thompson: Progestogens and cardiovascular reactions associated with oral contraceptives and a comparison of the safety of 50- and 35-mcg oestrogen preparations. *Brit. Med. J.,* 280(6224): 1157–1161, 1980.

39. Kay, C.R.: Progestogens and arterial disease: Evidence from the Royal College of General Practitioners' study. *Amer. J. Obstet. Gyn.,* 142:762–765, 1982.

40. Royal College of General Practitioners: Incidence of arterial disease among oral contraceptive users. *J. Coll. Gen. Pract.,* 33:75–82, 1983.

41. Ory, H.W.: Mortality associated with fertility and fertility control: 1983. *Family Planning Perspectives,* 15:50–56, 1983.

42. The Cancer and Steroid Hormone Study of the Centers for Disease Control and the National Institute of Child Health and Human Development: Oral-contraceptive use and the risk of breast cancer. *N.E.J.M.,* 315: 405–411, 1986.

43. Pike, M.C., B.E. Henderson, M.D. Krailo, A. Duke, and S. Roy: Breast cancer in young women and use of oral contraceptives: Possible modifying effect of formulation and age at use. *Lancet,* 2:926–929, 1983.

44. Paul, C., D.G. Skegg, G.F.S. Spears, and J.M. Kaldor: Oral contraceptives and breast cancer: A national study. *Brit. Med. J.,* 293:723–725, 1986.

45. Miller, D.R., L. Rosenberg, D.W. Kaufman, D. Schottenfeld, P.D. Stolley, and S. Shapiro: Breast cancer risk in relation to early oral contraceptive use. *Obstet. Gynec.,* 68:863–868, 1986.

46. Olson, H., K.L. Olson, T.R. Moller, J. Ranstam, P. Holm: Oral contraceptive use and breast cancer in young women in Sweden (letter). *Lancet,* 2:748–749, 1985.

47. McPherson, K., M. Vessey, A. Neill, R. Doll, L. Jones, and M. Roberts: Early contraceptive use and breast cancer: Results of another case-control study. *Brit. J. Cancer,* 56: 653–660, 1987.

48. Huggins, G.R., and P.F. Zucker: Oral contraceptives and neoplasia: 1987 update. *Fertil. Steril.,* 47:733–761, 1987.

49. McPherson, K., and J.O. Drife: The pill and breast cancer; Why the uncertainty? *Brit. Med. J.,* 293:709–710, 1986.

50. Shapiro, S.: Oral contraceptives: Time to take stock. *N.E.J.M.,* 315:450–451, 1987.

51. Ory, H., Z. Naib, S.B. Conger, R.A. Hatcher, and C.W. Tyler: Contraceptive choice and prevalence of cervical dysplasia and carcinoma in situ. *Am. J. Obstet. Gynec.,* 124:573–577, 1976.

52. Vessey, M.P., M. Lawless, K. McPherson, D. Yeates: Neoplasia of the cervix uteri and contraception: A possible adverse effect of the pill. *Lancet,* 2:930, 1983.

53. Brinton, L.A., G.R. Huggins, H.F. Lehman, K. Malii, D.A. Savitz, E. Trapido, J. Rosenthal, and R. Hoover: Long-term use of oral contraceptives and risk of invasive cervical cancer. *Int. J. Cancer,* 38:339–344, 1986.

54. WHO Collaborative Study of Neoplasia and Steroid Contraceptives: Invasive cervical cancer and combined oral contraceptives. *Brit. Med. J.,* 290:961–965, 1985.

55. Rooks, J.B., H.W. Ory, K.G. Ishak, L.T. Strauss, J.R. Greenspan, A.P. Hill, and C.W. Tyler: Epidemiology of hepatocellular adenoma: The role of oral contraceptive use. *J.A.M.A.,* 242:644–648, 1979.

56. Bein, N.N., and H.S. Goldsmith: Recurrent massive hemorrhage from benign hepatic tumors secondary to oral contraceptives. *Brit. J. Surg.,* 64:433–435, 1977.

57. Klatskin, G.: Hepatic tumors: Possible relationship to use of oral contraceptives. *Gastroenterology,* 73:386–394, 1977.

58. Henderson, B.E., S. Preston-Martin, H.A. Edmondson, R.L. Peters, and M.C. Pike: Hepatocellular carcinoma and oral contraceptives. *Brit. J. Cancer,* 48:437–440, 1983.

59. Neuberger, J., D. Forman, R. Doll, and R. Williams: Oral contraceptives and hepatocellular carcinoma. *Brit. Med. J.,* 292:1355–1357, 1986.

60. Forman, D., T.J. Vincent, and R. Doll: Cancer of the liver and oral contraceptives. *Brit. Med. J.,* 292:1357–1361, 1986.

61. Harlap, S., and J. Eldor: Births following oral contraceptive failures. *Obstet Gynec.,* 55:447–452, 1980.

62. Savolainen, E., E. Saksela, and L. Saxen: Teratogenic hazards of oral contraceptives analyzed in a national malformation register. *J. Obstet Gynec.,* 140:521–524, 1981.

63. Janerich, D.T., J.M. Piper, and D.M. Glebatis: Oral contraceptives and birth defects. *Am. J. Epidemiology,* 112:73–79, 1980.

64. Ferencz, C., G.M. Matanoski, P.D. Wilson, J.D. Rubin, C.A. Neill, and R. Gutberlet: Maternal hormone therapy and congenital heart disease. *Teratology,* 21:225–239, 1980.

65. Rothman, K.J., D.C. Fyler, A. Goldblatt, and M.B. Kreidberg: Exogenous hormones and other drug exposures of children with congenital heart disease. *Am. J. Epidemiology,* 109:433–439, 1979.

66. Boston Collaborative Drug Surveillance Program: Oral contraceptives and venous thromboembolic disease, surgically confirmed gallbladder disease, and breast tumors. *Lancet,* 1:1399–1404, 1973.

67. Royal College of General Practitioners: *Oral Contraceptives and Health.* New York, Pittman, 1974, 100p.

68. Layde, P.M., M.P. Vessey, and D. Yeates: Risk of gallbladder disease: A cohort study of young women attending family planning clinics. *J. Epidemiol. and Comm. Health*, 36:274–278, 1982.
69. Rome Group for the Epidemiology and Prevention of Cholelithiasis (GREPCO): Prevalence of gallstone disease in an Italian adult female population. *Am. J. Epidemiol.*, 119:796–805, 1984.
70. Strom, B.L., R.T. Tamragouri, M.L. Morse, E.L. Lazar, S.L. West, P.D. Stolley, and J.K. Jones: Oral contraceptives and other risk factors for gallbladder disease. *Clin. Pharmacol. Ther.*, 39:335–341, 1986.
71. Wynn, V., P.W. Adams, I.F. Goldsland, J. Melrose, R. Niththyananthan, N.W. Oakley, and A. Seedj: Comparison of effects of different combined oral-contraceptive formulations on carbohydrate and lipid metabolism. *Lancet*, 1:1045–1049, 1979.
72. Wynn, V.: Effect of progesterone and progestins on carbohydrate metabolism. In *Progesterone and Progestin*. Edited by C.W. Bardin, E. Milgrom, P. Mauvis-Jarvis. New York, Raven Press, 395–410, 1983.
73. Perlman, J.A., R.G. Roussell-Briefel, T.M. Ezzati, and G. Lieberknecht: Oral glucose tolerance and the potency of oral contraceptive progestogens. *J. Chronic Dis.*, 38: 857–864, 1985.
74. Royal College of General Practitioners' Oral Contraception Study: Effect on hypertension and benign breast disease of progestogen component in combined oral contraceptives. *Lancet*, 1:624, 1977.
75. Fisch, I.R., and J. Frank: Oral contraceptives and blood pressure. *J.A.M.A.*, 237:2499–2503, 1977.
76. Laragh, A.J.: Oral contraceptive induced hypertension: Nine years later. *Amer. J. Obstet. Gynecol.*, 126:141–147, 1976.
77. Ramcharan, S., E. Peritz, F.A. Pellegrin, and W.T. Williams: Incidence of hypertension in the Walnut Creek Contraceptive Drug Study cohort. In *Pharmacology of Steroid Contraceptive drugs*. Edited by S. Garattini and H.W. Berendes. New York, Raven Press, 277–288, 1977. (Monographs of the Mario Negri Institute for Pharmacological Research, Milan.)
78. Back DJ, Orme ML'E. Drug interactions, in Pharmacology of the contraceptive steroids, Goldzieher JW, Fotherby K (eds), Raven Press, Ltd., New York, 1994, 407–425.
79. The Cancer and Steroid Hormone Study of the Centers for Disease Control and the National Institute of Child Health and Human Development: Oral contraceptive use and the risk of ovarian cancer. *J.A.M.A.*, 249: 1596–1599, 1983.
80. The Cancer and Steroid Hormone Study of the Centers for Disease Control and the National Institute of Child Health and Human Development: Combination oral contraceptive use and the risk of endometrial cancer. *J.A.M.A.*, 257:796–800, 1987.
81. Ory, H.W.: Functional ovarian cysts and oral contraceptives: Negative association confirmed surgically. *J.A.M.A.*, 228:68–69, 1974.
82. Ory, H.W., P. Cole, B. Macmahon, and R. Hoover: Oral contraceptives and reduced risk of benign breast disease. *N.E.J.M.*, 294:41–422, 1976.
83. Ory, H.W.: The noncontraceptive health benefits from oral contraceptive use. *Fam. Plann. Perspectives*, 14:182–184, 1982.
84. Ory, H.W., J.D. Forrest, and R. Lincoln: Making Choices: Evaluating the health risks and benefits of birth control methods. New York, The Alan Guttmacher Institute, 1, 1983.
85. Miller, D.R., L. Rosenberg , D.W. Kaufman, P. Stolley, M.E. Warshauer, and S. Shapiro: Breast cancer before age 45 and oral contraceptive use: new findings. *Am. J. Epidemiol.*, 129:269–280, 1989.
86. Kay, C.R., and P.C. Hannaford: Breast cancer and the pill: a further report from the Royal College of General Practitioners Oral Contraception Study. *Br. J. Cancer*, 58: 675–680, 1988.
87. Stadel, B.V., S. Lai, J.J. Schlesselman, and P. Murray: Oral contraceptives and premenopausal breast cancer in nulliparous women. *Contraception*, 38:287–299, 1988.
88. UK National Case-Control Study Group: Oral contraceptive use and breast cancer risk in young women. *Lancet*, 973–982, 1989.
89. Romieu, I., W.C. Willett, G.A. Colditz, M.J. Stampfer, B. Rosner, C.H. Hennekens, and F.E. Speizer: Prospective study of oral contraceptive use and risk of breast cancer in women. *J. Natl. Cancer Inst.*, 81:1313–1321, 1989.

The patient labeling for oral contraceptive drug products is set forth below:

This product (like all oral contraceptives) is intended to prevent pregnancy. It does not protect against HIV infection (AIDS) and other sexually transmitted diseases.

BRIEF SUMMARY PATIENT PACKAGE INSERT

Oral contraceptives, also known as "birth control pills" or "the pill," are taken to prevent pregnancy and, when taken correctly, have a failure rate of about 1% per year when used without missing any pills. The typical failure rate of large numbers of pill users is less than 3% per year when women who miss pills are included. For most women oral contraceptives are also free of serious or unpleasant side effects. However, forgetting to take pills considerably increases the chances of pregnancy.

For the majority of women, oral contraceptives can be taken safely. But there are some women who are at high risk of developing certain serious diseases that can be life-threatening or may cause temporary or permanent disability. The risks associated with taking oral contraceptives increase significantly if you:

- Smoke
- Have high blood pressure, diabetes, high cholesterol
- Have or have had clotting disorders, heart attack, stroke, angina pectoris, cancer of the breast or sex organs, jaundice, or malignant or benign liver tumors.

You should not take the pill if you suspect you are pregnant or have unexplained vaginal bleeding.

> Cigarette smoking increases the risk of serious cardiovascular side effects from oral contraceptive use. This risk increases with age and with heavy smoking (15 or more cigarettes per day) and is quite marked in women over 35 years of age. Women who use oral contraceptives are strongly advised not to smoke.

Most side effects of the pill are not serious. The most common side effects are nausea, vomiting, bleeding between menstrual periods, weight gain, breast tenderness, and difficulty wearing contact lenses. These side effects, especially nausea, vomiting, and breakthrough bleeding, may subside within the first three months of use.

The serious side effects of the pill occur very infrequently, especially if you are in good health and are young. However, you should know that the following medical conditions have been associated with or made worse by the pill:

1. Blood clots in the legs (thrombophlebitis), lungs (pulmonary embolism), stoppage or rupture of a blood vessel in the brain (stroke), blockage of blood vessels in the heart (heart attack or angina pectoris), or other organs of the body. As mentioned above, smoking increases the risk of heart attacks and strokes and subsequent serious medical consequences.
2. Liver tumors, which may rupture and cause severe bleeding. A possible but not definite association has been found with the pill and liver cancer. However, liver cancers are extremely rare. The chance of developing liver cancer from using the pill is thus even rarer.
3. High blood pressure, although blood pressure usually returns to normal when the pill is stopped.

The symptoms associated with these serious side effects are discussed in the detailed leaflet given to you with your supply of pills. Notify your doctor or health care provider if you notice any unusual physical disturbances while taking the pill. In addition, drugs such as rifampin, as well as some anticonvulsants and some antibiotics, may decrease oral contraceptive effectiveness.

Most of the studies to date on breast cancer and pill use have found no increase in the risk of developing breast cancer, although some studies have reported an increased risk of developing breast cancer in certain groups of women. However, some studies have found an increase in the risk of developing cancer of the cervix in women taking the pill, but this finding may be related to differences in sexual behavior or other factors not related to use of the pill. Therefore, there is insufficient evidence to rule out the possibility that the pill may cause cancer of the breast or cervix.

Taking the pill provides some important non-contraceptive benefits. These include less painful menstruation, less menstrual blood loss and anemia, fewer pelvic infections, and fewer cancers of the ovary and the lining of the uterus.

Be sure to discuss any medical condition you may have with your health care provider. Your health care provider will take a medical and family history and examine you before prescribing oral contraceptives. The physical examination may be delayed to another time if you request it and your health care provider believes that it is a good medical practice to postpone it. You should be reexamined at least once a year while taking oral contraceptives. The detailed patient information leaflet gives you further information which you should read and discuss with your health care provider.

This product (like all oral contraceptives) is intended to prevent pregnancy. It does not protect against transmission of HIV (AIDS) and other sexually transmitted diseases such as chlamydia, genital herpes, genital warts, gonorrhea, hepatitis B, and syphilis.

INSTRUCTIONS TO PATIENT
TABLET DISPENSER

The Estrostep tablet dispenser has been designed to make oral contraceptive dosing as easy and as convenient as possible. The tablets are arranged in either three or four rows of seven tablets each with the days of the week appearing above the first row of tablets.

If your TABLET DISPENSER contains:	You are taking:
21 white tablets	ESTROSTEP 21
21 white tablets and 7 brown tablets	ESTROSTEP Fe

Each *triangle* tablet contains 1 mg norethindrone acetate and 20 mcg ethinyl estradiol.

Each *square* tablet contains 1 mg norethindrone acetate and 30 mcg ethinyl estradiol.

Each *round* tablet contains 1 mg norethindrone acetate and 35 mcg ethinyl estradiol.

Each *brown* tablet contains 75 mg ferrous fumarate and is intended to help you remember to take the tablets correctly. These brown tablets are not intended to have any health benefit.

DIRECTIONS

To remove a tablet, press down on it with your thumb or finger. The tablet will drop through the back of the tablet dispenser. Do not press with your thumbnail, fingernail, or any other sharp object.

HOW TO TAKE THE PILL

IMPORTANT POINTS TO REMEMBER

BEFORE YOU START TAKING YOUR PILLS:

1. BE SURE TO READ THESE DIRECTIONS:
Before you start taking your pills.
Anytime you are not sure what to do.
2. THE RIGHT WAY TO TAKE THE PILL IS TO TAKE ONE PILL EVERY DAY AT THE SAME TIME. If you miss pills you could get pregnant. This includes starting the pack late. The more pills you miss, the more likely you are to get pregnant.
3. MANY WOMEN HAVE SPOTTING OR LIGHT BLEEDING, OR MAY FEEL SICK TO THEIR STOMACH, DURING THE FIRST 1–3 PACKS OF PILLS. If you do have spotting or light bleeding or feel sick to your stomach, do not stop taking the pill. The problem will usually go away. If it doesn't go away, check with your doctor or clinic.
4. MISSING PILLS CAN ALSO CAUSE SPOTTING OR LIGHT BLEEDING, even when you make up these missed pills. On the days you take 2 pills to make up for missed pills, you could also feel a little sick to your stomach.
5. IF YOU HAVE VOMITING OR DIARRHEA, for any reason, or IF YOU TAKE SOME MEDICINES, including some antibiotics, your birth control pills may not work as well. Use a back-up birth control method (such as condoms or foam) until you check with your doctor or clinic.
6. IF YOU HAVE TROUBLE REMEMBERING TO TAKE THE PILL, talk to your doctor or clinic about how to make pill-taking easier or about using another method of birth control.
7. IF YOU HAVE ANY QUESTIONS OR ARE UNSURE ABOUT THE INFORMATION IN THIS LEAFLET, call your doctor or clinic.

BEFORE YOU START TAKING YOUR PILLS

1. DECIDE WHAT TIME OF DAY YOU WANT TO TAKE YOUR PILL. It is important to take it at about the same time every day.
2. LOOK AT YOUR PILL PACK TO SEE IF IT HAS 21 OR 28 PILLS:
The 21-pill pack has 21 "active" white pills (with hormones) to take for 3 weeks, followed by 1 week without pills.
The 28-pill pack has 21 "active" white pills (with hormones) to take for 3 weeks, followed by 1 week of reminder brown pills (without hormones).
3. ALSO FIND:
1) where on the pack to start taking pills,
2) in what order to take the pills (follow the arrows), and
3) the week numbers as shown in the following pictures:

Each Estrostep 21 tablet dispenser contains five white triangular tablets, seven white square tablets, and nine white round tablets. These tablets are to be taken in the following order: one triangular tablet each day for five days, followed by one square tablet each day for seven days, and then one round tablet each day for nine days.

Estrostep 21 will contain:

ALL WHITE PILLS

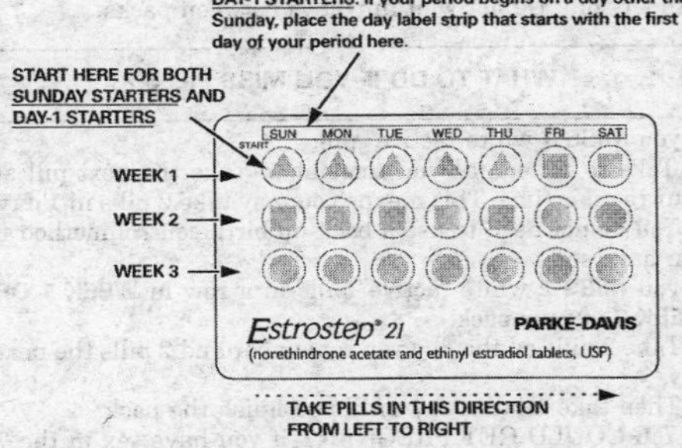
DAY-1 STARTERS: If your period begins on a day other than Sunday, place the day label strip that starts with the first day of your period here.
START HERE FOR BOTH SUNDAY STARTERS AND DAY-1 STARTERS
START
SUN
MON
TUE
WED
THU
FRI
SAT
WEEK 1
WEEK 2
WEEK 3
Estrostep® 21
PARKE-DAVIS
(norethindrone acetate and ethinyl estradiol tablets, USP)
TAKE PILLS IN THIS DIRECTION FROM LEFT TO RIGHT

Each Estrostep Fe tablet dispenser contains five white triangular tablets, seven white square tablets, nine white round tablets, and seven brown tablets. These tablets are to be taken in the following order: one triangular tablet each day for five days, then one square tablet each day for seven days, followed by one round tablet each day for nine days, and then one brown tablet each day for seven days.

Continued on next page

This product information was prepared in June 2000. On these and other Parke-Davis Products, information may be obtained by addressing PARKE-DAVIS, a Warner-Lambert Division, Morris Plains, New Jersey 07950.

Estrostep—Cont.

Estrostep Fe will contain:
21 WHITE PILLS for WEEKS 1, 2, and 3. WEEK 4 will contain BROWN PILLS ONLY.

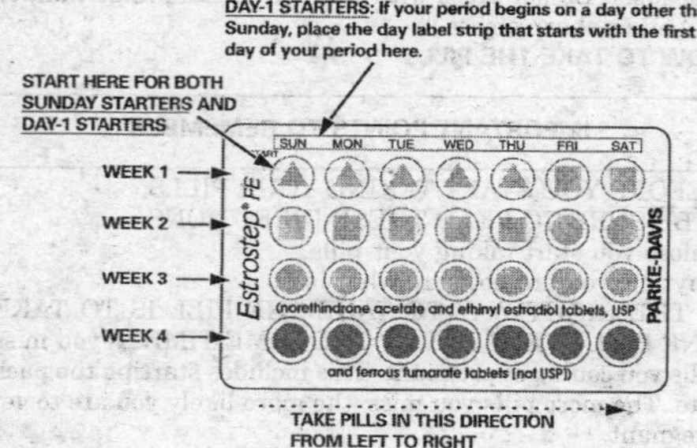
DAY-1 STARTERS: If your period begins on a day other than Sunday, place the day label strip that starts with the first day of your period here.
START HERE FOR BOTH SUNDAY STARTERS AND DAY-1 STARTERS
SUN MON TUE WED THU FRI SAT
WEEK 1
WEEK 2
WEEK 3
WEEK 4
Estrostep® Fe
PARKE-DAVIS
(norethindrone acetate and ethinyl estradiol tablets, USP
and ferrous fumarate tablets (not USP))
TAKE PILLS IN THIS DIRECTION FROM LEFT TO RIGHT

4. BE SURE YOU HAVE READY AT ALL TIMES: ANOTHER KIND OF BIRTH CONTROL (such as condoms or foam) to use as a back-up in case you miss pills. An EXTRA, FULL PILL PACK.

WHEN TO START THE FIRST PACK OF PILLS

You have a choice of which day to start taking your first pack of pills. Decide with your doctor or clinic which is the best day for you. Pick a time of day which will be easy to remember.

DAY-1 START:
1. Pick the day label strip that starts with the first day of your period. (This is the day you start bleeding or spotting, even if it is almost midnight when the bleeding begins.)
2. Place this day label strip on the tablet dispenser over the area that has the days of the week (starting with Sunday) printed on the plastic.
3. Take the first "active" white pill of the first pack during the first 24 hours of your period.
4. You will not need to use a back-up method of birth control, since you are starting the pill at the beginning of your period.

SUNDAY START:
1. Take the first "active" white pill of the first pack on the Sunday after your period starts, even if you are still bleeding. If your period begins on Sunday, start the pack that same day.
2. Use another method of birth control as a back-up method if you have sex anytime from the Sunday you start your first pack until the next Sunday (7 days). Condoms or foam are good back-up methods of birth control.

WHAT TO DO DURING THE MONTH

1. TAKE ONE PILL AT THE SAME TIME EVERY DAY UNTIL THE PACK IS EMPTY.
Do not skip pills even if you are spotting or bleeding between monthly periods or feel sick to your stomach (nausea).
Do not skip pills even if you do not have sex very often.
2. WHEN YOU FINISH A PACK OR SWITCH YOUR BRAND OF PILLS:
21 pills: Wait 7 days to start the next pack. You will probably have your period during that week. Be sure that no more than 7 days pass between 21-day packs.
28 pills: Start the next pack on the day after your last "reminder" pill. Do not wait any days between packs.

WHAT TO DO IF YOU MISS PILLS

If you **MISS 1** white "active" pill:
1. Take it as soon as you remember. Take the next pill at your regular time. This means you may take 2 pills in 1 day.
2. You do not need to use a back-up birth control method if you have sex.

If you **MISS 2** white "active" pills in a row in **WEEK 1 OR WEEK 2** of your pack:
1. Take 2 pills on the day you remember and 2 pills the next day.
2. Then take 1 pill a day until you finish the pack.
3. You COULD GET PREGNANT if you have sex in the 7 days after you miss pills. You MUST use another birth control method (such as condoms or foam) as a back-up method of birth control until you have taken a white "active" pill every day for 7 days.

If you **MISS 2** white "active" pills in a row in **THE 3rd WEEK:**
1. **If you are a Day-1 Starter:**
THROW OUT the rest of the pill pack and start a new pack that same day.
If you are a Sunday Starter:
Keep taking 1 pill every day until Sunday. On Sunday, THROW OUT the rest of the pack and start a new pack of pills that same day.
2. You may not have your period this month, but this is expected. However, if you miss your period 2 months in a row, call your doctor or clinic because you might be pregnant.
3. You COULD GET PREGNANT if you have sex in the 7 days after you miss pills. You MUST use another birth control method (such as condoms or foam) as a back-up method of birth control until you have taken a white "active" pill every day for 7 days.

If you **MISS 3 OR MORE** white "active" pills in a row (during the first 3 weeks):
1. **If you are a Day-1 Starter:**
THROW OUT the rest of the pill pack and start a new pack that same day.
If you are a Sunday Starter:
Keep taking 1 pill every day until Sunday. On Sunday, THROW OUT the rest of the pack and start a new pack of pills that same day.
2. You may not have your period this month, but this is expected. However, if you miss your period 2 months in a row, call your doctor or clinic because you might be pregnant.
3. You COULD GET PREGNANT if you have sex in the 7 days after you miss pills. You MUST use another birth control method (such as condoms or foam) as a back-up method of birth control until you have taken a white "active" pill every day for 7 days.

A REMINDER FOR THOSE ON 28-DAY PACKS:
IF YOU FORGET ANY OF THE 7 BROWN "REMINDER" PILLS IN WEEK 4:
THROW AWAY THE PILLS YOU MISSED.
KEEP TAKING 1 PILL EACH DAY UNTIL THE PACK IS EMPTY.
YOU DO NOT NEED A BACK-UP METHOD.

FINALLY, IF YOU ARE STILL NOT SURE WHAT TO DO ABOUT THE PILLS YOU HAVE MISSED:
Use a BACK-UP METHOD anytime you have sex.
KEEP TAKING ONE WHITE "ACTIVE" PILL EACH DAY until you can reach your doctor or clinic.

Based on his or her assessment of your medical needs, your doctor or health care provider has prescribed this drug for you. Do not give this drug to anyone else.
Keep this and all drugs out of the reach of children.
Rx only
Storage—Do not store above 25° C (77° F).
Protect from light.
Store tablets inside pouch when not in use.
This product (like all oral contraceptives) is intended to prevent pregnancy. It does not protect against HIV infection (AIDS) and other sexually transmitted diseases.

DETAILED PATIENT PACKAGE INSERT

What You Should Know About Oral Contraceptives
Any woman who considers using oral contraceptives (the "birth control pill" or "the pill") should understand the benefits and risk of using this form of birth control. This leaflet will give you much of the information you will need to make this decision and will also help you determine if you are at risk of developing any of the serious side effects of the pill. It will tell you how to use the pill properly so that it will be as effective as possible. However, this leaflet is not a replacement for a careful discussion between you and your health care provider. You should discuss the information provided in this leaflet with him or her, both when your first start taking the pill and during your revisits. You should also follow your health care provider's advice with regard to regular check-ups while you are on the pill.

EFFECTIVENESS OF ORAL CONTRACEPTIVES
Oral contraceptives or "birth control pills" or "the pill" are used to prevent pregnancy and are more effective than other nonsurgical methods of birth control. When they are taken correctly, the chance of becoming pregnant is less than 1% (1 pregnancy per 100 women per year of use) when used perfectly, without missing any pills. Typical failure rates are actually 3% per year. The chance of becoming pregnant increases with each missed pill during a menstrual cycle.
In comparison, typical failure rates for other methods of birth control during the first year of use are as follows:
Implant: <1%
Injection: <1%
IUD: <1% to 2%
Diaphragm with spermicides: 20%
Spermicides alone: 26%
Vaginal Sponge: 20 to 40%
Female sterilization: <1%
Male sterilization: <1%
Cervical Cap: 20 to 40%
Condom alone (male): 14%
Condom alone (female): 21%
Periodic abstinence: 25%
Withdrawal: 19%
No method: 85%

WHO SHOULD NOT TAKE ORAL CONTRACEPTIVES

Cigarette smoking increases the risk of serious cardiovascular side effects from oral contraceptive use. This risk increases with age and with heavy smoking (15 to more cigarettes per day) and is quite marked in women over 35 years of age. Women who use oral contraceptives are strongly advised not to smoke.

Some women should not use the pill. For example, you should not take the pill if you are pregnant or think you may be pregnant. You should also not use the pill if you have any of the following conditions:

- A history of heart attack or stroke
- Blood clots in the legs (thrombophlebitis), lungs (pulmonary embolism), or eyes
- A history of blood clots in the deep veins of your legs
- Chest pain (angina pectoris)
- Known or suspected breast cancer or cancer of the lining of the uterus, cervix, or vagina
- Unexplained vaginal bleeding (until a diagnosis is reached by your doctor)
- Yellowing of the whites of the eyes or the skin (jaundice) during pregnancy of during previous use of the pill
- Liver tumor (benign or cancerous)
- Known or suspected pregnancy

Tell your health care provider if you have ever had any of these conditions. Your health care provider can recommended a safer method of birth control.

OTHER CONSIDERATIONS BEFORE TAKING ORAL CONTRACEPTIVES
Tell your health care provider if you have:
- Breast nodules, fibrocystic disease of the breast, an abnormal breast x-ray or mammogram
- Diabetes
- Elevated cholesterol or triglycerides
- High blood pressure
- Migraine or other headaches or epilepsy
- Mental depression
- Gallbladder, heart, or kidney disease
- History of scanty or irregular menstrual periods

Women with any of these conditions should be checked often by their health care provider if they choose to use oral contraceptives.
Also, be sure to inform your doctor or health care provider if you smoke or are on any medications.

RISKS OF TAKING ORAL CONTRACEPTIVES
1. Risk of Developing Blood Clots
Blood clots and blockage of blood vessels are the most serious side effects of taking oral contraceptives; in particular, a clot in the leg can cause thrombophlebitis, and a clot that travels to the lungs can cause a sudden blocking of the vessel carrying blood to the lungs. Rarely, clots occur in the blood vessels of the eye and may cause blindness, double vision, or impaired vision.
If you take oral contraceptives and need elective surgery, need to stay in bed for a prolonged illness, or have recently delivered a baby, you may be at risk of developing blood clots. You should consult your doctor about stopping oral contraceptives three to four weeks before surgery and not taking oral contraceptives for two weeks after surgery or during bed rest. You should also not take oral contraceptives soon after delivery of a baby. It is advisable to wait for at least four weeks after delivery if you are not breast feeding. If you are breast feeding, you should wait until you have weaned your child before using the pill. (See also the section on Breast Feeding in GENERAL PRECAUTIONS.)
2. Heart Attacks and Strokes
Oral contraceptives may increase the tendency to develop strokes (stoppage or rupture of blood vessels in the brain) and angina pectoris and heart attacks (blockage of blood vessels in the heart). Any of these conditions can cause death or disability.
Smoking greatly increases the possibility of suffering heart attacks and strokes. Furthermore, smoking and the use of oral contraceptives greatly increase the chances of developing and dying of heart disease.
3. Gallbladder Disease
Oral contraceptive users probably have a greater risk than nonusers of having gallbladder disease, although this risk may be related to pills containing high doses of estrogens.
4. Liver Tumors
In rare cases, oral contraceptives can cause benign but dangerous liver tumors. These benign liver tumors can rupture and cause fatal internal bleeding. In addition, a possible but not definite association has been found with the pill and liver cancers in two studies, in which a few women who developed these very rare cancers were found to have used oral contraceptives for long periods. However, liver cancers are extremely rare. The change of developing liver cancer from using the pill is thus even rarer.
5. Cancer of the Reproductive Organs and Breasts
There is, at present, no confirmed evidence that oral contraceptives use increases the risk of developing cancer of the reproductive organs. Studies to date of women taking the pill have reported conflicting findings on whether pill use increases the risk of developing cancer of the breast or cervix. Most of the studies on breast cancer and pill use have found no overall increase in the risk of developing breast cancer, although some studies have reported an increased risk of developing breast cancer in certain groups of women. Women who use oral contraceptives and have a strong family history of breast cancer or who have breast nodules or abnormal mammograms should closely followed by their doctors.
Some studies have found an increase in the incidence of cancer of the cervix in women who use oral contraceptives. However, this finding may be related to factors other than the use of oral contraceptives.

ESTIMATED RISK OF DEATH FROM A BIRTH CONTROL METHOD OF PREGNANCY
All methods of birth control and pregnancy are associated with a risk of developing certain diseases which may lead to disability or death. An estimate of the number of deaths associated with different methods of birth control and pregnancy has been calculated and is shown in the following table.
[See table at bottom of next page]

In the above table, the risk of death from any birth control method is less than the risk of childbirth, except for oral contraceptive users over the age of 35 who smoke and pill users over the age of 40 even if they do not smoke. It can been seen in the table that for women aged 15 to 39, the risk of death was highest with pregnancy (7 to 26 deaths per 100,000 women, depending on age). Among pill users who do not smoke, the risk of death was always lower than that associated with pregnancy for any age group, although over the age of 40, the risk increases to 32 deaths per 100,000 women, compared to 28 associated with pregnancy at that age. However, for pill users who smoke and are over the age of 35, the estimated number of deaths exceeds those for other methods of birth control. If a woman is over the age of 40 and smokes, her estimated risk of death is four times higher (117/100,000 women) than the estimated risk associated with pregnancy (28/100,000 women) in that age group. The suggestion that women over 40 who don't smoke should not take oral contraceptives is based on information from older higher dose pills and on less selective use of pills than is practiced today. An Advisory Committee of the FDA discussed this issue in 1989 and recommended that the benefits of oral contraceptive use by healthy, non-smoking women over 40 years of age may outweigh the possible risks. However, all women, especially older women, are cautioned to use the lowest dose pill that is effective.

WARNING SIGNALS

If any of these adverse effects occur while you are taking oral contraceptives, call your doctor immediately:

- Sharp chest pain, coughing of blood, or sudden shortness of breath (indicating a possible clot in the lung)
- Pain in the calf (indicating a possible clot in the leg)
- Crushing chest pain or heaviness in the chest (indicating a possible heart attack)
- Sudden severe headache or vomiting, dizziness or fainting, disturbances of vision or speech, weakness, or numbness in an arm or leg (indicating a possible stroke)
- Sudden partial or complete loss of vision (indicating a possible clot in the eye)
- Breast lumps (indicating possible breast cancer or fibrocystic disease of the breast; ask your doctor or health care provider to show you how to examine your breasts)
- Severe pain or tenderness in the stomach area (indicating a possible ruptured liver tumor)
- Difficulty in sleeping, weakness, lack of energy, fatigue, or change in mood (possibly indicating severe depression)
- Jaundice or a yellowing of the skin or eyeballs, accompanied frequently by fever, fatigue, loss of appetite, dark colored urine, or light colored bowel movements (indicating possible liver problems)

SIDE EFFECTS OF ORAL CONTRACEPTIVES

1. Vaginal Bleeding

Irregular vaginal bleeding or spotting may occur while you are taking the pills. Irregular bleeding may vary from slight staining between menstrual periods to breakthrough bleeding which is a flow much like a regular period. Irregular bleeding occurs most often during the first few months of oral contraceptive use, but may also occur after you have been taking the pill for some time. Such bleeding may be temporary and usually does not indicate serious problems. It is important to continue taking your pills on schedule. If the bleeding occurs in more than one cycle or last for more than a few days, talk to your doctor or health care provider.

2. Contact Lenses

If you wear contact lenses and notice a change in vision or an inability to wear your lenses, contact your doctor or health care provider.

3. Fluid Retention

Oral contraceptives may cause edema (fluid retention) with swelling of the fingers or ankles and may raise your blood pressure. If you experienced fluid retention, contact your doctor or health care provider.

4. Melasma

A spotty darkening of the skin is possible, particularly of the face.

5. Other Side Effects

Other side effects may include change in appetite, headache, nervousness, depression, dizziness, loss of scalp hair, rash, and vaginal infections.

If any of these side effects bother you, call your doctor or health care provider.

GENERAL PRECAUTIONS

1. Missed Periods and Use of Oral Contraceptives Before or During Early Pregnancy

There may be times when your may not menstruate regularly after you have completed taking a cycle of pills. If you have taken your pills regularly and miss one menstrual period, continue taking your pills for the next cycle but be sure to inform your health care provider before doing so. If you have not taken the pills daily as instructed and missed a menstrual period, or if you missed two consecutive menstrual periods, you may be pregnant. Check with your health care provider immediately to determine whether you are pregnant. Do not continue to take oral contraceptives until you are sure you are not pregnant. But continue to use another method of contraception.

There is no conclusive evidence that oral contraceptive use is associated with an increase in birth defects, when taken inadvertently during early pregnancy. Previously, a few studies had reported that oral contraceptives might be associated with birth defects, but these studies have not been confirmed. Nevertheless, oral contraceptives or any other drugs should not be used during pregnancy unless clearly necessary and prescribed by your doctor. You should check with your doctor about risks to your unborn child of any medication taken during pregnancy.

2. While Breast Feeding

If you are breast feeding, consult your doctor before starting oral contraceptives. Some of the drug will be passed on to the child in the milk. A few adverse effects on the child have been reported, including yellowing of the skin (jaundice) and breast enlargement. In addition, oral contraceptives may decrease the amount and quality of your milk. If possible, do not use oral contraceptives while breast feeding. You should use another method of contraception since breast feeding provides only partial protection from becoming pregnant, and this partial protection decreases significantly as you breast feed for longer periods of time. You should consider starting oral contraceptives only after you have weaned your child completely.

3. Laboratory Tests

If you are scheduled for any laboratory tests, tell your doctor you are taking birth control pills. Certain blood tests may be affected by birth control pills.

4. Drug Interactions

Certain drugs may interact with birth control pills to make them less effective in preventing pregnancy or cause an increase in breakthrough bleeding. Such drugs include rifampin; drugs used for epilepsy such as barbiturates (for example, phenobarbital), carbamazepine, and phenytoin (Dilantin® is one brand of this drug); troglitazone; phenylbutazone; and possibly certain antibiotics. You may need to use additional contraception when you take drugs which can make oral contraceptives less effective.

Birth control pills interact with certain drugs. These drugs include acetaminophen, clofibric acid, cyclosporine, morphine, prednisolone, salicylic acid, temazepam, theophylline. You should tell your doctor if you are taking any of these medications.

5. This product (like all oral contraceptives) is intended to prevent pregnancy. It does not protect against transmission of HIV (AIDS) and other sexually transmitted diseases such as chlamydia, genital herpes, genital warts, gonorrhea, hepatitis B, and syphilis.

INSTRUCTIONS TO PATIENT

TABLET DISPENSER

The Estrostep tablet dispenser has been designed to make oral contraceptive dosing as easy and as convenient as possible. The tablets are arranged in either three or four rows of seven tablets each, with the days of the week appearing above the first row of tablets.

If your TABLET DISPENSER contains:	You are taking:
21 white tablets	ESTROSTEP 21
21 white tablets and 7 brown tablets	ESTROSTEP Fe

Each *triangle* tablet contains 1 mg norethindrone acetate and 20 mcg ethinyl estradiol.

Each *square* tablet contains 1 mg norethindrone acetate and 30 mcg ethinyl estradiol.

Each *round* tablet contains 1 mg norethindrone acetate and 35 mcg ethinyl estradiol.

Each *brown* tablet contains 75 mg ferrous fumarate and is intended to help you remember to take the tablets correctly. These brown tablets are not intended to have any health benefit.

DIRECTIONS

To remove a tablet, press down on it with your thumb or finger. The tablet will drop through the back of the tablet dispenser. Do not press with your thumbnail, fingernail, or any other sharp object.

HOW TO TAKE THE PILL

IMPORTANT POINTS TO REMEMBER

BEFORE YOU START TAKING YOUR PILLS:

1. BE SURE TO READ THESE DIRECTIONS:
Before you start taking your pills.
Anytime you are not sure what to do.

2. THE RIGHT WAY TO TAKE THE PILL IS TO TAKE ONE PILL EVERY DAY AT THE SAME TIME. If you miss pills you could get pregnant. This includes starting the pack late. The more pills you miss, the more likely you are to get pregnant.

3. MANY WOMEN HAVE SPOTTING OR LIGHT BLEEDING, OR MAY FEEL SICK TO THEIR STOMACH, DURING THE FIRST 1–3 PACKS OF PILLS. If you do have spotting or light bleeding or feel sick to your stomach, do not stop taking the pill. The problem will usually go away. If it doesn't go away, check with your doctor or clinic.

4. MISSING PILLS CAN ALSO CAUSE SPOTTING OR LIGHT BLEEDING, even when you make up these missed pills. On the days you take 2 pills to make up for missed pills, you could also feel a little sick to your stomach.

5. IF YOU HAVE VOMITING OR DIARRHEA, for any reason, or IF YOU TAKE SOME MEDICINES, including some antibiotics, your birth control pills may not work as well. Use a back-up birth control method (such as condoms or foam) until you check with your doctor or clinic.

6. IF YOU HAVE TROUBLE REMEMBERING TO TAKE THE PILL, talk to your doctor or clinic about how to make pill-taking easier or about using another method of birth control.

7. IF YOU HAVE ANY QUESTIONS OR ARE UNSURE ABOUT THE INFORMATION IN THIS LEAFLET, call your doctor or clinic.

BEFORE YOU START TAKING YOUR PILLS

1. DECIDE WHAT TIME OF DAY YOU WANT TO TAKE YOUR PILL. It is important to take it at about the same time every day.

2. LOOK AT YOUR PILL PACK TO SEE IF IT HAS 21 OR 28 PILLS:
The 21-pill pack has 21 "active" white pills (with hormones) to take for 3 weeks, followed by 1 week without pills.
The 28-pill pack has 21 "active" white pills (with hormones) to take for 3 weeks, followed by 1 week of reminder brown pills (without hormones).

3. ALSO FIND:
1) where on the pack to start taking pills,
2) in what order to take the pills (follow the arrows), and
3) the week numbers as shown in the following pictures:

Each Estrostep 21 tablet dispenser contains five white triangular tablets, seven white square tablets, and nine white round tablets. These tablets are to be taken in the following order: one triangular tablet each day for five days, followed by one square tablet each day for seven days, and then one round tablet each day for nine days.

Estrostep 21 will contain:

ALL WHITE PILLS

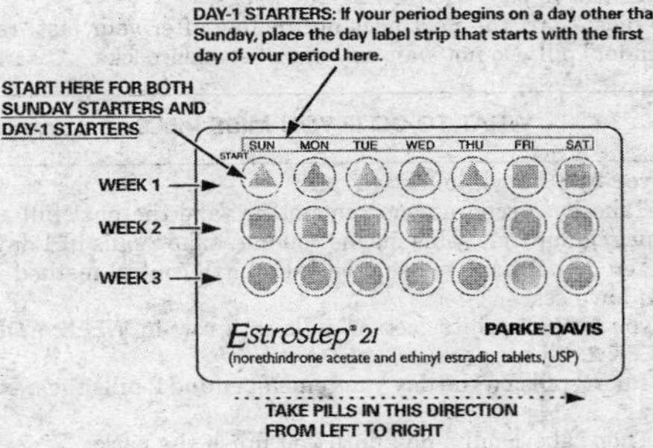
DAY-1 STARTERS: If your period begins on a day other than Sunday, place the day label strip that starts with the first day of your period here.
START HERE FOR BOTH SUNDAY STARTERS AND DAY-1 STARTERS
START
SUN MON TUE WED THU FRI SAT
WEEK 1
WEEK 2
WEEK 3
Estrostep® 21
PARKE-DAVIS
(norethindrone acetate and ethinyl estradiol tablets, USP)
TAKE PILLS IN THIS DIRECTION FROM LEFT TO RIGHT

Each Estrostep Fe tablet dispenser contains five white triangular tablets, seven white square tablets, nine white round tablets, and seven brown tablets. These tablets are to be taken in the following order: one triangular tablet each day for five days, then one square tablet each day for seven days, followed by one round tablet each day for nine days, and then one brown tablet each day for seven days.

Continued on next page

ANNUAL NUMBER OF BIRTH-RELATED OR METHOD-RELATED DEATHS ASSOCIATED WITH CONTROL OF FERTILITY PER 100,000 NONSTERILE WOMEN BY FERTILITY CONTROL METHOD ACCORDING TO AGE

Method of control and outcome	15–19	20–24	25–29	30–34	35–39	40–44
No fertility control methods*	7.0	7.4	9.1	14.8	25.7	28.2
Oral contraceptives non-smoker**	0.3	0.5	0.9	1.9	13.8	31.6
Oral contraceptives smoker**	2.2	3.4	6.6	13.5	51.1	117.2
IUD**	0.8	0.8	1.0	1.0	1.4	1.4
Condom*	1.1	1.6	0.7	0.2	0.3	0.4
Diaphragm/spermicide*	1.9	1.2	1.2	1.3	2.2	2.8
Periodic abstinence*	2.5	1.6	1.6	1.7	2.9	3.6

*Deaths are birth related.
**Deaths are method related.

This product information was prepared in June 2000. On these and other Parke-Davis Products, information may be obtained by addressing PARKE-DAVIS, a Warner-Lambert Division, Morris Plains, New Jersey 07950.

Estrostep—Cont.

Estrostep Fe will contain:
21 WHITE PILLS for **WEEKS 1, 2, and 3. WEEK 4** will contain **BROWN PILLS ONLY.**

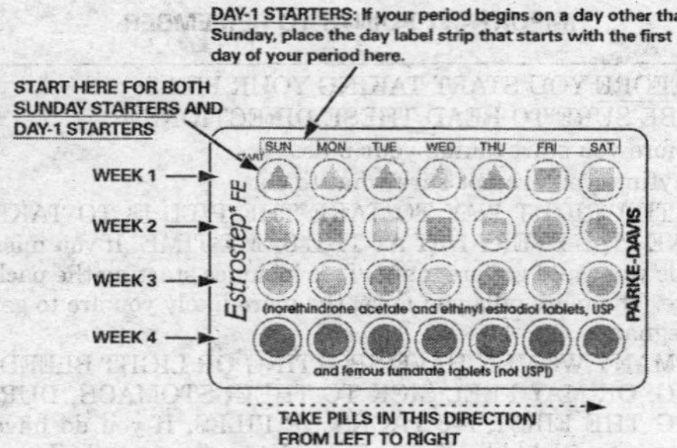
DAY-1 STARTERS: If your period begins on a day other than Sunday, place the day label strip that starts with the first day of your period here.
START HERE FOR BOTH SUNDAY STARTERS AND DAY-1 STARTERS
SUN MON TUE WED THU FRI SAT
WEEK 1
WEEK 2
WEEK 3
WEEK 4
Estrostep Fe
PARKE-DAVIS
(norethindrone acetate and ethinyl estradiol tablets, USP
and ferrous fumarate tablets (not USP))
TAKE PILLS IN THIS DIRECTION FROM LEFT TO RIGHT

4. BE SURE YOU HAVE READY AT ALL TIMES:
ANOTHER KIND OF BIRTH CONTROL (such as condoms or foam) to use as a back-up in case you miss pills.
An EXTRA, FULL PILL PACK.

WHEN TO START THE FIRST PACK OF PILLS

You have a choice of which day to start taking your first pack of pills. Decide with your doctor or clinic which is the best day for you. Pick a time of day which will be easy to remember.

DAY-1 START:
1. Pick the day label strip that starts with the first day of your period. (This is the day you start bleeding or spotting, even if it is almost midnight when the bleeding begins.)
2. Place this day label strip on the tablet dispenser over the area that has the days of the week (starting with Sunday) printed on the plastic.
3. Take the first "active" white pill of the first pack during the first 24 hours of your period.
4. You will not need to use a back-up method of birth control, since you are starting the pill at the beginning of your period.

SUNDAY START:
1. Take the first "active" white pill of the first pack on the Sunday after your period starts, even if you are still bleeding. If your period begins on Sunday, start the pack that same day.
2. Use another method of birth control as a back-up method if you have sex anytime from the Sunday you start your first pack until the next Sunday (7 days). Condoms or foam are good back-up methods of birth control.

WHAT TO DO DURING THE MONTH

1. TAKE ONE PILL AT THE SAME TIME EVERY DAY UNTIL THE PACK IS EMPTY.
Do not skip pills even if you are spotting or bleeding between monthly periods or feel sick to your stomach (nausea).
Do not skip pills even if you do not have sex very often.

2. WHEN YOU FINISH A PACK OR SWITCH YOUR BRAND OF PILLS:
21 pills: Wait 7 days to start the next pack. You will probably have your period during that week. Be sure that no more than 7 days pass between 21-day packs.
28 pills: Start the next pack on the day after your last "reminder" pill. Do not wait any days between packs.

WHAT TO DO IF YOU MISS PILLS

If you **MISS 1** white "active" pill:
1. Take it as soon as you remember. Take the next pill at your regular time. This means you may take 2 pills in 1 day.
2. You do not need to use a back-up birth control method if you have sex.

If you **MISS 2** white "active" pills in a row in **WEEK 1 OR WEEK 2** of your pack:
1. Take 2 pills on the day you remember and 2 pills the next day.
2. Then take 1 pill a day until you finish the pack.
3. You COULD GET PREGNANT if you have sex in the 7 days after you miss pills. You MUST use another birth control method (such as condoms or foam) as a back-up method of birth control until you have taken a white "active" pill every day for 7 days.

If you **MISS 2** white "active" pills in a row in **THE 3rd WEEK:**
1. **If you are a Day-1 Starter:**
THROW OUT the rest of the pill pack and start a new pack that same day.
If you are a Sunday Starter:
Keep taking 1 pill every day until Sunday. On Sunday, THROW OUT the rest of the pack and start a new pack of pills that same day.
2. You may not have your period this month, but this is expected. However, if you miss your period 2 months in a row, call your doctor or clinic because you might be pregnant.
3. You COULD GET PREGNANT if you have sex in the 7 days after you miss pills. You MUST use another birth control method (such as condoms or foam) as a back-up method of birth control until you have taken a white "active" pill every day for 7 days.

If you **MISS 3 OR MORE** white "active" pills in a row (during the first 3 weeks):
1. **If you are a Day-1 Starter:**
THROW OUT the rest of the pill pack and start a new pack that same day.
If you are a Sunday Starter:
Keep taking 1 pill every day until Sunday. On Sunday, THROW OUT the rest of the pack and start a new pack of pills that same day.
2. You may not have your period this month, but this is expected. However, if you miss your period 2 months in a row, call your doctor or clinic because you might be pregnant.
3. You COULD GET PREGNANT if you have sex in the 7 days after you miss pills. You MUST use another birth control method (such as condoms or foam) as a back-up method of birth control until you have taken a white "active" pill every day for 7 days.

A REMINDER FOR THOSE ON 28-DAY PACKS:
IF YOU FORGET ANY OF THE 7 BROWN "REMINDER" PILLS IN WEEK 4:
THROW AWAY THE PILLS YOU MISSED.
KEEP TAKING 1 PILL EACH DAY UNTIL THE PACK IS EMPTY.
YOU DO NOT NEED A BACK-UP METHOD.

FINALLY, IF YOU ARE STILL NOT SURE WHAT TO DO ABOUT THE PILLS YOU HAVE MISSED:
Use a BACK-UP METHOD anytime you have sex.
KEEP TAKING ONE WHITE "ACTIVE" PILL EACH DAY until you can reach your doctor or clinic.

PREGNANCY DUE TO PILL FAILURE
The incidence of pill failure resulting in pregnancy is approximately 1% (ie, one pregnancy per 100 women per year) if taken every day as directed, but more typical failure rates are about 3%. If failure does occur, the risk to the fetus is minimal.

PREGNANCY AFTER STOPPING THE PILL
There may be some delay in becoming pregnant after you stop using oral contraceptives, especially if you had irregular menstrual cycles before you used oral contraceptives. It may be advisable to postpone conception until you begin menstruating regularly once you have stopped taking the pill and desire pregnancy.
There does not appear to be any increase in birth defects in newborn babies when pregnancy occurs soon after stopping the pill.

OVERDOSAGE
Serious ill effects have not been reported following ingestion of large doses of contraceptives by young children. Overdosage may cause nausea and withdrawal bleeding in females. In case of overdosage, contact your health care provider or pharmacist.

OTHER INFORMATION
Your health care provider will take a medical and family history and examine you before prescribing oral contraceptives. The physical examination may be delayed to another time if you request it and your health care provider believes that it is a good medical practice to postpone it. You should be reexamined at least once a year. Be sure to inform your health care provider it there is a family history of any of the conditions listed previously in this leaflet. Be sure to keep all appointments with your health care provider, because this is a time to determine if there are early signs of side effects of oral contraceptive use.
Do not use the drug for any condition other than the one for which it was prescribed. This drug has been prescribed specifically for you; do not give it to others who may want birth control pills.

HEALTH BENEFITS FROM ORAL CONTRACEPTIVES
In addition to preventing pregnancy, use of oral contraceptives may provide certain benefits. They are:
- Menstrual cycles may become more regular.
- Blood flow during menstruation may be lighter and less iron may be lost. Therefore, anemia due to iron deficiency is less likely to occur.
- Pain or other symptoms during menstruation may be encountered less frequently.
- Ectopic (tubal) pregnancy may occur less frequently.
- Noncancerous cysts or lumps in the breast may occur less frequently.
- Acute pelvic inflammatory disease may occur less frequently.
- Oral contraceptive use may provide some protection against developing two forms of cancer: cancer of the ovaries and cancer of the lining of the uterus.

If you want more information about birth control pills, ask your doctor or pharmacist. They have a more technical leaflet called the "Physician Insert," which you may wish to read.
Remembering to take tablets according to schedule is stressed because of its importance in providing you the greatest degree of protection.

MISSED MENSTRUAL PERIODS FOR BOTH DOSAGE REGIMENS
At times there may be no menstrual period after a cycle of pills. Therefore, if you miss one menstrual period but have taken the pills *exactly as you were supposed to,* continue as usual into the next cycle. If you have not taken the pills correctly and miss a menstrual period, *you may be pregnant* and should stop taking oral contraceptives until your doctor or health care provider determines whether or not you are pregnant. Until you can get to your doctor or health care provider, use another form of contraception. If two consecutive menstrual periods are missed, you should stop taking pills until it is determined whether or not you are pregnant. Although there does not appear to be any increase in birth defects in newborn babies, if you become pregnant while using oral contraceptives, you should discuss the situation with your doctor or health care provider.

Periodic Examination
Your doctor or health care provider will take a complete medical and family history before prescribing oral contraceptives. At that time and about once a year therefore, he or she will generally examine your blood pressure, breasts, abdomen, and pelvic organs (including a Papanicolaou smear, ie, test for cancer).

Keep this and all drugs out of the reach of children.
Rx only
Storage: Do not store above 25°C (77°F).
Protect from light.
Store tablets inside pouch when not in use.
Revised November 1999
PARKE-DAVIS
Div. of Warner-Lambert Co ©1997-'99
Morris Plains, NJ 07950 USA
Direct Medical Inquiries to:
Parke-Davis
Warner-Lambert Company
201 Tabor Road, Morris Plains, NJ 07950
Attn: Medical Affairs Department 0928G254
Shown in Product Identification Guide, page 329

FEMHRT™ ℞
[fĕm-härt]
(norethindrone acetate/ethinyl estradiol tablets)

DESCRIPTION
femhrt™ 1/5 is a continuous dosage regimen of a progestin-estrogen combination for oral administration.
Each white D-shaped tablet contains 1 **mg** norethindrone acetate [(17-alpha)-17-(acetyloxy)-19-norpregna-4-en-20-yn-3-one] and 5 **mcg** ethinyl estradiol [(17-alpha)-19-norpregna-1,3,5(10)-trien-20-yn-2, 17-diol]. Each tablet also contains calcium stearate, lactose monohydrate, microcrystalline cellulose, and cornstarch.
The structural formulas are as follows:

Ethinyl Estradiol
Molecular Weight: 296.41
Molecular Formula: $C_{20}H_{24}O_2$

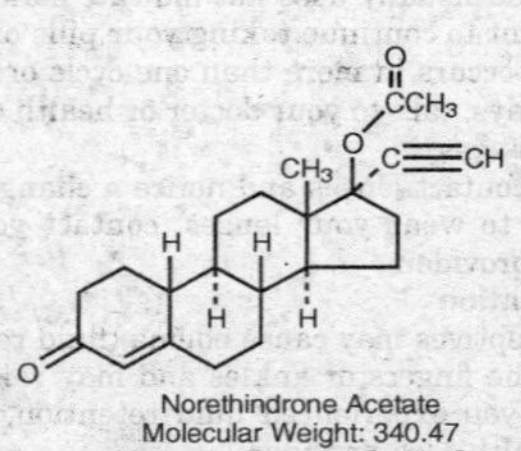

Norethindrone Acetate
Molecular Weight: 340.47
Molecular Formula: $C_{22}H_{28}O_3$

CLINICAL PHARMACOLOGY
Estrogens are largely responsible for the development and maintenance of the female reproductive system and secondary sex characteristics. Although circulating estrogens exist in a dynamic equilibrium of metabolic interconversions, estradiol is the principal intracellular human estrogen and is substantially more potent than estrone and estriol at the receptor level. The primary source of estrogen in normally cycling adult women is the ovarian follicle, which secretes 70 to 500 mcg of estradiol daily, depending on the phase of the menstrual cycle. After menopause, most endogenous estrogen is produced by conversion of androstenedione, secreted by the adrenal cortex, to estrone by peripheral tissues. Thus, estrone and the sulphate conjugated form, estrone sulphate, are the most abundant circulating estrogens in postmenopausal women. The pharmacologic effects of ethinyl estradiol are similar to those of endogenous estrogens.
Circulating estrogens modulate the pituitary secretion of the gonadotropins, luteinizing hormone (LH) and follicle stimulating hormone (FSH) through a negative feedback mechanism. Estrogen replacement therapy acts to reduce the elevated levels of these hormones seen in postmenopausal women.
Progestin compounds enhance cellular differentiation and generally oppose the actions of estrogens by decreasing estrogen receptor levels, increasing local metabolism of estrogens to less active metabolites, or inducing gene products that blunt cellular responses to estrogen. Progestins exert their effects in target cells by binding to specific progesterone receptors that interact with progesterone response ele-

ments in target genes. Progesterone receptors have been identified in the female reproductive tract, breast, pituitary, hypothalamus, bone, skeletal tissue and central nervous system. Progestins produce similar endometrial changes to those of the naturally occurring hormone progesterone.

The use of unopposed estrogen therapy has been associated with an increased risk of endometrial hyperplasia, a possible precursor of endometrial adenocarcinoma. The addition of continuous administration of progestin to an estrogen replacement regimen reduced the incidence of endometrial hyperplasia, and the attendant risk of carcinoma in women with intact uteri.

Pharmacokinetics

Absorption and Bioavailability

Norethindrone acetate (NA) is completely and rapidly deacetylated to norethindrone after oral administration, and the disposition of norethindrone acetate is indistinguishable from that of orally administered norethindrone. Norethindrone acetate and ethinyl estradiol (EE) are rapidly absorbed from *femhrt* 1/5 tablets, with maximum plasma concentrations of norethindrone and ethinyl estradiol generally occurring 1 to 2 hours postdose. Both are subject to first-pass metabolism after oral dosing, resulting in an absolute bioavailability of approximately 64% for norethindrone and 55% for ethinyl estradiol. Bioavailability of *femhrt* 1/5 tablets is similar to that from solution for norethindrone and slightly less for ethinyl estradiol. Administration of norethindrone acetate/ethinyl estradiol (NA/EE) tablets with a high fat meal decreases rate but not extent of ethinyl estradiol absorption. The extent of norethindrone absorption is increased by 27% following administration of NA/EE tablets with food.

The full pharmacokinetic profile of *femhrt* 1/5 (1 mg norethindrone acetate/5 mcg ethinyl estradiol) was not characterized due to assay sensitivity limitations. However, the multiple-dose pharmacokinetics were studied at a dose of 1 mg NA/10 mcg EE in 18 postmenopausal women. Mean plasma concentrations are shown below (Figure 1) and pharmacokinetic parameters are found in Table 1. Based on a population pharmacokinetic analysis, mean steady-state concentrations of norethindrone for 1 mg NA/5 mcg EE and 1/10 are slightly more than proportional to dose when compared to 0.5 mg NA/2.5 mcg EE tablets. It can be explained by higher sex hormone binding globulin (SHBG) concentrations. Mean steady-state plasma concentrations of ethinyl estradiol for the 0.5 mg NA/2.5 mcg EE tablets and *femhrt* 1/5 tablets are proportional to dose, but there is a less than proportional increase in steady-state concentrations for the NA/EE 1/10 tablet.

[See graphic above]

[See table 1 above]

Based on a population pharmacokinetic analysis, average steady-state concentrations (Css) of norethindrone and ethinyl estradiol for *femhrt* 1/5 (1 mg NA/5 mcg EE) are estimated to be 2.6 ng/mL and 11.4 pg/mL, respectively.

The pharmacokinetics of ethinyl estradiol and norethindrone acetate were not affected by age, (age range 40–62 years), in the postmenopausal population studied.

Distribution

Volume of distribution of norethindrone and ethinyl estradiol ranges from 2 to 4 L/kg. Plasma protein binding of both steroids is extensive (>95%); norethindrone binds to both albumin and sex hormone binding globulin (SHBG), whereas ethinyl estradiol binds only to albumin. Although ethinyl estradiol does not bind to SHBG, it induces SHBG synthesis.

Metabolism

Norethindrone undergoes extensive biotransformation, primarily via reduction, followed by sulfate and glucuronide conjugation. The majority of metabolites in the circulation are sulfates, with glucuronides accounting for most of the urinary metabolites. A small amount of norethindrone acetate is metabolically converted to ethinyl estradiol, such that exposure to ethinyl estradiol following administration of 1 mg of norethindrone acetate is equivalent to oral administration of 2.8 mcg ethinyl estradiol. Ethinyl estradiol is also extensively metabolized, both by oxidation and by conjugation with sulfate and glucuronide. Sulfates are the major circulating conjugates of ethinyl estradiol and glucuronides predominate in urine. The primary oxidative metabolite is 2-hydroxy ethinyl estradiol, formed by the CYP3A4 isoform of cytochrome P450. Part of the first-pass metabolism of ethinyl estradiol is believed to occur in gastrointestinal mucosa. Ethinyl estradiol may undergo enterohepatic circulation.

Excretion

Norethindrone and ethinyl estradiol are excreted in both urine and feces, primarily as metabolites. Plasma clearance values for norethindrone and ethinyl estradiol are similar (approximately 0.4 L/hr/kg). Steady-state elimination half-lives of norethindrone and ethinyl estradiol following administration of 1 mg NA/10 mcg EE tablets are approximately 13 hours and 24 hours, respectively.

Special Populations

Pediatric

femhrt 1/5 is not indicated in children.

Geriatrics

The pharmacokinetics of *femhrt* 1/5 have not been studied in a geriatric population.

Race

The effect of race on the pharmacokinetics of *femhrt* 1/5 has not been studied.

Patients with Renal Insufficiency

The effect of renal disease on the disposition of *femhrt* 1/5 has not been evaluated. In premenopausal women with

FIGURE 1. Mean Steady-State (Day 87) Plasma Norethindrone and Ethinyl Estradiol Concentrations Following Continuous Oral Administration of 1 mg NA/10 mcg EE Tablets

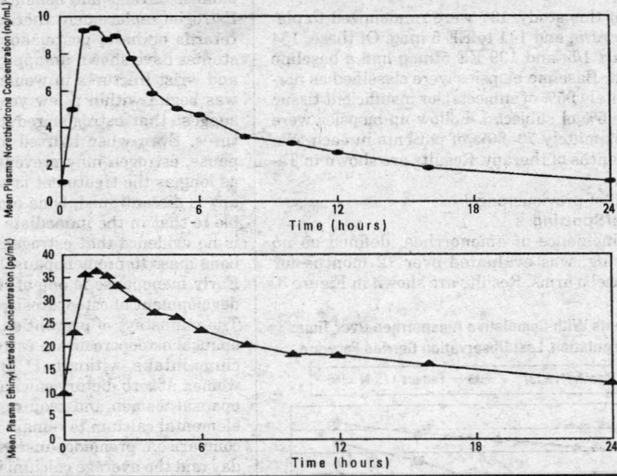

TABLE 1. Mean (SD) Single-Dose (Day 1) and Steady-State (Day 87) Pharmacokinetic Parameters[a] Following Administration of 1 mg NA/10 mcg EE Tablets

	C_{max}	t_{max}	AUC(0–24)	CL/F	$t_{½}$
Norethindrone	ng/mL	hr	ng•hr/mL	mL/min	hr
Day 1	6.0 (3.3)	1.8 (0.8)	29.7 (16.5)	588 (416)	10.3 (3.7)
Day 87	10.7 (3.6)	1.8 (0.8)	81.8 (36.7)	226 (139)	13.3 (4.5)
Ethinyl Estradiol	pg/mL	hr	pg•hr/mL	mL/min	hr
Day 1	33.5 (13.7)	2.2 (1.0)	339 (113)	ND[b]	ND[b]
Day 87	38.3 (11.9)	1.8 (0.7)	471 (132)	383 (119)	23.9 (7.1)

[a] C_{max} = Maximum plasma concentrations; t_{max} = time of C_{max}; AUC(0–24) = Area under the plasma concentration-time curve over the dosing interval; CL/F = Apparent oral clearance; $t_{½}$ = Elimination half-life

[b] ND = Not determined

Table 2. Endometrial Biopsy Results After 12 and 24 Months of Treatment

	Placebo	*femhrt* 1/5	5 mcg ethinyl estradiol
Number of Patients Biopsied at Baseline	N=134	N=143	N=139
MONTH 12			
Patients Biopsied (%)	113 (84)	110 (77)	114 (82)
Insufficient Tissue	30	45	20
Atrophic Tissue	60	41	2
Proliferative Tissue	23	24	91
Endometrial Hyperplasia[a]	0	0	1
MONTH 24			
Patients Biopsied (%)	94 (70)	102 (71)	107 (77)
Insufficient Tissue	35	37	17
Atrophic Tissue	38	33	2
Proliferative Tissue	20	32	86
Endometrial Hyperplasia[a]	1	0	2

[a]All patients with endometerial hyperplasia were carried forward for all time points.

chronic renal failure undergoing peritoneal dialysis who received multiple doses of an oral contraceptive containing ethinyl estradiol and norethindrone, plasma ethinyl estradiol concentrations were higher and norethindrone concentrations were unchanged compared to concentrations in premenopausal women with normal renal function (see **PRECAUTIONS, Fluid Retention**).

Patients With Hepatic Impairment

The effect of hepatic disease on the disposition of *femhrt* 1/5 has not been evaluated. However, ethinyl estradiol and norethindrone may be poorly metabolized in patients with impaired liver function (see **PRECAUTIONS**).

Drug Interactions

See **PRECAUTIONS, Drug Interactions.**

Clinical Studies

Effects of Vasomotor Symptoms

A 12-week placebo-controlled, multicenter, randomized clinical trial was conducted to determine the safety and efficacy of *femhrt* 1/5 for the treatment of vasomotor symptoms. The study assessed the efficacy of *femhrt* 1/5 in 266 symptomatic women who had at least 56 moderate to severe hot flashes during the week prior to randomization. On average, these patients had 12 hot flashes per day upon study entry.

The efficacy of *femhrt* 1/5 for the treatment of moderate to severe vasomotor symptoms (VMS) is demonstrated in Figure 2.

[See figure at top of next column]

Endometrial Hyperplasia

A 2-year, placebo-controlled, multicenter, randomized clinical trial was conducted to determine the safety and efficacy of *femhrt* 1/5 on maintaining bone mineral density, protecting the endometrium, and to determine effects on lipids. A total of 1265 women were enrolled and randomized to either placebo, 0.2 mg NA/1 mcg EE, 0.5 mg NA/2.5 mcg EE, *femhrt* 1/5 and 1 mg NA/10 mcg EE or matching unopposed EE

FIGURE 2. Mean Hot Flash Frequencies by Treatment Group: Baseline Through Week 12 (Intent-to-Treat Population, Last Observation Carried Forward)

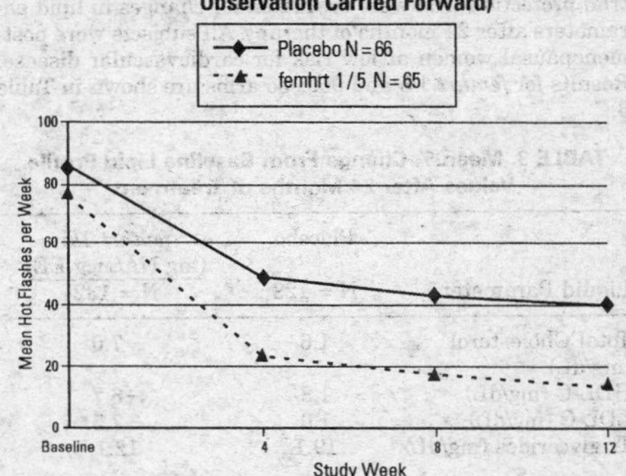

doses (1, 2.5, 5, or 10 mcg) for a total of 9 treatment groups. All participants received 1000 mg of calcium supplementation daily. Of the 1265 women randomized to the various

Continued on next page

This product information was prepared in June 2000. On these and other Parke-Davis Products, information may be obtained by addressing PARKE-DAVIS, a Warner-Lambert Division, Morris Plains, New Jersey 07950.

Femhrt—Cont.

treatment arms of this study, 137 were randomized to placebo, 146 to *femhrt* 1/5, and 141 to EE 5 **mcg**. Of these, 134 placebo, 143 *femhrt* 1/5, and 139 EE 5 **mcg** had a baseline endometrial result. Baseline biopsies were classified as normal (in approximately 95% of subjects), or insufficient tissue (in approximately 5% of subjects). Follow-up biopsies were obtained in approximately 70–80% of patients in each arm after 12 and 24 months of therapy. Results are shown in Table 2.

[See table 2 at top of previous page]

Irregular Bleeding/Spotting

The cumulative incidence of amenorrhea, defined as no bleeding or spotting, was evaluated over 12 months for *femhrt* 1/5 and placebo arms. Results are shown in Figure 3.

FIGURE 3. Patients With Cumulative Amenorrhea Over Time: Intent-to-Treat Population, Last Observation Carried Forward

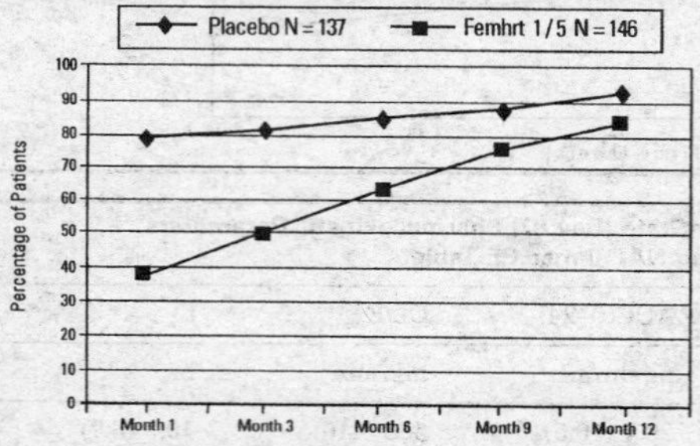

Effect on Bone Mineral Density

In the 2 year study, trabecular bone mineral density (BMD) was assessed at lumbar spine using quantitative computed tomography. A total of 283 postmenopausal women with intact uteri and normal baseline bone mineral density (124.14 mg/cc ± 9.60 mg/cc) were randomized to *femhrt* 1/5 (1 **mg** norethindrone acetate/5 **mcg** ethinyl estradiol) or placebo, and 87% contributed data to the Intent-to-Treat analysis. All patients received 1000 mg calcium in divided doses. Vitamin D was not supplemented. *femhrt* 1/5 resulted in significant increases in BMD at each assessment. There was a significant decrease in BMD in the placebo group (see Figure 4).

FIGURE 4. Mean Percent Change (±SE) From Baseline in Lumbar Spine BMD at Months 12 and 24 (Intent-to-Treat Population)

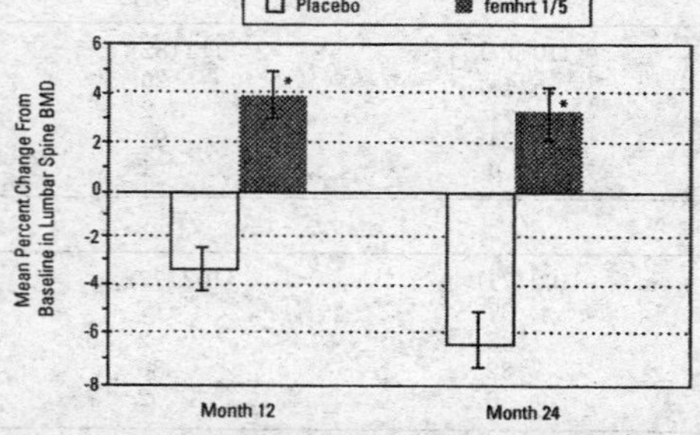

* Mean percent changes in BMD statistically significantly more positive than mean percent changes in placebo group at each time point.

Information Regarding Lipid Effects

Patients enrolled in the 2-year osteoporosis and endometrial protection trial were evaluated for changes in lipid parameters after 24 months of therapy. All subjects were postmenopausal women at low risk for cardiovascular disease. Results for *femhrt* 1/5 and placebo arms are shown in Table 3.

TABLE 3. Mean % Change From Baseline Lipid Profile. Values After 24 Months of Treatment

Liquid Parameter	Placebo N = 129	*femhrt* 1/5 (mg NA/mcg EE) N = 132
Total Cholesterol (mg/dL)	1.6	−7.0
HDL-C (mg/dL)	1.3	−6.7
LDL-C (mg/dL)	1.0	−7.5
Triglycerides (mg/dL)	19.1	12.1

NA = Norethindrone acetate. EE = Ethinyl estradiol.

INDICATIONS AND USAGE

femhrt 1/5 is indicated in women with an intact uterus for the:

1. Treatment of moderate to severe vasomotor symptoms associated with menopause.
2. Prevention of osteoporosis.

Since estrogen administration is associated with risks as well as benefits, selection of patients ideally should be based on prospective identification of risk factors for developing osteoporosis. Unfortunately, there is no certain way to identify those women who will develop osteoporotic fractures. Thus, patient selection must be individualized based on the balance of risks and benefits.

Estrogen replacement therapy reduces bone resorption and retards or halts postmenopausal bone loss. Case-control studies have shown an approximately 60% reduction in hip and wrist fractures in women whose estrogen replacement was begun within a few years of menopause. Studies also suggest that estrogen reduces the rate of vertebral fractures. Even when started as late as 6 years after menopause, estrogen may prevent further loss of bone mass for as long as the treatment is continued. When estrogen therapy is discontinued, bone mass declines at a rate comparable to that in the immediate postmenopausal period. There is no evidence that estrogen replacement therapy restores bone mass to premenopausal levels.

Early menopause is one of the strongest predictors for the development of osteoporosis.

The mainstays of prevention and management of postmenopausal osteoporosis are estrogen, an adequate lifetime calcium intake, vitamin D and exercise. Postmenopausal women absorb dietary calcium less efficiently than premenopausal women and require an average of 1500 mg/day of elemental calcium to remain in neutral calcium balance. By comparison, premenopausal women require about 1000 mg/day and the average calcium intake in the USA is 400 to 600 mg/day. Therefore, when not contraindicated, calcium supplementation and adequate daily intake of vitamin D (400 IU) may be helpful.

CONTRAINDICATIONS

Progestogens/estrogens should not be used in individuals with any of the following conditions or circumstances:

1. Known or suspected pregnancy, including use for missed abortion or as a diagnostic test for pregnancy. Progestin or estrogen may cause fetal harm when administered to a pregnant woman.
2. Known or suspected cancer of the breast.
3. Known or suspected estrogen-dependent neoplasia.
4. Undiagnosed abnormal genital bleeding.
5. Active or past history of thrombophlebitis or thromboembolic disorders.
6. Known sensitivity to *femhrt* 1/5 or other estrogen and progestin containing products.

WARNINGS

1. Induction of Malignant Neoplasms

Endometrial Cancer

The reported endometrial cancer risk among users of unopposed estrogen is about 2- to 12-fold greater than in nonusers, and appears dependent on duration of treatment and on estrogen dose. Most studies show no significant increased risk associated with the use of estrogens for less than 1 year. The greatest risk appears associated with prolonged use, with increased risks of 15- to 24-fold for use of 5 to 10 years or more, and this risk has been shown to persist for at least 15 years after cessation of estrogen treatment. Results from a 2-year clinical study of the effects of *femhrt* 1/5 on endometrial hyperplasia are shown in the **Clinical Studies** section of this label.

Clinical surveillance of all women taking progestin/estrogen combinations is important. Adequate diagnostic measures, including endometrial sampling when indicated, should be undertaken to rule out malignancy in all cases of undiagnosed persistent or recurring abnormal vaginal bleeding. There is no evidence that "natural" estrogens are more or less hazardous than "synthetic" estrogens at equivalent doses.

Breast Cancer

While the majority of studies have not shown an increased risk of breast cancer in women who have ever used estrogen replacement therapy, some have reported a moderately increased risk (relative risks of 1.3–2.0) in those taking higher doses or those taking lower doses for prolonged periods of time, especially in excess of 10 years.

The effect of added progestins on the risk of breast cancer is unknown.

2. Gallbladder Disease

A 2- to 4-fold increase in the risk of gallbladder disease requiring surgery in women receiving postmenopausal estrogen has been reported.

3. Hypercalcemia

Administration of estrogens may lead to severe hypercalcemia in patients with breast cancer and bone metastases (see **CONTRAINDICATIONS**). If this occurs, the drugs should be stopped and appropriate measures taken to reduce the serum calcium level.

4. Pregnancy

Use in pregnancy is not recommended (see **CONTRAINDICATIONS**).

5. Venous Thromboembolism

Five epidemiologic studies have found an increased risk of venous thromboembolism (VTE) in users of estrogen replacement therapy (ERT) who did not have predisposing conditions for VTE, such as a past history of cardiovascular disease or a recent history of pregnancy, surgery, trauma, or serious illness. The increased risk was found only in current ERT users; it did not persist in former users. The risk appeared to be higher in the first year of use and decreased thereafter. The findings were similar for ERT alone or with added progestin and pertain to commonly used oral and transdermal doses, with a possible dose-dependent effect on risk. The studies found the VTE risk to be about one case per 10,000 women per year among women not using ERT and without predisposing conditions. The risk in current ERT users was increased to 2–3 cases per 10,000 women per year.

6. Visual Disturbances

Medication should be discontinued pending examination if there is a sudden partial or complete loss of vision, or if there is a sudden onset of proptosis, diplopia or migraine. If examination reveals papilledema or retinal vascular lesions, medication should be withdrawn.

PRECAUTIONS

A. General

Based on experience with estrogens and/or progestins:

1. Cardiovascular Risk

A causal relationship between estrogen replacement therapy and reduction of cardiovascular disease in postmenopausal women has not been proven. Furthermore, the effect of added progestins on this putative benefit is not yet known.

In recent years many published studies have suggested that there may be a cause-effect relationship between postmenopausal oral estrogen replacement therapy without cyclical progestins and a decrease in cardiovascular disease in women. Although most of the observational studies which assessed this statistical association have reported a 20% to 50% reduction in coronary heart disease risk and associated mortality in estrogen takers, the following should be considered when interpreting these reports:

(1) Because only one of these studies was randomized and it was too small to yield statistically significant results, all relevant studies were subject to selection bias. Thus, the apparently reduced risk of coronary artery disease cannot be attributed with certainty to estrogen replacement therapy. It may instead have been caused by life-style and medical characteristics of the women studied with the result that healthier women were selected for estrogen therapy. In general, treated women were of higher socioeconomic and educational status, more slender, more physically active, more likely to have undergone surgical menopause, and less likely to have diabetes than the untreated women. Although some studies attempted to control for these selection factors, it is common for properly designed randomized trials to fail to confirm benefits suggested by less rigorous study designs. Ongoing and future large-scale randomized trials may help to clarify the apparent benefit.

(2) Current medical practice often includes the use of concomitant progestin therapy in women with intact uteri (see **PRECAUTIONS** and **WARNINGS**). While the effects of added progestins on the risk of ischemic heart disease are not known, all available progestins reverse at least some of the favorable effects of estrogens on HDL and LDL levels (see **Clinical Studies**).

(3) While the effects of added progestins on the risk of breast cancer are also unknown, available epidemiological evidence suggests that progestins do not reduce, and may enhance the moderately increased breast cancer incidence that has been reported with prolonged estrogen replacement therapy (see **WARNINGS**).

2. Elevated Blood Pressure

Occasional blood pressure increases during estrogen replacement therapy have been attributed to idiosyncratic reactions to estrogens. More often, blood pressure has remained the same or has dropped. One study showed that postmenopausal estrogen users have higher blood pressure than nonusers.

Two other studies showed slightly lower blood pressure among estrogen users compared to nonusers. The data on the risk of estrogen use in postmenopausal women and the risk of stroke have not been considered conclusive. Nonetheless, blood pressure should be monitored at regular intervals with estrogen use.

3. Use in Hysterectomized Women

Existing data do not support the use of the combination of progestin and estrogen in postmenopausal women without a uterus.

4. Physical Examination

A complete medical and family history should be taken prior to the initiation of *femhrt* 1/5 and annually thereafter. These examinations should include special reference to blood pressure, breasts, abdomen, and pelvic organs, and should include a Papanicolaou smear.

5. Fluid Retention

Progestin/estrogen therapy may cause some degree of fluid retention. Conditions which might be exacerbated by this factor such as asthma, epilepsy, migraine, and cardiac or renal dysfunction, require careful observation.

6. Uterine Bleeding and Mastodynia

Certain patients may develop undesirable manifestations of estrogenic stimulation, such as abnormal uterine bleeding, and mastodynia. In cases of undiagnosed abnormal uterine bleeding, adequate diagnostic measures are indicated (see **WARNINGS**).

7. Impaired Liver Function

Estrogens and progestins may be poorly metabolized in patients with impaired liver function. If needed, therapy should be administered with caution.

8. Pathology Specimens

The pathologist should be advised of progestin/estrogen therapy when relevant specimens are submitted.

9. Hypercoagulability

Some studies have shown that women taking estrogen replacement therapy have hypercoagulability, primarily related to decreased antithrombin activity. This effect appears dose- and duration-dependent and is less pronounced than that associated with oral contraceptive use. Also, postmenopausal women tend to have changes in coagulation parameters at baseline compared to premenopausal women. There is some suggestion that low dose postmenopausal mestranol may increase the risk of thromboembolism, although the majority of studies (of primarily conjugated estrogen users) report no such increase. There is insufficient information on hypercoagulability in women who have had previous thromboembolic disease, therefore, *femhrt* 1/5 is contraindicated in such women.

10. Familial Hyperlipoproteinemia
Estrogen therapy may be associated with massive elevations of plasma triglycerides leading to pancreatitis and other complications in patients with familial defects of lipoprotein metabolism.

11. Depression
Patients who have a history of depression should be carefully observed and the drug discontinued if the depression recurs to a serious degree.

12. Impaired Glucose Tolerance
Diabetic patients should be carefully observed while receiving progestin/estrogen therapy. The effects of *femhrt* 1/5 on glucose tolerance have not been studied.

13. Lipoprotein Metabolism
(See **Clinical Studies.**)

B. Information for Patients
See text of Patient Package Insert which appears after the **HOW SUPPLIED** section.

C. Drug/Laboratory Test Interactions
The following drug/laboratory interactions have been observed with estrogen therapy, and/or *femhrt* 1/5:

1. In a 12-week study, *femhrt* 1/5 decreased Factor VII and plasminogen activator inhibitor-1 from baseline in a dose-related manner, but remained within the laboratory reference range for postmenopausal women. Mean levels of fibrinogen and partial thromboplastin time did not change from baseline for *femhrt* 1/5.
2. Estrogen therapy may increase thyroxine-binding globulin (TBG), leading to increased circulating total thyroid hormone (T4) as measured by protein-bound iodine (PBI), T4 levels (by column or radioimmunoassay), or T3 levels by radioimmunoassay. T3 resin uptake is decreased, reflecting the elevated TBG. Free T4 and free T3 concentrations are unaltered.
3. Estrogen therapy may elevate other binding proteins in serum, ie, corticosteroid binding globulin (CBC), sex hormone-binding globulin (SHBG), leading to increased circulating corticosteroids and sex steroids, respectively. Free or biologically active hormone concentrations are unchanged. Other plasma proteins may be increased (angiotensinogen/renin substrate, alpha-1-antitrypsin, ceruloplasmin).
femhrt 1/5 was associated with a SHBG increase of 22%.
4. Estrogen therapy increases plasma HDL and HDL-2 subfraction concentrations, reduces LDL cholesterol concentration and increases triglyceride levels. (For effects during *femhrt* 1/5 treatment, see **Clinical Studies.**)
5. Estrogen therapy is associated with impaired glucose tolerance.
6. Estrogen therapy reduces response to metyrapone test.
7. Estrogen therapy reduces serum folate concentration.

D. Drug/Drug Interactions
No drug-drug interaction studies have been conducted with *femhrt* 1/5.
The following section contains information on drug interactions with ethinyl estradiol-containing products (specifically, oral contraceptives) that have been reported in the public literature. It is unknown whether such interactions occur with *femhrt* 1/5 or drug products containing other types of estrogens.

The Effects of Other Drugs on Ethinyl Estradiol
The metabolism of ethinyl estradiol is increased by rifampin and anticonvulsants such as phenobarbital, phenytoin, and carbamazepine. Coadministration of troglitazone and certain ethinyl-estradiol containing drug products (eg, oral contraceptives containing ethinyl estradiol) reduce the plasma concentrations of ethinyl estradiol by 30 percent.
Ascorbic acid and acetaminophen may increase AUC and/or plasma concentrations of ethinyl estradiol. Coadministration of atorvastatin and certain ethinyl-estradiol containing drug products (eg, oral contraceptives containing ethinyl estradiol) increase AUC values for ethinyl estradiol by 20 percent.
Clinical pharmacokinetic studies have not demonstrated any consistent effect of antibiotics (other than rifampin) on plasma concentrations of synthetic steroids.

The Effect of Ethinyl Estradiol on Other Drugs
Drug products containing ethinyl estradiol may inhibit the metabolism of other compounds. Increased plasma concentrations of cyclosporine, prednisolone, and theophylline have been reported with concomitant administration of certain drugs containing ethinyl estradiol (eg, oral contraceptives containing ethinyl estradiol). In addition, drugs containing ethinyl estradiol may induce the conjugation of other compounds.
Decreased plasma concentrations of acetaminophen and increased clearance of temazapam, salicylic acid, morphine, and clofibric acid have been noted when these drugs were administered with certain ethinyl-estradiol containing drug products (eg, oral contraceptives containing ethinyl estradiol).

E. Carcinogenesis, Mutagenesis, Impairment of Fertility
Long-term continuous administration of natural and synthetic estrogens in certain animal species increase the frequency of carcinomas of the breast, uterus, cervix, vagina, testis, and liver (see **CONTRAINDICATIONS** and **WARNINGS**).

F. Pregnancy Category X
Estrogens/progestins should not be used during pregnancy (see **CONTRAINDICATIONS** and **WARNINGS**).

G. Nursing Mothers
As a general principle, the administration of any drug to nursing mothers should be done only when clearly necessary since many drugs are excreted in human milk. Estrogen administration to nursing mothers has been shown to decrease the quantity and quality of the milk. Detectable amounts of drug have been identified in the milk of mothers receiving progestational drugs. The effect of this on the nursing infant has not been determined.

ADVERSE REACTIONS

Adverse events reported in controlled clinical studies of *femhrt* 1/5 are shown in Table 4 below.

TABLE 4. All Treatment-Emergent Adverse Events Reported at a Frequency of >5% of Patients with *femhrt* 1/5

	% of Patients	
BODY SYSTEM/ Adverse Event	Placebo N = 247	*femhrt* 1/5 N = 258
BODY AS A WHOLE	40.1	39.5
Headache	14.6	18.2
Back Pain	5.3	4.7
Pain	4.5	3.9
Viral Infection	7.7	7.0
Edema-Generalized	4.9	4.7
DIGESTIVE SYSTEM	24.4	33.0
Nausea and/or Vomiting	5.3	7.4
Abdominal Pain	4.5	8.1
Constipation	4.0	3.1
MUSCULOSKELETAL SYSTEM	21.7	20.4
Arthralgia	6.9	5.8
Myalgia	8.5	7.8
PSYCHOBIOLOGIC FUNCTION	8.3	14.1
Nervousness	1.6	5.4
Depression	3.6	5.8
RESPIRATORY SYSTEM	37.2	35.6
Rhinitis	15.4	15.1
Sinusitis	9.7	8.1
Upper Respiratory Infection	4.5	3.9
UROGENITAL SYSTEM	25.0	40.8
Breast Pain	5.3	8.1
Urinary Tract Infection	3.2	6.2
Vaginitis	4.9	5.4

The following adverse events have been reported with estrogen and/or progestin therapy:
Genitourinary system: changes in vaginal bleeding pattern and abnormal withdrawal bleeding or flow, breakthrough bleeding, spotting, increase in size of uterine leiomyomata, vaginal candidiasis, changes in amount of cervical secretion, premenstrual-like syndrome, cystitis-like syndrome.
Breasts: tenderness, enlargement, fibrocystic disease of the breast.
Gastrointestinal: cholestatic jaundice, pancreatitis, flatulence, bloating, abdominal cramps.
Skin: cholasma or melasma that may persist when drug is discontinued, erythema multiforme, erythema nodosum, hemorrhagic eruption, loss of scalp hair, hirsutism, itching, skin rash and pruritus.
CNS: headache, migraine, dizziness, chorea, insomnia.
Cardiovascular: changes in blood pressure, cerebrovascular accidents, deep venous thrombosis, and pulmonary embolism.
Eyes: intolerance to contact lenses, sudden partial or complete loss of vision, proptosis, diplopia, otosclerosis.
Miscellaneous: increase or decrease in weight, reduced carbohydrate tolerance, aggravation of porphyria, changes in libido, fatigue, allergic or anaphylactoid reactions, leiomyoma, fibromyoma of the uterus, endometriosis.

OVERDOSAGE
ACUTE OVERDOSAGE

Serious ill effects have not been reported following acute ingestion of large doses of progestin/estrogen-containing oral contraceptives by young children. Overdosage of estrogen may cause nausea and vomiting, and withdrawal bleeding may occur.

DOSAGE AND ADMINISTRATION

femhrt 1/5 therapy consists of a single tablet taken once daily.

1. For the Treatment of Vasomotor Symptoms
femhrt 1/5 should be given once daily for the treatment of moderate to severe vasomotor symptoms associated with the menopause. Patients should be reevaluated at 3 to 6 month intervals to determine if treatment is still necessary.

2. Prevention of Osteoporosis
femhrt 1/5 should be given once daily to prevent postmenopausal osteoporosis (see **Clinical Studies: Effect on Bone Mineral Density**). Response to therapy can be assessed by measurement of bone mineral density.
Treated patients with an intact uterus should be monitored closely for signs of endometrial cancer, and appropriate diagnostic measures should be taken to rule out malignancy in the event of persistent or recurring vaginal bleeding. Parents should be evaluated at least annually for breast abnormalities and more often if there are any symptoms.

HOW SUPPLIED

femhrt 1/5 tablets are white and available in the following strength and package sizes:
N 0071-0144-23 Bottle of 90 D-shaped tablets with 1 **mg** norethindrone acetate and 5 **mcg** ethinyl estradiol
N 0071-0144-45 Blister card of 28 D-shaped tablets with 1 **mg** norethindrone acetate and 5 **mcg** ethinyl estradiol
℞ only
Keep this drug and all drugs out of the reach of children. Store at 25°C (77°F); excursions permitted to 15–30°C (59–86°F) [see USP Controlled Room Temperature].

INFORMATION FOR THE PATIENT

What is *femhrt*™ 1/5?
Your healthcare provider has prescribed *femhrt* 1/5, a combination of two hormones, a progestin (1 mg norethindrone acetate) and an estrogen (5 mcg ethinyl estradiol) intended for use once a day. This insert describes the major benefits and risks of your treatment, as well as how and when treatment may be taken. If you have any questions, please contact your physician, nurse or pharmacist.

***femhrt* 1/5 is approved for use in the following ways:**

- **To reduce moderate to severe menopausal symptoms.** Estrogens are hormones produced by the ovaries of menstruating women. When a woman is between the ages of 45 and 55, the ovaries normally stop making estrogens. This drop in body estrogen levels causes the "change of life" or menopause, the end of monthly menstrual periods. When estrogen levels begin dropping, some women develop very uncomfortable symptoms, such as feelings of warmth in the face, neck, and chest, or sudden intense episodes of heat and sweating ("hot flashes" or "hot flushes"). In some women, the symptoms are mild; in others they can be severe. These symptoms may last only as few months or longer. Taking *femhrt* 1/5 can help reduce these symptoms. If you are not taking hormones for other reasons, such as the prevention of osteoporosis, you should take *femhrt* 1/5 only as long as you need it for relief from your menopausal symptoms.
- **To prevent thinning bones (osteoporosis).** Osteoporosis is a thinning of the bones that makes them weaker and allows them to break more easily. The bones of the spine, wrists, and hips may be affected by osteoporosis. *femhrt* 1/5 may be used as part of a program including weight-bearing exercise, such as walking or running, and calcium supplements.
  Women likely to develop osteoporosis often have the following characteristics: white or Asian race, slim, cigarette smokers, and a family history of osteoporosis in a mother, sister, or aunt. Women who have menopause at an earlier age, either naturally or because their ovaries were removed during an operation, are more like to develop osteoporosis than women whose menopause happens later in life.

Who should not take *femhrt* 1/5?
femhrt 1/5 should not be taken in the following situations:

- **During pregnancy.** If you think you may be pregnant, do not take *femhrt* 1/5. Taking estrogens while you are pregnant may cause your unborn child to have birth defects. Do not take *femhrt* 1/5 to prevent miscarriage.
- **If you have unusual vaginal bleeding that has not been checked by your healthcare provider.** Unusual vaginal bleeding can be a warning sign of a serious condition, including cancer of the uterus, especially if bleeding happens after menopause. Your doctor must find out of the cause of the bleeding to recommend the right treatment.
- **If you have had certain cancers.** Estrogens increase the risk of certain types of cancers, including cancer of the breast and uterus. If you have had cancer, talk with your doctor about whether you should take *femhrt* 1/5.
- **If you have any circulation problems.** Generally, estrogens should not be taken if you have ever had a blood-clotting condition or other circulatory problem. In special situations, some doctors may decide that estrogen therapy is so necessary that the risks of taking *femhrt* 1/5 are acceptable (see "What are the possible risks and side effects of *femhrt* 1/5").
- **After childbirth or when breast-feeding a baby.** *femhrt* 1/5 should not be used to try to stop the breasts from filling with milk after a baby is born. Taking *femhrt* 1/5 may increase your risk of developing blood clots (see "What are the possible risks and side effects of *femhrt* 1/5").
- **If you have had a hysterectomy (uterus removed).** *femhrt* 1/5 contains a progestin to decrease the risk of developing endometrial hyperplasia (an overgrowth of the lining of the uterus that may lead to cancer). If you do not have a uterus, you do not need a progestin, and you should not take *femhrt* 15.

How should I take *femhrt* 1/5?
Take your *femhrt* 1/5 pill once a day at about the same time each day. If you miss a dose, take it as soon as you remember. If it is almost time for your next dose, skip the missed dose and take only your next regularly scheduled dose. Do not take two doses at the same time.

Continued on next page

This product information was prepared in June 2000. On these and other Parke-Davis Products, information may be obtained by addressing PARKE-DAVIS, a Warner-Lambert Division, Morris Plains, New Jersey 07950.

Femhrt—Cont.

The length of treatment with estrogens varies from woman to woman. You and your healthcare provider should re-evaluate every 3 to 6 months whether or not your still need *femhrt* 1/5 to control your hot flashes.

What are the possible risks and side effects of *femhrt* 1/5?

- **Cancer of the uterus.** *femhrt* 1/5 has estrogen and progestin in it. If you take any drug that contains estrogen, including *femhrt* 1/5, you should see your doctor for regular check-ups and report any unusual vaginal bleeding right away. Vaginal bleeding after menopause may be a warning sign of a serious condition, including cancer of the uterus. Your doctor should identify the cause of any unusual vaginal bleeding.
  The risk of cancer of the uterus increases when estrogens are used without a progestin. The risk also increases the longer estrogens are taken and the larger the doses. You are more likely to get cancer of the uterus if you are overweight, diabetic, or have high blood pressure. *femhrt* 1/5, which contains a progestin, reduces the estrogen-related risk of getting a condition of the uterine lining called endometrial hyperplasia. This condition may lead to cancer of the uterus (see "Other Information").
- **Cancer of the breast.** Most studies have not shown a higher risk of breast cancer in women who have used estrogens. However, some studies report that breast cancer developed more often (up to twice the usual rate) in women who used estrogens for longer time periods, especially more than 10 years, or who used high doses for a shorter time period. The effects of added progestin on the risk of breast cancer are unknown. You should have regular breast examinations by a health professional and examine your own breasts monthly. Ask your healthcare provider to show you how to do a breast exam yourself. If you are over 50 years of age, you should have a mammogram every year.
- **Gallbladder disease.** Women who use estrogens after menopause are more likely to develop gallbladder disease that leads to surgery than women who do not use estrogens.
- **Abnormal blood clotting.** Taking estrogens may cause changes in your blood clotting system that allow the blood to clot more easily. If blood clots form in your bloodstream, they can cut off the blood supply to vital organs, causing serious problems. These problems may include a stroke (by cutting off blood to the brain), a heart attack (by cutting off blood of the heart), or a pulmonary embolus (by cutting off blood supply to the lungs). Any of these conditions may cause death or serious long-term disability.
- **Vaginal bleeding.** With *femhrt* 1/5, menstrual-like vaginal bleeding may occur. If bleeding occurs, it is frequently light spotting or bleeding, but it may be moderate or heavy. If you experience vaginal bleeding while taking *femhrt* 1/5, discuss your bleeding pattern with your healthcare provider.

In addition to the risks and side effects just listed, patients taking estrogen or progestin have reported the following side effects:

- nausea and vomiting
- breast tenderness or enlargement
- headache
- retention of extra fluid (edema), which may make some conditions worse, such as asthma, epilepsy, migraine, heart disease, or kidney disease
- runny nose
- abdominal pain
- enlargement of non-cancerous tumors (fibroids) of the uterus
- spotty darkening of the skin, particularly on the face; reddening of the skin; skin rashes

How can I reduce the risks associated with taking *femhrt* 1/5?

If you take *femhrt* 1/5, you can reduce your risks by carefully monitoring your treatment.

- **See your healthcare provider regularly.** While you take *femhrt* 1/5, see your doctor as least once a year for a checkup. If you develop vaginal bleeding while taking *femhrt* 1/5, you might need further evaluation. If members of your family have had breast cancer or if you have ever had breast lumps or an abnormal mammogram (breast x-ray), you may need more frequent breast examinations.
- **Reassess your need for treatment.** Every 3–6 months, you and your doctor should discuss whether or not you still need *femhrt* 1/5 for control of your hot flashes.
- **Be alert for signs of trouble.** If any of the following warning signs (or any other unusual symptoms) happen while you are taking *femhrt* 1/5, call your doctor right away:
  - pains in the calves or chest, sudden shortness of breath, or coughing blood (possible clots in the legs, heart, or lungs)
  - severe headache or vomiting, dizziness, faintness, or changes in vision or speech, weakness or numbness of an arm or leg (possible clots in the brain or eye)
  - breast lumps (possible breast cancer)
  - yellowing of the skin or whites of the eyes (possible liver problems)
  - pain, swelling, or tenderness in the abdomen (possible gallbladder problem)

Other Information

- Discuss carefully with your doctor or healthcare provider all the possible risks and benefits of long-term estrogen and progestin treatment as they affect you personally.
- If you take calcium supplements as part of your treatment to help prevent osteoporosis, ask your doctor about the amounts recommended. A daily intake of 1500 mg of calcium is often recommended for postmenopausal women. Vitamin D (400 IU daily) may help your body use more of the calcium.
- Taking estrogens with progestins may have unhealthy effects on blood sugar, which might make a diabetic condition worse.
- Your doctor has prescribed this drug for you and you alone. Do not give your *femhrt* 1/5 to anyone else. Do not take *femhrt* 1/5 for conditions for which it was not prescribed.
- Keep all drugs out of the reach of children. In case of overdose, call your doctor, hospital, or poison control center right away.

This leaflet provides the most important information about *femhrt* 1/5. If you want more information, ask your doctor or pharmacist for the professional labeling. The professional labeling is published in a book called "The Physicians' Desk Reference" or PDR, available in bookstores and public libraries.

October 1999

Manufactured by:
DURAMED PHARMACEUTICALS, INC.
CINCINNATI, OH 45213 USA

Distributed by:
PARKE-DAVIS
Div of Warner-Lambert Co
Morris Plains, NJ 07950 USA 0132G030

Shown in Product Identification Guide, page 329

LIPITOR® ℞
(Atorvastatin Calcium) Tablets

DESCRIPTION

Lipitor® (atorvastatin calcium) is a synthetic lipid-lowering agent. Atorvastatin is an inhibitor of 3-hydroxy-3-methylglutaryl-coenzyme A (HMG-CoA) reductase. This enzyme catalyzes the conversion of HMG-CoA to mevalonate, an early and rate-limiting step in cholesterol biosynthesis.

Atorvastatin calcium is [R-(R*,R*)]-2-(4-fluorophenyl)-β, δ-dihydroxy-5- (1-methylethyl) -3-phenyl-4- [(phenylamino)carbonyl]-1H-pyrrole-1-heptanoic acid, calcium salt (2:1) trihydrate. The empirical formula of atorvastatin calcium is $(C_{33}H_{34}FN_2O_5)_2Ca \bullet 3H_2O$ and its molecular weight is 1209.42. Its structural formula is:

Atorvastatin calcium is a white to off-white crystalline powder that is insoluble in aqueous solution of pH 4 and below. Atorvastatin calcium is very slightly soluble in distilled water, pH 7.4 phosphate buffer, and acetonitrile, slightly soluble in ethanol, and freely soluble in methanol.

Lipitor tablets for oral administration contain 10, 20, 40, or 80 mg atorvastatin and the following inactive ingredients: calcium carbonate, USP; candelilla wax, FCC; croscarmellose sodium, NF; hydroxypropyl cellulose, NF; lactose monohydrate, NF; magnesium stearate, NF; microcrystalline cellulose, NF; Opadry White YS-1-7040 (hydroxypropylmethylcellulose, polyethylene glycol, talc, titanium dioxide); polysorbate 80, NF; simethicone emulsion.

CLINICAL PHARMACOLOGY

Mechanism of Action

Atorvastatin is a selective, competitive inhibitor of HMG-CoA reductase, the rate-limiting enzyme that converts 3-hydroxy-3-methyl-glutaryl-coenzyme A to mevalonate, a precursor of sterols, including cholesterol. Cholesterol and triglycerides circulate in the bloodstream as part of lipoprotein complexes. With ultracentrifugation, these complexes separate into HDL (high-density lipoprotein), IDL (intermediate-density lipoprotein), LDL (low-density lipoprotein), and VLDL (very-low-density lipoprotein) fractions. Triglycerides (TG) and cholesterol in the liver are incorporated into VLDL and released into the plasma for delivery to peripheral tissues. LDL is formed from VLDL and is catabolized primarily through the high-affinity LDL receptor. Clinical and pathologic studies show that elevated plasma levels of total cholesterol (total-C), LDL-cholesterol (LDL-C), and apolipoprotein B (apo B) promote human atherosclerosis and are risk factors for developing cardiovascular disease, while increased levels of HDL-C are associated with a decreased cardiovascular risk.

In animal models, Lipitor lowers plasma cholesterol and lipoprotein levels by inhibiting HMG-CoA reductase and cholesterol synthesis in the liver and by increasing the number of hepatic LDL receptors on the cell-surface to enhance uptake and catabolism of LDL; Lipitor also reduces LDL production and the number of LDL particles. Lipitor reduces LDL-C in some patients with homozygous familial hypercholesterolemia (FH), a population that rarely responds to other lipid-lowering medication(s).

A variety of clinical studies have demonstrated that elevated levels of total-C, LDL-C, and apo B (a membrane complex for LDL-C) promote human atherosclerosis. Similarly, decreased levels of HDL-C (and its transport complex, apo A) are associated with the development of atherosclerosis. Epidemiologic investigations have established that cardiovascular morbidity and mortality vary directly with the level of total-C and LDL-C, and inversely with the level of HDL-C. The independent effect of raising HDL-C or lowering TG on the risk for coronary and cardiovascular morbidity and mortality has not been established.

Lipitor reduces total-C, LDL-C and apo B in patients with homozygous and heterozygous FH, nonfamilial forms of hypercholesterolemia, and mixed dyslipidemia. Lipitor also reduced VLDL-C and TG and produces variable increases in HDL-C and apolipoprotein A-1. Lipitor reduces total-C, LDL-C, VLDL-C, apo B, TG, and non-HDL-C, and increases HDL-C in patients with isolated hypertriglyceridemia. Lipitor reduces intermediate density lipoprotein cholesterol (IDL-C) in patients with dysbetalipoproteinemia. The effect of Lipitor on cardiovascular morbidity and mortality has not been determined.

Like LDL, cholesterol-enriched triglyceride-rich lipoproteins, including VLDL, intermediate density lipoprotein (IDL), and remnants, can also promote atherosclerosis. Elevated plasma triglycerides are frequently found in a triad with low HDL-C levels and small LDL particles, as well as in association with non-lipid metabolic risk factors for coronary heart disease. As such, total plasma TG has not consistently been shown to be an independent risk factor for CHD. Furthermore, the independent effect of raising HDL or lowering TG on the risk of coronary and cardiovascular morbidity and mortality has not been determined.

Pharmacodynamics

Atorvastatin as well as some of its metabolites are pharmacologically active in humans. The liver is the primary site of action and the principal site of cholesterol synthesis and LDL clearance. Drug dosage rather than systemic drug concentration correlates better with LDL-C reduction. Individualization of drug dosage should be based on therapeutic response (see DOSAGE AND ADMINISTRATION).

Pharmacokinetics and Drug Metabolism

Absorption: Atorvastatin is rapidly absorbed after oral administration; maximum plasma concentrations occur within 1 to 2 hours. Extent of absorption increases in proportion to atorvastatin dose. The absolute bioavailability of atorvastatin (parent drug) is approximately 14% and the systemic availability of HMG-CoA reductase inhibitory activity is approximately 30%. The low systemic availability is attributed to presystemic clearance in gastrointestinal mucosa and/or hepatic first-pass metabolism. Although food decreases the rate and extent of drug absorption by approximately 25% and 9%, respectively, as assessed by Cmax and AUC, LDL-C reduction is similar whether atorvastatin is given with or without food. Plasma atorvastatin concentrations are lower (approximately 30% for Cmax and AUC) following evening drug administration compared with morning. However, LDL-C reduction is the same regardless of the time of day of drug administration (see DOSAGE AND ADMINISTRATION).

Distribution: Mean volume of distribution of atorvastatin is approximately 381 liters. Atorvastatin is ≥98% bound to plasma proteins. A blood/plasma ratio of approximately 0.25 indicates poor drug penetration into red blood cells. Based on observation in rats, atorvastatin is likely to be secreted in human milk (see CONTRAINDICATIONS, Pregnancy and Lactation, and PRECAUTIONS, Nursing Mothers).

Metabolism: Atorvastatin is extensively metabolized to ortho- and parahydroxylated derivatives and various beta-oxidation products. *In vitro* inhibition of HMG-CoA reductase by ortho- and parahydroxylated metabolites is equivalent to that of atorvastatin. Approximately 70% of circulating inhibitory activity for HMG-CoA reductase is attributed to active metabolites. *In vitro* studies suggest the importance of atorvastatin metabolism by cytochrome P450 3A4, consistent with increased plasma concentrations of atorvastatin in humans following coadministration with erythromycin, a known inhibitor of this isozyme (see PRECAUTIONS, Drug Interactions). In animals, the ortho-hydroxy metabolite undergoes further glucuronidation.

Excretion: Atorvastatin and its metabolites are eliminated primarily in bile following hepatic and/or extrahepatic metabolism; however, the drug does not appear to undergo enterohepatic recirculation. Mean plasma elimination half-life of atorvastatin in humans is approximately 14 hours, but the half-life of inhibitory activity for HMG-CoA reductase is 20 to 30 hours due to the contribution of active metabolites. Less than 2% of a dose of atorvastatin is recovered in urine following oral administration.

Special Populations

Geriatric: Plasma concentrations of atorvastatin are higher (approximately 40% for Cmax and 30% for AUC) in healthy elderly subjects (age ≥65 years) than in young adults. LDL-C reduction is comparable to that seen in younger patient populations given equal doses of Lipitor.

Pediatric: Pharmacokinetic data in the pediatric population are not available.

Gender: Plasma concentrations of atorvastatin in women differ from those in men (approximately 20% higher for Cmax and 10% lower for AUC); however, there is no clinically significant difference in LDL-C reduction with Lipitor between men and women.

Renal Insufficiency: Renal disease has no influence on the plasma concentrations or LDL-C reduction of atorvastatin; thus, dose adjustment in patients with renal dysfunction is not necessary (see DOSAGE AND ADMINISTRATION).

Hemodialysis: While studies have not been conducted in patients with end-stage renal disease, hemodialysis is not expected to significantly enhance clearance of atorvastatin since the drug is extensively bound to plasma proteins.

Hepatic Insufficiency: In patients with chronic alcoholic liver disease, plasma concentrations of atorvastatin are markedly increased Cmax and AUC are each 4-fold greater in patients with Childs-Pugh A disease. Cmax and AUC are approximately 16-fold and 11-fold increased, respectively, in patients with Childs-Pugh B disease (see CONTRAINDICATIONS).

Clinical Studies

Hypercholesterolemia (Heterozygous Familial and Nonfamilial and Mixed Dyslipidemia (*Fredrickson* Types IIa and IIb)

Lipitor reduces total-C, LDL-C, VLDL-C, apo B, and TG, and increases HDL-C in patients with hypercholesterolemia and mixed dyslipidemia. Therapeutic response is seen within 2 weeks, and maximum response is usually achieved within 4 weeks and maintained during chronic therapy.

Lipitor is effective in a wide variety of patient populations with hypercholesterolemia, with and without hypertriglyceridemia, in men and women, and in the elderly. Experience in pediatric patients has been limited to patients with homozygous FH.

In two multicenter, placebo-controlled, dose-response studies in patients with hypercholesterolemia. Lipitor given as a single dose over 6 weeks significantly reduced total-C, LDL-C, apo B, and TG (Pooled results are provided in Table 1).

[See table 1 above]

TABLE 1. Dose-Response in Patients With Primary Hypercholesterolemia (Adjusted Mean % Change From Baseline)[a]

Dose	N	TC	LDL-C	Apo B	TG	HDL-C	Non-HDL-C/ HDL-C
Placebo	21	4	4	3	10	−3	7
10	22	−29	−39	−32	−19	6	−34
20	20	−33	−43	−35	−26	9	−41
40	21	−37	−50	−42	−29	6	−45
80	23	−45	−60	−50	−37	5	−53

[a] Results are pooled from 2 dose-response studies

In patients with *Fredrickson* Types IIa and IIb hyperlipoproteinemia pooled from 24 controlled trials, the median (25th and 75th percentile) percent changes from baseline in HDL-C for atorvastatin 10, 20, 40, and 80 mg were 6.4 (−1.4, 14), 8.7 (0, 17), 7.8 (0, 16), and 5.1 (−2.7, 15), respectively. Additionally, analysis of the pooled data demonstrated consistent and significant decreases in total-C, LDL-C, TG, total-C/HDL-C, and LDL-C/HDL-C.

In three multicenter, double-blind studies in patients with hypercholesterolemia, Lipitor was compared to other HMG-CoA reductase inhibitors. After randomization, patients were treated for 16 weeks with either Lipitor 10 mg per day or a fixed dose of the comparative agent (Table 2).

[See table 2 above]

TABLE 2. Mean Percent Change From Baseline at End Point (Double-Blind, Randomized, Active-Controlled Trials)

Treatment (Daily Dose)	N	Total-C	LDL-C	Apo B	TG	HDL-C	Non-HDL-C/ HDL-C
Study 1							
Atorvastatin 10 mg	707	−27[a]	−36[a]	−28[a]	−17[a]	+7	−37[a]
Lovastatin 20 mg	191	−19	−27	−20	−6	+7	−28
95% CI for Diff[1]		−9.2, −6.5	−10.7, −7.1	−10.0, −6.5	−15.2, −7.1	−1.7, −2.0	−11.1, −7.1
Study 2							
Atorvastatin 10 mg	222	−25[b]	−35[b]	−27[b]	−17[b]	+6	−36[b]
Pravastatin 20 mg	77	−17	−23	−17	−9	+8	−28
95% CI for Diff[1]		−10.8, −6.1	−14.5, −8.2	−13.4, −7.4	−14.1, −0.7	−4.9, −1.6	−11.5, −4.1
Study 3							
Atorvastatin 10 mg	132	−29[c]	−37[c]	−34[c]	−23[c]	+7	−39[c]
Simvastatin 10 mg	45	−24	−30	−30	−15	+7	−33
95% CI for Diff[1]		−8.7, −2.7	−10.1, −2.6	−8.0, −1.1	−15.1, −0.7	−4.3, −3.9	−9.6, −1.9

[1] A negative value for the 95% CI for the difference between treatment favors atorvastatin for all except HDL-C, for which a positive value favors atorvastatin. If the range does not include 0, this indicates a statistically significant difference.
[a] Significantly different from lovastatin, ANCOVA, $p \leq 0.05$
[b] Significantly different from pravastatin, ANCOVA, $p \leq 0.05$
[c] Significantly different from simvastatin, ANCOVA, $p \leq 0.05$

The impact on clinical outcomes of the differences in lipid-altering effects between treatments shown in Table 2 is not known. Table 2 does not contain data comparing the effects of atorvastatin 10 mg and higher doses of lovastatin, pravastatin, and simvastatin. The drugs compared in the studies summarized in the table are not necessarily interchangeable.

In a large clinical study, the number of patients meeting their National Cholesterol Education Program-Adult Treatment Panel (NCEP-ATP) II target LDL-C levels on 10 mg of Lipitor daily was assessed. After 16 weeks, 156/167 (93%) of patients with less than 2 risk factors for CHD and baseline LDL-C ≥ 190 mg/dL reached a target of ≤ 160 mg/dL; 141/218 (65%) of patients with 2 or more risk factors for CHD and LDL-C ≥ 160 mg/dL achieved a level of ≤130 mg/dL LDL-C, and 21/113 (19%) of patients with CHD and LDL-C ≥130 mg/dL reached a target level of ≤100 mg/dL LDL-C.

Hypertriglyceridemia (*Fredrickson* Type IV)

The response to atorvastatin in 64 patients with isolated hypertriglyceridemia treated across several clinical trials is shown in the table below. For the atorvastatin-treated patients, median (min, max) baseline TG level was 565 (267–1502).

[See table 3 above]

TABLE 3. Combined Patients With Isolated Elevated TG: Median (min, max) Percent Changes From Baseline

	Placebo (N=12)	Atorva 10 mg (N=37)	Atorva 20 mg (N=13)	Atorva 80 mg (N=14)
Triglycerides	−12.4 (−36.6, 82.7)	−41.0 (−76.2, 49.4)	−38.7 (−62.7, 29.5)	−51.8 (−82.8, 41.3)
Total-C	−2.3 (−15.5, 24.4)	−28.2 (−44.9, −6.8)	−34.9 (−49.6, −15.2)	−44.4 (−63.5, −3.8)
LDL-C	3.6 (−31.3, 31.6)	−26.5 (−57.7, 9.8)	−30.4 (−53.9, 0.3)	−40.5 (−60.6, −13.8)
HDL-C	3.8 (−18.6, 13.4)	13.8 (−9.7, 61.5)	11.0 (−3.2, 25.2)	7.5 (−10.8, 37.2)
VLDL-C	−1.0 (−31.9, 53.2)	−48.8 (−85.8, 57.3)	−44.6 (−62.2, −10.8)	−62.0 (−88.2, 37.6)
non-HDL-C	−2.8 (−17.6, 30.0)	−33.0 (−52.1, −13.3)	−42.7 (−53.7, −17.4)	−51.5 (−72.9, −4.3)

Dysbetalipoproteinemia (*Fredrickson* Type III)

The results of an open-label crossover study of 16 patients genoteypes: 14 apo E2/E2 and 2 apo E3/E2) with dysbetalipoprotein (*Fredrickson* Type III) are shown in the table below.

[See table 4 above]

TABLE 4. Open-Label Crossover Study of 16 Patients With Dysbetalipoproteinemia (Fredrickson Type III)

	Median (min, max) at baseline (mg/dL)	median % change (min, max) Atorva 10 mg	Atorva 80 mg
Total-C	442 (225, 1320)	−37 (−85, 17)	−58 (−90, −31)
Triglycerides	678 (273, 5990)	−39 (−92, −8)	−53 (−95, −30)
IDL-C + VLDL-C	215 (111, 613)	−32 (−76, 9)	−63 (−90, −8)
non-HDL-C	411 (218, 1272)	−43 (−87, −19)	−64 (−92, −36)

Homozygous Familial Hypercholesterolemia

In a study without a concurrent control group, 29 patients ages 6 to 37 years with homozygous FH received maximum daily doses of 20 to 80 mg of Lipitor. The mean LDL-C reduction in this study was 18%. Twenty-five patients with a reduction in LDL-C had a mean response of 20% (range of 7% to 53%, median of 24%); the remaining 4 patients had 7% to 24% increases in LDL-C. Five of the 29 patients had absent LDL-receptor function. Of these, 2 patients also had a portacaval shunt and had no significant reduction in LDL-C. The remaining 3 receptor-negative patients had a mean LDL-C reduction of 22%.

INDICATIONS AND USAGE

Lipitor is indicated:

1. as an adjunct to diet to reduce elevated total-C, LDL-C, apo B, and TG levels and to increase HDL-C in patients with primary hypercholesterolemia (heterozygous familial and nonfamilial) and mixed dyslipidemia (*Fredrickson* Types IIa and IIb);
2. as an adjunct to diet for the treatment of patients with elevated serum TG levels (*Fredrickson* Type IV);
3. for the treatment of patients with primary dysbetalipoproteinemia (*Fredrickson* Type III) who do not respond adequately to diet;
4. to reduce total-C and LDL-C in patients with homozygous familial hypercholesterolemia as an adjunct to other lipid-lowering treatments (eg, LDL apheresis) or if such treatments are unavailable.

Therapy with lipid-altering agents should be a component of multiple-risk-factor intervention in individuals at increased risk for atherosclerotic vascular disease due to hypercholesterolemia. Lipid-altering agents should be used in addition to a diet restricted in saturated fat and cholesterol only when the response to diet and other nonpharmacological measures has been inadequate (see *National Cholesterol Education Program (NCEP) Guidelines,* summarized in Table 5).

[See table 5 at top of next page]

At the time of hospitalization for an acute coronary event, consideration can be given to initiating drug therapy at discharge if the LDL-C level is ≥130 mg/dL (NCEP-ATP II).

Prior to initiating therapy with Lipitor, secondary causes for hypercholesterolemia (eg, poorly controlled diabetes mellitus, hypothyroidism, nephrotic syndrome, dysproteinemias, obstructive liver disease, other drug therapy, and alcoholism) should be excluded, and a lipid profile performed to measure total-C, LDL-C, HDL-C, and TG. For patients with TG <400 mg/dL (<4.5 mmol/L), LDL-C can be estimated using the following equation: LDL-C = total-C − (0.20 × [TG] + HDL-C). For TG levels >400 mg/dL (>4.5 mmol/L), this equation is less accurate and LDL-C concentrations should be determined by ultracentrifugation.

Lipitor has not been studied in conditions where the major lipoprotein abnormality is elevation of chylomicrons (*Fredrickson* Types I and V).

CONTRAINDICATIONS

Active liver disease or unexplained persistent elevations of serum transaminases.

Hypersensitivity to any component of this medication.

Pregnancy and Lactation

Atherosclerosis is a chronic process and discontinuation of lipid-lowering drugs during pregnancy should have little impact on the outcome of long-term therapy of primary hypercholesterolemia. Cholesterol and other products of cholesterol biosynthesis are essential components for fetal development (including synthesis of steroids and cell membranes). Since HMG-CoA reductase inhibitors decrease cholesterol synthesis and possibly the synthesis of other biologically active substances derived from cholesterol, they may cause fetal harm when administered to pregnant

Continued on next page

This product information was prepared in June 2000. On these and other Parke-Davis Products, information may be obtained by addressing PARKE-DAVIS, a Warner-Lambert Division, Morris Plains, New Jersey 07950.

Lipitor—Cont.

women. Therefore, HMG-CoA reductase inhibitors are contraindicated during pregnancy and in nursing mothers. ATORVASTATIN SHOULD BE ADMINISTERED TO WOMEN OF CHILDBEARING AGE ONLY WHEN SUCH PATIENTS ARE HIGHLY UNLIKELY TO CONCEIVE AND HAVE BEEN INFORMED OF THE POTENTIAL HAZARDS. If the patient becomes pregnant while taking this drug, therapy should be discontinued and the patient apprised of the potential hazard to the fetus.

WARNINGS

Liver Dysfunction

HMG-CoA reductase inhibitors, like some other lipid-lowering therapies, have been associated with biochemical abnormalities of liver function. **Persistent elevations (>3 times the upper limit of normal [ULN] occurring on 2 or more occasions) in serum transaminases occurred in 0.7% of patients who received atorvastatin in clinical trials. The incidence of these abnormalities was 0.2%, 0.2%, 0.6%, and 2.3% for 10, 20, 40, and 80 mg, respectively.**

One patient in clinical trials developed jaundice. Increases in liver function tests (LFT) in other patients were not associated with jaundice or other clinical signs or symptoms. Upon dose reduction, drug interruption, or discontinuation, transaminase levels returned to or near pretreatment levels without sequelae. Eighteen of 30 patients with persistent LFT elevations continued treatment with a reduced dose of atorvastatin.

It is recommended that liver function tests be performed prior to and at 12 weeks following both the initiation of therapy and any elevation of dose, and periodically (e.g., semiannually) thereafter. Liver enzyme changes generally occur in the first 3 months of treatment with atorvastatin. Patients who develop increased transaminase levels should be monitored until the abnormalities resolve. Should an increase in ALT or AST of >3 times ULN persist, reduction of dose or withdrawal of atorvastatin is recommended.

Atorvastatin should be used with caution in patients who consume substantial quantities of alcohol and/or have a history of liver disease. Active liver disease or unexplained persistent transaminase elevations are contraindications to the use of atorvastatin (see CONTRAINDICATIONS).

Skeletal Muscle

Rare cases of rhabdomyolysis with acute renal failure secondary to myoglobinuria have been reported with atorvastatin and with drugs in this class.

Uncomplicated myalgia has been reported in atorvastatin-treated patients (see ADVERSE REACTIONS). Myopathy, defined as muscle aches or muscle weakness in conjunction with increases in creatine phosphokinase (CPK) values >10 times ULN, should be considered in any patient with diffuse myalgias, muscle tenderness or weakness, and/or marked elevation of CPK. Patients should be advised to report promptly unexplained muscle pain, tenderness or weakness, particularly if accompanied by malaise or fever. Atorvastatin therapy should be discontinued if markedly elevated CPK levels occur or myopathy is diagnosed or suspected.

The risk of myopathy during treatment with other drugs in this class is increased with concurrent administration of cyclosporine, fibric acid derivatives, erythromycin, niacin, or azole antifungals. Physicians considering combined therapy with atorvastatin and fibric acid derivatives, erythromycin, immunosuppressive drugs, azole antifungals, or lipid-lowering doses of niacin should carefully weigh the potential benefits and risks and should carefully monitor patients for any signs or symptoms of muscle pain, tenderness, or weakness, particularly during the initial months of therapy and during any periods of upward dosage titration of either drug. Periodic creatine phosphokinase (CPK) determinations may be considered in such situations, but there is no assurance that such monitoring will prevent the occurrence of severe myopathy.

Atorvastatin therapy should be temporarily withheld or discontinued in any patient with an acute, serious condition suggestive of a myopathy or having a risk factor predisposing to the development of renal failure secondary to rhabdomyolysis (eg, severe acute infection, hypotension, major surgery, trauma, severe metabolic, endocrine and electrolyte disorders, and uncontrolled seizures).

PRECAUTIONS

General

Before instituting therapy with atorvastatin, an attempt should be made to control hypercholesterolemia with appropriate diet, exercise, and weight reduction in obese patients, and to treat other underlying medical problems (see INDICATIONS AND USAGE).

Information for Patients

Patients should be advised to report promptly unexplained muscle pain, tenderness, or weakness, particularly if accompanied by malaise or fever.

Drug Interactions

The risk of myopathy during treatment with drugs of this class is increased with concurrent administration of cyclosporine, fibric acid derivatives, niacin (nicotinic acid), erythromycin, azole antifungals (see WARNINGS, Skeletal Muscle).

Antacid: When atorvastatin and Maalox® TC suspension were coadministered, plasma concentrations of atorvastatin decreased approximately 35%. However, LDL-C reduction was not altered.

TABLE 5. NCEP Guidelines for Lipid Management

Definite Atherosclerotic Disease[a]	Two or More Other Risk Factors[b]	LDL-Cholesterol mg/dL (mmol/L) Initiation Level	Minimum Goal
No	No	≥190 (≥4.9)	<160 (<4.1)
No	Yes	≥160 (≥4.1)	<130 (<3.4)
Yes	Yes or No	≥130[c] (≥3.4)	≤100 (≤2.6)

[a] Coronary heart disease or peripheral vascular disease (including symptomatic carotid artery disease).
[b] Other risk factors for coronary heart disease (CHD) include: age (males: ≥45 years; females: ≥55 years or premature menopause without estrogen replacement therapy); family history of premature CHD; current cigarette smoking; hypertension; confirmed HDL-C <35 mg/dL (<0.91 mmol/L); and diabetes mellitus. Subtract 1 risk factor if HDL-C is ≥60 mg/dL (≥1.6 mmol/L).
[c] In CHD patients with LDL-C levels 100 to 129 mg/dL, the physician should exercise clinical judgment in deciding whether to initiate drug treatment.

Antipyrine: Because atorvastatin does not affect the pharmacokinetics of antipyrine, interactions with other drugs metabolized via the same cytochrome isozymes are not expected.

Colestipol: Plasma concentrations of atorvastatin decreased approximately 25% when colestipol and atorvastatin were coadministered. However, LDL-C reduction was greater when atorvastatin and colestipol were coadministered than when either drug was given alone.

Cimetidine: Atorvastatin plasma concentrations and LDL-C reduction were not altered by coadministration of cimetidine.

Digoxin: When multiple doses of atorvastatin and digoxin were coadministered, steady-state plasma digoxin concentrations increased by approximately 20%. Patients taking digoxin should be monitored appropriately.

Erythromycin: In healthy individuals, plasma concentrations of atorvastatin increased approximately 40% with coadministration of atorvastatin and erythromycin, a known inhibitor of cytochrome P450 3A4 (see WARNINGS, Skeletal Muscle).

Oral Contraceptives: Coadministration of atorvastatin and an oral contraceptive increased AUC values for norethindrone and ethinyl estradiol by approximately 30% and 20%. These increases should be considered when selecting an oral contraceptive for a woman taking atorvastatin.

Warfarin: Atorvastatin had no clinically significant effect on prothrombin time when administered to patients receiving chronic warfarin treatment.

Endocrine Function

HMG-CoA reductase inhibitors interfere with cholesterol synthesis and theoretically might blunt adrenal and/or gonadal steroid production. Clinical studies have shown that atorvastatin does not reduce basal plasma cortisol concentration or impair adrenal reserve. The effects of HMG-CoA reductase inhibitors on male fertility have not been studied in adequate numbers of patients. The effects, if any, on the pituitary-gonadal axis in premenopausal women are unknown. Caution should be exercised if an HMG-CoA reductase inhibitor is administered concomitantly with drugs that may decrease the levels or activity of endogenous steroid hormones, such as ketoconazole, spironolactone, and cimetidine.

CNS Toxicity

Brain hemorrhage was seen in a female dog treated for 3 months at 120 mg/kg/day. Brain hemorrhage and optic nerve vacuolation were seen in another female dog that was sacrificed in moribund condition after 11 weeks of escalating doses up to 280 mg/kg/day. The 120 mg/kg dose resulted in a systemic exposure approximately 16 times the human plasma area-under-the curve (AUC, 0–24 hours) based on the maximum human dose of 80 mg/day. A single tonic convulsion was seen in each of 2 male dogs (one treated at 10 mg/kg/day and one at 120 mg/kg/day) in a 2-year study. No CNS lesions have been observed in mice after chronic treatment for up to 2 years at doses up to 400 mg/kg/day or in rats at doses up to 100 mg/kg/day. These doses were 6 to 11 times (mouse) and 8 to 16 times (rat) the human AUC (0–24) based on the maximum recommended human dose of 80 mg/day.

CNS vascular lesions, characterized by perivascular hemorrhages, edema, and mononuclear cell infiltration of perivascular spaces, have been observed in dogs treated with other members of this class. A chemically similar drug in this class produced optic nerve degeneration (Wallerian degeneration of retinogeniculate fibers) in clinically normal dogs in a dose-dependent fashion at a dose that produced plasma drug levels about 30 times higher than the mean drug level in humans taking the highest recommended dose.

Carcinogenesis, Mutagenesis, Impairment of Fertility

In a 2-year carcinogenicity study in rats at dose levels of 10, 30, and 100 mg/kg/day, 2 rare tumors were found in muscle in high-dose females: in one, there was a rhabdomyosarcoma and, in another, there was a fibrosarcoma. This dose represents a plasma AUC (0–24) value of approximately 16 times the mean human plasma drug exposure after an 80 mg oral dose.

A 2-year carcinogenicity study in mice given 100, 200, or 400 mg/kg/day resulted in a significant increase in liver adenomas in high-dose males and liver carcinomas in high-dose females. These findings occurred at plasma AUC (0–24) values of approximately 6 times the mean human plasma drug exposure after an 80 mg oral dose.

In vitro, atorvastatin was not mutagenic or clastogenic in the following tests with and without metabolic activation: the Ames test with *Salmonella-typhimurium* and *Escherichia coli*, the HGPRT forward mutation assay in Chinese hamster lung cells, and the chromosomal aberration assay in Chinese hamster lung cells. Atorvastatin was negative in the *in vivo* mouse micronucleus test.

Studies in rats performed at doses up to 175 mg/kg (15 times the human exposure) produced no changes in fertility. There was aplasia and aspermia in the epididymis of 2 of 10 rats treated with 100 mg/kg/day of atorvastatin for 3 months (16 times the human AUC at the 80 mg dose); testis weights were significantly lower at 30 and 100 mg/kg and epididymal weight was lower at 100 mg/kg. Male rats given 100 mg/kg/day for 11 weeks prior to mating had decreased sperm motility, spermatid head concentration, and increased abnormal sperm. Atorvastatin caused no adverse effects on semen parameters, or reproductive organ histopathology in dogs given doses of 10, 40, or 120 mg/kg for two years.

Pregnancy

Pregnancy Category X

See CONTRAINDICATIONS

Safety in pregnant women has not been established. Atorvastatin crosses the rat placenta and reaches a level in fetal liver equivalent to that of maternal plasma. Atorvastatin was not teratogenic in rats at doses up to 300 mg/kg/day or in rabbits at doses up to 100 mg/kg/day. These doses resulted in multiples of about 30 times (rat) or 20 times (rabbit) the human exposure based on surface area (mg/m^2).

In a study in rats given 20, 100, or 225 mg/kg/day, from gestation day 7 through to lactation day 21 (weaning), there was decreased pup survival at birth, neonate, weaning, and maturity in pups of mothers dosed with 225 mg/kg/day. Body weight was decreased on days 4 and 21 in pups of mothers dosed at 100 mg/kg/day; pup body weight was decreased at birth and at days 4, 21, and 91 at 225 mg/kg/day. Pup development was delayed (rotorod performance at 100 mg/kg/day and acoustic startle at 225 mg/kg/day; pinnae detachment and eye opening at 225 mg/kg/day). These doses correspond to 6 times (100 mg/kg) and 22 times (225 mg/kg) the human AUC at 80 mg/day.

Rare reports of congenital anomalies have been received following intrauterine exposure to HMG-CoA reductase inhibitors. There has been one report of severe congenital bony deformity, tracheo-esophageal fistula, and anal atresia (VATER association) in a baby born to a woman who took lovastatin with dextroamphetamine sulfate during the first trimester of pregnancy. Lipitor should be administered to women of child-bearing potential only when such patients are highly unlikely to conceive and have been informed of the potential hazards. If the woman becomes pregnant while taking Lipitor, it should be discontinued and the patient advised again as to the potential hazards to the fetus.

Nursing Mothers

Nursing rat pups had plasma and liver drug levels of 50% and 40%, respectively, of that in their mother's milk. Because of the potential for adverse reactions in nursing infants, women taking Lipitor should not breast-feed (see CONTRAINDICATIONS).

Pediatric Use

Treatment experience in a pediatric population is limited to doses of Lipitor up to 80 mg/day for 1 year in 8 patients with homozygous FH. No clinical or biochemical abnormalities were reported in these patients. None of these patients was below 9 years of age.

Geriatric Use

Treatment experience in adults age ≥70 years with doses of Lipitor up to 80 mg/day has been evaluated in 221 patients. The safety and efficacy of Lipitor in this population were similar to those of patients <70 years of age.

ADVERSE REACTIONS

Lipitor is generally well-tolerated. Adverse reactions have usually been mild and transient. In controlled clinical studies of 2502 patients, <2% of patients were discontinued due to adverse experiences attributable to atorvastatin. The most frequent adverse events thought to be related to atorvastatin were constipation, flatulence, dyspepsia, and abdominal pain.

TABLE 6. Adverse Events in Placebo-Controlled Studies (% of Patients)

BODY SYSTEM/ Adverse Event	Placebo N = 270	Atorvastatin 10 mg N = 863	Atorvastatin 20 mg N = 36	Atorvastatin 40 mg N = 79	Atorvastatin 80 mg N = 94
BODY AS A WHOLE					
Infection	10.0	10.3	2.8	10.1	7.4
Headache	7.0	5.4	16.7	2.5	6.4
Accidental Injury	3.7	4.2	0.0	1.3	3.2
Flu Syndrome	1.9	2.2	0.0	2.5	3.2
Abdominal Pain	0.7	2.8	0.0	3.8	2.1
Back Pain	3.0	2.8	0.0	3.8	1.1
Allergic Reaction	2.6	0.9	2.8	1.3	0.0
Asthenia	1.9	2.2	0.0	3.8	0.0
DIGESTIVE SYSTEM					
Constipation	1.8	2.1	0.0	2.5	1.1
Diarrhea	1.5	2.7	0.0	3.8	5.3
Dyspepsia	4.1	2.3	2.8	1.3	2.1
Flatulence	3.3	2.1	2.8	1.3	1.1
RESPIRATORY SYSTEM					
Sinusitis	2.6	2.8	0.0	2.5	6.4
Pharyngitis	1.5	2.5	0.0	1.3	2.1
SKIN AND APPENDAGES					
Rash	0.7	3.9	2.8	3.8	1.1
MUSCULOSKELETAL SYSTEM					
Arthralgia	1.5	2.0	0.0	5.1	0.0
Myalgia	1.1	3.2	5.6	1.3	0.0

Clinical Adverse Experiences

Adverse experiences reported in ≥2% of patients in placebo-controlled clinical studies of atorvastatin, regardless of causality assessment, are shown in Table 6.

[See table 6 above]

The following adverse events were reported, regardless of causality assessment in patients treated with atorvastatin in clinical trials. The events in italics occurred in ≥2% of patients and the events in plain type occurred in <2% of patients.

Body as a Whole: *Chest pain*, face edema, fever, neck rigidity, malaise, photosensitivity reaction, generalized edema.

Digestive System: *Nausea*, gastroenteritis, liver function tests abnormal, colitis, vomiting, gastritis, dry mouth, rectal hemorrhage, esophagitis, eructation, glossitis, mouth ulceration, anorexia, increased appetite, stomatitis, biliary pain, cheilitis, duodenal ulcer, dysphagia, enteritis, melena, gum hemorrhage, stomach ulcer, tenesmus, ulcerative stomatitis, hepatitis, pancreatitis, cholestatic jaundice.

Respiratory System: *Bronchitis, rhinitis*, pneumonia, dyspnea, asthma, epistaxis.

Nervous System: *Insomnia, dizziness*, paresthesia, somnolence, amnesia, abnormal dreams, libido decreased, emotional lability, incoordination, peripheral neuropathy, torticollis, facial paralysis, hyperkinesia, depression, hypesthesia, hypertonia.

Musculoskeletal System: *Arthritis*, leg cramps, bursitis, tenosynovitis, myasthenia, tendinous contracture, myositis.

Skin and Appendages: Pruritus, contact dermatitis, alopecia, dry skin, sweating, acne, urticaria, eczema, seborrhea, skin ulcer.

Urogenital System: *Urinary tract infection*, urinary frequency, cystitis, hematuria, impotence, dysuria, kidney calculus, nocturia, epididymitis, fibrocystic breast, vaginal hemorrhage, albuminuria, breast enlargement, metrorrhagia, nephritis, urinary incontinence, urinary retention, urinary urgency, abnormal ejaculation, uterine hemorrhage.

Special Senses: Amblyopia, tinnitus, dry eyes, refraction disorder, eye hemorrhage, deafness, glaucoma, parosmia, taste loss, taste perversion.

Cardiovascular System: Palpitation, vasodilatation, syncope, migraine, postural hypotension, phlebitis, arrhythmia, angina pectoris, hypertension.

Metabolic and Nutritional Disorders: *Peripheral edema*, hyperglycemia, creatine phosphokinase increased, gout, weight gain, hypoglycemia.

Hemic and Lymphatic System: Ecchymosis, anemia, lymphadenopathy, thrombocytopenia, petechia.

Postintroduction Reports

Adverse events associated with Lipitor therapy reported since market introduction, that are not listed above, regardless of causality assessment, include the following: anaphylaxis, angioneurotic edema, bullous rashes (including erythema multiforme, Stevens-Johnson syndrome and toxic epidermal necrolysis), and rhabdomyolysis.

OVERDOSAGE

There is no specific treatment for atorvastatin overdosage. In the event of an overdose, the patient should be treated symptomatically, and supportive measures instituted as required. Due to extensive drug binding to plasma proteins, hemodialysis is not expected to significantly enhance atorvastatin clearance.

DOSAGE AND ADMINISTRATION

The patient should be placed on a standard cholesterol-lowering diet before receiving Lipitor and should continue on this diet during treatment with Lipitor.

Hypercholesterolemia (Heterozygous Familial and Nonfamilial) and Mixed Dyslipidemia (*Frederickson* Types IIa and IIb)

The recommended starting dose of Lipitor is 10 mg once daily. The dosage range is 10 to 80 mg once daily. Lipitor can be administered as a single dose at any time of the day, with or without food. Therapy should be individualized according to goal of therapy and response (see *NCEP Guidelines*, summarized in Table 5). After initiation and/or upon titration of Lipitor, lipid levels should be analyzed within 2 to 4 weeks and dosage adjusted accordingly.

Since the goal of treatment is to lower LDL-C, the NCEP recommends that LDL-C levels be used to initiate and assess treatment response. Only if LDL-C levels are not available, should total-C be used to monitor therapy.

Homozygous Familial Hypercholesterolemia

The dosage of Lipitor in patients with homozygous FH is 10 to 80 mg daily. Lipitor should be used as an adjunct to other lipid-lowering treatments (eg, LDL apheresis) in these patients or if such treatments are unavailable.

Concomitant Therapy

Atorvastatin may be used in combination with a bile acid binding resin for additive effect. The combination of HMG-CoA reductase inhibitors and fibrates should generally be avoided (see WARNINGS, Skeletal Muscle, and PRECAUTIONS, Drug Interactions for other drug-drug interactions).

Dosage in Patients With Renal Insufficiency

Renal disease does not affect the plasma concentrations nor LDL-C reduction of atorvastatin; thus, dosage adjustment in patients with renal dysfunction is not necessary (see CLINICAL PHARMACOLOGY, Pharmacokinetics).

HOW SUPPLIED

Lipitor is supplied as white, elliptical, film-coated tablets of atorvastatin calcium containing 10, 20, 40, and 80 mg atorvastatin.

10 mg tablets: coded "PD 155" on one side and "10" on the other.

N0071-0155-23 bottles of 90
N0071-0155-34 bottles of 5000
N0071-0155-40 10 × 10 unit dose blisters

20 mg tablets: coded "PD 156" on one side and "20" on the other.

N0071-0156-23 bottles of 90
N0071-0156-40 10 × 10 unit dose blisters

40 mg tablets: coded "PD 157" on one side and "40" on the other.

N0071-0157-23 bottles of 90

80 mg tablets: coded "PD 158" on one side and "80" on the other.

N0071-0158-23 bottles of 90

Storage

Store at controlled room temperature 20° to 25°C (68° to 77°F) [see USP].

Rx only

Revised March 2000

Manufactured by:
Warner-Lambert Export, Ltd. © 1998–'00
Dublin, Ireland

Distributed by:
PARKE-DAVIS
Div of Warner-Lambert Co
Morris Plains, NJ 07950 USA
MADE IN GERMANY

Marketed by:
PARKE-DAVIS
Div of Warner-Lambert Co and
PFIZER Inc.
New York, NY 10017

0155G610

Shown in Product Identification Guide, page 329

LOESTRIN® 21 ℞
(Norethindrone Acetate and Ethinyl Estradiol Tablets, USP)

LOESTRIN® 21 1/20 ℞
(Each white tablet contains 1 mg norethindrone acetate and 20 mcg ethinyl estradiol.)

LOESTRIN® 21 1.5/30 ℞
(Each green tablet contains 1.5 mg norethindrone acetate and 30 mcg ethinyl estradiol.)

LOESTRIN® Fe ℞
(Norethindrone Acetate and Ethinyl Estradiol Tablets, USP and Ferrous Fumarate Tablets*)
***Ferrous fumarate tablets are not USP for dissolution and assay**

LOESTRIN® Fe 1/20 ℞
(Each white tablet contains 1 mg norethindrone acetate and 20 mcg ethinyl estradiol.
Each brown tablet contains 75 mg ferrous fumarate.)

LOESTRIN® Fe 1.5/30 ℞
(Each green tablet contains 1 mg norethindrone acetate and 30 mcg ethinyl estradiol.
Each brown tablet contains 75 mg ferrous fumarate.)

Patients should be counseled that this product does not protect against HIV infection (AIDS) and other sexually transmitted diseases.

DESCRIPTION

Loestrin **21** and Loestrin **Fe** are progestogen-estrogen combinations.

Loestrin **Fe** 1/20 and 1.5/30: Each provides a continuous dosage regimen consisting of 21 oral contraceptive tablets and seven ferrous fumarate tablets. The ferrous fumarate tablets are present to facilitate ease of drug administration via a 28-day regimen, are non-hormonal, and do not serve any therapeutic purpose.

Each white tablet contains norethindrone acetate (17 alpha-ethinyl-19-nortestosterone acetate), 1 mg; ethinyl estradiol (17 alpha-ethinyl-1,3,5(10)-estratriene-3, 17 beta-diol), 20 mcg. Also contains acacia, NF; lactose, NF; magnesium stearate, NF; starch, NF; confectioner's sugar, NF; talc, USP.

Each green tablet contains norethindrone acetate (17 alpha-ethinyl-19-nortestosterone acetate), 1.5 mg; ethinyl estradiol (17 alpha-ethinyl-1,3,5(10)-estratriene-3, 17 beta-diol), 30 mcg. Also contains acacia, NF; lactose, NF; magnesium stearate, NF; starch, NF; confectioner's sugar, NF; talc, USP; D&C yellow No. 10; FD&C yellow No. 6; FD&C blue No. 1.

The structural formulas are as follows:

Norethindrone Acetate

Ethinyl Estradiol

Each brown tablet contains microcrystalline cellulose, NF; ferrous fumarate, USP; magnesium stearate, NF; povidone, USP; sodium starch glycolate, NF; sucrose with modified dextrins.

CLINICAL PHARMACOLOGY

Combination oral contraceptives act by suppression of gonadotropins. Although the primary mechanism of this action is inhibition of ovulation, other alterations include changes in the cervical mucus (which increase the difficulty of sperm entry into the uterus) and the endometrium (which reduce the likelihood of implantation).

Pharmacokinetics

The pharmacokinetics of Loestrin have not been characterized; however, the following pharmacokinetic information regarding norethindrone acetate and ethinyl estradiol is taken from the literature.

Absorption

Norethindrone acetate appears to be completely and rapidly deacetylated to norethindrone after oral administration, since the disposition of norethindrone acetate is indistin-

Continued on next page

This product information was prepared in June 2000. On these and other Parke-Davis Products, information may be obtained by addressing PARKE-DAVIS, a Warner-Lambert Division, Morris Plains, New Jersey 07950.

Loestrin—Cont.

guishable from that of orally administered norethindrone (1). Norethindrone acetate and ethinyl estradiol are subject to first-pass metabolism after oral dosing, resulting in an absolute bioavailability of approximately 64% for norethindrone and 43% for ethinyl estradiol (1–3).

Distribution

Volume of distribution of norethindrone and ethinyl estradiol ranges from 2 to 4 L/kg (1–3). Plasma protein binding of both steroids is extensive (>95%); norethindrone binds to both albumin and sex hormone binding globulin, whereas ethinyl estradiol binds only to albumin (4).

Metabolism

Norethindrone undergoes extensive biotransformation, primarily via reduction, followed by sulfate and glucuronide conjugation. The majority of metabolites in the circulation are sulfates, with glucuronides accounting for most of the urinary metabolites (5). A small amount of norethindrone acetate is metabolically converted to ethinyl estradiol. Ethinyl estradiol is also extensively metabolized, both by oxidation and by conjugation with sulfate and glucuronide. Sulfates are the major circulating conjugates of ethinyl estradiol and glucuronides predominate in urine. The primary oxidative metabolite is 2-hydroxy ethinyl estradiol, formed by the CYP3A4 isoform of cytochrome P450. Part of the first-pass metabolism of ethinyl estradiol is believed to occur in gastrointestinal mucosa. Ethinyl estradiol may under enterohepatic circulation (6).

Excretion

Norethindrone and ethinyl estradiol are excreted in both urine and feces, primarily as metabolites (5,6). Plasma clearance values for norethindrone and ethinyl estradiol are similar (approximately 0.4 L/hr/kg) (1–3).

Special Population

Race:

The effect of race on the disposition of Loestrin has not been evaluated.

Renal Insufficiency

The effect of renal disease on the disposition of Loestrin has not been evaluated. In premenopausal women with chronic renal failure undergoing peritoneal dialysis who received multiple doses of an oral contraceptive containing ethinyl estradiol and norethindrone, plasma ethinyl estradiol concentrations were higher and norethindrone concentrations were unchanged compared to concentrations in premenopausal women with normal renal function.

Hepatic Insufficiency

The effect of hepatic disease on the disposition of Loestrin has not been evaluated. However, ethinyl estradiol and norethindrone may be poorly metabolized in patients with impaired liver function.

Drug-Drug Interactions

Numerous drug-drug interactions have been reported for oral contraceptives. A summary of these is found under PRECAUTIONS, Drug Interactions.

INDICATIONS AND USAGE

Loestrin **21** and Loestrin **Fe** are indicated for the prevention of pregnancy in women who elect to use oral contraceptives as a method of contraception.

Oral contraceptives are highly effective. Table 1 lists the typical accidental pregnancy rates for users of combination oral contraceptives and other methods of contraception. The efficacy of these contraceptive methods, except sterilization, depends upon the reliability with which they are used. Correct and consistent use of methods can result in lower failure rates.

[See table below]

TABLE I

LOWEST EXPECTED AND TYPICAL FAILURE RATES DURING THE FIRST YEAR OF CONTINUOUS USE OF A METHOD

% of Women Experiencing an Unintended Pregnancy in the First Year of Continuous Use

Method	Lowest Expected*	Typical**
(No contraception)	(85)	(85)
Oral contraceptives		3
combined	0.1	N/A***
progestin only	0.5	N/A***
Diaphragm with spermicidal cream or jelly	6	20
Spermicides alone (foam, creams, gels, vaginal suppositories, and vaginal film)	6	26
Vaginal Sponge		
nulliparous	9	20
parous	20	40
Implant	0.05	0.05
Injection: depot medroxyprogesterone acetate	0.3	0.3
IUD		
progesterone T	1.5	2.0
copper T 380A	0.6	0.8
LNg 20	0.1	0.1
Condom without spermicides		
female	5	21
male	3	14
Cervical Cap with spermicidal cream or jelly		
nulliparous	9	20
parous	26	40
Periodic abstinence (all methods)	1–9	25
Withdrawal	4	19
Female sterilization	0.5	0.5
Male sterilization	0.10	0.15

Adapted from RA Hatcher et al, Reference 7.

*The authors' best guess of the percentage of women expected to experience an accidental pregnancy among couples who initiate a method (not necessarily for the first time) and who use it consistently and correctly during the first year if they do not stop for any other reason.

**This term represents "typical" couples who initiate use of a method (not necessarily for the first time), who experience an accidental pregnancy during the first year if they do not stop use for any other reason.

***N/A—Data not available.

CONTRAINDICATIONS

Oral contraceptives should not be used in women who currently have the following conditions:

- Thrombophlebitis or thromboembolic disorders
- A past history of deep vein thrombophlebitis or thromboembolic disorders
- Cerebral vascular or coronary artery disease
- Known or suspected carcinoma of the breast
- Carcinoma of the endometrium or other known or suspected estrogen-dependent neoplasia
- Undiagnosed abnormal genital bleeding
- Cholestatic jaundice of pregnancy or jaundice with prior pill use
- Hepatic adenomas or carcinomas
- Known or suspected pregnancy

WARNINGS

Cigarette smoking increases the risk of serious cardiovascular side effects from oral contraceptive use. This risk increases with age and with heavy smoking (15 or more cigarettes per day) and is quite marked in women over 35 years of age. Women who use oral contraceptives should be strongly advised not to smoke.

The use of oral contraceptives is associated with increased risks of several serious conditions including myocardial infarction, thromboembolism, stroke, hepatic neoplasia, and gallbladder disease, although the risk of serious morbidity or mortality is very small in healthy women without underlying risk factors. The risk of morbidity and mortality increases significantly in the presence of other underlying risk factors such as hypertension, hyperlipidemias, obesity, and diabetes.

Practitioners prescribing oral contraceptives should be familiar with the following information relating to these risks. The information contained in this package insert is principally based on studies carried out in patients who used oral contraceptives with higher formulations of estrogens and progestogens than those in common use today. The effect of long-term use of the oral contraceptives with lower formulations of both estrogens and progestogens remains to be determined.

Throughout this labeling, epidemiological studies reported are of two types: retrospective or case control studies and prospective or cohort studies. Case control studies provide a measure of the relative risk of a disease, namely, a *ratio* of the incidence of a disease among oral contraceptive users to that among nonusers. The relative risk does not provide information on the actual clinical occurrence of a disease. Cohort studies provide a measure of attributable risk, which is the *difference* in the incidence of disease between oral contraceptive users and nonusers. The attributable risk does not provide information about the actual occurrence of a disease in the population (adapted from References 8 and 9 with the author's permission). For further information, the reader is referred to a text on epidemiological methods.

1. Thromboembolic Disorders and Other Vascular Problems

a. Myocardial infarction

An increased risk of myocardial infarction has been attributed to oral contraceptive use. This risk is primarily in smokers or women with other underlying risk factors for coronary artery disease such as hypertension, hypercholesterolemia, morbid obesity, and diabetes. The relative risk of heart attack for current oral contraceptive users has been estimated to be two to six (10–16). The risk is very low under the age of 30.

Smoking in combination with oral contraceptive use has been shown to contribute substantially to the incidence of myocardial infarctions in women in their mid-thirties or older with smoking accounting for the majority of excess cases (17). Mortality rates associated with circulatory disease have been shown to increase substantially in smokers over the age of 35 and non-smokers over the age of 40 (Table II) among women who use oral contraceptives.

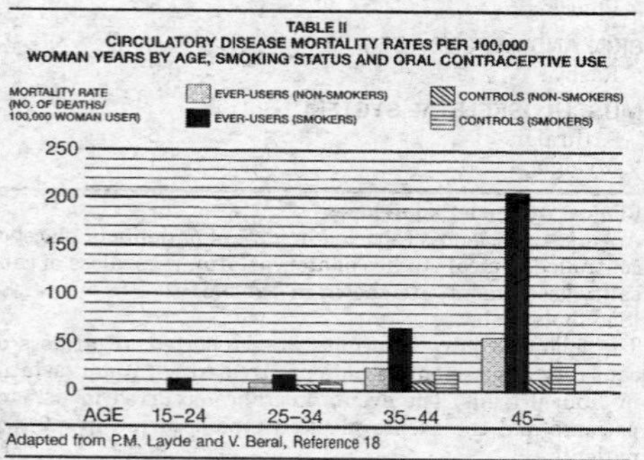

Adapted from P.M. Layde and V. Beral, Reference 18

Oral contraceptives may compound the effects of well-known risk factors, such as hypertension, diabetes, hyperlipidemias, age and obesity (19). In particular, some progestogens are known to decrease HDL cholesterol and cause glucose intolerance, while estrogens may create a state of hyperinsulinism (20–24). Oral contraceptives have been shown to increase blood pressure among users (see section 9 in WARNINGS). Similar effects on risk factors have been associated with an increased risk of heart disease. Oral contraceptives must be used with caution in women with cardiovascular disease risk factors.

b. Thromboembolism

An increased risk of thromboembolic and thrombotic disease associated with the use of oral contraceptives is well established. Case control studies have found the relative risk of users compared to non-users to be 3 for the first episode of superficial venous thrombosis, 4 to 11 for deep vein thrombosis or pulmonary embolism, and 1.5 to 6 for women with predisposing conditions for venous thromboembolic disease (9,10,25–30). Cohort studies have shown the relative risk to be somewhat lower, about 3 for new cases and about 4.5 for new cases requiring hospitalization (31). The risk of thromboembolic disease due to oral contraceptives is not related to length of use and disappears after pill use is stopped (8).

A two- to four-fold increase in relative risk of postoperative thromboembolic complications has been reported with the use of oral contraceptives (15,32). The relative risk of venous thrombosis in women who have predisposing conditions is twice that of women without such medical conditions (15,32). If feasible, oral contraceptives should be discontinued at least four weeks prior to and for two weeks after elective surgery of a type associated with an increase in risk of thromboembolism and during and following prolonged immobilization. Since the immediate postpartum period is also associated with an increased risk of thromboembolism, oral contraceptives should be started no earlier than four to six weeks after delivery in women who elect not to breast feed.

c. Cerebrovascular diseases

Oral contraceptives have been shown to increase both the relative and attributable risks of cerebrovascular events (thrombotic and hemorrhagic strokes), although, in general, the risk is greatest among older (>35 years), hypertensive women who also smoke. Hypertension was found to be a risk factor for both users and nonusers, for both types of strokes, while smoking interacted to increase the risk for hemorrhagic strokes (33–35).

In a large study, the relative risk of thrombotic strokes has been shown to range from 3 for normotensive users to 14 for users with severe hypertension (36). The relative risk of hemorrhagic stroke is reported to be 1.2 for non-smokers who used oral contraceptives, 2.6 for smokers who did not use oral contraceptives, 7.6 for smokers who used oral contraceptives, 1.8 for normotensive users, and 25.7 for users with severe hypertension (36). The attributable risk is also greater in older women (9).

d. Dose-related risk of vascular disease from oral contraceptives

A positive association has been observed between the amount of estrogen and progestogen in oral contraceptives and the risk of vascular disease (37–39). A decline in serum high-density lipoproteins (HDL) has been reported with many progestational agents (20–22). A decline in serum high-density lipoproteins has been associated with an increased incidence of ischemic heart disease. Because estrogens increase HDL cholesterol, the net effect of an oral contraceptive depends on a balance achieved between doses of estrogen and progestin and the nature of the progestin used in the contraceptives. The amount and activity of both hormones should be considered in the choice of an oral contraceptive.

Minimizing exposure to estrogen and progestogen is in keeping with good principles of therapeutics. For any particular oral contraceptive, the dosage regimen prescribed should be one which contains the least amount of estrogen and progestogen that is compatible with the needs of the individual patient. New acceptors of oral contraceptive agents should be started on preparations containing the lowest dose of estrogen which produces satisfactory results for the patient.

e. Persistence of risk of vascular disease

There are two studies which have shown persistence of risk of vascular disease for ever-users of oral contraceptives. In a study in the United States, the risk of developing myocardial infarction after discontinuing oral contraceptives persists for at least 9 years for women 40–49 years who had used oral contraceptives for 5 or more years, but this increased risk was not demonstrated in other age groups (14). In another study in Great Britain, the risk of developing cerebrovascular disease persisted for at least 6 years after discontinuation of oral contraceptives, although excess risk was very small (40). However, both studies were performed with oral contraceptive formulations containing 50 mcg or higher of estrogens.

2. Estimates of Mortality from Contraceptive Use

One study gathered data from a variety of sources which have estimated the mortality rate associated with different methods of contraception at different ages (Table III). These estimates include the combined risk of death associated with contraceptive methods plus the risk attributable to pregnancy in the event of method failure. Each method of contraception has its specific benefits and risks. The study concluded that with the exception of oral contraceptive users 35 and older who smoke and 40 and older who do not smoke, mortality associated with all methods of birth control is low and below that associated with childbirth. The observation of a possible increase in risk of mortality with age for oral contraceptive users is based on data gathered in the 1970's but not reported until 1983 (41). However, current clinical practice involves the use of lower estrogen dose formulations combined with careful restriction of oral contraceptive use to women who do not have the various risk factors listed in this labeling.

Because of these changes in practice and, also, because of some limited new data which suggest that the risk of cardiovascular disease with the use of oral contraceptives may now be less than previously observed (Porter JB, Hunter J, Jick H, et al. Oral contraceptives and nonfatal vascular disease. Obstet Gynecol 1985;66:1–4; and Porter JB, Hershel J, Walker AM. Mortality among oral contraceptive users. Obstet Gynecol 1987;70:29–32), the Fertility and Maternal Health Drugs Advisory Committee was asked to review the topic in 1989. The Committee concluded that although cardiovascular disease risks may be increased with oral contraceptive use after age 40 in healthy non-smoking women (even with the newer low-dose formulations), there are greater potential health risks associated with pregnancy in older women and with the alternative surgical and medical procedures which may be necessary if such women do not have access to effective and acceptable means of contraception.

Therefore, the Committee recommended that the benefits of oral contraceptive use by healthy non-smoking women over age 40 may outweigh the possible risks. Of course, older women, as all women who take oral contraceptives, should take the lowest possible dose formulation that is effective. [See table above]

TABLE III
ANNUAL NUMBER OF BIRTH-RELATED OR METHOD-RELATED DEATHS ASSOCIATED WITH CONTROL OF FERTILITY PER 100,000 NONSTERILE WOMEN BY FERTILITY CONTROL METHOD ACCORDING TO AGE

Method of control and outcome	15–19	20–24	25–29	30–34	35–39	40–44
No fertility control methods*	7.0	7.4	9.1	14.8	25.7	28.2
Oral contraceptives non-smoker**	0.3	0.5	0.9	1.9	13.8	31.6
Oral contraceptives smoker**	2.2	3.4	6.6	13.5	51.1	117.2
IUD**	0.8	0.8	1.0	1.0	1.4	1.4
Condom*	1.1	1.6	0.7	0.2	0.3	0.4
Diaphragm/spermicide*	1.9	1.2	1.2	1.3	2.2	2.8
Periodic abstinence*	2.5	1.6	1.6	1.7	2.9	3.6

*Deaths are birth related.
**Deaths are method related.

Adapted from H.W. Ory, Reference 41.

3. Carcinoma of the Reproductive Organs

Numerous epidemiological studies have been performed on the incidence of breast, endometrial, ovarian, and cervical cancer in women using oral contraceptives. Most of the studies on breast cancer and oral contraceptive use report that the use of oral contraceptives is not associated with an increase in the risk of developing breast cancer (42,44,89). Some studies have reported an increased risk of developing breast cancer in certain subgroups of oral contraceptive users, but the findings reported in these studies are not consistent (43,45–49,85–88).

Some studies suggest that oral contraceptive use has been associated with an increase in the risk of cervical intraepithelial neoplasia in some populations of women (51–54). However, there continues to be controversy about the extent to which such findings may be due to differences in sexual behavior and other factors.

In spite of many studies of the relationship between oral contraceptive use and breast and cervical cancers, a cause and effect relationship has not been established.

4. Hepatic Neoplasia

Benign hepatic adenomas are associated with oral contraceptive use, although the incidence of benign tumors is rare in the United States. Indirect calculations have estimated the attributable risk to be in the range of 3.3 cases/100,000 for users, a risk that increases after four or more years of use (55). Rupture of rare, benign, hepatic adenomas may cause death through intra-abdominal hemorrhage (56–57).

Studies from Britain have shown an increased risk of developing hepatocellular carcinoma (58–60) in long-term (>8 years) oral contraceptive users. However, these cancers are extremely rare in the U.S., and the attributable risk (the excess incidence) of liver cancers in oral contraceptive users approaches less than one per million users.

5. Ocular Lesions

There have been clinical case reports of retinal thrombosis associated with the use of oral contraceptives. Oral contraceptives should be discontinued if there is unexplained partial or complete loss of vision; onset of proptosis or diplopia; papilledema; or retinal vascular lesions. Appropriate diagnostic and therapeutic measures should be undertaken immediately.

6. Oral Contraceptive User Before and During Early Pregnancy

Extensive epidemiological studies have revealed no increased risk of birth defects in women who have used oral contraceptives prior to pregnancy (61–63). Studies also do not suggest a teratogenic effect, particularly insofar as cardiac anomalies and limb reduction defects are concerned (61,62,64,65) when taken inadvertently during early pregnancy.

The administration of oral contraceptives to induce withdrawal bleeding should not be used as a test for pregnancy. Oral contraceptives should not be used during pregnancy to treat threatened or habitual abortion.

It is recommended that for any patient who has missed two consecutive periods, pregnancy should be ruled out before continuing oral contraceptive use. If the patient has not adhered to the prescribed schedule, the possibility of pregnancy should be considered at the time of the first missed period. Oral contraceptive use should be discontinued if pregnancy is confirmed.

7. Gallbladder Disease

Earlier studies have reported an increased lifetime relative risk of gallbladder surgery in users of oral contraceptives and estrogens (66,67). More recent studies, however, have shown that the relative risk of developing gallbladder disease among oral contraceptive users may be minimall (68–70). The recent findings of minimal risk may be related to the use of oral contraceptive formulations containing lower hormonal doses of estrogens and progestogens.

8. Carbohydrate and Lipid Metabolic Effects

Oral contraceptives have shown to cause glucose intolerance in a significant percentage of users (23). Oral contraceptives containing greater than 75 mcg of estrogens cause hyperinsulinism, while lower doses of estrogen cause less glucose intolerance (71). Progestogens increase insulin secretion and create insulin resistance, this effect varying with different progestational agents (23,72). However, in the non-diabetic woman, oral contraceptives appear to have no effect on fasting blood glucose (73). Because of these demonstrated effects, prediabetic and diabetic women should be carefully observed while taking oral contraceptives.

A small proportion of women will have persistent hypertriglyceridemia while on the pill. As discussed earlier (see WARNINGS 1a. and 1d.), changes in serum triglycerides and lipoprotein levels have been reported in oral contraceptive users.

9. Elevated Blood Pressure

An increase in blood pressure has been reported in women taking oral contraceptives (74) and this increase is more likely in older oral contraceptive users (75) and with continued use (74). Data from the Royal College of General Practitioners (18) and subsequent randomized trials have shown that the incidence of hypertension increases with increasing concentrations of progestogens.

Women with a history of hypertension or hypertension-related diseases or renal disease (76) should be encouraged to use another method of contraception. If women elect to use oral contraceptives, they should be monitored closely, and if significant elevation of blood pressure occurs, oral contraceptives should be discontinued. For most women, elevated blood pressure will return to normal after stopping oral contraceptives (75), and there is no difference in the occurrence of hypertension among ever and never users (74,76,77).

10. Headache

The onset of exacerbation of migraine or development of headache with a new pattern which is recurrent, persistent, or severe requires discontinuation of oral contraceptives and evaluation of the cause.

11. Bleeding Irregularities

Breakthrough bleeding and spotting are sometimes encountered in patients on oral contraceptives, especially during the first three months of use. Non-hormonal causes should be considered, and adequate diagnostic measures taken to rule out malignancy or pregnancy in the event of breakthrough bleeding, as in the case of any abnormal vaginal bleeding. If pathology has been excluded, time or a change to another formulation may solve the problem. In the event of amenorrhea, pregnancy should be ruled out.

Some women may encounter post-pill amenorrhea or oligomenorrhea, especially when such a condition was preexistent.

PRECAUTIONS

1. Patients should be counseled that this product does not protect against HIV infection (AIDS) and other sexually transmitted diseases.

2. Physical Examination and Follow-Up

It is good medical practice for all women to have annual history and physical examinations, including women using oral contraceptives. The physical examination, however, may be deferred until after initiation of oral contraceptives if requested by the woman and judged appropriate by the clinician. The physical examination should include special reference to blood pressure, breasts, abdomen and pelvic organs, including cervical cytology, and relevant laboratory tests. In case of undiagnosed, persistent or recurrent abnormal vaginal bleeding, appropriate measures should be conducted to rule out malignancy. Women with a strong family history of breast cancer or who have breast nodules should be monitored with particular care.

3. Lipid Disorders

Women who are being treated for hyperlipidemia should be followed closely if they elect to use oral contraceptives. Some progestogens may elevate LDL levels and may render the control of hyperlipidemias more difficult.

4. Liver Function

If jaundice develops in any woman receiving such drugs, the medication should be discontinued. Steroid hormones may be poorly metabolized in patients with conditions with impaired liver function.

5. Fluid Retention

Oral contraceptives may cause some degree of fluid retention. They should be prescribed with caution, and only with careful monitoring, in patients which might be aggravated by fluid retention.

6. Emotional Disorders

Women with a history of depression should be carefully observed and the drug discontinued if depression recurs to a serious degree.

7. Contact Lenses

Contact lens wearers who develop visual changes or changes in lens tolerance should be assessed by an ophthalmologist.

8. Drug Interactions

Effects of Other Drugs on Oral Contraceptives (78)

Rifampin: Metabolism of both norethindrone and ethinyl estradiol is increased by rifampin. A reduction in contraceptive effectiveness and increased incidence of breakthrough bleeding and menstrual irregularities have been associated with concomitant use of rifampin.

Anticonvulsants: Anticonvulsants such as phenobarbital, phenytoin, and carbamazepine, have been shown to increase the metabolism of ethinyl estradiol and/or norethindrone, which could result in a reduction in contraceptive effectiveness.

Troglitazone: Administration of troglitazone with an oral contraceptive containing ethinyl estradiol and norethindrone reduced the plasma concentrations of both by approximately 30%, which could result in a reduction in contraceptive effectiveness.

Antibiotics: Pregnancy while taking oral contraceptives has been reported when the oral contraceptives were administered with antimicrobials such as ampicillin, tetracycline, and griseofulvin. However, clinical pharmacokinetic studies

Continued on next page

This product information was prepared in June 2000. On these and other Parke-Davis Products, information may be obtained by addressing PARKE-DAVIS, a Warner-Lambert Division, Morris Plains, New Jersey 07950.

Loestrin—Cont.

have not demonstrated any consistent effect of antibiotics (other than rifampin) on plasma concentrations of synthetic steroids.

Atorvastatin: Coadministration of atorvastatin and an oral contraceptive increased AUC values for norethindrone and ethinyl estradiol by approximately 30% and 20%, respectively.

Other: Ascorbic acid and acetaminophen may increase plasma ethinyl estradiol concentrations, possibly by inhibition of conjugation. A reduction in contraceptive effectiveness and increased incidence of breakthrough bleeding has been suggested with phenylbutazone.

Effects of Oral Contraceptives on Other Drugs

Oral contraceptive combinations containing ethinyl estradiol may inhibit the metabolism of other compounds. Increased plasma concentrations of cyclosporine, prednisolone, and theophylline have been reported with concomitant administration of oral contraceptives. In addition, oral contraceptives may induce the conjugation of other compounds. Decreased plasma concentrations of acetaminophen and increased clearance of temazepam, salicylic acid, morphine, and clofibric acid have been noted when these drugs were administered with oral contraceptives.

9. Interactions With Laboratory Tests

Certain endocrine and liver function tests and blood components may be affected by oral contraceptives:

a. Increased prothrombin and factors VII, VIII, IX, and X; decreased antithrombin 3; increased norepinephrine-induced platelet aggregability.

b. Increased thyroid binding globulin (TBG) leading to increased circulating total thyroid hormone, as measured by protein-bound iodine (PBI), T_4 by column or by radioimmunoassay. Free T_3 resin uptake is decreased, reflecting the elevated TBG; free T_4 concentration is unaltered.

c. Other binding proteins may be elevated in serum.

d. Sex-binding globulins are increased and result in elevated levels of total circulating sex steroids and corticoids; however, free or biologically active levels remain unchanged.

e. Triglycerides may be increased.

f. Glucose tolerance may be decreased.

g. Serum folate levels may be depressed by oral contraceptive therapy. This may be of clinical significance if a woman becomes pregnant shortly after discontinuing oral contraceptives.

10. Carcinogenesis

See **WARNINGS** section.

11. Pregnancy

Pregnancy Category X. See **CONTRAINDICATIONS** and **WARNINGS** sections.

12. Nursing Mothers

Small amounts of oral contraceptive steroids have been identified in the milk of nursing mothers and a few adverse effects on the child have been reported, including jaundice and breast enlargement. In addition, oral contraceptives given in the postpartum period may interfere with lactation by decreasing the quantity and quality of breast milk. If possible, the nursing mother should be advised not to use oral contraceptives but to use other forms of contraception until she has completely weaned her child.

13. Pediatric Use

Safety and efficacy of Loestrin have been established in women of reproductive age. Safety and efficacy are expected to be the same for postpubertal adolescents under the age of 16 and for users 16 years and older. Use of this product before menarche is not indicated.

INFORMATION FOR THE PATIENT

See patient labeling printed below.

ADVERSE REACTIONS

An increased risk of the following serious adverse reactions has been associated with the use of oral contraceptives (see **WARNINGS** section):

- Thrombophlebitis
- Arterial thromboembolism
- Pulmonary embolism
- Myocardial infarction
- Cerebral hemorrhage
- Cerebral thrombosis
- Hypertension
- Gallbladder disease
- Hepatic adenomas or benign liver tumors

There is evidence of an association between the following conditions and the use of oral contraceptives, although additional confirmatory studies are needed:

- Mesenteric thrombosis
- Retinal thrombosis

The following adverse reactions have been reported in patients receiving oral contraceptives and are believed to be drug-related:

- Nausea
- Vomiting
- Gastrointestinal symptoms (such as abdominal cramps and bloating)
- Breakthrough bleeding
- Spotting
- Change in menstrual flow
- Amenorrhea
- Temporary infertility after discontinuation of treatment
- Edema
- Melasma which may persist
- Breast changes: tenderness, enlargement, secretion
- Change in weight (increase or decrease)
- Change in cervical erosion and secretion
- Diminution in lactation when given immediately postpartum
- Cholestatic jaundice
- Migraine
- Rash (allergic)
- Mental depression
- Reduced tolerance to carbohydrates
- Vaginal candidiasis
- Change in corneal curvature (steepening)
- Intolerance to contact lenses

The following adverse reactions have been reported in users of oral contraceptives and the association has been neither confirmed nor refuted:

- Pre-menstrual syndrome
- Cataracts
- Changes in appetite
- Cystitis-like syndrome
- Headache
- Nervousness
- Dizziness
- Hirsutism
- Loss of scalp hair
- Erythema multiforme
- Erythema nodosum
- Hemorrhagic eruption
- Vaginitis
- Porphyria
- Impaired renal function
- Hemolytic uremic syndrome
- Budd-Chiari syndrome
- Acne
- Changes in libido
- Colitis

OVERDOSAGE

Serious ill effects have not been reported following acute ingestion of large doses of oral contraceptives by young children. Overdosage may cause nausea, and withdrawal bleeding may occur in females.

NON-CONTRACEPTIVE HEALTH BENEFITS

The following non-contraceptive health benefits related to the use of oral contraceptives are supported by epidemiological studies which largely utilized oral contraceptive formulations containing estrogen doses exceeding 0.035 mg of ethinyl estradiol or 0.05 mg of mestranol (79–84).

Effects on menses:

- Increased menstrual cycle regularity
- Decreased blood loss and decreased incidence of iron deficiency anemia
- Decreased incidence of dysmenorrhea

Effects related to inhibition of ovulation:

- Decreased incidence of functional ovarian cysts
- Decreased incidence of ectopic pregnancies

Effects from long-term use:

- Decreased incidence of fibroadenomas and fibrocystic disease of the breast
- Decreased incidence of acute pelvic inflammatory disease
- Decreased incidence of endometrial cancer
- Decreased incidence of ovarian cancer

DOSAGE AND ADMINISTRATION

The tablet dispenser has been designed to make oral contraceptive dosing as easy and as convenient as possible. The tablets are arranged in either three or four rows of seven tablets each, with the days of the week appearing on the tablet dispenser above the first row of tablets.

Note: Each tablet dispenser has been preprinted with the days of the week, starting with Sunday, to facilitate a Sunday-Start regimen. Six different day label strips have been provided with the Detailed Patient & Brief Summary Patient Package Insert in order to accommodate a Day-1 Start regimen. If the patient is using the Day-1 Start regimen, she should place the self-adhesive day label strip that corresponds to her starting day over the preprinted days.

Important: The patient should be instructed to use an additional method of protection until after the first week of administration in the initial cycle when utilizing the Sunday-Start regimen.

The possibility of ovulation and conception prior to initiation of use should be considered.

Dosage and Administration for 21-Day Dosage Regimen

To achieve maximum contraceptive effectiveness, Loestrin **21** must be taken exactly as directed and at intervals not exceeding 24 hours. Loestrin **21** provides the patient with a convenient tablet schedule of "3 weeks on—1 week off." Two dosage regimens are described, one of which may be more convenient or suitable than the other for an individual patient. For the initial cycle of therapy, the patient begins her tablets according to the Day-1 Start or Sunday-Start regimen. With either regimen, the patient takes one tablet daily for 21 consecutive days followed by one week of no tablets.

A. Sunday-Start Regimen: The patient begins taking tablets from the top row on the first Sunday after menstrual flow begins. When menstrual flow begins on Sunday, the first tablet is taken on the same day. The last tablet in the dispenser will then be taken on a Saturday, followed by no tablets for a week (7 days). For all subsequent cycles, the patient then begins a new 21-tablet regimen on the eighth day, Sunday, after taking her last tablet. Following this regimen of 21 days on—7 days off, the patient will start all subsequent cycles on a Sunday.

B. Day-1 Start Regimen: The first day of menstrual flow is Day 1. The patient places the self-adhesive day label strip that corresponds to her starting day over the preprinted days on the tablet dispenser. She starts taking one tablet daily, beginning with the first tablet in the top row. The patient completes her 21-tablet regimen when she has taken the last tablet in the tablet dispenser. She will then take no tablets for a week (7 days). For all subsequent cycles, the patient begins a new 21-tablet regimen on the eighth day after taking her last tablet, again starting with the first tablet in the top row after placing the appropriate day label strip over the preprinted days on the tablet dispenser. Following this regimen of 21 days on—7 days off, the patient will start all subsequent cycles on the same day of the week as the first course. Likewise, the interval of no tablets will always start on the same day of the week.

Tablets should be taken regularly with a meal or at bedtime. It should be stressed that efficacy of medication depends on strict adherence to the dosage schedule.

Special Notes on Administration

Menstruation usually begins two or three days, but may begin as late as the fourth or fifth day, after discontinuing medication. If spotting occurs while on the usual regimen of one tablet daily, the patient should continue medication without interruption.

If a patient forgets to take one or more tablets, the following is suggested:

One tablet is missed

- take tablet as soon as remembered
- take next tablet at the regular time

Two consecutive tablets are missed (week 1 or week 2)

- take *two* tablets as soon as remembered
- take *two* tablets the next day
- use another birth control method for seven days following the missed tablets

Two consecutive tablets are missed (week 3)

Sunday-Start Regimen:

- take *one* tablet daily until Sunday
- discard remaining tablets
- start new pack of tablets immediately (Sunday)
- use another birth control method for seven days following the missed tablets

Day-1 Start Regimen:

- discard remaining tablets
- start new pack of tablets that same day
- use another birth control method for seven days following the missed tablets

Three (or more) consecutive tablets are missed

Sunday-Start Regimen:

- take *one* tablet daily until Sunday
- discard remaining tablets
- start new pack of tablets immediately (Sunday)
- use another birth control method for seven days following the missed tablets

Day-1 Start Regimen:

- discard remaining tablets
- start new pack of tablets that same day
- use another birth control method for seven days following the missed tablets

The possibility of ovulation occurring increases with each successive day that scheduled tablets are missed. While there is little likelihood of ovulation occurring if only one tablet is missed, the possibility of spotting or bleeding is increased. This is particularly likely to occur if two or more consecutive tablets are missed.

In the rare case of bleeding which resembles menstruation, the patient should be advised to discontinue medication and then begin taking tablets from a new tablet dispenser on the next Sunday or the first day (Day 1), depending on her regimen. Persistent bleeding which is not controlled by this method indicates the need for reexamination of the patient, at which time nonfunctional causes should be considered.

Dosage and Administration for 28-Day Dosage Regimen

To achieve maximum contraceptive effectiveness, Loestrin **Fe** should be taken exactly as directed and at intervals not exceeding 24 hours.

Loestrin **Fe** provides a continuous administration regimen consisting of 21 light-colored (white or green) tablets of Loestrin and 7 brown non-hormone containing tablets of ferrous fumarate. The ferrous fumarate tablets are present to facilitate ease of drug administration via a 28-day regimen and do not serve any therapeutic purpose. There is no need for the patient to count days between cycles because there are no "off-tablet days."

A. Sunday-Start Regimen: The patient begins taking the first light-colored tablet from the top row of the dispenser (labeled Sunday) on the first Sunday after menstrual flow begins. When the menstrual flow begins on Sunday, the first light-colored tablet is taken on the same day. The patient takes one light-colored tablet daily for 21 days. The last light-colored tablet in the dispenser will be taken on a Saturday. Upon completion of all 21 light-colored tablets, and without interruption, the patient takes one brown tablet daily for 7 days. Upon completion of this first course of tablets, the patient begins a second course of 28-day tablets, without interruption, the next day (Sunday), starting with the Sunday light-colored tablet in the top row. Adhering to this regimen of one light-colored tablet daily for 21 days, followed without interruption by one brown tablet daily for seven days, the patient will start all subsequent cycles on a Sunday.

B. Day-1 Start Regimen: The first day of menstrual flow is Day 1. The patient places the self-adhesive day label strip that corresponds to her starting day over the preprinted days on the tablet dispenser. She starts taking one light-colored tablet daily, beginning with the first light-colored tablet in the top row. After the last light-colored tablet (at the end of the third row) has been taken, the patient will then take the brown tablets for a week (7 days). For all subsequent cycles, the patient begins a new 28 tablet regimen on the eighth day after taking her last light-colored tablet, again starting with the first tablet in the top row after placing the appropriate day label strip over the preprinted days on the tablet dispenser. Following this regimen of 21 light-colored tablets and 7 brown tablets, the patient will start all subsequent cycles on the same day of the week as the first source.

Tablets should be taken regularly with a meal or at bedtime. It should be stressed that efficacy of medication depends on strict adherence to the dosage schedule.

Special Notes on Administration

Menstruation usually begins two or three days, but may begin as late as the fourth or fifth day, after the brown tablets have been started. In any event, the next course of tablets should be started without interruption. If spotting occurs while the patient is taking light-colored tablets, continue medication without interruption.

If the patient forgets to take one or more *light-colored* tablets, the following is suggested:

One tablet is missed

- take tablet as soon as remembered
- take next tablet at the regular time

Two consecutive tablets are missed (week 1 or week 2)

- take *two* tablets as soon as remembered
- take *two* tablets the next day
- use another birth control method for seven days following the missed tablets

Two consecutive tablets are missed (week 3)

Sunday-Start Regimen:

- take *one* tablet daily until Sunday
- discard remaining tablets
- start new pack of tablets immediately (Sunday)
- use another birth control method for seven days following missed tablets

Day-1 Start Regimen:

- discard remaining tablets
- start new pack of tablets that same day
- use another birth control method for seven days following missed tablets

Three (or more) consecutive tablets are missed

Sunday-Start Regimen:

- take *one* tablet daily until Sunday
- discard remaining tablets
- start new pack of tablets immediately (Sunday)
- use another birth control method for seven days following missed tablets

Day-1 Start Regimen:

- discard remaining tablets
- start new pack of tablets that same day
- use another birth control method for seven days following missed tablets

The possibility of ovulation occurring increases with each successive day that scheduled light-colored tablets are missed. While there is little likelihood of ovulation occurring if only one light-colored tablet is missed, the possibility of spotting or bleeding is increased. This is particularly likely to occur if two or more consecutive light-colored tablets are missed.

If the patient forgets to take any of the seven brown tablets in week four, those brown tablets that were missed are discarded and one brown tablet is taken each day until the pack is empty. A back-up birth control method is not required during this time. A new pack of tablets should be started no later than the eighth day after the last light-colored tablet was taken.

In the rare case of bleeding which resembles menstruation, the patient should be advised to discontinue medication and then begin taking tablets from a new tablet dispenser on the next Sunday or the first day (Day-1), depending on her regimen. Persistent bleeding which is not controlled by this method indicates the need for reexamination of the patient, at which time nonfunctional causes should be considered.

Use of Oral Contraceptives in the Event of a Missed Menstrual Period

1. If the patient has not adhered to the prescribed dosage regimen, the possibility of pregnancy should be considered after the first missed period and oral contraceptives should be withheld until pregnancy has been ruled out.
2. If the patient has adhered to the prescribed regimen and misses two consecutive periods, pregnancy should be ruled out before continuing the contraceptive regimen.

After several months on treatment, bleeding may be reduced to a point of virtual absence. This reduced flow may occur as a result of medication, in which event it is not indicative of pregnancy.

HOW SUPPLIED

Loestrin **21** 1/20 is available in dispensers each containing 21 tablets. Each tablet contains 1 mg of norethindrone acetate and 20 mcg of ethinyl estradiol. Available in packages of five dispensers.

Loestrin **Fe** 1/20 is available in dispensers each containing 21 white tablets and 7 brown tablets. Each white tablet contains 1 mg of norethindrone acetate and 20 mcg of ethinyl estradiol. Each brown tablets contains 75 mg ferrous fumarate. Available in packages of five dispensers.

Loestrin **21** 1.5/30 is available in dispensers each containing 21 tablets. Each tablet contains 1.5 mg of norethindrone acetate and 30 mcg of ethinyl estradiol. Available in packages of five dispensers.

Loestrin **Fe** 1.5/30 is available in dispensers each containing 21 green tablets and 7 brown tablets. Each green tablet contains 1.5 mg of norethindrone acetate and 30 mcg of ethinyl estradiol. Each brown tablet contains 75 mg ferrous fumarate. Available in packages of five dispensers.

Store below 30°C (86°F).

REFERENCES

1. Back DJ, Breckenridge AM, Crawford FE, McIver M, Orme ML'E, Rowe PH and Smith E: Kinetics of norethindrone in women II. Single-dose kinetics. Clin Pharmacol Ther 1978;24:448–453.
2. Hümpel M, Nieuweboer B, Wendt H and Speck U: Investigations of pharmacokinetics of ethinyloestradiol to specific consideration of a possible first-pass effect in women. Contraception 1979;19:421–432.
3. Back DJ, Breckenridge AM, Crawford FE, MacIver M, Orme ML'E, Rowe PH and Watts MJ. An investigation of the pharmacokinetics of ethynylestradiol in women using radioimmunoassay. Contraception 1979;20:263–273.
4. Hammond GL, Lähteenmäki PLA, Lähteenmäki P and Luukkainen T. Distribution and percentages of non-protein bound contraceptive steroids in human serum. J Steroid Biochem 1982;17:375–380.
5. Fotherby K. Pharmacokinetics and metabolism of progestins in humans, in Pharmacology of the contraceptive steroids, Goldzieher JW, Fotherby K (eds), Raven Press, Ltd., New York, 1994; 99–126.
6. Goldzieher JW. Pharmacokinetics and metabolism of ethynyl estrogens, in Pharmacology of the contraceptive steroids, Goldzieher JW, Fotherby K (eds), Raven Press Ltd., New York, 1994; 127–151.
7. Hatcher RA, et al. 1998. Contraceptive Technology, Seventeenth Edition. New York: Irvington Publishers.
8. Stadel, B.V.: Oral contraceptives and cardiovascular disease. (Pt. 1). *New England Journal of Medicine*, 305:612–618, 1981.
9. Stadel, B.V.: Oral contraceptives and cardiovascular disease. (Pt. 2). *New England Journal of Medicine*, 305:672–677, 1981.
10. Adam S.A., and M. Thorogood: Oral contraception and myocardial infarction revisited: The effects of new preparations and prescribing patterns. *Brit. J. Obstet. and Gynec.*, 88:838–845, 1981.
11. Mann, J.I., and W.H, Inman: Oral contraceptives and death from myocardial infarction. *Brit. Med. J.*, 2(5965): 245–248, 1975.
12. Mann, J.I., M.P. Vessey, M. Thorogood, and R. Doll: Myocardial infarction in young women with special reference to oral contraceptive practice. *Brit. Med. J.*, 2(5956):241–245, 1975.
13. Royal College of General Practitioners' Oral Contraception Study: Further analyses of mortality in oral contraceptive users. *Lancet*, 1:541–546, 1981.
14. Slone, D., S. Shapiro, D.W. Kaufman, L. Rosenberg, O.S. Miettinen, and P.D. Stolley: Risk of myocardial infarction in relation to current and discontinued use of oral contraceptives. *N.E.J.M.*, 305:420–424, 1981.
15. Vessey, M.P.: Female hormones and vascular disease: An epidemiological overview. *Brit. J. Fam. Plann.*, 6:1–12, 1980.
16. Russell-Briefel, R.G., T.M. Ezzati, R. Fulwood, J.A. Perlman, and R.S. Murphy: Cardiovascular risk status and oral contraceptive use, United States, 1976–80. *Preventive Medicine*, 15:352–362, 1986.
17. Goldbaum, G.M., J.S. Kendrick, C.G. Hogelin, and E.M. Gentry: The relative impact of smoking and oral contraceptive use on women in the United States. *J.A.M.A.*, 258: 1339–1342, 1987.
18. Layde, P.M., and V. Beral: Further analyses of mortality in oral contraceptive users: Royal College General Practitioners' Oral Contraception Study. (Table 5) *Lancet*, 1:541–546, 1981.
19. Knopp, R.H.: Arteriosclerosis risk: The roles of oral contraceptives and postmenopausal estrogens. *J. of Reprod. Med.*, 31(9)(Supplement): 913–921, 1986.
20. Krauss, R.M., S. Roy, D.R. Mishell, J. Casagrande, and M.C. Pike: Effects of two low-dose oral contraceptives on serum lipids and lipoproteins: Differential changes in high-density lipoproteins subclasses. *Am. J. Obstet. Gyn.*, 145: 446–452, 1983.
21. Wahl, P., C. Walden, R. Knopp, J. Hoover, R. Wallace, G. Heiss, and B. Rifkind: Effect of estrogen/progestin potency on lipid/lipoprotein cholesterol. *N.E.J.M.*, 308:862–867, 1983.
22. Wynn, V., and R. Niththyananthan: The effect of progestin in combined oral contraceptives on serum lipids with special reference to high-density lipoproteins. Am. J. Obstet. and Gyn., 142:766–771, 1982.
23. Wynn, V., and I. Godsland: Effects of oral contraceptives on carbohydrate metabolism. *J. Reprod. Medicine*, 31 (9)(Supplement): 892–897, 1986.
24. LaRosa, J.C.: Atherosclerotic risk factors in cardiovascular disease. *J. Reprod. Med.*, 31(9)(Supplement): 906–912, 1986.
25. Inman, W.H., and M.P. Vessey: Investigations of death from pulmonary, coronary, and cerebral thrombosis and embolism in women of child-bearing age. *Brit. Med. J.*, 2(5599): 193–199, 1968.
26. Maguire, M.G., J. Tonascia, P.E. Sartwell, P.D. Stolley, and M.S. Tockman: Increased risk of thrombosis due to oral contraceptives: A further report. *Am. J. Epidemiology*, 110(2): 188–195, 1979.
27. Pettiti, D.B., J. Wingerd, F. Pelligrin, and S. Ramacharan: Risk of vascular disease in women: Smoking, oral contraceptives, noncontraceptive estrogens, and other factors. *J.A.M.A.*, 242:1150–1154, 1979.
28. Vessey, M.P., and R. Doll: Investigation of relation between use of oral contraceptives and thromboembolic disease. *Brit. Med. J.*, 2(5599): 199–205, 1968.
29. Vessey, M.P., and R. Doll: Investigation of relation between use of oral contraceptives and thromboembolic disease: A further report. *Brit. Med. J.*, 2(5658): 651–657, 1969.
30. Porter, J.B., J.R. Hunter, D.A. Danielson, H. Jick, and A. Stergachis: Oral contraceptives and non-fatal vascular disease: Recent experience. *Obstet. and Gyn.*, 59(3):299–302, 1982.
31. Vessey, M., R. Doll, R. Peto, B. Johnson, and P. Wiggins: A long-term follow-up study of women using different methods of contraception: An interim report. *J. Biosocial. Sci.*, 8:375–427, 1976.
32. Royal College of General Practitioners: Oral contraceptives, venous thrombosis, and varicose veins. *J. of Royal College of General Practitioners*, 28:393–399, 1978.
33. Collaborative Group for the study of stroke in young women: Oral contraception and increased risk of cerebral ischemia or thrombosis. *N.E.J.M.*, 288:871–878, 1973.
34. Petitti, D.B., and J. Wingerd: Use of oral contraceptives, cigarette smoking, and risk of subarachnoid hemorrhage. *Lancet*, 2:234–236, 1978.
35. Inman, W.H.: Oral contraceptives and fatal subarachnoid hemorrhage. *Brit. Med. J.*, 2(6203): 1468–70, 1979.
36. Collaborative Group for the study of stroke in young women: Oral contraceptives and stroke in young women: Associated risk factors. *J.A.M.A.*, 231:718–722, 1975.
37. Inman, W.H., M.P. Vessey, B. Westerholm, and A. Engelund: Thromboembolic disease and the steroidal content of oral contraceptives. A report to the Committee on Safety of Drugs. *Brit. Med. J.*, 2:203–209, 1970.
38. Meade, T.W., G. Greenberg, and S.G. Thompson: Progestogens and cardiovascular reactions associated with oral contraceptives and a comparison of the safety of 50- and 35-mcg oestrogen preparations. *Brit. Med. J.*, 280(6224): 1157–1161, 1980.
39. Kay, C.R.: Progestogens and arterial disease: Evidence from the Royal College of General Practitioners' study. *Amer. J. Obstet. Gyn.*, 142:762–765, 1982.
40. Royal College of General Practitioners: Incidence of arterial disease among oral contraceptive users. *J. Coll. Gen. Pract.*, 33:75–82, 1983.
41. Ory, H.W.: Mortality associated with fertility and fertility control:1983. *Family Planning Perspectives*, 15:50–56, 1983.
42. The Cancer and Steroid Hormone Study of the Centers for Disease Control and the National Institute of Child Health and Human Development: Oral-contraceptive user and the risk of breast cancer. *N.E.J.M.*, 315: 405–411, 1986.
43. Pike, M.C., B.E. Henderson, M.D. Krailo, A. Duke, and S. Roy: Breast cancer in young women and use of oral contraceptives: Possible modifying effect of formulation and age at use. *Lancet*, 2:926–929, 1983.
44. Paul, C., D.G. Skegg, G.F.S. Spears, and J.M. Kaldor: Oral contraceptives and breast cancer: A national study. *Brit. Med. J.*, 293:723–725, 1986.
45. Miller, D.R., L. Rosenberg, D.W. Kaufman, D. Schottenfeld, O.D. Stolley, and S. Shapiro: Breast cancer risk in relation to early oral contraceptive use. *Obstet. Gynec.*, 68: 863–868, 1986.
46. Olson, H., K.L. Olson, T.R. Moller, J. Ranstam, P. Holm: Oral contraceptive use and breast cancer in young women in Sweden (letter). *Lancet*, 2:748–749, 1985.
47. McPherson, K., M. Vessey, A. Neil, R. Doll, L. Jones, and M. Roberts: Early contraceptive use and breast cancer: Results of another case-control study. *Brit. J. Cancer*, 56: 653–660, 1987.
48. Huggins, G.R., and P.F. Zucker: Oral contraceptives and neoplasia: 1987 update. *Fertil. Steril.*, 47:733–761, 1987.
49. McPherson, K., and J.O. Drife: The pill and breast cancer: Why the uncertainty? *Brit. Med. J.*, 293:709–710, 1986.
50. Shapiro, S.: Oral contraceptives: Time to take stock. *N.E.J.M.*, 315:450–451, 1987.
51. Ory, H., Z. Naib, S.B. Conger, R.A. Hatcher, and C.W. Tyler: Contraceptive choice and prevalence of cervical dysplasia and carcinoma in situ. *Am. J. Obstet. Gynec.*, 124: 573–577, 1976.
52. Vessey, M.P., M. Lawless, K. McPherson, D. Yeates: Neoplasia of the cervix uteri and contraception: A possible adverse effect of the pill. *Lancet*, 2:930, 1983.
53. Brinton, L.A., G.R. Huggins, H.F. Lehman, K. Malli, D.A. Savitz, E. Trapido, J. Rosenthal, and R. Hoover: Long-term use of oral contraceptives and risk of invasive cervical cancer. *Int. J. Cancer*, 38:339–344, 1986.

Continued on next page

This product information was prepared in June 2000. On these and other Parke-Davis Products, information may be obtained by addressing PARKE-DAVIS, a Warner-Lambert Division, Morris Plains, New Jersey 07950.

Loestrin—Cont.

54. WHO Collaborative Study of Neoplasia and Steroid Contraceptives: Invasive cervical cancer and combined oral contraceptives. *Brit. Med. J.*, 290:961–965, 1985.
55. Rooks, J.B., H.W. Ory, K.G. Ishak, L.T. Strauss, J.R. Greenspan, A.P. Hill, and C.W. Tyler: Epidemiology of hepatocellular adenoma: The role of oral contraceptive use. *J.A.M.A.*, 242:644–648, 1979.
56. Bein, N.N., and H.S. Goldsmith: Recurrent massive hemorrhage from benign hepatic tumors secondary to oral contraceptives. *Brit. J. Surg.*, 64:433–435, 1977.
57. Klatskin, G.: Hepatic tumors: Possible relationship to use of oral contraceptives. *Gastroenterology*, 73:386–194, 1977.
58. Henderson, B.E., S. Preston-Martin, H.A. Edmondson, R.L. Peters, and M.C. Pike: Hepatocellular carcinoma and oral contraceptives. *Brit. J. Cancer*, 48:437–440. 1983.
59. Neuberger, J., D. Forman, R. Doll, and R. Williams: Oral contraceptives and hepatocellular carcinoma. *Brit. Med. J.*, 292:1355–1357, 1986.
60. Forman, D., T.J. Vincent, and R. Doll: Cancer of the liver and oral contraceptives. *Brit. Med. J.*, 292: 1357–1361, 1986.
61. Harlap, S., and J. Eldor: Births following oral contraceptive failures. *Obstet. Gynec.*, 55:447–452, 1980.
62. Savolainen, E., E. Saksela, and L. Saxen: Teratogenic hazards of oral contraceptives analyzed in a national malformation register. *Amer. J. Obstet. Gynec.*, 140:521–524, 1981.
63. Janerich, D.T., J.M. Piper, and D.M. Glebatis: Oral contraceptives and birth defects. *Am. J. Epidemiology*, 112:73–79, 1980.
64. Ferencz, C., G.M. Matanoski, P.D. Wilson, J.D. Rubin, C.A. Neill, and R. Gutberlet: Maternal hormone therapy and congenital heart disease. *Teratology*, 21:225–239, 1980.
65. Rothman, K.J., D.C. Fyler, A. Goldblatt, and M.B. Kreidberg: Exogenous hormones and other drug exposures of children with congenital heart disease. *Am. J. Epidemiology*, 109:433–439, 1979.
66. Boston Collaborative Drug Surveillance Program: Oral contraceptives and venous thromboembolic disease, surgically confirmed gallbladder disease, and breast tumors. *Lancet*, 1:1399–1404, 1973.
67. Royal College of General Practitioners: *Oral Contraceptives and Health*. New York, Pittman, 1974, 100p.
68. Layde, P.M., M.P. Vessey, and D. Yeates: Risk of gallbladder disease: A cohort study of young women attending family planning clinics. *J. of Epidemiol. and Comm. Health*, 36: 274–278, 1982.
69. Rome Group for the Epidemiology and Prevention of Cholelithiasis (GREPCO): Prevalence of gallstone disease in an Italian adult female population. *Am. J. Epidemiol.*, 119: 796–805, 1984.
70. Strom, B.L., R.T. Tamragouri, M.L. Morse, E.L. Lazar, S.L. West, P. D. Stolley, and J.K. Jones: Oral contraceptives and other risk factors for gallbladder disease. *Clin. Pharmacol. Ther.*, 39:335–341, 1986.
71. Wynn, V., P.W. Adams, I.F. Godsland, J. Melrose, R. Niththyananthan, N.W. Oakley, and A. Seedj: Comparison of effects of different combined oral-contraceptive formulations on carbohydrate and lipid metabolism. *Lancet*, 1:1045–1049, 1979.
72. Wynn, V.: effect of progesterone and progestins on carbohydrate metabolism. In Progesterone and Progestin. Edited by C.W. Bardin, E. Milgrom, P. Mauvis-Jarvis. New York, *Raven Press*, pp. 395–410. 1983.
73. Perlman, J.A., R.G. Roussell-Briefel, T.M. Ezzati, and G. Lieberknecht: Oral glucose tolerance and the potency of oral contraceptive progestogens. *J. Chronic. Dis.*, 38:857–864, 1985.
74. Royal College of General Practitioners' Oral Contraception Study: Effect on hypertension and benign breast disease of progestogen component in combined oral contraceptives. *Lancet*, 1:624, 1977.
75. Fisch, I.R., and J. Frank: Oral contraceptives and blood pressure. *J.A.M.A.*, 237:2499–2503, 1977.
76. Laragh, A.J.: Oral contraceptive induced hypertension: Nine years later. *Amer. J. Obstet. Gynecol.*, 126:141–147, 1976.
77. Ramcharan, S., E. Peritz, F.A. Pellegrin, and W.T. Williams: Incidence of hypertension in the Walnut Creek Contraceptive Drug Study cohort. In Pharmacology of Steroid Contraceptive Drugs. Edited by S. Garattini and H.W. Berendes. New York, *Raven Press*, pp. 277–288, 1977. (Monographs of the Mario Negri Institute for Pharmacological Research, Milan.)
78. Back DJ, Orme ML'E. Drug interactions, in Pharmacology of the contraceptive steroids, Goldzieher JW, Fotherby K (eds), Raven Press, Ltd., New York, 1994, 407–425.
79. The Cancer and Steroid Hormone Study of the Centers for Disease Control and the National Institute of Child Health and Human Development: Oral contraceptive use and the risk of ovarian cancer. *J.A.M.A.*, 249:1596–1599, 1983.
80. The Cancer and Steroid Hormone Study of the Centers for Disease Control and the National Institute of Child Health and Human Development: Combination oral contraceptive use and the risk of endometrial cancer. *J.A.M.A.*, 257:796–800. 1987.
81. Ory, H.W.: Functional ovarian cysts and oral contraceptives: Negative association confirmed surgically. *J.A.M.A.*, 228:68–69, 1974.
82. Ory, H.W., P. Cole, B. Macmahon, and R. Hoover: Oral contraceptives and reduced risk of benign breast disease. *N.E.J.M.*, 294:41–422, 1976.
83. Ory, H.W.: The noncontraceptive health benefits from oral contraceptive use. *Fam. Plann. Perspectives*, 14:182–184, 1982.
84. Ory, H.W., J.D. Forrest, and R. Lincoln: Making Choices: Evaluating the health risks and benefits of birth control methods. New York, The Alan Guttmacher Institute, p.1, 1983.
85. Miller, D.R., L. Rosenberg, D.W. Kaufman, P. Stolley, M.E. Warshauer, and S. Shapiro: Breast cancer before age 45 and oral contraceptive use: new findings. *Am. J. Epidemiol.*, 129:269–280, 1989.
86. Kay, C.R., and P.C. Hannaford: Breast cancer and the pill: a further report from the Royal College of General Practitioners Oral Contraception Study. *Br. J. Cancer*, 58: 675–680, 1988.
87. Stadel, B.V., S. Lai, J.J. Schlesselman, and P. Murray: Oral contraceptives and premenopausal breast cancer in nulliparous women. *Contraception*, 38:287–299, 1988.
88. UK National Case—Control Study Group: Oral contraceptive use and breast cancer risk in young women. *Lancet*, 973–982, 1989.
89. Romieu, I., W.C. Willett, G.A. Colditz, M.J. Stampfer, B. Rosner, C.H. Hennekens, and F.E. Speizer: Prospective study of oral contraceptive use and risk of breast cancer in women. *J. Natl. Cancer Inst.*, 81:1313–1321, 1989.

The patient labeling for oral contraceptive drug products is set forth below.

This product (like all oral contraceptives) is intended to prevent pregnancy. It does not protect against HIV infection (AIDS) and other sexually transmitted diseases.

BRIEF SUMMARY PATIENT PACKAGE INSERT

Oral contraceptives, also known as "birth control pills" or "the pill," are taken to prevent pregnancy and, when taken correctly, have a failure rate of about 1% per year when used without missing any pills. The typical failure rate of large numbers of pill users is less than 3% per year when women who miss pills are included. For most women oral contraceptives are also free of serious or unpleasant side effects. However, forgetting to take pills considerably increases the chances of pregnancy.

For the majority of women, oral contraceptives can be taken safely. But there are some women who are at high risk of developing certain serious diseases that can be life-threatening or may cause temporary or permanent disability. The risks associated with taking oral contraceptives increase significantly if you:

- Smoke
- Have high blood pressure, diabetes, high cholesterol
- Have or have had clotting disorders, heart attack, stroke, angina pectoris, cancer of the breast or sex organs, jaundice, or malignant or benign liver tumors.

You should not take the pill if you suspect you are pregnant or have unexplained vaginal bleeding.

Cigarette smoking increases the risk of serious cardiovascular side effects from oral contraceptive use. This risk increases with age and with heavy smoking (15 or more cigarettes per day) and is quite marked in women over 35 years of age. Women who use oral contraceptives are strongly advised not to smoke.

Most side effects of the pill are not serious. The most common side effects are nausea, vomiting, bleeding between menstrual periods, weight gain, breast tenderness, and difficulty wearing contact lenses. These side effects, especially nausea, vomiting, and breakthrough bleeding, may subside within the first three months of use.

The serious side effects of the pill occur very infrequently, especially if you are in good health and are young. However, you should know that the following medical conditions have been associated with or made worse by the pill:

1. Blood clots in the legs (thrombophlebitis), lungs (pulmonary embolism), stoppage or rupture of a blood vessel in the brain (stroke), blockage of blood vessels in the heart (heart attack or angina pectoris) or other organs of the body. As mentioned above, smoking increases the risk of heart attacks and strokes and subsequent serious medical consequences.
2. Liver tumors, which may rupture and cause severe bleeding. A possible but not definite association has been found with the pill and liver cancer. However, liver cancers are extremely rare. The chance of developing liver cancer from using the pill is thus even rarer.
3. High blood pressure, although blood pressure usually returns to normal when the pill is stopped.

The symptoms associated with these serious side effects are discussed in the detailed leaflet given to you with your supply of pills. Notify your doctor or health care provider if you notice any unusual physical disturbances while taking the pill. In addition, drugs such as rifampin, as well as some anticonvulsants and some antibiotics, may decrease oral contraceptive effectiveness.

Most of the studies to date on breast cancer and pill use have found no increase in the risk of developing breast cancer, although some studies have reported an increased risk of developing breast cancer in certain groups of women. However, some studies have found an increase in the risk of developing cancer of the cervix in women using the pill, but this finding may be related to differences in sexual behavior or other factors not related to use of the pill. Therefore, there is insufficient evidence to rule out the possibility that the pill may cause cancer of the breast or cervix.

Taking the pill provides some important non-contraceptive benefits. These include less painful menstruation, less menstrual blood loss and anemia, fewer pelvic infections, and fewer cancers of the ovary and the lining of the uterus.

Be sure to discuss any medical condition you may have with your health care provider. Your health care provider will take a medical and family history and examine you before prescribing oral contraceptives. The physical examination may be delayed to another time if you request it and your health care provider believes that it is a good medical practice to postpone it. You should be reexamined at least once a year while taking oral contraceptives. The detailed patient information leaflet gives you further information which you should read and discuss with your health care provider.

This product (like all oral contraceptives) is intended to prevent pregnancy. It does not protect against transmission of HIV (AIDS) and other sexually transmitted diseases such as chlamydia, genital herpes, genital warts, gonorrhea, hepatitis B and syphilis.

INSTRUCTIONS TO PATIENT
TABLET DISPENSER

The Loestrin tablet dispenser has been designed to make oral contraceptive dosing as easy and as convenient as possible. The tablets are arranged in either three or four rows of seven tablets each with the days of the week appearing above the first row of tablets.

[See table below]

Each *white* tablet contains 1 mg norethindrone acetate and 20 mcg ethinyl estradiol.

Each *green* tablet contains 1.5 mg norethindrone acetate and 30 mcg ethinyl estradiol.

Each *brown* tablet contains 75 mg ferrous fumarate, and is intended to help you remember to take the tablets correctly. These brown tablets are not intended to have any health benefit.

DIRECTIONS

To remove a tablet, press down on it with your thumb or finger. The tablet will drop through the back of the tablet dispenser. Do not press with your thumbnail, fingernail, or any other sharp object.

HOW TO TAKE THE PILL

IMPORTANT POINTS TO REMEMBER

BEFORE YOU START TAKING YOUR PILLS:

1. BE SURE TO READ THESE DIRECTIONS:
Before you start taking your pills.
Anytime you are not sure what to do.
2. THE RIGHT WAY TO TAKE THE PILL IS TO TAKE ONE PILL EVERY DAY AT THE SAME TIME. If you miss pills you could get pregnant. This includes starting the pack late. The more pills you miss, the more likely you are to get pregnant.
3. MANY WOMEN HAVE SPOTTING OR LIGHT BLEEDING, OR MAY FEEL SICK TO THEIR STOMACH, DURING THE FIRST 1–3 PACKS OF PILLS. If you do have spotting or light bleeding or feel sick to your stomach, do not stop taking the pill. The problem will usually go away. If it doesn't go away, check with your doctor or clinic.
4. MISSING PILLS CAN ALSO CAUSE SPOTTING OR LIGHT BLEEDING, even when you make up these missed pills. On the days you take 2 pills to make up for missed pills, you could also feel a little sick to your stomach.
5. IF YOU HAVE VOMITING OR DIARRHEA, for any reason, or IF YOU TAKE SOME MEDICINES, including some antibiotics, your birth control pills may not work as well. Use a back-up birth control method (such as condoms or foam) until you check with your doctor or clinic.
6. IF YOU HAVE TROUBLE REMEMBERING TO TAKE THE PILL, talk to your doctor or clinic about how to make pill-taking easier or about using another method of birth control.
7. IF YOU HAVE ANY QUESTIONS OR ARE UNSURE ABOUT THE INFORMATION IN THIS LEAFLET, call your doctor or clinic.

If your TABLET DISPENSER contains:	You are taking:
21 white tablets	LOESTRIN 21 1/20
21 green tablets	LOESTRIN 21 1.5/30
21 white tablets and 7 brown tablets	LOESTRIN Fe 1/20
21 green tablets and 7 brown tablets	LOESTRIN Fe 1.5/30

BEFORE YOU START TAKING YOUR PILLS

1. DECIDE WHAT TIME OF DAY YOU WANT TO TAKE YOUR PILL. It is important to take it at about the same time every day.
2. LOOK AT YOUR PILL PACK TO SEE IF IT HAS 21 OR 28 PILLS:
The 21-pill pack has 21 "active" white or green pills (with hormones) to take for 3 weeks, followed by 1 week without pills.
The 28-pill pack has 21 "active" white or green pills (with hormones) to take for 3 weeks, followed by 1 week of reminder brown pills (without hormones).
3. ALSO FIND:
1) where on the pack to start taking pills,
2) in what order to take the pills (follow the arrows), and
3) the week numbers as shown in the following pictures:

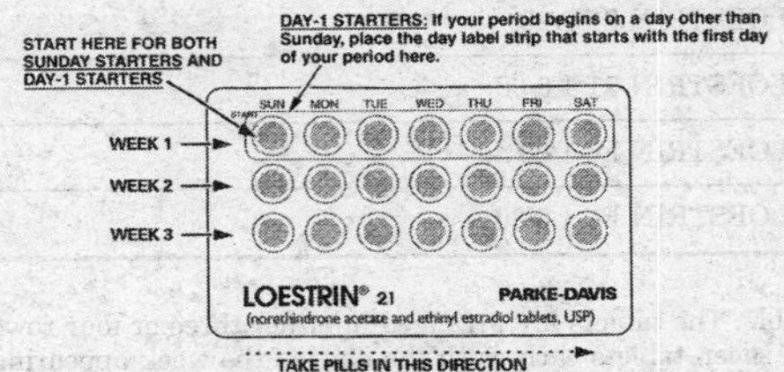
START HERE FOR BOTH SUNDAY STARTERS AND DAY-1 STARTERS
DAY-1 STARTERS: If your period begins on a day other than Sunday, place the day label strip that starts with the first day of your period here.
SUN MON TUE WED THU FRI SAT
WEEK 1
WEEK 2
WEEK 3
LOESTRIN® 21
PARKE-DAVIS
(norethindrone acetate and ethinyl estradiol tablets, USP)
TAKE PILLS IN THIS DIRECTION FROM LEFT TO RIGHT EACH WEEK.

Loestrin 21 1/20 will contain: **ALL WHITE PILLS**
Loestrin 21 1.5/30 will contain: **ALL GREEN PILLS**

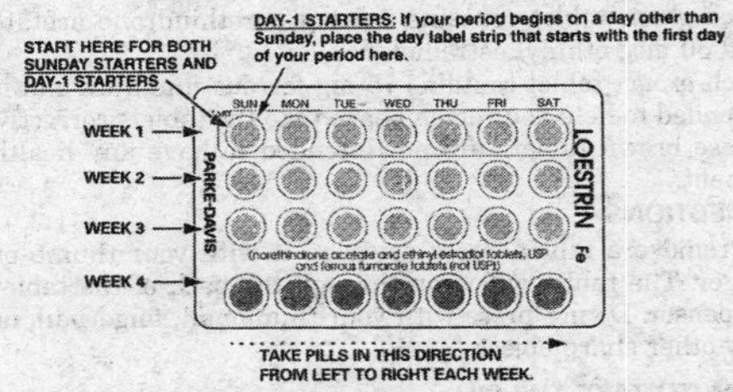
START HERE FOR BOTH SUNDAY STARTERS AND DAY-1 STARTERS
DAY-1 STARTERS: If your period begins on a day other than Sunday, place the day label strip that starts with the first day of your period here.
SUN MON TUE WED THU FRI SAT
WEEK 1
WEEK 2
WEEK 3
WEEK 4
PARKE-DAVIS
LOESTRIN Fe
(norethindrone acetate and ethinyl estradiol tablets, USP and ferrous fumarate tablets (not USP))
TAKE PILLS IN THIS DIRECTION FROM LEFT TO RIGHT EACH WEEK.

Loestrin Fe 1/20 will contain: **21 WHITE PILLS** for **WEEKS 1, 2 and 3. WEEK 4** will contain **BROWN PILLS ONLY.**
Loestrin Fe 1.5/30 will contain: **21 GREEN PILLS** for **WEEKS 1, 2 and 3. WEEK 4** will contain **BROWN PILLS ONLY.**
4. BE SURE YOU HAVE READY AT ALL TIMES:
ANOTHER KIND OF BIRTH CONTROL (such as condoms or foam) to use as a back-up in case you miss pills.
An EXTRA, FULL PILL PACK.

WHEN TO START THE FIRST PACK OF PILLS

You have a choice of which day to start taking your first pack of pills. Decide with your doctor or clinic which is the best day for you. Pick a time of day which will be easy to remember.

DAY-1 START:
1. Pick the day label strip that starts with the first day of your period. (This is the day you start bleeding or spotting, even if it is almost midnight when the bleeding begins.)
2. Place this day label strip on the tablet dispenser over the area that has the days of the week (starting with Sunday) printed on the plastic.
3. Take the first "active" white or green pill of the first pack during the first 24 hours of your period.
4. You will not need to use a back-up method of birth control, since you are starting the pill at the beginning of your period.

SUNDAY START:
1. Take the first "active" white or green pill of the first pack on the Sunday after your period starts, even if you are still bleeding. If your period begins on Sunday, start the pack that same day.
2. Use another method of birth control as a back-up method if you have sex anytime from the Sunday you start your first pack until the next Sunday (7 days). Condoms or foam are good back-up methods of birth control.

WHAT TO DO DURING THE MONTH

1. TAKE ONE PILL AT THE SAME TIME EVERY DAY UNTIL THE PACK IS EMPTY.
Do not skip pills even if you are spotting or bleeding between monthly periods or feel sick to your stomach (nausea).
Do not skip pills even if you do not have sex very often.
2. WHEN YOU FINISH A PACK OR SWITCH YOUR BRAND OF PILLS:
21 pills: Wait 7 days to start the next pack. You will probably have your period during that week. Be sure that no more than 7 days pass between 21-day packs.
28 pills: Start the next pack on the day after your last "reminder" pill. Do not wait any days between packs.

WHAT TO DO IF YOU MISS PILLS

If you **MISS 1** white or green "active" pill:
1. Take it as soon as you remember. Take the next pill at your regular time. This means you may take 2 pills in 1 day.
2. You do not need to use a back-up birth control method if you have sex.
If you **MISS 2** white or green "active" pills in a row in **WEEK 1 OR WEEK 2** of your pack:
1. Take 2 pills on the day you remember and 2 pills the next day.
2. Then take 1 pill a day until you finish the pack.
3. You COULD GET PREGNANT if you have sex in the 7 days after you miss pills. You MUST use another birth control method (such as condoms or foam) as a back-up method of birth control until you have taken a white or green "active" pill every day for 7 days.
If you **MISS 2** white or green "active" pills in a row in **THE 3rd WEEK:**
1. If you are a Day-1 Starter:
THROW OUT the rest of the pill pack and start a new pack that same day.
If you are a Sunday Starter:
Keep taking 1 pill every day until Sunday. On Sunday, THROW OUT the rest of the pack and start a new pack of pills that same day.
2. You may not have your period this month, but this is expected. However, if you miss your period 2 months in a row, call your doctor or clinic because you might be pregnant.
3. You COULD GET PREGNANT if you have sex in the 7 days after you miss pills. You MUST use another birth control method (such as condoms or foam) as a back-up method of birth control until you have taken a white or green "active" pill every day for 7 days.
If you **MISS 3 OR MORE** white or green "active" pills in a row (during the first 3 weeks).
1. If you are a Day-1 Starter:
THROW OUT the rest of the pill pack and start a new pack that same day.
If you are a Sunday Starter:
Keep taking 1 pill every day until Sunday. On Sunday, THROW OUT the rest of the pack and start a new pack of pills that same day.
2. You may not have your period this month, but this is expected. However, if you miss your period 2 months in a row, call your doctor or clinic because you might be pregnant.
3. You COULD GET PREGNANT if you have sex in the 7 days after you miss pills. You MUST use another birth control method (such as condoms or foam) as a back-up method of birth control until you have taken a white or green "active" pill every day for 7 days.

A REMINDER FOR THOSE ON 28-DAY PACKS:
IF YOU FORGET ANY OF THE 7 BROWN "REMINDER" PILLS IN WEEK 4:
THROW AWAY THE PILLS YOU MISSED.
KEEP TAKING 1 PILL EACH DAY UNTIL THE PACK IS EMPTY.
YOU DO NOT NEED A BACK-UP METHOD.

FINALLY, IF YOU ARE STILL NOT SURE WHAT TO DO ABOUT THE PILLS YOU HAVE MISSED:
Use a BACK-UP METHOD anytime you have sex.
KEEP TAKING ONE WHITE OR GREEN "ACTIVE" PILL EACH DAY until you can reach your doctor or clinic.

Based on his or her assessment of your medical needs, your doctor or health care provider has prescribed this drug for you. Do not give this drug to anyone else.
Keep this and all drugs out of the reach of children.
Rx only
Store below 30°C (86°F).
This product (like all oral contraceptives) is intended to prevent pregnancy. It does not protect against HIV infection (AIDS) and other sexually transmitted diseases.

DETAILED PATIENT PACKAGE INSERT

What You Should Know About Oral Contraceptives
Any woman who considers using oral contraceptives (the "birth control pill" or "the pill") should understand the benefits and risks of using this form of birth control. This leaflet will give you much of the information you will need to make this decision and will also help you determine if you are at risk of developing any of the serious effects of the pill. It will tell you how to use the pill properly so that it will be as effective as possible. However, this leaflet is not a replacement for a careful discussion between you and your health care provider. You should discuss the information provided in this leaflet with him or her, both when you first start taking the pill and during your revisits. You should also follow your health care provider's advice with regard to regular check-ups while you are on the pill.

EFFECTIVENESS OF ORAL CONTRACEPTIVES
Oral contraceptives or "birth control pills" or "the pill" are used to prevent pregnancy and are more effective than other non-surgical methods of birth control. When they are taken correctly, the chance of becoming pregnant is less than 1% (1 pregnancy per 100 women per year of use) when used perfectly, without missing any pills. Typical failure rates are actually 3% per year. The chance of becoming pregnant increases with each missed pill during a menstrual cycle.
In comparison, typical failure rates for other methods of birth control during the first year of use are as follows:
Implant: <1%
Injection: <1%
IUD: <1 to 2%
Diaphragm with spermicides: 20%
Spermicides alone: 26%
Vaginal Sponge: 20 to 40%
Female sterilization: <1%
Male sterilization: <1%
Cervical Cap: 20 to 40%
Condom alone (male): 14%
Condom alone (female): 21%
Periodic abstinence: 25%
Withdrawal: 19%
No method: 85%

WHO SHOULD NOT TAKE ORAL CONTRACEPTIVES

Cigarette smoking increases the risk of serious cardiovascular side effects from oral contraceptive use. This risk increases with age and with heavy smoking (15 or more cigarettes per day) and is quite marked in women over 35 years of age. Women who use oral contraceptives are strongly advised not to smoke.

Some women should not use the pill. For example, you should not take the pill if you are pregnant or think you may be pregnant. You should also not use the pill if you have any of the following conditions.
- A history of heart attack or stroke
- Blood clots in the legs (thrombophlebitis), lungs (pulmonary embolism), or eyes
- A history of blood clots in the deep veins of your legs
- Chest pain (angina pectoris)
- Known or suspected breast cancer or cancer of the lining of the uterus, cervix or vagina
- Unexplained vaginal bleeding (until a diagnosis is reached by your doctor)
- Yellowing of the whites of the eyes or of the skin (jaundice) during pregnancy or during previous use of the pill
- Liver tumor (benign or cancerous)
- Known or suspected pregnancy

Tell your health care provider if you have ever had any of these conditions. Your health care provider can recommend a safer method of birth control.

OTHER CONSIDERATIONS BEFORE TAKING ORAL CONTRACEPTIVES
Tell your health care provider if you have:
- Breast nodules, fibrocystic disease of the breast, an abnormal breast x-ray or mammogram
- Diabetes
- Elevated cholesterol or triglycerides
- High blood pressure
- Migraine or other headaches or epilepsy
- Mental depression
- Gallbladder, heart, or kidney disease
- History of scanty or irregular menstrual periods

Women with any of these conditions should be checked often by their health care provider if they choose to use oral contraceptives.
Also, be sure to inform your doctor or health care provider if you smoke or are on any medications.

RISKS OF TAKING ORAL CONTRACEPTIVES

1. Risk of Developing Blood Clots
Blood clots and blockage of blood vessels are the most serious side effects of taking oral contraceptives; in particular, a clot in the legs can cause thrombophlebitis, and a clot that travels to the lungs can cause a sudden blocking of the vessel carrying blood to the lungs. Rarely, clots occur in the blood vessels of the eye and may cause blindness, double vision, or impaired vision.
If you take oral contraceptives and need elective surgery, need to stay in bed for a prolonged illness, or have recently delivered a baby, you may be at risk of developing blood clots. You should consult your doctor about stopping oral contraceptives three to four weeks before surgery and not taking oral contraceptives for two weeks after surgery or during bed rest. You should also not take oral contraceptives soon after delivery of a baby. It is advisable to wait for at least four weeks after delivery if you are not breast feeding. If you are breast feeding, you should wait until you have weaned your child before using the pill. (See also the section on Breast Feeding in GENERAL PRECAUTIONS.)

2. Heart Attacks and Strokes
Oral contraceptives may increase the tendency to develop strokes (stoppage or rupture of blood vessels in the brain) and angina pectoris and heart attacks (blockage of blood vessels in the heart). Any of these conditions can cause death or disability.
Smoking greatly increases the possibility of suffering heart attacks and strokes. Furthermore, smoking and the use of oral contraceptives greatly increase the chances of developing and dying of heart disease.

3. Gallbladder Disease
Oral contraceptive users probably have a greater risk than nonusers of having gallbladder disease, although the risk may be related to pills containing high doses of estrogens.

4. Liver Tumors
In rare cases, oral contraceptives can cause benign but dangerous liver tumors. These benign liver tumors can rupture and cause fatal internal bleeding. In addition, a possible but not definite association has been found with the pill and liver cancers in two studies, in which a few women who developed these very rare cancers were found to have used oral contraceptives for long periods. However, liver cancers

Continued on next page

This product information was prepared in June 2000. On these and other Parke-Davis Products, information may be obtained by addressing PARKE-DAVIS, a Warner-Lambert Division, Morris Plains, New Jersey 07950.

Loestrin—Cont.

are extremely rare. The chance of developing liver cancer from using the pill is thus even rarer.

5. Cancer of the Reproductive Organs and Breasts

There is, at present, no confirmed evidence that oral contraceptive use increases the risk of developing cancer of the reproductive organs. Studies to date of women taking the pill have reported conflicting findings on whether pill use increases the risk of developing cancer of the breast or cervix. Most of the studies on breast cancer and pill use have found no overall increase in the risk of developing breast cancer, although some studies have reported an increased risk of developing breast cancer in certain groups of women. Women who use oral contraceptives and have a strong family history of breast cancer or who have breast nodules or abnormal mammograms should be closely followed by their doctors.

Some studies have found an increase in the incidence of cancer of the cervix in women who use oral contraceptives. However, this finding may be related to factors other than the use of oral contraceptives.

ESTIMATED RISK OF DEATH FROM A BIRTH CONTROL METHOD OR PREGNANCY

All methods of birth control and pregnancy are associated with a risk of developing certain diseases which may lead to disability or death. An estimate of the number of deaths associated with different methods of birth control and pregnancy has been calculated and is shown in the following table.

[See first table above]

In the above table, the risk of death from any birth control method is less than the risk of childbirth, except for oral contraceptive users over the age of 35 who smoke and pill users over the age of 40 even if they do not smoke. It can be seen in the table that for women aged 15 to 39, the risk of death was highest with pregnancy (7–26 deaths per 100,000 women, depending on age). Among pill users who do not smoke, the risk of death was always lower than that associated with pregnancy for any age group, although over the age of 40, the risk increases to 32 deaths per 100,000 women, compared to 28 associated with pregnancy at that age. However, for pill users who smoke and are over the age of 35, the estimated number of deaths exceeds those for other methods of birth control. If a woman is over the age of 40 and smokes, her estimated risk of death is four times higher (117/100,000 women) than the estimated risk associated with pregnancy (28/100,000 women) in that age group.

The suggestion that women over 40 who don't smoke should not take oral contraceptives is based on information from older higher dose pills and on less selective use of pills than is practiced today. An Advisory Committee of the FDA discussed this issue in 1989 and recommended that the benefits of oral contraceptive use by healthy, non-smoking women over 40 years of age may outweigh the possible risks. However, all women, especially older women, are cautioned to use the lowest dose pill that is effective.

WARNING SIGNALS

If any of these adverse effects occur while you are taking oral contraceptives, call your doctor immediately:

- Sharp chest pain, coughing of blood, or sudden shortness of breath (indicating a possible clot in the lung)
- Pain in the calf (indicating a possible clot in the leg)
- Crushing chest pain or heaviness in the chest (indicating a possible heart attack)
- Sudden severe headache or vomiting, dizziness or fainting, disturbances of vision or speech, weakness, or numbness in an arm or leg (indicating a possible stroke)
- Sudden partial or complete loss of vision (indicating a possible clot in the eye)
- Breast lumps (indicating possible breast cancer or fibrocystic disease of the breast; ask your doctor or health care provider to show you how to examine your breasts)
- Severe pain or tenderness in the stomach area (indicating a possibly ruptured liver tumor)
- Difficulty in sleeping, weakness, lack of energy, fatigue, or change in mood (possibly indicating severe depression)
- Jaundice or a yellowing of the skin or eyeballs, accompanied frequently by fever, fatigue, loss of appetite, dark colored urine, or light colored bowel movements (indicating possible liver problems)

SIDE EFFECTS OF ORAL CONTRACEPTIVES

1. Vaginal Bleeding

Irregular vaginal bleeding or spotting may occur while you are taking the pills. Irregular bleeding may vary from slight staining between menstrual periods to breakthrough bleeding which is a flow much like a regular period. Irregular bleeding occurs most often during the first few months of oral contraceptive use, but may also occur after you have been taking the pill for some time. Such bleeding may be temporary and usually does not indicate serious problems. It is important to continue taking your pills on schedule. If the bleeding occurs in more than one cycle or lasts for more than a few days, talk to your doctor or health care provider.

2. Contact Lenses

If you wear contact lenses and notice a change in vision or an inability to wear your lenses, contact your doctor or health care provider.

3. Fluid Retention

Oral contraceptives may cause edema (fluid retention) with swelling of the fingers or ankles and may raise your blood pressure. If you experience fluid retention, contact your doctor or health care provider.

ANNUAL NUMBER OF BIRTH-RELATED OR METHOD-RELATED DEATHS ASSOCIATED WITH CONTROL OF FERTILITY PER 100,000 NONSTERILE WOMEN BY FERTILITY CONTROL METHOD ACCORDING TO AGE

Method of control and outcome	15–19	20–24	25–29	30–34	35–39	40–44
No fertility control methods*	7.0	7.4	9.1	14.8	25.7	28.2
Oral contraceptives non-smoker**	0.3	0.5	0.9	1.9	13.8	31.6
Oral contraceptives smoker**	2.2	3.4	6.6	13.5	51.1	117.2
IUD**	0.8	0.8	1.0	1.0	1.4	1.4
Condom*	1.1	1.6	0.7	0.2	0.3	0.4
Diaphragm/spermicide*	1.9	1.2	1.2	1.3	2.2	2.8
Periodic abstinence*	2.5	1.6	1.6	1.7	2.9	3.6

*Deaths are birth related.
**Deaths are method related.

If your TABLET DISPENSER contains:	You are taking:
21 white tablets	LOESTRIN 21 1/20
21 green tablets	LOESTRIN 21 1.5/30
21 white tablets and 7 brown tablets	LOESTRIN Fe 1/20
21 green tablets and 7 brown tablets	LOESTRIN Fe 1.5/30

4. Melasma

A spotty darkening of the skin is possible, particularly of the face.

5. Other Side Effects

Other side effects may include change in appetite, headache, nervousness, depression, dizziness, loss of scalp hair, rash, and vaginal infections.

If any of these side effects bother you, call your doctor or health care provider.

GENERAL PRECAUTIONS

1. Missed Periods and Use of Oral Contraceptives Before or During Early Pregnancy

There may be times when you may not menstruate regularly after you have completed taking a cycle of pills. If you have taken your pills regularly and miss one menstrual period, continue taking your pills for the next cycle but be sure to inform your health care provider before doing so. If you have not taken the pills daily as instructed and missed a menstrual period, or if you missed two consecutive menstrual periods, you may be pregnant. Check with your health care provider immediately to determine whether you are pregnant. Do not continue to take oral contraceptives until you are sure you are not pregnant, but continue to use another method of contraception.

There is no conclusive evidence that oral contraceptive use is associated with an increase in birth defects, when taken inadvertently during early pregnancy. Previously, a few studies had reported that oral contraceptives might be associated with birth defects, but these studies have not been confirmed. Nevertheless, oral contraceptives or any other drugs should not be used during pregnancy unless clearly necessary and prescribed by your doctor. You should check with your doctor about risks to your unborn child of any medication taken during pregnancy.

2. While Breast Feeding

If you are breast feeding, consult your doctor before starting oral contraceptives. Some of the drug will be passed on to the child in the milk. A few adverse effects on the child have been reported, including yellowing of the skin (jaundice) and breast enlargement. In addition, oral contraceptives may decrease the amount and quality of your milk. If possible, do not use oral contraceptives while breast feeding. You should use another method of contraception since breast feeding provides only partial protection from becoming pregnant and this partial protection decreases significantly as you breast feed for longer periods of time. You should consider starting oral contraceptives only after you have weaned your child completely.

3. Laboratory Tests

If you are scheduled for any laboratory tests, tell your doctor you are taking birth control pills. Certain blood tests may be affected by birth control pills.

4. Drug Interactions

Certain drugs may interact with birth control pills to make them less effective in preventing pregnancy or cause an increase in breakthrough bleeding. Such drugs include rifampin; drugs used for epilepsy such as barbiturates (for example, phenobarbital), carbamazepine, and phenytoin (Dilantin® is one brand of this drug); troglitazone; phenylbutazone; and possibly certain antibiotics. You may need to use additional contraception when you take drugs which can make oral contraceptives less effective.

Birth control pills interact with certain drugs. These drugs include acetaminophen, clofibric acid, cyclosporine, morphine, prednisolone, salicylic acid, temazepam, and theophylline. You should tell your doctor if you are taking any of these medications.

5. This product (like all oral contraceptives) is intended to prevent pregnancy. It does not protect against transmission of HIV (AIDS) and other sexually transmitted diseases such as chlamydia, genital herpes, genital warts, gonorrhea, hepatitis B, and syphilis.

INSTRUCTIONS TO PATIENT

TABLET DISPENSER

The Loestrin tablet dispenser has been designed to make oral contraceptive dosing as easy and as convenient as possible. The tablets are arranged in either three or four rows of seven tablets each, with the days of the week appearing above the first row of tablets.

[See second table above]

Each *white* tablet contains 1 mg norethindrone acetate and 20 mcg ethinyl estradiol.

Each *green* tablet contains 1.5 mg norethindrone acetate and 30 mcg ethinyl estradiol.

Each *brown* tablet contains 75 mg ferrous fumarate and is intended to help you remember to take the tablets correctly. These brown tablets are not intended to have any health benefit.

DIRECTIONS

To remove a tablet, press down on it with your thumb or finger. The tablet will drop through the back of the tablet dispenser. Do not press with your thumbnail, fingernail, or any other sharp object.

HOW TO TAKE THE PILL

IMPORTANT POINTS TO REMEMBER

BEFORE YOU START TAKING YOUR PILLS:

1. BE SURE TO READ THESE DIRECTIONS:
Before you start taking your pills.
Anytime you are not sure what to do.

2. THE RIGHT WAY TO TAKE THE PILL IS TO TAKE ONE PILL EVERY DAY AT THE SAME TIME. If you miss pills you could get pregnant. This includes starting the pack late. The more pills you miss, the more likely you are to get pregnant.

3. MANY WOMEN HAVE SPOTTING OR LIGHT BLEEDING, OR MAY FEEL SICK TO THEIR STOMACH, DURING THE FIRST 1–3 PACKS OF PILLS. If you do have spotting or light bleeding or feel sick to your stomach, do not stop taking the pill. The problem will usually go away. If it doesn't go away, check with your doctor or clinic.

4. MISSING PILLS CAN ALSO CAUSE SPOTTING OR LIGHT BLEEDING, even when you make up these missed pills. On the days you take 2 pills to make up for missed pills, you could also feel a little sick to your stomach.

5. IF YOU HAVE VOMITING OR DIARRHEA, for any reason, of IF YOU TAKE SOME MEDICINES, including some antibiotics, your birth control pills may not work as well. Use a back-up birth control method (such as condoms or foam) until you check with your doctor or clinic.

6. IF YOU HAVE TROUBLE REMEMBERING TO TAKE THE PILL, talk to your doctor or clinic about how to make pill-taking easier or about using another method of birth control.

7. IF YOU HAVE ANY QUESTIONS OR ARE UNSURE ABOUT THE INFORMATION IN THIS LEAFLET, call your doctor or clinic.

BEFORE YOU START TAKING YOUR PILLS

1. DECIDE WHAT TIME OF DAY YOU WANT TO TAKE YOUR PILL. It is important to take it at about the same time every day.

2. LOOK AT YOUR PILL PACK TO SEE IF IT HAS 21 OR 28 PILLS:
The 21-pill pack has 21 "active" white or green pills (with hormones) to take for 3 weeks, followed by 1 week without pills.
The 28-pill pack has 21 "active" white or green pills (with hormones) to take for 3 weeks, followed by 1 week of reminder brown pills (without hormones).

3. ALSO FIND:
1) where on the pack to start taking pills,
2) in what order to take the pills (follow the arrows), and
3) the week numbers as shown in the following pictures:

[See figure at top of next column]

Loestrin 21 1/20 will contain: **ALL WHITE PILLS**
Loestrin 21 1.5/30 will contain: **ALL GREEN PILLS**

[See figure at top of next column]

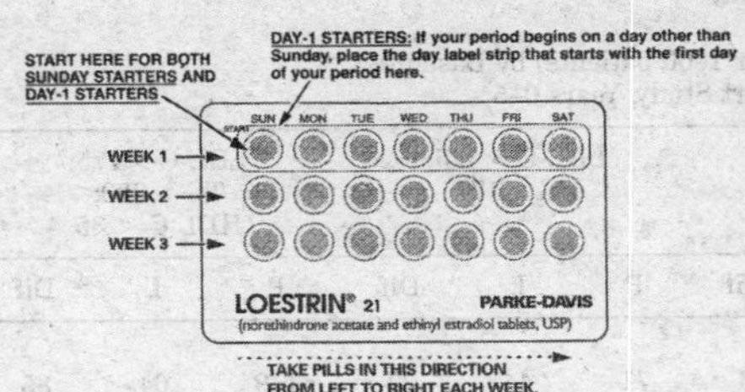
START HERE FOR BOTH SUNDAY STARTERS AND DAY-1 STARTERS
DAY-1 STARTERS: If your period begins on a day other than Sunday, place the day label strip that starts with the first day of your period here.
SUN MON TUE WED THU FRI SAT
WEEK 1
WEEK 2
WEEK 3
LOESTRIN® 21
PARKE-DAVIS
(norethindrone acetate and ethinyl estradiol tablets, USP)
TAKE PILLS IN THIS DIRECTION FROM LEFT TO RIGHT EACH WEEK.

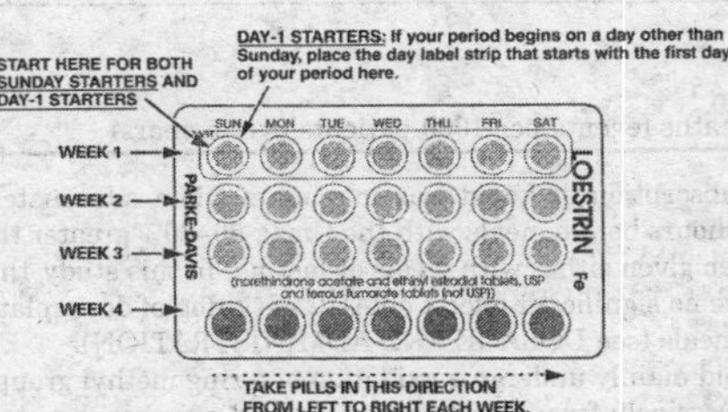
START HERE FOR BOTH SUNDAY STARTERS AND DAY-1 STARTERS
DAY-1 STARTERS: If your period begins on a day other than Sunday, place the day label strip that starts with the first day of your period here.
SUN MON TUE WED THU FRI SAT
WEEK 1
WEEK 2
WEEK 3
WEEK 4
PARKE-DAVIS
LOESTRIN Fe
TAKE PILLS IN THIS DIRECTION FROM LEFT TO RIGHT EACH WEEK.

Loestrin Fe 1/20 will contain: **21 WHITE PILLS** for **WEEKS 1, 2, and 3. WEEK 4** will contain **BROWN PILLS ONLY.**
Loestrin Fe 1.5/30 will contain: **21 GREEN PILLS** for **WEEKS 1, 2, and 3. WEEK 4** will contain **BROWN PILLS ONLY.**
4. BE SURE YOU HAVE READY AT ALL TIMES:
ANOTHER KIND OF BIRTH CONTROL (such as condoms or foam) to use as a back-up in case you miss pills.
An EXTRA, FULL PILL PACK.

WHEN TO START THE FIRST PACK OF PILLS

You have a choice of which day to start taking your first pack of pills. Decide with your doctor or clinic which is the best day for you. Pick a time of day which will be easy to remember.

DAY-1 START:
1. Pick the day label strip that starts with the first day of your period. (This is the day you start bleeding or spotting, even if it is almost midnight when the bleeding begins.)
2. Place this day label strip on the tablet dispenser over the area that has the days of the week (starting with Sunday) printed on the plastic.
3. Take the first "active" white or green pill of the first pack during the first 24 hours of your period.
4. You will not need to use a back-up method of birth control, since you are starting the pill at the beginning of your period.

SUNDAY START:
1. Take the first "active" white or green pill of the first pack on the Sunday after your period starts, even if you are still bleeding. If your period begins on Sunday, start the pack that same day.
2. Use another method of birth control as a back-up method if you have sex anytime from the Sunday you start your first pack until the next Sunday (7 days). Condoms or foam are good back-up methods of birth control.

WHAT TO DO DURING THE MONTH

1. TAKE ONE PILL AT THE SAME TIME EVERY DAY UNTIL THE PACK IS EMPTY.
Do not skip pills even if you are spotting or bleeding between monthly periods or feel sick to your stomach (nausea).
Do not skip pills even if you do not have sex very often.
2. WHEN YOU FINISH A PACK OR SWITCH YOUR BRAND OF PILLS:
21 pills: Wait 7 days to start the next pack. You will probably have your period during that week. Be sure that no more than 7 days pass between 21-day packs.
28 pills: Start the next pack on the day after your last "reminder" pill. Do not wait any days between packs.

WHAT TO DO IF YOU MISS PILLS

If you **MISS 1** white or green "active" pill:
1. Take it as soon as you remember. Take the next pill at your regular time. This means you may take 2 pills in 1 day.
2. You do not need to use a back-up birth control method if you have sex.
If you **MISS 2** white or green "active" pills in a row in **WEEK 1 OR WEEK 2** of your pack:
1. Take 2 pills on the day you remember and 2 pills the next day.
2. Then take 1 pill a day until you finish the pack.
3. You COULD GET PREGNANT if you have sex in the 7 days after you miss pills. You MUST use another birth control method (such as condoms or foam) as a back-up method of birth control until you have taken a white or green "active" pill every day for 7 days.
If you **MISS 2** white or green "active" pills in row in **THE 3rd WEEK:**
1. If you are a Day-1 Starter:
THROW OUT the rest of the pill pack and start a new pack that same day.
If you are a Sunday Starter:
Keep taking 1 pill every day until Sunday. On Sunday, THROW OUT the rest of the pack and start a new pack of pills that same day.
2. You may not have your period this month, but this is expected. However, if you miss your period 2 months in a row, call your doctor or clinic because you might be pregnant.
3. You COULD GET PREGNANT if you have sex in the 7 days after you miss pills. You MUST use another birth control method (such as condoms or foam) as a back-up method of birth control until you have taken a white or green "active" pill every day for 7 days.
If you **MISS 3 OR MORE** white or green "active" pills in row (during the first 3 weeks):
1. If you are a Day-1 Starter:
THROW OUT the rest of the pill pack and start a new pack that same day.
If you are a Sunday Starter:
Keep taking 1 pill every day until Sunday. On Sunday, THROW OUT the rest of the pack and start a new pack of pills that same day.
2. You may not have your period this month, but this is expected. However, if you miss your period 2 months in a row, call your doctor or clinic because you might be pregnant.
3. You COULD GET PREGNANT if you have sex in the 7 days after you miss pills. You MUST use another birth control method (such as condoms or foam) as a back-up method of birth control until you have taken a white or green "active" pill every day for 7 days.

A REMINDER FOR THOSE ON 28-DAY PACKS:
IF YOU FORGET ANY OF THE 7 BROWN "REMINDER" PILLS IN WEEK 4:
THROW AWAY THE PILLS YOU MISSED.
KEEP TAKING 1 PILL EACH DAY UNTIL THE PACK IS EMPTY.
YOU DO NOT NEED A BACK-UP METHOD.

FINALLY, IF YOU ARE STILL NOT SURE WHAT TO DO ABOUT THE PILLS YOU HAVE MISSED:
Use a BACK-UP METHOD anytime you have sex.
KEEP TAKING ONE WHITE OR GREEN "ACTIVE" PILL EACH DAY until you can reach your doctor or clinic.

PREGNANCY DUE TO PILL FAILURE
The incidence of pill failure resulting in pregnancy is approximately 1% (ie, one pregnancy per 100 women per year) if taken every day as directed, but more typical failure rates are about 3%. If failure does occur, the risk to the fetus is minimal.

PREGNANCY AFTER STOPPING THE PILL
There may be some delay in becoming pregnant after you stop using oral contraceptives, especially if you had irregular menstrual cycles before you used oral contraceptives. It may be advisable to postpone conception until you begin menstruating regularly once you have stopped taking the pill and desire pregnancy.
There does not appear to be any increase in birth defects in newborn babies when pregnancy occurs soon after stopping the pill.

OVERDOSAGE
Serious ill effects have not been reported following ingestion of large doses of oral contraceptives by young children. Overdosage may cause nausea and withdrawal bleeding in females. In case of overdosage, contact your health care provider or pharmacist.

OTHER INFORMATION
Your health care provider will take a medical and family history and examine you before prescribing oral contraceptives. The physical examination may be delayed to another time if you request it and your health care provider believes that it is a good medical practice to postpone it. You should be reexamined at least once a year. Be sure to inform your health care provider if there is a family history of any of the conditions listed previously in this leaflet. Be sure to keep all appointments with your health care provider, because this is a time to determine if there are early signs of side effects of oral contraceptive use.
Do not use the drug for any condition other than the one for which it was prescribed. This drug has been prescribed specifically for you; do not give it to others who may want birth control pills.

HEALTH BENEFITS FROM ORAL CONTRACEPTIVES
In addition to preventing pregnancy, use of oral contraceptives may provide certain benefits. They are:
- Menstrual cycles may become more regular
- Blood flow during menstruation may be lighter and less iron may be lost. Therefore, anemia due to iron deficiency is less likely to occur
- Pain or other symptoms during menstruation may be encountered less frequently
- Ectopic (tubal) pregnancy may occur less frequently
- Noncancerous cysts or lumps in the breast may occur less frequently
- Acute pelvic inflammatory disease may occur less frequently
- Oral contraceptive use may provide some protection against developing two forms of cancer: cancer of the ovaries and cancer of the lining of the uterus.

If you want more information about birth control pills, ask your doctor or pharmacist. They have a more technical leaflet called the "Physician Insert," which you may wish to read.
Remembering to take tablets according to schedule is stressed because of its importance in providing you the greatest degree of protection.

MISSED MENSTRUAL PERIODS FOR BOTH DOSAGE REGIMENS
At times there may be no menstrual period after a cycle of pills. Therefore, if you miss one menstrual period but have taken the pills *exactly as you were supposed to*, continue as usual into the next cycle. If you have not taken the pills correctly and miss a menstrual period, *you may be pregnant* and should stop taking oral contraceptives until your doctor or health care provider determines whether or not you are pregnant. Until you can get to your doctor or health care provider, use another form of contraception. If two consecutive menstrual periods are missed, you should stop taking pills until it is determined whether or not you are pregnant. Although there does not appear to be any increase in birth defects in newborn babies, if you become pregnant while using oral contraceptives you should discuss the situation with your doctor or health care provider.

Periodic Examination
Your doctor or health care provider will take a complete medical and family history before prescribing oral contraceptives. At that time and about once a year thereafter, he or she will generally examine your blood pressure, breasts, abdomen, and pelvic organs (including a Papanicolaou smear, ie, test for cancer).
Keep this and all drugs out of the reach of children.
Rx only
Store below 30°C (86°F).
Revised November 1999

PARKE-DAVIS
Div of Warner-Lambert Co ©1997-'99
Morris Plains, NJ 07950 USA

Direct Medical Inquiries to:
Parke-Davis
Warner-Lambert Company
201 Tabor Road, Morris Plains, NJ 07950
Attn: Medical Affairs Department
0913G515

LOPID® ℞
[lō ′pĭd]
(Gemfibrozil Tablets, USP)

DESCRIPTION
Lopid® (gemfibrozil tablets, USP) is a lipid regulating agent. It is available as tablets for oral administration. Each tablet contains 600 mg gemfibrozil. Each also contains calcium stearate, NF; candelilla wax FCC; microcrystalline cellulose, NF; hydroxypropyl cellulose, NF: hydroxypropyl methylcellulose, USP; methylparaben, NF; Opaspray white; polyethylene glycol, NF; polysorbate 80, NF; propylparaben, NF; colloidal silicon dioxide, NF; pregelatinized starch, NF. The chemical name is 5-(2,5-dimethylphenoxy)-2,2-dimethylpentanoic acid with the following structural formula:

[Structural formula: CH3, CH3 on ring; O–CH2–CH2–CH2–C(CH3)(CH3)–COOH]

The empirical formula is $C_{15}H_{22}O_3$ and the molecular weight is 250.35; the solubility in water and acid is 0.0019% and in dilute base it is greater than 1%. The melting point is 58°–61°C. Gemfibrozil is a white solid which is stable under ordinary conditions.

CLINICAL PHARMACOLOGY
Lopid (gemfibrozil tablets, USP) is a lipid regulating agent which decreases serum triglycerides and very low density lipoprotein (VLDL) cholesterol, and increases high density lipoprotein (HDL) cholesterol. While modest decreases in total and low density lipoprotein (LDL) cholesterol may be observed with Lopid therapy, treatment of patients with elevated triglycerides due to Type IV hyperlipoproteinemia often results in a rise in LDL-cholesterol. LDL-cholesterol levels in Type IIb patients with elevations of both serum LDL-cholesterol and triglycerides are, in general, minimally affected by Lopid treatment; however, Lopid usually raises HDL-cholesterol significantly in this group. Lopid increases levels of high density lipoprotein (HDL) subfractions HDL_2 and HDL_3, as well as apolipoproteins AI and AII. Epidemiological studies have shown that both low HDL-cholesterol and high LDL-cholesterol are independent risk factors for coronary heart disease.
In the primary prevention component of the Helsinki Heart Study (refs. 1,2), in which 4081 male patients between the ages of 40 and 55 were studied in a randomized, double-blind, placebo-controlled fashion, Lopid therapy was associated with significant reductions in total plasma triglycerides and a significant increase in high density lipoprotein cholesterol. Moderate reductions in total plasma cholesterol and low density lipoprotein cholesterol were observed for

Continued on next page

This product information was prepared in June 2000. On these and other Parke-Davis Products, information may be obtained by addressing PARKE-DAVIS, a Warner-Lambert Division, Morris Plains, New Jersey 07950.

Lopid—Cont.

the Lopid treatment group as a whole, but the lipid response was heterogeneous, especially among different Fredrickson types. The study involved subjects with serum non-HDL-cholesterol of over 200 mg/dL and no previous history of coronary heart disease. Over the 5-year study period, the Lopid group experienced a 1.4% absolute (34% relative) reduction in the rate of serious coronary events (sudden cardiac deaths plus fatal and nonfatal myocardial infarctions) compared to placebo, p = 0.04 (see Table I). There was a 37% relative reduction in the rate of nonfatal myocardial infarction compared to placebo, equivalent to a treatment-related difference of 13.1 events per thousand persons. Deaths from any cause during the double-blind portion of the study totaled 44 (2.2%) in the Lopid randomization group and 43 (2.1%) in the placebo group.

[See table above]

Table I
Reduction in CHD Rates (events per 1000 patients) by Baseline Lipids[1] in the Helsinki Heart Study, Years 0–5[2]

	All Patients			LDL-C > 175; HDL-C > 46.4			LDL-C > 175; TG > 177			LDL-C > 175; TG > 200; HDL-C < 35		
	P	L	Dif[3]	P	L	Dif	P	L	Dif	P	L	Dif
Incidence of Evidents[4]	41	27	14	32	29	3	71	44	27	149	64	85

[1] lipid values in mg/dL at baseline
[2] P=placebo group; L=Lopid group
[3] difference in rates between placebo and Lopid groups
[4] fatal and nonfatal myocardial infarctions plus sudden cardiac deaths (events per 1000 patients over 5 years)

Among Fredrickson types, during the 5-year double-blind portion of the primary prevention component of the Helsinki Heart Study, the greatest reduction in the incidence of serious coronary events occurred in Type IIb patients who had elevations of both LDL-cholesterol and total plasma triglycerides. This subgroup of Type IIb gemfibrozil group patients had a lower mean HDL-cholesterol level at baseline than the Type IIa subgroup that had elevations of LDL-cholesterol and normal plasma triglycerides. The mean increase in HDL-cholesterol among the Type IIb patients in this study was 12.6% compared to placebo. The mean change in LDL-cholesterol among Type IIb patients was −4.1% with Lopid compared to a rise of 3.9% in the placebo subgroup. The Type IIb subjects in the Helsinki Heart Study had 26 fewer coronary events per thousand persons over 5 years in the gemfibrozil group compared to placebo. The difference in coronary events was substantially greater between Lopid and placebo for that subgroup of patients with the triad of LDL-cholesterol >175 mg/dL (>4.5 mmol), triglycerides >200 mg/dL (>2.2 mmol), and HDL-cholesterol <35 mg/dL (<0.90 mmol) (see Table I).

Further information is available from a 3.5 year (8.5 year cumulative) follow-up of all subjects who had participated in the Helsinki Heart Study. At the completion of the Helsinki Heart study, subjects could choose to start, stop, or continue to receive Lopid; without knowledge of their own lipid values or double-blind treatment, 60% of patients originally randomized to placebo began therapy with Lopid and 60% of patients originally randomized to Lopid continued medication. After approximately 6.5 years following randomization, all patients were informed of their original treatment group and lipid values during the 5 years of the double-blind treatment. After further elective changes in Lopid treatment status, 61% of patients in the group originally randomized to Lopid were taking drug; in the group originally randomized to placebo, 65% were taking Lopid. The event rate per 1000 occurring during the open-label follow-up period is detailed in Table II.

Table II
Cardiac Events and All-Cause Mortality (events per 1000 patients) Occurring During the 3.5 Year Open-Label Follow-up to the Helsinki Heart Study[1]

Group:	PDrop N=215	PN N=494	PL N=1283	LDrop N=221	LN N=574	LL N=1207
Cardiac Events	38.8	22.9	22.5	37.2	28.3	25.4
All-Cause Mortality	41.9	22.3	15.6	72.3	19.2	24.9

[1] The six open-label groups are designated first by the original randomization (P = placebo, L = Lopid) and then by the drug taken in the follow-up period (N = Attend clinic but took no drug, L = Lopid, Drop = No attendance at clinic during open-label).

Cumulative mortality through 8.5 years showed a 20% relative excess of deaths in the group originally randomized to Lopid versus the originally randomized placebo group and a 20% relative decrease in cardiac events in the group originally randomized to Lopid versus the originally randomized placebo group (see Table III). This analysis of the originally randomized "intent-to-treat" population neglects the possible complicating effects of treatment switching during the open-label phase. Adjustment of hazard ratios taking into account open-label treatment status from years 6.5 to 8.5 could change the reported hazard ratios for mortality toward unity.

Table III
Cardiac Events, Cardiac Deaths, Non-Cardiac Deaths and All-Cause Mortality in the Helsinki Heart Study, Year 0–8.5.[1]

Event	Lopid at Study Start	Placebo at Study Start	Lopid: Placebo Hazard Ratio[2]	Cl Hazard[3] Ratio
Cardiac Events[4]	110	131	0.80	0.62–1.03
Cardiac Deaths	36	38	0.98	0.63–1.54
Non-Cardiac Deaths	65	45	1.40	0.95–2.05
All-Cause Mortality	101	83	1.20	0.90–1.61

[1] Intention-to-Treat Analysis of originally randomized patients neglecting the open-label treatment switches and exposure to study conditions.
[2] Hazard ratio for risk of event in the group originally randomized to Lopid compared to the group originally randomized to placebo neglecting open-label treatment switch and exposure to study condition.
[3] 95% confidence intervals of Lopid:placebo group hazard ratio.
[4] Fatal and non-fatal myocardial infarctions plus sudden cardiac deaths over the 8.5 year period.

It is not clear to what extent the findings of the primary prevention component of the Helsinki Heart Study can be extrapolated to other segments of the dyslipidemic population not studied (such as women, younger or older males, or those with lipid abnormalities limited solely to HDL-cholesterol) or to other lipid-altering drugs.

The secondary prevention component of the Helsinki Heart Study was conducted over 5 years in parallel and at the same centers in Finland in 628 middle-aged males excluded from the primary prevention component of the Helsinki Heart Study because of a history of angina, myocardial infarction or unexplained ECG changes (ref. 3). The primary efficacy endpoint of the study was cardiac events (the sum of fatal and non-fatal myocardial infarctions and sudden cardiac deaths). The hazard ratio (Lopid:placebo) for cardiac events was 1.47 (95% confidence limits 0.88–2.48, p = 0.14). Of the 35 patients in the Lopid group who experienced cardiac events, 12 patients suffered events after discontinuation from the study. Of the 24 patients in the placebo group with cardiac events, 4 patients suffered events after discontinuation from the study. There were 17 cardiac deaths in the Lopid group and 8 in the placebo group (hazard ratio 2.18; 95% confidence limits 0.94–5.05, p = 0.06). Ten of these deaths in the Lopid group and 3 in the placebo group occurred after discontinuation from therapy. In this study of patients with known or suspected coronary heart disease, no benefit from Lopid treatment was observed in reducing cardiac events or cardiac deaths. Thus, Lopid has shown benefit only in selected dyslipidemic patients *without* suspected or established coronary heart disease. Even in patients with coronary heart disease and the triad of elevated LDL-cholesterol, elevated triglycerides, plus low HDL-cholesterol, the possible effect of Lopid on coronary events has not been adequately studied.

No efficacy in the patients with established coronary heart disease was observed during the Coronary Drug Project with the chemically and pharmacologically related drug, clofibrate. The Coronary Drug Project was a 6-year randomized, double-blind study involving 1000 clofibrate, 1000 nicotinic acid, and 3000 placebo patients with known coronary heart disease. A clinically and statistically significant reduction in myocardial infarctions was seen in the concurrent nicotinic acid group compared to placebo; no reduction was seen with clofibrate.

The mechanism of action of gemfibrozil has not been definitely established. In man, Lopid has been shown to inhibit peripheral lipolysis and to decrease the hepatic extraction of free fatty acids, thus reducing hepatic triglyceride production. Lopid inhibits synthesis and increases clearance of VLDL carrier apolipoprotein B, leading to a decrease in VLDL production.

Animal studies suggest that gemfibrozil may, in addition to elevating HDL-cholesterol, reduce incorporation of long-chain fatty acids into newly formed triglycerides, accelerate turnover and removal of cholesterol from the liver, and increase excretion of cholesterol in the feces. Lopid is well absorbed from the gastrointestinal tract after oral administration. Peak plasma levels occur in 1 to 2 hours with a plasma half-life of 1.5 hours following multiple doses.

Gemfibrozil is completely absorbed after oral administration of Lopid tablets, reaching peak plasma concentrations 1 to 2 hours after dosing. Gemfibrozil pharmacokinetics are affected by the timing of meals relative to time of dosing. In one study (ref. 4), both the rate and extent of absorption of the drug were significantly increased when administered 0.5 hours before meals. Average AUC was reduced by 14–44% when Lopid was administered after meals compared to 0.5 hours before meals. In a subsequent study (ref. 4), rate of absorption of Lopid was maximum when administered 0.5 hours before meals with the Cmax 50–60% greater than when given either with meals or fasting. In this study, there were no significant effects on AUC of timing of dose relative to meals (see DOSAGE AND ADMINISTRATION).

Lopid mainly undergoes oxidation of a ring methyl group to successively form a hydroxymethyl and a carboxyl metabolite. Approximately seventy percent of the administered human dose is excreted in the urine, mostly as the glucuronide conjugate, with less than 2% excreted as unchanged gemfibrozil. Six percent of the dose is accounted for in the feces. Gemfibrozil is highly bound to plasma proteins and there is potential for displacement interactions with other drugs (see PRECAUTIONS).

INDICATIONS AND USAGE

Lopid (gemfibrozil tablets, USP) is indicated as adjunctive therapy to diet for:

1. Treatment of adult patients with very high elevations of serum triglyceride levels (Types IV and V hyperlipidemia) who present a risk of pancreatitis and who do not respond adequately to a determined dietary effort to control them. Patients who present such risk typically have serum triglycerides over 2000 mg/dL and have elevations of VLDL-cholesterol as well as fasting chylomicrons (Type V hyperlipidemia). Subjects who consistently have total serum or plasma triglycerides below 1000 mg/dL are unlikely to present a risk of pancreatitis. Lopid therapy may be considered for those subjects with triglyceride elevations between 1000 and 2000 mg/dL who have a history of pancreatitis or of recurrent abdominal pain typical of pancreatitis. It is recognized that some Type IV patients with triglycerides under 1000 mg/dL may, through dietary or alcoholic indiscretion, convert to a Type V pattern with massive triglyceride elevations accompanying fasting chylomicronemia, but the influence of Lopid therapy on the risk of pancreatitis in such situations has not been adequately studied. Drug therapy is not indicated for patients with Type I hyperlipoproteinemia, who have elevations of chylomicrons and plasma triglycerides, but who have normal levels of very low density lipoprotein (VLDL). Inspection of plasma refrigerated for 14 hours is helpful in distinguishing Types I, IV, and V hyperlipoproteinemia (ref. 5).
2. Reducing the risk of developing coronary heart disease **only** in Type IIb patients without history of or symptoms of existing coronary heart disease who have had an inadequate response to weight loss, dietary therapy, exercise, and other pharmacologic agents (such as bile acid sequestrants and nicotinic acid, known to reduce LDL- and raise HDL-cholesterol **and** who have the following triad of lipid abnormalities: low HDL-cholesterol levels in addition to elevated LDL-cholesterol and elevated triglycerides (see WARNINGS, PRECAUTIONS, and CLINICAL PHARMACOLOGY). The National Cholesterol Education Program has defined a serum HDL-cholesterol value that is consistently below 35 mg/dL as constituting an independent risk factor for coronary heart disease (ref. 6). Patients with significantly elevated triglycerides should be closely observed when treated with gemfibrozil. In some patients with high triglyceride levels, treatment with gemfibrozil is associated with a significant increase in LDL-cholesterol. BECAUSE OF POTENTIAL TOXICITY SUCH AS MALIGNANCY, GALLBLADDER DISEASE, ABDOMINAL PAIN LEADING TO APPENDECTOMY AND OTHER ABDOMINAL SURGERIES, AN INCREASED INCIDENCE IN NONCORONARY MORTALITY, AND THE 44% RELATIVE INCREASE DURING THE TRIAL PERIOD IN AGE-ADJUSTED ALL-CAUSE MORTALITY SEEN WITH THE CHEMICALLY AND PHARMACOLOGICALLY RELATED DRUG, CLOFIBRATE, THE POTENTIAL BENEFIT OF GEMFIBROZIL IN TREATING TYPE IIA PATIENTS WITH ELEVATIONS OF LDL-CHOLESTEROL ONLY IS NOT LIKELY TO OUTWEIGH THE RISKS. LOPID IS ALSO NOT INDICATED FOR THE TREATMENT OF PATIENTS WITH LOW HDL-CHOLESTEROL AS THEIR ONLY LIPID ABNORMALITY.

In a subgroup analysis of patients in the Helsinki Heart Study with above-median HDL-cholesterol values at baseline (greater than 46.4 mg/dL), the incidence of serious coronary events was similar for gemfibrozil and placebo subgroups (see Table I).

The initial treatment for dyslipidemia is dietary therapy specific for the type of lipoprotein abnormality. Excess body weight and excess alcohol intake may be important factors in hypertriglyceridemia and should be managed prior to any drug therapy. Physical exercise can be an important ancillary measure, and has been associated with rises in HDL-cholesterol. Diseases contributory to hyperlipidemia such as hypothyroidism or diabetes mellitus should be looked for and adequately treated. Estrogen therapy is sometimes associated with massive rises in plasma triglycerides, especially in subjects with familial hypertriglyceridemia. In such cases, discontinuation of estrogen therapy may obviate the need for specific drug therapy of hypertriglyceridemia. The use of drugs should be considered only when reasonable attempts have been made to obtain satisfactory results with nondrug methods. If the decision is made to use drugs, the patient should be instructed that this does not reduce the importance of adhering to diet.

CONTRAINDICATIONS

1. Hepatic or severe renal dysfunction, including primary biliary cirrhosis.
2. Preexisting gallbladder disease (see WARNINGS).
3. Hypersensitivity to gemfibrozil.

WARNINGS

1. Because of chemical, pharmacological, and clinical similarities between gemfibrozil and clofibrate, the adverse findings with clofibrate in two large clinical studies may also apply to gemfibrozil. In the first of those studies, the Coronary Drug Project, 1000 subjects with previous myocardial infarction were treated for 5 years with clofibrate. There was no difference in mortality between the clofibrate-treated subjects and 3000 placebo-treated subjects, but twice as many clofibrate-treated subjects developed cholelithiasis and cholecystitis requiring surgery. In the other study, conducted by the World Health Organization (WHO), 5000 subjects without known coronary heart disease were treated with clofibrate for 5 years and followed one year beyond. There was a statistically significant, 44%, higher age-adjusted total mortality in the clofibrate-treated than in a comparable placebo-treated control group during the trial period. The excess mortality was due to a 33% increase in noncardiovascular causes, including malignancy, post-cholecystectomy complications, and pancreatitis. The higher risk of clofibrate-treated subjects for gallbladder disease was confirmed.
   Because of the more limited size of the Helsinki Heart Study, the observed difference in mortality from any cause between the Lopid and placebo group is not statistically significantly different from the 29% excess mortality reported in the clofibrate group in the separate WHO study at the 9 year follow-up (see CLINICAL PHARMACOLOGY). Noncoronary heart disease related mortality showed an excess in the group originally randomized to Lopid primarily due to cancer deaths observed during the open-label extension.
   During the 5 year primary prevention component of the Helsinki Heart Study mortality from any cause was 44 (2.2%) in the Lopid group and 43 (2.1%) in the placebo group; including the 3.5 year follow-up period since the trial was completed, cumulative mortality from any cause was 101 (4.9%) in the Lopid group and 83 (4.1%) in the group originally randomized to placebo (hazard ratio 1.20 in favor of placebo). Because of the more limited size of the Helsinki Heart Study, the observed difference in mortality from any cause between the Lopid and placebo groups at year-5 or at year-8.5 is not statistically significantly different from the 29% excess mortality reported in the clofibrate group in the separate WHO study at the 9 year follow-up. Noncoronary heart disease related mortality showed an excess in the group originally randomized to Lopid at the 8.5 year follow-up (65 Lopid versus 45 placebo noncoronary deaths).
   The incidence of cancer (excluding basal cell carcinoma) discovered during the trial and in the 3.5 years after the trial was completed was 51 (2.5%) in both originally randomized groups. In addition, there were 16 basal cell carcinomas in the group originally randomized to Lopid and 9 in the group randomized to placebo (p = 0.22). There were 30 (1.5%) deaths attributed to cancer in the group originally randomized to Lopid and 18 (0.9%) in the group originally randomized to placebo (p = 0.11). Adverse outcomes, including coronary events, were higher in gemfibrozil patients in a corresponding study in men with a history of known or suspected coronary heart disease in the secondary prevention component of the Helsinki Heart Study. (See CLINICAL PHARMACOLOGY.)
   A comparative carcinogenicity study was also done in rats comparing three drugs in this class: fenofibrate (10 and 60 mg/kg; 0.3 and 1.6 times the human dose), clofibrate (400 mg/kg; 1.6 times the human dose), and gemfibrozil (250 mg/kg; 1.7 times the human dose). Pancreatic acinar adenomas were increased in males and females on fenofibrate; hepatocellular carcinoma and pancreatic acinar adenomas were increased in males and hepatic neoplastic nodules in females treated with clofibrate; hepatic neoplastic nodules were increased in males and females treated with gemfibrozil while testicular interstitial cell (Leydig cell) tumors were increased in males on all three drugs.
2. A gallstone prevalence substudy of 450 Helsinki Heart Study participants showed a trend toward a greater prevalence of gallstones during the study within the Lopid treatment group (7.5% vs 4.9% for the placebo group, a 55% excess for the gemfibrozil group). A trend toward a greater incidence of gallbladder surgery was observed for the Lopid group (17 vs 11 subjects, a 54% excess). This result did not differ statistically from the increased incidence of cholecystectomy observed in the WHO study in the group treated with clofibrate. Both clofibrate and gemfibrozil may increase cholesterol excretion into the bile leading to cholelithiasis. If cholelithiasis is suspected, gallbladder studies are indicated. Lopid therapy should be discontinued if gallstones are found.
3. Since a reduction of mortality from coronary heart disease has not been demonstrated and because liver and interstitial cell testicular tumors were increased in rats, Lopid should be administered only to those patients described in the INDICATIONS AND USAGE section. If a significant serum lipid response is not obtained, Lopid should be discontinued.
4. Concomitant Anticoagulants—Caution should be exercised when anticoagulants are given in conjunction with Lopid. The dosage of the anticoagulant should be reduced to maintain the prothrombin time at the desired level to prevent bleeding complications. Frequent prothrombin determinations are advisable until it has been definitely determined that the prothrombin level has stabilized.
5. Concomitant therapy with Lopid and Mevacor® (lovastatin) has been associated with rhabdomyolysis, markedly elevated creatine kinase (CK) levels and myoglobinuria, leading in a high proportion of cases to acute renal failure. IN VIRTUALLY ALL PATIENTS WHO HAVE HAD AN UNSATISFACTORY LIPID RESPONSE TO EITHER DRUG ALONE, ANY POTENTIAL LIPID BENEFIT OF COMBINED THERAPY WITH LOVASTATIN AND GEMFIBROZIL DOES NOT OUTWEIGH THE RISKS OF SEVERE MYOPATHY, RHABDOMYOLYSIS, AND ACUTE RENAL FAILURE (see Drug Interactions). The use of fibrates alone, including Lopid, may occasionally be associated with myositis. Patients receiving Lopid and complaining of muscle pain, tenderness, or weakness should have prompt medical evaluation for myositis, including serum creatine kinase level determination. If myositis is suspected or diagnosed, Lopid therapy should be withdrawn.
6. Cataracts—Subcapsular bilateral cataracts occurred in 10% and unilateral in 6.3% of male rats treated with gemfibrozil at 10 times the human dose.

	CAUSAL RELATIONSHIP PROBABLE	CAUSAL RELATIONSHIP NOT ESTABLISHED
General:		weight loss
Cardiac:		extrasystoles
Gastrointestinal:	cholestatic jaundice	pancreatitis hepatoma colitis
Central Nervous System:	dizziness somnolence paresthesia peripheral neuritis decreased libido depression headache	confusion convulsions syncope
Eye:	blurred vision	retinal edema
Genitourinary:	impotence	decreased male fertility renal dysfunction
Musculoskeletal:	myopathy myasthenia myalgia painful extremities arthralgia synovitis rhabdomyolysis (see WARNINGS and Drug Interactions under PRECAUTIONS)	
Clinical Laboratory:	increased creatine phosphokinase increased bilirubin increased liver transaminases (AST [SGOT], ALT [SGPT]) increased alkaline phosphatase	positive antinuclear antibody
Hematopoietic:	anemia leukopenia bone marrow hypoplasia eosinophilia	thrombocytopenia
Immunologic:	angioedema laryngeal edema urticaria	anaphylaxis Lupus-like syndrome vasculitis
Integumentary:	exfoliative dermatitis rash dermatitis pruritus	alopecia photosensitivity

PRECAUTIONS

1. **Initial Therapy**—Laboratory studies should be done to ascertain that the lipid levels are consistently abnormal. Before instituting Lopid therapy, every attempt should be made to control serum lipids with appropriate diet, exercise, weight loss in obese patients, and control of any medical problems such as diabetes mellitus and hypothyroidism that are contributing to the lipid abnormalities.
2. **Continued Therapy**—Periodic determination of serum lipids should be obtained, and the drug withdrawn if lipid response is inadequate after 3 months of therapy.
3. **Drug Interactions—(A) HMG-CoA reductase inhibitors:** Rhabdomyolysis has occurred with combined gemfibrozil and lovastatin therapy. It may be seen as early as 3 weeks after initiation of combined therapy or after several months. In most subjects who have had an unsatisfactory lipid response to either drug alone, the possible benefit of combined therapy with lovastatin (or other HMG-CoA reductase inhibitors) and gemfibrozil does not outweigh the risks of severe myopathy, rhabdomyolysis, and acute renal failure. There is no assurance that periodic monitoring of creatine kinase will prevent the occurrence of severe myopathy and kidney damage.
   (B) **Anticoagulants:** CAUTION SHOULD BE EXERCISED WHEN ANTICOAGULANTS ARE GIVEN IN CONJUNCTION WITH LOPID. THE DOSAGE OF THE ANTICOAGULANT SHOULD BE REDUCED TO MAINTAIN THE PROTHROMBIN TIME AT THE DESIRED LEVEL TO PREVENT BLEEDING COMPLICATIONS. FREQUENT PROTHROMBIN DETERMINATIONS ARE ADVISABLE UNTIL IT HAS BEEN DEFINITELY DETERMINED THAT THE PROTHROMBIN LEVEL HAS STABILIZED.
4. **Carcinogenesis, Mutagenesis, Impairment of Fertility**—Long-term studies have been conducted in rats at 0.2 and 1.3 times the human exposure (based on AUC). Based on two-week toxicokinetic studies, exposure (AUC) of the dose groups was estimated to be 0.2 and 1.3 times the human exposure. The incidence of benign liver nodules and liver carcinomas was significantly increased in high dose male rats. The incidence of liver carcinomas increased also in low dose males, but this increase was not statistically significant (p=0.1). Male rats had a dose-related and statistically significant increase of benign Leydig cell tumors. The higher dose female rats had a significant increase in the combined incidence of benign and malignant liver neoplasms.
   Long-term studies have been conducted in mice at 0.1 and 0.7 times the human exposure (based on AUC). There were no statistically significant differences from controls in the incidence of liver tumors, but the doses tested were lower than those shown to be carcinogenic with other fibrates.
   Electron microscopy studies have demonstrated a florid hepatic peroxisome proliferation following Lopid administration to the male rat. An adequate study to test

Continued on next page

This product information was prepared in June 2000. On these and other Parke-Davis Products, information may be obtained by addressing PARKE-DAVIS, a Warner-Lambert Division, Morris Plains, New Jersey 07950.

Lopid—Cont.

for peroxisome proliferation has not been done in humans, but changes in peroxisome morphology have been observed. Peroxisome proliferation has been shown to occur in humans with either of two other drugs of the fibrate class when liver biopsies were compared before and after treatment in the same individual.

Administration of approximately 0.6 and 2 times the human dose (based on surface area) to male rats for 10 weeks resulted in a dose-related decrease of fertility. Subsequent studies demonstrated that this effect was reversed after a drug-free period of about eight weeks, and it was not transmitted to the offspring.

5. **Pregnancy Category C**—Lopid has been shown to produce adverse effects in rats and rabbits at doses between 0.5 and 3 times the human dose (based on surface area). There are no adequate and well-controlled studies in pregnant women. Lopid should be used during pregnancy only if the potential benefit justifies the potential risk to the fetus.

   Administration of Lopid to female rats at 0.6 and 2 times the human dose (based on surface area) before and throughout gestation caused a dose-related decrease in conception rate and, at the high dose, an increase in stillborns and a slight reduction in pup weight during lactation. There were also dose-related increased skeletal variations. Anophthalmia occurred, but rarely.

   Administration of 0.6 and 2 times the human dose (based on surface area) of Lopid to female rats from gestation day 15 through weaning caused dose-related decreases in birth weight and suppressions of pup growth during lactation.

   Administration of 1 and 3 times the human dose (based on surface area) of Lopid to female rabbits during organogenesis caused a dose-related decrease in litter size and, at the high dose, an increased incidence of parietal bone variations.
6. **Nursing Mothers**—It is not known whether this drug is excreted in human milk. Because many drugs are excreted in human milk and because of the potential for tumorigenicity shown for Lopid in animal studies, a decision should be made whether to discontinue nursing or to discontinue the drug, taking into account the importance of the drug to the mother.
7. **Hematologic Changes**—Mild hemoglobin, hematocrit and white blood cell decreases have been observed in occasional patients following initiation of Lopid therapy. However, these levels stabilize during long-term administration. Rarely, severe anemia, leukopenia, thrombocytopenia, and bone marrow hypoplasia have been reported. Therefore, periodic blood counts are recommended during the first 12 months of Lopid administration.
8. **Liver Function**—Abnormal liver function tests have been observed occasionally during Lopid administration, including elevations of AST (SGOT), ALT (SGPT), LDH, bilirubin, and alkaline phosphatase. These are usually reversible when Lopid is discontinued. Therefore periodic liver function studies are recommended and Lopid therapy should be terminated if abnormalities persist.
9. **Kidney Function**—There have been reports of worsening renal insufficiency upon the addition of Lopid therapy in individuals with baseline plasma creatinine >2.0 mg/dL. In such patients, the use of alternative therapy should be considered against the risks and benefits of a lower dose of Lopid.
10. **Use in Pediatric Patients**—Safety and efficacy in pediatric patients have not been established.

ADVERSE REACTIONS

In the double-blind controlled phase of the primary prevention component of the Helsinki Heart Study, 2046 patients received Lopid for up to 5 years. In that study, the following adverse reactions were statistically more frequent in subjects in the Lopid group:

	LOPID (N=2046)	PLACEBO (N=2035)
	Frequency in percent of subjects	
Gastrointestinal reactions	34.2	23.8
Dyspepsia	19.6	11.9
Abdominal pain	9.8	5.6
Acute appendicitis (histologically confirmed in most cases where data were available)	1.2	0.6
Atrial fibrillation	0.7	0.1

Adverse events reported by more than 1% of subjects, but without a significant difference between groups:

Diarrhea	7.2	6.5
Fatigue	3.8	3.5
Nausea/Vomiting	2.5	2.1
Eczema	1.9	1.2
Rash	1.7	1.3
Vertigo	1.5	1.3
Constipation	1.4	1.3
Headache	1.2	1.1

Gallbladder surgery was performed in 0.9% of Lopid and 0.5% of placebo subjects in the primary prevention component, a 64% excess, which is not statistically different from the excess of gallbladder surgery observed in the clofibrate compared to the placebo group of the WHO study. Gallbladder surgery was also performed more frequently in the Lopid group compared to placebo (1.9% vs 0.3%, p = 0.07) in the secondary prevention component. A statistically significant increase in appendectomy in the gemfibrozil group was seen also in the secondary prevention component (6 on gemfibrozil vs 0 on placebo, p = 0.014).

Nervous system and special senses adverse reactions were more common in the Lopid group. These included hypesthesia, paresthesias, and taste perversion. Other adverse reactions that were more common among Lopid treatment group subjects but where a causal relationship was not established include cataracts, peripheral vascular disease, and intracerebral hemorrhage.

From other studies it seems probable that Lopid is causally related to the occurrence of MUSCULOSKELETAL SYMPTOMS (see WARNINGS), and to ABNORMAL LIVER FUNCTION TESTS and HEMATOLOGIC CHANGES (see PRECAUTIONS).

Reports of viral and bacterial infections (common cold, cough, urinary tract infections) were more common in gemfibrozil treated patients in other controlled clinical trials of 805 patients. Additional adverse reactions that have been reported for gemfibrozil are listed below by system. These are categorized according to whether a causal relationship to treatment with Lopid is probable or not established:

[See table at top of previous page]

DOSAGE AND ADMINISTRATION

The recommended dose for adults is 1200 mg administered in two divided doses 30 minutes before the morning and evening meal (see CLINICAL PHARMACOLOGY).

OVERDOSAGE

There have been reported cases of overdosage with Lopid. In one case a 7 year old child recovered after ingesting up to 9 grams of Lopid. Symptomatic supportive measures should be taken should an overdose occur.

HOW SUPPLIED

Lopid (Tablet 737), white, elliptical, film-coated, scored tablets, each containing 600 mg gemfibrozil, are available as follows:

N 0071-0737-20: Bottles of 60
N 0071-0737-30: Bottles of 500
Parcode No. 737

Storage: Store at controlled room temperature 20°–25° C (68°–77° F) [see USP]. Protect from light and humidity.

REFERENCES

1. Frick MH, Elo O, Haapa K, et al: Helsinki Heart Study: Primary prevention trial with gemfibrozil in middle-aged men with dyslipidemia. *N Engl J Med* 1987; 317:1237-1245.
2. Manninen V, Elo O, Frick MH, et al: Lipid alterations and decline in the incidence of coronary heart disease in the Helsinki Heart Study. *JAMA* 1988; 260:641-651.
3. Frick MH, Heinonen OP, et al: Efficacy of Gemfibrozil in Dyslipidemic Subjects with Suspected Heart Disease. An Ancillary Study in the Helsinki Heart Study Frame Population. *Annals of Medicine* 1993; 25:41–45.
4. Data on file. Parke-Davis; Morris Plains, NJ
5. Nikkila EA: Familial lipoprotein lipase deficiency and related disorders of chylomicron metabolism. In Stanbury J.B. et al. (eds.): *The Metabolic Basis of Inherited Disease,* 5th ed., McGraw-Hill, 1983, Chap. 30, pp. 622-642.
6. Report of the National Cholesterol Education Program Expert Panel on Detection, Evaluation, and Treatment of High Blood Cholesterol. *Arch Int Med* 1988;148:36-69.

℞ only

Revised May 1999
Manufactured by:
Parke Davis Pharmaceuticals, Ltd.
Vega Baja, PR 00694
Distributed by:
PARKE-DAVIS
Div of Warner-Lambert Co
Morris Plains, NJ 07950 USA

0737G303

Shown in Product Identification Guide, page 329

NARDIL® ℞

(Phenelzine Sulfate Tablets, USP)

DESCRIPTION

Nardil® (phenelzine sulfate) is a potent inhibitor of monoamine oxidase (MAO). Phenelzine sulfate is a hydrazine derivative. It is a molecular weight of 234.27 and is chemically described as $C_8H_{12}N_2{\cdot}N_2SO_4$. Its chemical structure is shown below:

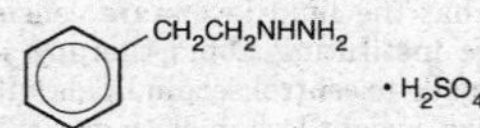

Molecular weight: 234.27

Each Nardil tablet for oral administration contains phenelzine sulfate equivalent to 15 mg of phenelzine base. Inactive ingredients include: acacia NF; calcium carbonate; carnauba wax, NF; corn-starch, NF; FD and C yellow No. 6; gelatin, NF; kaolin, USP; magnesium stearate, NF; mannitol, USP; pharmaceutical glaze, NF; povidone, USP; sucrose, NF; talc, USP; white wax, NF; white wheat flour.

CLINICAL PHARMACOLOGY

Monoamine oxidase is a complex enzyme system, widely distributed throughout the body. Drugs that inhibit monoamine oxidase in the laboratory are associated with a number of clinical effects. Thus, it is unknown whether MAO inhibition per se, other pharmacologic actions, or an interaction of both is responsible for the clinical effects observed. Therefore, the physician should become familiar with all the effects produced by drugs of this class.

INDICATIONS AND USAGE

Nardil has been found to be effective in depressed patients clinically characterized as "atypical," "nonendogenous," or "neurotic." These patients often have mixed anxiety and depression and phobic or hypochondriacal features. There is less conclusive evidence of its usefulness with severely depressed patients with endogenous features.

Nardil should rarely be the first antidepressant drug used. Rather, it is more suitable for use with patients who have failed to respond to the drugs more commonly used for these conditions.

CONTRAINDICATIONS

Nardil should not be used in patients who are hypersensitive to the drug or its ingredients, with pheochromocytoma, congestive heart failure, a history of liver disease, or abnormal liver function tests.

The potentiation of sympathomimetic substances and related compounds by MAO inhibitors may result in hypertensive crises (see WARNINGS). Therefore, patients being treated with Nardil should not take sympathomimetic drugs (including amphetamines, cocaine, methylphenidate, dopamine, epinephrine and norepinephrine) or related compounds (including methyldopa, L-dopa, L-tryptophan, L-tyrosine, and phenylalanine). Hypertensive crises during Nardil therapy may also be caused by the ingestion of foods with a high concentration of tyramine or dopamine. Therefore, patients being treated with Nardil should avoid high protein food that has undergone protein breakdown by aging, fermentation, pickling, smoking, or bacterial contamination. Patients should also avoid cheeses (especially aged varieties), pickled herring, beer, wine, liver, yeast extract (including brewer's yeast in large quantities), dry sausage (including Genoa salami, hard salami, pepperoni, and Lebanon bologna), pods of broad beans (fava beans), and yogurt. Excessive amounts of caffeine and chocolate may also cause hypertensive reactions.

Nardil should not be used in combination with dextromethorphan or with CNS depressants such as alcohol and certain narcotics. Excitation, seizures, delirium, hyperpyrexia, circulatory collapse, coma, and death have been reported in patients receiving MAOI therapy who have been given a single dose of meperidine. Nardil should not be administered together with or in rapid succession to other MAO inhibitors because HYPERTENSIVE CRISES and convulsive seizures, fever, marked sweating, excitation, delirium, tremor, coma, and circulatory collapse may occur.

A List of MAO Inhibitors by generic name follows:

pargyline hydrochloride
pargyline hydrochloride
  and methylclothiazide
furazolidone
isocarboxazid
procarbazine
tranylcypromine

Nardil should also not be used in combination with buspirone HCl, since several cases of elevated blood pressure have been reported in patients taking MAO inhibitors who were then given buspirone HCl. At least 10 days should elapse between the discontinuation of Nardil and the institution of another antidepressant or buspirone HCl, or the discontinuation of another MAO inhibitor and the institution of Nardil.

There have been reports of serious reactions (including hyperthermia, rigidity, myoclonic movements and death) when serotoninergic drugs (e.g., dexfenfluramine, fluoxetine, fluvoxamine, paroxetine, sertraline, venlafaxine) have been combined with an MAO inhibitor. Therefore the concomitant use of Nardil with serotoninergic agents is contraindicated (see PRECAUTIONS—*Drug Interactions*). Allow at least five weeks between discontinuation of fluoxetine and initiation of Nardil and at least 10 days between discontinuation of Nardil and initiation of fluoxetine, or other serotoninergic agents. Before initiating Nardil after using other serotoninergic agents, a sufficient amount of time must be allowed for clearance of the serotoninergic agent and its active metabolites.

The combination of MAO inhibitors and tryptophan has been reported to cause behavioral and neurologic syndromes including disorientation, confusion, amnesia, delirium, agitation, hypomanic signs, ataxia, myoclonus, hyperreflexia, shivering, ocular oscillations, and Babinski signs.

The concurrent administration of an MAO inhibitor and bupropion hydrochloride (Wellbutrin®) is contraindicated. At least 14 days should elapse between discontinuation of an MAO inhibitor and initiation of treatment with bupropion hydrochloride.

Patients taking Nardil should not undergo elective surgery requiring general anesthesia. Also, they should not be given cocaine or local anesthesia containing sympathomimetic vasoconstrictors. The possible combined hypotensive effects

of Nardil and spinal anesthesia should be kept in mind. Nardil should be discontinued at least 10 days prior to elective surgery.
MAO inhibitors, including Nardil, are contraindicated in patients receiving guanethidine.

WARNINGS

The most serious reactions to Nardil involve changes in blood pressure.
Hypertensive Crises: The most important reaction associated with Nardil administration is the occurrence of hypertensive crises, which have sometimes been fatal.
These crises are characterized by some or all of the following symptoms: occipital headache which may radiate frontally, palpitation, neck stiffness or soreness, nausea, vomiting, sweating (sometimes with fever and sometimes with cold, clammy skin), dilated pupils, and photophobia. Either tachycardia or bradycardia may be present and can be associated with constricting chest pain.
NOTE: Intracranial bleeding has been reported in association with the increase in blood pressure.
Blood pressure should be observed frequently to detect evidence of any pressor response in all patients receiving Nardil. Therapy should be discontinued immediately upon the occurrence of palpitation or frequent headaches during therapy.
Recommended treatment in hypertensive crisis: If a hypertensive crisis occurs, Nardil should be discontinued immediately and therapy to lower blood pressure should be instituted immediately. On the basis of present evidence, phentolamine is recommended. (The dosage reported for phentolamine is 5 mg intravenously.) Care should be taken to administer this drug slowly in order to avoid producing an excessive hypotensive effect. Fever should be managed by means of external cooling.
Warning to the Patient: All patients should be warned that the following foods, beverages, and medications must be avoided while taking Nardil, and for two weeks after discontinuing use.
Foods and Beverages To Avoid
Meat and Fish
Pickled herring
Liver
Dry sausage (including Genoa salami, hard salami, pepperoni, and Lebanon bologna)
Vegetables
Broad bean pods (fava bean pods)
Sauerkraut
Dairy Products
Cheese (cottage cheese and cream cheese are allowed)
Yogurt
Beverages
Beer and wine
Alcohol-free and reduced-alcohol beer and wine products
Miscellaneous
Yeast extract (including brewer's yeast in large quantities)
Meat extract
Excessive amounts of chocolate and caffeine
Also, any spoiled or improperly refrigerated, handled, or stored protein-rich foods such as meats, fish, and dairy products, including foods that may have undergone protein changes by aging, pickling, fermentation, or smoking to improve flavor should be avoided.
OTC Medications To Avoid
Cold and cough preparations (including those containing dextromethorphan)
Nasal decongestants (tablets, drops, or spray)
Hay-fever medications
Sinus medications
Asthma inhalant medications
Antiappetite medicines
Weight-reducing preparations
"Pep" pills
L-tryptophan containing preparations
Also, certain prescription drugs should be avoided. Therefore, patients under the care of another physician or dentist should inform him/her they are taking Nardil.
Patients should be warned that the use of the above foods, beverages, or medications may cause a reaction characterized by headache and other serious symptoms due to a rise in blood pressure, with the exception of dextromethorphan which may cause reactions similar to those seen with meperidine. Also, there has been a report of an interaction between Nardil and dextromethorphan (ingested as a lozenge) causing drowsiness and bizarre behavior.
Patients should be instructed to report promptly the occurrence of headache or other unusual symptoms.
Concomitant Use with Dibenzazepine Derivative Drugs
If the decision is made to administer Nardil concurrently with other antidepressant drugs, or within less than 10 days after discontinuation of antidepressant therapy, the patient should be cautioned by the physician regarding the possibility of adverse drug interaction.
A List of Dibenzazepine Derivative Drugs by generic name follows:
nortriptyline hydrochloride
amitriptyline hydrochloride
amitriptyline hydrochloride
perphenazine and amitriptyline hydrochloride
perphenazine and amitriptyline hydrochloride
clomipramine hydrochloride
desipramine hydrochloride
desipramine hydrochloride
imipramine hydrochloride
doxepin
doxepin
carbamazepine
cyclobenzaprine HCl
amoxapine
maprotiline HCl
trimipremine maleate
protriptyline HCl
mirtazapine

Nardil should be used with caution in combination with antihypertensive drugs, including thiazide diuretics and β-blockers, since exaggerated hypotensive effects may result.
Use in Pregnancy: The safe use of Nardil during pregnancy or lactation has not been established. The potential benefit of this drug, if used during pregnancy, lactation, or in women of childbearing age, should be weighed against the possible hazard to the mother or fetus.
Doses of Nardil in pregnant mice well exceeding the maximum recommended human dose have caused a significant decrease in the number of viable offspring per mouse. In addition, the growth of young dogs and rats has been retarded by doses exceeding the maximum human dose.
Use in Pediatric Patients: Nardil is not recommended for pediatric patients under 16 years of age, since there are no controlled studies of safety in this age group. Nardil, as with other hydrazine derivatives, has been reported to induce pulmonary and vascular tumors in an uncontrolled lifetime study in mice.

PRECAUTIONS

In depressed patients, the possibility of suicide should always be considered and adequate precautions taken. It is recommended that careful observations of patients undergoing Nardil treatment be maintained until control of depression is achieved. If necessary, additional measures (ECT, hospitalization, etc) should be instituted.
All patients undergoing treatment with Nardil should be closely followed for symptoms of postural hypotension. Hypotensive side effects have occurred in hypertensive as well as normotensive and hypotensive patients. Blood pressure usually returns to pretreatment levels rapidly when the drug is discontinued or the dosage is reduced.
Because the effect of Nardil on the convulsive threshold may be variable, adequate precautions should be taken when treating epileptic patients.
Of the more severe side effects that have been reported with any consistency, hypomania has been the most common. This reaction has been largely limited to patients in whom disorders characterized by hyperkinetic symptoms coexist with, but are obscured by, depressive affect; hypomania usually appeared as depression improved. If agitation is present, it may be increased with Nardil. Hypomania and agitation have also been reported at higher than recommended doses or following long-term therapy.
Nardil may cause excessive stimulation in schizophrenic patients; in manic-depressive states it may result in a swing from a depressive to a manic phase.
MAO inhibitors, including Nardil, potentiate hexobarbital hypnosis in animals. Therefore, barbiturates should be given at a reduced dose with Nardil.
MAO inhibitors inhibit the destruction of serotonin and norepinephrine, which are believed to be released from tissue stores by rauwolfia alkaloids. Accordingly, caution should be exercised when rauwolfia is used concomitantly with an MAO inhibitor, including Nardil.
There is conflicting evidence as to whether or not MAO inhibitors affect glucose metabolism or potentiate hypoglycemic agents. This should be kept in mind if Nardil is administered to diabetics.

Drug Interactions

In patients receiving nonselective monoamine oxidase (MOA) inhibitors in combination with serotoninergic agents (e.g., dexfenfluramine, fluoxetine, fluvoxamine, paroxetine, sertraline, venlafexine) there have been reports of serious, sometimes fatal, reactions. Because Nardil is a monoamine oxidase (MAO) inhibitor, Nardil should not be used concomitantly with a serotoninergic agent (See CONTRAINDICATIONS).

Geriatric Use

Clinical studies of Nardil did not include sufficient numbers of subjects aged 65 and over to determine whether they respond differently from younger subjects. Other reported clinical experience has not identified differences in responses between the elderly and younger patients. In general, dose selection for an elderly patient should be cautious, usually starting at the low end of the dosing range, reflecting the greater frequency of decreased hepatic, renal, or cardiac function, and of concomitant disease or other drug therapy.

ADVERSE REACTIONS

Nardil is a potent inhibitor of monoamine oxidase. Because this enzyme is widely distributed throughout the body, diverse pharmacologic effects can be expected to occur. When they occur, such effects tend to be mild or moderate in severity (see below), often subside as treatment continues, and can be minimized by adjusting dosage; rarely is it necessary to institute counteracting measures or to discontinue Nardil.
Common side effects include:
Nervous System —Dizziness, headache, drowsiness, sleep disturbances (including insomnia and hypersomnia), fatigue, weakness, tremors, twitching, myoclonic movements, hyperreflexia.
Gastrointestinal —Constipation, dry mouth, gastrointestinal disturbances, elevated serum transaminases (without accompanying signs and symptoms).
Metabolic —Weight gain.
Cardiovascular —Postural hypotension, edema.
Genitourinary —Sexual disturbances, eg, anorgasmia and ejaculatory disturbances and impotence.
Less common mild to moderate side effects (some of which have been reported in a single patient or by a single physician) include:
Nervous System —Jitteriness, palilalia, euphoria, nystagmus, paresthesias.
Genitourinary —Urinary retention.
Metabolic—Hypernatremia.
Dermatologic —Pruritus, Skin rash, sweating.
Special Senses —Blurred vision, glaucoma.
Although reported less frequently, and sometimes only once, additional severe side effects include:
Nervous System —Ataxia, shock-like coma, toxic delirium, manic reaction, convulsions, acute anxiety reaction, precipitation of schizophrenia, transient respiratory and cardiovascular depression following ECT.
Gastrointestinal —To date, fatal progressive necrotizing hepatocellular damage has been reported in a very few patients. Reversible jaundice.
Hematologic —Leukopenia.
Immunologic —Lupus-like syndrome.
Metabolic —Hypermetabolic syndrome (which may include, but is not limited to, hyperpyrexia, tachycardia, tachypnea, muscular rigidity, elevated CK levels, metabolic acidosis, hypoxia, coma and may resemble an overdose).
Respiratory —Edema of the glottis.
General —Fever associated with increased muscle tone.
Withdrawal may be associated with nausea, vomiting, and malaise.
An uncommon withdrawal syndrome following abrupt withdrawal of Nardil has been infrequently reported. Signs and symptoms of this syndrome generally commence 24 to 72 hours after drug discontinuation and may range from vivid nightmares with agitation to frank psychosis and convulsions. This syndrome generally responds to reinstitution of low-dose Nardil therapy followed by cautious downward titration and discontinuation.

DOSAGE AND ADMINISTRATION

Initial dose: The usual starting dose of Nardil is one tablet (15 mg) three times a day.
Early phase treatment: Dosage should be increased to at least 60 mg per day at a fairly rapid pace consistent with patient tolerance. It may be necessary to increase dosage up to 90 mg per day to obtain sufficient MAO inhibition. Many patients do not show a clinical response until treatment at 60 mg has been continued for at least 4 weeks.
Maintenance dose: After maximum benefit from Nardil is achieved, dosage should be reduced slowly over several weeks. Maintenance dose may be as low as one tablet, 15 mg, a day or every other day, and should be continued for as long as is required.

OVERDOSAGE

Note—For management of *hypertensive crises* see WARNINGS section.
Accidental or intentional overdosage may be more common in patients who are depressed. It should be remembered that multiple drugs and/or alcohol may have been ingested. Depending on the amount of overdosage with Nardil, a varying and mixed clinical picture may develop, including signs and symptoms of central nervous system and cardiovascular stimulation and/or depression. Signs and symptoms may be absent or minimal during the initial 12-hour period following ingestion and may develop slowly thereafter, reaching a maximum in 24–48 hours. Death has been reported following overdosage. Therefore, immediate hospitalization, with continuous patient observation and monitoring throughout this period, is essential.
Signs and symptoms of overdosage may include, alone or in combination, any of the following: drowsiness, dizziness, faintness, irritability, hyperactivity, agitation, severe headache, hallucinations, trismus, opisthotonus, rigidity, convulsions, and coma; rapid and irregular pulse, hypertension, hypotension, and vascular collapse; precordial pain, respiratory depression and failure, hyperpyrexia, diaphoresis, and cool, clammy skin.
Treatment: Intensive symptomatic and supportive treatment may be required. Induction of emesis or gastric lavage with instillation of charcoal slurry may be helpful in early poisoning, provided the airway has been protected against aspiration. Signs and symptoms of central nervous system stimulation, including convulsions, should be treated with diazepam, given slowly intravenously. Phenothiazine de-

Continued on next page

This product information was prepared in June 2000. On these and other Parke-Davis Products, information may be obtained by addressing PARKE-DAVIS, a Warner-Lambert Division, Morris Plains, New Jersey 07950.

Nardil—Cont.

rivatives and central nervous system stimulants should be avoided. Hypotension and vascular collapse should be treated with intravenous fluids and, if necessary, blood pressure titration with an intravenous infusion of dilute pressor agent. It should be noted that adrenergic agents may produce a markedly increased pressor response.

Respiration should be supported by appropriate measures, including management of the airway, use of supplemental oxygen, and mechanical ventilatory assistance, as required. Body temperature should be monitored closely. Intensive management of hyperpyrexia may be required. Maintenance of fluid and electrolyte balance is essential.

There are no data on the lethal dose in man. The pathophysiologic effects of massive overdosage may persist for several days, since the drug acts by inhibiting physiologic enzyme systems. With symptomatic and supportive measures, recovery from *mild* overdosage may be expected within 3 to 4 days.

Hemodialysis, peritoneal dialysis, and charcoal hemoperfusion may be of value in massive overdosage, but sufficient data are not available to recommend their routine use in these cases.

Toxic blood levels of phenelzine have not been established, and assay methods are not practical for clinical or toxicological use.

HOW SUPPLIED

Each Nardil tablet is orange, biconvex, glossy sugar-coated, and imprinted with "P-D 270" in brown ink and contains phenelzine sulfate equivalent to 15 mg of phenelzine base.

N 0071-0270-24 Bottles of 100

Storage: Store between 15°–30° C (59°–86°F).

Rx only

US Patent 3,314,855

Revised August 1998 0270G081

Shown in Product Identification Guide, page 329

NEURONTIN® ℞
(Gabapentin) Capsules

DESCRIPTION

Neurontin® (gabapentin) capsules and Neurontin® (gabapentin) tablets is supplied as imprinted hard shell capsules containing

100 mg, 300 mg, and 400 mg or elliptical film-coated tablets containing 600 mg and 800 mg of gabapentin.

The inactive ingredients for the capsules are lactose, cornstarch, and talc. The 100-mg capsule shell contains gelatin and titanium dioxide. The 300-mg capsule shell contains gelatin, titanium dioxide, and yellow iron oxide. The 400-mg capsules shell contains gelatin, red iron oxide, titanium dioxide, and yellow iron oxide. The imprinting ink contains FD&C Blue No. 2 and titanium dioxide.

The inactive ingredients for the tablets are poloxamer 407, copolyvidonium, cornstarch, magnesium stearate, hydroxypropyl cellulose, talc, candelilla wax and purified water. The imprinting ink for the 600 mg tablets contains synthetic black iron oxide, pharmaceutical shellac, pharmaceutical glaze, propylene glycol, ammonium hydroxide, isopropyl alcohol and n-butyl alcohol. The imprinting ink for the 800 mg tablets contains synthetic yellow iron oxide, synthetic red iron oxide, hydroxypropyl methylcellulose, propylene glycol, methanol, isopropyl alcohol and deionized water.

Gabapentin is described as 1-(aminomethyl)cyclohexaneacetic acid with an empirical formula of $C_9H_{17}NO_2$ and a molecular weight of 171.24. The molecular structure of gabapentin is:

CH_2NH_2

CH_2CO_2H

Gabapentin is a white to off-white crystalline solid. It is freely soluble in water and both basic and acidic aqueous solutions.

CLINICAL PHARMACOLOGY

Mechanism of Action

The mechanism by which gabapentin exerts its anticonvulsant action is unknown, but in animal test systems designed to detect anticonvulsant activity, gabapentin prevents seizures as do other marketed anticonvulsants. Gabapentin exhibits antiseizure activity in mice and rats in both the maximal electroshock and pentylenetetrazole seizure models and other preclinical models (e.g., strains with genetic epilepsy, etc.). The relevance of these models to human epilepsy is not known.

Gabapentin is structurally related to the neurotransmitter GABA (gamma-aminobutyric acid) but it does not interact with GABA receptors, it is not converted metabolically into GABA or a GABA agonist, and it is not an inhibitor of GABA uptake or degradation. Gabapentin was tested in radioligand binding assays at concentrations up to 100 µM and did not exhibit affinity for a number of other common receptor sites, including benzodiazepine, glutamate, N-methyl-D-aspartate (NMDA), quisqualate, kainate, strychnine-insensitive or strychnine-sensitive glycine, alpha 1, alpha 2, or beta adrenergic, adenosine A1 or A2, cholinergic muscarinic or nicotinic, dopamine D1 or D2, histamine H1, serotonin S1 or S2, opiate mu, delta or kappa, voltage-sensitive calcium channel sites labeled with nitrendipine or diltiazem, or at voltage-sensitive sodium channel sites with batrachotoxinin A 20-alpha-benzoate.

Several test systems ordinarily used to assess activity at the NMDA receptor have been examined. Results are contradictory. Accordingly, no general statement about the effects, if any, of gabapentin at the NMDA receptor can be made.

In vitro studies with radiolabeled gabapentin have revealed a gabapentin binding site in areas of rat brain including neocortex and hippocampus. The identity and function of this binding site remain to be elucidated.

Pharmacokinetics and Drug Metabolism

All pharmacological actions following gabapentin administration are due to the activity of the parent compound; gabapentin is not appreciably metabolized in humans.

Oral Bioavailability: Gabapentin bioavailability is not dose proportional; i.e., as dose is increased, bioavailability decreases. A 400-mg dose, for example, is about 25% less bioavailable than a 100-mg dose. Over the recommended dose range of 300 to 600 mg T.I.D., however, the differences in bioavailability are not large, and bioavailability is about 60 percent. Food has no effect on the rate and extent of absorption of gabapentin.

Distribution: Gabapentin circulates largely unbound (<3%) to plasma protein. The apparent volume of distribution of gabapentin after 150 mg intravenous administration is 58±6 L (Mean ±SD). In patients with epilepsy, steady-state predose (Cmin) concentrations of gabapentin in cerebrospinal fluid were approximately 20% of the corresponding plasma concentrations.

Elimination: Gabapentin is eliminated from the systemic circulation by renal excretion as unchanged drug. Gabapentin is not appreciably metabolized in humans.

Gabapentin elimination half-life is 5 to 7 hours and is unaltered by dose or following multiple dosing. Gabapentin elimination rate constant, plasma clearance, and renal clearance are directly proportional to creatinine clearance (see Special Populations: Patients With Renal Insufficiency, below). In elderly patients, and in patients with impaired renal function, gabapentin plasma clearance is reduced. Gabapentin can be removed from plasma by hemodialysis.

Dosage adjustment in patients with compromised renal function or undergoing hemodialysis is recommended (see DOSAGE AND ADMINISTRATION, Table 2).

Special Populations: *Patients With Renal Insufficiency:* Subjects (N = 60) with renal insufficiency (mean creatinine clearance ranging from 13–114 mL/min) were administered single 400-mg oral doses of gabapentin. The mean gabapentin half-life ranged from about 6.5 hours (patients with creatinine clearance >60 mL/min) to 52 hours (creatinine clearance <30 mL/min) and gabapentin renal clearance from about 90 mL/min (>60 mL/min group) to about 10 mL/min (<30 mL/min). Mean plasma clearance (CL/F) decreased from approximately 190 mL/min to 20 mL/min.

Dosage adjustment in patients with compromised renal function is necessary (see DOSAGE AND ADMINISTRATION).

Hemodialysis: In a study in anuric subjects (N = 11), the apparent elimination half-life of gabapentin on nondialysis days was about 132 hours; dialysis three times a week (4 hours duration) lowered the apparent half-life of gabapentin by about 60%, from 132 hours to 51 hours. Hemodialysis thus has a significant effect on gabapentin elimination in anuric subjects.

Dosage adjustment in patients undergoing hemodialysis is necessary (see DOSAGE AND ADMINISTRATION).

Hepatic Disease: Because gabapentin is not metabolized, no study was performed in patients with hepatic impairment.

Age: The effect of age was studied in subjects 20–80 years of age. Apparent oral clearance (CL/F) of gabapentin decreased as age increased, from about 225 mL/min in those under 30 years of age to about 125 mL/min in those over 70 years of age. Renal clearance (CLr) and CLr adjusted for body surface area also declined with age; however, the decline in the renal clearance of gabapentin with age can largely be explained by the decline in renal function. Reduction of gabapentin dose may be required in patients who have age related compromised renal function. (See PRECAUTIONS, Geriatric Use, and DOSAGE AND ADMINISTRATION.)

Pediatric: No pharmacokinetic data are available in pediatric patients below the age of 18 years.

Gender: Although no formal study has been conducted to compare the pharmacokinetics of gabapentin in men and women, it appears that the pharmacokinetic parameters for males and females are similar and there are no significant gender differences.

Race: Pharmacokinetic differences due to race have not been studied. Because gabapentin is primarily renally excreted and there are no important racial differences in creatinine clearance, pharmacokinetic differences due to race are not expected.

Clinical Studies

The effectiveness of Neurontin® as adjunctive therapy (added to other antiepileptic drugs) was established in three multicenter placebo-controlled, double-blind, parallel-group clinical trials in 705 adults with refractory partial seizures. The patients enrolled had a history of at least 4 partial seizures per month in spite of receiving one or more antiepileptic drugs at therapeutic levels and were observed on their established antiepileptic drug regimen during a 12-week baseline period. In patients continuing to have at least 2 (or 4 in some studies) seizures per month, Neurontin® or placebo was then added on to the existing therapy during a 12-week treatment period. Effectiveness was assessed primarily on the basis of the percent of patients with a 50% or greater reduction in seizure frequency from baseline to treatment (the "responder rate") and a derived measure called response ratio, a measure of change defined as (T − B)/(T + B), where B is the patient's baseline seizure frequency and T is the patient's seizure frequency during treatment. Response ratio is distributed within the range −1 to +1. A zero value indicates no change while complete elimination of seizures would give a value of −1; increased seizure rates would give positive values. A response ratio of −0.33 corresponds to a 50% reduction in seizure frequency. The results given below are for all partial seizures in the intent-to-treat (all patients who received any doses of treatment) population in each study, unless otherwise indicated.

One study compared Neurontin® 1200 mg/day T.I.D. with placebo. Responder rate was 23% (14/61) in the Neurontin® group and 9% (6/66) in the placebo group; the difference between groups was statistically significant. Response ratio was also better in the Neurontin® group (−0.199) than in the placebo group (−0.044), a difference that also achieved statistical significance.

A second study compared primarily 1200 mg/day T.I.D. Neurontin® (N = 101) with placebo (N = 98). Additional smaller Neurontin® dosage groups (600 mg/day, N = 53; 1800 mg/day, N = 54) were also studied for information regarding dose response. Responder rate was higher in the Neurontin® 1200 mg/day group (16%) than in the placebo group (8%), but the difference was not statistically significant. The responder rate at 600 mg (17%) was also not significantly higher than in the placebo, but the responder rate in the 1800 mg group (26%) was statistically significantly superior to the placebo rate. Response ratio was better in the Neurontin® 1200 mg/day group (−0.103) than in the placebo group (−0.022); but this difference was also not statistically significant (p = 0.224). A better response was seen in the Neurontin® 600 mg/day group (−0.105) and 1800 mg/day group (−0.222) than in the 1200 mg/day group, with the 1800 mg/day group achieving statistical significance compared to the placebo group.

A third study compared Neurontin® 900 mg/day T.I.D. (N = 111) and placebo (N = 109). An additional Neurontin® 1200 mg/day dosage group (N = 52) provided dose-response data. A statistically significant difference in responder rate was seen in the Neurontin® 900 mg/day group (22%) compared to that in the placebo group (10%). Response ratio was also statistically significantly superior in the Neurontin®

900 mg/day group (−0.119) compared to that in the placebo group (−0.027), as was response ratio in 1200 mg/day Neurontin® (−0.184) compared to placebo.

Analyses were also performed in each study to examine the effect of Neurontin® on preventing secondarily generalized tonic-clonic seizures. Patients who experienced a secondarily generalized tonic-clonic seizure in either the baseline or in the treatment period in all three placebo-controlled studies were included in these analyses. There were several response ratio comparisons that showed a statistically significant advantage for Neurontin® compared to placebo and favorable trends for almost all comparisons.

Analysis of responder rate using combined data from all three studies and all doses (N = 162, Neurontin®; N = 89, placebo) also showed a significant advantage for Neurontin® over placebo in reducing the frequency of secondarily generalized tonic-clonic seizures.

In two of the three controlled studies, more than one dose of Neurontin® was used. Within each study the results did not show a consistently increased response to dose. However, looking across studies, a trend toward increasing efficacy with increasing dose is evident (see Figure 1).

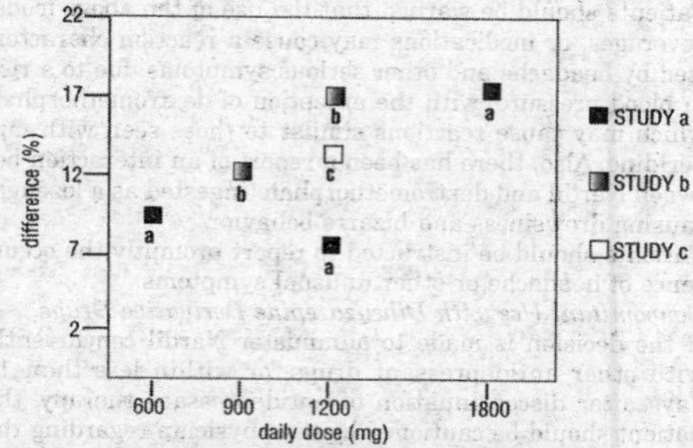

FIGURE 1. Responder Rate in Patients Receiving Neurontin® Expressed as a Difference from Placebo by Dose and Study

In the figure, treatment effect magnitude, measured on the Y axis in terms of the difference in the proportion of gabapentin and placebo assigned patients attaining a 50% or greater reduction in seizure frequency from baseline, is plotted against the daily dose of gabapentin administered (X axis).

Although no formal analysis by gender has been performed, estimates of response (Response Ratio) derived from clinical trials (398 men, 307 women) indicate no important gender differences exist. There was no consistent pattern indicating that age had any effect on the response to Neurontin®. There were insufficient numbers of patients of races other than Caucasian to permit a comparison of efficacy among racial groups.

INDICATIONS AND USAGE

Neurontin® (gabapentin) is indicated as adjunctive therapy in the treatment of partial seizures with and without secondary generalization in adults with epilepsy.

CONTRAINDICATIONS

Neurontin® is contraindicated in patients who have demonstrated hypersensitivity to the drug or its ingredients.

WARNINGS

Withdrawal Precipitated Seizure, Status Epilepticus

Antiepileptic drugs should not be abruptly discontinued because of the possibility of increasing seizure frequency.

In the placebo-controlled studies, the incidence of status epilepticus in patients receiving Neurontin® was 0.6% (3 of 543) versus 0.5% in patients receiving placebo (2 of 378). Among the 2074 patients treated with Neurontin® across all studies (controlled and uncontrolled) 31 (1.5%) had status epilepticus. Of these, 14 patients had no prior history of status epilepticus either before treatment or while on other medications. Because adequate historical data are not available, it is impossible to say whether or not treatment with Neurontin® is associated with a higher or lower rate of status epilepticus than would be expected to occur in a similar population not treated with Neurontin®.

Tumorigenic Potential

In standard preclinical *in vivo* lifetime carcinogenicity studies, an unexpectedly high incidence of pancreatic acinar adenocarcinomas was identified in male, but not in female, rats. (See PRECAUTIONS: Carcinogenesis, Mutagenesis, Impairment of Fertility.) The clinical significance of this finding is unknown. Clinical experience during gabapentin's premarketing development provides no direct means to assess its potential for inducing tumors in humans.

In clinical studies comprising 2085 patient-years of exposure, new tumors were reported in 10 patients (2 breast, 3 brain, 2 lung, 1 adrenal, 1 non-Hodgkin's lymphoma, 1 endometrial carcinoma *in situ*), and preexisting tumors worsened in 11 patients (9 brain, 1 breast, 1 prostate) during or up to 2 years following discontinuation of Neurontin®. Without knowledge of the background incidence and recurrence in a similar population not treated with Neurontin®, it is impossible to know whether the incidence seen in this cohort is or is not affected by treatment.

Sudden and Unexplained Deaths

During the course of premarketing development of Neurontin®, 8 sudden and unexplained deaths were recorded among a cohort of 2203 patients treated (2103 patient-years of exposure).

Some of these could represent seizure-related deaths in which the seizure was not observed, e.g., at night. This represents an incidence of 0.0038 deaths per patient-year. Although this rate exceeds that expected in a healthy population matched for age and sex, it is within the range of estimates for the incidence of sudden unexplained deaths in patients with epilepsy not receiving Neurontin® (ranging from 0.0005 for the general population of epileptics, to 0.003 for a clinical trial population similar to that in the Neurontin® program, to 0.005 for patients with refractory epilepsy). Consequently, whether these figures are reassuring or raise further concern depends on comparability of the populations reported upon to the Neurontin® cohort and the accuracy of the estimates provided.

PRECAUTIONS

Information for Patients

Patients should be instructed to take Neurontin® only as prescribed.

Patients should be advised that Neurontin® may cause dizziness, somnolence and other symptoms and signs of CNS depression. Accordingly, they should be advised neither to drive a car nor to operate other complex machinery until they have gained sufficient experience on Neurontin® to gauge whether or not it affects their mental and/or motor performance adversely.

Laboratory Tests

Clinical trials data do not indicate that routine monitoring of clinical laboratory parameters is necessary for the safe use of Neurontin®. The value of monitoring Neurontin® blood concentrations has not been established. Neurontin® may be used in combination with other antiepileptic drugs without concern for alteration of the blood concentrations of gabapentin or of other antiepileptic drugs.

Drug Interactions

Gabapentin is not appreciably metabolized nor does it interfere with the metabolism of commonly coadministered antiepileptic drugs.

The drug interaction data described in this section were obtained from studies involving healthy adults and patients with epilepsy.

Phenytoin: In a single and multiple dose study of Neurontin® (400 mg T.I.D.) in epileptic patients (N = 8) maintained on phenytoin monotherapy for at least 2 months, gabapentin had no effect on the steady-state trough plasma concentrations of phenytoin and phenytoin had no effect on gabapentin pharmacokinetics.

Carbamazepine: Steady-state trough plasma carbamazepine and carbamazepine 10, 11 epoxide concentrations were not affected by concomitant gabapentin (400 mg T.I.D.; N = 12) administration. Likewise, gabapentin pharmacokinetics were unaltered by carbamazepine administration.

Valproic Acid: The mean steady-state trough serum valproic acid concentrations prior to and during concomitant gabapentin administration (400 mg T.I.D.; N = 17) were not different and neither were gabapentin pharmacokinetic parameters affected by valproic acid.

Phenobarbital: Estimates of steady-state pharmacokinetic parameters for phenobarbital or gabapentin (300 mg T.I.D.; N = 12) are identical whether the drugs are administered alone or together.

Cimetidine: In the presence of cimetidine at 300 mg Q.I.D. (N = 12) the mean apparent oral clearance of gabapentin fell by 14% and creatinine clearance fell by 10%. Thus cimetidine appeared to alter the renal excretion of both gabapentin and creatinine, an endogenous marker of renal function. This small decrease in excretion of gabapentin by cimetidine is not expected to be of clinical importance. The effect of gabapentin on cimetidine was not evaluated.

Oral Contraceptive: Based on AUC and half-life, multiple-dose pharmacokinetic profiles of norethindrone and ethinyl estradiol following administration of tablets containing 2.5 mg of norethindrone acetate and 50 mcg of ethinyl estradiol were similar with and without coadministration of gabapentin (400 mg T.I.D.; N = 13). The Cmax of norethindrone was 13% higher when it was coadministered with gabapentin; this interaction is not expected to be of clinical importance.

Antacid (Maalox®): Maalox reduced the bioavailability of gabapentin (N = 16) by about 20%. This decrease in bioavailability was about 5% when gabapentin was administered

2 hours after Maalox. It is recommended that gabapentin be taken at least 2 hours following Maalox administration.

Effect of Probenecid: Probenecid is a blocker of renal tubular secretion. Gabapentin pharmacokinetic parameters without and with probenecid were comparable. This indicates that gabapentin does not undergo renal tubular secretion by the pathway that is blocked by probenecid.

Drug/Laboratory Tests Interactions

Because false positive readings were reported with the Ames N-Multistix SG® dipstick test for urinary protein when gabapentin was added to other antiepileptic drugs, the more specific sulfosalicylic acid precipitation procedure is recommended to determine the presence of urine protein.

Carcinogenesis, Mutagenesis, Impairment of Fertility

Gabapentin was given in the diet to mice at 200, 600, and 2000 mg/kg/day and to rats at 250, 1000, and 2000 mg/kg/day for 2 years. A statistically significant increase in the incidence of pancreatic acinar cell adenomas and carcinomas was found in male rats receiving the high dose; the no-effect dose for the occurrence of carcinomas was 1000 mg/kg/day. Peak plasma concentrations of gabapentin in rats receiving the high dose of 200 mg/kg were 10 times higher than plasma concentrations in humans receiving 3600 mg per day, and in rats receiving 1000 mg/kg/day peak plasma concentrations were 6.5 times higher than in humans receiving 3600 mg/day. The pancreatic acinar cell carcinomas did not affect survival, did not metastasize and were not locally invasive. Studies to attempt to define a mechanism by which this relatively rare tumor type is occurring are in progress. The relevance of this finding to carcinogenic risk in humans is unclear.

Gabapentin did not demonstrate mutagenic or genotoxic potential in three *in vitro* and two *in vivo* assays. It was negative in the Ames test and the *in vitro* HGPRT forward mutation assay in Chinese hamster lung cells; it did not produce significant increases in chromosomal aberrations in the *in vitro* Chinese hamster lung cell assay; it was negative in the *in vivo* chromosomal aberration assay and in the *in vivo* micronucleus test in Chinese hamster bone marrow.

No adverse effects on fertility or reproduction were observed in rats at doses up to 2000 mg/kg (approximately 5 times the maximum recommended human dose on an mg/m^2 basis).

Pregnancy

Pregnancy Category C: Gabapentin has been shown to be fetotoxic in rodents, causing delayed ossification of several bones in the skull, vertebrae, forelimbs, and hindlimbs. These effects occurred when pregnant mice received oral doses of 1000 or 3000 mg/kg/day during the period of organogenesis, or approximately 1 to 4 times the maximum dose of 3600 mg/day given to epileptic patients on a mg/m^2 basis. The no-effect level was 500 mg/kg/day or approximately $^1/_2$ of the human dose on a mg/m^2 basis.

When rats were dosed prior to and during mating, and throughout gestation, pups from all dose groups (500, 1000 and 2000 mg/kg/day) were affected. These doses are equivalent to less than approximately 1 to 5 times the maximum human dose on a mg/m^2 basis. There was an increased incidence of hydroureter and/or hydronephrosis in rats in a study of fertility and general reproductive performance at 2000 mg/kg/day with no effect at 1000 mg/kg/day, in a teratology study at 1500 mg/kg/day with no effect at 300 mg/kg/day, and in a perinatal and postnatal study at all doses studied (500, 1000 and 2000 mg/kg/day). The doses at which the effects occurred are approximately 1 to 5 times the maximum human dose of 3600 mg/day on a mg/m^2 basis; the no-effect doses were approximately 3 times (Fertility and General Reproductive Performance study) and approximately equal to (Teratogenicity study) the maximum human dose on a mg/m^2 basis. Other than hydroureter and hydronephrosis, the etiologies of which are unclear, the incidence of malformations was not increased compared to controls in offspring of mice, rats, or rabbits given doses up to 50 times (mice), 30 times (rats), and 25 times (rabbits) the human daily dose on a mg/kg basis, or 4 times (mice), 5 times (rats), or 8 times (rabbits) the human daily dose on a mg/m^2 basis.

In a teratology study in rabbits, an increased incidence of postimplantation fetal loss occurred in dams exposed to 60, 300 and 1500 mg/kg/day, or less than approximately $^1/_4$ to 8 times the maximum human dose on a mg/m^2 basis. There are no adequate and well-controlled studies in pregnant women. Because animal reproduction studies are not always predictive of human response, this drug should be used during pregnancy only if the potential benefit justifies the potential risk to the fetus.

Use in Nursing Mothers

It is not known if gabapentin is excreted in human milk and the effect on the nursing infant is unknown. However, because many drugs are excreted in human milk, Neurontin® should be used in women who are nursing only if the benefits clearly outweigh the risks.

Pediatric Use

Safety and effectiveness in pediatric patients below the age of 12 years have not been established.

Geriatric Use

No systemic studies in geriatric patients have been conducted. Adverse clinical events reported among 59 Neurontin® exposed patients over age 65 did not differ in kind from those reported for younger individuals. The small number of older individuals evaluated, however, limits the strength of any conclusions reached about the influence, if any, of age on the kind and incidence of adverse events or laboratory abnormality associated with the use of Neurontin®.

Because Neurontin® is eliminated primarily by renal excretion, the dose of Neurontin® should be adjusted as noted in DOSAGE AND ADMINISTRATION (Table 2) for elderly patients with compromised renal function. Creatinine clearance is difficult to measure in outpatients and serum creatinine may be reduced in the elderly because of decreased muscle mass. Creatinine clearance (C_{Cr}) can be reasonably well estimated using the equation of Cockcroft and Gault:

for females $C_{Cr} = (0.85)(140\text{-age})(wt)/[(72)(S_{Cr})]$

for males $C_{Cr} = (140\text{-age})(wt)/[(72)(S_{Cr})]$

where age is in years, wt is in kilograms and S_{Cr} is serum creatinine in mg/dL.

ADVERSE REACTIONS

The most commonly observed adverse events associated with the use of Neurontin® in combination with other antiepileptic drugs, not seen at an equivalent frequency among placebo-treated patients, were somnolence, dizziness, ataxia, fatigue, and nystagmus.

Approximately 7% of the 2074 individuals who received Neurontin® in premarketing clinical trials discontinued treatment because of an adverse event. The adverse events most commonly associated with withdrawal were somnolence (1.2%), ataxia (0.8%), fatigue (0.6%), nausea and/or vomiting (0.6%), and dizziness (0.6%).

Incidence in Controlled Clinical Trials

Table 1 lists treatment-emergent signs and symptoms that occurred in at least 1% of Neurontin®-treated patients with epilepsy participating in placebo-controlled trials and were numerically more common in the Neurontin® group. In these studies, either Neurontin® or placebo was added to the patient's current antiepileptic drug therapy. Adverse events were usually mild to moderate in intensity.

The prescriber should be aware that these figures, obtained when Neurontin® was added to concurrent antiepileptic drug therapy, cannot be used to predict the frequency of adverse events in the course of usual medical practice where patient characteristics and other factors may differ from those prevailing during clinical studies. Similarly, the cited frequencies cannot be directly compared with figures obtained from other clinical investigations involving different treatments, uses, or investigators. An inspection of these frequencies, however, does provide the prescribing physician with one basis to estimate the relative contribution of drug and nondrug factors to the adverse event incidences in the population studied.

[See table at top of next page]

Other events in more than 1% of patients but equally or more frequent in the placebo group included: headache, viral infection, fever, nausea and/or vomiting, abdominal pain, diarrhea, convulsions, confusion, insomnia, emotional lability, rash, acne.

Among the treatment-emergent adverse events occurring at an incidence of at least 10% of Neurontin-treated patients, somnolence and ataxia appeared to exhibit a positive dose-response relationship.

The overall incidence of adverse events and the types of adverse events seen were similar among men and women treated with Neurontin®. The incidence of adverse events increased slightly with increasing age in patients treated with either Neurontin® or placebo. Because only 3% of patients (28/921) in placebo-controlled studies were identified

Continued on next page

This product information was prepared in June 2000. On these and other Parke-Davis Products, information may be obtained by addressing PARKE-DAVIS, a Warner-Lambert Division, Morris Plains, New Jersey 07950.

Neurontin—Cont.

as nonwhite (black or other), there are insufficient data to support a statement regarding the distribution of adverse events by race.

Other Adverse Events Observed During All Clinical Trials
Neurontin® has been administered to 2074 individuals during all clinical trials, only some of which were placebo-controlled. During these trials, all adverse events were recorded by the clinical investigators using terminology of their own choosing. To provide a meaningful estimate of the proportion of individuals having adverse events, similar types of events were grouped into a smaller number of standardized categories using modified COSTART dictionary terminology. These categories are used in the listing below. The frequencies presented represent the proportion of the 2074 individuals exposed to Neurontin® who experienced an event of the type cited on at least one occasion while receiving Neurontin®. All reported events are included except those already listed in the previous table, those too general to be informative, and those not reasonably associated with the use of the drug.

Events are further classified within body system categories and enumerated in order of decreasing frequency using the following definitions: frequent adverse events are defined as those occurring in at least 1/100 patients; infrequent adverse events are those occurring in 1/100 to 1/1000 patients; rare events are those occurring in fewer than 1/1000 patients.

Body As A Whole: *Frequent:* asthenia, malaise, face edema; *Infrequent:* allergy, generalized edema, weight decrease, chill; *Rare:* strange feelings, lassitude, alcohol intolerance, hangover effect.

Cardiovascular System: *Frequent:* hypertension; *Infrequent:* hypotension, angina pectoris, peripheral vascular disorder, palpitation, tachycardia, migraine, murmur; *Rare:* atrial fibrillation, heart failure, thrombophlebitis, deep thrombophlebitis, myocardial infarction, cerebrovascular accident, pulmonary thrombosis, ventricular extrasystoles, bradycardia, premature atrial contraction, pericardial rub, heart block, pulmonary embolus, hyperlipidemia, hypercholesterolemia, pericardial effusion, pericarditis.

Digestive System: *Frequent:* anorexia, flatulence, gingivitis; *Infrequent:* glossitis, gum hemorrhage, thirst, stomatitis, increased salivation, gastroenteritis, hemorrhoids, bloody stools, fecal incontinence, hepatomegaly; *Rare:* dysphagia, eructation, pancreatitis, peptic ulcer, colitis, blisters in mouth, tooth discolor, perleche, salivary gland enlarged, lip hemorrhage, esophagitis, hiatal hernia, hematemesis, proctitis, irritable bowel syndrome, rectal hemorrhage, esophageal spasm.

Endocrine System: *Rare:* hyperthyroid, hypothyroid, goiter, hypoestrogen, ovarian failure, epididymitis, swollen testicle, cushingoid appearance.

Hematologic and Lymphatic System: *Frequent:* purpura most often described as bruises resulting from physical trauma; *Infrequent:* anemia, thrombocytopenia, lymphadenopathy; *Rare:* WBC count increased, lymphocytosis, non-Hodgkin's lymphoma, bleeding time increased.

Musculoskeletal System: *Frequent:* arthralgia; *Infrequent:* tendinitis, arthritis, joint stiffness, joint swelling, positive Romberg test; *Rare:* costochondritis, osteoporosis, bursitis, contracture.

Nervous System: *Frequent:* vertigo, hyperkinesia, paresthesia, decreased or absent reflexes, increased reflexes, anxiety, hostility; *Infrequent:* CNS tumors, syncope, dreaming abnormal, aphasia, hypesthesia, intracranial hemorrhage, hypotonia, dysesthesia, paresis, dystonia, hemiplegia, facial paralysis, stupor, cerebellar dysfunction, positive Babinski sign, decreased position sense, subdural hematoma, apathy, hallucination, decrease or loss of libido, agitation, paranoia, depersonalization, euphoria, feeling high, doped-up sensation, suicidal, psychosis; *Rare:* choreoathetosis, orofacial dyskinesia, encephalopathy, nerve palsy, personality disorder, increased libido, subdued temperament, apraxia, fine motor control disorder, meningismus, local myoclonus, hyperesthesia, hypokinesia, mania, neurosis, hysteria, antisocial reaction, suicide gesture.

Respiratory System: *Frequent:* pneumonia; *Infrequent:* epistaxis, dyspnea, apnea, *Rare:* mucositis, aspiration pneumonia, hyperventilation, hiccup, laryngitis, nasal obstruction, snoring, bronchospasm, hypoventilation, lung edema.

Dermatological: *Infrequent:* alopecia, eczema, dry skin, increased sweating, urticaria, hirsutism, seborrhea, cyst, herpes simplex; *Rare:* herpes zoster, skin discolor, skin papules, photosensitive reaction, leg ulcer, scalp seborrhea, psoriasis, desquamation, maceration, skin nodules, subcutaneous nodule, melanosis, skin necrosis, local swelling.

Urogenital System: *Infrequent:* hematuria, dysuria, urination frequency, cystitis, urinary retention, urinary incontinence, vaginal hemorrhage, amenorrhea, dysmenorrhea, menorrhagia, breast cancer, unable to climax, ejaculation abnormal; *Rare:* kidney pain, leukorrhea, pruritus genital, renal stone, acute renal failure, anuria, glycosuria, nephrosis, nocturia, pyuria, urination urgency, vaginal pain, breast pain, testicle pain.

Special Senses: *Frequent:* abnormal vision; *Infrequent:* cataract, conjunctivitis, eyes dry, eye pain, visual field defect, photophobia, bilateral or unilateral ptosis, eye hemorrhage, hordeolum, hearing loss, earache, tinnitus, inner ear infection, otitis, taste loss, unusual taste, eye twitching, ear fullness; *Rare:* eye itching, abnormal accomodation, perforated ear drum, sensitivity to noise, eye focusing problem, watery eyes, retinopathy, glaucoma, iritis, corneal disorders, lacrimal dysfunction, degenerative eye changes, blindness, retinal degeneration, miosis, chorioretinitis, strabismus, eustachian tube dysfunction, labyrinthitis, otitis externa, odd smell.

TABLE 1. Treatment-Emergent Adverse Event Incidence in Controlled Add-On Trials (Events in at least 1% of Neurontin patients and numerically more frequent than in the placebo group)

Body System/ Adverse Event	Neurontin®[a] N = 543 %	Placebo[a] N = 378 %
Body As A Whole		
Fatigue	11.0	5.0
Weight Increase	2.9	1.6
Back Pain	1.8	0.5
Peripheral Edema	1.7	0.5
Cardiovascular		
Vasodilatation	1.1	0.3
Digestive System		
Dyspepsia	2.2	0.5
Mouth or Throat Dry	1.7	0.5
Constipation	1.5	0.8
Dental Abnormalities	1.5	0.3
Increased Appetite	1.1	0.8
Hematologic and Lymphatic Systems		
Leukopenia	1.1	0.5
Musculoskeletal System		
Myalgia	2.0	1.9
Fracture	1.1	0.8
Nervous System		
Somnolence	19.3	8.7
Dizziness	17.1	6.9
Ataxia	12.5	5.6
Nystagmus	8.3	4.0
Tremor	6.8	3.2
Nervousness	2.4	1.9
Dysarthria	2.4	0.5
Amnesia	2.2	0.0
Depression	1.8	1.1
Thinking Abnormal	1.7	1.3
Twitching	1.3	0.5
Coordination Abnormal	1.1	0.3
Respiratory System		
Rhinitis	4.1	3.7
Pharyngitis	2.8	1.6
Coughing	1.8	1.3
Skin and Appendages		
Abrasion	1.3	0.0
Pruritus	1.3	0.5
Urogenital System		
Impotence	1.5	1.1
Special Senses		
Diplopia	5.9	1.9
Amblyopia[b]	4.2	1.1
Laboratory Deviations		
WBC Decreased	1.1	0.5

[a] Plus background antiepileptic drug therapy
[b] Amblyopia was often described as blurred vision.

Postmarketing and Other Experience
In addition to the adverse experiences reported during clinical testing of Neurontin®, the following adverse experiences have been reported in patients receiving marketed Neurontin®. These adverse experiences have not been listed above and data are insufficient to support an estimate of their incidence or to establish causation. The listing is alphabetized: angioedema, blood glucose fluctuation, erythema multiforme, elevated liver function tests, fever, jaundice, Stevens-Johnson syndrome.

DRUG ABUSE AND DEPENDENCE

The abuse and dependence potential of Neurontin® has not been evaluated in human studies.

OVERDOSAGE

A lethal dose of gabapentin was not identified in mice and rats receiving single oral doses as high as 8000 mg/kg. Signs of acute toxicity in animals included ataxia, labored breathing, ptosis, sedation, hypoactivity, or excitation.

Acute oral overdoses of Neurontin® up to 49 grams have been reported. In these cases, double vision, slurred speech, drowsiness, lethargy and diarrhea were observed. All patients recovered with supportive care.

Gabapentin can be removed by hemodialysis. Although hemodialysis has not been performed in the few overdose cases reported, it may be indicated by the patient's clinical state or in patients with significant renal impairment.

DOSAGE AND ADMINISTRATION

Neurontin® is recommended for add-on therapy in patients over 12 years of age. Evidence bearing on its safety and effectiveness in pediatric patients below the age of 12 is not available.

Neurontin® is given orally with or without food.

The effective dose of Neurontin® is 900 to 1800 mg/day and given in divided doses (three times a day) using 300- or 400-mg capsules or 600- or 800-mg tablets. The starting dose is 300 mg three times a day. If necessary, the dose may be increased using 300- or 400-mg capsules or 600- or 800-mg tablets three times a day up to 1800 mg/day. Dosages up to 2400 mg/day have been well tolerated in long-term clinical studies. Doses of 3600 mg/day have also been administered to a small number of patients for a relatively short duration, and have been well tolerated. The maximum time between doses in the T.I.D. schedule should not exceed 12 hours.

It is not necessary to monitor gabapentin plasma concentrations to optimize Neurontin® therapy. Further, because there are no significant pharmacokinetic interactions among Neurontin® and other commonly used antiepileptic drugs, the addition of Neurontin® does not alter the plasma levels of these drugs appreciably.

If Neurontin® is discontinued and/or an alternate anticonvulsant medication is added to the therapy, this should be done gradually over a minimum of 1 week.

Dosage adjustment in patients with compromised renal function or undergoing hemodialysis is recommended as follows:

TABLE 2. Neurontin® Dosage Based on Renal Function

Renal Function Creatinine Clearance (mL/min)	Total Daily Dose (mg/day)	Dose Regimen (mg)
>60	1200	400 T.I.D.
30—60	600	300 B.I.D.
15—30	300	300 Q.D.
<15	150	300 Q.O.D.[a]
Hemodialysis	—	300-300[b]

[a] Every other day
[b] Loading dose of 300 to 400 mg in patients who have never received Neurontin®, then 200 to 300 mg Neurontin® following each 4 hours of hemodialysis

HOW SUPPLIED

Neurontin® (gabapentin capsules and gabapentin tablets) are supplied as follows:

100-mg capsules;
White hard gelatin capsules printed with "PD" on one side and "Neurontin®/100 mg" on the other; available in:
Bottles of 100: N 0071-0803-24
Unit dose 50's: N 0071-0803-40

300-mg capsules;
Yellow hard gelatin capsules printed with "PD" on one side and "Neurontin®/300 mg" on the other; available in:
Bottles of 100: N 0071-0805-24
Unit dose 50's: N 0071-0805-40

400-mg capsules;
Orange hard gelatin capsules printed with "PD" on one side and "Neurontin®/400 mg" on the other; available in:
Bottles of 100: N 0071-0806-24
Unit dose 50's: N 0071-0806-40
600-mg tablets;
White elliptical film-coated tablets printed in black ink with "Neurontin® 600" on one side; available in:
Bottles of 100: N 0071-0416-24
Bottles of 500: N 0071-0416-30
Unit dose 50's: N 0071-0416-40
800-mg tablets;
White elliptical film-coated tablets printed in orange with "Neurontin® 800" on one side; available in:
Bottles of 100: N 0071-0426-24
Bottles of 500: N 0071-0426-30
Unit dose 50's: N 0071-0426-40

Storage (Capsules)
Store at controlled room temperature 15°–30°C (59°–86°F).
Storage (Tablets)
Store at 25°C (77°F); excursions permitted to 15°–30°C (59°–86°F) [see USP Controlled Room Temperature].

℞ only
Revised February 1999
Manufactured by:
Parke Davis Pharmaceuticals, Ltd.
Vega Baja, PR 00694
Distributed by:
PARKE-DAVIS
Div of Warner-Lambert Co
Morris Plains, NJ 07950 USA
 0416G031
Shown in Product Identification Guide, page 329

NITROSTAT® ℞
(Nitroglycerin Tablets, USP)

DESCRIPTION

Nitrostat is a stabilized sublingual compressed nitroglycerin tablet that contains 0.3 mg (1/200 grain), 0.4 mg (1/150 grain), or 0.6 mg (1/100 grain) nitroglycerin; as well as lactose monohydrate, NF; glyceryl monostearate, NF; pregelatinized starch, NF; calcium stearate, NF powder; and silicon dioxide, colloidal, NF.
Nitroglycerin, an organic nitrate, is a vasodilating agent. The chemical name for nitroglycerin is 1,2,3 propanetriol trinitrate and the chemical structure is:

$$O_2N-O-CH_2CH(O-NO_2)CH_2-O-NO_2$$

$C_3H_5N_3O_9$

Molecular weight: 227.09

CLINICAL PHARMACOLOGY

The principal pharmacological action of nitroglycerin is relaxation of vascular smooth muscle. Although venous effects predominate, nitroglycerin produces, in a dose-related manner, dilation of both arterial and venous beds. Dilation of postcapillary vessels, including large veins, promotes peripheral pooling of blood, decreases venous return to the heart, and reduces left ventricular end-diastolic pressure (preload). Nitroglycerin also produces arteriolar relaxation, thereby reducing peripheral vascular resistance and arterial pressure (afterload), and dilates large epicardial coronary arteries; however, the extent to which this latter effect contributes to the relief of exertional angina is unclear.
Therapeutic doses of nitroglycerin may reduce systolic, diastolic, and mean arterial blood pressure. Effective coronary perfusion pressure is usually maintained, but can be compromised if blood pressure falls excessively or increased heart rate decreases diastolic filling time.
Elevated central venous and pulmonary capillary wedge pressures, and pulmonary and systemic vascular resistance are also reduced by nitroglycerin therapy. Heart rate is usually slightly increased, presumably due to a compensatory response to the fall in blood pressure. Cardiac index may be increased, decreased, or unchanged. Myocardial oxygen consumption or demand (as measured by the pressure-rate product, tension-time index, and stroke-work index) is decreased and a more favorable supply-demand ratio can be achieved. Patients with elevated left ventricular filling pressures and increased systemic vascular resistance in association with a depressed cardiac index are likely to experience an improvement in cardiac index. In contrast, when filling pressures and cardiac index are normal, cardiac index may be slightly reduced following nitroglycerin administration.
Mechanism of Action: Nitroglycerin forms free radical nitric oxide (NO) which activates guanylate cyclase, resulting in an increase of guanosine 3'5' monophosphate (cyclic GMP) in smooth muscle and other tissues. These events lead to dephosphorylation of myosin light chains, which regulate the contractile state in smooth muscle, and result in vasodilatation.
Pharmacodynamics: Consistent with the symptomatic relief of angina, digital plethysmography indicates that onset of the vasodilatory effect occurs approximately 1 to 3 minutes after sublingual nitroglycerin administration and reaches a maximum by 5 minutes postdose. Effects persist for at least 25 minutes following Nitrostat administration.
Pharmacokinetics and Drug Metabolism Absorption: Nitroglycerin is rapidly absorbed following sublingual administration of Nitrostat tablets. Mean peak nitroglycerin plasma concentrations occur at a mean time of approximately 6 to 7 minutes postdose (Table 1). Maximum plasma nitroglycerin concentrations (Cmax) and area under the plasma concentration-time curves (AUC) increase dose-proportionally following 0.3 to 0.6 mg Nitrostat. The absolute bioavailability of nitroglycerin from Nitrostat tablets is approximately 40% but tends to be variable due to factors influencing drug absorption such as sublingual hydration and mucosal metabolism.

Table 1

	Mean Nitroglycerin (SD) Values	
	2 x 0.3 mg	1 x 0.6 mg
Parameter	Nitrostat Tablets	Nitrostat Tablets
Cmax, ng/mL	2.3 (1.7)	2.1 (1.5)
tmax, min	6.4 (2.5)	7.2 (3.2)
AUC (0–∞), min	14.9 (8.2)	14.9 (11.4)
$t_{1/2}$, min	2.8 (1.1)	2.6 (0.6)

Distribution: The volume of distribution (V_{Area}) of nitroglycerin following intravenous administration is 3.3 L/kg. At plasma concentrations between 50 and 500 ng/mL, the binding of nitroglycerin to plasma proteins is approximately 60%, while that of 1,2- and 1,3-dinitroglycerin is 60% and 30%, respectively.
Metabolism: A liver reductase enzyme is of primary importance in the metabolism of nitroglycerin to glycerol di- and mononitrate metabolites and ultimately to glycerol and organic nitrate. Known sites of extrahepatic metabolism include red blood cells and vascular walls. In addition to nitroglycerin, 2 major metabolites 1,2- and 1,3-dinitroglycerin, are found in plasma. Mean peak 1,2- and 1,3-dinitroglycerin plasma concentrations occur at approximately 15 minutes postdose. The elimination half-life of 1,2- and 1,3-dinitroglycerin is 36 and 32 minutes, respectively. The 1,2- and 1,3-dinitroglycerin metabolites have been reported to possess approximately 2% and 10% of the pharmacological activity of nitroglycerin. Higher plasma concentrations of the dinitro metabolites, along with their nearly 10-fold longer elimination half-lives, may contribute significantly to the duration of pharmacologic effect. Glycerol mononitrate metabolites of nitroglycerin are biologically inactive.
Elimination: Nitroglycerin plasma concentrations decrease rapidly with a mean elimination half-life of 2 to 3 minutes. Half-life values range from 1.5 to 7.5 minutes. Clearance (13.6 L/min) greatly exceeds hepatic blood flow. Metabolism is the primary route of drug elimination.

INDICATIONS AND USAGE

Nitroglycerin is indicated for the acute relief of an attack or acute prophylaxis of angina pectoris due to coronary artery disease.

CONTRAINDICATIONS

Allergic reactions to organic nitrates are extremely rare, but they do occur. Nitroglycerin is contraindicated in patients who are allergic to it.
Sublingual nitroglycerin therapy is contraindicated in patients with early myocardial infarction, severe anemia, increased intracranial pressure, and those with a known hypersensitivity to nitroglycerin.
Administration of Nitrostat (nitroglycerin tablets, USP) is contraindicated in patients who are using Viagra® since Viagra has been shown to potentiate the hypotensive effects of organic nitrates.

WARNINGS

The benefits of sublingual nitroglycerin in patients with acute myocardial infarction or congestive heart failure have not been established. If one elects to use nitroglycerin in these conditions, careful clinical or hemodynamic monitoring must be used because of the possibility of hypotension and tachycardia.

PRECAUTIONS

General: Only the smallest dose required for effective relief of the acute anginal attack should be used. Excessive use may lead to the development of tolerance. Nitrostat tablets are intended for sublingual or buccal administration and should not be swallowed.
Severe hypotension, particularly with upright posture, may occur with small doses of nitroglycerin. This drug should therefore be used with caution in patients who may be volume-depleted or who, for whatever reason, are already hypotensive. Hypotension induced by nitroglycerin may be accompanied by paradoxical bradycardia and increased angina pectoris.
Nitrate therapy may aggravate the angina caused by hypertrophic cardiomyopathy.
As tolerance to other forms of nitroglycerin develops, the effects of sublingual nitroglycerin on exercise tolerance, although still observable, is blunted.
In industrial workers who have had long-term exposure to unknown (presumably high) doses of organic nitrates, tolerance rarely occurs. Chest pain, acute myocardial infarction, and even sudden death have occurred during temporary withdrawal of nitrates from these workers, demonstrating the existence of true physical dependence.
Several clinical trials of nitroglycerin patches or infusions in patients with angina pectoris have evaluated regimens which incorporated a 10 to 12 hour nitrate free interval. In some of these trials, an increase in the frequency of anginal attacks during the nitrate free interval was observed in a small number of patients. In one trial, patients had decreased exercise tolerance at the end of the nitrate interval. Hemodynamic rebound has been observed only rarely; on the other hand, few studies were so designed that rebound, if it had occurred, would have been detected.
Nitrate tolerance as a result of sublingual nitroglycerin administration is probably possible, but only in patients who maintain high continuous nitrate levels for more than 10 or 12 hours daily. Such use of sublingual nitroglycerin would entail administration of scores of tablets daily and is not recommended.
The drug should be discontinued if blurring of vision or drying of the mouth occurs. Excessive dosage of nitroglycerin may produce severe headaches.
Information for Patients: If possible, patients should sit down when taking Nitrostat tablets. This eliminates the possibility of falling due to lightheadedness or dizziness.
Nitroglycerin may produce a burning or tingling sensation when administered sublingually; however, the ability to produce a burning or tingling sensation should not be considered a reliable method for determining the potency of the tablets.
Headaches can sometimes accompany treatment with nitroglycerin. In patients who get these headaches, the headaches may be a marker of the activity of the drug.
Treatment with nitroglycerin may be associated with lightheadedness on standing, especially just after rising from a recumbent or seated position. This effect may be more frequent in patients who have also consumed alcohol.
Nitroglycerin should be kept in the original glass container, tightly capped.
Drug Interactions: Patients receiving antihypertensive drugs, beta-adrenergic blockers, or phenothiazines and nitrates should be observed for possible additive hypotensive effects. Marked orthostatic hypotension has been reported when calcium channel blockers and organic nitrates were used concomitantly.
Concomitant use of nitrates and alcohol may cause hypotension.
The vasodilatory and hemodynamic effects of nitroglycerin may be enhanced by concomitant administration of aspirin.
Intravenous administration of nitroglycerin decreases the thrombolytic effect of alteplase. Therefore, caution should be observed in patients receiving sublingual nitroglycerin during alteplase therapy.
Intravenous nitroglycerin reduces the anticoagulant effect of heparin and activated partial thromboplastin times (APTT) should be monitored in patients receiving heparin and intravenous nitroglycerin. It is not known if this effect occurs following single sublingual nitroglycerin doses.
Tricyclic antidepressants, (amitriptyline, desipramine, doxepin, others) and anticholinergic drugs may cause dry mouth and diminished salivary secretions. This may make dissolution of sublingual nitroglycerin difficult. Increasing salivation with chewing gum or artificial saliva products may prove useful in aiding dissolution of sublingual nitroglycerin.
Oral administration of nitroglycerin markedly decreases the first-pass metabolism of dihydroergotamine and subsequently increases its oral bioavailability. Ergotamine is known to precipitate angina pectoris. Therefore, patients receiving sublingual nitroglycerin should avoid ergotamine and related drugs or be monitored for symptoms of ergotism if this is not possible.
Administration of nitroglycerin is contraindicated in patients who are using Viagra (sildenafil citrate). Viagra has been shown to potentiate the hypotensive effects of organic nitrates.
A decrease in therapeutic effect of sublingual nitroglycerin may result from use of long-acting nitrates.
Drug/Laboratory Test Interactions: Nitrates may interfere with the Zlatkis-Zak color reaction causing a false report of decreased serum cholesterol.
Carcinogenesis, Mutagenesis, Impairment of Fertility: Animal carcinogenesis studies with sublingually administered nitroglycerin have not been performed.
Rats receiving up to 434 mg/kg/day of dietary nitroglycerin for 2 years developed dose-related fibrotic and neoplastic changes in liver, including carcinomas, and interstitial cell tumors in testes. At high dose, the incidences of hepatocellular carcinomas in males was 48% and in females was 33% compared to 0% in untreated controls. Incidences of testicular tumors were 52% vs 8% in controls. Lifetime dietary administration of up to 1058 mg/kg/day of nitroglycerin was not tumorigenic in mice.
Nitroglycerin was weakly mutagenic in Ames tests performed in 2 different laboratories. Nevertheless, there was no evidence of mutagenicity in an *in vivo* dominant lethal assay with male rats treated with doses up to about 363 mg/kg/day, PO, or in *ex vivo* cytogenetic tests in rat and dog tissues.

Continued on next page

This product information was prepared in June 2000. On these and other Parke-Davis Products, information may be obtained by addressing PARKE-DAVIS, a Warner-Lambert Division, Morris Plains, New Jersey 07950.

Nitrostat—Cont.

In a 3-generation reproduction study, rats received dietary nitroglycerin at doses up to about 434 mg/kg/day for 6 months prior to mating of the F_0 generation with treatment continuing through successive F_1 and F_2 generations. The high dose was associated with decreased feed intake and body weight gain in both sexes at all matings. No specific effect on the fertility of the F_0 generation was seen. Infertility noted in subsequent generations, however, was attributed to increased interstitial cell tissue and aspermatogenesis in the high-dose males. In this 3-generation study there was no clear evidence of teratogenicity.

Pregnancy Category C: Animal reproduction and teratogenicity studies have not been conducted with nitroglycerin sublingual tablets. Teratology studies in rats and rabbits, however, were conducted with topically applied nitroglycerin ointment at doses up to 80 mg/kg/day and 240 mg/kg/day, respectively. No toxic effects on dams or fetuses were seen at any dose tested.

There are no adequate and well-controlled studies in pregnant women. Nitroglycerin should be given to a pregnant woman only if clearly needed.

Nursing Mothers: It is not known whether nitroglycerin is excreted in human milk. Because many drugs are excreted in human milk, caution should be exercised when nitroglycerin is administered to a nursing woman.

Pediatric Use: The safety and effectiveness of nitroglycerin in pediatric patients have not been established.

Geriatric Use: Clinical studies of Nitrostat did not include sufficient numbers of subjects age 65 and over to determine whether they respond differently from younger subjects. Other reported clinical experience has not identified differences in responses between the elderly and younger patients. In general, dose selection for an elderly patient should be cautious, usually starting at the low end of the dosing range, reflecting the greater frequency of decreased hepatic, renal, or cardiac function, and of concomitant disease or other drug therapy.

ADVERSE REACTIONS

Headache which may be severe and persistent may occur immediately after use. Vertigo, dizziness, weakness, palpitation, and other manifestations of postural hypotension may develop occasionally, particularly in erect, immobile patients. Marked sensitivity to the hypotensive effects of nitrates (manifested by nausea, vomiting, weakness, diaphoresis, pallor, and collapse) may occur at therapeutic doses. Syncope due to nitrate vasodilatation has been reported. Flushing, drug rash, and exfoliative dermatitis have been reported in patients receiving nitrate therapy.

OVERDOSAGE

HEMODYNAMIC EFFECTS: The effects of nitroglycerin overdose are generally the results of nitroglycerin's capacity to induce vasodilatation, venous pooling, reduced cardiac output, and hypotension. These hemodynamic changes may have protean manifestations, including increased intracranial pressure, with any or all of persistent throbbing headache, confusion, and moderate fever; vertigo; palpitations; tachycardia; visual disturbances; nausea and vomiting (possibly with colic and even bloody diarrhea); syncope (especially in the upright posture); dyspnea, later followed by reduced ventilatory effort, diaphoresis, with the skin either flushed or cold and clammy; heart block and bradycardia; paralysis; coma; seizures; and death.

No specific antagonist to the vasodilator effects of nitroglycerin is known, and no intervention has been subject to controlled study as a therapy of nitroglycerin overdose. Because the hypotension associated with nitroglycerin overdose is the result of venodilatation and arterial hypovolemia, prudent therapy in this situation should be directed toward increase in central fluid volume. Passive elevation of the patient's legs may be sufficient, but intravenous infusion of normal saline or similar fluid may also be necessary.

The use of epinephrine or other arterial vasoconstrictors in this setting is likely to do more harm than good.

In patients with renal disease or congestive heart failure, therapy resulting in central volume expansion is not without hazard. Treatment of nitroglycerin overdose in these patients may be subtle and difficult, and invasive monitoring may be required.

METHEMOGLOBINEMIA: Methemoglobinemia has been rarely reported in association with organic nitrates. The diagnosis should be suspected in patients who exhibit signs of impaired oxygen delivery despite adequate cardiac output and adequate arterial PO_2. Classically, methemoglobinemic blood is described as chocolate brown, without color change on exposure to air.

If methemoglobinemia is present, intravenous administration of methylene blue, 1 to 2 mg/kg of body weight, may be required.

DOSAGE AND ADMINISTRATION

One tablet should be dissolved under the tongue or in the buccal pouch at the first sign of an acute anginal attack. The dose may be repeated approximately every 5 minutes, until relief is obtained. If the pain persists after a total of 3 tablets in a 15-minute period, prompt medical attention is recommended. Nitrostat may be used prophylactically 5 to 10 minutes prior to engaging in activities which might precipitate an acute attack.

During administration the patient should rest, preferably in the sitting position.

No dosage adjustment is required in patients with renal failure.

HOW SUPPLIED

Nitrostat is supplied as white, round, flat-faced tablets in 3 strengths (0.3 mg, 0.4 mg, and 0.6 mg) in bottles containing 100 tablets each, with color-coded labels, and in color-coded Patient Convenience Packages of 4 bottles of 25 tablets each.

0.3 mg (1/200 grain):	Coded "N" on one side and "3" on the other.
	N 0071-0417-24—Bottle of 100 tablets
0.4 mg (1/150 grain):	Coded "N" on one side and "4" on the other.
	N 0071-0418-13—Convenience Package
	N 0071-0418-24—Bottle of 100 tablets
0.6 mg (1/100 grain):	Coded "N" on one side and "6" on the other.
	N 0071-0419-24—Bottle of 100 tablets

Store at Controlled Room Temperature 20°–25°C (68°–77°F) [see USP].

℞ only

March 2000

Manufactured by:
Parke Davis
Pharmaceuticals, Ltd.
Vega Baja, PR 00694
Distributed by:
PARKE-DAVIS
Div of Warner-Lambert Co
Morris Plains, NJ 07950 USA
©1999-'00, PDPL

Shown in Product Identification Guide, page 330

ZARONTIN® ℞

[ză ˈrŏn ˈtĭn]
(ethosuximide, USP)
Capsules

DESCRIPTION

Zarontin (ethosuximide) is an anticonvulsant succinimide, chemically designated as alpha-ethyl-alpha-methyl-succinimide, with the following structural formula:

Each Zarontin capsule contains 250 mg ethosuximide, USP. Also contains: polyethylene glycol 400, NF. The capsule contains D&C yellow No. 10; FD&C red No. 3; gelatin, NF; glycerin, USP; and sorbitol.

CLINICAL PHARMACOLOGY

Ethosuximide suppresses the paroxysmal three cycle per second spike and wave activity associated with lapses of consciousness which is common in absence (petit mal) seizures. The frequency of epileptiform attacks is reduced, apparently by depression of the motor cortex and elevation of the threshold of the central nervous system to convulsive stimuli.

INDICATIONS AND USAGE

Zarontin is indicated for the control of absence (petit mal) epilepsy.

CONTRAINDICATION

Ethosuximide should not be used in patients with a history of hypersensitivity to succinimides.

WARNINGS

Blood dyscrasias, including some with fatal outcome, have been reported to be associated with the use of ethosuximide; therefore, periodic blood counts should be performed. Should signs and/or symptoms of infection (eg, sore throat, fever) develop, blood counts should be considered at that point.

Ethosuximide is capable of producing morphological and functional changes in the animal liver. In humans, abnormal liver and renal function studies have been reported.

Ethosuximide should be administered with extreme caution to patients with known liver or renal diseases. Periodic urinalysis and liver function studies are advised for all patients receiving the drug.

Cases of systemic lupus erythematosus have been reported with the use of ethosuximide. The physician should be alert to this possibility.

Usage in Pregnancy: Reports suggest an association between the use of anticonvulsant drugs by women with epilepsy and an elevated incidence of birth defects in children born to these women. Data are more extensive with respect to phenytoin and phenobarbital, but these are also the most commonly prescribed anticonvulsants; less systematic or anecdotal reports suggest a possible similar association with the use of all known anticonvulsant drugs.

The reports suggesting an elevated incidence of birth defects in children of drug-treated epileptic women cannot be regarded as adequate to prove a definite cause and effect relationship. There are intrinsic methodological problems in obtaining adequate data on drug teratogenicity in humans; the possibility also exists that other factors, eg, genetic factors or the epileptic condition itself, may be more important than drug therapy in leading to birth defects. The great majority of mothers on anticonvulsant medication deliver normal infants. It is important to note that anticonvulsant drugs should not be discontinued in patients in whom the drug is administered to prevent major seizures because of the strong possibility of precipitating status epilepticus with attendant hypoxia and threat to life. In individual cases where the severity and frequency of the seizure disorder are such that the removal of medication does not pose a serious threat to the patient, discontinuation of the drug may be considered prior to and during pregnancy, although it cannot be said with any confidence that even minor seizures do not pose some hazard to the developing embryo or fetus.

The prescribing physician will wish to weigh these considerations in treating or counseling epileptic women of childbearing potential.

PRECAUTIONS

General

Ethosuximide, when used alone in mixed types of epilepsy, may increase the frequency of grand mal seizures in some patients.

As with other anticonvulsants, it is important to proceed slowly when increasing or decreasing dosage, as well as when adding or eliminating other medication. Abrupt withdrawal of anticonvulsant medication may precipitate absence (petit mal) status.

Information for Patients

Ethosuximide may impair the mental and/or physical abilities required for the performance of potentially hazardous tasks, such as driving a motor vehicle or other such activity requiring alertness; therefore, the patient should be cautioned accordingly.

Patients taking ethosuximide should be advised of the importance of adhering strictly to the prescribed dosage regimen.

Patients should be instructed to promptly contact their physician if they develop signs and/or symptoms (eg, sore throat, fever) suggesting an infection.

Drug Interactions

Since Zarontin (ethosuximide) may interact with concurrently administered antiepileptic drugs, periodic serum level determinations of these drugs may be necessary (eg, ethosuximide may elevate phenytoin serum levels and valproic acid has been reported to both increase and decrease ethosuximide levels).

Pregnancy

See WARNINGS.

Pediatric Use

Safety and effectiveness in pediatric patients below the age of 3 years have not been established. (See DOSAGE AND ADMINISTRATION section)

ADVERSE REACTIONS

Gastrointestinal System: Gastrointestinal symptoms occur frequently and include anorexia, vague gastric upset, nausea and vomiting, cramps, epigastric and abdominal pain, weight loss, and diarrhea. There have been reports of gum hypertrophy and swelling of the tongue.

Hemopoietic System: Hemopoietic complications associated with the administration of ethosuximide have included leukopenia, agranulocytosis, pancytopenia, with or without bone marrow suppression, and eosinophilia.

Nervous System: Neurologic and sensory reactions reported during therapy with ethosuximide have included drowsiness, headache, dizziness, euphoria, hiccups, irritability, hyperactivity, lethargy, fatigue, and ataxia. Psychiatric or psychological aberrations associated with ethosuximide administration have included disturbances of sleep, night terrors, inability to concentrate, and aggressiveness. These effects may be noted particularly in patients who have previously exhibited psychological abnormalities. There have been rare reports of paranoid psychosis, increased libido, and increased state of depression with overt suicidal intentions.

Integumentary System: Dermatologic manifestations which have occurred with the administration of ethosuximide have included urticaria, Stevens-Johnson syndrome, systemic lupus erythematosus, pruritic erythematous rashes, and hirsutism.

Special Senses: Myopia.

Genitourinary System: Vaginal bleeding, microscopic hematuria.

OVERDOSAGE

Acute overdoses may produce nausea, vomiting, and CNS depression including coma with respiratory depression. A relationship between ethosuximide toxicity and its plasma levels has not been established. The therapeutic range of serum levels is 40 mcg/mL to 100 mcg/mL, although levels as high as 150 mcg/mL have been reported without signs of toxicity.

Treatment:

Treatment should include emesis (unless the patient is or could rapidly become obtunded, comatose, or convulsing) or gastric lavage, activated charcoal, cathartics and general supportive measures. Hemodialysis may be useful to treat ethosuximide overdose. Forced diuresis and exchange transfusions are ineffective.

DOSAGE AND ADMINISTRATION

Zarontin is administered by the oral route. The *initial* dose for patients 3 to 6 years of age is one capsule (250 mg) per day; for patients 6 years of age and older, 2 capsules (500 mg) per day. The dose thereafter must be individualized according to the patient's response. Dosage should be increased by small increments. One useful method is to increase the daily dose by 250 mg every four to seven days until control is achieved with minimal side effects. Dosages exceeding 1.5 g daily, in divided doses, should be administered only under the strictest supervision of the physician. The *optimal* dose for most pediatric patients is 20 mg/kg/day. This dose has given average plasma levels within the accepted therapeutic range of 40 to 100 mcg/mL. Subsequent dose schedules can be based on effectiveness and plasma level determinations.

Zarontin may be administered in combination with other anticonvulsants when other forms of epilepsy coexist with absence (petit mal). The *optimal* dose for most pediatric patients is 20 mg/kg/day.

HOW SUPPLIED

Zarontin is supplied as:

N 0071-0237-24 Bottles of 100. Each capsule contains 250 mg ethosuximide.

Store at controlled room temperature 15°–30°C (59°–86°F).

Zarontin is also supplied as:

N 0071-2418-23—1 pint bottles. Each 5 mL of syrup contains 250 mg ethosuximide in a raspberry flavored base.

Rx only

Revised September 1998 **0237G202**

©1997–'98, Warner-Lambert Co.

Shown in Product Identification Guide, page 330

ZARONTIN® ℞

[*ză "rŏn 'tĭn*]

(ethosuximide)

Syrup

DESCRIPTION

Zarontin (ethosuximide) is an anticonvulsant succinimide, chemically designated as alpha-ethyl-alpha-methyl-succinimide, with the following structural formula:

Each teaspoonful (5 mL), for oral administration, contains 250 mg ethosuximide, USP. Also contains citric acid; anhydrous, USP; FD&C red No. 40; FD&C yellow No. 6; flavor; glycerin, USP; purified water, USP; saccharin sodium, USP; sodium benzoate, NF; sodium citrate, USP; sucrose, NF.

CLINICAL PHARMACOLOGY

Ethosuximide suppresses the paroxysmal three cycle per second spike and wave activity associated with lapses of consciousness which is common in absence (petit mal) seizures. The frequency of epileptiform attacks is reduced, apparently by depression of the motor cortex and elevation of the threshold of the central nervous system to convulsive stimuli.

INDICATION AND USAGE

Zarontin is indicated for the control of absence (petit mal) epilepsy.

CONTRAINDICATIONS

Ethosuximide should not be used in patients with a history of hypersensitivity to succinimides.

WARNINGS

Blood dyscrasias, including some with fatal outcome, have been reported to be associated with the use of ethosuximide; therefore, periodic blood counts should be performed. Should signs and/or symptoms of infection (eg, sore throat, fever) develop, blood counts should be considered at that point. Ethosuximide is capable of producing morphological and functional change in the animal liver. In humans, abnormal liver and renal function studies have been reported. Ethosuximide should be administered with extreme caution to patients with known liver or renal disease. Periodic urinalysis and liver function studies are advised for all patients receiving the drug.

Cases of systemic lupus erythematosus have been reported with the use of ethosuximide. The physician should be alert to this possibility.

Usage in Pregnancy: Reports suggest an association between the use of anticonvulsant drugs by women with epilepsy and an elevated incidence of birth defects in children born to these women. Data are more extensive with respect to phenytoin and phenobarbital, but these are also the most commonly prescribed anticonvulsants; less systematic or anecdotal reports suggest a possible similar association with the use of all known anticonvulsant drugs.

The reports suggesting an elevated incidence of birth defects in children of drug-treated epileptic women cannot be regarded as adequate to prove a definite cause and effect relationship. There are intrinsic methodologic problems in obtaining adequate data on drug teratogenicity in humans; the possibility also exists that other factors, eg. genetic factors or the epileptic condition itself, may be more important than drug therapy in leading to birth defects. The great majority of mothers on anticonvulsant medication deliver normal infants. It is important to note that anticonvulsant drugs should not be discontinued in patients in whom the drug is administered to prevent major seizures because of the strong possibility of precipitating status epilepticus with attendant hypoxia and threat to life. In individual cases where the severity and frequency of the seizure disorder are such that the removal of medication does not pose a serious threat to the patient, discontinuation of the drug may be considered prior to and during pregnancy, although it cannot be said with any confidence that even minor seizures do not pose some hazard to the developing embryo or fetus.

The prescribing physician will wish to weigh these considerations in treating or counseling epileptic women of childbearing potential.

PRECAUTIONS

General: Ethosuximide, when used alone in mixed types of epilepsy, may increase the frequency of grand mal seizures in some patients.

As with other anticonvulsants, it is important to proceed slowly when increasing or decreasing dosage, as well as when adding or eliminating other medication. Abrupt withdrawal of anticonvulsant medication may precipitate absence (petit mal) status.

Information for Patients: Ethosuximide may impair the mental and/or physical abilities required for the performance of potentially hazardous tasks such as driving a motor vehicle or other such activity requiring alertness; therefore, the patient should be cautioned accordingly.

Patients taking ethosuximide should be advised of the importance of adhering strictly to the prescribed dosage regimen. Patients should be instructed to promptly contact their physician when they develop signs and/or symptoms suggesting an infection (eg, sore throat, fever).

Drug Interactions: Since Zarontin (ethosuximide) may interact with concurrently administered antiepileptic drugs, periodic serum level determinations of both drugs are recommended (ethosuximide may elevate phenytoin serum levels and valproic acid has been reported to both increase and decrease ethosuximide levels).

Pregnancy: See WARNINGS

ADVERSE REACTIONS

Gastrointestinal System: Gastrointestinal symptoms occur frequently and include anorexia, vague gastric upset, nausea and vomiting, cramps, epigastric and abdominal pain, weight loss, and diarrhea. There have been reports of gum hypertrophy and swelling of the tongue.

Hemopoietic System: Hemopoietic complications associated with the administration of ethosuximide have included leukopenia, agranulocytosis, pancytopenia with or without bone marrow suppression, and eosinophilia.

Nervous System: Neurologic and sensory reactions reported during therapy with ethosuximide have included drowsiness, headache, dizziness, euphoria, hiccups, irritability, hyperactivity, lethargy, fatigue, and ataxia.

Psychiatric or psychological aberrations associated with ethosuximide administration have included disturbances of sleep, night terrors, inability to concentrate, and aggressiveness. These effects may be noted particularly in patients who have previously exhibited psychological abnormalities. There have been rare reports of paranoid psychosis, increased libido, and increased state of depression with overt suicidal intentions.

Integumentary System: Dermatologic manifestations which have occurred with the administration of ethosuximide have included urticaria, Stevens-Johnson syndrome, systemic lupus erythematosus, pruritic erythematous rashes, and hirsutism.

Special Senses: Myopia.

Genitourinary System: Vaginal bleeding, microscopic hematuria.

DOSAGE AND ADMINISTRATION

Zarontin is administered by the oral route. The *initial* dose for patients 3 to 6 years of age is one teaspoonful (250 mg) per day; for patients 6 years of age and older, 2 teaspoonfuls (500 mg) per day. The dose thereafter must be individualized according to the patient's response. Dosage should be increased by small increments. One useful method is to increase the daily dose by 250 mg every four to seven days until control is achieved with minimal side effects. Dosages exceeding 1.5 g daily, in divided doses, should be administered only under the strictest supervision of the physician. The *optimal* dose for most pediatric patients is 20 mg/kg/day. This dose has given average plasma levels within the accepted therapeutic range of 40 to 100 mcg/mL. Subsequent dose schedules can be based on effectiveness and plasma level determinations.

Zarontin may be administered in combination with other anticonvulsants when other forms of epilepsy coexist with absence (petit mal). The optimal dose for most pediatric patients is 20 mg/kg/day.

OVERDOSAGE

Acute overdoses produce CNS depression including coma with respiratory depression. A relationship between ethosuximide toxicity and its plasma levels has not been established. The therapeutic range of serum levels is 40 mcg/mL to 100 mcg/mL, although levels as high as 150 mcg/mL have been reported without signs of toxicity.

Treatment: Treatment should include emesis (unless the patient is, or could rapidly become, obtunded, comatose, or convulsing) or gastric lavage, activated charcoal, cathartics, and general supportive measures. Hemodialysis may be useful to treat ethosuximide overdose. Forced diuresis and exchange transfusions are ineffective.

HOW SUPPLIED

Zarontin is supplied as:

N0071-2418-23—1 pint bottles. Each 5 ml of syrup contains 250 mg ethosuximide in a raspberry flavored base.

Store below 30°C (86°F). Protect from freezing and light.

Zarontin is also supplied in the following form:

N0071-0237-24—Bottles of 100. Each capsule contains 250 mg ethosuximide.

Store at controlled room temperature 15°–30°C (59°–86°F).

Rx only

Revised December 1998 **2418G029**

©1996–'98, Warner-Lambert Co.

Pasteur Mérieux Connaught

SWIFTWATER, PA 18370

For product information see Aventis Pasteur Inc.

PathoGenesis Corporation

201 ELLIOTT AVENUE WEST
SEATTLE, WA 98119

Direct Inquiries to:

Ph. 1-888-508-TOBI (8624)

TOBI ℞

Tobramycin Solution for Inhalation
Nebulizer Solution—For Inhalation Use Only

PRESCRIBING INFORMATION

DESCRIPTION

TOBI® is a tobramycin solution for inhalation. It is a sterile, clear, slightly yellow, non-pyrogenic, aqueous solution with the pH and salinity adjusted specifically for administration by a compressed air driven reusable nebulizer. The chemical formula for tobramycin is $C_{18}H_{37}N_5O_9$ and the molecular weight is 467.52. Tobramycin is *O*-3-amino-3-deoxy-α-D-glucopyranosyl-(1→4)-*O*-[2,6-diamino-2,3,6-trideoxy-α-D-*ribo*-hexopyranosyl-(1→6)]-2-deoxy-L-streptamine. The structural formula for tobramycin is:

Each single-use 5 mL ampule contains 300 mg tobramycin and 11.25 mg sodium chloride in sterile water for injection. Sulfuric acid and sodium hydroxide are added to adjust the pH to 6.0. Nitrogen is used for sparging. All ingredients meet USP requirements. The formulation contains no preservatives.

CLINICAL PHARMACOLOGY

TOBI is specifically formulated for administration by inhalation. When inhaled, tobramycin is concentrated in the airways.

Pharmacokinetics

TOBI contains tobramycin, a cationic polar molecule that does not readily cross epithelial membranes.[1] The bioavailability of TOBI may vary because of individual differences in nebulizer performance and airway pathology.[2] Following administration of TOBI, tobramycin remains concentrated primarily in the airways.

Sputum Concentrations: Ten minutes after inhalation of the first 300 mg dose of TOBI, the average concentration of tobramycin was 1237 μg/g (ranging from 35 to 7414 μg/g) in sputum. Tobramycin does not accumulate in sputum; after 20 weeks of therapy with the TOBI regimen, the average concentration of tobramycin at ten minutes after inhalation was 1154 μg/g (ranging from 39 to 8085 μg/g) in sputum. High variability of tobramycin concentration in sputum was observed. Two hours after inhalation, sputum concentrations declined to approximately 14% of tobramycin levels at ten minutes after inhalation.

Serum Concentrations: The average serum concentration of tobramycin one hour after inhalation of a single 300 mg dose of TOBI by cystic fibrosis patients was 0.95 μg/mL. Af-

Continued on next page

TOBI—Cont.

ter 20 weeks of therapy on the TOBI regimen, the average serum tobramycin concentration one hour after dosing was 1.05 µg/mL.

Elimination: The elimination half-life of tobramycin from serum is approximately 2 hours after intravenous (IV) administration. Assuming tobramycin absorbed following inhalation behaves similarly to tobramycin following IV administration, systemically absorbed tobramycin is eliminated principally by glomerular filtration. Unabsorbed tobramycin, following TOBI administration, is probably eliminated primarily in expectorated sputum.

Microbiology

Tobramycin is an aminoglycoside antibiotic produced by *Streptomyces tenebrarius*.[1] It acts primarily by disrupting protein synthesis, leading to altered cell membrane permeability, progressive disruption of the cell envelope, and eventual cell death.[3]

Tobramycin has *in vitro* activity against a wide range of gram-negative organisms including *Pseudomonas aeruginosa*. It is bactericidal at concentrations equal to or slightly greater than inhibitory concentrations.

Susceptibility Testing

A single sputum sample from a cystic fibrosis patient may contain multiple morphotypes of *Pseudomonas aeruginosa* and each morphotype may have a different level of *in vitro* susceptibility to tobramycin. Treatment for 6 months with TOBI in two clinical studies did not affect the susceptibility of the majority of *P. aeruginosa* isolates tested; however, increased minimum inhibitory concentrations (MICs) were noted in some patients. The clinical significance of this information has not been clearly established in the treatment of *P. aeruginosa* in cystic fibrosis patients. For additional information regarding the effects of TOBI on *P. aeruginosa* MIC values and bacterial sputum density, please refer to the **CLINICAL STUDIES** section.

The *in vitro* antimicrobial susceptibility test methods used for parenteral tobramycin therapy can be used to monitor the susceptibility of *P. aeruginosa* isolated from cystic fibrosis patients. If decreased susceptibility is noted, the results should be reported to the clinician.

Susceptibility breakpoints established for parenteral administration of tobramycin do not apply to aerosolized administration of TOBI. The relationship between *in vitro* susceptibility test results and clinical outcome with TOBI therapy is not clear.

INDICATIONS AND USAGE

TOBI is indicated for the management of cystic fibrosis patients with *P. aeruginosa*.

Safety and efficacy have not been demonstrated in patients under the age of 6 years, patients with FEV_1 <25% or >75% predicted, or patients colonized with *Burkholderia cepacia* (see **CLINICAL STUDIES**).

CONTRAINDICATIONS

TOBI is contraindicated in patients with a known hypersensitivity to any aminoglycoside.

WARNINGS

Caution should be exercised when prescribing TOBI to patients with known or suspected renal, auditory, vestibular, or neuromuscular dysfunction. Patients receiving concomitant parenteral aminoglycoside therapy should be monitored as clinically appropriate.

Aminoglycosides can cause fetal harm when administered to a pregnant woman. Aminoglycosides cross the placenta, and streptomycin has been associated with several reports of total, irreversible, bilateral congenital deafness in pediatric patients exposed *in utero*. Patients who use TOBI during pregnancy, or become pregnant while taking TOBI should be apprised of the potential hazard to the fetus.

Ototoxicity

Ototoxicity, as measured by complaints of hearing loss or by audiometric evaluations, did not occur with TOBI therapy during clinical studies. However, transient tinnitus occurred in eight TOBI-treated patients versus no placebo patients in the clinical studies. Tinnitus is a sentinel symptom of ototoxicity, and therefore the onset of this symptom warrants caution (see **ADVERSE REACTIONS**). **In postmarketing experience, some patients receiving TOBI and extensive previous or concomitant parenteral aminoglycosides have reported hearing loss.** Ototoxicity, manifested as both auditory and vestibular toxicity, has been reported with parenteral aminoglycosides. Vestibular toxicity may be manifested by vertigo, ataxia or dizziness.

Nephrotoxicity

Nephrotoxicity was not seen during TOBI clinical studies but has been associated with aminoglycosides as a class. If nephrotoxicity occurs in a patient receiving TOBI, tobramycin therapy should be discontinued until serum concentrations fall below 2 µg/mL.

Muscular Disorders

TOBI should be used cautiously in patients with muscular disorders, such as myasthenia gravis or Parkinson's disease, since aminoglycosides may aggravate muscle weakness because of a potential curare-like effect on neuromuscular function.

Bronchospasm

Bronchospasm can occur with inhalation of TOBI. In clinical studies of TOBI, changes in FEV_1 measured after the inhaled dose were similar in the TOBI and placebo groups. Bronchospasm should be treated as medically appropriate.

PRECAUTIONS

Information for Patients

NOTE: In addition to information provided below, a Patient Medication Guide providing instructions for proper use of TOBI is contained inside the package.

Safety Information

TOBI is in a class of antibiotics that have caused hearing loss, dizziness, kidney damage, and harm to a fetus. Ringing in the ears and hoarseness were two symptoms that were seen in more patients taking TOBI than placebo in research studies. Patients with cystic fibrosis can have many symptoms. Some of these symptoms may be related to your medications. If you have new or worsening symptoms, you should tell your doctor.

Hearing: You should tell your doctor if you have ringing in the ears, dizziness, or any changes in hearing.

Kidney Damage: Inform your doctor if you have any history of kidney problems.

Pregnancy: If you want to become pregnant or are pregnant while on TOBI, you should talk with your doctor about the possibility of TOBI causing any harm.

Nursing Mothers: If you are nursing a baby, you should talk with your doctor before using TOBI.

TOBI Packaging

TOBI comes in a single dose, ready-to-use ampule containing 300 mg tobramycin. Each box of TOBI contains a 28-day supply - 56 ampules packaged in 14 foil pouches. Each foil pouch contains four ampules, for two days of TOBI therapy.

Dosage

The 300 mg dose of TOBI is the same for patients regardless of age or weight. TOBI has not been studied in patients less than six years old. Doses should be inhaled as close to 12 hours apart as possible and not less than six hours apart. You should not mix TOBI with dornase alfa (PULMOZYME®, Genentech) in the nebulizer.

If you are taking several medications the recommended order is as follows: bronchodilator first, followed by chest physiotherapy, then other inhaled medications and, finally, TOBI.

Treatment Schedule

You should take TOBI in repeated cycles of 28 days on drug followed by 28 days off drug. You should take TOBI twice a day during the 28 day period on drug.

How to Administer TOBI

THIS INFORMATION IS NOT INTENDED TO REPLACE CONSULTATION WITH YOUR PHYSICIAN AND CF CARE TEAM ABOUT PROPERLY TAKING MEDICATION OR USING INHALATION EQUIPMENT.

TOBI is specially formulated for inhalation using a PARI LC PLUS™ Reusable Nebulizer and a DeVilbiss Pulmo-Aide® air compressor. TOBI can be taken at home, school, or at work. The following are instructions on how to use the DeVilbiss Pulmo-Aide air-compressor and PARI LC PLUS Reusable Nebulizer to administer TOBI.

You will need the following supplies:

- TOBI plastic ampule (vial)
- DeVilbiss Pulmo-Aide air compressor
- PARI LC PLUS Reusable Nebulizer
- Tubing to connect the nebulizer and compressor
- Clean paper or cloth towels
- Nose clips (optional)

It is important that your nebulizer and compressor function properly before starting your TOBI therapy.

Note: Please refer to the manufacturers' care and use instructions for important information.

Preparing Your TOBI for Inhalation

1. Wash your hands thoroughly with soap and water.

2a. TOBI is packaged with four ampules per pouch

2b. Separate one ampule by gently pulling apart at the bottom tabs. Store all remaining ampules in the refrigerator as directed.

3. Lay out the contents of a PARI LC PLUS Reusable Nebulizer package on a clean, dry paper or cloth towel. You should have the following parts:

- Nebulizer Top and Bottom (Nebulizer Cup) Assembly
- Inspiratory Valve Cap
- Mouthpiece with Valve
- Tubing

4. Remove the Nebulizer Top from the Nebulizer Cup by twisting the Nebulizer Top counter-clock-wise, and then lifting. Place the Nebulizer Top on the clean paper towel or cloth towel. Stand the Nebulizer Cup upright on the towel.

5. Connect one end of the tubing to the compressor air outlet. The tubing should fit snugly. Plug in your compressor to an electrical outlet.

6. Open the TOBI ampule by holding the bottom tab with one hand and twisting off the top of the ampule with the other hand. Be careful not to squeeze the ampule until you are ready to empty its contents into the Nebulizer Cup.

7. Squeeze all the contents of the ampule into the Nebulizer Cup.

8. Replace the Nebulizer Top. Note: In order to insert the Nebulizer Top into the Nebulizer Cup, the semi-circle halfway down the stem of the Nebulizer Top should face the Nebulizer Outlet.

9. Attach the Mouthpiece to the Nebulizer Outlet. Then firmly push the Inspiratory Valve Cap in place on the Nebulizer Top. Note: the Inspiratory Valve Cap will fit snugly.

10. Connect the free end of the tubing to the Air Intake on the bottom of the nebulizer, making sure to keep the nebulizer upright. Press the tubing on the Air Intake firmly.

TOBI Treatment

1. Turn on the compressor.
2. Check for a steady mist from the Mouthpiece. If there is no mist, check all tubing connections and confirm that the compressor is working properly.
3. Sit or stand in an upright position that will allow you to breathe normally.
4. Place Mouthpiece between your teeth and on top of your tongue and breathe normally only through your mouth. Nose clips may help you breathe through your mouth and not through your nose. Do not block airflow with your tongue.
5. Continue treatment until all your TOBI is gone, and there is no longer any mist being produced. You may hear a sputtering sound when the Nebulizer Cup is empty. The entire TOBI treatment should take approximately 15 minutes to complete. Note: if you are interrupted, need to cough or rest during your TOBI treatment, turn off the compressor to save your medication. Turn the compressor back on when you are ready to resume your therapy.
6. Follow the nebulizer cleaning and disinfecting instructions after completing therapy.

Cleaning Your Nebulizer

To reduce the risk of infection, illness or injury from contamination, you must thoroughly clean all parts of the nebulizer as instructed after each treatment. Never use a nebulizer with a clogged nozzle. If the nozzle is clogged, no aerosol mist is produced, which will alter the effectiveness of the treatment. Replace the nebulizer if clogging occurs.

1. Remove tubing from nebulizer and disassemble nebulizer parts.
2. Wash all parts (except tubing) with warm water and liquid dish soap.
3. Rinse thoroughly with warm water and shake out water.
4. Air dry or hand dry nebulizer parts on a clean, lint-free cloth. Reassemble nebulizer when dry, and store.
5. You can also wash all parts of the nebulizer in a dishwasher (except tubing). Place the nebulizer parts in a dishwasher basket, then place on the top rack of the dishwasher. Remove and dry the parts when the cycle is complete.

Disinfecting Your Nebulizer

Your nebulizer is for your use only—Do not share your nebulizer with other people. You must regularly disinfect the nebulizer. Failure to do so could lead to serious or fatal illness.

1. Clean the nebulizer as described above. Every other treatment day, soak all parts of the nebulizer (except tubing) in a solution of 1 part distilled white vinegar and 3 parts hot tap water for 1 hour. You can substitute respiratory equipment disinfectants (such as Control III®) for distilled white vinegar (follow manufacturer's instructions for mixing). Rinse all parts of the nebulizer thoroughly with warm tap water and dry with a clean, lint-free cloth. Discard the vinegar solution when disinfection is complete.
2. The nebulizer parts (except tubing) may also be disinfected by boiling them in water for a full 10 minutes. Dry parts on a clean, lint-free cloth.

Care and Use of Your Pulmo-Aide Compressor

Follow the manufacturer's instructions for care and use of your compressor.

<u>Filter Change:</u>

1. DeVilbiss Compressor filters should be changed every six months or sooner if filter turns completely gray in color.

<u>Compressor Cleaning:</u>

1. With power switch in the "Off" position, unplug power cord from wall outlet.
2. Wipe outside of the compressor cabinet with a clean, damp cloth every few days to keep dust free.

Caution: Do not submerge in water: doing so will result in compressor damage.

Storage Instructions

You should store TOBI ampules in a refrigerator (2–8°C or 36–46°F). However, when you don't have a refrigerator available (e.g., transporting your TOBI), you may store the foil pouches (opened or unopened) at room temperature (up to 25°C/77°F) for up to 28 days.

Avoid exposing TOBI ampules to intense light.

Unrefrigerated TOBI, which is normally slightly yellow, may darken with age; however, the color change does not indicate any change in the quality of the product.

You should not use TOBI if it is cloudy, if there are particles in the solution, or if it has been stored at room temperature for more than 28 days. You should not use TOBI beyond the expiration date stamped on the ampule.

Additional Information

Nebulizer: 1-800-327-8632
Compressor: 1-800-338-1988
TOBI: 1-888-508-TOBI (8624)

Laboratory Tests

Audiograms

Clinical studies of TOBI did not identify hearing loss using audiometric tests which evaluated hearing up to 8000 Hz. **Physicians should consider an audiogram for patients who show any evidence of auditory dysfunction, or who are at increased risk for auditory dysfunction.** Tinnitus may be a sentinel symptom of ototoxicity, and therefore the onset of this symptom warrents caution.

Serum Concentrations

In patients with normal renal function treated with TOBI, serum tobramycin concentrations are approximately 1 µg/mL one hour after dose administration and do not require routine monitoring. Serum concentrations of tobramycin in patients with renal dysfunction or patients treated with concomitant parenteral tobramycin should be monitored at the discretion of the treating physician.

Renal Function

The clinical studies of TOBI did not reveal any imbalance in the percentage of patients in the TOBI and placebo groups who experienced at least a 50% rise in serum creatinine from baseline (see **ADVERSE REACTIONS**). Laboratory tests of urine and renal function should be conducted at the discretion of the treating physician.

Drug Interactions

In clinical studies of TOBI, patients taking TOBI concomitantly with dornase alfa (PULMOZYME®, Genentech), β-agonists, inhaled corticosteroids, other anti-pseudomonal antibiotics, or parenteral aminoglycosides demonstrated adverse experience profiles similar to the study population as a whole.

Concurrent and/or sequential use of TOBI with other drugs with neurotoxic or ototoxic potential should be avoided. Some diuretics can enhance aminoglycoside toxicity by altering antibiotic concentrations in serum and tissue. TOBI should not be administered concomitantly with ethacrynic acid, furosemide, urea, or mannitol.

Carcinogenesis, Mutagenesis, Impairment of Fertility

A two-year rat inhalation toxicology study to assess carcinogenic potential of TOBI is in progress.

TOBI has been evaluated for genotoxicity in a battery of *in vitro* and *in vivo* tests. The Ames bacterial reversion test, conducted with five tester strains, failed to show a significant increase in revertants with or without metabolic activation in all strains. Tobramycin was negative in the mouse lymphoma forward mutation assay, did not induce chromosomal aberrations in Chinese hamster ovary cells, and was negative in the mouse micronucleus test.

Subcutaneous administration of up to 100 mg/kg of tobramycin did not affect mating behavior or cause impairment of fertility in male or female rats.

Pregnancy

Teratogenic Effects—Pregnancy Category D

(See **WARNINGS**).

No reproduction toxicology studies have been conducted with TOBI. However, subcutaneous administration of tobramycin at doses of 100 or 20 mg/kg/day during organogenesis was not teratogenic in rats or rabbits, respectively. Doses of tobramycin ≥40 mg/kg/day were severely maternally toxic to rabbits and precluded the evaluation of teratogenicity.

Aminoglycosides can cause fetal harm (e.g., congenital deafness) when administered to a pregnant woman. Ototoxicity was not evaluated in offspring during nonclinical reproduction toxicity studies with tobramycin. If TOBI is used during pregnancy, or if the patient becomes pregnant while taking TOBI, the patient should be apprised of the potential hazard to the fetus.

Nursing Mothers

It is not known if TOBI will reach sufficient concentrations after administration by inhalation to be excreted in human breast milk. Because of the potential for ototoxicity and nephrotoxicity in infants, a decision should be made whether to terminate nursing or discontinue TOBI.

Pediatric Use

The safety and efficacy of TOBI have not been studied in pediatric patients under 6 years of age.

ADVERSE REACTIONS

TOBI was generally well tolerated during two clinical studies in 258 cystic fibrosis patients ranging in age from 6 to 48 years. Patients received TOBI in alternating periods of 28 days on and 28 days off drug in addition to their standard cystic fibrosis therapy for a total of 24 weeks.

Voice alteration and tinnitus were the only adverse experiences reported by significantly more TOBI-treated patients. Thirty-three patients (13%) treated with TOBI complained of voice alteration compared to 17 (7%) placebo patients. Voice alteration was more common in the on-drug periods. Eight patients from the TOBI group (3%) reported tinnitus compared to no placebo patients. All episodes were transient, resolved without discontinuation of the TOBI treatment regimen, and were not associated with loss of hearing in audiograms. Tinnitus is one of the sentinel symptoms of cochlear toxicity, and patients with this symptom should be carefully monitored for high frequency hearing loss. The numbers of patients reporting vestibular adverse experiences such as dizziness were similar in the TOBI and placebo groups.

Nine (3%) patients in the TOBI group and nine (3%) patients in the placebo group had increases in serum creatinine of at least 50% over baseline. In all nine patients in the TOBI group, creatinine decreased at the next visit.

Table 1 lists the percent of patients with treatment-emergent adverse experiences (spontaneously reported and solicited) that occurred in >5% of TOBI patients during the two Phase III studies.

Table 1: Percent of Patients With Treatment Emergent Adverse Experiences Occurring in >5% of TOBI Patients

Adverse Event	TOBI (n=258) %	(n=262) Placebo %
Cough increased	46.1	47.3
Pharyngitis	38.0	39.3
Sputum increased	37.6	39.7
Asthenia	35.7	39.3
Rhinitis	34.5	33.6
Dyspnea	33.7	38.5
Fever[1]	32.9	43.5
Lung Disorder	31.4	31.3
Headache	26.7	32.1
Chest pain	26.0	29.8
Sputum discoloration	21.3	19.8
Hemoptysis	19.4	23.7
Anorexia	18.6	27.9
Lung Function decreased[2]	16.3	15.3
Asthma	15.9	20.2
Vomiting	14.0	22.1
Abdominal pain	12.8	23.7
Voice alteration	12.8	6.5
Nausea	11.2	16.0
Weight loss	10.1	15.3
Pain	8.1	12.6
Sinusitis	8.1	9.2
Ear pain	7.4	8.8
Back pain	7.0	8.0
Epistaxis	7.0	6.5
Taste perversion	6.6	6.9
Diarrhea	6.2	10.3
Malaise	6.2	5.3
Lower Resp. Tract Infection	5.8	8.0
Dizziness	5.8	7.6
Hyperventilation	5.4	9.9
Rash	5.4	6.1

[1] Includes subjective complaints of fever.

[2] Includes reported decreases in pulmonary function tests or decreased lung volume on chest radiograph associated with intercurrent illness or study drug administration.

Table 2: Dosing Regimens in Clinical Studies

	Cycle 1		Cycle 2		Cycle 3	
	28 days	**28 days**	**28 days**	**28 days**	**28 days**	**28 days**
TOBI regimen n=258	**TOBI** 300 mg BID	no drug	**TOBI** 300 mg BID	no drug	**TOBI** 300 mg BID	no drug
Placebo regimen n=262	placebo BID	no drug	placebo BID	no drug	placebo BID	no drug

OVERDOSAGE

Signs and symptoms of acute toxicity from overdosage of IV tobramycin might include dizziness, tinnitus, vertigo, loss of high-tone hearing acuity, respiratory failure, and neuromuscular blockade. Administration by inhalation results in low systemic bioavailability of tobramycin. Tobramycin is not significantly absorbed following oral administration. Tobramycin serum concentrations may be helpful in monitoring overdosage.

In all cases of suspected overdosage, physicians should contact the Regional Poison Control Center for information about effective treatment. In the case of any overdosage, the possibility of drug interactions with alterations in drug disposition should be considered.

DOSAGE AND ADMINISTRATION

The recommended dosage for both adults and pediatric patients 6 years of age and older is one single-use ampule (300 mg) administered BID for 28 days. Dosage is not adjusted by weight. All patients should be administered 300 mg BID. The doses should be taken as close to 12 hours apart as possible; they should not be taken less than six hours apart.

TOBI is inhaled while the patient is sitting or standing upright and breathing normally through the mouthpiece of the nebulizer. Nose clips may help the patient breathe through the mouth.

TOBI is administered BID in alternating periods of 28 days. After 28 days of therapy, patients should stop TOBI therapy for the next 28 days, and then resume therapy for the next 28 day on/28 day off cycle.

TOBI is supplied as a single-use ampule and is administered by inhalation, using a hand-held PARI LC PLUS Reusable Nebulizer with a DeVilbiss Pulmo-Aide compressor. TOBI is not for subcutaneous, intravenous or intrathecal administration.

Usage

TOBI is administered by inhalation over an approximately 15 minute period, using a hand-held PARI LC PLUS Reusable Nebulizer with a DeVilbiss Pulmo-Aide compressor. TOBI should not be diluted or mixed with dornase alfa (PULMOZYME®, Genentech) in the nebulizer.

During clinical studies, patients on multiple therapies were instructed to take them first, followed by TOBI.

HOW SUPPLIED

TOBI is supplied in single-use, low-density polyethylene plastic 5 mL ampules. TOBI is packaged in boxes of 56 ampules (14 flexible, laminated foil over-pouches, each containing 4 ampules).

NDC 63430-065-01

Storage

TOBI should be stored under refrigeration at 2–8°C/36–46°F. Upon removal from the refrigerator, or if refrigeration is unavailable, TOBI pouches (opened or unopened) may be stored at room temperature (up to 25°C/77°F) for up to 28 days. TOBI should not be used beyond the expiration date stamped on the ampule when stored under refrigeration (2–8°C/36–46°F) or beyond 28 days when stored at room temperature (25°C/77°F).

TOBI ampules should not be exposed to intense light. The solution in the ampule is slightly yellow, but may darken with age if not stored in the refrigerator; however, the color change does not indicate any change in the quality of the product as long as it is stored within the recommended storage conditions.

CLINICAL STUDIES

Two identically designed, double-blind, randomized, placebo-controlled, parallel group, 24-week clinical studies (Study 1 and Study 2) at a total of 69 cystic fibrosis centers in the United States were conducted in cystic fibrosis patients with *P. aeruginosa*. Subjects who were less than six years of age, had a baseline creatinine of > 2 mg/dL, or had *Burkholderia cepacia* isolated from sputum were excluded. All subjects had baseline FEV_1 % predicted between 25% and 75%. In these clinical studies, 258 patients received TOBI therapy on an outpatient basis (see Table 2) using a hand-held PARI LC PLUS reusable nebulizer with a DeVilbiss Pulmo-Aide compressor.

[See table above]

All patients received either TOBI or placebo (saline with 1.25 mg quinine for flavoring) in addition to standard treatment recommended for cystic fibrosis patients, which included oral and parenteral anti-pseudomonal therapy, β_2-agonists, cromolyn, inhaled steroids, and airway clearance techniques. In addition, approximately 77% of patients were concurrently treated with dornase alfa (PULMOZYME®, Genentech).

In each study, TOBI-treated patients experienced significant improvement in pulmonary function. Improvement was demonstrated in the TOBI group in Study 1 by an average increase in FEV_1% predicted of about 11% relative to baseline (Week 0) during 24 weeks compared to no average change in placebo patients. In Study 2, TOBI treated patients had an average increase of about 7% compared to an average decrease of about 1% in placebo patients. Figure 1 shows the average relative change in FEV_1% predicted over 24 weeks for both studies.

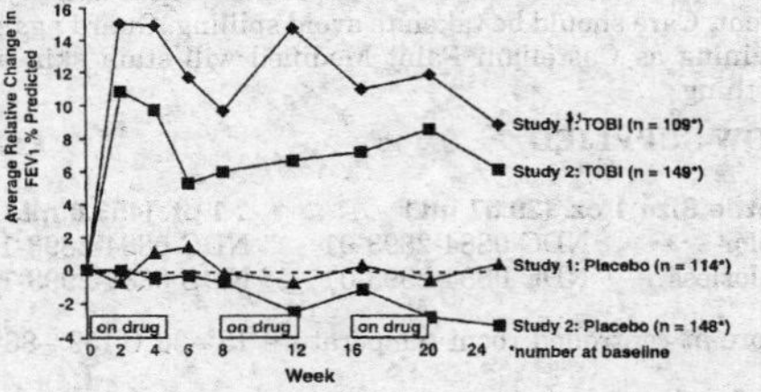

Figure 1: Relative Change From Baseline in FEV_1% Predicted

In each study, TOBI therapy resulted in a significant reduction in the number of *P. aeruginosa* colony forming units (CFUs) in sputum during the on-drug periods. Sputum bacterial density returned to baseline during the off-drug periods. Reductions in sputum bacterial density were smaller in each successive cycle (see Figure 2).

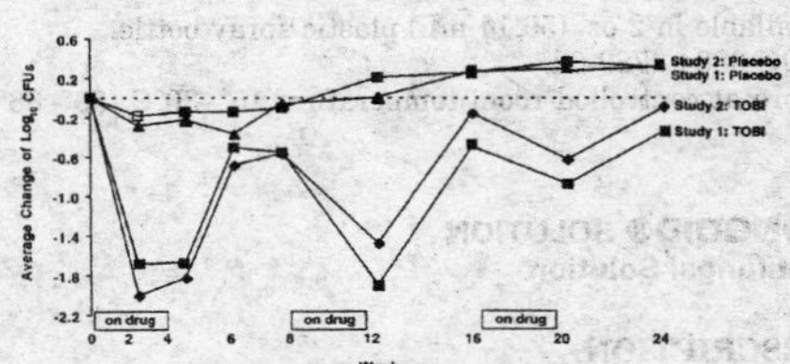

Figure 2: Absolute Change From Baseline in Log_{10} CFUs

Patients treated with TOBI were hospitalized for an average of 5.1 days compared to 8.1 days for placebo patients. Patients treated with TOBI required an average of 9.6 days of parenteral anti-pseudomonal antibiotic treatment compared to 14.1 days for placebo patients. During the six months of treatment, 40% of TOBI patients and 53% of placebo patients were treated with parenteral anti-pseudomonal antibiotics.

Continued on next page

TOBI—Cont.

The relationship between *in vitro* susceptibility test results and clinical outcome with TOBI therapy is not clear. However, four TOBI patients who began the clinical trial with *P. aeruginosa* isolates having MIC values ≥128 µg/mL did not experience an improvement in FEV_1 or a decrease in sputum bacterial density.
Treatment with TOBI did not affect the susceptibility of the majority of *P. aeruginosa* isolates during the six month studies. However, some *P. aeruginosa* isolates did exhibit increased tobramycin MICs. The percentage of patients with *P. aeruginosa* isolates with tobramycin MICs ≥ 16 µg/mL was 13% at the beginning, and 23% at the end of six months of the TOBI regimen.

REFERENCES

1. Neu HC. Tobramycin: an overview. [Review]. J Infect Dis 1976; Suppl 134:S3-19.
2. Weber A, Smith A, Williams-Warren J et al. Nebulizer delivery of tobramycin to the lower respiratory tract. Pediatr Pulmonol 1994; 17 (5):331-9.
3. Bryan LE. Aminoglycoside resistance. Bryan LE, Ed. Antimicrobial drug resistance. Orlando, FL: Academic Press, 1984: 241-77.

Rx Only

Manufactured for
PathoGenesis Corporation
201 Elliott Avenue West, Seattle, WA 98119
by Automatic Liquid Packaging, Inc.,
Woodstock, IL 60098
Packaged by Packaging Coordinators Inc.,
Philadelphia, PA 19114-1123

DATE OF ISSUANCE 4/99

Shown in Product Identification Guide, page 330

Pedinol Pharmacal Inc.

30 BANFI PLAZA NORTH
FARMINGDALE, N.Y. 11735

Direct Inquiries to:
Director of Professional Services
(631) 293-9500

CASTELLANI PAINT Modified — OTC
CASTELLANI PAINT Modified–Colorless — OTC

DESCRIPTION

Castellani Paint Modified is a first aid antiseptic and drying agent. Care should be taken to avoid spilling. Guard against staining as Castellani Paint Modified will stain skin and clothing.

HOW SUPPLIED

Bottle Size	1 oz. (29.57 mL)	1 pt. (453.6 mL)
Color	NDC 0884-2893-01	NDC 0884-2893-16
Colorless	NDC 0884-2993-01	NDC 0884-2993-16

Store at controlled room temperature 15°–30°C (59°–86°F)

FORMALYDE-10® SPRAY — ℞

DESCRIPTION

Formalyde-10 Spray is a topical solution containing Formaldehyde 10% to safeguard against offensive odor and dry excessive moisture of the feet. Drying agent for pre & post-surgical removal of warts where dryness is required.

HOW SUPPLIED

Available in 2 oz. (59.14 mL) plastic spray bottle.
NDC 0884-4789-02
Store at controlled room temperature 15°–30°C (59°–86°F)

FUNGOID® SOLUTION — ℞
Antifungal Solution

DESCRIPTION

Fungoid Solution (Clotrimazole Topical Solution USP, 1%) contains 10 mg Clotrimazole USP, a synthetic antifungal agent having the chemical name 1-(o-Chloro-a, α-diphenybenyzl) imidazole.
Clotrimazole is an odorless, white crystalline substance. It is practically insoluble in water, sparingly soluble in ether and very soluble in polyethylene glycol 400, ethanol and chloroform. Each mL of Fungoid Solution (Clotrimazole Topical Solution USP, 1%) contains 10 mg Clotrimazole USP in a nonaqueous vehicle of Polyethylene Glycol 400.
Prescription Fungoid Solution (Clotrimazole Topical Solution USP, 1%) product is indicated for the topical treatment of candidiasis due to *Candida albicans* and tinea versicolor due to *Malassezia furfur.*

HOW SUPPLIED

NDC 0884-3197-01
Available in a 1 oz (29.57 mL) plastic bottle with controlled dropper.
Store at controlled room temperature 15°–30°C (59°–86°F).

FUNGOID® TINCTURE — OTC

DESCRIPTION

A topical antifungal which is applied as a thin application twice a day (morning and night), to the affected area using the attached brush, **or as recommended by your physician.** Remove Fungoid Tincture from any untreated areas.

HOW SUPPLIED

1 oz. (29.57 mL) bottle with brush applicator NDC 0884-0293-01, 1 pt. (473.12 mL) bottle NDC 0884-0293-16.
FUNGOID TINCTURE TOPICAL ANTIFUNGAL TREATMENT KIT includes: 1 oz. (29.57 mL) FUNGOID TINCTURE, 2 oz. (56.7g) NAIL SCRUB, nail brush. NDC 0884-5493-01.
Store at controlled room temperature 15°–30°C (59°–86°F). Protect from freezing.

Gris-PEG® — ℞
(griseofulvin ultramicrosize)
Tablets, USP
125 mg; 250 mg

DESCRIPTION

Gris-PEG® Tablets contain ultramicrosize crystals of griseofulvin, an antibiotic derived from a species of *Penicillium.* Each Gris-PEG® contains:
Active Ingredient: griseofulvin ultramicrosize .... 125 mg
Inactive Ingredients: colloidal silicon dioxide, lactose, magnesium stearate; methylcellulose; methylparaben; polyethylene glycol 400 and 8000, polyvinylpyrrolidone; and titanium dioxide.
or
Active Ingredient: grisefulvin ultramicrosize ..... 250 mg
Inactive Ingredients: colloidal silicon dioxide; magnesium stearate; methylcellulose; methylparaben; polyethylene glycol 400 and 8000; povidone, sodium lauryl sulfate; and titanium dioxide.

ACTION

Microbiology – Griseofulvin in fungistatic with *in vitro* activity against various species of *Microsporum, Epidermophyton* and *Trichophyton.* It has no effect on bacteria or other genera of fungi.
Human Pharmacology – Following oral administration, griseofulvin is deposited in the keratin precursor cells and has a greater affinity for diseased tissue. The drug is tightly bound to the new keratin which becomes highly resistant to fungal invasions.
The efficiency of gastrointestinal absorption of ultramicrocrystalline griseofulvin is approximately one and one-half times that of the conventional microsize griseofulvin. This factor permits the oral intake of two-thirds as much ultramicrocrystalline griseofulvin as the microsize form. However, there is currently no evidence that this lower dose confers any significant clinical differences with regard to safety and/or efficacy.

INDICATIONS

Gris-PEG® (griseofulvin ultramicrosize) is indicated for the treatment of the following ringworm infections; tinea corporis (ringworm of the body), tinea pedis (athlete's foot), tinea cruris (ringworm of the groin and thigh); tinea barbae (barber's itch), tinea capitis (ringworm of the scalp), and tinea unguium (onychomycosis, ringworm of the nails), when caused by one or more of the following genera of fungi: *Trichophyton rubrum, Trichophyton tonsurans, Trichophyton mentagrophytes, Trichophyton interdigitalis, Trichophyton verrucosum, Trichophyton megnini, Trichophyton gallinae, Trichophyton crateriform, Trichophyton sulphureum, Trichophyton schoenleini, Microsporum audouini, Microsporum canis, Microsporum gypseum* and *Epidermophyton floccosum.* Note: Prior to therapy, the type of fungi responsible for the infection should be identified. The use of the drug is not justified in minor or trivial infections which will respond to topical agents alone. Griseofulvin in *not* effective in the following: bacterial infections, candidiasis (moniliasis), histoplasmosis, actinomycosis, sporotrichosis, chromoblastomycosis, coccidioidomycosis, North American blastomycosis, cryptococcosis (torulosis), tinea versicolor and nocardiosis.

CONTRAINDICATIONS

Two cases of conjoined twins have been reported since 1977 in patients taking griseofulvin during the first trimester of pregnancy. Griseofulvin should not be prescribed to pregnant patients. If the patient becomes pregnant while taking this drug, the patient should be apprised of the potential hazard to the fetus. This drug is contraindicated in patients with porphyria or hepatocellular failure and in individuals with a history of hypersensitivity to griseofulvin.

WARNINGS

Prophylactic Usage – Safety and efficacy of griseofulvin for prophylaxis of fungal infections have not been established.
Animal Toxicology – Chronic feeding of griseofulvin, at levels ranging from 0.5%–2.5% of the diet resulted in the development of liver tumors in several strains of mice, particularly in males. Smaller particle sizes result in an enhanced effect. Lower oral dosage levels have not been tested. Subcutaneous administration of relatively small doses of griseofulvin once a week during the first three weeks of life has also been reported to induce hepatomata in mice. Thyroid tumors, mostly adenomas but some carcinomas, have been reported in male rats receiving griseofulvin at levels of 2.0%, 1.0% and 0.2% of the diet, and in female rats receiving the two higher dose levels. Although studies in other animal species have not yielded evidence of tumorigenicity, these studies were not of adequate design to form a basis for conclusion in this regard. In subacute toxicity studies, orally administered griseofulvin produced hepatocellular necrosis in mice, but this has not been seen in other species. Disturbances in porphyrin metabolism have been reported in griseofulvin-treated laboratory animals. Griseofulvin has been reported to have a colchicine-like effect on mitosis and cocarcinogenicity with methylcholanthrene in cutaneous tumor induction in laboratory animals.
Usage in Pregnancy – see CONTRAINDICATIONS section.
Animal Reproduction Studies – It has been reported in the literature that griseofulvin was found to be embryotoxic and teratogenic on oral administration to pregnant rats. Pups with abnormalities have been reported in the litters of a few bitches treated with griseofulvin. Suppression of spermatogenesis has been reported to occur in rats, but investigation in man failed to confirm this.

PRECAUTIONS

Patients on prolonged therapy with any potent medication should be under close observation. Periodic monitoring of organ system function, including renal, hepatic and hematopoietic, should be done. Since griseofulvin is derived from species of *Penicillium,* the possibility of cross-sensitivity with penicillin exists; however, known penicillin-sensitive patients have been treated without difficulty. Since a photosensitivity reaction is occasionally associated with griseofulvin therapy, patients should be warned to avoid exposure to intense natural or artificial sunlight. Lupus erythematosus or lupus-like syndromes have been reported in patients receiving griseofulvin. Griseofulvin decreases the activity of warfarin-type anticoagulants so that patients receiving these drugs concomitantly may require dosage adjustment of the anticoagulant during and after griseofulvin therapy. Barbiturates usually depress griseofulvin activity and concomitant administration may require a dosage adjustment of the antifungal agent. There have been reports in the literature of possible interactions between griseofulvin and oral contraceptives. The effect of alcohol may be potentiated by griseofulvin, procuding such effects as tachycardia and flush.

ADVERSE REACTIONS

When adverse reactions occur, they are most commonly of the hypersensitivity type such as skin rashes, urticaria, erythema multiforme-like drug reactions, and rarely, angioneurotic edema, and may necessitate withdrawal of therapy and appropriate countermeasures. Paresthesias of the hands and feet have been reported rarely after extended therapy. Other side effects reported occasionally are oral thrush, nausea, vomiting, epigastric distress, diarrhea, headache, fatigue, dizziness, insomnia, mental confusion, and impairment of performance of routine activities. Proteinuria and leukopenia have been reported rarely. Administration of the drug should be discontinued if granulocytopenia occurs. When rare, serious reactions occur with griseofulvin, they are usually associated with high dosages, long periods of therapy, or both.

DOSAGE AND ADMINISTRATION

Accurate diagnosis of infecting organism is essential. Identification would be made either by direct microscopic examination of a mounting of infected tissue in a solution of potassium hydroxide or by culture on an appropriate medium. Medication must be continued until the infecting organism is completely eradicated as indicated by appropriate clinical or laboratory examination. Representative treatment periods are tinea capitis, 4 to 6 weeks; tinea corporis, 2 to 4 weeks; tinea pedis, 4 to 8 weeks; tinea unguium-depending on rate of growth-fingernails, at least 4 months; toenails, at least 6 months. General measures in regard to hygiene should be observed to control sources of infection or reinfection. Concomitant use of appropriate topical agents is usually required, particularly in treatment of tinea pedis. In some forms of athlete's foot, yeasts and bacteria may be involved as well as fungi. Griseofulvin will not eradicate the bacterial or monilial infection.
Adults: Daily administration of 375 mg (as a single dose or in divided doses) will give a satisfactory response in most patients with tinea corporis, tinea crurirs, and tinea capitis. For those fungal infections more difficult to eradicate, such as tinea pedis and tinea unguium, a divided dose of 750 mg is recommended.
Pediatric Use: Approximately 3.3 mg per pound of body weight per day of ultramicrosize griseofulvin is an effective dose for most pediatric patients. On this basis, the following dosage schedule is suggested:
Children weighing 35–60 pounds-125 mg to 187.5mg daily.
Children weighing over 60 pounds-187.5 mg to 375 mg daily.
Children and infants 2 years of age and younger-dosage has not been established. Clinical experience with griseofulvin in children with tinea capitis indicates that a single daily dose is effective. Clinical relapse will occur if the medication is not continued until the infecting organism is eradicated.

HOW SUPPLIED

Gris-PEG® (griseofulvin ultramicrosize) Tablets, 125 mg, white scored, elliptical-shaped, embossed "Gris-PEG" on one side and "125" on the other. Gris-PEG® (griseofulvin ultramicrosize) Tablets, 250 mg, white scored, capsule-shaped, embossed "Gris-PEG" on one side and "250" on the other. The 125 mg strength is available in bottles of 100 (NDC 0023-0763-04). The 250 mg strength is available in bottles of 100, and 500 (NDC 0023-0773-04, and NDC 0023-0773-50 respectively). Both strengths are film-coated.

Rx only

STORAGE

Store Gris-PEG® tablets at controlled room temperature 15°–30°C (59°–86°F) in tight, light-resistant containers.

Manufactured for:
PEDINOL PHARMACAL INC.
30 Banfi Plaza North, Farmingdale, NY 11735 U.S.A.
By:
NOVARTIS CONSUMER HEALTH INC.

LACTINOL-E® CREME ℞
LACTINOL® LOTION ℞

DESCRIPTION

Lactic acid has been reported as an effective naturally occurring humectant in the skin. It has beneficial effects on dry skin and on severe hyperkeratotic conditions. Vitamin E has been used as an aid to control dry or chapped skin. Vitamin E has also found application as an aid in the relief of minor skin disorders such as burns, sunburn, and irritated skin. It has antioxidant properties thus protecting the skin. Lactinol-E Creme and Lactinol Lotion which contain Lactic Acid 10%, is indicated for moisturizing and softening dry, scaly skin (xerosis), ichthyosis vulgaris and itching associated with these conditions.

HOW SUPPLIED

Lactinol-E Creme is available in a 4 oz. (113.4g) plastic jar.
NDC 0884-4990-04
Lactinol Lotion is available in a 12 oz. (354.84 mL) bottle w/pump.
NDC 0884-5292-12
Store at controlled room temperature 15°–30°C (59°–86°F).

LAZERFORMALYDE® SOLUTION ℞

DESCRIPTION

Lazerformalyde Solution is a topical solution containing Formaldehyde 10% as a drying agent for pre and post surgical removal of warts or for cryosurgical treatment of warts where dryness is required. Safeguards against offensive odor and dries excessive moisture of feet.

HOW SUPPLIED

Available in 3 oz. (88.71 mL) plastic bottle with roll-on applicator. NDC 0884-3986-03
Store at controlled room temperature 15°–30°C (59°–86°F).

PEDI–BORO® SOAK PAKS OTC

DESCRIPTION

Pedi-Boro makes a soothing wet dressing of a modified Burow's Solution, Buffered. A mild astringent solution to aid in the relief of minor skin irritations due to allergies, poison ivy, insect bites, or athlete's foot, and as an aid in the relief of swelling associated with minor bruises. Dissolve one or two paks in a pint of water and prepare fresh daily.

HOW SUPPLIED

Box of 12 NDC 0884-1773-27
Box of 100 NDC 0884-1773-10

PEDI–DRI® TOPICAL POWDER ℞

DESCRIPTION

Pedi-Dri Topical Powder provides in each gram 100,000 USP nystatin units dispersed in talc.
Nystatin is an antibiotic which is both fungistatic and fungicidal *in vitro* against a wide variety of yeasts and yeast-like fungi, including *Candida albicans, C. parapsilosis, C. tropicalis, C. guilliermondi, C. pseudotropicalis, C. krusei, Torulopsis glabrata, Tricophyton rubrum, T. mentagrophytes.*
Nystatin acts by binding to sterols in the cell membrane of susceptible species resulting in a change in membrane permeability and the subsequent leakage of intracellular components. Nystatin is a polyene antibiotic of undetermined structural formula that is obtained from Streptomyces noursei, and is the first well tolerated antifungal antibiotic of dependable efficacy for the treatment of cutaneous, oral and intestinal infections caused by Candida (Monilia) albicans and other candida species. It exhibits no appreciable activity against bacteria. Nystatin provides specific therapy for all localized forms of candidiasis. Symptomatic relief is rapid, often occurring within 24 to 48 hours after the initiation of treatment.
Pedi-Dri Topical Powder (Nystatin) is a topical preparation indicated in the treatment of cutaneous or mucocutaneous mycotic infections caused by Candida albicans and other Candida species.

HOW SUPPLIED

Available in a 2 oz. plastic bottle (56.7g) with shaker cap.
NDC 0884-0396-02
Store at controlled room temperature 15°–30°C (59°–86°F).

TI-SCREEN® OTC
SPF 15
SPF 16 (NATURAL AND BABY)
SPF 20 with Parsol® 1789
SPF 23
SPF 30 with Parsol® 1789
LIP PROTECTANT SPF 15

DESCRIPTION

SPF 15 and SPF 30 with Parsol® 1789 are moisturizing sunscreen lotions.
SPF 20 with Parsol® 1789 is a sportsgel. SPF 16 with titanium dioxide is a natural moisturizing sunblock. SPF 23 is a cooling sunscreen spray.
SPF 15 lip protectant sunscreen.

HOW SUPPLIED

TI-SCREEN SPF 15 Lotion 4 oz. bottle NDC 0884-1596-04
SPF 16 Lotion, 4 oz. bottle NDC 0884-1696-04
SPF 16 Baby 4 oz. bottle NDC 0884-6196-04
SPF 20 with Parsol® 1789 Gel 4 oz. bottle NDC 0884-2099-04
SPF 23 Spray, 4 oz. pump bottle, NDC 0884-2396-04
SPF 30 with Parsol® 1789 Lotion 4 oz. bottle NDC 0884-3099-04
SPF 15 Lip Prot. 0.15 oz. stick NDC 0884-1096-01

UREACIN–10® LOTION OTC
UREACIN–20® CREME OTC

DESCRIPTION

Ureacin-10 Lotion and Ureacin-20 Creme are topical treatments for rough, dry, cracked, calloused skin.

HOW SUPPLIED

Ureacin-10®, 8 oz. (226.8g) plastic bottle w/pump. 0884-3249-08.
Ureacin-20®, 4 oz. (113.4g) plastic jar 0884-0449-04.
Store at controlled room temperature 15°–30°C (59°–86°F)

Persōn & Covey, Inc.

616 ALLEN AVENUE
P.O. BOX 25018
GLENDALE, CA 91221-5018

For Additional Information:
(818) 240-1030
(800) 423-2341
FAX (818) 547-9821
E-Mail helpdesk@personandcovey.com

AQUANIL™ Lotion OTC

DESCRIPTION

A gentle, soapless lipid-free cleanser for non-irritating cleansing and moisturizing of sensitive skin.
Non-comedogenic, hypoallergenic and fragrance free. Can be used with or without water.

HOW SUPPLIED

8 oz Plastic bottle (NDC 0096-0724-08)
16 oz Plastic bottle (NDC 0096-0724-16)

AQUANIL HC™ LOTION OTC

DESCRIPTION

Contains 1.0% Hydrocortisone; an effective anti-itch compound; in a gentle, free flowing, lipid free (Oil Free) Lotion that is non-comedogenic.

INDICATIONS

For the temporary relief of minor skin irritations, inflammations, itches and rashes due to seborrheic dermatitis, insect bites, eczema, psoriasis, soaps, detergents, cosmetics, jewelry, poison oak, poison ivy and poison sumac. Other uses of this product should be only under the advice and supervision of a phyisican.

HOW SUPPLIED

118.3 ml (4 fluid oz.) Plastic bottle, (NDC 0096-0732-04)

DHS™ Tar Shampoo OTC
DHS™ Tar Gel Shampoo (Scented)
Tar, equivalent to 0.5% coal tar.

DESCRIPTION

Controls scalp itching and flaking symptomatic of psoriasis, seborrhea and dandruff.

HOW SUPPLIED

4 oz DHS Tar Shampoo Plastic bottle (NDC 0096-0728-04)
8 oz DHS Tar Shampoo Plastic bottle (NDC 0096-0728-08)
16 oz DHS Tar Shampoo Plastic bottle (NDC 0096-0728-16)
8 oz DHS Tar Gel Shampoo Plastic bottle (NDC 0096-0730-08)

DHS™ Zinc Shampoo – 2% Zinc Pyrithione OTC

DESCRIPTION

Controls the symptoms of dandruff, seborrheic dermatitis and psoriasis.

HOW SUPPLIED

8 oz Plastic bottle (NDC 0096-0729-08)
12 oz Plastic bottle (NDC 0096-0729-12)

DHS™ SAL SHAMPOO – 3% Salicylic Acid U.S.P. OTC

DESCRIPTION

A fragrance-free, color-free medication that controls symptoms of psoriasis, dandruff and seborrheic dermatitis. Particularly effective for controlling crusty scalp buildup, and relieving the itching and flaking of severe scalp conditions.

HOW SUPPLIED

4 oz Plastic bottle (NDC 0096-0731-04)

DHS™ SHAMPOO OTC

DESCRIPTION

A gentle foaming cleanser for routine daily hair and scalp cleaning.

HOW SUPPLIED

8 oz Plastic bottle (NDC 0096-0727-08)
16 oz Plastic bottle (NDC 0096-0727-16)

DHS™ CLEAR SHAMPOO OTC

DESCRIPTION

Contains a unique blend of cleansing agents that can be used daily on all hair types. Especially formulated for ph balance.

HOW SUPPLIED

8 oz Plastic bottle (NDC 0096-0725-08)
16 oz Plastic bottle (NDC 0096-0725-16)

DML™ FACIAL MOISTURIZER OTC

INDICATION

Contains special ingredients that help soothe dry, sensitive skin plus sunscreen agents with an SPF of 15 to protect from damaging effects of sunlight (UVA & UVB). Contains Hyaluronic Acid, is non-comedogenic and fragrance free.

HOW SUPPLIED

1.5 oz. Plastic tube, (NDC 0096-0721-45)

DML™-FORTE OTC

DESCRIPTION

Superior moisturizing cream for prolonged relief of severe dry chapped skin on hands, face and body. Fragrance free, hypoallergenic and non-comedogenic.

HOW SUPPLIED

4 oz Plastic Tube NDC 0096-0720-04

DML™-LOTION OTC

DESCRIPTION

Moisturizing lotion for daily care of dry, sensitive skin. It is non-sticky, non greasy, contains no irritants or potential sensitizers. It is a fast absorbing lotion which is fragrance free, non-comedogenic and hypoallergenic and leaves the skin soft and smooth.

HOW SUPPLIED

8 oz Plastic bottle NDC 0096-0722-08
16 oz Plastic bottle NDC 0096-0722-16

DRYSOL™ ℞

DESCRIPTION

A Solution of Aluminum Chloride (Hexahydrate) 20% w/v in Anhydrous Ethyl Alcohol (S.D. Alcohol 40) 93% v/v.

INDICATION

An aid in the management of hyperhidrosis.

Continued on next page

Drysol—Cont.

DIRECTIONS

Apply Drysol to the affected area once a day, **only at bedtime.** Wash the treated area the following morning. To help prevent irritation, the area should be completely dry prior to application. Do not apply Drysol to broken, irritated or recently shaved skin. Keep container tightly closed to prevent evaporation. Excessive sweating may stop after two or more treatments. Thereafter, apply Drysol once or twice weekly or as needed.

ADVERSE REACTIONS

Transient stinging or itching may occur. If intense, remove with soap and water.

WARNING

For external use only. Keep out of the reach of children. Avoid contact with the eyes. If irritation or sensitization occurs, discontinue use or consult with a physician. Drysol may be harmful to certain metals and fabrics. Keep away from open flame.

HOW SUPPLIED

37.5cc Plastic bottle (NDC 0096-0707-37)
35cc Plastic dab-O-Matic (NDC 0096-0707-35)
60cc Plastic dab-O-Matic (NDC 0096-0707-60)

SOLBAR® AVO SPF 32 OTC

CONTAINS

PARSOL® 1789 (Avobenzone)
Homosalate, Octyl Methoxycinnamate, Oxybenzone

INDICATIONS

Solbar-AVO lotion is specifically formulated to offer maximum protection from UVA & UVB radiation. It is non-comedogenic, paba and fragrance free and very water resistant.

HOW SUPPLIED

4oz. Plastic bottle (NDC 0096-0687-04)

SOLBAR® PF CREAM SPF 50 OTC

CONTAINS

Oxybenzone, Octyl Methoxycinnamate, Octocrylene

INDICATIONS

SOLBAR PF 50 Cream is specially formulated for ultra protection from the sun's burning and tanning rays (UVA/UVB). It is paba free, fragrance free, non-comedogenic and very water resistant.

HOW SUPPLIED

4oz. Plastic bottle, (NDC 0096-0686-04).

SOLBAR® PF LIQUID SPF 30 OTC

Ultra protection sunscreen
Broad Spectrum UVA and UVB protection

CONTAINS

Octocrylene, Octyl Methoxycinnamate, Oxybenzone and SD Alcohol 40.

INDICATIONS

SOLBAR PF 30 LIQUID is specially formulated for oily, acne prone skin. It is non-comedogenic, paba and fragrance free. A broad spectrum UVA/UVB sunscreen
WARNING: Keep away from open flame.

HOW SUPPLIED

3.8 oz. Plastic bottle, (NDC 0096-0685-04)

XERAC™ AC ℞

DESCRIPTION

A solution of Aluminum Chloride (Hexahydrate) 6.25% (w/v) in Anhydrous Ethyl Alcohol (S.D. Alcohol 40) 96% (v/v).

INDICATION

For topical application as an antiperspirant (anhidrotic).

DIRECTIONS

Apply Xerac AC to the axillae at bedtime or as directed by physician. To help prevent irritation, the area should be completely dry prior to application. Do not apply Xerac AC to broken or irritated skin. Keep container tightly closed.

ADVERSE REACTIONS

Transient stinging or itching may occur. It is not evidence of contact sensitivity and may be prevented or reduced by applying Xerac AC only to skin which is completely dry or by removing the solution with soap and water.

WARNING

For external use only. Some users of this product will experience skin irritation. If this occurs, discontinue use. Avoid contact with the eyes. This product may be harmful to certain metals and fabrics. Keep the container tightly closed when not in use to prevent evaporation. Keep this and all medication out of the reach of children. Do not use near open flame.

HOW SUPPLIED

35cc bottle/Dab-O-Matic head (NDC 0096-0709-35)
60cc bottle/Dab-O-Matic head (NDC 0096-0709-60)

Pfizer Inc

235 EAST 42nd STREET
NEW YORK, NY 10017–5755

For Medical Information Contact:
(800) 438-1985
24 hours a day, seven days a week.

Product Identification Codes

To provide quick and positive identification of Pfizer Inc products, we have either a unique identifying number of the National Drug Code or the product name on all tablets or capsules.
In order that you may quickly identify a product by its code number, we have compiled below a numerical list of code numbers with their corresponding product names. We are also listing the code numbers by alphabetical order of products.

Numerical Listing

Product Ident. Number	Product
092	**Urobiotic®-250 (oxytetracycline HCl 250 mg with sulfamethizole 250 mg and phenazopyridine 50 mg) Capsules**
094	**Vibramycin® Hyclate (doxycycline hyclate) Capsules 50 mg**
095	**Vibramycin® Hyclate (doxycycline hyclate) Capsules 100 mg**
099	**Vibra-Tabs® (doxycycline hyclate) Film Coated Tablets 100 mg**
143	**Geocillin® (carbenicillin indanyl sodium) Tablets, equivalent to 382 mg carbenicillin**
152	**Norvasc® (amlodipine besylate) Tablets 2.5 mg**
153	**Norvasc® (amlodipine besylate) Tablets 5 mg**
154	**Norvasc® (amlodipine besylate) Tablets 10 mg**
155	**Glucotrol XL® (glipizide) Extended Release Tablets, 5 mg GITS**
156	**Glucotrol XL® (glipizide) Extended Release Tablets, 10 mg GITS**
PD155	**Lipitor® (atorvastatin calcium) Tablets, 10 mg**
PD156	**Lipitor® (atorvastatin calcium) Tablets, 20 mg**
PD157	**Lipitor® (atorvastatin calcium) Tablets, 40 mg**
159	**TAO® (troleandomycin) Capsules, 250 mg**
210	**Antivert® (meclizine HCl) Tablets, 12.5 mg**
211	**Antivert® /25 (meclizine HCl) Tablets, 25 mg**
214	**Antivert® /50 (meclizine HCl) Tablets, 50 mg**
E245	**Aricept® (donepezil HCl) Tablets, 5 mg**
E246	**Aricept® (donepezil HCl) Tablets, 10 mg**
260	**Procardia® (nifedipine) Capsules, 10 mg**
261	**Procardia® (nifedipine) Capsules, 20 mg**
265	**Procardia XL® (nifedipine) Extended Release Tablets, 30 mg GITS**
266	**Procardia XL® (nifedipine) Extended Release Tablets, 60 mg GITS**
267	**Procardia XL® (nifedipine) Extended Release Tablets, 90 mg GITS**
275	**Cardura® (doxazosin mesylate) Tablets, 1 mg**
276	**Cardura® (doxazosin mesylate) Tablets, 2 mg**
277	**Cardura® (doxazosin mesylate) Tablets, 4 mg**
278	**Cardura® (doxazosin mesylate) Tablets, 8 mg**
	Celebrex™ (celecoxib) 7767, 1520 Capsule 100 mg 7767, 1525 Capsule 200 mg
305	**Zithromax® (azithromycin) Capsules 250 mg**
306	**Zithromax® (azithromycin) Z-Pak™(6 × 250-mg Tablets)**
306	**Zithromax® (azithromycin) Tablets, 250 mg**
308	**Zithromax® (azithromycin) Tablets 600 mg**
311	**Zithromax® (azithromycin for oral suspension) 300 mg (100 mg/5 mL)**
312	**Zithromax® (azithromycin for oral suspension) 600 mg (200 mg/5 mL)**
313	**Zithromax® (azithromycin for oral suspension) 900 mg (200 mg/5 mL)**
314	**Zithromax® (azithromycin for oral suspension) 1200 mg (200 mg/5 mL)**
315	**Zithromax® (azithromycin) for injection, 500 mg vial**
322	**Feldene® (piroxicam) Capsules 10 mg**
323	**Feldene® (piroxicam) Capsules 20 mg**
341	**Diflucan® (fluconazole) Tablets, 50 mg**
342	**Diflucan® (fluconazole) Tablets, 100 mg**
343	**Diflucan® (fluconazole) Tablets, 200 mg**
350	**Diflucan® (fluconazole) Tablets, 150 mg**
375	**Renese® (polythiazide) Tablets, 1 mg**
376	**Renese® (polythiazide) Tablets, 2 mg**
377	**Renese® (polythiazide) Tablets, 4 mg**
378	**Trovan® (trovafloxacin mesylate) Tablets, 100 mg**
379	**Trovan® (trovafloxacin mesylate) Tablets 200 mg**
389	**Trovan® I.V. (alatrofloxacin mesylate injection) 200 mg for intravenous infusion**
390	**Trovan® I.V. (alatrofloxacin mesylate injection) 300 mg for intravenous infusion**
393	**Diabinese® (chlorpropamide) Tablets 100 mg**
394	**Diabinese® (chlorpropamide) Tablets 250 mg**
411	**Glucotrol® (glipizide) Tablets, 5 mg**
412	**Glucotrol® (glipizide) Tablets, 10 mg**
420	**Viagra® (sildenafil citrate) Tablets, 25 mg**
421	**Viagra® (sildenafil citrate) Tablets, 50 mg**
422	**Viagra® (sildenafil citrate) Tablets, 100 mg**
430	**Minizide® 1 Capsules (1 mg prazosin HCl and 0.5 mg polythiazide)**
431	**Minipress® (prazosin HCl) Capsules 1 mg**
432	**Minizide® 2 Capsules (2 mg prazosin HCl and 0.5 mg polythiazide)**
436	**Minizide® 5 Capsules (5 mg prazosin HCl and 0.5 mg polythiazide)**
437	**Minipress® (prazosin HCl) Capsules 2 mg**
438	**Minipress® (prazosin HCl) Capsules 5 mg**
490	**Zoloft® (sertraline HCl) Tablets, 50 mg**
491	**Zoloft® (sertraline HCl) Tablets, 100 mg**
496	**Zoloft® (sertraline HCl) Tablets, 25 mg**
534	**Sinequan® (doxepin HCl) Capsules 10 mg**
535	**Sinequan® (doxepin HCl) Capsules 25 mg**
536	**Sinequan® (doxepin HCl) Capsules 50 mg**
537	**Sinequan® (doxepin HCl) Capsules 150 mg**
538	**Sinequan® (doxepin HCl) Capsules 100 mg**
539	**Sinequan® (doxepin HCl) Capsules 75 mg**
541	**Vistaril® (hydroxyzine pamoate) Capsules 25 mg**
542	**Vistaril® (hydroxyzine pamoate) Capsules 50 mg**
543	**Vistaril® (hydroxyzine pamoate) Capsules 100 mg**
550	**Zyrtec® (cetirizine hydrochloride) Tablets 5 mg**
551	**Zyrtec® (cetirizine hydrochloride) Tablets 10 mg**
553	**Zyrtec® (cetirizine hydrochloride) Syrup, 5 mg/5 mL**
560	**Atarax® (hydroxyzine HCl) Tablets, 10 mg**
561	**Atarax® (hydroxyzine HCl) Tablets, 25 mg**
562	**Atarax® (hydroxyzine HCl) Tablets, 50 mg**
563	**Atarax® (hydroxyzine HCl) Tablets, 100 mg**
571	**Navane® (thiothixene) Capsules, 1 mg**
572	**Navane® (thiothixene) Capsules, 2 mg**
573	**Navane® (thiothixene) Capsules, 5 mg**
574	**Navane® (thiothixene) Capsules, 10 mg**
577	**Navane® (thiothixene) Capsules, 20 mg**

Alphabetical Listing

Prod. Ident. Number	Product
210	**Antivert® (meclizine HCl) Tablets, 12.5 mg**

211 Antivert® /25 (meclizine HCl) Tablets, 25 mg
214 Antivert® /50 (meclizine HCl) Tablets, 50 mg
E245 Aricept® (donepezil HCl) Tablets, 5 mg
E246 Aricept® (donepezil HCl) Tablets, 10 mg
560 Atarax® (hydroxyzine HCl) Tablets, 10 mg
561 Atarax® (hydroxyzine HCl) Tablets, 25 mg
562 Atarax® (hydroxyzine HCl) Tablets, 50 mg
563 Atarax® (hydroxyzine HCl) Tablets, 100 mg
275 Cardura® (doxazosin mesylate) Tablets, 1 mg
276 Cardura® (doxazosin mesylate) Tablets, 2 mg
277 Cardura® (doxazosin mesylate) Tablets, 4 mg
278 Cardura® (doxazosin mesylate) Tablets, 8 mg
Celebrex™ (celecoxib)
7767, 1520 Capsule 100 mg
7767, 1525 Capsule 200 mg
393 Diabinese® (chlorpropamide) Tablets 100 mg
394 Diabinese® (chlorpropamide) Tablets 250 mg
341 Diflucan® (fluconazole) Tablets 50 mg
342 Diflucan® (fluconazole) Tablets 100 mg
350 Diflucan® (fluconazole) Tablets 150 mg
343 Diflucan® (fluconazole) Tablets 200 mg
344 Diflucan® (fluconazole for oral suspension) 10 mg/mL
345 Diflucan® (fluconazole for oral suspension) 40 mg/mL
322 Feldene® (piroxicam) Capsules 10 mg
323 Feldene® (piroxicam) Capsules 20 mg
143 Geocillin® (carbenicillin indanyl sodium) Tablets equivalent to 382 mg carbenicillin
411 Glucotrol® (glipizide) Tablets 5 mg
412 Glucotrol® (glipizide) Tablets 10 mg
155 Glucotrol XL® (glipizide) Extended Release Tablets 5 mg GITS
156 Glucotrol XL® (glipizide) Extended Release Tablets 10 mg GITS
PD155 Lipitor® (atorvastatin calcium) Tablets, 10 mg
PD156 Lipitor® (atorvastatin calcium) Tablets, 20 mg
PD157 Lipitor® (atorvastatin calcium) Tablets, 40 mg
431 Minipress® (prazosin HCl) Capsules 1 mg
437 Minipress® (prazosin HCl) Capsules 2 mg
438 Minipress® (prazosin HCl) Capsules 5 mg
430 Minizide® 1 Capsules (1 mg prazosin HCl and 0.5 mg polythiazide)
432 Minizide® 2 Capsules (2 mg prazosin HCl and 0.5 mg polythiazide)
436 Minizide® 5 Capsules (5 mg prazosin HCl and 0.5 mg polythiazide)
571 Navane® (thiothixene) Capsules, 1 mg
572 Navane® (thiothixene) Capsules, 2 mg
573 Navane® (thiothixene) Capsules, 5 mg
574 Navane® (thiothixene) Capsules, 10 mg
577 Navane® (thiothixene) Capsules, 20 mg
152 Norvasc® (amlodipine besylate) Tablets 2.5 mg
153 Norvasc® (amlodipine besylate) Tablets 5 mg
154 Norvasc® (amlodipine besylate) Tablets 10 mg
260 Procardia® (nifedipine) Capsules, 10 mg
261 Procardia® (nifedipine) Capsules, 20 mg
265 Procardia XL® (nifedipine) Extended Release Tablets, 30 mg GITS
266 Procardia XL® (nifedipine) Extended Release Tablets, 60 mg GITS
267 Procardia XL® (nifedipine) Extended Release Tablets, 90 mg GITS
375 Renese® (polythiazide) Tablets, 1 mg
376 Renese® (polythiazide) Tablets, 2 mg
377 Renese® (polythiazide) Tablets, 4 mg
378 Trovan® (trovafloxacin mesylate) Tablets, 100 mg
379 Trovan® (trovafloxacin mesylate) Tablets, 200 mg
389 Trovan® I.V. (alatrofloxacin mesylate injection) 200 mg for intravenous infusion
390 Trovan® I.V. (alatrofloxacin mesylate injection) 300 mg for intravenous infusion
420 Viagra® (sildenafil citrate) Tablets, 25 mg
421 Viagra® (sildenafil citrate) Tablets, 50 mg
422 Viagra® (sildenafil citrate) Tablets, 100 mg
534 Sinequan® (doxepin HCl) Capsules 10 mg
535 Sinequan® (doxepin HCl) Capsules 25 mg
536 Sinequan® (doxepin HCl) Capsules 50 mg
539 Sinequan® (doxepin HCl) Capsules 75 mg
538 Sinequan® (doxepin HCl) Capsules 100 mg
537 Sinequan® (doxepin HCl) Capsules 150 mg
159 TAO® (troleandomycin) Capsules, 250 mg
092 Urobiotic®-250 (oxytetracycline HCl 250 mg with sulfamethizole 250 mg and phenazopyridine 50 mg) Capsules
094 Vibramycin® Hyclate (doxycycline hyclate) Capsules 50 mg
095 Vibramycin® Hyclate (doxycycline hyclate) Capsules 100 mg
099 Vibra-Tabs® (doxycycline hyclate) Film Coated Tablets 100 mg
541 Vistaril® (hydroxyzine pamoate) Capsules 25 mg
542 Vistaril® (hydroxyzine pamoate) Capsules 50 mg
543 Vistaril® (hydroxyzine pamoate) Capsules 100 mg
305 Zithromax® (azithromycin) Capsules 250 mg
306 Zithromax® (azithromycin) Z-PAK™(6 × 250-mg Tablets)
306 Zithromax® (azithromycin) Tablets, 250-mg
308 Zithromax® (azithromycin) 600 mg Tablets
311 Zithromax® (azithromycin for oral suspension) 300 mg (100 mg/5 mL)
312 Zithromax® (azithromycin for oral suspension) 600 mg (200 mg/5 mL)
313 Zithromax® (azithromycin for oral suspension) 900 mg (200 mg/5 mL)
314 Zithromax® (azithromycin for oral suspension) 1200 mg (200 mg/5 mL)
315 Zithromax® Injection (azithromycin) 500 mg Vial
496 Zoloft® (sertraline HCl) Tablets, 25 mg
490 Zoloft® (sertraline HCl) Tablets, 50 mg
491 Zoloft® (sertraline HCl) Tablets, 100 mg
550 Zyrtec® (cetirizine hydrochloride) Tablets 5 mg
551 Zyrtec® (cetirizine hydrochloride) Tablets 10 mg
553 Zyrtec® (cetirizine hydrochloride) Syrup, 5 mg/5 mL

ANTIVERT® TABLETS ℞
[*ăn'tĭ-vert"*]
(12.5 mg meclizine HCl)

ANTIVERT®/25 TABLETS ℞
(25 mg meclizine HCl)

ANTIVERT®/50 TABLETS ℞
(50 mg meclizine HCl)

DESCRIPTION

Chemically, Antivert® (meclizine HCl) is 1-(*p*-chloro-α-phenylbenzyl) -4- (*m* -methylbenzyl) piperazine dihydrochloride monohydrate.

Inert ingredients for the tablets are: dibasic calcium phosphate; magnesium stearate; polyethylene glycol; starch; sucrose. The 12.5 mg tablets also contain: Blue 1. The 25 mg tablets also contain: Yellow 6 Lake; Yellow 10 Lake. The 50 mg tablets also contain: Blue 1 Lake; Yellow 10 Lake.

ACTIONS

Antivert is an antihistamine which shows marked protective activity against nebulized histamine and lethal doses of intravenously injected histamine in guinea pigs. It has a marked effect in blocking the vasodepressor response to histamine, but only a slight blocking action against acetylcholine. Its activity is relatively weak in inhibiting the spasmogenic action of histamine on isolated guinea pig ileum.

INDICATIONS

Based on a review of this drug by the National Academy of Sciences-National Research Council and/or other information, FDA has classified the indications as follows:
Effective: Management of nausea and vomiting, and dizziness associated with motion sickness.
Possibly Effective: Management of vertigo associated with diseases affecting the vestibular system.
Final classification of the less than effective indications requires further investigation.

CONTRAINDICATIONS

Meclizine HCl is contraindicated in individuals who have shown a previous hypersensitivity to it.

WARNINGS

Since drowsiness may, on occasion, occur with use of this drug, patients should be warned of this possibility and cautioned against driving a car or operating dangerous machinery.
Patients should avoid alcoholic beverages while taking this drug. Due to its potential anticholinergic action, this drug should be used with caution in patients with asthma, glaucoma, or enlargement of the prostate gland.

USAGE IN CHILDREN
Clinical studies establishing safety and effectiveness in children have not been done; therefore, usage is not recommended in children under 12 years of age.

USAGE IN PREGNANCY
Pregnancy Category B. Reproduction studies in rats have shown cleft palates at 25–50 times the human dose. Epidemiological studies in pregnant women, however, do not indicate that meclizine increases the risk of abnormalities when administered during pregnancy. Despite the animal findings, it would appear that the possibility of fetal harm is remote. Nevertheless, meclizine, or any other medication, should be used during pregnancy only if clearly necessary.

ADVERSE REACTIONS

Drowsiness, dry mouth and, on rare occasions, blurred vision have been reported.

DOSAGE AND ADMINISTRATION

Vertigo:
For the control of vertigo associated with diseases affecting the vestibular system, the recommended dose is 25 to 100 mg daily, in divided dosage, depending upon clinical response.
Motion Sickness:
The initial dose of 25 to 50 mg of Antivert should be taken one hour prior to embarkation for protection against motion sickness. Thereafter, the dose may be repeated every 24 hours for the duration of the journey.

HOW SUPPLIED

Antivert®—12.5 mg tablets:
Bottles of 100 (NDC 0662-2100-66), (NDC 0049-2100-66)
Bottles of 1000 (NDC 0662-2100-82), (NDC 0049-2100-82)
Antivert®/25—25 mg tablets:
Bottles of 100 (NDC 0662-2110-66), (NDC 0049-2110-66)
Bottles of 1000 (NDC 0662-2110-82), (NDC 0049-2110-82)
Antivert®/50—50 mg tablets:
Bottles of 100 (NDC 0662-2140-66), (NDC 0049-2140-66)
Revised June 1996 69-2148-00-8

ARICEPT® ℞
(Donepezil Hydrochloride Tablets)

DESCRIPTION

ARICEPT® (donepezil hydrochloride) is a reversible inhibitor of the enzyme acetylcholinesterase, known chemically as (±)-2,3-dihydro-5,6-dimethoxy-2-[[1-(phenylmethyl)-4-piperidinyl]methyl]-1*H*-inden-1-one hydrochloride. Donepezil hydrochloride is commonly referred to in the pharmacological literature as E2020. It has an empirical formula of $C_{24}H_{29}NO_3HCl$ and a molecular weight of 415.96. Donepezil hydrochloride is a white crystalline powder and is freely soluble in chloroform, soluble in water and in glacial acetic acid, slightly soluble in ethanol and in acetonitrile and practically insoluble in ethyl acetate and in n-hexane.

ARICEPT® is available for oral administration in film-coated tablets containing 5 or 10 mg of donepezil hydrochloride. Inactive ingredients are lactose monohydrate, corn starch, microcrystalline cellulose, hydroxypropyl cellulose,

Continued on next page

Aricept—Cont.

and magnesium stearate. The film coating contains talc, polyethylene glycol, hydroxypropyl methylcellulose and titanium dioxide. Additionally, the 10 mg tablet contains yellow iron oxide (synthetic) as a coloring agent.

CLINICAL PHARMACOLOGY

Current theories on the pathogenesis of the cognitive signs and symptoms of Alzheimer's Disease attribute some of them to a deficiency of cholinergic neurotransmission. Donepezil hydrochloride is postulated to exert its therapeutic effect by enhancing cholinergic function. This is accomplished by increasing the concentration of acetylcholine through reversible inhibition of its hydrolysis by acetylcholinesterase. If this proposed mechanism of action is correct, donepezil's effect may lessen as the disease process advances and fewer cholinergic neurons remain functionally intact. There is no evidence that donepezil alters the course of the underlying dementing process.

Clinical Trial Data

The effectiveness of ARICEPT® as a treatment for Alzheimer's Disease is demonstrated by the results of two randomized, double-blind, placebo-controlled clinical investigations in patients with Alzheimer's Disease (diagnosed by NINCDS and DSM III-R criteria, Mini-Mental State Examination ≥10 and ≤26 and Clinical Dementia Rating of 1 or 2). The mean age of patients participating in ARICEPT® trials was 73 years with a range of 50 to 94. Approximately 62% of patients were women and 38% were men. The racial distribution was white 95%, black 3% and other races 2%.

Study Outcome Measures: In each study, the effectiveness of treatment with ARICEPT® was evaluated using a dual outcome assessment strategy.

The ability of ARICEPT® to improve cognitive performance was assessed with the cognitive subscale of the Alzheimer's Disease Assessment Scale (ADAS-cog), a multi-item instrument that has been extensively validated in longitudinal cohorts of Alzheimer's Disease patients. The ADAS-cog examines selected aspects of cognitive performance including elements of memory, orientation, attention, reasoning, language and praxis. The ADAS-cog scoring range is from 0 to 70, with higher scores indicating greater cognitive impairment. Elderly normal adults may score as low as 0 or 1, but it is not unusual for non-demented adults to score slightly higher.

The patients recruited as participants in each study had mean scores on the Alzheimer's Disease Assessment Scale (ADAS-cog) of approximately 26 units, with a range from 4 to 61. Experience gained in longitudinal studies of ambulatory patients with mild to moderate Alzheimer's Disease suggest that they gain 6 to 12 units a year on the ADAS-cog. However, lesser degrees of change are seen in patients with very mild or very advanced disease because the ADAS-cog is not uniformly sensitive to change over the course of the disease. The annualized rate of decline in the placebo patients participating in ARICEPT® trials was approximately 2 to 4 units per year.

The ability of ARICEPT® to produce an overall clinical effect was assessed using a Clinician's Interview Based Impression of Change that required the use of caregiver information, the CIBIC plus. The CIBIC plus is not a single instrument and is not a standardized instrument like the ADAS-cog. Clinical trials for investigational drugs have used a variety of CIBIC formats, each different in terms of depth and structure. As such, results from a CIBIC plus reflect clinical experience from the trial or trials in which it was used and cannot be compared directly with the results of CIBIC plus evaluations from other clinical trials. The CIBIC plus used in ARICEPT® trials was a semi-structured instrument that was intended to examine four major areas of patient function: General, Cognitive, Behavioral and Activities of Daily Living. It represents the assessment of a skilled clinician based upon his/her observations at an interview with the patient, in combination with information supplied by a caregiver familiar with the behavior of the patient over the interval rated. The CIBIC plus is scored as a seven point categorical rating, ranging from a score of 1, indicating "markedly improved," to a score of 4, indicating "no change" to a score of 7, indicating "markedly worse." The CIBIC plus has not been systematically compared directly to assessments not using information from caregivers (CIBIC) or other global methods.

Thirty-Week Study

In a study of 30 weeks' duration, 473 patients were randomized to receive single daily doses of placebo, 5 mg/day or 10 mg/day of ARICEPT®. The 30-week study was divided into a 24-week double-blind active treatment phase followed by a 6-week single-blind placebo washout period. The study was designed to compare 5 mg/day or 10 mg/day fixed doses of ARICEPT® to placebo. However, to reduce the likelihood of cholinergic effects, the 10 mg/day treatment was started following an initial 7-day treatment with 5 mg/day doses.

Effects on the ADAS-cog: Figure 1 illustrates the time course for the change from baseline in ADAS-cog scores for all three dose groups over the 30 weeks of the study. After 24 weeks of treatment, the mean differences in the ADAS-cog change scores for ARICEPT® treated patients compared to the patients on placebo were 2.8 and 3.1 units for the 5 mg/day and 10 mg/day treatments, respectively. These differences were statistically significant. While the treatment effect size may appear to be slightly greater for the 10 mg/day treatment, there was no statistically significant difference between the two active treatments.

Following 6 weeks of placebo washout, scores on the ADAS-cog for both the ARICEPT® treatment groups were indistinguishable from those patients who had received only placebo for 30 weeks. This suggests that the beneficial effects of ARICEPT® abate over 6 weeks following discontinuation of treatment and do not represent a change in the underlying disease. There was no evidence of a rebound effect 6 weeks after abrupt discontinuation of therapy.

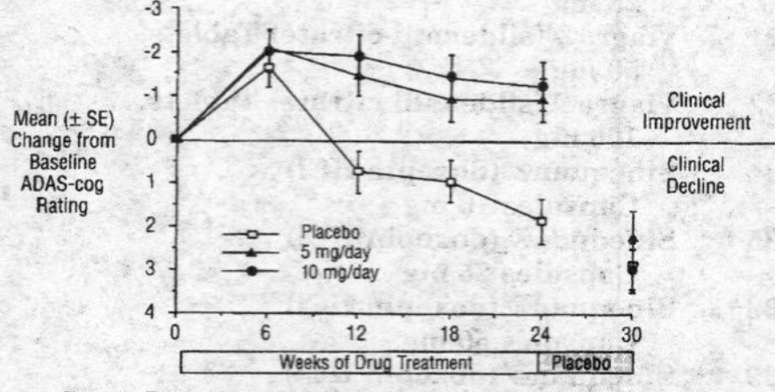

Figure 1. Time-course of the Change from Baseline in ADAS-cog Score for Patients Completing 24 Weeks of Treatment.

Figure 2 illustrates the cumulative percentages of patients from each of the three treatment groups who had attained the measure of improvement in ADAS-cog score shown on the X axis. Three change scores, (7-point and 4-point reductions from baseline or no change in score) have been identified for illustrative purposes and the percent of patients in each group achieving that result is shown in the inset table. The curves demonstrate that both patients assigned to placebo and ARICEPT® have a wide range of responses, but that the active treatment groups are more likely to show the greater improvements. A curve for an effective treatment would be shifted to the left of the curve for placebo, while an ineffective or deleterious treatment would be superimposed upon or shifted to the right of the curve for placebo, respectively.

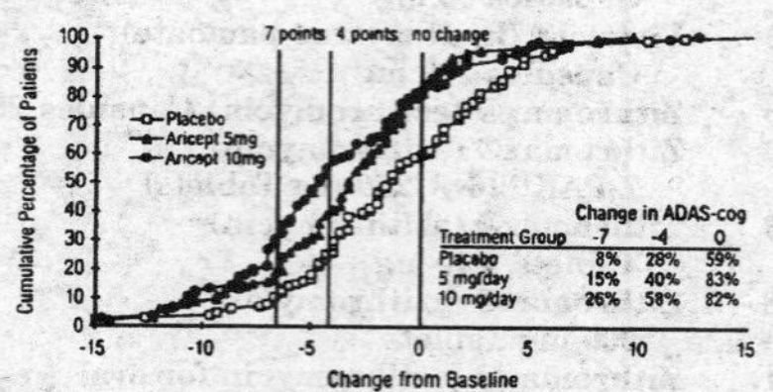

Figure 2 Cumulative Percentage of Patients Completing 24 Weeks of Double-blind Treatment with Specified Changes from Baseline ADAS-cog Scores. The Percentages of Randomized Patients who Completed the Study were: Placebo 80%, 5 mg/day 85% and 10 mg/day 68%

Effects on the CIBIC plus: Figure 3 is a histogram of the frequency distribution of CIBIC plus scores attained by patients assigned to each of the three treatment groups who completed 24 weeks of treatment. The mean drug-placebo differences for these groups of patients were 0.35 units and 0.39 units for 5 mg/day and 10 mg/day of ARICEPT®, respectively. These differences were statistically significant. There was no statistically significant difference between the two active treatments.

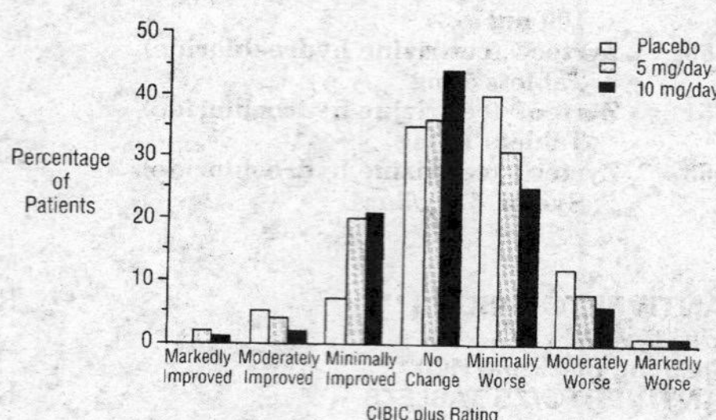

Figure 3. Frequency Distribution of CIBIC plus Scores at Week 24

Fifteen-Week Study

In a study of 15 weeks' duration, patients were randomized to receive single daily doses of placebo or either 5 mg/day or 10 mg/day of ARICEPT® for 12 weeks, followed by a 3-week placebo washout period. As in the 30-week study, to avoid acute cholinergic effects, the 10 mg/day treatment followed an initial 7-day treatment with 5 mg/day doses.

Effects on the ADAS-Cog: Figure 4 illustrates the time course of the change from baseline in ADAS-cog scores for all three dose groups over the 15 weeks of the study. After 12 weeks of treatment, the differences in mean ADAS-cog change scores for the ARICEPT® treated patients compared to the patients on placebo were 2.7 and 3.0 units each, for the 5 and 10 mg/day ARICEPT® treatment groups, respectively. These differences were statistically significant. The effect size for the 10 mg/day group may appear to be slightly larger than that for 5 mg/day. However, the differences between active treatments were not statistically significant.

[See figure at top of next column]

Following 3 weeks of placebo washout, scores on the ADAS-cog for both the ARICEPT® treatment groups increased, in-

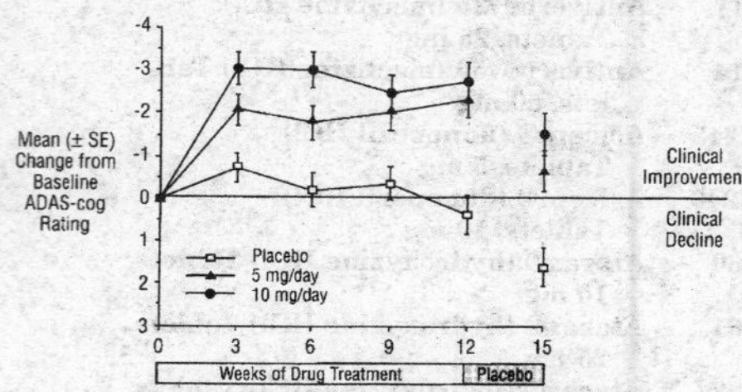

Figure 4. Time-course of the Change from Baseline in ADAS-cog Score for Patients Completing the 15-week Study.

dicating that discontinuation of ARICEPT® resulted in a loss of its treatment effect. The duration of this placebo washout period was not sufficient to characterize the rate of loss of the treatment effect, but, the 30-week study (see above) demonstrated that treatment effects associated with the use of ARICEPT® abate within 6 weeks of treatment discontinuation.

Figure 5 illustrates the cumulative percentages of patients from each of the three treatment groups who attained the measure of improvement in ADAS-cog score shown on the X axis. The same three change scores, (7-point and 4-point reductions from baseline or no change in score) as selected for the 30-week study have been used for this illustration. The percentages of patients achieving those results are shown in the inset table.

As observed in the 30-week study, the curves demonstrate that patients assigned to either placebo or to ARICEPT® have a wide range of responses, but that the ARICEPT® treated patients are more likely to show the greater improvements in cognitive performance.

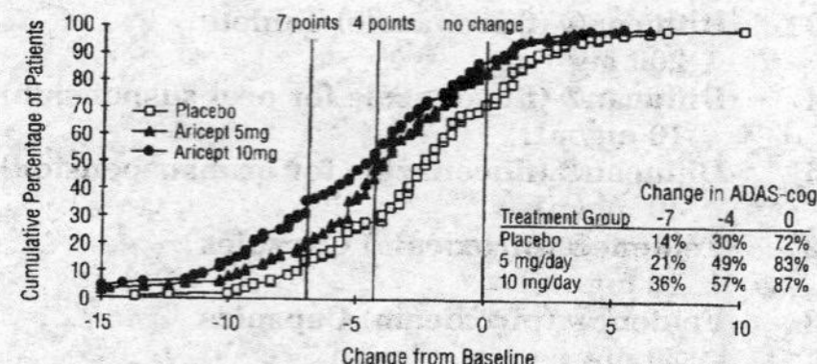

Figure 5. Cumulative Percentage of Patients with Specified Changes from Baseline ADAS-cog Scores. The Percentages of Randomized Patients Within Each Treatment Group Who Completed the Study Were: Placebo 93%, 5 mg/day 90% and 10 mg/day 82%.

Effects on the CIBIC plus: Figure 6 is a histogram of the frequency distribution of CIBIC plus scores attained by patients assigned to each of the three treatment groups who completed 12 weeks of treatment. The differences in mean scores for ARICEPT® treated patients compared to the patients on placebo at Week 12 were 0.36 and 0.38 units for the 5 mg/day and 10 mg/day treatment groups, respectively. These differences were statistically significant.

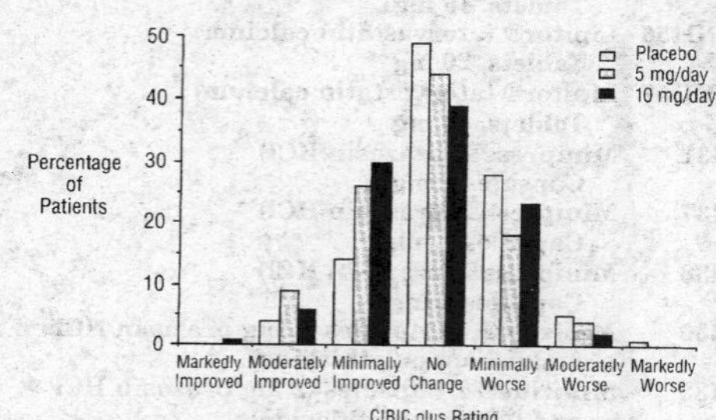

Figure 6. Frequency Distribution of CIBIC plus Scores at Week 12

In both studies, patient age, sex and race were not found to predict the clinical outcome of ARICEPT® treatment.

Clinical Pharmacokinetics

Donepezil is well absorbed with a relative oral bioavailability of 100% and reaches peak plasma concentrations in 3 to 4 hours. Pharmacokinetics are linear over a dose range of 1–10 mg given once daily. Neither food nor time of administration (morning vs. evening dose) influences the rate or extent of absorption. The elimination half life of donepezil is about 70 hours and the mean apparent plasma clearance (Cl/F) is 0.13 L/hr/kg. Following multiple dose administration, donepezil accumulates in plasma by 4–7 fold and steady state is reached within 15 days. The steady state volume of distribution is 12 L/kg. Donepezil is approximately 96% bound to human plasma proteins, mainly to albumins (about 75%) and alpha$_1$-acid glycoprotein (about 21%) over the concentration range of 2-1000 ng/mL.

Donepezil is both excreted in the urine intact and extensively metabolized to four major metabolites, two of which are known to be active, and a number of minor metabolites, not all of which have been identified. Donepezil is metabolized by CYP 450 isoenzymes 2D6 and 3A4 and undergoes glucuronidation. Following administration of ^{14}C-labeled donepezil, plasma radioactivity, expressed as a percent of the administered dose, was present primarily as intact donepezil (53%) and as 6-O-desmethyl donepezil (11%), which has been reported to inhibit AChE to the same extent as donepezil *in vitro* and was found in plasma at concentrations equal to about 20% of donepezil. Approximately 57% and 15% of the total radioactivity was recovered in urine and feces, respectively, over a period of 10 days, while 28% remained unrecovered, with about 17% of the donepezil dose recovered in the urine as unchanged drug.

Special Populations:

Hepatic Disease: In a study of 10 patients with stable alcoholic cirrhosis, the clearance of ARICEPT® was decreased by 20% relative to 10 healthy age and sex matched subjects.

Renal Disease: In a study of 4 patients with moderate to severe renal impairment (Cl_{Cr} <22 mL/min/1.73 m^2) the clearance of ARICEPT® did not differ from 4 age and sex matched healthy subjects.

Age: No formal pharmacokinetic study was conducted to examine age related differences in the pharmacokinetics of ARICEPT®. However, mean plasma ARICEPT® concentrations measured during therapeutic drug monitoring of elderly patients with Alzheimer's Disease are comparable to those observed in young healthy volunteers.

Gender and Race: No specific pharmacokinetic study was conducted to investigate the effects of gender and race on the disposition of ARICEPT®. However, retrospective pharmacokinetic analysis indicates that gender and race (Japanese and Caucasians) did not affect the clearance of ARICEPT®.

Drug-Drug Interactions

Drugs Highly Bound to Plasma Proteins: Drug displacement studies have been performed *in vitro* between this highly bound drug (96%) and other drugs such as furosemide, digoxin, and warfarin. ARICEPT® at concentrations of 0.3–10 μg/mL did not affect the binding of furosemide (5 μg/mL), digoxin (2 ng/mL), and warfarin (3 μg/mL) to human albumin. Similarly, the binding of ARICEPT® to human albumin was not affected by furosemide, digoxin and warfarin.

Effect of ARICEPT® on the Metabolism of Other Drugs: No *in vivo* clinical trials have investigated the effect of ARICEPT® on the clearance of drugs metabolized by CYP 3A4 (e.g. cisapride, terfenadine) or by CYP 2D6 (e.g. imipramine). However, *in vitro* studies show a low rate of binding to these enzymes (mean K_i about 50–130 μM), that, given the therapeutic plasma concentrations of donepezil (164 nM), indicates little likelihood of interference.

Whether ARICEPT® has any potential for enzyme induction is not known.

Formal pharmacokinetic studies evaluated the potential of ARICEPT® for interaction with theophylline, cimetidine, warfarin and digoxin. No significant effects on the pharmacokinetics of these drugs were observed.

Effect of Other Drugs on the Metabolism of ARICEPT®: Ketoconazole and quinidine, inhibitors of CYP450, 3A4 and 2D6, respectively, inhibit donepezil metabolism *in vitro*. Whether there is a clinical effect of these inhibitors is not known. Inducers of CYP 2D6 and CYP 3A4 (e.g., phenytoin, carbamazepine, dexamethasone, rifampin, and phenobarbital) could increase the rate of elimination of ARICEPT®.

Formal pharmacokinetic studies demonstrated that the metabolism of ARICEPT® is not significantly affected by concurrent administration of digoxin or cimetidine.

INDICATIONS AND USAGE

ARICEPT® is indicated for the treatment of mild to moderate dementia of the Alzheimer's type.

CONTRAINDICATIONS

ARICEPT® is contraindicated in patients with known hypersensitivity to donepezil hydrochloride or to piperidine derivatives.

WARNINGS

Anesthesia: ARICEPT®, as a cholinesterase inhibitor, is likely to exaggerate succinylcholine-type muscle relaxation during anesthesia.

Cardiovascular Conditions: Because of their pharmacological action, cholinesterase inhibitors may have vagotonic effects on heart rate (e.g., bradycardia). The potential for this action may be particularly important to patients with "sick sinus syndrome" or other supraventricular cardiac conduction conditions. Syncopal episodes have been reported in association with the use of ARICEPT®.

Gastrointestinal Conditions: Through their primary action, cholinesterase inhibitors may be expected to increase gastric acid secretion due to increased cholinergic activity. Therefore, patients should be monitored closely for symptoms of active or occult gastrointestinal bleeding, especially those at increased risk for developing ulcers, e.g., those with a history of ulcer disease or those receiving concurrent nonsteroidal anti-inflammatory drugs (NSAIDS). Clinical studies of ARICEPT® have shown no increase, relative to placebo, in the incidence of either peptic ulcer disease or gastrointestinal bleeding.

ARICEPT®, as a predictable consequence of its pharmacological properties, has been shown to produce diarrhea, nausea and vomiting. These effects, when they occur, appear more frequently with the 10 mg/day dose than with the 5 mg/day dose. In most cases, these effects have been mild and transient, sometimes lasting one to three weeks, and have resolved during continued use of ARICEPT®.

Genitourinary: Although not observed in clinical trials of ARICEPT®, cholinomimetics may cause bladder outflow obstruction.

Neurological Conditions: Seizures: Cholinomimetics are believed to have some potential to cause generalized convulsions. However, seizure activity also may be a manifestation of Alzheimer's Disease.

Table 1. Most Frequent Adverse Events Leading to Withdrawal from Controlled Clinical Trials by Dose Group

Dose Group	Placebo	5 mg/day ARICEPT®	10 mg/day ARICEPT®
Patients Randomized	355	350	315
Event/% Discontinuing			
Nausea	1%	1%	3%
Diarrhea	0%	<1%	3%
Vomiting	<1%	<1%	2%

Table 2. Comparison of rates of adverse events in patients titrated to 10 mg/day over 1 and 6 weeks

	No titration		One week titration	Six week titration
Adverse Event	Placebo (n=315)	5 mg/day (n=311)	10 mg/day (n=315)	10 mg/day (n=269)
Nausea	6%	5%	19%	6%
Diarrhea	5%	8%	15%	9%
Insomnia	6%	6%	14%	6%
Fatigue	3%	4%	8%	3%
Vomiting	3%	3%	8%	5%
Muscle cramps	2%	6%	8%	3%
Anorexia	2%	3%	7%	3%

Pulmonary Conditions: Because of their cholinomimetic actions, cholinesterase inhibitors should be prescribed with care to patients with a history of asthma or obstructive pulmonary disease.

PRECAUTIONS

Drug-Drug Interactions (see Clinical Pharmacology: Clinical Pharmacokinetics: Drug-drug Interactions)

Effect of ARICEPT® on the Metabolism of Other Drugs: No *in vivo* clinical trials have investigated the effect of ARICEPT® on the clearance of drugs metabolized by CYP 3A4 (e.g. cisapride, terfenadine) or by CYP 2D6 (e.g. imipramine). However, *in vitro* studies show a low rate of binding to these enzymes (mean K_i about 50–130 μM), that, given the therapeutic plasma concentrations of donepezil (164 nM), indicates little likelihood of interference.

Whether ARICEPT® has any potential for enzyme induction is not known.

Effect of Other Drugs on the Metabolism of ARICEPT®: Ketoconazole and quinidine, inhibitors of CYP450, 3A4 and 2D6, respectively, inhibit donepezil metabolism *in vitro*. Whether there is a clinical effect of these inhibitors is not known. Inducers of CYP 2D6 and CYP 3A4 (e.g., phenytoin, carbamazepine, dexamethasone, rifampin, and phenobarbital) could increase the rate of elimination of ARICEPT®.

Use with Anticholinergics: Because of their mechanism of action, cholinesterase inhibitors have the potential to interfere with the activity of anticholinergic medications.

Use with Cholinomimetics and Other Cholinesterase Inhibitors: A synergistic effect may be expected when cholinesterase inhibitors are given concurrently with succinylcholine, similar neuromuscular blocking agents or cholinergic agonists such as bethanechol.

Carcinogenesis, Mutagenesis, Impairment of Fertility

Carcinogenicity studies of donepezil have not been completed.

Donepezil was not mutagenic in the Ames reverse mutation assay in bacteria. In the chromosome aberration test in cultures of Chinese hamster lung (CHL) cells, some clastogenic effects were observed. Donepezil was not clastogenic in the *in vivo* mouse micronucleus test.

Donepezil had no effect on fertility in rats at doses up to 10 mg/kg/day (approximately 8 times the maximum recommended human dose on a mg/m^2 basis).

Pregnancy

Pregnancy Category C: Teratology studies conducted in pregnant rats at doses up to 16 mg/kg/day (approximately 13 times the maximum recommended human dose on a mg/m^2 basis) and in pregnant rabbits at doses up to 10 mg/kg/day (approximately 16 times the maximum recommended human dose on a mg/m^2 basis) did not disclose any evidence for a teratogenic potential of donepezil. However, in a study in which pregnant rats were given up to 10 mg/kg/day (approximately 8 times the maximum recommended human dose on a mg/m^2 basis) from day 17 of gestation through day 20 postpartum, there was a slight increase in still births and a slight decrease in pup survival through day 4 postpartum at this dose; the next lower dose tested was 3 mg/kg/day. There are no adequate or well-controlled studies in pregnant women. ARICEPT® should be used during pregnancy only if the potential benefit justifies the potential risk to the fetus.

Nursing Mothers

It is not known whether donepezil is excreted in human breast milk. ARICEPT® has no indication for use in nursing mothers.

Pediatric Use

There are no adequate and well-controlled trials to document the safety and efficacy of ARICEPT® in any illness occurring in children.

ADVERSE REACTIONS

Adverse Events Leading to Discontinuation

The rates of discontinuation from controlled clinical trials of ARICEPT® due to adverse events for the ARICEPT® 5 mg/day treatment groups were comparable to those of placebo-treatment groups at approximately 5%. The rate of discontinuation of patients who received 7-day escalations from 5 mg/day to 10 mg/day, was higher at 13%.

The most common adverse events leading to discontinuation, defined as those occurring in at least 2% of patients and at twice the incidence seen in placebo patients, are shown in Table 1.

[See table 1 above]

Most Frequent Adverse Clinical Events Seen in Association with the Use of ARICEPT®

The most common adverse events, defined as those occurring at a frequency of at least 5% in patients receiving 10 mg/day and twice the placebo rate, are largely predicted by ARICEPT®'s cholinomimetic effects. These include nausea, diarrhea, insomnia, vomiting, muscle cramp, fatigue and anorexia. These adverse events were often of mild intensity and transient, resolving during continued ARICEPT® treatment without the need for dose modification.

There is evidence to suggest that the frequency of these common adverse events may be affected by the rate of titration. An open-label study was conducted with 269 patients who received placebo in the 15 and 30-week studies. These patients were titrated to a dose of 10 mg/day over a 6-week period. The rates of common adverse events were lower than those seen in patients titrated to 10 mg/day over one week in the controlled clinical trials and were comparable to those seen in patients on 5 mg/day.

See Table 2 for a comparison of the most common adverse events following one and six week titration regimens.

[See table 2 above]

Adverse Events Reported in Controlled Trials

The events cited reflect experience gained under closely monitored conditions of clinical trials in a highly selected patient population. In actual clinical practice or in other clinical trials, these frequency estimates may not apply, as the conditions of use, reporting behavior, and the kinds of patients treated may differ. Table 3 lists treatment emergent signs and symptoms that were reported in at least 2% of patients in placebo-controlled trials who received ARICEPT® and for which the rate of occurrence was greater for ARICEPT® assigned than placebo assigned patients. In general, adverse events occurred more frequently in female patients and with advancing age.

[See table 3 at top of next page]

Other Adverse Events Observed During Clinical Trials

ARICEPT® has been administered to over 1700 individuals during clinical trials worldwide. Approximately 1200 of these patients have been treated for at least 3 months and more than 1000 patients have been treated for at least 6 months. Controlled and uncontrolled trials in the United States included approximately 900 patients. In regards to the highest dose of 10 mg/day, this population includes 650 patients treated for 3 months, 475 patients treated for 6 months and 116 patients treated for over 1 year. The range of patient exposure is from 1 to 1214 days.

Continued on next page

Aricept—Cont.

Treatment emergent signs and symptoms that occurred during 3 controlled clinical trials and two open-label trials in the United States were recorded as adverse events by the clinical investigators using terminology of their own choosing. To provide an overall estimate of the proportion of individuals having similar types of events, the events were grouped into a smaller number of standardized categories using a modified COSTART dictionary and event frequencies were calculated across all studies. These categories are used in the listing below. The frequencies represent the proportion of 900 patients from these trials who experienced that event while receiving ARICEPT®. All adverse events occurring at least twice are included, except for those already listed in Tables 2 or 3, COSTART terms too general to be informative, or events less likely to be drug caused. Events are classified by body system and listed using the following definitions: *frequent adverse events*—those occurring in at least 1/100 patients; *infrequent adverse events*—those occurring in 1/100 to 1/1000 patients. These adverse events are not necessarily related to ARICEPT® treatment and in most cases were observed at a similar frequency in placebo-treated patients in the controlled studies. No important additional adverse events were seen in studies conducted outside the United States.

Body as a Whole: *Frequent:* influenza, chest pain, toothache; *Infrequent:* fever, edema face, periorbital edema, hernia hiatal, abscess, cellulitis, chills, generalized coldness, head fullness, listlessness.

Cardiovascular System: *Frequent:* hypertension, vasodilation, atrial fibrillation, hot flashes, hypotension; *Infrequent:* angina pectoris, postural hypotension, myocardial infarction, AV block (first degree), congestive heart failure, arteritis, bradycardia, peripheral vascular disease, supraventricular tachycardia, deep vein thrombosis.

Digestive System: *Frequent:* fecal incontinence, gastrointestinal bleeding, bloating, epigastric pain; *Infrequent:* eructation, gingivitis, increased appetite, flatulence, periodontal abscess, cholelithiasis, diverticulitis, drooling, dry mouth, fever sore, gastritis, irritable colon, tongue edema, epigastric distress, gastroenteritis, increased transaminases, hemorrhoids, ileus, increased thirst, jaundice, melena, polydipsia, duodenal ulcer, stomach ulcer.

Endocrine System: *Infrequent:* diabetes mellitus, goiter.

Hemic and Lymphatic System: *Infrequent:* anemia, thrombocythemia, thrombocytopenia, eosinophilia, erythrocytopenia.

Metabolic and Nutritional Disorders: *Frequent:* dehydration; *Infrequent:* gout, hypokalemia, increased creatine kinase, hyperglycemia, weight increase, increased lactate dehydrogenase.

Musculoskeletal System: *Frequent:* bone fracture; *Infrequent:* muscle weakness, muscle fasciculation.

Nervous System: *Frequent:* delusions, tremor, irritability, paresthesia, aggression, vertigo, ataxia, increased libido, restlessness, abnormal crying, nervousness, aphasia; *Infrequent:* cerebrovascular accident, intracranial hemorrhage, transient ischemic attack, emotional lability, neuralgia, coldness (localized), muscle spasm, dysphoria, gait abnormality, hypertonia, hypokinesia, neurodermatitis, numbness (localized), paranoia, dysarthria, dysphasia, hostility, decreased libido, melancholia, emotional withdrawal, nystagmus, pacing.

Respiratory System: *Frequent:* dyspnea, sore throat, bronchitis; *Infrequent:* epistaxis, post nasal drip, pneumonia, hyperventilation, pulmonary congestion, wheezing, hypoxia, pharyngitis, pleurisy, pulmonary collapse, sleep apnea, snoring.

Skin and Appendages: *Frequent:* pruritus, diaphoresis, urticaria; *Infrequent:* dermatitis, erythema, skin discoloration, hyperkeratosis, alopecia, fungal dermatitis, herpes zoster, hirsutism, skin striae, night sweats, skin ulcer.

Special Senses: *Frequent:* cataract, eye irritation, vision blurred; *Infrequent:* dry eyes, glaucoma, earache, tinnitus, blepharitis, decreased hearing, retinal hemorrhage, otitis externa, otitis media, bad taste, conjunctival hemorrhage, ear buzzing, motion sickness, spots before eyes.

Urogenital System: *Frequent:* urinary incontinence, nocturia; *Infrequent:* dysuria, hematuria, urinary urgency, metrorrhagia, cystitis, enuresis, prostate hypertrophy, pyelonephritis, inability to empty bladder, breast fibroadenosis, fibrocystic breast, mastitis, pyuria, renal failure, vaginitis.

Postintroduction Reports

Voluntary reports of adverse events temporally associated with ARICEPT® that have been received since market introduction that are not listed above, and that there is inadequate data to determine the causal relationship with the drug include the following: abdominal pain, agitation, cholecystitis, confusion, convulsions, hallucinations, heart block (all types), hemolytic anemia, hepatitis, hyponatremia, pancreatitis, and rash.

OVERDOSAGE

Because strategies for the management of overdose are continually evolving, it is advisable to contact a Poison Control Center to determine the latest recommendations for the management of an overdose of any drug.

As in any case of overdose, general supportive measures should be utilized. Overdosage with cholinesterase inhibitors can result in cholinergic crisis characterized by severe nausea, vomiting, salivation, sweating, bradycardia, hypotension, respiratory depression, collapse and convulsions.

Table 3. Adverse Events Reported in Controlled Clinical Trials in at Least 2% of Patients Receiving ARICEPT® and at a Higher Frequency than Placebo-treated Patients

Body System/Adverse Event	Placebo (n=355)	ARICEPT® (n=747)
Percent of Patients with any Adverse Event	72	74
Body as a Whole		
Headache	9	10
Pain, various locations	8	9
Accident	6	7
Fatigue	3	5
Cardiovascular System		
Syncope	1	2
Digestive System		
Nausea	6	11
Diarrhea	5	10
Vomiting	3	5
Anorexia	2	4
Hemic and Lymphatic System		
Ecchymosis	3	4
Metabolic and Nutritional Systems		
Weight Decrease	1	3
Musculoskeletal System		
Muscle Cramps	2	6
Arthritis	1	2
Nervous System		
Insomnia	6	9
Dizziness	6	8
Depression	<1	3
Abnormal Dreams	0	3
Somnolence	<1	2
Urogenital System		
Frequent Urination	1	2

Increasing muscle weakness is a possibility and may result in death if respiratory muscles are involved. Tertiary anticholinergics such as atropine may be used as an antidote for ARICEPT® overdosage. Intravenous atropine sulfate titrated to effect is recommended: an initial dose of 1.0 to 2.0 mg IV with subsequent doses based upon clinical response. Atypical responses in blood pressure and heart rate have been reported with other cholinomimetics when co-administered with quaternary anticholinergics such as glycopyrrolate. It is not known whether ARICEPT® and/or its metabolites can be removed by dialysis (hemodialysis, peritoneal dialysis, or hemofiltration).

Dose-related signs of toxicity in animals included reduced spontaneous movement, prone position, staggering gait, lacrimation, clonic convulsions, depressed respiration, salivation, miosis, tremors, fasciculation and lower body surface temperature.

DOSAGE AND ADMINISTRATION

The dosages of ARICEPT® shown to be effective in controlled clinical trials are 5 mg and 10 mg administered once per day.

The higher dose of 10 mg did not provide a statistically significantly greater clinical benefit than 5 mg. There is a suggestion, however, based upon order of group mean scores and dose trend analyses of data from these clinical trials, that a daily dose of 10 mg of ARICEPT® might provide additional benefit for some patients. Accordingly, whether or not to employ a dose of 10 mg is a matter of prescriber and patient preference.

Evidence from the controlled trials indicates that the 10 mg dose, with a one week titration, is likely to be associated with a higher incidence of cholinergic adverse events than the 5 mg dose. In open label trials using a 6 week titration, the frequency of these same adverse events was similar between the 5 mg and 10 mg dose groups. Therefore, because steady state is not achieved for 15 days and because the incidence of untoward effects may be influenced by the rate of dose escalation, treatment with a dose of 10 mg should not be contemplated until patients have been on a daily dose of 5 mg for 4 to 6 weeks.

ARICEPT® should be taken in the evening, just prior to retiring. ARICEPT® can be taken with or without food.

HOW SUPPLIED

ARICEPT® is supplied as film-coated, round tablets containing either 5 mg or 10 mg of donepezil hydrochloride.

The 5 mg tablets are white. The strength, in mg (5), is debossed on one side and ARICEPT is debossed on the other side.

The 10 mg tablets are yellow. The strength, in mg (10), is debossed on one side and ARICEPT is debossed on the other side.

5 mg (White)	Bottles of 30 (NDC# 62856-245-30)
	Bottles of 90 (NDC# 62856-245-90)
	Unit Dose Blister Package 100 (10×10) (NDC# 62856-245-41)
10 mg (Yellow)	Bottles of 30 (NDC# 62856-246-30)
	Bottles of 90 (NDC# 62856-246-90)
	Unit Dose Blister Package 100 (10×10) (NDC# 62856-246-41)

Storage: Store at controlled room temperature, 15°C to 30°C (59°F to 86°F).

Rx only

ARICEPT® is a registered trademark of Eisai Co., Ltd., Tokyo, Japan
Manufactured and Marketed by
Eisai Inc., Teaneck, NJ 07666
Distributed/Marketed by
Roerig Division of Pfizer Inc, New York, NY 10017

200142 Revised February 2000

Shown in Product Identification Guide, page 330

ATARAX® ℞

[ăt ʹă-raks ʺ]
(hydroxyzine hydrochloride)
TABLETS AND SYRUP

DESCRIPTION

Hydroxyzine hydrochloride is designated chemically as 1-(p-chlorobenzhydryl) 4-[2-(2-hydroxyethoxy)-ethyl] piperazine dihydrochloride.

Inert ingredients for the tablets are: acacia; carnauba wax; dibasic calcium phosphate; gelatin; lactose; magnesium stearate; precipitated calcium carbonate; shellac; sucrose; talc; white wax. The 10 mg tablets also contain: sodium hydroxide; starch; titanium dioxide; Yellow 6 Lake. The 25 mg tablets also contain: starch, velo dark green. The 50 mg tablets also contain: starch; velo yellow. The 100 mg tablets also contain: alginic acid; Blue 1; polyethylene glycol; Red 3. The inert ingredients for the syrup are: alcohol; menthol; peppermint oil; sodium benzoate; spearmint oil; sucrose; water.

CLINICAL PHARMACOLOGY

Atarax is unrelated chemically to the phenothiazines, reserpine, meprobamate, or the benzodiazepines.
Atarax is not a cortical depressant, but its action may be due to a suppression of activity in certain key regions of the subcortical area of the central nervous system. Primary skeletal muscle relaxation has been demonstrated experimentally. Bronchodilator activity, and antihistaminic and analgesic effects have been demonstrated experimentally and confirmed clinically. An antiemetic effect, both by the apomorphine test and the veriloid test, has been demonstrated. Pharmacological and clinical studies indicate that hydroxyzine in therapeutic dosage does not increase gastric secretion or acidity and in most cases has mild antisecretory activity. Hydroxyzine is rapidly absorbed from the gastrointestinal tract and Atarax's clinical effects are usually noted within 15 to 30 minutes after oral administration.

INDICATIONS

For symptomatic relief of anxiety and tension associated with psychoneurosis and as an adjunct in organic disease states in which anxiety is manifested.
Useful in the management of pruritus due to allergic conditions such as chronic urticaria and atopic and contact dermatoses, and in histamine-mediated pruritus.
As a sedative when used as premedication and following general anesthesia, **Hydroxyzine may potentiate meperidine (Demerol®) and barbiturates,** so their use in pre-anesthetic adjunctive therapy should be modified on an individual basis. Atropine and other belladonna alkaloids are not affected by the drug. Hydroxyzine is not known to interfere with the action of digitalis in any way and it may be used concurrently with this agent.
The effectiveness of hydroxyzine as an antianxiety agent for long term use, that is more than 4 months, has not been assessed by systematic clinical studies. The physician should reassess periodically the usefulness of the drug for the individual patient.

CONTRAINDICATIONS

Hydroxyzine, when administered to the pregnant mouse, rat, and rabbit, induced fetal abnormalities in the rat and mouse at doses substantially above the human therapeutic range. Clinical data in human beings are inadequate to establish safety in early pregnancy. Until such data are available, hydroxyzine is contraindicated in early pregnancy.
Hydroxyzine is contraindicated for patients who have shown a previous hypersensitivity to it.

WARNINGS

Nursing Mothers: It is not known whether this drug is excreted in human milk. Since many drugs are so excreted, hydroxyzine should not be given to nursing mothers.
For Tablets Only: This product is manufactured with 1,1,1-trichloroethane, a substance which harms public health and the environment by destroying ozone in the upper atmosphere.

PRECAUTIONS

THE POTENTIATING ACTION OF HYDROXYZINE MUST BE CONSIDERED WHEN THE DRUG IS USED IN CONJUNCTION WITH CENTRAL NERVOUS SYSTEM DEPRESSANTS SUCH AS NARCOTICS, NON-NARCOTIC ANALGESICS AND BARBITURATES. Therefore when central nervous system depressants are administered concomitantly with hydroxyzine their dosage should be reduced.
Since drowsiness may occur with use of this drug, patients should be warned of this possibility and cautioned against driving a car or operating dangerous machinery while taking Atarax. Patients should be advised against the simultaneous use of other CNS depressant drugs, and cautioned that the effect of alcohol may be increased.

ADVERSE REACTIONS

Side effects reported with the administration of Atarax (hydroxyzine hydrochloride) are usually mild and transitory in nature.
Anticholinergic: Dry mouth.
Central Nervous System: Drowsiness is usually transitory and may disappear in a few days of continued therapy or upon reduction of the dose. Involuntary motor activity including rare instances of tremor and convulsions have been reported, usually with doses considerably higher than those recommended. Clinically significant respiratory depression has not been reported at recommended doses.

OVERDOSAGE

The most common manifestation of Atarax overdosage is hypersedation. As in the management of overdosage with any drug, it should be borne in mind that multiple agents may have been taken.
If vomiting has not occurred spontaneously, it should be induced. Immediate gastric lavage is also recommended. General supportive care, including frequent monitoring of the vital signs and close observation of the patient, is indicated. Hypotension, though unlikely, may be controlled with intravenous fluids and Levophed® (levarterenol), or Aramine® (metaraminol). Do not use epinephrine as Atarax counteracts its pressor action.
There is no specific antidote. It is doubtful that hemodialysis would be of any value in the treatment of overdosage with hydroxyzine. However, if other agents such as barbiturates have been ingested concomitantly, hemodialysis may be indicated. There is no practical method to quantitate hydroxyzine in body fluids or tissue after its ingestion or administration.

DOSAGE

For symptomatic relief of anxiety and tension associated with psychoneurosis and as an adjunct in organic disease states in which anxiety is manifested: in adults, 50–100 mg q.i.d.; children under 6 years, 50 mg daily in divided doses and over 6 years, 50–100 mg daily in divided doses.
For use in the management of pruritus due to allergic conditions such as chronic urticaria and atopic and contact dermatoses, and in histamine-mediated pruritus: in adults, 25 mg t.i.d. or q.i.d.; children under 6 years, 50 mg daily in divided doses and over 6 years, 50–100 mg daily in divided doses.
As a sedative when used as a premedication and following general anesthesia: 50–100 mg in adults, and 0.6 mg/kg in children.
When treatment is initiated by the intramuscular route of administration, subsequent doses may be administered orally.
As with all medications, the dosage should be adjusted according to the patient's response to therapy.

SUPPLY

Atarax Tablets
10 mg—orange tablets: 100's (NDC 0049-5600-66), 500's (NDC 0049-5600-73) Unit Dose 10 × 10's (NDC 0049-5600-41), and Unit of Use 40's (NDC 0049-5600-43)
25 mg—green tablets: 100's (NDC 0049-5610-66), 500's (NDC 0049-5610-73) Unit Dose 10 × 10's (NDC 0049-5610-41), and Unit of Use 40's (NDC 0049-5610-43)
50 mg—yellow tablets: 100's (NDC 0049-5620-66), 500's (NDC 0049-5620-73) and Unit Dose 10 × 10's (NDC 0049-5620-41)
100 mg—red tablets: 100's (NDC 0049-5630-66) and Unit Dose 10 × 10's (NDC 0049-5630-41)
Atarax Syrup
10 mg per teaspoon (5 ml): 1 pint bottles (NDC 0049-5590-93)
Alcohol Content—Ethyl Alcohol—0.5% v/v

BIBLIOGRAPHY

Available on request.
69-0618-00-5 Revised Dec. 1993

CARDURA® ℞
(doxazosin mesylate)
Tablets

DESCRIPTION

CARDURA® (doxazosin mesylate) is a quinazoline compound that is a selective inhibitor of the $alpha_1$ subtype of alpha adrenergic receptors. The chemical name of doxazosin mesylate is 1-(4-amino-6,7-dimethoxy-2-quinazolinyl)-4-(1,4-benzodioxan-2-ylcarbonyl) piperazine methanesulfonate. The empirical formula for doxazosin mesylate is $C_{23}H_{25}N_5O_5 \bullet CH_4O_3S$ and the molecular weight is 547.6. It has the following structure:

[Structure: H_3CO, H_3CO, NH_2, N–C(=O), • CH_3SO_3H]

CARDURA® (doxazosin mesylate) is freely soluble in dimethylsulfoxide, soluble in dimethylformamide, slightly soluble in methanol, ethanol, and water (0.8% at 25°C), and very slightly soluble in acetone and methylene chloride. CARDURA® is available as colored tablets for oral use and contains 1 mg (white), 2 mg (yellow), 4 mg (orange) and 8 mg (green) of doxazosin as the free base.
The inactive ingredients for all tablets are: microcrystalline cellulose, lactose, sodium starch glycolate, magnesium stearate and sodium lauryl sulfate. The 2 mg tablet contains D & C yellow 10 and FD & C yellow 6; the 4 mg tablet contains FD & C yellow 6; the 8 mg tablet contains FD & C blue 10 and D & C yellow 10.

CLINICAL PHARMACOLOGY

Pharmacodynamics
A. Benign Prostatic Hyperplasia (BPH)
Benign prostatic hyperplasia (BPH) is a common cause of urinary outflow obstruction in aging males. Severe BPH may lead to urinary retention and renal damage. A static and a dynamic component contribute to the symptoms and reduced urinary flow rate associated with BPH. The static component is related to an increase in prostate size caused, in part, by a proliferation of smooth muscle cells in the prostatic stroma. However, the severity of BPH symptoms and the degree of urethral obstruction do not correlate well with the size of the prostate. The dynamic component of BPH is associated with an increase in smooth muscle tone in the prostate and bladder neck. The degree of tone in this area is mediated by the $alpha_1$ adrenoceptor, which is present in high density in the prostatic stroma, prostatic capsule and bladder neck. Blockade of the $alpha_1$ receptor decreases urethral resistance and may relieve the obstruction and BPH symptoms. In the human prostate, CARDURA® antagonizes phenylephrine ($alpha_1$ agonist)-induced contractions, *in vitro*, and binds with high affinity to the $alpha_{1c}$ adrenoceptor. The receptor subtype is thought to be the predominant functional type in the prostate. CARDURA® acts within 1-2 weeks to decrease the severity of BPH symptoms and improve urinary flow rate. Since $alpha_1$ adrenoceptors are of low density in the urinary bladder (apart from the bladder neck), CARDURA® should maintain bladder contractility.
The efficacy of CARDURA® was evaluated extensively in over 900 patients with BPH in double-blind, placebo-controlled trials. CARDURA® treatment was superior to placebo in improving patient symptoms and urinary flow rate. Significant relief with CARDURA® was seen as early as one week into the treatment regimen, with CARDURA® treated patients (N=173) showing a significant ($p<0.01$) increase in maximum flow rate of 0.8 mL/sec compared to a decrease of 0.5 mL/sec in the placebo group (N=41). In long-term studies improvement was maintained for up to 2 years of treatment. In 66–71% of patients, improvements above baseline were seen in both symptoms and maximum urinary flow rate.
In three placebo-controlled studies of 14–16 weeks duration obstructive symptoms (hesitation, intermittency, dribbling, weak urinary stream, incomplete emptying of the bladder) and irritative symptoms (nocturia, daytime frequency, urgency, burning) of BPH were evaluated at each visit by patient-assessed symptom questionnaires. The bothersomeness of symptoms was measured with a modified Boyarsky questionnaire. Symptom severity/frequency was assessed using a modified Boyarsky questionnaire or an AUA-based questionnaire. Uroflowmetric evaluations were performed at times of peak (2–6 hours post-dose) and/or trough (24 hours post-dose) plasma concentrations of CARDURA®.
The results from the three placebo-controlled studies (N=609) showing significant efficacy with 4 mg and 8 mg doxazosin are summarized in Table 1. In all three studies, CARDURA® resulted in statistically significant relief of obstructive and irritative symptoms compared to placebo. Statistically significant improvements of 2.3–3.3 mL/sec in maximum flow rate were seen with CARDURA® in Studies 1 and 2, compared to 0.1–0.7 mL/sec with placebo.
[See table 1 at top of next page]
In one fixed dose study (study 2) CARDURA® (doxazosin mesylate) therapy (4–8 mg, once daily) resulted in a significant and sustained improvement in maximum urinary flow rate of 2.3–3.3 mL/sec (Table 1) compared to placebo (0.1 mL/sec). In this study, the only study in which weekly evaluations were made, significant improvement with CARDURA® vs. placebo was seen after one week. The proportion of patients who responded with a maximum flow rate improvement of ≥ 3 mL/sec was significantly larger with CARDURA® (34–42%) than placebo (13–17%). A significantly greater improvement was also seen in average flow rate with CARDURA® (1.6 mL/sec) than with placebo (0.2 mL/sec). The onset and time course of symptom relief and increased urinary flow from study 1 are illustrated in Figure 1.

Figure 1–Study 1

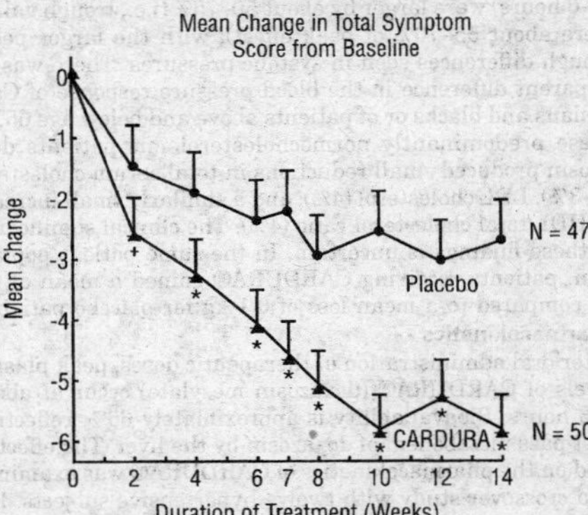

[See figure at top of next column]
In BPH patients (N=450) treated for up to 2 years in open-label studies, CARDURA® therapy resulted in significant improvement above baseline in urinary flow rates and BPH symptoms. The significant effects of CARDURA® were maintained over the entire treatment period.
Although blockade of $alpha_1$ adrenoceptors also lowers blood pressure in hypertensive patients with increased pe-

Continued on next page

Cardura—Cont.

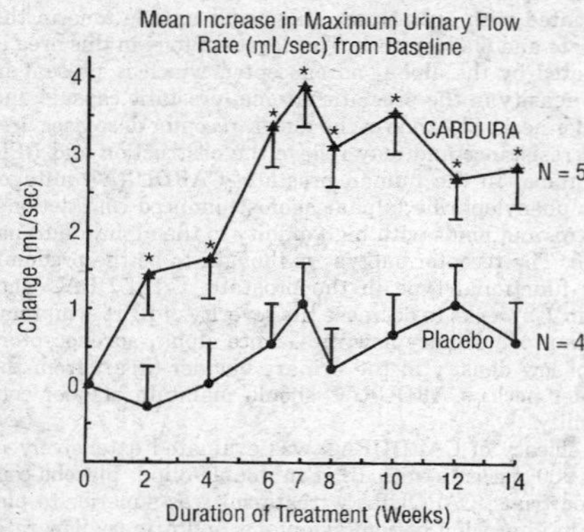

* p < 0.05 Compared to Placebo; + p < 0.05 Compared to Baseline; Doxazosin Titration to Maximum of 8 mg.

TABLE 1
SUMMARY OF EFFECTIVENESS DATA IN PLACEBO-CONTROLLED TRIALS

	SYMPTOM SCORE[a]			MAXIMUM FLOW RATE (mL/sec)		
	N	MEAN BASELINE	MEAN[b] CHANGE	N	MEAN BASELINE	MEAN[c] CHANGE
STUDY 1 (Titration to maximum dose of 8 mg)[e]						
Placebo	47	15.6	-2.3	41	9.7	+0.7
CARDURA	49	14.5	-4.9**	41	9.8	+2.9**
STUDY 2 (Titration to fixed dose–14 weeks)[d]						
Placebo	37	20.7	-2.5	30	10.6	+0.1
CARDURA 4 mg	38	21.2	-5.0**	32	9.8	+2.3*
CARDURA 8 mg	42	19.9	-4.2*	36	10.5	+3.3**
STUDY 3 (Titration to fixed dose–12 weeks)						
Placebo	47	14.9	-4.7	44	9.9	+2.1
CARDURA 4 mg	46	16.6	-6.1*	46	9.6	+2.6

[a] AUA questionnaire (range 0-30) in studies 1 and 3.
Modified Boyarsky Questionnaire (range 7-39) in study 2.
[b] Change is to endpoint.
[c] Change is to fixed-dose efficacy phase, 22-26 hours post-dose for studies 1 and 3 and 2-6 hours post-dose for study 2.
[d] Study in hypertensives with BPH
[e] 36 patients received a dose of 8 mg CARDURA®
*(**) $p < 0.05$ (0.01) compared to placebo mean change.

STUDY 2
Maximum Flow Rate
Placebo 0.1, -2.5; 4 mg 2.3*, -5.0**; 8 mg 3.3**, -4.2*
Symptom Score

TABLE 2
Mean Changes in Blood Pressure from Baseline to the Mean of the Final Efficacy Phase in Normotensives (Diastolic BP <90 mmHg) in Two Double-blind, Placebo-controlled U.S. Studies with CARDURA® 1-8 mg once daily.

	PLACEBO (N=85)		CARDURA® (N=183)	
Sitting BP (mmHg)	**Baseline**	**Change**	**Baseline**	**Change**
Systolic	128.4	−1.4	128.8	−4.9*
Diastolic	79.2	−1.2	79.6	−2.4*
Standing BP (mmHg)	**Baseline**	**Change**	**Baseline**	**Change**
Systolic	128.5	−0.6	128.5	−5.3*
Diastolic	80.5	−0.7	80.4	−2.6*

*p ≤0.05 compared to placebo

ripheral vascular resistance, CARDURA® treatment of normotensive men with BPH did not result in a clinically significant blood pressure lowering effect (Table 2). The proportion of normotensive patients with a sitting systolic blood pressure less than 90 mmHg and/or diastolic blood pressure less than 60 mmHg at any time during treatment with CARDURA® 1–8 mg once daily was 6.7% with doxazosin and not significantly different (statistically) from that with placebo (5%).

[See table 2 above]

B. *Hypertension*

The mechanism of action of CARDURA® (doxazosin mesylate) is selective blockade of the $alpha_1$ (postjunctional) subtype of adrenergic receptors. Studies in normal human subjects have shown that doxazosin competitively antagonized the pressor effects of phenylephrine (an $alpha_1$ agonist) and the systolic pressor effect of norepinephrine. Doxazosin and prazosin have similar abilities to antagonize phenylephrine. The antihypertensive effect of CARDURA® results from a decrease in systemic vascular resistance. The parent compound doxazosin is primarily responsible for the antihypertensive activity. The low plasma concentrations of known active and inactive metabolites of doxazosin (2-piperazinyl, 6′- and 7′-hydroxy and 6- and 7-O-desmethyl compounds) compared to parent drug indicate that the contribution of even the most potent compound (6′-hydroxy) to the antihypertensive effect of doxazosin in man is probably small. The 6′- and 7′-hydroxy metabolites have demonstrated antioxidant properties at concentrations of 5 μM, *in vitro*.

Administration of CARDURA® results in a reduction in systemic vascular resistance. In patients with hypertension there is little change in cardiac output. Maximum reductions in blood pressure usually occur 2–6 hours after dosing and are associated with a small increase in standing heart rate. Like other $alpha_1$-adrenergic blocking agents, doxazosin has a greater effect on blood pressure and heart rate in the standing position.

In a pooled analysis of placebo-controlled hypertension studies with about 300 hypertensive patients per treatment group, doxazosin, at doses of 1–16 mg given once daily, lowered blood pressure at 24 hours by about 10/8 mmHg compared to placebo in the standing position and about 9/5 mmHg in the supine position. Peak blood pressure effects (1–6 hours) were larger by about 50–75% (i.e., trough values were about 55–70% of peak effect), with the larger peak-trough differences seen in systolic pressures. There was no apparent difference in the blood pressure response of Caucasians and blacks or of patients above and below age 65. In these predominantly normocholesterolemic patients doxazosin produced small reductions in total serum cholesterol (2–3%), LDL cholesterol (4%), and a similarly small increase in HDL/total cholesterol ratio (4%). The clinical significance of these findings is uncertain. In the same patient population, patients receiving CARDURA® gained a mean of 0.6 kg compared to a mean loss of 0.1 kg for placebo patients.

Pharmacokinetics

After oral administration of therapeutic doses, peak plasma levels of CARDURA® (doxazosin mesylate) occur at about 2–3 hours. Bioavailability is approximately 65%, reflecting first pass metabolism of doxazosin by the liver. The effect of food on the pharmacokinetics of CARDURA® was examined in a crossover study with twelve hypertensive subjects. Reductions of 18% in mean maximum plasma concentration and 12% in the area under the concentration-time curve occurred when CARDURA® was administered with food. Neither of these differences was statistically or clinically significant.

CARDURA® is extensively metabolized in the liver, mainly by O-demethylation of the quinazoline nucleus or hydroxylation of the benzodioxan moiety. Although several active metabolites of doxazosin have been identified, the pharmacokinetics of these metabolites have not been characterized. In a study of two subjects administered radiolabelled doxazosin 2 mg orally and 1 mg intravenously on two separate occasions, approximately 63% of the dose was eliminated in the feces and 9% of the dose was found in the urine. On average only 4.8% of the dose was excreted as unchanged drug in the feces and only a trace of the total radioactivity in the urine was attributed to unchanged drug. At the plasma concentrations achieved by therapeutic doses approximately 98% of the circulating drug is bound to plasma proteins.

Plasma elimination of doxazosin is biphasic, with a terminal elimination half-life of about 22 hours. Steady-state studies in hypertensive patients given doxazosin doses of 2–16 mg once daily showed linear kinetics and dose proportionality. In two studies, following the administration of 2 mg orally once daily, the mean accumulation ratios (steady-state AUC vs. first dose AUC) were 1.2 and 1.7. Enterohepatic recycling is suggested by secondary peaking of plasma doxazosin concentrations.

In a crossover study in 24 normotensive subjects, the pharmacokinetics and safety of doxazosin were shown to be similar with morning and evening dosing regimens. The area under the curve after morning dosing was, however, 11% less than that after evening dosing and the time to peak concentration after evening dosing occurred significantly later than that after morning dosing (5.6 hr vs. 3.5 hr).

The pharmacokinetics of CARDURA® (doxazosin mesylate) in young (<65 years) and elderly (≥65 years) subjects were similar for plasma half-life values and oral clearance. Pharmacokinetic studies in elderly patients and patients with renal impairment have shown no significant alterations compared to younger patients with normal renal function. Administration of a single 2 mg dose to patients with cirrhosis (Child-Pugh Class A) showed a 40% increase in exposure to doxazosin. There are only limited data on the effects of drugs known to influence the hepatic metabolism of doxazosin [e.g., cimetidine (see PRECAUTIONS)]. As with any drug wholly metabolized by the liver, use of CARDURA® in patients with altered liver function should be undertaken with caution.

In two placebo-controlled studies, of normotensive and hypertensive BPH patients, in which doxazosin was administered in the morning and the titration interval was two weeks and one week, respectively, trough plasma concentrations of CARDURA® were similar in the two populations. Linear kinetics and dose proportionality were observed.

INDICATIONS AND USAGE

A. *Benign Prostatic Hyperplasia (BPH).* CARDURA® is indicated for the treatment of both the urinary outflow obstruction and obstructive and irritative symptoms associated with BPH: obstructive symptoms (hesitation, intermittency, dribbling, weak urinary stream, incomplete emptying of the bladder) and irritative symptoms (nocturia, daytime frequency, urgency, burning). CARDURA® may be used in all BPH patients whether hypertensive or normotensive. In patients with hypertension and BPH, both conditions were effectively treated with CARDURA® monotherapy. CARDURA® provides rapid improvement in symptoms and urinary flow rate in 66–71% of patients. Sustained improvements with CARDURA® were seen in patients treated for up to 14 weeks in double-blind studies and up to 2 years in open-label studies.

B. *Hypertension.* CARDURA® (doxazosin mesylate) is also indicated for the treatment of hypertension. CARDURA® may be used alone or in combination with diuretics, beta-adrenergic blocking agents, calcium channel blockers or angiotensin-converting enzyme inhibitors.

CONTRAINDICATIONS

CARDURA® is contraindicated in patients with a known sensitivity to quinazolines (e.g., prazosin, terazosin).

WARNINGS

Syncope and "First-dose" Effect: Doxazosin, like other alpha-adrenergic blocking agents, can cause marked hypotension, especially in the upright position, with syncope and other postural symptoms such as dizziness. Marked orthostatic effects are most common with the first dose but can also occur when there is a dosage increase, or if therapy is interrupted for more than a few days. To decrease the likelihood of excessive hypotension and syncope, it is essential that treatment be initiated with the 1 mg dose. The 2, 4, and 8 mg tablets are not for initial therapy. Dosage should then be adjusted slowly (see DOSAGE AND ADMINISTRATION section) with evaluations and increases in dose every two weeks to the recommended dose. Additional antihypertensive agents should be added with caution.

Patients being titrated with doxazosin should be cautioned to avoid situations where injury could result should syncope occur, during both the day and night.

In an early investigational study of the safety and tolerance of increasing daily doses of doxazosin in normotensives beginning at 1 mg/day, only 2 of 6 subjects could tolerate more than 2 mg/day without experiencing symptomatic postural hypotension. In another study of 24 healthy normotensive male subjects receiving initial doses of 2 mg/day of doxazosin, seven (29%) of the subjects experienced symptomatic postural hypotension between 0.5 and 6 hours after the first dose necessitating termination of the study. In this study, 2 of the normotensive subjects experienced syncope. Subsequent trials in hypertensive patients always began doxazosin dosing at 1 mg/day resulting in a 4% incidence of postural side effects at 1 mg/day with no cases of syncope.

In multiple dose clinical trials in hypertension involving over 1500 hypertensive patients with dose titration every one to two weeks, syncope was reported in 0.7% of patients. None of these events occurred at the starting dose of 1 mg and 1.2% (8/664) occurred at 16 mg/day.

In placebo-controlled, clinical trials in BPH, 3 out of 665 patients (0.5%) taking doxazosin reported syncope. Two of the patients were taking 1 mg doxazosin, while one patient was taking 2 mg doxazosin when syncope occurred. In the open-label, long-term extension follow-up of approximately 450 BPH patients, there were 3 reports of syncope (0.7%). One patient was taking 2 mg, one patient was taking 8 mg and one patient was taking 12 mg when syncope occurred. In a clinical pharmacology study, one subject receiving 2 mg experienced syncope.

If syncope occurs, the patient should be placed in a recumbent position and treated supportively as necessary.

Priapism: Rarely (probably less frequently than once in every several thousand patients), $alpha_1$ antagonists such as doxazosin have been associated with priapism (painful penile erection, sustained for hours and unrelieved by sexual intercourse or masturbation). Because this condition can lead to permanent impotence if not promptly treated, patients must be advised about the seriousness of the condition (see **PRECAUTIONS: Information for Patients**).

PRECAUTIONS

General:

Prostate Cancer: Carcinoma of the prostate causes many of the symptoms associated with BPH and the two disorders frequently co-exist. Carcinoma of the prostate should therefore be ruled out prior to commencing therapy with CARDURA®.

Orthostatic Hypotension: While syncope is the most severe orthostatic effect of CARDURA®, other symptoms of lowered blood pressure, such as dizziness, lightheadedness, or vertigo can occur, especially at initiation of therapy or at the time of dose increases.

a) Hypertension

These symptoms were common in clinical trials in hypertension, occurring in up to 23% of all patients treated and causing discontinuation of therapy in about 2%.

In placebo-controlled titration trials in hypertension, orthostatic effects were minimized by beginning therapy at 1 mg per day and titrating every two weeks to 2, 4, or 8 mg per day. There was an increased frequency of orthostatic effects in patients given 8 mg or more, 10%, compared to 5% at 1–4 mg and 3% in the placebo group.

b) Benign Prostatic Hyperplasia

In placebo-controlled trials in BPH, the incidence of orthostatic hypotension with doxazosin was 0.3% and did not increase with increasing dosage (to 8 mg/day). The incidence of discontinuations due to hypotensive or orthostatic symptoms was 3.3% with doxazosin and 1% with placebo. The titration interval in these studies was one to two weeks.

Patients in occupations in which orthostatic hypotension could be dangerous should be treated with particular caution. As $alpha_1$ antagonists can cause orthostatic effects, it is important to evaluate standing blood pressure two minutes after standing and patients should be advised to exercise care when arising from a supine or sitting position.

If hypotension occurs, the patient should be placed in the supine position and, if this measure is inadequate, volume expansion with intravenous fluids or vasopressor therapy may be used. A transient hypotensive response is not a contraindication to further doses of CARDURA® (doxazosin mesylate).

Information for Patients (See Patient Package Insert): Patients should be made aware of the possibility of syncopal and orthostatic symptoms, especially at the initiation of therapy, and urged to avoid driving or hazardous tasks for 24 hours after the first dose, after a dosage increase, and after interruption of therapy when treatment is resumed. They should be cautioned to avoid situations where injury could result should syncope occur during initiation of doxazosin therapy. They should also be advised of the need to sit or lie down when symptoms of lowered blood pressure occur, although these symptoms are not always orthostatic, and to be careful when rising from a sitting or lying position. If dizziness, lightheadedness, or palpitations are bothersome they should be reported to the physician, so that dose adjustment can be considered. Patients should also be told that drowsiness or somnolence can occur with CARDURA® (doxazosin mesylate) or any selective $alpha_1$ adrenoceptor antagonist, requiring caution in people who must drive or operate heavy machinery.

Patients should be advised about the possibility of priapism as a result of treatment with $alpha_1$ antagonists. Patients should know that this adverse event is very rare. If they experience priapism, it should be brought to immediate medical attention for if not treated promptly it can lead to permanent erectile dysfunction (impotence).

Drug/Laboratory Test Interactions: CARDURA® does not affect the plasma concentration of prostate specific antigen in patients treated for up to 3 years. Both doxazosin, an $alpha_1$ inhibitor, and finasteride, a 5-alpha reductase inhibitor, are highly protein bound and hepatically metabolized. There is no definitive controlled clinical experience on the concomitant use of $alpha_1$ inhibitors and 5-alpha reductase inhibitors at this time.

Impaired Liver Function: CARDURA® should be administered with caution to patients with evidence of impaired hepatic function or to patients receiving drugs known to influence hepatic metabolism (see CLINICAL PHARMACOLOGY).

Leukopenia/Neutropenia: Analysis of hematologic data from hypertensive patients receiving CARDURA® in controlled hypertension clinical trials showed that the mean WBC (N=474) and mean neutrophil counts (N=419) were decreased by 2.4% and 1.0%, respectively, compared to placebo, a phenomenon seen with other alpha blocking drugs. In BPH patients the incidence of clinically significant WBC abnormalities was 0.4% (2/459) with CARDURA® and 0% (0/147) with placebo, with no statistically significant difference between the two treatment groups. A search through a data base of 2400 hypertensive patients and 665 BPH patients revealed 4 hypertensives in which drug-related neutropenia could not be ruled out and one BPH patient in which drug related leukopenia could not be ruled out. Two hypertensives had a single low value on the last day of treatment. Two hypertensives had stable, non-progressive neutrophil counts in the 1000/mm³ range over periods of 20 and 40 weeks. One BPH patient had a decrease from a WBC count of 4800/mm³ to 2700/mm³ at the end of the study; there was no evidence of clinical impairment. In cases where follow-up was available the WBCs and neutrophil counts returned to normal after discontinuation of CARDURA®. No patients became symptomatic as a result of the low WBC or neutrophil counts.

Drug Interactions: Most (98%) of plasma doxazosin is protein bound. *In vitro* data in human plasma indicate that CARDURA® has no effect on protein binding of digoxin, warfarin, phenytoin or indomethacin. There is no information on the effect of other highly plasma protein bound drugs on doxazosin binding. CARDURA® has been administered without any evidence of an adverse drug interaction to patients receiving thiazide diuretics, beta-blocking agents, and nonsteroidal anti-inflammatory drugs. In a placebo-controlled trial in normal volunteers, the administration of a single 1 mg dose of doxazosin on day 1 of a four-day regimen of oral cimetidine (400 mg twice daily) resulted in a 10% increase in mean AUC of doxazosin (p=0.006), and a slight but not statistically significant increase in mean C_{max} and mean half-life of doxazosin. The clinical significance of this increase in doxazosin AUC is unknown.

In clinical trials, CARDURA® tablets have been administered to patients on a variety of concomitant medications; while no formal interaction studies have been conducted, no interactions were observed. CARDURA® tablets have been used with the following drugs or drug classes: 1) analgesic/anti-inflammatory (e.g., acetaminophen, aspirin, codeine and codeine combinations, ibuprofen, indomethacin); 2) antibiotics (e.g., erythromycin, trimethoprim and sulfamethoxazole, amoxicillin); 3) antihistamines (e.g., chlorpheniramine); 4) cardiovascular agents (e.g., atenolol, hydrochlorothiazide, propranolol); 5) corticosteroids); 6) gastrointestinal agents (e.g., antacids); 7) hypoglycemics and endocrine drugs; 8) sedatives and tranquilizers (e.g., diazepam); 9) cold and flu remedies.

Cardiac Toxicity in Animals: An increased incidence of myocardial necrosis or fibrosis was displayed by Sprague-Dawley rats after 6 months of dietary administration at concentrations calculated to provide 80 mg doxazosin/kg/day and after 12 months of dietary administration at concentrations calculated to provide 40 mg doxazosin/kg/day (AUC exposure in rats 8 times the human AUC exposure with a 12 mg/day therapeutic dose). Myocardial fibrosis was observed in both rats and mice treated in the same manner with 40 mg doxazosin/kg/day for 18 months (exposure 8 times human AUC exposure in rats and somewhat equivalent to human C_{max} exposure in mice). No cardiotoxicity was observed at lower doses (up to 10 or 20 mg/kg/day, depending on the study) in either species. These lesions were not observed after 12 months of oral dosing in dogs at maximum doses of 20 mg/kg/day [maximum plasma concentrations (C_{max}) in dogs 14 times the C_{max} exposure in humans receiving a 12 mg/day therapeutic dose] and in Wistar rats at doses of 100 mg/kg/day (C_{max} exposures 15 times human C_{max} exposure with a 12 mg/day therapeutic dose). There is no evidence that similar lesions occur in humans.

Carcinogenesis, Mutagenesis, Impairment of Fertility: Chronic dietary administration (up to 24 months) of doxazosin mesylate at maximally tolerated doses of 40 mg/kg/day in rats and 120 mg/kg/day in mice revealed no evidence of carcinogenic potential. The highest doses evaluated in the rat and mouse studies are associated with AUCs (a measure of systemic exposure) that are 8 times and 4 times, respectively, the human AUC at a dose of 16 mg/day.

Mutagenicity studies revealed no drug- or metabolite-related effects at either chromosomal or subchromosomal levels.

Studies in rats showed reduced fertility in males treated with doxazosin at oral doses of 20 (but not 5 or 10) mg/kg/day, about 4 times the AUC exposures obtained with a 12 mg/day human dose. This effect was reversible within two weeks of drug withdrawal. There have been no reports of any effects of doxazosin on male fertility in humans.

Pregnancy: Teratogenic Effects, Pregnancy Category C. Studies in pregnant rabbits and rats at daily oral doses of up to 41 and 20 mg/kg, respectively (plasma drug concentrations 10 and 4 times human C_{max} and AUC exposures with a 12 mg/day therapeutic dose), have revealed no evidence of harm to the fetus. A dosage regimen of 82 mg/kg/day in the rabbit was associated with reduced fetal survival. There are no adequate and well-controlled studies in pregnant women. Because animal reproduction studies are not always predictive of human response, CARDURA® should be used during pregnancy only if clearly needed.

Radioactivity was found to cross the placenta following oral administration of labelled doxazosin to pregnant rats.

Nonteratogenic Effects. In peri-postnatal studies in rats, postnatal development at maternal doses of 40 or 50 mg/kg/day of doxazosin (8 times human AUC exposure with a 12 mg/day therapeutic dose) was delayed as evidenced by slower body weight gain and slightly later appearance of anatomical features and reflexes.

Nursing Mothers: Studies in lactating rats given a single oral dose of 1 mg/kg of [2-^{14}C]-CARDURA® indicate that doxazosin accumulates in rat breast milk with a maximum concentration about 20 times greater than the maternal plasma concentration. It is not known whether this drug is excreted in human milk. Because many drugs are excreted in human milk, caution should be exercised when CARDURA® is administered to a nursing mother.

Pediatric Use: The safety and effectiveness of CARDURA® as an antihypertensive agent have not been established in children.

Use in Elderly: The safety and effectiveness profile of CARDURA® in BPH was similar in the elderly (age ≥65 years) and younger (age <65 years) patients.

ADVERSE REACTIONS

A. Benign Prostatic Hyperplasia

The incidence of adverse events has been ascertained from worldwide clinical trials in 965 BPH patients. The incidence rates presented below (Table 3) are based on combined data from seven placebo-controlled trials involving once daily administration of CARDURA® (doxazosin mesylate) in doses of 1–16 mg in hypertensives and 0.5–8 mg in normotensives. The adverse events when the incidence in the CARDURA® group was at least 1% are summarized in Table 3. No significant difference in the incidence of adverse events compared to placebo was seen except for dizziness, fatigue, hypotension, edema and dyspnea. Dizziness and dyspnea appeared to be dose-related.

TABLE 3
ADVERSE REACTIONS DURING
PLACEBO-CONTROLLED STUDIES
BENIGN PROSTATIC HYPERPLASIA

Body System	CARDURA® (N=665)	PLACEBO (N=300)
BODY AS A WHOLE		
Back pain	1.8%	2.0%
Chest pain	1.2%	0.7%
Fatigue	8.0%*	1.7%
Headache	9.9%	9.0%
Influenza-like symptoms	1.1%	1.0%
Pain	2.0%	1.0%
CARDIOVASCULAR SYSTEM		
Hypotension	1.7%*	0.0%
Palpitation	1.2%	0.3%
DIGESTIVE SYSTEM		
Abdominal Pain	2.4%	2.0%
Diarrhea	2.3%	2.0%
Dyspepsia	1.7%	1.7%
Nausea	1.5%	0.7%
METABOLIC AND NUTRITIONAL DISORDERS		
Edema	2.7%*	0.7%
NERVOUS SYSTEM		
Dizziness†	15.6%*	9.0%
Mouth Dry	1.4%	0.3%
Somnolence	3.0%	1.0%
RESPIRATORY SYSTEM		
Dyspnea	2.6%*	0.3%
Respiratory Disorder	1.1%	0.7%
SPECIAL SENSES		
Vision Abnormal	1.4%	0.7%
UROGENITAL SYSTEM		
Impotence	1.1%	1.0%
Urinary Tract Infection	1.4%	2.3%
SKIN & APPENDAGES		
Sweating Increased	1.1%	1.0%
PSYCHIATRIC DISORDERS		
Anxiety	1.1%	0.3%
Insomnia	1.2%	0.3%

*p ≤0.05 for treatment differences †Includes vertigo

In these placebo-controlled studies of 665 CARDURA® (doxazosin mesylate) patients, treated for a mean of 85 days, additional adverse reactions have been reported. These are less than 1% and not distinguishable from those that occurred in the placebo group. Adverse reactions with an incidence of less than 1% but of clinical interest are (CARDURA® vs. placebo): *Cardiovascular System:* angina pectoris (0.6% vs. 0.7%), postural hypotension (0.3% vs. 0.3%), syncope (0.5% vs. 0.0%), tachycardia (0.9% vs. 0.0%); *Urogenital System:* dysuria (0.5% vs. 1.3%), and *Psychiatric Disorders:* libido decreased (0.8% vs. 0.3%). The safety profile in patients treated for up to three years was similar to that in the placebo-controlled studies.

The majority of adverse experiences with CARDURA® were mild.

B. Hypertension

CARDURA® (doxazosin mesylate) has been administered to approximately 4000 hypertensive patients, of whom 1679 were included in the hypertension clinical development program. In that program, minor adverse effects were frequent, but led to discontinuation of treatment in only 7% of patients. In placebo-controlled studies adverse effects occurred in 49% and 40% of patients in the doxazosin and placebo groups, respectively, and led to discontinuation in 2% of patients in each group. The major reasons for discontinuation were postural effects (2%), edema, malaise/fatigue, and some heart rate disturbance, each about 0.7%.

Continued on next page

Cardura—Cont.

In controlled hypertension clinical trials directly comparing CARDURA® to placebo there was no significant difference in the incidence of side effects, except for dizziness (including postural), weight gain, somnolence and fatigue/malaise. Postural effects and edema appeared to be dose related. The prevalence rates presented below are based on combined data from placebo-controlled studies involving once daily administration of doxazosin at doses ranging from 1–16 mg. Table 4 summarizes those adverse experiences (possibly/probably related) reported for patients in these hypertension studies where the prevalence rate in the doxazosin group was at least 0.5% or where the reaction is of particular interest.

TABLE 4
ADVERSE REACTIONS DURING PLACEBO-CONTROLLED STUDIES

	HYPERTENSION	
	DOXAZOSIN (N=339)	PLACEBO (N=336)
CARDIOVASCULAR SYSTEM		
Dizziness	19%	9%
Vertigo	2%	1%
Postural Hypotension	0.3%	0%
Edema	4%	3%
Palpitation	2%	3%
Arrhythmia	1%	0%
Hypotension	1%	0%
Tachycardia	0.3%	1%
Peripheral Ischemia	0.3%	0%
SKIN & APPENDAGES		
Rash	1%	1%
Pruritus	1%	1%
MUSCULOSKELETAL SYSTEM		
Arthralgia/Arthritis	1%	0%
Muscle Weakness	1%	0%
Myalgia	1%	0%
CENTRAL & PERIPHERAL N.S.		
Headache	14%	16%
Paresthesia	1%	1%
Kinetic Disorders	1%	0%
Ataxia	1%	0%
Hypertonia	1%	0%
Muscle Cramps	1%	0%
AUTONOMIC		
Mouth Dry	2%	2%
Flushing	1%	0%
SPECIAL SENSES		
Vision Abnormal	2%	1%
Conjuncitivitis/Eye Pain	1%	1%
Tinnitus	1%	0.3%
PSYCHIATRIC		
Somnolence	5%	1%
Nervousness	2%	2%
Depression	1%	1%
Insomnia	1%	1%
Sexual Dysfunction	2%	1%
GASTROINTESTINAL		
Nausea	3%	4%
Diarrhea	2%	3%
Constipation	1%	1%
Dyspepsia	1%	1%
Flatulence	1%	1%
Abdominal Pain	0%	2%
Vomiting	0%	1%
RESPIRATORY		
Rhinitis	3%	1%
Dyspnea	1%	1%
Epistaxis	1%	0%
URINARY		
Polyuria	2%	0%
Urinary Incontinence	1%	0%
Micturition Frequency	0%	2%
GENERAL		
Fatigue/Malaise	12%	6%
Chest Pain	2%	2%
Asthenia	1%	1%
Face Edema	1%	0%
Pain	2%	2%

Additional adverse reactions have been reported, but these are, in general, not distinguishable from symptoms that might have occurred in the absence of exposure to doxazosin. The following adverse reactions occurred with a frequency of between 0.5% and 1%: syncope, hypoesthesia, increased sweating, agitation, increased weight. The following additional adverse reactions were reported by <0.5% of 3960 patients who received doxazosin in controlled or open, short- or long-term clinical studies, including international studies. *Cardiovascular System:* angina pectoris, myocardial infarction, cerebrovascular accident; *Autonomic Nervous System:* pallor; *Metabolic:* thirst, gout, hypokalemia; *Hematopoietic:* lymphadenopathy, purpura; *Reproductive System:* breast pain; *Skin Disorders:* alopecia, dry skin, eczema; *Central Nervous System:* paresis, tremor, twitching, confusion, migraine, impaired concentration; *Psychiatric:* paroniria, amnesia, emotional lability, abnormal thinking, depersonalization; *Special Senses:* parosmia, earache, taste perversion, photophobia, abnormal lacrimation; *Gastrointestinal System:* increased appetite, anorexia, fecal incontinence, gastroenteritis; *Respiratory System:* bronchospasm, sinusitis, coughing, pharyngitis; *Urinary System:* renal calculus; *General Body System:* hot flushes, back pain, infection, fever/rigors, decreased weight, influenza-like symptoms.

CARDURA® (doxazosin mesylate) has not been associated with any clinically significant changes in routine biochemical tests. No clinically relevant adverse effects were noted on serum potassium, serum glucose, uric acid, blood urea nitrogen, creatinine or liver function tests. CARDURA® has been associated with decreases in white blood cell counts (see PRECAUTIONS).

OVERDOSAGE

Experience with CARDURA® overdosage is limited. Two adolescents who each intentionally ingested 40 mg CARDURA® with diclofenac or paracetamol, were treated with gastric lavage with activated charcoal and made full recoveries. A two-year-old child who accidently ingested 4 mg CARDURA® was treated with gastric lavage and remained normotensive during the five-hour emergency room observation period. A six-month-old child accidentally received a crushed 1 mg tablet of CARDURA® and was reported to have been drowsy. A 32-year-old female with chronic renal failure, epilepsy and depression intentionally ingested 60 mg CARDURA® (blood level 0.9 μg/mL; normal values in hypertensives=0.02 μg/mL); death was attributed to a grand mal seizure resulting from hypotension. A 39-year-old female who ingested 70 mg CARDURA®, alcohol and Dalmane® (flurazepam) developed hypotension which responded to fluid therapy.

The oral LD_{50} of doxazosin is greater than 1000 mg/kg in mice and rats. The most likely manifestation of overdosage would be hypotension, for which the usual treatment would be intravenous infusion of fluid. As doxazosin is highly protein bound, dialysis would not be indicated.

DOSAGE AND ADMINISTRATION

DOSAGE MUST BE INDIVIDUALIZED. The initial dosage of CARDURA® in patients with hypertension and/or BPH is 1 mg given once daily in the a.m. or p.m. This starting dose is intended to minimize the frequency of postural hypotension and first dose syncope associated with CARDURA®. Postural effects are most likely to occur between 2 and 6 hours after a dose. Therefore blood pressure measurements should be taken during this time period after the first dose and with each increase in dose. If CARDURA® administration is discontinued for several days, therapy should be restarted using the initial dosing regimen.

A. ***BENIGN PROSTATIC HYPERPLASIA 1-8 mg once daily.*** The initial dosage of CARDURA® is 1 mg, given once daily in the a.m. or p.m. Depending on the individual patient's urodynamics and BPH symptomatology, dosage may then be increased to 2 mg and thereafter to 4 mg and 8 mg once daily, the maximum recommended dose for BPH. The recommended titration interval is 1-2 weeks. Blood pressure should be evaluated routinely in these patients.

B. ***HYPERTENSION 1-16 mg once daily.*** The initial dosage of CARDURA® is 1 mg given once daily. Depending on the individual patient's standing blood pressure response (based on measurements taken at 2-6 hours post-dose and 24 hours post-dose), dosage may then be increased to 2 mg and thereafter if necessary to 4 mg, 8 mg and 16 mg to achieve the desired reduction in blood pressure. **Increases in dose beyond 4 mg increase the likelihood of excessive postural effects including syncope, postural dizziness/vertigo and postural hypotension. At a titrated dose of 16 mg once daily the frequency of postural effects is about 12% compared to 3% for placebo.**

HOW SUPPLIED

CARDURA® (doxazosin mesylate) is available as colored tablets for oral administration. Each tablet contains doxazosin mesylate equivalent to 1 mg (white), 2 mg (yellow), 4 mg (orange) or 8 mg (green) of the active constituent, doxazosin.

CARDURA® TABLETS (doxazosin mesylate) are available as 1 mg (white), 2 mg (yellow), 4 mg (orange) and 8 mg (green) scored tablets.

Bottles of 100:	1 mg (NDC 0049-2750-66)
	2 mg (NDC 0049-2760-66)
	4 mg (NDC 0049-2770-66)
	8 mg (NDC 0049-2780-66)
Unit Dose Packages of 100:	1 mg (NDC 0049-2750-41)
	2 mg (NDC 0049-2760-41)
	4 mg (NDC 0049-2770-41)
	8 mg (NDC 0049-2780-41)

Recommended Storage: Store below 86°F (30°C).

CAUTION: Federal law prohibits dispensing without prescription.

70-4538-00-6 Revised June 1997

PATIENT INFORMATION ABOUT CARDURA®

Generic Name:
doxazosin mesylate
FOR BENIGN PROSTATIC HYPERPLASIA (BPH)

Read this leaflet:

- before you start taking CARDURA®
- each time you get a new prescription.

You and your doctor should discuss this treatment and your BPH symptoms before you start taking CARDURA® and at your regular checkups. This leaflet does NOT take the place of discussions with your doctor.

CARDURA® is used to treat both benign prostatic hyperplasia (BPH) and high blood pressure (hypertension). This leaflet describes CARDURA® as treatment for BPH (although you may be taking CARDURA® for both your BPH and high blood pressure).

What is BPH?

BPH is an enlargement of the prostate gland. This gland surrounds the tube that drains the urine from the bladder. The symptoms of BPH can be caused by a tensing of the enlarged muscle in the prostate gland which blocks the passage of urine. This can lead to such symptoms as:

- a weak or start-and-stop stream when urinating
- a feeling that the bladder is not completely emptied after urination
- a delay or difficulty in the beginning of urination
- a need to urinate often during the day and especially at night
- a feeling that you must urinate immediately.

Treatment Options for BPH

The four main treatment options for BPH are:

- If you are not bothered by your symptoms, you and your doctor may decide on a program of "watchful waiting." It is not an active treatment like taking medication or surgery but involves having regular checkups to see if your condition is getting worse or causing problems.
- Treatment with CARDURA® or other similar drugs. CARDURA® is the medication your doctor has prescribed for you. See "What CARDURA® Does," below.
- Treatment with the medication class of 5-alpha reductase inhibitors (e.g., Proscar®). It can cause the prostate to shrink. It may take 6 months or more for the full benefit of finasteride to be seen.
- Various surgical procedures. Your doctor can describe these procedures to you. The best procedure for you depends on your BPH symptoms and medical condition.

What CARDURA® Does

CARDURA® works on a specific type of muscle found in the prostate, causing it to relax. This in turn decreases the pressure within the prostate, thus improving the flow of urine and your symptoms.

- CARDURA® (doxazosin mesylate) helps relieve the symptoms of BPH (weak stream, start-and-stop stream, a feeling that your bladder is not completely empty, delay in beginning of urination, need to urinate often during the day and especially at night, and feeling that you must urinate immediately). It does not change the size of the prostate. The prostate may continue to grow; however, a larger prostate is not necessarily related to more symptoms or to worse symptoms. CARDURA® can decrease your symptoms and improve urinary flow, without decreasing the size of the prostate.
- If CARDURA® is helping you, you should notice an effect within 1 to 2 weeks after you start your medication. CARDURA® has been studied in over 900 patients for up to 2 years and the drug has been shown to continue to work during long-term treatment. Even though you take CARDURA® and it may help you, CARDURA® may not prevent the need for surgery in the future.
- CARDURA® does not affect PSA levels. PSA is the abbreviation for Prostate Specific Antigen. Your doctor may have done a blood test called PSA. You may want to ask your doctor more about this if you have had a PSA test done.

Other Important Facts

- You should see an improvement of your symptoms within 1 to 2 weeks. In addition to your other regular checkups you will need to continue seeing your doctor regularly to check your progress regarding your BPH and to monitor your blood pressure.
- CARDURA® (doxazosin mesylate) is not a treatment for prostate cancer. Your doctor has prescribed CARDURA® for your BPH and not for prostate cancer; however, a man can have BPH and prostate cancer at the same time. Doctors usually recommend that men be checked for prostate cancer once a year when they turn 50 (or 40 if a family member has had prostate cancer). A higher incidence of prostate cancer has been noted in men of African-American descent. These checks should continue even if you are taking CARDURA®.

How To Take CARDURA® and What You Should Know While Taking CARDURA® for BPH

CARDURA® Can Cause a Sudden Drop in Blood Pressure After the VERY FIRST DOSE. You may feel dizzy, faint or "light-headed," especially after you stand up from a lying or sitting position. This is more likely to occur after you've taken the first few doses or if you increase your dose, but can occur at any time while you are taking the drug. It can also occur if you stop taking the drug and then restart treatment. If you feel very dizzy, faint or "light-headed" you should contact your doctor. Your doctor will discuss with you how often you need to visit and how often your blood pressure should be checked.

Your blood pressure should be checked when you start taking CARDURA® even if you do not have high blood pressure (hypertension). Your doctor will discuss with you the details of how blood pressure is measured.

Blood Pressure Measurement: Whatever equipment is used, it is usual for your blood pressure to be measured in the following way: measure your blood pressure after lying quietly on your back for five minutes. Then, after standing for two minutes measure your blood pressure again. Your doctor will discuss with you what other times during the day your blood pressure should be taken, such as two to six hours after a dose, before bedtime or after waking up in the morning. Note that moderate to high-intensity exercise can, over a period of time, lower your average blood pressure.

You can take CARDURA® either in the morning or at bedtime and it will be equally effective. If you take CARDURA® at bedtime but need to get up from bed to go to the bathroom, get up slowly and cautiously until you are sure how the medication affects you. It is important to get up slowly from a chair or bed at any time until you learn how you react to CARDURA®. You should not drive or do any hazardous tasks until you are used to the effects of the medication. If you begin to feel dizzy, sit or lie down until you feel better.

- You will start with a 1 mg dose of CARDURA® once daily. Then the once daily dose will be increased as your body gets used to the effects of the medication. Follow your doctor's instructions about how to take CARDURA®. You must take it every day at the dose prescribed. Talk with your doctor if you don't take it for a few days for some reason; you may then need to restart the medication at a 1 mg dose, increase your dose gradually and again be cautious about possible dizziness. Do not share CARDURA® with anyone else; it was prescribed only for you.
- Other side effects you could have while taking CARDURA® (doxazosin mesylate), in addition to lowering of the blood pressure, include dizziness, fatigue (tiredness), swelling of the feet and shortness of breath. Most side effects are mild. However, you should discuss any unexpected effects you notice with your doctor.
- **WARNING:** Extremely rarely, CARDURA® and similar medications have caused painful erection of the penis, sustained for hours and unrelieved by sexual intercourse or masturbation. This condition is serious, and if untreated it can be followed by permanent inability to have an erection. If you have a prolonged abnormal erection, call your doctor or go to an emergency room as soon as possible.
- Keep CARDURA® and all medicines out of the reach of children.

FOR MORE INFORMATION ABOUT CARDURA® AND BPH TALK WITH YOUR DOCTOR, NURSE, PHARMACIST OR OTHER HEALTH CARE PROVIDER.

70-5039-00-1

Revised May 1997

Shown in Product Identification Guide, page 330

CEFOBID® ℞

[*sĕf ′ō-bĭd*]

(sterile cefoperazone)

Formerly known as sterile cefoperazone sodium

For Intravenous or Intramuscular Use

CEFOBID® ℞

(cefoperazone injection)

Formerly known as cefoperazone sodium injection in Galaxy® Plastic Container (PL 2040)

For Intravenous Use

DESCRIPTION

CEFOBID® (sterile cefoperazone), formerly known as sterile cefoperazone sodium, and CEFOBID (cefoperazone injection), formerly known as cefoperazone sodium injection in Galaxy® plastic container (PL 2040) contain cefoperazone as cefoperazone sodium. It is a semisynthetic, broad-spectrum, cephalosporin antibiotic. Chemically, cefoperazone sodium is sodium (6*R*, 7*R*)-7-[(*R*)-2-(4-ethyl-2,3-dioxo-1-piperazinecarboxamido)-2- (*p*-hydroxyphenyl)-acetamido)-3-[[(1-methyl- 1*H*- tetrazol-5-yl)thio] methyl]-8-oxo-5-thia-1-azabicyclo[4.2.0]oct-2-ene-2-carboxylate. Its molecular formula is $C_{25}H_{26}N_9NaO_8S_2$ with a molecular weight of 667.65. The structural formula is given below:

CEFOBID (sterile cefoperazone) contains 34 mg sodium (1.5 mEq) per gram. CEFOBID is a white powder which is freely soluble in water. The pH of a 25% (w/v) freshly reconstituted solution varies between 4.5–6.5 and the solution ranges from colorless to straw yellow depending on the concentration.

CEFOBID (sterile cefoperazone) in crystalline form is supplied in vials containing 1 g or 2 g cefoperazone as cefoperazone sodium for intravenous or intramuscular administration.

CEFOBID (sterile cefoperazone) is also supplied in Piggy Back Units for intravenous administration only.

TABLE 1. Cefoperazone Serum Concentrations

	Mean Serum Concentrations (mcg/mL)						
Dose/Route	**0***	**0.5 hr**	**1 hr**	**2 hr**	**4 hr**	**8 hr**	**12 hr**
1 g IV	153	114	73	38	16	4	0.5
2 g IV	252	153	114	70	32	8	2
3 g IV	340	210	142	89	41	9	2
4 g IV	506	325	251	161	71	19	6
1 g IM	32 **	52	65	57	33	7	1
2 g IM	40 **	69	93	97	58	14	4

* Hours post-administration, with 0 time being the end of the infusion.
** Values obtained 15 minutes post-injection.

CEFOBID (cefoperazone injection) in Galaxy® plastic container (PL 2040) is a frozen, iso-osmotic, sterile, non-pyrogenic premixed 50 mL solution containing 1 g or 2 g of cefoperazone as cefoperazone sodium. Dextrose hydrous, USP, has been added to adjust the osmolality to approximately 300 mOsmol/kg (approximately 2.3 g and 1.8 g to the 1 g and 2 g dosages, respectively). The pH may have been adjusted with sodium hydroxide and/or hydrochloric acid. After thawing to room temperature, it is intended for intravenous use only.

The Galaxy® container is fabricated from a specially designed multilayer plastic (PL 2040). Solutions are in contact with the polyethylene layer of this container and can leach out certain chemical components of the plastic in very small amounts within the expiration dating period. The suitability of the plastic has been confirmed in test in animals according to the USP biological tests for plastic containers, as well as by tissue culture toxicity studies.

CLINICAL PHARMACOLOGY

High serum and bile levels of CEFOBID are attained after a single dose of the drug. Table 1 demonstrates the serum concentrations of CEFOBID in normal volunteers following either a single 15-minute constant rate intravenous infusion of 1, 2, 3 or 4 grams of the drug, or a single intramuscular injection of 1 or 2 grams of the drug.

[See table above]

The mean serum half-life of CEFOBID is approximately 2.0 hours, independent of the route of administration.

In vitro studies with human serum indicate that the degree of CEFOBID reversible protein binding varies with the serum concentration from 93% at 25 mcg/mL of CEFOBID to 90% at 250 mcg/mL and 82% at 500 mcg/mL.

CEFOBID achieves therapeutic concentrations in the following body tissues and fluids:

Tissue or Fluid	**Dose**	**Concentration**
Ascitic Fluid	2 g	64 mcg/mL
Cerebrospinal Fluid (in patients with inflamed meninges)	50 mg/kg	1.8 mcg/mL to 8.0 mcg/mL
Urine	2 g	3,286 mcg/mL
Sputum	3 g	6.0 mcg/mL
Endometrium	2 g	74 mcg/g
Myometrium	2 g	54 mcg/g
Palatine Tonsil	1 g	8 mcg/g
Sinus Mucous Membrane	1 g	8 mcg/g
Umbilical Cord Blood	1 g	25 mcg/mL
Amniotic Fluid	1 g	4.8 mcg/mL
Lung	1 g	28 mcg/g
Bone	2 g	40 mcg/g

CEFOBID is excreted mainly in the bile. Maximum bile concentrations are generally obtained between one and three hours following drug administration and exceed concurrent serum concentrations by up to 100 times. Reported biliary concentrations of CEFOBID range from 66 mcg/mL at 30 minutes to as high as 6000 mcg/mL at 3 hours after an intravenous bolus injection of 2 grams.

Following a single intramuscular or intravenous dose, the urinary recovery of CEFOBID over a 12-hour period averages 20–30%. No significant quantity of metabolites has been found in the urine. Urinary concentrations greater than 2200 mcg/mL have been obtained following a 15-minute infusion of a 2 g dose. After an IM injection of 2 g, peak urine concentrations of almost 1000 mcg/mL have been obtained, and therapeutic levels are maintained for 12 hours.

Repeated administration of CEFOBID at 12-hour intervals does not result in accumulation of the drug in normal subjects. Peak serum concentrations, areas under the curve (AUC's), and serum half-lives in patients with severe renal insufficiency are not significantly different from those in normal volunteers. In patients with hepatic dysfunction, the serum half-life is prolonged and urinary excretion is increased. In patients with combined renal and hepatic insufficiencies, CEFOBID may accumulate in the serum.

CEFOBID has been used in pediatrics, but the safety and effectiveness in children have not been established. The half-life of CEFOBID in serum is 6–10 hours in low birth-weight neonates.

Microbiology

CEFOBID is active *in vitro* against a wide range of aerobic and anaerobic, gram-positive and gram-negative pathogens. The bactericidal action of CEFOBID results from the inhibition of bacterial cell wall synthesis. CEFOBID has a high degree of stability in the presence of beta-lactamases produced by most gram-negative pathogens. CEFOBID is usually active against organisms which are resistant to other beta-lactam antibiotics because of beta-lactamase production. CEFOBID is usually active against the following organisms *in vitro* and in clinical infections:

Gram-Positive Aerobes:

Staphylococcus aureus, penicillinase and non-penicillinase-producing strains
Staphylococcus epidermidis
Streptococcus pneumoniae (formerly *Diplococcus pneumoniae*)
Streptococcus pyogenes (Group A beta-hemolytic streptococci)
Streptococcus agalactiae (Group B beta-hemolytic streptococci)
Enterococcus (*Streptococcus faecalis, S. faecium* and *S. durans*)

Gram-Negative Aerobes:

Escherichia coli
Klebsiella species (including *K. pneumoniae*)
Enterobacter species
Citrobacter species
Haemophilus influenzae
Proteus mirabilis
Proteus vulgaris
Morganella morganii (formerly *Proteus morganii*)
Providencia stuartii
Providencia rettgeri (formerly *Proteus rettgeri*)
Serratia marcescens
Pseudomonas aeruginosa
Pseudomonas species
Some strains of *Acinetobacter calcoaceticus*
Neisseria gonorrhoeae

Anaerobic Organisms:

Gram-positive cocci (including *Peptococcus* and *Peptostreptococcus*)
Clostridium species
Bacteroides fragilis
Other *Bacteroides* species

CEFOBID is also active *in vitro* against a wide variety of other pathogens although the clinical significance is unknown. These organisms include: *Salmonella* and *Shigella* species, *Serratia liquefaciens, N. meningitidis, Bordetella pertussis, Yersinia enterocolitica, Clostridium difficile, Fusobacterium* species, *Eubacterium* species and beta-lactamase producing strains of *H. influenzae* and *N. gonorrhoeae.*

Susceptibility Testing:

Diffusion Technique. For the disk diffusion method of susceptibility testing, a 75 mcg CEFOBID diffusion disk should be used. Organisms should be tested with the CEFOBID 75 mcg disk since CEFOBID has been shown *in vitro* to be active against organisms which are found to be resistant to other beta-lactam antibiotics.

Tests should be interpreted by the following criteria:

Zone Diameter	**Interpretation**
Greater than or equal to 21 mm	Susceptible
16–20 mm	Moderately Susceptible
Less than or equal to 15 mm	Resistant

Quantitative procedures that require measurement of zone diameters give the most precise estimate of susceptibility. One such method which has been recommended for use with the CEFOBID 75 mcg disk is the NCCLS approved standard. (Performance Standards for Antimicrobic Disk Susceptibility Tests. Second Information Supplement Vol. 2 No. 2 pp. 49–69. Publisher—National Committee for Clinical Laboratory Standards, Villanova, Pennsylvania.)

A report of "susceptible" indicates that the infecting organism is likely to respond to CEFOBID therapy and a report of "resistant" indicates that the infecting organism is not likely to respond to therapy. A "moderately susceptible" report suggests that the infecting organism will be susceptible to CEFOBID if a higher than usual dosage is used or if the infection is confined to tissues and fluids (e.g., urine or bile) in which high antibiotic levels are attained.

Dilution Techniques. Broth or agar dilution methods may be used to determine the minimal inhibitory concentration (MIC) of CEFOBID. Serial twofold dilutions of CEFOBID should be prepared in either broth or agar. Broth should be inoculated to contain 5×10^5 organisms/mL and agar "spotted" with 10^4 organisms.

MIC test results should be interpreted in light of serum, tissue, and body fluid concentrations of CEFOBID. Organisms inhibited by CEFOBID at 16 mcg/mL or less are considered susceptible, while organisms with MIC's of 17–63 mcg/mL are moderately susceptible. Organisms inhibited at CEFO-

Continued on next page

Cefobid IV/IM—Cont.

BID concentrations of greater than or equal to 64 mcg/mL are considered resistant, although clinical cures have been obtained in some patients infected by such organisms.

INDICATIONS AND USAGE

CEFOBID is indicated for the treatment of the following infections when caused by susceptible organisms:

Respiratory Tract Infections caused by *S. pneumoniae, H. influenzae, S. aureus* (penicillinase and non-penicillinase producing strains), *S. pyogenes** (Group A beta-hemolytic streptococci), *P. aeruginosa, Klebsiella pneumoniae, E. coli, Proteus mirabilis,* and *Enterobacter* species.

Peritonitis and Other Intra-abdominal Infections caused by *E. coli, P. aeruginosa,** and anaerobic gram-negative bacilli (including *Bacteroides fragilis*).

Bacterial Septicemia caused by *S. pneumoniae, S. agalactiae*, S. aureus, Pseudomonas aeruginosa*, E. coli, Klebsiella* spp.,* *Klebsiella pneumoniae** , *Proteus* species* (indole-positive and indole-negative), *Clostridium* spp.* and anaerobic gram-positive cocci.*

Infections of the Skin and Skin Structures caused by *S. aureus* (penicillinase and non-penicillinase producing strains), *S. pyogenes**, and *P. aeruginosa*.

Pelvic Inflammatory Disease, Endometritis, and Other Infections of the Female Genital Tract caused by *N. gonorrhoeae, S. epidermidis*, S. agalactiae, E. coli, Clostridium* spp.,* *Bacteroides* species (including *Bacteroides fragilis*) and anaerobic gram-positive cocci.

Urinary Tract Infections caused by *Escherichia coli* and *Pseudomonas aeruginosa*.

Enterococcal Infections: Although cefoperazone has been shown to be clinically effective in the treatment of infections caused by enterococci in cases of **peritonitis and other intra-abdominal infections, infections of the skin and skin structures, pelvic inflammatory disease, endometritis and other infections of the female genital tract, and urinary tract infection,*** the majority of clinical isolates of enterococci tested are not susceptible to cefoperazone but fall just at or in the intermediate zone of susceptibilty, and are moderately resistant to cefoperazone. However, *in vitro* susceptibility testing may not correlate directly with *in vivo* results. Despite this, cefoperazone therapy has resulted in clinical cures of enterococcal infections, chiefly in polymicrobial infections. Cefoperazone should be used in enterococcal infections with care and at doses that achieve satisfactory serum levels of cefoperazone.

*Efficacy of this organism in this organ system was studied in fewer than 10 infections.

Susceptibility Testing

Before instituting treatment with CEFOBID, appropriate specimens should be obtained for isolation of the causative organism and for determination of its susceptibility to the drug. Treatment may be started before results of susceptibility testing are available.

Combination Therapy

Synergy between CEFOBID and aminoglycosides has been demonstrated with many gram-negative bacilli. However, such enhanced activity of these combinations is not predictable. If such therapy is considered, *in vitro* susceptibility tests should be performed to determine the activity of the drugs in combination, and renal function should be monitored carefully. (See PRECAUTIONS, and DOSAGE AND ADMINISTRATION sections).

CONTRAINDICATIONS

CEFOBID is contraindicated in patients with known allergy to the cephalosporin-class of antibiotics.

WARNINGS

BEFORE THERAPY WITH CEFOBID IS INSTITUTED, CAREFUL INQUIRY SHOULD BE MADE TO DETERMINE WHETHER THE PATIENT HAS HAD PREVIOUS HYPERSENSITIVITY REACTIONS TO CEPHALOSPORINS, PENICILLINS OR OTHER DRUGS. THIS PRODUCT SHOULD BE GIVEN CAUTIOUSLY TO PENICILLIN-SENSITIVE PATIENTS. ANTIBIOTICS SHOULD BE ADMINISTERED WITH CAUTION TO ANY PATIENT WHO HAS DEMONSTRATED SOME FORM OF ALLERGY, PARTICULARLY TO DRUGS. SERIOUS ACUTE HYPERSENSITIVITY REACTIONS MAY REQUIRE THE USE OF SUBCUTANEOUS EPINEPHRINE AND OTHER EMERGENCY MEASURES.

PSEUDOMEMBRANOUS COLITIS HAS BEEN REPORTED WITH THE USE OF CEPHALOSPORINS (AND OTHER BROAD-SPECTRUM ANTIBIOTICS); THEREFORE, IT IS IMPORTANT TO CONSIDER ITS DIAGNOSIS IN PATIENTS WHO DEVELOP DIARRHEA IN ASSOCIATION WITH ANTIBIOTIC USE.

Treatment with broad-spectrum antibiotics alters normal flora of the colon and may permit overgrowth of clostridia. Studies indicate a toxin produced by *Clostridium difficile* is one primary cause of antibiotic-associated colitis. Cholestyramine and colestipol resins have been shown to bind the toxin *in vitro*.

Mild cases of colitis may respond to drug discontinuance alone.

Moderate to severe cases should be managed with fluid, electrolyte, and protein supplementation as indicated.

When the colitis is not relieved by drug discontinuance or when it is severe, oral vancomycin is the treatment of choice for antibiotic-associated pseudomembranous colitis produced by *C. difficile*. Other causes of colitis should also be considered.

PRECAUTIONS

Although transient elevations of the BUN and serum creatinine have been observed, CEFOBID alone does not appear to cause significant nephrotoxicity. However, concomitant administration of aminoglycosides and other cephalosporins has caused nephrotoxicity.

CEFOBID is extensively excreted in bile. The serum half-life of CEFOBID is increased 2–4 fold in patients with hepatic disease and/or biliary obstruction. In general, total daily dosage above 4 g should not be necessary in such patients. If higher dosages are used, serum concentrations should be monitored.

Because renal excretion is not the main route of elimination of CEFOBID (see CLINICAL PHARMACOLOGY), patients with renal failure require no adjustment in dosage when usual doses are administered. When high doses of CEFOBID are used, concentrations of drug in the serum should be monitored periodically. If evidence of accumulation exists, dosage should be decreased accordingly.

The half-life of CEFOBID is reduced slightly during hemodialysis. Thus, dosing should be scheduled to follow a dialysis period. In patients with both hepatic dysfunction and significant renal disease, CEFOBID dosage should not exceed 1–2 g daily without close monitoring of serum concentrations.

As with other antibiotics, vitamin K deficiency has occurred rarely in patients treated with CEFOBID. The mechanism is most probably related to the suppression of gut flora which normally synthesize this vitamin. Those at risk include patients with a poor nutritional status, malabsorption states (e.g., cystic fibrosis), alcoholism, and patients on prolonged hyper-alimentation regimens (administered either intravenously or via a naso-gastric tube). Prothrombin time should be monitored in these patients and exogenous vitamin K administered as indicated.

A disulfiram-like reaction characterized by flushing, sweating, headache, and tachycardia has been reported when alcohol (beer, wine) was ingested within 72 hours after CEFOBID administration. Patients should be cautioned about the ingestion of alcoholic beverages following the administration of CEFOBID. A similar reaction has been reported with other cephalosporins.

Prolonged use of CEFOBID may result in the overgrowth of nonsusceptible organisms. Careful observation of the patient is essential. If superinfection occurs during therapy, appropriate measures should be taken.

CEFOBID should be prescribed with caution in individuals with a history of gastrointestinal disease, particularly colitis.

Drug Laboratory Test Interactions

A false-positive reaction for glucose in the urine may occur with Benedict's or Fehling's solution.

Carcinogenesis, Mutagenesis, Impairment of Fertility

Long term studies in animals have not been performed to evaluate carcinogenic potential. The maximum duration of CEFOBID animal toxicity studies is six months. In none of the *in vivo* or *in vitro* genetic toxicology studies did CEFOBID show any mutagenic potential at either the chromosomal or subchromosomal level. CEFOBID produced no impairment of fertility and had no effects on general reproductive performance or fetal development when administered subcutaneously at daily doses up to 500 to 1000 mg/kg prior to and during mating, and to pregnant female rats during gestation. These doses are 10 to 20 times the estimated usual single clinical dose. CEFOBID had adverse effects on the testes of prepubertal rats at all doses tested. Subcutaneous administration of 1000 mg/kg per day (approximately 16 times the average adult human dose) resulted in reduced testicular weight, arrested spermatogenesis, reduced germinal cell population and vacuolation of Sertoli cell cytoplasm. The severity of lesions was dose dependent in the 100 to 1000 mg/kg per day range; the low dose caused a minor decrease in spermatocytes. This effect has not been observed in adult rats. Histologically the lesions were reversible at all but the highest dosage levels. However, these studies did not evaluate subsequent development of reproductive function in the rats. The relationship of these findings to humans is unknown.

Usage in Pregnancy

Pregnancy Category B: Reproduction studies have been performed in mice, rats, and monkeys at doses up to 10 times the human dose and have revealed no evidence of impaired fertility or harm to the fetus due to CEFOBID. There are, however, no adequate and well controlled studies in pregnant women. Because animal reproduction studies are not always predictive of human response, this drug should be used during pregnancy only if clearly needed.

Usage in Nursing Mothers

Only low concentrations of CEFOBID are excreted in human milk. Although CEFOBID passes poorly into breast milk of nursing mothers, caution should be exercised when CEFOBID is administered to a nursing woman.

Pediatric Use

Safety and effectiveness in children have not been established. For information concerning testicular changes in prepubertal rats (see Carcinogenesis, Mutagenesis, Impairment of Fertility).

ADVERSE REACTIONS

In clinical studies the following adverse effects were observed and were considered to be related to CEFOBID therapy or of uncertain etiology:

Hypersensitivity: As with all cephalosporins, hypersensitivity manifested by skin reactions (1 patient in 45), drug fever (1 in 260), or a change in Coombs' test (1 in 60) has been reported. These reactions are more likely to occur in patients with a history of allergies, particularly to penicillin.

Hematology: As with other beta-lactam antibiotics, reversible neutropenia may occur with prolonged administration. Slight decreases in neutrophil count (1 patient in 50) have been reported. Decreased hemoglobins (1 in 20) or hematocrits (1 in 20) have been reported, which is consistent with published literature on other cephalosporins. Transient eosinophilia has occurred in 1 patient in 10.

Hepatic: Of 1285 patients treated with cefoperazone in clinical trials, one patient with a history of liver disease developed significantly elevated liver function enzymes during CEFOBID therapy. Clinical signs and symptoms of nonspecific hepatitis accompanied these increases. After CEFOBID therapy was discontinued, the patient's enzymes returned to pre-treatment levels and the symptomatology resolved. As with other antibiotics that achieve high bile levels, mild transient elevations of liver function enzymes have been observed in 5–10% of the patients receiving CEFOBID therapy. The relevance of these findings, which were not accompanied by overt signs or symptoms of hepatic dysfunction, has not been established.

Gastrointestinal: Diarrhea or loose stools has been reported in 1 in 30 patients. Most of these experiences have been mild or moderate in severity and self-limiting in nature. In all cases, these symptoms responded to symptomatic therapy or ceased when cefoperazone therapy was stopped. Nausea and vomiting have been reported rarely. Symptoms of pseudomembranous colitis can appear during or for several weeks subsequent to antibiotic therapy (see WARNINGS).

Renal Function Tests: Transient elevations of the BUN (1 in 16) and serum creatinine (1 in 48) have been noted.

Local Reactions: CEFOBID is well tolerated following intramuscular administration. Occasionally, transient pain (1 in 140) may follow administration by this route. When CEFOBID is administered by intravenous infusion some patients may develop phlebitis (1 in 120) at the infusion site.

DOSAGE AND ADMINISTRATION

The usual adult daily dose of CEFOBID (sterile cefoperazone) is 2 to 4 grams per day administered in divided doses every 12 hours.

In severe infections or infections caused by less sensitive organisms, the total daily dose and/or frequency may be increased. Patients have been successfully treated with a total daily dosage of 6–12 grams divided into 2, 3 or 4 administrations ranging from 1.5 to 4 grams per dose.

In a pharmacokinetic study, a total daily dose of 16 grams was administered to severely immunocompromised patients by constant infusion without complications. Steady state serum concentrations were approximately 150 mcg/mL in these patients.

When treating infections caused by *Streptococcus pyogenes*, therapy should be continued for at least 10 days.

Solutions of CEFOBID and aminoglycoside should not be directly mixed, since there is a physical incompatibility between them. If combination therapy with CEFOBID and an aminoglycoside is contemplated (see INDICATIONS) this can be accomplished by sequential intermittent intravenous infusion provided that separate secondary intravenous tubing is used, and that the primary intravenous tubing is adequately irrigated with an approved diluent between doses. It is also suggested that CEFOBID be administered prior to the aminoglycoside. *In vitro* testing of the effectiveness of drug combination(s) is recommended.

RECONSTITUTION

The following solutions may be used for the initial reconstitution of CEFOBID (sterile cefoperazone).

Table 1. Solutions for Initial Reconstitution.

- 5% Dextrose Injection (USP)
- 5% Dextrose and 0.9% Sodium Chloride Injection (USP)
- 5% Dextrose and 0.2% Sodium Chloride Injection (USP)
- 10% Dextrose Injection (USP)
- Bacteriostatic Water for Injection [Benzyl Alcohol or Parabens] (USP)*†
- 0.9% Sodium Chloride Injection (USP)
- Normosol® M and 5% Dextrose Injection
- Normosol® R
- Sterile Water for Injection*

* Not to be used as a vehicle for intravenous infusion

† Preparations containing Benzyl Alcohol should not be used in neonates.

General Reconstitution Procedures

CEFOBID (sterile cefoperazone) for intravenous or intramuscular use may be initially reconstituted with any compatible solution mentioned above in Table 1. Solutions should be allowed to stand after reconstitution to allow any foaming to dissipate to permit visual inspection for complete solubilization. Vigorous and prolonged agitation may be necessary to solubilize CEFOBID in higher concentrations (above 333 mg cefoperazone/mL). The maximum solubility of CEFOBID (sterile cefoperazone) is approximately 475 mg cefoperazone/mL of compatible diluent.

	Final Cefoperazone Concentration	Step 1 Volume of Sterile Water	Step 2 Volume of 2% Lidocaine	Withdrawable Volume*†
1 g vial	333 mg/mL	2.0 mL	0.6 mL	3 mL
	250 mg/mL	2.8 mL	1.0 mL	4 mL
2 g vial	333 mg/mL	3.8 mL	1.2 mL	6 mL
	250 mg/mL	5.4 mL	1.8 mL	8 mL

When a diluent other than Lidocaine HCl Injection (USP) is used reconstitute as follows:

	Cefoperazone Concentration	Volume of Diluent to be Added	Withdrawable Volume*
1 g vial	333 mg/mL	2.6 mL	3 mL
	250 mg/mL	3.8 mL	4 mL
2 g vial	333 mg/mL	5.0 mL	6 mL
	250 mg/mL	7.2 mL	8 mL

* There is sufficient excess present to allow for withdrawal of the stated volume.
† Final lidocaine concentration will approximate that obtained if a 0.5% Lidocaine Hydrochloride Solution is used as diluent.

Room Temperature (15°–25°C/59°–77°F) **24 Hours**	**Approximate Concentrations**
Bacteriostatic Water for Injection [Benzyl Alcohol or Parabens] (USP)	300 mg/mL
5% Dextrose Injection (USP)	2 mg to 50 mg/mL
5% Dextrose and Lactated Ringer's Injection	2 mg to 50 mg/mL
5% Dextrose and 0.9% Sodium Chloride Injection (USP)	2 mg to 50 mg/mL
5% Dextrose and 0.2% Sodium Chloride Injection (USP)	2 mg to 50 mg/mL
10% Dextrose Injection (USP)	2 mg to 50 mg/mL
Lactated Ringer's Injection (USP)	2 mg/mL
0.5% Lidocaine Hydrochloride Injection (USP)	300 mg/mL
0.9% Sodium Chloride Injection (USP)	2 mg to 300 mg/mL
Normosol® M and 5% Dextrose Injection	2 mg to 50 mg/mL
Normosol® R	2 mg to 50 mg/mL
Sterile Water for Injection	300 mg/mL

Reconstituted CEFOBID solutions may be stored in glass or plastic syringes, or in glass or flexible plastic parenteral solution containers.

Refrigerator Temperature (2°–8°C/36°–46°F) **5 Days**	**Approximate Concentrations**
Bacteriostatic Water for Injection [Benzyl Alcohol or Parabens] (USP)	300 mg/mL
5% Dextrose Injection (USP)	2 mg to 50 mg/mL
5% Dextrose and 0.9% Sodium Chloride Injection (USP)	2 mg to 50 mg/mL
5% Dextrose and 0.2% Sodium Chloride Injection (USP)	2 mg to 50 mg/mL
Lactated Ringer's Injection (USP)	2 mg/mL
0.5% Lidocaine Hydrochloride Injection (USP)	300 mg/mL
0.9% Sodium Chloride Injection (USP)	2 mg to 300 mg/mL
Normosol® M and 5% Dextrose Injection	2 mg to 50 mg/mL
Normosol® R	2 mg to 50 mg/mL
Sterile Water for Injection	300 mg/mL

Reconstituted CEFOBID solutions may be stored in glass or plastic syringes, or in glass or flexible plastic parenteral solution containers.

Freezer Temperature (−20° to −10°C/−4° to 14°F) **3 Weeks**	**Approximate Concentrations**
5% Dextrose Injection (USP)	50 mg/mL
5% Dextrose and 0.9% Sodium Chloride Injection (USP)	2 mg/mL
5% Dextrose and 0.2% Sodium Chloride Injection (USP)	2 mg/mL
5 Weeks	
0.9% Sodium Chloride Injection (USP)	300 mg/mL
Sterile Water for Injection	300 mg/mL

Reconstituted CEFOBID solutions may be stored in plastic syringes, or in flexible plastic parenteral solution containers.

Preparation For Intravenous Use

General. CEFOBID (sterile cefoperazone) concentrations between 2 mg/mL and 50 mg/mL are recommended for intravenous administration.

Preparation of Vials. Vials of CEFOBID (sterile cefoperazone) may be initially reconstituted with a minimum of 2.8 mL per gram of cefoperazone of any compatible reconstituting solution appropriate for intravenous administration listed above in Table 1. For ease of reconstitution the use of 5 mL of compatible solution per gram of CEFOBID is recommended. The entire quantity of the resulting solution should then be withdrawn for further dilution and administration using any of the following vehicles for intravenous infusion:

Table 2. Vehicles for Intravenous Infusion

- 5% Dextrose Injection (USP)
- 5% Dextrose and Lactated Ringer's Injection
- 5% Dextrose and 0.9% Sodium Chloride Injection (USP)
- 5% Dextrose and 0.2% Sodium Chloride Injection (USP)
- 10% Dextrose Injection (USP)
- Lactated Ringer's Injection (USP)
- 0.9% Sodium Chloride Injection (USP)
- Normosol® M and 5% Dextrose Injection
- Normosol® R

Preparation of Piggy Back Units. CEFOBID (sterile cefoperazone) in Piggy Back Units for intravenous use may be prepared by adding between 20 mL and 40 mL of any appropriate diluent listed in Table 2 per gram of cefoperazone. If 5% Dextrose and Lactated Ringer's Injection or Lactated Ringer's Injection (USP) is the chosen vehicle for administration the CEFOBID (sterile cefoperazone) should initially be reconstituted using 2.8–5 mL per gram of any compatible reconstituting solution listed in Table 1 prior to the final dilution.

The resulting intravenous solution should be administered in one of the following manners:

Intermittent Infusion: Solutions of CEFOBID should be administered over a 15–30 minute time period.

Continuous Infusion: CEFOBID can be used for continuous infusion after dilution to a final concentration of between 2 and 25 mg cefoperazone per mL.

Preparation For Intramuscular Injection

Any suitable solution listed above may be used to prepare CEFOBID (sterile cefoperazone) for intramuscular injection. When concentrations of 250 mg/mL or more are to be administered, a lidocaine solution should be used. These solutions should be prepared using a combination of Sterile Water for Injection and 2% Lidocaine Hydrochloride Injection (USP) that approximates a 0.5% Lidocaine Hydrochloride Solution. A two-step dilution process as follows is recommended: First, add the required amount of Sterile Water for Injection and agitate until CEFOBID powder is completely dissolved. Second, add the required amount of 2% lidocaine and mix.

[See first table above]

STORAGE AND STABILITY

CEFOBID (sterile cefoperazone) is to be stored at or below 25°C (77°F) and protected from light prior to reconstitution. After reconstitution, protection from light is not necessary. The following parenteral diluents and approximate concentrations of CEFOBID provide stable solutions under the following conditions for the indicated time periods. (After the indicated time periods, unused portions of solutions should be discarded.)

[See second table above]

DIRECTIONS FOR USE OF CEFOBID® (cefoperazone injection) IN GALAXY® PLASTIC CONTAINER (PL 2040)

CEFOBID in Galaxy® Container (PL 2040 Plastic) is to be administered either as a continuous or intermittent infusion.

Storage

Store in a freezer capable of maintaining a temperature of −20°C/−4°F.

Thawing of Plastic Container

Thaw frozen container at room temperature (25°C/77°F) or under refrigeration (5°C/41°F). [DO NOT FORCE THAW BY IMMERSION IN WATER BATHS OR BY MICROWAVE IRRADIATION.]

Check for minute leaks by squeezing container firmly. If leaks are detected, discard solution as sterility may be impaired.

DO NOT ADD SUPPLEMENTARY MEDICATION.

Preparation for Intravenous Administration (Use Aseptic Technique).

1. Suspend container from eyelet support
2. Remove protector from outlet port at bottom of container.
3. Attach administration set. Refer to complete directions accompanying set.

Caution: Do not use plastic containers in series connections. Such use could result in an embolism due to residual air being drawn from the primary container before administration of the fluid from the secondary container is complete.

HOW SUPPLIED

CEFOBID® (sterile cefoperazone) is available in vials containing cefoperazone sodium equivalent to 1 g cefoperazone × 10 (NDC 0049-1201-83), and 2 g cefoperazone × 10 (NDC 0049-1202-83) for intramuscular and intravenous administration.

CEFOBID® (sterile cefoperazone) is available in Piggy Back Units containing cefoperazone sodium equivalent to 1 g cefoperazone × 10 (NDC 0049-1211-83), and 2 g cefoperazone × 10 (NDC 0049-1212-83), and 10 g (NDC 0049-1219-28) Pharmacy Bulk Package for intravenous administration.

CEFOBID® (sterile cefoperazone) is supplied as a frozen, iso-osmotic, pre-mixed solution in a single dose Galaxy® plastic container (PL 2040) as follows:

1 g/50 mL .... NDC 0049–1216–18
2 g/50 mL .... NDC 0049–1215–18

Store container(s) at or below −20°C/−4°F.

See DIRECTIONS FOR USE OF CEFOBID® (cefoperazone injection) IN GALAXY® PLASTIC CONTAINER (PL 2040).

CEFOBID® (cefoperazone injection) in Galaxy® plastic container (PL 2040) is manufactured for Roerig Division of Pfizer Pharmaceuticals by Baxter Healthcare Corporation, Deerfield, IL 60015.

CEFOBID® is a registered trademark of Pfizer Inc. Galaxy® is a registered trademark of Baxter International Inc.

Rx only.

70–4169–00–8 Revised November 1999

CEFOBID® ℞

[*sĕf΄ō-bĭd*]

Formerly Known As Sterile Cefoperazone Sodium, USP
Sterile Cefoperazone, USP
PHARMACY BULK PACKAGE
NOT FOR DIRECT INFUSION

DESCRIPTION

CEFOBID (cefoperazone), formerly known as cefoperazone sodium, is a sterile, semisynthetic, broad-spectrum, parenteral cephalosporin antibiotic for intravenous or intramuscular administration. It is the sodium salt of 7-[(*R*)-2-(4-ethyl -2,3- dioxo -1- piperazinecarboxamido) -2- (*p* -hydroxy phenyl) acetamido-3- [[(1-methyl-*H* -tetrazol-5-yl) thio] methyl]-8-oxo-5-thia-1-azabicyclo[4.2.0]oct-2-ene-2-carboxylate. Its chemical formula is $C_{25}H_{26}N_9NaO_8S_2$ with a molecular weight of 667.65. The structural formula is given below:

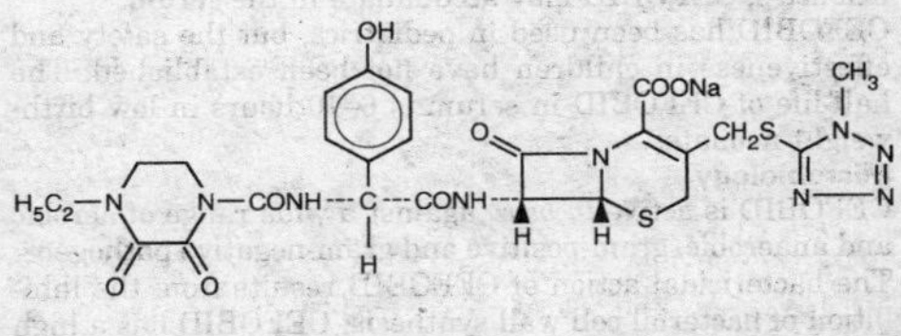

CEFOBID contains 34 mg sodium (1.5 mEq) per gram. CEFOBID is a white powder which is freely soluble in water. The pH of a 25% (w/v) freshly reconstituted solution varies between 4.5–6.5 and the solution ranges from colorless to straw yellow depending on the concentration.

CEFOBID in crystalline form is supplied in vials equivalent to 1 g or 2 g of cefoperazone and in Piggyback Units for intravenous administration equivalent to 1 g or 2 g cefoperazone. CEFOBID is also supplied premixed as a frozen, sterile, nonpyrogenic, iso-osmotic solution equivalent to 1 g or 2 g cefoperazone in plastic containers. After thawing, the solution is intended for intravenous use.

The plastic container is fabricated from specially formulated polyvinyl chloride. Solutions in contact with the plastic container can leach out certain of its chemical components in very small amounts within the expiration period, e.g., di 2-ethylhexyl phthalate (DEHP), up to 5 parts per million. However, the safety of the plastic has been confirmed in tests in animals according to the USP biological tests for plastic containers, as well as by tissue culture toxicity studies.

A pharmacy bulk package is a container of a sterile preparation for parenteral use that contains many single doses. This Pharmacy Bulk Package is for use in a pharmacy admixture service; it provides many single doses of cefoperazone for addition to suitable parenteral fluids in the preparation of admixtures for intravenous infusion. (See DOSAGE AND ADMINISTRATION, and DIRECTIONS FOR PROPER USE OF PHARMACY BULK PACKAGE).

CLINICAL PHARMACOLOGY

High serum and bile levels of CEFOBID are attained after a single dose of the drug. Table 1 demonstrates the serum

Continued on next page

Cefobid Pharmacy Bulk—Cont.

concentrations of CEFOBID in normal volunteers following either a single 15-minute constant rate intravenous infusion of 1, 2, 3 or 4 grams of the drug, or a single intramuscular injection of 1 or 2 grams of the drug.
[See table below]
The mean serum half-life of CEFOBID is approximately 2.0 hours, independent of the route of administration.
In vitro studies with human serum indicate that the degree of CEFOBID reversible protein binding varies with the serum concentration from 93% at 25 mcg/mL of CEFOBID to 90% at 250 mcg/mL and 82% at 500 mcg/mL.
CEFOBID achieves therapeutic concentrations in the following body tissues and fluids:

Tissue or Fluid	Dose		Concentration	
Ascitic Fluid	2	g	64	mcg/mL
Cerebrospinal Fluid (in patients with inflamed meninges)	50	mg/kg	1.8 8.0	mcg/mL to mcg/mL
Urine	2	g	3,286	mcg/mL
Sputum	3	g	6.0	mcg/mL
Endometrium	2	g	74	mcg/g
Myometrium	2	g	54	mcg/g
Palatine Tonsil	1	g	8	mcg/g
Sinus Mucous Membrane	1	g	8	mcg/g
Umbilical Cord Blood	1	g	25	mcg/mL
Amniotic Fluid	1	g	4.8	mcg/mL
Lung	1	g	28	mcg/g
Bone	2	g	40	mcg/g

CEFOBID is excreted mainly in the bile. Maximum bile concentrations are generally obtained between one and three hours following drug administration and exceed concurrent serum concentrations by up to 100 times. Reported biliary concentrations of CEFOBID range from 66 mcg/mL at 30 minutes to as high as 6000 mcg/mL at 3 hours after an intravenous bolus injection of 2 grams.
Following a single intramuscular or intravenous dose, the urinary recovery of CEFOBID over a 12-hour period averages 20–30%. No significant quantity of metabolites has been found in the urine. Urinary concentrations greater than 2200 mcg/mL have been obtained following a 15-minute infusion of a 2 g dose. After an IM injection of 2 g, peak urine concentrations of almost 1000 mcg/mL have been obtained, and therapeutic levels are maintained for 12 hours.
Repeated administration of CEFOBID at 12-hour intervals does not result in accumulation of the drug in normal subjects. Peak serum concentrations, areas under the curve (AUC's), and serum half-lives in patients with severe renal insufficiency are not significantly different from those in normal volunteers. In patients with hepatic dysfunction, the serum half-life is prolonged and urinary excretion is increased. In patients with combined renal and hepatic insufficiencies, CEFOBID may accumulate in the serum.
CEFOBID has been used in pediatrics, but the safety and effectiveness in children have not been established. The half-life of CEFOBID in serum is 6–10 hours in low birth-weight neonates.

Microbiology
CEFOBID is active *in vitro* against a wide range of aerobic and anaerobic, gram-positive and gram-negative pathogens. The bactericidal action of CEFOBID results from the inhibition of bacterial cell wall synthesis. CEFOBID has a high degree of stability in the presence of beta-lactamases produced by most gram-negative pathogens. CEFOBID is usually active against organisms which are resistant to other beta-lactam antibiotics because of beta-lactamase production. CEFOBID is usually active against the following organisms *in vitro* and in clinical infections:

Gram-Positive Aerobes:
Staphylococcus aureus, penicillinase and non-penicillinase-producing strains.
Staphylococcus epidermidis
Streptococcus pneumoniae (formerly *Diplococcus pneumoniae*)
Streptococcus pyogenes (Group A beta-hemolytic streptococci)
Streptococcus agalactiae (Group B beta-hemolytic streptococci)
Enterococcus (*Streptococcus faecalis, S. faecium* and *S. durans*)

Gram-Negative Aerobes:
Escherichia coli
Klebsiella species (including *K. pneumoniae*)
Enterobacter species
Citrobacter species
Haemophilus influenzae
Proteus mirabilis
Proteus vulgaris
Morganella morganii (formerly *Proteus morganii*)
Providencia stuartii
Providencia rettgeri (formerly *Proteus rettgeri*)
Serratia marcescens
Pseudomonas aeruginosa
Pseudomonas species
Some strains of *Acinetobacter calcoaceticus*
Neisseria gonorrhoeae

Anaerobic Organisms:
Gram-positive cocci (including *Peptococcus* and *Peptostreptococcus*)
Clostridium species
Bacteroides fragilis
Other *Bacteroides* species
CEFOBID is also active *in vitro* against a wide variety of other pathogens although the clinical significance is unknown. These organisms include: *Salmonella* and *Shigella* species, *Serratia liquefaciens, N. meningitidis, Bordetella pertussis, Yersinia enterocolitica, Clostridium difficile, Fusobacterium* species, *Eubacterium* species and beta-lactamase producing strains of *H. influenzae* and *N. gonorrhoeae.*

SUSCEPTIBILITY TESTING

Diffusion Technique. For the disk diffusion method of susceptibility testing, a 75 mcg CEFOBID diffusion disk should be used. Organisms should be tested with the CEFOBID 75 mcg disk since CEFOBID has been shown *in vitro* to be active against organisms which are found to be resistant to other beta-lactam antibiotics.
Tests should be interpreted by the following criteria:

Zone Diameter	Interpretation
Greater than or equal to 21 mm	Susceptible
16–20 mm	Moderately Susceptible
Less than or equal to 15 mm	Resistant

Quantitative procedures that require measurement of zone diameters give the most precise estimate of susceptibility. One such method which has been recommended for use with the CEFOBID 75 mcg disk is the NCCLS approved standard. (Performance Standards for Antimicrobic Disk Susceptibility Tests. Second Information Supplement Vol. 2 No. 2 pp. 49–69. Publisher—National Committee for Clinical Laboratory Standards, Villanova, Pennsylvania.)
A report of "susceptible" indicates that the infecting organism is likely to respond to CEFOBID therapy and a report of "resistant" indicates that the infecting organism is not likely to respond to therapy. A "moderately susceptible" report suggests that the infecting organism will be susceptible to CEFOBID if a higher than usual dosage is used or if the infection is confined to tissues and fluids (e.g., urine or bile) in which high antibiotic levels are attained.
Dilution Techniques. Broth or agar dilution methods may be used to determine the minimal inhibitory concentration (MIC) of CEFOBID. Serial twofold dilutions of CEFOBID should be prepared in either broth or agar. Broth should be inoculated to contain 5×10^5 organisms/mL and agar "spotted" with 10^4 organisms.
MIC test results should be interpreted in light of serum, tissue, and body fluid concentrations of CEFOBID. Organisms inhibited by CEFOBID at 16 mcg/mL or less are considered susceptible, while organisms with MIC's of 17–63 mcg/mL are moderately susceptible. Organisms inhibited at CEFOBID concentrations of greater than or equal to 64 mcg/mL are considered resistant, although clinical cures have been obtained in some patients infected by such organisms.

INDICATIONS AND USAGE

CEFOBID is indicated for the treatment of the following infections when caused by susceptible organisms:
Respiratory Tract Infections caused by *S. pneumoniae, H. influenzae, S. aureus* (penicillinase and non-penicillinase producing strains), *S. pyogenes** (Group A beta-hemolytic streptococci), *P. aeruginosa, Klebsiella pneumoniae, E. coli, Proteus mirabilis,* and *Enterobacter* species.
Peritonitis and Other Intra-abdominal Infections caused by *E. coli, P. aeruginosa,** and anaerobic gram-negative bacilli (including *Bacteroides fragilis*).
Bacterial Septicemia caused by *S. pneumoniae, S. agalactiae,** *S. aureus, Pseudomonas aeruginosa,** *E. coli, Klebsiella* spp.,* *Klebsiella pneumoniae,** *Proteus* species* (indole-positive and indole-negative), *Clostridium* spp.* and anaerobic gram-positive cocci.*
Infections of the Skin and Skin Structures caused by *S. aureus* (penicillinase and non-penicillinase producing strains), *S. pyogenes,** and *P. aeruginosa.*
Pelvic Inflammatory Disease, Endometritis, and Other Infections of the Female Genital Tract caused by *N. gonorrhoeae, S. epidermidis,** *S. agalactiae, E. coli, Clostridium* spp.,* *Bacteroides* species (including *Bacteroides fragilis*) and anaerobic gram-positive cocci.
Cefobid®, like other cephalosporins, has no activity against *Chlamydia trachomatis.* Therefore, when cephalosporins are used in the treatment of patients with pelvic inflammatory disease and *C. trachomatis* is one of the suspected pathogens, appropriate anti-chlamydial coverage should be added.
Urinary Tract Infections caused by *Escherichia coli* and *Pseudomonas aeruginosa.*
Enterococcal Infections: Although cefoperazone has been shown to be clinically effective in the treatment of infections caused by enterococci in cases of **peritonitis and other intra-abdominal infections, infections of the skin and skin structures, pelvic inflammatory disease, endometritis and other infections of the female genital tract, and urinary tract infections,*** the majority of clinical isolates of enterococci tested are not susceptible to cefoperazone but fall just at or in the intermediate zone of susceptibilty, and are moderately resistant to cefoperazone. However, *in vitro* susceptibility testing may not correlate directly with *in vivo* results. Despite this, cefoperazone therapy has resulted in clinical cures of enterococcal infections, chiefly in polymicrobial infections. Cefoperazone should be used in enterococcal infections with care and at doses that achieve satisfactory serum levels of cefoperazone.

*Efficacy of this organism in this organ system was studied in fewer than 10 infections.

Susceptibility Testing
Before instituting treatment with CEFOBID, appropriate specimens should be obtained for isolation of the causative organism and for determination of its susceptibility to the drug. Treatment may be started before results of susceptibility testing are available.
Combination Therapy
Synergy between CEFOBID and aminoglycosides has been demonstrated with many gram-negative bacilli. However, such enhanced activity of these combinations is not predictable. If such therapy is considered, *in vitro* susceptibility tests should be performed to determine the activity of the drugs in combination, and renal function should be monitored carefully. (See PRECAUTIONS, and DOSAGE AND ADMINISTRATION sections).

CONTRAINDICATIONS

CEFOBID is contraindicated in patients with known allergy to the cephalosporin-class of antibiotics.

WARNINGS

BEFORE THERAPY WITH CEFOBID IS INSTITUTED, CAREFUL INQUIRY SHOULD BE MADE TO DETERMINE WHETHER THE PATIENT HAS HAD PREVIOUS HYPERSENSITIVITY REACTIONS TO CEPHALOSPORINS, PENICILLINS OR OTHER DRUGS. THIS PRODUCT SHOULD BE GIVEN CAUTIOUSLY TO PENICILLIN-SENSITIVE PATIENTS. ANTIBIOTICS SHOULD BE ADMINISTERED WITH CAUTION TO ANY PATIENT WHO HAS DEMONSTRATED SOME FORM OF ALLERGY, PARTICULARLY TO DRUGS. SERIOUS ACUTE HYPERSENSITIVITY REACTIONS MAY REQUIRE THE USE OF SUBCUTANEOUS EPINEPHRINE AND OTHER EMERGENCY MEASURES.
PSEUDOMEMBRANOUS COLITIS HAS BEEN REPORTED WITH THE USE OF CEPHALOSPORINS (AND OTHER BROAD-SPECTRUM ANTIBIOTICS); THEREFORE, IT IS IMPORTANT TO CONSIDER ITS DIAGNOSIS IN PATIENTS WHO DEVELOP DIARRHEA IN ASSOCIATION WITH ANTIBIOTIC USE.
Treatment with broad-spectrum antibiotics alters normal flora of the colon and may permit overgrowth of clostridia. Studies indicate a toxin produced by *Clostridium difficile* is one primary cause of antibiotic-associated colitis. Cholestyramine and colestipol resins have been shown to bind the toxin *in vitro.*
Mild cases of colitis may respond to drug discontinuance alone.
Moderate to severe cases should be managed with fluid, electrolyte, and protein supplementation as indicated.
When the colitis is not relieved by drug discontinuance or when it is severe, oral vancomycin is the treatment of choice for antibiotic-associated pseudomembranous colitis produced by *C. difficile.* Other causes of colitis should also be considered.

PRECAUTIONS

Although transient elevations of the BUN and serum creatinine have been observed, CEFOBID alone does not appear to cause significant nephrotoxicity. However, concomitant administration of aminoglycosides and other cephalosporins has caused nephrotoxicity.
CEFOBID is extensively excreted in bile. The serum half-life of CEFOBID is increased 2–4 fold in patients with hepatic disease and/or biliary obstruction. In general, total

TABLE 1. Cefoperazone Serum Concentrations

	Mean Serum Concentrations (mcg/mL)						
Dose/Route	0*	0.5 hr	1 hr	2 hr	4 hr	8 hr	12 hr
1 g IV	153	114	73	38	16	4	0.5
2 g IV	252	153	114	70	32	8	2
3 g IV	340	210	142	89	41	9	2
4 g IV	506	325	251	161	71	19	6
1 g IM	32 **	52	65	57	33	7	1
2 g IM	40 **	69	93	97	58	14	4

* Hours post-administration, with 0 time being the end of the infusion.
** Values obtained 15 minutes post-injection.

daily dosage above 4 g should not be necessary in such patients. If higher dosages are used, serum concentrations should be monitored.

Because renal excretion is not the main route of elimination of CEFOBID (see CLINICAL PHARMACOLOGY), patients with renal failure require no adjustment in dosage when usual doses are administered. When high doses of CEFOBID are used, concentrations of drug in the serum should be monitored periodically. If evidence of accumulation exists, dosage should be decreased accordingly.

The half-life of CEFOBID is reduced slightly during hemodialysis. Thus, dosing should be scheduled to follow a dialysis period. In patients with both hepatic dysfunction and significant renal disease, CEFOBID dosage should not exceed 1–2 g daily without close monitoring of serum concentrations.

As with other antibiotics, vitamin K deficiency has occurred rarely in patients treated with CEFOBID. The mechanism is most probably related to the suppression of gut flora which normally synthesize this vitamin. Those at risk include patients with a poor nutritional status, malabsorption states (e.g., cystic fibrosis), alcoholism, and patients on prolonged hyper-alimentation regimens (administered either intravenously or via a naso-gastric tube). Prothrombin time should be monitored in these patients and exogenous vitamin K administered as indicated.

A disulfiram-like reaction characterized by flushing, sweating, headache, and tachycardia has been reported when alcohol (beer, wine) was ingested within 72 hours after CEFOBID administration. Patients should be cautioned about the ingestion of alcoholic beverages following the administration of CEFOBID. A similar reaction has been reported with other cephalosporins.

Prolonged use of CEFOBID may result in the overgrowth of nonsusceptible organisms. Careful observation of the patient is essential. If superinfection occurs during therapy, appropriate measures should be taken.

CEFOBID should be prescribed with caution in individuals with a history of gastrointestinal disease, particularly colitis.

Drug Laboratory Test Interactions

A false-positive reaction for glucose in the urine may occur with Benedict's or Fehling's solution.

Carcinogenesis, Mutagenesis, Impairment of Fertility

Long-term studies in animals have not been performed to evaluate carcinogenic potential. The maximum duration of CEFOBID animal toxicity studies is six months. In none of the *in vivo* or *in vitro* genetic toxicology studies did CEFOBID show any mutagenic potential at either the chromosomal or subchromosomal level. CEFOBID produced no impairment of fertility and had no effects on general reproductive performance or fetal development when administered subcutaneously at daily doses up to 500 to 1000 mg/kg prior to and during mating, and to pregnant female rats during gestation. These doses are 10 to 20 times the estimated usual single clinical dose. CEFOBID had adverse effects on the testes of prepubertal rats at all doses tested. Subcutaneous administration of 1000 mg/kg per day (approximately 16 times the average adult human dose) resulted in reduced testicular weight, arrested spermatogenesis, reduced germinal cell population and vacuolation of Sertoli cell cytoplasm. The severity of lesions was dose dependent in the 100 to 1000 mg/kg per day range; the low dose caused a minor decrease in spermatocytes. This effect has not been observed in adult rats. Histologically the lesions were reversible at all but the highest dosage levels. However, these studies did not evaluate subsequent development of reproductive function in the rats. The relationship of these findings to humans is unknown.

Usage in Pregnancy

Pregnancy Category B: Reproduction studies have been performed in mice, rats, and monkeys at doses up to 10 times the human dose and have revealed no evidence of impaired fertility or harm to the fetus due to CEFOBID. There are, however, no adequate and well controlled studies in pregnant women. Because animal reproduction studies are not always predictive of human response, this drug should be used during pregnancy only if clearly needed.

Usage in Nursing Mothers

Only low concentrations of CEFOBID are excreted in human milk. Although CEFOBID passes poorly into breast milk of nursing mothers, caution should be exercised when CEFOBID is administered to a nursing woman.

Pediatric Use

Safety and effectiveness in children have not been established. For information concerning testicular changes in prepubertal rats, see Carcinogenesis, Mutagenesis, Impairment of Fertility.

ADVERSE REACTIONS

In clinical studies the following adverse effects were observed and were considered to be related to CEFOBID therapy or of uncertain etiology:

Hypersensitivity: As with all cephalosporins, hypersensitivity manifested by skin reactions (1 patient in 45), drug fever (1 in 260), or a change in Coombs' test (1 in 60) has been reported. These reactions are more likely to occur in patients with a history of allergies, particularly to penicillin.

Hematology: As with other beta-lactam antibiotics, reversible neutropenia may occur with prolonged administration. Slight decreases in neutrophil count (1 patient in 50) have been reported. Decreased hemoglobins (1 in 20) or hematocrits (1 in 20) have been reported, which is consistent with published literature on other cephalosporins. Transient eosinophilia has occurred in 1 patient in 10.

Controlled Room Temperature (15°–25°C/59°–77°F) 24 Hours	**Approximate Concentrations**
Bacteriostatic Water for Injection [Benzyl Alcohol or Parabens] (USP)	300 mg/mL
5% Dextrose Injection (USP)	2 mg to 50 mg/mL
5% Dextrose and Lactated Ringer's Injection	2 mg to 50 mg/mL
5% Dextrose and 0.9% Sodium Chloride Injection (USP)	2 mg to 50 mg/mL
5% Dextrose and 0.2% Sodium Chloride Injection (USP)	2 mg to 50 mg/mL
10% Dextrose Injection (USP)	2 mg to 50 mg/mL
Lactated Ringer's Injection (USP)	2 mg/mL
0.5% Lidocaine Hydrochloride Injection (USP)	300 mg/mL
0.9% Sodium Chloride Injection (USP)	2 mg to 300 mg/mL
Normosol® M and 5% Dextrose Injection	2 mg to 50 mg/mL
Normosol® R	2 mg to 50 mg/mL
Sterile Water for Injection	100 mg to 300 mg/mL

Reconstituted CEFOBID solutions may be stored in glass or plastic syringes, or in glass or flexible plastic parenteral solution containers.

Refrigerator Temperature (2°–8°C/36°–46°F) 5 Days	**Approximate Concentrations**
Bacteriostatic Water for Injection [Benzyl Alcohol or Parabens] (USP)	300 mg/mL
5% Dextrose Injection (USP)	2 mg to 50 mg/mL
5% Dextrose and 0.9% Sodium Chloride Injection (USP)	2 mg to 50 mg/mL
5% Dextrose and 0.2% Sodium Chloride Injection (USP)	2 mg to 50 mg/mL
Lactated Ringer's Injection (USP)	2 mg/mL
0.5% Lidocaine Hydrochloride Injection (USP)	300 mg/mL
0.9% Sodium Chloride Injection (USP)	2 mg to 300 mg/mL
Normosol® M and 5% Dextrose Injection	2 mg to 50 mg/mL
Normosol® R	2 mg to 50 mg/mL
Sterile Water for Injection	100 mg to 300 mg/mL

Reconstituted CEFOBID solutions may be stored in glass or plastic syringes, or in glass or flexible plastic parenteral solution containers.

Freezer Temperature (−20° to −10°C/−4° to 14°F)	**Approximate Concentrations**
3 Weeks	
5% Dextrose Injection (USP)	50 mg/mL
5% Dextrose and 0.9% Sodium Chloride Injection (USP)	2 mg/mL
5% Dextrose and 0.2% Sodium Chloride Injection (USP)	2 mg/mL
5 Weeks	
0.9% Sodium Chloride Injection (USP)	300 mg/mL
Sterile Water for Injection	300 mg/mL

Reconstituted CEFOBID solutions may be stored in plastic syringes, or in flexible plastic parenteral solution containers. Frozen samples should be thawed at room temperature before use. After thawing, unused portions should be discarded. Do not refreeze.

Hepatic: Of 1285 patients treated with cefoperazone in clinical trials, one patient with a history of liver disease developed significantly elevated liver function enzymes during CEFOBID therapy. Clinical signs and symptoms of nonspecific hepatitis accompanied these increases. After CEFOBID therapy was discontinued, the patient's enzymes returned to pre-treatment levels and the symptomatology resolved. As with other antibiotics that achieve high bile levels, mild transient elevations of liver function enzymes have been observed in 5–10% of the patients receiving CEFOBID therapy. The relevance of these findings, which were not accompanied by overt signs or symptoms of hepatic dysfunction, has not been established.

Gastrointestinal: Diarrhea or loose stools has been reported in 1 in 30 patients. Most of these experiences have been mild or moderate in severity and self-limiting in nature. In all cases, these symptoms responded to symptomatic therapy or ceased when cefoperazone therapy was stopped. Nausea and vomiting have been reported rarely. Symptoms of pseudomembranous colitis can appear during or for several weeks subsequent to antibiotic therapy (see WARNINGS).

Renal Function Tests: Transient elevations of the BUN (1 in 16) and serum creatinine (1 in 48) have been noted.

Local Reactions: CEFOBID is well tolerated following intramuscular administration. Occasionally, transient pain (1 in 140) may follow administration by this route. When CEFOBID is administered by intravenous infusion some patients may develop phlebitis (1 in 120) at the infusion site.

DOSAGE AND ADMINISTRATION

Sterile cefoperazone sodium can be administered by IM or IV injection (following dilution). However, the intent of this pharmacy bulk package is for the preparation of solutions for IV infusion only.

The usual adult daily dose of CEFOBID is 2 to 4 grams per day administered in equally divided doses every 12 hours. In severe infections or infections caused by less sensitive organisms, the total daily dose and/or frequency may be increased. Patients have been successfully treated with a total daily dosage of 6–12 grams divided into 2, 3 or 4 administrations ranging from 1.5 to 4 grams per dose.

When treating infections caused by *Streptococcus pyogenes,* therapy should be continued for at least 10 days.

If *C. trachomatis* is a suspected pathogen, appropriate antichlamydial coverage should be added, because cefoperazone has no activity against this organism.

Solutions of CEFOBID and aminoglycoside should not be directly mixed, since there is a physical incompatibility between them. If combination therapy with CEFOBID and an aminoglycoside is contemplated (see INDICATIONS) this can be accomplished by sequential intermittent intravenous infusion provided that separate secondary intravenous tubing is used, and that the primary intravenous tubing is adequately irrigated with an approved diluent between doses. It is also suggested that CEFOBID be administered prior to the aminoglycoside. *In vitro* testing of the effectiveness of drug combination(s) is recommended.

In a pharmacokinetic study, a total daily dose of 16 grams was administered to severely immunocompromised patients by constant infusion without complications. Steady state serum concentrations were approximately 150 mcg/mL in these patients.

RECONSTITUTION

The following solutions may be used for the initial reconstitution of CEFOBID sterile powder:

Table 1. Solutions for Initial Reconstitution

- 5% Dextrose Injection (USP)
- 5% Dextrose and 0.9% Sodium Chloride Injection (USP)
- 5% Dextrose and 0.2% Sodium Chloride Injection (USP)
- 10% Dextrose Injection (USP)
- Bacteriostatic Water for Injection [Benzyl Alcohol or Parabens] (USP)*†
- 0.9% Sodium Chloride Injection (USP)
- Normosol® M and 5% Dextrose Injection
- Normosol® R
- Sterile Water for Injection*

* Not to be used as a vehicle for intravenous infusion.

† Preparations containing Benzyl Alcohol should not be used in neonates.

General Reconstitution Procedures

CEFOBID sterile powder for intravenous or intramuscular use may be initially reconstituted with any compatible solution mentioned above in Table 1. Solutions should be allowed to stand after reconstitution to allow any foaming to dissipate to permit visual inspection for complete solubilization. Vigorous and prolonged agitation may be necessary to solubilize CEFOBID in higher concentrations (above 333 mg cefoperazone/mL). The maximum solubility of CEFOBID sterile powder is approximately 475 mg cefoperazone/mL of compatible diluent.

Preparation For Intravenous Use

General. CEFOBID concentrations between 2 mg/mL and 50 mg/mL are recommended for intravenous administration.

Table 2. Vehicles for Intravenous Infusion

- 5% Dextrose Injection (USP)
- 5% Dextrose and Lactated Ringer's Injection
- 5% Dextrose and 0.9% Sodium Chloride Injection (USP)
- 5% Dextrose and 0.2% Sodium Chloride Injection (USP)
- 10% Dextrose Injection (USP)
- Lactated Ringer's Injection (USP)
- 0.9% Sodium Chloride Injection (USP)
- Normosol® M and 5% Dextrose Injection
- Normosol® R

DIRECTIONS FOR PROPER USE OF PHARMACY BULK PACKAGE

The 10 gram vial should be reconstituted with 95 mL of sterile water for injection in two separate aliquots in a suitable work area such as a laminar flow hood. Add 45 mL of solution, shake to dissolve and add 50 mL, shake for final solution. The resulting solution will contain 100 mg/mL of cefoperazone. This closure may be penetrated only one time after reconstitution, if needed, using a suitable sterile transfer device or dispensing set which allows measured dispensing of the contents.

Discard unused solution within 24 hours of initial entry.

Continued on next page

Cefobid Pharmacy Bulk—Cont.

Reconstituted Bulk Solutions Should Not Be Used For Direct Infusion.

Although after reconstitution of the Pharmacy Bulk Package, no significant loss of potency occurs for 24 hours at room temperature and for 5 days if refrigerated, transfer individual dose to appropriate intravenous infusion solutions as soon as possible following reconstituion of the bulk package. Discard unused portions of solution held longer than these recommended periods at room temperature or under refrigeration. The stability of the solution which has been transferred into a container varies according to diluent and concentration. (See STORAGE AND STABILITY.)

The 10 gram vials may be further diluted with the parenteral diluents listed under **Table 2. Vehicles for Intravenous Infusion.** The parenteral diluents and approximate concentrations of CEFOBID that provide stable solutions are presented under STORAGE AND STABILITY.

Parenteral drug products should be inspected visually for particulate matter and discoloration prior to administration, whenever solution and container permit.

DIRECTIONS FOR USE OF CEFOBID (cefoperazone) INJECTION IN PLASTIC CONTAINERS

CEFOBID supplied premixed as a frozen, sterile, iso-osmotic solution in plastic containers is to be administered either as continuous or intermittent infusion.

Thaw container at room temperature. After thawing, check for minute leaks by squeezing bag firmly. If leaks are found, discard solution as sterility may be impaired. Additives should not be introduced into this solution. Do not use if the solution is cloudy or precipitated or if the seal is not intact. After thawing, the solution is stable for 10 days if stored under refrigeration (5°C) and for 48 hours at room temperature. DO NOT REFREEZE. Use sterile equipment.

CAUTION: Do not use plastic container in series connections. Such use could result in air embolism due to residual air being drawn from the primary container before administration of the fluid from the secondary container is complete.

Preparation for Administration

1. Suspend container from eyelet support.
2. Remove plastic protector from outlet port at bottom of container.
3. Attach administration set. Refer to complete directions accompanying set.

STORAGE AND STABILITY

CEFOBID sterile powder is to be stored at or below 25°C (77°F) and protected from light prior to reconstitution. After reconstitution, protection from light is not necessary.

The following parenteral diluents and approximate concentrations of CEFOBID provide stable solutions under the following conditions for the indicated time periods. (After the indicated time periods, unused portions of solutions should be discarded.)

[See table at top of previous page]

HOW SUPPLIED

CEFOBID sterile powder is available in Pharmacy Bulk Package containing cefoperazone sodium equivalent to 10 g cefoperazone × 1 (NDC 0049-1219-28).

OTHER SIZE PACKAGES AVAILABLE

CEFOBID sterile powder is available in vials containing cefoperazone sodium equivalent to 1 g cefoperazone × 10 (NDC 0049-1201-83) and 2 g cefoperazone × 10 (NDC 0049-1202-83) for intramuscular and intravenous administration.

CEFOBID sterile powder is available in Piggyback Units containing cefoperazone sodium equivalent to 1 g cefoperazone × 10 (NDC 0049-1211-83), and 2 g cefoperazone × 10 (NDC 0049-1212-83).

CEFOBID (cefoperazone) injection is supplied premixed as a frozen, sterile, nonpyrogenic, iso-osmotic solution in plastic containers. Each 50 mL unit contains cefoperazone sodium equivalent to 1 g cefoperazone with approximately 2.3 g dextrose hydrous USP added (NDC 0049-1216-18) or 2 g cefoperazone with approximately 1.8 g dextrose hydrous USP added (NDC 0049-1215-18). The solution is iso-osmotic (approximately 300 mOsmol/L), and solution pH may have been adjusted with sodium hydroxide and/or hydrochloric acid. Do not store above −20°C.

CEFOBID supplied as a frozen, sterile, nonpyrogenic, iso-osmotic solution in 50 ml plastic containers is manufactured for Roerig Division of Pfizer Pharmaceuticals by Baxter Healthcare Corporation, Deerfield, IL 60015.

Rx only.

70-4482-00-6 Revised November 1999

CELEBREX™ ℞
(celecoxib capsules)

DESCRIPTION

CELEBREX (celecoxib) is chemically designated as 4-[5-(4-methylphenyl)-3-(trifluoromethyl)-1H-pyrazol-1-yl] benzenesulfonamide and is a diaryl substituted pyrazole. It has the following chemical structure:

[See chemical structure at top of next column]

The empirical formula for celecoxib is $C_{17}H_{14}F_3N_3O_2S$, and the molecular weight is 381.38.

NH2 O=S=O ... N—N ... CF3 ... CH3

CELEBREX oral capsules contain 100 mg and 200 mg of celecoxib.

The inactive ingredients in CELEBREX capsules include: croscarmellose sodium, edible inks, gelatin, lactose monohydrate, magnesium stearate, povidone, sodium lauryl sulfate and titanium dioxide.

CLINICAL PHARMACOLOGY

Mechanism of Action: CELEBREX is a nonsteroidal anti-inflammatory drug that exhibits anti-inflammatory, analgesic, and antipyretic activities in animal models. The mechanism of action of CELEBREX is believed to be due to inhibition of prostaglandin synthesis, primarily via inhibition of cyclooxygenase-2 (COX-2), and at therapeutic concentrations in humans, CELEBREX does not inhibit the cyclooxygenase-1 (COX-1) isoenzyme. In animal colon tumor models, celecoxib reduced the incidence and multiplicity of tumors.

Pharmacokinetics:

Absorption

Peak plasma levels of celecoxib occur approximately 3 hrs after an oral dose. Under fasting conditions, both peak plasma levels (C_{max}) and area under the curve (AUC) are roughly dose proportional up to 200 mg BID; at higher doses there are less than proportional changes in C_{max} and AUC (see Food Effects). Absolute bioavailability studies have not been conducted. With multiple dosing, steady state conditions are reached on or before day 5.

The pharmacokinetic parameters of celecoxib in a group of healthy subjects are shown in Table 1.

[See table below]

Food Effects

When CELEBREX capsules were taken with a high fat meal, peak plasma levels were delayed for about 1 to 2 hours with an increase in total absorption (AUC) of 10% to 20%. Under fasting conditions, at doses above 200 mg, there is less than a proportional increase in C_{max} and AUC, which is thought to be due to the low solubility of the drug in aqueous media. Coadministration of CELEBREX with an aluminum- and magnesium-containing antacid resulted in a reduction in plasma celecoxib concentrations with a decrease of 37% in C_{max} and 10% in AUC. CELEBREX, at doses up to 200 mg BID can be administered without regard to the timing of meals. Higher doses (400 mg BID) should be administered with food.

Distribution

In healthy subjects, celecoxib is highly protein bound (~97%) within the clinical dose range. *In vitro* studies indicate that celecoxib binds primarily to albumin and, to a lesser extent, α_1-acid glycoprotein. The apparent volume of distribution at steady state (V_{ss}/F) is approximately 400 L, suggesting extensive distribution into the tissues. Celecoxib is not preferentially bound to red blood cells.

Metabolism

Celecoxib metabolism is primarily mediated via cytochrome P450 2C9. Three metabolites, a primary alcohol, the corresponding carboxylic acid and its glucuronide conjugate, have been identified in human plasma. These metabolites are inactive as COX-1 or COX-2 inhibitors. Patients who are known or suspected to be P450 2C9 poor metabolizers based on a previous history should be administered celecoxib with caution as they may have abnormally high plasma levels due to reduced metabolic clearance.

Excretion

Celecoxib is eliminated predominantly by hepatic metabolism with little (<3%) unchanged drug recovered in the urine and feces. Following a single oral dose of radiolabeled drug, approximately 57% of the dose was excreted in the feces and 27% was excreted into the urine. The primary metabolite in both urine and feces was the carboxylic acid metabolite (73% of dose) with low amounts of the glucuronide also appearing in the urine. It appears that the low solubility of the drug prolongs the absorption process making terminal half-life ($t_{1/2}$) determinations more variable. The effective half-life is approximately 11 hours under fasted conditions. The apparent plasma clearance (CL/F) is about 500 mL/min.

Special Populations

Geriatric: At steady state, elderly subjects (over 65 years old) had a 40% higher C_{max} and a 50% higher AUC compared to the young subjects. In elderly females, celecoxib C_{max} and AUC are higher than those for elderly males, but these increases are predominantly due to lower body weight in elderly females. Dose adjustment in the elderly is not generally necessary. However, for patients of less than 50 kg in body weight, initiate therapy at the lowest recommended dose.

Pediatric: CELEBREX capsules have not been investigated in pediatric patients below 18 years of age.

Races: Meta-analysis of pharmacokinetic studies has suggested an approximately 40% higher AUC of celecoxib in Blacks compared to Caucasians. The cause and clinical significance of this finding is unknown.

Hepatic Insufficiency: A pharmacokinetic study in subjects with mild (Child-Pugh Class I) and moderate (Child-Pugh Class II) hepatic impairment has shown that steady-state celecoxib AUC is increased about 40% and 180%, respectively, above that seen in healthy control subjects. Therefore, the daily recommended dose of CELEBREX capsules should be reduced by approximately 50% in patients with moderate (Child-Pugh Class II) hepatic impairment. Patients with severe hepatic impairment have not been studied. The use of CELEBREX in patients with severe hepatic impairment is not recommended.

Renal Insufficiency: In a cross-study comparison, celecoxib AUC was approximately 40% lower in patients with chronic renal insufficiency (GFR 35–60 mL/min) than that seen in subjects with normal renal function. No significant relationship was found between GFR and celecoxib clearance. Patients with severe renal insufficiency have not been studied.

Drug Interactions

Also see PRECAUTIONS —Drug Interactions.

General: Significant interactions may occur when celecoxib is administered together with drugs that inhibit P450 2C9. *In vitro* studies indicate that celecoxib is not an inhibitor of cytochrome P450 2C9, 2C19 or 3A4.

Clinical studies with celecoxib have identified potentially significant interactions with fluconazole and lithium. Experience with nonsteroidal anti-inflammatory drugs (NSAIDs) suggests the potential for interactions with furosemide and ACE inhibitors. The effects of celecoxib on the pharmacokinetics and/or pharmacodynamics of glyburide, ketoconazole, methotrexate, phenytoin, and tolbutamide have been studied *in vivo* and clinically important interactions have not been found.

CLINICAL STUDIES

Osteoarthritis (OA): CELEBREX has demonstrated significant reduction in joint pain compared to placebo. CELEBREX was evaluated for treatment of the signs and the symptoms of OA of the knee and hip in approximately 4,200 patients in placebo- and active-controlled clinical trials of up to 12 weeks duration. In patients with OA, treatment with CELEBREX 100 mg BID or 200 mg QD resulted in improvement in WOMAC (Western Ontario and McMaster Universities) osteoarthritis index, a composite of pain, stiffness, and functional measures in OA. In three 12-week studies of pain accompanying OA flare, CELEBREX doses of 100 mg BID and 200 mg BID provided significant reduction of pain within 24–48 hours of initiation of dosing. At doses of 100 mg BID or 200 mg BID the effectiveness of CELEBREX was shown to be similar to that of naproxen 500 mg BID. Doses of 200 mg BID provided no additional benefit above that seen with 100 mg BID. A total daily dose of 200 mg has been shown to be equally effective whether administered as 100 mg BID or 200 mg QD.

Rheumatoid Arthritis (RA): CELEBREX has demonstrated significant reduction in joint tenderness/pain and joint swelling compared to placebo. CELEBREX was evaluated for treatment of the signs and symptoms of RA in approximately 2,100 patients in placebo- and active-controlled clinical trials of up to 24 weeks in duration. CELEBREX was shown to be superior to placebo in these studies, using the ACR20 Responder Index, a composite of clinical, laboratory, and functional measures in RA. CELEBREX doses of 100 mg BID and 200 mg BID were similar in effectiveness and both were comparable to naproxen 500 mg BID.

Although CELEBREX 100 mg BID and 200 mg BID provided similar overall effectiveness, some patients derived additional benefit from the 200 mg BID dose. Doses of 400 mg BID provided no additional benefit above that seen with 100–200 mg BID.

Familial Adenomatous Polyposis (FAP): CELEBREX was evaluated to reduce the number of adenomatous colorectal polyps. A randomized double-blind placebo-controlled study was conducted in 83 patients with FAP. The study population included 58 patients with a prior subtotal or total colectomy and 25 patients with an intact colon. Thirteen patients had the attenuated FAP phenotype.

One area in the rectum and up to four areas in the colon were identified at baseline for specific follow-up, and polyps were counted at baseline and following six months of treatment. The mean reduction in the number of colorectal polyps was 28% for CELEBREX 400 mg BID, 12% for CELEBREX 100 mg BID, and 5% for placebo. The reduction in polyps observed with CELEBREX 400 mg BID was statisti-

Table 1
Summary of Single Dose (200 mg) Disposition Kinetics of Celecoxib in Healthy Subjects[1]
Mean (%CV) PK Parameter Values

C_{max}, ng/mL	T_{max}, hr	Effective $t_{1/2}$, hr	Vss/F, L	CL/F, L/hr
705 (38)	2.8 (37)	11.2 (31)	429 (34)	27.7 (28)

[1]Subjects under fasting conditions (n=36, 19–52 yrs.)

cally superior to placebo at the six-month timepoint (p=0.003). (See Figure 1.)

Figure 1
Percent Change from Baseline in Number of Colorectal Polyps (FAP Patients)

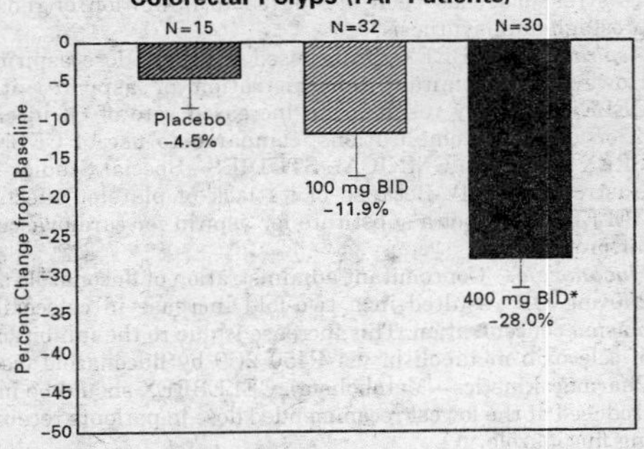

*p=0.003 versus placebo.

Special Studies

Gastrointestinal: Scheduled upper GI endoscopic evaluations were performed in over 4,500 arthritis patients who were enrolled in five controlled randomized 12–24 week trials using active comparators, two of which also included placebo controls. Twelve-week endoscopic ulcer data are available on approximately 1,400 patients and 24 week endoscopic ulcer data are available on 184 patients on CELEBREX at doses ranging from 50–400 mg BID. In all three studies that included naproxen 500 mg BID, and in the study that included ibuprofen 800 mg TID, CELEBREX was associated with a statistically significantly lower incidence of endoscopic ulcers over the study period. Two studies compared CELEBREX with diclofenac 75 mg BID; one study revealed a statistically significantly higher prevalence of endoscopic ulcers in the diclofenac group at the study endpoint (6 months on treatment), and one study revealed no statistically significant difference between cumulative endoscopic ulcer incidence rates in the diclofenac and CELEBREX groups after 1, 2, and 3 months of treatment. There was no consistent relationship between the incidence of gastroduodenal ulcers and the dose of CELEBREX over the range studied.

Figure 2 and Table 2 summarize the incidence of endoscopic ulcers in two 12-week studies that enrolled patients in whom baseline endoscopies revealed no ulcers.

Figure 2
Incidence of Endoscopically Observed Gastroduodenal Ulcers after Twelve Weeks of Treatment

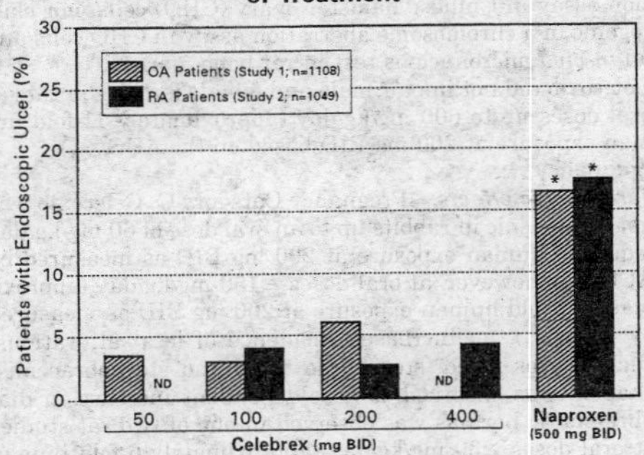

ND=Not Done

*Significantly different from all other treatments; p<0.05.

Celebrex 100 mg BID and 200 mg QD, BID are the recommended doses.

These studies were not powered to compare the endoscopic ulcer rates of Celebrex vs. placebo.

Study 1: placebo ulcer rate = 2.3%

Study 2: placebo ulcer rate = 2.0%

[See table 2 above]

Figure 3 and Table 3 summarize data from two 12-week studies that enrolled patients in whom baseline endoscopies revealed no ulcers. Patients underwent interval endoscopies every 4 weeks to give information on ulcer risk over time.

[See figure 3 at top of next column]

[See table 3 above]

One randomized and double-blinded 6-month study in 430 RA patients was conducted in which an endoscopic examination was performed at 6 months. The results are shown in Figure 4.

[See figure 4 at top of next column]

The correlation between findings of endoscopic studies, and the relative incidence of clinically serious upper GI events that may be observed with different products, has not been fully established. Serious clinically significant upper GI bleeding has been observed in patients receiving CELEBREX in controlled and open-labeled trials, albeit infrequently (see WARNINGS—Gastrointestinal [GI] Effects). Prospective, long-term studies required to compare the incidence of serious, clinically significant upper GI adverse events in patients taking CELEBREX vs. comparator NSAID products have not been performed.

Use with Aspirin: Approximately 11% of patients (440/4,000) enrolled in 4 of the 5 endoscopic studies were taking

Table 2
Incidence of Gastroduodenal Ulcers from Endoscopic Studies in OA and RA Patients

	3 Month Studies	
	Study 1 (n=1108)	**Study 2 (n=1049)**
Placebo	2.3% (5/217)	2.0% (4/200)
Celebrex 50 mg BID	3.4% (8/233)	—
Celebrex 100 mg BID	3.1% (7/227)	4.0% (9/223)
Celebrex 200 mg BID	5.9% (13/221)	2.7% (6/219)
Celebrex 400 mg BID	—	4.1% (8/197)
Naproxen 500 mg BID	16.2% (34/210)*	17.6% (37/210)*

*p≤0.05 vs all other treatments

Table 3
Incidence of Gastroduodenal Ulcers from 3-Month Serial Endoscopy Studies in OA and RA Patients

	Week 4	Week 8	Week 12	Final
Study 3 (n=523)				
Celebrex 200 mg BID	4.0% (10/252)*	2.2% (5/227)*	1.5% (3/196)*	7.5% (20/266)*
Naproxen 500 mg BID	19.0% (47/247)	14.2% (26/182)	9.9% (14/141)	34.6% (89/257)
Study 4 (n=1062)				
Celebrex 200 mg BID	3.9% (13/337)†	2.4% (7/296)†	1.8% (5/274)†	7.0% (25/356)†
Diclofenac 75 mg BID	5.1% (18/350)	3.3% (10/306)	2.9% (8/278)	9.7% (36/372)
Ibuprofen 800 mg TID	13.0% (42/323)	6.2% (15/241)	9.6% (21/219)	23.3% (78/334)

*p≤0.05 Celebrex vs. naproxen based on interval and cumulative analyses

†p≤0.05 Celebrex vs. ibuprofen based on interval and cumulative analyses

Figure 3
Cumulative Incidence of Gastroduodenal Ulcers Based on 4 Serial Endoscopies over 12 Weeks

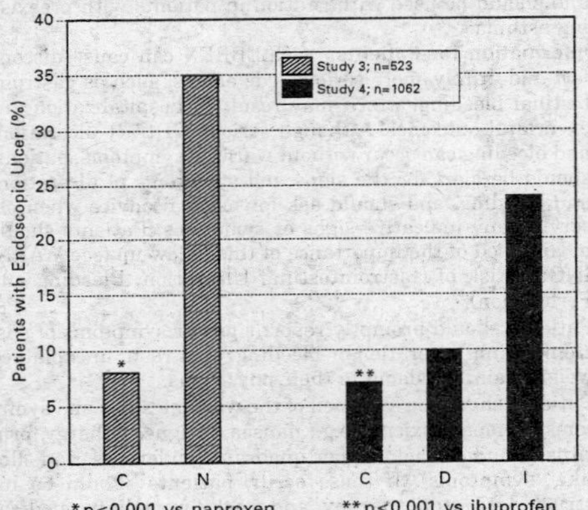

*p<0.001 vs naproxen **p<0.001 vs ibuprofen

C=Celecoxib 200 mg BID D=Diclofenac 75 mg BID
N=Naproxen 500 mg BID I=Ibuprofen 800 mg TID

Figure 4
Prevalence of Endoscopically Observed Gastroduodenal Ulcers after Six Months of Treatment in Patients with Rheumatoid Arthritis

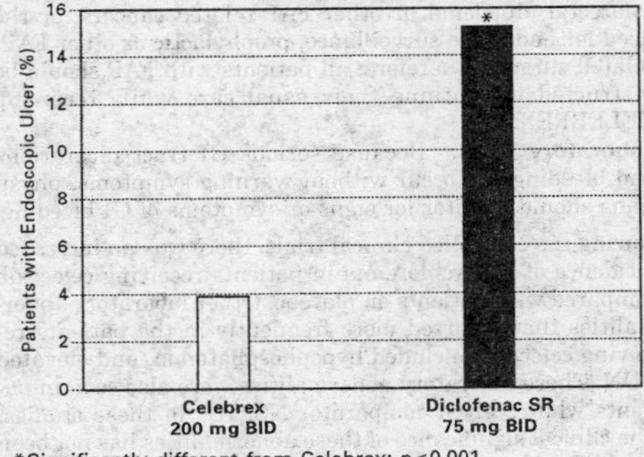

*Significantly different from Celebrex; p<0.001

aspirin (≤325 mg/day). In the CELEBREX groups, the endoscopic ulcer rate appeared to be higher in aspirin users than in non-users. However, the increased rate of ulcers in these aspirin users was less than the endoscopic ulcer rates observed in the active comparator groups, with or without aspirin.

Platelets: In clinical trials, CELEBREX at single doses up to 800 mg and multiple doses of 600 mg BID for up to 7 days duration (higher than recommended therapeutic doses) had no effect on platelet aggregation and bleeding time. Comparators (naproxen 500 mg BID, ibuprofen 800 mg TID, diclofenac 75 mg BID) significantly reduced platelet aggregation and prolonged bleeding time.

INDICATIONS AND USAGE

CELEBREX is indicated:

1) For relief of the signs and symptoms of osteoarthritis.
2) For relief of the signs and symptoms of rheumatoid arthritis in adults.
3) To reduce the number of adenomatous colorectal polyps in familial adenomatous polyposis (FAP), as an adjunct to usual care (e.g., endoscopic surveillance, surgery). It is not known whether there is a clinical benefit from a reduction in the number of colorectal polyps in FAP patients. It is also not known whether the effects of CELEBREX treatment will persist after CELEBREX is discontinued. The efficacy and safety of CELEBREX treatment in patients with FAP beyond six months have not been studied (see CLINICAL STUDIES, WARNINGS, and PRECAUTIONS sections).

CONTRAINDICATIONS

CELEBREX is contraindicated in patients with known hypersensitivity to celecoxib.

CELEBREX should not be given to patients who have demonstrated allergic-type reactions to sulfonamides.

CELEBREX should not be given to patients who have experienced asthma, urticaria, or allergic-type reactions after taking aspirin or other NSAIDs. Severe, rarely fatal, anaphylactic-like reactions to NSAIDs have been reported in such patients (see WARNINGS—Anaphylactoid Reactions, and PRECAUTIONS—Preexisting Asthma).

WARNINGS

Gastrointestinal (GI) Effects—Risk of GI Ulceration, Bleeding, and Perforation

Serious gastrointestinal toxicity such as bleeding, ulceration, and perforation of the stomach, small intestine or large intestine, can occur at any time, with or without warning symptoms, in patients treated with nonsteroidal anti-inflammatory drugs (NSAIDs). Minor upper gastrointestinal problems, such as dyspepsia, are common and may also occur at any time during NSAID therapy. Therefore, physicians and patients should remain alert for ulceration and bleeding, even in the absence of previous GI tract symptoms. Patients should be informed about the signs and/or symptoms of serious GI toxicity and the steps to take if they occur. The utility of periodic laboratory monitoring has not been demonstrated, nor has it been adequately assessed. Only one in five patients who develop a serious upper GI adverse event on NSAID therapy is symptomatic. It has been demonstrated that upper GI ulcers, gross bleeding or perforation, caused by NSAIDs, appear to occur in approximately 1% of patients treated for 3–6 months, and in about 2–4% of patients treated for one year. These trends continue thus, increasing the likelihood of developing a serious GI event at some time during the course of therapy. However, even short-term therapy is not without risk.

It is unclear, at the present time, how the above rates apply to CELEBREX (See CLINICAL STUDIES—Special Studies). Among 5,285 patients who received CELEBREX in controlled clinical trials of 1 to 6 months duration (most were 3

Continued on next page

Celebrex—Cont.

month studies) at a daily dose of 200 mg or more, 2 (0.04%) experienced significant upper GI bleeding, at 14 and 22 days after initiation of dosing. Approximately 40% of these 5,285 patients were in studies that required them to be free of ulcers by endoscopy at study entry. Thus it is unclear if this study population is representative of the general population. Prospective, long-term studies required to compare the incidence of serious, clinically significant upper GI adverse events in patients taking CELEBREX vs. comparator NSAID products have not been performed.

NSAIDs should be prescribed with extreme caution in patients with a prior history of ulcer disease or gastrointestinal bleeding. Most spontaneous reports of fatal GI events are in elderly or debilitated patients and therefore special care should be taken in treating this population. **To minimize the potential risk for an adverse GI event, the lowest effective dose should be used for the shortest possible duration.** For high risk patients, alternate therapies that do not involve NSAIDs should be considered.

Studies have shown that patients with a *prior history of peptic ulcer disease and/or gastrointestinal bleeding* and who use NSAIDs, have a greater than 10-fold higher risk for developing a GI bleed than patients with neither of these risk factors. In addition to a past history of ulcer disease, pharmacoepidemiological studies have identified several other co-therapies or co-morbid conditions that may increase the risk for GI bleeding such as: treatment with oral corticosteroids, treatment with anticoagulants, longer duration of NSAID therapy, smoking, alcoholism, older age, and poor general health status.

Anaphylactoid Reactions

As with NSAIDs in general, anaphylactoid reactions have occurred in patients without known prior exposure to CELEBREX. In post-marketing experience, rare cases of anaphylactoid reactions and angioedema have been reported in patients receiving CELEBREX. CELEBREX should not be given to patients with the aspirin triad. This symptom complex typically occurs in asthmatic patients who experience rhinitis with or without nasal polyps, or who exhibit severe, potentially fatal bronchospasm after taking aspirin or other NSAIDs (see CONTRAINDICATIONS and PRECAUTIONS—Preexisting Asthma). Emergency help should be sought in cases where an anaphylactoid reaction occurs.

Advanced Renal Disease

No information is available regarding the use of CELEBREX in patients with advanced kidney disease. Therefore, treatment with CELEBREX is not recommended in these patients. If CELEBREX therapy must be initiated, close monitoring of the patient's kidney function is advisable (see PRECAUTIONS—Renal Effects).

Pregnancy

In late pregnancy CELEBREX should be avoided because it may cause premature closure of the ductus arteriosus.

Familial Adenomatous Polyposis (FAP): Treatment with CELEBREX in FAP has not been shown to reduce the risk of gastrointestinal cancer or the need for prophylactic colectomy or other FAP-related surgeries. Therefore, the usual care of FAP patients should not be altered because of the concurrent administration of CELEBREX. In particular, the frequency of routine endoscopic surveillance should not be decreased and prophylactic colectomy or other FAP-related surgeries should not be delayed.

PRECAUTIONS

General: CELEBREX cannot be expected to substitute for corticosteroids or to treat corticosteroid insufficiency. Abrupt discontinuation of corticosteroids may lead to exacerbation of corticosteroid-responsive illness. Patients on prolonged corticosteroid therapy should have their therapy tapered slowly if a decision is made to discontinue corticosteroids.

The pharmacological activity of CELEBREX in reducing inflammation, and possibly fever, may diminish the utility of these diagnostic signs in detecting infectious complications of presumed noninfectious, painful conditions.

Hepatic Effects: Borderline elevations of one or more liver tests may occur in up to 15% of patients taking NSAIDs, and notable elevations of ALT or AST (approximately three or more times the upper limit of normal) have been reported in approximately 1% of patients in clinical trials with NSAIDs. These laboratory abnormalities may progress, may remain unchanged, or may be transient with continuing therapy. Rare cases of severe hepatic reactions, including jaundice and fatal fulminant hepatitis, liver necrosis and hepatic failure (some with fatal outcome) have been reported with NSAIDs, including CELEBREX. (See ADVERSE REACTIONS—post-marketing experience.) In controlled clinical trials of CELEBREX, the incidence of borderline elevations of liver tests was 6% for CELEBREX and 5% for placebo, and approximately 0.2% of patients taking CELEBREX and 0.3% of patients taking placebo had notable elevations of ALT and AST.

A patient with symptoms and/or signs suggesting liver dysfunction, or in whom an abnormal liver test has occurred, should be monitored carefully for evidence of the development of a more severe hepatic reaction while on therapy with CELEBREX. If clinical signs and symptoms consistent with liver disease develop, or if systemic manifestations occur (e.g., eosinophilia, rash, etc.), CELEBREX should be discontinued.

Renal Effects: Long-term administration of NSAIDs has resulted in renal papillary necrosis and other renal injury. Renal toxicity has also been seen in patients in whom renal prostaglandins have a compensatory role in the maintenance of renal perfusion. In these patients, administration of a nonsteroidal anti-inflammatory drug may cause a dose-dependent reduction in prostaglandin formation and, secondarily, in renal blood flow, which may precipitate overt renal decompensation. Patients at greatest risk of this reaction are those with impaired renal function, heart failure, liver dysfunction, those taking diuretics and ACE inhibitors, and the elderly. Discontinuation of NSAID therapy is usually followed by recovery to the pretreatment state. Clinical trials with CELEBREX have shown renal effects similar to those observed with comparator NSAIDs.

Caution should be used when initiating treatment with CELEBREX in patients with considerable dehydration. It is advisable to rehydrate patients first and then start therapy with CELEBREX. Caution is also recommended in patients with pre-existing kidney disease (see WARNINGS–Advanced Renal Disease).

Hematological Effects: Anemia is sometimes seen in patients receiving CELEBREX. In controlled clinical trials the incidence of anemia was 0.6% with CELEBREX and 0.4% with placebo. Patients on long-term treatment with CELEBREX should have their hemoglobin or hematocrit checked if they exhibit any signs or symptoms of anemia or blood loss. CELEBREX does not generally affect platelet counts, prothrombin time (PT), or partial thromboplastin time (PTT), and does not appear to inhibit platelet aggregation at indicated dosages (See CLINICAL STUDIES—Special Studies—Platelets).

Fluid Retention and Edema: Fluid retention and edema have been observed in some patients taking CELEBREX (see ADVERSE REACTIONS). Therefore, CELEBREX should be used with caution in patients with fluid retention, hypertension, or heart failure.

Preexisting Asthma: Patients with asthma may have aspirin-sensitive asthma. The use of aspirin in patients with aspirin-sensitive asthma has been associated with severe bronchospasm which can be fatal. Since cross reactivity, including bronchospasm, between aspirin and other nonsteroidal anti-inflammatory drugs has been reported in such aspirin-sensitive patients, CELEBREX should not be administered to patients with this form of aspirin sensitivity and should be used with caution in patients with preexisting asthma.

Information for Patients: CELEBREX can cause discomfort and, rarely, more serious side effects, such as gastrointestinal bleeding, which may result in hospitalization and even fatal outcomes. Although serious GI tract ulcerations and bleeding can occur without warning symptoms, patients should be alert for the signs and symptoms of ulcerations and bleeding, and should ask for medical advice when observing any indicative signs or symptoms. Patients should be apprised of the importance of this follow-up (see WARNINGS—Risk of Gastrointestinal Ulceration, Bleeding and Perforation).

Patients should promptly report signs or symptoms of gastrointestinal ulceration or bleeding, skin rash, unexplained weight gain, or edema to their physicians.

Patients should be informed of the warning signs and symptoms of hepatotoxicity (e.g., nausea, fatigue, lethargy, pruritus, jaundice, right upper quadrant tenderness, and "flu-like" symptoms). If these occur, patients should be instructed to stop therapy and seek immediate medical therapy.

Patients should also be instructed to seek immediate emergency help in the case of an anaphylactoid reaction (see WARNINGS).

In late pregnancy CELEBREX should be avoided because it may cause premature closure of the ductus arteriosus.

Patients with familial adenomatous polyposis (FAP) should be informed that CELEBREX has not been shown to reduce colorectal, duodenal or other FAP-related cancers, or the need for endosopic surveillance, prophylactic or other FAP-related surgery. Therefore, all patients with FAP should be instructed to continue their usual care while receiving CELEBREX.

Laboratory Tests: Because serious GI tract ulcerations and bleeding can occur without warning symptoms, physicians should monitor for signs or symptoms of GI bleeding.

During the controlled clinical trials, there was an increased incidence of hyperchloremia in patients receiving celecoxib compared with patients on placebo. Other laboratory abnormalities that occurred more frequently in the patients receiving celecoxib included hypophosphatemia, and elevated BUN. These laboratory abnormalities were also seen in patients who received comparator NSAIDs in these studies. The clinical significance of these abnormalities has not been established.

Drug Interactions

General: Celecoxib metabolism is predominantly mediated via cytochrome P450 2C9 in the liver. Co-administration of celecoxib with drugs that are known to inhibit 2C9 should be done with caution.

In vitro studies indicate that celecoxib, although not a substrate, is an inhibitor of cytochrome P450 2D6. Therefore, there is a potential for an *in vivo* drug interaction with drugs that are metabolized by P450 2D6.

ACE-inhibitors: Reports suggest that NSAIDs may diminish the antihypertensive effect of Angiotensin Converting Enzyme (ACE) inhibitors. This interaction should be given consideration in patients taking CELEBREX concomitantly with ACE-inhibitors.

Furosemide: Clinical studies, as well as post marketing observations, have shown that NSAIDs can reduce the natriuretic effect of furosemide and thiazides in some patients. This response has been attributed to inhibition of renal prostaglandin synthesis.

Aspirin: CELEBREX can be used with low dose aspirin. However, concomitant administration of aspirin with CELEBREX may result in an increased rate of GI ulceration or other complications, compared to use of CELEBREX alone (see CLINICAL STUDIES—Special Studies—Gastrointestinal). Because of its lack of platelet effects, CELEBREX is not a substitute for aspirin for cardiovascular prophylaxis.

Fluconazole: Concomitant administration of fluconazole at 200 mg QD resulted in a two-fold increase in celecoxib plasma concentration. This increase is due to the inhibition of celecoxib metabolism via P450 2C9 by fluconazole (see Pharmacokinetics—Metabolism). CELEBREX should be introduced at the lowest recommended dose in patients receiving fluconazole.

Lithium: In a study conducted in healthy subjects, mean steady-state lithium plasma levels increased approximately 17% in subjects receiving lithium 450 mg BID with CELEBREX 200 mg BID as compared to subjects receiving lithium alone. Patients on lithium treatment should be closely monitored when CELEBREX is introduced or withdrawn.

Methotrexate: In an interaction study of rheumatoid arthritis patients taking methotrexate, CELEBREX did not have a significant effect on the pharmacokinetics of methotrexate.

Warfarin: Anticoagulant activity should be monitored, particularly in the first few days, after initiating or changing CELEBREX therapy in patients receiving warfarin or similar agents, since these patients are at an increased risk of bleeding complications. The effect of celecoxib on the anticoagulant effect of warfarin was studied in a group of healthy subjects receiving daily doses of 2 to 5 mg of warfarin. In these subjects, celecoxib did not alter the anticoagulant effect of warfarin as determined by prothrombin time. However, in post-marketing experience, bleeding events have been reported, predominantly in the elderly, in association with increases in prothrombin time in patients receiving CELEBREX concurrently with warfarin.

Carcinogenesis, mutagenesis, impairment of fertility: Celecoxib was not carcinogenic in rats given oral doses up to 200 mg/kg for males and 10 mg/kg for females (approximately 2- to 4-fold the human exposure as measured by the AUC_{0-24} at 200 mg BID) or in mice given oral doses up to 25 mg/kg for males and 50 mg/kg for females (approximately equal to human exposure as measured by the AUC_{0-24} at 200 mg BID) for two years.

Celecoxib was not mutagenic in an Ames test and a mutation assay in Chinese hamster ovary (CHO) cells, nor clastogenic in a chromosome aberration assay in CHO cells and an *in vivo* micronucleus test in rat bone marrow.

Celecoxib did not impair male and female fertility in rats at oral doses up to 600 mg/kg/day (approximately 11-fold human exposure at 200 mg BID based on the AUC_{0-24}).

Pregnancy

Teratogenic effects: Pregnancy Category C. Celecoxib was not teratogenic in rabbits up to an oral dose of 60 mg/kg/day (equal to human exposure at 200 mg BID as measured by AUC_{0-24}); however, at oral doses ≥150 mg/kg/day (approximately 2-fold human exposure at 200 mg BID as measured by AUC_{0-24}), an increased incidence of fetal alterations, such as ribs fused, sternebrae fused and sternebrae misshapen, was observed. A dose-dependent increase in diaphragmatic hernias was observed in one of two rat studies at oral doses ≥30 mg/kg/day (approximately 6-fold human exposure based on the AUC_{0-24} at 200 mg BID). There are no studies in pregnant women. CELEBREX should be used during pregnancy only if the potential benefit justifies the potential risk to the fetus.

Nonteratogenic effects: Celecoxib produced pre-implantation and post-implantation losses and reduced embryo/fetal survival in rats at oral dosages ≥50 mg/kg/day (approximately 6-fold human exposure based on the AUC_{0-24} at 200 mg BID). These changes are expected with inhibition of prostaglandin synthesis and are not the result of permanent alteration of female reproductive function, nor are they expected at clinical exposures. No studies have been conducted to evaluate the effect of celecoxib on the closure of the ductus arteriosus in humans. Therefore, use of CELEBREX during the third trimester of pregnancy should be avoided.

Labor and delivery: Celecoxib produced no evidence of delayed labor or parturition at oral doses up to 100 mg/kg in rats (approximately 7-fold human exposure as measured by the AUC_{0-24} at 200 mg BID). The effects of CELEBREX on labor and delivery in pregnant women are unknown.

Nursing mothers: Celecoxib is excreted in the milk of lactating rats at concentrations similar to those in plasma. It is not known whether this drug is excreted in human milk. Because many drugs are excreted in human milk and because of the potential for serious adverse reactions in nursing infants from CELEBREX, a decision should be made whether to discontinue nursing or to discontinue the drug, taking into account the importance of the drug to the mother.

Pediatric Use

Safety and effectiveness in pediatric patients below the age of 18 years have not been evaluated.

Geriatric Use
Of the total number of patients who received CELEBREX in clinical trials, more than 2,100 were 65–74 years of age, while approximately 800 additional patients were 75 years and over. While the incidence of adverse experiences tended to be higher in elderly patients, no substantial differences in safety and effectiveness were observed between these subjects and younger subjects. Other reported clinical experience has not identified differences in response between the elderly and younger patients, but greater sensitivity of some older individuals cannot be ruled out.
In clinical studies comparing renal function as measured by the GFR, BUN and creatinine, and platelet function as measured by bleeding time and platelet aggregation, the results were not different between elderly and young volunteers.

ADVERSE REACTIONS

Of the CELEBREX treated patients in controlled trials, approximately 4,250 were patients with OA, approximately 2,100 were patients with RA, and approximately 1,050 were patients with post-surgical pain. More than 8,500 patients have received a total daily dose of CELEBREX of 200 mg (100 mg BID or 200 mg QD) or more, including more than 400 treated at 800 mg (400 mg BID). Approximately 3,900 patients have received CELEBREX at these doses for 6 months or more; approximately 2,300 of these have received it for 1 year or more and 124 of these have received it for 2 years or more.
Adverse events from controlled trials: Table 4 lists all adverse events, regardless of causality, occurring in ≥2% of patients receiving CELEBREX from 12 controlled studies conducted in patients with OA or RA that included a placebo and/or a positive control group.
[See table above]

Table 4
Adverse Events Occurring in ≥2% of Celebrex Patients From Controlled Arthritis Trials

	Celebrex (100–200 mg BID or 200 mg QD) (N=4146)	Placebo (N=1864)	Naproxen 500 mg BID (N=1366)	Ibuprofen 800 mg TID (N=387)	Diclofenac 75 mg BID (N=345)
Gastrointestinal					
Abdominal pain	4.1%	2.8%	7.7%	9.0%	9.0%
Diarrhea	5.6%	3.8%	5.3%	9.3%	5.8%
Dyspepsia	8.8%	6.2%	12.2%	10.9%	12.8%
Flatulence	2.2%	1.0%	3.6%	4.1%	3.5%
Nausea	3.5%	4.2%	6.0%	3.4%	6.7%
Body as a whole					
Back pain	2.8%	3.6%	2.2%	2.6%	0.9%
Peripheral edema	2.1%	1.1%	2.1%	1.0%	3.5%
Injury-accidental	2.9%	2.3%	3.0%	2.6%	3.2%
Central and peripheral nervous system					
Dizziness	2.0%	1.7%	2.6%	1.3%	2.3%
Headache	15.8%	20.2%	14.5%	15.5%	15.4%
Psychiatric					
Insomnia	2.3%	2.3%	2.9%	1.3%	1.4%
Respiratory					
Pharyngitis	2.3%	1.1%	1.7%	1.6%	2.6%
Rhinitis	2.0%	1.3%	2.4%	2.3%	0.6%
Sinusitis	5.0%	4.3%	4.0%	5.4%	5.8%
Upper respiratory tract infection	8.1%	6.7%	9.9%	9.8%	9.9%
Skin					
Rash	2.2%	2.1%	2.1%	1.3%	1.2%

In placebo- or active-controlled clinical trials, the discontinuation rate due to adverse events was 7.1% for patients receiving CELEBREX and 6.1% for patients receiving placebo. Among the most common reasons for discontinuation due to adverse events in the CELEBREX treatment groups were dyspepsia and abdominal pain (cited as reasons for discontinuation in 0.8% and 0.7% of CELEBREX patients, respectively). Among patients receiving placebo, 0.6% discontinued due to dyspepsia and 0.6% withdrew due to abdominal pain.
The following adverse events occurred in 0.1–1.9% of patients regardless of causality.
Celebrex
(100–200 mg BID or 200 mg QD)
Gastrointestinal: Constipation, diverticulitis, dysphagia, eructation, esophagitis, gastritis, gastroenteritis, gastroesophageal reflux, hemorrhoids, hiatal hernia, melena, dry mouth, stomatitis, tenesmus, tooth disorder, vomiting
Cardiovascular: Aggravated hypertension, angina pectoris, coronary artery disorder, myocardial infarction
General: Allergy aggravated, allergic reaction, asthenia, chest pain, cyst NOS, edema generalized, face edema, fatigue, fever, hot flushes, influenza-like symptoms, pain, peripheral pain
Resistance mechanism disorders: Herpes simplex, herpes zoster, infection bacterial, infection fungal, infection soft tissue, infection viral, moniliasis, moniliasis genital, otitis media
Central, peripheral nervous system: Leg cramps, hypertonia, hypoesthesia, migraine, neuralgia, neuropathy, paresthesia, vertigo
Female reproductive: Breast fibroadenosis, breast neoplasm, breast pain, dysmenorrhea, menstrual disorder, vaginal hemorrhage, vaginitis
Male reproductive: Prostatic disorder
Hearing and vestibular: Deafness, ear abnormality, earache, tinnitus
Heart rate and rhythm: Palpitation, tachycardia
Liver and biliary system: Hepatic function abnormal, SGOT increased, SGPT increased
Metabolic and nutritional: BUN increased, CPK increased, diabetes mellitus, hypercholesterolemia, hyperglycemia, hypokalemia, NPN increase, creatinine increased, alkaline phosphatase increased, weight increase
Musculoskeletal: Arthralgia, arthrosis, bone disorder, fracture accidental, myalgia, neck stiffness, synovitis, tendinitis
Platelets (bleeding or clotting): Ecchymosis, epistaxis, thrombocythemia
Psychiatric: Anorexia, anxiety, appetite increased, depression, nervousness, somnolence
Hemic: Anemia
Respiratory: Bronchitis, bronchospasm, bronchospasm aggravated, coughing, dyspnea, laryngitis, pneumonia
Skin and appendages: Alopecia, dermatitis, nail disorder, photosensitivity reaction, pruritus, rash erythematous, rash maculopapular, skin disorder, skin dry, sweating increased, urticaria
Application site disorders: Cellulitis, dermatitis contact, injection site reaction, skin nodule
Special senses: Taste perversion
Urinary system: Albuminuria, cystitis, dysuria, hematuria, micturition frequency, renal calculus, urinary incontinence, urinary tract infection
Vision: Blurred vision, cataract, conjunctivitis, eye pain, glaucoma
Other serious adverse reactions which occur rarely (estimated <0.1%), regardless of causality: The following serious adverse events have occurred rarely in patients, taking CELEBREX. Cases reported only in the post-marketing experience are indicated in italics.
Cardiovascular: Syncope, congestive heart failure, ventricular fibrillation, pulmonary embolism, cerebrovascular accident, peripheral gangrene, thrombophlebitis, vasculitis
Gastrointestinal: Intestinal obstruction, intestinal perforation, gastrointestinal bleeding, colitis with bleeding, esophageal perforation, pancreatitis, cholelithiasis, ileus
Liver and biliary system: Cholelithiasis, *hepatitis, jaundice, liver failure*
Hemic and lymphatic: Thrombocytopenia *agranulocytosis, aplastic anemia, pancytopenia, leukopenia*
Metabolic: *Hypoglycemia*
Nervous system: Ataxia
Renal: Acute renal failure, *interstitial nephritis*
Skin: *Erythemia multiforme, exfoliative dermatitis, Stevens-Johnson syndrome, toxic epidermal necrolysis*
General: Sepsis, sudden death, *anaphylactoid reaction, angioedema.*
Adverse events from the controlled trial in familial adenomatous polyposis: The adverse event profile reported for the 83 patients with familial adenomatous polyposis enrolled in the randomized, controlled clinical trial was similar to that reported for patients in the arthritis controlled trials. Intestinal anastomotic ulceration was the only new adverse event reported in the FAP trial, regardless of causality, and was observed in 3 of 58 patients (one at 100 mg BID, and two at 400 mg BID) who had prior intestinal surgery.

OVERDOSAGE

Symptoms following acute NSAID overdoses are usually limited to lethargy, drowsiness, nausea, vomiting, and epigastric pain, which are generally reversible with supportive care. Gastrointestinal bleeding can occur. Hypertension, acute renal failure, respiratory depression and coma may occur, but are rare. Anaphylactoid reactions have been reported with therapeutic ingestion of NSAIDs, and may occur following an overdose.
Patients should be managed by symptomatic and supportive care following an NSAID overdose. There are no specific antidotes. No information is available regarding the removal of celecoxib by hemodialysis, but based on its high degree of plasma protein binding (>97%) dialysis is unlikely to be useful in overdose. Emesis and/or activated charcoal (60 to 100 g in adults, 1 to 2 g/kg in children) and/or osmotic cathartic may be indicated in patients seen within 4 hours of ingestion with symptoms or following a large overdose. Forced diuresis, alkalinization of urine, hemodialysis, or hemoperfusion may not be useful due to high protein binding.

DOSAGE AND ADMINISTRATION

For osteoarthritis and rheumatoid arthritis, the lowest dose of CELEBREX should be sought for each patient. These doses can be given witout regard to the timing of meals.
Osteoarthritis: For relief of the signs and symptoms of osteoarthritis the recommended oral dose is 200 mg per day administered as a single dose or as 100 mg twice per day.
Rheumatoid arthritis: For relief of the signs and symptoms of rheumatoid arthritis the recommended oral dose is 100 to 200 mg twice per day.
Familial adenomatous polyposis (FAP): Usual medical care for FAP patients should be continued while on CELEBREX. To reduce the number of adenomatous colorectal polyps in patients with FAP, the recommended oral dose is 400 mg (2 × 200 mg capsules) twice per day to be taken with food.
Hepatic Insufficiency: The daily recommended dose of CELEBREX capsules in patients with moderate hepatic impairment (Child-Pugh Class II) should be reduced by approximately 50% (see CLINICAL PHARMACOLOGY—Special populations).

HOW SUPPLIED

CELEBREX 100-mg capsules are white, reverse printed white on blue band of body and cap with markings of 7767 on the cap and 100 on the body, supplied as:

NDC Number	Size
0025-1520-31	bottle of 100
0025-1520-51	bottle of 500
0025-1520-34	carton of 100 unit dose

CELEBREX 200-mg capsules are white, with reverse printed white on gold band with markings of 7767 on the cap and 200 on the body, supplied as:

NDC Number	Size
0025-1525-31	bottle of 100
0025-1525-51	bottle of 500
0025-1525-34	carton of 100 unit dose

Store at 25°C (77°F); excursions permitted to 15–30°C (59–86°F). [See USP Controlled Room Temperature]
Rx only **A05264-5 • 12/23/99**
Mfd. for Searle Ltd.
Caguas PR 00725

Marketed by:
G.D. Searle & Co.
Chicago IL 60680 USA
Pfizer Inc.
New York NY 10017 USA

Address medical inquiries to:
G.D. Searle & Co.
Healthcare Information Services
5200 Old Orchard Rd.
Skokie IL 60077

Shown in Product Identification Guide, page 330

DIABINESE® ℞
[dī-ab 'in-ees]
(chlorpropamide)
Tablets, USP
For Oral Use

DESCRIPTION

DIABINESE® (chlorpropamide), is an oral blood-glucose-lowering drug of the sulfonylurea class. Chlorpropamide is 1-[(p-Chlorophenyl) sulfonyl]-3-propylurea, $C_{10}H_{13}ClN_2O_3S$, and has the structural formula:

$$Cl-C_6H_4-SO_2-NH-\overset{O}{\overset{\|}{C}}-NH-CH_2CH_2CH_3$$

Chlorpropamide is a white crystalline powder, that has a slight odor. It is practically insoluble in water at pH 7.3 (solubility at pH 6 is 2.2 mg/ml). It is soluble in alcohol and moderately soluble in chloroform. The molecular weight of chlorpropamide is 276.74. DIABINESE is available as 100 mg and 250 mg tablets.
Inert ingredients are: alginic acid; Blue 1 Lake; hydroxypropyl cellulose; magnesium stearate; precipitated calcium carbonate; sodium lauryl sulfate; starch.

CLINICAL PHARMACOLOGY

DIABINESE appears to lower the blood glucose acutely by stimulating the release of insulin from the pancreas, an effect dependent upon functioning beta cells in the pancreatic islets. The mechanism by which DIABINESE lowers blood glucose during long-term administration has not been

Continued on next page

Diabinese—Cont.

clearly established. Extra-pancreatic effects may play a part in the mechanism of action of oral sulfonylurea hypoglycemic drugs. While chlorpropamide is a sulfonamide derivative, it is devoid of antibacterial activity.
DIABINESE may also prove effective in controlling certain patients who have experienced primary or secondary failure to other sulfonylurea agents.
A method developed which permits easy measurement of the drug in blood is available on request.
Chlorpropamide does not interfere with the usual tests to detect albumin in the urine.
DIABINESE is absorbed rapidly from the gastrointestinal tract. Within one hour after a single oral dose, it is readily detectable in the blood, and the level reaches a maximum within two to four hours. It undergoes metabolism in humans and it is excreted in the urine as unchanged drug and as hydroxylated or hydrolyzed metabolites. The biological half-life of chlorpropamide averages about 36 hours. Within 96 hours, 80–90% of a single oral dose is excreted in the urine. However, long-term administration of therapeutic doses does not result in undue accumulation in the blood, since absorption and excretion rates become stabilized in about 5 to 7 days after the initiation of therapy.
DIABINESE exerts a hypoglycemic effect in normal humans within one hour, becoming maximal at 3 to 6 hours and persisting for at least 24 hours. The potency of chlorpropamide is approximately six times that of tolbutamide. Some experimental results suggest that its increased duration of action may be the result of slower excretion and absence of significant deactivation.

INDICATIONS AND USAGE

DIABINESE is indicated as an adjunct to diet to lower the blood glucose in patients with non-insulin-dependent diabetes mellitus (type II) whose hyperglycemia cannot be controlled by diet alone.
In initiating treatment for non-insulin-dependent diabetes, diet should be emphasized as the primary form of treatment. Caloric restriction and weight loss are essential in the obese diabetic patient. Proper dietary management alone may be effective in controlling the blood glucose and symptoms of hyperglycemia. The importance of regular physical activity should also be stressed, and cardiovascular risk factors should be identified and corrective measures taken where possible.
If this treatment program fails to reduce symptoms and/or blood glucose, the use of an oral sulfonylurea or insulin should be considered. Use of DIABINESE must be viewed by both the physician and patient as a treatment in addition to diet, and not as a substitute for diet or as a convenient mechanism for avoiding dietary restraint. Furthermore, loss of blood glucose control on diet alone may be transient, thus requiring only short-term administration of DIABINESE.
During maintenance programs, DIABINESE should be discontinued if satisfactory lowering of blood glucose is no longer achieved. Judgments should be based on regular clinical and laboratory evaluations.
In considering the use of DIABINESE in asymptomatic patients, it should be recognized that controlling the blood glucose in non-insulin-dependent diabetes, has not been definitely established to be effective in preventing the long-term cardiovascular or neural complications of diabetes.

CONTRAINDICATIONS

DIABINESE is contraindicated in patients with:

1. Known hypersensitivity to the drug.
2. Diabetic ketoacidosis, with or without coma. This condition should be treated with insulin.

WARNINGS

SPECIAL WARNING ON INCREASED RISK OF CARDIOVASCULAR MORTALITY

The administration of oral hypoglycemic drugs has been reported to be associated with increased cardiovascular mortality as compared to treatment with diet alone or diet plus insulin. This warning is based on the study conducted by the University Group Diabetes Program (UGDP), a long-term prospective clinical trial designed to evaluate the effectiveness of glucose-lowering drugs in preventing or delaying vascular complications in patients with non-insulin-dependent diabetes. The study involved 823 patients who were randomly assigned to one of four treatment groups (*Diabetes*, 19 (supp. 2): 747–830, 1970.)

UGDP reported that patients treated for 5 to 8 years with diet plus a fixed dose of tolbutamide (1.5 grams per day) had a rate of cardiovascular mortality approximately $2^1/_2$ times that of patients treated with diet alone. A significant increase in total mortality was not observed, but the use of tolbutamide was discontinued based on the increase in cardiovascular mortality, thus limiting the opportunity for the study to show an increase in over-all mortality. Despite controversy regarding the interpretation of these results, the findings of the UGDP study provide an adequate basis for this warning. The patient should be informed of the potential risks and advantages of DIABINESE and of alternative modes of therapy.

Although only one drug in the sulfonylurea class (tolbutamide) was included in this study, it is prudent from a safety standpoint to consider that this warning may also apply to other oral hypoglycemic drugs in this class, in view of their close similarities in mode of action and chemical structure.

Strength	Tablet Description	Tablet Code	NDC	Package Size
DIABINESE (chlorpropamide) 100 mg	Blue, D-shaped, scored	393	0663-3930-66	100's
			0069-3930-66	
			0663-3930-73	500's
			0069-3930-73	
			0663-3930-41	100 (10 × 10) unit dose
			0069-3930-41	
DIABINESE (chlorpropamide) 250 mg	Blue, D-shaped, scored	394	0663-3940-66	100's
			0069-3940-66	
			0663-3940-71	250's
			0069-3940-71	
			0663-3940-82	1000's
			0069-3940-82	
			0663-3940-41	100 (10 × 10) unit dose
			0069-3940-41	

PRECAUTIONS

General

Hypoglycemia: All sulfonylurea drugs are capable of producing severe hypoglycemia. Proper patient selection, dosage, and instructions are important to avoid hypoglycemic episodes. Renal or hepatic insufficiency may cause elevated blood levels of DIABINESE and the latter may also diminish gluconeogenic capacity, both of which increase the risk of serious hypoglycemic reactions. Elderly, debilitated or malnourished patients, and those with adrenal or pituitary insufficiency are particularly susceptible to the hypoglycemic action of glucose-lowering drugs. Hypoglycemia may be difficult to recognize in the elderly, and in people who are taking beta-adrenergic blocking drugs. Hypoglycemia is more likely to occur when caloric intake is deficient, after severe or prolonged exercise, when alcohol is ingested, or when more than one glucose-lowering drug is used.
Because of the long half-life of chlorpropamide, patients who become hypoglycemic during therapy require careful supervision of the dose and frequent feedings for at least 3 to 5 days. Hospitalization and intravenous glucose may be necessary.
Loss of control of blood glucose: When a patient stabilized on any diabetic regimen is exposed to stress such as fever, trauma, infection, or surgery, a loss of control may occur. At such times, it may be necessary to discontinue DIABINESE and administer insulin.
The effectiveness of any oral hypoglycemic drug, including DIABINESE, in lowering blood glucose to a desired level decreases in many patients over a period of time, which may be due to progression of the severity of the diabetes or to diminished responsiveness to the drug. This phenomenon is known as secondary failure, to distinguish it from primary failure in which the drug is ineffective in an individual patient when first given.

INFORMATION FOR PATIENTS

Patients should be informed of the potential risks and advantages of DIABINESE and of alternative modes of therapy. They should also be informed about the importance of adherence to dietary instructions, of a regular exercise program, and of regular testing of urine and/or blood glucose.
The risks of hypoglycemia, its symptoms and treatment, and conditions that predispose to its development should be explained to patients and responsible family members. Primary and secondary failure should also be explained.
Patients should be instructed to contact their physician promptly if they experience symptoms of hypoglycemia or other adverse reactions.

LABORATORY TESTS

Blood and urine glucose should be monitored periodically. Measurement of glycosylated hemoglobin may be useful.

DRUG INTERACTIONS

The hypoglycemic action of sulfonylurea may be potentiated by certain drugs including nonsteroidal anti-inflammatory agents and other drugs that are highly protein bound, salicylates, sulfonamides, chloramphenicol, probenecid, coumarins, monoamine oxidase inhibitors, and beta adrenergic blocking agents. When such drugs are administered to a patient receiving DIABINESE, the patient should be observed closely for hypoglycemia. When such drugs are withdrawn from a patient receiving DIABINESE, the patient should be observed closely for loss of control.
Certain drugs tend to produce hyperglycemia and may lead to loss of control. These drugs include the thiazides and other diuretics, corticosteroids, phenothiazines, thyroid products, estrogens, oral contraceptives, phenytoin, nicotinic acid, sympathomimetics, calcium channel blocking drugs, and isoniazid. When such drugs are administered to a patient receiving DIABINESE, the patient should be closely observed for loss of control. When such drugs are withdrawn from a patient receiving DIABINESE, the patient should be observed closely for hypoglycemia.
Since animal studies suggest that the action of barbiturates may be prolonged by therapy with chlorpropamide, barbiturates should be employed with caution. In some patients, a disulfiram-like reaction may be produced by the ingestion of alcohol.
A potential interaction between oral miconazole and oral hypoglycemic agents leading to severe hypoglycemia has been reported. Whether this interaction also occurs with the intravenous, topical, or vaginal preparations of miconazole is not known.
Carcinogenesis, Mutagenesis, Impairment of Fertility: Chronic toxicity studies have been carried out in dogs and rats. Dogs treated for 6, 13, or 20 months with doses of DIABINESE greater than 20 times the human dose, have not shown any gross histological or pathological abnormalities. After treatment with 100 mg/kg of DIABINESE for 20 months, a dog showed no histopathological liver changes.
Rats treated with continuous DIABINESE therapy for 6 to 12 months showed varying degrees of suppression of spermatogenesis at higher dosage levels (up to 125 mg/kg). The extent of suppression seemed to follow that of growth retardation associated with chronic administration of high-dose DIABINESE in rats.

Pregnancy

Teratogenic Effects:
Pregnancy Category C. Animal reproductive studies have not been conducted with DIABINESE. It is also not known whether DIABINESE can cause fetal harm when administered to a pregnant woman or can affect reproduction capacity. DIABINESE should be given to a pregnant woman only if clearly needed.
Because recent information suggests that abnormal blood glucose levels during pregnancy are associated with a higher incidence of congenital abnormalities, many experts recommend that insulin be used during pregnancy to maintain blood glucose levels as close to normal as possible.
Nonteratogenic Effects:
Prolonged severe hypoglycemia (4 to 10 days) has been reported in neonates born to mothers who were receiving a sulfonylurea drug at the time of delivery. This has been reported more frequently with the use of agents with prolonged half-lives. If DIABINESE is used during pregnancy, it should be discontinued at least one month before the expected delivery date.
Nursing Mothers: An analysis of a composite of two samples of human breast milk, each taken five hours after ingestion of 500 mg of chlorpropamide by a patient, revealed a concentration of 5 mcg/ml. For reference, the normal peak blood level of chlorpropamide after a single 250 mg dose is 30 mcg/ml. Therefore, it is not recommended that a woman breast feed while taking this medication.
Use in Children: Safety and effectiveness in children have not been established.

ADVERSE REACTIONS

Hypoglycemia: See PRECAUTIONS and OVERDOSAGE sections.
Gastrointestinal Reactions: Cholestatic jaundice may occur rarely; DIABINESE should be discontinued if this occurs. Gastrointestinal disturbances are the most common reactions; nausea has been reported in less than 5% of patients, and diarrhea, vomiting, anorexia, and hunger in less than 2%. Other gastrointestinal disturbances have occurred in less than 1% of patients including proctocolitis. They tend to be dose related and may disappear when dosage is reduced.
Dermatologic Reactions: Pruritus has been reported in less than 3% of patients. Other allergic skin reactions, e.g., urticaria and maculopapular eruptions have been reported in approximately 1% or less of patients. These may be transient and may disappear despite continued use of DIABINESE; if skin reactions persist the drug should be discontinued.
Porphyria cutanea tarda and photosensitivity reactions have been reported with sulfonylureas.
Skin eruptions rarely progressing to erythema multiforme and exfoliative dermatitis have also been reported.
Hematologic Reactions: Leukopenia, agranulocytosis, thrombocytopenia, hemolytic anemia, aplastic anemia, pancytopenia, and eosinophilia have been reported with sulfonylureas.
Metabolic Reactions: Hepatic porphyria and disulfiram-like reactions have been reported with DIABINESE. See DRUG INTERACTIONS section.
Endocrine Reactions: On rare occasions, chlorpropamide has caused a reaction identical to the syndrome of inappropriate antidiuretic hormone (ADH) secretion. The features of this syndrome result from excessive water retention and include hyponatremia, low serum osmolality, and high urine osmolality. This reaction has also been reported for other sulfonylureas.

OVERDOSAGE

Overdosage of sulfonylureas including DIABINESE can produce hypoglycemia. Mild hypoglycemic symptoms without loss of consciousness or neurologic findings should be treated aggressively with oral glucose and adjustments in drug dosage and/or meal patterns. Close monitoring should continue until the physician is assured that the patient is out of danger. Severe hypoglycemic reactions with coma, seizure, or other neurological impairment occur infrequently, but constitute medical emergencies requiring immediate hospitalization. If hypoglycemic coma is diagnosed or suspected, the patient should be given a rapid intravenous injection of concentrated (50%) glucose solution. This should be followed by a continuous infusion of a more dilute (10%) glucose solution at a rate that will maintain the blood glucose at a level above 100 mg/dL. Patients should be closely monitored for a minimum of 24 to 48 hours since hypoglycemia may recur after apparent clinical recovery.

DOSAGE AND ADMINISTRATION

There is no fixed dosage regimen for the management of diabetes mellitus with DIABINESE or any other hypoglycemic agent. In addition to the usual monitoring of urinary glucose, the patient's blood glucose must also be monitored periodically to determine the minimum effective dose for the patient; to detect primary failure, i.e., inadequate lowering of blood glucose at the maximum recommended dose of medication; and to detect secondary failure, i.e., loss of an adequate blood glucose lowering response after an initial period of effectiveness. Glycosylated hemoglobin levels may also be of value in monitoring the patient's response to therapy.
Short-term administration of DIABINESE may be sufficient during periods of transient loss of control in patients usually controlled well on diet.
The total daily dosage is generally taken at a single time each morning with breakfast. Occasionally cases of gastrointestinal intolerance may be relieved by dividing the daily dosage. A LOADING OR PRIMING DOSE IS NOT NECESSARY AND SHOULD NOT BE USED.

Initial Therapy: 1. The mild to moderately severe, middle-aged, stable, non-insulin-dependent diabetic patient should be started on 250 mg daily. In elderly patients, debilitated or malnourished patients, and patients with impaired renal or hepatic function, the initial and maintenance dosing should be conservative to avoid hypoglycemic reactions (see PRECAUTIONS section). Older patients should be started on smaller amounts of DIABINESE, in the range of 100 to 125 mg daily.
2. No transition period is necessary when transferring patients from other oral hypoglycemic agents to DIABINESE. The other agent may be discontinued abruptly and chlorpropamide started at once. In prescribing chlorpropamide, due consideration must be given to its greater potency.
Many mild to moderately severe, middle-aged, stable non-insulin-dependent diabetic patients receiving insulin can be placed directly on the oral drug and their insulin abruptly discontinued. For patients requiring more than 40 units of insulin daily, therapy with DIABINESE may be initiated with a 50 per cent reduction in insulin for the first few days, with subsequent further reductions dependent upon the response.
During the initial period of therapy with chlorpropamide, hypoglycemic reactions may occasionally occur, particularly during the transition from insulin to the oral drug. Hypoglycemia within 24 hours after withdrawal of the intermediate or long-acting types of insulin will usually prove to be the result of insulin carry-over and not primarily due to the effect of chlorpropamide.
During the insulin withdrawal period, the patient should test his urine for sugar and ketone bodies at least three times daily and report the results frequently to his physician. If they are abnormal, the physician should be notified immediately. In some cases, it may be advisable to consider hospitalization during the transition period.
Five to seven days after the initial therapy, the blood level of chlorpropamide reaches a plateau. Dosage may subsequently be adjusted upward or downward by increments of not more than 50 to 125 mg at intervals of three to five days to obtain optimal control. More frequent adjustments are usually undesirable.

Maintenance Therapy: Most moderately severe, middle-aged, stable non-insulin-dependent diabetic patients are controlled by approximately 250 mg daily. Many investigators have found that some milder diabetics do well on daily doses of 100 mg or less. Many of the more severe diabetics may require 500 mg daily for adequate control. PATIENTS WHO DO NOT RESPOND COMPLETELY TO 500 MG DAILY WILL USUALLY NOT RESPOND TO HIGHER DOSES. MAINTENANCE DOSES ABOVE 750 mg DAILY SHOULD BE AVOIDED.

HOW SUPPLIED

[See table at top of previous page]

RECOMMENDED STORAGE

Store below 86°F (30°C).

CAUTION

Federal law prohibits dispensing without prescription.
69-2141-00-1 Revised April 1995

DIFLUCAN® ℞
(fluconazole tablets)
(fluconazole injection-
for intravenous infusion only)
(fluconazole for oral suspension)

DESCRIPTION

DIFLUCAN® (fluconazole), the first of a new subclass of synthetic triazole antifungal agents, is available as tablets for oral administration, as a powder for oral suspension and as a sterile solution for intravenous use in glass and in Viaflex® Plus plastic containers.
Fluconazole is designated chemically as 2,4-difluoro-α,α[1]-bis(1H-1,2,4-triazol-l-ylmethyl) benzyl alcohol with an empirical formula of $C_{13}H_{12}F_2N_6O$ and molecular weight 306.3. The structural formula is:

Fluconazole is a white crystalline solid which is slightly soluble in water and saline.
DIFLUCAN tablets contain 50, 100, 150, or 200 mg of fluconazole and the following inactive ingredients: microcrystalline cellulose, dibasic calcium phosphate anhydrous, povidone, croscarmellose sodium, FD&C Red No. 40 aluminum lake dye, and magnesium stearate.
DIFLUCAN for oral suspension contains 350 mg or 1400 mg of fluconazole and the following inactive ingredients: sucrose, sodium citrate dihydrate, citric acid anhydrous, sodium benzoate, titanium dioxide, colloidal silicon dioxide, xanthan gum and natural orange flavor. After reconstitution with 24 mL of distilled water or Purified Water (USP), each mL of reconstituted suspension contains 10 mg or 40 mg of fluconazole.
DIFLUCAN injection is an iso-osmotic, sterile, nonpyrogenic solution of fluconazole in a sodium chloride or dextrose diluent. Each mL contains 2 mg of fluconazole and 9 mg of sodium chloride or 56 mg of dextrose, hydrous. The pH ranges from 4.0 to 8.0 in the sodium chloride diluent and from 3.5 to 6.5 in the dextrose diluent. Injection volumes of 100 mL and 200 mL are packaged in glass and in Viaflex® Plus plastic containers.
The Viaflex® Plus plastic container is fabricated from a specially formulated polyvinyl chloride (PL 146® Plastic) (Viaflex and PL 146 are registered trademarks of Baxter International, Inc.). The amount of water that can permeate from inside the container into the overwrap is insufficient to affect the solution significantly. Solutions in contact with the plastic container can leach out certain of its chemical components in very small amounts within the expiration period, e.g., di-2-ethylhexylphthalate (DEHP), up to 5 parts per million. However, the suitability of the plastic has been confirmed in tests in animals according to USP biological tests for plastic containers as well as by tissue culture toxicity studies.

CLINICAL PHARMACOLOGY

Mode of Action

Fluconazole is a highly selective inhibitor of fungal cytochrome P-450 sterol C-14 alpha-demethylation. Mammalian cell demethylation is much less sensitive to fluconazole inhibition. The subsequent loss of normal sterols correlates with the accumulation of 14 alpha-methyl sterols in fungi and may be responsible for the fungistatic activity of fluconazole.

Pharmacokinetics and Metabolism

The pharmacokinetic properties of fluconazole are similar following administration by the intravenous or oral routes.
In normal volunteers, the bioavailability of orally administered fluconazole is over 90% compared with intravenous administration. Bioequivalence was established between the 100 mg tablet and both suspension strengths when administered as a single 200 mg dose.
Peak plasma concentrations (Cmax) in fasted normal volunteers occur between 1 and 2 hours with a terminal plasma elimination half-life of approximately 30 hours (range: 20–50 hours) after oral administration.
In fasted normal volunteers, administration of a single oral 400 mg dose of DIFLUCAN (fluconazole) leads to a mean Cmax of 6.72 μg/mL (range: 4.12 to 8.08 μg/mL) and after single oral doses of 50–400 mg, fluconazole plasma concentrations and AUC (area under the plasma concentration-time curve) are dose proportional.
Administration of a single oral 150 mg tablet of DIFLUCAN (fluconazole) to ten lactating women resulted in a mean Cmax of 2.61 μg/mL (range: 1.57 to 3.65 μg/mL).
Steady-state concentrations are reached within 5–10 days following oral doses of 50–400 mg given once daily. Administration of a loading dose (on day 1) of twice the usual daily dose results in plasma concentrations close to steady-state by the second day. The apparent volume of distribution of fluconazole approximates that of total body water. Plasma protein binding is low (11–12%). Following either single- or multiple-oral doses for up to 14 days, fluconazole penetrates into all body fluids studied (see table below). In normal volunteers, saliva concentrations of fluconazole were equal to or slightly greater than plasma concentrations regardless of dose, route, or duration of dosing. In patients with bronchiectasis, sputum concentrations of fluconazole following a single 150 mg oral dose were equal to plasma concentrations at both 4 and 24 hours post dose. In patients with fungal meningitis, fluconazole concentrations in the CSF are approximately 80% of the corresponding plasma concentrations.
A single oral 150 mg dose of fluconazole administered to 27 patients penetrated into vaginal tissue, resulting in tissue: plasma ratios ranging from 0.94 to 1.14 over the first 48 hours following dosing.
A single oral 150 mg dose of fluconazole administered to 14 patients penetrated into vaginal fluid, resulting in fluid: plasma ratios ranging from 0.36 to 0.71 over the first 72 hours following dosing.

Tissue or Fluid	Ratio of Fluconazole Tissue (Fluid)/Plasma Concentration*
Cerebrospinal fluid†	0.5–0.9
Saliva	1
Sputum	1
Blister fluid	1
Urine	10
Normal skin	10
Nails	1
Blister skin	2
Vaginal tissue	1
Vaginal fluid	0.4–0.7

*Relative to concurrent concentrations in plasma in subjects with normal renal function.
†Independent of degree of meningeal inflammation.

In normal volunteers, fluconazole is cleared primarily by renal excretion, with approximately 80% of the administered dose appearing in the urine as unchanged drug. About 11% of the dose is excreted in the urine as metabolites.
The pharmacokinetics of fluconazole are markedly affected by reduction in renal function. There is an inverse relationship between the elimination half-life and creatinine clearance. The dose of DIFLUCAN may need to be reduced in patients with impaired renal function. (See **DOSAGE AND ADMINISTRATION**.) A 3-hour hemodialysis session decreases plasma concentrations by approximately 50%.
In normal volunteers, DIFLUCAN administration (doses ranging from 200 mg to 400 mg once daily for up to 14 days) was associated with small and inconsistent effects on testosterone concentrations, endogenous corticosteroid concentrations, and the ACTH-simulated cortisol response.

Pharmacokinetics in Children

In children, the following pharmacokinetic data {Mean(%cv)} have been reported:
[See table above]

Age Studied	Dose (mg/kg)	Clearance (mL/min/kg)	Half-life (Hours)	Cmax (μg/mL)	Vdss (L/kg)
9 Months-13 years	Single-Oral 2 mg/kg	0.40 (38%) N=14	25.0	2.9 (22%) N=16	—
9 Months-13 years	Single-Oral 8 mg/kg	0.51 (60%) N=15	19.5	9.8 (20%) N=15	—
5–15 years	Multiple IV 2 mg/kg	0.49 (40%) N=4	17.4	5.5 (25%) N=5	0.722 (36%) N=4
5–15 years	Multiple IV 4 mg/kg	0.59 (64%) N=5	15.2	11.4 (44%) N=6	0.729 (33%) N=5
5–15 years	Multiple IV 8 mg/kg	0.66 (31%) N=7	17.6	14.1 (22%) N=8	1.069 (37%) N=7

Clearance corrected for body weight was not affected by age in these studies. Mean body clearance in adults is reported to be 0.23 (17%) mL/min/kg.
In premature newborns (gestational age 26 to 29 weeks), the mean (%cv) clearance within 36 hours of birth was 0.180 (35%, N=7) mL/min/kg, which increased with time to a mean of 0.218 (31%, N=9) mL/min/kg six days later and 0.333 (56%, N=4) mL/min/kg 12 days later. Similarly, the half-life was 73.6 hours, which decreased with time to a mean of 53.2 hours six days later and 46.6 hours 12 days later.

Drug Interaction Studies

Oral contraceptives: Oral contraceptives were administered as a single dose both before and after the oral administration of DIFLUCAN 50 mg once daily for 10 days in 10 healthy women. There was no significant difference in ethinyl estradiol or levonorgestrel AUC after the administration of 50 mg of DIFLUCAN. The mean increase in ethinyl estradiol AUC was 6% (range: –47 to 108%) and levonorgestrel AUC increased 17% (range: –33 to 141%).

Continued on next page

Diflucan—Cont.

In a second study, twenty-five normal females received daily doses of both 200 mg DIFLUCAN tablets or placebo for two, ten-day periods. The treatment cycles were one month apart with all subjects receiving DIFLUCAN during one cycle and placebo during the other. The order of study treatment was random. Single doses of an oral contraceptive tablet containing levonorgestrel and ethinyl estradiol were administered on the final treatment day (day 10) of both cycles. Following administration of 200 mg of DIFLUCAN, the mean percentage increase of AUC for levonorgestrel compared to placebo was 25% (range: -12 to 82%) and the mean percentage increase for ethinyl estradiol compared to placebo was 38% (range: -11 to 101%). Both of these increases were statistically significantly different from placebo.

Cimetidine: DIFLUCAN 100 mg was administered as a single oral dose alone and two hours after a single dose of cimetidine 400 mg to six healthy male volunteers. After the administration of cimetidine, there was a significant decrease in fluconazole AUC and Cmax. There was a mean ±SD decrease in fluconazole AUC of 13% ± 11% (range: –3.4 to –31%) and Cmax decreased 19% ± 14% (range: –5 to –40%). However, the administration of cimetidine 600 mg to 900 mg intravenously over a four-hour period (from one hour before to 3 hours after a single oral dose of DIFLUCAN 200 mg) did not affect the bioavailability or pharmacokinetics of fluconazole in 24 healthy male volunteers.

Antacid: Administration of Maalox® (20 mL) to 14 normal male volunteers immediately prior to a single dose of DIFLUCAN 100 mg had no effect on the absorption or elimination of fluconazole.

Hydrochlorothiazide: Concomitant oral administration of 100 mg DIFLUCAN and 50 mg hydrochlorothiazide for 10 days in 13 normal volunteers resulted in a significant increase in fluconazole AUC and Cmax compared to DIFLUCAN given alone. There was a mean ± SD increase in fluconazole AUC and Cmax of 45% ± 31% (range: 19 to 114%) and 43% ± 31% (range: 19 to 122%), respectively. These changes are attributable to a mean ± SD reduction in renal clearance of 30% ± 12% (range: –10 to –50%).

Rifampin: Administration of a single oral 200 mg dose of DIFLUCAN after 15 days of rifampin administered as 600 mg daily in eight healthy male volunteers resulted in a significant decrease in fluconazole AUC and a significant increase in apparent oral clearance of fluconazole. There was a mean ± SD reduction in fluconazole AUC of 23% ± 9% (range: –13 to –42%). Apparent oral clearance of fluconazole increased 32% ± 17% (range: 16 to 72%). Fluconazole half-life decreased from 33.4 ± 4.4 hours to 26.8 ± 3.9 hours. (See **PRECAUTIONS**.)

Warfarin: There was a significant increase in prothrombin time response (area under the prothrombin time-time curve) following a single dose of warfarin (15 mg) administered to 13 normal male volunteers following oral DIFLUCAN 200 mg administered daily for 14 days as compared to the administration of warfarin alone. There was a mean ± SD increase in the prothrombin time response (area under the prothrombin time-time curve) of 7% ± 4% (range: –2 to 13%). (See **PRECAUTIONS**.) Mean is based on data from 12 subjects as one of 13 subjects experienced a 2-fold increase in his prothrombin time response.

Phenytoin: Phenytoin AUC was determined after 4 days of phenytoin dosing (200 mg daily, orally for 3 days followed by 250 mg intravenously for one dose) both with and without the administration of fluconazole (oral DIFLUCAN 200 mg daily for 16 days) in 10 normal male volunteers. There was a significant increase in phenytoin AUC. The mean ± SD increase in phenytoin AUC was 88% ± 68% (range: 16 to 247%). The absolute magnitude of this interaction is unknown because of the intrinsically nonlinear disposition of phenytoin. (See **PRECAUTIONS**.)

Cyclosporine: Cyclosporine AUC and Cmax were determined before and after the administration of fluconazole 200 mg daily for 14 days in eight renal transplant patients who had been on cyclosporine therapy for at least 6 months and on a stable cyclosporine dose for at least 6 weeks. There was a significant increase in cyclosporine AUC, Cmax, Cmin (24-hour concentration), and a significant reduction in apparent oral clearance following the administration of fluconazole. The mean ± SD increase in AUC was 92% ± 43% (range: 18 to 147%). The Cmax increased 60% ± 48% (range: –5 to 133%). The Cmin increased 157% ± 96% (range: 33 to 360%). The apparent oral clearance decreased 45% ± 15% (range: –15 to –60%). (See **PRECAUTIONS**.)

Zidovudine: Plasma zidovudine concentrations were determined on two occasions (before and following fluconazole 200 mg daily for 15 days) in 13 volunteers with AIDS or ARC who were on a stable zidovudine dose for at least two weeks. There was a significant increase in zidovudine AUC following the administration of fluconazole. The mean ± SD increase in AUC was 20% ± 32% (range: –27 to 104%). The metabolite, GZDV, to parent drug ratio significantly decreased after the administration of fluconazole, from 7.6 ± 3.6 to 5.7 ± 2.2.

Theophylline: The pharmacokinetics of theophylline were determined from a single intravenous dose of aminophylline (6 mg/kg) before and after the oral administration of fluconazole 200 mg daily for 14 days in 16 normal male volunteers. There were significant increases in theophylline AUC, Cmax, and half-life with a corresponding decrease in clearance. The mean ± SD theophylline AUC increased 21% ± 16% (range: –5 to 48%). The Cmax increased 13% ± 17% (range: –13 to 40%). Theophylline clearance decreased 16% ± 11% (range: –32 to 5%). The half-life of theophylline increased from 6.6 ± 1.7 hours to 7.9 ± 1.5 hours. (See **PRECAUTIONS**.)

Terfenadine: Six healthy volunteers received terfenadine 60 mg BID for 15 days. Fluconazole 200 mg was administered daily from days 9 through 15. Fluconazole did not affect terfenadine plasma concentrations. Terfenadine acid metabolite AUC increased 36% ± 36% (range: 7 to 102%) from day 8 to day 15 with the concomitant administration of fluconazole. There was no change in cardiac repolarization as measured by Holter QTc intervals. Another study at a 400-mg and 800-mg daily dose of fluconazole demonstrated that DIFLUCAN taken in doses of 400 mg per day or greater significantly increases plasma levels of terfenadine when taken concomitantly. (See **CONTRAINDICATIONS** and **PRECAUTIONS**.)

Oral hypoglycemics: The effects of fluconazole on the pharmacokinetics of the sulfonylurea oral hypoglycemic agents tolbutamide, glipizide, and glyburide were evaluated in three placebo-controlled studies in normal volunteers. All subjects received the sulfonylurea alone as a single dose and again as a single dose following the administration of DIFLUCAN 100 mg daily for 7 days. In these three studies 22/46 (47.8%) of DIFLUCAN treated patients and 9/22 (40.1%) of placebo treated patients experienced symptoms consistent with hypoglycemia. (See **PRECAUTIONS**.)

Tolbutamide: In 13 normal male volunteers, there was significant increase in tolbutamide (500 mg single dose) AUC and Cmax following the administration of fluconazole. There was a mean ± SD increase in tolbutamide AUC of 26% ± 9% (range: 12 to 39%). Tolbutamide Cmax increased 11% ± 9% (range: –6 to 27%). (See **PRECAUTIONS**.)

Glipizide: The AUC and Cmax of glipizide (2.5 mg single dose) were significantly increased following the administration of fluconazole in 13 normal male volunteers. There was a mean ± SD increase in AUC of 49% ± 13% (range: 27 to 73%) and an increase in Cmax of 19% ± 23% (range: –11 to 79%). (See **PRECAUTIONS**.)

Glyburide: The AUC and Cmax of glyburide (5 mg single dose) were significantly increased following the administration of fluconazole in 20 normal male volunteers. There was a mean ± SD increase in AUC of 44% ± 29% (range: –13 to 115%) and Cmax increased 19% ± 19% (range: –23 to 62%). Five subjects required oral glucose following the ingestion of glyburide after 7 days of fluconazole administration. (See **PRECAUTIONS**.)

Rifabutin: There have been published reports that an interaction exists when fluconazole is administered concomitantly with rifabutin, leading to increased serum levels of rifabutin. (See **PRECAUTIONS**.)

Tacrolimus: There have been published reports that an interaction exists when fluconazole is administered concomitantly with tacrolimus, leading to increased serum levels of tacrolimus. (See **PRECAUTIONS**.)

Cisapride: A preliminary report from a placebo-controlled, randomized multiple-dose study in subjects given fluconazole 200 mg daily and cisapride 20 mg four times daily starting after 7 days of fluconazole dosing found that fluconazole significantly increased the AUC and Cmax of cisapride both after single (AUC 102% and Cmax 92% increases) and multiple (AUC 192% and Cmax 153% increases) dosing of cisapride. Fluconazole significantly increased the QTc interval in subjects receiving cisapride 20 mg four times for 5 days. (See **CONTRAINDICATIONS** and **PRECAUTIONS**.)

Microbiology

Fluconazole exhibits *in vitro* activity against *Cryptococcus neoformans* and *Candida* spp. Fungistatic activity has also been demonstrated in normal and immunocompromised animal models for systemic and intracranial fungal infections due to *Cryptococcus neoformans* and for systemic infections due to *Candida albicans*.

In common with other azole antifungal agents, most fungi show a higher apparent sensitivity to fluconazole *in vivo* than *in vitro*. Fluconazole administered orally and/or intravenously was active in a variety of animal models of fungal infection using standard laboratory strains of fungi. Activity has been demonstrated against fungal infections caused by *Aspergillus flavus* and *Aspergillus fumigatus* in normal mice. Fluconazole has also been shown to be active in animal models of endemic mycoses, including one model of *Blastomyces dermatitidis* pulmonary infections in normal mice; one model of *Coccidioides immitis* intracranial infections in normal mice; and several models of *Histoplasma capsulatum* pulmonary infection in normal and immunosuppressed mice. The clinical significance of results obtained in these studies is unknown.

Oral fluconazole has been shown to be active in an animal model of vaginal candidiasis.

Concurrent administration of fluconazole and amphotericin B in infected normal and immunosuppressed mice showed the following results: a small additive antifungal effect in systemic infection with *C. albicans*, no interaction in intracranial infection with *Cr. neoformans*, and antagonism of the two drugs in systemic infection with *Asp. fumigatus*. The clinical significance of results obtained in these studies is unknown.

There have been reports of cases of superinfection with *Candida* species other than *C. albicans*, which are often inherently not susceptible to DIFLUCAN (e.g., *Candida krusei*). Such cases may require alternative antifungal therapy.

INDICATIONS AND USAGE

DIFLUCAN (fluconazole) is indicated for the treatment of:

1. Vaginal candidiasis (vaginal yeast infections due to *Candida*).
2. Oropharyngeal and esophageal candidiasis. In open noncomparative studies of relatively small numbers of patients, DIFLUCAN was also effective for the treatment of *Candida* urinary tract infections, peritonitis, and systemic *Candida* infections including candidemia, disseminated candidiasis, and pneumonia.
3. Cryptococcal meningitis. Before prescribing DIFLUCAN (fluconazole) for AIDS patients with cryptococcal meningitis, please see **CLINICAL STUDIES** section. Studies comparing DIFLUCAN to amphotericin B in non-HIV infected patients have not been conducted.

Prophylaxis. DIFLUCAN is also indicated to decrease the incidence of candidiasis in patients undergoing bone marrow transplantation who receive cytotoxic chemotherapy and/or radiation therapy.

Specimens for fungal culture and other relevant laboratory studies (serology, histopathology) should be obtained prior to therapy to isolate and identify causative organisms. Therapy may be instituted before the results of the cultures and other laboratory studies are known; however, once these results become available, anti-infective therapy should be adjusted accordingly.

CLINICAL STUDIES

Cryptococcal meningitis: In a multicenter study comparing DIFLUCAN (200 mg/day) to amphotericin B (0.3 mg/kg/day) for treatment of cryptococcal meningitis in patients with AIDS, a multivariate analysis revealed three pretreatment factors that predicted death during the course of therapy: abnormal mental status, cerebrospinal fluid cryptococcal antigen titer greater than 1:1024, and cerebrospinal fluid white blood cell count of less than 20 cells/mm^3. Mortality among high risk patients was 33% and 40% for amphotericin B and DIFLUCAN patients, respectively (p=0.58), with overall deaths 14% (9 of 63 subjects) and 18% (24 of 131 subjects) for the 2 arms of study (p=0.48). Optimal doses and regimens for patients with acute cryptococcal meningitis and at high risk for treatment failure remain to be determined. (Saag, *et al*. N Engl J Med 1992; 326:83-9.)

Vaginal candidiasis: Two adequate and well-controlled studies were conducted in the U.S. using the 150 mg tablet. In both, the results of the fluconazole regimen were comparable to the control regimen (clotrimazole or miconazole intravaginally for 7 days) both clinically and statistically at the one month post-treamtent evaluation.

The therapeutic cure rate, defined as a complete resolution of signs and symptoms of vaginal candidiasis (clinical cure), along with a negative KOH examination and negative culture for *Candida* (microbiologic eradication), was 55% in both the fluconazole group and the vaginal products group. [See first table above]

	Fluconazole PO 150 mg tablet	Vaginal Product qhs × 7 days
Enrolled	448	422
Evaluable at Late Follow-Up	347 (77%)	327 (77%)
Clinical cure	239/347 (69%)	235/327 (72%)
Mycologic erad.	213/347 (61%)	196/327 (60%)
Therapeutic cure	190/347 (55%)	179/327 (55%)

Parameter	Fluconazole PO	Vaginal Products
Evaluable patients	448	422
With any adverse event	141 (31%)	112 (27%)
Nervous System	90 (20%)	69 (16%)
Gastrointestinal	73 (16%)	18 (4%)
With drug-related event	117 (26%)	67 (16%)
Nervous System	61 (14%)	29 (7%)
Headache	58 (13%)	28 (7%)
Gastrointestinal	68 (15%)	13 (3%)
Abdominal pain	25 (6%)	7 (2%)
Nausea	30 (7%)	3 (1%)
Diarrhea	12 (3%)	2 (<1%)
Application site event	0 (0%)	19 (5%)
Taste Perversion	6 (1%)	0 (0%)

Approximately three-fourths of the enrolled patients had acute vaginitis (<4 episodes/12 months) and achieved 80% clinical cure, 67% mycologic eradication and 59% therapeu-

tic cure when treated with a 150 mg DIFLUCAN tablet administered orally. These rates were comparable to control products. The remaining one-fourth of enrolled patients had recurrent vaginitis (≥4 episodes/12 months) and achieved 57% clinical cure, 47% mycologic eradication and 40% therapeutic cure. The numbers are too small to make meaningful clinical or statistical comparisons with vaginal products in the treatment of patients with recurrent vaginitis.
Substantially more gastrointestinal events were reported in the fluconazole group compared to the vaginal product group. Most of the events were mild to moderate. Because fluconazole was given as a single dose, no discontinuations occurred.
[See second table at top of previous page]

Pediatric Studies

Oropharyngeal candidiasis: An open-label, comparative study of the efficacy and safety of DIFLUCAN (2–3 mg/kg/day) and oral nystatin (400,000 I.U. 4 times daily) in immunocompromised children with oropharyngeal candidiasis was conducted. Clinical and mycological response rates were higher in the children treated with fluconazole.
Clinical cure at the end of treatment was reported for 86% of fluconazole treated patients compared to 46% of nystatin treated patients. Mycologically, 76% of fluconazole treated patients had the infecting organism eradicated compared to 11% for nystatin treated patients.
[See table above]

	Fluconazole	Nystatin
Enrolled	96	90
Clinical Cure	76/88 (86%)	36/78 (46%)
Mycological eradication*	55/72 (76%)	6/54 (11%)

*Subjects without follow-up cultures for any reason were considered nonevaluable for mycological response.

The proportion of patients with clinical relapse 2 weeks after the end of treatment was 14% for subjects receiving DIFLUCAN and 16% for subjects receiving nystatin. At 4 weeks after the end of treatment the percentages of patients with clinical relapse were 22% for DIFLUCAN and 23% for nystatin.

CONTRAINDICATIONS

DIFLUCAN (fluconazole) is contraindicated in patients who have shown hypersensitivity to fluconazole or to any of its excipients. There is no information regarding cross-hypersensitivity between fluconazole and other azole antifungal agents. Caution should be used in prescribing DIFLUCAN to patients with hypersensitivity to other azoles. Coadministration of terfenadine is contraindicated in patients receiving DIFLUCAN (fluconazole) at multiple doses of 400 mg or higher based upon results of a multiple dose interaction study. Coadministration of cisapride is contraindicated in patients receiving DIFLUCAN (fluconazole). (See **CLINICAL PHARMACOLOGY: Drug Interaction Studies** and **PRECAUTIONS.**)

WARNINGS

(1) Hepatic injury: DIFLUCAN has been associated with rare cases of serious hepatic toxicity, including fatalities primarily in patients with serious underlying medical conditions. In cases of DIFLUCAN-associated hepatotoxicity, no obvious relationship to total daily dose, duration of therapy, sex or age of the patient has been observed.
DIFLUCAN hepatotoxicity has usually, but not always, been reversible on discontinuation of therapy. Patients who develop abnormal liver function tests during DIFLUCAN therapy should be monitored for the development of more severe hepatic injury. DIFLUCAN should be discontinued if clinical signs and symptoms consistent with liver disease develop that may be attributable to DIFLUCAN.
(2) Anaphylaxis: In rare cases, anaphylaxis has been reported.
(3) Dermatologic: Patients have rarely developed exfoliative skin disorders during treatment with DIFLUCAN. In patients with serious underlying diseases (predominantly AIDS and malignancy), these have rarely resulted in a fatal outcome. Patients who develop rashes during treatment with DIFLUCAN should be monitored closely and the drug discontinued if lesions progress.

PRECAUTIONS

General

Single Dose

The convenience and efficacy of the single dose oral tablet of fluconazole regimen for the treatment of vaginal yeast infections should be weighed against the acceptability of a higher incidence of drug related adverse events with DIFLUCAN (26%) versus intravaginal agents (16%) in U.S. comparative clinical studies. (See **ADVERSE REACTIONS** and **CLINICAL STUDIES.**)

Drug Interactions:

(See **CLINICAL PHARMACOLOGY: Drug Interaction Studies** and **CONTRAINDICATIONS.**) Clinically or potentially significant drug interactions between DIFLUCAN and the following agents/classes have been observed. These are described in greater detail below:

- Oral hypoglycemics
- Coumarin-type anticoagulants
- Phenytoin
- Cyclosporine
- Rifampin
- Theophylline
- Terfenadine
- Cisapride
- Astemizole
- Rifabutin
- Tacrolimus

Oral hypoglycemics: Clinically significant hypoglycemia may be precipitated by the use of DIFLUCAN with oral hypoglycemic agents; one fatality has been reported from hypoglycemia in association with combined DIFLUCAN and glyburide use. DIFLUCAN reduces the metabolism of tolbutamide, glyburide, and glipizide and increases the plasma concentration of these agents. When DIFLUCAN is used concomitantly with these or other sulfonylurea oral hypoglycemic agents, blood glucose concentrations should be carefully monitored and the dose of the sulfonylurea should be adjusted as necessary. (See **CLINICAL PHARMACOLOGY: Drug Interaction Studies.**)
Coumarin-type anticoagulants: Prothrombin time may be increased in patients receiving concomitant DIFLUCAN and coumarin-type anticoagulants. Careful monitoring of prothrombin time in patients receiving DIFLUCAN and coumarin-type anticoagulants is recommended. (See **CLINICAL PHARMACOLOGY: Drug Interaction Studies.**)
Phenytoin: DIFLUCAN increases the plasma concentrations of phenytoin. Careful monitoring of phenytoin concentrations in patients receiving DIFLUCAN and phenytoin is recommended. (See **CLINICAL PHARMACOLOGY: Drug Interaction Studies.**)
Cyclosporine: DIFLUCAN may significantly increase cyclosporine levels in renal transplant patients with or without renal impairment. Careful monitoring of cyclosporine concentrations and serum creatinine is recommended in patients receiving DIFLUCAN and cyclosporine. (See **CLINICAL PHARMACOLOGY: Drug Interaction Studies.**)
Rifampin: Rifampin enhances the metabolism of concurrently administered DIFLUCAN. Depending on clinical circumstances, consideration should be given to increasing the dose of DIFLUCAN when it is administered with rifampin. (See **CLINICAL PHARMACOLOGY: Drug Interaction Studies.**)
Theophylline: DIFLUCAN increases the serum concentrations of theophylline. Careful monitoring of serum theophylline concentrations in patients receiving DIFLUCAN and theophylline is recommended. (See **CLINICAL PHARMACOLOGY: Drug Interaction Studies.**)
Terfenadine: Because of the occurrence of serious cardiac dysrhythmias secondary to prolongation of the QTc interval in patients receiving azole antifungals in conjunction with terfenadine, interaction studies have been performed. One study at a 200-mg daily dose of fluconazole failed to demonstrate a prolongation in QTc interval. Another study at a 400-mg and 800-mg daily dose of fluconazole demonstrated that DIFLUCAN taken in doses of 400 mg per day or greater significantly increases plasma levels of terfenadine when taken concomitantly. The combined use of fluconazole at doses of 400 mg or greater with terfenadine is contraindicated. (See **CONTRAINDICATIONS** and **CLINICAL PHARMACOLOGY: Drug Interaction Studies.**) The coadministration of fluconazole at doses lower than 400 mg/day with terfenadine should be carefully monitored.
Cisapride: There have been reports of cardiac events, including torsade de pointes in patients to whom fluconazole and cisapride were coadministered. The combined use of fluconazole with cisapride is contraindicated. (See **CONTRAINDICATIONS** and **CLINICAL PHARMACOLOGY: Drug Interaction Studies.**)
Astemizole: The use of fluconazole in patients concurrently taking astemizole or other drugs metabolized by the cytochrome P450 system may be associated with elevations in serum levels of these drugs. In the absence of definitive information, caution should be used when coadministering fluconazole. Patients should be carefully monitored.
Rifabutin: There have been reports of uveitis in patients to whom fluconazole and rifabutin were coadministered. Patients receiving rifabutin and fluconazole concomitantly should be carefully monitored. (See **CLINICAL PHARMACOLOGY: Drug Interaction Studies.**)
Tacrolimus: There have been reports of nephrotoxicity in patients to whom fluconazole and tacrolimus were coadministered. Patients receiving tacrolimus and fluconazole concomitantly should be carefully monitored. (See **CLINICAL PHARMACOLOGY: Drug Interaction Studies.**)
Fluconazole tablets coadministered with ethinyl estradiol- and levonorgestrel-containing oral contraceptives produced an overall mean increase in ethinyl estradiol and levonorgestrel levels; however, in some patients there were decreases up to 47% and 33% of ethinyl estradiol and levonorgestrel levels. (See **CLINICAL PHARMACOLOGY: Drug Interaction Studies.**) The data presently available indicate that the decreases in some individual ethinyl estradiol and levonorgestrel AUC values with fluconazole treatment are likely the result of random variation. While there is evidence that fluconazole can inhibit the metabolism of ethinyl estradiol and levonorgestrel, there is no evidence that fluconazole is a net inducer of ethinyl estradiol or levonorgestrel metabolism. The clinical significance of these effects is presently unknown.
Physicians should be aware that interaction studies with medications other than those listed in the **CLINICAL PHARMACOLOGY** section have not been conducted, but such interactions may occur.

Carcinogenesis, Mutagenesis and Impairment of Fertility

Fluconazole showed no evidence of carcinogenic potential in mice and rats treated orally for 24 months at doses of 2.5, 5 or 10 mg/kg/day (approximately 2–7× the recommended human dose). Male rats treated with 5 and 10 mg/kg/day had an increased incidence of hepatocellular adenomas.
Fluconazole, with or without metabolic activation, was negative in tests for mutagenicity in 4 strains of *S. typhimurium*, and in the mouse lymphoma L5178Y system. Cytogenetic studies *in vivo* (murine bone marrow cells, following oral administration of fluconazole) and *in vitro* (human lymphocytes exposed to fluconazole at 1000 μg/mL) showed no evidence of chromosomal mutations.
Fluconazole did not affect the fertility of male or female rats treated orally with daily doses of 5, 10 or 20 mg/kg or with parenteral doses of 5, 25 or 75 mg/kg, although the onset of parturition was slightly delayed at 20 mg/kg PO. In an intravenous perinatal study in rats at 5, 20 and 40 mg/kg, dystocia and prolongation of parturition were observed in a few dams at 20 mg/kg (approximately 5–15× the recommended human dose) and 40 mg/kg, but not at 5 mg/kg. The disturbances in parturition were reflected by a slight increase in the number of still-born pups and decrease of neonatal survival at these dose levels. The effects on parturition in rats are consistent with the species specific estrogen-lowering property produced by high doses of fluconazole. Such a hormone change has not been observed in women treated with fluconazole. (See **CLINICAL PHARMACOLOGY.**)

Pregnancy

Teratogenic Effects. Pregnancy Category C: Fluconazole was administered orally to pregnant rabbits during organogenesis in two studies, at 5, 10 and 20 mg/kg and at 5, 25, and 75 mg/kg, respectively. Maternal weight gain was impaired at all dose levels, and abortions occurred at 75 mg/kg (approximately 20–60× the recommended human dose); no adverse fetal effects were detected. In several studies in which pregnant rats were treated orally with fluconazole during organogenesis, maternal weight gain was impaired and placental weights were increased at 25 mg/kg. There were no fetal effects at 5 or 10 mg/kg; increases in fetal anatomical variants (supernumerary ribs, renal pelvis dilation) and delays in ossification were observed at 25 and 50 mg/kg and higher doses. At doses ranging from 80 mg/kg (approximately 20–60× the recommended human dose) to 320 mg/kg embryolethality in rats was increased and fetal abnormalities included wavy ribs, cleft palate and abnormal cranio-facial ossification. These effects are consistent with the inhibition of estrogen synthesis in rats and may be a result of known effects of lowered estrogen on pregnancy, organogenesis and parturition.
There are no adequate and well controlled studies in pregnant women. There have been reports of multiple congenital abnormalities in infants whose mothers were being treated for 3 or more months with high dose (400–800 mg/day) fluconazole therapy for coccidioidomycosis (an unindicated use). The relationship between fluconazole use and these events is unclear. DIFLUCAN should be used in pregnancy only if the potential benefit justifies the possible risk to the fetus.

Nursing Mothers

Fluconazole is secreted in human milk at concentrations similar to plasma. Therefore, the use of DIFLUCAN in nursing mothers is not recommended.

Pediatric Use

An open-label, randomized, controlled trial has shown DIFLUCAN to be effective in the treatment of oropharyngeal candidiasis in children 6 months to 13 years of age. (See **CLINICAL STUDIES.**)
The use of DIFLUCAN in children with cryptococcal meningitis, *Candida* esophagitis, or systemic *Candida* infections is supported by the efficacy shown for these indications in adults and by the results from several small noncomparative pediatric clinical studies. In addition, pharmacokinetic studies in children (see **CLINICAL PHARMACOLOGY**) have established a dose proportionality between children and adults. (See **DOSAGE AND ADMINISTRATION.**)
In a noncomparative study of children with serious systemic fungal infections, most of which were candidemia, the effectiveness of DIFLUCAN was similar to that reported for the treatment of candidemia in adults. Of 17 subjects with culture-confirmed candidemia, 11 of 14 (79%) with baseline symptoms (3 were asymptomatic) had a clinical cure; 13/15 (87%) of evaluable patients had a mycologic cure at the end of treatment but two of these patients relapsed at 10 and 18 days, respectively, following cessation of therapy.
The efficacy of DIFLUCAN for the suppression of cryptococcal meningitis was successful in 4 of 5 children treated in a compassionate-use study of fluconazole for the treatment of life-threatening or serious mycosis. There is no information regarding the efficacy of fluconazole for primary treatment of cryptococcal meningitis in children.
The safety profile of DIFLUCAN in children has been studied in 577 children ages 1 day to 17 years who received doses ranging from 1 to 15 mg/kg/day for 1 to 1,616 days. (See **ADVERSE REACTIONS.**)
Efficacy of DIFLUCAN has not been established in infants less than 6 months of age. (See **CLINICAL PHARMACOLOGY.**) A small number of patients (29) ranging in age from 1 day to 6 months have been treated safely with DIFLUCAN.

Continued on next page

Diflucan—Cont.

ADVERSE REACTIONS

In Patients Receiving a Single Dose for Vaginal Candidiasis: During comparative clinical studies conducted in the United States, 448 patients with vaginal candidiasis were treated with DIFLUCAN, 150 mg single dose. The overall incidence of side effects possibly related to DIFLUCAN was 26%. In 422 patients receiving active comparative agents, the incidence was 16%. The most common treatment-related adverse events reported in the patients who received 150 mg single dose fluconazole for vaginitis were headache (13%), nausea (7%), and abdominal pain (6%). Other side effects reported with an incidence equal to or greater than 1% included diarrhea (3%), dyspepsia (1%), dizziness (1%), and taste perversion (1%). Most of the reported side effects were mild to moderate in severity. Rarely, angioedema and anaphylactic reaction have been reported in marketing experience.

In Patients Receiving Multiple Doses for Other Infections: Sixteen percent of over 4000 patients treated with DIFLUCAN (fluconazole) in clinical trials of 7 days or more experienced adverse events. Treatment was discontinued in 1.5% of patients due to adverse clinical events and in 1.3% of patients due to laboratory test abnormalities.

Clinical adverse events were reported more frequently in HIV infected patients (21%) than in non-HIV infected patients (13%); however, the patterns in HIV infected and non-HIV infected patients were similar. The proportions of patients discontinuing therapy due to clinical adverse events were similar in the two groups (1.5%).

The following treatment-related clinical adverse events occurred at an incidence of 1% or greater in 4048 patients receiving DIFLUCAN for 7 or more days in clinical trials: nausea 3.7%, headache 1.9%, skin rash 1.8%, vomiting 1.7%, abdominal pain 1.7%, and diarrhea 1.5%.

The following adverse events have occurred under conditions where a causal association is probable:

Hepatobiliary: In combined clinical trials and marketing experience, there have been rare cases of serious hepatic reactions during treatment with DIFLUCAN. (See **WARNINGS**.) The spectrum of these hepatic reactions has ranged from mild transient elevations in transaminases to clinical hepatitis, cholestasis and fulminant hepatic failure, including fatalities. Instances of fatal hepatic reactions were noted to occur primarily in patients with serious underlying medical conditions (predominantly AIDS or malignancy) and often while taking multiple concomitant medications. Transient hepatic reactions, including hepatitis and jaundice, have occurred among patients with no other identifiable risk factors. In each of these cases, liver function returned to baseline on discontinuation of DIFLUCAN.

In two comparative trials evaluating the efficacy of DIFLUCAN for the suppression of relapse of cryptococcal meningitis, a statistically significant increase was observed in median AST (SGOT) levels from a baseline value of 30 IU/L to 41 IU/L in one trial and 34 IU/L to 66 IU/L in the other. The overall rate of serum transaminase elevations of more than 8 times the upper limit of normal was approximately 1% in fluconazole-treated patients in clinical trials. These elevations occurred in patients with severe underlying disease, predominantly AIDS or malignancies, most of whom were receiving multiple concomitant medications, including many known to be hepatotoxic. The incidence of abnormally elevated serum transaminases was greater in patients taking DIFLUCAN concomitantly with one or more of the following medications: rifampin, phenytoin, isoniazid, valproic acid, or oral sulfonylurea hypoglycemic agents.

Immunologic: In rare cases, anaphylaxis has been reported.

The following adverse events have occurred under conditions where a causal association is uncertain:

Central Nervous System: Seizures.

Dermatologic: Exfoliative skin disorders including Stevens-Johnson syndrome and toxic epidermal necrolysis (see **WARNINGS**), alopecia.

Hematopoietic and *Lymphatic:* Leukopenia, including neutropenia and agranulocytosis, thrombocytopenia.

Metabolic: Hypercholesterolemia, hypertriglyceridemia, hypokalemia.

Adverse Reactions in Children:

In Phase II/III clinical trials conducted in the United States and in Europe, 577 pediatric patients, ages 1 day to 17 years were treated with DIFLUCAN at doses up to 15 mg/kg/day for up to 1,616 days. Thirteen percent of children experienced treatment related adverse events. The most commonly reported events were vomiting (5%), abdominal pain (3%), nausea (2%), and diarrhea (2%). Treatment was discontinued in 2.3% of patients due to adverse clinical events and in 1.4% of patients due to laboratory test abnormalities. The majority of treatment-related laboratory abnormalities were elevations of transaminases or alkaline phosphatase.

[See first table above]

Percentage of Patients With Treatment-Related Side Effects

	Fluconazole (N=577)	Comparative Agents (N=451)
With any side effect	13.0	9.3
Vomiting	5.4	5.1
Abdominal pain	2.8	1.6
Nausea	2.3	1.6
Diarrhea	2.1	2.2

Fluconazole Content per Bottle	Concentration of Reconstituted Suspension
350 mg	10 mg/mL
1400 mg	40 mg/mL

OVERDOSAGE

There has been one reported case of overdosage with DIFLUCAN (fluconazole). A 42-year-old patient infected with human immunodeficiency virus developed hallucinations and exhibited paranoid behavior after reportedly ingesting 8200 mg of DIFLUCAN. The patient was admitted to the hospital, and his condition resolved within 48 hours. In the event of overdose, symptomatic treatment (with supportive measures and gastric lavage if clinically indicated) should be instituted.

Fluconazole is largely excreted in urine. A three-hour hemodialysis session decreases plasma levels by approximately 50%.

In mice and rats receiving very high doses of fluconazole, clinical effects in both species included decreased motility and respiration, ptosis, lacrimation, salivation, urinary incontinence, loss of righting reflex and cyanosis; death was sometimes preceded by clonic convulsions.

DOSAGE AND ADMINISTRATION

Dosage and Administration in Adults:

Single Dose

Vaginal candidiasis: The recommended dosage of DIFLUCAN for vaginal candidiasis is 150 mg as a single oral dose.

Multiple Dose

SINCE ORAL ABSORPTION IS RAPID AND ALMOST COMPLETE, THE DAILY DOSE OF DIFLUCAN (FLUCONAZOLE) IS THE SAME FOR ORAL (TABLETS AND SUSPENSION) AND INTRAVENOUS ADMINISTRATION. In general, a loading dose of twice the daily dose is recommended on the first day of therapy to result in plasma concentrations close to steady-state by the second day of therapy.

The daily dose of DIFLUCAN for the treatment of infections other than vaginal candidiasis should be based on the infecting organism and the patient's response to therapy. Treatment should be continued until clinical parameters or laboratory tests indicate that active fungal infection has subsided. An inadequate period of treatment may lead to recurrence of active infection. Patients with AIDS and cryptococcal meningitis or recurrent oropharyngeal candidiasis usually require maintenance therapy to prevent relapse.

Oropharyngeal candidiasis: The recommended dosage of DIFLUCAN for oropharyngeal candidiasis is 200 mg on the first day, followed by 100 mg once daily. Clinical evidence of oropharyngeal candidiasis generally resolves within several days, but treatment should be continued for at least 2 weeks to decrease the likelihood of relapse.

Esophageal candidiasis: The recommended dosage of DIFLUCAN for esophageal candidiasis is 200 mg on the first day, followed by 100 mg once daily. Doses up to 400 mg/day may be used, based on medical judgment of the patient's response to therapy. Patients with esophageal candidiasis should be treated for a minimum of three weeks and for at least two weeks following resolution of symptoms.

Systemic Candida infections: For systemic *Candida* infections including candidemia, disseminated candidiasis, and pneumonia, optimal therapeutic dosage and duration of therapy have not been established. In open, noncomparative studies of small numbers of patients, doses of up to 400 mg daily have been used.

Urinary tract infections and peritonitis: For the treatment of *Candida* urinary tract infections and peritonitis, daily doses of 50–200 mg have been used in open, noncomparative studies of small numbers of patients.

Cryptococcal meningitis: The recommended dosage for treatment of acute cryptococcal meningitis is 400 mg on the first day, followed by 200 mg once daily. A dosage of 400 mg once daily may be used, based on medical judgment of the patient's response to therapy. The recommended duration of treatment for initial therapy of cryptococcal meningitis is 10–12 weeks after the cerebrospinal fluid becomes culture negative. The recommended dosage of DIFLUCAN for suppression of relapse of crytpococcal meningitis in patients with AIDS is 200 mg once daily.

Prophylaxis in patients undergoing bone marrow transplantation: The recommended DIFLUCAN daily dosage for the prevention of candidiasis of patients undergoing bone marrow transplantation is 400 mg, once daily. Patients who are anticipated to have severe granulocytopenia (less than 500 neutrophils per cu mm) should start DIFLUCAN prophylaxis several days before the anticipated onset of neutropenia, and continue for 7 days after the neutrophil count rises above 1000 cells per cu mm.

Dosage and Administration in Children:

The following dose equivalency scheme should generally provide equivalent exposure in pediatric and adult patients:

Pediatric Patients	Adults
3 mg/kg	100 mg
6 mg/kg	200 mg
12* mg/kg	400 mg

*Some older children may have clearances similar to that of adults. Absolute doses exceeding 600 mg/day are not recommended.

Experience with DIFLUCAN in neonates is limited to pharmacokinetic studies in premature newborns. (See **CLINICAL PHARMACOLOGY**.) Based on the prolonged half-life seen in premature newborns (gestational age 26 to 29 weeks), these children, in the first two weeks of life, should receive the same dosage (mg/kg) as in older children, but administered every 72 hours. After the first two weeks, these children should be dosed once daily. No information regarding DIFLUCAN pharmacokinetics in full-term newborns is available.

Oropharyngeal candidiasis: The recommended dosage of DIFLUCAN for oropharyngeal candidiasis in children is 6 mg/kg on the first day, followed by 3 mg/kg once daily. Treatment should be administered for at least 2 weeks to decrease the likelihood of relapse.

Esophageal candidiasis: For the treatment of esophageal candidiasis, the recommended dosage of DIFLUCAN in children is 6 mg/kg on the first day, followed by 3 mg/kg once daily. Doses up to 12 mg/kg/day may be used based on medical judgment of the patient's response to therapy. Patients with esophageal candidiasis should be treated for a minimum of three weeks and for at least 2 weeks following the resolution of symptoms.

Systemic Candida infections: For the treatment of candidemia and disseminated *Candida* infections, daily doses of 6–12 mg/kg/day have been used in an open, noncomparative study of a small number of children.

Cryptococcal meningitis: For the treatment of acute cryptococcal meningitis, the recommended dosage is 12 mg/kg on the first day, followed by 6 mg/kg once daily. A dosage of 12 mg/kg once daily may be used, based on medical judgment of the patient's response to therapy. The recommended duration of treatment for initial therapy of cryptococcal meningitis is 10–12 weeks after the cerebrospinal fluid becomes culture negative. For suppression of relapse of cryptococcal meningitis in children with AIDS, the recommended dose of DIFLUCAN is 6 mg/kg once daily.

Dosage In Patients With Impaired Renal Function:

Fluconazole is cleared primarily by renal excretion as unchanged drug. There is no need to adjust single dose therapy for vaginal candidiasis because of impaired renal function. In patients with impaired renal function who will receive multiple doses of DIFLUCAN, an initial loading dose of 50 to 400 mg should be given. After the loading dose, the daily dose (according to indication) should be based on the following table:

Creatinine Clearance (mL/min)	Percent of Recommended Dose
>50	100%
≤50 (no dialysis)	50%
Regular dialysis	100% after each dialysis

These are suggested dose adjustments based on pharmacokinetics following administration of multiple doses. Further adjustment may be needed depending upon clinical condition.

When serum creatinine is the only measure of renal function available, the following formula (based on sex, weight, and age of the patient) should be used to estimate the creatinine clearance in adults:

Males: $$\frac{\text{Weight (kg)} \times (140\text{-age})}{72 \times \text{serum creatinine (mg/100 mL)}}$$

Females: $0.85 \times$ above value

Although the pharmacokinetics of fluconazole has not been studied in children with renal insufficiency, dosage reduction in children with renal insufficiency should parallel that recommended for adults. The following formula may be used to estimate creatinine clearance in children:

$$K\times \frac{\text{linear length or height (cm)}}{\text{serum creatinine (mg/100 mL)}}$$

(Where K=0.55 for children older than 1 year and 0.45 for infants.)

Administration

DIFLUCAN may be administered either orally or by intravenous infusion. DIFLUCAN injection has been used safely for up to fourteen days of intravenous therapy. The intravenous infusion of DIFLUCAN should be administered at a maximum rate of approximately 200 mg/hour, given as a continuous infusion.

DIFLUCAN injections in glass and Viaflex® Plus plastic containers are intended only for intravenous administration using sterile equipment.

Parenteral drug products should be inspected visually for particulate matter and discoloration prior to administration whenever solution and container permit.

Do not use if the solution is cloudy or precipitated or if the seal is not intact.

Directions for Mixing the Oral Suspension

Prepare a suspension at time of dispensing as follows: tap bottle until all the powder flows freely. To reconstitute, add 24 mL of distilled water or Purified Water (USP) to fluconazole bottle and shake vigorously to suspend powder. Each bottle will deliver 35 mL of suspension. The concentrations of the reconstituted suspensions are as follows:

[See second table at top of previous page]

Note: Shake oral suspension well before using. Store reconstituted suspension between 86°F (30°C) and 41°F (5°C) and discard unused portion after 2 weeks. Protect from freezing.

Directions for IV Use of DIFLUCAN in Viaflex® Plus Plastic Containers

Do not remove unit from overwrap until ready for use. The overwrap is a moisture barrier. The inner bag maintains the sterility of the product.

CAUTION: Do not use plastic containers in series connections. Such use could result in air embolism due to residual air being drawn from the primary container before administration of the fluid from the secondary container is completed.

To Open

Tear overwrap down side at slit and remove solution container. Some opacity of the plastic due to moisture absorption during the sterilization process may be observed. This is normal and does not affect the solution quality or safety. The opacity will diminish gradually. After removing overwrap, check for minute leaks by squeezing inner bag firmly. If leaks are found, discard solution as sterility may be impaired.

DO NOT ADD SUPPLEMENTARY MEDICATION.

Preparation for Administration:

1. Suspend container from eyelet support.
2. Remove plastic protector from outlet port at bottom of container.
3. Attach administration set. Refer to complete directions accompanying set.

HOW SUPPLIED

DIFLUCAN® Tablets: Pink trapezoidal tablets containing 50, 100 or 200 mg of fluconazole are packaged in bottles or unit dose blisters. The 150 mg fluconazole tablets are pink and oval shaped, packaged in a single dose unit blister.

DIFLUCAN® Tablets are supplied as follows:

DIFLUCAN® 50 mg Tablets: Engraved with "DIFLUCAN" and "50" on the front and "ROERIG" on the back.

NDC 0049-3410-30 Bottles of 30

DIFLUCAN® 100 mg Tablets: Engraved with "DIFLUCAN" and "100" on the front and "ROERIG" on the back.

NDC 0049-3420-30 Bottles of 30
NDC 0049-3420-41 Unit dose package of 100

DIFLUCAN® 150 mg Tablets: Engraved with "DIFLUCAN" and "150" on the front and "ROERIG" on the back.

NDC 0049-3500-79 Unit dose package of 1

DIFLUCAN® 200 mg Tablets: Engraved with "DIFLUCAN" and "200" on the front and "ROERIG" on the back.

NDC 0049-3430-30 Bottles of 30
NDC 0049-3430-41 Unit dose package of 100

Storage: Store tablets below 86°F (30°C).

DIFLUCAN® for Oral Suspension: DIFLUCAN® for oral suspension is supplied as an orange-flavored powder to provide 35 mL per bottle as follows:

NDC 0049-3440-19 Fluconazole 350 mg per bottle
NDC 0049-3450-19 Fluconazole 1400 mg per bottle

Storage: Store dry powder below 86°F (30°C). Store reconstituted suspension between 86°F (30°C) and 41°F (5°C) and discard unused portion after 2 weeks. Protect from freezing.

DIFLUCAN® Injections: DIFLUCAN® injections for intravenous infusion administration are formulated as sterile iso-osmotic solutions containing 2 mg/mL of fluconazole. They are supplied in glass bottles or in Viaflex® Plus plastic containers containing volumes of 100 mL or 200 mL affording doses of 200 mg and 400 mg of fluconazole, respectively. DIFLUCAN® injections in Viaflex® Plus plastic containers are available in both sodium chloride and dextrose diluents.

DIFLUCAN® Injections in Glass Bottles:

NDC 0049-3371-26 Fluconazole in Sodium Chloride Diluent 200 mg/100 mL × 6

NDC 0049-3372-26 Fluconazole in Sodium Chloride Diluent 400 mg/200 mL × 6

Storage: Store between 86°F (30°C) and 41°F (5°C). Protect from freezing.

DIFLUCAN® Injections in Viaflex® Plus Plastic Containers:

NDC 0049-3435-26 Fluconazole in Sodium Chloride Diluent 200 mg/100 mL × 6

NDC 0049-3436-26 Fluconazole in Sodium Chloride Diluent 400 mg/200 mL × 6

NDC 0049-3437-26 Fluconazole in Dextrose Diluent 200 mg/100 mL × 6

NDC 0049-3438-26 Fluconazole in Dextrose Diluent 400 mg/200 mL × 6

Storage: Store between 77°F (25°C) and 41°F (5°C). Brief exposure up to 104°F (40°C) does not adversely affect the product. Protect from freezing.

Roerig
Division of Pfizer Inc, NY, NY 10017

70-4526-00-7 Revised June 1998

Shown in Product Identification Guide, page 330

FELDENE® ℞

[fēl 'deen]
(piroxicam)
CAPSULES
10 mg and 20 mg
For Oral Use

DESCRIPTION

FELDENE® contains piroxicam which is a member of the oxicam group of nonsteroidal anti-inflammatory drugs (NSAIDSs). Each maroon and blue capsule contains 10 mg piroxicam, each maroon capsule contains 20 mg piroxicam for oral administration. The chemical name for piroxicam is 4-hydroxyl-2-methyl-*N*-2-pyridinyl-2*H*-1,2-benzothiazine-3-carboxamide 1,1-dioxide. Piroxicam occurs as a white crystalline solid, sparingly soluble in water, dilute acid and most organic solvents. It is slightly soluble in alcohol and in aqueous solutions. It exhibits a weakly acidic 4-hydroxy proton (pKa 5.1) and a weakly basic pyridyl nitrogen (pKa 1.8). The molecular weight of piroxicam is 331.35. Its molecular formula is $C_{15}H_{13}N_3O_4S$ and it has the following structural formula:

The inactive ingredients in FELDENE capsules include: Blue 1, Red 3, lactose, magnesium stearate, sodium lauryl sulfate, starch.

CLINICAL PHARMACOLOGY

Pharmacodynamics

FELDENE is a nonsteroidal anti-inflammatory drug (NSAID) that exhibits anti-inflammatory, analgesic, and antipyretic activities in animal models. The mechanism of action of FELDENE, like that of other NSAIDS, is not completely understood but may be related to prostaglandin synthetase inhibition.

Pharmacokinetics

Absorption: FELDENE is well absorbed following oral administration. Drug plasma concentrations are proportional for 10 and 20 mg doses and generally peak within three to five hours after medication. The prolonged half-life (50 hours) results in the maintenance of relatively stable plasma concentrations throughout the day on once daily doses and to significant accumulation upon multiple dosing. A single 20-mg dose generally produces peak piroxicam plasma levels of 1.5 to 2 mcg/mL, while maximum drug plasma concentrations, after repeated daily ingestion of 20 mg FELDENE, usually stabilize at 3–8 mcg/mL. Most patients approximate steady state plasma levels within 7–12 days. Higher levels, which approximate steady state at two to three weeks, have been observed in patients in whom longer plasma half-lives of piroxicam occurred.

With food there is a slight delay in the rate but not the extent of absorption following oral administration. The concomitant administration of antacids (aluminum hydroxide or aluminum hydroxide with magnesium hydroxide) have been shown to have no effect on the plasma levels of orally administered piroxicam.

Distribution: The apparent volume of distribution of piroxicam is approximately 0.14 L/kg. Ninety-nine percent of plasma piroxicam is bound to plasma proteins. Piroxicam is excreted into human milk. The presence in breast milk has been determined during initial and long-term conditions (52 days). Piroxicam appeared in breast milk at about 1% to 3% of the maternal concentration. No accumulation of piroxicam occurred in milk relative to that in plasma during treatment.

Metabolism: Metabolism of piroxicam occurs by hydroxylation at the 5 position of the pyridyl side chain and conjugation of this product; by cyclodehydration; and by a sequence of reactions involving hydrolysis of the amide linkage, decarboxylation, ring contraction and N-demethylation. The biotransformation products of piroxicam metabolism are reported to not have any anti-inflammatory activity.

Excretion: FELDENE and its biotransformation products are excreted in urine and feces, with about twice as much appearing in the urine as in the feces. Approximately 5% of a FELDENE dose is excreted unchanged. The plasma half-life ($T_{½}$) for piroxicam is approximately 50 hours.

Special Populations

Pediatric: FELDENE has not been investigated in pediatric patients.

Race: Pharmacokinetic differences due to race have not been identified.

Hepatic Insufficiency: The effects of hepatic disease on FELDENE pharmacokinetics have not been established. However, a substantial portion of FELDENE elimination occurs by hepatic metabolism. Consequently, patients with hepatic disease may require reduced doses of FELDENE as compared to patients with normal hepatic function.

Renal Insufficiency: FELDENE pharmacokinetics have been investigated in patients with renal insufficiency. Studies indicate patients with mild to moderate renal impairment may not require dosing adjustments. However, the pharmacokinetic properties of FELDENE in patients with severe renal insufficiency or those receiving hemodialysis are not known.

Other Information

In controlled clinical trials, the effectiveness of FELDENE has been established for both acute exacerbations and long-term management of rheumatoid arthritis and osteoarthritis.

The therapeutic effects of FELDENE are evident early in the treatment of both diseases with a progressive increase in response over several (8–12) weeks. Efficacy is seen in terms of pain relief and, when present, subsidence of inflammation.

Doses of 20 mg/day FELDENE display a therapeutic effect comparable to therapeutic doses of aspirin, with a lower incidence of minor gastrointestinal effects and tinnitus.

FELDENE has been administered concomitantly with fixed doses of gold and corticosteroids. The existence of a "steroid-sparing" effect has not been adequately studied to date.

INDICATIONS AND USAGE

FELDENE is indicated for acute or long-term use in the relief of signs and symptoms of the following:

1. Osteoarthritis.
2. Rheumatoid arthritis.

CONTRAINDICATIONS

FELDENE is contraindicated in patients with known hypersensitivity to piroxicam. FELDENE should not be given to patients who have experienced asthma, urticaria or allergic-type reactions after taking aspirin or other NSAIDs. Severe, rarely fatal, anaphylactic-like reactions to NSAIDs have been reported in such patients (see **WARNINGS: Anaphylactoid Reactions** and **PRECAUTIONS: Preexisting Asthma**).

WARNINGS

Gastrointestinal (GI) Effects—Risk of GI Ulceration, Bleeding and Perforation

Serious gastrointestinal toxicity, such as inflammation, bleeding, ulceration, and perforation of the stomach, small intestine or large intestine, can occur at any time, with or without warning symptoms, in patients treated with nonsteroidal anti-inflammatory drugs (NSAIDs). Minor upper gastrointestinal problems, such as dyspepsia, are common and may also occur at any time during NSAID therapy. Therefore, physicians and patients should remain alert for ulceration and bleeding, even in the absence of previous GI tract symptoms. Patients should be informed about the signs and/or symptoms of serious GI toxicity and the steps to take if they occur. The utility of periodic laboratory monitoring has not been demonstrated, nor has it been adequately assessed. Only one in five patients who develop a serious upper GI adverse event on NSAID therapy is symptomatic. It has been demonstrated that upper GI ulcers, gross bleeding or perforation, caused by NSAIDs, appear to occur in approximately 1% of patients treated for 3–6 months, and in about 2%–4% of patients treated for one year. These trends continue thus, increasing the likelihood of developing a serious GI event at some time during the course of therapy. However, even short-term therapy is not without risk.

NSAIDs should be prescribed with extreme caution in those with a prior history of ulcer disease or gastrointestinal bleeding. Most spontaneous reports of fatal GI events are in elderly or debilitated patients and, therefore, special care should be taken in treating this population. To minimize the potential risk for an adverse GI event, the lowest effective dose should be used for the shortest possible duration. For high risk patients, alternate therapies that do not involve NSAIDs should be considered.

Studies have shown that patients with *a prior history of peptic ulcer disease and/or gastrointestinal bleeding* and who use NSAIDs, have a greater than 10-fold risk for developing a GI bleed than patients with neither of these risk factors. In addition to a past history of ulcer disease, pharmacoepidemiological studies have identified several other cotherapies or comorbid conditions that may increase the risk for GI bleeding such as: treatment with oral corticosteroids, treatment with anticoagulants, longer duration of NSAID therapy, smoking, alcoholism, older age, and poor general health status.

Anaphylactoid Reactions

As with other NSAIDs, anaphylactoid reactions may occur in patients without known prior exposure to FELDENE. FELDENE should not be given to patients with the aspirin triad. This symptom complex typically occurs in asthmatic patients who experience rhinitis with or without nasal polyps, or who exhibit severe, potentially fatal bronchospasm after taking aspirin or other NSAIDs (see **CONTRAINDICATIONS** and **PRECAUTIONS: Preexisting Asthma**). Emergency help should be sought in cases where an anaphylactoid reaction occurs.

Advanced Renal Disease

In cases with advanced kidney disease, treatment with FELDENE is not recommended. If NSAID therapy, however, must be initiated, close monitoring of the patient's kidney function is advisable (see **PRECAUTIONS: Renal Effects**).

Pregnancy

In late pregnancy, as with other NSAIDs, FELDENE should be avoided because it may cause premature closure of the ductus arteriosus.

PRECAUTIONS

General

FELDENE cannot be expected to substitute for corticosteroids or to treat corticosteroid insufficiency. Abrupt discontinuation of corticosteroids may lead to disease exacerbation.

Continued on next page

Feldene—Cont.

Patients on prolonged corticosteroid therapy should have their therapy tapered slowly if a decision is made to discontinue corticosteroids.
The pharmacological activity of FELDENE in reducing fever and inflammation may diminish the utility of these diagnostic signs in detecting complications of presumed noninfectious, painful conditions.

Hepatic Effects
Borderline elevations of one or more liver tests may occur in up to 15% of patients taking NSAIDs including FELDENE. These laboratory abnormalities may progress, may remain unchanged, or may be transient with continuing therapy. Notable elevations of ALT or AST (approximately three or more times the upper limit of normal) have been reported in approximately 1% of patients in clinical trials with NSAIDs. In addition, rare cases of severe hepatic reactions, including jaundice and fatal fulminant hepatitis, liver necrosis and hepatic failure, some of them with fatal outcomes have been reported.
A patient with symptoms and/or signs suggesting liver dysfunction, or in whom an abnormal liver test has occurred, should be evaluated for evidence of the development of more severe hepatic reaction while on therapy with FELDENE. If clinical signs and symptoms consistent with liver disease develop, or if systemic manifestations occur (e.g., eosinophilia, rash, etc.), FELDENE should be discontinued (see **ADVERSE REACTIONS**).

Renal Effects
Caution should be used when initiating treatment with FELDENE in patients with considerable dehydration. It is advisable to rehydrate patients first and then start therapy with FELDENE. Caution is also recommended in patients with preexisting kidney disease (see **WARNINGS: Advanced Renal Disease**).
As with other NSAIDs, long-term administration of FELDENE has resulted in renal papillary necrosis and other renal medullary changes. In humans, there have been reports of acute interstitial nephritis with hematuria, proteinuria and occasionally, nephrotic syndrome. Renal toxicity has also been seen in patients in which renal prostaglandins have a compensatory role in the maintenance of renal perfusion. In these patients, administration of nonsteroidal anti-inflammatory drug may cause a dose-dependent reduction in prostaglandin formation and, secondarily, in renal blood flow, which may precipitate overt renal decompensation. Patients at greatest risk of this reaction are those with impaired renal function, heart failure, liver dysfunction, those taking diuretics and ACE inhibitors, and the elderly. Discontinuation of nonsteroidal anti-inflammatory drug therapy is usually followed by recovery to the pretreatment state.
Because of extensive renal excretion of piroxicam and its biotransformation products less than 5% of the daily dose is excreted unchanged (see **CLINICAL PHARMACOLOGY**), lower doses of piroxicam should be anticipated in patients with impaired renal function, and they should be carefully monitored.

Hematological Effects
Anemia is sometimes seen in patients receiving NSAIDs, including FELDENE. This may be due to fluid retention, GI blood loss, or an incompletely described effect upon erythropoiesis. Patients on long-term treatment with NSAIDs, including FELDENE, should have their hemoglobin or hematocrit checked if they exhibit any signs or symptoms of anemia.
All drugs which inhibit the biosynthesis of prostaglandins may interfere to some extent with platelet function and vascular responses to bleeding.
NSAIDs inhibit platelet aggregation and have been shown to prolong bleeding time in some patients. Unlike aspirin, their effect on platelet function is quantitatively less, of shorter duration, and reversible. FELDENE does not generally affect platelet counts, prothrombin time (PT), or partial thromboplastin time (PTT). Patients receiving FELDENE who may be adversely affected by alterations in platelet function, such as those with coagulation disorders or patients receiving anticoagulants, should be carefully monitored.

Ophthalmologic Effects
Because of reports of adverse eye findings with nonsteroidal anti-inflammatory agents, it is recommended that patients who develop visual complaints during treatment with FELDENE have ophthalmic evaluations.

Fluid Retention and Edema
Fluid retention and edema have been observed in some patients taking NSAIDs. Therefore, as with other NSAIDs, FELDENE should be used with caution in patients with fluid retention, hypertension, or heart failure.

Preexisting Asthma
Patients with asthma may have aspirin-sensitive asthma. The use of aspirin in patients with aspirin-sensitive asthma has been associated with severe bronchospasm which can be fatal. Since cross-reactivity, including bronchospasm, between aspirin and other nonsteroidal anti-inflammatory drugs has been reported in such aspirin-sensitive patients, FELDENE should not be administered to patients with this form of aspirin sensitivity and should be used with caution in patients with preexisting asthma.

Other Hypersensitivity Reactions
A combination of dermatological and/or allergic signs and symptoms suggestive of serum sickness have occasionally occurred in conjunction with the use of FELDENE. These include arthralgias, pruritus, fever, fatigue, and rash including vesiculobullous reactions and exfoliative dermatitis.

Information for Patients
FELDENE, like other drugs of its class, can cause discomfort and, rarely, more serious side effects, such as gastrointestinal bleeding, which may result in hospitalization and even fatal outcomes. Although serious GI tract ulceration and bleeding can occur without warning symptoms, patients should be alert for the signs and symptoms of ulceration and bleeding, and should ask for medical advice when observing any indicative sign or symptom. Patients should be apprised of the importance of this follow-up (see **WARNINGS: Gastrointestinal (GI) Effects—Risk of GI Ulceration, Bleeding and Perforation**).
Patients should report to their physicians, signs or symptoms of gastrointestinal ulceration or bleeding, skin rash, weight gain, or edema.
Patients should be informed of the warning signs and symptoms of hepatotoxicity (e.g., nausea, fatigue, lethargy, pruritus, jaundice, right upper quadrant tenderness and "flu-like" symptoms). If these occur, patients should be instructed to stop therapy and seek immediate medical therapy.
Patients should also be instructed to seek immediate emergency help in the case of an anaphylactoid reaction (see **WARNINGS**).
In late pregnancy, as with other NSAIDs, FELDENE should be avoided because it will cause premature closure of the ductus arteriosus.

Laboratory Tests
Patients on long-term treatment with NSAIDs should have their CBC and a chemistry profile checked periodically. If clinical signs and symptoms consistent with liver or renal disease develop, systemic manifestations occur (e.g., eosinophilia, rash, etc.) or if abnormal liver tests persist or worsen, FELDENE should be discontinued.

Drug Interactions
Highly Protein Bound Drugs: FELDENE is highly protein bound and, therefore, might be expected to displace other protein bound drugs. Physicians should closely monitor patients for a change in dosage requirements when administering FELDENE to patients on other highly protein bound drugs.
Aspirin: Plasma levels of piroxicam are depressed to approximately 80% of their normal values when FELDENE is administered (20 mg/day) in conjunction with aspirin (3900 mg/day). As with other NSAIDs, concomitant administration of piroxicam and aspirin is not generally recommended because of the potential for increased adverse effects.
Methotrexate: NSAIDs have been reported to competitively inhibit methotrexate accumulation in rabbit kidney slices. This may indicate that they could enhance the toxicity of methotrexate. Caution should be used when NSAIDs are administered concomitantly with methotrexate.
ACE Inhibitors: Reports suggest that NSAIDs may diminish the antihypertensive effect of ACE inhibitors. This interaction should be given consideration in patients taking NSAIDs concomitantly with ACE inhibitors.
Furosemide: Clinical studies, as well as post-marketing observations, have shown that FELDENE can reduce the natriuretic effect of furosemide and thiazides in some patients. This response has been attributed to inhibition of renal prostaglandin synthesis. During concomitant therapy with NSAIDs, the patient should be observed closely for signs of renal failure (see **PRECAUTIONS: Renal Effects**), as well as to assure diuretic efficacy.
Lithium: NSAIDs have produced an elevation of plasma lithium levels and a reduction in renal lithium clearance. The mean minimum lithium concentration increased 15% and the renal clearance was decreased by approximately 20%. These effects have been attributed to inhibition of renal prostaglandin synthesis by the NSAID. Thus, when NSAIDs and lithium are administered concurrently, subjects should be observed carefully for signs of lithium toxicity.
Warfarin: The effects of warfarin and NSAIDs on GI bleeding are synergistic, such that users of both drugs together have a risk of serious GI bleeding higher than users of either drug alone.

Carcinogenesis, Mutagenesis, Impairment of Fertility
Subacute, acute and chronic toxicity studies have been carried out in rats, mice, dogs and monkeys. The pathology most often seen was that characteristically associated with the animal toxicology of anti-inflammatory agents: renal papillary necrosis (see **PRECAUTIONS**) and gastrointestinal lesions.
Reproductive studies revealed no impairment of fertility in animals.

Pregnancy
Teratogenic Effects: Pregnancy Category C—Reproductive studies conducted in rats and rabbits have not demonstrated evidence of developmental abnormalities. However, animal reproduction studies are not always predictive of human response. There are no adequate and well-controlled studies in pregnant women. FELDENE is not recommended for use in pregnant women since safety has not been established in humans.
Nonteratogenic Effects: Because of the known effects of nonsteroidal anti-inflammatory drugs on the fetal cardiovascular system (closure of ductus arteriosus), use during pregnancy (particularly late pregnancy) should be avoided. In animal studies, gastrointestinal tract toxicity was increased in pregnant females in the last trimester of pregnancy compared to nonpregnant females or females in earlier trimesters of pregnancy.

Labor and Delivery
In rat studies with NSAIDs, as with other drugs known to inhibit prostaglandin synthesis, an increased incidence of dystocia, delayed parturition, and decreased pup survival occurred. The effects of FELDENE on labor and delivery in pregnant women are unknown.

Nursing Mothers
Piroxicam is excreted into human milk. The presence in breast milk has been determined during initial and long-term conditions (52 days). Piroxicam appeared in breast milk at about 1% to 3% of the maternal concentration. No accumulation of piroxicam occurred in milk relative to that in plasma during treatment. FELDENE is not recommended for use in nursing mothers.

Pediatric Use
Safety and effectiveness in pediatric patients have not been established.

Geriatric Use
As with any NSAIDs, caution should be exercised in treating the elderly (65 years and older).

ADVERSE REACTIONS

In patients taking FELDENE or other NSAIDs, the most frequently reported adverse experiences occurring in approximately 1–10% of patients are:
Cardiovascular System: Edema.
Digestive System: Anorexia, abdominal pain, constipation, diarrhea, dyspepsia, elevated liver enzymes, flatulence, gross bleeding/perforation, heartburn, nausea, ulcers (gastric/duodenal), vomiting.
Hemic and Lymphatic System: Anemia, increased bleeding time.
Nervous System: Dizziness, headache.
Skin and Appendages: Pruritus, rash.
Special Senses: Tinnitus.
Urogenital System: Abnormal renal function.
Additional adverse experiences reported occasionally include:
Body As a Whole: Fever, infection, sepsis.
Cardiovascular System: Congestive heart failure, hypertension, tachycardia, syncope.
Digestive System: Dry mouth, esophagitis, gastritis, glossitis, hematemesis, hepatitis, jaundice, melena, rectal bleeding, stomatitis.
Hemic and Lymphatic System: Ecchymosis, eosinophilia, epistaxis, leukopenia, purpura, petechial rash, thrombocytopenia.
Metabolic and Nutritional: Weight changes.
Nervous System: Anxiety, asthenia, confusion, depression, dream abnormalities, drowsiness, insomnia, malaise, nervousness, paresthesia, somnolence, tremors, vertigo.
Respiratory System: Asthma, dyspnea.
Skin and Appendages: Alopecia, bruising, desquamation, erythema, photosensitivity, sweat.
Special Senses: Blurred vision.
Urogenital System: Cystitis, dysuria, hematuria, hyperkalemia, interstitial nephritis, nephrotic syndrome, oliguria/polyuria, proteinuria, renal failure.
Other adverse reactions which occur rarely are:
Body As a Whole: Anaphylactic reactions, appetite changes, death, flu-like syndrome, pain (colic), serum sickness.
Cardiovascular System: Arrhythmia, exacerbation of angina, hypotension, myocardial infarction, palpitations, vasculitis.
Digestive System: Eructation, liver failure, pancreatitis.
Hemic and Lymphatic System: Agranulocytosis, hemolytic anemia, aplastic anemia, lymphadenopathy, pancytopenia.
Hypersensitivity: Positive ANA.
Metabolic and Nutritional: Hyperglycemia, hypoglycemia.
Nervous System: Akathisia, convulsions, coma, hallucinations, meningitis, mood alterations.
Respiratory: Respiratory depression, pneumonia.
Skin and Appendages: Angioedema, toxic epidermal necrosis, erythema multiforme, exfoliative dermatitis, onycholysis, Stevens-Johnson syndrome, urticaria, vesiculobullous reaction.
Special Senses: Conjunctivitis, hearing impairment, swollen eyes.

OVERDOSAGE

Symptoms following acute NSAID overdoses are usually limited to lethargy, drowsiness, nausea, vomiting, and epigastric pain, which are generally reversible with supportive care. Gastrointestinal bleeding can occur. Hypertension, acute renal failure, respiratory depression and coma may occur, but are rare. Anaphylactoid reactions have been reported with therapeutic ingestion of NSAIDs, and may occur following an overdose.
Patients should be managed by symptomatic and supportive care following an NSAID overdose. There are no specific antidotes. Emesis and/or activated charcoal (60–100 g in adults, 1–2 g/kg in children) and/or osmotic cathartic may be indicated. The long plasma half-life of piroxicam should be considered when treating an overdose with piroxicam. Experiments in dogs have demonstrated that the use of multiple-dose treatments with activated charcoal could reduce the half-life of piroxicam by more than 50% and systemic bioavailability by as much as 37% when activated charcoal is given as late as 6 hours after ingestion of piroxicam. Forced diuresis, alkalinization of urine, hemodialysis, or hemoperfusion may not be useful due to high protein binding.

DOSAGE AND ADMINISTRATION

As with other NSAIDs, the lowest dose should be sought for each patient. Therefore, after observing the response to initial therapy with FELDENE, the dose and frequency should be adjusted to suit an individual patient's needs.

For the relief of rheumatoid arthritis and osteoarthritis, the recommended dose is 20 mg given orally once per day. If desired, the daily dose may be divided. Because of the long-half-life of FELDENE, steady-state blood levels are not reached for 7–12 days. Therefore, although the therapeutic effects of FELDENE are evident early in treatment, there is a progressive increase in response over several weeks and the effect of therapy should not be assessed for two weeks.

HOW SUPPLIED

FELDENE® Capsules for oral administration:
Bottles of 100: 10 mg (NDC 0069-3220-66) maroon and blue #322,
20 mg (NDC 0069-3230-66) maroon #323.
Bottles of 500: 20 mg (NDC 0069-3230-73) maroon #323.
Rx only.

Pfizer Labs
Division of Pfizer Inc, NY, NY 10017

65-4100-00-6

Revised June 1999

Shown in Product Identification Guide, page 330

GEOCILLIN® ℞

[gē ′ō-sil-ĭn]
(carbenicillin indanyl sodium)
TABLETS
For Oral Use

DESCRIPTION

Geocillin, a semisynthetic penicillin, is the sodium salt of the indanyl ester of Geopen® (carbenicillin disodium). The chemical name is:
1-(5-Indanyl)-N-(2-carboxy-3,3-dimethyl-7-oxo-4-thia-1-azabicyclo[3.2.0]hept-6-yl)-2-phenylmalonamate monosodium salt.
The structural formula is:

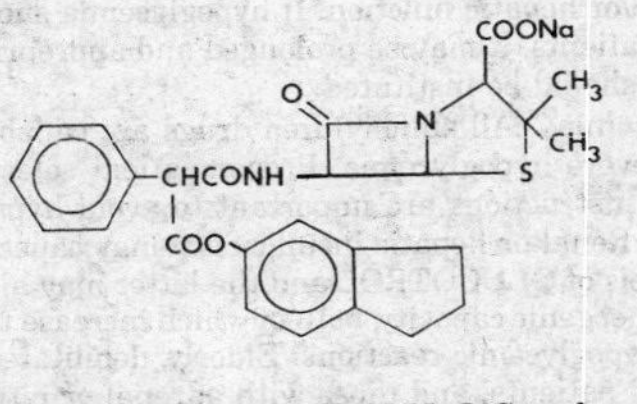

The empirical formula is: $C_{26}H_{25}N_2NaO_6S$ and mol. wt. is 516.55.

Geocillin tablets are yellow, capsule-shaped and film-coated, made of a white crystalline solid. Carbenicillin is freely soluble in water. Each Geocillin tablet contains 382 mg of carbenicillin, 118 mg of indanyl sodium ester. Each Geocillin tablet contains 23 mg of sodium.

Inert ingredients are: glycine; magnesium stearate and sodium lauryl sulfate. May also include the following: hydroxypropyl cellulose; hydroxypropyl methylcellulose; opaspray (which may include Blue 2 Lake, Yellow 6 Lake, Yellow 10 Lake, and other inert ingredients); opadry light yellow (which may contain D&C Yellow 10 Lake, FD&C Yellow 6 Lake and other inert ingredients); opadry clear (which may contain other inert ingredients).

CLINICAL PHARMACOLOGY

Free carbenicillin is the predominant pharmacologically active fraction of Geocillin. Carbenicillin exerts its antibacterial activity by interference with final cell wall synthesis of susceptible bacteria.

Geocillin is acid stable, and rapidly absorbed from the small intestine following oral administration. It provides relatively low plasma concentrations of antibiotic and is primarily excreted in the urine. After absorption, Geocillin is rapidly converted to carbenicillin by hydrolysis of the ester linkage. Following ingestion of a single 500 mg tablet of Geocillin, a peak carbenicillin plasma concentration of approximately 6.5 mcg/ml is reached in 1 hour. About 30% of this dose is excreted in the urine unchanged within 12 hours, with another 6% excreted over the next 12 hours.

In a multiple dose study utilizing volunteers with normal renal function, the following mean urine and serum levels of carbenicillin were achieved:

[See table above]

Microbiology

The antibacterial activity of Geocillin is due to its rapid conversion to carbenicillin by hydrolysis after absorption. Though Geocillin provides substantial *in vitro* activity against a variety of both gram-positive and gram-negative microorganisms, the most important aspect of its profile is in its antipseudomonal and antiproteal activity. Because of the high urine levels obtained following administration, Geocillin has demonstrated clinical efficacy in urinary infections due to susceptible strains of:

Escherichia coli
Proteus mirabilis
Proteus vulgaris

Mean Urine Concentration of Carbenicillin mcg/ml Hours After Initial Dose

DRUG	DOSE	0–3	3–6	6–24
Geocillin	1 tablet q.6 hr	1130	352	292
Geocillin	2 tablets q.6 hr	1428	789	809

Mean serum concentrations of carbenicillin in this study for these dosages are:

Mean Serum Concentration mcg/ml Hours After Initial Dose

DRUG	DOSE	$\frac{1}{2}$	1	2	4	6	24	25	26	28
Geocillin	1 tablet q.6 hr	5.1	6.5	3.2	1.9	0.0	0.4	8.8	5.4	0.4
Geocillin	2 tablets q.6 hr	6.1	9.6	7.9	2.6	0.4	0.8	13.2	12.8	3.8

Morganella morganii (formerly *Proteus morganii*)
Pseudomonas species
Providencia rettgeri (formerly *Proteus rettgeri*)
Enterobacter species
Enterococci (*S. faecalis*)

In addition, *in vitro* data, not substantiated by clinical studies, indicate the following pathogens to be usually susceptible to Geocillin:

Staphylococcus species (nonpenicillinase producing)
Streptococcus species

Resistance

Most *Klebsiella* species are usually resistant to the action of Geocillin. Some strains of *Pseudomonas* species have developed resistance to carbenicillin.

Susceptibility Testing

Geopen (carbenicillin disodium) Susceptibility Powder or 100 ug Geopen Susceptibility Discs may be used to determine microbial susceptibility to Geocillin using one of the following standard methods recommended by the National Committee for Clinical Laboratory Standards:
M2-A3, "Performance Standards for Antimicrobial Disk Susceptibility Tests"
M7-A, "Methods for Dilution Antimicrobial Susceptibility Tests for Bacteria that Grow Aerobically"
M11-A, "Reference Agar Dilution Procedure for Antimicrobial Susceptibility Testing of Anaerobic Bacteria"
M17-P, "Alternative Methods for Antimicrobial Susceptibility Testing of Anaerobic Bacteria"
Tests should be interpreted by the following criteria:

Disk Diffusion Zone diameter (mm)

Organisms	Suscept.	Intermed.	Resist.
Enterobacter	≥23	18–22	≤17
Pseudomonas sp.	≥17	14–16	≤13

Dilution MIC (μ/ml)

Organisms	Suscept.	Moderately Suscept.	Resist.
Enterobacter	≤16	32	≥64
Pseudomonas sp.	≥128	—	≥156

Interpretations of susceptible, intermediate, and resistant correlate zone size diameters with MIC values. A laboratory report of "susceptible" indicates that the suspected causative microorganism most likely will respond to therapy with carbenicillin. A laboratory report of "resistant" indicates that the infecting microorganism most likely will not respond to therapy. A laboratory report of "moderately susceptible" indicates that the microorganism is most likely susceptible if a high dosage of carbenicillin is used, or if the infection is such that high levels of carbenicillin may be attained as in urine. A report of "intermediate" using the disk diffusion method may be considered an equivocal result, and dilution tests may be indicated.

INDICATIONS AND USAGE

Geocillin (carbenicillin indanyl sodium) is indicated in the treatment of acute and chronic infections of the upper and lower urinary tract and in asymptomatic bacteriuria due to susceptible strains of the following organisms:

Escherichia coli
Proteus mirabilis
Morganella morganii
(formerly *Proteus morganii*)
Providencia rettgeri
(formerly *Proteus rettgeri*)
Proteus vulgaris
Pseudomonas
Enterobacter
Enterococci

Geocillin is also indicated in the treatment of prostatitis due to susceptible strains of the following organisms:

Escherichia coli
Enterococcus (*S. faecalis*)
Proteus mirabilis
Enterobacter sp.

WHEN HIGH AND RAPID BLOOD AND URINE LEVELS OF ANTIBIOTIC ARE INDICATED, THERAPY WITH GEOPEN (CARBENICILLIN DISODIUM) SHOULD BE INITIATED BY PARENTERAL ADMINISTRATION FOLLOWED, AT THE PHYSICIAN'S DISCRETION, BY ORAL THERAPY.

NOTE: Susceptibility testing should be performed prior to and during the course of therapy to detect the possible emergence of resistant organisms which may develop.

CONTRAINDICATIONS

Geocillin is ordinarily contraindicated in patients who have a known penicillin allergy.

WARNINGS

Serious and occasionally fatal hypersensitivity (anaphylactic) reactions have been reported in patients on oral penicillin therapy. Although anaphylaxis is more frequent following parenteral therapy, it has occurred in patients on oral penicillins. These reactions are more apt to occur in individuals with a history of penicillin hypersensitivity and/or a history of sensitivity to multiple allergens.

There have been reports of individuals with a history of penicillin hypersensitivity who have experienced severe hypersensitivity reactions when treated with a cephalosporin, and vice versa. Before initiating therapy with a penicillin, careful inquiry should be made concerning previous hypersensitivity reactions to penicillins, cephalosporins, or other allergens. If an allergic reaction occurs, the drug should be discontinued and the appropriate therapy instituted.

SERIOUS ANAPHYLACTOID REACTIONS REQUIRE IMMEDIATE EMERGENCY TREATMENT WITH EPINEPHRINE. OXYGEN, INTRAVENOUS STEROIDS AND AIRWAY MANAGEMENT, INCLUDING INTUBATION, SHOULD ALSO BE ADMINISTERED AS INDICATED.

PRECAUTIONS

General: As with any penicillin preparation, an allergic response, including anaphylaxis, may occur particularly in a hypersensitive individual.

Long term use of Geocillin may result in the overgrowth of nonsusceptible organisms. If superinfection occurs during therapy, appropriate measures should be taken.

Since carbenicillin is primarily excreted by the kidney, patients with severe renal impairment (creatinine clearance of less than 10 ml/min) will not achieve therapeutic urine levels of carbenicillin.

In patients with creatinine clearance of 10–20 ml/min it may be necessary to adjust dosage to prevent accumulation of drug.

Laboratory Tests: As with other penicillins, periodic assessment of organ system function including renal, hepatic, and hematopoietic systems is recommended during prolonged therapy.

Drug Interactions: Geocillin (carbenicillin indanyl sodium) blood levels may be increased and prolonged by concurrent administration of probenecid.

Carcinogenesis, Mutagenesis, Impairment of Fertility: There are no long-term animal or human studies to evaluate carcinogenic potential. Rats fed 250–1000 mg/kg/day for 18 months developed mild liver pathology (e.g., bile duct hyperplasia) at all dose levels, but there was no evidence of drug-related neoplasia. Geocillin administered at daily doses ranging to 1000 mg/kg had no apparent effect on the fertility or reproductive performance of rats.

Pregnancy Category B: Reproduction studies have been performed at dose levels of 1000 or 500 mg/kg in rats, 200 mg/kg in mice, and at 500 mg/kg in monkeys with no harm to fetus due to Geocillin. There are, however, no adequate and well controlled studies in pregnant women. Because animal reproduction studies are not always predictive of human response, this drug should be used during pregnancy only if clearly needed.

Labor and Delivery: It is not known whether the use of Geocillin in humans during labor or delivery has immediate or delayed adverse effects on the fetus, prolongs the duration of labor, or increases the likelihood that forceps delivery or other obstetrical intervention or resuscitation of the newborn will be necessary.

Nursing Mothers: Carbenicillin class antibiotics are excreted in milk although the amounts excreted are unknown; therefore, caution should be exercised if administered to a nursing woman.

Pediatric Use: Since only limited clinical data is available to date in children, the safety of Geocillin administration in this age group has not yet been established.

Continued on next page

Geocillin—Cont.

ADVERSE REACTIONS

The following adverse reactions have been reported as possibly related to Geocillin administration in controlled studies which include 344 patients receiving Geocillin.

Gastrointestinal: The most frequent adverse reactions associated with Geocillin therapy are related to the gastrointestinal tract. Nausea, bad taste, diarrhea, vomiting, flatulence, and glossitis were reported. Abdominal cramps, dry mouth, furry tongue, rectal bleeding, anorexia, and unspecified epigastric distress were rarely reported.

Dermatologic: Hypersensitivity reactions such as skin rash, urticaria, and less frequently pruritus.

Hematologic: As with other penicillins, anemia, thrombocytopenia, leukopenia, neutropenia, and eosinophilia have infrequently been observed. The clinical significance of these abnormalities is not known.

Miscellaneous: Other reactions rarely reported were hyperthermia, headache, itchy eyes, vaginitis, and loose stools.

Abnormalities of Hepatic Function Tests: Mild SGOT elevations have been observed following Geocillin administration.

OVERDOSAGE

Geocillin is generally nontoxic. Geocillin when taken in excessive amounts may produce mild gastrointestinal irritation. The drug is rapidly excreted in the urine and symptoms are transitory. The usual symptoms of anaphylaxis may occur in hypersensitive individuals.

Carbenicillin blood levels achievable with Geocillin are very low, and toxic reactions as a function of overdosage should not occur systematically. The oral LD_{50} in mice is 3,600 mg/kg, in rats 2,000 mg/kg, and in dogs is in excess of 500 mg/kg. The lethal human dose is not known.

Although never reported, the possibility of accumulation of indanyl should be considered when large amounts of Geocillin are ingested. Free indole, which is a phenol derivative, may be potentially toxic. In general 8–15 grams of phenol, and presumably a similar amount of indole, are required orally before toxicity (peripheral vascular collapse) may occur. The metabolic by-products of indole are nontoxic. In patients with hepatic failure it may be possible for unmetabolized indole to accumulate.

The metabolic by-products of Geocillin, indanyl sulfate and glucuronide, as well as free carbenicillin, are dialyzable.

DOSAGE AND ADMINISTRATION

Geocillin is available as a coated tablet to be administered orally.

Usual Adult Dose

URINARY TRACT INFECTIONS	
Escherichia coli, Proteus species, and *Enterobacter*	1–2 tablets 4 times daily
Pseudomonas and *Enterococcus*	2 tablets 4 times daily
PROSTATITIS	
Escherichia coli, Proteus mirabilis, Enterobacter and *Enterococcus*	2 tablets 4 times daily

HOW SUPPLIED

Geocillin is available as film-coated tablets in bottles of 100's (NDC 0049-1430-66), and unit-dose packages of 100 (10 × 10's) (NDC 0049-1430-41). Each tablet contains carbenicillin indanyl sodium equivalent to 382 mg of carbenicillin.

Revised Sept. 1991 69-1970-00-2

GLUCOTROL® ℞

[glū 'kă-trōl]
(glipizide)
TABLETS
For Oral Use

DESCRIPTION

GLUCOTROL (glipizide) is an oral blood-glucose-lowering drug of the sulfonylurea class.

The Chemical Abstracts name of glipizide is 1-cyclohexyl-3-[[p- [2-(5-methylpyrazinecarboxamido)ethyl]phenyl] sulfonyl]urea. The molecular formula is $C_{21}H_{27}N_5O_4S$; the molecular weight is 445.55; the structural formula is shown below:

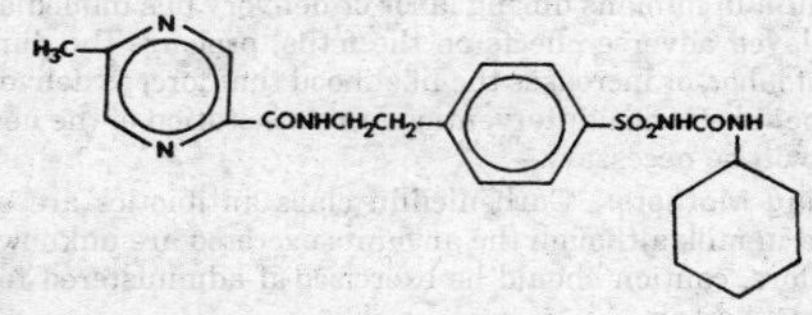

Glipizide is a whitish, odorless powder with a pKa of 5.9. It is insoluble in water and alcohols, but soluble in 0.1 *N* NaOH; it is freely soluble in dimethylformamide. GLUCOTROL tablets for oral use are available in 5 and 10 mg strengths.

Inert ingredients are: colloidal silicon dioxide; lactose; microcrystalline cellulose; starch; stearic acid.

CLINICAL PHARMACOLOGY

Mechanism of Action: The primary mode of action of GLUCOTROL in experimental animals appears to be the stimulation of insulin secretion from the beta cells of pancreatic islet tissue and is thus dependent on functioning beta cells in the pancreatic islets. In humans GLUCOTROL appears to lower the blood glucose acutely by stimulating the release of insulin from the pancreas, an effect dependent upon functioning beta cells in the pancreatic islets. The mechanism by which GLUCOTROL lowers blood glucose during long-term administration has not been clearly established. In man, stimulation of insulin secretion by GLUCOTROL in response to a meal is undoubtedly of major importance. Fasting insulin levels are not elevated even on long-term GLUCOTROL administration, but the postprandial insulin response continues to be enhanced after at least 6 months of treatment. The insulinotropic response to a meal occurs within 30 minutes after an oral dose of GLUCOTROL in diabetic patients, but elevated insulin levels do not persist beyond the time of the meal challenge. Extrapancreatic effects may play a part in the mechanism of action of oral sulfonylurea hypoglycemic drugs.

Blood sugar control persists in some patients for up to 24 hours after a single dose of GLUCOTROL, even though plasma levels have declined to a small fraction of peak levels by that time (see Pharmacokinetics below).

Some patients fail to respond initially, or gradually lose their responsiveness to sulfonylurea drugs, including GLUCOTROL. Alternatively, GLUCOTROL may be effective in some patients who have not responded or have ceased to respond to other sulfonylureas.

Other Effects: It has been shown that GLUCOTROL therapy was effective in controlling blood sugar without deleterious changes in the plasma lipoprotein profiles of patients treated for NIDDM.

In a placebo-controlled, crossover study in normal volunteers, GLUCOTROL had no antidiuretic activity, and, in fact, led to a slight increase in free water clearance.

Pharmacokinetics: Gastrointestinal absorption of GLUCOTROL in man is uniform, rapid, and essentially complete. Peak plasma concentrations occur 1–3 hours after a single oral dose. The half-life of elimination ranges from 2–4 hours in normal subjects, whether given intravenously or orally. The metabolic and excretory patterns are similar with the two routes of administration, indicating that first-pass metabolism is not significant. GLUCOTROL does not accumulate in plasma on repeated oral administration. Total absorption and disposition of an oral dose was unaffected by food in normal volunteers, but absorption was delayed by about 40 minutes. Thus GLUCOTROL was more effective when administered about 30 minutes before, rather than with, a test meal in diabetic patients. Protein binding was studied in serum from volunteers who received either oral or intravenous GLUCOTROL and found to be 98–99% one hour after either route of administration. The apparent volume of distribution of GLUCOTROL after intravenous administration was 11 liters, indicative of localization within the extracellular fluid compartment. In mice no GLUCOTROL or metabolites were detectable autoradiographically in the brain or spinal cord of males or females, nor in the fetuses of pregnant females. In another study, however, very small amounts of radioactivity were detected in the fetuses of rats given labelled drug.

The metabolism of GLUCOTROL is extensive and occurs mainly in the liver. The primary metabolites are inactive hydroxylation products and polar conjugates and are excreted mainly in the urine. Less than 10% unchanged GLUCOTROL is found in the urine.

INDICATIONS AND USAGE

GLUCOTROL is indicated as an adjunct to diet for the control of hyperglycemia and its associated symptomatology in patients with non-insulin-dependent diabetes mellitus (NIDDM; type II), formerly known as maturity-onset diabetes, after an adequate trial of dietary therapy has proved unsatisfactory.

In initiating treatment for non-insulin-dependent diabetes, diet should be emphasized as the primary form of treatment. Caloric restriction and weight loss are essential in the obese diabetic patient. Proper dietary management alone may be effective in controlling the blood glucose and symptoms of hyperglycemia. The importance of regular physical activity should also be stressed, and cardiovascular risk factors should be identified, and corrective measures taken where possible.

If this treatment program fails to reduce symptoms and/or blood glucose, the use of an oral sulfonylurea or insulin should be considered. Use of GLUCOTROL must be viewed by both the physician and patient as a treatment in addition to diet, and not as a substitute for diet or as a convenient mechanism for avoiding dietary restraint. Furthermore, loss of blood glucose control on diet alone also may be transient, thus requiring only short-term administration of GLUCOTROL.

During maintenance programs, GLUCOTROL should be discontinued if satisfactory lowering of blood glucose is no longer achieved. Judgments should be based on regular clinical and laboratory evaluations.

In considering the use of GLUCOTROL in asymptomatic patients, it should be recognized that controlling blood glucose in non-insulin-dependent diabetes has not been definitely established to be effective in preventing the long-term cardiovascular or neural complications of diabetes.

CONTRAINDICATIONS

GLUCOTROL is contraindicated in patients with:

1. Known hypersensitivity to the drug.
2. Diabetic ketoacidosis, with or without coma. This condition should be treated with insulin.

WARNINGS

SPECIAL WARNING ON INCREASED RISK OF CARDIOVASCULAR MORTALITY: The administration of oral hypoglycemic drugs has been reported to be associated with increased cardiovascular mortality as compared to treatment with diet alone or diet plus insulin. This warning is based on the study conducted by the University Group Diabetes Program (UGDP), a long-term prospective clinical trial designed to evaluate the effectiveness of glucose-lowering drugs in preventing or delaying vascular complications in patients with non-insulin-dependent diabetes. The study involved 823 patients who were randomly assigned to one of four treatment groups (*Diabetes,* 19, supp. 2: 747–830, 1970). UGDP reported that patients treated for 5 to 8 years with diet plus a fixed dose of tolbutamide (1.5 grams per day) had a rate of cardiovascular mortality approximately $2^1/_2$ times that of patients treated with diet alone. A significant increase in total mortality was not observed, but the use of tolbutamide was discontinued based on the increase in cardiovascular mortality, thus limiting the opportunity for the study to show an increase in overall mortality. Despite controversy regarding the interpretation of these results, the findings of the UGDP study provide an adequate basis for this warning. The patient should be informed of the potential risks and advantages of GLUCOTROL and of alternative modes of therapy.

Although only one drug in the sulfonylurea class (tolbutamide) was included in this study, it is prudent from a safety standpoint to consider that this warning may also apply to other oral hypoglycemic drugs in this class, in view of their close similarities in mode of action and chemical structure.

PRECAUTIONS

General

Renal and Hepatic Disease: The metabolism and excretion of GLUCOTROL may be slowed in patients with impaired renal and/or hepatic function. If hypoglycemia should occur in such patients, it may be prolonged and appropriate management should be instituted.

Hypoglycemia: All sulfonylurea drugs are capable of producing severe hypoglycemia. Proper patient selection, dosage, and instructions are important to avoid hypoglycemic episodes. Renal or hepatic insufficiency may cause elevated blood levels of GLUCOTROL and the latter may also diminish gluconeogenic capacity, both of which increase the risk of serious hypoglycemic reactions. Elderly, debilitated or malnourished patients, and those with adrenal or pituitary insufficiency are particularly susceptible to the hypoglycemic action of glucose-lowering drugs. Hypoglycemia may be difficult to recognize in the elderly, and in people who are taking beta-adrenergic blocking drugs. Hypoglycemia is more likely to occur when caloric intake is deficient, after severe or prolonged exercise, when alcohol is ingested, or when more than one glucose-lowering drug is used.

Loss of Control of Blood Glucose: When a patient stabilized on any diabetic regimen is exposed to stress such as fever, trauma, infection, or surgery, a loss of control may occur. At such times, it may be necessary to discontinue GLUCOTROL and administer insulin.

The effectiveness of any oral hypoglycemic drug, including GLUCOTROL, in lowering blood glucose to a desired level decreases in many patients over a period of time, which may be due to progression of the severity of the diabetes or to diminished responsiveness to the drug. This phenomenon is known as secondary failure, to distinguish it from primary failure in which the drug is ineffective in an individual patient when first given.

Laboratory Tests: Blood and urine glucose should be monitored periodically. Measurement of glycosylated hemoglobin may be useful.

Information for Patients: Patients should be informed of the potential risks and advantages of GLUCOTROL and of alternative modes of therapy. They should also be informed about the importance of adhering to dietary instructions, of a regular exercise program, and of regular testing of urine and/or blood glucose.

The risks of hypoglycemia, its symptoms and treatment, and conditions that predispose to its development should be explained to patients and responsible family members. Primary and secondary failure should also be explained.

Drug Interactions: The hypoglycemic action of sulfonylureas may be potentiated by certain drugs including nonsteroidal anti-inflammatory agents, some azoles, and other drugs that are highly protein bound, salicylates, sulfonamides, chloramphenicol, probenecid, coumarins, monoamine oxidase inhibitors, and beta adrenergic blocking agents. When such drugs are administered to a patient receiving GLUCOTROL, the patient should be observed closely for hypoglycemia. When such drugs are withdrawn from a patient receiving GLUCOTROL, the patient should be observed closely for loss of control. *In vitro* binding studies with human serum proteins indicate that GLUCOTROL binds differently than tolbutamide and does not interact with salicylate or dicumarol. However, caution must be ex-

ercised in extrapolating these findings to the clinical situation and in the use of GLUCOTROL with these drugs.
Certain drugs tend to produce hyperglycemia and may lead to loss of control. These drugs include the thiazides and other diuretics, corticosteroids, phenothiazines, thyroid products, estrogens, oral contraceptives, phenytoin, nicotinic acid, sympathomimetics, calcium channel blocking drugs, and isoniazid. When such drugs are administered to a patient receiving GLUCOTROL, the patient should be closely observed for loss of control. When such drugs are withdrawn from a patient receiving GLUCOTROL, the patient should be observed closely for hypoglycemia.
A potential interaction between oral miconazole and oral hypoglycemic agents leading to severe hypoglycemia has been reported. Whether this interaction also occurs with the intravenous, topical, or vaginal preparations of miconazole is not known. The effect of concomitant administration of DIFLUCAN (fluconazole) and GLUCOTROL has been demonstrated in a placebo-controlled crossover study in normal volunteers. All subjects received GLUCOTROL alone and following treatment with 100 mg of DIFLUCAN as a single daily oral dose for 7 days. The mean percentage increase in the GLUCOTROL AUC after fluconazole administration was 56.9% (range: 35 to 81).
Carcinogenesis, Mutagenesis, Impairment of Fertility: A twenty month study in rats and an eighteen month study in mice at doses up to 75 times the maximum human dose revealed no evidence of drug-related carcinogenicity. Bacterial and *in vivo* mutagenicity tests were uniformly negative. Studies in rats of both sexes at doses up to 75 times the human dose showed no effects on fertility.
Pregnancy: Pregnancy Category C: GLUCOTROL (glipizide) was found to be mildly fetotoxic in rat reproductive studies at all dose levels (5–50 mg/kg). This fetotoxicity has been similarly noted with other sulfonylureas, such as tolbutamide and tolazamide. The effect is perinatal and believed to be directly related to the pharmacologic (hypoglycemic) action of GLUCOTROL. In studies in rats and rabbits no teratogenic effects were found. There are no adequate and well controlled studies in pregnant women. GLUCOTROL should be used during pregnancy only if the potential benefit justifies the potential risk to the fetus.
Because recent information suggests that abnormal blood glucose levels during pregnancy are associated with a higher incidence of congenital abnormalities, many experts recommend that insulin be used during pregnancy to maintain blood glucose levels as close to normal as possible.
Nonteratogenic Effects: Prolonged severe hypoglycemia (4 to 10 days) has been reported in neonates born to mothers who were receiving a sulfonylurea drug at the time of delivery. This has been reported more frequently with the use of agents with prolonged half-lives. If GLUCOTROL is used during pregnancy, it should be discontinued at least one month before the expected delivery date.
Nursing Mothers: Although it is not known whether GLUCOTROL is excreted in human milk, some sulfonylurea drugs are known to be excreted in human milk. Because the potential for hypoglycemia in nursing infants may exist, a decision should be made whether to discontinue nursing or to discontinue the drug, taking into account the importance of the drug to the mother. If the drug is discontinued and if diet alone is inadequate for controlling blood glucose, insulin therapy should be considered.
Pediatric Use: Safety and effectiveness in children have not been established.

ADVERSE REACTIONS

In U.S. and foreign controlled studies, the frequency of serious adverse reactions reported was very low. Of 702 patients, 11.8% reported adverse reactions and in only 1.5% was GLUCOTROL discontinued.
Hypoglycemia: See PRECAUTIONS and OVERDOSAGE sections.
Gastrointestinal: Gastrointestinal disturbances are the most common reactions. Gastrointestinal complaints were reported with the following approximate incidence: nausea and diarrhea, one in seventy; constipation and gastralgia, one in one hundred. They appear to be dose-related and may disappear on division or reduction of dosage. Cholestatic jaundice may occur rarely with sulfonylureas: GLUCOTROL should be discontinued if this occurs.
Dermatologic: Allergic skin reactions including erythema, morbilliform or maculopapular eruptions, urticaria, pruritus, and eczema have been reported in about one in seventy patients. These may be transient and may disappear despite continued use of GLUCOTROL; if skin reactions persist, the drug should be discontinued. Porphyria cutanea tarda and photosensitivity reactions have been reported with sulfonylureas.
Hematologic: Leukopenia, agranulocytosis, thrombocytopenia, hemolytic anemia, aplastic anemia, and pancytopenia have been reported with sulfonylureas.
Metabolic: Hepatic porphyria and disulfiram-like reactions have been reported with sulfonylureas. In the mouse, GLUCOTROL pretreatment did not cause an accumulation of acetaldehyde after ethanol administration. Clinical experience to date has shown that GLUCOTROL has an extremely low incidence of disulfiram-like alcohol reactions.
Endocrine Reactions: Cases of hyponatremia and the syndrome of inappropriate antidiuretic hormone (SIADH) secretion have been reported with this and other sulfonylureas.
Miscellaneous: Dizziness, drowsiness, and headache have each been reported in about one in fifty patients treated with GLUCOTROL. They are usually transient and seldom require discontinuance of therapy.
Laboratory Tests: The pattern of laboratory test abnormalities observed with GLUCOTROL was similar to that for other sulfonylureas. Occasional mild to moderate elevations of SGOT, LDH, alkaline phosphatase, BUN and creatinine were noted. One case of jaundice was reported. The relationship of these abnormalities to GLUCOTROL is uncertain, and they have rarely been associated with clinical symptoms.

OVERDOSAGE

There is no well documented experience with GLUCOTROL overdosage. The acute oral toxicity was extremely low in all species tested (LD_{50} greater than 4 g/kg).
Overdosage of sulfonylureas including GLUCOTROL can produce hypoglycemia. Mild hypoglycemic symptoms without loss of consciousness or neurologic findings should be treated aggressively with oral glucose and adjustments in drug dosage and/or meal patterns. Close monitoring should continue until the physician is assured that the patient is out of danger. Severe hypoglycemic reactions with coma, seizure, or other neurological impairment occur infrequently, but constitute medical emergencies requiring immediate hospitalization. If hypoglycemic coma is diagnosed or suspected, the patient should be given a rapid intravenous injection of concentrated (50%) glucose solution. This should be followed by a continuous infusion of a more dilute (10%) glucose solution at a rate that will maintain the blood glucose at a level above 100 mg/dL. Patients should be closely monitored for a minimum of 24 to 48 hours since hypoglycemia may recur after apparent clinical recovery. Clearance of GLUCOTROL from plasma would be prolonged in persons with liver disease. Because of the extensive protein binding of GLUCOTROL, dialysis is unlikely to be of benefit.

DOSAGE AND ADMINISTRATION

There is no fixed dosage regimen for the management of diabetes mellitus with GLUCOTROL or any other hypoglycemic agent. In addition to the usual monitoring of urinary glucose, the patient's blood glucose must also be monitored periodically to determine the minimum effective dose for the patient; to detect primary failure, i.e., inadequate lowering of blood glucose at the maximum recommended dose of medication; and to detect secondary failure, i.e., loss of an adequate blood-glucose-lowering response after an initial period of effectiveness. Glycosylated hemoglobin levels may also be of value in monitoring the patient's response to therapy.
Short-term administration of GLUCOTROL may be sufficient during periods of transient loss of control in patients usually controlled well on diet.
In general, GLUCOTROL should be given approximately 30 minutes before a meal to achieve the greatest reduction in postprandial hyperglycemia.
Initial Dose: The recommended starting dose is 5 mg, given before breakfast. Geriatric patients or those with liver disease may be started on 2.5 mg.
Titration: Dosage adjustments should ordinarily be in increments of 2.5–5 mg, as determined by blood glucose response. At least several days should elapse between titration steps. If response to a single dose is not satisfactory, dividing that dose may prove effective. The maximum recommended once daily dose is 15 mg. Doses above 15 mg should ordinarily be divided and given before meals of adequate caloric content. The maximum recommended total daily dose is 40 mg.
Maintenance: Some patients may be effectively controlled on a once-a-day regimen, while others show better response with divided dosing. Total daily doses above 15 mg should ordinarily be divided. Total daily doses above 30 mg have been safely given on a b.i.d. basis to long-term patients.
In elderly patients, debilitated or malnourished patients, and patients with impaired renal or hepatic function, the initial and maintenance dosing should be conservative to avoid hypoglycemic reactions (see PRECAUTIONS section).
Patients Receiving Insulin: As with other sulfonylurea-class hypoglycemics, many stable non-insulin-dependent diabetic patients receiving insulin may be safely placed on GLUCOTROL. When transferring patients from insulin to GLUCOTROL, the following general guidelines should be considered:

For patients whose daily insulin requirement is 20 units or less, insulin may be discontinued and GLUCOTROL therapy may begin at usual dosages. Several days should elapse between GLUCOTROL titration steps.

For patients whose daily insulin requirement is greater than 20 units, the insulin dose should be reduced by 50% and GLUCOTROL therapy may begin at usual dosages. Subsequent reductions in insulin dosage should depend on individual patient response. Several days should elapse between GLUCOTROL titration steps.

During the insulin withdrawal period, the patient should test urine samples for sugar and ketone bodies at least three times daily. Patients should be instructed to contact the prescriber immediately if these tests are abnormal. In some cases, especially when patient has been receiving greater than 40 units of insulin daily, it may be advisable to consider hospitalization during the transition period.
Patients Receiving Other Oral Hypoglycemic Agents: As with other sulfonylurea-class hypoglycemics, no transition period is necessary when transferring patients to GLUCOTROL. Patients should be observed carefully (1–2 weeks) for hypoglycemia when being transferred from longer half-life sulfonylureas (e.g., chlorpropamide) to GLUCOTROL due to potential overlapping of drug effect.

HOW SUPPLIED

GLUCOTROL tablets are white, dye-free, scored, diamond-shaped, and imprinted as follows:
5 mg–Pfizer 411; 10 mg–Pfizer 412.
5 mg Bottles: 100's (NDC 0049-4110-66) (NDC 59012-411-66);
500's (NDC 0049-4110-73) (NDC 59012-411-73);
UNIT DOSE 100's (NDC 0049-4110-41) (NDC 59012-411-41).
10 mg Bottles: 100's (NDC 0049-4120-66) (NDC 59012-412-66);
500's (NDC 0049-4120-73) (NDC 59012-412-73);
UNIT DOSE 100's (NDC 0049-4120-41) (NDC 59012-412-41).
RECOMMENDED STORAGE: Store below 86°F (30°C).
CAUTION: Federal law prohibits dispensing without a prescription.
Rev. Jan 1993 69-4856-00-9

Shown in Product Identification Guide, page 330

GLUCOTROL XL® ℞
(glipizide)
Extended Release Tablets
For Oral Use

DESCRIPTION

Glipizide is an oral blood-glucose-lowering drug of the sulfonylurea class.
The Chemical Abstracts name of glipizide is 1-cyclo-hexyl-3-[[p-[2-(5-methylpyrazinecarboxamido)-ethyl]-phenyl]sulfonyl]urea. The molecular formula is $C_{21}H_{27}N_5O_4S$; the molecular weight is 445.55; the structural formula is shown below:

Glipizide is a whitish, odorless powder with a pKa of 5.9. It is insoluble in water and alcohols, but soluble in 0.1 N NaOH; it is freely soluble in dimethylformamide. GLUCOTROL XL® is a registered trademark for glipizide GITS. Glipizide GITS (Gastrointestinal Therapeutic System) is formulated as a once-a-day controlled release tablet for oral use and is designed to deliver 2.5, 5, or 10 mg of glipizide. Inert ingredients in the 2.5 mg, 5 mg and 10 mg formulations are: polyethylene oxide, hydroxpropyl methylcellulose, magnesium stearate, sodium chloride, red ferric oxide, cellulose acetate, polyethylene glycol, opadry blue (OY-LS-20921) (2.5 mg tablets), opadry white (YS-2-7063) (5 mg and 10 mg tablet) and black ink (S-1-8106).
System Components and Performance
GLUCOTROL XL Extended Release Tablet is similar in appearance to a conventional tablet. It consists, however, of an osmotically active drug core surrounded by a semipermeable membrane. The core itself is divided into two layers: an "active" layer containing the drug, and a "push" layer containing pharmacologically inert (but osmotically active) components. The membrane surrounding the tablet is permeable to water but not to drug or osmotic excipients. As water from the gastrointestinal tract enters the tablet, pressure increases in the osmotic layer and "pushes" against the drug layer, resulting in the release of drug through a small, laser-drilled orifice in the membrane on the drug side of the tablet.
The GLUCOTROL XL Extended Release Tablet is designed to provide a controlled rate of delivery of glipizide into the gastrointestinal lumen which is independent of pH or gastroinestinal motility. The function of the GLUCOTROL XL Extended Release Tablet depends upon the existence of an osmotic gradient between the contents of the bi-layer core and fluid in the GI tract. Drug delivery is essentially constant as long as the osmotic gradient remains constant, and then gradually falls to zero. The biologically inert components of the tablet remain intact during GI transit and are eliminated in the feces as an insoluble shell.

CLINICAL PHARMACOLOGY

Mechanism of Action: Glipizide appears to lower blood glucose acutely by stimulating the release of insulin from the pancreas, an effect dependent upon functioning beta cells in the pancreatic islets. Extrapancreatic effects also may play a part in the mechanism of action of oral sulfonylurea hypoglycemic drugs. Two extrapancreatic effects shown to be important in the action of glipizide are an increase in insulin sensitivity and a decrease in hepatic glucose production. However, the mechanism by which glipizide lowers blood glucose during long-term administration has not been clearly established. Stimulation of insulin secretion by glipizide in response to a meal is of major importance. The insulinotropic response to a meal is enhanced with GLUCOTROL XL administration in diabetic patients. The postprandial insulin and C-peptide responses continue to be enhanced after at least 6 months of treatment. In 2 randomized, double-blind, dose-response studies comprising a total of 347 patients, there was no significant increase in fasting insulin in all GLUCOTROL XL-treated patients

Continued on next page

Glucotrol XL—Cont.

combined compared to placebo, although minor elevations were observed at some doses. There was no increase in fasting insulin over the long term.

Some patients fail to respond initially, or gradually lose their responsiveness to sulfonylurea drugs, including glipizide. Alternatively, glipizide may be effective in some patients who have not responded or have ceased to respond to other sulfonylureas.

Effects on Blood Glucose

The effectiveness of GLUCOTROL XL Extended Release Tablets in type 2 diabetes at doses from 5–60 mg once daily has been evaluated in 4 therapeutic clinical trials each with long-term open extensions involving a total of 598 patients. Once daily administration of 5, 10 and 20 mg produced statistically significant reductions from placebo in hemoglobin A_{1C}, fasting plasma glucose and postprandial glucose in patients with mild to severe type 2 diabetes. In a pooled analysis of the patients treated with 5 mg and 20 mg, the relationship between dose and GLUCOTROL XL's effect of reducing hemoglobin A_{1C} was not established. However, in the case of fasting plasma glucose patients treated with 20 mg had a statistically significant reduction of fasting plasma glucose compared to the 5 mg-treated group.

The reductions in hemoglobin A_{1C} and fasting plasma glucose were similar in younger and older patients. Efficacy of GLUCOTROL XL was not affected by gender, race or weight (as assessed by body mass index). In long term extension trials, efficacy of GLUCOTROL XL was maintained in 81% of patients for up to 12 months.

In an open, two-way crossover study 132 patients were randomly assigned to either GLUCOTROL XL or Glucotrol® for 8 weeks and then crossed over to the other drug for an additional 8 weeks. GLUCOTROL XL administration resulted in significantly lower fasting plasma glucose levels and equivalent hemoglobin A_{1C} levels, as compared to Glucotrol.

Other Effects: It has been shown that GLUCOTROL XL therapy is effective in controlling blood glucose without deleterious changes in the plasma lipoprotein profiles of patients treated for type 2 diabetes.

In a placebo-controlled, crossover study in normal volunteers, glipizide had no antidiuretic activity, and, in fact, led to a slight increase in free water clearance.

Pharmacokinetics and Metabolism: Glipizide is rapidly and completely absorbed following oral administration in an immediate release dosage form. The absolute bioavailability of glipizide was 100% after single oral doses in patients with type 2 diabetes. Beginning 2 to 3 hours after administration of GLUCOTROL XL Extended Release Tablets, plasma drug concentrations gradually rise reaching maximum concentrations within 6 to 12 hours after dosing. With subsequent once daily dosing of GLUCOTROL XL Extended Release Tablets, effective plasma glipizide concentrations are maintained throughout the 24 hour dosing interval with less peak to trough fluctuation than that observed with twice daily dosing of immediate release glipizide. The mean relative bioavailability of glipizide in 21 males with type 2 diabetes after administration of 20 mg GLUCOTROL XL Extended Release Tablets, compared to immediate release Glucotrol (10 mg given twice daily), was 90% at steady-state. Steady-state plasma concentrations were achieved by at least the fifth day of dosing with GLUCOTROL XL Extended Release Tablets in 21 males with type 2 diabetes and patients younger than 65 years. Approximately 1 to 2 days longer were required to reach steady-state in 24 elderly (≥65 years) males and females with type 2 diabetes. No accumulation of drug was observed in patients with type 2 diabetes during chronic dosing with GLUCOTROL XL Extended Release Tablets. Administration of GLUCOTROL XL with food has no effect on the 2 to 3 hour lag time in drug absorption. In a single dose, food effect study in 21 healthy male subjects, the administration of GLUCOTROL XL immediately before a high fat breakfast resulted in a 40% increase in the glipizide mean Cmax value, which was significant, but the effect on the AUC was not significant. There was no change in glucose response between the fed and fasting state. Markedly reduced GI retention times of the GLUCOTROL XL tablets over prolonged periods (e.g., short bowel syndrome) may influence the pharmacokinetic profile of the drug and potentially result in lower plasma concentrations. In a multiple dose study in 26 males with type 2 diabetes, the pharmacokinetics of glipizide were linear over the dose range of 5 to 60 mg of GLUCOTROL XL in that the plasma drug concentrations increased proportionately with dose. In a single dose study in 24 healthy subjects, four 5 mg, two 10 mg, and one 20 mg GLUCOTROL XL Extended Release Tablets were bioequivalent. In a separate single dose study in 36 healthy subjects, four 2.5-mg GLUCOTROL XL Extended Release Tablets were bioequivalent to one 10-mg GLUCOTROL XL Extended Release Tablet.

Glipizide is eliminated primarily by hepatic biotransformation: less than 10% of a dose is excreted as unchanged drug in urine and feces; approximately 90% of a dose is excreted as biotransformation products in urine (80%) and feces (10%). The major metabolites of glipizide are products of aromatic hydroxylation and have no hypoglycemic activity. A minor metabolite which accounts for less than 2% of a dose, an acetylaminoethyl benzene derivative, is reported to have $^1/_{10}$ to $^1/_3$ as much hypoglycemic activity at the parent compound. The mean total body clearance of glipizide was approximately 3 liters per hour after single intravenous doses in patients with type 2 diabetes. The mean apparent volume of distribution was approximately 10 liters. Glipizide is 98–99% bound to serum proteins, primarily to albumin. The mean terminal elimination half-life of glipizide ranged from 2 to 5 hours after single or multiple doses in patients with type 2 diabetes. There were no significant differences in the pharmacokinetics of glipizide after single dose administration to older diabetic subjects compared to younger healthy subjects. There is only limited information regarding the effects of renal impairment on the disposition of glipizide, and no information regarding the effects of hepatic disease. However, since glipizide is highly protein bound and hepatic biotransformation is the predominant route of elimination, the pharmacokinetics and/or pharmacodynamics of glipizide may be altered in patients with renal or hepatic impairment.

In mice no glipizide or metabolites were detectable autoradiographically in the brain or spinal cord of males or females, nor in the fetuses of pregnant females. In another study, however, very small amounts of radioactivity were detected in the fetuses of rats given labelled drug.

INDICATIONS AND USAGE

GLUCOTROL XL is indicated as an adjunct to diet for the control of hyperglycemia and its associated symptomatology in patients with type 2 diabetes formerly known as non-insulin-dependent diabetes mellitus (NIDDM) or maturity-onset diabetes, after an adequate trial of dietary therapy has proved unsatisfactory. GLUCOTROL XL is indicated when diet alone has been unsuccessful in correcting hyperglycemia, but even after the introduction of the drug in the patient's regimen, dietary measures should continue to be considered as important. In 12 week, well-controlled studies there was a maximal average net reduction in hemoglobin A_{1C} of 1.7% in absolute units between placebo-treated and GLUCOTROL XL-treated patients.

In initiating treatment for type 2 diabetes, diet should be emphasized as the primary form of treatment. Caloric restriction and weight loss are essential in the obese diabetic patient. Proper dietary management alone may be effective in controlling blood glucose and symptoms of hyperglycemia. The importance of regular physical activity should also be stressed, cardiovascular risk factors should be identified, and corrective measures taken where possible.

If this treatment program fails to reduce symptoms and/or blood glucose, the use of an oral sulfonylurea should be considered. If additional reduction of symptoms and/or blood glucose is required, the addition of insulin to the treatment regimen should be considered. Use of GLUCOTROL XL must be viewed by both the physician and patient as a treatment in addition to diet, and not as a substitute for diet or as a convenient mechanism for avoiding dietary restraint. Furthermore, loss of blood glucose control on diet alone also may be transient, thus requiring only short-term administration of glipizide.

Some patients fail to respond initially or gradually lose their responsiveness to sulfonylurea drugs, including GLUCOTROL XL. In these cases, the addition of another oral blood glucose-lowering agent to GLUCOTROL XL therapy can be considered. Other approaches that can be considered include substitution of GLUCOTROL XL therapy with that of another oral blood glucose-lowering agent or insulin. GLUCOTROL XL should be discontinued if it no longer contributes to glucose lowering. Judgment of response to therapy should be based on regular clinical and laboratory evaluations.

In considering the use of GLUCOTROL XL in asymptomatic patients, it should be recognized that controlling blood glucose in type 2 diabetes has not been definitely established to be effective in preventing the long-term cardiovascular or neural complications of diabetes. However, in insulin-dependent diabetes mellitus controlling blood glucose has been effective in slowing the progression of diabetic retinopathy, nephropathy, and neuropathy.

CONTRAINDICATIONS

Glipizide is contraindicated in patients with:

1. Known hypersensitivity to the drug.
2. Diabetic ketoacidosis, with or without coma. This condition should be treated with insulin.

WARNINGS

SPECIAL WARNING ON INCREASED RISK OF CARDIOVASCULAR MORTALITY: The administration of oral hypoglycemic drugs has been reported to be associated with increased cardiovascular mortality as compared to treatment with diet alone or diet plus insulin. This warning is based on the study conducted by the University Group Diabetes Program (UGDP), a long-term prospective clinical trial designed to evaluate the effectiveness of glucose-lowering drugs in preventing or delaying vascular complications in patients with type 2 diabetes. The study involves 823 patients who were randomly assigned to one of four treatment groups (Diabetes, 19, SUPP. 2: 747-830, 1970).

UGDP reported that patients treated for 5 to 8 years with diet plus a fixed dose of tolbutamide (1.5 grams per day) had a rate of cardiovascular mortality approximately 2½ times that of patients treated with diet alone. A significant increase in total mortality was not observed, but the use of tolbutamide was discontinued based on the increase in cardiovascular mortality, thus limiting the opportunity for the study to show an increase in overall mortality. Despite controversy regarding the interpretation of these results, the findings of the UGDP study provide an adequate basis for this warning. The patient should be informed of the potential risks and advantages of glipizide and of alternative modes of therapy.

Although only one drug in the sulfonylurea class (tolbutamide) was included in this study, it is prudent from a safety standpoint to consider that this warning may also apply to other oral hypoglycemic drugs in this class, in view of their close similarities in mode of action and chemical structure.

As with any other non-deformable material, caution should be used when administering GLUCOTROL XL Extended Release Tablets in patients with preexisting severe gastrointestinal narrowing (pathologic or iatrogenic). There have been rare reports of obstructive symptoms in patients with known strictures in association with the ingestion of another drug in this non-deformable sustained release formulation.

PRECAUTIONS

General

Renal and Hepatic Disease: The pharmacokinetics and/or pharmacodynamics of glipizide may be affected in patients with impaired renal or hepatic function. If hypoglycemia should occur in such patients, it may be prolonged and appropriate management should be instituted.

GI Disease: Markedly reduced GI retention times of the GLUCOTROL XL Extended Release Tablets may influence the pharmacokinetic profile and hence the clinical efficacy of the drug.

Hypoglycemia: All sulfonylurea drugs are capable of producing severe hypoglycemia. Proper patient selection, dosage, and instructions are important to avoid hypoglycemic episodes. Renal or hepatic insufficiency may affect the disposition of glipizide and the latter may also diminish gluconeogenic capacity, both of which increase the risk of serious hypoglycemic reactions. Elderly, debilitated or malnourished patients, and those with adrenal or pituitary insufficiency are particularly susceptible to the hypoglycemic action of glucose-lowering drugs. Hypoglycemia may be difficult to recognize in the elderly, and in people who are taking beta-adrenergic blocking drugs. Hypoglycemia is more likely to occur when caloric intake is deficient, after severe or prolonged exercise, when alcohol is ingested, or when more than one glucose-lowering drug is used. Therapy with a combination of glucose-lowering agents may increase the potential for hypoglycemia.

Loss of Control of Blood Glucose: When a patient stabilized on any diabetic regimen is exposed to stress such as fever, trauma, infection, or surgery, a loss of control may occur. At such times, it may be necessary to discontinue glipizide and administer insulin.

The effectiveness of any oral hypoglycemic drug, including glipizide, in lowering blood glucose to a desired level decreases in many patients over a period of time, which may be due to progression of the severity of the diabetes or to diminished responsiveness to the drug. This phenomenon is known as secondary failure, to distinguish it from primary failure in which the drug is ineffective in an individual patient when first given. Adequate adjustment of dose and adherence to diet should be assessed before classifying a patient as a secondary failure.

Laboratory Tests: Blood and urine glucose should be monitored periodically. Measurement of hemoglobin A_{1C} may be useful.

Information for Patients: Patients should be informed that GLUCOTROL XL Extended Release Tablets should be swallowed whole. Patients should not chew, divide or crush tablets. Patients should not be concerned if they occasionally notice in their stool something that looks like a tablet. In the GLUCOTROL XL Extended Release Tablet, the medication is contained within a nonabsorbable shell that has been specially designed to slowly release the drug so the body can absorb it. When this process is completed, the empty tablet is eliminated from the body.

Patients should be informed of the potential risks and advantages of GLUCOTROL XL and of alternative modes of therapy. They should also be informed about the importance of adhering to dietary instructions, of a regular exercise program, and of regular testing of urine and/or blood glucose. The risks of hypoglycemia, its symptoms and treatment, and conditions that predispose to its development should be explained to patients and responsible family members. Primary and secondary failure also should be explained.

Drug Interactions: The hypoglycemic action of sulfonylureas may be potentiated by certain drugs including nonsteroidal anti-inflammatory agents and other drugs that are highly protein bound, salicylates, sulfonamides, chloramphenicol, probenecid, coumarins, monoamine oxidase inhibitors, and beta-adrenergic blocking agents. When such drugs are administered to a patient receiving glipizide, the patient should be observed closely for hypoglycemia. When such drugs are withdrawn from a patient receiving glipizide, the patient should be observed closely for loss of control. In vitro binding studies with human serum proteins indicate that glipizide binds differently than tolbutamide and does not interact with salicylate or dicumarol. However, caution must be exercised in extrapolating these findings to the clinical situation and in the use of glipizide with these drugs.

Certain drugs tend to produce hyperglycemia and may lead to loss of control. These drugs include the thiazides and other diuretics, corticosteroids, phenothiazines, thyroid products, estrogens, oral contraceptives, phenytoin, nicotinic acid, sympathomimetics, calcium channel blocking drugs, and isoniazid. When such drugs are administered to a patient receiving glipizide, the patient should be closely observed for loss of control. When such drugs are withdrawn from a patient receiving glipizide, the patient should be observed closely for hypoglycemia.

A potential interaction between oral miconazole and oral hypoglycemic agents leading to severe hypoglycemia has been reported. Whether this interaction also occurs with the intravenous, topical, or vaginal preparations of miconazole is not known. The effect of concomitant administration of Diflucan® (fluconazole) and Glucotrol has been demonstrated in a placebo-controlled crossover study in normal volunteers. All subjects received Glucotrol alone and following treatment with 100 mg of Diflucan® as a single daily oral dose for 7 days. The mean percentage increase in the Glucotrol AUC after fluconazole administration was 56.9% (range: 35 to 81%).

Carcinogenesis, Mutagenesis, Impairment of Fertility: A twenty month study in rats and an eighteen month study in mice at doses up to 75 times the maximum human dose revealed no evidence of drug-related carcinogenicity. Bacterial and in vivo mutagenicity tests were uniformly negative. Studies in rats of both sexes at doses up to 75 times the human dose showed no effects on fertility.

Pregnancy: Pregnancy Category C: Glipizide was found to be mildly fetotoxic in rat reproductive studies at all dose levels (5–50 mg/kg). This fetotoxicity has been similarly noted with other sulfonylureas, such as tolbutamide and tolazamide. The effect is perinatal and believed to be directly related to the pharmacologic (hypoglycemic) action of glipizide. In studies in rats and rabbits no teratogenic effects were found. There are no adequate and well controlled studies in pregnant women. Glipizides should be used during pregnancy only if the potential benefit justifies the potential risk to the fetus.

Because recent information suggests that abnormal blood glucose levels during pregnancy are associated with a higher incidence of congenital abnormalities, many experts recommend that insulin be used during pregnancy to maintain blood glucose levels as close to normal as possible.

Nonteratogenic Effects: Prolonged severe hypoglycemia (4 to 10 days) has been reported in neonates born to mothers who were receiving a sulfonylurea drug at the time of delivery. This has been reported more frequently with the use of agents with prolonged half-lives. If glipizide is used during pregnancy, it should be discontinued at least one month before the expected delivery date.

Nursing Mothers: Although it is not known whether glipizide is excreted in human milk, some sulfonylurea drugs are known to be excreted in human milk. Because the potential for hypoglycemia in nursing infants may exist, a decision should be made whether to discontinue nursing or to discontinue the drug, taking into account the importance of the drug to the mother. If the drug is discontinued and if diet alone is inadequate for controlling blood glucose, insulin therapy should be considered.

Pediatric Use: Safety and effectiveness in children have not been established.

Geriatric Use: Of the total number of patients in clinical studies of GLUCOTROL XL, 33 percent were 65 and over. No overall differences in effectiveness or safety were observed between these patients and younger patients, but greater sensitivity of some individuals cannot be ruled out. Approximately 1–2 days longer were required to reach steady-state in the elderly. (See CLINICAL PHARMACOLOGY and DOSAGE AND ADMINISTRATION).

ADVERSE REACTIONS

In U.S. controlled studies the frequency of serious adverse experiences reported was very low and causal relationship has not been established.

The 580 patients from 31 to 87 years of age who received GLUCOTROL XL Extended Release Tablets in doses from 5 mg to 60 mg in both controlled and open trials were included in the evaluation of adverse experiences. All adverse experiences reported were tabulated independently of their possible causal relation to medication.

Hypoglycemia: See PRECAUTIONS and OVERDOSAGE sections.

Only 3.4% of patients receiving GLUCOTROL XL Extended Release Tablets had hypoglycemia documented by a blood glucose measurement < 60 mg/dL and/or symptoms believed to be associated with hypoglycemia. In a comparative efficacy study of GLUCOTROL XL and Glucotrol, hypoglycemia occurred rarely with an incidence of less than 1% with both drugs.

In double-blind, placebo-controlled studies the adverse experiences reported with an incidence of 3% or more in GLUCOTROL XL-treated patients include:

Adverse Effect	GLUCOTROL XL (%) (N=278)	Placebo (%) (N=69)
Asthenia	10.1	13.0
Headache	8.6	8.7
Dizziness	6.8	5.8
Nervousness	3.6	2.9
Tremor	3.6	0.0
Diarrhea	5.4	0.0
Flatulence	3.2	1.4

The following adverse experiences occurred with an incidence of less than 3% in GLUCOTROL XL-treated patients:

Body as a whole—pain

Nervous system—insomnia, paresthesia, anxiety, depression and hypesthesia

Gastrointestinal—nausea, dyspepsia, constipation and vomiting

Metabolic—hypoglycemia

Musculoskeletal—arthralgia, leg cramps and myalgia

Cardiovascular—syncope

Skin—sweating and pruritus

Respiratory—rhinitis

Special senses—blurred vision

Urogenital—polyuria

Other adverse experiences occurred with an incidence of less than 1% in GLUCOTROL XL-treated patients:

Body as a whole—chills

Nervous system—hypertonia, confusion, vertigo, somnolence, gait abnormality and decreased libido

Gastrointestinal—anorexia and trace blood in stool

Metabolic—thirst and edema

Cardiovascular—arrhythmia, migraine, flushing and hypertension

Skin—rash and urticaria

Respiratory—pharyngitis and dyspnea

Special senses—pain in the eye, conjunctivitis and retinal hemorrhage

Urogenital—dysuria

Although these adverse experiences occurred in patients treated with GLUCOTROL XL, a causal relationship to the medication has not been established in all cases.

There have been rare reports of gastrointestinal irritation and gastrointestinal bleeding with use of another drug in this non-deformable sustained release formulation, although causal relationship to the drug is uncertain.

The following are adverse experiences reported with immediate release glipizide and other sulfonylureas, but have not been observed with GLUCOTROL XL:

Hematologic: Leukopenia, agranulocytosis, thrombocytopenia, hemolytic anemia, aplastic anemia, and pancytopenia have been reported with sulfonylureas.

Metabolic: Hepatic porphyria and disulfiram-like reactions have been reported with sulfonylureas. In the mouse, glipizide pretreatment did not cause an accumulation of acetaldehyde after ethanol administration. Clinical experience to date has shown that glipizide has an extremely low incidence of disulfiram-like alcohol reactions.

Endocrine Reactions: Cases of hyponatremia and the syndrome of inappropriate antidiuretic hormone (SIADH) secretion have been reported with glipizide and other sulfonylureas.

Laboratory Tests: The pattern of laboratory test abnormalities observed with glipizide was similar to that for other sulfonylureas. Occasional mild to moderate elevations of SGOT, LDH, alkaline phosphatase. BUN and creatinine were noted. One case of jaundice was reported. The relationship of these abnormalities to glipizide is uncertain, and they have rarely been associated with clinical symptoms.

OVERDOSAGE

There is no well-documented experience with GLUCOTROL XL overdosage in humans. There have been no known suicide attempts associated with purposeful overdosing with GLUCOTROL XL. In nonclinical studies the acute oral toxicity of glipizide was extremely low in all species tested (LD_{50} greater than 4 g/kg). Overdosage of sulfonylureas including glipizide can produce hypoglycemia. Mild hypoglycemic symptoms without loss of consciousness or neurologic findings should be treated aggressively with oral glucose and adjustments in drug dosage and/or meal patterns. Close monitoring should continue until the physician is assured that the patient is out of danger. Severe hypoglycemic reactions with coma, seizure, or other neurological impairment occur infrequently, but constitute medical emergencies requiring immediate hospitalization. If hypoglycemic coma is diagnosed or suspected, the patient should be given rapid intravenous injection of concentrated (50%) glucose solution. This should be followed by a continuous infusion of a more dilute (10%) glucose solution at a rate that will maintain the blood glucose at a level above 100 mg/dL. Patients should be closely monitored for a minimum of 24 to 48 hours since hypoglycemia may recur after apparent clinical recovery. Clearance of glipizide from plasma may be prolonged in persons with liver disease. Because of the extensive protein binding of glipizide, dialysis is unlikely to be of benefit.

DOSAGE AND ADMINISTRATION

There is no fixed dosage regimen for the management of diabetes mellitus with GLUCOTROL XL Extended Release Tablet or any other hypoglycemic agent. Glycemic control should be monitored with hemoglobin A_{1C} and/or blood glucose levels to determine the minimum effective dose for the patient; to detect primary failure, i.e., inadequate lowering of blood glucose at the maximum recommended dose of medication; and to detect secondary failure, i.e., loss of an adequate blood-glucose-lowering response after an initial period of effectiveness. Home blood glucose monitoring may also provide useful information to the patient and physician. Short-term administration of GLUCOTROL XL Extended Release Tablet may be sufficient during periods of transient loss of control in patients usually controlled on diet.

In general, GLUCOTROL XL should be given with breakfast.

Recommended Dosing: The recommended starting dose of GLUCOTROL XL is 5 mg per day, given with breakfast. The recommended dose for geriatric patients is also 5 mg per day.

Dosage adjustment should be based on laboratory measures of glycemic control. While fasting blood glucose levels generally reach steady-state following initiation or change in GLUCOTROL XL dosage, a single fasting glucose determination may not accurately reflect the response to therapy. In most cases, hemoglobin A_{1C} level measured at three month intervals is the preferred means of monitoring response to therapy.

Hemoglobin A_{1C} should be measured as GLUCOTROL XL therapy is initiated at the 5 mg dose and repeated approximately three months later. If the result of this test suggests that glycemic control over the preceding three months was inadequate, the GLUCOTROL XL dose may be increased. Subsequent dosage adjustments should be made on the basis of hemoglobin A_{1C} levels measured at three month intervals. If no improvement is seen after three months of therapy with a higher dose, the previous dose should be resumed. Decisions which utilize fasting blood glucose to adjust GLUCOTROL XL therapy should be based on at least two or more similar, consecutive values obtained seven days or more after the previous dose adjustment.

Most patients will be controlled with 5 mg to 10 mg taken once daily. However, some patients may require up to the maximum recommended daily dose of 20 mg. While the glycemic control of selected patients may improve with doses which exceed 10 mg, clinical studies conducted to date have not demonstrated an additional group average reduction of hemoglobin A_{1C} beyond what was achieved with the 10 mg dose.

Based on the results of a randomized crossover study, patients receiving immediate release glipizide may be switched safely to GLUCOTROL XL Extended Release Tablets once-a-day at the nearest equivalent total daily dose. Patients receiving immediate release Glucotrol also may be titrated to the appropriate dose of GLUCOTROL XL starting with 5 mg once daily. The decision to switch to the nearest equivalent dose or to titrate should be based on clinical judgment.

In elderly patients, debilitated or malnourished patients, and patients with impaired renal or hepatic function, the initial and maintenance dosing should be conservative to avoid hypoglycemic reactions (see PRECAUTIONS section).

When GLUCOTROL XL is used in combination with other oral blood glucose-lowering agents, the second agent should be added at the lowest recommended dose and patients should be observed carefully. Titration of the added oral agent should be based on clinical judgment.

Patients Receiving Insulin: As with other sulfonylurea-class hypoglycemics, many patients with stable type 2 diabetes receiving insulin may be transferred safely to treatment with GLUCOTROL XL Extended Release Tablets. When transferring patients from insulin to GLUCOTROL XL, the following general guidelines should be considered:

For patients whose daily insulin requirement is 20 units or less, insulin may be discontinued and GLUCOTROL XL therapy may begin at usual dosages. Several days should elapse between titration steps.

For patients whose daily insulin requirement is greater than 20 units, the insulin dose should be reduced by 50% and GLUCOTROL XL therapy may begin at usual dosages. Subsequent reductions in insulin dosage should depend on individual patient response. Several days should elapse between titration steps.

During the insulin withdrawal period, the patient should test urine samples for sugar and ketone bodies at least three times daily. Patients should be instructed to contact the prescriber immediately if these tests are abnormal. In some cases, especially when the patient has been receiving greater than 40 units of insulin daily, it may be advisable to consider hospitalization during the transition period.

Patients Receiving Other Oral Hypoglycemic Agents: As with other sulfonylurea-class hypoglycemics, no transition period is necessary when transferring patients to GLUCOTROL XL Extended Release Tablets. Patients should be observed carefully (1–2 weeks) for hypoglycemia when being transferred from longer half-life sulfonylureas (e.g., chlorpropamide) to GLUCOTROL XL due to potential overlapping of drug effect.

HOW SUPPLIED

GLUCOTROL XL® (glipizide) Extended Release Tablets are supplied as 2.5 mg, 5 mg, and 10 mg round, biconvex tablets and imprinted with black ink as follows:

2.5 mg tablets are blue and imprinted with "GLUCOTROL XL 2.5" on one side.
Bottles of 30: NDC 0049-1620-30

5 mg tablets are white and imprinted with "GLUCOTROL XL 5" on one side.
Bottles of 100: NDC 0049-1550-66
Bottles of 500: NDC 0049-1550-73

10 mg tablets are white and imprinted with "GLUCOTROL XL 10" on one side.
Bottles of 100: NDC 0049-1560-66
Bottles of 500: NDC 0049-1560-73

Recommended Storage: The tablets should be protected from moisture and humidity and stored at controlled room temperature, 59° to 86°F (15° to 30°C).

Rx only

65-4951-00-5 Revised August 1999

Shown in Product Identification Guide, page 330

Continued on next page

LIPITOR®
(Atorvastatin Calcium) Tablets ℞

DESCRIPTION

Lipitor® (atorvastatin calcium) is a synthetic lipid-lowering agent. Atorvastatin is an inhibitor of 3-hydroxy-3-methylglutaryl-coenzyme A (HMG-CoA) reductase. This enzyme catalyzes the conversion of HMG-CoA to mevalonate, an early and rate-limiting step in cholesterol biosynthesis.
Atorvastatin calcium is [R-(R*, R*)]-2-(4-fluorophenyl)-β, δ-dihydroxy-5-(1-methylethyl)-3-phenyl-4-[(phenylamino) carbonyl]-1H-pyrrole-1-heptanoic acid, calcium salt (2:1) trihydrate. The empirical formula of atorvastatin calcium is $(C_{33}H_{34}FN_2O_5)_2Ca \bullet 3H_2O$ and its molecular weight is 1209.42. Its structural formula is:

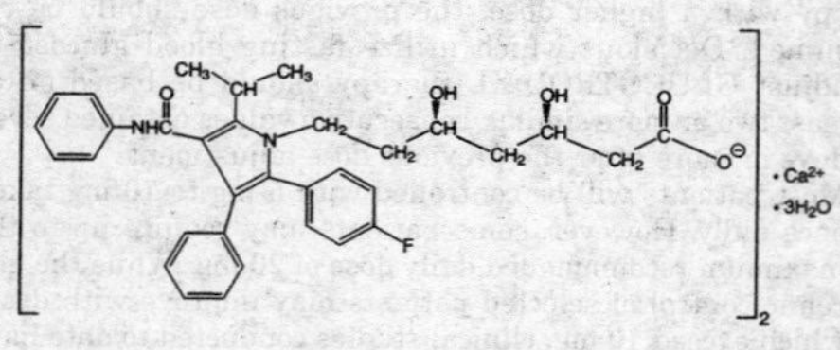

Atorvastatin calcium is a white to off-white crystalline powder that is insoluble in aqueous solutions of pH 4 and below. Atorvastatin calcium is very slightly soluble in distilled water, pH 7.4 phosphate buffer, and acetonitrile, slightly soluble in ethanol, and freely soluble in methanol.
Lipitor tablets for oral administration contain 10, 20, 40, or 80 mg atorvastatin and the following inactive ingredients: calcium carbonate, USP; candelilla wax, FCC; croscarmellose sodium, NF; hydroxypropyl cellulose, NF; lactose monohydrate, NF; magnesium stearate, NF; microcrystalline cellulose, NF; Opadry White YS-1-7040 (hydroxypropylmethylcellulose, polyethylene glycol, talc, titanium dioxide); polysorbate 80, NF; simethicone emulsion.

CLINICAL PHARMACOLOGY

Mechanism of Action
Atorvastatin is a selective, competitive inhibitor of HMG-CoA reductase, the rate-limiting enzyme that converts 3-hydroxy-3-methylglutaryl-coenzyme A to mevalonate, a precursor of sterols, including cholesterol. Cholesterol and triglycerides circulate in the bloodstream as part of lipoprotein complexes. With ultracentrifugation, these complexes separate into HDL (high-density lipoprotein), IDL (intermediate-density lipoprotein), LDL (low-density lipoprotein), and VLDL (very-low-density lipoprotein) fractions. Triglycerides (TG) and cholesterol in the liver are incorporated into VLDL and released into the plasma for delivery to peripheral tissues. LDL is formed from VLDL and is catabolized primarily through the high-affinity LDL receptor. Clinical and pathologic studies show that elevated plasma levels of total cholesterol (total-C), LDL-cholesterol (LDL-C), and apolipoprotein B (apo B) promote human atherosclerosis and are risk factors for developing cardiovascular disease, while increased levels of HDL-C are associated with a decreased cardiovascular risk.
In animal models, Lipitor lowers plasma cholesterol and lipoprotein levels by inhibiting HMG-CoA reductase and cholesterol synthesis in the liver and by increasing the number of hepatic LDL receptors on the cell-surface to enhance uptake and catabolism of LDL; Lipitor also reduces LDL production and the number of LDL particles. Lipitor reduces LDL-C in some patients with homozygous familial hypercholesterolemia (FH), a population that rarely responds to other lipid-lowering medication(s).
A variety of clinical studies have demonstrated that elevated levels of total-C, LDL-C, and apo B (a membrane complex for LDL-C) promote human atherosclerosis. Similarly, decreased levels of HDL-C (and its transport complex, apo A) are associated with the development of atherosclerosis. Epidemiologic investigations have established that cardiovascular morbidity and mortality vary directly with the level of total-C and LDL-C, and inversely with the level of HDL-C.
Lipitor reduces total-C, LDL-C, and apo B in patients with homozygous and heterozygous FH, nonfamilial forms of hypercholesterolemia, and mixed dyslipidemia. Lipitor also reduces VLDL-C and TG and produces variable increases in HDL-C and apolipoprotein A-1. Lipitor reduces total-C, LDL-C, VLDL-C, apo B, TG, and non-HDL-C, and increases HDL-C in patients with isolated hypertriglyceridemia. Lipitor reduces intermediate density lipoprotein cholesterol (IDL-C) in patients with dysbetalipoproteinemia. The effect of Lipitor on cardiovascular morbidity and mortality has not been determined.
Like LDL, cholesterol-enriched triglyceride-rich lipoproteins, including VLDL, intermediate density lipoprotein (IDL), and remnants, can also promote atherosclerosis. Elevated plasma triglycerides are frequently found in a triad with low HDL-C levels and small LDL particles, as well as in association with non-lipid metabolic risk factors for coronary heart disease. As such, total plasma TG has not consistently been shown to be an independent risk factor for CHD. Furthermore, the independent effect of raising HDL or lowering TG on the risk of coronary and cardiovascular morbidity and mortality has not been determined.

Pharmacodynamics
Atorvastatin as well as some of its metabolites are pharmacologically active in humans. The liver is the primary site of action and the principal site of cholesterol synthesis and LDL clearance. Drug dosage rather than systemic drug concentration correlates better with LDL-C reduction. Individualization of drug dosage should be based on therapeutic response (see DOSAGE AND ADMINISTRATION).

TABLE 1. Dose-Response in Patients With Primary Hypercholesterolemia (Adjusted Mean % Change From Baseline)[a]

Dose	N	TC	LDL-C	Apo B	TG	HDL-C	Non-HDL-C/ HDL-C
Placebo	21	4	4	3	10	−3	7
10	22	−29	−39	−32	−19	6	−34
20	20	−33	−43	−35	−26	9	−41
40	21	−37	−50	−42	−29	6	−45
80	23	−45	−60	−50	−37	5	−53

[a]Results are pooled from 2 dose-response studies

TABLE 2. Mean Percent Change From Baseline at End Point (Double-Blind, Randomized, Active-Controlled Trials)

Treatment (Daily Dose)	N	Total-C	LDL-C	Apo B	TG	HDL-C	Non-HDL-C/ HDL-C
Study 1							
Atorvastatin 10 mg	707	−27[a]	−36[a]	−28[a]	−17[a]	+7	−37[a]
Lovastatin 20 mg	191	−19	−27	−20	−6	+7	−28
95% CI for Diff[1]		−9.2, −6.5	−10.7, −7.1	−10.0, −6.5	−15.2, −7.1	−1.7, 2.0	−11.1, −7.1
Study 2							
Atorvastatin 10 mg	222	−25[b]	−35[b]	−27[b]	−17[b]	+6	−36[b]
Pravastatin 20 mg	77	−17	−23	−17	−9	+8	−28
95% CI for Diff[1]		−10.8, −6.1	−14.5, −8.2	−13.4, −7.4	−14.1, −0.7	−4.9, 1.6	−11.5, −4.1
Study 3							
Atorvastatin 10 mg	132	−29[c]	−37[c]	−34[c]	−23[c]	+7	−39[c]
Simvastatin 10 mg	45	−24	−30	−30	−15	+7	−33
95% CI for Diff[1]		−8.7, −2.7	−10.1, −2.6	−8.0, −1.1	−15.1, −0.7	−4.3, 3.9	−9.6, −1.9

[1] A negative value for the 95% CI for the difference between treatments favors atorvastatin for all except HDL-C, for which a positive value favors atorvastatin. If the range does not include 0, this indicates a statistically significant difference.
[a] Significantly different from lovastatin, ANCOVA, $p \leq 0.05$
[b] Significantly different from pravastatin, ANCOVA, $p \leq 0.05$
[c] Significantly different from simvastatin, ANCOVA, $p \leq 0.05$

Pharmacokinetics and Drug Metabolism
Absorption: Atorvastatin is rapidly absorbed after oral administration; maximum plasma concentrations occur within 1 to 2 hours. Extent of absorption increases in proportion to atorvastatin dose. The absolute bioavailability of atorvastatin (parent drug) is approximately 14% and the systemic availability of HMG-CoA reductase inhibitory activity is approximately 30%. The low systemic availability is attributed to presystemic clearance in gastrointestinal mucosa and/or hepatic first-pass metabolism. Although food decreases the rate and extent of drug absorption by approximately 25% and 9%, respectively, as assessed by Cmax and AUC, LDL-C reduction is similar whether atorvastatin is given with or without food. Plasma atorvastatin concentrations are lower (approximately 30% for Cmax and AUC) following evening drug administration compared with morning. However, LDL-C reduction is the same regardless of the time of day of drug administration (see DOSAGE AND ADMINISTRATION).
Distribution: Mean volume of distribution of atorvastatin is approximately 381 liters. Atorvastatin is ≥98% bound to plasma proteins. A blood/plasma ratio of approximately 0.25 indicates poor drug penetration into red blood cells. Based on observations in rats, atorvastatin is likely to be secreted in human milk (see CONTRAINDICATIONS, Pregnancy and Lactation, and PRECAUTIONS, Nursing Mothers).
Metabolism: Atorvastatin is extensively metabolized to ortho- and parahydroxylated derivatives and various beta-oxidation products. *In vitro* inhibition of HMG-CoA reductase by ortho- and parahydroxylated metabolites is equivalent to that of atorvastatin. Approximately 70% of circulating inhibitory activity for HMG-CoA reductase is attributed to active metabolites. *In vitro* studies suggest the importance of atorvastatin metabolism by cytochrome P450 3A4, consistent with increased plasma concentrations of atorvastatin in humans following coadministration with erythromycin, a known inhibitor of this isozyme (see PRECAUTIONS, Drug Interactions). In animals, the ortho-hydroxy metabolite undergoes further glucuronidation.
Excretion: Atorvastatin and its metabolites are eliminated primarily in bile following hepatic and/or extrahepatic metabolism; however, the drug does not appear to undergo enterohepatic recirculation. Mean plasma elimination half-life of atorvastatin in humans is approximately 14 hours, but the half-life of inhibitory activity for HMG-CoA reductase is 20 to 30 hours due to the contribution of active metabolites. Less than 2% of a dose of atorvastatin is recovered in urine following oral administration.

Special Populations
Geriatric: Plasma concentrations of atorvastatin are higher (approximately 40% for Cmax and 30% for AUC) in healthy elderly subjects (age ≥65 years) than in young adults. LDL-C reduction is comparable to that seen in younger patient populations given equal doses of Lipitor.
Pediatric: Pharmacokinetic data in the pediatric population are not available.
Gender: Plasma concentrations of atorvastatin in women differ from those in men (approximately 20% higher for Cmax and 10% lower for AUC); however, there is no clinically significant difference in LDL-C reduction with Lipitor between men and women.
Renal Insufficiency: Renal disease has no influence on the plasma concentrations or LDL-C reduction of atorvastatin; thus, dose adjustment in patients with renal dysfunction is not necessary (see DOSAGE AND ADMINISTRATION).
Hemodialysis: While studies have not been conducted in patients with end-stage renal disease, hemodialysis is not expected to significantly enhance clearance of atorvastatin since the drug is extensively bound to plasma proteins.
Hepatic Insufficiency: In patients with chronic alcoholic liver disease, plasma concentrations of atorvastatin are markedly increased. Cmax and AUC are each 4-fold greater in patients with Childs-Pugh A disease. Cmax and AUC are approximately 16-fold and 11-fold increased, respectively, in patients with Childs-Pugh B disease (see CONTRAINDICATIONS).

Clinical Studies
Hypercholesterolemia (Heterozygous Familial and Nonfamilial) and Mixed Dyslipidemia (*Fredrickson* Types IIa and IIb)
Lipitor reduces total-C, LDL-C, VLDL-C, apo B, and TG, and increases HDL-C in patients with hypercholesterolemia and mixed dyslipidemia. Therapeutic response is seen within 2 weeks, and maximum response is usually achieved within 4 weeks and maintained during chronic therapy.
Lipitor is effective in a wide variety of patient populations with hypercholesterolemia, with and without hypertriglyceridemia, in men and women, and in the elderly. Experience in pediatric patients has been limited to patients with homozygous FH.
In two multicenter, placebo-controlled, dose-response studies in patients with hypercholesterolemia, Lipitor given as a single dose over 6 weeks significantly reduced total-C, LDL-C, apo B, and TG (Pooled results are provided in Table 1).
[See table 1 above]
In patients with *Fredrickson* Types IIa and IIb hyperlipoproteinemia pooled from 24 controlled trials, the median (25th and 75th percentile) percent changes from baseline in HDL-C for atorvastatin 10, 20, 40, and 80 mg were 6.4 (−1.4, 14), 8.7 (0, 17), 7.8 (0, 16), and 5.1 (−2.7, 15), respectively. Additionally, analysis of the pooled data demonstrated consistent and significant decreases in total-C, LDL-C, TG, total-C/HDL-C, and LDL-C/HDL-C.
In three multicenter, double-blind studies in patients with hypercholesterolemia, Lipitor was compared to other HMG-CoA reductase inhibitors. After randomization, patients were treated for 16 weeks with either Lipitor 10 mg per day or a fixed dose of the comparative agent (Table 2).
[See table 2 above]
The impact on clinical outcomes of the differences in lipid-altering effects between treatments shown in Table 2 is not known. Table 2 does not contain data comparing the effects of atorvastatin 10 mg and higher doses of lovastatin, pravastatin, and simvastatin. The drugs compared in the studies summarized in the table are not necessarily interchangeable.
In a large clinical study, the number of patients meeting their National Cholesterol Education Program-Adult Treatment Panel (NCEP-ATP) II target LDL-C levels on 10 mg of Lipitor daily was assessed. After 16 weeks, 156/167 (93%) of

patients with less than 2 risk factors for CHD and baseline LDL-C ≥190 mg/dL reached a target of ≤160 mg/dL; 141/218 (65%) of patients with 2 or more risk factors for CHD and LDL-C ≥160 mg/dL achieved a level of ≤130 mg/dL LDL-C; and 21/113 (19%) of patients with CHD and LDL-C ≥130 mg/dL reached a target level of ≤100 mg/dL LDL-C.

Hypertriglyceridemia (*Fredrickson* Type IV)

The response to Lipitor in 64 patients with isolated hypertriglyceridemia treated across several clinical trials is shown in the table below. For the atorvastatin-treated patients, median (min, max) baseline TG level was 565 (267–1502).

[See table 3 above]

Dysbetalipoproteinemia (*Fredrickson* Type III)

The results of an open-label crossover study of 16 patients (genotypes: 14 apo E2/E2 and 2 apo E3/E2) with dysbetalipoproteinemia (*Fredrickson* Type III) are shown in the table below.

[See table 4 above]

Homozygous Familial Hypercholesterolemia

In a study without a concurrent control group, 29 patients ages 6 to 37 years with homozygous FH received maximum daily doses of 20 to 80 mg of Lipitor. The mean LDL-C reduction in this study was 18%. Twenty-five patients with a reduction in LDL-C had a mean response of 20% (range of 7% to 53%, median of 24%); the remaining 4 patients had 7% to 24% increases in LDL-C. Five of the 29 patients had absent LDL-receptor function. Of these, 2 patients also had a portacaval shunt and had no significant reduction in LDL-C. The remaining 3 receptor-negative patients had a mean LDL-C reduction of 22%.

TABLE 3. Combined Patients With Isolated Elevated TG: Median (min, max) Percent Changes From Baseline

	Placebo (N=12)	Atorvastatin 10 mg (N=37)	Atorvastatin 20 mg (N=13)	Atorvastatin 80 mg (N=14)
Triglycerides	−12.4 (−36.6, 82.7)	−41.0 (−76.2 49.4)	−38.7 (−62.7, 29.5)	−51.8 (−82.8, 41.3)
Total-C	−2.3 (−15.5, 24.4)	−28.2 (−44.9, −6.8)	−34.9 (−49.6, −15.2)	−44.4 (−63.5, −3.8)
LDL-C	3.6 (−31.3, 31.6)	−26.5 (−57.7, 9.8)	−30.4 (−53.9, 0.3)	−40.5 (−60.6, −13.8)
HDL-C	3.8 (−18.6, 13.4)	13.8 (−9.7, 61.5)	11.0 (−3.2, 25.2)	7.5 (−10.8, 37.2)
VLDL-C	−1.0 (−31.9, 53.2)	−48.8 (−85.8, 57.3)	−44.6 (−62.2, −10.8)	−62.0 (−88.2, 37.6)
non-HDL-C	−2.8 (−17.6, 30.0)	−33.0 (−52.1, −13.3)	−42.7 (−53.7, −17.4)	−51.5 (−72.9, −4.3)

TABLE 4. Open-Label Crossover Study of 16 Patients With Dysbetalipoproteinemia (*Fredrickson* Type III)

	Median (min, max) at Baseline (mg/dL)	Median % Change (min, max)	
		Atorvastatin 10 mg	Atorvastatin 80 mg
Total-C	442 (225, 1320)	−37 (−85, 17)	−58 (−90, −31)
Triglycerides	678 (273, 5990)	−39 (−92, −8)	−53 (−95, −30)
IDL-C + VLDL-C	215 (111, 613)	−32 (−76, 9)	−63 (−90, −8)
non-HDL-C	411 (218, 1272)	−43 (−87, −19)	−64 (−92, −36)

INDICATIONS AND USAGE

Lipitor is indicated:

1. as an adjunct to diet to reduce elevated total-C, LDL-C, apo B, and TG levels and to increase HDL-C in patients with primary hypercholesterolemia (heterozygous familial and nonfamilial) and mixed dyslipidemia (*Fredrickson* Types IIa and IIb);
2. as an adjunct to diet for the treatment of patients with elevated serum TG levels (*Fredrickson* Type IV);
3. for the treatment of patients with primary dysbetalipoproteinemia (*Fredrickson* Type III) who do not respond adequately to diet;
4. to reduce total-C and LDL-C in patients with homozygous familial hypercholesterolemia as an adjunct to other lipid-lowering treatments (eg, LDL apheresis) or if such treatments are unavailable.

Therapy with lipid-altering agents should be a component of multiple-risk-factor intervention in individuals at increased risk for atherosclerotic vascular disease due to hypercholesterolemia. Lipid-altering agents should be used in addition to a diet restricted in saturated fat and cholesterol only when the response to diet and other nonpharmacological measures has been inadequate (see *National Cholesterol Education Program (NCEP) Guidelines*, summarized in Table 5).

TABLE 5. NCEP Guidelines for Lipid Management

Definite Atherosclerotic Disease[a]	Two or More Other Risk Factors[b]	LDL-Cholesterol mg/dL (mmol/L) Initiation Level	Minimum Goal
No	No	≥190 (≥4.9)	<160 (<4.1)
No	Yes	≥160 (≥4.1)	<130 (<3.4)
Yes	Yes or No	≥130[c] (≥3.4)	≤100 (≤2.6)

[a] Coronary heart disease or peripheral vascular disease (including symptomatic carotid artery disease).

[b] Other risk factors for coronary heart disease (CHD) include: age (males: ≥45 years; females: ≥55 years or premature menopause without estrogen replacement therapy); family history of premature CHD; current cigarette smoking; hypertension; confirmed HDL-C <35 mg/dL (<0.91 mmol/L); and diabetes mellitus. Subtract 1 risk factor if HDL-C is ≥60 mg/dL (≥1.6 mmol/L).

[c] In CHD patients with LDL-C levels 100 to 129 mg/dL, the physician should exercise clinical judgment in deciding whether to initiate drug treatment.

At the time of hospitalization for an acute coronary event, consideration can be given to initiating drug therapy at discharge if the LDL-C level is ≥130 mg/dL (NCEP-ATP II).

Prior to initiating therapy with Lipitor, secondary causes for hypercholesterolemia (eg, poorly controlled diabetes mellitus, hypothyroidism, nephrotic syndrome, dysproteinemias, obstructive liver disease, other drug therapy, and alcoholism) should be excluded, and a lipid profile performed to measure total-C, LDL-C, HDL-C, and TG. For patients with TG <400 mg/dL (<4.5 mmol/L), LDL-C can be estimated using the following equation: LDL-C = total-C - (0.20 × [TG] + HDL-C). For TG levels >400 mg/dL (>4.5 mmol/L), this equation is less accurate and LDL-C concentrations should be determined by ultracentrifugation.

Lipitor has not been studied in conditions where the major lipoprotein abnormality is elevation of chylomicrons (*Fredrickson* Types I and V).

CONTRAINDICATIONS

Active liver disease or unexplained persistent elevations of serum transaminases.

Hypersensitivity to any component of this medication.

Pregnancy and Lactation

Atherosclerosis is a chronic process and discontinuation of lipid-lowering drugs during pregnancy should have little impact on the outcome of long-term therapy of primary hypercholesterolemia. Cholesterol and other products of cholesterol biosynthesis are essential components for fetal development (including synthesis of steroids and cell membranes). Since HMG-CoA reductase inhibitors decrease cholesterol synthesis and possibly the synthesis of other biologically active substances derived from cholesterol, they may cause fetal harm when administered to pregnant women. Therefore, HMG-CoA reductase inhibitors are contraindicated during pregnancy and in nursing mothers. ATORVASTATIN SHOULD BE ADMINISTERED TO WOMEN OF CHILDBEARING AGE ONLY WHEN SUCH PATIENTS ARE HIGHLY UNLIKELY TO CONCEIVE AND HAVE BEEN INFORMED OF THE POTENTIAL HAZARDS. If the patient becomes pregnant while taking this drug, therapy should be discontinued and the patient apprised of the potential hazard to the fetus.

WARNINGS

Liver Dysfunction

HMG-CoA reductase inhibitors, like some other lipid-lowering therapies, have been associated with biochemical abnormalities of liver function. **Persistent elevations (>3 times the upper limit of normal [ULN] occurring on 2 or more occasions) in serum transaminases occurred in 0.7% of patients who received atorvastatin in clinical trials. The incidence of these abnormalities was 0.2%, 0.2%, 0.6%, and 2.3% for 10, 20, 40, and 80 mg, respectively.**

One patient in clinical trials developed jaundice. Increases in liver function tests (LFT) in other patients were not associated with jaundice or other clinical signs or symptoms. Upon dose reduction, drug interruption, or discontinuation, transaminase levels returned to or near pretreatment levels without sequelae. Eighteen of 30 patients with persistent LFT elevations continued treatment with a reduced dose of atorvastatin.

It is recommended that liver function tests be performed prior to and at 12 weeks following both the initiation of therapy and any elevation of dose, and periodically (eg, semiannually) thereafter. Liver enzyme changes generally occur in the first 3 months of treatment with atorvastatin. Patients who develop increased transaminase levels should be monitored until the abnormalities resolve. Should an increase in ALT or AST of >3 times ULN persist, reduction of dose or withdrawal of atorvastatin is recommended.

Atorvastatin should be used with caution in patients who consume substantial quantities of alcohol and/or have a history of liver disease. Active liver disease or unexplained persistent transaminase elevations are contraindications to the use of atorvastatin (see CONTRAINDICATIONS).

Skeletal Muscle

Rare cases of rhabdomyolysis with acute renal failure secondary to myoglobinuria have been reported with atorvastatin and with other drugs in this class.

Uncomplicated myalgia has been reported in atorvastatin-treated patients (see ADVERSE REACTIONS). Myopathy, defined as muscle aches or muscle weakness in conjunction with increases in creatine phosphakinase (CPK) values >10 times ULN, should be considered in any patient with diffuse myalgias, muscle tenderness or weakness, and/or marked elevation of CPK. Patients should be advised to report promptly unexplained muscle pain, tenderness or weakness, particularly if accompanied by malaise or fever. Atorvastatin therapy should be discontinued if markedly elevated CPK levels occur or myopathy is diagnosed or suspected.

The risk of myopathy during treatment with drugs in this class is increased with concurrent administration of cyclosporine, fibric acid derivatives, erythromycin, niacin, or azole antifungals. Physicians considering combined therapy with atorvastatin and fibric acid derivatives, erythromycin, immunosuppressive drugs, azole antifungals, or lipid-lowering doses of niacin should carefully weigh the potential benefits and risks and should carefully monitor patients for any signs or symptoms of muscle pain, tenderness, or weakness, particularly during the initial months of therapy and during any periods of upward dosage titration of either drug. Periodic creatine phosphokinase (CPK) determinations may be considered in such situations, but there is no assurance that such monitoring will prevent the occurrence of severe myopathy.

Atorvastatin therapy should be temporarily withheld or discontinued in any patient with an acute, serious condition suggestive of a myopathy or having a risk factor predisposing to the development of renal failure secondary to rhabdomyolysis (eg, severe acute infection, hypotension, major surgery, trauma, severe metabolic, endocrine and electrolyte disorders, and uncontrolled seizures).

PRECAUTIONS

General

Before instituting therapy with atorvastatin, an attempt should be made to control hypercholesterolemia with appropriate diet, exercise, and weight reduction in obese patients, and to treat other underlying medical problems (see INDICATIONS AND USAGE).

Information for Patients

Patients should be advised to report promptly unexplained muscle pain, tenderness, or weakness, particularly if accompanied by malaise or fever.

Drug Interactions

The risk of myopathy during treatment with drugs of this class is increased with concurrent administration of cyclosporine, fibric acid derivatives, niacin (nicotinic acid), erythromycin, azole antifungals (see WARNINGS, Skeletal Muscle).

Antacid: When atorvastatin and Maalox® TC suspension were coadministered, plasma concentrations of atorvastatin decreased approximately 35%. However, LDL-C reduction was not altered.

Antipyrine: Because atorvastatin does not affect the phamacokinetics of antipyrine, interactions with other drugs metabolized via the same cytochrome isozymes are not expected.

Colestipol: Plasma concentrations of atorvastatin decreased approximately 25% when colestipol and atorvastatin were coadministered. However, LDL-C reduction was greater when atorvastatin and colestipol were coadministered than when either drug was given alone.

Cimetidine: Atorvastatin plasma concentrations and LDL-C reduction were not altered by coadministration of cimetidine.

Digoxin: When multiple doses of atorvastatin and digoxin were coadministered, steady-state plasma digoxin concentrations increased by approximately 20%. Patients taking digoxin should be monitored appropriately.

Erythromycin: In healthy individuals, plasma concentrations of atorvastatin increased approximately 40% with coadministration of atorvastatin and erythromycin, a known inhibitor of cytochrome P450 3A4 (see WARNINGS, Skeletal Muscle).

Continued on next page

Lipitor—Cont.

Oral Contraceptives: Coadministration of atorvastatin and an oral contraceptive increased AUC values for norethindrone and ethinyl estradiol by approximately 30% and 20%. These increases should be considered when selecting an oral contraceptive for a woman taking atorvastatin.

Warfarin: Atorvastatin had no clinically significant effect on prothrombin time when administered to patients receiving chronic warfarin treatment.

Endocrine Function

HMG-CoA reductase inhibitors interfere with cholesterol synthesis and theoretically might blunt adrenal and/or gonadal steroid production. Clinical studies have shown that atorvastatin does not reduce basal plasma cortisol concentration or impair adrenal reserve. The effects of HMG-CoA reductase inhibitors on male fertility have not been studied in adequate numbers of patients. The effects, if any, on the pituitary-gonadal axis in premenopausal women are unknown. Caution should be exercised if an HMG-CoA reductase inhibitor is administered concomitantly with drugs that may decrease the levels or activity of endogenous steroid hormones, such as ketoconazole, spironolactone, and cimetidine.

CNS Toxicity

Brain hemorrhage was seen in a female dog treated for 3 months at 120 mg/kg/day. Brain hemorrhage and optic nerve vacuolation were seen in another female dog that was sacrificed in moribund condition after 11 weeks of escalating doses up to 280 mg/kg/day. The 120 mg/kg dose resulted in a systemic exposure approximately 16 times the human plasma area-under-the-curve (AUC, 0–24 hours) based on the maximum human dose of 80 mg/day. A single tonic convulsion was seen in each of 2 male dogs (one treated at 10 mg/kg/day and one at 120 mg/kg/day) in a 2-year study. No CNS lesions have been observed in mice after chronic treatment for up to 2 years at doses up to 400 mg/kg/day or in rats at doses up to 100 mg/kg/day. These doses were 6 to 11 times (mouse) and 8 to 16 times (rat) the human AUC (0–24) based on the maximum recommended human dose of 80 mg/day.

CNS vascular lesions, characterized by perivascular hemorrhages, edema, and mononuclear cell infiltration of perivascular spaces, have been observed in dogs treated with other members of this class. A chemically similar drug in this class produced optic nerve degeneration (Wallerian degeneration of retinogeniculate fibers) in clinically normal dogs in a dose-dependent fashion at a dose that produced plasma drug levels about 30 times higher than the mean drug level in humans taking the highest recommended dose.

Carcinogenesis, Mutagenesis, Impairment of Fertility

In a 2-year carcinogenicity study in rats at dose levels of 10, 30, and 100 mg/kg/day, 2 rare tumors were found in muscle in high-dose females: in one, there was a rhabdomyosarcoma and, in another, there was a fibrosarcoma. This dose represents a plasma AUC (0–24) value of approximately 16 times the mean human plasma drug exposure after an 80 mg oral dose.

A 2-year carcinogenicity study in mice given 100, 200, or 400 mg/kg/day resulted in a significant increase in liver adenomas in high-dose males and liver carcinomas in high-dose females. These findings occurred at plasma AUC (0–24) values of approximately 6 times the mean human plasma drug exposure after an 80 mg oral dose.

In vitro, atorvastatin was not mutagenic or clastogenic in the following tests with and without metabolic activation: the Ames test with *Salmonella typhimurium* and *Escherichia coli*, the HGPRT forward mutation assay in Chinese hamster lung cells, and the chromosomal aberration assay in Chinese hamster lung cells. Atorvastatin was negative in the *in vivo* mouse micronucleus test.

Studies in rats performed at doses up to 175 mg/kg (15 times the human exposure) produced no changes in fertility. There was aplasia and aspermia in the epididymis of 2 of 10 rats treated with 100 mg/kg/day of atorvastatin for 3 months (16 times the human AUC at the 80 mg dose); testis weights were significantly lower at 30 and 100 mg/kg and epididymal weight was lower at 100 mg/kg. Male rats given 100 mg/kg/day for 11 weeks prior to mating had decreased sperm motility, spermatid head concentration, and increased abnormal sperm. Atorvastatin caused no adverse effects on semen parameters, or reproductive organ histopathology in dogs given doses of 10, 40, or 120 mg/kg for two years.

Pregnancy

Pregnancy Category X

See CONTRAINDICATIONS

Safety in pregnant women has not been established. Atorvastatin crosses the rat placenta and reaches a level in fetal liver equivalent to that of maternal plasma. Atorvastatin was not teratogenic in rats at doses up to 300 mg/kg/day or in rabbits at doses up to 100 mg/kg/day. These doses resulted in multiples of about 30 times (rat) or 20 times (rabbit) the human exposure based on surface area (mg/m^2).

In a study in rats given 20, 100, or 225 mg/kg/day, from gestation day 7 through to lactation day 21 (weaning), there was decreased pup survival at birth, neonate, weaning, and maturity in pups of mothers dosed with 225 mg/kg/day. Body weight was decreased on days 4 and 21 in pups of mothers dosed at 100 mg/kg/day; pup body weight was decreased at birth and at days 4, 21, and 91 at 225 mg/kg/day. Pup development was delayed (rotorod performance at 100 mg/kg/day and acoustic startle at 225 mg/kg/day; pinnae detachment and eye opening at 225 mg/kg/day). These doses correspond to 6 times (100 mg/kg) and 22 times (225 mg/kg) the human AUC at 80 mg/day.

Rare reports of congenital anomalies have been received following intrauterine exposure to HMG-CoA reductase inhibitors. There has been one report of severe congenital bony deformity, tracheo-esophageal fistula, and anal atresia (VATER association) in a baby born to a woman who took lovastatin with dextroamphetamine sulfate during the first trimester of pregnancy. Lipitor should be administered to women of child-bearing potential only when such patients are highly unlikely to conceive and have been informed of the potential hazards. If the woman becomes pregnant while taking Lipitor, it should be discontinued and the patient advised again as to the potential hazards to the fetus.

Nursing Mothers

Nursing rat pups had plasma and liver drug levels of 50% and 40%, respectively, of that in their mother's milk. Because of the potential for adverse reactions in nursing infants, women taking Lipitor should not breast-feed (see CONTRAINDICATIONS).

Pediatric Use

Treatment experience in a pediatric population is limited to doses of Lipitor up to 80 mg/day for 1 year in 8 patients with homozygous FH. No clinical or biochemical abnormalities were reported in these patients. None of these patients was below 9 years of age.

Geriatric Use

Treatment experience in adults age ≥70 years with doses of Lipitor up to 80 mg/day has been evaluated in 221 patients. The safety and efficacy of Lipitor in this population were similar to those of patients <70 years of age.

ADVERSE REACTIONS

Lipitor is generally well-tolerated. Adverse reactions have usually been mild and transient. In controlled clinical studies of 2502 patients, <2% of patients were discontinued due to adverse experiences attributable to atorvastatin. The most frequent adverse events thought to be related to atorvastatin were constipation, flatulence, dyspepsia, and abdominal pain.

Clinical Adverse Experiences

Adverse experiences reported in ≥2% of patients in placebo-controlled clinical studies of atorvastatin, regardless of causality assessment, are shown in Table 6.

[See table 6 below]

The following adverse events were reported, regardless of causality assessment in patients treated with atorvastatin in clinical trials. The events in italics occurred in ≥2% of patients and the events in plain type occurred in <2% of patients.

Body as a Whole: *Chest pain*, face edema, fever, neck rigidity, malaise, photosensitivity reaction, generalized edema.

Digestive System: *Nausea*, gastroenteritis, liver function tests abnormal, colitis, vomiting, gastritis, dry mouth, rectal hemorrhage, esophagitis, eructation, glossitis, mouth ulceration, anorexia, increased appetite, stomatitis, biliary pain, chelitis, duodenal ulcer, dysphagia, enteritis, melena, gum hemorrhage, stomach ulcer, tenesmus, ulcerative stomatitis, hepatitis, pancreatitis, cholestatic jaundice.

Respiratory System: *Bronchitis, rhinitis*, pneumonia, dyspnea, asthma, epistaxis.

Nervous System: *Insomnia, dizziness*, paresthesia, somnolence, amnesia, abnormal dreams, libido decreased, emotional lability, incoordination, peripheral neuropathy, torticollis, facial paralysis, hyperkinesia, depression, hypesthesia, hypertonia.

Musculoskeletal System: *Arthritis*, leg cramps, bursitis, tenosynovitis, myasthenia, tendinous contracture, myositis.

Skin and Appendages: Pruritus, contact dermatitis, alopecia, dry skin, sweating, acne, urticaria, eczema, seborrhea, skin ulcer.

Urogenital System: *Urinary tract infection*, urinary frequency, cystitis, hematuria, impotence, dysuria, kidney calculus, nocturia, epididymitis, fibrocystic breast, vaginal hemorrhage, albuminuria, breast enlargement, metrorrhagia, nephritis, urinary incontinence, urinary retention, urinary urgency, abnormal ejaculation, uterine hemorrhage.

Special Senses: Amblyopia, tinnitus, dry eyes, refraction disorder, eye hemorrhage, deafness, glaucoma, parosmia, taste loss, taste perversion.

Cardiovascular System: Palpitation, vasodilatation, syncope, migraine, postural hypotension, phlebitis, arrhythmia, angina pectoris, hypertension.

Metabolic and Nutritional Disorders: *Peripheral edema*, hyperglycemia, creatine phosphokinase increased, gout, weight gain, hypoglycemia.

Hemic and Lymphatic System: Ecchymosis, anemia, lymphadenopathy, thrombocytopenia, petechia.

Postintroduction Reports

Adverse events associated with Lipitor therapy reported since market introduction, that are not listed above, regardless of causality assessment, include the following: anaphylaxis, angioneurotic edema, bullous rashes (including erythema multiforme, Stevens-Johnson syndrome, and toxic epidermal necrolysis), and rhabdomyolysis.

OVERDOSAGE

There is no specific treatment for atorvastatin overdosage. In the event of an overdose, the patient should be treated symptomatically, and supportive measures instituted as required. Due to extensive drug binding to plasma proteins, hemodialysis is not expected to significantly enhance atorvastatin clearance.

DOSAGE AND ADMINISTRATION

The patient should be placed on a standard cholesterol-lowering diet before receiving Lipitor and should continue on this diet during treatment with Lipitor.

Hypercholesterolemia (Heterozygous Familial and Nonfamilial) and Mixed Dyslipidemia (*Fredrickson* Types IIa and IIb)

The recommended starting dose of Lipitor is 10 mg once daily. The dosage range is 10 to 80 mg once daily. Lipitor can be administered as a single dose at any time of the day, with or without food. Therapy should be individualized according to goal of therapy and response (see *NCEP Guidelines*, summarized in Table 5). After initiation and/or upon titration of Lipitor, lipid levels should be analyzed within 2 to 4 weeks and dosage adjusted accordingly.

Since the goal of treatment is to lower LDL-C, the NCEP recommends that LDL-C levels be used to initiate and assess treatment response. Only if LDL-C levels are not available, should total-C be used to monitor therapy.

Homozygous Familial Hypercholesterolemia

The dosage of Lipitor in patients with homozygous FH is 10 to 80 mg daily. Lipitor should be used as an adjunct to other lipid-lowering treatments (eg, LDL apheresis) in these patients or if such treatments are unavailable.

Concomitant Therapy

Atorvastatin may be used in combination with a bile acid binding resin for additive effect. The combination of HMG-CoA reductase inhibitors and fibrates should generally be avoided (see WARNINGS, Skeletal Muscle, and PRECAUTIONS, Drug Interactions for other drug-drug interactions).

Dosage in Patients With Renal Insufficiency

Renal disease does not affect the plasma concentrations nor LDL-C reduction of atorvastatin; thus, dosage adjustment in patients with renal dysfunction is not necessary (see CLINICAL PHARMACOLOGY, Pharmacokinetics).

HOW SUPPLIED

Lipitor is supplied as white, elliptical, film-coated tablets of atorvastatin calcium containing 10, 20, 40, and 80 mg atorvastatin.

TABLE 6. Adverse Events in Placebo-Controlled Studies (% of Patients)

BODY SYSTEM/ Adverse Event	Placebo N = 270	Atorvastatin 10 mg N = 863	Atorvastatin 20 mg N = 36	Atorvastatin 40 mg N = 79	Atorvastatin 80 mg N = 94
BODY AS A WHOLE					
Infection	10.0	10.3	2.8	10.1	7.4
Headache	7.0	5.4	16.7	2.5	6.4
Accidental Injury	3.7	4.2	0.0	1.3	3.2
Flu Syndrome	1.9	2.2	0.0	2.5	3.2
Abdominal Pain	0.7	2.8	0.0	3.8	2.1
Back Pain	3.0	2.8	0.0	3.8	1.1
Allergic Reaction	2.6	0.9	2.8	1.3	0.0
Asthenia	1.9	2.2	0.0	3.8	0.0
DIGESTIVE SYSTEM					
Constipation	1.8	2.1	0.0	2.5	1.1
Diarrhea	1.5	2.7	0.0	3.8	5.3
Dyspepsia	4.1	2.3	2.8	1.3	2.1
Flatulence	3.3	2.1	2.8	1.3	1.1
RESPIRATORY SYSTEM					
Sinusitis	2.6	2.8	0.0	2.5	6.4
Pharyngitis	1.5	2.5	0.0	1.3	2.1
SKIN AND APPENDAGES					
Rash	0.7	3.9	2.8	3.8	1.1
MUSCULOSKELETAL SYSTEM					
Arthralgia	1.5	2.0	0.0	5.1	0.0
Myalgia	1.1	3.2	5.6	1.3	0.0

10 mg tablets: coded "PD 155" on one side and "10" on the other.
N0071-0155-23 bottles of 90
N0071-0155-34 bottles of 5000
N0071-0155-40 10 × 10 unit dose blisters
20 mg tablets: coded "PD 156" on one side and "20" on the other.
N0071-0156-23 bottles of 90
N0071-0156-40 10 × 10 unit dose blisters
40 mg tablets: coded "PD 157" on one side and "40" on the other.
N0071-0157-23 bottles of 90
80 mg tablets: coded "PD 158" on one side and "80" on the other.
N0071-0158-23 bottles of 90

Storage
Store at controlled room temperature 20°–25°C (68°–77°F) [see USP].

Rx only 0155G247
Revised March 2000
Manufactured by:
Warner-Lambert Export, Ltd. © 1998–'00
Dublin, Ireland
Distributed by:
PARKE-DAVIS
Div of Warner-Lambert Co
Morris Plains, NJ 07950 USA
MADE IN PUERTO RICO
Marketed by:
PARKE-DAVIS
Div of Warner-Lambert Co and **PFIZER** Inc.
New York, NY 10017
Shown in Product Identification Guide, page 330

MINIPRESS® CAPSULES ℞

[*mĭn 'ē-prĕs*]
(prazosin hydrochloride)
For Oral Use

DESCRIPTION

MINIPRESS® (prazosin hydrochloride), a quinazoline derivative, is the first of a new chemical class of antihypertensives. It is the hydrochloride salt of 1-(4-amino-6,7-dimethoxy-2-quinazolinyl)-4-(2-furoyl) piperazine and its structural formula is:

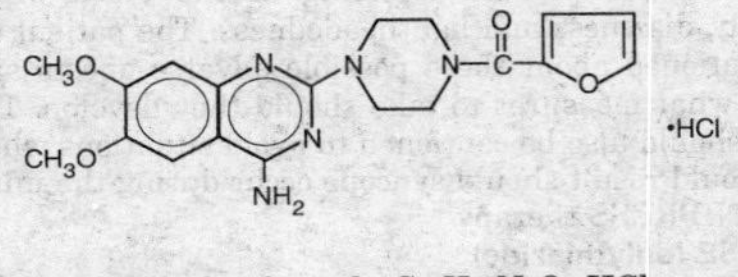

Molecular formula $C_{19}H_{21}N_5O_4 \cdot HCl$

It is a white, crystalline substance, slightly soluble in water and isotonic saline, and has a molecular weight of 419.87. Each 1 mg capsule of MINIPRESS for oral use contains drug equivalent to 1 mg free base.

Inert ingredients in the formulations are: hard gelatin capsules (which may contain Blue 1, Red 3, Red 28, Red 40, and other inert ingredients); magnesium stearate; sodium lauryl sulfate; starch; sucrose.

CLINICAL PHARMACOLOGY

The exact mechanism of the hypotensive action of prazosin is unknown. Prazosin causes a decrease in total peripheral resistance and was originally thought to have a direct relaxant action on vascular smooth muscle. Recent animal studies, however, have suggested that the vasodilator effect of prazosin is also related to blockade of postsynaptic *alpha*-adrenoceptors. The results of dog forelimb experiments demonstrate that the peripheral vasodilator effect of prazosin is confined mainly to the level of the resistance vessels (arterioles). Unlike conventional *alpha*-blockers, the antihypertensive action of prazosin is usually not accompanied by a reflex tachycardia. Tolerance has not been observed to develop in long term therapy.

Hemodynamic studies have been carried out in man following acute single dose administration and during the course of long term maintenance therapy. The results confirm that the therapeutic effect is a fall in blood pressure unaccompanied by a clinically significant change in cardiac output, heart rate, renal blood flow and glomerular filtration rate. There is no measurable negative chronotropic effect.

In clinical studies to date, MINIPRESS (prazosin hydrochloride) has not increased plasma renin activity.

In man, blood pressure is lowered in both the supine and standing positions. This effect is most pronounced on the diastolic blood pressure.

Following oral administration, human plasma concentrations reach a peak at about three hours with a plasma half-life of two to three hours. The drug is highly bound to plasma protein. Bioavailability studies have demonstrated that the total absorption relative to the drug in a 20% alcoholic solution is 90%, resulting in peak levels approximately 65% of that of the drug in solution. Animal studies indicate that MINIPRESS (prazosin hydrochloride) is extensively metabolized, primarily by demethylation and conjugation, and excreted mainly via bile and feces. Less extensive human studies suggest similar metabolism and excretion in man.

Strength	Capsule Color	Capsule Code	NDC	Package Size
MINIPRESS® 1 mg	White	431	0069-4310-71	250's
			0069-4310-82	1000's
			0063-4310-82	
			0069-4310-41	100 (10×10)
			0663-4310-41	Unit Dose
MINIPRESS® 2 mg	Pink and White	437	0069-4370-71	250's
			0663-4370-71	
			0069-4370-82	1000's
			0663-4370-82	
			0069-4370-41	100 (10×10)
			0663-4370-41	Unit Dose
MINIPRESS® 5 mg	Blue and White	438	0069-4380-71	250's
			0663-4380-71	
			0069-4380-73	500's
			0663-4380-73	
			0069-4380-41	100 (10×10)
			0663-4380-41	Unit Dose

In clinical studies in which lipid profiles were followed, there were generally no adverse changes noted between pre- and post-treatment lipid levels.

INDICATIONS AND USAGE

MINIPRESS (prazosin hydrochloride) is indicated in the treatment of hypertension. It can be used alone or in combination with other antihypertensive drugs such as diuretics or beta-adrenergic blocking agents.

CONTRAINDICATIONS

None known.

WARNINGS

MINIPRESS (prazosin hydrochloride) may cause syncope with sudden loss of consciousness. In most cases this is believed to be due to an excessive postural hypotensive effect, although occasionally the syncopal episode has been preceded by a bout of severe tachycardia with heart rates of 120–160 beats per minute. Syncopal episodes have usually occurred within 30 to 90 minutes of the initial dose of the drug; occasionally they have been reported in association with rapid dosage increases or the introduction of another antihypertensive drug into the regimen of a patient taking high doses of MINIPRESS (prazosin hydrochloride). The incidence of syncopal episodes is approximately 1% in patients given an initial dose of 2 mg or greater. Clinical trials conducted during the investigational phase of this drug suggest that syncopal episodes can be minimized by limiting the initial dose of the drug to 1 mg, by subsequently increasing the dosage slowly, and by introducing any additional antihypertensive drugs into the patient's regimen with caution (see DOSAGE AND ADMINISTRATION). Hypotension may develop in patients given MINIPRESS who are also receiving a beta-blocker such as propranolol.

If syncope occurs, the patient should be placed in the recumbent position and treated supportively as necessary. This adverse effect is self-limiting and in most cases does not recur after the initial period of therapy or during subsequent dose titration.

Patients should always be started on the 1 mg capsules of MINIPRESS (prazosin hydrochloride). The 2 and 5 mg capsules are not indicated for initial therapy.

More common than loss of consciousness are the symptoms often associated with lowering of the blood pressure, namely, dizziness and lightheadedness. The patient should be cautioned about these possible adverse effects and advised what measures to take should they develop. The patient should also be cautioned to avoid situations where injury could result should syncope occur during the initiation of MINIPRESS (prazosin hydrochloride) therapy.

PRECAUTIONS

Information for Patients: Dizziness or drowsiness may occur after the first dose of this medicine. Avoid driving or performing hazardous tasks for the first 24 hours after taking this medicine or when the dose is increased. Dizziness, lightheadedness or fainting may occur, especially when rising from a lying or sitting position. Getting up slowly may help lessen the problem. These effects may also occur if you drink alcohol, stand for long periods of time, exercise, or if the weather is hot. While taking MINIPRESS, be careful in the amount of alcohol you drink. Also, use extra care during exercise or hot weather, or if standing for long periods. Check with your physician if you have any questions.

Drug Interactions
MINIPRESS (prazosin hydrochloride) has been administered without any adverse drug interaction in limited clinical experience to date with the following: (1) cardiac glycosides—digitalis and digoxin; (2) hypoglycemics—insulin, chlorpropamide, phenformin, tolazamide, and tolbutamide; (3) tranquilizers and sedatives—chlordiazepoxide, diazepam, and phenobarbital; (4) antigout—allopurinol, colchicine, and probenecid; (5) antiarrhythmics—procainamide, propranolol (see WARNINGS however), and quinidine; and (6) analgesics, antipyretics and anti-inflammatories—propoxyphene, aspirin, indomethacin, and phenylbutazone.

Addition of a diuretic or other antihypertensive agent to MINIPRESS has been shown to cause an additive hypotensive effect. This effect can be minimized by reducing the MINIPRESS dose to 1 to 2 mg three times a day, by introducing additional antihypertensive drugs cautiously and then by retitrating MINIPRESS based on clinical response.

Drug/Laboratory Test Interactions
In a study on five patients given from 12 to 24 mg of prazosin per day for 10 to 14 days, there was an average increase of 42% in the urinary metabolite of norepinephrine and an average increase in urinary VMA of 17%. Therefore, false positive results may occur in screening tests for pheochromocytoma in patients who are being treated with prazosin. If an elevated VMA is found, prazosin should be discontinued and the patient retested after a month.

Laboratory Tests
In clinical studies in which lipid profiles were followed, there were generally no adverse changes noted between pre- and post-treatment lipid levels.

Carcinogenesis, Mutagenesis, Impairment of Fertility: No carcinogenic potential was demonstrated in an 18 month study in rats with MINIPRESS at dose levels more than 225 times the usual maximum recommended human dose of 20 mg per day. MINIPRESS was not mutagenic in *in vivo* genetic toxicology studies. In a fertility and general reproductive performance study in rats, both males and females, treated with 75 mg/kg (225 times the usual maximum recommended human dose), demonstrated decreased fertility while those treated with 25 mg/kg (75 times the usual maximum recommended human dose) did not.

In chronic studies (one year or more) of MINIPRESS in rats and dogs, testicular changes consisting of atrophy and necrosis occurred at 25 mg/kg/day (75 times the usual maximum recommended human dose). No testicular changes were seen in rats or dogs at 10 mg/kg/day (30 times the usual maximum recommended human dose). In view of the testicular changes observed in animals, 105 patients on long term MINIPRESS therapy were monitored for 17-ketosteroid excretion and no changes indicating a drug effect were observed. In addition, 27 males on MINIPRESS for up to 51 months did not have changes in sperm morphology suggestive of drug effect.

Usage in Pregnancy: Pregnancy Category C. MINIPRESS has been shown to be associated with decreased litter size at birth, 1, 4, and 21 days of age in rats when given doses more than 225 times the usual maximum recommended human dose. No evidence of drug-related external, visceral, or skeletal fetal abnormalities were observed. No drug-related external, visceral, or skeletal abnormalities were observed in fetuses of pregnant rabbits and pregnant monkeys at doses more than 225 times and 12 times the usual maximum recommended human dose respectively.

The use of prazosin and a beta-blocker for the control of severe hypertension in 44 pregnant women revealed no drug-related fetal abnormalities or adverse effects. Therapy with prazosin was continued for as long as 14 weeks.[1]

Prazosin has also been used alone or in combination with other hypotensive agents in severe hypertension of pregnancy by other investigators. No fetal or neonatal abnormalities have been reported with the use of prazosin.[2]

There are no adequate and well controlled studies which establish the safety of MINIPRESS (prazosin HCl) in pregnant women. MINIPRESS should be used during pregnancy only if the potential benefit justifies the potential risk to the mother and fetus.

Nursing Mothers: MINIPRESS has been shown to be excreted in small amounts in human milk. Caution should be exercised when MINIPRESS is administered to a nursing woman.

Usage in Children: Safety and effectiveness in children have not been established.

ADVERSE REACTIONS

Clinical trials were conducted on more than 900 patients. During these trials and subsequent marketing experience, the most frequent reactions associated with MINIPRESS therapy are: dizziness 10.3%, headache 7.8%, drowsiness 7.6%, lack of energy 6.9%, weakness 6.5%, palpitations 5.3%, and nausea 4.9%. In most instances side effects have disappeared with continued therapy or have been tolerated with no decrease in dose of drug.

Less frequent adverse reactions which are reported to occur in 1–4% of patients are:

Continued on next page

Minipress—Cont.

Gastrointestinal: vomiting, diarrhea, constipation.
Cardiovascular: edema, orthostatic hypotension, dyspnea, syncope.
Central Nervous System: vertigo, depression, nervousness.
Dermatologic: rash.
Genitourinary: urinary frequency.
EENT: blurred vision, reddened sclera, epistaxis, dry mouth, nasal congestion.

In addition, fewer than 1% of patients have reported the following (in some instances, exact causal relationships have not been established):

Gastrointestinal: abdominal discomfort and/or pain, liver function abnormalities, pancreatitis.
Cardiovascular: tachycardia.
Central Nervous System: paresthesia, hallucinations.
Dermatologic: pruritus, alopecia, lichen planus.
Genitourinary: incontinence, impotence, priapism.
EENT: tinnitus.
Other: diaphoresis, fever, positive ANA titer, arthralgia.

Single reports of pigmentary mottling and serous retinopathy, and a few reports of cataract development or disappearance have been reported. In these instances, the exact causal relationship has not been established because the baseline observations were frequently inadequate.

In more specific slit-lamp and funduscopic studies, which included adequate baseline examinations, no drug-related abnormal ophthalmological findings have been reported.

Literature reports exist associating MINIPRESS therapy with a worsening of pre-existing narcolepsy. A causal relationship is uncertain in these cases.

OVERDOSAGE

Accidental ingestion of at least 50 mg of MINIPRESS (prazosin hydrochloride) in a two year old child resulted in profound drowsiness and depressed reflexes. No decrease in blood pressure was noted. Recovery was uneventful.

Should overdosage lead to hypotension, support of the cardiovascular system is of first importance. Restoration of blood pressure and normalization of heart rate may be accomplished by keeping the patient in the supine position. If this measure is inadequate, shock should first be treated with volume expanders. If necessary, vasopressors should then be used. Renal function should be monitored and supported as needed. Laboratory data indicate MINIPRESS is not dialysable because it is protein bound.

DOSAGE AND ADMINISTRATION

The dose of MINIPRESS should be adjusted according to the patient's individual blood pressure response. The following is a guide to its administration:

Initial Dose

1 mg two or three times a day. (See WARNINGS)

Maintenance Dose

Dosage may be slowly increased to a total daily dose of 20 mg given in divided doses. The therapeutic dosages most commonly employed have ranged from 6 mg to 15 mg daily given in divided doses. Doses higher than 20 mg usually do not increase efficacy, however a few patients may benefit from further increases up to a daily dose of 40 mg given in divided doses. After initial titration some patients can be maintained adequately on a twice daily dosage regimen.

Use With Other Drugs

When adding a diuretic or other antihypertensive agent, the dose of MINIPRESS should be reduced to 1 mg or 2 mg three times a day and retitration then carried out.

HOW SUPPLIED

[See table at top of previous page]

References

1. Lubbe, WF, and Hodge, JV: *New Zealand Med J* **94** (691) 169–172, 1981.
2. Davey, DA, and Dommisse, J: *S.A. Med J*, Oct 4, 1980 (551–556).

69-2318-00-3 Revised June 1996

MINIZIDE® CAPSULES ℞

[*mĭn 'ē-zīd*]

(prazosin hydrochloride/polythiazide)

FOR ORAL ADMINISTRATION

This fixed combination drug is not indicated for initial therapy of hypertension. Hypertension requires therapy titrated to the individual patient. If the fixed combination represents the dose so determined, its use may be more convenient in patient management. The treatment of hypertension is not static, but must be reevaluated as conditions in each patient warrant.

DESCRIPTION

MINIZIDE® is a combination of MINIPRESS® (prazosin hydrochloride) plus RENESE® (polythiazide).

MINIPRESS (prazosin hydrochloride), a quinazoline derivative, is the first of that chemical class of antihypertensives. It is the hydrochloride salt of 1-(4-amino-6, 7-dimethoxy-2-quinazolinyl)-4-(2-furoyl) piperazine and its structural formula is:

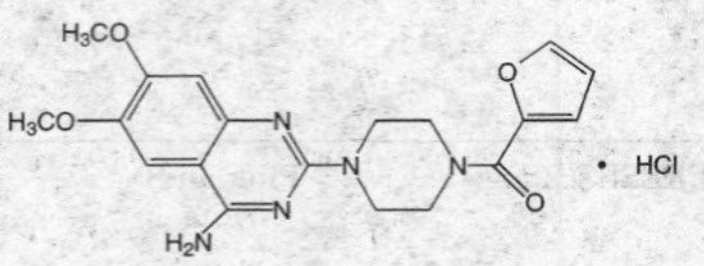

[structural formula: H_3CO, H_3CO, H_2N, N, N, O, • HCl]

It is a white, crystalline substance, slightly soluble in water and isotonic saline, and has a molecular weight of 419.87. Each 1 mg capsule of MINIPRESS (prazosin hydrochloride) contains drug equivalent to 1 mg free base.

RENESE (polythiazide) is an orally effective, nonmercurial diuretic, saluretic, and antihypertensive agent.

It is designated chemically as 2*H*-1,2,4-Benzothiadiazine-7-sulfonamide,6-chloro-3,4-dihydro -2- methyl -3-[[(2,2,2-trifluoroethyl) thio]methyl]-,1,1-dioxide, and has the following structural formula:

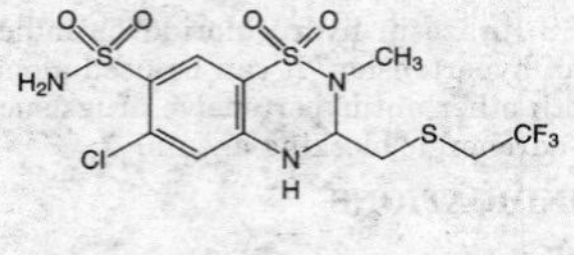

[structural formula: H_2N, S, O, O, CH_3, Cl, N, H, S, CF_3]

It is a white, crystalline substance insoluble in water, but readily soluble in alkaline solution.

Inert ingredients in the formulations are: hard gelatin capsules (which may contain Blue 1, Green 3, Red 3 and other inert ingredients); magnesium stearate; sodium lauryl sulfate; starch; sucrose.

CLINICAL PHARMACOLOGY

MINIZIDE (prazosin hydrochloride/polythiazide)

Minizide produces a more pronounced antihypertensive response than occurs after either prazosin hydrochloride or polythiazide alone in equivalent doses.

MINIPRESS (prazosin hydrochloride)

The exact mechanism of the hypotensive action of prazosin is unknown. Prazosin causes a decrease in total peripheral resistance and was originally thought to have a direct relaxant action on vascular smooth muscle. Recent animal studies, however, have suggested that the vasodilator effect of prazosin is also related to blockade of postsynaptic *alpha* -adrenoceptors. The results of dog forelimb experiments demonstrate that the peripheral vasodilator effect of prazosin is confined mainly to the level of the resistance vessels (arterioles). Unlike conventional *alpha* -blockers, the antihypertensive action of prazosin is usually not accompanied by a reflex tachycardia. Tolerance has not been observed to develop in long term therapy.

Hemodynamic studies have been carried out in man following acute single dose administration and during the course of long term maintenance therapy. The results confirm that the therapeutic effect is a fall in blood pressure unaccompanied by a clinically significant change in cardiac output, heart rate, renal blood flow, and glomerular filtration rate. There is no measurable negative chronotropic effect.

In clinical studies to date, MINIPRESS has not increased plasma renin activity.

In man, blood pressure is lowered in both the supine and standing positions. This effect is most pronounced on the diastolic blood pressure.

Following oral administration, human plasma concentrations reach a peak at about three hours with a plasma half-life of two to three hours. The drug is highly bound to plasma protein. Bioavailability studies have demonstrated that the total absorption relative to the drug in a 20% alcoholic solution is 90%, resulting in peak levels approximately 65% of that of the drug in solution. Animal studies indicate that MINIPRESS is extensively metabolized, primarily by demethylation and conjugation, and excreted mainly via bile and feces. Less extensive human studies suggest similar metabolism and excretion in man.

MINIPRESS has been administered without any adverse drug interaction in limited clinical experience to date with the following: (1) cardiac glycosides—digitalis and digoxin; (2) hypoglycemics—insulin, chlorpropamide, phenformin, tolazamide, and tolbutamide; (3) tranquilizers and sedatives—chlordiazepoxide, diazepam, and phenobarbital; (4) antigout—allopurinol, colchicine, and probenecid; (5) antiarrhythmics—procainamide, propranolol (see WARNINGS however), and quinidine; and (6) analgesics, antipyretics and anti-inflammatories—propoxyphene, aspirin, indomethacin, and phenylbutazone.

RENESE (polythiazide)

RENESE is a member of the benzothiadiazine (thiazide) family of diuretic/antihypertensive agents. Its mechanism of action results in an interference with the renal tubular mechanism of electrolyte reabsorption. At maximal therapeutic dosage all thiazides are approximately equal in their diuretic potency. The mechanism whereby thiazides function in the control of hypertension is unknown. Renese is well absorbed, giving peak human plasma concentrations about 5 hours after oral administration. Drug is removed slowly thereafter with a plasma elimination half-life of approximately 27 hours. One fifth of the drug is recovered unchanged in human urine; the remainder is cleared via feces and as metabolites. Animal studies indicate metabolism occurs by rupture of the thiadiazine ring and loss of the side chain.

INDICATIONS AND USAGE

MINIZIDE is indicated in the treatment of hypertension. (See box warning.)

CONTRAINDICATIONS

RENESE is contraindicated in patients with anuria, and in patients known to be sensitive to thiazides or to other sulfonamide derivatives.

WARNINGS

MINIPRESS (prazosin hydrochloride)

MINIPRESS may cause syncope with sudden loss of consciousness. In most cases this is believed to be due to an excessive postural hypotensive effect, although occasionally the syncopal episode has been preceded by a bout of severe tachycardia with heart rates of 120–160 beats per minute. Syncopal episodes have usually occurred within 30 to 90 minutes of the initial dose of the drug; occasionally they have been reported in association with rapid dosage increases or the introduction of another antihypertensive drug into the regimen of a patient taking high doses of MINIPRESS. The incidence of syncopal episodes is approximately 1% in patients given an initial dose of 2 mg or greater. Clinical trials conducted during the investigational phase of this drug suggest that syncopal episodes can be minimized by limiting the initial dose of the drug to 1 mg, by subsequently increasing the dosage slowly, and by introducing any additional antihypertensive drugs into the patient's regimen with caution (see DOSAGE AND ADMINISTRATION). Hypotension may develop in patients given MINIPRESS who are also receiving a beta-blocker such as propranolol.

If syncope occurs, the patient should be placed in the recumbent position and treated supportively as necessary. This adverse effect is self-limiting and in most cases does not recur after the initial period of therapy or during subsequent dose titration.

Patients should always be started on the 1 mg capsules of MINIPRESS (prazosin hydrochloride). The 2 and 5 mg capsules are not indicated for initial therapy.

More common than loss of consciousness are the symptoms often associated with lowering of the blood pressure, namely, dizziness and lightheadedness. The patient should be cautioned about these possible adverse effects and advised what measures to take should they develop. The patient should also be cautioned to avoid situations where injury could result should syncope occur during the initiation of MINIPRESS therapy.

RENESE (polythiazide)

RENESE should be used with caution in severe renal disease. In patients with renal disease, thiazides may precipitate azotemia. Cumulative effects of the drug may develop in patients with impaired renal function.

Thiazides should be used with caution in patients with impaired hepatic function or progressive liver disease, since minor alterations of fluid and electrolyte balance may precipitate hepatic coma.

Sensitivity reactions may occur in patients with a history of allergy or bronchial asthma.

The possibility of exacerbation or activation of systemic lupus erythematosus has been reported.

Thiazides may be additive or potentiative of the action of other antihypertensive drugs.

Potentiation occurs with ganglionic or peripheral adrenergic blocking drugs.

Periodic determinations of serum electrolytes to detect possible electrolyte imbalance should be performed at appropriate intervals.

All patients receiving thiazide therapy should be observed for clinical signs of fluid or electrolyte imbalance, namely, hyponatremia, hypochloremic alkalosis, and hypokalemia. Serum and urine electrolyte determinations are particularly important when the patient is vomiting excessively or receiving parenteral fluids. Medications such as digitalis may also influence serum electrolytes. Warning signs, irrespective of cause, are: dryness of mouth, thirst, weakness, lethargy, drowsiness, restlessness, muscle pains or cramps, muscular fatigue, hypotension, oliguria, tachycardia, and gastrointestinal disturbances such as nausea and vomiting.

Hypokalemia may develop with thiazides as with any potent diuretic, especially with brisk diuresis, when severe cirrhosis is present, or during concomitant use of corticosteroids or ACTH.

Interference with adequate oral electrolyte intake will also contribute to hypokalemia. Digitalis therapy may exaggerate the metabolic effects of hypokalemia, especially with reference to myocardial activity.

Any chloride deficit is generally mild and usually does not require specific treatment except under extraordinary circumstances (as in hepatic or renal disease). Dilutional hyponatremia may occur in edematous patients in hot weather; appropriate therapy is water restriction rather than administration of salt, except in rare instances when the hyponatremia is life-threatening. In actual salt depletion, appropriate replacement is the therapy of choice.

Hyperuricemia may occur or frank gout may be precipitated in certain patients receiving thiazide therapy.

STRENGTH	COMPONENTS	COLOR	CAPSULE CODE	PKG. SIZE
MINIZIDE® 1	1 mg prazosin + 0.5 mg polythiazide (NDC 0663-4300-66) (NDC 0069-4300-66)	Blue-Green	430	100's
MINIZIDE® 2	2 mg prazosin + 0.5 mg polythiazide (NDC 0663-4320-66) (NDC 0069-4320-66)	Blue-Green/Pink	432	100's
MINIZIDE® 5	5 mg prazosin + 0.5 mg polythiazide (NDC 0663-4360-66) (NDC 0069-4360-66)	Blue-Green/Blue	436	100's

Insulin requirements in diabetic patients may be either increased, decreased, or unchanged. Latent diabetes mellitus may become manifest during thiazide administration.
Thiazide drugs may increase responsiveness to tubocurarine.
The antihypertensive effects of the drug may be enhanced in the post-sympathectomy patient.
Thiazides may decrease arterial responsiveness to norepinephrine. This diminution is not sufficient to preclude effectiveness of the pressor agent for therapeutic use.
If progressive renal impairment becomes evident, as indicated by a rising nonprotein nitrogen or blood urea nitrogen, a careful reappraisal of therapy is necessary with consideration given to withholding or discontinuing diuretic therapy.
Thiazides may decrease serum protein-bound iodine levels without signs of thyroid disturbance.

PRECAUTIONS

Drug/Laboratory Test Interactions: In a study on five patients given from 12 to 24 mg of prazosin per day for 10 to 14 days, there was an average increase of 42% in the urinary metabolite of norepinephrine and an average increase in urinary VMA of 17%. Therefore, false positive results may occur in screening tests for pheochromocytoma in patients who are being treated with prazosin. If an elevated VMA is found, prazosin should be discontinued and the patient retested after a month.

Carcinogenesis, Mutagenesis, Impairment of Fertility: No carcinogenic or mutagenic studies have been conducted with MINIZIDE. However, no carcinogenic potential was demonstrated in 18 month studies in rats with either MINIPRESS or RENESE at dose levels more than 100 times the usual maximum human doses. MINIPRESS was not mutagenic in *in vivo* genetic toxicology studies.
MINIZIDE produced no impairment of fertility in male or female rats at 50 and 25 mg/kg/day of MINIPRESS and RENESE respectively. In chronic studies (one year or more) of MINIPRESS in rats and dogs, testicular changes consisting of atrophy and necrosis occurred at 25 mg/kg/day (60 times the usual maximum recommended human dose). No testicular changes were seen in rats or dogs at 10 mg/kg/day (24 times the usual maximum recommended human dose). In view of the testicular changes observed in animals, 105 patients on long term MINIPRESS therapy were monitored for 17-ketosteroid excretion and no changes indicating a drug effect were observed. In addition, 27 males on MINIPRESS alone for up to 51 months did not have changes in sperm morphology suggestive of drug effect.

Use in Pregnancy: Pregnancy Category C. MINIZIDE was not teratogenic in either rats or rabbits when administered in oral doses more than 100 times the usual maximum human dose. Studies in rats indicated that the combination of RENESE (40 times the usual maximum recommended human dose) and MINIPRESS (8 times the usual maximum recommended human dose) caused a greater number of stillbirths, a more prolonged gestation, and a decreased survival of pups to weaning than that caused by MINIPRESS alone. There are no adequate and well controlled studies in pregnant women. Therefore, MINIZIDE should be used in pregnancy only if the potential benefit justifies the potential risk to the fetus.

Nursing Mothers: It is not known whether MINIPRESS or RENESE is excreted in human milk. Thiazides appear in breast milk. Thus, if use of the drug is deemed essential the patient should stop nursing.

Pediatric Use: Safety and effectiveness in children has not been established.

ADVERSE REACTIONS

MINIPRESS (prazosin hydrochloride)

The most common reactions associated with MINIPRESS therapy are: dizziness 10.3%, headache 7.8%, drowsiness 7.6%, lack of energy 6.9%, weakness 6.5%, palpitations 5.3%, and nausea 4.9%. In most instances side effects have disappeared with continued therapy or have been tolerated with no decrease in dose of drug.
The following reactions have been associated with MINIPRESS, some of them rarely. (In some instances exact causal relationships have not been established.)

Gastrointestinal: vomiting, diarrhea, constipation, abdominal discomfort and/or pain, liver function abnormalities, pancreatitis.
Cardiovascular: edema, dyspnea, syncope, tachycardia.
Central Nervous System: nervousness, vertigo, depression, paresthesia, hallucinations.
Dermatologic: rash, pruritus, alopecia, lichen planus.
Genitourinary: urinary frequency, incontinence, impotence, priapism.
EENT: blurred vision, reddened sclera, epistaxis, tinnitus, dry mouth, nasal congestion.
Other: diaphoresis, fever.

Single reports of pigmentary mottling and serous retinopathy, and a few reports of cataract development or disappearance have been reported. In these instances, the exact causal relationship has not been established because the baseline observations were frequently inadequate.
In more specific slit-lamp and funduscopic studies, which included adequate baseline examinations, no drug-related abnormal ophthalmological findings have been reported.
Literature reports exist associating MINIPRESS therapy with a worsening of pre-existing narcolepsy. A causal relationship is uncertain in these cases.

RENESE (polythiazide)

Gastrointestinal: anorexia, gastric irritation, nausea, vomiting, cramping, diarrhea, constipation, jaundice (intrahepatic cholestatic jaundice), pancreatitis.
Central Nervous System: dizziness, vertigo, paresthesia, headache, xanthopsia.
Hematologic: leukopenia, agranulocytosis, thrombocytopenia, aplastic anemia.
Dermatologic: purpura, photosensitivity, rash, urticaria, necrotizing angiitis, (vasculitis) (cutaneous vasculitis).
Cardiovascular: Orthostatic hypotension may occur and be aggravated by alcohol, barbiturates, or narcotics.
Other: hyperglycemia, glycosuria, hyperuricemia, muscle spasm, weakness, restlessness.

OVERDOSAGE

MINIPRESS (prazosin hydrochloride)

Accidental ingestion of at least 50 mg of MINIPRESS in a two year old child resulted in profound drowsiness and depressed reflexes. No decrease in blood pressure was noted. Recovery was uneventful.
Should overdosage lead to hypotension, support of the cardiovascular system is of first importance. Restoration of blood pressure and normalization of heart rate may be accomplished by keeping the patient in the supine position. If this measure is inadequate, shock should first be treated with volume expanders. If necessary, vasopressors should then be used. Renal function should be monitored and supported as needed. Laboratory data indicate that MINIPRESS is not dialyzable because it is protein bound.

RENESE (polythiazide)

Should overdosage with RENESE occur, electrolyte balance and adequate hydration should be maintained. Gastric lavage is recommended, followed by supportive treatment. Where necessary, this may include intravenous dextrose and saline with potassium and other electrolyte therapy, administered with caution as indicated by laboratory testing at appropriate intervals.

DOSAGE AND ADMINISTRATION

MINIZIDE (prazosin hydrochloride/polythiazide)

Dosage: as determined by individual titration of MINIPRESS (prazosin hydrochloride) and RENESE (polythiazide). (See box warning.)
Usual MINIZIDE dosage is one capsule two or three times daily, the strength depending upon individual requirement following titration.
The following is a general guide to the administration of the individual components of MINIZIDE:

MINIPRESS (prazosin hydrochloride)

Initial Dose: 1 mg two or three times a day. (See WARNINGS.)

Maintenance Dose: Dosage may be slowly increased to a total daily dose of 20 mg given in divided doses. The therapeutic dosages most commonly employed have ranged from 6 mg to 15 mg daily given in divided doses. Doses higher than 20 mg usually do not increase efficacy, however a few patients may benefit from further increases up to a daily dose of 40 mg given in divided doses. After initial titration some patients can be maintained adequately on a twice daily dosage regimen.

Use With Other Drugs: When adding a diuretic or other antihypertensive agent, the dose of MINIPRESS should be reduced to 1 mg or 2 mg three times a day and retitration then carried out.

RENESE (polythiazide)

The usual dose of RENESE for antihypertensive therapy is 2 to 4 mg daily.

HOW SUPPLIED

[See table above]
#69-2463-00-7 Revised Oct. 1995

NAVANE® ℞
[*nah 'vān*]
(thiothixene) CAPSULES

NAVANE® ℞
(thiothixene hydrochloride) CONCENTRATE

DESCRIPTION

Navane® (thiothixene) is a thioxanthene derivative. Specifically, it is the *cis* isomer of N,N-dimethyl-9-[3-(4-methyl-1-piperazinyl)-propylidene] thioxanthene-2-sulfonamide.

S
$SO_2N(CH_3)_2$
H — C — CH_2CH_2N N-CH_3

The thioxanthenes differ from the phenothiazines by the replacement of nitrogen in the central ring with a carbon-linked side chain fixed in space in a rigid structural configuration. An N,N-dimethyl sulfonamide functional group is bonded to the thioxanthene nucleus.
Inert ingredients for the capsule formulations are: hard gelatin capsules (which contain gelatin and titanium dioxide; may contain Yellow 10, Yellow 6, Blue 1, Green 3, Red 3, and other inert ingredients); lactose; magnesium stearate; sodium lauryl sulfate; starch.
Inert ingredients for the oral concentrate formulation are: alcohol; cherry flavor; dextrose; passion fruit flavor; sorbitol solution; water.

ACTIONS

Navane is a psychotropic agent of the thioxanthene series. Navane possesses certain chemical and pharmacological similarities to the piperazine phenothiazines and differences from the aliphatic group of phenothiazines.

INDICATIONS

Navane is effective in the management of manifestations of psychotic disorders. Navane has not been evaluated in the management of behavioral complications in patients with mental retardation.

CONTRAINDICATIONS

Navane is contraindicated in patients with circulatory collapse, comatose states, central nervous system depression due to any cause, and blood dycrasias. Navane is contraindicated in individuals who have shown hypersensitivity to the drug. It is not known whether there is a cross sensitivity between the thioxanthenes and the phenothiazine derivatives, but this possibility should be considered.

WARNINGS

Tardive Dyskinesia—Tardive dyskinesia, a syndrome consisting of potentially irreversible, involuntary, dyskinetic movements may develop in patients treated with neuroleptic (antipsychotic) drugs. Although the prevalence of the syndrome appears to be highest among the elderly, especially elderly women, it is impossible to rely upon prevalence estimates to predict, at the inception of neuroleptic treatment, which patients are likely to develop the syndrome. Whether neuroleptic drug products differ in their potential to cause tardive dyskinesia is unknown.
Both the risk of developing the syndrome and the likelihood that it will become irreversible are believed to increase as the duration of treatment and the total cumulative dose of neuroleptic drugs administered to the patient increase. However, the syndrome can develop, although much less commonly, after relatively brief treatment periods at low doses.
There is no known treatment for established cases of tardive dyskinesia, although the syndrome may remit, partially or completely, if neuroleptic treatment is withdrawn. Neuroleptic treatment, itself, however, may suppress (or partially suppress) the signs and symptoms of the syndrome and thereby may possibly mask the underlying disease process. The effect that symptomatic suppression has upon the long-term course of the syndrome is unknown.
Given these considerations, neuroleptics should be prescribed in a manner that is most likely to minimize the occurrence of tardive dyskinesia. Chronic neuroleptic treatment should generally be reserved for patients who suffer from a chronic illness that, 1) is known to respond to neuroleptic drugs, and, 2) for whom alternative, equally effective, but potentially less harmful treatments are not available or appropriate. In patients who do require chronic treatment, the smallest dose and the shortest duration of treatment producing a satisfactory clinical response should be sought. The need for continued treatment should be reassessed periodically.
If signs and symptoms of tardive dyskinesia appear in a patient on neuroleptics, drug discontinuation should be considered. However, some patients may require treatment despite the presence of the syndrome. (For further information about the description of tardive dyskinesia and its clinical detection, please refer to "Information for Patients" in the PRECAUTIONS section, and to the ADVERSE REACTIONS section.)

Neuroleptic Malignant Syndrome (NMS)—A potentially fatal symptom complex sometimes referred to as Neuroleptic Malignant Syndrome (NMS) has been reported in association with antipsychotic drugs. Clinical manifestations of

Continued on next page

Navane Caps/Conc.—Cont.

NMS are hyperpyrexia, muscle rigidity, altered mental status and evidence of autonomic instability (irregular pulse or blood pressure, tachycardia, diaphoresis, and cardiac dysrhythmias).
The diagnostic evaluation of patients with this syndrome is complicated. In arriving at a diagnosis, it is important to identify cases where the clinical presentation includes both serious medical illness (e.g., pneumonia, systemic infection, etc.) and untreated or inadequately treated extrapyramidal signs and symptoms (EPS). Other important considerations in the differential diagnosis include central anticholinergic toxicity, heat stroke, drug fever and primary central nervous system (CNS) pathology.
The management of NMS should include 1) immediate discontinuation of antipsychotic drugs and other drugs not essential to concurrent therapy, 2) intensive symptomatic treatment and medical monitoring, and 3) treatment of any concomitant serious medical problems for which specific treatments are available. There is no general agreement about specific pharmacological treatment regimens for uncomplicated NMS.
If a patient requires antipsychotic drug treatment after recovery from NMS, the potential reintroduction of drug therapy should be carefully considered. The patient should be carefully monitored, since recurrences of NMS have been reported.
Usage in Pregnancy—Safe use of Navane during pregnancy has not been established. Therefore, this drug should be given to pregnant patients only when, in the judgment of the physician, the expected benefits from the treatment exceed the possible risks to mother and fetus. Animal reproduction studies and clinical experience to date have not demonstrated any teratogenic effects.
In the animal reproduction studies with Navane, there was some decrease in conception rate and litter size, and an increase in resorption rate in rats and rabbits. Similar findings have been reported with other psychotropic agents. After repeated oral administration of Navane to rats (5 to 15 mg/kg/day), rabbits (3 to 50 mg/kg/day), and monkeys (1 to 3 mg/kg/day) before and during gestation, no teratogenic effects were seen.
Usage in Children—The use of Navane in children under 12 years of age is not recommended because safe conditions for its use have not been established.
As is true with many CNS drugs, Navane may impair the mental and/or physical abilities required for the performance of potentially hazardous tasks such as driving a car or operating machinery, especially during the first few days of therapy. Therefore, the patient should be cautioned accordingly.
As in the case of other CNS-acting drugs, patients receiving Navane (thiothixene) should be cautioned about the possible additive effects (which may include hypotension) with CNS depressants and with alcohol.

PRECAUTIONS

An antiemetic effect was observed in animal studies with Navane; since this effect may also occur in man, it is possible that Navane may mask signs of overdosage of toxic drugs and may obscure conditions such as intestinal obstruction and brain tumor.
In consideration of the known capability of Navane and certain other psychotropic drugs to precipitate convulsions, extreme caution should be used in patients with a history of convulsive disorders or those in a state of alcohol withdrawal, since it may lower the convulsive threshold. Although Navane potentiates the actions of the barbiturates, the dosage of the anticonvulsant therapy should not be reduced when Navane is administered concurrently.
Though exhibiting rather weak anticholinergic properties, Navane should be used with caution in patients who might be exposed to extreme heat or who are receiving atropine or related drugs.
Use with caution in patients with cardiovascular disease.
Caution as well as careful adjustment of the dosages is indicated when Navane is used in conjunction with other CNS depressants.
Also, careful observation should be made for pigmentary retinopathy and lenticular pigmentation (fine lenticular pigmentation has been noted in a small number of patients treated with Navane for prolonged periods). Blood dyscrasias (agranulocytosis, pancytopenia, thrombocytopenic purpura), and liver damage (jaundice, biliary stasis) have been reported with related drugs.
Neuroleptic drugs elevate prolactin levels; the elevation persists during chronic administration. Tissue culture experiments indicate that approximately one-third of human breast cancers are prolactin dependent *in vitro*, a factor of potential importance if the prescription of these drugs is contemplated in a patient with a previously detected breast cancer. Although disturbances such as galactorrhea, amenorrhea, gynecomastia, and impotence have been reported, the clinical significance of elevated serum prolactin levels is unknown for most patients. An increase in mammary neoplasms has been found in rodents after chronic administration of neuroleptic drugs. Neither clinical studies nor epidemiologic studies conducted to date, however, have shown an association between chronic administration of these drugs and mammary tumorigenesis; the available evidence is considered too limited to be conclusive at this time.

Information for Patients: Given the likelihood that some patients exposed chronically to neuroleptics will develop tardive dyskinesia, it is advised that all patients in whom chronic use is contemplated be given, if possible, full information about this risk. The decision to inform patients and/or their guardians must obviously take into account the clinical circumstances and the competency of the patient to understand the information provided.

ADVERSE REACTIONS

NOTE: Not all of the following adverse reactions have been reported with Navane. However, since Navane has certain chemical and pharmacologic similarities to the phenothiazines, all of the known side effects and toxicity associated with phenothiazine therapy should be borne in mind when Navane is used.
Cardiovascular Effects: Tachycardia, hypotension, lightheadedness, and syncope. In the event hypotension occurs, epinephrine should not be used as a pressor agent since a paradoxical further lowering of blood pressure may result. Nonspecific EKG changes have been observed in some patients receiving Navane. These changes are usually reversible and frequently disappear on continued Navane therapy. The incidence of these changes is lower than that observed with some phenothiazines. The clinical significance of these changes is not known.
CNS Effects: Drowsiness, usually mild, may occur although it usually subsides with continuation of Navane therapy. The incidence of sedation appears similar to that of the piperazine group of phenothiazines but less than that of certain aliphatic phenothiazines. Restlessness, agitation and insomnia have been noted with Navane. Seizures and paradoxical exacerbation of psychotic symptoms have occurred with Navane infrequently.
Hyperreflexia has been reported in infants delivered from mothers having received structurally related drugs.
In addition, phenothiazine derivatives have been associated with cerebral edema and cerebrospinal fluid abnormalities.
Extrapyramidal symptoms, such as pseudoparkinsonism, akathisia and dystonia have been reported. Management of these extrapyramidal symptoms depends upon the type and severity. Rapid relief of acute symptoms may require the use of an injectable antiparkinson agent. More slowly emerging symptoms may be managed by reducing the dosage of Navane and/or administering an oral antiparkinson agent.
Persistent Tardive Dyskinesia: As with all antipsychotic agents, tardive dyskinesia may appear in some patients on long-term therapy or may occur after drug therapy has been discontinued. The syndrome is characterized by rhythmical involuntary movements of the tongue, face, mouth or jaw (e.g., protrusion of tongue, puffing of cheeks, puckering of mouth, chewing movements). Sometimes these may be accompanied by involuntary movements of extremities.
Since early detection of tardive dyskinesia is important, patients should be monitored on an ongoing basis. It has been reported that fine vermicular movement of the tongue may be an early sign of the syndrome. If this or any other presentation of the syndrome is observed, the clinician should consider possible discontinuation of neuroleptic medication. (See WARNINGS section.)
Hepatic Effects: Elevations of serum transaminase and alkaline phosphatase, usually transient, have been infrequently observed in some patients. No clinically confirmed cases of jaundice attributable to Navane (thiothixene) have been reported.
Hematologic Effects: As is true with certain other psychotropic drugs, leukopenia and leucocytosis, which are usually transient, can occur occasionally with Navane. Other antipsychotic drugs have been associated with agranulocytosis, eosinophilia, hemolytic anemia, thrombocytopenia and pancytopenia.
Allergic Reactions: Rash, pruritus, urticaria, photosensitivity and rare cases of anaphylaxis have been reported with Navane. Undue exposure to sunlight should be avoided. Although not experienced with Navane, exfoliative dermatitis and contact dermatitis (in nursing personnel) have been reported with certain phenothiazines.
Endocrine Disorders: Lactation, moderate breast enlargement and amenorrhea have occurred in a small percentage of females receiving Navane. If persistent, this may necessitate a reduction in dosage or the discontinuation of therapy. Phenothiazines have been associated with false positive pregnancy tests, gynecomastia, hypoglycemia, hyperglycemia and glycosuria.
Autonomic Effects: Dry mouth, blurred vision, nasal congestion, constipation, increased sweating, increased salivation and impotence have occurred infrequently with Navane therapy. Phenothiazines have been associated with miosis, mydriasis, and adynamic ileus.
Other Adverse Reactions: Hyperpyrexia, anorexia, nausea, vomiting, diarrhea, increase in appetite and weight, weakness or fatigue, polydipsia, and peripheral edema.
Although not reported with Navane, evidence indicates there is a relationship between phenothiazine therapy and the occurrence of a systemic lupus erythematosus-like syndrome.
Neuroleptic Malignant Syndrome (NMS): Please refer to the text regarding NMS in the WARNINGS section.
NOTE: Sudden deaths have occasionally been reported in patients who have received certain phenothiazine derivatives. In some cases the cause of death was apparently cardiac arrest or asphyxia due to failure of the cough reflex. In others, the cause could not be determined nor could it be established that death was due to phenothiazine administration.

DOSAGE AND ADMINISTRATION

Dosage of Navane should be individually adjusted depending on the chronicity and severity of the condition. In general, small doses should be used initially and gradually increased to the optimal effective level, based on patient response.
Some patients have been successfully maintained on once-a-day Navane therapy.
The use of Navane in children under 12 years of age is not recommended because safe conditions for its use have not been established.
In milder conditions, an initial dose of 2 mg three times daily. If indicated, a subsequent increase to 15 mg/day total daily dose is often effective.
In more severe conditions, an initial dose of 5 mg twice daily.
The usual optimal dose is 20 to 30 mg daily. If indicated, an increase to 60 mg/day total daily dose is often effective. Exceeding a total daily dose of 60 mg rarely increases the beneficial response.

OVERDOSAGE

Manifestations include muscular twitching, drowsiness and dizziness. Symptoms of gross overdosage may include CNS depression, rigidity, weakness, torticollis, tremor, salivation, dysphagia, hypotension, disturbances of gait, or coma.
Treatment: Essentially symptomatic and supportive. Early gastric lavage is helpful. Keep patient under careful observation and maintain an open airway, since involvement of the extrapyramidal system may produce dysphagia and respiratory difficulty in severe overdosage. If hypotension occurs, the standard measures for managing circulatory shock should be used (I.V. fluids and/or vasoconstrictors).
If a vasoconstrictor is needed, levarterenol and phenylephrine are the most suitable drugs. Other pressor agents, including epinephrine, are not recommended, since phenothiazine derivatives may reverse the usual pressor action of these agents and cause further lowering of blood pressure.
If CNS depression is marked, symptomatic treatment is indicated. Extrapyramidal symptoms may be treated with antiparkinson drugs.
There are no data on the use of peritoneal or hemodialysis, but they are known to be of little value in phenothiazine intoxication.

HOW SUPPLIED

Navane® (thiothixene) Capsules

Bottles of 100's:	1 mg (NDC 0049-5710-66)
	2 mg (NDC 0049-5720-66)
	5 mg (NDC 0049-5730-66)
	10 mg (NDC 0049-5740-66)
	20 mg (NDC 0049-5770-66)
1000's:	2 mg (NDC 0049-5720-82)
	5 mg (NDC 0049-5730-82)
	10 mg (NDC 0049-5740-82)
500's:	20 mg (NDC 0049-5770-73).
Unit Doses of:	1 mg (NDC 0049-5710-41)
	2 mg (NDC 0049-5720-41)
	5 mg (NDC 0049-5730-41)
	10 mg (NDC 0049-5740-41)
	20 mg (NDC 0049-5770-41)

Navane® (thiothixene hydrochloride) Concentrate is available in 120 mL (4 oz) bottles (NDC 0049-5750-47), with an accompanying dropper calibrated at 2 mg, 3 mg, 4 mg, 5 mg, 6 mg, 8 mg, and 10 mg; in 30 mL (1 oz) bottles (NDC 0049-5750-51), with an accompanying dropper calibrated at 2 mg, 3 mg, 4 mg, and 5 mg. Each mL contains thiothixene hydrochloride equivalent to 5mg of thiothixene. Contains alcohol U.S.P. 7.0% v/v (small loss unavoidable).

69-1655-00-8 Revised January 1997

Shown in Product Identification Guide, page 330

NAVANE® ℞

[*nah 'vān*]
(thiothixene hydrochloride)
Intramuscular For Injection
STERILE

DESCRIPTION

Navane (thiothixene hydrochloride) is a thioxanthene derivative. Specifically, thiothixene is the *cis* isomer of N,N-dimethyl-9-[3-(4-methyl-1-piperazinyl)-propylidene] thioxanthene-2-sulfonamide.
The thioxanthenes differ from the phenothiazines by the replacement of nitrogen in the central ring with a carbon-linked side chain fixed in space in a rigid structural configuration. An N,N-dimethyl sulfonamide functional group is bonded to the thioxanthene nucleus.

$SO_2N(CH_3)_2 \cdot 2HCl \cdot 2H_2O$

thiothixene hydrochloride

Inert ingredients for the intramuscular for injection formulation are: water; mannitol.

ACTIONS

Navane is a psychotropic agent of the thioxanthene series. Navane possesses certain chemical and pharmacological similarities to the piperazine phenothiazines and differences from the aliphatic group of phenothiazines. Navane's mode of action has not been clearly established.

INDICATIONS

Navane is effective in the management of manifestations of psychotic disorders. Navane has not been evaluated in the management of behavioral complications in patients with mental retardation.

CONTRAINDICATIONS

Navane is contraindicated in patients with circulatory collapse, comatose states, central nervous system depression due to any cause, and blood dyscrasias. Navane is contraindicated in individuals who have shown hypersensitivity to the drug. It is not known whether there is a cross sensitivity between the thioxanthenes and the phenothiazine derivatives, but this possibility should be considered.

WARNINGS

Tardive Dyskinesia—Tardive dyskinesia, a syndrome consisting of potentially irreversible, involuntary, dyskinetic movements may develop in patients treated with neuroleptic (antipsychotic) drugs. Although the prevalence of the syndrome appears to be highest among the elderly, especially elderly women, it is impossible to rely upon prevalence estimates to predict, at the inception of neuroleptic treatment, which patients are likely to develop the syndrome. Whether neuroleptic drug products differ in their potential to cause tardive dyskinesia is unknown.

Both the risk of developing the syndrome and the likelihood that it will become irreversible are believed to increase as the duration of treatment and the total cumulative dose of neuroleptic drugs administered to the patient increase. However, the syndrome can develop, although much less commonly, after relatively brief treatment periods at low doses.

There is no known treatment for established cases of tardive dyskinesia, although the syndrome may remit, partially or completely, if neuroleptic treatment is withdrawn. Neuroleptic treatment, itself, however, may suppress (or partially suppress) the signs and symptoms of the syndrome and thereby may possibly mask the underlying disease process. The effect that symptomatic suppression has upon the long-term course of the syndrome is unknown.

Given these considerations, neuroleptics should be prescribed in a manner that is most likely to minimize the occurrence of tardive dyskinesia. Chronic neuroleptic treatment should generally be reserved for patients who suffer from a chronic illness that, 1) is known to respond to neuroleptic drugs, and, 2) for whom alternative, equally effective, but potentially less harmful treatments are *not* available or appropriate. In patients who do require chronic treatment, the smallest dose and the shortest duration of treatment producing a satisfactory clinical response should be sought. The need for continued treatment should be reassessed periodically.

If signs and symptoms of tardive dyskinesia appear in a patient on neuroleptics, drug discontinuation should be considered. However, some patients may require treatment despite the presence of the syndrome.

(For further information about the description of tardive dyskinesia and its clinical detection, please refer to "Information for Patients" in the PRECAUTIONS section, and to the ADVERSE REACTIONS section.)

Neuroleptic Malignant Syndrome (NMS)—A potentially fatal symptom complex sometimes referred to as Neuroleptic Malignant Syndrome (NMS) has been reported in association with antipsychotic drugs. Clinical manifestations of NMS are hyperpyrexia, muscle rigidity, altered mental status and evidence of autonomic instability (irregular pulse or blood pressure, tachycardia, diaphoresis, and cardiac dysrhythmias).

The diagnostic evaluation of patients with this syndrome is complicated. In arriving at a diagnosis, it is important to identify cases where the clinical presentation includes both serious medical illness (e.g., pneumonia, systemic infection, etc.) and untreated or inadequately treated extrapyramidal signs and symptoms (EPS). Other important considerations in the differential diagnosis include central anticholinergic toxicity, heat stroke, drug fever and primary central nervous system (CNS) pathology.

The management of NMS should include 1) immediate discontinuation of antipsychotic drugs and other drugs not essential to concurrent therapy, 2) intensive symptomatic treatment and medical monitoring, and 3) treatment of any concomitant serious medical problems for which specific treatments are available. There is no general agreement about specific pharmacological treatment regimens for uncomplicated NMS.

If a patient requires antipsychotic drug treatment after recovery from NMS, the potential reintroduction of drug therapy should be carefully considered. The patient should be carefully monitored, since recurrences of NMS have been reported.

Usage in Pregnancy—Safe use of Navane during pregnancy has not been established. Therefore, this drug should be given to pregnant patients only when, in the judgment of the physician, the expected benefits from treatment exceed the possible risks to mother and fetus. Animal reproductive studies and clinical experience to date have not demonstrated any teratogenic effects.

In the animal reproduction studies with Navane, there was some decrease in conception rate and litter size, and an increase in resorption rate in rats and rabbits, changes which have been similarly reported with other psychotropic agents. After repeated oral administration of Navane to rats (5 to 15 mg/kg/day), rabbits (3 to 50 mg/kg/day), and monkeys (1 to 3 mg/kg/day) before and during gestation, no teratogenic effects were seen. (See Precautions)

Usage in Children—The use of Navane in children under 12 years of age is not recommended because safety and efficacy in the pediatric age group have not been established.

As is true with many CNS drugs, Navane may impair the mental and/or physical abilities required for the performance of potentially hazardous tasks such as driving a car or operating machinery, especially during the first few days of therapy. Therefore, the patient should be cautioned accordingly.

As in the case of other CNS-acting drugs, patients receiving Navane should be cautioned about the possible additive effects (which may include hypotension) with CNS depressants and with alcohol.

PRECAUTIONS

General: An antiemetic effect was observed in animal studies with Navane (thiothixene hydrochloride); since this effect may also occur in man, it is possible that Navane may mask signs of overdosage of toxic drugs and may obscure conditions such as intestinal obstruction and brain tumor.

In consideration of the known capability of Navane and certain other psychotropic drugs to precipitate convulsions, extreme caution should be used in patients with a history of convulsive disorders, or those in a state of alcohol withdrawal since it may lower the convulsive threshold. Although Navane potentiates the actions of the barbiturates, the dosage of the anticonvulsant therapy should not be reduced when Navane is administered concurrently.

Caution as well as careful adjustment of the dosage is indicated when Navane is used in conjunction with other CNS depressants other than anticonvulsant drugs.

Though exhibiting rather weak anticholinergic properties, Navane should be used with caution in patients who are known or suspected to have glaucoma, or who might be exposed to extreme heat, or who are receiving atropine or related drugs.

Use with caution in patients with cardiovascular disease.

Also, careful observation should be made for pigmentary retinopathy, and lenticular pigmentation (fine lenticular pigmentation has been noted in a small number of patients treated with Navane for prolonged periods). Blood dyscrasias (agranulocytosis, pancytopenia, thrombocytopenic purpura), and liver damage (jaundice, biliary stasis), have been reported with related drugs.

Undue exposure to sunlight should be avoided. Photosensitive reactions have been reported in patients on Navane.

As with all intramuscular preparations, Navane Intramuscular For Injection should be injected well within the body of a relatively large muscle. The preferred sites are the upper outer quadrant of the buttock (i.e., gluteus maximus) and the mid-lateral thigh.

The deltoid area should be used only if well developed such as in certain adults and older children, and then only with caution to avoid radial nerve injury. Intramuscular injections should not be made into the lower and mid-thirds of the upper arm. As with all intramuscular injections, aspiration is necessary to help avoid inadvertent injection into a blood vessel.

Neuroleptic drugs elevate prolactin levels; the elevation persists during chronic administration. Tissue culture experiments indicate that approximately one-third of human breast cancers are prolactin dependent *in vitro,* a factor of potential importance if the prescription of these drugs is contemplated in a patient with a previously detected breast cancer. Although disturbances such as galactorrhea, amenorrhea, gynecomastia, and impotence have been reported, the clinical significance of elevated serum prolactin levels is unknown for most patients. An increase in mammary neoplasms has been found in rodents after chronic administration of neuroleptic drugs. Neither clinical studies nor epidemiologic studies conducted to date, however, have shown an association between chronic administration of these drugs and mammary tumorigenesis; the available evidence is considered too limited to be conclusive at this time.

Information for Patients: Given the likelihood that some patients exposed chronically to neuroleptics will develop tardive dyskinesia, it is advised that all patients in whom chronic use is contemplated be given, if possible, full information about this risk. The decision to inform patients and/or their guardians must obviously take into account the clinical circumstances and the competency of the patient to understand the information provided.

ADVERSE REACTIONS

NOTE: Not all of the following adverse reactions have been reported with Navane. However, since Navane has certain chemical and pharmacologic similarities to the phenothiazines, all of the known side effects and toxicity associated with phenothiazine therapy should be borne in mind when Navane is used.

Cardiovascular Effects: Tachycardia, hypotension, lightheadedness, and syncope. In the event hypotension occurs, epinephrine should not be used as a pressor agent since a paradoxical further lowering of blood pressure may result. Nonspecific EKG changes have been observed in some patients receiving Navane. These changes are usually reversible and frequently disappear on continued Navane therapy. The clinical significance of these changes is not known.

CNS Effects: Drowsiness, usually mild, may occur although it usually subsides with continuation of Navane therapy. The incidence of sedation appears similar to that of the piperazine group of phenothiazines, but less than that of certain aliphatic phenothiazines. Restlessness, agitation and insomnia have been noted with Navane. Seizures and paradoxical exacerbation of psychotic symptoms have occurred with Navane infrequently.

Hyperreflexia has been reported in infants delivered from mothers having received structurally related drugs.

In addition, phenothiazine derivatives have been associated with cerebral edema and cerebrospinal fluid abnormalities.

Extrapyramidal symptoms, such as pseudo-parkinsonism, akathisia, and dystonia have been reported. Management of these extrapyramidal symptoms depends upon the type and severity. Rapid relief of acute symptoms may require the use of an injectable antiparkinson agent. More slowly emerging symptoms may be managed by reducing the dosage of Navane and/or administering an oral antiparkinson agent.

Persistent Tardive Dyskinesia: As with all antipsychotic agents tardive dyskinesia may appear in some patients on long term therapy or may occur after drug therapy has been discontinued. The syndrome is characterized by rhythmical involuntary movements of the tongue, face, mouth or jaw (e.g., protrusion of tongue, puffing of cheeks, puckering of mouth, chewing movements). Sometimes these may be accompanied by involuntary movements of extremities.

Since early detection of tardive dyskinesia is important, patients should be monitored on an ongoing basis. It has been reported that fine vermicular movement of the tongue may be an early sign of the syndrome. If this or any other presentation of the syndrome is observed, the clinician should consider possible discontinuation of neuroleptic medication. (See WARNINGS section.)

Hepatic Effects: Elevations of serum transaminase and alkaline phosphatase, usually transient, have been infrequently observed in some patients. No clinically confirmed cases of jaundice attributable to Navane (thiothixene hydrochloride) have been reported.

Hematologic Effects: As is true with certain other psychotropic drugs, leukopenia and leucocytosis, which are usually transient, can occur occasionally with Navane. Other antipsychotic drugs have been associated with agranulocytosis, eosinophilia, hemolytic anemia, thrombocytopenia and pancytopenia.

Allergic Reactions: Rash, pruritus, urticaria, and rare cases of anaphylaxis have been reported with Navane. Undue exposure to sunlight should be avoided. Although not experienced with Navane, exfoliative dermatitis, contact dermatitis (in nursing personnel), have been reported with certain phenothiazines.

Endocrine Disorders: Lactation, moderate breast enlargement and amenorrhea have occurred in a small percentage of females receiving Navane. If persistent, this may necessitate a reduction in dosage or the discontinuation of therapy. Phenothiazines have been associated with false positive pregnancy tests, gynecomastia, hypoglycemia, hyperglycemia, and glycosuria.

Autonomic Effects: Dry mouth, blurred vision, nasal congestion, constipation, increased sweating, increased salivation, and impotence have occurred infrequently with Navane therapy. Phenothiazines have been associated with miosis, mydriasis, and adynamic ileus.

Other Adverse Reactions: Hyperpyrexia, anorexia, nausea, vomiting, diarrhea, increase in appetite and weight, weakness or fatigue, polydipsia and peripheral edema.

Although not reported with Navane, evidence indicates there is a relationship between phenothiazine therapy and the occurrence of a systemic lupus erythematosus-like syndrome.

Neuroleptic Malignant Syndrome (NMS): Please refer to the text regarding NMS in the WARNINGS section.

NOTE: Sudden deaths have occasionally been reported in patients who have received certain phenothiazine derivatives. In some cases the cause of death was apparently cardiac arrest or asphyxia due to failure of the cough reflex. In others, the cause could not be determined nor could it be established that death was due to phenothiazine administration.

DOSAGE AND ADMINISTRATION

Preparation

Navane (thiothixene hydrochloride) Intramuscular For Injection must be reconstituted with 2.2 ml of sterile water for injection.

For Intramuscular Use Only

Dosage of Navane should be individually adjusted depending on the chronicity and severity of the condition. In general, small doses should be used initially and gradually increased to the optimal effective level, based on patient response.

Usage in children under 12 years of age is not recommended.

Where more rapid control and treatment of acute behavior is desirable, the intramuscular form of Navane may be indicated. It is also of benefit where the very nature of the patient's symptomatology, whether acute or chronic, renders oral administration impractical or even impossible.

Continued on next page

Navane IM—Cont.

For treatment of acute symptomatology or in patients unable or unwilling to take oral medication, the usual dose is 4 mg of Navane Intramuscular For Injection administered 2 to 4 times daily. Dosage may be increased or decreased depending on response. Most patients are controlled on a total daily dosage of 16 to 20 mg. The maximum recommended dosage is 30 mg/day. An oral form should supplant the injectable form as soon as possible. It may be necessary to adjust the dosage when changing from the intramuscular to oral dosage forms. Dosage recommendations for Navane Capsules and Concentrate can be found in the Navane oral package insert.

OVERDOSAGE

Manifestations include muscular twitching, drowsiness, and dizziness. Symptoms of gross overdosage may include CNS depression, rigidity, weakness, torticollis, tremor, salivation, dysphagia, hypotension, disturbances of gait, or coma.

Treatment: Essentially symptomatic and supportive. Keep patient under careful observation and maintain an open airway, since involvement of the extrapyramidal system may produce dysphagia and respiratory difficulty in severe overdosage. If hypotension occurs, the standard measures for managing circulatory shock should be used (I.V. fluids and/ or vasoconstrictors).

If a vasoconstrictor is needed, levarterenol and phenylephrine are the most suitable drugs. Other pressor agents, including epinephrine, are not recommended, since phenothiazine derivatives may reverse the usual pressor elevating action of these agents and cause further lowering of blood pressure.

If CNS depression is marked, symptomatic treatment is indicated. Extrapyramidal symptoms may be treated with antiparkinson drugs.

There are no data on the use of peritoneal or hemodialysis, but they are known to be of little value in phenothiazine intoxication.

HOW SUPPLIED

Navane (thiothixene hydrochloride) Intramuscular For Injection is available in amber glass vials in packages of 10 vials (NDC 0049-5765-83). When reconstituted with 2.2 ml of STERILE WATER FOR INJECTION, each ml contains thiothixene hydrochloride equivalent to 5 mg of thiothixene, and 59.6 mg of mannitol. The reconstituted solution of Navane Intramuscular For Injection may be stored for 48 hours at room temperature before discarding.

70-4177-00-4
Revised January 1988

NORVASC® ℞

[*nor 'vask*]
(amlodipine besylate)
Tablets

DESCRIPTION

NORVASC® is the besylate salt of amlodipine, a long-acting calcium channel blocker.

NORVASC is chemically described as (R.S.) 3-ethyl-5-methyl-2-(2-aminoethoxymethyl)-4-(2-chlorophenyl)-1,4-dihydro-6-methyl-3,5-pyridinedicarboxylate benzenesulphonate. Its empirical formula is $C_{20}H_{25}ClN_2O_5 \cdot C_6H_6O_3S$, and its structural formula is:

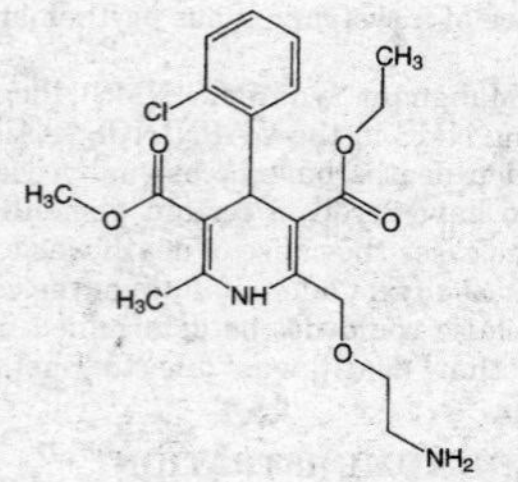

$C_6H_6O_3S$

Amlodipine besylate is a white crystalline powder with a molecular weight of 567.1. It is slightly soluble in water and sparingly soluble in ethanol. NORVASC (amlodipine besylate) tablets are formulated as white tablets equivalent to 2.5, 5 and 10 mg of amlodipine for oral administration. In addition to the active ingredient, amlodipine besylate, each tablet contains the following inactive ingredients: microcrystalline cellulose, dibasic calcium phosphate anhydrous, sodium starch glycolate, and magnesium stearate.

CLINICAL PHARMACOLOGY

Mechanism of Action: NORVASC is a dihydropyridine calcium antagonist (calcium ion antagonist or slow-channel blocker) that inhibits the transmembrane influx of calcium ions into vascular smooth muscle and cardiac muscle. Experimental data suggest that NORVASC binds to both dihydropyridine and nondihydropyridine binding sites. The contractile processes of cardiac muscle and vascular smooth muscle are dependent upon the movement of extracellular calcium ions into these cells through specific ion channels. NORVASC inhibits calcium ion influx across cell membranes selectively, with a greater effect on vascular smooth muscle cells than on cardiac muscle cells. Negative inotropic effects can be detected *in vitro* but such effects have not been seen in intact animals at therapeutic doses. Serum calcium concentration is not affected by NORVASC. Within the physiologic pH range, NORVASC is an ionized compound (pKa=8.6), and its kinetic interaction with the calcium channel receptor is characterized by a gradual rate of association and dissociation with the receptor binding site, resulting in a gradual onset of effect.

NORVASC is a peripheral arterial vasodilator that acts directly on vascular smooth muscle to cause a reduction in peripheral vascular resistance and reduction in blood pressure.

The precise mechanisms by which NORVASC relieves angina have not been fully delineated, but are thought to include the following:

Exertional Angina: In patients with exertional angina, NORVASC reduces the total peripheral resistance (afterload) against which the heart works and reduces the rate pressure product, and thus myocardial oxygen demand, at any given level of exercise.

Vasospastic Angina: NORVASC has been demonstrated to block constriction and restore blood flow in coronary arteries and arterioles in response to calcium, potassium epinephrine, serotonin, and thromboxane A_2 analog in experimental animal models and in human coronary vessels *in vitro*. This inhibition of coronary spasm is responsible for the effectiveness of NORVASC in vasospastic (Prinzmetal's or variant) angina.

Pharmacokinetics and Metabolism: After oral administration of therapeutic doses of NORVASC, absorption produces peak plasma concentrations between 6 and 12 hours. Absolute bioavailability has been estimated to be between 64 and 90%. The bioavailability of NORVASC is not altered by the presence of food.

NORVASC is extensively (about 90%) converted to inactive metabolites via hepatic metabolism with 10% of the parent compound and 60% of the metabolites excreted in the urine. *Ex vivo* studies have shown that approximately 93% of the circulating drug is bound to plasma proteins in hypertensive patients. Elimination from the plasma is biphasic with a terminal elimination half-life of about 30–50 hours. Steady-state plasma levels of NORVASC are reached after 7 to 8 days of consecutive daily dosing.

The pharmacokinetics of NORVASC are not significantly influenced by renal impairment. Patients with renal failure may therefore receive the usual initial dose.

Elderly patients and patients with hepatic insufficiency have decreased clearance of amlodipine with a resulting increase in AUC of approximately 40–60%, and a lower initial dose may be required. A similar increase in AUC was observed in patients with moderate to severe heart failure.

Pharmacodynamics: *Hemodynamics* Following administration of therapeutic doses to patients with hypertension, NORVASC produces vasodilation resulting in a reduction of supine and standing blood pressures. These decreases in blood pressure are not accompanied by a significant change in heart rate or plasma catecholamine levels with chronic dosing. Although the acute intravenous administration of amlodipine decreases arterial blood pressure and increases heart rate in hemodynamic studies of patients with chronic stable angina, chronic administration of oral amlodipine in clinical trials did not lead to clinically significant changes in heart rate or blood pressures in normotensive patients with angina.

With chronic once daily oral administration, antihypertensive effectiveness is maintained for at least 24 hours. Plasma concentrations correlate with effect in both young and elderly patients. The magnitude of reduction in blood pressure with NORVASC is also correlated with the height of pretreatment elevation; thus, individuals with moderate hypertension (diastolic pressure 105–114 mmHg) had about a 50% greater response than patients with mild hypertension (diastolic pressure 90–104 mmHg). Normotensive subjects experienced no clinically significant change in blood pressures (+1/–2 mmHg).

In hypertensive patients with normal renal function, therapeutic doses of NORVASC resulted in a decrease in renal vascular resistance and an increase in glomerular filtration rate and effective renal plasma flow without change in filtration fraction or proteinuria.

As with other calcium channel blockers, hemodynamic measurements of cardiac function at rest and during exercise (or pacing) in patients with normal ventricular function treated with NORVASC have generally demonstrated a small increase in cardiac index without significant influence on dP/dt or on left ventricular end diastolic pressure or volume. In hemodynamic studies, NORVASC has not been associated with a negative inotropic effect when administered in the therapeutic dose range to intact animals and man, even when co-administered with beta-blockers to man. Similar findings, however, have been observed in normals or well-compensated patients with heart failure with agents possessing significant negative inotropic effects.

Studies in Patients with Congestive Heart Failure: NORVASC has been compared to placebo in four 8–12 week studies of patients with NYHA class II/III heart failure, involving a total of 697 patients. In these studies, there was no evidence of worsened heart failure based on measures of exercise tolerance, NYHA classification, symptoms, or LVEF. In a long-term (follow-up at least 6 months, mean 13.8 months) placebo-controlled mortality/morbidity study of NORVASC 5–10 mg in 1153 patients with NYHA classes III (n=931) or IV (n=222) heart failure on stable doses of diuretics, digoxin, and ACE inhibitors, NORVASC had no effect on the primary endpoint of the study which was the combined endpoint of all-cause mortality and cardiac morbidity (as defined by life-threatening arrhythmia, acute myocardial infarction, or hospitalization for worsened heart failure), or on NYHA classification, or symptoms of heart failure. Total combined all-cause mortality and cardiac morbidity events were 222/571 (39%) for patients on NORVASC and 246/583 (42%) for patients on placebo; the cardiac morbid events represented about 25% of the endpoints in the study.

Electrophysiologic Effects: NORVASC does not change sinoatrial nodal function or atrioventricular conduction in intact animals or man. In patients with chronic stable angina, intravenous administration of 10 mg did not significantly alter A-H and H-V conduction and sinus node recovery time after pacing. Similar results were obtained in patients receiving NORVASC and concomitant beta blockers. In clinical studies in which NORVASC was administered in combination with beta-blockers to patients with either hypertension or angina, no adverse effects on electrocardiographic parameters were observed. In clinical trials with angina patients alone, NORVASC therapy did not alter electrocardiographic intervals or produce higher degrees of AV blocks.

Effects in Hypertension: The antihypertensive efficacy of NORVASC has been demonstrated in a total of 15 double-blind, placebo-controlled, randomized studies involving 800 patients on NORVASC and 538 on placebo. Once daily administration produced statistically significant placebo-corrected reductions in supine and standing blood pressures at 24 hours postdose, averaging about 12/6 mmHg in the standing position and 13/7 mmHg in the supine position in patients with mild to moderate hypertension. Maintenance of the blood pressure effect over the 24-hour dosing interval was observed, with little difference in peak and trough effect. Tolerance was not demonstrated in patients studied for up to 1 year. The 3 parallel, fixed dose, dose response studies showed that the reduction in supine and standing blood pressures was dose-related within the recommended dosing range. Effects on diastolic pressure were similar in young and older patients. The effect on systolic pressure was greater in older patients, perhaps because of greater baseline systolic pressure. Effects were similar in black patients and in white patients.

Effects in Chronic Stable Angina: The effectiveness of 5–10 mg/day of NORVASC in exercise-induced angina has been evaluated in 8 placebo-controlled, double-blind clinical trials of up to 6 weeks duration involving 1038 patients (684 NORVASC, 354 placebo) with chronic stable angina. In 5 of the 8 studies significant increases in exercise time (bicycle or treadmill) were seen with the 10 mg dose. Increases in symptom-limited exercise time averaged 12.8% (63 sec) for NORVASC 10 mg, and averaged 7.9% (38 sec) for NORVASC 5 mg. NORVASC 10 mg also increased time to 1 mm ST segment deviation in several studies and decreased angina attack rate. The sustained efficacy of NORVASC in angina patients has been demonstrated over long-term dosing. In patients with angina there were no clinically significant reductions in blood pressures (4/1 mmHg) or changes in heart rate (+0.3 bpm).

Effects in Vasospastic Angina: In a double-blind, placebo-controlled clinical trial of 4 weeks duration in 50 patients, NORVASC therapy decreased attacks by approximately 4/week compared with a placebo decrease of approximately 1/week ($p<0.01$). Two of 23 NORVASC and 7 of 27 placebo patients discontinued from the study due to lack of clinical improvement.

INDICATIONS AND USAGE

1. Hypertension

NORVASC is indicated for the treatment of hypertension. It may be used alone or in combination with other antihypertensive agents.

2. Chronic Stable Angina

NORVASC is indicated for the treatment of chronic stable angina. NORVASC may be used alone or in combination with other antianginal agents.

3. Vasospastic Angina (Prinzmetal's or Variant Angina)

NORVASC is indicated for the treatment of confirmed or suspected vasospastic angina. NORVASC may be used as monotherapy or in combination with other antianginal drugs.

CONTRAINDICATIONS

NORVASC is contraindicated in patients with known sensitivity to amlodipine.

WARNINGS

Increased Angina and/or Myocardial Infarction: Rarely, patients, particularly those with severe obstructive coronary artery disease, have developed documented increased frequency, duration and/or severity of angina or acute myocardial infarction on starting calcium channel blocker therapy or at the time of dosage increase. The mechanism of this effect has not been elucidated.

PRECAUTIONS

General: Since the vasodilation induced by NORVASC is gradual in onset, acute hypotension has rarely been reported after oral administration of NORVASC. Nonetheless, caution should be exercised when administering NORVASC as with any other peripheral vasodilator particularly in patients with severe aortic stenosis.

Use in Patients with Congestive Heart Failure: In general, calcium channel blockers should be used with caution in patients with heart failure. NORVASC (5–10 mg per day) has been studied in a placebo-controlled trial of 1153 patients with NYHA Class III or IV heart failure (see CLINICAL PHARMACOLOGY) on stable doses of ACE inhibitor, digoxin, and diuretics. Follow-up was at least 6 months, with a mean of about 14 months. There was no overall adverse effect on survival or cardiac morbidity (as defined by life-threatening arrhythmia, acute myocardial infarction, or hospitalization for worsened heart failure). NORVASC has been compared to placebo in four 8–12 week studies of patients with NYHA class II/III heart failure, involving a total of 697 patients. In these studies, there was no evidence of worsened heart failure based on measures of exercise tolerance, NYHA classification, symptoms, or LVEF.

Beta-Blocker Withdrawal: NORVASC is not a beta-blocker and therefore gives no protection against the dangers of abrupt beta-blocker withdrawal; any such withdrawal should be by gradual reduction of the dose of beta-blocker.

Patients with Hepatic Failure: Since NORVASC is extensively metabolized by the liver and the plasma elimination half-life (t 1/2) is 56 hours in patients with impaired hepatic function, caution should be exercised when administering NORVASC to patients with severe hepatic impairment.

Drug Interactions: *In vitro* data in human plasma indicate that NORVASC has no effect on the protein binding of drugs tested (digoxin, phenytoin, warfarin, and indomethacin).

Special Studies: Effect of other agents on NORVASC

CIMETIDINE. Co-administration of NORVASC with cimetidine did not alter the pharmacokinetics of NORVASC.

GRAPEFRUIT JUICE: Co-administration of 240 mL of grapefruit juice with a single oral dose of amlodipine 10 mg in 20 healthy volunteers had no significant effect on the pharmacokinetics of amlodipine.

MAALOX (antacid): Co-administration of the antacid Maalox with a single dose of NORVASC had no significant effect on the pharmacokinetics of NORVASC.

SILDENAFIL. A single 100 mg dose of sildenafil (Viagra®) in subjects with essential hypertension had no effect on the pharmacokinetic parameters of NORVASC. When NORVASC and sildenafil were used in combination, each agent independently exerted its own blood pressure lowering effect.

Special Studies: Effect of NORVASC on other agents.

ATORVASTATIN: Co-administration of multiple 10 mg doses of NORVASC with 80 mg of atorvastatin resulted in no significant change in the steady state pharmacokinetic parameters of atorvastatin.

DIGOXIN: Co-administration of NORVASC with digoxin did not change serum digoxin levels or digoxin renal clearance in normal volunteers.

ETHANOL (alcohol): Single and multiple 10 mg doses of NORVASC had no significant effect on the pharmacokinetics of ethanol.

WARFARIN: Co-administration of NORVASC with warfarin did not change the warfarin prothrombin response time.

In clinical trials, NORVASC has been safely administered with thiazide diuretics, beta-blockers, angiotensin-converting enzyme inhibitors, long-acting nitrates, sublingual nitroglycerin, digoxin, warfarin, non-steroidal anti-inflammatory drugs, antibiotics, and oral hypoglycemic drugs.

Drug/Laboratory Test Interactions: None known.

Carcinogenesis, Mutagenesis, Impairment of Fertility: Rats and mice treated with amlodipine in the diet for two years, at concentrations calculated to provide daily dosage levels of 0.5, 1.25, and 2.5 mg/kg/day showed no evidence of carcinogenicity. The highest dose (for mice, similar to, and for rats twice* the maximum recommended clinical dose of 10 mg on a mg/m^2 basis) was close to the maximum tolerated dose for mice but not for rats.

Mutagenicity studies revealed no drug related effects at either the gene or chromosome levels.

There was no effect on the fertility of rats treated with amlodipine (males for 64 days and females 14 days prior to mating) at doses up to 10 mg/kg/day (8 times* the maximum recommended human dose of 10 mg on a mg/m^2 basis).

Pregnancy Category C: No evidence of teratogenicity or other embryo/fetal toxicity was found when pregnant rats or rabbits were treated orally with up to 10 mg/kg amlodipine (respectively 8 times* and 23 times* the maximum recommended human dose of 10 mg on a mg/m^2 basis) during their respective periods of major organogenesis. However, litter size was significantly decreased (by about 50%) and the number of intrauterine deaths was significantly increased (about 5-fold) in rats administered 10 mg/kg amlodipine for 14 days before mating and throughout mating and gestation. Amlodipine has been shown to prolong both the gestation period and the duration of labor in rats at this dose. There are no adequate and well-controlled studies in pregnant women. Amlodipine should be used during pregnancy only if the potential benefit justifies the potential risk to the fetus.

*Based on patient weight of 50 kg.

Nursing Mothers: It is not known whether amlodipine is excreted in human milk. In the absence of this information, it is recommended that nursing be discontinued while NORVASC is administered.

Pediatric Use: Safety and effectiveness of NORVASC in children have not been established.

Geriatric Use: Clinical studies of NORVASC did not include sufficient numbers of subjects aged 65 and over to determine whether they respond differently from younger subjects. Other reported clinical experience has not identified differences in responses between the elderly and younger patients. In general, dose selection for an elderly patient should be cautious, usually starting at the low end of the dosing range, reflecting the greater frequency of decreased hepatic, renal, or cardiac function, and of concomitant disease or other drug therapy. Elderly patients have decreased clearance of amlodipine with a resulting increase of AUC of approximately 40–60%, and a lower initial dose may be required (see **DOSAGE AND ADMINISTRATION**).

ADVERSE REACTIONS

NORVASC has been evaluated for safety in more than 11,000 patients in U.S. and foreign clinical trials. In general, treatment with NORVASC was well-tolerated at doses up to 10 mg daily. Most adverse reactions reported during therapy with NORVASC were of mild or moderate severity. In controlled clinical trials directly comparing NORVASC (N=1730) in doses up to 10 mg to placebo (N=1250), discontinuation of NORVASC due to adverse reactions was required in only about 1.5% of patients and was not significantly different from placebo (about 1%). The most common side effects are headache and edema. The incidence (%) of side effects which occurred in a dose related manner are as follows:

Adverse Event	2.5 mg N=275	5.0 mg N=296	10.0 mg N=268	Placebo N=520
Edema	1.8	3.0	10.8	0.6
Dizziness	1.1	3.4	3.4	1.5
Flushing	0.7	1.4	2.6	0.0
Palpitation	0.7	1.4	4.5	0.6

Other adverse experiences which were not clearly dose related but which were reported with an incidence greater than 1.0% in placebo-controlled clinical trials include the following:

Placebo-Controlled Studies

	NORVASC (%) (N=1730)	PLACEBO (%) (N=1250)
Headache	7.3	7.8
Fatigue	4.5	2.8
Nausea	2.9	1.9
Abdominal Pain	1.6	0.3
Somnolence	1.4	0.6

For several adverse experiences that appear to be drug and dose related, there was a greater incidence in women than men associated with amlodipine treatment as shown in the following table:

ADR	NORVASC M=% (N=1218)	NORVASC F=% (N=512)	PLACEBO M=% (N=914)	PLACEBO F=% (N=336)
Edema	5.6	14.6	1.4	5.1
Flushing	1.5	4.5	0.3	0.9
Palpitations	1.4	3.3	0.9	0.9
Somnolence	1.3	1.6	0.8	0.3

The following events occurred in ≤1% but >0.1% of patients in controlled clinical trials or under conditions of open trials or marketing experience where a causal relationship is uncertain; they are listed to alert the physician to a possible relationship:

Cardiovascular: arrhythmia (including ventricular tachycardia and atrial fibrillation), bradycardia, chest pain, hypotension, peripheral ischemia, syncope, tachycardia, postural dizziness, postural hypotension, vasculitis.

Central and Peripheral Nervous System: hypoesthesia, neuropathy peripheral, paresthesia, tremor, vertigo.

Gastrointestinal: anorexia, constipation, dyspepsia,** dysphagia, diarrhea, flatulence, pancreatitis, vomiting, gingival hyperplasia.

General: allergic reaction, asthenia,** back pain, hot flushes, malaise, pain, rigors, weight gain.

Musculoskeletal System: arthralgia, arthrosis, muscle cramps,** myalgia.

Psychiatric: sexual dysfunction (male** and female), insomnia, nervousness, depression, abnormal dreams, anxiety, depersonalization.

Respiratory System: dyspnea,** epistaxis.

Skin and Appendages: angioedema, erythema multiforme, pruritus,** rash,** rash erythematous, rash maculopapular.

**These events occurred in less than 1% in placebo-controlled trials, but the incidence of these side effects was between 1% and 2% in all multiple dose studies.

Special Senses: abnormal vision, conjunctivitis, diplopia, eye pain, tinnitus.

Urinary System: micturition frequency, micturition disorder, nocturia.

Autonomic Nervous System: dry mouth, sweating increased.

Metabolic and Nutritional: hyperglycemia, thirst.

Hemopoietic: leukopenia, purpura, thrombocytopenia.

The following events occurred in ≤0.1% of patients: cardiac failure, pulse irregularity, extrasystoles, skin discoloration, urticaria, skin dryness, alopecia, dermatitis, muscle weakness, twitching, ataxia, hypertonia, migraine, cold and clammy skin, apathy, agitation, amnesia, gastritis, increased appetite, loose stools, coughing, rhinitis, dysuria, polyuria, parosmia, taste perversion, abnormal visual accommodation, and xerophthalmia.

Other reactions occurred sporadically and cannot be distinguished from medications or concurrent disease states such as myocardial infarction and angina.

NORVASC therapy has not been associated with clinically significant changes in routine laboratory tests. No clinically relevant changes were noted in serum potassium, serum glucose, total triglycerides, total cholesterol, HDL cholesterol, uric acid, blood urea nitrogen, or creatinine.

The following postmarketing event has been reported infrequently where a causal relationship is uncertain: gynecomastia. In postmarketing experience, jaundice and hepatic enzyme elevations (mostly consistent with cholestasis or hepatitis) in some cases severe enough to require hospitalization have been reported in association with use of amlodipine.

NORVASC has been used safely in patients with chronic obstructive pulmonary disease, well-compensated congestive heart failure, peripheral vascular disease, diabetes mellitus, and abnormal lipid profiles.

OVERDOSAGE

Single oral doses of 40 mg/kg and 100 mg/kg in mice and rats, respectively, caused deaths. A single oral dose of 4 mg/kg or higher in dogs caused a marked peripheral vasodilation and hypotension.

Overdosage might be expected to cause excessive peripheral vasodilation with marked hypotension and possibly a reflex tachycardia. In humans, experience with intentional overdosage of NORVASC is limited. Reports of intentional overdosage include a patient who ingested 250 mg and was asymptomatic and was not hospitalized; another (120 mg) was hospitalized, underwent gastric lavage and remained normotensive; the third (105 mg) was hospitalized and had hypotension (90/50 mmHg) which normalized following plasma expansion. A patient who took 70 mg amlodipine and an unknown quantity of benzodiazepine in a suicide attempt developed shock which was refractory to treatment and died the following day with abnormally high benzodiazepine plasma concentration. A case of accidental drug overdose has been documented in a 19-month-old male who ingested 30 mg amlodipine (about 2mg/kg). During the emergency room presentation, vital signs were stable with no evidence of hypotension, but a heart rate of 180 bpm. Ipecac was administered 3.5 hours after ingestion and on subsequent observation (overnight) no sequelae were noted.

If massive overdose should occur, active cardiac and respiratory monitoring should be instituted. Frequent blood pressure measurements are essential. Should hypotension occur, cardiovascular support including elevation of the extremities and the judicious administration of fluids should be initiated. If hypotension remains unresponsive to these conservative measures, administration of vasopressors (such as phenylephrine) should be considered with attention to circulating volume and urine output. Intravenous calcium gluconate may help to reverse the effects of calcium entry blockade. As NORVASC is highly protein bound, hemodialysis is not likely to be of benefit.

DOSAGE AND ADMINISTRATION

The usual initial antihypertensive oral dose of NORVASC is 5 mg once daily with a maximum dose of 10 mg once daily. Small, fragile, or elderly individuals, or patients with hepatic insufficiency may be started on 2.5 mg once daily and this dose may be used when adding NORVASC to other antihypertensive therapy.

Dosage should be adjusted according to each patient's need. In general, titration should proceed over 7 to 14 days so that the physician can fully assess the patient's response to each dose level. Titration may proceed more rapidly, however, if clinically warranted, provided the patient is assessed frequently.

The recommended dose for chronic stable or vasospastic angina is 5–10 mg, with the lower dose suggested in the elderly and in patients with hepatic insufficiency. Most patients will require 10 mg for adequate effect. See ADVERSE REACTIONS section for information related to dosage and side effects.

Co-administration with Other Antihypertensive and/or Antianginal Drugs: NORVASC has been safely administered with thiazides, ACE inhibitors, beta-blockers, long-acting nitrates, and/or sublingual nitroglycerin.

HOW SUPPLIED

NORVASC®–2.5 mg Tablets (amlodipine besylate equivalent to 2.5 mg of amlodipine per tablet) are supplied as white, diamond, flat-faced, beveled edged engraved with "NORVASC" on one side and "2.5" on the other side and supplied as follows:

NDC 0069-1520-68	Bottle of 90
NDC 0069-1520-66	Bottle of 100

NORVASC®–5 mg Tablets (amlodipine besylate equivalent to 5 mg of amlodipine per tablet) are white, elongated octagon, flat-faced, beveled edged engraved with both "NORVASC" and "5" on one side and plain on the other side and supplied as follows:

NDC 0069-1530-68	Bottle of 90
NDC 0069-1530-66	Bottle of 100
NDC 0069-1530-41	Unit Dose package of 100
NDC 0069-1530-72	Bottle of 300

NORVASC®–10 mg Tablets (amlodipine besylate equivalent to 10 mg of amlodipine per tablet) are white, round, flat-

Continued on next page

Norvasc—Cont.

faced, beveled edged engraved with both "NORVASC" and "10" on one side and plain on the other side and supplied as follows:

NDC 0069-1540-68	Bottle of 90
NDC 0069-1540-66	Bottle of 100
NDC 0069-1540-41	Unit Dose package of 100

Store bottles at controlled room temperature, 59° to 86°F (15° to 30°C) and dispense in tight, light-resistant containers (USP).

65-4782-00-9 Revised April 2000

Shown in Product Identification Guide, page 330

PERMAPEN® *ISOJECT®* ℞

(Penicillin G Benzathine)
Injectable Suspension
1,200,000 units
For Intramuscular Use Only
STORE BETWEEN 2°–8°C (36°–46°F)
SHAKE WELL BEFORE USING

DESCRIPTION

Permapen® (Penicillin G Benzathine) Injectable Suspension, a sterile antibacterial agent, is a repository penicillin compound which provides blood levels for long periods following its intramuscular injection. This property is the result of its extremely low solubility in water. Each milliliter contains 600,000 units of penicillin G benzathine; 0.006 grams sodium citrate; 0.003 grams polyvinylpyrrolidone; 0.010 grams lecithin, and 0.003 grams sodium carboxymethylcellulose in an aqueous suspension. Permapen also contains methylparaben 0.09% and propylparaben 0.01% as preservatives.

Chemically, Permapen is 3,3-dimethyl-7-oxo-6-(2-phenylacetamido)-4-thia-l-azabicyclo [3.2.0] heptane-2-carboxylic acid compound with N,N′-dibenzylethylenediamine (2:1) tetrahydrate. It is prepared by the reaction of dibenzyltetrahydrate-ethylenediamine with 2 molecules of penicillin G.

It has a molecular weight of 981.19 and the following chemical structure:

Formula

$$C_{16}H_{20}N_2{\cdot}2C_{16}H_{18}N_2O_4S{\cdot}4H_2O$$

Penicillin G benzathine occurs as a white crystalline powder and is very slightly soluble in water.

The pH of the injectable suspension is between 5.0–7.5.

CLINICAL PHARMACOLOGY

Intramuscular penicillin G benzathine is absorbed very slowly into the blood stream from the intramuscular site and converted by hydrolysis to penicillin G. This combination of hydrolysis and slow absorption results in blood serum levels much lower than those of other parenteral penicillins.

Approximately 60% of penicillin G is bound to serum protein. The drug is distributed throughout the body tissues in widely varying amounts. Highest levels are found in the kidneys with lesser amounts in the liver, skin, and intestines. Penicillin G penetrates into all other tissues and the spinal fluid to a lesser degree. With normal kidney function the drug is excreted rapidly by tubular excretion. A small amount is secreted into the bile. In neonates and young infants, and in individuals with impaired kidney function, excretion is considerably delayed.

Microbiology: Penicillin G exerts a bactericidal action against penicillin-susceptible microorganisms during the stage of active multiplication. It acts through the inhibition of biosynthesis of cell wall mucopeptide. It is not active against the penicillinase-producing bacteria, which includes many strains of staphylococci.

While *in vitro* studies have demonstrated the susceptibility of most strains of the following organisms, clinical efficacy for infections other than those included in the INDICATIONS AND USAGE section has not been documented. Penicillin G exerts high *in vitro* activity against staphylococci (except penicillinase-producing strains), streptococci (groups A, C, G, H, L, and M), and pneumococci. Other organisms sensitive to penicillin G are: *Corynebacterium diphtheriae, Bacillus anthracis,* Clostridia, *Actinomyces bovis, Streptobacillus moniliformis, Listeria monocytogenes,* and Leptospira. *Treponema pallidum* is extremely sensitive to the bactericidal action of penicillin G.

Penicillin acts synergistically with gentamicin or tobramycin against many strains of enterococci.

INDICATIONS AND USAGE

Intramuscular penicillin G benzathine is indicated in the treatment of infections in both children and adults due to penicillin G-susceptible microorganisms that are susceptible to the low and very prolonged serum levels common to this particular dosage form in the indications listed below. Therapy should be guided by clinical response.

Note: When high sustained serum levels are required, injectable penicillin G either IM or IV should be used.

The following infections will usually respond to adequate dosages of intramuscular penicillin G benzathine:

Upper Respiratory Tract (pharyngitis): streptococci (group A – without bacteremia).

Venereal Infections: Syphilis Yaws, bejel, and pinta.

Medical Conditions in Which Penicillin G Benzathine Therapy is Indicated As Prophylaxis: *rheumatic fever and/or chorea:* Prophylaxis with penicillin G benzathine has proven effective in preventing recurrence of these conditions. It has also been used as follow-up prophylactic therapy for rheumatic heart disease and acute glomerulonephritis.

CONTRAINDICATIONS

A history of a previous hypersensitivity reaction to any penicillin is a contraindication.

WARNINGS

Serious and occasionally fatal hypersensitivity (anaphylactoid) reactions have been reported in patients on penicillin therapy. These reactions are more likely to occur in individuals with a history of penicillin hypersensitivity and/or a history of sensitivity to multiple allergens. There have been reports of individuals with a history of penicillin hypersensitivity who have experienced severe reactions when treated with cephalosporins. Before initiating therapy with any penicillin, careful inquiry should be made concerning previous hypersensitivity reactions to penicillin, cephalosporins, and other allergens. If an allergic reaction occurs, the drug should be discontinued and the appropriate therapy instituted. Serious anaphylactoid reactions require immediate emergency treatment with epinephrine. Oxygen, intravenous steroids, and airway management—including intubation, should be administered as indicated.

PRECAUTIONS

General: Penicillin should be used with caution in individuals with histories of significant allergies and/or asthma.

Intramuscular therapy: Care should be taken to avoid intravenous administration, accidental intraarterial administration, or injection into or near major peripheral nerves or blood vessels, since many injections may produce neurovascular damage.

As with all intramuscular preparations, penicillin G benzathine should be injected well within the body of a relatively large muscle.

ADULTS: The preferred site is the upper outer quadrant of the buttock (i.e., gluteus maximus), or the mid-lateral thigh.

CHILDREN: It is recommended that intramuscular injections be given preferably in the mid-lateral muscles of the thigh. In infants and small children the periphery of the upper outer quadrant of the gluteal region should be used only when necessary, such as in burn patients, in order to minimize the possibility of damage to the sciatic nerve.

The deltoid area should be used only if well developed such as in certain adults and older children, and then only with caution to avoid radial nerve injury. Intramuscular injections should not be made into the lower and mid-third of the upper arm. As with all intramuscular injections, aspiration is necessary to help avoid inadvertent injection into a blood vessel.

Irritation at the site of injection may occur. In addition, subcutaneous and fat-layer injections should be avoided since they may cause pain and induration. If these occur, they may be relieved by the application of an ice pack.

In streptococcal infections, therapy must be sufficient to eliminate the organism (10 days minimum), otherwise the sequelae of streptococcal disease may occur. Cultures should be taken following completion of treatment to determine whether streptococci have been eradicated.

The use of antibiotics may result in overgrowth of nonsusceptible organisms. Constant observation of the patient is essential. If new infections due to bacteria or fungi appear during therapy, the drug should be discontinued and appropriate measures taken. Whenever allergic reactions occur, penicillin should be withdrawn unless, in the opinion of the physician, the condition being treated is life threatening and amenable only to penicillin therapy.

Laboratory Tests: In prolonged therapy with penicillin, periodic evaluation of the renal, hepatic and hematopoietic systems for organ dysfunction is recommended. This is particularly important in prematures, neonates and other infants, and when high doses are used.

When treating gonococcal infections in which primary and secondary syphilis are suspected, proper diagnostic procedures, including dark field examinations, should be done before receiving penicillin and monthly serological tests made for at least four months. All cases of penicillin-treated syphilis should receive clinical and serological examinations every six months for two to three years.

In streptococcal infections, cultures should be taken following completion of treatment to determine whether streptococci have been eradicated.

Drug Interactions: Concurrent administration of bacteriostatic antibiotics (e.g., erythromycin, tetracycline) may diminish the bactericidal effects of penicillins by slowing the rate of bacterial growth. Bactericidal agents work most effectively against the immature cell wall of rapidly proliferating microorganisms. This has been demonstrated *in vitro*; however, the clinical significance of this interaction is not well documented. There are few clinical situations in which the concurrent use of "static" and "cidal" antibiotics are indicated. However, in selected circumstances in which such therapy is appropriate, using adequate doses of antibacterial agents and beginning penicillin therapy first, should minimize the potential for interaction.

Penicillin blood levels may be prolonged by concurrent administration of probenecid which blocks the renal tubular secretion of penicillins.

Displacement of penicillins from plasma protein binding sites will elevate the level of free penicillin in the serum.

Carcinogenesis, Mutagenesis, Impairment of Fertility: No information or long term studies are available on the carcinogenesis, mutagenesis, or impairment of fertility with the use of penicillins.

Pregnancy

Pregnancy Category B—*Teratogenic Effects:* Reproduction studies in the mouse, rat and rabbit have revealed no evidence of impaired fertility or harm to the fetus due to penicillin G. Human experience with the penicillins during pregnancy has not shown any positive evidence of adverse effects on the fetus. There are, however, no adequate and well controlled studies in pregnant women showing conclusively that harmful effects of these drugs on the fetus can be excluded. Because animal reproduction studies are not always predictive of human response, this drug should be used during pregnancy only if clearly needed.

Nursing Mothers: Penicillin G benzathine has been reported in milk. Caution should be exercised when penicillin G benzathine is administered to a nursing woman.

Pediatric Use: Penicillins are excreted largely unchanged by the kidney. Because of incompletely developed renal function in infants, the rate of elimination will be slow. Use caution in administering to newborns and evaluate organ system function frequently.

ADVERSE REACTIONS

The hypersensitivity reactions reported are skin eruptions (maculopapular to exfoliative dermatitis), urticaria and other serum sickness reactions, laryngeal edema and anaphylaxis. Fever and eosinophilia may frequently be the only reaction observed. Hemolytic anemia, leucopenia, thrombocytopenia, neuropathy, and nephropathy are infrequent reactions and usually associated with high doses of parenteral penicillin.

OVERDOSAGE

Penicillin in overdosage has the potential to cause neuromuscular hyperirritability. In case of overdosage discontinue medication, treat symptomatically, and institute supportive measures as required.

Penicillin G is hemodialyzable.

DOSAGE AND ADMINISTRATION

Administer by deep IM injection in the upper outer quadrant of the buttock. In infants and small children, the midlateral aspect of the thigh may be preferable. When doses are repeated, vary the injection site (see PRECAUTIONS).

Pediatric Dosage Schedule: In children under 12 years of age, dosage should be adjusted in accordance with the age and weight of the child and the severity of the infection. Under 2 years of age, the dose may be divided between the two buttocks if necessary.

Streptococcal Infections (group A) pharyngitis: A single injection of 900,000 units for older children; 1,200,000 units for adults.

Venereal Infections

Syphilis—Primary, secondary, and latent: 2.4 million units (1 dose).

Late Syphilis (tertiary and neurosyphilis): 3 million units at 7 day intervals for a total of 6–9 million units.

Congenital Syphilis (asymptomatic with normal cerebrospinal fluid): Under 2 years of age—50,000 units/kg body weight in a single dose; ages 2–12 years—adjust dosage based on adult dosage schedule.

Yaws, Bejel, and Pinta: 1.2 million units (1 injection).

Prophylaxis: For rheumatic fever and glomerulonephritis. Following an acute attack, penicillin G benzathine (parenteral) may be given in doses of 1,200,000 units once a month or 600,000 units every 2 weeks.

Parenteral drug products should be visually inspected for particulate matter and discoloration prior to administration, whenever solution and container permit.

HOW SUPPLIED

Permapen® (Penicillin G Benzathine) Injectable Suspension is supplied in an ISOJECT syringe: 1,200,000 units in packages of 10 (NDC 0049-0210-35). ISOJECT is a pre-filled disposable syringe unit with a 20-gauge, $1^1/_4$ inch needle. Each 2 mL contains 1,200,000 units penicillin G benzathine; 0.012 g sodium citrate; 0.006 g polyvinylpyrrolidone; 0.020 g lecithin, and 0.006 g sodium carboxymethylcellulose. Preservatives: methylparaben 0.09%, propylparaben 0.01%.

The product should be stored between 2°–8°C (36°–46°F). Keep from freezing.

℞ **only**

***Pfizer* Roerig**
Division of Pfizer Inc, NY, NY 10017

23-1173-00-3 Revised March 1999

Buffered PFIZERPEN® ℞

(penicillin G potassium)
for Injection

DESCRIPTION

Buffered Pfizerpen® (penicillin G potassium) for Injection is a sterile, pyrogen-free powder for reconstitution. Buffered Pfizerpen for Injection is an antibacterial agent for intramuscular, continuous intravenous drip, intrapleural or other local infusion, and intrathecal administration.

Each million units contains approximately 6.8 milligrams of sodium (0.3 mEq) and 65.6 milligrams of potassium (1.68 mEq).

Chemically, Pfizerpen is monopotassium 3,3-dimethyl-7-oxo-6-(2-phenylacetamido)-4-thia-1-azabicyclo (3.2.0) heptane-2-carboxylate. It has a molecular weight of 372.48 and the following chemical structure:

Formula
$C_{16}H_{17}KN_2O_4S$

Penicillin G potassium is a colorless or white crystal, or a white crystalline powder which is odorless, or practically so, and moderately hygroscopic. Penicillin G potassium is very soluble in water. The pH of the reconstituted product is between 6.0–8.5.

CLINICAL PHARMACOLOGY

Aqueous penicillin G is rapidly absorbed following both intramuscular and subcutaneous injection. Initial blood levels following parenteral administration are high but transient. Penicillins bind to serum proteins, mainly albumin. Therapeutic levels of the penicillins are easily achieved under normal circumstances in extracellular fluid and most other body tissues. Penicillins are distributed in varying degrees into pleural, pericardial, peritoneal, ascitic, synovial, and interstitial fluids. Penicillins are excreted in breast milk. Penetration into the cerebrospinal fluid, eyes, and prostate is poor. Penicillins are rapidly excreted in the urine by glomerular filtration and active tubular secretion, primarily as unchanged drug. Approximately 60 percent of the total dose of 300,000 units is excreted in the urine within this 5-hour period. For this reason, high and frequent doses are required to maintain the elevated serum levels desirable in treating certain severe infections in individuals with normal kidney function. In neonates and young infants, and in individuals with impaired kidney function, excretion is considerably delayed.

Microbiology

Penicillin G exerts a bactericidal action against penicillin-susceptible microorganisms during the stage of active multiplication. It acts through the inhibition of biosynthesis of cell wall mucopeptide rendering the cell wall osmotically unstable. It is not active against the penicillinase-producing bacteria, which include many strains of staphylococci. While *in vitro* studies have demonstrated that susceptibility of most strains of the following organisms, clinical efficacy for infections other than those included in the INDICATIONS AND USAGE section has not been documented. Penicillin G exerts high *in vitro* activity against staphylococci (except penicillinase-producing strains), streptococci (groups A, C, G, H, L, and M), and pneumococci. Other organisms susceptible to penicillin G are *N. gonorrhoeae, Corynebacterium diphtheriae, Bacillus anthracis,* Clostridia, *Actinomyces bovis, Streptobacillus moniliformis, Listeria monocytogenes* and Leptospira. *Treponema pallidum* is extremely sensitive to the bactericidal action of penicillin G. Some species of gram-negative bacilli are sensitive to moderate to high concentrations of the drug obtained with intravenous administration. These include most strains of *Escherichia coli;* all strains of *Proteus mirabilis,* Salmonella and Shigella; and some strains of *Aerobacter aerogenes* and *Alcaligenes faecalis.*

Penicillin acts synergistically with gentamicin or tobramycin against many strains of enterococci.

Susceptibility Testing: Penicillin G Susceptibility Powder or 10 units Penicillin G Susceptibility Discs may be used to determine microbial susceptibility to penicillin G using one of the following standard methods recommended by the National Committee for Laboratory Standards:

M2-A3, "Performance Standards for Antimicrobial Disk Susceptibility Tests"

M7-A, "Methods for Dilution Antimicrobial Susceptibility Tests for Bacteria that Grow Aerobically"

M11-A, "Reference Agar Dilution Procedure for Antimicrobial Susceptibility Testing of Anaerobic Bacteria"

M17-P, "Alternative Methods for Antimicrobial Susceptibility Testing of Anaerobic Bacteria"

Tests should be interpreted by the following criteria:

[See first table above]

[See second table above]

Interpretations of susceptible, intermediate, and resistant correlate zone size diameters with MIC values. A laboratory report of "susceptible" indicates that the suspected causative microorganism most likely will respond to therapy with penicillin G. A laboratory report of "resistant" indicates that the infecting microorganism most likely will not respond to therapy. A laboratory report of "moderately susceptible" indicates that the microorganism is most likely susceptible if a high dosage of penicillin G is used, or if the infection is such that high levels of penicillin G may be attained, as in urine. A report of "intermediate" using the disk diffusion method may be considered an equivocal result, and dilution tests may be indicated.

Control organisms are recommended for susceptibility testing. Each time the test is performed the following organisms should be included. The range for zones of inhibition is shown below:

Control Organism	Zone of Inhibition Range
Staphylococcus aureus (ATCC 25923)	27–35

Zone Diameter, nearest whole mm

	Susceptible	Moderately Susceptible	Resistant
Staphylococci	≥29	—	≤28
N. gonorrhoeae	≥20	—	≤19
Enterococci	—	≥15	≤14
Non-enterococcal streptococci and *L. monocytogenes*	≥28	20–27	≤19

Approximate MIC Correlates

	Susceptible	Resistant
Staphylococci	≤0.1 µg/mL	β-lactamase
N. gonorrhoeae	≤0.1 µg/mL	β-lactamase
Enterococci	—	≥16 µg/mL
Non-enterococcal streptococci and *L. monocytogenes*	≤0.12 µg/mL	≥ 4 µg/mL

INDICATIONS AND USAGE

Aqueous penicillin G (parenteral) is indicated in the therapy of severe infections caused by penicillin G-susceptible microorganisms when rapid and high penicillin levels are required in the conditions listed below. Therapy should be guided by bacteriological studies (including susceptibility tests) and by clinical response.

The following infections will usually respond to adequate dosage of penicillin G (parenteral):

Streptococcal infections.

NOTE: Streptococci in groups A, C, H, G, L, and M are very sensitive to penicillin G. Some group D organisms are sensitive to the high serum levels obtained with aqueous penicillin G.

Aqueous penicillin G (parenteral) is the penicillin dosage form of choice for bacteremia, empyema, severe pneumonia, pericarditis, endocarditis, meningitis, and other severe infections caused by sensitive strains of the gram-positive species listed above.

Pneumococcal infections.

Staphylococcal infections—penicillin G sensitive.

Other infections:

Anthrax.

Actinomycosis.

Clostridial infections (including tetanus).

Diphtheria (to prevent carrier state).

Erysipeloid *(Erysipelothrix insidiosa)* endocarditis.

Fusospirochetal infections—severe infections of the oropharynx (Vincent's), lower respiratory tract and genital area due to *Fusobacterium fusiformisans* spirochetes.

Gram-negative bacillary infections (bacteremias)–*(E. coli, A. aerogenes, A. faecalis,* Salmonella, Shigella and *P. mirabilis).*

Listeria infections *(Listeria monocytogenes).*

Meningitis and endocarditis.

Pasteurella infections *(Pasteurella multocida).*

Bacteremia and meningitis.

Rat-bite fever *(Spirillum minus* or *Streptobacillus moniliformis).*

Gonorrheal endocarditis and arthritis *(N. gonorrhoeae).*

Syphilis *(T. pallidum)* including congenital syphilis.

Meningococcic meningitis.

Although no controlled clinical efficacy studies have been conducted, aqueous crystalline penicillin G for injection and penicillin G procaine suspension have been suggested by the American Heart Association and the American Dental Association for use as part of a combined parenteral-oral regimen for prophylaxis against bacterial endocarditis in patients with congenital heart disease or rheumatic, or other acquired valvular heart disease when they undergo dental procedures and surgical procedures of the upper respiratory tract.[1] Since it may happen that *alpha* hemolytic streptococci relatively resistant to penicillin may be found when patients are receiving continuous oral penicillin for secondary prevention of rheumatic fever, prophylactic agents other than penicillin may be chosen for these patients and prescribed in addition to their continuous rheumatic fever prophylactic regimen.

NOTE: When selecting antibiotics for the prevention of bacterial endocarditis, the physician or dentist should read the full joint statement of the American Heart Association and the American Dental Association.[1]

CONTRAINDICATIONS

A history of a previous hypersensitivity reaction to any penicillin is a contraindication.

WARNINGS

Serious and occasionally fatal hypersensitivity (anaphylactoid) reactions have been reported in patients on penicillin therapy. These reactions are more likely to occur in individuals with a history of penicillin hypersensitivity and/or a history of sensitivity to multiple allergens. There have been reports of individuals with a history of penicillin hypersensitivity who have experienced severe reactions when treated with cephalosporins. Before initiating therapy with any penicillin, careful inquiry should be made concerning previous hypersensitivity reactions to penicillin, cephalosporins, or other allergens. If an allergic reaction occurs, the drug should be discontinued and the appropriate therapy instituted. Serious anaphylactoid reactions require immediate emergency treatment with epinephrine. Oxygen, intravenous steroids, and airway management including intubation, should also be administered as indicated.

PRECAUTIONS

General: Penicillin should be used with caution in individuals with histories of significant allergies and/or asthma.

Intramuscular Therapy: Care should be taken to avoid intravenous or accidental intraarterial administration, or injection into or near major peripheral nerves or blood vessels, since such injections may produce neurovascular damage.

Particular care should be taken with IV administration because of the possibility of thrombophlebitis.

In streptococcal infections, therapy must be sufficient to eliminate the organism (10 days minimum), otherwise the sequelae of streptococcal disease may occur. Cultures should be taken following the completion of treatment to determine whether streptococci have been eradicated.

The use of antibiotics may result in overgrowth of nonsusceptible organisms. Constant observation of the patient is essential. If new infections due to bacteria or fungi appear during therapy, the drug should be discontinued and appropriate measures taken. Whenever allergic reactions occur, penicillin should be withdrawn unless, in the opinion of the physician, the condition being treated is life threatening and amenable only to penicillin therapy.

Aqueous penicillin G by the intravenous route in high doses (above 10 million units) should be administered slowly because of the adverse effects of electrolyte imbalance from either the potassium or sodium content of the penicillin. Penicillin G potassium contains 1.7 mEq potassium and 0.3 mEq sodium per million units. The patient's renal, cardiac, and vascular status should be evaluated and if impairment of function is suspected or known to exist a reduction in the total dosage should be considered. Frequent evaluation of electrolyte balance, renal and hematopoietic function is recommended during therapy when high doses of intravenous aqueous penicillin G are used.

Laboratory Tests: In prolonged therapy with penicillin, periodic evaluation of the renal, hepatic, and hematopoietic systems is recommended for organ system dysfunction. This is particularly important in prematures, neonates and other infants, and when high doses are used.

Positive Coomb's tests have been reported after large intravenous doses.

Monitor serum potassium and implement corrective measures when necessary.

When treating gonococcal infections in which primary and secondary syphilis are suspected, proper diagnostic procedures, including dark field examinations, should be done before receiving penicillin and monthly serological tests made for at least four months. All cases of penicillin treated syphilis should receive clinical and serological examinations every six months for two to three years.

In suspected staphylococcal infections, proper laboratory studies, including susceptibility tests, should be performed.

In streptococcal infections, cultures should be taken following completion of treatment to determine whether streptococci have been eradicated. Therapy must be sufficient to eliminate the organism (a minimum of 10 days), otherwise the sequelae of streptococcal disease (e.g., endocarditis, rheumatic fever) may occur.

Drug Interactions: Concurrent administration of bacteriostatic antibiotics (e.g., erythromycin, tetracycline) may diminish the bactericidal effects of penicillins by slowing the rate of bacterial growth. Bactericidal agents work most effectively against the immature cell wall of rapidly proliferating microorganisms. This has been demonstrated *in vitro;* however, the clinical significance of this interaction is not well documented. There are few clinical situations in which the concurrent use of "static" and "cidal" antibiotics are indicated. However, in selected circumstances in which such therapy is appropriate, using adequate doses of antibacterial agents and beginning penicillin therapy first, should minimize the potential for interaction.

Penicillin blood levels may be prolonged by concurrent administration of probenecid which blocks the renal tubular secretion of penicillins.

Displacement of penicillin from plasma protein binding sites will elevate the level of free penicillin in the serum.

Carcinogenesis, Mutagenesis, Impairment of Fertility: No information on long-term studies are available on the carcinogenesis, mutagenesis, or the impairment of fertility with the use of penicillins.

Continued on next page

Pfizerpen—Cont.

Pregnancy Category B–*Teratogenic Effects:* Reproduction studies performed in the mouse, rat, and rabbit have revealed no evidence of impaired fertility or harm to the fetus due to penicillin G. Human experience with the penicillins during pregnancy has not shown any positive evidence of adverse effects on the fetus. There are, however, no adequate and well controlled studies in pregnant women showing conclusively that harmful effects of these drugs on the fetus can be excluded. Because animal reproduction studies are not always predictive of human response, this drug should be used during pregnancy only if clearly needed.

Nursing Mothers: Penicillins are excreted in human milk. Caution should be exercised when penicillin G is administered to a nursing woman.

Pediatric Use: Penicillins are excreted largely unchanged by the kidney. Because of incompletely developed renal function in infants, the rate of elimination will be slow. Use caution in administering to newborns and evaluate organ system function frequently.

ADVERSE REACTIONS

Penicillin is a substance of low toxicity but does have a significant index of sensitization. The following hypersensitivity reactions have been reported: skin rashes ranging from maculopapular eruptions to exfoliative dermatitis; urticaria; and reactions resembling serum sickness, including chills, fever, edema, arthralgia and prostration. Severe and occasionally fatal anaphylaxis has occurred (see WARNINGS).

Hemolytic anemia, leucopenia, thrombocytopenia, nephropathy, and neuropathy are rarely observed adverse reactions and are usually associated with high intravenous dosage.

Patients given continuous intravenous therapy with penicillin G potassium in high dosage (10 million to 100 million units daily) may suffer severe or even fatal potassium poisoning, particularly if renal insufficiency is present. Hyperreflexia, convulsions, and coma may be indicative of this syndrome.

Cardiac arrhythmias and cardiac arrest may also occur. (High dosage of penicillin G sodium may result in congestive heart failure due to high sodium intake.)

The Jarisch-Herxheimer reaction has been reported in patients treated for syphilis.

OVERDOSAGE

Neurological adverse reactions, including convulsions, may occur with the attainment of high CSF levels of beta-lactams. In case of overdosage, discontinue medication, treat symptomatically, and institute supportive measures as required.

Penicillin G potassium is hemodialyzable.

DOSAGE AND ADMINISTRATION

Severe infections due to Susceptible Strains of Streptococci, Pneumococci, and Staphylococci—bacteremia, pneumonia, endocarditis, pericarditis, empyema, meningitis, and other severe infections—a minimum of 5 million units daily.

Syphilis—Aqueous penicillin G may be used in the treatment of acquired and congenital syphilis, but because of the necessity of frequent dosage, hospitalization is recommended. Dosage and duration of therapy will be determined by age of patient and stage of the disease.

Gonorrheal endocarditis—a minimum of 5 million units daily.

Meningococcic meningitis—1–2 million units intramuscularly every 2 hours, or continuous IV drip of 20–30 million units/day.

Actinomycosis—1–6 million units/day for cervicofacial cases; 10–20 million units/day for thoracic and abdominal disease.

Clostridial infections—20 million units/day; penicillin is adjunctive therapy to antitoxin.

Fusospirochetal infections—severe infections of oropharynx, lower respiratory tract, and genital area–5–10 million units/day.

Rat-bite fever (Spirillum minus or *Streptobacillus moniliformis)*—12–15 million units/day for 3–4 weeks.

Listeria infections (Listeria monocytogenes)

Neonates—500,000 to 1 million units/day.

Adults with meningitis—15–20 million units/day for 2 weeks.

Adults with endocarditis—15–20 million units/day for 4 weeks.

Pasteurella infections (Pasteurella multocida)

Bacteremia and meningitis—4–6 million units/day for 2 weeks.

Erysipeloid (Erysipelothrix insidiosa)

Endocarditis—2–20 million units/day for 4–6 weeks.

Gram-negative bacillary infections (E. coli, Enterobacter aerogenes, A. faecalis, Salmonella, Shigella and *Proteus mirabilis)*

Bacteremia—20–80 million units/day.

Diphtheria (carrier state)—300,000–400,000 units of penicillin/day in divided doses for 10–12 days.

Anthrax—A minimum of 5 million units of penicillin/day in divided doses until cure is effected.

For prophylaxis against bacterial endocarditis[1] in patients with congenital heart disease or rheumatic or other acquired valvular heart disease, when undergoing dental procedures or surgical procedures of the upper respiratory tract, use a combined parenteral-oral regimen. One million units of aqueous crystalline penicillin G (30,000 units/kg in children) intramuscularly, mixed with 600,000 units procaine penicillin G (600,000 units for children) should be given one-half to one hour before the procedure. Oral penicillin V (phenoxymethyl penicillin), 500 mg for adults or 250 mg for children less than 60 lb, should be given every 6 hours for 8 doses. Doses for children should not exceed recommendations for adults for a single dose or for a 24 hour period.

Reconstitution

The following table shows the amount of solvent required for solution of various concentrations:

[See table below]

When the required volume of solvent is greater than the capacity of the vial, the penicillin can be dissolved by first injecting only a portion of the solvent into the vial, then withdrawing the resultant solution and combining it with the remainder of the solvent in a larger sterile container.

Buffered Pfizerpen (penicillin G potassium) for Injection is highly water soluble. It may be dissolved in small amounts of Water for Injection, or Sterile Isotonic Sodium Chloride Solution for Parenteral Use. All solutions should be stored in a refrigerator. When refrigerated, penicillin solutions may be stored for seven days without significant loss of potency.

Buffered Pfizerpen for Injection may be given intramuscularly or by continuous intravenous drip for dosages of 500,000, 1,000,000, or 5,000,000 units. It is also suitable for intrapleural, intraarticular, and other local instillations.

THE 20,000,000 UNIT DOSAGE MAY BE ADMINISTERED BY INTRAVENOUS INFUSION ONLY.

(1) Intramuscular Injection: Keep total volume of injection small. The intramuscular route is the preferred route of administration. Solutions containing up to 100,000 units of penicillin per mL of diluent may be used with a minimum of discomfort. Greater concentration of penicillin G per mL is physically possible and may be employed where therapy demands. When large dosages are required, it may be advisable to administer aqueous solutions of penicillin by means of continuous intravenous drip.

(2) Continuous Intravenous Drip: Determine the volume of fluid and rate of its administration required by the patient in a 24 hour period in the usual manner for fluid therapy, and add the appropriate daily dosage of penicillin to this fluid. For example, if an adult patient requires 2 liters of fluid in 24 hours and a daily dosage of 10 million units of penicillin, add 5 million units to 1 liter and adjust the rate of flow so the liter will be infused in 12 hours.

(3) Intrapleural or Other Local Infusion: If fluid is aspirated, give infusion in a volume equal to ¼ or ½ the amount of fluid aspirated, otherwise, prepare as for intramuscular injection.

(4) Intrathecal Use: The intrathecal use of penicillin in meningitis must be highly individualized. It should be employed only with full consideration of the possible irritating effects of penicillin when used by this route. The preferred route of therapy in bacterial meningitides is intravenous, supplemented by intramuscular injection.

Parenteral drug products should be inspected visually for particulate matter and discoloration prior to administration, whenever solution and container permit.

Sterile solution may be left in refrigerator for one week without significant loss of potency.

HOW SUPPLIED

Buffered Pfizerpen® (penicillin G potassium) for Injection is available in vials containing respectively 1,000,000 units × 10's (NDC 0049-0510-83), 1,000,000 units × 100's (NDC 0049-0510-95), 5,000,000 units × 10's (NDC 0049-0520-83), 5,000,000 units × 100's (NDC 0049-0520-95), 20,000,000 units × 1's (NDC 0049-0530-28), and a bulk pharmacy package of 20,000,000 units × 10's (NDC 0049-0530-83) of dry powder for reconstitution; buffered with sodium citrate and citric acid to an optimum pH.

Each million units contains approximately 6.8 milligrams of sodium (0.3 mEq) and 65.6 milligrams of potassium (1.68 mEq).

Store the dry powder below 86°F (30°C).

Reference

1. American Heart Association, 1977. Prevention of bacterial endocarditis. Circulation. **56**:139A–143A.

Approx. Desired Concentration (units/mL)	Approx. Volume (mL) 1,000,000 units	Solvent for Vial of 5,000,000 units	Infusion Only 20,000,000 units
50,000	20.0	—	—
100,000	10.0	—	—
250,000	4.0	18.2	75.0
500,000	1.8	8.2	33.0
750,000	—	4.8	—
1,000,000	—	3.2	11.5

©1997 PFIZER INC

Roerig
Division of Pfizer Inc, NY, NY 10017
70-4209-00-6 Revised January 1997

PROCARDIA® ℞

[*pro-car 'dē-ă*]
nifedipine
CAPSULES
For Oral Use

DESCRIPTION

PROCARDIA® (nifedipine) is an antianginal drug belonging to a class of pharmacological agents, the calcium channel blockers. Nifedipine is 3,5-pyridinedicarboxylic acid, 1,4-dihydro-2, 6-dimethyl-4-(2-nitrophenyl)-, dimethyl ester, $C_{17}H_{18}N_2O_6$, and has the structural formula:

Nifedipine is a yellow crystalline substance, practically insoluble in water but soluble in ethanol. It has a molecular weight of 346.3. PROCARDIA capsules are formulated as soft gelatin capsules for oral administration each containing 10 mg or 20 mg nifedipine.

Inert ingredients in the formulations are: glycerin; peppermint oil; polyethylene glycol; soft gelatin capsules (which contain Yellow 6, and may contain Red Ferric Oxide and other inert ingredients), and water. The 10 mg capsules also contain saccharin sodium.

CLINICAL PHARMACOLOGY

PROCARDIA is a calcium ion influx inhibitor (slow-channel blocker or calcium ion antagonist) and inhibits the transmembrane influx of calcium ions into cardiac muscle and smooth muscle. The contractile processes of cardiac muscle and vascular smooth muscle are dependent upon the movement of extracellular calcium ions into these cells through specific ion channels. PROCARDIA selectively inhibits calcium ion influx across the cell membrane of cardiac muscle and vascular smooth muscle without changing serum calcium concentrations.

Mechanism of Action

The precise means by which this inhibition relieves angina has not been fully determined, but includes at least the following two mechanisms:

1) Relaxation and Prevention of Coronary Artery Spasm

PROCARDIA dilates the main coronary arteries and coronary arterioles, both in normal and ischemic regions, and is a potent inhibitor of coronary artery spasm, whether spontaneous or ergonovine-induced. This property increases myocardial oxygen delivery in patients with coronary artery spasm, and is responsible for the effectiveness of PROCARDIA in vasospastic (Prinzmetal's or variant) angina. Whether this effect plays any role in classical angina is not clear, but studies of exercise tolerance have not shown an increase in the maximum exercise rate-pressure product, a widely accepted measure of oxygen utilization. This suggests that, in general, relief of spasm or dilation of coronary arteries is not an important factor in classical angina.

2) Reduction of Oxygen Utilization

PROCARDIA regularly reduces arterial pressure at rest and at a given level of exercise by dilating peripheral arterioles and reducing the total peripheral resistance (afterload) against which the heart works. This unloading of the heart reduces myocardial energy consumption and oxygen requirements and probably accounts for the effectiveness of PROCARDIA in chronic stable angina.

Pharmacokinetics and Metabolism

PROCARDIA is rapidly and fully absorbed after oral administration. The drug is detectable in serum 10 minutes after oral administration, and peak blood levels occur in approximately 30 minutes. Bioavailability is proportional to dose from 10 to 30 mg; half-life does not change significantly with dose. There is little difference in relative bioavailability when PROCARDIA capsules are given orally and either swallowed whole, bitten and swallowed, or, bitten and held sublingually. However, biting through the capsule prior to swallowing does result in slightly earlier plasma concentrations (27 ng/mL 10 minutes after 10 mg) than if capsules are swallowed intact. It is highly bound by serum proteins. PROCARDIA is extensively converted to inactive metabolites and approximately 80 percent of PROCARDIA and metabolites are eliminated via the kidneys. The half-life of nifedipine in plasma is approximately two hours. Since hepatic biotransformation is the predominant route for the disposition of nifedipine, the pharmacokinetics may be altered in patients with chronic liver disease. Patients with hepatic impairment (liver cirrhosis) have a longer disposition half-life and higher bioavailability of nifedipine than healthy volunteers. The degree of serum protein binding of nifedipine is high (92–98%). Protein binding may be greatly reduced in patients with renal or hepatic impairment.

Hemodynamics

Like other slow channel blockers, PROCARDIA exerts a negative inotropic effect on isolated myocardial tissue. This is rarely, if ever, seen in intact animals or man, probably because of reflex responses to its vasodilating effects. In man, PROCARDIA causes decreased peripheral vascular resistance and a fall in systolic and diastolic pressure, usually modest (5–10mm Hg systolic), but sometimes larger. There is usually a small increase in heart rate, a reflex response to vasodilation. Measurements of cardiac function in patients with normal ventricular function have generally found a small increase in cardiac index without major effects on ejection fraction, left ventricular end diastolic pressure (LVEDP) or volume (LVEDV). In patients with impaired ventricular function, most acute studies have shown some increase in ejection fraction and reduction in left ventricular filling pressure.

Electrophysiologic Effects

Although, like other members of its class, PROCARDIA decreases sinoatrial node function and atrioventricular conduction in isolated myocardial preparations, such effects have not been seen in studies in intact animals or in man. In formal electrophysiologic studies, predominantly in patients with normal conduction systems, PROCARDIA has had no tendency to prolong atrioventricular conduction, prolong sinus node recovery time, or slow sinus rate.

INDICATIONS AND USAGE

I. Vasospastic Angina

PROCARDIA (nifedipine) is indicated for the management of vasospastic angina confirmed by any of the following criteria: 1) classical pattern of angina at rest accompanied by ST segment elevation, 2) angina or coronary artery spasm provoked by ergonovine, or 3) angiographically demonstrated coronary artery spasm. In those patients who have had angiography, the presence of significant fixed obstructive disease is not incompatible with the diagnosis of vasospastic angina, provided that the above criteria are satisfied. PROCARDIA may also be used where the clinical presentation suggests a possible vasospastic component but where vasospasm has not been confirmed, e.g., where pain has a variable threshold on exertion or when angina is refractory to nitrates and/or adequate doses of beta blockers.

II. Chronic Stable Angina
(Classical Effort-Associated Angina)

PROCARDIA is indicated for the management of chronic stable angina (effort-associated angina) without evidence of vasospasm in patients who remain symptomatic despite adequate doses of beta blockers and/or organic nitrates or who cannot tolerate those agents.

In chronic stable angina (effort-associated angina) PROCARDIA has been effective in controlled trials of up to eight weeks duration in reducing angina frequency and increasing exercise tolerance, but confirmation of sustained effectiveness and evaluation of long term safety in these patients are incomplete.

Controlled studies in small numbers of patients suggest concomitant use of PROCARDIA and beta-blocking agents may be beneficial in patients with chronic stable angina, but available information is not sufficient to predict with confidence the effects of concurrent treatment, especially in patients with compromised left ventricular function or cardiac conduction abnormalities. When introducing such concomitant therapy, care must be taken to monitor blood pressure closely since severe hypotension can occur from the combined effects of the drugs. (See WARNINGS.)

CONTRAINDICATIONS

Known hypersensitivity reaction to PROCARDIA.

WARNINGS

Excessive Hypotension

Although in most patients, the hypotensive effect of PROCARDIA is modest and well tolerated, occasional patients have had excessive and poorly tolerated hypotension. These responses have usually occurred during initial titration or at the time of subsequent upward dosage adjustment. Although patients have rarely experienced excessive hypotension on PROCARDIA alone, this may be more common in patients on concomitant beta-blocker therapy. Although not approved for this purpose, PROCARDIA and other immediate-release nifedipine capsules have been used (orally and sublingually) for acute reduction of blood pressure. Several well-documented reports describe cases of profound hypotension, myocardial infarction, and death when immediate-release nifedipine was used in this way. **PROCARDIA capsules should not be used for the acute reduction of blood pressure.**

PROCARDIA and other immediate-release nifedipine capsules have also been used for the long-term control of essential hypertension, although no properly-controlled studies have been conducted to define an appropriate dose or dose interval for such treatment. **PROCARDIA capsules should not be used for the control of essential hypertension.**

Several well-controlled, randomized trials studied the use of immediate-release nifedipine in patients who had just sustained myocardial infarctions. In none of these trials did immediate-release nifedipine appear to provide any benefit. In some of the trials, patients who received immediate-release nifedipine had significantly worse outcomes than patients who received placebo. **PROCARDIA capsules should not be administered within the first week or two after myocardial infarction, and they should also be avoided in the setting of acute coronary syndrome (when infarction may be imminent).**

Severe hypotension and/or increased fluid volume requirements have been reported in patients receiving PROCARDIA together with a beta blocking agent who underwent coronary artery bypass surgery using high dose fentanyl anesthesia. The interaction with high dose fentanyl appears to be due to the combination of PROCARDIA and a beta-blocker, but the possibility that it may occur with PROCARDIA alone, with low doses of fentanyl, in other surgical procedures, or with other narcotic analgesics cannot be ruled out. In PROCARDIA treated patients where surgery using high dose fentanyl anesthesia is contemplated, the physician should be aware of these potential problems and, if the patient's condition permits, sufficient time (at least 36 hours) should be allowed for PROCARDIA to be washed out of the body prior to surgery.

Increased Angina and/or Myocardial Infarction

Rarely, patients, particularly those who have severe obstructive coronary artery disease, have developed well documented increased frequency, duration and/or severity of angina or acute myocardial infarction on starting PROCARDIA or at the time of dosage increase. The mechanism of this effect is not established.

Beta Blocker Withdrawal

Patients recently withdrawn from beta blockers may develop a withdrawal syndrome with increased angina, probably related to increased sensitivity to catecholamines. Initiation of PROCARDIA treatment will not prevent this occurrence and might be expected to exacerbate it by provoking reflex catecholamine release. There have been occasional reports of increased angina in a setting of beta blocker withdrawal and PROCARDIA initiation. It is important to taper beta blockers if possible, rather than stopping them abruptly before beginning PROCARDIA.

Congestive Heart Failure

Rarely, patients, usually receiving a beta blocker, have developed heart failure after beginning PROCARDIA. Patients with tight aortic stenosis may be at greater risk for such an event, as the unloading effect of PROCARDIA would be expected to be of less benefit to these patients, owing to their fixed impedance to flow across the aortic valve.

PRECAUTIONS

General: Hypotension: Because PROCARDIA decreases peripheral vascular resistance, careful monitoring of blood pressure during the initial administration and titration of PROCARDIA is suggested. Close observation is especially recommended for patients already taking medications that are known to lower blood pressure. (See WARNINGS.)

Peripheral Edema: Mild to moderate peripheral edema, typically associated with arterial vasodilation and not due to left ventricular dysfunction, occurs in about one in ten patients treated with PROCARDIA (nifedipine). This edema occurs primarily in the lower extremities and usually responds to diuretic therapy. With patients whose angina is complicated by congestive heart failure, care should be taken to differentiate this peripheral edema from the effects of increasing left ventricular dysfunction.

Laboratory Tests: Rare, usually transient, but occasionally significant elevations of enzymes such as alkaline phosphatase, CPK, LDH, SGOT and SGPT have been noted. The relationship to PROCARDIA therapy is uncertain in most cases, but probable in some. These laboratory abnormalities have rarely been associated with clinical symptoms; however, cholestasis with or without jaundice has been reported. Rare instances of allergic hepatitis have been reported.

PROCARDIA, like other calcium channel blockers, decreases platelet aggregation *in vitro*. Limited clinical studies have demonstrated a moderate but statistically significant decrease in platelet aggregation and an increase in bleeding time in some PROCARDIA patients. This is thought to be a function of inhibition of calcium transport across the platelet membrane. No clinical significance for these findings has been demonstrated.

Positive direct Coombs Test with/without hemolytic anemia has been reported but a causal relationship between PROCARDIA administration and positivity of this laboratory test, including hemolysis, could not be determined.

Although PROCARDIA has been used safely in patients with renal dysfunction and has been reported to exert a beneficial effect in certain cases, rare, reversible elevations in BUN and serum creatinine have been reported in patients with pre-existing chronic renal insufficiency. The relationship to PROCARDIA therapy is uncertain in most cases but probable in some.

Drug Interactions: Beta-adrenergic blocking agents: (See INDICATIONS AND USAGE and WARNINGS.) Experience in over 1400 patients in a non-comparative clinical trial has shown that concomitant administration of PROCARDIA and beta-blocking agents is usually well tolerated, but there have been occasional literature reports suggesting that the combination may increase the likelihood of congestive heart failure, severe hypotension or exacerbation of angina.

Long-acting nitrates: PROCARDIA may be safely co-administered with nitrates, but there have been no controlled studies to evaluate the antianginal effectiveness of this combination.

Digitalis: Since there have been isolated reports of patients with elevated digoxin levels, and there is a possible interaction between digoxin and nifedipine, it is recommended that digoxin levels be monitored when initiating, adjusting, and discontinuing nifedipine to avoid possible over- or under-digitalization.

Quinidine: There have been rare reports of an interaction between quinidine and nifedipine (with a decreased plasma level of quinidine).

Coumarin anticoagulants: There have been rare reports of increased prothrombin time in patients taking coumarin anticoagulants to whom PROCARDIA was administered. However, the relationship to PROCARDIA therapy is uncertain.

Cimetidine: A study in six healthy volunteers has shown a significant increase in peak nifedipine plasma levels (80%) and area-under-the-curve (74%) after a one week course of cimetidine at 1000 mg per day and nifedipine at 40 mg per day. Ranitidine produced smaller, non-significant increases. The effect may be mediated by the known inhibition of cimetidine on hepatic cytochrome P-450, the enzyme system probably responsible for the first-pass metabolism of nifedipine. If nifedipine therapy is initiated in a patient currently receiving cimetidine, cautious titration is advised.

Carcinogenesis, Mutagenesis, Impairment of Fertility: Nifedipine was administered orally to rats for two years and was not shown to be carcinogenic. When given to rats prior to mating, nifedipine caused reduced fertility at a dose approximately 30 times the maximum recommended human dose. There is a literature report of reversible reduction in the ability of human sperm obtained from a limited number of infertile men taking recommended doses of nifedipine to bind to and fertilize an ovum *in vitro*. *In vivo* mutagenicity studies were negative.

Pregnancy: Pregnancy Category C: Nifedipine has been shown to produce teratogenic findings in rats and rabbits, including digital anomalies similar to those reported for phenytoin. Digital anomalies have been reported to occur with other members of the dihydropyridine class and are possibly a result of compromised uterine blood flow. Nifedipine administration was associated with a variety of embryotoxic, placentotoxic, and fetotoxic effects, including stunted fetuses (rats, mice, rabbits), rib deformities (mice), cleft palate (mice), small placentas and underdeveloped chorionic villi (monkeys), embryonic and fetal deaths (rats, mice, rabbits), and prolonged pregnancy/decreased neonatal survival (rats; not evaluated in other species). On a mg/kg basis, all of the doses associated with the teratogenic embryotoxic or fetotoxic effects in animals were higher (3.5 to 42 times) than the maximum recommended human dose of 120 mg/day. On a mg/m^2 basis, some doses were higher and some were lower than the maximum recommended human dose but all are within an order of magnitude of it. The doses associated with placentotoxic effects in monkeys were equivalent to or lower than the maximum recommended human dose on mg/m^2 basis.

There are no adequate and well-controlled studies in pregnant women. PROCARDIA should be used during pregnancy only if the potential benefit justifies the potential risk to the fetus.

Pediatric Use: Safety and effectiveness in pediatric patients have not been established. Use in pediatric population is not recommended.

ADVERSE REACTIONS

In multiple-dose U.S. and foreign controlled studies in which adverse reactions were reported spontaneously, adverse effects were frequent but generally not serious and rarely required discontinuation of therapy or dosage adjustment. Most were expected consequences of the vasodilator effects of PROCARDIA.

Adverse Effect	PROCARDIA CAPSULES (%) (N=226)	Placebo (%) (N=235)
Dizziness, lightheadedness, giddiness	27	15
Flushing, heat sensation	25	8
Headache	23	20
Weakness	12	10
Nausea, heartburn	11	8
Muscle cramps, tremor	8	3
Peripheral edema	7	1
Nervousness, mood changes	7	4
Palpitation	7	5
Dyspnea, cough, wheezing	6	3
Nasal congestion, sore throat	6	8

There is also a large uncontrolled experience in over 2100 patients in the United States. Most of the patients had vasospastic or resistant angina pectoris, and about half had concomitant treatment with beta-adrenergic blocking agents. The most common adverse events were:

Incidence Approximately 10%

Cardiovascular: peripheral edema
Central Nervous System: dizziness or lightheadedness
Gastrointestinal: nausea
Systemic: headache and flushing, weakness

Incidence Approximately 5%

Cardiovascular: transient hypotension

Incidence 2% or Less

Cardiovascular: palpitation
Respiratory: nasal and chest congestion, shortness of breath
Gastrointestinal: diarrhea, constipation, cramps, flatulence
Musculoskeletal: inflammation, joint stiffness, muscle cramps
Central Nervous System: shakiness, nervousness, jitteriness, sleep disturbances, blurred vision, difficulties in balance

Continued on next page

Procardia—Cont.

Other: dermatitis, pruritus, urticaria, fever, sweating, chills, sexual difficulties

Incidence Approximately 0.5%

Cardiovascular: syncope (mostly with initial dosing and/or an increase in dose), erythromelalgia.

Incidence Less Than 0.5%

Hematologic: thrombocytopenia, anemia, leukopenia, purpura

Gastrointestinal: allergic hepatitis

Face and Throat: angioedema (mostly oropharyngeal edema with breathing difficulty in a few patients), gingival hyperplasia.

CNS: depression, paranoid syndrome

Special Senses: transient blindness at the peak of plasma level, tinnitus

Urogenital: nocturia, polyuria

Other: arthritis with ANA (+), exfoliative dermatitis, gynecomastia

Musculoskeletal: myalgia

Several of these side effects appear to be dose related. Peripheral edema occurred in about one in 25 patients at doses less than 60 mg per day and in about one patient in eight at 120 mg per day or more. Transient hypotension, generally of mild to moderate severity and seldom requiring discontinuation of therapy, occurred in one of 50 patients at less than 60 mg per day and in one of 20 patients at 120 mg per day or more.

Very rarely, introduction of PROCARDIA therapy was associated with an increase in anginal pain, possibly due to associated hypotension. Transient unilateral loss of vision has also occurred.

In addition, more serious adverse events were observed, not readily distinguishable from the natural history of the disease in these patients. It remains possible, however, that some or many of these events were drug related. Myocardial infarction occurred in about 4% of patients and congestive heart failure or pulmonary edema in about 2%. Ventricular arrhythmias or conduction disturbances each occurred in fewer than 0.5% of patients.

In a subgroup of over 1000 patients receiving PROCARDIA with concomitant beta blocker therapy, the pattern and incidence of adverse experiences was not different from that of the entire group of PROCARDIA (nifedipine) treated patients. (See PRECAUTIONS.)

In a subgroup of approximately 250 patients with a diagnosis of congestive heart failure as well as angina pectoris (about 10% of the total patient population), dizziness or lightheadedness, peripheral edema, headache or flushing each occurred in one in eight patients. Hypotension occurred in about one in 20 patients. Syncope occurred in approximately one patient in 250. Myocardial infarction or symptoms of congestive heart failure each occurred in about one patient in 15. Atrial or ventricular dysrhythmias each occurred in about one patient in 150.

In post-marketing experience, there have been rare reports of exfoliative dematitis caused by nifedipine.

There have been rare reports of exfoliative or bullous skin adverse events (such as exfoliative dermatitis, erythema mutiforme, Stevens-Johnson Syndrome, and toxic epidermal necrolysis) and photosensitivity reactions.

OVERDOSAGE

Experience with nifedipine overdosage is limited. Generally, overdosage with nifedipine leading to pronounced hypotension calls for active cardiovascular support including monitoring of cardiovascular and respiratory function, elevation of extremities, and judicious use of calcium infusion, pressor agents and fluids. Clearance of nifedipine would be expected to be prolonged in patients with impaired liver function. Since nifedipine is highly protein bound, dialysis is not likely to be of any benefit; however, plasmapheresis may be beneficial.

DOSAGE AND ADMINISTRATION

The dosage of PROCARDIA needed to suppress angina and that can be tolerated by the patient must be established by titration. Excessive doses can result in hypotension.

Therapy should be initiated with the 10 mg capsule. The starting dose is one 10 mg capsule, swallowed whole, 3 times/day. The usual effective dose range is 10–20 mg three times daily. Some patients, especially those with evidence of coronary artery spasm, respond only to higher doses, more frequent administration, or both. In such patients, doses of 20–30 mg three or four times daily may be effective. Doses above 120 mg daily are rarely necessary. More than 180 mg per day is not recommended.

In most cases, PROCARDIA titration should proceed over a 7–14 day period so that the physician can assess the response to each dose level and monitor the blood pressure before proceeding to higher doses.

If symptoms so warrant, titration may proceed more rapidly provided that the patient is assessed frequently. Based on the patient's physical activity level, attack frequency, and sublingual nitroglycerin consumption, the dose of PROCARDIA may be increased from 10 mg t.i.d. to 20 mg t.i.d. and then to 30 mg t.i.d. over a three-day period.

In hospitalized patients under close observation, the dose may be increased in 10 mg increments over four- to six-hour periods as required to control pain and arrhythmias due to ischemia. A single dose should rarely exceed 30 mg.

No "rebound effect" has been observed upon discontinuation of PROCARDIA. However, if discontinuation of PROCARDIA is necessary, sound clinical practice suggests that the dosage should be decreased gradually with close physician supervision.

Co-Administration with Other Antianginal Drugs

Sublingual nitroglycerin may be taken as required for the control of acute manifestations of angina, particularly during PROCARDIA titration. See **PRECAUTIONS, Drug Interactions**, for information on co-administration of PROCARDIA with beta blockers or long-acting nitrates.

HOW SUPPLIED

PROCARDIA® soft gelatin capsules are supplied in:

Bottles of 100:

10 mg (NDC 0069-2600-66) (NDC 59012-260-66) orange #260;

20 mg (NDC 0069-2610-66) (NDC 59012-261-66) orange and light brown #261

Bottles of 300:

10 mg (NDC 0069-2600-72) (NDC 59012-260-72) orange #260;

20 mg (NDC 0069-2610-72) (NDC 59012-261-72) orange and light brown #261

Unit dose packages of 100:

10 mg (NDC 0069-2600-41) (NDC 59012-260-41) orange #260;

20 mg (NDC 0069-2610-41) (NDC 59012-261-41) orange and light brown #261

The capsules should be protected from light and moisture and stored at controlled room temperature 59° to 77°F (15° to 25°C) in the manufacturer's original container.

Manufactured by Pfizer Inc. Encapsulated by R.P. Scherer, Clearwater, FL 33518

69-4990-00-9 Revised March 1997

Shown in Product Identification Guide, page 330

PROCARDIA XL® ℞

[pro-car ' dē-ă]

(nifedipine)

Extended Release Tablets

For Oral Use

DESCRIPTION

Nifedipine is a drug belonging to a class of pharmacological agents known as the calcium channel blockers. Nifedipine is 3,5-pyridinedicarboxylic acid, 1,4-dihydro-2,6-dimethyl-4-(2-nitrophenyl)-, dimethyl ester, $C_{17}H_{18}N_2O_6$, and has the structural formula:

Nifedipine is a yellow crystalline substance, practically insoluble in water but soluble in ethanol. It has a molecular weight of 346.3. PROCARDIA XL is a registered trademark for Nifedipine GITS. Nifedipine GITS (Gastrointestinal Therapeutic System) Tablet is formulated as a once-a-day controlled-release tablet for oral administration designed to deliver 30, 60, or 90 mg of nifedipine.

Inert ingredients in the formulations are: cellulose acetate; hydroxypropyl cellulose; hydroxypropyl methylcellulose; magnesium stearate; polyethylene glycol; polyethylene oxide; red ferric oxide; sodium chloride; titanium dioxide.

System Components and Performance

PROCARDIA XL Extended Release Tablet is similar in appearance to a conventional tablet. It consists, however, of a semipermeable membrane surrounding an osmotically active drug core. The core itself is divided into two layers: an "active" layer containing the drug, and a "push" layer containing pharmacologically inert (but osmotically active) components. As water from the gastrointestinal tract enters the tablet, pressure increases in the osmotic layer and "pushes" against the drug layer, releasing drug through the precision laser-drilled tablet orifice in the active layer.

PROCARDIA XL Extended Release Tablet is designed to provide nifedipine at an approximately constant rate over 24 hours. This controlled rate of drug delivery into the gastrointestinal lumen is independent of pH or gastrointestinal motility. PROCARDIA XL depends for its action on the existence of an osmotic gradient between the contents of the bi-layer core and fluid in the GI tract. Drug delivery is essentially constant as long as the osmotic gradient remains constant, and then gradually falls to zero. Upon swallowing, the biologically inert components of the tablet remain intact during GI transit and are eliminated in the feces as an insoluble shell.

CLINICAL PHARMACOLOGY

Nifedipine is a calcium ion influx inhibitor (slow-channel blocker or calcium ion antagonist) and inhibits the transmembrane influx of calcium ions into cardiac muscle and smooth muscle. The contractile processes of cardiac muscle and vascular smooth muscle are dependent upon the movement of extracellular calcium ions into these cells through specific ion channels. Nifedipine selectively inhibits calcium ion influx across the cell membrane of cardiac muscle and vascular smooth muscle without altering serum calcium concentrations.

Mechanism of Action

A) Angina

The precise mechanisms by which inhibition of calcium influx relieves angina has not been fully determined, but includes at least the following two mechanisms:

1) Relaxation and Prevention of Coronary Artery Spasm

Nifedipine dilates the main coronary arteries and coronary arterioles, both in normal and ischemic regions, and is a potent inhibitor of coronary artery spasm, whether spontaneous or ergonovine-induced. This property increases myocardial oxygen delivery in patients with coronary artery spasm, and is responsible for the effectiveness of nifedipine in vasospastic (Prinzmetal's or variant) angina. Whether this effect plays any role in classical angina is not clear, but studies of exercise tolerance have not shown an increase in the maximum exercise rate-pressure product, a widely accepted measure of oxygen utilization. This suggests that, in general, relief of spasm or dilation of coronary arteries is not an important factor in classical angina.

2) Reduction of Oxygen Utilization

Nifedipine regularly reduces arterial pressure at rest and at a given level of exercise by dilating peripheral arterioles and reducing the total peripheral vascular resistance (afterload) against which the heart works. This unloading of the heart reduces myocardial energy consumption and oxygen requirements, and probably accounts for the effectiveness of nifedipine in chronic stable angina.

B) Hypertension

The mechanism by which nifedipine reduces arterial blood pressure involves peripheral arterial vasodilatation and the resulting reduction in peripheral vascular resistance. The increased peripheral vascular resistance that is an underlying cause of hypertension results from an increase in active tension in the vascular smooth muscle. Studies have demonstrated that the increase in active tension reflects an increase in cytosolic free calcium.

Nifedipine is a peripheral arterial vasodilator which acts directly on vascular smooth muscle. The binding of nifedipine to voltage-dependent and possibly receptor-operated channels in vascular smooth muscle results in an inhibition of calcium influx through these channels. Stores of intracellular calcium in vascular smooth muscle are limited and thus dependent upon the influx of extracellular calcium for contraction to occur. The reduction in calcium influx by nifedipine causes arterial vasodilation and decreased peripheral vascular resistance which results in reduced arterial blood pressure.

Pharmacokinetics and Metabolism

Nifedipine is completely absorbed after oral administration. Plasma drug concentrations rise at a gradual, controlled rate after a PROCARDIA XL Extended Release Tablet dose and reach a plateau at approximately six hours after the first dose. For subsequent doses, relatively constant plasma concentrations at this plateau are maintained with minimal fluctuations over the 24-hour dosing interval. About a four-fold higher fluctuation index (ratio of peak to trough plasma concentration) was observed with the conventional immediate-release Procardia® capsule at t.i.d. dosing than with once daily PROCARDIA XL Extended Release Tablet. At steady-state the bioavailability of the PROCARDIA XL Extended Release Tablet is 86% relative to Procardia capsules. Administration of the PROCARDIA XL Extended Release Tablet in the presence of food slightly alters the early rate of drug absorption, but does not influence the extent of drug bioavailability. Markedly reduced GI retention time over prolonged periods (i.e., short bowel syndrome), however, may influence the pharmacokinetic profile of the drug which could potentially result in lower plasma concentrations. Pharmacokinetics of PROCARDIA XL Extended Release Tablets are linear over the dose range of 30 to 180 mg in that plasma drug concentrations are proportional to dose administered. There was no evidence of dose dumping either in the presence or absence of food for over 150 subjects in pharmacokinetic studies.

Nifedipine is extensively metabolized to highly water-soluble, inactive metabolites accounting for 60 to 80% of the dose excreted in the urine. The elimination half-life of nifedipine is approximately two hours. Only traces (less than 0.1% of the dose) of unchanged form can be detected in the urine. The remainder is excreted in the feces in metabolized form, most likely as a result of biliary excretion. Thus, the pharmacokinetics of nifedipine are not significantly influenced by the degree of renal impairment. Patients in hemodialysis or chronic ambulatory peritoneal dialysis have not reported significantly altered pharmacokinetics of nifedipine. Since hepatic biotransformation is the predominant route for the disposition of nifedipine, the pharmacokinetics may be altered in patients with chronic liver disease. Patients with hepatic impairment (liver cirrhosis) have a longer disposition half-life and higher bioavailability of nifedipine than healthy volunteers. The degree of serum protein binding of nifedipine is high (92–98%). Protein binding may be greatly reduced in patients with renal or hepatic impairment.

Hemodynamics

Like other slow-channel blockers, nifedipine exerts a negative inotropic effect on isolated myocardial tissue. This is rarely, if ever, seen in intact animals or man, probably because of reflex responses to its vasodilating effects. In man, nifedipine decreases peripheral vascular resistance which leads to a fall in systolic and diastolic pressures, usually minimal in normotensive volunteers (less than 5–10 mm Hg systolic), but sometimes larger. With PROCARDIA XL Extended Release Tablets, these decreases in blood pressure are not accompanied by any significant change in heart rate. Hemodynamic studies in patients with normal ventricular function have generally found a small increase in cardiac index without major effects on ejection fraction, left ventricular end diastolic pressure (LVEDP) or volume (LVEDV). In patients with impaired ventricular function, most acute studies have shown some increase in ejection fraction and reduction in left ventricular filling pressure.

Electrophysiologic Effects

Although, like other members of its class, nifedipine causes a slight depression of sinoatrial node function and atrioventricular conduction in isolated myocardial preparations, such effects have not been seen in studies in intact animals or in man. In formal electrophysiologic studies, predominantly in patients with normal conduction systems, nifedipine has had no tendency to prolong atrioventricular conduction or sinus node recovery time, or to slow sinus rate.

INDICATIONS AND USAGE

I. Vasospastic Angina

PROCARDIA XL is indicated for the management of vasospastic angina confirmed by any of the following criteria: 1) classical pattern of angina at rest accompanied by ST segment elevation, 2) angina or coronary artery spasm provoked by ergonovine, or 3) angiographically demonstrated coronary artery spasm. In those patients who have had angiography, the presence of significant fixed obstructive disease is not incompatible with the diagnosis of vasospastic angina, provided that the above criteria are satisfied. PROCARDIA XL may also be used where the clinical presentation suggests a possible vasospastic component but where vasospasm has not been confirmed, e.g., where pain has a variable threshold on exertion or in unstable angina where electrocardiographic findings are compatible with intermittent vasospasm, or when angina is refractory to nitrates and/or adequate doses of beta blockers.

II. Chronic Stable Angina
(Classical Effort-Associated Angina)

PROCARDIA XL is indicated for the management of chronic stable angina (effort-associated angina) without evidence of vasospasm in patients who remain symptomatic despite adequate doses of beta blockers and/or organic nitrates or who cannot tolerate those agents.

In chronic stable angina (effort-associated angina) nifedipine has been effective in controlled trials of up to eight weeks duration in reducing angina frequency and increasing exercise tolerance, but confirmation of sustained effectiveness and evaluation of long-term safety in these patients is incomplete.

Controlled studies in small numbers of patients suggest concomitant use of nifedipine and beta-blocking agents may be beneficial in patients with chronic stable angina, but available information is not sufficient to predict with confidence the effects of concurrent treatment, especially in patients with compromised left ventricular function or cardiac conduction abnormalities. When introducing such concomitant therapy, care must be taken to monitor blood pressure closely since severe hypotension can occur from the combined effects of the drugs. (See WARNINGS.)

III. Hypertension

PROCARDIA XL is indicated for the treatment of hypertension. It may be used alone or in combination with other antihypertensive agents.

CONTRAINDICATIONS

Known hypersensitivity reaction to nifedipine.

WARNINGS

Excessive Hypotension

Although in most angina patients the hypotensive effect of nifedipine is modest and well tolerated, occasional patients have had excessive and poorly tolerated hypotension. These responses have usually occurred during initial titration or at the time of subsequent upward dosage adjustment, and may be more likely in patients on concomitant beta blockers.

Severe hypotension and/or increased fluid volume requirements have been reported in patients receiving nifedipine together with a beta-blocking agent who underwent coronary artery bypass surgery using high dose fentanyl anesthesia. The interaction with high dose fentanyl appears to be due to the combination of nifedipine and a beta blocker, but the possibility that it may occur with nifedipine alone, with low doses of fentanyl, in other surgical procedures, or with other narcotic analgesics cannot be ruled out. In nifedipine-treated patients where surgery using high dose fentanyl anesthesia is contemplated, the physician should be aware of these potential problems and if the patient's condition permits, sufficient time (at least 36 hours) should be allowed for nifedipine to be washed out of the body prior to surgery.

The following information should be taken into account in those patients who are being treated for hypertension as well as angina:

Increased Angina and/or Myocardial Infarction

Rarely, patients, particularly those who have severe obstructive coronary artery disease, have developed well documented increased frequency, duration and/or severity of angina or acute myocardial infarction on starting nifedipine or at the time of dosage increase. The mechanism of this effect is not established.

Beta Blocker Withdrawal

It is important to taper beta blockers if possible, rather than stopping them abruptly before beginning nifedipine. Patients recently withdrawn from beta blockers may develop a withdrawal syndrome with increased angina, probably related to increased sensitivity to catecholamines. Initiation of nifedipine treatment will not prevent this occurrence and on occasion has been reported to increase it.

Congestive Heart Failure

Rarely, patients, usually receiving a beta blocker, have developed heart failure after beginning nifedipine. Patients with tight aortic stenosis may be at greater risk for such an event, as the unloading effect of nifedipine would be expected to be of less benefit to those patients, owing to their fixed impedance to flow across the aortic valve.

PRECAUTIONS

General—Hypotension: Because nifedipine decreases peripheral vascular resistance, careful monitoring of blood pressure during the initial administration and titration of nifedipine is suggested. Close observation is especially recommended for patients already taking medications that are known to lower blood pressure. (See WARNINGS.)

Peripheral Edema: Mild to moderate peripheral edema occurs in a dose dependent manner with an incidence ranging from approximately 10% to about 30% at the highest dose studied (180 mg). It is a localized phenomenon thought to be associated with vasodilation of dependent arterioles and small blood vessels and not due to left ventricular dysfunction or generalized fluid retention. With patients whose angina or hypertension is complicated by congestive heart failure, care should be taken to differentiate this peripheral edema from the effects of increasing left ventricular dysfunction.

Other: As with any other non-deformable material, caution should be used when administering PROCARDIA XL in patients with preexisting severe gastrointestinal narrowing (pathologic or iatrogenic). There have been rare reports of obstructive symptoms in patients with known strictures in association with the ingestion of PROCARDIA XL.

Information for Patients: PROCARDIA XL Extended Release Tablets should be swallowed whole. Do not chew, divide or crush tablets. Do not be concerned if you occasionally notice in your stool something that looks like a tablet. In PROCARDIA XL, the medication is contained within a nonabsorbable shell that has been specially designed to slowly release the drug for your body to absorb. When this process is completed, the empty tablet is eliminated from your body.

Laboratory Tests: Rare, usually transient, but occasionally significant elevations of enzymes such as alkaline phosphatase, CPK, LDH, SGOT, and SGPT have been noted. The relationship to nifedipine therapy is uncertain in most cases, but probable in some. These laboratory abnormalities have rarely been associated with clinical symptoms; however, cholestasis with or without jaundice has been reported. A small (5.4%) increase in mean alkaline phosphatase was noted in patients treated with PROCARDIA XL. This was an isolated finding not associated with clinical symptoms and it rarely resulted in values which fell outside the normal range. Rare instances of allergic hepatitis have been reported. In controlled studies, PROCARDIA XL did not adversely affect serum uric acid, glucose, or cholesterol. Serum potassium was unchanged in patients receiving PROCARDIA XL in the absence of concomitant diuretic therapy, and slightly decreased in patients receiving concomitant diuretics.

Nifedipine, like other calcium channel blockers, decreases platelet aggregation *in vitro*. Limited clinical studies have demonstrated a moderate but statistically significant decrease in platelet aggregation and an increase in bleeding time in some nifedipine patients. This is thought to be a function of inhibition of calcium transport across the platelet membrane. No clinical significance for these findings has been demonstrated.

Positive direct Coombs test with/without hemolytic anemia has been reported but a causal relationship between nifedipine administration and positivity of this laboratory test, including hemolysis, could not be determined.

Although nifedipine has been used safely in patients with renal dysfunction and has been reported to exert a beneficial effect, in certain cases, rare, reversible elevations in BUN and serum creatinine have been reported in patients with pre-existing chronic renal insufficiency. The relationship to nifedipine therapy is uncertain in most cases but probable in some.

Drug Interactions: Beta-adrenergic blocking agents: (See INDICATIONS AND USAGE and WARNINGS.) Experience in over 1400 patients with Procardia capsules in a noncomparative clinical trial has shown that concomitant administration of nifedipine and beta-blocking agents is usually well tolerated, but there have been occasional literature reports suggesting that the combination may increase the likelihood of congestive heart failure, severe hypotension, or exacerbation of angina.

Long-acting Nitrates: Nifedipine may be safely co-administered with nitrates, but there have been no controlled studies to evaluate the antianginal effectiveness of this combination.

Digitalis: Administration of nifedipine with digoxin increased digoxin levels in nine of twelve normal volunteers. The average increase was 45%. Another investigator found no increase in digoxin levels in thirteen patients with coronary artery disease. In an uncontrolled study of over two hundred patients with congestive heart failure during which digoxin blood levels were not measured, digitalis toxicity was not observed. Since there have been isolated reports of patients with elevated digoxin levels, it is recommended that digoxin levels be monitored when initiating, adjusting, and discontinuing nifedipine to avoid possible over- or under-digitalization.

Coumarin Anticoagulants: There have been rare reports of increased prothrombin time in patients taking coumarin anticoagulants to whom nifedipine was administered. However, the relationship to nifedipine therapy is uncertain.

Cimetidine: A study in six healthy volunteers has shown a significant increase in peak nifedipine plasma levels (80%) and area-under-the-curve (74%), after a one week course of cimetidine at 1000 mg per day and nifedipine at 40 mg per day. Ranitidine produced smaller, non-significant increases. The effect may be mediated by the known inhibition of cimetidine on hepatic cytochrome P-450, the enzyme system probably responsible for the first-pass metabolism of nifedipine. If nifedipine therapy is initiated in a patient currently receiving cimetidine, cautious titration is advised.

Carcinogenesis, Mutagenesis, Impairment of Fertility: Nifedipine was administered orally to rats for two years and was not shown to be carcinogenic. When given to rats prior to mating, nifedipine caused reduced fertility at a dose approximately 30 times the maximum recommended human dose. There is a literature report of reversible reduction in the ability of human sperm obtained from a limited number of infertile men taking recommended doses of nifedipine to bind to and fertilize an ovum *in vitro*. *In vivo* mutagenicity studies were negative.

Pregnancy: Pregnancy Category C: Nifedipine has been shown to produce teratogenic findings in rats and rabbits, including digital anomalies similar to those reported for phenytoin. Digital anomalies have been reported to occur with other members of the dihydropyridine class and are possibly a result of compromised uterine blood flow. Nifedipine administration was associated with a variety of embryotoxic, placentotoxic, and fetotoxic effects, including stunted fetuses (rats, mice, rabbits), rib deformities (mice), cleft palate (mice), small placentas and underdeveloped chorionic villi (monkeys), embryonic and fetal deaths (rats, mice, rabbits), and prolonged pregnancy/decreased neonatal survival (rats; not evaluated in other species). On a mg/kg basis, all of the doses associated with the teratogenic embryotoxic or fetotoxic effects in animals were higher (3.5 to 42 times) than the maximum recommended human dose of 120 mg/day. On a mg/m^2 basis, some doses were higher and some were lower than the maximum recommended human dose but all are within an order of magnitude of it. The doses associated with placentotoxic effects in monkeys were equivalent to or lower than the maximum recommended human dose on a mg/m^2 basis.

There are no adequate and well-controlled studies in pregnant women. PROCARDIA XL Extended Release Tablets should be used during pregnancy only if the potential benefit justifies the potential risk to the fetus.

Pediatric Use: Safety and effectiveness in pediatric patients have not been established.

ADVERSE EXPERIENCES

Over 1000 patients from both controlled and open trials with PROCARDIA XL Extended Release Tablets in hypertension and angina were included in the evaluation of adverse experiences. All side effects reported during PROCARDIA XL Extended Release Tablet therapy were tabulated independent of their causal relation to medication. The most common side effect reported with PROCARDIA XL was edema which was dose related and ranged in frequency from approximately 10% to about 30% at the highest dose studied (180 mg). Other common adverse experiences reported in placebo-controlled trials include:

Adverse Effect	PROCARDIA XL (%) (N=707)	Placebo (%) (N=266)
Headache	15.8	9.8
Fatigue	5.9	4.1
Dizziness	4.1	4.5
Constipation	3.3	2.3
Nausea	3.3	1.9

Of these, only edema and headache were more common in PROCARDIA XL patients than placebo patients.

The following adverse reactions occurred with an incidence of less than 3.0%. With the exception of leg cramps, the incidence of these side effects was similar to that of placebo alone.

Body as a Whole/Systemic: asthenia, flushing, pain
Cardiovascular: palpitations
Central Nervous System: insomnia, nervousness, paresthesia, somnolence
Dermatologic: pruritus, rash
Gastrointestinal: abdominal pain, diarrhea, dry mouth, dyspepsia, flatulence
Musculoskeletal: arthralgia, leg cramps
Respiratory: chest pain (nonspecific), dyspnea
Urogenital: impotence, polyuria

Other adverse reactions were reported sporadically with an incidence of 1.0% or less. These include:

Body as a Whole/Systemic: face edema, fever, hot flashes, malaise, periorbital edema, rigors
Cardiovascular: arrhythmia, hypotension, increased angina, tachycardia, syncope

Continued on next page

Procardia XL—Cont.

Central Nervous System: anxiety, ataxia, decreased libido, depression, hypertonia, hypoesthesia, migraine, paroniria, tremor, vertigo
Dermatologic: alopecia, increased sweating, urticaria, purpura
Gastrointestinal: eructation, gastroesophageal reflux, gum hyperplasia, melena, vomiting, weight increase
Musculoskeletal: back pain, gout, myalgias
Respiratory: coughing, epistaxis, upper respiratory tract infection, respiratory disorder, sinusitis
Special Senses: abnormal lacrimation, abnormal vision, taste perversion, tinnitus
Urogenital/Reproductive: breast pain, dysuria, hematuria, nocturia

Adverse experiences which occurred in less than 1 in 1000 patients cannot be distinguished from concurrent disease states or medications.

The following adverse experiences, reported in less than 1% of patients, occurred under conditions (e.g., open trials, marketing experience) where a causal relationship is uncertain: gastrointestinal irritation, gastrointestinal bleeding, gynecomastia.

In multiple-dose U.S. and foreign controlled studies with nifedipine capsules in which adverse reactions were reported spontaneously, adverse effects were frequent but generally not serious and rarely required discontinuation of therapy or dosage adjustment. Most were expected consequences of the vasodilator effects of nifedipine.

Adverse Effect	PROCARDIA CAPSULES (%) (N=226)	Placebo (%) (N=235)
Dizziness, lightheadedness, giddiness	27	15
Flushing, heat sensation	25	8
Headache	23	20
Weakness	12	10
Nausea, heartburn	11	8
Muscle cramps, tremor	8	3
Peripheral edema	7	1
Nervousness, mood changes	7	4
Palpitation	7	5
Dyspnea, cough, wheezing	6	3
Nasal congestion, sore throat	6	8

There is also a large uncontrolled experience in over 2100 patients in the United States. Most of the patients had vasospastic or resistant angina pectoris, and about half had concomitant treatment with beta-adrenergic blocking agents. The relatively common adverse events were similar in nature to those seen with PROCARDIA XL.

In addition, more serious adverse events were observed, not readily distinguishable from the natural history of the disease in these patients. It remains possible, however, that some or many of these events were drug related. Myocardial infarction occurred in about 4% of patients and congestive heart failure or pulmonary edema in about 2%. Ventricular arrhythmias or conduction disturbances each occurred in fewer than 0.5% of patients.

In a subgroup of over 1000 patients receiving PROCARDIA with concomitant beta blocker therapy, the pattern and incidence of adverse experiences was not different from that of the entire group of PROCARDIA (nifedipine) treated patients. (See PRECAUTIONS.)

In a subgroup of approximately 250 patients with a diagnosis of congestive heart failure as well as angina, dizziness, or lightheadedness, peripheral edema, headache or flushing each occurred in one in eight patients. Hypotension occurred in about one in 20 patients. Syncope occurred in approximately one patient in 250. Myocardial infarction or symptoms of congestive heart failure each occurred in about one patient in 15. Atrial or ventricular dysrhythmias each occurred in about one patient in 150.

In post-marketing experience, there have been rare reports of exfoliative dermatitis caused by nifedipine.

There have been rare reports of exfoliative or bullous skin adverse events (such as exfoliative dermatitis, erythema multiforme, Stevens-Johnson Syndrome, and toxic epidermal necrolysis) and photosensitivity reactions.

OVERDOSAGE

Experience with nifedipine overdosage is limited. Generally, overdosage with nifedipine leading to pronounced hypotension calls for active cardiovascular support including monitoring of cardiovascular and respiratory function, elevation of extremities, judicious use of calcium infusion, pressor agents and fluids. Clearance of nifedipine would be expected to be prolonged in patients with impaired liver function. Since nifedipine is highly protein-bound, dialysis is not likely to be of any benefit.

There has been one reported case of massive overdosage with PROCARDIA XL Extended Release Tablets. The main effects of ingestion of approximately 4800 mg of PROCARDIA XL in a young man attempting suicide as a result of cocaine-induced depression was initial dizziness, palpitations, flushing, and nervousness. Within several hours of ingestion, nausea, vomiting, and generalized edema developed. No significant hypotension was apparent at presentation, 18 hours post-ingestion. Electrolyte abnormalities consisted of a mild, transient elevation of serum creatinine, and modest elevations of LDH and CPK, but normal SGOT. Vital signs remained stable, no electrocardiographic abnormalities were noted and renal function returned to normal within 24 to 48 hours with routine supportive measures alone. No prolonged sequelae were observed.

The effect of a single 900 mg ingestion of Procardia capsules in a depressed anginal patient also on tricyclic antidepressants was loss of consciousness within 30 minutes of ingestion, and profound hypotension, which responded to calcium infusion, pressor agents, and fluid replacement. A variety of ECG abnormalities were seen in this patient with a history of bundle branch block, including sinus bradycardia and varying degrees of AV block. These dictated the prophylactic placement of a temporary ventricular pacemaker, but otherwise resolved spontaneously. Significant hyperglycemia was seen initially in this patient, but plasma glucose levels rapidly normalized without further treatment.

A young hypertensive patient with advanced renal failure ingested 280 mg of Procardia capsules at one time, with resulting marked hypotension responding to calcium infusion and fluids. No AV conduction abnormalities, arrhythmias, or pronounced changes in heart rate were noted, nor was there any further deterioration in renal function.

DOSAGE AND ADMINISTRATION

Dosage must be adjusted according to each patient's needs. Therapy for either hypertension or angina should be initiated with 30 or 60 mg once daily. PROCARDIA XL Extended Release Tablets should be swallowed whole and should not be bitten or divided. In general, titration should proceed over a 7–14 day period so that the physician can fully assess the response to each dose level and monitor blood pressure before proceeding to higher doses. Since steady-state plasma levels are achieved on the second day of dosing, if symptoms so warrant, titration may proceed more rapidly provided the patient is assessed frequently. Titration to doses above 120 mg are not recommended.

Angina patients controlled on Procardia capsules alone or in combination with other antianginal medications may be safely switched to PROCARDIA XL Extended Release Tablets at the nearest equivalent total daily dose (e.g., 30 mg t.i.d. of Procardia capsules may be changed to 90 mg once daily of PROCARDIA XL Extended Release Tablets). Subsequent titration to higher or lower doses may be necessary and should be initiated as clinically warranted. Experience with doses greater than 90 mg in patients with angina is limited. Therefore, doses greater than 90 mg should be used with caution and only when clinically warranted.

No "rebound effect" has been observed upon discontinuation of PROCARDIA XL Extended Release Tablets. However, if discontinuation of nifedipine is necessary, sound clinical practice suggests that the dosage should be decreased gradually with close physician supervision.

Care should be taken when dispensing PROCARDIA XL to assure that the extended release dosage form has been prescribed.

Co-Administration with Other Antianginal Drugs

Sublingual nitroglycerin may be taken as required for the control of acute manifestations of angina, particularly during nifedipine titration. See PRECAUTIONS, Drug Interactions, for information on co-administration of nifedipine with beta blockers or long-acting nitrates.

HOW SUPPLIED

PROCARDIA XL® Extended Release Tablets are supplied as 30 mg, 60 mg and 90 mg round, biconvex, rose-pink, film-coated tablets in:

Bottles of 100: 30 mg (NDC 0069-2650-66)
(NDC 59012-265-66)
60 mg (NDC 0069-2660-66)
(NDC 59012-266-66)
90 mg (NDC 0069-2670-66)
(NDC 59012-267-66)

Bottles of 300: 30 mg (NDC 0069-2650-72)
(NDC 59012-265-72)
60 mg (NDC 0069-2660-72)
(NDC 59012-266-72)

Bottles of 5000: 30 mg (NDC 0069-2650-94)
(NDC 59012-265-94)
60 mg (NDC 0069-2660-94)
(NDC 59012-266-94)

Unit dose packages of 100: 30 mg (NDC 0069-2650-41)
(NDC 59012-265-41)
60 mg (NDC 0069-2660-41)
(NDC 59012-266-41)
90 mg (NDC 0069-2670-41)
(NDC 59012-267-41)

Store below 86°F (30°C).
Protect from moisture and humidity.

69-4467-00-6 Revised March 1997

Shown in Product Identification Guide, page 330

RENESE® ℞

[rĕ-nēs]
(polythiazide)
TABLETS
for Oral Administration

DESCRIPTION

Renese® is designated generically as polythiazide, and chemically as 2*H*-1,2,4-Benzothiadiazine-7-sulfonamide, 6-chloro-3,4-dihydro-2-methyl-3-[[(2,2,2-trifluoroethyl)thio]methyl]-, 1,1-dioxide. It is a white crystalline substance, insoluble in water but readily soluble in alkaline solution.

Inert Ingredients: dibasic calcium phosphate; lactose; magnesium stearate; polyethylene glycol; sodium lauryl sulfate; starch; vanillin. The 2 mg tablets also contain: Yellow 6; Yellow 10.

ACTION

The mechanism of action results in an interference with the renal tubular mechanism of electrolyte reabsorption. At maximal therapeutic dosage all thiazides are approximately equal in their diuretic potency. The mechanism whereby thiazides function in the control of hypertension is unknown.

INDICATIONS

Renese is indicated as adjunctive therapy in edema associated with congestive heart failure, hepatic cirrhosis, and corticosteroid and estrogen therapy.

Renese has also been found useful in edema due to various forms of renal dysfunction as: Nephrotic syndrome; Acute glomerulonephritis; and Chronic renal failure.

Renese is indicated in the management of hypertension either as the sole therapeutic agent or to enhance the effectiveness of other antihypertensive drugs in the more severe forms of hypertension.

Usage in Pregnancy. The routine use of diuretics in an otherwise healthy woman is inappropriate and exposes mother and fetus to unnecessary hazard. Diuretics do not prevent development of toxemia of pregnancy, and there is no satisfactory evidence that they are useful in the treatment of developed toxemia.

Edema during pregnancy may arise from pathological causes or from the physiologic and mechanical consequences of pregnancy. Thiazides are indicated in pregnancy when edema is due to pathologic causes, just as they are in the absence of pregnancy (however, see Warnings, below). Dependent edema in pregnancy, resulting from restriction of venous return by the expanded uterus, is properly treated through elevation of the lower extremities and use of support hose; use of diuretics to lower intravascular volume in this case is illogical and unnecessary. There is hypervolemia during normal pregnancy which is harmful to neither the fetus nor the mother (in the absence of cardiovascular disease), but which is associated with edema, including generalized edema, in the majority of pregnant women. If this edema produces discomfort, increased recumbency will often provide relief. In rare instances, this edema may cause extreme discomfort which is not relieved by rest. In these cases, a short course of diuretics may provide relief and may be appropriate.

CONTRAINDICATIONS

Anuria. Hypersensitivity to this or other sulfonamide derived drugs.

WARNINGS

Thiazides should be used with caution in severe renal disease. In patients with renal disease, thiazides may precipitate azotemia. Cumulative effects of the drug may develop in patients with impaired renal function.

Thiazides should be used with caution in patients with impaired hepatic function or progressive liver disease, since minor alterations of fluid and electrolyte balance may precipitate hepatic coma.

Thiazides may add to or potentiate the action of other antihypertensive drugs. Potentiation occurs with ganglionic or peripheral adrenergic blocking drugs.

Sensitivity reactions may occur in patients with a history of allergy or bronchial asthma.

The possibility of exacerbation or activation of systemic lupus erythematosus has been reported.

Usage in Pregnancy. Thiazides cross the placental barrier and appear in cord blood. The use of thiazides in pregnant women requires that the anticipated benefit be weighed against possible hazards to the fetus. These hazards include fetal or neonatal jaundice, thrombocytopenia, and possibly other adverse reactions which have occurred in the adult.

Nursing Mothers. Thiazides appear in breast milk. If use of the drug is deemed essential, the patient should stop nursing.

PRECAUTIONS

Periodic determination of serum electrolytes to detect possible electrolyte imbalance should be performed at appropriate intervals.

All patients receiving thiazide therapy should be observed for clinical signs of fluid or electrolyte imbalance; namely, hyponatremia, hypochloremic alkalosis, and hypokalemia. Serum and urine electrolyte determinations are particularly important when the patient is vomiting excessively or receiving parenteral fluids. Medication such as digitalis may also influence serum electrolytes. Warning signs, irrespective of cause, are: dryness of mouth, thirst, weakness, lethargy, drowsiness, restlessness, muscle pains or cramps, muscular fatigue, hypotension, oliguria, tachycardia, and gastrointestinal disturbances such as nausea and vomiting.

Hypokalemia may develop with thiazides as with any other potent diuretic, especially with brisk diuresis, when severe cirrhosis is present, or during concomitant use of corticosteroids or ACTH.

Interference with adequate oral electrolyte intake will also contribute to hypokalemia. Digitalis therapy may exaggerate metabolic effects of hypokalemia especially with reference to myocardial activity.

Any chloride deficit is generally mild and usually does not require specific treatment except under extraordinary cir-

cumstances (as in liver disease or renal disease). Dilutional hyponatremia may occur in edematous patients in hot weather; appropriate therapy is water restriction, rather than administration of salt except in rare instances when the hyponatremia is life threatening. In actual salt depletion, appropriate replacement is the therapy of choice.
Hyperuricemia may occur or frank gout may be precipitated in certain patients receiving thiazide therapy.
Insulin requirements in diabetic patients may be increased, decreased, or unchanged. Latent diabetes mellitus may become manifest during thiazide administration.
Thiazide drugs may increase the responsiveness to tubocurarine.
The antihypertensive effects of the drug may be enhanced in the postsympathectomy patient.
Thiazides may decrease arterial responsiveness to norepinephrine. This diminution is not sufficient to preclude effectiveness of the pressor agent for therapeutic use.
If progressive renal impairment becomes evident, as indicated by a rising nonprotein nitrogen or blood urea nitrogen, a careful reappraisal of therapy is necessary with consideration given to withholding or discontinuing diuretic therapy.
Thiazides may decrease serum PBI levels without signs of thyroid disturbance.
Pediatric Use: Safety and effectiveness in pediatric patients have not been established.

ADVERSE REACTIONS

A. GASTROINTESTINAL SYSTEM REACTIONS
1. anorexia
2. gastric irritation
3. nausea
4. vomiting
5. cramping
6. diarrhea
7. constipation
8. jaundice (intrahepatic cholestatic jaundice)
9. pancreatitis

B. CENTRAL NERVOUS SYSTEM REACTIONS
1. dizziness
2. vertigo
3. paresthesias
4. headache
5. xanthopsia

C. HEMATOLOGIC REACTIONS
1. leukopenia
2. agranulocytosis
3. thrombocytopenia
4. aplastic anemia

D. DERMATOLOGIC—HYPERSENSITIVITY REACTIONS
1. purpura
2. photosensitivity
3. rash
4. urticaria
5. necrotizing angiitis
(vasculitis)
(cutaneous vasculitis)

E. CARDIOVASCULAR REACTION
Orthostatic hypotension may occur and may be aggravated by alcohol, barbiturates or narcotics.

F. OTHER
1. hyperglycemia
2. glycosuria
3. hyperuricemia
4. muscle spasm
5. weakness
6. restlessness

Whenever adverse reactions are moderate or severe, thiazide dosage should be reduced or therapy withdrawn.

DOSAGE AND ADMINISTRATION

Therapy should be individualized according to patient response. This therapy should be titrated to gain maximal therapeutic response as well as the minimal dose possible to maintain that therapeutic response. The usual dose of Renese tablets for diuretic therapy is 1 to 4 mg daily, and for antihypertensive therapy is 2 to 4 mg daily.

HOW SUPPLIED

RENESE® (polythiazide) Tablets are available as:
1 mg white, scored tablets in bottles of 100 (NDC 0069-3750-66).
2 mg yellow, scored tablets in bottles of 100 (NDC 0069-3760-66).
4 mg white, scored tablets in bottles of 100 (NDC 0069-3770-66).

Pfizer Labs
Division of Pfizer Inc, NY, NY 10017
69-1116-00-6 Revised April 1997

SINEQUAN® ℞

[sin 'a-kwon]
(doxepin HCl)
Capsules
Oral Concentrate

DESCRIPTION

SINEQUAN® (doxepin hydrochloride) is one of a class of psychotherapeutic agents known as dibenzoxepin tricyclic compounds. The molecular formula of the compound is $C_{19}H_{21}NO{\cdot}HCl$ having a molecular weight of 316. It is a white crystalline solid readily soluble in water, lower alcohols and chloroform.
Inert ingredients for the capsule formulations are: hard gelatin capsules (which may contain Blue 1, Red 3, Red 40, Yellow 10, and other inert ingredients); magnesium stearate; sodium lauryl sulfate; starch.
Inert ingredients for the oral concentrate formulation are: glycerin; methylparaben; peppermint oil; propylparaben; water.

CHEMISTRY

SINEQUAN (doxepin HCl) is a dibenzoxepin derivative and is the first of a family of tricyclic psychotherapeutic agents. Specifically, it is an isomeric mixture of: 1-Propanamine, 3-dibenz[*b,e*]oxepin-11(6*H*)ylidene-*N,N*-dimethyl-, hydrochloride.

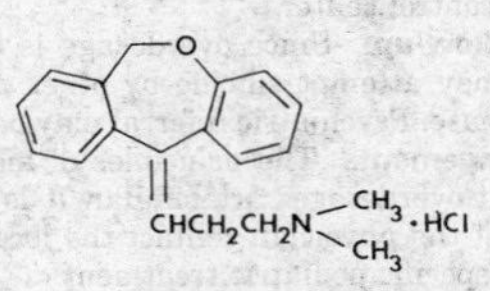

SINEQUAN (doxepin HCl)

ACTIONS

The mechanism of action of SINEQUAN (doxepin HCl) is not definitely known. It is not a central nervous system stimulant nor a monoamine oxidase inhibitor. The current hypothesis is that the clinical effects are due, at least in part, to influences on the adrenergic activity at the synapses so that deactivation of norepinephrine by reuptake into the nerve terminals is prevented. Animal studies suggest that doxepin HCl does not appreciably antagonize the antihypertensive action of guanethidine. In animal studies anticholinergic, antiserotonin and antihistamine effects on smooth muscle have been demonstrated. At higher than usual clinical doses, norepinephrine response was potentiated in animals. This effect was not demonstrated in humans.
At clinical dosages up to 150 mg per day, SINEQUAN can be given to man concomitantly with guanethidine and related compounds without blocking the antihypertensive effect. At dosages above 150 mg per day blocking of the antihypertensive effect of these compounds has been reported.
SINEQUAN is virtually devoid of euphoria as a side effect. Characteristic of this type of compound, SINEQUAN has not been demonstrated to produce the physical tolerance or psychological dependence associated with addictive compounds.

INDICATIONS

SINEQUAN is recommended for the treatment of:
1. Psychoneurotic patients with depression and/or anxiety.
2. Depression and/or anxiety associated with alcoholism (not to be taken concomitantly with alcohol).
3. Depression and/or anxiety associated with organic disease (the possibility of drug interaction should be considered if the patient is receiving other drugs concomitantly).
4. Psychotic depressive disorders with associated anxiety including involutional depression and manic-depressive disorders.

The target symptoms of psychoneurosis that respond particularly well to SINEQUAN include anxiety, tension, depression, somatic symptoms and concerns, sleep disturbances, guilt, lack of energy, fear, apprehension and worry.
Clinical experience has shown that SINEQUAN is safe and well tolerated even in the elderly patient. Owing to lack of clinical experience in the pediatric population, SINEQUAN is not recommended for use in children under 12 years of age.

CONTRAINDICATIONS

SINEQUAN is contraindicated in individuals who have shown hypersensitivity to the drug. Possibility of cross sensitivity with other dibenzoxepines should be kept in mind.
SINEQUAN is contraindicated in patients with glaucoma or a tendency to urinary retention. These disorders should be ruled out, particularly in older patients.

WARNINGS

The once-a-day dosage regimen of SINEQUAN in patients with intercurrent illness or patients taking other medications should be carefully adjusted. This is especially important in patients receiving other medications with anticholinergic effects.
Usage in Geriatrics: The use of SINEQUAN on a once-a-day dosage regimen in geriatric patients should be adjusted carefully based on the patient's condition.
Usage in Pregnancy: Reproduction studies have been performed in rats, rabbits, monkeys and dogs and there was no evidence of harm to the animal fetus. The relevance to humans is not known. Since there is no experience in pregnant women who have received this drug, safety in pregnancy has not been established. There has been a report of apnea and drowsiness occurring in a nursing infant whose mother was taking SINEQUAN.
Usage in Children: The use of SINEQUAN in children under 12 years of age is not recommended because safe conditions for its use have not been established.

PRECAUTIONS

Drug Interactions: *Drugs Metabolized by P450 2D6:* The biochemical activity of the drug metabolizing isozyme cytochrome P450 2D6 (debrisoquin hydroxylase) is reduced in a subset of the Caucasian population (about 7–10% of Caucasians are so-called "poor metabolizers"); reliable estimates of the prevalence of reduced P450 2D6 isozyme activity among Asian, African and other populations are not yet available. Poor metabolizers have higher than expected plasma concentrations of tricyclic antidepressants (TCAs) when given usual doses. Depending on the fraction of drug metabolized by P450 2D6, the increase in plasma concentration may be small, or quite large (8-fold increase in plasma AUC of the TCA).
In addition, certain drugs inhibit the activity of this isozyme and make normal metabolizers resemble poor metabolizers. An individual who is stable on a given dose of TCA may become abruptly toxic when given one of these inhibiting drugs as concomitant therapy. The drugs that inhibit cytochrome P450 2D6 include some that are not metabolized by the enzyme (quinidine; cimetidine) and many that are substrates for P450 2D6 (many other antidepressants, phenothiazines, and the Type 1C antiarrythmics propafenone and flecainide). While all the selective serotonin reuptake inhibitors (SSRIs), e.g., fluoxetine, sertraline, and paroxetine, inhibit P450 2D6, they may vary in the extent of inhibition. The extent to which SSRI-TCA interactions may pose clinical problems will depend on the degree of inhibition and the pharmacokinetics of the SSRI involved. Nevertheless, caution is indicated in the co-administration of TCAs with any of the SSRIs and also in switching from one class to the other. Of particular importance, sufficient time must elapse before initiating TCA treatment in a patient being withdrawn from fluoxetine, given the long half-life of the parent and active metabolite (at least 5 weeks may be necessary).
Concomitant use of tricyclic antidepressants with drugs that can inhibit cytochrome P450 2D6 may require lower doses than usually prescribed for either the tricyclic antidepressant or the other drug. Furthermore, whenever one of these other drugs is withdrawn from co-therapy, an increased dose of tricyclic antidepressant may be required. It is desirable to monitor TCA plasma levels whenever a TCA is going to be coadministered with another drug known to be an inhibitor of P450 2D6.
MAO Inhibitors: Serious side effects and even death have been reported following the concomitant use of certain drugs with MAO inhibitors. Therefore, MAO inhibitors should be discontinued at least two weeks prior to the cautious initiation of therapy with SINEQUAN. The exact length of time may vary and is dependent upon the particular MAO inhibitor being used, the length of time it has been administered, and the dosage involved.
Cimetidine: Cimetidine has been reported to produce clinically significant fluctuations in steady-state serum concentrations of various tricyclic antidepressants. Serious anticholinergic symptoms (i.e., severe dry mouth, urinary retention and blurred vision) have been associated with elevations in the serum levels of tricyclic antidepressant when cimetidine therapy is initiated. Additionally, higher than expected tricyclic antidepressant levels have been observed when they are begun in patients already taking cimetidine. In patients who have been reported to be well controlled on tricyclic antidepressants receiving concurrent cimetidine therapy, discontinuation of cimetidine has been reported to decrease established steady-state serum tricyclic antidepressant levels and compromise their therapeutic effects.
Alcohol: It should be borne in mind that alcohol ingestion may increase the danger inherent in any intentional or unintentional SINEQUAN overdosage. This is especially important in patients who may use alcohol excessively.
Tolazamide: A case of severe hypoglycemia has been reported in a type II diabetic patient maintained on tolazamide (1 gm/day) 11 days after the addition of doxepin (75 mg/day).
Drowsiness: Since drowsiness may occur with the use of this drug, patients should be warned of the possibility and cautioned against driving a car or operating dangerous machinery while taking the drug. Patients should also be cautioned that their response to alcohol may be potentiated.
Suicide: Since suicide is an inherent risk in any depressed patient and may remain so until significant improvement has occurred, patients should be closely supervised during the early course of therapy. Prescriptions should be written for the smallest feasible amount.
Psychosis: Should increased symptoms of psychosis or shift to manic symptomatology occur, it may be necessary to reduce dosage or add a major tranquilizer to the dosage regimen.

ADVERSE REACTIONS

NOTE: Some of the adverse reactions noted below have not been specifically reported with SINEQUAN use. However, due to the close pharmacological similarities among the tricyclics, the reactions should be considered when prescribing SINEQUAN (doxepin HCl).
Anticholinergic Effects: Dry mouth, blurred vision, constipation, and urinary retention have been reported. If they do not subside with continued therapy, or become severe, it may be necessary to reduce the dosage.
Central Nervous System Effects: Drowsiness is the most commonly noticed side effect. This tends to disappear as therapy is continued. Other infrequently reported CNS side effects are confusion, disorientation, hallucinations, numbness, paresthesias, ataxia, extrapyramidal symptoms, seizures, tardive dyskinesia, and tremor.

Continued on next page

Sinequan—Cont.

Cardiovascular: Cardiovascular effects including hypotension, hypertension, and tachycardia have been reported occasionally.
Allergic: Skin rash, edema, photosensitization, and pruritus have occasionally occurred.
Hematologic: Eosinophilia has been reported in a few patients. There have been occasional reports of bone marrow depression manifesting as agranulocytosis, leukopenia, thrombocytopenia, and purpura.
Gastrointestinal: Nausea, vomiting, indigestion, taste disturbances, diarrhea, anorexia, and aphthous stomatitis have been reported. (See Anticholinergic Effects.)
Endocrine: Raised or lowered libido, testicular swelling, gynecomastia in males, enlargement of breasts and galactorrhea in the female, raising or lowering of blood sugar levels, and syndrome of inappropriate antidiuretic hormone secretion have been reported with tricyclic administration.
Other: Dizziness, tinnitus, weight gain, sweating, chills, fatigue, weakness, flushing, jaundice, alopecia, headache, exacerbation of asthma, and hyperpyrexia (in association with chlorpromazine) have been occasionally observed as adverse effects.
Withdrawal Symptoms: The possibility of development of withdrawal symptoms upon abrupt cessation of treatment after prolonged SINEQUAN administration should be borne in mind. These are not indicative of addiction and gradual withdrawal of medication should not cause these symptoms.

DOSAGE AND ADMINISTRATION

For most patients with illness of mild to moderate severity, a starting daily dose of 75 mg is recommended. Dosage may subsequently be increased or decreased at appropriate intervals and according to individual response. The usual optimum dose range is 75 mg/day to 150 mg/day.
In more severely ill patients higher doses may be required with subsequent gradual increase to 300 mg/day if necessary. Additional therapeutic effect is rarely to be obtained by exceeding a dose of 300 mg/day.
In patients with very mild symptomatology or emotional symptoms accompanying organic disease, lower doses may suffice. Some of these patients have been controlled on doses as low as 25-50 mg/day.
The total daily dosage of SINEQUAN may be given on a divided or once-a-day dosage schedule. If the once-a-day schedule is employed, the maximum recommended dose is 150 mg/day. This dose may be given at bedtime. **The 150 mg capsule strength is intended for maintenance therapy only and is not recommended for initiation of treatment.**
Anti-anxiety effect is apparent before the antidepressant effect. Optimal antidepressant effect may not be evident for two to three weeks.

OVERDOSAGE

Deaths may occur from overdosage with this class of drugs. Multiple drug ingestion (including alcohol) is common in deliberate tricyclic antidepressant overdose. As the management is complex and changing, it is recommended that the physician contact a poison control center for current information on treatment. Signs and symptoms of toxicity develop rapidly after tricyclic antidepressant overdose; therefore, hospital monitoring is required as soon as possible.
Manifestations: Critical manifestations of overdose include: cardiac dysrhythmias, severe hypotension, convulsions, and CNS depression, including coma. Changes in the electrocardiogram, particularly in QRS axis or width, are clinically significant indicators of tricyclic antidepressant toxicity.
Other signs of overdose may include: confusion, disturbed concentration, transient visual hallucinations, dilated pupils, agitation, hyperactive reflexes, stupor, drowsiness, muscle rigidity, vomiting, hypothermia, hyperpyrexia, or any of the symptoms listed under ADVERSE REACTIONS.
General Recommendations:
General: Obtain an ECG and immediately initiate cardiac monitoring. Protect the patient's airway, establish an intravenous line and initiate gastric decontamination. A minimum of six hours of observation with cardiac monitoring and observation for signs of CNS or respiratory depression, hypotension, cardiac dysrhythmias and/or conduction blocks, and seizures is strongly advised. If signs of toxicity occur at any time during this period, extended monitoring is recommended. There are case reports of patients succumbing to fatal dysrhythmias late after overdose; these patients had clinical evidence of significant poisoning prior to death and most received inadequate gastrointestinal decontamination. Monitoring of plasma drug levels should not guide management of the patient.
Gastrointestinal Decontamination: All patients suspected of tricyclic antidepressant overdose should receive gastrointestinal decontamination. This should include large volume gastric lavage followed by activated charcoal. If consciousness is impaired, the airway should be secured prior to lavage. Emesis is contraindicated.
Cardiovascular: A maximal limb-lead QRS duration of ≥0.10 seconds may be the best indication of the severity of the overdose. Intravenous sodium bicarbonate should be used to maintain the serum pH in the range of 7.45 to 7.55. If the pH response is inadequate, hyperventilation may also be used. Concomitant use of hyperventilation and sodium bicarbonate should be done with extreme caution, with frequent pH monitoring. A pH >7.60 or a pCO_2 <20 mm Hg is undesirable. Dysrhythmias unresponsive to sodium bicarbonate therapy/hyperventilation may respond to lidocaine, bretylium or phenytoin. Type 1A and 1C antiarrhythmics are generally contraindicated (e.g., quinidine, disopyramide, and procainamide).
In rare instances, hemoperfusion may be beneficial in acute refractory cardiovascular instability in patients with acute toxicity. However, hemodialysis, peritoneal dialysis, exchange tranfusions, and forced diuresis generally have been reported as ineffective in tricyclic antidepressant poisoning.
CNS: In patients with CNS depression, early intubation is advised because of the potential for abrupt deterioration. Seizures should be controlled with benzodiazepines, or if these are ineffective, other anticonvulsants (e.g., phenobarbital, phenytoin). Physostigmine is not recommended except to treat life-threatening symptoms that have been unresponsive to other therapies, and then only in consultation with a poison control center.
Psychiatric Follow-up: Since overdosage is often deliberate, patients may attempt suicide by other means during the recovery phase. Psychiatric referral may be appropriate.
Pediatric Management: The principles of management of child and adult overdosages are similar. It is strongly recommended that the physician contact the local poison control center for specific pediatric treatment.

HOW SUPPLIED

SINEQUAN® is available as capsules containing doxepin HCl equivalent to:
10 mg—100's (NDC 0049-5340-66) (NDC 0662-5340-66),
1000's (NDC 0049-5340-82) (NDC 0662-5340-82)
25 mg—100's (NDC 0049-5350-66) (NDC 0662-5350-66),
1000's (NDC 0049-5350-82) (NDC 0662-5350-82),
5000's (NDC 0049-5350-94) (NDC 0662-5350-94)
50 mg—100's (NDC 0049-5360-66) (NDC 0662-5360-66),
1000's (NDC 0049-5360-82) (NDC 0662-5360-82),
5000's (NDC 0049-5360-94) (NDC 0662-5360-94)
75 mg—100's (NDC 0049-5390-66) (NDC 0662-5390-66),
1000's (NDC 0049-5390-82) (NDC 0662-5390-82)
100 mg—100's (NDC 0049-5380-66) (NDC 0662-5380-66),
1000's (NDC 0049-5380-82) (NDC 0662-5380-82)
150 mg—50's (NDC 0049-5370-50) (NDC 0662-5370-50),
500's (NDC 0049-5370-73) (NDC 0062-5370-73)
SINEQUAN® Oral Concentrate is available in 120 mL bottles (NDC 0049-5100-47) (NDC 0662-5100-47) with an accompanying dropper calibrated at 5 mg, 10 mg, 15 mg, 20 mg, and 25 mg. Each mL contains doxepin HCl equivalent to 10 mg doxepin. Just prior to administration, SINEQUAN® Oral Concentrate should be diluted with approximately 120 mL of water, whole or skimmed milk, or orange, grapefruit, tomato, prune or pineapple juice. SINEQUAN® Oral Concentrate is not physically compatible with a number of carbonated beverages. For those patients requiring antidepressant therapy who are on methadone maintenance, SINEQUAN® Oral Concentrate and methadone syrup can be mixed together with Gatorade®, lemonade, orange juice, sugar water, Tang®, or water; but not with grape juice. Preparation and storage of bulk dilutions is not recommended.

69-2135-00-0 Revised May 1996
Shown in Product Identification Guide, page 330

STREPTOMYCIN SULFATE Injection, USP ℞

1 g/2.5 mL Ampules
For Intramuscular Use Only

WARNING
THE RISK OF SEVERE NEUROTOXIC REACTIONS IS SHARPLY INCREASED IN PATIENTS WITH IMPAIRED RENAL FUNCTION OR PRE-RENAL AZOTEMIA. THESE INCLUDE DISTURBANCES OF VESTIBULAR AND COCHLEAR FUNCTION. OPTIC NERVE DYSFUNCTION, PERIPHERAL NEURITIS, ARACHNOIDITIS, AND ENCEPHALOPATHY MAY ALSO OCCUR. THE INCIDENCE OF CLINICALLY DETECTABLE, IRREVERSIBLE VESTIBULAR DAMAGE IS PARTICULARLY HIGH IN PATIENTS TREATED WITH STREPTOMYCIN.
RENAL FUNCTION SHOULD BE MONITORED CAREFULLY; PATIENTS WITH RENAL IMPAIRMENT AND/OR NITROGEN RETENTION SHOULD RECEIVE REDUCED DOSAGES. THE PEAK SERUM CONCENTRATION IN INDIVIDUALS WITH KIDNEY DAMAGE SHOULD NOT EXCEED 20 TO 25 MCG/ML.
THE CONCURRENT OR SEQUENTIAL USE OF OTHER NEUROTOXIC AND/OR NEPHROTOXIC DRUGS WITH STREPTOMYCIN SULFATE, INCLUDING NEOMYCIN, KANAMYCIN, GENTAMICIN, CEPHALORIDINE, PAROMOMYCIN, VIOMYCIN, POLYMYXIN B, COLISTIN, TOBRAMYCIN AND CYCLOSPORINE SHOULD BE AVOIDED.
THE NEUROTOXICITY OF STREPTOMYCIN CAN RESULT IN RESPIRATORY PARALYSIS FROM NEUROMUSCULAR BLOCKAGE, ESPECIALLY WHEN THE DRUG IS GIVEN SOON AFTER THE USE OF ANESTHESIA OR OF MUSCLE RELAXANTS.
THE ADMINISTRATION OF STREPTOMYCIN IN PARENTERAL FORM SHOULD BE RESERVED FOR PATIENTS WHERE ADEQUATE LABORATORY AND AUDIOMETRIC TESTING FACILITIES ARE AVAILABLE DURING THERAPY.

DESCRIPTION

Streptomycin is a water-soluble aminoglycoside derived from *Streptomyces griseus*. It is marketed as the sulfate salt of streptomycin. The chemical name of streptomycin sulfate is D-Streptamine, *O*-2-deoxy-2-(methylamino)-α-L-glucopyranosyl-(1→2)-*O*-5-deoxy-3-*C*-formyl-α-L-lyxofuranosyl-(1→4)-*N,N*′-bis(aminoiminomethyl)-, sulfate (2:3) (salt). The empirical formula for Streptomycin Sulfate is $(C_{21}H_{39}N_7O_{12})_2 \cdot 3H_2SO_4$ and the molecular weight is 1457.38. It has the following structure:

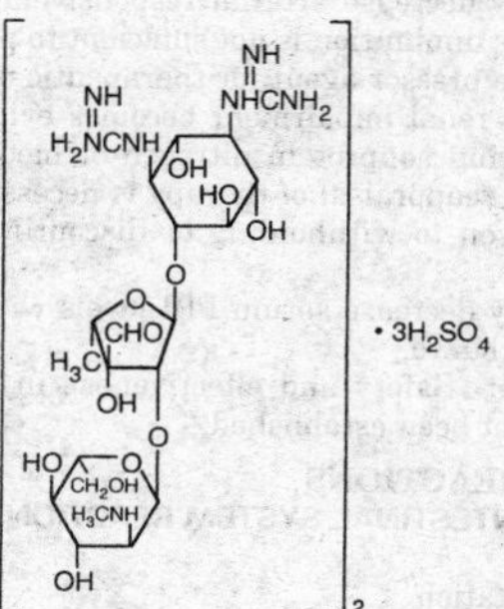

Streptomycin Sulfate Injection, 1 g/2.5 mL (400 mg/mL), is supplied as a sterile, nonpyrogenic solution for intramuscular use.
Each mL contains: Streptomycin sulfate equivalent to 400 mg of streptomycin, sodium citrate dihydrate 12 mg, phenol 0.25% w/v as preservative, sodium metabisulfite 2 mg in Water for Injection. pH range 5.0 to 8.0.

CLINICAL PHARMACOLOGY

Following intramuscular injection of 1 g of streptomycin, as the sulfate, a peak serum level of 25 to 50 mcg/mL is reached within 1 hour, diminishing slowly to about 50 percent after 5 to 6 hours.
Appreciable concentrations are found in all organ tissues except the brain. Significant amounts have been found in pleural fluid and tuberculous cavities. Streptomycin passes through the placenta with serum levels in the cord blood similar to maternal levels. Small amounts are excreted in milk, saliva, and sweat.
Streptomycin is excreted by glomerular filtration. In patients with normal kidney function, between 29% and 89% of a single 600 mg dose is excreted in the urine within 24 hours. Any reduction of glomerular function results in decreased excretion of the drug and concurrent rise in serum and tissue levels.

Microbiology
Streptomycin sulfate is a bactericidal antibiotic. It acts by interfering with normal protein synthesis.
Streptomycin has been shown to be active against most strains of the following organisms both *in vitro* and in clinical infection. (See INDICATIONS AND USAGE.):
Brucella (brucellosis),
Calymmatobacterium granulomatis (donovanosis, granuloma inguinale),
Escherichia coli, Proteus spp., Aerobacter aerogenes, Klebsiella pneumoniae, and *Enterococcus faecalis* in urinary tract infections,
Francisella tularensis,
Haemophilus ducreyi (chancroid),
Haemophilus influenzae (in respiratory, endocardial, and meningeal infections—concomitantly with another antibacterial agent),
Klebsiella pneumoniae pneumonia (concomitantly with another antibacterial agent),
Mycobacterium tuberculosis,
Pasteurella pestis
Streptococcus viridans, *Enterococcus faecalis* (in endocardial infections—concomitantly with penicillin).
SUSCEPTIBILITY TESTS: Diffusion Techniques
Quantitative methods that require measurement of zone diameters give the most precise estimate of the susceptibility of bacteria to antimicrobial agents. One such standard procedure[1] which has been recommended for use with disks to test susceptibility of organisms to streptomycin uses the 10 mcg streptomycin disk. Interpretation involves the correlation of the diameter obtained in the disk test with the minimum inhibitory concentration (MIC) for streptomycin.
Reports from the laboratory giving results of the standard single disk susceptibility test with a 10 mcg streptomycin disk should be interpreted according to the following criteria:

Zone Diameter (mm)	Interpretation
≥15	(S) Susceptible
11–12	(I) Intermediate
≤10	(R) Resistant

A report of "Susceptible" indicates that the pathogen is likely to respond to monotherapy with streptomycin. A report of "Intermediate" indicates that the result be considered equivocal, and, if the organism is not fully susceptible

to alternative clinically feasible drugs, the test should be repeated. This category provides a buffer zone which prevents small uncontrolled technical factors from causing major discrepancies in interpretations. A report of "Resistant" indicates that achievable drug concentrations are unlikely to be inhibitory and other therapy should be selected.
Standardized procedures require the use of laboratory control organisms. The 10 mcg streptomycin disk should give the following zone diameter:

Organism	Zone diameter (mm)
E. coli ATCC 25922	12–20
S. aureus ATCC 25923	14–22

Methods Section:
Two standardized *in vitro* susceptibility methods are available for testing streptomycin against *Mycobacterium tuberculosis* organisms. The agar proportion method (CDC or NCCLS M24–P) utilizes middlebrook 7H10 medium impregnated with streptomycin at two final concentrations, 2.0 and 10.0 mcg/mL. MIC_{90} values are calculated by comparing the quantity of organisms growing in the medium containing drug to the control cultures. Mycobacterial growth in the presence of drug ≥ 1% of the control indicates resistance.
The radiometric broth method employs the BACTEC 460 machine to compare the growth index from untreated control cultures to cultures grown in the presence of 6.0 mcg/mL of streptomycin. Strict adherence to the manufacturer's instructions for sample processing and data interpretation is required for this assay.
Susceptibility test results obtained by these two different methods cannot be compared unless equivalent drug concentrations are evaluated.
The clinical relevance of *in vitro* susceptibility test results for mycobacterial species other than *M. tuberculosis* using either the BACTEC or the proportion method has not been determined.

INDICATIONS AND USAGE

Streptomycin is indicated for the treatment of individuals with moderate to severe infections caused by susceptible strains of microorganisms in the specific conditions listed below:

1. Mycobacterium tuberculosis: The Advisory Council for the Elimination of Tuberculosis, the American Thoracic Society, and the Center for Disease Control recommend that either streptomycin or ethambutol be added as a fourth drug in a regimen containing isoniazid (INH), rifampin and pyrazinamide for initial treatment of tuberculosis unless the likelihood of INH or rifampin resistance is very low. The need for a fourth drug should be reassessed when the results of susceptibility testing are known. In the past when the national rate of primary drug resistance to isoniazid was known to be less than 4% and was either stable or declining, therapy with two and three drug regimens was considered adequate. If community rates of INH resistance are currently less than 4%, an initial treatment regimen with less than four drugs may be considered.

Streptomycin is also indicated for therapy of tuberculosis when one or more of the above drugs is contraindicated because of toxicity or intolerance. The management of tuberculosis has become more complex as a consequence of increasing rates of drug resistance and concomitant HIV infection. Additional consultation from experts in the treatment of tuberculosis may be desirable in those settings.

2. Non-tuberculosis infections: The use of streptomycin should be limited to the treatment of infections caused by bacteria which have been shown to be susceptible to the antibacterial effects of streptomycin and which are not amenable to therapy with less potentially toxic agents.

a. *Pasteurella pestis* (plague),
b. *Francisella tularensis* (tularemia),
c. *Brucella,*
d. *Calymmatobacterium granulomatis* (donovanosis, granuloma inguinale),
e. *H. ducreyi* (chancroid),
f. *H. influenzae* (in respiratory, endocardial, and meningeal infections—concomitantly with another antibacterial agent),
g. *K. pneumoniae* pneumonia (concomitantly with another antibacterial agent),
h. *E. coli, Proteus, A. aerogenes, K. pneumoniae,* and *Enterococcus faecalis* in urinary tract infections,
i. *Streptococcus* viridans, *Enterococcus faecalis* (in endocardial infections—concomitantly with penicillin),
j. Gram-negative bacillary bacteremia (concomitantly with another antibacterial agent).

CONTRAINDICATIONS

A history of clinically significant hypersensitivity to streptomycin is a contraindication to its use. Clinically significant hypersensitivity to other aminoglycosides may contraindicate the use of streptomycin because of the known cross-sensitivity of patients to drugs in this class.

WARNINGS

Ototoxicity: Both vestibular and auditory dysfunction can follow the administration of streptomycin. The degree of impairment is directly proportional to the dose and duration of streptomycin administration, to the age of the patient, to the level of renal function and to the amount of underlying existing auditory dysfunction. The ototoxic effects of the aminoglycosides, including streptomycin, are potentiated by the co-administration of ethacrynic acid, mannitol, furosemide and possibly other diuretics.
The vestibulotoxic potential of streptomycin exceeds that of its capacity for cochlear toxicity. Vestibular damage is heralded by headache, nausea, vomiting and disequilibrium. Early cochlear injury is demonstrated by the loss of high frequency hearing. Appropriate monitoring and early discontinuation of the drug may permit recovery prior to irreversible damage to the sensorineural cells.
Sulfites: Streptomycin contains sodium metabisulfite, a sulfite that may cause allergic type reactions including anaphylactic symptoms and life-threatening or less severe asthmatic episodes in certain susceptible people. The overall prevalence of sulfite sensitivity in the general population is unknown and probably low. Sulfite sensitivity is seen more frequently in asthmatic than in non-asthmatic people.
Pregnancy: Streptomycin can cause fetal harm when administered to a pregnant woman. Because streptomycin readily crosses the placental barrier, caution in use of the drug is important to prevent ototoxicity in the fetus. If this drug is used during pregnancy, or if the patient becomes pregnant while taking this drug, the patient should be apprised of the potential hazard to the fetus.

PRECAUTIONS

General: Baseline and periodic caloric stimulation tests and audiometric tests are advisable with extended streptomycin therapy. Tinnitus, roaring noises, or a sense of fullness in the ears indicates need for audiometric examination or termination of streptomycin therapy or both.
Care should be taken by individuals handling streptomycin for injection to avoid skin sensitivity reactions. As with all intramuscular preparations, Streptomycin Sulfate Injection should be injected well within the body of a relatively large muscle and care should be taken to minimize the possibility of damage to peripheral nerves. (See DOSAGE AND ADMINISTRATION.)
Extreme caution must be exercised in selecting a dosage regimen in the presence of pre-existing renal insuffiency. In severely uremic patients a single dose may produce high blood levels for several days and the cumulative effect may produce ototoxic sequelae. When streptomycin must be given for prolonged periods of time alkalinization of the urine may minimize or prevent renal irritation.
A syndrome of apparent central nervous system depression, characterized by stupor and flaccidity, occasionally coma and deep respiratory depression, has been reported in very young infants in whom streptomycin dosage had exceeded the recommended limits. Thus, infants should not receive streptomycin in excess of the recommended dosage.
In the treatment of venereal infections such as granuloma inguinale, and chancroid, if concomitant syphilis is suspected, suitable laboratory procedures such as a dark field examination should be performed before the start of treatment, and monthly serologic tests should be done for at least four months.
As with other antibiotics, use of this drug may result in overgrowth of nonsusceptible organisms, including fungi. If superinfection occurs, appropriate therapy should be instituted.
Drug Interactions: The ototoxic effects of the aminoglycosides, including streptomycin, are potentiated by the co-administration of ethacrynic acid, furosemide, mannitol and possibly other diuretics.
Pregnancy: Category D: See WARNINGS section.
Nursing Mothers: Because of the potential for serious adverse reactions in nursing infants from streptomycin, a decision should be made whether to discontinue nursing or to discontinue the drug, taking into account the importance of the drug to the mother.
Pediatric Use: (See DOSAGE AND ADMINISTRATION.)

ADVERSE REACTIONS

The following reactions are common: vestibular ototoxicity (nausea, vomiting, and vertigo); paresthesia of face; rash; fever; urticaria; angioneurotic edema; and eosinophilia.
The following reactions are less frequent: cochlear ototoxicity (deafness); exfoliative dermatitis; anaphylaxis; azotemia; leucopenia; thrombocytopenia, pancytopenia; hemolytic anemia; muscular weakness; and amblyopia.
Vestibular dysfunction resulting from the parenteral administration of streptomycin is cumulatively related to the total daily dose. When 1.8 to 2 g/day are given, symptoms are likely to develop in the large percentage of patients—especially in the elderly or patients with impaired renal function—within four weeks. Therefore, it is recommended that caloric and audiometric tests be done prior to, during, and following intensive therapy with streptomycin in order to facilitate detection of any vestibular dysfunction and/or impairment of hearing which may occur.
Vestibular symptoms generally appear early and usually are reversible with early detection and cessation of streptomycin administration. Two to three months after stopping the drug, gross vestibular symptoms usually disappear, except for the relative inability to walk in total darkness or on very rough terrain.
Although streptomycin is the least nephrotoxic of the aminoglycosides, nephrotoxicity does occur rarely.
Clinical judgment as to termination of therapy must be exercised when side effects occur.

DOSAGE AND ADMINISTRATION

Intramuscular Route Only
Adults: The preferred site is the upper outer quadrant of the buttock, (*i.e.,* gluteus maximus), or the mid-lateral thigh.
Children: It is recommended that intramuscular injections be given preferably in the mid-lateral muscles of the thigh. In infants and small children the periphery of the upper outer quadrant of the gluteal region should be used only when necessary, such as in burn patients, in order to minimize the possibility of damage to the sciatic nerve.
The deltoid area should be used only if well developed such as in certain adults and older children, and then only with caution to avoid radial nerve injury. Intramuscular injections should not be made into the lower and mid-third of the upper arm. As with all intramuscular injections, aspiration is necessary to help avoid inadvertent injection into a blood vessel.
Injection sites should be alternated. As higher doses or more prolonged therapy with streptomycin may be indicated for more severe or fulminating infections (endocarditis, meningitis, etc.), the physician should always take adequate measures to be immediately aware of any toxic signs or symptoms occurring in the patient as a result of streptomycin therapy.

1. TUBERCULOSIS: The standard regimen for the treatment of drug susceptible tuberculosis has been two months of INH, rifampin and pyrazinamide followed by four months of INH and rifampin (patients with concomitant infection with tuberculosis and HIV may require treatment for a longer period). When streptomycin is added to this regimen because of suspected or proven drug resistance (see **INDICATIONS AND USAGE** section), the recommended dosing for streptomycin is as follows:

	Daily	*Twice Weekly*	*Thrice Weekly*
Children	20–40 mg/kg	25–30 mg/kg	25–30 mg/kg
	Max 1 g	Max 1.5 g	Max 1.5 g
Adults	15 mg/kg	25–30 mg/kg	25–30 mg/kg
	Max 1 g	Max 1.5 g	Max 1.5 g

Streptomycin is usually administered daily as a single intramuscular injection. A total dose of not more than 120 g over the course of therapy should be given unless there are no other therapeutic options. In patients older than 60 years of age the drug should be used at a reduced dosage due to the risk of increased toxicity. (See **BOXED WARNING**).
Therapy with streptomycin may be terminated when toxic symptoms have appeared, when impending toxicity is feared, when organisms become resistant, or when full treatment effect has been obtained. The total period of drug treatment of tuberculosis is a minimum of 1 year; however, indications for terminating therapy with streptomycin may occur at any time as noted above.

2. TULAREMIA: One to 2 g daily in divided doses for 7 to 14 days until the patient is afebrile for 5 to 7 days.
3. PLAGUE: Two grams of streptomycin daily in two divided doses should be administered intramuscularly. A minimum of 10 days of therapy is recommended.
4. BACTERIAL ENDOCARDITIS:
   a. *Streptococcal endocarditis:* In penicillin-sensitive alpha and non-hemolytic streptococcal endocarditis (penicillin MIC≤0.1 mcg/mL), streptomycin may be used for 2-week treatment concomitantly with penicillin. The streptomycin regimen is 1 g b.i.d. for the first week, and 500 mg b.i.d. for the second week. If the patient is over 60 years of age, the dosage should be 500 mg b.i.d. for the entire 2-week period.
   b. *Enterococcal endocarditis:* Streptomycin in doses of 1 g b.i.d. for 2 weeks and 500 mg b.i.d. for an additional 4 weeks is given in combination with penicillin. Ototoxicity may require termination of the streptomycin prior to completion of the 6-week course of treatment.
5. CONCOMITANT USE WITH OTHER AGENTS: For concomitant use with other agents to which the infecting organism is also sensitive: Streptomycin is considered a second-line agent for the treatment of gram-negative bacillary bacteremia, meningitis, and pneumonia; brucellosis; granuloma inguinale; chancroid, and urinary tract infection.

For adults: 1 to 2 grams in divided doses every six to twelve hours for moderate to severe infections. Doses should generally not exceed 2 grams per day.
For children: 20 to 40 mg/kg/day (8 to 20 mg/lb/day) in divided doses every 6 to 12 hours. (Particular care should be taken to avoid excessive dosage in children.)
Parenteral drug products should be inspected visually for particulate matter and discoloration prior to administration, whenever solution and container permit.

HOW SUPPLIED

Streptomycin Sulfate Injection, USP is supplied in packages of 10 ampules (NDC 0049-0620-33). Each ampule contains streptomycin sulfate equivalent to 1 g of streptomycin in 2.5 mL.
Store under refrigeration at 36° to 46°F (2° to 8°C).

REFERENCES

[1] National Committee for Clinical Laboratory Standards. Performance Standards for Antimicrobial Disk Susceptibility Tests—Fourth Edition. Approved Standard NCCLS Document M2-A4. Vol. 10, No. 7. NCCLS, Villanova, PA 1990.

70-4895-00-0 Issued April 1993

Continued on next page

TAO® ℞
[tā 'ō]
(troleandomycin)
Capsules

DESCRIPTION

TAO (troleandomycin) is a synthetically derived acetylated ester of oleandomycin, an antibiotic elaborated by a species of *Streptomyces antibioticus*. It is a white crystalline compound, insoluble in water, but readily soluble and stable in the presence of gastric juice. The compound has a molecular weight of 814 and corresponds to the empirical formula $C_{41}H_{67}NO_{15}$.
Inert ingredients in the formulation are: hard gelatin capsules (which may contain inert ingredients); lactose; magnesium stearate; sodium lauryl sulfate; starch.

ACTIONS

TAO is an antibiotic shown to be active *in vitro* against the following gram-positive organisms:
Streptococcus pyogenes
Diplococcus pneumoniae
Susceptibility plate testing: If the Kirby-Bauer method of disc sensitivity is used, a 15 mcg. oleandomycin disc should give a zone of over 18 mm when tested against a troleandomycin sensitive bacterial strain.

INDICATIONS

Diplococcus pneumoniae
Pneumococcal pneumonia due to susceptible strains.
Streptococcus pyogenes
Group A beta-hemolytic streptococcal infections of the upper respiratory tract.
Injectable benzathine penicillin G is considered by the American Heart Association to be the drug of choice in the treatment and prevention of streptococcal pharyngitis and in long term prophylaxis of rheumatic fever.
Troleandomycin is generally effective in the eradication of streptococci from the nasopharynx. However, substantial data establishing the efficacy of TAO in the subsequent prevention of rheumatic fever are not available at present.

CONTRAINDICATIONS

Troleandomycin is contraindicated in patients with known hypersensitivity to this antibiotic.

WARNINGS

Usage in Pregnancy: Safety for use in pregnancy has not been established.
The administration of troleandomycin has been associated with an allergic type of cholestatic hepatitis. Some patients receiving troleandomycin for more than two weeks or in repeated courses have shown jaundice accompanied by right upper quadrant pain, fever, nausea, vomiting, eosinophilia, and leukocytosis. These changes have been reversible on discontinuance of the drug. Liver function tests should be monitored in patients on such dosage, and the drug discontinued if abnormalities develop. Reports in the literature have suggested that the concurrent use of ergotamine-containing drugs and troleandomycin may induce ischemic reactions. Therefore, the concurrent use of ergotamine-containing drugs and troleandomycin should be avoided. Troleandomycin should be administered with caution to patients concurrently receiving estrogen containing oral contraceptives.
Studies in chronic asthmatic patients have suggested that the concurrent use of theophylline and troleandomycin may result in elevated serum concentrations of theophylline. Therefore, it is recommended that patients receiving such concurrent therapy be observed for signs of theophylline toxicity, and that therapy be appropriately modified if such signs develop.

PRECAUTIONS

Troleandomycin is principally excreted by the liver.
Caution should be exercised in administering the antibiotic to patients with impaired hepatic function.

ADVERSE REACTIONS

The most frequent side effects of troleandomycin preparations are gastrointestinal, such as abdominal cramping and discomfort, and are dose related. Nausea, vomiting, and diarrhea occur infrequently with usual oral doses.
During prolonged or repeated therapy, there is a possibility of overgrowth of nonsusceptible bacteria or fungi. If such infections occur, the drug should be discontinued and appropriate therapy instituted.
Mild allergic reactions such as urticaria and other skin rashes have occurred. Serious allergic reactions, including anaphylaxis, have been reported.

DOSAGE AND ADMINISTRATION

Clinical judgment based on the type of infection and its severity should determine dosage within the below listed ranges.
Adults: 250 to 500 mg 4 times a day
Children: 125 to 250 mg (3-5 mg/lb or 6.6 to 11 mg/kg) every 6 hours
When used in streptococcal infection, therapy should be continued for ten days.

HOW SUPPLIED

TAO is supplied as:
Capsules 250 mg: Each capsule contains troleandomycin equivalent to 250 mg of oleandomycin; bottles of 100 (NDC 0049-1590-66).
Revised July 1995 69-1800-00-8

TERRA-CORTRIL® ℞
Terramycin ® (oxytetracycline HCl)
—Cortril® (hydrocortisone acetate)
OPHTHALMIC SUSPENSION

DESCRIPTION

Terra-Cortril suspension combines the antibiotic, oxytetracycline HCl ($C_{22}H_{24}N_2O_9{\cdot}HCl$) and the adrenocorticoid, hydrocortisone acetate ($C_{23}H_{32}O_6$). **Each ml of Terra-Cortril contains Terramycin (oxytetracycline HCl) equivalent to 5 mg of oxytetracycline, and 15 mg of Cortril (hydrocortisone acetate) incorporated in mineral oil with aluminum tristearate.**

For Ophthalmic Use Only.

CLINICAL PHARMACOLOGY

Corticosteroids suppress the inflammatory response to a variety of agents and they probably delay or slow healing. Since corticoids may inhibit the body's defense mechanism against infection, a concomitant antimicrobial drug may be used when this inhibition is considered to be clinically significant in a particular case.
The anti-infective component in the combination is included to provide action against specific organisms susceptible to it.
Terramycin is considered active against the following microorganisms:
Rickettsiae (Rocky Mountain spotted fever, typhus fever and the typhus group, Q fever, rickettsialpox and tick fevers),
Mycoplasma pneumoniae (PPLO, Eaton Agent),
Agents of psittacosis and ornithosis,
Agents of lymphogranuloma venereum and granuloma inguinale,
The spirochetal agent of relapsing fever (*Borrelia recurrentis*).
The following gram-negative microorganisms:
Haemophilus ducreyi (chancroid),
Pasteurella pestis and *Pasteurella tularensis,*
Bartonella bacilliformis,
Bacteroides species,
Vibrio comma and *Vibrio fetus,*
Brucella species (in conjunction with streptomycin).
Because many strains of the following groups of microorganisms have been shown to be resistant to tetracyclines, culture and susceptibility testing are recommended.
Oxytetracycline is indicated for treatment of infections caused by the following gram-negative microorganisms, when bacteriologic testing indicates appropriate susceptibility to the drug:
Escherichia coli,
Enterobacter aerogenes (formerly *Aerobacter aerogenes*),
Shigella species,
Mima species and *Herellea* species,
Haemophilus influenzae (respiratory infections),
Klebsiella species (respiratory and urinary infections).
Oxytetracycline is indicated for treatment of infections caused by the following gram-positive microorganisms when bacteriologic testing indicates appropriate susceptibility to the drug:
Streptococcus species:
Up to 44 percent of strains of *Streptococcus pyogenes* and 74 percent of *Streptococcus faecalis* have been found to be resistant to tetracycline drugs. Therefore, tetracyclines should not be used for streptococcal disease unless the organism has been demonstrated to be sensitive.
For upper respiratory infections due to Group A beta-hemolytic streptococci, pencillin is the usual drug of choice, including prophylaxis of rheumatic fever.
Diplococcus pneumoniae,
Staphylococcus aureus, skin and soft tissue infections. Oxytetracycline is not the drug of choice in the treatment of any type of staphylococcal infections.
When penicillin is contraindicated, tetracyclines are alternative drugs in the treatment of infections due to:
Neisseria gonorrhoeae,
Treponema pallidum and *Treponema pertenue* (syphilis and yaws),
Listeria monocytogenes,
Clostridium species,
Bacillus anthracis,
Fusobacterium fusiforme (Vincent's infection),
Actinomyces species.
Tetracyclines are indicated in the treatment of trachoma, although the infectious agent is not always eliminated, as judged by immunofluorescence.
Inclusion conjunctivitis may be treated with oral tetracyclines or with a combination of oral and topical agents.
When a decision to administer both a corticoid and an antimicrobial is made, the administration of such drugs in combination has the advantage of greater patient compliance and convenience, with the added assurance that the appropriate dosage of both drugs is administered, plus assured compatibility of ingredients when both types of drug are in the same formulation and, particularly, that the correct volume of drug is delivered and retained.
The relative potency of corticosteroids depends on the molecular structure, concentration, and release from the vehicle.

INDICATIONS AND USAGE

For steroid-responsive inflammatory ocular conditions for which a corticosteroid is indicated and where bacterial infection or risk of bacterial ocular infection exists.
Ocular steroids are indicated in inflammatory conditions of the palpebral and bulbar conjunctiva, cornea, and anterior segment of the globe where the inherent risk of steroid use in certain infective conjunctivitides is accepted to obtain a diminution in edema and inflammation. They are also indicated in chronic anterior uveitis and corneal injury from chemical radiation, thermal burns, or penetration of foreign bodies.
The use of a combination drug with an anti-infective component is indicated where the risk of infection is high or where there is an expectation that potentially dangerous numbers of bacteria will be present in the eye.
The particular anti-infective drug in this product is active against the following common bacterial eye pathogens:
Staphylococcus aureus
Streptococci, including *Streptococcus pneumoniae*
Escherichia coli
Neisseria species
The product does not provide adequate coverage against:
Haemophilus influenzae
Klebsiella / Enterobacter species
Pseudomonas aeruginosa
Serratia marcescens

CONTRAINDICATIONS

Epithelial herpes simplex keratitis (dendritic keratitis), vaccinia, varicella, and many other viral diseases of the cornea and conjunctiva. Mycobacterial infection of the eye. Fungal diseases of ocular structures. Hypersensitivity to a component of the medication. (Hypersensitivity to the antibiotic component occurs at a higher rate than for other components.)
The use of these combinations is always contraindicated after uncomplicated removal of a corneal foreign body.

WARNINGS

Prolonged use may result in glaucoma, with damage to the optic nerve, defects in visual acuity and fields of vision, and posterior subcapsular cataract formation. Prolonged use may suppress the host response and thus increase the hazard of secondary ocular infections. In those diseases causing thinning of the cornea or sclera, perforations have been known to occur with the use of topical steroids. In acute purulent conditions of the eye, steroids may mask infection or enhance existing infection. If these products are used for 10 days or longer, intraocular pressure should be routinely monitored even though it may be difficult in children and uncooperative patients.
Employment of steroid medication in the treatment of herpes simplex requires great caution.

PRECAUTIONS

The initial prescription and renewal of the medication order beyond 20 milliliters should be made by a physician only after examination of the patient with the aid of magnification, such as slit lamp biomicroscopy and, where appropriate, fluorescein staining.
The possibility of persistent fungal infections of the cornea should be considered after prolonged steroid dosing.

ADVERSE REACTIONS

Adverse reactions have occurred with steroid/anti-infective combination drugs which can be attributed to the steroid component, the anti-infective component, or the combination. Exact incidence figures are not available since no denominator of treated patients is available.
Reactions occurring most often from the presence of the anti-infective ingredient are allergic sensitizations. The reactions due to the steroid component in decreasing order of frequency are: elevation of intraocular pressure (IOP) with possible development of glaucoma, and infrequent optic nerve damage; posterior subcapsular cataract formation; and delayed wound healing.
Secondary Infection: The development of secondary infection has occurred after use of combinations containing steroids and antimicrobials. Fungal infections of the cornea are particularly prone to develop coincidentally with long-term applications of steroid. The possibility of fungal invasion must be considered in any persistent corneal ulceration where steroid treatment has been used.
Secondary bacterial ocular infection following suppression of host responses also occurs.

DOSAGE AND ADMINISTRATION

Instill 1 or 2 drops of Terra-Cortril Ophthalmic Suspension into the affected eye three times daily.
Not more than 20 milliliters should be prescribed initially and the prescription should not be refilled without further evaluation as outlined in "Precautions" above.

HOW SUPPLIED

Terra-Cortril Ophthalmic Suspension (NDC 0049-0670-48) is supplied in 5 ml vials with separate sterile dropper.
Revised August 1987 60-2323-00-3

TERRAMYCIN® ℞
(oxytetracycline)
INTRAMUSCULAR SOLUTION*
FOR INTRAMUSCULAR USE ONLY
contains 2% lidocaine

DESCRIPTION

Oxytetracycline is a product of the metabolism of *Streptomyces rimosus* and is one of the family of tetracycline antibiotics.
Oxytetracycline diffuses readily through the placenta into the fetal circulation, into the pleural fluid and, under some circumstances, into the cerebrospinal fluid. It appears to be

concentrated in the hepatic system and excreted in the bile, so that it appears in the feces, as well as in the urine, in a biologically active form.

COMPOSITION

[See table above]

ACTIONS

Oxytetracycline is primarily bacteriostatic and is thought to exert its antimicrobial effect by the inhibition of protein synthesis. Oxytetracycline is active against a wide range of gram-negative and gram-positive organisms.

The drugs in the tetracycline class have closely similar antimicrobial spectra, and cross resistance among them is common. Microorganisms may be considered susceptible if the M.I.C. (minimum inhibitory concentration) is not more than 4.0 mcg/ml and intermediate if the M.I.C. is 4.0 to 12.5 mcg/ml.

Susceptibility plate testing: A tetracycline disc may be used to determine microbial susceptibility to drugs in the tetracycline class. If the Kirby-Bauer method of disc susceptibility testing is used, a 30 mcg tetracycline disc should give a zone of at least 19 mm when tested against an oxytetracycline-susceptible bacterial strain.

Tetracyclines are readily absorbed and are bound to plasma proteins in varying degree. They are concentrated by the liver in the bile, and excreted in the urine and feces at high concentrations and in a biologically active form.

INDICATIONS

Oxytetracycline is indicated in infections caused by the following microorganisms:

Rickettsiae (Rocky Mountain spotted fever, typhus fever and the typhus group, Q fever, rickettsialpox and tick fevers),

Mycoplasma pneumoniae (PPLO, Eaton Agent),

Agents of psittacosis and ornithosis,

Agents of lymphogranuloma venereum and granuloma inguinale,

The spirochetal agent of relapsing fever *(Borrelia recurrentis).*

The following gram-negative microorganisms:

Haemophilus ducreyi (chancroid),

Pasteurella pestis, and *Pasteurella tularensis,*

Bartonella bacilliformis,

Bacteroides species,

Vibrio comma and *Vibrio fetus,*

Brucella species (in conjunction with streptomycin).

Because many strains of the following groups of microorganisms have been shown to be resistant to tetracyclines, culture and susceptibility testing are recommended.

Oxytetracycline is indicated for treatment of infections caused by the following gram-negative microorganisms, when bacteriologic testing indicates appropriate susceptibility to the drug:

Escherichia coli,

Enterobacter aerogenes (formerly *Aerobacter aerogenes*),

Shigella species,

Mima species and *Herellea* species,

Haemophilus influenzae (respiratory infections),

Klebsiella species (respiratory and urinary infections).

Oxytetracycline is indicated for treatment of infections caused by the following gram-positive microorganisms when bacteriologic testing indicates appropriate susceptibility to the drug:

Streptococcus species:

Up to 44 percent of strains of *Streptococcus pyogenes* and 74 percent of *Streptococcus faecalis* have been found to be resistant to tetracycline drugs. Therefore, tetracyclines should not be used for streptococcal disease unless the organism has been demonstrated to be sensitive.

For upper respiratory infections due to Group A beta-hemolytic streptococci, penicillin is the usual drug of choice, including prophylaxis of rheumatic fever.

Diplococcus pneumoniae,

Staphylococcus aureus, skin and soft tissue infections. Oxytetracycline is not the drug of choice in the treatment of any type of staphylococcal infections.

When penicillin is contraindicated, tetracyclines are alternative drugs in the treatment of infections due to:

Neisseria gonorrhoeae,

Treponema pallidum and *Treponema pertenue* (syphilis and yaws),

Listeria monocytogenes,

Clostridium species,

Bacillus anthracis,

Fusobacterium fusiforme (Vincent's infection),

Actinomyces species.

In acute intestinal amebiasis, the tetracyclines may be a useful adjunct to amebicides.

Tetracyclines are indicated in the treatment of trachoma, although the infectious agent is not always eliminated, as judged by immunofluorescence.

Inclusion conjunctivitis may be treated with oral tetracyclines or with a combination of oral and topical agents.

CONTRAINDICATIONS

This drug is contraindicated in persons who have shown hypersensitivity to any of the tetracyclines.

WARNINGS

THE USE OF TETRACYCLINES DURING TOOTH DEVELOPMENT (LAST HALF OF PREGNANCY, INFANCY, AND CHILDHOOD TO THE AGE OF 8 YEARS) MAY CAUSE PERMANENT DISCOLORATION OF THE TEETH (YELLOW-GRAY-BROWN). This adverse reaction is more common during long term use of the drugs but has been observed following repeated short term courses. Enamel hypoplasia has also been reported. *TETRACYCLINES, THEREFORE, SHOULD NOT BE USED IN THIS AGE GROUP UNLESS OTHER DRUGS ARE NOT LIKELY TO BE EFFECTIVE OR ARE CONTRAINDICATED.*

Terramycin Intramuscular
contents per ml (m/v)

Ingredient	2 ml Single Dose Ampules		10 ml Vial Multidose
	100 mg/2 ml	250 mg/2 ml	50 mg/ml 10 ml (5 × 2 ml Doses)
oxytetracycline	50 mg	125 mg	50 mg
lidocaine	2.0%	2.0%	2.0%
magnesium chloride hexahydrate	2.5%	6.0%	2.5%
sodium formaldehyde sulfoxylate	0.5%	0.5%	0.3%
α-monothioglycerol	—	—	1.0%
monoethanolamine	approx. 1.7%	approx. 4.2%	approx. 2.6%
citric acid	—	—	1.0%
propyl gallate	—	—	0.02%
propylene glycol	75.2%	67.0%	74.1%
water	18.8%	16.8%	18.5%

If renal impairment exists, even usual oral or parenteral doses may lead to excessive systemic accumulation of the drug and possible liver toxicity. Under such conditions, lower than usual total doses are indicated and, if therapy is prolonged, serum level determinations of the drug may be advisable. This hazard is of particular importance in the parenteral administration of tetracyclines to pregnant or postpartum patients with pyelonephritis. When used under these circumstances, the blood level should not exceed 15 mcg/ml and liver function tests should be made at frequent intervals. Other potentially hepatotoxic drugs should not be prescribed concomitantly.

(In the presence of renal dysfunction, particularly in pregnancy, intravenous tetracycline therapy in daily doses exceeding 2 grams has been associated with deaths due to liver failure.)

Photosensitivity manifested by an exaggerated sunburn reaction has been observed in some individuals taking tetracyclines. Patients apt to be exposed to direct sunlight or ultraviolet light should be advised that this reaction can occur with tetracycline drugs, and treatment should be discontinued at the first evidence of skin erythema.

The antianabolic action of the tetracyclines may cause an increase in BUN. While this is not a problem in those with normal renal function, in patients with significantly impaired function, higher serum levels of this drug may lead to azotemia, hyperphosphatemia, and acidosis.

The product contains sodium formaldehyde sulfoxylate which serves as an antioxidant. Upon oxidation, this compound can form a potential sulfiting agent. Sulfiting agents may cause allergic-type reactions including anaphylactic symptoms and life-threatening or less severe asthmatic episodes in certain susceptible people. The over-all prevalence of sulfite sensitivity in the general population is unknown and probably low. Sulfite sensitivity is seen more frequently in asthmatic than in nonasthmatic people.

Usage in pregnancy. (See above "Warnings" about use during tooth development.)

Results of animal studies indicate that tetracyclines cross the placenta, are found in fetal tissues and can have toxic effects on the developing fetus (often related to retardation of skeletal development). Evidence of embryotoxicity has also been noted in animals treated early in pregnancy.

Usage in newborns, infants, and children. (See above "Warnings" about use during tooth development).

All tetracyclines form a stable calcium complex in any bone-forming tissue. A decrease in the fibula growth rate has been observed in prematures given oral tetracycline in doses of 25 mg/kg every 6 hours. This reaction was shown to be reversible when the drug was discontinued.

Tetracyclines are present in the milk of lactating women who are taking a drug in this class.

PRECAUTIONS

As with all intramuscular preparations, Terramycin (oxytetracycline) Intramuscular Solution should be injected well within the body of a relatively large muscle. ADULTS: The preferred sites are the upper outer quadrant of the buttock, (i.e., gluteus maximus), and the mid-lateral thigh. CHILDREN: It is recommended that intramuscular injections be given preferably in the mid-lateral muscles of the thigh. In infants and small children the periphery of the upper outer quadrant of the gluteal region should be used only when necessary, such as in burn patients, in order to minimize the possibility of damage to the sciatic nerve.

The deltoid area should be used only if well developed such as in certain adults and older children, and then only with caution to avoid radial nerve injury. Intramuscular injections should not be made into the lower and mid-thirds of the upper arm. As with all intramuscular injections, aspiration is necessary to help avoid inadvertent injection into a blood vessel.

As with other antibiotic preparations, use of this drug may result in overgrowth of nonsusceptible organisms, including fungi. If superinfection occurs, the antibiotic should be discontinued and appropriate therapy instituted.

In venereal diseases when coexistent syphilis is suspected, a dark field examination should be done before treatment is started and the blood serology repeated monthly for at least 4 months.

Because tetracyclines have been shown to depress plasma prothrombin activity, patients who are on anticoagulant therapy may require downward adjustment of their anticoagulant dosage.

In long term therapy, periodic laboratory evaluation of organ systems, including hematopoietic, renal and hepatic studies should be performed.

All infections due to Group A beta-hemolytic streptococci should be treated for at least 10 days.

Since bacteriostatic drugs may interfere with the bactericidal action of penicillin, it is advisable to avoid giving tetracycline in conjunction with penicillin.

ADVERSE REACTIONS

Local irritation may be present after intramuscular injection. The injection should be deep, with care taken not to injure the sciatic nerve nor inject intravascularly.

Gastrointestinal: anorexia, nausea, vomiting, diarrhea, glossitis, dysphagia, enterocolitis, and inflammatory lesions (with monilial overgrowth) in the anogenital region. These reactions have been caused by both the oral and parenteral administration of tetracyclines.

Skin: maculopapular and erythematous rashes. Exfoliative dermatitis has been reported but is uncommon. Photosensitivity is discussed above. (See "Warnings").

Renal toxicity: Rise in BUN has been reported and is apparently dose related. (See "Warnings").

Hypersensitivity reactions: Urticaria, angioneurotic edema, anaphylaxis, anaphylactoid purpura, pericarditis, and exacerbation of systemic lupus erythematosus.

Bulging fontanels in infants and benign intracranial hypertension in adults have been reported in individuals receiving full therapeutic dosages. These conditions disappeared rapidly when the drug was discontinued.

Blood: Hemolytic anemia, thrombocytopenia, neutropenia, and eosinophilia have been reported.

When given over prolonged periods, tetracyclines have been reported to produce brown-black microscopic discoloration of thyroid glands. No abnormalities of thyroid function studies are known to occur.

DOSAGE AND ADMINISTRATION

Intramuscular Administration:

Adults: The usual daily dose is 250 mg administered once every 24 hours or 300 mg given in divided doses at 8 to 12 hour intervals.

For children above eight years of age: 15–25 mg/kg of body weight up to a maximum of 250 mg per single daily injection. Dosage may be divided and given at 8 to 12 hour intervals.

Intramuscular therapy should be reserved for situations in which oral therapy is not feasible.

The intramuscular administration of oxytetracycline produces lower blood levels than oral administration in the recommended dosages. Patients placed on intramuscular oxytetracycline should be changed to the oral dosage form as soon as possible. If rapid, high blood levels are needed, oxytetracycline should be administered intravenously.

In patients with renal impairment: (See "Warnings") Total dosage should be decreased by reduction of recommended individual doses and/or by extending time intervals between doses.

HOW SUPPLIED

Terramycin (oxytetracycline) Intramuscular Solution is available as follows:

250 mg/2ml—in 2 ml pre-scored glass ampules, packages of 5 (NDC 0049–0770–09).

100 mg/2ml—in 2 ml pre-scored glass ampules, packages of 5 (NDC 0049–0760–09).

50 mg/ml—in 10 ml multiple dose vials, packages of 5 (NDC 0049-0750-77).

*U.S. Pat. Nos. 3,017,323 and 3,026,248

Revised March 1987 70-1051-00-2

Continued on next page

TERRAMYCIN® ℞

(oxytetracycline HCl with polymyxin B sulfate)
OPHTHALMIC OINTMENT
STERILE

DESCRIPTION

Each gram of sterile ointment contains oxytetracycline HCl equivalent to 5 mg oxytetracycline, 10,000 units of polymyxin B sulfate, white petrolatum, and liquid petrolatum.

ACTIONS

Terramycin is a widely used antibiotic with clinically proved activity against gram-positive and gram-negative bacteria, rickettsiae, spirochetes, large viruses, and certain protozoa. Polymyxin B Sulfate, one of a group of related antibiotics derived from *Bacillus polymyxa*, is rapidly bactericidal. This action is exclusively against gram-negative organisms. It is particularly effective against *Pseudomonas aeruginosa (B. pyocyaneus)* and Koch-Weeks bacillus, frequently found in local infections of the eye.

There is thus made available a particularly effective antimicrobial combination of the broad-spectrum antibiotic Terramycin as well as polymyxin B sulfate against primarily causative or secondarily infecting organisms.

INDICATIONS

The sterile preparation, Terramycin with Polymyxin B Sulfate Ophthalmic Ointment, is indicated for the treatment of superficial ocular infections involving the conjunctiva and/or cornea caused by Terramycin with Polymyxin B Sulfate-susceptible organisms.

It may be administered topically alone, or as an adjunct to systemic therapy.

It is effective in infections caused by susceptible strains of staphylococci, streptococci, pneumococci, *Haemophilus influenzae, Pseudomonas aeruginosa,* Koch-Weeks bacillus, and *Proteus.*

CONTRAINDICATIONS

This drug is contraindicated in individuals who have shown hypersensitivity to any of its components.

PRECAUTIONS

As with all antibiotic preparations, use of this drug may result in overgrowth of nonsusceptible organisms, including fungi. If superinfection occurs, the antibiotic should be discontinued and appropriate specific therapy should be instituted.

ADVERSE REACTIONS

Terramycin with Polymyxin B Sulfate Ophthalmic Ointment is well tolerated by the epithelial membranes and other tissues of the eye. Allergic or inflammatory reactions due to individual hypersensitivity are rare.

DOSAGE AND ADMINISTRATION

Approximately $^1/_2$ inch of the ointment is squeezed from the tube onto the lower lid of the affected eye two to four times daily.

The patient should be instructed to avoid contamination of the tip of the tube when applying the ointment.

HOW SUPPLIED

Terramycin with Polymyxin B Sulfate Ophthalmic Ointment is supplied in $^1/_8$ oz (3.5 g) tubes (NDC 0049-0801-08).

August 1987 60-2324-00-1

TIKOSYN™ ℞

[*tĭk-ō-sĭn*]
(dofetilide)
Capsules

> To minimize the risk of induced arrhythmia, patients initiated or re-initiated on TIKOSYN should be placed for a minimum of 3 days in a facility that can provide calculations of creatinine clearance, continuous electrocardiographic monitoring, and cardiac resuscitation. For detailed instructions regarding dose selection, see **DOSAGE AND ADMINISTRATION**. TIKOSYN is available only to hospitals and prescribers who have received appropriate TIKOSYN dosing and treatment initiation education, see **DOSAGE AND ADMINISTRATION.**

DESCRIPTION

TIKOSYN (dofetilide) is an antiarrhythmic drug with Class III (cardiac action potential duration prolonging) properties. Its empirical formula is $C_{19}H_{27}N_3O_5S_2$ and it has a molecular weight of 441.6. The structural formula is

CH_3SO_2HN H_3C N O $NHSO_2CH_3$

The chemical name for dofetilide is *N*-[4-[2-[methyl[2-[4-[(methylsulfonyl)amino]phenoxy]ethyl]amino]ethyl]phenyl]- methanesulfonamide.

Dofetilide is a white to off-white powder. It is very slightly soluble in water and propan-2-ol and is soluble in 0.1M aqueous sodium hydroxide, acetone and aqueous 0.1M hydrochloric acid.

TIKOSYN capsules contain the following inactive ingredients: microcrystalline cellulose, corn starch, colloidal silicon dioxide and magnesium stearate. TIKOSYN is supplied for oral administration in three dosage strengths: 125 mcg (0.125 mg) orange and white capsules, 250 mcg (0.25 mg) peach capsules, and 500 mcg (0.5 mg) peach and white capsules.

CLINICAL PHARMACOLOGY

Mechanism of Action

TIKOSYN (dofetilide) shows Vaughan Williams Class III antiarrhythmic activity. The mechanism of action is blockade of the cardiac ion channel carrying the rapid component of the delayed rectifier potassium current, I_{Kr}. At concentrations covering several orders of magnitude, dofetilide blocks only I_{Kr} with no relevant block of the other repolarizing potassium currents (e.g., I_{Ks}, I_{K1}). At clinically relevant concentrations, dofetilide has no effect on sodium channels (associated with Class I effect), adrenergic alpha-receptors, or adrenergic beta-receptors.

Electrophysiology

TIKOSYN (dofetilide) increases the monophasic action potential duration in a predictable, concentration-dependent manner, primarily due to delayed repolarization. This effect, and the related increase in effective refractory period, is observed in the atria and ventricles in both resting and paced electrophysiology studies. The increase in QT interval observed on the surface ECG is a result of prolongation of both effective and functional refractory periods in the His-Purkinje system and the ventricles.

Dofetilide did not influence cardiac conduction velocity and sinus node function in a variety of studies in patients with or without structural heart disease. This is consistent with a lack of effect of dofetilide on the PR interval and QRS width in patients with pre-existing heart block and/or sick sinus syndrome.

In patients, dofetilide terminates induced re-entrant tachyarrhythmias (e.g., atrial fibrillation/flutter and ventricular tachycardia) and prevents their re-induction. TIKOSYN does not increase the electrical energy required to convert electrically-induced ventricular fibrillation, and it significantly reduces the defibrillation threshold in patients with ventricular tachycardia and ventricular fibrillation undergoing implantation of a cardioverter-defibrillator device.

Hemodynamic Effects

In hemodynamic studies, TIKOSYN had no effect on cardiac output, cardiac index, stroke volume index, or systemic vascular resistance in patients with ventricular tachycardia, mild to moderate congestive heart failure or angina and either normal or low left ventricular ejection fraction. There was no evidence of a negative inotropic effect related to TIKOSYN therapy in patients with atrial fibrillation. There was no increase in heart failure in patients with significant left ventricular dysfunction (see **Safety in Patients with Structural Heart Disease: DIAMOND Studies**). In the overall clinical program, TIKOSYN did not affect blood pressure. Heart rate was decreased by 4–6 bpm in studies in patients.

Pharmacokinetics, General

Absorption and Distribution: The oral bioavailability of dofetilide is >90%, with maximal plasma concentrations occurring at about 2–3 hours in the fasted state. Oral bioavailability is unaffected by food or antacid. The terminal half life of TIKOSYN is approximately 10 hours; steady state plasma concentrations are attained within 2–3 days, with an accumulation index of 1.5 to 2.0. Plasma concentrations are dose proportional. Plasma protein binding of dofetilide is 60–70%, is independent of plasma concentration, and is unaffected by renal impairment. Volume of distribution is 3 L/kg.

Metabolism and Excretion: Approximately 80% of a single dose of dofetilide is excreted in urine, of which approximately 80% is excreted as unchanged dofetilide with the remaining 20% consisting of inactive or minimally active metabolites. Renal elimination involves both glomerular filtration and active tubular secretion (via the cation transport system, a process that can be inhibited by cimetidine, trimethoprim, prochlorperazine, megestrol and ketoconazole). *In vitro* studies with human liver microsomes show that dofetilide can be metabolized by CYP3A4, but it has a low affinity for this isoenzyme. Metabolites are formed by N-dealkylation and N-oxidation. There are no quantifiable metabolites circulating in plasma, but 5 metabolites have been identified in urine.

Pharmacokinetics in Special Populations

Renal Impairment: In volunteers with varying degrees of renal impairment and patients with arrhythmias, the clearance of dofetilide decreases with decreasing creatinine clearance. As a result, and as seen in clinical studies, the half-life of dofetilide is longer in patients with lower creatinine clearances. **Because increase in QT interval and the risk of ventricular arrhythmias are directly related to plasma concentrations of dofetilide, dosage adjustment based on calculated creatinine clearance is critically important** (see **DOSAGE AND ADMINISTRATION**). Patients with severe renal impairment (creatinine clearance <20 mL/min) were not included in clinical or pharmacokinetic studies (see **CONTRAINDICATIONS**).

Hepatic Impairment: There was no clinically significant alteration in the pharmacokinetics of dofetilide in volunteers with mild to moderate hepatic impairment (Child-Pugh class A and B) compared to age- and weight-matched healthy volunteers. Patients with severe hepatic impairment were not studied.

Patients with Heart Disease: Population pharmacokinetic analyses indicate that the plasma concentration of dofetilide in patients with supraventricular and ventricular arrhythmias, ischemic heart disease, or congestive heart failure are similar to those of healthy volunteers, after adjusting for renal function.

Elderly: After correction for renal function, clearance of dofetilide is not related to age.

Women: A population pharmacokinetic analysis showed that women have approximately 12–18% lower dofetilide oral clearances than men (14–22% greater plasma dofetilide levels), after correction for weight and creatinine clearance. In females, as in males, renal function was the single most important factor influencing dofetilide clearance. In normal female volunteers, hormone replacement therapy (a combination of conjugated estrogens and medroxyprogesterone) did not increase dofetilide exposure.

Drug-Drug Interactions (see PRECAUTIONS)

Dose-Response and Concentration Response for Increase in QT Interval

Increase in QT interval is directly related to dofetilide dose and plasma concentration. Figure 1 shows that the relationship in normal volunteers between dofetilide plasma concentrations and change in QTc is linear, with a positive slope of approximately 15–25 msec/(ng/mL) after the first dose and approximately 10–15 msec/(ng/mL) at Day 23 (reflecting a steady state of dosing). A linear relationship between mean QTc increase and dofetilide dose was also seen in patients with renal impairment, in patients with ischemic heart disease, and in patients with supraventricular and ventricular arrhythmias.

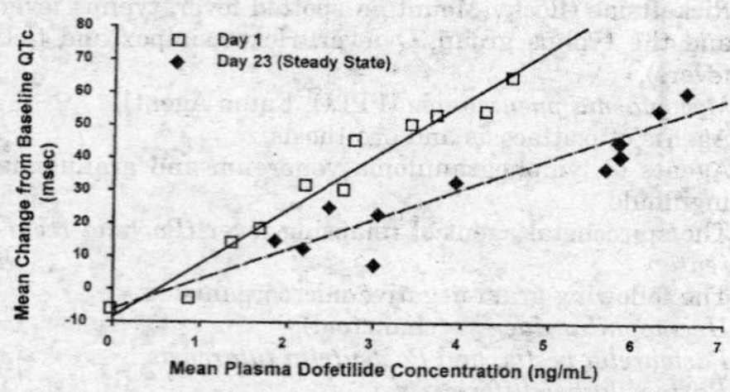

Figure 1: Mean QTc-Concentration Relationship in Young Volunteers Over 24 Days.
Note: The range of dofetilide plasma concentrations achieved with the 500 mcg BID dose adjusted for creatinine clearance is 1-3.5 ng/mL.

The relationship between dose, efficacy and the increase in QTc from baseline at steady state for the two randomized, placebo-controlled studies (described further below) is shown in Figure 2. The studies examined the effectiveness of TIKOSYN in conversion to sinus rhythm and maintenance of normal sinus rhythm after conversion in patients with atrial fibrillation/flutter of >1 week duration. As shown, both the probability of a patient's remaining in sinus rhythm at six months and the change in QTc from baseline at steady state of dosing increased in an approximately linear fashion with increasing dose of TIKOSYN.

Note that in these studies doses were modified by results of creatinine clearance measurement and in-hospital QTc prolongation.

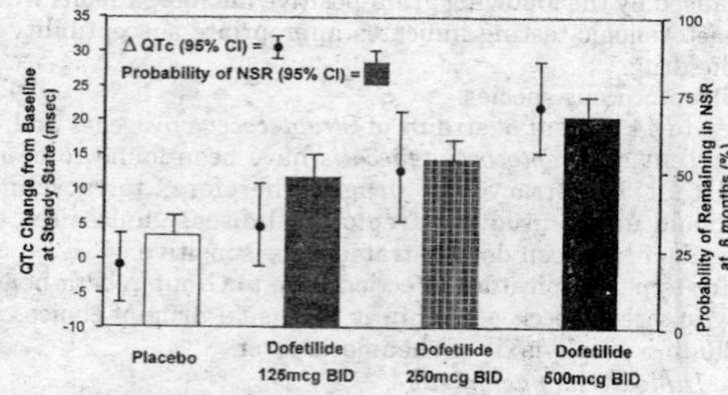

Number of patients evaluated for maintenance of NSR: 503 TIKOSYN, 174 placebo.
Number of patients evaluated for QTc change: 478 TIKOSYN, 167 placebo.

Figure 2: Relationship Between TIKOSYN Dose, QTc Increase and Maintenance of NSR.

CLINICAL STUDIES

Chronic Atrial Fibrillation and/or Atrial Flutter

Two randomized, parallel, double-blind, placebo controlled, dose-response trials evaluated the ability of TIKOSYN 1) to convert patients with atrial fibrillation or atrial flutter (AF/AFl) of more than 1 week duration to normal sinus rhythm (NSR) and 2) to maintain NSR (delay time to recurrence of AF/AFl) after drug-induced or electrical cardioversion. A total of 996 patients with a one week to two year history of atrial fibrillation/atrial flutter were enrolled. Both studies randomized patients to placebo or to doses of TIKOSYN 125 mcg, 250 mcg, 500 mcg or in one study a comparator drug, given twice a day (these doses were lowered based on calculated creatinine clearance and, in one of the studies, for QT interval or QTc). **All patients were started on therapy in a hospital where their ECG was monitored (see DOSAGE AND ADMINISTRATION).**

Patients were excluded from participation if they had had syncope within the past 6 months, AV block greater than first degree, MI or unstable angina within 1 month, cardiac surgery within 2 months, history of QT interval prolongation or polymorphic ventricular tachycardia associated with use of anti-arrhythmic drugs, QT interval or QTc >440 msec, serum creatinine >2.5 mg/mL, significant diseases of other organ systems; used cimetidine; or used drugs known to prolong the QT interval.

Both studies enrolled mostly Caucasians (over 90%), males (over 70%) and patients ≥65 years of age (over 50%). Most (>90%) were NYHA Functional Class I or II. Approximately one-half had structural heart disease (including ischemic heart disease, cardiomyopathies, and valvular disease) and about one-half were hypertensive. A substantial proportion of patients were on concomitant therapy, including digoxin (over 60%), diuretics (over 20%) and ACE inhibitors (over 30%). About 90% were on anticoagulants.
Acute conversion rates are shown in Table 1 for randomized doses (doses were adjusted for calculated creatinine clearance and, in Study 1, for QT interval or QTc). Of patients who converted pharmacologically, approximately 70% converted within 24–36 hours.

Table 1: Conversion of Atrial Fibrillation/Flutter to Normal Sinus Rhythm

	TIKOSYN Dose			
	125 mcg BID	250 mcg BID	500 mcg BID	Placebo
Study 1	5/82(6%)	8/82(10%)	23/77(30%)	1/84(1%)
Study 2	8/135(6%)	14/ 133(11%)	38/ 129(29%)	2/137(1%)

Patients who did not convert to NSR with randomized therapy within 48–72 hours had electrical cardioversion. Those patients remaining in NSR after conversion in hospital were continued on randomized therapy as outpatients (maintenance period) for up to one year unless they experienced a recurrence of atrial fibrillation/atrial flutter or withdrew for other reasons.
Table 2 shows, by randomized dose, the percentage of patients at 6 and 12 months in both studies, who remained on treatment in NSR and the percentage of patients who withdrew because of recurrence of AF/AFl or adverse events.
[See table 2 above]
Table 3 and Figures 3 and 4 show, by randomized dose, the effectiveness of TIKOSYN in maintaining NSR using Kaplan Meier analysis, which shows patients remaining on treatment.
[See table 3 at right]

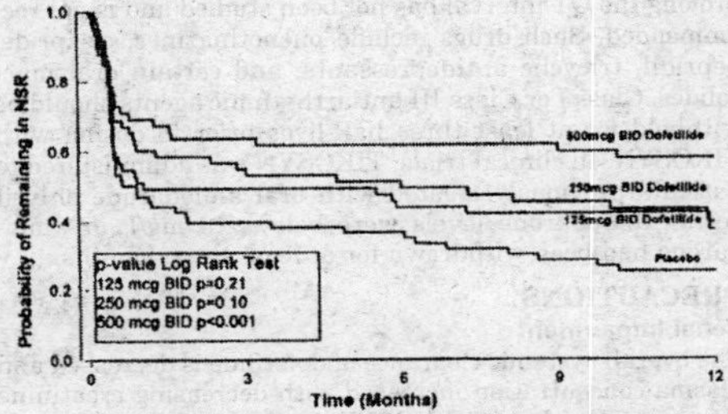

Figure 3: Maintenance of Normal Sinus Rhythm, TIKOSYN Regimen vs. Placebo (Study 1).

The point estimates of the probabilities of remaining in NSR at 6 and 12 months were 62% and 58% respectively for TIKOSYN 500 mcg BID, 50% and 37% for TIKOSYN 250 mcg BID, and 37% and 25% respectively on placebo.

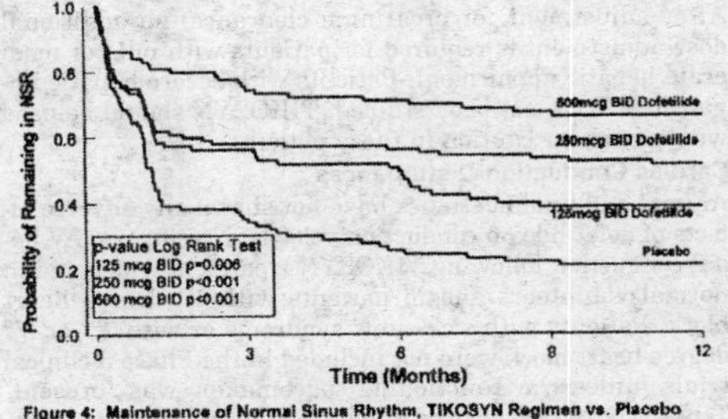

Figure 4: Maintenance of Normal Sinus Rhythm, TIKOSYN Regimen vs. Placebo (Study 2).

The point estimates of the probabilities of remaining in NSR at 6 and 12 months were 71% and 66% respectively for TIKOSYN 500 mcg BID, 56% and 51% for TIKOSYN 250 mcg BID, and 26% and 21% respectively on placebo.
In both studies, TIKOSYN resulted in a dose-related increase in the number of patients maintained in NSR at all time periods and delayed the time of recurrence of sustained AF. Data pooled from both studies show that there is a positive relationship between the probability of staying in NSR, TIKOSYN dose, and increase in QTc (see Figure 2 in **CLINICAL PHARMACOLOGY: Dose-Response and Concentration Response for QT Interval**).
Analysis of pooled data for patients randomized to a TIKOSYN dose of 500 mcg twice daily showed that maintenance of NSR was similar in both males and females, in both patients aged <65 years and patients ≥65 years of age, and in both patients with atrial flutter as a primary diagnosis and those with a primary diagnosis of atrial fibrillation.
During the period of in-hospital initiation of dosing, 23% of patients in Studies 1 and 2 had their dose adjusted downward on the basis of their calculated creatinine clearance, and 3% had their dose down-titrated due to increased QT interval or QTc. Increased QT interval or QTc led to discontinuation of therapy in 3% of patients.

Table 2: Patient Status at 6 and 12 Months Post Randomization

	TIKOSYN Dose			
	125 mcg BID	250 mcg BID	500 mcg BID	Placebo
Study 1				
Randomized	82	82	77	84
Achieved NSR	60	61	61	68
6 months				
Still on treatment in NSR	38%	44%	52%	32%
D/C for recurrence	55%	49%	33%	63%
D/C for AEs	3%	3%	8%	4%
12 months				
Still on treatment in NSR	32%	26%	46%	22%
D/C for recurrence	58%	57%	36%	72%
D/C for AEs	7%	11%	8%	6%
Study 2				
Randomized	135	133	129	137
Achieved NSR	103	118	100	106
6 months				
Still on treatment in NSR	41%	49%	57%	22%
D/C for recurrence	48%	42%	27%	72%
D/C for AEs	9%	6%	10%	4%
12 months				
Still on treatment in NSR	25%	42%	49%	16%
D/C for recurrence	59%	47%	32%	76%
D/C for AEs	11%	6%	12%	5%

Please note that columns do not add up to 100% due to discontinuations for "other" reasons

Table 3: P-Values and Median Time (days) to Recurrence of AF/AFl

	TIKOSYN Dose			
	125 mcg BID	250 mcg BID	500 mcg BID	Placebo
Study 1				
p-value vs placebo	P=0.21	P=0.10	P<0.001	
Median time to recurrence (days)	31	179	>365	27
Study 2				
p-value vs placebo	P=0.006	P<0.001	P<0.001	
Median time to recurrence (days)	182	>365	>365	34

Median time to recurrence of AF/AFl could not be estimated accurately for the 250 mcg BID treatment group in Study 2 and the 500 mcg BID treatment groups in Studies 1 and 2 because TIKOSYN maintained >50% of patients (51%, 58% and 66%, respectively) in NSR for the 12 months duration of the studies.

Safety in Patients with Structural Heart Disease: DIAMOND Studies (The Danish Investigations of Arrhythmia and Mortality on Dofetilide)
The two DIAMOND studies were 3-year trials comparing the effects of TIKOSYN and placebo on mortality and morbidity in patients with impaired left ventricular function (ejection fraction ≤35%). Patients were treated for at least one year. One study was in patients with moderate to severe (60% NYHA Class III or IV) congestive heart failure (DIAMOND CHF) and the other was in patients with recent myocardial infarction (DIAMOND MI) (of whom 40% had NYHA Class III or IV heart failure). Both groups were at relatively high risk of sudden death. The DIAMOND trials were intended to determine whether TIKOSYN could reduce that risk. The trials did not demonstrate a reduction in mortality; however, they provide reassurance that, when initiated carefully, in a hospital or equivalent setting, TIKOSYN did not increase mortality in patients with structural heart disease, an important finding because other antiarrhythmics [notably the Class IC antiarrhythmics studied in the Cardiac Arrhythmia Suppression Trial (CAST) and a pure Class III antiarrhythmic, d-sotalol (SWORD)] have increased mortality in post-infarction populations. The DIAMOND trials therefore provide evidence of a method of safe use of TIKOSYN in a population susceptible to ventricular arrhythmias. In addition, the subset of patients with AF in the DIAMOND trials provide further evidence of safety in a population of patients with structural heart disease accompanying the AF. Note, however, that this AF population was given a lower (250 mcg BID) dose (see DIAMOND Patients with Atrial Fibrillation).
In both DIAMOND studies, patients were randomized to 500 mcg BID of TIKOSYN, but this was reduced to 250 mcg BID if calculated creatinine clearance was 40–60 mL/min, if patients had AF, or if QT interval prolongation (>550 msec or >20% increase from baseline) occurred after dosing. Dose reductions for reduced calculated creatinine clearance occurred in 47% and 45% of DIAMOND CHF and MI patients. Dose reductions for increased QT interval or QTc occurred in 5% and 7% of DIAMOND CHF and MI patients, respectively. Increased QT interval or QTc (>550 msec or >20% increase from baseline) resulted in discontinuation of 1.8% of patients in DIAMOND CHF and 2.5% of patients in DIAMOND MI.
In the DIAMOND studies all patients were hospitalized for at least 3 days after treatment was initiated and monitored by telemetry. Patients with QTc greater than 460 msec, second or third degree AV block (unless with pacemaker), resting heart rate <50 bpm, or prior history of polymorphic ventricular tachycardia were excluded.
DIAMOND CHF studied 1518 patients hospitalized with severe CHF who had confirmed impaired left ventricular function (ejection fraction ≤35%). Patients received a median duration of therapy of greater than one year. There were 311 deaths from all causes in patients randomized to TIKOSYN (n=762) and 317 deaths in patients randomized to placebo (n=756). The probability of survival at one year was 73% (95% CI: 70% – 76%) in the TIKOSYN group and 72%

Continued on next page

Tikosyn—Cont.

(95% CI: 69% – 75%) in the placebo group. Similar results were seen for cardiac deaths and arrhythmic deaths. Torsade de pointes occurred in 25/762 patients (3.3%) receiving TIKOSYN. The majority of cases (76%) occurred within the first 3 days of dosing. In all, 437/762 (57%) of patients on TIKOSYN and 459/756 (61%) on placebo required hospitalization. Of these, 229/762 (30%) of patients on TIKOSYN and 290/756 (38%) on placebo required hospitalization because of worsening heart failure.

DIAMOND MI studied 1510 patients hospitalized with recent myocardial infarction (2–7 days) who had confirmed impaired left ventricular function (ejection fraction ≤35%). Patients received a median duration of therapy of greater than one year. There were 230 deaths in patients randomized to TIKOSYN (n=749) and 243 deaths in patients randomized to placebo (n=761). The probability of survival at one year was 79% (95% CI: 76% – 82%) in the TIKOSYN group and 77% (95% CI: 74% – 80%) in the placebo group. Cardiac and arrhythmic mortality showed a similar result. Torsade de pointes occurred in 7/749 patients (0.9%) receiving TIKOSYN. Of these, 4 cases occurred within the first 3 days of dosing and 3 cases occurred between Day 4 and the conclusion of the study. In all, 371/749 (50%) of patients on TIKOSYN and 419/761 (55%) on placebo required hospitalization. Of these, 200/749 (27%) of patients on TIKOSYN and 205/761 (27%) on placebo required hospitalization because of worsening heart failure.

DIAMOND Patients with Atrial Fibrillation(the DIAMOND AF subpopulation). There were 506 patients in the two DIAMOND studies who had atrial fibrillation (AF) at entry to the studies (249 randomized to TIKOSYN and 257 randomized to placebo). DIAMOND AF patients randomized to TIKOSYN received 250 mcg BID; 65% of these patients had impaired renal function, so that 250 mcg BID represents the dose they would have received in the AF trials, which would give drug exposure similar to a person with normal renal function given 500 mcg BID. In the DIAMOND AF subpopulation there were 111 deaths (45%) in the 249 patients in the TIKOSYN group and 116 deaths (45%) in the 257 patients in the placebo group. Hospital readmission rates for any reason were 125/249 or 50% on TIKOSYN and 156/257 or 61% for placebo. Of these, readmission rates for worsening heart failure were 73/249 or 29% on TIKOSYN and 102/257 or 40% for placebo.

Of the 506 patients in the DIAMOND studies who had atrial fibrillation or flutter at baseline, 12% of patients in the TIKOSYN group and 2% of patients in the placebo group had converted to normal sinus rhythm after one month. In those patients converted to normal sinus rhythm, 79% of the TIKOSYN group and 42% of the placebo group remained in normal sinus rhythm for one year.

In the DIAMOND studies, although torsade de pointes occurred more frequently in the TIKOSYN-treated patients (see **ADVERSE REACTIONS**), TIKOSYN, given with an initial 3-day hospitalization and with dose modified for reduced creatinine clearance and increased QT interval, was not associated with an excess risk of mortality in these populations with structural heart disease in the individual studies or in an analysis of the combined studies. The presence of atrial fibrillation did not affect outcome.

INDICATIONS AND USAGE

Maintenance of Normal Sinus Rhythm (Delay in AF/AFl Recurrence)

TIKOSYN is indicated for the maintenance of normal sinus rhythm (delay in time to recurrence of atrial fibrillation/atrial flutter [AF/AFl]) in patients with atrial fibrillation/atrial flutter of greater than one week duration who have been converted to normal sinus rhythm. Because TIKOSYN can cause life threatening ventricular arrhythmias, it should be reserved for patients in whom atrial fibrillation/atrial flutter is highly symptomatic.

In general, antiarrhythmic therapy for atrial fibrillation/atrial flutter aims to prolong the time in normal sinus rhythm. Recurrence is expected in some patients. (See **CLINICAL TRIALS**.)

Conversion of Atrial Fibrillation/Flutter

TIKOSYN is indicated for the conversion of atrial fibrillation and atrial flutter to normal sinus rhythm.

TIKOSYN has not been shown to be effective in patients with paroxysmal atrial fibrillation.

CONTRAINDICATIONS

TIKOSYN is contraindicated in patients with congenital or acquired long QT syndromes. TIKOSYN should not be used in patients with a baseline QT interval or QTc >440 msec (500 msec in patients with ventricular conduction abnormalities). TIKOSYN is also contraindicated in patients with severe renal impairment (calculated creatinine clearance <20 mL/min).

The concomitant use of verapamil or the cation transport system inhibitors cimetidine, trimethoprim (alone or in combination with sulfamethoxazole) or ketoconazole with TIKOSYN is contraindicated (see **PRECAUTIONS, Drug-Drug Interactions**), as each of these drugs cause a substantial increase in dofetilide plasma concentrations. In addition, other known inhibitors of the renal cation transport system such as prochlorperazine and megestrol should not be used in patients on TIKOSYN.

TIKOSYN is also contraindicated in patients with a known hypersensitivity to the drug.

Table 4: Summary of Torsade de Pointes in Patients Randomized to Dofetilide by Dose; Patients with Supraventricular Arrhythmias

	TIKOSYN Dose				
	<250 mcg BID	250 mcg BID	>250-500 mcg BID	>500 mcg BID	All Doses
Number of Patients	217	388	703	38	1346
Torsade de Pointes	0	1 (0.3%)	6 (0.9%)	4 (10.5%)	11 (0.8%)

Table 5: Incidence of Torsade de Pointes Before and After Introduction of Dosing According to Renal Function

	Total	Before	After
Population:	n/N %	n/N %	n/N %
Supraventricular Arrhythmias	11/1346 (0.8%)	6/193 (3.1%)	5/1153 (0.4%)
DIAMOND CHF	25/762 (3.3%)	7/148 (4.7%)	18/614 (2.9%)
DIAMOND MI	7/749 (0.9%)	3/101 (3.0%)	4/648 (0.6%)
DIAMOND AF	4/249 (1.6%)	0/43 (0%)	4/206 (1.9%)

WARNINGS

Ventricular Arrhythmia: TIKOSYN (dofetilide) can cause serious ventricular arrhythmias, primarily torsade de pointes (TdP) type ventricular tachycardia, a polymorphic ventricular tachycardia associated with QT interval prolongation. QT interval prolongation is directly related to dofetilide plasma concentration. Factors such as reduced creatinine clearance or certain dofetilide drug interactions will increase dofetilide plasma concentration. The risk of TdP can be reduced by controlling the plasma concentration through adjustment of the initial dofetilide dose according to creatinine clearance and by monitoring the ECG for excessive increases in the QT interval.

Treatment with dofetilide must therefore be started only in patients placed for a minimum of three days in a facility that can provide electrocardiographic monitoring and in the presence of personnel trained in the management of serious ventricular arrhythmias. Calculation of the creatinine clearance for all patients must precede administration of the first dose of dofetilide. For detailed instructions regarding dose selection, see DOSAGE AND ADMINISTRATION.

The risk of dofetilide induced ventricular arrhythmia was assessed in three ways in clinical studies: 1) by description of the QT interval and its relation to the dose and plasma concentration of dofetilide; 2) by observing the frequency of TdP in TIKOSYN treated patients according to dose; 3) by observing the overall mortality rate in patients with atrial fibrillation and in patients with structural heart disease.

Relation of QT Interval to Dose: The QT interval increases linearly with increasing TIKOSYN dose (see Figures 1 and 2 in **CLINICAL PHARMACOLOGY: Dose-Response and Concentration Response for Increase in QT Interval**).

Frequency of Torsade de Pointes: In the supraventricular arrhythmia population (patients with AF and other supraventricular arrhythmias) the overall incidence of torsade de pointes was 0.8%. The frequency of TdP by dose is shown in Table 4. There were no cases of TdP on placebo.

[See table 4 above]

As shown in Table 5, the rate of TdP was reduced when patients were dosed according to their renal function (see **CLINICAL PHARMACOLOGY: Pharmacokinetics in Special Populations: Renal Impairment**, and **DOSAGE AND ADMINISTRATION**).

[See table 5 above]

The majority of the episodes of TdP occurred within the first three days of TIKOSYN therapy (10/11 events in the studies of patients with supraventricular arrhythmias; 19/25 and 4/7 events in DIAMOND CHF and DIAMOND MI, respectively; 2/4 events in the DIAMOND AF subpopulation).

Mortality: In a pooled survival analysis of patients in the supraventricular arrhythmia population (low prevalence of structural heart disease), deaths occurred in 0.9% (12/1346) of patients receiving TIKOSYN and 0.4% (3/677) in the placebo group. Adjusted for duration of therapy, primary diagnosis, age, gender, and prevalence of structural heart disease, the point estimate of the hazard ratio for the pooled studies (TIKOSYN/placebo) was 1.1 (95% CI: 0.3, 4.3). The DIAMOND CHF and MI trials examined mortality in patients with structural heart disease (ejection fraction ≤35%). In these large, double-blind studies, deaths occurred in 36% (541/1511) of TIKOSYN patients and 37% (560/1517) of placebo patients. In an analysis of 506 DIAMOND patients with atrial fibrillation/flutter at baseline, one year mortality on TIKOSYN was 31% vs. 32% on placebo (see **CLINICAL STUDIES**).

Because of the small number of events, an excess mortality due to TIKOSYN cannot be ruled out with confidence in the pooled survival analysis of placebo-controlled trials in patients with supraventricular arrhythmias. However, it is reassuring that in two large placebo-controlled mortality studies in patients with significant heart disease (DIAMOND CHF/MI), there were no more deaths in TIKOSYN-treated patients than in patients given placebo (see **CLINICAL STUDIES**).

Drug-Drug Interactions (see CONTRAINDICATIONS)

Because there is a linear relationship between dofetilide plasma concentration and QTc, concomitant drugs that interfere with the metabolism or renal elimination of dofetilide may increase the risk of arrhythmia (torsade de pointes). TIKOSYN is metabolized to a small degree by the CYP3A4 isoenzyme of the cytochrome P450 system and an inhibitor of this system could increase systemic dofetilide exposure. More important, dofetilide is eliminated by cationic renal secretion, and three inhibitors of this process have been shown to increase systemic dofetilide exposure. The magnitude of the effect on renal elimination by cimetidine, trimethoprim and ketoconazole (all contraindicated concomitant uses with dofetilide) suggests that all renal cation transport inhibitors should be contraindicated.

Use with Drugs that Prolong QT Interval and Antiarrhythmic Agents

The use of TIKOSYN in conjunction with other drugs that prolong the QT interval has not been studied and is not recommended. Such drugs include phenothiazines, cisapride, bepridil, tricyclic antidepressants, and certain oral macrolides. Class I or Class III antiarrhythmic agents should be withheld for at least three half-lives prior to dosing with TIKOSYN. In clinical trials, TIKOSYN was administered to patients previously treated with oral amiodarone only if serum amiodarone levels were below 0.3 mg/L or amiodarone had been withdrawn for at least three months.

PRECAUTIONS

Renal Impairment

The overall systemic clearance of dofetilide is decreased and plasma concentration increased with decreasing creatinine clearance. The dose of TIKOSYN must be adjusted based on creatinine clearance (see **DOSAGE AND ADMINISTRATION**). Patients undergoing dialysis were not included in clinical studies, and appropriate dosing recommendations for these patients are unknown. There is no information about the effectiveness of hemodialysis in removing dofetilide from plasma.

Hepatic Impairment

After adjustment for creatinine clearance, no additional dose adjustment is required for patients with mild or moderate hepatic impairment. Patients with severe hepatic impairment have not been studied. TIKOSYN should be used with particular caution in these patients.

Cardiac Conduction Disturbances

Animal and human studies have not shown any adverse effects of dofetilide on conduction velocity. No effect on AV nodal conduction following TIKOSYN treatment was noted in normal volunteers and in patients with 1st degree heart block. Patients with sick sinus syndrome or with 2nd or 3rd degree heart block were not included in the Phase 3 clinical trials unless a functioning pacemaker was present. TIKOSYN has been used safely in conjunction with pacemakers (53 patients in DIAMOND studies, 136 in trials in patients with ventricular and supraventricular arrhythmias).

Potassium-Depleting Diuretics

Hypokalemia or hypomagnesemia may occur with administration of potassium-depleting diuretics, increasing the potential for torsade de pointes. Potassium levels should be within the normal range prior to administration of TIKOSYN and maintained in the normal range during administration of TIKOSYN.

Information for Patients

Please refer patient to the patient package insert.

Prior to initiation of TIKOSYN therapy, the patient should be advised to read the patient package insert and reread it each time therapy is renewed in case the patient's status has changed. The patient should be fully instructed on the need for compliance with the recommended dosing of TIKOSYN and the potential for drug interactions, and the need for periodic monitoring of QTc and renal function to minimize the risk of serious abnormal rhythms.

Medications and Supplements: Assessment of patients' medication history should include all over-the-counter, prescription and herbal/natural preparations with emphasis on preparations that may affect the pharmacokinetics of TIKOSYN such as cimetidine (see **CONTRAINDICATIONS**), trimethoprim alone or in combination with sulfamethoxazole (see **CONTRAINDICATIONS**), prochlorperazine (see **CONTRAINDICATIONS**), megestrol (see **CONTRAINDICATIONS**), ketoconazole (see **CONTRAINDICATIONS**), other cardiovascular drugs (especially verapamil—see **CONTRAINDICATIONS**), phenothiazines, and tricyclic antidepressants (see **WARNINGS**). If a patient is taking TIKOSYN and requires anti-ulcer therapy, omeprazole, ranitidine or antacids (aluminum and magnesium hydroxides) should be used as alternatives to cimetidine, as these agents have no effect on the pharmacokinetics of TIKOSYN. Patients should be instructed to notify their health care providers of any change in over-the-counter, prescription or supplement use. If a patient is hospitalized or is prescribed a new medication for any condition, the patient must inform the health care provider of ongoing TIKOSYN therapy. Patients should also check with their health care provider and/or pharmacist prior to taking a new over-the-counter preparation.

Electrolyte Imbalance: If patients experience symptoms that may be associated with altered electrolyte balance, such as excessive or prolonged diarrhea, sweating, or vomiting or loss of appetite or thirst, these conditions should immediately be reported to their health care provider.

Dosing Schedule: Patients should be instructed NOT to double the next dose if a dose is missed. The next dose should be taken at the usual time.

Drug/Laboratory Test Interactions

None known.

Drug-Drug Interactions

Cimetidine: (see **CONTRAINDICATIONS**) Concomitant use of cimetidine is contraindicated. Cimetidine at 400 mg BID (the usual prescription dose) co-administered with TIKOSYN (500 mcg BID) for 7 days has been shown to increase dofetilide plasma levels by 58%. Cimetidine at doses of 100 mg BID (OTC dose) resulted in a 13% increase in dofetilide plasma levels (500 mcg single dose). No studies have been conducted at intermediate doses of cimetidine. If a patient requires TIKOSYN and anti-ulcer therapy, it is suggested that omeprazole, ranitidine, or antacids (aluminum and magnesium hydroxides) be used as alternatives to cimetidine, as these agents have no effect on the pharmacokinetic profile of TIKOSYN.

Verapamil: (see **CONTRAINDICATIONS**) Concomitant use of verapamil is contraindicated. Co-administration of TIKOSYN with verapamil resulted in increases in dofetilide peak plasma levels of 42%, although overall exposure to dofetilide was not significantly increased. In an analysis of the supraventricular arrhythmia and DIAMOND patient populations, the concomitant administration of verapamil with dofetilide was associated with a higher occurrence of torsade de pointes.

Ketoconazole: (see **CONTRAINDICATIONS**) Concomitant use of ketoconazole is contraindicated. Ketoconazole at 400 mg daily (the maximum approved prescription dose) co-administered with TIKOSYN (500 mcg BID) for 7 days has been shown to increase dofetilide Cmax by 53% in males and 97% in females, and AUC by 41% in males and 69% in females.

Trimethoprim Alone or in Combination with Sulfamethoxazole: (see **CONTRAINDICATIONS**) Concomitant use of trimethoprim alone or in combination with sulfamethoxazole is contraindicated. Trimethoprim 160 mg in combination with 800 mg sulfamethoxazole co-administered BID with TIKOSYN (500 mcg BID) for 4 days has been shown to increase dofetilide AUC by 103% and Cmax by 93%.

Potential Drug Interactions

Dofetilide is eliminated in the kidney by cationic secretion. Inhibitors of renal cationic secretion are contraindicated with TIKOSYN. In addition, drugs that are actively secreted via this route (e.g., triamterene, metformin and amiloride) should be co-administered with care as they might increase dofetilide levels.

Dofetilide is metabolized to a small extent by the CYP3A4 isoenzyme of the cytochrome P450 system. Inhibitors of the CYP3A4 isoenzyme could increase systemic dofetilide exposure. Inhibitors of this isoenzyme (e.g., macrolide antibiotics, azole antifungal agents, protease inhibitors, serotonin reuptake inhibitors, amiodarone, cannabinoids, diltiazem, grapefruit juice, nefazadone, norfloxacin, quinine, zafirlukast) should be cautiously coadministered with TIKOSYN as they can potentially increase dofetilide levels. Dofetilide is not an inhibitor of CYP3A4 nor of other cytochrome P450 isoenzymes (e.g., CYP2C9, CYP2D6) and is not expected to increase levels of drugs metabolized by CYP3A4.

Other Drug Interaction Information

Digoxin: Studies in healthy volunteers have shown that TIKOSYN does not affect the pharmacokinetics of digoxin. In patients, the concomitant administration of digoxin with dofetilide was associated with a higher occurrence of torsade de pointes. It is not clear whether this represents an interaction with TIKOSYN or the presence of more severe structural heart disease in patients on digoxin; structural heart disease is a known risk factor for arrhythmia. No increase in mortality was observed in patients taking digoxin as concomitant medication.

Other Drugs: In healthy volunteers, amlodipine, phenytoin, glyburide, ranitidine, omeprazole, hormone replacement therapy (a combination of conjugated estrogens and medroxyprogesterone), antacid (aluminum and magnesium

Table 6: Incidence of Serious Arrhythmias and Conduction Disturbances in Patients with Supraventricular Arrhythmias

	TIKOSYN Dose				Placebo
Arrhythmia event:	<250 mcg BID N=217	250 mcg BID N=388	>250-500 mcg BID N=703	>500 mcg BID N=38	N=677
Ventricular arrhythmias* ^	3.7%	2.6%	3.4%	15.8%	2.7%
Ventricular fibrillation	0	0.3%	0.4%	2.6%	0.1%
Ventricular tachycardia^	3.7%	2.6%	3.3%	13.2%	2.5%
Torsade de pointes	0	0.3%	0.9%	10.5%	0
Various forms of block					
AV block	0.9%	1.5%	0.4%	0	0.3%
Bundle branch block	0	0.5%	0.1%	0	0.1%
Heart block	0	0.5%	0.1%	0	0.1%

* Patients with more than one arrhythmia are counted only once in this category.

^ Ventricular arrhythmias and ventricular tachycardia include all cases of torsade de pointes.

Table 7: Incidence of Serious Arrhythmias and Conduction Disturbances in Patients with AF at Entry to the DIAMOND Studies

	TIKOSYN	Placebo
	N=249	N=257
Ventricular arrhythmias*^	14.5%	13.6%
Ventricular fibrillation	4.8%	3.1%
Ventricular tachycardia^	12.4%	11.3%
Torsade de pointes	1.6%	0
Various forms of block		
AV block	0.8%	2.7%
(Left) bundle branch block	0	0.4%
Heart block	1.2%	0.8%

* Patients with more than one arrhythmia are counted only once in this category.

^ Ventricular arrhythmias and ventricular tachycardia include all cases of torsade de pointes.

hydroxides) and theophylline did not affect the pharmacokinetics of TIKOSYN. In addition, studies in healthy volunteers have shown that TIKOSYN does not affect the pharmacokinetics or pharmacodynamics of warfarin, or the pharmacokinetics of propranolol (40 mg twice daily), phenytoin, theophylline, or oral contraceptives.

Population pharmacokinetic analyses were conducted on plasma concentration data from 1445 patients in clinical trials to examine the effects of concomitant medications on clearance or volume of distribution of dofetilide. Concomitant medications were grouped as ACE inhibitors, oral anticoagulants, calcium channel blockers, beta blockers, cardiac glycosides, inducers of CYP3A4, substrates and inhibitors of CYP3A4, substrates and inhibitors of P-glycoprotein, nitrates, sulphonylureas, loop diuretics, potassium sparing diuretics, thiazide diuretics, substrates and inhibitors of tubular organic cation transport, and QTc-prolonging drugs. Differences in clearance between patients on these medications (at any occasion in the study) and those off medications varied between -16% and +3%. The mean clearances of dofetilide were 16% and 15% lower in patients on thiazide diuretics and inhibitors of tubular organic cation transport, respectively.

Carcinogenesis, Mutagenesis, Impairment of Fertility

Dofetilide had no genotoxic effects, with or without metabolic activation, based on the bacterial mutation assay and tests of cytogenetic aberrations *in vivo* in mouse bone marrow and *in vitro* in human lymphocytes. Rats and mice treated with dofetilide in the diet for two years showed no evidence of an increased incidence of tumors compared to controls. The highest dofetilide dose administered for 24 months was 10 mg/kg/day to rats and 20 mg/kg/day to mice. Mean dofetilide AUCs$_{(0-24hr)}$ at these doses were about 26 and 10 times, respectively, the maximum likely human AUC.

There was no effect on mating or fertility when dofetilide was administered to male and female rats at doses as high as 1.0 mg/kg/day, a dose that would be expected to provide a mean dofetilide AUC $_{(0-24hr)}$ about 3 times the maximum likely human AUC. Increased incidences of testicular atrophy and epididymal oligospermia and a reduction in testicular weight were, however, observed in other studies in rats. Reduced testicular weight and increased incidence of testicular atrophy were also consistent findings in dogs and mice. The no effect doses for these findings in chronic administration studies in these 3 species (3, 0.1 and 6 mg/kg/day) were associated with mean dofetilide AUCs that were about 4, 1.3 and 3 times the maximum likely human AUC, respectively.

Pregnancy Category C

Dofetilide has been shown to adversely affect *in utero* growth and survival of rats and mice when orally administered during organogenesis at doses of 2 or more mg/kg/day.

Other than an increased incidence of non-ossified 5th metacarpal, and the occurrence of hydroureter and hydronephroses at doses as low as 1 mg/kg/day in the rat, structural anomalies associated with drug treatment were not observed in either species at doses below 2 mg/kg/day. The clearest drug-effect associations were for sternebral and vertebral anomalies in both species; cleft palate, adactyly, levocardia, dilation of cerebral ventricles, hydroureter, hydronephroses, and unossified metacarpal in the rat; and increased incidence of unossified calcaneum in the mouse. The "no observed adverse effect dose" in both species was 0.5 mg/kg/day. The mean dofetilide AUCs$_{(0-24hr)}$ at this dose in the rat and mouse are estimated to be about equal to the maximum likely human AUC and about half the likely human AUC, respectively. There are no adequate and well controlled studies in pregnant women. Therefore, dofetilide should only be administered to pregnant women where the benefit to the patient justifies the potential risk to the fetus.

Nursing Mothers

There is no information on the presence of dofetilide in breast milk. Patients should be advised not to breast feed an infant if they are taking TIKOSYN.

Geriatric Use

Of the total number of patients in clinical studies of TIKOSYN, 46% were 65 to 89 years old. No overall differences in safety, effect on QTc, or effectiveness were observed between elderly and younger patients. Because elderly patients are more likely to have decreased renal function with a reduced creatinine clearance, care must be taken in dose selection. (See **DOSAGE AND ADMINISTRATION**.)

Use in Women

Female patients constituted 32% of the patients in the placebo-controlled trials of TIKOSYN. As with other drugs that cause torsade de pointes, TIKOSYN was associated with a greater risk of torsade de pointes in female patients than in male patients. During the TIKOSYN clinical development program the risk of torsade de pointes in females was approximately 3 times the risk in males. Unlike torsade de pointes, the incidence of other ventricular arrhythmias was similar in female patients receiving TIKOSYN and patients receiving placebo. Although no study specifically investigated this risk, in post-hoc analyses, no increased mortality was observed in females on TIKOSYN compared to females on placebo.

Pediatric Use

The safety and effectiveness of TIKOSYN in children (<18 years old) has not been established.

ADVERSE REACTIONS

The TIKOSYN clinical program involved approximately 8,600 patients in 130 clinical studies of normal volunteers and patients with supraventricular and ventricular arrhythmias. TIKOSYN was administered to 5,194 patients,

Continued on next page

Tikosyn—Cont.

including two large, placebo-controlled mortality trials (DIAMOND CHF and DIAMOND MI) in which 1,511 patients received TIKOSYN for up to three years.

In the following section, adverse reaction data for cardiac arrhythmias and non-cardiac adverse reactions are presented separately for patients included in the supraventricular arrhythmia development program and for patients included in the DIAMOND CHF and MI mortality trials (see **CLINICAL STUDIES: Safety in Patients with Structural Heart Disease—DIAMOND Studies**, for a description of these trials).

In studies of patients with supraventricular arrhythmias a total of 1346 and 677 patients were exposed to TIKOSYN and placebo for 551 and 207 patient years, respectively. A total of 8.7% of patients in the dofetilide groups were discontinued from clinical trials due to adverse events compared to 8.0% in the placebo groups. The most frequent reason for discontinuation (>1%) was ventricular tachycardia (2.0% on dofetilide vs. 1.3% on placebo). The most frequent adverse events were headache, chest pain, and dizziness.

Serious Arrhythmias and Conduction Disturbances: Torsade de pointes is the only arrhythmia that showed a dose-response relationship to TIKOSYN treatment. It did not occur in placebo treated patients. The incidence of torsade de pointes in patients with supraventricular arrhythmias was 0.8% (11/1346) (see **WARNINGS**). The incidence of torsade de pointes in patients who were dosed according to the recommended dosing regimen (see **DOSAGE AND ADMINISTRATION**) was 0.8% (4/525). Table 6 shows the frequency by randomized dose of serious arrhythmias and conduction disturbances reported as adverse events in patients with supraventricular arrhythmias.

[See table 6 at top of previous page]

In the DIAMOND trials a total of 1511 patients were exposed to TIKOSYN for 1757 patient years. The incidence of torsade de pointes was 3.3% in CHF patients and 0.9% in patients with a recent MI.

Table 7 shows the incidence of serious arrhythmias and conduction disturbances reported as adverse events in the DIAMOND subpopulation that had AF at entry to these trials.

[See table 7 at top of previous page]

Other Adverse Reactions: Table 8 presents other adverse events reported with a frequency of >2% on TIKOSYN and reported numerically more frequently on TIKOSYN than on placebo in the studies of patients with supraventricular arrhythmias.

Table 8: Frequency of Adverse Events Occurring at >2% on TIKOSYN, and Numerically More Frequently on TIKOSYN than Placebo in Patients with Supraventricular Arrhythmias

	TIKOSYN	Placebo
Adverse Event	%	%
headache	11	9
chest pain	10	7
dizziness	8	6
respiratory tract infection	7	5
dyspnea	6	5
nausea	5	4
flu syndrome	4	2
insomnia	4	3
accidental injury	3	1
back pain	3	2
procedure (medical/surgical/health service)	3	2
diarrhea	3	2
rash	3	2
abdominal pain	3	2

Adverse events reported at a rate >2% but no more frequently on TIKOSYN than on placebo were: angina pectoris, anxiety, arthralgia, asthenia, atrial fibrillation, complications (application, injection, incision, insertion, or device), hypertension, pain, palpitation, peripheral edema, supraventricular tachycardia, sweating, urinary tract infection, ventricular tachycardia.

The following adverse events have been reported with a frequency of ≤2% and numerically more frequently with TIKOSYN than placebo in patients with supraventricular arrhythmias: angioedema, bradycardia, cerebral ischemia, cerebrovascular accident, edema, facial paralysis, flaccid paralysis, heart arrest, increased cough, liver damage, migraine, myocardial infarct, paralysis, paresthesia, sudden death, and syncope.

The incidences of clinically significant laboratory test abnormalities in patients with supraventricular arrhythmias were similar for patients on TIKOSYN and those on placebo. No clinically relevant effects were noted in serum alkaline phosphatase, serum GGT, LDH, AST, ALT, total bilirubin, total protein, blood urea nitrogen, creatinine, serum electrolytes (calcium, chloride, glucose, magnesium, potassium, sodium) or creatine kinase. Similarly, no clinically relevant effects were observed in hematologic parameters.

In the DIAMOND population, adverse events other than those related to the post-infarction and heart failure patient population were generally similar to those seen in the supraventricular arrhythmia groups.

OVERDOSAGE

There is no known antidote to TIKOSYN; treatment of overdose should therefore be symptomatic and supportive. The most prominent manifestation of overdosage is likely to be excessive prolongation of the QT interval.

In cases of overdose cardiac monitoring should be initiated. Charcoal slurry may be given soon after overdosing but has been useful only when given within 15 minutes of TIKOSYN administration. Treatment of torsade de pointes or overdose may include administration of isoproterenol infusion, with or without cardiac pacing. Administration of intravenous magnesium sulfate may be effective in the management of torsade de pointes. Close medical monitoring and supervision should continue until the QT interval returns to normal levels.

Isoproterenol infusion into anesthetized dogs with cardiac pacing rapidly attenuates the dofetilide-induced prolongation of atrial and ventricular effective refractory periods in a dose-dependent manner. Magnesium sulfate, administered prophylactically either intravenously or orally in a dog model, was effective in the prevention of dofetilide-induced torsade de pointes ventricular tachycardia. Similarly, in man, intravenous magnesium sulfate may terminate torsade de pointes, irrespective of cause.

TIKOSYN overdose was rare in clinical studies; there were two reported cases of TIKOSYN overdose in the oral clinical program. One patient received very high multiples of the recommended dose (28 capsules), was treated with gastric aspiration 30 minutes later, and experienced no events. One patient inadvertently received two 500 mcg doses one hour apart and experienced ventricular fibrillation and cardiac arrest 2 hours after the second dose.

In the supraventricular arrhythmia population only 38 patients received doses greater than 500 mcg BID, all of whom received 750 mcg BID irrespective of creatinine clearance. In this very small patient population the incidence of torsade de pointes was 10.5% (4/38 patients), and the incidence of new ventricular fibrillation was 2.6% (1/38 patients).

DOSAGE AND ADMINISTRATION

- Therapy with TIKOSYN must be initiated (and, if necessary, re-initiated) in a setting that provides continuous electrocardiographic (ECG) monitoring and in the presence of personnel trained in the management of serious ventricular arrhythmias. Patients should continue to be monitored in this way for a minimum of three days. Additionally, patients should not be discharged within 12 hours of electrical or pharmacological conversion to normal sinus rhythm.
- **The dose of TIKOSYN must be individualized according to calculated creatinine clearance and QTc. (QT interval should be used if the heart rate is <60 beats per minute. There are no data on use of TIKOSYN when the heart rate is <50 beats per minute.)** The usual recommended dose of TIKOSYN is 500 mcg BID, as modified by the dosing algorithm described below. For consideration of a lower dose, see **Special Considerations** below.
- Patients with atrial fibrillation should be anticoagulated according to usual medical practice prior to electrical or pharmacological cardioversion. Anticoagulant therapy may be continued after cardioversion according to usual medical practice for the treatment of people with AF. Hypokalemia should be corrected before initiation of TIKOSYN therapy (see **WARNINGS, Ventricular Arrhythmia**).
- Patients to be discharged on TIKOSYN therapy from an in-patient setting as described above must have an adequate supply of TIKOSYN, at the patient's individualized dose, to allow uninterrupted dosing until the patient receives the first outpatient supply.
- TIKOSYN is distributed only to those hospitals and other appropriate institutions confirmed to have received applicable dosing and treatment initiation education programs. Inpatient and subsequent outpatient discharge and refill prescriptions are filled only upon confirmation that the prescribing physician has received applicable dosing and treatment initiation education programs. For this purpose, a list for use by pharmacists is maintained containing hospitals and physicians who have received one of the education programs.

Instructions for Individualized Dose Initiation

Initiation of TIKOSYN Therapy

Step 1. Electrocardiographic assessment: Prior to administration of the first dose, the QTc must be determined using an average of 5–10 beats. If the QTc is greater than 440 msec (500 msec in patients with ventricular conduction abnormalities), TIKOSYN is contraindicated. If heart rate is less than 60 beats per minute, QT interval should be used. Patients with heart rates <50 beats per minute have not been studied.

$$\text{creatinine clearance (male)} = \frac{(140\text{-age}) \times \text{body weight in kg}}{72 \times \text{serum creatinine (mg/dL)}}$$

$$\text{creatinine clearance (female)} = \frac{(140\text{-age}) \times \text{body weight in kg} \times 0.85}{72 \times \text{serum creatinine (mg/dL)}}$$

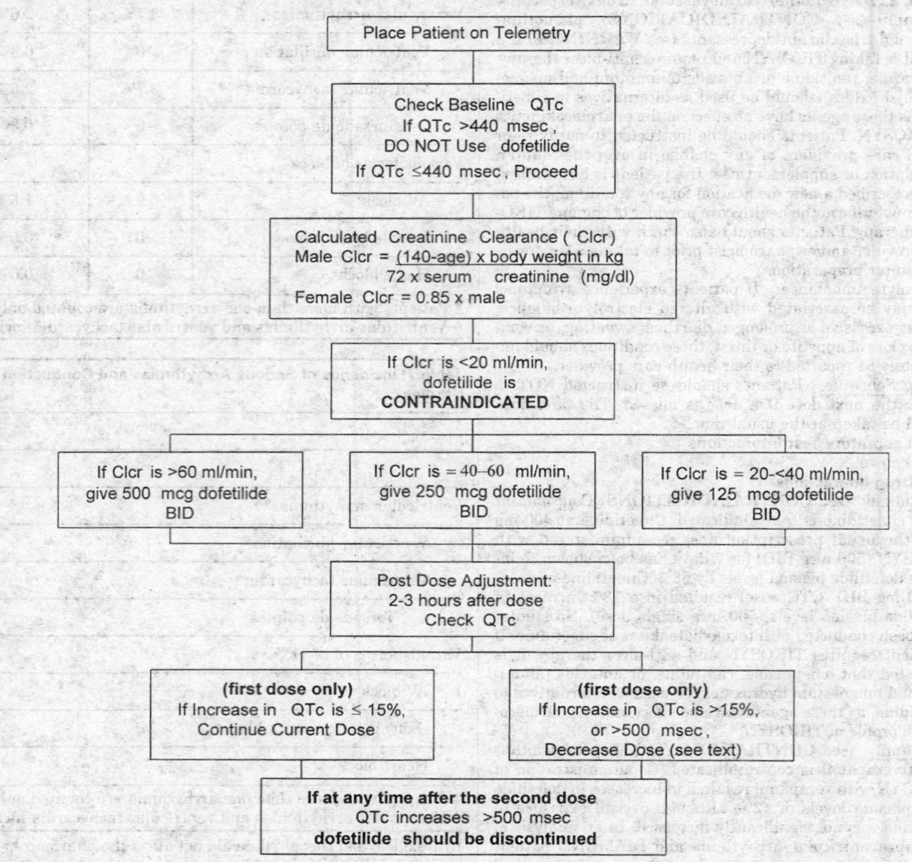

	125 mcg (0.125 mg)	250 mcg (0.25 mg)	500 mcg (0.5 mg)
Observe:	TKN 125	TKN 250	TKN 500
Reverse	PFIZER	PFIZER	PFIZER
Bottle of 14	0069-5800-61	0069-5810-61	0069-5820-61
Bottle of 60	0069-5800-60	0069-5810-60	0069-5820-60
Unit dose / 40	0069-5800-43	0069-5810-43	0069-5820-43

Step 2. Calculation of creatinine clearance: Prior to the administration of the first dose, the patient's creatinine clearance must be calculated using the following formula:
[See table at top of previous page]
When serum creatinine is given in μmol/L, divide the value by 88.4 (1 mg/dL = 88.4 μmol/L).
Step 3. Starting Dose: The starting dose of TIKOSYN is determined as follows:

Calculated Creatinine Clearance	TIKOSYN Dose
>60 mL/min	500 mcg twice daily
40–60 mL/min	250 mcg twice daily
20–<40 mL/min	125 mcg twice daily
<20 mL/min	Dofetilide is contraindicated in these patients

Step 4. Administer the adjusted TIKOSYN dose and begin continuous ECG monitoring.
Step 5. At 2–3 hours after administering the first dose of TIKOSYN, determine the QTc. If the QTc has increased by greater than 15% compared to the baseline established in Step 1 OR if the QTc is greater than 500 msec (550 msec in patients with ventricular conduction abnormalities), subsequent dosing should be adjusted as follows:

If the Starting Dose Based on Creatinine Clearance is:	Then the Adjusted Dose (for QTc Prolongation) is:
500 mcg twice daily	250 mcg twice daily
250 mcg twice daily	125 mcg twice daily
125 mcg twice daily	125 mcg once a day

Step 6. At 2–3 hours after each subsequent dose of TIKOSYN, determine the QTc (for in-hospital doses 2–5). No further down titration of TIKOSYN based on QTc is recommended.
NOTE: If at any time after the second dose of TIKOSYN is given, the QTc is greater than 500 msec (550 msec in patients with ventricular conduction abnormalities) TIKOSYN should be discontinued.
Step 7. Patients are to be continuously monitored by ECG for a minimum of three days, or for a minimum of 12 hours after electrical or pharmacological conversion to normal sinus rhythm, whichever is greater.
The steps described above are summarized in the following diagram:
[See graphic at top of previous page]

Maintenance of TIKOSYN Therapy
Renal function and QTc should be re-evaluated every three months or as medically warranted. If QTc exceeds 500 milliseconds (550 msec in patients with ventricular conduction abnormalities), TIKOSYN therapy should be discontinued and patients should be carefully monitored until QTc returns to baseline levels. If renal function deteriorates, adjust dose as described in **Initiation of TIKOSYN Therapy, Step 3.**

Special Considerations
Consideration of a Dose Lower than that Determined by the Algorithm: The dosing algorithm shown above should be used to determine the individualized dose of TIKOSYN. In clinical trials (see **CLINICAL STUDIES**), the highest dose of 500 mcg BID of TIKOSYN as modified by the dosing algorithm led to greater effectiveness than lower doses of 125 or 250 mcg BID as modified by the dosing algorithm. The risk of torsade de pointes, however, is related to dose as well as to patient characteristics (see **WARNINGS**). Physicians, in consultation with their patients, may therefore in some cases choose doses lower than determined by the algorithm. It is critically important that if at any time this lower dose is increased, the patient needs to be rehospitalized for three days. Previous toleration of higher doses does not eliminate the need for rehospitalization.
The maximum recommended dose in patients with a calculated creatinine clearance greater than 60 mL/min is 500 mcg BID; doses greater than 500 mcg BID have been associated with an increased incidence of torsade de pointes.
A patient who misses a dose should NOT double the next dose. The next dose should be taken at the usual time.
Cardioversion: If patients do not convert to normal sinus rhythm within 24 hours of initiation of TIKOSYN therapy, electrical conversion should be considered. Patients continuing on TIKOSYN after successful electrical cardioversion should continue to be monitored by electrocardiography for 12 hours post cardioversion, or a minimum of 3 days after initiation of TIKOSYN therapy, whichever is greater.

Switch to TIKOSYN from Class I or other Class III Antiarrhythmic Therapy
Before initiating TIKOSYN therapy, previous antiarrhythmic therapy should be withdrawn under careful monitoring for a minimum of three (3) plasma half-lives. Because of the unpredictable pharmacokinetics of amiodarone, TIKOSYN should not be initiated following amiodarone therapy until amiodarone plasma levels are below 0.3 mcg/mL or until amiodarone has been withdrawn for at least three months.

Stopping TIKOSYN Prior to Administration of Potentially Interacting Drugs
If TIKOSYN needs to be discontinued to allow dosing of other potentially interacting drug(s), a washout period of at least two days should be followed before starting the other drug(s).

HOW SUPPLIED
TIKOSYN™ 125 mcg (0.125 mg) capsules are supplied as No. 4 capsules with a light orange cap and white body, printed with TKN 125 PFIZER, and are available in:
TIKOSYN 250 mcg (0.25 mg) capsules are supplied as No. 4 capsules, peach cap and body, printed with TKN 250 PFIZER, and are available in:
TIKOSYN 500 mcg (0.5 mg) capsules are supplied as No. 2 capsules, peach cap and white body, printed with TKN 500 PFIZER, and are available in:
[See table above]
Store at controlled room temperature, 15° to 30°C (59° to 86°F).
PROTECT FROM MOISTURE AND HUMIDITY.
Dispense in tight containers (USP).
Rx only
Pfizer Labs
Division of Pfizer Inc, NY, NY 10017
69-5549-00-2 Issued December 1999
Shown in Product Identification Guide, page 330

TROVAN® Tablets ℞
[trō-văn]
(trovafloxacin mesylate)
TROVAN® I.V. ℞
(alatrofloxacin mesylate injection)
For Intravenous Infusion

TROVAN® HAS BEEN ASSOCIATED WITH SERIOUS LIVER INJURY LEADING TO LIVER TRANSPLANTATION AND/OR DEATH. TROVAN-ASSOCIATED LIVER INJURY HAS BEEN REPORTED WITH BOTH SHORT-TERM AND LONG-TERM DRUG EXPOSURE. TROVAN USE EXCEEDING 2 WEEKS IN DURATION IS ASSOCIATED WITH A SIGNIFICANTLY INCREASED RISK OF SERIOUS LIVER INJURY. LIVER INJURY HAS ALSO BEEN REPORTED FOLLOWING TROVAN RE-EXPOSURE. TROVAN SHOULD BE RESERVED FOR USE IN PATIENTS WITH SERIOUS, LIFE- OR LIMB-THREATENING INFECTIONS WHO RECEIVE THEIR INITIAL THERAPY IN AN IN-PATIENT HEALTH CARE FACILITY (I.E., HOSPITAL OR LONG-TERM NURSING CARE FACILITY). TROVAN SHOULD NOT BE USED WHEN SAFER, ALTERNATIVE ANTIMICROBIAL THERAPY WILL BE EFFECTIVE. (SEE WARNINGS.)

TROVAN® is available as TROVAN Tablets (trovafloxacin mesylate) for oral administration and as TROVAN I.V. (alatrofloxacin mesylate injection), a prodrug of trovafloxacin, for intravenous administration.

DESCRIPTION

TROVAN Tablets
TROVAN Tablets contain trovafloxacin mesylate, a synthetic broad-spectrum antibacterial agent for oral administration. Chemically, trovafloxacin mesylate, a fluoronaphthyridone related to the fluoroquinolone antibacterials, is (1α, 5α, 6α)-7-(6-amino-3-azabicyclo[3.1.0]hex-3-yl)-1-(2,4-difluorophenyl)-6-fluoro-1,4-dihydro-4-oxo-1,8-naphthyridine-3-carboxylic acid, monomethanesulfonate. Trovafloxacin mesylate differs from other quinolone derivatives by having a 1,8-naphthyridine nucleus.
The chemical structure is:

Its empirical formula is $C_{20}H_{15}F_3N_4O_3 \cdot CH_3SO_3H$ and its molecular weight is 512.46.
Trovafloxacin mesylate is a white to off-white powder.
Trovafloxacin mesylate is available in 100 mg and 200 mg (trovafloxacin equivalent) blue, film-coated tablets. TROVAN Tablets contain microcrystalline cellulose, cross-linked sodium carboxymethylcellulose and magnesium stearate. The tablet coating is a mixture of hydroxypropylcellulose, hydroxypropylmethylcellulose, titanium dioxide, polyethylene glycol and FD&C blue #2 aluminum lake.

TROVAN I.V.
TROVAN I.V. contains alatrofloxacin mesylate, the L-alanyl-L-alanyl prodrug of trovafloxacin mesylate. Chemically, alatrofloxacin mesylate is (1α, 5α, 6α)-L-alanyl-*N*-[3-[6-carboxy-8-(2,4-difluorophenyl)-3-fluoro-5,8-dihydro-5-oxo-1,8-naphthyridine-2-yl]-3-azabicyclo[3.1.0]hex-6-yl]-L-alaninamide, monomethanesulfonate. It is intended for administration by intravenous infusion.
Following intravenous administration, the alanine substituents in alatrofloxacin are rapidly hydrolyzed *in vivo* to yield trovafloxacin. (See **CLINICAL PHARMACOLOGY**.)
The chemical structure is:

Its empirical formula is $C_{26}H_{25}F_3N_6O_5 \bullet CH_3SO_3H$ and its molecular weight is 654.62.
Alatrofloxacin mesylate is a white to light yellow powder.
TROVAN I.V. is available in 40 mL and 60 mL single use vials as a sterile, preservative-free aqueous concentrate of 5 mg trovafloxacin/mL as alatrofloxacin mesylate intended for dilution prior to intravenous administration of doses of 200 mg or 300 mg of trovafloxacin, respectively. (See **HOW SUPPLIED**.)
The formulation contains Water for Injection, and may contain sodium hydroxide or hydrochloric acid for pH adjustment. The pH range for the 5 mg/mL aqueous concentrate is 3.5 to 4.3.

CLINICAL PHARMACOLOGY
After intravenous administration, alatrofloxacin is rapidly converted to trovafloxacin. Plasma concentrations of alatrofloxacin are below quantifiable levels within 5 to 10 minutes of completion of a 1 hour infusion.

Absorption
Trovafloxacin is well-absorbed from the gastrointestinal tract after oral administration. The absolute bioavailability is approximately 88%. For comparable dosages, no dosage adjustment is necessary when switching from parenteral to oral administration (Figure 1). (See **DOSAGE AND ADMINISTRATION**.)

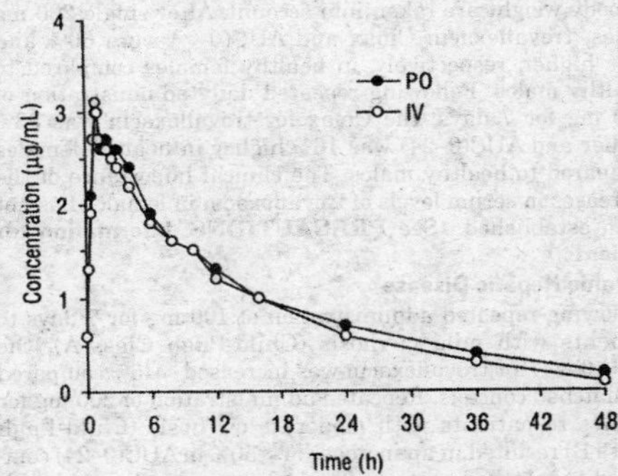

Figure 1. Mean trovafloxacin serum concentrations determined following 1 hour intravenous infusions of alatrofloxacin at daily doses of 200 mg (trovafloxacin equivalents) to healthy male volunteers and following daily oral administration of 200 mg trovafloxacin for 7 days to six male and six female healthy young volunteers.

Pharmacokinetics
The mean pharmacokinetic parameters (±SD) of trovafloxacin after single and multiple 100 mg and 200 mg oral doses and 1 hour intravenous infusions of alatrofloxacin in doses of 200 and 300 mg (trovafloxacin equivalents) appear in the chart below.
[See first table at top of next page]
Serum concentrations of trovafloxacin are dose-proportional after oral administration of trovafloxacin in the dose range of 30 to 1000 mg or after intravenous administration of alatrofloxacin in the dose range of 30 to 400 mg (trovafloxacin equivalents). Steady state concentrations are achieved by the third daily oral or intravenous dose of trovafloxacin with an accumulation factor of approximately 1.3 times the single dose concentrations.
Oral absorption of trovafloxacin is not altered by concomitant food intake; therefore, it can be administered without regard to food.
The systemic exposure to trovafloxacin ($AUC_{0-\infty}$) administered as crushed tablets via nasogastric tube into the stomach was identical to that of orally administered intact tab-

Continued on next page

Trovan—Cont.

lets. Administration of concurrent enteral feeding solutions had no effect on the absorption of trovafloxacin given via nasogastric tube into the stomach. When trovafloxacin was administered as crushed tablets into the duodenum via nasogastric tube, the $AUC_{0-\infty}$ and peak serum concentration (C_{max}) were reduced by 30% relative to the orally administered intact tablets. Time to peak serum level (T_{max}) was also decreased from 1.7 hrs to 1.1 hrs.

Distribution

The mean plasma protein bound fraction is approximately 76%, and is concentration-independent. Trovafloxacin is widely distributed throughout the body. Rapid distribution of trovafloxacin into tissues results in significantly higher trovafloxacin concentrations in most target tissues than in plasma or serum.

[See second table at right]

Presence in Breast Milk

Trovafloxacin was found in measurable concentrations in the breast milk of three lactating subjects. The average measurable breast milk concentration was 0.8 µg/mL (range: 0.3–2.1 µg/mL) after single I.V. alatrofloxacin (300 mg trovafloxacin equivalents) and repeated oral trovafloxacin (200 mg) doses.

Metabolism

Trovafloxacin is metabolized by conjugation (the role of cytochrome P_{450} oxidative metabolism of trovafloxacin is minimal). Thirteen percent of the administered dose appears in the urine in the form of the ester glucuronide and 9% appears in the feces as the N-acetyl metabolite (2.5% of the dose is found in the serum as the active N-acetyl metabolite). Other minor metabolites (diacid, sulfamate, hydroxycarboxylic acid) have been identified in both urine and feces in small amounts (<4% of the administered dose).

Excretion

Approximately 50% of an oral dose is excreted unchanged (43% in the feces and 6% in the urine).

After multiple 200 mg doses, to healthy subjects, mean (±SD) cumulative urinary trovafloxacin concentrations were 12.1±3.4 µg/mL. With these levels of trovafloxacin in urine, crystals of trovafloxacin have not been observed in the urine of human subjects.

Special Populations

Geriatric

In adult subjects, the pharmacokinetics of trovafloxacin are not affected by age (range 19–78 years).

Pediatric

Limited information is available in the pediatric population (see **Distribution**). The pharmacokinetics of trovafloxacin have not been fully characterized in pediatric populations less than 18 years of age.

Gender

There are no significant differences in trovafloxacin pharmacokinetics between males and females when differences in body weight are taken into account. After single 200 mg doses, trovafloxacin Cmax and AUC(0–∞) were 60% and 32% higher, respectively, in healthy females compared to healthy males. Following repeated daily administration of 200 mg for 7 days, the Cmax for trovafloxacin was 38% higher and AUC(0–24) was 16% higher in healthy females compared to healthy males. The clinical importance of the increases in serum levels of trovafloxacin in females has not been established. (See **PRECAUTIONS: Information for Patients.**)

Chronic Hepatic Disease

Following repeated administration of 100 mg for 7 days to patients with mild cirrhosis (Child-Pugh Class A), the AUC(0–24) for trovafloxacin was increased ~45% compared to matched controls. Repeated administration of 200 mg for 7 days to patients with moderate cirrhosis (Child-Pugh Class B) resulted in an increase of ~50% in AUC(0–24) compared to matched controls. There appeared to be no significant effect on trovafloxacin Cmax for either group. The oral clearance of trovafloxacin was reduced ~30% in both cirrhosis groups, which corresponded to prolongation of half-life by 2–2.5 hours (25–30% increase) compared to controls. There are no data in patients with severe cirrhosis (Child-Pugh Class C). Dosage adjustment is recommended in patients with mild to moderate cirrhosis. (See **DOSAGE AND ADMINISTRATION.**)

Renal Insufficiency

The pharmacokinetics of trovafloxacin are not affected by renal impairment. Trovafloxacin serum concentrations are not significantly altered in subjects with severe renal insufficiency (creatinine clearance <20 mL/min), including patients on hemodialysis.

Photosensitivity Potential

In a study of the skin response to ultraviolet and visible radiation conducted in 48 healthy volunteers (12 per group), the minimum erythematous dose (MED) was measured for ciprofloxacin, lomefloxacin, trovafloxacin and placebo before and after drug administration for 5 days. In this study, trovafloxacin (200 mg q.d.) was shown to have a lower potential for producing delayed photosensitivity skin reactions than ciprofloxacin (500 mg b.i.d.) or lomefloxacin (400 mg q.d.), although greater than placebo. (See **PRECAUTIONS: Information for Patients.**)

Drug-drug Interactions

The systemic availability of trovafloxacin following oral tablet administration is significantly reduced by the concomitant administration of antacids containing aluminum and magnesium salts, sucralfate, vitamins or minerals containing iron, and concomitant intravenous morphine administration.

TROVAFLOXACIN PHARMACOKINETIC PARAMETERS

	C_{max} (µg/mL)	T_{max} (hrs)	$AUC^{1,2}$ (µg•h/mL)	$T_{1/2}$ (hrs)	Vd_{ss} (L/Kg)	CL (mL/hr/Kg)	CL_1 (mL/hr/Kg)
Trovafloxacin 100 mg							
Single dose	1.0±0.3	0.9±0.4	11.2±2.2	9.1	—	—	—
Multiple dose	1.1±0.2	1.0±0.5	11.8±1.8	10.5	—	—	—
Trovafloxacin 200 mg							
Single dose	2.1±0.5	1.8±0.9	26.7±7.5	9.6	—	—	—
Multiple dose	3.1±1.0	1.2±0.5	34.4±5.7	12.2	—	—	—
Alatrofloxacin 200 mg*							
Single dose	2.7±0.4	1.0±0.0	28.1±5.1	9.4	1.2±0.2	93.0±17.4	6.5±3.5
Multiple dose	3.1±0.6	1.0±0.0	32.2±7.3	11.7	1.3±0.1	81.7±17.8	8.6±2.4
Alatrofloxacin 300 mg*							
Single dose	3.6±0.6	1.3±0.4	46.1±5.2	11.2	1.2±0.1	84.6±6.0	6.9±0.5
Multiple dose	4.4±0.6	1.2±0.2	46.3±3.9	12.7	1.4±0.1	84.5±11.1	8.4±1.8

* trovafloxacin equivalents

[1,2]Single dose: AUC(0-∞), multiple dose: AUC(0-24)

C_{max}= Maximum serum concentration; T_{max}=Time to C_{max}; AUC=Area under concentration vs. time curve; $T_{1/2}$=serum half-life; Vd_{ss}=Volume of distribution; CI=Total clearance; CI_r=Renal clearance

Fluid or Tissue	Tissue-Fluid/Serum Ratio* (Range)
Respiratory	
bronchial macrophages	
(multiple dose)	24.1 (9.6–41.8)
lung mucosa	1.1 (0.7–1.5)
lung epithelial lining fluid	
(multiple dose)	5.8 (1.1–17.5)
whole lung	2.1 (0.42–5.03)
Skin, Musculoskeletal	
skin	1.0 (0.20–1.88)
subcutaneous tissue	0.4 (0.15–0.68)
skin blister fluid	0.7–0.9 (blister/plasma)
skeletal muscle	1.5 (0.50–2.90)
bone	1.0 (0.55–1.67)
Gastrointestinal	
colonic tissue	0.7 (0.0–1.47)
peritoneal fluid	0.4 (0.0–1.25)
bile	15.4 (11.9–21.0)
Central Nervous System	
cerebrospinal fluid (CSF), adults	0.25 (0.03–0.33)
cerebrospinal fluid (CSF), children	0.28**
Reproductive	
prostatic tissue	1.0 (0.5–1.6)
cervix (multiple dose)	0.6 (0.5–0.7)
ovary	1.6 (0.3–2.2)
fallopian tube	0.7 (0.2–1.1)
myometrium (multiple dose)	0.6 (0.4–0.8)
uterus	0.6 (0.3–0.8)
vaginal fluid (multiple dose)	4.7 (0.8–20.8)

*Mean values in adults over 2–29 hours following drug administration, except individual lung tissues, which were single time points of 6 hours following drug administration

**Ratio of composite AUC(0–24) in CSF/composite AUC (0–24) in serum in 22 pediatric patients aged 1 to 12 years after 1 hour I.V. infusion of single dose alatrofloxacin (equivalent trovafloxacin dose range: 4.5–9.9 mg/kg)

Administration of trovafloxacin (300 mg p.o.) 30 minutes after administration of an antacid containing magnesium hydroxide and aluminum hydroxide resulted in reductions in systemic exposure to trovafloxacin (AUC) of 66% and peak serum concentration (Cmax) of 60%. (See **PRECAUTIONS: Drug Interactions, DOSAGE AND ADMINISTRATION.**)

Concomitant sucralfate administration (1g) with trovafloxacin 200 mg p.o. resulted in a 70% decrease in trovafloxacin systemic exposure (AUC) and a 77% reduction in peak serum concentration (Cmax). (See **PRECAUTIONS: Drug Interactions, DOSAGE AND ADMINISTRATION.**)

Concomitant administration of ferrous sulfate (120 mg elemental iron) with trovafloxacin 200 mg p.o. resulted in a 40% reduction in trovafloxacin systemic exposure (AUC) and a 48% decrease in trovafloxacin Cmax. (See **PRECAUTIONS: Drug Interactions, DOSAGE AND ADMINISTRATION.**)

Concomitant administration of intravenous morphine (0.15 mg/kg) with oral trovafloxacin (200 mg) resulted in a 36% reduction in trovafloxacin AUC and a 46% decrease in trovafloxacin Cmax. Trovafloxacin administration had no effect on the pharmacokinetics of morphine or its pharmacologically active metabolite, morphine-6-b-glucuronide. (See **PRECAUTIONS: Drug Interactions, DOSAGE AND ADMINISTRATION.**)

Minor pharmacokinetic interactions that are most likely without clinical significance include calcium carbonate, omeprazole and caffeine.

Concomitant administration of calcium carbonate (1000 mg) with trovafloxacin 200 mg p.o. resulted in a 20% reduction in trovafloxacin AUC and a 17% reduction in peak serum trovafloxacin concentration (Cmax).

A 40 mg dose of omeprazole given 2 hours prior to trovafloxacin (300 mg p.o.) resulted in a 17% reduction in trovafloxacin AUC and a 17% reduction in trovafloxacin peak serum concentration (Cmax).

Administration of trovafloxacin (200 mg) concomitantly with caffeine (200 mg) resulted in a 17% increase in caffeine AUC and a 15% increase in caffeine Cmax. These changes in caffeine exposure are not considered clinically significant.

No significant pharmacokinetic interactions were seen when TROVAN was co-administered with cimetidine, theophylline, digoxin, warfarin and cyclosporine.

Cimetidine co-administration (400 mg twice daily for 5 days) with trovafloxacin (200 mg p.o. daily for 3 days) resulted in changes in trovafloxacin AUC and Cmax of less than 5%.

Trovafloxacin (200 mg p.o. daily for 7 days) co-administration with theophylline (300 mg twice daily for 14 days) resulted in no change in theophylline AUC and Cmax.

Trovafloxacin (200 mg p.o. daily for 10 days) co-administration with digoxin (0.25 mg daily for 20 days) did not significantly alter systemic exposure (AUC) to digoxin or the renal clearance of digoxin.

Trovafloxacin (200 mg p.o. daily for 7 days) did not interfere with either the pharmacokinetics or the pharmacodynamics of warfarin (daily for 21 days).

Concomitant oral administration of trovafloxacin did not affect the systemic exposure (AUC) or peak plasma concentrations (Cmax) of the S or R isomers of warfarin, nor did it influence prothrombin times. (See **PRECAUTIONS: Drug Interactions**.)

Trovafloxacin (200 mg p.o. daily for 7 days) co-administration with cyclosporine (daily doses from 150–450 mg for 7 days) resulted in decreases of 10% or less in systemic exposure to cyclosporine (AUC) and in the peak blood concentrations of cyclosporine.

Microbiology

Trovafloxacin is a fluoronaphthyridone related to the fluoroquinolones with *in vitro* activity against a wide range of gram-negative and gram-positive aerobic, and anaerobic microorganisms. The bactericidal action of trovafloxacin results from inhibition of DNA gyrase and topoisomerase IV. DNA gyrase is an essential enzyme that is involved in the replication, transcription and repair of bacterial DNA. Topoisomerase IV is an enzyme known to play a key role in the partitioning of the chromosomal DNA during bacterial cell division. Mechanism of action of fluoroquinolones including trovafloxacin is different from that of penicillins, cephalosporins, aminoglycosides, macrolides, and tetracyclines. Therefore, fluoroquinolones may be active against pathogens that are resistant to these antibiotics. There is no cross-resistance between trovafloxacin and the mentioned classes of antibiotics. The overall results obtained from *in vitro* synergy studies, testing combinations of trovafloxacin with beta-lactams and aminoglycosides, indicate that synergy is strain specific and not commonly encountered. This agrees with results obtained previously with other fluoroquinolones. Resistance to trovafloxacin *in vitro* develops slowly via multiple-step mutation in a manner similar to other fluoroquinolones. Resistance to trovafloxacin *in vitro* occurs at a general frequency of between 1×10^{-7} to 10^{-10}. Although cross-resistance has been observed between trovafloxacin and some other fluoroquinolones, some microorganisms resistant to other fluoroquinolones may be susceptible to trovafloxacin.

Trovafloxacin has been shown to be active against most strains of the following microorganisms, both *in vitro* and in clinical infections as described in the **INDICATIONS AND USAGE** section:

Aerobic gram-positive microorganisms

Enterococcus faecalis (many strains are only moderately susceptible)
Staphylococcus aureus (methicillin-susceptible strains)
Streptococcus agalactiae
Streptococcus pneumoniae (penicillin-susceptible strains)
Viridans group streptococci

Aerobic gram-negative microorganisms

Escherichia coli
Gardnerella vaginalis
Haemophilus influenzae
Klebsiella pneumoniae
Moraxella catarrhalis
Proteus mirabilis
Pseudomonas aeruginosa

Anaerobic microorganisms

Bacteroides fragilis
Peptostreptococcus species
Prevotella species

Other microorganisms

Chlamydia pneumoniae
Legionella pneumophila
Mycoplasma pneumoniae

The following *in vitro* data are available, **but their clinical significance is unknown**.

Trovafloxacin exhibits *in vitro* minimum inhibitory concentrations (MICs) of ≤2 µg/mL against most (90%) strains of the following microorganisms; however, the safety and effectiveness of trovafloxacin in treating clinical infections due to these microorganisms have not been established in adequate and well-controlled clinical trials.

Aerobic gram-positive microorganisms

Streptococcus pneumoniae (penicillin-resistant strains)

Microorganism	MIC Range (µg/mL)
Escherichia coli ATCC 25922	0.004–0.016
Staphylococcus aureus ATCC 29213	0.008–0.03
Pseudomonas aeruginosa ATCC 27853	0.25–2.0
Enterococcus faecalis ATCC 29212	0.06–0.25
Haemophilus influenzae[d] ATCC 49247	0.004–0.016
Streptococcus pneumoniae[e] ATCC 49619	0.06–0.25

[d] This quality control range is applicable to only *H. influenzae* ATCC 49247 tested by a microdilution procedure using HTM[1].
[e] This quality control range is applicable to only *S. pneumoniae* ATCC 49619 tested by a microdilution procedure using cation-adjusted Mueller-Hinton broth with 2–5% lysed horse blood.

Microorganism	Zone Diameter Range (µg/mL)
Escherichia coli ATCC 25922	29–36
Staphylococcus aureus ATCC 25923	29–35
Pseudomonas aeruginosa ATCC 27853	21–27
Haemophilus influenzae[i] ATCC 49247	32–39
Streptococcus pneumoniae[j] ATCC 49619	25–32

[i] This quality control limit applies to tests conducted with *Haemophilus influenzae* ATCC 49247 using HTM[2].
[j] This quality control range is applicable only to tests performed by disk diffusing using Mueller-Hinton agar supplemented with 5% defibrinated sheep blood.

Aerobic gram-negative microorganisms

Citrobacter freundii
Enterobacter aerogenes
Morganella morganii
Proteus vulgaris

Anaerobic microorganisms

Bacteroides distasonis
Bacteroides ovatus
Clostridium perfringens

Other microorganisms

Mycoplasma hominis
Ureaplasma urealyticum

NOTE: *Mycobacterium tuberculosis* and *Mycobacterium avium-intracellulare* complex organisms are commonly resistant to trovafloxacin.

NOTE: The activity of trovafloxacin against *Treponema pallidum* has not been evaluated; however, other quinolones are not active against *Treponema pallidum*. (See **WARNINGS**.)

Susceptibility Tests:

Dilution Techniques: Quantitative methods are used to determine antimicrobial minimum inhibitory concentrations (MICs). These MICs provide estimates of the susceptibility of bacteria to antimicrobial compounds. The MICs should be determined using a standardized procedure. Standardized procedures are based on dilution methods[1] (broth or agar) or equivalent with standardized inoculum concentrations and standardized concentrations of trovafloxacin mesylate powder. The MIC values should be interpreted according to the following criteria:

For testing non-fastidious aerobic organisms:

MIC (µg/mL)	Interpretation
≤2.0	Susceptible (S)
4.0	Intermediate (I)
≥8.0	Resistant (R)

For testing *Haemophilus* spp.[a]:

MIC (µg/mL)	Interpretation[b]
≤1.0	Susceptible (S)

[a] This interpretive standard is applicable only to broth microdilution susceptibility tests with *Haemophilus* spp. using Haemophilus Test Medium (HTM)[1].
[b] The current absence of data on resistant strains precludes defining any results other than "Susceptible". Strains yielding MIC results suggestive of a "nonsusceptible" category should be submitted to a reference laboratory for further testing.

For testing *Streptococcus* spp. including *Streptococcus pneumoniae*[c]:

MIC (µg/mL)	Interpretation
≤1.0	Susceptible (S)
2.0	Intermediate (I)
≥4.0	Resistant (R)

[c] These interpretive standards are applicable only to broth microdilution susceptibility tests using cation-adjusted Mueller-Hinton broth with 2–5% lysed horse blood.

A report of "Susceptible" indicates that the pathogen is likely to be inhibited if the antimicrobial compound in the blood reaches the concentration usually achievable. A report of "Intermediate" indicates that the result should be considered equivocal, and, if the microorganism is not fully susceptible to alternative, clinically feasible drugs, the test should be repeated. This category implies possible clinical applicability in body sites where the drug is physiologically concentrated or in situations where high dosage of drug can be used. This category also provides a buffer zone which prevents small uncontrolled technical factors from causing major discrepancies in interpretation. A report of "Resistant" indicates that the pathogen is not likely to be inhibited if the antimicrobial compound in the blood reaches the concentration usually achievable; other therapy should be selected.

Standardized susceptibility test procedures require the use of laboratory control microorganisms to control the technical aspects of the laboratory procedures. Standard trovafloxacin mesylate powder should provide the following MIC values:

[See first table above]

Diffusion Techniques: Quantitative methods that require measurement of zone diameters also provide reproducible estimates of the susceptibility of bacteria to antimicrobial compounds. One such standardized procedure[2] requires the use of standardized inoculum concentrations. This procedure uses paper disks impregnated with trovafloxacin mesylate equivalent to 10 µg trovafloxacin to test the susceptibility of microorganisms to trovafloxacin.

Reports from the laboratory providing results of the standard single-disk susceptibility test with a trovafloxacin mesylate disk (equivalent to 10 µg trovafloxacin) should be interpreted according to the following criteria:

The following zone diameter interpretive criteria should be used for testing non-fastidious aerobic organisms:

Zone Diameter (mm)	Interpretation
≥17	Susceptible (S)
14–16	Intermediate (I)
≤13	Resistant (R)

For testing *Haemophilus* spp.[f]:

Zone Diameter (mm)	Interpretation[g]
≥22	Susceptible (S)

[f] This zone diameter standard is applicable only to tests with *Haemophilus* spp. using HTM[2].
[g] The current absence of data on resistant strains precludes defining any results other than "Susceptible". Strains yielding MIC results suggestive of a "nonsusceptible" category should be submitted to a reference laboratory for further testing.

For testing *Streptococcus* spp. including *Streptococcus pneumoniae*[h]:

Zone Diameter (mm)	Interpretation
≥19	Susceptible (S)
18–16	Intermediate (I)
≤15	Resistant (R)

[h] These zone diameter standards only apply to tests performed using Mueller-Hinton agar supplemented with 5% sheep blood incubated in 5% CO_2.

Interpretation should be as stated above for results using dilution techniques. Interpretation involves correlation of the diameter obtained in the disk test with the MIC for trovafloxacin.

As with standardized dilution techniques, diffusion methods require the use of laboratory control microorganisms that are used to control the technical aspects of the laboratory procedures. For the diffusion technique, the trovafloxacin mesylate equivalent to 10-µg trovafloxacin disk should provide the following zone diameters in these laboratory quality control strains:

[See second table above]

Anaerobic Techniques: For anaerobic bacteria, the susceptibility to trovafloxacin as MICs can be determined by standardized test methods[3]. The MIC values obtained should be interpreted according to the following criteria:

MIC (µg/mL)	Interpretation
≤2.0	Susceptible (S)
4.0	Intermediate (I)
≥8.0	Resistant (R)

Interpretation is identical to that stated above for results using dilution techniques.

As with other susceptibility techniques, the use of laboratory control microorganisms is required to control the technical aspects of the laboratory standardized procedures. Standardized trovafloxacin mesylate powder should provide the following MIC values:

Microorganism	MIC[k] (µg/mL)
Bacteroides fragilis ATCC 25285	0.125–0.5
*Bacteroides thetaiotamicron*ATCC 29741	0.25–1.0
Eubacterium lentum ATCC 43055	0.25–1.0

[k] These quality control ranges were derived from tests performed in the broth formulation of Wilkins-Chalgren agar.

Continued on next page

Trovan—Cont.

INDICATIONS AND USAGE

TROVAN is indicated for the treatment of patients initiating therapy in in-patient health care facilities (i.e., hospitals and long term nursing care facilities) with serious, life- or limb-threatening infections caused by susceptible strains of the designated microorganisms in the conditions listed below. (See **DOSAGE AND ADMINISTRATION**.)

Nosocomial pneumonia caused by *Escherichia coli, Pseudomonas aeruginosa, Haemophilus influenzae*, or *Staphylococcus aureus*. As with other antimicrobials, where *Pseudomonas aeruginosa* is a documented or presumptive pathogen, combination therapy with either an aminoglycoside or aztreonam may be clinically indicated.

Community acquired pneumonia caused by *Streptococcus pneumoniae, Haemophilus influenzae, Klebsiella pneumoniae, Staphylococcus aureus, Mycoplasma pneumoniae, Moraxella catarrhalis, Legionella pneumophila*, or *Chlamydia pneumoniae*.

Complicated intra-abdominal infections, including post-surgical infections caused by *Escherichia coli, Bacteroides fragilis*, viridans group streptococci, *Pseudomonas aeruginosa, Klebsiella pneumoniae, Peptostreptococcus* species, or *Prevotella species*.

Gynecologic and pelvic infections including endomyometritis, parametritis, septic abortion and post-partum infections caused by *Escherichia coli, Bacteroides fragilis*, viridans group streptococci, *Enterococcus faecalis, Streptococcus agalactiae, Peptostreptococcus* species, *Prevotella* species, or *Gardnerella vaginalis*.

Complicated skin and skin structure infections, including diabetic foot infections, caused by *Staphylococcus aureus, Streptococcus agalactiae, Pseudomonas aeruginosa, Enterococcus faecalis, Escherichia coli*, or *Proteus mirabilis*. **NOTE:** TROVAN has not been studied in the treatment of osteomyelitis.(See **WARNINGS**.)

CONTRAINDICATIONS

TROVAN is contraindicated in persons with a history of hypersensitivity to trovafloxacin, alatrofloxacin, quinolone antimicrobial agents or any other components of these products.

WARNINGS

(See boxed **WARNING**.) **TROVAN-ASSOCIATED LIVER ENZYME ABNORMALITIES, SYMPTOMATIC HEPATITIS, JAUNDICE, AND LIVER FAILURE (INCLUDING RARE REPORTS OF ACUTE HEPATIC NECROSIS WITH EOSINOPHILIC INFILTRATION, LIVER TRANSPLANTATION AND/OR DEATH) HAVE BEEN REPORTED WITH BOTH SHORT-TERM AND LONG-TERM DRUG EXPOSURE IN MEN AND WOMEN. TROVAN USE EXCEEDING 2 WEEKS IN DURATION IS ASSOCIATED WITH A SIGNIFICANTLY INCREASED RISK OF SERIOUS LIVER INJURY. LIVER INJURY HAS ALSO BEEN REPORTED FOLLOWING TROVAN RE-EXPOSURE. CLINICIANS SHOULD MONITOR LIVER FUNCTION TESTS (e.g., AST, ALT, BILIRUBIN) IN TROVAN RECIPIENTS WHO DEVELOP SIGNS OR SYMPTOMS CONSISTENT WITH HEPATITIS. CLINICIANS SHOULD CONSIDER DISCONTINUING TROVAN IN THOSE PATIENTS WHO DEVELOP LIVER FUNCTION TEST ABNORMALITIES.**

THE SAFETY AND EFFECTIVENESS OF TROVAFLOXACIN IN PEDIATRIC PATIENTS AND ADOLESCENTS LESS THAN 18 YEARS OF AGE, PREGNANT WOMEN, AND NURSING WOMEN HAVE NOT BEEN ESTABLISHED. (See **PRECAUTIONS: Pediatric Use, Pregnancy,** and **Nursing Mothers** subsections.)

As with other members of the quinolone class, trovafloxacin has caused arthropathy and/or chondrodysplasia in immature rats and dogs. The significance of these findings to humans is unknown. (See **ANIMAL PHARMACOLOGY**.)

Convulsions, increased intracranial pressure and psychosis have been reported in patients receiving quinolones. Quinolones may also cause central nervous system stimulation which may lead to tremors, restlessness, lightheadedness, confusion, hallucinations, paranoia, depression, nightmares and insomnia. These reactions may occur following the first dose. If these reactions occur in patients receiving trovafloxacin or alatrofloxacin, the drug should be discontinued and appropriate measures instituted. (See **PRECAUTIONS: General, Information for Patients, Drug Interactions** and **ADVERSE REACTIONS.)**

As with other quinolones, TROVAN should be used with caution in patients with known or suspected CNS disorders, such as severe cerebral atherosclerosis, epilepsy, and other factors that predispose to seizures. (See **ADVERSE REACTIONS**.)

Serious and occasionally fatal hypersensitivity and/or anaphylactic reactions have been reported in patients receiving therapy with TROVAN. These reactions may occur following the first dose. Some reactions have been accompanied by cardiovascular collapse, hypotension/shock, seizure, loss of consciousness, tingling, angioedema (including tongue, laryngeal, throat or facial edema/swelling), airway obstruction (including bronchospasm, shortness of breath and acute respiratory distress), dyspnea, urticaria, itching and other serious skin reactions, including generalized erythema.

Life-threatening hypotension has been reported with alatrofloxacin administration. This has occurred in patients receiving alatrofloxacin at either the recommended rate of infusion or if given more rapidly. Hypotension may be potentiated with the concomitant administration of anesthetic agents. Alatrofloxacin should only be administered by slow intravenous infusion over a period of 60 minutes. Blood pressure should be monitored closely during infusion.

TROVAN should be discontinued at the first appearance of a skin rash or any other sign of hypersensitivity. Serious acute hypersensitivity reactions may require treatment with epinephrine and other resuscitative measures, including oxygen, intravenous fluids, antihistamines, corticosteroids, pressor amines and airway management, as clinically indicated. (See **PRECAUTIONS** and **ADVERSE REACTIONS**.)

Serious and sometimes fatal events, some due to hypersensitivity and some due to uncertain etiology, have been reported in patients receiving therapy with all antibiotics. These events may be severe and generally occur following the administration of multiple doses. Clinical manifestations may include one or more of the following: fever, rash or severe dermatologic reactions (e.g., toxic epidermal necrolysis, Stevens-Johnson syndrome); vasculitis, arthralgia, myalgia, serum sickness; allergic pneumonitis, interstitial nephritis; acute renal insufficiency or failure; hepatitis, jaundice, acute hepatic necrosis or failure; anemia, including hemolytic and aplastic; thrombocytopenia, including thrombotic thrombocytopenic purpura; leukopenia; agranulocytosis; pancytopenia; and/or other hematologic abnormalities.

Pseudomembranous colitis has been reported with nearly all antibacterial agents, including TROVAN, and may range in severity from mild to life-threatening. Therefore, it is important to consider this diagnosis in patients who present with diarrhea subsequent to the administration of any antibacterial agent.

Treatment with antibacterial agents alters the flora of the colon and may permit overgrowth of clostridia. Studies indicate that a toxin produced by *Clostridium difficile* is the primary cause of "antibiotic-associated colitis."

After the diagnosis of pseudomembranous colitis has been established, therapeutic measures should be initiated. Mild cases of pseudomembranous colitis usually respond to drug discontinuation alone. In moderate to severe cases, consideration should be given to management with fluids and electrolytes, protein supplementation, and treatment with an antibacterial drug clinically effective against *C. difficile* colitis. (See **ADVERSE REACTIONS**.)

Although not seen in TROVAN clinical trials, ruptures of the shoulder, hand, and Achilles tendons that required surgical repair or resulted in prolonged disability have been reported in patients receiving quinolones. TROVAN should be discontinued if the patient experiences pain, inflammation or rupture of a tendon. Patients should rest and refrain from exercise until the diagnosis of tendinitis or tendon rupture has been confidently excluded. Tendon rupture can occur during or after therapy with quinolones.

Trovafloxacin has not been shown to be effective in the treatment of syphilis. Antimicrobial agents used in high doses for short periods of time to treat gonorrhea may mask or delay the symptoms of incubating syphilis. All patients with gonorrhea should have a serologic test for syphilis at the time of diagnosis.

PRECAUTIONS

General:

Moderate to severe phototoxicity reactions have been observed in patients who are exposed to direct sunlight while receiving some drugs in this class. Therapy should be discontinued if phototoxicity (e.g., a skin eruption, etc.) occurs. The safety and efficacy of TROVAN in patients with severe cirrhosis (Child-Pugh Class C) have not been studied.

Symptomatic pancreatitis has been reported on therapy. Clinicians should monitor pancreatic tests in patients who develop symptoms consistent with pancreatitis as clinically indicated.

Because a rapid or bolus intravenous injection may result in life-threatening hypotension, alatrofloxacin should only be administered by slow intravenous infusion over a period of 60 minutes. Profound hypotension has also been reported in patients receiving alatrofloxacin at the recommended rate of infusion. (See **WARNINGS** and **DOSAGE AND ADMINISTRATION: Intravenous Administration**.)

Information for Patients:

Patients should be advised:

- to discontinue therapy and to inform their physician immediately if they develop symptoms suggestive of hepatic dysfunction including fatigue, anorexia, vomiting, abdominal pain, jaundice, dark urine or pale stool. (See **WARNINGS**.)
- to inform their physician if they develop symptoms suggestive of pancreatitis including abdominal pain and/or nausea and vomiting. (See **PRECAUTIONS: General**.)
- that TROVAN Tablets may be taken without regard to meals;
- that vitamins or minerals containing iron, aluminum- or magnesium-base antacids, antacids containing citric acid buffered with sodium citrate, or sucralfate or Videx®, (Didanosine), chewable/buffered tablets or the pediatric powder for oral solution, should be taken at least 2 hours before or 2 hours after taking TROVAN tablets. (See **PRECAUTIONS: Drug Interactions**.);
- that TROVAN may cause lightheadedness and/or dizziness. Dizziness and/or lightheadedness was the most common adverse reaction reported, and for females under 45 years, it was reported significantly more frequently than in other groups. The incidence of dizziness may be substantially reduced if TROVAN Tablets are taken at bedtime or with food. Patients should know how they react to trovafloxacin before they operate an automobile or machinery or engage in activities requiring mental alertness and coordination. (See **WARNINGS** and **ADVERSE REACTIONS**.);
- to discontinue treatment and inform their physician if they experience pain, inflammation or rupture of a tendon, and to rest and refrain from exercise until the diagnosis of tendinitis or tendon rupture has been confidently excluded;
- that TROVAN may be associated with hypersensitivity reactions, even following the first dose, and to discontinue the drug at the first sign of a skin rash, hives or other skin reactions, difficulty in swallowing or breathing, any swelling suggesting angioedema (e.g., swelling of the lips, tongue, face, tightness of the throat, hoarseness), or other symptoms of an allergic reaction. (See **WARNINGS** and **ADVERSE REACTIONS**.);
- to avoid excessive sunlight or artificial ultraviolet light (e.g., tanning beds) while taking TROVAN and to discontinue therapy if phototoxicity (e.g., sunburn-like reaction or skin eruption) occurs.
- that convulsions have been reported in patients taking quinolones, including trovafloxacin, and to notify their physician before taking this drug if there is a history of this condition.

Drug Interactions:

Antacids, Sucralfate, and Iron: The absorption of oral trovafloxacin is significantly reduced by the concomitant administration of some antacids containing magnesium or aluminum, citric acid/sodium citrate (Bicitra®), as well as sucralfate and iron (ferrous ions). These agents as well as formulations containing divalent and trivalent cations such as Videx®, (Didanosine), chewable/buffered tablets or the pediatric powder for oral solution, should be taken at least 2 hours before or 2 hours after oral trovafloxacin administration. (See **CLINICAL PHARMACOLOGY**.)

Morphine: Co-administration of intravenous morphine significantly reduces the absorption of oral trovafloxacin. Intravenous morphine should be administered at least 2 hours after oral TROVAN dosing in the fasted state and at least 4 hours after oral TROVAN is taken with food. Trovafloxacin administration had no effect on the pharmacokinetics of morphine or its metabolite, morphine-6-β-glucuronide. (See **CLINICAL PHARMACOLOGY**.)

Warfarin: There have been reports during the post-marketing experience that trovafloxacin/alatrofloxacin enhance the effects of warfarin, including cases of bleeding. The mechanism for this reaction is unknown. Prothrombin time, International Normalized Ratio (INR) or other suitable anticoagulation tests should be closely monitored if trovafloxacin/alatrofloxacin is administered concomitantly with warfarin. Patients should also be monitored for evidence of bleeding.

Minor pharmacokinetic interactions without clinical significance have been observed with co-administration of TROVAN Tablets with caffeine, omeprazole and calcium carbonate. (See **CLINICAL PHARMACOLOGY**.)

No significant pharmacokinetic interactions with theophylline, cimetidine, digoxin, warfarin, or cyclosporine have been observed with TROVAN Tablets. (See **CLINICAL PHARMACOLOGY**.)

Alatrofloxacin should not be co-administered with any solution containing multivalent cations, e.g., magnesium, through the same intravenous line. (See **DOSAGE AND ADMINISTRATION**.)

Laboratory Test Interactions:

There are no reported laboratory test interactions.

Carcinogenesis, Mutagenesis, Impairment of Fertility:

Long term studies in animals to determine the carcinogenic potential of trovafloxacin or alatrofloxacin have not been conducted.

TROVAN did not shorten the time to development of UV-induced skin tumors in hairless albino (Skh-1) mice; thus, it was not photo co-carcinogenic in this model. These mice received oral trovafloxacin and concurrent irradiation with simulated sunlight 5 days per week for 40 weeks followed by a 12-week treatment-free observation period. The daily dose of UV radiation used in this study was approximately 30% of the minimal dose of UV radiation that would induce erythema in Caucasian humans. The median time to the development of skin tumors in the hairless mice (42–43 weeks) was similar in the vehicle control group and those given 10 or 30 mg/kg of trovafloxacin daily. At a dose level of 30 mg/kg/day, the mice had skin trovafloxacin concentrations of approximately 7 μg/g. Following multiple 200 mg daily doses of trovafloxacin, the amount in human skin is estimated to be about 3 μg/g, based upon plasma concentrations measured at this dose level.

Trovafloxacin was not mutagenic in the Ames Salmonella reversion assay or CHO/HGPRT mammalian cell gene mutation assay and it was not clastogenic in mitogen-stimulated human lymphocytes or mouse bone marrow cells. A mouse micronucleus test conducted with alatrofloxacin was also negative. The positive response observed in the *E. coli* bacterial mutagenicity assay may be due to the inhibition of DNA gyrase by trovafloxacin.

Trovafloxacin and alatrofloxacin did not affect the fertility of male or female rats at oral and I.V. doses of 75 mg/kg/day and 50 mg/kg/day, respectively. These doses are 15 and 10 times the recommended maximum human dose based on mg/kg or approximately 2 times based on mg/m^2. However, oral doses of trovafloxacin at 200 mg/kg/day (40 times the recommended maximum human dose based on mg/kg or about 6 times based on mg/m^2) were associated with increased preimplantation loss in rats.

Pregnancy: Teratogenic Effects. Pregnancy Category C:
An increase in skeletal variations was observed in rat fetuses after daily oral 75 mg/kg maternal doses of trovafloxacin (approximately 15 times the highest recommended human dose based on mg/kg or 2 times based upon body surface area) were administered during organogenesis. However, fetal skeletal variations were not observed in rats dosed orally with 15 mg/kg trovafloxacin. Evidence of fetotoxicity (increased perinatal mortality and decreased body weights) was also observed in rats at 75 mg/kg. Daily oral doses of trovafloxacin at 45 mg/kg (approximately 9 times the highest recommended human dose based on mg/kg or 2.7 times based upon body surface area) in the rabbit were not associated with an increased incidence of fetal skeletal variations or malformations.
An increase in skeletal variations and malformations was observed in rat fetuses after daily intravenous doses of alatrofloxacin at ≥20 mg/kg/day (approximately 4 times the highest recommended human dose based on mg/kg or 0.6 times based upon body surface area) were administered to dams during organogenesis. In the rabbit, an increase in fetal skeletal malformations was also observed when 20 mg/kg/day (approximately equal to the highest recommended human dose based upon body surface area) of alatrofloxacin was given intravenously during the period of organogenesis. Intravenous dosing of alatrofloxacin at 6.5 mg/kg in the rat or rabbit was not associated with an increased incidence of skeletal variations or malformations. Fetotoxicity and fetal skeletal malformations have been associated with other quinolones.
Oral doses of trovafloxacin >5 mg/kg were associated with an increased gestation time in rats, and several dams at 75 mg/kg experienced uterine dystocia.
There are no adequate and well-controlled studies in pregnant women. TROVAN should be used during pregnancy only if the potential benefit justifies the potential risk to the fetus. (See **WARNINGS**.)

Nursing Mothers:
Trovafloxacin is excreted in human milk and was found in measurable concentrations in the breast milk of lactating subjects. (See **CLINICAL PHARMACOLOGY, Distribution**.)
Because of the potential for unknown effects from trovafloxacin in nursing infants from mothers taking trovafloxacin, a decision should be made either to discontinue nursing or to discontinue the drug, taking into account the importance of the drug to the mother.

Pediatric Use:
The safety and effectiveness of trovafloxacin in pediatric patients and adolescents less than 18 years of age have not been established. Quinolones, including trovafloxacin, cause arthropathy and osteochondrosis in juvenile animals of several species. (See **WARNINGS**.)

Geriatric Use:
In multiple-dose clinical trials of trovafloxacin, 27% of patients were ≥65 years of age and 12% of patients were ≥75 years of age. The overall incidence of drug-related adverse reactions, including central nervous system and gastrointestinal side effects, was less in the ≥65 year group than the other age groups.

ADVERSE REACTIONS

Over 6000 patients have been treated with TROVAN in multidose clinical efficacy trials worldwide.
In TROVAN studies the majority of adverse reactions were described as mild in nature (over 90% were described as mild or moderate). TROVAN was discontinued for adverse events thought related to drug in 5% of patients (dizziness 2.4%, nausea 1.9%, headache 1.1%, and vomiting 1.0%).
[See first table above]

TROVAN Drug-Related Adverse Reactions (frequency ≥1%) in Multiple-Dose Clinical Trials

	200 mg oral qd (N=3259)	200 mg I.V.→ 200 mg oral qd (N=634)	300 mg I.V.→ 200 mg oral qd (N=623)
Dizziness	11%	2%	2%
Lightheadedness	4%	2%	<1%
Nausea	8%	5%	4%
Headache	5%	5%	1%
Vomiting	3%	1%	3%
Diarrhea	2%	2%	2%
Abdominal Pain	1%	1%	0%
Application/injection/ insertion site reaction	n/a	5%	2%
Vaginitis	2%	2%	<1%
Pruritus	<1%	2%	2%
Rash	<1%	2%	2%

DOSAGE GUIDELINES

INFECTION*/LOCATION AND TYPE	DAILY UNIT DOSE AND ROUTE OF ADMINISTRATION	TOTAL DURATION (See **WARNINGS**.)
Nosocomial Pneumonia (See NOTE 1 below.)	300 mg I.V.† followed by 200 mg oral	10–14 days
Community Acquired Pneumonia	200 mg oral or 200 mg I.V. followed by 200 mg oral	7–14 days
Complicated Intra-Abdominal Infections, including post-surgical infections	300 mg I.V.† followed by 200 mg oral	7–14 days
Gynecologic and Pelvic Infections	300 mg I.V.† followed by 200 mg oral	7–14 days
Skin and Skin Structure Infections, Complicated, including diabetic foot infections	200 mg oral or 200 mg I.V. followed by 200 mg oral	10–14 days

*due to the designated pathogens (See **INDICATIONS AND USAGE**.)
† Where the 300 mg TROVAN I.V. dose is indicated, therapy should be decreased to the 200 mg dose as soon as clinically indicated.

Dizziness/lightheadedness on TROVAN is generally mild, lasts for a few hours following a dose, and in most cases, resolves with continued dosing. The incidence of dizziness and lightheadedness in TROVAN patients over 65 years is 3.1% and 0.6%, respectively. (See **PRECAUTIONS: Information for Patients**.)
TROVAN appears to have a low potential for phototoxicity. In clinical trials with TROVAN, only mild, treatment-related phototoxicity was observed in less than 0.03% (2/7096) of patients.
Additional reported drug-related events in clinical trials (remotely, possibly, probably or unknown) that occurred in <1% of TROVAN-treated patients are:
APPLICATION/INJECTION/INSERTION SITE: Application/injection/insertion site device complications, inflammation, pain, edema
AUTONOMIC NERVOUS: flushing, increased sweating, dry mouth, cold clammy skin, increased saliva
CARDIOVASCULAR: peripheral edema, chest pain, thrombophlebitis, hypotension, palpitation, periorbital edema, hypertension, syncope, tachycardia, angina pectoris, bradycardia, peripheral ischemia, edema, dizziness postural
CENTRAL & PERIPHERAL NERVOUS SYSTEM: confusion, paresthesia, vertigo, hypoesthesia, ataxia, convulsions, dysphonia, hypertonia, migraine, involuntary muscle contractions, speech disorder, encephalopathy, abnormal gait, hyperkinesia, hypokinesia, tongue paralysis, abnormal coordination, tremor, dyskinesia
GASTROINTESTINAL: altered bowel habit, constipation, diarrhea-*Clostridium difficile*, dyspepsia, flatulence, loose stools, gastritis, dysphagia, increased appetite, gastroenteritis, rectal disorder, colitis, pseudomembranous colitis, enteritis, eructation, gastrointestinal disorder, melena, hiccup
ORAL CAVITY: gingivitis, stomatitis, altered saliva, tongue disorder, tongue edema, tooth disorder, cheilitis, halitosis
GENERAL/OTHER: fever, fatigue, pain, asthenia, moniliasis, hot flushes, back pain, chills, infection (bacterial, fungal), malaise, sepsis, alcohol intolerance, allergic reaction, anaphylactoid reaction, drug (other) toxicity/reaction, weight increase, weight decrease
HEMATOPOIETIC: anemia, granulocytopenia, hemorrhage unspecified, leukopenia, prothrombin decreased, thrombocythemia, thrombocytopenia
LIVER/BILIARY: increased hepatic enzymes, hepatic function abnormal, bilirubinemia, discolored feces, jaundice
METABOLIC/NUTRITIONAL: hyperglycemia, thirst
MUSCULOSKELETAL: arthralgia, muscle cramps, myalgia, muscle weakness, skeletal pain, tendinitis, arthropathy
PSYCHIATRIC: anxiety, anorexia, agitation, nervousness, somnolence, insomnia, depression, amnesia, concentration impaired, depersonalization, dreaming abnormal, emotional lability, euphoria, hallucination, impotence, libido decreased-male, paroniria, thinking abnormal
REPRODUCTIVE: Female: leukorrhea, menstrual disorder; Male: balanoposthitis
RESPIRATORY: dyspnea, rhinitis, sinusitis, bronchospasm, coughing, epistaxis, respiratory insufficiency, upper respiratory tract infection, respiratory disorder, asthma, hemoptysis, hypoxia, stridor
SKIN/APPENDAGES: pruritus ani, skin disorder, skin ulceration, angioedema, dermatitis, dermatitis fungal, photosensitivity skin reaction, seborrhea, skin exfoliation, urticaria
SPECIAL SENSES: taste perversion, eye pain, abnormal vision, conjunctivitis, photophobia, conjuctival hemorrhage, hyperacusis, scotoma, tinnitus, visual field defect, diplopia, xerophthalmia
URINARY SYSTEM: dysuria, face edema, micturition frequency, interstitial nephritis, renal failure acute, renal function abnormal, urinary incontinence
LABORATORY CHANGES: Changes in laboratory parameters, without regard to drug relationship, occurring in ≥1% of TROVAN-treated patients were: decreased hemoglobin and hematocrit; increased platelets; decreased and increased WBC; eosinophilia; increased ALT (SGPT), AST (SGOT), and alkaline phosphatase; decreased protein and albumin; increased BUN and creatinine; decreased sodium; and bicarbonate. It is not known whether these abnormalities were caused by the drug or the underlying condition being treated.
The incidence and magnitude of liver function abnormalities with TROVAN were the same as comparator agents except in the only study in which oral TROVAN was administered for 28 days. In this study (chronic bacterial prostatitis) nine percent (13/140) of TROVAN-treated patients experienced elevations of serum transaminases (AST and/or ALT) of ≥3 times the upper limit of normal. These liver function test abnormalities generally developed at the end of, or following completion of, the planned 28-day course of therapy, but were not associated with concurrent elevations of related laboratory measures of hepatic function (such as serum bilirubin, alkaline phosphatase, or lactate dehydrogenase). Patients were asymptomatic with these abnormalities, which generally returned to normal within 1-2 months after discontinuation of therapy. (See **ADVERSE REACTIONS: POST-MARKETING EXPERIENCE** subsection.)
POST-MARKETING EXPERIENCE: Adverse reactions reported with TROVAN during the post-marketing period include:
GASTROINTESTINAL: symptomatic pancreatitis.
GENERAL/OTHER: anaphylaxis, Stevens-Johnson syndrome.
HEMATOPOIETIC: agranulocytosis, aplastic anemia, pancytopenia.
LIVER/BILIARY: symptomatic hepatitis (some patients experienced an associated peripheral eosinophilia), liver failure (including acute hepatic necrosis with eosinophilic infiltration). TROVAN-associated liver enzyme abnormalities and/or symptomatic hepatitis have occurred during short-term or long-term therapy. (See **WARNINGS**.)

OVERDOSAGE

Trovafloxacin has a low order of acute toxicity. The minimum lethal oral dose in mice and rats was 2000 mg/kg or greater. The minimum lethal I.V. dose for the prodrug, alatrofloxacin, was 50–125 mg/kg for mice and greater than 75 mg/kg for rats. Clinical signs observed included decreased activity and respiration, ataxia, ptosis, tremors and convulsions.
In the event of acute oral overdosage, the stomach should be emptied by inducing vomiting or by gastric lavage. The pa-

Continued on next page

Trovan—Cont.

tient should be carefully observed and given symptomatic and supportive treatment. Adequate hydration should be maintained. Trovafloxacin is not efficiently removed from the body by hemodialysis.

DOSAGE AND ADMINISTRATION

The recommended dosage for TROVAN for the treatment of serious, life- or limb-threatening infections is described in the table below. Doses of TROVAN are administered once every 24 hours. TROVAN should not usually be administered for more than 2 weeks. It should only be administered for longer than 2 weeks if the treating physician believes the benefits to the individual patients clearly outweigh the risks of such longer-term treatment. (See boxed **WARNING**.)

Oral doses should be administered at least 2 hours before or 2 hours after antacids containing magnesium or aluminum, as well as sucralfate, citric acid buffered with sodium citrate (e.g., Bicitra®), metal cations (e.g., ferrous sulfate) and Videx®, (Didanosine), chewable/buffered tablets or the pediatric powder for oral solution.

Intravenous morphine should be administered at least 2 hours after oral TROVAN dosing in the fasted state and at least 4 hours after oral TROVAN is taken with food.

Patients whose therapy is started with TROVAN I.V. may be switched to TROVAN Tablets to complete the course of therapy, if deemed appropriate by the treating physician. In certain patients with serious and life- or limb-threatening infections as described in the **INDICATIONS AND USAGE** Section, TROVAN Tablets may be considered appropriate initial therapy, when the treating physician believes that the benefit of the product for the patient outweighs the potential risk.

TROVAN I.V. (alatrofloxacin mesylate injection) should only be administered by INTRAVENOUS infusion. It is not for intramuscular, intrathecal, intraperitoneal, or subcutaneous administration.

Single-use vials require dilution prior to administration. (See **PREPARATION OF ALATROFLOXACIN MESYLATE INJECTION FOR ADMINISTRATION**.)

[See second table at top of previous page]

NOTE: As with other antimicrobials, where *Pseudomonas aeruginosa* is a documented or presumptive pathogen, combination therapy with either an aminoglycoside or aztreonam may be clinically indicated.

IMPAIRED RENAL FUNCTION: No adjustment in the dosage of TROVAN is necessary in patients with impaired renal function. Trovafloxacin is eliminated primarily by biliary excretion. Trovafloxacin is not efficiently removed from the body by hemodialysis.

CHRONIC HEPATIC DISEASE (cirrhosis): The following table provides dosing guidelines for patients with mild or moderate cirrhosis (Child-Pugh Class A and B). There are no data in patients with severe cirrhosis (Child-Pugh Class C).

INDICATED DOSE (Normal hepatic function)	CHRONIC HEPATIC DISEASE DOSE
300 mg I.V.	200 mg I.V.
200 mg I.V. or oral	100 mg I.V. or oral

INTRAVENOUS ADMINISTRATION

AFTER DILUTION WITH AN APPROPRIATE DILUENT, TROVAN I.V. SHOULD BE ADMINISTERED BY INTRAVENOUS INFUSION OVER A PERIOD OF 60 MINUTES. CAUTION: RAPID OR BOLUS INTRAVENOUS INFUSION SHOULD BE AVOIDED. (See **PRECAUTIONS**.)

TROVAN I.V. is supplied in single-use vials containing a concentrated solution of alatrofloxacin mesylate in Water for Injection (equivalent of 200 mg or 300 mg as trovafloxacin). Each mL contains alatrofloxacin mesylate equivalent to 5 mg trovafloxacin. (See **HOW SUPPLIED** for container sizes.) THESE TROVAN I.V. SINGLE-USE VIALS MUST BE FURTHER DILUTED WITH AN APPROPRIATE SOLUTION PRIOR TO INTRAVENOUS ADMINISTRATION. This parenteral drug product should be inspected visually for discoloration and particulate matter prior to dilution and administration. Since no preservative or bacteriostatic agent is present in this product, aseptic technique must be used in preparation of the final parenteral solution.

PREPARATION OF ALATROFLOXACIN MESYLATE INJECTION FOR ADMINISTRATION

The intravenous dose should be prepared by aseptically withdrawing the appropriate volume of concentrate from the vials of TROVAN I.V. This should be diluted with a suitable intravenous solution to a final concentration of 1-2 mg/mL. (See **Compatible Intravenous Solutions.**) The resulting solution should be infused over a period of 60 minutes by direct infusion or through a Y-type intravenous infusion set which may already be in place.

Since the vials are for single use only, any unused portion should be discarded.

Since only limited data are available on the compatibility of alatrofloxacin intravenous injection with other intravenous substances, additives or other medications should not be added to TROVAN I.V. in single-use vials or infused simultaneously through the same intravenous line.

DOSAGE STRENGTH (mg) (trovafloxacin equivalent)	VOLUME TO WITHDRAW (mL)	DILUENT VOLUME (mL)	TOTAL VOLUME (mL)	INFUSION CONC (mg/mL)
100 mg	20	30	50	2
100 mg	20	80	100	1
200 mg	40	60	100	2
200 mg	40	160	200	1
300 mg	60	90	150	2
300 mg	60	240	300	1

	End of Treatment		End of Study	
Pathogen	TROVAN	Comparators	TROVAN	Comparators
S. pneumoniae	89% (63/71)	95% (62/65)	87% (55/63)	91% (50/55)
H. influenzae	97% (35/36)	94% (46/49)	90% (28/31)	94% (44/47)
M. catarrhalis	100% (8/8)	100% (4/4)	100% (6/6)	100% (4/4)
S. aureus	100% (8/8)	93% (13/14)	100% (6/6)	91% (10/11)
K. pneumoniae	100% (3/3)	89% (8/9)	100% (3/3)	86% (6/7)
L. pneumophila	77% (10/13)	86% (12/14)	75% (9/12)	86% (12/14)
M. pneumoniae	100% (20/20)	87% (13/15)	94% (17/18)	79% (11/14)
C. pneumoniae	75% (6/8)	100% (18/18)	67% (4/6)	94% (16/17)

	End of Treatment		End of Study	
Pathogen	TROVAN	Ciprofloxacin	TROVAN	Ciprofloxacin
P. aeruginosa	67% (10/15)	55% (6/11)	62% (8/13)	25% (2/8)
H. influenzae	88% (7/8)	89% (8/9)	83% (5/6)	86% (6/7)
E. coli	71% (5/7)	80% (4/5)	50% (3/6)	80% (4/5)
S. aureus	64% (7/11)	80% (8/10)	50% (4/8)	67% (4/6)

If the same intravenous line is used for sequential infusion of several different drugs, the line should be flushed before and after infusion of TROVAN I.V. with an infusion solution compatible with TROVAN I.V. and with any other drug(s) administered via this common line.

If TROVAN I.V. is to be given concomitantly with another drug, each drug should be given separately in accordance with the recommended dosage and route of administration for each drug.

The desired dosage of TROVAN I.V. may be prepared according to the following chart:

[See first table above]

For example, to prepare a 200 mg dose at an infusion concentration of 2 mg/mL (as trovafloxacin), 40 mL of TROVAN I.V. is withdrawn from a vial and diluted with 60 mL of a compatible intravenous fluid to produce a total infusion solution volume of 100 mL.

Compatible Intravenous Solutions:

5% Dextrose Injection, USP
0.45% Sodium Chloride Injection, USP
5% Dextrose and 0.45% Sodium Chloride Injection, USP
5% Dextrose and 0.2% Sodium Chloride Injection, USP
Lactated Ringer's and 5% Dextrose Injection, USP

TROVAN I.V. should not be diluted with 0.9% Sodium Chloride Injection, USP (normal saline), alone or in combination with other diluents. A precipitate may form under these conditions. In addition, TROVAN I.V. should not be diluted with Lactated Ringer's, USP.

Normal saline, 0.9% Sodium Chloride Injection, USP can be used for flushing I.V. lines prior to or after administration of TROVAN I.V.

Stability of TROVAN I.V. as Supplied:

When stored under recommended conditions, TROVAN I.V., as supplied in 40 mL or 60 mL vials, is stable through the expiration date printed on the label.

Stability of TROVAN I.V. Following Dilution:

TROVAN I.V., when diluted with compatible intravenous solutions to concentrations of 0.5 to 2.0 mg/mL (as trovafloxacin), is physically and chemically stable for up to 7 days when refrigerated or up to 3 days at room temperature stored in glass bottles or plastic (PVC type) intravenous containers.

HOW SUPPLIED

Trovan Tablets and Injection are being distributed only to hospitals and long term nursing care facilities for patients initiating therapy in these facilities.

Tablets

TROVAN® (trovafloxacin mesylate) Tablets are available as blue, film-coated tablets. The 100 mg tablets are round and contain trovafloxacin mesylate equivalent to 100 mg trovafloxacin. The 200 mg tablets are modified oval-shaped and contain trovafloxacin mesylate equivalent to 200 mg trovafloxacin.

TROVAN Tablets are packaged and in unit dose blister strips in the following configurations:

100-mg tablets: color: blue; shape: round; debossing: "PFIZER" on one side and "378" on the other
  Bottles of 30 (NDC 0049-3780-30)
  Unit Dose/40 tablets (NDC 0049-3780-43)

200-mg tablets: color: blue; shape: modified oval; debossing: "PFIZER" on one side and "379" on the other
  Bottles of 30 (NDC 0049-3790-30)
  Unit Dose/40 tablets (NDC 0049-3790-43)

Storage

TROVAN Tablets should be stored at 15°C to 30°C (59°F to 86°F) in airtight containers (USP).

Injection

TROVAN is also available for intravenous administration as the prodrug, TROVAN® I.V. (alatrofloxacin mesylate injection), in the following configurations:

Single-use vials containing a clear, colorless to pale-yellow concentrated solution of alatrofloxacin mesylate equivalent to 5 mg trovafloxacin/mL.
  5 mg/mL, 40 mL, 200 mg
  Unit dose package (NDC 0049-3890-28)
  5 mg/mL, 60 mL, 300 mg
  Unit dose package (NDC 0049-3900-28)

Storage

TROVAN I.V. should be stored at 15°C to 30°C (59°F to 86°F). Protect From Light. Do Not Freeze.

ANIMAL PHARMACOLOGY

Quinolones have been shown to cause arthropathy in immature animals.

Arthropathy and chondrodysplasia were observed in immature animals given trovafloxacin. (See **WARNINGS**.)

At doses from 10 to 15 times the human dose based on mg/kg or approximately 3 to 5 times based on mg/m^2, trovafloxacin has been shown to cause arthropathy in immature rats and dogs. In addition, these drugs are associated with an increased incidence of chondrodysplasia in rats compared to controls. There is no evidence of arthropathies in fully mature rats and dogs at doses from 40 or 10 times the human dose based on mg/kg or approximately 5 times based on mg/m^2 for a 6 month exposure period.

Unlike some other members of the quinolone class, crystalluria and ocular toxicity were not observed in chronic safety studies with rats or dogs with either trovafloxacin or its prodrug, alatrofloxacin.

Quinolones have been reported to have proconvulsant activity that is exacerbated with concomitant use of non-steroidal anti-inflammatory drugs (NSAIDS). Neither trovafloxacin administered orally at 500 mg/kg, nor alatrofloxacin administered intravenously at 75 mg/kg, showed an increase in measures of seizure activity in mice at doses when used in combination with the active metabolite of the NSAID, fenbufen.

As with other members of the quinolone class, trovafloxacin at doses 5 to 10 times the human dose based on mg/kg or 1 to 5 times the human dose based on mg/m^2 produces testicular degeneration in rats and dogs dosed for 6 months.

Pathogen	End of Treatment		End of Study	
	TROVAN	Imipenem/Cila Amox/Clav	TROVAN	Imipenem/Cila Amox/Clav
E. coli	94% (72/77)	90% (52/58)	86% (66/77)	86% (51/59)
Bacteroides fragilis	97% (30/31)	82% (28/34)	84% (26/31)	75% (27/36)
viridans group streptococci	90% (18/20)	83% (19/23)	90% (18/20)	78% (18/23)
Pseudomonas aeruginosa	94% (15/16)	82% (14/17)	88% (14/16)	83% (15/18)
Klebsiella pneumoniae	80% (12/15)	71% (10/14)	67% (10/15)	71% (10/14)
Peptostreptococcus spp.	86% (12/14)	88% (7/8)	79% (11/14)	75% (6/8)
Prevotella spp.	77% (10/13)	50% (2/4)	77% (10/13)	60% (3/5)

At a dose of trovafloxacin 10 times the highest human dose based on mg/kg or approximately 5 times based on mg/m^2, elevated liver enzyme levels which correlated with centrilobular hepatocellular vacuolar degeneration and necrosis were observed in dogs in a 6 month study. A subsequent study demonstrated reversibility of these effects when trovafloxacin was discontinued.

CLINICAL STUDIES

Hospitalized Community Acquired Pneumonia

Adult patients with clinically and radiologically documented community acquired pneumonia, requiring hospitalization and initial intravenous therapy, participated in two randomized, multicenter, double-blind, double-dummy trials. The first trial compared intravenous alatrofloxacin (200 mg once daily for 2 to 7 days) followed by oral trovafloxacin (200 mg once daily) for a total of 7 to 14 days of therapy to intravenous ciprofloxacin (400 mg BID) plus ampicillin (500 mg QID) for 2 to 7 days followed by oral ciprofloxacin (500 mg BID) plus amoxicillin (500 mg TID) for a total of 7 to 14 days of therapy. The second study compared intravenous alatrofloxacin (200 mg once daily for 2 to 7 days) followed by oral trovafloxacin (200 mg once daily) for a total of 7 to 14 days of therapy to intravenous ceftriaxone (1000 mg once daily for 2 to 7 days) followed by oral cefpodoxime (400 mg BID) for 7 to 14 days of total therapy with optional blinded erythromycin added to the ceftriaxone/cefpodoxime arm if an atypical pneumonia was suspected.

The clinical success rate (cure + improvement with no need for further antibiotic therapy) at the End of Treatment was 90% (311/346) and 90% (325/363) for TROVAN and the comparator agents, respectively. The clinical success rate at the End of Study (Day 30) was 86% (256/299) and 85% (283/334) for TROVAN and the comparator agents, respectively. All cause mortality (Day 1-35) was 2.45% (10/408) on TROVAN and 5.45% (23/422) on the comparator agents.

The following outcomes are the clinical success rates for the clinically evaluable patient groups by pathogen in these two studies:

[See second table at top of previous page]

Of the above patients with clinical failure at end of treatment or study, only one alatrofloxacin patient (*H. influenzae* + *S. pneumoniae*) and one ceftriaxone + erythromycin patient (*Legionella*) had a microbiologically confirmed persistent pathogen at the time of failure with no emergence of resistance in either study.

Nosocomial Pneumonia

Adult patients with clinically and radiologically documented nosocomial pneumonia participated in a randomized, multicenter, double-blind, double-dummy trial comparing intravenous alatrofloxacin (300 mg once daily for 2 to 7 days) followed by oral trovafloxacin (200 mg once daily) for a total of 7 to 14 days of therapy to intravenous ciprofloxacin (400 mg BID) for 2 to 7 days followed by oral ciprofloxacin (750 mg BID) for a total of 7 to 14 days of therapy with optional blinded clindamycin or metronidazole added to the ciprofloxacin arm if an anaerobic pneumonia was suspected. In subjects with documented Pseudomonas infection or methicillin-resistant *S. aureus*, aztreonam or vancomycin, respectively, could have been added to either treatment regimen.

The clinical success rate (cure + improvement with no need for further antibiotic therapy) at the End of Treatment was 77% (68/88) and 78% (79/101) for TROVAN and ciprofloxacin, respectively. The clinical success rate at the End of Study (Day 30) was 69% (50/72) and 68% (54/79) for TROVAN and ciprofloxacin, respectively.

The following outcomes are the clinical success rates for the clinically evaluable patient groups by pathogen:

[See third table at top of previous page]

Of the above patients with clinical failure at end of treatment or study, 2 alatrofloxacin patients (*S. aureus, P. aeruginosa*) and 4 ciprofloxacin patients (all *P. aeruginosa*) had a microbiologically confirmed persistent pathogen at the time of failure. Three of the 4 ciprofloxacin patients with clinical failure and persistence had emergence of resistance with none on alatrofloxacin.

Complicated Intra-Abdominal Infections

Patients hospitalized with clinically documented, complicated intra-abdominal infections, including post-surgical infections, participated in a randomized, double-blind, multicenter trial comparing intravenous alatrofloxacin (300 mg once daily) followed by oral trovafloxacin (200 mg once daily) to intravenous imipenem/cilastatin (1g q8h) followed by oral amoxicillin/clavulanic acid (500 mg TID) for a maximum of 14 days of therapy. The clinical success rate (cure + improvement) at the End of Treatment was 88% (136/155) and 86% (122/142) for alatrofloxacin→trovafloxacin and imipenem/cilastatin→amoxicillin/clavulanic acid, respectively. The clinical success rate at the End of Study (Day 30) was 83% (129/156) and 84% (127/152) for alatrofloxacin→trovafloxacin and imipenem/cilastatin→amoxicillin/clavulanic acid, respectively.

The following are the clinical success rates for the clinically evaluable patient groups by pathogen:

[See table above]

Of patients with a baseline pathogen and a clinical response of failure at the End of Study, 9 of 26 on TROVAN and 10 of 21 on imipenem/cilastatin had microbiologically-confirmed persistence of the baseline pathogen with no emergence of resistance in either group.

REFERENCES

1. National Committee for Clinical Laboratory Standards, Methods for Dilution Antimicrobial Susceptibility Tests for Bacteria That Grow Aerobically – Fourth Edition; Approved Standard, NCCLS Document M7-A4, Vol. 17, No. 2, NCCLS, Wayne, PA, January, 1997.
2. National Committee for Clinical Laboratory Standards. Performance Standards for Antimicrobial Disk Susceptibility Tests – Sixth Edition; Approved Standard, NCCLS Document M2-A6, Vol. 17, No. 1, NCCLS, Wayne, PA, January, 1997.
3. National Committee for Clinical Laboratory Standards. Methods for Antimicrobial Susceptibility Testing of Anaerobic Bacteria – Fourth Edition; Approved Standard, NCCLS Document M11-A4, Vol. 17, No. 22, NCCLS, Wayne, PA, December, 1997.

R_x only

U.S. Patent No. 5,164,402

Shown in Product Identification Guide, page 330

UNASYN® ℞

(ampicillin sodium/sulbactam sodium)

DESCRIPTION

UNASYN is an injectable antibacterial combination consisting of the semisynthetic antibiotic ampicillin sodium and the beta-lactamase inhibitor sulbactam sodium for intravenous and intramuscular administration.

Ampicillin sodium is derived from the penicillin nucleus, 6-aminopenicillanic acid. Chemically, it is monosodium (2S, 5R, 6R)-6-[(R)-2-amino-2-phenylacetamido]-3,3-dimethyl-7-oxo-4-thia-1-azabicyclo[3.2.0]heptane-2-carboxylate and has a molecular weight of 371.39. Its chemical formula is $C_{16}H_{18}N_3NaO_4S$. The structural formula is:

Sulbactam sodium is a derivative of the basic penicillin nucleus. Chemically, sulbactam sodium is sodium penicillinate sulfone; sodium (2S, 5R)-3,3-dimethyl-7-oxo-4-thia-1-azabicyclo[3.2.0]heptane-2-carboxylate 4,4-dioxide. Its chemical formula is $C_8H_{10}NNaO_5S$ with a molecular weight of 255.22. The structural formula is:

UNASYN, ampicillin sodium/sulbactam sodium parenteral combination, is available as a white to off-white dry powder for reconstitution. UNASYN dry powder is freely soluble in aqueous diluents to yield pale yellow to yellow solutions containing ampicillin sodium and sulbactam sodium equivalent to 250 mg ampicillin per mL and 125 mg sulbactam per mL. The pH of the solutions is between 8.0 and 10.0.

Dilute solutions (up to 30 mg ampicillin and 15 mg sulbactam per mL) are essentially colorless to pale yellow. The pH of dilute solutions remains the same.

1.5 g of UNASYN (1 g ampicillin as the sodium salt plus 0.5 g sulbactam as the sodium salt) parenteral contains approximately 115 mg (5 mEq) of sodium.

3 g of UNASYN (2 g ampicillin as the sodium salt plus 1 g sulbactam as the sodium salt) parenteral contains approximately 230 mg (10 mEq) of sodium.

CLINICAL PHARMACOLOGY

General: Immediately after completion of a 15-minute intravenous infusion of UNASYN, peak serum concentrations of ampicillin and sulbactam are attained. Ampicillin serum levels are similar to those produced by the administration of equivalent amounts of ampicillin alone. Peak ampicillin serum levels ranging from 109 to 150 mcg/mL are attained after administration of 2000 mg of ampicillin plus 1000 mg sulbactam and 40 to 71 mcg/mL after administration of 1000 mg ampicillin plus 500 mg sulbactam. The corresponding mean peak serum levels for sulbactam range from 48 to 88 mcg/mL and 21 to 40 mcg/mL, respectively. After an intramuscular injection of 1000 mg ampicillin plus 500 mg sulbactam, peak ampicillin serum levels ranging from 8 to 37 mcg/mL and peak sulbactam serum levels ranging from 6 to 24 mcg/mL are attained.

The mean serum half-life of both drugs is approximately 1 hour in healthy volunteers.

Approximately 75 to 85% of both ampicillin and sulbactam are excreted unchanged in the urine during the first 8 hours after administration of UNASYN to individuals with normal renal function. Somewhat higher and more prolonged serum levels of ampicillin and sulbactam can be achieved with the concurrent administration of probenecid.

In patients with impaired renal function the elimination kinetics of ampicillin and sulbactam are similarly affected, hence the ratio of one to the other will remain constant whatever the renal function. The dose of UNASYN in such patients should be administered less frequently in accordance with the usual practice for ampicillin (see Dosage and Administration).

Ampicillin has been found to be approximately 28% reversibly bound to human serum protein and sulbactam approximately 38% reversibly bound.

The following average levels of ampicillin and sulbactam were measured in the tissues and fluids listed:

TABLE A
Concentration of UNASYN in Various Body Tissues and Fluids

Fluid or Tissue	Dose (grams) Ampicillin/ Sulbactam	Concentration (mcg/mL or mcg/g) Ampicillin Sulbactam
Peritoneal Fluid	0.5/0.5 IV	7/14
Blister Fluid (Cantharides)	0.5/0.5 IV	8/20
Tissue Fluid	1/0.5 IV	8/4
Intestinal Mucosa	0.5/0.5 IV	11/18
Appendix	2/1 IV	3/40

Penetration of both ampicillin and sulbactam into cerebrospinal fluid in the presence of inflamed meninges has been demonstrated after IV administration of UNASYN.

MICROBIOLOGY

Ampicillin is similar to benzyl penicillin in its bactericidal action against susceptible organisms during the stage of active multiplication. It acts through the inhibition of cell wall mucopeptide biosynthesis. Ampicillin has a broad spectrum of bactericidal activity against many gram-positive and gram-negative aerobic and anaerobic bacteria. (Ampicillin is, however, degraded by beta-lactamases and therefore the spectrum of activity does not normally include organisms which produce these enzymes.)

A wide range of beta-lactamases found in microorganisms resistant to penicillins and cephalosporins have been shown in biochemical studies with cell free bacterial systems to be irreversibly inhibited by sulbactam. Although sulbactam alone possesses little useful antibacterial activity except against the *Neisseriaciae*, whole organism studies have shown that sulbactam restores ampicillin activity against beta-lactamase producing strains. In particular, sulbactam has good inhibitory activity against the clinically important plasmid mediated beta-lactamases most frequently responsible for transferred drug resistance. Sulbactam has no effect on the activity of ampicillin against ampicillin susceptible strains.

The presence of sulbactam in the UNASYN formulation effectively extends the antibiotic spectrum of ampicillin to include many bacteria normally resistant to it and to other beta-lactam antibiotics. Thus, UNASYN possesses the properties of a broad-spectrum antibiotic and a beta-lactamase inhibitor.

While *in vitro* studies have demonstrated the susceptibility of most strains of the following organisms, clinical efficacy for infections other than those included in the indications section has not been documented.

Continued on next page

Unasyn—Cont.

Gram-Positive Bacteria: *Staphylococcus aureus* (beta-lactamase and non-beta-lactamase producing), *Staphylococcus epidermidis* (beta-lactamase and non-beta-lactamase producing), *Staphylococcus saprophyticus* (beta-lactamase and non-beta-lactamase producing), *Streptococcus faecalis*† (Enterococcus), *Streptococcus pneumoniae*† (formerly *D. pneumoniae), Streptococcus pyogenes*†, *Streptococcus viridans*†.
Gram-Negative Bacteria: *Hemophilus influenzae* (beta-lactamase and non-beta-lactamase producing). *Moraxella (Branhamella) catarrhalis* (beta-lactamase and non-beta-lactamase producing). *Escherichia coli* (beta-lactamase and non-beta-lactamase producing). *Klebsiella* species (all known strains are beta-lactamase producing). *Proteus mirabilis* (beta-lactamase and non-beta-lactamase producing). *Proteus vulgaris, Providencia rettgeri, Providencia stuartii, Morganella morganii,* and *Neisseria gonorrhoeae* (beta-lactamase and non-beta-lactamase producing).
Anaerobes: *Clostridium* species†, *Peptococcus* species†, *Peptostreptococcus* species, *Bacteroides* species, including *B. fragilis.*
†These are not beta-lactamase producing strains and, therefore, are susceptible to ampicillin alone.
Susceptibility Testing
Diffusion Technique: For the Kirby-Bauer method of susceptibility testing, a 20 mcg (10 mcg ampicillin + 10 mcg sulbactam) diffusion disk should be used. The method is one outlined in the NCCLS publication M2-A4.[1] With this procedure, a report from the laboratory of "Susceptible" indicates that the infecting organism is likely to respond to UNASYN therapy and a report of "Resistant" indicates that the infecting organism is not likely to respond to therapy. An "Intermediate" susceptibility report suggests that the infecting organism would be susceptible to UNASYN if a higher dosage is used or if the infection is confined to tissues or fluids (e.g., urine) in which high antibiotic levels are attained.
Dilution Techniques: Broth or agar dilution methods may be used to determine the minimal inhibitory concentration (MIC) value for susceptibility of bacterial isolates to ampicillin/sulbactam. The method used is one outlined in the NCCLS publication M7-A2.[2] Tubes should be inoculated to contain 10^5 to 10^6 organisms/mL or plates "spotted" with 10^4 organisms.
The recommended dilution method employs a constant ampicillin/sulbactam ratio of 2:1 in all tubes with increasing concentrations of ampicillin. MIC's are reported in terms of ampicillin concentration in the presence of sulbactam at a constant 2 parts ampicillin to 1 part sulbactam.
[See table below]

INDICATIONS AND USAGE

UNASYN is indicated for the treatment of infections due to susceptible strains of the designated microorganisms in the conditions listed below.
Skin and Skin Structure Infections caused by beta-lactamase producing strains of *Staphylococcus aureus, Escherichia coli,* Klebsiella* spp.* (including *K. pneumoniae*), Proteus mirabilis,* Bacteroides fragilis,* Enterobacter* spp.,* and *Acinetobacter calcoaceticus.**
NOTE: For information on use in pediatric patients see PRECAUTIONS—Pediatric Use and CLINICAL STUDIES sections.
Intra-Abdominal Infections caused by beta-lactamase producing strains of *Escherichia coli, Klebsiella* spp. (including *K. pneumoniae*), Bacteroides* spp. (including *B. fragilis*), and *Enterobacter* spp.*
Gynecological Infections caused by beta-lactamase producing strains of *Escherichia coli,** and *Bacteroides* spp.* (including *B. fragilis**).
*Efficacy for this organism in this organ system was studied in fewer than 10 infections.
While UNASYN is indicated only for the conditions listed above, infections caused by ampicillin-susceptible organisms are also amenable to treatment with UNASYN due to its ampicillin content. Therefore, mixed infections caused by ampicillin-susceptible organisms and beta-lactamase producing organisms susceptible to UNASYN should not require the addition of another antibiotic.
Appropriate culture and susceptibility tests should be performed before treatment in order to isolate and identify the organisms causing infection and to determine their susceptibility to UNASYN.
Therapy may be instituted prior to obtaining the results from bacteriological and susceptibility studies, when there is reason to believe the infection may involve any of the beta-lactamase producing organisms listed above in the indicated organ systems. Once the results are known, therapy should be adjusted if appropriate.

CONTRAINDICATIONS

The use of UNASYN is contraindicated in individuals with a history of hypersensitivity reactions to any of the penicillins.

WARNINGS

SERIOUS AND OCCASIONALLY FATAL HYPERSENSITIVITY (ANAPHYLACTIC) REACTIONS HAVE BEEN REPORTED IN PATIENTS ON PENICILLIN THERAPY. THESE REACTIONS ARE MORE APT TO OCCUR IN INDIVIDUALS WITH A HISTORY OF PENICILLIN HYPERSENSITIVITY AND/OR HYPERSENSITIVITY REACTIONS TO MULTIPLE ALLERGENS. THERE HAVE BEEN REPORTS OF INDIVIDUALS WITH A HISTORY OF PENICILLIN HYPERSENSITIVITY WHO HAVE EXPERIENCED SEVERE REACTIONS WHEN TREATED WITH CEPHALOSPORINS. BEFORE THERAPY WITH A PENICILLIN, CAREFUL INQUIRY SHOULD BE MADE CONCERNING PREVIOUS HYPERSENSITIVITY REACTIONS TO PENICILLINS, CEPHALOSPORINS, AND OTHER ALLERGENS. IF AN ALLERGIC REACTION OCCURS, UNASYN SHOULD BE DISCONTINUED AND THE APPROPRIATE THERAPY INSTITUTED.
SERIOUS ANAPHYLACTOID REACTIONS REQUIRE IMMEDIATE EMERGENCY TREATMENT WITH EPINEPHRINE. OXYGEN, INTRAVENOUS STEROIDS, AND AIRWAY MANAGEMENT, INCLUDING INTUBATION, SHOULD ALSO BE ADMINISTERED AS INDICATED.
Pseudomembranous colitis has been reported with nearly all antibacterial agents, including UNASYN, and has ranged in severity from mild to life-threatening. Therefore, it is important to consider this diagnosis in patients who present with diarrhea subsequent to the administration of antibacterial agents.
Treatment with antibacterial agents alters the normal flora of the colon and may permit overgrowth of clostridia. Studies indicate that toxin produced by *Clostridium difficile* is one primary cause of "antibiotic-associated colitis."
Mild cases of pseudomembranous colitis usually respond to drug discontinuation alone. In moderate to severe cases, consideration should be given to management with fluids and electrolytes, protein supplementation and treatment with an antibacterial drug clinically effective against *C. difficile* colitis.

PRECAUTIONS

General: A high percentage of patients with mononucleosis who receive ampicillin develop a skin rash. Thus, ampicillin class antibiotics should not be administered to patients with mononucleosis. In patients treated with UNASYN the possibility of superinfections with mycotic or bacterial pathogens should be kept in mind during therapy. If superinfections occur (usually involving *Pseudomonas* or *Candida*), the drug should be discontinued and/or appropriate therapy instituted.
Drug Interactions: Probenecid decreases the renal tubular secretion of ampicillin and sulbactam. Concurrent use of probenecid with UNASYN may result in increased and prolonged blood levels of ampicillin and sulbactam. The concurrent administration of allopurinol and ampicillin increases substantially the incidence of rashes in patients receiving both drugs as compared to patients receiving ampicillin alone. It is not known whether this potentiation of ampicillin rashes is due to allopurinol or the hyperuricemia present in these patients. There are no data with UNASYN and allopurinol administered concurrently. UNASYN and aminoglycosides should not be reconstituted together due to the *in vitro* inactivation of aminoglycosides by the ampicillin component of UNASYN.
Drug/Laboratory Test Interactions: Administration of UNASYN will result in high urine concentration of ampicillin. High urine concentrations of ampicillin may result in false positive reactions when testing for the presence of glucose in urine using Clinitest™, Benedict's Solution or Fehling's Solution. It is recommended that glucose tests based on enzymatic glucose oxidase reactions (such as Clinistix™ or Testape™) be used. Following administration of ampicillin to pregnant women, a transient decrease in plasma concentration of total conjugated estriol, estriol-glucuronide, conjugated estrone and estradiol has been noted. This effect may also occur with UNASYN.
Carcinogenesis, Mutagenesis, Impairment of Fertility: Long-term studies in animals have not been performed to evaluate carcinogenic or mutagenic potential.
Pregnancy
Pregnancy Category B: Reproduction studies have been performed in mice, rats, and rabbits at doses up to ten (10) times the human dose and have revealed no evidence of impaired fertility or harm to the fetus due to UNASYN. There are, however, no adequate and well controlled studies in pregnant women. Because animal reproduction studies are not always predictive of human response, this drug should be used during pregnancy only if clearly needed. (See—Drug/Laboratory Test Interactions.)
Labor and Delivery: Studies in guinea pigs have shown that intravenous administration of ampicillin decreased the uterine tone, frequency of contractions, height of contractions, and duration of contractions. However, it is not known whether the use of UNASYN in humans during labor or delivery has immediate or delayed adverse effects on the fetus, prolongs the duration of labor, or increases the likelihood that forceps delivery or other obstetrical intervention or resuscitation of the newborn will be necessary.
Nursing Mothers: Low concentrations of ampicillin and sulbactam are excreted in the milk; therefore, caution should be exercised when UNASYN is administered to a nursing woman.
Pediatric Use: The safety and effectiveness of UNASYN have been established for pediatric patients one year of age and older for skin and skin structure infections as approved in adults. Use of UNASYN in pediatric patients is supported by evidence from adequate and well-controlled studies in adults with additional data from pediatric pharmacokinetic studies, a controlled clinical trial conducted in pediatric patients and post-marketing adverse events surveillance. (See **CLINICAL PHARMACOLOGY, INDICATIONS AND USAGE, ADVERSE REACTIONS, DOSAGE AND ADMINISTRATION,** and **CLINICAL STUDIES** sections.)
The safety and effectiveness of UNASYN have not been established for pediatric patients for intra-abdominal infections.

ADVERSE REACTIONS

UNASYN is generally well tolerated. The following adverse reactions have been reported.
Local Adverse Reactions
Pain at IM injection site—16%
Pain at IV injection site—3%
Thrombophlebitis—3%
Systemic Adverse Reactions
The most frequently reported adverse reactions were diarrhea in 3% of the patients and rash in less than 2% of the patients.
Additional systemic reactions reported in less than 1% of the patients were: itching, nausea, vomiting, candidiasis, fatigue, malaise, headache, chest pain, flatulence, abdominal distension, glossitis, urine retention, dysuria, edema, facial swelling, erythema, chills, tightness in throat, substernal pain, epistaxis and mucosal bleeding.
Pediatric Patients: Available safety data for pediatric patients treated with UNASYN demonstrate a similar adverse events profile to those observed in adult patients. Additionally, atypical lymphocytosis has been observed in one pediatric patient receiving UNASYN.
Adverse Laboratory Changes
Adverse laboratory changes without regard to drug relationship that were reported during clinical trials were:
Hepatic: Increased AST (SGOT), ALT (SGPT), alkaline phosphatase, and LDH.
Hematologic: Decreased hemoglobin, hematocrit, RBC, WBC, neutrophils, lymphocytes, platelets and increased lymphocytes, monocytes, basophils, eosinophils, and platelets.
Blood Chemistry: Decreased serum albumin and total proteins.
Renal: Increased BUN and creatinine.
Urinalysis: Presence of RBC's and hyaline casts in urine.
The following adverse reactions have been reported with ampicillin-class antibiotics and can also occur with UNASYN.
Gastrointestinal: Gastritis, stomatitis, black "hairy" tongue, and enterocolitis. Onset of pseudomembranous colitis symptoms may occur during or after antibiotic treatment. (See WARNINGS.)
Hypersensitivity Reactions: Urticaria, erythema multiforme, and an occasional case of exfoliative dermatitis have

Recommended ampicillin/sulbactam, Susceptibility Ranges [1,2,3]

	Resistant	Intermediate	Susceptible
Gram(−) and Staphylococcus			
Bauer/Kirby Zone Sizes	≤11 mm	12–13 mm	≥14 mm
MIC (mcg of ampicillin/mL)	≥32	16	≤ 8
Hemophilus influenzae			
Bauer/Kirby Zone Sizes	≤19	—	≥20
MIC (mcg of ampicillin/mL)	≥ 4	—	≤ 2

[1]The non-beta-lactamase producing organisms which are normally susceptible to ampicillin, such as *Streptococci,* will have similar zone sizes as for ampicillin disks.
[2]*Staphylococci* resistant to methicillin, oxacillin, or nafcillin must be considered resistant to UNASYN.
[3]The quality control cultures should have the following assigned daily ranges for ampicillin/sulbactam:

		Disks	Mode MIC (mcg/mL ampicillin/mcg/mL sulbactam)
E. coli	(ATCC 25922)	20–24 mm	2/1
S. aureus	(ATCC 25923)	29–37 mm	0.12/0.06
E. coli	(ATCC 35218)	13–19 mm	8/4

been reported. These reactions may be controlled with antihistamines and, if necessary, systemic corticosteroids. Whenever such reactions occur, the drug should be discontinued, unless the opinion of the physician dictates otherwise. Serious and occasional fatal hypersensitivity (anaphylactic) reactions can occur with a penicillin. (See WARNINGS.)

Hematologic: In addition to the adverse laboratory changes listed above for UNASYN, agranulocytosis has been reported during therapy with penicillins. All of these reactions are usually reversible on discontinuation of therapy and are believed to be hypersensitivity phenomena. Some individuals have developed positive direct Coombs Tests during treatment with UNASYN, as with other beta-lactam antibiotics.

OVERDOSAGE

Neurological adverse reactions, including convulsions, may occur with the attainment of high CSF levels of beta-lactams. Ampicillin may be removed from circulation by hemodialysis. The molecular weight, degree of protein binding and pharmacokinetics profile of sulbactam suggest that this compound may also be removed by hemodialysis.

CLINICAL STUDIES

Skin and Skin Structure Infections in Pediatric Patients: Data from a controlled clinical trial conducted in pediatric patients provided evidence supporting the safety and efficacy of UNASYN for the treatment of skin and skin structure infections. Of 99 pediatric patients evaluable for clinical efficacy, 60 patients received a regimen containing intravenous UNASYN, and 39 patients received a regimen containing intravenous cefuroxime. This trial demonstrated similar outcomes (assessed at an appropriate interval after discontinuation of all antimicrobial therapy) for UNASYN- and cefuroxime-treated patients:

Therapeutic Regimen	Clinical Success	Clinical Failure
UNASYN	51/60 (85%)	9/60 (15%)
Cefuroxime	34/39 (87%)	5/39 (13%)

Most patients received a course of oral antimicrobials following initial treatment with intravenous administration of parenteral antimicrobials. The study protocol required that the following three criteria be met prior to transition from intravenous to oral antimicrobial therapy: 1) receipt of a minimum of 72 hours of intravenous therapy; 2) no documented fever for prior 24 hours; and 3) improvement or resolution of the signs and symptoms of infection.

The choice of oral antimicrobial agent used in this trial was determined by susceptibility testing of the original pathogen, if isolated, to oral agents available. The course of oral antimicrobial therapy should not routinely exceed 14 days.

DOSAGE AND ADMINISTRATION

UNASYN may be administered by either the IV or the IM routes.

For IV administration, the dose can be given by slow intravenous injection over at least 10–15 minutes or can also be delivered, in greater dilutions with 50–100 mL of a compatible diluent as an intravenous infusion over 15–30 minutes.

UNASYN may be administered by deep intramuscular injection. (See Preparation for Intramuscular Injection.)

The recommended adult dosage of UNASYN is 1.5 g (1 g ampicillin as the sodium salt plus 0.5 g sulbactam as the sodium salt) to 3 g (2 g ampicillin as the sodium salt plus 1 g sulbactam as the sodium salt) every six hours. This 1.5 to 3 g range represents the total of ampicillin content plus the sulbactam content of UNASYN, and corresponds to a range of 1 g ampicillin/0.5 g sulbactam to 2 g ampicillin/1 g sulbactam. The total dose of sulbactam should not exceed 4 grams per day.

Impaired Renal Function

In patients with impairment of renal function the elimination kinetics of ampicillin and sulbactam are similarly affected, hence the ratio of one to the other will remain constant whatever the renal function. The dose of UNASYN in such patients should be administered less frequently in accordance with the usual practice for ampicillin and according to the following recommendations:

UNASYN Dosage Guide For Patients With Renal Impairment

Creatinine Clearance (mL/min/1.73m²)	Ampicillin/Sulbactam Half-Life (Hours)	Recommended UNASYN Dosage
≥30	1	1.5–3.0 g q 6h–q 8h
15–29	5	1.5–3.0 g q 12h
5–14	9	1.5–3.0 g q 24h

When only serum creatinine is available, the following formula (based on sex, weight, and age of the patient) may be used to convert this value into creatinine clearance. The serum creatinine should represent a steady state of renal function.

$$\text{Males} \quad \frac{\text{weight (kg)} \times (140-\text{age})}{72 \times \text{serum creatinine}}$$

Females 0.85 × above value

COMPATABILITY, RECONSTITUTION AND STABILITY

UNASYN sterile powder is to be stored at or below 30°C (86°F) prior to reconstitution.

When concomitant therapy with aminoglycosides is indicated, UNASYN and aminoglycosides should be reconstituted and administered separately, due to the *in vitro* inactivation of aminoglycosides by any of the aminopenicillins.

Diluent	Maximum Concentration (mg/mL) UNASYN (Ampicillin/Sulbactam)	Use Periods
Sterile Water for Injection	45 (30/15)	8 hrs @ 25°C
	45 (30/15)	48 hrs @ 4°C
	30 (20/10)	72 hrs @ 4°C
0.9% Sodium Chloride Injection	45 (30/15)	8 hrs @ 25°C
	45 (30/15)	48 hrs @ 4°C
	30 (20/10)	72 hrs @ 4°C
5% Dextrose Injection	30 (20/10)	2 hrs @ 25°C
	30 (20/10)	4 hrs @ 4°C
	3 (2/1)	4 hrs @ 25°C
Lactated Ringer's Injection	45 (30/15)	8 hrs @ 25°C
	45 (30/15)	24 hrs @ 4°C
M/6 Sodium Lactate Injection	45 (30/15)	8 hrs @ 25°C
	45 (30/15)	8 hrs @ 4°C
5% Dextrose in 0.45% Saline	3 (2/1)	4 hrs @ 25°C
	15 (10/5)	4 hrs @ 4°C
10% Invert Sugar	3 (2/1)	4 hrs @ 25°C
	30 (20/10)	3 hrs @ 4°C

DIRECTIONS FOR USE

General Dissolution Procedures: UNASYN sterile powder for intravenous and intramuscular use may be reconstituted with any of the compatible diluents described in this insert. Solutions should be allowed to stand after dissolution to allow any foaming to dissipate in order to permit visual inspection for complete solubilization.

Preparation for Intravenous Use

1.5 g and 3.0 g Bottles: UNASYN sterile powder in piggyback units may be reconstituted directly to the desired concentrations using any of the following parenteral diluents. Reconstitution of UNASYN, at the specified concentrations, with these diluents provide stable solutions for the time periods indicated in the following table: (After the indicated time periods, any unused portions of solutions should be discarded.)

[See table above]

If piggyback bottles are unavailable, standard vials of UNASYN sterile powder may be used. Initially, the vials may be reconstituted with Sterile Water for Injection to yield solutions containing 375 mg UNASYN per mL (250 mg ampicillin/125 mg sulbactam per mL). An appropriate volume should then be immediately diluted with a suitable parenteral diluent to yield solutions containing 3 to 45 mg UNASYN per mL (2 to 30 mg ampicillin/1 to 15 mg sulbactam per mL).

1.5 g ADD-Vantage® Vials: UNASYN in the ADD-Vantage® system is intended as a single dose for intravenous administration after dilution with the ADD-Vantage® Flexible Diluent Container containing 50 mL, 100 mL or 250 mL of 0.9% Sodium Chloride Injection, USP.

3 g ADD-Vantage® Vials: UNASYN in the ADD-Vantage® system is intended as a single dose for intravenous administration after dilution with the ADD-Vantage® Flexible Diluent Container containing 100 mL or 250 mL of 0.9% Sodium Chloride Injection, USP.

UNASYN in the ADD-Vantage® system is to be reconstituted with 0.9% Sodium Chloride Injection, USP only. See INSTRUCTIONS FOR USE OF THE ADD-Vantage® VIAL. Reconstitution of UNASYN, at the specified concentration, with 0.9% Sodium Chloride Injection, USP provides stable solutions for the time period indicated below:

Diluent	Maximum Concentration (mg/mL) UNASYN (Ampicillin/Sulbactam)	Use Period
0.9% Sodium Chloride Injection	30 (20/10)	8 hrs @ 25°C

In 0.9% Sodium Chloride Injection, USP

The final diluted solution of UNASYN should be completely administered *within 8 hours* in order to assure proper potency.

Preparation for Intramuscular Injection

1.5 g and 3.0 g Standard Vials: Vials for intramuscular use may be reconstituted with Sterile Water for Injection USP, 0.5% Lidocaine Hydrochloride Injection USP or 2% Lidocaine Hydrochloride Injection USP. Consult the following table for recommended volumes to be added to obtain solutions containing 375 mg UNASYN per mL (250 mg ampicillin/125 mg sulbactam per mL). Note: *Use only freshly prepared solutions and administer within one hour after preparation.*

UNASYN Vial Size	Volume of Diluent to be Added	Withdrawal Volume*
1.5 g	3.2 mL	4.0 mL
3.0 g	6.4 mL	8.0 mL

*There is sufficient excess present to allow withdrawal and administration of the stated volumes.

Animal Pharmacology: While reversible glycogenosis was observed in laboratory animals, this phenomenon was dose- and time-dependent and is not expected to develop at the therapeutic doses and corresponding plasma levels attained during the relatively short periods of combined ampicillin/sulbactam therapy in man.

HOW SUPPLIED

UNASYN (ampicillin sodium/sulbactam sodium) is supplied as a sterile off-white dry powder in glass vials and piggyback bottles. The following packages are available:

Vials containing 1.5 g (NDC 0049-0013-83) equivalent of UNASYN (1 g ampicillin as the sodium salt plus 0.5 g sulbactam as the sodium salt)

Vials containing 3 g (NDC 0049-0014-83) equivalent of UNASYN (2 g ampicillin as the sodium salt plus 1 g sulbactam as the sodium salt)

Bottles containing 1.5 g (NDC 0049-0022-83) equivalent of UNASYN (1 g ampicillin as the sodium salt plus 0.5 g sulbactam as the sodium salt)

Bottles containing 3 g (NDC 0049-0023-83) equivalent of UNASYN (2 g ampicillin as the sodium salt plus 1 g sulbactam as the sodium salt)

Pharmacy Bulk Package containing 15 g (NDC 0049-0024-28) equivalent of UNASYN (10 g ampicillin as the sodium salt plus 5 g sulbactam as the sodium salt)

ADD-Vantage® vials containing 1.5 g (NDC 0049-0031-83) equivalent of UNASYN (1 g ampicillin as the sodium salt plus 0.5 g sulbactam as the sodium salt) are distributed by Pfizer Inc.

ADD-Vantage® vials containing 3 g (NDC 0049-0032-83) equivalent of UNASYN (2 g ampicillin as the sodium salt plus 1 g sulbactum as the sodium salt) are distributed by Pfizer Inc.

The 1.5 g UNASYN ADD-Vantage® vials are only to be used with Abbott Laboratories' ADD-Vantage® Flexible Diluent Container containing 0.9% Sodium Chloride Injection, USP, 50 mL, 100 mL, or 250 mL sizes.

The 3 g UNASYN ADD-Vantage® vials are only to be used with Abbott Laboratories' ADD-Vantage® Flexible Diluent Container containing 0.9% Sodium Chloride Injection, USP, 100 mL or 250 mL sizes.

INSTRUCTIONS FOR USE OF THE ADD-Vantage® VIAL

To Open Diluent Container: Peel overwrap from the corner and remove container. Some opacity of the plastic due to moisture absorption during the sterilization process may be observed. This is normal and does not affect the solution quality or safety. The opacity will diminish gradually.

To Assemble Vial and Flexible Diluent Container: (Use Aseptic Technique)

1. Remove the protective covers from the top of the vial and the vial port on the diluent container as follows:
   a. To remove the breakaway vial cap, swing the pull ring over the top of the vial and pull down far enough to start the opening (see Figure 1), pull the ring approximately half way around the cap and then pull straight up to remove the cap (see Figure 2).

NOTE: Do not access vial with syringe.

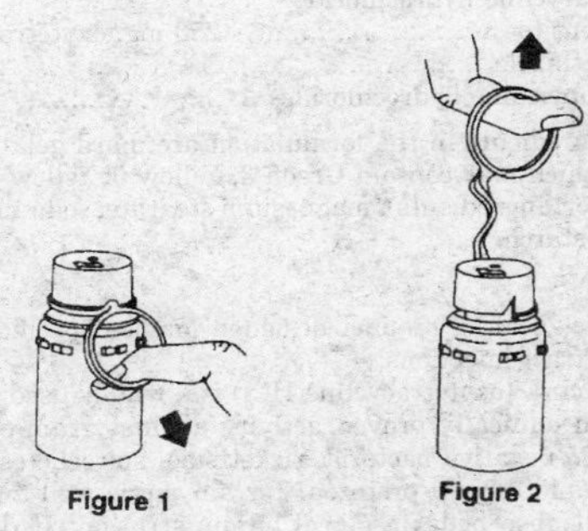

Figure 1 Figure 2

   b. To remove the vial port cover, grasp the tab on the pull ring, pull up to break the three tie strings, then pull back to remove the cover. (See Figure 3.)
2. Screw the vial into the vial port until it will go no further. THE VIAL MUST BE SCREWED IN TIGHTLY TO ASSURE A SEAL. This occurs approximately $^1/_2$ turn (180°) after the first audible click. (See Figure 4.) The clicking sound does not assure a seal, the vial must be turned as far as it will go.

Continued on next page

Unasyn—Cont.

NOTE: Once vial is sealed, do not attempt to remove. (See Figure 4.)

3. Recheck the vial to assure that it is tight by trying to turn it further in the direction of assembly.
4. Label appropriately.

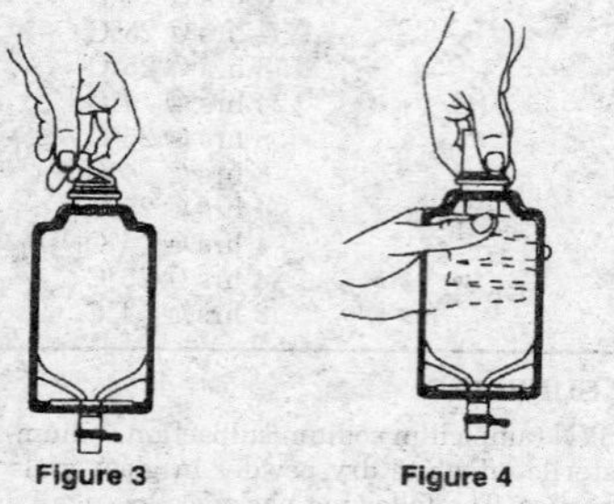

Figure 3 Figure 4

To Prepare Admixture

1. Squeeze the bottom of the diluent container gently to inflate the portion of the container surrounding the end of the drug vial.
2. With the other hand, push the drug vial down into the container telescoping the walls of the container. Grasp the inner cap of the vial through the walls of the container. (See Figure 5.)
3. Pull the inner cap from the drug vial. (See Figure 6.) Verify that the rubber stopper has been pulled out, allowing the drug and diluent to mix.
4. Mix container contents thoroughly and use within the specified time.

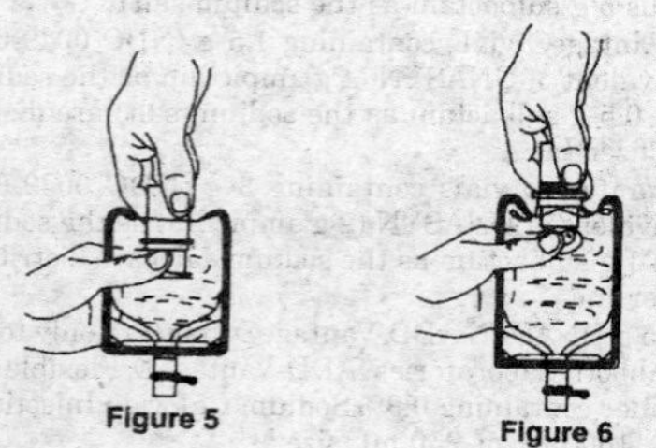

Figure 5 Figure 6

REFERENCES

1. National Committee for Clinical Laboratory Standards, *Performance Standards for Antimicrobial Disk Susceptibility Tests*—Fourth Edition. Approved Standard NCCLS Document M2-A4, Vol. 10, No. 7 NCCLS. Villanova, PA. April 1990.
2. National Committee for Clinical Laboratory Standards, *Methods for Dilution Antimicrobial Susceptibility Tests for Bacteria that Grow Aerobically.* Second Edition. Approved Standard NCCLS Document M7-A2. Vol. 10, No. 8 NCCLS. Villanova, PA. April 1990.

69-4361-00-3 Rev. March 1997

Shown in Product Identification Guide, page 330

UROBIOTIC®-250 ℞

[*u "rō-bī-ot 'ik*]
CAPSULES

Each capsule contains
Oxytetracycline hydrochloride
equivalent to .... 250 mg. oxytetracycline
Sulfamethizole .... 250 mg
Phenazopyridine hydrochloride .... 50 mg

Inert ingredients in the formulation are: hard gelatin capsules (which may contain Green 3, Yellow 6, Yellow 10 and other inert ingredients); magnesium stearate; sodium lauryl sulfate; starch.

ACTIONS

Urobiotic-250 is a product designed for use specifically in urinary tract infections.

Terramycin® (oxytetracycline HCl) is a widely used antibiotic with clinically proved activity against gram-positive and gram-negative bacteria, rickettsiae, spirochetes, large viruses, and certain protozoa. Terramycin is well tolerated and well absorbed after oral administration. It diffuses readily through the placenta and is present in the fetal circulation. It diffuses into the pleural fluid, and under some circumstances, into the cerebrospinal fluid. Oxytetracycline HCl appears to be concentrated in the hepatic system and is excreted in the bile. It is excreted in the urine and in the feces, in high concentrations, in a biologically active form.

Sulfamethizole is a chemotherapeutic agent active against a number of important gram-positive and gram-negative bacteria. This sulfonamide is well absorbed, has a low degree of acetylation, and is extremely soluble. Because of these features and its rapid renal excretion, sulfamethizole has a low order of toxicity and provides prompt and high concentrations of the active drug in the urinary tract.

Phenazopyridine is an orally absorbed agent which produces prompt and effective local analgesia and relief of urinary symptoms by virtue of its rapid excretion in the urinary tract. These effects are confined to the genitourinary system and are not accompanied by generalized sedation or narcosis.

INDICATIONS

Based on a review of this drug by the National Academy of Sciences-National Research Council and/or other information, FDA has classified the indications as follows:

"Lacking substantial evidence of effectiveness as a fixed combination":

Urobiotic-250 is indicated in the therapy of a number of genitourinary infections caused by susceptible organisms. These infections include the following: pyelonephritis, pyelitis, ureteritis, cystitis, prostatitis, and urethritis.

Since both Terramycin and sulfamethizole provide effective levels in blood, tissue, and urine, Urobiotic-250 provides a multiple antimicrobial approach at the site of infection. Both antibacterial components are active against the most common urinary pathogens, including *Escherichia coli, Pseudomonas aeruginosa, Aerobacter aerogenes, Streptococcus faecalis, Streptococcus hemolyticus,* and *Micrococcus pyogenes.* Urobiotic-250 is particularly useful in the treatment of infections caused by bacteria more sensitive to the combination than to either component alone. The combination is also of value in those cases with mixed infections, and in those instances where the causative organism is unknown pending laboratory isolation. **Final classification of the less than effective indications requires further investigation. Clinical studies to substantiate the efficacy of Urobiotic-250 are ongoing. Completion of these ongoing studies will provide data for final classification of these indications.**

CONTRAINDICATIONS

This drug is contraindicated in individuals who have shown hypersensitivity to any of its components.

This drug, because of the sulfonamide component, should not be used in patients with a history of sulfonamide sensitivities, and in pregnant females at term.

WARNINGS

If renal impairment exists, even usual oral or parenteral doses may lead to excessive systemic accumulation of the drug and possible liver toxicity. Under such conditions, lower than usual doses are indicated and if therapy is prolonged, tetracycline serum level determinations may be advisable.

Oxytetracycline HCl, which is one of the ingredients of Urobiotic-250, may form a stable calcium complex in any bone-forming tissue with no serious harmful effects reported thus far in humans. However, use of oxytetracycline during tooth development (last trimester of pregnancy, neonatal period and early childhood) may cause discoloration of the teeth (yellow-grey-brownish). This effect occurs mostly during long term use of the drug but it also has been observed in usual short treatment courses.

Because of its sulfonamide content, this drug should be used only after critical appraisal in patients with liver damage, renal damage, urinary obstruction, or blood dyscrasias. Deaths have been reported from hypersensitivity reactions, agranulocytosis, aplastic anemia, and other blood dyscrasias associated with sulfonamide administration. When used intermittently, or for a prolonged period, blood counts and liver and kidney function tests should be performed.

Certain hypersensitive individuals may develop a photodynamic reaction precipitated by exposure to direct sunlight during the use of this drug. This reaction is usually of the photoallergic type which may also be produced by other tetracycline derivatives. Individuals with a history of photosensitivity reactions should be instructed to avoid exposure to direct sunlight while under treatment with this or other tetracycline drugs, and treatment should be discontinued at first evidence of skin discomfort.

NOTE: Reactions of a photoallergic nature are exceedingly rare with Terramycin (oxytetracycline HCl). Phototoxic reactions are not believed to occur with Terramycin.

PRECAUTIONS

As with all antibiotic preparations, use of this drug may result in overgrowth of nonsusceptible organisms, including fungi. If superinfection occurs, the antibiotic should be discontinued and appropriate specific therapy should be instituted. This drug should be used with caution in persons having histories of significant allergies and/or asthma.

ADVERSE REACTIONS

Glossitis, stomatitis, proctitis, nausea, diarrhea, vaginitis, and dermatitis, as well as reactions of an allergic nature, may occur during oxytetracycline HCl therapy, but are rare. If adverse reactions, individual idiosyncrasy, or allergy occur, discontinue medication. Rare instances of esophagitis and esophageal ulcerations have been reported in patients receiving capsule forms of drugs in the tetracycline class. Most of these patients took medications immediately before going to bed. (See Dosage and Administration.)

With oxytetracycline therapy bulging fontanels in infants and benign intracranial hypertension in adults have been reported in individuals receiving full therapeutic dosages. These conditions disappeared rapidly when the drug was discontinued.

As in all sulfonamide therapy, the following reactions may occur: nausea, vomiting, diarrhea, hepatitis, pancreatitis, blood dyscrasias, neuropathy, drug fever, skin rash, infection of the conjunctiva and sclera, petechiae, purpura, hematuria and crystalluria. The dosage should be decreased or the drug withdrawn, depending upon the severity of the reaction.

DOSAGE AND ADMINISTRATION

Urobiotic-250 is recommended in adults only. A dose of 1 capsule four times daily is suggested. In refractory cases 2 capsules four times a day may be used.

Therapy should be continued for a minimum of seven days or until bacteriologic cure in acute urinary tract infections.

Administration of adequate amounts of fluid along with capsule forms of drugs in the tetracycline class is recommended to wash down the drugs and reduce the risk of esophageal irritation and ulceration. (See Adverse Reactions.)

To aid absorption of the drug, it should be given at least one hour before or two hours after eating. Aluminum hydroxide gel given with antibiotics has been shown to decrease their absorption and is contraindicated.

SUPPLY

Urobiotic-250 capsules: bottles of 50 (NDC 0049-0920-50), and unit dose packages of 100 (10 × 10's) (NDC 0049-0920-41).

LITERATURE AVAILABLE

Yes.

70-1636-00-9
Revised Dec. 1986

VIAGRA® ℞

[*vī agra*]
(sildenafil citrate)
Tablets

DESCRIPTION

VIAGRA®, an oral therapy for erectile dysfunction, is the citrate salt of sildenafil, a selective inhibitor of cyclic guanosine monophosphate (cGMP)-specific phosphodiesterase type 5 (PDE5).

Sildenafil citrate is designated chemically as 1-[[3-(6,7-dihydro-1-methyl-7-oxo-3-propyl-1*H*-pyrazolo[4,3-*d*]pyrimidin-5-yl)-4-ethoxyphenyl]sulfonyl]-4-methylpiperazine citrate and has the following structural formula:

[structural formula: CH_3CH_2O, HN, O, CH_3, N, $CH_2CH_2CH_3$, O_2S, N, CH_3; HOOC, CO_2H, OH, CO_2H]

Sildenafil citrate is a white to off-white crystalline powder with a solubility of 3.5 mg/mL in water and a molecular weight of 666.7. VIAGRA (sildenafil citrate) is formulated as blue, film-coated rounded-diamond-shaped tablets equivalent to 25 mg, 50 mg and 100 mg of sildenafil for oral administration. In addition to the active ingredient, sildenafil citrate, each tablet contains the following inactive ingredients: microcrystalline cellulose, anhydrous dibasic calcium phosphate, croscarmellose sodium, magnesium stearate, hydroxypropyl methylcellulose, titanium dioxide, lactose, triacetin, and FD & C Blue #2 aluminum lake.

CLINICAL PHARMACOLOGY

Mechanism of Action

The physiologic mechanism of erection of the penis involves release of nitric oxide (NO) in the corpus cavernosum during sexual stimulation. NO then activates the enzyme guanylate cyclase, which results in increased levels of cyclic guanosine monophosphate (cGMP), producing smooth muscle relaxation in the corpus cavernosum and allowing inflow of blood. Sildenafil has no direct relaxant effect on isolated human corpus cavernosum, but enhances the effect of nitric oxide (NO) by inhibiting phosphodiesterase type 5 (PDE5), which is responsible for degradation of cGMP in the corpus cavernosum. When sexual stimulation causes local release of NO, inhibition of PDE5 by sildenafil causes increased levels of cGMP in the corpus cavernosum, resulting in smooth muscle relaxation and inflow of blood to the corpus cavernosum. Sildenafil at recommended doses has no effect in the absence of sexual stimulation.

Studies *in vitro* have shown that sildenafil is selective for PDE5. Its effect is more potent on PDE5 than on other known phosphodiesterases (>80-fold for PDE1, >1,000-fold for PDE2, PDE3, and PDE4). The approximately 4,000-fold selectivity for PDE5 versus PDE3 is important because that PDE is involved in control of cardiac contractility. Sildenafil is only about 10-fold as potent for PDE5 compared to PDE6, an enzyme found in the retina; this lower selectivity is thought to be the basis for abnormalities related to color vision observed with higher doses or plasma levels (see **Pharmacodynamics**).

In addition to human corpus cavernosum smooth muscle, PDE5 is also found in lower concentrations in other tissues including platelets, vascular and visceral smooth muscle, and skeletal muscle. The inhibition of PDE5 in these tissues by sildenafil may be the basis for the enhanced platelet antiaggregatory activity of nitric oxide observed *in vitro*, an inhibition of platelet thrombus formation *in vivo* and peripheral arterial-venous dilatation *in vivo*.

Pharmacokinetics and Metabolism

VIAGRA is rapidly absorbed after oral administration, with absolute bioavailability of about 40%. Its pharmacokinetics are dose-proportional over the recommended dose range. It is eliminated predominantly by hepatic metabolism (mainly cytochrome P450 3A4) and is converted to an active metabolite with properties similar to the parent, sildenafil. The concomitant use of potent cytochrome P450 3A4 inhibitors (e.g., erythromycin, ketoconazole, itraconazole) as well as the nonspecific CYP inhibitor, cimetidine, is associated with increased plasma levels of sildenafil (see **DOSAGE AND ADMINISTRATION**). Both sildenafil and the metabolite have terminal half lives of about 4 hours.

Mean sildenafil plasma concentrations measured after the administration of a single oral dose of 100 mg to healthy male volunteers is depicted below:

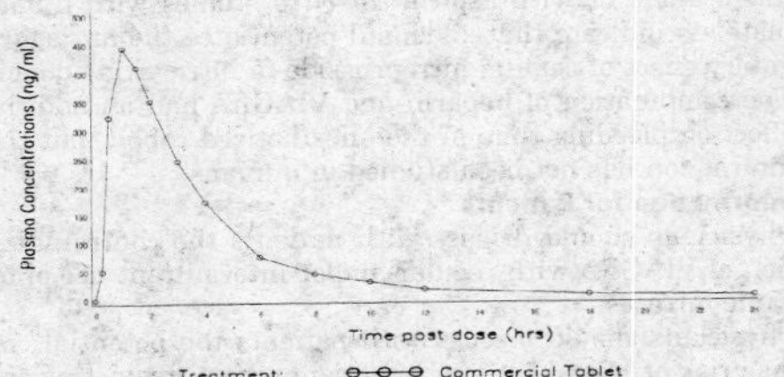

Figure 1: Mean Sildenafil Plasma Concentrations in Healthy Male Volunteers.

Absorption and Distribution: VIAGRA is rapidly absorbed. Maximum observed plasma concentrations are reached within 30 to 120 minutes (median 60 minutes) of oral dosing in the fasted state. When VIAGRA is taken with a high fat meal, the rate of absorption is reduced, with a mean delay in T_{max} of 60 minutes and a mean reduction in C_{max} of 29%. The mean steady state volume of distribution (Vss) for sildenafil is 105 L, indicating distribution into the tissues. Sildenafil and its major circulating N-desmethyl metabolite are both approximately 96% bound to plasma proteins. Protein binding is independent of total drug concentrations.

Based upon measurements of sildenafil in semen of healthy volunteers 90 minutes after dosing, less than 0.001% of the administered dose may appear in the semen of patients.

Metabolism and Excretion: Sildenafil is cleared predominantly by the CYP3A4 (major route) and CYP2C9 (minor route) hepatic microsomal isoenzymes. The major circulating metabolite results from N-desmethylation of sildenafil, and is itself further metabolized. This metabolite has a PDE selectivity profile similar to sildenafil and an *in vitro* potency for PDE5 approximately 50% of the parent drug. Plasma concentrations of this metabolite are approximately 40% of those seen for sildenafil, so that the metabolite accounts for about 20% of sildenafil's pharmacologic effects.

After either oral or intravenous administration, sildenafil is excreted as metabolites predominantly in the feces (approximately 80% of administered oral dose) and to a lesser extent in the urine (approximately 13% of administered oral dose). Similar values for pharmacokinetic parameters were seen in normal volunteers and in the patient population, using a population pharmacokinetic approach.

Pharmacokinetics in Special Populations

Geriatrics: Healthy elderly volunteers (65 years or over) had a reduced clearance of sildenafil, with free plasma concentrations approximately 40% greater than those seen in healthy younger volunteers (18–45 years).

Renal Insufficiency: In volunteers with mild (CLcr=50–80 mL/min) and moderate (CLcr=30–49 mL/min) renal impairment, the pharmacokinetics of a single oral dose of VIAGRA (50 mg) were not altered. In volunteers with severe (CLcr=<30 mL/min) renal impairment, sildenafil clearance was reduced, resulting in approximately doubling of AUC and C_{max} compared to age-matched volunteers with no renal impairment.

Hepatic Insufficiency: In volunteers with hepatic cirrhosis (Child-Pugh A and B), sildenafil clearance was reduced, resulting in increases in AUC (84%) and C_{max} (47%) compared to age-matched volunteers with no hepatic impairment.

Therefore, age >65, hepatic impairment and severe renal impairment are associated with increased plasma levels of sildenafil. A starting oral dose of 25 mg should be considered in those patients (see **DOSAGE AND ADMINISTRATION**).

Pharmacodynamics

Effects of VIAGRA on Erectile Response: In eight double-blind, placebo-controlled crossover studies of patients with either organic or psychogenic erectile dysfunction, sexual stimulation resulted in improved erections, as assessed by an objective measurement of hardness and duration of erections (RigiScan®), after VIAGRA administration compared with placebo. Most studies assessed the efficacy of VIAGRA approximately 60 minutes post dose. The erectile response, as assessed by RigiScan®, generally increased with increasing sildenafil dose and plasma concentration. The time course of effect was examined in one study, showing an effect for up to 4 hours but the response was diminished compared to 2 hours.

TABLE 1. HEMODYNAMIC DATA IN PATIENTS WITH STABLE ISCHEMIC HEART DISEASE AFTER IV ADMINISTRATION OF 40 MG SILDENAFIL

Means ± SD	At rest				After 4 minutes of exercise			
	n	Baseline (B2)	n	Sildenafil (D1)	n	Baseline	n	Sildenafil
PAOP (mmHg)	8	8.1 ± 5.1	8	6.5 ± 4.3	8	36.0 ± 13.7	8	27.8 ± 15.3
Mean PAP (mmHg)	8	16.7 ± 4	8	12.1 ± 3.9	8	39.4 ± 12.9	8	31.7 ± 13.2
Mean RAP (mmHg)	7	5.7 ± 3.7	8	4.1 ± 3.7	–	–	–	–
Systolic SAP (mmHg)	8	150.4 ± 12.4	8	140.6 ± 16.5	8	199.5 ± 37.4	8	187.8 ± 30.0
Diastolic SAP (mmHg)	8	73.6 ± 7.8	8	65.9 ± 10	8	84.6 ± 9.7	8	79.5 ± 9.4
Cardiac output (L/min)	8	5.6 ± 0.9	8	5.2 ± 1.1	8	11.5 ± 2.4	8	10.2 ± 3.5
Heart rate (bpm)	8	67 ± 11.1	8	66.9 ± 12	8	101.9 ± 11.6	8	99.0 ± 20.4

Effects of VIAGRA on Blood Pressure: Single oral doses of sildenafil (100 mg) administered to healthy volunteers produced decreases in supine blood pressure (mean maximum decrease of 8.4/5.5 mmHg). The decrease in blood pressure was most notable approximately 1–2 hours after dosing, and was not different than placebo at 8 hours. Similar effects on blood pressure were noted with 25 mg, 50 mg and 100 mg of VIAGRA, therefore the effects are not related to dose or plasma levels. Larger effects were recorded among patients receiving concomitant nitrates (see **CONTRAINDICATIONS**).

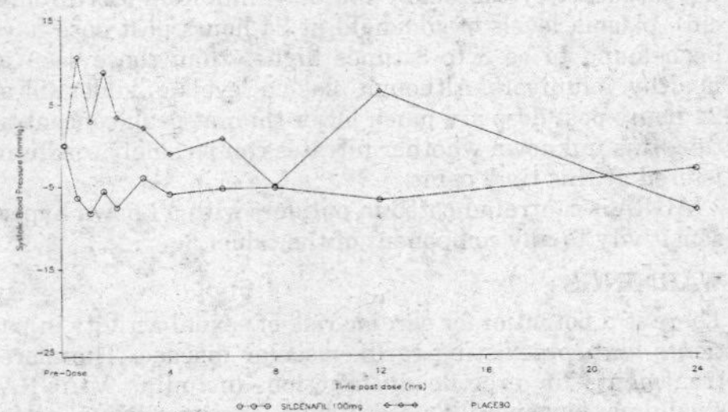

Figure 2: Mean Change from Baseline in Sitting Systolic Blood Pressure, Healthy Volunteers.

Effects of VIAGRA on Cardiac Parameters: Single oral doses of sildenafil up to 100 mg produced no clinically relevant changes in the ECGs of normal male volunteers.

Studies have produced relevant data on the effects of VIAGRA on cardiac output. In one small, open-label, uncontrolled, pilot study, eight patients with stable ischemic heart disease underwent Swan-Ganz catheterization. A total dose of 40 mg sildenafil was administered by four intravenous infusions.

The results from this pilot study are shown in Table 1; the mean resting systolic and diastolic blood pressures decreased by 7% and 10% compared to baseline in these patients. Mean resting values for right atrial pressure, pulmonary artery pressure, pulmonary artery occluded pressure and cardiac output decreased by 28%, 28%, 20% and 7% respectively. Even though this total dosage produced plasma sildenafil concentrations which were approximately 2 to 5 times higher than the mean maximum plasma concentrations following a single oral dose of 100 mg in healthy male volunteers, the hemodynamic response to exercise was preserved in these patients.

[See table above]

Effects of VIAGRA on Vision: At single oral doses of 100 mg and 200 mg, transient dose-related impairment of color discrimination (blue/green) was detected using the Farnsworth-Munsell 100-hue test, with peak effects near the time of peak plasma levels. This finding is consistent with the inhibition of PDE6, which is involved in phototransduction in the retina. An evaluation of visual function at doses up to twice the maximum recommended dose revealed no effects of VIAGRA on visual acuity, intraocular pressure, or pupillometry.

Clinical Studies

In clinical studies, VIAGRA was assessed for its effect on the ability of men with erectile dysfunction (ED) to engage in sexual activity and in many cases specifically on the ability to achieve and maintain an erection sufficient for satisfactory sexual activity. VIAGRA was evaluated primarily at doses of 25 mg, 50 mg and 100 mg in 21 randomized, double-blind, placebo-controlled trials of up to 6 months in duration, using a variety of study designs (fixed dose, titration, parallel, crossover). VIAGRA was administered to more than 3,000 patients aged 19 to 87 years, with ED of various etiologies (organic, psychogenic, mixed) with a mean duration of 5 years. VIAGRA demonstrated statistically significant improvement compared to placebo in all 21 studies. The studies that established benefit demonstrated improvements in success rates for sexual intercourse compared with placebo.

The effectiveness of VIAGRA was evaluated in most studies using several assessment instruments. The primary measure in the principal studies was a sexual function questionnaire (the International Index of Erectile Function—IIEF) administered during a 4-week treatment-free run-in period, at baseline, at follow-up visits, and at the end of double-blind, placebo-controlled, at-home treatment. Two of the questions from the IIEF served as primary study endpoints; categorical responses were elicited to questions about (1) the ability to achieve erections sufficient for sexual intercourse and (2) the maintenance of erections after penetration. The patient addressed both questions at the final visit for the last 4 weeks of the study. The possible categorical responses to these questions were (0) no attempted intercourse, (1) never or almost never, (2) a few times, (3) sometimes, (4) most times, and (5) almost always or always. Also collected as part of the IIEF was information about other aspects of sexual function, including information on erectile function, orgasm, desire, satisfaction with intercourse, and overall sexual satisfaction. Sexual function data were also recorded by patients in a daily diary. In addition, patients were asked a global efficacy question and an optional partner questionnaire was administered.

The effect on one of the major end points, maintenance of erections after penetration, is shown in Figure 3, for the pooled results of 5 fixed-dose, dose-response studies of greater than one month duration, showing response according to baseline function. Results with all doses have been pooled, but scores showed greater improvement at the 50 and 100 mg doses than at 25 mg. The pattern of responses was similar for the other principal question, the ability to achieve an erection sufficient for intercourse. The titration studies, in which most patients received 100 mg, showed similar results. Figure 3 shows that regardless of the baseline levels of function, subsequent function in patients treated with VIAGRA was better than that seen in patients treated with placebo. At the same time, on-treatment function was better in treated patients who were less impaired at baseline.

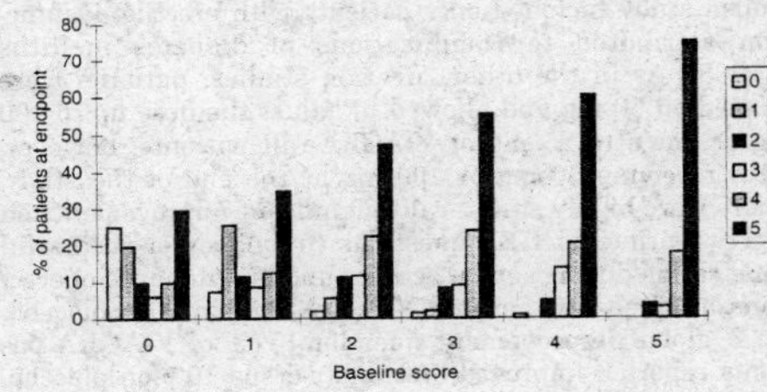

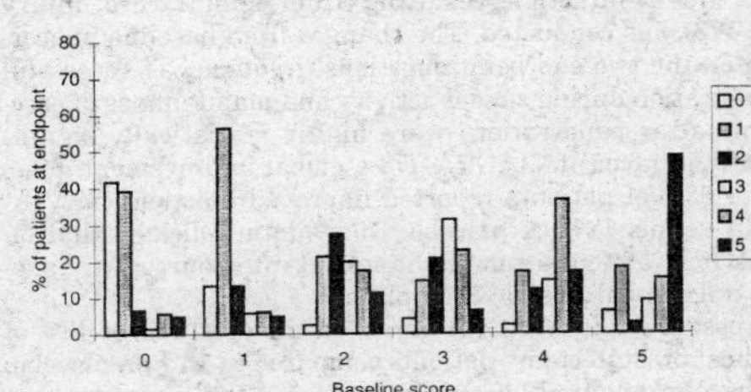

Figure 3. Effect of VIAGRA and Placebo on Maintenance of Erection by Baseline Score.

Continued on next page

Viagra—Cont.

The frequency of patients reporting improvement of erections in response to a global question in four of the randomized, double-blind, parallel, placebo-controlled fixed dose studies (1797 patients) of 12 to 24 weeks duration is shown in Figure 4. These patients had erectile dysfunction at baseline that was characterized by median categorical scores of 2 (a few times) on principal IIEF questions. Erectile dysfunction was attributed to organic (58%; generally not characterized, but including diabetes and excluding spinal cord injury), psychogenic (17%), or mixed (24%) etiologies. Sixty-three percent, 74%, and 82% of the patients on 25 mg, 50 mg and 100 mg of VIAGRA, respectively, reported an improvement in their erections, compared to 24% on placebo. In the titration studies (n=644) (with most patients eventually receiving 100 mg), results were similar.

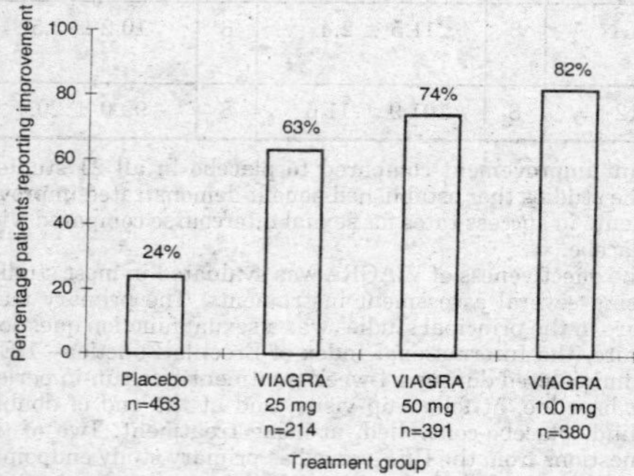

Overall treatment p<0.0001

Figure 4. Percentage of Patients Reporting an Improvement in Erections.

The patients in studies had varying degrees of ED. One-third to one-half of the subjects in these studies reported successful intercourse at least once during a 4-week, treatment-free run-in period.

In many of the studies, of both fixed dose and titration designs, daily diaries were kept by patients. In these studies, involving about 1600 patients, analyses of patient diaries showed no effect of VIAGRA on rates of attempted intercourse (about 2 per week), but there was clear treatment-related improvement in sexual function: per patient weekly success rates averaged 1.3 on 50–100 mg of VIAGRA vs 0.4 on placebo; similarly, group mean success rates (total successes divided by total attempts) were about 66% on VIAGRA vs about 20% on placebo.

During 3 to 6 months of double-blind treatment or longer-term (1 year), open-label studies, few patients withdrew from active treatment for any reason, including lack of effectiveness. At the end of the long-term study, 88% of patients reported that VIAGRA improved their erections.

Men with untreated ED has relatively low baseline scores for all aspects of sexual function measured (again using a 5-point scale) in the IIEF. VIAGRA improved these aspects of sexual function: frequency, firmness and maintenance of erections; frequency of orgasm; frequency and level of desire; frequency, satisfaction and enjoyment of intercourse; and overall relationship satisfaction.

One randomized, double-blind, flexible-dose, placebo-controlled study included only patients with erectile dysfunction attributed to complications of diabetes mellitus (n=268). As in the other titration studies, patients were started on 50 mg and allowed to adjust the dose up to 100 mg or down to 25 mg of VIAGRA; all patients, however, were receiving 50 mg or 100 mg at the end of the study. There were highly statistically significant improvements on the two principal IIEF questions (frequency of successful penetration during sexual activity and maintenance of erections after penetration) on VIAGRA compared to placebo. On a global improvement question, 57% of VIAGRA patients reported improved erections versus 10% on placebo. Diary data indicated that on VIAGRA, 48% of intercourse attempts were successful versus 12% on placebo.

One randomized, double-blind, placebo-controlled, crossover, flexible-dose (up to 100 mg) study of patients with erectile dysfunction resulting from spinal cord injury (n=178) was conducted. The changes from baseline in scoring on the two end point questions (frequency of successful penetration during sexual activity and maintenance of erections after penetration) were highly statistically significantly in favor of VIAGRA. On a global improvement question, 83% of patients reported improved erections on VIAGRA versus 12% on placebo. Diary data indicated that on VIAGRA, 59% of attempts at sexual intercourse were successful compared to 13% on placebo.

Across all trials, VIAGRA improved the erections of 43% of radical prostatectomy patients compared to 15% on placebo.

Subgroup analyses of responses to a global improvement question in patients with psychogenic etiology in two fixed-dose studies (total n=179) and two titration studies (total n=149) showed 84% of VIAGRA patients reported improvement in erections compared with 26% of placebo. The changes from baseline in scoring on the two end point questions (frequency of successful penetration during sexual activity and maintenance of erections after penetration) were highly statistically significantly in favor of VIAGRA. Diary data in two of the studies (n=178) showed rates of successful intercourse per attempt of 70% for VIAGRA and 29% for placebo.

A review of population subgroups demonstrated efficacy regardless of baseline severity, etiology, race and age. VIAGRA was effective in a broad range of ED patients, including those with a history of coronary artery disease, hypertension, other cardiac disease, peripheral vascular disease, diabetes mellitus, depression, coronary artery bypass graft (CABG), radical prostatectomy, transurethral resection of the prostate (TURP) and spinal cord injury, and in patients taking antidepressants/antipsychotics and antihypertensives/diuretics.

Analysis of the safety database showed no apparent difference in the side effect profile in patients taking VIAGRA with and without antihypertensive medication. This analysis was performed retrospectively, and was not powered to detect any pre-specified difference in adverse reactions.

INDICATION AND USAGE

VIAGRA is indicated for the treatment of erectile dysfunction.

CONTRAINDICATIONS

Consistent with its known effects on the nitric oxide/cGMP pathway (see **CLINICAL PHARMACOLOGY**), VIAGRA was shown to potentiate the hypotensive effects of nitrates, and its administration to patients who are using organic nitrates, either regularly and/or intermittently, in any form is therefore contraindicated.

After patients have taken VIAGRA, it is unknown when nitrates, if necessary, can be safely administered. Based on the pharmacokinetic profile of a single 100 mg oral dose given to healthy normal volunteers, the plasma levels of sildenafil at 24 hours post dose are approximately 2 ng/mL (compared to peak plasma levels of approximately 440 ng/mL) (see **CLINICAL PHARMACOLOGY: Pharmacokinetics and Metabolism**). In the following patients: age >65, hepatic impairment (e.g., cirrhosis), severe renal impairment (e.g., creatinine clearance <30 mL/min), and concomitant use of potent cytochrome P450 3A4 inhibitors (erythromycin), plasma levels of sildenafil at 24 hours post dose have been found to be 3 to 8 times higher than those seen in healthy volunteers. Although plasma levels of sildenafil at 24 hours post dose are much lower than at peak concentration, it is unknown whether nitrates can be safely coadministered at this time point.

VIAGRA is contraindicated in patients with a known hypersensitivity to any component of the tablet.

WARNINGS

There is a potential for cardiac risk of sexual activity in patients with preexisting cardiovascular disease. Therefore, treatments for erectile dysfunction, including VIAGRA, should not be generally used in men for whom sexual activity is inadvisable because of their underlying cardiovascular status.

VIAGRA has systemic vasodilatory properties that resulted in transient decreases in supine blood pressure in healthy volunteers (mean maximum decrease of 8.4/5.5 mmHg), (see **CLINICAL PHARMACOLOGY: Pharmacodynamics**). While this normally would be expected to be of little consequence in most patients, prior to prescribing VIAGRA, physicians should carefully consider whether their patients with underlying cardiovascular disease could be affected adversely by such vasodilatory effects, especially in combination with sexual activity.

There is no controlled clinical data on the safety or efficacy of VIAGRA in the following groups; if prescribed, this should be done with caution.

- Patients who have suffered a myocardial infarction, stroke, or life-threatening arrhythmia within the last 6 months;
- Patients with resting hypotension (BP <90/50) or hypertension (BP >170/110);
- Patients with cardiac failure or coronary artery disease causing unstable angina;
- Patients with retinitis pigmentosa (a minority of these patients have genetic disorders of retinal phosphodiesterases).

Prolonged erection greater than 4 hours and priapism (painful erections greater than 6 hours in duration) have been reported infrequently since market approval of VIAGRA. In the event of an erection that persists longer than 4 hours, the patient should seek immediate medical assistance. If priapism is not treated immediately, penile tissue damage and permanent loss of potency could result.

The concomitant administration of the protease inhibitor ritonavir substantially increases serum concentrations of sildenafil (**11-fold increase in AUC**). If VIAGRA is prescribed to patients taking ritonavir, caution should be used. Data from subjects exposed to high systemic levels of sildenafil are limited. Visual disturbances occurred more commonly at higher levels of sildenafil exposure. Decreased blood pressure, syncope, and prolonged erection were reported in some healthy volunteers exposed to high doses of sildenafil (200–800 mg). To decrease the chance of adverse events in patients taking ritonavir, a decrease in sildenafil dosage is recommended (see **Drug Interactions, ADVERSE REACTIONS,** and **DOSAGE AND ADMINISTRATION**).

PRECAUTIONS

General

The evaluation of erectile dysfunction should include a determination of potential underlying causes and the identification of appropriate treatment following a complete medical assessment.

Before prescribing VIAGRA, it is important to note the following:

Patients on multiple antihypertensive medications were included in the pivotal clinical trials for VIAGRA. In a separate drug interaction study, when amlodipine, 5 mg or 10 mg, and VIAGRA, 100 mg were orally administered concomitantly to hypertensive patients mean additional blood pressure reduction of 8 mmHg systolic and 7 mmHg diastolic were noted (see **Drug Interactions**). Controlled studies of drug interactions between VIAGRA and other antihypertensive medications have not been performed.

The safety of VIAGRA is unknown in patients with bleeding disorders and patients with active peptic ulceration.

VIAGRA should be used with caution in patients with anatomical deformation of the penis (such as angulation, cavernosal fibrosis or Peyronie's disease), or in patients who have conditions which may predispose them to priapism (such as sickle cell anemia, multiple myeloma, or leukemia).

The safety and efficacy of combinations of VIAGRA with other treatments for erectile dysfunction have not been studied. Therefore, the use of such combinations is not recommended.

In humans, VIAGRA has no effect on bleeding time when taken alone or with aspirin. *In vitro* studies with human platelets indicate that sildenafil potentiates the antiaggregatory effect of sodium nitroprusside (a nitric oxide donor). The combination of heparin and VIAGRA had an additive effect on bleeding time in the anesthetized rabbit, but this interaction has not been studied in humans.

Information for Patients

Physicians should discuss with patients the contraindication of VIAGRA with regular and/or intermittent use of organic nitrates.

Physicians should discuss with patients the potential cardiac risk of sexual activity in patients with preexisting cardiovascular risk factors. Patients who experience symptoms (e.g., angina pectoris, dizziness, nausea) upon initiation of sexual activity should be advised to refrain from further activity and should discuss the episode with their physician.

Physicians should warn patients that prolonged erections greater than 4 hours and priapism (painful erections greater than 6 hours in duration) have been reported infrequently since market approval of VIAGRA. In the event of an erection that persists longer than 4 hours, the patient should seek immediate medical assistance. If priapism is not treated immediately, penile tissue damage and permanent loss of potency may result.

The use of VIAGRA offers no protection against sexually transmitted diseases. Counseling of patients about the protective measures necessary to guard against sexually transmitted diseases, including the Human Immunodeficiency Virus (HIV), may be considered.

Drug Interactions

Effects of Other Drugs on VIAGRA

***In vitro* studies:** Sildenafil metabolism is principally mediated by the cytochrome P450 (CYP) isoforms 3A4 (major route) and 2C9 (minor route). Therefore, inhibitors of these isoenzymes may reduce sildenafil clearance.

***In vivo* studies:** Cimetidine (800 mg), a nonspecific CYP inhibitor, caused a 56% increase in plasma sildenafil concentrations when coadministered with VIAGRA (50 mg) to healthy volunteers.

When a single 100 mg dose of VIAGRA was administered with erythromycin, a specific CYP3A4 inhibitor, at steady state (500 mg bid for 5 days), there was a 182% increase in sildenafil systemic exposure (AUC). In addition, in a study performed in healthy male volunteers, coadministration of the HIV protease inhibitor saquinavir, also a CYP3A4 inhibitor, at steady state (1200 mg tid) with VIAGRA (100 mg single dose) resulted in a 140% increase in sildenafil C_{max} and a 210% increase in sildenafil AUC. VIAGRA had no effect on saquinavir pharmacokinetics. Stronger CYP3A4 inhibitors such as ketoconazole or itraconazole would be expected to have still greater effects, and population data from patients in clinical trials did indicate a reduction in sildenafil clearance when it was coadministered with CYP3A4 inhibitors (such as ketoconazole, erythromycin, or cimetidine). (see **DOSAGE AND ADMINISTRATION**).

In another study in healthy male volunteers, coadministration with the HIV protease inhibitor ritonavir, which is a highly potent P450 inhibitor, at steady state (500 mg bid) with VIAGRA (100 mg single dose) resulted in a 300% (4-fold) increase in sildenafil C_{max} and a 1000% (11-fold) increase in sildenafil plasma AUC. At 24 hours the plasma levels of sildenafil were still approximately 200 ng/mL, compared to approximately 5 ng/mL when sildenafil was dosed alone. This is consistent with ritonavir's marked effects on a broad range of P450 substrates. VIAGRA had no effect on ritonavir pharmacokinetics (see **DOSAGE AND ADMINISTRATION**).

Although the interaction between other protease inhibitors and sildenafil has not been studied, their concomitant use is expected to increase sildenafil levels.

It can be expected that concomitant administration of CYP3A4 inducers, such as rifampin, will decrease plasma levels of sildenafil.

Single doses of antacid (magnesium hydroxide/aluminum hydroxide) did not affect the bioavailability of VIAGRA.

Pharmacokinetic data from patients in clinical trials showed no effect on sildenafil pharmacokinetics of CYP2C9 inhibitors (such as tolbutamide, warfarin), CYP2D6 inhibitors (such as selective serotonin reuptake inhibitors, tricy-

	25 mg	50 mg	100 mg
Obverse	VGR25	VGR50	VGR100
Reverse	PFIZER	PFIZER	PFIZER
Bottle of 30	NDC-0069-4200-30	NDC-0069-4210-30	NDC-0069-4220-30
Bottle of 100	N/A	NDC-0069-4210-66	NDC-0069-4220-66

clic antidepressants), thiazide and related diuretics, ACE inhibitors, and calcium channel blockers. The AUC of the active metabolite, N-desmethyl sildenafil, was increased 62% by loop and potassium-sparing diuretics and 102% by nonspecific beta-blockers. These effects on the metabolite are not expected to be of clinical consequence.

Effects of VIAGRA on Other Drugs

***In vitro* studies:** Sildenafil is a weak inhibitor of the cytochrome P450 isoforms 1A2, 2C9, 2C19, 2D6, 2E1 and 3A4 (IC50 >150 µM). Given sildenafil peak plasma concentrations of approximately 1 µM after recommended doses, it is unlikely that VIAGRA will alter the clearance of substrates of these isoenzymes.

***In vivo* studies:** When VIAGRA 100 mg oral was coadministered with amlodipine, 5 mg or 10 mg oral, to hypertensive patients, the mean additional reduction on supine blood pressure was 8 mmHg systolic and 7 mmHg diastolic.

No significant interactions were shown with tolbutamide (250 mg) or warfarin (40 mg), both of which are metabolized by CYP2C9.

VIAGRA (50 mg) did not potentiate the increase in bleeding time caused by aspirin (150 mg).

VIAGRA (50 mg) did not potentiate the hypotensive effect of alcohol in healthy volunteers with mean maximum blood alcohol levels of 0.08%.

In a study of healthy male volunteers, sildenafil (100 mg) did not affect the steady state pharmacokinetics of the HIV protease inhibitors, saquinavir and ritonavir, both of which are CYP3A4 substrates.

Carcinogenesis, Mutagenesis, Impairment of Fertility

Sildenafil was not carcinogenic when administered to rats for 24 months at a dose resulting in total systemic drug exposure (AUCs) for unbound sildenafil and its major metabolite of 29- and 42-times, for male and female rats, respectively, the exposures observed in human males given the Maximum Recommended Human Dose (MRHD) of 100 mg. Sildenafil was not carcinogenic when administered to mice for 18–21 months at dosages up to the Maximum Tolerated Dose (MTD) of 10 mg/kg/day, approximately 0.6 times the MRHD on a mg/m^2 basis.

Sildenafil was negative in *in vitro* bacterial and Chinese hamster ovary cell assays to detect mutagenicity, and *in vitro* human lymphocytes and *in vivo* mouse micronucleus assays to detect clastogenicity.

There was no impairment of fertility in rats given sildenafil up to 60 mg/kg/day for 36 days to females and 102 days to males, a dose producing an AUC value of more than 25 times the human male AUC.

There was no effect on sperm motility or morphology after single 100 mg oral doses of VIAGRA in healthy volunteers.

Pregnancy, Nursing Mothers and Pediatric Use

VIAGRA is not indicated for use in newborns, children, or women.

Pregnancy Category B. No evidence of teratogenicity, embryotoxicity or fetotoxicity was observed in rats and rabbits which received up to 200 mg/kg/day during organogenesis. These doses represent, respectively, about 20 and 40 times the MRHD on a mg/m^2 basis in a 50 kg subject. In the rat pre- and postnatal development study, the no observed adverse effect dose was 30 mg/kg/day given for 36 days. In the nonpregnant rat the AUC at this dose was about 20 times human AUC. There are no adequate and well-controlled studies of sildenafil in pregnant women.

Geriatric Use: Healthy elderly volunteers (65 years or over) had a reduced clearance of sildenafil (see **CLINICAL PHARMACOLOGY: Pharmacokinetics in Special Populations**). Since higher plasma levels may increase both the efficacy and incidence of adverse events, a starting dose of 25 mg should be considered (see **DOSAGE AND ADMINISTRATION**).

ADVERSE REACTIONS

PRE-MARKETING EXPERIENCE:

VIAGRA was administered to over 3700 patients (aged 19–87 years) during clinical trials worldwide. Over 550 patients were treated for longer than one year.

In placebo-controlled clinical studies, the discontinuation rate due to adverse events for VIAGRA (2.5%) was not significantly different from placebo (2.3%). The adverse events were generally transient and mild to moderate in nature.

In trials of all designs, adverse events reported by patients receiving VIAGRA were generally similar. In fixed-dose studies, the incidence of some adverse events increased with dose. The nature of the adverse events in flexible-dose studies, which more closely reflect the recommended dosage regimen, was similar to that for fixed-dose studies.

When VIAGRA was taken as recommended (on an as-needed basis) in flexible-dose, placebo-controlled clinical trials, the following adverse events were reported:

TABLE 2. ADVERSE EVENTS REPORTED BY ≥2% OF PATIENTS TREATED WITH VIAGRA AND MORE FREQUENT ON DRUG THAN PLACEBO IN PRN FLEXIBLE-DOSE PHASE II/III STUDIES

Adverse Event	Percentage of Patients Reporting Event	
	VIAGRA N = 734	PLACEBO N = 725
Headache	16%	4%
Flushing	10%	1%
Dyspepsia	7%	2%
Nasal Congestion	4%	2%
Urinary Tract Infection	3%	2%
Abnormal Vision[†]	3%	0%
Diarrhea	3%	1%
Dizziness	2%	1%
Rash	2%	1%

[†] Abnormal Vision: Mild and transient, predominantly color tinge to vision, but also increased sensitivity to light or blurred vision. In these studies, only one patient discontinued due to abnormal vision.

Other adverse reactions occurred at a rate of >2%, but equally common on placebo: respiratory tract infection, back pain, flu syndrome, and arthralgia.

In fixed-dose studies, dyspepsia (17%) and abnormal vision (11%) were more common at 100 mg than at lower doses. At doses above the recommended dose range, adverse events were similar to those detailed above but generally were reported more frequently.

The following events occurred in <2% of patients in controlled clinical trials; a causal relationship to VIAGRA is uncertain. Reported events include those with a plausible relation to drug use; omitted are minor events and reports too imprecise to be meaningful:

Body as a whole: face edema, photosensitivity reaction, shock, asthenia, pain, chills, accidental fall, abdominal pain, allergic reaction, chest pain, accidental injury.

Cardiovascular: angina pectoris, AV block, migraine, syncope, tachycardia, palpitation, hypotension, postural hypotension, myocardial ischemia, cerebral thrombosis, cardiac arrest, heart failure, abnormal electrocardiogram, cardiomyopathy.

Digestive: vomiting, glossitis, colitis, dysphagia, gastritis, gastroenteritis, esophagitis, stomatitis, dry mouth, liver function tests abnormal, rectal hemorrhage, gingivitis.

Hemic and Lymphatic: anemia and leukopenia.

Metabolic and Nutritional: thirst, edema, gout, unstable diabetes, hyperglycemia, peripheral edema, hyperuricemia, hypoglycemic reaction, hypernatremia.

Musculoskeletal: arthritis, arthrosis, myalgia, tendon rupture, tenosynovitis, bone pain, myasthenia, synovitis.

Nervous: ataxia, hypertonia, neuralgia, neuropathy, paresthesia, tremor, vertigo, depression, insomnia, somnolence, abnormal dreams, reflexes decreased, hypesthesia.

Respiratory: asthma, dyspnea, laryngitis, pharyngitis, sinusitis, bronchitis, sputum increased, cough increased.

Skin and Appendages: urticaria, herpes simplex, pruritus, sweating, skin ulcer, contact dermatitis, exfoliative dermatitis.

Special Senses: mydriasis, conjunctivitis, photophobia, tinnitus, eye pain, deafness, ear pain, eye hemorrhage, cataract, dry eyes.

Urogenital: cystitis, nocturia, urinary frequency, breast enlargement, urinary incontinence, abnormal ejaculation, genital edema and anorgasmia.

POST-MARKETING EXPERIENCE:

Cardiovascular

Serious cardiovascular events, including myocardial infarction, sudden cardiac death, ventricular arrhythmia, cerebrovascular hemorrhage, transient ischemic attack and hypertension, have been reported post-marketing in temporal association with the use of VIAGRA. Most, but not all, of these patients had preexisting cardiovascular risk factors. Many of these events were reported to occur during or shortly after sexual activity, and a few were reported to occur shortly after the use of VIAGRA without sexual activity. Others were reported to have occurred hours to days after the use of VIAGRA and sexual activity. It is not possible to determine whether these events are related directly to VIAGRA, to sexual activity, to the patient's underlying cardiovascular disease, to a combination of these factors, or to other factors (see **WARNINGS** for further important cardiovascular information).

Other events

Other events reported post-marketing to have been observed in temporal association with VIAGRA and not listed in the pre-marketing adverse reactions section above include:

Nervous: seizure and anxiety.

Urogenital: prolonged erection, priapism (see **WARNINGS**) and hematuria.

Ocular: diplopia, temporary vision loss/decreased vision, ocular redness or bloodshot appearance, ocular burning, ocular swelling/pressure, increased intraocular pressure, retinal vascular disease or bleeding, vitreous detachment/traction and paramacular edema.

OVERDOSAGE

In studies with healthy volunteers of single doses up to 800 mg, adverse events were similar to those seen at lower doses but incidence rates were increased.

In cases of overdose, standard supportive measures should be adopted as required. Renal dialysis is not expected to accelerate clearance as sildenafil is highly bound to plasma proteins and it is not eliminated in the urine.

DOSAGE AND ADMINISTRATION

For most patients, the recommended dose is 50 mg taken, as needed, approximately 1 hour before sexual activity. However, VIAGRA may be taken anywhere from 4 hours to 0.5 hour before sexual activity. Based on effectiveness and toleration, the dose may be increased to a maximum recommended dose of 100 mg or decreased to 25 mg. The maximum recommended dosing frequency is once per day.

The following factors are associated with increased plasma levels of sildenafil: age >65 (40% increase in AUC), hepatic impairment (e.g., cirrhosis, 80%), severe renal impairment (creatinine clearance <30 mL/min, 100%), and concomitant use of potent cytochrome P450 3A4 inhibitors [ketoconazole, itraconazole, erythromycin (182%), saquinavir (210%)]. Since higher plasma levels may increase both the efficacy and incidence of adverse events, a starting dose of 25 mg should be considered in these patients.

Ritonavir greatly increased the systemic level of sildenafil in a study of healthy, non-HIV infected volunteers (11-fold increase in AUC, see **Drug Interactions.**) Based on these pharmacokinetic data, it is recommended not to exceed a maximum single dose of 25 mg of VIAGRA in a 48 hour period.

VIAGRA was shown to potentiate the hypotensive effects of nitrates and its administration in patients who use nitric oxide donors or nitrates in any form is therefore contraindicated.

HOW SUPPLIED

VIAGRA® (sildenafil citrate) is supplied as blue, film-coated, rounded-diamond-shaped tablets containing sildenafil citrate equivalent to the nominally indicated amount of sildenafil as follows:

[See table above]

Recommended Storage: Store at controlled room temperature, 15° to 30°C (59° to 86°F)

Rx only

Distributed by

Pfizer Labs

Division of Pfizer Inc, NY, NY 10017

69-5485-00-6 Revised January 2000

Shown in Product Identification Guide, page 330

VIBRAMYCIN® Calcium ℞

[*vī-brə 'mīs-ən*]

doxycycline calcium
oral suspension
SYRUP

VIBRAMYCIN® Hyclate

[*vī-brə 'mīs-ən*]

doxycycline hyclate
CAPSULES

VIBRAMYCIN® Monohydrate

[*vī-brə 'mīs-ən*]

doxycycline monohydrate
for ORAL SUSPENSION

VIBRA–TABS®

[*vī-brə 'mīs-ən*]

doxycycline hyclate
FILM COATED TABLETS

DESCRIPTION

Vibramycin is a broad-spectrum antibiotic synthetically derived from oxytetracycline, and is available as Vibramycin Monohydrate (doxycycline monohydrate); Vibramycin Hyclate and Vibra-Tabs (doxycycline hydrochloride hemiethanolate hemihydrate); and Vibramycin Calcium (doxycycline calcium) for oral administration.

The structural formula of doxycycline monohydrate is

OH O OH OH O CONH₂ · H₂O OH H H H CH₃ OH N(CH₃)₂ H H H

with a molecular formula of $C_{22}H_{24}N_2O_8 \cdot H_2O$ and a molecular weight of 462.46. The chemical designation for doxycy-

Continued on next page

Vibramycin/Vibra-Tabs—Cont.

cline is 4-(Dimethylamino)-1, 4, 4a, 5, 5a, 6, 11, 12a-octahydro-3, 5, 10, 12, 12a-pentahydroxy-6-methyl-1, 11-dioxo-2-naphthacenecarboxamide monohydrate. The molecular formula for doxycycline hydrochloride hemiethanolate hemihydrate is $(C_{22}H_{24}N_2O_8{\cdot}HCl)_2{\cdot}C_2H_6O{\cdot}H_2O$ and the molecular weight is 1025.89. Doxycycline is a light-yellow crystalline powder. Doxycycline hyclate is soluble in water, while doxycycline monohydrate is very slightly soluble in water.

Doxycycline has a high degree of lipoid solubility and a low affinity for calcium binding. It is highly stable in normal human serum. Doxycycline will not degrade into an epianhydro form.

Inert ingredients in the syrup formulation are: apple flavor; butylparaben; calcium chloride; carmine; glycerin; hydrochloric acid; magnesium aluminum silicate; povidone; propylene glycol; propylparaben; raspberry flavor; simethicone emulsion; sodium hydroxide; sodium metabisulfite; sorbitol solution; water.

Inert ingredients in the capsule formulations are: hard gelatin capsules (which may contain Blue 1 and other inert ingredients); magnesium stearate; microcrystalline cellulose; sodium lauryl sulfate.

Inert ingredients for the oral suspension formulation are: carboxymethylcellulose sodium; Blue 1; methylparaben; microcrystalline cellulose; propylparaben; raspberry flavor; Red 28; simethicone emulsion; sucrose.

Inert ingredients for the tablet formulation are: ethylcellulose; hydroxypropyl methylcellulose; magnesium stearate; microcrystalline cellulose; propylene glycol; sodium lauryl sulfate; talc; titanium dioxide; Yellow 6 Lake.

CLINICAL PHARMACOLOGY

Tetracyclines are readily absorbed and are bound to plasma proteins in varying degree. They are concentrated by the liver in the bile, and excreted in the urine and feces at high concentrations and in a biologically active form. Doxycycline is virtually completely absorbed after oral administration.

Following a 200 mg dose, normal adult volunteers averaged peak serum levels of 2.6 mcg/mL of doxycycline at 2 hours decreasing to 1.45 mcg/mL at 24 hours. Excretion of doxycycline by the kidney is about 40%/72 hours in individuals with normal function (creatinine clearance about 75 mL/min.). This percentage excretion may fall as low as 1–5%/72 hours in individuals with severe renal insufficiency (creatinine clearance below 10 mL/min.). Studies have shown no significant difference in serum half-life of doxycycline (range 18–22 hours) in individuals with normal and severely impaired renal function.

Hemodialysis does not alter serum half-life.

Results of animal studies indicate that tetracyclines cross the placenta and are found in fetal tissues.

Microbiology

The tetracyclines are primarily bacteriostatic and are thought to exert their antimicrobial effect by the inhibition of protein synthesis. The tetracyclines, including doxycycline, have a similar antimicrobial spectrum of activity against a wide range of gram-positive and gram-negative organisms. Cross-resistance of these organisms to tetracyclines is common.

Gram-Negative Bacteria

Neisseria gonorrhoeae
Calymmatobacterium granulomatis
Haemophilus ducreyi
Haemophilus influenzae
Yersinia pestis (formerly *Pasteurella pestis*)
Francisella tularensis (formerly *Pasteurella tularensis*)
Vibrio cholera (formerly *Vibrio comma*)
Bartonella bacilliformis
Brucella species

Because many strains of the following groups of gram-negative microorganisms have been shown to be resistant to tetracyclines, culture and susceptibility testing are recommended:

Escherichia coli
Klebsiella species
Enterobacter aerogenes
Shigella species
Acinetobacter species (formerly *Mima* species and *Herellea* species)
Bacteroides species

Gram-Positive Bacteria

Because many strains of the following groups of gram-positive microorganisms have been shown to be resistant to tetracycline, culture and susceptibility testing are recommended. Up to 44 percent of strains of *Streptococcus pyogenes* and 74 percent of *Streptococcus faecalis* have been found to be resistant to tetracycline drugs. Therefore, tetracycline should not be used for streptococcal disease unless the organism has been demonstrated to be susceptible.

Streptococcus pyogenes
Streptococcus pneumoniae
Enterococcus group (*Streptococcus faecalis* and *Streptococcus faecium*)
Alpha-hemolytic streptococci (viridans group)

Other Microorganisms

Rickettsiae
Chlamydia psittaci
Chlamydia trachomatis
Mycoplasma pneumoniae
Ureaplasma urealyticum
Borrelia recurrentis
Treponema pallidum
Treponema pertenue
Clostridium species
Fusobacterium fusiforme
Actinomyces species
Bacillus anthracis
Propionbacterium acnes
Entamoeba species
Balantidium coli
Plasmodium falciparum

Doxycycline has been found to be active against the asexual erythrocytic forms of *Plasmodium falciparum* but not against the gametocytes of *P. falciparum*. The precise mechanism of action of the drug is not known.

Susceptibility tests: Diffusion techniques: Quantitative methods that require measurement of zone diameters give the most precise estimate of the susceptibility of bacteria to antimicrobial agents. One such standard procedure[1] which has been recommended for use with disks to test susceptibility of organisms to doxycycline uses the 30-mcg tetracycline-class disk or the 30-mcg doxycycline disk. Interpretation involves the correlation of the diameter obtained in the disk test with the minimum inhibitory concentration (MIC) for tetracycline or doxycycline, respectively.

Reports from the laboratory giving results of the standard single-disk susceptibility test with a 30-mcg tetracycline-class disk or the 30-mcg doxycycline disk should be interpreted according to the following criteria:

Zone Diameter (mm)		Interpretation
tetracycline	doxycycline	
≥19	≥16	Susceptible
15–18	13–15	Intermediate
≤14	≤12	Resistant

A report of "Susceptible" indicates that the pathogen is likely to be inhibited by generally achievable blood levels. A report of "Intermediate" suggests that the organism would be susceptible if a high dosage is used or if the infection is confined to tissues and fluids in which high antimicrobial levels are attained. A report of "Resistant" indicates that achievable concentrations are unlikely to be inhibitory, and other therapy should be selected.

Standardized procedures require the use of laboratory control organisms. The 30-mcg tetracycline-class disk or the 30-mcg doxycycline disk should give the following zone diameters:

Organism	Zone Diameter (mm)	
	tetracycline	doxycycline
E. coli ATCC 25922	18–25	18–24
S. aureus ATCC 25923	19–28	23–29

Dilution techniques: Use a standardized dilution method[2] (broth, agar, microdilution) or equivalent with tetracycline powder. The MIC values obtained should be interpreted according to the following criteria:

MIC (mcg/mL)	Interpretation
≤4	Susceptible
8	Intermediate
≥16	Resistant

As with standard diffusion techniques, dilution methods require the use of laboratory control organisms. Standard tetracycline powder should provide the following MIC values:

Organism	MIC (mcg/mL)
E. coli ATCC 25922	1.0–4.0
S. aureus ATCC 29213	0.25–1.0
E. faecalis ATCC 29212	8–32
P. aeruginosa ATCC 27853	8–32

INDICATIONS AND USAGE

Treatment:

Doxycycline is indicated for the treatment of the following infections:

Rocky mountain spotted fever, typhus fever and the typhus group, Q fever, rickettsialpox, and tick fevers caused by Rickettsiae.

Respiratory tract infections caused by *Mycoplasma pneumoniae*.

Lymphogranuloma venereum caused by *Chlamydia trachomatis*.

Psittacosis (ornithosis) caused by *Chlamydia psittaci*.

Trachoma caused by *Chlamydia trachomatis,* although the infectious agent is not always eliminated as judged by immunofluorescence.

Inclusion conjunctivitis caused by *Chlamydia trachomatis*.

Uncomplicated urethral, endocervical or rectal infections in adults caused by *Chlamydia trachomatis*.

Nongonococcal urethritis caused by *Ureaplasma urealyticum*.

Relapsing fever due to *Borrelia recurrentis*.

Doxycycline is also indicated for the treatment of infections caused by the following gram-negative microorganisms:

Chancroid caused by *Haemophilus ducreyi*.

Plague due to *Yersinia pestis* (formerly *Pasteurella pestis*).

Tuleremia due to *Francisella tulerensis* (formerly *Pasteurella tulerensis*).

Cholera caused by *Vibrio cholerae* (formerly *Vibrio comma*).

Campylobacter fetus infections caused by *Campylobacter fetus* (formerly *Vibrio fetus*).

Brucellosis due to *Brucella* species (in conjunction with streptomycin).

Bartonellosis due to *Bartonella bacilliformis*.

Granuloma inguinale caused by *Calymmatobacterium granulomatis*.

Because many strains of the following groups of microorganisms have been shown to be resistant to doxycycline, culture and susceptibility testing are recommended.

Doxycycline is indicated for treatment of infections caused by the following gram-negative microorganisms, when bacteriologic testing indicates appropriate susceptibility to the drug:

Escherichia coli.

Enterobacter aerogenes (formerly *Aerobacter aerogenes*).

Shigella species.

Acinetobacter species (formerly *Mima* species and *Herellea* species).

Respiratory tract infections caused by *Haemophilus influenzae*.

Respiratory tract and urinary tract infections caused by *Klebsiella* species.

Doxycycline is indicated for treatment of infections caused by the following gram-positive microorganisms when bacteriologic testing indicates appropriate susceptibility to the drug:

Upper respiratory infections caused by *Streptococcus pneumoniae* (formerly *Diplococcus pneumoniae*).

When penicillin is contraindicated, doxycycline is an alternative drug in the treatment of the following infections:

Uncomplicated gonorrhea caused by *Neisseria gonorrhoeae*.

Syphilis caused by *Treponema pallidum*.

Yaws caused by *Treponema pertenue*.

Listeriosis due to *Listeria monocytogenes*.

Anthrax due to *Bacillus anthracis*.

Vincent's infection caused by *Fusobacterium fusiforme*.

Actinomycosis caused by *Actinomyces israelii*.

Infections caused by *Clostridium* species.

In acute intestinal amebiasis, doxycycline may be a useful adjunct to amebicides.

In severe acne, doxycycline may be useful adjunctive therapy.

Prophylaxis:

Doxycycline is indicated for the prophylaxis of malaria due to *Plasmodium falciparum* in short-term travelers (<4 months) to areas with chloroquine and/or pyrimethamine-sulfadoxine resistant strains. See DOSAGE AND ADMINISTRATION section and Information for Patients subsection of the PRECAUTIONS section.

CONTRAINDICATIONS

This drug is contraindicated in persons who have shown hypersensitivity to any of the tetracyclines.

WARNINGS

THE USE OF DRUGS OF THE TETRACYCLINE CLASS DURING TOOTH DEVELOPMENT (LAST HALF OF PREGNANCY, INFANCY AND CHILDHOOD TO THE AGE OF 8 YEARS) MAY CAUSE PERMANENT DISCOLORATION OF THE TEETH (YELLOW-GRAY-BROWN).

This adverse reaction is more common during long-term use of the drugs, but has been observed following repeated short-term courses. Enamel hypoplasia has also been reported. TETRACYCLINE DRUGS, THEREFORE, SHOULD NOT BE USED IN THIS AGE GROUP UNLESS OTHER DRUGS ARE NOT LIKELY TO BE EFFECTIVE OR ARE CONTRAINDICATED.

All tetracyclines form a stable calcium complex in any bone-forming tissue. A decrease in fibula growth rate has been observed in prematures given oral tetracycline in doses of 25 mg/kg every 6 hours. This reaction was shown to be reversible when the drug was discontinued.

Results of animal studies indicate that tetracyclines cross the placenta, are found in fetal tissues, and can have toxic effects on the developing fetus (often related to retardation of skeletal development). Evidence of embryotoxicity has also been noted in animals treated early in pregnancy. If any tetracycline is used during pregnancy or if the patient becomes pregnant while taking this drug, the patient should be apprised of the potential hazard to the fetus.

The antianabolic action of the tetracyclines may cause an increase in BUN. Studies to date indicate that this does not occur with the use of doxycycline in patients with impaired renal function.

Photosensitivity manifested by an exaggerated sunburn reaction has been observed in some individuals taking tetracyclines. Patients apt to be exposed to direct sunlight or ultraviolet light should be advised that this reaction can occur with tetracycline drugs, and treatment should be discontinued at the first evidence of skin erythema.

Vibramycin Syrup contains sodium metabisulfite, a sulfite that may cause allergic-type reactions including anaphylactic symptoms and life-threatening or less severe asthmatic episodes in certain susceptible people. The over-all prevalence of sulfite sensitivity in the general population is unknown and probably low. Sulfite sensitivity is seen more frequently in asthmatic than in non-asthmatic people.

PRECAUTIONS

General

As with other antibiotic preparations, use of this drug may result in overgrowth of nonsusceptible organisms, including fungi. If superinfection occurs, the antibiotic should be discontinued and appropriate therapy instituted.

Bulging fontanels in infants and benign intracranial hypertension in adults have been reported in individuals receiving tetracyclines. These conditions disappeared when the drug was discontinued.

Incision and drainage or other surgical procedures should be performed in conjunction with antibiotic therapy, when indicated.
Doxycycline offers substantial but not complete suppression of the asexual blood stages of *Plasmodium* strains.
Doxycycline does not suppress *P. falciparum's* sexual blood stage gametocytes. Subjects completing this prophylactic regimen may still transmit the infection to mosquitoes outside endemic areas.

Information for Patients
Patients taking doxycycline for malaria prophylaxis should be advised:
—that no present-day antimalarial agent, including doxycycline, guarantees protection against malaria.
—to avoid being bitten by mosquitoes by using personal protective measures that help avoid contact with mosquitoes, especially from dusk to dawn (e.g., staying in well-screened areas, using mosquito nets, covering the body with clothing, and using an effective insect repellent.)
—that doxycycline prophylaxis:
—should begin 1–2 days before travel to the malarious area,
—should be continued daily while in the malarious area and after leaving the malarious area,
—should be continued for 4 further weeks to avoid development of malaria after returning from an endemic area,
—should not exceed 4 months.
All patients taking doxycycline should be advised:
—to avoid excessive sunlight or artificial ultraviolet light while receiving doxycycline and to discontinue therapy if phototoxicity (e.g., skin eruption, etc.) occurs. Sunscreen or sunblock should be considered. (See WARNINGS.)
—to drink fluids liberally along with doxycycline to reduce the risk of esophageal irritation and ulceration. (See ADVERSE REACTIONS.)
—that the absorption of tetracyclines is reduced when taken with foods, especially those which contain calcium. However, the absorption of doxycycline is not markedly influenced by simultaneous ingestion of food or milk. (See DRUG INTERACTIONS.)
—that the absorption of tetracyclines is reduced when taking bismuth subsalicylate. (See DRUG INTERACTIONS.)
—that the use of doxycycline might increase the incidence of vaginal candidiasis.

Laboratory Tests
In venereal disease, when co-existent syphilis is suspected, dark field examinations should be done before treatment is started and the blood serology repeated monthly for at least 4 months.
In long-term therapy, periodic laboratory evaluation of organ systems, including hematopoietic, renal, and hepatic studies, should be performed.

Drug Interactions
Because tetracyclines have been shown to depress plasma prothrombin activity, patients who are on anticoagulant therapy may require downward adjustment of their anticoagulant dosage.
Since bacteriostatic drugs may interfere with the bactericidal action of penicillin, it is advisable to avoid giving tetracyclines in conjunction with penicillin.
Absorption of tetracyclines is impaired by antacids containing aluminum, calcium, or magnesium, and iron-containing preparations.
Absorption of tetracyclines is impaired by bismuth subsalicylate.
Barbiturates, carbamazepine, and phenytoin decrease the half-life of doxycycline.
The concurrent use of tetracycline and Penthrane (methoxyflurane) has been reported to result in fatal renal toxicity.
Concurrent use of tetracycline may render oral contraceptives less effective.

Drug/Laboratory Test Interactions
False elevations of urinary catecholamine levels may occur due to interference with the fluorescence test.

Carcinogenesis, Mutagenesis, Impairment of Fertility
Long-term studies in animals to evaluate carcinogenic potential of doxycycline have not been conducted. However, there has been evidence of oncogenic activity in rats in studies with the related antibiotics, oxytetracycline (adrenal and pituitary tumors), and minocycline (thyroid tumors).
Likewise, although mutagenicity studies of doxycycline have not been conducted, positive results in *in vitro* mammalian cell assays have been reported for related antibiotics (tetracycline, oxytetracycline).
Doxycycline administered orally at dosage levels as high as 250 mg/kg/day had no apparent effect on the fertility of female rats. Effect on male fertility has not been studied.

Pregnancy Category
Teratogenic effects: Category "D" — (See WARNINGS).
Nonteratogenic effects: (See WARNINGS).

Labor and Delivery
The effect of tetracyclines on labor and delivery is unknown.

Nursing Mothers
Tetracyclines are excreted in human milk. Because of the potential for serious adverse reactions in nursing infants from doxycycline, a decision should be made whether to discontinue nursing or to discontinue the drug, taking into account the importance of the drug to the mother. (See WARNINGS).

Pediatric Use
See WARNINGS and DOSAGE AND ADMINISTRATION.

ADVERSE REACTIONS

Due to oral doxycycline's virtually complete absorption, side effects of the lower bowel, particularly diarrhea, have been infrequent. The following adverse reactions have been observed in patients receiving tetracyclines:
Gastrointestinal: anorexia, nausea, vomiting, diarrhea, glossitis, dysphagia, enterocolitis, and inflammatory lesions (with monilial overgrowth) in the anogenital region. Hepatotoxicity has been reported rarely. These reactions have been caused by both the oral and parenteral administration of tetracyclines. Rare instances of esophagitis and esophageal ulcerations have been reported in patients receiving capsule and tablet forms of the drugs in the tetracycline class. Most of these patients took medications immediately before going to bed. (See DOSAGE AND ADMINISTRATION.)
Skin: maculopapular and erythematous rashes. Exfoliative dermatitis has been reported but is uncommon. Photosensitivity is discussed above. (See WARNINGS.)
Renal toxicity: Rise in BUN has been reported and is apparently dose related. (See WARNINGS.)
Hypersensitivity reactions: urticaria, angioneurotic edema, anaphylaxis, anaphylactoid purpura, serum sickness, pericarditis, and exacerbation of systemic lupus erythematosus.
Blood: Hemolytic anemia, thrombocytopenia, neutropenia, and eosinophilia have been reported.
Other: bulging fontanels in infants and intracranial hypertension in adults. (See PRECAUTIONS—General.)
When given over prolonged periods, tetracyclines have been reported to produce brown-black microscopic discoloration of the thyroid gland. No abnormalities of thyroid function studies are known to occur.

OVERDOSAGE

In case of overdosage, discontinue medication, treat symptomatically and institute supportive measures. Dialysis does not alter serum half-life and thus would not be of benefit in treating cases of overdosage.

DOSAGE AND ADMINISTRATION

THE USUAL DOSAGE AND FREQUENCY OF ADMINISTRATION OF DOXYCYCLINE DIFFERS FROM THAT OF THE OTHER TETRACYCLINES. EXCEEDING THE RECOMMENDED DOSAGE MAY RESULT IN AN INCREASED INCIDENCE OF SIDE EFFECTS. Adults: The usual dose of oral doxycycline is 200 mg on the first day of treatment (administered 100 mg every 12 hours) followed by a maintenance dose of 100 mg/day. The maintenance dose may be administered as a single dose or as 50 mg every 12 hours.
In the management of more severe infections (particularly chronic infections of the urinary tract), 100 mg every 12 hours is recommended.
For children above eight years of age: The recommended dosage schedule for children weighing 100 pounds or less is 2 mg/lb of body weight divided into two doses on the first day of treatment, followed by 1 mg/lb of body weight given as a single daily dose or divided into two doses, on subsequent days. For more severe infections up to 2 mg/lb of body weight may be used. For children over 100 lb the usual adult dose should be used.
The therapeutic antibacterial serum activity will usually persist for 24 hours following recommended dosage.
When used in streptococcal infections, therapy should be continued for 10 days.
Administration of adequate amounts of fluid along with capsule and tablet forms of drugs in the tetracycline class is recommended to wash down the drugs and reduce the risk of esophageal irritation and ulceration. (See ADVERSE REACTIONS.)
If gastric irritation occurs, it is recommended that doxycycline be given with food or milk. The absorption of doxycycline is not markedly influenced by simultaneous ingestion of food or milk.
Studies to date have indicated that administration of doxycycline at the usual recommended doses does not lead to excessive accumulation of the antibiotic in patients with renal impairment.
Uncomplicated gonococcal infections in adults (except anorectal infections in men): 100 mg, by mouth, twice a day for 7 days. As an alternate single visit dose, administer 300 mg stat followed in one hour by a second 300 mg dose. The dose may be administered with food, including milk or carbonated beverage, as required.
Uncomplicated urethral, endocervical, or rectal infection in adults caused by *Chlamydia trachomatis:* 100 mg by mouth twice a day for 7 days.
Nongonococcal urethritis (NGU) caused by *C. trachomatis* or *U. urealyticum:* 100 mg by mouth twice a day for 7 days.
Syphilis—early: Patients who are allergic to penicillin should be treated with doxycycline 100 mg by mouth twice a day for 2 weeks.
Syphilis of more than one year's duration: Patients who are allergic to penicillin should be treated with doxycycline 100 mg by mouth twice a day for 4 weeks.
Acute epididymo-orchitis caused by *N. gonorrhoeae:* 100 mg, by mouth, twice a day for at least 10 days.
Acute epididymo-orchitis caused by *C. trachomatis:* 100 mg, by mouth, twice a day for at least 10 days.
For prophylaxis of malaria: For adults, the recommended dose is 100 mg daily. For children over 8 years of age, the recommended dose is 2 mg/kg given once daily up to the adult dose. Prophylaxis should begin 1–2 days before travel to the malarious area. Prophylaxis should be continued daily during travel in the malarious area and for 4 weeks after the traveler leaves the malarious area.

HOW SUPPLIED

Vibramycin Hyclate (doxycycline hyclate) is available in capsules containing doxycycline hyclate equivalent to:
50 mg doxycycline
bottles of 50 (NDC 0069-0940-50),
unit-dose pack of 100 (10 × 10's) (NDC 0069-0940-41).
The capsules are white and light blue and are imprinted with "VIBRA" on one half and "PFIZER 094" on the other half.
100 mg doxycycline
bottles of 50 (NDC 0069-0950-50) and 500 (NDC 0069-0950-73),
unit-dose pack of 100 (10 × 10's) (NDC 0069-0950-41).
The capsules are light blue and are imprinted with "VIBRA" on one half and "PFIZER 095" on the other half.
Vibra-Tabs (doxycycline hyclate) is available in salmon colored film-coated tablets containing doxycycline hyclate equivalent to:
100 mg doxycycline
bottles of 50 (NDC 0069-0990-50) and 500 (NDC 0069-0990-73),
The tablets are imprinted on one side with "VIBRA-TABS" and "PFIZER 099" on the other side.
Vibramycin Calcium Syrup (doxycycline calcium oral suspension) is available as a raspberry-apple flavored oral suspension. Each teaspoonful (5 mL) contains doxycycline calcium equivalent to 50 mg of doxycycline: bottles of 1 oz (30 mL) (NDC 0069-0971-51), and 1 pint (473 mL) (NDC 0069-0971-93).
Vibramycin Monohydrate (doxycycline monohydrate) for Oral Suspension is available as a raspberry-flavored, dry powder for oral suspension. When reconstituted, each teaspoonful (5 mL) contains doxycycline monohydrate equivalent to 25 mg of doxycycline: 2 oz (60 mL) bottles (NDC 0069-0970-65).
All products are to be stored below 86°F (30°C) and dispensed in tight, light-resistant containers (USP). The unit dose packs should also be stored in a dry place.

ANIMAL PHARMACOLOGY AND ANIMAL TOXICOLOGY

Hyperpigmentation of the thyroid has been produced by members of the tetracycline class in the following species: in rats by oxytetracycline, doxycycline, tetracycline PO_4, and methacycline; in minipigs by doxycycline, minocycline, tetracycline PO_4, and methacycline; in dogs by doxycycline and minocycline; in monkeys by minocycline.
Minocycline, tetracycline PO_4, methacycline, doxycycline, tetracycline base, oxytetracycline HCl, and tetracycline HCl were goitrogenic in rats fed a low iodine diet. This goitrogenic effect was accompanied by high radioactive iodine uptake. Administration of minocycline also produced a large goiter with high radioiodine uptake in rats fed a relatively high iodine diet.
Treatment of various animal species with this class of drugs has also resulted in the induction of thyroid hyperplasia in the following: in rats and dogs (minocycline); in chickens (chlortetracycline); and in rats and mice (oxytetracycline). Adrenal gland hyperplasia has been observed in goats and rats treated with oxytetracycline.

REFERENCES

1. National Committee for Clinical Laboratory Standards, *Performance Standards for Antimicrobial Disk Susceptibility Tests,* Fourth Edition. Approved Standard NCCLS Document M2-A4, Vol. 10, No. 7 NCCLS, Villanova, PA, April 1990.
2. National Committee for Clinical Laboratory Standards, *Methods for Dilution Antimicrobial Susceptibility Tests for Bacteria that Grow Aerobically,* Second Edition. Approved Standard NCCLS Document M7-A2, Vol. 10, No. 8 NCCLS, Villanova, PA, April 1990.

69-1680-00-5 Revised April 1993

VIBRAMYCIN® Hyclate ℞
[*vī "bra-mī 'sin*]
doxycycline hyclate for injection
INTRAVENOUS
For Intravenous Use Only

DESCRIPTION

Vibramycin (doxycycline hyclate for injection) Intravenous is a broad–spectrum antibiotic synthetically derived from oxytetracycline, and is available as Vibramycin Hyclate (doxycycline hydrochloride hemiethanolate hemihydrate). The chemical designation of this light-yellow crystalline powder is alpha-6-deoxy-5-oxytetracycline. Doxycycline has a high degree of lipoid solubility and a low affinity for calcium binding. It is highly stable in normal human serum.

ACTIONS

Doxycycline is primarily bacteriostatic and thought to exert its antimicrobial effect by the inhibition of protein synthesis. Doxycycline is active against a wide range of gram-positive and gram-negative organisms.
The drugs in the tetracycline class have closely similar antimicrobial spectra and cross resistance among them is

Continued on next page

Vibramycin Intravenous—Cont.

common. Microorganisms may be considered susceptible to doxycycline (likely to respond to doxycycline therapy) if the minimum inhibitory concentration (M.I.C.) is not more than 4.0 mcg/mL. Microorganisms may be considered intermediate (harboring partial resistance) if the M.I.C. is 4.0 to 12.5 mcg/mL and resistant (not likely to respond to therapy) if the M.I.C. is greater than 12.5 mcg/mL.

Susceptibility plate testing: If the Kirby-Bauer method of disc susceptibility testing is used, a 30 mcg doxycycline disc should give a zone of at least 16 mm when tested against a doxycycline-susceptible bacterial strain. A tetracycline disc may be used to determine microbial susceptibility. If the Kirby-Bauer method of disc susceptibility testing is used, a 30 mcg tetracycline disc should give a zone of at least 19 mm when tested against a tetracycline-susceptible bacterial strain.

Tetracyclines are readily absorbed and are bound to plasma proteins in varying degree. They are concentrated by the liver in the bile, and excreted in the urine and feces at high concentrations and in a biologically active form.

Following a single 100 mg dose administered in a concentration of 0.4 mg/mL in a one-hour infusion, normal adult volunteers average a peak of 2.5 mcg/mL, while 200 mg of a concentration of 0.4 mg/mL administered over two hours averaged a peak of 3.6 mcg/mL.

Excretion of doxycycline by the kidney is about 40 percent/72 hours in individuals with normal function (creatinine clearance about 75 mL/min.). This percentage excretion may fall as low as 1-5 percent/72 hours in individuals with severe renal insufficiency (creatinine clearance below 10 mL/min.). Studies have shown no significant difference in serum half-life of doxycycline (range 18-22 hours) in individuals with normal and severely impaired renal function. Hemodialysis does not alter this serum half-life of doxycycline.

INDICATIONS

Doxycycline is indicated in infections caused by the following microorganisms:

Rickettsiae (Rocky Mountain spotted fever, typhus fever, and the typhus group, Q fever, rickettsialpox and tick fevers).

Mycoplasma pneumoniae (PPLO, Eaton Agent).

Agents of psittacosis and ornithosis.

Agents of lymphogranuloma venereum and granuloma inguinale.

The spirochetal agent of relapsing fever *(Borrelia recurrentis).*

The following gram-negative microorganisms:

Haemophilus ducreyi (chancroid),
Pasteurella pestis and *Pasteurella tularensis,*
Bartonella bacilliformis,
Bacteroides species,
Vibrio comma and *Vibrio fetus,*
Brucella species (in conjunction with streptomycin).

Because many strains of the following groups of microorganisms have been shown to be resistant to tetracyclines, culture and susceptibility testing are recommended. Doxycycline is indicated for treatment of infections caused by the following gram-negative microorganisms when bacteriologic testing indicates appropriate susceptibility to the drug:

Escherichia coli,
Enterobacter aerogenes (formerly *Aerobacter aerogenes*),
Shigella species,
Mima species and *Herellea* species,
Haemophilus influenzae (respiratory infections),
Klebsiella species (respiratory and urinary infections).

Doxycycline is indicated for treatment of infections caused by the following gram-positive microorganisms when bacteriologic testing indicates appropriate susceptibility to the drug:

Streptococcus species:

Up to 44 percent of strains of *Streptococcus pyogenes* and 74 percent of *Streptococcus faecalis* have been found to be resistant to tetracycline drugs. Therefore, tetracyclines should not be used for streptococcal disease unless the organism has been demonstrated to be sensitive.

For upper respiratory infections due to group A beta-hemolytic streptococci, penicillin is the usual drug of choice, including prophylaxis of rheumatic fever.

Diplococcus pneumoniae,

Staphylococcus aureus, respiratory, skin and soft tissue infections. Tetracyclines are not the drugs of choice in the treatment of any type of staphylococcal infections.

When penicillin is contraindicated, doxycycline is an alternative drug in the treatment of infections due to:

Neisseria gonorrhoeae and *N. meningitidis,*
Treponema pallidum and *Treponema pertenue* (syphilis and yaws),
Listeria monocytogenes,
Clostridium species,
Bacillus anthracis,
Fusobacterium fusiforme (Vincent's infection),
Actinomyces species.

In acute intestinal amebiasis, doxycycline may be a useful adjunct to amebicides.

Doxycycline is indicated in the treatment of trachoma, although the infectious agent is not always eliminated, as judged by immunofluorescence.

CONTRAINDICATIONS

This drug is contraindicated in persons who have shown hypersensitivity to any of the tetracyclines.

WARNINGS

THE USE OF DRUGS OF THE TETRACYCLINE CLASS DURING TOOTH DEVELOPMENT (LAST HALF OF PREGNANCY, INFANCY AND CHILDHOOD TO THE AGE OF 8 YEARS) MAY CAUSE PERMANENT DISCOLORATION OF THE TEETH (YELLOW-GRAY-BROWN). This adverse reaction is more common during long-term use of the drugs but has been observed following repeated short-term courses. Enamel hypoplasia has also been reported. *TETRACYCLINE DRUGS, THEREFORE, SHOULD NOT BE USED IN THIS AGE GROUP UNLESS OTHER DRUGS ARE NOT LIKELY TO BE EFFECTIVE OR ARE CONTRAINDICATED.*

Photosensitivity manifested by an exaggerated sunburn reaction has been observed in some individuals taking tetracyclines. Patients apt to be exposed to direct sunlight or ultraviolet light should be advised that this reaction can occur with tetracycline drugs, and treatment should be discontinued at the first evidence of skin erythema.

The antianabolic action of the tetracyclines may cause an increase in BUN. Studies to date indicate that this does not occur with the use of doxycycline in patients with impaired renal function.

Usage in Pregnancy

(See above WARNINGS about use during tooth development.)

Vibramycin Intravenous has not been studied in pregnant patients. It should not be used in pregnant women unless, in the judgment of the physician, it is essential for the welfare of the patient.

Results of animal studies indicate that tetracyclines cross the placenta, are found in fetal tissues and can have toxic effects on the developing fetus (often related to retardation of skeletal development). Evidence of embryotoxicity has also been noted in animals treated early in pregnancy.

Usage in Children

The use of Vibramycin Intravenous in children under 8 years is not recommended because safe conditions for its use have not been established.

(See above WARNINGS about use during tooth development.)

As with other tetracyclines, doxycycline forms a stable calcium complex in any bone-forming tissue. A decrease in the fibula growth rate has been observed in prematures given oral tetracycline in doses of 25 mg/kg every 6 hours. This reaction was shown to be reversible when the drug was discontinued.

Tetracyclines are present in the milk of lactating women who are taking a drug in this class.

PRECAUTIONS

As with other antibiotic preparations, use of this drug may result in overgrowth of nonsusceptible organisms, including fungi. If superinfection occurs, the antibiotic should be discontinued and appropriate therapy instituted.

In venereal diseases when coexistent syphilis is suspected, a dark field examination should be done before treatment is started and the blood serology repeated monthly for at least 4 months.

Because tetracyclines have been shown to depress plasma prothrombin activity, patients who are on anticoagulant therapy may require downward adjustment of their anticoagulant dosage.

In long-term therapy, periodic laboratory evaluation of organ systems, including hematopoietic, renal, and hepatic studies should be performed.

All infections due to group A beta-hemolytic streptococci should be treated for at least 10 days.

Since bacteriostatic drugs may interfere with the bactericidal action of penicillin, it is advisable to avoid giving tetracycline in conjunction with penicillin.

ADVERSE REACTIONS

Gastrointestinal: anorexia, nausea, vomiting, diarrhea, glossitis, dysphagia, enterocolitis, and inflammatory lesions (with monilial overgrowth) in the anogenital region. Hepatotoxicity has been reported rarely. These reactions have been caused by both the oral and parenteral administration of tetracyclines.

Skin: maculopapular and erythematous rashes. Exfoliative dermatitis has been reported but is uncommon. Photosensitivity is discussed above. (See WARNINGS.)

Renal toxicity: Rise in BUN has been reported and is apparently dose related. (See WARNINGS.)

Hypersensitivity reactions: urticaria, angioneurotic edema, anaphylaxis, anaphylactoid purpura, pericarditis and exacerbation of systemic lupus erythematosus.

Bulging fontanels in infants and benign intracranial hypertension in adults have been reported in individuals receiving full therapeutic dosages. These conditions disappeared rapidly when the drug was discontinued.

Blood: Hemolytic anemia, thrombocytopenia, neutropenia and eosinophilia have been reported.

When given over prolonged periods, tetracyclines have been reported to produce brown-black microscopic discoloration of thyroid glands. No abnormalities of thyroid function studies are known to occur.

DOSAGE AND ADMINISTRATION

Note: Rapid administration is to be avoided. Parenteral therapy is indicated only when oral therapy is not indicated. Oral therapy should be instituted as soon as possible. If intravenous therapy is given over prolonged periods of time, thrombophlebitis may result.

THE USUAL DOSAGE AND FREQUENCY OF ADMINISTRATION OF VIBRAMYCIN I.V. (100-200 MG/DAY) DIFFERS FROM THAT OF THE OTHER TETRACYCLINES (1-2 G/DAY). EXCEEDING THE RECOMMENDED DOSAGE MAY RESULT IN AN INCREASED INCIDENCE OF SIDE EFFECTS.

Studies to date have indicated that Vibramycin at the usual recommended doses does not lead to excessive accumulation of the antibiotic in patients with renal impairment.

Adults: The usual dosage of Vibramycin I.V. is 200 mg on the first day of treatment administered in one or two infusions. Subsequent daily dosage is 100 to 200 mg depending upon the severity of infection, with 200 mg administered in one or two infusions.

In the treatment of primary and secondary syphilis, the recommended dosage is 300 mg daily for at least 10 days.

For children above eight years of age: The recommended dosage schedule for children weighing 100 pounds or less is 2 mg/lb of body weight on the first day of treatment, administered in one or two infusions. Subsequent daily dosage is 1 to 2 mg/lb of body weight given as one or two infusions, depending on the severity of the infection. For children over 100 pounds the usual adult dose should be used. (See WARNINGS Section for Usage in Children.)

General: The duration of infusion may vary with the dose (100 to 200 mg per day), but is usually one to four hours. A recommended minimum infusion time for 100 mg of a 0.5 mg/mL solution is one hour. Therapy should be continued for at least 24-48 hours after symptoms and fever have subsided. The therapeutic antibacterial serum activity will usually persist for 24 hours following recommended dosage. Intravenous solutions should not be injected intramuscularly or subcutaneously. Caution should be taken to avoid the inadvertent introduction of the intravenous solution into the adjacent soft tissue.

PREPARATION OF SOLUTION

To prepare a solution containing 10 mg/mL, the contents of the vial should be reconstituted with 10 mL (for the 100 mg/vial container) or 20 mL (for the 200 mg/vial container) of Sterile Water for Injection or any of the ten intravenous infusion solutions listed below. Each 100 mg of Vibramycin (i.e., withdraw entire solution from the 100 mg vial) is further diluted with 100 mL to 1000 mL of the intravenous solutions listed below. Each 200 mg of Vibramycin (i.e., withdraw entire solution from the 200 mg vial) is further diluted with 200 mL to 2000 mL of the following intravenous solutions:

1. Sodium Chloride Injection, USP
2. 5% Dextrose Injection, USP
3. Ringer's Injection, USP
4. Invert Sugar, 10% in Water
5. Lactated Ringer's Injection, USP
6. Dextrose 5% in Lactated Ringer's
7. Normosol-M® in D5-W (Abbott)
8. Normosol-R® in D5-W (Abbott)
9. Plasma-Lyte® 56 in 5% Dextrose (Travenol)
10. Plasma-Lyte® 148 in 5% Dextrose (Travenol)

This will result in desired concentrations of 0.1 to 1.0 mg/mL. Concentrations lower than 0.1 mg/mL or higher than 1.0 mg/mL are not recommended.

Stability

Vibramycin IV is stable for 48 hours in solution when diluted with Sodium Chloride Injection, USP, or 5% Dextrose Injection, USP, to concentrations between 1.0 mg/mL and 0.1 mg/ mL and stored at 25°C. Vibramycin IV in these solutions is stable under fluorescent light for 48 hours, but must be protected from direct sunlight during storage and infusion. Reconstituted solutions (1.0 to 0.1 mg/mL) may be stored up to 72 hours prior to start of infusion if refrigerated and protected from sunlight and artificial light. Infusion must then be completed within 12 hours. Solutions must be used within these time periods or discarded.

Vibramycin IV, when diluted with Ringer's Injection, USP, or Invert Sugar, 10% in Water, or Normosol-M® in D5-W (Abbott), or Normosol-R®in D5-W (Abbott), or Plasma-Lyte® 56 in 5% Dextrose (Travenol), or Plasma-Lyte® 148 in 5% Dextrose (Travenol) to a concentration between 1.0 mg/mL and 0.1 mg/mL, must be completely infused within 12 hours after reconstitution to ensure adequate stability. During infusion, the solution must be protected from direct sunlight. Reconstituted solutions (1.0 to 0.1 mg/mL) may be stored up to 72 hours prior to start of infusion if refrigerated and protected from sunlight and artifical light. Infusion must then be completed within 12 hours. Solutions must be used within these time periods or discarded.

When diluted with Lactated Ringer's Injection, USP, or Dextrose 5% in Lactated Ringer's, infusion of the solution (ca. 1.0 mg/mL) or lower concentrations (not less than 0.1 mg/mL) must be completed within six hours after reconstitution to ensure adequate stability. During infusion, the solution must be protected from direct sunlight. Solutions must be used within this time period or discarded.

Solutions of Vibramycin (doxycycline hyclate for injection) at a concentration of 10 mg/mL in Sterile Water for Injection, when frozen immediately after reconstitution are stable for 8 weeks when stored at −20°C. If the product is warmed, care should be taken to avoid heating it after the thawing is complete. Once thawed the solution should not be refrozen.

HOW SUPPLIED

Vibramycin (doxycycline hyclate for injection) Intravenous is available as a sterile powder in a vial containing doxycycline hyclate equivalent to 100 mg of doxycycline with 480 mg of ascorbic acid, packages of 5 (NDC 0049-0960-77), and in individually packaged vials containing doxycycline hyclate equivalent to 200 mg of doxycycline with 960 mg of ascorbic acid (0049–0980–81).

65-1940-00-2

LITERATURE AVAILABLE

Yes.

Revised March 1991

VISTARIL® ℞

[*vĭs 'tăr-ĭl*]

(hydroxyzine pamoate)

Capsules and Oral Suspension

DESCRIPTION

Hydroxyzine pamoate is designated chemically as 1-(p-chlorobenzhydryl) 4- [2- (2-hydroxyethoxy) ethyl] diethylenediamine salt of 1,1'- methylene bis (2 hydroxy-3-naphthalene carboxylic acid).

Inert ingredients for the capsule formulations are: hard gelatin capsules (which may contain Yellow 10, Green 3, Yellow 6, Red 33, and other inert ingredients); magnesium stearate; sodium lauryl sulfate; starch; sucrose.

Inert ingredients for the oral suspension formulation are: carboxymethylcellulose sodium; lemon flavor; propylene glycol; sorbic acid; sorbitol solution; water.

CLINICAL PHARMACOLOGY

Vistaril® (hydroxyzine pamoate) is unrelated chemically to the phenothiazines, reserpine, meprobamate, or the benzodiazepines.

Vistaril is not a cortical depressant, but its action may be due to a suppression of activity in certain key regions of the subcortical area of the central nervous system. Primary skeletal muscle relaxation has been demonstrated experimentally. Bronchodilator activity, and antihistaminic and analgesic effects have been demonstrated experimentally and confirmed clinically. An antiemetic effect, both by the apomorphine test and the veriloid test, has been demonstrated. Pharmacological and clinical studies indicate that hydroxyzine in therapeutic dosage does not increase gastric secretion or acidity and in most cases has mild antisecretory activity. Hydroxyzine is rapidly absorbed from the gastrointestinal tract and Vistaril's clinical effects are usually noted within 15 to 30 minutes after oral administration.

INDICATIONS

For symptomatic relief of anxiety and tension associated with psychoneurosis and as an adjunct in organic disease states in which anxiety is manifested.

Useful in the management of pruritus due to allergic conditions such as chronic urticaria and atopic and contact dermatoses, and in histamine-mediated pruritus.

As a sedative when used as premedication and following general anesthesia, **Hydroxyzine may potentiate meperidine (Demerol®) and barbiturates,** so their use in pre-anesthetic adjunctive therapy should be modified on an individual basis. Atropine and other belladonna alkaloids are not affected by the drug. Hydroxyzine is not known to interfere with the action of digitalis in any way and it may be used concurrently with this agent.

The effectiveness of hydroxyzine as an antianxiety agent for long–term use, that is, more than 4 months, has not been assessed by systematic clinical studies. The physician should reassess periodically the usefulness of the drug for the individual patient.

CONTRAINDICATIONS

Hydroxyzine, when administered to the pregnant mouse, rat, and rabbit, induced fetal abnormalities in the rat and mouse at doses substantially above the human therapeutic range. Clinical data in human beings are inadequate to establish safety in early pregnancy. Until such data are available, hydroxyzine is contraindicated in early pregnancy.

Hydroxyzine pamoate is contraindicated for patients who have shown a previous hypersensitivity to it.

WARNINGS

Nursing Mothers: It is not known whether this drug is excreted in human milk. Since many drugs are so excreted, hydroxyzine should not be given to nursing mothers.

PRECAUTIONS

THE POTENTIATING ACTION OF HYDROXYZINE MUST BE CONSIDERED WHEN THE DRUG IS USED IN CONJUNCTION WITH CENTRAL NERVOUS SYSTEM DEPRESSANTS SUCH AS NARCOTICS, NON-NARCOTIC ANALGESICS AND BARBITURATES. Therefore, when central nervous system depressants are administered concomitantly with hydroxyzine, their dosage should be reduced. Since drowsiness may occur with use of the drug, patients should be warned of this possibility and cautioned against driving a car or operating dangerous machinery while taking Vistaril (hydroxyzine pamoate). Patients should be advised against the simultaneous use of other CNS depressant drugs, and cautioned that the effect of alcohol may be increased.

ADVERSE REACTIONS

Side effects reported with the administration of Vistaril are usually mild and transitory in nature.

Anticholinergic: Dry mouth.

Central Nervous System: Drowsiness is usually transitory and may disappear in a few days of continued therapy or upon reduction of the dose. Involuntary motor activity, including rare instances of tremor and convulsions, has been reported, usually with doses considerably higher than those recommended. Clinically significant respiratory depression has not been reported at recommended doses.

OVERDOSAGE

The most common manifestation of overdosage of Vistaril is hypersedation. As in the management of overdosage with any drug, it should be borne in mind that multiple agents may have been taken.

If vomiting has not occurred spontaneously, it should be induced. Immediate gastric lavage is also recommended. General supportive care, including frequent monitoring of the vital signs and close observation of the patient, is indicated. Hypotension, though unlikely, may be controlled with intravenous fluids and Levophed® (levarterenol) or Aramine® (metaraminol). Do not use epinephrine, as Vistaril counteracts its pressor action. Caffeine and Sodium Benzoate Injection, USP, may be used to counteract central nervous system depressant effects.

There is no specific antidote. It is doubtful that hemodialysis would be of any value in the treatment of overdosage with hydroxyzine. However, if other agents such as barbiturates have been ingested concomitantly, hemodialysis may be indicated. There is no practical method to quantitate hydroxyzine in body fluids or tissue after its ingestion or administration.

DOSAGE

For symptomatic relief of anxiety and tension associated with psychoneurosis and as an adjunct in organic disease states in which anxiety is manifested: in adults, 50–100 mg q.i.d.; children under 6 years, 50 mg daily in divided doses and over 6 years, 50–100 mg daily in divided doses.

For use in the management of pruritus due to allergic conditions such as chronic urticaria and atopic and contact dermatoses, and in histamine-mediated pruritus: in adults, 25 mg t.i.d. or q.i.d.; children under 6 years, 50 mg daily in divided doses and over 6 years, 50–100 mg daily in divided doses.

As a sedative when used as a premedication and following general anesthesia: 50–100 mg in adults, and 0.6 mg/kg in children.

When treatment is initiated by the intramuscular route of administration, subsequent doses may be administered orally.

As with all medications, the dosage should be adjusted according to the patient's response to therapy.

HOW SUPPLIED

Vistaril® Capsules (hydroxyzine pamoate equivalent to hydroxyzine hydrochloride)

25 mg:	100's (NDC 0069-5410-66), 500's (NDC 0069-5410-73), and Unit Dose (10 × 10's) (NDC 0069-5410-41) two-tone green capsules
50 mg:	100's (NDC 0069-5420-66), 500's (NDC 0069-5420-73), and Unit Dose (10 × 10's) (NDC 0069-5420-41) green and white capsules
100 mg:	100's (NDC 0069-5430-66), 500's (NDC 0069-5430-73), and Unit Dose (10 × 10's) (NDC 0069-5430-41) green and gray capsules

Vistaril® Oral Suspension (hydroxyzine pamoate equivalent to 25 mg hydroxyzine hydrochloride per teaspoonful-5 mL): 1 pint (473 mL) bottles (NDC 0069-5440-93) and 4 ounce (120 mL) bottles (NDC 0069-5440-97) in packages of 4.

Shake vigorously until product is completely resuspended.

BIBLIOGRAPHY

Available on request.

69-0846-00-1 Revised November 1994

VISTARIL® ℞

hydroxyzine hydrochloride

Intramuscular Solution

For Intramuscular Use Only

CHEMISTRY

Hydroxyzine hydrochloride is designated chemically as 1-(p-chlorobenzhydryl) 4-[2-(2-hydroxyethoxy) ethyl] piperazine dihydrochloride.

ACTIONS

VISTARIL (hydroxyzine hydrochloride) is unrelated chemically to phenothiazine, reserpine, and meprobamate. Hydroxyzine has demonstrated its clinical effectiveness in the chemotherapeutic aspect of the total management of neuroses and emotional disturbances manifested by anxiety, tension, agitation, apprehension or confusion.

Hydroxyzine has been shown clinically to be a rapid-acting true ataraxic with a wide margin of safety. It induces a calming effect in anxious, tense, psychoneurotic adults and also in anxious, hyperkinetic children without impairing mental alertness. It is not a cortical depressant, but its action may be due to a suppression of activity in certain key regions of the subcortical area of the central nervous system.

Primary skeletal muscle relaxation has been demonstrated experimentally.

Hydroxyzine has been shown experimentally to have antispasmodic properties, apparently mediated through interference with the mechanism that responds to spasmogenic agents such as serotonin, acetylcholine, and histamine. Antihistaminic effects have been demonstrated experimentally and confirmed clinically.

An antiemetic effect, both by the apomorphine test and the veriloid test, has been demonstrated. Pharmacological and clinical studies indicate that hydroxyzine in therapeutic dosage does not increase gastric secretion or acidity and in most cases provides mild antisecretory benefits.

INDICATIONS

The total management of anxiety, tension, and psychomotor agitation in conditions of emotional stress requires in most instances a combined approach of psychotherapy and chemotherapy. Hydroxyzine has been found to be particularly useful for this latter phase of therapy in its ability to render the disturbed patient more amenable to psychotherapy in long term treatment of the psychoneurotic and psychotic, although it should not be used as the sole treatment of psychosis or of clearly demonstrated cases of depression.

Hydroxyzine is also useful in alleviating the manifestations of anxiety and tension as in the preparation for dental procedures and in acute emotional problems. It has also been recommended for the management of anxiety associated with organic disturbances and as adjunctive therapy in alcoholism and allergic conditions with strong emotional overlay, such as in asthma, chronic urticaria, and pruritus.

VISTARIL (hydroxyzine hydrochloride) Intramuscular Solution is useful in treating the following types of patients when intramuscular administration is indicated:

1. The acutely disturbed or hysterical patient.
2. The acute or chronic alcoholic with anxiety withdrawal symptoms or delirium tremens.
3. As pre- and postoperative and pre- and postpartum adjunctive medication to permit reduction in narcotic dosage, allay anxiety and control emesis.

VISTARIL (hydroxyzine hydrochloride) has also demonstrated effectiveness in controlling nausea and vomiting, excluding nausea and vomiting of pregnancy. (See Contraindications.)

In prepartum states, the reduction in narcotic requirement effected by hydroxyzine is of particular benefit to both mother and neonate.

Hydroxyzine benefits the cardiac patient by its ability to allay the associated anxiety and apprehension attendant to certain types of heart disease. Hydroxyzine is not known to interfere with the action of digitalis in any way and may be used concurrently with this agent.

The effectiveness of hydroxyzine in long term use, that is, more than 4 months, has not been assessed by systematic clinical studies. The physician should reassess periodically the usefulness of the drug for the individual patient.

CONTRAINDICATIONS

Hydroxyzine hydrochloride intramuscular solution is intended only for intramuscular administration and should not, under any circumstances, be injected subcutaneously, intra-arterially, or intravenously.

This drug is contraindicated for patients who have shown a previous hypersensitivity to it.

Hydroxyzine, when administered to the pregnant mouse, rat, and rabbit, induced fetal abnormalities in the rat at doses substantially above the human therapeutic range. Clinical data in human beings are inadequate to establish safety in early pregnancy. Until such data are available, hydroxyzine is contraindicated in early pregnancy.

PRECAUTIONS

THE POTENTIATING ACTION OF HYDROXYZINE MUST BE CONSIDERED WHEN THE DRUG IS USED IN CONJUNCTION WITH CENTRAL NERVOUS SYSTEM DEPRESSANTS SUCH AS NARCOTICS, BARBITURATES, AND ALCOHOL. Rarely, cardiac arrests and death have been reported in association with the combined use of hydroxyzine hydrochloride IM and other CNS depressants. Therefore when central nervous system depressants are administered concomitantly with hydroxyzine their dosage should be reduced up to 50 per cent. The efficacy of hydroxyzine as adjunctive pre- and postoperative sedative medication has also been well established, especially as regards its ability to allay anxiety, control emesis, and reduce the amount of narcotic required.

HYDROXYZINE MAY POTENTIATE NARCOTICS AND BARBITURATES, so their use in preanesthetic adjunctive therapy should be modified on an individual basis. Atropine and other belladonna alkaloids are not affected by the drug. When hydroxyzine is used preoperatively or prepartum, narcotic requirements may be reduced as much as 50 per cent. Thus, when 50 mg of VISTARIL (hydroxyzine hydrochloride) Intramuscular Solution is employed, meperidine dosage may be reduced from 100 mg to 50 mg. The administration of meperidine may result in severe hypotension in the postoperative patient or any individual whose ability to maintain blood pressure has been compromised by a depleted blood volume. Meperidine should be used with great caution and in reduced dosage in patients who are receiving other pre- and/or postoperative medications and in whom there is a risk of respiratory depression, hypotension, and profound sedation or coma occurring. Before using any medications concomitant with hydroxyzine, the manufacturer's prescribing information should be read carefully.

Since drowsiness may occur with the use of this drug, patients should be warned of this possibility and cautioned against driving a car or operating dangerous machinery while taking this drug.

Continued on next page

Vistaril—Cont.

As with all intramuscular preparations, VISTARIL Intramuscular Solution should be injected well within the body of a relatively large muscle. Inadvertent subcutaneous injection may result in significant tissue damage.
ADULTS: The preferred site is the upper outer quadrant of the buttock, (i.e., gluteus maximus), or the mid-lateral thigh.
CHILDREN: It is recommended that intramuscular injections be given preferably in the mid-lateral muscles of the thigh. In infants and small children the periphery of the upper outer quadrant of the gluteal region should be used only when necessary, such as in burn patients, in order to minimize the possibility of damage to the sciatic nerve.
The deltoid area should be used only if well developed such as in certain adults and older children, and then only with caution to avoid radial nerve injury. Intramuscular injections should not be made into the lower and mid-third of the upper arm. As with all intramuscular injections, aspiration is necessary to help avoid inadvertent injection into a blood vessel.

ADVERSE REACTIONS

Therapeutic doses of hydroxyzine seldom produce impairment of mental alertness. However, drowsiness may occur; if so, it is usually transitory and may disappear in a few days of continued therapy or upon reduction of the dose. Dryness of the mouth may be encountered at higher doses. Extensive clinical use has substantiated the absence of toxic effects on the liver or bone marrow when administered in the recommended doses for over four years of uninterrupted therapy. The absence of adverse effects has been further demonstrated in experimental studies in which excessively high doses were administered.
Involuntary motor activity, including rare instances of tremor and convulsions, has been reported, usually with doses considerably higher than those recommended. Continuous therapy with over one gram per day has been employed in some patients without these effects having been encountered.

DOSAGE AND ADMINISTRATION

The recommended dosages for VISTARIL (hydroxyzine hydrochloride) Intramuscular Solution are:

For adult psychiatric and emotional emergencies, including acute alcoholism.	IM: 50–100 mg stat., and q. 4–6h., p.r.n.
Nausea and vomiting excluding nausea and vomiting of pregnancy.	Adults: 25–100 mg IM Children: 0.5 mg/lb body weight IM
Pre- and postoperative adjunctive medication.	Adults: 25–100 mg IM Children: 0.5 mg/lb body weight IM
Pre- and postpartum adjunctive therapy.	25–100 mg IM

As with all potent medications, the dosage should be adjusted according to the patient's response to therapy.
FOR ADDITIONAL INFORMATION OF THE ADMINISTRATION AND SITE OF SELECTION SEE PRECAUTIONS SECTION. NOTE: VISTARIL (hydroxyzine hydrochloride) Intramuscular Solution may be administered without further dilution.
Patients may be started on intramuscular therapy when indicated. They should be maintained on oral therapy whenever this route is practicable.

HOW SUPPLIED

VISTARIL (hydroxyzine hydrochloride) Intramuscular Solution
Multi-Dose Vials
25 mg/mL: 10 mL vials (NDC 0049-5450-74)
50 mg/mL: 10 mL vials (NDC 0049-5460-74)
Unit Dose Vials
50 mg/mL–1 mL fill: packages of 25 vials (NDC 0049-5462-76)
100 mg/2 mL–2 mL fill: packages of 25 vials (NDC 0049-5460-76)

STORAGE

Store below 86° F (30 ° C).
Protect from freezing.

FORMULA

Dosage Strength	25 mg/1 mL	50 mg/1 mL 100 mg/2 mL
Hydroxyzine hydrochloride	25 mg/mL	50 mg/mL
Benzyl Alcohol	0.9%	0.9%
Sodium hydroxide	to adjust to optimum pH	

70-0843-00-5
Revised May 1993

ZITHROMAX® ℞
(azithromycin tablets)
(azithromycin capsules)
and
(azithromycin for oral suspension)

DESCRIPTION

ZITHROMAX® (azithromycin tablets, azithromycin capsules and azithromycin for oral suspension) contain the active ingredient azithromycin, an azalide, a subclass of macrolide antibiotics, for oral administration. Azithromycin has the chemical name (*2R, 3S, 4R, 5R, 8R, 10R, 11R, 12S, 13S, 14R*)-13-[(2,6-dideoxy-3-*C*-methyl-3-*O*-methyl-α-*L*-*ribo*-hexopyranosyl)oxy]-2-ethyl-3,4,10-trihydroxy-3,5,6,8,10,12,14-heptamethyl-11-[[3,4,6-trideoxy-3-(dimethylamino)-β-*D*-*xylo*-hexopyranosyl]oxy]-1-oxa-6-azacyclopentadecan-15-one. Azithromycin is derived from erythromycin; however, it differs chemically from erythromycin in that a methyl-substituted nitrogen atom is incorporated into the lactone ring. Its molecular formula is $C_{38}H_{72}H_2O_{12}$, and its molecular weight is 749.00. Azithromycin has the following structural formula:

Azithromycin, as the dihydrate, is a white crystalline powder with a molecular formula of $C_{38}H_{72}N_2O_{12}\bullet 2H_2O$ and a molecular weight of 785.0.
ZITHROMAX® is supplied for oral administration as film-coated, modified capsular shaped tablets containing azithromycin dihydrate equivalent to 250 mg azithromycin and the following inactive ingredients: dibasic calcium phosphate anhydrous, pregelatinized starch, sodium croscarmellose, magnesium stearate, sodium lauryl sulfate, hydroxypropyl methylcellulose, lactose, titanium dioxide, triacetin and D&C Red #30 aluminum lake.
ZITHROMAX® capsules contain azithromycin dihydrate equivalent to 250 mg of azithromycin. The capsules are supplied in red opaque hard-gelatin capsules (containing FD&C Red #40). They also contain the following inactive ingredients: anhydrous lactose, corn starch, magnesium stearate, and sodium lauryl sulfate.
It is also supplied as a powder for oral suspension.
ZITHROMAX® for oral suspension is supplied in bottles containing azithromycin dihydrate powder equivalent to 300 mg, 600 mg, 900 mg, or 1200 mg azithromycin per bottle and the following inactive ingredients: sucrose; sodium phosphate, tribasic, anhydrous; hydroxypropyl cellulose; xanthan gum; FD&C Red #40; and spray dried artificial cherry, creme de vanilla and banana flavors. After constitution, each 5 mL of suspension contains 100 mg or 200 mg of azithromycin.

CLINICAL PHARMACOLOGY

Adult Pharmacokinetics: Following oral administration, azithromycin is rapidly absorbed and widely distributed throughout the body. Rapid distribution of azithromycin into tissues and high concentration within cells result in significantly higher azithromycin concentrations in tissues than in plasma or serum.
The pharmacokinetic parameters of azithromycin capsules in plasma after a loading dose of 500 mg (2–250 mg capsules) on day one followed by 250 mg (1–250 mg capsule) q.d. on days two through five in healthy young adults (age 18–40 years old) are portrayed in the following chart:

Pharmacokinetic Parameters (Mean)	Total n = 12 Day 1	Day 5
C_{max} (µg/mL)	0.41	0.24
T_{max} (h)	2.5	3.2
AUC_{0-24} (µg•h/mL)	2.6	2.1
C_{min} (µg/mL)	0.05	0.05
Urinary Excret. (% dose)	4.5	6.5

In this study, there was no significant difference in the disposition of azithromycin between male and female subjects. Plasma concentrations of azithromycin following single 500 mg oral and i.v. doses declined in a polyphasic pattern resulting in an average terminal half-life of 68 hours. With a regimen of 500 mg on Day 1 and 250 mg/day on Days 2–5, C_{min} and C_{max} remained essentially unchanged from Day 2 through Day 5 of therapy. However, without a loading dose, azithromycin C_{min} levels required 5 to 7 days to reach steady-state.
In an open, randomized, two-way crossover study, pharmacokinetic parameters (AUC_{0-72}, C_{max}, T_{max}) determined from 36 fasted healthy male volunteers who received two 250-mg commercial capsules and two 250-mg tablets were:

	Capsule	Tablet	90% CI
AUC_{0-72} (µg•h/mL)	4.1 (1.2)	4.3 (1.2)	(99-113%)
C_{max} (µg/mL)	0.5 (0.2)	0.5 (0.2)	(96-121%)
T_{max} (hours)	2.1 (0.8)	2.2 (0.9)	

When azithromycin capsules were administered with food to 11 adult healthy male subjects, the rate of absorption (C_{max}) of azithromycin from the capsule formulation was reduced by 52% and the extent of absorption (AUC) by 43%. In an open label, randomized, two-way crossover study in 12 healthy subjects to assess the effect of a high fat standard meal on the serum concentrations of azithromycin resulting from the oral administration of two 250-mg film-coated tablets, it was shown that food increased C_{max} by 23% while there was no change in AUC.
When azithromycin suspension was administered with food to 28 adult healthy male subjects, the rate of absorption (C_{max}) was increased by 56% while the extent of absorption (AUC) was unchanged.
The AUC of azithromycin was unaffected by co-administration of an antacid containing aluminum and magnesium hydroxide with ZITHROMAX® capsules (azithromycin); however, the C_{max} was reduced by 24%. Administration of cimetidine (800 mg) two hours prior to azithromycin had no effect on azithromycin absorption.
When studied in healthy elderly subjects from age 65 to 85 years, the pharmacokinetic parameters of azithromycin in elderly men were similar to those in young adults; however, in elderly women, although higher peak concentrations (increased by 30 to 50%) were observed, no significant accumulation occurred.
The high values in adults for apparent steady-state volume of distribution (31.1 L/kg) and plasma clearance (630 mL/min) suggest that the prolonged half-life is due to extensive uptake and subsequent release of drug from tissues.
The serum protein binding of azithromycin is variable in the concentration range approximating human exposure, decreasing from 51% at 0.02 µg/mL to 7% at 2 µg/mL.
Biliary excretion of azithromycin, predominantly as unchanged drug, is a major route of elimination. Over the course of a week, approximately 6% of the administered dose appears as unchanged drug in urine.
There are no pharmacokinetic data available from studies in hepatically- or renally-impaired individuals.
The effect of azithromycin on the plasma levels or pharmacokinetics of theophylline administered in multiple doses adequate to reach therapeutic steady-state plasma levels is not known. (See **PRECAUTIONS.**)
Selected tissue (or fluid) concentration and tissue (or fluid) to plasma/serum concentration ratios are shown in the following table:
[See table at top of next page]
The extensive tissue distribution was confirmed by examination of additional tissues and fluids (bone, ejaculum, prostate, ovary, uterus, salpinx, stomach, liver, and gallbladder). As there are no data from adequate and well-controlled studies of azithromycin treatment of infections in these additional body sites, the clinical significance of these tissue concentration data is unknown.
Following a regimen of 500 mg on the first day and 250 mg daily for 4 days, only very low concentrations were noted in cerebrospinal fluid (less than 0.01 µg/mL) in the presence of non-inflamed meninges.

Pediatric Pharmacokinetics:
In two clinical studies, azithromycin for oral suspension was dosed at 10 mg/kg on day 1, followed by 5 mg/kg on days 2 through 5 to two groups of children (aged 1–5 years and 5–15 years, respectively). The mean pharmacokinetic parameters at Day 5 were C_{max} = 0.216 µg/mL, T_{max} = 1.9 hours, and AUC_{0-24} = 1.822 µg•hr/mL for the 1- to 5-year-old group and were C_{max} = 0.383 µg/mL, T_{max} = 2.4 hours, and AUC_{0-24} = 3.109 µg•hr/mL for the 5- to 15-year-old group.
There are no pharmacokinetic data on azithromycin suspension when administered at a dose of 12 mg/kg/day in the presence or absence of food. (For the pediatric pharyngitis/tonsillitis dose, see **DOSAGE AND ADMINISTRATION.**)
Microbiology: Azithromycin acts by binding to the 50S ribosomal subunit of susceptible microorganisms and, thus, interfering with microbial protein synthesis. Nucleic acid synthesis is not affected.
Azithromycin concentrates in phagocytes and fibroblasts as demonstrated by *in vitro* incubation techniques. Using such methodology, the ratio of intracellular to extracellular concentration was > 30 after one hour incubation. *In vivo* studies suggest that concentration in phagocytes may contribute to drug distribution to inflamed tissues.
Azithromycin has been shown to be active against most strains of the following microorganisms, both *in vitro* and in clinical infections as described in the **INDICATIONS AND USAGE** section.

Aerobic gram-positive microorganisms
Staphylococcus aureus
Streptococcus agalactiae
Streptococcus pneumoniae
Streptococcus pyogenes
NOTE: Azithromycin demonstrates cross-resistance with erythromycin-resistant gram-positive strains. Most strains of *Enterococcus faecalis* and methicillin-resistant staphylococci are resistant to azithromycin.

Aerobic gram-negative microorganisms
Haemophilus ducreyi
Haemophilus influenzae
Moraxella catarrhalis
Neisseria gonorrhoeae

"Other" microorganisms
Chlamydia pneumoniae
Chlamydia trachomatis
Mycoplasma pneumoniae
Beta-lactamase production should have no effect on azithromycin activity.
The following *in vitro* data are available, **but their clinical significance is unknown.**
Azithromycin exhibits *in vitro* minimum inhibitory concentrations (MIC's) of 0.5 µg/mL or less against most (≥90%)

strains of streptococci and MIC's of 2.0 μg/mL or less against most (≥90%) strains of other listed microorganisms. However, the safety and effectiveness of azithromycin in treating clinical infections due to these microorganisms have not been established in adequate and well-controlled trials.

Aerobic gram-positive microorganisms
Streptococci (Groups C, F, G)
Viridans group streptococci

Aerobic gram-negative microorganisms
Bordetella pertussis
Legionella pneumophila

Anaerobic microorganisms
Peptostreptococcus species
Prevotella bivia

"Other" microorganisms
Ureaplasma urealyticum

Susceptibility Tests

Azithromycin can be solubilized for *in vitro* susceptibility testing using dilution techniques by dissolving in a minimum amount of 95% ethanol and diluting to the working stock concentration with broth. Further dilutions may be made in water.

Dilution Techniques:

Quantitative methods are used to determine antimicrobial minimum inhibitory concentrations (MIC's). These MIC's provide estimates of the susceptibility of bacteria to antimicrobial compounds. The MIC's should be determined using a standardized procedure. Standardized procedures are based on a dilution method[1] (broth or agar) or equivalent with standardized inoculum concentrations and standardized concentrations of azithromycin powder. The MIC values should be interpreted according to the following criteria:

For testing aerobic microorganisms other than *Haemophilus* species, *Neisseria gonorrhoeae*, and streptococci:

MIC (μg/mL)	Interpretation
≤ 2	Susceptible (S)
4	Intermediate (I)
≥ 8	Resistant (R)

For testing *Haemophilus* species:[a]

MIC (μg/mL)	Interpretation
≤ 4	Susceptible (S)

[a]These interpretive standards are applicable only to broth microdilution susceptibility testing with *Haemophilus* species using Haemophilus Test Medium.[1]

The current absence of data on resistant strains precludes defining any categories other than "Susceptible." Strains yielding MIC results suggestive of a "nonsusceptible" category should be submitted to a reference laboratory for further testing.

For testing Streptococci including *S. pneumoniae:*[b]

MIC (μg/mL)	Interpretation
≤ 0.5	Susceptible (S)
1	Intermediate (I)
≥ 2	Resistant (R)

[b]These interpretive standards are applicable only to broth microdilution susceptibility tests using cation-adjusted Mueller-Hinton broth with 2–5% lysed horse blood.

No interpretive criteria have been established for testing *Neisseria gonorrhoeae*. This species is not usually tested.

A report of "Susceptible" indicates that the pathogen is likely to respond to monotherapy with azithromycin. A report of "Intermediate" indicates that the result should be considered equivocal, and, if the microorganism is not fully susceptible to alternative, clinically feasible drugs, the test should be repeated. This category implies possible clinical applicability in body sites where the drug is physiologically concentrated or in situations where high dosage of drug can be used. This category also provides a buffer zone which prevents small uncontrolled technical factors from causing major discrepancies in interpretation. A report of "Resistant" indicates that achievable drug concentrations are unlikely to be inhibitory; other therapy should be selected.

Standardized susceptibility test procedures require the use of laboratory control microorganisms to control the technical aspects of the laboratory procedures. Standard azithromycin powder should provide the following MIC values:

Microorganism	MIC (μg/mL)
Haemophilus influenzae ATCC 49247[a]	1.0-4.0
Staphylococcus aureus ATCC 29213	0.5-2.0
Streptococcus pneumoniae ATCC 49619[b]	0.06-0.25

[a]This quality control range is applicable to only *H. influenzae* ATCC 49247 tested by a broth microdilution procedure using Haemophilus Test Medium (HTM).[1]

[b]This quality control range is applicable to only *S. pneumoniae* ATCC 49619 tested by a broth microdilution procedure using cation-adjusted Mueller-Hinton broth with 2-5% lysed horse blood.

No interpretive criteria have been established for testing *Neisseria gonorrhoeae*. This species is not usually tested.

Diffusion Techniques:

Quantitative methods that require measurement of zone diameters also provide reproducible estimates of the susceptibility of bacteria to antimicrobial compounds. One such

AZITHROMYCIN CONCENTRATIONS FOLLOWING TWO-250 mg (500 mg) CAPSULES IN ADULTS

TISSUE OR FLUID	TIME AFTER DOSE (h)	TISSUE OR FLUID CONCENTRATION (μg/g or μg/mL)[1]	CORRESPONDING PLASMA OR SERUM LEVEL (μg/mL)	TISSUE (FLUID) PLASMA (SERUM) RATIO[1]
SKIN	72-96	0.4	0.012	35
LUNG	72-96	4.0	0.012	>100
SPUTUM*	2-4	1.0	0.64	2
SPUTUM**	10-12	2.9	0.1	30
TONSIL***	9-18	4.5	0.03	>100
TONSIL***	180	0.9	0.006	>100
CERVIX****	19	2.8	0.04	70

[1] High tissue concentrations should not be interpreted to be quantitatively related to clinical efficacy. The antimicrobial activity of azithromycin is pH related. Azithromycin is concentrated in cell lysosomes which have a low intraorganelle pH, at which the drug's activity is reduced. However, the extensive distribution of drug to tissues may be relevant to clinical activity.
* Sample was obtained 2-4 hours after the first dose.
** Sample was obtained 10-12 hours after the first dose.
*** Dosing regimen of 2 doses of 250 mg each, separated by 12 hours.
**** Sample was obtained 19 hours after a single 500 mg dose.

standardized procedure[2] requires the use of standardized inoculum concentrations. This procedure uses paper disks impregnated with 15-μg azithromycin to test the susceptibility of microorganisms to azithromycin.

Reports from the laboratory providing results of the standard single-disk susceptibility test with a 15-μg azithromycin disk should be interpreted according to the following criteria:

For testing aerobic microorganisms (including streptococci)[a] except *Haemophilus* species and *Neisseria gonorrhoeae:*

Zone Diameter (mm)	Interpretation
≥ 18	Susceptible (S)
14-17	Intermediate (I)
≤ 13	Resistant (R)

[a]These zone diameter standards for streptococci apply only to tests performed using Mueller-Hinton agar supplemented with 5% sheep blood and incubated in 5% CO_2.

For testing *Haemophilus* species:[b]

Zone Diameter (mm)	Interpretation
≥ 12	Susceptible (S)

[b]These zone diameter standards apply only to tests with *Haemophilus* species using Haemophilus Test Medium (HTM).[2]

The current absence of data on resistant strains precludes defining any categories other than "Susceptible." Strains yielding zone diameter results suggestive of a "nonsusceptible" category should be submitted to a reference laboratory for further testing.

No interpretive criteria have been established for testing *Neisseria gonorrhoeae*. This species is not usually tested.

Interpretation should be as stated above for results using dilution techniques. Interpretation involves correlation of the diameter obtained in the disk test with the MIC for azithromycin.

As with standardized dilution techniques, diffusion methods require the use of laboratory control microorganisms that are used to control the technical aspects of the laboratory procedures. For the diffusion technique, the 15-μg azithromycin disk should provide the following zone diameters in these laboratory test quality control strains:

Microorganism	Zone Diameter (mm)
Haemophilus influenzae ATCC 49247[a]	13-21
Staphylococcus aureus ATCC 25923	21-26
Streptococcus pneumoniae ATCC 49619[b]	19-25

[a]These quality control limits apply only to tests conducted with *H. influenzae* ATCC 49247 using Haemophilus Test Medium (HTM).[2]

[b]These quality control limits apply only to tests conducted with *S. pneumoniae* ATCC 49619 using Mueller-Hinton agar supplemented with 5% sheep blood incubated in 5% CO_2.

INDICATIONS AND USAGE

ZITHROMAX® (azithromycin) is indicated for the treatment of patients with mild to moderate infections (pneumonia: see **WARNINGS**) caused by susceptible strains of the designated microorganisms in the specific conditions listed below. As recommended dosages, durations of therapy, and applicable patient populations vary among these infections, please see **DOSAGE AND ADMINISTRATION** for specific dosing recommendations.

Adults:

Acute bacterial exacerbations of chronic obstructive pulmonary disease due to *Haemophilus influenzae, Moraxella catarrhalis*, or *Streptococcus pneumoniae*.

Community-acquired pneumonia due to *Chlamydia pneumoniae, Haemophilus influenzae, Mycoplasma pneumoniae*, or *Streptococcus pneumoniae* in patients appropriate for oral therapy.

NOTE: Azithromycin should not be used in patients with pneumonia who are judged to be inappropriate for oral therapy because of moderate to severe illness or risk factors such as any of the following:
patients with cystic fibrosis,
patients with nosocomially acquired infections,
patients with known or suspected bacteremia,
patients requiring hospitalization,
elderly or debilitated patients, or
patients with significant underlying health problems that may compromise their ability to respond to their illness (including immunodeficiency or functional asplenia).

Pharyngitis/tonsillitis caused by *Streptococcus pyogenes* as an alternative to first-line therapy in individuals who cannot use first-line therapy.

NOTE: Penicillin by the intramuscular route is the usual drug of choice in the treatment of *Streptococcus pyogenes* infection and the prophylaxis of rheumatic fever. ZITHROMAX® is often effective in the eradication of susceptible strains of *Streptococcus pyogenes* from the nasopharynx. Because some strains are resistant to ZITHROMAX®, susceptibility tests should be performed when patients are treated with ZITHROMAX®. Data establishing efficacy of azithromycin in subsequent prevention of rheumatic fever are not available.

Uncomplicated skin and skin structure infections due to *Staphylococcus aureus, Streptococcus pyogenes*, or *Streptococcus agalactiae*. Abscesses usually require surgical drainage.

Urethritis and cervicitis due to *Chlamydia trachomatis* or *Neisseria gonorrhoeae*.

Genital ulcer disease in men due to *Haemophilus ducreyi* (chancroid). Due to the small number of women included in clinical trials, the efficacy of azithromycin in the treatment of chancroid in women has not been established.

ZITHROMAX®, at the recommended dose, should not be relied upon to treat syphilis. Antimicrobial agents used in high doses for short periods of time to treat non-gonococcal urethritis may mask or delay the symptoms of incubating syphilis. All patients with sexually-transmitted urethritis or cervicitis should have a serologic test for syphilis and appropriate cultures for gonorrhea performed at the time of diagnosis. Appropriate antimicrobial therapy and follow-up tests for these diseases should be initiated if infection is confirmed.

Appropriate culture and susceptibility tests should be performed before treatment to determine the causative organism and its susceptibility to azithromycin. Therapy with ZITHROMAX® may be initiated before results of these tests are known; once the results become available, antimicrobial therapy should be adjusted accordingly.

Children: (See **Pediatric Use** and **CLINICAL STUDIES IN PEDIATRIC PATIENTS.**)

Acute otitis media caused by *Haemophilus influenzae, Moraxella catarrhalis*, or *Streptococcus pneumoniae*. (For specific dosage recommendation, see **DOSAGE AND ADMINISTRATION.**)

Community-acquired penumonia due to *Chlamydia pneumoniae, Haemophilus influenzae, Mycoplasma pneumoniae*, or *Streptococcus pneumoniae* in patients appropriate for oral therapy. (For specific dosage recommendation, see **DOSAGE AND ADMINISTRATION.**)

NOTE: Azithromycin should not be used in pediatric patients with pneumonia who are judged to be inappropriate for oral therapy because of moderate to severe illness or risk factors such as any of the following:
patients with cystic fibrosis,
patients with nosocomially acquired infections,

Continued on next page

Zithromax—Cont.

patients with known or suspected bacteremia, patients requiring hospitalization, or patients with significant underlying health problems that may compromise their ability to respond to their illness (including immunodeficiency or functional asplenia).

Pharyngitis/tonsillitis caused by *Streptococcus pyogenes* as an alternative to first-line therapy in individuals who cannot use first-line therapy. (For specific dosage recommendation, see **DOSAGE AND ADMINISTRATION.**)

NOTE: Penicillin by the intramuscular route is the usual drug of choice in the treatment of *Streptococcus pyogenes* infection and the prophylaxis of rheumatic fever. ZITHROMAX® is often effective in the eradication of susceptible strains of *Streptococcus pyogenes* from the nasopharynx. Because some strains are resistant to ZITHROMAX®, susceptibility tests should be performed when patients are treated with ZITHROMAX®. Data establishing efficacy of azithromycin in subsequent prevention of rheumatic fever are not available.

Appropriate culture and susceptibility tests should be performed before treatment to determine the causative organism and its susceptibility to azithromycin. Therapy with ZITHROMAX® may be initiated before results of these tests are known; once the results become available, antimicrobial therapy should be adjusted accordingly.

CONTRAINDICATIONS

ZITHROMAX® is contraindicated in patients with known hypersensitivity to azithromycin, erythromycin, or any macrolide antibiotic.

WARNINGS

Serious allergic reactions, including angioedema, anaphylaxis, and dermatologic reactions including Stevens Johnson Syndrome and toxic epidermal necrolysis have been reported rarely in patients on azithromycin therapy. Although rare, fatalities have been reported. (See **CONTRAINDICATIONS.**) Despite initially successful symptomatic treatment of the allergic symptoms, when symptomatic therapy was discontinued, the allergic symptoms **recurred soon thereafter in some patients without further azithromycin exposure.** These patients required prolonged periods of observation and symptomatic treatment. The relationship of these episodes to the long tissue half-life of azithromycin and subsequent prolonged exposure to antigen is unknown at present.

If an allergic reaction occurs, the drug should be discontinued and appropriate therapy should be instituted. Physicians should be aware that reappearance of the allergic symptoms may occur when symptomatic therapy is discontinued.

In the treatment of pneumonia, azithromycin has only been shown to be safe and effective in the treatment of community-acquired pneumonia due to *Chlamydia pneumoniae, Haemophilus influenzae, Mycoplasma pneumoniae,* or *Streptococcus pneumoniae* in patients appropriate for oral therapy. Azithromycin should not be used in patients with pneumonia who are judged to be inappropriate for oral therapy because of moderate to severe illness or risk factors such as any of the following: patients with cystic fibrosis, patients with nosocomially acquired infections, patients with known or suspected bacteremia, patients requiring hospitalization, elderly or debilitated patients, or patients with significant underlying health problems that may compromise their ability to respond to their illness (including immunodeficiency or functional asplenia).

Pseudomembranous colitis has been reported with nearly all antibacterial agents and may range in severity from mild to life-threatening. Therefore, it is important to consider this diagnosis in patients who present with diarrhea subsequent to the administration of antibacterial agents.

Treatment with antibacterial agents alters the normal flora of the colon and may permit overgrowth of clostridia. Studies indicate that a toxin produced by *Clostridium difficile* is a primary cause of "antibiotic-associated colitis."

After the diagnosis of pseudomembranous colitis has been established, therapeutic measures should be initiated. Mild cases of pseudomembranous colitis usually respond to discontinuation of the drug alone. In moderate to severe cases, consideration should be given to management with fluids and electrolytes, protein supplementation, and treatment with an antibacterial drug clinically effective against *Clostridium difficile* colitis.

PRECAUTIONS

General: Because azithromycin is principally eliminated via the liver, caution should be exercised when azithromycin is administered to patients with impaired hepatic function. There are no data regarding azithromycin usage in patients with renal impairment; thus, caution should be exercised when prescribing azithromycin in these patients.

The following adverse events have not been reported in clinical trials with azithromycin, an azalide; however, they have been reported with macrolide products: ventricular arrhythmias, including ventricular tachycardia and *torsade de pointes*, in individuals with prolonged QT intervals.

There has been a spontaneous report from the post-marketing experience of a patient with previous history of arrhythmias who experienced *torsade de pointes* and subsequent myocardial infarction following a course of azithromycin therapy.

Information for Patients:

Patients should be cautioned to take ZITHROMAX® capsules and ZITHROMAX® suspension at least one hour prior to a meal or at least two hours after a meal. These medications should not be taken with food.

ZITHROMAX® tablets can be taken with or without food.

Patients should also be cautioned not to take aluminum- and magnesium-containing antacids and azithromycin simultaneously.

The patient should be directed to discontinue azithromycin immediately and contact a physician if any signs of an allergic reaction occur.

Drug Interactions: Aluminum- and magnesium-containing antacids reduce the peak serum levels (rate) but not the AUC (extent) of azithromycin absorption.

Administration of cimetidine (800 mg) two hours prior to azithromycin had no effect on azithromycin absorption.

Azithromycin did not affect the plasma levels or pharmacokinetics of theophylline administered as a single intravenous dose. The effect of azithromycin on the plasma levels or pharmacokinetics of theophylline administered in multiple doses resulting in therapeutic steady-state levels of theophylline is not known. However, concurrent use of macrolides and theophylline has been associated with increases in the serum concentrations of theophylline. Therefore, until further data are available, prudent medical practice dictates careful monitoring of plasma theophylline levels in patients receiving azithromycin and theophylline concomitantly.

Azithromycin did not affect the prothrombin time response to a single dose of warfarin. However, prudent medical practice dictates careful monitoring of prothrombin time in all patients treated with azithromycin and warfarin concomitantly. Concurrent use of macrolides and warfarin in clinical practice has been associated with increased anticoagulant effects.

The following drug interactions have not been reported in clinical trials with azithromycin; however, no specific drug interaction studies have been performed to evaluate potential drug-drug interaction. Nonetheless, they have been observed with macrolide products. Until further data are developed regarding drug interactions when azithromycin and these drugs are used concomitantly, careful monitoring of patients is advised:

Digoxin—elevated digoxin levels.

Ergotamine or dihydroergotamine-acute ergot toxicity characterized by severe peripheral vasospasm and dysesthesia.

Triazolam—decrease the clearance of triazolam and thus may increase the pharmacologic effect of triazolam.

Drugs metabolized by the cytochrome P^{450} system—elevations of serum carbamazepine, terfenadine, cyclosporine, hexobarbital, and phenytoin levels.

Laboratory Test Interactions: There are no reported laboratory test interactions.

Carcinogenesis, Mutagenesis, Impairment of Fertility: Long-term studies in animals have not been performed to evaluate carcinogenic potential. Azithromycin has shown no mutagenic potential in standard laboratory tests: mouse lymphoma assay, human lymphocyte clastogenic assay, and mouse bone marrow clastogenic assay. No evidence of impaired fertility due to azithromycin was found.

Pregnancy: Teratogenic Effects. Pregnancy Category B: Reproduction studies have been performed in rats and mice at doses up to moderately maternally toxic dose levels (i.e., 200 mg/kg/day). These doses, based on a mg/m^2 basis, are estimated to be 4 and 2 times, respectively, the human daily dose of 500 mg. In the animal studies, no evidence of harm to the fetus due to azithromycin was found. There are, however, no adequate and well-controlled studies in pregnant women. Because animal reproduction studies are not always predictive of human response, azithromycin should be used during pregnancy only if clearly needed.

Nursing Mothers: It is not known whether azithromycin is excreted in human milk. Because many drugs are excreted in human milk, caution should be exercised when azithromycin is administered to a nursing woman.

Pediatric Use: (See **CLINICAL PHARMACOLOGY, INDICATIONS AND USAGE,** and **DOSAGE AND ADMINISTRATION.**)

Acute Otitis Media (dosage regimen: 10 mg/kg on Day 1 followed by 5 mg/kg on Days 2–5): Safety and effectiveness in the treatment of children with otitis media under 6 months of age have not been established.

Community-Acquired Pneumonia (dosage regimen: 10 mg/kg on Day 1 followed by 5 mg/kg on Days 2–5): Safety and effectiveness in the treatment of children with community-acquired pneumonia under 6 months of age have not been established. Safety and effectiveness for pneumonia due to *Chlamydia pneumoniae* and *Mycoplasma pneumoniae* were documented in pediatric clinical trials. Safety and effectiveness for pneumonia due to *Haemophilus infuenzae* and *Streptococcus pneumoniae* were not documented bacteriologically in the pediatric clinical trial due to difficulty in obtaining specimens. Use of azithromycin for these two microorganisms is supported, however, by evidence from adequate and well-controlled studies in adults.

Pharyngitis/Tonsillitis (dosage regimen: 12 mg/kg on Days 1–5): Safety and effectiveness in the treatment of children with pharyngitis/tonsillitis under 2 years of age have not been established.

Studies evaluating the use of repeated courses of therapy have not been conducted. (See CLINICAL PHARMACOLOGY and ANIMAL TOXICOLOGY.)

Geriatric Use: Pharmacokinetic parameters in older volunteers (65–85 years old) were similar to those in younger volunteers (18–40 years old) for the 5-day therapeutic regimen. Dosage adjustment does not appear to be necessary for older patients with normal renal and hepatic function receiving treatment with this dosage regimen. (See **CLINICAL PHARMACOLOGY.**)

ADVERSE REACTIONS

In clinical trials, most of the reported side effects were mild to moderate in severity and were reversible upon discontinuation of the drug. Approximately 0.7% of the patients (adults and children) from the multiple-dose clinical trials discontinued ZITHROMAX® (azithromycin) therapy because of treatment-related side effects. Most of the side effects leading to discontinuation were related to the gastrointestinal tract, e.g., nausea, vomiting, diarrhea, or abdominal pain. Potentially serious side effects of angioedema and cholestatic jaundice were reported rarely.

Clinical:

Adults:

Multiple-dose regimen: Overall, the most common side effects in adult patients receiving a multiple-dose regimen of ZITHROMAX® were related to the gastrointestinal system with diarrhea/loose stools (5%), nausea (3%), and abdominal pain (3%) being the most frequently reported.

No other side effects occurred in patients on the multiple-dose regimen of ZITHROMAX® with a frequency greater than 1%. Side effects that occurred with a frequency of 1% or less included the following:

Cardiovascular: Palpitations, chest pain.

Gastrointestinal: Dyspepsia, flatulence, vomiting, melena, and cholestatic jaundice.

Genitourinary: Monilia, vaginitis, and nephritis.

Nervous System: Dizziness, headache, vertigo, and somnolence.

General: Fatigue.

Allergic: Rash, photosensitivity, and angioedema.

Single 1-gram dose regimen: Overall, the most common side effects in patients receiving a single-dose regimen of 1 gram of ZITHROMAX® were related to the gastrointestinal system and were more frequently reported in patients receiving the multiple-dose regimen.

Side effects that occurred in patients on the single one-gram dosing regimen of ZITHROMAX® with a frequency of 1% or greater included diarrhea/loose stools (7%), nausea (5%), abdominal pain (5%), vomiting (2%), dyspepsia (1%), and vaginitis (1%).

Singe 2-gram dose regimen: Overall, the most common side effects in patients receiving a single 2-gram dose of ZITHROMAX® were related to the gastrointestinal system. Side effects that occurred in patients in this study with a frequency of 1% or greater included nausea (18%), diarrhea/loose stools (14%), vomiting (7%), abdominal pain (7%), vaginitis (2%), dyspepsia (1%), and dizziness (1%). The majority of these complaints were mild in nature.

Children:

Multiple-dose regimens: The types of side effects in children were comparable to those seen in adults, with different incidence rates for the two dosage regimens recommended in children.

Acute Otitis Media: For the recommended dosage regimen of 10 mg/kg on Day 1 followed by 5 mg/kg on Days 2–5, the most frequent side effects attributed to treatment were diarrhea/loose stools (2%), abdominal pain (2%), vomiting (1%), and nausea (1%).

Community-Acquired Pneumonia: For the recommended dosage regimen of 10 mg/kg on Day 1 followed by 5 mg/kg on Days 2–5, the most frequent side effects attributed to treatment were diarrhea/loose stools (5.8%), abdominal pain, vomiting, and nausea (1.9% each), and rash (1.6%).

Pharyngitis/tonsillitis: For the recommended dosage regimen of 12 mg/kg on Days 1–5, the most frequent side effects attributed to treatment were diarrhea/loose stools (6%), vomiting (5%), abdominal pain (3%), nausea (2%), and headache (1%).

With either treatment regimen, no other side effects occurred in children treated with ZITHROMAX® with a frequency greater than 1%. Side effects that occurred with a frequency of 1% or less included the following:

Cardiovascular: Chest pain.

Gastrointestinal: Dyspepsia, constipation, anorexia, flatulence, and gastritis.

Nervous System: Headache (otitis media dosage), hyperkinesia, dizziness, agitation, nervousness, insomnia.

General: Fever, fatigue, malaise.

Allergic: Rash.

Skin and Appendages: Pruritus, urticaria.

Special Senses: Conjunctivitis.

Post-Marketing Experience:

Adverse events reported with azithromycin during the post-marketing period in adult and/or pediatric patients for which a causal relationship may not be established include:

Allergic: Arthralgia, edema, urticaria, angioedema.

Cardiovascular: Arrhythmias including ventricular tachycardia.

Gastrointestinal: Anorexia, constipation, dyspepsia, flatulence, vomiting/diarrhea rarely resulting in dehydration, pseudomembranous colitis and rare reports of tongue discoloration.

General: Asthenia, paresthesia and anaphylaxis (rarely fatal).

Genitourinary: Interstitial nephritis and acute renal failure, moniliasis, vaginitis.

Hematopoietic: Thrombocytopenia.
Liver/Biliary: Abnormal liver function including hepatitis and cholestatic jaundice, as well as rare cases of hepatic necrosis and hepatic failure, which have rarely resulted in death.
Nervous System: Convulsions, dizziness/vertigo, headache, somnolence, hyperactivity, nervousness, and agitation.
Psychiatric: Aggressive reaction and anxiety.
Skin/Appendages: Pruritus, rarely serious skin reactions including erythema multiforme, Stevens Johnson Syndrome, and toxic epidermal necrolysis.
Special Senses: Hearing disturbances including hearing loss, deafness, and/or tinnitus, rare reports of taste perversion.

Laboratory Abnormalities:

Adults:

Significant abnormalities (irrespective of drug relationship) occurring during the clinical trials were reported as follows: with an incidence of 1–2%, elevated serum creatine phosphokinase, potassium, ALT (SGPT), GGT, and AST (SGOT); with an incidence of less than 1%, leukopenia, neutropenia, decreased platelet count, elevated serum alkaline phosphatase, bilirubin, BUN, creatinine, blood glucose, LDH, and phosphate.
When follow-up was provided, changes in laboratory tests appeared to be reversible.
In multiple-dose clinical trials involving more than 3000 patients, 3 patients discontinued therapy because of treatment-related liver enzyme abnormalities and 1 because of a renal function abnormality.

Children:

Significant abnormalities (irrespective of drug relationship) occurring during clinical trials were all reported at a frequency of less than 1%, but were similar in type to the adult pattern.
In multiple-dose clinical trials involving almost 3300 pediatric patients, no patients discontinued therapy because of treatment-related laboratory abnormalities.

DOSAGE AND ADMINISTRATION

(See INDICATIONS AND USAGE and CLINICAL PHARMACOLOGY.)

Adults:

The recommended dose of ZITHROMAX® for the treatment of mild to moderate acute bacterial exacerbations of chronic obstructive pulmonary disease, community-acquired pneumonia of mild severity, pharyngitis/tonsillitis (as second-line therapy), and uncomplicated skin and skin structure infections due to the indicated organisms is: 500 mg as a single dose on the first day followed by 250 mg once daily on days 2 through 5.
ZITHROMAX® capsules should be given at least 1 hour before or 2 hours after a meal. ZITHROMAX® capsules should not be taken with food.
ZITHROMAX® tablets can be taken with or without food.
The recommended dose of ZITHROMAX® for the treatment of genital ulcer disease due to *Haemophilus ducreyi* (chancroid), non-gonococcal urethritis and cervicitis due to *C. trachomatis* is: a single 1 gram (1000 mg) dose of ZITHROMAX®.
The recommended dose of ZITHROMAX® for the treatment of urethritis and cervicitis due to *Neisseria gonorrhoeae* is a single 2 gram (2000 mg) dose of ZITHROMAX®.

Children:

Acute Otitis Media and Community-Acquired Pneumonia: The recommended dose of ZITHROMAX® for oral suspension for the treatment of children with acute otitis media and community-acquired pneumonia is 10 mg/kg as a single dose on the first day (not to exceed 500 mg/day) followed by 5 mg/kg on days 2 through 5 (not to exceed 250 mg/day). (See chart below.)
ZITHROMAX® for oral suspension should be given at least 1 hour before or 2 hours after a meal.
ZITHROMAX® for oral suspension should not be taken with food.
[See first table above]
Pharyngitis/Tonsillitis: The recommended dose for children with pharyngitis/tonsillitis is 12 mg/kg once a day for 5 days (not to exceed 500 mg/day). (See chart below.)
ZITHROMAX® for oral suspension should be given at least 1 hour before or 2 hours after a meal.
ZITHROMAX® for oral suspension should not be taken with food.
[See second table above]
Constituting instructions for ZITHROMAX® Oral Suspension, 300, 600, 900, 1200 mg bottles. The table below indicates the volume of water to be used for constitution:
[See third table above]
Shake well before each use. Oversized bottle provides shake space. Keep tightly closed.
After mixing, store at 5° to 30°C (41° to 86°F) and use within 10 days. Discard after full dosing is completed.

HOW SUPPLIED

ZITHROMAX® tablets are supplied as red modified capsular shaped, engraved, film-coated tablets containing azithromycin dihydrate equivalent to 250 mg of azithromycin.
ZITHROMAX® tablets are engraved with "PFIZER" on one side and "306" on the other. These are packaged in bottles and blister cards of 6 tablets (Z-PAKS®) as follows:

Bottles of 30	NDC 0069-3060-30
Boxes of 3 (Z-PAKS® of 6)	NDC 0069-3060-75
Unit Dose package of 50	NDC 0069-3060-86

PEDIATRIC DOSAGE GUIDELINES FOR OTITIS MEDIA AND COMMUNITY-ACQUIRED PNEUMONIA
(Age 6 months and above, see Pediatric Use.)
Based on Body Weight

OTITIS MEDIA AND COMMUNITY-ACQUIRED PNEUMONIA

Dosing Calculated on 10 mg/kg on Day 1 dose, followed by 5 mg/kg on Days 2 to 5.

Weight Kg	Weight lbs	100 mg/5 mL Suspension Day 1	100 mg/5 mL Suspension Days 2-5	200 mg/5 mL Suspension Day 1	200 mg/5 mL Suspension Days 2-5	Total mL per Treatment Course
10	22	5 mL (1 tsp)	2.5 mL (1/2 tsp)			15 mL
20	44			5 mL (1 tsp)	2.5 mL (1/2 tsp)	15 mL
30	66			7.5 mL (1 1/2tsp)	3.75 mL (3/4 tsp)	22.5 mL
40	88			10 mL (2 tsp)	5 mL (1 tsp)	30 mL

PEDIATRIC DOSAGE GUIDELINES FOR PHARYNGITIS/TONSILLITIS
(Age 2 years and above, see Pediatric Use.)
Based on Body Weight

PHARYNGITIS/TONSILLITIS

Dosing Calculated on 12 mg/kg once daily Days 1 to 5.

Weight Kg	Weight lbs	200 mg/5 mL Suspension Day 1-5	Total mL per Treatment Course
8	18	2.5 mL (1/2 tsp)	12.5 mL
17	37	5 mL (1 tsp)	25 mL
25	55	7.5 mL (1 1/2 tsp)	37.5 mL
33	73	10 mL (2 tsp)	50 mL
40	88	12.5 mL (2 1/2 tsp)	62.5 mL

Amount of water to be added	Total volume after constitution (azithromycin content)	Azithromycin concentration after constitution
9 mL (300 mg)	15 mL (300 mg)	100 mg/5 mL
9 mL (600 mg)	15 mL (600 mg)	200 mg/5 mL
12 mL (900 mg)	22.5 mL (900 mg)	200 mg/5 mL
15 mL (1200 mg)	30 mL (1200 mg)	200 mg/5 mL

	Day 11 Azithromycin	Day 30 Azithromycin
S. pneumoniae	61/74 (82%)	40/56 (71%)
H. influenzae	43/54 (80%)	30/47 (64%)
M. catarrhalis	28/35 (80%)	19/26 (73%)
S. pyogenes	11/11 (100%)	7/7
Overall	177/217 (82%)	97/137 (73%)

	Day 11 Azithromycin	Day 11 Control	Day 30 Azithromycin	Day 30 Control
S. pneumoniae	25/29 (86%)	26/26 (100%)	22/28 (79%)	18/22 (82%)
H. influenzae	9/11 (82%)	9/9	8/10 (80%)	6/8
M. catarrhalis	7/7	5/5	5/5	2/3
S. pyogenes	2/2	5/5	2/2	4/4
Overall	43/49 (88%)	45/45 (100%)	37/45 (82%)	30/37 (81%)

Three U.S. Streptococcal Pharyngitis Studies
Azithromycin vs. Penicillin V
EFFICACY RESULTS

	Day 14	Day 30
Bacteriologic Eradication:		
Azithromycin	323/340 (95%)	255/330 (77%)
Penicillin V	242/332 (73%)	206/325 (63%)
Clinical Success (Cure plus improvement):		
Azithromycin	336/343 (98%)	310/330 (94%)
Penicillin V	284/338 (84%)	241/325 (74%)

ZITHROMAX® tablets should be stored between 15° to 30°C (59° to 86°F).
ZITHROMAX® for oral suspension after constitution contains a flavored suspension.
ZITHROMAX® for oral suspension is supplied in bottles with accompanying calibrated dropper as follows:

Azithromycin contents per bottle	NDC
300 mg	0069-3110-19
600 mg	0069-3120-19
900 mg	0069-3130-19
1200 mg	0069-3140-19

Storage: Store dry powder below 30°C (86°F). Store constituted suspension between 5° to 30°C (41° to 86°F) and discard when full dosing is completed.

CLINICAL STUDIES IN PEDIATRIC PATIENTS

(See INDICATIONS AND USAGE and Pediatric Use.)

From the perspective of evaluating pediatric clinical trials, Days 11–14 (6–9 days after completion of the five-day regimen) were considered on-therapy evaluations because of the extended half-life of azithromycin. Day 11–14 data are provided for clinical guidance. Day 30 evaluations were considered the primary test of cure endpoint.

Acute Otitis Media

Efficacy Protocol 1

In a double-blind, controlled clinical study of acute otitis media performed in the United States, azithromycin (10 mg/kg on Day 1 followed by 5 mg/kg on Days 2–5) was compared to an antimicrobial/beta-lactamase inhibitor. In this study, very strict evaluability criteria were used to determine clinical response and safety results were obtained. For the 553 patients who were evaluated for clinical efficacy, the clinical success rate (i.e., cure plus improvement) at the Day 11 visit was 88% for azithromycin and 88% for the control agent. For the 521 patients who were evaluated at the Day 30 visit, the clinical success rate was 73% for azithromycin and 71% for the control agent.
In the safety analysis of the above study, the incidence of adverse events, primarily gastrointestinal, in all patients treated was 9% with azithromycin and 31% with the control agent. The most common side effects were diarrhea/loose stools (4% azithromycin vs. 20% control), vomiting (2% azithromycin vs. 7% control), and abdominal pain (2% azithromycin vs. 5% control).

Continued on next page

Zithromax—Cont.

Efficacy Protocol 2
In a noncomparative clinical and microbiologic trial performed in the United States, where significant rates of beta-lactamase producing organisms (35%) were found, 131 patients were evaluable for clinical efficacy. The combined clinical success rate (i.e., cure and improvement) at the Day 11 visit was 84% for azithromycin. For the 122 patients who were evaluated at the Day 30 visit, the clinical success rate was 70% for azithromycin.
Microbiologic determinations were made at the pre-treatment visit. Microbiology was not reassessed at later visits. The following presumptive bacterial/clinical cure outcomes (i.e., clinical success) were obtained from the evaluable group:
Bacteriologic Eradication:
[See fourth table at top of previous page]
In the safety analysis of this study, the incidence of adverse events, primarily gastrointestinal, in all patients treated was 9%. The most common side effect was diarrhea (4%).
Efficacy Protocol 3
In another controlled comparative clinical and microbiologic study of otitis media performed in the United States, azithromycin was compared to an antimicrobial/beta-lactamase inhibitor. This study utilized two of the same investigators as Efficacy Protocol 2 (above), and these two investigators enrolled 90% of the patients in Efficacy Protocol 3. For this reason, Efficacy Protocol 3 was not considered to be an independent study. Significant rates of beta-lactamase producing organisms (20%) were found. Ninety-two (92) patients were evaluable for clinical and microbiologic efficacy. The combined clinical success rate (i.e., cure and improvement) of those patients with a baseline pathogen at the Day 11 visit was 88% for azithromycin vs. 100% for control; at the Day 30 visit, the clinical success rate was 82% for azithromycin vs. 80% for control.
Microbiologic determinations were made at the pre-treatment visit. Microbiology was not reassessed at later visits. At the Day 11 and Day 30 visits, the following presumptive bacterial/clinical cure outcomes (i.e., clinical success) were obtained from the evaluable group:
Bacteriologic Eradication:
[See fifth table at top of previous page]
In the safety analysis of the above study, the incidence of adverse events, primarily gastrointestinal, in all patients treated was 4% with azithromycin and 31% with the control agent. The most common side effect was diarrhea/loose stools (2% azithromycin vs. 29% control).

Pharyngitis/Tonsillitis
In 3 double-blind controlled studies, conducted in the United States, azithromycin (12 mg/kg once a day for 5 days) was compared to penicillin V (250 mg three times a day for 10 days) in the treatment of pharyngitis due to documented Group A β-hemolytic streptococci (GABHS or *S. pyogenes*). Azithromycin was clinically and microbiologically statistically superior to penicillin at Day 14 and Day 30 with the following clinical success (i.e., cure and improvement) and bacteriologic efficacy rates (for the combined evaluable patient with documented GABHS):
[See sixth table at top of previous page]
Approximately 1% of azithromycin-susceptible *S. pyogenes* isolates were resistant to azithromycin following therapy.
The incidence of adverse events, primarily gastrointestinal, in all patients treated was 18% on azithromycin and 13% on penicillin. The most common side effects were diarrhea/loose stools (6% azithromycin vs. 2% penicillin), vomiting (6% azithromycin vs. 4% penicillin), and abdominal pain (3% azithromycin vs. 1% penicillin).

ANIMAL TOXICOLOGY

Phospholipidosis (intracellular phospholipid accumulation) has been observed in some tissues of mice, rats, and dogs given multiple doses of azithromycin. It has been demonstrated in numerous organ systems (e.g., eye, dorsal root ganglia, liver, gallbladder, kidney, spleen, and pancreas) in dogs treated with azithromycin at doses which, expressed on a mg/kg basis, are only 2 times greater than the recommended adult human dose and in rats at doses comparable to the recommended adult human dose. This effect has been reversible after cessation of azithromycin treatment. Phospholipidosis has been observed to a similar extent in the tissues of neonatal rats and dogs given daily doses of azithromycin ranging from 10 days to 30 days. Based on pharmacokinetic data, phospholipidosis has been seen in the rat (30 mg/kg dose) at observed C_{max} value of 1.3 μg/mL (6 times greater than the observed C_{max} of 0.216 μg/mL at the pediatric dose of 10 mg/kg). Similarly, it has been shown in the dog (10 mg/kg dose) at observed C_{max} value of 1.5 μg/mL (7 times greater than the observed same C_{max} and drug dose in the studied pediatric population). On mg/m^2 basis, 30 mg/kg dose in the rat (135 mg/m^2) and 10 mg/kg dose in the dog (79 mg/m^2) or approximately 0.4 and 0.6 times, respectively, the recommended dose in the pediatric patients with an average body weight of 25 kg. This effect, similar to that seen in the adult animals, is reversible after cessation of azithromycin treatment. The significance of these findings for animals and for humans is unknown.

REFERENCES:

1. National Committee for Clinical Laboratory Standards. Methods for Dilution Antimicrobial Susceptibility Tests for Bacteria that Grow Aerobically—Third Edition. Approved Standard NCCLS Document M7–A3, Vol. 13, No. 25, NCCLS, Villanova, PA, December 1993.
2. National Committee for Clinical Laboratory Standards. Performance Standards for Antimicrobial Disk Susceptibility Tests—Fifth Edition. Approved Standard NCCLS Document M2–A5, Vol. 13, No. 24, NCCLS, Villanova, PA, December 1993.

Rx only
Licensed from Pliva
Pfizer Labs
Division of Pfizer Inc, NY, NY 10017
70-5179-00-7 Revised September 1999
Shown in Product Identification Guide, page 330

ZITHROMAX® ℞

(azithromycin capsules)
(azithromycin tablets)
and
(azithromycin for oral suspension)

DESCRIPTION

ZITHROMAX® (azithromycin capsules, azithromycin tablets and azithromycin for oral suspension) contain the active ingredient azithromycin, an azalide, a subclass of macrolide antibiotics, for oral administration. Azithromycin has the chemical name *(2R, 3S, 4R, 5R, 8R, 10R, 11R, 12S, 13S, 14R)*-13-[(2,6-dideoxy-3-*C*-methyl-3-*O*-methyl-α-*L-ribo*-hexopyranosyl)oxy]-2-ethyl-3,4,10-trihydroxy-3,5,6,8,10,12,14-heptamethyl-11- [[3,4,6-trideoxy-3- (dimethylamino) -β-*D-xylo*-hexopyranosyl] oxy] -1-oxa-6-azacyclopentadecan-15-one. Azithromycin is derived from erythromycin; however, it differs chemically from erythromycin in that a methyl-substituted nitrogen atom is incorporated into the lactone ring. Its molecular formula is $C_{38}H_{72}N_2O_{12}$, and its molecular weight is 749.0. Azithromycin has the following structural formula:

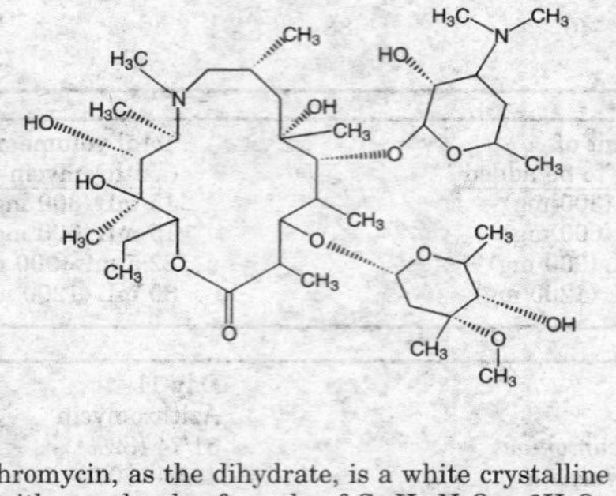

Azithromycin, as the dihydrate, is a white crystalline powder with a molecular formula of $C_{38}H_{72}N_2O_{12}•2H_2O$ and a molecular weight of 785.0
ZITHROMAX® capsules contain azithromycin dihydrate equivalent to 250 mg of azithromycin. The capsules are supplied in red opaque hard-gelatin capsules (containing FD&C Red #40). They also contain the following inactive ingredients: anhydrous lactose, corn starch, magnesium stearate, and sodium lauryl sulfate.
ZITHROMAX® tablets contain azithromycin dihydrate equivalent to 600 mg azithromycin. The tablets are supplied as white, modified oval-shaped, film-coated tablets. They also contain the following inactive ingredients: dibasic calcium phosphate anhydrous, pregelatinized starch, sodium croscarmellose, magnesium stearate, sodium lauryl sulfate and an aqueous film coat consisting of hydroxypropyl methyl cellulose, titanium dioxide, lactose and triacetin.
ZITHROMAX® for oral suspension is supplied in a single dose packet containing azithromycin dihydrate equivalent to 1 g azithromycin. It also contains the following inactive ingredients: colloidal silicon dioxide, sodium phosphate tribasic, anhydrous; spray dried artificial banana flavor, spray dried artificial cherry flavor, and sucrose.

CLINICAL PHARMACOLOGY

Pharmacokinetics: Following oral administration, azithromycin is rapidly absorbed and widely distributed throughout the body. Rapid distribution of azithromycin into tissues and high concentration within cells result in significantly higher azithromycin concentrations in tissues than in plasma or serum. The 1 g single dose packet is bioequivalent to four 250 mg capsules.
The pharmacokinetic parameters of azithromycin in plasma after dosing as per labeled recommendations in healthy young adults (age 18–40 years old) are portrayed in the following chart:
[See table below]
In these studies (500 mg Day 1, 250 mg Day 2–5), there was no significant difference in the disposition of azithromycin between male and female subjects. Plasma concentrations of azithromycin following single 500 mg oral and i.v. doses declined in a polyphasic pattern resulting in an average terminal half-life of 68 hours. With a regimen of 500 mg on Day 1 and 250 mg/day on Days 2–5, C_{min} and C_{max} remained essentially unchanged from Day 2 through Day 5 of therapy. However, without a loading dose, azithromycin C_{min} levels required 5 to 7 days to reach steady-state.
When azithromycin capsules were administered with food, the rate of absorption (C_{max}) of azithromycin was reduced by 52% and the extent of absorption (AUC) by 43%.
When the oral suspension of azithromycin was administered with food, the C_{max} increased by 46% and the AUC by 14%.
The absolute bioavailability of two 600 mg tablets was 34% (CV=56%). Administration of two 600 mg tablets with food increased C_{max} by 31% (CV=43%) while the extent of absorption (AUC) was unchanged (mean ratio of AUCs=1.00; CV=55%).
The AUC of azithromycin in 250 mg capsules was unaffected by coadministration of an antacid containing aluminum and magnesium hydroxide with ZITHROMAX® (azithromycin); however, the C_{max} was reduced by 24%. Administration of cimetidine (800 mg) two hours prior to azithromycin had no effect on azithromycin absorption.
When studied in healthy elderly subjects from age 65 to 85 years, the pharmacokinetic parameters of azithromycin (500 mg Day 1, 250 mg Days 2–5) in elderly men were similar to those in young adults; however, in elderly women, although higher peak concentrations (increased by 30 to 50%) were observed, no significant accumulation occurred.
The high values in adults for apparent steady-state volume of distribution (31.1 L/kg) and plasma clearance (630 mL/min) suggest that the prolonged half-life is due to extensive uptake and subsequent release of drug from tissues. Selected tissue (or fluid) concentration and tissue (or fluid) to plasma/serum concentration ratios are shown in the following table:
[See table at bottom of next page]
The extensive tissue distribution was confirmed by examination of additional tissues and fluids (bone, ejaculum, prostate, ovary, uterus, salpinx, stomach, liver, and gallbladder). As there are no data from adequate and well-controlled studies of azithromycin treatment of infections in these additional body sites, the clinical significance of these tissue concentration data is unknown.
Following a regimen of 500 mg on the first day and 250 mg daily for 4 days, only very low concentrations were noted in cerebrospinal fluid (less than 0.01 μg/mL) in the presence of non-inflamed meninges.
Following oral administration of a single 1200 mg dose (two 600 mg tablets), the mean maximum concentration in peripheral leukocytes was 140 μg/mL. Concentrations remained above 32 μg/mL for approximately 60 hr. The mean half-lives for 6 males and 6 females were 34 hr and 57 hr, respectively. Leukocyte to plasma C_{max} ratios for males and females were 258 (±77%) and 175 (±60%), respectively, and the AUC ratios were 804 (±31%) and 541 (±28%), respectively. The clinical relevance of these findings is unknown.
The serum protein binding of azithromycin is variable in the concentration range approximating human exposure, decreasing from 51% at 0.02 μg/mL to 7% at 2 μg/mL. Biliary excretion of azithromycin, predominantly as unchanged drug, is a major route of elimination. Over the course of a week, approximately 6% of the administered dose appears as unchanged drug in urine.
There are no pharmacokinetic data available from studies in hepatically- or renally-impaired individuals.
The effect of azithromycin on the plasma levels or pharmacokinetics of theophylline administered in multiple doses adequate to reach therapeutic steady-state plasma levels is not known. (See PRECAUTIONS.)

Mechanism of Action: Azithromycin acts by binding to the 50S ribosomal subunit of susceptible microorganisms and, thus, interfering with microbial protein synthesis. Nucleic acid synthesis is not affected.
Azithromycin concentrates in phagocytes and fibroblasts as demonstrated by *in vitro* incubation techniques. Using such methodology, the ratio of intracellular to extracellular concentration was >30 after one hour incubation. *In vivo* studies suggest that concentration in phagocytes may contribute to drug distribution to inflamed tissues.

Microbiology:
Azithromycin has been shown to be active against most strains of the following microorganisms, both *in vitro* and in clinical infections as described in the INDICATIONS AND USAGE section.

Aerobic Gram-Positive Microorganisms
Staphylococcus aureus
Streptococcus agalactiae

MEAN (CV%) PK PARAMETER

DOSE/DOSAGE FORM	Subjects	Day No.	C_{max} (μg/ml)	T_{max} (hr)	C_{24} (μg/mL)	AUC (μg•hr/ml)	$T_{½}$ (hr)	Urinary Excretion (% of dose)
500 mg/250 mg capsule	12	Day 1	0.41	2.5	0.05	2.6[a]	—	4.5
and 250 mg on Days 2–5	12	Day 5	0.24	3.2	0.05	2.1[a]	—	6.5
1200 mg/600 mg tablets	12	Day 1	0.66	2.5	0.074	6.8[b]	40	—
			(62%)	(79%)	(49%)	(64%)	(33%)	

[a]0–24 hr; [b]0–last.

Streptococcus pneumoniae
Streptococcus pyogenes

Note: Azithromycin demonstrates cross-resistance with erythromcyin-resistant gram-positive strains. Most strains of *Enterococcus faecalis* and methicillin-resistant staphylococci are resistant to azithromycin.

Aerobic Gram-Negative Microorganisms

Haemophilus influenzae
Moraxella catarrhalis

"Other" MIcroorganisms

Chlamydia trachomatis

Beta-lactamase production should have no effect on azithromycin activity.

Azithromycin has been shown to be active *in vitro* and in the prevention of disease caused by the following microorganisms:

Mycobacteria

Mycobacterium avium complex (MAC) consisting of:
Mycobacterium avium
Mycobacterium intracellulare.

The following *in vitro* data are available, *but their clinical significance is unknown.*

Azithromycin exhibits *in vitro* minimal inhibitory concentrations (MICs) of 2.0 μg/mL or less against most (≥90%) strains of the following microorganisms; however, the safety and effectiveness of azithromycin in treating clinical infections due to these microorganisms have not been established in adequate and well-controlled trials.

Aerobic Gram-Positive Microorganisms

Streptococci (Groups C, F, G)
Viridans group streptococci

Aerobic Gram-Negative Microorganisms

Bordetella pertussis
Campylobacter jejuni
Haemophilus ducreyi
Legionella pneumophila

Anaerobic Microorganisms

Bacteroides bivius
Clostridium perfringens
Peptostreptococcus species

"Other" Microorganisms

Borrelia burgdorferi
Mycoplasma pneumoniae
Treponema pallidum
Ureaplasma urealyticum

Susceptibility Testing of Bacteria Excluding Mycobacteria

The *in vitro* potency of azithromycin is markedly affected by the pH of the microbiological growth medium during incubation. Incubation in a 10% CO_2 atmosphere will result in lowering of media pH (7.2 to 6.6) within 18 hours and in an apparent reduction of the *in vitro* potency of azithromycin. Thus, the initial pH of the growth medium should be 7.2–7.4, and the CO_2 content of the incubation atmosphere should be as low as practical.

Azithromycin can be solubilized for *in vitro* susceptibility testing by dissolving in a minimum amount of 95% ethanol and diluting to working concentration with water.

Dilution Techniques:

Quantitative methods are used to determine minimal inhibitory concentrations that provide reproducible estimates of the susceptibility of bacteria to antimicrobial compounds. One such standardized procedure uses a standardized dilution method[1] (broth, agar or microdilution) or equivalent with azithromycin powder. The MIC values should be interpreted according to the following criteria:

MIC (μg/mL)	Interpretation
≤ 2	Susceptible (S)
4	Intermediate (I)
≥ 8	Resistant (R)

A report of "Susceptible" indicates that the pathogen is likely to respond to monotherapy with azithromycin. A report of "Intermediate" indicates that the result should be considered equivocal, and, if the microorganism is not fully susceptible to alternative, clinically feasible drugs, the test should be repeated. This category also provides a buffer zone which prevents small uncontrolled technical factors from causing major discrepancies in interpretation. A report of "Resistant" indicates that usually achievable drug concentrations are unlikely to be inhibitory and that other therapy should be selected.

Measurement of MIC or MBC and achieved antimicrobial compound concentrations may be appropriate to guide therapy in some infections. (See CLINICAL PHARMACOLOGY section for further information on drug concentrations achieved in infected body sites and other pharmacokinetic properties of this antimicrobial drug product.)

Standardized susceptibility test procedures require the use of laboratory control microorganisms.

Standard azithromycin powder should provide the following MIC values:

Microorganism	MIC (μg/mL)
Escherichia coli ATCC 25922	2.0–8.0
Enterococcus faecalis ATCC 29212	1.0–4.0
Staphylococcus aureus ATCC 29213	0.25–1.0

Diffusion Techniques:

Quantitative methods that require measurement of zone diameters also provide reproducible estimates of the susceptibility of bacteria to antimicrobial compounds. One such standardized procedure[2] that has been recommended for use with disks to test the susceptibility of microorganisms to azithromycin uses the 15-μg azithromycin disk. Interpretation involves the correlation of the diameter obtained in the disk test with the minimal inhibitory concentration (MIC) for azithromycin.

Reports from the laboratory providing results of the standard single-disk susceptiblity test with a 15 μg azithromycin disk should be interpreted according to the following criteria:

Zone Diameter (mm)	Interpretation
≥ 18	(S) Susceptible
14–17	(I) Intermediate
≤ 13	(R) Resistant

Interpretation should be as stated above for results using dilution techniques.

As with standardized dilution techniques, diffusion methods require the use of laboratory control microorganisms. The 15-μg azithromycin disk should provide the following zone diameters in these laboratory test quality control strains:

Microorganism	Zone Diameter (mm)
Staphylococcus aureus ATCC 25923	21–26

***In Vitro* Activity of Azithromycin Against Mycobacteria.**

Azithromycin has demonstrated *in vitro* activity against *Mycobacterium avium* complex (MAC) organisms. While gene probe techniques may be used to distinguish *M. avium* species from *M. intracellulare,* many studies only report results on *M. avium* complex (MAC) isolates. Azithromycin has also been shown to be active against phagocytized *M. avium* complex (MAC) organisms in mouse and human macrophage cell cultures as well as in the beige mouse infection model.

Various *in vitro* methodologies employing broth or solid media at different pHs, with and without oleic acid-albumin dextrose-catalase (OADC), have been used to determine azithromycin MIC values for *Mycobacterium avium* complex strains. In general, MIC values decreased 4 to 8 fold as the pH of middlebrook 7H11 agar media increased from 6.6 to 7.4. At pH 7.4, MIC values determined with Mueller-Hinton agar were 4 fold higher than that observed with middlebrook 7H12 media at the same pH. Utilization of oleic acid-albumin-dextrose-catalase (OADC) in these assays has been shown to further alter MIC values. The ability to correlate MIC values and plasma drug levels is difficult as azithromycin concentrates in macrophages and tissues.

A cross resistance relationship between azithromycin and clarithromycin has been observed with some *Mycobacterium avium* complex (MAC) isolates. The various mechanisms of cross resistance between azithromycin and clarithromycin for *M. avium* complex organism have not been fully characterized. The clinical significance of azithromycin and clarithromycin cross resistance is unknown.

Susceptibility testing for *Mycobacterium avium* complex (MAC):

The disk diffusion techniques and dilution methods for susceptibility testing against gram-positive and gram-negative bacteria should not be used for determining azithromycin MIC values against mycobacteria. *In vitro* susceptibility testing methods and diagnostic products currently available for determining minimal inhibitory concentration (MIC) values against *Mycobacterium avium* complex (MAC) organisms have not been established or validated. Azithromycin MIC values will vary depending on the susceptibility testing method employed, composition and pH of media and the utilization of nutritional supplements. Breakpoints to determine whether clinical isolates of *M. avium* or *M. intracellulare* are susceptible to azithromycin have not been established.

INDICATIONS AND USAGE

ZITHROMAX® (azithromycin) is indicated for the treatment of patients with mild to moderate infections (pneumonia: see WARNINGS) caused by susceptible strains of the designated microorganisms in the specific conditions listed below.

Lower Respiratory Tract:

Acute bacterial exacerbations of chronic obstructive pulmonary disease due to *Haemophilus influenzae, Moraxella catarrhalis,* or *Streptococcus pneumoniae.*

Community-acquired pneumonia of mild severity due to *Streptococcus pneumoniae* or *Haemophilus influenzae* in patients appropriate for outpatient oral therapy.

NOTE: Azithromycin should not be used in patients with pneumonia who are judged to be inappropriate for outpatient oral therapy because of moderate to severe illness or risk factors such as any of the following:

patients with nosocomially acquired infections,
patients with known or suspected bacteremia,
patients requiring hospitalization,
elderly or debilitated patients, or
patients with significant underlying health problems that may compromise their ability to respond to their illness (including immunodeficiency or functional asplenia).

Upper Respiratory Tract:

Streptococcal pharyngitis/tonsillitis—As an alternative to first line therapy of acute pharyngitis/tonsillitis due to *Streptococcus pyogenes* occurring in individuals who cannot use first line therapy.

NOTE: Penicillin is the usual drug of choice in the treatment of *Streptococcus pyogenes* infection and the prophylaxis of rheumatic fever. ZITHROMAX® is often effective in the eradication of susceptible strains of *Streptococcus pyogenes* from the nasopharynx. Data establishing efficacy of azithromycin in subsequent prevention of rheumatic fever are not available.

Skin and Skin Structure

Uncomplicated skin and skin structure infections due to *Staphylococcus aureus, Streptococcus pyogenes,* or *Streptococcus agalactiae.* Abscesses usually require surgical drainage.

Sexually Transmitted Diseases

Non-gonococcal urethritis and cervicitis due to *Chlamydia trachomatis.*

ZITHROMAX®, at the recommended dose, should not be relied upon to treat gonorrhea or syphilis. Antimicrobial agents used in high doses for short periods of time to treat non-gonococcal urethritis may mask or delay the symptoms of incubating gonorrhea or syphilis. All patients with sexually-transmitted urethritis or cervicitis should have a serologic test for syphilis and appropriate cultures for gonorrhea performed at the time of diagnosis. Appropriate antimicrobial therapy and follow-up tests for these diseases should be initiated if infection is confirmed.

Appropriate culture and susceptibility tests should be performed before treatment to determine the causative organism and its susceptibility to azithromycin. Therapy with ZITHROMAX® may be initiated before results of these tests are known; once the results become available, antimicrobial therapy should be adjusted accordingly.

Disseminated *Mycobacterium Avium* Complex (MAC) Disease

ZITHROMAX®, taken alone or in combination with rifabutin at its approved dose, is indicated for the prevention of disseminated *Mycobacterium avium* complex (MAC) disease in persons with advanced HIV infection. (See Clinical Trials section.)

CONTRAINDICATIONS

ZITHROMAX® is contraindicated in patients with known hypersensitivity to azithromycin, erythromycin, or any macrolide antibiotic.

WARNINGS

Rare serious allergic reactions, including angioedema and anaphylaxis, have been reported rarely in patients on azithromycin therapy. (See **CONTRAINDICATIONS.**) Despite initially successful symptomatic treatment of the al-

Continued on next page

AZITHROMYCIN CONCENTRATIONS FOLLOWING TWO 250 MG (500 MG) CAPSULES IN ADULTS

TISSUE OR FLUID	TIME AFTER DOSE (h)	TISSUE OR FLUID CONCENTRATION (μg/g or μg/mL)[1]	CORRESPONDING PLASMA OR SERUM LEVEL (μg/mL)	TISSUE (FLUID) PLASMA (SERUM) RATIO[1]
SKIN	72–96	0.4	0.012	35
LUNG	72–96	4.0	0.012	>100
SPUTUM*	2–4	1.0	0.64	2
SPUTUM**	10–12	2.9	0.1	30
TONSIL***	9–18	4.5	0.03	>100
TONSIL***	180	0.9	0.006	>100
CERVIX****	19	2.8	0.04	70

[1] High tissue concentrations should not be interpreted to be quantitatively related to clinical efficacy. The antimicrobial activity of azithromycin is pH related. Azithromycin is concentrated in cell lysosomes which have a lower intraorganelle pH, at which the drug's activity is reduced. However, the extensive distribution of drug to tissues may be relevant to clinical activity.

* Sample was obtained 2–4 hours after the first dose.
** Sample was obtained 10–12 hours after the first dose.
*** Dosing regimen of 2 doses of 250 mg each, separated by 12 hours.
**** Sample was obtained 19 hours after a single 500 mg dose.

Zithromax—Cont.

lergic symptoms, when symptomatic therapy was discontinued, the allergic symptoms **recurred soon thereafter in some patients without further azithromycin exposure.** These patients required prolonged periods of observation and symptomatic treatment. The relationship of these episodes to the long tissue half-life of azithromycin and subsequent prolonged exposure to antigen is unknown at present. If an allergic reaction occurs, the drug should be discontinued and appropriate therapy should be instituted. Physicians should be aware that reappearance of the allergic symptoms may occur when symptomatic therapy is discontinued.

In the treatment of pneumonia, azithromycin has only been shown to be safe and effective in the treatment of community-acquired pneumonia of mild severity due to *Streptococcus pneumonia* or *Haemophilus influenzae* in patients appropriate for outpatient oral therapy. Azithromycin should not be used in patients with pneumonia who are judged to be inappropriate for outpatient oral therapy because of moderate to severe illness or risk factors such as any of the following: patients with nosocomially acquired infections, patients with known or suspected bacteremia, patients requiring hospitalization, elderly or debilitated patients, or patients with significant underlying health problems that may compromise their ability to respond to their illness (including immunodeficiency or functional asplenia).

Pseudomembranous colitis has been reported with nearly all antibacterial agents and may range in severity from mild to life-threatening. Therefore, it is important to consider this diagnosis in patients who present with diarrhea subsequent to the administration of antibacterial agents.

Treatment with antibacterial agents alters the normal flora of the colon and may permit overgrowth of clostridia. Studies indicate that a toxin produced by *Clostridium difficile* is a primary cause of "antibiotic-associated colitis."

After the diagnosis of pseudomembranous colitis has been established, therapeutic measures should be initiated. Mild cases of pseudomembranous colitis usually respond to discontinuation of the drug alone. In moderate to severe cases, consideration should be given to management with fluids and electrolytes, protein supplementation, and treatment with an antibacterial drug clinically effective against *Clostridium difficile* colitis.

PRECAUTIONS

General: Because azithromycin is principally eliminated via the liver, caution should be exercised when azithromycin is administered to patients with impaired hepatic function. There are no data regarding azithromycin usage in patients with renal impairment; thus, caution should be exercised when prescribing azithromycin in these patients.

The following adverse events have not been reported in clinical trials with azithromycin, an azalide; however, they have been reported with macrolide products: ventricular arrhythmias, including ventricular tachycardia and *torsade de pointes,* in individuals with prolonged QT intervals.

Information for Patients:

Patients should be cautioned to take ZITHROMAX® capsules at least one hour prior to a meal or at least two hours after a meal. Azithromycin capsules should not be taken with food.

ZITHROMAX® tablets may be taken with or without food. However, increased tolerability has been observed when tablets are taken with food.

ZITHROMAX® for oral suspension in single 1 g packets can be taken with or without food after constitution.

Patients should also be cautioned not to take aluminum- and magnesium-containing antacids and azithromycin simultaneously.

The patient should be directed to discontinue azithromycin immediately and contact a physician if any signs of an allergic reaction occur.

Drug Interactions: Aluminum- and magnesium-containing antacids reduce the peak serum levels (rate) but not the AUC (extent) of azithromycin (500 mg) absorption.

Administration of cimetidine (800 mg) two hours prior to azithromycin had no effect on azithromycin (500 mg) absorption.

Azithromycin (500 mg Day 1, 250 mg Days 2–5) did not affect the plasma levels or pharmacokinetics of theophylline administered as a single intravenous dose. The effect of azithromycin on the plasma levels or pharmacokinetics of theophylline administered in multiple doses resulting in therapeutic steady-state levels of theophylline is not known. However, concurrent use of macrolides and theophylline has been associated with increases in the serum concentrations of theophylline. Therefore, until further data are available, prudent medical practice dictates careful monitoring of plasma theophylline levels in patients receiving azithromycin and theophylline concomitantly.

Azithromycin (500 mg Day 1, 250 mg Days 2–5) did not affect the prothrombin time response to a single dose of warfarin. However, prudent medical practice dictates careful monitoring of prothrombin time in all patients treated with azithromycin and warfarin concomitantly. Concurrent use of macrolides and warfarin in clinical practice has been associated with increased anticoagulant effects.

Dose adjustments are not indicated when azithromycin and zidovudine are coadministered. When zidovudine (100 mg q3h x5) was coadministered with daily azithromycin (600 mg, n=5 or 1200 mg, n=7), mean C_{max}, AUC and Clr in-

Cumulative Incidence Rate, %: Placebo (n=89)

Month	MAC Free and Alive	MAC	Adverse Experience	Lost to Follow-up
6	69.7	13.5	6.7	10.1
12	47.2	19.1	15.7	18.0
18	37.1	22.5	18.0	22.5

Cumulative Incidence Rate, %: Azithromycin (n=85)

Month	MAC Free and Alive	MAC	Adverse Experience	Lost to Follow-up
6	84.7	3.5	9.4	2.4
12	63.5	8.2	16.5	11.8
18	44.7	11.8	25.9	17.6

Cumulative Incidence Rate, %: Rifabutin (n=223)

Month	MAC Free and Alive	MAC	Adverse Experience	Lost to Follow-up
6	83.4	7.2	8.1	1.3
12	60.1	15.2	16.1	8.5
18	40.8	21.5	24.2	13.5

Cumulative Incidence Rate, %: Azithromycin (n=223)

Month	MAC Free and Alive	MAC	Adverse Experience	Lost to Follow-up
6	85.2	3.6	5.8	5.4
12	65.5	7.6	16.1	10.8
18	45.3	12.1	23.8	18.8

Cumulative Incidence Rate, %: Azithromycin/Rifabutin Combination (n=218)

Month	MAC Free and Alive	MAC	Adverse Experience	Lost to Follow-up
6	89.4	1.8	5.5	3.2
12	71.6	2.8	15.1	10.6
18	49.1	6.4	29.4	15.1

creased by 26% (CV 54%), 10% (CV 26%) and 38% (CV 114%), respectively. The mean AUC of phosphorylated zidovudine increased by 75% (CV 95%), while zidovudine glucuronide C_{max} and AUC increased by less than 10%. In another study, addition of 1 gram azithromycin per week to a regimen of 10 mg/kg daily zidovudine resulted in 25% (CV 70%) and 13% (CV 37%) increases in zidovudine C_{max} and AUC, respectively. Zidovudine glucuronide mean C_{max} and AUC increased by 16% (CV 61%) and 8.0% (CV 32%), respectively.

Doses of 1200 mg/day azithromycin for 14 days in 6 subjects increased C_{max} of concurrently administered didanosine (200 mg *q.* 12h) by 44% (54% CV) and AUC by 14% (23% CV). However, none of these changes were significantly different from those produced in a parallel placebo control group of subjects.

Preliminary data suggest that coadministration of azithromycin and rifabutin did not markedly affect the mean serum concentrations of either drug. Administration of 250 mg azithromycin daily for 10 days (500 mg on the first day) produced mean concentrations of azithromycin 1 day after the last dose of 53 ng/ml when coadministered with 300 mg daily rifabutin and 49 mg/ml when coadministered with placebo. Mean concentrations 5 days after the last dose were 23 ng/ml and 21 ng/ml in the two groups of subjects. Administration of 300 mg rifabutin for 10 days produced mean concentrations of rifabutin one half day after the last dose of 60 mg/ml when coadministered with daily 250 mg azithromycin and 71 ng/ml when coadministered with placebo. Mean concentrations 5 days after the last dose with 8.1 ng/ml and 9.2 ng/ml in the two groups of subjects.

The following drug interactions have not been reported in clinical trials with azithromycin; however, no specific drug interaction studies have been performed to evaluate potential drug-drug interaction. Nonetheless, they have been observed with macrolide products. Until further data are developed regarding drug interactions when azithromycin and these drugs are used concomitantly, careful monitoring of patients is advised:

Digoxin-elevated digoxin levels.

Ergotamine or dihydroergotamine-acute ergot toxicity characterized by severe peripheral vasospasm and dysesthesia.

Triazolam-decrease the clearance of triazolam and thus may increase the pharmacologic effect of triazolam.

Drugs metabolized by the cytochrome P^{450} system-elevations of serum carbamazepine, cyclosporine, hexobarbital, and phenytoin levels.

Laboratory Test Interactions: There are no reported laboratory test interactions.

Carcinogenesis, Mutagenesis, Impairment of Fertility: Long-term studies in animals have not been performed to evaluate carcinogenic potential. Azithromycin has shown no mutagenic potential in standard laboratory tests: mouse lymphoma assay, human lymphocyte clastogenic assay, and mouse bone marrow clastogenic assay.

Pregnancy: Teratogenic Effects. Pregnancy Category B: Reproduction studies have been performed in rats and mice at doses up to moderately maternally toxic dose levels (i.e., 200 mg/kg/day). These doses, based on a mg/m^2 basis, are estimated to be 4 and 2 times, respectively, the human daily dose of 500 mg.

With regard to the MAC prophylaxis dose of 1200 mg weekly, on a mg/m^2/day basis, the doses in rats and mice are approximately 2 and 1 times the human dose, respectively. No evidence of impaired fertility or harm to the fetus due to azithromycin was found. There are, however, no adequate and well-controlled studies in pregnant women. Because animal reproduction studies are not always predictive of human response, azithromycin should be used during pregnancy only if clearly needed.

Nursing Mothers: It is not known whether azithromycin is excreted in human milk. Because many drugs are excreted in human milk, caution should be exercised when azithromycin is administered to a nursing woman.

Pediatric Use: In controlled clinical studies, azithromycin has been administered to pediatric patients ranging in age from 6 months to 12 years. For information regarding the use of ZITHROMAX (azithromycin for oral suspension) in the treatment of pediatric patients, please refer to the INDICATIONS AND USAGE and DOSAGE AND ADMINISTRATION sections of the prescribing information for ZITHROMAX (azithromycin for oral suspension) 100 mg/5 mL and 200 mg/5 mL bottles.

Prevention of Disseminated *Mycobacterium avium* complex (MAC) Disease: Safety and efficacy of azithromycin for the prevention of MAC in children have not been established. Limited safety data are available for 24 children 5 months to 14 years of age (mean 4.6 years) who received azithromycin for treatment of opportunistic infections. The mean duration of therapy was 186.7 days (range 13–710 days) at doses of <5 to 20 mg/kg/day. Three children were treated for 6 months or more and 4 children were treated for 1 month or more with a dose of >10 mg/kg/day. Adverse events were similar to those observed in the adult population, most of which involved the gastrointestinal tract. While none of these children prematurely discontinued treatment due to a side effect, one child discontinued due to a laboratory abnormality (eosinophilia). The protocols upon which these data are based specified a daily dose of 10–20 mg/kg/day of azithromycin.

Geriatric Use: Pharmacokinetic parameters in older volunteers (65–85 years old) were similar to those in younger volunteers (18–40 years old) for the 5-day therapeutic regimen. Dosage adjustment does not appear to be necessary for older patients with normal renal and hepatic function receiving treatment with this dosage regimen. (See CLINICAL PHARMACOLOGY.)

ADVERSE REACTIONS

In clinical trials, most of the reported side effects were mild to moderate in severity and were reversible upon discontinuation of the drug. Approximately 0.7% of the patients from the multiple-dose clinical trials discontinued ZITHROMAX® (azithromycin) therapy because of treatment-related side effects. Most of the side effects leading to discontinuation were related to the gastrointestinal tract, e.g., nausea, vomiting, diarrhea, or abdominal pain. Rarely but potentially serious side effects were angioedema and cholestatic jaundice.

Clinical:

Multiple-dose regimen:

Overall, the most common side effects in adult patients receiving a multiple-dose regimen of ZITHROMAX® were related to the gastrointestinal system with diarrhea/loose stools (5%), nausea (3%), and abdominal pain (3%) being the most frequently reported.

No other side effects occurred in patients on the multiple-dose regimen of ZITHROMAX® with a frequency greater than 1%. Side effects that occurred with a frequency of 1% or less included the following:

Cardiovascular: Palpitations, chest pain.

Gastrointestinal: Dyspepsia, flatulence, vomiting, melena, and cholestatic jaundice.

Genitourinary: Monilia, vaginitis, and nephritis.

Nervous System: Dizziness, headache, vertigo, and somnolence.

General: Fatigue.

Allergic: Rash, photosensitivity, and angioedema.

Chronic therapy with 1200 mg weekly regimen: The nature of side effects seen with the 1200 mg weekly dosing regimen for the prevention of *Mycobacterium avium* infection in severely immunocompromised HIV-infected patients were similar to those seen with short term dosing regimens. (See CLINICAL TRIALS.)

Single 1-gram dose regimen: Overall, the most common side effects in patients receiving a single-dose regimen of 1 gram of ZITHROMAX® were related to the gastrointestinal system and were more frequently reported than in patients receiving the multiple-dose regimen.

Side effects that occurred in patients on the single one-gram dosing regimen of ZITHROMAX® with a frequency of 1% or greater included diarrhea/loose stools (7%), nausea (5%), abdominal pain (5%), vomiting (2%), dyspepsia (1%), and vaginitis (1%).

Post-Marketing Experience:

Adverse events reported with azithromycin during the post-marketing period in adult and/or pediatric patients for which a causal relationship may not be established include:

Allergic: Arthralgia, edema, urticaria, angioedema.

Cardiovascular: Arrhythmias including ventricular tachycardia.

Gastrointestinal: Anorexia, constipation, dyspepsia, flatulence, vomiting/diarrhea rarely resulting in dehydration, pseudomembranous colitis and rare reports of tongue discoloration.

General: Asthenia, paresthesia and anaphylaxis (rarely fatal).

Genitourinary: Interstitial nephritis and acute renal failure, moniliasis, vaginitis.

Hematopoietic: Thrombocytopenia.

Liver/Biliary: Abnormal liver function including hepatitis and cholestatic jaundice, as well as rare cases of hepatic necrosis and hepatic failure, which have rarely resulted in death.

Nervous System: Convulsions, dizziness/vertigo, headache, somnolence, hyperactivity, nervousness, and agitation.

Psychiatric: Aggressive reaction and anxiety.

Skin/Appendages: Pruritus, rarely serious skin reactions including erythema multiforme, Stevens Johnson Syndrome, and toxic epidermal necrolysis.

Special Senses: Hearing disturbances including hearing loss, deafness, and/or tinnitus, rare reports of taste perversion.

Laboratory Abnormalities:

Significant abnormalities (irrespective of drug relationship) occurring during the clinical trials were reported as follows:

With an incidence of 1–2%, elevated serum creatine phosphokinase, potassium, ALT (SGPT), GGT, and AST (SGOT).

With an incidence of less than 1%, leukopenia, neutropenia, decreased platelet count, elevated serum alkaline phosphatase, bilirubin, BUN, creatinine, blood glucose, LDH, and phosphate.

When follow-up was provided, changes in laboratory tests appeared to be reversible.

In multiple-dose clinical trials involving more than 3000 patients, 3 patients discontinued therapy because of treatment-related liver enzyme abnormalities and 1 because of a renal function abnormality.

In a phase I drug interaction study performed in normal volunteers, 1 of 6 subjects given the combination of azithromycin and rifabutin, 1 of 7 given rifabutin alone and 0 of 6 given azithromycin alone developed a clinically significant neutropenia (<500 cells/mm^3).

Laboratory abnormalities seen in clinical trials for the prevention of disseminated *Mycobacterium avium* disease in severely immunocompromised HIV-infected patients are presented in the CLINICAL TRIALS section.

INCIDENCE OF ONE OR MORE TREATMENT RELATED* ADVERSE EVENTS IN HIV INFECTED PATIENTS RECEIVING PROPHYLAXIS FOR DISSEMINATED MAC OVER APPROXIMATELY 1 YEAR**

	Study 155		Study 174		
	Placebo (N=91)	Azithromycin 1200 mg weekly (N=89)	Azithromycin 1200 mg weekly (N=233)	Rifabutin 300 mg daily (N=236)	Azithromycin + Rifabutin (N=224)
Mean Duration of Therapy (days)	303.8	402.9	315	296.1	344.4
Discontinuation of Therapy	2.3	8.2	13.5	15.9	22.7
Autonomic Nervous System					
Mouth Dry	0	0	0	3.0	2.7
Central Nervous System					
Dizziness	0	1.1	3.9	1.7	0.4
Headache	0	0	3.0	5.5	4.5
Gastrointestinal					
Diarrhea	15.4	52.8	50.2	19.1	50.9
Loose Stools	6.6	19.1	12.9	3.0	9.4
Abdominal Pain	6.6	27	32.2	12.3	31.7
Dyspepsia	1.1	9	4.7	1.7	1.8
Flatulence	4.4	9	10.7	5.1	5.8
Nausea	11	32.6	27.0	16.5	28.1
Vomiting	1.1	6.7	9.0	3.8	5.8
General					
Fever	1.1	0	2.1	4.2	4.9
Fatigue	0	2.2	3.9	2.1	3.1
Malaise	0	1.1	0.4	0	2.2
Musculoskeletal					
Arthralgia	0	0	3.0	4.2	7.1
Psychiatric					
Anorexia	1.1	0	2.1	2.1	3.1
Skin & Appendages					
Pruritus	3.3	0	3.9	3.4	7.6
Rash	3.2	3.4	8.1	9.4	11.1
Skin discoloration	0	0	0	2.1	2.2
Special Senses					
Tinnitus	4.4	3.4	0.9	1.3	0.9
Hearing Decreased	2.2	1.1	0.9	0.4	0
Uveitis	0	0	0.4	1.3	1.8
Taste Perversion	0	0	1.3	2.5	1.3

* Includes those events considered possibly or probably related to study drug

** >2% adverse event rates for any group (except uveitis).

Prophylaxis Against Disseminated MAC Abnormal Laboratory Values*

		Placebo	Azithromycin 1200 mg weekly	Rifabutin 300 mg daily	Azithromycin & Rifabutin
Hemoglobin	<8 g/dl	1/51 2%	4/170 2%	4/114 4%	8/107 8%
Platelet Count	$<50 \times 10^3/mm^3$	1/71 1%	4/260 2%	2/182 1%	6/181 3%
WBC Count	$<1 \times 10^3/mm^3$	0/8 0%	2/70 3%	2/47 4%	0/43 0%
Neutrophils	$<500/mm^3$	0/26 0%	4/106 4%	3/82 4%	2/78 3%
SGOT	>5 × ULN[a]	1/41 2%	8/158 5%	3/121 3%	6/114 5%
SGPT	>5 × ULN	0/49 0%	8/166 5%	3/130 2%	5/117 4%
Alk Phos	>5 × ULN	1/80 1%	4/247 2%	2/172 1%	3/164 2%

[a]=Upper Limit of Normal

*excludes subjects outside of the relevant normal range at baseline

DOSAGE AND ADMINISTRATION
(See INDICATIONS AND USAGE.)

ZITHROMAX® capsules should be given at least 1 hour before or 2 hours after a meal. ZITHROMAX® capsules should not be mixed with or taken with food.

ZITHROMAX® for oral suspension (single dose 1 g packet) can be taken with or without food after constitution. Not for pediatric use. For pediatric suspension, please refer to the INDICATIONS AND USAGE and DOSAGE AND ADMINISTRATION sections of the prescribing information for ZITHROMAX (azithromycin for oral suspension) 100 mg/5 mL and 200 mg/5 mL bottles.

ZITHROMAX® tablets may be taken without regard to food. However, increased tolerability has been observed when tablets are taken with food.

The recommended dose of ZITHROMAX® or the treatment of individuals 16 years of age and older with mild to moderate acute bacterial exacerbations of chronic obstructive pulmonary disease, pneumonia, pharyngitis/tonsillitis (as second line therapy), and uncomplicated skin and skin structure infections due to the indicated organisms is: 500 mg as a single dose on the first day followed by 250 mg once daily on Days 2 through 5 for a total dose of 1.5 grams of ZITHROMAX®.

The recommended dose of ZITHROMAX® for the prevention of disseminated *Mycobacterium avium* complex (MAC) disease is: 1200 mg taken once weekly. This dose of ZITHROMAX® may be combined with the approved dosage regimen of rifabutin.

The recommended dose of ZITHROMAX® for the treatment of non-gonococcal urethritis and cervicitis due to *C. trachomatis* is: a single 1 gram (1000 mg) dose of ZITHROMAX®. This dose can be administered as four 250 mg capsules or as one single dose packet (1 g).

DIRECTIONS FOR ADMINISTRATION OF ZITHROMAX® for oral suspension in the single dose packet (1 g): The entire contents of the packet should be mixed thoroughly with two ounces (approximately 60 mL) of water. Drink the entire contents immediately; add an additional two ounces of water, mix, and drink to assure complete consumption of dosage. **The single dose packet should not be used to administer doses other than 1000 mg of azithromycin. This packet not for pediatric use.**

HOW SUPPLIED

ZITHROMAX® capsules (imprinted with "Pfizer 305") are supplied in red opaque hard-gelatin capsules containing azithromycin dihydrate equivalent to 250 mg of azithromycin. These are packaged in bottles and blister cards of 6 capsules (Z-PAKS™) as follows:

Bottles of 50	NDC 0069-3050-50
Boxes of 3 (Z-PAKS™ of 6)	NDC 0069-3050-34
Unit Dose package of 50	NDC 0069-3050-86

Store capsules below 30°C (86°F).

ZITHROMAX® 600 mg tablets (engraved on front with "PFIZER" and on back with "308") are supplied as white, modified oval-shaped, film-coated tablets containing azithromycin dihydrate equivalent to 600 mg azithromycin. These are packaged in bottles of 30 tablets. ZITHROMAX® tablets are supplied as follows:

Bottles of 30	NDC 0069-3080-30

Tablets should be stored at or below 30°C (86°F).

ZITHROMAX® for oral suspension is supplied in single dose packets containing azithromycin dihydrate equivalent to 1 gram of azithromycin as follows:

Bottles of 10 Single Dose Packets (1 g)	NDC 0069-3051-07
Boxes of 3 Single Dose Packets (1 g)	NDC 0069-3051-75

Store single dose packets between 5° and 30°C (41° and 86°F).

Continued on next page

Zithromax—Cont.

CLINICAL STUDIES IN PATIENTS WITH ADVANCED HIV INFECTION FOR THE PREVENTION OF DISEASE DUE TO DISSEMINATED *MYCOBACTERIUM AVIUM* COMPLEX (MAC)
(See INDICATIONS AND USAGE):

Two randomized, double blind clinical trials were performed in patients with CD4 counts <100 cells/µL. The first study (155) compared azithromycin (1200 mg once weekly) to placebo and enrolled 182 patients with a mean CD4 count of 35 cells/µL. The second study (174) randomized 723 patients to either azithromycin (1200 mg once weekly), rifabutin (300 mg daily) or the combination of both. The mean CD4 count was 51 cells/µL. The primary endpoint in these studies was disseminated MAC disease. Other endpoints included the incidence of clinically significant MAC disease and discontinuations from therapy for drug-related side effects.

MAC bacteremia

In trial 155, 85 patients randomized to receive azithromycin and 89 patients randomized to receive placebo met study entrance criteria. Cumulative incidences at 6, 12 and 18 months of the possible outcomes are in the following table:

[See first table at top of page 2548]

The difference in the one year cumulative incidence rates of disseminated MAC disease (placebo-azithromycin) is 10.9%. This difference is statistically significant (p=0.037) with a 95% confidence interval for this difference of (0.8%, 20.9%). The comparable number of patients experiencing adverse events and the fewer number of patients lost to follow-up on azithromycin should be taken into account when interpreting the significance of this difference.

In trial 174, 223 patients randomized to receive rifabutin, 223 patients randomized to receive azithromycin, and 218 patients randomized to receive both rifabutin and azithromycin met study entrance criteria. Cumulative incidences at 6, 12 and 18 months of the possible outcomes are recorded in the following table:

[See second table at top of page 2548]

Comparing the cumulative one year incidence rates, azithromycin monotherapy is at least as effective as rifabutin monotherapy. The difference (rifabutin-azithromycin) in the one year rates (7.6%) is statistically significant (p=0.022) with an adjusted 95% confidence interval (0.9%, 14.3%). Additionally, azithromycin/rifabutin combination therapy is more effective than rifabutin alone. The difference (rifabutin-azithromycin/rifabutin) in the cumulative one year incidence rates (12.5%) is statistically significant (p<0.001) with an adjusted 95% confidence interval of (6.6%, 18.4%). The comparable number of patients experiencing adverse events and the fewer number of patients lost to follow-up on rifabutin should be taken into account when interpreting the significance of this difference.

In Study 174, sensitivity testing* was performed on all available MAC isolates from subjects randomized to either azithromycin, rifabutin or the combination. The distribution of MIC values for azithromycin from susceptibility testing of the breakthrough isolates was similar between study arms. As the efficacy of azithromycin in the treatment of disseminated MAC has not been established, the clinical relevance of these *in vitro* MICs as an indicator of susceptibility or resistance is not known. (*Methodology per Inderlied CB, et al. Determination of *In Vitro* Susceptibility of *Mycobacterium avium* Complex Isolates to Antimicrobial Agents by Various Methods. Antimicrob. Agents Chemother 1987; 31: 1697–1702.)

Clinically Significant Disseminated MAC Disease

In association with the decreased incidence of bacteremia, patients in the groups randomized to either azithromycin alone or azithromycin in combination with rifabutin showed reductions in the signs and symptoms of disseminated MAC disease, including fever or night sweats, weight loss and anemia.

Discontinuations From Therapy For Drug-Related Side Effects

In Study 155, discontinuations for drug-related toxicity occurred in 8.2% of subjects treated with azithromycin and 2.3% of those given placebo (p=0.121). In Study 174, more subjects discontinued from the combination of azithromycin and rifabutin (22.7%) than from azithromycin alone (13.5%; p=0.026) or rifabutin alone (15.9%; p=0.209).

Safety

As these patients with advanced HIV disease were taking multiple concomitant medications and experienced a variety of intercurrent illnesses, it was often difficult to attribute adverse events to study medication. Overall, the nature of side effects seen on the weekly dosage regimen of azithromycin over a period of approximately one year in patients with advanced HIV disease was similar to that previously reported for shorter course therapies.

[See first table at top of previous page]

Side effects related to the gastrointestinal tract were seen more frequently in patients receiving azithromycin than in those receiving placebo or rifabutin. In study 174, 86% of diarrheal episodes were mild to moderate in nature with discontinuation of therapy for this reason occurring in only 9/233 (3.8%) of patients.

Changes in Laboratory Values

In these immunocompromised patients with advanced HIV infection, it was necessary to assess laboratory abnormalities developing on study with additional criteria if baseline values were outside the relevant normal range.

[See second table at top of previous page]

ANIMAL TOXICOLOGY

Phospholipidosis (intracellular phospholipid binding) has been observed in some tissues of mice, rats, and dogs given multiple doses of azithromycin. It has been demonstrated in numerous organ systems (e.g., eye, dorsal root ganglia, liver, gallbladder, kidney, spleen, and pancreas) in dogs administered doses which, based on pharmacokinetics, are as low as 2 times greater than the recommended adult human dose and in rats at doses comparable to the recommended adult human dose. This effect has been reversible after cessation of azithromycin treatment. The significance of these findings for humans is unknown.

REFERENCES:

1. National Committee for Clinical Laboratory Standards. Methods for Dilution Antimicrobial Susceptibility Tests for Bacteria that Grow Aerobically—Third Edition. Approved Standard NCCLS Document M7–A3, Vol. 13, No. 25, NCCLS, Villanova, PA, December 1993
2. National Committee for Clinical Laboratory Standards. Performance Standards for Antimicrobial Disk Susceptibility Tests—Fifth Edition. Approved Standard NCCLS Document M2–A5, Vol 13, No. 24, NCCLS, Villanova, PA, December 1993.

Rx only

Licensed from Pliva

Pfizer Labs

Division of Pfizer Inc, NY, NY 10017

69-4763-00-3 Revised September 1999

Shown in Product Identification Guide, page 330

ZITHROMAX® ℞

(azithromycin for injection)

For IV infusion only

DESCRIPTION

ZITHROMAX® (azithromycin for injection) contains the active ingredient azithromycin, an azalide, a subclass of macrolide antibiotics, for intravenous injection. Azithromycin has the chemical name (*2R,3S,4R,5R,8R,10R,11R,12S,13S,14R*)-13-[(2,6-dideoxy-3-*C*-methyl-3-*O*-methyl-α-*L*-*ribo*-hexopyranosyl)oxy]-2-ethyl-3,4,10-trihydroxy-3,5,6,8,10,12,14-hepta-methyl-11-[[3,4,6-trideoxy-3-(dimethylamino)-β-*D*-*xylo*-hexopyranosyl]oxy]-1-oxa-6-azacyclopentadecan-15-one. Azithromycin is derived from erythromycin; however, it differs chemically from erythromycin in that a methyl-substituted nitrogen atom is incorporated into the lactone ring. Its molecular formula is $C_{38}H_{72}N_2O_{12}$, and its molecular weight is 749.00. Azithromycin has the following structural formula:

[See chemical structure at top of next column]

Azithromycin, as the dihydrate, is a white crystalline powder with a molecular formula of $C_{38}H_{72}N_2O_{12} \bullet 2H_2O$ and a molecular weight of 785.0.

ZITHROMAX® (azithromycin for injection) consists of azithromycin dihydrate and the following inactive ingredients: citric acid and sodium hydroxide. ZITHROMAX® (azithromycin for injection) is supplied in lyophilized form in a 10-mL vial equivalent to 500 mg of azithromycin for intravenous administration. Reconstitution, according to label directions, results in approximately 5 mL of ZITHROMAX® for intravenous injection with each mL containing azithromycin dihydrate equivalent to 100 mg of azithromycin.

CLINICAL PHARMACOLOGY

In patients hospitalized with community-acquired pneumonia receiving single daily one-hour intravenous infusions for 2 to 5 days of 500 mg azithromycin at a concentration of 2 mg/mL, the mean C_{max} ± S.D. achieved was 3.63 ± 1.60 µg/mL, while the 24-hour trough level was 0.20 ± 0.15 µg/mL, and the AUC_{24} was 9.60 ± 4.80 µg•h/mL.

The mean C_{max}, 24-hour trough and AUC_{24} values were 1.14 ± 0.14 µg/mL, 0.18 ± 0.02 µg/mL, and 8.03 ±0.86 µg•h/mL, respectively, in normal volunteers receiving a 3-hour intravenous infusion of 500 mg azithromycin at a concentration of 1 mg/mL. Similar pharmacokinetic values were obtained in patients hospitalized with community-acquired pneumonia that received the same 3-hour dosage regimen for 2-5 days.

[See table below]

The average CL_t and V_d values were 10.18 mL/min/kg and 33.3 L/kg, respectively, in 18 normal volunteers receiving 1000 to 4000-mg doses given as 1 mg/mL over 2 hours.

Comparison of the plasma pharmacokinetic parameters following the 1st and 5th daily doses of 500 mg intravenous azithromycin showed only an 8% increase in C_{max} but a 61% increase in AUC_{24} reflecting a threefold rise in C_{24} trough levels.

Following single oral doses of 500 mg azithromycin to 12 healthy volunteers, C_{max}, trough level, and AUC_{24} were reported to be 0.41 µg/mL, 0.05 µg/mL, and 2.6 µg•h/mL, respectively. These oral values are approximately 38%, 83%, and 52% of the values observed following a single 500-mg I.V. 3-hour infusion (C_{max}: 1.08 µg/mL, trough: 0.06 µg/mL, and AUC^{24}: 5.0 µg•h/mL). Thus, plasma concentrations are higher following the intravenous regimen throughout the 24-hour interval. The pharmacokinetic parameters on day 5 of azithromycin 250-mg capsules following a 500-mg oral loading dose to healthy young adults (age 18-40 years old) were as follows: C_{max}: 0.24 µg/mL, AUC_{24}: 2.1 µg•h/mL. Tissue levels have not been obtained following intravenous infusions of azithromycin. Selected tissue (or fluid) concentration and tissue (or fluid) to plasma/serum concentration ratios following oral administration of azithromycin are shown in the following table:

[See table at top of next page]

Tissue levels were determined following a single oral dose of 500 mg azithromycin in 7 gynecological patients. Approximately 17 hours after dosing, azithromycin concentrations were 2.7 µg/g in ovarian tissue, 3.5 µg/g in uterine tissue, and 3.3 µg/g in salpinx. Tissue levels have not been obtained following intravenous infusion of azithromycin.

In a multiple-dose study in 12 normal volunteers utilizing a 500-mg (1 mg/mL) one-hour intravenous-dosage regimen for five days, the amount of administered azithromycin dose excreted in urine in 24 hours was about 11% after the 1st dose and 14% after the 5th dose. These values are greater than the reported 6% excreted unchanged in urine after oral administration of azithromycin. Biliary excretion is a major route of elimination for unchanged drug, following oral administration.

The serum protein binding of azithromycin is variable in the concentration range approximating human exposure decreasing from 51% at 0.02 µg/mL to 7% at 2 µg/mL.

Microbiology: Azithromycin acts by binding to the 50S ribosomal subunit of susceptible microorganisms and, thus, interfering with microbial protein synthesis. Nucleic acid synthesis is not affected.

Azithromycin concentrates in phagocytes and fibroblasts as demonstrated by *in vitro* incubation techniques. Using such methodology, the ratio of intracellular to extracellular concentration was >30 after one hour incubation. *In vivo* studies suggest that concentration in phagocytes may contribute to drug distribution to inflamed tissues.

Azithromycin has been shown to be active against most strains of the following microorganisms, both *in vitro* and in clinical infections as described in the **INDICATIONS AND USAGE** section of the package insert for ZITHROMAX® (azithromycin for injection).

Aerobic gram-positive microorganisms

Staphylococcus aureus
Streptococcus pneumoniae

NOTE: Azithromycin demonstrates cross-resistance with erythromycin-resistant gram-positive strains. Most strains of *Enterococcus faecalis* and methicillin-resistant staphylococci are resistant to azithromycin.

Aerobic gram-negative microorganisms

Haemophilus influenzae
Moraxella catarrhalis
Neisseria gonorrhoeae

"Other" microorganisms

Chlamydia pneumoniae
Chlamydia trachomatis
Legionella pneumophila
Mycoplasma hominis
Mycoplasma pneumoniae

Beta-lactamase production should have no effect on azithromycin activity.

Plasma concentrations (µg/mL ± S.D.) after the last daily intravenous infusion of 500 mg azithromycin

Infusion Concentration, Duration	Time after starting the infusion (hr)								
	0.5	1	2	3	4	6	8	12	24
2 mg/mL, 1 hr[a]	2.98 ±1.12	3.63 ±1.73	0.60 ±0.31	0.40 ±0.23	0.33 ±0.16	0.26 ±0.14	0.27 ±0.15	0.20 ±0.12	0.20 ±0.15
1 mg/mL, 3 hr[b]	0.91 ±0.13	1.02 ±0.11	1.14 ±0.13	1.13 ±0.16	0.32 ±0.05	0.28 ±0.04	0.27 ±0.03	0.22 ±0.02	0.18 ±0.02

a= 500 mg (2 mg/mL) for 2–5 days in Community-acquired pneumonia patients.
b= 500 mg (1 mg/mL) for 5 days in healthy subjects.

Azithromycin has been shown to be active against most strains of the following microorganisms, both *in vitro* and in clinical infections as described in the **INDICATIONS AND USAGE** section of the package insert for ZITHROMAX® (azithromycin tablets) and ZITHROMAX® (azithromycin for oral suspension).

Aerobic gram-positive microorganisms
Staphylococcus aureus
Streptococcus agalactiae
Streptococcus pneumoniae
Streptococcus pyogenes

Aerobic gram-negative microorganisms
Haemophilus ducreyi
Haemophilus influenzae
Moraxella catarrhalis
Neisseria gonorrhoeae

"Other" microorganisms
Chlamydia pneumoniae
Chlamydia trachomatis
Mycoplasma pneumoniae

The following *in vitro* data are available, **but their clinical significance is unknown.**

Azithromycin exhibits *in vitro* minimum inhibitory concentrations (MIC's) of 0.5 μg/mL or less against most (≥90%) strains of streptococci listed below and MIC's of 2.0 μg/mL or less against most (≥90%) strains of other listed microorganisms. However, the safety and effectiveness of azithromycin in treating clinical infections due to these microorganisms have not been established in adequate and well-controlled clinical trials.

Aerobic gram-positive microorganisms
Streptococci (Groups C, F, G)
Viridans group streptococci

Aerobic gram-negative microorganisms
Bordetella pertussis

Anaerobic microorganisms
Peptostreptococcus species
Prevotella bivia

"Other" microorganisms
Ureaplasma urealyticum

Susceptibility Tests

Azithromycin can be solubilized for *in vitro* susceptibility testing using dilution techniques by dissolving in a minimum amount of 95% ethanol and diluting to the working stock concentration with broth.

Dilution Techniques:

Quantitative methods are used to determine antimicrobial minimum inhibitory concentrations (MIC's). These MIC's provide estimates of the susceptibility of bacteria to antimicrobial compounds. The MIC's should be determined using a standardized procedure. Standardized procedures are based on a dilution method[1] (broth or agar) or equivalent with standardized inoculum concentrations and standardized concentrations of azithromycin powder. The MIC values should be interpreted according to the following criteria:

For testing aerobic microorganisms other than *Haemophilus* species, *Neisseria gonorrhoeae,* and streptococci:

MIC (μg/mL)	Interpretation
≤ 2	Susceptible (S)
4	Intermediate (I)
≥ 8	Resistant (R)

For testing *Haemophilus* species:[a]

MIC (μg/mL)	Interpretation
≤ 4	Susceptible (S)

[a] This interpretive standard is applicable only to broth microdilution susceptibility testing with *Haemophilus* species using *Haemophilus* Test Medium (HTM)[1].

The current absence of data on resistant strains precludes defining any categories other than "Susceptible". Strains yielding MIC results suggestive of a "nonsusceptible" category should be submitted to a reference laboratory for further testing.

For testing streptococci including *S. pneumoniae:*[b]

MIC (μg/mL)	Interpretation
≤ 0.5	Susceptible (S)
1	Intermediate (I)
≥ 2	Resistant (R)

[b] These interpretive standards are applicable only to broth microdilution susceptibility tests using cation-adjusted Mueller-Hinton broth with 2–5% lysed horse blood.[1]

No interpretive criteria have been established for testing *Neisseria gonorrhoeae*. This species is not usually tested.

A report of "Susceptible" indicates that the pathogen is likely to respond to monotherapy with azithromycin. A report of "Intermediate" indicates that the result should be considered equivocal, and, if the microorganism is not fully susceptible to alternative, clinically feasible drugs, the test should be repeated. This category implies possible clinical applicability in body sites where the drug is physiologically concentrated or in situations where high dosage of drug can be used. This category also provides a buffer zone which prevents small uncontrolled technical factors from causing major discrepancies in interpretation. A report of "Resistant" indicates that achievable drug concentrations are unlikely to be inhibitory; other therapy should be selected.

Standardized susceptibility test procedures require the use of laboratory control microorganisms to control the technical aspects of the laboratory procedures. Standard azithromycin powder should provide the following MIC values:

AZITHROMYCIN CONCENTRATIONS FOLLOWING
TWO – 250 mg (500 mg) CAPSULES IN ADULTS

TISSUE OR FLUID	TIME AFTER DOSE (h)	TISSUE OR FLUID CONCENTRATION (μg/g or μg/mL)[1]	CORRESPONDING PLASMA OR SERUM LEVEL (μg/mL)	TISSUE (FLUID) PLASMA (SERUM) RATIO[1]
SKIN	72–96	0.4	0.012	35
LUNG	72–96	4.0	0.012	>100
SPUTUM*	2–4	1.0	0.64	2
SPUTUM**	10–12	2.9	0.1	30
TONSIL***	9–18	4.5	0.03	>100
TONSIL***	180	0.9	0.006	>100
CERVIX****	19	2.8	0.04	70

[1]High tissue concentrations should not be interpreted to be quantitatively related to clinical efficacy. The antimicrobial activity of azithromycin is pH related. Azithromycin is concentrated in cell lysosomes which have a low intraorganelle pH, at which the drug's activity is reduced. However, the extensive distribution of drug to tissues may be relevant to clinical activity.

* Sample was obtained 2–4 hours after the first dose.
** Sample was obtained 10–12 hours after the first dose.
*** Dosing regimen of 2 doses of 250 mg each, separated by 12 hours.
**** Sample was obtained 19 hours after a single 500 mg dose.

Microorganism	MIC (μg/mL)
Haemophilus influenzae ATCC 49247[a]	1.0–4.0
Staphylococcus aureus ATCC 29213	0.5–2.0
Streptococcus pneumoniae ATCC 49619[b]	0.06–0.25

[a] This quality control range is applicable to only *H. influenzae* ATCC 49247 tested by a broth microdilution procedure using *Haemophilus* Test Medium (HTM)[1].

[b] This quality control range is applicable to only *S. pneumoniae* ATCC 49619 tested by a broth microdilution procedure using cation-adjusted Mueller-Hinton broth with 2–5% lysed horse blood.[1]

Diffusion Techniques:

Quantitative methods that require measurement of zone diameters also provide reproducible estimates of the susceptibility of bacteria to antimicrobial compounds. One such standardized procedure[2] requires the use of standardized inoculum concentrations. This procedure uses paper disks impregnated with 15-μg azithromycin to test the susceptibility of microorganisms to azithromycin.

Reports from the laboratory providing results of the standard single-disk susceptibility test with a 15-μg azithromycin disk should be interpreted according to the following criteria:

For testing aerobic microorganisms (including streptococci)[a] except *Haemophilus* species and *Neisseria gonorrhoeae:*

Zone Diameter (mm)	Interpretation
≥ 18	Susceptible (S)
14–17	Intermediate (I)
≤ 13	Resistant (R)

[a] These zone diameter standards for streptococci apply only to tests performed using Mueller-Hinton agar supplemented with 5% sheep blood and incubated in 5% CO_2[2].

For testing *Haemophilus* species:[b]

Zone Diameter (mm)	Interpretation
≥ 12	Susceptible (S)

[b] This zone diameter standard is applicable only to tests with *Haemophilus* species using *Haemophilus* Test Medium (HTM)[2].

The current absence of data on resistant strains precludes defining any categories other than "Susceptible". Strains yielding zone diameter results suggestive of a "nonsusceptible" category should be submitted to a reference laboratory for further testing.

No interpretive criteria have been established for testing *Neisseria gonorrhoeae*. This species is not usually tested.

Interpretation should be as stated above for results using dilution techniques. Interpretation involves correlation of the diameter obtained in the disk test with the MIC for azithromycin.

As with standardized dilution techniques, diffusion methods require the use of laboratory control microorganisms that are used to control the technical aspects of the laboratory procedures. For the diffusion technique, the 15-μg azithromycin disk should provide the following zone diameters in these laboratory test quality control strains:

Microorganism	Zone Diameter (mm)
Haemophilus influenzae ATCC 49247[a]	13–21
Staphylococcus aureus ATCC 25923	21–26
Streptococcus pneumoniae ATCC 49619[b]	19–25

[a] These quality control limits are applicable only to tests conducted with *H. influenzae* ATCC 49247 using *Haemophilus* Test Medium (HTM)[2].

[b] These quality control limits are applicable only to tests conducted with *S. pneumoniae* ATCC 49619 using Mueller-Hinton agar supplemented with 5% sheep blood incubated in 5% CO_2[2].

INDICATIONS AND USAGE

ZITHROMAX® (azithromycin for injection) is indicated for the treatment of patients with infections caused by susceptible strains of the designated microorganisms in the conditions listed below. As recommended dosages, durations of therapy, and applicable patient populations vary among these infections, please see **DOSAGE AND ADMINISTRATION** for dosing recommendations.

Community-acquired pneumonia due to *Chlamydia pneumoniae, Haemophilus influenzae, Legionella pneumophila, Moraxella catarrhalis, Mycoplasma pneumoniae, Staphylococcus aureus,* or *Streptococcus pneumoniae* in patients who require initial intravenous therapy.

Pelvic inflammatory disease due to *Chlamydia trachomatis, Neisseria gonorrhoeae,* or *Mycoplasma hominis* in patients who require initial intravenous therapy. If anaerobic microorganisms are suspected of contributing to the infection, an antimicrobial agent with anaerobic activity should be administered in combination with ZITHROMAX®.

ZITHROMAX® (azithromycin for injection) should be followed by ZITHROMAX® by the oral route as required. (See **DOSAGE AND ADMINISTRATION.**)

Appropriate culture and susceptibility tests should be performed before treatment to determine the causative microorganism and its susceptibility to azithromycin. Therapy with ZITHROMAX® may be initiated before results of these tests are known; once the results become available, antimicrobial therapy should be adjusted accordingly.

CONTRAINDICATIONS

ZITHROMAX® is contraindicated in patients with known hypersensitivity to azithromycin, erythromycin, or any macrolide antibiotic.

WARNINGS

Serious allergic reactions, including angioedema, anaphylaxis, and dermatologic reactions including Stevens Johnson Syndrome and toxic epidermal necrolysis have been reported rarely in patients on azithromycin therapy. Although rare, fatalities have been reported. (See **CONTRAINDICATIONS.**) Despite initially successful symptomatic treatment of the allergic symptoms, when symptomatic therapy was discontinued, the allergic symptoms **recurred soon thereafter in some patients without further azithromycin exposure**. These patients required prolonged periods of observation and symptomatic treatment. The relationship of these episodes to the long tissue half-life of azithromycin and subsequent prolonged exposure to antigen is unknown at present.

If an allergic reaction occurs, the drug should be discontinued and appropriate therapy should be instituted. Physicians should be aware that reappearance of the allergic symptoms may occur when symptomatic therapy is discontinued.

Pseudomembranous colitis has been reported with nearly all antibacterial agents and may range in severity from mild to life-threatening. Therefore, it is important to consider this diagnosis in patients who present with diarrhea subsequent to the administration of antibacterial agents.

Treatment with antibacterial agents alters the normal flora of the colon and may permit overgrowth of clostridia. Studies indicate that a toxin produced by *Clostridium difficile* is a primary cause of "antibiotic-associated colitis."

After the diagnosis of pseudomembranous colitis has been established, therapeutic measures should be initiated. Mild cases of pseudomembranous colitis usually respond to discontinuation of the drug alone. In moderate to severe cases,

Continued on next page

Zithromax—Cont.

consideration should be given to management with fluids and electrolytes, protein supplementation, and treatment with an antibacterial drug clinically effective against *Clostridium difficile* colitis.

PRECAUTIONS

General: Because azithromycin is principally eliminated via the liver, caution should be exercised when azithromycin is administered to patients with impaired hepatic function. There are no data regarding azithromycin usage in patients with renal impairment; therefore, caution should be exercised when prescribing azithromycin in these patients.

ZITHROMAX® (azithromycin for injection) should be reconstituted and diluted as directed and administered as an intravenous infusion over not less than 60 minutes. (See **DOSAGE AND ADMINISTRATION**.)

Local I.V. site reactions have been reported with the intravenous administration of azithromycin. The incidence and severity of these reactions were the same when 500 mg azithromycin were given over 1 hour (2 mg/mL as 250 mL infusion) or over 3 hours (1 mg/mL as 500 mL infusion). (See **ADVERSE REACTIONS**.) All volunteers who received infusate concentrations above 2.0 mg/mL experienced local I.V. site reactions and, therefore, higher concentrations should be avoided.

The following adverse events have not been reported in clinical trials with azithromycin; however, they have been reported with macrolide products: ventricular arrhythmias, including ventricular tachycardia, and *torsades de pointes*, in individuals with prolonged QT intervals. There has been a spontaneous report from the post-marketing experience of a patient with previous history of arrhythmias who experienced *torsades de pointes* and subsequent myocardial infarction following a course of oral azithromycin therapy.

Information for Patients:

Patients should be cautioned not to take aluminum- and magnesium-containing antacids and azithromycin by the oral route simultaneously.

Patients should be directed to discontinue azithromycin and contact a physician if any signs of an allergic reaction occur.

Drug Interactions: Aluminum- and magnesium-containing antacids reduce the peak serum levels (rate) but not the AUC (extent) of orally administered azithromycin.

Administration of cimetidine (800 mg) two hours prior to orally administered azithromycin had no effect on azithromycin absorption.

Azithromycin given by the oral route did not affect the plasma levels or pharmacokinetics of theophylline administered as a single intravenous dose. The effect of azithromycin on the plasma levels or pharmacokinetics of theophylline administered in multiple doses resulting in therapeutic steady-state levels of theophylline is not known. However, concurrent use of macrolides and theophylline has been associated with increases in the serum concentrations of theophylline. Therefore, until further data are available, prudent medical practice dictates careful monitoring of plasma theophylline levels in patients receiving azithromycin and theophylline concomitantly.

Azithromycin given by the oral route did not affect the prothrombin time response to a single dose of warfarin. However, prudent medical practice dictates careful monitoring of prothrombin time in all patients treated with azithromycin and warfarin concomitantly. Concurrent use of macrolides and warfarin in clinical practice has been associated with increased anticoagulant effects.

The following drug interactions have not been reported in clinical trials with azithromycin; however, no specific drug interaction studies have been performed to evaluate potential drug-drug interaction. Nonetheless, they have been observed with macrolide products. Until further data are developed regarding drug interactions when azithromycin and these drugs are used concomitantly, careful monitoring of patients is advised:

Digoxin—elevated digoxin levels.

Ergotamine or dihydroergotamine—acute ergot toxicity characterized by severe peripheral vasospasm and dysesthesia.

Triazolam—Increased pharmacologic effect of triazolam by decreasing the clearance of triazolam.

Drugs metabolized by the cytochrome P^{450} system—elevations of serum carbamazepine, terfenadine, cyclosporine, hexobarbital, and phenytoin levels.

Laboratory Test Interactions: There are no reported laboratory test interactions.

Carcinogenesis, Mutagenesis, Impairment of Fertility: Long-term studies in animals have not been performed to evaluate carcinogenic potential. Azithromycin has shown no mutagenic potential in standard laboratory tests: mouse lymphoma assay, human lymphocyte clastogenic assay, and mouse bone marrow clastogenic assay. No evidence of impaired fertility due to azithromycin was found.

Pregnancy: Teratogenic Effects. Pregnancy Category B: Reproduction studies have been performed in rats and mice at doses up to moderately maternally toxic dose levels (i.e., 200 mg/kg/day by the oral route). These doses, based on a mg/m^2 basis, are estimated to be 4 and 2 times, respectively, the human daily dose of 500 mg by the oral route. In the animal studies, no evidence of harm to the fetus due to azithromycin was found. There are, however, no adequate and well-controlled studies in pregnant women. Because animal reproduction studies are not always predictive of human response, azithromycin should be used during pregnancy only if clearly needed.

Nursing Mothers: It is not known whether azithromycin is excreted in human milk. Because many drugs are excreted in human milk, caution should be exercised when azithromycin is administered to a nursing woman.

Pediatric Use: Safety and effectiveness of azithromycin for injection in children or adolescents under 16 years have not been established. In controlled clinical studies, azithromycin has been administered to pediatric patients (age 6 months to 16 years) by the oral route. For information regarding the use of ZITHROMAX® (azithromycin for oral suspension) in the treatment of pediatric patients, refer to the **INDICATIONS AND USAGE** and **DOSAGE AND ADMINISTRATION** sections of the prescribing information for ZITHROMAX® (azithromycin for oral suspension) 100 mg/5 mL and 200 mg/5 mL bottles.

Geriatric Use: Pharmacokinetic studies with intravenous azithromycin have not been performed in older volunteers. Pharmacokinetics of azithromycin following oral administration in older volunteers (65–85 years old) were similar to those in younger volunteers (18–40 years old) for the 5-day therapeutic regimen.

ADVERSE REACTIONS

In clinical trials of intravenous azithromycin for community-acquired pneumonia, in which 2–5 I.V. doses were given, most of the reported side effects were mild to moderate in severity and were reversible upon discontinuation of the drug. The majority of patients in these trials had one or more comorbid diseases and were receiving concomitant medications. Approximately 1.2% of the patients discontinued intravenous ZITHROMAX® therapy, and a total of 2.4% discontinued azithromycin therapy by either the intravenous or oral route because of clinical or laboratory side effects.

In clinical trials conducted in patients with pelvic inflammatory disease, in which 1-2 I.V. doses were given, 2% of women who received monotherapy with azithromycin and 4% who received azithromycin plus metronidazole discontinued therapy due to clinical side effects.

Clinical side effects leading to discontinuations from these studies were most commonly gastrointestinal (abdominal pain, nausea, vomiting, diarrhea), and rashes; laboratory side effects leading to discontinuation were increases in transaminase levels and/or alkaline phosphatase levels.

Clinical:

Overall, the most common side effects associated with treatment in adult patients who received I.V./P.O. ZITHROMAX® in studies of community-acquired pneumonia were related to the gastrointestinal system with diarrhea/loose stools (4.3%), nausea (3.9%), abdominal pain (2.7%), and vomiting (1.4%) being the most frequently reported. Approximately 12% of patients experienced a side effect related to the intravenous infusion; most common were pain at the injection site (6.5%) and local inflammation (3.1%).

The most common side effects associated with treatment in adult women who received I.V./P.O. ZITHROMAX® in studies of pelvic inflammatory disease were related to the gastrointestinal system. Diarrhea (8.5%) and nausea (6.6%) were most commonly reported, followed by vaginitis (2.8%), abdominal pain (1.9%), anorexia (1.9%), rash and pruritus (1.9%). When azithromycin was co-administered with metronidazole in these studies, a higher proportion of women experienced side effects of nausea (10.3%), abdominal pain (3.7%), vomiting (2.8%), application site reaction, stomatitis, dizziness, or dyspnea (all at 1.9%).

No other side effects occurred in patients on the multiple dose I.V./P.O. regimen of ZITHROMAX® in these studies with a frequency greater than 1%.

Side effects that occurred with a frequency of 1% or less including the following:

Gastrointestinal: dyspepsia, flatulence, mucositis, oral moniliasis, and gastritis

Nervous System: headache, somnolence

Allergic: bronchospasm

Special Senses: taste perversion

Post-Marketing Experience:

Adverse events reported with orally administered azithromycin during the post-marketing period in adult and/or pediatric patients for which a causal relationship could not be established include:

Allergic: arthralgia, edema, urticaria, angioedema

Cardiovascular: arrhythmias, including ventricular tachycardia

Gastrointestinal: anorexia, constipation, dyspepsia, flatulence, vomiting/diarrhea rarely resulting in dehydration, pseudomembranous colitis and rare reports of tongue discoloration

General: asthenia, paresthesia and anaphylaxis (rarely fatal)

Genitourinary: interstitial nephritis and acute renal failure, moniliasis, vaginitis

Hematopoietic: thrombocytopenia

Liver/Biliary: abnormal liver function including hepatitis and cholestatic jaundice, as well as rare cases of hepatic necrosis and hepatic failure, which have rarely resulted in death

Nervous System: convulsions, dizziness/vertigo, headache, somnolence, hyperactivity, nervousness, and agitation

Psychiatric: aggressive reaction and anxiety

Skin/Appendages: pruritus, rarely serious skin reactions including erythema multiforme, Stevens Johnson Syndrome, and toxic epidermal necrolysis

Special Senses: hearing disturbances including hearing loss, deafness, and/or tinnitus, rare reports of taste perversion

Laboratory Abnormalities:

Significant abnormalities (irrespective of drug relationship) occurring during the clinical trials were reported as follows: with an incidence of 4–6%, elevated ALT (SGPT), AST (SGOT), creatinine with an incidence of 1–3%, elevated LDH, bilirubin with an incidence of less than 1%, leukopenia, neutropenia, decreased platelet count, and elevated serum alkaline phosphatase

When follow-up was provided, changes in laboratory tests appeared to be reversible.

In multiple-dose clinical trials involving more than 750 patients treated with ZITHROMAX® (I.V./P.O.), less than 2% of patients discontinued azithromycin therapy because of treatment-related liver enzyme abnormalities.

DOSAGE AND ADMINISTRATION

(See INDICATIONS AND USAGE and CLINICAL PHARMACOLOGY.)

The recommended dose of ZITHROMAX® (azithromycin for injection) for the treatment of adult patients with community-acquired pneumonia due to the indicated organisms is: 500 mg as a single daily dose by the intravenous route for at least two days. Intravenous therapy should be followed by azithromycin by the oral route at a single, daily dose of 500 mg, administered as two 250-mg tablets to complete a 7- to 10-day course of therapy. The timing of the switch to oral therapy should be done at the discretion of the physician and in accordance with clinical response.

The recommended dose of ZITHROMAX® (azithromycin) for the treatment of adult patients with pelvic inflammatory disease due to the indicated organisms is: 500 mg as a single daily dose by the intravenous route for one or two days. Intravenous therapy should be followed by azithromycin by the oral route at a single, daily dose of 250 mg to complete a 7-day course of therapy. The timing of the switch to oral therapy should be done at the discretion of the physician and in accordance with clinical response. If anaerobic microorganisms are suspected of contributing to the infection, an antimicrobial agent with anaerobic activity should be administered in combination with ZITHROMAX®.

The infusate concentration and rate of infusion for ZITHROMAX® (azithromycin for injection) should be either 1 mg/mL over 3 hours or 2 mg/mL over 1 hour.

Preparation of the solution for intravenous administration is as follows:

Reconstitution

Prepare the initial solution of ZITHROMAX® (azithromycin for injection) by adding 4.8 mL of Sterile Water For Injection to the 500 mg vial and shaking the vial until all of the drug is dissolved. Since ZITHROMAX® (azithromycin for injection) is supplied under vacuum, it is recommended that a standard 5 mL (non-automated) syringe be used to ensure that the exact amount of 4.8 mL of Sterile Water is dispensed. Each mL of reconstituted solution contains 100 mg azithromycin. Reconstituted solution is stable for 24 hours when stored below 30°C or 86°F.

Parenteral drug products should be inspected visually for particulate matter prior to administration. If particulate matter is evident in reconstituted fluids, the drug solution should be discarded.

Dilute this solution further prior to administration as instructed below.

Dilution

To provide azithromycin over a concentration range of 1.0-2.0 mg/mL, transfer 5 mL of the 100 mg/mL azithromycin solution into the appropriate amount of any of the diluents listed below:

Normal Saline (0.9% sodium chloride)
1/2 Normal Saline (0.45% sodium chloride)
5% Dextrose in Water
Lactated Ringer's Solution
5% Dextrose in 1/2 Normal Saline (0.45% sodium chloride) with 20 mEq KCl
5% Dextrose in Lactated Ringer's Solution
5% Dextrose in 1/3 Normal Saline (0.3% sodium chloride)
5% Dextrose in 1/2 Normal Saline (0.45% sodium chloride)
Normosol®-M in 5% Dextrose
Normosol®-R in 5% Dextrose

Final Infusion Solution Concentration (mg/mL)	Amount of Diluent (mL)
1.0 mg/mL	500 mL
2.0 mg/mL	250 mL

It is recommended that a 500-mg dose of ZITHROMAX® (azithromycin for injection), diluted as above, be infused over a period of not less than 60 minutes.

ZITHROMAX® (azithromycin for injection) should not be given as a bolus or as an intramuscular injection.

Storage

When diluted according to the instructions (1.0 mg/mL to 2.0 mg/mL), ZITHROMAX® (azithromycin for injection) is stable for 24 hours at or below room temperature (30°C or 86°F), or for 7 days if stored under refrigeration (5°C or 41°F).

HOW SUPPLIED

ZITHROMAX® (azithromycin for injection) is supplied in lyophilized form under a vacuum in a 10-mL vial equivalent to 500 mg of azithromycin for intravenous administration. Each vial also contains sodium hydroxide and 413.6 mg citric acid.

Evidence of Infection	Total	Cure	Improved	Cure + Improved
Mycoplasma pneumoniae	18	11 (61%)	5 (28%)	16 (89%)
Chlamydia pneumoniae	34	15 (44%)	13 (38%)	28 (82%)
Legionella pneumophila	16	5 (31%)	8 (50%)	13 (81%)

These are packaged as follows:
10 vials of 500 mg NDC 0069-3150-83

CLINICAL STUDIES

Community-Acquired Pneumonia

In a controlled study of community-acquired pneumonia performed in the U.S., azithromycin (500 mg as a single daily dose by the intravenous route for 2–5 days, followed by 500 mg/day by the oral route to complete 7–10 days therapy) was compared to cefuroxime (2250 mg/day in three divided doses by the intravenous route for 2–5 days followed by 1000 mg/day in two divided doses by the oral route to complete 7–10 days therapy), with or without erythromycin. For the 291 patients who were evaluable for clinical efficacy, the clinical outcome rates, i.e., cure, improved, and success (cure + improved) among the 277 patients seen at 10–14 days post-therapy were as follows:

Clinical Outcome	Azithromycin	Comparator
Cure	46%	44%
Improved	32%	30%
Success (Cure + Improved)	78%	74%

In a separate, uncontrolled clinical and microbiological trial performed in the U.S., 94 patients with community-acquired pneumonia who received azithromycin in the same regimen were evaluable for clinical efficacy. The clinical outcome rates, i.e., cure, improved, and success (cure + improved) among the 84 patients seen at 10–14 days post-therapy were as follows:

Clinical Outcome	Azithromycin
Cure	60%
Improved	29%
Success (Cure + Improved)	89%

Microbiological determinations in both trials were made at the pre-treatment visit and, where applicable, were reassessed at later visits. Serological testing was done on baseline and final visit specimens. The following combined presumptive bacteriological eradication rates were obtained from the evaluable groups:

Combined Bacteriological Eradication Rates for Azithromycin:

(at last completed visit)	Azithromycin
S. pneumoniae	64/67 (96%)[a]
H. influenzae	41/43 (95%)
M. catarrhalis	9/10
S. aureus	9/10

[a] Nineteen of twenty-four patients (79%) with positive blood cultures for *S. pneumoniae* were cured (intent to treat analysis) with eradication of the pathogen.

The presumed bacteriological outcomes at 10–14 days post-therapy for patients treated with azithromycin with evidence (serology and/or culture) of atypical pathogens for both trials were as follows:
[See table above]

ANIMAL TOXICOLOGY

Phospholipidosis (intracellular phospholipid accumulation) has been observed in some tissues of mice, rats, and dogs given multiple doses of azithromycin. It has been demonstrated in numerous organ systems (e.g., eye, dorsal root ganglia, liver, gallbladder, kidney, spleen, and pancreas) in dogs treated with azithromycin at doses which, expressed on a mg/kg basis, are only 2 times greater than the recommended adult human dose and in rats at doses comparable to the recommended adult human dose. This effect has been reversible after cessation of azithromycin treatment. Phospholipidosis has been observed to a similar extent in the tissues of neonatal rats and dogs given daily doses of azithromycin ranging from 10 days to 30 days. Based on the pharmacokinetic data, phospholipidosis has been seen in the rat (30 mg/kg dose) at observed C_{max} value of 1.3 µg/mL (6 times greater than the observed C_{max} of 0.216 µg/mL at the pediatric dose of 10 mg/kg). Similarly, it has been shown in the dog (10 mg/kg dose) at observed C_{max} value of 1.5 µg/mL (7 times greater than the observed same C_{max} and drug dose in the studied pediatric population). On mg/m^2 basis, 30 mg/kg dose in the rat (135 mg/m^2) and 10 mg/kg dose in the dog (79 mg/m^2) are approximately 0.4 and 0.6 times, respectively, the recommended dose in the pediatric patients with an average body weight of 25 kg. This effect, similar to that seen in the adult animals, is reversible after cessation of azithromycin treatment. The significance of these findings for animals and for humans is unknown.

REFERENCES:

1. National Committee for Clinical Laboratory Standards. Methods for Dilution Antimicrobial Susceptibility Tests for Bacteria that Grow Aerobically—Third Edition. Approved Standard NCCLS Document M7-A3, Vol. 13, No. 25, NCCLS, Villanova, PA, December, 1993.
2. National Committee for Clinical Laboratory Standards. Performance Standards for Antimicrobial Disk Susceptibility Tests—Fifth Edition. Approved Standard NCCLS Document M2-A5, Vol. 13, No. 24, NCCLS, Villanova, PA, December, 1993.

Rx only

Licensed from Pliva

Pfizer Labs
Division of Pfizer Inc
NY, NY 10017
70-5191-00-3

Revised September 1999

Shown in Product Identification Guide, page 331

ZOLOFT® ℞

(sertraline hydrochloride)
Tablets and Oral Concentrate

DESCRIPTION

ZOLOFT® (sertraline hydrochloride) is a selective serotonin reuptake inhibitor (SSRI) for oral administration. It is chemically unrelated to other SSRIs, tricyclic, tetracyclic, or other available antidepressant agents. It has a molecular weight of 342.7. Sertraline hydrochloride has the following chemical name: (1S-cis)-4-(3,4-dichlorophenyl)-1,2,3,4-tetrahydro-N-methyl-1-naphthalenamine hydrochloride. The empirical formula $C_{17}H_{17}NCl_2 \bullet HCl$ is represented by the following structural formula:

NHCH$_3$•HCl
Cl
Cl

Sertraline hydrochloride is a white crystalline powder that is slightly soluble in water and isopropyl alcohol, and sparingly soluble in ethanol.

ZOLOFT is supplied for oral administration as scored tablets containing sertraline hydrochloride equivalent to 25, 50 and 100 mg of sertraline and the following inactive ingredients: dibasic calcium phosphate dihydrate, D & C Yellow #10 aluminum lake (in 25 mg tablet), FD & C Blue #1 aluminum lake (in 25 mg tablet), FD & C Red #40 aluminum lake (in 25 mg tablet), FD & C Blue #2 aluminum lake (in 50 mg tablet), hydroxypropyl cellulose, hydroxypropyl methylcellulose, magnesium stearate, microcrystalline cellulose, polyethylene glycol, polysorbate 80, sodium starch glycolate, synthetic yellow iron oxide (in 100 mg tablet), and titanium dioxide.

ZOLOFT oral concentrate is available in a multidose 60 mL bottle. Each mL of solution contains sertraline hydrochloride equivalent to 20 mg of sertraline. The solution contains the following inactive ingredients: glycerin, alcohol (12%), menthol, butylated hydroxytoluene (BHT). The oral concentrate must be diluted prior to administration (see PRECAUTIONS, Information for Patients and DOSAGE AND ADMINISTRATION).

CLINICAL PHARMACOLOGY

Pharmacodynamics

The mechanism of action of sertraline is presumed to be linked to its inhibition of CNS neuronal uptake of serotonin (5HT). Studies at clinically relevant doses in man have demonstrated that sertraline blocks the uptake of serotonin into human platelets. *In vitro* studies in animals also suggest that sertraline is a potent and selective inhibitor of neuronal serotonin reuptake and has only very weak effects on norepinephrine and dopamine neuronal reuptake. *In vitro* studies have shown that sertraline has no significant affinity for adrenergic (alpha$_1$, alpha$_2$, beta), cholinergic, GABA, dopaminergic, histaminergic, serotonergic ($5HT_{1A}$, $5HT_{1B}$, $5HT_2$), or benzodiazepine receptors; antagonism of such receptors has been hypothesized to be associated with various anticholinergic, sedative, and cardiovascular effects for other psychotropic drugs. The chronic administration of sertraline was found in animals to downregulate brain norepinephrine receptors, as has been observed with other clinically effective antidepressants. Sertraline does not inhibit monoamine oxidase.

Pharmacokinetics

Systemic Bioavailability—In man, following oral once-daily dosing over the range of 50 to 200 mg for 14 days, mean peak plasma concentrations (C_{max}) of sertraline occurred between 4.5 to 8.4 hours post-dosing. The average terminal elimination half-life of plasma sertraline is about 26 hours. Based on this pharmacokinetic parameter, steady-state sertraline plasma levels should be achieved after approximately one week of once-daily dosing. Linear dose-proportional pharmacokinetics were demonstrated in a single dose study in which the C_{max} and area under the plasma concentration time curve (AUC) of sertraline were proportional to dose over a range of 50 to 200 mg. Consistent with the terminal elimination half-life, there is an approximately two-fold accumulation, compared to a single dose, of sertraline with repeated dosing over a 50 to 200 mg dose range. The single dose bioavailability of sertraline tablets is approximately equal to an equivalent dose of solution.

In a relative bioavailability study comparing the pharmacokinetics of 100 mg sertraline as the oral solution to a 100 mg sertraline tablet in 16 healthy adults, the solution to tablet ratio of geometric mean AUC and C_{max} values were 114.8% and 120.6%, respectively. 90% confidence intervals (CI) were within the range of 80–125% with the exception of the upper 90% CI limit for C_{max} which was 126.5%.

The effects of food on the bioavailability of the sertraline tablet and oral concentrate were studied in subjects administered a single dose with and without food. For the tablet, AUC was slightly increased when drug was administered with food but the C_{max} was 25% greater, while the time to reach peak plasma concentration (T_{max}) decreased from 8 hours post-dosing to 5.5 hours. For the oral concentrate, T_{max} was slightly prolonged from 5.9 hours to 7.0 hours with food.

Metabolism—Sertraline undergoes extensive first pass metabolism. The principal initial pathway of metabolism for sertraline is N-demethylation. N-desmethylsertraline has a plasma terminal elimination half-life of 62 to 104 hours. Both *in vitro* biochemical and *in vivo* pharmacological testing have shown N-desmethylsertraline to be substantially less active than sertraline. Both sertraline and N-desmethylsertraline undergo oxidative deamination and subsequent reduction, hydroxylation, and glucuronide conjugation. In a study of radiolabeled sertraline involving two healthy male subjects, sertraline accounted for less than 5% of the plasma radioactivity. About 40–45% of the administered radioactivity was recovered in urine in 9 days. Unchanged sertraline was not detectable in the urine. For the same period, about 40–45% of the administered radioactivity was accounted for in feces, including 12–14% unchanged sertraline.

Desmethylsertraline exhibits time-related, dose dependent increases in AUC (0–24 hour), C_{max} and C_{min}, with about a 5–9 fold increase in these pharmacokinetic parameters between day 1 and day 14.

Protein Binding—*In vitro* protein binding studies performed with radiolabeled ^{3}H-sertraline showed that sertraline is highly bound to serum proteins (98%) in the range of 20 to 500 ng/mL. However, at up to 300 and 200 ng/mL concentrations, respectively, sertraline and N-desmethylsertraline did not alter the plasma protein binding of two other highly protein bound drugs, viz., warfarin and propranolol (see PRECAUTIONS).

Pediatric Pharmacokinetics—Sertraline pharmacokinetics were evaluated in a group of 61 pediatric patients (29 aged 6–12 years, 32 aged 13–17 years) with a DSM-III-R diagnosis of depression or obsessive-compulsive disorder. Patients included both males (N=28) and females (N=33). During 42 days of chronic sertraline dosing, sertraline was titrated up to 200 mg/day and maintained at that dose for a minimum of 11 days. On the final day of sertraline 200 mg/day, the 6–12 year old group exhibited a mean sertraline AUC (0–24 hr) of 3107 ng-hr/mL, mean C_{max} of 165 ng/mL, and mean half-life of 26.2 hr. The 13–17 year old group exhibited a mean sertraline AUC (0–24 hr) of 2296 ng-hr/mL, mean C_{max} of 123 ng/mL, and mean half-life of 27.8 hr. Higher plasma levels in the 6–12 year old group were largely attributable to patients with lower body weights. No gender associated differences were observed. By comparison, a group of 22 separately studied adults between 18 and 45 years of age (11 male, 11 female) received 30 days of 200 mg/day sertraline and exhibited a mean sertraline AUC (0–24 hr) of 2570 ng-hr/mL, mean C_{max} of 142 ng/mL, and mean half-life of 27.2 hr. Relative to the adults, both the 6–12 year olds and the 13–17 years olds showed about 22% lower AUC (0–24 hr) and C_{max} values when plasma concentration was adjusted for weight. These data suggest that pediatric patients metabolize sertraline with slightly greater efficiency than adults. Nevertheless, lower doses may be advisable for pediatric patients given their lower body weights, especially in very young patients, in order to avoid excessive plasma levels (see DOSAGE AND ADMINISTRATION).

Age—Sertraline plasma clearance in a group of 16 (8 male, 8 female) elderly patients treated for 14 days at a dose of 100 mg/day was approximately 40% lower than in a similarly studied group of younger (25 to 32 y.o.) individuals. Steady-state, therefore, should be achieved after 2 to 3 weeks in older patients. The same study showed a decreased clearance of desmethylsertraline in older males, but not in older females.

Liver Disease—As might be predicted from its primary site of metabolism, liver impairment can affect the elimination of sertraline. In patients with chronic mild liver impairment (N=10, 8 patients with Child-Pugh scores of 5–6 and 2 patients with Child-Pugh scores of 7–8) who received 50 mg sertraline per day maintained for 21 days, sertraline clearance was reduced, resulting in approximately 3-fold greater exposure compared to age-matched volunteers with no hepatic impairment (N=10). The exposure to desmethylsertraline was approximately 2-fold greater compared to age-matched volunteers with no hepatic impairment. There were no significant differences in plasma protein binding observed between the two groups. The effects of sertraline in patients with moderate and severe hepatic impairment have not been studied. The results suggest that the use of sertraline in patients with liver disease must be approached with caution. If sertraline is administered to patients with liver impairment, a lower or less frequent dose should be used (see PRECAUTIONS and DOSAGE AND ADMINISTRATION).

Continued on next page

Zoloft—Cont.

Renal Disease—Sertraline is extensively metabolized and excretion of unchanged drug in urine is a minor route of elimination. In volunteers with mild to moderate (CLcr=30–60 mL/min), moderate to severe (CLcr=10–29 mL/min) or severe (receiving hemodialysis) renal impairment (N=10 each group), the pharmacokinetics and protein binding of 200 mg sertraline per day maintained for 21 days were not altered compared to age-matched volunteers (N=12) with no renal impairment. Thus sertraline multiple dose pharmacokinetics appear to be unaffected by renal impairment (see PRECAUTIONS).

Clinical Trials

Depression—The efficacy of ZOLOFT as a treatment for depression was established in two placebo-controlled studies in adult outpatients meeting DSM-III criteria for major depression. Study 1 was an 8-week study with flexible dosing of ZOLOFT in a range of 50 to 200 mg/day; the mean dose for completers was 145 mg/day. Study 2 was a 6-week fixed-dose study, including ZOLOFT doses of 50, 100, and 200 mg/day. Overall, these studies demonstrated ZOLOFT to be superior to placebo on the Hamilton Depression Rating Scale and the Clinical Global Impression Severity and Improvement scales. Study 2 was not readily interpretable regarding a dose response relationship for effectiveness.

Study 3 involved depressed outpatients who had responded by the end of an initial 8-week open treatment phase on ZOLOFT 50–200 mg/day. These patients (N=295) were randomized to continuation for 44 weeks on double-blind ZOLOFT 50–200 mg/day or placebo. A statistically significantly lower relapse rate was observed for patients taking ZOLOFT compared to those on placebo. The mean dose for completers was 70 mg/day.

Analyses for gender effects on outcome did not suggest any differential responsiveness on the basis of sex.

Obsessive-Compulsive Disorder (OCD)—The effectiveness of ZOLOFT in the treatment of OCD was demonstrated in three multicenter placebo-controlled studies of adult outpatients (Studies 1–3). Patients in all studies had moderate to severe OCD (DSM-III or DSM-III-R) with mean baseline ratings on the Yale Brown Obsessive-Compulsive Scale (YBOCS) total score ranging from 23 to 25.

Study 1 was an 8-week study with flexible dosing of ZOLOFT in a range of 50 to 200 mg/day; the mean dose for completers was 186 mg/day. Patients receiving ZOLOFT experienced a mean reduction of approximately 4 points on the YBOCS total score which was significantly greater than the mean reduction of 2 points in placebo-treated patients.

Study 2 was a 12-week fixed-dose study, including ZOLOFT doses of 50, 100, and 200 mg/day. Patients receiving ZOLOFT doses of 50 and 200 mg/day experienced mean reductions of approximately 6 points on the YBOCS total score which were significantly greater than the approximately 3 point reduction in placebo-treated patients.

Study 3 was a 12-week study with flexible dosing of ZOLOFT in a range of 50 to 200 mg/day; the mean dose for completers was 185 mg/day. Patients receiving ZOLOFT experienced a mean reduction of approximately 7 points on the YBOCS total score which was significantly greater than the mean reduction of approximately 4 points in placebo-treated patients.

Analyses for age and gender effects on outcome did not suggest any differential responsiveness on the basis of age or sex.

The effectiveness of ZOLOFT for the treatment of OCD was also demonstrated in a 12-week, multicenter, parallel group study in a pediatric outpatient population (children and adolescents, ages 6–17). Patients in this study were initiated at doses of either 25 mg/day (children, ages 6–12) or 50 mg/day (adolescents, ages 13–17), and then titrated over the next four weeks to a maximum dose of 200 mg/day, as tolerated. The mean dose for completers was 178 mg/day. Dosing was once a day in the morning or evening. Patients in this study had moderate to severe OCD (DSM-III-R) with mean baseline ratings on the Children's Yale-Brown Obsessive-Compulsive Scale (CYBOCS) total score of 22. Patients receiving sertraline experienced a mean reduction of approximately 7 units on the CYBOCS total score which was significantly greater than the 3 unit reduction for placebo patients. Analyses for age and gender effects on outcome did not suggest any differential responsiveness on the basis of age or sex.

Panic Disorder—The effectiveness of ZOLOFT in the treatment of panic disorder was demonstrated in three double-blind, placebo-controlled studies (Studies 1–3) of adult outpatients who had a primary diagnosis of panic disorder (DSM-III-R), with or without agoraphobia.

Studies 1 and 2 were 10-week flexible dose studies. ZOLOFT was initiated at 25 mg/day for the first week, and then patients were dosed in a range of 50–200 mg/day on the basis of clinical response and toleration. The mean ZOLOFT doses for completers to 10 weeks were 131 mg/day and 144 mg/day, respectively, for Studies 1 and 2. In these studies, ZOLOFT was shown to be significantly more effective than placebo on change from baseline in panic attack frequency and on the Clinical Global Impression Severity of Illness and Global Improvement scores. The difference between ZOLOFT and placebo in reduction from baseline in the number of full panic attacks was approximately 2 panic attacks per week in both studies.

Study 3 was a 12-week fixed-dose study, including ZOLOFT doses of 50, 100, and 200 mg/day. Patients receiving ZOLOFT experienced a significantly greater reduction in panic attack frequency than patients receiving placebo. Study 3 was not readily interpretable regarding a dose response relationship for effectiveness.

Subgroup analyses did not indicate that there were any differences in treatment outcomes as a function of age, race, or gender.

Posttraumatic Stress Disorder (PTSD)—The effectiveness of ZOLOFT in the treatment of PTSD was established in two multicenter placebo-controlled studies (Studies 1–2) of adult outpatients who met DSM-III-R criteria for PTSD. The mean duration of PTSD for these patients was 12 years (Studies 1 and 2 combined) and 44% of patients (169 of the 385 patients treated) had secondary depressive disorder.

Studies 1 and 2 were 12-week flexible dose studies. ZOLOFT was initiated at 25 mg/day for the first week, and patients were then dosed in the range of 50–200 mg/day on the basis of clinical response and toleration. The mean ZOLOFT dose for completers was 146 mg/day and 151 mg/day, respectively for Studies 1 and 2. Study outcome was assessed by the Clinician-Administered PTSD Scale Part 2 (CAPS) which is a multi-item instrument that measures the three PTSD diagnostic symptom clusters of reexperiencing/intrusion, avoidance/numbing, and hyperarousal as well as the patient-rated Impact of Event Scale (IES) which measures intrusion and avoidance symptoms. ZOLOFT was shown to be significantly more effective than placebo on change from baseline to endpoint on the CAPS, IES and on the Clinical Global Impressions (CGI) Severity of Illness and Global Improvement scores. In two additional placebo-controlled PTSD trials, the difference in response to treatment between patients receiving ZOLOFT and patients receiving placebo was not statistically significant. One of these additional studies was conducted in patients similar to those recruited for Studies 1 and 2, while the second additional study was conducted in predominantly male veterans.

As PTSD is a more common disorder in women than men, the majority (76%) of patients in these trials were women (152 and 139 women on sertraline and placebo versus 39 and 55 men on sertraline and placebo; Studies 1 and 2 combined). Post hoc exploratory analyses revealed a significant difference between ZOLOFT and placebo on the CAPS, IES and CGI in women, regardless of baseline diagnosis of comorbid depression, but essentially no effect in the relatively smaller number of men in these studies. The clinical significance of this apparent gender interaction is unknown at this time. There was insufficient information to determine the effect of race or age on outcome.

INDICATIONS AND USAGE

Depression—ZOLOFT® (sertraline hydrochloride) is indicated for the treatment of depression.

The efficacy of ZOLOFT in the treatment of a major depressive episode was established in six to eight week controlled trials of outpatients whose diagnoses corresponded most closely to the DSM-III category of major depressive disorder (see Clinical Trials under CLINICAL PHARMACOLOGY).

A major depressive episode implies a prominent and relatively persistent depressed or dysphoric mood that usually interferes with daily functioning (nearly every day for at least 2 weeks); it should include at least 4 of the following 8 symptoms: change in appetite, change in sleep, psychomotor agitation or retardation, loss of interest in usual activities or decrease in sexual drive, increased fatigue, feelings of guilt or worthlessness, slowed thinking or impaired concentration, and a suicide attempt or suicidal ideation.

The antidepressant action of ZOLOFT in hospitalized depressed patients has not been adequately studied.

The efficacy of ZOLOFT in maintaining an antidepressant response for up to 44 weeks following 8 weeks of open-label acute treatment (52 weeks total) was demonstrated in a placebo-controlled trial. The usefulness of the drug in patients receiving ZOLOFT for extended periods should be reevaluated periodically (see Clinical Trials under CLINICAL PHARMACOLOGY).

Obsessive-Compulsive Disorder—ZOLOFT is indicated for the treatment of obsessions and compulsions in patients with obsessive-compulsive disorder (OCD), as defined in the DSM-III-R; i.e., the obsessions or compulsions cause marked distress, are time-consuming, or significantly interfere with social or occupational functioning.

The efficacy of ZOLOFT was established in 12-week trials with obsessive-compulsive outpatients having diagnoses of obsessive-compulsive disorder as defined according to DSM-III or DSM-III-R criteria (see Clinical Trials under CLINICAL PHARMACOLOGY).

Obsessive-compulsive disorder is characterized by recurrent and persistent ideas, thoughts, impulses, or images (obsessions) that are ego-dystonic and/or repetitive, purposeful, and intentional behaviors (compulsions) that are recognized by the person as excessive or unreasonable.

The effectiveness of ZOLOFT in long-term use for OCD, i.e., for more than 12 weeks, has not been systematically evaluated in placebo-controlled trials. Therefore, the physician who elects to use ZOLOFT for extended periods should periodically reevaluate the long-term usefulness of the drug for the individual patient (see DOSAGE AND ADMINISTRATION).

Panic Disorder—ZOLOFT is indicated for the treatment of panic disorder, with or without agoraphobia, as defined in DSM-IV. Panic disorder is characterized by the occurrence of unexpected panic attacks and associated concern about having additional attacks, worry about the implications or consequences of the attacks, and/or a significant change in behavior related to the attacks.

The efficacy of ZOLOFT was established in three 10-12 week trials in panic disorder patients whose diagnoses corresponded to the DSM-III-R category of panic disorder (see Clinical Trials under CLINICAL PHARMACOLOGY).

Panic disorder (DSM-IV) is characterized by recurrent unexpected panic attacks, i.e., a discrete period of intense fear or discomfort in which four (or more) of the following symptoms develop abruptly and reach a peak within 10 minutes: (1) palpitations, pounding heart, or accelerated heart rate; (2) sweating; (3) trembling or shaking; (4) sensations of shortness of breath or smothering; (5) feeling of choking; (6) chest pain or discomfort; (7) nausea or abdominal distress; (8) feeling dizzy, unsteady, lightheaded, or faint; (9) derealization (feelings of unreality) or depersonalization (being detached from oneself); (10) fear of losing control; (11) fear of dying; (12) paresthesias (numbness or tingling sensations); (13) chills or hot flushes.

The effectiveness of ZOLOFT® (sertraline hydrochloride) in long-term use, that is, for more than 12 weeks, has not been systematically evaluated in controlled trials. Therefore, the physician who elects to use ZOLOFT for extended periods should periodically re-evaluate the long-term usefulness of the drug for the individual patient (see DOSAGE AND ADMINISTRATION).

Posttraumatic Stress Disorder (PTSD)—ZOLOFT (sertraline hydrochloride) is indicated for the treatment of posttraumatic stress disorder.

The efficacy of ZOLOFT in the treatment of PTSD was established in two 12-week placebo-controlled trials of outpatients whose diagnosis met criteria for the DSM-III-R category of PTSD (see Clinical Trials under CLINICAL PHARMACOLOGY).

PTSD, as defined by DSM-III-R/IV, requires exposure to a traumatic event that involved actual or threatened death or serious injury, or threat to the physical integrity of self or others, and a response which involves intense fear, helplessness, or horror. Symptoms that occur as a result of exposure to the traumatic event include reexperiencing of the event in the form of intrusive thoughts, flashbacks or dreams, and intense psychological distress and physiological reactivity on exposure to cues to the event; avoidance of situations reminiscent of the traumatic event, inability to recall details of the event, and/or numbing of general responsiveness manifested as diminished interest in significant activities, estrangement from others, restricted range of affect, or sense of foreshortened future; and symptoms of autonomic arousal including hypervigilance, exaggerated startle response, sleep disturbance, impaired concentration, and irritability or outbursts of anger. A PTSD diagnosis requires that the symptoms are present for at least a month and that they cause clinically significant distress or impairment in social, occupational, or other important areas of functioning.

The effectiveness of ZOLOFT in long-term use for PTSD, i.e., for more than 12 weeks, has not been systematically evaluated in placebo-controlled trials; therefore, the physician who elects to use ZOLOFT for extended periods should periodically reevaluate the long-term usefulness of the drug for the individual patient (see DOSAGE AND ADMINISTRATION).

CONTRAINDICATIONS

All Dosage Forms of ZOLOFT:

Concomitant use in patients taking monoamine oxidase inhibitors (MAOIs) is contraindicated (see WARNINGS).

Oral Concentrate:

ZOLOFT oral concentrate is contraindicated with ANTABUSE (disulfiram) due to the alcohol content of the concentrate.

WARNINGS

Cases of serious sometimes fatal reactions have been reported in patients receiving ZOLOFT® (sertraline hydrochloride), a selective serotonin reuptake inhibitor (SSRI), in combination with a monoamine oxidase inhibitor (MAOI). Symptoms of a drug interaction between an SSRI and an MAOI include: hyperthermia, rigidity, myoclonus, autonomic instability with possible rapid fluctuations of vital signs, mental status changes that include confusion, irritability, and extreme agitation progressing to delirium and coma. These reactions have also been reported in patients who have recently discontinued an SSRI and have been started on an MAOI. Some cases presented with features resembling neuroleptic malignant syndrome. Therefore, ZOLOFT should not be used in combination with an MAOI, or within 14 days of discontinuing treatment with an MAOI. Similarly, at least 14 days should be allowed after stopping ZOLOFT before starting an MAOI.

PRECAUTIONS

General

Activation of Mania/Hypomania—During premarketing testing, hypomania or mania occurred in approximately 0.4% of ZOLOFT® (sertraline hydrochloride) treated patients.

Weight Loss—Significant weight loss may be an undesirable result of treatment with sertraline for some patients, but on average, patients in controlled trials had minimal, 1 to 2 pound weight loss, versus smaller changes on placebo. Only rarely have sertraline patients been discontinued for weight loss.

Seizure—ZOLOFT has not been evaluated in patients with a seizure disorder. These patients were excluded from clinical studies during the product's premarket testing. No seizures were observed among approximately 3000 patients treated with ZOLOFT in the development program for depression. However, 4 patients out of approximately 1800 (220 <18 years of age) exposed during the development program for obsessive-compulsive disorder experienced seizures, representing a crude incidence of 0.2%. Three of these patients were adolescents, two with a seizure disorder and one with a family history of seizure disorder, none of whom were receiving anticonvulsant medication. Accordingly, ZOLOFT should be introduced with care in patients with a seizure disorder.

Suicide—The possibility of a suicide attempt is inherent in depression and may persist until significant remission occurs. Close supervision of high risk patients should accompany initial drug therapy. Prescriptions for ZOLOFT should be written for the smallest quantity of tablets consistent with good patient management, in order to reduce the risk of overdose.

Because of the well-established comorbidity between OCD and depression, panic disorder and depression, and PTSD and depression, the same precautions observed when treating patients with depression should be observed when treating patients with OCD, panic disorder or PTSD.

Weak Uricosuric Effect—ZOLOFT® (sertraline hydrochloride) is associated with a mean decrease in serum uric acid of approximately 7%. The clinical significance of this weak uricosuric effect is unknown, and there have been no reports of acute renal failure with ZOLOFT.

Use in Patients with Concomitant Illness—Clinical experience with ZOLOFT in patients with certain concomitant systemic illness is limited. Caution is advisable in using ZOLOFT in patients with diseases or conditions that could affect metabolism or hemodynamic responses.

ZOLOFT has not been evaluated or used to any appreciable extent in patients with a recent history of myocardial infarction or unstable heart disease. Patients with these diagnoses were excluded from clinical studies during the product's premarket testing. However, the electrocardiograms of 774 patients who received ZOLOFT in double-blind trials were evaluated and the data indicate that ZOLOFT is not associated with the development of significant ECG abnormalities.

ZOLOFT is extensively metabolized by the liver. In patients with chronic mild liver impairment, sertraline clearance was reduced, resulting in increased AUC, C_{max} and elimination half-life. The effects of sertraline in patients with moderate and severe hepatic impairment have not been studied. The use of sertraline in patients with liver disease must be approached with caution. If sertraline is administered to patients with liver impairment, a lower or less frequent dose should be used (see CLINICAL PHARMACOLOGY and DOSAGE AND ADMINISTRATION).

Since ZOLOFT is extensively metabolized, excretion of unchanged drug in urine is a minor route of elimination. A clinical study comparing sertraline pharmacokinetics in healthy volunteers to that in patients with renal impairment ranging from mild to severe (requiring dialysis) indicated that the pharmacokinetics and protein binding are unaffected by renal disease. Based on the pharmacokinetic results, there is no need for dosage adjustment in patients with renal impairment (see CLINICAL PHARMACOLOGY).

Interference with Cognitive and Motor Performance—In controlled studies, ZOLOFT did not cause sedation and did not interfere with psychomotor performance.

Hyponatremia—Several cases of hyponatremia have been reported and appeared to be reversible when ZOLOFT was discontinued. Some cases were possibly due to the syndrome of inappropriate antidiuretic hormone secretion. The majority of these occurrences have been in elderly individuals, some in patients taking diuretics or who were otherwise volume depleted.

Platelet Function—There have been rare reports of altered platelet function and/or abnormal results from laboratory studies in patients taking ZOLOFT. While there have been reports of abnormal bleeding or purpura in several patients taking ZOLOFT, it is unclear whether ZOLOFT had a causative role.

Information for Patients

Physicians are advised to discuss the following issues with patients for whom they prescribe ZOLOFT:

Patients should be told that although ZOLOFT has not been shown to impair the ability of normal subjects to perform tasks requiring complex motor and mental skills in laboratory experiments, drugs that act upon the central nervous system may affect some individuals adversely.

Patients should be told that although ZOLOFT has not been shown in experiments with normal subjects to increase the mental and motor skill impairments caused by alcohol, the concomitant use of ZOLOFT and alcohol is not advised.

Patients should be told that while no adverse interaction of ZOLOFT with over-the-counter (OTC) drug products is known to occur, the potential for interaction exists. Thus, the use of any OTC product should be initiated cautiously according to the directions of use given for the OTC product.

Patients should be advised to notify their physician if they become pregnant or intend to become pregnant during therapy.

Patients should be advised to notify their physician if they are breast feeding an infant.

TABLE 1
MOST COMMON TREATMENT-EMERGENT ADVERSE EVENTS: INCIDENCE IN PLACEBO-CONTROLLED CLINICAL TRIALS

	Percentage of Patients Reporting Event							
	Depression/Other*		OCD		Panic Disorder		PTSD	
Body System/ Adverse Event	ZOLOFT (N=861)	Placebo (N=853)	ZOLOFT (N=533)	Placebo (N=373)	ZOLOFT (N=430)	Placebo (N=275)	ZOLOFT (N=374)	Placebo (N=376)
Autonomic Nervous System Disorders								
Ejaculation Failure[(1)]	7	<1	17	2	19	1	11	1
Mouth Dry	16	9	14	9	15	10	11	6
Sweating Increased	8	3	6	1	5	1	4	2
Centr. & Periph. Nerv. System Disorders								
Somnolence	13	6	15	8	15	9	13	9
Tremor	11	3	8	1	5	1	5	1
General								
Fatigue	11	8	14	10	11	6	10	5
Gastrointestinal Disorders								
Anorexia	3	2	11	2	7	2	8	2
Constipation	8	6	6	4	7	3	3	3
Diarrhea/Loose Stools	18	9	24	10	20	9	24	15
Dyspepsia	6	3	10	4	10	8	6	6
Nausea	26	12	30	11	29	18	21	11
Psychiatric Disorders								
Agitation	6	4	6	3	6	2	5	5
Insomnia	16	9	28	12	25	18	20	11
Libido Decreased	1	<1	11	2	7	1	7	2

[(1)]Primarily ejaculatory delay. Denominator used was for male patients only (N=271 ZOLOFT depression/other*; N=271 placebo depression/other*; N=296 ZOLOFT OCD; N=219 placebo OCD; N=216 ZOLOFT panic disorder; N=134 placebo panic disorder; N=130 ZOLOFT PTSD; N=149 placebo PTSD).
*Depression and other premarketing controlled trials.

ZOLOFT oral concentrate is contraindicated with ANTABUSE (disulfiram) due to the alcohol content of the concentrate.

ZOLOFT Oral Concentrate contains 20 mg/mL of sertraline (as the hydrochloride) as the active ingredient and 12% alcohol. ZOLOFT Oral Concentrate must be diluted before use. Just before taking, use the dropper provided to remove the required amount of ZOLOFT Oral Concentrate and mix with 4 oz (1/2 cup) of water, ginger ale, lemon/lime soda, lemonade or orange juice ONLY. Do not mix ZOLOFT Oral Concentrate with anything other than the liquids listed. The dose should be taken immediately after mixing. Do not mix in advance. At times, a slight haze may appear after mixing; this is normal. Note that caution should be exercised for persons with latex sensitivity, as the dropper dispenser contains dry natural rubber.

Laboratory Tests

None.

Drug Interactions

Potential Effects of Coadministration of Drugs Highly Bound to Plasma Proteins—Because sertraline is tightly bound to plasma protein, the administration of ZOLOFT® (sertraline hydrochloride) to a patient taking another drug which is tightly bound to protein (e.g., warfarin, digitoxin) may cause a shift in plasma concentrations potentially resulting in an adverse effect. Conversely, adverse effects may result from displacement of protein bound ZOLOFT by other tightly bound drugs.

In a study comparing prothrombin time AUC (0–120 hr) following dosing with warfarin (0.75 mg/kg) before and after 21 days of dosing with either ZOLOFT (50–200 mg/day) or placebo, there was a mean increase in prothrombin time of 8% relative to baseline for ZOLOFT compared to a 1% decrease for placebo ($p<0.02$). The normalization of prothrombin time for the ZOLOFT group was delayed compared to the placebo group. The clinical significance of this change is unknown. Accordingly, prothrombin time should be carefully monitored when ZOLOFT therapy is initiated or stopped.

Cimetidine—In a study assessing disposition of ZOLOFT (100 mg) on the second of 8 days of cimetidine administration (800 mg daily), there were significant increases in ZOLOFT mean AUC (50%), C_{max} (24%) and half-life (26%) compared to the placebo group. The clinical significance of these changes is unknown.

CNS Active Drugs—In a study comparing the disposition of intravenously administered diazepam before and after 21 days of dosing with either ZOLOFT (50 to 200 mg/day escalating dose) or placebo, there was a 32% decrease relative to baseline in diazepam clearance for the ZOLOFT group compared to a 19% decrease relative to baseline for the placebo group ($p<0.03$). There was a 23% increase in T_{max} for desmethyldiazepam in the ZOLOFT group compared to a 20% decrease in the placebo group ($p<0.03$). The clinical significance of these changes is unknown.

In a placebo-controlled trial in normal volunteers, the administration of two doses of ZOLOFT did not significantly alter steady-state lithium levels or the renal clearance of lithium.

Nonetheless, at this time, it is recommended that plasma lithium levels be monitored following initiation of ZOLOFT therapy with appropriate adjustments to the lithium dose.

The risk of using ZOLOFT in combination with other CNS active drugs has not been systematically evaluated. Consequently, caution is advised if the concomitant administration of ZOLOFT and such drugs is required.

There is limited controlled experience regarding the optimal timing of switching from other antidepressants to ZOLOFT. Care and prudent medical judgment should be exercised when switching, particularly from long-acting agents. The duration of an appropriate washout period which should intervene before switching from one selective serotonin reuptake inhibitor (SSRI) to another has not been established.

Monoamine Oxidase Inhibitors—See CONTRAINDICATIONS and WARNINGS.

Drugs Metabolized by P450 3A4—In two separate *in vivo* interaction studies, sertraline was co-administered with cytochrome P450 3A4 substrates, terfenadine or carbamazepine, under steady-state conditions. The results of these studies demonstrated that sertraline co-administration did not increase plasma concentrations of terfenadine or carbamazepine. These data suggest that sertraline's extent of inhibition of P450 3A4 activity is not likely to be of clinical significance.

Drugs Metabolized by P450 2D6—Many antidepressants, e.g., the SSRIs, including sertraline, and most tricyclic antidepressants inhibit the biochemical activity of the drug metabolizing isozyme cytochrome P450 2D6 (debrisoquin hydroxylase), and, thus, may increase the plasma concentrations of co-administered drugs that are metabolized by P450 2D6. The drugs for which this potential interaction is of greatest concern are those metabolized primarily by 2D6 and which have a narrow therapeutic index, e.g., the tricyclic antidepressants and the Type 1C antiarrhythmics propafenone and flecainide. The extent to which this interac-

Continued on next page

Zoloft—Cont.

tion is an important clinical problem depends on the extent of the inhibition of P450 2D6 by the antidepressant and the therapeutic index of the co-administered drug. There is variability among the antidepressants in the extent of clinically important 2D6 inhibition, and in fact sertraline at lower doses has a less prominent inhibitory effect on 2D6 than some others in the class. Nevertheless, even sertraline has the potential for clinically important 2D6 inhibition. Consequently, concomitant use of a drug metabolized by P450 2D6 with ZOLOFT may require lower doses than usually prescribed for the other drug. Furthermore, whenever ZOLOFT is withdrawn from co-therapy, an increased dose of the co-administered drug may be required (see Tricyclic Antidepressants under PRECAUTIONS).

Sumatriptan—There have been rare postmarketing reports describing patients with weakness, hyperreflexia, and incoordination following the use of a selective serotonin reuptake inhibitor (SSRI) and sumatriptan. If concomitant treatment with sumatriptan and an SSRI (e.g., citalopram, fluoxetine, fluvoxamine, paroxetine, sertraline) is clinically warranted, appropriate observation of the patient is advised.

Tricyclic Antidepressants (TCAs)—The extent to which SSRI-TCA interactions may pose clinical problems will depend on the degree of inhibition and the pharmacokinetics of the SSRI involved. Nevertheless, caution is indicated in the co-administration of TCAs with ZOLOFT, because sertraline may inhibit TCA metabolism. Plasma TCA concentrations may need to be monitored, and the dose of TCA may need to be reduced, if a TCA is co-administered with ZOLOFT (see Drugs Metabolized by P450 2D6 under PRECAUTIONS).

Hypoglycemic Drugs—In a placebo-controlled trial in normal volunteers, administration of ZOLOFT for 22 days (including 200 mg/day for the final 13 days) caused a statistically significant 16% decrease from baseline in the clearance of tolbutamide following an intravenous 1000 mg dose. ZOLOFT administration did not noticeably change either the plasma protein binding or the apparent volume of distribution of tolbutamide, suggesting that the decreased clearance was due to a change in the metabolism of the drug. The clinical significance of this decrease in tolbutamide clearance is unknown.

Atenolol—ZOLOFT (100 mg) when administered to 10 healthy male subjects had no effect on the beta-adrenergic blocking ability of atenolol.

Digoxin—In a placebo-controlled trial in normal volunteers, administration of ZOLOFT for 17 days (including 200 mg/day for the last 10 days) did not change serum digoxin levels or digoxin renal clearance.

Microsomal Enzyme Induction—Preclinical studies have shown ZOLOFT to induce hepatic microsomal enzymes. In clinical studies, ZOLOFT was shown to induce hepatic enzymes minimally as determined by a small (5%) but statistically significant decrease in antipyrine half-life following administration of 200 mg/day for 21 days. This small change in antipyrine half-life reflects a clinically insignificant change in hepatic metabolism.

Electroconvulsive Therapy—There are no clinical studies establishing the risks or benefits of the combined use of electroconvulsive therapy (ECT) and ZOLOFT.

Alcohol—Although ZOLOFT did not potentiate the cognitive and psychomotor effects of alcohol in experiments with normal subjects, the concomitant use of ZOLOFT and alcohol is not recommended.

Carcinogenesis—Lifetime carcinogenicity studies were carried out in CD-1 mice and Long-Evans rats at doses up to 40 mg/kg/day. These doses correspond to 1 times (mice) and 2 times (rats) the maximum recommended human dose (MRHD) on a mg/m^2 basis. There was a dose-related increase of liver adenomas in male mice receiving sertraline at 10–40 mg/kg (0.25-1.0 times the MRHD on a mg/m^2 basis). No increase was seen in female mice or in rats of either sex receiving the same treatments, nor was there an increase in hepatocellular carcinomas. Liver adenomas have a variable rate of spontaneous occurrence in the CD-1 mouse and are of unknown significance to humans. There was an increase in follicular adenomas of the thyroid in female rats receiving sertraline at 40 mg/kg (2 times the MRHD on a mg/m^2 basis); this was not accompanied by thyroid hyperplasia. While there was an increase in uterine adenocarcinomas in rats receiving sertraline at 10–40 mg/kg (0.5–2.0 times the MRHD on a mg/m^2 basis) compared to placebo controls, this effect was not clearly drug related.

Mutagenesis—Sertraline had no genotoxic effects, with or without metabolic activation, based on the following assays: bacterial mutation assay; mouse lymphoma mutation assay; and tests for cytogenetic aberrations *in vivo* in mouse bone marrow and *in vitro* in human lymphocytes.

Impairment of Fertility—A decrease in fertility was seen in one of two rat studies at a dose of 80 mg/kg (4 times the maximum recommended human dose on a mg/m^2 basis).

Pregnancy-Pregnancy Category C—Reproduction studies have been performed in rats and rabbits at doses up to 80 mg/kg/day and 40 mg/kg/day, respectively. These doses correspond to approximately 4 times the maximum recommended human dose (MRHD) on a mg/m^2 basis. There was no evidence of teratogenicity at any dose level. When pregnant rats and rabbits were given sertraline during the period of organogenesis, delayed ossification was observed in fetuses at doses of 10 mg/kg (0.5 times the MRHD on a mg/m^2 basis) in rats and 40 mg/kg (4 times the MRHD on a mg/m^2 basis) in rabbits. When female rats received sertraline during the last third of gestation and throughout lactation, there was an increase in the number of stillborn pups and in the number of pups dying during the first 4 days after birth. Pup body weights were also decreased during the first four days after birth. These effects occurred at a dose of 20 mg/kg (1 times the MRHD on a mg/m^2 basis). The no effect dose for rat pup mortality was 10 mg/kg (0.5 times the MRHD on a mg/m^2 basis). The decrease in pup survival was shown to be due to *in utero* exposure to sertraline. The clinical significance of these effects is unknown. There are no adequate and well-controlled studies in pregnant women. ZOLOFT® (sertraline hydrochloride) should be used during pregnancy only if the potential benefit justifies the potential risk to the fetus.

Labor and Delivery—The effect of ZOLOFT on labor and delivery in humans is unknown.

Nursing Mothers—It is not known whether, and if so in what amount, sertraline or its metabolites are excreted in human milk. Because many drugs are excreted in human milk, caution should be exercised when ZOLOFT is administered to a nursing woman.

Pediatric Use—The efficacy of ZOLOFT for the treatment of obsessive-compulsive disorder was demonstrated in a 12-week, multicenter, placebo-controlled study with 187 outpatients ages 6–17 (see Clinical Trials under CLINICAL PHARMACOLOGY). The effectiveness of ZOLOFT in pediatric patients with depression or panic disorder has not been systematically evaluated.

Sertraline pharmacokinetics were evaluated in 61 pediatric patients between 6 and 17 years of age with depression or OCD and revealed similar drug exposures to those of adults when plasma concentration was adjusted for weight (see Pharmacokinetics under CLINICAL PHARMACOLOGY).

More than 250 patients with depression or OCD between 6 and 17 years of age have received ZOLOFT in clinical trials. The adverse event profile observed in these patients was generally similar to that observed in adult studies with ZOLOFT (see ADVERSE REACTIONS). As with other SSRIs, decreased appetite and weight loss have been observed in association with the use of ZOLOFT. Consequently, regular monitoring of weight and growth is recommended if treatment of a child with an SSRI is to be continued long term. Safety and effectiveness in pediatric patients below the age of 6 have not been established.

The risks, if any, that may be associated with sertraline's extended use in children and adolescents with OCD have not been systematically assessed. The prescriber should be mindful that the evidence relied upon to conclude that sertraline is safe for use in children and adolescents derives from relatively short-term clinical studies and from extrapolation of experience gained with adult patients. In particular, there are no studies that directly evaluate the effects of long-term sertraline use on the growth, development, and maturation of children and adolescents. Although there is

TABLE 2
TREATMENT-EMERGENT ADVERSE EVENTS: INCIDENCE IN PLACEBO-CONTROLLED CLINICAL TRIALS
Percentage of Patients Reporting Event
Depression/Other*, OCD, Panic Disorder and PTSD combined

Body System/Adverse Event**	ZOLOFT (N=2198)	Placebo (N=1877)
Autonomic Nervous System Disorders		
Ejaculation Failure(1)	14	1
Mouth Dry	15	9
Sweating Increased	6	2
Centr. & Periph. Nerv. System Disorders		
Somnolence	14	7
Dizziness	12	7
Headache	26	24
Paresthesia	3	2
Tremor	8	2
Disorders of Skin and Appendages		
Rash	3	2
Gastrointestinal Disorders		
Anorexia	6	2
Constipation	7	5
Diarrhea/Loose Stools	21	11
Dyspepsia	8	4
Flatulence	4	3
Nausea	27	13
Vomiting	4	2
General		
Fatigue	11	7
Hot Flushes	2	1
Psychiatric Disorders		
Agitation	6	4
Anxiety	4	3
Insomnia	22	11
Libido Decreased	6	1
Nervousness	6	4
Special Senses		
Vision Abnormal	4	2

(1)Primarily ejaculatory delay. Denominator used was for male patients only (N=913 ZOLOFT; N=773 placebo).
*Depression and other premarketing controlled trials.
**Included are events reported by at least 2% of patients taking ZOLOFT except the following events, which had an incidence on placebo greater than or equal to ZOLOFT: abdominal pain and pharyngitis.

no affirmative finding to suggest that sertraline possesses a capacity to adversely affect growth, development or maturation, the absence of such findings is not compelling evidence of the absence of the potential of sertraline to have adverse effects in chronic use.

Geriatric Use—Several hundred elderly patients have participated in clinical studies with ZOLOFT. The pattern of adverse reactions in the elderly was similar to that in younger patients.

ADVERSE REACTIONS

During its premarketing assessment, multiple doses of ZOLOFT were administered to over 4000 adult subjects as of February 26, 1998. The conditions and duration of exposure to ZOLOFT varied greatly, and included (in overlapping categories) clinical pharmacology studies, open and double-blind studies, uncontrolled and controlled studies, inpatient and outpatient studies, fixed-dose and titration studies, and studies for multiple indications, including depression, OCD, panic disorder and PTSD.

Untoward events associated with this exposure were recorded by clinical investigators using terminology of their own choosing. Consequently, it is not possible to provide a meaningful estimate of the proportion of individuals experiencing adverse events without first grouping similar types of untoward events into a smaller number of standardized event categories. In the tabulations that follow, a World Health Organization dictionary of terminology has been used to classify reported adverse events. The frequencies presented, therefore, represent the proportion of the over 4000 adult individuals exposed to multiple doses of ZOLOFT who experienced a treatment-emergent adverse event of the type cited on at least one occasion while receiving ZOLOFT. An event was considered treatment-emergent if it occurred for the first time or worsened while receiving therapy following baseline evaluation. It is important to emphasize that events reported during therapy were not necessarily caused by it.

The prescriber should be aware that the figures in the tables and tabulations cannot be used to predict the incidence of side effects in the course of usual medical practice where patient characteristics and other factors differ from those that prevailed in the clinical trials. Similarly, the cited frequencies cannot be compared with figures obtained from other clinical investigations involving different treatments, uses, and investigators. The cited figures, however, do provide the prescribing physician with some basis for estimating the relative contribution of drug and nondrug factors to the side effect incidence rate in the population studied.

Incidence in Placebo-Controlled Trials—Table 1 enumerates the most common treatment-emergent adverse events associated with the use of ZOLOFT (incidence of at least 5% for ZOLOFT and at least twice that for placebo within at least one of the indications) for the treatment of adult patients with depression/other*, OCD, panic disorder and PTSD in placebo-controlled clinical trials. Most patients received doses of 50 to 200 mg/day. Table 2 enumerates treatment-emergent adverse events that occurred in 2% or more of adult patients treated with ZOLOFT and with incidence greater than placebo who participated in controlled clinical trials comparing ZOLOFT with placebo in the treatment of depression/other*, OCD, panic disorder and PTSD. Table 2 provides combined data for the pool of studies that are provided separately by indication in Table 1.

[See table 1 at top of page 2555]

[See table 2 at top of previous page]

Associated with Discontinuation in Placebo-Controlled Clinical Trials

Table 3 lists the adverse events associated with discontinuation of ZOLOFT® (sertraline hydrochloride) treatment (incidence at least twice that for placebo and at least 1% for ZOLOFT in clinical trials) in depression/other*, OCD, panic disorder and PTSD.

[See table 3 above]

Male and Female Sexual Dysfunction with SSRIs

Although changes in sexual desire, sexual performance and sexual satisfaction often occur as manifestations of a psychiatric disorder, they may also be a consequence of pharmacologic treatment. In particular, some evidence suggests that selective serotonin reuptake inhibitors (SSRIs) can cause such untoward sexual experiences. Reliable estimates of the incidence and severity of untoward experiences involving sexual desire, performance and satisfaction are difficult to obtain, however, in part because patients and physicians may be reluctant to discuss them. Accordingly, estimates of the incidence of untoward sexual experience and performance cited in product labeling, are likely to underestimate their actual incidence.

Table 4 below displays the incidence of sexual side effects reported by at least 2% of patients taking ZOLOFT in placebo-controlled trials.

[See table 4 above]

There are no adequate and well-controlled studies examining sexual dysfunction with sertraline treatment.

Priapism has been reported with all SSRIs.

While it is difficult to know the precise risk of sexual dysfunction associated with the use of SSRIs, physicians should routinely inquire about such possible side effects.

Other Adverse Events in Pediatric Patients—In approximately N=250 pediatric patients treated with ZOLOFT, the overall profile of adverse events was generally similar to that seen in adult studies, as shown in Tables 1 and 2. However, the following adverse events, not appearing in Tables 1 and 2, were reported at an incidence of at least 2% and occurred at a rate of at least twice the placebo rate in a controlled trial (N=187): hyperkinesia, twitching, fever, malaise, purpura, weight decrease, concentration impaired, manic reaction, emotional lability, thinking abnormal, and epistaxis.

TABLE 3
MOST COMMON ADVERSE EVENTS ASSOCIATED WITH DISCONTINUATION IN PLACEBO-CONTROLLED CLINICAL TRIALS

Adverse Event	Depression/Other*, OCD, Panic Disorder and PTSD combined (N=2198)	Depression/Other* (N=861)	OCD (N=533)	Panic Disorder (N=430)	PTSD (N=374)
Agitation	1%	1%	—	2%	—
Diarrhea	2%	2%	2%	1%	—
Dizziness	1%	—	1%	—	—
Dry Mouth	—	1%	—	—	—
Dyspepsia	—	—	—	1%	—
Ejaculation Failure[1]	1%	1%	1%	2%	—
Headache	1%	2%	—	—	1%
Insomnia	2%	1%	3%	2%	—
Nausea	3%	4%	3%	3%	2%
Nervousness	—	—	—	2%	—
Somnolence	2%	1%	2%	2%	—
Tremor	—	2%	—	—	—

[1]Primarily ejaculatory delay. Denominator used was for male patients only (N=271 depression/other*; N=296 OCD; N=216 panic disorder; N=130 PTSD).

*Depression and other premarketing controlled trials.

TABLE 4

Treatment	Ejaculation failure (primarily delayed ejaculation)		Decreased libido	
	N (males only)	Incidence	N (males and females)	Incidence
ZOLOFT	913	14%	2198	6%
Placebo	773	1%	1877	1%

Other Events Observed During the Premarketing Evaluation of ZOLOFT® (sertraline hydrochloride)—Following is a list of treatment-emergent adverse events reported during premarketing assessment of ZOLOFT in clinical trials (over 4000 adult subjects) except those already listed in the previous tables or elsewhere in labeling.

In the tabulations that follow, a World Health Organization dictionary of terminology has been used to classify reported adverse events. The frequencies presented, therefore, represent the proportion of the over 4000 adult individuals exposed to multiple doses of ZOLOFT who experienced an event of the type cited on at least one occasion while receiving ZOLOFT. All events are included except those already listed in the previous tables or elsewhere in labeling and those reported in terms so general as to be uninformative and those for which a causal relationship to ZOLOFT treatment seemed remote. It is important to emphasize that although the events reported occurred during treatment with ZOLOFT, they were not necessarily caused by it.

Events are further categorized by body system and listed in order of decreasing frequency according to the following definitions: frequent adverse events are those occurring on one or more occasions in at least 1/100 patients; infrequent adverse events are those occurring in 1/100 to 1/1000 patients; rare events are those occurring in fewer than 1/1000 patients. Events of major clinical importance are also described in the PRECAUTIONS section.

Autonomic Nervous System Disorders—*Frequent:* impotence; *Infrequent:* flushing, increased saliva, cold clammy skin, mydriasis; *Rare:* pallor, glaucoma, priapism, vasodilation.

Body as a Whole—General Disorders—*Rare:* allergic reaction, allergy.

Cardiovascular—*Frequent:* palpitations, chest pain; *Infrequent:* hypertension, tachycardia, postural dizziness, postural hypotension, periorbital edema, peripheral edema, hypotension, peripheral ischemia, syncope, edema, dependent edema; *Rare:* precordial chest pain, substernal chest pain, aggravated hypertension, myocardial infarction, cerebrovascular disorder.

Central and Peripheral Nervous System Disorders—*Frequent:* hypertonia, hypoesthesia; *Infrequent:* twitching, confusion, hyperkinesia, vertigo, ataxia, migraine, abnormal coordination, hyperesthesia, leg cramps, abnormal gait, nystagmus, hypokinesia; *Rare:* dysphonia, coma, dyskinesia, hypotonia, ptosis, choreoathetosis, hyporeflexia.

Disorders of Skin and Appendages—*Infrequent:* pruritus, acne, urticaria, alopecia, dry skin, erythematous rash, photosensitivity reaction, maculopapular rash; *Rare:* follicular rash, eczema, dermatitis, contact dermatitis, bullous eruption, hypertrichosis, skin discoloration, pustular rash.

Endocrine Disorders—*Rare:* exophthalmos, gynecomastia.

Gastrointestinal Disorders—*Frequent:* appetite increased; *Infrequent:* dysphagia, tooth caries aggravated, eructation, esophagitis, gastroenteritis; *Rare:* melena, glossitis, gum hyperplasia, hiccup, stomatitis, tenesmus, colitis, diverticulitis, fecal incontinence, gastritis, rectum hemorrhage, hemorrhagic peptic ulcer, proctitis, ulcerative stomatitis, tongue edema, tongue ulceration.

General—*Frequent:* back pain, asthenia, malaise, weight increase; *Infrequent:* fever, rigors, generalized edema; *Rare:* face edema, aphthous stomatitis.

Hearing and Vestibular Disorders—*Rare:* hyperacusis, labyrinthine disorder.

Hematopoietic and Lymphatic—*Rare:* anemia, anterior chamber eye hemorrhage.

Liver and Biliary System Disorders—*Rare:* abnormal hepatic function.

Metabolic and Nutritional Disorders—*Infrequent:* thirst; *Rare:* hypoglycemia, hypoglycemia reaction.

Musculoskeletal System Disorders—*Frequent:* myalgia; *Infrequent:* arthralgia, dystonia, arthrosis, muscle cramps, muscle weakness.

Psychiatric Disorders—*Frequent:* yawning, other male sexual dysfunction, other female sexual dysfunction; *Infrequent:* depression, amnesia, paroniria, teeth-grinding, emotional lability, apathy, abnormal dreams, euphoria, paranoid reaction, hallucination, aggressive reaction, aggravated depression, delusions; *Rare:* withdrawal syndrome, suicide ideation, libido increased, somnambulism, illusion.

Reproductive—*Infrequent:* menstrual disorder, dysmenorrhea, intermenstrual bleeding, vaginal hemorrhage, amenorrhea, leukorrhea; *Rare:* female breast pain, menorrhagia, balanoposthitis, breast enlargement, atrophic vaginitis, acute female mastitis.

Respiratory System Disorders—*Frequent:* rhinitis; *Infrequent:* coughing, dyspnea, upper respiratory tract infection, epistaxis, bronchospasm, sinusitis; *Rare:* hyperventilation, bradypnea, stridor, apnea, bronchitis, hemoptysis, hypoventilation, laryngismus, laryngitis.

Special Senses—*Frequent:* tinnitus; *Infrequent:* conjunctivitis, earache, eye pain, abnormal accommodation; *Rare:* xerophthalmia, photophobia, diplopia, abnormal lacrimation, scotoma, visual field defect.

Urinary System Disorders—*Infrequent:* micturition frequency, polyuria, urinary retention, dysuria, nocturia, urinary incontinence; *Rare:* cystitis, oliguria, pyelonephritis, hematuria, renal pain, strangury.

Laboratory Tests—In man, asymptomatic elevations in serum transaminases (SGOT [or AST] and SGPT [or ALT]) have been reported infrequently (approximately 0.8%) in association with ZOLOFT® (sertraline hydrochloride) administration. These hepatic enzyme elevations usually occurred

Continued on next page

Zoloft—Cont.

within the first 1 to 9 weeks of drug treatment and promptly diminished upon drug discontinuation.
ZOLOFT therapy was associated with small mean increases in total cholesterol (approximately 3%) and triglycerides (approximately 5%), and a small mean decrease in serum uric acid (approximately 7%) of no apparent clinical importance.
The safety profile observed with ZOLOFT treatment in patients with depression, OCD, panic disorder and PTSD is similar.
Other Events Observed During the Postmarketing Evaluation of ZOLOFT—Reports of adverse events temporally associated with ZOLOFT that have been received since market introduction, that are not listed above and that may have no causal relationship with the drug, include the following: increased coagulation times, bradycardia, AV block, atrial arrhythmias, hypothyroidism, leukopenia, thrombocytopenia, hyperglycemia, priapism, galactorrhea, hyperprolactinemia, neuroleptic malignant syndrome-like events, psychosis, severe skin reactions, which potentially can be fatal, such as Stevens-Johnson syndrome, vasculitis, photosensitivity and other severe cutaneous disorders, rare reports of pancreatitis, and liver events—clinical features (which in the majority of cases appeared to be reversible with discontinuation of ZOLOFT) occurring in one or more patients include: elevated enzymes, increased bilirubin, hepatomegaly, hepatitis, jaundice, abdominal pain, vomiting, liver failure and death.

DRUG ABUSE AND DEPENDENCE

Controlled Substance Class—ZOLOFT® (sertraline hydrochloride) is not a controlled substance.
Physical and Psychological Dependence—In a placebo-controlled, double-blind, randomized study of the comparative abuse liability of ZOLOFT, alprazolam, and d-amphetamine in humans, ZOLOFT did not produce the positive subjective effects indicative of abuse potential, such as euphoria or drug liking, that were observed with the other two drugs. Premarketing clinical experience with ZOLOFT did not reveal any tendency for a withdrawal syndrome or any drug-seeking behavior. In animal studies ZOLOFT does not demonstrate stimulant or barbiturate-like (depressant) abuse potential. As with any CNS active drug, however, physicians should carefully evaluate patients for history of drug abuse and follow such patients closely, observing them for signs of ZOLOFT misuse or abuse (e.g., development of tolerance, incrementation of dose, drug-seeking behavior).

OVERDOSAGE

Human Experience—As of November 1992, there were 79 reports of non-fatal acute overdoses involving ZOLOFT, of which 28 were overdoses of ZOLOFT alone and the remainder involved a combination of other drugs and/or alcohol in addition to ZOLOFT. In those cases of overdose involving only ZOLOFT, the reported doses ranged from 500 mg to 6000 mg. In a subset of 18 of these patients in whom ZOLOFT blood levels were determined, plasma concentrations ranged from <5 ng/mL to 554 ng/mL. Symptoms of overdose with ZOLOFT alone included somnolence, nausea, vomiting, tachycardia, ECG changes, anxiety and dilated pupils. Treatment was primarily supportive and included monitoring and use of activated charcoal, gastric lavage or cathartics and hydration. Although there were no reports of death when ZOLOFT was taken alone, there were 4 deaths involving overdoses of ZOLOFT in combination with other drugs and/or alcohol. Therefore, any overdosage should be treated aggressively.
Overdose Management—Treatment should consist of those general measures employed in the management of overdosage with any antidepressant.
Ensure an adequate airway, oxygenation and ventilation. Monitor cardiac rhythm and vital signs. General supportive and symptomatic measures are also recommended. Induction of emesis is not recommended. Gastric lavage with a large-bore orogastric tube with appropriate airway protection, if needed, may be indicated if performed soon after ingestion, or in symptomatic patients.
Activated charcoal should be administered. Due to large volume of distribution of this drug, forced diuresis, dialysis, hemoperfusion and exchange transfusion are unlikely to be of benefit. No specific antidotes for sertraline are known.
In managing overdosage, consider the possibility of multiple drug involvement. The physician should consider contacting a poison control center on the treatment of any overdose. Telephone numbers for certified poison control centers are listed in the *Physicians' Desk Reference*® (PDR®).

DOSAGE AND ADMINISTRATION

Initial Treatment
Dosage for Adults
Depression and Obsessive-Compulsive Disorder—ZOLOFT treatment should be administered at a dose of 50 mg once daily.
Panic Disorder and Posttraumatic Stress Disorder—ZOLOFT treatment should be initiated with a dose of 25 mg once daily. After one week, the dose should be increased to 50 mg once daily.
While a relationship between dose and effect has not been established for depression, OCD, panic disorder or PTSD, patients were dosed in a range of 50–200 mg/day in the clinical trials demonstrating the effectiveness of ZOLOFT for the treatment of these indications. Consequently, a dose of 50 mg, administered once daily, is recommended as the initial dose. Patients not responding to a 50 mg dose may benefit from dose increases up to a maximum of 200 mg/day. Given the 24 hour elimination half-life of ZOLOFT, dose changes should not occur at intervals of less than 1 week.
ZOLOFT should be administered once daily, either in the morning or evening.
Dosage for Pediatric Population (Children and Adolescents)
Obsessive-Compulsive Disorder—ZOLOFT treatment should be initiated with a dose of 25 mg once daily in children (ages 6–12) and at a dose of 50 mg once daily in adolescents (ages 13–17).
While a relationship between dose and effect has not been established for OCD, patients were dosed in a range of 25–200 mg/day in the clinical trials demonstrating the effectiveness of ZOLOFT for pediatric patients (6–17 years) with OCD. Patients not responding to an initial dose of 25 or 50 mg/day may benefit from dose increases up to a maximum of 200 mg/day. For children with OCD, their generally lower body weights compared to adults should be taken into consideration in advancing the dose, in order to avoid excess dosing. Given the 24 hour elimination half-life of ZOLOFT, dose changes should not occur at intervals of less than 1 week.
ZOLOFT should be administered once daily, either in the morning or evening.
Dosage for Hepatically Impaired Patients
The use of sertraline in patients with liver disease should be approached with caution. The effects of sertraline in patients with moderate and severe hepatic impairment have not been studied. If sertraline is administered to patients with liver impairment, a lower or less frequent dose should be used (see CLINICAL PHARMACOLOGY and PRECAUTIONS).
Maintenance/Continuation/Extended Treatment
Depression—It is generally agreed that acute episodes of depression require several months or longer of sustained pharmacologic therapy. Whether the dose of antidepressant needed to induce remission is identical to the dose needed to maintain and/or sustain euthymia is unknown. Systematic evaluation of ZOLOFT has shown that its antidepressant efficacy is maintained for periods of up to 44 weeks following 8 weeks of open-label acute treatment (52 weeks total) at a dose of 50–200 mg/day (mean dose of 70 mg/day) (see Clinical Trials under CLINICAL PHARMACOLOGY).
Obsessive-Compulsive Disorder, Panic Disorder and Posttraumatic Stress Disorder—Although the efficacy of ZOLOFT beyond 10–12 weeks of dosing for OCD, panic disorder and PTSD has not been documented in controlled trials, all are chronic conditions, and it is reasonable to consider continuation of a responding patient. Dosage adjustments may be needed to maintain the patient on the lowest effective dosage, and patients should be periodically reassessed to determine the need for continued treatment.
Switching Patients to or from a Monoamine Oxidase Inhibitor—At least 14 days should elapse between discontinuation of an MAOI and initiation of therapy with ZOLOFT. In addition, at least 14 days should be allowed after stopping ZOLOFT before starting an MAOI (see CONTRAINDICATIONS and WARNINGS).
ZOLOFT Oral Concentrate
ZOLOFT Oral Concentrate contains 20 mg/mL of sertraline (as the hydrochloride) as the active ingredient and 12% alcohol. ZOLOFT Oral Concentrate must be diluted before use. Just before taking, use the dropper provided to remove the required amount of ZOLOFT Oral Concentrate and mix with 4 oz (1/2 cup) of water, ginger ale, lemon/lime soda, lemonade or orange juice ONLY. Do not mix ZOLOFT Oral Concentrate with anything other than the liquids listed. The dose should be taken immediately after mixing. Do not mix in advance. At times, a slight haze may appear after mixing; this is normal. Note that caution should be exercised for patients with latex sensitivity, as the dropper dispenser contains dry natural rubber.
ZOLOFT oral concentrate is contraindicated with ANTABUSE (disulfiram) due to the alcohol content of the concentrate.

HOW SUPPLIED

ZOLOFT® (sertraline hydrochloride) capsular-shaped scored tablets, containing sertraline hydrochloride equivalent to 25, 50 and 100 mg of sertraline, are packaged in bottles.
ZOLOFT® 25 mg Tablets: light green film coated tablets engraved on one side with ZOLOFT and on the other side scored and engraved with 25 mg.
NDC 0049-4960-50 Bottles of 50
ZOLOFT® 50 mg Tablets: light blue film coated tablets engraved on one side with ZOLOFT and on the other side scored and engraved with 50 mg.
NDC 0049-4900-66 Bottles of 100
NDC 0049-4900-73 Bottles of 500
NDC 0049-4900-94 Bottles of 5000
NDC 0049-4900-41 Unit Dose Packages of 100
ZOLOFT® 100 mg Tablets: light yellow film coated tablets engraved on one side with ZOLOFT and on the other side scored and engraved with 100 mg.
NDC 0049-4910-66 Bottles of 100
NDC 0049-4910-73 Bottles of 500
NDC 0049-4910-94 Bottles of 5000
NDC 0049-4910-41 Unit Dose Packages of 100
Store at controlled room temperature, 59° to 86°F (15° to 30°C).
ZOLOFT®, Oral Concentrate: ZOLOFT Oral Concentrate is a clear, colorless solution with a menthol scent containing sertraline hydrochloride equivalent to 20 mg of sertraline per mL and 12% alcohol. It is supplied as a 60 mL bottle with an accompanying calibrated dropper.
NDC 0049-4940-23 Bottles of 60 mL
Store at controlled room temperature, 59° to 86°F (15° to 30°C).
℞ only

Distributed by
Roerig
Division of Pfizer Inc, NY, NY 10017
69-4721-00-6 Revised January 2000
Shown in Product Identification Guide, page 331

ZYRTEC® ℞

(cetirizine hydrochloride)
Tablets and Syrup
For Oral Use

DESCRIPTION

Cetirizine hydrochloride, the active component of ZYRTEC® tablets and syrup, is an orally active and selective H_1-receptor antagonist. The chemical name is (±) - [2- [4- [(4-chlorophenyl)phenylmethyl] -1- piperazinyl] ethoxy] acetic acid, dihydrochloride. Cetirizine hydrochloride is a racemic compound with an empirical formula of $C_{21}H_{25}ClN_2O_3 \cdot 2HCl$. The molecular weight is 461.82 and the chemical structure is shown below:

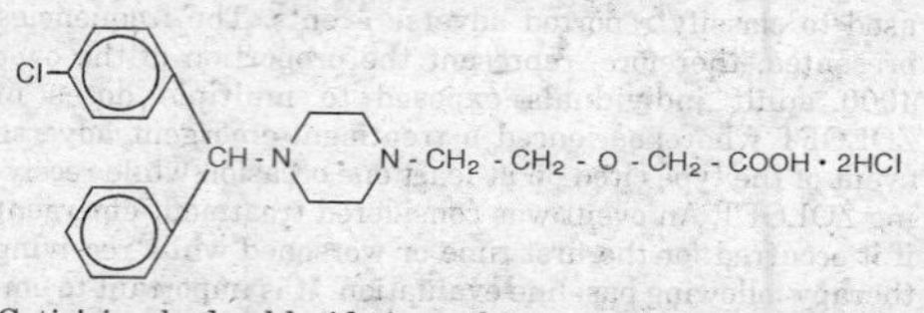

Cl — CH - N N - CH_2 - CH_2 - O - CH_2 - COOH • 2HCl

Cetirizine hydrochloride is a white, crystalline powder and is water soluble. ZYRTEC tablets are formulated as white, film-coated, rounded-off rectangular shaped tablets for oral administration and are available in 5 and 10 mg strengths. Inactive ingredients are: lactose; magnesium stearate; povidone; titanium dioxide; hydroxypropyl methylcellulose; polyethylene glycol; and corn starch.
ZYRTEC syrup is a colorless to slightly yellow syrup containing cetirizine hydrochloride at a concentration of 1 mg/mL (5 mg/5 mL) for oral administration. The pH is between 4 and 5. The inactive ingredients of the syrup are: banana flavor; glacial acetic acid; glycerin; grape flavor; methylparaben; propylene glycol; propylparaben; sodium acetate; sugar syrup; and water.

CLINICAL PHARMACOLOGY

Mechanism of Actions: Cetirizine, a human metabolite of hydroxyzine, is an antihistamine; its principal effects are mediated via selective inhibition of peripheral H_1 receptors. The antihistaminic activity of cetirizine has been clearly documented in a variety of animal and human models. *In vivo* and *ex vivo* animal models have shown negligible anticholinergic and antiserotonergic activity. In clinical studies, however, dry mouth was more common with cetirizine than with placebo. *In vitro* receptor binding studies have shown no measurable affinity for other than H_1 receptors. Autoradiographic studies with radiolabeled cetirizine in the rat have shown negligible penetration into the brain. *Ex vivo* experiments in the mouse have shown that systemically administered cetirizine does not significantly occupy cerebral H_1 receptors.
Pharmacokinetics:
Absorption: Cetirizine was rapidly absorbed with a time to maximum concentration (T_{max}) of approximately 1 hour following oral administration of tablets or syrup in adults. Comparable bioavailability was found between the tablet and syrup dosage forms. When healthy volunteers were administered multiple doses of cetirizine (10 mg tablets once daily for 10 days), a mean peak plasma concentration (C_{max}) of 311 ng/mL was observed. No accumulation was observed. Cetirizine pharmacokinetics were linear for oral doses ranging from 5 to 60 mg. Food had no effect on the extent of cetirizine exposure (AUC) but T_{max} was delayed by 1.7 hours and C_{max} was decreased by 23% in the presence of food.
Distribution: The mean plasma protein binding of cetirizine is 93%, independent of concentration in the range of 25–1000 ng/mL, which includes the therapeutic plasma levels observed.
Metabolism: A mass balance study in 6 healthy male volunteers indicated that 70% of the administered radioactivity was recovered in the urine and 10% in the feces. Approximately 50% of the radioactivity was identified in the urine as unchanged drug. Most of the rapid increase in peak plasma radioactivity was associated with parent drug, suggesting a low degree of first-pass metabolism. Cetirizine is metabolized to a limited extent by oxidative O-dealkylation to a metabolite with negligible antihistaminic activity. The enzyme or enzymes responsible for this metabolism have not been identified.
Elimination: The mean elimination half-life in 146 healthy volunteers across multiple pharmacokinetic studies was 8.3 hours and the apparent total body clearance for cetirizine was approximately 53 mL/min.
Interaction Studies
Pharmacokinetic interaction studies with cetirizine in adults were conducted with pseudoephedrine, antipyrine, ketoconazole, erythromycin and azithromycin. No interactions were observed. In a multiple dose study of theophylline (400 mg once daily for 3 days) and cetirizine (20 mg once daily for 3 days), a 16% decrease in the clearance of cetirizine was observed. The disposition of theophylline was not altered by concomitant cetirizine administration.

Special Populations

Pediatric Patients: When pediatric patients aged 7 to 12 years received a single, 5-mg oral cetirizine capsule, the mean C_{max} was 275 ng/mL. Based on cross-study comparisons, the weight-normalized, apparent total body clearance was 33% greater and the elimination half-life was 33% shorter in this pediatric population than in adults. In pediatric patients aged 2 to 5 years who received 5 mg of cetirizine, the mean C_{max} was 660 ng/mL. Based on cross-study comparisons, the weight-normalized apparent total body clearance was 81 to 111% greater and the elimination half-life was 33 to 41% shorter in this pediatric population than in adults.

Geriatric Patients: Following a single, 10-mg oral dose, the elimination half-life was prolonged by 50% and the apparent total body clearance was 40% lower in 16 geriatric subjects with a mean age of 77 years compared to 14 adult subjects with a mean age of 53 years. The decrease in cetirizine clearance in these elderly volunteers may be related to decreased renal function.

Effect of Gender: The effect of gender on cetirizine pharmacokinetics has not been adequately studied.

Effect of Race: No race-related differences in the kinetics of cetirizine have been observed.

Renal Impairment: The kinetics of cetirizine were studied following multiple, oral, 10-mg daily doses of cetirizine for 7 days in 7 normal volunteers (creatinine clearance 89–128 mL/min), 8 patients with mild renal function impairment (creatinine clearance 42–77 mL/min) and 7 patients with moderate renal function impairment (creatinine clearance 11–31 mL/min). The pharmacokinetics of cetirizine were similar in patients with mild impairment and normal volunteers. Moderately impaired patients had a 3-fold increase in half-life and a 70% decrease in clearance compared to normal volunteers.

Patients on hemodialysis (n=5) given a single, 10-mg dose of cetirizine had a 3-fold increase in half-life and a 70% decrease in clearance compared to normal volunteers. Less than 10% of the administered dose was removed during the single dialysis session.

Dosing adjustment is necessary in patients with moderate or severe renal impairment and in patients on dialysis (see **DOSAGE AND ADMINISTRATION**).

Hepatic Impairment: Sixteen patients with chronic liver diseases (hepatocellular, cholestatic, and biliary cirrhosis), given 10 to 20 mg of cetirizine as a single, oral dose had a 50% increase in half-life along with a corresponding 40% decrease in clearance compared to 16 healthy subjects.

Dosing adjustment may be necessary in patients with hepatic impairment (see **DOSAGE AND ADMINISTRATION**).

Pharmacodynamics: Studies in 69 adult normal volunteers (aged 20 to 61 years) showed that ZYRTEC at doses of 5 and 10 mg strongly inhibited the skin wheal and flare caused by the intradermal injection of histamine. The onset of this activity after a single 10-mg dose occurred within 20 minutes in 50% of subjects and within one hour in 95% of subjects; this activity persisted for at least 24 hours. ZYRTEC at doses of 5 and 10 mg also strongly inhibited the wheal and flare caused by intradermal injection of histamine in 19 pediatric volunteers (aged 5 to 12 years) and the activity persisted for at least 24 hours. In a 35-day study in children aged 5 to 12, no tolerance to the antihistaminic (suppression of wheal and flare response) effects of ZYRTEC was found. The effects of intradermal injection of various other mediators or histamine releasers were also inhibited by cetirizine, as was response to a cold challenge in patients with cold-induced urticaria. In mildly asthmatic subjects, ZYRTEC at 5 to 20 mg blocked bronchoconstriction due to nebulized histamine, with virtually total blockade after a 20-mg dose. In studies conducted for up to 12 hours following cutaneous antigen challenge, the late phase recruitment of eosinophils, neutrophils and basophils, components of the allergic inflammatory response, was inhibited by ZYRTEC at a dose of 20 mg.

In four clinical studies in healthy adult males, no clinically significant mean increases in QTc were observed in ZYRTEC treated subjects. In the first study, a placebo-controlled crossover trial, ZYRTEC was given at doses up to 60 mg per day, 6 times the maximum clinical dose, for 1 week, and no significant mean QTc prolongation occurred. In the second study, a crossover trial, ZYRTEC 20 mg and erythromycin (500 mg every 8 hours) were given alone and in combination. There was no significant effect on QTc with the combination or with ZYRTEC alone. In the third trial, also a crossover study, ZYRTEC 20 mg and ketoconazole (400 mg per day) were given alone and in combination. ZYRTEC caused a mean increase in QTc of 9.1 msec from baseline after 10 days of therapy. Ketoconazole also increased QTc by 8.3 msec. The combination caused an increase of 17.4 msec, equal to the sum of the individual effects. Thus, there was no significant drug interaction on QTc with the combination of ZYRTEC and ketoconazole. In the fourth study, a placebo-controlled parallel trial, ZYRTEC 20 mg was given alone or in combination with azithromycin (500 mg as a single dose on the first day followed by 250 mg once daily). There was no significant increase in OTc with ZYRTEC 20 mg alone or in combination with azithromycin.

In a four-week clinical trial in pediatric patients aged 6 to 11 years, results of randomly obtained ECG measurements before treatment and after 2 weeks of treatment showed that ZYRTEC 5 or 10 mg did not significantly increase QTc versus placebo. The effects of ZYRTEC on the QTc interval at doses higher than the 10 mg dose have not been studied in children less than 12 years of age. The effect of ZYRTEC on the QTc interval in children less than 6 years of age has not been studied.

In a six-week, placebo-controlled study of 186 patients (aged 12 to 64 years) with allergic rhinitis and mild to moderate asthma, ZYRTEC 10 mg once daily improved rhinitis symptoms and did not alter pulmonary function. In a two-week, placebo-controlled clinical trial, a subset analysis of 65 pediatric (aged 6 to 11 years) allergic rhinitis patients with asthma showed ZYRTEC did not alter pulmonary function. These studies support the safety of administering ZYRTEC to pediatric and adult allergic rhinitis patients with mild to moderate asthma.

Clinical Studies: Nine multicenter, randomized, double-blind, clinical trials comparing cetirizine 5 to 20 mg to placebo in patients 12 years and older with seasonal or perennial allergic rhinitis were conducted in the United States. Five of these showed significant reductions in symptoms of allergic rhinitis, 3 in seasonal allergic rhinitis (1 to 4 weeks in duration) and 2 in perennial allergic rhinitis for up to 8 weeks in duration. Two 4-week multicenter, randomized, double-blind, clinical trials comparing cetirizine 5 to 20 mg to placebo in patients with chronic idiopathic urticaria were also conducted and showed significant improvement in symptoms of chronic idiopathic urticaria. In general, the 10-mg dose was more effective than the 5-mg dose and the 20-mg dose gave no added effect. Some of these trials included pediatric patients aged 12 to 16 years. In addition, four multicenter, randomized, placebo-controlled, double-blind 2–4 week trials in 534 pediatric patients aged 6 to 11 years with seasonal allergic rhinitis were conducted in the United States at doses up to 10 mg.

INDICATIONS AND USAGE

Seasonal Allergic Rhinitis: ZYRTEC is indicated for the relief of symptoms associated with seasonal allergic rhinitis due to allergens such as ragweed, grass and tree pollens in adults and children 2 years of age and older. Symptoms treated effectively include sneezing, rhinorrhea, nasal pruritus, ocular pruritus, tearing, and redness of the eyes.

Perennial Allergic Rhinitis: ZYRTEC is indicated for the relief of symptoms associated with perennial allergic rhinitis due to allergens such as dust mites, animal dander and molds in adults and children 2 years of age and older. Symptoms treated effectively include sneezing, rhinorrhea, postnasal discharge, nasal pruritus, ocular pruritus, and tearing.

Chronic Urticaria: ZYRTEC is indicated for the treatment of the uncomplicated skin manifestations of chronic idiopathic urticaria in adults and children 2 years of age and older. It significantly reduces the occurrence, severity, and duration of hives and significantly reduces pruritus.

CONTRAINDICATIONS

ZYRTEC is contraindicated in those patients with a known hypersensitivity to it or any of its ingredients or hydroxyzine.

PRECAUTIONS

Activities Requiring Mental Alertness: In clinical trials, the occurrence of somnolence has been reported in some patients taking ZYRTEC; due caution should therefore be exercised when driving a car or operating potentially dangerous machinery. Concurrent use of ZYRTEC with alcohol or other CNS depressants should be avoided because additional reductions in alertness and additional impairment of CNS performance may occur.

Drug-Drug Interactions: No clinically significant drug interactions have been found with theophylline at a low dose, azithromycin, pseudoephedrine, ketoconazole, or erythromycin. There was a small decrease in the clearance of cetirizine caused by a 400-mg dose of theophylline; it is possible that larger theophylline doses could have a greater effect.

Carcinogenesis, Mutagenesis and Impairment of Fertility: In a 2-year carcinogenicity study in rats, cetirizine was not carcinogenic at dietary doses up to 20 mg/kg (approximately 15 times the maximum recommended daily oral dose in adults on a mg/m^2 basis, or approximately 10 times the maximum recommended daily oral dose in children on a mg/m^2 basis). In a 2-year carcinogenicity study in mice, cetirizine caused an increased incidence of benign liver tumors in males at a dietary dose of 16 mg/kg (approximately 6 times the maximum recommended daily oral dose in adults on a mg/m^2 basis, or approximately 4 times the maximum recommended daily oral dose in children on a mg/m^2 basis). No increase in the incidence of liver tumors was observed in mice at a dietary dose of 4 mg/kg (approximately 2 times the maximum recommended daily oral dose in adults on a mg/m^2 basis, or approximately equal to the maximum recommended daily oral dose in children on a mg/m^2 basis). The clinical significance of these findings during long-term use of ZYRTEC is not known.

Cetirizine was not mutagenic in the Ames test, and not clastogenic in the human lymphocyte assay, the mouse lymphoma assay, and *in vivo* micronucleus test in rats.

In a fertility and general reproductive performance study in mice, cetirizine did not impair fertility at an oral dose of 64 mg/kg (approximately 25 times the maximum recommended daily oral dose in adults on a mg/m^2 basis).

Pregnancy Category B: In mice, rats, and rabbits, cetirizine was not teratogenic at oral doses up to 96, 225, and 135 mg/kg, respectively (approximately 40, 180 and 220 times the maximum recommended daily oral dose in adults on a mg/m^2 basis). There are no adequate and well-controlled studies in pregnant women. Because animal studies are not always predictive of human response, ZYRTEC should be used in pregnancy only if clearly needed.

Nursing Mothers: In mice, cetirizine caused retarded pup weight gain during lactation at an oral dose in dams of 96 mg/kg (approximately 40 times the maximum recommended daily oral dose in adults on a mg/m^2 basis). Studies in beagle dogs indicated that approximately 3% of the dose was excreted in milk. Cetirizine has been reported to be excreted in human breast milk. Because many drugs are excreted in human milk, use of ZYRTEC in nursing mothers is not recommended.

Geriatric Use: Of the total number of patients in clinical studies of ZYRTEC, 186 patients were 65 years and older, and 39 patients were 75 years and older. No overall differences in safety were observed between these patients and younger patients, but greater sensitivity of some older individuals cannot be ruled out. With regard to efficacy, clinical studies of ZYRTEC for each approved indication did not include sufficient numbers of patients aged 65 years and older to determine whether they respond differently than younger patients.

ZYRTEC is known to be substantially excreted by the kidney, and the risk of toxic reactions to this drug may be greater in patients with impaired renal function. Because elderly patients are more likely to have decreased renal function, care should be taken in dose selection, and it may be useful to monitor renal function. (See Geriatric Patients and Renal Impairment subsections in CLINICAL PHARMACOLOGY).

Pediatric Use: The safety of ZYRTEC, at daily doses of 5 or 10 mg, has been demonstrated in 376 pediatric patients aged 6 to 11 years in placebo-controlled trials lasting up to four weeks and in 254 patients in a non-placebo-controlled 12-week trial. The safety of cetirizine has been demonstrated in 168 patients aged 2 to 5 years in placebo-controlled trials of up to 4 weeks duration. On a mg/kg basis, most of the 168 patients received between 0.2 and 0.4 mg/kg of cetirizine HCl.

The effectiveness of ZYRTEC for the treatment of seasonal and perennial allergic rhinitis and chronic idiopathic urticaria in pediatric patients aged 2 to 11 years is based on an extrapolation of the demonstrated efficacy of ZYRTEC in adults in these conditions and the likelihood that the disease course, pathophysiology and the drug's effect are substantially similar between these two populations. The recommended doses for the pediatric population are based on cross-study comparisons of the pharmacokinetics and pharmacodynamics of cetirizine in adult and pediatric subjects and on the safety profile of cetirizine in both adult and pediatric patients at doses equal to or higher than the recommended doses. The cetirizine AUC and C_{max} in pediatric subjects aged 2 to 5 years who received a single dose of 5 mg of cetirizine syrup and in pediatric subjects aged 6 to 11 years who received a single dose of 10 mg of cetirizine syrup were estimated to be intermediate between that observed in adults who received a single dose of 10 mg of cetirizine tablets and those who received a single dose of 20 mg of cetirizine tablets.

The safety and effectiveness of cetirizine in pediatric patients under the age of 2 years have not yet been established.

ADVERSE REACTIONS

Controlled and uncontrolled clinical trials conducted in the United States and Canada included more than 6000 patients aged 12 years and older, with more than 3900 receiving ZYRTEC at doses of 5 to 20 mg per day. The duration of treatment ranged from 1 week to 6 months, with a mean exposure of 30 days.

Most adverse reactions reported during therapy with ZYRTEC were mild or moderate. In placebo-controlled trials, the incidence of discontinuations due to adverse reactions in patients receiving ZYRTEC 5 or 10 mg was not significantly different from placebo (2.9% vs. 2.4%, respectively).

The most common adverse reaction in patients aged 12 years and older that occurred more frequently on ZYRTEC than placebo was somnolence. The incidence of somnolence associated with ZYRTEC was dose related, 6% in placebo, 11% at 5 mg and 14% at 10 mg. Discontinuations due to somnolence for ZYRTEC was uncommon (1.0% on ZYRTEC vs. 0.6% on placebo). Fatigue and dry mouth also appeared to be treatment-related adverse reactions. There were no differences by age, race, gender or by body weight with regard to the incidence of adverse reactions.

Table 1 lists adverse experiences in patients aged 12 years and older which were reported for ZYRTEC 5 and 10 mg in controlled clinical trials in the United States and that were more common with ZYRTEC than placebo.

Table 1.
Adverse Experiences Reported in Patients Aged 12 Years and Older in Placebo-Controlled United States ZYRTEC Trials (Maximum Dose of 10 mg) at Rates of 2% or Greater (Percent Incidence)

Adverse Experience	ZYRTEC (N=2034)	Placebo (N=1612)
Somnolence	13.7	6.3
Fatigue	5.9	2.6
Dry Mouth	5.0	2.3

Continued on next page

Zyrtec—Cont.

Pharyngitis	2.0	1.9
Dizziness	2.0	1.2

In addition, headache and nausea occurred in more than 2% of the patients, but were more common in placebo patients.
Pediatric studies were also conducted with ZYRTEC. More than 1300 pediatric patients aged 6 to 11 years with more than 900 treated with ZYRTEC at doses of 1.25 to 10 mg per day were included in controlled and uncontrolled clinical trials conducted in the United States. The duration of treatment ranged from 2 to 12 weeks. Placebo-controlled trials up to 4 weeks duration included 168 pediatric patients aged 2 to 5 years who received cetirizine, the majority of whom received single daily doses of 5 mg.
The majority of adverse reactions reported in pediatric patients aged 2 to 11 years with ZYRTEC were mild or moderate. In placebo-controlled trials, the incidence of discontinuations due to adverse reactions in pediatric patients receiving up to 10 mg of ZYRTEC was uncommon (0.4% on ZYRTEC vs. 1.0% on placebo).
Table 2 lists adverse experiences which were reported for ZYRTEC 5 and 10 mg in pediatric patients aged 6 to 11 years in placebo-controlled clinical trials in the United States and were more common with ZYRTEC than placebo. Of these, abdominal pain was considered treatment-related and somnolence appeared to be dose-related, 1.3% in placebo, 1.9% at 5 mg and 4.2% at 10 mg. The adverse experiences reported in pediatric patients aged 2 to 5 years in placebo-controlled trials were qualitatively similar in nature and generally similar in frequency to those reported in trials with children aged 6 to 11 years.

Table 2.
Adverse Experiences Reported in Pediatric Patients Aged 6 to 11 Years in Placebo-Controlled United States ZYRTEC Trials (5 or 10 mg Dose) Which Occurred at a Frequency of ≥2% in Either the 5-mg or the 10-mg ZYRTEC Group, and More Frequently Than in the Placebo Group

Adverse Experiences	Placebo (N=309)	ZYRTEC 5 mg (N=161)	ZYRTEC 10 mg (N=215)
Headache	12.3%	11.0%	14.0%
Pharyngitis	2.9%	6.2%	2.8%
Abdominal pain	1.9%	4.4%	5.6%
Coughing	3.9%	4.4%	2.8%
Somnolence	1.3%	1.9%	4.2%
Diarrhea	1.3%	3.1%	1.9%
Epistaxis	2.9%	3.7%	1.9%
Bronchospasm	1.9%	3.1%	1.9%
Nausea	1.9%	1.9%	2.8%
Vomiting	1.0%	2.5%	2.3%

The following events were observed infrequently (less than 2%), in either 3982 adults and children 12 years and older or in 659 pediatric patients aged 6 to 11 years who received ZYRTEC in U.S. trials, including an open adult study of six months duration. A causal relationship of these infrequent events with ZYRTEC administration has not been established.
Autonomic Nervous System: anorexia, flushing, increased salivation, urinary retention.
Cardiovascular: cardiac failure, hypertension, palpitation, tachycardia.
Central and Peripheral Nervous Systems: abnormal coordination, ataxia, confusion, dysphonia, hyperesthesia, hyperkinesia, hypertonia, hypoesthesia, leg cramps, migraine, myelitis, paralysis, paresthesia, ptosis, syncope, tremor, twitching, vertigo, visual field defect.
Gastrointestinal: abnormal hepatic function, aggravated tooth caries, constipation, dyspepsia, eructation, flatulence, gastritis, hemorrhoids, increased appetite, melena, rectal hemorrhage, stomatitis including ulcerative stomatitis, tongue discoloration, tongue edema.
Genitourinary: cystitis, dysuria, hematuria, micturition frequency, polyuria, urinary incontinence, urinary tract infection.
Hearing and Vestibular: deafness, earache, ototoxicity, tinnitus.
Metabolic/Nutritional: dehydration, diabetes mellitus, thirst.
Musculoskeletal: arthralgia, arthritis, arthrosis, muscle weakness, myalgia.
Psychiatric: abnormal thinking, agitation, amnesia, anxiety, decreased libido, depersonalization, depression, emotional lability, euphoria, impaired concentration, insomnia, nervousness, paroniria, sleep disorder.
Respiratory System: bronchitis, dyspnea, hyperventilation, increased sputum, pneumonia, respiratory disorder, rhinitis, sinusitis, upper respiratory tract infection.
Reproductive: dysmenorrhea, female breast pain, intermenstrual bleeding, leukorrhea, menorrhagia, vaginitis.
Reticuloendothelial: lymphadenopathy.
Skin: acne, alopecia, angioedema, bullous eruption, dermatitis, dry skin, eczema, erythematous rash, furunculosis, hyperkeratosis, hypertrichosis, increased sweating, maculopapular rash, photosensitivity reaction, photosensitivity toxic reaction, pruritus, purpura, rash, seborrhea, skin disorder, skin nodule, urticaria.
Special Senses: parosmia, taste loss, taste perversion.
Vision: blindness, conjunctivitis, eye pain, glaucoma, loss of accommodation, ocular hemorrhage, xerophthalmia.
Body as a Whole: accidental injury, asthenia, back pain, chest pain, enlarged abdomen, face edema, fever, generalized edema, hot flashes, increased weight, leg edema, malaise, nasal polyp, pain, pallor, periorbital edema, peripheral edema, rigors.
Occasional instances of transient, reversible hepatic transaminase elevations have occurred during cetirizine therapy. Hepatitis with significant transaminase elevation and elevated bilirubin in association with the use of ZYRTEC has been reported.
In foreign marketing experience the following additional rare, but potentially severe adverse events have been reported: anaphylaxis, cholestasis, glomerulonephritis, hemolytic anemia, hepatitis, orofacial dyskinesia, severe hypotension, stillbirth, and thrombocytopenia.

DRUG ABUSE AND DEPENDENCE

There is no information to indicate that abuse or dependency occurs with ZYRTEC.

OVERDOSAGE

Overdosage has been reported with ZYRTEC. In one adult patient who took 150 mg of ZYRTEC, the patient was somnolent but did not display any other clinical signs or abnormal blood chemistry or hematology results. In an 18 month old pediatric patient who took an overdose of ZYRTEC (approximately 180 mg), restlessness and irritability were observed initially; this was followed by drowsiness. Should overdose occur, treatment should be symptomatic or supportive, taking into account any concomitantly ingested medications. There is no known specific antidote to ZYRTEC. ZYRTEC is not effectively removed by dialysis, and dialysis will be ineffective unless a dialyzable agent has been concomitantly ingested. The acute minimal lethal oral doses were 237 mg/kg in mice (approximately 95 times the maximum recommended daily oral dose in adults on a mg/m^2 basis, or approximately 55 times the maximum recommended daily oral dose in children on a mg/m^2 basis) and 562 mg/kg in rats (approximately 460 times the maximum recommended daily oral dose in adults on a mg/m^2 basis, or approximately 270 times the maximum recommended daily oral dose in children on a mg/m^2 basis). In rodents, the target of acute toxicity was the central nervous system, and the target of multiple-dose toxicity was the liver.

DOSAGE AND ADMINISTRATION

Adults and Children 12 Years and Older: The recommended initial dose of ZYRTEC is 5 or 10 mg per day in adults and children 12 years and older, depending on symptom severity. Most patients in clinical trials started at 10 mg. ZYRTEC is given as a single daily dose, with or without food. The time of administration may be varied to suit individual patient needs.
Children 6 to 11 Years: The recommended initial dose of ZYRTEC in children aged 6 to 11 years is 5 or 10 mg (1 or 2 teaspoons) once daily depending on symptom severity. The time of administration may be varied to suit individual patient needs.
Children 2 to 5 Years: The recommended initial dose of ZYRTEC syrup in children aged 2 to 5 years is 2.5 mg (½ teaspoon) once daily. The dosage in this age group can be increased to a maximum dose of 5 mg per day given as 1 teaspoon (5 mg) once daily, or as ½ teaspoon (2.5 mg) given every 12 hours, depending on symptom severity and patient response.
Dose Adjustment for Renal and Hepatic Impairment: In patients 12 years of age and older with decreased renal function (creatinine clearance 11–31 mL/min), patients on hemodialysis (creatinine clearance less than 7 mL/min), and in hepatically impaired patients, a dose of 5 mg once daily is recommended. Similarly, pediatric patients aged 6 to 11 years with impaired renal or hepatic function should use the lower recommended dose. Because of the difficulty in reliably administering doses of less than 2.5 mg (½ teaspoon) of ZYRTEC syrup and in the absence of pharmacokinetic and safety information for cetirizine in children below the age of 6 years with impaired renal or hepatic function, its use in this impaired patient population is not recommended.

HOW SUPPLIED

ZYRTEC® tablets are white, film-coated, rounded-off rectangular shaped containing 5 mg or 10 mg cetirizine hydrochloride.
5 mg tablets are engraved with "ZYRTEC" on one side and "5" on the other.
Bottles of 100: NDC 0069-5500-66
10 mg tablets are engraved with "ZYRTEC" on one side and "10" on the other.
Bottles of 100: NDC 0069-5510-66
STORAGE: Store at room temperature 59° to 86°F (15° to 30°C).
ZYRTEC® syrup is colorless to slightly yellow with a banana-grape flavor. Each teaspoonful (5 mL) contains 5 mg cetirizine hydrochloride. ZYRTEC® syrup is supplied as follows:
120 mL amber glass bottles NDC 0069-5530-47
1 pint amber glass bottles NDC 0069-5530-93
STORAGE: Store at 41° to 86°F (5° to 30°C).
Cetirizine is licensed from UCB Pharma, Inc.

Manufactured/Marketed by
Pfizer Labs
Division of Pfizer Inc, NY, NY 10017
Marketed by
UCB Pharma, Inc.
Smyrna, GA 30080
70-4573-00-4 Revised March 2000

Shown in Product Identification Guide, page 331

Pfizer Labs Division

235 EAST 42ND STREET
NEW YORK, NY 10017-5755

For Medical Information Contact:
24 hours a day, seven days a week:
(800) 438-1985

Distribution:
1855 Shelby Oaks Drive North
Memphis, TN 38134
(901) 387-5200
Customer Service:
(800) 533-4535

EXPORT INQUIRIES:
Pfizer International Inc.
(212) 573-2323

(See Pfizer Inc.)

Pharmaceutical Associates, Inc.

A Subsidiary of Beach Products, Inc.
201 DELAWARE STREET
GREENVILLE, SC 29605

Direct Inquiries to:
Clete Harmon, Director of Q.A.
PH: (800) 845-8210
(864) 277-7282
FAX: (864) 277-8045

HOSPITAL UNIT DOSE / TRADE PACKAGE

NDC Prefix: 00121-

PRODUCT LISTING

ACETAMINOPHEN ORAL SOLUTION USP OTC
(160 mg per 5 mL)
Unit Dose 10.15 mL and 20.3 mL

ACETAMINOPHEN and CODEINE PHOSPHATE ORAL SOLUTION USP ©℞
(120 mg/12 mg per 5 mL)
Unit Dose 5 mL, 10 mL, 12.5 mL, and 15 mL
Bottles of 4 fl oz and 16 fl oz

ALUMINUM HYDROXIDE GEL USP OTC
(320 mg per 5 mL)
Unit Dose 30 mL
Bottles of 12 fl oz and 16 fl oz

ALUMINUM HYDROXIDE GEL CONCENTRATE OTC
(600 mg per 5 mL)
Bottles of 12 fl oz

AMANTADINE HYDROCHLORIDE SYRUP USP ℞
(50 mg per 5 mL)
Unit Dose 10 mL and 20 mL
Bottles of 16 fl oz

AROMATIC CASCARA FLUIDEXTRACT USP OTC
Unit Dose 5 mL

CHLORAL HYDRATE SYRUP USP ©℞
(500 mg per 5 mL)
Unit Dose 5 mL

CIMETIDINE HYDROCHLORIDE ORAL SOLUTION ℞
(300 mg per 5 mL)
Bottles of 8 fl oz

DIPHENHYDRAMINE HYDROCHLORIDE ELIXIR USP ℞
(12.5 mg per 5 mL)
Unit Dose 5 mL, 10 mL, and 20 mL

DOCUSATE SODIUM LIQUID OTC
(50 mg per 5 mL)
Unit Dose 10 mL and 25 mL
Bottles of 16 fl oz

DOCUSATE SODIUM SYRUP USP OTC
(20 mg per 5 mL)
Unit Dose 25 ml
Bottles of 16 fl oz

DOCUSATE SODIUM with CASANTHRANOL OTC
(20 mg/10 mg per 5 mL)
Unit Dose 15 mL and 30 mL
Bottles of 16 fl oz

FERROUS SULFATE LIQUID OTC
(300 mg per 5 mL)
Unit Dose 5 mL

FLUPHENAZINE HYDROCHLORIDE ELIXIR USP ℞
(2.5 mg per 5 mL)
Bottles of 60 mL and 16 fl oz

FLUPHENAZINE HYDROCHLORIDE ORAL SOLUTION USP Concentrate ℞
(5 mg per 1 mL)
Bottles of 4 fl oz

GUAIFENESIN SYRUP USP OTC
(100 mg per 5 mL)
Unit Dose 5 mL, 10 mL, and 15 mL
Bottles of 4 fl oz

GUAIFENESIN SYRUP with CODEINE CV OTC
(100 mg/10 mg per 5 mL)
Unit Dose 5 mL and 10 mL
Bottles of 4 fl oz and 16 fl oz

GUAIFENESIN SYRUP and DEXTROMETHORPHAN OTC
(100 mg/10 mg per 5 mL)
Unit Dose 5 mL and 10 mL
Bottles of 4 fl oz

HALOPERIDOL ORAL SOLUTION USP Concentrate ℞
(2 mg per 1 mL)
Unit Dose 5 mL and 10 mL
Bottles of 4 fl oz

HYDROCODONE BITARTRATE and ACETAMINOPHEN ELIXIR CIII ℞
(7.5 mg/500 mg per 15 mL)
Unit Dose 15 mL
Bottles of 4 fl oz and 16 fl oz

HYDROCODONE BITARTRATE and GUAIFENESIN EXPECTORANT CIII ℞
(5 mg/100 mg per 5 mL)
Bottles of 16 fl oz

LACTULOSE SOLUTION USP ℞
(10 g per 15 mL)
Unit Dose 30 mL

METOCLOPRAMIDE ORAL SOLUTION USP ℞
(5 mg per 5 mL)
Unit Dose 10 mL
Bottles of 16 fl oz

MILK OF MAGNESIA USP OTC
(400 mg per 5 mL)
Unit Dose 30 mL

MILK OF MAGNESIA CONCENTRATE OTC
(2400 mg per 10 mL)
Unit Dose 10 mL

MILK OF MAGNESIA CASCARA SUSPENSION OTC
(2400 mg/5 mL per 30 mL)
Unit Dose 15 mL and 30 mL
Bottles of 4 fl oz

MINERAL OIL OTC
Unit Dose 30 mL

OXYBUTYNIN CHLORIDE SYRUP USP ℞
(5 mg per 5 mL)
Unit Dose 5 mL
Bottles of 16 fl oz

PHENOBARBITAL ELIXIR CIV ℞
(20 mg per 5 mL)
Unit Dose 5 mL, 7.5 mL, and 15 mL

POTASSIUM CHLORIDE ORAL SOLUTION USP 10% ℞
(20 mEq per 15 mL)
Unit Dose 15 mL and 30 mL

POTASSIUM CHLORIDE ORAL SOLUTION USP 20% ℞
(40 mEq per 15 mL)
Unit Dose 15 mL

POTASSIUM CITRATE and CITRIC ACID ORAL SOLUTION USP ℞
(1100 mg/334 mg per 5 mL)
Bottles of 16 fl oz

PROMETHAZINE HYDROCHLORIDE and CODEINE PHOSPHATE SYRUP CV ℞
(6.25 mg/10 mg per 5 mL)
Unit Dose 5 mL

PSEUDOEPHEDRINE HYDROCHLORIDE SYRUP USP OTC
(30 mg per 5 mL)
Bottles of 4 fl oz

SODIUM CITRATE and CITRIC ACID ORAL SOLUTION USP ℞
(500 mg/334 mg per 5 mL)
Unit Dose 15 mL and 30 mL
Bottles of 16 fl oz

SORBITOL SOLUTION USP OTC
(70% w/w)
Unit Dose 30 mL
Bottles of 16 fl oz

SORE THROAT SPRAY OTC
(Phenol 1.4%) Cherry
Bottles of 6 fl oz

THIORIDAZINE HYDROCHLORIDE ORAL SOLUTION USP Concentrate ℞
(30 mg per 1 mL)
Bottles of 4 fl oz
(100 mg per 1 mL)
Bottles of 4 fl oz

TRICITRATES ORAL SOLUTION ℞
(550 mg/500 mg/334 mg per 5 mL)
Bottles of 16 fl oz

TRIHEXYPHENIDYL HYDROCHLORIDE ELIXIR USP ℞
(2 mg per 5 mL)
Unit Dose 5 mL
Bottles of 16 fl oz

Pharmacia & Upjohn

100 ROUTE 206 NORTH
PEAPACK, NEW JERSEY 07977

Direct Inquiries to:
1-888-768-5501

For Medical and Pharmaceutical Information, Including Emergencies, Contact:
(616) 833-8244

PRODUCT IDENTIFICATION
Prescription capsules and tablets manufactured by Pharmacia & Upjohn Company are imprinted with one or a combination of the following: (1) Product trademark, (2) Dosage strength, (3) "Adria," "Pharmacia," "Upjohn," "U," or the code "KP." That portion of the National Drug Code (NDC) number that indicates product and strength.
A list of oral solid dosage forms with NDC product identification numbers is provided below.

Code #	Product	Strength
01	**DOSTINEX®** Tablets (carbergoline tablets)	0.5 mg
02	**MIRAPEX®** Tablets (pramipexole dihydrochloride tablets) *See Product Identification Guide*	0.125 mg
04	**MIRAPEX®** Tablets (pramipexole dihydrochloride tablets) *See Product Identification Guide*	0.25 mg
06	**MIRAPEX®** Tablets (pramipexole dihydrochloride tablets) *See Product Identification Guide*	1 mg
08	**MIRAPEX®** Tablets (pramipexole dihydrochloride tablets) *See Product Identification Guide*	0.5 mg
10	**HALCION®**Tablets (triazolam tablets, USP) *See Product Identification Guide*	0.125 mg
12	**CORTEF®** Tablets (hydrocortisone tablets, USP)	5 mg
14	**HALOTESTIN®** Tablets (fluoxymesterone tablets, USP)	2 mg
15	**CORTISONE ACETATE** Tablets, USP	5 mg
17	**HALCION®** Tablets (triazolam tablets, USP) *See Product Identification Guide*	0.25 mg
18	**DIDREX®** Tablets (benzphetamine hydrochloride tablets)	50 mg
19	**HALOTESTIN®** Tablets (fluoxymesterone tablets, USP)	5 mg
23	**CORTISONE ACETATE** Tablets, USP	10 mg
29	**XANAX®** Tablets (alprazolam tablets, USP) *See Product Identification Guide*	0.25 mg
31	**CORTEF®** Tablets (hydrocortisone tablets, USP)	10 mg
32	**DELTASONE®** Tablets (prednisone tablets, USP)	2.5 mg
32	**EMCYT** Capsules (estramustine phosphate sodium)	140 mg
34	**CORTISONE ACETATE** Tablets, USP	25 mg
36	**HALOTESTIN®** Tablets (fluoxymesterone tablets, USP)	10 mg
37	**MIRAPEX®** Tablets (pramipexole dihydrochloride tablets) *See Product Identification Guide*	1.5 mg
41	**DETROL®** Tablets (tolterodine tartrate tablets) *See Product Identification Guide*	2 mg
44	**CORTEF®** Tablets (hydrocortisone tablets, USP)	20 mg
45	**DELTASONE®** Tablets (prednisone tablets, USP)	5 mg
49	**MEDROL®** Tablets (methylprednisolone tablets, USP)	2 mg
50	**PROVERA®** Tablets (medroxyprogesterone acetate tablets, USP) *See Product Identification Guide*	10 mg
55	**XANAX®** Tablets (alprazolam tablets, USP) *See Product Identification Guide*	0.5 mg
64	**PROVERA®** Tablets (medroxyprogesterone acetate tablets, USP) *See Product Identification Guide*	2.5 mg
90	**XANAX®** Tablets (alprazolam tablets, USP) *See Product Identification Guide*	1 mg
94	**XANAX®** Tablets (alprazolam tablets, USP) *See Product Identification Guide*	2 mg
100	**ORINASE®** Tablets (tolbutamide tablets, USP)	500 mg
101	**ALBAMYCIN®** Capsules (novobiocin sodium capsules)	250 mg
101	**AZULFIDINE** Tablets (sulfasalazine)	500 mg
102	**AZULFIDINE EN-tabs** (sulfasalazine delayed release) *See Product Identification Guide*	500 mg
105	**DIPENTUM** Capsules (olsalazine sodium)	250 mg
121	**LONITEN®** Tablets (minoxidil tablets, USP)	2.5 mg
131	**MICRONASE®** Tablets (glyburide tablets)	1.25 mg
137	**LONITEN®** Tablets (minoxidil tablets, USP)	10 mg
141	**MICRONASE®** Tablets (glyburide tablets)	2.5 mg
165	**DELTASONE®** Tablets (prednisone tablets, USP)	20 mg
171	**MICRONASE®**Tablets (glyburide tablets)	5 mg
193	**DELTASONE®** Tablets (prednisone tablets, USP)	10 mg
225	**CLEOCIN HCl®** Capsules (clindamycin hydrochloride capsules, USP)	150 mg
286	**PROVERA®** Tablets (medroxyprogesterone acetate tablets, USP) *See Product Identification Guide*	5 mg
301	**MYCOBUTIN** (rifabutin capsules) *See Product Identification Guide*	150 mg
331	**CLEOCIN HCl®** Capsules (clindamycin hydrochloride capsules, USP)	75 mg
341	**GLYNASE®** PresTab® Tablets (micronized glyburide tablets)	1.5 mg
352	**GLYNASE®** PresTab® Tablets (micronized glyburide tablets)	3 mg
388	**DELTASONE®** Tablets (prednisone tablets, USP)	50 mg
395	**CLEOCIN HCl®** Capsules (clindamycin hydrochloride capsules, USP)	300 mg
450	**COLESTID®** Tablets (micronized colestipol hydrochloride)	1 g
500	**LINCOCIN®** Capsules (lincomycin hydrochloride capsules, USP)	500 mg
617	**VANTIN®** Tablets (cefpodoxime proxetil tablets) *See Product Identification Guide*	100 mg
618	**VANTIN®** Tablets (cefpodoxime proxetil tablets) *See Product Identification Guide*	200 mg
3449	**GLYNASE®** PresTab Tablets (micronized glyburide tablets)	6 mg
3772	**OGEN®** Tablets (estropipate tablets, USP)	0.75 mg
3773	**OGEN®** Tablets (estropipate tablets, USP)	1.5 mg
3774	**OGEN®** Tablets (estropipate tablets, USP)	3 mg

ACTIVELLA™ ℞

estradiol/norethindrone acetate tablets
1 mg estradiol
0.5 mg norethindrone acetate

DESCRIPTION

Activella™ is a single tablet containing an estrogen, estradiol (E_2), and a progestin, norethindrone acetate (NETA),

Continued on next page

Information on these Pharmacia & Upjohn products is based on labeling in effect June 1, 2000. Further information concerning these and other Pharmacia & Upjohn products may be obtained by direct inquiry to Medical Information, Pharmacia & Upjohn, Kalamazoo, MI 49001.

Activella—Cont.

for oral administration. Each tablet contains 1 mg estradiol and 0.5 mg norethindrone acetate and the following excipients: lactose monohydrate, starch (corn), copovidone, talc, magnesium stearate, hydroxypropyl methylcellulose and triacetin.

Estradiol (E_2) is a white or almost white crystalline powder. Its chemical name is estra-1, 3, 5 (10)-triene-3, 17β-diol hemihydrate with the empirical formula of $C_{18}H_{24}O_2$, 1/2 H_2O and a molecular weight of 281.4. The structural formula of E_2 is as follows:

Estradiol

Norethindrone acetate (NETA) is a white or yellowish-white crystalline powder. Its chemical name is 17β-acetoxy-19-nor-17α-pregn-4-en-20-yn-3-one with the empirical formula of $C_{22}H_{28}O_3$ and a molecular weight of 340.5. The structural formula of NETA is as follows:

Norethindrone Acetate

CLINICAL PHARMACOLOGY

Estrogen drug products act by regulating the transcription of a limited number of genes. Estrogens diffuse through cell membranes and bind to and activate the nuclear estrogen receptor, a DNA-binding protein that is found in estrogen-responsive tissues. The activated estrogen receptor binds to specific DNA sequences, or hormone-response elements, that enhance the transcription of adjacent genes and in turn lead to the observed effects. Estrogen receptors have been identified in tissues of the reproductive tract, breast, pituitary, hypothalamus, liver, and bone in women.

Estrogens are largely responsible for the development and maintenance of the female reproductive system and secondary sexual characteristics. Although circulating estrogens exist in a dynamic equilibrium of metabolic interconversions, estradiol is the principal intracellular human estrogen and is substantially more potent than its metabolites, estrone and estriol, at the receptor level. The primary source of estrogen is normally cycling adult women is the ovarian follicle, which secretes 70 to 500 µg of estradiol daily, depending on the phase of the menstrual cycle. After menopause, most endogenous estrogen is produced by conversion in peripheral tissues of androstenedione which is secreted by the adrenal cortex, to estrone. Thus, estrone and the sulfate conjugated form, estrone sulfate, are the most abundant circulating estrogens in postmenopausal women.

Circulating estrogens modulate the pituitary secretion of the gonadotropins, luteinizing hormone (LH), and follicle-stimulating hormone (FSH) through a negative feedback mechanism, and estrogen replacement therapy acts to reduce the elevated levels of these hormones seen in postmenopausal women. Progestin compounds enhance cellular differentiation and generally oppose the actions of estrogens by decreasing estrogen receptor levels, increasing local metabolism of estrogens to less active metabolites, or inducing gene products that blunt cellular responses to estrogen.

Progestins exert their effects in target cells by binding to specific progesterone receptors that interact with progesterone response elements in target genes. Progesterone receptors have been identified in the female reproductive tract, breast, pituitary, hypothalamus, and central nervous system. Progestins produce similar endometrial changes to those of the naturally occurring hormone progesterone.

The use of unopposed estrogen therapy has been associated with an increased risk of endometrial hyperplasia, a possible precursor of endometrial adenocarcinoma. The addition of a progestin, in adequate doses and appropriate duration, to an estrogen replacement regimen reduces the incidence of endometrial hyperplasia, and the attendant risk of carcinoma in women with intact uterus.

PHARMACOKINETICS

ABSORPTION

Estradiol is well absorbed through the gastrointestinal tract. Following oral administration of Activella™ (estradiol/norethindrone acetate tablets), peak plasma estradiol concentrations are reached slowly within 5–8 hours. When given orally, estradiol is extensively metabolized (first-pass effect) to estrone sulfate, with smaller amounts of other conjugated and unconjugated estrogens. After oral administration, norethindrone acetate is rapidly absorbed and transformed to norethindrone. It undergoes first-pass metabolism in the liver and other enteric organs, and reaches a peak plasma concentration within 0.5–1.5 hours. The oral bioavailability of estradiol and norethindrone following administration of Activella™ when compared to a combination oral solution is 53% and 100%, respectively. The pharmacokinetic parameters of estradiol (E_2). estrone (E_1), and norethindrone (NET) following single oral administration of Activella™ in 25 volunteers are summarized in TABLE 1.

TABLE 1
PHARMACOKINETIC PARAMETERS AFTER A SINGLE DOSE OF ACTIVELLA™ IN HEALTHY POSTMENOPAUSAL WOMEN

	Activella™ (n=25) Mean[c] ± SD
Estradiol [a] (E_2)	
AUC (0–72h)(pg/ml*h)	1053 ± 310
C_{max} (pg/ml)	34.6 ± 10.8
t_{max} (h)	6.8 ± 2.9
$t_{1/2}$ (h) [d]	13.2 ± 4.7
Estrone [a] (E_1)	
AUC (0–72h)(pg/ml*h)	5223 ± 1618
C_{max} (pg/ml)	251.1 ± 91.0
t_{max} (h)	5.7 ± 1.4
$t_{1/2}$ (h) [d]	12.2 ± 4.6
Norethindrone (NET)	
AUC (0–72h)(pg/ml*h)	23681 ± 9023[b]
C_{max} (pg/ml)	5308 ± 1510
t_{max} (h)	1.0 ± 0.0
$t_{1/2}$ (h)	11.4 ± 2.7

AUC = area under the curve,
C_{max} = maximum plasma concentration,
t_{max} = time at maximum plasma concentration,
$t_{1/2}$ = half-life,
SD = standard deviation
[a] baseline unadjusted data; [b] (n=23); [c] arithmetic mean;
[d] baseline adjusted data

Following continuous dosing with once-daily administration of Activella™ (estradiol/norethindrone acetate tablets), serum levels of estradiol, estrone, and norethindrone reached steady-state within two weeks with an accumulation of 33–47% above levels following single dose adminstration. Unadjusted circulating levels of E_2, E_1, and NET during Activella™ treatment at steady state (dosing at time 0) are provided in Figures 1a and 1b.

Figure 1a
Levels of Estradiol and Estrone at Steady State during Continuous Dosing with Activella™ (n=24)

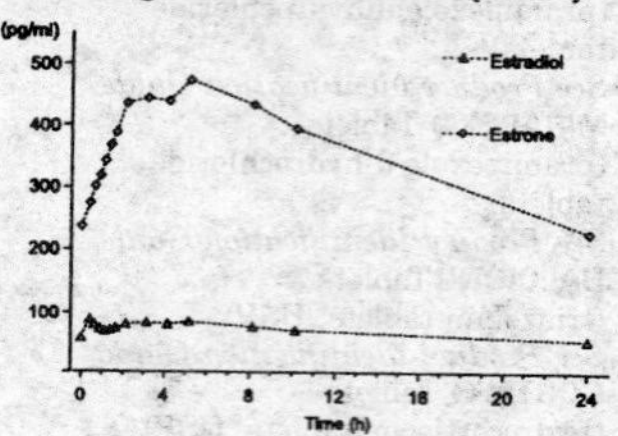

Figure 1b
Levels of Norethindrone at Steady State during Continuous Dosing with Activella™ (n=24)

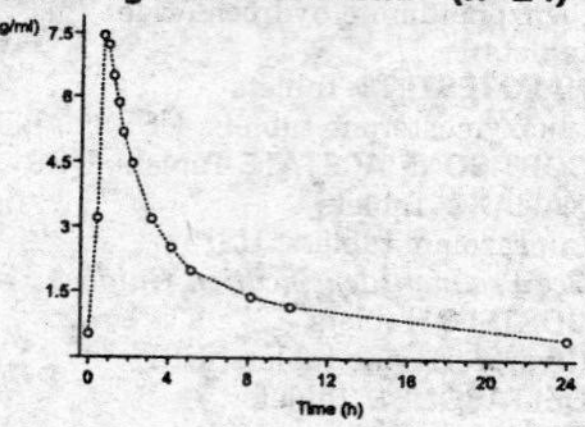

DISTRIBUTION

The distribution of exogenous estrogens is similar to that of endogenous estrogens. Estrogens are widely distributed in the body and are generally found in higher concentrations in the sex hormone target organs. Estradiol circulates in the blood bound to sex-hormone-binding globulin (SHBG) (37%) and to albumin (61%), while only approximately 1–2% is unbound. Norethindrone also binds to a similar extent to SHBG (36%) and to albumin (61%).

METABOLISM AND EXCRETION

Estradiol: Exogenous estrogens are metabolized in the same manner as endogenous estrogens. Circulating estrogens exist in a dynamic equilibrium of metabolic interconversions. These transformations take place mainly in the liver. Estradiol is converted reversibly to estrone, and both can be converted to estriol, which is the major urinary metabolite.

Estrogens also undergo enterohepatic recirculation via sulfate and glucuronide conjugation in the liver, biliary secretion of conjugates into the intestine, and hydrolysis in the gut followed by reabsorption. In postmenopausal women, a significant portion of the circulating estrogens exist as sulfate conjugates, especially estrone sulfate, which serves as a circulating reservoir for the formation of more active estrogens. The half-life of estradiol following single dose administration of Activella™ (estradiol/norethindrone acetate tablets) is 12–14 hours.

Norethindrone Acetate: The most important metabolites of norethindrone are isomers of 5α-dihydro-norethindrone and tetrahydro-norethindrone, which are excreted mainly in the urine as sulfate or glucuronide conjugates. The terminal half-life of norethindrone is about 8–11 hours.

DRUG-DRUG INTERACTIONS

Coadministration of estradiol with norethindrone acetate did not elicit any apparent influence on the pharmacokinetics of norethindrone. Similarly, no relevant interaction of norethindrone on the pharmacokinetics of estradiol was found within the NETA dose range investigated in a single dose study.

FOOD-DRUG INTERACTIONS

A single-dose study in 24 healthy postmenopausal women was conducted to investigate any potential impact of administration of Activella™ with and without food. Administration of Activella™ with food did not modify the bioavailability of estradiol. although increases in AUC_{0-72} of 19% and decreases in C_{max} of 36% for norethindrone were seen.

CLINICAL STUDIES

VASOMOTOR SYMPTOMS

Activella™ is effective in reducing the number of moderate-to-severe vasomotor symptoms in postmenopausal women. In a 12-week radomized clinical trial involving 92 subjects, Activella™ was compared to 1 mg of estradiol and to placebo. The mean number and intensity of hot flushes were significantly reduced from baseline to week 12 in both the Activella™ and the 1 mg estradiol group compared to placebo (see Figure 2).

Figure 2
Mean Weekly Number of Moderate and Severe Hot Flushes in a 12-Week Study

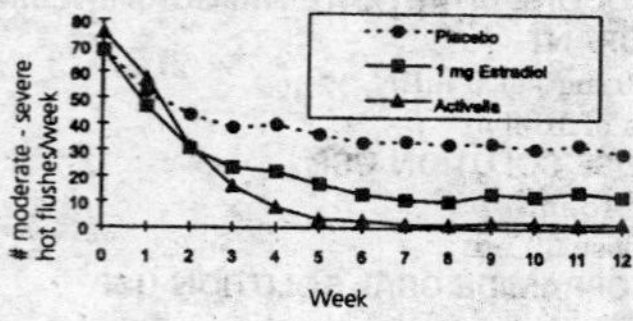

ENDOMETRIAL HYPERPLASIA

Activella™ (estradiol/norethindrone acetate tablets) reduced the incidence of estrogen-induced endometrial hyperplasia at 1 year in a randomized, controlled clinical trial. This trial enrolled 1,176 subjects who were randomized to one of 4 arms: 1 mg estradiol unopposed (n=296), 1 mg E_2 + 0.1 mg NETA (n=294), 1 mg E_2 + 0.25 mg NETA (n=291), and Activella™ [1 mg E_2 + 0.5 mg NETA] (n=295). At the end of the study, endometrial biopsy results were available for 988 subjects. The results of the 1 mg estradiol unopposed arm compared to Activella™ are shown in TABLE 2.

TABLE 2
INCIDENCE OF ENDOMETRIAL HYPERPLASIA WITH UNOPPOSED ESTRADIOL AND ACTIVELLA™ IN A 12–MONTH STUDY

	1 mg E_2 (n=296)	Activella™ (n=295)
No. of subjects with histological evaluation at the end of the study	247	241
No. (%) of subjects with endometrial hyperplasia at the end of the study	36 (14.6%)	1 (0.4%)

During the initial months of therapy, irregular bleeding or spotting occurred with Activella™ treatment. However, bleeding tended to decrease over time, and after 12 months of treatment with Activella™ , fewer than 3% of women reported bleeding (see Figure 3).

[See figure 3 at top of next column]

INFORMATION REGARDING LIPID EFFECTS

A 12-month, placebo-controlled clinical trial in 80 postmenopausal Caucasian women at low risk for cardiovascular disease compared the effects of Activella™ to placebo on lipid parameters. These results are shown in TABLE 3.

TABLE 3
PERCENTAGE CHANGE FROM BASELINE IN SELECTED LIPID PARAMETERS WITH ACTIVELLA™ IN A 12–MONTH PLACEBO-CONTROLLED STUDY

Lipid Parameter %	Activella™ (n=35)	Placebo (n=34)
Total Cholesterol	−10.5%	−0.8%
HDL-C[1]	−12.4%	−6.1%
LDL-C[2]	−10.8%	0.8%
LDL: HDL Ratio	0.1%	9.2%
Triglycerides	2.2%	4.4%

[1] High density lipoprotein-cholesterol
[2] Low density lipoprotein-cholesterol

Figure 3
Percentage of Women Bleeding at Each Month in a 12-Month Study

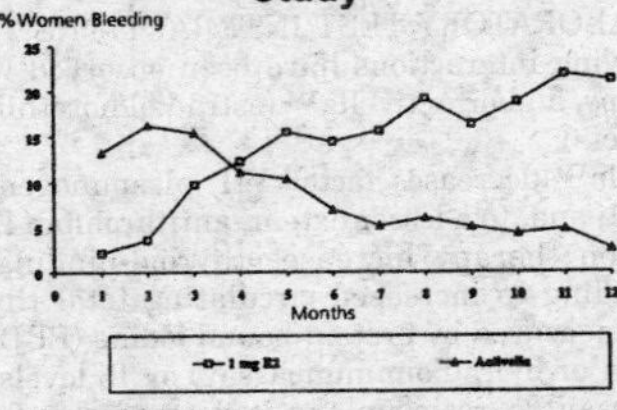

n=number of women
1 mg E2 (3, 6, 9 and 12 months): n=278, 255, 226, 212
Activella™ (3, 6, 9 and 12 months): n=273, 246, 238, 232

EFFECT ON BONE MINERAL DENSITY

The results of two randomized, multicenter, calcium-supplemented (500–1000 mg/day), placebo-controlled, 2 year clinical trials have shown that Activella™ (estradiol/norethindrone acetate tablets) is effective in preventing bone loss in postmenopausal women. A total of 462 postmenopausal women with intact uteri and baseline BMD values for lumbar spine within 2 standard deviations of the mean in healthy young women were enrolled. In a US trial, 327 postmenopausal women (mean time from menopause 2.5 to 3.1 years) with a mean age of 53 years were randomized to 7 groups (0.25 mg, 0.5 mg, and 1 mg of estradiol alone, 1 mg estradiol with 0.25 mg norethindrone acetate, 1 mg estradiol with 0.5 mg norethindrone acetate, and 2 mg estradiol with 1 mg norethindrone acetate, and placebo. In a European trial, 135 postmenopausal women (mean time from menopause 8.4 to 9.3 years) with a mean age of 58 years were randomized to 1 mg estradiol with 0.25 mg norethindrone acetate, 1 mg estradiol with 0.5 mg norethindrone acetate, and placebo.

Approximately 58% and 67% of the randomized subjects in the two clinical trials, respectively, completed the two clinical trials. BMD was measured using dual-energy x-ray absorptiometry (DEXA).

A summary of the results comparing Activella™ and placebo from the two prevention trials is shown in Table 4.

[See table 4 above]

TABLE 4
PERCENTAGE CHANGE (MEAN±SEM) IN BONE MINERAL DENSITY (BMD)
(Intent to Treat Analysis, Last Observation Carried Forward)

	US Trial		EU Trial	
	Placebo (n=37)	Activella™ (n=37)	Placebo (n=40)	Activella™ (n=38)
Lumbar spine	−2.1±0.5	3.8±0.5*	−0.9±0.6	5.4±0.8*
Femoral neck	−2.3±0.6	1.8±0.7*	−1.0±0.7	0.7±0.9
Femoral trochanter	−2.0±0.7	3.7±0.7*	0.8±1.1	6.3±1.2*
Ward's triangle	–	–	−1.6±1.3	2.7±1.7
Distal radius	–	–	−0.7±0.5	2.1±0.5*
Total body	–	–	0.4±0.4	3.0±0.5*

US = United States, EU = European
* Significantly (p<0.001) different from placebo

The overall difference in mean percentage change in BMD at the lumbar spine between Activella™ and placebo was 5.9% in the US trial (1000 mg/day calcium) and 6.3% in the European trial (500 mg/day calcium). Activella™ also increased BMD at the femoral neck and femoral trochanter compared to placebo. The increase in lumbar spine BMD in the US and European clinical trials is displayed in Figure 4.

FIGURE 4
Percentage Change in Bone Mineral Density (BMD) of the Lumbar Spine (L1-L4) (Intent to Treat Analysis with Last Observation Carried Forward)

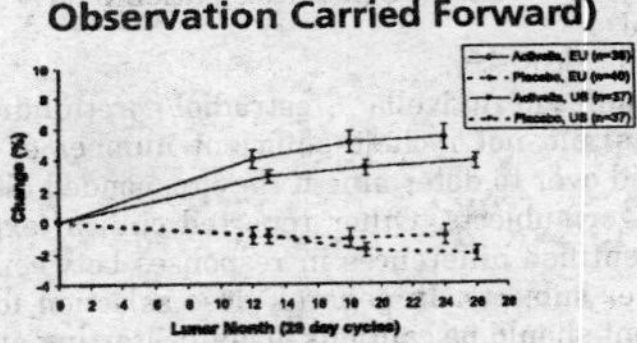

EFFECT ON BONE TURNOVER

Activella™ (estradiol/norethindrone acetate tablets) significantly reduced serum and urine markers of bone turnover with a marked decrease in bone resorption makers (e.g., urinary pyridinoline crosslinks Type 1 collagen C-telopeptide, pyridinoline, deoxypyridinoline) and to a lesser extent in bone formation markers (e.g., serum osteocalcin, bone-specific alkaline phosphatase, C-terminal propetide of Type 1 collagen). The suppression of bone turnover markers was evident by 3 months and persisted throughout the 24-month treatment period.

INDICATIONS AND USAGE

Activella™ therapy is indicated in women with an intact uterus for the:

1. Treatment of moderate to severe vasomotor symptoms associated with the menopause. There is no adequate evidence that estrogens are effective for nervous symptoms or depression that might occur during menopause and they should not be used to treat these conditions.
2. Treatment of vulvar and vaginal atrophy.
3. Prevention of postmenopausal osteoporosis.

Most prospective studies of efficacy for the osteoporosis prevention indication have been carried out in white postmenopausal women, without stratification by other risk factors, and tend to show a universally beneficial effect on bone. Since estrogen administration is associated with risk, patient selection must be individualized based on the balance of risks and benefits.

Case-control studies have shown an approximately 60-percent reduction in hip and wrist fractures in women whose estrogen replacement was begun within a few years after menopause. Studies also suggest that estrogen reduces the rate of vertebral fractures. When estrogen therapy is discontinued, bone mass declines at a rate comparable to the immediate postmenopausal period. White and Asian women are at higher risk for osteoporosis than black women, and thin women are at a higher risk than heavier women, who generally have higher endogenous estrogen levels. Early menopause is one of the strongest predictors for the development of osteoporosis. Other factors associated with osteoporosis include genetic factors (small build, family history), lifestyle (cigarette smoking, alcohol abuse, sedentary exercise habits) and nutrition (below average body weight and dietary calcium intake).

The mainstays of prevention and management of osteoporosis are weight-bearing exercise, adequate calcium intake, and, when indicated, estrogen. Postmenopausal women absorb dietary calcium less efficiently than premenopausal women and require an average of 1500 mg/day of elemental calcium to remain in neutral calcium balance. The average calcium intake in the USA is 400–600 mg/day. Therefore, when not contraindicated, calcium supplementation may be helpful for women with suboptimal dietary intake.

CONTRAINDICATIONS

Estrogens/progestins combined should not be used in women under any of the following conditions or circumstances.

1. Known or suspected pregnancy, including use for missed abortions or as a diagnostic test for pregnancy. Estrogen or progestin may cause fetal harm when administered to a pregnant woman.
2. Known or suspected breast cancer, or past history of breast cancer associated with the use of estrogens.
3. Known or suspected estrogen-dependent neoplasia, e.g., endometrial cancer.
4. Abnormal genital bleeding unknown etiology.
5. Known or suspected active deep venous thrombosis, thromboembolic disorders or stroke or past history of these conditions associated with estrogen use.
6. Liver dysfunction or disease.
7. Hypersensitivity to any of the components of Activella™ (estradiol/norethindrone acetate tablets).

WARNINGS

ALL WARNINGS BELOW PERTAIN TO THE USE OF THIS COMBINATION PRODUCT.

Based on experience with estrogens and/or progestins:

1. Induction of malignant neoplasms

Endometrial cancer. The reported endometrial cancer risk among unopposed estrogen users is about 2- to 12-fold greater than in non-users, and appears dependent on duration of treatment and on estrogen dose. There is no significant increased risk associated with the use of estrogens for less than one year. The greatest risk appears to be associated with prolonged use with increased risks of 15- to 24-fold with five or more years of use. In three studies, persistence of risk was demonstrated for 8 to over 15 years after cessation of estrogen treatment. In one study, a significant decrease in the incidence of endometrial cancer occurred six months after withdrawal. Progestins taken with estrogens have been shown to significantly reduce, but not eliminate, the risk of endometrial cancer associated with estrogen use. In a large clinical trial, the incidence of endometrial hyperplasia with Activella™ was 0.4% (one simple hyperplasia without atypia) compared to 14.6% with 1 mg estradiol unopposed (see CLINICAL STUDIES).

Clinical surveillance of all women taking estrogen/progestin combinations is important. Adequate diagnostic measures, including endometrial sampling when indicated, should be undertaken to rule out malignancy in all cases of undiagnosed persistent or recurring abnormal vaginal bleeding. There is no evidence that "natural" estrogens are more or less hazardous than "synthetic" estrogens at equivalent estrogen doses.

Brerast cancer. While the majority of studies have not shown an increased risk of breast cancer in women who have ever used estrogen replacement therapy, some have reported a moderately increased risk (relative risks of 1.3–2.0) in those taking higher doses, or in those taking lower doses for prolonged periods of time, especially in excess of 10 years.

While the effects of added progestins on the risk of breast cancer are also unknown, available epidemiological evidence suggest that progestins do not reduce, and may enhance, the moderately increased breast cancer risk that has been reported with prolonged estrogen replacement therapy.

In a one-year trial among 1,176 women who received either unopposed 1 mg estradiol or a combination of 1 mg estradiol plus one of three different doses of NETA (0.1, 0.25 and 0.5 mg), seven new cases of breast cancer were diagnosed, two of which occurred among the group of 295 Activella™ (estradiol/norethindrone acetate tablets) treated women.

Women on hormone replacement therapy should have regular breast examinations and should be instructed in breast self-examination, and women over the age of 40 should have regular mammograms.

2. Congenital lesions with malignant potential. Estrogen therapy during pregnancy is associated with an increased risk of fetal congential reproductive tract disorders, and possible other birth defects.

Studies of women who received diethylstilbestrol (DES) during pregnancy have shown that female offspring have an increased risk of vaginal adenosis, squamous cell dysplasia of the uterine cervix, and clear cell vaginal cancer later in life; male offspring have an increased risk of urogenital abnormalities and possibly testicular cancer later in life. Although some of these changes are benign, others are precursors of malignancy.

3. Cardiovascular disease. Large doses of estrogens (5 mg conjugated estrogen per day), comparable to those used to treat cancer of the prostate and breast, have been shown in a large prospective clinical trial in men to increase the risk of nonfatal myocardial infarction, pulmonary embolism, and thrombophlebitis.

These risks cannot necessarily be extrapolated from men to women or from unopposed estrogen to combination estrogen/progestin therapy. However, to avoid the theoretical cardiovascular risk to women caused by high estrogen doses, the dose for estrogen replacement therapy should not exceed the lowest effective dose.

4. Hypercalcemia. Administration of estrogens may lead to severe hypercalcemia in patients with breast cancer and bone metastases. If this occurs, the drugs should be stopped and appropriate measures taken to reduce the serum calcium level.

5. Effects during pregnancy. Use in pregnancy is not recommended.

6. Gallbladder disease. Two studies have reported a 2- to 4-fold increase in the risk of surgically confirmed gallbladder disease in women receiving postmenopausal estrogens. Among the 1,516 women treated in clinical trials with 1 mg estradiol alone or in combination with several doses of NETA, 3 women had surgically confirmed cholelithiasis, none of them on Activella™ (estradiol/norethindrone acetate tablets) treatment.

7. Elevated blood pressure. Occasional blood pressure increases during estrogen replacement therapy have been attributed to idiosyncratic reactions to estrogens. More often, blood pressure has remained the same or has dropped. One study showed that postmenopausal estrogen users have higher blood pressure than non-users. Two other studies showed slightly lower blood pressure among estrogen users compared to non-users. Postmenopausal estrogen use does not increase the risk of stroke. Nonetheless, blood pressure should be monitored at regular intervals with estrogen use.

8. Thromboembolic disorders. The physician should be alert to the earliest manifestations of thrombotic disorders (thrombophlebitis, cerebrovascular disorders, pulmonary embolism, and retinal thrombosis). Should any of these occur or be suspected, the drugs should be discontinued immediately. In a one-year study where 295 women were exposed to Activella™, there were two cases of deep vein thromboses reported.

9. Visual abnormalities. Discontinue medication pending examination if there is a sudden partial or complete loss of vision, or a sudden onset of proptosis, diplopia, or migraine. If examinations reveal papilledema or retinal vascular lesions, medication should be withdrawn.

PRECAUTIONS

GENERAL

Based on experience with estrogens and/or progestins:

1. Cardiovascular risk. A causal relationship between estrogen replacement therapy and reduction of cardiovascular

Continued on next page

Information on these Pharmacia & Upjohn products is based on labeling in effect June 1, 2000. Further information concerning these and other Pharmacia & Upjohn products may be obtained by direct inquiry to Medical Information, Pharmacia & Upjohn, Kalamazoo, MI 49001.

Activella—Cont.

disease in postmenopausal women has not been proven. Furthermore, the effect of added progestins on this putative benefit is not yet known.

In recent years, many published studies have suggested that there may be a cause-effect relationship between postmenopausal oral estrogen replacement therapy without added progestins and a decrease in cardiovascular disease in women. Although most of the observational studies that assessed this statistical association have reported a 20% to 50% reduction in coronary heart disease risk and associated mortality in estrogen takers, the following should be considered when interpreting these reports. Because only one of these studies was randomized and it was too small to yield statistically significant results, all relevant studies were subject to selection bias. Thus, the apparently reduced risk of coronary artery disease cannot be attributed with certainty to estrogen replacement therapy. It may instead have been caused by life-style and medical characteristics of the women studied with the result that healthier women were selected for estrogen therapy. In general, treated women were of higher socioeconomic and educational status, more slender, more physically active, more likely to have undergone surgical menopause, and less likely to have diabetes than the untreated women. Although some studies attempted to control for these selection factors, it is common for properly designed randomized trials to fail to confirm benefits suggested by less rigorous study designs. Thus, ongoing and future large-scale randomized trials may fail to confirm this apparent benefit.

Current medical practice often includes the use of concomitant progestin therapy in women with intact uterus. While the effects of added progestins on the risk of ischemic heart disease are not known, all available progestins attenuate at least some of the favorable effects of estrogens on HDL levels, although they maintain the favorable effect of estrogens on LDL levels.

The safety data regarding Activella™ (estradiol/norethindrone acetate tablets) were obtained primarily from clinical trials and epidemiologic studies of postmenopausal Caucasian women, who were at generally low risk of cardiovascular disease and higher than average risk for osteoporosis. The safety profile of Activella™ derived from these study populations cannot necessarily be extrapolated to other populations of diverse racial and/or demographic composition. When considering prescribing Activella™, physicians are advised to weigh the potential benefits and risks of therapy as applicable to each individual patient.

2. Use in hysterectomized women. Existing data do not support the use of the combination of estrogen and progestin in postmenopausal women without a uterus. Risks that may be associated with the inclusion of progestin in estrogen replacement regimens include deterioration in glucose tolerance, and less favorable effects on lipid metabolism compared to the effects of estrogen alone.

The effects of Activella™ on glucose tolerance and lipid metabolism have been studied (see CLINICAL PHARMACOLOGY, Clinical Studies, and PRECAUTIONS, Drug/Laboratory Test Interactions).

3. Physical examination. A complete medical and family history should be taken prior to the initiation of any estrogen/progestin therapy. The pretreatment and periodic physical examinations should include special reference to blood pressure, breasts, abdomen, and pelvic organs, and should include a Papanicolaou smear. As a general rule, estrogen should not be prescribed for longer than one year without another physical examination being performed.

4. Fluid retention. Because estrogens/progestins may cause some degree of fluid retention, conditions that might be influenced by this factor, such as asthma, epilepsy, migraine, and cardiac or renal dysfunction, require careful observation.

5. Uterine bleeding. Certain patients may develop abnormal uterine bleeding. In cases of undiagnosed abnormal uterine bleeding, adequate diagnostic measures are indicated (see WARNINGS).

6. The pathologist should be advised of estrogen/progestin therapy when relevant specimens are submitted.

Based on experience with estrogens:

1. Familial hyperlipoproteinemia. Estrogen therapy may be associated with massive elevations of plasma triglycerides leading to pancreatitis and other complications in patients with familial defects in lipoprotein metabolism.

2. Hypercoagulability. Some studies have shown that women taking estrogen replacement therapy have hypercoagulability primarily related to decreased antithrombin activity. This effect appears dose- and duration-dependent and is less pronounced than that associated with oral contraceptive use. Also, postmenopausal women tend to have changes in levels of coagulation parameters at baseline compared to premenopausal women. Epidemiological studies have suggested that estrogen use is associated with a higher relative risk of developing venous thromboembolism, i.e., deep vein thrombosis or pulmonary embolism. The studies found a 2-3- fold higher risk for estrogen users compared to non-users. There is insufficient information on hypercoagulability in women who have had previous thromboembolic disease. The effects of Activella™ (estradiol/norethindrone acetate tablets) (n=40) compared to placebo (n=40) on selected clotting factors were evaluated in a 12-month study with postmenopausal women.

Activella™ decreased factor VII, plasminogen activator inhibitor-1, and, to a lesser extent, antithrombin III activity, compared to placebo. Fibrinogen remained unchanged during Activella™ treatment in comparison with an increase over time in the placebo group.

3. Mastodynia. Certain patients may develop undesirable manifestations of estrogenic stimulation such as mastodynia. In clinical trials, less than one-fifth of the women treated with Activella™ reported breast tenderness or breast pain. The majority of the cases were reported as breast tenderness, primarily during the initial months of the treatment.

Based on experience with progestins:

1. Lipoprotein metabolism. (see CLINICAL STUDIES)

2. Impaired glucose tolerance. Diabetic patients should be carefully observed while receiving estrogen/progestin therapy.

The effects of Activella™ on glucose tolerance have been studied (see PRECAUTIONS, Drug/Laboratory Test Interactions).

TABLE 5

ALL TREATMENT-EMERGENT ADVERSE EVENTS REGARDLESS OF RELATIONSHIP REPORTED AT A FREQUENCY OF ≥5% WITH ACTIVELLA™

	Endometrial Hyperplasia Study (12-Months)		Vasomotor Symptoms Study (3-Months)		Osteoporosis Study (2 Years)	
	Activella™ (n=295)	1 mg E2 (n=296)	Activella™ (n=29)	Placebo (n=34)	Activella™ (n=47)	Placebo (n=48)
Body as a Whole						
Back Pain	6%	5%	3%	3%	6%	4%
Headache	16%	16%	17%	18%	11%	6%
Digestive System						
Nausea	3%	5%	10%	0%	11%	0%
Gastroenteritis	2%	2%	0%	0%	6%	4%
Nervous System						
Insomnia	6%	4%	3%	3%	0%	8%
Emotional Lability	1%	1%	0%	0%	6%	0%
Respiratory System						
Upper Respiratory Tract Infection	18%	15%	10%	6%	15%	19%
Sinusitis	7%	11%	7%	0%	15%	10%
Metabolic and Nutritional						
Weight increase	0%	0%	0%	0%	9%	6%
Urogenital System						
Breast Pain	24%	10%	21%	0%	17%	8%
Post-Menopausal Bleeding	5%	15%	10%	3%	11%	0%
Uterine Fibroid	5%	4%	0%	0%	4%	8%
Ovarian Cyst	3%	2%	7%	0%	0%	8%
Resistance Mechanism						
Infection Viral	4%	6%	0%	3%	6%	6%
Moniliasis Genital	4%	7%	0%	0%	6%	0%
Secondary Terms						
Injury Accidental	4%	3%	3%	0%	17%*	4%*
Other Events	2%	3%	3%	0%	6%	4%

* including one upper extremity fracture in each group

3. Depression. Patients who have a history of depression should be observed and the drugs discontinued if the depression recurs to a serious degree.

INFORMATION FOR THE PATIENT

See text of Patient Package Insert which appears after the **How Supplied** section.

DRUG/LABORATORY TEST INTERACTIONS

The following interactions have been observed with estrogen therapy, and/or Activella™ (estradiol/norethindrone acetate tablets):

1. Activella™ decreases factor VII, plasminogen activator inhibitor-1, and, to a lesser extent, antithrombin III activity.
2. Estrogen therapy increases thyroid-binding globulin (TBG) leading to increased circulating total thyroid hormone, as measured by protein-bound iodine (PBI), T_4 levels (by column or by radioimmunoassay) or T_3 levels by radioimmunoassay. T_3 resin uptake is decreased, reflecting the elevated TBG. Free T_4 and free T_3 concentrations are unaltered.
3. Estrogen therapy may elevate other binding proteins in serum i.e., corticosteroid-binding globulin (CBG), sex-hormone-binding globulin (SHBG), leading to increased circulating corticosteroids and sex steroids respectively. Free or biologically active hormone concentrations are unchanged. Other plasma proteins may be increased (angiotensinogen/renin substrate, alpha-1-antitrypsin, ceruloplasmin). In a 12-month clinical trial, SHBG was found to increase with Activella™.
4. Estrogen therapy increases plasma HDL and HDL-2 subfraction concentrations, reduces LDL cholesterol concentration, and increases triglyceride levels. (For effects during Activella™ treatment, see CLINICAL PHARMACOLOGY, Clinical Studies).
5. Activella™ treatment of healthy postmenopausal women does not decrease glucose tolerance when assessed by an oral glucose tolerance test; the insulin response decreases without any increase in the glucose serum levels. Activella™ treatment does not deteriorate insulin sensitivity in healthy postmenopausal women when assessed by an hyperinsulinemic euglycemic clamp.
6. Estrogen therapy reduces response to metyrapone test.
7. Estrogen therapy reduces serum folate concentration.

CARCINOGENESIS, MUTAGENESIS, and IMPAIRMENT OF INFERTILITY

Long-term continuous administration of natural and synthetic estrogens in certain animal species increases the frequency of carcinomas of the breast, uterus, cervix, vagina, testis, and liver. (See CONTRAINDICATIONS and WARNINGS.)

PREGNANCY CATEGORY X:

Estrogens/progestins should not be used during pregnancy. (See CONTRAINDICATIONS and WARNINGS.)

NURSING MOTHERS:

Detectable amounts of estradiol and norethindrone acetate have been identified in the milk of mothers receiving these products and has been reported to decrease the quantity and the quality of the milk.

As a general principle, the administration of any drug to nursing mothers should be done only when clearly necessary since many drugs are excreted in human milk.

PEDIATRIC USE:

Safety and effectiveness in pediatric patients have not been established.

GERIATRIC USE:

Clinical studies of Activella™ (estradiol/norethindrone acetate tablets) did not include sufficient number of subjects aged 65 and over to determine if they responded differently from younger subjects. Other reported clinical experience has not identified differences in responses between elderly and younger subjects. In general, dose selection for an elderly patient should be cautious, usually starting at the low end of the dosing range, reflecting the greater frequency of decreased hepatic, renal, or cardiac function, and of concomitant disease or other drug therapy.

ADVERSE REACTIONS

(See WARNINGS regarding induction of neoplasia, adverse effects on the fetus, increased incidence of gallbladder disease, elevated blood pressure, thromboembolic disorders, cardiovascular disease, visual abnormalities, and hypercalcemia and PRECAUTIONS regarding cardiovascular disease.)

Adverse events reported by investigators in the Phase 3 studies regardless of causality assessment are shown in TABLE 5.

[See table 5 at left]

The following adverse reactions have been reported with estrogen and/or progestin therapy:

Genitourinary system: changes in vaginal bleeding pattern and abnormal withdrawal bleeding or flow, breakthrough bleeding, spotting, increase in size of uterine leiomyomata, vaginal candidiasis, changes in amount of cervical secretion, premenstrual-like syndrome, cystitis-like syndrome.

Breasts: tenderness, enlargement.

Gastrointestinal: nausea, vomiting, changes in appetite, cholestatic jaundice, abdominal pain, flatulence, bloating, increased incidence of gallbladder disease.

Skin: chloasma or melasma that may persist when drug is discontinued, erythema multiforme, erythema nodosum, hemorrhagic eruption, loss of scalp hair, hirsutism, itching, skin rash and pruritus.

Cardiovascular: changes in blood pressure, cerebrovascular accidents, deep venous thrombosis and pulmonary embolism.

CNS: headache, migraine, dizziness, depression, chorea, insomnia, nervousness.
Eyes: steepening of corneal curvature, intolerance to contact lenses.
Miscellaneous: increase or decrease in weight, aggravation of porphyria, edema, changes in libido, fatigue, allergic reactions, back pain, arthralgia, myalgia.

OVERDOSAGE

Acute Overdose: Serious ill effects have not been reported following acute ingestion of large doses of estrogen/progestin-containing oral contraceptives by young children. Overdosage may cause nausea and vomiting and withdrawal bleeding may occur in females.

DOSAGE AND ADMINISTRATION

Activella™ (estradiol/norethindrone acetate tablets) therapy consists of a single tablet to be taken once daily. For the treatment of moderate to severe vasomotor symptoms associated with the menopause, treatment of vulvar and vaginal atrophy, and the prevention of postmenopausal osteoporosis – Activella™ 1 mg E_2 / 0.5 mg NETA daily. the doses of 17beta-estradiol and norethindrone acetate in Activella™ may not be the lowest effective dose-combination for the prevention of osteoporosis.
Treated patients with an intact uterus should be monitored closely for signs of endometrial cancer, and appropriate diagnostic measures should be taken to rule out malignancy in the event of persistent or recurring abnormal vaginal bleeding.

HOW SUPPLIED

Activella™, 1 mg estradiol and 0.5 mg norethindrone acetate, is a white, film-coated tablet, engraved with NOVO 288 on one side and the APIS bull on the other. It is round, 6 mm in diameter and bi-convex.
Activella™ is supplied as:
28 tablets in a calendar dial pack dispenser NDC 0009-5174-02.
Store in a dry place protected from light. Store at 25°C (77°F); excursions permitted to 15–30°C (59–86°F).
[See USP Controlled Room Temperature]

Rx only
Activella™ is a trademark owned by
Novo Nordisk A/S
Revised May 2000
818 163 001
Manufactured for
Pharmacia & Upjohn Company
Kalamazoo, MI 49001, USA
By
Novo Nordisk A/S
2880 Bagsværd, Denmark

ADRIAMYCIN RDF® ℞
doxorubicin hydrochloride
for injection, USP

ADRIAMYCIN PFS® ℞
doxorubicin hydrochloride
injection, USP
FOR INTRAVENOUS USE ONLY

WARNING

1. Severe local tissue necrosis will occur if there is extravasation during administration (see DOSAGE AND ADMINISTRATION). Doxorubicin must not be given by the intramuscular or subcutaneous route.
2. Myocardial toxicity manifested in its most severe form by potentially fatal congestive heart failure may occur either during therapy or months to years after termination of therapy. The probability of developing impaired myocardial function based on a combined index of signs, symptoms and decline in left ventricular ejection fraction (LVEF) is estimated to be 1 to 2% at a total cumulative dose of 300 mg/m² of doxorubicin, 3 to 5% at a dose of 400 mg/m², 5 to 8% at 450 mg/m² and 6 to 20% at 500 mg/m².* The risk of developing CHF increases rapidly with increasing total cumulative doses of doxorubicin in excess of 450 mg/m². This toxicity may occur at lower cumulative doses in patients with prior mediastinal irradiation or on concurrent cyclophosphamide therapy or with pre-existing heart disease. Pediatric patients are at increased risk for developing delayed cardiotoxicity.
3. Dosage should be reduced in patients with impaired hepatic function.
4. Severe myelosuppression may occur.
5. Doxorubicin should be administered only under the supervision of a physician who is experienced in the use of cancer chemotherapeutic agents.

* Data on file at Pharmacia & Upjohn

DESCRIPTION

Doxorubicin is a cytotoxic anthracycline antibiotic isolated from cultures of *Streptomyces peucetius* var. *caesius*.
Doxorubicin consists of a naphthacenequinone nucleus linked through a glycosidic bond at ring atom 7 to an amino sugar, daunosamine.
Chemically, doxorubicin hydrochloride is: 5,12-Naphthacenedione, 10-[(3-amino-2,3,6-trideoxy-α-L-*lyxo*-hexopyranosyl)oxy]-7,8,9,10-tetrahydro-6,8,11-trihydroxy-8-(hydroxylacetyl)-1-(methoxy-, hydrochloride (8*S*-*cis*)-. The structural formula is as follows:

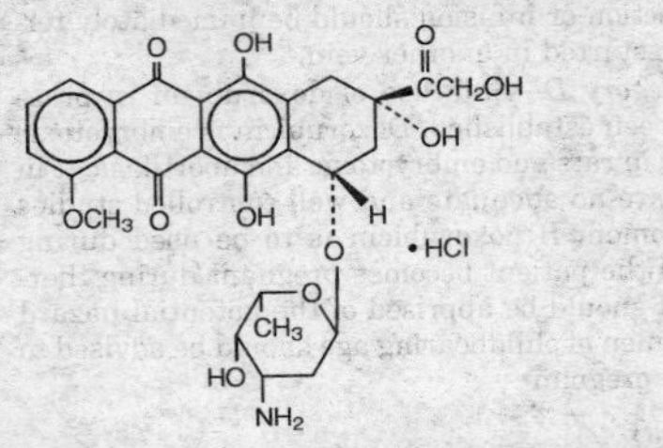

$C_{27}H_{29}NO_{11}$ • HCl
M.W.—579.99

Doxorubicin binds to nucleic acids, presumably by specific intercalation of the planar anthracycline nucleus with the DNA double helix. The anthracycline ring is lipophilic, but the saturated end of the ring system contains abundant hydroxyl groups adjacent to the amino sugar, producing a hydrophilic center. The molecule is amphoteric, containing acidic functions in the ring phenolic groups and a basic function in the sugar amino group. It binds to cell membranes as well as plasma proteins.
ADRIAMYCIN RDF® (doxorubicin hydrochloride for injection, USP) a sterile red-orange lyophilized powder for intravenous use only, is available in 10, 20 and 50 mg single dose vials and a 150 mg multidose vial.
Each 10 mg single dose vial contains 10 mg of doxorubicin HCl, USP, 50 mg of lactose, NF (hydrous) and 1 mg of methylparaben, NF (added to enhance dissolution) as a sterile red-orange lyophilized powder.
Each 20 mg single dose vial contains 20 mg of doxorubicin HCl, USP, 100 mg of lactose, NF (hydrous) and 2 mg of methylparaben, NF (added to enhance dissolution) as a sterile red-orange lyophilized powder.
Each 50 mg single dose vial contains 50 mg of doxorubicin HCl, USP, 250 mg of lactose, NF (hydrous) and 5 mg of methylparaben, NF (added to enhance dissolution) as a sterile red-orange lyophilized powder.
Each 150 mg multidose vial contains 150 mg of doxorubicin HCl, USP, 750 mg of lactose, NF (hydrous) and 15 mg of methylparaben, NF (added to enhance dissolution) as a sterile red-orange lyophilized powder.
ADRIAMYCIN PFS® (doxorubicin hydrochloride injection, USP) is a sterile parenteral, isotonic solution for intravenous use only, containing no preservative, available in 5 mL (10 mg), 10 mL (20 mg), 25 mL (50 mg), and 37.5 mL (75 mg) single dose vials and a 100 mL (200 mg) multidose vial.
Each mL contains doxorubicin HCl 2 mg, USP and the following inactive ingredients: sodium chloride 0.9% and water for injection q.s. Hydrochloric acid is used to adjust the pH to a target pH of 3.0.

CLINICAL PHARMACOLOGY

The cytotoxic effect of doxorubicin on malignant cells and its toxic effects on various organs are thought to be related to nucleotide base intercalation and cell membrane lipid binding activities of doxorubicin. Intercalation inhibits nucleotide replication and action of DNA and RNA polymerases. The interaction of doxorubicin with topoisomerase II to form DNA-cleavable complexes appears to be an important mechanism of doxorubicin cytocidal activity. Doxorubicin cellular membrane binding may effect a variety of cellular functions. Enzymatic electron reduction of doxorubicin by a variety of oxidases, reductases and dehydrogenases generate highly reactive species including the hydroxyl free radical OH•. Free radical formation has been implicated in doxorubicin cardiotoxicity by means of Cu (II) and Fe (III) reduction at the cellular level. Cells treated with doxorubicin have been shown to manifest the characteristic morphologic changes associated with apoptosis or programmed cell death. Doxorubicin-induced apoptosis may be an integral component of the cellular mechanism of action relating to therapeutic effects, toxicities, or both.
Animal studies have shown activity in a spectrum of experimental tumors, immunosuppression, carcinogenic properties in rodents, induction of a variety of toxic effects, including delayed and progressive cardiac toxicity, myelosuppression in all species and atrophy to testes in rats and dogs.
Pharmacokinetic studies, determined in patients with various types of tumors undergoing either single or multi-agent therapy have shown that doxorubicin follows a multiphasic disposition after intravenous injection. The initial distributive half-life of approximately 5.0 minutes suggests rapid tissue uptake of doxorubicin, while its slow elimination from tissues is reflected by a terminal half-life of 20 to 48 hours. Steady-state distribution volumes exceed 20 to 30 L/kg and are indicative of extensive drug uptake into tissues. Plasma clearance is in the range of 8 to 20 mL/min/kg and is predominately by metabolism and biliary excretion. Approximately 40% of the dose appears in the bile in 5 days, while only 5 to 12% of the drug and its metabolites appear in the urine during the same time period. Binding of doxorubicin and its major metabolite, doxorubicinol to plasma proteins is about 74 to 76% and is independent of plasma concentration of doxorubicin up to 2 μM. Enzymatic reduction at the 7 position and cleavage of the daunosamine sugar yields aglycones which are accompanied by free radical formation, the local production of which may contribute to the cardiotoxic activity of doxorubicin. Disposition of doxorubicinol (DOX-OL) in patients is formation rate limited. The terminal half-life of DOX-OL is similar to doxorubicin. The relative exposure of DOX-OL, compared to doxorubicin ranges between 0.4 to 0.6. In urine, <3% of the dose was recovered as DOX-OL over 7 days.
A published clinical study involving 6 men and 21 women with no prior anthracycline therapy reported a significantly higher median doxorubicin clearance in the men compared to the women (113 versus 45 L/hr). However, the terminal half-life of doxorubicin was longer in men compared to the women (54 versus 35 hrs.).
In four patients, dose-independent pharmacokinetics have been shown for doxorubicin in the dose range of 30 to 70 mg/m². Systemic clearance of doxorubicin is significantly reduced in obese women with ideal body weight greater than 130%. There was a significant reduction in clearance without any change in volume of distribution in obese patients when compared with normal patients with less than 115% ideal body weight. The clearance of doxorubicin and doxorubicinol was also reduced in patients with impaired hepatic function. Doxorubicin was excreted in the milk of one lactating patient, with peak milk concentration at 24 hours after treatment being approximately 4.4 -fold greater than the corresponding plasma concentration. Doxorubicin was detectable in the milk up to 72 hours after therapy with 70 mg/m² of doxorubicin given as a 15 minute intravenous infusion and 100 mg/m² of cisplatin as a 26 hour intravenous infusion. The peak concentration of doxorubicinol in milk at 24 hours was 0.2 μM and AUC up to 24 hours was 16.5 μM.hr while the AUC for doxorubicin was 9.9 μM.hr.
Following administration of 10 to 75-mg/m² doses of doxorubicin to 60 children and adolescents ranging from 2 months to 20 years of age, doxorubicin clearance average 1443 ± 114 mL/min/m². Further analysis demonstrated that clearance in 52 children greater than 2 years of age (1540 mL/min/m²) was increased compared with adults. However, clearance in infants younger than 2 years of age (813 mL/min/m²) was decreased compared with older children and approached the range of clearance values determined in adults.
Doxorubicin does not cross the blood brain barrier.

INDICATIONS AND USAGE

ADRIAMYCIN PFS and ADRIAMYCIN RDF have been used successfully to produce regression in disseminated neoplastic conditions such as acute lymphoblastic leukemia, acute myeloblastic leukemia, Wilms' tumor, neuroblastoma, soft tissue and bone sarcomas, breast carcinoma, ovarian carcinoma, transitional cell bladder carinoma, thyroid carcinoma, gastric carcinoma, Hodgkin's disease, malignant lymphoma and bronchogenic carcinoma in which the small cell histologic type is the most responsive compared to other cell types.

CONTRAINDICATIONS

Doxorubicin therapy should not be started in patients who have marked myelosuppression induced by previous treatment with other antitumor agents or by radiotherapy. Doxorubicin treatment is contraindicated in patients who received previous treatment with complete cumulative doses of doxorubicin, daunorubicin, idarubicin, and/or other anthracyclines and anthracenes.

WARNINGS

Special attention must be given to the cardiotoxicity induced by doxorubicin. Irreversible myocardial toxicity, manifested in its most severe form by life-threatening or fatal congestive heart failure, may occur either during therapy or months to years after termination of therapy. The probability of developing impaired myocardial function, based on a combined index of signs, symptoms and decline in left ventricular ejection fraction (LVEF) is estimated to be 1 to 2% at a total cumulative dose of 300 mg/m² of doxorubicin, 3 to 5% at a dose of 400 mg/m², 5 to 8% at a dose of 450 mg/m² and 6 to 20% at a dose of 500 mg/m² given in a schedule of a bolus injection once every 3 weeks (data on file at Pharmacia & Upjohn). In a retrospective review by Von Hoff et al, the probability of developing congestive heart failure was reported to be 5/168 (3%) at a cumulative dose of 430 mg/m² of doxorubicin, 8/110 (7%) at 575 mg/m² and 3/14 (21%) at 728 mg/m². The cumulative incidence of CHF was 2.2%. In a prospective study of doxorubicin in combination with cyclophosphamide, fluorouracil and/or vincristine in patients with breast cancer or small cell lung cancer, the cumulative incidence of congestive heart failure was 5 to 6%. The probability of CHF at various cumulative doses of doxorubicin was 1.5% at 300 mg/m², 4.9% at 400 mg/m², 7.7% at 450 mg/m² and 20.5% at 500 mg/m².
Cardiotoxicity may occur at lower doses in patients with prior mediastinal irradiation, concurrent cyclophosphamide therapy exposure at an early age and advanced age. Data also suggest that pre-existing heart disease is a co-factor for increased risk of doxorubicin cadiotoxicity. In such cases, cardiac toxicity may occur at doses lower than the respective recommended cumulative dose of doxorubicin. Studies have suggested that concomitant administration of doxoru-

Continued on next page

Information on these Pharmacia & Upjohn products is based on labeling in effect June 1, 2000. Further information concerning these and other Pharmacia & Upjohn products may be obtained by direct inquiry to Medical Information, Pharmacia & Upjohn, Kalamazoo, MI 49001.

Adriamycin RDF & PFS—Cont.

bicin and calcium channel entry blockers may increase the risk of doxorubicin cardiotoxicity. The total dose of doxorubicin administered to the individual patient should also take into account previous or concomitant therapy with related compounds such as daunorubicin, idarubicin and mitoxantrone. Cardiomyopathy and/or congestive heart failure may be encountered several months or years after discontinuation of doxorubicin therapy.

The risk of congestive heart failure and other acute manifestations of doxorubicin cardiotoxicity in pediatric patients may be as much or lower than in adults. Pediatric patients appear to be at particular risk for developing delayed cardiac toxicity in that doxorubicin induced cardiomyopathy impairs myocardial growth as pediatric patients mature, subsequently leading to possible development of congestive heart failure during early adulthood. As many as 40% of pediatric patients may have subclinical cardiac dysfunction and 5 to 10% of pediatric patients may develop congestive heart failure on long term follow-up. This late cardiac toxicity may be related to the dose of doxorubicin. The longer the length of follow-up the greater the increase in the detection rate.

Treatment of doxorubicin induced congestive heart failure includes the use of digitalis, diuretics, after load reducers such as angiotensin I converting enzyme (ACE) inhibitors, low salt diet, and bed rest. Such intervention may relieve symptoms and improve the functional status of the patient.

Monitoring Cardiac Function

In adult patients severe cardiac toxicity may occur precipitously without antecedent ECG changes. Cardiomyopathy induced by anthracyclines is usually associated with very characteristic histopathologic changes on an endomyocardial biopsy (EM biopsy), and a decrease of left ventricular ejection fraction (LVEF), as measured by multi-gated radionuclide angiography (MUGA scans) and/or echocardiogram (ECHO), from pretreatment baseline values. However, it has not been demonstrated that monitoring of the ejection fraction will predict when individual patients are approaching their maximally tolerated cumulative dose of doxorubicin. Cardiac function should be carefully monitored during treatment to minimize the risk of cardiac toxicity. A baseline cardiac evaluation with an ECG, LVEF, and/or an echocardiogram (ECHO) is recommended especially in patients with risk factors for increased cardiac toxicity (pre-existing heart disease mediastinal irradiation, or concurrent cyclophosphamide therapy). Subsequent evaluations should be obtained at a cumulative dose of doxorubicin of at least 400 mg/m^2 and periodically thereafter during the course of therapy. Pediatric patients are at increased risk for developing delayed cardiotoxicity following doxorubicin administration and therefore at follow-up cardiac evaluation is recommended periodically to monitor for this delayed cardiotoxicity.

In adults, a 10% decline in LVEF to below the lower limit of normal or an absolute LVEF of 45%, or a 20% decline in LVEF at any level is indicative of deterioration in cardiac function. In pediatric patients, deterioration in cardiac function during or after the completion of therapy with doxorubicin is indicated by a drop in fractional shortening (FS) by an absolute value of ≥10 percentile units or below 29%, and a decline in LVEF of 10 percentile units or an LVEF below 55%. In general, if test results indicate deterioration in cardiac function associated with doxorubicin, the benefit of continued therapy should be carefully evaluated against the risk of producing irreversible cardiac damage.

Acute life-threatening arrhythmias have been reported to occur during or within a few hours after doxorubicin administration.

There is a high incidence of bone marrow depression, primarily of leukocytes, requiring careful hematologic monitoring. With the recommended dose schedule, leukopenia is usually transient, reaching its nadir 10 to 14 days after treatment with recovery usually occurring by the 21st day. White blood counts as low as $1000/mm^3$ are to be expected during treatment with appropriate doses of doxorubicin. Red blood cell and platelet levels should also be monitored since they may also be depressed. Hematologic toxicity may require dose reduction or suspension or delay of doxorubicin therapy. Persistent severe myelosuppression may result in superinfection or hemorrhage.

Doxorubicin may potentiate the toxicity of other anticancer therapies. Exacerbation of cyclophosphamide induced hemorrhagic cystitis and enhancement of the hepatotoxicity of 6-mercaptopurine have been reported. Radiation induced toxicity to the myocardium, mucosae, skin and liver have been reported to be increased by the administration of doxorubicin. Pediatric patients receiving concomitant doxorubicin and actinomycin-D have manifested acute "recall" pneumonitis at variable times after local radiation therapy.

Since metabolism and excretion of doxorubicin occurs predominantly by the hepatobiliary route, toxicity to recommended doses of doxorubicin can be enhanced by hepatic impairment; therefore, prior to the individual dosing, evaluation of hepatic function is recommended using conventional laboratory tests such as SGOT, SGPT, alkaline phosphatase and bilirubin (see DOSAGE AND ADMINISTRATION).

Necrotizing colitis manifested by typhlitis (cecal inflammation), bloody stools and severe and sometimes fatal infections have been associated with a combination of doxorubicin given by i.v. push daily for 3 days and cytarabine given by continuous infusion daily for 7 or more days.

On intravenous administration of doxorubicin, extravasation may occur with or without an accompanying stinging or burning sensation, even if blood returns well on aspiration of the infusion needle (see DOSAGE AND ADMINISTRATION). If any signs or symptoms of extravasation have occurred, the injection or infusion should be immediately terminated and restarted in another vein.

Pregnancy Category D—Safe use of doxorubicin in pregnancy has not been established. Doxorubicin is embryotoxic and teratogenic in rats and embryotoxic and abortifacient in rabbits. There are no adequate and well-controlled studies in pregnant women. If doxorubicin is to be used during pregnancy, or if the patient becomes pregnant during therapy, the patient should be apprised of the potential hazard to the fetus. Women of childbearing age should be advised to avoid becoming pregnant.

PRECAUTIONS

General

Doxorubicin is not an anti-microbial agent.

Information for Patients

ADRIAMYCIN PFS and ADRIAMYCIN RDF impart a red coloration to the urine for 1 to 2 days after administration, and patients should be advised to expect this during active therapy.

Drug Interactions

Paclitaxel: Two published studies report that initial administration of paclitaxel infused over 24 hours followed by doxorubicin administered over 48 hours resulted in a significant decrease in doxorubicin clearance with more profound neutropenic and stomatitis episodes than the reverse sequence of administration.

Progesterone: In a published study, progesterone was given intravenously to patients with advanced malignancies (ECOG PS<2) at high doses (up to 10 g over 24 hours) concomitantly with a fixed doxorubicin dose (60 mg/m^2) via bolus. Enhanced doxorubicin-induced neutropenia and thrombocytopenia were observed.

Verapamil: A study of the effects of verapamil on the acute toxicity of doxorubicin in mice revealed higher initial peak concentrations of doxorubicin in the heart with a higher incidence and severity of degenerative changes in cardiac tissue resulting in a shorter survival.

Cyclosporine: The addition of cyclosporine to doxorubicin may result in increases in AUC for both doxorubicin and doxorubicinol possibly due to a decrease in clearance of parent drug and a decrease in metabolism of doxorubicinol. Literature reports suggest that adding cyclosporine to doxorubicin results in more profound and prolonged hematologic toxicity than doxorubicin alone. Coma and/or seizures have also been described.

Drug Interactions: Literature reports have also described the following drug interactions: phenobarbital increases the elimination of doxorubicin, phenytoin levels may be decreased by doxorubicin, streptozocin (Zanosar®) may inhibit hepatic metabolism of doxorubicin, and administration of live vaccines to immunosuppressed patients including those undergoing cytotoxic chemotherapy may be hazardous.

Laboratory Tests

Initial treatment with doxorubicin requires observation of the patient and periodic monitoring of complete blood counts, hepatic function tests, and radionuclide left ventricular ejection fraction. (See WARNINGS).

Like other cytotoxic drugs, doxorubicin may induce "tumor lysis syndrome" and hyperuricemia in patients with rapidly growing tumors. Appropriate supportive and pharmacologic measures may prevent or alleviate this complication.

Carcinogenesis, Mutagenesis, Impairment of Fertility

Formal long-term carcinogenicity studies have not been conducted with doxorubicin. Doxorubicin and related compounds have been shown to have mutagenic and carcinogenic properties when tested in experimental models (including bacterial systems, mammalian cells in culture, and female Sprague-Dawley rats).

The possible adverse effect on fertility in males and females in humans or experimental animals have not been adequately evaluated. Testicular atrophy was observed in rats and dogs.

A variant of chemotherapy-related acute non-lymphocytic leukemia has been reported to occur infrequently a few years after multiple drug treatment of some neoplasms, which sometimes included doxorubicin. The exact role of doxorubicin has not been elucidated. Pediatric patients treated with doxorubicin or other topoisomerase II inhibitors are at a risk for developing acute myelogenous leukemia and other neoplasms. The extent of increased risk associated with doxorubicin has not been precisely quantified.

Pregnancy Category D

(See **WARNINGS**.)

Nursing Mothers:

Because of the potential for serious adverse reactions in nursing infants from doxorubicin, mothers should be advised to discontinue nursing during doxorubicin therapy.

Pediatric Use:

Pediatric patients are at increased risk for developing delayed cardiotoxicity. Follow-up cardiac evaluations are recommended periodically to monitor for this delayed cardiotoxicity (see WARNINGS).

Doxorubicin, as a component of intensive chemotherapy regimens administered to pediatric patients, may contribute to prepubertal growth failure. It may also contribute to gonadal impairment, which is usually temporary.

ADVERSE REACTIONS

Dose limiting toxicities of therapy are myelosuppression and cardiotoxicity. Other reactions reported are:

Cardiotoxicity—(See **WARNINGS**.)

Cutaneous—Reversible complete alopecia occurs in most cases. Hyperpigmentation of nailbeds and dermal crease, primarily in pediatric patients, and onycholysis have been reported in a few cases. Recall of skin reaction due to prior radiotherapy has occurred with doxorubicin administration.

Gastrointestinal—Acute nausea and vomiting occurs frequently and may be severe. This may be alleviated by antiemetic therapy. Mucositis (stomatitis and esophagitis) may occur 5 to 10 days after administration. The effect may be severe leading to ulceration and represents a site of origin for severe infections. The dosage regimen consisting of administration of doxorubicin on three successive days results in greater incidence and severity of mucositis. Ulceration and necrosis of the colon, especially the cecum, may occur leading to bleeding or severe infections which can be fatal. This reaction has been reported in patients with acute nonlymphocytic leukemia treated with a 3-day course of doxorubicin combined with cytarabine. Anorexia and diarrhea have been occasionally reported.

Vascular—Phlebosclerosis has been reported especially when small veins are used or a single vein is used for repeated administration. Facial flushing may occur if the injection is given too rapidly.

Local—Severe cellulitis, vesication and tissue necrosis will occur if extravasation of doxorubicin occurs during administration. Erythematous streaking along the vein proximal to the site of injection had been reported (see **DOSAGE AND ADMINISTRATION**).

Hematologic—The occurrence of secondary acute myeloid leukemia with or without a preleukemic phase has been reported rarely in patients concurrently treated with doxorubicin in association with DNA-damaging antineoplastic agents. Such cases could have a short (1–3 years) latency period. Pediatric patients are also at risk of developing secondary acute myeloid leukemia.

Hypersensitivity—Fever, chills and urticaria have been reported occasionally. Anaphylaxis may occur. A case of apparent cross sensitivity to lincomycin has been reported.

Neurological—Peripheral neurotoxicity in the form of local-regional sensory and/or disturbances have been reported in patients treated intra-arterially with doxorubicin, mostly in combination with cisplatin. Animal studies have demonstrated seizures and coma in rodents and dogs treated with intra-carotid doxorubicin. Seizures and coma have been reported in patients treated with doxorubicin in combination with cisplatin or vincristine.

Other—Conjunctivitis and lacrimation occur rarely.

OVERDOSAGE

Acute overdosage with doxorubicin enhances the toxic effect of mucositis, leukopenia and thrombocytopenia. Treatment of acute overdosage consists of treatment of the severely myelosuppressed patient with hospitalization, antimicrobials, platelet transfusions and symptomatic treatment of mucositis. Use of hemopoietic growth factor (G-CSF, GM-CSF) may be considered.

The 150 mg ADRIAMYCIN RDF and the 100 mL (2 mg/mL) ADRIAMYCIN PFS vials are packaged as multiple dose vials and caution should be exercised to prevent inadvertent overdosage.

Cumulative dosage with doxorubicin increases the risk of cardiomyopathy and resultant congestive heart failure (see **WARNINGS**). Treatment consists of vigorous management of congestive heart failure with digitalis preparations, diuretics, and after-load reducers such as ACE inhibitors.

DOSAGE AND ADMINISTRATION

Care in the administration of ADRIAMYCIN PFS and ADRIAMYCIN RDF will reduce the chance of perivenous infiltration (see **WARNINGS**). It may also decrease the change of local reactions such as urticaria and erythematous streaking. On intravenous administration of doxorubicin, extravasation may occur with or without an accompanying burning or stinging sensation, even if blood returns well on aspiration of the infusion needle. If any signs or symptoms of extravasation have occurred, the injection or infusion should be immediately terminated and restarted in another vein. If extravasation is suspected, intermittent application of ice to the site for 15 min. q.i.d. × 3 days may be useful. The benefit of local administration of drugs has not been clearly established. Because of the progressive nature of extravasation reactions, close observation and plastic surgery consultation is recommended. Blistering, ulceration and/or persistent pain are indications for wide excision surgery, followed by split-thickness skin grafting.

The most commonly used dose schedule when used as a single agent is 60 to 75 mg/m^2 as a single intravenous injection administered at 21-day intervals. The lower dosage should be given to patients with inadequate marrow reserves due to old age, or prior therapy, or neoplastic marrow infiltration. ADRIAMYCIN PFS and ADRIAMYCIN RDF have been used concurrently with other approved chemotherapeutic agents. Evidence is available that in some types of neoplastic disease combination chemotherapy is superior to single agents. The benefits and risks of such therapy continue to be elucidated. When used in combination with other chemotherapy drugs, the most commonly used dosage of doxorubicin is 40 to 60 mg/m^2 given as a single intravenous injection every 21 to 28 days. Doxorubicin dosage must be reduced in case of hyperbilirubinemia as follows:

Plasma bilirubin concentration (mg/dL)	Dosage reduction (%)
1.2 – 3.0	50
3.1 – 5.0	75

Reconstitution Directions: ADRIAMYCIN RDF 10 mg, 20 mg, 50 mg, and 150 mg vials should be reconstituted with 5 mL, 10 mL, 25 mL, and 75 mL, respectively, of Sodium Chloride Injection, USP (0.9%), to give a final concentration of 2 mg/mL of doxorubicin hydrochloride. An appropriate volume of air should be withdrawn from the vial during reconstitution to avoid excessive pressure buildup. Bacteriostatic diluents are not recommended.

After adding the diluent, the vial should be shaken and the contents allowed to dissolve. The reconstituted solution is stable for 7 days at room temperature and under normal room light (100 foot-candles) and 15 days under refrigeration (2° to 8°C). It should be protected from exposure to sunlight. Discard any of the unused solution from the 10 mg, 20 mg, and 50 mg single dose vials. Unused solutions of the multiple dose vial remaining beyond the recommended storage times should be discarded.

It is recommended that ADRIAMYCIN PFS and ADRIAMYCIN RDF be slowly administered into the tubing of a freely running intravenous infusion of Sodium Chloride Injection, USP, or 5% Dextrose Injection, USP. The tubing should be attached to a Butterfly® needle inserted preferably into a large vein. If possible, avoid veins over joints or in extremities with compromised venous or lymphatic drainage. The rate of administration is dependent on the size of the vein, and the dosage. However, the dose should be administered in not less than 3 to 5 minutes. Local erythematous streaking along the vein as well as facial flushing may be indicated of too rapid an administration. A burning or stinging sensation may be indicative of perivenous infiltration and the infusion should be immediately terminated and restarted in another vein. Perivenous infiltration may occur painlessly.

Doxorubicin should not be mixed with heparin or fluorouracil since it has been reported that these drugs are incompatible to the extent that a precipitate may form. Until specific compatibility data are available, it is not recommended that doxorubicin be mixed with other drugs.

Parenteral drug products should be inspected visually for particulate matter and discoloration prior to administration, whenever solution and container permit.

Handling and Disposal: Skin reactions associated with doxorubicin have been reported. Skin accidentally exposed to doxorubicin should be rinsed copiously with soap and warm water, and if the eyes are involved, standard irrigation techniques should be used immediately. The use of goggles, gloves, and protective gowns is recommended during preparation and administration of the drug.

Procedures for proper handling and disposal of anti-cancer drugs should be considered. Several guidelines on this subject have been published.[1–7] There is no general agreement that all the procedures recommended in the guidelines are necessary or appropriate.

Caregivers of pediatric patients receiving doxorubicin should be counseled to take precautions (such as wearing latex gloves) to prevent contact with the patient's urine and other body fluids for at least 5 days after each treatment.

HOW SUPPLIED

ADRIAMYCIN RDF® Powder for Injection (doxorubicin hydrochloride for injection, USP) is available as follows:

NDC 0013-1086-91	10 mg single dose vial, 10 vial packs
NDC 0013-1096-91	20 mg single dose vial, 10 vial packs
NDC 0013-1106-79	50 mg single dose vial, single packs

Store at controlled room temperature, 15° to 30°C (59° to 86°F). Protect from light.

Retain in carton until time of use. Contains no preservative. Discard unused portion.

MULTIDOSE VIAL:

NDC 0013-1116-83	150 mg multidose vial, single packs

Store at controlled room temperature, 15° to 30°C (59° to 86°F). Protect from light.

Retain in carton until time of use.

RECONSTITUTED SOLUTION STABILITY:

After adding the diluent, the vial should be shaken and the contents allowed to dissolve. The reconstituted solution is stable for 7 days at room temperature and under normal room light (100 foot-candles) and 15 days under refrigeration (2° to 8°C). It should be protected from exposure to sunlight. Discard any unused solution from the 10 mg, 20 mg and 50 mg single dose vials. Unused solutions of the multiple dose vial remaining beyond the recommended storage times should be discarded.

MANUFACTURER:

Pharmacia & Upjohn S.p.A.
Milan, Italy

HOW SUPPLIED

ADRIAMYCIN PFS® Injection (doxorubicin hydrochloride injection, USP)

SINGLE DOSE VIALS:

Sterile single use only, contains no preservative.

NDC 0013-1136-91	10 mg vial, 2 mg/mL, 5 mL, 10 vial packs
NDC 0013-1146-91	20 mg vial, 2 mg/mL, 10 mL, 10 vial packs
NDC 0013-1156-79	50 mg vial, 2 mg/mL, 25 mL, single vial packs
NDC 0013-1176-87	75 mg vial, 2 mg/mL, 37.5 mL, single vial packs

Store refrigeration, 2° to 8°C (36° to 46°F). Protect from light. Retain in carton until time of use. Discard unused portion.

MULTIDOSE VIAL:

Sterile multidose vial, contains no preservative.

NDC 0013-1166-83	200 mg, 2 mg/mL, 100 mL, multidose vial, single vial packs

Store refrigeration, 2° to 8°C (36° to 46°F). Protect from light. Retain in carton until contents are used.

MANUFACTURERS:

Pharmacia & Upjohn S.p.A.
Milan, Italy
SP Pharmaceuticals LLC
Albuquerque, NM 87109, USA

Rx only

REFERENCES

1. Recommendations for the Safe Handling of Parenteral Antineoplastic Drugs, NIH Publication No. 83–2621. For sale by the Superintendent of Documents, U.S. Government Printing Office, Washington, DC 20402.
2. AMA Council Report. Guidelines for Handling Parenteral Antineoplastics. JAMA 1985; 2.53(11):1590–1592.
3. National Study Commission on Cytotoxic Exposure-Recommendations for Handling of Cytotoxic Agents. Available from Louis P. Jeffrey, ScD., Chairman, National Study Commission on Cytotoxic Exposure, Massachusetts College of Pharmacy and Allied Health Sciences, 179 Longwood Avenue, Boston, MA 02115.
4. Clinical Oncology Society of Australia, Guidelines and Recommendations for Safe Handling of Antineoplastic Agents. Med J Australia 1983; 1:426–428.
5. Jones RB, et al. Safe Handling of Chemotherapeutic Agents: A Report from the Mount Sinai Medical Center. CA-A Cancer Journal for Clinicians 1983; (Sept/Oct): 258–263.
6. American Society of Hospital Pharmacists Technical Assistance Bulletin on Handling Cytotoxic and Hazardous Drugs. Am J Hosp Pharm 1990; 47:1033–1049.
7. Controlling Occupational Exposure to Hazardous Drugs (OSHA Work-Practice Guidelines). Am J Health-Syst Pharm 1996; 53:1669–1685.

DISTRIBUTED BY:

Pharmacia & Upjohn Company, Kalamazoo, MI 49001, USA
817 336 203 Revised April 2000

AROMASIN® ℞
exemestane tablets

DESCRIPTION

AROMASIN® Tablets for oral administration contain 25 mg of exemestane, an irreversible, steroidal aromatase inactivator. Exemestane is chemically described as 6-methylenandrosta-1,4-diene-3,17-dione. Its molecular formula is $C_{20}H_{24}O_2$ and its structural formula is as follows:

CH3 O CH3 H H H O CH2

The active ingredient is a white to slightly yellow crystalline powder with a molecular weight of 296.41. Exemestane is freely soluble in N, N-dimethylformamide, soluble in methanol, and practically insoluble in water.

Each AROMASIN Tablet contains the following inactive ingredients: mannitol, crospovidone, polysorbate 80, hydroxypropyl methylcellulose, colloidal silicon dioxide, microcrystalline cellulose, sodium starch glycolate, magnesium stearate, simethicone, polyethylene glycol 6000, sucrose, magnesium carbonate, titanium dioxide, methylparaben, and polyvinyl alcohol.

CLINICAL PHARMACOLOGY

Mechanism of Action

Breast cancer cell growth may be estrogen-dependent. Aromatase is the principal enzyme that converts androgens to estrogens both in pre- and postmenopausal women. While the main source of estrogen (primarily estradiol) is the ovary in premenopausal women, the principal source of circulating estrogens in postmenopausal women is from conversion of adrenal and ovarian androgens (androstenedione and testosterone) to estrogens (estrone and estradiol) by the aromatase enzyme in peripheral tissues. Estrogen deprivation through aromatase inhibition is an effective and selective treatment for some postmenopausal patients with hormone-dependent breast cancer.

Exemestane is an irreversible, steroidal aromatase inactivator, structurally related to the natural substrate androstenedione. It acts as a false substrate for the aromatase enzyme, and is processed to an intermediate that binds irreversibly to the active site of the enzyme causing its inactivation, an effect also known as "suicide inhibition." Exemestane significantly lowers circulating estrogen concentrations in postmenopausal women, but has no detectable effect on adrenal biosynthesis of corticosteroids or aldosterone. Exemestane has no effect on other enzymes involved in the steroidogenic pathway up to a concentration at least 600 times higher than that inhibiting the aromatase enzyme.

Pharmacokinetics

Following oral administration to healthy postmenopausal women, exemestane is rapidly absorbed. After maximum plasma concentration is reached, levels decline polyexponentially with a mean terminal half-life of about 24 hours. Exemestane is extensively distributed and is cleared from the systemic circulation primarily by metabolism. The pharmacokinetics of exemestane are dose proportional after single (10 to 200 mg) or repeated oral doses (0.5 to 50 mg). Following repeated daily doses of exemestane 25 mg, plasma concentrations of unchanged drug are similar to levels measured after a single dose.

Pharmacokinetic parameters in postmenopausal women with advanced breast cancer following single or repeated doses have been compared with those in healthy, postmenopausal women. Exemestane appeared to be more rapidly absorbed in the women with breast cancer than in the healthy women, with a mean t_{max} of 1.2 hours in the women with breast cancer and 2.9 hours in the healthy women. After repeated dosing, the average oral clearance in women with advanced breast cancer was 45% lower than the oral clearance in healthy postmenopausal women, with corresponding higher systemic exposure. Mean AUC values following repeated doses in women with breast cancer (75.4 ng•h/mL) were about twice those in healthy women (41.4 ng•h/mL).

Absorption: Following oral administration of radiolabeled exemestane, at least 42% of radioactivity was absorbed from the gastrointestinal tract. Exemestane plasma levels increased by approximately 40% after a high-fat breakfast.

Distribution: Exemestane is distributed extensively into tissues. Exemestane is 90% bound to plasma proteins and the fraction bound is independent of the total concentration. Albumin and α_1-acid glycoprotein both contribute to the binding. The distribution of exemestane and its metabolites into blood cells is negligible.

Metabolism and Excretion: Following administration of radiolabeled exemestane to healthy postmenopausal women, the cumulative amounts of radioactivity excreted in urine and feces were similar (42 ± 3% in urine and 42 ± 6% in feces over a 1-week collection period). The amount of drug excreted unchanged in urine was less than 1% of the dose. Exemestane is extensively metabolized, with levels of the unchanged drug in plasma accounting for less than 10% of the total radioactivity. The initial steps in the metabolism of exemestane are oxidation of the methylene group in position 6 and reduction of the 17-keto group with subsequent formation of many secondary metabolites. Each metabolite accounts for only a limited amount of drug-related material. The metabolites are inactive or inhibit aromatase with decreased potency compared with the parent drug. One metabolite may have androgenic activity (see Pharmacodynamics, Other Endocrine Effects). Studies using human liver preparations indicate that cytochrome P-450 3A4 (CYP 3A4) is the principal isoenzyme involved in the oxidation of exemestane.

Special Populations:

Geriatric: Healthy postmenopausal women aged 43 to 68 years were studied in the pharmacokinetic trials. Age-related alterations in exemestane pharmacokinetics were not seen over this age range.

Gender: The pharmacokinetics of exemestane following administration of a single, 25-mg tablet to fasted healthy males (mean age 32 years) were similar to the pharmacokinetics of exemestane in fasted healthy postmenopausal women (mean age 55 years).

Race: The influence of race on exemestane pharmacokinetics has not been evaluated.

Hepatic Insufficiency: The pharmacokinetics of exemestane have been investigated in subjects with moderate or severe hepatic insufficiency (Childs-Pugh B or C). Following a single 25-mg oral dose, the AUC of exemestane was approximately 3 times higher than that observed in healthy volunteers (see PRECAUTIONS).

Renal Insufficiency: The AUC of exemestane after a single 25-mg dose was approximately 3 times higher in subjects with moderate or severe renal insufficiency (creatinine clearance <35 mL/min/1.73m²) compared with the AUC in healthy volunteers (see PRECAUTIONS).

Pediatric: The pharmacokinetics of exemestane have not been studied in pediatric patients.

Continued on next page

Information on these Pharmacia & Upjohn products is based on labeling in effect June 1, 2000. Further information concerning these and other Pharmacia & Upjohn products may be obtained by direct inquiry to Medical Information, Pharmacia & Upjohn, Kalamazoo, MI 49001.

Aromasin—Cont.

Drug-Drug Interactions

Exemestane is metabolized by cytochrome P-450 3A4 (CYP 3A4) and aldoketoreductases. It does not inhibit any of the major CYP isoenzymes, including CYP 1A2, 2C9, 2D6, 2E1, and 3A4. In a clinical pharmacokinetic study, ketoconazole showed no significant influence on the pharmacokinetics of exemestane. Although no other formal drug-drug interaction studies have been conducted, significant effects on exemestane clearance by CYP isoenzymes inhibitors appear unlikely. However, a possible decrease of exemestane plasma levels by known inducers of CYP 3A4 cannot be excluded.

Pharmacodynamics

Effect on Estrogens: Multiple doses of exemestane ranging from 0.5 to 600 mg/day were administered to postmenopausal women with advanced breast cancer. Plasma estrogen (estradiol, estrone, and estrone sulfate) suppression was seen starting at a 5-mg daily dose of exemestane, with a maximum suppression of at least 85% to 95% achieved at a 25-mg dose. Exemestane 25 mg daily reduced whole body aromatization (as measured by injecting radiolabeled androstenedione) by 98% in postmenopausal women with breast cancer. After a single dose of exemestane 25 mg, the maximal suppression of circulating estrogens occurred 2 to 3 days after dosing and persisted for 4 to 5 days.

Effect on Corticosteroids: In multiple-dose trials of doses up to 200 mg daily, exemestane selectivity was assessed by examining its effect on adrenal steroids. Exemestane did not affect cortisol or aldosterone secretion at baseline or in response to ACTH at any dose. Thus, no glucocorticoid or mineralocorticoid replacement therapy is necessary with exemestane treatment.

Other Endocrine Effects: Exemestane does not bind significantly to steroidal receptors, except for a slight affinity for the androgen receptor (0.28% relative to dihydrotestosterone). The binding affinity of its 17-dihydrometabolite for the androgen receptor, however, is 100-times that of the parent compound. Daily doses of exemestane up to 25 mg had no significant effect on circulating levels of testosterone, androstenedione, dehydroepiandrosterone sulfate, or 17-hydroxyprogesterone. Increases in testosterone and androstenedione levels have been observed at daily doses of 200 mg or more. A dose-dependent decrease in sex hormone binding globulin (SHBG) has been observed with daily exemestane doses of 2.5 mg or higher. Slight, nondose-dependent increases in serum lutenizing hormone (LH) and follicle-stimulating hormone (FSH) levels have been observed even at low doses as a consequence of feedback at the pituitary level.

CLINICAL STUDIES

Exemestane 25 mg administered once daily was evaluated in a randomized double-blind, multicenter, multinational comparative study and in two multicenter single-arm studies of postmenopausal women with advanced breast cancer who had disease progression after treatment with tamoxifen for metastatic disease or as adjuvant therapy. Some patients also have received prior cytotoxic therapy, either as adjuvant treatment or for metastatic disease.

The primary purpose of the three studies was evaluation of objective response rate (complete response [CR] and partial response [PR]). Time to tumor progression and overall survival were also assessed in the comparative trial. Response rates were assessed based on World Health Organization (WHO) criteria, and in the comparative study, were submitted to an external review committee that was blinded to patient treatment. In the comparative study, 769 patients were randomized to receive AROMASIN (exemestane tablets) 25 mg once daily (N = 366) or megestrol acetate 40 mg four times daily (N = 403). Demographics and baseline characteristics are presented in Table 1.

[See table 1 above]

The efficacy results from the comparative study are shown in Table 2. The objective response rates observed in the two treatment arms showed that AROMASIN was not different from megestrol acetate. Response rates for exemestane from the two single-arm trials were 23.4% and 28.1%.

[See table 2 above]

There were too few deaths occurring across treatment groups to draw conclusions on overall survival differences. The Kaplan-Meier curve for time to tumor progression in the comparative study is shown in Figure 1.

Figure 1. Time to Tumor Progression in the Comparative Study of Postmenopausal Women With Advanced Breast Cancer Whose Disease Had Progressed After Tamoxifen Therapy

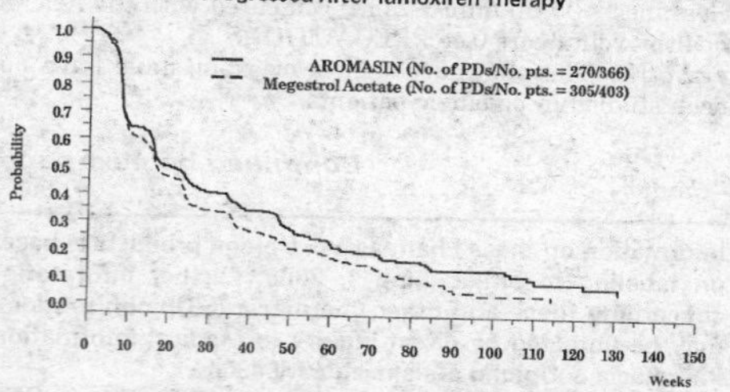

Table 1. Demographics and Baseline Characteristics from the Comparative Study of Postmenopausal Women with Advanced Breast Cancer Whose Disease Had Progressed after Tamoxifen Therapy

Parameter	AROMASIN (N = 366)	Megestrol Acetate (N = 403)
Median Age (range)	65 (35–89)	65 (30–91)
ECOG Performance Status		
0	167 (46%)	187 (46%)
1	162 (44%)	172 (43%)
2	34 (9%)	42 (10%)
Receptor Status		
ER and/or PgR +	246 (67%)	274 (68%)
ER and PgR unknown	116 (32%)	128 (32%)
Responders to prior tamoxifen	68 (19%)	85 (21%)
NE for response to prior tamoxifen	46 (13%)	41 (10%)
Site of Metastasis		
Visceral ± other sites	207 (57%)	239 (59%)
Bone only	61 (17%)	73 (18%)
Soft tissue only	54 (15%)	51 (13%)
Bone & soft tissue	43 (12%)	38 (9%)
Measurable Disease	287 (78%)	314 (78%)
Prior Tamoxifen Therapy		
Adjuvant or Neoadjuvant	145 (40%)	152 (38%)
Advanced Disease, Outcome		
CP, PR or SD≥ 6 months	179 (49%)	210 (52%)
SD< 6 months, PD or NE	42 (12%)	41 (10%)
Prior Chemotherapy		
For advanced disease ± adjuvant	58 (16%)	67 (17%)
Adjuvant only	104 (28%)	108 (27%)
No chemotherapy	203 (56%)	226 (56%)

Table 2. Efficacy Results from the Comparative Study of Postmenopausal Women with Advanced Breast Cancer Whose Disease Had Progressed after Tamoxifen Therapy

Response Characteristics	AROMASIN (N=366)		Megestrol Acetate (N=403)
Objective Response Rate = CR+ PR (%)	15.0		12.4
Difference in Response Rate (AR-MA)		2.6	
95% C. I.		7.5, -2.3	
CR (%)	2.2		1.2
PR (%)	12.8		11.2
SD ≥ 24 Weeks (%)	21.3		21.1
Median Duration of Response (weeks)	76.1		71.0
Median TTP (weeks)	20.3		16.6
Hazard Ratio (AR-MA)		0.84	

Abbreviations: CR = complete response, PR = partial response, SD = stable disease (no change), TTP = time to tumor progression, C. I. = confidence interval, MA = megestrol acetate, AR = AROMASIN

INDICATIONS AND USAGE

AROMASIN Tablets are indicated for the treatment of advanced breast cancer in postmenopausal women whose disease has progressed following tamoxifen therapy.

CONTRAINDICATIONS

AROMASIN Tablets are contraindicated in patients with a known hypersensitivity to the drug or to any of the excipients.

WARNINGS

AROMASIN Tablets may cause fetal harm when administered to a pregnant woman. Radioactivity related to ^{14}C-exemestane crossed the placenta of rats following oral administration of 1 mg/kg exemestane. The concentration of exemestane and its metabolites was approximately equivalent in maternal and fetal blood. When rats were administered exemestane from 14 days prior to mating until either days 15 or 20 of gestation, and resuming for the 21 days of lactation, an increase in placental weight was seen at 4 mg/kg/day (approximately 1.5 times the recommended human daily dose on a mg/m^2 basis). Prolonged gestation and abnormal or difficult labor was observed at doses equal to or greater than 20 mg/kg/day. Increased resorption, reduced number of live fetuses, decreased fetal weight, and retarded ossification were also observed at these doses. No malformations were noted when exemestane was administered to pregnant rats during the organogenesis period at doses up to 810 mg/kg/day (approximately 320 times the recommended human dose on a mg/m^2 basis). Daily doses of exemestane, given to rabbits during organogenesis caused a decrease in placental weight at 90 mg/kg/day (approximately 70 times the recommended human daily dose on a mg/m^2 basis). Abortions, an increase in resorptions, and a reduction in fetal body weight were seen at 270 mg/kg/day. There was no increase in the incidence of malformations in rabbits at doses up to 270 mg/kg/day (approximately 210 times the recommended human dose on a mg/m^2 basis).

There are no studies in pregnant women using AROMASIN. AROMASIN is indicated for postmenopausal women. If there is exposure to AROMASIN during pregnancy, the patient should be apprised of the potential hazard to the fetus and potential risk for loss of the pregnancy.

PRECAUTIONS

General. AROMASIN Tablets should not be administered to premenopausal women. AROMASIN should not be coadministered with estrogen-containing agents as these could interfere with its pharmacologic action.

Hepatic Insufficiency. The pharmacokinetics of exemestane have been investigated in subjects with moderate or severe hepatic insufficiency (Childs-Pugh B or C). Following a single 25-mg oral dose, the AUC of exemestane was approximately 3 times higher than that observed in healthy volunteers. The safety of chronic dosing in patients with moderate or severe hepatic impairment has not been studied. Based on experience with exemestane at repeated doses up to 200 mg daily that demonstrated a moderate increase in non-life threatening adverse events, dosage adjustment does not appear to be necessary.

Renal Insufficiency. The AUC of exemestane after a single 25-mg dose was approximately 3 times higher in subjects with moderate or severe renal insufficiency (creatinine clearance <35 mL/min/1.73m^2) compared with the AUC in healthy volunteers. The safety of chronic dosing in patients with moderate or severe renal impairment has not been studied. Based on experience with exemestane at repeated doses up to 200 mg daily that demonstrated a moderate increase in non-life threatening adverse events, dosage adjustment does not appear to be necessary.

Laboratory Tests. Approximately 20% of patients receiving exemestane in clinical studies, experienced Common Toxicity Criteria (CTC) grade 3 or 4 lymphocytopenia. Of these patients, 89% had a pre-existing lower grade lymphopenia. Forty percent of patients either recovered or improved to a lesser severity while on treatment. Patients did not have a significant increase in viral infections, and no opportunistic infections were observed. Elevations or serum levels of AST, ALT, alkaline phosphatase and gamma glutamyl transferase > 5 times the upper value of the normal range (i.e., ≥CTC grade 3) have been rarely reported but appear mostly attributable to the underlying presence of liver and/or bone metastases. In the comparative study, CTC grade 3 or 4 elevation of gamma glutamyl transferase without documented evidence of liver metatasis was reported in 2.7% of patients treated with AROMASIN and in 1.8% of patients treated with megestrol acetate.

Drug Interactions. Exemestane is extensively metabolized by CYP 3A4, but coadministration of ketoconazole, a potent inhibitor of CYP 3A4, has no significant effect on exemestane pharmacokinetics. Significant pharmacokinetic interactions mediated by inhibition of CYP isoenzymes therefore appear unlikely; however, a possible decrease of exemestane plasma levels by known inducers of CYP 3A4 cannot be excluded (see CLINICAL PHARMACOLOGY, Pharmacokinetics).

Table 3. Incidence (%) of Adverse Events of all Grades* and Causes Occurring in ≥5% of Patients in Each Treatment in the Comparative Study

Event	AROMASIN 25 mg once daily (N=358)	Megestrol Acetate 40 mg QID (N=400)
Autonomic Nervous		
Increased sweating	6	9
Body as a Whole		
Fatigue	22	29
Hot flashes	13	6
Pain	13	13
Influenza-like symptoms	6	5
Edema (includes edema, peripheral edema, leg edema)	7	6
Cardiovascular		
Hypertension	5	6
Nervous		
Depression	13	9
Insomnia	11	9
Anxiety	10	11
Dizziness	8	6
Headache	8	7
Gastrointestinal		
Nausea	18	12
Vomiting	7	4
Abdominal pain	6	11
Anorexia	6	5
Constipation	5	8
Diarrhea	4	5
Increased appetite	3	6
Respiratory		
Dyspnea	10	15
Coughing	6	7

* Graded according to Common Toxicity Criteria

Drug/Laboratory Tests Interactions. No clinically relevant changes in the results of clinical laboratory tests have been observed.

Carcinogenesis, Mutagenesis, Impairment of Fertility. Carcinogenicity studies have not been conducted with exemestane. Exemestane was not mutagenic in bacteria (Ames test) or mammalian cells (V79 Chinese hamster lung cells). Exemestane was clastogenic in human lymphocytes in vitro without metabolic activation but was not clastogenic in vivo (micronucleus assay in mouse bone marrow). Exemestane did not increase unscheduled DNA synthesis in rat hepatocytes.

Untreated female rats showed reduced fertility when mated to males treated with 500 mg/kg/day exemestane (approximately 200 times the recommended human dose on a mg/m^2 basis) for 63 days prior to and during cohabitation. Exemestane given to female rats 14 days prior to mating and through day 15 or 20 of gestation increased the placental weights at 4 mg/kg/day (approximately 1.5 times the human dose on a mg/m^2 basis). Exemestane showed no effects on female fertility parameters (e.g., ovarian function, mating behavior conception rate) in rats given doses up to 20 mg/kg/day (approximately 8 times the human dose on a mg/m^2 basis), but mean litter size was decreased at this dose. In general toxicology studies, changes in the ovary, including hyperplasia, an increase in ovarian cysts and a decrease in corpora lutea were observed with variable frequency in mice, rats and dogs at doses that ranged from 3–20 times the human dose on a mg/m^2 basis.

Pregnancy. Pregnancy Category D. See WARNINGS.

Nursing Mothers. AROMASIN is only indicated in postmenopausal women. However, radioactivity related to exemestane appeared in rat milk within 15 minutes of oral administration of radiolabeled exemestane. Concentrations of exemestane and its metabolites were approximately equivalent in the milk and plasma of rats for 24 hours after a single oral dose of 1 mg/kg ^{14}C-exemestane. It is not known whether exemestane is excreted in human milk. Because many drugs are excreted in human milk, caution should be exercised if a nursing mother is inadvertently exposed to AROMASIN (see WARNINGS).

Pediatric Use. The safety and effectiveness of AROMASIN in pediatric patients have not been established.

Geriatric Use. The use of AROMASIN in geriatric patients does not require special precautions.

ADVERSE REACTIONS

A total of 1058 patients were treated with exemestane 25 mg once daily in the clinical trials program. Exemestane was generally well tolerated, and adverse events were usually mild to moderate. Only one death was considered possibly related to treatment with exemestane; an 80-year-old woman with known coronary artery disease had a myocardial infarction with multiple organ failure after 9 weeks on study treatment. In the clinical trials program, only 3% of the patients discontinued treatment with exemestane because of adverse events, mainly within the first 10 weeks of treatment; late discontinuations because of adverse events were uncommon (0.3%).

In the comparative study, adverse reactions were assessed for 358 patients with AROMASIN and 400 patients treated with megestrol acetate. Fewer patients receiving AROMASIN discontinued treatment because of adverse events than those treated with megestrol acetate (2% vs. 5%). Adverse events that were considered drug related or of interdeterminate cause included hot flashes (13% vs. 5%), nausea (9% vs. 5%), fatigue (8% vs. 10%), increased sweating (4% vs. 8%), and increased appetite (3% vs. 6%). The proportion of patients experiencing an excessive weight gain (>10% of their baseline weight) was significantly higher with megestrol acetate than with AROMASIN (17% vs. 8%). Table 3 shows the adverse events of all CTC grades, regardless of causality, reported in 5% or greater of patients in the study treated either with AROMASIN or megestrol acetate.

[See table 3 above]

Less frequent adverse events of any cause (from 2% to 5%) reported in the comparative study for patients receiving AROMASIN 25 mg once daily were fever, generalized weakness, paresthesia, pathological fracture, bronchitis, sinusitis, rash, itching, urinary tract infection, and lymphedema.

Additional adverse events of any cause observed in the overall clinical trials program (N = 1058) in 5% or greater of patients treated with exemestane 25 mg once daily but not in the comparative study included pain at tumor sites (8%), asthenia (6%) and fever (5%). Adverse events of any cause reported in 2% to 5% of all patients treated with exemestane 25 mg in the overall clinical trials program but not in the comparative study included chest pain, hypoesthesia, confusion, dyspepsia, arthralgia, back pain, skeletal pain, infection, upper respiratory tract infection, pharyngitis, rhinitis, and alopecia.

OVERDOSAGE

Clinical trials have been conducted with exemestane given as a single dose to healthy female volunteers at doses as high as 800 mg daily for 12 weeks to postmenopausal women with advanced breast cancer at doses as high as 600 mg. These dosages were well tolerated. There is no specific antidote to overdosage and treatment must be symptomatic. General supportive care, including frequent monitoring of vital signs and close observation of the patient, is indicated.

A male child (age unknown) accidentally ingested a 25-mg tablet of exemestane. The initial physical examination was normal, but blood tests performed 1 hour after ingestion indicated leucocytosis (WBC 25000/mm^3 with 90% neutrophils). Blood tests were repeated 4 days after the incident and were normal. No treatment was given.

In mice, mortality was observed after a single oral dose of exemestane of 3200 mg/kg, the lowest dose tested (about 640 times the recommended human dose on a mg/m^2 basis). In rats and dogs, mortality was observed after single oral doses of exemestane of 5000 mg/kg (about 2000 times the recommended human dose on a mg/m^2 basis) and of 3000 mg/kg (about 4000 times the recommended human dose on a mg/m^2 basis), respectively.

Convulsions were observed after single doses of exemestane of 400 mg/kg and 3000 mg/kg in mice and dogs (approximately 80 and 4000 times the recommended human dose on a mg/m^2 basis), respectively.

DOSAGE AND ADMINISTRATION

The recommended dose of AROMASIN Tablets is 25 mg once daily after a meal. Treatment with AROMASIN should continue until tumor progression is evident.

The safety of chronic closing in patients with moderate or severe hepatic or renal impairment has not been studied. Based on experience with exemestane at repeated doses up to 200 mg daily that demonstrated a moderate increase in non-life threatening adverse events, dosage adjustment does not appear to be necessary (see CLINICAL PHARMACOLOGY, Special Populations and PRECAUTIONS).

HOW SUPPLIED

AROMASIN Tablets are round, bioconvex, and off-white to slightly gray. Each tablet contains 25 mg of exemestane. The tablets are printed on one side with the number "7663" in black. AROMASIN is packaged in HDPE bottles with a child-resistant screw cap, supplied in packs of 30 tablets.

30-tablet HDPE bottle NDC 0009-7663-04

Store at 25°C (77°F); excursions permitted to 15°–30°C (59°–86°F) [see USP Controlled Room Temperature].

℞ only

Manufactured for: Pharmacia & Upjohn Company, Kalamazoo, Michigan 49001, USA

By: Pharmacia & Upjohn S.p.A., Ascoli Piceno, Italy

October 1999 100000665 00 817 885 000

AZULFIDINE EN-tabs® ℞

[*azul' fidīne*]

sulfasalazine delayed release tablets, USP

Prescribing Information

Enteric-coated Tablets

DESCRIPTION

AZULFIDINE EN-tabs Tablets contain sulfasalazine, formulated in a delayed release tablet (enteric-coated), 500 mg, for oral administration.

AZULFIDINE EN-tabs Tablets are film coated with cellulose acetate phthalate to retard disintegration of the tablet in the stomach and reduce potential irritation of the gastric mucosa.

Therapeutic Classification: Anti-inflammatory agent and/or immunomodulatory agent.

Chemical Designation: 5-([p-(2-pyridylsulfamoyl)phenyl]azo) salicylic acid.

Chemical Structure:

Molecular Formula: $C_{18}H_{14}N_4O_5S$

CLINICAL PHARMACOLOGY

Pharmacodynamics

The mode of action of sulfasalazine (SSZ) or its metabolites, 5-aminosalicylic acid (5-ASA) and sulfapyridine (SP), is still under investigation, but may be related to the anti-inflammatory and/or immunomodulatory properties that have been observed in animal and in vitro models, to its affinity for connective tissue, and/or to the relatively high concentration it reaches in serous fluids, the liver and intestinal walls, as demonstrated in autoradiographic studies in animals. In ulcerative colitis, clinical studies utilizing rectal administration of SSZ, SP and 5-ASA have indicated that the major therapeutic action may reside in the 5-ASA moiety. The relative contribution of the parent drug and the major metabolites in rheumatoid arthritis remains under investigation.

Pharmacokinetics

In vivo studies have indicated that the absolute bioavailability of orally administered SSZ is less than 15% for parent drug. In the intestine, SSZ is metabolized by intestinal bacteria to SP and 5-ASA. Of the two species, SP is relatively well absorbed from the intestine and highly metabolized, while 5-ASA is much less well absorbed.

Absorption: Following oral administration of 1 g of SSZ to 9 healthy males, less than 15% of a dose of SSZ is absorbed as parent drug. Detectable serum concentrations of SSZ have been found in healthy subjects within 90 minutes after the ingestion. Maximum concentrations of SSZ occur between 3 and 12 hours post-ingestion, with the mean peak concentration (6 μg/mL) occurring at 6 hours.

In comparison, peak plasma levels of both SP and 5-ASA occur approximately 10 hours after dosing. This longer time to peak is indicative of gastrointestinal transit to the lower intestine, where bacteria-mediated-metabolism occurs. SP apparently is well absorbed from the colon, with an estimated bioavailability of 60%. In this same study 5-ASA is much less well absorbed from the gastrointestinal tract, with an estimated bioavailability of from 10% to 30%.

Distribution: Following intravenous injection, the calculated volume of distribution (Vdss) for SSZ was 7.5 ± 1.6 L.

Continued on next page

Information on these Pharmacia & Upjohn products is based on labeling in effect June 1, 2000. Further information concerning these and other Pharmacia & Upjohn products may be obtained by direct inquiry to Medical Information, Pharmacia & Upjohn, Kalamazoo, MI 49001.

Azulfidine—Cont.

SSZ is highly bound to albumin (>99.3%), while SP is only about 70% bound to albumin. Acetylsulfapyridine (AcSP), the principal metabolite of SP, is approximately 90% bound to plasma proteins.

Metabolism: As mentioned above, SSZ is metabolized by intestinal bacteria to SP and 5-ASA. Approximately 15% of a dose of SSZ is absorbed as parent and is metabolized to some extent in the liver to the same two species. The observed plasma half-life for intravenous sulfasalazine is 7.6 ± 3.4 hrs. The primary route of metabolism of SP is via acetylation to form AcSP. The rate of metabolism of SP to AcSP is dependent upon acetylator or phenotype. In fast acetylators, the mean plasma half-life of SP is 10.4 hrs, while in slow acetylators it is 14.8 hrs. SP can also be metabolized to 5-hydroxy-sulfapyridine (SPOH) and N-acetyl-5-hydroxy-sulfapyridine. 5-ASA is primarily metabolized in both the liver and intestine to N-acetyl-5-aminosalicylic acid via a non-acetylation phenotype dependent route Due to low plasma levels produced by 5-ASA after oral administration, reliable estimates of plasma half-life are not possible.

Excretion: Absorbed SP and 5-ASA and their metabolites are primarily eliminated in the urine either as free metabolites or as glucuronide conjugates. The majority of 5-ASA stays within the colonic lumen and is excreted as 5-ASA and acetyl-5-ASA with the feces. The calculated clearance of SSZ following intravenous administration was 1 L/hr. Renal clearance was estimated to account for 37% of total clearance.

Special Populations

Elderly: Elderly patients with rheumatoid arthritis showed a prolonged plasma half-life for SSZ, SP, and their metabolites. The clinical impact of this is unknown.

Acetylator Status: The metabolism of SP to AcSP is mediated by polymorphic enzymes such that two distinct populations of slow and fast metabolizers exist. Approximately 60% of the Caucasian population can be classified as belonging to the slow acetylator phenotype. These subjects will display a prolonged plasma half-life for SP (14.8 hrs vs 10.4 hrs) and an accumulation of higher plasma levels of SP than fast acetylators. The clinical implication of this is unclear; however, in a small pharmacokinetic trial where acetylator status was determined, subjects who were slow acetylators of SP showed a higher incidence of adverse events.

Gender: Gender appears not to have an effect on either the rate or the pattern of metabolites of SSZ, SP, or 5-ASA.

INDICATIONS AND USAGE

AZULFIDINE EN-tabs Tablets are indicated:

a) in the treatment of mild to moderate ulcerative colitis, and as adjunctive therapy in severe ulcerative colitis;
b) for the prolongation of the remission period between acute attacks of ulcerative colitis; and
c) in the treatment of patients with rheumatoid arthritis who have responded inadequately to salicylates or other nonsteroidal anti-inflammatory drugs.

AZULFIDINE EN-tabs is particularly indicated in patients with ulcerative colitis who cannot take uncoated sulfasalazine tablets because of gastrointestinal intolerance, and in whom there is evidence that this intolerance is not primarily the result of high blood levels of sulfapyridine and its metabolites, e.g., patients experiencing nausea and vomiting with the first few doses of the drug, or patients in whom a reduction in dosage does not alleviate the adverse gastrointestinal effects.

AZULFIDINE EN-tabs is recommended in the management of adults with active, classic, and definitive rheumatoid arthritis who have had an insufficient therapeutic response to, or are intolerant of, an adequate trial of full doses of one or more nonsteroidal anti-inflammatory drugs. In rheumatoid arthritis, concurrent treatment with analgesics and/or nonsteroidal anti-inflammatory drugs is recommended at least until the effect of AZULFIDINE EN-tabs is apparent. Rest and physiotherapy as indicated should be continued. Unlike anti-inflammatory drugs, AZULFIDINE EN-tabs does not produce an immediate response.

CONTRAINDICATIONS

AZULFIDINE EN-tabs Tablets are contraindicated in:

Hypersensitivity to sulfasalazine, its metabolites, sulfonamides or salicylates,

Pediatric patients under two years of age,

Patients with intestinal or urinary obstruction,

Patients with porphyria, as the sulfonamides have been reported to precipitate an acute attack.

WARNINGS

Only after critical appraisal should AZULFIDINE EN-tabs Tablets be given to patients with hepatic or renal damage or blood dyscrasias. Deaths associated with the administration of sulfasalazine have been reported from hypersensitivity reactions, agranulocytosis, aplastic anemia, other blood dyscrasias, renal and liver damage, irreversible neuromuscular and central nervous system changes, and fibrosing alveolitis. The presence of clinical signs such as sore throat, fever, pallor, purpura or jaundice may be indications of serious blood disorders. Complete blood counts, as well as urinalysis with careful microscopic examination, should be done frequently in patients receiving AZULFIDINE EN-tabs (see Laboratory Tests). Oligospermia and infertility have been observed in men treated with sulfasalazine. Withdrawal of the drug appears to reverse these effects.

PRECAUTIONS

General: AZULFIDINE EN-tabs Tablets should be given with caution to patients with severe allergy or bronchial asthma. Adequate fluid intake must be maintained in order to prevent crystalluria and stone formation. Patients with glucose-6-phosphate dehydrogenase deficiency should be observed closely for signs of hemolytic anemia. This reaction is frequently dose related. If toxic or hypersensitivity reactions occur, AZULFIDINE EN-tabs should be discontinued immediately.

Isolated instances have been reported when AZULFIDINE EN-tabs Tablets have passed undisintegrated. If this is observed, the administration of AZULFIDINE EN-tabs should be discontinued immediately.

Information for Patients: Patients should be informed of the possibility of adverse effects and of the need for careful medical supervision. The occurrence of sore throat, fever, pallor, purpura or jaundice may indicate a serious blood disorder. Should any of these occur, the patient should seek medical advice.

Patients should be instructed to take AZULFIDINE EN-tabs in evenly divided doses, preferably after meals, and to swallow the tablets whole. Additionally, patients should be advised that sulfasalazine may produce an orange-yellow discoloration of the urine or skin.

Ulcerative Colitis: Patients with ulcerative colitis should be made aware that ulcerative colitis rarely remits completely, and that the risk of relapse can be substantially reduced by continued administration of AZULFIDINE EN-tabs at a maintenance dosage.

Rheumatoid Arthritis: Rheumatoid arthritis rarely remits. Therefore, continued administration of AZULFIDINE EN-tabs is indicated. Patients requiring sulfasalazine should follow up with their physicians to determine the need for continued administration.

Laboratory Tests: Complete blood counts, including differential white cell count and liver function tests, should be performed before starting AZULFIDINE EN-tabs and every second week during the first three months of therapy. During the second three months, the same tests should be done once monthly and thereafter once every three months, and as clinically indicated. Urinalysis and an assessment of renal function should also be done periodically during treatment with AZULFIDINE EN-tabs.

The determination of serum sulfapyridine levels may be useful since concentrations greater than 50 µg/mL appear to be associated with an increased incidence of adverse reactions.

Drug Interactions: Reduced absorption of folic acid and digoxin have been reported when those agents were administered concomitantly with sulfasalazine.

Carcinogenesis, Mutagenesis, Impairment of Fertility: Two year oral carcinogenicity studies were conducted in male and female F344/N rats and B6C3F1 mice. Sulfasalazine was tested at 84 (496 mg/m^2), 168 (991 mg/m^2) and 337.5 (1991 mg/m^2) mg/kg/day doses in rats. A statistically significant increase in the incidence of urinary bladder transitional cell papillomas was observed in male rats. In female rats, two (4%) of the 337.5 mg/kg rats had transitional cell papilloma of the kidney. The increased incidence of neoplasms in the urinary bladder and kidney of rats was also associated with an increase in the renal calculi formation and hyperplasia of transitional cell epithelium. For the mouse study, sulfasalazine was tested at 675 (2025 mg/m^2), 1350 (4050 mg/m^2) and 2700 (8100 mg/m^2) mg/kg/day. The incidence of hepatocellular adenoma or carcinoma in male and female mice was significantly greater than the control at all doses tested.

Sulfasalazine did not show mutagenicity in the bacterial reverse mutation assay (Ames test) or in the L51784 mouse lymphoma cell assay at the HGPRT gene. However, sulfasalazine showed equivocal mutagenic response in the micronucleus assay of mouse and rat bone marrow and mouse peripheral RBC and the sister chromatid exchange, chromosomal aberration, and micronucleus assays in lymphocytes obtained from humans.

Impairments of male fertility was observed in reproductive studies performed in rats at a dose of 800 mg/kg/day (4800 mg/m^2). Oligospermia and infertility have been described in men treated with sulfasalazine. Withdrawal of the drug appears to reverse these effects.

Pregnancy:

Teratogenic Effects: Pregnancy Category B. Reproduction studies have been performed in rats and rabbits at doses up to 6 times the human dose and have revealed no evidence if impaired female fertility or harm to the fetus due to sulfasalazine. There are, however, no adequate and well-controlled studies in pregnant women. Because animal reproduction studies are not always predictive of human response, this drug should be used during pregnancy only if clearly needed.

A national survey evaluated the outcome of pregnancies associated with inflammatory bowel disease (IBD). In 186 pregnancies in women treated with sulfasalazine alone or sulfasalazine and concomitant steroid therapy, the incidence of fetal morbidity and mortality was comparable both to that of 245 untreated IBD pregnancies, and to pregnancies in the general population.[1]

A study of 1455 pregnancies associated with exposure to sulfonamides including sulfasalazine, indicated that this group of drugs did not appear to be associated with fetal malformation.[2] A review of the medical literature covering 1155 pregnancies in women with ulcerative colitis suggested that the outcome was similar to that expected in the general population.[3]

No clinical studies have been performed to evaluate the effect of sulfasalazine on the growth development and functional maturation of children whose mothers received the drug during pregnancy.

Nonteratogenic Effects: Sulfasalazine and sulfapyridine pass the placental barrier. Although sulfapyridine has been shown to have poor bilirubin-displacing capacity, the potential for kernicterus in newborns should be kept in mind.

A case of agranulocytosis has been reported in an infant whose mother was taking both sulfasalazine and prednisone throughout pregnancy.

Nursing Mothers: Caution should be exercised when AZULFIDINE EN-tabs is administered to a nursing mother. Sulfonamides are excreted in the milk. In the newborn, they compete with bilirubin for binding sites on the plasma proteins and may cause kernicterus. Insignificant amounts of uncleaved sulfasalazine have been found in milk, whereas the sulfapyridine levels in milk are about 30% to 60% of those in the maternal serum. Sulfapyridine has been shown to have a poor bilirubin-displacing capacity.

Pediatric Use: The safety and effectiveness of AZULFIDINE EN-tabs in pediatric patients below the age of two years with ulcerative colitis have not been established. The safety and effectiveness in juvenile rheumatoid arthritis have not been established. It has been reported that the frequency of adverse events in patients with systemic onset of juvenile arthritis is high.[4]

ADVERSE REACTIONS

Clinical experience to data has indicated that patients with rheumatoid arthritis treated with AZULFIDINE EN-tabs Tablets appear to have a similar profile and incidence of adverse effects to patients with ulcerative colitis. There are no known adverse effects that are specific to patients with rheumatoid arthritis treated with sulfasalazine with the possible exception of skin rash, which was seen in 13% of patients in rheumatoid arthritis clinical trials, but in about 1 in 30 patients or less in ulcerative colitis studies. The estimated incidence of adverse effects other than skin rash in patients treated with sulfasalazine is as follows for both ulcerative colitis and rheumatoid arthritis.

The most common adverse reactions associated with sulfasalazine are anorexia, headache, nausea, vomiting, gastric distress, and apparently reversible oligospermia. These occur in about one-third of the patients. Less frequent adverse reactions are pruritus, urticaria, fever, Heinz body anemia, hemolytic anemia and cyanosis, which may occur at a frequency of 1 in 30 patients or less. Experience suggests that with a daily dose of 4 g or more, or total serum sulfapyridine levels above 50 µg/mL, the incidence of adverse reactions tends to increase.

Although the listing which follows includes a few adverse reactions which have not been reported with this specific drug, the pharmacological similarities among the sulfonamides require that each of these reactions be considered when AZULFIDINE EN-tabs is administered.

Other adverse reactions which occur rarely, in approximately 1 in 1000 patients or less are:

Blood dyscrasias: aplastic anemia, agranulocytosis, leukopenia, megaloblastic (macrocytic) anemia, purpura, thrombocytopenia, hypoprotherombinemia, methemoglobinemia, congenital neutropenia, and myelodysplastic syndrome.

Hypersensitivity reactions: erythema multiforme (Stevens-Johnson syndrome), exfoliative dermatitis, epidermal necrolysis (Lyell's syndrome) with corneal damage, anaphylaxis, serum sickness syndrome, pneumonitis with or without eosinophilia, vasculitis, fibrosing alveolitis, pleuritis, pericarditis with or without tamponade, allergic myocarditis, polyarteritis nodosa, lupus erythematosus-like syndrome, hepatitis and hepatic necrosis with or without immune complexes, fulminant hepatitis, sometimes leading to liver transplantation, parapsoriasis varioliformis acuta (Mucha-Haberman syndrome), rhabdomyolysis, photosensitization, arthralgia, periorbital edema, conjunctival and scleral injection and alopecia.

Gastrointestinal reactions: hepatitis, pancreatitis, bloody diarrhea, impaired folic acid absorption, impaired digoxin absorption, stomatitis, diarrhea, abdominal pains, and neutropenic enterocolitis.

Central Nervous System reactions: transverse myelitis, convulsions, meningitis, transient lesions of the posterior spinal column, cauda equina syndrome, Guillain-Barre syndrome, peripheral neuropathy, mental depression, vertigo, hearing loss, insomnia, ataxia, hallucinations, tinnitus and drowsiness.

Renal reactions: toxic nephrosis with liguria and anuria, nephritis, nephrotic syndrome, hematuria, crystalluria, proteinuria, and hemolytic-uremic syndrome.

Other reactions: urine discoloration and skin discoloration.

The sulfonamides bear certain chemical similarities to some goitrogens, diuretics (acetazolamide and the thiazides), and oral hypoglycemic agents. Goiter production, diuresis and hypoglycemia have occurred rarely in patients receiving sulfonamides. Cross-sensitivity may exist with these agents. Rats appear to be especially susceptible to the goitrogenic effects of sulfonamides and long-term administration has produced thyroid maligancies in this species.

Postmarketing Reports

The following events have been identified during post-approval use of products which contain (or are metabolized to)

Suggested Dosing Schedule:

Week of Treatment	Number of Azulfidine EN-tabs Tablets Morning	Evening
1	-	One
2	One	One
3	One	Two
4	Two	Two

mesalamine in clinical practice. Because they are reported voluntarily from a population of unknown size, estimates of frequency cannot be made. These events have been chosen for inclusion due to a combination of seriousness, frequency of reporting, or potential causal connection to mesalamine:
Gastrointestinal: Reports of hepatotoxicity, including elevated liver function tests (SGOT/AST, SGPT/ALT, GGT, LDH, alkaline phosphatase, bilirubin), jaundice, cholestatic jaundice, cirrhosis, and possible hepatocellular damage including liver necrosis and liver failure. Some of these cases were fatal. One case of Kawasaki-like syndrome, which included hepatic function changes, was also reported.

DRUG ABUSE AND DEPENDENCE

None reported.

OVERDOSAGE

There is evidence that the incidence and severity of toxicity following overdosage is directly related to the total serum sulfapyridine concentration. Symptoms of overdosage may include nausea, vomiting, gastric distress and abdominal pains. In more advanced cases, central nervous system symptoms such as drowsiness, convulsions, etc, may be observed. Serum sulfapyridine concentrations may be used to monitor the progress of recovery from overdosage.
There are no documented reports of deaths due to ingestion of large single doses of sulfasalazine.
It has not been possible to determine the LD_{50} in laboratory animals such as mice, since the highest oral daily dose of sulfasalazine which can be given (12 g/kg) is not lethal. Doses of regular sulfasalazine tablets of 16 g per day have been given to patients without mortality.
Instructions for Overdosage: Gastric lavage or emesis plus catharsis as indicated. Alkalinizeurine. If kidney function is normal, force fluids. If anuria is present, restrict fluids and salt, and treat appropriately. Catheterization of the ureters may be indicated for complete renal blockage by crystals. The low molecular weight of sulfasalazine and its metabolites may facilitate their removal by dialysis. For agranulocytosis, discontinue the drug immediately, hospitalize the patient, and institute appropriate therapy. For hypersensitivity reactions, discontinue treatment immediately. Such reactions may be controlled with antihistamines and, if necessary, systemic corticosteroids. When, in the physican's opinion, reinstitution of AZULFIDINE EN-tabs Tablets is warranted, regimens modeled upon recommended desensitization procedures may be attempted approximately two weeks after treatment has been discontinued and symptoms have disappeared (see DOSAGE AND ADMINISTRATION).

DOSAGE AND ADMINISTRATION

The dosage of AZULFIDINE EN-tabs Tablets should be adjusted to each individual's response and tolerance. The drug should be given in evenly divided doses over each 24-hour period; intervals between nighttime doses should not exceed 8 hours, with administration after meals recommended when feasible. Experience suggests that with daily dosages of 4 g or more, the incidence of adverse effects tends to increase; hence, patients receiving these dosages should be instructed about, and carefully observed for, the appearance of adverse effects.
Some patients may be sensitive to treatment with sulfasalazine. Various desensitization-like regimens have been reported to be effective in 34 of 53 patients,[5] 7 of 8 patients,[6] and 19 of 20 patients.[7] These regimens suggest starting with a total daily dose of 50 to 250 mg sulfasalazine initially, and doubling it every 4 to 7 days until the desired therapeutic level is achieved. If the symptoms of sensitivity recur, AZULFIDINE EN-tabs should be discontinued. Desensitization should not be attempted in patients who have a history of agranulocytosis, or who have experienced an anaphylactoid reaction while previously receiving sulfasalazine.
Usual Dosage
Patients should be instructed to take AZULFIDINE EN-tabs in evenly divided doses, preferably after meals, and to swallow the tablets whole.
Ulcerative Colitis:
Initial Therapy:
Adults: 3 to 4 g daily in evenly divided doses. It may be advisable to initiate therapy with a lower dosage, eg, 1 to 2 g daily, to reduce possible gastrointestinal intolerance. If daily doses exceeding 4 g are required to achieve the desired therapeutic effect, the increased risk of toxicity should be kept in mind.
Children two years of age and older: 40 to 60 mg/kg of body weight in each 24-hour period, divided into 3 to 6 doses.
Maintenance Therapy:
Adults: 2 g daily.
Children, two years of age and older: 30 mg/kg of body weight in each 24-hour period, divided into 4 doses. The response of acute ulcerative colitis to AZULFIDINE EN-tabs can be evaluated by clinical criteria, including the presence of fever, weight changes, and degree and frequency of diarrhea and bleeding, as well as by sigmoidoscopy and the evaluation of biopsy samples. It is often necessary to continue medication even when clinical symptoms, including diarrhea, have been controlled. When endoscopic examination confirms satisfactory improvement, dosage of AZULFIDINE EN-tabs should be reduced to a maintenance level. If diarrhea recurs, dosage should be increased to previously effective levels.
AZULFIDINE EN-tabs is particularly indicated in patients who cannot take uncoated sulfasalazine tablets because of gastrointestinal intolerance (eg, anorexia, nausea). If symptoms of gastric intolerance (anorexia, nausea, vomiting, etc.) occur after the first few doses of AZULFIDINE EN-tabs, they are probably due to increased serum levels of total sulfapyridine, and may be alleviated by halving the daily dose of AZULFIDINE EN-tabs and subsequently increasing it gradually over several days. If gastric intolerance continues, the drug should be stopped for 5 to 7 days, then reintroduced at a lower daily dose.
Rheumatoid Arthritis:
Adults: 2 g daily in evenly divided doses. It is advisable to initiate therapy with a lower dosage of AZULFIDINE EN-tabs, eg, 0.5 to 1.0 g daily, to reduce possible gastrointestinal intolerance. A suggested dosing schedule is given below.
In rheumatoid arthritis, the effect of AZULFIDINE EN-tabs can be assessed by the degree of improvement in the number and extent of actively inflamed joints. A therapeutic response has been observed as early as 4 weeks after starting treatment with AZULFIDINE EN-tabs, but treatment for 12 weeks may be required in some patients before clinical benefit is noted. Consideration can be given to increasing the daily dose of AZULFIDINE EN-tabs to 3 g if the clinical response after 12 weeks is inadequate. Careful monitoring is recommended for doses over 2 g per day.
[See table above]

HOW SUPPLIED

AZULFIDINE EN-tabs Tablets, 500 mg, are elliptical, gold-colored, film enteric-coated tablets, monogrammed "102" on one side and "KPh" on the other. They are available in the following package sizes:

Bottles of 100	NDC 0013-0102-01
Bottles of 300	NDC 0013-0102-20

Storage: Store at 25 °C (77° F); excursions permitted to 15–30° C (59–86° F) [see USP Controlled Room Temperature]
Rx only
Instructions for Converting the Child-resistant Safeguard Cap to an Easy-Open Cap
NOTE: When the locking ring of the child-resistant safeguard cap has been removed, this bottle of AZULFIDINE EN-tabs Tablets should be kept out of the reach of children.
1. After the child-resistant safeguard cap has been removed, it may be reapplied as is, so that the bottle remains child resistant, or it may be converted to an easy-open cap.
2. To convert to an easy-open cap, remove the child-resistant safeguard cap and turn it upside down. The inner rim of the transparent cap is the child-resistant locking ring mechanism. Take a sharply pointed utensil (eg, scissors or a knife tip) and carefully pry off the locking ring. Once the locking ring is removed, the transparent cap should slide off the orange cap. Replace the orange cap on the bottle. It has now been converted to an easy-open cap.

REFERENCES

1. Mogadam M, et al. Pregnancy in inflammatory bowel disease: effect of sulfasalazine and corticosteroids on fetal outcome. Gastroenterology 1981;80:726.
2. Kaufman, DW, editor. Birth defects and drugs during pregnancy. Littleton, MA: Publishing Sciences Group, Inc. 1977:296–313.
3. Jarnerot G. Fertility, sterility and pregnancy in chronic inflammatory bowel disease. Scand J Gastroenterol 1982;17:1–4.
4. Hertzberger-ten Cate R, Cats A. Toxicity of sulfasalazine in systemic juvenile chronic arthritis. Clin Exp Rheumatol 1991;9:85–8.
5. Korelitz B, et al. Desensitization to sulfasalazine in allergic patients with IBD: an important therapeutic modality. Gastroenterology 1982;82:1104.
6. Holdworth CG, Sulphasalazine desensitization. Br Med J 1981;282:110.
7. Taffet SL, Das KM. Desensitization of patients with inflammatory bowel disease to sulfasalazine. Am J Med 1982;73:520–4.

Mfd for: Pharmacia & Upjohn Company
Kalamazoo, MI 49001, USA
by: Pharmacia & Upjohn AB
Stockholm, Sweden
103010599
Revised: May 1999

Shown in Product Identification Guide, page 331

CAMPTOSAR® ℞

Irinotecan hydrochloride injection
For Intravenous Use Only

WARNINGS

CAMPTOSAR Injection should be administered only under the supervision of a physician who is experienced in the use of cancer chemotherapeutic agents. Appropriate management of complications is possible only when adequate diagnostic and treatment facilities are readily available.
CAMPTOSAR can induce both early and late forms of diarrhea that appear to be mediated by different mechanisms. Both forms of diarrhea may be severe. Early diarrhea (occurring during or shortly after infusion of CAMPTOSAR) may be accompanied by cholinergic symptoms of rhinitis, increased salivation, miosis, lacrimation, diaphoresis, flushing, and intestinal hyperperistalsis that can cause abdominal cramping. Early diarrhea and other cholinergic symptoms may be prevented or ameliorated by atropine (see PRECAUTIONS, General). Late diarrhea (generally occurring more than 24 hours after administration of CAMPTOSAR) can be prolonged, may lead to dehydration and electrolyte imbalance, and can be life threatening. Late diarrhea should be treated promptly with loperamide; patients with severe diarrhea should be carefully monitored and given fluid and electrolyte replacement if they become dehydrated (see WARNINGS). Administration of CAMPTOSAR should be interrupted and subsequent doses reduced if severe diarrhea occurs (see DOSAGE AND ADMINISTRATION).
Severe myelosuppression may occur (see WARNINGS).

DESCRIPTION

CAMPTOSAR Injection (irinotecan hydrochloride injection) is an antineoplastic agent of the topoisomerase I inhibitor class. Irinotecan hydrochloride was clinically investigated as CPT-11.
CAMPTOSAR is supplied as a sterile, pale yellow, clear, aqueous solution. It is available in two single-dose sizes: 2 mL-fill vials contain 40 mg irinotecan hydrochloride and 5 mL-fill vials contain 100 mg irinotecan hydrochloride. Each milliliter of solution contains 20 mg of irinotecan hydrochloride (on the basis of the trihydrate salt), 45 mg of sorbitol NF powder, and 0.9 mg of lactic acid, USP. The pH of the solution has been adjusted to 3.5 (range, 3.0 to 3.8) with sodium hydroxide or hydrochloric acid. CAMPTOSAR is intended for dilution with 5% Dextrose Injection, USP (D5W), or 0.9% Sodium Chloride Injection, USP, prior to intravenous infusion. The preferred diluent is 5% Dextrose Injection, USP.
Irinotecan hydrochloride is a semisynthetic derivative of camptothecin, an alkaloid extract from plants such as *Camptotheca acuminata*. The chemical name is (*S*)-4,11-diethyl-3,4,12,14-tetrahydro-4-hydroxy-3,14-dioxo-1*H*-pyrano[3',4':6,7] -indolizino[1,2-b]quinolin-9-yl- [1,4'-bipiperidine]-1'-carboxylate, monohydrochloride, trihydrate. Its structural formula is as follows:

Irinotecan Hydrochloride

Irinotecan hydrochloride is a pale yellow to yellow crystalline powder, with the empirical formula $C_{33}H_{38}N_4O_6 \cdot HCl \cdot 3H_2O$ and a molecular weight of 677.19. It is slightly soluble in water and organic solvents.

CLINICAL PHARMACOLOGY

Irinotecan is a derivative of camptothecin. Camptothecins interact specifically with the enzyme topoisomerase I which relieves torsional strain in DNA by inducing reversible single-strand breaks. Irinotecan and its active metabolite SN-38 bind to the topoisomerase I-DNA complex and prevent religation of these single-strand breaks. Current research suggests that the cytotoxicity of irinotecan is due to double-strand DNA damage produced during DNA synthesis when replication enzymes interact with the ternary complex formed by topoisomerase I, DNA, and either irinotecan or SN-38. Mammalian cells cannot efficiently repair these double-strand breaks.
Irinotecan serves as a water-soluble precursor of the lipophilic metabolite SN-38. SN-38 is formed from irinotecan by carboxylesterase-mediated cleavage of the carbamate bond between the camptothecin moiety and the dipiperidino side chain. SN-38 is approximately 1000 times as potent as

Continued on next page

Information on these Pharmacia & Upjohn products is based on labeling in effect June 1, 2000. Further information concerning these and other Pharmacia & Upjohn products may be obtained by direct inquiry to Medical Information, Pharmacia & Upjohn, Kalamazoo, MI 49001.

Camptosar—Cont.

irinotecan as an inhibitor of topoisomerase I purified from human and rodent tumor cell lines. In vitro cytotoxicity assays show that the potency of SN-38 relative to irinotecan varies from 2- to 2000-fold. However, the plasma area under the concentration versus time curve (AUC) values for SN-38 are 2% to 8% of irinotecan and SN-38 is 95% bound to plasma proteins compared to approximately 50% bound to plasma proteins for irinotecan (see Pharmacokinetics). The precise contribution of SN-38 to the activity of CAMPTOSAR is thus unknown. Both irinotecan and SN-38 exist in an active lactone form and an inactive hydroxy acid anion form. A pH-dependent equilibrium exists between the two forms such that an acid pH promotes the formation of the lactone, while a more basic pH favors the hydroxy acid anion form.

Administration of irinotecan has resulted in antitumor activity in mice bearing cancers of rodent origin and in human carcinoma xenografts of various histological types.

Pharmacokinetics

After intravenous infusion of irinotecan in humans, irinotecan plasma concentrations decline in a multiexponential manner, with a mean terminal elimination half-life of about 6 to 12 hours. The mean terminal elimination half-life of the active metabolite SN-38 is about 10 to 20 hours. The half-lives of the lactone (active) forms of irinotecan and SN-38 are similar to those of total irinotecan and SN-38, as the lactone and hydroxy acid forms are in equilibrium.

Over the recommended dose range of 50 to 350 mg/m^2, the AUC of irinotecan increases linearly with dose; the AUC of SN-38 increases less than proportionally with dose. Maximum concentrations of the active metabolite SN-38 are generally seen within 1 hour following the end of a 90-minute infusion of irinotecan. Pharmacokinetic parameters for irinotecan and SN-38 following a 90-minute infusion of irinotecan at dose levels of 125 and 340 mg/m^2 determined in two clinical studies in patients with solid tumors are summarized in Table 1.

[See table 1 above]

Irinotecan exhibits moderate plasma protein binding (30% to 68% bound). SN-38 is highly bound to human plasma proteins (approximately 95% bound). The plasma protein to which irinotecan and SN-38 predominantly binds is albumin.

Metabolism and Excretion: The metabolic conversion of irinotecan to the active metabolite SN-38 is mediated by carboxylesterase enzymes and primarily occurs in the liver. SN-38 subsequently undergoes conjugation to form a glucuronide metabolite. SN-38 glucuronide had 1/50 to 1/100 the activity of SN-38 in cytotoxicity assays using two cell lines in vitro. The disposition of irinotecan has not been fully elucidated in humans. The urinary excretion of irinotecan is 11% to 20%; SN-38, <1%; and SN-38 glucuronide, 3%. The cumulative biliary and urinary excretion of irinotecan and its metabolites (SN-38 and SN-38 glucuronide) over a period of 48 hours following administration of irinotecan in two patients ranged from approximately 25% (100 mg/m^2) to 50% (300 mg/m^2).

Pharmacokinetics in Special Populations

Geriatric: In studies using the weekly schedule, the terminal half-life of irinotecan was 6.0 hours in patients who were 65 years or older and 5.5 hours in patients younger than 65 years. Dose-normalized AUC_{0-24} for SN-38 in patients who were at least 65 years of age was 11% higher than in patients younger than 65 years. No change in the starting dose is recommended for geriatric patients receiving the weekly dosage schedule of irinotecan. The pharmacokinetics of irinotecan given once every 3 weeks has not been studied in the geriatric population; a lower starting dose is recommended in patients 70 years or older based on clinical toxicity experience with this schedule (see DOSAGE AND ADMINISTRATION).

Pediatric: Information regarding the pharmacokinetics of irinotecan is not available.

Gender: The pharmacokinetics of irinotecan do not appear to be influenced by gender.

Race: The influence of race on the pharmacokinetics of irinotecan has not been evaluated.

Hepatic Insufficiency: The influence of hepatic insufficiency on the pharmacokinetic characteristics of irinotecan and its metabolites has not been formally studied. Among patients with known hepatic tumor involvement (a majority of patients), irinotecan and SN-38 AUC values were somewhat higher than values for patients without liver metastases (see PRECAUTIONS).

Renal Insufficiency: The influence of renal insufficiency on the pharmacokinetics of irinotecan has not been evaluated.

Drug-Drug Interactions

In a phase 1 clinical study involving irinotecan, 5-fluorouracil (5-FU), and leucovorin (LV) in 26 patients with solid tumors, the disposition of irinotecan was not substantially altered when the drugs were co-administered. Although the C_{max} and AUC_{0-24} of SN-38, the active metabolite, were reduced (by 14% and 8%, respectively) when irinotecan was followed by 5-FU and LV administration compared with when irinotecan was given alone, this sequence of administration was used in the combination trials and is recommended (see DOSAGE AND ADMINISTRATION). Formal in vivo or in vitro drug interaction studies to evaluate the influence of irinotecan on the disposition of 5-FU and LV have not been conducted.

Table 1. Summary of Mean (± Standard Deviation) Irinotecan and SN-38 Pharmacokinetic Parameters in Patients With Solid Tumors

Dose (mg/m^2)	Irinotecan					SN-38		
	C_{max} (ng/mL)	AUC_{0-24} (ng•h/mL)	$t_{1/2}$ (h)	V_Z (L/m^2)	CL (L/h/m^2)	C_{max} (ng/mL)	AUC_{0-24} (ng•h/mL)	$t_{1/2}$ (h)
125 (N=64)	1,660 ±797	10,200 ±3,270	5.8[a] ±0.7	110 ±48.5	13.3 ±6.01	26.3 ±11.9	229 ±108	10.4[a] ±3.1
340 (N=6)	3,392 ±874	20,604 ±6,027	11.7[b] ±1.0	234 ±69.6	13.9 ±4.00	56.0 ±28.2	474 ±245	21.0[b] ±4.3

C_{max} - Maximum plasma concentration
AUC_{0-24} - Area under the plasma concentration-time curve from time 0 to 24 hours after the end of the 90-minute infusion
$t_{1/2}$ - Terminal elimination half-life
V_Z - Volume of distribution of terminal elimination phase
CL - Total systemic clearance
[a] Plasma specimens collected for 24 hours following the end of the 90-minute infusion.
[b] Plasma specimens collected for 48 hours following the end of the 90-minute infusion. Because of the longer collection period, these values provide a more accurate reflection of the terminal elimination half-lives of irinotecan and SN-38.

Table 2. Combination Dosage Schedule: Study Results

	Study 1			Study 2	
	Irinotecan + Bolus 5-FU/LV weekly x 4 q 6 weeks	Bolus 5-FU/LV daily x 5 q 4 weeks	Irinotecan weekly x 4 q 6 weeks	Irinotecan + Infusional 5-FU/LV	Infusional 5-FU/LV
Number of Patients	231	226	226	198	187
Demographics and Treatment Administration					
Female/Male (%)	34/65	45/54	35/64	33/67	47/53
Median Age in years (range)	62 (25–85)	61 (19–85)	61 (30–87)	62 (27–75)	59 (24–75)
Performance Status (%)					
0	39	41	46	51	51
1	46	45	46	42	41
2	15	13	8	7	8
Primary Tumor (%)					
Colon	81	85	84	55	65
Rectum	17	14	15	45	35
Median Time from Diagnosis to Randomization (months, range)	1.9 (0–161)	1.7 (0–203)	1.8 (0.1–185)	4.5 (0–88)	2.7 (0–104)
Prior Adjuvant 5-FU Therapy (%)					
No	89	92	90	74	76
Yes	11	8	10	26	24
Median Duration of Study Treatment[a] (months)	5.5	4.1	3.9	5.6	4.5
Median Relative Dose Intensity (%)[a]					
Irinotecan	72	—	75	87	—
5-FU	71	86	—	86	93
Efficacy Results					
Confirmed Objective Tumor Response Rate[b] (%)	39	21 (p<0.0001)[c]	18	35	22 (p<0.005)[c]
Median Time to Tumor Progression[d] (months)	7.0	4.3 (p=0.004)[d]	4.2	6.7	4.4 (p<0.001)[d]
Median Survival (months)	14.8	12.6 (p<0.05)[d]	12.0	17.4	14.1 (p<0.05)[d]

[a] Study 1: N=225 (irinotecan/5-FU/LV), N=219 (5-FU/LV), N=223 (irinotecan)
Study 2: N=199 (irinotecan/5-FU/LV), N=186 (5-FU/LV)
[b] Confirmed ≥4 to 6 weeks after first evidence of objective response
[c] Chi-square test
[d] Log-rank test

Possible pharmacokinetic interactions of CAMPTOSAR with other concomitantly administered medications have not been formally investigated.

CLINICAL STUDIES

Irinotecan has been studied in clinical trials in combination with 5-fluorouracil (5-FU) and leucovorin (LV) and as a single agent) see DOSAGE AND ADMINISTRATION). When given as a component of combination-agent treatment, irinotecan was either given with a weekly schedule of bolus 5-FU/LV or with an every-2-week schedule of infusional 5-FU/LV. Weekly and a once-every-3-week dosage schedules were used for the single-agent irinotecan studies. Clinical studies of combination and single-agent use are described below.

First-Line Therapy in Combination with 5-FU/LV for the Treatment of Metastatic Colorectal Cancer

Two phase 3, randomized, controlled, multinational clinical trials support the use of CAMPTOSAR Injection as first-line treatment of patients with metastatic carcinoma of the colon or rectum. In each study, combinations of irinotecan with 5-FU and LV were compared with 5-FU and LV alone. Study 1 compared combination irinotecan/bolus 5-FU/LV therapy given weekly with a standard bolus regimen of 5-FU/LV alone given daily for 5 days every 4 weeks; an irinotecan-alone treatment arm given on a weekly schedule was also included. Study 2 evaluated two different methods of administering infusional 5-FU/LV, with or without irinotecan.

In both studies, the combination of irinotecan/5-FU/LV therapy resulted in significant improvements in objective tumor response rates, time to tumor progression, and survival when compared with 5-FU/LV alone. These differences in survival were observed in spite of second-line therapy in a majority of patients on both arms, including crossover to irinotecan-containing regimens in the control arm. Patient characteristics and major efficacy results are shown in Table 2.

[See table 2 above]

Improvement was noted with irinotecan-based combination therapy relative to 5-FU/LV when response rates and time to tumor progression were examined across the following demographic and disease-related subgroups (age, gender, ethnic origin, performance status, extent of organ involvement with cancer, time from diagnosis of cancer, prior adjuvant therapy, and baseline laboratory abnormalities). Figures 1 and 2 illustrate the Kaplan-Meier survival curves for the comparison of irinotecan/5-FU/LV versus 5-FU/LV in Studies 1 and 2, respectively.

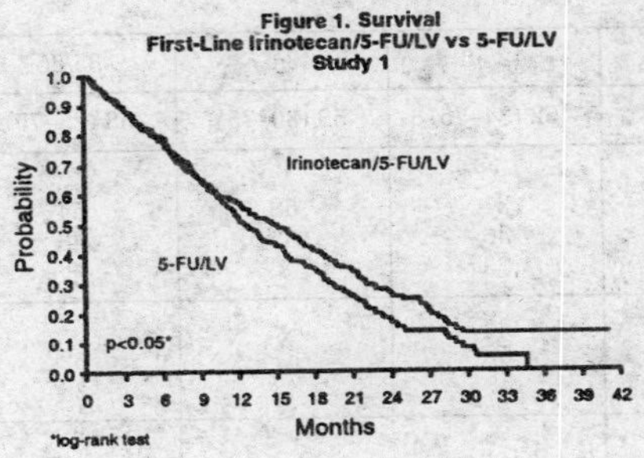

Figure 1. Survival First-Line Irinotecan/5-FU/LV vs 5-FU/LV Study 1

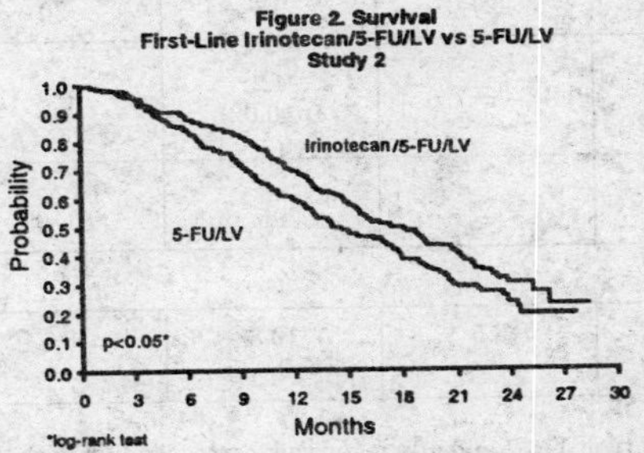

Figure 2. Survival First-Line Irinotecan/5-FU/LV vs 5-FU/LV Study 2

Second-Line Treatment for Recurrent or Progressive Metastatic Colorectal Cancer After 5-FU-Based Treatment

Weekly Dosage Schedule

Data from three open-label, single-agent, clinical studies, involving a total of 304 patients in 59 centers, support the use of CAMPTOSAR in the treatment of patients with metastatic cancer of the colon or rectum that has recurred or progressed following treatment with 5-FU-based therapy. These studies were designed to evaluate tumor response rate and do not provide information on actual clinical benefit, such as effects on survival and disease-related symptoms. In each study, CAMPTOSAR was administered in repeated 6-week courses consisting of a 90-minute intravenous infusion once weekly for 4 weeks, followed by a 2-week rest period. Starting doses of CAMPTOSAR in these trials were 100, 125, or 150 mg/m^2, but the 150-mg/m^2 dose was poorly tolerated (due to unacceptably high rates of grade 4 late diarrhea and febrile neutropenia). Study 1 enrolled 48 patients and was conducted by a single investigator at several regional hospitals. Study 2 was a multicenter study conducted by the North Central Cancer Treatment Group. All 90 patients enrolled in Study 2 received a starting dose of 125 mg/m^2. Study 3 was a multicenter study that enrolled 166 patients from 30 institutions. The initial dose in Study 3 was 125 mg/m^2 but was reduced to 100 mg/m^2 because the toxicity seen at the 125-mg/m^2 dose was perceived to be greater than that seen in previous studies. All patients in these studies had metastatic colorectal cancer, and the majority had disease that recurred or progressed following a 5-FU-based regimen administered for metastatic disease. The results of the individual studies are shown in Table 3.

[See table 3 above]

Table 3. Weekly Dosage Schedule: Study Results

	Study			
	1	2	3	
Number of Patients	48	90	64	102
Starting Dose (mg/m^2/wk × 4)	125[a]	125	125	100
Demographics and Treatment Administration				
Female/Male (%)	46/54	36/64	50/50	51/49
Median Age in years (range)	63 (29–78)	63 (32–81)	61 (42–84)	64 (25–84)
Ethnic Origin (%)				
White	79	96	81	91
African American	12	4	11	5
Hispanic	8	0	8	2
Oriental/Asian	0	0	0	2
Performance Status (%)				
0	60	38	59	44
1	38	48	33	51
2	2	14	8	5
Primary Tumor (%)				
Colon	100	71	89	87
Rectum	0	29	11	8
Unknown	0	0	0	5
Prior 5-FU Therapy (%)				
For Metastatic Disease	81	66	73	68
≤6 months after Adjuvant	15	7	27	28
>6 months after Adjuvant	2	16	0	2
Classification Unknown	2	12	0	3
Prior Pelvic/Abdominal Irradiation (%)				
Yes	3	29	0	0
Other	0	9	2	4
None	97	62	98	96
Duration of Treatment with CAMPTOSAR (median, months)	5	4	4	3
Relative Dose Intensity[b] (median %)	74	67	73	81
Efficacy				
Confirmed Objective Response Rate (%)[c] (95% CI)	21 (9.3–32.3)	13 (6.3–20.4)	14 (5.5–22.6)	9 (3.3–14.3)
Time to Response (median, months)	2.6	1.5	2.8	2.8
Response Duration (median, months)	6.4	5.9	5.6	6.4
Survival (median, months)	10.4	8.1	10.7	9.3
1-Year Survival (%)	46	31	45	43

[a] Nine patients received 150 mg/m^2 as a starting dose; two (22.2%) responded to CAMPTOSAR.
[b] Relative dose intensity for CAMPTOSAR based on planned dose intensity of 100, 83.3, and 66.7 mg/m^2/wk corresponding with 150, 125, and 100 mg/m^2 starting doses, respectively.
[c] Confirmed ≥ 4 to 6 weeks after first evidence of objective response.

In the intent-to-treat analysis of the pooled data across all three studies, 193 of the 304 patients began therapy at the recommended starting dose of 125 mg/m^2. Among these 193 patients, 2 complete and 27 partial responses were observed, for an overall response rate of 15.0% (95% Confidence Interval [CI], 10.0% to 20.1%) at this starting dose. A considerably lower response rate was seen with a starting dose of 100 mg/m^2. The majority of responses were observed within the first two courses of therapy, but responses did occur in later courses of treatment (one response was observed after the eighth course). The median response duration for patients beginning therapy at 125 mg/m^2 was 5.8 months (range, 2.6 to 15.1 months). Of the 304 patients treated in the three studies, response rates to CAMPTOSAR were similar in males and females and among patients older and younger than 65 years. Rates were also similar in patients with cancer of the colon or cancer of the rectum and in patients with single and multiple metastatic sites. The response rate was 18.5% in patients with a performance status of 0 and 8.2% in patients with a performance status of 1 or 2. Patients with a performance status of 3 or 4 have not been studied. Over half of the patients responding to CAMPTOSAR had not responded to prior 5-FU. Patients who had received previous irradiation to the pelvis responded to CAMPTOSAR at approximately the same rate as those who had not previously received irradiation.

Once-Every-3-Week Dosage Schedule

Single-Arm Studies: Data from an open-label, single-agent, single-arm, multicenter, clinical study involving a total of 132 patients support a once every-3-week dosage schedule of irinotecan in the treatment of patients with metastatic cancer of the colon or rectum that recurred or progressed following treatment with 5-FU. Patients received a starting dose of 350 mg/m^2 given by 30-minute intravenous infusion once every 3 weeks. Among the 132 previously treated patients in this trial, the intent-to-treat response rate was 12.1% (95% CI, 7.0% to 18.1%).

Randomized Trials: Two multicenter, randomized, clinical studies further support the use of irinotecan given by the once-every-3-week dosage schedule in patients with metastatic colorectal cancer whose disease has recurred or progressed following prior 5-FU therapy. In the first study, second-line irinotecan therapy plus best supportive care was compared with best supportive care alone. In the second study, second-line irinotecan therapy was compared with infusional 5-FU-based therapy. In both studies, irinotecan was administered intravenously at a starting dose of 350 mg/m^2 over 90 minutes once every 3 weeks. The starting dose was 300 mg/m^2 for patients who were 70 years and older or who had a performance status of 2. The highest total dose permitted was 700 mg. Dose reductions and/or administration delays were permitted in the event of severe hematologic and/or nonhematologic toxicities while on treatment. Best supportive care was provided to patients in both arms of Study 1 and included antibiotics, analgesics, corticosteroids, transfusions, psychotherapy, or any other symptomatic therapy as clinically indicated. Concomitant medications such as antiemetics, atropine, and loperamide were given to patients in the irinotecan arm for prophylaxis and/or management of symptoms from treatment. If late diarrhea persisted for greater than 24 hours despite loperamide, a 7-day course of fluoroquinolone antibiotic prophylaxis was given. Patients in the control arm of the second study received one of the following 5-FU regimens: (1) LV, 200 mg/m^2 IV over 2 hours; followed by 5 FU, 400 mg/m^2 IV bolus; followed by 5-FU, 600 mg/m^2 continuous IV infusion over 22 hours on days 1 and 2 every 2 weeks; (2) 5-FU, 250 to 300 mg/m^2/day protracted continuous IV infusion until toxicity; (3) 5-FU, 2.6 to 3 g/m^2 IV over 24 hours every week for 6 weeks with or without LV, 20 to 500 mg/m^2/day every week IV for 6 weeks with 2-week rest between courses. Patients were to be followed every 3 to 6 weeks for 1 year.

A total of 535 patients were randomized in the two studies at 94 centers. The primary endpoint in both studies was survival. The studies demonstrated a significant overall survival advantage for irinotecan compared with best supportive care (p=0.0001) and infusional 5-FU-based therapy (p=0.035) as shown in Figures 3 and 4. In Study 1, median survival for patients treated with irinotecan was 9.2 months compared with 6.5 months for patients receiving best supportive care. In Study 2, median survival for patients treated with irinotecan was 10.8 months compared with 8.5 months for patients receiving infusional 5-FU-based therapy. Multiple regression analyses determined that patients' baseline characteristics also had a significant effect on survival. When adjusted for performance status and other baseline prognostic factors, survival among patients treated with irinotecan remained significantly longer than in the control populations (p=0.001) for Study 1 and p=0.017 for Study 2). Measurements of pain, performance status, and

Continued on next page

Information on these Pharmacia & Upjohn products is based on labeling in effect June 1, 2000. Further information concerning these and other Pharmacia & Upjohn products may be obtained by direct inquiry to Medical Information, Pharmacia & Upjohn, Kalamazoo, MI 49001.

Camptosar—Cont.

weight loss were collected prospectively in the two studies; however, the plan for the analysis of these data was defined retrospectively. When comparing irinotecan with best supportive care in Study 1, this analysis showed a statistically significant advantage for irinotecan, with longer time to development of pain (6.9 months versus 2.0 months), time to performance status deterioration (5.7 months versus 3.3 months), and time to > 5% weight loss (6.4 months versus 4.2 months). Additionally, 33.3% (33/99) of patients with a baseline performance status of 1 or 2 showed an improvement in performance status when treated with irinotecan versus 11.3% (7/62) of patients receiving best supportive care (p=0.002). Because of the inclusion of patients with non-measurable disease, intent-to-treat response rates could not be assessed.

Figure 3. Survival
Second-Line Irinotecan vs Best Supportive Care (BSC)
Study 1

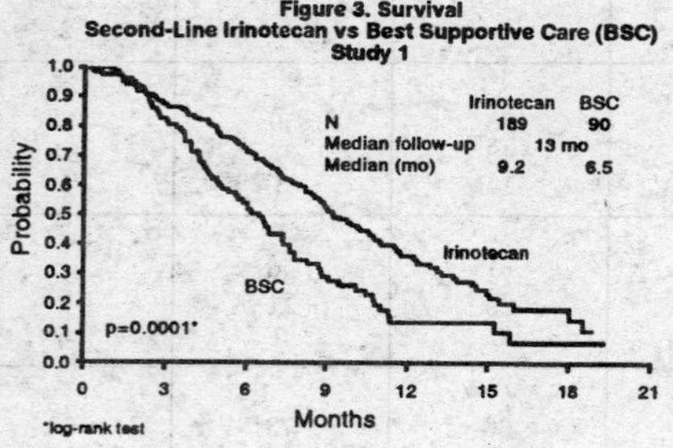

Figure 4. Survival
Second-Line Irinotecan vs Infusional 5-FU
Study 2

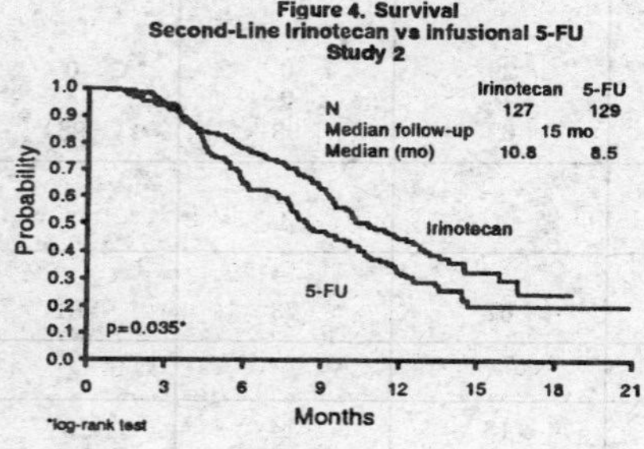

[See table 4 above]

In the two randomized studies, the EORTC QLQ-C30 instrument was utilized. At the start of each course of therapy, patients completed a questionnaire consisting of 30 questions, such as "Did pain interfere with daily activities?" (1 = Not at All, to 4 = Very Much) and "Do you have any trouble taking a long walk?" (Yes or No). The answers from the 30 questions were converted into 15 subscales, that were scored from 0 to 100, and the global health status subscale that was derived from two questions about the patient's sense of general well being in the past week. In addition to the global health status subscale, there were five functional (i.e., cognitive, emotional, social, physical, role) and nine symptom (i.e., fatigue, appetite loss, pain assessment, insomnia, constipation, dyspnea, nausea/vomiting, financial impact, diarrhea) subscales. The results as summarized in Table 5 are based on patients' worst post-baseline scores. In Study 1, a multivariate analysis and univariate analyses of the individual subscales were performed and corrected for multivariate testing. Patients receiving irinotecan reported significantly better results for the global health status, on two of five functional subscales, and on four of nine symptom subscales. As expected, patients receiving irinotecan noted significantly more diarrhea than those receiving best supportive care. In Study 2, the multivariate analysis on all 15 subscales did not indicate a statistically significant difference between irinotecan and infusional 5-FU.

[See table 5 above]

Table 4. Once-Every-3-Week Dosage Schedule: Study Results

	Study 1		Study 2	
	Irinotecan	BSC[a]	Irinotecan	5-FU
Number of Patients	189	90	127	129
Demographics and Treatment Administration				
Female/Male (%)	32/68	42/58	43/57	35/65
Median Age in years (range)	59 (22–75)	62 (34–75)	58 (30–75)	58 (25–75)
Performance Status (%)				
0	47	31	58	54
1	39	46	35	43
2	14	23	8	3
Primary Tumor (%)				
Colon	55	52	57	62
Rectum	45	48	43	38
Prior 5-FU Therapy (%)				
For Metastatic Disease	70	63	58	68
As Adjuvant Treatment	30	37	42	32
Prior Irradiation (%)	26	27	18	20
Duration of Study Treatment (median, months) (Log-rank Test)	4.1	—	4.2 (p=0.02)	2.8
Relative Dose Intensity (median %)[b]	94	—	95	81–99
Survival				
Survival (median, months) (Log-rank Test)	9.2 (p=0.0001)	6.5	10.8 (p=0.035)	8.5

[a] BSC = best supportive care
[b] Relative dose intensity for irinotecan based on planned dose intensity of 116.7 and 100 mg/m²/wk corresponding with 350 and 300 mg/m² starting doses, respectively.

Table 5. EORTC QLQ-C30: Mean Worst Post-Baseline Score[a]

QLQ-C30 Subscale	Study 1			Study 2		
	Irinotecan	BSC	p-value	Irinotecan	5-FU	p-value
Global Health Status	47	37	0.03	5.3	52	0.9
Functional Scales						
Cognitive	77	68	0.07	79	83	0.9
Emotional	68	64	0.4	64	68	0.9
Social	58	47	0.06	65	67	0.9
Physical	60	40	0.0003	66	66	0.9
Role	53	35	0.02	54	57	0.9
Symptom Scales						
Fatigue	51	63	0.03	47	46	0.9
Appetite Loss	37	57	0.0007	35	38	0.9
Pain Assessment	41	56	0.009	38	34	0.9
Insomnia	39	47	0.3	39	33	0.9
Constipation	28	41	0.03	25	19	0.9
Dyspnea	31	40	0.2	25	24	0.9
Nausea/Vomiting	27	29	0.5	25	16	0.09
Financial Impact	22	26	0.5	24	15	0.3
Diarrhea	32	19	0.01	32	22	0.2

[a] For the five functional subscales and global health status subscale, higher scores imply better functioning, whereas, on the nine symptom subscales, higher scores imply more severe symptoms. The subscale scores of each patient were collected at each visit until the patient dropped out of the study.

INDICATIONS AND USAGE

CAMPTOSAR Injection is indicated as a component of first-line therapy in combination with 5-fluorouracil and leucovorin for patients with metastatic carcinoma of the colon or rectum. CAMPTOSAR is also indicated for patients with metastatic carcinoma of the colon or rectum whose disease has recurred or progressed following initial fluorouracil-based therapy.

CONTRAINDICATIONS

CAMPTOSAR Injection is contraindicated in patients with a known hypersensitivity to the drug.

WARNINGS

General

Outside of a well-designed clinical study, CAMPTOSAR Injection should not be used in combination with the "Mayo Clinic" regimen of 5-FU/LV (administration for 4–5 consecutive days every 4 weeks) because of reports of increased toxicity, including toxic deaths. CAMPTOSAR should be used as recommended (see DOSAGE AND ADMINISTRATION, Table 10).

Diarrhea

CAMPTOSAR can induce both early and late forms of diarrhea that appear to be mediated by different mechanisms. Early diarrhea (occurring during or shortly after infusion of CAMPTOSAR) is cholinergic in nature. It is usually transient and only infrequently is severe. It may be accompanied by symptoms of rhinitis, increased salivation, miosis, lacrimation, diaphoresis, flushing, and intestinal hyperperistalsis that can cause abdominal cramping. Early diarrhea and other cholinergic symptoms may be prevented or ameliorated by administration of atropine (see PRECAUTIONS, General, for dosing recommendations for atropine).

Late diarrhea (generally occurring more than 24 hours after administration of CAMPTOSAR) can be prolonged, may lead to dehydration and electrolyte imbalance, and can be life threatening. Late diarrhea should be treated promptly with loperamide (see PRECAUTIONS, Information for Patients, for dosing recommendations for loperamide). Patients with severe diarrhea should be carefully monitored and given fluid and electrolyte replacement if they become dehydrated. National Cancer Institute (NCI) grade 3 diarrhea is defined as an increase of 7 to 9 stools daily, or incontinence, or severe cramping and NCI grade 4 diarrhea is defined as an increase of ≥10 stools daily, or grossly bloody stool, or need for parenteral support. If grade 3 or 4 late diarrhea occurs, administration of CAMPTOSAR should be delayed until the patient recovers and subsequent doses should be decreased (see DOSAGE AND ADMINISTRATION).

Myelosuppression

Deaths due to sepsis following severe myelosuppression have been reported in patients treated with CAMPTOSAR. Therapy with CAMPTOSAR should be temporarily omitted during a course of therapy if neutropenic fever occurs or if the absolute neutrophil count drops below 1000/mm³. After the patient recovers to an absolute neutrophil count ≥1000/

Table 6. Study 1: Percent (%) of Patients Experiencing Clinically Relevant Adverse Events in Combination Therapies

Adverse Event	Study 1					
	Irinotecan + Bolus 5-FU/LV weekly × 4 q 6 weeks N=225		Bolus 5-FU/LV daily × 5 q 4 weeks N=219		Irinotecan weekly × 4 q 6 weeks N=223	
	Grade 1–4	Grade 3&4	Grade 1–4	Grade 3&4	Grade 1–4	Grade 3&4
TOTAL Adverse Events	100	53.3	100	45.7	99.6	45.7
GASTROINTESTINAL						
Diarrhea						
late	84.9	22.7	69.4	13.2	83.0	31.0
grade 3	—	15.1	—	5.9	—	18.4
grade 4	—	7.6	—	7.3	—	12.6
early	45.8	4.9	31.5	1.4	43.0	6.7
Nausea	79.1	15.6	67.6	8.2	81.6	16.1
Abdominal pain	63.1	14.6	50.2	11.5	67.7	13.0
Vomiting	60.4	9.7	46.1	4.1	62.8	12.1
Anorexia	34.2	5.8	42.0	3.7	43.9	7.2
Constipation	41.3	3.1	31.5	1.8	32.3	0.4
Mucositis	32.4	2.2	76.3	16.9	29.6	2.2
HEMATOLOGIC						
Neutropenia	96.9	53.8	98.6	66.7	96.4	31.4
grade 3	—	29.8	—	23.7	—	19.3
grade 4	—	24.0	—	42.5	—	12.1
Leukopenia	96.9	37.8	98.6	23.3	96.4	21.5
Anemia	96.9	8.4	98.6	5.5	98.9	4.5
Neutropenic fever	—	7.1	—	14.6	—	5.8
Thrombocytopenia	96.0	2.6	98.6	2.7	96.0	1.7
Neutropenic infection	—	1.8	—	0	—	2.2
BODY AS A WHOLE						
Asthenia	70.2	19.5	64.4	11.9	69.2	13.9
Pain	30.7	3.1	26.9	3.6	22.9	2.2
Fever	42.2	1.7	32.4	3.6	43.5	0.4
Infection	22.2	0	16.0	1.4	13.9	0.4
METABOLIC & NUTRITIONAL						
↑ Bilirubin	87.6	7.1	92.2	8.2	83.9	7.2
DERMATOLOGIC						
Exfoliative dermatitis	0.9	0	3.2	0.5	0	0
Rash	19.1	0	26.5	0.9	14.3	0.4
Alopecia[a]	43.1	—	26.5	—	46.1	—
RESPIRATORY						
Dyspnea	27.6	6.3	16.0	0.5	22.0	2.2
Cough	26.7	1.3	18.3	0	20.2	0.4
Pneumonia	6.2	2.7	1.4	1.0	3.6	1.3
NEUROLOGIC						
Dizziness	23.1	1.3	16.4	0	21.1	1.8
Somnolence	12.4	1.8	4.6	1.8	9.4	1.3
Confusion	7.1	1.8	4.1	0	2.7	0
CARDIOVASCULAR						
Vasodilation	9.3	0.9	5.0	0	9.0	0
Hypotension	5.8	1.3	2.3	0.5	5.8	1.7
Thrombophlebitis	5.3	2.7	6.8	3.2	3.1	1.8
Pulmonary embolus	2.7	2.7	1.4	1.4	0.9	0.4
Myocardial infarction	1.3	1.3	0	0	0.4	0.4

[a]Complete hair loss = Grade 2

Table 7. Study 2: Percent (%) of Patients Experiencing Clinically Relevant Adverse Events in Combination Therapies

Adverse Event	Study 2			
	Irinotecan + 5-FU/LV Infusional at 1&2 q 2 weeks N=145		5-FU/LV Infusional at 1&2 q 2 weeks N=143	
	Grade 1–4	Grade 3&4	Grade 1–4	Grade 3&4
TOTAL Adverse Events	100	72.4	100	39.2
GASTROINTESTINAL				
Diarrhea				
late	68.3	14.5	44.8	6.3
grade 3	—	10.3	—	4.2
grade 4	—	4.1	—	2.1
Cholinergic syndrome[a]	28.3	1.4	0.7	0
Nausea	66.9	2.1	55.2	3.5
Abdominal pain	17.2	2.1	16.8	0.7
Vomiting	44.1	3.5	32.2	2.8
Anorexia	35.2	2.1	18.9	0.7
Constipation	30.3	0.7	25.2	1.4
Mucositis	40.0	4.1	26.7	2.8
HEMATOLOGIC				
Neutropenia	82.5	46.2	47.9	13.4
grade 3	—	36.4	—	12.7
grade 4	—	9.8	—	0.7
Leukopenia	81.3	17.4	42.0	3.5
Anemia	97.2	2.1	90.0	2.1
Neutropenic fever	—	9.3	—	2.3
Thrombocytopenia	32.6	0	32.2	0
Neutropenic infection	—	2.1	—	0

Continued on next page

mm^3, subsequent doses of CAMPTOSAR should be reduced depending upon the level of myelosuppression observed (see DOSAGE AND ADMINISTRATION).

Routine administration of a colony-stimulating factor (CSF) is not necessary, but physicians may wish to consider CSF use in individual patients experiencing significant neutropenia.

Hypersensitivity

Hypersensitivity reactions including severe anaphylactic or anaphylactoid reactions have been observed.

Colitis/Ileus

Cases of colitis complicated by ulceration, bleeding, ileus or what was described as toxic megacolon have been observed rarely. Cases of ileus without preceding colitis have also been observed rarely.

Renal Impairment/Renal Failure

Rare cases of renal impairment and acute renal failure have been identified, usually in patients who became volume depleted from severe vomiting and/or diarrhea.

Pregnancy

CAMPTOSAR may cause fetal harm when administered to a pregnant woman. Radioactivity related to ^{14}C-irinotecan crosses the placenta of rats following intravenous administration of 10 mg/kg (which in separate studies produced an irinotecan C_{max} and AUC about 3 and 0.5 times, respectively, the corresponding values in patients administered 125 mg/m^2). Administration of 6 mg/kg/day intravenous irinotecan to rats (which in separate studies produced an irinotecan C_{max} and AUC about 2 and 0.2 times, respectively, the corresponding values in patients administered 125 mg/m^2) and rabbits (about one-half the recommended human weekly starting dose on a mg/m^2 basis) during the period of organogenesis, is embryotoxic as characterized by increased post-implantation loss and decreased numbers of live fetuses. Irinotecan was teratogenic in rats at doses greater than 1.2 mg/kg/day (which in separate studies produced an irinotecan C_{max} and AUC about 2/3 and 1/40th, respectively, of the corresponding values in patients administered 125 mg/m^2) and in rabbits at 6.0 mg/kg/day (about one-half the recommended human weekly starting dose on a mg/m^2 basis). Teratogenic effects included a variety of external, visceral, and skeletal abnormalities. Irinotecan administered to rat dams for the period following organogenesis through weaning at doses of 6 mg/kg/day caused decreased learning ability and decreased female body weights in the offspring. There are no adequate and well-controlled studies of irinotecan in pregnant women. If the drug is used during pregnancy, or if the patient becomes pregnant while receiving this drug, the patient should be apprised of the potential hazard to the fetus. Women of childbearing potential should be advised to avoid becoming pregnant while receiving treatment with CAMPTOSAR.

PRECAUTIONS

General

Care of Intravenous Site: CAMPTOSAR Injection is administered by intravenous infusion. Care should be taken to avoid extravasation, and the infusion site should be monitored for signs of inflammation. Should extravasation occur, flushing the site with sterile water and applications of ice are recommended.

Premedication with Antiemetics: Irinotecan is emetigenic. It is recommended that patients receive premedication with antiemetic agents. In clinical studies of the weekly dosage schedule, the majority of patients received 10 mg of dexamethasone given in conjunction with another type of antiemetic agents, such as a 5-HT^3 blocker (e.g., odansetron or granisetron). Antiemetic agents should be given on the day of treatment, starting at least 30 minutes before administration of CAMPTOSAR. Physicians should also consider providing patients with an antiemetic regimen (e.g., prochlorperazine) for subsequent use as needed.

Treatment of Cholinergic Symptoms: Prophylactic or therapeutic administration of 0.25 to 1 mg of intravenous or subcutaneous atropine should be considered (unless clinically contraindicated) in patients experiencing rhinitis, increased salivation, miosis, lacrimation, diaphoresis, flushing, abdominal cramping, or diarrhea (occurring during or shortly after infusion of CAMPTOSAR). These symptoms are expected to occur more frequently with higher irinotecan doses.

Patients at Particular Risk: Physicians should exercise particular caution in monitoring the effects of CAMPTOSAR in the elderly (≥65 years) and in patients who had previously received pelvic/abdominal irradiation (see ADVERSE REACTIONS).

The use of CAMPTOSAR in patients with significant hepatic dysfunction has not been established. In clinical trials of either dosing schedule, irinotecan was not administered to patients with serum bilirubin >2.0 mg/dL, or transaminase >3 times the upper limit of normal if no liver metastasis, or transaminase >5 times the upper limit of normal with liver metastasis.

However in clinical trials of the weekly dosage schedule, it has been noted in patients with modestly elevated baseline

Continued on next page

Information on these Pharmacia & Upjohn products is based on labeling in effect June 1, 2000. Further information concerning these and other Pharmacia & Upjohn products may be obtained by direct inquiry to Medical Information, Pharmacia & Upjohn, Kalamazoo, MI 49001.

Camptosar—Cont.

serum total bilirubin levels (1.0 to 2.0 mg/dL) have had a significantly greater likelihood of experiencing first-course grade 3 or 4 neutropenia than those with bilirubin levels that were less than 1.0 mg/dL (50.0% [19/38] versus 17.7% [47/226]; $p<0.001$). Patients with abnormal glucuronidation of bilirubin, such as those with Gilbert's syndrome, may also be at greater risk of myelosuppression when receiving therapy with CAMPTOSAR. An association between baseline bilirubin elevations and an increased risk of late diarrhea has not been observed in studies of the weekly dosage schedule.

Information for Patients

Patients and patients' caregivers should be informed of the expected toxic effects of CAMPTOSAR, particularly of its gastrointestinal manifestations, such as nausea, vomiting, and diarrhea. Each patient should be instructed to have loperamide readily available and to begin treatment for late diarrhea (generally occurring more than 24 hours after administration of CAMPTOSAR) at the first episode of poorly formed or loose stools or the earliest onset of bowel movements more frequent than normally expected for the patient. One dosage regimen for loperamide used in clinical trials consisted of the following (Note: This dosage regimen exceeds the usual dosage recommendations for loperamide.): 4 mg at the first onset of late diarrhea and then 2 mg every 2 hours until the patient is diarrhea-free for at least 12 hours. During the night, the patient may take 4 mg of loperamide every 4 hours. The patient should also be instructed to notify the physician if diarrhea occurs. Premedication with loperamide is not recommended.

The use of drugs with laxative properties should be avoided because of the potential for exacerbation of diarrhea. Patients should be advised to contact their physician to discuss any laxative use.

Patients should consult their physician if vomiting occurs, fever or evidence of infection develops, or if symptoms of dehydration, such as fainting, light-headedness, or dizziness, are noted following therapy with CAMPTOSAR.

Patients should be alerted to the possibility of alopecia.

Laboratory Tests

Careful monitoring of the white blood cell count with differential, hemoglobin, and platelet count is recommended before each dose of CAMPTOSAR.

Drug Interactions

The adverse effects of CAMPTOSAR, such as myelosuppression and diarrhea, would be expected to be exacerbated by other antineoplastic agents having similar adverse effects.

Patients who have previously received pelvic/abdominal irradiation are at increased risk of severe myelosuppression following the administration of CAMPTOSAR. The concurrent administration of CAMPTOSAR with irradiation has not been adequately studied and is not recommended.

Lymphocytopenia has been reported in patients receiving CAMPTOSAR, and it is possible that the administration of dexamethasone as antiemetic prophylaxis may have enhanced the likelihood of this effect. However, serious opportunistic infections have not been observed, and no complications have specifically been attributed to lymphocytopenia.

Hyperglycemia has also been reported in patients receiving CAMPTOSAR. Usually, this has been observed in patients with a history of diabetes mellitus or evidence of glucose intolerance prior to administration of CAMPTOSAR. It is probable that dexamethasone, given as antiemetic prophylaxis, contributed to hyperglycemia in some patients.

The incidence of akathisia in clinical trials of the weekly dosage schedule was greater (8.5%, 4/47 patients) when prochlorperazine was administered on the same day as CAMPTOSAR than when these drugs were given on separate days (1.3%, 1/80 patients). The 8.5% incidence of akathisia, however, is within the range reported for use of prochlorperazine when given as a premedication for other chemotherapies.

It would be expected that laxative use during therapy with CAMPTOSAR would worsen the incidence or severity of diarrhea, but this has not been studied.

In view of the potential risk of dehydration secondary to vomiting and/or diarrhea induced by CAMPTOSAR, the physician may wish to withhold diuretics during dosing with CAMPTOSAR and, certainly, during periods of active vomiting or diarrhea.

Drug-Laboratory Test Interactions

There are no known interactions between CAMPTOSAR and laboratory tests.

Carcinogenesis, Mutagenesis & Impairment of Fertility

Long-term carcinogenicity studies with irinotecan were not conducted. Rats were, however, administered intravenous doses of 2 mg/kg or 25 mg/kg irinotecan once per week for 13 weeks (in separate studies, the 25 mg/kg dose produced an irinotecan C_{max} and AUC that were about 7.0 times and 1.3 times the respective values in patients administered 125 mg/m^2 weekly) and were then allowed to recover for 91 weeks. Under these conditions, there was a significant linear trend with dose for the incidence of combined uterine horn endometrial stromal polyps and endometrial stromal sarcomas. Neither irinotecan or SN-38 was mutagenic in the in vitro Ames assay. Irinotecan was clastogenic both in vitro (chromosome aberrations in Chinese hamster ovary cells) and in vivo (micronucleus test in mice). No significant adverse effects on fertility and general reproductive perfor-

Table 7. Study 2: Percent (%) of Patients Experiencing Clinically Relevant Adverse Events in Combination Therapies

Adverse Event	Study 2: Irinotecan + 5-FU/LV Infusional at 1&2 q 2 weeks N=145		5-FU/LV Infusional at 1&2 q 2 weeks N=143	
	Grade 1–4	Grade 3&4	Grade 1–4	Grade 3&4
TOTAL Adverse Events	100	72.4	100	39.2
BODY AS A WHOLE				
Asthenia	57.9	9.0	48.3	4.2
Pain	64.1	9.7	61.5	8.4
Fever	22.1	0.7	25.9	0.7
Infection	35.9	7.6	33.6	3.5
METABOLIC & NUTRITIONAL				
↑ Bilirubin	19.1	3.5	35.9	10.6
DERMATOLOGIC				
Hand & foot syndrome	10.3	0.7	12.6	0.7
Cutaneous signs	17.2	0.7	20.3	0
Alopecia[b]	56.6	—	16.8	—
RESPIRATORY				
Dyspnea	9.7	1.4	4.9	0
CARDIOVASCULAR				
Hypotension	3.4	1.4	0.7	0

[a] Includes rhinitis, increased salivation, miosis, lacrimation, diaphoresis, flushing, abdominal cramping or diarrhea (occurring during or shortly after infusion of irinotecan)

[b] Complete hair loss = Grade 2

Table 8. Adverse Events Occurring in >10% of 304 Previously Treated Patients with Metastatic Carcinoma of the Colon or Rectum

Body System & Event	% of Patients Reporting: NCI Grades 1–4	NCI Grades 3 & 4
GASTROINTESTINAL		
Diarrhea (late)[a]	88	31
7–9 stools/day (grade 3)	—	(16)
≥10 stools/day (grade 4)	—	(14)
Nausea	86	17
Vomiting	67	12
Anorexia	55	6
Diarrhea (early)[b]	51	8
Constipation	30	2
Flatulence	12	0
Stomatitis	12	1
Dyspepsia	10	0
HEMATOLOGIC		
Leukopenia	63	28
Anemia	60	7
Neutropenia	54	26
500 to <1000/mm^3 (grade 3)	—	(15)
<500/mm^3 (grade 4)	—	(12)
BODY AS A WHOLE		
Asthenia	76	12
Abdominal cramping/pain	57	16
Fever	45	1
Pain	24	2
Headache	17	1
Back pain	14	2
Chills	14	0
Minor Infection[c]	14	0
Edema	10	1
Abdominal Enlargement	10	0
METABOLIC & NUTRITIONAL		
↓ Body weight	30	1
Dehydration	15	4
↑ Alkaline phosphatase	13	4
↑ SGOT	10	1
DERMATOLOGIC		
Alopecia	60	NA[d]
Sweating	16	0
Rash	13	1
RESPIRATORY		
Dyspnea	22	4
↑ Coughing	17	0
Rhinitis	16	0
NEUROLOGIC		
Insomnia	19	0
Dizziness	15	0
CARDIOVASCULAR		
Vasodilation (Flushing)	11	0

[a] Occurring >24 hours after administration of CAMPTOSAR

[b] Occurring ≤24 hours after administration of CAMPTOSAR

[c] Primarily upper respiratory infections

[d] Not applicable; complete hair loss = NCI grade 2

Table 9. Percent of Patients Experiencing Grade 3 & 4 Adverse Events in Comparative Studies of Once-Every-3-Week Irinotecan Therapy

	Study 1		Study 2	
Adverse Event	**Irinotecan N=189**	**BSC[a] N=90**	**Irinotecan N=127**	**5-FU N=129**
TOTAL Grade 3/4 Adverse Events	79	67	69	54
GASTROINTESTINAL				
Diarrhea	22	6	22	11
Vomiting	14	8	14	5
Nausea	14	3	11	4
Abdominal pain	14	16	9	8
Constipation	10	8	8	6
Anorexia	5	7	6	4
Mucositis	2	1	2	5
HEMATOLOGIC				
Leukopenia/Neutropenia	22	0	14	2
Anemia	7	6	6	3
Hemorrhage	5	3	1	3
Thrombocytopenia	1	0	4	2
Infection				
without grade 3/4 neutropenia	8	3	1	4
with grade 3/4 neutropenia	1	0	2	0
Fever				
without grade 3/4 neutropenia	2	1	2	0
with grade 3/4 neutropenia	2	0	4	2
BODY AS A WHOLE				
Pain	19	22	17	13
Asthenia	15	19	13	12
METABOLIC & NUTRITIONAL				
Hepatic[b]	9	7	9	6
DERMATOLOGIC				
Hand & foot syndrome	0	0	0	5
Cutaneous signs[c]	2	0	1	3
RESPIRATORY[d]	10	8	5	7
NEUROLOGIC[e]	12	13	9	4
CARDIOVASCULAR[f]	9	3	4	2
OTHER[g]	32	28	12	14

[a] BSC = best supportive care
[b] Hepatic includes events such as ascites and jaundice
[c] Cutaneous signs include events such as rash
[d] Respiratory includes events such as dyspnea and cough
[e] Neurologic includes events such as somnolence
[f] Cardiovascular includes events such as dysrhythmias, ischemia, and mechanical cardiac dysfunction
[g] Other includes events such as accidental injury, hepatomegaly, syncope, vertigo, and weight loss

Table 10. Combination-Agent Dosage Regimens & Dose Modifications[a]

Regimen 1 6-wk course with bolus 5-FU/LV (next course begins on day 43)	CAMPTOSAR LV 5-FU	125 mg/m² IV over 90 min, d 1, 8, 15, 22 20 mg/m² IV bolus, d 1, 8, 15, 22 500 mg/m² IV bolus, d 1, 8, 15, 22		
		Starting Dose & Modified Dose Levels (mg/m²)		
		Starting Dose	Dose Level - 1	Dose Level - 2
	CAMPTOSAR LV 5-FU	125 20 500	100 20 400	75 20 300
Regimen 2 6-wk course with infusional 5-FU/LV (next course begins on day 43)	CAMPTOSAR LV 5-FU Bolus 5-FU Infusion[b]	180 mg/m² IV over 90 min, d 1, 15, 29 200 mg/m² IV over 2 h, d 1, 2, 15, 16, 29, 30 400 mg/m² IV bolus, d 1, 2, 15, 16, 29, 30 600 mg/m² over 22 h, d 1, 2, 15, 16, 29, 30		
		Starting Dose & Modified Dose Levels (mg/m²)		
		Starting Dose	Dose Level - 1	Dose Level - 2
	CAMPTOSAR LV 5-FU Bolus 5-FU Infusion[b]	180 200 400 600	150 200 320 480	120 200 240 360

[a] Dose reductions beyond dose level −2 by decrements of ≈20% may be warranted for patients continuing to experience toxicity. Provided intolerable toxicity does not develop, treatment with additional courses may be continued indefinitely as long as patients continue to experience clinical benefit.
[b] Infusion follows bolus administration.

mance was observed after intravenous administration of irinotecan in doses of up to 6 mg/kg/day to rats and rabbits. However, atrophy of male reproductive organs was observed after multiple daily irinotecan doses both in rodents at 20 mg/kg (which in separate studies produced an irinotecan C_{max} and AUC about 5 and 1 times, respectively, the corresponding values in patients administered 125 mg/m² weekly) and dogs at 0.4 mg/kg (which in separate studies produced an irinotecan C_{max} and AUC about one-half and 1/15th, respectively, the corresponding values in patients administered 125 mg/m² weekly).

Pregnancy
Pregnancy Category D—see WARNINGS.

Nursing Mothers
Radioactivity appeared in rat milk within 5 minutes of intravenous administration of radiolabeled irinotecan and was concentrated up to 65-fold at 4 hours after administration relative to plasma concentrations. Because many drugs are excreted in human milk and because of the potential for serious adverse reactions in nursing infants, it is recommended that nursing be discontinued when receiving therapy with CAMPTOSAR.

Pediatric Use
The safety and effectiveness of CAMPTOSAR in pediatric patients have not been established.

Geriatric Use
Patients greater than 65 years of age should be closely monitored because of a greater risk of late diarrhea in this population (see CLINICAL PHARMACOLOGY, Pharmacokinetics in Special Populations and ADVERSE REACTIONS, Overview of Adverse Events). The starting dose of CAMPTOSAR in patients 70 years and older for the once-every-3-week-dosage schedule should be 300 mg/m² (see DOSAGE AND ADMINISTRATION).

ADVERSE REACTIONS

First-Line Combination Therapy
A total of 955 patients with metastatic colorectal cancer received the recommended regimens of irinotecan in combination with 5-FU/LV, 5-FU/LV alone, or irinotecan alone. In the two phase 3 studies, 370 patients received irinotecan in combination with 5-FU/LV, 362 patients received 5-FU/LV alone, and 223 patients received irinotecan alone. (See Table 10 in DOSAGE AND ADMINISTRATION for recommended combination-agent regimens.)

In Study 1, 49 (7.3%) patients died, within 30 days of study treatment: 21 (9.3%) received irinotecan in combination with 5-FU/LV, 15 (6.8%) received 5-FU/LV alone, and 13 (5.8%) received irinotecan alone. Deaths potentially related to treatment occurred in 2 (0.9%) patients who received irinotecan in combination with 5-FU/LV (2 neutropenic fever/sepsis), 3 (1.4%) patients who received 5-FU/LV alone (1 neutropenic fever/sepsis, 1 CNS bleeding during thrombocytopenia, 1 unknown) and 2 (0.9%) patients who received irinotecan alone (2 neutropenic fever). Discontinuations due to adverse events were reported for 17 (7.6%) patients who received irinotecan in combination with 5-FU/LV, 14 (6.4%) patients who received 5-FU/LV alone, and 26 (11.7%) patients who received irinotecan alone.

In Study 2, 10 (3.5%) patients died within 30 days of study treatment: 6 (4.1%) received irinotecan in combination with 5-FU/LV and 4 (2.8%) received 5-FU/LV alone. There was one potentially treatment-death, which occurred in a patient who received irinotecan in combination with 5-FU/LV (0.7%, neutropenic sepsis). Discontinuations due to adverse events were reported for 9 (6.2%) patients who received irinotecan in combination with 5-FU/LV and 1 (0.7%) patients who received 5-FU/LV alone.

The most clinically significant adverse events (all grades 1–4) for patients receiving irinotecan-based therapy were diarrhea, nausea, vomiting, neutropenia, and alopecia. The most clinically significant adverse events for patients receiving 5-FU/LV therapy were diarrhea, neutropenia, neutropenic fever, and mucositis. In Study 1, grade 4 neutropenia, neutropenic fever (defined as grade 2 fever and grade 4 neutropenia), and mucositis were observed less often with weekly irinotecan/5-FU/LV than with monthly administration of 5-FU/LV.

Tables 6 and 7 list the clinically relevant adverse events reported in Studies 1 and 2, respectively.
[See table 6 at top of page 2575]
[See table 7 at bottom of page 2575 and top of page 2576]

Second-Line Single-Agent Therapy
Weekly Dosage Schedule
In three clinical studies evaluating the weekly dosage schedule, 304 patients with metastatic carcinoma of the colon or rectum that had recurred or progressed following 5-FU-based therapy were treated with CAMPTOSAR. Seventeen of the patients died within 30 days of the administration of CAMPTOSAR; in five cases (1.6%, 5/304), the deaths were potentially drug-related. These five patients experienced a constellation of medical events that included known effects of CAMPTOSAR. One of these patients died of neutropenic sepsis without fever. Neutropenic fever occurred in nine (3.0%) other patients; these patients recovered with supportive care.

One hundred nineteen (39.1%) of the 304 patients were hospitalized a total of 156 times because of adverse events; 81 (26.6%) patients were hospitalized for events judged to be related to administration of CAMPTOSAR. The primary reasons for drug-related hospitalization were diarrhea, with or without nausea and/or vomiting (18.4%); neutropenia/leukopenia, with or without diarrhea and/or fever (8.2%); and nausea and/or vomiting (4.9%).

Adjustments in the dose of CAMPTOSAR were made during the course of treatment and for subsequent courses based on individual patient tolerance. The first dose of at least one course of CAMPTOSAR was reduced for 67% of patients who began the studies at the 125 mg/m² starting dose. Within-course dose reductions were required for 32% of the courses initiated at the 125 mg/m² dose level. The most common reasons for dose reduction were late diarrhea, neutropenia, and leukopenia. Thirteen (4.3%) patients discontinued treatment with CAMPTOSAR because of adverse events. The adverse events in Table 8 are based on the ex-

Continued on next page

Information on these Pharmacia & Upjohn products is based on labeling in effect June 1, 2000. Further information concerning these and other Pharmacia & Upjohn products may be obtained by direct inquiry to Medical Information, Pharmacia & Upjohn, Kalamazoo, MI 49001.

Camptosar—Cont.

perience of the 304 patients enrolled in the three studies described in the CLINICAL STUDIES, Studies Evaluating the Weekly Dosage Schedule, section.

[See table 8 at bottom of page 2576]

Once-Every-3-Week Dosage Schedule

A total of 535 patients with metastatic colorectal cancer whose disease had recurred or progressed following prior 5-FU therapy participated in the two phase 3 studies: 316 received irinotecan, 129 received 5-FU, and 90 received best supportive care. Eleven (3.5%) patients treated with irinotecan died within 30 days of treatment. In three cases (1%, 3/316), the deaths were potentially related to irinotecan treatment and were attributed to neutropenic infection, grade 4 diarrhea, and asthenia, respectively. One (0.8%, 1/129) patient treated with 5-FU died within 30 days of treatment; this death was attributed to grade 4 diarrhea.

Hospitalizations due to serious adverse events (whether or not related to study treatment) occurred at least once in 60% (188/316) of patients who received irinotecan, 63% (57/90) who received best supportive care, and 39% (50/129) who received 5-FU based therapy. Eight percent of patients treated with irinotecan and 7% treated with 5-FU based therapy discontinued treatment due to adverse events.

Of the 316 patients treated with irinotecan, the most clinically significant adverse events (all grades, 1–4) were diarrhea (84%), alopecia (72%), nausea (70%), vomiting (62%), cholinergic symptoms (47%), and neutropenia (30%). Table 9 lists the grade 3 and 4 adverse events reported in the patients enrolled to all treatment arms of the two studies described in the CLINICAL STUDIES, Studies Evaluating the Once-Every-3-Week Dosage Schedule, section.

[See table 9 at top of previous page]

Overview of Adverse Events

Gastrointestinal: Nausea, vomiting, and diarrhea are common adverse events following treatment with CAMPTOSAR and can be severe. When observed, nausea and vomiting usually occur during or shortly after infusion of CAMPTOSAR. In the clinical studies testing the every 3-week-dosage schedule, the median time to the onset of late diarrhea was 5 days after irinotecan infusion. In the clinical studies evaluating the weekly dosage schedule, the median time to onset of late diarrhea was 11 days following administration of CAMPTOSAR. For patients starting treatment at the 125 mg/m^2 weekly dose, the median duration of any grade of late diarrhea was 3 days. Among those patients treated at the 125 mg/m^2 weekly dose who experienced grade 3 or 4 late diarrhea, the median duration of the entire episode of diarrhea was 7 days. The frequency of grade 3 or 4 late diarrhea was somewhat greater in patients starting treatment at 125 mg/m^2 than in patients given a 100 mg/m^2 weekly starting dose (34% [65/193] versus 23% [24/102]; p=0.08). The frequency of grade 3 and 4 late diarrhea by age was significantly greater in patients ≥65 years than in patients <65 years (40% [53/133] versus 23% [40/171]; p=0.002). In one study of the weekly dosage treatment, the frequency of grade 3 and 4 late diarrhea was significantly greater in male than in female patients (43% [25/58] versus 16% [5/32]; p=0.01), but there were no gender differences in the frequency of grade 3 and 4 late diarrhea in the other two studies of the weekly dosage treatment schedule. Colonic ulceration, sometimes with gastrointestinal bleeding, has been observed in association with administration of CAMPTOSAR.

Hematology: CAMPTOSAR commonly causes neutropenia, leukopenia (including lymphocytopenia), and anemia. Serious thrombocytopenia is uncommon. When evaluated in the trials of weekly administration, the frequency of grade 3 and 4 neutropenia was significantly higher in patients who received previous pelvic/abdominal irradiation than in those who had not received such irradiation (48% [13/27] versus 24% [67/277]; p=0.04). In these same studies, patients with baseline serum total bilirubin levels of 1.0 mg/dL or more also had a significantly greater likelihood of experiencing first-course grade 3 or 4 neutropenia than those with bilirubin levels that were less than 1.0 mg/dL (50% [19/38] versus 18% [47/266]; p<0.001). There were no significant differences in the frequency of grade 3 and 4 neutropenia by age or gender. In the clinical studies evaluating the weekly dosage schedule, neutropenic fever (concurrent NCl grade 4 neutropenia and fever of grade 2 or greater) occurred in 3% of the patients; 6% of patients received G-CSF for the treatment of neutropenia. NCl grade 3 or 4 anemia was noted in 7% of the patients receiving weekly treatment; blood transfusions were given to 10% of the patients in these trials.

Body as a Whole: Asthenia, fever, and abdominal pain are generally the most common events of this type.

Cholinergic Symptoms: Patients may have cholinergic symptoms of rhinitis, increased salivation, miosis, lacrimation, diaphoresis, flushing, and intestinal hyperperistalsis that can cause abdominal cramping and early diarrhea. If these symptoms occur, they manifest during or shortly after drug infusion. They are thought to be related to the anticholinesterase activity of the irinotecan parent compound and are expected to occur more frequently with higher irinotecan doses.

Hepatic: In the clinical studies evaluating the weekly dosage schedule, NCl grade 3 or 4 liver enzyme abnormalities were observed in fewer than 10% of patients. These events typically occur in patients with known hepatic metastases.

Dermatologic: Alopecia has been reported during treatment with CAMPTOSAR. Rashes have also been reported but did not result in discontinuation of treatment.

Table 11. Recommended Dose Modifications for CAMPTOSAR/5-Fluorouracil (5-FU)/Leucovorin (LV) Combination Schedules

A new course of therapy should not begin until the granulocyte count has recovered to ≥1500/mm^3, and the platelet count has recovered to ≥100,000/mm^3, and treatment-related diarrhea is fully resolved. Treatment should be delayed 1 to 2 weeks to allow for recovery from treatment-related toxicities. If the patient has not recovered after a 2-week delay, consideration should be given to discontinuing therapy.

Toxicity NCI CTC grade[a] (Value)	During a Course of Therapy	At the Start of Subsequent Courses of Therapy[b]
No toxicity	Maintain dose level	Maintain dose level
Neutropenia		
1 (1500 to 1999/mm^3)	Maintain dose level	Maintain dose level
2 (1000 to 1499/mm^3)	↓ 1 dose level	Maintain dose level
3 (500 to 999/mm^3)	Omit dose, then ↓ 1 dose level when resolved to ≤ grade 2	↓ 1 dose level
4 (< 500/mm^3)	Omit dose, then ↓ 2 dose levels when resolved to ≤ grade 2	↓ 2 dose levels
Neutropenic fever (grade 4 neutropenia & ≥ grade 2 fever)	Omit dose, then ↓ 2 dose levels when resolved	↓ 2 dose levels
Other hematologic toxicities	Dose modifications for leukopenia or thrombocytopenia during a course of therapy and at the start of subsequent courses of therapy are also based on NCl toxicity criteria and are the same as recommended for neutropenia above.	
Diarrhea		
1 (2–3 stools/day > pretx[c])	Maintain dose level	Maintain dose level
2 (4–6 stools/day > pretx)	↓ 1 dose level	Maintain dose level
3 (7–9 stools/day > pretx)	Omit dose, then ↓ 1 dose level when resolved to ≤ grade 2	↓ 1 dose level
4 (≥10 stools/day > pretx)	Omit dose, then ↓ 2 dose levels when resolved to ≤ grade 2	↓ 2 dose levels
Other nonhematologic toxicities		
1	Maintain dose level	Maintain dose level
2	↓ 1 dose level	Maintain dose level
3	Omit dose, then ↓ 1 dose level when resolved to ≤ grade 2	↓ 1 dose level
4	Omit dose, then ↓ 2 dose levels when resolved to ≤ grade 2	↓ 2 dose levels
	For mucositis/stomatitis decrease only 5-FU, not CAMPTOSAR	*For mucositis/stomatitis decrease only 5-FU, not CAMPTOSAR*

[a]National Cancer Institute Common Toxicity Criteria
[b]Relative to the starting dose used in the previous course
[c]Pretreatment

Table 12. Single-Agent Regimens of CAMPTOSAR and Dose Modifications

Weekly Regimen[a]	125 mg/m^2 IV over 90 min, d 1, 8, 15, 22 then 2-wk rest		
	Starting Dose & Modified Dose Levels[c] (mg/m^2)		
	Starting Dose	Dose Level −1	Dose Level −2
	125	100	75
Once-Every-3-Week Regimen[b]	350 mg/m^2 IV over 90 min, once every 3 wks[c]		
	Starting Dose & Modified Dose Levels (mg/m^2)		
	Starting Dose	Dose Level −1	Dose Level −2
	350	300	250

[a] Subsequent doses may be adjusted as high at 150 mg/m^2 or to as low as 50 mg/m^2 in 25 to 50 mg/m^2 decrements depending upon individual patient tolerance.
[b] Subsequent doses may be adjusted as low as 200 mg/m^2 in 50 mg/m^2 decrements depending upon individual patient tolerance.
[c] Provided intolerable toxicity does not develop, treatment with additional courses may be continued indefinitely as long as patients continue to experience clinical benefit.

Respiratory: Severe pulmonary events are infrequent. In the clinical studies evaluating the weekly dosage schedule, NCl grade 3 or 4 dyspnea was reported in 4% of patients. Over half the patients with dyspnea had lung metastases; the extent to which malignant pulmonary involvement or other preexisting lung disease may have contributed to dyspnea in these patients is unknown.

Neurologic: Insomnia and dizziness can occur, but are not usually considered to be directly related to the administration of CAMPTOSAR. Dizziness may sometimes represent symptomatic evidence of orthostatic hypotension in patients with dehydration.

Cardiovascular: Vasodilation (flushing) may occur during administration of CAMPTOSAR. Bradycardia may also occur, but has not required intervention. These effects have been attributed to the cholinergic syndrome sometimes observed during or shortly after infusion of CAMPTOSAR.

Other Non-U.S. Clinical Trials

Irinotecan has been studied in over 1100 patients in Japan. Patients in these studies had a variety of tumor types, including cancer of the colon or rectum, and were treated with several different doses and schedules. In general, the types of toxicities observed were similar to those seen in U.S. trials with CAMPTOSAR. There is some information from Japanese trials that patients with considerable ascites or pleural effusions were at increased risk for neutropenia or diarrhea. A potentially life-threatening pulmonary syndrome, consisting of dyspnea, fever, and a reticulonodular pattern on chest x-ray, was observed in a small percentage of patients in early Japanese studies. The contribution of irinotecan to these preliminary events was difficult to assess because these patients also had lung tumors and some had preexisting nonmalignant pulmonary disease. As a result of these observations, however, clinical studies in the United States have enrolled few patients with compromised pulmonary function, significant ascites, or pleural effusions.

Post-Marketing Experience

The following events have been identified during post-marketing use of CAMPTOSAR in clinical practice. The events, which have been chosen for inclusion due to either their seriousness, frequency of reporting, possible causal connection to CAMPTOSAR, or a combination of these factors, include: rare cases of colitis complicated by ulceration, bleeding, ileus, or what was described as toxic megacolon; rare cases of ileus without preceding colitis; and rare cases of renal impairment and acute renal failure, generally in patients who became volume depleted from severe vomiting and/or diarrhea (see WARNINGS).

Hypersensitivity reactions including severe anaphylactic or anaphylactoid reactions have been observed (see WARNINGS).

OVERDOSAGE

In U.S. phase 1 trials, single doses of up to 345 mg/m^2 of irinotecan were administered to patients with various cancers. Single doses of up to 750 mg/m^2 of irinotecan have been given in non-U.S. trials. The adverse events in these patients were similar to those reported with the recommended dosage and regimen. There is no known antidote for overdosage of CAMPTOSAR. Maximum supportive care should be instituted to prevent dehydration due to diarrhea and to treat any infectious complications.

DOSAGE AND ADMINISTRATION

Combination-Agent Dosage

Dosage Regimens:

CAMPTOSAR Injection in Combination with 5-Fluorouracil (5-FU) and Leucovorin (LV)

CAMPTOSAR should be administered as an intravenous infusion over 90 minutes (see Preparation of Infusion Solution). For all regimens, the dose of LV should be administered immediately after CAMPTOSAR, with the administration of 5-FU to occur immediately after receipt of LV. CAMPTOSAR should be used as recommended; the currently recommended regimens are shown in Table 10.

Dosing for patients with bilirubin >2 mg/dL cannot be recommended since such patients were not included in clinical studies. It is recommended that patients receive premedication with antiemetic agents. Prophylactic or therapeutic administration of atropine should be considered in patients experiencing cholinergic symptoms. See PRECAUTIONS, General.

Dose Modifications

Patients should be carefully monitored for toxicity, and doses of CAMPTOSAR and 5-FU should be modified as necessary to accommodate individual patient tolerance to treatment. Based on the recommended dose-levels described in Table 10, Combination-Agent Dosage Regimens & Dose Modifications, subsequent doses should be adjusted as suggested in Table 11, Recommended Dose Modifications for Combination Schedules. All dose modifications should be based on the worst preceding toxicity.

A new course of therapy should not begin until the toxicity has recovered to NCI grade 1 or less. Treatment may be delayed 1 to 2 weeks to allow for recovery from treatment-related toxicity. If the patient has not recovered, consideration should be given to discontinuing therapy. Provided intolerable toxicity does not develop, treatment with additional courses of CAMPTOSAR/5-FU/LV may be continued indefinitely as long as patients continue to experience clinical benefit.

[See table 10 at top of page 2577]

[See table 11 at top of previous page]

Single-Agent Dosage Schedules

Dosage Regimens

CAMPTOSAR should be administered as an intravenous infusion over 90 minutes for both the weekly and once-every-3-week dosage schedules (see Preparation of Infusion Solution). Single-agent dosage regimens are shown in Table 12.

A reduction in the starting dose by one dose level of CAMPTOSAR may be considered for patients with any of the following conditions: age ≥65 years, prior pelvic/abdominal radiotherapy, performance status of 2, or increased bilirubin levels. Dosing for patients with bilirubin >2 mg/dL cannot be recommended since such patients were not included in clinical studies.

It is recommended that patients receive premedication with antiemetic agents. Prophylactic or therapeutic administration of atropine should be considered in patients experiencing cholinergic symptoms. See PRECAUTIONS, General.

Dose Modifications

Patients should be carefully monitored for toxicity and doses of CAMPTOSAR should be modified as necessary to accommodate individual patient tolerance to treatment. Based on recommended dose-levels described in Table 12, Single-Agent Regimens of CAMPTOSAR and Dose Modifications, subsequent doses should be adjusted as suggested in Table 13, Recommended Dose Modifications for Single-Agent Schedules. All dose modifications should be based on the worst preceding toxicity.

A new course of therapy should not begin until the toxicity has recovered to NCI grade 1 or less. Treatment may be delayed 1 to 2 weeks to allow for recovery from treatment-related toxicity. If the patient has not recovered, consideration should be given to discontinuing this combination therapy. Provided intolerable toxicity does not develop, treatment with additional courses of CAMPTOSAR may be continued indefinitely as long as patients continue to experience clinical benefit.

[See table 12 at top of previous page]

[See table 13 above]

Table 13. Recommended Dose Modifications for Single-Agent Schedules[a]

A new course of therapy should not begin until the granulocyte count has recovered to ≥1500/mm³, and the platelet count has recovered to ≥100,000/mm³, and treatment-related diarrhea is fully resolved. Treatment should be delayed 1 to 2 weeks to allow for recovery from treatment-related toxicities. If the patient has not recovered after a 2-week delay, consideration should be given to discontinuing CAMPTOSAR.

Worst Toxicity NCI Grade[b] (Value)	During a Course of Therapy	At the Start of the Next Courses of Therapy (After Adequate Recovery), Compared with the Starting Dose in the Previous Course[a]	
	Weekly	Weekly	Once Every 3 Weeks
No toxicity	Maintain dose level	↑ 25 mg/m² up to a maximum dose of 150 mg/m²	Maintain dose level
Neutropenia			
1 (1500 to 1999/mm³)	Maintain dose level	Maintain dose level	Maintain dose level
2 (1000 to 1499/mm³)	↓ 25 mg/m²	Maintain dose level	Maintain dose level
3 (500 to 999/mm³)	Omit dose, then ↓ 25 mg/m² when resolved to ≤ grade 2	↓ 25 mg/m²	↓ 50 mg/m²
4 (<500/mm³)	Omit dose, then ↓ 50 mg/m² when resolved to ≤ grade 2	↓ 50 mg/m²	↓ 50 mg/m²
Neutropenic fever (grade 4 neutropenia & ≥ grade 2 fever)	Omit dose, then ↓ 50 mg/m² when resolved	↓ 50 mg/m²	↓ 50 mg/m²
Other hematologic toxicities	Dose modifications for leukopenia, thrombocytopenia, and anemia during a course of therapy and at the start of subsequent courses of therapy are also based on NCI toxicity criteria and are the same as recommended for neutropenia above.		
Diarrhea			
1 (2–3 stools/day > pretx[c])	Maintain dose level	Maintain dose level	Maintain dose level
2 (4–6 stools/day > pretx)	↓ 25 mg/m²	Maintain dose level	Maintain dose level
3 (7–9 stools/day > pretx)	Omit dose, then ↓ 25 mg/m² when resolved to ≤ grade 2	↓ 25 mg/m²	↓ 50 mg/m²
4 (≥ 10 stools/day > pretx)	Omit dose, then ↓ 50 mg/m² when resolved to ≤ grade 2	↓ 50 mg/m²	↓ 50 mg/m²
Other nonhematologic toxicities			
1	Maintain dose level	Maintain dose level	Maintain dose level
2	↓ 25 mg/m²	↓ 25 mg/m²	↓ 50 mg/m²
3	Omit dose, then ↓ 25 mg/m² when resolved to ≤ grade 2	↓ 25 mg/m²	↓ 50 mg/m²
4	Omit dose, then ↓ 50 mg/m² when resolved to ≤ grade 2	↓ 50 mg/m²	↓ 50 mg/m²

[a] All dose modifications should be based on the worst preceding toxicity

[b] National Cancer Institute Common Toxicity Criteria

[c] Pretreatment

Preparation & Administration Precautions

As with other potentially toxic anticancer agents, care should be exercised in the handling and preparation of infusion solutions prepared from CAMPTOSAR Injection. The use of gloves is recommended. If a solution of CAMPTOSAR contacts the skin, wash the skin immediately and thoroughly with soap and water. If CAMPTOSAR contacts the mucous membranes, flush thoroughly with water. Several published guidelines for handling and disposal of anticancer agents are available.[1–7]

Preparation of Infusion Solution

Inspect vial contents for particulate matter and repeat inspection when drug product is withdrawn from vial into syringe.

CAMPTOSAR Injection must be diluted prior to infusion. CAMPTOSAR should be diluted in 5% Dextrose Injection, USP, (preferred) or 0.9% Sodium Chloride Injection, USP, to a final concentration range of 0.12 to 2.8 mg/mL. In most clinical trials, CAMPTOSAR was administered in 250 mL to 500 mL of 5% Dextrose Injection, USP.

The solution is physically and chemically stable for up to 24 hours at room temperature (approximately 25°C) and in ambient fluorescent lighting. Solutions diluted in 5% Dextrose Injection, USP, and stored at refrigerated temperatures (approximately 2° to 8°C), and protected from light are physically and chemically stable for 48 hours. Refrigeration of admixtures using 0.9% Sodium Chloride Injection, USP, is not recommended due to a low and sporadic incidence of visible particulates. Freezing CAMPTOSAR and admixtures of CAMPTOSAR may result in precipitation of the drug and should be avoided. Because of possible microbial contamination during dilution, it is advisable to use the admixture prepared with 5% Dextrose Injection, USP, within 24 hours of refrigerated (2° to 8°C, 36° to 46°F). In the case of admixtures prepared with 5% Dextrose Injection, USP, or Sodium Chloride Injection, USP, the solutions should be used within 6 hours if kept at room temperature (15° to 30°C, 59° to 86°F).

Other drugs should not be added to the infusion solution. Parenteral drug products should be inspected visually for particulate matter and discoloration prior to administration whenever solution and container permit.

HOW SUPPLIED

Each mL of CAMPTOSAR Injection contains 20 mg irinotecan (on the basis of the trihydrate salt); 45 mg sorbitol; and 0.9 mg lactic acid. When necessary, pH has been adjusted to 3.5 (range, 3.0 to 3.8) with sodium hydroxide or hydrochloric acid.

CAMPTOSAR Injection is available in single-dose amber glass vials in the following package sizes:

2 mL	NDC 0009-7529-02
5 mL	NDC 0009-7529-01

This is packaged in a backing/plastic blister to protect against inadvertent breakage and leakage. The vial should be inspected for damage and visible signs of leaks before removing the backing/plastic blister. If damaged, incinerate the unopened package.

Store at controlled room temperature 15° to 30°C (59° to 86°F). Protect from light. It is recommended that the vial (and backing/plastic blister) should remain in the carton until the time of use.

℞ only

REFERENCES

1. Recommendations for the Safe Handling of Parenteral Antineoplastic Drugs. NIH Publication No. 83-2621. For sale by the Superintendent of Documents, U.S. Government Printing Office, Washington, DC 20402.
2. AMA Council Report. Guidelines for handling parenteral antineoplastics. JAMA 1985; 253(11): 1590–2.
3. National Study Commission of Cytotoxic Exposure. Recommendations for handling cytotoxic agents. Available from Louis P. Jeffrey, ScD, Chairman, National Study Commission on Cytotoxic Exposure, Massachusetts College of Pharmacy and Allied Health Sciences, 179 Longwood Avenue, Boston, MA 02115.
4. Clinical Oncological Society of Australia. Guidelines and recommendations for safe handling of antineoplastic agents. Med J Australia 1983;1:426–8.
5. Jones RB, et. al. Safe handling of chemotherapeutic agents: a report from the Mount Sinai Medical Center. CA-A Cancer J for Clinicians, 1983; Sept./Oct., 258–63.
6. American Society of Hospital Pharmacists Technical Assistance Bulletin on handling cytotoxic and hazardous drugs. Am J Hosp Pharm 1990; 47:1033–49.
7. OSHA work-practice guidelines for personnel dealing with cytotoxic (antineoplastic) drugs. Am J Hosp Pharm 1986;43:1193–1204.

Manufactured by Pharmacia & Upjohn Company
Kalamazoo, Michigan 49001, USA
Licensed from Yakult Honsha Co., LTD, Japan, and Daiichi Pharmaceutical Co., LTD, Japan
Revised April 2000 816 907 111
692839

CAVERJECT®
Sterile Powder ℞
alprostadil for injection
For Intracavernosal Use

DESCRIPTION

CAVERJECT Sterile Powder contains alprostadil as the naturally occurring form of prostaglandin E_1 (PGE_1) and is designated chemically as (11α, 13E, 15S)-11,15-dihydroxy-9-oxoprost-13-en-1-oic acid. The molecular weight is 354.49. Alprostadil is a white to off-white crystalline powder with a melting point between 115° and 116°C. Its solubility at 35°C is 8000 micrograms per 100 milliliter double distilled water. CAVERJECT is available as a sterile freeze-dried powder

Continued on next page

Information on these Pharmacia & Upjohn products is based on labeling in effect June 1, 2000. Further information concerning these and other Pharmacia & Upjohn products may be obtained by direct inquiry to Medical Information, Pharmacia & Upjohn, Kalamazoo, MI 49001.

Caverject—Cont.

for intracavernosal use in four sizes: 5, 10, 20 and 40 micrograms per vial—When reconstituted as directed with 1 milliliter of bacteriostatic water for injection or sterile water, both preserved with benzyl alcohol 0.945% w/v, gives 1.13 milliliters of reconstituted solution. Each milliliter of CAVERJECT contains 5.4, 10.5, 20.5 or 41.1 micrograms of alprostadil depending on vial strength, 172 milligrams of lactose, 47 micrograms of sodium citrate and 8.4 milligrams of benzyl alcohol. The deliverable amount of alprostadil is 5, 10, 20 or 40 micrograms per milliliter because approximately 0.4 microgram for the 5 microgram strength, 0.5 microgram for the 10 and 20 microgram strengths and 1.1 microgram for the 40 microgram strength is lost due to adsorption to the vial and syringe. When necessary, the pH of alprostadil for injection was adjusted with hydrochloric acid and/or sodium hydroxide before lyophilization.

The structural formula of alprostadil is represented below:

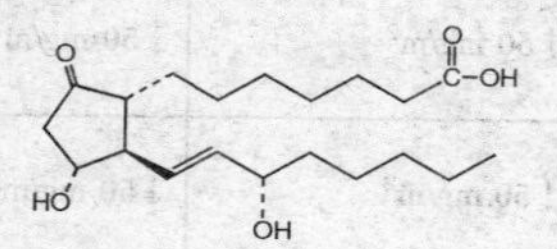

CLINICAL PHARMACOLOGY

Alprostadil has a wide variety of pharmacological actions; vasodilation and inhibition of platelet aggregation are among the most notable of these effects. In most animal species tested, alprostadil relaxed retractor penis and corpus cavernosum urethrae *in vitro*. Alprostadil also relaxed isolated preparations of human corpus cavernosum and spongiosum, as well as cavernous arterial segments contracted by either noradrenaline or $PGF_{2\alpha}$ *in vitro*. In pigtail monkeys (*Macaca nemestrina*), alprostadil increased cavernous arterial blood flow *in vivo*. The degree and duration of cavernous smooth muscle relaxation in this animal model was dose-dependent.

Alprostadil induces erection by relaxation of trabecular smooth muscle and by dilation of cavernosal arteries. This leads to expansion of lacunar spaces and entrapment of blood by compressing the venules against the tunica albuginea, a process referred to as the corporal veno-occlusive mechanism.

Pharmacokinetics:

Absorption: For the treatment of erectile dysfunction, alprostadil is administered by injection into the corpora cavernosa. The absolute bioavailability of alprostadil has not been determined.

Distribution: Following intracavernosal injection of 20 micrograms alprostadil, mean peripheral plasma concentrations of alprostadil at 30 and 60 minutes after injection (89 and 102 picograms/milliliter, respectively) were not significantly greater than baseline levels of endogenous alprostadil (96 picograms/milliliter). Alprostadil is bound in plasma primarily to albumin (81% bound) and to a lesser extent α-globulin IV-4 fraction (55% bound). No significant binding to erythrocytes or white blood cells was observed.

Metabolism: Alprostadil is rapidly converted to compounds which are further metabolized prior to excretion. Following intravenous administration, approximately 80% of circulating alprostadil is metabolized in one pass through the lungs, primarily by *beta*- and *omega*-oxidation. Hence, any alprostadil entering the systemic circulation following intracavernosal injection is very rapidly metabolized. Following intracavernosal injection of 20 micrograms alprostadil, peripheral levels of the major circulating metabolite, 13,14-dihydro-15-oxo-PGE_1, increased to reach a peak 30 minutes after injection and returned to pre-dose levels by 60 minutes after injection.

Excretion: The metabolites of alprostadil are excreted primarily by the kidney, with almost 90% of an administered intravenous dose excreted in urine within 24 hours post-dose. The remainder of the dose is excreted in the feces. There is no evidence of tissue retention of alprostadil or its metabolites following intravenous administration.

Pharmacokinetics in Special Populations:

Geriatric: The potential effect of age on the pharmacokinetics of alprostadil has not been formally evaluated. In patients with acute respiratory distress syndrome (ARDS), the mean (± SD), pulmonary extraction of alprostadil was 72% ± 15% in 11 elderly patients aged 65 years or older (mean, 71 ± 6 years) and 65% ± 20% in 6 young patients aged 35 years or younger (mean, 28 ± 5 years).

Pediatric: Alprostadil plasma concentrations were measured in 10 neonates (gestational age of 34 weeks in 2 infants and 38 to 40 weeks in 8 infants) receiving steady-state intravenous infusions of alprostadil to treat underlying cardiac malformations. Infusion rates of alprostadil ranged from 5 to 50 (median, 45) nanograms/kilogram/minute, resulting in alprostadil plasma concentrations ranging between 22 and 530 (median, 56) picograms/milliliter. The wide range of alprostadil plasma concentrations in neonates reflects high variability in individual clearances of alprostadil in this patient population.

Gender: The potential influence of gender on the pharmacokinetics of alprostadil has not been formally studied in healthy subjects. Two studies determined the pulmonary extraction of alprostadil following intravascular administration in 23 patients with ARDS. The mean (± SD) pulmonary extraction was 66% ± 20% in 17 male patients and 69% ± 18% in 6 female patients, suggesting that the pharmacokinetics of alprostadil are not influenced by gender.

Race: The potential influence of race on the pharmacokinetics of alprostadil has not been formally evaluated.

Renal and Hepatic Insufficiency: The pharmacokinetics of alprostadil have not been formally examined in patients with renal or hepatic insufficiency.

Pulmonary Disease: The pulmonary extraction of alprostadil following intravascular administration was reduced by 15% (66 ± 3.2% vs 78 ± 2.4%) in patients with ARDS compared with a control group of patients with normal respiratory function who were undergoing cardiopulmonary bypass surgery. Pulmonary clearance was found to vary as a function of cardiac output and pulmonary intrinsic clearance in a group of 14 patients with ARDS or at risk of developing ARDS following trauma or sepsis. In this study, the extraction efficiency of alprostadil ranged from subnormal (11%) to normal (90%), with an overall mean of 67%.

Drug-Drug Interactions:

The potential for pharmacokinetic drug-drug interactions between alprostadil and other agents has not been formally studied.

INDICATION AND USAGE

CAVERJECT is indicated for the treatment of erectile dysfunction due to neurogenic, vasculogenic, psychogenic, or mixed etiology.

Intracavernosal CAVERJECT may be a useful adjunct to other diagnostic tests in the diagnosis of erectile dysfunction.

CONTRAINDICATIONS

CAVERJECT should not be used in patients who have a known hypersensitivity to the drug, in patients who have conditions that might predispose them to priapism, such as sickle cell anemia or trait, multiple myeloma, or leukemia, or in patients with anatomical deformation of the penis, such as angulation, cavernosal fibrosis, or Peyronie's disease. Patients with penile implants should not be treated with CAVERJECT

CAVERJECT should not be used in women or children and is not for use in newborns.

CAVERJECT should not be used in men for whom sexual activity is inadvisable or contraindicated.

PRECAUTIONS

General Precautions: Prolonged erection (erection lasting 4 to 6 hours) and priapism (erection lasting over 6 hours) are known to occur following intracavernosal administration of vasoactive substances, including CAVERJECT. The patient should be instructed to immediately report to his physician or, if unavailable, to seek immediate medical assistance for any erection that persists for longer than 4 hours. Treatment of priapism should be according to established medical practice.

The overall incidence of penile fibrosis, including Pyronie's disease, reported in clinical studies with CAVERJECT was 3%. In one self-injection clinical study where duration of use was up to 18 months, the incidence of fibrosis was 7.8%. Regular follow-up of patients, with careful examination of the penis, is strongly recommended to detect signs of penile fibrosis. Treatment with CAVERJECT should be discontinued in patients who develop penile angulation, cavernosal fibrosis, or Peyronie's disease.

Patients on anticoagulants, such as warfarin or heparin, may have increased propensity for bleeding after intracavernosal injection.

Underlying treatable medical causes of erectile dysfunction should be diagnosed and treated prior to initiation of therapy with CAVERJECT.

The safety and efficacy of combinations of CAVERJECT and other vasoactive agents have not been systematically studied. Therefore, the use of such combinations is not recommended.

The patient should be instructed not to re-use or to share needles or syringes. As with all prescription medicines, the patient should not allow anyone else to use his medicine.

Information for the Patient:

To ensure safe and effective use of CAVERJECT, the patient should be thoroughly instructed and trained in the self-injection technique before he begins intracavernosal treatment with CAVERJECT at home. The desirable dose should be established in the physician's office. The instructions for preparation of the solution of CAVERJECT should be carefully followed. Vials with precipitates or discoloration should be discarded. The reconstituted vial is designed for one use only and should be discarded after withdrawal of proper volume of the solution. The content of the reconstituted vial should not be shaken. The needle must be properly discarded after use; it must not be re-used or shared with other persons. Patient instructions for administration are included in each package of CAVERJECT.

The dose of CAVERJECT that is established in the physician's office should not be changed by the patient without consulting the physician. The patient may expect an erection to occur within 5 to 20 minutes. A standard treatment goal is to produce an erection lasting no longer than 1 hour. Generally, CAVERJECT should be used no more than 3 times per week, with at least 24 hours between each use. Patients should be aware of possible side effects of therapy with CAVERJECT; the most frequently occurring is penile pain after injection, usually mild to moderate in severity. A potentially serious adverse reaction with intracavernosal therapy is priapism. Accordingly, the patient should be instructed to contact the physician's office immediately or, if unavailable, to seek immediate medical assistance if an erection persists for longer than 4 hours.

The patient should report any penile pain that was not present before or that increased in intensity, as well as the occurrence of nodules or hard tissue in the penis to his physician as soon as possible. As with any intravenous injection, an infection is a possibility. Patients should be instructed to report to the physician any penile redness, swelling, tenderness or curvature of the erect penis. The patient must visit the physician's office for regular checkups for assessment of the therapeutic benefit and safety of treatment with CAVERJECT.

Note: Use of intracavernosal CAVERJECT offers no protection from the transmission of sexually transmitted diseases. Individuals who use CAVERJECT should be counseled about the protective measures that are necessary to guard against the spread of sexually transmitted diseases, including the human immunodeficiency virus (HIV).

The injection of CAVERJECT can induce a small amount of bleeding at the site of injection (see ADVERSE REACTIONS section—hematoma, ecchymosis, hemorrhage at the site of injection). In patients infected with blood-borne diseases, this could increase the risk of transmission of blood-borne diseases between partners.

In clinical trials, concomitant use of agents such as antihypertensive drugs, diuretics, antidiabetic agents (including insulin), or non-steroidal anti-inflammatory drugs had no effect on the efficacy or safety of CAVERJECT.

Carcinogenesis, Mutagenesis, and Impairment of Fertility:

Long-term carcinogenicity studies have not been conducted. Rat reproductive studies indicate that alprostadil at doses of up to 0.2 milligram/kilogram/day does not adversely affect or alter rat spermatogenesis, providing a 200-fold margin of safety compared with the usual human doses. The following battery of mutagenicity assays revealed no potential for mutagenesis: bacterial mutation (Ames), alkaline elution, rat micronucleus, sister chromatid exchange, CHO/HGPRT mammalian cell forward gene mutation, and unscheduled DNA synthesis (UDS).

A 1-year irritancy study was conducted in three groups of 5 male Cynomolgus monkeys injected intracavernosally twice weekly with either vehicle or 3 or 8.25 micrograms of alprostadil per injection. An additional two groups of 6 monkeys each were injected with vehicle or with 8.25 micrograms/injection twice weekly as described previously plus they received multiple doses during weeks 44, 48, and 52. Three monkeys from each group were retained for a 4-week recovery period. There was no evidence of drug-related penile irritancy or nonpenile tissue lesions, which could be directly related to alprostadil. The irritancy which was noted for control and treated monkeys was considered to be a result of the injection procedure itself, and any lesions noted were shown to be reversible. At the end of the 4-week recovery period, the histological changes in the penis had regressed.

Pregnancy, Nursing Mothers, and Pediatric Use:

CAVERJECT is not indicated for use in newborns, children, or women.

ADVERSE REACTIONS

Local Adverse Reactions: The following local adverse reaction information was derived from controlled and uncontrolled studies, including an uncontrolled 18-month safety study.

[See table below]

Penile Pain: Penile pain after intracavernosal administration of CAVERJECT was reported at least once by 37% of patients in clinical studies of up to 18 months in duration. In the majority of the cases, penile pain was rated mild or moderate in intensity. Three percent of patients discontinued treatment because of penile pain. The frequency of penile pain was 2% in 294 patients who received 1 to 3 injections of placebo.

Prolonged Erection/Priapism: In clinical trials, prolonged erection was defined as an erection that lasted for 4 to 6 hours; priapism was defined as erection that lasted 6 hours or longer. The frequency of prolonged erection after intrac-

Local Adverse Reactions Reported by ≥ 1% of Patients Treated with CAVERJECT for up to 18 Months*

Event	CAVERJECT N = 1861	Event	CAVERJECT N = 1861
Penile pain	37%	Penis disorder***	3%
Prolonged erection	4%	Injection site ecchymosis	2%
Penile fibrosis**	3%	Penile rash	1%
Injection site hematoma	3%	Penile edema	1%

* Except for penile pain (2%), no significant local adverse reactions were reported by 294 patients who received 1 to 3 injections of placebo.

** See General Precautions.

*** Includes numbness, yeast infection, irritation, sensitivity, phimosis, pruritus, erythema, venous leak, penile skin tear, strange feeling of penis, discoloration of penile head, itch at tip of penis.

avernosal administration of CAVERJECT was 4%, while the frequency of priapism was 0.4%. In the majority of cases, spontaneous detumescence occurred. To minimize the chances of prolonged erection or priapism, CAVERJECT should be titrated slowly to the lowest effect dose (see DOSAGE AND ADMINISTRATION section). The patient must be instructed to immediately report to his physician or, if unavailable, to seek immediate medical assistance for any erection that persists for longer than 4 hours. If priapism is not treated immediately, penile tissue damage and permanent loss of potency may result.

Hematoma/Ecchymosis: The frequency of hematoma and ecchymosis was 3% and 2%, respectively. In most cases, hematoma/ecchymosis was judged to be a complication of a faulty injection technique. Accordingly, proper instruction of the patient in self-injection is of importance to minimize the potential of hematoma/ecchymosis (see DOSAGE AND ADMINISTRATION).

The following local adverse reactions were reported by fewer than 1% of patients after injection of CAVERJECT: balanitis, injection site hemorrhage, injection site inflammation, injection site itching, injection site swelling, injection site edema, urethral bleeding, penile warmth, numbness, yeast infection, irritation, sensitivity, phimosis, pruritus, erythema, venous leak, painful erection, and abnormal ejaculation.

Systemic Adverse Events: The following systemic adverse event information was derived from controlled and uncontrolled studies, including an uncontrolled 18-month safety study.

[See table above]

Systemic Adverse Events Reported by ≥ 1% of Patients Treated with CAVERJECT for up to 18 Months*

Body System/Reaction	CAVERJECT N = 1861
Cardiovascular System	
Hypertension	2%
Central Nervous System	
Headache	2%
Dizziness	1%
Musculoskeletal System	
Back pain	1%
Respiratory System	
Upper respiratory infection	4%
Flu syndrome	2%
Sinusitis	2%
Nasal congestion	1%
Cough	1%

Body System/Reaction *(continued)*	CAVERJECT N = 1861
Urogenital System	
Prostatic Disorder**	2%
Miscellaneous	
Localized pain***	2%
Trauma****	2%

* No significant adverse events were reported by 294 patients who received 1 to 3 injections of placebo.
** prostatitis, pain, hypertrophy, enlargement
*** pain in various anatomical structures other than injection site
**** injuries, fractures, abrasions, lacerations, dislocations

The following systemic events, which were reported for < 1% of patients in clinical studies, were judged by investigators to be possibly related to use of CAVERJECT: testicular pain, scrotal disorder, scrotal edema, hematuria, testicular disorder, impaired urination, urinary frequency, urinary urgency, pelvic pain, hypotension, vasodilation, peripheral vascular disorder, supraventricular extrasystoles, vasovagal reactions, hypesthesia, non-generalized weakness, diaphoresis, rash, non-application site pruritus, skin neoplasm, nausea, dry mouth, increased serum creatinine, leg cramps, and mydriasis.

Hemodynamic changes, manifested as decreases in blood pressure and increases in pulse rate, were observed during clinical studies, principally at doses above 20 micrograms and above 30 micrograms of alprostadil, respectively, and appeared to be dose-dependent. However, these changes were usually clinically unimportant; only three patients discontinued the treatment because of symptomatic hypotension.

CAVERJECT had no clinically important effect on serum or urine laboratory tests.

OVERDOSAGE

Overdosage was not observed in clinical trials with CAVERJECT. If intracavernous overdose of CAVERJECT occurs, the patient should be under medical supervision until any systemic effects have resolved and/or until penile detumescence has occurred. Symptomatic treatment of any systemic symptoms would be appropriate.

DOSAGE AND ADMINISTRATION

The dose of CAVERJECT should be individualized for each patient by careful titration under supervision by the physician. In clinical studies, patients were treated with CAVERJECT in doses ranging from 0.2 to 140 micrograms; however, since 99% of patients received doses of 60 micrograms or less, doses of greater than 60 micrograms are not recommended. In general, the lowest possible effective dose should always be employed. In clinical studies, over 80% of patients experienced an erection sufficient for sexual intercourse after intracavernosal injection of CAVERJECT. A 1/2-inch, 27- to 30-gauge needle is generally recommended.

Initial Titration in Physician's Office:

Erectile Dysfunction of Vasculogenic, Psychogenic, or Mixed Etiology. Dosage titration should be initiated at 2.5 micrograms of alprostadil. If there is a partial response, the dose may be increased by 2.5 micrograms to a dose of 5 micrograms and then in increments of 5 to 10 micrograms, depending upon erectile response, until the dose that produces an erection suitable for intercourse and not exceeding a duration of 1 hour is reached. If there is no response to the initial 2.5-microgram dose, the second dose may be increased to 7.5 micrograms, followed by increments of 5 to 10 micrograms. The patient must stay in the physician's office until complete detumescence occurs. If there is no response, then the next higher dose may be given within 1 hour. If there is a response, then there should be at least a 1-day interval before the next dose is given.

Erectile Dysfunction of Pure Neurogenic Etiology (Spinal Cord Injury). Dosage titration should be initiated at 1.25 micrograms of alprostadil. The dose may be increased by 1.25 micrograms to a dose of 2.5 micrograms, followed by an increment of 2.5 micrograms to a dose of 5 micrograms, and then in 5-microgram increments until the dose that produces an erection suitable for intercourse and not exceeding a duration of 1 hour is reached. The patient must stay in the physician's office until complete detumescence occurs. If there is no response, then the next higher dose may be given within 1 hour. If there is a response, then there should be at least a 1-day interval before the next dose is given.

The majority of patients (56%) in one clinical study involving 579 patients were titrated to doses of greater than 5 micrograms but less than or equal to 20 micrograms. The mean dose at the end of the titration phase was 17.8 micrograms of alprostadil.

Maintenance Therapy:

The first injections of CAVERJECT must be done at the physician's office by medically trained personnel. Self-injection therapy by the patient can be started only after the patient is properly instructed and well trained in the self-injection technique. The physician should make a careful assessment of the patient's skills and competence with this procedure. The intracavernosal injection must be done under sterile conditions. The site of injection is usually along the dorso-lateral aspect of the proximal third of the penis. Visible veins should be avoided. The side of the penis that is injected and the site of injection must be alternated; the injection site must be cleansed with an alcohol swab.

The dose of CAVERJECT that is selected for self-injection treatment should provide the patient with an erection that is satisfactory for sexual intercourse and that is maintained for no longer than 1 hour. If the duration of erection is longer than 1 hour, the dose of CAVERJECT should be reduced. Self-injection therapy for use at home should be initiated at the dose that was determined in the physician's office; however, dose adjustment, if required (up to 57% of patients in one clinical study), should be made only after consultation with the physician. The dose should be adjusted in accordance with the titration guidelines described above. The effectiveness of CAVERJECT for long-term use of up to 6 months has been documented in an uncontrolled, self-injection study. The mean dose of CAVERJECT at the end of 6 months was 20.7 micrograms in this study.

Careful and continuous follow-up of the patient while in the self-injection program must be exercised. This is especially true for the initial self-injections, since adjustments in the dose of CAVERJECT may be needed. The recommended frequency of injection is no more than 3 times weekly, with at least 24 hours between each dose. The reconstituted vial of CAVERJECT is intended for single use only and should be discarded after use. The user should be instructed in the proper disposal of the syringe, needle, and vial.

While on self-injection treatment, it is recommended that the patient visit the prescribing physician's office every 3 months. At that time, the efficacy and safety of the therapy should be assessed, and the dose of CAVERJECT should be adjusted, if needed.

CAVERJECT as an Adjunct to the Diagnosis of Erectile Dysfunction:

In the simplest diagnostic test for erectile dysfunction (pharmacologic testing), patients are monitored for the occurrence of an erection after an intracavernosal injection of CAVERJECT. Extensions of this testing are the use of CAVERJECT as an adjunct to laboratory investigations, such as duplex or Doppler imaging. ^{133}Xenon washout tests, radioisotope penogram, and penile arteriography, to allow visualization and assessment of penile vasculature. For any of these tests, a single dose of CAVERJECT that induces an erection with firm rigidity should be used.

General Procedure for Solution Preparation:

CAVERJECT is packaged in a 5-milliliter glass vial. Bacteriostatic water for injection or sterile water, both preserved with benzyl alcohol 0.945% w/v, must be used as the diluent for reconstitution. After reconstitution with 1 milliliter of diluent, the volume of the resulting solution is 1.13 milliliters. One milliliter of this solution will contain 5.4, 10.5, 20.5 or 41.1 micrograms of alprostadil depending on vial strength, 172 milligrams of lactose, 47 micrograms of sodium citrate and 8.4 milligrams of benzyl alcohol. The deliverable amount of alprostadil is 5, 10, 20 or 40 micrograms per milliliter because approximately 0.4 microgram for the 5 microgram strength, 0.5 microgram for the 10 and 20 microgram strengths and 1.1 microgram for the 40 microgram strength is lost due to adsorption to the vial and syringe. After reconstitution, the solution of CAVERJECT should be used within 24 hours when stored at or below 25°C (77°F) and not refrigerated or frozen. Parenteral drug products should be inspected visually for particulate matter and discoloration prior to administration whenever the solution and container permit.

HOW SUPPLIED

CAVERJECT is a dry lyophilized powder and is supplied in vials containing 6.15, 11.9, 23.2 or 46.4 micrograms of alprostadil for intracavernosal administration. Store the 5, 10 and 20 microgram strengths at or below 25°C (77°F).

Store the 40 microgram strength at 2° to 8°C (36° to 46°F) until dispensed. After dispensing, the CAVERJECT 40 microgram strength may be stored at or below 25°C (77°F) for 3 months or until expiration date, whichever occurs first.

When reconstituted and used as directed, the deliverable amount of alprostadil is 5, 10, 20 or 40 micrograms, respectively. The reconstituted solution should be used within 24 hours when stored at or below 25°C (77°F) and not refrigerated or frozen. Only the accompanying diluent or bacteriostatic water for injection with benzyl alcohol should be used when reconstituting CAVERJECT.

CAVERJECT is available in the following packages:

6–10 microgram vials
NDC 0009-3778-05
6–20 microgram vials
NDC 0009-3701-05
6–40 microgram vials
NDC 0009-7686-04

Other available packages:

6–5 microgram vials with diluent syringes
NDC 0009-7212-03
6–10 microgram vials with diluent syringes
NDC 0009-3778-08
6–20 microgram vials with diluent syringes
NDC 0009-3701-01

PATIENT INSTRUCTIONS FOR Caverject®

alprostadil for injection

IMPOTENCE: CAUSES AND TREATMENTS

There are several causes of impotence, a condition known medically as erectile dysfunction. These include: medications that you may be taking for other conditions, impaired blood circulation in the penis, nerve damage, emotional problems, excessive smoking or alcohol use, use of street drugs, and hormonal imbalances. Often, impotence is due to more than one cause.

Treatments for impotence include: switching medications (if you are taking a medication that causes impotence), administration of hormones, penile injections, use of medical devices that produce an erection, surgical procedures to correct blood flow in the penis, penile implants, and psychological counseling. Your doctor has selected CAVERJECT for injection to treat your impotence. Your doctor can also discuss other available treatments. You should not stop taking any prescription medications, unless told to do so by your doctor.

USE OF CAVERJECT

CAVERJECT is injected into a specific area of the penis and should produce an erection in 5 to 20 minutes. The erection should last for about 1 hour. Generally, you should not use CAVERJECT more than 3 times a week, with at least 24 hours between uses.

Who Should Not Use CAVERJECT?

Men who have conditions that might result in long-lasting erections should not use CAVERJECT. Some of these conditions include: sickle cell anemia or trait, leukemia, and tumor of the bone marrow (multiple myeloma). Men with penile implants, or an abnormally formed penis, or who have been advised not to engage in sexual activity should not use CAVERJECT. CAVERJECT should not be used by women or children.

What Are The Risks Of Using CAVERJECT?

Erections that last more than 4 hours can cause serious and permanent damage. **Call your doctor or seek professional helf immediately if you still have an erection 4 hours after injection.**

The most common side effect of CAVERJECT is mild to moderate pain after injection. About one-third of patients report this effect.

Call your doctor if you notice any redness, lumps, swelling, tenderness, or curving of the erect penis.

A small amount of bleeding at the injection site may occur. Tell your doctor if you have a condition or are taking a medicine that interferes with blood clotting.

NOTE: CAVERJECT offers no protection from the transmission of sexually transmitted diseases such as HIV (the virus

Continued on next page

Information on these Pharmacia & Upjohn products is based on labeling in effect June 1, 2000. Further information concerning these and other Pharmacia & Upjohn products may be obtained by direct inquiry to Medical Information, Pharmacia & Upjohn, Kalamazoo, MI 49001.

Caverject—Cont.

that causes AIDS). Small amounts of bleeding at the injection site can increase the risk of transmission of blood-borne diseases between partners.

There is no approved injectable treatment using multiple drug components or "cocktails" for erectile dysfunction. Moreover, there are no data on the efficacy and safety of these combinations.

STORAGE

1. Unused packs of 5, 10 and 20 microgram vials of CAVERJECT may be stored at or below 25°C (77°F). **Unused packs of the 40 microgram vial may be stored at or below 25°C (77°F) for 3 months or until expiration date, whichever occurs first.** Do not freeze.
2. After reconstitution, the solution of CAVERJECT should be used within 24 hours when stored at or below 25°C (77°F) and not refrigerated or frozen.
3. During travel, care should be taken to avoid allowing the product to freeze or be stored at temperatures above 25°C (77°F). Therefore, do not store in checked luggage during air travel or leave in a closed automobile.

ADDITIONAL INFORMATION

There is a technical leaflet discussion of CAVERJECT written for health-care professionals that your pharmacist can let you read.

More information about erectile dysfunction and its treatment is available from the National Institutes of Health (Washington, DC), the American Foundation for Urological Diseases (Baltimore, MD), or the Impotence Institute of America (Washington, DC).

PREPARING AND INJECTING CAVERJECT

You must be properly instructed and trained in the injection technique by your doctor before using CAVERJECT.

Before using CAVERJECT, talk to your doctor about what to expect when using it, possible side effects, and what to do if side effects occur. Your dose has been selected for your individual needs. Do not change your dose without consulting your doctor. If your are not sure of the volume or dose to be used, talk to your doctor or pharmacist.

Follow these instructions exactly to prepare and inject a sterile dose of CAVERJECT.

If the needle is severely bent at any time, do not use it for injecting CAVERJECT and do not attempt to straighten it prior to injecting CAVERJECT. A severely bent and re-straightened needle may be predisposed to breakage. Needle breakage, with a portion of the needle remaining in the penis, has been reported and, in some cases, required hospitalization and surgical removal. If the needle is severely bent while preparing the injection, remove it from the syringe, discard, and attach a new, unused sterile needle to the syringe as described under "Prepare the Dose" below.

Use the needle, syringe, alcohol swabs, and vials **only once** then safely discard the supplies and any unused solution. Discard your needle/syringe, and alcohol swabs in a special container for disposal of sharp medical supplies. Ask your doctor or pharmacist where you can get these special containers.

Supplies Needed

To prepare and inject CAVERJECT you will need a vial of CAVERJECT Sterile Powder, a vial of diluent (bacteriostatic water for injection or sterile water, both preserved with benzyl alcohol 0.945% w/v), a disposable sterile 3-milliliter (3-cc) syringe, a 1/2-inch 27-gauge sterile needle, and two alcohol swabs (Figure A).

CAVERJECT comes in 5, 10, 20 or 40 microgram strengths. **MAKE SURE YOU HAVE THE RIGHT STRENGTH VIAL OF CAVERJECT.**

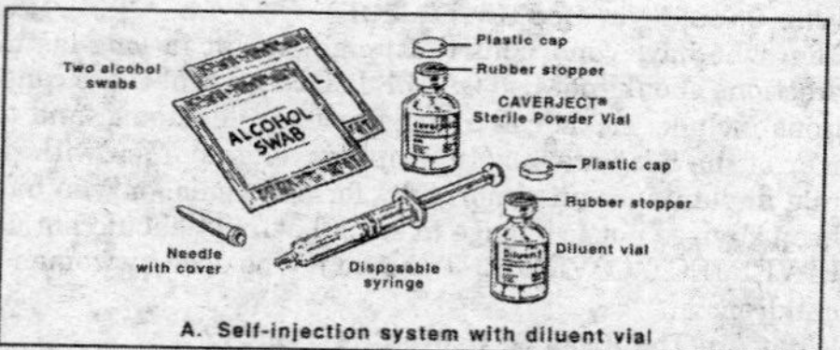

A. Self-injection system with diluent vial

Prepare the Dose

1. Wash your hands thoroughly, and dry them with a clean towel.
2. Assemble the needle and syringe as follows:
   a. Remove the syringe from its sterile wrapping.
   b. To remove the sterile needle from its wrapping, carefully pull the wrapper tabs back enough to expose the sterile open end of the needle assembly. Do not touch the open end of the needle (Figure B).

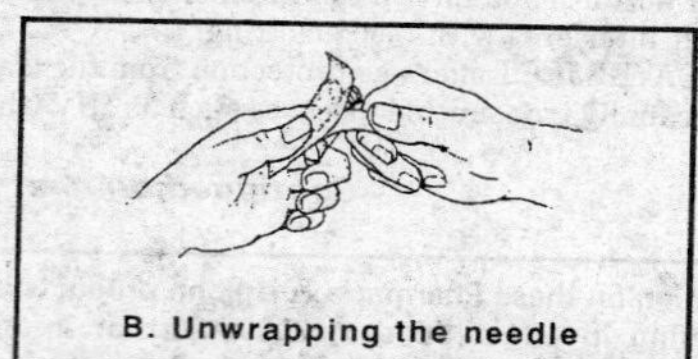

B. Unwrapping the needle

   c. While holding the sterile needle assembly between the thumb and forefinger, pick up syringe with other hand. With same two fingers, remove the plastic syringe cap (Figure C). Do not touch the syringe tip.

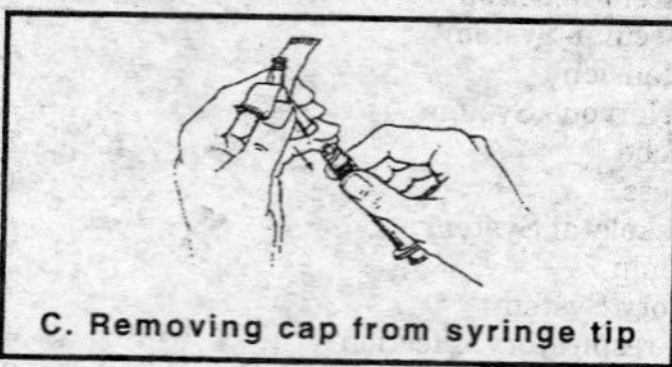

C. Removing cap from syringe tip

   d. Without removing the plastic needle cover, firmly attach the needle to the syringe tip (twist to tighten) (Figure D).

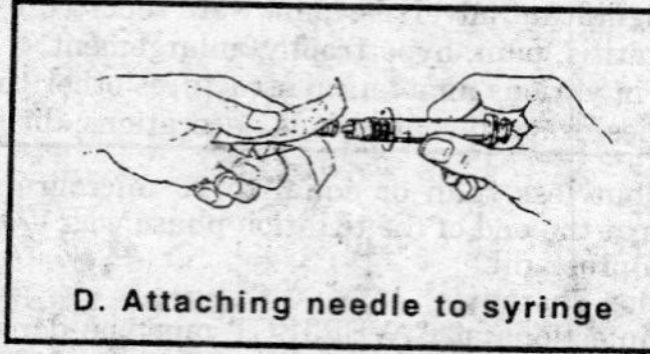

D. Attaching needle to syringe

   e. With the needle cover in place, set the syringe and needle down on a clean, level surface.
3. Remove the plastic caps from the vials of CAVERJECT and diluent.
4. Wipe the rubber stoppers on the vials of CAVERJECT and diluent with one alcohol swab. Discard this alcohol swab.
5. Grasp the syringe barrel (not the plunger) and remove the needle cover. Do not discard the needle cover, you will need to use it again (see step 16). Do not touch the exposed needle. Holding the syringe/needle in a straight line with the diluent vial to avoid bending the needle, push the needle through the center of the diluent vial's rubber stopper.
6. Keeping the needle in the vial, firmly hold the vial and syringe upside down in one hand (see Figure E).

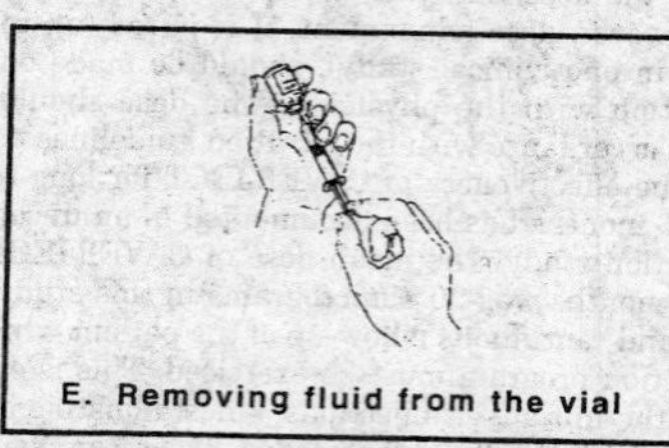

E. Removing fluid from the vial

7. Keeping the needle tip below the level of fluid, pull back on the syringe plunger until all the diluent is removed from vial.
8. Push the syringe plunger to the 1-cc (mL) mark on the syringe. This will expel air and excess diluent back into the vial.
9. Grasp the side of syringe barrel (not the plunger) and pull the needle/syringe from the diluent vial in a straight line to avoid bending the needle.
10. Holding the syringe/needle in a straight line with the vial of CAVERJECT to avoid bending the needle, push the needle through the center of the rubber stopper of the vial of CAVERJECT and push the syringe plunger all the way down to expel all the diluent into the vial. Proceed immediately to step 11.
11. Without removing the needle or touching the needle or stopper, **gently** swirl (do not shake) the vial until all the powder is dissolved in the diluent. Then turn the vial and needle/syringe upside down and **gently** swirl the vial to dissolve any powder in the neck of the vial. **DO NOT USE THE SOLUTION IF IT IS CLOUDY, COLORED OR CONTAINS PARTICLES.**
12. Keeping the needle in the vial, firmly hold the vial and syringe upside down in one hand (see Figure E).
13. Keeping the needle tip below the level of fluid, slowly pull back on the syringe plunger until all the fluid is removed from the vial.
14. If there are air bubbles, gently tap the syringe barrel until they float to the top of the solution (see Figure F). Holding the syringe upright, push the syringe plunger to the correct volume mark for the dose prescribed by your doctor. This will expel any air and excess solution into the vial.

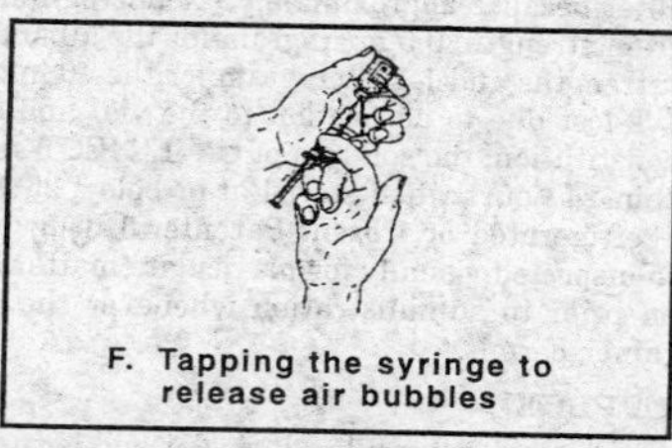

F. Tapping the syringe to release air bubbles

15. Grasp the syringe barrel (not the plunger) and pull the needle/syringe from the vial of CAVERJECT in a straight line to avoid bending the needle.
16. Place the needle cover over the needle and set the syringe down on a level surface.

Select Injection Site

1. CAVERJECT will be injected into a corpus cavernosum (spongy tissue) of the penis. One corpus cavernosum runs the length of the right side of the penis. Another corpus cavernosum runs the length of the left side of the penis (see Figures G and H).

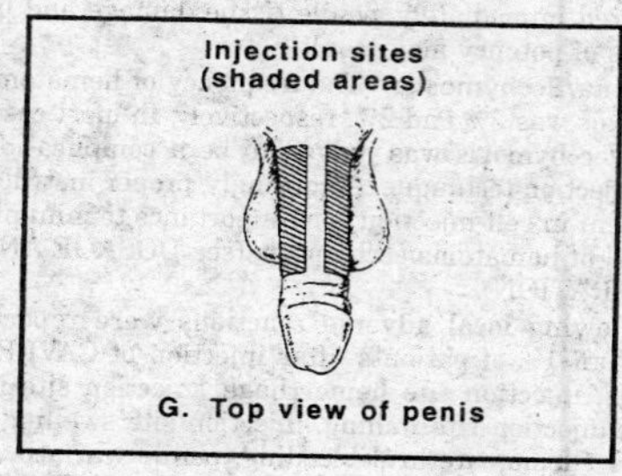

G. Top view of penis

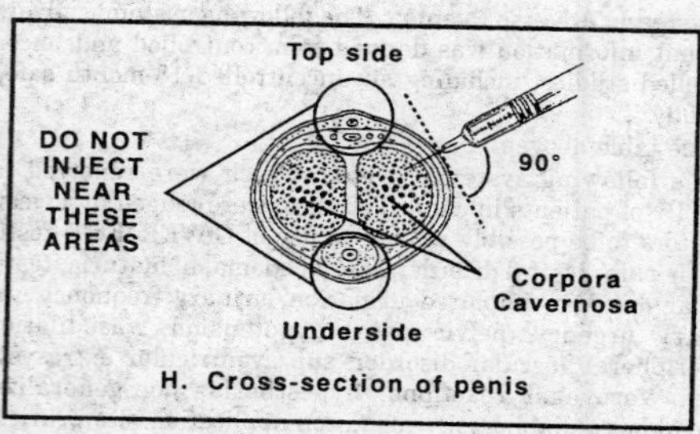

H. Cross-section of penis

2. Choose an injection site on one side of the shaft of the penis as shown in Figure G. AVOID VISIBLE BLOOD VESSELS.
3. WITH EACH USE OF CAVERJECT, ALTERNATE THE SIDE OF THE PENIS AND VARY THE SITE OF THE INJECTION.

Inject Your Dose of CAVERJECT

1. You should be sitting upright or slightly reclined when injecting CAVERJECT.
2. If your penis is not circumcised, pull the foreskin back. Holding the head of your penis with your thumb and forefinger, stretch it lengthwise along your thigh so that you can clearly see the selected injection site.
3. Clean the injection site with a new alcohol swab. Do not discard this swab, you will need to use it again (see step 7).
4. Remove the cover from the needle. Reposition the penis firmly against your thigh as in step 2 to keep it from moving during the injection.
5. Hold the syringe between your thumb and index finger (Figure 1). Using a steady motion, push the needle straight into the selected site until the metal part of the needle is almost entirely in the penis.

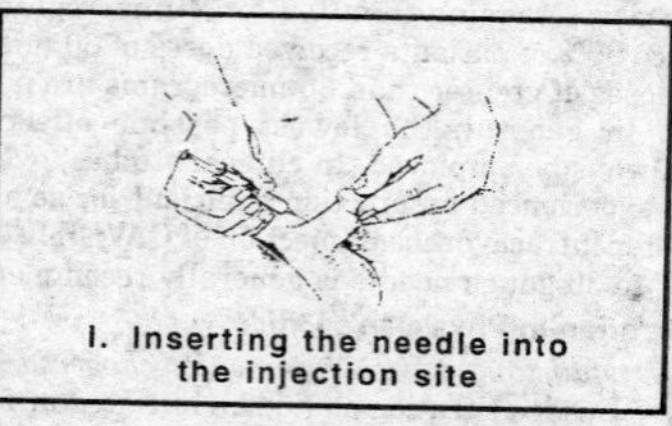

I. Inserting the needle into the injection site

6. Holding the syringe barrel between two fingers, move your thumb or finger to the top of the plunger and, with a steady motion, push down on the plunger so that the entire volume of CAVERJECT is slowly injected (Figure J).

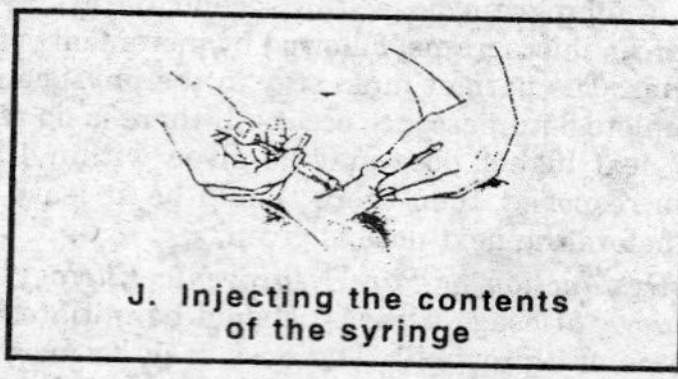

J. Injecting the contents of the syringe

7. Grasp the syringe barrel and pull the needle out of your penis. **APPLY PRESSURE TO THE INJECTION SITE WITH THE ALCOHOL SWAB FOR ABOUT 5 MINUTES OR UNTIL BLEEDING STOPS.**

Disposal of Injection Materials

1. Discard your needle, syringe, and alcohol swabs in a special container for disposal of sharp medical supplies. Ask your doctor or pharmacist where you can obtain these special containers. Follow the directions on your disposal container for proper disposal procedures.

2. **Do not re-use or share needles or syringes. As with all prescription medicines, do not allow anyone else to use your medicine.**

℞ only

Pharmacia & Upjohn Company • Kalamazoo, MI 49001, USA

Revised February 1999 816 176 0007 691800

Shown in Product Identification Guide, page 331

CLEOCIN HCl ℞

[clēō-sĭn]

brand of clindamycin hydrochloride capsules, USP

> **WARNING**
>
> **Pseudomembranous colitis has been reported with nearly all antibacterial agents, including clindamycin, and may range in severity from mild to life-threatening. Therefore, it is important to consider this diagnosis in patients who present with diarrhea subsequent to the administration of antibacterial agents.**
>
> Because clindamycin therapy has been associated with severe colitis which may end fatally, it should be reserved for serious infections where less toxic antimicrobial agents are inappropriate, as described in the **INDICATIONS AND USAGE** section. It should not be used in patients with nonbacterial infections such as most upper respiratory tract infections. Treatment with antibacterial agents alters the normal flora of the colon and may permit overgrowth of clostridia. Studies indicate that a toxin produced by *Clostridium difficile* is one primary cause of "antibiotic-associated colitis".
>
> After the diagnosis of pseudomembranous colitis has been established, therapeutic measures should be initiated. Mild cases of pseudomembranous colitis usually respond to drug discontinuation alone. In moderate to severe cases, consideration should be given to management with fluids and electrolytes, protein supplementation, and treatment with an antibacterial drug clinically effective against *C. difficile* colitis.
>
> Diarrhea, colitis, and pseudomembranous colitis have been observed to begin up to several weeks following cessation of therapy with clindamycin.

DESCRIPTION

Clindamycin hydrochloride is the hydrated hydrochloride salt of clindamycin. Clindamycin is a semisynthetic antibiotic produced by a 7(S)-chloro-substitution of the 7(R)-hydroxyl group of the parent compound lincomycin.

CLEOCIN HCl Capsules contain clindamycin hydrochloride equivalent to 75 mg, 150 mg or 300 mg of clindamycin.

Inactive ingredients: **75 mg**—corn starch, FD&C blue no. 1, FD&C yellow no. 5, gelatin, lactose, magnesium stearate and talc; **150 mg**—corn starch, FD&C blue no. 1, FD&C yellow no. 5, gelatin, lactose, magnesium stearate, talc and titanium dioxide; **300 mg**—corn starch, FD&C blue no. 1, gelatin, lactose, magnesium stearate, talc and titanium dioxide.

The structural formula is represented below:

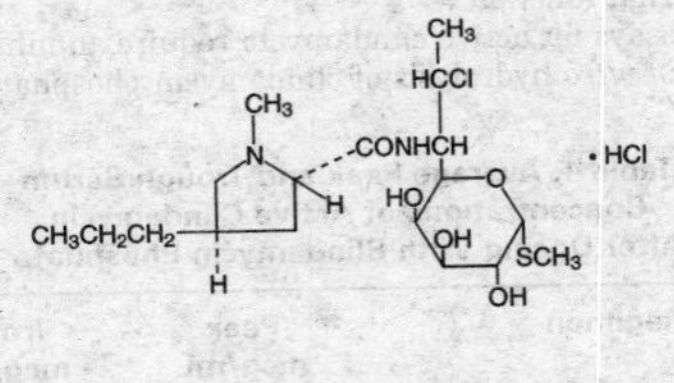

The chemical name for clindamycin hydrochloride is Methyl 7-chloro-6,7,8-trideoxy-6-(1-methyl-*trans*-4-propyl-L-2-pyrrolidinecarboxamido)-1-thio-L-*threo*-α-D-*galacto*-octopyranoside monohydrochloride.

CLINICAL PHARMACOLOGY

Microbiology: Clindamycin has been shown to have *in vitro* activity against isolates of the following organisms:

Aerobic gram-positive cocci, including:

Staphylococcus aureus

Staphylococcus epidermidis

(penicillinase and nonpenicillinase producing strains). When tested by *in vitro* methods some staphylococcal strains originally resistant to erythromycin rapidly develop resistance to clindamycin.

Streptococci (except *Streptococcus faecalis*)

Pneumococci

Anaerobic gram-negative bacilli, including:

Bacteroides species (including *Bacteroides fragilis* group and *Bacteroides melaninogenicus* group)

Fusobacterium species

Anaerobic gram-positive nonsporeforming bacilli, including:

Propionibacterium

Eubacterium

Actinomyces species

Anaerobic and microaerophilic gram-positive cocci, including:

Peptococcus species

Peptostreptococcus species

Microaerophilic streptococci

Clostridia: Clostridia are more resistant than most anaerobes to clindamycin. Most *Clostridium perfringens* are susceptible, but other species, eg, *Clostridium sporogenes* and *Clostridium tertium* are frequently resistant to clindamycin. Susceptibility testing should be done.

Cross resistance has been demonstrated between clindamycin and lincomycin.

Antagonism has been demonstrated between clindamycin and erythromycin.

Human Pharmacology: Serum level studies with a 150 mg oral dose of clindamycin hydrochloride in 24 normal adult volunteers showed that clindamycin was rapidly absorbed after oral administration. An average peak serum level of 2.50 mcg/mL was reached in 45 minutes; serum levels averaged 1.51 mcg/mL at 3 hours and 0.70 mcg/mL at 6 hours. Absorption of an oral dose is virtually complete (90%), and the concomitant administration of food does not appreciably modify the serum concentrations; serum levels have been uniform and predictable from person to person and dose to dose. Serum level studies following multiple doses of CLEOCIN HCl for up to 14 days show no evidence of accumulation or altered metabolism of drug.

Serum half-life of clindamycin is increased slightly in patients with markedly reduced renal function. Hemodialysis and peritoneal dialysis are not effective in removing clindamycin from the serum.

Concentrations of clindamycin in the serum increased linearly with increased dose. Serum levels exceed the MIC (minimum inhibitory concentration) for most indicated organisms for at least six hours following administration of the usually recommended doses. Clindamycin is widely distributed in body fluids and tissues (including bones). The average biological half-life is 2.4 hours. Approximately 10% of the bioactivity is excreted in the urine and 3.6% in the feces; the remainder is excreted as bioinactive metabolites.

Doses of up to 2 grams of clindamycin per day for 14 days have been well tolerated by healthy volunteers, except that the incidence of gastrointestinal side effects is greater with the higher doses.

No significant levels of clindamycin are attained in the cerebrospinal fluid, even in the presence of inflamed meninges.

Pharmacokinetic studies in elderly volunteers (61–79 years) and younger adults (18–39 years) indicate that age alone does not alter clindamycin pharmacokinetics (clearance, elimination half-life, volume of distribution, and area under the serum concentration-time curve) after IV administration of clindamycin phosphate. After oral administration of clindamycin hydrochloride, elimination half-life is increased to approximately 4.0 hours (range 3.4–5.1 h) in the elderly compared to 3.2 hours (range 2.1–4.2 h) in younger adults. The extent of absorption, however, is not different between age groups and no dosage alteration is necessary for the elderly with normal hepatic function and normal (age-adjusted) renal function[1].

INDICATIONS AND USAGE

Clindamycin is indicated in the treatment of serious infections caused by susceptible anaerobic bacteria.

Clindamycin is also indicated in the treatment of serious infections due to susceptible strains of streptococci, pneumococci, and staphylococci. Its use should be reserved for penicillin-allergic patients or other patients for whom, in the judgment of the physician, a penicillin is inappropriate. Because of the risk of colitis, as described in the WARNING box, before selecting clindamycin the physician should consider the nature of the infection and the suitability of less toxic alternatives (eg, erythromycin).

Anaerobes: Serious respiratory tract infections such as empyema, anaerobic pneumonitis and lung abscess; serious skin and soft tissue infections; septicemia; intra-abdominal infections such as peritonitis and intra-abdominal abscess (typically resulting from anaerobic organisms resident in the normal gastrointestinal tract); infections of the female pelvis and genital tract such as endometritis, nongonococcal tubo-ovarian abscess, pelvic cellulitis and postsurgical vaginal cuff infection.

Streptococci: Serious respiratory tract infections; serious skin and soft tissue infections.

Staphylococci: Serious respiratory tract infections; serious skin and soft tissue infections.

Pneumococci: Serious respiratory tract infections.

Bacteriologic studies should be performed to determine the causative organisms and their susceptibility to clindamycin.

***In Vitro* Susceptibility Testing:** A standardized disk testing procedure* is recommended for determining susceptibility of aerobic bacteria to clindamycin. A description is contained in the CLEOCIN® Susceptibility Disk insert. Using this method, the laboratory can designate isolates as resistant, intermediate, or susceptible. Tube or agar dilution methods may be used for both anaerobic and aerobic bacteria. When the directions in the CLEOCIN® Susceptibility Powder insert are followed, an MIN of 1.6 mcg/mL may be considered susceptible; MICs of 1.6 to 4.8 mcg/mL may be considered intermediate and MICs greater than 4.8 mcg/mL may be considered resistant.

*Bauer AW, Kirby WMM, Sherris JC, et al: Antibiotic susceptibility testing by a standardized single disc method. *Am J Clin Pathol* **45**:493–496, 1966. Standardized disc susceptibility test. *Federal Register* **37**:20527–29, 1972.

CLEOCIN Susceptibility Disks 2 mcg. See package insert for use.

CLEOCIN Susceptibility Powder 20 mg. See package insert for use.

For anaerobic bacteria the minimal inhibitory concentration (MIC) of clindamycin can be determined by agar dilution and broth dilution (including microdilution) techniques. If MICs are not determined routinely, the disk broth method is recommended for routine use. THE KIRBY-BAUER DISK DIFFUSION METHOD AND ITS INTERPRETIVE STANDARDS ARE NOT RECOMMENDED FOR ANAEROBES.

CONTRAINDICATIONS

CLEOCIN HCl is contraindicated in individuals with a history of hypersensitivity to preparations containing clindamycin or lincomycin.

WARNINGS

See WARNING box.

Pseudomembranous colitis has been reported with nearly all antibacterial agents, including clindamycin, and may range in severity from mild to life-threatening. Therefore, it is important to consider this diagnosis in patients who present with diarrhea subsequent to the administration of antibacterial agents.

Treatment with antibacterial agents alters the normal flora of the colon and may permit overgrowth of clostridia. Studies indicate that a toxin produced by *Clostridium difficile* is one primary cause of "antibiotic associated colitis".

After the diagnosis of pseudomembranous colitis has been established, therapeutic measures should be initiated. Mild cases of pseudomembranous colitis usually respond to drug discontinuation alone. In moderate to severe cases, consideration should be given to management with fluids and electrolytes, protein supplementation, and treatment with an antibacterial drug clinically effective against *C. difficile* colitis.

A careful inquiry should be made concerning previous sensitivities to drugs and other allergens.

Usage in Meningitis—Since clindamycin does not diffuse adequately into the cerebrospinal fluid, the drug should not be used in the treatment of meningitis.

PRECAUTIONS

General

Review of experience to date suggests that a subgroup of older patients with associated severe illness may tolerate diarrhea less well. When clindamycin is indicated in these patients, they should be carefully monitored for change in bowel frequency.

CLEOCIN HCl should be prescribed with caution in individuals with a history of gastrointestinal disease, particularly colitis.

CLEOCIN HCl should be prescribed with caution in atopic individuals.

Indicated surgical procedures should be performed in conjunction with antibiotic therapy.

The use of CLEOCIN HCl occasionally results in overgrowth of nonsusceptible organisms—particularly yeasts. Should superinfections occur, appropriate measures should be taken as indicated by the clinical situation.

Clindamycin dosage modification may not be necessary in patients with renal disease. In patients with moderate to severe liver disease, prolongation of clindamycin half-life has been found. However, it was postulated from studies that when given every eight hours, accumulation should rarely occur. Therefore, dosage modification in patients with liver disease may not be necessary. However, period liver enzyme determinations should be made when treating patients with severe liver disease.

The 75 mg and 150 mg capsules contain FD&C yellow no. 5 (tartrazine) which may cause allergic-type reactions (including bronchial asthma) in certain susceptible individuals. Although the overall incidence of FD&C yellow no. 5 (tartrazine) sensitivity in the general population is low, it is frequently seen in patients who also have aspirin hypersensitivity.

Laboratory Tests

During prolonged therapy, periodic liver and kidney function tests and blood counts should be performed.

Drug Interactions

Clindamycin has been shown to have neuromuscular blocking properties that may enhance the action of other neuromuscular blocking agents. Therefore, it should be used with caution in patients receiving such agents.

Antagonism has been demonstrated between clindamycin and erythromycin *in vitro*. Because of possible clinical significance, these two drugs should not be administered concurrently.

Carcinogenesis, Mutagenesis, Impairment of Fertility

Long term studies in animals have not been performed with clindamycin to evaluate carcinogenic potential. Genotoxicity tests performed included a rat micronucleus test and an Ames Salmonella reversion test. Both tests were negative. Fertility studies in rats treated orally with up to 300 mg/kg/day (approximately 1.6 times the highest recommended adult human dose based on mg/m^2) revealed no effects on fertility or mating ability.

Continued on next page

Information on these Pharmacia & Upjohn products is based on labeling in effect June 1, 2000. Further information concerning these and other Pharmacia & Upjohn products may be obtained by direct inquiry to Medical Information, Pharmacia & Upjohn, Kalamazoo, MI 49001.

Cleocin HCL—Cont.

Pregnancy: Teratogenic effects
Pregnancy category B
Reproduction studies performed in rats and mice using oral doses of clindamycin up to 600 mg/kg/day (3.2 and 1.6 times the highest recommended adult human dose based on mg/m^2, respectively) or subcutaneous doses of clindamycin up to 250 mg/kg/day (1.3 and 0.7 times the highest recommended adult human dose based on mg/m^2, respectively) revealed no evidence of teratogenicity.
There are, however, no adequate and well-controlled studies in pregnant women. Because animal reproduction studies are not always predictive of the human response, this drug should be used during pregnancy only if clearly needed.
Nursing Mothers
Clindamycin has been reported to appear in breast milk in the range of 0.7 to 3.8 mcg/mL.
Pediatric Use
When CLEOCIN HCl is administered to the pediatric population (birth to 16 years), appropriate monitoring of organ system functions is desirable.
Geriatric Use
Clinical studies of clindamycin did not include sufficient numbers of patients age 65 and over to determine whether they respond differently from younger patients. However, other reported clinical experience indicates that antibiotic-associated colitis and diarrhea (due to *Clostridium difficile*) seen in association with most antibiotics occur more frequently in the elderly (>60 years) and may be more severe. These patients should be carefully monitored for the development of diarrhea.
Pharmacokinetic studies with clindamycin have shown no clinically important differences between young and elderly subjects with normal hepatic function and normal (age-adjusted) renal function after oral or intravenous administration.

ADVERSE REACTIONS

The following reactions have been reported with the use of clindamycin.
Gastrointestinal: Abdominal pain, pseudomembranous colitis, esophagitis, nausea, vomiting and diarrhea (see **WARNING** box). The onset of pseudomembranous colitis symptoms may occur during or after antibacterial treatment (see **WARNINGS**).
Hypersensitivity Reactions: Generalized mild to moderate morbilliform-like (maculopapular) skin rashes are the most frequently reported adverse reactions. Vesiculobullous rashes, as well as urticaria, have been observed during drug therapy. Rare instances of erythema multiforme, some resembling Stevens-Johnson syndrome, and a few cases of anaphylactoid reactions have also been reported.
Skin and Mucous Membranes: Pruritus, vaginitis, and rare instances of exfoliative dermatitis have been reported. (see *Hypersensitivity Reactions*.)
Liver: Jaundice and abnormalities in liver function tests have been observed during clindamycin therapy.
Renal: Although no direct relationship of clindamycin to renal damage has been established, renal dysfunction as evidenced by azotemia, oliguria, and/or proteinuria has been observed in rare instances.
Hematopoietic: Transient neutropenia (leukopenia) and eosinophilia have been reported. Reports of agranulocytosis and thrombocytopenia have been made. No direct etiologic relationship to concurrent clindamycin therapy could be made in any of the foregoing.
Musculoskeletal: Rare instances of polyarthritis have been reported.

OVERDOSAGE

Significant mortality was observed in mice at an intravenous dose of 855 mg/kg and in rats at an oral or subcutaneous dose of approximately 2618 mg/kg. In the mice, convulsions and depression were observed.
Hemodialysis and peritoneal dialysis are not effective in removing clindamycin from the serum.

DOSAGE AND ADMINISTRATION

If significant diarrhea occurs during therapy, this antibiotic should be discontinued (see **WARNING** box).
Adults: *Serious infections*—150 to 300 mg every 6 hours. *More severe infections*—300 to 450 mg every 6 hours. **Pediatric Patients:** *Serious infections*—8 to 16 mg/kg/day (4 to 8 mg/lb/day) divided into three or four equal doses. *More severe infections*—16 to 20 mg/kg/day (8 to 10 mg/lb/day) divided into three or four equal doses.
To avoid the possibility of esophageal irritation, CLEOCIN HCl Capsules should be taken with a full glass of water.
Serious infections due to anaerobic bacteria are usually treated with CLEOCIN PHOSPHATE® Sterile Solution. However, in clinically appropriate circumstances, the physician may elect to initiate treatment or continue treatment with CLEOCIN HCl Capsules.
In cases of β-hemolytic streptococcal infections, treatment should continue for at least 10 days.

HOW SUPPLIED

CLEOCIN HCl Capsules are available in the following strengths, colors and sizes:

75 mg Green
Bottles of 100 NDC 0009-0331-02
150 mg Light Blue and Green
Bottles of 16 NDC 0009-0225-01
Bottles of 100 NDC 0009-0225-02
Unit dose package of 100 NDC 0009-0225-03
300 mg Light Blue
Bottles of 16 NDC 0009-0395-13
Bottles of 100 NDC 0009-0395-14
Unit dose package of 100 NDC 0009-0395-02

Store at controlled room temperature 20° to 25° C (68° to 77° F) [see USP].

ANIMAL TOXICOLOGY

One year oral toxicity studies in Spartan Sprague-Dawley rats and beagle dogs at dose levels up to 300 mg/kg/day (approximately 1.6 and 5.4 times the highest recommended adult human dose based on mg/m^2, respectively) have shown clindamycin to be well tolerated. No appreciable difference in pathological findings has been observed between groups of animals treated with clindamycin and comparable control groups. Rats receiving clindamycin hydrochloride at 600 mg/kg/day (approximately 3.2 times the highest recommended adult human dose based on mg/m^2) for 6 months tolerated the drug well; however, dogs dosed at this level (approximately 10.8 times the highest recommended adult human dose based on mg/m^2) vomited, would not eat, and lost weight.
Rx only

REFERENCES

1. Smith RB, Phillips JP: Evaluation of CLEOCIN HCl and CLEOCIN Phosphate in an Aged Population. Upjohn TR 8147-82-9122-021, December 1982.

Made in Canada for
Pharmacia & Upjohn Company
Kalamazoo, MI 49001, USA
By Global Pharm Inc.
Don Mills, Ontario M3B 1Y5
Canada
Revised November 1998 810 570 625
692166

CLEOCIN PHOSPHATE® ℞

[*clēō-sĭn*]
clindamycin injection, USP and
clindamycin injection in 5% dextrose
Sterile Solution is for Intramuscular and Intravenous Use
CLEOCIN PHOSPHATE in the ADD-Vantage™ Vial is For Intravenous Use Only

WARNING
Pseudomembranous colitis has been reported with nearly all antibacterial agents, including clindamycin, and may range in severity from mild to life-threatening. Therefore, it is important to consider this diagnosis in patients who present with diarrhea subsequent to the administration of antibacterial agents.
Because clindamycin therapy has been associated with severe colitis which may end fatally, it should be reserved for serious infections where less toxic antimicrobial agents are inappropriate, as described in the **INDICATIONS AND USAGE** section. It should not be used in patients with nonbacterial infections such as most upper respiratory tract infections. Treatment with antibacterial agents alters the normal flora of the colon and may permit overgrowth of clostridia. Studies indicate that a toxin produced by *Clostridium difficile* is one primary cause of "antibiotic-associated colitis".
After the diagnosis of pseudomembranous colitis has been established, therapeutic measures should be initiated. Mild cases of pseudomembranous colitis usually respond to drug discontinuation alone. In moderate to severe cases, consideration should be given to management with fluids and electrolytes, protein supplementation, and treatment with an antibacterial drug clinically effective against *C. difficile* colitis.
Diarrhea, colitis, and pseudomembranous colitis have been observed to begin up to several weeks following cessation of therapy with clindamycin.

DESCRIPTION

CLEOCIN PHOSPHATE Sterile Solution in vials contains clindamycin phosphate, a water soluble ester of clindamycin and phosphoric acid. Each mL contains the equivalent of 150 mg clindamycin, 0.5 mg disodium edetate and 9.45 mg benzyl alcohol added as preservative in each mL. Clindamycin is a semisynthetic antibiotic produced by a 7(S)-chloro-substitution of the 7(R)-hydroxyl group of the parent compound lincomycin.
The chemical name of clindamycin phosphate is L-*threo*-α-D-*galacto*-Octopyranoside, methyl 7-chloro-6,7,8-trideoxy-6-[[(1-methyl-4-propyl-2-pyrrolidinyl) carbonyl] amino]-1-thio-, 2-(dihydrogen phosphate), (2*S*-*trans*)-.
The molecular formula is $C_{18}H_{34}ClN_2O_8PS$ and the molecular weight is 504.96.
The structural formula is represented below:
[See chemical structure at top of next column]
CLEOCIN PHOSPHATE in the ADD-Vantage Vial is intended for intravenous use only after further dilution with appropriate volume of ADD-Vantage diluent base solution.
CLEOCIN PHOSPHATE IV Solution in the Galaxy® plastic container for intravenous use is composed of clindamycin phosphate equivalent to 300, 600 and 900 mg of clindamycin premixed with 5% dextrose as a sterile solution. Disodium edetate has been added at a concentration of 0.04 mg/mL. The pH has been adjusted with sodium hydroxide and/or hydrochloric acid.
The plastic container is fabricated from a specially designed multilayer plastic, PL 2501. Solutions in contact with the plastic container can leach out certain of its chemical components in very small amounts within the expiration period. The suitability of the plastic has been confirmed in tests in animals according to the USP biological tests for plastic containers, as well as by tissue culture toxicity studies.

CLINICAL PHARMACOLOGY

Biologically inactive clindamycin phosphate is rapidly converted to active clindamycin.
By the end of short-term intravenous infusion, peak serum levels of active clindamycin are reached. Biologically inactive clindamycin phosphate disappears rapidly from the serum; the average elimination half-life is 6 minutes; however, the serum elimination half-life of active clindamycin is about 3 hours in adults and 2½ hours in pediatric patients.
After intramuscular injection of clindamycin phosphate, peak levels of active clindamycin are reached within 3 hours in adults and 1 hour in pediatric patients. Serum level curves may be constructed from IV peak serum levels as given in Table 1 by application of elimination half-lives listed above.
Serum levels of clindamycin can be maintained above the *in vitro* minimum inhibitory concentrations for most indicated organisms by administration of clindamycin phosphate every 8 to 12 hours in adults and every 6 to 8 hours in pediatric patients, or by continuous intravenous infusion. An equilibrium state is reached by the third dose.
The elimination half-life of clindamycin is increased slightly in patients with markedly reduced renal or hepatic function. Hemodialysis and peritoneal dialysis are not effective in removing clindamycin from the serum. Dosage schedules need not be modified in the presence of mild or moderate renal or hepatic disease.
No significant levels of clindamycin are attained in the cerebrospinal fluid even in the presence of inflamed meninges.
Pharmacokinetic studies in elderly volunteers (61–79 years) and younger adults (18–39 years) indicate that age alone does not alter clindamycin pharmacokinetics (clearance, elimination half-life, volume of distribution, and area under the serum concentration-time curve) after IV administration of clindamycin phosphate. After oral administration of clindamycin hydrochloride, elimination half-life is increased to approximately 4.0 hours (range 3.4–5.1 h) in the elderly compared to 3.2 hours (range 2.1–4.2 h) in younger adults. The extent of absorption, however, is not different between age groups and no dosage alteration is necessary for the elderly with normal hepatic function and normal (age-adjusted) renal function[1].
Serum assays for active clindamycin require an inhibitor to prevent *in vitro* hydrolysis of clindamycin phosphate.

Table 1. Average Peak and Trough Serum Concentrations of Active Clindamycin After Dosing With Clindamycin Phosphate

Dosage Regimen	Peak mcg/mL	Trough mcg/mL9
Healthy Adult Males (Post equilibrium)		
600 mg IV in 30 min q6h	10.9	2.0
600 mg IV in 30 min q8h	10.8	1.1
900 mg IV in 30 min q8h	14.1	1.7
600 mg IM q12h*	9	
Pediatric Patients (first dose)*		
5–7 mg/kg IV in 1 hour	10	
5–7 mg/kg IM	8	
3–5 mg/kg IM	4	

*Data in this group from patients being treated for infection.

Microbiology: Although clindamycin phosphate is inactive *in vitro*, rapid *in vivo* hydrolysis converts this compound to the antibacterially active clindamycin.
Clindamycin has been shown to have *in vitro* activity against isolates of the following organisms:
Aerobic gram positive cocci, including:

Staphylococcus aureus Staphylococcus epidermidis	(penicillinase and non-penicillinase producing strains). When tested by *in vitro* methods, some staphylococcal strains originally resistant to erythromycin rapidly develop resistance to clindamycin.

Streptococci (except *Enterococcus faecalis*)
Pneumococci
Anaerobic gram negative bacilli, including:
Bacteroides species (including *Bacteroides fragilis* group and *Bacteroides melaninogenicus* group)
Fusobacterium species
Anaerobic gram positive nonsporeforming bacilli, including:
Propionibacterium
Eubacterium
Actinomyces species
Anaerobic and *microaerophilic gram positive cocci*, including:
Peptococcus species
Peptostreptococcus species
Microaerophilic streptococci

Clostridia: Clostridia are more resistant than most anaerobes to clindamycin. Most *Clostridium perfringens* are susceptible, but other species, e.g., *Clostridium sporogenes* and *Clostridium tertium* are frequently resistant to clindamycin. Susceptibility testing should be done.

Cross resistance has been demonstrated between clindamycin and lincomycin.

Antagonism has been demonstrated between clindamycin and erythromycin.

***In vitro* Susceptibility Testing:**

Disk diffusion technique-Quantitative methods that require measurement of zone diameters give the most precise estimates of antibiotic susceptibility. One such procedure[2] has been recommended for use with disks to test susceptibility to clindamycin.

Reports from a laboratory using the standardized single-disk susceptibility test[1] with a 2 mcg clindamycin disk should be interpreted according to the following criteria:

Susceptible organisms produce zones of 17 mm or greater, indicating that the testes organism is likely to respond to therapy.

Organisms of intermediate susceptibility produce zones of 15–16 mm, indicating that the tested organism would be susceptible if a high dosage is used or if the infection is confined to tissues and fluids (e.g., urine), in which high antibiotic levels are attained.

Resistant organisms produce zones of 14 mm or less, indicating that other therapy should be selected.

Standardized procedures require the use of control organisms. The 2 mcg clindamycin disk should givea zone diameter between 24 and 30 mm for *S. aureus* ATCC 25923.

Dilution techniques—A bacterial isolate may be considered susceptible if the minimum inhibitory (MIC) for clindamycin is not more than 1.6 mcg/mL. Organisms are considered moderately susceptible if the MIC is greater than 1.6 mcg/mL and less than or equal to 4.8 mcg/mL. Organisms are considered resistant if the MIC is greater than 4.8 mcg per mL.

The range of MICs for the control strains are as follows:
S. aureus ATCC 29213, 0.06–0.25 mcg/mL.
E. faecalis ATCC 29212, 4.0–16 mcg/mL.

For anaerobic bacteria the minimum inhibitory concentration (MIC) of clindamycin can be determined by agar dilution and broth dilution (including microdilution) techniques.[3] Ig MICs are not determined routinely, the disk broth method is recommended for routine use. THE KIRBY-BAUER DISK DIFFUSION METHOD AND ITS INTERPRETIVE STANDARDS ARE NOT RECOMMENDED FOR ANAEROBES.

INDICATIONS AND USAGE

CLEOCIN PHOSPHATE products are indicated in the treatment of serious infections caused by susceptible anaerobic bacteria.

CLEOCIN PHOSPHATE products are also indicated in the treatment of serious infections due to susceptible strains of streptococci, pneumococci, and staphylococci. Its use should be reversed for penicillin-allergic patients or other patients for whom, in the judgment of the physician, a penicillin is inappropriate. Because of the risk of antibiotic-associated pseudomembranous colitis, as described in the WARNING box, before selecting clindamycin the physician should consider the nature of the infection and the suitability of less toxic alternatives (e.g., erythromycin).

Bacteriologic studies should be performed to determine the causative organisms and their susceptibility to clindamycin.

Indicated surgical procedures should be performed in conjunction with antibiotic therapy.

CLEOCIN PHOSPHATE is indicated in the treatment of serious infections caused by susceptible strains of the designated organisms in the conditions listed below:

Lower respiratory tract infections including pneumonia, empyema, and lung abscess caused by anaerobes, *Streptococcus pneumoniae*, other strepcococci (except *E. faecalis*), and *Staphylococcus aureus*.

Skin and skin structure infections caused by *Streptococcus pyogenes*, *Staphylococcus aureus*, and anaerobes.

Gynecological infections including endometritis, nongonococcal tubo-ovarian abscess, pelvic cellulitis, and postsurgical vaginal cuff infection caused by susceptible anaerobes.

Intra-abdominal infections including peritonitis and intra-abdominal abscess caused by susceptible anaerobic organisms.

Septicemia caused by *Staphylococcus aureus*, streptococci (except *Enterococcus faecalis*), and susceptible anaerobes.

Bone and joint infections including acute hematogenous osteomyelitis caused by *Staphylococcus aureus* and as adjunctive therapy in the surgical treatment of chronic bone and joint infections due to susceptible organisms.

CONTRAINDICATIONS

This drug is contraindicated in individuals with a history of hypersensitivity to preparations containing clindamycin or lincomycin.

WARNINGS

See **WARNING** box.

Pseudomembranous colitis has been reported with nearly all antibacterial agents, including clindamycin, and may range in severity from mild to life-threatening. Therefore, it is important to consider this diagnosis in patients who present with diarrhea subsequent to the administration of antibacterial agents.

Treatment with antibacterial agents alters the normal flora of the colon and may permit overgrowth of clostridia. Studies indicate that a toxin produced by *clostridium difficile* is one primary cause of "antibiotic-associated colitis".

After diagnosis of pseudomembranous colitis has been established, therapeutic measures should be initiated. Mild cases of pseudomembranous colitis usually respond to drug discontinuation alone. In moderate to severe cases, consideration should be given to management with fluids and electrolytes, protein supplementation, and treatment with an antibacterial drug clinically effective against *C. difficile* colitis.

A careful inquiry should be made concerning previous sensitivities to drugs and other allergens.

This product contains benzyl alcohol as a preservative. Benzyl alcohol has been associated with a fatal "Gasping Syndrome" in premature infants. (See **PRECAUTIONS—Pediatric Use.**)

Usage in Meningitis—Since clindamycin does not diffuse adequately into the cerebrospinal fluid, the drug should not be used in the treatment of meningitis.

SERIOUS ANAPHYLACTOID REACTIONS REQUIRE IMMEDIATE EMERGENCY TREATMENT WITH EPINEPHRINE. OXYGEN AND INTRAVENOUS CORTICOSTEROIDS SHOULD ALSO BE ADMINISTERED AS INDICATED.

PRECAUTIONS

General

Review of experience to date suggests that a subgroup of older patients with associated severe illness may tolerate diarrhea less well. When clindamycin is indicated in these patients, thy should be carefully monitored for change in bowel frequency.

CLEOCIN PHOSPHATE products should be prescribed with caution in individuals with a history of gastrointestinal disease, particularly colitis.

CLEOCIN PHOSPHATE should be prescribed with caution in atopic individuals.

Certain infections may require incision and drainage or other indicated surgical procedures in addition to antibiotic therapy.

The use of CLEOCIN PHOSPHATE may result in overgrowth of nonsusceptible organisms—particularly yeasts. Should superinfections occur, appropriate measures should be taken as indicated by the clinical situation.

CLEOCIN PHOSPHATE should not be injected intravenously undiluted as a bolus, but should be infused over at least 10–60 minutes as directed in the DOSAGE AND ADMINISTRATION section.

Clindamycin dosage modification may not be necessary in patients with renal disease. In patients with moderate to severe liver disease, prolongation of clindamycin half-life has been found. However, it was postulated from studies that when given every eight hours, accumulation should rarely occur. Therefore, dosage modification in patients with liver disease may not be necessary. However, periodic liver enzyme determinations should be made when treating patients with severe liver disease.

Laboratory Tests

During prolonged therapy periodic liver and kidney function tests and blood counts should be performed.

Drug Interactions

Clindamycin has been shown to have neuromuscular blocking properties that may enhance the action of other neuromuscular blocking agents. Therefore, it should be used with caution in patients receiving such agents.

Antagonism has been demonstrated between clindamycin and erythromycin *in vitro*. Because of possible clinical significance, the two drugs should not be administered concurrently.

Carcinogenesis, Mutagenesis, Impairment of Fertility

Long term studies in animals have not been performed with clindamycin to evaluate carcinogenic potential. Genotoxicity tests performed included a rat micronucleus test and an Ames Salmonella reversion test. Both tests were negative.

Fertility studies in rats treated orally with up to 300 mg/kg/day (approximately 1.1 times the highest recommended adult human dose based on mg/m^2) revealed no effects on fertility or mating ability.

Pregnancy: Teratogenic effects

Pregnancy category B

Reproduction studies performed in rats and mice using oral doses of clindamycin up to 600 mg/kg/day (2.1 and 1.1 times the highest recommended adults human dose based on mg/m^2, respectively) or subcutaneous doses of clindamycin up to 250 mg/kg/day (0.9 and 0.5 times the highest recommended adult human dose based on mg/m^2, respectively) revealed no evidence of teratogenicity.

There are, however, no adequate and well-controlled studies in pregnant women. Because animal reproduction studies are not always predictive of the human response, this drug should be used during pregnancy only if clearly needed.

Nursing Mothers

Clindamycin has been reported to appear in breast milk in the range of 0.7 to 3.8 mcg/mL at dosages of 150 mg orally to 600 mg intravenously. Because of the potential for adverse reactions due to clindamycin in neonates (see **Pediatric Use**), the decision to discontinue the drug should be made, taking into account the importance of the drug to the mother.

Pediatric Use

When CLEOCIN PHOSPHATE Sterile Solution is administered to the pediatric population (birth to 16 years) appropriate monitoring of organ system functions is desirable.

Usage in Newborns and Infants

This product contains benzyl alcohol as a preservative. Benzyl alcohol has been associated with a fatal "Gasping Syndrome" in premature infants.

The potential for the toxic effect in the pediatric population from chemicals that may leach from the single dose premixed IV preparation in plastic has not been evaluated.

Geriatric Use

Clinical studies of clindamycin did not include sufficient numbers of patients age 65 and over to determine whether they respond differently from younger patients. However, other reported clinical experience indicates that antibiotic-associated colitis and diarrhea (due to *Clostridium difficile*) seen in association with most antibiotics occur more frequently in the elderly (>60 years) and may be more severe. These patients should be carefully monitored for the development of diarrhea.

Pharmacokinetic studies with clindamycin have shown no clinically important differences between young and elderly subjects with normal hepatic function and normal (age-adjusted) renal function after oral or intravenous administration.

ADVERSE REACTIONS

The following reactions have been reported with the use of clindamycin.

Gastrointestinal: Antibiotic-associated colitis (see **WARNINGS**), pseudomembranous colitis, abdominal pain, nausea, and vomiting. The onset of pseudomembranous colitis symptoms may occur during or after antibacterial treatment (see **WARNINGS**). An unpleasant or metallic taste occasionally has been reported after intravenous administration of the higher doses of clindamycin phosphate.

Hypersensitivity Reactions: Maculopapular rash and urticaria have been observed during drug therapy. Generalized mild to moderate morbilliform-like skin rashes are the most frequently reported of all adverse reactions. Rare instances of erythema multiforme, some resembling Steven-Johnson syndrome, have been associated with clindamycin. A few cases of anaphylactoid reactions have been reported. If a hypersensitivity reaction occurs, the drug should be discontinued. The usual agents (epinephrine, corticosteroids, antihistamines) should be available for emergency treatment of serious reactions.

Skin and Mucous Membranes: Pruritus, vaginitis, and rare instances of exfoliative dermatitis have been reported (see *Hypersensitivity Reactions*).

Liver: Jaundice and abnormalities in liver function tests have been observed during clindamycin therapy.

Renal: Although no direct relationship of clindamycin to renal damage has been established, renal dysfunction as evidenced by azotemia, oliguria, and/or protein-uria has been observed in rate instances.

Hematopoietic: Transient neutropenia (leukopenia) and eosinophilia have been reported. Reports of agranulocytosis and thrombocytopenia have been made. No direct etiologic relationship to concurrent clindamycin therapy could be made in any of the foregoing.

Local Reactions: Pain, induration and sterile abscess have been reported after intramuscular injection and thrombophlebitis after intravenous infusion. Reactions can be minimized or avoided by giving deep intramuscular injections and avoiding prolonged use of indwelling intravenous catheters.

Musculoskeletal: Rare instances of polyarthritis have been reported.

Cardiovascular: Rare instances of cardiopulmonary arrest and hypotension have been reported following too rapid intravenous administration. (See **DOSAGE AND ADMINISTRATION** section.)

OVERDOSAGE

Significant mortality was observed in mice at an intravenous dose of 855 mg/kg and in rats at an oral or subcutaneous dose of approximately 2618 mg/kg. In the mice, convulsions and depression were observed.

Hemodialysis and peritoneal dialysis are not effective in removing clindamycin from the serum.

Continued on next page

Information on these Pharmacia & Upjohn products is based on labeling in effect June 1, 2000. Further information concerning these and other Pharmacia & Upjohn products may be obtained by direct inquiry to Medical Information, Pharmacia & Upjohn, Kalamazoo, MI 49001.

Cleocin Phosphate—Cont.

DOSAGE AND ADMINISTRATION

If diarrhea occurs during therapy, this antibiotic should be discontinued (see **WARNING** box).

Adults: Parenteral (IM or IV Administration): Serious infections due to aerobic gram-positive cocci and the more susceptible anaerobes (NOT generally including *Bacteroides fragilis, Peptococcus* species and *Clostridium* species other than *Clostridium perfringens*):

600–1200 mg/day in 2, 3 or 4 equal doses.

More severe infections, particularly those due to proven or suspected *Bacteroides fragilis, Peptococcus* species, or *Clostridium* species other than *Clostridium perfringens*:

1200–2700 mg/day in 2, 3 or 4 equal doses.

For more serious infections, these doses may have to be increased. In life-threatening situations due to either aerobes or anaerobes these doses may be increased. Doses of as much as 4800 mg daily have been given intravenously to adults. See **Dilution and Infusion Rates** section below.

Single intramuscular injections of greater than 600 mg are not recommended.

Alternatively, drug may be administered in the form of a single rapid infusion of the first dose followed by continuous IV infusion as follows:

[See table at bottom of page]

Neonates (less than 1 month):

15 to 20 mg/kg/day in 3 to 4 equal doses. The lower dosage may be adequate for small prematures.

Pediatric patients 1 month of age to 16 years: Parenteral (IM or IV) administration: 20 to 40 mg/kg/day in 3 or 4 equal doses. The higher doses would be used for more severe infections. As an alternative to dosing on a body weight basis, pediatric patients may be dosed on the basis of square meters body surface: 350mg/m^2/day for serious infections and 450 mg/m^2/day for more severe infections.

Parenteral therapy may be changed to oral CLEOCIN PEDIATRIC® Flavored Granules (clindamycin palmitate hydrochloride) or CLEOCIN HCl® Capsules (clindamycin hydrochloride) when the condition warrants and at the discretion of the physician.

In cases of β-hemolytic streptococcal infections, treatment should be continued for at least 10 days.

Dilution and Infusion Rates: Clindamycin phosphate must be diluted prior to IV administration. The concentration of clindamycin in diluent for infusion should not exceed 18 mg per mL. Infusion rates should not exceed 30 mg per minute. The usual infusion dilutions and rates are as follows:

Dose	Diluent	Time
300 mg	50 mL	10 min
600 mg	50 mL	20 min
900 mg	50–100 mL	30 min
1200 mg	100 mL	40 min

Administration of more than 1200 mg in a single 1-hour infusion is not recommended.

Parenteral drug products should be inspected visually for particulate matter and discoloration prior to administration, whenever solution and container permit.

Dilution and Compatibility: Physical and biological compatibility studies monitored for 24 hours at room temperature have demonstrated no inactivation or incompatibility with the use of CLEOCIN PHOSPHATE Sterile Solution (clindamycin phosphate) in IV solutions containing sodium chloride, glucose, calcium or potassium, and solutions containing vitamin B complex in concentrations usually used clinically. No incompatibility has been demonstrated with the antibiotics cephalothin, kanamycin, gentamicin, penicillin or carbenicillin.

The following drugs are physically incompatible with clindamycin phosphate: ampicillin sodium, phenytoin sodium, barbiturates, aminophylline, calcium gluconate, and magnesium sulfate.

The compatibility and duration of stability of drug admixtures will vary depending on concentration and other conditions. For current information regarding compatibilities of clindamycin phosphate under specific conditions, please contact the Medical and Drug Information Unit, Pharmacia & Upjohn Company.

Physico-Chemical Stability of diluted solutions of CLEOCIN PHOSPHATE

Room temperature: 6, 9 and 12 mg/mL (equivalent to clindamycin base) in dextrose injection 5%, sodium chloride injection 0.9%, or Lactated Ringers Injection in glass bottles or minibags, demonstrated physical and chemical stability for at least 16 days at 25°C. Also, 18 mg/mL (equivalent to clindamycin base) in dextrose injection 5%, in minibags, demonstrated physical and chemical stability for at least 16 days at 25°C.

Refrigeration: 6, 9 and 12 mg/mL (equivalent to clindamycin base) in dextrose injection 5%, sodium chloride injection 0.9%, or Lactated Ringers Injection in glass bottles or minibags, demonstrated physical and chemical stability for at least 32 days at 4°C.

IMPORTANT: This chemical stability information in no way indicates that it would be acceptable practice to use this product well after the preparation time. Good professional practice suggests that compounded admixtures should be administered as soon after preparation as is feasible.

Frozen: 6, 9 and 12 mg/mL (equivalent to clindamycin base) in dextrose injection 5%, sodium chloride injection 0.9%, or Lactated Ringers Injection in minibags demonstrated physical and chemical stability for at least eight weeks at -10°C. Frozen solutions should be thawed at room temperature and not refrozen.

DIRECTIONS FOR DISPENSING

Pharmacy Bulk Package—Not for Direct Infusion

The Pharmacy Bulk Package is for use in a Pharmacy Admixture Service only under a laminar flow hood. Entry into the vial should be made with a small diameter sterile transfer set or other small diameter sterile dispensing device, and contents dispensed in aliquots using aseptic technique. Multiple entries with a needle and syringe are not recommended. AFTER ENTRY USE ENTIRE CONTENTS OF VIAL PROMPTLY. ANY UNUSED PORTION MUST BE DISCARDED WITHIN 24 HOURS AFTER INITIAL ENTRY.

DIRECTIONS FOR USE

CLEOCIN PHOSPHATE IV Solution in Galaxy Plastic Container

Premixed CLEOCIN PHOSPHATE IV Solution is for intravenous administration using sterile equipment. Check for minute leaks prior to use by squeezing bag firmly. If leaks re found, discard solution as sterility may be impaired. Do not add supplementary medication. Parenteral drug products should be inspected visually for particulate matter and discoloration prior to administration whenever solution and container permit. Do not use unless solution is clear and seal is intact.

Caution: Do not use plastic containers in series connections. Such use could result in air embolism due to residual air being drawn from the primary container before administration of the fluid from the secondary container is complete.

Preparation for Administration:

1. Suspend container from eyelet support.
2. Remove protector from outlet port at bottom of container.
3. Attach administration set. Refer to complete directions accompanying set.

Preparation of CLEOCIN PHOSPHATE in ADD-Vantage System—For IV Use Only. CLEOCIN PHOSPHATE 600 mg and 900 mg may be reconstituted in 50 mL or 100 mL, respectively, of Dextrose Injection 5% or Sodium Chloride Injection 0.9% in the ADD-diluent container. Refer to separate instructions for ADD-Vantage‡ System.

HOW SUPPLIED

Each mL of CLEOCIN PHOSPHATE Sterile Solution contains clindamycin phosphate equivalent to 150 mg clindamycin; 0.5 mg disodium edetate; 9.45 mg benzyl alcohol added as preservative. When necessary, pH is adjusted with sodium hydroxide and/or hydrochloric acid. CLEOCIN PHOSPHATE is available in the following packages:

25–2 mL vials	NDC 0009-0870-21
25–4 mL vials	NDC 0009-0775-26
25–6 mL vials	NDC 0009-0902-11
1–60 mL Pharmacy Bulk Package	NDC 0009-0728-05

CLEOCIN PHOSPHATE is supplied in ADD-Vantage vials as follows:

NDC	Vial Size	Total Clindamycin Phosphate/vial	Amount of Diluent
0009-3124-01	4 mL	600 mg	50 mL
0009-3447-01	6 mL	900 mg	100 mL

Store at controlled room temperature 20° to 25°C (68° to 77°F) [see USP].

CLEOCIN PHOSPHATE IV Solution in Galaxy plastic containers is a sterile solution of clindamycin phosphate with 5% dextrose. The single dose Galaxy plastic containers are available as follows:

24-300 mg/50 mL containers	NDC 0009-3381-01
24-600 mg/50 mL containers	NDC 0009-3375-01
24-900 mg/50 mL containers	NDC 0009-3382-01

Exposure of pharmaceutical products to heat should be minimized. It is recommended that Galaxy plastic containers be stored at room temperature (25°C). Avoid temperatures above 30°C.

ANIMAL TOXICOLOGY

One year oral toxicity studies in Spartan Sprague-Dawley rats and beagle dogs at dose levels up to 300 mg/kg/day (approximately 1.1 and 3.6 times the highest recommended adult human dose based on mg/m^2, respectively) have shown clindamycin to be well tolerated. No appreciable difference in pathological findings has been observed between groups of animals treated with clindamycin and comparable control groups. Rats receiving clindamycin hydrochloride at 600 mg/kg/day (approximately 2.1 times the highest recommended adult human dose based on mg/m^2) for 6 months tolerated the drug well; however, dogs dosed at this level (approximately 7.2 times the highest recommended adult human dose based on mg/m^2) vomited, would not eat, and lost weight.

Rx only

Pharmacia & Upjohn Company • Kalamazoo, MI 49001, USA

Revised June 1999 810 020 137 691273

REFERENCES

1. Smith RB, Phillips JP: Evaluation of CLEOCIN HCl and CLEOCIN Phosphate in an Aged Population. Upjohn TR 8147-82-9122-021, December 1982.
2. Bauer AW, Kirby WMM, Sherris JC, Turck M; Antibiotic susceptibility testing by a standardized single disk method. *Am. J. Clin. Path.*, **45**:493–496, 1966. Standardized Disk Susceptibility Test, *Federal Register*, 37:20527–29, 1972.
3. National Committee for Clinical Lab. Standards. Methods for Antimicrobial Susceptibility Testing of Anaerobic Bacteria—Second Edition; Tentative Standard. NCCLS publication M11-T2. Villanova, PA; NCCLS; 1988.

‡ADD-Vantage is a registered trademark of Abbott Laboratories.

CLEOCIN PHOSPHATE IV Solution in the Galaxy plastic containers is manufactured for Pharmacia & Upjohn Company by Baxter Healthcare Corporation, Deerfield, IL 60015.

Galaxy® is a registered trademark of Baxter International, Inc.

CLEOCIN® ℞

[*clēō-sĭn*]

clindamycin phosphate vaginal cream, USP

FOR INTRAVAGINAL USE ONLY
NOT FOR OPHTHALMIC, DERMAL, OR ORAL USE

DESCRIPTION

Clindamycin phosphate is a water soluble ester of the semi-synthetic antibiotic produced by a 7(S)-chloro-substitution of the 7(R)-hydroxyl group of the parent antibiotic lincomycin. The chemical name for clindamycin phosphate is methyl 7-chloro-6,7,8-trideoxy-6-(1-methyl-*trans*-4-propyl-L-2-pyrrolidinecarboxamido)-1-thio-L-*threo*-α-*D*-*galacto*-octopyranoside 2-(dihydrogen phosphate). It has a molecular weight of 504.96, and the molecular formula is $C_{18}H_{34}ClN_2O_8PS$. The structural formula is represented at right:

CLEOCIN Vaginal Cream 2%, is a semi-solid, white cream, which contains 2% clindamycin phosphate, USP, at a concentration equivalent to 20 g clindamycin per gram. The pH of the cream is between 3.0 and 6.0. The cream also contains benzyl alcohol, cetostearyl alcohol, cetyl palmitate, mineral oil, polysorbate 60, propylene glycol, purified water, sorbitan monostearate, and stearic acid.

Each applicatorful of 5 grams of vaginal cream contains approximately 100 mg of clindamycin phosphate.

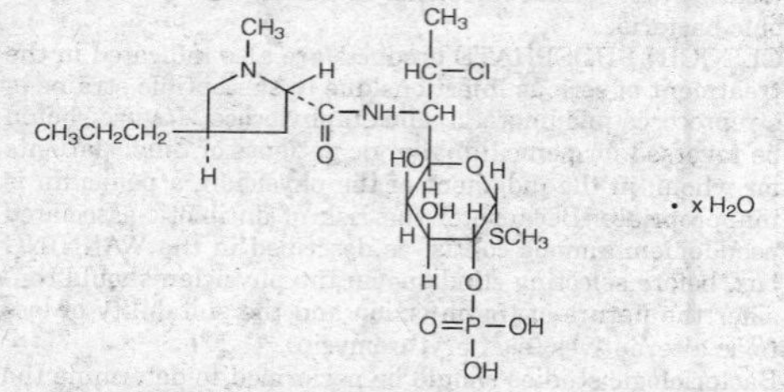

CLINICAL PHARMACOLOGY

Following a once a day intravaginal dose of 100 mg of clindamycin vaginal cream 2%, administered to 6 healthy female volunteers for 7 days, approximately 5% (range 0.6% to 11%) of the administered dose was absorbed systemically. The peak serum clindamycin concentration observed on the first day averaged 18 ng/mL (range 4 to 47 ng/mL) and on day 7 it averaged 25 ng/mL (range 6 to 61 ng/mL). These peak concentrations were attained approximately 10 hours post-dosing (range 4–24 hours).

Following a once a day intravaginal dose of 100 mg of clindamycin phosphate vaginal cream 2%, administered for 7 consecutive days to 5 women with bacterial vaginosis, absorption was slower and less variable than that observed in healthy females. Approximately 5% (range 2% to 8%) of the dose was absorbed systemically. The peak serum clindamycin concentration observed on the first day averaged 13 ng/mL (range 6 to 34 ng/mL) and on day 7 it averaged 16 ng/mL (range 7 to 26 ng/mL). These peak concentrations were attained approximately 14 hours post-dosing (range 4–24 hours).

There was little or no systemic accumulation of clindamycin after repeated vaginal dosing of clindamycin phosphate vaginal cream 2%. The systemic half-life was 1.5 to 2.6 hours.

To maintain serum clindamycin levels	Rapid infusion rate	Maintenance infusion rate
Above 4 mcg/mL	10 mg/min for 30 min	0.75 mg/min
Above 5 mcg/mL	15 mg/min for 30 min	1.00 mg/min
Above 6 mcg/mL	20 mg/min for 30 min	1.25 mg/min

MICROBIOLOGY

Clindamycin inhibits bacterial protein synthesis at the level of the bacterial ribosome. The antibiotic binds preferentially to the 50S ribosomal subunit and affects the process of peptide chain initiation. Although clindamycin phosphate is inactive *in vitro*, rapid *in vivo* hydrolysis converts this compound to the antibacterially active clindamycin.

Culture and sensitivity testing of bacteria are not routinely performed to establish the diagnosis of bacterial vaginosis. (See INDICATIONS AND USAGE.) Standard methodology for the susceptibility testing of the potential bacterial vaginosis pathogens, *Gardnerella vaginalis, Mobiluncus* spp., or *Mycoplasma hominis*, has not been defined. Nonetheless, clindamycin is an antimicrobial agent active *in vitro* against most strains of the following organisms that have been reported to be associated with bacterial vaginosis:

Bacteroides spp.
Gardnerella vaginalis
Mobiluncus spp.
Mycoplasma hominis
Peptostreptococcus spp.

INDICATIONS AND USAGE

CLEOCIN Vaginal Cream 2%, is indicated in the treatment of bacterial vaginosis (formerly referred to as *Haemophilus* vaginitis, *Gardnerella* vaginitis, nonspecific vaginitis, *Corynebacterium* vaginitis, or anaerobic vaginosis). CLEOCIN Vaginal Cream 2%, can be used to treat non-pregnant women and pregnant women during the second and third trimester. (See CLINICAL STUDIES.)

NOTE: For purposes of this indication, a clinical diagnosis of bacterial vaginosis is usually defined by the presence of a homogeneous vaginal discharge that (a) has a pH of greater than 4.5, (b) emits a "fishy" amine odor when mixed with a 10% KOH solution, and (c) contains clue cells on microscopic examination. Gram's stain results consistent with a diagnosis of bacterial vaginosis include (a) markedly reduced or absent *Lactobacillus* morphology, (b) predominance of *Gardnerella* morphotype, and (c) absent or few white blood cells.

Other pathogens commonly associated with vulvovaginitis, eg, *Trichomonas vaginalis, Chlamydia trachomatis, N. gonorrhoeae, Candida albicans*, and *Herpes simplex* virus should be ruled out.

CONTRAINDICATIONS

CLEOCIN Vaginal Cream 2%, is contraindicated in individuals with a history of hypersensitivity to clindamycin, lincomycin, or any of the components of this vaginal cream. CLEOCIN Vaginal Cream 2%, is also contraindicated in individuals with a history of regional enteritis, ulcerative colitis, or a history of "antibiotic-associated" colitis.

WARNINGS

Pseudomembranous colitis has been reported with nearly all antibacterial agents, including clindamycin, and may range in severity from mild to life-threatening. Orally and parenterally administered clindamycin has been associated with severe colitis which may end fatally. Diarrhea, bloody diarrhea, and colitis (including pseudomembranous colitis) have been reported with the use of orally and parenterally administered clindamycin, as well as with topical (dermal) formulations of clindamycin. Therefore, it is important to consider this diagnosis in patients who present with diarrhea subsequent to the administration of clindamycin, even when administered by the vaginal route, because approximately 5% of the clindamycin dose is systemically absorbed from the vagina.

Treatment with antibacterial agents alters the normal flora of the colon and may permit overgrowth of clostridia. Studies indicate that a toxin produced by *Clostridium difficile* is a primary cause of "antibiotic-associated" colitis.

After the diagnosis of pseudomembranous colitis has been established, therapeutic measures should be initiated. Mild cases of pseudomembranous colitis usually respond to discontinuation of the drug alone. In moderate to severe cases, consideration should be given to management with fluids and electrolytes, protein supplementation, and treatment with an antibacterial drug clinically effective against *Clostridium difficile* colitis.

Onset of pseudomembranous colitis symptoms may occur during or after antimicrobial treatment.

PRECAUTIONS

General

CLEOCIN Vaginal Cream 2%, contains ingredients that will cause burning and irritation of the eye. In the event of accidental contact with the eye, rinse the eye with copious amounts of cool tap water.

The use of CLEOCIN Vaginal Cream 2% may result in the overgrowth of nonsusceptible organisms in the vagina. In clinical studies involving 600 non-pregnant women who received treatment for 3 days, *Candida albicans* was detected, either symptomatically or by culture, in 8.8% of patients. In 9% of the patients, vaginitis was recorded. In clinical studies involving 1325 non-pregnant women who received treatment for 7 days, *Candida albicans* was detected, either symptomatically or by culture, in 10.5% of patients. Vaginitis was recorded in 10.7% of the patients. In 180 pregnant women who received treatment for 7 days, *Candida albicans* was detected, either symptomatically or by culture, in 13.3% of patients. In 7.2% of the patients, vaginitis was recorded. *Candida albicans*, as reported here, includes the terms: vaginal moniliasis and moniliasis (body as a whole). Vaginitis includes the terms: vulvo-vaginal disorder, vulvovaginitis, vaginal discharge, trichomonal vaginitis, and vaginitis.

Information for the Patient:

The patient should be instructed not to engage in vaginal intercourse, or use other vaginal products (such as tampons or douches) during treatment with this product.

The patient should also be advised that this cream contains mineral oil that may weaken latex or rubber products such as condoms or vaginal contraceptive diaphragms. Therefore, use of such products within 72 hours following treatment with CLEOCIN Vaginal Cream 2%, is not recommended.

Drug Interactions

Clindamycin has been shown to have neuromuscular blocking properties that may enhance the action of other neuromuscular blocking agents. Therefore, it should be used with caution in patients receiving such agents.

Carcinogenesis, Mutagenesis, Impairment of Fertility

Long term studies in animals have not been performed with clindamycin to evaluate carcinogenic potential. Genotoxicity tests performed included a rat micronuculeus test and an Ames test. Both tests were negative. Fertility studies in rats treated orally with up to 300 mg/kg/day (31 times the human exposure based on mg/m^2) revealed no effects on fertility or mating ability.

Pregnancy: Teratogenic effects

Pregnancy Category B

There are no adequate and well-controlled studies in pregnant women during the first trimester of pregnancy. This drug should be used during the first trimester of pregnancy only if clearly needed.

CLEOCIN Vaginal Cream 2% has been studied in pregnant women during the second trimester. In women treated for seven days, abnormal labor was reported in 1.1% of patients who received clindamycin vaginal cream 2% compared with 0.5% of patients who received placebo.

Reproduction studies have been performed in rats and mice using oral and parenteral doses of clindamycin up to 600 mg/kg/day (62 and 25 times, respectively, the maximum human exposure based on mg/m^2) and have revealed no evidence of harm to the fetus due to clindamycin. In one mouse strain, cleft palates were observed in treated fetuses; this outcome was not produced in other mouse strains or in other species and is, therefore, considered to be a strain specific effect.

See INDICATIONS AND USAGE; PRECAUTIONS, General; and ADVERSE REACTIONS.

Nursing Mothers

Clindamycin has been detected in human milk after oral or parenteral administration. It is not known if clindamycin is excreted in human milk following the use of vaginally administered clindamycin phosphate.

Because of the potential for serious adverse reactions in nursing infants from clindamycin phosphate, a decision should be made whether to discontinue nursing or to discontinue the drug, taking into account the importance of the drug to the mother.

Pediatric Use

Safety and effectiveness in pediatric patients have not been established.

ADVERSE REACTIONS

Clinical trials

Non-pregnant Women: In clinical trials involving non-pregnant women, 1.8% of 600 patients who received treatment with CLEOCIN Vaginal Cream 2% for 3 days and 2.7% of 1325 patients who received treatment for 7 days discontinued therapy due to drug-related adverse events. Medical events judged to be related, probably related, possibly related, or of unknown relationship to vaginally administered clindamycin phosphate vaginal cream 2%, were reported for 20.7% of the patients receiving treatment for 3 days and 21.3% of the patients receiving treatment for 7 days. Events occurring in ≥1% of patients receiving clindamycin phosphate vaginal cream 2% are shown in Table 1.

TABLE 1—Events Occurring in ≥1% of Non-pregnant Patients Receiving Clindamycin Phosphate Vaginal Cream 2%

Event	CLEOCIN Vaginal Cream	
	3 Day n=600	7 Day n=1325
Urogenital		
Vaginal moniliasis	7.7	10.4
Vulvovaginitis	6.0	4.4
Vulvovaginal disorder	3.2	5.3
Trichomonal vaginitis	0	1.3
Body as a Whole		
Moniliasis (body)	1.3	0.2

Other events occurring in <1% of the clindamycin vaginal cream 2% groups include:

Urogenital system: vaginal discharge, metrorrhagia, urinary tract infection, endometriosis, menstrual disorder, vaginitis/vaginal infection, and vaginal pain.

Body as a whole: localized abdominal pain, generalized abdominal pain, abdominal cramps, halitosis, headache, bacterial infection, inflammatory swelling, allergic reaction, and fungal infection.

Digestive system: nausea, vomiting, constipation, dyspepsia, flatulence, diarrhea, and gastrointestinal disorder.

Endocrine system: hyperthyroidism.

Central nervous system: dizziness and vertigo.

Respiratory system: epistaxis.

Skin: pruritus (non-application site), moniliasis, rash, maculopapular rash, erythema, and urticaria.

Special senses: taste perversion.

Pregnant Women: In a clinical trial involving pregnant women during the second trimester, 1.7% of 180 patients who received treatment for 7 days discontinued therapy due to drug-related adverse events. Medical events judged to be related, probably related, possibly related, or of unknown relationship to vaginally administered clindamycin phosphate vaginal cream 2%, were reported for 22.8% of pregnant patients. Events occurring in ≥1% of patients receiving either clindamycin phosphate vaginal cream 2% or placebo are shown in Table 2.

TABLE 2—Events Occurring in ≥1% of Pregnant Patients Receiving Clindamycin Phosphate Vaginal Cream 2% or Placebo

Event	CLEOCIN Vaginal Cream	Placebo
	7 Day n=180	7 Day n=184
Urogenital		
Vaginal moniliasis	13.3	7.1
Vulvovaginal disorder	6.7	7.1
Abnormal labor	1.1	0.5
Body as a Whole		
Fungal infection	1.7	0
Skin		
Pruritus, non-application site	1.1	0

Other events occurring in <1% of the clindamycin vaginal cream 2% group include:

Urogenital system: dysuria, metrorrhagia, vaginal pain, and trichomonal vaginitis.

Body as a whole: upper respiratory infection.

Skin: pruritus (topical application site) and erythema.

Other clindamycin formulations:

Clindamycin vaginal cream affords minimal peak serum levels and systemic exposure (AUCs) of clindamycin compared to 100 mg oral clindamycin dosing. Although these lower levels of exposure are less likely to produce the common reactions seen with oral clindamycin, the possibility of these and other reactions cannot be excluded presently. Data from well-controlled trials directly comparing clindamycin orally to clindamycin administered vaginally are not available.

The following adverse reactions and altered laboratory tests have been reported with the **oral or parenteral** use of clindamycin.

Gastrointestinal: Abdominal pain, esophagitis, nausea, vomiting, and diarrhea. (See WARNINGS.)

Hematopoietic: Transient neutropenia (leukopenia), eosinophilia, agranulocytosis, and thrombocytopenia have been reported. No direct etiologic relationship to concurrent clindamycin therapy could be made in any of these reports.

Hypersensitivity Reactions: Maculopapular rash and urticaria have been observed during drug therapy. Generalized mild to moderate morbilliform-like skin rashes are the most frequently reported of all adverse reactions. Rare instances of erythema multiforme, some resembling Stevens-Johnson syndrome, have been associated with clindamycin. A few cases of anaphylactoid reactions have been reported. If a hypersensitivity reaction occurs, the drug should be discontinued.

Liver: Jaundice and abnormalities in liver function tests have been observed during clindamycin therapy.

Musculoskeletal: Rare instances of polyarthritis have been reported

Renal: Although no direct relationship of clindamycin to renal damage has been established, renal dysfunction as evidenced by azotemia, oliguria, and/or proteinuria has been observed in rare instances.

OVERDOSAGE

Vaginally applied clindamycin phosphate vaginal cream 2% could be absorbed in sufficient amounts to produce systemic effects (See WARNINGS.)

DOSAGE AND ADMINISTRATION

The recommended dose is one applicatorful of clindamycin phosphate vaginal cream 2%, (5 grams containing approximately 100 mg of clindamycin phosphate) intravaginally,

Continued on next page

Information on these Pharmacia & Upjohn products is based on labeling in effect June 1, 2000. Further information concerning these and other Pharmacia & Upjohn products may be obtained by direct inquiry to Medical Information, Pharmacia & Upjohn, Kalamazoo, MI 49001.

Cleocin Vaginal Cream—Cont.

preferably at bedtime, for 3 or 7 consecutive days in non-pregnant patients and for 7 consecutive days in pregnant patients. (See CLINICAL STUDIES.)

HOW SUPPLIED

CLEOCIN Vaginal Cream 2%, (clindamycin phosphate vaginal cream) is supplied as follows:

40 g tube
(with 7 disposable applicators) NDC 0009-3448-01

Store at controlled room temperature 20° to 25° C (68° to 77° F) [see USP]. Protect from freezing.

CLINICAL STUDIES

In two clinical studies involving 674 evaluable non-pregnant women with bacterial vaginosis comparing CLEOCIN Vaginal Cream 2% for 3 or 7 days, the clinical cure rates, determined at 1 month posttherapy, ranged from 72% to 81% for the 3-day treatment and 84% to 86% for the 7-day treatment.

	CLEOCIN 3 Day		CLEOCIN 7 Day	
US Study	94/131	72%	110/128	86%
European Study	161/199	81%	181/216	84%

In a clinical study involving 249 evaluable pregnant patients in the second and third trimester treated for 7 days, the clinical cure rate, determined at 1 month posttherapy, was 60% (77/129) in the clindamycin arm and 9% (11/120) for the vehicle arm. The determination of clinical cure was based on the absence of a "fishy" amine odor when the vaginal discharge was mixed with a 10% KOH solution and the absence of clue cells on microscopic examination.

℞ only

Pharmacia & Upjohn Company
Kalamazoo, Michigan 49001, USA
Revised June 2000

815 255 5507
692116

DIRECTIONS FOR USE

Disposable plastic applicators are provided with this package. They are designed to allow proper vaginal administration of the cream.

Remove cap from cream tube. Screw a plastic applicator on the threaded end of the tube.

Rolling tube from the bottom, squeeze gently and force the medication into the applicator. The applicator is filled when the plunger reaches its predetermined stopping point.

Unscrew the applicator from the tube and replace the cap.

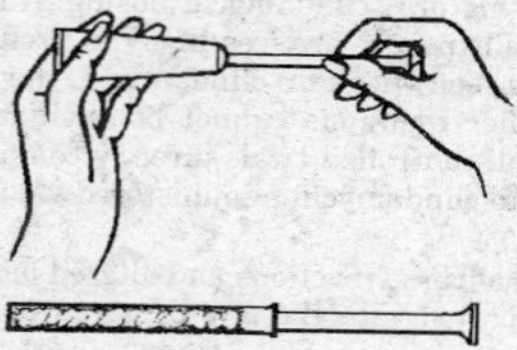

While lying on your back, firmly grasp the applicator barrel and insert into vagina as far as possible without causing discomfort.

Slowly push the plunger until it stops.

Carefully withdraw applicator from vagina, and discard applicator.

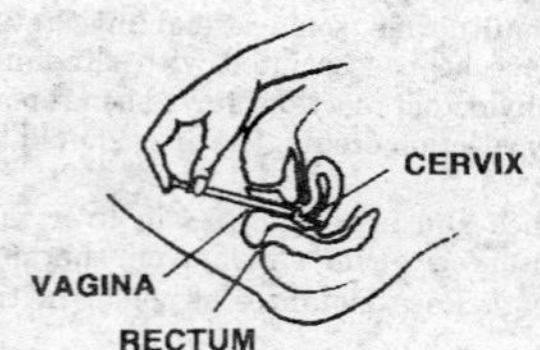

REMEMBER TO APPLY ONE APPLICATORFUL EACH NIGHT BEFORE BEDTIME, OR AS PRESCRIBED BY YOUR DOCTOR.

CLEOCIN® VAGINAL OVULES ℞

[*clēō-sĭn*]

clindamycin phosphate vaginal suppositories
FOR INTRAVAGINAL USE ONLY

DESCRIPTION

Clindamycin phosphate is a water-soluble ester of the semi-synthetic antibiotic produced by a 7(S)-chloro-substitution of the 7(R)-hydroxyl group of the parent antibiotic lincomycin. The chemical name for clindamycin phosphate is methyl 7-chloro-6,7,8-trideoxy-6-(1-methyl-*trans*-4-propyl-L-2-pyrrolidinecarboxamido)-1-thio-L-*threo*-α-D-*galacto*-octopyranoside 2-(dihydrogen phosphate). The monohydrate form has a molecular weight of 522.98, and the molecular formula is $C_{18}H_{34}ClN_2O_8PS \bullet H_2O$. The structural formula is represented below:

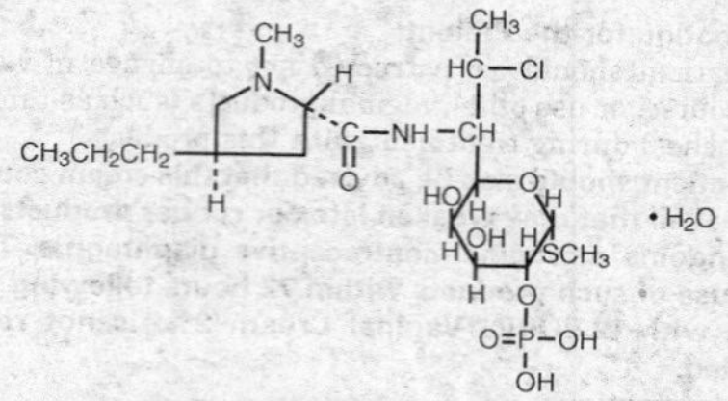

CLEOCIN Vaginal Ovules are semisolid, white to off-white suppositories for intravaginal administration. Each 2.5 g suppository contains clindamycin phosphate equivalent to 100 mg clindamycin in a base consisting of a mixture of glycerides of saturated fatty acids.

CLINICAL PHARMACOLOGY

Systemic absorption of clindamycin was estimated following a once-a-day intravaginal dose of one clindamycin phosphate vaginal suppository (equivalent to 100 mg clindamycin) administered to 11 healthy female volunteers for 3 days. Approximately 30% (range 6% to 70%) of the administered dose was absorbed systemically on day 3 of dosing based on area under the concentration-time curve (AUC). Systemic absorption was estimated using a subtherapeutic 100 mg intravenous dose of clindamycin phosphate as a comparator in the same volunteers. The mean AUC following day 3 of dosing with the suppository was 3.2 μg•hr/mL (range 0.42 to 11 μg•hr/mL). The C_{max} observed on day 3 of dosing with the suppository averaged 0.27 μg/mL (range 0.03 to 0.67 μg/mL) and was observed about 5 hours after dosing (range 1 to 10 hours). In contrast, the AUC and C_{max} after the single intravenous dose averaged 11 μg•hr/mL (range 5.1 to 26 μg•hr/mL) and 3.7 μg/mL (range 2.4 to 5.0 μg/mL), respectively. The mean apparent elimination half-life after dosing with the suppository was 11 hours (range 4 to 35 hours) and is considered to be limited by the absorption rate.

The results from this study showed that systemic exposure to clindamycin (based on AUC) from the suppository was, on average, three-fold lower than that from a single subtherapeutic 100 mg intravenous dose of clindamycin. In addition, the recommended daily and total doses of intravaginal clindamycin suppository are far lower than those typically administered in oral or parenteral clindamycin therapy (100 mg of clindamycin per day for 3 days equivalent to about 30 mg absorbed per day from the ovule relative to 600 to 2700 mg/day for up to 10 days or more, orally or parenterally).

The overall systemic exposure to clindamycin form Cleocin Vaginal Ovules is substantially lower than the systemic exposure from therapeutic doses of oral clindamycin hydrochloride (two-fold to 20-fold lower) or parenteral clindamycin phosphate (40-fold to 50-fold lower).

MICROBIOLOGY

Clindamycin inhibits bacterial protein synthesis at the level of the bacterial ribosome. The antibiotic binds preferentially to the 50S ribosomal subunit and affects the process of peptide chain initiation. Although clindamycin phosphate is inactive in vitro, rapid in vivo hydrolysis converts this compound to the antibacterially active clindamycin.

Culture and sensitivity testing of bacteria are not routinely performed to establish the diagnosis of bacterial vaginosis. (See INDICATIONS AND USAGE.) Standard methodology for the susceptibility testing of the potential bacterial vaginosis pathogens, *Gardnerella vaginalis, Mobiluncus* spp, or *Mycoplasma hominis*, has not been defined. Nonetheless, clindamycin is an antimicrobial agent active in vitro against most strains of the following organisms that have been reported to be associated with bacterial vaginosis.

Bacteroides spp
Gardnerella vaginalis
Mobiluncus spp
Mycoplasma hominis
Peptostreptococcus spp

INDICATIONS AND USAGE

CLEOCIN Vaginal Ovules are indicated for 3-day treatment of bacterial vaginosis in non-pregnant women. There are no adequate and well-controlled studies of CLEOCIN Vaginal Ovules in pregnant women.

NOTE: For purposes of this indication, a clinical diagnosis of bacterial vaginosis is usually defined by the presence of a homogenous vaginal discharge that (a) has a pH of greater than 4.5, (b) emits a "fishy" amine odor when mixed with a 10% KOH solution, and (c) contains clue cells on microscopic examination. Gram's stain results consistent with a diagnosis of bacterial vaginosis include (a) markedly reduced or absent *Lactobacillus* morphology, (b) predominance of *Gardnerella* morphotype, and (c) absent or few white blood cells. Other pathogens commonly associated with vulvovaginitis, eg, *Trichomonas vaginalis, Chlamydia trachomatis, Neisseria gonorrhoeae, Candida albicans,* and herpes simplex virus, should be ruled out.

CONTRAINDICATIONS

CLEOCIN Vaginal Ovules are contraindicated in individuals with a history of hypersensitivity to clindamycin, lincomycin, or any of the components of this vaginal suppository. CLEOCIN Vaginal Ovules are also contraindicated in individuals with a history of regional enteritis, ulcerative colitis, or a history of "antibiotic-associated" colitis.

WARNINGS

Pseudomembranous colitis has been reported with nearly all antibacterial agents, including clindamycin, and may range in severity from mild to life-threatening. Orally and parenterally administered clindamycin has been associated with severe colitis, which may end fatally, Diarrhea, bloody diarrhea, and colitis (including pseudomembranous colitis) have been reported with the use of orally and parenterally administered clindamycin, as well as with topical (dermal) formulations of clindamycin. Therefore, it is important to consider this diagnosis in patients who present with diarrhea subsequent to the administration of CLEOCIN Vaginal Ovules, because approximately 30% of the clindamycin dose is systemically absorbed from the vagina.

Treatment with antibacterial agents alters the normal flora of the colon and may permit overgrowth of clostridia. Studies indicate that a toxin produced by *Clostridium difficile* is a primary cause of "antibiotic-associated" colitis.

After the diagnosis of pseudomembranous colitis has been established, therapeutic measures should be initiated. Mild cases of pseudomembranous colitis usually respond to discontinuation of the drug alone. In moderate to severe cases, consideration should be given to management with fluids and electrolytes, protein supplementation, and treatment with an antibacterial drug clinically effective against *Clostridium difficile* colitis.

Onset of pseudomembranous colitis symptoms may occur during or after antimicrobial treatment.

PRECAUTIONS

General

The use of CLEOCIN Vaginal Ovules may result in the overgrowth of nonsusceptible organisms in the vagina. In clinical studies using CLEOCIN Vaginal Ovules, treatment-related moniliasis was reported in 2.7% and vaginitis in 3.6% of 589 nonpregnant women. Moniliasis, as reported here, includes the terms: vaginal or nonvaginal moniliasis and fungal infection. Vaginitis includes the terms: vulvovaginal disorder, vaginal discharge, and vaginitis/vaginal infection.

Information for the Patient

The patient should be instructed not to engage in vaginal intercourse or use other vaginal products (such as tampons or douches) during treatment with this product.

The patient should also be advised that these suppositories use an oleaginous base that may weaken latex or rubber products such as condoms or vaginal contraceptive diaphragms. Therefore, the use of such products within 72 hours following treatment with CLEOCIN Vaginal Ovules is not recommended.

Drug Interactions

Clindamycin has been shown to have neuromuscular blocking properties that may enhance the action of other neuromuscular blocking agents. Therefore, it should be used with caution in patients receiving such agents.

Carcinogenesis, Mutagenesis, Impairment of Fertility

Long-term studies in animals have not been performed with clindamycin to evaluate carcinogenic potential. Genotoxicity tests performed included a rat micronucleus test and an Ames test. Both tests were negative. Fertility studies in rats treated orally with up to 300 mg/kg/day (31 times the human exposure based on mg/m^2) revealed no effects on fertility or mating ability.

Pregnancy: Teratogenic effects

Pregnancy Category B

There are no adequate and well-controlled studies of CLEOCIN Vaginal Ovules in pregnant women.

CLEOCIN Vaginal Cream, 2%, has been studied in pregnant women during the second trimester. In women treated for 7 days, abnormal labor was reported more frequently in patients who received CLEOCIN Vaginal Cream compared to those receiving placebo (1.1% vs. 0.5% of patients, respectively).

Reproduction studies have been performed in rats and mice using oral and parenteral doses of clindamycin up to 600 mg/kg/day (62 and 25 times, respectively, the maximum human dose based on mg/m^2) and have revealed no evidence of harm to the fetus due to clindamycin. Cleft palates were observed in fetuses from one mouse strain treated intraperitoneally with clindamycin at 200 mg/kg/day (about 10 times the recommended dose based on body surface area conversions). Since this effect was not observed in other mouse strains or in other species, the effect may be strain specific. CLEOCIN Vaginal Ovules should be used during pregnancy only if the potential benefit justifies the potential risk to the fetus.

Nursing Mothers

Clindamycin has been detected in human milk after oral or parenteral administration. It is not known if clindamycin is excreted in human milk following the use of vaginally administered clindamycin phosphate.

Because of the potential for serious adverse reactions in nursing infants from clindamycin phosphate, a decision should be made whether to discontinue nursing or to discontinue the drug, taking into account the importance of the drug to the mother.

Pediatric Use

The safety and efficacy of CLEOCIN Vaginal Ovules in the treatment of bacterial vaginosis in post-menarchal females have been established on the extrapolation of clinical trial data from adult women. When a post-menarchal adolescent presents to a health professional with bacterial vaginosis symptoms, a careful evaluation for sexually transmitted diseases and other risk factors for bacterial vaginosis should be considered. The safety and efficacy of CLEOCIN Vaginal Ovules in pre-menarchal females have not been established.

Geriatric Use

Clinical studies of CLEOCIN Vaginal Ovules did not include sufficient numbers of subjects aged 65 and over to determine whether they respond differently from younger subjects.

ADVERSE REACTIONS

Clinical Trials

In clinical trials, 3 (0.5%) of 589 nonpregnant women who received treatment with CLEOCIN Vaginal Ovules discontinued therapy due to drug-related adverse events. Adverse events judged to have a reasonable possibility of having been caused by clindamycin phosphate vaginal suppositories were reported for 10.5% of patients. Events reported by 1% or more of patients receiving CLEOCIN Vaginal Ovules were as follows:

Urogenital system: Vulvovaginal disorder (3.4%), vaginal pain (1.9%), and vaginal moniliasis (1.5%).

Body as a whole: Fungal infection (1.0%).

Other events reported by <1% of patients included:

Urogenital system: Menstrual disorder, dysuria, pyelonephritis, vaginal discharge, and vaginitis/vaginal infection.

Body as a whole: Abdominal cramps, localized abdominal pain, fever, flank pain, generalized pain, headache, localized edema, and moniliasis.

Digestive system: Diarrhea, nausea, and vomiting.

Skin: Nonapplication-site pruritis, rash, application-site pain, and application-site pruritis.

Other clindamycin formulations:

The overall systemic exposure to clindamycin from CLEOCIN Vaginal Ovules is substantially lower than the systemic exposure for therapeutic doses of oral clindamycin hydrochloride (two-fold to 20-fold lower) or parenteral clindamycin phosphate (40-fold to 50-fold lower) (see CLINICAL PHARMACOLOGY). Although these lower levels of exposure are less likely to produce the common reactions seen with oral or parenteral clindamycin, the possibility of these and other reactions cannot be excluded.

The following adverse reactions and altered laboratory tests have been reported with the **oral or parenteral** use of clindamycin and may also occur following administration of CLEOCIN Vaginal Ovules:

Gastrointestinal: Abdominal pain, esophagitis, nausea, vomiting, and diarrhea. (See WARNINGS.)

Hematopoietic: Transient neutropenia (leukopenia), eosinophilia, agranulocytosis, and thrombocytopenia have been reported. No direct etiologic relationship to concurrent clindamycin therapy could be made in any of these reports.

Hypersensitivity Reactions: Maculopapular rash and urticaria have been observed during drug therapy. Generalized mild to moderate morbilliform-like skin rashes are the most frequently reported of all adverse reactions. Rare instances of erythema multiforme, some resembling Stevens-Johnson syndrome, have been associated with clindamycin. A few cases of anaphylactoid reactions have been reported. If a hypersensitivity reaction occurs, the drug should be discontinued.

Liver: Jaundice and abnormalities in liver function tests have been observed during clindamycin therapy.

Musculoskeletal: Rare instances of polyarthritis have been reported.

Renal: Although no direct relationship of clindamycin to renal damage has been established, renal dysfunction as evidenced by azotemia, oliguria, and/or proteinuria has been observed in rare instances.

OVERDOSAGE

Vaginally applied clindamycin phosphate contained in CLEOCIN Vaginal Ovules could be absorbed in sufficient amounts to produce systemic effects (see WARNINGS and ADVERSE REACTIONS).

DOSAGE AND ADMINISTRATION

The recommended dose is one CLEOCIN Vaginal Ovule (containing clindamycin phosphate equivalent to 100 mg clindamycin per 2.5 g suppository) intravaginally per day, preferably at bedtime, for 3 consecutive days.

HOW SUPPLIED

CLEOCIN Vaginal Ovules are supplied as follows:

Carton of three suppositories with one applicator ..... NDC 0009-7667-01

Important Information: Store at 25 °C (77 °F); excursions permitted to 15–30 °C (59–86 °F) [see USP Controlled Room Temperature]. **Caution:** Avoid high humidity. See end of carton for the lot number and expiration date.

Rx only

Pharmacia & Upjohn Company
Kalamazoo, Michigan 49001, USA
August 1999 817 946 000
692166

Cleocin® Vaginal Ovules
clindamycin phosphate
vaginal suppositories
DIRECTIONS FOR USE

How do I use CLEOCIN Vaginal Ovules?

For vaginal use only. Do not take by mouth.

Use one CLEOCIN Vaginal Ovule daily, preferably at bedtime for 3 days in a row.

Read the full directions below before using.

Insertion with the applicator:

1. Remove the vaginal ovule from its packaging. (See Figure 1.)

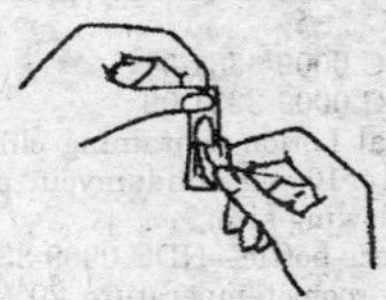

Figure 1

2. Pull back the plunger about an inch and place the vaginal ovule in the wider end of the applicator barrel. (See Figure 2.)

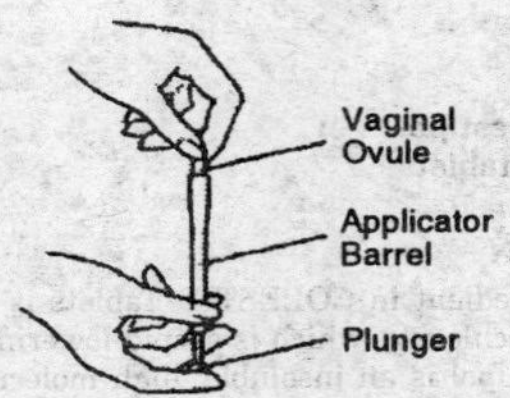

Figure 2

3. Hold the applicator as shown and gently insert the end of the applicator into the vagina as far as it will go comfortably. This can be done while lying on your back with your knees bent (as shown in Figure 3), or while standing with your feet apart and your knees bent.

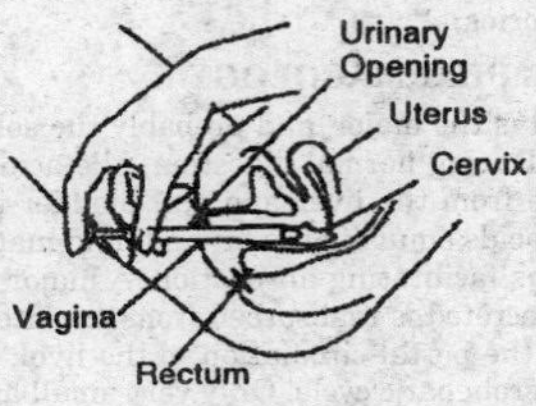

Figure 3

4. While holding the barrel of the applicator in place, push the plunger in until it stops to release the vaginal ovule. Remove the applicator form the vagina.
5. Clean the applicator after each use. Pull the two pieces apart and wash them with soap and warm water. Rinse well and dry. Put the two pieces back together and store in a clean, dry place.
6. Once inside the vagina, the ovule melts. Lie down as soon as possible. This will keep leakage to a minimum.
7. Repeat steps 1 through 6, before bedtime, for the next 2 days.

Insertion without the applicator:

1. Remove the vaginal ovule from its packaging. (See Figure 1.)
2. Holding the ovule with your thumb and a finger, insert it into the vagina.
3. Using your finger, gently push the ovule into the vagina as far as it will comfortably go.
4. Once inside the vagina, the ovule melts. Lie down as soon as possible. This will keep leakage to a minimum.
5. Repeat steps 1 through 4, before bedtime, for the next 2 days.

STORAGE CONDITIONS:

Store at 25 °C (77 °F); excursions permitted to 15–30 °C (59–86 °F) [see USP Controlled Room Temperature]. **Caution:** Avoid high humidity. See end of carton for the lot number and expiration date.

CLEOCIN T® ℞

[*clēō-sĭn*]

clindamycin phosphate topical solution, USP, topical gel, and topical lotion

For External Use

DESCRIPTION

CLEOCIN T Topical Solution and CLEOCIN T Topical Lotion contain clindamycin phosphate, USP, at a concentration equivalent to 10 mg clindamycin per milliliter. CLEOCIN T Topical Gel contains clindamycin phosphate, USP, at a concentration equivalent to 10 mg clindamycin per gram. Each CLEOCIN T Topical Solution pledget applicator contains approximately 1 mL of topical solution.

Clindamycin phosphate is a water soluble ester of the semi-synthetic antibiotic produced by a 7(S)-chloro-substitution of the 7(R)-hydroxyl group of the parent antibiotic lincomycin.

The solution contains isopropyl alcohol 50% v/v, propylene glycol, and water.

The gel contains allantoin, carbomer 934P, methylparaben, polyethylene glycol 400, propylene glycol, sodium hydroxide, and purified water.

The lotion contains cetostearyl alcohol (2.5%); glycerin; glyceryl stearate SE (with potassium monostearate); isostearyl alcohol (2.5%); methylparaben (0.3%); sodium lauroyl sarcosinate; stearic acid; and purified water.

The structural formula is represented below:

The chemical name for clindamycin phosphate is Methyl 7-chloro-6,7,8-trideoxy-6-(1-methyl-*trans*-4-propyl-L-2-pyrrolidinecarboxamido)-1-thio-L-*threo*-α-D-*galacto*-octopyranoside 2-(dihydrogen phosphate).

CLINICAL PHARMACOLOGY

Although clindamycin phosphate is inactive *in vitro*, rapid *in vivo* hydrolysis converts this compound to the antibacterially active clindamycin.

Cross resistance has been demonstrated between clindamycin and lincomycin.

Antagonism has been demonstrated between clindamycin and erythromycin.

Following multiple topical applications of clindamycin phosphate at a concentration equivalent to 10 mg clindamycin per mL in an isopropyl alcohol and water solution, very low levels of clindamycin are present in the serum (0–3 ng/mL) and less than 0.2% of the dose is recovered in urine as clindamycin.

Clindamycin activity has been demonstrated in comedones from acne patients. The mean concentration of antibiotic activity in extracted comedones after application of CLEOCIN T Topical Solution for 4 weeks was 597 mcg/g of comedonal material (range 0–1490). Clindamycin *in vitro* inhibits all *Propionibacterium acnes* cultures tested (MICs 0.4 mcg/mL). Free fatty acids on the skin surface have been decreased from approximately 14% to 2% following application of clindamycin.

INDICATIONS AND USAGE

CLEOCIN T Topical Solution, CLEOCIN T Topical Gel and CLEOCIN T Topical Lotion are indicated in the treatment of acne vulgaris. In view of the potential for diarrhea, bloody diarrhea and pseudomembranous colitis, the physician should consider whether other agents are more appropriate. (See CONTRAINDICATIONS, WARNINGS and ADVERSE REACTIONS.)

CONTRAINDICATIONS

CLEOCIN T Topical Solution, CLEOCIN T Topical Gel and CLEOCIN T Topical Lotion are contraindicated in individuals with a history of hypersensitivity to preparations containing clindamycin or lincomycin, a history of regional enteritis or ulcerative colitis, or a history of antibiotic-associated colitis.

WARNINGS

Orally and parenterally administered clindamycin has been associated with severe colitis which may result in patient death. Use of the topical formulation of clindamycin results in absorption of the antibiotic from the skin surface. Diarrhea, bloody diarrhea, and colitis (including pseudomembranous colitis) have been reported with the use of topical and systemic clindamycin.

Studies indicate a toxin(s) produced by clostridia is one primary cause of antibiotic-associated colitis. The colitis is usually characterized by severe persistent diarrhea and severe abdominal cramps and may be associated with the passage of blood and mucus. Endoscopic examination may reveal pseudomembranous colitis. Stool culture for *Clostridium difficile* and stool assay for *C. difficile* toxin may be helpful diagnostically.

When significant diarrhea occurs, the drug should be discontinued. Large bowel endoscopy should be considered to establish a definitive diagnosis in cases of severe diarrhea.

Antiperistaltic agents such as opiates and diphenoxylate with atropine may prolong and/or worsen the condition.

Continued on next page

Information on these Pharmacia & Upjohn products is based on labeling in effect June 1, 2000. Further information concerning these and other Pharmacia & Upjohn products may be obtained by direct inquiry to Medical Information, Pharmacia & Upjohn, Kalamazoo, MI 49001.

Cleocin T—Cont.

Vancomycin has been found to be effective in the treatment of antibiotic-associated pseudomembranous colitis produced by *Clostridium difficile*. The usual adult dosage is 500 milligrams to 2 grams of vancomycin orally per day in three to four divided doses administered for 7 to 10 days. Cholestyramine or colestipol resins bind vancomycin *in vitro*. If both a resin and vancomycin are to be administered concurrently, it may be advisable to separate the time of administration of each drug.
Diarrhea, colitis, and pseudomembranous colitis have been observed to begin up to several weeks following cessation of oral and parenteral therapy with clindamycin.

PRECAUTIONS

General
CLEOCIN T Topical Solution contains an alcohol base which will cause burning and irritation of the eye. In the event of accidental contact with sensitive surfaces (eye, abraded skin, mucous membranes), bathe with copious amounts of cool tap water. The solution has an unpleasant taste and caution should be exercised when applying medication around the mouth.
CLEOCIN T should be prescribed with caution in atopic individuals.
Drug Interactions
Clindamycin has been shown to have neuromuscular blocking properties that may enhance the action of other neuromuscular blocking agents. Therefore it should be used with caution in patients receiving such agents.
Pregnancy: Teratogenic effects—Pregnancy Category B
Reproduction studies have been performed in rats and mice using subcutaneous and oral doses of clindamycin ranging from 100 to 600 mg/kg/day and have revealed no evidence of impaired fertility or harm to the fetus due to clindamycin. There are, however, no adequate and well-controlled studies in pregnant women. Because animal reproduction studies are not always predictive of human response, this drug should be used during pregnancy only if clearly needed.
Nursing Mothers
It is not known whether clindamycin is excreted in human milk following use of CLEOCIN T. However, orally and parenterally administered clindamycin has been reported to appear in breast milk. Because of the potential for serious adverse reactions in nursing infants, a decision should be made whether to discontinue nursing or to discontinue the drug, taking into account the importance of the drug to the mother.
Pediatric Use
Safety and effectiveness is pediatric patients under the age of 12 have not been established.

ADVERSE REACTIONS

In 18 clinical studies of various formulations of CLEOCIN T using placebo vehicle and/or active comparator drugs as controls, patients experienced a number of treatment emergent adverse dermatologic events [see table below].

Number of Patients Reporting Events

Treatment Emergent Adverse Event	Solution n=553 (%)	Gel n=148 (%)	Lotion n=160 (%)
Burning	62 (11)	15 (10)	17 (11)
Itching	36 (7)	15 (10)	17 (11)
Burning/Itching	60 (11)	# (—)	# (—)
Dryness	105 (19)	34 (23)	29 (18)
Erythema	86 (16)	10 (7)	22 (14)
Oiliness/Oily Skin	8 (1)	26 (18)	12* (10)
Peeling	61 (11)	# (—)	11 (7)

\# not recorded
* of 126 subjects

Orally and parenterally administered clindamycin has been associated with severe colitis which may end fatally.
Cases of diarrhea, bloody diarrhea and colitis (including pseudomembranous colitis) have been reported as adverse reactions in patients treated with oral and parenteral formulations of clindamycin and rarely with topical clindamycin (see WARNINGS).
Abdominal pain and gastrointestinal disturbances as well as gram-negative folliculitis have also been reported in association with the use of topical formulations of clindamycin.

OVERDOSAGE

Topically applied CLEOCIN T can be absorbed in sufficient amounts to produce systemic effects. (See WARNINGS.)

DOSAGE AND ADMINISTRATION

Apply a thin film of CLEOCIN T Topical Solution, CLEOCIN T Topical Lotion, CLEOCIN T Topical Gel, or use a CLEOCIN T Topical Solution pledget for the application of CLEOCIN T twice daily to affected area. More than one pledget may be used. Each pledget should be used only once and then be discarded.
Lotion: Shake well immediately before using.
Pledget: Remove pledget from foil just before use. Do not use if the seal is broken. Discard after single use.
Keep all liquid dosage forms in containers tightly closed.

HOW SUPPLIED

CLEOCIN T Topical Solution containing clindamycin phosphate equivalent to 10 mg clindamycin per milliliter is available in the following sizes:
30 mL applicator bottle—NDC 0009-3116-01
60 mL applicator bottle—NDC 0009-3116-02
Carton of 60 single-use pledget applicators—NDC 0009-3116-14
CLEOCIN T Topical Gel containing clindamycin phosphate equivalent to 10 mg clindamycin per gram is available in the following sizes:
60 gram tube—NDC 0009-3331-01
30 gram tube—NDC 0009-3331-02
CLEOCIN T Topical Lotion containing clindamycin phosphate equivalent to 10 mg clindamycin per milliliter is available in the following size:
60 mL plastic squeeze bottle—NDC 0009-3329-01
Store at controlled room temperature 20° to 25°C (68° to 77°F) [see USP].
Protect from freezing.
Rx only
Pharmacia & Upjohn Company, Kalamazoo, MI 49001, USA
Revised March 1999 811 373 430
691223

Shown in Product Identification Guide, page 331

COLESTID® ℞

[*kō-less-tĭd*]
micronized colestipol hydrochloride tablets

DESCRIPTION

The active ingredient in COLESTID Tablets is micronized colestipol hydrochloride, which is a lipid lowering agent for oral use. Colestipol is an insoluble, high molecular weight basic anion-exchange copolymer of diethylenetriamine and 1-chloro-2, 3-epoxypropane, with approximately 1 out of 5 amine nitrogens protonated (chloride form). It is a light yellow water-insoluble resin which is hygroscopic and swells when suspended in water or aqueous fluids.
Each COLESTID Tablet contains one gram of micronized colestipol hydrochloride. COLESTID Tablets are light yellow in color and are tasteless and odorless. Inactive ingredients: cellulose acetate phthalate, glyceryl triacetate, carnauba wax, hydroxypropyl methylcellulose, magnesium stearate, povidone, silicon dioxide. COLESTID Tablets contain no calories.

CLINICAL PHARMACOLOGY

Cholesterol is the major, and probably the sole precursor of bile acids. During normal digestion, bile acids are secreted via the bile from the liver and gall bladder into the intestines. Bile acids emulsify the fat and lipid materials present in food, thus facilitating absorption. A major portion of the bile acids secreted is reabsorbed from the intestines and returned via the portal circulation to the liver, thus completing the enterohepatic cycle. Only very small amounts of bile acids are found in normal serum.
Colestipol hydrochloride binds bile acids in the intestine forming a complex that is excreted in the feces. This nonsystemic action results in a partial removal of the bile acids from the enterohepatic circulation, preventing their reabsorption. Since colestipol hydrochloride is an anion exchange resin, the chloride anions of the resin can be replaced by other anions, usually those with a greater affinity for the resin than the chloride ion.
Colestipol hydrochloride is hydrophilic, but it is virtually water insoluble (99.75%) and it is not hydrolyzed by digestive enzymes. The high molecular weight polymer in colestipol hydrochloride apparently is not absorbed. In humans, less than 0.17% of a single ^{14}C-labeled colestipol hydrochloride dose is excreted in the urine when given following 60 days of dosing of 20 grams of colestipol hydrochloride per day.
The increased fecal loss of bile acids due to colestipol hydrochloride administration leads to an increased oxidation of cholesterol to bile acids. This results in an increase in the number of low-density lipoprotein (LDL) receptors, increased hepatic uptake of LDL and a decrease in beta lipoprotein or LDL serum levels, and a decrease in serum cholesterol levels. Although colestipol hydrochloride produces an increase in the hepatic synthesis of cholesterol in man, serum cholesterol levels fall.
There is evidence to show that this fall in cholesterol is secondary to an increased rate of clearance of cholesterol-rich lipoproteins (beta or low-density lipoproteins) from the plasma. Serum triglyceride levels may increase or remain unchanged in colestipol hydrochloride treated patients.
The decline in serum cholesterol levels with colestipol hydrochloride treatment is usually evident by one month. When colestipol hydrochloride is discontinued, serum cholesterol levels usually return to baseline levels within one month. Periodic determinations of serum cholesterol levels as outlined in the National Cholesterol Education Program (NCEP) guidelines, should be done to confirm a favorable initial and long-term response.[1]
In a large, placebo-controlled, multiclinic study, the LRC-CPPT[2], hypercholesterolemic subjects treated with cholestyramine, a bile-acid sequestrant with a mechanism of action and an effect on serum cholesterol similar to that of colestipol hydrochloride, had reductions in total and LDL-C. Over the 7-year study period the cholestyramine group experienced a 19% reduction (relative to the incidence in the placebo group) in the combined rate of coronary heart disease (CHD) death plus nonfatal myocardial infarction (cumulative incidences of 7% cholestyramine and 8.6% placebo). The subjects included in the study were middle-aged men (aged 35–59) with serum cholesterol levels above 265 mg/dL, LDL-C above 175 mg/dL on a moderate cholesterol-lowering diet, and no history of heart disease. It is not clear to what extent these findings can be extrapolated to other segments of the hypercholesterolemic population not studied.
Treatment with colestipol results in a significant increase in lipoprotein LpAI. Lipoprotein LpAI is one of the two major lipoprotein particles within the high-density lipoprotein (HDL) density range[3], and has been shown in cell culture to promote cholesterol efflux or removal from cells[4]. Although the significance of this finding has not been established in clinical studies, the elevation of the lipoprotein LpAI patients within the HDL fraction is consistent with an anti-atherogenic effect of colestipol hydrochloride, even though little change is observed in HDL cholesterol (HDL-C).
In patients with heterozygous familial hypercholesterolemia who have not obtained an optimal response to colestipol hydrochloride alone in maximal doses, the combination of colestipol hydrochloride and nicotinic acid has been shown to further lower serum cholesterol, triglyceride, and LDL-cholesterol (LDL-C) values. Simultaneously, HDL-C values increased significantly. In many such patients it is possible to normalize serum lipid values.[5–7]
Preliminary evidence suggests that the cholesterol-lowering effects of lovastatin and the bile acid sequestrant, colestipol hydrochloride, are additive.
The effect of intensive lipid-lowering therapy on coronary atherosclerosis has been assessed by arteriography in hyperlipidemic patients. In these randomized, controlled clinical trials, patients were treated for two to four years by either conventional measures (diet, placebo, or in some cases low-dose resin), or with intensive combination therapy using diet and COLESTID Granules plus either nicotinic acid or lovastatin. When compared to conventional measures, intensive lipid-lowering combination therapy significantly reduced the frequency of progression and increased the frequency of regeression of coronary atherosclerotic lesions in patients with or at risk for coronary artery disease.[8–11]

INDICATIONS AND USAGE

Since no drug is innocuous, strict attention should be paid to the indications and contraindications, particularly when selecting drugs for chronic long-term use.
COLESTID Tablets are indicated as adjunctive therapy to diet for the reduction of elevated serum total and LDL-C in patients with primary hypercholesterolemia (elevated LDL-C) who do not respond adequately to diet. Generally, COLESTID Tablets have no clinically significant effect on serum triglycerides, but with their use, triglyceride levels may be raised in some patients.
Therapy with lipid-altering agents should be a component of multiple risk factor intervention in those individuals at significantly increased risk for atherosclerotic vascular disease due to hypercholesterolemia. Treatment should begin and continue with dietary therapy (see NCEP guidelines). A minimum of six months of intensive dietary therapy and counseling should be carried out prior to initiation of drug therapy. Shorter periods may be considered in patients with severe elevations of LDL-C or with definite CHD.
According to the NCEP guidelines, the goal of treatment is to lower LDL-C, and LDL-C is to be used to initiate and assess treatment response. Only if LDL-C levels are not available, should the Total-C be used to monitor therapy. The NCEP treatment guidelines are shown below.

		LDL-Cholesterol mg/dL (mmol/L)	
Definite Atherosclerotic Disease*	Two or More Other Risk Factors**	Initiation Level	Goal
No	No	≥190 (≥4.9)	<160 (<4.1)
No	Yes	≥160 (≥4.1)	<130 (<3.4)
Yes	Yes or No	≥130 (≥3.4)	≤100 (≤2.6)

*Coronary heart disease or peripheral vascular disease (including symptomatic carotid artery disease).
**Other risk factors for coronary heart disease (CHD) include: age (males: ≥45 years; female: ≥55 years or premature monopause without estrogen replacement therapy); family history of premature CHD; current cigarette smoking; hypertension; confirmed HDL-C <35 mg/dL (0.91 mmol/L); and diabetes mellitus. Subtract one risk factor if HDL-C is ≥60 mg/dL (1.6 mmol/L).

CONTRAINDICATIONS

COLESTID Tablets are contraindicated in those individuals who have shown hypersensitivity to any of their components.

PRECAUTIONS

Prior to initiating therapy with COLESTID Tablets, secondary causes of hypercholesterolemia (e.g., poorly controlled diabetes mellitus, hypothyroidism, nephrotic syndrome, dysproteinemias, obstructive liver disease, other drug therapy, alcoholism), should be excluded, and a lipid profile performed to assess total cholesterol, HDL-C and triglycerides

(TG). For individuals with TG less than 400 mg/dL (<4.5 mmol/L), LDL-C can be estimated using the following equation:

LDL-C = Total cholesterol – [(Triglycerides/5) + HDL-C]

For TG levels >400 mg/dL, this equation is less accurate and LDL-C concentrations should be determined by ultracentrifiguation. In hypertriglyceridemic patients, LDL-C may be low or normal despite elevated Total-C. In such cases COLESTID Tablets may not be indicated.

Because it sequesters bile acids, colestipol hydrochloride may interfere with normal fat absorption and, thus, may reduce absorption of folic acid and fat soluble vitamins such as A, D and K.

Chronic use of colestipol hydrochloride may be associated with an increased bleeding tendency due to hypoprothrombinemia from vitamin K deficiency. This will usually respond promptly to parenteral vitamin K_1 and recurrences can be prevented by oral administration of vitamin K_1.

Serum cholesterol and triglyceride levels should be determined periodically based on NCEP guidelines to confirm a favorable initial and adequate long-term response.

COLESTID Tablets may produce or severely worsen pre-existing constipation. The dosage should be increased gradually in patients to minimize the risk of developing fecal impaction. In patients with pre-existing constipation, the starting dose should be 2 grams once or twice a day. Increased fluid and fiber intake should be encouraged to alleviate constipation and a stool softener may occasionally be indicated. If the initial dose is well tolerated, the dose may be increased as needed by a further 2 to 4 grams/day (at monthly intervals) with periodic monitoring of serum lipoproteins. If constipation worsens or the desired therapeutic response is not achieved at 2 to 16 grams/day, combination therapy or alternate therapy should be considered. Particular effort should be made to avoid constipation in patients with symptomatic coronary artery disease. Constipation associated with COLESTID tablets may aggravate hemorrhoids.

While there have been no reports of hypothyroidism induced in individuals with normal thyroid function, the theoretical possibility exists, particularly in patients with limited thyroid reserve.

Since colestipol hydrochloride is a chloride form of an anion exchange resin, there is a possibility that prolonged use may lead to the development of hypercholeremia acidosis.

Carcinogenesis, Mutagenesis and Impairment of Fertility

In studies conducted in rats in which cholestyramine resin (a bile acid sequestering agent similar to colestipol hydrochloride) was used as a tool to investigate the role of various intstinal factors, such as fat, bile salts, and microbial flora, in the development of intestinal tumors induced by potent carcinogens, the incidence of such tumors was observed to be greater in cholestyramine resin treated rats than in control rats.

The relevance of this laboratory observation from studies in rats with cholestyramine resin to the clinical use of COLESTID Tablets is not known. In the LRC-CPPT study referred to above, the total incidence of fatal and nonfatal neoplasms was similar in both treatment groups. When the many different categories of tumors are examined, various alimentary system cancers were somewhat more prevalent in the cholestyramine group. The small numbers and the multiple categories prevent conclusions from being drawn. Further follow-up of the LRC-CPPT participants by the sponsors of that study is planned for cause-specific mortality and cancer morbidity. When colestipol hydrochloride was administered in the diet to rats for 18 months, there was no evidence of any drug related intestinal tumor formation. In the Ames assay, colestipol hydrochloride was not mutagenic.

Use in Pregnancy

Since colestipol hydrochloride is essentially not absorbed systemically (less than 0.17% of the dose), it is not expected to cause fetal harm when administered during pregnancy in recommended dosages. There are no adequate and well-controlled studies in pregnant women, and the known interference with absorption of fat-soluble vitamins may be detrimental even in the presence of supplementation.

Nursing Mothers: Caution should be exercised when COLESTID Tablets are administered to a nursing mother. The possible lack of proper vitamin absorption described in the "Pregnancy" section may have an effect on nursing infants.

Pediatric Use

Safety and effectiveness in the pediatric population have not been established.

Information for Patients

COLESTID Tablets may be larger than pills you have taken before. If you have had swallowing problems or choking with food, liquids or other tablets or capsules in the past, you should discuss this with your doctor before taking COLESTID Tablets.

It is important that you take COLESTID Tablets correctly:

1. Always take one tablet at a time and swallow promptly.
2. Swallow each tablet whole. Do not cut, crush, or chew the tablets.
3. COLESTID Tablets must be taken with water or another liquid that you prefer. Swallowing the tablets will be easier if you drink plenty of liquid as you swallow each tablet.

Difficulty swallowing and temporary obstruction of the esophagus (the tube between your mouth and stomach) have been rarely reported in patients taking COLESTID Tablets. If a tablet does get stuck after you swallow it, you may notice pressure or discomfort. If this happens to you, you should contact your doctor. Do not take COLESTID Tablets again without your doctor's advice.

If you are taking other medications, you should take them at least one hour before or four hours after taking COLESTID Tablets.

DRUG INTERACTIONS

Since colestipol hydrochloride is an anion exchange resin, it may have a strong affinity for anions other than the bile acids. *In vitro* studies have indicated that colestipol hydrochloride binds a number of drugs. Therefore, COLESTID Tablets may delay or reduce the absorption of concomitant oral medication. The interval between the administration of COLESTID Tablets and any other medication should be as long as possible. Patients should take other drugs at least one hour before or four hours after COLESTID Tablets to avoid impeding their absorption.

Repeating doses of colestipol hydrochloride given prior to a single dose of propranolol in human trials have been reported to decrease propranolol absorption. However, in a follow-up study in normal subjects, single-dose administration of colestipol hydrochloride and propranolol and twice-a-day administration for 5 days of both agents did not affect the extent of propranolol absorption, but had a small yet statistically significant effect on its rate of absorption; the time to reach maximum concentration was delayed approximately 30 minutes. Effects on the absorption of the other beta-blockers have not been determined. Therefore, patients on propranolol should be observed when COLESTID Tablets are either added or deleted from a therapeutic regimen.

Studies in human show that the absorption of chlorothiazide as reflected in urinary excretion is markedly decreased even when administered one hour before colestipol hydrochloride. The absorption of tetracycline, furosemide, penicillin G, hydrochlorothiazide, and gemfibrozil was significantly decreased when given simultaneously with colestipol hydrochloride; these drugs were not tested to determine the effect of administration one hour before colestipol hydrochloride.

No depressant effect on blood levels in humans was noted when colestipol hydrochloride was administered with any of the following drugs: aspirin, clindamycin, clofibrate, methyldopa, nicotinic acid (niacin), tolbutamide, phentyoin or warfarin. Particular caution should be observed with digitalis preparations since there are conflicting results for the effect of colestipol hydrochloride on the availability of digoxin and digitoxin. The potential for binding of these drugs if given concomitantly is present. Discontinuing colestipol hydrochloride could pose a hazard to health if a potentially toxic drug that is significantly bound to the resin has been titrated to a maintenance level while the patient was taking colestipol hydrochloride.

Bile acid binding resins may also interfere with the absorption of oral phosphate supplements and hydrocortisone.

ADVERSE EVENTS

Gastrointestinal

The most common adverse reactions are confined to the gastrointestinal tract. To achieve minimal GI disturbance with an optimal LDL-C lowering effect, a gradual increase of dosage starting with 2 grams, once or twice daily is recommended. Constipation is the major single complaint and at times is severe. Most instances of constipation are mild, transient, and controlled with standard treatment. Increased fluid intake and inclusion of additional dietary fiber should be the first step; a stool softener may be added if needed. Some patients require decreased dosage or discontinuation of therapy. Hemmorhoids may be aggravated.

Other, less frequent gastrointestinal complaints consist of abdominal discomfort (abdominal pain and cramping), intestinal gas (bloating and flatulence), indigestion and heartburn, diarrhea and loose stools, and nausea and vomiting. Bleeding hemorrhoids and blood in the stool have been infrequently reported. Peptic ulceration, cholecystitis, and cholelithiasis have been rarely reported in patients receiving colestipol hydrochloride granules, and are not necessarily drug related.

Difficulty swallowing and transient esophageal obstruction have been rarely reported in patients taking COLESTID Tablets.

Transient and modest elevations of aspartate aminotransferase (AST, SGOT), alanine aminotransferase (ALT, SGPT) and alkaline phosphatase were observed on one or more occasions in various patients treated with colestipol hydrochloride.

The following nasogastrointestinal adverse reactions have been reported with generally equal frequency in patients receiving COLESTID Tablets, colestipol granules, or placebo in clinical studies.

Cardiovascular

Chest pain, angina, and tachycardia have been infrequently reported.

Hypersensitivity

Rash has been infrequently reported. Urticaria and dermatitis have been rarely noted in patients receiving colestipol hydrochloride granules.

Musculoskeletal

Musculoskeletal pain, aches and pains in the extremities, joint pain and arthritis, and backache have been reported.

Neurologic

Headache, migraine headache, and sinus headache have been reported. Other infrequently reported complaints include dizziness, light-headedness, and insomnia.

Miscellaneous

Anorexia, fatigue, weakness, shortness of breath, and swelling of the hands or feet, have been infrequently reported.

OVERDOSAGE

Overdosage of COLESTID Tablets has not been reported. Should overdosage occur, however, the chief potential harm would be obstruction of the gastrointestinal tract. The location of such potential obstruction, the degree of obstruction and the presence or absence of normal gut motility would determine treatment.

DOSAGE AND ADMINISTRATION

For adults, COLESTID Tablets are recommended in doses of 2 to 16 grams/day once or in divided doses. The starting dose should be 2 grams once or twice daily. Dosage increases of 2 grams, once or twice daily should occur at 1- or 2-month intervals. Appropriate use of lipid profiles as per NCEP guidelines including LDL-C and triglycerides, is advised so that optimal but not excessive doses are used to obtain the desired therapeutic effect on LDL-C level. If the desired therapeutic effect is not obtained at a dose of 2 to 16 grams/day with good compliance and acceptable side effects, combined therapy or alternate treatment should be considered.

COLESTID Tablets must be taken one at a time and be promptly swallowed whole, using plenty of water or other appropriate liquid. Do not cut, crush, or chew the tablets. Patients should take other drugs at least one hour before or four hours after COLESTID Tablets to minimize possible interference iwth their absorption. (See DRUG INTERACTIONS.)

Before Administration of COLESTID Tablets

1. Define the type of hyperlipoproteinemia, as described in NCEP guidelines.
2. Institute a trial of diet and weight reduction.
3. Establish baseline serum total and LDL-C and triglyceride levels.

During Administration of COLESTID Tablets

1. The patient should be carefully monitored clinically, including serum cholesterol and triglyceride levels. Periodic determinations of serum cholesterol levels as outlined in the NCEP guidelines should be done to confirm a favorable initial and long-term response.
2. Failure of total or LDL-C to fall within the desired range should lead one to first examine dietary and drug compliance. If these are deemed acceptable, combined therapy or alternate treatment should be considered.
3. Significant rise in triglyceride level should be considered as indication for dose reduction, drug discontinuation, or combined or alternate therapy.

HOW SUPPLIED

COLESTID Tablets are yellow, elliptical, imprinted U, and are supplied as follows:

Bottles of 120	NDC 0009-0450-03
Bottles of 500	NDC 0009-0450-04

Each tablet contains 1 gram of colestipol hydrochloride.

Store at controlled room temperature 20° to 25° C (68° to 77° F) [see USP].

REFERENCES

1. Summary of the Second Report of the National Cholesterol Education Program (NCEP) Expert Panel on Detection, Evaluation, and Treatment of High Blood Cholesterol in Adults (Adult Treatment Panel II). *JAMA* 1993; 269(23):3015–3023.
2. Lipid Metabolism-Atherogenesis Branch, National Heart, Lung, and Blood Institute, Bethesda, MD: The Lipid Research Clinics Coronary Primary Prevention Trial Results. I. Reduction in Incidence of Coronary Heart Disease. *JAMA* 1984; 251:351–364.
3. Parra HJ, et al. Differential electroimmunoassay of human LpA-I lipoprotein particles on ready-to-use plates. *Clin. Chem.* 1990; 36(8):1431–1435.
4. Barbaras R, et al. Cholesterol efflux from cultured adipose cells is mediated by LpAl particles but not by LpAl: All particles. *Biochem. Biophys. Res. Comm.* 1987; 142(1):63–69.
5. Kane JP, et al. Normalization of low-density-lipoprotein levels in heterozygous familial hypercholesterolemia with a combined drug regimen. *N Engl J. Med.* 1981; 305:251–258.
6. Illingworth DR, et al. Colestipol plus nicotinic acid in treatment of heterozygous familial hypercholesterolemia. *Lancet* 1981; 1:296–298.
7. Kuo PT, et al. Familial type II hyperlipoprotenemia with coronary heart disease: Effect of diet-cholestipol-nicotinic acid treatment. *Chest* 1981; 79:286–291.
8. Blankenhorn DH, et al. Beneficial Effects of Combined Colestipol-Niacin Therapy on Coronary Atherosclerosis and Coronary Venous Bypass Grafts. *JAMA* 1987; 257(23):3233–3240.
9. Cashin-Hemphill L, et al. Beneficial Effects of Colestipol-Niacin on Coronary Atherosclerosis: A 4-Year Follow-up. *JAMA* 1990; 264:3013–3017.

Continued on next page

Information on these Pharmacia & Upjohn products is based on labeling in effect June 1, 2000. Further information concerning these and other Pharmacia & Upjohn products may be obtained by direct inquiry to Medical Information, Pharmacia & Upjohn, Kalamazoo, MI 49001.

Colestid—Cont.

10. Brown G. et al. Regression of Coronary Artery Disease as a Result of Intensive Lipid-Lowering Therapy in Men with High Levels of Apolipoprotein B. *N. Engl. J. Med.* 1990; 323:1289–1298.
11. Kane JP, et al. Regression of Coronary Atherosclerosis During Treatment of Familial Hypercholesterolemia with Combined Drug Regimens. *JAMA* 1990; 264:3007–3012.

Rx only
Pharmacia & Upjohn Company
Kalamazoo, MI 49001, USA
Revised February 1999 815 838 205
692166

CORVERT® ℞

[cŏr-vĕrt]
ibutilide fumarate injection
For intravenous infusion only

DESCRIPTION

CORVERT Injection (ibutilide fumarate injection) is an antiarrhythmic drug with predominantly class III (cardiac action potential prolongation) properties according to the Vaughan Williams Classification. Each milliliter of CORVERT Injection contains 0.1 mg of ibutilide fumarate (equivalent to 0.087 mg ibutilide free base), 0.189 mg sodium acetate trihydrate, 8.90 mg sodium chloride, hydrochloric acid to adjust pH to approximately 4.6, and Water for Injection.
CORVERT Injection is an isotonic, clear, colorless, sterile aqueous solution.
Ibutilide fumarate has one chiral center, and exists as a racemate of the (+) and (−) enantiomers.
The chemical name for ibutilide fumarate is Methanesulfonamide, N-{4-{4-(ethylheptylamino)-1-hydroxybutyl]-phenyl}, (+) (−), (E)-2-butenedioate (1:0.5) (hemifumarate salt). Its molecular formula is $C_{22}H_{38}N_2O_5S$, and its molecular weight is 442.62.
Ibutilide fumarate is a white to off-white powder with an aqueous solubility of over 100 mg/mL at pH 7 or lower.
The structural formula is represented below:

$CH_3-SO_2-NH-C_6H_4-CH(OH)-CH_2CH_2CH_2-N(CH_2CH_3)(CH_2(CH_2)_5CH_3)$ · 0.5 $HOOC-CH=CH-COOH$

Ibutilide Fumarate

CLINICAL PHARMACOLOGY

Mechanism of Action: CORVERT Injection prolongs action potential duration in isolated adult cardiac myocytes and increases both atrial and ventricular refractoriness *in vivo*, ie, class III electrophysiologic effects. Voltage clamp studies indicate that CORVERT, at nanomolar concentrations, delays repolarization by activation of a slow, inward current (predominantly sodium), rather than by blocking outward potassium currents, which is the mechanism by which most other class III antiarrhythmics act. These effects lead to prolongation of atrial and ventricular action potential duration and refractoriness, the predominant electrophysiologic properties of CORVERT in humans that are thought to be the basis for its antiarrhythmic effect.
Electrophysiologic Effects: CORVERT produces mild slowing of the sinus rate and atrioventricular conduction. CORVERT produces no clinically significant effect on QRS duration at intravenous doses up to 0.03 mg/kg administered over a 10-minute period. Although there is no established relationship between plasma concentration and antiarrhythmic effect, CORVERT produces dose-related prolongation of the QT interval, which is thought to be associated with its antiarrhythmic activity. (See WARNINGS for relationship between QTc prolongation and torsades de pointes-type arrhythmias.) In a study in healthy volunteers, intravenous infusions of CORVERT resulted in prolongation of the QT interval that was directly correlated with ibutilide plasma concentration during and after 10-minute and 8-hour infusions. A steep ibutilide concentration/response (QT prolongation) relationship was shown. The maximum effect was a function of both the dose of CORVERT and the infusion rate.
Hemodynamic Effects: A study of hemodynamic function in patients with ejection fractions both above and below 35% showed no clinically significant effects on cardiac output, mean pulmonary arterial pressure, or pulmonary capillary wedge pressure at doses of CORVERT up to 0.03 mg/kg.
Pharmacokinetics: After intravenous infusion, ibutilide plasma concentrations rapidly decrease in a multiexponential fashion. The pharmacokinetics of ibutilide are highly variable among subjects. Ibutilide has a high systemic plasma clearance that approximates liver blood flow (about 29 mL/min/kg), a large steady-state volume of distribution (about 11 L/kg) in healthy volunteers, and minimal (about 40%) protein binding. Ibutilide is also cleared rapidly and highly distributed in patients being treated for atrial flutter or atrial fibrillation. The elimination half-life averages about 6 hours (range from 2 to 12 hours). The pharmacokinetics of ibutilide are linear with respect to the dose of CORVERT over the dose range of 0.01 mg/kg to 0.10 mg/kg. The enantiomers of ibutilide fumarate have pharmacokinetic properties similar to each other and to ibutilide fumarate. The pharmacokinetics of CORVERT Injection in patients with atrial flutter or atrial fibrillation are similar regardless of the type of arrhythmia, patient age, sex, or the concomitant use of digoxin, calcium channel blockers, or beta blockers.
Metabolism and elimination: In healthy male volunteers, about 82% of a 0.01 mg/kg dose of [^{14}C] ibutilide fumarate was excreted in the urine (about 7% of the dose as unchanged ibutilide) and the remainder (about 19%) was recovered in the feces.
Eight metabolites of ibutilide were detected in metabolic profiling of urine. These metabolites are thought to be formed primarily by ω-oxidation followed by sequential β-oxidation of the heptyl side chain of ibutilide. Of the eight metabolites, only the ω-hydroxy metabolite possesses class III electrophysiologic properties similar to that of ibutilide in an *in vitro* isolated rabbit myocardium model. The plasma concentrations of this active metabolite, however, are less than 10% of that of ibutilide.
Clinical Studies: Treatment with intravenous ibutilide fumarate for acute termination of recent onset atrial flutter/fibrillation was evaluated in 466 patients participating in two randomized, double-blind, placebo-controlled clinical trials. Patients had had their arrhythmias for 3 hours to 90 days, were anticoagulated for at least 2 weeks if atrial fibrillation was present more than 3 days, had serum potassium of at lest 4.0 mEq/L and QTc below 440 msec, and were monitored by telemetry for at least 24 hours. Patients could not be on class I or other class III antiarrhythmics (these had to be discontinued at least 5 half-lives prior to infusion) but could be on calcium channel blockers, beta blockers, or digoxin. In one trial, single 10-minute infusions of 0.005 to 0.025 mg/kg were tested in parallel groups (0.3 to 1.5 mg in a 60 kg person). In the second trial, up to two infusions of ibutilide fumarate were evaluated—the first 1.0 mg, the second given 10 minutes after completion of the first infusion, either 0.5 or 1.0 mg. In a third double-blind study, 319 patients with atrial fibrillation or atrial flutter of 3 hours to 45 days duration were randomized to receive single, 10-minute intravenous infusions of either sotalol (1.5 mg/kg) or CORVERT (1 mg or 2 mg). Among patients with atrial flutter, 53% receiving 1 mg ibutilide fumarate and70% receiving 2 mg ibutilide fumarate converted, compared to 18% of those receiving sotalol. In patients with atrial fibrillation, 22% receiving 1 mg ibutilide fumarate and 43% receiving 2 mg ibutilide fumarate converted compared to 10% of patients receiving sotalol.
Patients in registration trials were hemodynamically stable. Patients with specific cardiovascular conditions such as symptomatic heart failure, recent acute myocardial infarction, and angina were excluded. About two thirds had cardiovascular symptoms, and the majority of patients had left atrial enlargement, decreased left ventricular ejection fraction, a history of valvular disease, or previous history of atrial fibrillation or flutter. Electrical cardioversion was allowed 90 minutes after the infusion was complete. Patients could be given other antiarrhythmic drugs 4 hours postinfusion.
Results of the first two studies are shown in the tables below. Conversion of atrial flutter/fibrillation usually (70% of those who converted) occurred within 30 minutes of the start of infusion and was dose related. The latest conversion seen was at 90 minutes after the start of the infusion. Most converted patients remained in normal sinus rhythm for 24 hours. Overall responses in these patients, defined as termination of arrhythmias for any length of time during or within 1 hour following completed infusion of randomized dose, were in the range of 43% to 48% at doses above 0.0125 mg/kg (vs 2% for placebo). Twenty-four hour responses were similar. For these atrial arrhythmias, ibutilide was more effective in patients with flutter than fibrillation (≥48% vs ≤40%).

PERCENT OF PATIENTS WHO CONVERTED (First Trial)

			Ibutilide			
		Placebo	0.005 mg/kg	0.01 mg/kg	0.015 mg/kg	0.025 mg/kg
	n	41	41	40	38	40
Both	Initially*	2	12	33	45	48
	At 24 hours†	2	12	28	42	43
Atrial flutter	Initially*	0	14	30	58	55
	At 24 hours†	0	14	30	58	50
Atrial fibrillation	Initially*	5	10	35	32	40
	At 24 hours†	5	10	25	26	35

* Percent of patients who converted within 70 minutes after the start of infusion.
† Percent of patients who remained in sinus rhythm 24 hours after dosing.

PERCENT OF PATIENTS WHO CONVERTED (Second Trial)

			Ibutilide	
		Placebo	1.0 mg/0.5 mg	1.0 mg/1.0 mg
	n	86	86	94
Both	Initially*	2	43	44
	At 24 hours†	2	34	37
Atrial flutter	Initially*	2	48	63
	At 24 hours†	2	45	59
Atrial fibrillation	Initially*	2	38	25
	At 24 hours†	2	21	17

* Percent of patients who converted within 90 minutes after the start of infusion.
† Percent of patients who remained in sinus rhythm 24 hours after dosing.

[See first table above]
[See second table above]
The numbers of patients who remained in the converted rhythm at the end of 24 hours were slightly less than those patients who converted initially, but the difference between conversion rates for ibutilide compared to placebo was still statistically significant. In long-term follow-up, approximately 40% of all patients remained recurrence free, usually with chronic prophylactic treatment, 400 to 500 days after acute treatment, regardless of the method of conversion.
Patients with more recent onset of arrhythmia had a higher rate of conversion. Response rates were 42% and 50% for patients with onset of atrial fibrillation/flutter for less than 30 days in the two efficacy studies compared to 16% and 31% in those with more chronic arrhythmias.
Ibutilide was equally effective in patients below and above 65 years of age and in men and women. Female patients constituted about 20% of patients in controlled studies.
Post-cardiac Surgery: In a double-blind, parallel group study, 302 patients with atrial fibrillation (n=201) or atrial flutter (n=101) that occurred 1 to 7 days after coronary artery bypass graft or valvular surgery and lasted 1 hour to 3 days were randomized to receive two 10-minute infusions of placebo, or 0.25, 0.5 or 1 mg of ibutilide fumarate. Among patients with atrial flutter, conversion rates at 1.5 hours were: placebo, 4%; 0.25 mg ibutilide fumarate, 56%; 0.5 ibutilide fumarate, 61%; and 1 mg ibutilide fumarate, 78%. Among patients with atrial fibrillation, conversion rates at 1.5 hours were: placebo, 20%; 0.25 mg ibutilide fumarate, 28%; 0.5 mg ibutilide fumarate, 42%, and 1 mg ibutilide fumarate, 44%. The majority of patients (53% and 72% in the 0.5-mg and 1-mg dose groups, respectively) converted to sinus rhythm remained in sinus rhythm for 24 hours. Patients were not given other antiarrhythmic drugs within 24 hours of ibutilide fumarate infusion in this study.

INDICATIONS AND USAGE

CORVERT Injection is indicated for the rapid conversion of atrial fibrillation or atrial flutter of recent onset to sinus rhythm. Patients with atrial arrhythmias of longer duration are less likely to respond to CORVERT. The effectiveness of ibutilide has not been determined in patients with arrhythmias of more than 90 days in duration.

LIFE-THREATENING ARRHYTHMIAS—APPROPRIATE TREATMENT ENVIRONMENT
CORVERT can cause potentially fatal arrhythmias, particularly sustained polymorphic ventricular tachycardia, usually in association with QT prolongation (torsades de pointes), but sometimes without documented QT prolongation. In registration studies, these arrhythmias, which require cardioversion, occurred in 1.7% of treated patients during, or within a number of hours of, use of CORVERT. These arrhythmias can be reversed if treated promptly (see WARNINGS, Proarrhythmia). It is essential that CORVERT be administered in a setting of continuous ECG monitoring and by personnel trained in identification and treatment of acute ventricular arrhythmias, particularly polymorphic ventricular tachycardia. *Patients with atrial fibrillation of more than 2 to 3 days' duration must be adequately anticoagulated, generally for at least 2 weeks.*

CHOICE OF PATIENTS
Patients with chronic atrial fibrillation have a strong tendency to revert after conversion to sinus rhythm (see CLINICAL STUDIES) and treatments to maintain sinus rhythm carry risks. Patients to be treated with CORVERT, therefore, should be carefully selected such that the expected benefits of maintaining sinus rhythm outweigh the immediate risks of CORVERT, and the risks of maintenance therapy, and are likely to offer an advantage compared with alternative management.

CONTRAINDICATIONS

CORVERT Injection is contraindicated in patients who have previously demonstrated hypersensitivity to ibutilide fumarate or any of the other product components.

WARNINGS

Proarrhythmia: Like other antiarrhythmic agents, CORVERT Injection can induce or worsen ventricular arrhythmias in some patients. This may have potentially fatal consequences. Torsades de pointes, a polymorphic ventricular tachycardia that develops in the setting of a prolonged QT interval, may occur because of the effect CORVERT has on cardiac repolarization, but CORVERT can also cause polymorphic VT in the absence of excessive prolongation of the QT interval. In general, with drugs that prolong the QT interval, the risk of torsades de pointes is thought to increase progressively as the QT interval is prolonged and may be worsened with bradycardia, a varying heart rate, and hypokalemia. In clinical trials conducted in patients with atrial fibrillation and atrial flutter, those with QTc intervals >440 msec were not usually allowed to participate, and serum potassium had to be above 4.0 mEq/L. Although change in QTc was dose dependent for ibutilide, there was no clear relationship between risk of serious proarrhythmia and dose in clinical studies, possibly due to the small number of events. In clinical trials of intravenous ibutilide, patients with a history of congestive heart failure (CHF) or low left ventricular ejection fraction appeared to have a higher incidence of sustained polymorphic ventricular tachycardia (VT), than those without such underlying conditions; for sustained polymorphic VT the rate was 5.4% in patients with a history of CHF and 0.8% without it. There was also a suggestion that women had a higher risk of proarrhythmia, but the sex difference was not observed in all studies and was most prominent for nonsustained ventricular tachycardia. The incidence of sustained ventricular arrhythmias was similar in male (1.8%) and female (1.5%) patients, possibly due to the small number of events. CORVERT is not recommended in patients who have previously demonstrated polymorphic ventricular tachycardia (eg, torsades de pointes).

During reigstration trials, 1.7% of patients with atrial flutter or atrial fibrillation treated with CORVERT developed sustained polymorphic ventricular tachycardia requiring cardioversion. In these clinical trials, many initial episodes of polymorphic ventricular tachycardia occurred after the infusion of CORVERT was stopped but generally not more than 40 minutes after the start of the first infusion. There were, however, instances of recurrent polymorphic VT that occurred about 3 hours after the initial infusion. In two cases, the VT degenerated into ventricular fibrillation, requiring immediate defibrillation. Other cases were managed with cardiac pacing and magnesium sulfate infusions. Nonsustained polymorphic ventricular tachycardia occurred in 2.7% of patients and nonsustained monomorphic ventricular tachycardias occurred in 4.9% of the patients (see ADVERSE REACTIONS).

Proarrhythmic events must be anticipated. Skilled personnel and proper equipment, including cardiac monitoring equipment, intracardiac pacing facilities, a cardioverter/defibrillator, and medication for treatment of sustained ventricular tachycardia, including polymorphic ventricular tachycardia, must be available during and after administration of CORVERT. Before treatment with CORVERT, hypokalemia and hypomagnesemia should be corrected to reduce the potential for proarrhythmia. Patients should be observed with continuous ECG monitoring for at least 4 hours following infusion or until QTc has returned to baseline. Longer monitoring is required if any arrhythmic activity is noted. Management of polymorphic ventricular tachycardia includes discontinuation of ibutilide, correction of electrolyte abnormalities, especially potassium and magnesium, and overdrive cardiac pacing, electrical cardioversion, or defibrillation. Pharmacologic therapies include magnesium sulfate infusions. Treatment with antiarrhythmics should generally be avoided.

Recommended Dose of CORVERT Injection

Patient Weight	*Initial Infusion (over 10 minutes)*	*Second Infusion*
60 kg (132 lb) or more	*One vial (1 mg ibutilide fumarate)*	*If the arrhythmia does not terminate within 10 minutes after the end of the initial infusion, a second 10-minute infusion of equal strength may be administered 10 minutes after completion of the first infusion.*
Less than 60 kg (132 lb)	*0.1 mL/kg (0.01 mg/kg ibutilide fumarate)*	

PRECAUTIONS

General

Antiarrhythmics: Class Ia antiarrhythmic drugs (Vaughan Williams Classification), such as disopyramide, quinidine, and procainamide, and other class III drugs, such as amiodarone and sotalol, should not be given concomitantly with CORVERT Injection or within 4 hours postinfusion because of their potential to prolong refractoriness. In the clinical trials, class I or other class III antiarrhythmic agents were withheld for at least 5 half-lives prior to ibutilide infusion and for 4 hours after dosing, but thereafter were allowed at the physician's discretion.

Other drugs that prolong the QT interval: The potential for proarrhythmia may increase with the administration of CORVERT Injection to patients who are being treated with drugs that prolong the QT interval, such as phenothiazines, tricyclic antidepressants, tetracyclic antidepressants, and certain antihistamine drugs (H_1 receptor antagonists).

Heart block: Of the nine (1.5%) ibutilide-treated patients with reports of reversible heart block, five had first degree, three had second degree, and one had complete heart block.

Laboratory Test Interactions: None known.

Drug Interactions: No specific pharmacokinetic or other formal drug interaction studies were conducted.

Digoxin: Supraventricular arrhythmias may mask the cardiotoxicity associated with excessive digoxin levels. Therefore, it is advisable to be particularly cautious in patients whose plasma digoxin levels are above or suspected to be above the usual therapeutic range. Coadministration of digoxin did not have effects on either the safety or efficacy of ibutilide in the clinical trials.

Calcium channel blocking agents: Coadministration of calcium channel blockers did not have any effect on either the safety or efficacy of ibutilide in the clinical trials.

Beta-adrenergic blocking agents: Coadministration of beta-adrenergic blocking agents did not have any effect on either the safety or efficacy of ibutilide in the clinical trials.

Carcinogenesis, Mutagenesis, Impairment of Fertility: No animal studies have been conducted to determine the carcinogenic potential of CORVERT; however, it was not genotoxic in a battery of assays, (Ames assay, mammalian cell forward gene mutation assay, unscheduled DNA synthesis assay, and mouse micronucleus assay). Similarly, no drug-related effects on fertility or mating were noted in a reproductive study in rats in which ibutilide was administered orally to both sexes up to doses of 20 mg/kg/day. On a mg/m^2 basis, corrected for 3% bioavailability, the highest dose tested was approximately four times the maximum recommended human dose (MRHD).

Pregnancy: Pregnancy Category C. Ibutilide administered orally was teratogenic (abnormalities included adactyly, interventricular septal defects, and scoliosis) and embryocidal in reproduction studies in rats. On a mg/m^2 basis, corrected for the 3% oral bioavailability, the "no adverse effect dose" (5 mg/kg/day given orally) was approximately the same as the maximum recommended human dose (MRHD); the teratogenic dose (20 mg/kg/day given orally) was about four times the MRHD on a mg/m^2 basis, or 16 times the MRHD on a mg/kg basis. CORVERT should not be administered to a pregnant woman unless clinical benefit outweighs potential risk to the fetus.

Nursing Mothers: The excretion of ibutilide into breast milk has not been studied; accordingly, breastfeeding should be discouraged during therapy with CORVERT.

Pediatric Use: Clinical trials with CORVERT in patients with atrial fibrillation and atrial flutter did not include anyone under the age of 18. Safety and effectiveness of ibutilide in pediatric patients has not been established.

Geriatric Use: The mean age of patients in clinical trials was 65. No age-related differences were observed in pharmacokinetic, efficacy, or safety parameters for patients less than 65 compared to patients 65 years and older.

Use in Patients With Hepatic or Renal Dysfunction: The safety, effectiveness, and pharmacokinetics of CORVERT have not been established in patients with hepatic or renal dysfunction. However, it is unlikely that dosing adjustments would be necessary in patients with compromised renal or hepatic function based on the following considerations: (1) CORVERT is indicated for rapid intravenous therapy (duration ≤30 minutes) and is dosed to a known, well-defined pharmacologic action (termination of arrhythmia) or to a maximum of two 10-minute infusions; (2) less than 10% of the dose of CORVERT is excreted unchanged in the urine; and (3) drug distribution appears to be one of the primary mechanisms responsible for termination of the pharmacologic effect. Nonetheless, patients with abnormal liver function should be monitored by telemetry for more than the 4-hour period generally recommended.

In 285 patients with atrial fibrillation or atrial flutter who were treated with CORVERT, the clearance of ibutilide was independent of renal function, as assessed by creatinine clearance (range 21 to 140 mL/min).

ADVERSE REACTIONS

CORVERT Injection was generally well tolerated in clinical trials. Of the 586 patients with atrial fibrillation or atrial flutter who received CORVERT in phase II/III studies, 149 (25%) reported medical events related to the cardiovascular system, including sustained polymorphic ventricular tachycardia (1.7%) and nonsustained polymorphic ventricular tachycardia (2.7%).

Other clinically important adverse events with an uncertain relationship to CORVERT include the following (0.2% represents one patient): sustained monomorphic ventricular tachycardia (0.2%), nonsustained monomorphic ventricular tachycardia (4.9%), AV block (1.5%), bundle branch block (1.9%), ventricular extrasystoles (5.1%), supraventricular extrasystoles (0.9%), hypotension/postural hypotension (2.0%), bradycardia/sinus bradycardia (1.2%), nodal arrhythmia (0.7%), congestive heart failure (0.5%), tachycardia/sinus tachycardia/supraventricular tachycardia (2.7%), idioventricular rhythm (0.2%), syncope (0.3%), and renal failure (0.3%). The incidence of these events, except for syncope, was greater in the group treated with CORVERT than in the placebo group.

Another adverse reaction that may be associated with the administration of CORVERT was nausea, which occurred with a frequency greater than 1% more in ibutilide-treated patients than those treated with placebo.

The medical events reported for more than 1% of the placebo- and ibutilide-treated patients are shown in the following Table.

Treatment-Emergent Medical Events With Frequency of More Than 1% and Higher Than That of Placebo

Event	Placebo N=127		All Ibutilide N=586	
	Patients		Patients	
	n	%	n	%
CARDIOVASCULAR				
Ventricular extrasystoles	1	0.8	30	5.1
Nonsustained monomorphic VT	1	0.8	29	4.9
Nonsustained polymorphic VT	—	—	16	2.7
Hypotension	2	1.6	12	2.0
Bundle branch block	—	—	11	1.9
Sustained polymorphic VT	—	—	10	1.7
AV block	1	0.8	9	1.5
Hypertension	—	—	7	1.2
QT segment prolonged	—	—	7	1.2
Bradycardia	1	0.8	7	1.2
Palpitation	1	0.8	6	1.0
Tachycardia	1	0.8	16	2.7
GASTROINTESTINAL				
Nausea	1	0.8	11	1.9
CENTRAL NERVOUS SYSTEM				
Headache	4	3.1	21	3.6

In the post-cardiac surgery study (see CLINICAL STUDIES), similar types of medical events were reported. In the 1 mg ibutilide fumarate treatment group (N=70), 2 patients (2.9%) developed sustained polymorphic ventricular tachycardia and 2 other patients (2.9%) developed nonsustained polymorphic ventricular tachycardia. Polymorphic ventricular tachycardia was not reported in the 73 patients in the 0.5 mg dose group or in the 75 patients in the 0.25 mg dose group.

OVERDOSAGE

Acute Experience in Animals: Acute overdose in animals results in CNS toxicity; notably, CNS depression, rapid gasping breathing, and convulsions. The intravenous median lethal dose in the rat was more than 50 mg/kg which is, on a mg/m^2 basis, at least 250 times the maximum recommended human dose.

Human Experience: In the registration trials with COVERT injection, four patients were unintentionally overdosed. The largest dose was 3.4 mg administered over 15

Continued on next page

Information on these Pharmacia & Upjohn products is based on labeling in effect June 1, 2000. Further information concerning these and other Pharmacia & Upjohn products may be obtained by direct inquiry to Medical Information, Pharmacia & Upjohn, Kalamazoo, MI 49001.

Corvert—Cont.

minutes. One patient (0.025 mg/kg) developed increased ventricular ectopy and monomorphic ventricular tachycardia, another patient (0.032 mg/kg) developed AV block—3rd degree and nonsustained polymorphic VT, and two patients (0.038 and 0.020 mg/kg) had no medical event reports. Based on known pharmacology, the clinical effects of an overdosage with ibutilide could exaggerate the expected prolongation of repolarization seen at usual clinical doses. Medical events (eg, proarrhythmia, AV block) that occur after the overdosage should be treated with measures appropriate for that condition.

DOSAGE AND ADMINISTRATION

The recommended dose based on controlled trials (see CLINICAL STUDIES) is outlined in the Table below. Ibutilide infusion should be stopped as soon as the presenting arrhythmia is terminated or in the event of sustained or nonsustained ventricular tachycardia, or marked prolongation of QT or QTc.

[See table at top of previous page]

In a trial comparing ibutilide and sotalol (see CLINICAL STUDIES), 2 mg ibutilide fumarate administered as a single infusion to patients weighing more than 60 kg was also effective in terminating atrial fibrillation or atrial flutter.

In the post-cardiac surgery study (see CLINICAL STUDIES), one or two intravenous infusions of 0.5 mg (0.005 mg/kg per dose for patients weighing less than 60 kg) was effective in terminating atrial fibrillation or atrial flutter.

Patients should be observed with continuous ECG monitoring for at least 4 hours following infusion or until QTc has returned to baseline. Longer monitoring is required if any arrhythmic activity is noted. Skilled personnel and proper equipment (see WARNINGS, Proarrhythmia), such as a cardioverter/defibrillator, and medication for treatment of sustained ventricular tachycardia, including polymorphic ventricular tachycardia, must be available during administration of CORVERT and subsequent monitoring of the patient.

Dilution: CORVERT Injection may be administered undiluted or diluted in 50 mL of diluent. CORVERT may be added to 0.9% Sodium Chloride Injection or 5% Dextrose Injection before infusion. The contents of one 10 mL vial (0.1 mg/mL) may be added to a 50 mL infusion bag to form an admixture of approximately 0.017 mg/mL ibutilide fumarate. Parenteral drug products should be inspected visually for particulate matter and discoloration prior to administration whenever solution and container permit.

Compatibility and Stability: The following diluents are compatible with CORVERT Injection (0.1 mg/mL):

5% Dextrose Injection

0.9% Sodium Chloride Injection

The following intravenous solution containers are compatible with admixtures of CORVERT Injection (0.1 mg/mL):

polyvinyl chloride plastic bags

polyolefin bags

Admixtures of the product, with approved diluents, are chemically and physically stable for 24 hours at room temperature (15° to 30° C or 59° to 86° F) and for 48 hours at refrigerated temperatures (2° to 8°C or 36° to 46°F). Strict adherence to the use of aseptic technique during the preparation of the admixture is recommended in order to maintain sterility.

HOW SUPPLIED

CORVERT Injection (ibutilide fumarate injection) is supplied as an acetate-buffered isotonic solution at a concentration of 0.1 mg/mL that has been adjusted to approximately pH 4.6 in 10 mL clear glass, single-dose, flip-top vials.

Single-dose 10 mL vial,
1 mg/10 mL (0.1 mg/mL) NDC 0009-3794-01

Store at controlled room temperature 20° to 25°C (68° to 77°F) [see USP]. Store vial in carton until used.

Rx only

Pharmacia & Upjohn Company • Kalamazoo, Michigan 49001, USA

Revised May 1999 816 418 003
691659

DEPO-MEDROL® ℞

[depō' mĕ-drōl]

methylprednisolone acetate injectable suspension, USP

Not For Intravenous Use

DESCRIPTION

DEPO-MEDROL Sterile Aqueous Suspension contains methylprednisolone acetate which is the 6-methyl derivative of prednisolone. Methylprednisolone acetate is a white or practically white, odorless, crystalline powder which melts at about 215° with some decomposition. It is soluble in dioxane, sparingly soluble in acetone, in alcohol, in chloroform, and in methanol, and slightly soluble in ether. It is practically insoluble in water. The chemical name for methylprednisolone acetate is pregna-1,4-diene-3,20-dione, 21-(acetyloxy)-11,17-dihydroxy-6-methyl-, (6α, 11β)-and the molecular weight is 416.51. The structural formula is represented below:

DEPO-MEDROL is an anti-inflammatory glucocorticoid for intramuscular, intrasynovial, soft tissue or intralesional injection. It is available in three strengths: 20 mg/mL; 40 mg/mL; 80 mg/mL.

Each mL of these preparations contains:

Methylprednisolone acetate	20 mg	40 mg	80 mg
Polyethylene glycol 3350	29.5 mg	29.1 mg	28.2 mg
Polysorbate 80	1.97 mg	1.94 mg	1.88 mg
Monobasic sodium phosphate	6.9 mg	6.8 mg	6.59 mg
Dibasic sodium phosphate USP	1.44 mg	1.42 mg	1.37 mg
Benzyl alcohol added as a preservative	9.3 mg	9.16 mg	8.88 mg

Sodium Chloride was added to adjust tonicity.

When necessary, pH was adjusted with sodium hydroxide and/or hydrochloric acid.

The pH of the finished product remains within the USP specified range; ie, 3.5 to 7.0.

ACTIONS

Naturally occurring glucocorticoids (hydrocortisone), which also have salt retaining properties, are used in replacement therapy in adrenocortical deficiency states. Their synthetic analogs are used primarily for their potent anti-inflammatory effects in disorders of many organ systems.

Glucocorticoids cause profound and varied metabolic effects. In addition, they modify the body's immune response to diverse stimuli.

As of November, 1990, the formulation for DEPO-MEDROL Sterile Aqueous Suspension was revised. In a bioavailability study with thirty subjects, the new formulation was found to be more bioavailable than the previous formulation. An increase in the extent of methylprednisolone absorption was observed for the new formulation as indicated by significantly increased values for area under the serum methylprednisolone concentration curve and maximum serum methylprednisolone concentration (see table below). No difference in elimination half-life ($t_{1/2}$, calculated from the mean terminal elimination rate) was observed between the two formulations. No medically meaningful differences between the two formulations were seen in relation to vital signs, safety laboratory analyses, formulation effects, local tolerance, or side effects. This increase in absorption is not considered clinically significant.

	Previous Formulation	*Current Formulation*
AUC 0–240 hrs (ng × hr/mL)	1053 (47.3)* [133–2297]**	1286 (39.2) [208–2225]
C_{MAX} (ng/mL)	8.98 (65.9) [0–28.5]	11.8 (44.1) [3.37–23.4]
$t_{1/2}$ (hr)	139 [46–990]	139 [58–866]

* Coefficient of variation (%)
** Range of values

INDICATIONS

A. FOR INTRAMUSCULAR ADMINISTRATION

When oral therapy is not feasible and the strength, dosage form, and route of administration of the drug reasonably lend the preparation to the treatment of the condition, the intramuscular use of DEPO-MEDROL Sterile Aqueous Suspension is indicated as follows:

1. **Endocrine Disorders**
   Primary or secondary adrenocortical insufficiency (hydrocortisone or cortisone is the drug of choice; synthetic analogs may be used in conjunction with mineralocorticoids where applicable; in infancy, mineralocorticoid supplementation is of particular importance)
   Acute adrenocortical insufficiency (hydrocortisone or cortisone is the drug of choice; mineralocorticoid supplementation may be necessary, particularly when synthetic analogs are used)
   Preoperatively and in the event of serious trauma or illness, in patients with known adrenal insufficiency or when adrenocortical reserve is doubtful:
   Congenital adrenal hyperplasia
   Hypercalcemia associated with cancer
   Nonsuppurative thyroiditis
2. **Rheumatic Disorders**
   As adjunctive therapy for short-term administration (to tide the patient over an acute episode or exacerbation) in:
   Post-traumatic osteoarthritis
   Synovitis of osteoarthritis
   Rheumatoid arthritis, including juvenile rheumatoid arthritis (selected cases may require low-dose maintenance therapy)
   Acute and subacute bursitis
   Epicondylitis
   Acute nonspecific tenosynovitis
   Acute gouty arthritis
   Psoriatic arthritis
   Ankylosing spondylitis
3. **Collagen Diseases**
   During an exacerbation or as maintenance therapy in selected cases of:
   Systemic lupus erythematosus
   Systemic dermatomyositis (polymyositis)
   Acute rheumatic carditis
4. **Dermatologic Diseases**
   Pemphigus
   Severe erythema multiforme (Stevens-Johnson syndrome)
   Exfoliative dermatitis
   Bullous dermatitis herpetiformis
   Severe seborrheic dermatitis
   Severe psoriasis
   Mycosis fungoides
5. **Allergic States**
   Control of severe or incapacitating allergic conditions intractable to adequate trials of conventional treatment in:
   Bronchial asthma
   Contact dermatitis
   Atopic dermatitis
   Serum sickness
   Seasonal or perennial allergic rhinitis
   Drug hypersensitivity reactions
   Urticarial transfusion reactions
   Acute noninfectious laryngeal edema (epinephrine is the drug of first choice)
6. **Ophthalmic Diseases**
   Severe acute and chronic allergic and inflammatory processes involving the eye, such as:
   Herpes zoster ophthalmicus
   Iritis, iridocyclitis
   Chorioretinitis
   Diffuse posterior uveitis and choroiditis
   Optic neuritis
   Sympathetic ophthalmia
   Anterior segment inflammation
   Allergic conjunctivitis
   Allergic corneal marginal ulcers
   Keratitis
7. **Gastrointestinal Diseases**
   To tide the patient over in a critical period of the disease in:
   Ulcerative colitis (systemic therapy)
   Regional enteritis (systemic therapy)
8. **Respiratory Diseases**
   Symptomatic sarcoidosis
   Berylliosis
   Fulminating or disseminated pulmonary tuberculosis when used concurrently with appropriate antituberculous chemotherapy
   Loeffler's syndrome not manageable by other means
   Aspiration pneumonitis
9. **Hematologic Disorders**
   Acquired (autoimmune) hemolytic anemia
   Secondary thrombocytopenia in adults
   Erythroblastopenia (RBC anemia)
   Congenital (erythroid) hypoplastic anemia
10. **Neoplastic Diseases**
   For palliative management of:
   Leukemias and lymphomas in adults
   Acute leukemia of childhood
11. **Edematous States**
   To induce diuresis or remission of proteinuria in the nephrotic syndrome, without uremia, of the idiopathic type or that due to lupus erythematosus
12. **Nervous System**
   Acute exacerbations of multiple sclerosis
13. **Miscellaneous**
   Tuberculous meningitis with subarachnoid block or impending block when used concurrently with appropriate antituberculous chemotherapy
   Trichinosis with neurologic or myocardial involvement

B. FOR INTRASYNOVIAL OR SOFT TISSUE ADMINISTRATION (See WARNINGS).

DEPO-MEDROL is indicated as adjunctive therapy for short-term administration (to tide the patient over an acute episode or exacerbation) in:
Synogitis of osteoarthritis
Rheumatoid arthritis
Acute and subacute bursitis
Acute gouty arthritis
Epicondylitis
Acute nonspecific tenosynovitis
Post-traumatic osteoarthritis

C. FOR INTRALESIONAL ADMINISTRATION

DEPO-MEDROL is indicated for intralesional use in the following conditions:
Keloids

Localized hypertrophic, infiltrated, inflammatory lesions of:
lichen planus, psoriatic plaques, granuloma annulare, and lichen simplex chronicus (neurodermatitis)
Discoid lupus erythematosus
Necrobiosis lipoidica diabetirocum
Alopecia areata
DEPO-MEDROL also may be useful in cystic tumors of an aponeurosis or tendon (ganglia).

CONTRAINDICATIONS

DEPO-MEDROL Sterile Aqueous Suspension is contraindicated for intrathecal administration. Reports of severe medical events have been associated with this route of administration. DEPO-MEDROL is contraindicated for use in premature infants because the formulation contains benzyl alcohol. Benzyl alcohol has been reported to be associated with a fatal "gasping syndrome" in premature infants. DEPO-MEDROL is also contraindicated in systemic fungal infections and patients with known hypersensitivity to the product and its constitutents.

WARNINGS

This product contains benzyl alcohol which is potentially toxic when administered locally to neural tissue.

Multidose use of DEPO-MEDROL Sterile Aqueous Suspension from a single vial requires special care to avoid contamination. Although initially sterile, any multidose use of vials may lead to contamination unless strict aseptic technique is observed. Particular care, such as use of disposable sterile syringes and needles is necessary.

While crystals of adrenal steroids in the dermis suppress inflammatory reactions, their presence may cause disintegration of the cellular elements and physiochemical changes in the ground substance of the connective tissue. The resultant infrequently occurring dermal and/or subdermal changes may form depressions in the skin at the injection site. The degree to which this reaction occurs will vary with the amount of adrenal steroid injected. Regeneration is usually complete within a few months or after all crystals of the adrenal steroid have been absorbed.

In order to minimize the incidence of dermal and subdermal atrophy, care must be exercised not to exceed rcommended doses in injections. Multiple small injections into the area of the lesion should be made whenever possible. The technique of intrasynovial and intramuscular injection should include precautions against injection or leakage into the dermis. Injection into the deltoid muscle should be avoided because of a high incidence of subcutaneous atrophy.

It is critital that, during administration of DEPO-MEDROL, appropriate technique be used and care taken to assure proper placement of drug.

In patients on corticosteroid therapy subjected to any unusual stress, increased dosage of rapidly acting corticosteroids before, during, and after the stressful situation is indicated.

Corticosteroids may mask some signs of infection, and new infections may appear during their use. There may be decreased resistance and inability to localize infection when corticosteroids are used. Infections with any pathogen including viral, bacterial, fungal, protozoan or helminthic infections, in any location of the body, may be associated with the use of corticosteroids alone or in combination with other immunosuppressive agents that affect cellular immunity, humoral immunity, or neutrophil function.[1]

These infections may be mild, but can be severe and at times fatal. With increasing doses of corticosteroids, the rate of occurrence of infectious complications increases.[2] Do not use intra-articularly, intrabursally or for intratendinous administration for *local* effect in the presence of acute infection.

Prolonged use of corticosteroids may produce posterior subcapsular cataracts, glaucoma with possible damage to the optic nerves, and may enhance the establishment of secondary ocular infections due to fungi or viruses.

Usage in pregnancy. Since adequate human reproduction studies have not been done with corticosteroids, the use of these drugs in pregnancy, nursing mothers, or women of childbearing potential requires that the possible benefits of the drug be weighed against the potential hazards to the mother and embryo or fetus. Infants born of mothers who have received substantial doses of corticosteroids during pregnancy should be carefully observed for signs of hypoadrenalism.

Average and large doses of cortisone or hydrocortisone can cause elevation of blood pressure, salt and water retention, and increased excretion of potassium. These effects are less likely to occur with the synthetic derivatives except when used in large doses. Dietary salt and restriction and potassium supplementation may be necessary. All corticosteroids increase calcium excretion.

Administration of live or live, attenuated vaccines is contraindicated in patients receiving immunosuppressive doses of corticosteroids. Killed or inactivated vacines may be administrated to patients receiving immunosuppressive doses of corticosteroids; however, the response to such vaccines may be diminished. Indicated immunization procedures may be undertaken in patients receiving nonimmunosuppressive doses of corticosteroids.

The use of DEPO-MEDROL in active tuberculosis should be restricted to those cases of fulminating or disseminated tuberculosis in which the corticosteroid is used for the management of the disease in conjunction with appropriate antituberculous regimen.

If corticosteroids are indicated in patients with latent tuberculosis or tuberculin reactivity, close observation is necessary as a reactivation of the disease may occur. During prolonged corticosteroids therapy, these patients should receive chemoprophylaxis.

Because rare instances of anaphylactoid reactions have occurred in patients receiving prenatal corticosteroid therapy, appropriate precautionary measures should be taken prior to administration, especially when the patient has a history of allergy to any drug.

Patients who are on drugs which suppress the immune system are more susceptible to infections than healthy individuals. Chicken pox and measles, for example, can have a more serious or even fatal course in non-immune children or adults on corticosteroids. In such children or adults who have not had these diseases, particular care should be taken to avoid exposure. How the dose, route and duration of corticosteroid administration affects the risk of developing a disseminated infection is not known. The contribution of the underlying disease and/or prior corticosteroid treatment to the risk is also not known. If exposed to chicken pox, prophylaxis with varicella zoster immune globulin (VZIG) may be indicated. If exposed to measles, prophylaxis with pooled intramuscular immunoglobulin (IG) may be indicated. (See the respective package inserts for complete VZIG and IG prescribing information.) If chicken pox develops, treatment with antiviral agents may be considered. Similarly, corticosteroids should be used with great care in patients with known or suspected Strongyloides (threadworm) infection. In such patients, corticosteroid-inuced immunosuppression may lead to Strongyloides hyperinfection and dissemination with widespread larval migration, often accompanied by severe enterocolitis and potentially fatal gram-negative septicemia.

PRECAUTIONS

General precautions

Drug-induced secondary adrenocortical insufficiency may be minimized by gradual reducton of dosage. This type of relative insufficiency may persist for months after discontinuation of therapy; therefore, in any situation of stress occurring during that period, hormone therapy should be reinstituted. Since mineralocorticoid secretion may be impaired, salt and/or a mineralocorticoid should be administered concurrently.

When multidose vials are used, special care to prevent contamination of the contents is essential. There is some evidence that benzalkonium chloride is not an adequate antiseptic for sterilizing DEPO-MEDROL Sterile Aqueous Suspension multidose vials. A povidone-iodine solution or similar product is recommended to cleanse the vial top prior to aspiration of contents (See WARNINGS.)

There is an enhanced effect of corticosteroids in patients with hypothyroidism and in those with cirrhosis.

Corticosteroids should be used cautiously in patients with ocular herpes simplex for fear of corneal perforation.

The lowest possible dose of corticosteroid should be used to control the condition under treatment, and when reduction in dosage is possible, the reduction must be gradual.

Psychic derangements may appear when corticosteroids are used, ranging from euphoria, insomnia, mood swings, personality changes, and severe depression to frank psychotic manifestations. Also, existing emotional instability or psychotic tendencies may be aggravated by corticosteroids.

Steroids should be used with caution in nonspecific ulcerative colitis, if there is a probability of impending perforation, abscess or other pyogenic infection. Caution must also be used in diverticulitis, fresh intestinal anastomoses, active or latent peptic ulcer, renal insufficiency, hyertension, osteoprosis, and myasthenia gravis, when steroids are used as direct or adjunctive therapy.

Growth and development of infants and children on prolonged corticosteroid therapy should be carefully followed.

Kaposi's sarcoma has been reported to occur in patients receiving corticosteroid therapy. Discontinuation of corticosteroids may result in clinical remission.

The following additional precautions apply for parenteral corticosteroids. Intrasynovial injection of a corticosteroid may produce systemic as well as local effects.

Appropriate examination of any joint fluid present is necessary to exclude a septic process.

A marked increse in pain accompanied by local swelling, further restriction of joint motion, fever, and malaise are suggestive of septic arthritis. If this complication occurs and the diagnosis of sepsis is confirmed, appropriate antimicrobial therapy should be instituted.

Local injection of a steroid into a previously infected joint is to be avoided.

Corticosteroids should not be injected into unstable joints.

The slower rate of absorption by intramuscular administration should be recognized.

Although controlled clinical trials have shown corticosteroids to be effective in speeding the resolution of acute exacerbations of multiple sclerosis, they do not show that corticosteroids affect the ultimate outcome or natural history of the disease. The studies do show that relatively high doses of corticosteroids are necessary to demonstrate a significant effect. (See DOSAGE AND ADMINISTRATION.)

Since complications of treatment with glucocorticoids are dependent on the size of the dose and the duration of treatment, a risk/benefit decision must be made in each individual case as to dose and duration of treatment and as to whether daily or intermittent therapy should be used.

DRUG INTERACTIONS:

The pharmacokinetic interactions listed below are potentially clinically important. Mutual inhibition of metabolism occurs with concurrent use of cyclosporin and methylprednisolone; therefore, it is possible that adverse events associated with the individual use of either drug may be more apt to occur. Convulsions have been reported with concurrent use of methylprednisolone and cyclosporin. Drugs that induce hepatic enzymes such as phenobarbital, phenytoin and rifampin may increase the clearance of methylprednisolone and may require increases in methylprednisolone dose to achieve the desired response. Drugs such as troleandomycin and ketoconazole may inhibit the metabolism of methylprednisolone and thus decrease its clearance. Therefore, the dose of methylprednisolone should be titrated to avoid steroid toxicity.

Methylprednisolone may increase the clearance of chronic high dose aspirin. This could lead to decreased salicylate serum levels or increase the risk of salicylate toxicity when methylprednisolone is withdrawn. Aspirin should be used cautiously in conjunction with corticosteroids in patients suffering from hypoprothrombinemia.

The effect of methylprednisolone on oral anticoagulants is variable. There are reprots of enhanced as well as diminished effects of anticoagulant when given concurrently with corticosteroids. Therefore, coagulation indices should be monitored to maintain the desired anticoagulant effect.

Information for the Patient

Persons who are on immunosuppressant doses of corticosteroids should be warned to avoid exposure to chicken pox or measles. Patients should also be advised that if they are exposed, medical advice should be sought without delay.

ADVERSE REACTIONS

Fluid and electrolyte disturbances
Sodium retention
Fluid retention
Congestive heart failure in susceptible patients
Potassium loss
Hypokalemic alkalosis
Hypertension

Musculoskeletal
Muscle weakness
Steroid myopathy
Loss of muscle mass
Osteoporosis
Tendon rupture, particularly of the Achilles tendon
Vertebral compression fractures
Aseptic necrosis of femoral and humeral heads
Pathologic fracture of long bones

Gastrointestinal
Peptic ulcer with possible subsequent perforation and hemorrhage
Pancreatitis
Abdominal distention
Ulcerative esophagitis
Increases in alanine transaminase (ALT, SGPT), aspartate transaminase (AST, SGOT), and alkaline phosphatase have been observed following corticosteroid treatment. These changes are usually small, not associated with any clinical syndrome and are reversible upon discontinuation.

Dermatologic
Impaired wound healing
Thin fragile skin
Petehiae and ecchymoses
Facial erythema
Increased sweating
May suppress reactions to skin tests

Neurological
Convulsions
Increased intracranial pressure with papilledema (pseudotumor cerebri) usually after treatment
Vertigo
Headache

Endocrine
Menstrual irregularities
Development of Cushingoid state
Suppression of growth in children
Secondary adrenocortical and pituitary unresponsiveness, particularly in times of stress, as in trauma, surgery or illness
Decreased carbohydrate tolerance
Manifestations of latent diabetes mellitus
Increased requirements for insulin or oral hypoglycemic agents in diabetes

Ophthalmic
Posterior subcapsular cataracts
Increased intraocular pressure
Glaucoma
Exophthalmos

Metabolic
Negative nitrogen balance due to protein catabolism

The following *additional* adverse reactions are related to parenteral corticosteroid therapy:
Anaphylactic reaction

Continued on next page

Information on these Pharmacia & Upjohn products is based on labeling in effect June 1, 2000. Further information concerning these and other Pharmacia & Upjohn products may be obtained by direct inquiry to Medical Information, Pharmacia & Upjohn, Kalamazoo, MI 49001.

Depo-Medrol—Cont.

Allergic or hypersensitivity reactions
Urticaria
Hyperpigmentation or hypopigmentation
Subcutaneous and cutaneous atrophy
Sterile abscess
Injection site infections following non-sterile administration (see WARNINGS)
Postinjection flare, following intrasynovial use
Charcot-like atrophy

Adverse Reactions Reported with the Following Routes of Administration

Intrathecal/Epidural
Arachnoiditis
Meningitis
Paraparesis/paraplegia
Sensory disturbances
Bowel/bladder dysfunction
Headaches
Seizures

Intranasal
Temporary/permanent visual impairment including blindness
Allergic reactions
Rhinitis

Ophthalmic
Temporary/permanent visual impairment including blindness
Increased intraocular pressure
Ocular and periocular inflammation including allergic reactions
Infection
Residue or slough at injection site

Miscellaneous injection sites (scalp, tonsillar fauces, sphenopalatine ganglion)-blindness

DOSAGE AND ADMINISTRATION

Because of possible physical incompatibilities, DEPO-MEDROL Sterile Aqueous Suspension should not be diluted or mixed with other solutions.

A. Administration for Local Effect

Therapy with DEPO-MEDROL does not obviate the need for the conventional measures usually employed. Although this method of treatment will ameliorate symptoms, it is in no sense a cure and the hormone has no effect on the cause of the inflammation.

1. Rheumatoid and Osteoarthritis. The dose for intra-articular administration depends upon the size of the joint and varies with the severity of the condition in the individual patient. In chronic cases, injections may be repeated at intervals ranging from one to five or more weeks depending upon the degree of relief obtained from the initial injection. The doses in the following table are given as a general guide:

Size of Joint	*Examples*	*Range of Dosage*
Large	Knees Ankles Shoulders	20 to 80 mg
Medium	Elbows Wrists	10 to 40 mg
Small	Metacarpophalangeal Interphalangeal Sternoclavicular Acromioclavicular	4 to 10 mg

Procedure: It is recommended that the anatomy of the joint involved be reviewed before attempting intra-articular injection. In order to obtain the full anti-inflammatory effect it is important that the injection be made into the synovial space. Employing the same sterile technique as for a lumbar puncture, a sterile 20 to 24 gauge needle (on a dry syringe) is quickly inserted into the synovial cavity. Procaine infiltration is elective. The aspiration of only a few drops of joint fluid proves the joint space has been entered by the needle. *The injection site for each joint is determined by that location where the synovial cavity is most superficial and most free of large vessels and nerves.* With the needle in place, the aspirating syringe is removed and replaced by a second syringe containing the desired amount of DEPO-MEDROL. The plunger is then pulled outward slightly to aspirate synovial fluid and to make sure the needle is still in the synovial space. After injection, the joint is moved gently a few times to aid mixing of the synovial fluid and the suspension. The site is covered with a small sterile dressing.

Suitable sites for intra-articular injection are the knee, ankle, wrist, elbow, shoulder, phalangeal, and hip joints. Since difficulty is not infrequently encountered in entering the hip joint, precautions should be taken to avoid any large blood vessels in the area. Joints not suitable for injection are those that are anatomically inaccessible such as the spinal joints and those like the sacroiliac joints that are devoid of synovial space. Treatment failures are most frequently the result of failure to enter the joint space. Little or no benefit follows injection into surrounding tissue. If failures occur when injections into the synovial spaces are certain, as determined by aspiration of fluid, repeated injections are usually futile. Local therapy does not alter the underlying disease process, and whenever possible comprehensive therapy including physiotherapy and orthopedic correction should be employed.

Following intra-articular steroid therapy, care should be taken to avoid overuse of joints in which symptomatic benefit has been obtained. Negligence in this matter may permit an increase in joint deterioration that will more than offset the beneficial effects of the steroid.

Unstable joints should not be injected. Repeated intra-articular injection may in some cases result in instability of the joint. X-ray follow-up is suggested in selected cases to detect deterioration.

If a local anesthetic is used prior to injection of DEPO-MEDROL, the anesthetic package insert should be read carefully and all the precautions observed.

2. Bursitis. The area around the injection site is prepared in a sterile way and a wheal at the site made with 1 percent procaine hydrochloride solution. A 20 to 24 gauge needle attached to a dry syringe is inserted into the bursa and the fluid aspirated. The needle is left in place and the aspirating syringe changed for a small syringe containing the desired dose. After injection, the needle is withdrawn and a small dressing applied.

3. Miscellaneous: Ganglion, Tendinitis, Epicondylitis. In the treatment of conditions such as tendinitis or tenosynovitis, care should be taken, following application of a suitable antiseptic to the overlying skin, to inject the suspension into the tendon sheath rather than into the substance of the tendon. The tendon may be readily palpated when placed on a stretch. When treating conditions such as epicondylitis, the area of the greatest tenderness should be outlined carefully and the suspension infiltrated into the area. For ganglia of the tendon sheaths, the suspension is injected directly into the cyst. In many cases, a single injection causes a marked decrease in the size of the cystic tumor and may effect disappearance. The usual sterile precautions should be observed, of course, with each injection.

The dose in the treatment of the various conditions of the tendinous or bursal structures listed above varies with the condition being treated and ranges from 4 to 30 mg. In recurrent or chronic conditions, repeated injections may be necessary.

4. Injections for Local Effect in Dermatologic Conditions. Following cleansing with an appropriate antiseptic such as 70% alcohol, 20 to 60 mg of the suspension is injected into the lesion. It may be necessary to distribute doses ranging from 20 to 40 mg by repeated local injections in the case of large lesions. Care should be taken to avoid injection of sufficient material to cause blanching since this may be followed by a small slough. One to four injections are usually employed, the intervals between injections varying with the type of lesion being treated and the duration of improvement produced by the initial injection.

When multidose vials are used, special care to prevent contamination of the contents is essential. (See WARNINGS.)

B. Administration for Systemic Effect.

The intramuscular dosage will vary with the condition being treated. When employed as a temporary substitute for oral therapy, a single injection during each 24-hour period of a dose of the suspension equal to the total daily oral dose of MEDROL® Tablets (methylprednisolone) is usually sufficient. When a prolonged effect is desired, the weekly dose may be calculated by multiplying the daily oral dose by 7 and given as a single intramuscular injection.

Dosage must be individualized according to the severity of the disease and response of the patient. For infants and children, the recommended dosage will have to be reduced, but dosage should be governed by the severity of the condition rather than by strict adherence to the ratio indicated by age or body weight.

Hormone therapy is an adjunct to, and not a replacement for, conventional therapy. Dosage must be decreased or discontinued gradually when the drug has been administered for more than a few days. The severity, prognosis and expected duration of the disease and the reaction of the patient to medication are primary factors in determining dosage. If a period of spontaneous remission occurs in a chronic condition, treatment should be discontinued. Routine laboratory studies, such as urinalysis, two-hour postprandial blood sugar, determination of blood pressure and body weight, and a chest X-ray should be made at regular intervals during prolonged therapy. Upper GI X-rays are desirable in patients with an ulcer history or significant dyspepsia.

In patients with the **adrenogenital syndrome,** a single intramuscular injection of 40 mg every two weeks may be adequate. For maintenance of patients with **rheumatoid arthritis,** the weekly intramuscular dose will vary from 40 to 120 mg. The usual dosage for patients with **dermatologic lesions** benefited by systemic corticoid therapy is 40 to 120 mg of methylprednisolone acetate administered intramuscularly at weekly intervals for one to four weeks. In acute severe dermatitis due to poison ivy, relief may result within 8 to 12 hours following intramuscular administration of a single dose of 80 to 120 mg. In chronic contact dermatitis repeated injections at 5 to 10 day intervals may be necessary. In seborrheic dermatitis, a weekly dose of 80 mg may be adequate to control the condition.

Following intramuscular administration of 80 to 120 mg to asthmatic patients, relief may result within 6 to 48 hours and persist for several days to two weeks. Similarly in patients with allergic rhinitis (hay fever) an intramuscular dose of 80 to 120 mg may be followed by relief of coryzal symptoms within six hours persisting for several days to three weeks.

If signs of stress are associated with the condition being treated, the dosage of the suspension should be increased. If a rapid hormonal effect of maximum intensity is required, the intravenous administration of highly soluble methylprednisolone sodium succinate is indicated.

Multiple Sclerosis

In the treatment of acute exacerbations of multiple sclerosis daily doses of 200 mg of prednisolone for a week followed by 80 mg every other day for 1 month have been shown to be effective (4 mg of methylprednisolone is equivalent to 5 mg of presnisolone).

HOW SUPPLIED

DEPO-MEDROL Sterile Aqueous Suspension is available in the following strengths and package sizes:

20 mg per mL	
5 mL vials	NDC 0009-0274-01
40 mg per mL	
5 mL vials	NDC 0009-0280-02
25 × 5 mL vials	NDC 0009-0280-51
10 mL vials	NDC 0009-0280-03
25 × 10 mL vials	NDC 0009-0280-52
80 mg per mL	
5 mL vials	NDC 0009-0306-02
25 × 5 mL vials	NDC 0009-0306-12

Store at controlled room temperature 20° to 25°C (68° to 77°F) [see USP].

REFERENCES

[1]Fekety R. Infections associated with corticosteroids and immunosuppressive therapy. In: Gorbach SL, Bartlett JG, Blacklow NR, eds. *Infectious Diseases.* Philadelphia: WBSaunders Company 1992:1050–1.

[2]Stuck AE, Minder CE, Frey FJ. Risk of infectious complications in patients taking glucocorticoids. *Rev Infect Dis* 1989:11(6):954–63.

Rx only

Pharmacia & Upjohn Company • Kalamazoo, Michigan 49001, USA

810 341 327

Revised March 1999 691211

DEPO-PROVERA® ℞

[*dep-ō-prō-vera*]

Contraceptive Injection
medroxyprogesterone acetate injectable suspension, USP

Patients should be counseled that this product does not protect against HIV infection (AIDS) and other sexually transmitted diseases.

DESCRIPTION

DEPO-PROVERA Contraceptive Injection contains medroxyprogesterone acetate, a derivative of progesterone, as its active ingredient. Medroxyprogesterone acetate is active by the parenteral and oral routes of administration. It is a white to off-white, odorless crystalline powder that is stable in air and that melts between 200°C and 210°C. It is freely soluble in chloroform, soluble in acetone and dioxane, sparingly soluble in alcohol and methanol, slightly soluble in ether, and insoluble in water.

The chemical name for medroxyprogesterone acetate is pregn-4-ene-3,20-dione, 17-(acetyloxy)-6-methyl-, (6α)-. The structural formula is as follows:

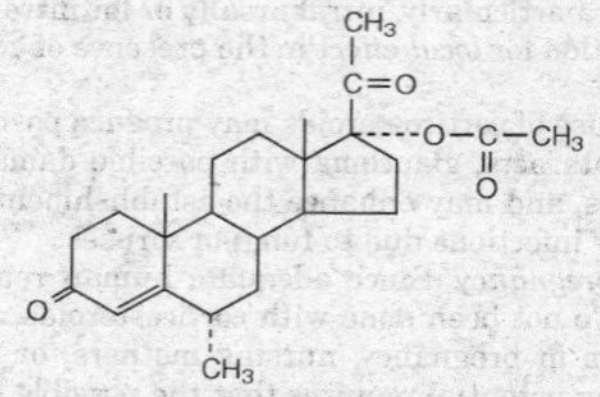

DEPO-PROVERA Contraceptive Injection for intramuscular (IM) injection is available in vials and prefilled syringes, each containing 1 mL of medroxyprogesterone acetate sterile aqueous suspension 150 mg/mL.

Each mL contains:	
Medroxyprogesterone acetate	150 mg
Polyethylene glycol 3350	28.9 mg
Polysorbate 80	2.41 mg
Sodium chloride	8.68 mg
Methylparaben	1.37 mg
Propylparaben	0.150 mg
Water for injection	qs

When necessary, pH is adjusted with sodium hydroxide or hydrochloric acid, or both.

CLINICAL PHARMACOLOGY

DEPO-PROVERA Contraceptive Injection (medroxyprogesterone acetate), when administered at the recommended dose to women every 3 months, inhibits the secretion of gonadotropins which, in turn, prevents follicular maturation and ovulation and results in endometrial thinning. These actions produce its contraceptive effect.

Following a single 150 mg IM dose of DEPO-PROVERA Contraceptive Injection, medroxyprogesterone acetate concentrations, measured by an extracted radioimmunoassay procedure, increase for approximately 3 weeks to reach peak plasma concentrations of 1 to 7 ng/mL. The levels then decrease exponentially until they become undetectable (<100 pg/mL) between 120 to 200 days following injection. Using an unextracted radioimmunoassay procedure for the assay of medroxyprogesterone acetate in serum, the apparent half-life for medroxyprogesterone acetate following IM administration of DEPO-PROVERA Contraceptive Injection is approximately 50 days.

Women with lower body weights conceive sooner than women with higher body weights after discontinuing DEPO-PROVERA Contraceptive Injection.

The effect of hepatic and/or renal disease on the pharmacokinetics of DEPO-PROVERA Contraceptive Injection is unknown.

INDICATIONS AND USAGE

DEPO-PROVERA Contraceptive Injection is indicated only for the prevention of pregnancy. To ensure that DEPO-PROVERA Contraceptive Injection is not administered inadvertently to a pregnant woman, the first injection must be given **ONLY** during the first 5 days of a normal menstrual period; **ONLY** within the first 5-days postpartum if not breast-feeding, and if exclusively breast-feeding, **ONLY** at the sixth postpartum week. The efficacy of DEPO-PROVERA Contraceptive Injection depends on adherence to the recommended dosage schedule (see DOSAGE AND ADMINISTRATION). It is a long-term injectable contraceptive in women when administered at 3-month (13-week) intervals. Dosage does not need to be adjusted for body weight.

In five clinical studies using DEPO-PROVERA Contraceptive Injection, the 12-month failure rate for the group of women treated with DEPO-PROVERA Contraceptive Injection was zero (no pregnancies reported) to 0.7 by Life-Table method. Pregnancy rates with contraceptive measures are typically reported for only the first year of use as shown in Table 1. Except for intrauterine devices (IUD), implants, sterilization, and DEPO-PROVERA Contraceptive Injection, the efficacy of these contraceptive measures depends in part on the reliability of use. The effectiveness of DEPO-PROVERA Contraceptive Injection is dependent on the patient returning every 3 months (13 weeks) for reinjection.

[See table above]

Table 1
Lowest Expected and Typical Failure Rates*
Expressed as Percent of Women Experiencing an Accidental Pregnancy in the First Year of Continuous Use

Method	Lowest Expected	Typical
Injectable progestogen		
DEPO-PROVERA	0.3	0.3
Implants		
Norplant (6 capsules)	0.2†	0.2†
Female sterilization	0.2	0.4
Male sterilization	0.1	0.15
Pill		3
Combined	0.1	
Progestogen only	0.5	
IUD		3
Progestasert	2	
Copper T 380A	0.8	
Condom	2	12
Diaphragm	6	18
Cap	6	18
Spermicides	3	21
Sponge		
Parous women	9	28
Nulliparous women	6	18
Periodic abstinence	1–9	20
Withdrawal	4	18
No method	85	85

Source: Trussell et al[1]

*Lowest expected - when used exactly as directed.
Typical - includes those not following directions exactly.
†from Norplant® package insert.

CONTRAINDICATIONS

1. Known or suspected pregnancy or as a diagnostic test for pregnancy.
2. Undiagnosed vaginal bleeding.
3. Known or suspected malignancy of breast.
4. Active thrombophlebitis, or current or past history of thromboembolic disorders, or cerebral vascular disease.
5. Liver dysfunction or disease.
6. Known hypersensitivity to DEPO-PROVERA Contraceptive Injection (medroxyprogesterone acetate or any of its other ingredients).

WARNINGS

1. Bleeding Irregularities

Most women using DEPO-PROVERA Contraceptive Injection experience disruption of menstrual bleeding patterns. Altered menstrual bleeding patterns include irregular or unpredictable bleeding or spotting, or rarely, heavy or continuous bleeding. If abnormal bleeding persists or is severe, appropriate investigation should be instituted to rule out the possibility or organic pathology, and appropriate treatment should be instituted when necessary.

As women continue using DEPO-PROVERA Contraceptive Injection, fewer experience irregular bleeding and more experience amenorrhea. By month 12 amenorrhea was reported by 55% of women, and by month 24 amenorrhea was reported by 68% of women using DEPO-PROVERA Contraceptive Injection.[2]

2. Bone Mineral Density Changes

Use of DEPO-PROVERA Contraceptive Injection may be considered among the risk factors for development of osteoporosis. The rate of bone loss is greatest in the early years of use and then subsequently approaches the normal rate of age related fall.

3. Cancer Risks

Long-term case-controlled surveillance of users of DEPO-PROVERA Contraceptive Injection found slight or no increased overall risk of breast cancer[3] and no overall increased risk of ovarian,[4] liver,[5] or cervical[6] cancer and a prolonged, protective effect of reducing the risk of endometrial[7] cancer in the population of users.

A pooled analysis[14] from two case-control studies, the World Health Organization Study[3] and the New Zealand Study[13], reported the relative risk (RR) of breast cancer for women who had ever used DEPO-PROVERA Contraceptive Injection as 1.1 (95% confidence interval (Cl) 0.97 to 1.4). Overall, there was no increase in risk with increasing duration of use of DEPO-PROVERA Contraceptive Injection. The RR of breast cancer for women of all ages who had initiated use of DEPO-PROVERA Contraceptive Injection within the previous 5 years was estimated to be 2.0 (95% Cl 1.5 to 2.8).

The World Health Organization Study[3], a component of the pooled analysis[14] described above, showed an increased RR of 2.19 (95% Cl 1.23 to 3.89) of breast cancer associated with use of DEPO-PROVERA Contraceptive Injection in women whose first exposure to drug was within the previous 4 years and who were under 35 years of age. However, the overall RR for ever-users of DEPO-PROVERA Contraceptive Injection was only 1.2 (95% Cl 0.96 to 1.52).

[**NOTE:** A RR of 1.0 indicates neither an increased nor a decreased risk of cancer associated with the use of the drug, relative to no use of the drug. In the case of the subpopulation with a RR of 2.19, the 95% Cl is fairly wide and does not include the value of 1.0, thus inferring an increased risk of breast cancer in the defined subgroup relative to nonusers. The value of 2.19 means that women whose first exposure to drug was within the previous 4 years and who are under 35 years of age have a 2.19-fold (95% Cl 1.23 to 3.89-fold) increased risk of breast cancer relative to nonusers. The National Cancer Institute[8] reports an average annual incidence rate for breast cancer for US women, all races, age 30 to 34 years of 26.7 per 100,000. A RR of 2.19, thus, increases the possible risk from 26.7 to 58.5 cases per 100,000 women. The attributable risk, thus, is 31.8 per 100,000 women per year.]

A statistically insignificant increase in RR estimates of invasive squamous-cell cervical cancer has been associated with the use of DEPO-PROVERA Contraceptive Injection in women who were first exposed before the age of 35 years (RR 1.22 to 1.28 and 95% Cl 0.93 to 1.70). The overall, non-significant relative rate of invasive squamous-cell cervical cancer in women who ever used DEPO-PROVERA Contraceptive Injection was estimated to be 1.11 (95% Cl 0.96 to 1.29). No trends in risk with duration of use or times since initial or most recent exposure were observed.

4. Thromboembolic Disorders

The physician should be alert to the earliest manifestations of thrombotic disorders (thrombophlebitis, pulmonary embolism, cerebrovascular disorders, and retinal thrombosis). Should any of these occur or be suspected, the drug should not be readministered.

5. Ocular Disorders

Medication should not be readministered pending examination if there is a sudden partial or complete loss of vision or if there is a sudden onset of proptosis, diplopia, or migraine. If examination reveals papilledema or retinal vascular lesions, medication should not be readministered.

6. Unexpected Pregnancies

To ensure that DEPO-PROVERA Contraceptive Injection is not administered inadvertently to a pregnant woman, the first injection must be given **ONLY** during the first 5 days of a normal menstrual period; **ONLY** within the first 5-days postpartum if not breast-feeding, and if exclusively breast-feeding, **ONLY** at the sixth postpartum week (see DOSAGE AND ADMINISTRATION).

Neonates from unexpected pregnancies that occur 1 to 2 months after injection of DEPO-PROVERA Contraceptive Injection may be at an increased risk of low birth weight, which, in turn, is associated with an increased risk of neonatal death. The attributable risk is low because such pregnancies are uncommon.[9,10]

A significant increase in incidence of polysyndactyly and chromosomal anomalies was observed among infants of users of DEPO-PROVERA Contraceptive Injection, the former being most pronounced in women under 30 years of age. The unrelated nature of these defects, the lack of confirmation from other studies, the distant preconceptual exposure to DEPO-PROVERA Contraceptive Injection, and the chance effects due to multiple statistical comparisons, make a causal association unlikely.[11]

Neonates exposed to medroxyprogesterone acetate *in utero* and followed to adolescence, showed no evidence of any adverse effects on their health including their physical, intellectual, sexual, or social development.

Several reports suggest an association between intrauterine exposure to progestational drugs in the first trimester of pregnancy and genital abnormalities in male and female fetuses. The risk of hypospadias (five to eight per 1,000 male births in the general population) may be approximately doubled with exposure to these drugs. There are insufficient data to quantify the risk to exposed female fetuses, but because some of these drugs induce mild virilization of the external genitalia of the female fetus and because of the increased association of hypospadias in the male fetus, it is prudent to avoid the use of these drugs during the first trimester of pregnancy.

To ensure that DEPO-PROVERA Contraceptive Injection is not administered inadvertently to a pregnant woman, it is important that the first injection be given only during the first 5 days after the onset of a normal menstrual period within 5 days postpartum if not breast-feeding and if breast-feeding, at the sixth week postpartum (see DOSAGE AND ADMINISTRATION).

7. Ectopic Pregnancy

Health-care providers should be alert to the possibility of an ectopic pregnancy among women using DEPO-PROVERA Contraceptive Injection who become pregnant or complain of severe abdominal pain.

8. Lactation

Detectable amounts of drug have been identified in the milk of mothers receiving DEPO-PROVERA Contraceptive Injec-

Continued on next page

Information on these Pharmacia & Upjohn products is based on labeling in effect June 1, 2000. Further information concerning these and other Pharmacia & Upjohn products may be obtained by direct inquiry to Medical Information, Pharmacia & Upjohn, Kalamazoo, MI 49001.

Depo-Provera Injection—Cont.

tion. In nursing mothers treated with DEPO-PROVERA Contraceptive Injection, milk composition, quality, and amount are not adversely affected. Neonates and infants exposed to medroxyprogesterone from breast milk have been studied for developmental and behavioral effects through puberty. No adverse effects have been noted.

9. Anaphylaxis and Anaphylactoid Reaction

Anaphylaxis and anaphylactoid reaction have been reported with the use of DEPO-PROVERA Contraceptive Injection. If an anaphylactic reaction occurs appropriate therapy should be instituted. Serious anaphylactic reactions require emergency medical treatment.

PRECAUTIONS

GENERAL

1. Physical Examination

It is good medical practice for all women to have annual history and physical examinations, including women using DEPO-PROVERA Contraceptive Injection. The physical examination, however, may be deferred until after initiation of DEPO-PROVERA if requested by the woman and judged appropriate by the clinician. The physical examination should include special reference to blood pressure, breasts, abdomen and pelvic organs, including cervical cytology and relevant laboratory tests. In case of undiagnosed, persistent or recurrent abnormal vaginal bleeding, appropriate measures should be conducted to rule out malignancy. Women with a strong family history of breast cancer or who have breast nodules should be monitored with particular care.

2. Fluid Retention

Because progestational drugs may cause some degree of fluid retention, conditions that might be influenced by this condition, such as epilepsy, migraine, asthma, and cardiac or renal dysfunction, require careful observation.

3. Weight Changes

There is a tendency for women to gain weight while on therapy with DEPO-PROVERA Contraceptive Injection. From an initial average body weight of 136 lb, women who completed 1 year of therapy with DEPO-PROVERA Contraceptive Injection gained an average of 5.4 lb. Women who completed 2 years of therapy gained an average of 8.1 lb.
Women who completed 4 years gained an average of 13.8 lb.
Women who completed 6 years gained an average of 16.5 lb.
Two percent of women withdrew from a large-scale clinical trial because of excessive weight gain.

4. Return of Fertility

DEPO-PROVERA Contraceptive Injection has a prolonged contraceptive effect. In a large US study of women who discontinued use of DEPO-PROVERA Contraceptive Injection to become pregnant, data are available for 61% of them. Based on Life-Table analysis of these data, it is expected that 68% of women who do become pregnant may conceive within 12 months, 83% may conceive within 15 months, and 93% may conceive within 18 months from the last injection. The median time to conception for those who do conceive is 10 months following the last injection with a range of 4 to 31 months, and is unrelated to the duration of use. No data are available for 39% of the patients who discontinued DEPO-PROVERA Contraceptive Injection to become pregnant and who were lost to follow-up or changed their mind.

5. CNS Disorders and Convulsions

Patients who have a history of psychic depression should be carefully observed and the drug not be readministered if the depression recurs.
There have been a few reported cases of convulsions in patients who were treated with DEPO-PROVERA Contraceptive Injection. Association with drug use or pre-existing conditions is not clear.

6. Carbohydrate Metabolism

A decrease in glucose tolerance has been observed in some patients on DEPO-PROVERA Contraceptive Injection treatment. The mechanism of this decrease is obscure. For this reason, diabetic patients should be carefully observed while receiving such therapy.

7. Liver Function

If jaundice develops, consideration should be given to not readministering the drug.

8. Protection Against Sexually Transmitted Diseases

Patients should be counseled that this product does not protect against HIV infection (AIDS) and other sexually transmitted diseases.

DRUG INTERACTIONS

Aminoglutethimide administered concomitantly with the DEPO-PROVERA Contraceptive Injection may significantly depress the serum concentrations of medroxyprogesterone acetate.[12] Users of DEPO-PROVERA Contraceptive Injection should be warned of the possibility of decreased efficacy with the use of this or any related drugs.

LABORATORY TEST INTERACTIONS

The pathologist should be advised of progestin therapy when relevant specimens are submitted.
The following laboratory tests may be affected by progestins including DEPO-PROVERA Contraceptive Injection:

(a) Plasma and urinary steroid levels are decreased (eg, progesterone, estradiol, pregnanediol, testosterone, cortisol).
(b) Gonadotropin levels are decreased.
(c) Sex-hormone-binding-globulin concentrations are decreased.
(d) Protein-bound iodine and butanol extractable protein-bound iodine may increase.
T_3-uptake values may decrease.
(e) Coagulation test values for prothrombin (Factor II), and Factors VII, VIII, IX, and X may increase.
(f) Sulfobromopthalein and other liver function test values may be increased.
(g) The effects of medroxyprogesterone acetate on lipid metabolism are inconsistent. Both increases and decreases in total cholesterol, triglycerides, low-density lipoprotein (LDL) cholesterol, and high-density lipoprotein (HDL) cholesterol have been observed in studies.

CARCINOGENESIS

See "WARNINGS" section 3.

PREGNANCY

Pregnancy Category X. See "WARNINGS" section 6.

NURSING MOTHERS

See "WARNINGS" section 8.

PEDIATRIC USE

Safety and effectiveness in pediatric patients have not been established. See "WARNINGS" section 6.

INFORMATION FOR THE PATIENT

See Patient Labeling.
Patient labeling is included with each single-dose vial and prefilled syringe of DEPO-PROVERA Contraceptive Injection to help describe its characteristics to the patient. It is recommended that prospective users be given this labeling and be informed about the risks and benefits associated with the use of DEPO-PROVERA Contraceptive Injection, as compared with other forms of contraception or with no contraception at all. It is recommended that physicians or other health-care providers responsible for those patients advise them at the beginning of treatment that their menstrual cycle may be disrupted and that irregular and unpredictable bleeding or spotting results, and that this usually decreases to the point of amenorrhea as treatment with DEPO-PROVERA Contraceptive Injection continues, without other therapy being required.

ADVERSE REACTIONS

In the largest clinical trial with DEPO-PROVERA Contraceptive Injection, over 3,900 women, who were treated for up to 7 years, reported the following adverse reactions, which may or may not be related to the use of DEPO-PROVERA Contraceptive Injection.
The following adverse reactions were reported by more than 5% of subjects:

Menstrual irregularities
(bleeding or amenorrhea, or both)
Weight changes
Headache
Nervousness
Abdominal pain or discomfort
Dizziness
Asthenia (weakness or fatigue)

Adverse reactions reported by 1% to 5% of subjects using DEPO-PROVERA Contraceptive Injection were:

Decreased libido or anorgasmia
Backache
Leg cramps
Depression
Nausea
Insomnia
Leukorrhea
Acne
Vaginitis
Pelvic pain
Breast pain
No hair growth or alopecia
Bloating
Rash
Edema
Hot flashes
Arthralgia

Events reported by fewer than 1% of subjects included: galactorrhea, melasma, chloasma, convulsions, changes in appetite, gastrointestinal disturbances, jaundice, genitourinary infections, vaginal cysts, dyspareunia, paresthesia, chest pain, pulmonary embolus, allergic reactions, anemia, drowsiness, syncope, dyspnea and asthma, tachycardia, fever, excessive sweating and body odor, dry skin, chills, increased libido, excessive thirst, hoarseness, pain at injection site, blood dyscrasia, rectal bleeding, changes in breast size, breast lumps or nipple bleeding, axillary swelling, breast cancer, prevention of lactation, sensation of pregnancy, lack of return to fertility, paralysis, facial palsy, scleroderma, osteoporosis, uterine hyperplasia, cervical cancer, varicose veins, dysmenorrhea, hirsutism, unexpected pregnancy, thrombophlebitis, deep vein thrombosis.
In addition, voluntary reports have been received of anaphylaxis and anaphylactoid reaction with use of DEPO-PROVERA Contraceptive Injection.

DOSAGE AND ADMINISTRATION

Both the 1 mL vial and the 1 mL prefilled syringe of DEPO-PROVERA Contraceptive Injection should be vigorously shaken just before use to ensure that the dose being administered represents a uniform suspension.
The recommended dose is 150 mg of DEPO-PROVERA Contraceptive Injection every 3 months (13 weeks) administered by deep, IM injection in the gluteal or deltoid muscle. To ensure the patient is not pregnant at the time of the first injection, the first injection **MUST** be given **ONLY** during the first 5 days of a normal menstrual period; **ONLY** within the first 5-days postpartum if not breast-feeding; and if exclusively breast-feeding, **ONLY** at the sixth postpartum week.
If the time interval between injections is greater than 13 weeks, the physician should determine that the patient is not pregnant before administering the drug. The efficacy of DEPO-PROVERA Contraceptive Injection depends on adherence to the dosage schedule of administration.

HOW SUPPLIED

DEPO-PROVERA Contraceptive Injection (medroxyprogesterone acetate injectable suspension 150 mg/mL) is available as:

NDC 0009-0746-30	1 mL vial
NDC 0009-0746-34	5 × 1 mL vials
NDC 0009-0746-35	25 × 1 mL vials
NDC 0009-7376-01	1 mL prefilled syringe
NDC 0009-7376-02	6 × 1 mL prefilled syringes
NDC 0009-7376-03	24 × 1 mL prefilled syringes

Store at controlled room temperature 20° to 25° C (68° to 77° F) [see USP].

REFERENCES

1. Trussell J. Hatcher RA, Cates W Jr, Stewart FH, Kost K. A guide to interpreting contraceptive efficacy studies. Obstet Gynecol. 1990; *76*:558–567.
2. Schwallie PC, Assenzo JR. Contraceptive use-efficacy study utilizing medroxyprogesterone acetate administered as an intramuscular injection once every 90 days. Fertil Steril. 1973; *24*:331–339.
3. WHO Collaborative Study of Neoplasia and Steroid Contraceptives. Breast cancer and depot-medroxyprogesterone acetate: a multi-national study. Lancet. 1991; *338*:833–838.
4. WHO Collaborative Study of Neoplasia and Steroid Contraceptives. Depot-medroxyprogesterone acetate (DMPA) and risk of epithelial ovarian cancer. Int J Cancer. 1991; *49*:191–195.
5. WHO Collaborative Study of Neoplasia and Steroid Contraceptives. Depot-medroxyprogesterone acetate (DMPA) and risk of liver cancer. Int J Cancer. 1991; *49*:182–185.
6. WHO Collaborative Study of Neoplasia and Steroid Contraceptives. Depot-medroxyprogesterone acetate (DMPA) and risk of invasive squamous-cell cervical cancer. Contraception. 1992; *45*:299–312.
7. WHO Collaborative Study of Neoplasia and Steroid Contraceptives. Depot-medroxyprogesterone acetate (DMPA) and risk of endometrial cancer. Int J Cancer. 1991; *49*:186–190.
8. Surveillance, Epidemiology, and End Results: Incidence and Mortality Data, 1973–1977. National Cancer Institute Monograph, 57: June 1981. (NIH publication No. 81-2330).
9. Gray RH, Pardthaisong T. *In Utero* exposure to steroid contraceptives and survival during infancy. Am J Epidemiol. 1991; *134*:804–811.
10. Pardthaisong T, Gray RH. *In Utero* exposure to steroid contraceptives and outcome of pregnancy. Am J Epidemiol. 1991; *134*:795–803.
11. Pardthaisong T, Gray RH, McDaniel EB, Chandacham A. Steroid contraceptive use and pregnancy outcome. Teratology. 1988; *38*:51–58.
12. Van Deijk WA, Biljham GH, Mellink WAM, Meulenberg PMM. Influence of aminoglutethimide on plasma levels of medroxyprogesterone acetate: its correlation with serum cortisol. Cancer Treatment Reports. 1985; *69*:1, 85–90.
13. Paul C, Skegg DCG, Spears GFS. Depot medroxyprogesterone (Depo-Provera) and risk of breast cancer. Br Med J. 1989; *299*:759–762.
14. Skegg DCG, Noonan EA, Paul C, Spears GFS, Meirik O, Thomas DB. Depot Medroxyprogesterone Acetate and Breast Cancer: A Pooled Analysis from the World Health Organization and New Zealand Studies. JAMA. 1995; *273(10)*:799–804.

Rx only

DEPO-PROVERA Contraceptive Injection 1 mL vials are manufactured by
Pharmacia & Upjohn Company, Kalamazoo, MI 49001, USA
DEPO-PROVERA Contraceptive Injection 1 mL prefilled syringes are manufactured by
Pharmacia & Upjohn N.V./S.A., Puurs, Belgium for Pharmacia & Upjohn Company, Kalamazoo, MI 49001, USA
Revised March 1999 815 459 414A
691400

DEPO-PROVERA®
Contraceptive Injection
medroxyprogesterone acetate
injectable suspension, USP

This product is intended to prevent pregnancy. It does not protect against HIV infection (AIDS) and other sexually transmitted diseases.

Patient Labeling

Introduction

Every woman who considers using DEPO-PROVERA Contraceptive Injection needs to understand the benefits and risks of this form of birth control and to discuss them with her health-care provider. This leaflet is intended to give you much of the information you will need in order to decide if DEPO-PROVERA Contraceptive Injection is the right choice for you. Your health-care provider will help you to compare DEPO-PROVERA Contraceptive Injection with other contraceptive methods and will answer any questions you have after you have read this information.
DEPO-PROVERA Contraceptive Injection is given as an intramuscular injection (a shot) in the buttock or upper arm

once every 3 months (13 weeks). Promptly at the end of the 3-month interval, you will need to return to your health-care provider for your next injection in order to continue your contraceptive protection.
DEPO-PROVERA Contraceptive Injection contains medroxyprogesterone acetate, a chemical similar to (but not the same as) the natural hormone progesterone that is produced by your ovaries during the second half of your menstrual cycle. DEPO-PROVERA Contraceptive Injection acts by preventing your egg cells from ripening. If an egg is not released from the ovaries during your menstrual cycle, it cannot become fertilized by sperm and result in pregnancy. DEPO-PROVERA Contraceptive Injection also causes changes in the lining of your uterus that make it less likely for pregnancy to occur.

Effectiveness of DEPO-PROVERA Contraceptive Injection

To ensure that DEPO-PROVERA Contraceptive Injection is not administered inadvertently to a pregnant woman, the first injection must be given **ONLY** during the first 5 days of a normal menstrual period; **ONLY** within the first 5-days postpartum if not breast-feeding, and if exclusively breast-feeding, **ONLY** at the sixth postpartum week (see **Administration of DEPO-PROVERA Contraceptive Injection**). The efficacy of DEPO-PROVERA Contraceptive Injection depends on adherence to the recommended dosage schedule.
DEPO-PROVERA Contraceptive Injection is over 99% effective, making it one of the most reliable methods of birth control available. This means that the average annual pregnancy rate is less than one for every 100 women who use DEPO-PROVERA Contraceptive Injection. The effectiveness of most contraceptive methods depends, in part, on how reliably each woman uses the method. The effectiveness of DEPO-PROVERA Contraceptive Injection depends only on the patient returning every 3 months (13 weeks) for her next injection.
The following table shows the percent of women who become pregnant while using different kinds of contraceptive methods. It gives both the lowest expected rate of pregnancy (the rate expected in women who use each method exactly as it should be used) and the typical rate of pregnancy (which includes women who became pregnant because they forgot to use their birth control or because they did not follow the directions exactly).

Percent of Women Experiencing an Accidental Pregnancy in the First Year of Continuous Use

Method	Lowest Expected	Typical
DEPO-PROVERA	0.3	0.3
Implants (Norplant)	0.2*	0.2*
Female sterilization	0.2	0.4
Male sterilization	0.1	0.15
Oral contraceptives (pill)	–	3
Combined	0.1	–
Progestogen only	0.5	–
IUD		
Progestasert	2	–
Copper T 380A	0.8	–
Condom (without spermicide)	2	12
Diaphragm (with spermicide)	6	18
Cervical cap	6	18
Withdrawal	4	18
Periodic abstinence	1–9	20
Spermicide alone	3	21
Vaginal sponge	–	–
used before childbirth	6	18
used after childbirth	9	28
No method	85	85

Source: Trussell et al; Obstet Gynecol 1990;76:558–567.

* From Norplant® package insert.

Who Should Not Use DEPO-PROVERA Contraceptive Injection

Certain women should not use DEPO-PROVERA Contraceptive Injection. You should not use DEPO-PROVERA Contraceptive Injection if you have any of the following conditions:

- if you think you might be pregnant
- if you have any vaginal bleeding without a known reason
- if you have had cancer of the breast
- if you have had a stroke
- if you have or have had blood clots (phlebitis) in your legs
- if you have problems with your liver or liver disease
- if you are allergic to DEPO-PROVERA Contraceptive Injection (medroxyprogesterone acetate or any of its other ingredients)

Other Things to Consider Before Choosing DEPO-PROVERA Contraceptive Injection

Before your doctor prescribes DEPO-PROVERA Contraceptive Injection, you will have a physical examination. It is important to tell your doctor or health-care provider if you have any of the following:

- a family history of cancer of the breast
- an abnormal mammogram (breast X-ray), fibrocystic breast disease, breast nodules or lumps, or bleeding from your nipples
- kidney disease
- irregular or scanty menstrual periods
- high blood pressure
- migraine headaches
- asthma
- epilepsy (convulsions or seizures)
- diabetes or a family history of diabetes
- a history of depression
- if you are taking any prescription or over-the-counter medications

This product is intended to prevent pregnancy. It does not protect against transmission of HIV (AIDS) and other sexually transmitted diseases such as chlamydia, genital herpes, genital warts, gonorrhea, hepatitis B, and syphilis.

Return of Fertility

Because DEPO-PROVERA Contraceptive Injection is a long-acting birth control method, it takes some time after your last injection for its effect to wear off. Based on the results from a large study done in the United States, of those women who stop using DEPO-PROVERA Contraceptive Injection in order to become pregnant, about half of those who become pregnant do so in about 10 months after their last injection; about two-thirds of those who become pregnant do so in about 12 months, about 83% of those who become pregnant do so in about 15 months, and about 93% of those who become pregnant do so in about 18 months after their last injection. The length of time you use DEPO-PROVERA Contraceptive Injection has no effect on how long it takes you to become pregnant after you stop using it.

Risks of Using DEPO-PROVERA Contraceptive Injection

1. Irregular Menstrual Bleeding

The side effect reported most frequently by women who use DEPO-PROVERA Contraceptive Injection for contraception is a change in their normal menstrual cycle. During the first year of using DEPO-PROVERA Contraceptive Injection, you might have one or more of the following changes:

- irregular or unpredictable bleeding or spotting,
- an increase or decrease in menstrual bleeding, or
- no bleeding at all.

Unusually heavy or continuous bleeding, however, is not a usual effect of DEPO-PROVERA Contraceptive Injection and if this happens you should see your health-care provider right away.
With continued use of DEPO-PROVERA Contraceptive Injection, bleeding usually decreases and many women stop having periods completely. In clinical studies of DEPO-PROVERA Contraceptive Injection, 55% of the women studied reported no menstrual bleeding (amenorrhea) after 1 year of use and 68% of the women studied reported no menstrual bleeding after 2 years of use.
The reason that your periods stop is because DEPO-PROVERA Contraceptive Injection causes a resting state in your ovaries. When your ovaries do not release an egg monthly, the regular monthly growth of the lining of your uterus does not occur and, therefore, the bleeding that comes with your normal menstruation does not take place. When you stop using DEPO-PROVERA Contraceptive Injection your menstrual period will usually, in time, return to its normal cycle.

2. Bone Mineral Changes

Use of DEPO-PROVERA Contraceptive Injection may be associated with a decrease in the amount of mineral stored in your bones. This could increase your risk of developing bone fractures. The rate of bone mineral loss is greatest in the early years of DEPO-PROVERA Contraceptive Injection use but, after that, it begins to resemble the normal rate of age-related bone mineral loss.

3. Cancer

Studies of women who have used different forms of contraception found that women who used DEPO-PROVERA Contraceptive Injection for contraception had no increased overall risk of developing cancer of the breast, ovary, uterus, cervix, or liver. However, women under 35 years of age whose first exposure to DEPO-PROVERA Contraceptive Injection was within the previous 4 to 5 years may have a slightly increased risk of developing breast cancer similar to that seen with oral contraceptives. You should discuss this with your health-care provider.

4. Unexpected Pregnancy

Because DEPO-PROVERA Contraceptive Injection is such an effective contraceptive method, the risk of unexpected pregnancy for women who get their shots regularly (every 3 months [13 weeks]) is very low. While there have been reports of an increased risk of low birth weight and neonatal infant death or other health problems in infants conceived close to the time of injection, such pregnancies are uncommon. If you think you may have become pregnant while using DEPO-PROVERA Contraceptive Injection for contraception, see your health-care provider as soon as possible.

5. Allergic Reactions

Severe allergic reactions known as anaphylaxis and anaphylactoid reactions have also been reported in some women using DEPO-PROVERA Contraceptive Injection.

6. Other Risks

Women who use hormone-based contraceptives may have an increased risk of blood clots or stroke. Also, if a contraceptive method fails, there is a possibility that the fertilized egg will begin to develop outside of the uterus (ectopic pregnancy). While these events are rare, you should tell your health-care provider if you have any of the Warning Signals listed in the next section.

Warning Signals

If any of these problems occur following an injection of DEPO-PROVERA Contraceptive Injection, call your health-care provider immediately:

- Sharp chest pain, coughing up of blood, or sudden shortness of breath (indicating a possible clot in the lung)
- Sudden severe headache or vomiting, dizziness or fainting, problems with your eyesight or speech, weakness, or numbness in an arm or leg (indicating a possible stroke)
- Severe pain or swelling in the calf (indicating a possible clot in the leg)
- Unusually heavy vaginal bleeding
- Severe pain or tenderness in the lower abdominal area
- Persistent pain, pus, or bleeding at the injection site

Side Effects of DEPO-PROVERA Contraceptive Injection

1. Weight Gain

You may experience a weight gain while you are using DEPO-PROVERA Contraceptive Injection. About two-thirds of the women who used DEPO-PROVERA Contraceptive Injection in the clinical trials reported a weight gain of about 5 pounds during the first year of use. You may continue to gain weight after the first year. Women in one large study who used DEPO-PROVERA Contraceptive Injection for 2 years gained an average total of 8.1 pounds over those 2 years, or approximately 4 pounds per year. Women who continued for 4 years gained an average total of 13.8 pounds over those 4 years, or approximately 3.5 pounds per year. Women who continued for 6 years gained an average total of 16.5 pounds over those 6 years, or approximately 2.75 pounds per year.

2. Other Side Effects

In a clinical study of over 3,900 women who used DEPO-PROVERA Contraceptive Injection for up to 7 years, some women reported the following effects that may or may not have been related to their use of DEPO-PROVERA Contraceptive Injection:

- irregular menstrual bleeding
- amenorrhea
- headache
- nervousness
- abdominal cramps
- dizziness
- weakness or fatigue
- decreased sexual desire
- leg cramps
- nausea
- vaginal discharge or irritation
- breast swelling and tenderness
- bloating
- swelling of the hands or feet
- backache
- depression
- insomnia
- acne
- pelvic pain
- no hair growth or excessive hair loss
- rash
- hot flashes
- joint pain

Other problems were reported by very few of the women in the clinical trials, but some of these could be serious. These include: convulsions, jaundice, urinary tract infections, allergic reactions, fainting, paralysis, osteoporosis, lack of return to fertility, deep vein thrombosis, pulmonary embolus, breast cancer, or cervical cancer. If these or any other problems occur during your use of DEPO-PROVERA Contraceptive Injection, discuss them with your health-care provider.

General Precautions

1. Missed Periods

During the time you are using DEPO-PROVERA Contraceptive Injection for contraception, you may skip a period, or your periods may stop completely. If you have been receiving your injection of DEPO-PROVERA Contraceptive Injection regularly every 3 months (13 weeks), then you are probably not pregnant. However, if you think that you may be pregnant, see your health-care provider.

2. Laboratory Test Interactions

If you are scheduled for any laboratory tests, tell your health-care provider that you are using DEPO-PROVERA Contraceptive Injection for contraception. Certain blood tests are affected by hormones such as DEPO-PROVERA Contraceptive Injection.

3. Drug Interactions

Cytadren (aminoglutethimide) is an anticancer drug that may significantly decrease the effectiveness of DEPO-PROVERA Contraceptive Injection if the two drugs are given during the same time.

4. Nursing Mothers

Although DEPO-PROVERA Contraceptive Injection can be passed to the nursing infant in the breast milk, no harmful effects have been found in these children. DEPO-PROVERA Contraceptive Injection does not prevent the breasts from producing milk, so it can be used by nursing mothers. However, to minimize the amount of DEPO-PROVERA Contraceptive Injection that is passed to the infant in the first weeks after birth, you should wait until 6 weeks after childbirth before you start using DEPO-PROVERA Contraceptive Injection for contraception.

Continued on next page

Information on these Pharmacia & Upjohn products is based on labeling in effect June 1, 2000. Further information concerning these and other Pharmacia & Upjohn products may be obtained by direct inquiry to Medical Information, Pharmacia & Upjohn, Kalamazoo, MI 49001.

Depo-Provera Injection—Cont.

Administration of DEPO-PROVERA Contraceptive Injection
The recommended dose of DEPO-PROVERA Contraceptive Injection is 150 mg every 3 months (13 weeks) given in a single intramuscular injection in the buttock or upper arm. To ensure that you are not pregnant at the time of the first injection, it is essential that the injection be given **ONLY** during the first 5 days of a normal menstrual period. If used following the delivery of a child, the first injection of DEPO-PROVERA Contraceptive Injection **MUST** be given within 5 days after childbirth if you are not breast-feeding, or if you are exclusively breast-feeding, the injection **MUST** be given 6 weeks after childbirth. If you wait longer than 3 months (13 weeks) between injections, or longer than 6 weeks after delivery, your health-care provider should determine that you are not pregnant before giving you your injection of DEPO-PROVERA Contraceptive Injection.

Rx only

Pharmacia & Upjohn Company
Kalamazoo, MI 49001, USA
Revised March 1999 815 459 414
691400

Shown in Product Identification Guide, page 331

DETROL™
[dē trōl]
tolterodine tartrate tablets ℞

DESCRIPTION

DETROL Tablets contain tolterodine tartrate. The active moiety, tolterodine, is a muscarinic receptor antagonist. The chemical name of tolterodine tartrate is (R)-N,N-diisopropyl-3-(2-hydroxy-5-methylphenyl)-3-phenylpropanamine L-hydrogen tartrate. The empirical formula of tolterodine tartrate is $C_{26}H_{37}NO_7$, and its molecular weight is 475.6. The structural formula of tolterodine tartrate is represented below:

Tolterodine tartrate is a white, crystalline powder. It is soluble at 12 mg/mL in water at room temperature and is soluble in methanol, slightly soluble in ethanol, and practically insoluble in toluene.

DETROL Tablets for oral administration contain 1 or 2 mg of tolterodine tartrate. The inactive ingredients are colloidal anhydrous silica, calcium hydrogen phosphate dihydrate, cellulose microcrystalline, hydroxypropyl methylcellulose, magnesium stearate, sodium starch glycolate (pH 3.0 to 5.0), stearic acid, and titanium dioxide.

CLINICAL PHARMACOLOGY

Tolterodine is a competitive muscarinic receptor antagonist. Both urinary bladder contraction and salivation are mediated via cholinergic muscarinic receptors. In the anesthetized cat, tolterodine shows a selectivity for the urinary bladder over salivary glands; however, the clinical relevance of this finding has not been established.

After oral administration, tolterodine is metabolized in the liver, resulting in the formation of the 5-hydroxymethyl derivative, a major pharmacologically active metabolite. The 5-hydroxymethyl metabolite, which exhibits an antimuscarinic activity similar to that of tolterodine, contributes significantly to the therapeutic effect. Both tolterodine and the 5-hydroxymethyl metabolite exhibit a high specificity for muscarinic receptors, since both show negligible activity or affinity for other neurotransmitter receptors and other potential cellular targets, such as calcium channels.

Tolterodine has a pronounced effect on bladder function in healthy volunteers. The main effects following a 6.4-mg single dose of tolterodine were an increase in residual urine, reflecting an incomplete emptying of the bladder, and a decrease in detrusor pressure. These findings are consistent with a potent antimuscarinic action on the lower urinary tract.

Pharmacokinetics

Absorption: In a study of ^{14}C-tolterodine in healthy volunteers who received a 5-mg oral dose, at least 77% of the radiolabeled dose was absorbed. Tolterodine is rapidly absorbed, and maximum serum concentrations (C_{max}) typically occur within 1 to 2 hours after dose administration. The pharmacokinetics of tolterodine, based on C_{max} and area under the concentration-time curve (AUC) determinations, are dose-proportional over the range of 1 to 4 mg.

Effect of Food: Food intake increases the bioavailability of tolterodine (average increase 53%) and does not affect the levels of the 5-hydroxymethyl metabolite in extensive metabolizers. This change is not expected to be a safety concern and adjustment of dose in not needed.

Distribution: Tolterodine is highly bound to plasma proteins, primarily α_1-acid glycoprotein. Unbound concentrations of tolterodine average 3.7% ± 0.13% over the concentration range achieved in clinical studies. The 5-hydroxymethyl metabolite is not extensively protein bound, with

Phenotype (CYP2D6)	Tolterodine t_{max} (h)	Tolterodine C_{max}* (μg/L)	Tolterodine C_{avg}* (μg/L)	Tolterodine $t_{1/2}$ (h)	Tolterodine CL/F (L/h)	5-Hydroxymethyl Metabolite t_{max} (h)	5-Hydroxymethyl Metabolite C_{max}* (μg/L)	5-Hydroxymethyl Metabolite C_{avg}* (μg/L)	5-Hydroxymethyl Metabolite $t_{1/2}$ (h)
Single-dose									
EM	1.6±1.5	1.6±1.2	0.50±0.35	2.0±0.7	534±697	1.8±1.4	1.8±0.7	0.62±0.26	3.1±0.7
PM	1.4±0.5	10±4.9	8.3±4.3	6.5±1.6	17±7.3	—†	—	—	—
Multiple-dose									
EM	1.2±0.5	2.6±2.8	0.58±0.54	2.2±0.4	415±377	1.2±0.5	2.4±1.3	0.92±0.46	2.9±0.4
PM	1.9±1.0	19±7.5	12±5.1	9.6±1.5	11±4.2	—	—	—	—

* Parameter was dose-normalized from 4 mg to 2 mg.
C_{max} = Maximum plasma concentration; t_{max} = Time of occurrence of C_{max};
C_{avg} = Average plasma concentration; $t_{1/2}$ = Terminal elimination half-life; CL/F = Apparent oral clearance.
†— = not applicable.

95% Confidence Intervals for the Difference between DETROL (2 mg bid) and Placebo for the Median Change at Week 12 from Baseline

Number of Micturitions per 24 Hours

Study		DETROL	Placebo
008	number of patients	118	56
	median baseline	10.5	10.6
	median (SD) change from baseline	-2.2 (3.8)	-1.1 (3.6)
009	number of patients	128	64
	median baseline	10.4	10.4
	median (SD) change from baseline	-2.2 (2.1)	-1.2 (2.3)
010	number of patients	108	56
	median baseline	11.0	10.9
	median (SD) change from baseline	-1.6 (2.3)	-1.1 (2.8)

Between Treatment Difference in Change from Baseline
Favors DETROL Favors Placebo
−2 −1 0 1 2

Number of Incontinence Episodes per 24 Hours

Study		DETROL	Placebo
008	number of patients	93	40
	median baseline	2.4	2.5
	median (SD) change from baseline	-1.2 (3.2)	-0.8 (1.5)
009	number of patients	116	55
	median baseline	2.5	3.2
	median (SD) change from baseline	-1.4 (2.5)	-1.1 (2.5)
010	number of patients	90	50
	median baseline	2.7	2.2
	median (SD) change from baseline	-1.5 (2.4)	-0.9 (2.1)

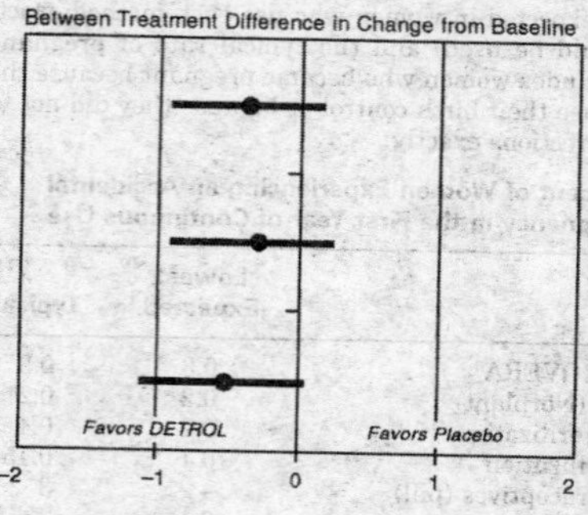

Volume Voided per Micturition (mL)

Study		DETROL	Placebo
008	number of patients	118	56
	median baseline	156	155
	median (SD) change from baseline	34 (54)	5 (42)
009	number of patients	128	64
	median baseline	149	157
	median (SD) change from baseline	34 (50)	8 (47)
010	number of patients	108	56
	median baseline	148	164
	median (SD) change from baseline	27 (45)	10 (52)

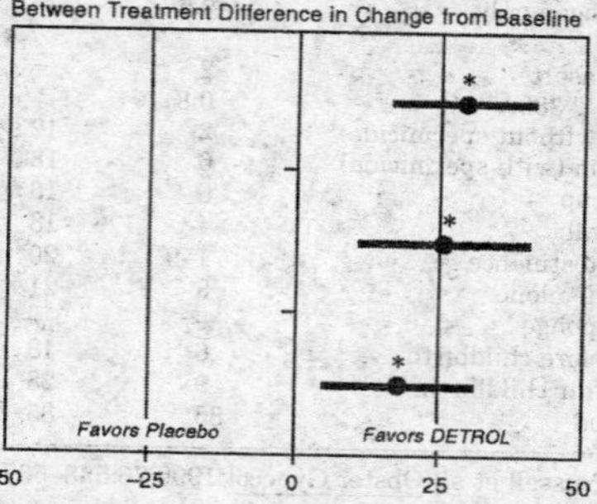

*The difference between DETROL and placebo was statistically significant.

unbound fraction concentrations averaging 36% ± 4.0%. The blood to serum ratio of tolterodine and the 5-hydroxymethyl metabolite averages 0.6 and 0.8, respectively, indicating that these compounds do not distribute extensively into erythrocytes. The volume of distribution of tolterodine following administration of a 1.28-mg intravenous dose is 113 ± 26.7 L.

Metabolism: Tolterodine is extensively metabolized by the liver following oral dosing. The primary metabolic route involves the oxidation of the 5-methyl group and is mediated by the cytochrome P450 2D6 and leads to the formation of a pharmacologically active 5-hydroxymethyl metabolite. Further metabolism leads to formation of the 5-carboxylic acid and N-dealkylated 5-carboxylic acid metabolites, which account for 51% ± 14% and 29% ± 6.3% of the metabolites recovered in the urine, respectively.

Variability in Metabolism: A subset (about 7%) of the population is devoid of cytochrome P450 2D6, the enzyme responsible for the formation of the 5-hydroxymethyl metabolite of tolterodine. The identified pathway of metabolism for these individuals, referred to as "poor metabolizers," is dealkylation via cytochrome P450 3A4 to N-dealkylated tolterodine. The remainder of the population is referred to as "extensive metabolizers." Pharmacokinetic studies revealed that tolterodine is metabolized at a slower rate in poor metabolizers than in extensive metabolizers; this results in significantly higher serum concentrations of tolterodine and in negligible concentrations of the 5-hydroxymethyl metabolite. Because of differences in the protein-binding characteristics of tolterodine and the 5-hydroxymethyl metabolite, the sum of unbound serum concentrations of tolterodine and the 5-hydroxymethyl metabolite is similar in extensive and poor metabolizers at steady state. Since tolterodine and the 5-hydroxymethyl metabolite have similar antimuscarinic effects, the net activity of DETROL Tablets is expected to be similar in extensive and poor metabolizers.

Excretion: Following administration of a 5-mg oral dose of ^{14}C-tolterodine to healthy volunteers, 77% of radioactivity was recovered in urine and 17% was recovered in feces. Less than 1% (<2.5% in poor metabolizers) of the dose was recovered as intact tolterodine, and 5% to 14% (<1% in poor metajbolizers) was recovered as the active 5-hydroxymethyl metabolite. Most of the radioactivity was recovered within the first 24 hours, which is consistent with the apparent half-life of tolterodine: 1.9 to 3.7 hours in pharmacokinetic studies.

A summary of mean (± standard deviation) pharmacokinetic parameters of tolterodine and the 5-hydroxymethyl metabolite in extensive (EM) and poor (PM) metabolizers is provided in the following table. These data were obtained following single- and multiple-doses of tolterodine 4 mg administered twice daily to 16 healthy male subjects (8 EM, 8 PM).

[See first table above]

Pharmacokinetics in Special Populations

Age: In Phase 1, multiple-dose studies in which tolterodine 2 mg was administered twice daily, serum concentrations of tolterodine and of the 5-hydroxymethyl metabolite were similar in healthy elderly volunteers (aged 64 through

80 years) and healthy young volunteers (aged less than 40 years). In another Phase 1 study, elderly volunteers (aged 71 through 81 years) were given tolterodine 1 or 2 mg twice daily. Mean serum concentrations of tolterodine and the 5-hydroxymethyl metabolite in these elderly volunteers were approximately 20% and 50% higher, respectively, than reported in young healthy volunteers. However, no overall differences were observed in safety between older and younger patients in Phase 3, 12-week, controlled clinical studies; therefore, no dosage adjustment is recommended (see PRECAUTIONS, Geriatric Use).

Pediatric: The pharmacokinetics of tolterodine have not been established in pediatric patients.

Gender: The pharmacokinetics of tolterodine and the 5-hydroxymethyl metabolite are not influenced by gender. Mean C_{max} of tolterodine (1.6 µg/L in males versus 2.2 µg/L in females) and the active 5-hydroxymethyl metabolite (2.2 µg/L in males versus 2.5 µg/L in females) are similar in males and females who were administered tolterodine 2 mg. Mean AUC values of tolterodine (6.7 µg•h/L in males versus 7.8 µg•h/L in females) and the 5-hydroxymethyl metabolite (10 µg•h/L in males versus 11 µg•h/L in females) are also similar. The elimination half-life of tolterodine for both males and females is 2.4 hours, and the half-life of the 5-hydroxymethyl metabolite is 3.0 hours in females and 3.3 hours in males.

Race: Pharmacokinetic differences due to race have not been established.

Renal Insufficiency: The pharmacokinetics of tolterodine in patients with renal insufficiency have not been evaluated. The renal excretion of tolterodine and the 5-hydroxymethyl metabolite are negligible, and a decrease in total body clearance is not expected in patients with renal insufficiency. However, patients with renal impairment should be treated with caution.

Hepatic Insufficiency: Liver impairment can significantly alter the disposition of tolterodine. In a study conducted in cirrhotic patients, the elimination half-life to tolterodine was longer in cirrhotic patients (mean, 8.7 hours) than in healthy, young and elderly volunteers (mean, 2 to 4 hours). The clearance of orally administered tolterodine was substantially lower in cirrhotic patients (1.1 ± 1.7 L/h/kg) than in the healthy volunteers (5.7 ± 3.8 L/h/kg). Patients with significantly reduced hepatic function should not receive doses of DETROL greater than 1 mg twice daily (see PRECAUTIONS, General).

Drug-Drug Interactions

Fluoxetine: Fluoxetine is a selective serotonin reuptake inhibitor and a potent inhibitor of cytochrome P450 2D6 activity. In a study to assess the effect of fluoxetine on the pharmacokinetics of tolterodine and its metabolites, it was observed that fluoxetine significantly inhibited the metabolism of tolterodine in extensive metabolizers, resulting in a 4.8-fold increase in tolterodine AUC. There was a 52% decrease in C_{max} and a 20% decrease in AUC of the 5-hydroxymethyl metabolite. Fluoxetine thus alters the pharmacokinetics in patients who would otherwise be extensive metabolizers of tolterodine to resemble the pharmacokinetics profile in poor metabolizers. The sums of unbound serum concentrations of tolterodine and the 5-hydroxymethyl metabolite are only 25% higher during the interaction. No dose adjustment is required when DETROL and fluoxetine are coadministered.

Other Drugs Metabolized by Cytochrome P450 2D6: Tolterodine is not expected to influence the pharmacokinetics of drugs that are metabolized by cytochrome P450 2D6, such as flecainide, vinblastine, carbamazepine, and tricyclic antidepressants; however, the potential effect of tolterodine on the pharmacokinetics of these drugs has not been formally evaluated.

Warfarin: In healthy volunteers, coadministration of tolterodine 2 mg twice daily for 7 days and a single 25-mg dose of warfarin on day 4 had no effect on prothrombin time, Factor VII suppression, or on the pharmacokinetics of warfarin.

Oral Contraceptives: Tolterodine 2 mg twice daily had no effect on the pharmacokinetics of an oral contraceptive (ethinyl estradiol 30 µg/levonorgestrel 150 µg) as evidenced by the monitoring of ethinyl estradiol and levonorgestrel over a 2-month cycle in healthy female volunteers.

Diuretics: Coadministration of tolterodine up to 4 mg twice daily for up to 12 weeks with diuretic agents, such as indapamide, hydrochlorothiazide, triamterene, bendroflumethiazide, chlorothiazide, methylchlorothiazide, of furosemide, did not cause any adverse electrocardiographic (ECG) effects.

CLINICAL STUDIES

DETROL Tablets were evaluated for the treatment of patients with an overactive bladder with symptoms of urinary frequency, urgency, or urge incontinence in three placebo-controlled, 12-week studies. A total of 339 patients received DETROL 2 mg twice daily and 177 patients received placebo. The majority of patients were Caucasian (95%) and female (75%), with a mean age of 60 years (range, 19 to 91 years). At study entry, nearly all patients perceived they had urgency (98%) and most patients had increased frequency of micturitions (89%) and urge incontinence (83%). These characteristics were well balanced across treatment groups for the three studies.

The efficacy endpoints included the change from baseline for:

- number of micturitions per 24 hours (averaged over 7 days)

Incidence (%) of Adverse Events Reported in ≥1% of Patients Treated with DETROL (2 mg bid) in 12-Week, Phase 3 Clinical Studies

Body System	Adverse Event*	DETROL 2 mg bid N=474	Placebo N=176
% Patients Reporting Adverse Events		75.5	77.8
% Patients Reporting Serious Adverse Events		3.7	3.4
% Patients Discontinuing due to Adverse Events		8.0	5.7
Autonomic Nervous	dry mouth	39.5	15.9
General	back pain	2.7	3.4
	chest pain	3.4	1.7
	fatigue	6.8	7.4
	headache	11.0	7.4
	influenza-like symptoms	4.4	6.3
	fall	1.3	0.6
Central/ Peripheral Nervous	paresthesia	1.1	0.6
	vertigo/dizziness	8.6	9.1
Gastrointestinal	abdominal pain	7.6	6.3
	constipation	6.5	4.5
	diarrhea	4.0	6.3
	dyspepsia	5.9	1.7
	flatulence	1.3	0.6
	nausea	4.2	5.7
	vomiting/nausea	1.7	0.6
Respiratory	bronchitis	2.1	0.6
	coughing	2.1	1.7
	pharyngitis	1.5	2.3
	rhinitis	1.1	1.1
	sinusitis	1.1	5.7
	URI	5.9	9.1
Urinary	dysuria	2.5	4.0
	micturition frequency	1.1	1.7
	urinary retention/mict dis	1.7	2.8
	UTI	5.5	7.4
Skin/ Appendages	pruritus	1.3	1.1
	rash/erythema	1.9	2.8
	skin dry	1.7	0.6
Musculoskeletal	arthralgia	2.3	2.8
Vision	vision abnormal (including accommodation)	4.7	4.0
	xerophthalmia (dry eyes)	3.8	1.7
Psychiatric	nervousness	1.1	0.6
	somnolence	3.0	1.7
Metabolic/Nutritional	weight gain	1.5	1.1
Cardiovascular	hypertension	1.5	0.6
Resistance Mechanism	infection	2.1	1.1
	infection fungal	1.1	0.0

*Abbreviations: URI = upper respiratory infection, UTI = urinary tract infection, mict dis = micturition disorders.

- number of incontinence episodes per 24 hours (averaged over 7 days)
- volume of urine voided per micturition (averaged over 2 days)

Efficacy results for the three placebo-controlled, 12-week studies are presented in the following figures:

[See graphic at top of previous page]

INDICATIONS AND USAGE

DETROL Tablets are indicated for the treatment of patients with an overactive bladder with symptoms of urinary frequency, urgency, or urge incontinence.

CONTRAINDICATIONS

DETROL Tablets are contraindicated in patients with urinary retention, gastric retention, or uncontrolled narrow-angle glaucoma. DETROL is also contraindicated in patients who have demonstrated hypersensitivity to the drug or its ingredients.

PRECAUTIONS

General

Risk of Urinary Retention and Decreased Gastrointestinal Motility: DETROL Tablets should be administered with caution to patients with clinically significant bladder outflow obstruction because of the risk of urinary retention and to patients with gastrointestinal obstructive disorders, such as pyloric stenosis, because of the risk of gastric retention (see CONTRAINDICATIONS).

Controlled Narrow-Angle Glaucoma: DETROL should be used with caution in patients being treated for narrow-angle glaucoma.

Reduced Hepatic and Renal Function: Patients with signfiicantly reduced hepatic function should not receive doses of DETROL greater than 1 mg twice daily. Patients with renal impairment should be treated with caution (see CLINICAL PHARMACOLOGY, Pharmacokinetics in Special Populations).

Information for Patients

Patients should be informed that antimuscarinic agents such as tolterodine may produce the following effects: blurred vision, dizziness, or drowsiness.

Drug Interactions

Cytochrome P450 3A4 Inhibitors: Pharmacokinetic studies with patients concomitantly receiving cytochrome P450 3A4 inhibitors, such as macrolide antibiotics (erythromycin and clarithromycin) or antifungal agents (ketoconazole, itraconazole, and miconazole), have not been performed. Patients receiving cytochrome P450 3A4 inhibitors should not receive doses of DETROL greater than 1 mg twice daily.

Drug-Laboratory-Test Interactions

Interactions between tolterodine and laboratory tests have not been studied.

Carcinogenesis, Mutagenesis, Impairment of Fertility

Carcinogenicity studies with tolterodine were conducted in mice and rats. At the maximum tolterated dose in mice (30 mg/kg/day), female rats (20 mg/kg/day), and male rats (30 mg/kg/day), AUC values obtained for tolterodine were 355, 291, and 462 µg•h/L, respectively. In comparison, the human AUC value for a 2-mg dose administered twice daily is estimated at 34 µg•h/L. Thus, tolterodine exposure in the carcinogenicity studies was 9- to 14-fold higher than expected in humans. No increase in tumors was found in either mice or rats.

No mutagenic effects of tolterodine were detected in a battery of in vitro tests, including bacterial mutation assays

Continued on next page

Information on these Pharmacia & Upjohn products is based on labeling in effect June 1, 2000. Further information concerning these and other Pharmacia & Upjohn products may be obtained by direct inquiry to Medical Information, Pharmacia & Upjohn, Kalamazoo, MI 49001.

Detrol—Cont.

(Ames test) in four strains of *Salmonella typhimurium* and in two strains of *Escherichia coil,* a gene mutation assay in L5178Y mouse lymphoma cells, and chromosomal aberration tests in human lymphocytes. Tolterodine was also negative in vivo in the bone marrow micronucleus test in the mouse.
In female mice treated for 2 weeks before mating and during gestation with 20 mg/kg/day (corresponding to AUC valve of about 500 µg•h/L), neither effects on reproductive performance or fertility were seen. Based on AUC values, the systemic exposure was about 15-fold higher in animals than in humans. In male mice, a dose of 30 mg/kg/day did not induce any adverse effects on fertility.

Pregnancy

Pregnancy Category C. At oral doses of 20 mg/kg/day (approximately 14 times the human exposure), no anomalies or malformations were observed in mice. When given at doses of 30 to 40 mg/kg/day, tolterodine has been shown to be embryolethal and reduce fetal weight, and increase the incidence of fetal abnormalities (cleft palate, digital abnormalities, intra-abdominal hemorrhage, and various skeletal abnormalities, primarily reduced ossification) in mice. At these doses, the AUC values were about 20- to 25-fold higher than in humans. Rabbits treated subcutaneously at a dose of 0.8 mg/kg/day achieved an AUC of 100 µg•h/L, which is about three-fold higher than that resulting from the human dose. This dose did not result in any embryotoxicity or teratogenicity. There at no studies of tolterodine in pregnant women. Therefore, DETROL should be used during pregnancy only if the potential benefit for the mother justifies the potential risk for the fetus.

Nursing Mothers

Tolterodine is excreted into the milk in mice. Offspring of female mice treated with tolterodine 20 mg/kg/day during the lactation period had slightly reduced body-weight gain. The offspring regained the weight during the maturation phase. It is not known whether tolterodine is excreted in human milk; therefore, administration of DETROL should be discontinued during nursing.

Pediatric Use

The safety and effectiveness of DETROL in pediatric patients have not been established.

Geriatric Use

Of the 1120 patients who were treated in the four, Phase 3, 12-week clinical studies of DETROL, 474 (42%) were 65 to 91 years of age. No overall differences in safety were observed between the older and younger patients (see CLINICAL PHARMACOLOGY, Pharmacokinetics in Special Populations).

ADVERSE REACTIONS

The Phase 2 and 3 clinical trial program for DETROL Tablets included 2049 patients who were treated with DETROL (N=1619) or placebo (N=430). No differences in the safety profile of tolterodine were identified based on age, gender, race, or metabolism. Four Phase 3, 12-week, controlled clinical studies form the basis for the main evaluation of safety, and the results are summarized below.
Adverse events considered to be treatment-related were dry mouth, dyspepsia, headache, constipation, and dry eyes. Dry mouth, constipation, abnormal vision (accommodation abnormalities), dry eyes, and urinary retention are expected side effects of antimuscarinic agents.
Dry mouth was the most frequently reported adverse event for patients treated with DETROL 2 mg twice daily in the Phase 3 clinical studies, occurring in 39.5% of patients treated with DETROL and 15.9% of placebo-treated patients; 0.8% of patients treated with DETROL discontinued treatment due to dry mouth.
The frequency of discontinuation due to adverse events was highest during the first 4 weeks of treatment. Eight percent of patients treated with DETROL 2 mg twice daily discontinued treatment due to adverse events; the most common adverse events leading to discontinuation were dizziness and headache.
The following table lists the adverse events reported in 1% or more of the patients treated with DETROL 2 mg twice daily in the 12-week studies. The adverse events are reported regardless of causality.
[See table at top of previous page]
Expected adverse effects of antimuscarinic agents reported in less than 1% of patients treated with DETROL in 12-week controlled clinical studies were confusion, gastroesophageal reflux, and flushed skin.

Postmarketing Surveillance

The following events have been reported in association with tolterodine use in clinical practice: anaphylactoid reactions, tachycardia, peripheral edema.

OVERDOSAGE

A 27-month-old child who ingested 5 to 7 DETROL Tablets 2 mg was treated with a suspension of activated charcoal and was hospitalized overnight with symptoms of dry mouth. The child fully recovered.

Management of Overdosage

Overdosage with DETROL can potentially result in severe central anticholinergic effects and should be treated accordingly.
ECG monitoring is recommended in the event of overdosage. In dogs, changes in the QT interval (slight prolongation of 10% to 20%) were observed at a suprapharmacologic dose of 4.5 mg/kg, which is about 68 times higher than the recommended human dose. In clinical trials of normal volunteers and patients, QT interval prolongation was not observed at doses up to 4 mg twice daily of tolterodine (higher doses were not evaluated).

DOSAGE AND ADMINISTRATION

The initial recommended dose is 2 mg twice daily. The dose may be lowered to 1 mg twice daily based on individual response and tolerability. For patients with significantly reduced hepatic function or who are currently taking drugs that are inhibitors of cytochrome P450 3A4, the recommended dose is 1 mg twice daily (see PRECAUTIONS, General).

HOW SUPPLIED

DETROL Tablets 1 mg (white, round, biconvex, film-coated tablets engraved with arcs above and below the letters "TO") and **DETROL Tablets 2 mg** (white, round, biconvex, film-coated tablets engraved with arcs above and below the letters "DT") are supplied as follows:

Bottles of 60
1 mg NDC 0009-4541-02
2 mg NDC 0009-4544-02
Bottles of 500
1 mg NDC 0009-4541-03
2 mg NDC 0009-4544-03
Unit Dose Pack of 140
1 mg NDC 0009-4541-01
2 mg NDC 0009-4544-01

Store at controlled room temperature 20° to 25° C (68° to 77° F) [see USP].

Rx only

US Patent No. 5,382,600
Pharmacia & Upjohn Company
Kalamazoo, MI 49001, USA
June 2000 817 413 002
692167

Shown in Product Identification Guide, page 331

DIPENTUM® ℞

[dī-pent 'um]
olsalazine sodium capsules

DESCRIPTION

The active ingredient in DIPENTUM Capsules (olsalazine sodium) is the sodium salt of a salicylate, disodium 3,3'-azobis (6-hydroxybenzoate) a compound that is effectively bioconverted to 5-aminosalicylic acid (5- ASA), which has anti-inflammatory activity in ulcerative colitis. Its empirical formula is $C_{14}H_8N_2Na_2O_6$ with a molecular weight of 346.21.
The structural formula is:

NaOOC
HO— —N = N— —OH
COONa

Olsalazine sodium is a yellow crystalline powder which melts with decomposition at 240°C. It is the sodium salt of a weak acid, soluble in water and DMSO, and practically insoluble in ethanol, chloroform and ether. Olsalazine sodium has acceptable stability under acidic or basic conditions.
DIPENTUM is supplied in hard gelatin capsules for oral administration. The inert ingredient in each 250 mg capsule of olsalazine sodium is magnesium stearate. The capsule shell has the following inactive ingredients: black iron oxide, caramel, gelatin, and titanium dioxide.

CLINICAL PHARMACOLOGY

After oral administration, olsalazine has limited systemic bioavailability. Based on oral and intravenous dosing studies, approximately 2.4% of a single 1.0 g oral dose is absorbed. Less than 1% of olsalazine is recovered in the urine. The remaining 98 to 99% of an oral dose will reach the colon where each molecule is rapidly converted into two molecules of 5-aminosalicylic acid (5-ASA) by colonic bacteria and the low prevailing redox potential found in this environment. The liberated 5-ASA is absorbed slowly resulting in very high local concentrations in the colon.
The conversion of olsalazine to mesalamine (5-ASA) in the colon is similar to that of sulfasalazine, which is converted into sulfapyridine and mesalamine. It is thought that the mesalamine component is therapeutically active in ulcerative colitis (A.K. Azad-Kahn et al, *LANCET,* 2:892–895, 1977). The usual dose of sulfasalazine for maintenance of remission in patients with ulcerative colitis is 2 grams daily, which would provide approximately 0.8 gram of mesalamine to the colon. More than 0.9 gram of mesalamine would usually be made available in the colon from 1 gram of olsalazine.
The mechanism of action of mesalamine (and sulfalazine) is unknown, but appears to be topical rather than systemic. Mucosal production of arachidonic acid (AA) metabolites, both through the cyclooxygenase pathways, i.e., prostanoids, and through the lipoxygenase pathways, i.e., leukotrienes (LTs) and hydroxyiecosatetraenoic acids (HETEs) is increased in patients with chronic inflammatory bowel disease, and it is possible that mesalamine diminishes inflammation by blocking cyclooxygenase and inhibiting prostaglandin (PG) production in the colon.

<u>Pharmacokinetics</u>
The pharmacokinetics of olsalazine are similar in both healthy volunteers and in patients with ulcerative colitis. Maximum serum concentrations of olsalazine appear after approximately 1 hour, and, even after a 1.0 g single dose, are low, e.g., 1.6 to 6.2 µmol/L. Olsalazine has a very short serum half-life, approximately 0.9 hours. Olsalazine is more than 99% bound to plasma proteins. It does not interfere with protein binding of warfarin. The urinary recovery of olsalazine is below 1%. Total recovery of oral ^{14}C-labeled olsalazine in animals and humans ranging from 90 to 97%.
Approximately 0.1% of an oral dose of olsalazine is metabolized in the liver to olsalazine-O-sulfate (olsalazine-S). Olsalasine-S, in contrast to olsalazine has a half-life of 7 days. Olsalazine-S accumulates to steady state within 2 to 3 weeks.
Patients on daily doses of 1.0 g olsalazine for 2 to 4 years show a stable plasma concentration of olsalazine-S (3.3 to 12.4 µmol/L). Olsalazine-S is more than 99% bound to plasma proteins. Its long half-life is mainly due to slow dissociation from the protein binding site. Less than 1% of both olsalazine and olsalazine-S appears undissociated in plasma.
5-aminosalicylic acid (5-ASA): Serum concentrations of 5-ASA are detected after 4 to 8 hours. The peak levels of 5-ASA after an oral dose of 1.0 g olsalazine are low, i.e., 0 to 4.3 µmol/L. Of the total 5-ASA found in the urine, more than 90% is in the form of N-acetyl-5-ASA (Ac-5-ASA). Only small amounts of 5-ASA are detected.
N-acetyl-5-ASA (Ac-5-ASA), the major metabolite of 5-ASA found in plasma and urine, is acetylated (deactivated) in at least two sites, the colonic epithelium and the liver. Ac-5-ASA is found in the serum, with peak values of 1.7 to 8.7 µmol/L after a single 1.0 g dose. Approximately 20% of the total 5-ASA is recovered in the urine, where it is found almost exclusively as Ac-5-ASA. The remaining 5-ASA is partially acetylated and is excreted in the feces. From fecal dialysis, the concentration of 5-ASA in the colon following olsalazine has been calculated to be 18 to 49 mmol/L. No accumulation of 5-ASA or Ac-5-ASA in plasma has been detected. 5-ASA and Ac-5-ASA are 74 and 81%, respectively, bound to plasma proteins.

ANIMAL TOXICOLOGY

Preclinical subacute and chronic toxicity studies in rats have shown the kidney to be the major target organ of olsalazine toxicity. At an oral daily dose of 400 mg/kg or higher, olsalazine treatment produced nephritis and tubular necrosis in a 4-week study; interstitial nephritis and tubular calcinosis in a 6-month study, and renal fibrosis, mineralization and transitional cell hyperplasia in a 1-year study.

CLINICAL STUDIES

Two controlled studies have demonstrated the efficacy of olsalazine as maintenance therapy in patients with ulcerative colitis. In the first, ulcerative colitis patients in remission were randomized to olsalazine 500 mg B.I.D. or placebo, and relapse rates for a six month period of time were compared. For the 52 patients randomized to olsalazine, 12 relapses occurred, while for the 49 placebo patients, 22 relapses occurred. This difference in relapse rates was significant ($p<.02$).
In the second study, 164 ulcerative colitis patients in remission were randomized to olsalazine 500 mg B.I.D. or sulfasalazine 1 gram B.I.D., and relapse rates were compared after six months. The relapse rate for olsalazine was 19.5% while that for sulfasalazine was 12.2%, a non-significant difference.

INDICATIONS AND USAGE

Olsalazine is indicated for the maintenance of ulcerative colitis in patients who are intolerant of sulfasalazine.

CONTRAINDICATIONS

Hypersensitivity to salicylates.

PRECAUTIONS

<u>General</u>
Overall, approximately 17% of subjects receiving olsalazine in clinical studies reported diarrhea sometime during therapy. This diarrhea resulted in withdrawal of treatment in 6% of patients. This diarrhea appears to be dose related, although it may be difficult to distinguish from the underlying symptoms of the disease.
Exacerbation of the symptoms of colitis thought to have been caused by mesalamine or sulfasalazine has been noted. Although renal abnormalities were not reported in clinical trials with olsalazine, there have been rare reports from post-marketing experience (see under ADVERSE REACTIONS). Therefore, the possibility of renal tubular damage due to absorbed mesalamine or its n-acetylated metabolite, as noted in the ANIMAL TOXICOLOGY section must be kept in mind, particularly for patients with pre-existing renal disease. In these patients, monitoring with urinalysis, BUN and creatinine determinations is advised.

<u>Information for Patients</u>
Patients should be instructed to take olsalazine with food. The drug should be taken in evenly divided doses. Patients should be informed that about 17% of subjects receiving olsalazine during clinical studies reported diarrhea sometime during therapy. If diarrhea occurs, patients should contact their physician.

<u>Drug Interactions:</u> Increased prothrombin time in patients taking concomitant warfarin has been reported.

<u>Drug/Laboratory Test Interactions:</u> None known.

<u>Carcinogenesis, Mutagenesis, Impairment of Fertility</u>
In a two year oral rat carcinogenicity study, olsalazine was tested in male and female Wistar rats at daily doses of 200,

TABLE 1
Adverse Reactions Resulting in Withdrawal From Controlled Studies

	Total	
	Olsalazine (N = 441)	Placebo (N = 208)
Diarrhea/Loose Stools	26 (5.9%)	10 (4.8%)
Nausea	3	2
Abdominal Pain	5 (1.1%)	0
Rash/Itching	5 (1.1%)	0
Headache	3	0
Heartburn	2	0
Rectal Bleeding	1	0
Insomnia	1	0
Dizziness	1	0
Anorexia	1	0
Light Headedness	1	0
Depression	1	0
Miscellaneous	4 (0.9%)	3 (1.4%)
Total Number of Patients Withdrawn	46 (10.4%)	14 (6.7%)

TABLE 2: COMPARATIVE INCIDENCE (%) OF ADVERSE EFFECTS REPORTED BY ONE PERCENT OR MORE OF ULCERATIVE COLITIS PATIENTS TREATED WITH OLSALAZINE OR PLACEBO IN DOUBLE BLIND CONTROLLED STUDIES

ADVERSE EVENT	Olsalazine (N = 441) %	Placebo (N = 208) %
Digestive System		
Diarrhea	11.1	6.7
Abdominal Pain/Cramps	10.1	7.2
Nausea	5.0	3.9
Dyspepsia	4.0	4.3
Bloating	1.5	1.4
Anorexia	1.3	1.9
Vomiting	1.0	–
Stomatitis	1.0	–
Increased Blood in Stool	–	3.4
CNS/Psychiatric		
Headache	5.0	4.8
Fatigue/Drowsiness/Lethargy	1.8	2.9
Depression	1.5	–
Vertigo/Dizziness	1.0	–
Insomnia	–	2.4
Skin		
Rash	2.3	1.4
Itching	1.3	–
Musculoskeletal		
Arthralgia/Joint Pain	4.0	2.9
Miscellaneous		
Upper Respiratory Infection	1.5	–

400 and 800 mg/kg/day (approximately 10 to 40 times the human maintenance dose, based on a patient weight of 50 kg and a human dose of 1 g). Urinary bladder transitional cell carcinomas were found in three male rats (6%, p=0.022, exact trend test) receiving 40 times the human dose and were not found in untreated male controls. In the same study, urinary bladder transitional cell carcinoma and papilloma occurred in 2 untreated control female rats (2%). No such tumors were found in any of the female rats treated at doses up to 40 times the human dose.

In an eighteen month oral mouse carcinogenicity study, olsalazine was tested in male and female CD-1 mice at daily doses of 500, 1000 and 2000 mg/kg/day (approximately 25 to 100 times the human maintenance dose). Liver hemangiosarcomata were found in two male mice (4%) receiving olsalazine at 100 times the human dose, while no such tumor occurred in the other treated male mice groups or any of the treated female mice. The observed incidence of this tumor is within the 4% incidence in historical controls.

Olsalazine was not mutagenic in *in vitro* Ames tests, mouse lymphoma cell mutation assays, human lymphocyte chromosomal aberration tests and the *in vivo* rat bone marrow cell chromosomal aberration test.

Olsalazine in a dose range of 100 to 400 mg/kg/day (approximately 5 to 20 times the human maintenance dose) did not influence the fertility of male or female rats. The oligospermia and infertility in men associated with sulfasalazine have not been reported with olsalazine.

Pregnancy. Teratogenic Effects. Pregnancy Category C.

Olsalazine has been shown to produce fetal developmental toxicity as indicated by reduced fetal weights, retarded ossifications and immaturity of the fetal visceral organs when given during organogenesis to pregnant rats in doses 5 to 20 times the human dose (100 to 400 mg/kg). There are no adequate and well-controlled studies in pregnant women. Olsalazine should be used during pregnancy only if the potential benefit justifies the potential risk to the fetus.

Nursing Mothers

Oral administration of olsalazine to lactating rats in doses 5 to 20 times the human dose produced growth retardation in their pups. It is not known whether this drug is excreted in human milk. Because many drugs are excreted in human milk, caution should be exercised when olsalazine is administered to a nursing woman.

Pediatric Use

Safety and effectiveness in a pediatric population have not been established.

ADVERSE REACTIONS

Olsalazine has been evaluated in ulcerative colitis patients in remission as well as those with acute disease. Both sulfasalazine-tolerant and intolerant patients have been studied in controlled clinical trials. Overall, 10.4% of patients discontinued olsalazine because of an adverse experience compared with 6.7% of placebo patients. The most commonly reported adverse reactions leading to treatment withdrawal were diarrhea or loose stools (olsalazine 5.9%; placebo 4.8%), abdominal pain and rash or itching (slightly more than 1% of patients receiving olsalazine). Other adverse reactions to olsalazine leading to withdrawal occurred in fewer than 1% of patients (TABLE 1).

[See table 1 above]

For those controlled studies, the comparative incidences of adverse reactions reported in 1% or more patients treated with olsalazine or placebo are provided in TABLE 2.

[See table 2 above]

Over 2,500 patients have been treated with olsalazine in various controlled and uncontrolled clinical studies. In these as well as in the post-marketing experience, olsalazine was administered mainly to patients intolerant to sulfasalazine. There have been rare reports of the following adverse effects in patients receiving olsalazine. These were often difficult to distinguish from possible symptoms of the underlying disease or from the effects of prior and/or concomitant therapy. A causal relationship to the drug has not been demonstrated for some of these reactions.

Digestive: Pancreatitis, diarrhea with dehydration, increased blood in stool, rectal bleeding, flare in symptoms, rectal discomfort, epigastric discomfort, flatulence.

Rare cases of granulomatous hepatitis and nonspecific, reactive hepatitis have been reported in patients receiving olsalazine. Additionally, a patient developed mild cholestatic hepatitis during treatment with sulfasalazine and experienced the same symptoms two weeks later after the treatment was changed to olsalazine. Withdrawal of olsalazine led to complete recovery in these cases.

Neurologic: Paresthesia, tremors, insomnia, mood swings, irritability, fever chills, rigors.

Dermatologic: Erythema nodosum, photosensitivity, erythema, hot flashes, alopecia.

Musculoskeletal: Muscle cramps.

Cardiovascular/Pulmonary: Pericarditis, second degree heart block, interstitial pulmonary disease, hypertension, orthostatic hypotension, peripheral edema, chest pains, tachycardia, palpitations, bronchospasm, shortness of breath.

A patient who developed thyroid disease 9 days after starting DIPENTUM Capsules was given propranolol and radioactive iodine and subsequently developed shortness of breath and nausea. The patient died 5 days later with signs and symptoms of acute diffuse myocarditis.

Genitourinary: Frequency, dysuria, hematuria, proteinuria, nephrotic syndrome, interstitial nephritis, impotence, menorrhagia.

Hematologic: Leucopenia, neutropenia, lymphopenia, eosinophilia, thrombocytopenia, anemia, hemolytic anemia, reticulocytosis.

Laboratory: ALT (SGPT) or AST (SGOT) elevated beyond the normal range.

Special Senses: Tinnitus, dry mouth, dry eyes, watery eyes, blurred vision.

Postmarketing Reports

The following events have been identified during post-approval use of products which contain (or are metabolized to) mesalamine in clinical practice. Because they are reported voluntarily from a population of unknown size, estimates of frequency cannot be made. These events have been chosen for inclusion due to a combination of seriousness, frequency of reporting, or potential causal connection to mesalamine:

Gastrointestinal: Reports of hepatotoxicity, including elevated liver function tests (SGOT/AST, SGPT/ALT, GGT, LDH, alkaline phosphatase, bilirubin), jaundice, cholestatic jaundice, cirrhosis, and possible hepatocellular damage including liver necrosis and liver failure. Some of these cases were fatal. One case of Kawasaki-like syndrome, which included hepatic function changes, was also reported.

DRUG ABUSE AND DEPENDENCY

Abuse: None reported.

Dependence: Drug dependence has not been reported with chronic administration of olsalazine.

OVERDOSAGE

No overdosage has been reported in humans. Maximum single oral doses of 5 g/kg in mice and rats and 2 g/kg in dogs were not lethal. Symptoms of acute toxicity were decreased motor activity and diarrhea in all species tested and in addition, vomiting in dogs.

DOSAGE AND ADMINISTRATION

The usual dosage in adults for maintenance of remission is 1.0 g/day in two divided doses.

HOW SUPPLIED

Beige colored capsules, containing 250 mg olsalazine sodium imprinted with "DIPENTUM® 250 mg" on the capsule shell. Packaged in bottles of 100 (NDC 0013-0105-01) and 300 (NDC 0013-0105-20).

Storage

Store at 25°C (77°F). Excursions permitted to 15° to 30°C (59° to 86°F) [see USP Controlled Room Temperature].

℞ only

Manufactured for: Pharmacia & Upjohn Company, Kalamazoo, MI 49001, USA
by: Pharmacia & Upjohn AB, Stockholm, Sweden

111010799 Revised: July 1999

DOSTINEX® ℞
cabergoline tablets

DESCRIPTION

DOSTINEX Tablets contain cabergoline, a dopamine receptor agonist. The chemical name for cabergoline is 1-[(6-allylergolin-8β-yl)-carbonyl]-1-[3-(dimethylamino)propyl]-3-ethylurea. Its empirical formula is $C_{26}H_{37}N_5O_2$, and its molecular weight is 451.62. The structural formula is as follows:

Cabergoline is a white powder soluble in ethyl alcohol, chloroform, and N, N-dimethylformamide (DMF); slightly soluble in 0.1N hydrochloric acid; very slightly soluble in n-hexane; and insoluble in water.

Continued on next page

Information on these Pharmacia & Upjohn products is based on labeling in effect June 1, 2000. Further information concerning these and other Pharmacia & Upjohn products may be obtained by direct inquiry to Medical Information, Pharmacia & Upjohn, Kalamazoo, MI 49001.

Dostinex—Cont.

DOSTINEX Tablets, for oral administration, contain 0.5 mg of cabergoline. Inactive ingredients consist of leucine, USP, and lactose, NF.

CLINICAL PHARMACOLOGY

Mechanism of Action: The secretion of prolactin by the anterior pituitary is mainly under hypothalmic inhibitory control, likely exerted through release of dopamine by tuberoinfundibular neurons. Cabergoline is a long-acting dopamine receptor agonist with a high affinity for D_2 receptors. Results of in vitro studies demonstrate that cabergoline exerts a direct inhibitory effect on the secretion of prolactin by rat pituitary lactotrophs. Cabergoline decreased serum prolactin levels in reserpinized rats. Receptor-binding studies indicate that cabergoline has low affinity for dopamine D_1, α_1- and α_2-adrenergic, and 5-HT_1- and 5-HT_2-serotonin receptors.

Clinical Studies: The prolactin-lowering efficacy of DOSTINEX was demonstrated in hyperprolactinemic women in two randomized, double-blind, comparative studies, one with placebo and the other with bromocriptine. In the placebo-controlled study (placebo n=20; cabergoline n=168), DOSTINEX produced a dose-related decrease in serum prolactin levels with prolactin normalized after 4 weeks of treatment in 29%, 76%, 74% and 95% of the patients receiving 0.125, 0.5, 0.75, and 1.0 mg twice weekly respectively.

In the 8-week, double-blind period of the comparative trial with bromocriptine (cabergoline n=223; bromocriptine n=236 in the intent-to-treat analysis), prolactin was normalized in 77% of the patients treated with DOSTINEX at 0.5 mg twice weekly compared with 59% of those treated with bromocriptine at 2.5 mg twice daily. Restoration of menses occurred in 77% of the women treated with DOSTINEX, compared with 70% of those treated with bromocriptine. Among patients with galactorrhea, this symptom disappeared in 73% of those treated with DOSTINEX compared with 56% of those treated with bromocriptine.

Pharmacokinetics

Absorption: Following single oral doses of 0.5 mg to 1.5 mg given to 12 healthy adult volunteers, mean peak plasma levels of 30 to 70 picograms (pg)/mL of cabergoline were observed within 2 to 3 hours. Over the 0.5-to-7 mg dose range, cabergoline plasma levels appeared to be dose-proportional in 12 healthy adult volunteers and nine adult parkinsonian patients. A repeat-dose study in 12 healthy volunteers suggests that steady-state levels following a once-weekly dosing schedule are expected to be twofold to threefold higher than after a single dose. The absolute bioavailability of cabergoline is unknown. A significant fraction of the administered dose undergoes a first-pass effect. The elimination half-life of cabergoline estimated from urinary data of 12 healthy subjects ranged between 63 to 69 hours. The prolonged prolactin-lowering effect of cabergoline may be related to its slow elimination and long half-life.

Distribution: In animals, based on total radioactivity, cabergoline (and/or its metabolites) has shown extensive tissue distribution. Radioactivity in the pituitary exceeded that in plasma by >100-fold and was eliminated with a half-life of approximately 60 hours. This finding is consistent with the long-lasting prolactin-lowering effect of the drug. Whole body autoradiography studies in pregnant rats showed no fetal uptake but high levels in the uterine wall. Significant radioactivity (parent plus metabolites) detected in the milk of lactating rats suggests a potential for exposure to nursing infants. The drug is extensively distributed throughout the body. Cabergoline is moderately bound (40% to 42%) to human plasma proteins in a concentration-independent manner. Concomitant dosing of highly protein-bound drugs is unlikely to affect its disposition.

Metabolism: In both animals and humans, cabergoline is extensively metabolized, predominately via hydrolysis of the acylurea bond or the urea moiety. Cytochrome P-450 mediated metabolism appears to be minimal. Cabergoline does not cause enzyme induction and/or inhibition in the rat. Hydrolysis of the acylurea or urea moiety abolishes the prolactin-lowering effect of cabergoline, and major metabolites identified thus far do not contribute to the therapeutic effect.

Excretion: After oral dosing of radioactive cabergoline to five healthy volunteers, approximately 22% and 60% of the dose was excreted within 20 days in the urine and feces, respectively. Less than 4% of the dose was excreted unchanged in the urine. Nonrenal and renal clearances for cabergoline are about 3.2 L/min and 0.08 L/min, respectively. Urinary excretion in hyperprolactinemic patients was similar.

Special Populations

Renal Insufficiency: The pharmacokinetics of cabergoline were not altered in 12 patients with moderate-to-severe renal insufficiency as assessed by creatinine clearance.

Hepatic Insufficiency: In 12 patients with mild-to-moderate hepatic dysfunction (Child-Pugh score ≤10), no effect on mean cabergoline C_{max} or area under the plasma concentration curve (AUC) was observed. However, patients with severe insufficiency (Child-Pugh score >10) show a substantial increase in the mean cabergoline C_{max} and AUC, and thus necessitate caution.

Elderly: Effect of age on the pharmacokinetics of cabergoline has not been studied.

Food-Drug Interaction

In 12 healthy adult volunteers, food did not alter cabergoline kinetics.

Pharmacodynamics

Dose response with inhibition of plasma prolactin, onset of maximal effect, and duration of effect has been documented following single cabergoline doses to healthy volunteers (0.05 to 1.5 mg) and hyperprolactinemic patients (0.3 to 1 mg). In volunteers, prolactin inhibition was evident at doses >0.2 mg, while doses ≥0.5 mg caused maximal suppression in most subjects. Higher doses produce prolactin suppression in a greater proportion of subjects and with an earlier onset and longer duration of action. In 12 healthy volunteers, 0.5, 1, and 1.5 mg doses resulted in complete prolactin inhibition, with a maximum effect within 3 hours in 92% to 100% of subjects after the 1 and 1.5 mg doses compared with 50% of subjects after the 0.5 mg dose.

In hyperprolactinemic patients (N=51), the maximal prolactin decrease after a 0.6 mg single dose of cabergoline was comparable to 2.5 mg bromocriptine; however, the duration of effect was markedly longer (14 days vs 24 hours). The time to maximal effect was shorter for bromocriptine than cabergoline (6 hours vs 48 hours).

In 72 healthy volunteers, single or multiple doses (up to 2 mg) of cabergoline resulted in selective inhibition of prolactin with no apparent effect on other anterior pituitary hormones (GH, FSH, LH, ACTH, and TSH) or cortisol.

INDICATIONS AND USAGE

DOSTINEX Tablets are indicated for the treatment of hyperprolactinemic disorders, either idiopathic or due to pituitary adenomas.

CONTRAINDICATIONS

DOSTINEX Tablets are contraindicated in patients with uncontrolled hypertension or known hypersensitivity to ergot derivatives.

WARNINGS

Dopamine agonists in general should not be used in patients with pregnancy-induced hypertension, for example, preeclampsia and eclampsia, unless the potential benefit is judged to outweigh the possible risk.

PRECAUTIONS

General: Initial doses higher than 1.0 mg may produce orthostatic hypotension. Care should be exercised when administering DOSTINEX with other medications known to lower blood pressure.

Postpartum Lactation Inhibition or Suppression: DOSTINEX is not indicated for the inhibition or suppression of physiologic lactation. Use of bromocriptine, another dopamine agonist for this purpose, has been associated with cases of hypertension, stroke, and seizures.

Hepatic Impairment: Since cabergoline is extensively metabolized by the liver, caution should be used, and careful monitoring exercised, when administering DOSTINEX to patients with hepatic impairment.

Information for Patients: A patient should be instructed to notify her physician if she suspects she is pregnant, becomes pregnant, or intends to become pregnant during therapy. A pregnancy test should be done if there is any suspicion of pregnancy and continuation of treatment should be discussed with her physician.

Drug Interactions: DOSTINEX should not be administered concurrently with D_2-antagonists, such as phenothiazines, butyrophenones, thioxanthines, or metoclopramide.

Carcinogenesis, Mutagenesis, Impairment of Fertility: Carcinogenicity studies were conducted in mice and rats with cabergoline given by gavage at doses up to 0.98 mg/kg/day and 0.32 mg/kg/day, respectively. These doses are 7 times and 4 times the maximum recommended human dose calculated on a body surface area basis using total mg/m^2/week in rodents and mg/m^2/week for a 50 kg human.

There was a slight increase in the incidence of cervical and uterine leiomyomas and uterine leiomyosarcomas in mice. In rats, there was a slight increase in malignant tumors of the cervix and uterus and interstitial cell adenomas. The occurrence of tumors in female rodents may be related to the prolonged suppression of prolactin secretion because prolactin is needed in rodents for the maintenance of the corpus luteum. In the absence of prolactin, the estrogen/progesterone ratio is increased, thereby increasing the risk for uterine tumors. In male rodents, the decrease in serum prolactin levels was associated with an increase in serum luteinizing hormone, which is thought to be a compensatory effect to maintain testicular steroid synthesis. Since these hormonal mechanisms are thought to be species-specific, the relevance of these tumors to humans is not known.

The mutagenic potential of cabergoline was evaluated and found to be negative in a battery of in vitro tests. These tests included the bacterial mutation (Ames) test with *Salmonella typhimurium*, the gene mutation assay with *Schizosaccharomyces pombe P* $_1$ and V79 Chinese hamster cells, DNA damage and repair in *Saccharomyces cerevisiae D* $_4$, and chromosomal aberrations in human lymphocytes. Cabergoline was also negative in the bone marrow micronucleus test in the mouse.

In female rats, a daily dose of 0.003 mg/kg for 2 weeks prior to mating and throughout the mating period inhibited conception. This dose represents approximately 1/28 the maximum recommended human dose calculated on a body surface area basis using total mg/m^2/week in rats and mg/m^2/week for a 50 kg human.

Pregnancy: Teratogenic Effects: Category B. Reproduction studies have been performed with cabergoline in mice, rats, and rabbits administered by gavage.

(Multiples of the maximum recommended human dose in this section are calculated on a body surface area basis using total mg/m^2/week for animals and mg/m^2/week for a 50 kg human.)

There were maternotoxic effects but no teratogenic effects in mice given cabergoline at doses up to 8 mg/kg/day (approximately 55 times the maximum recommended human dose) during the period of organogenesis.

A dose of 0.012 mg/kg/day (approximately 1/7 the maximum recommended human dose) during the period of organogenesis in rats caused an increase in post-implantation embryofetal losses. These losses could be due to the prolactin inhibitory properties of cabergoline in rats. At daily doses of 0.5 mg/kg/day (approximately 19 times the maximum recommended human dose) during the period of organogenesis in the rabbit, cabergoline caused maternotoxicity characterized by a loss of body weight and decreased food consumption. Doses of 4 mg/kg/day (approximately 150 times the maximum recommended human dose) during the period of organogenesis in the rabbit caused an increased occurrence of various malformations. However, in another study in rabbits, no treatment-related malformations or embryofetotoxicity were observed at doses up to 8 mg/kg/day (approximately 300 times the maximum recommended human dose).

In rats, doses higher than 0.003 mg/kg/day (approximately 1/28 the maximum recommended human dose) from 6 days before parturition and throughout the lactation period inhibited growth and caused death of offspring due to decreased milk secretion.

There are, however, no adequate and well-controlled studies in pregnant women. Because animal reproduction studies are not always predictive of human response, this drug should be used during pregnancy only if clearly needed.

Nursing Mothers: It is not known whether this drug is excreted in human milk. Because many drugs are excreted in human milk and because of the potential for serious adverse reactions in nursing infants from cabergoline, a decision should be made whether to discontinue nursing or to discontinue the drug, taking into account the importance of the drug to the mother. Use of DOSTINEX for the inhibition or suppression of physiologic lactation is not recommended (see PRECAUTIONS section).

The prolactin-lowering action of cabergoline suggests that it will interfere with lactation. Due to this interference with lactation, DOSTINEX should not be given to women postpartum who are breastfeeding or who are planning to breastfeed.

Pediatric Use: Safety and effectiveness of DOSTINEX in pediatric patients have not been established.

Geriatric Use: Clinical studies of DOSTINEX did not include sufficient numbers of subjects aged 65 and over to determine whether they respond differently from younger patients. Other reported clinical experience has not identified differences in responses between the elderly and younger patients. In general, dose selection for an elderly patient should be cautious, usually starting at the low end of the dosing range, reflecting the greater frequency of decreased hepatic, renal, or cardiac function, and of concomitant disease or other drug therapy.

ADVERSE REACTIONS

The safety of DOSTINEX Tablets has been evaluated in more than 900 patients with hyperprolactinemic disorders. Most adverse events were mild or moderate in severity.

In a 4-week, double-blind, placebo-controlled study, treatment consisted of placebo or cabergoline at fixed doses of 0.125, 0.5, 0.75, or 1.0 mg twice weekly. Doses were halved during the first week. Since a possible dose-related effect was observed for nausea only, the four cabergoline treatment groups have been combined. The incidence of the most common adverse events during the placebo-controlled study is presented in the following table.

Incidence of Reported Adverse Events During the 4-Week, Double-Blind, Placebo-Controlled Trial

Adverse Event*	Cabergoline (n=168) 0.125 to 1 mg two times a week	Placebo (n=20)
	Number (percent)	
Gastrointestinal		
Nausea	45 (27)	4 (20)
Constipation	16 (10)	0
Abdominal pain	9 (5)	1 (5)
Dyspepsia	4 (2)	0
Vomiting	4 (2)	0
Central and Peripheral Nervous System		
Headache	43 (26)	5 (25)
Dizziness	25 (15)	1 (5)
Paresthesia	2 (1)	0
Vertigo	2 (1)	0
Body As a Whole		
Asthenia	15 (9)	2 (10)
Fatigue	12 (7)	0
Hot flashes	2 (1)	1 (5)
Psychiatric		
Somnolence	9 (5)	1 (5)
Depression	5 (3)	1 (5)
Nervousness	4 (2)	0

Autonomic Nervous System		
Postural hypotension	6 (4)	0
Reproductive—Female		
Breast pain	2 (1)	0
Dysmenorrhea	2 (1)	0
Vision		
Abnormal vision	2 (1)	0

*Reported at ≥1% for cabergoline

In the 8-week, double-blind period of the comparative trial with bromocriptine, DOSTINEX (at a dose of 0.5 mg twice weekly) was discontinued because of an adverse event in 4 of 221 patients (2%) while bromocriptine (at a dose of 2.5 mg two times a day) was discontinued in 14 of 231 patients (6%). The most common reasons for discontinuation from DOSTINEX were headache, nausea and vomiting (3, 2 and 2 patients respectively); the most common reasons for discontinuation from bromocriptine were nausea, vomiting, headache, and dizziness or vertigo (10, 3, 3, and 3 patients respectively). The incidence of the most common adverse events during the double-blind portion of the comparative trial with bromocriptine is presented in the following table.

Incidence of Reported Adverse Events During the 8-week, Double-Blind Period of the Comparative Trial With Bromocriptine

Adverse Event*	Cabergoline (n=221)	Placebo (n=231)
	Number (percent)	
Gastrointestinal		
Nausea	63 (29)	100 (43)
Constipation	15 (7)	21 (9)
Abdominal pain	12 (5)	19 (8)
Dyspepsia	11 (5)	16 (7)
Vomiting	9 (4)	16 (7)
Dry mouth	5 (2)	2 (1)
Diarrhea	4 (2)	7 (3)
Flatulence	4 (2)	3 (1)
Throat irritation	2 (1)	0
Toothache	2 (1)	0
Central and Peripheral Nervous System		
Headache	58 (26)	62 (27)
Dizziness	38 (17)	42 (18)
Vertigo	9 (4)	10 (4)
Paresthesia	5 (2)	6 (3)
Body As a Whole		
Asthenia	13 (6)	15 (6)
Fatigue	10 (5)	18 (8)
Syncope	3 (1)	3 (1)
Influenza-like symptoms	2 (1)	0
Malaise	2 (1)	0
Periorbital edema	2 (1)	2 (1)
Peripheral edema	2 (1)	1
Psychiatric		
Depression	7 (3)	5 (2)
Somnolence	5 (2)	5 (2)
Anorexia	3 (1)	3 (1)
Anxiety	3 (1)	3 (1)
Insomnia	3 (1)	2 (1)
Impaired concentration	2 (1)	1
Nervousness	2 (1)	5 (2)
Cardiovascular		
Hot flashes	6 (3)	3 (1)
Hypotension	3 (1)	4 (2)
Dependent edema	2 (1)	1
Palpitation	2 (1)	5 (2)
Reproductive—Female		
Breast pain	5 (2)	8 (3)
Dysmenorrhea	2 (1)	1
Skin and Appendages		
Acne	3 (1)	0
Pruritus	2 (1)	1
Musculoskeletal		
Pain	4 (2)	6 (3)
Arthralgia	2 (1)	0
Respiratory		
Rhinitis	2 (1)	9 (4)
Vision		
Abnormal vision	2 (1)	2 (1)

*Reported at ≥1% for cabergoline

Other adverse events that were reported at an incidence of <1.0% in the overall clinical studies follow.

Body As a Whole: facial edema, influenza-like symptoms, malaise

Cardiovascular System: hypotension, syncope, palpitations

Digestive System: dry mouth, flatulence, diarrhea, anorexia

Metabolic and Nutritional System: weight loss, weight gain

Nervous System: somnolence, nervousness, paresthesia, insomnia, anxiety

Respiratory System: nasal stuffiness, epistaxis

Skin and Appendages: acne, pruritus

Special Senses: abnormal vision

Urogenital System: dysmenorrhea, increased libido

The safety of cabergoline has been evaluated in approximately 1,200 patients with Parkinson's disease in controlled and uncontrolled studies at dosages of up to 11.5 mg/day which greatly exceeds the maximum recommended dosage of cabergoline for hyperprolactinemic disorders. In addition to the adverse events that occurred in the patients with hyperprolactinemic disorders, the most common adverse events in patients with Parkinson's disease were dyskinesia, hallucinations, confusion, and peripheral edema. Heart failure, pleural effusion, pulmonary fibrosis, and gastric or duodenal ulcer occurred rarely. One case of constrictive pericarditis has been reported.

OVERDOSAGE

Overdosage might be expected to produce nasal congestion, syncope, or hallucinations. Measures to support blood pressure should be taken if necessary.

DOSAGE AND ADMINISTRATION

The recommended dosage of DOSTINEX Tablets for initiation of therapy is 0.25 mg twice a week. Dosage may be increased by 0.25 mg twice weekly up to a dosage of 1 mg twice a week according to the patient's serum prolactin level.

Dosage increases should not occur more rapidly than every 4 weeks, so that the physician can assess the patient's response to each dosage level. If the patient does not respond adequately, and no additional benefit is observed with higher doses, the lowest dose that achieved maximal response should be used and other therapeutic approaches considered.

After a normal serum prolactin level has been maintained for 6 months, DOSTINEX may be discontinued, with periodic monitoring of the serum prolactin level to determine whether or when treatment with DOSTINEX should be reinstituted. The durability of efficacy beyond 24 months of therapy with DOSTINEX has not been established.

HOW SUPPLIED

DOSTINEX Tablets are white, scored, capsule-shaped tablets containing 0.5 mg cabergoline. Each tablet is scored on one side and has the letter P and the letter U on either side of the breakline. The other side of the tablet is engraved with the number 700.

DOSTINEX is available as follows:

Bottles of 8 tablets NDC 0013-7001-12

STORAGE

Store at controlled room temperature 20° to 25° C (68° to 77° F) [see USP].

℞ only

U.S. Patent No. 4,526, 892.

Manufactured for: Pharmacia & Upjohn Company
Kalamazoo, MI 49001, USA
by: Pharmacia & Upjohn S.p.A.
Milan, Italy

816 989 102 N. 320000700.00.8 Revised August 1999

ELLENCE™ ℞

epirubicin hydrochloride injection

WARNING

1. Severe local tissue necrosis will occur if there is extravasation during administration (See PRECAUTIONS). Epirubicin must not be given by the intramuscular or subcutaneous route.
2. Myocardial toxicity, manifested in its most severe form by potentially fatal congestive heart failure (CHF), may occur either during therapy with epirubicin or months to years after termination of therapy. The probability of developing clinically evident CHF is estimated as approximately 0.9% at a cumulative dose of 550 mg/m^2, 1.6% at 700 mg/m^2, and 3.3% at 900 mg/m^2. In the adjuvant treatment of breast cancer, the maximum cumulative dose used in clinical trials was 720 mg/m^2. The risk of developing CHF increases rapidly with increasing total cumulative doses of epirubicin in excess of 900 mg/m^2; this cumulative dose should only be exceeded with extreme caution. Active or dormant cardiovascular disease, prior or concomitant radiotherapy to the mediastinal/pericardial area, previous therapy with other anthracyclines or anthracenediones, or concomitant use of other cardiotoxic drugs may increase the risk of cardiac toxicity. Cardiac toxicity with ELLENCE may occur at lower cumulative doses whether or not cardiac risk factors are present.
3. Secondary acute myelogenous leukemia (AML) has been reported in patients with breast cancer treated with anthracyclines, including epirubicin. The occurrence of refractory secondary leukemia is more common when such drugs are given in combination with DNA-damaging anti-neoplastic agents, when patients have been heavily pretreated with cytotoxic drugs, or when doses of anthracyclines have been escalated. The cumulative risk of developing treatment-related AML, in 3844 patients with breast cancer who received adjuvant treatment with epirubicin-containing regimens, was estimated as 0.2% at 3 years and 0.8% at 5 years.
4. Dosage should be reduced in patients with impaired hepatic function (see DOSAGE AND ADMINISTRATION).
5. Severe myelosuppression may occur.
6. Epirubicin should be administered only under the supervision of a physician who is experienced in the use of cancer chemotherapeutic agents.

DESCRIPTION

ELLENCE Injection (epirubicin hydrochloride injection) is an anthracycline cytotoxic agent, intended for intravenous administration. ELLENCE is supplied as a sterile, clear, red solution and is available in polypropylene vials containing 50 and 200 mg of epirubicin hydrochloride as a preservative-free, ready-to-use solution. Each milliliter of solution contains 2 mg of epirubicin hydrochloride. Inactive ingredients include sodium chloride, USP, and water for injection, USP. The pH of the solution has been adjusted to 3.0 with hydrochloric acid, NF.

Epirubicin hydrochloride is the 4-epimer of doxorubicin and is a semi-synthetic, derivative of daunoru-bicin. The chemical name is (8S- *cis*)-10-[(3-amino-2,3,6-trideoxy-α-L- ***arabino***-hexopyranosyl)oxy]-7,8,9,10- tetrahydro-6,8,11-trihydroxy-8-(hydroxyacetyl)-1-methoxy-5,12-naphthacenedione hydrochloride. The active ingredient is a red-orange hygroscopic powder, with the empirical formula $C_{27}H_{29}NO_{11}HCl$ and a molecular weight of 579.95. The structural formula is as follows:

CLINICAL PHARMACOLOGY

Epirubicin is an anthracycline cytotoxic agent. Although it is known that anthracyclines can interfere with a number of biochemical and biological functions within eukaryotic cells, the precise mechanisms of epirubicin's cytotoxic and/or antiproliferative properties have not been completely elucidated.

Epirubicin forms a complex with DNA by intercalation of its planar rings between nucleotide base pairs, with consequent inhibition of nucleic acid (DNA and RNA) and protein synthesis. Such intercalation triggers DNA cleavage by topoisomerase II, resulting in cytocidal activity. Epirubicin also inhibits DNA helicase activity, preventing the enzymatic separation of double-stranded DNA and interfering with replication and transcription. Epirubicin is also involved in oxidation/reduction reactions by generating cytotoxic free radicals. The antiproliferative and cytotoxic activity of epirubicin is thought to result from these or other possible mechanisms.

Epirubicin is cytotoxic in vitro to a variety of established murine and human cell lines and primary cultures of human tumors. It is also active in vivo against a variety of murine tumors and human xenografts in athymic mice, including breast tumors.

Pharmacokinetics

Epirubicin pharmacokinetics are linear over the dose range of 60 to 150 mg/m^2 and plasma clearance is not affected by the duration of infusion or administration schedule. Pharmacokinetic parameters for epirubicin following 6- to 10-minute, single-dose intravenous infusions of epirubicin at doses of 60 to 150 mg/m^2 in patients with solid tumors are shown in Table 1. The plasma concentration declined in a triphasic manner with mean half-lives for the alpha, beta, and gamma phases of about 3 minutes, 2.5 hours and 33 hours, respectively.

[See table 1 at top of next page]

Distribution. Following intravenous administration, epirubicin is rapidly and widely distributed into the tissues. Binding of epirubicin to plasma proteins, predominantly albumin, is about 77% and is not affected by drug concentration. Epirubicin also appears to concentrate in red blood cells; whole blood concentrations are approximately twice those of plasma.

Metabolism. Epirubicin is extensively and rapidly metabolized by the liver and is also metabolized by other organs and cells, including red blood cells. Four main metabolic routes have been identified:

(1) reduction of the C-13 keto-group with the formation of the 13(S)-dihydro derivative epirubicinol;

Continued on next page

Information on these Pharmacia & Upjohn products is based on labeling in effect June 1, 2000. Further information concerning these and other Pharmacia & Upjohn products may be obtained by direct inquiry to Medical Information, Pharmacia & Upjohn, Kalamazoo, MI 49001.

Ellence—Cont.

(2) conjugation of both the unchanged drug and epirubicinol with glucuronic acid; (3) loss of the amino sugar moiety through a hydrolytic process with the formation of the doxorubicin and doxorubicinol aglycones; and (4) loss of the amino sugar moiety through a redox process with the formation of the 7-deoxy-doxorubicin aglycone and 7-deoxydoxorubicinol aglycone. Epirubicinol has in vitro cytotoxic activity one-tenth that of epirubicin. As plasma levels of epirubicinol are lower than those of the unchanged drug, they are unlikely to reach in vivo concentrations sufficient for cytotoxicity. No significant activity or toxicity has been reported for the other metabolites.

Excretion. Epirubicin and its major metabolites are eliminated through biliary excretion and, to a lesser extent, by urinary excretion. Mass-balance data from one patient found about 60% of the total radioactive dose in feces (34%) and urine (27%). These data are consistent with those from 3 patients with extrahepatic obstruction and percutaneous drainage, in whom approximately 35% and 20% of the administered dose were recovered as epirubicin or its major metabolites in bile and urine, respectively, in the 4 days after treatment.

Pharmacokinetics in Special Populations

Age. A population analysis of plasma data from 36 cancer patients (13 males and 23 females, 20 to 73 years) showed that age affects plasma clearance of epirubicin in female patients. The predicted plasma clearance for a female patient of 70 years of age was about 35% lower than that for a female patient of 25 years of age. An insufficient number of males > 50 years of age were included in the study to draw conclusions about age-related alterations in clearance in males. Although a lower epirubicin starting dose does not appear necessary in elderly female patients, and was not used in clinical trials, particular care should be taken in monitoring toxicity when epirubicin is administered to female patients > 70 years of age. (See PRECAUTIONS).

Gender. In patients ≤ 50 years of age, mean clearance values in adult male and female patients were similar. The clearance of epirubicin is decreased in elderly women (See Pharmacokinetics in Special Populations—Age).

Pediatric. The pharmacokinetics of epirubicin in pediatric patients have not been evaluated.

Race. The influence of race on the pharmacokinetics of epirubicin has not been evaluated.

Hepatic Impairment. Epirubicin is eliminated by both hepatic metabolism and biliary excretion and clearance is reduced in patients with hepatic dysfunction. In a study of the effect of hepatic dysfunction, patients with solid tumors were classified into 3 groups. Patients in Group 1 (n=22) had serum AST (SGOT) levels above the upper limit of normal (median: 93 IU/L) and normal serum bilirubin levels (median: 0.5 mg/dL) and were given epirubicin doses of 12.5 to 90 mg/m². Patients in Group 2 had alterations in both serum AST (median: 175 IU/L) and bilirubin levels (median: 2.7 mg/dL) and were treated with an epirubicin dose of 25 mg/m² (n=8). Their pharmacokinetics were compared to those of patients with normal serum AST and bilirubin values, who received epirubicin doses of 12.5 to 120 mg/m². The median plasma clearance of epirubicin was decreased compared to patients with normal hepatic function by about 30% in patients in Group 1 and by 50% in patients in Group 2. Patients with more severe hepatic impairment have not been evaluated. (See WARNINGS and DOSAGE AND ADMINISTRATION.)

Renal Impairment. No significant alterations in the pharmacokinetics of epirubicin or its major metabolite, epirubicinol, have been observed in patients with serum creatinine (< 5 mg/dL. A 50% reduction in plasma clearance was reported in four patients with serum creatinine ≥ 5 mg/dL (see WARNINGS and DOSAGE AND ADMINISTRATION). Patients on dialysis have not been studied.

Drug-Drug Interactions

Taxanes. Coadministration of paclitaxel or docetaxel did not affect the pharmacokinetics of epirubicin when given immediately following the taxane.

Cimetidine. Coadministration of cimetidine (400 mg twice daily for 7 days starting 5 days before chemotherapy) increased the mean AUC of epirubicin (100 mg/m² by 50% and decreased its plasma clearance by 30% (see PRECAUTIONS).

Drugs metabolized by cytochrome P-450 enzymes. No systematic in vitro or in vivo evaluation has been performed to examine the potential for inhibition or induction by epirubicin of oxidative cytochrome P-450 isoenzymes.

Table 1. Summary of Mean (±SD) Pharmacokinetic Parameters in Patients[1] with Solid Tumors Receiving Intravenous Epirubicin 60 to 150 mg/m²

Dose[2] (mg/m²)	C_{max}[3] (μg/mL)	AUC[4] (μg • h/mL)	t ½[5] (hours)	CL[6] (L/hour)	Vss[7] (L/kg)
60	5.7 ± 1.6	1.6 ± 0.2	35.3 ± 9	65 ± 8	21 ± 2
75	5.3 ± 1.5	1.7 ± 0.3	32.1 ± 5	83 ± 14	27 ± 11
120	9.0 ± 3.5	3.4 ± 0.7	33.7 ± 4	65 ± 13	23 ± 7
150	9.3 ± 2.9	4.2 ± 0.8	31.1 ± 6	69 ± 13	21 ± 7

[1] Advanced solid tumor cancers, primarily of the lung
[2] N=6 patients per dose level
[3] Plasma concentration at the end of 6 to 10 minute infusion
[4] Area under the plasma concentration curve
[5] Half-life terminal phase
[6] Plasma clearance
[7] Steady state volume of distribution

Table 2. Treatment Regimens Used in Phase 3 Studies of Patients with Early Breast Cancer

	Treatment Groups	Agent	Regimen
MA-5[1] N=716	**CEF-120** (total, 6 cycles)[2] N=356	Cyclophosphamide ELLENCE Fluorouracil	75 mg/m² PO, d 1-14, q 28 days 60 mg/m² IV, d 1 & 8, q 28 days 500 mg/m² IV, d 1 & 8, q 28 days
	CMF (total, 6 cycles) N=360	Cyclophosphamide Methotrexate Fluorouracil	100 mg/m²PO, d 1-14, q 28 days 40 mg/m² IV, d 1 & 8, q 28 days 600 mg/m² IV, d 1 & 8, q 28 days
GFEA-05[3] N=565	**FEC-100** (total, 6 cycles) N=276	Fluorouracil ELLENCE Cyclophosphamide	500 mg/m²IV, d 1, q 21 days 100 mg/m² IV, d 1, q 21 days 500 mg/m² IV, d 1, q 21 days
	FEC-50 (total, 6 cycles) N=289	Fluorouracil ELLENCE Cyclophosphamide	500 mg/m²IV, d 1, q 21 days 50 mg/m² IV, d 1, q 21 days 500 mg/m² IV, d 1, 21 days
	Tamoxifen 30 mg daily × 3 years, postmenopausal women, any receptor status		

[1] In women who underwent lumpectomy, breast irradiation was to be administered after completion of study chemotherapy.
[2] Patients also received prophylactic antibiotic therapy with trimethoprim-sulfamethoxazole or fluroquinolone for the duration of their chemotherapy.
[3] All women were to receive breast irradiation after the completion of chemotherapy.

Table 3. Efficacy Results from Phase 3 Studies of Patients with Early Breast Cancer*

	MA-5 Study		GFEA-05 Study	
	CEF-120 N=356	CMF N=360	FEC-100 N=276	FEC-50 N=289
RFS at 5 yrs (%)	62	53	65	52
Log-rank Test	(stratified p=0.013)		(p=0.007)	
OS at 5 yrs	77	70	76	65
Log-rank Test	(stratified p=0.043) (unstratified p=0.13)		(p=0.007)	

*Based on Kaplan-Meier estimates

CLINICAL STUDIES

Two randomized, open-label, multicenter studies evaluated the use of ELLENCE Injection 100 to 120 mg/m² in combination with cyclophosphamide and fluorouracil for the adjuvant treatment of patients with axiliary-node-positive breast cancer and no evidence of distant metastatic disease (Stage II or III). Study MA-5 evaluated 120 mg/m² of epirubicin per course in combination with cyclophosphamide and fluorouracil (CEF-120 regimen). This study randomized premenopausal and perimenopausal women with one or more positive lymph nodes to an epirubicin-containing CEF-120 regimen or to a CMF regimen. Study GFEA-05 evaluated the use of 100 mg/m² of epirubicin per course in combination with fluorouracil and cyclophosphamide (FEC-100). This study randomized pre- and postmenopausal women to the FEC-100 regimen or to a lower-dose FEC-50 regimen. In the GFEA-05 study, eligible patients were either required to have ≥ 4 nodes involved with tumor or, if only 1 to 3 nodes were positive, to have negative estrogen- and progesterone-receptors and a histologic tumor grade of 2 or 3. A total of 1281 women participated in these studies. Patients with T4 tumors were not eligible for either study. Table 2 shows the treatment regimens that the patients received.

[See table 2 above]

In the MA-5 trial, the median age of the study population was 45 years. Approximately 60% of patients had 1 to 3 involved nodes and approximately 40% had ≥ 4 nodes involved with tumor. In the GFEA-05 study, the median age was 51 years and approximately half of the patients were postmenopausal. About 17% of the study population had 1 to 3 positive nodes and 80% of patients had ≥ 4 involved lymph nodes. Demographic and tumor characteristics were well-balanced between treatment arms in each study.

The efficacy endpoints of relapse-free survival (RFS) and overall survival (OS) were analyzed using Kaplan-Meier methods in the intent-to-treat (ITT) patient populations in each study. Results for end-points are described in terms of the outcomes at 5 years. In Study MA-5, epirubicin-containing combination therapy (CEF-120) showed significantly longer 5-year RFS than CMF (62% versus 53%; stratified logrank p=0.013). The overall reduction in risk of relapse was 24%. The 5-year OS was also greater for the epirubicin-containing CEF-120 regimen than for the CMF regimen (77% versus 70%; stratified logrank p=0.043; non-stratified logrank p=0.13). The overall relative reduction in the risk of death was 29%.

In Study GFEA-05, patients treated with the higher-dose epirubicin regimen (FEC-100) had a significantly longer 5-year RFS (65% versus 52%, logrank p=0.007) and OS (76% versus 65%, logrank p=0.007) than patients given the lower dose regimen (FEC-50). The overall reduction in risk of relapse was 32%. The relative reduction in the risk of death was 31%.

Although the trials were not powered for subset analyses, improvement in RFS, and OS were observed both in patients with 1–3 nodes positive and those with ≥ 4 nodes positive for tumor involvement when comparing the CEF-120 or FEC-100 groups with the control groups. In addition, in the GFEA-05 study, similar improvements in RFS and OS were observed in both pre- and postmenopausal women treated with FEC-100 compared to FEC-50. Efficacy results for the two studies are shown in Table 3.

[See table 3 above]

The Kaplan-Meier curves for RFS and OS from Study MA-5 are shown in Figures 1 and 2 and those for Study GFEA-05 are shown in Figures 3 and 4.

[See graphic at top of next page]

INDICATIONS AND USAGE

ELLENCE Injection is indicated as a component of adjuvant therapy in patients with evidence of axillary node tumor involvement following resection of primary breast cancer.

CONTRAINDICATIONS

Patients should not be treated with ELLENCE Injection if they have any of the following conditions: baseline neutrophil count < 1500 cells/mm³; severe myocardial insufficiency or recent myocardial infarction; previous treatment with anthracyclines up to the maximum cumulative dose; hypersensitivity to epirubicin, other anthracyclines, or anthracenediones; or severe hepatic dysfunction (see WARNINGS and DOSAGE AND ADMINISTRATION).

WARNINGS

ELLENCE Injection should be administered only under the supervision of qualified physicians experienced in the use of cytotoxic therapy. Initial treatment with ELLENCE should be preceded by a careful baseline assessment of blood counts; serum levels of total bilirubin, AST, and creatinine; and cardiac function as measured by left ventricular ejection function (LVEF). Patients should be carefully monitored during treatment for possible clinical complications due to myelosuppression. Supportive care may be necessary for the treatment of severe neutropenia and severe infectious complications. Monitoring for potential cardiotoxicity is also important, especially with greater cumulative exposure to epirubicin.

Hematologic Toxicity. A dose-dependent, reversible leukopenia and/or neutropenia is the predominant manifestation of hematologic toxicity associated with epirubicin and represents the most common acute dose-limiting toxicity of this drug. In most cases, the white blood cell (WBC) nadir is reached 10 to 14 days from drug administration. Leukopenia/neutropenia is usually transient, with WBC and neutrophil counts generally returning to normal values by Day 21 after drug administration. As with other cytotoxic agents, ELLENCE at the recommended dose in combination with cyclophosphamide and fluorouracil can produce severe leukopenia and neutropenia. Severe thrombocytopenia and anemia may also occur. Clinical consequences of severe myelosuppression include fever, infection, septicemia, septic shock, hemorrhage, tissue hypoxia, symptomatic anemia, or death. If myelosuppressive complications occur, appropriate supportive measures (e.g., intravenous antibiotics, colony-stimulating factors, transfusions) may be required. Myelosuppression requires careful monitoring. Total and differential WBC, red blood cell (RBC), and platelet counts should be assessed before and during each cycle of therapy with ELLENCE.

Cardiac Function. Cardiotoxicity is a known risk of anthracycline treatment. Anthracycline-induced cardiac toxicity may be manifested by early (or acute) or late (delayed) events. Early cardiac toxicity of epirubicin consists mainly of sinus tachycardia and/or ECG abnormalities such as non-specific ST-T wave changes, but tachyarrhythmias, including premature ventricular contractions and ventricular tachycardia, bradycardia, as well as atrioventricular and bundle-branch block have also been reported. These effects do not usually predict subsequent development of delayed cardiotoxicity, are rarely of clinical importance, and are generally not considered an indication for the suspension of epirubicin treatment. Delayed cardiac toxicity results from a characteristic cardiomyopathy that is manifested by reduced LVEF and/or signs and symptoms of congestive heart failure (CHF) such as tachycardia, dyspnea, pulmonary edema, dependent edema, hepatomegaly, ascites, pleural effusion, gallop rhythm. Life-theatening CHF is the most severe form of anthracycline-induced cardiomyopathy. This toxicity appears to be dependent on the cumulative dose of ELLENCE and represents the cumulative dose-limiting toxicity of the drug. If it occurs, delayed cardiotoxicity usually develops late in the course of therapy with ELLENCE or within 2 to 3 months after completion of treatment, but later events (several months to years after treatment termination) have been reported.

In a retrospective survey, including 9144 patients, mostly with solid tumors in advanced stages, the probability of developing CHF increased with increasing cumulative doses of ELLENCE (Figure 5). The estimated risk of epirubicin-treated patients developing clinically evident CHF was 0.9% at a cumulative dose of 500 mg/m^2, 1.6% at 700 mg/m^2, and 3.3% at 900 mg/m^2. The risk of developing CHF in the absence of other cardiac risk factors increased steeply after an epirubicin cumulative dose of 900 mg/m^2.

Figure 5. Risk of CHF in 9144 Patients Treated with Epirubicin

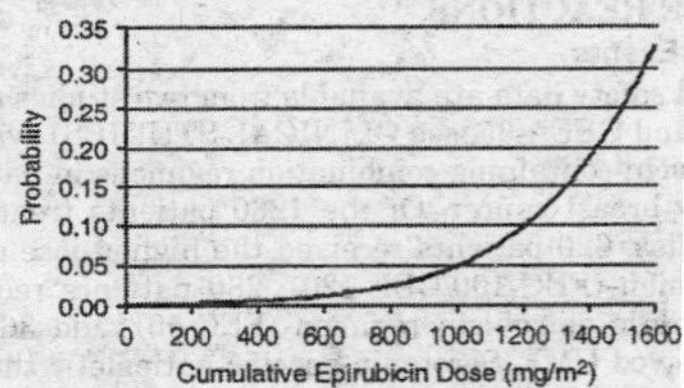

In another retrospective survey of 469 epirubicin-treated patients with metastatic or early breast cancer, the reported risk of CHF was comparable to that observed in the larger study of over 9000 patients.

Given the risk of cardiomyopathy, a cumulative dose of 900 mg/m^2 ELLENCE should be exceeded only with extreme caution. Risk factors (active or dormant cardiovascular disease, prior or concomitant radiotherapy to the mediastinal/pericardial area, previous therapy with other anthracyclines or anthracenediones, concomitant use of other drugs with the ability to suppress cardiac contractility) may increase the risk of cardiac toxicity. Although not formally tested, it is probable that the toxicity of epirubicin and other anthracyclines or anthracenediones is additive. Cardiac toxicity with ELLENCE may occur at lower cumulative doses whether or not cardiac risk factors are present.

Although endomyocardial biopsy is recognized as the most sensitive diagnostic tool to detect anthracycline-induced cardiomyopathy, this invasive examination is not practically performed on a routine basis. Electrocardiogram (ECG) changes such as dysrhythmias, a reduction of the QRS voltage, or a prolongation beyond normal limits of the systolic time interval may be indicative of anthracycline-induced cardiomyopathy, but ECG is not a sensitive or specific method for following anthracycline-related cardiotoxicity. The risk of serious cardiac impairment may be decreased through regular monitoring of LVEF during the course of treatment with prompt discontinuation of ELLENCE at the first sign of impaired function. The preferred method for repeated assessment of cardiac function is evaluation of LVEF measured by multi-gated radionuclide angiography (MUGA) or echocardiography (ECHO). A baseline cardiac evaluation with an ECG and a MUGA scan or an ECHO is recommended, especially in patients with risk factors for increased cardiac toxicity. Repeated MUGA or ECHO determinations of LVEF should be performed, particularly with higher, cumulative anthracycline doses. The technique used for assessment should be consistent through follow-up. In patients with risk factors, particularly prior anthracycline or anthracenedione use, the monitoring of cardiac function must be particularly strict and the risk-benefit of continuing treatment with ELLENCE in patients with impaired cardiac function must be carefully evaluated.

Figure 1. Relapse-Free Survival in Study MA-5

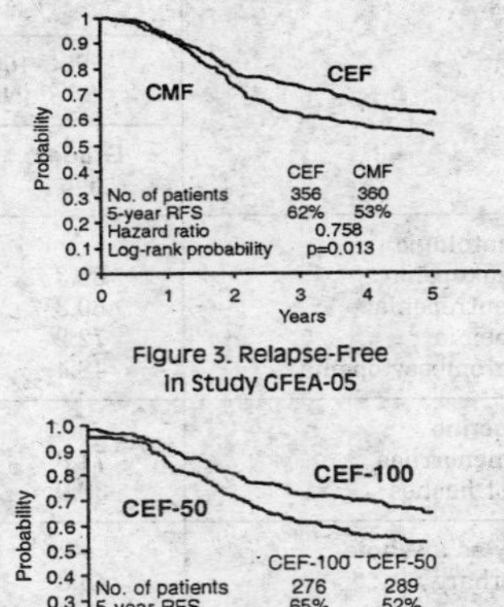

Figure 2. Overall Survival in Study MA-5

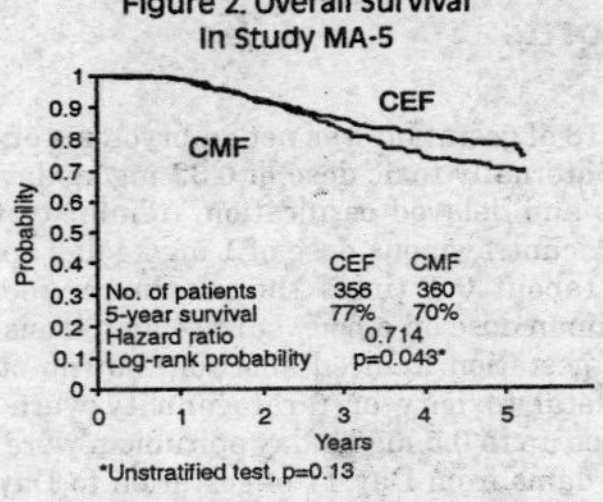

Figure 3. Relapse-Free Survival Figure 4. Overall Survival in Study GFEA-05 in Study GFEA-0

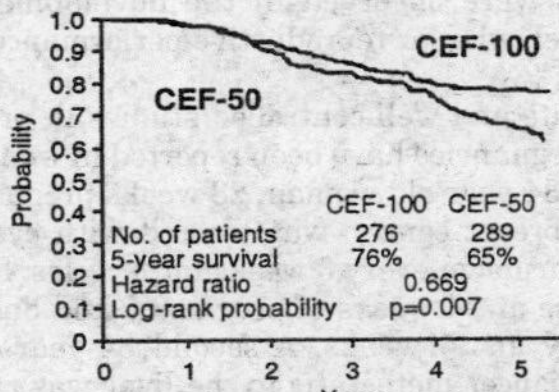

Secondary Leukemia. The occurrence of secondary acute myelogenous leukemia, with or without a preleukemic phase, has been reported in patients treated with anthracyclines. Secondary leukemia is more common when such drugs are given in combination with DNA-damaging antineoplastic agents, when patients have been heavily pretreated with cytotoxic drugs, or when doses of the anthracyclines have been escalated. These leukemias can have a short 1- to 3- year latency period. An analysis of 3844 patients who received adjuvant treatment with epirubicin in controlled clinical trials, showed a cumulative risk of secondary acute myelogenous leukemia of about 0.2% (approximate 95% Cl, 0.05–0.4) at 3 years and approximately 0.8% (approximate 95% Cl, 0.3–1.2) at 5 years. ELLENCE is mutagenic, clastogenic, and carcinogenic in animals (see next section, Carcinogenesis, Mutagenesis, and Impairment of Fertility).

Carcinogenesis, Mutagenesis & Impairment of Fertility. Treatment-related acute myelogenous leukemia has been reported in women treated with epirubicin-based adjuvant chemotherapy regimens (see above section, WARNINGS, Secondary Leukemia). Conventional long-term animal studies to evaluate the carcinogenic potential of epirubicin have not been conducted, but intravenous administration of a single 3.6 mg/kg epirubicin dose to female rats (about 0.2 times the maximum recommended human dose on a body surface area basis) approximately doubled the incidence of mammary tumors (primarily fibroadenomas) observed at 1 year. Administration of 0.5 mg/kg epirubicin intravenously to rats (about 0.025 times the maximum recommended human dose on a body surface area basis) every 3 weeks for ten doses increased the incidences of subcutaneous fibromas in males over an 18-month observation period. In addition, subcutaneous administration of 0.75 or 1.0 mg/kg/day (about 0.015 times the maximum recommended human dose on a body surface area basis) to newborn rats for 4 days on both the first and tenth day after birth for a total of eight doses increased the incidence of animals with tumors compared to controls during a 24-month observation period.

Epirubicin was mutagenic in vitro to bacteria (Ames test) either in the presence or absence of metabolic activation and to mammalian cells (HGPRT assay in V79 Chinese hamster lung fibroblasts) in the absence but not in the presence of metabolic activation. Epirubicin was clastogenic in vitro (chromosome aberrations in human lymphocytes) both in the presence and absence of metabolic activation and was also clastogenic in vivo (chromosome aberration in mouse bone marrow).

In fertility studies in rats, males were given epirubicin daily for 9 weeks and mated with females that were given epirubicin daily for 2 weeks prior to mating and through day 7 of gestation. When 0.3 mg/kg/day (about 0.015 times the maximum recommended human single dose on a body surface area basis) was administered to both sexes, no pregnancies resulted. No effects on mating behavior or fertility were observed at 0.1 mg/kg/day, but male rats had atrophy of the testes and epididymis, and reduced spermatogenesis. The 0.1 mg/kg/day dose also caused embryolethality. An increased incidence of fetal growth retardation was observed in these studies at 0.03 mg/kg/day (about 0.0015 times the maximum recommended human single dose on a body surface area basis). Multiple daily doses of epirubicin to rabbits and dogs also caused atrophy or male reproduction organs. Single 20.5 and 12 mg/kg doses of intravenous epirubicin caused testicular atrophy in mice and rats, respectively (both approximately 0.5 times the maximum recommended human dose on a body surface area basis). A single dose of 16.7 mg/kg epirubicin caused uterine atrophy in rats.

Although experimental data are not available, ELLENCE could induce chromosomal damage in human spermatozoa due to its genotoxic potential. Men undergoing treatment with ELLENCE should use effective contraceptive methods.

ELLENCE may cause irreversible amenorrhea (premature menopause) in premenopausal women.

Liver Function. The major route of elimination of epirubicin is the hepatobiliary system (see CLINICAL PHARMACOLOGY, Pharmacokinetics in Special Populations). Serum total bilirubin and AST levels should be evaluated before and during treatment with ELLENCE. Patients with elevated bilirubin or AST may experience slower clearance of drug with an increase in overall toxicity. Lower doses are recommended in these patients (see DOSAGE AND ADMINISTRATION). Patients with severe hepatic impairment have not been evaluated; therefore, epirubicin should not be used in this patient population.

Renal Function. Serum creatinine should be assessed before and during therapy. Dosage adjustment is necessary in patients with serum creatinine >5 mg/dL (see DOSAGE AND ADMINISTRATION). Patients undergoing dialysis have not been studied.

Tumor-Lysis Syndrome. As with other cytotoxic agents, ELLENCE may induce hyperuricemia as a consequence of the extensive purine catabolism that accompanies drug-induced rapid lysis of highly chemosensitive neoplastic cells (tumor lysis syndrome). Other metabolic abnormalities may also occur. While not generally a problem in patients with breast cancer, physicians should consider the potential for tumor-lysis syndrome in potentially susceptible patients and should consider monitoring serum uric acid, potassium, calcium phosphate, and creatinine immediately after initial chemotherapy administration. Hydration, urine alkalinization, and prophylaxis with allopurinol to prevent hyperuricemia may minimize potential complications of tumor-lysis syndrome.

Pregnancy—Category D. ELLENCE may cause fetal harm when administered to a pregnant woman. Administration of 0.8 mg/kg/day intravenously of epirubicin to rats (about 0.04 times the maximum recommended single human dose on a body surface area basis) during Days 5 to 15 of gestation was embryotoxic (increased resorptions and post-implantation loss) and caused fetal growth retardation (decreased body weight), but was not teratogenic up to this dose. Administration of 2 mg/kg/day intravenously of epirubicin to rats (about 0.1 times the maximum recommended single human dose on a body surface area basis) on Days 9 and 10 of gestation was embryotoxic (increased late resorptions, post-implantation losses, and dead fetuses; and decreased live fetuses), retarded fetal growth (decreased body weight), and caused decreased placental weight. This dose was also teratogenic, causing numerous external (anal atresia, misshapen tail, abnormal genital tubercle), visceral (primarily gastrointestinal, urinary, and cardiovascular systems), and skeletal (deformed long bones and girdles, rib abnormalities, irregular spinal ossification) malformations. Administration of intravenous epirubicin to rabbits at doses up to 0.2 mg/kg/day (about 0.02 times the maximum recommended single human dose on a body surface area basis)

Continued on next page

Information on these Pharmacia & Upjohn products is based on labeling in effect June 1, 2000. Further information concerning these and other Pharmacia & Upjohn products may be obtained by direct inquiry to Medical Information, Pharmacia & Upjohn, Kalamazoo, MI 49001.

Ellence—Cont.

during Days 6 to 18 of gestation was not embryotoxic or teratogenic, but a maternally toxic dose of 0.32 mg/kg/day increased abortions and delayed ossification. Administration of a maternity toxic intravenous dose of 1 mg/kg/day epirubicin to rabbits (about 0.1 times the maximum recommended single human dose on a body surface area basis) on Days 10 to 12 of gestation induced abortion, but no other signs of embryofetal toxicity or teratogenicity were observed. When doses up to 0.5 mg/kg/day epirubicin were administered to rat dams from Day 17 of gestation to Day 21 after delivery (about 0.025 times the maximum recommended single human dose on a body surface area basis), no permanent changes were observed in the development, functional activity, behavior, or reproductive performance of the offspring.
There are no adequate and well-controlled studies in pregnant women. Two pregnancies have been reported in women taking epirubicin. A 34-year-old woman, 28 weeks pregnant at her diagnosis of breast cancer, was treated with cyclophosphamide and epirubicin every 3 weeks for 3 cycles. She received the last dose at 34 weeks of pregnancy and delivered a healthy baby at 35 weeks. A second 34-year-old woman with breast cancer metastatic to the liver was randomized to FEC-50 but was removed from study because of pregnancy. She experienced a spontaneous abortion. If epirubicin is used during pregnancy, or if the patient becomes pregnant while taking this drug, the patient should be apprised of the potential hazard to the fetus. Women of childbearing potential should be advised to avoid becoming pregnant.

PRECAUTIONS

General

ELLENCE Injection is administered by intravenous infusion. Venous sclerosis may result from an injection into a small vessel or from repeated injections into the same vein. Extravasation of epirubicin during the infusion may cause local pain, severe tissue lesions and necrosis. It is recommended that ELLENCE be slowly administered into the tubing of a freely running intravenous infusion. If possible, veins over joints or in extremities with compromised venous or lymphatic drainage should be avoided. The dose should be administered over 3 to 5 minutes. A burning or stinging sensation may be indicative of perivenous infiltration, and the infusion should be immediately terminated and restarted in another vein. Perivenous infiltration may occur without causing pain.
Facial flushing, as well as local erythematous streaking along the vein, may be indicative of excessively rapid administration. It may precede local phlebitis or thrombophlebitis.
Patients administered the 120-mg/m^2 regimen of ELLENCE as a component of combination chemotherapy should also receive prophylactic antibiotic therapy with trimethoprim-sulfamethoxazole (e.g., Septra®, Bactrim®) or a fluoroquinolone (see CLINICAL STUDIES, Early Breast Cancer, and DOSAGE AND ADMINISTRATION).
Epirubicin is emetigenic. Antiemetics may reduce nausea and vomiting; prophylactic use of antiemetics should be considered before administration of ELLENCE, particularly when given in conjunction with other emetigenic drugs.
As with other anthracyclines, administration of ELLENCE after previous radiation therapy may induce an inflammatory recall reaction at the site of irradiation.

Information for Patients

Patients should be informed of the expected adverse effects of epirubicin, including gastrointestinal symptoms (nausea, vomiting, diarrhea, and stomatitis) and potential neutropenic complications. Patients should consult their physician if vomiting, dehydration, fever, evidence of infection, symptoms of CHF, or injection-site pain occurs following therapy with ELLENCE. Patients should be informed that they will almost certainly develop alopecia. Patients should be advised that their urine may appear red for 1 to 2 days after administration of ELLENCE and that they should not be alarmed. Patients should understand that there is a risk of irreversible myocardial damage associated with treatment with ELLENCE, as well as a risk of treatment-related leukemia. Because epirubicin may induce chromosomal damage in sperm, men undergoing treatment with ELLENCE should use effective contraceptive methods. Women treated with ELLENCE may develop irreversible amenorrhea, or premature menopause.

Laboratory Testing

See WARNINGS. Blood counts, including absolute neutrophil counts and liver function should be assessed before and during each cycle of therapy with epirubicin. Repeated evaluations of LVEF should be performed during therapy.

Drug Interactions

ELLENCE when used in combination with other cytotoxic drugs may show on-treatment additive toxicity, especially hematologic and gastrointestinal effects.
Concomitant use of ELLENCE with other cardioactive compounds that could cause heart failure (e.g., calcium channel blockers), requires close monitoring of cardiac function throughout treatment.
There are few data regarding the coadministration of radiation therapy and epirubicin. In adjuvant trials of epirubicin-containing CEF-120 or FEC-100 chemotherapies, breast irradiation was delayed until after chemotherapy was completed. This practice resulted in no apparent increase in local breast cancer recurrence relative to published accounts in the literature. A small number of patients received epirubicin-based chemotherapy concomitantly with radiation therapy but had chemotherapy interrupted in order to avoid potential overlapping toxicities. It is likely that use of epirubicin with radiotherapy may sensitize tissues to the cytotoxic actions of irradiation. Administration of ELLENCE after previous radiation therapy may induce an inflammatory recall reaction at the site of irradiation.
Epirubicin is extensively metabolized by the liver. Changes in hepatic function induced by concomitant therapies may affect epirubicin metabolism, pharmacokinetics, therapeutic efficacy, and/or toxicity.
Cimetidine increased the AUC of epirubicin by 50%. Cimetidine treatment should be stopped during treatment with ELLENCE (see CLINICAL PHARMACOLOGY).

Drug-Laboratory Test Interactions

There are no known interactions between ELLENCE and laboratory tests.

Carcinogenesis, Mutagenesis & Impairment of Fertility

See WARNINGS.

Pregnancy

Pregnancy Category D—see WARNINGS.

Nursing Mothers

Epirubicin was excreted into the milk of rats treated with 0.50 mg/kg/day of epirubicin during peri- and postnatal periods. It is not known whether epirubicin is excreted in human milk. Because many drugs, including other anthracyclines, are excreted in human milk and because of the potential for serious adverse reactions in nursing infants from epirubicin, mothers should discontinue nursing prior to taking this drug.

Geriatric Use

Although a lower starting dose of ELLENCE was not used in trials in elderly female patients, particular care should be taken in monitoring toxicity when ELLENCE is administered to female patients ≥ 70 years of age. (See CLINICAL PHARMACOLOGY, Pharmacokinetics in Special Populations).

Pediatric Use

The safety and effectiveness of epirubicin in pediatric patients have not been established in adequate and well-controlled clinical trials. Pediatric patients may be at greater risk for anthracycline-induced acute manifestations of cardiotoxicity and for chronic CHF.

ADVERSE REACTIONS

On-Study Events

Integrated safety data are available from two studies (studies MA-5 and GFEA-05, see CLINICAL STUDIES) evaluating epirubicin-containing combination regimens in patients with early breast cancer. Of the 1260 patients treated in these studies, 620 patients received the higher-dose epirubicin regimen (FEC-100/CEF-120), 280 patients received the lower-dose epirubicin regimen (FEC-50), and 360 patients received CMF. Serotonin-specific antiemetic therapy and colony-stimulating factors were not used in these trials. Clinically relevant acute adverse events are summarized in Table 4.
[See table 4 above]

Table 4. Clinically Relevant Acute Adverse Events in Patients with Early Breast Cancer

Event	% of Patients					
	FEC-100/CEF-120 (N=620)		FEC-50 (N=280)		CMF (N=360)	
	Grades 1–4	Grades 3/4	Grades 1–4	Grades 3/4	Grades 1–4	Grades 3/4
Hematologic						
Leukopenia	80.3	58.6	49.6	1.5	98.1	60.3
Neutropenia	80.3	67.2	53.9	10.5	95.8	78.1
Anemia	72.2	5.8	12.9	0	70.9	0.9
Thrombocytopenia	48.4	5.4	4.6	0	51.4	3.6
Endocrine						
Amenorrhea	71.8	0	69.3	0	67.7	0
Hot flashes	38.9	4.0	5.4	0	69.1	6.4
Body as a Whole						
Lethargy	45.8	1.9	1.1	0	72.7	0.3
Fever	5.2	0	1.4	0	4.5	0
Gastrointestinal						
Nausea/vomiting	92.4	25.0	83.2	22.1	85.0	6.4
Mucositis	58.5	8.9	9.3	0	52.9	1.9
Diarrhea	24.8	0.8	7.1	0	50.7	2.8
Anorexia	2.9	0	1.8	0	5.8	0.3
Infection						
Infection	21.5	1.6	15.0	0	25.9	0.6
Febrile neutropenia	N/A	6.1	0	0	NA	1.1
Ocular						
Conjunctivitis/keratitis	14.8	0	1.1	0	38.4	0
Skin						
Alopecia	95.5	56.6	69.6	19.3	84.4	6.7
Local toxicity	19.5	0.3	2.5	0.4	8.1	0
Rash/itch	8.9	0.3	1.4	0	14.2	0
Skin changes	4.7	0	0.7	0	7.2	0

FEC & CEF = cyclophosphamide + epirubicin + fluorouracil; CMF = cyclophosphamide + methotrexate + flurouracil
NA = not available

Grade 1 or 2 changes in transaminase levels were observed but were more frequently seen with CMF than with CEF.

Delayed Events

Table 5 describes the incidence of delayed adverse events in patients participating in the MA-5 and GFEA-05 trials.
[See table 5 above]

Table 5. Long-Term Adverse Events in Patients with Early Breast Detection

Event	% of Patients		
	FEC-100/CEF-120 (N=620)	FEC-50 (N=280)	CMF (N=360)
Cardiac toxicity			
Asymptomatic drops in LVEF	1.8	1.4	0.8
CHF	1.5	0.4	0.3
Leukemia			
AML	0.8	0	0.3

Two cases of acute lymphoid leukemia (ALL) were also observed in patients receiving epirubicin. However, an association between anthracyclines such as epirubicin and ALL has not been clearly established.

Overview of Acute and Delayed Toxicities

Hematologic—See WARNINGS.

Gastrointestinal. A dose-dependent mucositis (mainly oral stomatitis, less often esophagitis) may occur in patients treated with epirubicin. Clinical manifestations of mucositis may include a pain or burning sensation, erythema, erosions, ulcerations, bleeding, or infections. Mucositis generally appears early after drug administration and, if severe, may progress over a few days to mucosal ulcerations; most patients recover from this adverse event by the third week of therapy. Hyperpigmentation of the oralmucosa may also occur.
Nausea, vomiting, and occasionally diarrhea and abdominal pain can also occur. Severe vomiting and diarrhea may pro-

CEF-120:	Cyclophosphamide	75 mg/m^2 PO D 1–14
	ELLENCE	60 mg/m^2 IV D 1, 8
	5-Fluorouracil	500 mg/m^2 IV D 1, 8
	Repeated every 28 days for 6 cycles	
FEC-100:	5-Fluorouracil	500 mg/m^2
	ELLENCE	100 mg/m^2
	Cyclophosphamide	500 mg/m^2
	All drugs administered intravenously on Day 1 and repeated every 21 days for 6 cycles	

duce dehydration. Antiemetics may reduce nausea and vomiting; prophylactic use of antiemetics should be considered before therapy (see PRECAUTIONS).

Cutaneous and Hypersensitivity Reactions. Alopecia occurs frequently, but is usually reversible, with hair regrowth occurring within 2 to 3 months from the termination of therapy. Flushes, skin and nail hyperpigmentation, photosensitivity, and hypersensitivity to irradiated skin (radiation-recall reaction) have been observed. Urticaria and anaphylaxis have been reported in patients treated with epirubicin; signs and symptoms of these reactions may vary from skin rash and pruritus to fever, chills, and shock.

Cardiovascular—See WARNINGS.

Secondary Leukemia—See WARNINGS.

Injection-Site Reactions—See PRECAUTIONS.

OVERDOSAGE

A 36-year-old man with non-Hodgkin's lymphoma received a daily 95 mg/m^2 dose of ELLENCE Injection for 5 consecutive days. Five days later, he developed bone marrow aplasia, grade 4 mucositis, and gastrointestinal bleeding. No signs of acute cardiac toxicity were observed. He was treated with antibiotics, colony-stimulating factors, and antifungal agents, and recovered completely. A 63-year-old woman with breast cancer and liver metastasis received a single 320 mg/m^2 dose of ELLENCE. She was hospitalized with hyperthermia and developed multiple organ failure (respiratory and renal), with lactic acidosis, increased lactate dehydrogenase, and anuria. Death occurred within 24 hours after administration of ELLENCE. Additional instances of administration of doses higher than recommended have been reported at doses ranging from 150 to 250 mg/m^2. The observed adverse events in these patients were qualitatively similar to known toxicities of epirubicin. Most of the patients recovered with appropriate supportive care.

If an overdose occurs, supportive treatment (including antibiotic therapy, blood and platelet transfusions, colony-stimulating factors, and intensive care as needed) should be provided until the recovery of toxicities. Delayed CHF has been observed months after anthracycline administration. Patients must be observed carefully over time for signs of CHF and provided with appropriate supportive therapy.

DOSAGE AND ADMINISTRATION

ELLENCE Injection is administered to patients by intravenous infusion. ELLENCE is given in repeated 3- to 4-week cycles. The total dose of ELLENCE may be given on Day 1 of each cycle or divided equally and given on Days 1 and 8 of each cycle. The recommended dosage of ELLENCE are as follows:

Starting Doses

The recommended starting dose of ELLENCE is 100 to 120 mg/m^2. The following regimens were used in the trials supporting use of ELLENCE as a component of adjuvant therapy in patients with axillary-node positive breast cancer:

[See table above]

Patients administered the 120-mg/m^2 regimen of ELLENCE also received prophylactic antibiotic therapy with trimethoprim-sulfamethoxazole (e.g., Septra®, Bactrim®) or a fluoroquinolone.

Bone Marrow Dysfunction. Consideration should be given to administration of lower starting doses (75–90 mg/m^2) for heavily pretreated patients, patients with pre-existing bone marrow depression, or in the presence of neoplastic bone marrow infiltration (see WARNINGS and PRECAUTIONS).

Hepatic Dysfunction. Definitive recommendation regarding use of ELLENCE in patients with hepatic dysfunction are not available because patients with hepatic abnormalities were excluded from participation in adjuvant trials of FEC-100/CEF-120 therapy. In patients with elevated serum AST or serum total bilirubin concentrations, the following dose reductions were recommended in clinical trials, although few patients experienced hepatic impairment:

- Bilirubin 1.2 to 3 mg/dL or AST 2 to 4 times upper limit of normal
  1/2 of recommended starting dose
- Bilirubin > 3 mg/dL or AST > 4 times upper limit of normal
  1/4 of recommended starting dose

Information regarding experience in patients with hepatic dysfunction is provided in CLINICAL PHARMACOLOGY, Pharmacokinetics in Special Populations.

Renal Dysfunction. While no specific dose recommendation can be made based on the limited available data in patients with renal impairment, lower doses should be considered in patients with severe renal impairment (serum creatinine > 5 mg/dL).

Dose Modifications

Dosage adjustments after the first treatment cycle should be made on hematologic and non-hematologic toxicities. Patients experiencing during treatment cycle nadir platelet counts <50,000/mm^3, absolute neutrophil counts (ANC) <250/mm^3, neutropenic fever, or Grades 3/4 nonhematologic toxicity should have the Day 1 dose in subsequent cycles reduced to 75% of the Day 1 dose given in the current cycle. Day 1 chemotherapy in subsequent courses of treatment should be delayed until platelet counts are ≥100,000/mm^3, ANC ≥1500/mm^3, and nonhematologic toxicities have recovered to ≤Grade 1.

For patients receiving a divided dose of ELLENCE (Day 1 and Day 8), the Day 8 dose should be 75% of Day 1 if platelet counts are 75,000–100,000/mm^3 and ANC is 1000 to 1499/mm^3. If Day 8 platelet counts are <75,000/mm^3, ANC <1000/mm^3, or Grade 3/4 nonhematologic toxicity has occurred, the Day 8 dose should be omitted.

Preparation & Administration Precautions

Parenteral drug products should be inspected visually for particulate matter and discoloration prior to administration, whenever solution and container permit.

Protective measures. The following protective measures should be taken when handling ELLENCE:

- Personnel should be trained in appropriate techniques for reconstitution and handling.
- Pregnant staff should be excluded from working with this drug.
- Personnel handling ELLENCE should wear protective clothing: goggles, gowns and disposable gloves and masks.
- A designated area should be defined for syringe preparation (preferably under a laminar flow system), with the work surface protected by disposable, plastic-backed, absorbent paper.
- All items used for reconstitution, administration or cleaning (including gloves) should be placed in high-risk, waste-disposable bags for high temperature incineration.

Spillage or leakage should be treated with dilute sodium hypochlorite (1% available chlorine) solution, preferably by soaking, and then water. All contaminated and cleaning materials should be placed in high-risk, waste-disposal bags for incineration. Accidental contact with the skin or eyes should be treated immediately by copious lavage with water, or soap and water, or sodium bicarbonate solution; medical attention should be sought.

Incompatibilities. Prolonged contact with any solution of an alkaline pH should be avoided as it will result in hydrolysis of the drug. ELLENCE should not be mixed with heparin or fluorouracil due to chemical incompatibility that may lead to precipitation.

ELLENCE can be used in combination with other antitumor agents, but it is not recommended that it be mixed with other drugs in the same syringe.

Preparation of Infusion Solution

ELLENCE is provided as a preservative-free, ready-to-use solution.

Intravenous administration of ELLENCE should be performed with caution. It is recommended that ELLENCE be administered into the tubing of a freely flowing intravenous infusion (0.9% sodium chloride or 5% glucose solution) over a period of 3 to 5 minutes. This technique is intended to minimize the risk of thrombosis or perivenous extravasation, which could lead to severe cellulitis, vesication, or tissue necrosis. A direct push injection is not recommended due to the risk of extravasation, which may occur even in the presence of adequate blood return upon needle aspiration. Venous sclerosis may result from injection into small vessels or repeated injections into the same vein (see PRECAUTIONS). ELLENCE should be used within 24 hours of first penetration of the rubber stopper. Discard any unused solution.

HOW SUPPLIED

ELLENCE Injection is available in polypropylene single-use vials containing 2 mg epirubicin hydrochloride per mL as a sterile, preservative-free, ready-to-use solution in the following strengths.

50 mg/25 mL single-use vial	NDC 0009-5091-01
200 mg/100 mL single-use vial	NDC 0009-5093-01

Store refrigerated between 2°C and 8°C (36°F and 46°F). Do not freeze. Protect from light. Discard unused portion.

Rx only

US Patent No. 5,977,082

Manufactured for: Pharmacia & Upjohn Company, Kalamazoo, MI 49001 USA

By: Pharmacia & Upjohn (Perth) Pty Limited, Bentley WA 6102 Australia

September 1999 817 911 101
692532

EMCYT® ℞

[em 'cyt]

estramustine phosphate sodium capsules

DESCRIPTION

Estramustine phosphate sodium, an antineoplastic agent, is an off-white powder readily soluble in water. EMCYT Capsules are white and opaque, each containing estramustine phosphate sodium as the disodium salt monohydrate equivalent to 140 mg estramustine phosphate, for oral administration. Each capsule also contains magnesium stearate, silicon dioxide, sodium lauryl sulfate, and talc. Gelatin capsule shells contain the following pigment: titanium dioxide. Chemically, estramustine phosphate sodium is estra-1,3,5(10)-triene-3,17-diol(17β)-, 3-[bis(2-chloroethyl)carbamate] 17-(dihydrogen phosphate), disodium salt, monohydrate. It is also referred to as estradiol 3-[bis(2-chloroethyl)carbamate] 17-(dihydrogen phosphate), disodium salt, monohydrate.

Estramustine phosphate sodium has an empiric formula of $C_{23}H_{30}Cl_2NNa_2O_6P \bullet H_2O$, a calculated molecular weight of 582.4, and the following structural formula:

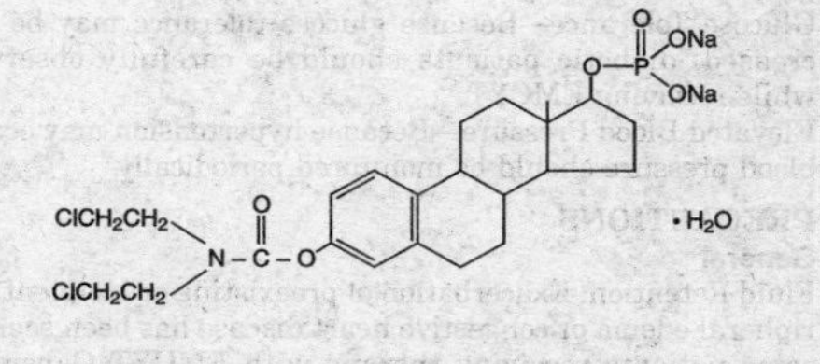

CLINICAL PHARMACOLOGY

Estramustine phosphate (Figure 1) is a molecule combining estradiol and nornitrogen mustard by a carbamate link. The molecule is phosphorylated to make it water soluble.

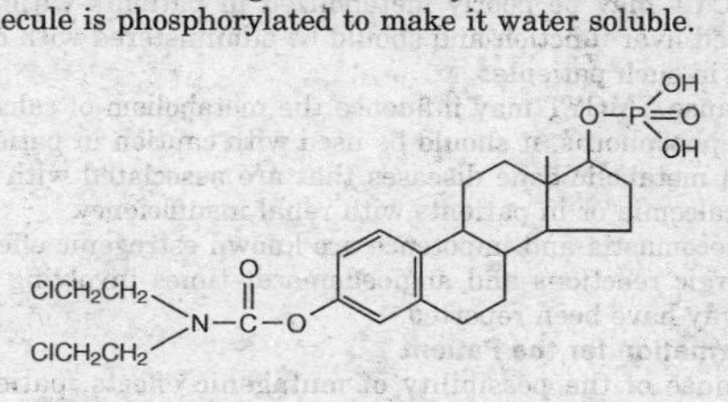

Figure 1. Estramustine Phosphate

Estramustine phosphate taken orally is readily dephosphorylated during absorption, and the major metabolites in plasma are estramustine (Figure 2), the estrone analog (Figure 3), estradiol, and estrone.

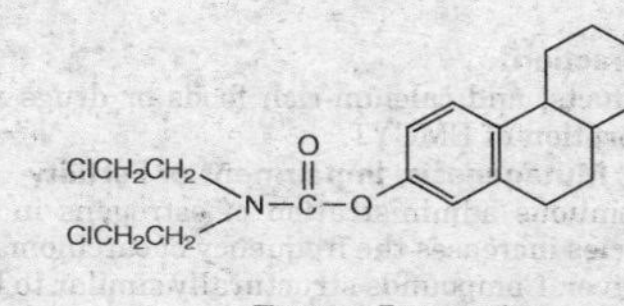

Figure 2. Estramustine

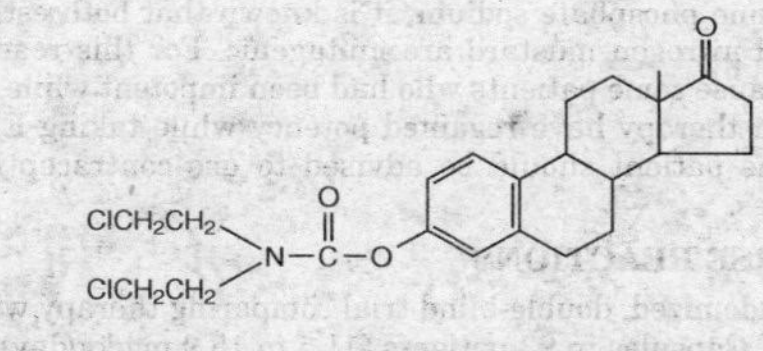

Figure 3. Estrone Analog of Estramustine

Prolonged treatment with estramustine phosphate produces elevated total plasma concentrations of estradiol that fall within ranges similar to the elevated estradiol levels found in prostatic cancer patients given conventional estradiol therapy. Estrogenic effects, as demonstrated by changes in circulating levels of steroids and pituitary hormones, are similar in patients treated with either estramustine phosphate or conventional estradiol.

The metabolic urinary patterns of the estradiol moiety of estramustine phosphate and estradiol itself are very similar, although the metabolites derived from estramustine phosphate are excreted at a slower rate.

INDICATIONS AND USAGE

EMCYT Capsules are indicated in the palliative treatment of patients with metastatic and/or progressive carcinoma of the prostate.

CONTRAINDICATIONS

EMCYT Capsules should not be used in patients with any of the following conditions:

1) Known hypersensitivity to either estradiol or to nitrogen mustard.
2) Active thrombophlebitis or thromboembolic disorders, except in those cases where the actual tumor mass is the

Continued on next page

Information on these Pharmacia & Upjohn products is based on labeling in effect June 1, 2000. Further information concerning these and other Pharmacia & Upjohn products may be obtained by direct inquiry to Medical Information, Pharmacia & Upjohn, Kalamazoo, MI 49001.

Emcyt—Cont.

cause of the thromboembolic phenomenon and the physician feels the benefits of therapy may outweigh the risks.

WARNINGS

It has been shown that there is an increased risk of thrombosis, including fatal and nonfatal myocardial infarction, in men receiving estrogens for prostatic cancer. EMCYT Capsules should be used with caution in patients with a history of thrombophlebitis, thrombosis, or thromboembolic disorders, especially if they were associated with estrogen therapy. Caution should also be used in patients with cerebral vascular or coronary artery disease.
Glucose Tolerance—Because glucose tolerance may be decreased, diabetic patients should be carefully observed while receiving EMCYT.
Elevated Blood Pressure—Because hypertension may occur, blood pressure should be monitored periodically.

PRECAUTIONS

General

Fluid Retention. Exacerbation of preexisting or incipient peripheral edema or congestive heart disease has been seen in some patients receiving therapy with EMCYT Capsules. Other conditions which might be influenced by fluid retention, such as epilepsy, migraine, or renal dysfunction, require careful observation.
EMCYT may be poorly metabolized in patients with impaired liver function and should be administered with caution in such patients.
Because EMCYT may influence the metabolism of calcium and phosphorus, it should be used with caution in patients with metabolic bone diseases that are associated with hypercalcemia or in patients with renal insufficiency.
Gynecomastia and impotence are known estrogenic effects. Allergic reactions and angioedema at times involving the airway have been reported.

Information for the Patient

Because of the possibility of mutagenic effects, patients should be advised to use contraceptive measures.

Laboratory Tests

Certain endocrine and liver function tests may be affected by estrogen-containing drugs. EMCYT may depress testosterone levels. Abnormalities of hepatic enzymes and of bilirubin have occurred in patients receiving EMCYT. Such tests should be done at appropriate intervals during therapy and repeated after the drug has been withdrawn for two months.

Food/Drug Interaction

Milk, milk products, and calcium-rich foods or drugs may impair the absorption of EMCYT.

Carcinogenesis, Mutagenesis, Impairment of Fertility

Long-term continuous administration of estrogens in certain animal species increases the frequency of carcinomas of the breast and liver. Compounds structurally similar to EMCYT are carcinogenic in mice. Carcinogenic studies of EMCYT have not been conducted in man. Although testing by the Ames method failed to demonstrate mutagenicity for estramustine phosphate sodium, it is known that both estradiol and nitrogen mustard are mutagenic. For this reason and because some patients who had been impotent while on estrogen therapy have regained potency while taking EMCYT, the patient should be advised to use contraceptive measures.

ADVERSE REACTIONS

In a randomized, double-blind trial comparing therapy with EMCYT Capsules in 93 patients (11.5 to 15.9 mg/kg/day) or diethylstilbestrol (DES) in 93 patients (3.0 mg/day), the following adverse effects were reported:

	EMCYT n=93	DES n=93
CARDIOVASCULAR-RESPIRATORY		
Cardiac Arrest	0	2
Cerebrovascular Accident	2	0
Myocardial Infarction	3	1
Thrombophlebitis	3	7
Pulmonary Emboli	2	5
Congestive Heart Failure	3	2
Edema	19	17
Dyspnea	11	3
Leg Cramps	8	11
Upper Respiratory Discharge	1	1
Hoarseness	1	0
GASTROINTESTINAL		
Nausea	15	8
Diarrhea	12	11
Minor Gastrointestinal Upset	11	6
Anorexia	4	3
Flatulence	2	0
Vomiting	1	1
Gastrointestinal Bleeding	1	0
Burning Throat	1	0
Thirst	1	0
INTEGUMENTARY		
Rash	1	4
Pruritus	2	2
Dry Skin	2	0
Pigment Changes	0	3
Easy Bruising	3	0
Flushing	1	0
Night Sweats	0	1
Fingertip—Peeling Skin	1	0
Thinning Hair	1	1
BREAST CHANGES		
Tenderness	66	64
Enlargement		
Mild	60	54
Moderate	10	16
Marked	0	5
MISCELLANEOUS		
Lethargy Alone	4	3
Depression	0	2
Emotional Lability	2	0
Insomnia	3	0
Headache	1	1
Anxiety	1	0
Chest Pain	1	1
Hot Flashes	0	1
Pain in Eyes	0	1
Tearing of Eyes	1	1
Tinnitus	0	1
LABORATORY ABNORMALITIES		
Hematologic		
Leukopenia	4	2
Thrombopenia	1	2
Hepatic		
Bilirubin Alone	1	5
Bilirubin and LDH	0	1
Bilirubin and SGOT	2	1
Bilirubin, LDH and SGOT	2	0
LDH and/or SGOT	31	28
Miscellaneous		
Hypercalcemia—Transient	0	1

OVERDOSAGE

Although there has been no experience with overdosage to date, it is reasonable to expect that such episodes may produce pronounced manifestations of the known adverse reactions. In the event of overdosage, the gastric contents should be evacuated by gastric lavage and symptomatic therapy should be initiated. Hematologic and hepatic parameters should be monitored for at least 6 weeks after overdosage of EMCYT Capsules

DOSAGE AND ADMINISTRATION

The recommended daily dose is 14 mg per kg of body weight (ie, one 140 mg capsule for each 10 kg or 22 lb of body weight), given in 3 or 4 divided doses. Most patients in studies in the United States have been treated at a dosage range of 10 to 16 mg per kg per day.
Patients should be instructed to take EMCYT Capsules at least 1 hour before or 2 hours after meals. EMCYT should be swallowed with water. Milk, milk products, and calcium-rich foods or drugs (such as calcium-contraining antacids) must not be taken simultaneously with EMCYT.
Patients should be treated for 30 to 90 days before the physician determines the possible benefits of continued therapy. Therapy should be continued as long as the favorable response lasts. Some patients have been maintained on therapy for more than 3 years at doses ranging from 10 to 16 mg per kg of body weight per day.
Procedures for proper handling and disposal of anticancer drugs should be considered. Several guidelines on this subject have been published.[1-7] There is no general agreement that all of the procedures recommended in the guidelines are necessary or appropriate.

HOW SUPPLIED

White opaque capsules, each containing estramustine phosphate sodium as the disodium salt monohydrate equivalent to 140 mg estramustine phosphate—bottle of 100 (NDC 0013-0132-02).

NOTE

EMCYT Capsules should be stored at 36° to 46°F (2° to 8°C).

REFERENCES

1. Recommendations for the Safe Handling of Parenteral Antineoplastic Drugs. NIH Publication No. 83–2621. For sale by the Superintendent of Documents, U.S. Government Printing Office, Washington, DC, 20402.
2. AMA Council Report, Guidelines for Handling Parenteral Antineoplastics, JAMA. 1985; 253 (11):1590–1592.
3. National Study Commission on Cytotoxic Exposure-Recommendations for Handling Cytotoxic Agents. Available from Louis P. Jeffrey, Sc.D., Chairman, National Study Commission on Cytotoxic Exposure, Massachusetts College of Pharmacy and Allied Health Sciences, 179 Longwood Avenue, Boston, Massachusetts 02115.
4. Clinical Oncological Society of Australia. Guidelines and Recommendations for Safe Handling of Antineoplastic Agents. Med J Australia. 1983; 1:426–428.
5. Jones RB, et al. Safe Handling of Chemotherapeutic Agents: A Report from the Mount Sinai Medical Center. CA-A Cancer Journal for Clinicians. 1983; (Sept/Oct) 258–263.
6. American Society of Hospital Pharmacists Technical Assistance Bulletin on Handling Cytotoxic and Hazardous Drugs. Am J Hosp Pharm. 1990; 47:1033–1049.
7. OSHA Work-Practice Guidelines for Personnel Dealing with Cytotoxic (Antineoplastic) Drugs. Am J Hosp Pharm. 1986; 43:1193–1204.

℞ only
Manufactured for: Pharmacia & Upjohn Company, Kalamazoo, MI 49001, USA
by: Pharmacia & Upjohn S.p.A., Ascoli Piceno, Italy
108010299 Revised: February 1999

ESTRING® ℞

estradiol vaginal ring
2 mg

1. ESTROGENS HAVE BEEN REPORTED TO INCREASE THE RISK OF ENDOMETRIAL CARCINOMA IN POSTMENOPAUSAL WOMEN.
   Close clinical surveillance of all women taking estrogens is important. Adequate diagnostic measures, including endometrial sampling when indicated, should be undertaken to rule out malignancy in all cases of undiagnosed persistent or recurring abnormal vaginal bleeding. There is no evidence that "natural" estrogens are more or less hazardous than "synthetic" estrogens at equi-estrogenic doses.
2. ESTROGENS SHOULD NOT BE USED DURING PREGNANCY.
   There is no indication for estrogen therapy during pregnancy or during immediate postpartum period. Estrogens are ineffective for the prevention or treatment of threatened or habitual abortion. Estrogens are not indicated for the prevention of postpartum breast engorgement.
   Estrogen therapy during pregnancy is associated with an increased risk of congenital defects in the reproductive organs of the fetus, and possibly other birth defects. Studies of women who received diethylstilbestrol (DES) during pregnancy have shown that female offspring have an increased risk of vaginal adenosis, squamous cell dysplasia of the uterine cervix, and clear cell vaginal cancer later in life; male offspring have an increased risk of urogenital abnormalities and possibly testicular cancer later in life. The 1985 DES Task Force concluded that the use of DES during pregnancy is associated with a subsequent increased risk of breast cancer in the mothers, although a causal relationship remains unproven and the observed level of excess risk is similar to that for a number of other breast cancer risk factors.

DESCRIPTION

ESTRING (estradiol vaginal ring) is a slightly opaque ring with a whitish core containing a drug reservoir of 2 mg estradiol. Estradiol, silicone polymers and barium sulfate are combined to form the ring. When placed in the vagina, ESTRING releases estradiol approximately 7.5 µg/24 hours, in a consistent stable manner over 90 days. ESTRING has the following dimensions: outer diameter 55 mm; cross-sectional diameter 9 mm; core diameter 2 mm. One ESTRING should be inserted into the upper third of the vaginal vault, to be worn continuously for three months.
Estradiol is chemically described as estra-1,3,5(10)-triene-3,17β-diol. The molecular formula of estradiol is $C_{18}H_{24}O_2$ and the structural formula is:

CH3 OH HO

The molecular weight of estradiol is 272.39.

CLINICAL PHARMACOLOGY

Pharmacokinetics

ABSORPTION

Estrogens used in therapeutics are well absorbed through the skin, mucous membranes, and the gastrointestinal (GI) tract. The vaginal delivery of estrogens circumvents first-pass metabolism possibly reducing the induction of several other hepatic proteins.
In a Phase I study of 14 postmenopausal women, the insertion of ESTRING (estradiol vaginal ring) rapidly increased serum estradiol (E_2) levels attesting to the rapid absorption of estradiol via the vaginal mucosa. The time to attain peak serum estradiol levels (T_{max}) was 0.5 to 1 hour. Peak serum estradiol concentrations post-initial burst declined rapidly over the next 24 hours and were virtually indistinguishable from the baseline mean (range: 5 to 22 pg/mL). Serum levels of estradiol and estrone (E_1) over the following 12 weeks during which the ring was maintained in the vaginal vault remained relatively unchanged (see Table 1).
The initial estradiol peak post-application of the second ring in the same women resulted in ~ 38% lower C_{max}, apparently due to reduced systemic absorption via the revitalized vaginal epithelium. The relative systemic exposure from the initial peak of ESTRING accounted for approximately 4% of the total estradiol exposure over the 12 week period.
The constant and stable release of estradiol from ESTRING was demonstrated in a Phase II study of 166–222 postmenopausal women who inserted up to four rings consecutively at three month intervals. Low dose systemic delivery of estradiol from ESTRING resulted in mean steady state serum estradiol estimates of 7.8, 7.0, 7.0, 8.1 pg/mL at weeks 12, 24, 36, and 48, respectively. Similar reproducibility is also seen in levels of estrone. Lower systemic exposure to estradiol and estrone is further supported by serum levels measured during a pivotal Phase III study.

In post-menopausal women, mean dose of estradiol systemicaly absorbed unchanged from ESTRING is ~ 8% [95% CI: 2.8–12.8%] of the daily amount released locally. Low systemic exposure to estradiol and estrone resulting from ESTRING should elicit lower estrogen-dependent effects.

DISTRIBUTION

Circulating, unbound estrogens are known to modulate pharmacologic response. Estrogens circulate in blood bound to sex-hormone binding globulin (SHBG) and albumin. A dynamic equilibrium exists between the conjugated and the unconjugated forms of estradiol and estrone, which undergo rapid interconversion.

METABOLISM

Exogenously delivered or endogenously derived estrogens are primarily metabolized in the liver to estrone and estriol, which are also found in the systemic circulation. Estrogen metabolites are primarily excreted in the urine as glucuronides and sulphates. Of the several estrogen metabolites, urinary estrone and estrone sulphate (E_1S), post-ESTRING use, are in the normal post-menopausal range.

EXCRETION

Mean percent dose excreted in the 24-hour urine as estradiol, 4 and 12 weeks post-application of ESTRING in a Phase I study was 5% and 8%, respectively, of the daily released amount.

Drug-Drug Interactions

No formal *drug-drug* interactions studies have been done with ESTRING. It is anticipated that lower exposure to systemic estrogens may reduce the potential for drug interactions thus maintaining the benefit to risk ratio of concomitant drugs.

TABLE 1: PHARMACOKINETIC MEAN ESTIMATES FOLLOWING ESTRING APPLICATION

Estrogen	C_{max} (pg/mL)	$C_{ss-48\,hr}$ (pg/mL)	C_{ss-4w} (pg/mL)	C_{ss-12w} (pg/mL)
Estradiol (E_2)	63.2[a]	11.2	9.5	8.0
Baseline-adjusted E_2[b]	55.6	3.6	2.0	0.4
Estrone (E_1)	66.3	52.5	43.8	47.0
Baseline-adjusted E_1	20.0	6.2	−2.4	0.8

[a] n=14 [b] Based on means

Pharmacodynamics

In vivo, estrogens diffuse through cell membranes, distribute throughout the cell, bind to and activate the estrogen receptors, thereby eliciting their biological effects. Estrogen receptors have been identified in tissues of the reproductive tract, breast, pituitary, hypothalamus, liver and bone of women. ESTRING delivers estradiol constantly at a mean rate of ~ 7.5 μg/24 hours for a period of 24 days. Its use in post-menopausal patients in Phase I and II studies showed no apparent effects on systemic levels of hepatic protein SHBG, or FSH. Lowering of the pretreatment vaginal pH from a mean of 6.0 to a mean of 4.6 (as found in fertile women) over the 12 to 48 week treatment period, and improvements evident in the vaginal mucosal epithelium seen in all studies attest to the local dynamic effects of estrogen.

INDICATIONS AND USAGE

ESTRING (estradiol vaginal ring) is indicated for the treatment of urogenital symptoms associated with post-menopausal atrophy of the vagina (such as dryness, burning, pruritus and dyspareunia) and/or the lower urinary tract (urinary urgency and dysuria).

CLINICAL STUDIES

Two pivotal controlled studies have demonstrated the efficacy of ESTRING (estradiol vaginal ring) in the treatment of post-menopausal urogenital symptoms due to estrogen deficiency.

In a U.S. study where ESTRING was compared with conjugated estrogens vaginal cream, no difference in efficacy between the treatment groups was found with respect to improvement in the physician's global assessment of vaginal symptoms (83% and 82% of patients receiving ESTRING and cream, respectively) and in the patient's global assessment of vaginal symptoms (83% and 82% of patients receiving ESTRING and cream, respectively) after 12 weeks of treatment. In an Australian study, ESTRING was also compared with conjugated estrogens vaginal cream and no difference in the physician's assessment of improvement of vaginal mucosal atrophy (79% and 75% for ESTRING and cream, respectively) or in the patient's assessment of improvement in vaginal dryness (82% and 76% for ESTRING and cream, respectively) after 12 weeks of treatment.

In the U.S. study, symptoms of dysuria and urinary urgency improved in 74% and 65%, respectively, of patients receiving ESTRING as assessed by the patient. In the Australian study, symptoms of dysuria and urinary urgency improved in 90% and 71%, respectively, of patients receiving ESTRING as assessed by the patient.

In both studies, ESTRING and conjugated estrogens vaginal cream had a similar ability to reduce vaginal pH levels and to mature the vaginal mucosa (as measured cytologically using the maturation index and/or the maturation value) after 12 weeks of treatment. In supportive studies, ESTRING was also shown to have a similar significant treatment effect on the maturation of the urethral mucosa.

Endometrial overstimulation, as evaluated in non-hysterectomized patients participating in the U.S. study by the progestogen challenge test and pelvic sonogram, was reported for none of the 58 (0%) patients receiving ESTRING and 4 of the 35 patients (11%) receiving conjugated estrogens vaginal cream.

Of the U.S. women who completed 12 weeks of treatment, 95% rated product comfort for ESTRING as excellent or very good compared with 65% of patients receiving conjugated estrogens vaginal cream, 95% of ESTRING patients judged the product to be very easy or easy to use compared with 88% of cream patients, and 82% gave ESTRING an overall rating of excellent or very good compared with 58% for the cream.

CONTRAINDICATIONS

1. Estrogens should not be used in women with any of the following conditions:
   a. Known or suspected pregnancy (see **BOXED WARNING**).
   b. Undiagnosed abnormal genital bleeding.
   c. Known or suspected cancer of the breast.
   d. Known or suspected estrogen-dependent neoplasia.
2. ESTRING (estradiol vaginal ring) should not be used in patients hypersensitive to any of its ingredients.

WARNINGS

1. **Breast cancer.**
   While the majority of studies have not shown an increased risk of breast cancer in women who have ever used estrogen replacement therapy, some have reported a moderately increased risk (relative risks of 1.3 to 2.0) in those taking higher doses or those taking lower doses for prolonged period of time, especially in excess of ten years. Other studies have not shown this relationship.
2. **Other.**
   Congenital lesions with malignant potential, gallbladder disease, cardiovascular disease, elevated blood pressure and hypercalcemia have been associated with systemic estrogen treatment.

PRECAUTIONS

A. General

1. **Use of Progestins.**
   It is common practice with systemic administration of estrogen to add progestin for ten or more days during a cycle to lower the incidence of endometrial proliferation or hyperplasia. From the available clinical data, it seems unlikely that ESTRING would have adverse effects on the endometrium. Furthermore, addition of progestins to a patient being treated with ESTRING is not expected to result in vaginal bleeding.
2. **Physical Examination.**
   A complete medical and family history should be taken prior to the initiation of any estrogen therapy. The pretreatment and periodic physical examinations should include special reference to blood pressure, breasts, abdomen, and pelvic organs and should include a Papanicolaou smear. As a general rule, estrogen should not be prescribed for longer than one year without reexamining the patient.
3. **Uterine Bleeding and Mastodynia.**
   Although uncommon with ESTRING, certain patients may develop undesirable manifestations of estrogenic stimulation, such as abnormal uterine bleeding and mastodynia.
4. **Liver Disease.**
   ESTRING should be used with caution in patients with impaired liver function.
5. **Location of ESTRING.**
   Some women have experienced moving or gliding of ESTRING within the vagina. Instances of ESTRING being expelled from the vagina in connection with moving the bowels, strain, or constipation have been reported. If this occurs, ESTRING can be rinsed in lukewarm water and reinserted into the vagina by the patient.
6. **Vaginal Irritation.**
   ESTRING may not be suitable for women with narrow, short, or stenosed vaginas. Narrow vagina, vaginal stenosis, prolapse, and vaginal infections are conditions that make the vagina more susceptible to ESTRING-caused irritation or ulceration. Women with signs or symptoms of vaginal irritation should alert their physician.
7. **Vaginal Infection.**
   Vaginal infection is generally more common in post-menopausal women due to the lack of the normal flora of fertile women, especially lactobacillus, and the subsequent higher pH. Vaginal infections should be treated with appropriate antimicrobial therapy before initiation of ESTRING. If a vaginal infection develops during use of ESTRING, then ESTRING should be removed and reinserted only after the infection has been appropriately treated.
8. **Other.**
   Hypercoagulability and hyperlipidemia have been reported in women on other types of estrogen replacement therapy but, these have not been seen with ESTRING patients.
   Fluid retention is another known risk factor with estrogen therapy and may be harmful to patients with asthma, epilepsy, migraine and cardiac or renal dysfunction.
   ESTRING treatment has not been associated with any indication of increase in body weight up to 48 weeks of treatment.

B. Information for the Patient.

See text of **Information for Patients** which appears at the end of this insert.

C. Drug-Drug and Drug-Laboratory Interactions.

It is recommended that ESTRING be removed during treatment with other vaginally administered preparations.

Drug-drug and drug-laboratory interactions have been reported with estrogen administration overall, but were not observed in clinical trials with ESTRING. However, the possibility of the following interactions should be considered when treating patients with ESTRING.

1. Accelerated prothrombin time, partial thromboplastin time, and platelet aggregation time; increased platelet count; increased factors II, VII antigen, VIII antigen, VIII coagulant activity, IX, X, XII, VII-X complex, II-VII-X complex, and beta-thromboglobulin; decreased levels of anti-factor Xa and antithrombin III, decreased antithrombin III activity; increased levels of fibrinogen and fibrinogen activity; increased plasminogen antigen and activity.
2. Increased plasma HDL and HDL-2 subfraction concentrations, reduced LDL cholesterol concentration, increased triglycerides levels.

D. Carcinogenesis, Mutagenesis, and Impairment of Fertility.

Long term continuous administration of natural and synthetic estrogens in certain animal species increases the frequency of carcinomas of the breast, uterus, cervix, vagina, and liver (see **CONTRAINDICATIONS** and **BOXED WARNING**).

E. Pregnancy Category X.

Estrogens should not be used during pregnancy (see **CONTRAINDICATIONS** and **BOXED WARNING**).

F. Nursing Mothers.

This product is not intended for nursing mothers. As a general principle, the administration of any drug to nursing mothers should be done only when clearly necessary since many drugs are excreted in human milk. In addition, estrogen administration to nursing mothers has been shown to decrease the quantity and quality of the milk.

G. Geriatric Use.

Of the total number of subjects in clinical studies of ESTRING (including subjects treated with ESTRING, placebo, and comparator drug; n=951), 25% were 65 and over, while 4% were 75 and over. No overall differences in safety or effectiveness were observed between these subjects and younger subjects, and other reported clinical experience has not identified differences in responses between the elderly and younger patients, but greater sensitivity of some older individuals cannot be ruled out.

ADVERSE REACTIONS

The biological safety of the silicone elastomer has been studied in various *in vitro* and *in vivo* test models. The results show that the silicone elastomer is non-toxic, non-pyrogenic, non-irritating, and non-sensitizing. Long-term implantation induced encapsulation equal to or less than the negative control (polyethylene) used in the USP test. No toxic reaction or tumor formation was observed with the silicone elastomer.

In general, ESTRING (estradiol vaginal ring) was well tolerated. In the two pivotal controlled studies, discontinuation of treatment due to an adverse event was required by 5.4% of patients receiving ESTRING and 3.9% of patients receiving conjugated estrogens vaginal cream. The most common reasons for withdrawal from ESTRING treatment due to an adverse event were vaginal discomfort and gastrointestinal symptoms.

The adverse events reported with a frequency of 3% or greater in the two pivotal controlled studies by patients receiving ESTRING or conjugated estrogens vaginal cream are listed in Table 2.

Table 2: Adverse Events Reported by 3% or More of Patients Receiving Either ESTRING or Conjugated Estrogens Vaginal Cream in Two Pivotal Controlled Studies

ADVERSE EVENT	Estring (n=257) %	Conjugated Estrogens Vaginal Cream (n=129) %
Musculoskeletal		
Back Pain	6	8
Arthritis	4	2
Arthralgia	3	5
Skeletal Pain	2	4
CNS/Peripheral Nervous System		
Headache	13	16
Psychiatric		
Insomnia	4	0
Gastrointestinal		
Abdominal Pain	4	2
Nausea	3	2
Respiratory		
Upper Respiratory Tract Infection	5	6

Continued on next page

Information on these Pharmacia & Upjohn products is based on labeling in effect June 1, 2000. Further information concerning these and other Pharmacia & Upjohn products may be obtained by direct inquiry to Medical Information, Pharmacia & Upjohn, Kalamazoo, MI 49001.

Estring—Cont.

Sinusitis	4	3
Pharyngitis	1	3
Urinary		
Urinary Tract Infection	2	7
Female Reproductive		
Leukorrhea	7	3
Vaginitis	5	2
Vaginal Discomfort/Pain	5	5
Vaginal Hemorrhage	4	5
Asymptomatic Genital Bacterial Growth	4	6
Breast Pain	1	7
Resistance Mechanisms		
Genital Moniliasis	6	7
Body as a Whole		
Flu-Like Symptoms	3	2
Hot Flushes	2	3
Allergy	1	4
Miscellaneous		
Family Stress	2	3

Other adverse events (listed alphabetically) occurring at a frequency of 1 to 3% in the two pivotal controlled studies by patients receiving ESTRING include: anxiety, bronchitis, chest pain, cystitis, dermatitis, diarrhea, dyspepsia, dysuria, flatulence, gastritis, genital eruption, genital pruritus, hemorrhoids, leg edema, migraine, otitis media, skin hypertrophy, syncope, toothache, tooth disorder, urinary incontinence.

The following additional adverse events were reported at least once by patients receiving ESTRING in the worldwide clinical program, which includes controlled and uncontrolled studies. A causal relationship with ESTRING has not been established.

Body as a Whole: allergic reaction

CNS/Peripheral Nervous System: dizziness

Gastrointestinal: enlarged abdomen, vomiting

Metabolic/Nutritional Disorders: weight decrease or increase

Psychiatric: depression, decreased libido, nervousness

Reproductive: breast engorgement, breast enlargement, intermenstrual bleeding, genital edema, vulval disorder

Skin/Appendages: pruritus, pruritus ani

Urinary: micturition frequency, urethral disorder

Vascular: thrombophlebitis

Vision: abnormal vision

OVERDOSAGE

Given the nature and design of ESTRING (estradiol vaginal ring), it is unlikely that overdosage will occur. However, should overdosage occur, it may manifest itself as nausea, vomiting, and/or vaginal bleeding. Serious ill effects have not been reported following acute ingestion of large doses of estrogen-containing oral contraceptives by young children.

DOSAGE AND ADMINISTRATION

One ESTRING (estradiol vaginal ring) is to be inserted as deeply as possible into the upper one-third of the vaginal vault. The ring is to remain in place continuously for three months, after which it is to be removed and, if appropriate, replaced by a new ring. The need to continue treatment should be assessed at 3 or 6 month intervals.

Should the ring be removed or fall out at any time during the 90-day treatment period, the ring should be rinsed in lukewarm water and re-inserted by the patient, or, if necessary, by a physician or nurse.

Retention of the ring for greater than 90 days does not represent overdosage but will result in progressively greater underdosage with the attendant risk of loss of efficacy and increasing risk of vaginal infections and/or erosions.

Instructions for Use

ESTRING (estradiol vaginal ring) insertion

The ring should be pressed into an oval and inserted into the upper third of the vaginal vault. The exact position is not critical. When ESTRING is in place, the patient should not feel anything. If the patient feels discomfort, ESTRING is probably not far enough inside. Gently push ESTRING further into the vagina.

ESTRING use

ESTRING should be left in place continuously for 90 days and then, if continuation of therapy is deemed appropriate, replaced by a new ESTRING.

The patient should not feel ESTRING when it is in place and it should not interfere with sexual intercourse. Straining at defecation may make ESTRING move down in the lower part of the vagina. If so, it may be pushed up again with a finger.

If ESTRING is expelled totally from the vagina, it should be rinsed in lukewarm water and reinserted by the patient (or doctor/nurse if necessary).

ESTRING removal

ESTRING may be removed by hooking a finger through the ring and pulling it out.

For patient instructions, see **Information for Patients**.

HOW SUPPLIED

Each ESTRING (estradiol vaginal ring) is individually packaged in a heat-sealed rectangular pouch consisting of three layers, from outside to inside: polyester, aluminum foil, and low density polyethylene, respectively. The pouch is provided with a tear-off notch on one side.

NDC 0013-2150-36 ESTRING (estradiol vaginal ring) 2 mg—available in single packs.

STORAGE—Store at controlled room temperature 15° to 30°C (59° to 86°F).

℞ only

INFORMATION FOR PATIENTS

INTRODUCTION

This leaflet describes when and how to use ESTRING (estradiol vaginal ring), and the risks and benefits of estrogen treatment. Please read this information carefully before starting treatment.

Estrogens have important benefits but also some risks. You must decide, with your doctor, whether the risks to you of estrogen use are acceptable because of their benefits. If you use estrogens, check with your doctor to be sure you are using the dose that is appropriate for you, and that you don't use them longer than necessary. How long you need to use estrogens should be decided by you and your doctor.

1. **ESTROGENS INCREASE THE RISK OF CANCER OF THE UTERUS IN WOMEN WHO HAVE HAD THEIR MENOPAUSE ("CHANGE OF LIFE")**
   If you use any estrogen-containing drug, it is important to visit your doctor regularly and report any unusual vaginal bleeding right away. Vaginal bleeding after menopause may be a warning sign of uterine cancer. Your doctor should evaluate any unusual vaginal bleeding to find out the cause.
2. **ESTROGENS SHOULD NOT BE USED DURING PREGNANCY**
   Estrogens do not prevent miscarriage (spontaneous abortion) and are not needed in the days following childbirth. If you take estrogens during pregnancy, your unborn child has a greater than usual chance of having birth defects. The risk of developing these defects is small, but clearly larger than the risk in children whose mothers did not take estrogens during pregnancy. These birth defects may affect the baby's urinary system and sex organs. Daughters born to mothers who took DES (an estrogen drug) have a higher than usual chance of developing cancer of the vagina or cervix when they become teenagers or young adults. Sons may have a higher than usual chance of developing cancer of the testicles when they become teenagers or young adults.

USES OF ESTROGEN

Estrogens are hormones made by the ovaries of women during their reproductive years. Between ages 45 and 55, the ovaries normally stop making estrogens. This leads to a drop in body estrogen levels which causes the "change of life" or menopause (the end of monthly menstrual periods). If both ovaries are removed during an operation before natural menopause takes place, the sudden drop in estrogen levels results in what is known as "surgically induced menopause".

When the estrogen levels begin dropping, some women develop very uncomfortable symptoms, such as feelings of warmth in the face, neck, and chest, or sudden intense episodes of heat and sweating ("hot flashes" or "hot flushes"). Using estrogen drugs can help the body adjust to lower estrogen levels and reduce these symptoms. ESTRING (estradiol vaginal ring) DOES NOT PROVIDE ENOUGH ESTROGEN TO REDUCE THESE SYMPTOMS.

The declining estrogen levels associated with advancing age after menopause may also result in thinning and drying of the tissue in the urinary tract and vagina (urogenital atrophy). Vaginal symptoms of this condition include dryness in the vagina (atrophic vaginitis), genital itching and burning, and pain with intercourse. Urinary symptoms may include urinary urgency and pain on urination. Small amounts of estrogen delivered directly to the local tissue can be used to help reduce these symptoms.

USE OF ESTRING (estradiol vaginal ring)

ESTRING is a local estrogen therapy designed to relieve vaginal and urinary symptoms of postmenopausal estrogen deficiency for a full 90 days. ESTRING exerts its effect locally in the lower urogenital tract and has not been shown to have significant effects in other estrogen-sensitive organs or tissues of the body. Consequently, ESTRING PROVIDES RELIEF OF LOCAL SYMPTOMS OF MENOPAUSE ONLY.

DESCRIPTION

ESTRING (estradiol vaginal ring) contains a drug reservoir of 2 mg of the estrogen, estradiol, in its core. ESTRING releases estradiol into the vagina in a consistent, stable manner for 90 days. The soft, flexible ring is placed in the upper third of the vagina (by the physician or the patient) and worn continuously for 90 days, then removed and replaced if continuation of therapy is indicated.

WHO SHOULD NOT USE ESTRING (estradiol vaginal ring)

ESTRING should not be used:

During pregnancy (see **BOXED WARNING**).

Women who are definitely postmenopausal cannot become pregnant. Women who believe they are postmenopausal because their menstrual cycles have recently stopped should confirm that they are not pregnant before using any form of estrogen-containing drug. Using estrogens while pregnant may cause the unborn child to have birth defects. Estrogens do not prevent miscarriage.

In the presence of unusual vaginal bleeding which has not been evaluated by a doctor (see **BOXED WARNING**).

Unusual vaginal bleeding after menopause can be a warning sign of cancer of the uterus. Estrogens may increase the risk of cancer of the uterus in women who have had their menopause ("change of life"). If you use any estrogen-containing drug, it is important to visit your doctor regularly and report any unusual vaginal bleeding right away. Your doctor should evaluate any unusual vaginal bleeding to find out the cause.

If there is a history of certain types of cancer.

Estrogens may increase the risk of certain types of cancer. In general, ESTRING should not be used in women who have ever had cancer of the breast or uterus.

During treatment for vaginal infection with vaginal antimicrobial therapy.

It is recommended that ESTRING be discontinued while other vaginal medications are being used to treat a vaginal infection. Use of ESTRING can be resumed after termination of the other vaginal medication, and after first consulting with a physician.

After childbirth or when breast-feeding a baby.

ESTRING should not be used to try to stop the breasts from filling with milk after a baby is born. Women who are breast-feeding should avoid using any drugs because many drugs pass through to the baby in the milk. While nursing a baby, drugs should only be taken on the advice of your healthcare giver.

POSSIBLE RISKS FROM TREATMENT WITH ESTROGENS

The following risk factors apply to estrogens in general:

Cancer of the uterus.

Estrogens increase the risk of developing a condition (endometrial hyperplasia) that may lead to cancer of the lining of the uterus (endometrial cancer). The risk of endometrial cancer is greater in estrogen users than nonusers. Studies have shown that this increased risk depends on estrogen dose, duration of treatment, and treatment regimen.

If the uterus has been removed (total hysterectomy), there is no danger of developing cancer of the uterus.

Cancer of the breast.

Most studies have not shown a higher risk of breast cancer in women who have ever used estrogens. However, some studies have reported that breast cancer developed more often (up to twice the usual rate) in women who used estrogens for long periods of time (especially more than 10 years), or who used higher doses for shorter time periods. Regular breast examinations by a health professional and monthly self-examination are recommended for all women.

Gallbladder disease and abnormal blood clotting.

Gallbladder disease and abnormal blood clotting are risk factors associated with medium to high doses of estrogen. Most studies of low dose estrogen usage by women do not show an increased risk of these complications, and to date have not been seen with ESTRING (estradiol vaginal ring) treatment.

SIDE EFFECTS

Like all medications, ESTRING (estradiol vaginal ring) may cause side effects. The most frequently reported side effect is increased vaginal secretions. Many of these vaginal secretions are like those that occur normally prior to menopause and indicate that ESTRING is working. Vaginal secretions that are associated with a bad odor, vaginal itching, or other signs of vaginal infection are NOT normal and may indicate a risk or a cause for concern. Other side effects may include vaginal discomfort, abdominal pain, or genital itching.

Estrogens in General

In addition to the risks listed above, the following side effects have been reported with estrogen use:

— Nausea and vomiting.

— Breast tenderness or enlargement.

— Enlargement of benign tumors ("fibroids") of the uterus.

— Retention of excess fluid. This may worsen some conditions, such as asthma, epilepsy, migraine, heart disease, or kidney disease.

— Spotty darkening of the skin, particularly on the face.

REDUCING RISK OF ESTROGEN USE

If you use estrogens, you may reduce your risks by doing these things:

See your doctor regularly.

While you are using estrogens, it is important to visit your doctor at least once a year for a check-up. If you develop vaginal bleeding while taking estrogens, call your doctor - you may need further evaluation. If members of your family have had breast cancer or if you have ever had breast lumps or an abnormal mammogram (breast X-ray), you may need to have more frequent breast examinations.

Reassess your need for estrogens.

You and your doctor should reevaluate whether or not you still need estrogens at least every 6 months.

Be alert for warning signs.

If any of these warning signals (or any other unusual symptoms) happen while you are using estrogens, call your doctor immediately:

— Abnormal bleeding from the vagina (possible uterine cancer).

— Pains in the calves or chest, sudden shortness of breath, or coughing blood (possible clot in the legs, heart, or lungs).

— Severe headache or vomiting, dizziness, faintness, changes in vision or speech, weakness or numbness of an arm or leg (possible clot in the brain or eye).

— Breast lumps (possible breast cancer; ask your doctor or health professional to show you how to examine your breasts monthly).

— Yellowing of skin or eyes (possible liver problem).

— Pain, swelling, or tenderness in the abdomen (possible gallbladder problem).

OTHER INFORMATION

1. Estrogens increase the risk of developing a condition (endometrial hyperplasia) that may lead to cancer of the lining of the uterus. Progestin, another hormone drug, is usually prescribed with higher-dose estrogen preparations to lower the risk of developing endometrial hyperplasia. Progestins are not usually needed for women using ESTRING (estradiol vaginal ring) alone.
2. Some women have experienced moving or sliding of ESTRING within the vagina. If this happens, ESTRING can be gently pushed back into position with a clean finger. Instances of ESTRING slipping out of the vagina have been infrequent and were usually associated with moving the bowels, straining, or constipation within the first few weeks of treatment. If this occurs, ESTRING can be washed with lukewarm (NOT hot) water and reinserted. If this happens repeatedly, you should consult with your doctor or healthcare giver and determine whether continued treatment is appropriate for you.
3. ESTRING may not be suitable for women with narrow, short, or stenosed (constricted) vaginas. A narrow vagina, vaginal stenosis (constriction), significant prolapse, and vaginal infections are conditions that make the vagina more susceptible to irritation or ulceration caused by ESTRING. Women with signs or symptoms of vaginal irritation should alert their doctor or healthcare giver.
4. Vaginal infection is generally more common in postmenopausal women. Vaginal infections should be treated with appropriate antimicrobial therapy before initiation of ESTRING. If a vaginal infection develops during use of ESTRING, then ESTRING should be removed and reinserted only after the infection has been appropriately treated. See your doctor or healthcare giver if you have vaginal discomfort or suspect you have a vaginal infection.
5. Your doctor has prescribed this drug for you and you alone. Do not give the drug to anyone else.
6. Keep this and all drugs out of the reach of children.
7. This leaflet provides a summary of important information about ESTRING. If you want more information, ask your doctor or pharmacist to show you the professional labeling. The professional labeling is also published in a book called the "Physicians' Desk Reference®," which is available in book stores and public libraries. Generic drugs carry virtually the same labeling information as their brand name versions.

HOW SUPPLIED

Each ESTRING (estradiol vaginal ring) is individually packaged in a heat-sealed rectangular pouch. The pouch is provided with a tear-off notch on one side.

NDC 0013-2150-36 ESTRING (estradiol vaginal ring) 2 mg available in single units.

Storage: Store at controlled room temperature 15° to 30° C (59° to 86°F).

℞ only

A Patient Guide to ESTRING
(estradiol vaginal ring) 2 mg
Insertion and Removal

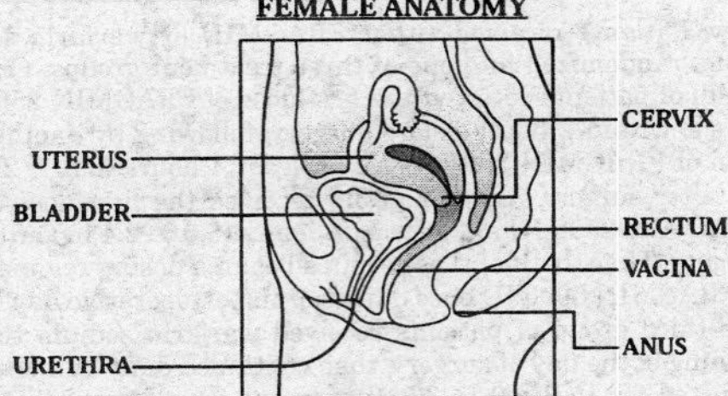

ESTRING INSERTION

ESTRING can be inserted and removed by you or your doctor. To insert ESTRING yourself, choose the position that is most comfortable for you: standing with one leg up, squatting, or lying down.

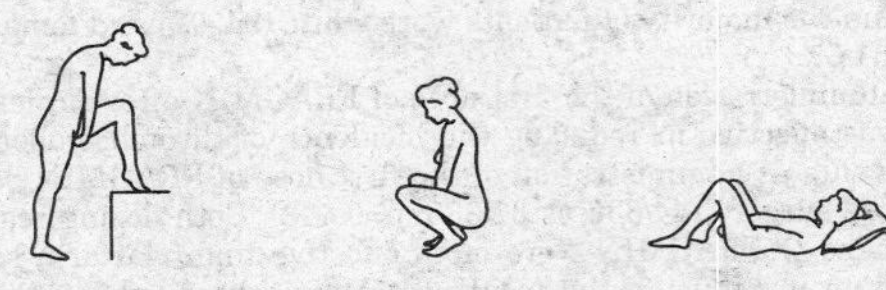

FRAGMIN® ℞
[frăg-mĭn]
dalteparin sodium injection
For *Subcutaneous* Use Only

SPINAL/EPIDURAL HEMATOMAS

When neuraxial anesthesia (epidural/spinal anesthesia) or spinal puncture is employed, patients anticoagulated or scheduled to be anticoagulated with low molecular weight heparins or heparinoids for prevention of thromboembolic complications are at risk of developing an epidural or spinal hematoma which can result in long-term or permanent paralysis.

The risk of these events is increased by the use of indwelling epidural catheters for administration of analgesia or by the concomitant use of drugs affecting hemostasis such as non steroidal anti-inflammatory drugs (NSAIDSs), platelet inhibitors, or other anticoagulants. The risk also appears to be increased by traumatic or repeated epidural or spinal puncture.

Patients should be frequently monitored for signs and symptoms of neurological impairment. If neurological compromise is noted, urgent treatment is necessary.

The physician should consider the potential benefit versus risk before neuraxial intervention in patients anticoagulated or to be anticoagulated for thromboprophylaxis (also see WARNINGS, Hemorrhage and PRECAUTIONS, Drug Interactions).

DESCRIPTION

FRAGMIN Injection (dalteparin sodium injection) is a sterile, low molecular weight heparin. It is available in single-dose, prefilled syringes and a multiple-dose vial. With reference to the W.H.O. First International Low Molecular Weight Heparin Reference Standard, each syringe contains 2500 (16 mg dalteparin sodium) or 5000 (32 mg dalteparin sodium) anti-Factor Xa international units (IU) in 0.2 mL. Each 9.5 mL vial contains 10,000 (64 mg dalteparin sodium) anti-Factor Xa IU per 1 mL, for a total of 95,000 anti-Factor Xa IU per vial.

Each prefilled syringe also contains Water for Injection and sodium chloride, when required, to maintain physiologic ionic strength. The prefilled syringes are preservative free. Each multiple-dose also contains Water for Injection and 14 mg of benzyl alcohol per mL as a preservative. The pH of both formulations is 5.0 to 7.5.

Dalteparin sodium is produced through controlled nitrous acid depolymerization of sodium heparin from porcine intestinal mucosa followed by a chromatographic purification process. It is composed of strongly acidic sulphated polysaccharide chains (oligosaccharide, containing 2,5-anhydro-D-mannitol residues as end groups) with an average molecular weight of 5000 and about 90% of the material within the range 2000–9000. The molecular weight distribution is:

Continued on next page

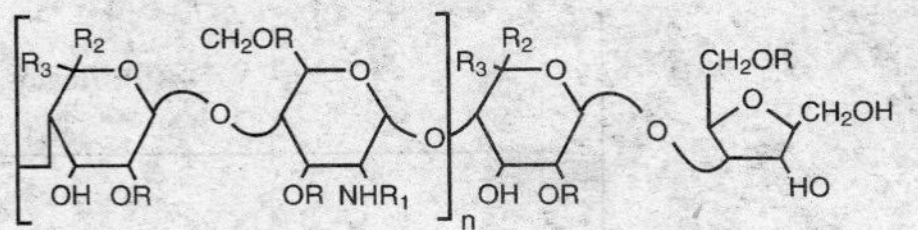

R = H or SO_3Na
R_1 = $COCH_3$ or SO_3Na
R_2 = H R_3 = COONa
R_2 = COONa R_3 = H
n = 3-20

Table 1
Efficacy of FRAGMIN in the Prophylaxis of Ischemic Complications in Unstable Angina and Non-Q-Wave Myocardial Infarction

Indication	Dosing Regimen	
	FRAGMIN 120 IU/kg/12 hr s.c.	Placebo q 12 hr s.c.
All treated Unstable Angina and Non-Q-wave MI Patients	746	760
Primary Endpoints—6 day timepoint Death, MI	13/741 (1.8%)[1]	36/757 (4.8%)
Secondary Endpoints—6 day timepoint Death, MI, i.v. heparin, i.v. nitroglycerin Revascularization	59/739 (8.0%)[1]	106/756 (14.0%)

[1] p-value = 0.001

Table 2
Efficacy of FRAGMIN in the Prophylaxis of Deep Vein Thrombosis Following Hip Replacement Surgery

Indication	Dosing Regimen	
	FRAGMIN 5000 IU qd[1] s.c.	Warfarin Sodium qd[2] oral
All Treated Hip Replacement Surgery Patients	271	279
Treatment Failures in Evaluable Patients DVT, Total	28/192 (14.6%)[3]	49/190 (25.8%)
Proximal DVT	10/192 (5.2%)[4]	16/190 (8.4%)
PE	2/271 (0.7%)	2/279 (0.7%)

[1] The daily dose on the day of surgery was divided: 2500 IU was given two hours before surgery and again in the evening of the day of surgery.
[2] Warfarin sodium dosage was adjusted to maintain a prothrombin time index of 1.4 to 1.5, corresponding to an International Normalized Ratio (INR) of approximately 2.5.
[3] p-value = 0.006
[4] p-value = 0.185

Table 3
Efficacy of FRAGMIN in the Prophylaxis of Deep Vein Thrombosis Following Abdominal Surgery

Indication	Dosing Regimen	
	FRAGMIN 2500 IU qd s.c.	Placebo qd s.c.
All Treated Abdominal Surgery Patients	102	102
Treatment Failures in Evaluable Patients Total Thromboembolic Events	4/91 (4.4%)[1]	16/91 (17.6%)
Proximal DVT	0	5/91 (5.5%)
Distal DVT	4/91 (4.4%)	11/91 (12.1%)
PE	0	2/91 (2.2%)[2]

[1] p-value = 0.008
[2] Both patients also had DVT, 1 proximal and 1 distal

Information on these Pharmacia & Upjohn products is based on labeling in effect June 1, 2000. Further information concerning these and other Pharmacia & Upjohn products may be obtained by direct inquiry to Medical Information, Pharmacia & Upjohn, Kalamazoo, MI 49001.

Fragmin—Cont.

< 3000 daltons	3.0–15.0%
3000 to 8000 daltons	65.0–78.0%
> 8000 daltons	14.0–26.0%

Structural Formula

[See chemical structure at top of previous page]

CLINICAL PHARMACOLOGY

Dalteparin is a low molecular weight heparin with antithrombotic properties. It acts by enhancing the inhibition of Factor Xa and thrombin by antithrombin. In man, dalteparin potentiates preferentially the inhibition of coagulation Factor Xa, while only slightly affecting clotting time, e.g., activated partial thromboplastin time (APTT).

Pharmacodynamics:
Doses of FRAGMIN Injection of up to 10,000 anti-Factor Xa IU administered subcutaneously as a single dose or two 5000 IU doses 12 hours apart to healthy subjects do not produce a significant change in platelet aggregation, fibrinolysis, or global clotting tests such as prothrombin time (PT), thrombin time (TT) or APTT. Subcutaneous (s.c.) administration of doses of 5000 IU bid of FRAGMIN for seven consecutive days to patients undergoing abdominal surgery did not markedly affect APTT, Platelet Factor 4 (PF4), or lipoprotein lipase.

Pharmacokinetics:
Mean peak levels of plasma anti-Factor Xa activity following single s.c. doses of 2500, 5000 and 10,000 IU were 0.19 ± 0.04, 0.41 ± 0.07 and 0.82 ± 0.10 IU/mL, respectively, and were attained in about 4 hours in most subjects. Absolute bioavailability in healthy volunteers, measured as the anti-Factor Xa activity, was 87 ± 6%. Increasing the dose from 2500 to 10,000 IU resulted in an overall increase in anti-Factor Xa AUC that was greater than proportional by about one-third.
Peak anti-Factor Xa activity increased more or less linearly with dose over the same dose range. There appeared to be no appreciable accumulation of anti-Factor Xa activity with twice-daily dosing of 100 IU/kg s.c. for up to 7 days.
The volume of distribution for dalteparin anti-Factor Xa activity was 40 to 60 mL/kg. The mean plasma clearances of dalteparin anti-Factor Xa activity in normal volunteers following single intravenous bolus doses of 30 and 120 anti-Factor Xa IU/kg were 24.6 ± 5.4 and 15.6 ± 2.4 mL/hr/kg, respectively. The corresponding mean disposition half-lives are 1.47 ± 0.3 and 2.5 ± 0.3 hours.
Following intravenous doses of 40 and 60 IU/kg, mean terminal half-lives were 2.1 ± 0.3 and 2.3 ± 0.4 hours, respectively. Longer apparent terminal half-lives (3 to 5 hours) are observed following s.c. dosing, possibly due to delayed absorption. In patients with chronic renal insufficiency requiring hemodialysis, the mean terminal half-life of anti-Factor Xa activity following a single intravenous dose of 5000 IU FRAGMIN was 5.7 ± 2.0 hours, i.e. considerably longer than values observed in healthy volunteers, therefore, greater accumulation can be expected in these patients.

CLINICAL TRIALS

Prophylaxis of Ischemic Complications in Unstable Angina and Non-Q-Wave Myocardial Infarction:
In a double-blind, randomized, placebo-controlled clinical trial, patients who recently experienced unstable angina with EKG changes or non-Q-wave myocardial infarction (MI) were randomized to FRAGMIN Injection 120 IU/kg every 12 hours subcutaneously (s.c.) or placebo every 12 hours s.c. In this trial, unstable angina was defined to include only angina with EKG changes. All patients, except when contraindicated, were treated concurrently with aspirin (75 mg once daily) and beta blockers. Treatment was initiated within 72 hours of the event (the majority of patients received treatment within 24 hours) and continued for 5 to 8 days. A total of 1506 patients were enrolled and treated; 746 received FRAGMIN and 760 received placebo. The mean age of the study population was 68 years (range 40 to 90 years) and the majority of patients were white (99.7%) and male (63.9%). The combined incidence of the double endpoint of death or myocardial infarction was lower for FRAGMIN compared with placebo at 6 days after initiation of therapy. These results were observed in an analysis of all-randomized and all-treated patients. The combined incidence of death, MI, need for intravenous (i.v.) heparin or i.v. nitroglycerin, and revascularization was also lower for FRAGMIN than for placebo (see Table 1).

[See table 1 at top of previous page]

In a second randomized, controlled trial designed to evaluate long-term treatment with FRAGMIN (days 6 to 45), data were also collected comparing 1-week (5 to 8 days) treatment of FRAGMIN 120 IU/kg every 12 hours s.c. with heparin at an APTT-adjusted dosage. All patients, except when contraindicated, were treated concurrently with aspirin (100 to 165 mg per day). Of the total enrolled study population of 1499 patients, 1482 patients were treated; 751 received FRAGMIN and 731 received heparin. The mean age of the study population was 64 years (range 25 to 92 years) and the majority of patients were white (96.0%) and male (64.2%). The incidence of the combined triple endpoint of death, myocardial infarction, or recurrent angina during this 1-week treatment period (5 to 8 days) was 9.3% for FRAGMIN and 7.6% for heparin (p=0.323).

Prophylaxis of Deep Vein Thrombosis in Patients Following Hip Replacement Surgery:
In an open-label randomized study, FRAGMIN 5000 IU administered once daily s.c. was compared with warfarin sodium, administered orally, in patients undergoing hip replacement surgery. Treatment with FRAGMIN was initiated with a 2500 IU dose s.c. within 2 hours before surgery, followed by a 2500 IU dose s.c. the evening of the day of surgery. Then, a dosing regimen of FRAGMIN 5000 IU s.c. once daily was initiated on the first postoperative day. The first dose of warfarin sodium was given the evening before surgery, then continued daily at a dose adjusted for INR 2.0 to 3.0. Treatment in both groups was then continued for 5 to 9 days postoperatively. Of the total enrolled study population of 580 patients, 553 were treated and 550 underwent surgery. Of those who underwent surgery, 271 received FRAGMIN and 279 received warfarin sodium. The mean age of the study population was 63 years (range 20 to 92 years) and the majority of patients were white (91.1%) and female (52.9%). The incidence of deep vein thrombosis (DVT), any vein, as determined by evaluable venography, was significantly lower for the group treated with FRAGMIN compared with patients treated with warfarin sodium (28/192 vs 49/190; p=0.006) [see Table 2].

[See table 2 at top of previous page]

In a second single-center, double-blind study of patients undergoing hip replacement surgery, FRAGMIN 5000 IU once daily s.c. starting the evening before surgery, was compared with heparin 5000 U s.c. tid, starting the morning of surgery. Treatment in both groups was continued for up to 9 days postoperatively. Of the total enrolled study population of 140 patients, 139 were treated and 136 underwent surgery. Of those who underwent surgery, 67 received FRAGMIN and 69 received heparin. The mean age of the study population was 69 years (range 42 to 87 years) and the majority of patients were female (58.8%). In the intent-to-treat analysis, the incidence of proximal DVT was significantly lower for patients treated with FRAGMIN compared with patients treated with heparin (6/67 vs 18/69; p=0.012). Further, the incidence of pulmonary embolism detected by lung scan was also significantly lower in the group treated with FRAGMIN (9/67 vs 19/69; p=0.032).
A third multi-center, double-blind, randomized study evaluated a postoperative dosing regimen of FRAGMIN for thromboprophylaxis following total hip replacement surgery. Patients received either FRAGMIN or warfarin sodium, randomized into one of three treatment groups. One group of patients received the first dose of FRAGMIN 2500 IU s.c. within 2 hours before surgery, following by another dose of FRAGMIN 2500 IU s.c. at least 4 hours (6.6 ± 2.3 hr) after surgery. Another group received the first dose of FRAGMIN 2500 IU s.c. at least 4 hours (6.6 ± 2.4 hr) after surgery. Then, both of these groups began a dosing regimen of FRAGMIN 5000 IU once daily s.c. on postoperative day 1. The third group of patients received warfarin sodium the evening of the day of surgery, then continued daily at a dose adjusted for INR 2.0 to 3.0. Treatment for all groups was continued for 4 to 8 days postoperatively, after which time all patients underwent bilateral venography.
In the total enrolled study population of 1501 patients, 1472 patients were treated; 496 received FRAGMIN (first dose before surgery), 487 received FRAGMIN (first dose after surgery) and 489 received warfarin sodium. The mean age of the study population was 63 years (range 18 to 91 years) and the majority of patients were white (94.4%) and female (51.8%).
Administration of the first dose of FRAGMIN after surgery was effective in reducing the incidence of thromboembolic events as administration of the first dose of FRAGMIN before surgery (44/336 vs 37/338; p=0.448). Both dosing regimens of FRAGMIN were more effective than warfarin sodium in reducing the incidence of thromboembolic events following hip replacement surgery.

Prophylaxis of Deep Vein Thrombosis Following Abdominal Surgery in Patients at Risk for Thromboemoblic Complications:
Abdominal surgery patients at risk include those who are over 40 years of age, obese, undergoing surgery under general anesthesia lasting longer than 30 minutes, or who have additional risk factors such as malignancy or a history of deep vein thrombosis or pulmonary embolism.
FRAGMIN administered once daily s.c. beginning prior to surgery and continuing for 5 to 10 days after surgery, was shown to reduce the risk of DVT in patients at risk for thromboembolic complications in two double-blind, randomized, controlled clinical trials performed in patients under-

Table 4
Efficacy of FRAGMIN in the Prophylaxis of Deep Vein Thrombosis Following Abdominal Surgery

Indication	Dosing Regimen	
	FRAGMIN 2500 IU qd s.c.	Heparin 5000 U bid s.c.
All Treated Abdominal Surgery Patients	195	196
Treatment Failures in Evaluable Patients Total Thromboembolic Events	7/178 (3.9%)[1]	7/174 (4.0%)
Proximal DVT	3/178 (1.7%)	4/174 (2.3%)
Distal DVT	3/178 (1.7%)	3/174 (1.7%)
PE	1/178 (0.6%)	0

[1] p-value = 0.74

Table 5
Efficacy of FRAGMIN in Abdominal Surgery Patients with Malignancy

Indication	Dosing Regimen	
	FRAGMIN 2500 IU qd s.c.	FRAGMIN 5000 IU qd s.c.
All Treated Abdominal Surgery Patients[1]	696	679
Treatment Failures in Evaluable Patients Total Thromboembolic Events	99/ 656 (15.1%)[2]	60/645 (9.3%)
Proximal DVT	18/657 (2.7%)	14/646 (2.2%)
Distal DVT	80/657 (12.2%)	41/646 (6.3%)
PE		
Fatal	1/674 (0.1%)	1/669 (0.1%)
Non-fatal	2	4

[1] Major abdominal surgery with malignancy
[2] p-value = 0.001

Table 6
Major Bleeding Events in Unstable Angina and Non-Q-Wave Myocardial Infarction

Indication	Dosing Regimen		
Unstable Angina and Non-Q-wave MI	FRAGMIN 120 IU/kg/12 hr s.c.[1]	Heparin i.v. and s.c.[2]	Placebo q 12 hr s.c.
Major Bleeding Events[3,4]	15/1497 (1.0%)	7/731 (1.0%)	4/760 (0.5%)

[1] Treatment was administered for 5 to 8 days.
[2] Heparin i.v. infusion for at least 48 hours, APPT 1.5 to 2 times control, then 12,500 U s.c. every 12 hours for 5 to 8 days.
[3] Aspirin (75 to 165 mg per day) and beta blocker therapies were administered concurrently.
[4] Bleeding events were considered major if: 1) accompanied by a decrease in hemoglobin of ≥2 g/dL in connection with clinical symptoms; 2) a transfusion was required; 3) bleeding led to interruption of treatment or death; or 4) intracranial bleeding.

going major abdominal surgery. In the first study, a total of 204 patients were enrolled and treated; 102 received FRAGMIN and 102 received placebo. The mean age of the study population was 64 years (range 40 to 98 years) and the majority of patients were female (54.9%). In the second study, a total of 391 patients were enrolled and treated: 195 received FRAGMIN and 196 received heparin. The mean age of the study population was 59 years (range 30 to 88 years) and the majority of patients were female (51.9%). As summarized in the following tables, FRAGMIN 2500 IU was superior to placebo and similar to heparin in reducing the risk of DVT (see Tables 3 and 4).

[See table 3 at top of page 2613]
[See table 4 at top of previous page]

In a third double-blind, randomized study performed in patients undergoing major abdominal surgery with malignancy, FRAGMIN 5000 IU once daily was compared with FRAGMIN 2500 IU once daily. Treatment was continued for 6 to 8 days. A total of 1375 patients were enrolled and treated; 679 received FRAGMIN 5000 IU and 696 received 2500 IU. The mean age of the combined groups was 71 years (range 40 to 95 years). The majority of patients were female (51.0%). The study showed that FRAGMIN 5000 IU once daily was more effective than FRAGMIN 2500 IU once daily in reducing the risk of DVT in patients undergoing abdominal surgery with malignancy (see Table 5).

[See table 5 at top of previous page]

INDICATIONS AND USAGE

FRAGMIN Injection is indicated for the prophylaxis of ischemic complications in unstable angina and non-Q-wave myocardial infarction, when concurrently administered with aspirin therapy (as described in CLINICAL TRIALS, Prophylaxis of Ischemic Complications in Unstable Angina and Non-Q-Wave Myocardial Infarction).

FRAGMIN is also indicated for the prophylaxis of deep vein thrombosis (DVT), which may lead to pulmonary embolism (PE):

- In patients undergoing hip replacement surgery:
- In patients undergoing abdominal surgery who are at risk for thromboembolic complications.

CONTRAINDICATIONS

FRAGMIN Injection is contraindicated in patients with known hypersensitivity to the drug, active major bleeding, or thrombocytopenia associated with positive ***in vitro*** tests for anti-platelet antibody in the presence of FRAGMIN.

Patients undergoing regional anesthesia should not receive FRAGMIN for unstable angina or non-Q-wave myocardial infarction due to an increased risk of bleeding associated with the dosage of FRAGMIN recommended for unstable anginal and non-Q-wave myocardial infarction.

Patients with known hypersensitivity to heparin or pork products should not be treated with FRAGMIN.

WARNINGS

FRAGMIN Injection is not intended for intramuscular administration.

FRAGMIN cannot be used interchangeably (unit for unit) with unfractionated heparin or other low molecular weight heparins.

FRAGMIN should be used with extreme caution in patients with history of heparin-induced thrombocytopenia.

Hemorrhage:

FRAGMIN, like other anticoagulants, should be used with extreme caution in patients who have an increased risk of hemorrhage, such as those with severe uncontrolled hypertension, bacterial endocarditis, congenital or acquired bleeding disorders, active ulceration and angiodysplastic gastrointestinal disease, hemorrhagic stroke, or shortly after brain, spinal or ophthalmological surgery.

Spinal or epidural hematomas can occur with the associated use of low molecular weight heparins or heparinoids and neuraxial (spinal/epidural) anesthesia or spinal puncture, which can result in long-term or permanent paralysis. The risk of these events is higher with the use of indwelling epidural catheters or concomitant use of additional drugs affecting hemostasis such as NSAIDs (see boxed WARNING and ADVERSE REACTIONS, Ongoing Safety Surveillance).

As with other anticoagulants, bleeding can occur at any site during therapy with FRAGMIN. An unexpected drop in hematocrit or blood pressure should lead to a search for a bleeding site.

Thrombocytopenia:

In clinical trials, thrombocytopenia with platelet counts of $<100{,}000/mm^3$ and $<50{,}000/mm^3$ occurred in <1% and <1%, respectively. In clinical practice, rare cases of thrombocytopenia with thrombosis have also been observed.

Thrombocytopenia of any degree should be monitored closely. Heparin-induced thrombocytopenia can occur with the administration of FRAGMIN. The incidence of this complication is unknown at present.

Miscellaneous:

The multiple-dose vial of FRAGMIN contains benzyl alcohol as a preservative. Benzyl alcohol has been reported to be associated with a fatal "Gasping Syndrome" in premature infants. Because benzyl alcohol may cross the placenta, FRAGMIN preserved with benzyl alcohol should not be used in pregnant women (see PRECAUTIONS, Pregnancy Category B., Nonteratogenic Effects).

PRECAUTIONS

General:

FRAGMIN Injection should not be mixed with other injections or infusions unless specific compatibility data are available that support such mixing.

Table 7
Bleeding Events Following Hip Replacement Surgery

Indication	FRAGMIN vs Warfarin Sodium		FRAGMIN vs Heparin	
	Dosing Regimen		Dosing Regimen	
Hip Replacement Surgery	FRAGMIN 5000 IU qd s.c. (n=274[2])	Warfarin Sodium[1] oral (n=279)	FRAGMIN 5000 IU qd s.c. (n=69[4])	Heparin 5000 U tid s.c. (n=69)
Major Bleeding Events[3]	7/274 (2.6%)	1/279 (0.4%)	0	3/69 (4.3%)
Other Bleeding Events[5] Hematuria	8/274 (2.9%)	5/279 (1.8%)	0	0
Wound Hematoma	6/274 (2.2%)	0	0	0
Injection Site Hematoma	3/274 (1.1%)	NA	2/69 (2.9%)	7/69 (10.1%)

[1] Warfarin sodium dosage was adjusted to maintain a prothrombin time index of 1.4 to 1.5, corresponding to an International Normalized Ratio (INR) of approximately 2.5.
[2] Includes three treated patients who did not undergo a surgical procedure.
[3] A bleeding event was considered major if: 1) hemorrhage caused a significant clinical event, 2) it was associated with a hemoglobin decrease of ≥2 g/dL or transfusion of 2 or more units of blood products, 3) it resulted in reoperation due to bleeding, or 4) it involved retroperitoneal or intracranial hemorrhage.
[4] Includes two treated patients who did not undergo a surgical procedure.
[5] Occurred at a rate of at least 2% in the group treated with FRAGMIN 5000 IU once daily.

Table 8
Bleeding Events Following Abdominal Surgery

Indication	FRAGMIN vs Heparin				FRAGMIN vs Placebo		FRAGMIN vs FRAGMIN	
	Dosing Regimen				Dosing Regimen		Dosing Regimen	
Abdominal Surgery	FRAGMIN 2500 IU qd s.c.	Heparin 5000 U bid s.c.	FRAGMIN 5000 IU qd s.c.	Heparin 5000 U bid s.c.	FRAGMIN 2500 IU qd s.c.	Placebo qd s.c.	FRAGMIN 2500 IU qd s.c.	FRAGMIN 5000 IU qd s.c.
Postoperative Transfusions	26/459 (5.7%)	36/454 (7.9%)	81/508 (15.9%)	63/498 (12.7%)	14/182 (7.7%)	13/182 (7.1%)	89/1025 (8.7%)	125/1033 (12.1%)
Wound Hematoma	16/467 (3.4%)	18/467 (3.9%)	12/508 (2.4%)	6/498 (1.2%)	2/79 (2.5%)	2/77 (2.6%)	1/1030 (0.1%)	4/1039 (0.4%)
Reoperation Due to Bleeding	2/392 (0.5%)	3/392 (0.8%)	4/508 (0.8%)	2/498 (0.4%)	1/79 (1.3%)	1/78 (1.3%)	2/1030 (0.2%)	13/1038 (1.3%)
Injection Site Hematoma	1/466 (0.2%)	5/464 (1.1%)	36/506 (7.1%)	47/493 (9.5%)	8/172 (4.7%)	2/174 (1.1%)	36/1026 (3.5%)	57/1035 (5.5%)

Table 9
Volume of FRAGMIN to be Administered by Patient Weight

Patient weight (lb)	<110	110 to 131	132 to 153	154 to 175	176 to 197	≥198
Patient weight (kg)	<50	50 to 59	60 to 69	70 to 79	80 to 89	≥90
Volume of FRAGMIN (mL)[1]	0.55	0.65	0.75	0.90	1.00	1.00

[1] Calculated volume based on the 9.5 mL multiple-dose vial (10,000 anti-Factor Xa IU/mL)

FRAGMIN should be used with caution in patients with bleeding diathesis, thrombocytopenia or platelet defects; severe liver or kidney insufficiency, hypertensive or diabetic retinopathy, and recent gastrointestinal bleeding.

If a thromboembolic events should occur despite dalteparin prophylaxis, FRAGMIN should be discontinued and appropriate therapy initiated.

Drug Interactions:

FRAGMIN should be used with care in patients receiving oral anticoagulants, platelet inhibitors, and thrombolytic agents because of increased risk of bleeding (see PRECAUTIONS, Laboratory Tests). Aspirin, unless contraindicated, is recommended in patients treated for unstable angina or non-Q-wave myocardial infarction (see DOSAGE AND ADMINISTRATION).

Laboratory Tests:

Periodic routine complete blood counts, including platelet count, and stool occult blood tests are recommended during the course of treatment with FRAGMIN. No special monitoring of blood clotting times (e.g., APTT) is needed.

When administered at recommended prophylaxis doses, routine coagulation tests such as Prothrombin Time (PT) and Activated Partial Thromboplastin Time (APTT) are relatively insensitive measure of FRAGMIN activity and, therefore, unsuitable for monitoring.

Drug/Laboratory Test Interactions:

Elevations of Serum Transaminases:

Asymptomatic increases in transaminase levels (SGOT/AST and SGPT/ALT) greater than three times the upper limit of normal of the laboratory reference range have been reported in 1.7 and 4.3%, respectively, of patients during treatment with FRAGMIN. Similar significant increases in transaminase levels have also been observed in patients treated with heparin and other low molecular weight heparins. Such elevations are fully reversible and are rarely associated with increases in bilirubin. Since transaminase determinations are important in the differential diagnosis of myocardial infarction, liver disease and pulmonary emboli, elevations that might be caused by drugs like FRAGMIN should be interpreted with caution.

Carcinogenicity, Mutagenesis, Impairment of Fertility:

Dalteparin sodium has not been tested for its carcinogenic potential in long-term animal studies. It was not mutagenic in the ***in vitro*** Ames Test, mouse lymphoma cell forward mutation test and human lymphocyte chromosomal aberration test and in the ***in vivo*** mouse micronucleus test. Dalteparin sodium at subcutaneous doses up to 1200 IU/kg (7080 IU/m^2) did not affect the fertility or reproductive performance of male and female rats.

Pregnancy: Pregnancy Category B.

Teratogenic Effects:

Reproduction studies with dalteparin sodium at intravenous doses up to 2400 IU/kg (14,160 IU/m^2) in pregnant rats and 4800 IU/kg (40,800 IU/m^2) in pregnant rabbits did not produce any evidence of impaired fertility or harm to the fetuses. There are, however, no adequate and well-con-

Continued on next page

Information on these Pharmacia & Upjohn products is based on labeling in effect June 1, 2000. Further information concerning these and other Pharmacia & Upjohn products may be obtained by direct inquiry to Medical Information, Pharmacia & Upjohn, Kalamazoo, MI 49001.

Fragmin—Cont.

trolled studies in pregnant women. Because animal reproduction studies are not always predictive of human response, this drug should be used during pregnancy only if clearly needed.

Nonteratogenic Effects:

Cases of "Gasping Syndrome" have occurred when large amounts of benzyl alcohol have been administered (99–404 mg/kg/day). The 9.5 mL multiple-dose vials of FRAGMIN contains 14 mg/mL of benzyl alcohol.

Nursing Mothers:

It is not known whether dalteparin sodium is excreted in human milk. Because many drugs are excreted in human milk, caution should be exercised when FRAGMIN is administered to a nursing mother.

Pediatric Use:

Safety and effectiveness in pediatric patients have not been established.

ADVERSE REACTIONS

Hemorrhage:

The incidence of hemorrhagic complications during treatment with FRAGMIN Injection has been low. The most commonly reported side effect is hematoma at the injection site. The incidence of bleeding may increase with higher doses; however, in abdominal surgery patients with malignancy, no significant increase in bleeding was observed when comparing FRAGMIN 5000 IU to either FRAGMIN 2500 IU or low dose heparin.

In a trial comparing FRAGMIN 5000 IU once daily to FRAGMIN 2500 IU once daily in patients undergoing surgery for malignancy, the incidence of bleeding events was 4.6% and 3.6%, respectively (n.s.). In a trial comparing FRAGMIN 5000 IU once daily to heparin 5000 U twice daily, the incidence of bleeding events was 3.2% and 2.7%, respectively (n.s.) in the malignancy subgroup.

Unstable Angina and Non-Q-Wave Myocardial Infarction:

Table 6 summarizes major bleeding events that occurred with FRAGMIN, heparin, and placebo in clinical trials of unstable angina and non-Q-wave myocardial infarction.

[See table 6 at top of page 2614]

Hip Replacement Surgery:

Table 7 summarizes: 1) all major bleeding events and, 2) other bleeding events possibly or probably related to treatment with FRAGMIN (preoperative dosing regimen), warfarin sodium, or heparin in two hip replacement surgery clinical trials.

[See table 7 at top of previous page]

Six of the patients treated with FRAGMIN experienced seven major bleeding events. Two of the events were wound hematoma (one requiring reoperation), three were bleeding from the operative site, one was intraoperative bleeding due to vessel damage, and one was gastrointestinal bleeding. None of the patients experienced retroperitoneal or intracranial hemorrhage nor died of bleeding complications.

In the third hip replacement surgery clinical trial, the incidence of major bleeding events was similar in all three treatment groups: 3.6% (18/496) for patients who started FRAGMIN before surgery; 2.5% (12/487) for patients who started FRAGMIN after surgery; and 3.1% (45/489) for patients treated with warfarin sodium.

Abdominal Surgery:

Table 8 summarizes bleeding events that occurred in clinical trials which studied FRAGMIN 2500 and 5000 IU administered once daily to abdominal surgery patients.

[See table 8 at top of previous page]

Thrombocytopenia: See WARNINGS: Thrombocytopenia.

Other:

Allergic Reactions:

Allergic reactions (i.e., pruritus, rash, fever, injection site reaction, bulleous eruption) and skin necrosis have occurred rarely. A few cases of anaphylactoid reactions have been reported.

Local Reactions:

Pain at the injection site, the only non-bleeding event determined to be possibly or probably related to treatment with FRAGMIN and reported at a rate of at least 2% in the group treated with FRAGMIN, was reported in 4.5% of patients treated with FRAGMIN 5000 IU qd vs 11.8% of patients treated with heparin 5000 U bid in the abdominal surgery trials. In the hip replacement trials, pain at injection site was reported in 12% of patients treated with FRAGMIN 5000 IU qd vs 13% of patients treated with heparin 5000 U tid.

Ongoing Safety Surveillance:

Since first international market introduction in 1985, there have been six reports of epidural or spinal hematoma formation with concurrent use of dalteparin sodium and spinal/epidural anesthesia or spinal puncture. Five of the six patients had post-operative indwelling epidural catheters placed for analgesia or received additional drugs affecting hemostasis. The hematomas caused long-term or permanent paralysis (partial or complete) in four of these cases. The sixth patient experienced temporary paraplegia but made a full recovery. Because these events were reported voluntarily from a population of unknown size, estimates of frequency cannot be made.

OVERDOSAGE

Symptoms/Treatment:

An excessive dosage of FRAGMIN Injection may lead to hemorrhagic complications. These may generally be stopped by the slow intravenous injection of protamine sulfate (1% solution), at a dose of 1 mg protamine for every 100 anti-Xa IU of FRAGMIN given. A second infusion of 0.5 mg protamine sulfate per 100 anti-Xa IU of FRAGMIN may be administered if the APTT measured 2 to 4 hours after the first infusion remains prolonged. Even with these additional doses of protamine, the APTT may remain more prolonged than would usually be found following administration of conventional heparin. In all cases, the anti-Factor Xa activity is never completely neutralized (maximum about 60 to 75%).

Particular care should be taken to avoid overdosage with protamine sulfate. Administration of protamine sulfate can cause severe hypotensive and anaphylactoid reactions. Because fatal reactions, often resembling anaphylaxis, have been reported with protamine sulfate, it should be given only when resuscitation techniques and treatment of anaphylactic shock are readily available. For additional information, consult the labeling of Protamine Sulfate Injection, USP, products. A single subcutaneous dose of 100,000 IU/kg of FRAGMIN to mice caused a mortality of 8% (1/12) whereas 50,000 IU/kg was a non-lethal dose. The observed sign was hematoma at the site of injection.

DOSAGE AND ADMINISTRATION

Unstable Angina and Non-Q-Wave Myocardial Infarction:

In patients with unstable angina or non-Q-wave myocardial infarction, the recommended dose of FRAGMIN Injection is 120 IU/kg of body weight, but not more than 10,000 IU, subcutaneously (s.c.) every 12 hours with concurrent oral aspirin (75 to 165 mg once daily) therapy. Treatment should be continued until the patient is clinically stabilized. The usual duration of administration is 5 to 8 days. Concurrent aspirin therapy is recommended except when contraindicated. Table 9 lists the volume of FRAGMIN to be administered for a range of patient weights.

[See table 9 at top of previous page]

Hip Replacement Surgery:

Table 10 presents the dosing options for patients undergoing hip replacement surgery. The usual duration of administration is 5 to 10 days after surgery; up to 14 days of treatment with FRAGMIN have been well tolerated in clinical trials.

[See table 10 below]

Abdominal Surgery:

In patients undergoing abdominal surgery with a risk of thromboembolic complications, the recommended dose of FRAGMIN is 2500 IU administered by s.c. injection once daily, starting 1 to 2 hours prior to surgery and repeated once daily postoperatively. The usual duration of administration is 5 to 10 days.

In patients undergoing abdominal surgery associated with a high risk of thromboembolic complications, such as malignant disorder, the recommended dose of FRAGMIN is 5000 IU s.c. the evening before surgery, then once daily postoperatively. The usual duration of administration is 5 to 10 days. Alternatively, in patients with malignancy, 2500 IU of FRAGMIN can be administered s.c. 1 to 2 hours before surgery followed by 2500 IU s.c. 12 hours later, and then 5000 IU once daily postoperatively. The usual duration of administration is 5 to 10 days.

Dosage adjustment and routine monitoring of coagulation parameters are not required if the dosage and administration recommendations specified above are followed.

Administration:

FRAGMIN is administered by subcutaneous injection. It must not be administered by intramuscular injection.

Subcutaneous injection technique: Patients should be sitting or lying down and FRAGMIN administered by deep s.c. injection. FRAGMIN may be injected in a U-shape area around the navel, the upper outer side of the thigh or the upper outer quadrangle of the buttock. The injection site should be varied daily. When the area around the navel or the thigh is used, using the thumb and forefinger, you **must** lift up a fold of skin while giving the injection. The entire length of the needle should be inserted at a 45 to 90 degree angle.

Parenteral drug products should be inspected visually for particulate matter and discoloration prior to administration, whenever solution and container permit.

Table 10
Dosing Options for Patients Undergoing Hip Replacement Surgery

Timing of First Dose of FRAGMIN	Dose of FRAGMIN to be Given Subcutaneously: 10 to 14 Hours Before Surgery	Within 2 Hours Before Surgery	4 to 8 Hours After Surgery[1]	Postoperative Period[2]
Postoperative Start	—	—	2500 IU[3]	5000 IU qd
Preoperative Start - Day of Surgery	—	2500 IU	2500 IU[3]	5000 IU qd
Preoperative Start - Evening Before Surgery[4]	5000 IU	—	5000 IU	5000 IU qd

[1] Or later, if hemostasis has not been achieved.
[2] Up to 14 days of treatment was well tolerated in controlled clinical trials, where the usual duration of treatment was 5 to 10 days postoperatively.
[3] Allow a minimum of 6 hours between this dose and the dose to be given on Postoperative Day 1. Adjust the timing of the dose on Postoperative Day 1 accordingly.
[4] Allow approximately 24 hours between doses.

HOW SUPPLIED

FRAGMIN Injection is available in the following strengths and package sizes:

0.2 mL single-dose prefilled syringe, affixed with a 27-gauge × 1/2 inch needle.

Package of 10:

2500 anti-Factor Xa IU	NDC 0013-2406-91
5000 anti-Factor Xa IU	NDC 0013-2426-91
9.5 mL multiple-dose vial:	
10,000 anti-Factor Xa IU/mL (95,000 anti-Factor Xa IU/vial)	NDC 0013-2436-06

Store at controlled room temperature 20° to 25°C (68° to 77°F) [see USP].

℞ only

U.S. Patent 4,303,651

Manufactured for: Pharmacia & Upjohn Company
Kalamazoo, MI 49001, USA
by: Vetter Pharma-Fertigung
Ravensburg, Germany
(prefilled syringes)
Pharmacia & Upjohn N.V./S.A.
Puurs, Belgium
(multiple-dose vial)

KV0404-09
818 312 001 Revised August 2000

GENOTROPIN® ℞

[gen-ō″ trō-pin]

somatropin [rDNA origin] for injection

In a Two-Chamber Cartridge

DESCRIPTION

GENOTROPIN Lyophilized Powder contains somatropin [rDNA origin], which is a polypeptide hormone of recombinant DNA origin. It has 191 amino acid residues and a molecular weight of 22,124 daltons. The amino acid sequence of the product is identical to that of human growth hormone of pituitary origin (somatropin). GENOTROPIN is synthesized in a strain of ***Escherichia coli*** that has been modified by the addition of the gene for human growth hormone. GENOTROPIN is a sterile white lyophilized powder intended for subcutaneous injection.

GENOTROPIN 1.5 mg is dispensed in a two-chamber cartridge. The front chamber contains recombinant somatropin 1.5 mg (approximately 4.5 IU), glycine 27.6 mg, sodium dihydrogen phosphate anhydrous 0.3 mg, and disodium phosphate anhydrous 0.3 mg; the rear chamber contains 1.13 mL water for injection.

GENOTROPIN 5.8 mg is dispensed in a two-chamber cartridge. The front chamber contains recombinant somatropin 5.8 mg (approximately 17.4 IU), glycine 2.2 mg, mannitol 1.8 mg, sodium dihydrogen phosphate anhydrous 0.32 mg, and disodium phosphate anhydrous 0.31 mg; the rear chamber contains 0.3% m-Cresol (as a preservative) and mannitol 45 mg in 1.14 mL water for injection.

GENOTROPIN 13.8 mg is dispensed in a two-chamber cartridge. The front chamber contains recombinant somatropin 13.8 mg (approximately 41.4 IU), glycine 2.3 mg, mannitol 14.0 mg, sodium dihydrogen phosphate anhydrous 0.47 mg, and disodium phosphate anhydrous 0.46 mg; the rear chamber contains 0.3% m-Cresol (as a preservative) and mannitol 32 mg in 1.13 mL water for injection.

GENOTROPIN MINIQUICK® is dispensed as a single-use syringe device containing a two-chamber cartridge. GENOTROPIN MINIQUICK is available as individual doses of 0.2 mg to 2.0 mg in 0.2-mg increments. The front chamber contains recombinant somatropin 0.22 to 2.2 mg (approximately 0.66 to 6.6 IU), glycine 0.23 mg, mannitol 1.14 mg, sodium dihydrogen phosphate 0.05 mg, and disodium phosphate anhydrous 0.027 mg; the rear chamber contains mannitol 12.6 mg in water for injection 0.275 mL.

GENOTROPIN is a highly purified preparation. The reconstituted recombinant somatropin solution has an osmolality of approximately 300 mOsm/kg, and a pH of approximately

6.7. The concentration of the reconstituted solution varies by strength and presentation (see HOW SUPPLIED section).

CLINICAL PHARMACOLOGY

In vitro, preclinical, and clinical tests have demonstrated that GENOTROPIN Lyophilized Powder is therapeutically equivalent to human growth hormone of pituitary origin and achieves similar pharmacokinetic profiles in normal adults. In pediatric patients who have growth hormone deficiency (GHD) or Prader-Willi syndrome (PWS), treatment with GENOTROPIN stimulates linear growth and normalizes concentrations of IGF-I (Insulin-like Growth Factor/Somatomedin-C). In adults with GHD, treatment with GENOTROPIN results in reduced fat mass, increased lean body mass, metabolic alterations that include beneficial changes in lipid metabolism, and normalization of IGF-I concentrations.

In addition, the following actions have been demonstrated for GENOTROPIN and/or somatropin.

1. Tissue Growth

A. ***Skeletal Growth:*** GENOTROPIN stimulates skeletal growth in pediatric patients with GHD or PWS. The measurable increase in body length after administration of GENOTROPIN results from an effect on the epiphyseal plates of long bones. Concentrations of IGF-I, which may play a role in skeletal growth, are generally low in the serum of pediatric patients with GHD or PWS, but tend to increase during treatment with GENOTROPIN. Elevations in mean serum alkaline phosphatase concentration are also seen.

B. ***Cell Growth:*** It has been shown that there are fewer skeletal muscle cells in short-statured pediatric patients who lack endogenous growth hormone as compared with the normal pediatric population. Treatment with somatropin results in an increase in both the number and size of muscle cells.

2. Protein Metabolism

Linear growth is facilitated in part by increased cellular protein synthesis. Nitrogen retention, as demonstrated by decreased urinary nitrogen excretion and serum urea nitrogen, follows the initiation of therapy with GENOTROPIN.

3. Carbohydrate Metabolism

Pediatric patients with hypopituitarism sometimes experience fasting hypoglycemia that is improved by treatment with GENOTROPIN. Large doses of growth hormone may impair glucose tolerance.

4. Lipid Metabolism

In GHD patients, administration of somatropin has resulted in lipid mobilization, reduction in body fat stores, and increased plasma fatty acids.

5. Mineral Metabolism

Somatropin induces retention of sodium, potassium, and phosphorus. Serum concentrations of inorganic phosphate are increased in patients with GHD after therapy with GENOTROPIN. Serum calcium is not significantly altered by GENOTROPIN. Growth hormone could increase calciuria.

6. Body Composition

Adult GHD patients treated with GENOTROPIN at the recommended adult dose (see DOSAGE AND ADMINISTRATION) demonstrate a decrease in fat mass and an increase in lean body mass. When these alterations are coupled with the increase in total body water, the overall effect of GENOTROPIN is to modify body composition, an effect that is maintained with continued treatment.

PHARMACOKINETICS

Absorption

Following a 0.03 mg/kg subcutaneous (SC) injection in the thigh of 1.3 mg/mL GENOTROPIN to adult GHD patients, approximately 80% of the dose was systemically available as compared with that available following intravenous dosing. Results were comparable in both male and female patients. Similar bioavailability has been observed in healthy adult male subjects.

In healthy adult males, following an SC injection in the thigh of 0.03 mg/kg, the extent of absorption (AUC) of a concentration of 5.3 mg/mL GENOTROPIN was 35% greater than that for 1.3 mg/mL GENOTROPIN. The mean (± standard deviation) peak (C_{max}) serum levels were 23.0 (± 9.4) ng/mL and 17.4 (± 9.2) ng/mL, respectively.

In a similar study involving pediatric GHD patients, 5.3 mg/mL GENOTROPIN yielded a mean AUC that was 17% greater than that for 1.3 mg/mL GENOTROPIN. The mean C_{max} levels were 21.0 ng/mL and 16.3 ng/mL, respectively.

Adult GHD patients received two single SC doses of 0.03 mg/kg of GENOTROPIN at a concentration of 1.3 mg/mL, with a one- to four-week washout period between injections. Mean C_{max} levels were 12.4 ng/mL (first injection) and 12.2 ng/mL (second injection), achieved at approximately six hours after dosing.

There are no data on the bioequivalence between the 12 mg/mL formulation and either the 1.3 mg/mL or the 5.3 mg/mL formulations.

Distribution

The mean volume of distribution of GENOTROPIN following administration to GHD adults was estimated to be 1.3 (± 0.8) L/kg.

Metabolism

The metabolic fate of GENOTROPIN involves classical protein catabolism in both the liver and kidneys. In renal cells, at least a portion of the breakdown products are returned to the systemic circulation. The mean terminal half-life of intravenous GENOTROPIN in normal adults is 0.4 hours, whereas subcutaneously administered GENOTROPIN has a half-life of 3.0 hours in GHD adults. The observed difference is due to slow absorption from the subcutaneous injection site.

Table 1
Mean SC Pharmacokinetic Parameters in Adult GHD Patients

	Bioavailability (%) (N=15)	T_{max} (hours) (N=16)	CL/F (L/hr × kg) (N=16)	Vss/F (L/kg) (N=16)	$T_{½}$ (hours) (N=16)
Mean (± SD)	80.5 *	5.9 (± 1.65)	0.3 (± 0.11)	1.3 (± 0.80)	3.0 (± 1.44)
95% Cl	70.5 – 92.1	5.0 – 6.7	0.2 – 0.4	0.9 – 1.8	2.2 – 3.7

T_{max} = time of maximum plasma concentration
CL/F = plasma clearance
Vss/F = volume of distribution
$T_{½}$ = terminal half-life
SD = standard deviation
Cl = confidence interval

* The absolute bioavailability was estimated under the assumption that the log-transformed data follow a normal distribution. The mean and standard deviation of the log-transformed data were mean = 0.22 (± 0.241).

Excretion

The mean clearance of subcutaneously administered GENOTROPIN in 16 GHD adult patients was 0.3 (± 0.11) L/hrs/kg.

Special Populations

Pediatric: The pharmacokinetics of GENOTROPIN are similar in GHD pediatric and adult patients.

Gender: No gender studies have been performed in pediatric patients; however, GHD adults, the absolute bioavailability of GENOTROPIN was similar in males and females.

Race: No studies have been conducted with GENOTROPIN to assess pharmacokinetic differences among races.

Renal or hepatic insufficiency: No studies have been conducted with GENOTROPIN in these patient populations.

[See table 1 above]

CLINICAL STUDIES

Adult Patients with Growth Hormone Deficiency (GHD)

GENOTROPIN Lyophilized Powder was compared with placebo in six randomized clinical trials involving a total of 172 adult GHD patients. These trials included a 6-month double-blind treatment period, during which 85 patients received GENOTROPIN and 87 patients received placebo, followed by an open-label treatment period in which participating patients received GENOTROPIN for up to a total of 24 months. GENOTROPIN was administered as a daily SC injection at a dose of 0.04 mg/kg week for the first month of treatment and 0.08 mg/kg/week for subsequent months.

Beneficial changes in body composition were observed at the end of the 6-month treatment period for the patients receiving GENOTROPIN as compared with the placebo patients. Lean body mass, total body water, and lean/fat ratio increased while total body fat mass and waist circumference decreased. These effects on body composition were maintained when treatment was continued beyond 6 months. Bone mineral density declined after 6 months of treatment but returned to baseline values after 12 months of treatment.

Pediatric Patients with Prader-Willi Syndrome (PWS)

The safety and efficacy of GENOTROPIN in the treatment of pediatric patients with Prader-Willi syndrome (PWS) were evaluated in two randomized, open-label, controlled clinical trials. Patients received either GENOTROPIN or no treatment for the first year of the studies, while all patients received GENOTROPIN during the second year. GENOTROPIN was administered as a daily SC injection, and the dose was calculated for each patient every 3 months. In Study 1, the treatment group received GENOTROPIN at a dose of 0.24 mg/kg/week during the entire study. During the second year, the control group received GENOTROPIN at a dose of 0.48 mg/kg/week. In Study 2, the treatment group received GENOTROPIN at a dose of 0.36 mg/kg/week during the entire study. During the second year, the control group received GENOTROPIN at a dose of 0.36 mg/kg/week.

Patients who received GENOTROPIN showed significant increases in linear growth during the first year of study, compared with patients who received no treatment (see Table 2). Linear growth continued to increase in the second year, when both groups received treatment with GENOTROPIN.

[See table 2 above]

Table 2
Efficacy of GENOTROPIN in Pediatric Patients with Prader-Willi Syndrome (Mean ± SD)

	Study 1		Study 2	
	GENOTROPIN (0.24 mg/kg/week) n=15	Untreated Control n=12	GENOTROPIN (0.36 mg/kg/week) n=7	Untreated Control n=9
Linear growth (cm) Baseline height	112.7 ± 14.9	109.5 ± 12.0	120.3 ± 17.5	120.5 ± 11.2
Growth from months 0 to 12	11.6* ± 2.3	5.0 ± 1.2	10.7* ± 2.3	4.3 ± 1.5
Height Standard Deviation Score (SDS) for age Baseline SDS	−1.6 ± 1.3	−1.8 ± 1.5	−2.6 ± 1.7	−2.1 ± 1.4
SDS at 12 months	−0.5† ± 1.3	−1.9 ± 1.4	−1.4† ± 1.5	−2.2 ± 1.4

* $p \le 0.001$
† $p \le 0.002$ (when comparing SDS change at 12 months)

Changes in body composition were also observed in the patients receiving GENOTROPIN (see Table 3). These changes included a decrease in the amount of fat mass, and increases in the amount of lean body mass and the ratio of lean-to-fat tissue, while changes in body weight were similar to those seen in patients who received no treatment. Treatment with GENOTROPIN did not accelerate bone age, compared with patients who received no treatment.

[See table 3 at top of next page]

INDICATIONS AND USAGE

GENOTROPIN Lyophilized Powder is indicated for:

- Long-term treatment of pediatric patients who have growth failure due to an inadequate secretion of endogenous growth hormone.
- Long-term treatment of pediatric patients who have growth failure due to Prader-Willi syndrome (PWS). The diagnosis of PWS should be confirmed by appropriate genetic testing.
  Other causes of short stature in pediatric patients should be excluded.
- Long-term replacement therapy in adults with growth hormone deficiency (GHD) of either childhood- or adult-onset etiology. GHD should be confirmed by an appropriate growth hormone stimulation test.

CONTRAINDICATIONS

GENOTROPIN Lyophilized Powder should not be used when there is any evidence of neoplastic activity. Intracranial lesions must be inactive and antitumor therapy complete prior to the institution of therapy. GENOTROPIN should be discontinued if there is evidence of tumor growth. Growth hormone should not be used for growth promotion in pediatric patients with fused epiphyses.

Growth hormone should not be initiated to treat patients with acute critical illness due to complications following open heart or abdominal surgery, multiple accidental trauma, or to patients having acute respiratory failure. Two placebo-controlled clinical trials in non-growth hormone deficient adult patients (n=522) with these conditions revealed a significant increase in mortality (41.9% vs 19.3%) among somatropin treated patients (doses 5.3 to 8 mg/day) compared to those receiving placebo (see WARNINGS).

WARNINGS

The 5.8 mg and 13.8 mg presentations of GENOTROPIN Lyophilized Powder contain m-Cresol as a preservative. These products should not be used by patients with a known

Continued on next page

Information on these Pharmacia & Upjohn products is based on labeling in effect June 1, 2000. Further information concerning these and other Pharmacia & Upjohn products may be obtained by direct inquiry to Medical Information, Pharmacia & Upjohn, Kalamazoo, MI 49001.

Genotropin—Cont.

sensitivity to this preservative. The GENOTROPIN 1.5 mg and GENOTROPIN MINIQUICK presentations are preservative-free. (See HOW SUPPLIED section.)

See CONTRAINDICATIONS for information on increased mortality in patients with acute critical illnesses in intensive care units due to complications following open heart or abdominal surgery, multiple accidental trauma, or with acute repiratory failure. The safety of continuing growth hormone treatment in patients receiving replacement doses for approved indications who concurrently develop these illnesses has not been established. Therefore, the potential benefit of treatment continuation with growth hormone in patients having acute critical illnesses should be weighed against the potential risk.

PRECAUTIONS

General

Treatment with GENOTROPIN Lyophilized Powder, as with other growth hormone preparations, should be directed by physicians who are experienced in the diagnosis and management of patients with GHD or Prader-Willi syndrome (PWS).

Patients and caregivers who will administer GENOTROPIN in medically unsupervised situations should receive appropriate training and instruction on the proper use of GENOTROPIN from the physician or other suitably qualified health professional.

Patients with GHD secondary to an intracranial lesion should be examined frequently for progression or recurrence of the underlying disease process. Review of literature reports of pediatric use of somatropin replacement therapy reveals no relationship between this therapy and recurrence of central nervous system (CNS) tumors. In adults, it is unknown whether there is any relationship between somatropin treatment and CNS tumor recurrence.

Patients should be monitored carefully for any malignant transformation of skin lesions.

Caution should be used if growth hormone is administered to patients with diabetes mellitus, and insulin dosage may need to be adjusted. Because growth hormone may induce a state of insulin resistance, patients should be observed for evidence of glucose intolerance. Patients with diabetes or glucose intolerance should be monitored closely during treatment with GENOTROPIN. Patients with risk factors for glucose intolerance, such as obesity (including obese patients with PWS) or a family history of Type II diabetes, should be monitored closely as well.

In patients with hypopituitarism (multiple hormonal deficiencies) standard hormonal replacement therapy should be monitored closely when treatment with GENOTROPIN is instituted. Hypothyroidism may develop during treatment with GENOTROPIN, and inadequate treatment of hypothyroidism may prevent optimal response to GENOTROPIN. Therefore, patients should have periodic thyroid function tests and be treated with thyroid hormone when indicated.

Pediatric patients with endocrine disorders, including GHD, have a higher incidence of slipped capital femoral epiphyses. Any pediatric patient with the onset of a limp or complaints of hip or knee pain during growth hormone therapy should be evaluated.

Progression of scoliosis can occur in patients who experience rapid growth. Because growth hormone increases growth rate, patients with a history of scoliosis who are treated with growth hormone should be monitored for progression of scoliosis. However, growth hormone has not been shown to increase the incidence of scoliosis. Scoliosis is commonly seen in untreated patients with PWS. Physicians should be alert to this abnormality, which may manifest during growth hormone therapy.

Intracranial hypertension (IH) with papilledema, visual changes, headache, nausea and/or vomiting has been reported in a small number of patients treated with growth hormone products. Symptoms usually occurred within the first 8 weeks of the initiation of growth hormone therapy. In all reported cases, IH-associated signs and symptoms resolved after termination of therapy or a reduction of the growth hormone dose. Funduscopic examination of patients is recommended at the initiation, and periodically during the course of, growth hormone therapy. Patients with PWS may be at increased risk for development of IH.

Before continuing treatment as an adult, a post-pubertal GHD patient who received growth hormone replacement therapy in childhood should be reevaluated with proper testing as described in INDICATIONS AND USAGE. If continued treatment is appropriate, GENOTROPIN should be administered at the reduced dose level recommended for adult GHD patients.

Drug Interactions

Concomitant glucocorticoid treatment may inhibit the growth-promoting effect of growth hormone. Pediatric GHD patients with coexisting ACTH deficiency should have their glucocorticoid replacement dose carefully adjusted to avoid an inhibitory effect on growth. See also PRECAUTIONS—General. Limited published data indicate that growth hormone treatment increases cytochrome P450 (CP450) mediated antipyrine clearance in man. These data suggest that growth hormone administration may alter the clearance of compounds known to be metabolized by CP450 liver enzymes (e.g., corticosteroids, sex steroids, anticonvulsants,

Table 3
Effect of GENOTROPIN on Body Composition
In Pediatric Patients with Prader-Willi Syndrome (Mean ± SD)

	GENOTROPIN n=14	Untreated Control n=10
Fat mass (kg)		
Baseline	12.3 ± 6.8	9.4 ± 4.9
Change from months 0 to 12	−0.9* ± 2.2	2.3 ± 2.4
Lean body mass (kg)		
Baseline	15.6 ± 5.7	14.3 ± 4.0
Change from months 0 to 12	4.7* ± 1.9	0.7 ± 2.4
Lean body mass/Fat mass		
Baseline	1.4 ± 0.4	1.8 ± 0.8
Change from months 0 to 12	1.0* ± 1.4	−0.1 ± 0.6
Body weight (kg)†		
Baseline	27.2 ± 12.0	23.2 ± 7.0
Change from months 0 to 12	3.7‡ ± 2.0	3.5 ± 1.9

* $p < 0.005$
† n=15 for the group receiving GENOTROPIN; n=12 for the Control group
‡ n.s.

Table 4
Adverse Events Reported by ≥ 5% of 1,145 Adult GHD Patients During Clinical Trials of GENOTROPIN and Placebo, Grouped by Duration of Treatment

Adverse Event	Double Blind Phase: Placebo 0–6 mo. n=572 % Patients	Double Blind Phase: GENOTROPIN 0–6 mo. n=573 % Patients	Open Label Phase GENOTROPIN: 6–12 mo. n=504 % Patients	Open Label Phase GENOTROPIN: 12–18 mo. n=63 % Patients	Open Label Phase GENOTROPIN: 18–24 mo. n=60 % Patients
Swelling, peripheral	5.1	17.5*	5.6	0	1.7
Arthralgia	4.2	17.3*	6.9	6.3	3.3
Upper respiratory infection	14.5	15.5	13.1	15.9	13.3
Pain, extremities	5.9	14.7*	6.7	1.6	3.3
Edema, peripheral	2.6	10.8*	3.0	0	0
Paresthesia	1.9	9.6*	2.2	3.2	0
Headache	7.7	9.9	6.2	0	0
Stiffness of extremities	1.6	7.9*	2.4	1.6	0
Fatigue	3.8	5.8	4.6	6.3	1.7
Myalgia	1.6	4.9*	2.0	4.8	6.7
Back pain	4.4	2.8	3.4	4.8	5.0

* increased significantly when compared to placebo, $P \leq .025$: Fisher's Exact Test (one-sided)
n = number of patients receiving treatment during the indicated period.
% = percentage of patients who reported the event during the indicated period.

cyclosporine). Careful monitoring is advisable when growth hormone is administered in combination with other drugs known to be metabolized by CP450 liver enzymes.

Carcinogenesis, Mutagenesis, Impairment of Fertility

Carcinogenicity studies have not been conducted with rhGH. No potential mutagenicity of rhGH was revealed in a battery of tests including induction of gene mutations in bacteria (the Ames test), gene mutations in mammalian cells grown in vitro (mouse L5178Y cells), and chromosomal damage in intact animals (bone marrow cells in rats). See PREGNANCY section for effect on fertility.

Pregnancy: Pregnancy Category B

Reproduction studies carried out with GENOTROPIN at doses of 0.3, 1, and 3.3 mg/kg/day administered SC in the rat and 0.08, 0.3, and 1.3 mg/kg/day administered intramuscularly in the rabbit (highest doses approximately 24 times and 19 times the recommended human therapeutic levels, respectively, based on body surface area) resulted in decreased maternal body weight gains but were not teratogenic. In rats receiving SC doses during gametogenesis and up to 7 days of pregnancy, 3.3 mg/kg/day (approximately 24 times human dose) produced anestrus or extended estrus cycles in females and fewer and less motile sperm in males. When given to pregnant female rats (days 1 to 7 of gestation) at 3.3 mg/kg/day a very slight increase in fetal deaths was observed. At 1 mg/kg/day (approximately seven times human dose) rats showed slightly extended estrus cycles, whereas at 0.3 mg/kg/day no effects were noted.

In perinatal and postnatal studies in rats, GENOTROPIN doses of 0.3, 1, and 3.3 mg/kg/day produced growth-promoting effects in the dams but not in the fetuses. Young rats at the highest dose showed increased weight gain during suckling but the effect was not apparent by 10 weeks of age. No adverse effects were observed on gestation, morphogenesis, parturition, lactation, postnatal development, or reproductive capacity of the offsprings due to GENOTROPIN. There are, however, no adequate and well-controlled studies in pregnant women. Because animal reproduction studies are not always predictive of human response, this drug should be used during pregnancy only if clearly needed.

Nursing Mothers

There have been no studies conducted with GENOTROPIN in nursing mothers. It is not known whether this drug is excreted in human milk. Because many drugs are excreted in human milk, caution should be exercised when GENOTROPIN is administered to a nursing woman.

ADVERSE REACTIONS

As with all protein drugs, a small number of patients may develop antibodies to the protein. Growth hormone antibody with binding lower than 2 mg/L has not been associated with growth attenuation. In some cases when binding capacity is > 2 mg/L, interference with growth response has been observed.

In 419 pediatric patients evaluated in clinical studies with GENOTROPIN Lyophilized Powder, 244 had been treated previously with GENOTROPIN or other growth hormone preparations and 175 had received no previous growth hormone therapy. Antibodies to growth hormone (anti-hGH antibodies) were present in six previously treated patients at baseline. Three of the six became negative for anti-hGH antibodies during 6 to 12 months of treatment with GENOTROPIN. Of the remaining 413 patients, eight (1.9%) developed detectable anti-hGH antibodies during treatment with GENOTROPIN; none had an antibody binding capacity > 2 mg/L. There was no evidence that the growth response to GENOTROPIN was affected in these antibody-positive patients.

Preparations of GENOTROPIN contain a small amount of periplasmic ***Escherichia coli*** peptides (PECP). Anti-PECP antibodies are found in a small number of patients treated with GENOTROPIN, but these appear to be of no clinical significance.

In clinical studies with GENOTROPIN in pediatric GHD patients, the following events were reported infrequently: injection site reactions, including pain or burning associated with the injection, fibrosis, nodules, rash, inflammation, pigmentation, or bleeding; lipoatrophy; headache; hematuria; hypothyroidism; and mild hyperglycemia.

Leukemia has been reported in a small number of pediatric patients who have been treated with growth hormone, including growth hormone of pituitary origin and recombinant somatropin. The relationship, if any, between leukemia and growth hormone therapy is uncertain.

In two clinical studies with GENOTROPIN in pediatric patients with Prader-Willi syndrome, the following drug-re-

0.2 mg	NDC 0013-2649-02	1.2 mg	NDC 0013-2654-02
0.4 mg	NDC 0013-2650-02	1.4 mg	NDC 0013-2655-02
0.6 mg	NDC 0013-2651-02	1.6 mg	NDC 0013-2656-02
0.8 mg	NDC 0013-2652-02	1.8 mg	NDC 0013-2657-02
1.0 mg	NDC 0013-2653-02	2.0 mg	NDC 0013-2658-02

lated events were reported: edema, aggressiveness, arthralgia, benign intracranial hypertension, hair loss, headache, and myalgia.

In clinical trials with GENOTROPIN in 1,145 GHD adults, the majority of the adverse events consisted of mild to moderate symptoms of fluid retention, including peripheral swelling, arthralgia, pain and stiffness of the extremities, peripheral edema, myalgia, paresthesia, and hypoesthesia. These events were reported early during therapy, and tended to be transient and/or responsive to dosage reduction.

Table 4 displays the adverse events reported by 5% or more of adult GHD patients in clinical trials after various durations of treatment with GENOTROPIN. Also presented are the corresponding incidence rates of these adverse events in placebo patients during the 6-month double-blind portion of the clinical trials.

[See table 4 at top of previous page]

In expanded post-trial extension studies, diabetes mellitus developed in 12 of 3,031 patients (0.4%) during treatment with GENOTROPIN. All 12 patients had predisposing factors, e.g., elevated glycated hemoglobin levels and/or marked obesity, prior to receiving GENOTROPIN. Of the 3,031 patients receiving GENOTROPIN, 61 (2%) developed symptoms of carpal tunnel syndrome, which lessened after dosage reduction or treatment interruption (52) or surgery (9). Other adverse events that have been reported include generalized edema and hypoesthesia.

OVERDOSAGE

There is little information on acute or chronic overdosage with GENOTROPIN Lyophilized Powder. Intravenously administered growth hormone has been shown to result in an acute decrease in plasma glucose. Subsequently, hyperglycemia was seen. It is thought that the same effect might occur on rare occasions with a high dosage of GENOTROPIN administered SC. Long-term overdosage may result in signs and symptoms of acromegaly consistent with overproduction of growth hormone.

DOSAGE AND ADMINISTRATION

The dosage of GENOTROPIN Lyophilized Powder must be adjusted for the individual patient. The weekly dose should be divided into 6 or 7 **subcutaneous** injections. GENOTROPIN may be given in the thigh, buttocks, or abdomen; the site of SC injections should be rotated daily to help prevent lipoatrophy.

Pediatric GHD Patients: Generally, a dose of 0.16 to 0.24 mg/kg body weight/week is recommended.

Pediatric PWS Patients: Generally, a dose of 0.24 mg/kg body weight/week is recommended.

Adult GHD Patients: The recommended dosage at the start of therapy is not more than 0.04 mg/kg/week. The dose may be increased at 4- to 8-week intervals according to individual patient requirements to a maximum of 0.08 mg/kg/week, depending upon patient tolerance of treatment. Clinical response, side effects, and determination of age-adjusted serum IGF-I may be used as guidance in dose titration. This approach will tend to result in weight-adjusted doses that are larger for women compared with men and smaller for older and obese patients.

GENOTROPIN must not be injected intravenously.

GENOTROPIN is supplied in a two-chamber cartridge, with the lyophilized powder in the front chamber and a diluent in the rear chamber. A reconstitution device is used to mix the diluent and powder.

Follow the directions for reconstitution provided with each device. **Do not shake**; shaking may cause denaturation of the active ingredient.

All parenteral drug products should be inspected visually for particulate matter and discoloration prior to administration, whenever solution and container permit. If the solution is cloudy, the contents **MUST NOT** be injected.

Patients and caregivers who will administer GENOTROPIN in medically unsupervised situations should receive appropriate training and instruction on the proper use of GENOTROPIN from the physician or other suitably qualified health professional.

STABILITY AND STORAGE

Except as noted below, store GENOTROPIN Lyophilized Powder under refrigeration at 2° to 8°C (36° to 46°F). Do not freeze. Protect from light.

The 1.5 mg cartridge of GENOTROPIN contains a diluent with no preservative. After reconstitution, the cartridge may be stored under refrigeration for up to 24 hours. Use once only and discard any remaining solution.

The 5.8 mg and 13.8 mg cartridges of GENOTROPIN contain a diluent with a preservative. Thus, after reconstitution, they may be stored under refrigeration for up to 21 days.

The GENOTROPIN MINIQUICK Growth Hormone Delivery Device should be refrigerated prior to dispensing, but may be stored at or below 25°C (77°F) for up to three months after dispensing. The diluent has no preservative. After reconstitution, the GENOTROPIN MINIQUICK may be stored under refrigeration for up to 24 hours before use. The GENOTROPIN MINIQUICK should be used only once and then discarded.

HOW SUPPLIED

GENOTROPIN Lyophilized Powder is available in the following packages:

1.5 mg two-chamber cartridge (without preservative)

concentration of 1.3 mg/mL (approximately 4 IU/mL)

Preassembled in a GENOTROPIN INTRA-MIX™ Growth Hormone Reconstitution Device and packaged with a pressure release needle

Package of 5 NDC 0013-2606-94

5.8 mg two-chamber cartridge (with preservative)

concentration of 5 mg/mL (approximately 15 IU/mL)

For use with the GENOTROPIN PEN® 5 Growth Hormone Delivery Device and/or the GENOTROPIN MIXER™ Growth Hormone Reconstitution Device

Package of 5 NDC 0013-2626-94
Package of 1 NDC 0013-2626-81

Preassembled in a GENOTROPIN INTRA-MIX Growth Hormone Reconstitution Device and packaged with a pressure release needle

Package of 5 NDC 0013-2616-94
Package of 1 NDC 0013-2616-81

13.8 mg two-chamber cartridge (with preservative)

concentration of 12 mg/mL (approximately 36 IU/mL)

For use with the GENOTROPIN PEN 12 Growth Hormone Delivery Device and/or the GENOTROPIN MIXER Growth Hormone Reconstitution Device

Package of 5 NDC 0013-2646-94
Package of 1 NDC 0013-2646-81

GENOTROPIN MINIQUICK Growth Hormone Delivery Device containing a two-chamber cartridge of GENOTROPIN (without preservative)

After reconstitution, each GENOTROPIN MINIQUICK delivers a fixed volume of 0.25 mL, regardless of strength. Available in the following strengths, each in a package of 7:

[See table above]

Please see accompanying directions for use of the reconstitution and/or delivery device.

Rx only

Manufactured for: Pharmacia & Upjohn Company
Kalamazoo, MI 49001, USA
By: Pharmacia & Upjohn AB
Stockholm, Sweden

Revised June 2000
818 279 000 420-665

Shown in Product Identification Guide, page 331

GLYSET™ ℞

[*glī-set*]
miglitol tablets

DESCRIPTION

GLYSET Tablets contain miglitol, an oral alpha-glucosidase inhibitor for use in the management of non-insulin-dependent diabetes mellitus (NIDDM). Miglitol is a desoxynojirimycin derivative, and is chemically known as 3,4,5-piperidinetriol, 1-(2-hydroxyethyl)-2-(hydroxymethyl)-, [2R-(2α,3β,4α,5β)]-. It is a white to pale-yellow powder with a molecular weight of 207.2 Miglitol is soluble in water and has a pK_a of 5.9. Its empirical formula is $C_8H_{17}NO_5$ and its chemical structure is as follows:

OH, N, OH, HO, HO, OH

GLYSET is available as 25 mg, 50 mg and 100 mg tablets for oral use. The inactive ingredients are starch, microcrystalline cellulose magnesium stearate, hydroxypropyl methylcellulose, polyethylene glycol, titanium dioxide, and polysorbate 80.

CLINICAL PHARMACOLOGY

Miglitol is a desoxynojirimycin derivative that delays the digestion of ingested carbohydrates, thereby resulting in a smaller rise in blood glucose concentration following meals. As a consequence of plasma glucose reduction, GLYSET Tablets reduce levels of glycosylated hemoglobin in patients with Type II (non-insulin-dependent) diabetes mellitus. Systemic nonenzymatic protein glycosylation, as reflected by levels of glycosylated hemoglobin, is a function of average blood glucose concentration over time.

Mechanism of Action

In contrast to sulfonylureas, GLYSET does not enhance insulin secretion. The antihyperglycemic action of miglitol results from a reversible inhibition of membrane-bound intestinal α-glucoside hydrolase enzymes. Membrane-bound intestinal α-glucosidases hydrolyze oligosaccharides and disaccharides to glucose and other monosaccharides in the brush border of the small intestine. In diabetic patients, this enzyme inhibition results in delayed glucose absorption and lowering of postprandial hyperglycemia.

Because its mechanism of action is different, the effect of GLYSET to enhance glycemic control is additive to that of sulfonylureas when used in combination. In addition, GLYSET diminishes the insulinotropic and weight-increasing effects of sulfonylureas.

Miglitol has minor inhibitory activity against lactase and consequently, at the recommended doses, would not be expected to induct lactose intolerance.

Pharmacokinetics

Absorption: Absorption of miglitol is saturable at high doses: a dose of 25 mg is completely absorbed, whereas a dose of 100 mg is only 50%–70% absorbed. For all doses, peak concentrations are reached in 2–3 hours. There is no evidence that systemic absorption of miglitol contributes to its therapeutic effect.

Distribution: The protein binding of miglitol is negligible (<4.0%). Miglitol has a volume of distribution of 0.18 L/kg, consistent with distribution primarily into the extracellular fluid.

Metabolism: Miglitol is not metabolized in man or in any animal species studied. No metabolites have been detected in plasma, urine, or feces, indicating a lack of either systemic or pre-systemic metabolism.

Excretion: Miglitol is eliminated by renal excretion as unchanged drug. Thus, following a 25-mg dose, over 95% of the dose is recovered in the urine within 24 hours. At higher doses, the cumulative recovery of drug from urine is somewhat lower due to the incomplete bioavailability. The elimination half-life of miglitol from plasma is approximately 2 hours.

Special Populations

Renal Impairment: Because miglitol is excreted primarily by the kidneys, accumulation of miglitol is expected in patients with renal impairment. Patients with creatinine clearance < 25 mL/min taking 25 mg 3 times daily exhibited a greater than two-fold increase in miglitol plasma levels as compared to subjects with creatinine clearance > 60 mL/min. Dosage adjustment to correct the increased plasma concentrations is not feasible because miglitol acts locally. Little information is available on the safety of miglitol in patients with creatinine clearance <25 mL/min.

Hepatic impairment: Miglitol pharmacokinetics were not altered in cirrhotic patients relative to healthy control subjects. Since miglitol is not metabolized, no influence of hepatic function on the kinetics of miglitol is expected.

Geriatric: The pharmacokinetics of miglitol were studied in elderly and young males (n = 8 per group). At a dosage of 100 mg 3 times daily for 3 days, no difference between the two groups were found.

Gender: No significant difference in the pharmacokinetics of miglitol was observed between elderly men and women when body weight was taken into account.

Race: Several pharmacokinetic studies were conducted in Japanese volunteers, with results similar to those observed in Caucasians. A study comparing the pharmacodynamic response to a single 50-mg dose in Black and Caucasian healthy volunteers indicated similar glucose and insulin responses in both populations.

CLINICAL STUDIES

Clinical Experience in Non-Insulin-Dependent Diabetes Mellitus (NIDDM) Patients on Dietary Treatment Only

GLYSET Tablets were evaluated in two U.S. and three non-U.S. controlled, fixed-dose, monotherapy studies, in which 735 patients treated with GLYSET were evaluated for efficacy analyses (see Table 1).

[See table 1 at top of next page]

In Study 1, a one-year study in which GLYSET was evaluated as monotherapy and also as combination therapy, there was a statistically significantly smaller increase in mean glycosylated hemoglobin (HbA1c) over time in the miglitol 50 mg 3 times daily monotherapy arm compared to placebo. Significant reductions in mean fasting and postprandial plasma glucose levels and in mean postprandial insulin levels were observed in patients treated with GLYSET compared with the placebo group.

In Study 2, a 14-week study, there was a significant decrease in HbA1c in patients receiving GLYSET 50 mg 3 times daily or 100 mg 3 times daily compared to placebo. In addition, there were significant reductions in postprandial plasma glucose and postprandial serum insulin levels compared to placebo.

Study 3 was a 6-month dose-ranging trial evaluating GLYSET at doses from 25 mg 3 times daily to 200 mg 3 times daily. GLYSET produced a greater reduction in HbA1c than placebo at all doses, although the effect was statistically significant only at the 100 mg 3 times daily and 200 mg 3 times daily doses. In addition, all doses of GLYSET produced significant reductions in postprandial plasma glucose and postprandial insulin levels compared to placebo.

Studies 4 and 5 were 6-month studies evaluating GLYSET at 50 and 100 mg 3 times daily, and 100 mg 3 times daily, respectively. As compared to placebo, GLYSET produced significant reductions in HbA1c, as well as a significant reduction in postprandial plasma glucose in both studies at the doses employed.

Continued on next page

Information on these Pharmacia & Upjohn products is based on labeling in effect June 1, 2000. Further information concerning these and other Pharmacia & Upjohn products may be obtained by direct inquiry to Medical Information, Pharmacia & Upjohn, Kalamazoo, MI 49001.

Glyset—Cont.

Clinical Experience in NIDDM Patients Receiving Sulfonylureas
GLYSET was studied as adjunctive therapy to a background of maximal or near-maximal sulfonylurea (SFU) treatment in three large, double-blind, randomized studies (two U.S. and one non-U.S.) in which 471 patients treated with GLYSET were evaluated for efficacy (see Table 2).
[See table 2 at right]
Study 6 included patients under treatment with maximal doses of SFU at entry. At the end of this 14-week study, the mean treatment effects on glycosylated hemoglobin (HbA1c) were -0.82% and -0.74% for patients receiving GLYSET 50 mg 3 times daily plus SFU, and GLYSET 100 mg 3 times daily plus SFU, respectively.
Study 7 was a one-year study in which GLYSET at 25, 50 or 100 mg 3 times daily was added to a maximal dose of glyburide (10 mg twice daily). At the end of this study, the mean treatment effects on HbA1c of GLYSET when added to maximum glyburide therapy were -0.30%, -0.62%, and -0.73% with the 25, 50 and 100 mg 3 times daily dosages of GLYSET, respectively.
In Study 8, the addition of GLYSET 100 mg 3 times daily to a background of treatment with glyburide produced an additional mean treatment effect on HbA1c of -0.66%.

Dose-Response
Results from controlled, fixed-dose studies of GLYSET as monotherapy or as combination treatment with a sulfonylurea were combined to derive a pooled estimate of the difference from placebo in the mean change from baseline in glycosylated hemoglobin (HbA1c) and postprandial plasma glucose as shown in Figures 1 and 2:

Figure 1
HbA1c (%)
Mean Change From Baseline:
Treatment Effect
Pooled Results from Controlled Fixed-Dose Studies in Tables 1 and 2

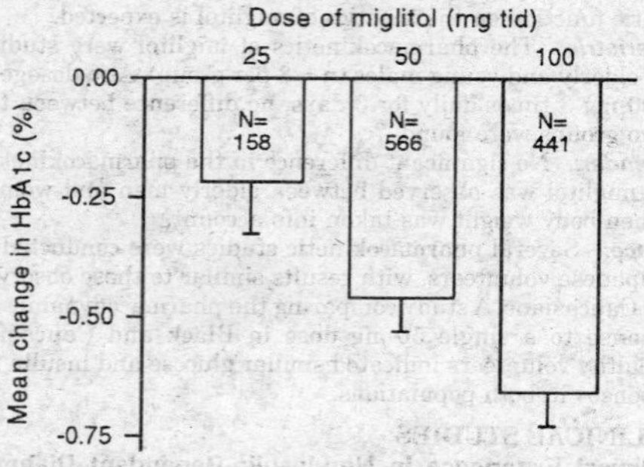

Figure 2
1-Hour Postprandial Plasma Glucose
Mean Change From Baseline:
Treatment Effect
Pooled Results from Controlled Fixed-Dose Studies in Tables 1 and 2

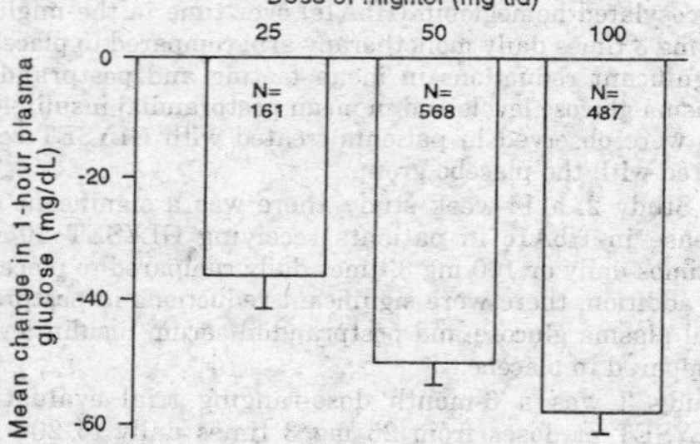

Because of its mechanism of action, the primary pharmacologic effect of miglitol is manifested as a reduction in postprandial plasma glucose, as shown previously in all of the major clinical trials. GLYSET was statistically significantly different from placebo at all doses, in each of the individual studies with respect to effect on mean one-hour postprandial plasma glucose, and there is a dose response from 25 to 100 mg 3 times daily for this efficacy parameter.

Table 1
Results of Monotherapy Study with GLYSET

Study	Treatment	HbA1c (%) Mean Change from Baseline*	HbA1c (%) Treatment Effect**	1-hour Postprandial Glucose (mg/dL) Mean Change from Baseline	1-hour Postprandial Glucose (mg/dL) Treatment Effect**
1 (U.S.)	Placebo	+0.71	—	+24	—
	GLYSET 50 mg t.i.d.***	+0.13	−0.58†	−39	−63†
2 (U.S.)	Placebo	+0.47	—	+15	—
	GLYSET 50 mg t.i.d.	−0.22	−0.69†	−52	−67†
	GLYSET 100 mg t.i.d.	−0.28	−0.75†	−59	−74†
3 (non-U.S.)	Placebo	+0.18	—	+2	—
	GLYSET 25 mg t.i.d.	−0.08	−0.26	−33	−35†
	GLYSET 50 mg t.i.d.	−0.22	−0.40	−45	−47†
	GLYSET 100 mg t.i.d.	−0.63	−0.81†	−62	−64†
	GLYSET 200 mg t.i.d.‡	−0.84	−1.02†	−85	−87†
4 (non-U.S.)	Placebo	+0.01	—	+8	—
	GLYSET 50 mg t.i.d.	−0.35	−0.36†	−20	−28†
	GLYSET 100 mg t.i.d.	−0.57	−0.58	−25	−33†
5 (non-U.S.)	Placbo	+0.32	—	+17	—
	GLYSET 100 mg t.i.d.	−0.43	−0.75†	−38	−55†

* Mean baseline ranged from 7.54 to 8.72% in these studies.
** The result of subtracting the placebo group average.
*** t.i.d. = 3 times daily
† p≤ 0.05
‡ Although results for the 200 mg 3 times daily are presented for completeness, the maximum recommended dosage of GLYSET is 100 mg 3 times daily.

Table 2
Results of Combination Therapy with GLYSET Plus Sulfonylurea (SFU)

Study	Treatment	HbA1c (%) Mean Change from Baseline*	HbA1c (%) Treatment Effect**	1-hour Postprandial Glucose (mg/dL) Mean Change from Baseline	1-hour Postprandial Glucose (mg/dL) Treatment Effect**
6 (U.S.)	Placebo + SFU	+0.33	—	−1	—
	GLYSET 50 mg t.i.d.*** + SFU	−0.49	−0.82†	−69	−68†
	GLYSET 100 mg t.i.d. + SFU	−0.41	−0.74†	−73	−72†
7 (U.S.)	Placebo + SFU	+1.01	—	48	—
	GLYSET 25 mg t.i.d. + SFU	+0.71	−0.30	−2	−50†
	GLYSET 50 mg t.i.d. + SFU	+0.39	−0.62†	−13	−61†
	GLYSET 100 mg t.i.d. + SFU	+0.28	−0.73†	−33	−81†
8 (non-U.S.)	Placebo + SFU	+0.16	—	+10	—
	GLYSET 100 mg t.i.d. + SFU	−0.50	−0.66†	−36	−46†

* Mean baseline ranged from 8.56 to 9.16% in these studies.
** The result of subtracting the placebo group average.
*** t.i.d. = 3 times daily
† p≤ 0.05

INDICATIONS AND USAGE

GLYSET Tablets, as monotherapy, are indicated as an adjunct to diet to improve glycemic control in patients with non-insulin-dependent diabetes mellitus (NIDDM) whose hyperglycemia cannot be managed with diet alone. GLYSET may also be used in combination with a sulfonylurea when diet plus either GLYSET or a sulfonylurea alone do not result in adequate glycemic control. The effect of GLYSET to enhance glycemic control is additive to that of sulfonylureas when used in combination, presumably because its mechanism of action is different.
In initiating treatment for NIDDM, diet should be emphasized as the primary form of treatment. Caloric restriction and weight loss are essential in the obese diabetic patient. Proper dietary management alone may be effective in controlling blood glucose and symptoms of hyperglycemia. The importance of regular physical activity when appropriate should also be stressed. If this treatment program fails to result in adequate glycemic control, the use of GLYSET should be considered. The use of GLYSET must be viewed by both the physician and patient as a treatment in addition to diet and not as a substitute for diet or as a convenient mechanism for avoiding dietary restraint.

CONTRAINDICATIONS

GLYSET Tablets are contraindicated in patients with:

- Diabetic ketoacidosis
- Inflammatory bowel disease, colonic ulceration, or partial intestinal obstruction, and in patients predisposed to intestinal obstruction
- Chronic intestinal diseases associated with marked disorders of digestion or absorption, or with conditions that may deteriorate as a result of increased gas formation in the intestine.
- Hypersensitivity to the drug or any of its components.

PRECAUTIONS

General
Hypoglycemia: Because of its mechanism of action, GLYSET when administered alone should not cause hypoglycemia in the fasted or postprandial state. Sulfonylurea agents may cause hypoglycemia. Because GLYSET Tablets given in combination with a sulfonylurea will cause a further lowering of blood glucose, it may increase the hypoglycemic potential of the sulfonylurea, although this was not observed in clinical trials. Oral glucose (dextrose), whose absorption is not delayed by GLYSET, should be used instead of sucrose (cane sugar) in the treatment of mild-to-moderate hypoglycemia. Sucrose, whose hydrolysis to glucose and fructose is inhibited by GLYSET, is unsuitable for the rapid correction of hypoglycemia. Severe hypoglycemia may require the use of either intravenous glucose infusion or glucagon injection.
Loss of Control of Blood Glucose: When diabetic patients are exposed to stress such as fever, trauma, infection, or surgery, a temporary loss of control of blood glucose may occur. At such times, temporary insulin therapy may be necessary.
Renal Impairment: Plasma concentrations of GLYSET in renally impaired volunteers were proportionally increased relative to the degree of renal dysfunction. Long-term clinical trials in diabetic patients with significant renal dysfunction (serum creatinine >2.0 mg/dL) have not been conducted. Therefore, treatment of these patients with GLYSET is not recommended.

Information for Patients
The following information should be provided to patients:

- GLYSET should be taken orally three times a day at the start (with the first bite) of each main meal. It is important to continue to adhere to dietary instructions, a regular exercise program, and regular testing of urine and/or blood glucose.
- GLYSET itself does not cause hypoglycemia even when administered to patients in the fasted state. Sulfonylurea drugs and insulin, however, can lower blood sugar levels enough to cause symptoms or sometimes lift-threatening hypoglycemia. Because GLYSET given in combination with a sulfonylurea or insulin will cause a further lower-

ing of blood sugar, it may increase the hypoglycemic potential of these agents. The risk of hypoglycemia, its symptoms and treatment, and conditions that predispose to its development should be well understood by patients and responsible family members. Because GLYSET prevents the breakdown of table sugar, a source of glucose (dextrose, D-glucose) should be readily available to treat symptoms of low blood sugar when taking GLYSET in combination with a sulfonylurea or insulin.

- If side effects occur with GLYSET, they usually develop during the first few weeks of therapy. They are most commonly mild-to-moderate does-related gastrointestinal effects, such as flatulence, soft stools, diarrhea, or abdominal discomfort, and they generally diminish in frequency and intensity with time. Discontinuation of drug usually results in rapid resolution of these gastrointestinal symptoms.

Laboratory Tests

Therapeutic response to GLYSET may be monitored by periodic blood glucose tests. Measurement of glycosylated hemoglobin levels is recommended for the monitoring of long-term glycemic control.

Drug Interactions

Several studies investigated the possible interaction between miglitol and glyburide. In six healthy volunteers given a single dose of 5-mg glyburide on a background of 6 days treatment with miglitol (50 mg 3 times daily for 4 days followed by 100 mg 3 times daily for 2 days) or placebo, the mean C_{max} and AUC values for glyburide were 17% and 25% lower, respectively, when glyburide was given with miglitol. In a study in diabetic patients in which the effects of adding miglitol 100 mg 3 times daily × 7 days or placebo to a background regimen of 3.5 mg glyburide daily were investigated, the mean AUC value for glyburide was 18% lower in the group treated with miglitol, although this difference was not statistically significant. Further information on a potential interaction with glyburide was obtained from one of the large U.S. clinical trials (Study 7) in which patients were dosed with either miglitol or placebo on a background of glyburide 10 mg twice daily. At the 6-month and 1-year clinic visits, patients taking concomitant miglitol 100 mg 3 times daily exhibited mean C_{max} values for glyburide that were 16% and 8% lower, respectively, compared to patients taking glyburide alone. However, these differences were not statistically significant. Thus, although there was a trend toward lower AUC and C_{max} values for glyburide when co-administered with GLYSET, no definitive statement regarding a potential interaction can be made based on the foregoing three studies.

The effect of miglitol (100 mg 3 times daily × 7 days) on the pharmacokinetics of a single 1000-mg dose of metformin was investigated in healthy volunteers. Mean AUC and C_{max} values for metformin were 12% to 13% lower when the volunteers were given miglitol as compared with placebo, but this difference was not statistically significant.

In a healthy volunteer study, co-administration of either 50 mg or 100 mg miglitol 3 times daily together with digoxin reduced the average plasma concentrations of digoxin by 19% and 28%, respectively. However, in diabetic patients under treatment with digoxin, plasma digoxin concentrations were not altered by co-administration of miglitol 100 mg 3 times daily × 14 days.

Other healthy volunteer studies have demonstrated that miglitol may significantly reduce the bioavailability of ranitidine and propranolol by 60% and 40%, respectively. No effect of miglitol was observed on the pharmacokinetics or pharmacodynamics of either warfarin or nifedipine.

Intestinal adsorbents (e.g., charcoal) and digestive enzyme preparations containing carbohydrate-splitting enzymes (e.g., amylase, pancreatin) may reduce the effect of GLYSET and should not be taken concomitantly.

In 12 healthy males, concomitantly administered antacid did not influence the pharmacokinetics of miglitol.

Carcinogenesis, Mutagenesis, and Impairment of Fertility

Miglitol was administered to mice by the dietary route at doses as high as approximately 500 mg/kg body weight (corresponding to greater than 5 times the exposure in humans based on AUC) for 21 months. In a two-year rat study, miglitol was administered in the diet at exposures comparable to the maximum human exposures based on AUC. There was no evidence of carcinogenicity resulting from dietary treatment with miglitol.

In vitro, miglitol was found to be non-mutagenic in the bacterial mutagenesis (Ames) assay and the eukaryotic forward mutation assay (CHO/HGPRT). Miglitol did not have any clastogenic effects *in vivo* in the mouse micronucleus test. There were no heritable mutations detected in dominant lethal assay.

A combined male and female fertility study conducted in Wistar rats treated orally with miglitol at dose levels of 300 mg/kg body weight (approximately 8 times the maximum human exposure based on body surface area) produced no untoward effect on reproductive performance or capability to reproduce. In addition, survival, growth, development, and fertility of the offspring were not compromised.

Pregnancy

Teratogenic Effects: Pregnancy Category B. The safety of GLYSET in pregnant women has not been established. Developmental toxicology studies have been performed in rats at doses of 50, 150 and 450 mg/kg, corresponding to levels of approximately 1.5, 4, and 12 times the maximum recommended human exposure based on body surface area. In rabbits, doses of 10, 45, and 200 mg/kg corresponding to levels of approximately 0.5, 3, and 10 times the human exposure were examined. These studies revealed no evidence of fetal malformations attributable to miglitol. Doses of miglitol up to 4 and 3 times the human dose (based on body surface area), for rats and rabbits, respectively, did not reveal evidence of impaired fertility or harm to the fetus. The highest doses tested in these studies, 450 mg/kg in the rat and 200 mg/kg in the rabbit promoted maternal and/or fetal toxicity. Fetotoxicity was indicated by a slight but significant reduction in fetal weight in the rat study and slight reduction in fetal weight, delayed ossification of the fetal skeleton and increase in the percentage of non-viable fetuses in the rabbit study. In the peri-postnatal study in rats, the NOAEL (No Observed Adverse Effect Level) was 100 mg/kg (corresponding to approximately four times the exposure to humans, based on body surface area). An increase in stillborn progeny was noted at the high dose (300 mg/kg) in the rat peri-postnatal study, but not at the high dose (450 mg/kg) in the delivery segment of the rat developmental toxicity study. Otherwise, there was no adverse effect on survival, growth, development, behavior, or fertility in either the rat developmental toxicity or peri-postnatal studies. There are, however, no adequate and well-controlled studies in pregnant women. Because animal reproduction studies are not always predictive of human response, this drug should be used during pregnancy only if clearly needed.

Nursing Mothers

Miglitol has been shown to be excreted in human milk to a very small degree. Total excretion into milk accounted for 0.02% of a 100-mg maternal dose. The estimated exposure to a nursing infant is approximately 0.4% of the maternal dose. Although the levels of miglitol reached in human milk are exceedingly low, it is recommended that GLYSET not be administered to a nursing woman.

Pediatric Use

Safety and effectiveness of GLYSET in pediatric patients have not been established.

Geriatric Use

Of the total number of subjects in clinical studies of GLYSET in the United States, patients valid for safety analyses included 24% over 65, and 3% over 75. No overall differences in safety and effectiveness were observed between these subjects and younger subjects. The pharmacokinetics of miglitol were studied in elderly and young males (n=8 per group). At the dosage of 100 mg 3 times daily for 3 days, no differences between the two groups were found.

ADVERSE REACTIONS

Gastrointestinal: Gastrointestinal symptoms are the most common reactions to GLYSET Tablets. In U.S. placebo-controlled trials, the incidences of abdominal pain, diarrhea, and flatulence were 11.7%, 28.7%, and 41.5% respectively in 962 patients treated with GLYSET 25-100 mg 3 times daily, whereas the corresponding incidences were 4.7%, 10.0%, and 12.0% in 603 placebo-treated patients. The incidence of diarrhea and abdominal pain tended to diminish considerably with continued treatment.

Dermatologic: Skin rash was reported in 4.3% of patients treated with GLYSET compared to 2.4% of placebo-treated patients. Rashes were generally transient and most were assessed as unrelated to GLYSET by physician-investigators.

Abnormal Laboratory Findings: Low serum iron occurred more often in patients treated with GLYSET (9.2%) than in placebo-treated patients (4.2%) but did not persist in the majority of cases and was not associated with reductions in hemoglobin or changes in other hematologic indices.

OVERDOSAGE

Unlike sulfonylureas or insulin, an overdose of GLYSET Tablets will not result in hypoglycemia. An overdose may result in transient increases in flatulence, diarrhea, and abdominal discomfort. Because of the lack of extraintestinal effects seen with GLYSET, no serious systemic reactions are expected in the event of an overdose.

DOSAGE AND ADMINISTRATION

There is no fixed dosage regimen for the management of diabetes mellitus with GLYSET Tablets or any other pharmacologic agent. Dosage of GLYSET must be individualized on the basis of both effectiveness and tolerance while not exceeding the maximum recommended dosage of 100 mg 3 times daily. GLYSET should be taken three times daily at the start (with the first bite) of each main meal. GLYSET should be started at 25 mg, and the dosage gradually increased as described below, both to reduce gastrointestinal adverse effects and to permit identification of the minimum dose required for adequate glycemic control of the patient. During treatment initiation and dose titration (see below), one-hour postprandial plasma glucose may be used to determine the therapeutic response to GLYSET and identify the minimum effective dose for the patient. Thereafter, glycosylated hemoglobin should be measured at intervals of approximately three months. The therapeutic goal should be to decrease both postprandial plasma glucose and glycosylated hemoglobin levels to normal or near normal by using the lowest effective dose of GLYSET, either as monotherapy or in combination with a sulfonylurea.

Initial Dosage: The recommended starting dosage of GLYSET is 25 mg, given orally three times daily at the start (with the first bite) of each main meal. However, some patients may benefit by starting at 25 mg once daily to minimize gastrointestinal adverse effects, and gradually increasing the frequency of administration to 3 times daily.

Maintenance Dosage: The usual maintenance dose of GLYSET is 50 mg 3 times daily, although some patients may benefit from increasing the dose to 100 mg 3 times daily. In order to allow adaptation to potential gastrointestinal adverse effects, it is recommended that GLYSET therapy be initiated at a dosage of 25 mg 3 times daily, the lowest effective dosage, and then gradually titrated upward to allow adaptation. After 4–8 weeks of the 25 mg 3 times daily regimen, the dosage should be increased to 50 mg 3 times daily for approximately three months, following which a glycosylated hemoglobin level should be measured to assess therapeutic response. If, at that time, the glycosylated hemoglobin level is not satisfactory, the dosage may be further increased to 100 mg 3 times daily, the maximum recommended dosage. Pooled data from controlled studies suggest a dose-response for both HbA1c and one-hour postprandial plasma glucose throughout the recommended dosage range. However, no single study has examined the effect on glycemic control of titrating patients' doses upwards within the same study. If no further reduction in postprandial glucose or glycosylated hemoglobin levels is observed with titration to 100 mg 3 times daily consideration should be given to lowering the dose. Once an effective and tolerated dosage is established, it should be maintained.

Maximum Dosage: The maximum recommended dosage of GLYSET is 100 mg 3 times daily. In one clinical trial, 200 mg 3 times daily gave additional improved glycemic control but increased the incidence of the gastrointestinal symptoms described above.

Patients Receiving Sulfonylureas: Sulfonylurea agents may cause hypoglycemia. There was no increased incidence of hypoglycemia in patients who took GLYSET in combination with sulfonylurea agents compared to the incidence of hypoglycemia in patients receiving sulfonylureas alone in any clinical trial. However, GLYSET given in combination with a sulfonylurea will cause a further lowering of blood glucose and may increase the risk of hypoglycemia due to the additive effects of the two agents. If hypoglycemia occurs, appropriate adjustments in the dosage of these agents should be made.

HOW SUPPLIED

GLYSET Tablets are available as 25 mg, 50 mg, and 100 mg white, round, film-coated tablets. The tablets are debossed with the word "GLYSET" on one side and the strength on the other side, as indicated below.

Strength	NDC	Table Identification Front	Back
Bottles of 100:			
25 mg	0009-5012-01	GLYSET	25
50 mg	0009-5013-01	GLYSET	50
100 mg	0009-5014-01	GLYSET	100

Store at 25°C; excursions permitted to 15°–30°C (59°–86°F) [see USP Controlled Room Temperature].

℞ only

U.S. Patent No. 4,639,436

Manufactured for:
Pharmacia & Upjohn Company
Kalamazoo, MI 49001, USA
By:
Bayer Corporation
West Haven, CT 06516, USA

GLYSET is a trademark of Bayer Corporation used under license.

Revised September 1999 817 700 202
PD500147 9305

HALCION® Ⓒ ℞
[*hăl-cĭon*]
triazolam tablets, USP

DESCRIPTION

HALCION Tablets contain triazolam, a triazolobenzodiazepine hypnotic agent.

Triazolam is a white crystalline powder, soluble in alcohol and poorly soluble in water. It has a molecular weight of 343.21.

The chemical name for triazolam is 8-chloro-6-(o-chlorophenyl)-1-methyl-4H-s-tria-zolo-[4,3-α][1,4] benzodiazepine.

The structural formula is represented below:

CH_3 N N N Cl N Cl

Each HALCION Tablet, for oral administration, contains 0.125 mg or 0.25 mg of triazolam. Inactive ingredients:

Continued on next page

Information on these Pharmacia & Upjohn products is based on labeling in effect June 1, 2000. Further information concerning these and other Pharmacia & Upjohn products may be obtained by direct inquiry to Medical Information, Pharmacia & Upjohn, Kalamazoo, MI 49001.

Halcion—Cont.

0.125 mg—cellulose, corn starch, docusate sodium, lactose, magnesium stearate, silicon dioxide, sodium benzoate; **0.25 mg**—cellulose, corn starch, docusate sodium, FD&C Blue No. 2, lactose, magnesium stearate, silicon dioxide, sodium benzoate.

CLINICAL PHARMACOLOGY

Triazolam is a hypnotic with a short mean plasma half-life reported to be in the range of 1.5 to 5.5 hours. In normal subjects treated for 7 days with four times the recommended dosage, there was no evidence of altered systemic bioavailability, rate of elimination, or accumulation. Peak plasma levels are reached within 2 hours following oral administration. Following recommended doses of HALCION, triazolam peak plasma levels in the range of 1 to 6 ng/mL are seen. The plasma levels achieved are proportional to the dose given.

Triazolam and its metabolites, principally as conjugated glucuronides, which are presumably inactive, are excreted primarily in the urine. Only small amounts of unmetabolized triazolam appear in the urine. The two primary metabolites accounted for 79.9% of urinary excretion. Urinary excretion appeared to be biphasic in its time course.

HALCION Tablets 0.5 mg, in two separate studies, did not affect the prothrombin times or plasma warfarin levels in male volunteers administered sodium warfarin orally.

Extremely high concentrations of triazolam do not displace bilirubin bound to human serum albumin *in vitro*.

Triazolam ^{14}C was administered orally to pregnant mice. Drug-related material appeared uniformly distributed in the fetus with ^{14}C concentrations approximately the same as in the brain of the mother.

In sleep laboratory studies, HALCION Tablets significantly decreased sleep latency, increased the duration of sleep, and decreased the number of nocturnal awakenings. After 2 weeks of consecutive nightly administration, the drug's effect on total wake time is decreased, and the values recorded in the last third of the night approach baseline levels. On the first and/or second night after drug discontinuance (first or second post-drug night), total time asleep, percentage of time spent sleeping, and rapidity of falling asleep frequently were significantly less than on baseline (predrug) nights. This effect is often called "rebound" insomnia.

The type and duration of hypnotic effects and the profile of unwanted effects during administration of benzodiazepine drugs may be influenced by the biologic half-life of administered drug and any active metabolites formed. When half-lives are long, the drug or metabolites may accumulate during periods of nightly administration and be associated with impairments of cognitive and motor performance during waking hours; the possibility of interaction with other psychoactive drugs or alcohol will be enhanced. In contrast, if half-lives are short, the drug and metabolites will be cleared before the next dose is ingested, and carry-over effects related to excessive sedation or CNS depression should be minimal or absent. However, during nightly use for an extended period pharmacodynamic tolerance or adaptation to some effects of benzodiazepine hypnotics may develop. If the drug has a short half-life of elimination, it is possible that a relative deficiency of the drug or its active metabolites (ie, in relationship to the receptor site) may occur at some point in the interval between each night's use. This sequence of events may account for two clinical findings reported to occur after several weeks of nightly use of rapidly eliminated benzodiazepine hypnotics: 1) increased wakefulness during the last third of the night and 2) the appearance of increased daytime anxiety after 10 days of continuous treatment.

INDICATIONS AND USAGE

HALCION is indicated for the short-term treatment of insomnia (generally 7–10 days). Use for more than 2–3 weeks requires complete reevaluation of the patient (see WARNINGS).

Prescriptions for HALCION should be written for short-term use (7–10 days) and it should not be prescribed in quantities exceeding a 1-month supply.

CONTRAINDICATIONS

HALCION Tablets are contraindicated in patients with known hypersensitivity to this drug or other benzodiazepines.

Benzodiazepines may cause fetal damage when administered during pregnancy. An increased risk of congenital malformations associated with the use of diazepam and chlordiazepoxide during the first trimester of pregnancy has been suggested in several studies. Transplacental distribution has resulted in neonatal CNS depression following the ingestion of therapeutic doses of a benzodiazepine hypnotic during the last weeks of pregnancy.

HALCION is contraindicated in pregnant women. If there is a likelihood of the patient becoming pregnant while receiving HALCION, she should be warned of the potential risk to the fetus. Patients should be instructed to discontinue the drug prior to becoming pregnant. The possibility that a woman of childbearing potential may be pregnant at the time of institution of therapy should be considered.

HALCION is contraindicated with ketoconazole, itraconazole, and nefazodone, medications that significantly impair the oxidative metabolism mediated by cytochrome P450 3A (CYP 3A) (see WARNINGS and PRECAUTIONS–Drug Interactions).

WARNINGS

Sleep disturbance may be the presenting manifestation of a physical and/or psychiatric disorder. Consequently, a decision to initiate symptomatic treatment of insomnia should only be made after the patient has been carefully evaluated. The failure of insomnia to remit after 7–10 days of treatment may indicate the presence of a primary psychiatric and/or medical illness.

Worsening of insomnia or the emergence of new abnormalities of thinking or behavior may be the consequence of an unrecognized psychiatric or physical disorder. These have also been reported to occur in association with the use of HALCION.

Because some of the adverse effects of HALCION appear to be dose related (see PRECAUTIONS and DOSAGE AND ADMINISTRATION), it is important to use the smallest possible effective dose. Elderly patients are especially susceptible to dose related adverse effects.

An increase in daytime anxiety has been reported for HALCION after as few as 10 days of continuous use. In some patients this may be a manifestation of interdose withdrawal (see CLINICAL PHARMACOLOGY). If increased daytime anxiety is observed during treatment, discontinuation of treatment may be advisable.

A variety of abnormal thinking and behavior changes have been reported to occur in association with the use of benzodiazepine hypnotics including HALCION. Some of these changes may be characterized by decreased inhibition, eg, aggressiveness and extroversion that seem excessive, similar to that seen with alcohol and other CNS depressants (eg, sedative/hypnotics). Other kinds of behavioral changes have also been reported, for example, bizarre behavior, agitation, hallucinations, depersonalization. In primarily depressed patients, the worsening of depression, including suicidal thinking, has been reported in association with the use of benzodiazepines.

It can rarely be determined with certainty whether a particular instance of the abnormal behaviors listed above is drug induced, spontaneous in origin, or a result of an underlying psychiatric or physical disorder. Nonetheless, the emergence of any new behavioral sign or symptom of concern requires careful and immediate evaluation.

Because of its depressant CNS effects, patients receiving triazolam should be cautioned against engaging in hazardous occupations requiring complete mental alertness such as operating machinery or driving a motor vehicle. For the same reason, patients should be cautioned about the concomitant ingestion of alcohol and other CNS depressant drugs during treatment with HALCION Tablets.

As with some, but not all benzodiazepines, anterograde amnesia of varying severity and paradoxical reactions have been reported following therapeutic doses of HALCION. Data from several sources suggest that anterograde amnesia may occur at a higher rate with HALCION than with other benzodiazepine hypnotics.

Triazolam interaction with drugs that inhibit metabolism via cytochrome P450 3A:

The initial step in triazolam metabolism is hydroxylation catalyzed by cytochrome P450 3A (CYP 3A). Drugs that inhibit this metabolic pathway may have a profound effect on the clearance of triazolam. Consequently, triazolam should be avoided in patients receiving very potent inhibitors of CYP 3A. With drugs inhibiting CYP 3A to a lesser but still significant degree, triazolam should be used only with caution and consideration of appropriate dosage reduction. For some drugs, an interaction with triazolam has been quantified with clinical data; for other drugs, interactions are predicted from *in vitro* data and/or experience with similar drugs in the same pharmacologic class.

The following are examples of drugs known to inhibit the metabolism of triazolam and/or related benzodiazepines, presumably through inhibition of CYP 3A.

Potent CYP 3A inhibitors: Potent inhibitors of CYP 3A that should not be used concomitantly with triazolam include ketoconazole, itraconazole, and nefazodone. Although data concerning the effects of azole-type antifungal agents other than ketoconazole and itraconazole on triazolam metabolism are not available, they should be considered potent CYP 3A inhibitors, and their coadministration with triazolam is not recommended (see CONTRAINDICATIONS).

Drugs demonstrated to be CYP 3A inhibitors on the basis of clinical studies involving triazolam (caution and consideration of dose reduction are recommended during coadministration with triazolam):

Macrolide Antibiotics—Coadministration of erythromycin increased the maximum plasma concentration of triazolam by 46%, decreased clearance by 53%, and increased half-life by 35%; caution and consideration of appropriate triazolam dose reduction are recommended. Similar caution should be observed during coadministration with clarithromycin and other macrolide antibiotics.

Cimetidine—Coadministration of cimetidine increased the maximum plasma concentration of triazolam by 51%, decreased clearance by 55%, and increased half-life by 68%; caution and consideration of appropriate triazolam dose reduction are recommended.

Other drugs possibly affecting triazolam metabolism: Other drugs possibly affecting triazolam metabolism by inhibition of CYP 3A are discussed in the PRECAUTIONS section (see PRECAUTIONS–Drug Interactions).

PRECAUTIONS

General: In elderly and/or debilitated patients it is recommended that treatment with HALCION Tablets be initiated at 0.125 mg to decrease the possibility of development of oversedation, dizziness, or impaired coordination.

Some side effects reported in association with the use of HALCION appear to be dose related. These include drowsiness, dizziness, light-headedness, and amnesia.

The relationship between dose and what may be more serious behavioral phenomena is less certain. Specifically, some evidence, based on spontaneous marketing reports, suggests that confusion, bizarre or abnormal behavior, agitation, and hallucinations may also be dose related, but this evidence is inconclusive. In accordance with good medical practice it is recommended that therapy be initiated at the lowest effective dose (see DOSAGE AND ADMINISTRATION).

Cases of "traveler's amnesia" have been reported by individuals who have taken HALCION to induce sleep while traveling, such as during an airplane flight. In some of these cases, insufficient time was allowed for the sleep period prior to awakening and before beginning activity. Also, the concomitant use of alcohol may have been a factor in some cases.

Caution should be exercised if HALCION is prescribed to patients with signs or symptoms of depression that could be intensified by hypnotic drugs. Suicidal tendencies may be present in such patients and protective measures may be required. Intentional overdosage is more common in these patients, and the least amount of drug that is feasible should be available to the patient at any one time.

The usual precautions should be observed in patients with impaired renal or hepatic function, chronic pulmonary insufficiency, and sleep apnea. In patients with compromised respiratory function, respiratory depression and apnea have been reported infrequently.

Information for patients: The text of a patient package insert is printed at the end of this insert. To assure safe and effective use of HALCION, the information and instructions provided in this patient package insert should be discussed with patients.

Laboratory tests: Laboratory tests are not ordinarily required in otherwise healthy patients.

Drug interactions: Both pharmacodynamic and pharmacokinetic interactions have been reported with benzodiazepines. In particular, triazolam produces additive CNS depressant effects when coadministered with other psychotropic medications, anticonvulsants, antihistamines, ethanol, and other drugs which themselves produce CNS depression.

Drugs that inhibit triazolam metabolism via cytochrome P450 3A: The initial step in triazolam metabolism is hydroxylation catalyzed by cytochrome P450 3A (CYP 3A). Drugs which inhibit this metabolic pathway may have a profound effect on the clearance of triazolam (see CONTRAINDICATIONS and WARNINGS for additional drugs of this type).

Drugs and other substances demonstrated to be CYP 3A inhibitors of possible clinical significance on the basis of clinical studies involving triazolam (caution is recommended during coadministration with triazolam):

Isoniazid—Coadministration of isoniazid increased the maximum plasma concentration of triazolam by 20%, decreased clearance by 42%, and increased half-life by 31%.

Oral contraceptives—Coadministration of oral contraceptives increased maximum plasma concentration by 6%, decreased clearance by 32%, and increased half-life by 16%.

Grapefruit juice—Coadministration of grapefruit juice increased the maximum plasma concentration of triazolam by 25%, increased the area under the concentration curve by 48%, and increased half-life by 18%.

Drugs demonstrated to be CYP 3A inhibitors on the basis of clinical studies involving benzodiazepines metabolized similarly to triazolam or on the basis of in vitro studies with triazolam or other benzodiazepines (caution is recommended during coadministration with triazolam): Available data from clinical studies of benzodiazepines other than triazolam suggest a possible drug interaction with triazolam for the following: fluvoxamine, diltiazem, and verapamil. Data from *in vitro* studies of triazolam suggest a possible drug interaction with triazolam for the following: sertraline and paroxetine. Data from *in vitro* studies of benzodiazepines other than triazolam suggest a possible drug interaction with triazolam for the following: ergotamine, cyclosporine, amiodarone, nicardipine, and nifedipine. Caution is recommended during coadministration of any of these drugs with triazolam (see WARNINGS).

Drugs that affect triazolam pharmacokinetics by other mechanisms:

Ranitidine—Coadministration of ranitidine increased the maximum plasma concentration of triazolam by 30%, increased the area under the concentration curve by 27%, and increased half-life by 3.3%. Caution is recommended during coadministration with triazolam.

Carcinogenesis, mutagenesis, impairment of fertility: No evidence of carcinogenic potential was observed in mice during a 24-month study with HALCION in doses up to 4,000 times the human dose.

Pregnancy:

1. Teratogenic effects: Pregnancy category X (see CONTRAINDICATIONS).

2. Non-teratogenic effects: It is to be considered that the child born of a mother who is on benzodiazepines may be at some risk for withdrawal symptoms from the drug, during

the postnatal period. Also, neonatal flaccidity has been reported in an infant born of a mother who had been receiving benzodiazepines.

Nursing mothers: Human studies have not been performed; however, studies in rats have indicated that HALCION and its metabolites are secreted in milk. Therefore, administration of HALCION to nursing mothers is not recommended.

Pediatric use: Safety and effectiveness of HALCION in individuals below 18 years of age have not been established.

ADVERSE REACTIONS

During placebo-controlled clinical studies in which 1,003 patients received HALCION Tablets, the most troublesome side effects were extensions of the pharmacologic activity of triazolam, eg, drowsiness, dizziness, or light-headedness.

The figures cited below are estimates of untoward clinical event incidence among subjects who participated in the relatively short duration (ie, 1 to 42 days) placebo-controlled clinical trials of HALCION. The figures cannot be used to predict precisely the incidence of untoward events in the course of usual medical practice where patient characteristics and other factors often differ from those in clinical trials. These figures cannot be compared with those obtained from other clinical studies involving related drug products and placebo, as each group of drug trials is conducted under a different set of conditions.

Comparison of the cited figures, however, can provide the prescriber with some basis for estimating the relative contributions of drug and nondrug factors to the untoward event incidence rate in the population studied. Even this use must be approached cautiously, as a drug may relieve a symptom in one patient while inducing it in others. (For example, an anticholinergic, anxiolytic drug may relieve dry mouth [a sign of anxiety] in some subjects but induce it [an untoward event] in others.)

	HALCION	PLACEBO
Number of Patients	1003	997
% Patients Reporting:		
Central Nervous System		
Drowsiness	14.0	6.4
Headache	9.7	8.4
Dizziness	7.8	3.1
Nervousness	5.2	4.5
Light-headedness	4.9	0.9
Coordination dis-orders/ataxia	4.6	0.8
Gastrointestinal		
Nausea/vomiting	4.6	3.7

In addition to the relatively common (ie, 1% or greater) untoward events enumerated above, the following adverse events have been reported less frequently (ie, 0.9% to 0.5%): euphoria, tachycardia, tiredness, confusional states/memory impairment, cramps/pain, depression, visual disturbances.

Rare (ie, less than 0.5%) adverse reactions included constipation, taste alterations, diarrhea, dry mouth, dermatitis/allergy, dreaming/nightmares, insomnia, paresthesia, tinnitus, dysesthesia, weakness, congestion, death from hepatic failure in a patient also receiving diuretic drugs.

In addition to these untoward events for which estimates of incidence are available, the following adverse events have been reported in association with the use of HALCION and other benzodiazepines: amnestic symptoms (anterograde amnesia with appropriate or inappropriate behavior), confusional states (disorientation, derealization, depersonalization, and/or clouding of consciousness), dystonia, anorexia, fatigue, sedation, slurred speech, jaundice, pruritus, dysarthria, changes in libido, menstrual irregularities, incontinence, and urinary retention. Other factors may contribute to some of these reactions, eg, concomitant intake of alcohol or other drugs, sleep deprivation, an abnormal premorbid state, etc.

Other events reported include: paradoxical reactions such as stimulation, mania, an agitational state (restlessness, irritability, and excitation), increased muscle spasticity, sleep disturbances, hallucinations, delusions, aggressiveness, falling, somnambulism, syncope, inappropriate behavior and other adverse behavioral effects. Should these occur, use of the drug should be discontinued.

The following events have also been reported: chest pain, burning tongue/glossitis/stomatitis.

Laboratory analyses were performed on all patients participating in the clinical program for HALCION. The following incidences of abnormalities were observed in patients receiving HALCION and the corresponding placebo group. None of these changes were considered to be of physiological significance.

	HALCION		PLACEBO	
Number of Patients	380		361	
% of Patients Reporting:	Low	High	Low	High
Hematology				
Hematocrit	*	*	*	*
Hemoglobin	*	*	*	*
Total WBC count	1.7	2.1	*	1.3
Neutrophil count	1.5	1.5	3.3	1.0
Lymphocyte count	2.3	4.0	3.1	3.8
Monocyte count	3.6	*	4.4	1.5
Eosinophil count	10.2	3.2	9.8	3.4
Basophil count	1.7	2.1	*	1.8
Urinalysis				
Albumin	–	1.1	–	*
Sugar	–	*	–	*
RBC/HPF	–	2.9	–	2.9
WBC/HPF	–	11.7	–	7.9
Blood chemistry				
Creatinine	2.4	1.9	3.6	1.5
Bilirubin	*	1.5	1.0	*
SGOT	*	5.3	*	4.5
Alkaline phosphatase	*	2.2	*	2.6

* Less than 1%

When treatment with HALCION is protracted, periodic blood counts, urinalysis, and blood chemistry analyses are advisable.

Minor changes in EEG patterns, usually low-voltage fast activity, have been observed in patients during therapy with HALCION and are of no known significance.

DRUG ABUSE AND DEPENDENCE

Controlled Substance: Triazolam is a controlled substance under the Controlled Substance Act, and HALCION Tablets have been assigned to Schedule IV.

Abuse, Dependence and Withdrawal: Withdrawal symptoms, similar in character to those noted with barbiturates and alcohol (convulsions, tremor, abdominal and muscle cramps, vomiting, sweating, dysphoria, perceptual disturbances and insomnia), have occurred following abrupt discontinuance of benzodiazepines, including HALCION. The more severe symptoms are usually associated with higher dosages and longer usage, although patients at therapeutic dosages given for as few as 1–2 weeks can also have withdrawal symptoms and in some patients there may be withdrawal symptoms (daytime anxiety, agitation) between nightly doses (see CLINICAL PHARMACOLOGY). Consequently, abrupt discontinuation should be avoided and a gradual dosage tapering schedule is recommended in any patient taking more than the lowest dose for more than a few weeks. The recommendation for tapering is particularly important in any patient with a history of seizure.

The risk of dependence is increased in patients with a history of alcoholism, drug abuse, or in patients with marked personality disorders. Such dependence-prone individuals should be under careful surveillance when receiving HALCION. As with all hypnotics, repeat prescriptions should be limited to those who are under medical supervision.

OVERDOSAGE

Because of the potency of triazolam, some manifestations of overdosage may occur at 2 mg, four times the maximum recommended therapeutic dose (0.5 mg).

Manifestations of overdosage with HALCION Tablets include somnolence, confusion, impaired coordination, slurred speech, and ultimately, coma. Respiratory depression and apnea have been reported with overdosages of HALCION. Seizures have occasionally been reported after overdosages. Death has been reported in association with overdoses of triazolam by itself, as it has with other benzodiazepines. In addition, fatalities have been reported in patients who have overdosed with a combination of a single benzodiazepine, including triazolam, and alcohol; benzodiazepine and alcohol levels seen in some of these cases have been lower than those usually associated with reports of fatality with either substance alone.

As in all cases of drug overdosage, respiration, pulse, and blood pressure should be monitored and supported by general measures when necessary. Immediate gastric lavage should be performed. An adequate airway should be maintained. Intravenous fluids may be administered.

Flumazenil, a specific benzodiazepine receptor antagonist, is indicated for the complete or partial reversal of the sedative effects of benzodiazepines and may be used in situations when an overdose with a benzodiazepine is known or suspected. Prior to the administration of flumazenil, necessary measures should be instituted to secure airway, ventilation and intravenous access. Flumazenil is intended as an adjunct to, not as a substitute for, proper management of benzodiazepine overdose. Patients treated with flumazenil should be monitored for re-sedation, respiratory depression, and other residual benzodiazepine effects for an appropriate period after treatment. **The prescriber should be aware of a risk of seizure in association with flumazenil treatment, particularly in long-term benzodiazepine users and in cyclic antidepressant overdose**. The complete flumazenil package insert including CONTRAINDICATIONS, WARNINGS and PRECAUTIONS should be consulted prior to use.

Experiments in animals have indicated that cardiopulmonary collapse can occur with massive intravenous doses of triazolam. This could be reversed with positive mechanical respiration and the intravenous infusion of norepinephrine bitartrate or metaraminol bitartrate. Hemodialysis and forced diuresis are probably of little value. As with the management of intentional overdosage with any drug, the physician should bear in mind that multiple agents may have been ingested by the patient.

The oral LD_{50} in mice is greater than 1,000 mg/kg and in rats is greater than 5,000 mg/kg.

DOSAGE AND ADMINISTRATION

It is important to individualize the dosage of HALCION Tablets for maximum beneficial effect and to help avoid significant adverse effects.

The recommended dose for most adults is 0.25 mg before retiring. A dose of 0.125 mg may be found to be sufficient for some patients (eg, low body weight). A dose of 0.5 mg should be used only for exceptional patients who do not respond adequately to a trial of a lower dose since the risk of several adverse reactions increases with the size of the dose administered. A dose of 0.5 mg should not be exceeded.

In geriatric and/or debilitated patients the recommended dosage range is 0.125 mg to 0.25 mg. Therapy should be initiated at 0.125 mg in this group and the 0.25 mg dose should be used only for exceptional patients who do not respond to a trial of the lower dose. A dose of 0.25 mg should not be exceeded in these patients.

As with all medications, the lowest effective dose should be used.

HOW SUPPLIED

HALCION Tablets are available in the following strengths and package sizes:

0.125 mg (white, elliptical, imprinted HALCION 0.125):

Reverse numbered	
Unit Dose (100)	NDC 0009-0010-32
10–10 Tablet Bottles	NDC 0009-0010-38
Bottles of 500	NDC 0009-0010-11

0.25 mg (powder blue, elliptical, scored, imprinted HALCION 0.25):

Reverse numbered	
Unit Dose (100)	NDC 0009-0017-55
10–10 Tablet Bottles	NDC 0009-0017-59
Bottles of 500	NDC 0009-0017-02

Store at controlled room temperature 20° to 25°C (68° to 77°F) [see USP].

Rx only

The text of the patient insert for HALCION is set forth below.

PATIENT INFORMATION

INTRODUCTION

HALCION is intended to help you sleep. It is one of several benzodiazepine sleeping pills that have generally similar properties. Anyone who is considering using one of these medications should be aware of both their benefits and several important risks and limitations, including diminishing effectiveness with continued use and the possible development of dependence (addiction) and possibly mental changes particularly when the drugs are used for more than a few days to a week. This patient information statement is intended to provide you with knowledge about this class of medications in general and about HALCION in particular that will be useful to guide you in the safe use of this product, BUT IT SHOULD NOT REPLACE A DISCUSSION BETWEEN YOU AND YOUR PHYSICIAN ABOUT THE RISKS AND BENEFITS OF HALCION.

This leaflet will focus on the beneficial and adverse effects of all members of this class of medications, as well as some specific information about HALCION. There are some differences among these products, and your physician may wish to discuss any specific advantages and disadvantages of particular members of this drug class with you.

EFFECTIVENESS OF BENZODIAZEPINE SLEEPING PILLS

Benzodiazepine sleeping pills are effective medications and are relatively free of serious problems when they are used for short-term management of sleep problems (insomnia). Insomnia is not always the same. It may be reflected in difficulty in falling asleep, frequent awakening during the night, and/or early morning awakening. Insomnia is often transient in nature, responding to brief treatment with sleeping pills. Use for more than a short while requires discussion with your physician about the risks and benefits of prolonged use.

SIDE EFFECTS

Common Side Effects

The most common side effects of benzodiazepine sleeping pills are related to the ability of the medications to make you sleepy; drowsiness, dizziness, light-headedness, and difficulty with coordination. Users must be cautious about engaging in hazardous activities requiring complete mental alertness, eg, operating machinery or driving a motor vehicle. Do not take alcohol while using HALCION. Benzodiazepine sleeping pills should not be used with other medications or substances that may cause drowsiness, without discussing said use with your physician.

How sleepy you are the day after you use one of these sleep medications depends on your individual response and on how quickly the product is eliminated from your body. The larger the dose, the more likely an individual will experience next day residual effects such as drowsiness. For this reason, it is important to use the lowest effective dose for each individual patient. Benzodiazepines that are eliminated rapidly, eg, HALCION, tend to cause less next day drowsiness but may cause more withdrawal problems the day after use (see below).

Special Concerns

Memory Problems

All benzodiazepine sleeping pills can cause a special type of amnesia (memory loss) in which a person may not recall

Continued on next page

Information on these Pharmacia & Upjohn products is based on labeling in effect June 1, 2000. Further information concerning these and other Pharmacia & Upjohn products may be obtained by direct inquiry to Medical Information, Pharmacia & Upjohn, Kalamazoo, MI 49001.

Halcion—Cont.

events occurring during some period of time, usually several hours, after taking a drug. This is ordinarily not a problem, because the person taking a sleeping pill intends to be asleep during this vulnerable period of time. It can be a problem when the drugs are taken to induce sleep while traveling, such as during an airplane flight, because the person may awake before the effect of the drug is gone. This has been called "traveler's amnesia". HALCION is more likely than other members of the class to cause this problem.

Tolerance/Withdrawal Phenomena

Some loss of effectiveness or adaptation to the sleep inducing effects of these medications may develop after nightly use for more than a few weeks and there may be a degree of dependence that develops. For the benzodiazepine sleeping pills that are eliminated quickly from the body, a relative deficiency of the drug may occur at some point in the interval between each night's use. This can lead to (1) increased wakefulness during the last third of the night, and (2) the appearance of increased signs of daytime anxiety or nervousness. These two events have been reported in particular for HALCION.

There can be more severe 'withdrawal' effects when a benzodiazepine sleeping pill is stopped. Such effects can occur after discontinuing these drugs following use for only a week or two, but may be more common and more severe after longer periods of continuous use. One type of withdrawal phenomenon is the occurrence of what is known as 'rebound insomnia'. That is, on the first few nights after the drug is stopped, insomnia is actually worse than before the sleeping pill was given. Other withdrawal phenomena following abrupt stopping of benzodiazepine sleeping pills range from mild unpleasant feelings to a major withdrawal syndrome which may include abdominal and muscle cramps, vomiting, sweating, tremor, and rarely, convulsions. These more severe withdrawal phenomena are uncommon.

Dependence/Abuse Phenomena

All benzodiazepine sleeping pills can cause dependence (addiction), especially when used regularly for more than a few weeks or at higher doses. Some people develop a need to continue taking these drugs, either at the prescribed dose or at increasing doses, not so much for continued therapeutic effect, but rather, to avoid withdrawal phenomena and/or to achieve nontherapeutic effects. Individuals who have been dependent on alcohol or other drugs may be at particular risk of becoming dependent on drugs in this class, but all people appear to be at some risk. This possibility must be considered before extending the use of these drugs for more than a few weeks.

Mental and Behavioral Changes

A variety of abnormal thinking and behavior changes have been reported to occur in association with the use of benzodiazepine sleeping pills. Some of these changes are like the release of inhibition seen in association with alcohol, eg, aggressiveness and extroversion that seem out of character. Others, however, can be more unusual and more extreme, such as confusion, bizarre behavior, agitation, hallucinations, depersonalization, and worsening of depression, including suicidal thinking. It is rarely clear whether such events are induced by the drug being taken, are caused by some underlying illness or are simply spontaneous happenings. In fact, worsened insomnia may in some cases be associated with illnesses that were present before the medication was used. In any event, the most important fact is to understand that regardless of the cause, users of these medications should promptly report any mental or behavioral changes to their doctor.

Effects on Pregnancy

Certain benzodiazepines have been linked to birth defects when administered during the early months of pregnancy. In addition, the administration of benzodiazepines during the last weeks of pregnancy has been associated with sedation of the fetus. Consequently, the use of this drug should be avoided at any time during pregnancy.

Interactions with Other Medications

HALCION should not be taken with ketoconazole, itraconazole and nefazodone. Taking HALCION with certain other medications may cause increased levels of the drug in the blood and result in an excessive effect. Always tell your doctor about all medications you are taking.

SAFE USE OF BENZODIAZEPINE SLEEPING PILLS

To assure the safe and effective use of HALCION, you should adhere to the following cautions:

1. HALCION is a prescription medication and, therefore, should be used only as directed by your doctor. Follow your doctor's advice about how to take it, when to take it, and how long to take it. As with other prescription medication, HALCION should be taken only by the individual for whom it is prescribed.
2. Do not extend your use of HALCION beyond 7–10 days without first consulting your physician.
3. If you develop any unusual and disturbing thoughts or behavior during treatment with HALCION, you should discuss such problems with your physician.
4. Inform your physician about any alcohol consumption and medicine you are taking now, including drugs you may buy without a prescription. Do not use alcohol while taking HALCION.
5. Do not take HALCION in circumstances where a full night's sleep and elimination of the drug from the body are not possible before you would again need to be active and functional, eg, an overnight flight of less than 7–8 hours, because amnestic episodes have been reported in such situations.
6. Do not increase the prescribed dose except on the advice of your physician.
7. Until you experience how this medication affects you, do not drive a car or operate potentially dangerous machinery, etc.
8. Be aware that you may experience an increase in sleep difficulties (rebound insomnia) on the first night or two after discontinuing HALCION.
9. Inform your physician if you are planning to become pregnant, if you are pregnant, or if you become pregnant while you are taking this medicine. The use of HALCION should be avoided at any time during pregnancy.
10. Always tell your doctor about all medications you are taking.

Pharmacia & Upjohn Company
Kalamazoo, Michigan 49001, USA
Revised May 1999 812 110 829
692167

Shown in Product Identification Guide, page 331

IDAMYCIN PFS ℞

[*eye-dă-mī-sin PFS*]

idarubicin hydrochloride injection

FOR INTRAVENOUS USE ONLY

WARNINGS

1. IDAMYCIN PFS Injection should be given slowly into a freely flowing intravenous infusion. It must *never* be given intramuscularly or subcutaneously. Severe local tissue necrosis can occur if there is extravasation during administration.
2. As is the case with other anthracyclines the use of IDAMYCIN PFS can cause myocardial toxicity leading to congestive heart failure. Cardiac toxicity is more common in patients who have received prior anthracyclines or who have pre-existing cardiac disease.
3. As is usual with antileukemic agents, severe myelosuppression occurs when IDAMYCIN PFS is used at effective therapeutic doses.
4. It is recommended that IDAMYCIN PFS be administered only under the supervision of a physician who is experienced in leukemia chemotherapy and in facilities with laboratory and supportive resources adequate to monitor drug tolerance and protect and maintain a patient compromised by drug toxicity. The physician and institution must be capable of responding rapidly and completely to severe hemorrhagic conditions and/or overwhelming infection.
5. Dosage should be reduced in patients with impaired hepatic or renal function. (See DOSAGE AND ADMINISTRATION.)

DESCRIPTION

IDAMYCIN PFS Injection contains idarubicin hydrochloride and is a sterile, semi-synthetic, preservative-free solution (PFS) antineoplastic anthracycline for intravenous use. Chemically, idarubicin hydrochloride is 5, 12-Naphthacenedione, 9-acetyl-7-[(3-amino-2,3,6-trideoxy-α-L-*lyxo*-hexopyranosyl)oxy]-7,8,9,10-tetrahydro-6,9,11-trihydroxyhydrochloride, (7S-*cis*). The structural formula is as follows:

O OH O CCH₃ OH H O OH O · HCl CH₃ HO NH₂

$C_{26}H_{27}NO_9 \cdot HCl$ M.W. 533.96

IDAMYCIN PFS is a sterile, red-orange, isotonic parenteral preservative-free solution, available in 5 mL (5 mg), 10 mL (10 mg) and 20 mL (20 mg) single use only vials.

Each mL contains Idarubicin HCl, USP 1 mg and the following inactive ingredients: Glycerin, USP 25 mg and Water for Injection, USP q.s. Hydrochloric Acid, NF is used to adjust the pH to a target of 3.5.

CLINICAL PHARMACOLOGY

Mechanism of Action

Idarubicin hydrochloride is a DNA-intercalating analog of daunorubicin which has an inhibitory effect on nucleic acid synthesis and interacts with the enzyme topoisomerase II. The absence of a methoxy group at position 4 of the anthracycline structure gives the compound a high lipophilicity which results in an increased rate of cellular uptake compared with other anthracyclines.

Pharmacokinetics

General Pharmacokinetics: Pharmacokinetic studies have been performed in adult leukemia patients with normal renal and hepatic function following intravenous administration of 10 to 12 mg/m^2 of idarubicin daily for 3 to 4 days as a single agent or combined with cytarabine. The plasma concentrations of idarubicin are best described by a two or three compartment open model. The elimination rate of idarubicin from plasma is slow with an estimated mean terminal half-life of 22 hours (range, 4 to 48 hours) when used as a single agent and 20 hours (range, 7 to 38 hours) when used in combination with cytarabine. The elimination of the primary active metabolite, idarubicinol, is considerably slower than that of the parent drug with an estimated mean terminal half-life that exceeds 45 hours; hence, its plasma levels are sustained for a period greater than 8 days.

Distribution: The disposition profile shows a rapid distributive phase with a very high volume of distribution presumably reflecting extensive tissue binding. Studies of cellular (nucleated blood and bone marrow cells) drug concentrations in leukemia patients have shown that peak cellular idarubicin concentrations are reached a few minutes after injection. Concentrations of idarubicin and idarubicinol in nucleated blood and bone marrow cells are more than a hundred times the plasma concentrations. Idarubicin disappearance rates in plasma and cells were comparable with a terminal half-life of about 15 hours. The terminal half-life of idarubicinol in cells was about 72 hours. The extent of drug and metabolite accumulation predicted in leukemia patients for Days 2 and 3 of dosing, based on the mean plasma levels and half-life obtained after the first dose, is 1.7- and 2.3-fold, respectively, and suggests no change in kinetics following a daily × 3 regimen. The percentages of idarubicin and idarubicinol bound to human plasma proteins averaged 97% and 94%, respectively, at concentrations similar to maximum plasma levels obtained in the pharmacokinetic studies. The binding is concentration independent. The plasma clearance is twice the expected hepatic plasma flow indicating extensive extrahepatic metabolism.

Metabolism: The primary active metabolite formed is idarubicinol. As idarubicinol has cytotoxic activity, it presumably contributes to the effects of idarubicin.

Elimination: The drug is eliminated predominately by biliary and to a lesser extent by renal excretion, mostly in the form of idarubicinol.

Pharmacokinetics in Special Populations

Pediatric Patients: Idarubicin studies in pediatric leukemia patients, at doses of 4.2 to 13.3 mg/m^2 /day × 3, suggest dose independent kinetics. There is no difference between the half-lives of the drug following daily × 3 or weekly × 3 administration. Cerebrospinal fluid (CSF) levels of idarubicin and idarubicinol were measured in pediatric leukemia patients treated intravenously. Idarubicin was detected in 2 of 21 CSF samples (0.14 and 1.57 ng/mL), while idarubicinol was detected in 20 of these 21 CSF samples obtained 18 to 30 hours after dosing (mean = 0.51 ng/mL; range, 0.22 to 1.05 ng/mL). The clinical relevance of these findings is unknown.

Hepatic and Renal Impairment: The pharmacokinetics of idarubicin have not been evaluated in leukemia patients with hepatic impairment. It is expected that in patients with moderate or severe hepatic dysfunction, the metabolism of idarubicin may be impaired and lead to higher systemic drug levels. The disposition of idarubicin may be also affected by renal impairment. Therefore, a dose reduction should be considered in patients with hepatic and/or renal impairment (see DOSAGE AND ADMINISTRATION).

Drug-Drug Interactions

No formal drug interaction studies have been performed.

CLINICAL STUDIES

Four prospective randomized studies, three U.S. and one Italian, have been conducted to compare the efficacy and safety of idarubicin (IDR) to that of daunorubicin (DNR), each in combination with cytarabine as induction therapy in previously untreated adult patients with acute myeloid leukemia (AML). These data are summarized in the following table and demonstrate significantly greater complete remission rates for the IDR regimen in two of the three U.S. studies and significantly longer overall survival for the IDR regimen in two of the three U.S. studies.

[See table at bottom of next page]

There is no consensus regarding optional regimens to be used for consolidation; however, the following consolidation regimens were used in U.S. controlled trials. Patients received the same anthracycline for consolidation as was used for induction.

Studies 1 and 3 utilized 2 courses of consolidation therapy consisting of idarubicin 12 or 13 mg/m^2 daily for 2 days, respectively (or DNR 50 or 45 mg/m^2 daily for 2 days), and cytarabine, either 25 mg/m^2 by IV bolus followed by 200 mg/m^2 daily by continuous infusion for 4 days (Study 1), or 100 mg/m^2 daily for 5 days by continuous infusion (Study 3). A rest period of 4 to 6 weeks is recommended prior to initiation of consolidation and between the courses. Hematologic recovery is mandatory prior to initiation of each consolidation course.

Study 2 utilized 3 consolidation courses, administered at intervals of 21 days or upon hematologic recovery. Each course consisted of idarubicin 15 mg/m^2 IV for 1 dose (or DNR 50 mg/m^2 IV for 1 dose), cytarabine 100 mg/m^2 every 12 hours for 10 doses and 6-thioguanine 100 mg/m^2 orally for 10 doses. If severe myelosuppression occurred, subsequent courses were given with 25% reduction in the doses of all drugs. In addition, this study included 4 courses of maintenance therapy (2 days of the same anthracycline as was used in induction and 5 days of cytarabine).

Toxicities and duration of aplasia were similar during induction on the 2 arms in the U.S. studies except for an increase in mucositis on the IDR arm in one study. During consolidation, duration of aplasia on the IDR arm was longer in all three studies and mucositis was more frequent in two studies. During consolidation, transfusion requirements were higher on the IDR arm in the two studies in which they were tabulated, and patients on the IDR arm in Study 3 spent more days on IV antibiotics (Study 3 used a higher dose of idarubicin).

The benefit of consolidation and maintenance therapy in prolonging the duration of remission and survival is not proven.

Intensive maintenance with idarubicin is not recommended in view of the considerable toxicity (including deaths in remission) experienced by patients during the maintenance phase of Study 2.

A higher induction death rate was noted in patients on the IDR arm in the Italian trial. Since this was not noted in patients of similar age in the U.S. trials, one may speculate that it was due to a difference in the level of supportive care.

INDICATIONS AND USAGE

IDAMYCIN PFS Injection in combination with other approved antileukemic drugs is indicated for the treatment of acute myeloid leukemia (AML) in adults. This includes French-American-British (FAB) classifications M1 through M7.

WARNINGS

Idarubicin is intended for administration under the supervision of a physician who is experienced in leukemia chemotherapy.

Idarubicin is a potent bone marrow suppressant. Idarubicin should not be given to patients with pre-existing bone marrow suppression induced by previous drug therapy or radiotherapy unless the benefit warrants the risk.

Severe myelosuppression will occur in all patients given a therapeutic dose of this agent for induction, consolidation or maintenance. Careful hematologic monitoring is required. Deaths due to infection and/or bleeding have been reported during the period of severe myelosuppression. Facilities with laboratory and supportive resources adequate to monitor drug tolerability and protect and maintain a patient compromised by drug toxicity should be available. It must be possible to treat rapidly and completely a severe hemorrhagic condition and/or a severe infection.

Pre-existing heart disease and previous therapy with anthracyclines at high cumulative doses or other potentially cardiotoxic agents are co-factors for increased risk of idarubicin-induced cardiac toxicity and the benefit to risk ratio of idarubicin therapy in such patients should be weighed before starting treatment with idarubicin.

Myocardial toxicity as manifested by potentially fatal congestive heart failure, acute life-threatening arrhythmias or other cardiomyopathies may occur following therapy with idarubicin. Appropriate therapeutic measures for the management of congestive heart failure and/or arrhythmias are indicated.

Cardiac function should be carefully monitored during treatment in order to minimize the risk of cardiac toxicity of the type described for other anthracycline compounds. The risk of such myocardial toxicity may be higher following concomitant or previous radiation to the mediastinal-pericardial area or in patients with anemia, bone marrow depression, infections, leukemic pericarditis and/or myocarditis. While there are no reliable means for predicting congestive heart failure, cardiomyopathy induced by anthracyclines is usually associated with a decrease of the left ventricular ejection fraction (LVEF) from pretreatment baseline values.

Since hepatic and/or renal function impairment can affect the disposition of idarubicin, liver and kidney function should be evaluated with conventional clinical laboratory tests (using serum bilirubin and serum creatinine as indicators) prior to and during treatment. In a number of Phase III clinical trials, treatment was not given if bilirubin and/or creatinine serum levels exceeded 2 mg%. However, in one Phase III trial, patients with bilirubin levels between 2.6 and 5 mg% received the anthracycline with a 50% reduction in dose. Dose reduction of idarubicin should be considered if the bilirubin and/or creatinine levels are above the normal range. (See DOSAGE AND ADMINISTRATION.)

Pregnancy Category D—Idarubicin was embryotoxic and teratogenic in the rat at a dose of 1.2 mg/m^2/day or one tenth the human dose, which was nontoxic to dams. Idarubicin was embryotoxic but not teratogenic in the rabbit even at a dose of 2.4 mg/m^2/day or two tenths the human dose, which was toxic to dams. There is no conclusive information about idarubicin adversely affecting human fertility or causing teratogenesis. There has been one report of a fetal fatality after maternal exposure to idarubicin during the second trimester.

There are no adequate and well-controlled studies in pregnant women. If idarubicin is to be used during pregnancy, or if the patient becomes pregnant during therapy, the patient should be apprised of the potential hazard to the fetus. Women of childbearing potential should be advised to avoid pregnancy.

PRECAUTIONS

General

Therapy with idarubicin requires close observation of the patient and careful laboratory monitoring. Hyperuricemia secondary to rapid lysis of leukemic cells may be induced. Appropriate measures must be taken to prevent hyperuricemia and to control any systemic infection before beginning therapy.

Extravasation of idarubicin can cause severe local tissue necrosis. Extravasation may occur with or without an accompanying stinging or burning sensation even if blood returns well on aspiration of the infusion needle. If signs or symptoms of extravasation occur the injection or infusion should be terminated immediately and restarted in another vein. (See DOSAGE AND ADMINISTRATION.)

Laboratory Tests

Frequent complete blood counts and monitoring of hepatic and renal function tests are recommended.

Carcinogenesis, Mutagenesis, Impairment of Fertility

Formal long-term carcinogenicity studies have not been conducted with idarubicin. Idarubicin and related compounds have been shown to have mutagenic and carcinogenic properties when tested in experimental models (including bacterial systems, mammalian cells in culture and female Sprague-Dawley rats).

In male dogs given 1.8 mg/m^2/day 3 times/week (about one seventh the weekly human dose on a mg/m^2 basis) for 13 weeks, or 3 times the human dose, testicular atrophy was observed with inhibition of spermatogenesis and sperm maturation with few or no mature sperm. These effects were not readily reversed after a recovery of 8 weeks.

Pregnancy Category D

(See WARNINGS.)

Nursing Mothers

It is not known whether this drug is excreted in human milk. Because many drugs are excreted in human milk and because of the potential for serious adverse reactions in nursing infants from idarubicin, mothers should discontinue nursing prior to taking this drug.

Pediatric Use

Safety and effectiveness in children have not been established.

ADVERSE REACTIONS

Approximately 550 patients with AML have received idarubicin in combination with cytarabine in controlled clinical trials worldwide. In addition, over 550 patients with acute leukemia have been treated in uncontrolled trials utilizing idarubicin as a single agent or in combination. The table below lists the adverse experiences reported in U.S. Study 2 (see CLINICAL STUDIES) and is representative of the experiences in other studies. These adverse experiences constitute all reported or observed experiences, including those not considered to be drug related. Patients undergoing induction therapy for AML are seriously ill due to their disease, are receiving multiple transfusions, and concomitant medications including potentially toxic antibiotics and antifungal agents. The contribution of the study drug to the adverse experience profile is difficult to establish.

Induction Phase	Percentage of Patients	
Adverse Experiences	IDR (N=110)	DNR (N=118)
Infection	95%	97%
Nausea & Vomiting	82%	80%
Hair Loss	77%	72%
Abdominal Cramps/Diarrhea	73%	68%
Hemorrhage	63%	65%
Mucositis	50%	55%
Dermatologic	46%	40%
Mental Status	41%	34%
Pulmonary-Clinical	39%	39%
Fever (not elsewhere classified)	26%	28%
Headache	20%	24%
Cardiac-Clinical	16%	24%
Neurologic-Peripheral Nerves	7%	9%
Pulmonary Allergy	2%	4%
Seizure	4%	5%
Cerebellar	4%	4%

The duration of aplasia and incidence of mucositis were greater on the IDR arm than the DNR arm, especially during consolidation in some U.S. controlled trials (see CLINICAL STUDIES).

The following information reflects experience based on U.S. controlled clinical trials.

Myelosuppression

Severe myelosuppression is the major toxicity associated with idarubicin therapy, but this effect of the drug is required in order to eradicate the leukemic clone. During the period of myelosuppression, patients are at risk of developing infection and bleeding which may be life-threatening or fatal.

Gastrointestinal

Nausea and/or vomiting, mucositis, abdominal pain and diarrhea were reported frequently, but were severe (equivalent to WHO Grade 4) in less than 5% of patients. Severe enterocolitis with perforation has been reported rarely. The risk of perforation may be increased by instrumental intervention. The possibility of perforation should be considered in patients who develop severe abdominal pain and appropriate steps for diagnosis and management should be taken.

Dermatologic

Alopecia was reported frequently and dermatologic reactions including generalized rash, urticaria and a bullous erythrodermatous rash of the palms and soles have occurred. The dermatologic reactions were usually attributed to concomitant antibiotic therapy. Local reactions including hives at the injection site have been reported. Recall of skin reaction due to prior radiotherapy has occurred with idarubicin administration.

Hepatic and Renal

Changes in hepatic and renal function tests have been observed. These changes were usually transient and occurred in the setting of sepsis and while patients were receiving potentially hepatotoxic and nephrotoxic antibiotics and antifungal agents. Severe changes in renal function (equivalent to WHO Grade 4) occurred in no more than 1% of patients, while severe changes in hepatic function (equivalent to WHO Grade 4) occurred in less than 5% of patients.

Cardiac

Congestive heart failure (frequently attributed to fluid overload), serious arrhythmias including atrial fibrillation, chest pain, myocardial infarction and asymptomatic declines in LVEF have been reported in patients undergoing induction therapy for AML. Myocardial insufficiency and arrhythmias were usually reversible and occurred in the setting of sepsis, anemia and aggressive intravenous fluid administration. The events were reported more frequently in patients over age 60 years and in those with pre-existing cardiac disease.

OVERDOSAGE

There is no known antidote to idarubicin. Two cases of fatal overdosage in patients receiving therapy for AML have been reported. The doses were 135 mg/m^2 over 3 days and 45 mg/m^2 of idarubicin and 90 mg/m^2 of daunorubicin over a three day period.

It is anticipated that overdosage with idarubicin will result in severe and prolonged myelosuppression and possibly in increased severity of gastrointestinal toxicity. Adequate supportive care including platelet transfusions, antibiotics and symptomatic treatment of mucositis is required. The effect of acute overdose on cardiac function is not fully known, but severe arrhythmia occurred in 1 of the 2 patients exposed. It is anticipated that very high doses of idarubicin may cause acute cardiac toxicity and may be associated with a higher incidence of delayed cardiac failure.

Disposition studies with idarubicin in patients undergoing dialysis have not been carried out. The profound multicompartment behavior, extensive extravascular distribution

Continued on next page

	Induction[a] Regimen Dose in mg/m^2- Daily × 3 Days		Complete Remission Rate, All Pts Randomized		Median Survival (Days) All Pts Randomized	
	IDR	DNR	IDR	DNR	IDR	DNR
U.S. (IND Studies)						
1. MSKCC* (Age ≤ 60 years)	12[b]	50[b]	51/65† (78%)	38/65 (58%)	508†	435
2. SEG** (Age ≥ 15 years)	12[c]	45[c]	76/111† (69%)	65/119 (55%)	328	277
3. U.S. Multicenter (Age ≥ 18 years)	13[c]	45[c]	68/101 (67%)	66/113 (58%)	393†	281
Foreign (non-IND study)						
GIMEMA*** (Age ≥ 55 years)	12[c]	45[c]	49/124 (40%)	49/125 (39%)	87	169

*Memorial Sloan Kettering Cancer Center
**Southeastern Cancer Study Group
***Gruppo Italiano Malattie Ematologiche Maligne dell' Adulto
†Overall $p < 0.05$, unadjusted for prognostic factors or multiple endpoints.
[a]Patients who had persistent leukemia after the first induction course received a second course.
[b]Cytarabine 25 mg/m^2 bolus IV followed by 200 mg/m^2 daily × 5 days by continuous infusion
[c]Cytarabine 100 mg/m^2 daily × 7 days by continuous infusion.

Information on these Pharmacia & Upjohn products is based on labeling in effect June 1, 2000. Further information concerning these and other Pharmacia & Upjohn products may be obtained by direct inquiry to Medical Information, Pharmacia & Upjohn, Kalamazoo, MI 49001.

Idamycin PFS—Cont.

and tissue binding, coupled with the low unbound fraction available in the plasma pool make it unlikely that therapeutic efficacy or toxicity would be altered by conventional peritoneal or hemodialysis.

DOSAGE AND ADMINISTRATION (See WARNINGS)

For induction therapy in adult patients with AML the following dose schedule is recommended:

IDAMYCIN PFS Injection 12 mg/m^2 daily for 3 days by slow (10 to 15 min) intravenous injection in combination with cytarabine. The cytarabine may be given as 100 mg/m^2 daily by continuous infusion for 7 days or as cytarabine 25 mg/m^2 intravenous bolus followed by cytarabine 200 mg/m^2 daily for 5 days continuous infusion. In patients with unequivocal evidence of leukemia after the first induction course, a second course may be administered. Administration of the second course should be delayed in patients who experience severe mucositis, until recovery from this toxicity has occurred, and a dose reduction of 25% is recommended. In patients with hepatic and/or renal impairment, a dose reduction of IDAMYCIN PFS should be considered. IDAMYCIN PFS should not be administered if the bilirubin level exceeds 5 mg%. (See WARNINGS.)

The benefit of consolidation in prolonging the duration of remissions and survival is not proven. There is no consensus regarding optional regimens to be used for consolidation. (See CLINICAL STUDIES for doses used in U.S. Clinical studies.)

Preparation and Administration Precautions

Caution in handling the solution must be exercised as skin reactions associated with IDAMYCIN PFS may occur. Skin accidentally exposed to IDAMYCIN PFS should be washed thoroughly with soap and water and if the eyes are involved, standard irrigation techniques should be used immediately. The use of goggles, gloves, and protective gowns is recommended during preparation and administration of the drug.

Care in the administration of IDAMYCIN PFS will reduce the chance of perivenous infiltration. It may also decrease the chance of local reactions such as urticaria and erythematous streaking. During intravenous administration of IDAMYCIN PFS extravasation may occur with or without an accompanying stinging or burning sensation even if blood returns well on aspiration of the infusion needle. If any signs or symptoms of extravasation have occurred, the injection or infusion should be immediately terminated and restarted in another vein. If it is known or suspected that subcutaneous extravasation has occurred, it is recommended that intermittent ice packs (1/2 hour immediately, then 1/2 hour 4 times per day for 3 days) be placed over the area of extravasation and that the affected extremity be elevated. Because of the progressive nature of extravasation reactions, the area of injection should be frequently examined and plastic surgery consultation obtained early if there is any sign of a local reaction such as pain, erythema, edema or vesication. If ulceration begins or there is severe persistent pain at the site of extravasation, early wide excision of the involved area should be considered.[1]

IDAMYCIN PFS should be administered slowly (over 10 to 15 minutes) into the tubing of a freely running intravenous infusion of Sodium Chloride Injection, USP (0.9%) or 5% Dextrose Injection, USP. The tubing should be attached to a Butterfly needle or other suitable device and inserted preferably into a large vein.

Incompatibility

Unless specific compatibility data are available, IDAMYCIN PFS should not be mixed with other drugs. Precipitation occurs with heparin. Prolonged contact with any solution of an alkaline pH will result in degradation of the drug. Parenteral drug products should be inspected visually for particulate matter and discoloration prior to administration whenever solution and containers permit.

Handling and Disposal—Procedures for handling and disposal of anticancer drugs should be considered. Several guidelines on this subject have been published.[2–8] There is no general agreement that all of the procedures recommended in the guidelines are necessary or appropriate.

HOW SUPPLIED

IDAMYCIN PFS Injection (idarubicin hydrochloride injection)

Single Dose Vials: Sterile single use only, contains no preservative.

NDC 0013-2536-78 5 mg vial, 1 mg/mL, 5 mL, 5 vial packs.
NDC 0013-2546-86 10 mg vial, 1 mg/mL, 10 mL, single vials.
NDC 0013-2556-67 20 mg vial, 1 mg/mL, 20 mL, single vials.

Single Dose Cytosafe™ Vials: Sterile single use only, contains no preservative.

NDC 0013-2576-91 5 mg vial, 1 mg/mL, 5 mL, single vials.
NDC 0013-2586-91 10 mg vial, 1 mg/mL, 10 mL, single vials.
NDC 0013-2596-91 20 mg vial, 1 mg/mL, 20 mL, single vials.

Store under refrigeration 2° to 8°C (36° to 46°F), and protect from light. Retain in carton until time of use.

Rx only

Manufactured by:
Pharmacia & Upjohn S.p.A.
Milan, Italy

For:
Pharmacia & Upjohn Company
Kalamazoo, MI 49001, USA

REFERENCES

1. Rudolph R, Larson DL: Etiology and Treatment of Chemotherapeutic Agent Extravasation Injuries: A Review. J Clin Oncol 5: 1116-1126, 1987.
2. Recommendations for the Safe Handling of Parenteral Antineoplastic Drugs. NIH Publication No. 83-2621. For sale by the Superintendent of Documents, US Government Printing Office, Washington, DC 20402.
3. AMA Council Report, Guidelines for Handling Parenteral Antineoplastics, JAMA. 1985; 253 (11): 1590-1592.
4. National Study Commission on Cytotoxic Exposure-Recommendations for Handling Cytotoxic Agents. Available from Louis P. Jeffrey, Sc.D., Chairman, National Study Commission on Cytotoxic Exposure, Massachusetts College of Pharmacy and Allied Health Sciences, 179 Longwood Avenue, Boston, Massachusetts 02115.
5. Clinical Oncological Society of Australia. Guidelines and Recommendations for Safe Handling of Antineoplastic Agents. Med J Australia. 1983; 1:426-428.
6. Jones RB, et al: Safe Handling of Chemotherapeutic Agents: A Report from the Mount Sinai Medical Center. CA-A Cancer Journal for Clinicians. 1983; (Sept/Oct) 258-263.
7. American Society of Hospital Pharmacists Technical Assistance Bulletin on Handling Cytotoxic and Hazardous Drugs. Am J Hosp Pharm. 1990; 47:1033-1049.
8. OSHA Work-Practice Guidelines for Personnel Dealing with Cytotoxic (Antineoplastic) Drugs. Am J Hosp Pharm. 1986; 43:1193-1204.

817 166 204 Revised June 2000
N.224295407.01.0

MIRAPEX® ℞

[*mĭr-ă-pex*]
pramipexole
dihydrochloride tablets

DESCRIPTION

MIRAPEX Tablets contain pramipexole, a dopamine agonist indicated for the treatment of the signs and symptoms of idiopathic Parkinson's disease. The chemical name of pramipexole dihydrochloride is (*S*)-2-amino-4,5,6,7-tetrahydro-6-(propylamino)benzothiazole dihydrochloride monohydrate. Its empirical formula is $C_{10}H_{17}N_3S \bullet 2\ HCl \bullet H_2O$, and its molecular weight is 302.27.

The structural formula is:

Pramipexole dihydrochloride is a white to off-white powder substance. Melting occurs in the range of 296°C to 301°C, with decomposition. Pramipexole dihydrochloride is more than 20% soluble in water, about 8% in methanol, about 0.5% in ethanol, and practically insoluble in dichloromethane.

MIRAPEX Tablets, for oral administration, contain 0.125 mg, 0.25 mg, 0.5 mg, 1.0 mg, or 1.5 mg of pramipexole dihydrochloride monohydrate. Inactive ingredients consist of mannitol, corn starch, colloidal silicon dioxide, povidone, and magnesium stearate.

CLINICAL PHARMACOLOGY

Pramipexole is a nonergot dopamine agonist with high relative in vitro specificity and full intrinsic activity at the D_2 subfamily of dopamine receptors, binding with higher affinity to D_3 than to D_2 or D_4 receptor subtypes. The relevance of D_3 receptor binding in Parkinson's disease is unknown.

The precise mechanism of action of pramipexole as a treatment for Parkinson's disease is unknown, although it is believed to be related to its ability to stimulate dopamine receptors in the striatum. This conclusion is supported by electrophysiologic studies in animals that have demonstrated that pramipexole influences striatal neuronal firing rates via activation of dopamine receptors in the striatum and the substantia nigra, the site of neurons that send projections to the striatum.

Pharmacokinetics

Pramipexole is rapidly absorbed, reaching peak concentrations in approximately 2 hours. The absolute bioavailability of pramipexole is greater than 90%, indicating that it is well absorbed an undergoes little presystemic metabolism. Food does not affect the extent of pramipexole absorption, although the time of maximum plasma concentration (T_{max}) is increased by about 1 hour when the drug is taken with a meal.

Pramipexole is extensively distributed, having a volume of distribution of about 500 L (coefficient of variation [CV]=20%). It is about 15% bound to plasma proteins. Pramipexole distributes into red blood cells as indicated by an erythrocyte-to-plasma ratio of approximately 2.

Pramipexole displays linear pharmacokinetics over the clinical dose range. Its terminal half-life is about 8 hours in young healthy volunteers and about 12 hours in elderly volunteers (see CLINICAL PHARMACOLOGY, Pharmacokinetics in Special Population). Steady-state concentrations are achieved within 2 days of dosing.

Metabolism and elimination: Urinary excretion is the major route of pramipexole elimination, with 90% of a pramipexole dose recovered in urine, almost all as unchanged drug. Nonrenal routes may contribute to a small extent to pramipexole elimination, although no metabolites have been identified in plasma or urine. The renal clearance of pramipexole is approximately 400 mL/min (CV=25%), approximately three times higher than the glomerular filtration rate. Thus, pramipexole is secreted by the renal tubules, probably by the organic cation transport system.

Pharmacokinetics in Special Populations

Because therapy with pramipexole is initiated at a subtherapeutic dosage and gradually titrated upward according to clinical tolerability to obtain the optimum therapeutic effect, adjustment of the initial dose based on gender, weight, or age is not necessary. However, renal insufficiency, which can cause a large decrease in the ability to eliminate pramipexole, may necessitate dosage adjustment (see CLINICAL PHARMACOLOGY, Renal Insufficiency).

Gender: Pramipexole clearance is about 30% lower in women than in men, but most of this difference can be accounted for by differences in body weight. There is no difference in half-life between males and females.

Age: Pramipexole clearance decreases with age as the half-life and clearance are about 40% longer and 30% lower, respectively, in elderly (aged 65 years or older) compared with young healthy volunteers (aged less than 40 years). This difference is most likely due to the well-known reduction in renal function with age, since pramipexole clearance is correlated with renal function, as measured by creatinine clearance (see CLINICAL PHARMACOLOGY, Renal Insufficiency).

Parkinson's disease patients: A cross-study comparison of data suggests that the clearance of pramipexole may be reduced by about 30% in Parkinson's disease patients compared with healthy elderly volunteers. The reason for this difference appears to be reduced renal function in Parkinson's disease patients, which may be related to their poorer general health. The pharmacokinetics of pramipexole were comparable between early and advanced Parkinson's disease patients.

Pediatric: The pharmacokinetics of pramipexole in the pediatric population have not been evaluated.

Hepatic insufficiency: The influence of hepatic insuffficency on pramipexole pharmacokinetics has not been evaluated. Because approximately 90% of the recovered dose is excreted in the urine as unchanged drug, hepatic impairment would not be expected to have a significant effect on pramipexole elimination.

Renal insufficiency: The clearance of pramipexole was about 75% lower in patients with severe renal impairment (creatinine clearance approximately 20 mL/min) and about 60% lower in patients with moderate impairment (creatinine clearance approximately 40 mL/min) compared with healthy volunteers. A lower starting and maintenance dose is recommended in these patients (see PRECAUTIONS and DOSAGE AND ADMINISTRATION). In patients with varying degrees of renal impairment, pramipexole clearance correlates well with creatinine clearance. Therefore, creatinine clearance can be used as a predictor of the extent of decrease in pramipexole clearance. Pramipexole clearance is extremely low in dialysis patients, as a negligible amount of pramipexole is removed by dialysis. Caution should be exercised when administering pramipexole to patients with renal disease.

CLINICAL STUDIES

The effectiveness of MIRAPEX Tablets in the treatment of Parkinson's disease was evaluated in a multinational drug development program consisting of seven randomized, controlled trials. Three were conducted in patients with early Parkinson's disease who were not receiving concomitant levodopa, and four were conducted in patients with advanced Parkinson's disease who were receiving concomitant levodopa. Among these seven studies, three studies provide the most persuasive evidence of pramipexole's effectiveness in the management of patients with Parkinson's disease who were and were not receiving concomitant levodopa. Two of these three trials enrolled patients with early Parkinson's disease (not receiving levodopa), and one enrolled patients with advanced Parkinson's disease who were receiving maximally tolerated doses of levodopa.

In all studies, the Unified Parkinson's Disease Rating Scale (UPDRS), or one or more of its subparts, served as the primary outcome assessment measure. The UPDRS in a four-part multi-item rating scale intended to evaluate mentation (part I), activities of daily living (part II), motor performance (part III), and complications of therapy (part IV).

Part II of the UPDRS contains 13 questions relating to activities of daily living (ADL), which are scored from 0 (normal) to 4 (maximal severity) for a maximum (worst) score of 52. Part III of the UPDRS contains 27 questions (for 14 items) and is scored as described for part II. It is designed to assess the severity of the cardinal motor findings in patients with Parkinson's disease (eg, tremor, rigidity, bradykinesia, postural instability, etc), scored for different body regions, and has a maximum (worst) score of 108.

Studies in Patients With Early Parkinson's Disease

Patients (N=599) in the two studies of early Parkinson's disease had a mean disease duration of 2 years, limited or no prior exposure to levodopa (generally none in the preceding 6 months), and were not experiencing the "on-off" phenomenon and dyskinesia characteristic of later stages of the disease.

One of the two early Parkinson's disease studies (N=335) was a double-blind, placebo-controlled, parallel trial consisting of a 7-week dose-escalation period and a 6-month maintenance period. Patients could be on selegiline, anticholinergics, or both, but could not be on levodopa products or amantadine. Patients were randomized to MIRAPEX or placebo. Patients treated with MIRAPEX had a starting daily dose of 0.375 mg were titrated to a maximally tolerated dose, but no higher than 4.5 mg/day in three divided doses. At the end of the 6-month maintenance period, the mean improvement from baseline on the UPDRS part II (ADL) total score was 1.9 in the group receiving MIRAPEX and -0.4 in the placebo group, a difference that was statistically significant. The mean improvement from baseline on the UPDRS part III total score was 5.0 in the group receiving MIRAPEX and -0.8 in the placebo group, a difference that was also statistically significant. A statistically significant difference between groups in favor of MIRAPEX was seen beginning at week 2 of the UPDRS part II (maximum dose 0.75 mg/day) and at week 3 of the UPDRS part III (maximum dose 1.5 mg/day).

The second early Parkinson's disease study (N=264) was a double-blind, placebo-controlled, parallel trial consisting of a 6-week dose-escalation period and a 4-week maintenance period. Patients could be on selegiline, anticholinergics, amantadine, or any combination of these, but could not be on levodopa products. Patients were randomized to 1 of 4 fixed doses of MIRAPEX (1.5 mg, 3.0 mg, 4.5 mg, or 6.0 mg per day) or placebo. At the end of the 4-week maintenance period, the mean improvement from baseline on the UPDRS part II total score was 1.8 in the patients treated with MIRAPEX, regardless of assigned dose group, and 0.3 in placebo-treated patients. The mean improvement from baseline on the UPDRS part III total score was 4.2 in patients treated with MIRAPEX and 0.6 in placebo-treated patients.

No dose-response relationship was demonstrated. The between-treated differences on both parts of the UPDRS were statistically significant in favor of MIRAPEX for all doses.

No differences in effectiveness based on age or gender were detected. There were too few non-Caucasian patients to evaluate the effect of race. Patients receiving selegiline or anticholinergics had responses similar to patients not receiving these drugs.

Studies in Patients With Advanced Parkinson's Disease

In the advanced Parkinson's disease study, the primary assessments were the UPDRS and daily diaries that quantified amounts of "on" and "off" time.

Patients in the advanced Parkinson's disease study (N=360) had a mean disease duration of 9 years, had been exposed to levodopa for long periods of time (mean 8 years), used concomitant levodopa during the trial, and had "on-off" periods.

The advanced Parkinson's disease study was a double-blind, placebo-controlled, parallel trial consisting of a 7-week dose-escalation period and a 6-month maintenance period. Patients were all treated with concomitant levodopa products and could additionally be on concomitant selegiline, anticholinergics, amantadine, or any combination. Patients treated with MIRAPEX had a starting dose of 0.375 mg/day and were titrated to a maximally tolerated dose, but no higher than 4.5 mg/day in three divided doses. At selected times during the 6-month maintenance period, patients were asked to record the amount of "off," "on," or "on with dyskinesia" time per day for several sequential days. At the end of the 6-month maintenance period, the mean improvement from baseline on the UPDRS part II total score was 2.7 in the group treated with MIRAPEX and 0.5 in the placebo group, a difference that was statistically significant. The mean improvement from baseline on the UPDRS part III total score was 5.6 in the group treated with MIRAPEX and 2.8 in the placebo group, a different that was statistically significant. A statistically significant difference between groups in favor of MIRAPEX was seen at week 3 of the UPDRS part II (maximum dose 1.5 mg/day) and at week 2 of the UPDRS part III (maximum dose 0.75 mg/day). Dosage reduction of levodopa was allowed during this study if dyskinesia (or hallucinations) developed; levodopa dosage reduction occurred in 76% of patients treated with MIRAPEX versus 54% of placebo patients. On average, the levodopa dose was reduced 27%.

The mean number of "off" hours per day during baseline was 6 hours for both treatment groups. Throughout the trial, patients treated with MIRAPEX had a mean of 4 "off" hours per day, while placebo-treated patients continued to experience 6 "off" hours per day.

No differences in effectiveness based on age or gender were detected. There were too few non-Caucasian patients to evaluate the effect of race.

INDICATIONS AND USAGE

MIRAPEX Tablets are indicated for the treatment of the signs and symptoms of idiopathic Parkinson's disease.

The effectiveness of MIRAPEX was demonstrated in randomized, controlled trials in patients with early Parkinson's disease who were not receiving concomitant levodopa therapy as well as in patients with advanced disease on concomitant levodopa (see CLINICAL STUDIES).

CONTRAINDICATIONS

MIRAPEX Tablets are contraindicated in patients who have demonstrated hypersensitivity to the drug or its ingredients.

WARNINGS

Falling Asleep During Activities of Daily Living:

Patients treated with MIRAPEX have reported falling asleep while engaged in activities of daily living, including the operation of motor vehicles which sometimes resulted in accidents. Although many of these patients reported somnolence while on MIRAPEX, some perceived that they had no warning signs such as excessive drowsiness, and believed that they were alert immediately prior to the event. Some of these events had been reported as late as one year after the initiation of treatment.

Somnolence is a common occurrence in patients receiving MIRAPEX at doses above 1.5 mg/day. Many clinical experts believe that falling asleep while engaged in activities of daily living always occurs in a setting of preexisting somnolence, although patients may not give such a history. For this reason, prescribers should continually reassess patients for drowsiness or sleepiness, especially since some of the events occur well after the start of treatment. Prescribers should also be aware that patients may not acknowledge drowsiness or sleepiness until directly questioned about drowsiness or sleepiness during specific activities.

Before initiating treatment with MIRAPEX, patients should be advised of the potential to develop drowsiness and specifically asked about factors that may increase the risk with MIRAPEX such as concomitant sedating medications, the presence of sleep disorders, and concomitant medications that increase pramipexole plasma levels (e.g., cimetidine—see PRECAUTIONS, Drug Interactions). If a patient develops significant daytime sleepiness or episodes of falling asleep during activities that require active participation (e.g., conversations, eating. etc.), MIRAPEX should ordinarily be discontinued. If a decision is made to continue MIRAPEX, patients should be advised to not drive and to avoid other potentially dangerous activities. While dose reduction clearly reduces the degree of somnolence, there is insufficient information to establish that dose reduction will eliminate episodes of falling asleep while engaged in activities of daily living.

Symptomatic Hypotension: Dopamine agonists, in clinical studies and clinical experience, appear to impair the systemic regulation of blood pressure, with resulting orthostatic hypotension, especially during dose escalation. Parkinson's disease patients, in addition, appear to have an impaired capacity to respond to an orthostatic challenge. For these reasons, Parkinson's disease patients being treated with dopaminergic agonists ordinarily require careful monitoring for signs and symptoms of orthostatic hypotension, especially during dose escalation, and should be informed of this risk (see PRECAUTIONS, Information for Patients).

In clinical trials of pramipexole, however, and despite clear orthostatic effects in normal volunteers, the reported incidence of clinically significant orthostatic hypotension was not greater among those assigned to MIRAPEX Tablets than among those assigned to placebo. This result is clearly unexpected in light of the previous experience with the risks of dopamine agonist therapy.

While this finding could result a unique property of pramipexole, it might also be explained by the conditions of the study and the nature of the population enrolled in the clinical trials. Patients were very carefully titrated, and patients with active cardiovascular disease or significant orthostatic hypotension at baseline were excluded.

Hallucinations: In the three double-blind, placebo-controlled trials in early Parkinson's disease, hallucinations were observed in 9% (35 of 388) of patients receiving MIRAPEX, compared with 2.6% (6 of 235) of patients receiving placebo. In the four double-blind, placebo-controlled trials in advanced Parkinson's disease, where patients received MIRAPEX and concomitant levodopa, hallucinations were observed in 16.5% (43 of 260) patients receiving MIRAPEX compared with 3.8% (10 of 264) of patients receiving placebo. Hallucinations were of sufficient severity to cause discontinuation of treatment in 3.1% of the early Parkinson's disease patients and 2.7% of the advanced Parkinson's disease patients compared with about 0.4% of placebo patients in both populations.

Age appears to increase the risk of hallucinations attributable to pramipexole. In the early Parkinson's disease patients, the risk of hallucinations was 1.9 times greater than placebo in patients younger than 65 years and 6.8 times greater than placebo in patients older than 65 years. In the advanced Parkinson's disease patients, the risk of hallucinations was 3.5 times greater than placebo in patients younger than 65 years and 5.2 times greater than placebo in patients older than 65 years.

PRECAUTIONS

Rhabdomyolysis: A single case of rhabdomyolysis occurred in a 49-year-old male with advanced Parkinson's disease treated with MIRAPEX Tablets. The patient was hospitalized with an elevated CPK (10,631 IU/L). The symptoms resolved with discontinuation of the medication.

Renal: Since pramipexole is eliminated through the kidneys, caution should be exercised when prescribing MIRAPEX to patients with renal insufficiency (see DOSAGE AND ADMINISTRATION).

Dyskinesia: MIRAPEX may potentiate the dopaminergic side effects of levodopa and may cause or exacerbate preexisting dyskinesia. Decreasing the dose of levodopa may ameliorate this side effect.

Retinal pathology in albino rats: Pathologic changes (degeneration and loss of photoreceptor cells) were observed in the retina of albino rats in the 2-year carcinogenicity study. Evaluation of the retinas of albino mice, pigmented rats, monkeys, and minipigs did not reveal similar changes. The potential significance of this effect in humans has not been established, but cannot be disregarded because disruption of a mechanism that is universally present in vertebrates (ie, disk shedding) may be involved (see ANIMAL TOXICOLOGY).

Events Reported With Dopaminergic Therapy

Although the events enumerated below have not been reported in association with the use of pramipexole in its development program, they are associated with the use of other dopaminergic drugs. The expected incidence of these events, however, is so low that even if pramipexole caused these events at rates similar to those attributable to other dopaminergic therapies, it would be unlikely that even a single case would have occurred in a cohort of the size exposed to pramipexole in studies to date.

Withdrawal-emergent hyperpyrexia and confusion: Although not reported with pramipexole in the clinical development program, a symptom complex resembling the neuroleptic malignant syndrome (characterized by elevated temperature, muscular rigidity, altered consciousness, and autonomic instability), with no other obvious etiology, has been reported in association with rapid dose reduction, withdrawal of, or changes in antiparkinsonian therapy.

Fibrotic complications: Although not reported with pramipexole in the clinical development program, cases of retroperitoneal fibrosis, pulmonary infiltrates, pleural effusion, and pleural thickening have been reported in some patients treated with ergot-derived dopaminergic agents. While these complications may resolve when the drug is discontinued, complete resolution does not always occur.

Although these adverse events are believed to be related to the ergoline structure to these compounds, whether other, nonergot derived dopamine agonists can cause them is unknown.

Information for Patients: Patients should be instructed to take MIRAPEX only as prescribed.

Patients should be alerted to the potential sedating effects associated with MIRAPEX, including somnolence and the possibility of falling asleep while engaged in activities of daily living. Since somnolence is a frequent adverse event with potentially serious consequences, patients should neither drive a car nor engage in other potentially dangerous activities until they have gained sufficient experience with MIRAPEX to gauge whether or not it affects their mental and/or motor performance adversely. Patients should be advised that if increased somnolence or new episodes of falling asleep during activities of daily living (e.g., watching television, passenger in a car, etc.) are experienced at any time during treatment, they should not drive or participate in potentially dangerous activities until they have contacted their physician. Because of possible additive effects, caution should be advised when patients are taking other sedating medications or alcohol in combination with MIRAPEX and when taking concomitant medications that increase plasma levels of pramipexole (e.g., cimetidine).

Patients should be informed that hallucinations can occur and that the elderly are at a higher risk than younger patients with Parkinson's disease.

Patients may develop postural (orthostatic) hypotension, with or without symptoms such as dizziness, nausea, fainting or blackouts, and sometimes, sweating. Hypotension may occur more frequently during initial therapy. Accordingly, patients should be cautioned against rising rapidly after sitting or lying down, especially if they have been doing so for prolonged periods and especially at the initiation of treatment with MIRAPEX.

Because the teratogenic potential of pramipexole has not been completely established in laboratory animals, and because experience in humans is limited, patients should be advised to notify their physicians if they become pregnant or intend to because pregnant during therapy (see PRECAUTIONS, Pregnancy).

Because of the possibility that pramipexole may be excreted in breast milk, patients should be advised to notify their physicians if they intend to breast-feed or are breast-feeding an infant.

If patients develop nausea, they should be advised that taking MIRAPEX with food may reduce the occurrence of nausea.

Laboratory Tests: During the development of MIRAPEX, no systematic abnormalities on routine laboratory testing were noted. Therefore, no specific guidance is offered regarding routine monitoring; the practitioner retains responsibility for determining how best to monitor the patient in his or her care.

Drug Interactions

Carbidopa/levodopa: Carbidopa/levodopa did not influence the pharmacokinetics of pramipexole in healthy volunteers (N=10). Pramipexole did not alter the extent of absorption (AUC) or the elimination of carbidopa/levodopa, although it caused an increase in levodopa C_{max} by about 40% and a decrease in T_{max} from 2.5 to 0.5 hours.

Selegiline: In healthy volunteers (N=11), selegiline did not influence the pharmacokinetics of pramipexole.

Amantadine: Population pharmacokinetic analysis suggests that amantadine is unlikely to alter the oral clearance of pramipexole (N=54).

Continued on next page

Information on these Pharmacia & Upjohn products is based on labeling in effect June 1, 2000. Further information concerning these and other Pharmacia & Upjohn products may be obtained by direct inquiry to Medical Information, Pharmacia & Upjohn, Kalamazoo, MI 49001.

Mirapex—Cont.

Cimetidine: Cimetidine, a known inhibitor of renal tubular secretion of organic bases via the cationic transport system, caused a 50% increase in pramipexole AUC and a 40% increase in half-life (N=12).

Probenecid: Probenecid, a known inhibitor of renal tubular secretion of organic acids via the anionic transporter, did not noticeably influence pramipexole pharmacokinetics (N=12).

Other drugs eliminated via renal secretion: Population pharmcokinetic analysis suggests that coadministration of drugs that are secreted by the cationic transport system (eg, cimetidine, ranitidine, diltiazem, triamterene, verapamil, quinidine, and quinine) decreases the oral clearance of pramipexole by about 20%, while those secreted by the anionic transport system (eg, cephalosporins, penicillins, indomethacin, hydrochlorothiazide, and chlorpropamide) are likely to have little effect on the oral clearance of pramipexole.

CYP interactions: Inhibitors of cytochrome P450 enzymes would not be expected to affect pramipexole elimination because pramipexole is not appreciably metabolized by these enzymes in vivo or in vitro. Pramipexole does not inhibit CYP enzymes CYP1A2, CYP2C9, CYP2C19, CYP2E1, and CYP3A4. Inhibition of CYP2D6 was observed with an apparent Ki of 30 µM, indicating that pramipexole will not inhibit CYP enzymes at plasma concentrations observed following the highest recommended clinical dose (1.5 mg tid).

Dopamine antagonists: Since pramipexole is a dopamine agonist, it is possible that dopamine antagonists, such as the neuroleptics (phenothiazines, butyrophenones, thioxanthenes) or metoclopramide, may diminish the effectiveness of MIRAPEX.

Drug/Laboratory Test Interactions: There are no known interactions between MIRAPEX and laboratory tests.

Carcinogenesis, Mutagenesis, Impairment of Fertility: Two-year carcinogenicity studies with pramipexole have been conducted in mice and rats. Pramipexole was administered in the diet to Chbb:NMRI mice at doses of 0.3, 2, and 10 mg/kg/day (0.3, 2.2, and 11 times the highest recommended clinical dose [1.5 mg tid] on a mg/m^2 basis). Pramipexole was administered in the diet to Wistar rats at 0.3, 2, and 8 mg/kg/day (plasma AUCs equal to 0.3, 2.5, and 12.5 times the AUC in humans receiving 1.5 mg tid). No significant increases in tumors occurred in either species.

Pramipexole was not mutagenic or clastogenic in a battery of assays, including the in vitro Ames assay, V79 gene mutation assay for HGPRT mutants, chromosomal aberration assay in Chinese hamster ovary cells, and in vivo mouse micronucleus assay.

In rat fertility studies, pramipexole at a dose of 2.5 mg/kg/day (5.4 times the highest clinical dose on a mg/m^2 basis), prolonged estrus cycles and inhibited implantation. These effects were associated with reductions in serum levels of prolactin, a hormone necessary for implantation and maintenance of early pregnancy in rats.

Pregnancy: Pregnancy Category C. When pramipexole was given to female rats throughout pregnancy, implantation was inhibited at a dose of 2.5 mg/kg/day (5.4 times the highest clinical dose on a mg/m^2 basis). Administration of 1.5 mg/kg/day of pramipexole to pregnant rats during the period of organogenesis (gestation days 7 through 16) resulted in a high incidence of total resorption of embryos. The plasma AUC in rats dosed at this level was 4.3 times the AUC in humans receiving 1.5 mg tid. These findings are thought to be due to the prolactin-lowering effect of pramipexole, since prolactin is necessary for implantation and maintenance of early pregnancy in rats (but not rabbits or humans). Because of pregnancy disruption and early embryonic loss in these studies, the teratogenic potential of pramipexole could not be adequately evaluated. There was no evidence of adverse effects on embryo-fetal development following administration of up to 10 mg/kg/day to pregnant rabbits during organogenesis (plasma AUC was 71 times that in humans receiving 1.5 tid). Postnatal growth was inhibited in the offspring of rats treated with 0.5 mg/kg/day (approximately equivalent to the highest clinical dose on a mg/m^2 basis) or greater during the latter part of pregnancy and throughout lactation.

There are no studies of pramipexole in human pregnancy. Because animal reproduction studies are not always predictive of human response, pramipexole should be used during pregnancy only if the potential benefit outweighs the potential risk to the fetus.

Nursing Mothers: A single-dose, radio-labeled study showed that drug-related materials were excreted into the breast milk of lactating rats. Concentrations of radioactivity in milk were three to six times higher than concentrations in plasma at equivalent time points.

Other studies have shown that pramipexole treatment resulted in an inhibition of prolactin secretion in humans and rats.

It is not known whether this drug is excreted in human milk. Because many drugs are excreted in human milk and because of the potential for serious adverse reactions in nursing infants from pramipexole, a decision should be made as to whether to discontinue nursing or to discontinue the drug, taking into account the importance of the drug to the mother.

Pediatric Use: The safety and efficacy of MIRAPEX in pediatric patients has not been established.

Geriatric Use: Pramipexole total oral clearance was approximately 30% lower in subjects older than 65 years compared with younger subjects, because of a decline in pramipexole renal clearance due to an age-related reduction in renal function. This resulted in an increase in elimination half-life from approximately 8.5 hours to 12 hours. In clinical studies, 38.7% of patients were older than 65 years. There were no apparent differences in efficacy or safety between older and younger patients, except that the relative risk of hallucination associated with the use of MIRAPEX was increased in the elderly.

ADVERSE EVENTS

During the premarketing development of pramipexole, patients with either early or advanced Parkinson's disease were enrolled in clinical trials. Apart from the severity and duration of their disease, the two populations differed in their use of concomitant levodopa therapy. Patients with early disease did not receive concomitant levodopa therapy during treatment with pramipexole; those with advanced Parkinson's disease all received concomitant levodopa treatment. Because these two populations may have differential risks for various adverse events, this section will, in general, present adverse-event data for these two populations separately.

Because the controlled trials performed during premarketing development all used a titration design, with a resultant confounding of time and dose, it was impossible to adequately evaluate the effects of dose on the incidence of adverse events.

Early Parkinson's Disease

In the three double-blind, placebo-controlled trials of patients with early Parkinson's disease, the most commonly observed adverse events (>5%) that were numerically more frequent in the group treated with MIRAPEX Tablets were nausea, dizziness, somnolence, insomnia, constipation, asthenia, and hallucinations.

Approximately 12% of 388 patients with early Parkinson's disease and treated with MIRAPEX who participated in the double-blind, placebo-controlled trials discontinued treatment due to adverse events compared with 11% of 235 patients who received placebo. The adverse events most commonly causing discontinuation of treatment were related to the nervous system (hallucinations [3.1% on MIRAPEX vs 0.4% on placebo]; dizziness [2.1% on MIRAPEX vs 1% on placebo]; somnolence [1.6% on MIRAPEX vs 0% on placebo]; extrapyramidal syndrome [1.6% on MIRAPEX vs 6.4% on placebo]; headache and confusion [1.3% and 1.0%, respectively, on MIRAPEX vs 0% on placebo]); and gastrointestinal system (nausea [2.1% on MIRAPEX vs 0.4% on placebo]).

Adverse-event incidence in controlled clinical studies in early Parkinson's disease: Table 1 lists treatment-emergent adverse events that occurred in the double-blind, placebo-controlled studies in early Parkinson's disease that were reported by ≥1% of patients treated with MIRAPEX and were numerically more frequent than in the placebo group. In these studies, patients did not receive concomitant levodopa. Adverse events were usually mild or moderate in intensity.

The prescriber should be aware that these figures cannot be used to predict the incidence of adverse events in the course of usual medical practice where patient characteristics and other factors differ from those that prevailed in the clinical studies. Similarly, the cited frequencies cannot be compared with figures obtained from other clinical investigations involving different treatments, uses, and investigators. However, the cited figures do provide the prescribing physician with some basis for estimating the relative contribution of drug and nondrug factors to the adverse-event incidence rate in the population studied.

Table 1
Treatment-Emergent Adverse-Event* Incidence in Double-Blind, Placebo-Controlled Trials in Early Parkinson's Disease (Events ≥1% of Patients Treated With MIRAPEX and Numerically More Frequent Than in the Placebo Group)

Body System/ Adverse Event	MIRAPEX N=388	Placebo N=235
Body as a Whole		
Asthenia	14	12
General edema	5	3
Malaise	2	1
Reaction unevaluable	2	1
Fever	1	0
Digestive System		
Nausea	28	18
Constipation	14	6
Anorexia	4	2
Dysphagia	2	0
Metabolic & Nutritional System		
Peripheral edema	5	4
Decreased weight	2	0
Nervous System		
Dizziness	25	24
Somnolence	22	9
Insomnia	17	12
Hallucinations	9	3
Confusion	4	1
Amnesia	4	2
Hypesthesia	3	1
Dystonia	2	1
Akathisia	2	0
Thinking abnormalities	2	0
Decreased libido	1	0
Myoclonus	1	0
Special Senses		
Vision abnormalities	3	0
Urogenital System		
Impotence	2	1

*Patients may have reported multiple adverse experiences during the study or at discontinuation; thus, patients may be included in more than one category.

Other events reported by 1% or more of patients with early Parkinson's disease and treated with MIRAPEX but reported equally or more frequently in the placebo group were infection, accidental injury, headache, pain, tremor, back pain, syncope, postural hypotension, hypertonia, depression, abdominal pain, anxiety, dyspepsia, flatulence, diarrhea, rash, ataxia, dry mouth, extrapyramidal syndrome, leg cramps, twitching, pharyngitis, sinusitis, sweating, rhinitis, urinary tract infection, vasodilation, flu syndrome, increased saliva, tooth disease, dyspnea, increased cough, gait abnormalities, urinary frequency, vomiting, allergic reaction, hypertension, pruritis, hypokinesia, increased creatine PK, nervousness, dream abnormalities, chest pain, neck pain, paresthesia, tachycardia, vertigo, voice alteration, conjunctivitis, paralysis, accommodation abnormalities, tinnitus, diplopia, and taste perversions.

In a fixed-dose study in early Parkinson's disease, occurrence of the following events increased in frequency as the dose increased over the range from 1.5 mg/day to 6 mg/day: postural hypotension, nausea, constipation, somnolence, and amnesia. The frequency of these events was generally 2-fold greater than placebo for pramipexole doses greater than 3 mg/day. The incidence of somnolence with pramipexole at a dose of 1.5 mg/day was comparable to that reported for placebo.

Advanced Parkinson's Disease

In the four double-blind, placebo-controlled trials of patients with advanced Parkinson's disease, the most commonly observed adverse events (>5%) that were numerically more frequent in the group treated with MIRAPEX and concomitant levodopa were postural (orthostatic) hypotension, dyskinesia, extrapyramidal syndrome, insomnia, dizziness, hallucinations, accidental injury; dream abnormalities, confusion, constipation, asthenia, somnolence, dystonia, gait abnormality, hypertonia, dry mouth, amnesia, and urinary frequency.

Approximately 12% of 260 patients with advanced Parkinson's disease who received MIRAPEX and concomitant levodopa in the double-blind, placebo-controlled trials discontinued treatment due to adverse events compared with 16% of 264 patients who received placebo and concomitant levodopa. The events most commonly causing discontinuation of treatment were related to the nervous system (hallucinations [2.7% on MIRAPEX vs 0.4% on placebo]; dyskinesia [1.9% on MIRAPEX vs 0.8% on placebo]; extrapyramidal syndrome [1.5% on MIRAPEX vs 4.9% on placebo]; dizziness [1.2% on MIRAPEX vs 1.5% on placebo]; confusion [1.2% on MIRAPEX vs 2.3% on placebo]; and cardiovascular system (postural [orthostatic] hypotension [2.3% on MIRAPEX vs 1.1% on placebo]).

Adverse-event incidence in controlled clinical studies in advanced Parkinson's disease: Table 2 lists treatment-emergent adverse events that occurred in the double-blind, placebo-controlled studies in advanced Parkinson's disease that were reported by ≥1% of patients treated with MIRAPEX and were numerically more frequent than in the placebo group. In these studies, MIRAPEX or placebo was administered to patients who were also receiving concomitant levodopa. Adverse events were usually mild to moderate in intensity.

The prescriber should be aware that these figures cannot be used to predict the incidence of adverse events in the course of usual medical practice where patient characteristics and other factors differ from those that prevailed in the clinical studies. Similarly, the cited frequencies cannot be compared with figures obtained from other clinical investigations involving different treatments, uses, and investigators. However, the cited figures do provide the prescribing physician with some basis for estimating the relative contribution of drug and nondrug factors to the adverse-events incidence rate in the population studied.

Table 2
Treatment-Emergent Adverse-Event* Incidence in Double-Blind, Placebo-Controlled Trials in Advanced Parkinson's Disease (Events ≥ 1% of Patients Treated With MIRAPEX and Numerically More Frequent Than in the Placebo Group)

Body System/ Adverse Event	MIRAPEX† N=260	Placebo† N=264
Body as a Whole		
Accidental injury	17	15
Asthenia	10	8
General edema	4	3
Chest pain	3	2
Malaise	3	2
Cardiovascular System		
Postural hypotension	53	48
Digestive System		
Constipation	10	9
Dry mouth	7	3
Metabolic & Nutritional System		
Peripheral edema	2	1
Increased creatine PK	1	0
Musculoskeletal System		
Arthritis	3	1
Twitching	2	0
Bursitis	2	0
Myasthenia	1	0
Nervous System		
Dyskinesia	47	31
Extrapyramidal syndrome	28	26
Insomnia	27	22
Dizziness	26	25
Hallucinations	17	4
Dream abnormalities	11	10
Confusion	10	7
Somnolence	9	6
Dystonia	8	7
Gait abnormalities	7	5
Hypertonia	7	6
Amnesia	6	4
Akathisia	3	2
Thinking abnormalities	3	2
Paranoid reaction	3	2
Delusions	1	0
Sleep disorders	1	0
Respiratory System		
Dyspnea	4	3
Rhinitis	3	1
Pneumonia	2	0
Skin & Appendages		
Skin disorders	2	1
Special Senses		
Accommodation abnormalities	4	2
Vision abnormalities	3	1
Diplopia	1	0
Urogenital System		
Urinary frequency	6	3
Urinary tract infection	4	3
Urinary incontinence	2	1

*Patients may have reported multiple adverse experiences during the study or at discontinuation; thus, patients may be included in more than one category.
†Patients received concomitant levodopa.

Other events reported by 1% or more of patients with advanced Parkinson's disease and treated with MIRAPEX but reported equally or more frequently in the placebo group were nausea, pain, infection, headache, depression, tremor, hypokinesia, anorexia, back pain, dyspepsia, flatulence, ataxia, flu syndrome, sinusitis, diarrhea, myalgia, abdominal pain, anxiety, rash, paresthesia, hypertension, increased saliva, tooth disorder, apathy, hypotension, sweating, vasodilation, vomiting, increased cough, nervousness, pruritus, hypesthesia, neck pain, syncope, arthralgia, dysphagia, palpitations, pharyngitis, vertigo, leg cramps, conjunctivitis, and lacrimation disorders.

Adverse Events; Relationship to Age, Gender, and Race: Among the treatment-emergent adverse events in patients treated with MIRAPEX, hallucination appeared to exhibit a positive relationship to age. No gender-related differences were observed. Only a small percentage (4%) of patients enrolled were non-Caucasian, therefore, an evaluation of adverse events related to race is not possible.

Other Adverse Events Observed During All Phase 2 and 3 Clinical Trials: MIRAPEX has been administered to 1,408 individuals during all clinical trials (Parkinson's disease and other patient populations), 648 of whom were in seven double-blind, placebo-controlled Parkinson's disease trials. During these trials, all adverse events were recorded by the clinical investigators using terminology of their own choosing. To provide a meaningful estimate of the proportion of individuals having adverse events, similar types of events were grouped into a smaller number of standardized categories using modified COSTART dictionary terminology. These categories are used in the listing below. The events listed below occurred in less than 1% of the 1,408 individuals exposed to MIRAPEX and occurred on at least two occasions (on one occasion if the event was serious). All reported events, except those already listed above, are included, without regard to determination of a causal relationship to MIRAPEX.

Events are listed within body-system categories in order of decreasing frequency.

Body as a whole: enlarged abdomen, death, fever, suicide attempt.

Cardiovascular system: peripheral vascular disease, myocardial infarction, angina pectoris, atrial fibrillation, heart failure, arrhythmia, atrial arrhythmia, pulmonary embolism.

Digestive system: thirst.

Musculoskeletal system: joint disorder, myasthenia.

Nervous system: agitation, CNS stimulation, hyperkinesia, psychosis, convulsions.

Respiratory system: pneumonia.

Special senses: cataract, eye disorder, glaucoma.

Urogenital system: dysuria, abnormal ejaculation, prostate cancer, hematuria, prostate disorder.

Falling Asleep During Activities of Daily Living: Patients treated with MIRAPEX have reported falling asleep while engaged in activities of daily living, including operation of a motor vehicle which sometimes resulted in accidents (see bolded WARNING).

DRUG ABUSE AND DEPENDENCE

Pramipexole is not a controlled substance.

Pramipexole has not been systematically studied in animals or humans for its potential for abuse, tolerance, physical dependence. However, in a rat model on cocaine self-administration, pramipexole had little or no effect.

OVERDOSAGE

There is no clinical experience with massive overdosage. One patient, with a 10-year history of schizophrenia, took 11 mg/day of pramipexole for 2 days; this is two to three times the protocol recommended daily dose. No adverse events were reported related to the increased dose. Blood pressure remained stable although pulse rate increased to between 100 and 120 beats/minute. The patient withdrew from the study at the end of week 2 due to lack of efficacy. There is no known antidote for overdosage of a dopamine agonist. If signs of central nervous system stimulation are present, a phenothiazine or other butyrophenone neuroleptic agent may be indicated; the efficacy of such drugs in reversing the effects of overdosage has not been assessed. Management of overdose may require general supportive measures along with gastric lavage, intravenous fluids, and electrocardiogram monitoring.

DOSAGE AND ADMINISTRATION

In all clinical studies, dosage was initiated at a subtherapeutic level to avoid intolerable adverse effects and orthostatic hypotension. MIRAPEX should be titrated gradually in all patients. The dosage should be increased to achieve a maximum therapeutic effect, balanced against the principal side effects of dyskinesia, hallucinations, somnolence, and dry mouth.

Dosing in Patients With Normal Renal Function

Initial Treatment: Dosages should be increased gradually from a starting dose of 0.375 mg/day given in three divided doses and should not be increased more frequently than every 5 to 7 days. A suggested ascending dosage schedule that was used in clinical studies is shown in the following table:

Ascending Dosage Schedule of MIRAPEX

Week	Dosage (mg)	Total Daily Dose (mg)
1	0.125 tid	0.375
2	0.25 tid	0.75
3	0.5 tid	1.50
4	0.75 tid	2.25
5	1.0 tid	3.0
6	1.25 tid	3.75
7	1.5 tid	4.50

Maintenance Treatment: MIRAPEX Tablets were effective and well tolerated over a dosage range of 1.5 to 4.5 mg/day administered in equally divided doses three times per day with or without concomitant levodopa (approximately 800 mg/day).

In a fixed-dose study in early Parkinson's disease patients, doses of 3 mg, 4.5 mg, and 6 mg per day of MIRAPEX were not shown to provide any significant benefit beyond that achieved at a daily dose of 1.5 mg/day However, in the same fixed-dose study, the following adverse events were dose related: postural hypotension, nausea, constipation, somnolence, and amnesia. The frequency of these events was generally 2-fold greater than placebo for pramipexole doses greater than 3 mg/day. The incidence of somnolence reported with pramipexole at a dose of 1.5 mg/day was comparable to placebo.

When MIRAPEX is used in combination with levodopa, a reduction of the levodopa dosage should be considered. In a controlled study in advanced Parkinson's disease, the dosage of levodopa was reduced by an average of 27% from baseline.

Patients with Renal Impairment

Pramipexole Dosage in the Renally Impaired

Renal Status	Starting Dose (mg)	Maximum Dose (mg)
Normal to mild impairment (creatinine Cl > 60 mL/min)	0.125 tid	1.5 tid
Moderate impairment (creatinine Cl = 35 to 59 mL/min)	0.125 bid	1.5 bid
Severe impairment (creatinine Cl = 15 to 34 mL/min)	0.125 qd	1.5 qd
Very severe impairment (creatinine Cl < 15 mL/min and hemodialysis patients)	The use of MIRAPEX has not been adequately studied in this group of patients.	

Discontinuation of Treatment: It is recommended that MIRAPEX be discontinued over a period of 1 week; in some studies, however, abrupt discontinuation was uneventful.

HOW SUPPLIED

MIRAPEX Tablets are available as follows:

0.125 mg: white, round tablet with "U" on one side and "2" on the reverse side.
Bottles of 63 NDC 0009-0002-02

0.25 mg: white, oval, scored tablet with "U" twice on one side and "4" twice on the reverse side.
Bottles of 90 NDC 0009-0004-02
Unit dose packages of 100 NDC 0009-0004-06

0.5 mg: white, oval, scored tablet with "U" twice on one side and "8" twice on the reverse side.
Bottles of 90 NDC 0009-0008-02
Unit dose packages of 100 NDC 0009-0008-03

1 mg: white, round, scored tablet with "U" twice on one side and "6" twice on the reverse side.
Bottles of 90 NDC 0009-0006-02
Unit dose packages of 100 NDC 0009-0006-06

1.5 mg: white, round, scored tablet with "U" twice on one side and "37" twice on the reverse side.
Bottles of 90 NDC 0009-0037-02
Unit dose packages of 100 NDC 0009-0037-06

Store at 25°C (77°F); excursions permitted to 15°–30°C (59°–86°F) [see USP Controlled Room Temperature]. Protect from light.

℞ only

ANIMAL TOXICOLOGY

Retinal Pathology in Albino Rats

Pathologic changes (degeneration and loss of photoreceptor cells) were observed in the retina of albino rats in the 2-year carcinogenicity study with pramipexole. These findings were first observed during week 76 and were dose dependent in animals receiving 2 or 8 mg/kg/day (plasma AUCs

Continued on next page

Information on these Pharmacia & Upjohn products is based on labeling in effect June 1, 2000. Further information concerning these and other Pharmacia & Upjohn products may be obtained by direct inquiry to Medical Information, Pharmacia & Upjohn, Kalamazoo, MI 49001.

Mirapex—Cont.

equal to 2.5 and 12.5 times the AUC in humans that received 1.5 mg tid). Similar findings were not present in rats receiving 0.3 mg/kg/day (plasma AUC equal to 0.3 times the AUC in humans that received 1.5 mg tid).
Investigative studies demonstrated that pramipexole reduced the rate of disk shedding from the photoreceptor rod cells of the retina in albino rats, which was associated with enhanced sensitivity to the damaging effects of light. In a comparative study, degeneration and loss of photoreceptor cells occurred in albino rats after 13 weeks of treatment with 25 mg/kg/day of pramipexole (54 times the highest clinical dose on a mg/m^2 basis) and constant light (100 lux) but not in pigmented rats exposed to the same dose and higher light intensities (500 lux). Thus, the retina of albino rats is considered to be uniquely sensitive to the damaging effects of pramipexole and light. Similar changes in the retina did not occur in a 2-year carcinogenicity study in albino mice treated with 0.3, 2, or 10 mg/kg/day (0.3, 2.2 and 11 times the highest clinical dose on a mg/m^2 basis). Evaluation of the retinas of monkeys given 0.1, 0.5, or 2.0 mg/kg/day of pramipexole (0.4, 2.2, and 8.6 times the highest clinical dose on a mg/m^2 basis) for 12 months and minipigs given 0.3, 1, or 5 mg/kg/day of pramipexole for 13 weeks also detected no changes.
The potential significance of this effect in humans has not been established, but cannot be disregarded because disruption of a mechanism that is universally present in vertebrates (ie, disk shedding) may be involved.

Fibro-osseous Proliferative Lesions in Mice

An increased incidence of fibro-osseous proliferative lesions occurred in the femurs of female mice treated for 2 years with 0.3, 2.0, or 10 mg/kg/day (0.3, 2.2, and 11 times the highest clinical dose on a mg/m^2 basis). Lesions occurred at a lower rate in control animals. Similar lesions were not observed in male mice or rats and monkeys of either sex that were treated chronically with pramipexole.
The significance of this lesion to humans is not known.
Pharmacia & Upjohn Company
Kalamazoo, Michigan 49001, USA
Revised August 1999 817 017 006
691439

Shown in Product Identification Guide, page 331

MYCOBUTIN® ℞

[*my-cō 'butin*]
rifabutin capsules, USP

DESCRIPTION

MYCOBUTIN Capsules contain the antimycobacterial agent rifabutin, which is a semisynthetic ansamycin antibiotic derived from rifamycin S. MYCOBUTIN Capsules for oral administration contain 150 mg of rifabutin, USP, per capsule, along with the inactive ingredients microcrystalline cellulose, magnesium stearate, red iron oxide, silica gel, sodium lauryl sulfate, titanium dioxide, and edible white ink.
The chemical name for rifabutin is 1',4-didehydro-1-deoxy-1,4-dihydro-5'-(2-methylpropyl)-1-oxorifamycin XIV (Chemical Abstracts Service, 9th Collective Index) or (9*S*, 12*E*, 14*S*, 15*R*, 16*S*, 17*R*, 18*R*, 19*R*, 20*S*, 21*S*, 22*E*, 24*Z*)-6,16,18,20-tetrahydroxy-1'-isobutyl-14-methoxy-7,9,15,17, 19,21,25-hepatmethyl-spiro[9,4-(epoxypentadecal[1,11,13] trienimino)-2*H*-furo[2',3':7,8]naphth[1,2-*d*]imidazole-2,4'-piperidine]-5,10,26-(3*H*,9*H*)-trione-16-acetate. Rifabutin has a molecular formula of $C_{46}H_{62}N_4O_{11}$, a molecular weight of 847.02 and the following structure:

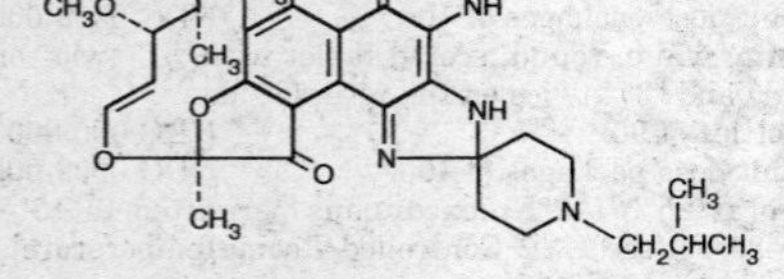

Rifabutin is a red-violet powder soluble in chloroform and methanol, sparingly soluble in ethanol, and very slightly soluble in water (0.19 mg/mL). Its log P value (the base 10 logarithm of the partition coefficient between n-octanol and water) is 3.2 (n-octanol/water).

CLINICAL PHARMACOLOGY

Pharmacokinetics

Following a single oral dose of 300 mg to nine healthy adult volunteers, rifabutin was readily absorbed from the gastrointestinal tract with mean (±SD) peak plasma levels (C_{max}) of 375 (±267) ng/mL (range: 141 to 1033 ng/mL) attained in 3.3 (±0.9) hours (T_{max} range: 2 to 4 hours). Plasma concentrations post -C_{max} declined in an apparent biphasic manner. Kinetic dose-proportionality has been established over the 300 to 600 mg dose range in nine healthy adult volunteers (crossover design) and in 16 early symptomatic human immunodeficiency virus (HIV)-positive patients over a 300 to 900 mg dose range. Rifabutin was slowly eliminated from plasma in seven healthy adult volunteers, presumably because of *distribution-limited elimination*, with a mean terminal half-life of 45 (±17) hours (range: 16 to 69 hours). Although the systemic levels of rifabutin following multiple dosing decreased by 38%, its terminal half-life remained unchanged. Rifabutin, due to its high lipophilicity, demonstrates a high propensity for distribution and intracellular tissue uptake. Estimates of apparent steady-state distribution volume (9.3 ± 1.5 L/kg) in five HIV-positive patients, following I.V. dosing, exceed total body water by approximately 15-fold. Substantially higher intracellular tissue levels than those seen in plasma have been observed in both rat and man. The lung to plasma concentration ratio, obtained at 12 hours, was found to be approximately 6.5 in four surgical patients administered an oral dose. Mean rifabutin steady-state trough levels ($C_{p\ min}$ ^{ss}; 24-hour post-dose) ranged from 50 to 65 ng/mL in HIV-positive patients and in healthy adult volunteers. About 85% of the drug is bound in a concentration-independent manner to plasma proteins over a concentration range of 0.05 to 1 µg/mL. Binding does not appear to be influenced by renal or hepatic dysfunction.
Mean systemic clearance (CL_s/F) in healthy adult volunteers following a single oral dose was 0.69 (±0.32) L/hr/kg (range: 0.46 to 1.34 L/hr/kg). Renal and biliary clearance of unchanged drug each contribute approximately 5% to CL_s/F. About 30% of the dose is excreted in the feces. A mass-balance study in three healthy adult volunteers with ^{14}C-labeled drug has shown that 53% of the oral dose was excreted in the urine, primarily as metabolites. Of the five metabolites that have been identified, 25-O-desacetyl and 31-hydroxy are the most predominant, and show a plasma metabolite:parent area under the curve ratio of 0.10 and 0.07, respectively. The former has an activity equal to the parent drug and contributes up to 10% to the total antimicrobial activity.
Absolute bioavailability assessed in five HIV-positive patients, who received both oral and I.V. doses, averaged 20%. Total recovery of radioactivity in the urine indicates that at least 53% of the orally administered rifabutin dose is absorbed from the G.I. tract. The bioavailability of rifabutin from the capsule dosage form, relative to a solution, was 85% in 12 healthy adult volunteers. High-fat meals slow the rate without influencing the extent of absorption from the capsule dosage form. The overall pharmacokinetics of rifabutin are modified only slightly by alterations in hepatic function or age. Rifabutin steady-state kinetics in early symptomatic HIV-positive patients are similar to healthy volunteers. Compared to healthy volunteers, steady-state kinetics of rifabutin are more variable in elderly patients (>70 years) and in symptomatic HIV-positive patients. Somewhat reduced drug distribution and faster elimination of rifabutin in patients with compromised renal function may result in decreased drug concentrations. The clinical implications of this are unknown.
No rifabutin disposition information is currently available in children or adolescents under 18 years of age.

Microbiology

Mechanism of Action

Rifabutin inhibits DNA-dependent RNA polymerase in susceptible strains of *Escherichia coli* and *Bacillus subtilis* but not in mammalian cells. In resistant strains of *E. coli*, rifabutin, like rifampin, did not inhibit this enzyme. It is not known whether rifabutin inhibits DNA-dependent RNA polymerase in *Mycobacterium avium* or in *M. intracellulare* which comprise *M. avium* complex (MAC).

Susceptibility Testing

In vitro susceptibility testing methods and diagnostic products used for determining minimum inhibitory concentration (MIC) values against *M. avium* complex (MAC) organisms have not been standardized. Breakpoints to determine whether clinical isolates of MAC and other mycobacterial species are susceptible or resistant to rifabutin have not been established.

In Vitro Studies

Rifabutin has demonstrated in vitro activity against *M. avium* complex (MAC) organisms isolated from both HIV-positive and HIV-negative people. While gene probe techniques may be used to identify these two organisms, many reported studies did not distinguish between these two species. The vast majority of isolates from MAC-infected. HIV-positive people are *M. avium*, whereas in HIV-negative people, about 40% of the MAC isolates are *M intracellulare*.
Various in vitro methodologies employing broth or solid media, with and without polysorbate 80 (Tween 80), have been used to determine rifabutin MIC values for mycobacterial species. In general, MIC values determined in broth are several fold lower than that observed with methods employing solid media. Utilization of Tween 80 in these assays has been shown to further lower MIC values. However, MIC values were substantially higher for egg based compared to agar based solid media.
Rifabutin activity against 211 MAC isolates from HIV-positive people was evaluated in vitro utilizing a radiometric broth and an agar dilution method. Results showed that 78% and 82% of these isolates had MIC_{99} values of ≤0.25 µg/mL and ≤1.0 µg/mL, respectively, when evaluated by these two methods. Rifabutin was also shown to be active against phagocytized, *M. avium* complex in a mouse macrophage cell culture model.
Rifabutin has in vitro activity against many strains of *Mycobacterium tuberculosis*. In one study, utilizing the radiometric broth method, each of 17 and 20 rifampin-naive clinical isolates tested from the United States and Taiwan, respectively, were shown to be susceptible to rifabutin concentrations of ≤0.125 µg/mL.
Cross-resistance between rifampin and rifabutin is commonly observed with *M. tuberculosis* and *M. avium* complex isolates. Isolates of *M. tuberculosis* resistant to rifampin are likely to be resistant to rifabutin. Rifampicin and rifabutin MIC_{99} values against 523 isolates of *M. avium* complex were determined utilizing the agar dilution method (Ref. Heifets, Leonid B, and Iseman, Michael D. 1985. Determination of in vitro susceptibility of Mycobacteria to Ansamycin. Am. Rev. Respir. Dis. 132 (3):710–711).
[See table above]

SUSCEPTIBILITY OF *M. AVIUM* COMPLEX STRAINS OF RIFAMPIN AND RIFABUTIN

Susceptibility to Rifampin (µg/mL)	Number of Strains	% of Strains Susceptible/Resistant to Different Concentrations of Rifabutin (µg/mL)			
		Susceptible to 0.5	Resistant to 0.5 only	Resistant to 1.0	Resistant to 2.0
Susceptible to 1.0	30	100.0	0.0	0.0	0.0
Resistant to 1.0 only	163	88.3	11.7	0.0	0.0
Resistant to 5.0	105	38.0	57.1	2.9	2.0
Resistant to 10.0	225	20.0	50.2	19.6	10.2
TOTAL	523	49.5	36.7	9.0	4.8

Rifabutin in vitro MIC_{99} values of ≤0.5 µg/mL, determined by the agar dilution method, for *M. kansasii*, *M. gordonae* and *M. marinum* have been reported; however, the clinical significance of these results is unknown.

INDICATIONS AND USAGE

MYCOBUTIN Capsules are indicated for the prevention of disseminated *Mycobacterium avium* complex (MAC) disease in patients with advanced HIV infection.

Clinical Studies

Two randomized, double-blind clinical trials (study 023 and study 027) compared MYCOBUTIN (300 mg/day) to placebo in patients with CDC-defined AIDS and CD4 counts ≤200 cells/µL. These studies accrued patients from 2/90 through 2/92. Study 023 enrolled 590 patients, with a median CD4 cell count at steady entry of 42 cells/µL (mean 61). Study 027 enrolled 556 patients with a median CD4 cell count at study entry of 40 cells/µL (mean 58).
Endpoints included the following:

(1) MAC bacteremia, defined as at least one blood culture positive for *M. avium* complex bacteria.
(2) Clinically significant disseminated MAC disease, defined as MAC bacteremia accompanied by signs or symptoms of serious MAC infection, including one or more of the following: fever, night sweats, rigors, weight loss, worsening anemia, and/or elevations in alkaline phosphatase.
(3) Survival

MAC bacteremia

Participants who received MYCOBUTIN were one-third to one-half as likely to develop MAC bacteremia as were participants who received placebo. These results were statistically significant (study 023: $p<0.001$; study 027: $p=0.002$).
In study 023, the one-year cumulative incidence of MAC bacteremia, on an intent to treat basis, was 9% for patients randomized to MYCOBUTIN and 22% for patients randomized to placebo. In study 027, these rates were 13% and 28% for patients receiving MYCOBUTIN and placebo, respectively.
Most cases of MAC bacteremia (approximately 90% in these studies) occurred among participants whose CD4 count at study entry was ≤100 cells/µL. The median and mean CD4 counts at onset of MAC bacteremia were 13 cells/µL and 24 cells/µL, respectively. These studies did not investigate the optimal time to begin MAC prophylaxis.

Clinically significant disseminated MAC disease

In association with the decreased incidence of bacteremia, patients on MYCOBUTIN showed reductions in the signs and symptoms or disseminated MAC disease, including fever, night sweats, weight loss, fatigue, abdominal pain, anemia, and hepatic dysfunction.

PERCENTAGE OF PATIENTS WITH LABORATORY ABNORMALITIES

LABORATORY ABNORMALITIES	MYCOBUTIN (n = 566) %	PLACEBO (n = 580) %
Chemistry:		
Increased Alkaline Phosphatase[1]	<1	3
Increased SGOT[2]	7	12
Increased SGPT[2]	9	11
Hematology:		
Anemia[3]	6	7
Eosinophilia	1	1
Leukopenia[4]	17	16
Neutropenia[5]	25	20
Thrombocytopenia [6]	5	4

INCLUDES GRADE 3 OR 4 TOXICITIES AS SPECIFIED:

1 all values >450 U/L
2 all values >150 U/L
3 all hemoglobin values < 8.0 g/dL
4 all WBC values < 1,500/mm^3
5 all ANC values < 750/mm^3
6 all platelet count values < 50,000/mm^3

Survival
The one year survival rates in study 023 were 77% for the group receiving MYCOBUTIN and 77% for the placebo group. In study 027, the one year survival rates were 77% for the group receiving MYCOBUTIN and 70% for the placebo group. These differences were not statistically significant.

CONTRAINDICATIONS
MYCOBUTIN Capsules are contraindicated in patients who have had clinically significant hypersensitivity to rifabutin or to any other rifamycins.

WARNINGS
MYCOBUTIN Capsules must not be administered for MAC prophylaxis to patients with active tuberculosis. Tuberculosis in HIV-positive patients is common and may present with atypical or extrapulmonary findings. Patients are likely to have a nonreactive purified protein derivative (PPD) despite active disease. In addition to chest X-ray and sputum culture, the following studies may be useful in the diagnosis of tuberculosis in the HIV-positive patient: blood culture, urine culture, or biopsy of a suspicious lymph node. Patients who develop complaints consistent with active tuberculosis while on prophylaxis with MYCOBUTIN should be evaluated immediately, so that those with active disease may be given an effective combination regimen of anti-tuberculosis medications. Administration of MYCOBUTIN as a single agent to patients with active tuberculosis is likely to lead to the development of tuberculosis that is resistant to MYCOBUTIN and to rifampin.
There is no evidence that MYCOBUTIN is effective prophylaxis against *M. tuberculosis*. Patients requiring prophylaxis against both *M. tuberculosis* and *Mycobacterium avium* complex may be given isoniazid and MYCOBUTIN concurrently.

PRECAUTIONS
Because treatment with MYCOBUTIN Capsules may be associated with neutropenia, and more rarely thrombocytopenia, physicians should consider obtaining hematologic studies periodically in patients receiving prophylaxis with MYCOBUTIN.
Information for Patients
Patients should be advised of the signs and symptoms of both MAC and tuberculosis, and should be instructed to consult their physicians if they develop new complaints consistent with either of these diseases. In addition, since MYCOBUTIN may rarely be associated with myositis and uveitis, patients should be advised to notify their physicians if they develop signs or symptoms suggesting either of these disorders.
Urine, feces, saliva, sputum, perspiration, tears, and skin may be colored brown-orange with rifabutin and some of its metabolites. Soft contact lenses may be permanently stained. Patients to be treated with MYCOBUTIN should be made aware of these possibilities.
Drug Interactions
In 10 healthy adult volunteers and 8 HIV-positive patients, steady-state plasma levels of zidovudine (ZDV), an antiretroviral agent which is metabolized mainly through glucuronidation, were decreased after repeated dosing with MYCOBUTIN; the mean decrease in C_{max} and AUC was decreased by 48% and 32%, respectively. In vitro studies have demonstrated that rifabutin does not affect the inhibition of HIV by ZDV.
Steady-state kinetics in 12 HIV-positive patients show that both the rate and extent of systemic availability of didanosine (ddI), was not altered after repeated dosing of MYCOBUTIN.
Rifabutin has liver enzyme-inducing properties. The related drug rifampin is known to reduce the activity of a number of other drugs, including dapsone, narcotics (including methadone), anticoagulants, corticosteroids, cyclosporine, cardiac glycoside preparations, quinidine, oral contraceptives, oral hypoglycemic agents (sulfonylureas), and analgesics. Rifampin has also been reported to decrease the effects of concurrently administered ketoconazole, barbiturates, diazepam, verapamil, beta-adrenergic blockers, clofibrate, progestins, disopyramide, mexiletine, theophylline, chloramphenicol, and anticonvulsants. Because of the structural similarity of rifabutin and rifampin, MYCOBUTIN may be expected to have some effect on these drugs as well. However, unlike rifampin, MYCOBUTIN appears not to affect the acetylation of isoniazid. When rifabutin was compared with rifampin in a study with 8 healthy normal volunteers, rifabutin appeared to be a less potent enzyme inducer than rifampin. The significance of this finding for clinical drug interactions is not known. Dosage adjustment of drugs listed above may be necessary if they are given concurrently with MYCOBUTIN. Patients using oral contraceptives should consider changing to nonhormonal methods of birth control.
Carcinogenesis, Mutagenesis, Impairment of Fertility:
Long term carcinogenicity studies were conducted with rifabutin in mice and in rats. Rifabutin was not carcinogenic in mice at doses up to 180 mg/kg/day, or approximately 36 times the recommended human daily dose. Rifabutin was not carcinogenic in the rat at doses up to 60 mg/kg/day, about 12 times the recommended human dose.
Rifabutin was not mutagenic in the bacterial mutation assay (Ames Test) using both rifabutin-susceptible and resistant strains. Rifabutin was not mutagenic in *Schizosaccharomyces pombe* P_1 and was not genotoxic in V-79 Chinese hamster cells, human lymphocytes in vitro, or mouse bone marrow cells in vivo.
Fertility was impaired in male rats given 160 mg/kg (32 times the recommended human daily dose).
Pregnancy:
Pregnancy Category B: Reproduction studies have been carried out in rats and rabbits given rifabutin using dose levels up to 200 mg/kg (40 times the recommended human daily dose). No teratogenicity was observed in either species. In rats, given 200 mg/kg/day, there was a decrease in fetal viability. In rats, at 40 mg/kg/day (8 times the recommended human daily dose), rifabutin caused an increase in fetal skeletal variants. In rabbits, at 80 mg/kg/day (16 times the recommended human daily dose), rifabutin caused maternotoxicity and increase in fetal skeletal anomalies. There are no adequate and well-controlled studies in pregnant women. Because animal reproduction studies are not always predictive of human response, rifabutin should be used in pregnant women only if the potential benefit justifies the potential risk to the fetus.
Nursing Mothers:
It is not known whether rifabutin is excreted in human milk. Because many drugs are excreted in human milk and because of the potential for serious adverse reactions in nursing infants, a decision should be made whether to discontinue nursing or discontinue the drug, taking into account the importance of the drug to the mother.
Pediatric Use:
Safety and effectiveness of rifabutin for prophylaxis of MAC in children have not been established. Limited safety data are available from treatment use in 22 HIV-positive children with MAC who received MYCOBUTIN in combination with at least two other antimycobacterials for periods from 1 to 183 weeks. Mean doses (mg/kg) for these children were: 18.5 (range 15.0 to 25.0) for infants one year of age; 8.6 (range 4.4 to 18.8) for children 2 to 10 years of age; and 4.0 (range 2.8 to 5.4) for adolescents 14 to 16 years of age. There is no evidence that doses greater than 5 mg/kg daily are useful. Adverse experiences were similar to those observed in the adult population, and included leukopenia, neutropenia and rash. Doses of MYCOBUTIN may be administered mixed with foods such as applesauce.
Geriatric Use
Clinical studies of MYCOBUTIN did not include sufficient numbers of subjects aged 65 and over to determine whether they respond differently from younger subjects. Other reported clinical experience has not identified differences in responses between the elderly and younger patients. In general, dose selection for an elderly patient should be cautious, usually starting at the low end of the dosing range, reflecting the greater frequency of decreased hepatic, renal, or cardiac function, and of concomitant disease or other drug therapy (see CLINICAL PHARMACOLOGY).

ADVERSE REACTIONS
MYCOBUTIN Capsules were generally well tolerated in the controlled clinical trials. Discontinuation of therapy due to an adverse event was required in 16% of patients receiving MYCOBUTIN compared to 8% of patients receiving placebo in these trials. Primary reasons for discontinuation of MYCOBUTIN were rash (4% of treated patients), gastrointestinal intolerance (3%), and neutropenia (2%).
The following table enumerates adverse experiences that occurred at a frequency of 1% or greater, among the patients treated with MYCOBUTIN in studies 023 and 027.

CLINICAL ADVERSE EXPERIENCES REPORTED IN ≥1% OF PATIENTS TREATED WITH MYCOBUTIN

ADVERSE EVENT	MYCOBUTIN (n=566) %	PLACEBO (n=580) %
BODY AS A WHOLE		
Abdominal Pain	4	3
Asthenia	1	1
Chest Pain	1	1
Fever	2	1
Headache	3	5
Pain	1	2
DIGESTIVE SYSTEM		
Anorexia	2	2
Diarrhea	3	3
Dyspepsia	3	1
Eructation	3	1
Flatulence	2	1
Nausea	6	5
Nausea and Vomiting	3	2
Vomiting	1	1
MUSCULOSKELETAL SYSTEM		
Myalgia	2	1
NERVOUS SYSTEM		
Insomnia	1	1
SKIN AND APPENDAGES		
Rash	11	8
SPECIAL SENSES		
Taste Perversion	3	1
UROGENITAL SYSTEM		
Discolored Urine	30	6

CLINICAL ADVERSE EVENTS REPORTED IN <1% OF PATIENTS WHO RECEIVED MYCOBUTIN
Considering data from the 023 and 027 pivotal trials, and from other clinical studies, MYCOBUTIN appears to be a likely cause of the following adverse events which occurred in less than 1% of treated patients: flu-like syndrome, hepatitis, hemolysis, arthralgia, myositis, chest pressure or pain with dyspnea, and skin discoloration.
The following adverse events have occurred in more than one patient receiving MYCOBUTIN, but an etiologic role has not been established: seizure, paresthesia, aphasia, confusion, and non-specific T wave changes on electrocardiogram.
When MYCOBUTIN was administered at doses from 1050 mg/day to 2400 mg/day, generalized arthralgia and uveitis were reported. These adverse experiences abated when MYCOBUTIN was discontinued.
The following table enumerates the changes in laboratory values that were considered as laboratory abnormalities in studies 023 and 027.
[See table at top of page]
The incidence of neutropenia in patients treated with MYCOBUTIN was significantly greater than in patients treated with placebo ($p = 0.03$). Although thrombocytopenia was not significantly more common among patients treated with MYCOBUTIN in these trials, MYCOBUTIN has been clearly linked to thrombocytopenia in rare cases. One patient in study 023 developed thrombotic thrombocytopenic purpura, which was attributed to MYCOBUTIN.
Uveitis is rare when MYCOBUTIN is used as a single agent at 300 mg/day for prophylaxis of MAC in HIV-infected persons, even with the concomitant use of fluconazole and/or macrolide antibiotics. However, if higher doses of MYCOBUTIN are administered in combination with these agents, the incidence of uveitis is higher.
Patients who developed uveitis had mild to severe symptoms that resolved after treatment with corticosteroids and/or mydriatic eye drops; in some severe cases, however, resolution of symptoms occurred after several weeks.
When uveitis occurs, temporary discontinuance of MYCOBUTIN and ophthalmic evaluation are recommended. In most mild cases, MYCOBUTIN may be restarted; however,

Continued on next page

Information on these Pharmacia & Upjohn products is based on labeling in effect June 1, 2000. Further information concerning these and other Pharmacia & Upjohn products may be obtained by direct inquiry to Medical Information, Pharmacia & Upjohn, Kalamazoo, MI 49001.

Mycobutin—Cont.

if signs or symptoms recur, use of MYCOBUTIN should be discontinued (Morbidity and Mortality Weekly Report, September 4, 1994).

ANIMAL TOXICOLOGY

Liver abnormalities (increased bilirubin and liver weight), occurred in all species tested, in rats at doses 5 times, in monkeys at doses 8 times, and in mice at doses 6 times the recommended human daily dose. Testicular atrophy occurred in baboons at doses 4 times the recommended human dose, and in rats at doses 40 times the recommended human daily dose.

OVERDOSAGE

No information is available on accidental overdosage in humans.

Treatment

While there is no experience in the treatment of overdose with MYCOBUTIN Capsules, clinical experience with rifamycins suggest that gastric lavage to evacuate gastric contents (within a few hours of overdose), followed by instillation of an activated charcoal slurry into the stomach, may help absorb any remaining drug from the gastrointestinal tract.

Rifabutin is 85% protein bound and distributed extensively into tissues (Vss:8 to 9 L/kg). It is not primarily excreted via the urinary route (less than 10% as unchanged drug), therefore, neither hemodialysis nor forced diuresis is expected to enhance the systemic elimination of unchanged rifabutin from the body in a patient with an overdose of MYCOBUTIN.

DOSAGE AND ADMINISTRATION

It is recommended that MYCOBUTIN Capsules be administered at a dose of 300 mg once daily. For those patients with propensity to nausea, vomiting, or other gastrointestinal upset, administration of MYCOBUTIN at doses of 150 mg twice daily taken with food may be useful.

HOW SUPPLIED

MYCOBUTIN Capsules (rifabutin capsules, USP) are supplied as hard gelatin capsules having an opaque red-brown cap and body, imprinted with MYCOBUTIN/PHARMACIA & UPJOHN in white ink, each containing 150 mg of rifabutin, USP.

MYCOBUTIN is available as follows:

NDC 0013-5301-17 Bottles of 100 capsules

Keep tightly closed and dispense in a tight container as defined in the USP. Store at 25°C (77°F); excursions permitted to 15°–30°C (59°–86°F) [see USP Controlled Room Temperature].

Rx only

Manufactured for: Pharmacia & Upjohn Company
Kalamazoo, MI 49001, USA

By: Pharmacia & Upjohn S.p.A.
Ascoli Piceno, Italy

Revised August 1999 10000035101

057020899

Shown in Product Identification Guide, page 331

OGEN® ℞

[ō-gĕn]

estropipate tablets, USP

WARNINGS:

1. ESTROGENS HAVE BEEN REPORTED TO INCREASE THE RISK OF ENDOMETRIAL CARCINOMA IN POSTMENOPAUSAL WOMEN.

Close clinical surveillance of all women taking estrogens is important. Adequate diagnostic measures, including endometrial sampling when indicated, should be undertaken to rule out malignancy in all cases of undiagnosed persistent or recurring abnormal vaginal bleeding. There is no evidence that "natural" estrogens are more or less hazardous than "synthetic" estrogens at equiestrogenic doses.

2. ESTROGENS SHOULD NOT BE USED DURING PREGNANCY.

There is no indication for estrogen therapy during pregnancy or during the immediate postpartum period. Estrogens are ineffective for the prevention or treatment of threatened, or habitual abortion. Estrogens are not indicated for the prevention of postpartum breast engorgement.

Estrogen therapy during pregnancy is associated with an increased risk of congenital defects in the reproductive organs of the fetus, and possibly other birth defects. Studies of women who received diethylstilbestrol (DES) during pregnancy have shown that female offspring have an increased risk of vaginal adenosis, squamous cell dysplasia of the uterine cervix, and clear cell vaginal cancer later in life; male offspring have an increased risk of urogenital abnormalities and possibly testicular cancer later in life. The 1985 DES Task Force concluded that use of DES during pregnancy is associated with a subsequent increased risk of breast cancer in the mothers, although a causal relationship remains unproven and the observed level of excess risk is similar to that for a number of other breast cancer risk factors.

DESCRIPTION

OGEN (estropipate tablets), (formerly piperazine estrone sulfate), is a natural estrogenic substance prepared from purified crystalline estrone, solubilized as the sulfate and stabilized with piperazine. It is appreciably soluble in water and has almost no odor or taste—properties which are ideally suited for oral administration. The amount of piperazine in OGEN is not sufficient to exert a pharmacological action. Its addition ensures solubility, stability, and uniform potency of the estrone sulfate. Chemically estropipate, molecular weight: 436.56, is represented by estra-1,3,5(10)-trien-17-one,3-(sulfooxy)-, compound with piperazine (1:1). The structural formula may be represented as follows:

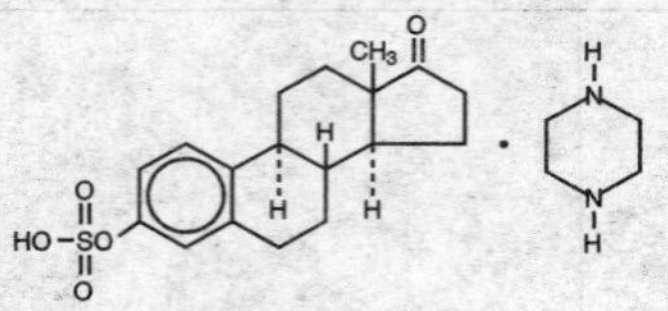

OGEN is available as tablets for oral administration containing either 0.75 mg (OGEN .625), 1.5 mg (OGEN 1.25), or 3 mg (OGEN 2.5) estropipate (Calculated as sodium estrone sulfate 0.625 mg, 1.25 mg, and 2.5 mg, respectively).

Inactive Ingredients

Each tablet contains: Colloidal silicon dioxide, dibasic potassium phosphate, hydrogenated vegetable oil wax, hydroxypropyl cellulose, lactose, magnesium stearate, microcrystalline cellulose, sodium starch glycolate and tromethamine.

OGEN .625 also contains: D&C Yellow No. 10 and FD&C Yellow No. 6.

OGEN 1.25 also contains: FD&C Yellow No. 6.

OGEN 2.5 also contains: FD&C Blue No. 2.

CLINICAL PHARMACOLOGY

Estrogen drug products act by regulating the transcription of a limited number of genes. Estrogens diffuse through cell membranes, distribute themselves throughout the cell, and bind to and activate the nuclear estrogen receptor, a DNA-binding protein which is found in estrogen-responsive tissues. The activated estrogen receptor binds to specific DNA sequences, or hormone-response elements, which enhance the transcription of adjacent genes and in turn lead to the observed effects. Estrogen receptors have been identified in tissues of the reproductive tract, breast, pituitary, hypothalamus, liver, and bone of women.

Estrogens are important in the development and maintenance of the female reproductive system and secondary sex characteristics. By a direct action, they cause growth and development of the uterus. Fallopian tubes, and vagina. With other hormones, such as pituitary hormones and progesterone, they cause enlargement of the breasts through promotion of ductal growth, stromal development, and the accretion of fat. Estrogens are intricately involved with other hormones, especially progesterone, in the processes of ovulatory menstrual cycle and pregnancy, and affect the release of pituitary gonadotropins. They also contribute to the shaping of the skeleton, maintenance of tone and elasticity of urogenital structures, changes in the epiphyses of the long bones that allow for the pubertal growth spurt and its termination, and pigmentation of the nipples and genitals. Estrogens occur naturally in several forms. The primary source of estrogen in normally cycling adult women is the ovarian follicle, which secretes 70 to 500 micrograms of estradiol daily, depending on the phase of the menstrual cycle. This is converted primarily to estrone, which circulates in roughly equal proportion to estradiol, and to small amounts of estriol. After menopause, most endogenous estrogen is produced by conversion of androstenedione, secreted by the adrenal cortex, to estrone by peripheral tissues. Thus, estrone—especially in its sulfate ester form—is the most abundant circulating estrogen in postmenopausal women. Although circulating estrogens exist in a dynamic equilibrium of metabolic interconversions, estradiol is the principal intracellular human estrogen and is substantially more potent than estrone or estriol at the receptor.

Estrogens used in therapy are well absorbed through the skin, mucous membranes, and gastrointestinal tract. When applied for a local action, absorption is usually sufficient to cause systemic effects. When conjugated with aryl and alkyl groups for parenteral administration, the rate of absorption of oily preparations is slowed with a prolonged duration of action, such that a single intramuscular injection of estradiol valerate or estradiol cypionate is absorbed over several weeks.

Administered estrogens and their esters are handled within the body essentially the same as the endogenous hormones. Metabolic conversion of estrogens occurs primarily in the liver (first pass effect), but also at local target tissue sites. Complex metabolic processes result in a dynamic equilibrium of circulating conjugated and unconjugated estrogenic forms which are continuously interconverted, especially between estrone and estradiol and between esterified and unesterified forms. Although naturally-occurring estrogens circulate in the blood largely bound to sex hormone-binding globulin and albumin, only unbound estrogens enter target tissue cells. A significant proportion of the circulating estrogen exists as sulfate conjugates, especially estrone sulfate, which serves as a circulating reservoir for the formation of more active estrogenic species. A certain proportion of the estrogen is excreted into the bile and then reabsorbed from the intestine. During this enterohepatic recirculation, estrogens are desulfated and resulfated and undergo degradation through conversion to less active estrogens (estriol and other estrogens), oxidation to nonestrogenic substances (catecholestrogens, which interact with catecholamine metabolism, especially in the central nervous system), and conjugation with glucuronic acids (which are then rapidly excreted in the urine).

When given orally, naturally-occurring estrogens and their esters are extensively metabolized (first pass effect) and circulate primarily as estrone sulfate, with smaller amounts of other conjugated and unconjugated estrogenic species. This results in limited oral potency. By contrast, synthetic estrogens, such as ethinyl estradiol and the nonsteroidal estrogens, are degraded very slowly in the liver and other tissues, which results in their high intrinsic potency. Estrogen drug products administered by non-oral routes are not subject to first-pass metabolism, but also undergo significant hepatic uptake, metabolism, and enterohepatic recycling.

INDICATIONS AND USAGE

Estrogen drug products are indicated in the:

1. Treatment of moderate to severe vasomotor symptoms associated with the menopause. There is no adequate evidence that estrogens are effective for nervous symptoms or depression which might occur during menopause and they should not be used to treat these conditions.
2. Treatment of vulval and vaginal atrophy.
3. Treatment of hypoestrogenism due to hypogonadism, castration or primary ovarian failure.
4. Prevention of osteoporosis.

Since estrogen administration is associated with risk, selection of patients should ideally be based on prospective identification of risk factors for developing osteoporosis. Unfortunately, there is no certain way to identify those women who will develop osteoporotic fractures. Most prospective studies of efficacy for this indication have been carried out in white menopausal women, without stratification by other risk factors, and tend to show a universally salutary effect on bone. Thus, patient selection must be individualized based on the balance of risks and benefits. A more favorable risk/benefit ratio exists in a hysterectomized woman because she has no risk of endometrial cancer (see **BOXED WARNINGS**).

Estrogen replacement therapy reduces bone resorption and retards or halts postmenopausal bone loss. Case-control studies have shown an approximately 60 percent reduction in hip and wrist fractures in women whose estrogen replacement was begun within a few years of menopause. Studies also suggest that estrogen reduces the rate of vertebral fractures. Even when started as late as 6 years after menopause, estrogen prevents further loss of bone mass for as long as the treatment is continued. The results of a double-blind, placebo-controlled two-year study have shown that treatment with one table of OGEN .625 daily for 25 days (of a 31-day cycle per month) prevents vertebral bone mass loss in postmenopausal women. When estrogen therapy is discontinued, bone mass declines at a rate comparable to the immediate postmenopausal period. There is no evidence that estrogen replacement therapy restores bone mass to premenopausal levels.

At skeletal maturity there are sex and race differences in both the total amount of bone present and its density, in favor of men and blacks. Thus, women are at higher risk than men because they start with less bone mass and, for several years following natural or induced menopause, the rate of bone mass decline is accelerated. White and Asian women are at higher risk than black women.

Early menopause is one of the strongest predictors for the development of osteoporosis. In addition, other factors affecting the skeleton which are associated with osteoporosis include genetic factors (small build, family history), endocrine factors (nulliparity, thyrotoxicosis, hyperparathyroidism, Cushing's syndrome, hyperprolactinemia, Type I diabetes), lifestyle (cigarette smoking, alcohol abuse, sedentary exercise habits) and nutrition (below average body weight, dietary calcium intake).

The mainstays of prevention and management of osteoporosis are estrogen, an adequate lifetime calcium intake, and exercise. Postmenopausal women absorb dietary calcium less efficiently than premenopausal women and require an average of 1500 mg/day of elemental calcium to remain in neutral calcium balance. By comparison, premenopausal women require about 1000 mg/day and the average calcium intake in the USA is 400–600 mg/day. Therefore, when not contraindicated, calcium supplementation may by helpful.

Weight-bearing exercise and nutrition may be important adjuncts to the prevention and management of osteoporosis. Immobilization and prolonged bed rest produce rapid bone loss, while weight-bearing exercise has been shown both to reduce bone loss and to increase bone mass. The optimal type and amount of physical activity that would prevent osteoporosis have not been established, however in two studies an hour of walking and running exercises twice or three times weekly significantly increased lumbar spine bone mass.

CONTRAINDICATIONS

Estrogens should not be used in individuals with any of the following conditions:

1. Known or suspected pregnancy (see **BOXED WARNINGS**). Estrogens may cause fetal harm when administered to a pregnant woman.

2. Undiagnosed abnormal genital bleeding.
3. Known or suspected cancer of the breast except in appropriately selected patients being treated for metastatic disease.
4. Known or suspected estrogen-dependent neoplasia.
5. Active thrombophlebitis or thromboembolic disorders.

WARNINGS

1. ***Induction of malignant neoplasms.***

Endometrial cancer. The reported endometrial cancer risk among unopposed estrogen users is about 2–12-fold greater than in nonusers, and appears dependent on duration of treatment and on estrogen dose. Most studies show no significant increased risk associated with use of estrogens for less than one year. The greatest risk appears associated with prolonged use—with increased risks of 15–24-fold for five to ten years of more. In three studies, persistence of risk was demonstrated for 8 to over 15 years after cessation of estrogen treatment. In one study a significant decrease in the incidence of endometrial cancer occurred six months after estrogen withdrawal. Concurrent progestin therapy may offset this risk but the overall health impact in post-menopausal women is not known (see **PRECAUTIONS**).

Breast Cancer. While the majority of studies have not shown an increased risk of breast cancer in women who have ever used estrogen replacement therapy, some have reported a moderately increased risk (relative risks of 1.3–2.0) in those taking higher doses or those taking lower doses for prolonged periods of time, especially in excess of 10 years. Other studies have not shown this relationship.

Congenital lesions with malignant potential. Estrogen therapy during pregnancy is associated with an increased risk of fetal congenital reproductive tract disorders, and possibly other birth defects. Studies of women who received DES during pregnancy have shown that female offspring have an increased risk of vaginal adenosis, squamous cell dysplasia of the uterine cervix, and clear cell vaginal cancer later in life; male offspring have an increased risk of urogenital abnormalities and possibly testicular cancer later in life. Although some of these changes are benign, others are precursors of malignancy.

2. ***Gallbladder disease.*** Two studies have reported a 2- to 4-fold increase in the risk of gallbladder disease requiring surgery in women receiving postmenopausal estrogens.
3. ***Cardiovascular disease.*** Large doses of estrogen (5 mg conjugated estrogens per day), comparable to those used to treat cancer of the prostate and breast, have been shown in a large prospective clinical trial in men to increase the risks of nonfatal myocardial infarction, pulmonary embolism, and thrombophlebitis. These risks cannot necessarily be extrapolated from men to women. However, to avoid the theoretical cardiovascular risk to women caused by high estrogen doses, the dose for estrogen replacement therapy should not exceed the lowest effective dose.
4. ***Elevated blood pressure.*** Occasional blood pressure increases during estrogen replacement therapy have been attributed to idiosyncratic reactions to estrogens. More often, blood pressure has remained the same or has dropped. One study showed that postmenopausal estrogen users have higher blood pressure than nonusers. Two other studies showed slightly lower blood pressure among estrogen users compared to nonusers. Postmenopausal estrogen use does not increase the risk of stroke. Nonetheless, blood pressure should be monitored at regular intervals with estrogen use.
5. ***Hypercalcemia.*** Administration of estrogens may lead to severe hypercalcemia in patients with breast cancer and bone metastases. If this occurs, the drug should be stopped and appropriate measures taken to reduce the serum calcium level.

PRECAUTIONS

A. *General*

1. **Addition of a progestin.** Studies of the addition of a progestin for seven or more days of a cycle of estrogen administration have reported a lowered incidence of endometrial hyperplasia which would otherwise be induced by estrogen treatment. Morphological and biochemical studies of endometrium suggest that 10 to 14 days of progestin are needed to provide maximal maturation of the endometrium and to eliminate any hyperplastic changes. There are possible additional risks which may be associated with the inclusion of progestins in estrogen replacement regimens. These include: (1) adverse effects on lipoprotein metabolism (lowering HDL and raising LDL) which may diminish the possible cardioprotective effect of estrogen therapy (see **PRECAUTIONS,** D.4., below); (2) impairment of glucose tolerance; and (3) possible enhancement of mitotic activity in breast epithelial tissue (although few epidemiological data are available to address this point). The choice of progestin, its dose, and its regimen may be important in minimizing these adverse effects, but these issues remain to be clarified.
2. **Physical examination.** A complete medical and family history should be taken prior to the initiation of any estrogen therapy. The pretreatment and periodic physical examinations should include special reference to blood pressure, breasts, abdomen, and pelvic organs, and should include a Papanicolaou smear. As a general rule, estrogen should not be prescribed for longer than one year without reexamining the patient.
3. **Hypercoagulability.** Some studies have shown that women taking estrogen replacement therapy have hypercoagulability, primarily related to decreased antithrombin activity. This effect appears dose- and duration-dependent and is less pronounced than that associated with oral contraceptive use. Also, postmenopausal women tend to have increased coagulation parameters at baseline compared to premenopausal women. There is some suggestion that low dose postmenopausal mestranol may increase the risk of thromboembolism, although the majority of studies (of primarily conjugated estrogen users) report no such increase. There is insufficient information on hypercoagulability in women who have had previous thromboembolic disease.
4. **Familial hyperlipoproteinemia.** Estrogen therapy may be associated with massive elevations of plasma triglycerides leading to pancreatitis and other complications in patients with familial defects of lipoprotein metabolism.
5. **Fluid retention.** Because estrogens may cause some degree of fluid retention, conditions which might be exacerbated by this factor, such as asthma, epilepsy, migraine, and cardiac or renal dysfunction, require careful observation.
6. **Uterine bleeding and mastodynia.** Certain patients develop undesirable manifestations of estrogenic stimulation, such as abnormal uterine bleeding and mastodynia.
7. **Impaired liver function.** Estrogen may be poorly metabolized in patients with impaired liver function and should be administered with caution.

B. *Information for the Patient.* See text of Patient Package Insert below.

C. *Laboratory Tests.* Estrogen administration should generally be guided by clinical response at the smallest dose, rather than laboratory monitoring, for relief of symptoms for those indications in which symptoms are observable. For prevention and treatment of osteoporosis, however, see **DOSAGE AND ADMINISTRATION** section.

D. *Drug/Laboratory Test Interactions.*

1. Accelerated prothrombin time, partial thromboplastin time, and platelet aggregation time; increased platelet count; increased factors II, VII antigen, VIII antigen, VIII coagulant activity, IX, X, XII, VII—X complex, II—VII—X complex, and beta-thromboglobulin; decreased levels of anti-factor Xa and antithrombin III, decreased antithrombin III activity; increased levels of fibrinogen and fibrinogen activity; increased plasminogen antigen and activity.
2. Increased thyroid-binding globulin (TBG) leading to increased circulating total thyroid hormone, as measured by protein-bound iodine (PBI), T4 levels (by column) or by radioimmunoassay) or T3 levels by radioimmunoassay. T3 resin uptake is decreased, reflecting the elevated TBG. Free T4 and free T3 concentrations are unaltered.
3. Other binding proteins may be elevated in serum, i.e., corticosteroid binding globulin (CBG), sex hormone-binding globulin (SHBG), leading to increased circulating corticosteroid and sex steroids respectively. Free or biologically active hormone concentrations are unchanged. Other plasma proteins may be increased (angiotensinogen/renin substrate, alpha-1-antitrypsin, ceruloplasmin).
4. Increased plasma HDL and HDL-2 subfraction concentrations, reduced LDL cholesterol concentration, increased triglycerides levels.
5. Impaired glucose tolerance.
6. Reduced response to metyrapone test.
7. Reduced serum folate concentration

E. *Carcinogenesis, Mutagenesis, and Impairment of Fertility.* Long term continuous administration of natural and synthetic estrogens in certain animal species increases the frequency of carcinomas of the breast, uterus, cervix, vagina, testis, and liver. See **"CONTRAINDICATIONS"** and **"WARNINGS"** sections.

F. *Pregnancy Category X.* Estrogens should not be used during pregnancy. See **"CONTRAINDICATIONS"** and **BOXED WARNINGS.**

G. *Nursing Mothers.* As a general principle, the administration of any drug to nursing mothers should be done only when clearly necessary since many drugs are excreted in human milk. In addition, estrogen administration to nursing mothers has been shown to decrease the quantity and quality of the milk.

ADVERSE REACTIONS

The following additional adverse reactions have been reported with estrogen therapy (see **WARNINGS** regarding induction of neoplasia, adverse effects on the fetus, increased incidence of gallbladder disease, cardiovascular disease, elevated blood pressure, and hypercalcemia).

1. *Genitourinary system.*
   Changes in vaginal bleeding pattern and abnormal withdrawal bleeding or flow; breakthrough bleeding, spotting.
   Increase in size of uterine leiomyomata.
   Vaginal candidiasis.
   Change in amount of cervical secretion.
2. *Breast.*
   Tenderness, enlargement.
3. *Gastrointestinal.*
   Nausea, vomiting.
   Abdominal cramps, bloating.
   Cholestatic jaundice.
   Increased incidence of gallbladder disease.
4. *Skin.*
   Chloasma or melasma that may persist when drug is discontinued.
   Erythema multiforme.
   Erythema nodosum.
   Hemorrhagic eruption.
   Loss of scalp hair.
   Hirsutism.
5. *Eyes.*
   Steepening of corneal curvature.
   Intolerance to contact lenses.
6. *Central Nervous System.*
   Headache, migraine, dizziness.
   Mental depression.
   Chorea.
7. *Miscellaneous.*
   Increase or decrease in weight.
   Reduced carbohydrate tolerance.
   Aggravation of porphyria.
   Edema.
   Changes in libido.

OVERDOSAGE

Serious ill effects have not been reported following acute ingestion of large doses of estrogen-containing oral contraceptives by young children. Overdosage of estrogen may cause nausea and vomiting, and withdrawal bleeding may occur in females.

DOSAGE AND ADMINISTRATION

1. For treatment of moderate to severe vasomotor symptoms, vulval and vaginal atrophy associated with the menopause, the lowest dose and regimen that will control symptoms should be chosen and medication should be discontinued as promptly as possible.
   Attempts to discontinue or taper medication should be made at 3-month to 6-month intervals.
   Usual dosage ranges:
   Vasomotor symptoms—One OGEN .625 (0.75 mg estropipate) tablet to two OGEN 2.5 (3 mg estropipate) tablets per day. The lowest dose that will control symptoms should be chosen. If the patient has not menstruated within the last two months or more, cyclic administration is started arbitrarily. If the patient is menstruating, cyclic administration is started on day 5 of bleeding.
   Vulval and vaginal atrophy—One OGEN .625 (0.75 mg estropipate) tablet to two OGEN 2.5 (3 mg estropipate) tablets daily, depending upon the tissue response of the individual patient. The lowest dose that will control symptoms should be chosen. Administer cyclically.
2. For treatment of female hypoestrogenism due to hypogonadism, castration, or primary ovarian failure.
   Usual dosage ranges:
   Female hypogonadism—A daily dose of one OGEN 1.25 (1.5 mg estropipate) tablet to three OGEN 2.5 (3 mg estropipate) tablets may be given for the first three weeks of a theoretical cycle, followed by a rest period of eight to ten days. The lowest dose that will control symptoms should be chosen. If bleeding does not occur by the end of this period, the same dosage schedule is repeated. The number of courses of estrogen therapy necessary to produce bleeding may vary depending on the responsiveness of the endometrium. If satisfactory withdrawal bleeding does not occur, an oral progestogen may be given in addition to estrogen during the third week of the cycle.
   Female castration or primary ovarian failure—A daily dose of one OGEN 1.25 (1.5 mg estropipate) tablet to three OGEN 2.5 (3 mg estropipate) tablets may be given for the first three weeks of a theoretical cycle, followed by a rest period of eight to ten days. Adjust dosage upward or downward according to severity of symptoms and response of the patient. For maintenance, adjust dosage to lowest level that will provide effective control.
   Treated patients with an intact uterus should be monitored closely for signs of endometrial cancer and appropriate diagnostic measures should be taken to rule out malignancy in the event of persistent or recurring abnormal vaginal bleeding.
3. For prevention of osteoporosis. A daily dose of OGEN .625 (0.75 mg estropipate) tablet for 25 days of a 31-day cycle per month.

HOW SUPPLIED

OGEN (estropipate tablets, USP) is supplied as OGEN .625 (0.75 mg estropipate; calculated as sodium estrone sulfate 0.625 mg), yellow, scored tablets, imprinted U 3772, **NDC** 0009-3772-01; OGEN 1.25 (1.5 mg estropipate; calculated as sodium estrone sulfate 1.25 mg), peach-colored, scored tablets, imprinted U 3773, **NDC** 0009-3773-01; and OGEN 2.5 (3 mg estropipate; calculated as sodium estrone sulfate 2.5 mg), blue, scored tablets, imprinted U 3774, **NDC** 0009-3774-01. Tablets of all three dosage levels are standardized to provide uniform estrone activity and are scored to provide dosage flexibility. All tablet sizes of OGEN are available in bottles of 100.

Continued on next page

Information on these Pharmacia & Upjohn products is based on labeling in effect June 1, 2000. Further information concerning these and other Pharmacia & Upjohn products may be obtained by direct inquiry to Medical Information, Pharmacia & Upjohn, Kalamazoo, MI 49001.

Ogen—Cont.

Recommended storage: Store below 77°F (25°C).
Rx only

PATIENT INFORMATION

WHAT YOU SHOULD KNOW ABOUT ESTROGENS

Ogen®
brand of estropipate tablets, USP

INTRODUCTION

This leaflet describes when and how to use estrogens, and the risks and benefits of estrogen treatment.

Estrogens have important benefits but also some risks. You must decide, with your doctor, whether the risks to you of estrogen use are acceptable because of their benefits. If you use estrogens, check with your doctor to be sure you are using the lowest possible dose that works, and that you don't use them longer than necessary. How long you need to use estrogens will depend on the reason for use.

WARNINGS

ESTROGENS INCREASE THE RISK OF CANCER OF THE UTERUS IN WOMEN WHO HAVE HAD THEIR MENOPAUSE ("CHANGE OF LIFE").

If you use any estrogen-containing drug, it is important to visit your doctor regularly and report any unusual vaginal bleeding right away. Vaginal bleeding after menopause may be a warning sign of uterine cancer. Your doctor should evaluate any unusual vaginal bleeding to find out the cause.

ESTROGENS SHOULD NOT BE USED DURING PREGNANCY.

Estrogens do not prevent miscarriage (spontaneous abortion) and are not needed in the days following childbirth. If you take estrogens during pregnancy, your unborn child has a greater than usual chance of having birth defects. The risk of developing these defects is small, but clearly larger than the risk in children whose mothers did not take estrogens during pregnancy. These birth defects may affect the baby's urinary system and sex organs. Daughters born to mothers who took DES (an estrogen drug) have a higher than usual chance of developing cancer of the vagina or cervix when they become teenagers or young adults. Sons may have a higher than usual chance of developing cancer of the testicles when they become teenagers or young adults.

USES OF ESTROGEN

(**Not every estrogen drug is approved for every use listed in this section.** If you want to know which of these possible uses are approved for the medicine prescribed for you, ask your doctor or pharmacist to show you the professional labeling. You can also look up the specific estrogen product in a book called the "Physicians' Desk Reference", which is available in many book stores and public libraries. Generic drugs carry virtually the same labeling information as their brand name versions.)

+ To reduce moderate or severe menopausal symptoms. Estrogens are hormones made by the ovaries of normal women. Between ages 45 and 55, the ovaries normally stop making estrogens. This leads to a drop in body estrogen levels which causes the "change of life" or menopause (the end of monthly menstrual periods). If both ovaries are removed during an operation before natural menopause takes place, the sudden drop in estrogen levels causes "surgical menopause".

When the estrogen levels begin dropping, some women develop very uncomfortable symptoms, such as feelings of warmth in the face, neck, and chest, or sudden intense episodes of heat and sweating ("hot flashes" or "hot flushes"). Using estrogen drugs can help the body adjust to lower estrogen levels and reduce these symptoms. Most women have only mild menopausal symptoms or none at all and do not need to use estrogen drugs for these symptoms. Others may need to take estrogens for a few months while their bodies adjust to lower estrogen levels. The majority of women do not need estrogen replacement for longer than six months for these symptoms.

+ To treat vulval and vaginal atrophy (itching, burning, dryness in or around the vagina, difficulty or burning on urination) associated with menopause.

+To treat certain conditions in which a young woman's ovaries do no produce enough estrogen naturally.

+ To treat certain types of abnormal vaginal bleeding due to hormonal imbalance when your doctor has found no serious cause of the bleeding.

+ To treat certain cancers in special situations, in men and women.

+ To prevent thinning of bones.

Osteoporosis is a thinning of the bones that makes them weaker and allows them to break more easily. The bones of the spine, wrists and hips break most often in osteoporosis. Both men and women start to lose bone mass after about age 40, but women lose bone mass faster after the menopause. Using estrogens after the menopause slows down bone thinning and may prevent bones from breaking. Lifelong adequate calcium intake, either in the diet (such as dairy products) or by calcium supplements (to reach a total daily intake of 1000 milligrams per day before menopause or 1500 milligrams per day after menopause), may help to prevent osteoporosis. Regular weight-bearing exercise (like walking and running for an hour, two or three times a week) may also help to prevent osteoporosis. Before you change you calcium intake or exercise habits, it is important to discuss these lifestyle changes with your doctor to find out if they are safe for you.

Since estrogen use has some risks, only women who are likely to develop osteoporosis should use estrogens for prevention. Women who are likely to develop osteoporosis often have the following characteristics: white or Asian race, slim, cigarette smokers, and a family history of osteoporosis in a mother, sister, or aunt. Women who have relatively early menopause, often because their ovaries are removed during an operation ("surgical menopause"), are more likely to develop osteoporosis than women whose menopause happens at the average age.

WHO SHOULD NOT USE ESTROGENS

Estrogens should not be used:

+ During pregnancy (see BOXED WARNINGS).

If you think you may be pregnant, do not use any form of estrogen-containing drug. Using estrogens while you are pregnant may cause your unborn child to have birth defects. Estrogens do not prevent miscarriage.

+ If you have unusual vaginal bleeding which has not been evaluated by your doctor (see BOXED WARNINGS).

Unusual vaginal bleeding can be a warning sign of cancer of the uterus, especially if it happens after menopause. Your doctor must find out the cause of the bleeding so that he or she can recommend the proper treatment. Taking estrogens without visiting your doctor can cause you serious harm if your vaginal bleeding is caused by cancer of the uterus.

+ If you have had cancer.

Since estrogens increase the risk of certain types of cancer, you should not use estrogens if you have ever had cancer of the breast or uterus, unless your doctor recommends that the drug may help in the cancer treatment. (For certain patients with breast cancer or prostate cancer, estrogens may help.)

+ If you have any circulation problems.

Estrogen drugs should not be used except in unusually special situations in which your doctor judges that you need estrogen therapy so much that the risks are acceptable. Men and women with abnormal blood clotting conditions should avoid estrogen use (see **DANGERS OF ESTROGENS,** below).

+ When they do not work.

During menopause, some women develop nervous symptoms or depression. Estrogens do not relieve these symptoms. You may have heard that taking estrogens for years after menopause will keep you skin soft and supple and keep you feeling young. There is no evidence for these claims and such long-term estrogen use may have serious risks.

+ After childbirth or when breastfeeding a baby.

Estrogens should not be used to try to stop the breasts from filling with milk after a baby is born. Such treatment may increase the risk of developing blood clots (see **DANGERS OF ESTROGENS,** below).

If you are breastfeeding, you should avoid using any drugs because many drugs pass through to the baby in the milk. While nursing a baby, you should take drugs only on the advice of your health care provider.

DANGERS OF ESTROGENS

+ Cancer of the uterus.

Your risk of developing cancer of the uterus gets higher the longer you use estrogens and the larger doses you use. One study showed that after women stop taking estrogens, this higher cancer risk quickly returns to the usual level of risk (as if you had never used estrogen therapy). Three other studies showed that the cancer risk stayed high for 8 to more than 15 years after stopping estrogen treatment. **Because of this risk, IT IS IMPORTANT TO TAKE THE LOWEST DOSE THAT WORKS AND TO TAKE IT ONLY AS LONG AS YOU NEED IT.**

Using progestin therapy together with estrogen therapy may reduce the higher risk of uterine cancer related to estrogen use (but see **OTHER INFORMATION,** below).

If you have had your uterus removed (total hysterectomy), there is no danger of developing cancer of the uterus.

+ Cancer of the breast.

Most studies have not shown a higher risk of breast cancer in women who have ever used estrogens. However, some studies have reported that breast cancer developed more often (up to twice the usual rate) in women who used estrogens for long periods of time (especially more than 10 years), or who used higher doses for shorter time periods.

Regular breast examinations by a health professional and monthly self-examination are recommended for all women.

+ Gallbladder disease.

Women who use estrogens after menopause are more likely to develop gallbladder disease needing surgery than women who do not use estrogens.

+ Abnormal blood clotting.

Taking estrogens may cause changes in you blood clotting system. These changes allow the blood to clot more easily, possibly allowing clots to form in you bloodstream. If blood clots do form in your bloodstream, they can cut off the blood supply to vital organs, causing serious problems. These problems may include a stroke (by cutting off blood to the brain), a heart attack (by cutting off blood to the heart), a pulmonary embolus (by cutting off blood to the lungs), or other problems. Any of these conditions may cause death or serious long term disability. However, most studies of low dose estrogen usage by women do not show an increased risk of these complications.

SIDE EFFECTS

In addition to the risks listed above, the following side effects have been reported with estrogen use:

Nausea and vomiting.

Breast tenderness or enlargement.

Enlargement of benign tumors ("fibroids") of the uterus.

Retention of excess fluid. This may make some conditions worsen, such as asthma, epilepsy, migraine, heart disease, or kidney disease.

A spotty darkening of the skin, particularly on the face.

REDUCING THE RISK OF ESTROGEN USE

If you use estrogens, you can reduce your risks by doing these things:

+ See your doctor regularly. While you are using estrogens, it is important to visit you doctor at least once a year for a check-up. If you develop vaginal bleeding while taking estrogens, you may need further evaluation. If members of your family have had breast cancer or if you have ever had breast lumps or an abnormal mammogram (breast x-ray), you may need to have more frequent breast examinations.

+ Reassess your need for estrogens. You and your doctor should reevaluate whether or not you still need estrogens at least every six months.

+ Be alert for signs of trouble. If any of these warning signals (or any other unusual symptoms) happen while you are using estrogens, call your doctor immediately:

Abnormal bleeding from the vagina (possible uterine cancer).

Pains in the calves or chest, sudden shortness of breath, or coughing blood (possible clot in the legs, heart, or lungs).

Severe headache or vomiting, dizziness, faintness, changes in vision or speech, weakness or numbness of an arm or leg (possible clot in the brain or eye).

Breast lumps (possible breast cancer: ask your doctor or health professional to show you how to examine your breasts monthly).

Yellowing of the skin or eyes (possible liver problem).

Pain, swelling, or tenderness in the abdomen (possible gallbladder problem).

OTHER INFORMATION

Some doctors may choose to prescribe a progestin, a different hormonal drug, for you to take together with your estrogen treatment. Progestins lower your risk of developing endometrial hyperplasia (a possible pre-cancerous condition of the uterus) while using estrogens. Taking estrogens and progestins together may also protect you from the higher risk of uterine cancer, but this has not been clearly established. Combined use of progestin and estrogen treatment may have additional risks, however. The possible risks include unhealthy effects on blood fats (especially a lowering of HDL cholesterol, the "good" blood fat which protects against heart disease risk), unhealthy effects on blood sugar (which might worsen a diabetic condition), and a possible further increase in the breast cancer risk which may be associated with long-term estrogen use. The type of progestin drug used and its dosage schedule may be important in minimizing these effects.

Your doctor has prescribed this drug for you and you alone. Do not give the drug to anyone else.

If you will be taking calcium supplements as part of the treatment to help prevent osteoporosis, check with your doctor about how much to take.

Keep this and all drugs out of the reach of children. In case of overdose, call your doctor, hospital or poison control center immediately.

This leaflet provides a summary of the most important information about estrogens. If you want more information, ask your doctor or pharmacist to show you the professional labeling. The professional labeling is also published in a book called the "Physicians' Desk Reference", which is available in book stores and public libraries. Generic drugs carry virtually the same labeling information as their brand name versions.

HOW SUPPLIED

OGEN (estropipate tablets, USP) is supplied as: OGEN .625 (0.75 mg estropipate), yellow tablets; OGEN 1.25 (1.5 mg estropipate), peach-colored tablets; OGEN 2.5 (3 mg estropipate), blue tablets.

Manufactured for
Pharmacia & Upjohn Company
Kalamazoo, MI 49001, USA
By Abbott Laboratories
North Chicago, IL 60064, USA
Revised April 1998 816 035 003

PLETAL® ℞

[PLAY-tal]
(cilostazol) (sil-OS-tah-zol)
Tablets

CONTRAINDICATION

Cilostazol and several of its metabolites are inhibitors of phosphodiesterase III. Several drugs with this pharmacologic effect have caused decreased survival compared to placebo in patients with class III-IV congestive heart failure. PLETAL is contraindicated in patients with congestive heart failure of any severity.

DESCRIPTION

PLETAL (cilostazol) is a quinolinone derivative that inhibits its cellular phosphodiesterase (more specific for phosphodi-

esterase III). The empirical formula of cilostazol is $C_{20}H_{27}N_5O_2$, and its molecular weight is 369.47. Cilostazol is 6-[4-(1-cyclohexyl-1*H*-tetrazol-5-yl)butoxy]-3,4-dihydro-2(1*H*)-quinolinone, CAS-73963-72-1.
The structural formula is:

CILOSTAZOL

Cilostazol occurs as white to off-white crystals or as a crystalline powder that is slightly soluble in methanol and ethanol, and is practically insoluble in water, 0.1 N HCl, and 0.1 N NaOH.
PLETAL (cilostazol) tablets for oral administration are available in 50 mg triangular and 100 mg round, white debossed tablets. Each tablet, in addition to the active ingredient, contains the following inactive ingredients: carboxymethylcellulose calcium, corn starch, hydroxypropyl methylcellulose 2910, magnesium stearate, and microcrystalline cellulose.

CLINICAL PHARMACOLOGY

Mechanism of Action:
The mechanism of the effects of PLETAL on the symptoms of intermittent claudication is not fully understood. PLETAL and several of its metabolites are cyclic AMP (cAMP) phosphodiesterase III inhibitors (PDE III inhibitors), inhibiting phosphodiesterase activity and suppressing cAMP degradation with a resultant increase in cAMP in platelets and blood vessels, leading to inhibition of platelet aggregation and vasodilation, respectively.
PLETAL reversibly inhibits platelet aggregation induced by a variety of stimuli, including thrombin, ADP, collagen, arachidonic acid, epinephrine, and shear stress. Effects on circulating plasma lipids have been examined in patients taking PLETAL. After 12 weeks, as compared to placebo, PLETAL 100 mg b.i.d. produced a reduction in triglycerides of 29.3 mg/dL (15%) and an increase in HDL-cholesterol of 4.0 mg/dL (≅10%).
Cardiovascular Effects:
Cilostazol affects both vascular beds and cardiovascular function. It produces non-homogenous dilation of vascular beds, with greater dilation in femoral beds than in vertebral, carotid, or superior mesenteric arteries. Renal arteries were not responsive to the effects of cilostazol.
In dogs or cynomolgous monkeys, cilostazol increased heart rate, myocardial contractile force, and coronary blood flow as well as ventricular automaticity, as would be expected for a PDE III inhibitor. Left ventricular contractility was increased at doses required to inhibit platelet aggregation. A-V conduction was accelerated. In humans, heart rate increased in a dose-proportional manner by a mean of 5.1 and 7.4 beats per minute in patients treated with 50 and 100 mg b.i.d., respectively. In 264 patients evaluated with Holter monitors, numerically more cilostazol-treated patients had increases in ventricular premature beats and non-sustained ventricular tachycardia events than did placebo-treated patients; the increases were not dose-related.

Pharmacokinetics:
PLETAL is absorbed after oral administration. A high fat meal increases absorption, with an approximately 90% increase in C_{max} and a 25% increase in AUC. Absolute bioavailability is not known. Cilostazol is extensively metabolized by hepatic cytochrome P-450 enzymes, mainly 3A4, with metabolites largely excreted in urine. Two metabolites are active, with one metabolite appearing to account for at least 50% of the pharmacologic (PDE III inhibition) activity after administration of PLETAL. Pharmacokinetics are approximately dose proportional. Cilostazol and its active metabolites have apparent elimination half-lives of about 11–13 hours. Cilostazol and its active metabolites accumulate about 2-fold with chronic administration and reach steady state blood levels within a few days. The pharmacokinetics of cilostazol and its two major active metabolites were similar in healthy normal subjects and patients with intermittent claudication due to peripheral arterial disease (PAD).
The mean ± SEM plasma concentration-time profile at steady state after multiple dosing of PLETAL 100 mg b.i.d. is shown below:
[See figure at top of next column]
Distribution:
Plasma Protein and Erythrocyte Binding:
Cilostazol is 95%–98% protein bound, predominantly to albumin. The mean percent binding for 3,4-dehydro-cilostazol is 97.4% and for 4′-trans-hydroxy-cilostazol is 66%. Mild hepatic impairment did not affect protein binding. The free fraction of cilostazol was 27% higher in subjects with renal impairment than in normal volunteers. The displacement of cilostazol from plasma proteins by erythromycin, quinidine, warfarin, and omeprazole was not clinically significant.
Metabolism and Excretion:
Cilostazol is eliminated predominately by metabolism and subsequent urinary excretion of metabolites. Based on *in vitro* studies, the primary isoenzymes involved in cilostazol's

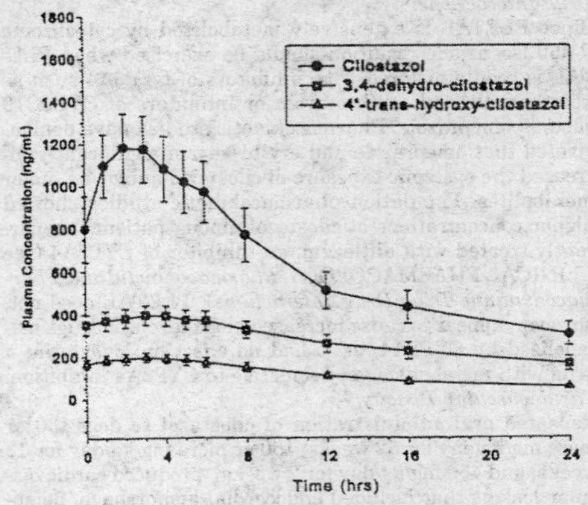

metabolism are CYP3A4 and, to a lesser extent, CYP2C19. The enzyme responsible for metabolism of 3,4-dehydro-cilostazol, the most active of the metabolites, is unknown.
Following oral administration of 100 mg radiolabeled cilostazol, 56% of the total analytes in plasma was cilostazol, 15% was 3,4-dehydro-cilostazol (4–7 times as active as cilostazol), and 4% was 4′-trans-hydroxy-cilostazol (one fifth as active as cilostazol). The primary route of elimination was via the urine (74%), with the remainder excreted in the feces (20%). No measurable amount of unchanged cilostazol was excreted in the urine, and less than 2% of the dose was excreted as 3,4-dehydro-cilostazol. About 30% of the dose was excreted in the urine as 4′-trans-hydroxy-cilostazol. The remainder was excreted as other metabolites, none of which exceeded 5%. There was no evidence of induction of hepatic microenzymes.
Special Populations:
Age and Gender:
The total and unbound oral clearances, adjusted for body weight, of cilostazol and its metabolites were not significantly different with respect to age and/or gender across a 50-to-80-year-old age range.
Smokers:
Population pharmacokinetic analysis suggests that smoking decreased cilostazol exposure by about 20%.
Hepatic Impairment:
The pharmacokinetics of cilostazol and its metabolites were similar in subjects with mild hepatic disease as compared to healthy subjects.
Patients with moderate or severe hepatic impairment have not been studied.
Renal Impairment:
The total pharmacologic activity of cilostazol and its metabolites was similar in subjects with mild to moderate renal impairment and in normal subjects. Severe renal impairment increases metabolite levels and alters protein binding of the parent and metabolites. The expected pharmacologic activity, however, based on plasma concentrations and relative PDE III inhibiting potency of parent drug and metabolites, appeared little changed. Patients on dialysis have not been studied, but, it is unlikely that cilostazol can be removed efficiently by dialysis because of its high protein binding (95%–98%).
Pharmacokinetic and Pharmacodynamic Drug-Drug Interactions:
Cilostazol could have pharmacodynamic interactions with other inhibitors of platelet function and pharmacokinetic interactions because of effects of other drugs on its metabolism by CYP3A4 or CYP2C19. Cilostazol does not appear to inhibit CYP3A4 (see *Pharmacokinetic and Pharmacodynamic Drug-Drug Interactions,* Lovastatin).
Aspirin:
Short-term (≤4 days) coadministration of aspirin with PLETAL showed a 23%–35% increase in inhibition of ADP-induced *ex vivo* platelet aggregation compared to aspirin alone; there was no clinically significant impact on PT, aPTT, or bleeding time compared to aspirin alone. There was no additive or synergistic effect on arachidonic acid-induced platelet aggregation. Effects of long-term coadministration in the general population are unknown. In eight randomized, placebo-controlled, double-blind clinical trials, aspirin was coadministered with cilostazol to 201 patients. The most frequent doses and mean durations of aspirin therapy were 75–81 mg daily for 137 days (107 patients) and 325 mg daily for 54 days (85 patients). There was no apparent greater incidence of hemorrhagic adverse effects in patients taking cilostazol and aspirin compared to patients taking placebo and equivalent doses of aspirin.
Warfarin:
The cytochrome P-450 isoenzymes involved in the metabolism of R-warfarin are CYP3A4, CYP1A2, and CYP2C19, and in the metabolism of S-warfarin, CYP2C9. Cilostazol did not inhibit either the metabolism or the pharmacologic effects (PT, aPTT, bleeding time, or platelet aggregation) of R- and S-warfarin after a single 25 mg dose of warfarin. The effect of concomitant multiple dosing of warfarin and PLETAL on the pharmacokinetics and pharmacodynamics of both drugs is unknown.
Omeprazole:
Coadministration of omeprazole did not significantly affect the metabolism of cilostazol, but the systemic exposure to 3,4-dehydro-cilostazol was increased by 69%, probably the result of omeprazole's potent inhibition of CYP2C19 (see DOSAGE AND ADMINISTRATION).
Erythromycin and other macrolide antibiotics:
Erythromycin is a moderately strong inhibitor of CYP3A4. Coadministration of erythromycin 500 mg q 8h with a single dose of cilostazol 100 mg increased cilostazol C_{max} by 47% and AUC by 73%. Inhibition of cilostazol metabolism by erythromycin increased the AUC of 4′-trans-hydroxy-cilostazol by 141%. Other macrolide antibiotics would be expected to have a similar effect (see DOSAGE AND ADMINISTRATION).
Diltiazem:
Diltiazem, a moderate inhibitor of CYP3A4, has been shown to increase cilostazol plasma concentrations by approximately 53% (see DOSAGE AND ADMINISTRATION).
This information was obtained from population pharmacokinetic analysis.
Quinidine:
Concomitant administration of quinidine with a single dose of cilostazol 100 mg did not alter cilostazol pharmacokinetics.
Strong Inhibitors of CYP3A4:
Strong inhibitors of CYP3A4, such as ketoconazole, itraconazole, fluconazole, miconazole, fluvoxamine, fluoxetine, nefazodone, and sertraline, have not been studied in combination with cilostazol but would be expected to cause a greater increase in plasma levels of cilostazol and its metabolites than erythromycin.
Lovastatin:
Coadministration of a single dose of lovastatin 80 mg with cilostazol at steady state did not result in clinically significant increases in lovastatin and its hydroxyacid metabolite plasma concentrations.
Clinical Efficacy:
The ability of PLETAL to improve walking distance in patients with stable intermittent claudication was studied in eight large, randomized, placebo-controlled, double-blind trials of 12 to 24 weeks' duration using dosages of 50 mg b.i.d. (n=303), 100 mg b.i.d. (n=998), and placebo (n=973). Efficacy was determined primarily by the change in maximal walking distance from baseline (compared to change on placebo) on one of several standardized exercise treadmill tests.
Compared to patients treated with placebo, patients treated with PLETAL 50 or 100 mg b.i.d. experienced statistically significant improvements in walking distances both for the distance before the onset of claudication pain and the distance before exercise-limiting symptoms supervened (maximal walking distance). The effect of PLETAL on walking distance was seen as early as the first on-therapy observation point of two or four weeks.
The following figure depicts the mean percentage improvement in maximal walking distance, respectively, at study end for each of the eight studies.

Mean Percentage Improvement in Maximal Walking Distance at Study End for the Eight Randomized, Double-Blind, Placebo-Controlled Clinical Trials
Placebo
PLETAL 50 mg b.i.d.
PLETAL 100 mg b.i.d.
Mean Percentage Improvement at Maximal Walking Distance
Trial: 1** N=419; 2** N=377; 3** N=245; 4** N=431; 5+ N=219; 6* N=77; 7* N=175; 8* N=126
**24 weeks' duration; +16 weeks' duration; *12 weeks' duration

Across the eight clinical trials, the range of improvement in maximal walking distance in patients treated with PLETAL 100 mg b.i.d., expressed as the percent mean change from baseline, was 28% to 100%.
The corresponding changes in the placebo group were −10% to 30%.
The Walking Impairment Questionnaire, which was administered in six of the eight clinical trials, assesses the impact of a therapeutic intervention on walking ability. In a pooled analysis of the six trials, patients treated with either PLETAL 100 mg b.i.d. or 50 mg b.i.d. reported improvements in their walking speed and walking distance as compared to placebo. Improvements in walking performance were seen in the various subpopulations evaluated, including those defined by gender, smoking status, diabetes mellitus, duration of peripheral artery disease, age, and concomitant use of beta blockers or calcium channel blockers. PLETAL has not been studied in patients with rapidly progressing claudication or in patients with leg pain at rest, ischemic leg ulcers, or gangrene. Its long-term effects on limb preservation and

Continued on next page

Information on these Pharmacia & Upjohn products is based on labeling in effect June 1, 2000. Further information concerning these and other Pharmacia & Upjohn products may be obtained by direct inquiry to Medical Information, Pharmacia & Upjohn, Kalamazoo, MI 49001.

Pletal—Cont.

hospitalization have not been evaluated. No reliable estimate of its effect on survival is available (see PRECAUTIONS).

INDICATIONS AND USAGE

PLETAL is indicated for the reduction of symptoms of intermittent claudication, as indicated by an increased walking distance.

CONTRAINDICATIONS

Cilostazol and several of its metabolites are inhibitors of phosphodiesterase III. Several drugs with this pharmacologic effect have caused decreased survival compared to placebo in patients with class III-IV congestive heart failure.

PLETAL is contraindicated in patients with congestive heart failure of any severity.

PLETAL is contraindicated in patients with known or suspected hypersensitivity to any of its components.

PRECAUTIONS

PLETAL is contraindicated in patients with congestive heart failure. In patients without congestive heart failure, the long-term effects of PDE III inhibitors (including PLETAL) are unknown. Patients in the 3–6 month placebo-controlled trials of PLETAL were relatively stable (no recent myocardial infarction or strokes, no rest pain or other signs of rapidly progressing disease) and only 19 patients died (0.7% in the placebo group and 0.8% in the PLETAL group). The calculated relative risk of death of 1.2 has a wide 95% confidence limit (0.5–3.1). There are no data as to longer-term risk or risk in patients with more severe underlying heart disease.

Use with Clopidogrel.

There is no information with respect to the efficacy or safety of the concurrent use of cilostazol and clopidogrel, a platelet-aggregation inhibiting drug indicated for use in patients with peripheral arterial disease. Studies of concomitant use of cilostazol and clopidogrel are planned.

Information for Patients:

Please refer to the patient package insert.

Patients should be advised:

- to read the patient package insert for PLETAL carefully before starting therapy and to reread it each time therapy is renewed in case the information has changed.
- to take PLETAL at least one-half hour before or two hours after food.
- that the beneficial effects of PLETAL on the symptoms of intermittent claudication may not be immediate. Although the patient may experience benefit in 2 to 4 weeks after initiation of therapy, treatment for up to 12 weeks may be required before a beneficial effect is experienced.
- about the uncertainty concerning cardiovascular risk in long-term use or in patients with severe underlying heart disease, as described under PRECAUTIONS.

Hepatic Impairment:

Patients with moderate or severe hepatic impairment have not been studied in clinical trials.

Drug Interactions:

Since PLETAL is extensively metabolized by cytochrome P-450 isoenzymes, caution should be exercised when PLETAL is coadministered with inhibitors of CYP3A4 such as ketoconazole and erythromycin or inhibitors of CYP2C19 such as omeprazole. Pharmacokinetic studies have demonstrated that omeprazole and erythromycin significantly increased the systemic exposure of cilostazol and/or its major metabolites. Population pharmacokinetic studies showed higher concentrations of cilostazol among patients concurrently treated with diltiazem, an inhibitor of CYP3A4 (see CLINICAL PHARMACOLOGY, *Pharmacokinetic and Pharmacodynamic Drug-Drug Interactions*). PLETAL does not, however, appear to cause increased blood levels of drugs metabolized by CYP3A4, as it had no effect on lovastatin, a drug with metabolism very sensitive to CYP3A4 inhibition.

Cardiovascular Toxicity:

Repeated oral administration of cilostazol to dogs (30 or more mg/kg/day for 52 weeks, 150 or more mg/kg/day for 13 weeks, and 450 mg/kg/day for 2 weeks), produced cardiovascular lesions that included endocardial hemorrhage, hemosiderin deposition and fibrosis in the left ventricle, hemorrhage in the right atrial wall, hemorrhage and necrosis of the smooth muscle in the wall of the coronary artery, intimal thickening of the coronary artery, and coronary arteritis and periarteritis. At the lowest dose associated with cardiovascular lesions in the 52-week study, systemic exposure (AUC) to unbound cilostazol was less than that seen in humans at the maximum recommended human dose (MRHD) of 100 mg b.i.d. Similar lesions have been reported in dogs following the administration of other positive inotropic agents (including PDE III inhibitors) and/or vasodilating agents. No cardiovascular lesions were seen in rats following 5 or 13 weeks of administration of cilostazol at doses up to 1500 mg/kg/day. At this dose, systemic exposures (AUCs) to unbound cilostazol were only about 1.5 and 5 times (male and female rats, respectively) the exposure seen in humans at the MRHD. Cardiovascular lesions were also not seen in rats following 52 weeks of administration of cilostazol at doses up to 150 mg/kg/day. At this dose, systemic exposures (AUCs) to unbound cilostazol were about 0.5 and 5 times (male and female rats, respectively) the exposure in humans at the MRHD. In female rats, cilostazol AUCs were similar at 150 and 1500 mg/kg/day.

Cardiovascular lesions were also not observed in monkeys after oral administration of cilostazol for 13 weeks at doses up to 1800 mg/kg/day. While this dose of cilostazol produced pharmacologic effects in monkeys, plasma cilostazol levels were less than those seen in humans given the MRHD, and those seen in dogs given doses associated with cardiovascular lesions.

Carcinogenesis, Mutagenesis, Impairment of Fertility:

Dietary administration of cilostazol to male and female rats and mice for up to 104 weeks, at doses up to 500 mg/kg/day in rats and 1000 mg/kg/day in mice, revealed no evidence of carcinogenic potential. The maximum doses administered in both rat and mouse studies were, on a systemic exposure basis, less than the human exposure at the MRHD of the drug. Cilostazol tested negative in bacterial gene mutation, bacterial DNA repair, mammalian cell gene mutation, and mouse *in vivo* bone marrow chromosomal aberration assays. It was, however, associated with a significant increase in chromosomal aberrations in the *in vitro* Chinese Hamster Ovary Cell assay.

Cilostazol did not affect fertility or mating performance of male and female rats at doses as high as 1000 mg/kg/day. At this dose, systemic exposures (AUCs) to unbound cilostazol were less than 1.5 times in males, and about 5 times in females, the exposure in humans at the MRHD.

Pregnancy:

Pregnancy Category C: In a rat developmental toxicity study, oral administration of 1000 mg cilostazol/kg/day was associated with decreased fetal weights, and increased incidences of cardiovascular, renal, and skeletal anomalies (ventricular septal, aortic arch and subclavian artery abnormalities; renal pelvic dilation; 14th rib; and retarded ossification). At this dose, systemic exposure to unbound cilostazol in nonpregnant rats was about 5 times the exposure in humans given the MRHD. Increased incidences of ventricular septal defect and retarded ossification were also noted at 150 mg/kg/day (5 times the MRHD on a systemic exposure basis). In a rabbit developmental toxicity study, an increased incidence of retardation of ossification of the sternum was seen at doses as low as 150 mg/kg/day. In nonpregnant rabbits given 150 mg/kg/day, exposure to unbound cilostazol was considerably lower than that seen in humans given the MRHD, and exposure to 3,4-dehydro-cilostazol was barely detectable.

When cilostazol was administered to rats during late pregnancy and lactation, an increased incidence of stillborn and decreased birth weights of offspring was seen at doses of 150 mg/kg/day (5 times the MRHD on a systemic exposure basis). There are no adequate and well-controlled studies in pregnant women.

Nursing Mothers:

Transfer of cilostazol into milk has been reported in experimental animals (rats). Because of the potential risk to nursing infants, a decision should be made to discontinue nursing or to discontinue PLETAL.

Pediatric Use:

The safety and effectiveness of PLETAL in pediatric patients have not been established.

Geriatric Use:

Of the total number of subjects (n = 2274) in clinical studies of PLETAL, 56 percent were 65-years-old and over, while 16 percent were 75-years-old and over. No overall differences in safety or effectiveness were observed between these subjects and younger subjects, and other reported clinical experience has not identified differences in responses between the elderly and younger patients, but greater sensitivity of some older individuals cannot be ruled out. Pharmacokinetic studies have not disclosed any age-related effects on the absorption, distribution, metabolism, and elimination of cilostazol and its metabolites.

ADVERSE REACTIONS

Adverse events were assessed in eight placebo-controlled clinical trials involving 2274 patients exposed to either 50 or 100 mg b.i.d. PLETAL (n=1301) or placebo (n=973), with a median treatment duration of 127 days for patients on PLETAL and 134 days for patients on placebo.

The only adverse event resulting in discontinuation of therapy in ≥3% of patients treated with PLETAL 50 or 100 mg b.i.d. was headache, which occurred with an incidence of 1.3%, 3.5%, and 0.3% in patients treated with PLETAL 50 mg b.i.d., 100 mg b.i.d, or placebo, respectively. Other frequent causes of discontinuation included palpitation and diarrhea, both 1.1% for cilostazol (all doses) versus 0.1% for placebo.

The most commonly reported adverse events, occurring in ≥2% of patients treated with PLETAL 50 or 100 mg b.i.d., are shown in the table (to the right).

Other events seen with an incidence of ≥2%, but occurring in the placebo group at least as frequently as in the 100 mg b.i.d. group, were: asthenia, hypertension, vomiting, leg cramps, hyperesthesia, paresthesia, dyspnea, rash, hematuria, urinary tract infection, flu syndrome, angina pectoris, arthritis, and bronchitis.

[See table below]

Less frequent adverse events (<2%) that were experienced by patients exposed to PLETAL 50 mg b.i.d. or 100 mg b.i.d. in the eight controlled clinical trials and that occurred at a frequency in the 100 mg b.i.d. group greater than in the placebo group, regardless of suspected drug relationship, are listed below.

Body as a whole: Chills, face edema, fever, generalized edema, malaise, neck rigidity, pelvic pain, retroperitoneal hemorrhage.

Cardiovascular: Atrial fibrillation, atrial flutter, cerebral infarct, cerebral ischemia, congestive heart failure, heart arrest, hemorrhage, hypotension, myocardial infarction, myocardial ischemia, nodal arrhythmia, postural hypotension, supraventricular tachycardia, syncope, varicose vein, vasodilation, ventricular extrasystoles, ventricular tachycardia.

Digestive: Anorexia, cholelithiasis, colitis, duodenal ulcer, duodenitis, esophageal hemorrhage, esophagitis, increased GGT, gastritis, gastroenteritis, gum hemorrhage, hematemesis, melena, peptic ulcer, periodontal abscess, rectal hemorrhage, stomach ulcer, tongue edema.

Endocrine: Diabetes mellitus.

Hemic and Lymphatic: Anemia, ecchymosis, iron deficiency anemia, polycythemia, purpura.

Most Commonly Reported AEs (Incidence ≥2%) in Patients on PLETAL (PLT) 50 mg b.i.d. or 100 mg b.i.d. and Occurring at a Rate in the 100 mg b.i.d. Group Higher Than in Patients on Placebo

Adverse Events (AEs) by Body System	PLT 50 mg b.i.d. (N=303) %	PLT 100 mg b.i.d. (N=998) %	Placebo (N=973) %
BODY AS A WHOLE			
Abdominal pain	4	5	3
Back pain	6	7	6
Headache	27	34	14
Infection	14	10	8
CARDIOVASCULAR			
Palpitation	5	10	1
Tachycardia	4	4	1
DIGESTIVE			
Abnormal stools	12	15	4
Diarrhea	12	19	7
Dyspepsia	6	6	4
Flatulence	2	3	2
Nausea	6	7	6
METABOLIC & NUTRITIONAL			
Peripheral edema	9	7	4
MUSCULO-SKELETAL			
Myalgia	2	3	2
NERVOUS			
Dizziness	9	10	6
Vertigo	3	1	1
RESPIRATORY			
Cough increased	3	4	3
Pharyngitis	7	10	7
Rhinitis	12	7	5

Metabolic and Nutritional: Increased creatinine, gout, hyperlipemia, hyperuricemia.
Musculo-skeletal: Arthralgia, bone pain, bursitis.
Nervous: Anxiety, insomnia, neuralgia.
Respiratory: Asthma, epistaxis, hemoptysis, pneumonia, sinusitis.
Skin and Appendages: Dry skin, furunculosis, skin hypertrophy, urticaria.
Special Senses: Amblyopia, blindness, conjunctivitis, diplopia, ear pain, eye hemorrhage, retinal hemorrhage, tinnitus.
Urogenital: Albuminuria, cystitis, urinary frequency, vaginal hemorrhage, vaginitis.

OVERDOSAGE

Information on acute overdosage with PLETAL in humans is limited. The signs and symptoms of an acute overdose can be anticipated to be those of excessive pharmacologic effect: severe headache, diarrhea, hypotension, tachycardia, and possibly cardiac arrhythmias. The patient should be carefully observed and given supportive treatment. Since cilostazol is highly protein-bound, it is unlikely that it can be efficiently removed by hemodialysis or peritoneal dialysis. The oral LD_{50} of cilostazol is >5.0 g/kg in mice and rats and >2.0 g/kg in dogs.

DOSAGE AND ADMINISTRATION

The recommended dosage of PLETAL is 100 mg b.i.d. taken at least half an hour before or two hours after breakfast and dinner. A dose of 50 mg b.i.d. should be considered during coadministration of such inhibitors of CYP3A4 as ketoconazole, itraconazole, erythromycin and diltiazem, and during coadministration of such inhibitors of CYP2C19 as omeprazole. CPY3A4 is also inhibited by grapefruit juice. Because the magnitude and timing of this interaction have not yet been investigated, patients receiving PLETAL should avoid consuming grapefruit juice.

Patients may respond as early as 2 to 4 weeks after the initiation of therapy, but treatment for up to 12 weeks may be needed before a beneficial effect is experienced.

Discontinuation of Therapy: The available data suggest that the dosage of PLETAL can be reduced or discontinued without rebound (i.e., platelet hyperaggregability).

HOW SUPPLIED

PLETAL is supplied as 50 mg and 100 mg tablets. The 50 mg tablets are white, triangular, debossed with PLETAL 50, and provided in bottles of 60 tablets (NDC #59148-003-16), and hospital unit dose packs of 100 tablets (NDC #59148-003-35). The 100 mg tablets are white, round, debossed with PLETAL 100, and provided in bottles of 60 tablets (NDC #59148-002-16), and hospital unit dose packs of 100 tablets (NDC #59148-002-35).

Rx ONLY.

STORAGE

Store PLETAL tablets at 25°C (77°F); excursions permitted to 15–30°C (59–86°F) [See USP Controlled Room Temperature].

Manufactured for
OTSUKA AMERICA PHARMACEUTICAL, INC.
Rockville, MD 20850
Copromoted with
PHARMACIA & UPJOHN
Kalamazoo, MI 49001
Manufactured by
OTSUKA PHARMACEUTICAL CO., LTD
Tokushima 771-0192, Japan
1073/01-99
U.S. Patent No. 4,277,479

Shown in Product Identification Guide, page 331

PREPIDIL® Gel ℞

[prĕp-ə-dĭl]
dinoprostone cervical gel
For Endocervical Use

DESCRIPTION

PREPIDIL Gel contains dinoprostone as the naturally occurring form of prostaglandin E_2 (PGE_2) and is designated chemically as (5Z, 11a, 13E, 15S) - 11,15 - Dihydroxy-9-oxoprosta-5, 13-dien-1-oic acid. The molecular formula is $C_{20}H_{32}O_5$ and the molecular weight is 352.5. Dinoprostone occurs as a white to off-white crystalline powder with a melting point within the range of 65° to 69°C. It is soluble in ethanol, in 25% ethanol in water, and in water to the extent of 130 mg/100 mL. The active constituent of PREPIDIL Gel is dinoprostone 0.5 mg/3 g (2.5 mL gel); other constituents are colloidal silicon dioxide NF (240 mg/3 g) and triacetin USP (2760 mg/3 g).

The structural formula is represented below:

CLINICAL PHARMACOLOGY

PREPIDIL Gel (dinoprostone) administered endocervically may stimulate the myometrium of the gravid uterus to contract in a manner similar to contractions seen in the term uterus during labor. Whether or not this action results from a direct effect of dinoprostone on the myometrium has not been determined. Dinoprostone is also capable of stimulating smooth muscle of the gastrointestinal tract in humans. This activity may be responsible for the vomiting and/or diarrhea that is occasionally seen when dinoprostone is used for preinduction cervical ripening.

In laboratory animals, and also in humans, large doses of dinoprostone can lower blood pressure, probably as a result of its effect on smooth muscle of the vascular system. With the doses of dinoprostone used for cervical ripening this effect has not been seen. In laboratory animals, and also in humans, dinoprostone can elevate body temperature; however, with the dosing used for cervical ripening this effect has not been seen.

In addition to an oxytocic effect, there is evidence suggesting that this agent has a local cervical effect in initiating softening, effacement, and dilation. These changes, referred to as cervical ripening, occur spontaneously as the normal pregnancy progresses toward term and allow evacuation of uterine contents by decreasing cervical resistance at the same time that myometrial activity increases. While not completely understood, biochemical changes within the cervix during natural cervical ripening are similar to those following PGE_2-induced ripening. Further, it has been shown that these changes can take place independent of myometrial activity; however, it is quite likely that PGE_2 administered endocervically produces effacement and softening by combined contraction-inducing and cervical-ripening properties. There is evidence to suggest that the changes that take place within the cervix are due to collagen degradation resulting from collagenase secretion as a response, at least in part, to PGE_2.

Using an unvalidated assay, the following information was determined. When PREPIDIL Gel was administered endocervically to women undergoing preinduction ripening, results from measurement of plasma levels of the metabolite 13,14-dihydro-15-keto-PGE_2 (DHK-PGE_2) showed that PGE_2 was relatively rapidly absorbed and the T_{max} was 0.5 to 0.75 hours. Plasma mean C_{max} for gel-treated subjects was 433 ± 51 pg/mL versus 137 ± 24 pg/mL for untreated controls. In those subjects in which a clinical response was observed, mean C_{max} was 484 ± 57 pg/mL versus 213 ± 69 pg/mL in nonresponders and 219 ± 92 pg/mL in control subjects who had positive clinical progression toward normal labor. These elevated levels in gel-treated subjects appear to be largely a result of absorption of PGE_2 from the gel rather than from endogenous sources.

PGE_2 is completely metabolized in humans. PGE_2 is extensively metabolized in the lungs, and the resulting metabolites are further metabolized in the liver and kidney. The major route of elimination of the products of PGE_2 metabolism is the kidneys.

INDICATIONS AND USAGE

PREPIDIL Gel is indicated for ripening an unfavorable cervix in pregnant women at or near term with a medical or obstetrical need for labor induction.

CONTRAINDICATIONS

Endocervically administered PREPIDIL Gel is not recommended for the following:

a. Patients in whom oxytocic drugs are generally contraindicated or where prolonged contractions of the uterus are considered inappropriate, such as:
   - cases with a history of cesarean section or major uterine surgery
   - cases in which cephalopelvic disproportion is present
   - cases in which there is a history of difficult labor and/or traumatic delivery
   - grand multiparae with six or more previous term pregnancies cases with non-vertex presentation
   - cases with hyperactive or hypertonic uterine patterns
   - cases of fetal distress where delivery is not imminent
   - in obstetric emergencies where the benefit-to-risk ratio for either the fetus or the mother favors surgical intervention

b. Patients with hypersensitivity to prostaglandins or constituents of the gel.

c. Patients with placenta previa or unexplained vaginal bleeding during this pregnancy.

d. Patients for whom vaginal delivery is not indicated, such as vasa previa or active herpes genitalia.

WARNINGS

FOR HOSPITAL USE ONLY

Dinoprostone, as with other potent oxytocic agents, should be used only with strict adherence to recommended dosages. Dinoprostone should be administered by physicians in a hospital that can provide immediate intensive care and acute surgical facilities.

PRECAUTIONS

1. General Precautions:

During use, uterine activity, fetal status, and character of the cervix (dilation and effacement) should be carefully monitored either by auscultation or electronic fetal monitoring to detect possible evidence of undesired responses, eg, hypertonus, sustained uterine contractility, or fetal distress. In cases where there is a history of hypertonic uterine contractility or tetanic uterine contractions, it is recommended that uterine activity and the state of the fetus should be continuously monitored. The possibility of uterine rupture should be borne in mind when high-tone myometrial contractions are sustained. Feto-pelvic relationships should be carefully evaluated before use of PREPIDIL Gel (see CONTRAINDICATIONS).

Caution should be exercised in administration of PREPIDIL Gel in patients with:
- asthma or history of asthma
- glaucoma or raised intraocular pressure

Caution should be taken so as not to administer PREPIDIL Gel above the level of the internal os. Careful vaginal examination will reveal the degree of effacement which will regulate the size of the shielded endocervical catheter to be used. That is, the 20 mm endocervical catheter should be used if no effacement is present, and the 10 mm catheter should be used if the cervix is 50% effaced. Placement of PREPIDIL Gel into the extra-amniotic space has been associated with uterine hyperstimulation.

As PREPIDIL Gel is extensively metabolized in the lung, liver, and kidney, and the major route of elimination is the kidney, PREPIDIL Gel should be used with caution in patients with renal and hepatic dysfunction.

2. Patients With Ruptured Membranes:

Caution should be exercised in the administration of PREPIDIL Gel in patients with ruptured membranes. The safety of use of PREPIDIL Gel in these patients has not been determined.

3. Drug Interactions:

PREPIDIL Gel may augment the activity of other oxytocic agents and their concomitant use is not recommended. For the sequential use of oxytocin following PREPIDIL Gel administration, a dosing interval of 6–12 hours is recommended.

4. Carcinogenesis, Mutagenesis, Impairment of Fertility:

Carcinogenic bioassay studies have not been conducted in animals with PREPIDIL Gel due to the limited indications for use and short duration of administration. No evidence of mutagenicity was observed in the Micronucleus Test or Ames Assay.

5. Pregnancy, Teratogenic Effects:

PREGNANCY CATEGORY C

Prostaglandin E_2 produced an increase in skeletal anomalies in rats and rabbits. No effect would be expected clinically, when used as indicated, since PREPIDIL Gel is administered after the period of organogenesis. PREPIDIL Gel has been shown to be embryotoxic in rats and rabbits, and any dose that produces sustained increased uterine tone could put the embryo or fetus at risk. See statements under General Precautions.

6. Pediatric Use:

Safety and effectiveness in pediatric patients have not been established.

ADVERSE REACTIONS

PREPIDIL Gel is generally well-tolerated. In controlled trials, in which 1731 women were entered, the following events were reported at an occurrence of ≥1%:

[See table above]

Adverse Reaction	PGE_2 (N=884)		Control* (N=847)	
	N	(%)	N	(%)
Maternal				
Uterine contractile abnormality	58	(6.6)	34	(4.0)
Any gastrointestinal effect	50	(5.7)	22	(2.6)
Back pain	27	(3.1)	0	(0)
Warm feeling in vagina	13	(1.5)	0	(0)
Fever	12	(1.4)	10	(1.2)
Fetal				
Any fetal heart rate abnormality	150	(17.0)	123	(14.5)
Bradycardia	36	(4.1)	26	(3.1)
Deceleration				
Late	25	(2.8)	18	(2.1)
Variable	38	(4.3)	29	(3.4)
Unspecified	19	(2.1)	19	(2.2)

*placebo gel or no treatment

In addition, in other trials amnionitis and intrauterine fetal sepsis have been associated with extra-amniotic intrauter-

Continued on next page

Information on these Pharmacia & Upjohn products is based on labeling in effect June 1, 2000. Further information concerning these and other Pharmacia & Upjohn products may be obtained by direct inquiry to Medical Information, Pharmacia & Upjohn, Kalamazoo, MI 49001.

Prepidil—Cont.

ine administration of PGE_2. Uterine rupture has been reported in association with the use of PREPIDIL Gel intracervically. Additional events reported in the literature, associated by the authors with the use of PREPIDIL Gel, included premature rupture of membranes, fetal depression (1 min Apgar <7), and fetal acidosis (umbilical artery pH <7.15).

DRUG ABUSE AND DEPENDENCE

No drug abuse or drug dependence has been seen with the use of PREPIDIL Gel.

OVERDOSAGE

Overdosage with PREPIDIL Gel may be expressed by uterine hypercontractility and uterine hypertonus. Because of the transient nature of PGE_2-induced myometrial hyperstimulation, nonspecific, conservative management was found to be effective in the vast majority of the cases; ie, maternal position change and administration of oxygen to the mother. β-adrenergic drugs may be used as a treatment of hyperstimulation following the administration of PGE_2 for cervical ripening.

DOSAGE AND ADMINISTRATION

NOTE: USE CAUTION IN HANDLING THIS PRODUCT TO PREVENT CONTACT WITH SKIN. WASH HANDS THOROUGHLY WITH SOAP AND WATER AFTER ADMINISTRATION.

PREPIDIL Gel should be brought to room temperature (59° to 86°F; 15° to 30°C) just prior to administration. Do not force the warming process by using a water bath or other source of external heat (eg, microwave oven).

To prepare the product for use, remove the peel-off seal from the end of the syringe. Then remove the protective end cap (to serve as plunger extension) and insert the protective end cap into the plunger stopper assembly in the barrel of syringe. Choose the appropriate length shielded catheter (10 mm or 20 mm) and aseptically remove the sterile shielded catheter from the package. Careful vaginal examination will reveal the degree of effacement which will regulate the size of the shielded endocervical catheter to be used. That is, the 20 mm endocervical catheter should be used if no effacement is present, and the 10 mm catheter should be used if the cervix is 50% effaced. Firmly attach the catheter hub to the syringe tip as evidenced by a distinct click. Fill the catheter with sterile gel by pushing the plunger assembly to expel air from the catheter prior to administration to the patient. Proper assembly of the dosing apparatus is shown below.

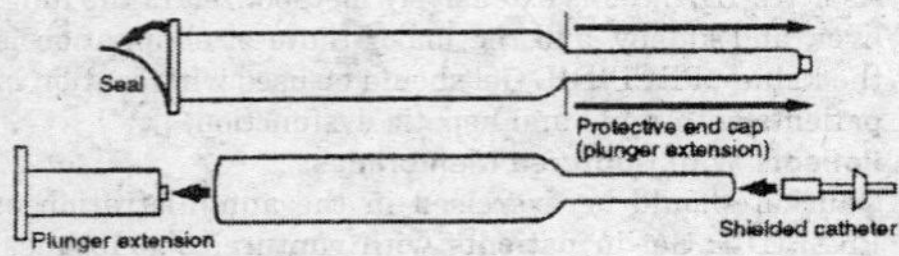

To properly administer the product, the patient should be in a dorsal position with the cervix visualized using a speculum. Using sterile technique, introduce the gel with the catheter provided into the cervical canal just below the level of the internal os. Administer the contents of the syringe by gentle expulsion and then remove the catheter. The gel is easily extrudable from the syringe. Use the contents of one syringe for one patient only. No attempt should be made to administer the small amount of gel remaining in the catheter. The syringe, catheter, and any unused package contents should be discarded after use. Following administration of PREPIDIL Gel, the patient should remain in the supine position for at least 15–30 minutes to minimize leakage from the cervical canal. If the desired response is obtained from PREPIDIL Gel, the recommended interval before giving intravenous oxytocin is 6–12 hours. If there is no cervical/uterine response to the initial dose of PREPIDIL Gel, repeat dosing may be given. The recommended repeat dose is 0.5 mg dinoprostone with a dosing interval of 6 hours. The need for additional dosing and the interval must be determined by the attending physician based on the course of clinical events. The maximum recommended cumulative dose for a 24-hour period is 1.5 mg of dinoprostone (7.5 mL PREPIDIL Gel).

HOW SUPPLIED

PREPIDIL Gel is available as a sterile semitranslucent viscous preparation for endocervical application: 0.5 mg PGE_2 per 3.0 g (2.5 mL) in syringe. In addition, each package contains two shielded catheters (10 mm and 20 mm tip) enclosed in sterile envelopes. The contents are not guaranteed sterile if envelopes are not intact.

Each 3 gram syringe applicator contains:
dinoprostone, 0.5 mg; colloidal silicon dioxide, 240 mg; triacetin, 2760 mg.

5 × 3 gram syringes NDC 0009-3359-02

PREPIDIL Gel has a shelf life of 24 months when stored under continuous refrigeration (36° to 46°F; 2° to 8°C).

Rx only

Manufactured by Pharmacia & Upjohn N.V. / S.A.,
Puurs-Belgium for
Pharmacia & Upjohn Company
Kalamazoo, MI 49001, USA
Revised April 1999 815 040 206

PROSTIN E2® ℞
dinoprostone vaginal suppository

DESCRIPTION

PROSTIN E2 Vaginal Suppository, an oxytocic, contains dinoprostone as the naturally occurring prostaglandin E2 (PGE2).

Its chemical name is (5Z,11α,13E,15S)-11,15-Dihydroxy-9-oxo-prosta-5,13-dien-1-oic acid and the structural formula is represented below:

The molecular formula is $C_{20}H_{32}O_5$. The molecular weight of dinoprostone is 352.5. Dinoprostone occurs as a white crystalline powder. It has a melting point within the range of 64° to 71° C. Dinoprostone is soluble in ethanol and in 25% ethanol in water. It is soluble in water to the extent of 130 mg/100 mL.

Each suppository contains 20 mg of dinoprostone in a mixture of glycerides of fatty acids.

CLINICAL PHARMACOLOGY

PROSTIN E2 Vaginal Suppository administered intravaginally stimulates the myometrium of the gravid uterus to contract in a manner that is similar to the contractions seen in the term uterus during labor. Whether or not this action results from a direct effect of dinoprostone on the myometrium has not been determined with certainty at this time. Nonetheless, the myometrial contractions induced by the vaginal administration of dinoprostone are sufficient to produce evacuation of the products of conception from the uterus in the majority of cases.

Dinoprostone is also capable of stimulating the smooth muscle of the gastrointestinal tract of man. This activity may be responsible for the vomiting and/or diarrhea that is not uncommon when dinoprostone is used to terminate pregnancy. In laboratory animals, and also in man, large doses of dinoprostone can lower blood pressure, probably as a consequence of its effect on the smooth muscle of the vascular system. With the doses of dinoprostone used for terminating pregnancy this effect has not been clinically significant. In laboratory animals, and also in man, dinoprostone can elevate body temperature. With the clinical doses of dinoprostone used for the termination of pregnancy some patients do exhibit temperature increases.

INDICATIONS AND USAGE

1. PROSTIN E2 Vaginal Suppository is indicated for the termination of pregnancy from the 12th through the 20th gestational week as calculated from the first day of the last normal menstrual period.
2. PROSTIN E2 is also indicated for evacuation of the uterine contents in the management of missed abortion or intrauterine fetal death up to 28 weeks of gestational age as calculated from the first day of the last normal menstrual period.
3. PROSTIN E2 is indicated in the management of nonmetastatic gestational trophoblastic disease (benign hydatidiform mole).

CONTRAINDICATIONS

1. Hypersensitivity to dinoprostone
2. Acute pelvic inflammatory disease
3. Patients with active cardiac, pulmonary, renal, or hepatic disease

WARNINGS

Dinoprostone, as with other potent oxytocic agents, should be used only with strict adherence to recommended dosages. Dinoprostone should be used by medically trained personnel in a hospital which can provide immediate intensive care and acute surgical facilities.

Dinoprostone does not appear to directly affect the fetoplacental unit. Therefore, the possibility does exist that the previable fetus aborted by dinoprostone could exhibit transient life signs. Dinoprostone is not indicated if the fetus in utero has reached the stage of viability. Dinoprostone should not be considered a feticidal agent.

Evidence from animal studies has suggested that certain prostaglandins may have some teratogenic potential. Therefore, any failed pregnancy termination with dinoprostone should be completed by some other means.

PROSTIN E2 Vaginal Suppository should not be used for extemporaneous preparation of any other dosage form. Neither the PROSTIN E2 Vaginal Suppository, as dispensed nor any extemporaneous formulation made from the PROSTIN E2 Vaginal Suppository should be used for cervical ripening or other indication in the patient with term pregnancy.

PRECAUTIONS

1. **General precautions**

Animal studies lasting several weeks at high doses have shown that prostaglandins of the E and F series can induce proliferation of bone. Such effects have also been noted in newborn infants who have received prostaglandin E1 during prolonged treatment. There is no evidence that short term administration of PROSTIN E2 Vaginal Suppository can cause similar bone effects.

As in spontaneous abortion, where the process is sometimes incomplete, abortion induced by PROSTIN E2 may sometimes be incomplete. In such cases, other measures should be taken to assure complete abortion.

In patients with a history of asthma, hypo- or hypertension, cardiovascular disease, renal disease, hepatic disease, anemia, jaundice, diabetes or history of epilepsy, dinoprostone should be used with caution.

Dinoprostone administered by the vaginal route should be used with caution in the presence of cervicitis, infected endocervical lesions, or acute vaginitis.

As with any oxytocic agent, dinoprostone should be used with caution in patients with compromised (scarred) uteri.

Dinoprostone vaginal therapy is associated with transient pyrexia that may be due to its effect on hypothalamic thermoregulation. In the patients studied, temperature elevations in excess of 2°F (1.1°C) were observed in approximately one-half of the patients on the recommended dosage regimen. In all cases, temperature returned to normal on discontinuation of therapy. Differentiation of post-abortion endometritis from drug-induced temperature elevations is difficult, but with increasing clinical exposure and experience with PGE2 vaginal therapy the distinctions become more obviously apparent and are summarized below:

[See table below]

In the absence of clinical or bacteriological evidence of intrauterine infection, supportive therapy for drug induced fevers includes the forcing of fluids. As all PGE2-induced fevers have been found to be transient or self-limiting, it is doubtful if any simple empirical measures for temperature reduction are indicated.

2. **Laboratory tests**

When a pregnancy diagnosed as missed abortion is electively interrupted with intravaginal administration of dinoprostone, confirmation of intrauterine fetal death

Endometritis pyrexia	PGE2 induced pyrexia
a. **Time of onset**: Typically, on third post-abortional day (38°C or higher).	Within 15–45 minutes of suppository administration.
b. **Duration**: Untreated pyrexia and infection continue and may give rise to other infective pelvic pathology.	Elevations revert to pretreatment levels within 2–6 hours after discontinuation of therapy or removal of suppository from vagina without any other treatment.
c. **Retention**: Products of conception are often retained in the cervical os or uterine cavity.	Elevation occurs irrespective of any retained tissue.
d. **Histology**: Endometrium shows evidence of inflammatory lymphocytic infiltration with areas of necrotic hemorrhagic tissue.	Although the endometrial stroma may be edematous and vascular, there is relative absence of inflammatory reaction.
e. **The uterus**: Often remains boggy and soft with tenderness over the fundus, and pain on moving the cervix, on bimanual examination.	Normal uterine involution not tender.
f. **Discharge**: Often associated foul-smelling lochia and leukorrhea.	Lochia normal.

g. **Cervical culture**
The culture of pathological organisms from the cervix or uterine cavity after abortion does not, of itself, warrant the diagnosis of septic abortion in the absence of clinical evidence of sepsis. It is not uncommon to culture pathogens from cases of recent abortion *not* clinically infected. Persistent positive culture with clear clinical signs of infection are significant in the differential diagnosis.

h. **Blood count**
Leukocytosis and differential white cell counts are not of major clinical importance in distinguishing between the two conditions, since total WBC's may be increased as a result of infection and transient leukocytosis may also be drug induced.

should be obtained in respect to a *negative pregnancy test* for chorionic gonadotropic activity (U.C.G. test or equivalent). When a pregnancy with late fetal intrauterine death is interrupted with intravaginal administration of dinoprostone, confirmation of intrauterine fetal death should be obtained prior to treatment.

3. **Drug interactions**
PROSTIN E2 may augment the activity of other oxytocic drugs. Concomitant use with other oxytocic agents is not recommended.
4. **Carcinogenesis, mutagenesis, impairment of fertility**
Carcinogenic bioassay studies have not been conducted in animals with PROSTIN E2 due to the limited indications for use and short duration of administration. No evidence of mutagenicity was observed in the Micronucleus Test or Ames Assay.
5. **Pregnancy:** Teratogenic Effects: Pregnancy Category C
Animal studies do not indicate that PROSTIN E2 is teratogenic, however, it has been shown to be embryotoxic in rats and rabbits and any dose which produces increased uterine tone could put the embryo or fetus at risk. See WARNINGS section.
6. **Pediatric use:** Safety and effectiveness in pediatric patients have not been established.

ADVERSE REACTIONS

The most frequent adverse reactions observed with the use of dinoprostone for abortion are related to its contractile effect on smooth muscle.

In the patients studied, approximately two-thirds experienced vomiting, one-half temperature elevations, two-fifths diarrhea, one-third some nausea, one-tenth headache and one-tenth shivering and chills.

In addition, approximately one-tenth of the patients studied exhibited transient diastolic blood pressure decreases of greater than 20 mmHg.

Two cases of myocardial infarction following the use of dinoprostone have been reported in patients with a history of cardiovascular disease.

It is not known whether these events were related to the administration of dinoprostone.

Adverse effects in decreasing order of their frequency, observed with the use of dinoprostone, not all of which are clearly drug related include:

Vomiting
Diarrhea
Nausea
Fever
Headache
Chills or shivering
Backache
Joint inflammation or pain new or exacerbated
Flushing or hot flashes
Dizziness
Arthralgia
Vaginal pain
Chest pain
Dyspnea
Endometritis
Syncope or fainting sensation
Vaginitis or vulvitis
Weakness
Muscle cramp or pain
Tightness in chest
Nocturnal leg cramps
Uterine rupture
Breast tenderness
Blurred vision
Coughing
Rash
Myalgia
Stiff neck
Dehydration
Tremor
Paresthesia
Hearing impairment
Urine retention
Pharyngitis
Laryngitis
Diaphoresis
Eye pain
Wheezing
Cardiac arrhythmia
Skin discoloration
Vaginismus
Tension

DOSAGE AND ADMINISTRATION

STORE IN A FREEZER NOT ABOVE –20°C (–4°F) BUT BRING TO ROOM TEMPERATURE JUST PRIOR TO USE. REMOVE FOIL BEFORE USE.

A suppository containing 20 mg of dinoprostone should be inserted high into the vagina. The patient should remain in the supine position for ten minutes following insertion.

Additional intravaginal administration of each subsequent suppository should be at 3- to 5-hour intervals until abortion occurs. Within the above recommended intervals administration time should be determined by abortifacient progress, uterine contractility response, and by patient tolerance. Continuous administration of the drug for more than 2 days is not recommended.

HOW SUPPLIED

PROSTIN E2 Vaginal Suppositories are available in foil strips of 5 individually sealed suppositories. Each suppository contains 20 mg of dinoprostone in a mixture of glycerides of fatty acids.

STORE IN A FREEZER NOT ABOVE –20°C (–4°F).

℞ only

Pharmacia & Upjohn Company
Kalamazoo, MI 49001, USA
Revised August 1999 810 994 514
692166

PROVERA® ℞
[*prō-vĕră*]
medroxyprogesterone acetate tablets, USP

DESCRIPTION

PROVERA Tablets contain medroxyprogesterone acetate, which is a derivative of progesterone. It is a white to off-white, odorless crystalline powder, stable in air, melting between 200 and 210°C. It is freely soluble in chloroform, soluble in acetone and in dioxane, sparingly soluble in alcohol and in methanol, slightly soluble in ether, and insoluble in water.

The chemical name for medroxyprogesterone acetate is Pregn-4-ene-3,20-dione, 17-(acetyloxy)-6-methyl-, (6α)-. The structural formula is:

Each PROVERA tablet for oral administration contains 2.5 mg, 5 mg or 10 mg of medroxyprogesterone acetate. Inactive ingredients: calcium stearate, corn starch, lactose, mineral oil, sorbic acid, sucrose, talc. The 2.5 mg tablet contains FD&C Yellow no. 6.

CLINICAL PHARMACOLOGY

Medroxyprogesterone acetate (MPA), administered orally or parenterally in the recommended doses to women with adequate endogenous estrogen, transforms proliferative into secretory endometrium. Androgenic and anabolic effects have been noted, but the drug is apparently devoid of significant estrogenic activity. While parenterally administered MPA inhibits gonadotropin production, which in turn prevents follicular maturation and ovulation, available data indicate that this does not occur when the usually recommended oral dosage is given as single daily doses.

Pharmacokinetics

The pharmacokinetics of MPA were determined in 20 postmenopausal women following a single-dose administration of eight PROVERA Tablets 2.5 mg or a single administration of two PROVERA Tablets 10 mg under fasting conditions. In another study, the steady-state pharmacokinetics of MPA were determined under fasting conditions in 30 postmenopausal women following daily adminstration of one PROVERA Tablet 10 mg for 7 days. In both studies, MPA was quantitated in serum using a validated gas chromatography-mass spectrometry (GC-MS) method. Estimates of the pharmacokinetic parameters of MPA after single and multiple doses of PROVERA Tablets were highly variable and are summarized in Table 1.

[See table above]

Table 1. Mean (SD) Pharmacokinetic Parameters for Medroxyprogesterone Acetate (MPA)

Tablet Strength	C_{max} (ng/mL)	T_{max} (h)	$Auc_{0-\infty}$ (ng•h/mL)	$t_{1/2}$ (h)	Vd/f (L)	CL/f (mL/min)
Single Dose						
2 × 10 mg	1.01 (0.599)	2.65 (1.41)	6.95 (3.39)	12.1 (3.49)	78024 (47220)	64110 (42662)
8 × 2.5 mg	0.805 (0.413)	2.22 (1.39)	5.62 (2.79)	11.6 (2.81)	62748 (40146)	74123 (35126)
Multiple Dose						
10 mg*	0.71 (0.35)	2.83 (1.83)	6.01 (3.16)	16.6 (15.0)	40564 (38256)	41963 (38402)

*Following Day 7 dose

Absorption: No specific investigation on the absolute bioavailability of MPA in humans has been conducted. MPA is rapidly absorbed from the gastrointestinal tract, and maximum MPA concentrations are obtained between 2 to 4 hours after oral administration.

Effect of Food: Administration of PROVERA with food increases the bioavailability of MPA. A 10-mg dose of PROVERA, taken immediately before or after a meal, increased MPA C_{max} (50 to 70%) and AUC (18 to 33%). The half-life of MPA was not changed with food.

Distribution: MPA is approximately 90% protein bound, primarily to albumin; no MPA binding occurs with sex-hormone binding globulin. The unbound MPA modulates pharmacologic responses.

Metabolism: Following oral dosing, MPS is extensively metabolized in the liver via ring A and/or side-chain hydroxylation, with subsequent conjugation and elimination in the urine. At least 16 MPA metabolites have been identified.

Excretion: Most MPA metabolites are excreted in the urine as glucuronide conjugates with only minor amounts excreted as sulfates. Mean percent dose excreted in the 24-hour urine of patients with fatty liver as intact MPA after a 10-mg or 100-mg dose was 7.3% and 6.4%, respectively.

Special Populations

Renal Insufficiency: The pharmacokinetics of MPA in patients with varying degrees of renal insufficiency have not been investigated. The renal clearance of MPA is negligible and a decrease in total body clearance is not expected in patients with renal insufficiency.

Hepatic Insufficiency: MPA is almost exclusively eliminated via hepatic metabolism. In 14 patients with advanced liver disease, MPA disposition was significantly altered (reduced elimination). As such, PROVERA is contraindicated in patients with severe hepatic disease (see CONTRAINDICATIONS). However, for patients with mild-moderate degree of hepatic impairment, a lower dose of PROVERA or a less frequent administration should be considered.

Drug-Drug Interactions

No formal pharmacokinetic drug-drug interaction studies have been conducted with PROVERA. However, published literature indicates that coadministration of conjugated estrogens with MPA does not affect the pharmacokinetic profile of MPA; similarly, MPA does not affect the pharmacokinetic profile of the conjugated or unconjugated estrogens. Literature data also indicate that concomitant administration with aminoglutethimide would significantly reduce serum concentrations of MPA, likely by increasing the clearance of the drug.

CLINICAL STUDIES

The use of unopposed estrogen therapy has been associated with an increased risk of endometrial hyperplasia, a possible precursor of endometrial carcinoma.[1] The incidence of estrogen-associated endometrial hyperplasia and endometrial cancer was assessed in two large, long-term, randomized clinical trials. The histological results of the clinical studies indicate that the addition of PROVERA to an estrogen replacement regimen for 12 to 14 days per cycle reduces the incidence of endometrial hyperplasia in women with intact uteri. The addition of a progestin to 0.625 mg conjugated estrogen has not been shown to interfere with the efficacy of 0.625 mg conjugated estrogen for its approved indications.[1–3]

A 3-year, double-blind, placebo-controlled study of nonhysterectomized, postmenopausal women between the ages of 45 and 64 years were randomized to receive placebo, conjugated estrogen only, or conjugated estrogen plus cyclic PROVERA. The treatment group receiving 10 mg PROVERA plus 0.625 mg conjugated estrogens showed a significantly lower rate of hyperplasia in comparison to the group given 0.625 mg conjugated estrogens only. The 3-year histological results are summarized in Table 2.

Table 2. Number (%) of Endometrial Biopsy Changes Since Baseline After 3 Years of Treatment*

Histological Results	Placebo (n=119)	CEE† (n=119)	PROVERA‡ + CEE (n=118)
Normal/No hyperplasia (%)	116 (97)	45 (38)	112 (95)
Simple (cystic) hyperplasia (%)	1 (1)	33 (28)	4 (3)
Complex (adenomatous) hyperplasia (%)	1 (1)	27 (22)	2 (2)
Atypia (%)	0	14 (12)	0
Adenocarcinoma (%)	1 (1)	0	0

* Includes most extreme abnormal result
† CEE = conjugated equine estrogens 0.625 mg/day
‡ PROVERA = medroxyprogesterone acetate tablets 10 mg/day for 12 days

In a second study, postmenopausal women between the ages of 45 and 65 years were enrolled in a 1-year, double-blind study. All patients received conjugated estrogen 0.625 mg every day of a 28-day cycle, and were randomized to receive cyclic MPA 5 mg, cyclic MPA 10 mg, or conjugated estrogen only. The treatment groups receiving MPA 5 or 10 mg plus conjugated estrogens showed a significantly lower rate of

Continued on next page

Information on these Pharmacia & Upjohn products is based on labeling in effect June 1, 2000. Further information concerning these and other Pharmacia & Upjohn products may be obtained by direct inquiry to Medical Information, Pharmacia & Upjohn, Kalamazoo, MI 49001.

Provera—Cont.

hyperplasia in comparison to the group given conjugated estrogens only. The incidence of endometrial hyperplasia is shown in Table 3.

Table 3. Number (%) of Women with Endometrial Hyperplasia at 1 Year

	CEE*	MPA† + CEE*	
	(n=283)	MPA 5 mg (n=277)	MPA 10 mg (n=272)
Cystic hyperplasia (%)	55 (19)	3 (1)	0
Adenomatous hyperplasia without atypia	2 (1)	0	0

* CEE = conjugated equine estrogen 0.625 mg every day of a 28-day cycle.
† Cyclic medroxyprogesterone acetate on days 15 to 28

INDICATIONS AND USAGE

PROVERA Tablets are indicated for secondary amenorrhea and for abnormal uterine bleeding due to hormonal imbalance in the absence of organic pathology, such as fibroids or uterine cancer. PROVERA Tablets are also indicated to reduce the incidence of endometrial hyperplasia in nonhysterectomized postmenopausal women receiving 0.625 mg conjugated estrogen.

CONTRAINDICATIONS

1. Thrombophlebitis, thromboemoblic disorders, cerebral apoplexy or patients with a past history of these conditions.
2. Liver dysfunction or disease.
3. Known or suspected malignancy of breast or genital organs.
4. Undiagnosed vaginal bleeding.
5. Missed abortion.
6. As a diagnostic test for pregnancy.
7. Known sensitivity to PROVERA Tablets.
8. Known or suspected pregnancy.

WARNINGS

1. The physician should be alert to the earliest manifestations of thrombotic disorders (thrombophlebitis, cerebrovascular disorders, pulmonary embolism, and retinal thrombosis). Should any of these occur or be suspected, the drug should be discontinued immediately.
2. Beagle dogs treated with medroxyprogesterone acetate developed mammary nodules some of which were malignant. Although nodules occasionally appeared in control animals, they were intermittent in nature, whereas the nodules in the drug-treated animals were larger, more numerous, persistent, and there were some breast malignancies with metastases. Their significance with respect to humans has not been established.
3. Discontinue medication pending examination if there is sudden partial or complete loss of vision, or if there is a sudden onset of proptosis, diplopia or migraine. If examination reveals papilledema or retinal vascular lesions, medication should be withdrawn.
4. Detectable amounts of progestin have been identified in the milk of mothers receiving the drug. The effect of this on the nursing neonate and infant has not been determined.
5. Usage in pregnancy is contraindicated.
6. Retrospective studies of morbidity and mortality in Great Britain and studies of morbidity in the United States have shown a statistically significant association between thrombophlebitis, pulmonary embolism, and cerebral thrombosis and emoblism and the use of oral contraceptives.[4–7] The estimate of the relative risk of thromboembolism in the study by Vessey and Doll[6] was about sevenfold, while Sartwell and associates[7] in the United States found a relative risk of 4.4, meaning that the users are several times as likely to undergo thromboemoblic disease without evident cause as nonusers. The American study also indicated that the risk did not persist after discontinuation of adminstration, and that it was not enhanced by long continued adminstration. The American study was not designed to evaluate a difference between products.

PRECAUTIONS

General

1. The pretreatment physical examination should include special reference to breast and pelvic organs, as well as Papanicolaou smear.
2. Because progestogens may cause some degree of fluid retention, conditions which might be influenced by this factor, such as epilepsy, migraine, asthma, cardiac or renal dysfunction, require careful observation.
3. In case of breakthrough bleeding, as in all cases of irregular bleeding via vaginam, nonfunctional causes should be borne in mind. In cases of undiagnosed vaginal bleeding, adequate diagnostic measures are indicated.
4. Patients who have a history of psychic depression should be carefully observed and the drug discontinued if the depression recurs to a serious degree.
5. Any possible influence of prolonged progestin therapy on pituitary, ovarian, adrenal, hepatic or uterine functions awaits further study.
6. Diabetic patients should be carefully observed while receiving progestin therapy.
7. The age of the patient constitutes no absolute limiting factor although treatment with progestins may mask the onset of the climacteric.
8. The pathologist should be advised of progestin therapy when relevant specimens are submitted.
9. Because of the occurrence of thrombotic disorders, (thrombophlebitis, pulmonary emoblism, retinal thrombosis, and cerebrovascular disorders) in patients taking estrogen-progestin combinations and since the mechanism is obscure, the physician should be alert to the earliest mainfestation of these disorders.

Carcinogenesis, Mutagenesis, Impairment of Fertility.

Long-term intramuscular administration of PROVERA has been shown to produce mammary tumors in beagle dogs. There was no evidence of a carcinogenic effect associated with the oral administration of PROVERA to rats and mice. Medroxyprogesterone acetate was not mutagenic in a battery of *in vitro* or *in vivo* genetic toxicity assays.
Medroxyprogesterone acetate at high doses is an antifertility drug and high doses would be expected to impair fertility until the cessation of treatment.

Information for the Patient

See Patient Information at end of insert.

Pregnancy

Pregnancy Category X—PROVERA Tablets are contraindicated during pregnancy. Several reports suggest an association between intrauterine exposure to progestational drugs in the first trimester of pregnancy and genital abnormalities in male and female fetuses. The risk of hypospadias in male fetuses may be doubled with exposure to these drugs. Some progestational drugs induce mild virilization of the external genitalia of female fetuses.

Nursing Mothers

The administration of any drug to nursing mothers should be done only when clearly necessary since many drugs are excreted in human milk. Detectable amounts of progestin have been identified in the milk of nursing mothers receiving progestins. The effect of this on the nursing infant has not been determined.

Pediatric Use

The safety and effectiveness of PROVERA Tablets in pediatric patients has not been established.

ADVERSE REACTIONS

Breast—Breast tenderness or galactorrhea has been reported.
Skin—Sensitivity reactions consisting of urticaria, pruritus, edema and generalized rash have occurred. Acne, alopecia and hirsutism have been reported.
Thromboembolic Phenomena—Thromboembolic phenomena including thrombophlebitis and pulmonary embolism have been reported.
Other—The following adverse reactions have been observed in women taking progestins, including PROVERA Tablets:
breakthrough bleeding
spotting
change in menstrual flow
amenorrhea
endema
change in weight (increase or decrease)
changes in cervical erosion and cervical secretions
cholestatic jaundice
anaphylactoid reactions and anaphylaxis rash (allergic) with and without pruritus
mental depression
pyrexia
insomnia
nausea
somnolence
Althouth available evidence is suggestive of an association, such a relationship has been neither confirmed nor refuted for the following serious adverse reactions:
neuro-ocular lesions, eg, retinal thrombosis and optic neuritis.
The following adverse reactions have been observed in patients receiving estrogen-progestin combination drugs:
rise in blood pressure in susceptible individuals
premenstrual-like syndrome
changes in libido
changes in appetite
cystitis-like syndrome headache
nervousness
fatigue
backache
hirsutism
loss of scalp hair
erythema multiforme
erythema nodosum
hemorrhagic eruption
itching
dizziness
Laboratory Tests—The following laboratory results may be altered by the use of estrogen-progestin combination drugs:
Increased sulfobromophthalein retention and other hepatic function tests.
Coagulation tests: increase in prothrombin factors VII, VIII, IX and X.
Metyrapone test.
Pregnanediol determination.
Thyroid function: increase in PBI, and butanol extractable protein bound iodine and decrease in T³uptake values.

DOSAGE AND ADMINISTRATION

Secondary Amenorrhea—PROVERA Tablets may be given in dosages of 5 or 10 mg daily for 5 to 10 days. A dose for inducing an optimum secretory transformation of an endometrium that has been adequately primed with either endogenous or exogenous estrogen is 10 mg of PROVERA daily for 10 days. In cases of secondary amenorrhea, therapy may be started at any time. Progestin withdrawal bleeding usually occurs within three to seven days after discontinuing PROVERA therapy.
Abnormal Uterine Bleeding Due to Hormonal Imbalance in the Absence of Organic Pathology—Beginning on the calculated 16th or 21st day of the menstrual cycle, 5 or 10 mg of medroxyprogesterone acetate may be given daily for 5 to 10 days. To produce an optimum secretory transformation of an endometrium that has been adequately primed with either endogenous or exogenous estrogen, 10 mg of medroxyprogesterone acetate daily for 10 days beginning on the 16th day of the cycle is suggested. Progestin withdrawal bleeding usually occurs within three to seven days after discontinuing therapy with PROVERA. Patients with a past history of recurrent episodes of abnormal uterine bleeding may benefit from planned menstrual cycling with PROVERA.
Reduction of endometrial hyperplasia in post-menopausal women receiving 0.625 mg conjugated estrogens—PROVERA Tablets may be given in dosages of 5 or 10 mg daily for 12 to 14 consecutive days per month, either beginning on the 1st day of the cycle or the 16th day of the cycle.

HOW SUPPLIED

PROVERA Tablets are available in the following strengths and package sizes:

2.5 mg (scored, round, orange)	
Bottles of 30	NDC 0009-0064-06
Bottles of 100	NDC 0009-0064-04
5 mg (scored, hexagonal, white)	
Bottles of 30	NDC 0009-0286-32
Bottles of 100	NDC 0009-0286-03
10 mg (scored, round, white)	
Bottles of 30	NDC 0009-0050-09
Bottles of 100	NDC 0009-0050-02
Bottles of 500	NDC 0009-0050-11

Store at controlled room temperature 20° to 25°C (68° to 77°F) [see USP].

REFERENCES

1. Writing Group for the PEPI Trial: Effects of hormone replacement therapy on endometrial histology in postmenopausal women. JAMA **275**:370–375, 1996.
2. Woodruff JD, Pickar JH: Incidence of endometrial hyperplasia in postmenopausal women taking conjugated estrogens (Premarin) with medroxyprogesterone acetate or conjugated estrogens alone (The Menopause Study Group). Am J Obstet Gynecol **170**:1213–1223, 1994.
3. Speroff L, Rowan J, Symons J, et al: The comparative effect on bone density, endometrium, and lipids of continuous hormones as replacement therapy (CHART Study) JAMA **276**:1397–1403, 1996.
4. Royal College of General Practitioners: Oral contraception and thromboembolic disease. J Coll Gen Pract **13**: 267–279, 1967.
5. Inman WHW, Vessey MP: Investigation of deaths from pulmonary, coronary, and cerebral thrombosis and embolism in women in child-bearing age. Br Med J **2**:193–199, 1968.
6. Vessey MP, Doll R: Investigation of relation between use of oral contraceptives and thromboembolic disease. A further report. Br Med J **2**:651–657, 1969.
7. Sartwell PE, Masi AT, Arthes FG, et al: Thromboembolism and oral contraceptives: An epidemiological case-control study. Am J Epidemiol **90**:365–380, 1969.

The text of the patient insert for progesterone and progesterone-like drugs is set forth below.

PATIENT INFORMATION

PROVERA Tablets contain medroxyprogesterone acetate, a progesterone. The information below is that which the U.S. Food and Drug Administration requires be provided for all patients taking progesterones. The information below relates only to the risk to the unborn child associated with use of progesterone during pregnancy. For further information on the use, side effects and other risks associated with this product, ask your doctor.

WARNING FOR WOMEN

Progesterone or progesterone-like drugs have been used to prevent miscarriage in the first few months of pregnancy. No adequate evidence is available to show that they are effective for this purpose. Furthermore, most cases of early miscarriage are due to causes which could not be helped by these drugs.
There is an increased risk of minor birth defects in children whose mothers take this drug during the first 4 months of pregnancy. Several reports suggest an association between mothers who take these drugs in the first trimester of pregnancy and genital abnormalities in male and female babies. The risk to the male baby is the possibility of being born with a condition in which the opening of the penis is on the underside rather than the tip of the penis (hypospadias).

Hypospadias occurs in about 5 to 8 per 1,000 male births and is about doubled with exposure to these drugs. There is not enough information to quantify the risk to exposed female fetuses, but enlargement of the clitoris and fusion of the labia may occur, although rarely.

Therefore, since drugs of this type may induce mild masculinization of the external genitalia of the female fetus, as well as hypospadias in the male fetus, it is wise to avoid using the drug during the first trimester of pregnancy.

These drugs have been used as a test for pregnancy but such use is no longer considered safe because of possible damage to a developing baby. Also, more rapid methods for testing for pregnancy are now available.

If you take PROVERA and later find you were pregnant when you took it, be sure to discuss this with your doctor as soon as possible.

Rx only

Pharmacia & Upjohn Company
Kalamazoo, MI 49001, USA
Revised August 1998 812 584 512
691015

Shown in Product Identification Guide, page 331

SOLU-MEDROL® ℞
[*sōlū-mĕdrōl*]
methylprednisolone sodium succinate
for injection, USP
For Intravenous or Intramuscular Administration

DESCRIPTION

SOLU-MEDROL Sterile Powder contains methylprednisolone sodium succinate as the active ingredient. Methylprednisolone sodium succinate, USP, occurs as a white, or nearly white, odorless hygroscopic, amorphous solid. It is very soluble in water and in alcohol; it is insoluble in chloroform and is very slightly soluble in acetone.

The chemical name for methylprednisolone sodium succinate is pregna-1,4-diene-3,20-dione,21-(3-carboxy-1-oxopropoxy)-11,17-dihydroxy-6-methyl-monosodium salt, (6α, 11β), and the molecular weight is 496.53.

The structural formula is represented below:

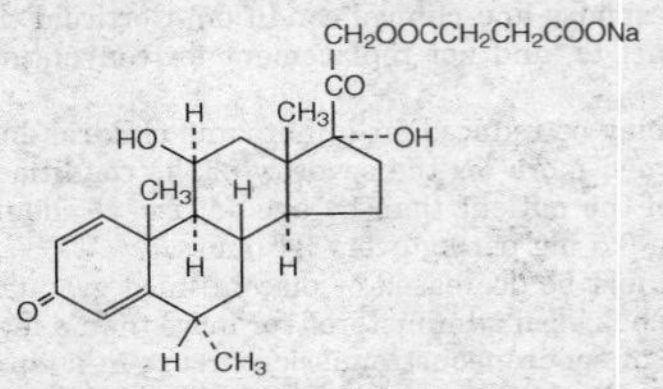

Methylprednisolone sodium succinate is so extremely soluble in water that it may be administered in a small volume of diluent and is especially well suited for intravenous use in situations in which high blood levels of methylprednisolone are required rapidly.

SOLU-MEDROL is available in several strengths and packages for intravenous or intramuscular administration.

40 mg Act-O-Vial® System (Single-Dose Vial)—Each mL (when mixed) contains methylprednisolone sodium succinate equivalent to 40 mg methylprednisolone; also 1.6 mg monobasic sodium phosphate anhydrous; 17.46 mg dibasic sodium phosphate dried; 25 mg lactose hydrous; 8.8 mg benzyl alcohol added as preservative.

125 mg Act-O-Vial System (Single-Dose Vial)—Each 2 mL (when mixed) contains methylprednisolone sodium succinate equivalent to 125 mg methylprednisolone; also 1.6 mg monobasic sodium phosphate anhydrous; 17.4 mg dibasic sodium phosphate dried; 17.6 mg benzyl alcohol added as preservative.

500 mg Vial—Each 8 mL (when mixed as directed) contains methylprednisolone sodium succinate equivalent to 500 mg methylprednisolone; also 6.4 mg monobasic sodium phosphate anhydrous; 69.6 mg dibasic sodium phosphate dried.

500 mg Vial with Diluent—Each 8 mL (when mixed as directed) contains methylprednisolone sodium succinate equivalent to 500 mg methylprednisolone; also 6.4 mg monobasic sodium phosphate anhydrous; 69.6 mg dibasic sodium phosphate dried; 70.2 mg benzyl alcohol added as preservative.

500 mg Act-O-Vial System (Single-Dose Vial)—Each 4 mL (when mixed) contains methylprednisolone sodium succinate equivalent to 500 mg methylprednisolone; also 6.4 mg monobasic sodium phosphate anhydrous; 69.6 mg dibasic sodium phosphate dried; 33.7 mg benzyl alcohol added as preservative.

1 gram Vial—Each 16 mL (when mixed as directed) contains methylprednisolone sodium succinate equivalent to 1 gram methylprednisolone; also 12.8 mg monobasic sodium phosphate anhydrous; 139.2 mg dibasic sodium phosphate dried.

1 gram Act-O-Vial System (Single-Dose Vial)—Each 8 mL (when mixed) contains methylprednisolone sodium succinate equivalent to 1 gram methylprednisolone; also 12.8 mg monobasic sodium phosphate anhydrous; 139.2 mg dibasic sodium phosphate dried; 66.8 mg benzyl alcohol added as preservative.

2 gram Vial—Each 30.6 mL (when mixed as directed) contains methylprednisolone sodium succinate equivalent to 2 grams methylprednisolone; also 25.6 mg monobasic sodium phosphate anhydrous; 278 mg dibasic sodium phosphate dried.

2 gram Vial with Diluent—Each 30.6 mL (when mixed as directed) contains methylprednisolone sodium succinate equivalent to 2 grams methylprednisolone; also 25.6 mg monobasic sodium phosphate anhydrous; 278 mg dibasic sodium phosphate dried; 273 mg benzyl alcohol added as preservative.

When necessary, the pH of each formula was adjusted with sodium hydroxide so that the pH of the reconstituted solution is within the USP specified range of 7 to 8 and the tonicities are, for the 40 mg per mL solution, 0.50 osmolar; for the 125 mg per 2 mL, 500 mg per 8 mL and 1 gram per 16 mL solutions, 0.40 osmolar; for the 1 gram per 8 mL solution, 0.44 osmolar; for the 2 gram per 30.6 mL solutions, 0.42 osmolar. (Isotonic saline = 0.28 osmolar).

IMPORTANT—Use only the accompanying diluent or Bacteriostatic Water For Injection with Benzyl Alcohol when reconstituting SOLU-MEDROL
Use within 48 hours after mixing.

ACTIONS

Naturally occurring glucocorticoids (hydrocortisone and cortisone), which also have salt-retaining properties, are used as replacement therapy in adrenocortical deficiency states. Their synthetic analogs are primarily used for their potent anti-inflammatory effects in disorders of many organ systems.

Glucocorticoids cause profound and varied metabolic effects. In addition, they modify the body's immune responses to diverse stimuli.

Methylprednisolone is a potent anti-inflammatory steroid with greater anti-inflammatory potency than prednisolone and even less tendency than prednisolone to induce sodium and water retention.

Methylprednisolone sodium succinate has the same metabolic and anti-inflammatory actions as methylprednisolone. When given parenterally and in equimolar quantities, the two compounds are equivalent in biologic activity. The relative potency of SOLU-MEDROL Sterile Powder and hydrocortisone sodium succinate, as indicated by depression of eosinophil count, following intravenous administration, is at least four to one. This is in good agreement with the relative oral potency of methylprednisolone and hydrocortisone.

INDICATIONS

When oral therapy is not feasible, and the strength, dosage form and route of administration of the drug reasonably lend the preparation to the treatment of the condition, SOLU-MEDROL Sterile Powder is indicated for intravenous or intramuscular use in the following conditions:

1. Endocrine Disorders
Primary or secondary adrenocortical insufficiency (hydrocortisone is the drug of choice; synthetic analogs may be used in conjunction with mineralocorticoids where applicable; in infancy, mineralocorticoid supplementation is of particular importance)
Acute adrenocortical insufficiency (hydrocortisone or cortisone is the drug of choice; mineralocorticoid supplementation may be necessary, particularly when synthetic analogs are used)
Preoperatively and in the event of serious trauma or illness, in patients with known adrenal insufficiency or when adrenocortical reserve is doubtful
Shock unresponsive to conventional therapy if adrenocortical insufficiency exists or is suspected
Congenital adrenal hyperplasia
Hypercalcemia associated with cancer
Nonsuppurative thyroiditis

2. Rheumatic Disorders
As adjunctive therapy for short-term administration (to tide the patient over an acute episode or exacerbation) in:
Post-traumatic osteoarthritis
Synovitis of osteoarthritis
Rheumatoid arthritis, including juvenile rheumatoid arthritis (selected cases may require low-dose maintenance therapy)
Acute and subacute bursitis
Epicondylitis
Acute nonspecific tenosynovitis
Acute gouty arthritis
Psoriatic arthritis
Ankylosing spondylitis

3. Collagen Diseases
During an exacerbation or as maintenance therapy in selected cases of:
Systemic lupus erythematosus
Systemic dermatomyositis (polymyositis)
Acute rheumatic carditis

4. Dermatologic Diseases
Pemphigus
Severe erythema multiforme (Stevens-Johnson syndrome)
Exfoliative dermatitis
Bullous dermatitis herpetiformis
Severe seborrheic dermatitis
Severe psoriasis
Mycosis fungoides

5. Allergic States
Control of severe or incapacitating allergic conditions intractable to adequate trials of conventional treatment in:
Bronchial asthma
Contact dermatitis
Atopic dermatitis
Serum sickness
Seasonal or perennial allergic rhinitis
Drug hypersensitivity reactions
Urticarial transfusion reactions
Acute noninfectious laryngeal edema (epinephrine is the drug of first choice)

6. Ophthalmic Diseases
Severe acute and chronic allergic and inflammatory processes involving the eye, such as:
Herpes zoster ophthalmicus
Iritis, iridocyclitis
Chorioretinitis
Diffuse posterior uveitis and choroiditis
Optic neuritis
Sympathetic ophthalmia
Anterior segment inflammation
Allergic conjunctivitis
Allergic corneal marginal ulcers
Keratitis

7. Gastrointestinal Diseases
To tide the patient over a critical period of the disease in:
Ulcerative colitis (systemic therapy)
Regional enteritis (systemic therapy)

8. Respiratory Diseases
Symptomatic sarcoidosis
Berylliosis
Fulminating or disseminated pulmonary tuberculosis when used concurrently with appropriate antituberculous chemotherapy
Loeffler's syndrome not manageable by other means
Aspiration pneumonitis

9. Hematologic Disorders
Acquired (autoimmune) hemolytic anemia
Idiopathic thrombocytopenic purpura in adults (IV only; IM administration is contraindicated)
Secondary thrombocytopenia in adults
Erythroblastopenia (RBC anemia)
Congenital (erythroid) hypoplastic anemia

10. Neoplastic Diseases
For palliative management of:
Leukemias and lymphomas in adults
Acute leukemia of childhood

11. Edematous States
To induce diuresis or remission of proteinuria in the nephrotic syndrome, without uremia, of the idiopathic type or that due to lupus erythematosus

12. Nervous System
Acute exacerbations of multiple sclerosis

13. Miscellaneous
Tuberculous meningitis with subarachnoid block or impending block when used concurrently with appropriate antituberculous chemotherapy
Trichinosis with neurologic or myocardial involvement

CONTRAINDICATIONS

The use of SOLU-MEDROL Sterile Powder is contraindicated in premature infants because the **40 mg Act-O-Vial**, the **125 mg Act-O-Vial**, the **500 mg Act-O-Vial**, the **1 gram Act-O-Vial** system, and the accompanying diluent for the 500 mg and 2 gram vials contain benzyl alcohol. Benzyl alcohol has been reported to be associated with a fatal "Gasping Syndrome" in premature infants. SOLU-MEDROL Sterile Powder is also contraindicated in systemic fungal infections, and patients with known hypersensitivity to the product and its constituents.

WARNINGS

In patients on corticosteroid therapy subjected to any unusual stress, increased dosage of rapidly acting corticosteroids before, during, and after the stressful situation is indicated.

Corticosteroids may mask some signs of infection, and new infections may appear during their use. There may be decreased resistance and inability to localize infection when corticosteroids are used. Infections with any pathogen including viral, bacterial, fungal, protozoan or helminthic infections, in any location of the body, may be associated with the use of corticosteroids alone or in combination with other immunosuppressive agents that affect cellular immunity, humoral immunity, or neutrophil function.[1]

These infections may be mild, but can be severe and at times fatal. With increasing doses of corticosteroids, the rate of occurrence of infectious complications increases.[2]

A study has failed to establish the efficacy of SOLU-MEDROL in the treatment of sepsis syndrome and septic shock. The study also suggests that treatment of these conditions with SOLU-MEDROL may increase the risk of mortality in certain patients (ie, patients with elevated serum creatinine levels or patients who develop secondary infections after SOLU-MEDROL).

Prolonged use of corticosteroids may produce posterior subcapsular cataracts, glaucoma with possible damage to the optic nerves, and may enhance the establishment of secondary ocular infections due to fungi or viruses.

Continued on next page

Information on these Pharmacia & Upjohn products is based on labeling in effect June 1, 2000. Further information concerning these and other Pharmacia & Upjohn products may be obtained by direct inquiry to Medical Information, Pharmacia & Upjohn, Kalamazoo, MI 49001.

Solu-Medrol—Cont.

Usage in pregnancy. Since adequate human reproduction studies have not been done with corticosteroids, the use of these drugs in pregnancy, nursing mothers, or women of childbearing potential requires that the possible benefits of the drug be weighed against the potential hazards to the mother and embryo or fetus. Infants born of mothers who have received substantial doses of corticosteroids during pregnancy should be carefully observed for signs of hypoadrenalism.

Average and large doses of cortisone or hydrocortisone can cause elevation of blood pressure, salt and water retention, and increased excretion of potassium. These effects are less likely to occur with the synthetic derivatives except when used in large doses. Dietary salt restriction and potassium supplementation may be necessary. All corticosteroids increase calcium excretion.

Administration of live or live, attenuated vaccines is contraindicated in patients receiving immunosuppressive doses of corticosteroids. Killed or inactivated vaccines may be administered to patients receiving immunosuppressive doses of corticosteroids; however, the response to such vaccines may be diminished. Indicated immunization procedures may be undertaken in patients receiving nonimmunosuppressive doses of corticosteroids.

The use of SOLU-MEDROL Sterile Powder in active tuberculosis should be restricted to those cases of fulminating or disseminated tuberculosis in which the corticosteroid is used for the management of the disease in conjunction with appropriate antituberculous regimen.

If corticosteroids are indicated in patients with latent tuberculosis or tuberculin reactivity, close observation is necessary as reactivation of the disease may occur. During prolonged corticosteroids therapy, these patients should receive chemoprophylaxis.

Because rare instances of anaphylactic (eg, bronchospasm) reactions have occurred in patients receiving parenteral corticosteroid therapy, appropriate precautionary measures should be taken prior to administration, especially when the patient has a history of allergy to any drug.

There are reports of cardiac arrhythmias and/or circulatory collapse and/or cardiac arrest following the rapid administration of large IV doses of SOLU-MEDROL (greater than 0.5 gram administered over a period of less than 10 minutes). Bradycardia has been reported during or after the administration of large doses of methylprednisolone sodium succinate, and may be unrelated to the speed or duration of infusion.

Persons who are on drugs which suppress the immune system are more susceptible to infections than healthy individuals. Chicken pox and measles, for example, can have a more serious or even fatal course in non-immune children or adults on corticosteroids. In such children or adults who have not had these diseases, particular care should be taken to avoid exposure. How the dose, route and duration of corticosteroid administration affects the risk of developing a disseminated infection is not known. The contribution of the underlying disease and/or prior corticosteroid treatment to the risk is also not known. If exposed to chicken pox, prophylaxis with varicella zoster immune globulin (VZIG) may be indicated. If exposed to measles, prophylaxis with pooled intramuscular immunoglobulin (IG) may be indicated. (See the respective package inserts for complete VZIG and IG prescribing information.) If chicken pox develops, treatment with antiviral agents may be considered. Similarly, corticosteroids should be used with great care in patients with known or suspected Strongyloides (thread-worm) infestation. In such patients, corticosteroid-induced immunosuppression may lead to Strongyloides hyperinfection and dissemination with widespread larval migration, often accompanied by severe enterocolitis and potentially fatal gram-negative septicemia.

PRECAUTIONS

General precautions

Drug-induced secondary adrenocortical insufficiency may be minimized by gradual reduction of dosage. This type of relative insufficiency may persist for months after discontinuation of therapy; therefore, in any situation of stress occurring during that period, hormone therapy should be reinstituted. Since mineralocorticoid secretion may be impaired, salt and/or a mineralocorticoid should be administered concurrently.

There is an enhanced effect of corticosteroids on patients with hypothyroidism and in those with cirrhosis.

Corticosteroids should be used cautiously in patients with ocular herpes simplex because of possible corneal perforation.

The lowest possible dose of corticosteroid should be used to control the condition under treatment, and when reduction in dosage is possible, the reduction should be gradual.

Psychic derangements may appear when corticosteroids are used, ranging from euphoria, insomnia, mood swings, personality changes, and severe depression, to frank psychotic manifestations. Also, existing emotional instability or psychotic tendencies may be aggravated by corticosteroids.

Steroids should be used with caution in nonspecific ulcerative colitis, if there is a probability of impending perforation, abscess or other pyogenic infection; diverticulitis; fresh intestinal anastomoses; active or latent peptic ulcer; renal insufficiency; hypertension; osteoporosis; and myasthenia gravis.

Growth and development of infants and children on prolonged corticosteroid therapy should be carefully observed.

Kaposi's sarcoma has been reported to occur in patients receiving corticosteroid therapy. Discontinuation of corticosteroids may result in clinical remission.

Although controlled clinical trials have shown corticosteroids to be effective in speeding the resolution of acute exacerbations of multiple sclerosis, they do not show that corticosteroids affect the ultimate outcome or natural history of the disease. The studies do show that relatively high doses of corticosteroids are necessary to demonstrate a significant effect. (See DOSAGE AND ADMINISTRATION.)

An acute myopathy has been observed with the use of high doses of corticosteroids, most often occurring in patients with disorders of neuromuscular transmission (eg, myasthenia gravis), or in patients receiving concomitant therapy with neuromuscular blocking drugs (eg, pancuronium). This acute myopathy is generalized, may involve ocular and respiratory muscles, and may result in quadriparesis. Elevations of creatine kinase may occur. Clinical improvement or recovery after stopping corticosteroids may require weeks to years.

Since complications of treatment with glucocorticoids are dependent on the size of the dose and the duration of treatment, a risk/benefit decision must be made in each individual case as to dose and duration of treatment and as to whether daily or intermittent therapy should be used.

DRUG INTERACTIONS

The pharmacokinetic interactions listed below are potentially clinically important. Mutual inhibition of metabolism occurs with concurrent use of cyclosporin and methylprednisolone; therefore, it is possible that adverse events associated with the individual use of either drug may be more apt to occur. Convulsions have been reported with concurrent use of methylprednisolone and cyclosporin. Drugs that include hepatic enzymes such as phenobarbital, phenytoin and rifampin may increase the clearance of methylprednisolone and may require increases in methylprednisolone dose to achieve the desired response. Drugs such as troleandomycin and ketoconazole may inhibit the metabolism of methylprednisolone and thus decrease its clearance. Therefore, the dose of methylprednisolone should be titrated to avoid steroid toxicity. Methylprednisolone may increase the clearance of chronic high dose aspirin. This could lead to decreased salicylate serum levels or increase the risk of salicylate toxicity when methylprednisolone is withdrawn. Aspirin should be used cautiously in conjunction with corticosteroids in patients suffering from hypoprothrombinemia. The effect of methylprednisolone on oral anticoagulants is variable. There are reports of enhanced as well as diminished effects of anticoagulant when given concurrently with corticosteroids. Therefore, coagulation indices should be monitored to maintain the desired anticoagulant effect.

Information for the Patient

Persons who are on immunosuppressant doses of corticosteroids should be warned to avoid exposure to chicken pox or measles. Patients should also be advised that if they are exposed, medical advice should be sought without delay.

ADVERSE REACTIONS

Fluid and Electrolyte Disturbances

Sodium retention
Fluid retention
Congestive heart failure in susceptible patients
Potassium loss
Hypokalemic alkalosis
Hypertension

Musculoskeletal

Muscle weakness
Steroid myopathy
Loss of muscle mass
Severe arthralgia
Vertebral compression fractures
Aseptic necrosis of femoral and humeral heads
Pathologic fracture of long bones
Osteoporosis
Tendon rupture, particularly of the Achilles tendon

Gastrointestinal

Peptic ulcer with possible perforation and hemorrhage
Pancreatitis
Abdominal distention
Ulcerative esophagitis
Increases in alanine transaminase (AST, SGPT), aspartate transaminase (AST, SGOT), and alkaline phosphatase have been observed following corticosteroid treatment. These changes are usually small, not associated with any clinical syndrome and are reversible upon discontinuation.

Dermatologic

Impaired wound healing
Thin fragile skin
Petechiae and ecchymoses
Facial erythema
Increased sweating
May suppress reactions to skin tests

Neurological

Increased intracranial pressure with papilledema (pseudotumor cerebri) usually after treatment
Convulsions
Vertigo
Headache

Endocrine

Development of Cushingoid state
Suppression of growth in children
Secondary adrenocortical and pituitary unresponsiveness, particularly in times of stress, as in trauma, surgery or illness
Menstrual irregularities
Decreased carbohydrate tolerance
Manifestations of latent diabetes mellitus
Increased requirements for insulin or oral hypoglycemic agents in diabetics

Ophthalmic

Posterior subcapsular cataracts
Increased intraocular pressure
Glaucoma
Exophthalmos

Metabolic

Negative nitrogen balance due to protein catabolism

The following *additional* adverse reactions are related to parenteral corticosteroid therapy:
Hyperpigmentation or hypopigmentation
Subcutaneous and cutaneous atrophy
Sterile abscess
Anaphylactic reaction with or without circulatory collapse, cardiac arrest, bronchospasm
Urticaria
Nausea and vomiting
Cardiac arrhythmias; hypotension or hypertension

DOSAGE AND ADMINISTRATION

When high dose therapy is desired, the recommended dose of SOLU-MEDROL Sterile Powder is 30 mg/kg administered intravenously over at least 30 minutes. This dose may be repeated every 4 to 6 hours for 48 hours.

In general, high dose corticosteroid therapy should be continued only until the patient's condition has stabilized; usually not beyond 48 to 72 hours.

Although adverse effects associated with high dose short-term corticoid therapy are uncommon, peptic ulceration may occur. Prophylactic antacid therapy may be indicated.

In other indications initial dosage will vary from 10 to 40 mg of methylprednisolone depending on the clinical problem being treated. The larger doses may be required for short-term management of severe, acute conditions. The initial dose usually should be given intravenously over a period of several minutes. Subsequent doses may be given intravenously or intramuscularly at intervals dictated by the patient's response and clinical condition. Corticoid therapy is an adjunct to, and not replacement for conventional therapy.

Dosage may be reduced for infants and children but should be governed more for the severity of the condition and response of the patient than by age or size. It should not be less than 0.5 mg per kg every 24 hours.

Dosage must be decreased or discontinued gradually when the drug has been administered for more than a few days. If a period of spontaneous remission occurs in a chronic condition, treatment should be discontinued. Routine laboratory studies, such as urinalysis, two-hour postprandial blood sugar, determination of blood pressure and body weight, and a chest X-ray should be made at regular intervals during prolonged therapy. Upper GI X-rays are desirable in patients with an ulcer history or significant dyspepsia.

SOLU-MEDROL may be administered by intravenous or intramuscular injection or by intravenous infusion, the preferred method for initial emergency use being intravenous injection. To administer by intravenous (or intramuscular) injection, prepare solution as directed. The desired dose may be administered intravenously over a period of several minutes. If desired, the medication may be administered in diluted solutions by adding Water for Injection or other suitable diluent (see below) to the **Act-O-Vial** and withdrawing the indicated dose.

To prepare solutions for intravenous infusion, first prepare the solution for injection as directed. This solution may then be added to indicated amounts of 5% dextrose in water, isotonic saline solution or 5% dextrose in isotonic saline solution.

Multiple Sclerosis

In treatment of acute exacerbations of multiple sclerosis, daily doses of 200 mg of prednisolone for a week followed by 80 mg every other day for 1 month have been shown to be effective (4 mg of methylprednisolone is equivalent to 5 mg of prednisolone).

DIRECTIONS FOR USING THE ACT-O-VIAL SYSTEM

1. Press down on plastic activator to force diluent into the lower compartment.
2. Gently agitate to effect solution.
3. Remove plastic tab covering center of stopper.
4. Sterilize top of stopper with a suitable germicide.
5. Insert needle **squarely through center** of stopper until tip is just visible. Invert vial and withdraw dose.

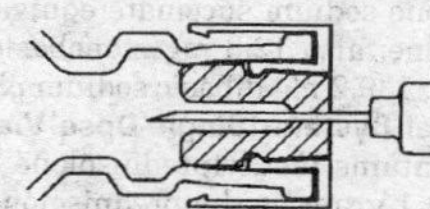

STORAGE CONDITIONS

Protect from light.
Store unreconstituted product at controlled room temperature 20° to 25°C (68° to 77°F) [see USP].
Store solution at controlled room temperature 20° to 25°C (68° to 77°F) [see USP].
Use solution within 48 hours after mixing.

HOW SUPPLIED

SOLU-MEDROL Sterile Powder is available in the following packages:

40 mg Act-O-Vial System (Single-Dose Vial)
1 mL NDC 0009-0113-12
25 × 1 mL NDC 0009-0113-19

125 mg Act-O-Vial System (Single-Dose Vial)
2 mL NDC 0009–0190–09
25 × 2 mL NDC 0009-0190-16

500 mg Vial NDC 0009-0758-01
500 mg Vial with Diluent NDC 0009-0887-01

500 mg Act-O-Vial System (Single-Dose Vial)
4 mL NDC 0009-0765-02

1 gram Vial NDC 0009-0698-01

1 gram Act-O-Vial System (Single-Dose Vial)
8 mL NDC 0009-3389-01

2 gram Vial with Diluent NDC 0009-0796-01

REFERENCES

1. Fekety R. Infections associated with corticosteroids and immunosuppressive therapy. In: Gorbach SL, Bartlett JG, Blacklow NR, eds. *Infectious Diseases.* Philadelphia: WBSaunders Company 1992:1050–1.
2. Stuck AE, Minder CE, Frey FJ. Risk of infectious complications in patients taking glucocorticoids. *Rev Infect Dis* 1989:11(6):954–63.

Rx only

Pharmacia & Upjohn Company • Kalamazoo, Michigan 49001, USA

Revised February 2000 810 431 235
691211

VAGIFEM® ℞

[văg ə' fĕm]

estradiol vaginal tablets
25μg
PHYSICIAN PACKAGE INSERT

ESTROGENS HAVE BEEN REPORTED TO INCREASE THE RISK OF ENDOMETRIAL CARCINOMA.

Three independent, case controlled studies have reported an increased risk of endometrial cancer in postmenopausal women exposed to exogenous estrogens for more than one year. This risk was independent of the other known risk factors for endometrial cancer. These studies are further supported by the finding that incident rates of endometrial cancer have increased sharply since 1969 in eight different areas of the United States with population-based cancer-reporting systems, an increase which may be related to the rapidly expanding use of estrogens during the last decade.

The three case-controlled studies reported that the risk of endometrial cancer in estrogen users was about 4.5 to 13.9 times greater than in nonusers. The risk appears to depend on both duration of treatment and on estrogen dose. In view of these findings, when estrogens are used for the treatment of menopausal symptoms, the lowest dose that will control symptoms should be utilized and medication should be discontinued as soon as possible. When prolonged treatment is medically indicated, the patient should be reassessed, on at least a semi-annual basis, to determine the need for continued therapy.

Close clinical surveillance of all women taking estrogens is important. In all cases of undiagnosed persistent or reoccurring abnormal vaginal bleeding, adequate diagnostic measures should be undertaken to rule out malignancy.

There is no evidence at present that "natural" estrogens are more or less hazardous than "synthetic" estrogens at equi-estrogenic doses.

DESCRIPTION

VAGIFEM® (estradiol vaginal tablets) are small, white, film-coated tabletes containing 25.8μg of estradiol hemihydrate equivalent to 25μg of estradiol.

Each tablet contains the following inactive ingredients: hydroxypropyl methylcellulose, lactose monohydrate, maize starch and magnesium stearate. The film coating contains hydroxypropyl methylcellulose and polyethylene glycol.

Each white tablet is 6 mm in diameter and is placed in a disposable applicator.

Each tablet-filled applicator is packaged separately in a blister pack. 17β-estradiol hemihydrate is a white, almost white or colorless crystalline solid, chemically described as estra-1,3,5 (10)-triene-3, 17 diol.

The chemical formula is $C_{18}H_{24}O_2 \cdot {}^1/_2\ H_2O$ with a molecular weight of 281.4.

The structural formula is:

OH
HO

CLINICAL PHARMACOLOGY

In vivo estrogens diffuse through cell membranes, distribute throughout the cell, bind to and activate the estrogen receptors, thereby eliciting their biological effects. Estrogen receptors have been identified in tissue of the reproductive tract, breast, pituitary, hypothalamus, liver and bone of women. The estrogen contained in VAGIFEM, 17 β-estradiol is chemically and biologically identical to the endogenous human 17 β-estradiol and is, therefore, classified as a human estrogen.

Estrogens regulate growth, differentiation and functioning of many different tissues within and outside of the reproductive system. Estrogens are intricately involved with other hormones, especially progesterone, and during the ovulatory phase of the menstrual cycle cause proliferation of the endometrium. Most of the activity of estrogens appear to be exerted via estrogen receptors in target cells of tissues of the woman's reproductive tract: breast, pituitary, hypothalamus, brain, liver, and bone.

The steroid-receptor complex is bound to the cell's DNA and induces synthesis of specific proteins.

Maturation of the vaginal epithelium is dependent on estrogen as it increases the number of superficial and intermediate cells as compared with basal cells. Estrogen keeps the pH of the vagina at approximately 4.5 which enhances normal bacteria flora, predominately, *Lactobacillus döderlein.*

Pharmacokinetics

Absorption

Estrogen drug products are well absorbed through the skin, mucous membranes, and the gastrointestinal (GI) tract. The vaginal delivery of estrogens circumvents first-pass metabolism.

A single-center, randomized, double-blind comparison study conducted in the U.S. showed that vaginal application of VAGIFEM® over a 12-week course demonstrated a mean C_{max} of estradiol of 50 pg/mL and that there was no significant accumulation of estradiol as measured by the AUC_{0-24} (See Table 1 below).

Table 1:
MEAN (±STANDARD DEVIATION) PHARMACOKINETIC PARAMETERS FOR ESTRADIOL
(Uncorrected for base line)

	Timepoint		
	Day 1	Day 14	Day 84
PK Parameter:			
AUC (pg.hr/mL)	538 (±265)	567 (±246)	563 (±341)
C_{max} (pg/mL)	51 (±34)	47 (±21)	49 (±27)

Distribution

Circulating, unbound estrogens are known to modulate pharmacological response. Estrogens circulate in the blood bound to sex-hormone binding globulin (SHBG) and albumin. A dynamic equilibrium exists between the conjugated and the unconjugated forms of estradiol and estrone, which undergo rapid interconversion.

Metabolism

Exogenously-delivered or endogenously-derived estrogens are primarily metabolized in the liver to estrone and estradiol, which are also found in the systemic circulation. VAGIFEM intravaginal administration voids first-pass metabolism that occurs with oral estrogens.

The levels of E_1 seen during 12 weeks of VAGIFEM administration do not show any accumulation of E_1, and the observed values are within the postmenopausal range. See Table 2 below.

Table 2:
MEAN
(±STANDARD DEVIATION)
PHARMACOKINETIC
PARAMETERS FOR ESTRONE
(Uncorrected for base line)

	Timepoint		
	Day 1	Day 14	Day 84
E1:			
AUC (pg.hr/mL)	649 (±230)	744 (±267)	681 (±271)
C_{max} (pg/mL)	35 (±12)	39 (±13)	35 (±12)

Excretion

Estrogen metabolites are primarily excreted in the urine as glucoronides and sulfates.

Drug-Drug Interactions

No formal drug-drug interaction studies have been done with VAGIFEM.

CLINICAL STUDIES

A placebo-controlled comparison study was done in the U.S., in which 230 patients were randomized to receive either placebo, VAGIFEM, or 10μg estradiol vaginal tablets.

Patients inserted one tablet intravaginally each day for 14 days, then one tablet twice weekly for the remaining 10 weeks. All patients were assessed for vaginal symptoms. VAGIFEM® was superior to placebo in the relief of symptoms of the dryness, soreness, and irritation associated with atrophic vaginitis. This change of symptoms was seen at Week 7 and was maintained throughout to Week 12. (See Figure 1)

An open, controlled comparison study was done in Canada in which 159 patients were randomized to receive either VAGIFEM or the conjugated estrogen vaginal cream, comparator drug. Two (2) grams (~ 1.25 mg conjugated estrogens) of the comparator drug, which is the highest approved dose, was given daily for 3 weeks, withheld for 1 week, then repeated cyclically (3 weeks on, 1 week off) for up to 24 weeks; VAGIFEM was administered daily for 2 weeks, then twice weekly for the remaining 22 weeks. Of all patients entering into treatment phase of the study 10% of patients discontinued their treatment in the VAGIFEM group and 32% discontinued their treatment in the comparator group. In this study, patients were assessed for relief of symptoms. VAGIFEM 25μg was not less effective than the approved comparator product at the 2.0 gm dose in the relief of symptoms.

Symptoms of dryness, soreness, and irritation were rated as 0 = none, 1 = mild, 2 = moderate and 3 = severe. The average severity score of the three symptoms over time for the placebo controlled and comparator studies are shown in the following figures:

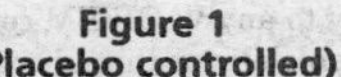

Figure 1
(Placebo controlled)

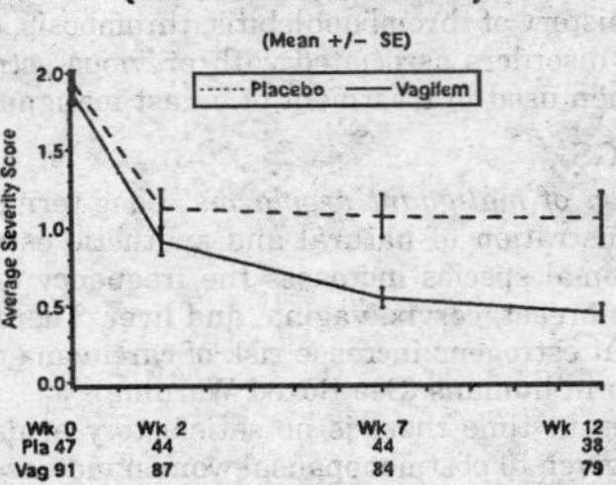

Figure 2
(Comparator)

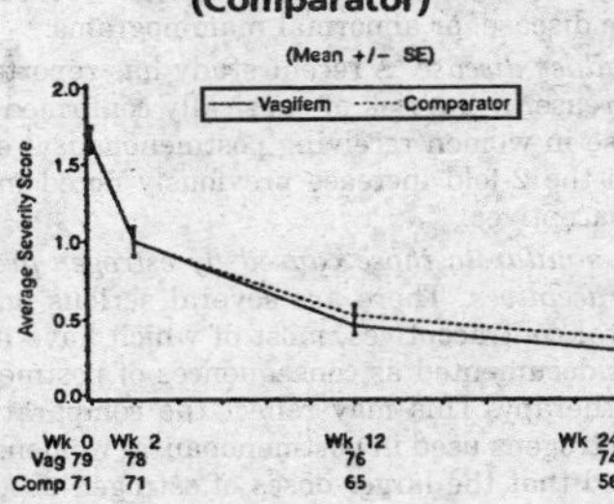

The endometrium was evaluated at the end of each study by endometrial biopsy. See Tables 3 & 4 below.

Table 3:
ENDOMETRIAL BIOPSY RESULTS COMPARING VAGIFEM WITH PLACEBO OVER 12 WEEKS OF TREATMENT
(US Trial)

	VAGIFEM	Placebo
Total Number of Patients enrolled	91	47
Patients with uterus (non-hysterectomized)	48	24
Total Biopsies	32	21
Atrophic Endometrium	27 (84%)	18 (86%)
Weakly Proliferative	0 (0%)	0 (0%)
Proliferative	1 (3%)	0 (0%)
Simple Hyperplasia	1 (3%)	0 (0%)
Complex Hyperplasia	0 (0%)	0 (0%)
Insufficient Tissue	3 (9%)	3 (14%)

Table 4:
ENDOMETRIAL BIOPSY RESULTS COMPARING VAGIFEM TO COMPARATOR GIVEN OVER 24 WEEKS

	VAGIFEM	Comparator
Total Number of Patients enrolled	80	79
Patients with uterus (non-hysterectomized)	80	79
Total Biopsies	49	49
Atrophic Endometrium	34 (68%)	15 (30%)
Weakly Proliferative	0 (0%)	4 (8%)
Proliferative	1 (2%)	7 (14%)
Simple Hyperplasia	0 (0%)	1 (2%)
Complex Hyperplasia	0 (0%)	1 (2%)
Insufficient Tissue	14 (28%)	21 (42%)

Continued on next page

Information on these Pharmacia & Upjohn products is based on labeling in effect June 1, 2000. Further information concerning these and other Pharmacia & Upjohn products may be obtained by direct inquiry to Medical Information, Pharmacia & Upjohn, Kalamazoo, MI 49001.

Vagifem—Cont.

INDICATIONS AND USE

VAGIFEM® is indicated for the treatment of atrophic vaginitis.

CONTRAINDICATIONS

The use of VAGIFEM is contraindicated in women who exhibit one or more of the following:
1. Known or suspected breast carcinoma.
2. Known or suspected estrogen-dependent neoplasia; e.g. endometrial carcinoma.
3. Abnormal genital bleeding of unknown etiology.
4. Known or suspected pregnancy. (See PRECAUTIONS)
5. Porphyria.
6. Hypersensitivity to any VAGIFEM constituents.
7. Active thrombophlebitis or thromboembolic disorders.
8. A past history of thrombophlebitis, thrombosis, or thromboembolic disorders associated with previous estrogen use (except when used in treatment of breast malignancy).

WARNINGS

1. *Induction of malignant neoplasms.* Long-term, continuous administration of natural and synthetic estrogens in certain animal species increases the frequency of carcinomas of the breast, cervix, vagina, and liver. There are now reports that estrogens increase risk of carcinoma of the endometrium in humans (See Boxed Warning).
At the present time there is no satisfactory evidence that estrogens given to postmenopausal women increase the risk of cancer of the breast, although a recent long-term follow-up of a single physician's practice has raised this possibility. Because of the animal data, there is a need for caution in prescribing estrogens for women with a strong family history of breast cancer or who have breast nodules, fibrocystic disease, or abnormal mammograms.
2. *Gallbladder disease.* A recent study has reported a 2- to 3-fold increase in the risk of surgically confirmed gallbladder disease in women receiving postmenopausal estrogens, similar to the 2-fold increase previously noted in users of oral contraceptives.
3. *Effects similar to those caused by estrogen-progestogen oral contraceptives.* There are several serious adverse effects of oral contraceptives, most of which have not, up to now, been documented as consequences of postmenopausal estrogen therapy. This may reflect the comparatively low doses of estrogens used in postmenopausal women. It would be expected that the larger doses of estrogen used to treat prostatic or breast cancer are more likely to result in these adverse effects, and, in fact, it has been shown that there is an increased risk of thrombosis in men receiving estrogens for prostatic cancer.
a. *Thromboembolic disease.* It is now well established that users of oral contraceptives have an increased risk of various thromboembolic and thrombotic vascular diseases, such at thrombophlebitis, pulmonary embolism, stroke, and myocardial infarction. Cases of retinal thrombosis, mesenteric thrombosis, and optic neuritis have been reported in oral-contraceptive users. There is evidence that the risk of several of these adverse reactions is related to the dose of the drug. An increased risk of postsurgery thromboembolic complications has also been reported in users of oral contraceptives. If feasible, estrogen should be discontinued at least 4 weeks before surgery of the type associated with an increased risk of thromboembolism, or during periods of prolonged immobilization.
While an increased rate of thromboembolism and thrombotic disease in postmenopausal users of estrogens has not been found, this does not rule out the possibility that such an increase may be present, or that subgroups of women who have underlying risk factors, or who are receiving large doses of estrogens, may have increased risk. Therefore, estrogens should not be used (except in treatment of malignancy) in a person with a history of such disorders in association with estrogen use. They should be used with caution in patients with cerebral vascular or coronary artery disease and only for those in whom estrogens are clearly needed.
Large doses of estrogens (5 mg conjugated estrogens per day), comparable to those used to treat cancer of the prostate and breast, have been shown in a large prospective clinical trial in men, to increase the risk of nonfatal myocardial infarction, pulmonary embolism, and thrombophlebitis. When estrogen doses of this size are used, any of the thromboembolic and thrombotic adverse effects associated with oral contraceptive use should be considered a clear risk.
b. *Hepatic adenoma.* Benign hepatic adenomas appear to be associated with the oral contraceptives.
Although benign, and rare, these may rupture and may cause death through intra-abdominal hemorrhage. Such lesions have not yet been reported in association with other estrogen or progestogen preparations but should be considered in estrogen users having abdominal pain and tenderness, abdominal mass, or hypovolemic shock.
Hepatocellular carcinoma has also been reported in women taking estrogen-containing oral contraceptives. The relationship of this malignancy to these drugs is not known at this time.
c. *Elevated blood pressure.* Women using oral contraceptives sometimes experience increased blood pressure which, in most cases, returns to normal on discontinuing the drug. There is now a report that this may occur with the use of estrogens in the menopause and blood pressure should be monitored with estrogen use, especially if high doses are used.
d. *Glucose tolerance.* A worsening of glucose tolerance has been observed in a significant percentage of patients on estrogen-containing oral contraceptives. For this reason, diabetic patients should be carefully observed while using estrogens.
4. *Hypercalcemia.* Administration of estrogens may lead to severe hypercalcemia in patients with breast cancer and bone metastases. If this occurs, the drug should be stopped and appropriate measures taken to reduce the serum calcium level.
5. *Rare Event:* Trauma induced by the VAGIFEM® applicator may occur, especially in patients with severely atrophic vaginal mucosa.

PRECAUTIONS

A. General Precautions.

1. A complete medical and family history should be taken prior to the initiation of any estrogen therapy.
The pretreatment and periodic physical examinations should include special references to blood pressure, breast, abdomen, and pelvic organs, and should include a Papanicolaou smear. As a general rule, estrogens should not be prescribed for longer than one year without another physical exam being performed.
2. Fluid retention—Because estrogens may cause some degree of fluid retention, conditions which might be influenced by this factor, such as asthma, epilepsy, migraine, and cardiac and renal dysfunction, require careful observation.
3. Familial Hyperlipoproteinemia—Estrogen therapy may be associated with massive elevations of plasma triglycerides leading to pancreatitis and other complications in patients with familial defects of lipoprotein metabolism.
4. Certain patients may develop undesirable manifestations of excessive estrogenic stimulation, such as abnormal or excessive uterine bleeding, mastodynia, etc.
5. Prolonged administration of unopposed estrogen therapy has been reported to increase the risk of endometrial hyperplasia in some patients.
6. Preexisting uterine leiomyomata may increase in size during estrogen use.
7. The pathologist should be advised of estrogen therapy when relevant specimens are submitted.
8. Patients with a history of jaundice during pregnancy have an increased risk of recurrence of jaundice while receiving estrogen-containing oral contraceptive therapy. If jaundice develops in any patient receiving estrogen, the medication should be discontinued while the cause is investigated.
9. Estrogens may be poorly metabolized in patients with impaired liver function and should be administered with caution in such patients.
10. Because estrogens influence the metabolism of calcium and phosphorus, they should be used with caution in patients with metabolic bone diseases that are associated with hypercalcemia or in patients with renal insufficiency.
11. Because of the effects of estrogens on epiphyseal closure, they should be used judiciously in young patients in whom bone growth is not yet complete.
12. Insertion of the VAGIFEM® applicator—Patients with severly atrophic vaginal mucosa should be instructed to exercise care during insertion of the applicator. After gynecological surgery, any vaginal applicator should be used with caution and only if clearly indicated.
13. Vaginal infection—Vaginal infection is generally more common in postmenopausal women due to the lack of normal flora seen in fertile women, especially lactobacilla; hence the subsequent higher pH. Vaginal infections should be treated with appropriate antimicrobial therapy before initiation of VAGIFEM therapy.

B. Information for the Patient

See text of patient Package Insert which appears above.

C. Drug/Laboratory Test Interactions

Certain endocrine and liver function tests may be affected by estrogen-containing oral contraceptives. The following similar changes may be expected with larger doses of estrogens:
a. Increased prothrombin and factors VII, VIII, IX, and X, decreased antithrombin III; increased norepinephrine induced platelet aggregability.
b. Increased thyroid binding globulin (TBG) leading to increased circulating total thyroid hormone, as measured by PBI, T_4 by column, or T_4 by radioimmunoassay. Free T_4 resin uptake is decreased, reflecting the elevated TBG, free T_4 concentration is unaltered.
c. Impaired glucose tolerance.
d. Reduced response to metyrapone test.
e. Reduced serum folate concentration.
f. Increased serum triglyceride and phospholipid concentration.

D. Carcinogenesis, Mutagenesis and Impairment of Fertility

Long term continuous administration of natural and synthetic estrogens in certain animal species increases the frequency of carcinomas of the breast, uterus, vagina and liver. (See CONTRAINDICATIONS AND WARNINGS)

E. Pregnancy Category X

Estrogens are not indicated for use during pregnancy or the immediate postpartum period. Estrogens are ineffective for the prevention or treatment of threatened or habitual abortion. Treatment with diethylstilbesterol (DES) during pregnancy has been associated with an increased risk of congenital defects and cancer in the reproductive organs of the fetus, and possibly other birth defects. The use of DES during pregnancy has also been associated with a subsequent increased risk of breast cancer in the mothers.

F. Nursing Mothers

As a general principle, administration of any drug to nursing mothers should be done only when clearly necessary since many drugs are excreted in human milk. In addition, estrogen administration to nursing mothers has been shown to decrease the quantity and quality of the milk. Estrogens are not indicated for the prevention of postpartum breast engorgement.

G. Pediatric Use

Safety and effectiveness in pediatric patients have not been established.

H. Geriatric Use

Clinical studies of VAGIFEM® did not include sufficient numbers of subjects aged 65 and over to determine whether they respond differently from younger subjects. Other reported clinical experience has not identified differences in responses between the elderly and younger patients. In general, dose selection for an elderly patient should be cautious, usually starting at the low end of the dosing range, reflecting the greater frequency of decreased hepatic, renal, or cardiac function, and of concomitant disease or other drug therapy.

ADVERSE EVENTS

Adverse events generally have been mild: vaginal spotting, vaginal discharge, allergic reaction and skin rash. Adverse events with an incidence of 5% or greater are reported for two comparative trials. Data for patients receiving either VAGIFEM or placebo in the double blind study are listed in Table 5, and data for patients receiving VAGIFEM in the open label comparator study are listed in Table 6.

Table 5:
ADVERSE EVENTS REPORTED IN 5% OR GREATER NUMBER OF PATIENTS RECEIVING VAGIFEM® IN THE PLACEBO CONTROLLED TRIAL.

	VAGIFEM	Placebo
	(n=91)	(n=47)
ADVERSE EVENT	%	%
HEADACHE	9	6
ABDOMINAL PAIN	7	4
UPPER RESPIRATORY TRACT INFECTION	5	4
MONILIASIS GENITAL	5	2
BACK PAIN	7	6

Table 6:
ADVERSE EVENTS REPORTED IN 5% OR GREATER NUMBER OF PATIENTS RECEIVING VAGIFEM® IN THE OPEN LABEL STUDY.

	VAGIFEM
	(n=80)
ADVERSE EVENT	%
PRURITUS GENITAL	6
HEADACHE	10
UPPER RESPIRATORY TRACT INFECTION	11

Other adverse events that occurred in 3–5% of VAGIFEM subjects included: allergy, bronchitis, dyspepsia, haematuria, hot flashes, insomnia, pain, sinusitis, vaginal discomfort, vaginitis. A causal relationship to VAGIFEM has not been established.

OVERDOSAGE

Numerous reports of ingestion of large doses of estrogen containing oral contraceptives by young children indicate that acute serious ill effects do not occur. Overdosage with estrogens may cause nausea, and withdrawal bleeding may occur in females.

DOSAGE AND ADMINISTRATION

VAGIFEM is gently inserted into the vagina as far as it can comfortably go without force, using the supplied applicator.

- Initial dose: One (1) VAGIFEM tablet, inserted vaginally, once daily for two (2) weeks. It is advisable to have the patient administer treatment at the same time each day.
- Maintenance dose: One (1) VAGIFEM tablet, inserted vaginally, twice weekly.

The need to continue therapy should be assessed by the physician with the patient. Attempts to discontinue or taper medication should be made at three to six month intervals.

HOW SUPPLIED

Each VAGIFEM® (estradiol vaginal tablets), 25µg is contained in a disposable, single-use applicator, packaged in a blister pack. Cartons contain 15 applicators with inset tablets.
NDC 0009-5173-02
STORAGE: Store at 25°C (77°F); excursions permitted to 15°C–30°C (59°F–86°F). [See USP Controlled Room Temperature.]
Rx only
818 280 000
Vagifem® is a trademark owned
by Novo Nordisk A/S
Revised June 2000

Manufactured for
Pharmacia & Upjohn Company
Kalamazoo, MI 49001, USA
By
Novo Nordisk A/S
2880 Bagsværd, Denmark

VAGIFEM®
estradiol vaginal tablets
25µg
INFORMATION FOR PATIENTS

Introduction

This leaflet describes when and how to use VAGIFEM® (estradiol vaginal tablets) and the risks and benefits of estrogen treatment. Please read this information carefully before starting treatment.

Estrogens have important benefits but also some risks. You must decide, with your doctor or health care provider, whether the risks to you of estrogen use are acceptable because of their benefits. If you use estrogens, check with your health care provider to be sure you are using the dose that is appropriate for you, and that you don't use them longer than necessary. How long you need to use estrogens should be decided by you and your health care provider. Estrogens are hormones made by the ovaries of normal women. Between ages 45 and 55, the ovaries normally stop making estrogens. This leads to a drop in body estrogen levels which causes the "change of life" or menopause (the end of monthly menstrual periods). If both ovaries are removed during an operation before natural menopause takes place, the sudden drop in estrogen levels causes "surgical menopause."

When the estrogen levels begin dropping, some women develop very uncomfortable symptoms, such as feeling of warmth in the face, neck, and chest, or sudden intense episodes of heat and sweating ("hot flashes" or "hot flushes"). Using estrogen drugs can help the body adjust to lower estrogen levels and reduce these symptoms. Most women have only mild menopausal symptoms or none at all and may not need to use estrogen drugs. VAGIFEM DOES NOT PROVIDE ENOUGH ESTROGEN TO REDUCE THESE SYMPTOMS.

The declining estrogen levels associated with advancing age after menopause may also result in thinning and drying of the tissue in the vagina and urinary tract (urogenital atrophy). Vaginal symptoms of this condition include dryness in the vagina (atrophic vaginitis), genital itching and burning, and pain with intercourse. Urinary symptoms may include urinary urgency and pain on urination. Small amounts of estrogens delivered directly to the local tissue can be used to help reduce these symptoms.

Use of VAGIFEM®
(estradiol vaginal tablets)

VAGIFEM is a local estrogen therapy designed to relieve vaginal symptoms, a major component of the urogenital symptoms found in post-menopausal estrogen deficiency. VAGIFEM® (estradiol vaginal tablets) exerts it effect locally in the lower urogenital tract, particularly the vagina, and has not been associated with significant effects in other estrogen-sensitive organs or tissues of the body. Consequently, VAGIFEM provides relief of local symptoms of menopause only.

Description

VAGIFEM® (estradiol vaginal tablets) contains 25µg (micrograms) of estrogen (estradiol). VAGIFEM releases estradiol into the vagina. A gel layer forms when the tablet comes in contact with the vagina. The estradiol is released from this gel layer. See Figure 1.

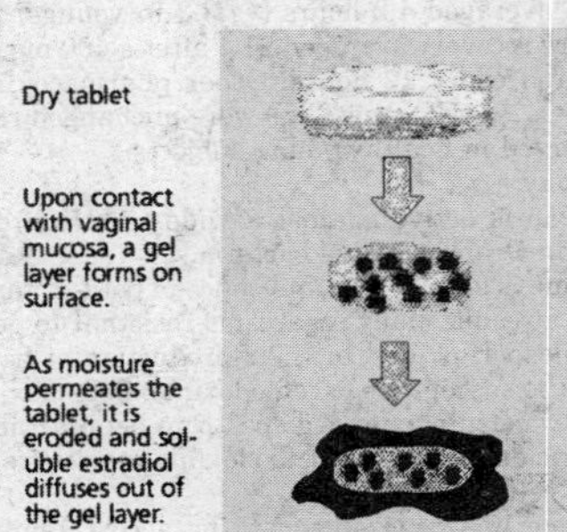
Dry tablet
Upon contact with vaginal mucosa, a gel layer forms on surface.
As moisture permeates the tablet, it is eroded and soluble estradiol diffuses out of the gel layer.

Fig.1

Dosage

One (1) VAGIFEM tablet inserted vaginally once daily for the first two (2) weeks. Then one (1) tablet twice weekly. (See table below).

Administration Regimen

Days:	1	2	3	4	5	6	7
Week 1 1 Vagifem tablet everyday	/	/	/	/	/	/	/
Week 2 1 Vagifem tablet everyday	/	/	/	/	/	/	/
Week 3 and Thereafter 1 Vagifem tablet twice weekly			/			/	

Directions for use of VAGIFEM®:

Step 1: Tear off a single applicator.

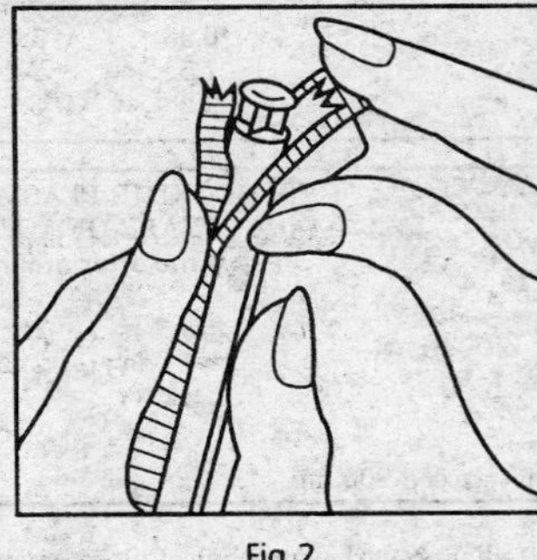

Fig.2

Step 2: Separate the plastic wrap and remove the applicator from the plastic wrap. See Figure 2.

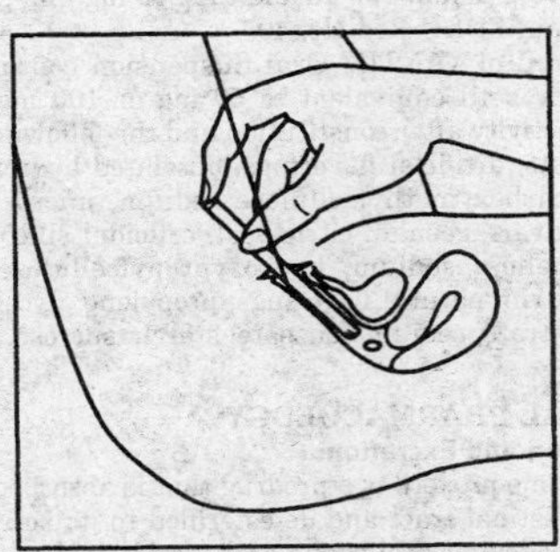

Fig.3

Step 3: First select the best position for vaginal insertion of VAGIFEM® (estradiol vaginal tablets) that is most comfortable for you. See suggested reclining Figure 3 or standing Figure 4 position illustrated below:

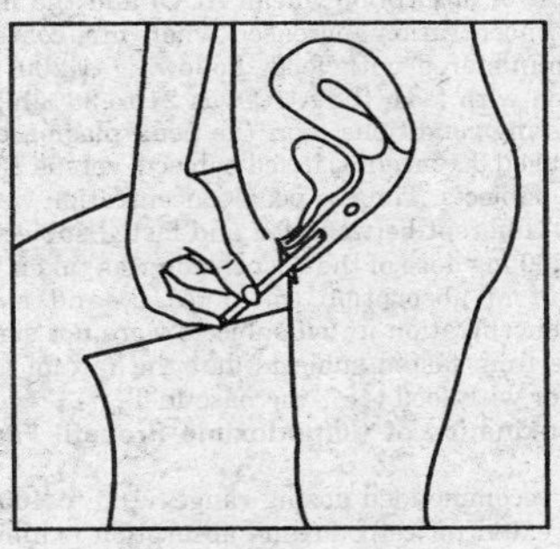

Fig.4

Step 4: The applicator should be held so that the finger of one hand can press the applicator plunger. See Figure 5.

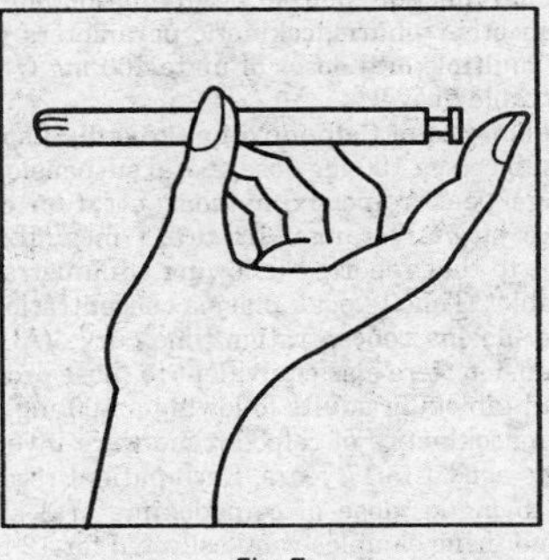

Fig.5

Step 5: The other hand should be used to guide the applicator gently and comfortably through the vaginal opening (see Figures 3 and 4 above). If the tablet has come out of the applicator prior to insertion, do not attempt to replace it. Use a fresh tablet-filled applicator.

Step 6: The applicator should be inserted (without forcing) as far as comfortably possible, or until half of the applicator is inside your vagina, whichever is less.

Step 7: Once the tablet-filled applicator has been inserted, gently press the plunger until a click is heard and the plunger is fully depressed. This will eject the tablet inside your vagina where it will dissolve slowly over several hours.

Step 8: After depressing the plunger, gently remove the applicator and dispose of it the same way you would a plastic tampon applicator. The applicator is of no further use and should be discarded properly. Insertion may be done at any time of the day. It is advisable to use the same time daily for all applications of VAGIFEM® (estradiol vaginal tablets). If you have any questions, please consult your health care provider or pharmacist.

Who Should Not Use VAGIFEM®
(estradiol vaginal tablets)

VAGIFEM should not be used:

During pregnancy—Women who are definitely postmenopausal cannot become pregnant. Women who believe they are postmenopausal because their menstrual cycles have recently stopped should confirm that they are not pregnant before using any form of estrogen-containing drug. Using estrogens while pregnant may cause the unborn child to have birth defects. Estrogens do not prevent miscarriage.

In the presence of unusual vaginal bleeding which has not been evaluated by a health care provider. Unusual vaginal bleeding after menopause can be a warning sign of cancer of the uterus. Estrogens may increase the risk of cancer of the uterus in women who have had their menopause ("change of life"). If you use any estrogen-containing drug, it is important to visit your health care provider regularly and report any unusual vaginal bleeding right away. Your health care provider should evaluate any unusual vaginal bleeding to find out the cause.

If there is a history of certain types of cancer—Estrogens may increase the risk of certain types of cancer, usually uterine or breast. VAGIFEM has not been associated with an increased risk of uterine cancer. Although there are reports of increased risk of breast cancer in women on hormone replacement therapy, VAGIFEM is administered locally and is not expected to pose an increased risk.

After childbirth or when breast-feeding a baby—VAGIFEM should not be used to try to stop the breasts from filling with milk after a baby is born. Women who are breast-feeding should avoid using any drugs because many drugs pass through to the baby in the milk. While nursing a baby, drugs should only be taken on the advice of your healthcare giver.

Possible Risks from Treatment with Estrogens

The following risk factors apply to estrogens in general:

Cancer of the uterus—Estrogens increase the risk of developing a condition (endometrial hyperplasia) that may lead to cancer of the lining of the uterus (endometrial cancer). The risk of endometrial cancer is greater in estrogen users than nonusers. Studies have shown that this increased risk depends on estrogen dose, duration of treatment, and treatment regimen.

Using progestin therapy together with estrogen therapy may reduce the higher risk of uterine cancer related to estrogen use.

If the uterus has been removed (total hysterectomy), there is no danger of developing cancer of the uterus.

Cancer of the breast—Most studies have not shown a higher risk of breast cancer in women who have ever used estrogens. However, some studies have reported that breast cancer developed more often (up to twice the usual rate) in women who used estrogens for long periods of time (especially more than 10 years) or who used higher doses for shorter time periods. VAGIFEM® (estradiol vaginal tablets) is not expected to increase the risk since it is a low dose, applied topically in the vagina, is minimally absorbed into the systemic circulation and is used for relatively short periods of time.

Regular breast examinations by a health professional and monthly self-examination are recommended for all women.

Gallbladder disease and abnormal blood clotting—Gallbladder disease and abnormal blood clotting are risk factors associated with medium to high doses of estrogen. Most studies of low-dose estrogen usage by women do not show an increased risk of these complications, and to date there have not been complications with VAGIFEM (estradiol vaginal tablets) treatment.

Side Effects

Few side effects have been reported: vaginal spotting, vaginal discharge, allergic reaction and skin rash.

Estrogens in General

In addition to the risks listed above, the following side effects have been reported with estrogen use:

Nausea and vomiting, breast tenderness or enlargement, enlargement of benign tumors ("fibroids") of the uterus, retention of excess fluid.

Estrogen may worsen some conditions, such as asthma, epilepsy, migraine, heart disease, or kidney disease. Spotty darkening of the skin, particularly on the face.

If you use estrogens, you may reduce your risks by doing these things: See your health care provider regularly. While you are using estrogens, it is important to visit your health care provider at least annually for a check-up. If you develop vaginal bleeding while taking estrogens, call your health care provider; you may need further evaluation. If members of your family have had breast cancer or if you have ever had breast lumps or an abnormal mammogram

Continued on next page

Information on these Pharmacia & Upjohn products is based on labeling in effect June 1, 2000. Further information concerning these and other Pharmacia & Upjohn products may be obtained by direct inquiry to Medical Information, Pharmacia & Upjohn, Kalamazoo, MI 49001.

Vagifem—Cont.

(breast X-ray), you may need to have more frequent breast examinations. Reassess your need for estrogens. You and your health care provider should reevaluate whether or not you still need estrogens at least every six months.

Be alert for warning signs. If any of these warning signals (or any other unusual symptoms) happen while you are using estrogens, call your health care provider immediately: Abnormal bleeding from the vagina (possible uterine cancer); pains in the calves or chest, sudden shortness of breath, or coughing blood (possible clot in the legs, heart, or lungs); severe headache or vomiting, dizziness, faintness, changes in vision or speech, weakness or numbness of an arm or leg (possible clot in the brain or eye); breast lumps (possible breast cancer; ask your health care provider to show you how to examine your breasts monthly); yellowing of skin or eyes (possible liver problem); pain, swelling, or tenderness in the abdomen (possible gallbladder problem).

1. Estrogens increase the risk of developing a condition called endometrial hyperplasia that may lead to cancer of the lining of the uterus. Progestin, another hormone drug, is usually prescribed with higher-dose estrogen preparations in order to lower the risk of developing endometrial hyperplasia. Progestins are not usually needed for women using VAGIFEM® (estradiol vaginal tablets) alone.

2. Vaginal infection is generally more common in postmenopausal women. Vaginal infections should be treated by your health care provider with the appropriate antimicrobial therapy before initiation of VAGIFEM. If a vaginal infection develops during use of VAGIFEM, it may be continued while the infection is being treated. See your health care provider if you have vaginal discomfort or suspect you have a vaginal infection.

3. Your health care provider has prescribed this drug for you and you alone. Do not give the drug to anyone else.

4. Keep this and all drugs out of the reach of children.

5. This leaflet provides a summary of important information about VAGIFEM. If you want more information, ask your health care provider or pharmacist to show you the professional labeling. The professional labeling is also published in a book called the "Physicians' Desk Reference" which is available in book stores and public libraries. Generic drugs carry virtually the same labeling information as their brand name versions.

HOW SUPPLIED

Each VAGIFEM® (estradiol vaginal tablets), 25μg is contained in a disposable, single-use applicator, packaged in a blister pack. Cartons contain 15 applicators with inset tablets.

NDC 0009-5173-02

STORAGE: Store at 25°C (77°F); excursions permitted to 15°C–30°C (59°F–86°F). [See USP Controlled Room Temperature.]

Rx only

Vagifem® is a trademark owned by Novo Nordisk A/S

Revised June 2000

Manufactured for
Pharmacia & Upjohn Company
Kalamazoo, MI 49001, USA
By
Novo Nordisk A/S
2880 Bagsværd, Denmark

VANTIN® ℞

[*văn-tĭn*]

Tablets and Oral Suspension
cefpodoxime proxetil tablets and
cefpodoxime proxetil for oral suspension
For Oral Use Only

DESCRIPTION

Cefpodoxime proxetil is an orally administered, extended spectrum, semi-synthetic antibiotic of the cephalosporin class. The chemical name is (RS)-1(isopropoxycarbonyloxy-)ethyl (+)-(6R,7R)-7-[2-(2-amino-4-thiazolyl)-2-{(Z)methoxy-imino}acetamido]-3-methoxymethyl-8-oxo-5-thia-1-azabicyclo [4.2.0] oct-2-ene-2-carboxylate.

Its empirical formula is $C_{21}H_{27}N_5O_9S_2$ and its structural formula is represented below:

The molcular weight of cefpodoxime proxetil is 557.6.

Cefpodoxime proxetil is a prodrug; its active metabolite is cefpodoxime. All doses of cefpodoxime proxetil in this insert are expressed in terms of the active cefpodoxime moiety. The drug is supplied both as film-coated tablets and as flavored granules for oral suspension.

VANTIN Tablets contain cefpodoxime proxetil equivalent to 100 mg or 200 mg of cefpodoxime activity and the following inactive ingredients: carboxymethylcellulose calcium, carnauba wax, FD&C Yellow No. 6, hydroxypropylcellulose, hydroxypropylmethylcellulose, lactose hydrous, magnesium stearate, propylene glycol, sodium lauryl sulfate and titanium dioxide. In addition, the 100 mg film-coated tablets contain D&C Yellow No. 10 and the 200 mg film-coated tablets contain FD&C Red No. 40.

Each 5 mL of VANTIN Oral Suspension contains cefpodoxime proxetil equivalent to 50 mg or 100 mg of cefpodoxime activity after constitution and the following inactive ingredients: artificial flavorings, butylated hydroxy anisole (BHA), carboxymethylcellulose sodium, microcrystalline cellulose, carrageenan, citric acid, colloidal silicon dioxide, croscarmellose sodium, hydroxypropylcellulose, lactose, maltodextrin, natural flavorings, propylene glycol alginate, sodium citrate, sodium benzoate, starch, sucrose, and vegetable oil.

CLINICAL PHARMACOLOGY

Absorption and Excretion:

Cefpodoxime proxetil is a prodrug that is absorbed from the gastrointestinal tract and de-esterified to its active metabolite, cefpodoxime. Following oral administration of 100 mg of cefpodoxime proxetil to fasting subjects, approximately 50% of the administered cefpodoxime dose was absorbed systemically. Over the recommended dosing range (100 to 400 mg), approximately 29 to 33% of the administered cefpodoxime dose was excreted unchanged in the urine in 12 hours. There is minimal metabolism of cefpodoxime *in vivo*.

Effects on Food:

The extent of absorption (mean AUC) and the mean peak plasma concentration increased when film-coated tablets were administered with food. Following a 200 mg tablet dose taken with food, the AUC was 21 to 33% higher than under fasting conditions, and the peak plasma concentration averaged 3.1 mcg/mL in fed subjects versus 2.6 mcg/mL in fasted subjects. Time to peak concentration was not significantly different between fed and fasted subjects.

When a 200 mg dose of the suspension was taken with food, the extent of absorption (mean AUC) and mean peak plasma concentration in fed subjects were not significantly difference from fasted subjects, but the rate of absorption was slower with food (48% increase in T_{max}).

Pharmacokinetics of Cefpodoxime Proxetil Film-coated Tablets:

Over the recommended dosing range, (100 to 400 mg), the rate and extent of cefpodoxime absorption exhibited dose-dependency; dose-normalized C_{max} and AUC decreased by up to 32% with increasing dose. Over the recommended dosing range, the T_{max} was approximately 2 to 3 hours and the $T_{1/2}$ ranged from 2.09 to 2.84 hours. Mean C_{max} was 1.4 mcg/mL for the 100 mg dose, 2.3 mcg/mL for the 200 mg dose, and 3.9 mcg/mL for the 400 mg dose. In patients with normal renal function, neither accumulation nor significant changes in other pharmacokinetic parameters were noted following multiple oral doses of up to 400 mg Q 12 hours. [See first table above]

CEFPODOXIME PLASMA LEVELS (mcg/mL) IN FASTED ADULTS AFTER FILM-COATED TABLET ADMINISTRATION (Single Dose)

Dose (cefpodoxime equivalents)	Time after oral ingestion						
	1hr	**2hr**	**3hr**	**4hr**	**6hr**	**8hr**	**12hr**
100 mg	0.98	1.4	1.3	1.0	0.59	0.29	0.08
200 mg	1.5	2.2	2.2	1.8	1.2	0.62	0.18
400 mg	2.2	3.7	3.8	3.3	2.3	1.3	0.38

Pharmacokinetics of Cefpodoxime Proxetil Suspension:

In adult subjects, a 100 mg dose of oral suspension produced an average peak cefpodoxime concentration of approximately 1.5 mcg/mL (range: 1.1 to 2.1 mcg/mL), which is equivalent to that reported following administration of the 100 mg tablet. Time to peak plasma concentration and area under the plasma concentration-time curve (AUC) for the oral suspension were also equivalent to those produced with film-coated tablets in adults following a 100 mg oral dose.

The pharmacokinetics of cefpodoxime were investigated in 29 patients aged 1 to 17 years. Each patient received a single, oral, 5 mg/kg dose of cefpodoxime oral suspension. Plasma and urine samples were collected for 12 hours after dosing. The plasma levels reported from this study are as follows:

[See second table above]

CEFPODOXIME PLASMA LEVELS (mcg/mL) IN FASTED PATIENTS (1 to 17 YEARS OF AGE) AFTER SUSPENSION ADMINISTRATION

Dose (cefpodoxime equivalents)	Time after oral ingestion						
	1hr	**2hr**	**3hr**	**4hr**	**6hr**	**8hr**	**12hr**
5 mg/kg[1]	1.4	2.1	2.1	1.7	0.90	0.40	0.090

[1] Dose did not exceed 200 mg.

Distribution:

Protein binding of cefpodoxime ranges from 22 to 33% in serum and from 21 to 29% in plasma.

Skin Blister:

Following multiple-dose administration every 12 hours for 5 days of 200 mg or 400 mg cefpodoxime proxetil, the mean maximum cefpodoxime concentration in skin blister fluid averaged 1.6 to 2.8 mcg/mL, respectively. Skin blister fluid cefpodoxime levels at 12 hours after dosing averaged 0.2 and 0.4 mcg/mL for the 200 mg and 400 mg multiple-dose regimens, respectively.

Tonsil Tissue:

Following a single, oral 100 mg cefpodoxime proxetil film-coated tablet, the mean maximum cefpodoxime concentration in tonsil tissue averaged 0.24 mcg/g at 4 hours post-dosing and 0.09 mcg/g at 7 hours post-dosing. Equilibrium was achieved between plasma and tonsil tissue within 4 hours of dosing. No detection of cefpodoxime in tonsillar tissue was reported 12 hours after dosing. These results demonstrated that concentrations of cefpodoxime exceeded the MIC_{90} of *S. pyogenes* for at least 7 hours after dosing of 100 mg of cefpodoxime proxetil.

Lung Tissue:

Following a single, oral 200 mg cefpodoxime proxetil film-coated tablet, the mean maximum cefpodoxime concentration in lung tissue averaged 0.63 mcg/g at 3 hours post-dosing, 0.52 mcg/g at 6 hours post-dosing, and 0.19 mcg/g at 12 hours post-dosing. The results of this study indicated that cefpodoxime penetrated into lung tissue and produced sustained drug concentrations for at least 12 hours after dosing at levels that exceeded the MIC_{90} for *S. pneumoniae* and *H. influenzae*.

CSF:

Adequate data on CSF levels of cefpodoxime are not available.

Effects of Decreased Renal Function:

Elimination of cefpodoxime is reduced in patients with moderate to severe renal impairment (<50 mL/min creatinine clearance). (See **PRECAUTIONS** and **DOSAGE AND ADMINISTRATION**.) In subjects with mild impairment of renal function (50 to 80 mL/min creatinine clearance), the average plasma half-life of cefpodoxime was 3.5 hours. In subjects with moderate (30 to 49 mL/min creatinine clearance) or severe renal impairment (5 to 29 mL/min creatinine clearance), the half-life increased to 5.9 to 9.8 hours, respectively. Approximately 23% of the administered dose was cleared from the body during a standard 3-hour hemodialysis procedure.

Effect of Hepatic Impairment (cirrhosis):

Absorption was somewhat diminished and elimination unchanged in patients with cirrhosis. The mean cefpodoxime $T_{1/2}$ and renal clearance in cirrhotic patients were similar to those derived in studies of healthy subjects. Ascites did not appear to affect values in cirrhotic subjects. No dosage adjustment is recommended in this patient population.

Pharmacokinetics in Elderly Subjects:

Elderly subjects do not require dosage adjustments unless they have diminished renal function. (See **PRECAUTIONS**.) In healthy geriatric subjects, cefpodoxime half-life in plasma averaged 4.2 hours (vs 3.3 in younger subjects) and urinary recovery averaged 21% after a 400 mg dose was administered every 12 hours. Other pharmacokinetic parameters (C_{max}, AUC, and T_{max}) were unchanged relative to those observed in healthy young subjects.

Microbiology:

Cefpodoxime is active against a wide-spectrum of Gram-positive and Gram-negative bacteria.

Cefpodoxime is stable in the presence of beta-lactamase enzymes. As a result, many organisms resistant to penicillins and cephalosporins, due to their production of beta lactamase, may be susceptible to cefpodoxime. Cefpodoxime is inactivated by certain extended spectrum beta-lactamases.

The bactericidal activity of cefpodoxime results from its inhibition of cell wall synthesis.

Cefpodoxime has been shown to be active against most strains of the following microorganisms, both *in vitro* and in clinical infections, as described in the **INDICATIONS AND USAGE** section.

Aerobic Gram-positive microorganisms:

Staphylococcus aureus (including penicillinase-producing strains)

NOTE: Cefpodoxime is inactive against methicillin-resistant staphylococci.

Staphylococcus saprophyticus

Streptococcus pneumoniae (excluding penicillin-resistant strains)

Streptococcus pyogenes

Aerobic Gram-negative microorgansims:

Escherichia coli

Klebsiella pneumoniae

Proteus mirabilis

Haemophilus influenzae (including beta-lactamase producing strains)

Moraxella (Branhamella) catarrhalis

Neisseria gonorrhoeae (including penicillinase-producing strains)

The following *in vitro* data are available, but their clinical significance is unknown. Cefpodoxime exhibits *in vitro* minimum inhibitory concentrations (MICs) of ≤ 2.0 mcg/mL against most (≥ 90%) of isolates of the following microorganisms. However, the safety and efficacy of cefpodoxime in treating clinical infections due to these microorganisms have not been established in adequate and well controlled clinical trials.

Aerobic Gram-positive microorganisms:
Streptococcus agalactiae
Streptococcus spp. (Groups C, F, G)
NOTE: Cefpodoxime is inactive against enterococci.

Aerobic Gram-negative microorganisms:
Citrobacter diversus
Klebsiella oxytoca
Proteus vulgaris
Providencia rettgeri
Haemophilus parainfluenzae
NOTE: Cefpodoxime is inactive against most strains of *Pseudomonas* and *Enterobacter*.

Anaerobic Gram-positive microorganisms:
Peptostreptococcus magnus

SUSCEPTIBILITY TESTING

Dilution Techniques: Quantitative methods are used to determine antimicrobial inhibitory concentrations (MICs). These MICs provide estimates of the suscpetibility of microorganisms to antimicrobial compounds. The MICs should be determined using a standardized procedure. Standardized procedures are based on dilution methods[1,2] (broth or agar) or equivalent using standardized inoculum concentrations, and standardized concentrations of cefpodoxime from a powder of known potency. The MIC values should be interpreted according to the following criteria:

For Susceptibility Testing of *Enterobacteriaceae*, and *Staphylococcus* spp.

MIC (mcg/mL)	Interpretation
≤2.0	Susceptible (S)
4.0	Intermediate (I)
≥8.0	Resistant (R)

For Susceptibility Testing of *Haemophilus* spp.[a]

MIC (mcg/mL)	Interpretation[b]
≤2.0	Susceptible (S)

[a] The interpretive criteria for *Haemophilus* spp. is applicable only to broth microdilution susceptibility testing done with Haemophilus Test Medium (HTM) broth.[2]
[b] "Intermediate" and "Resistant" categories have not been determined.

For Susceptibility Testing of *Neisseria gonorrhoeae*.[c]

MIC (mcg/mL)	Interpretation[d]
≤0.5	Susceptible (S)

[c] The interpretive value for *N. gonorroheae* is applicable only to agar dilution susceptibility testing done with *Neisseria gonorrhoeae* susceptibility test medium.[2]
[d] "Intermediate" and "Resistant" categories have not been determined.

For Susceptibility Testing of *Streptococcus pneumoniae*.

MIC (mcg/mL)	Interpretation[e]
≤0.5	Susceptible (S)
1.0	Intermediate (I)
≥2.0	Resistant (R)

[e] The interpretive value for *S. pneumoniae* is applicable only to broth microdilution susceptibility testing done with cation-adjusted Mueller-Hinton broth with lysed horse blood (LHB) (2–5% v/v).[2]

For Susceptibility Testing of *Streptococcus* spp. other than *Streptococcus pneumoniae*.[f]
A streptococcal isolate that is susceptible to penicillin (MIC ≤ 0.12 mcg/mL) can be considered susceptible to cefpodoxime for approved indications, and need not be tested against cefpodoxime.

[f] The interpretive value for Streptococcus spp. is applicable only to broth microdilution susceptibility testing done with cation-adjusted Mueller-Hinton broth with lysed horse blood (LHB) (2–5% v/v).[2]

A report of "Susceptible" indicates that the pathogen is likely to be inhibited if the concentration of the antimicrobial compound in the blood reaches usually achievable levels. A report of "Intermediate" indicates that the results should be considered equivocal, and, if the microorganism is not fully susceptible to alternative, clinically feasible drugs, the test should be repeated. This category implies possible clinical applicability in body sites where the drug is physiologically concentrated or in situations where high dosage of drug can be used. This category also provides a buffer zone which prevents small technical factors from causing major discrepancies in interpretation. A report of "Resistant" indicates that the pathogen is not likely to be inhibited if the antimicrobial compound in the blood reaches the concentrations usually achievable; other therapy should be selected.

Quality Control
A standardized susceptible test procedure requires the use of laboratory control organisms to control the technical aspects of the laboratory procedures. Standard cefpodoxime powder should provide the following MIC values with the indicated quality control strains:

Microorganism (ATCC®#)	MIC Range (mcg/mL)
Escherichia coli (25922)	0.25–1.0
Staphylococcus aureus (29213)	1.0–8.0
Haemophilus influenzae (49247)	0.25–1.0[g]
Neisseria gonorrhoeae (49226)	0.03–0.12[h]
Streptococcus pneumoniae(49619)[j]	0.03–0.12[i]

[g] These quality control ranges are applicable to tests performed by a broth microdilution procedure using Haemophilus Test Medium (HTM).
[h] These quality control ranges are applicable to tests performed by agar dilution only using GC agar base with 1% defined growth supplement.
[i] These quality control ranges are applicable to tests performed by the broth microdilution method only using cation-adjusted Mueller-Hinton broth with 2 to 5% lysed horse blood.
[j] When susceptibility testing *Streptococcus pneumoniae* or *Streptococcus* spp. this quality control strain should be tested.

Diffusion Techniques: Quantitative methods that require measurement of zone diameters also provide reproducible estimates of the susceptibility of bacteria to antimicrobial compounds. One such standardized procedure[3] requires the use of standardized inoculum concentrations. This procedure uses paper disks impregnated with 10 mcg cefpodoxime to test the susceptibility of microorganisms to cefpodoxime. Reports from the laboratory providing results of the standard single-disk susceptibility test with a 10 mcg cefpodoxime disk should be interpreted according the the following criteria:

For Susceptibility Testing of *Enterobacteriaceae*, and *Staphylococcus* spp.

Zone Diameter (mm)	Interpretation
≥21	Susceptible (S)
18–20	Intermediate (I)
≤17	Resistant (R)

For Susceptibility Testing of *Haemophilus* spp.[k]

Zone Diameter (mm)	Interpretation[l]
≥21	Susceptible (S)

[k] The zone diameter for *Haemophilus* spp. is applicable only to tests performed on Haemophilus Test Medium (HTM) agar incubated under 5% CO_2.[2]
[l] "Intermediate" and "Resistant" criteria have not been determined.

For Susceptibility Testing of *Neisseria gonorrhoeae*.[m]

Zone Diameter (mm)	Interpretation[n]
≥29	Susceptible (S)

[m] The zone diameter for *N. gonorrhoeae* is applicable only to tests performed on GC agar base and 1% defined growth supplement incubated under 5% CO_2.[2]
[n] "Intermediate" and "Resistant" categories have not been determined.

For Susceptibility Testing of *Streptococcus pneumoniae*.[o]
Isolates of pneumococci with oxacillin zone sizes of ≥20 mm are susceptible (MIC ≤0.06 mcg/mL) to penicillin and can be considered susceptible to cefpodoxime for approved indications, and cefpodoxime need not be tested.

[o] The zone diameter for *S. pneumoniae* is applicable only to tests performed on Mueller-Hinton agar with 5% sheep blood incubated in 5% CO_2.[2]

For Susceptibility Testing of *Streptococcus* spp. other than *Streptococcus pneumoniae*.[p]
A streptococcal isolate that is susceptible to penicillin (zone diameter ≥28 mm) can be considered susceptible to cefpodoxime for approved indications, and cefpodoxime need not be tested.

[p] The zone diameter for *Streptococcus* spp. is applicable only to tests performed on Mueller-Hinton agar with 5% sheep blood incubated in 5% CO_2.[2]

Quality Control
As with standardized dilution techniques, diffusion methods require the use of laboratory control microorganisms that are used to control the technical aspects of the laboratory procedures. For the diffusion technique, the 10 mcg cefpodoxime disk should provide the following zone diameters with the quality control strains listed below:

Microorganism (ATCC®#)	Zone Diameter Range (mm)
Escherichia coli (25922)	23–28
Staphylococcus aureus (25923)	19–25
Haemophilus influenzae (49247)	25–31[q]
Neisseria gonorrhoeae (49226)	35–43[r]
Streptococcus pneumoniae(49619)[t]	28–34[s]

[q] This zone diameter range is only applicable to tests performed on Haemophilus Test Medium (HTM) agar incubated in 5% CO_2.
[r] This zone diameter range is only applicable to tests performed on GC agar base and 1% defined growth supplement incubated in 5% CO_2.
[s] This zone diameter range is only applicable to tests performed on Mueller-Hinton agar supplemented with 5% defibrinated sheep blood, incubated in 5% CO_2.
[t] This organism is to be used for quality control testing for both *S. pneumoniae* and *Streptococcus* spp. ATCC® is a registered trademark of the American Type Culture Collection.

INDICATIONS AND USAGE

Cefpodoxime proxetil is indicated for the treatment of patients with mild to moderate infections caused by susceptible strains of the designated microorganisms in the conditions listed below. **Recommended dosages, durations of therapy, and applicable patient populations vary among these infections. Please see DOSAGE AND ADMINISTRATION for specific recommendations.**

Acute otitis media caused by *Streptococcus pneumoniae*, (excluding penicillin-resistant strains), *Streptococcus pyogenes*, *Haemophilus influenzae* (including beta-lactamase-producing strains), or *Moraxella (Branhamella) catarrhalis* (including beta-lactamase producing strains).

Pharyngitis and/or tonsillitis caused by *Streptococcus pyogenes*.

NOTE: Only penicillin by the intramuscular route of administration has been shown to be effective in the prophylaxis of rheumatic fever. Cefpodoxime proxetil is generally effective in the eradication of streptococci from the oropharynx. However, data establishing the efficacy of cefpodoxime proxetil for the prophylaxis of subsequent rheumatic fever are not available.

Community-acquired pneumonia caused by *S. pneumoniae* or *H. influenzae* (including beta-lactamase-producing strains).

Acute bacterial exacerbation of chronic bronchitis caused by *S. pneumoniae*, *H. influenzae* (non-beta-lactamase-producing strains only), or *M. catarrhalis*. Data are insufficient at this time to establish efficacy in patients with acute bacterial exacerbations of chronic bronchitis caused by beta-lactamase-producing strains of *H. influenzae*.

Acute, uncomplicated urethral and cervical gonorrhea caused by *Neisseria gonorrhoeae* (including penicillinase-producing strains).

Acute, uncomplicated ano-rectal infections in women due to *Neisseria gonorrhoeae* (including penicillinase-producing strains).

NOTE: The efficacy of cefpodoxime in treating male patients with rectal infections caused by *N. gonorrhoeae* has not been established. Data do not support the use of cefpodoxime proxetil in the treatment of pharyngeal infections due to *N. gonorrhoeae* in men or women.

Uncomplicated skin and skin structure infections caused by *Staphylococcus aureus* (including penicillinase-producing strains) or *Streptococcus pyogenes*. Abscesses should be surgically drained as clinically indicated.

NOTE: In clinical trials, successful treatment of uncomplicated skin and skin structure infections was dose-related. The effective therapeutic dose for skin infections was higher than those used in other recommended indications. (See **DOSAGE AND ADMINISTRATION.**)

Acute maxillary sinusitis caused by *Haemophilus influenzae* (including beta-lactamase producing strains), *Streptococcus pneumoniae*, and *Moraxella catarrhalis*.

Uncomplicated urinary tract infections (cystitis) caused by *Escherichia coli*, *Klebsiella pneumoniae*, *Proteus mirabilis*, or *Staphylococcus saprophyticus*.

NOTE: In considering the use of cefpodoxime proxetil in the treatment of cystitis, cefpodoxime proxetil's lower bacterial eradication rates should be weighed against the increased eradication rates and different safety profiles of some other classes of approved agents. (See **CLINICAL STUDIES** section.)

Appropriate specimens for bacteriological examination should be obtained in order to isolate and identify causative organisms and to determine their susceptibility to cefpodoxime. Therapy may be instituted while awaiting the results of these studies. Once these results become available, antimicrobial therapy should be adjusted accordingly.

CONTRAINDICATIONS

Cefpodoxime proxetil is contraindicated in patients with a known allergy to cefpodoxime or to the cephalosporin group of antibiotics.

WARNINGS

BEFORE THERAPY WITH CEFPODOXIME PROXETIL IS INSTITUTED, CAREFUL INQUIRY SHOULD BE MADE TO DETERMINE WHETHER THE PATIENT HAS HAD PREVIOUS HYPERSENSITIVITY REACTIONS TO CEFPODOXIME, OTHER CEPHALOSPORINS, PENICILLINS, OR OTHER DRUGS. IF CEFPODOXIME IS TO BE ADMINISTERED TO PENICILLIN SENSITIVE PATIENTS, CAUTION SHOULD BE EXERCISED BECAUSE CROSS HYPERSENSITIVITY AMONG BETA-LACTAM ANTIBIOTICS HAS BEEN CLEARLY DOCUMENTED AND MAY OCCUR IN UP TO 10% OF PA-

Continued on next page

Information on these Pharmacia & Upjohn products is based on labeling in effect June 1, 2000. Further information concerning these and other Pharmacia & Upjohn products may be obtained by direct inquiry to Medical Information, Pharmacia & Upjohn, Kalamazoo, MI 49001.

Vantin—Cont.

TIENTS WITH A HISTORY OF PENICILLIN ALLERGY. IF AN ALLERGIC REACTION TO CEFPODOXIME PROXETIL OCCURS, DISCONTINUE THE DRUG. SERIOUS ACUTE HYPERSENSITIVITY REACTIONS MAY REQUIRE TREATMENT WITH EPINEPHRINE AND OTHER EMERGENCY MEASURES, INCLUDING OXYGEN, INTRAVENOUS FLUIDS, INTRAVENOUS ANTIHISTAMINE, AND AIRWAY MANAGEMENT, AS CLINICALLY INDICATED. PSEUDOMEMBRANOUS COLITIS HAS BEEN REPORTED WITH NEARLY ALL ANTIBACTERIAL AGENTS, INCLUDING CEFPODOXIME, AND MAY RANGE IN SEVERITY FROM MILD TO LIFE-THREATENING. THEREFORE, IT IS IMPORTANT TO CONSIDER THIS DIAGNOSIS IN PATIENTS WHO PRESENT WITH DIARRHEA SUBSEQUENT TO THE ADMINISTRATION OF ANTIBACTERIAL AGENTS.

Extreme caution should be observed when using this product in patients at increased risk for antibiotic-induced, pseudomembranous colitis because of exposure to institutional settings, such as nursing homes or hospitals with endemic *C. difficile*.

Treatment with broad-spectrum antibiotics, including cefpodoxime proxetil, alters the normal flora of the colon and may permit overgrowth of clostridia. Studies indicate a toxin produced by *Clostridium difficile* is the primary cause of "antibiotic-associated colitis".

After the diagnosis of pseudomembranous colitis has been established, therapeutic measures should be initiated. Mild cases of pseudomembranous colitis usually respond to drug discontinuation alone. In moderate to severe cases, consideration should be given to management with fluids and electrolytes, protein supplementation, and treatment with an oral antibacterial drug effective against *C. difficile*.

A concerted effort to monitor for *C. difficile* in cefpodoxime-treated patients with diarrhea was undertaken because of an increased incidence of diarrhea associated with *C. difficile* in early trails in normal subjects. *C. difficile* organisms or toxin was reported in 10% of the cefpodoxime-treated adult patients with diarrhea; however, no specific diagnosis of pseudomembranous colitis was made in these patients.

In post-marketing experience outside the United States, reports of pseudomembranous colitis associated with the use of cefpodoxime proxetil have been received.

PRECAUTIONS

General:

In patients with transient or persistent reduction in urinary output due to renal insufficiency, the total daily dose of cefpodoxime proxetil should be reduced because high and prolonged serum antibiotic concentrations can occur in such individuals following usual doses. Cefpodoxime, like other cephalosporins, should be administered with caution to patients receiving concurrent treatment with potent diuretics. (See **DOSAGE AND ADMINISTRATION**.)

As with other antibiotics, prolonged use of cefpodoxime proxetil may result in overgrowth of non-susceptible organisms. Repeated evaluation of the patient's condition is essential. If superinfection occurs during therapy, appropriate measures should be taken.

Drug Interactions:

Antacids: Concomitant administration of high doses of antacids (sodium bicarbonate and aluminum hydroxide) or H_2 blockers reduces peak plasma levels by 24% to 42% and the extent of absorption by 27% to 32%, respectively. The rate of absorption is not altered by these concomitant medications. Oral anti-cholinergics (e.g., propantheline) delay peak plasma levels (47% increase in T_{max}), but do not affect the extent of absorption (AUC).

Probenecid: As with other beta-lactam antibiotics, renal excretion of cefpodoxime was inhibited by probenecid and resulted in an approximately 31% increase in AUC and 20% increase in peak cefpodoxime plasma levels.

Nephrotoxic drugs: Although nephrotoxicity has not been noted when cefpodoxime proxetil was given alone, close monitoring of renal function is advised when cefpodoxime proxetil is administered concomitantly with compounds of known nephrotoxic potential.

Drug/Laboratory Test Interactions:

Cephalosporins, including cefpodoxime proxetil, are known to occasionally induce a positive direct Coombs' test.

Carcinogenesis, Mutagenesis, Impairment of Fertility:

Long-term animal carcinogenesis studies of cefpodoxime proxetil have not been performed. Mutagenesis studies of cefpodoxime, including the Ames test both with and without metabolic activation, the chromosome aberration test, the unscheduled DNA synthesis assay, mitotic recombination and gene conversion, the forward gene mutation assay and the *in vivo* micronucleus test, were all negative. No untoward effects on fertility or reproduction were noted when 100 mg/kg/day or less (2 times the human dose based on mg/m^2) was administered orally to rats.

Pregnancy—Teratogenic Effects:

Pregnancy Category B

Cefpodoxime proxetil was neither teratogenic nor embryocidal when administered to rats during organogenesis at doses up to 100 mg/kg/day (2 times the human dose based on mg/m^2) or to rabbits at doses up to 30 mg/kg/day (1–2 times the human dose based on mg/m^2).

There are, however, no adequate and well-controlled studies of cefpodoxime proxetil use in pregnant women. Because animal reproduction studies are not always predictive of human response, this drug should be used during pregnancy only if clearly needed.

Adults and Adolescents (age 12 years and older):

Type of Infection	Total Daily Dose	Dose Frequency	Duration
Pharyngitis and/or tonsillitis	200 mg	100 mg Q 12 hours	5 to 10 days
Acute community-acquired pneumonia	400 mg	200 mg Q 12 hours	14 days
Acute bacterial exacerbations of chronic bronchitis	400 mg	200 mg Q 12 hours	10 days
Uncomplicated gonorrhea (men and women) and rectal gonococcal infections (women)	200 mg	single dose	
Skin and skin structures	800 mg	400 mg Q 12 hours	7 to 14 days
Acute maxillary sinusitis	400 mg	200 mg Q 12 hours	10 days
Uncomplicated urinary tract infection	200 mg	100 mg Q 12 hours	7 days

Adults and Adolescents (age 12 years and older):

Type of Infection	Total Daily Dose	Dose Frequency	Duration
Pharyngitis and/or tonsillitis	200 mg	100 mg Q 12 hours	5 to 10 days
Acute community-acquired pneumonia	400 mg	200 mg Q 12 hours	14 days
Uncomplicated gonorrhea (men and women) and rectal gonococcal infections (women)	200 mg	single dose	
Skin and skin structure	800 mg	400 mg Q 12 hours	7 to 14 days
Acute maxillary sinusitis	400 mg	200 mg Q 12 hours	10 days
Uncomplicated urinary tract infection	200 mg	100 mg Q 12 hours	7 days

Infants and Pediatric Patients (age 2 months through 12 years):

Type of Infection	Total Daily Dose	Dose Frequency	Duration
Acute otitis media	10 mg/kg/day (Max 400 mg/day)	5 mg/kg Q 12 h (Max 400 mg/dose)	5 days
Pharyngitis and/or tonsillitis	10 mg/kg/day (Max 200 mg/day)	5 mg/kg/dose Q 12 h (Max 100 mg/dose)	5 to 10 days
Acute maxillary sinusitis	10 mg/kg/day (Max 400 mg/kg/day)	5 mg/kg Q 12 hours (Max 200 mg/dose)	10 days

Labor and Delivery:

Cefpodoxime proxetil has not been studied for use during labor and delivery. Treatment should only be given if clearly needed.

Nursing Mothers:

Cefpodoxime is excreted in human milk. In a study of 3 lactating women, levels of cefpodoxime in human milk were 0%, 2% and 6% of concomitant serum levels at 4 hours following a 200 mg oral dose of cefpodoxime proxetil. At 6 hours post-dosing, levels were 0%, 9% and 16% of concomitant serum levels. Because of the potential for serious reactions in nursing infants, a decision should be made whether to discontinue nursing or to discontinue the drug, taking into account the importance of the drug to the mother.

Pediatric Use:

Safety and efficacy in infants less than 2 months of age have not been established.

Geriatric Use:

Of the 3338 patients in multiple-dose clinical studies of cefpodoxime proxetil film-coated tablets, 521 (16%) were 65 and over, while 214 (6%) were 75 and over. No overall differences in effectiveness or safety were observed between the elderly and young patients. In healthy geriatric subjects with normal renal function, cefpodoxime half-life in plasma averaged 4.2 hours and urinary recovery averaged 21% after a 400 mg dose was given every 12 hours for 15 days. Other pharmacokinetic parameters were unchanged relative to those observed in healthy younger subjects.

Dose adjustment in elderly patients with normal renal function is not necessary.

ADVERSE REACTIONS

Clinical Trials:

Film-coated Tablets (Multiple dose):

In clinical trials using multiple doses of cefpodoxime proxetil film-coated tablets, 4696 patients were treated with the recommended dosage of cefpodoxime (100 to 400 mg Q 12 hours). There were no deaths or permanent disabilities thought related to drug toxicity. One-hundred twenty-nine (2.7%) patients discontinued medication due to adverse events thought possibly- or probably-related to drug toxicity. Ninety-three (52%) of the 178 patients who discontinued therapy (whether thought related to drug therapy or not) did so because of gastrointestinal disturbances, nausea, vomiting, or diarrhea. The percentage of cefpodoxime proxetil-treated patients who discontinued study drug because of adverse events was significantly greater at a dose of 800 mg daily than at a dose of 400 mg daily or at a dose of 200 mg daily. Adverse events thought possibly- or probably-related to cefpodoxime in multiple dose clinical trials (N = 4696 cefpodoxime-treated patients) were:

Incidence Greater Than 1%:

Diarrhea	7.0%

Diarrhea or loose stools were dose related: decreasing from 10.4% of patients receiving 800 mg per day to 5.7% for those receiving 200 mg per day. Of patients with diarrhea, 10% had *C. difficile* organism or toxin in the stool (See **WARNINGS**.)

Nausea	3.3%
Vaginal Fungal Infections	1.0%
Vulvovaginal Infections	1.3%
Abdominal Pain	1.2%
Headache	1.0%

Incidence Less Than 1%: By body system in decreasing order:

Clinical Studies

Adverse events thought possibly or probably related to cefpodoxime proxetil that occurred in **less than 1%** of patients (N = 4696)

Body—fungal infections, abdominal distention, malaise, fatigue, asthenia, fever, chest pain, back pain, chills, generalized pain, abnormal microbiological tests, moniliasis, abscess, allergic reaction, facial edema, bacterial infections, parasitic infections, localized edema, localized pain.

Cardiovascular—congestive heart failure, migraine, palpitations, vasodilation, hematoma, hypertension, hypotension.

Digestive—vomiting, dyspepsia, dry mouth, flatulence, decreased appetite, constipation, oral moniliasis, anorexia, eructation, gastritis, mouth ulcers, gastrointestinal disorders, rectal disorders, tongue disorders, tooth disorders, increased thirst, oral lesions, tenesmus, dry throat, toothache.

Hemic and Lymphatic—anemia.

Metabolic and Nutritional—dehydration, gout, peripheral edema, weight increase.

Musculo-skeletal—myalgia.

Nervous—dizziness, insomnia, somnolence, anxiety, shakiness, nervousness, cerebral infarction, change in dreams, impaired concentration, confusion, nightmares, paresthesia, vertigo.

Respiratory—asthma, cough, epistaxis, rhinitis, wheezing, bronchitis, dyspnea, pleural effusion, pneumonia, sinusitis.

Skin—urticaria, rash, pruritus non-application site, diaphoresis, maculopapular rash, fungal dermatitis, desquamation, dry skin non-application site, hair loss, vesiculobullous rash, sunburn.

Special Senses—taste alterations, eye irritation, taste loss, tinnitus.

Urogenital—hematuria, urinary tract infections, metrorrhagia, dysuria frequency, nocturia, penile infection, proteinuria, vaginal pain.

Granules for Oral Suspension (Multiple dose):

In clinical trials using multiple doses of cefpodoxime proxetil granules for oral suspension, 2128 pediatric patients (93% of whom were less than 12 years of age) were treated with the recommended dosages of cefpodoxime (10 mg/kg/day Q 24 hours or divided Q 12 hours to a maximum equivalent adult dose). There were no deaths or permanent disabilities in any of the patients in these studies. Twenty-four patients (1.1%) discontinued medication due to adverse events thought possibly- or probably-related to study drug. Primarily, these discontinuations were for gastrointestinal disturbances, usually diarrhea, vomiting, or rashes.

Adverse events thought possibly- or probably-related, or of unknown relationship to cefpodoxime proxetil for oral suspension in multiple dose clinical trials (N = 2128 patients treated with cefpodoxime) were:

Incidence Greater Than 1%:

Diarrhea	6.0%

The incidence of diarrhea in infants and toddlers (age 1 month to 2 years) was 12.8%.

Diaper rash/Fungal skin rash:	2.0% (includes moniliasis).

The incidence of diaper rash in infants and toddlers was 8.5%

Other skin rashes: 1.8%

Vomiting: 2.3%

Incidence Less Than 1%:

Body: Localized abdominal pain, abdominal cramp, headache, monilia, generalized abdominal pain, asthenia, fever, fungal infection.

Digestive: Nausea, monilia, anorexia, dry mouth, stomatitis, pseudomembranous colitis.

Hemic & Lymphatic: Thrombocytopenia, positive direct Coombs' test, eosinophilia, leukocytosis, leukopenia, prolonged partial thromboplastin time, thrombocytopenic purpura.

Metabolic & Nutritional: Increased SGPT.

Musculo-Skeletal: Myalgia.

Nervous: Hallucination, hyperkinesia, nervousness, somnolence.

Respiratory: Epistaxis, rhinitis.

Skin: Skin moniliasis, urticaria, fungal dermatitis, acne, exfoliative dermatitis, maculopapular rash.

Special Senses: Taste perversion.

Film-coated Tablets (Single dose):

In clinical trials using a single dose of cefpodoxime proxetil film-coated tablets, 509 patients were treated with the recommended dosage of cefpodoxime (200 mg). There were no deaths or permanent disabilities thought related to drug toxicity in these studies.

Adverse events thought possibly- or probably-related to cefpodoxime in single dose clinical trials conducted in the United States were:

Incidence Greater Than 1%:

Nausea 1.4%

Diarrhea 1.2%

Incidence Less Than 1%

Central Nervous System: Dizziness, headache, syncope.

Dermatologic: Rash.

Genital: Vaginitis.

Gastrointestinal: Abdominal pain.

Psychiatric: Anxiety.

Laboratory Changes

Significant laboratory changes that have been reported in adult and pediatric patients in clinical trials of cefpodoxime proxetil, without regard to drug relationship, were:

Hepatic: Transient increases in AST (SGOT), ALT (SGPT), GGT, alkaline phosphatase, bilirubin, and LDH.

Hematologic: Eosinophilia, leukocytosis, lymphocytosis, granulocytosis, basophilia, monocytosis, thrombocytosis, decreased hemoglobin, decreased hematocrit, leukopenia, neutropenia, lymphocytopenia, thrombocytopenia, thrombocythemia, positive Coombs' test, and prolonged PT, and PTT.

Serum Chemistry: hyperglycemia, hypoglycemia, hypoalbuminemia, hypoproteinemia, hyperkalemia, and hyponatremia.

Renal: Increases in BUN and creatinine.

Most of these abnormalities were transient and not clinically significant.

Post-marketing Experience:

The following serious adverse experiences have been reported: allergic reactions including Stevens-Johnson syndrome, toxic epidermal necrolysis, erythema multiforme and serum sickness-like reactions, pseudomembranous colitis, bloody diarrhea with abdominal pain, ulcerative colitis, rectorrhagia with hypotension, anaphylactic shock, acute liver injury, *in utero* exposure with miscarriage, purpuric nephritis, pulmonary infiltrate with eosinophilia, and eyelid dermatitis.

One death was attributed to pseudomembranous colitis and disseminated intravascular coagulation.

Cephalosporin Class Labeling:

In addition to the adverse reactions listed above which have been observed in patients treated with cefpodoxime proxetil, the following adverse reactions and altered laboratory tests have been reported for cephalosporin class antibiotics:

Adverse Reactions and Abnormal Laboratory Tests: Renal dysfunction, toxic nephropathy, hepatic dysfunction including cholestasis, aplastic anemia, hemolytic anemia, serum sickness-like reaction, hemorrhage, agranulocytosis, and pancytopenia.

Several cephalosporins have been implicated in triggering seizures, particularly in patients with renal impairment when the dosage was not reduced. (See **DOSAGE AND ADMINISTRATION** and **OVERDOSAGE**.)

If seizures associated with drug therapy occur, the drug should be discontinued. Anticonvulsant therapy can be given if clinically indicated.

OVERDOSAGE

In acute rodent toxicity studies, a single 5 g/kg oral dose produced no adverse effects.

In the event of serious toxic reaction from overdosage, hemodialysis or peritoneal dialysis may aid in the removal of cefpodoxime from the body, particularly if renal function is compromised.

The toxic symptoms following an overdose of beta-lactam antibiotics may include nausea, vomiting, epigastric distress, and diarrhea.

DOSAGE AND ADMINISTRATION

(See INDICATIONS AND USAGE for indicated pathogens.)

Constitution Directions For Oral Suspension

Bottle Size	Final Concentration	Directions
50 mL	50 mg per 5 mL	Suspend in a total of 29 mL of distilled water. Method: First, shake the bottle to loosen granules. Then add the water in two approximately equal portions, shaking vigorously after each aliquot of water.
75 mL	50 mg per 5 mL	Suspend in a total of 44 mL of distilled water. Method: First, shake the bottle to loosen granules. Then add the water in two approximately equal portions, shaking vigorously after each aliquot of water.
100 mL	50 mg per 5 mL	Suspend in a total of 58 mL of distilled water. Method: First, shake the bottle to loosen granules. Then add the water in two approximately equal portions, shaking vigorously after each aliquot of water.
50 mL	100 mg per 5 mL	Suspend in a total of 29 mL of distilled water. Method: First, shake the bottle to loosen granules. Then add the water in two approximately equal portions, shaking vigorously after each aliquot of water.
75 mL	100 mg per 5 mL	Suspend in a total of 43 mL of distilled water. Method: First, shake the bottle to loosen granules. Then add the water in two approximately equal portions, shaking vigorously after each aliquot of water.
100 mL	100 mg per 5 mL	Suspend in a total of 57 mL of water. Method: First, shake the bottle to loosen granules. Then add the water in two approximately equal portions, shaking vigorously after each aliquot of water.

Pathogen	Cefpodoxime	Comparator
E. coli	200/243 (82%)	99/123 (80%)
Other pathogens	34/42 (81%)	23/28 (82%)
K. pneumoniae		
P. mirabilis		
S. saprophyticus		
TOTAL	234/285 (82%)	122/151 (81%)

Pathogen	Cefpodoxime Proxetil 5 mg/kg Q 12h × 5 d	Cefixime
S. pneumoniae	88/122 (72%)	72/124 (58%)
H. influenzae	50/76 (66%)	61/81 (75%)
M. catarrhalis	22/39 (56%)	23/41 (56%)
S. pyogenes	20/25 (80%)	13/23 (57%)
Clinical success rate	171/254 (67%)	165/258 (64%)

FILM-COATED TABLETS:

VANTIN Tablets should be administered orally with food to enhance absorption. (See **CLINICAL PHARMACOLOGY.**)

The recommended dosages, durations of treatment, and applicable patient population are as described in the following chart:

[See first table at top of previous page]

GRANULES FOR ORAL SUSPENSION:

VANTIN Oral Suspension may be given without regard to food. The recommended dosages, durations of treatment, and applicable patient populations are as described in the following chart:

[See second table at top of previous page]

Patients with Renal Dysfunction:

For patients with severe renal impairment (<30 mL/min creatinine clearance), the dosing intervals should be increased to Q 24 hours. In patients maintained on hemodialysis, the dose frequency should be 3 times/week after hemodialysis.

When only the serum creatinine level is available, the following formula (based on sex, weight, and age of the patient) may be used to estimate creatinine clearance (mL/min). For this estimate to be valid, the serum creatinine level should represent a steady state of renal function.

$$\text{Males: (mL/min)} \quad \frac{\text{Weight (kg)} \times (140 - \text{age})}{72 \times \text{serum creatinine (mg/100 mL)}}$$

Females: (mL/min) 0.85 × above value

Patients with Cirrhosis:

Cefpodoxime pharmacokinetics in cirrhotic patients (with or without ascites) are similar to those in healthy subjects. Dose adjustment is not necessary in this population.

Preparation of Suspension:

[See first table above]

After mixing, the suspension should be stored in a refrigerator, 2° to 8°C (36° to 46°F). Shake well before using. Keep container tightly closed. The mixture may be used for 14 days. Discard unused portion after 14 days.

HOW SUPPLIED

VANTIN Tablets are available in the following strengths (cefpodoxime equivalent), colors, and sizes:

100 mg, (light orange, elliptical, debossed with U3617)

Bottles of 20	NDC 0009-3617-01
Bottles of 100	NDC 0009-3617-02
Unit dose packs of 100	NDC 0009-3617-03

200 mg, (coral red, elliptical, debossed with U3618)

Bottles of 20	NDC 0009-3618-01
Bottles of 100	NDC 0009-3618-02
Unit dose packs of 100	NDC 0009-3618-03

Store tablets at controlled room temperature 20° to 25°C (68° to 77°F) [see USP]. Replace cap securely after each opening. Protect unit dose packs from excessive moisture.

VANTIN Oral Suspension is available in the following strengths (cefpodoxime equivalents when constituted according to directions), flavor, and size:

50 mg/5 mL, lemon creme flavor in 100 mL bottles NDC 0009-3531-01

50 mg/5 mL, lemon creme flavor in 75 mL bottles NDC 0009-3531-02

50 mg/5 mL, lemon creme flavor in 50 mL bottles NDC 0009-3531-03

100 mg/5 mL, lemon creme flavor in 100 mL bottles NDC 0009-3615-01

100 mg/5 mL, lemon creme flavor in 75 mL bottles NDC 0009-3615-02

100 mg/5 mL, lemon creme flavor in 50 mL bottles NDC 0009-3615-03

Store unsuspended granules at controlled room temperatures 20° to 25°C (68° to 77°F) [see USP].

Directions for mixing are included on the label. After mixing, suspension should be stored in a refrigerator, 2° to 8°C (36° to 46°F). Shake well before using. Keep container tightly closed. The mixture may be used for 14 days. Discard unused portion after 14 days.

REFERENCES

1. NCCLS. Methods for dilution antimicrobial susceptibility tests for bacteria that grow aerobically—fourth edition; Approved standard. NCCLS document M7-A4 (ISBN 1-56238-309-4). NCCLS, 940 West Valley Rd., Suite 1400, Wayne, PA 19087-1898, 1997.
2. NCCLS. Performance standards for antimicrobial susceptibility testing; Eighth informational supplement. NCCLS document M100-S8 (ISBN 1-56238-337-x). NCCLS, 940 West Valley Rd., Suite 1400, Wayne, PA 19087-1898, 1998.

Continued on next page

Information on these Pharmacia & Upjohn products is based on labeling in effect June 1, 2000. Further information concerning these and other Pharmacia & Upjohn products may be obtained by direct inquiry to Medical Information, Pharmacia & Upjohn, Kalamazoo, MI 49001.

Vantin—Cont.

3. NCCLS. Performance standards for antimicrobial disk susceptibility tests—sixth edition; Approved standard. NCCLS document M2-A6 (ISBN 1-56238-306-6). NCCLS, 940 West Valley Rd., Suite 1400, Wayne, PA 19087-1898, 1997.

CLINICAL TRIALS

Cystitis

In two double-blind, 2:1 randomized, comparative trials performed in adults in the United States, cefpodoxime proxetil was compared to other beta-lactam antibiotics. In these studies, the following bacterial eradication rates were obtained at 5 to 9 days after therapy:

[See second table at top of previous page]

In these studies, clinical cure rates and bacterial eradication rates for cefpodoxime proxetil were comparable to the comparator agents; however, the clinical cure rates and bacteriologic eradication rates were lower than those observed with some other classes of approved agents for cystitis.

Acute Otitis Media Studies

In controlled studies of acute otitis media performed in the United States, where significant rates of beta-lactamase-producing organisms were found, cefpodoxime proxetil was compared to cefixime. In these studies, using very strict evaluability criteria and microbiologic and clinical response criteria at the 4 to 21 day post-therapy follow-up, the following presumptive bacterial eradication/clinical success outcomes (cured and improved) were obtained.

[See third table at top of previous page]

Rx only

U.S. Patent Nos. 4,486,425; 4,409,215.
Licensed from Sankyo Company, Ltd., Japan
Mfd by: Pharmacia & Upjohn N.V./S.A., Puurs - Belgium
For: Pharmacia & Upjohn Company, Kalamazoo, Michigan 49001, USA
Revised December 1998 815 267 014

Shown in Product Identification Guide, page 331

XANAX® Ⓒ ℞

[*zăn-ăx*]

alprazolam tablets, USP

DESCRIPTION

XANAX Tablets contain alprazolam which is a triazolo analog of the 1,4 benzodiazepine class of central nervous system-active compounds.

The chemical name of alprazolam is 8-Chloro-1-methyl-6-phenyl-4H-s-triazolo [4,3-α] [1,4] benzodiazepine.

The structural formula is represented below:

Alprazolam is a white crystalline powder, which is soluble in methanol or ethanol but which has no appreciable solubility in water at physiological pH.

Each XANAX Tablet, for oral administration, contains 0.25, 0.5, 1 or 2 mg of alprazolam.

XANAX Tablets, 2 mg, are multi-scored and may be divided as shown below:

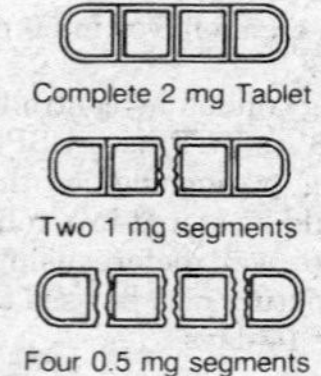

Complete 2 mg Tablet

Two 1 mg segments

Four 0.5 mg segments

Inactive ingredients: Cellulose, corn starch, docusate sodium, lactose, magnesium stearate, silicon dioxide and sodium benzoate. In addition, the 0.5 mg tablet contains FD&C Yellow No. 6 and the 1 mg tablet contains FD&C Blue No. 2.

CLINICAL PHARMACOLOGY

CNS agents of the 1,4 benzodiazepine class presumably exert their effects by binding at stereo specific receptors at several sites within the central nervous system. Their exact mechanism of action is unknown. Clinically, all benzodiazepines cause a dose-related central nervous system depressant activity varying from mild impairment of task performance to hypnosis.

Following oral administration, alprazolam is readily absorbed. Peak concentrations in the plasma occur in one to two hours following administration. Plasma levels are proportionate to the dose given; over the dose range of 0.5 to 3.0 mg, peak levels of 8.0 to 37 ng/mL were observed. Using a specific assay methodology, the mean plasma elimination half-life of alprazolam has been found to be about 11.2 hours (range: 6.3–26.9 hours) in healthy adults.

The predominant metabolites are α-hydroxy-alprazolam and a benzophenone derived from alprazolam. The biological activity of α-hydroxy-alprazolam is approximately one-half that of alprazolam. The benzophenone metabolite is essentially inactive. Plasma levels of these metabolites are extremely low, thus precluding precise pharmacokinetic description. However, their half-lives appear to be of the same order of magnitude as that of alprazolam. Alprazolam and its metabolites are excreted primarily in the urine.

The ability of alprazolam to induce human hepatic enzyme systems has not yet been determined. However, this is not a property of benzodiazepines in general. Further, alprazolam did not affect the prothrombin or plasma warfarin levels in male volunteers administered sodium warfarin orally.

In vitro, alprazolam is bound (80 percent) to human serum protein.

Changes in the absorption, distribution, metabolism and excretion of benzodiazepines have been reported in a variety of disease states including alcoholism, impaired hepatic function and impaired renal function. Changes have also been demonstrated in geriatric patients. A mean half-life of alprazolam of 16.3 hours has been observed in healthy elderly subjects (range: 9.0–26.9 hours, n=16) compared to 11.0 hours (range: 6.3–15.8 hours, n=16) in healthy adult subjects. In patients with alcoholic liver disease the half-life of alprazolam ranged between 5.8 and 65.3 hours (mean: 19.7 hours, n=17) as compared to between 6.3 and 26.9 hours (mean=11.4 hours, n=17) in healthy subjects. In an obese group of subjects the half-life of alprazolam ranged between 9.9 and 40.4 hours (mean=21.8 hours, n=12) as compared to between 6.3 and 15.8 hours (mean=10.6 hours, n=12) in healthy subjects.

Because of its similarity to other benzodiazepines, it is assumed that alprazolam undergoes transplacental passage and that it is excreted in human milk.

INDICATIONS AND USAGE

XANAX Tablets (alprazolam) are indicated for the management of anxiety disorder (a condition corresponding most closely to the APA Diagnostic and Statistical Manual [DSM-III-R] diagnosis of generalized anxiety disorder) or the short-term relief of symptoms of anxiety. Anxiety or tension associated with the stress of everyday life usually does not require treatment with an anxiolytic.

Generalized anxiety disorder is characterized by unrealistic or excessive anxiety and worry (apprehensive expectation) about two or more life circumstances, for a period of six months or longer, during which the person has been bothered more days than not by these concerns. At least 6 of the following 18 symptoms are often present in these patients: *Motor Tension* (trembling, twitching, or feeling shaky; muscle tension, aches, or soreness; restlessness; easy fatigability); *Autonomic Hyperactivity* (shortness of breath or smothering sensations; palpitations or accelerated heart rate; sweating, or cold clammy hands; dry mouth; dizziness or light-headedness; nausea, diarrhea, or other abdominal distress; flushes or chills; frequent urination; trouble swallowing or 'lump in throat'); *Vigilance and Scanning* (feeling keyed up or on edge; exaggerated startle response; difficulty concentrating or 'mind going blank' because of anxiety; trouble falling or staying asleep; irritability). These symptoms must not be secondary to another psychiatric disorder or caused by some organic factor.

Anxiety associated with depression is responsive to XANAX.

XANAX is also indicated for the treatment of panic disorder, with or without agoraphobia.

Studies supporting this claim were conducted in patients whose diagnoses corresponded closely to the DSM-III-R criteria for panic disorder (see CLINICAL STUDIES).

Panic disorder is an illness characterized by recurrent panic attacks. The panic attacks, at least initially, are unexpected. Later in the course of this disturbance certain situations, eg, driving a car or being in a crowded place, may become associated with having a panic attack. These panic attacks are not triggered by situations in which the person is the focus of others' attention (as in social phobia). The diagnosis requires four such attacks within a four week period, or one or more attacks followed by at least a month of persistent fear of having another attack. The panic attacks must be characterized by at least four of the following symptoms: dyspnea or smothering sensations; dizziness, unsteady feelings, or faintness; palpitations or tachycardia; trembing or shaking; sweating; choking; nausea or abdominal distress; depersonalization or derealization; paresthesias; hot flashes or chills; chest pain or discomfort; fear of dying; fear of going crazy or of doing something uncontrolled. At least some of the panic attack symptoms must develop suddenly, and the panic attack symptoms must not be attributable to some known organic factors. Panic disorder is frequently associated with some symptoms of agoraphobia.

Demonstrations of the effectiveness of XANAX by systematic clinical study are limited to four months duration for anxiety disorder and four to ten weeks duration for panic disorder; however, patients with panic disorder have been treated on an open basis for up to eight months without apparent loss of benefit. The physician should periodically reassess the usefulness of the drug for the individual patient.

CONTRAINDICATIONS

XANAX Tablets are contraindicated in patients with known sensitivity to this drug or other benzodiazepines. XANAX may be used in patients with open angle glaucoma who are receiving appropriate therapy, but is contraindicated in patients with acute narrow angle glaucoma.

XANAX is contraindicated with ketoconazole and itraconazole, since these medications significantly impair the oxidative metabolism mediated by cytochrome P450 3A (CYP 3A) (see WARNINGS and PRECAUTIONS - Drug Interactions).

WARNINGS

Dependence and withdrawal reactions, including seizures: Certain adverse clinical events, some life-threatening, are a direct consequence of physical dependence to XANAX. These include a spectrum of withdrawal symptoms; the most important is seizure (see DRUG ABUSE AND DEPENDENCE). Even after relatively short-term use at the doses recommended for the treatment of transient anxiety and anxiety disorder (ie, 0.75 to 4.0 mg per day), there is some risk of dependence. Spontaneous reporting system data suggest that the risk of dependence and its severity appear to be greater in patients treated with doses greater than 4 mg/day and for long periods (more than 12 weeks). However, in a controlled postmarketing discontinuation study of panic disorder patients, the duration of treatment (three months compared to six months) had no effect on the ability of patients to taper to zero dose. In contrast, patients treated with doses of XANAX greater than 4 mg/day had more difficulty tapering to zero than those treated with less than 4 mg/day.

The importance of dose and the risks of XANAX as a treatment for panic disorder:

Because of the management of panic disorder often requires the use of average daily doses of XANAX above 4 mg, the risk of dependence among panic disorder patients may be higher than that among those treated for less severe anxiety. Experience in randomized placebo-controlled discontinuation studies of patients with panic disorder showed a high rate of rebound and withdrawal symptoms in patients treated with XANAX compared to placebo treated patients.

Relapse or return of illness was defined as a return of symptoms characteristic of panic disorder (primarily panic attacks) to levels approximately equal to those seen at baseline before active treatment was initiated. Rebound refers to a return of symptoms of panic disorder to a level substantially greater in frequency, or more severe in intensity than seen at baseline. Withdrawal symptoms were identified as those which were generally not characteristic of panic disorder and which occurred for the first time more frequently during discontinuation than at baseline.

In a controlled clinical trial in which 63 patients were randomized to XANAX and where withdrawal symptoms were specifically sought, the following were identified as symptoms of withdrawal: heightened sensory perception, impaired concentration, dysosmia, clouded sensorium, paresthesias, muscle cramps, muscle twitch, diarrhea, blurred vision, appetite decrease and weight loss. Other symptoms, such as anxiety and insomnia, were frequently seen during discontinuation, but it could not be determined if they were due to return of illness, rebound or withdrawal.

In a larger database comprised of both controlled and uncontrolled studies in which 641 patients received XANAX, discontinuation-emergent symptoms which occurred at a rate of over 5% in patients treated with XANAX and at a greater rate than the placebo treated group were as follows:

DISCONTINUATION-EMERGENT SYMPTOM INCIDENCE
Percentage of 641 XANAX-Treated Panic Disorder Patients Reporting Events

Body System/Event		Body System/Event	
Neurologic		**Gastrointestinal**	
Insomnia	29.5	Nausea/Vomiting	16.5
Light-headedness	19.3	Diarrhea	13.6
Abnormal involuntary movement	17.3	Decreased salivation	10.6
Headache	17.0	**Metabolic-Nutritional**	
Muscular twitching	6.9	Weight loss	13.3
Impaired coordination	6.6	Decreased appetite	12.8
Muscle tone disorders	5.9		
Weakness	5.8	**Dermatological**	
Psychiatric		Sweating	14.4
Anxiety	19.2		
Fatigue and Tiredness	18.4	**Cardiovascular**	
Irritability	10.5	Tachycardia	12.2
Cognitive Disorder	10.3		
Memory impairment	5.5	**Special Senses**	
Depression	5.1	Blurred vision	10.0
Confusional state	5.0		

From the studies cited, it has not been determined whether these symptoms are clearly related to the dose and duration of therapy with XANAX in patients with panic disorder.

In two controlled trials of six to eight weeks duration where the ability of patients to discontinue medication was measured, 71%–93% of XANAX treated patients tapered completely off therapy compared to 89%–96% of placebo treated patients. In a controlled postmarketing discontinuation study of panic disorder patients, the duration of treatment (three months compared to six months) had no effect on the ability of patients to taper to zero dose.

Seizures attributable to XANAX were seen after drug discontinuance or dose reduction in 8 of 1980 patients with panic disorder or in patients participating in clinical trials where doses of XANAX greater than 4 mg/day for over 3 months were permitted. Five of these cases clearly occurred during abrupt dose reduction, or discontinuation from daily doses of 2 to 10 mg. Three cases occurred in situations where there was not a clear relationship to abrupt dose reduction or discontinuation. In one instance, seizure occurred after discontinuation from a single dose of 1 mg after tapering at a rate of 1 mg every three days from 6 mg daily. In two other instances, the relationship to taper is indeterminate; in both of these cases the patients had been receiving doses of 3 mg daily prior to seizure. The duration of use in the above 8 cases ranged from 4 to 22 weeks. There have been occasional voluntary reports of patients developing seizures while apparently tapering gradually from XANAX. The risk of seizure seems to be greatest 24–72 hours after discontinuation (see DOSAGE AND ADMINISTRATION for recommended tapering and discontinuation schedule.

Status epilepticus and its treatment:
The medical event voluntary reporting system shows that withdrawal seizures have been reported in association with the discontinuation of XANAX. In most cases, only a single seizure was reported; however, multiple seizures and status epilepticus were reported as well. Ordinarily, the treatment of status epilepticus of any etiology involves use of intravenous benzodiazepines plus phenytoin or barbiturates, maintenance of a patent airway and adequate hydration. For additional details regarding therapy, consultation with an appropriate specialist may be considered.

Interdose Symptoms:
Early morning anxiety and emergence of anxiety symptoms between doses of XANAX have been reported in patients with panic disorder taking prescribed maintenance doses of XANAX. These symptoms may reflect the development of tolerance or a time interval between doses which is longer than the duration of clinical action of the administered dose. In either case, it is presumed that the prescribed dose is not sufficient to maintain plasma levels above those needed to prevent relapse, rebound or withdrawal symptoms over the entire course of the interdosing interval. In these situations, it is recommended that the same total daily dose be given divided as more frequent administrations (see DOSAGE AND ADMINISTRATION).

Risk of dose reduction:
Withdrawal reactions may occur when dosage reduction occurs for any reason. This includes purposeful tapering, but also inadvertent reduction of dose (eg, the patient forgets, the patient is admitted to a hospital, etc.). Therefore, the dosage of XANAX should be reduced or discontinued gradually (see DOSAGE AND ADMINISTRATION).

XANAX Tablets are not of value in the treatment of psychotic patients and should not be employed in lieu of appropriate treatment for psychosis. Because of its CNS depressant effects, patients receiving XANAX should be cautioned against engaging in hazardous occupations or activities requiring complete mental alertness such as operating machinery or driving a motor vehicle. For the same reason, patients should be cautioned about the simultaneous ingestion of alcohol and other CNS depressant drugs during treatment with XANAX.

Benzodiazepines can potentially cause fetal harm when administered to pregnant women. If XANAX is used during pregnancy, or if the patient becomes pregnant while taking this drug, the patient should be apprised of the potential hazard to the fetus. Because of experience with other members of the benzodiazepine class, XANAX is assumed to be capable of causing an increased risk of congenital abnormalities when administered to a pregnant woman during the first trimester. Because use of these drugs is rarely a matter of urgency, their use during the first trimester should almost always be avoided. The possibility that a woman of childbearing potential may be pregnant at the time of institution of therapy should be considered. Patients should be advised that if they become pregnant during therapy or intend to become pregnant they should communicate with their physicians about the desirability of discontinuing the drug.

Alprazolam interaction with drugs that inhibit metabolism via cytochrome P450 3A: The initial step in alprazolam metabolism is hydroxylation catalyzed by cytochrome P450 3A (CYP 3A). Drugs that inhibit this metabolic pathway may have a profound effect on the clearance of alprazolam. Consequently, alprazolam should be avoided in patients receiving very potent inhibitors of CYP 3A. With drugs inhibiting CYP 3A to a lesser but still significant degree, alprazolam should be used only with caution and consideration of appropriate dosage reduction. For some drugs, an interaction with alprazolam has been quantified with clinical data; for other drugs, interactions are predicted from *in vitro* and/or experience with similar drugs in the same pharmacologic class.

The following are examples of drugs known to inhibit the metabolism of alprazolam and/or related benzodiazepines, presumably through inhibition of CYP 3A.

Potent CYP 3A inhibitors:
Azole antifungal agents—Although *in vivo* interaction data with alprazolam are not available, ketoconazole and itraconazole are potent CYP 3A inhibitors and the coadministration of alprazolam with them is not recommended. Other azole-type antifungal agents should also be considered potent CYP 3A inhibitors and the coadministration of alprazolam with them is not recommended (see CONTRAINDICATIONS).

Drugs demonstrated to be CYP 3A inhibitors on the basis of clinical studies involving alprazolam (caution and consideration of appropriate alprazolam dose reduction are recommended during coadministration with the following drugs):
Nefazodone—Coadministration of nefazodone increased alprazolam concentration two-fold.

Fluvoxamine—Coadministration of fluvoxamine approximately doubled the maximum plasma concentration of alprazolam, decreased clearance by 49%, increased half-life by 71%, and decreased measured psychomotor performance.

Cimetidine—Coadministration of cimetidine increased the maximum plasma concentration of alprazolam by 86%, decreased clearance by 42%, and increased half-life by 16%.

Other drugs possibly affecting alprazolam metabolism: Other drugs possibly affecting alprazolam metabolism by inhibition of CYP 3A are discussed in the PRECAUTIONS section (see PRECAUTIONS - Drug Interactions).

PRECAUTIONS

General: If XANAX Tablets are to be combined with other psychotropic agents or anticonvulsant drugs, careful consideration should be given to the pharmacology of the agents to be employed, particularly with compounds which might potentiate the action of benzodiazepines (see DRUG INTERACTIONS).

As with other psychotropic medications, the usual precautions with respect to administration of the drug and size of the prescription are indicated for severely depressed patients or those in whom there is reason to expect concealed suicidal ideation or plans.

It is recommended that the dosage be limited to the smallest effective dose to preclude the development of ataxia or oversedation which may be a particular problem in elderly or debilitated patients. (See DOSAGE AND ADMINISTRATION.) The usual precautions in treating patients with impaired renal, hepatic or pulmonary functions should be observed. There have been rare reports of death in patients with severe pulmonary disease shortly after the initiation of treatment with XANAX. A decreased systemic alprazolam elimination rate (eg, increased plasma half-life) has been observed in both alcoholic liver disease patients and obese patients receiving XANAX (see CLINICAL PHARMACOLOGY).

Episodes of hypomania and mania have been reported in association with the use of XANAX in patients with depression.

Alprazolam has a weak uricosuric effect. Although other medications with weak uricosuric effect have been reported to cause acute renal failure, there have been no reported instances of acute renal failure attributable to therapy with XANAX.

Information for Patients:
For all users of XANAX:
To assure safe and effective use of benzodiazepines, all patients prescribed XANAX should be provided with the following guidance. In addition, panic disorder patients, for whom doses greater than 4 mg/day are typically prescribed, should be advised about the risks associated with the use of higher doses.

1. Inform your physician about any alcohol consumption and medicine you are taking now, including medication you may buy without a prescription. Alcohol should generally not be used during treatment with benzodiazepines.
2. Not recommended for use in pregnancy. Therefore, inform your physician if you are pregnant, if you are planning to have a child, or if you become pregnant while you are taking this medication.
3. Inform your physician if you are nursing.
4. Until you experience how this medication affects you, do not drive a car or operate potentially dangerous machinery, etc.
5. Do not increase the dose even if you think the medication "does not work anymore" without consulting your physician. Benzodiazepines, even when used as recommended, may produce emotional and/or physical dependence.
6. Do not stop taking this medication abruptly or decrease the dose without consulting your physician, since withdrawal symptoms can occur.

Additional advice for panic disorder patients:
The use of XANAX at doses greater than 4 mg/day, often necessary to treat panic disorder, is accompanied by risks that you need to carefully consider. When used at doses greater than 4 mg/day, which may or may not be required for your treatment, XANAX has the potential to cause severe emotional and physical dependence in some patients and these patients may find it exceedingly difficult to terminate treatment. In two controlled trials of six to eight weeks duration where the ability of patients to discontinue medication was measured, 7 to 29% of patients treated with XANAX did not completely taper off therapy. In a controlled postmarketing discontinuation study of panic disorder patients, the patients treated with doses of XANAX greater than 4 mg/day had more difficulty tapering to zero dose than patients treated with less than 4 mg/day. In all cases, it is important that your physician help you discontinue this medication in a careful and safe manner to avoid overly extended use of XANAX.

In addition, the extended use at doses greater than 4 mg/day appears to increase the incidence and severity of withdrawal reactions when XANAX is discontinued. These are generally minor but seizure can occur, especially if you reduce the dose too rapidly or discontinue the medication abruptly. Seizure can be life-threatening.

Laboratory Tests: Laboratory tests are not ordinarily required in otherwise healthy patients.

Drug Interactions: The benzodiazepines, including alprazolam, produce additive CNS depressant effects when coadministered with other psychotropic medications, anticonvulsants, antihistaminics, ethanol and other drugs which themselves produce CNS depression.

The steady state plasma concentrations of imipramine and desipramine have been reported to be increased an average of 31% and 20%, respectively, by the concomitant administration of XANAX Tablets in doses up to 4 mg/day. The clinical significance of these changes is unknown.

Drugs that inhibit alprazolam metabolism via cytochrome P450 3A: The initial step in alprazolam metabolism is hydroxylation catalyzed by cytochrome P450 3A (CYP 3A). Drugs which inhibit this metabolic pathway may have a profound effect on the clearance of alprazolam (see CONTRAINDICATIONS and WARNINGS for additional drugs of this type.

Drugs demonstrated to be CYP 3A inhibitors of possible clinical significance on the basis of clinical studies involving alprazolam (caution is recommended during coadministration with alprazolam):
Fluoxetine—Coadministration of fluoxetine with alprazolam increased the maximum plasma concentration of alprazolam by 46%, decreased clearance by 21%, increased half-life by 17%, and decreased measured psychomotor performance.

Propoxyphene—Coadministration of propoxyphene decreased the maximum plasma concentration of alprazolam by 6%, decreased clearance by 38%, and increased half-life by 58%.

Oral Contraceptives—Coadministration of oral contraceptives increased the maximum plasma concentration of alprazolam by 18%, decreasd clearance by 22%, and increased half-life by 29%.

Drugs and other substances demonstrated to be CYP 3A inhibitors on the basis of clinical studies involving benzodiazepines metabolized similarly to alprazolam or on the basis of in vitro studies with alprazolam or other benzodiazepines (caution is recommended during coadministration): Available data from clinical studies of benzodiazepines other than alprazolam suggest a possible drug interaction with alprazolam for the following: diltiazem, isoniazid, macrolide antibiotics such as erythromycin and clarithromycin, and grapefruit juice. Data from *in vitro* studies of alprazolam suggest a possible drug interaction with alprazolam for the following: sertraline and paroxetine. Data from *in vitro* studies of benzodiazepines other than alprazolam suggest a possible drug interaction for the following: ergotamine, cyclosporine, amiodarone, nicradipine, and nifedipine. Caution is recommended during the coadministration of any of these with alprazolam (see WARNINGS).

Drug/Laboratory Test Interactions: Although interactions between benzodiazepines and commonly employed clinical laboratory tests have occasionally been reported, there is no consistent pattern for a specific drug or specific test.

Carcinogenesis, Mutagenesis, Impairment of Fertility: No evidence of carcinogenic potential was observed during 2-year bioassay studies of alprazolam in rats at doses up to 30 mg/kg/day (150 times the maximum recommended daily human dose of 10 mg/day) and in mice at doses up to 10 mg/kg/day (50 times the maximum recommended daily human dose).

Alprazolam was not mutagenic in the rat micronucleus test at doses up to 100 mg/kg, which is 500 times the maximum recommended daily human dose of 10 mg/day. Alprazolam also was not mutagenic *in vitro* in the DNA Damage/Alkaline Elution Assay or the Ames Assay.

Alprazolam produced no impairment of fertility in rats at doses up to 5 mg/kg/day, which is 25 times the maximum recommended daily human dose of 10 mg/day.

Pregnancy: Teratogenic Effects: Pregnancy Category D: (See WARNINGS Section).

Nonteratogenic Effects: It should be considered that the child born of a mother who is receiving benzodiazepines may be at some risk for withdrawal symptoms from the drug during the postnatal period. Also, neonatal flaccidity and respiratory problems have been reported in children born of mothers who have been receiving benzodiazepines.

Labor and Delivery: XANAX has no established use in labor or delivery.

Nursing Mothers: Benzodiazepines are known to be excreted in human milk. It should be assumed that alprazolam is as well. Chronic administration of diazepam to nursing mothers has been reported to cause their infants to become lethargic and to lose weight. As a general rule, nursing should not be undertaken by mothers who must use XANAX.

Pediatric Use: Safety and effectiveness of XANAX in individuals below 18 years of age have not been established.

Geriatric Use: The elderly may be more sensitive to the effects of benzodiazepines. They exhibit higher plasma alprazolam concentrations due to reduced clearance of the drug as compared with a younger population receiving the same doses. The smallest effective dose of XANAX should be used in the elderly to preclude the development of ataxia and oversedation (see CLINICAL PHARMACOLOGY and DOSAGE AND ADMINISTRATION).

ADVERSE REACTIONS

Side effects to XANAX Tablets, if they occur, are generally observed at the beginning of therapy and usually disappear

Continued on next page

Information on these Pharmacia & Upjohn products is based on labeling in effect June 1, 2000. Further information concerning these and other Pharmacia & Upjohn products may be obtained by direct inquiry to Medical Information, Pharmacia & Upjohn, Kalamazoo, MI 49001.

Xanax—Cont.

upon continued medication. In the usual patient, the most frequent side effects are likely to be an extension of the pharmacological activity of alprazolam, eg, drowsiness or light-headedness.

The data cited in the two tables below are estimates of untoward clinical event incidence among patients who participated under the following clinical conditions: relatively short duration (ie, four weeks) placebo-controlled clinical studies with dosages up to 4 mg/day of XANAX (for the management of anxiety disorders or for the short-term relief of the symptoms of anxiety) and short-term (up to ten weeks) placebo-controlled clinical studies with dosages up to 10 mg/day of XANAX in patients with panic disorder, with or without agoraphobia.

These data cannot be used to predict precisely the incidence of untoward events in the course of usual medical practice where patient characteristics, and other factors often differ from those in clinical trials. These figures cannot be compared with those obtained from other clinical studies involving related drug products and placebo as each group of drug trials are conducted under a different set of conditions.

Comparison of the cited figures, however, can provide the prescriber with some basis for estimating the relative contributions of drug and non-drug factors in the untoward event incidence in the population studied. Even this use must be approached cautiously, as a drug may relieve a symptom in one patient but induce it in others. For example, an anxiolytic drug may relieve dry mouth [a symptom of anxiety] in some subjects but induce it [an untoward event] in others.)

Additionally, for anxiety disorders the cited figures can provide the prescriber with an indication as to the frequency with which physician intervention (eg, increased surveillance, decreased dosage or discontinuation of drug therapy) may be necessary because of the untoward clinical event.

[See table above]

In addition to the relatively common (ie, greater than 1%) untoward event enumerated in the table above, the following adverse events have been reported in association with the use of benzodiazepines: dystonia, irritability, concentration difficulties, anorexia, transient amnesia or memory impairment, loss of coordination, fatigue, seizures, sedation, slurred speech, jaundice, musculoskeletal weakness, pruritus, diplopia, dysarthria, changes in libido, menstrual irregularities, incontinence and urinary retention.

[See table at bottom of next page]

In addition to the relatively common (ie, greater than 1%) untoward event enumerated in the table above, the following adverse events have been reported in association with the use of XANAX: seizures, hallucinations, depersonalization, taste alterations, diplopia, elevated bilirubin, elevated hepatic enzymes, and jaundice.

There have also been reports of withdrawal seizures upon rapid decrease or abrupt discontinuation of XANAX Tablets (see WARNINGS).

To discontinue treatment in patients taking XANAX, the dosage should be reduced slowly in keeping with good medical practice. It is suggested that the daily dosage of XANAX be decreased by no more than 0.5 mg every three days (see DOSAGE AND ADMINISTRATION). Some patients may benefit from an even slower dosage reduction. In a controlled postmarketing discontinuation study of panic disorder patients which compared this recommended taper schedule with a slower taper schedule, no difference was observed between the groups in the proportion of patients who tapered to zero dose; however, the slower schedule was associated with a reduction in symptoms associated with a withdrawal syndrome.

Panic disorder has been associated with primary and secondary major depressive disorders and increased reports of suicide among untreated patients. Therefore, the same precaution must be exercised when using doses of XANAX greater than 4 mg/day in treating patients with panic disorders as is exercised with the use of any psychotropic drug in treating depressed patients or those in whom there is reason to expect concealed suicidal ideation or plans.

As with all benzodiazepines, paradoxical reactions such as stimulation, increased muscle spasticity, sleep disturbances, hallucinations and other adverse behavioral effects such as agitation, rage, irritability, and aggressive or hostile behavior have been reported rarely. In many of the spontaneous case reports of adverse behavioral effects, patients were receiving other CNS drugs concomitantly and/or were described as having underlying psychiatric conditions. Should any of the above events occur, alprazolam should be discontinued. Isolated published reports involving small numbers of patients have suggested that patients who have borderline personality disorder, a prior history of violent or aggressive behavior, or alcohol or substance abuse may be at risk for such events. Instances of irritability, hostility, and intrusive thoughts have been reported during discontinuation of alprazolam in patients with post-traumatic stress disorder.

Laboratory analyses were performed on patients participating in the clinical program for XANAX. The following incidences of abnormalities shown below were observed in patients receiving XANAX and in patients in the corresponding placebo group. Few of these abnormalities were considered to be of physiological signficance.

ANXIETY DISORDERS

	Treatment-Emergent Symptom Incidence† XANAX	PLACEBO	Incidence of Intervention Because of Symptom XANAX
Number of Patients	565	505	565
% of Patients Reporting:			
Central Nervous System			
Drowsiness	41.0	21.6	15.1
Light-headedness	20.8	19.3	1.2
Depression	13.9	18.1	2.4
Headache	12.9	19.6	1.1
Confusion	9.9	10.0	0.9
Insomnia	8.9	18.4	1.3
Nervousness	4.1	10.3	1.1
Syncope	3.1	4.0	*
Dizziness	1.8	0.8	2.5
Akathisia	1.6	1.2	*
Tiredness/Sleepiness	*	*	1.8
Gastrointestinal			
Dry Mouth	14.7	13.3	0.7
Constipation	10.4	11.4	0.9
Diarrhea	10.1	10.3	1.2
Nausea/Vomiting	9.6	12.8	1.7
Increased Salivation	4.2	2.4	*
Cardiovascular			
Tachycardia/Palpitations	7.7	15.6	0.4
Hypotension	4.7	2.2	*
Sensory			
Blurred Vision	6.2	6.2	0.4
Musculoskeletal			
Rigidity	4.2	5.3	*
Tremor	4.0	8.8	0.4
Cutaneous			
Dermatitis/Allergy	3.8	3.1	0.6
Other			
Nasal Congestion	7.3	9.3	*
Weight Gain	2.7	2.7	*
Weight Loss	2.3	3.0	*

*None reported
†Events reported by 1% or more of XANAX patients are included.*

	XANAX Low	XANAX High	PLACEBO Low	PLACEBO High
Hematology				
Hematocrit	*	*	*	*
Hemoglobin	*	*	*	*
Total WBC Count	1.4	2.3	1.0	2.0
Neutrophil Count	2.3	3.0	4.2	1.7
Lymphocyte Count	5.5	7.4	5.4	9.5
Monocyte Count	5.3	2.8	6.4	*
Eosinophil Count	3.2	9.5	3.3	7.2
Basophil Count	*	*	*	*
Urinalysis				
Albumin	–	*	–	*
Sugar	–	*	–	*
RBC/HPF	–	3.4	–	5.0
WBC/HPF	–	25.7	–	25.9
Blood Chemistry				
Creatinine	2.2	1.9	3.5	1.0
Bilirubin	*	1.6	*	*
SGOT	*	3.2	1.0	1.8
Alkaline Phosphatase	*	1.7	*	1.8

Less than 1%

When treatment with XANAX is protracted, periodic blood counts, urinalysis and blood chemistry analyses are advisable.

Minor changes in EEG patterns, usually low-voltage fast activity have been observed in patients during therapy with XANAX and are of no known signficance.

Post Introduction Reports: Various adverse drug reactions have been reported in association with the use of XANAX since market introduction. The majority of these reactions were reported through the medical event voluntary reporting system. Because of the spontaneous nature of the reporting of medical events and the lack of controls, a causal relationship to the use of XANAX cannot be readily determined. Reported events include: liver enzyme elevations, hepatitis, hepatic failure, Stevens-Johnson syndrome, hyperprolactinemia, gynecomastia and galactorrhea.

DRUG ABUSE AND DEPENDENCE

Physical and Psychological Dependence: Withdrawal symptoms similar in character to those noted with sedative/hypnotics and alcohol have occurred following discontinuance of benzodiazepines, including XANAX. The symptoms can range from mild dysphoria and insomnia to a major syndrome that may include abdominal and muscle cramps, vomiting, sweating, tremors and convulsions. Distinguishing between withdrawal emergent signs and symptoms and the recurrence of illness is often difficult in patients undergoing dose reduction. The long term strategy for treatment of these phenomena will vary with their cause and the therapeutic goal. When necessary, immediate management of withdrawal symptoms requires re-institution of treatment at doses of XANAX sufficient to suppress symptoms. There have been reports of failure of other benzodiazepines to fully suppress these withdrawal symptoms. These failures have been attributed to incomplete cross-tolerance but may also reflect the use of inadequate dosing regimen of the substituted benzodiazepine or the effects of concomitant medications.

While it is difficult to distinguish withdrawal and recurrence for certain patients, the time course and the nature of the symptoms may be helpful. A withdrawal syndrome typically includes the occurrence of new symptoms, tends to appear toward the end of taper or shortly after discontinuation, and will decrease with time. In recurring panic disorder, symptoms similar to those observed before treatment may recur either early or late, and they will persist.

While the severity and incidence of withdrawal phenomena appear to be related to dose and duration of treatment, withdrawal symptoms, including seizures, have been reported after only brief therapy with XANAX at doses within the recommended range for the treatment of anxiety (eg, 0.75 to 4 mg/day). Signs and symptoms of withdrawal are often more prominent after rapid decrease of dosage or abrupt discontinuance. The risk of withdrawal seizures may be increased at doses above 4 mg/day (see WARNINGS).

Patients, especially individuals with a history of seizures or epilepsy, should not be abruptly discontinued from any CNS depressant agent, including XANAX. It is recommended that all patients on XANAX who require a dosage reduction be gradually tapered under close supervision (see WARNINGS and DOSAGE AND ADMINISTRATION).

Psychological dependence is a risk with all benzodiazepines, including XANAX. The risk of psychological dependence may also be increased at doses greater than 4 mg/day and with longer term use, and this risk is further increased in patients with a history of alcohol or drug abuse. Some patients have experienced considerable difficulty in tapering and discontinuing from XANAX, especially those receiving higher doses for extended periods. Addiction-prone individuals should be under careful surveillance when receiving XANAX. As with all anxiolytics, repeat prescriptions should be limited to those who are under medical supervision.

Controlled Substance Class: Alprazolam is a controlled substance under the Controlled Substance Act by the Drug Enforcement Administration and XANAX Tablets have been assigned to Schedule IV.

OVERDOSAGE

Manifestations of alprazolam overdosage include somnolence, confusion, impaired coordination, diminished reflexes and coma. Death has also been reported in association with overdoses of alprazolam by itself, as it has with other benzodiazepines. In addition, fatalities have been reported in patients who have overdosed with a combination of a single benzodiazepine, including alprazolam, and alcohol; alcohol levels seen in some of these patients have been lower than those usually associated with alcohol-induced fatality.

The acute oral LD_{50} in rats is 331–2171 mg/kg. Other experiments in animals have indicated that cardiopulmonary collapse can occur following massive intravenous doses of alprazolam (over 195 mg/kg; 975 times the maximum recommended daily human dose of 10 mg/day). Animals could be resuscitated with positive mechanical ventilation and the intravenous infusion of norepinephrine bitartrate.

Animal experiments have suggested that forced diuresis or hemodialysis are probably of little value in treating overdosage.

General Treatment of Overdose: Overdosage reports with XANAX Tablets are limited. As in all cases of drug overdosage, respiration, pulse rate, and blood pressure should be monitored. General supportive measures should be employed, along with immediate gastric lavage. Intravenous fluids should be administered and an adequate airway maintained. If hypotension occurs, it may be combated by the use of vasopressors. Dialysis is of limited value. As with the management of intentional overdosing with any drug, it should be borne in mind that multiple agents may have been ingested.

Flumazenil, a specific benzodiazepine receptor antagonist, is indicated for the complete or partial reversal of the sedative effects of benzodiazepines and may be used in situations when an overdose with a benzodiazepine is known or suspected. Prior to the administration of flumazenil, necessary measures should be instituted to secure airway, ventilation and intravenous access. Flumazenil is intended as an adjunct to, not as a substitute for, proper management of benzodiazepine overdosage. Patients treated with flumazenil should be monitored for re-sedation, respiratory depression, and other residual benzodiazepine effects for an appropriate period after treatment. **The prescriber should be aware of a risk of seizure in association with flumazenil treatment, particularly in long-term benzodiazepine users and in cyclic antidepressant overdose.** The complete flumazenil package insert including CONTRAINDICATIONS, WARNINGS and PRECAUTIONS should be consulted prior to use.

DOSAGE AND ADMINISTRATION

Dosage should be individualized for maximum beneficial effect. While the usual daily dosages given below will meet the needs of most patients, there will be some who require doses greater than 4 mg/day. In such cases, dosage should be increased cautiously to avoid adverse effects.

Anxiety disorders and transient symptoms of anxiety:

Treatment for patients with anxiety should be initiated with a dose of 0.25 to 0.5 mg given three times daily. The dose may be increased to achieve a maximum therapeutic effect, at intervals of 3 to 4 days, to a maximum daily dose of 4 mg, given in divided doses. The lowest possible effective dose should be employed and the need for continued treatment reassessed frequently. The risk of dependence may increase with dose and duration of treatment.

In elderly patients, in patients with advanced liver disease or in patients with debilitating disease, the usual starting dose is 0.25 mg, given two or three times daily. This may be gradually increased if needed and tolerated. The elderly may be especially sensitive to the effects of benzodiazepines. If side effects occur at the recommended starting dose, the dose may be lowered.

In all patients, dosage should be reduced gradually when discontinuing therapy or when decreasing the daily dosage.

Although there are no systematically collected data to support a specific discontinuation schedule, it is suggested that the daily dosage be decreased by no more than 0.5 mg every three days. Some patients may require an even slower dosage reduction.

Panic disorder:

The successful treatment of many panic disorder patients has required the use of XANAX at doses greater than 4 mg daily. In controlled trials conducted to establish the efficacy of XANAX in panic disorder, doses in the range of 1 to 10 mg daily were used. The mean dosage employed was approximately 5 to 6 mg daily. Among the approximately 1700 patients participating in the panic disorder development program, about 300 received XANAX in dosages of greater than 7 mg/day, including approximately 100 patients who received maximum dosages of greater than 9 mg/day. Occasional patients required as much as 10 mg a day to achieve a successful response.

Generally, therapy should be initiated at a low dose to minimize the risk of adverse responses in patients especially sensitive to the drug. Thereafter, the dose can be increased at intervals equal to at least 5 times the elimination half-life (about 11 hours in young patients, about 16 hours in elderly patients). Longer titration intervals should probably be used because the maximum therapeutic response may not occur until after the plasma levels achieve steady state. Dose should be advanced until an acceptable therapeutic response (ie, a substantial reduction in or total elimination of panic attacks) is achieved, intolerance occurs, or the maximum recommended dose is attained. For patients receiving doses greater than 4 mg/day, periodic reassessment and consideration of dosage reduction is advised. In a controlled postmarketing dose-response study, patients treated with doses of XANAX greater than 4 mg/day for three months were able to taper to 50% of their total maintenance dose without apparent loss of clinical benefit. Because of the danger of withdrawal, abrupt discontinuation of treatment should be avoided. (See WARNINGS, PRECAUTIONS, DRUG ABUSE AND DEPENDENCE).

The following regimen is one that follows the principles outlined above:

Treatment may be initiated with a dose of 0.5 mg three times daily. Depending on the response, the dose may be increased at intervals of 3 to 4 days in increments of no more than 1 mg per day. Slower titration to the dose levels greater than 4 mg/day may be advisable to allow full expression of the pharmacodynamic effect of XANAX. To lessen the possibility of interdose symptoms, the times of administration should be distributed as evenly as possible throughout the waking hours, that is, on a three or four times per day schedule.

The necessary duration of treatment for panic disorder patients responding to XANAX is unknown. After a period of extended freedom from attacks, a carefully supervised tapered discontinuation may be attempted, but there is evidence that this may often be difficult to accomplish without recurrence of symptoms and/or the manifestation of withdrawal phenomena.

In any case, reduction of dose must be undertaken under close supervision and must be gradual. If significant withdrawal symptoms develop, the previous dosing schedule should be reinstituted and, only after stabilization, should a less rapid schedule of discontinuation be attempted. In a controlled postmarketing discontinuation study of panic disorder patients which compared this recommended taper schedule with a slower taper schedule, no difference was observed between the groups in the proportion of patients who tapered to zero dose; however, the slower schedule was associated with a reduction in symptoms associated with a withdrawal syndrome. It is suggested that the dose be reduced by no more than 0.5 mg every three days, with the understanding that some patients may benefit from an even more gradual discontinuation. Some patients may prove resistant to all discontinuation regimens.

PANIC DISORDER

	Treatment-Emergent Symptom Incidence*	
	XANAX	**PLACEBO**
Number of Patients	1388	1231
% of Patients Reporting:		
Central Nervous System		
Drowsiness	76.8	42.7
Fatigue and Tiredness	48.6	42.3
Impaired Coordination	40.1	17.9
Irritability	33.1	30.1
Memory Impairment	33.1	22.1
Light-headedness/Dizziness	29.8	36.9
Insomnia	29.4	41.8
Headache	29.2	35.6
Cognitive Disorder	28.8	20.5
Dysarthria	23.3	6.3
Anxiety	16.6	24.9
Abnormal Involuntary Movement	14.8	21.0
Decreased Libido	14.4	8.0
Depression	13.8	14.0
Confusional State	10.4	8.2
Muscular Twitching	7.9	11.8
Increased Libido	7.7	4.1
Change in Libido (Not Specified)	7.1	5.6
Weakness	7.1	8.4
Muscle Tone Disorders	6.3	7.5
Syncope	3.8	4.8
Akathisia	3.0	4.3
Agitation	2.9	2.6
Disinhibition	2.7	1.5
Paresthesia	2.4	3.2
Talkativeness	2.2	1.0
Vasomotor Disturbances	2.0	2.6
Derealization	1.9	1.2
Dream Abnormalities	1.8	1.5
Fear	1.4	1.0
Feeling Warm	1.3	0.5
Gastrointestinal		
Decreased Salivation	32.8	34.2
Constipation	26.2	15.4
Nausea/Vomiting	22.0	31.8
Diarrhea	20.6	22.8
Abdominal Distress	18.3	21.5
Increased Salivation	5.6	4.4
Cardio-Respiratory		
Nasal Congestion	17.4	16.5
Tachycardia	15.4	26.8
Chest Pain	10.6	18.1
Hyperventilation	9.7	14.5
Upper Respiratory Infection	4.3	3.7
Sensory		
Blurred Vision	21.0	21.4
Tinnitus	6.6	10.4
Musculoskeletal		
Muscular Cramps	2.4	2.4
Muscle Stiffness	2.2	3.3
Cutaneous		
Sweating	15.1	23.5
Rash	10.8	8.1
Other		
Increased Appetite	32.7	22.8
Decreased Appetite	27.8	24.1
Weight Gain	27.2	17.9
Weight Loss	22.6	16.5
Micturition Difficulties	12.2	8.6
Menstrual Disorders	10.4	8.7
Sexual Dysfunction	7.4	3.7
Edema	4.9	5.6
Incontinence	1.5	0.6
Infection	1.3	1.7

**Events reported by 1% or more of XANAX patients are included.*

HOW SUPPLIED

XANAX Tablets are available as follows:

0.25 mg (white, oval, scored, imprinted "XANAX 0.25")
- Bottles of 100 — NDC 0009-0029-01
- Reversed Numbered Unit Dose (100) — NDC 0009-0029-46
- Bottles of 500 — NDC 0009-0029-02
- Bottles of 1000 — NDC 0009-0029-14

0.5 mg (peach, oval, scored, imprinted "XANAX 0.5")
- Bottles of 100 — NDC 0009-0055-01
- Reversed Numbered Unit Dose (100) — NDC 0009-0055-46
- Bottles of 500 — NDC 0009-0055-03
- Bottles of 1000 — NDC 0009-0055-15

1 mg (blue, oval, scored, imprinted "XANAX 1.0")
- Bottles of 100 — NDC 0009-0090-01
- Bottles of 500 — NDC 0009-0090-04
- Bottles of 1000 — NDC 0009-0090-13

2 mg (white, oblong, multi-scored, imprinted "XANAX" on one side and "2" on the reverse side)

Continued on next page

Information on these Pharmacia & Upjohn products is based on labeling in effect June 1, 2000. Further information concerning these and other Pharmacia & Upjohn products may be obtained by direct inquiry to Medical Information, Pharmacia & Upjohn, Kalamazoo, MI 49001.

Xanax—Cont.

Bottles of 100 NDC 0009-0094-01
Bottles of 500 NDC 0009-0094-03

Store at controlled room temperature 20° to 25°C (68° to 77°F) [see USP].

Rx only

ANIMAL STUDIES

When rats were treated with alprazolam at 3, 10, and 30 mg/kg/day (15 to 150 times the maximum recommended human dose) orally for 2 years, a tendency for a dose related increase in the number of cataracts was observed in females and a tendency for a dose related increase in corneal vascularization was observed in males. These lesions did not appear until after 11 months of treatment.

CLINICAL STUDIES

Anxiety Disorders:
XANAX Tablets were compared to placebo in double blind clinical studies (doses up to 4 mg/day) in patients with a diagnosis of anxiety or anxiety with associated depressive symptomatology. XANAX was significantly better than placebo at each of the evaluation periods of these four week studies as judged by the following psychometric instruments: Physician's Global Impressions, Hamilton Anxiety Rating Scale, Target Symptoms, Patient's Global Impressions and Self-Rating Symptom Scale.

Panic Disorder:
Support for the effectiveness of XANAX in the treatment of panic disorder came from three short-term, placebo-controlled studies (up to 10 weeks) in patients with diagnoses closely corresponding to DSM-III-R criteria for panic disorder.

The average dose of XANAX was 5–6 mg/day in two of the studies, and the doses of XANAX were fixed at 2 and 6 mg/day in the third study. In all three studies, XANAX was superior to placebo on a variable defined as "the number of patients with zero panic attacks" (range, 37–83% met this criterion), as well as on a global improvement score. In two of the three studies, XANAX was superior to placebo on a variable defined as "change from baseline on the number of panic attacks per week" (range, 3.3–5.2), and also on a phobia rating scale. A subgroup of patients who were improved on XANAX during short-term treatment in one of these trials was continued on an open basis up to eight months, without apparent loss of benefit.

Pharmacia & Upjohn Company
Kalamazoo, Michigan 49001, USA 811 557 928
Revised June 2000 692167

Shown in Product Identification Guide, page 331

ZINECARD® ℞

[*zĭn "ă card ' *]
dexrazoxane for injection

DESCRIPTION

ZINECARD® (dexrazoxane for injection) is a sterile, pyrogen-free lyophilizate intended for intravenous administration. It is a cardioprotective agent for use in conjunction with doxorubicin.

Chemically, dexrazoxane is (S)-4,4'-(1-methyl-1,2-ethanediyl)bis-2,6-piperazinedione. The structural formula is as follows:

$C_{11}H_{16}N_4O_4$ M.W. 268.28

Dexrazoxane, a potent intracellular chelating agent is a derivative of EDTA. Dexrazoxane is a whitish crystalline powder which melts at 191° to 197°C. It is sparingly soluble in water and 0.1 N HCl, slightly soluble in ethanol and methanol and practically insoluble in nonpolar organic solvents. The pK_a is 2.1. Dexrazoxane has an octanol/water partition coefficient of 0.025 and degrades rapidly above a pH of 7.0. ZINECARD is available in 250 mg and 500 mg single use only vials.

Each **250 mg vial** contains dexrazoxane hydrochloride equivalent to 250 mg dexrazoxane. Hydrochloric Acid, NF is added for pH adjustment. When reconstituted as directed with the 25 mL vial of 0.167 Molar (M/6) Sodium Lactate Injection, USP diluent provided, each mL contains: 10 mg dexrazoxane. The pH of the resultant solution is 3.5 to 5.5.

Each **500 mg vial** contains dexrazoxane hydrochloride equivalent to 500 mg dexrazoxane. Hydrochloric Acid, NF is added for pH adjustment. When reconstituted as directed with the 50 mL vial of 0.167 Molar (M/6) Sodium Lactate Injection, USP diluent provided, each mL contains: 10 mg dexrazoxane. The pH of the resultant solution is 3.5 to 5.5.

CLINICAL PHARMACOLOGY

Mechanism of Action: The mechanism by which ZINECARD exerts its cardioprotective activity is not fully understood. Dexrazoxane is a cyclic derivative of EDTA that readily penetrates cell membranes. Results of laboratory studies suggest that dexrazoxane is converted intracellularly to a ring-opened chelating agent that interferes with iron-mediated free radical generation thought to be responsible, in part, for anthracycline-induced cardiomyopathy.

Pharmacokinetics: The pharmacokinetics of dexrazoxane have been studied in advanced cancer patients with normal renal and hepatic function. Generally, the pharmacokinetics of dexrazoxane can be adequately described by a two-compartment open model with first-order elimination. Dexrazoxane has been administered as a 15 minute infusion over a dose-range of 60 to 900 mg/m² with 60 mg/m² of doxorubicin, and at a fixed dose of 500 mg/m² with 50 mg/m² doxorubicin. The disposition kinetics of dexrazoxane are dose-independent, as shown by linear relationship between the area under plasma concentration-time curves and administered doses ranging from 60 to 900 mg/m². The mean peak plasma concentration of dexrazoxane was 36.5 µg/mL at the end of the 15 minute infusion of a 500 mg/m² dose of ZINECARD administered 15 to 30 minutes prior to the 50 mg/m² doxorubicin dose. The important pharmacokinetic parameters of dexrazoxane are summarized in the following table.

[See table below]

Following a rapid distributive phase (~0.2 to 0.3 hours), dexrazoxane reaches post-distributive equilibrium within two to four hours. The estimated steady-state volume of distribution of dexrazoxane suggests its distribution primarily in the total body water (25 L/m²). The mean systemic clearance and steady-state volume of distribution of dexrazoxane in two Asian female patients at 500 mg/m² dexrazoxane along with 50 mg/m² doxorubicin were 15.15 L/h/m² and 36.27 L/m², respectively, but their elimination half-life and renal clearance of dexrazoxane were similar to those of the ten Caucasian patients from the same study. Qualitative metabolism studies with ZINECARD have confirmed the presence of unchanged drug, a diacid-diamide cleavage product, and two monoacid-monoamide ring products in the urine of animals and man. The metabolite levels were not measured in the pharmacokinetic studies.

Urinary excretion plays an important role in the elimination of dexrazoxane. Forty-two percent of the 500 mg/m² dose of ZINECARD was excreted in the urine.

Protein Binding: *In vitro* studies have shown that ZINECARD is not bound to plasma proteins.

Special Populations: The pharmacokinetics of ZINECARD have not been evaluated in pediatric populations nor in hepatic or renal insufficiency patients.

Drug Interactions: There was no significant change in the pharmacokinetics of doxorubicin (50 mg/m²) and its predominant metabolite, doxorubicinol, in the presence of dexrazoxane (500 mg/m²) in a crossover study in cancer patients.

Clinical Studies: The ability of ZINECARD to prevent/reduce the incidence and severity of doxorubicin-induced cardiomyopathy was demonstrated in three prospectively randomized placebo-controlled studies. In these studies, patients were treated with a doxorubicin-containing regimen and either ZINECARD or placebo starting with the first course of chemotherapy. There was no restriction on the cumulative dose of doxorubicin. Cardiac function was assessed by measurement of the left ventricular ejection fraction (LVEF), utilizing resting multigated nuclear medicine (MUGA) scans, and by clinical evaluations. Patients receiving ZINECARD had significantly smaller mean decreases from baseline in LVEF and lower incidences of congestive heart failure than the control group. The difference in decline from baseline in LVEF was evident beginning with a cumulative doxorubicin dose of 150 mg/m² and reached statistical significance in patients who received ≥400 mg/m² of doxorubicin. In addition to evaluating the effect of ZINECARD on cardiac function, the studies also assessed the effect of the addition of ZINECARD on the antitumor efficacy of the chemotherapy regimens. In one study (the largest of three breast cancer studies) patients with advanced breast cancer receiving fluorouracil, doxorubicin and cyclophosphamide (FAC) with ZINECARD had a lower response rate (48% vs 63%, p=0.007) and a shorter time to progression than patients who received FAC + placebo, although the survival of patients who did or did not receive ZINECARD with FAC was similar.

Two of the randomized breast cancer studies evaluating the efficacy and safety of FAC with either ZINECARD or placebo were amended to allow patients on the placebo arm who had attained a cumulative dose of doxorubicin of 300 mg/m² (six courses of FAC) to receive FAC with open-label ZINECARD for each subsequent course. This change in design allowed examination of whether there was a cardioprotective effect of ZINECARD even when it was started after substantial exposure to doxorubicin.

Retrospective historical analyses were then performed to compare the likelihood of heart failure in patients to whom ZINECARD was added to the FAC regimen after they had received six (6) courses of FAC (and who then continued treatment with FAC therapy) with the heart failure rate in patients who had received six (6) courses of FAC and continued to receive this regimen without added ZINECARD. These analyses showed that the risk of experiencing a cardiac event (see Table 1 for definition) at a given cumulative dose of doxorubicin above 300 mg/m² was substantially greater in the 99 patients who did *not* receive ZINECARD beginning with their seventh course of FAC than in the 102 patients who did receive ZINECARD (See Figure 1).

Table 1
The development of cardiac events is shown by:

1. Development of congestive heart failure, defined as having two or more of the following:
   a. Cardiomegaly by X-ray
   b. Basilar Rales
   c. S_3 Gallop
   d. Paroxysmal nocturnal dyspnea and/or orthopnea and/or significant dyspnea on exertion.
2. Decline from baseline in LVEF by ≥10% and to below the lower limit of normal for the institution.
3. Decline in LVEF by ≥20% from baseline value.
4. Decline in LVEF to ≥5% below lower limit of normal for the institution.

Figure 1 displays the risk of developing congestive heart failure by cumulative dose of doxorubicin in patients who received ZINECARD starting with their seventh course of FAC compared to patients who did not. Patients unprotected by ZINECARD had a 13 times greater risk of developing congestive heart failure. Overall, 3% of patients treated with ZINECARD developed CHF compared with 22% of patients not receiving ZINECARD.

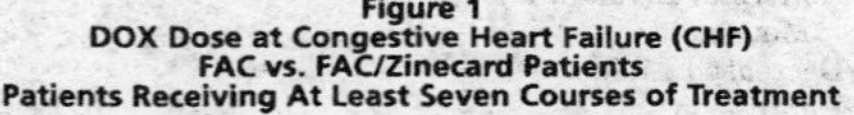

Figure 1
DOX Dose at Congestive Heart Failure (CHF)
FAC vs. FAC/Zinecard Patients
Patients Receiving At Least Seven Courses of Treatment

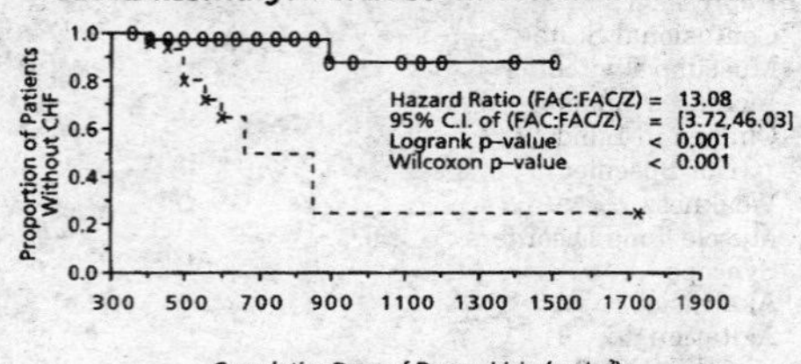

Because of its cardioprotective effect, ZINECARD permitted a greater percentage of patients to be treated with extended doxorubicin therapy. Figure 2 shows the number of patients still on treatment at increasing cumulative doses.

Figure 2
Cumulative Number of Patients On Treatment
FAC vs. FAC/Zinecard Patients
Patients Receiving at Least Seven Courses of Treatment

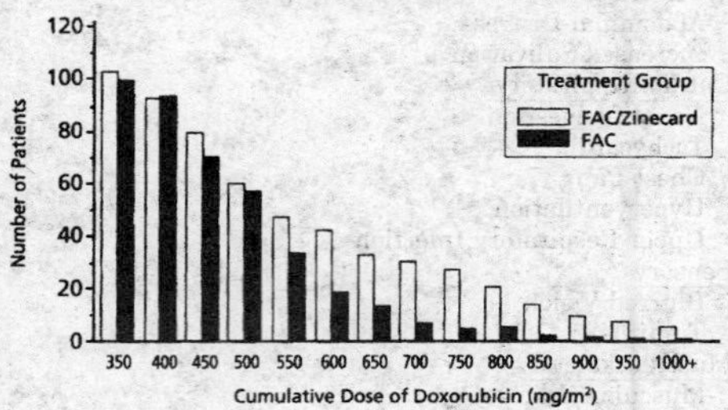

In addition to evaluating the cardioprotective efficacy of ZINECARD in this setting, the time to tumor progression and survival of these two groups of patients were also compared. There was a similar time to progression in the two groups and survival was at least as long for the group of patients that received ZINECARD starting with their seventh course, i.e., starting after a cumulative dose of doxorubicin of 300 mg/m_2. These time to progression and survival data should be interpreted with caution, however, because they are based on comparisons of groups entered sequentially in the studies and are not comparisons of prospectively randomized patients.

INDICATIONS AND USAGE

ZINECARD is indicated for reducing the incidence and severity of cardiomyopathy associated with doxorubicin ad-

SUMMARY OF MEAN (%CV[a]) DEXRAZOXANE
PHARMACOKINETIC PARAMETERS AT A DOSAGE RATIO OF
10:1 OF ZINECARD: DOXORUBICIN

Dose Doxorubicin (mg/m²)	Dose Zinecard (mg/m²)	Number of Subjects	Elimination Half-Life (h)	Plasma Clearance (L/h/m²)	Renal Clearance (L/h/m²)	[b]Volume of Distribution (L/m²)
50	500	10	2.5 (16)	7.88 (18)	3.35 (36)	22.4 (22)
60	600	5	2.1 (29)	6.25 (31)	—	22.0 (55)

[a] Coefficient of variation
[b] Steady-state volume of distribution

ministration in women with metastatic breast cancer who have received a cumulative doxorubicin dose of 300 mg/m$_2$ and who, in their physician's opinion, would benefit from continuing therapy with doxorubicin. It is not recommended for use with the initiation of doxorubicin therapy (see **WARNINGS**).

CONTRAINDICATIONS

ZINECARD should not be used with chemotherapy regimens that do not contain an anthracycline.

WARNINGS

ZINECARD may add to the myelosuppression caused by chemotherapeutic agents.

There is some evidence that the use of dexrazoxane concurrently with the initiation of fluorouracil, doxorubicin and cyclophosphamide (FAC) therapy interferes with the antitumor efficacy of the regimen, and this use is not recommended. In the largest of three breast cancer trials, patients who received dexrazoxane starting with their first cycle of FAC therapy had a lower response rate (48% vs 63%; p=0.007) and shorter time to progression than patients who did not receive dexrazoxane (see **Clinical Studies** section of **CLINICAL PHARMACOLOGY**). Therefore, ZINECARD should only be used in those patients who have received a cumulative doxorubicin dose of 300 mg/m$_2$ and are continuing with doxorubicin therapy.

Although clinical studies have shown that patients receiving FAC with ZINECARD may receive a higher cumulative dose of doxorubicin before experiencing cardiac toxicity than patients receiving FAC without ZINECARD, the use of ZINECARD in patients who have already received a cumulative dose of doxorubicin of 300 mg/m$_2$ without ZINECARD, does not eliminate the potential for anthracycline induced cardiac toxicity. Therefore, cardiac function should be carefully monitored.

Secondary malignancies (primarily acute myeloid leukemia) have been reported in patients treated chronically with oral razoxane. Razoxane is the racemic mixture, of which dexrazoxane is the S(+)-enantiomer. In these patients, the total cumulative dose of razoxane ranged from 26 to 480 grams and the duration of treatment was from 42 to 319 weeks. One case of T-cell lymphoma, a case of B-cell lymphoma and six to eight cases of cutaneous basal cell or squamous cell carcinoma have also been reported in patients treated with razoxane.

PRECAUTIONS

General

Doxorubicin should not be given prior to the intravenous injection of ZINECARD. ZINECARD should be given by slow I.V. push or rapid drip intravenous infusion from a bag. Doxorubicin should be given within 30 minutes after beginning the infusion with ZINECARD. (See **DOSAGE AND ADMINISTRATION**).

As ZINECARD will always be used with cytotoxic drugs, patients should be monitored closely. While the myelosuppressive effects of ZINECARD at the recommended dose are mild, additive effects upon the myelosuppressive activity of chemotherapeutic agents may occur.

Laboratory tests

As ZINECARD may add to the myelosuppressive effects of cytotoxic drugs, frequent complete blood counts are recommended. (See **ADVERSE REACTIONS**).

Drug Interactions

ZINECARD does not influence the pharmacokinetics of doxorubicin.

Carcinogenesis, Mutagenesis, Impairment of Fertility (see **WARNINGS** section for information on human carcinogenicity)—No long-term carcinogenicity studies have been carried out with dexrazoxane in animals. Dexrazoxane was not mutagenic in the Ames test but was found to be clastogenic to human lymphocytes *in vitro* and to mouse bone marrow erythrocytes *in vivo* (micronucleus test).

The possible adverse effects of ZINECARD on the fertility of humans and experimental animals, male or female, have not been adequately studied. Testicular atrophy was seen with dexrazoxane administration at doses as low as 30 mg/kg weekly for 6 weeks in rats (1/3 the human dose on a mg/m^2 basis) and as low as 20 mg/kg weekly for 13 weeks in dogs (approximately equal to the human dose on a mg/m^2 basis).

Pregnancy—*Pregnancy Category C*—Dexrazoxane was maternotoxic at doses of 2 mg/kg (1/40 the human dose on a mg/m^2 basis) and embryotoxic and terotogenic at 8 mg/kg (approximately 1/10 the human dose on a mg/m^2 basis) when given daily to pregnant rats during the period of organogenesis. Teratogenic effects in the rat included imperforate anus, microphthalmia, and anophthalmia. In offspring allowed to develop to maturity, fertility was impaired in the male and female rats treated in utero during organogenesis at 8 mg/kg. In rabbits, doses of 5 mg/kg (approximately 1/10 the human dose on a mg/m^2 basis) daily during the period of organogenesis were maternotoxic and dosages of 20 mg/kg (1/2 the human dose on a mg/m^2 basis) were embryotoxic and teratogenic. Teratogenic effects in the rabbit included several skeletal malformations such as short tail, rib and thoracic malformations, and soft tissue variations including subcutaneous, eye and cardiac hemorrhagic areas, as well as agenesis of the gallbladder and of the intermediate lobe of the lung. There are no adequate and well-controlled studies in pregnant women. ZINECARD should be used during pregnancy only if the potential benefit justifies the potential risk to the fetus.

TABLE 2

ADVERSE EXPERIENCE	PERCENTAGE (%) OF BREAST CANCER PATIENTS WITH ADVERSE EXPERIENCE			
	FAC + ZINECARD		FAC + PLACEBO	
	Courses 1–6 N = 413	Courses ≥ 7 N = 102	Courses 1–6 N = 458	Course ≥ 7 N = 99
Alopecia	94	100	97	98
Nausea	77	51	84	60
Vomiting	59	42	72	49
Fatigue/Malaise	61	48	58	55
Anorexia	42	27	47	38
Stomatitis	34	26	41	28
Fever	34	22	29	18
Infection	23	19	18	21
Diarrhea	21	14	24	7
Pain on Injection	12	13	3	0
Sepsis	17	12	14	9
Neurotoxicit	17	10	13	5
Streaking/ Erythema	5	4	4	2
Phlebitis	6	3	3	5
Esophagitis	6	3	7	4
Dysphagia	8	0	10	5
Hemorrhage	2	3	2	1
Extravasation	1	3	1	2
Urticaria	2	2	2	0
Recall Skin Reaction	1	1	2	0

Nursing Mothers—It is not known whether dexrazoxane is excreted in human milk. Because many drugs are excreted in human milk and because of the potential for serious adverse reactions in nursing infants exposed to dexrazoxane, mothers should be advised to discontinue nursing during dexrazoxane therapy.

Pediatric Use—Safety and effectiveness of dexrazoxane in pediatric patients have not been established.

ADVERSE REACTIONS

ZINECARD at a dose of 500 mg/m^2 has been administered in combination with FAC in randomized, placebo-controlled, double-blind studies to patients with metastatic breast cancer. The dose of doxorubicin was 50 mg/m^2 in each of the trials. Courses were repeated every three weeks, provided recovery from toxicity had occurred. Table 2 below lists the incidence of adverse experiences for patients receiving FAC with either ZINECARD or placebo in the breast cancer studies. Adverse experiences occurring during courses 1 through 6 are displayed for patients receiving ZINECARD or placebo with FAC beginning with their first course of therapy (column 1 & 3, respectively). Adverse experiences occurring at course 7 and beyond for patients who received placebo with FAC during the first six courses and who then received either ZINECARD or placebo with FAC are also displayed (column 2 & 4, respectively).

[See table above]

The adverse experiences listed above are likely attributable to the FAC regimen with the exception of pain on injection that was observed mainly on the ZINECARD arm.

Myelosuppression

Patients receiving FAC with ZINECARD experienced more severe leucopenia, granulocytopenia and thrombocytopenia at nadir than patients receiving FAC without ZINECARD, but recovery counts were similar for the two groups of patients.

Hepatic and Renal

Some patients receiving FAC + ZINECARD or FAC + placebo experienced marked abnormalities in hepatic or renal function tests, but the frequency and severity of abnormalities in bilirubin, alkaline phosphatase, BUN, and creatinine were similar for patients receiving FAC with or without ZINECARD.

OVERDOSAGE

There have been no instances of drug overdose in the clinical studies sponsored by either Pharmacia & Upjohn Company or the National Cancer Institute. The maximum dose administered during the cardioprotective trials was 1000 mg/m^2 every three weeks.

Disposition studies with ZINECARD have not been conducted in cancer patients undergoing dialysis, but retention of a significant dose fraction (>0.4) of the unchanged drug in the plasma pool, minimal tissue partitioning or binding, and availability of greater than 90% of the systemic drug levels in the inbound form suggest that it could be removed using conventional peritoneal or hemodialysis.

There is no known antidote for dexrazoxane. Instances of suspected overdose should be managed with good supportive care until resolution of myelosuppression and related conditions is complete. Management of overdose should include treatment of infections, fluid regulation, and maintenance of nutritional requirements.

DOSAGE AND ADMINISTRATION

The recommended dosage ratio of ZINECARD:DOX is 10:1 (eg, 500 mg/m^2 ZINECARD:50 mg/m^2 DOX). ZINECARD must be reconstituted with 0.167 Molar (M/6) Sodium Lactate Injection, USP, to give a concentration of 10 mg ZINECARD for each mL of sodium lactate. The reconstituted solution should be given by slow I.V. push or rapid drip intravenous infusion from a bag. After completing the infusion of ZINECARD, and prior to a total elapsed time of 30 minutes (from the beginning of the ZINECARD infusion), the intravenous injection of doxorubicin should be given.

Reconstituted ZINECARD, when transferred to an empty infusion bag, is stable for 6 hours from the time of reconstitution when stored at controlled room temperature, 15° to 30°C (59° to 86°F) or under refrigeration, 2° to 8°C (36° to 46°F). DISCARD UNUSED SOLUTIONS.

The reconstituted ZINECARD solution may be diluted with either 0.9% Sodium Chloride Injection, USP or 5.0% Dextrose Injection, USP to a concentration range of 1.3 to 5.0 mg/mL in intravenous infusion bags. The resultant solutions are stable for 6 hours when stored at controlled room temperature, 15° to 30°C (59° to 86°F) or under refrigeration, 2° to 8°C (36° to 46°F). DISCARD UNUSED SOLUTIONS.

Incompatibility

ZINECARD should not be mixed with other drugs.

Parenteral drug products should be inspected visually for particulate matter and discoloration prior to administration, whenever solution and container permit.

Handling and Disposal: Caution in the handling and preparation of the reconstituted solution must be exercised and the use of gloves is recommended. If ZINECARD powder or

Continued on next page

Information on these Pharmacia & Upjohn products is based on labeling in effect June 1, 2000. Further information concerning these and other Pharmacia & Upjohn products may be obtained by direct inquiry to Medical Information, Pharmacia & Upjohn, Kalamazoo, MI 49001.

Zinecard—Cont.

solutions contact the skin or mucosae, immediately wash thoroughly with soap and water.
Procedures normally used for proper handling and disposal of anticancer drugs should be considered for use with ZINECARD. Several guidelines on this subject have been published.[1–7] There is no general agreement that all of the procedures recommended in the guidelines are necessary or appropriate.

HOW SUPPLIED

ZINECARD® (dexrazoxane for injection) is available in the following strengths as sterile, pyrogen-free lyophilizates.

NDC 0013-8715-62 250 mg single dose vial with a red flip-top seal, packaged in single vial packs.
(This package also contains a 25 mL vial of 0.167 Molar (M/6) Sodium Lactate Injection, USP.)

NDC 0013-8725-89 500 mg single dose vial with a blue flip-top seal, packaged in single vial packs.
(This package also contains a 50 mL vial of 0.167 Molar (M/6) Sodium Lactate Injection, USP.)

Store at 25°C (77°F); excursions permitted to 15° to 30°C (59° to 86°F) [see USP Controlled Room Temperature]. Reconstituted solutions of ZINECARD are stable for 6 hours at controlled room temperature or under refrigeration, 2° to 8°C (36° to 46°F). DISCARD UNUSED SOLUTIONS.

Rx only

REFERENCES

1. Recommendations for the Safe Handling of Parenteral Antineoplastic Drugs. NIH Publication No. 83-2621. For sale by the Superintendent of Documents, U.S. Government Printing Office, Washington, DC 20402.
2. AMA Council Report. Guidelines for Handling Parenteral Antineoplastics JAMA. 1985 March 15.
3. National Study Commission on Cytotoxic Exposure-Recommendations for Handling Cytotoxic Agents. Available from Louis P. Jeffrey, Sc.D., Chairman, National Study Commission on Cytotoxic Exposure, Massachusetts College of Pharmacy and Allied Health Sciences, 179 Longwood Avenue, Boston, Massachusetts 02115.
4. Clinical Oncological Society of Australia, Guidelines and Recommendations for Safe Handling of Antineoplastic Agents. Med J Australia. 1983; 1:426–428.
5. Jones RB, et al. Safe handling of Chemotherapeutic Agents: A report from the Mount Sinai Medical Center. CA - A Cancer Journal for Clinicians. 1983; (Sept/Oct) 258–263.
6. American Society of Hospital Pharmacists Technical Assistance Bulletin on Handling Cytotoxic and Hazardous Drugs. Am J Hosp Pharm. 1990; 47:1033–1049.
7. OSHA Work-Practice Guidelines for Personnel Dealing with Cytotoxic (Antineoplastic) Drugs. Am J Hosp Pharm. 1986; 43:1193–1204.

Manufactered for: Pharmacia & Upjohn Company
Kalamazoo, MI 49001, USA
By: SP Pharmaceuticals LLC
Albuquerque, NM 87109, USA

August 1998 817 546 000

ZYVOX™ ℞

[zī-vŏx]

linezolid injection
linezolid tablets
linezolid for oral suspension

DESCRIPTION

ZYVOX I.V. Injection, ZYVOX Tablets, and ZYVOX for Oral Suspension contain linezolid, which is a synthetic antibacterial agent of the oxazolidinone class. The chemical name for linezolid is (S)-N-[[3-[3-Fluoro-4-(4-morpholinyl)phenyl]-2-oxo-5-oxazolidinyl] methyl]-acetamide.
The empirical formula is $C_{16}H_{20}FN_3O$. Its molecular weight is 337.35, and its chemical structure is represented below:

[chemical structure of linezolid]

ZYVOX I.V. Injection is supplied as a ready-to-use sterile isotonic solution for intravenous infusion. Each mL contains 2 mg of linezolid. Inactive ingredients are sodium citrate, citric acid, and dextrose in an aqueous vehicle for intravenous administration. The sodium (Na^+) content is 0.38 mg/mL (5 mEq per 300-mL bag; 3.3 mEq per 200-mL bag; and 1.7 mEq per 100-mL bag).
ZYVOX Tablets for oral administration contain 400 mg or 600 mg linezolid as film-coated compressed tablets. Inactive ingredients are corn starch, microcrystalline cellulose, hydroxypropylcellulose, sodium starch glycolate, magnesium stearate, hydroxypropyl methylcellulose, polyethylene glycol, titanium dioxide, and carnauba wax. The sodium (Na^+) content is 1.95 mg per 400-mg tablet and 2.92 mg per 600-mg tablet (0.1 mEq per tablet, regardless of strength).
ZYVOX for Oral Suspension is supplied as an orange-flavored granule/powder for constitution into a suspension for oral administration. Following constitution, each 5 mL contains 100 mg of linezolid. Inactive ingredients are sucrose, citric acid, sodium citrate, microcrystalline cellulose and carboxymethylcellulose sodium, aspartame, xanthan gum, mannitol, sodium benzoate, colloidal silicon dioxide, sodium chloride, and flavors (see **PRECAUTIONS, Information for Patients**). The sodium (Na^+) content is 8.52 mg per 5 mL (0.4 mEq per 5 mL).

Table 1. Mean (Standard Deviation) Pharmacokinetic Parameters of Linezolid

Dose of Linezolid	C_{max} µg/mL	C_{min} µg/mL	T_{max} hrs	AUC* µg • h/mL	$t_{1/2}$ hrs	CL mL/min
400 mg tablet						
single dose†	8.10 (1.83)	—	1.52 (1.01)	55.10 (25.00)	5.20 (1.50)	146 (67)
every 12 hours	11.00 (4.37)	3.08 (2.25)	1.12 (0.47)	73.40 (33.50)	4.69 (1.70)	110 (49)
600 mg tablet						
single dose	12.70 (3.96)	—	1.28 (0.66)	91.40 (39.30)	4.26 (1.65)	127 (48)
every 12 hours	21.20 (5.78)	6.15 (2.94)	1.03 (0.62)	138.00 (42.10)	5.40 (2.06)	80 (29)
600 mg IV injection‡						
single dose	12.90 (1.60)	—	0.50 (0.10)	80.20 (33.30)	4.40 (2.40)	138 (39)
every 12 hours	15.10 (2.52)	3.68 (2.36)	0.51 (0.03)	89.70 (31.00)	4.80 (1.70)	123 (40)
600 mg oral suspension						
single dose	11.00 (2.76)	—	0.97 (0.88)	80.80 (35.10)	4.60 (1.71)	141 (45)

* AUC for single dose = $AUC_{0-\infty}$; for multiple-dose = $AUC_{0-\tau}$
† Data dose-normalized from 375 mg
‡ Data dose-normalized from 625 mg, IV dose was given as 0.5-hour infusion.
C_{max} = Maximum plasma concentration; C_{min} = Minimum plasma concentration; T_{max} = Time to C_{max}; AUC = Area under concentration-time curve; $t_{1/2}$ = Elimination half-life; CL = Systemic clearance

CLINICAL PHARMACOLOGY

Pharmacokinetics

The mean pharmacokinetic parameters of linezolid after single and multiple oral and intravenous doses are summarized in Table 1. Plasma concentrations of linezolid at steady-state after oral doses of 600 mg given every 12 hours (q12h) are shown in Figure 1.
[See table 1 above]

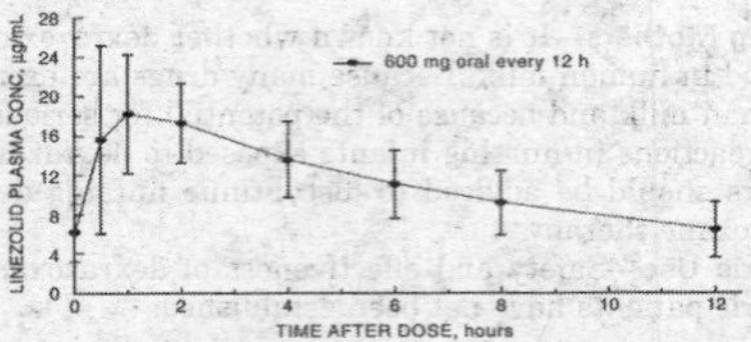

Figure 1. Plasma Concentrations of Linezolid at Steady-State Following Oral Dosing Every 12 Hours (Mean ± Standard Deviation, n=16)

Absorption: Linezolid is rapidly and extensively absorbed after oral dosing. Maximum plasma concentrations are reached approximately 1 to 2 hours after dosing, and the absolute bioavailability is approximately 100%. Therefore, linezolid may be given orally or intravenously without dose adjustment.
Linezolid may be administered without regard to the timing of meals. The time to reach the maximum concentration is delayed from 1.5 hours to 2.2 hours and C_{max} is decreased by about 17% when high fat food is given with linezolid. However, the total exposure measured as $AUC_{0-\infty}$ values is similar under both conditions.

Distribution: Animal and human pharmacokinetic studies have demonstrated that linezolid readily distributes to well-perfused tissues. The plasma protein binding of linezolid is approximately 31% and is concentration-independent. The volume of distribution of linezolid at steady-state averaged 40 to 50 liters in healthy adult volunteers.
Linezolid concentrations have been determined in various fluids from a limited number of subjects in Phase 1 volunteer studies following multiple dosing of linezolid. The ratio of linezolid in saliva relative to plasma was 1.2 to 1 and for sweat relative to plasma was 0.55 to 1.

Metabolism: Linezolid is primarily metabolized by oxidation of the morpholine ring, which results in two inactive ring-opened carboxylic acid metabolites: the aminoethoxyacetic acid metabolite (A), and the hydroxyethyl glycine metabolite (B). Formation of metabolite B is mediated by a non-enzymatic chemical oxidation mechanism in vitro. Linezolid is not an inducer of cytochrome P450 (CYP) in rats, and it has been demonstrated from in vitro studies that linezolid is not detectably metabolized by human cytochrome P450 and it does not inhibit the activities of clinically significant human CYP isoforms (1A2, 2C9, 2C19, 2D6, 2E1, 3A4).

Excretion: Nonrenal clearance accounts for approximately 65% of the total clearance of linezolid. Under steady-state conditions, approximately 30% of the dose appears in the urine as linezolid, 40% as metabolite B, and 10% as metabolite A. The renal clearance of linezolid is low (average 40 mL/min) and suggests net tubular reabsorption. Virtually no linezolid appears in the feces, while approximately 6% of the dose appears in the feces as metabolite B, and 3% as metabolite A.
A small degree of nonlinearity in clearance was observed with increasing doses of linezolid, which appears to be due to lower renal and nonrenal clearance of linezolid at higher concentrations. However, the difference in clearance was small and was not reflected in the apparent elimination half-life.

Special Populations

Geriatric: The pharmacokinetics of linezolid are not significantly altered in elderly patients (65 years or older). Therefore, dose adjustment for geriatric patients is not necessary.

Pediatric: Currently, there are limited data on the pharmacokinetics of linezolid during multiple dosing in pediatric patients of all ages. No data have been collected in infants younger than 3 months of age.
Pharmacokinetic information indicates that pediatric patients dosed with 10 mg/kg IV have a similar C_{max} but a higher average clearance when corrected by body weight, and shorter apparent elimination half-life than adults receiving 625 mg of linezolid. Pediatric dosing regimens that provide a pharmacokinetic profile similar to adults have not been determined. Studies using doses higher than 10 mg/kg or dosing more frequently than every 12 hours have not been conducted in pediatric patients.

Gender: Females have a slightly lower volume of distribution of linezolid than males. Plasma concentrations are higher in females than in males, which is partly due to body weight differences. After a 600-mg dose, mean oral clearance is approximately 38% lower in females than in males. However, there are no significant gender differences in mean apparent elimination-rate constant or half-life. Thus, drug exposure in females is not expected to substantially increase beyond levels known to be well tolerated. Therefore, dose adjustment by gender does not appear to be necessary.

Renal Insufficiency: The pharmacokinetics of the parent drug, linezolid, are not altered in patients with any degree of renal insufficiency; however, the two primary metabolites of linezolid may accumulate in patients with renal insufficiency, with the amount of accumulation increasing with the severity of renal dysfunction (see Table 2). The clinical significance of accumulation of these two metabolites has not been determined in patients with severe renal insufficiency. Because similar plasma concentrations of linezolid are achieved regardless of renal function, no dose adjustment is recommended for patients with renal insufficiency. However, given the absence of information on the clinical significance of accumulation of the primary metabolites, use of linezolid in patients with renal insufficiency should be weighed against the potential risks of accumulation of these metabolites. Both linezolid and the two metabolites are eliminated by dialysis. No information is available on the effect of peritoneal dialysis on the pharmacokinetics of linezolid. Approximately 30% of a dose was eliminated in a 3-hour dialysis session beginning 3 hours after the dose of linezolid was administered; therefore, linezolid should be given after hemodialysis.
[See table 2 at bottom of next page]

Hepatic Insufficiency: The pharmacokinetics of linezolid are not altered in patients (n=7) with mild-to-moderate hepatic insufficiency (Child-Pugh class A or B). On the basis of the available information, no dose adjustment is recommended for patients with mild-to-moderate hepatic insufficiency. The pharmacokinetics of linezolid in patients with severe hepatic insufficiency have not been evaluated.

Drug-Drug Interactions

Drugs Metabolized by Cytochrome P450: Linezolid is not an inducer of cytochrome P450 (CYP) in rats. It is not detectably metabolized by human cytochrome P450 and it does not inhibit the activities of clinically significant human CYP isoforms (1A2, 2C9, 2C19, 2D6, 2E1, 3A4). Therefore, no CYP450-induced drug interactions are expected with linezolid. Concurrent administration of linezolid does not substantially alter the pharmacokinetic characteristics of (S)-warfarin, which is extensively metabolized by CYP2C9. Drugs such as warfarin and phenytoin, which are CYP2C9 substrates, may be given with linezolid without changes in dosage regimen.

Antibiotics:

Aztreonam: The pharmacokinetics of linezolid or aztreonam are not altered when administered together.

Gentamicin: The pharmacokinetics of linezolid or gentamicin are not altered when administered together.

Monoamine Oxidase Inhibition: Linezolid is a reversible, nonselective inhibitor of monoamine oxidase. Therefore, linezolid has the potential for interaction with adrenergic and serotonergic agents.

Adrenergic Agents: A significant pressor response has been observed in normal adult subjects receiving linezolid and tyramine doses of more than 100 mg. Therefore, patients receiving linezolid need to avoid consuming large amounts of foods or beverages with high tyramine content (see **PRECAUTIONS, Information for Patients**).

A reversible enhancement of the pressor response of either pseudoephedrine HCl (PSE) or phenylpropanolamine HCl (PPA) is observed when linezolid is administered to healthy normotensive subjects (see **PRECAUTIONS, Drug Interactions**). A similar study has not been conducted in hypertensive patients. The interaction studies conducted in normotensive subjects evaluated the blood pressure and heart rate effects of placebo, PPA or PSE alone, linezolid alone, and the combination of steady-state linezolid (600 mg q12h for 3 days) with two doses of PPA (25 mg) or PSE (60 mg) given 4 hours apart. Heart rate was not affected by any of the treatments. Blood pressure was increased with both combination treatments. Maximum blood pressure levels were seen 2 to 3 hours after the second dose of PPA or PSE, and returned to baseline 2 to 3 hours after peak. The results of the PPA study follow, showing the mean (and range) maximum systolic blood pressure in mm Hg: placebo = 121 (103 to 158); linezolid alone = 120 (107 to 135); PPA alone = 125 (106 to 139); PPA with linezolid = 147 (129 to 176). The results from the PSE study were similar to those in the PPA study. The mean maximum increase in systolic blood pressure over baseline was 32 mm Hg (range: 20-52 mm Hg) and 38 mm Hg (range: 18-79 mm Hg) during co-administration of linezolid with pseudoephedrine or phenylpropanolamine, respectively.

Serotonergic Agents: The potential drug-drug interaction with dextromethorphan was studied in healthy volunteers. Subjects were administered dextromethorphan (two 20-mg doses given 4 hours apart) with or without linezolid. No serotonin syndrome effects (confusion, delirium, restlessness, tremors, blushing, diaphoresis, hyperpyrexia) have been observed in normal subjects receiving linezolid and dextromethorphan. The effects of other serotonin re-uptake inhibitors have not been studied.

MICROBIOLOGY

Linezolid is a synthetic antibacterial agent of a new class of antibiotics, the oxazolidinones, which has clinical utility in the treatment of infections caused by aerobic gram-positive bacteria. The in vitro spectrum of activity of linezolid also includes certain gram-negative bacteria and anaerobic bacteria. Linezolid inhibits bacterial protein synthesis through a mechanism of action different from that of other antibacterial agents; therefore, cross-resistance between linezolid and other classes of antibiotics is unlikely. Linezolid binds to a site on the bacterial 23S ribosomal RNA of the 50S subunit and prevents the formation of a functional 70S initiation complex, which is an essential component of the bacterial translation process. The results of time-kill studies have shown linezolid to be bacteriostatic against enterococci and staphylococci. For streptococci, linezolid was found to be bactericidal for the majority of strains.

In clinical trials, resistance to linezolid developed in 6 patients infected with *E. faecium* (4 patients received 200 mg q12h, lower than the recommended dose, and 2 patients received 600 mg q12h). In a compassionate use program, resistance to linezolid developed in 8 patients with *E. faecium* and in 1 patient with *E. faecalis*. All patients had either unremoved prosthetic devices or undrained abscesses. Resistance to linezolid occurs in vitro at a frequency of 1×10^{-9} to 1×10^{-11}. In vitro studies have shown that point mutations in the 23S rRNA are associated with linezolid resistance. Resistance to linezolid has not been seen in clinical trials in patients infected with *Staphylococcus* spp. or *Streptococcus* spp., including *S. pneumoniae*.

In vitro studies have demonstrated additivity or indifference between linezolid and vancomycin, gentamicin, rifampin, imipenem-cilastatin, aztreonam, ampicillin, or streptomycin.

Linezolid has been shown to be active against most isolates of the following microorganisms, both in vitro and in clinical infections, as described in the **INDICATIONS AND USAGE** section.

Aerobic and facultative Gram-positive microorganisms

Enterococcus faecium (vancomycin-resistant strains only)
Staphylococcus aureus (including methicillin-resistant strains)
Streptococcus agalactiae
Streptococcus pneumoniae (penicillin-susceptible strains only)
Streptococcus pyogenes

The following in vitro data are available, but their clinical significance is unknown. At least 90% of the following microorganisms exhibit an in vitro minimum inhibitory concentration (MIC) less than or equal to the susceptible breakpoint for linezolid. However, the safety and effectiveness of linezolid in treating clinical infections due to these microorganisms have not been established in adequate and well-controlled clinical trials.

Aerobic and facultative Gram-positive microorganisms

Enterococcus faecalis (including vancomycin-resistant strains)
Enterococcus faecium (vancomycin-susceptible strains)
Staphylococcus epidermidis (including methicillin-resistant strains)
Staphylococcus haemolyticus
Streptococcus pneumoniae (penicillin-resistant strains)
Viridans group streptococci

Aerobic and facultative Gram-negative microorganisms

Pasteurella multocida

Susceptibility Testing Methods

NOTE: Susceptibility testing by dilution methods requires the use of linezolid susceptibility powder.

When available, the results of in vitro susceptibility tests should be provided to the physician as periodic reports which describe the susceptibility profile of nosocomial and community-acquired pathogens. These reports should aid the physician in selecting the most effective antimicrobial.

Dilution Techniques: Quantitative methods are used to determine antimicrobial minimum inhibitory concentrations (MICs). These MICs provide estimates of the susceptibility of bacteria to antimicrobial compounds. The MICs should be determined using a standardized procedure. Standardized procedures are based on a dilution method [1,3] (broth or agar) or equivalent with standardized inoculum concentrations and standardized concentrations of linezolid powder. The MIC values should be interpreted according to criteria provided in Table 3.

Diffusion Techniques: Quantitative methods that require measurement of zone diameters also provide reproducible estimates of the susceptibility of bacteria to antimicrobial compounds. One such standardized procedure [2,3] requires the use of standardized inoculum concentrations. This procedure uses paper disks impregnated with 30 μg of linezolid to test the susceptibility of microorganisms to linezolid. The disk diffusion interpretive criteria are provided in Table 3.

Table 3. Susceptibility Interpretive Criteria for Linezolid

Pathogen	Susceptibility Interpretive Criteria: Minimal Inhibitory Concentrations (MIC in μg/mL) S	I	R	Disk Diffusion (Zone Diameters in mm) S	I	R
Enterococcus spp	≤2	4	≥8	≥23	21-22	≤20
Staphylococcus spp[a]	≤4	—	—	≥21	—	—
Streptococcus pneumoniae[a]	≤2[b]	—	—	≥21[c]	—	—
Streptococcus spp other than *S pneumoniae*[a]	≤2[b]	—	—	≥21[c]	—	—

[a] The current absence of data on resistant strains precludes defining any categories other than "Susceptible." Strains yielding test results suggestive of a "nonsusceptible" category should be retested, and if the result is confirmed, the isolate should be submitted to a reference laboratory for further testing.

[b] These interpretive standards for *S. pneumoniae* and *Streptococcus* spp. other than *S. pneumoniae* are applicable only to tests performed by broth microdilution using cation-adjusted Mueller-Hinton broth with 2 to 5% lysed horse blood inoculated with a direct colony suspension and incubated in ambient air at 35°C for 20 to 24 hours.

[c] These zone diameter interpretive standards are applicable only to tests performed using Mueller-Hinton agar supplemented with 5% defibrinated sheep blood inoculated with a direct colony suspension and incubated in 5% CO_2 at 35°C for 20 to 24 hours.

A report of "Susceptible" indicates that the pathogen is likely to be inhibited if the antimicrobial compound in the blood reaches the concentrations usually achievable. A report of "Intermediate" indicates that the result should be considered equivocal, and, if the microorganism is not fully susceptible to alternative, clinically feasible drugs, the test should be repeated. This category implies possible clinical applicability in body sites where the drug is physiologically concentrated or in situations where high dosage of drug can be used. This category also provides a buffer zone which prevents small uncontrolled technical factors from causing major discrepancies in interpretation. A report of "Resistant" indicates that the pathogen is not likely to be inhibited if the antimicrobial compound in the blood reaches the concentrations usually achievable; other therapy should be selected.

Quality Control

Standardized susceptibility test procedures require the use of quality control microorganisms to control the technical aspects of the test procedures Standard linezolid powder should provide the following range of values noted in Table 4. **NOTE:** Quality control microorganisms are specific strains of organisms with intrinsic biological properties relating to resistance mechanisms and their genetic expression within bacteria; the specific strains used for microbiological quality control are not clinically significant.

Table 4. Acceptable Quality Control Ranges for Linezolid to be Used in Validation of Susceptibility Test Results

QC Strain	Acceptable Quality Control Ranges: Minimum Inhibitory Concentration (MIC in μg/mL)	Disk Diffusion (Zone Diameters in mm)
Enterococcus faecalis ATCC 29212	1-4	Not applicable
Staphylococcus aureus ATCC 29213	1-4	Not applicable

Table 2. Mean (Standard Deviation) AUCs and Elimination Half-Lives of Linezolid and Metabolites A and B in Patients with Varying Degrees of Renal Insufficiency After a Single 600-mg Oral Dose of Linezolid

Parameter	Healthy Subjects	Moderate Renal Impairment	Severe Renal Impairment	Hemodialysis-Dependent: Off Dialysis*	On Dialysis
	CL_{CR}>80 mL/min	30 <CL_{CR} <80 mL/min	10 <CL_{CR} <30 mL/min		
Linezolid					
$AUC_{0-\infty}$, μg h/mL	110 (22)	128 (53)	127 (66)	141 (45)	83 (23)
$t_{1/2}$, hours	6.4 (2.2)	6.1 (1.7)	7.1 (3.7)	8.4 (2.7)	7.0 (1.8)
Metabolite A					
$AUC_{0-\infty}$, μg h/mL	7.6 (1.9)	11.7 (4.3)	56.5 (30.6)	185 (124)	68.8 (23.9)
$t_{1/2}$, hours	6.3 (2.1)	6.6 (2.3)	9.0 (4.6)	NA	NA
Metabolite B					
AUC_{0-48}, μg h/mL	30.5 (6.2)	51.1 (38.5)	203 (92)	467 (102)	239 (44)
$t_{1/2}$, hours	6.6 (2.7)	9.9 (7.4)	11.0 (3.9)	NA	NA

* between hemodialysis sessions
NA = Not applicable

Continued on next page

Information on these Pharmacia & Upjohn products is based on labeling in effect June 1, 2000. Further information concerning these and other Pharmacia & Upjohn products may be obtained by direct inquiry to Medical Information, Pharmacia & Upjohn, Kalamazoo, MI 49001.

Zyvox—Cont.

Staphylococcus aureus ATCC 25923	Not applicable	27-31
Streptococcus pneumoniae ATCC 49619[d]	0.50-2[e]	28-34[f]

[d] This organism may be used for validation of susceptibility test results when testing *Streptococcus* spp. other than *S. pneumoniae*.

[e] This quality control range for *S. pneumoniae* is applicable only to tests performed by broth microdilution using cation-adjusted Mueller-Hinton broth with 2 to 5% lysed horse blood inoculated with a direct colony suspension and incubated in ambient air at 35°C for 20 to 24 hours.

[f] This quality control zone diameter range is applicable only to tests performed using Mueller-Hinton agar supplemented with 5% defibrinated sheep blood inoculated with a direct colony suspension and incubated in 5% CO_2 at 35°C for 20 to 24 hours.

INDICATIONS AND USAGE

ZYVOX formulations are indicated for the treatment of adult patients with the following infections caused by susceptible strains of the designated microorganisms (see **DOSAGE AND ADMINISTRATION**).

Vancomycin-Resistant *Enterococcus faecium* infections, including cases with concurrent bacteremia (see **CLINICAL STUDIES**).

Nosocomial pneumonia caused by *Staphylococcus aureus* (methicillin-susceptible and -resistant strains), or *Streptococcus pneumoniae* (penicillin-susceptible strains only). Combination therapy may be clinically indicated if the documented or presumptive pathogens include gram-negative organisms (see **CLINICAL STUDIES**).

Complicated skin and skin structure infections caused by *Staphylococcus aureus* (methicillin-susceptible and -resistant strains), *Streptococcus pyogenes*, or *Streptococcus agalactiae*. ZYVOX has not been studied in the treatment of diabetic foot and decubitus ulcers. Combination therapy may be clinically indicated if the documented or presumptive pathogens include gram-negative organisms (see **CLINICAL STUDIES**).

Uncomplicated skin and skin structure infections caused by *Staphylococcus aureus* (methicillin-susceptible strains only) or *Streptococcus pyogenes*.

Community-acquired pneumonia caused by *Streptococcus pneumoniae* (penicillin-susceptible strains only), including cases with concurrent bacteremia, or *Staphylococcus aureus* (methicillin-susceptible strains only).

Due to concerns about inappropriate use of antibiotics leading to an increase in resistant organisms, prescribers should carefully consider alternatives before initiating treatment with ZYVOX in the outpatient setting.

Appropriate specimens for bacteriological examination should be obtained in order to isolate and identify the causative organisms and to determine their susceptibility to linezolid. Therapy may be instituted empirically while awaiting the results of these tests. Once these results become available, antimicrobial therapy should be adjusted accordingly.

CONTRAINDICATIONS

ZYVOX formulations are contraindicated for use in patients who have known hypersensitivity to linezolid or any of the other product components.

WARNINGS

Pseudomembranous colitis has been reported with nearly all antibacterial agents, including ZYVOX, and may range in severity from mild to life-threatening. Therefore, it is important to consider this diagnosis in patients who present with diarrhea subsequent to the administration of any antibacterial agent.

Treatment with antibacterial agents alters the normal flora of the colon and may permit overgrowth of clostridia. Studies indicated that a toxin produced by *Clostridium difficile* is a primary cause of "antibiotic-associated colitis."

After the diagnosis of pseudomembranous colitis has been established, appropriate therapeutic measures should be initiated. Mild cases of pseudomembranous colitis usually respond to drug discontinuation alone. In moderate to severe cases, consideration should be given to management with fluids and electrolytes, protein supplementation, and treatment with an antibacterial agent clinically effective against *Clostridium difficile*.

PRECAUTIONS

General

The use of antibiotics may promote the overgrowth of nonsusceptible organisms. Should superinfection occur during therapy, appropriate measures should be taken.

ZYVOX has not been studied in patients with uncontrolled hypertension, pheochromocytoma, carcinoid syndrome, or untreated hyperthyroidism.

The safety and efficacy of ZYVOX formulations given for longer than 28 days have not been evaluated in controlled clinical trials.

Thrombocytopenia

Thrombocytopenia has been reported in patients receiving linezolid (see **ADVERSE REACTIONS**). Platelet counts should be monitored in patients who are at increased risk for bleeding, who have pre-existing thrombocytopenia, who receive concomitant medications that may decrease platelet count or function, or who may require longer than 2 weeks of linezolid therapy.

Information for Patients

Patients should be advised that:

- ZYVOX may be taken with or without food.
- They should inform their physician if they have a history of hypertension.
- Large quantities of foods or beverages with high tyramine content should be avoided while taking ZYVOX. Quantities of tyramine consumed should be less than 100 mg per meal. Foods high in tyramine content include those that may have undergone protein changes by aging, fermentation, pickling, or smoking to improve flavor, such as aged cheeses (0 to 15 mg tyramine per ounce); fermented or air-dried meats (0.1 to 8 mg tyramine per ounce); sauerkraut (8 mg tyramine per 8 ounces); soy sauce (5 mg tyramine per 1 teaspoon); tap beers (4 mg tyramine per 12 ounces); red wines (0 to 6 mg tyramine per 8 ounces). The tyramine content of any protein-rich food may be increased if stored for long periods or improperly refrigerated.[4,5]
- They should inform their physician if taking medications containing pseudoephedrine HCl or phenylpropanolamine HCl, such as cold remedies and decongestants.
- They should inform their physician if taking serotonin re-uptake inhibitors or other antidepressants.
- *Phenylketonurics:* Each 5 mL of the 100 mg/5 mL ZYVOX for Oral Suspension contains 20 mg phenylalanine. The other ZYVOX formulations do not contain phenylalanine. Contact your physician or pharmacist.

Drug Interactions (see also CLINICAL PHARMACOLOGY, Drug-Drug Interactions)

Monoamine Oxidase Inhibition: Linezolid is a reversible, nonselective inhibitor of monoamine oxidase. Therefore, linezolid has the potential for interaction with adrenergic and serotonergic agents.

Adrenergic Agents: Some individuals receiving ZYVOX may experience a reversible enhancement of the pressor response to indirect-acting sympathomimetic agents, vasopressor or dopaminergic agents. Commonly used drugs such as phenylpropanolamine and pseudoephedrine have been specifically studied. Initial doses of adrenergic agents, such as dopamine or epinephrine, should be reduced and titrated to achieve the desired response.

Serotonergic Agents: Co-administration of linezolid and serotonergic agents was not associated with serotonin syndrome in phase 1, 2 or 3 studies. Since there is limited experience with concomitant administration of linezolid and serotonergic agents, physicians should be alert to the possibility of signs and symptoms of serotonin syndrome (e.g., hyperpyrexia, and cognitive dysfunction) in patients receiving such concomitant therapy.

Drug-Laboratory Test Interactions

There are no reported drug-laboratory test interactions.

Carcinogenesis, Mutagenesis, Impairment of Fertility

Although lifetime studies in animals have not been conducted to evaluate the carcinogenic potential of linezolid, no mutagenic or clastogenic potential was found in a battery of tests, including the Ames and AS52 assays, an in vitro unscheduled DNA synthesis (UDS) assay, an in vitro chromosome aberration assay in human lymphocytes, and an in vivo mouse micronucleus assay.

Linezolid did not affect the fertility or reproductive performance of adult female rats. It reversibly decreased fertility and reproductive performance in adult male rats when given at doses ≥ 50 mg/kg/day, with exposures approximately equal to or greater than the expected human exposure level (exposure comparisons are based on AUCs). Epithelial cell hypertrophy in the epididymis may have contributed to the decreased fertility by affecting sperm maturation. Similar epididymal changes were not seen in dogs. Although the concentrations of sperm in the testes were in the normal range, the concentrations in the cauda epididymis were decreased, and sperm from the vas deferens had decreased motility.

Mildly decreased fertility occurred in juvenile male rats treated with linezolid through most of their period of sexual development (50 mg/kg/day from days 7 to 36 of age, and 100 mg/kg/day from days 37 to 55 of age, with exposures ranging from 0.4-fold to 1.2-fold that expected in humans based on AUCs). No histopathological evidence of adverse effects was observed in the male reproductive tract.

Pregnancy

Teratogenic Effects. Pregnancy Category C: Linezolid was not teratogenic in mice or rats at exposure levels 4-fold (in mice) or equivalent to (in rats) the expected human exposure level, based on AUCs. However, embryo and fetal toxicities were seen (see **Non-teratogenic Effects**). There are no adequate and well-controlled studies in pregnant women. ZYVOX should be used during pregnancy only if the potential benefit justifies the potential risk to the fetus.

Non-teratogenic Effects

In mice, embryo and fetal toxicities were seen only at doses that caused maternal toxicity (clinical signs and reduced body weight gain). A dose of 450 mg/kg/day (4-fold the estimated human exposure level based on AUCs) correlated with increased postimplantational embryo death, including total litter loss, decreased fetal body weights, and an increased incidence of costal cartilage fusion.

In rats, mild fetal toxicity was observed at 15 and 50 mg/kg/day (exposure levels 0.13- to 0.64-fold the estimated human exposure, respectively based on AUCs). The effects consisted of decreased fetal body weights and reduced ossification of sternebrae, a finding often seen in association with decreased fetal body weights. Slight maternal toxicity, in the form of reduced body weight gain, was seen at 50 mg/kg/day.

When female rats were treated with 50 mg/kg/day (0.64-fold the estimated human exposure based on AUCs) of linezolid during pregnancy and lactation, survival of pups was decreased on postnatal days 1 to 4. Pups permitted to mature to reproductive age, when mated, showed an increase in preimplantation loss, with a corresponding decrease in fertility.

Nursing Mothers

Linezolid and its metabolites are excreted in the milk of lactating rats. Concentrations in milk were similar to those in maternal plasma. It is not known whether linezolid is excreted in human milk. Because many drugs are excreted in human milk, caution should be exercised when ZYVOX is administered to a nursing woman.

Pediatric Use

Although it may be possible to extrapolate adult efficacy to pediatric patients, the appropriate dose and safety of ZYVOX have not been established in this population. Drug clearance of ZYVOX is increased in pediatric patients compared to adults, resulting in a shorter half-life (see **CLINICAL PHARMACOLOGY, Pediatric**). Pediatric dosing regimens that provide a pharmacokinetic profile similar to adults have not been determined.

Geriatric Use

Of the 2046 patients treated with ZYVOX in phase 3 comparator-controlled clinical trials, 589 (29%) were 65 years or older and 253 (12%) were 75 years or older. No overall differences in safety or effectiveness were observed between these patients and younger patients.

ANIMAL PHARMACOLOGY

Dose- and time-dependent myelosuppression, as evidenced by bone marrow hypocellularity, decreased hematopoiesis, and decreased levels of circulating erythrocytes, leukocytes, and platelets, has been seen in animal studies. The hematopoietic effects occurred at doses of 40 and 80 mg/kg/day in dogs and rats, respectively (at exposures approximately 0.6 times in the dog and equal in the rat to the expected human exposure based on AUC). Hematopoietic effects were reversible, although in some studies reversal was incomplete within the duration of the recovery period.

ADVERSE REACTIONS

The safety of ZYVOX formulations was evaluated in 2046 patients enrolled in seven phase 3 comparator-controlled clinical trials, who were treated for up to 28 days. In these studies, 85% of the adverse events reported with ZYVOX were described as mild to moderate in intensity. Table 5 shows the incidence of adverse events reported in at least 2% of patients in these trials. The most common adverse events in patients treated with ZYVOX were diarrhea (incidence across studies: 2.8% to 11.0%), headache (incidence across studies: 0.5% to 11.3%), and nausea (incidence across studies: 3.4% to 9.6%).

Table 5. Incidence (%) of Adverse Events Reported in ≥2% of Patients in Comparator-Controlled Clinical Trials with ZYVOX

Event	ZYVOX (n = 2046)	All Comparators* (n = 2001)
Diarrhea	8.3	6.3
Headache	6.5	5.5
Nausea	6.2	4.6
Vomiting	3.7	2.0
Insomnia	2.5	1.7
Constipation	2.2	2.1
Rash	2.0	2.2
Dizziness	2.0	1.9
Fever	1.6	2.1

* Comparators included cefpodoxime proxetil 200 mg PO q12h; ceftriaxone 1 g IV q12h; clarithromycin 250 mg PO q12h; dicloxacillin 500 mg PO q6h; oxacillin 2 g IV q6h; vancomycin 1 g IV q12h.

Other adverse events reported in phase 2 and phase 3 studies included oral moniliasis, vaginal moniliasis, hypertension, dyspepsia, localized abdominal pain, pruritus, and tongue discoloration.

Table 6 shows the incidence of drug-related adverse events reported in at least 1% of patients in these trials by dose of ZYVOX.

[See table 6 at top of next page]

Laboratory Changes

ZYVOX has been associated with thrombocytopenia when used in doses up to and including 600 mg every 12 hours for up to 28 days. In phase 3 comparator-controlled trials, the percentage of patients who developed a substantially low platelet count (defined as less than 75% of lower limit of normal and/or baseline) was 2.4% (range among studies: 0.3 to 10.0%) with ZYVOX and 1.5% (range among studies: 0.4

Table 6. Incidence of Drug-Related Adverse Events Occurring in >1% of Patients Treated with ZYVOX in Comparator-Controlled Clinical Trials

Adverse Event	Uncomplicated Skin and Skin Structure Infections		All Other Indications	
	ZYVOX 400 mg PO q12h (n=548)	Clarithromycin 250 mg PO q12h (n=537)	ZYVOX 600 mg q12h (n=1498)	All Other Comparators* (n=1464)
% of patients with 1 drug-related adverse event	25.4	19.6	20.4	14.3
% of patients discontinuing due to drug-related adverse events†	3.5	2.4	2.1	1.7
Diarrhea	5.3	4.8	4.0	2.7
Nausea	3.5	3.5	3.3	1.8
Headache	2.7	2.2	1.9	1.0
Taste alteration	1.8	2.0	0.9	0.2
Vaginal moniliasis	1.6	1.3	1.0	0.4
Fungal infection	1.5	0.2	0.1	<0.1
Abnormal liver function tests	0.4	0	1.3	0.5
Vomiting	0.9	0.4	1.2	0.4
Tongue discoloration	1.1	0	0.2	0
Dizziness	1.1	1.5	0.4	0.3
Oral moniliasis	0.4	0	1.1	0.4

* Comparators included cefpodoxime proxetil 200 mg PO q12h; ceftriaxone 1 g IV q12h; dicloxacillin 500 mg PO q6h; oxacillin 2 g IV q6h; vancomycin 1 g IV q12h.
† The most commonly reported drug-related adverse events leading to discontinuation in patients treated with ZYVOX were nausea, headache, diarrhea, and vomiting.

Table 7. Percent of Patients who Experienced at Least One Substantially Abnormal* Hematology Laboratory Value in Comparator-Controlled Clinical Trials with ZYVOX

Laboratory Assay	Uncomplicated Skin and Skin Structure Infections		All Other Indications	
	ZYVOX 400 mg q12h	Clarithromycin 250 mg q12h	ZYVOX 600 mg q12h	All Other Comparators†
Hemoglobin (g/dL)	0.9	0.0	7.1	6.6
Platelet count ($\times 10^3$/mm^3)	0.7	0.8	3.0	1.8
WBC ($\times 10^3$/mm^3)	0.2	0.6	2.2	1.3
Neutrophils ($\times 10^3$/mm^3)	0.0	0.2	1.1	1.2

* <75% (<50% for neutrophils) of Lower Limit of Normal (LLN) for values normal at baseline;
<75% (<50% for neutrophils) of LLN and of baseline for values abnormal at baseline.
† Comparators included cefpodoxime proxetil 200 mg PO q12h; ceftriaxone 1 g IV q12h; dicloxacillin 500 mg PO q6h; oxacillin 2 g IV q6h; vancomycin 1 g IV q12h.

Table 8. Percent of Patients who Experienced at Least One Substantially Abnormal* Serum Chemistry Laboratory Value in Comparator-Controlled Clinical Trials with ZYVOX

Laboratory Assay	Uncomplicated Skin and Skin Structure Infections		All Other Indications	
	ZYVOX 400 mg q12h	Clarithromycin 250 mg q12h	ZYVOX 600 mg q12h	All Other Comparators†
AST (U/L)	1.7	1.3	5.0	6.8
ALT (U/L)	1.7	1.7	9.6	9.3
LDH (U/L)	0.2	0.2	1.8	1.5
Alkaline phosphatase (U/L)	0.2	0.2	3.5	3.1
Lipase (U/L)	2.8	2.6	4.3	4.2
Amylase (U/L)	0.2	0.2	2.4	2.0
Total bilirubin (mg/dL)	0.2	0.0	0.9	1.1
BUN (mg/dL)	0.2	0.0	2.1	1.5
Creatinine (mg/dL)	0.2	0.0	0.2	0.6

* >2 × Upper Limit of Normal (ULN) for values normal at baseline;
>2 × ULN and >2× baseline for values abnormal at baseline.
† Comparators included cefpodoxime proxetil 200 mg PO q12h; ceftriaxone 1 g IV q12h; dicloxacillin 500 mg PO q6h; oxacillin 2 g IV q6h; vancomycin 1 g IV q12h.

to 7.0%) with a comparator. Thrombocytopenia associated with the use of ZYVOX appears to be dependent on duration of therapy (generally greater than 2 weeks of treatment). The platelet counts for most patients returned to the normal range/baseline during the follow-up period. No related clinical adverse events were identified in phase 3 clinical trials in patients developing thrombocytopenia. Bleeding events were identified in thrombocytopenic patients in a compassionate use program for ZYVOX; the role of linezolid in these events cannot be determined (see **PRECAUTIONS**). Changes seen in other laboratory parameters, without regard to drug relationship, revealed no substantial differences between ZYVOX and the comparators. These changes were generally not clinically significant, did not lead to discontinuation of therapy, and were reversible. The incidence of patients with at least one substantially abnormal hematologic or serum chemistry value is presented in Tables 7 and 8.
[See tables 7 and 8 below]

OVERDOSAGE

In the event of overdosage, supportive care is advised, with maintenance of glomerular filtration. Hemodialysis may facilitate more rapid elimination of linezolid. In a phase 1 clinical trial, approximately 30% of a dose of linezolid was removed during a 3-hour hemodialysis session beginning 3 hours after the dose of linezolid was administered. Data are not available for removal of linezolid with peritoneal dialysis or hemoperfusion. Clinical signs of acute toxicity in animals were decreased activity and ataxia in rats and vomiting and tremors in dogs treated with 3000 mg/kg/day and 2000 mg/kg/day, respectively.

DOSAGE AND ADMINISTRATION

The recommended dosage for ZYVOX formulations for the treatment of infections is described in Table 9. Doses of ZYVOX are administered every twelve hours (q12h).
[See table 9 at top of next page]
Patients with infection due to MRSA should be treated with ZYVOX 600 mg q12h.
In controlled clinical trials, the protocol-defined duration of treatment for all infections ranged from 7 to 28 days. Total treatment duration was determined by the treating physician based on site and severity of the infection, and on the patient's clinical response.
No dose adjustment is necessary when switching from intravenous to oral administration. Patients whose therapy is started with ZYVOX I.V. Injection may be switched to either ZYVOX Tablets or Oral Suspension at the discretion of the physician, when clinically indicated.

Intravenous Administration

ZYVOX I.V. Injection is supplied in single-use, ready-to-use infusion bags (see **HOW SUPPLIED** for container sizes). Parenteral drug products should be inspected visually for particulate matter prior to administration. Check for minute leaks by firmly squeezing the bag. If leaks are detected, discard the solution, as sterility may be impaired.
ZYVOX I.V. Injection should be administered by intravenous infusion over a period of 30 to 120 minutes. **Do not use this intravenous infusion bag in series connections.** Additives should not be introduced into this solution. If ZYVOX I.V. Injection is to be given concomitantly with another drug, each drug should be given separately in accordance with the recommended dosage and route of administration for each product. In particular, physical incompatibilities resulted when ZYVOX I.V. Injection was combined with the following drugs during simulated Y-site administration: amphotericin B, chlorpromazine HCl, diazepam, pentamidine isothionate, erythromycin lactobionate, phenytoin sodium, and trimethoprim-sulfamethoxazole. Additionally, chemical incompatibility resulted when ZYVOX I.V. Injection was combined with ceftriaxone sodium.
If the same intravenous line is used for sequential infusion of several drugs, the line should be flushed before and after infusion of ZYVOX I.V. Injection with an infusion solution compatible with ZYVOX I.V. Injection and with any other drug(s) administered via this common line (see **Compatible Intravenous Solutions**).

Compatible Intravenous Solutions

5% Dextrose Injection, USP
0.9% Sodium Chloride Injection, USP
Lactated Ringer's Injection, USP
Keep the infusion bags in the overwrap until ready to use. Store at room temperature. Protect from freezing. ZYVOX I.V. Injection may exhibit a yellow color that can intensify over time without adversely affecting potency.

Constitution of Oral Suspension

ZYVOX for Oral Suspension is supplied as a powder/granule for constitution. Gently tap bottle to loosen powder. Add a total of 123 mL distilled water in two portions. After adding the first half, shake vigorously to wet all of the powder. Then add the second half of the water and shake vigorously to obtain a uniform suspension. After constitution, each 5 mL of the suspension contains 100 mg of linezolid. Before using, gently mix by inverting the bottle 3 to 5 times. **DO NOT SHAKE.** Store constituted suspension at room temperature. Use within 21 days after constitution.

HOW SUPPLIED

Injection

ZYVOX I.V. Injection is available in single-use, ready-to-use flexible plastic infusion bags in a foil laminate overwrap. The infusion bags and ports are latex-free. The infusion bags are available in the following package sizes:

100 mL bag (200 mg linezolid)	NDC 0009-5137-01
200 mL bag (400 mg linezolid)	NDC 0009-5139-01
300 mL bag (600 mg linezolid)	NDC 0009-5140-01

Tablets

ZYVOX Tablets are available as follows:
400 mg (white, oblong, film-coated tablets printed with "ZYVOX 400 mg")

100 tablets in HDPE bottle	NDC 0009-5134-01
20 tablets in HDPE bottle	NDC 0009-5134-02
Unit dose packages of 30 tablets	NDC 0009-5134-03

Continued on next page

Information on these Pharmacia & Upjohn products is based on labeling in effect June 1, 2000. Further information concerning these and other Pharmacia & Upjohn products may be obtained by direct inquiry to Medical Information, Pharmacia & Upjohn, Kalamazoo, MI 49001.

Zyvox—Cont.

600 mg (white, capsule-shaped, film-coated tablets printed with "ZYVOX 600 mg")

100 tablets in HDPE bottle	NDC 0009-5135-01
20 tablets in HDPE bottle	NDC 0009-5135-02
Unit dose packages of 30 tablets	NDC 0009-5135-03

Oral Suspension

ZYVOX for Oral Suspension is available as a dry, white to off-white, orange-flavored granule/powder. When constituted as directed, each bottle will contain 150 mL of a suspension providing the equivalent of 100 mg of linezolid per each 5 mL. ZYVOX for Oral Suspension is supplied as follows:

100 mg/5 mL in 240-mL glass bottles	NDC 0009-5136-01

Storage of ZYVOX Formulations

Store at 25°C (77°F); excursions permitted to 15-30°C (59-86°F) [see USP Controlled Room Temperature]. Protect from light. Keep bottles tightly closed to protect from moisture. It is recommended that the infusion bags be kept in the overwrap until ready to use. Protect infusion bags from freezing.

CLINICAL STUDIES

Vancomycin-Resistant Enterococcal Infections

Adult patients with documented or suspected vancomycin-resistant enterococcal infection were enrolled in a randomized, multi-center, double-blind trial comparing a high dose of ZYVOX (600 mg q12h IV or orally) with a low dose of ZYVOX (200 mg q12h IV or orally) for 7 to 28 days. Patients could receive concomitant aztreonam or aminoglycosides. There were 79 patients randomized to high-dose linezolid and 66 to low-dose linezolid. The intent-to-treat (ITT) population with documented vancomycin-resistant enterococcal infection at baseline consisted of 65 patients in the high-dose arm and 52 in the low-dose arm.

The cure rates for the ITT population with documented vancomycin-resistant enterococcal infection at baseline are presented in Table 10 by source of infection. These cure rates do not include patients with missing or indeterminate outcomes. The cure rate was higher in the high-dose arm than in the low-dose arm, although the difference was not statistically significant at the 0.05 level.

Table 10. Cure Rates at the Test-of-Cure Visit for ITT Patients with Documented Vancomycin-Resistant Enterococcal Infections at Baseline

Source of Infection	Cured	
	ZYVOX 600 mg q12h n/N (%)	ZYVOX 200 mg q12h n/N (%)
Any site	39/58 (67)	24/46 (52)
Any site with associated bacteremia	10/17 (59)	4/14 (29)
Bacteremia of unknown origin	5/10 (50)	2/7 (29)
Skin and skin structure	9/13 (69)	5/5 (100)
Urinary tract	12/19 (63)	12/20 (60)
Pneumonia	2/3 (67)	0/1 (0)
Other*	11/13 (85)	5/13 (39)

* Includes sources of infection such as hepatic abscess, biliary sepsis, necrotic gallbladder, pericolonic abscess, pancreatitis, and catheter-related infection.

Nosocomial Pneumonia

Adult patients with clinically and radiologically documented nosocomial pneumonia were enrolled in a randomized, multicenter, double-blind trial. Patients were treated for 7 to 21 days. One group received ZYVOX I.V. Injection 600 mg every twelve hours (q12h), and the other group received vancomycin 1 g q12h intravenously (IV). Both groups received concomitant aztreonam (1 to 2 every 8 hours IV), which could be continued if clinically indicated. There were 203 linezolid-treated and 193 vanocmycin-treated patients enrolled in the study. One hundred twenty-two (60%) linezolid-treated patients and 103 (53%) vancomycin-treated patients were clinically evaluable. The cure rates in clinically evaluable patients were 57% for linezolid-treated patients and 60% for vancomycin-treated patients. The cure rates in clinically evaluable patients with ventilator-associated pneumonia were 47% for linezolid-treated patients and 40% for vancomycin-treated patients. A modified intent-to-treat (MITT) analysis of 94 linezolid-treated patients and 83 vancomycin-treated patients included subjects who had a pathogen isolated before treatment. The cure rates in the MITT analysis were 57% in linezolid-treated patients and 46% in vancomycin-treated patients. The cure rates by pathogen for microbiologically evaluable patients are presented in Table 11.

Table 9. Dosage Guidelines for ZYVOX

Infection*	Dosage and Route of Administration	Recommended Duration of Treatment (consecutive days)
Vancomycin-resistant *Enterococcus faecium* infections, including concurrent bacteremia	600 mg IV or oral† q12h	14 to 28
Nosocomial pneumonia	600 mg IV or oral† q12h	10 to 14
Complicated skin and skin structure infections		
Community-acquired pneumonia, including concurrent bacteremia		
Uncomplicated skin and skin structure infections	400 mg oral† q12h	10 to 14

* due to the designated pathogens (see **INDICATIONS AND USAGE**)
† oral dosing using either ZYVOX Tablets or ZYVOX for Oral Suspension

Table 11. Cure Rates at the Test-of-Cure Visit for Microbiologically Evaluable Patients with Nosocomial Pneumonia

Pathogen	Cured	
	ZYVOX n/N (%)	Vancomycin n/N (%)
Staphylococcus aureus	23/38 (61)	14/23 (61)
Methicillin-resistant *S. aureus*	13/22 (59)	7/10 (70)
Streptococcus pneumoniae	9/9 (100)	9/10 (90)

Complicated Skin and Skin Structure Infections

Adult patients with clinically documented complicated skin and skin structure infections were enrolled in a randomized, multi-center, double-blind, double-dummy trial comparing study medications administered IV followed by medications given orally for a total of 10 to 21 days of treatment. One group of patients received ZYVOX I.V. Injection 600 mg q12h followed by ZYVOX Tablets 600 mg q12h; the other group received oxacillin 2 g every 6 hours (q6h) IV followed by dicloxacillin 500 mg q6h orally. Patients could receive concomitant aztreonam if clinically indicated. There were 400 linezolid-treated and 419 oxacillin-treated patients enrolled in the study. Two hundred forty-five (61%) linezolid-treated patients and 242 (58%) oxacillin-treated patients were clinically evaluable. The cure rates in clinically evaluable patients were 90% in linezolid-treated patients and 85% in oxacillin-treated patients. A modified intent-to-treat (MITT) analysis of 316 linezolid-treated patients and 313 oxacillin-treated patients included subjects who met all criteria for study entry. The cure rates in the MITT analysis were 86% in linezolid-treated patients and 82% in oxacillin-treated patients. The cure rates by pathogen for microbiologically evaluable patients are presented in Table 12.

Table 12. Cure Rates at the Test-of-Cure Visit for Microbiologically Evaluable Patients with Complicated Skin and Skin Structure Infections

Pathogen	Cured	
	ZYVOX n/N (%)	Oxacillin/ Dicloxacillin n/N (%)
Staphylococcus aureus	73/83 (88)	72/84 (86)
Methicillin-resistant *S. aureus*	2/3 (67)	0/0 (–)
Streptococcus agalactiae	6/6 (100)	3/6 (50)
Streptococcus pyogenes	18/26 (69)	21/28 (75)

A separate study provided additional experience with the use of linezolid in the treatment of methicillin-resistant *Staphylococcus aureus* (MRSA) infections. This was a randomized, open-label trial in hospitalized adult patients with documented or suspected MRSA infection.

One group of patients received ZYVOX I.V. Injection 600 mg q12h followed by ZYVOX Tablets 600 mg q12h. The other group of patients received vancomycin 1 g q12h IV. Both groups were treated for 7 to 28 days, and could receive concomitant aztreonam or gentamicin if clinically indicated. The cure rates in microbiologically evaluable patients with MRSA skin and skin structure infection were 26/33 (79%) for linezolid-treated patients and 24/33 (73%) for vancomycin-treated patients.

REFERENCES

1. National Committee for Clinical Laboratory Standards. Methods for Dilution Antimicrobial Susceptibility Tests for Bacteria that Grow Aerobically. Fifth Edition. Approved Standard NCCLS Document M7-A5, Vol. 20, No. 2, NCCLS, Wayne, PA, January 2000.
2. National Committee for Clinical Laboratory Standards. Performance Standards for Antimicrobial Disk Susceptibility Tests. Seventh Edition. Approved Standard NCCLS Document M2-A7, Vol. 20, No. 1, NCCLS, Wayne, PA, January 2000.
3. National Committee for Clinical Laboratory Standards. Tenth Informational Supplement. Approved NCCLS Document M100-S10, Vol. 20, No. 1, NCCLS, Wayne, PA, January 2000.
4. Walker, SE et al. Tyramine content of previously restricted foods in monoamine oxidase inhibitor diets. Journal of Clinical Psychopharmacology 1996; 16 (5):383-388.
5. DaPrada, M et al. On tyramine, food, beverages and the reversible MAO inhibitor moclobemide. 1988; [Supplement] 26:31-56.

℞ only

US Patent No. 5,688,792

Injection

Manufactured for: Pharmacia & Upjohn Company, Kalamazoo, Michigan 49001
By: Fresenius Kabi Norge AS, Halden, Norway

Tablets and Oral Suspension

Manufactured by: Pharmacia & Upjohn Company, Kalamazoo, Michigan 49001

April 2000 818 073 000

PolyMedica Pharmaceuticals (U.S.A.), Inc.

11 STATE STREET
WOBURN, MA 01801

For Medical Information Contact:
In Emergencies:
Peter Etzel or Arthur Siciliano
(781) 933-2020
FAX: (781) 933-7992

ANESTACON® ℞

(lidocaine hydrochloride jelly, USP) 2%

DESCRIPTION

Each mL contains: Active: Lidocaine Hydrochloride 20 mg/ml (2%). Vehicle: Hydroxypropyl Methylcellulose 10 mg (1%). Preservative: Benzalkonium Chloride 0.1 mg (0.01%). Inactive: Sodium Chloride, Hydrochloric Acid and/or Sodium Hydroxide (to adjust pH to 6.0–7.0), Purified Water. The resulting mixture maximizes contact with mucosa and provides lubrication for instrumentation.

HOW SUPPLIED

In 15 ml. unit-dose for **SINGLE PATIENT USE.**

B & O SUPPRETTES® CII ℞

No. 15A and No. 16A
(Belladonna and Opium) Rectal Suppositories

DESCRIPTION

Each B&O SUPPRETTE® contains (in the water-soluble NEOCERA® Suppository Base for rectal administration):

B&O No. 15A: Powdered opium* 30 mg (0.46 gr) and Powdered Belladonna Extract 16.2 mg (equivalent to 0.21 mg or 0.0032 gr belladonna alkaloids).

B&O No. 16A: Powdered opium* 60 mg (0.92 gr) and Powdered Belladonna Extract 16.2 mg (equivalent to 0.21 mg or 0.0032 gr belladonna alkaloids).

Store at room temperature. DO NOT REFRIGERATE.

HOW SUPPLIED

In strip packaged units of 12 and 144.

CYSTOSPAZ® ℞
(hyoscyamine) Tablets

CYSTOSPAZ–M® ℞
(hyoscyamine sulfate) Timed-Release Capsules

DESCRIPTION

CYSTOSPAZ® is a pale blue uncoated compressed tablet for oral administration. It contains the parasympatholytic agent hyoscyamine as the free base. Each tablet contains: hyoscyamine 0.15 mg.
CYSTOSPAZ-M® is a light blue timed-release capsule containing hyoscyamine sulfate 0.375 mg.

CLINICAL PHARMACOLOGY

Through its parasympatholytic action, hyoscyamine relaxes smooth muscle spasm resulting from parasympathetic stimulation. It inhibits gastrointestinal propulsive motility and decreases gastric acid secretion. It also controls excessive pharyngeal, tracheal and bronchial secretions. It is theλ-isomer of atropine and therefore exhibits the same clinical effects as atropine. It is, however, approximately twice as active peripherally as atropine, since the latter is the racemic (dλ) form of hyoscyamine and d-hyoscyamine possesses only a very weak anti-cholinergic action. Since only one-half the atropine dose is required for λ-hyoscyamine, it has only one-half the unwanted central effects of atropine.

INDICATIONS AND USAGE

In the management of disorders of the lower urinary tract associated with hypermotility. Although specific therapy is often required to remove the underlying cause of spasm, CYSTOSPAZ Tablets and CYSTOSPAZ-M Capsules are offered as antispasmodic agent dosage forms which may be combined with other forms of therapy where indicated.
CYSTOSPAZ Tablets and CYSTOSPAZ-M capsules are effective as adjunctive therapy in the treatment of peptic ulcer and irritable bowel syndrome (irritable colon, spastic colon, mucous colitis), acute entercolitis and other functional gastrointestinal disorders.
CYSTOSPAZ Tablets and CYSTOSPAZ-M Capsules can also be used to control gastric secretion, visceral spasm and hypermotility in cystitis, pylorospasm and associated abdominal cramps. May be used in functional intestinal disorders to reduce symptoms such as those seen in mild dysenteries and diverticulitis. They are indicated (along with appropriate analgesics) in symptomatic relief of biliary and renal colic.

CONTRAINDICATIONS

Glaucoma, obstructive uropathy (for example, bladder neck obstruction due to prostatic hypertrophy); obstructive disease of the gastrointestinal tract (as in achalasia, pyloroduodenal stenosis); paralytic ileus, intestinal atony of elderly or debilitated patients; unstable cardiovascular status in acute hemorrhage; severe ulcerative colitis; toxic megacolon complicating ulcerative colitis; myasthenia gravis. Hypersensitivity to any of the ingredients.

WARNINGS

In the presence of high environmental temperature, heat prostration can occur with drug use (fever and heat stroke due to decreased sweating). Diarrhea may be an early symptom of incomplete intestinal obstruction, especially in patients with ileostomy or colostomy. In this instance, treatment with this drug would be inappropriate and possibly harmful. Like other anticholinergic agents, these products may produce drowsiness or blurred vision. In this event, the patient should be warned not to engage in activities requiring mental alertness such as operating a motor vehicle or other machinery or to perform hazardous work while taking this drug.

PRECAUTIONS

General: Use with caution in patients with autonomic neuropathy, hyperthyroidism, coronary heart disease, congestive heart failure, cardiac arrhythmias, and hypertension. Investigate any tachycardia before giving any anticholinergic drug since they may increase the heart rate. Use with caution in patients with hiatal hernia associated with reflux esophagitis.
Information for Patients: CYSTOSPAZ Tablets and CYSTOSPAZ-M Capsules may cause drowsiness, dizziness or blurred vision; patients should observe caution before driving, using machinery or performing other tasks requiring mental alertness. Use of CYSTOSPAZ Tablets or CYSTOSPAZ-M Capsules may decrease sweating resulting in heat prostration, fever or heat stroke; febrile patients or those who may be exposed to elevated environmental temperatures should use caution. Prolonged use of CYSTOSPAZ Tablets or CYSTOSPAZ-M Capsules may decrease or inhibit salivary flow, thus contributing to the development of caries, periodontal disease, oral candidiasis, and discomfort.

DRUG INTERACTIONS

Additive adverse effects resulting from cholinergic blockade may occur when CYSTOSPAZ® Tablets or CYSTOSPAZ-M Capsules are administered concomitantly with other antimuscarinics, amanatadine, haloperidol, phenothiazines, monoamine oxidase (MAO) inhibitors, tricyclic antidepressants or some antihistamines. Antacids may interfere with the absorption of CYSTOSPAZ Tablets or CYSTOSPAZ-M Capsules; take CYSTOSPAZ Tablets or CYSTOSPAZ-M Capsules before meals and antacids after meals.

Carcinogenesis, Mutagenesis, Impairment Of Fertility: No long term studies in animals have been performed to determine the carcinogenic, mutagenic or impairment of fertility potential of CYSTOSPAZ Tablets or CYSTOSPAZ-M Capsules.
Pregnancy Category C—Animal reproduction studies have not been conducted with CYSTOSPAZ Tablets or CYSTOSPAZ-M Capsules. It is also not known whether CYSTOSPAZ Tablets or CYSTOSPAZ-M Capsules can cause fetal harm when administered to a pregnant woman or can affect reproduction capacity. CYSTOSPAZ Tablets or CYSTOSPAZ-M Capsules should be taken by a pregnant woman only if clearly needed.
Nursing Mothers—Hyoscyamine is excreted in human milk. Caution should be exercised when CYSTOSPAZ Tablets or CYSTOSPAZ-M Capsules are administered to a nursing woman.

ADVERSE REACTIONS

Adverse reactions may include dryness of the mouth; urinary hesitancy and retention; blurred vision; tachycardia; palpitations; mydriasis; cycloplegia; increased ocular tension; headache; nervousness; drowsiness; weakness; suppression of lactation; allergic reactions or drug idiosyncrasies; urticaria and other dermal manifestations; and decreased sweating. **Note:** Slight dryness of the mouth is an indication that parasympathetic blockage is effective.

DRUG ABUSE AND DEPENDENCE

A dependence on the use of CYSTOSPAZ Tablets or CYSTOSPAZ-M Capsules has not been reported and due to the nature of their ingredients, abuse of CYSTOSPAZ Tablets or CYSTOSPAZ-M Capsules is not expected.

OVERDOSAGE

Symptoms of overdosage include severe dryness of the mouth, nose, throat, and hot dry flushed skin, hyperpyrexia (especially in children), difficulty or inability to swallow, difficult speech, dilated pupils until iris almost disappears, restlessness and garrulity indicating an irritability of the brain, marked tremors, convulsions, respiratory failure, death. In adults, symptoms of overdosage may begin in the range of ingestion of 0.6 to 1 mg with doses exceeding 1–2 mg eliciting more profound toxicity. Measures to be taken are immediate lavage of the stomach and injection of physostigmine 0.5 to 2 mg intravenously and repeated as necessary up to a total of 5 mg. Fever may be treated symptomatically (tepid water sponge baths, hypothermic blanket). Excitement to a degree which demands attention may be managed with sodium thiopental 2% solution given slowly intravenously or chloral hydrate (100–200 ml. of a 2% solution) by rectal infusion.

DOSAGE AND ADMINISTRATION

Adults: CYSTOSPAZ Tablets—One or two tablets four times daily or fewer if needed. CYSTOSPAZ-M Capsules—One capsule every twelve hours.
Children (12 and under): Reduce dosage in proportion to age and weight.

HOW SUPPLIED

CYSTOSPAZ Tablets— Bottles of 100 light blue tablets. Tablets are imprinted with a "**W** 2225". CYSTOSPAZ-M Capsules—Bottles of 100 light blue timed-release capsules. Capsules are identified with "**W** 2260" printed in black.

URISED® ℞

DESCRIPTION

URISED® is a dark blue, round, tablet for oral administration. It is a combination of antiseptics (Methenamine, Methylene Blue, Phenyl Salicylate, Benzoic Acid) and parasympatholytics (Atropine Sulfate, Hyoscyamine).
Each tablet contains: Methenamine 40.8 mg, Phenyl Salicylate 18.1 mg, Methylene Blue 5.4 mg, Benzoic Acid 4.5 mg, Atropine Sulfate 0.03 mg and Hyoscyamine (as the sulfate) 0.03 mg.

CLINICAL PHARMACOLOGY

Methenamine itself does not have antiseptic, irritant, or toxic properties in the urine. Methenamine, in an acid urine (pH 6 or below), hydrolyzes into formaldehyde within the urinary tract providing mild antiseptic activity. When given as directed and the daily urine volume is 1000 to 1500 mL, a daily dose of 2 grams will yield a urinary concentration of 18–60 mcg/mL of free formaldehyde in the urine. This is more than the minimal inhibitory dose of formaldehyde which must be available for most urinary tract pathogens. Methenamine is readily absorbed from the gastrointestinal tract and is rapidly excreted almost entirely in the urine. Methylene Blue and Benzoic Acid are mild but effective antiseptics which contribute to the antiseptic properties of Methenamine. Phenyl Salicylate is a mild analgesic and antipyretic with weak antiseptic activity. All of these compounds are readily absorbed from the gastrointestinal tract and excreted in the urine. Through parasympatholytic action, atropine and hyoscyamine relax smooth muscle spasms resulting from parasympathetic stimulation.

INDICATIONS AND USAGE

URISED is indicated for the relief of discomfort of the lower urinary tract caused by hypermotility resulting from inflammation or diagnostic procedures and in the treatment of cystitis, urethritis, and trigonitis when caused by organisms which maintain or produce an acid urine and are susceptible to formaldehyde.

CONTRAINDICATIONS

Glaucoma, urinary bladder neck obstruction, pyloric or duodenal obstruction, or cardiospasm. Hypersensitivity to any of the ingredients.

WARNINGS

Do not exceed recommended dose. Methenamine may combine with sulfonamides in the urine to give mutual antagonism and should not be used with sulfonamides.

PRECAUTIONS

Administer with caution to persons with known idiosyncrasy to atropine-like compounds and to patients suffering from cardiac disease. Bacteriological studies of the urine may be helpful in following the patient response. Methylene Blue interferes with the analysis for some urinary components such as free formaldehyde. Drugs and/or foods which produce an alkaline urine should be restricted.
Patient should be advised that the urine may become blue to blue-green and the feces may be discolored as a result of excretion of Methylene Blue, so care should be taken to avoid staining clothing or other items. To avoid Methylene Blue stains on the skin, mouth or teeth, patients should be sure their hands are dry and that the tablets are swallowed quickly followed with liberal fluid intake. Methenamine preparations should not be given to patients taking sulfonamides since insoluble precipitates may form with formaldehyde in the urine. No known long-term animal studies have been performed to evaluate carcinogenic potential. The precautions related to drug interaction, diagnostic interference, medical problems and side effects to use of belladonna alkaloids, should be observed.
Pregnancy Category C. Animal reproduction studies have not been conducted with URISED® tablets. It is also not known whether URISED tablets can cause fetal harm when administered to a pregnant woman or can affect reproduction capacity. URISED tablets should be given to a pregnant woman only if clearly needed.
Nursing Mothers: It is not known whether this drug is excreted in human milk. Because many drugs are excreted in human milk, caution should be exercised when URISED tablets are administered to a nursing woman.
Prolonged Use: There have been no studies to establish the safety of prolonged use in humans.

ADVERSE REACTIONS

Prolonged use may result in a generalized skin rash, pronounced dryness of the mouth, flushing, difficulty in initiating micturition, rapid pulse, dizziness or blurring of vision. If any of these reactions occurs, discontinue use immediately. Acute urinary retention may be precipitated in prostatic hypertrophy. See "OVERDOSAGE."

DRUG ABUSE AND DEPENDENCE

A dependence on the use of URISED has not been reported and due to the nature of its ingredients, abuse of URISED is not expected.

OVERDOSAGE

By exceeding the recommended dosage of URISED, symptomology related to the overdose of its individual active ingredients may be expected as follows:
Atropine Sulfate, Hyoscyamine: Symptoms associated with an overdosage of URISED will most probably be manifested in the symptoms related to overdosage of the alkaloids Atropine Sulfate and Hyoscyamine. Such symptoms as dryness of mucous membranes; dilatation of pupils; hot, dry, flushed skin; hyperpyrexia; tachycardia; palpitations; elevated blood pressure; coma; circulatory collapse and death from respiratory failure can occur due to overdosage of these alkaloids.
Methenamine: If large amounts of the drug (2–8 gm daily) are used over extended periods (3–4 weeks), bladder and gastrointestinal irritation, painful and frequent micturition, albuminuria and gross hematuria may be expected.
Methylene Blue: Symptoms of Methylene Blue overdosage associated with the overdosage of URISED are not expected to be discernible from those associated with the other active ingredients in URISED.
Benzoic Acid: Symptoms of Benzoic Acid overdosage associated with the overdosage of URISED are not expected to be discernible from those associated with the other active ingredients in URISED.
Phenyl Salicylate: Symptoms of Phenyl Salicylate overdosage include burning pain in throat and mouth, white necrotic lesions in the mouth, abdominal pain, vomiting, bloody diarrhea, pallor, sweating, weakness, headache, dizziness and tinnitus. The symptoms, however, are not expected to be discernible from those associated with the other active ingredients in URISED.

DOSAGE AND ADMINISTRATION

Adults: Two tablets four times daily. See "PRECAUTIONS."
Usual pediatric dosage: Children up to 6 years of age—Use is not recommended. Children 6 years of age and older—Dosage must be individualized by physician.

HOW SUPPLIED

Bottles of 100 and 500 tablets imprinted "**W** 2183".

Procter & Gamble
P.O. BOX 5516
CINCINNATI, OH 45201

Direct Inquiries to:
Charles Lambert
(800) 358-8707

For Medical Emergencies:
Call Collect: (513) 558-4422

CHILDREN'S VICKS® NYQUIL® OTC
COLD/COUGH RELIEF
Antihistamine/Nasal Decongestant/Cough Suppressant

(See PDR For Nonprescription Drugs.)

HEAD & SHOULDERS® DANDRUFF SHAMPOO OTC

Head & Shoulders Dandruff Shampoo for Normal hair offers effective control of persistent dandruff, and beautiful hair from a pleasant-to-use formula. Double-blind and expert-graded testing have proven that Head & Shoulders Dandruff Shampoo reduces dandruff. It is also gentle enough to use every day for clean, manageable hair.

ACTIVE INGREDIENT

1% pyrithione zinc suspended in a mild surfactant base. Shampoo also includes mild conditioning agents.

INDICATIONS

For effective control of dandruff of the scalp.

ACTIONS

Head & Shoulders reduces the flaking and itching caused by dandruff. The pyrithione zinc active helps kill the microscopic fungus associated with dandruff.

WARNINGS

For external use only. Avoid contact with eyes. If contact occurs, rinse eyes thoroughly with water. If condition worsens or does not improve after regular use of this product as directed, consult a doctor. Keep this and all drugs out of the reach of children.

DOSAGE AND ADMINISTRATION

For best results, use Head & Shoulders at least twice a week or as directed by a doctor. It is gentle enough to use for every shampoo.

INGREDIENTS

Pyrithione zinc in a shampoo base of water, ammonium laureth sulfate, ammonium lauryl sulfate, sodium lauroyl sarcosinate, glycol distearate, sodium sulfate, dimethicone, fragrance, DMDM hydantoin, disodium phosphate, sodium phosphate, lauryl alcohol, PEG-600, sodium chloride, polyquaternium-10 and FD&C Blue No. 1.

HOW SUPPLIED

Head & Shoulders Dandruff Shampoo is available in 2 FL OZ, 6.8 FL OZ, 15.2 FL OZ and 25.4 FL OZ unbreakable plastic bottles.

HEAD & SHOULDERS® DANDRUFF SHAMPOO DRY SCALP OTC

Head & Shoulders Dandruff Shampoo Dry Scalp offers effective control of persistent dandruff, and beautiful hair from a pleasant-to-use formula. Double-blind and expert-graded testing have proven that Head & Shoulders Dandruff Shampoo reduces dandruff. It is also gentle enough to use every day for clean, manageable hair.

ACTIVE INGREDIENT

1% pyrithione zinc suspended in a mild surfactant base. Shampoo also includes mild conditioning agents.

INDICATIONS

For effective control of dandruff of the scalp.

ACTIONS

Head & Shoulders reduces the flaking and itching caused by dandruff. The pyrithione zinc active helps kill the microscopic fungus associated with dandruff.

WARNINGS

For external use only. Avoid contact with eyes. If contact occurs, rinse eyes thoroughly with water. If condition worsens or does not improve after regular use of this product as directed, consult a doctor. Keep this and all drugs out of the reach of children.

DOSAGE AND ADMINISTRATION

For best results, use Head & Shoulders at least twice a week or as directed by a doctor. It is gentle enough to use for every shampoo.

INGREDIENTS

Pyrithione zinc in a shampoo base of water, ammonium laureth sulfate, ammonium lauryl sulfate, sodium lauroyl sarcosinate, glycol distearate, sodium sulfate, dimethicone, fragrance, DMDM hydantoin, disodium phosphate, sodium phosphate, lauryl alcohol, PEG-600, sodium chloride polyquaternium-10 and FD&C Blue No. 1.

HOW SUPPLIED

Head & Shoulders Dandruff Shampoo Dry Scalp is available in 2 FL OZ, 6.8 FL OZ, 15.2 FL OZ and 25.4 FL OZ unbreakable plastic bottles.

HEAD & SHOULDERS® INTENSIVE TREATMENT DANDRUFF AND SEBORRHEIC DERMATITIS SHAMPOO OTC

Head & Shoulders Intensive Treatment Dandruff and Seborrheic Dermatitis Shampoo offers effective control of persistent dandruff, and beautiful hair from a pleasant-to-use formula. Double-blind and expert-graded testing have proven that Intensive Treatment Dandruff and Seborrheic Dermatitis Shampoo reduces persistent dandruff. It is also gentle enough to use every day for clean, manageable hair.

Active Ingredient 1% selenium sulfide suspended in a mild surfactant base. Shampoo also includes mild conditioning agents.

INDICATIONS

For effective control of seborrheic dermatitis and dandruff of the scalp.

ACTIONS

Selenium sulfide is substantive to the scalp and remains after rinsing. Its mechanism is believed to be antiproliferative, and to also control the microorganisms associated with persistent dandruff flaking and itching.

WARNINGS

For external use only. Avoid contact with the eyes. If contact occurs, rinse eyes thoroughly with water. If condition worsens or does not improve after regular use of this product as directed, consult a doctor. Keep this and all drugs out of the reach of children.

CAUTION

If used on bleached, tinted, grey, or permed hair, rinse for 5 minutes.

DOSAGE AND ADMINISTRATION

For best results, use at least twice a week or as directed by a doctor. It is gentle enough to use for every shampoo.

INGREDIENTS

Selenium sulfide in a shampoo base of water, ammonium laureth sulfate, ammonium lauryl sulfate, cocamide MEA, glycol distearate, ammonium xylenesulfonate, dimethicone, fragrance, tricetylmonium chloride, cetyl alcohol, DMDM hydantoin, sodium chloride, stearyl alcohol, hydroxypropyl methylcellulose, FD&C Red No. 4.

HOW SUPPLIED

Intensive Treatment Dandruff and Seborrheic Dermatitis Shampoo is available in 15 FL OZ unbreakable plastic bottles.

METAMUCIL® FIBER LAXATIVE OTC
[*met uh-mü sil*]
(psyllium husk)
Also see ***Metamucil Dietary Fiber Supplement*** *in PDR for Nonprescription Drugs*

DESCRIPTION

Metamucil contains psyllium husk (from the plant *Plantago ovata*), a bulk forming, natural therapeutic fiber for restoring and maintaining regularity when recommended by a physician. Metamucil contains no chemical stimulants and does not disrupt normal bowel function. Each dose contains approximately 3.4 grams of psyllium husk (or about 2.3 grams of soluble fiber). Inactive ingredients, sodium, calcium, potassium, calories, carbohydrate, and dietary fiber content are shown in the following table for all versions and flavors. Metamucil Smooth Texture Sugar-Free Regular flavor contains no sugar and no artificial sweeteners; Metamucil Smooth Texture Sugar-Free Orange Flavor contains aspartame (phenylalanine content per dose is 25 mg). Metamucil powdered products are gluten-free. Metamucil Fiber Wafers contain gluten: Apple Crisp contains 0.7g/dose, Cinnamon Spice contains 0.5g/dose. Each two-wafer dose contains 5 grams of fat.

ACTIONS

The active ingredient in Metamucil is psyllium husk, a natural fiber which promotes elimination due to its bulking effect in the colon. This bulking effect is due to both the water-holding capacity of undigested fiber and the increased bacterial mass following partial fiber digestion. These actions result in enlargement of the lumen of the colon and softer

Metamucil®

Fiber Laxative/Dietary Fiber Supplement

Versions/Flavors	Ingredients	Sodium mg/dose	Calcium mg/dose	Potassium mg/dose	Calories kcal/dose	Total Carbohydrate g/dose	Dietary Fiber/ (Soluble)g per dose	Dosage (Weight in gms)	How Supplied
Smooth Texture Orange Flavor Metamucil Powder	Citric Acid, F D & C Yellow #6, Natural and Artificial Flavor, Psyllium Husk, Sucrose	5	7	30	45	12	3 (2.3)	1 rounded tablespoon ~ 12g	Canisters: Doses: 48, 72, 114; Cartons: 30 single-dose packets.
Smooth Texture Sugar-Free Orange Flavor Metamucil Powder	Aspartame, Citric Acid, FD&C Yellow #6, Maltodextrin, Natural and Artificial Flavor, Psyllium Husk	5	7	30	20	5	3 (2.3)	1 rounded teaspoon ~5.8g	Canisters: Doses: 48, 72 114, 180; Cartons:30 single-dose packets
Smooth Texture Sugar-Free Regular Flavor Metamucil Powder	Citric Acid, Maltodextrin, Psyllium Husk	4	7	30	20	5	3 (2.3)	1 rounded teaspoon ~5.4g	Canisters: Doses: 48, 72 114
Original Texture Regular Flavor Metamucil Powder	Psyllium Husk, Sucrose	3	6	30	25	6	3 (2.3)	1 rounded teaspoon ~7g	Canisters: Doses: 48, 72 114
Original Texture Orange Flavor Metamucil Powder	Citric Acid, FD&C Yellow #6, Natural and Artificial Flavor, Psyllium Husk, Sucrose	5	6	30	40	10	3 (2.3)	1 rounded tablespoon ~11g	Canisters: Doses: 48, 72 114
Fiber Laxative									
Apple Crisp Metamucil Wafers	(1)	20	14	60	120	17	6	2 wafers 24 g	Cartons: 12 doses
Cinnamon Spice Metamucil Wafers	(2)	20	14	60	120	17	6	2 wafers 24g	Cartons: 12 doses

(1) Ascorbic Acid, Brown Sugar, Cinnamon, Corn Oil, Flavoring, Fructose, Lecithin, Modified Food Starch, Molasses, Oat Hull Fiber, Sodium Bicarbonate, Sucrose, Wate, Wheat Flour
(2) Ascorbic Acid, Cinnamon, Corn Oil, Flavoring, Fructose, Lecithin, Modified Food Starch, Molasses, Nutmeg, Oat Hull Fiber, Oats, Sodium Bicarbonate, Sucrose,, Water, Wheat Flour

stool, thereby decreasing intraluminal pressure and straining, and speeding colonic transit in constipated patients.

INDICATIONS

Metamucil is indicated for the treatment of occasional constipation, and when recommended by a physician, for chronic constipation and constipation associated with irritable bowel syndrome, diverticulosis, hemorrhoids, convalescence, senility and pregnancy. Pregnancy: Category B. If considering use of Metamucil as part of a cholesterol-lowering program, see **Metamucil Dietary Fiber Supplement** in Dietary Supplement Section.

CONTRAINDICATIONS

Intestinal obstruction, fecal impaction, allergy to any component.

WARNINGS

Patients are advised they should consult a doctor before using this product if they have abdominal pain, nausea, vomiting or rectal bleeding, if they have noticed a sudden change in bowel habits that persists over a period of two weeks, or if they are considering use of this product as part of a cholesterol-lowering program. Patients are advised to consult a physician if constipation persists for longer than one week, as this may be a sign of serious medical condition. **Patients are cautioned that taking this product without adequate fluid may cause it to swell and block the throat or esophagus and may cause choking. They should not take the product if they have difficulty in swallowing. If they experience chest pain, vomiting, or difficulty in swallowing or breathing after taking this product, they are advised to seek immediate medical attention.** Psyllium products may cause allergic reaction in people sensitive to inhaled or ingested psyllium. Keep out of the reach of children. In case of accidental overdose, seek professional assistance or contact a poison control center immediately.

PRECAUTION

Notice to Health Care Professional: To minimize the potential for allergic reaction, health care professionals who frequently dispense powdered psyllium products should avoid inhaling airborne dust while dispensing these products. Handling and Dispensing: To minimize generating airborne dust, spoon product from the canister into a glass according to label directions.

DOSAGE AND ADMINISTRATION

The usual adult dosage is one rounded teaspoon, or tablespoon, depending on the product version. Some versions are available in single-dose packets. For children (6 to 12 years old) use ½ the adult dose; for children under 6, consult a doctor. The appropriate dose should be mixed with 8 oz. of liquid (e.g., cool water, fruit juice, milk) following the label instructions. Metamucil Fiber Wafers should be consumed with 8 oz. of liquid. **The product (child or adult dose) should be taken with at least 8 oz. (a full glass) of water or other fluid. Taking this product without enough liquid may cause choking (see warnings).** Metamucil can be taken one to three times per day, depending on the need and response. It may require continued use for 2 to 3 days to provide optimal benefit. Generally produces effect in 12–72 hours.

Laxatives, including bulk fibers, may affect how well other medicines work. If you are taking a prescription medicine by mouth, take this product at least 2 hours before or 2 hours after the prescribed medicine. As your body adjusts to increased fiber intake, you may experience changes in bowel habits or minor bloating.

HOW SUPPLIED

Powder: canisters and cartons of single-dose packets. Wafers: cartons of single dose packets. (See Table 1)

[See table at bottom of previous page]

PEDIATRIC VICKS® 44e — OTC
COUGH & CHEST CONGESTION RELIEF
Cough Suppressant/Expectorant

(See PDR For Nonprescription Drugs.)

PEDIATRIC VICKS® 44m — OTC
COUGH & COLD RELIEF
Cough Suppressant/Nasal Decongestant/Antihistamine

(See PDR For Nonprescription Drugs.)

PEPTO-BISMOL® — OTC
ORIGINAL LIQUID, ORIGINAL AND CHERRY TABLETS AND EASY-TO-SWALLOW CAPLETS
For upset stomach, indigestion, diarrhea, heartburn and nausea.

Multi-symptom Pepto-Bismol contains bismuth subsalicylate and is the only leading OTC stomach remedy clinically proven effective for both upper and lower GI symptoms. Pepto-Bismol is in more households than any other stomach remedy, making it a convenient recommendation with a name your patients will know. It has been clinically proven in double-blind placebo-controlled trials for relief of upset stomach symptoms and diarrhea.

DESCRIPTION

Each tablespoon (15 ml) of Pepto-Bismol Liquid contains 262 mg bismuth subsalicylate. Each tablespoonful of liquid contains a total of 130 mg non-aspirin salicylate. Pepto-Bismol liquid contains no sugar and is low in sodium (less than 5 mg/tablespoonful). Inactive ingredients: benzoic acid, D&C Red No. 22, D&C Red No. 28, flavor, magnesium aluminum silicate, methylcellulose, saccharin sodium, salicylic acid, sodium salicylate, sorbic acid and water.

Each Pepto-Bismol Tablet contains 262 mg bismuth subsalicylate. Each tablet contains a total of 102 mg non-aspirin salicylate (99 mg non-aspirin salicylate for Cherry). Pepto-Bismol tablets contain no sugar and are very low in sodium (less than 2 mg/tablet). Inactive ingredients include: adipic acid (in Cherry only), calcium carbonate, D&C Red No. 27, FD&C Red No. 40 (in Cherry only), flavors, magnesium stearate, mannitol, povidone, saccharin sodium and talc.

Each Pepto-Bismol Caplet contains 262 mg bismuth subsalicylate. Each caplet contains a total of 99 mg non-aspirin salicylate. Caplets contain no sugar and are low in sodium (less than 3 mg/caplet). Inactive ingredients include: calcium carbonate, D&C Red No. 27, magnesium stearate, mannitol, microcrystalline cellulose, polysorbate 80, povidone, silicon dioxide, and sodium starch glycolate.

INDICATIONS

Pepto-Bismol controls diarrhea within 24 hours, relieving associated abdominal cramps; soothes heartburn and indigestion without constipating; and relieves nausea and upset stomach.

ACTIONS

For upset stomach symptoms (i.e., indigestion, heartburn, nausea and fullness caused by over-indulgence), the active ingredient is believed to work via a topical effect on the stomach mucosa. For diarrhea, it is believed to work by several mechanisms in the gastrointestinal tract, including: 1) normalizing fluid movement via an antisecretory mechanism, 2) binding bacterial toxins and 3) antimicrobial activity.

WARNINGS

Children and teenagers who have or are recovering from chicken pox or flu should not use this medicine to treat nausea or vomiting. If nausea or vomiting is present, patients are advised to consult a doctor because this could be an early sign of Reye syndrome, a rare but serious illness.

This product contains non-aspirin salicylates. If taken with aspirin and ringing in the ears occurs, discontinue use. This product does not contain aspirin, but should not be administered to those patients who have a known allergy to aspirin or non-aspirin salicylates as an adverse reaction may occur. Caution is advised in the administration to patients taking medication for anticoagulation, diabetes and gout.

If diarrhea is accompanied by a high fever or continues more than 2 days, patients are advised to consult a physician. As with any drug, caution is advised in the administration to pregnant or nursing women.

Keep all medicine out of the reach of children.

Note: This medication may cause a temporary and harmless darkening of the tongue and/or stool. Stool darkening should not be confused with melena.

OVERDOSAGE

In case of overdose, patients are advised to contact a physician or Poison Control Center. Emesis induced by ipecac syrup is indicated in large ingestions provided ipecac can be administered within one hour of ingestion. Activated charcoal should be administered after gastric emptying. Patients should be evaluated for signs and symptoms of salicylate toxicity.

DOSAGE AND ADMINISTRATION

Liquid: Shake well before using.

Adults— 2 tablespoonsful (1 dose cup, 30 ml)

Children (according to age)—

9–12 yrs.	1 tablespoonful ($^1/_2$ dose cup, 15 ml)
6–9 yrs.	2 teaspoonsful ($^1/_3$ dose cup, 10 ml)
3–6 yrs.	1 teaspoonful ($^1/_6$ dose cup, 5 ml)

Repeat dosage every $^1/_2$ to 1 hour, if needed, to a maximum of 8 doses in a 24-hour period. Drink plenty of clear fluids to help prevent dehydration which may accompany diarrhea. For children under 3 years of age, consult a physician.

Tablets:

Adults—Two tablets

Children (according to age)—

9–12 yrs.	1 tablet
6–9 yrs.	$^2/_3$ tablet
3–6 yrs.	$^1/_3$ tablet

Chew or dissolve in mouth. Repeat every $^1/_2$ to 1 hour as needed, to a maximum of 8 doses in a 24-hour period. Drink plenty of clear fluids to help prevent dehydration, which may accompany diarrhea. For children under 3 years of age, consult a physician.

Caplets:

Adults—Two caplets

Children (according to age)—

9–12 yrs.	1 caplet
6–9 yrs.	$^2/_3$ caplet
3–6 yrs.	$^1/_3$ caplet

Swallow caplet(s) with water, do not chew. Repeat every $^1/_2$ to 1 hour as needed, to a maximum of 8 doses in a 24-hour period. Drink plenty of clear fluids to help prevent dehydration, which may accompany diarrhea. For children under 3 years of age, consult a physician.

HOW SUPPLIED

Pepto-Bismol Liquid is available in: 4, 8, 12, and 16 FL OZ bottles. Pepto-Bismol Tablets are pink, round, chewable tablets imprinted with a debossed triangle and "Pepto-Bismol" on one side. Tablets are available in: boxes of 30 and 48. Caplets are available in bottles of 24 and 40. Caplets are imprinted with "Pepto-Bismol" on one side.

PEPTO-BISMOL® — OTC
MAXIMUM STRENGTH LIQUID
For upset stomach, indigestion, diarrhea, heartburn and nausea.

Multi-symptom Pepto-Bismol contains bismuth subsalicylate and is the only leading OTC stomach remedy clinically proven effective for both upper and lower GI symptoms. Pepto-Bismol is in more households than any other stomach remedy, making it a convenient recommendation with a name your patients will know. It has been clinically-proven in double-blind placebo-controlled trials for relief of upset stomach symptoms and diarrhea.

DESCRIPTION

Each tablespoonful (15 ml) of Maximum Strength Pepto-Bismol Liquid contains 525 mg bismuth subsalicylate (236 mg non-aspirin salicylate). Maximum Strength Pepto-Bismol Liquid contains no sugar and is low in sodium (less than 5 mg/tablespoonful). Inactive ingredients include: benzoic acid, D&C Red No. 22, D&C Red No. 28, flavor, magnesium aluminum silicate, methylcellulose, saccharin sodium, salicylic acid, sodium salicylate, sorbic acid and water.

INDICATIONS

Maximum Strength Pepto-Bismol soothes upset stomach and indigestion without constipating; controls diarrhea within 24 hours, relieving associated abdominal cramps; and relieves heartburn and nausea.

ACTIONS

For upset stomach symptoms (i.e. indigestion, heartburn, nausea and fullness caused by over-indulgence), the active ingredient is believed to work via a topical effect on the stomach mucosa. For diarrhea, it is believed to work by several mechanisms in the gastrointestinal tract, including: 1) normalizing fluid movement via an antisecretory mechanism, 2) binding bacterial toxins, and 3) antimicrobial activity.

WARNINGS

Children and teenagers who have or are recovering from chicken pox or flu should not use this medicine to treat nausea or vomiting. If nausea or vomiting is present, patients are advised to consult a doctor because this could be an early sign of Reye syndrome, a rare but serious illness.

This product contains non-aspirin salicylates. If taken with aspirin and ringing in the ears occurs, discontinue use. This product does not contain aspirin, but should not be administered to those patients who have a known allergy to aspirin or other non-aspirin salicylates as an adverse reaction may occur. Caution is advised in the administration to patients taking medication for anticoagulation, diabetes and gout.

If diarrhea is accompanied by a high fever or continues more than 2 days, patients are advised to consult a physician. As with any drug, caution is advised in the administration to pregnant or nursing women.

Keep all medicine out of the reach of children.

Note: This medication may cause a temporary and harmless darkening of the tongue and/or stool. Stool darkening should not be confused with melena.

OVERDOSAGE

In case of overdose, patients are advised to contact a physician or Poison Control Center. Emesis induced by ipecac syrup is indicated in large ingestions provided ipecac can be administered within one hour of ingestion. Activated charcoal should be administered after gastric emptying. Patients should be evaluated for signs and symptoms of salicylate toxicity.

DOSAGE AND ADMINISTRATION

Shake well before using.

Adults— 2 tablespoonsful (1 dose cup, 30 ml)

Children (according to age)—

9–12 yrs.	1 tablespoonful ($^1/_2$ dose cup, 15 ml)
6–9 yrs.	2 teaspoonsful ($^1/_3$ dose cup, 10 ml)
3–6 yrs.	1 teaspoonful ($^1/_6$ dose cup, 5 ml)

Repeat dosage every hour, if needed, to a maximum of 4 doses in a 24-hour period. Drink plenty of clear fluids to help prevent dehydration, which may accompany diarrhea.

Continued on next page

Pepto-Bismol Maximum—Cont.

HOW SUPPLIED

Maximum Strength Pepto-Bismol is available in: 4, 8, and 12 FL OZ bottles.

VICKS® COUGH DROPS OTC
ORIGINAL VICKS® COUGH DROPS OTC
Menthol Cough Suppressant/Oral Anesthetic
Menthol & Cherry Flavors

(See PDR For Nonprescription Drugs.)

VICKS® DAYQUIL® OTC
VICKS® DAYQUIL® LIQUICAPS® OTC
MULTI-SYMPTOM COLD/FLU RELIEF
Nasal Decongestant/Pain Reliever
Cough Suppressant/Fever Reducer

(See PDR For Nonprescription Drugs.)

VICKS® DAYQUIL® OTC
SINUS PRESSURE & PAIN RELIEF
WITH IBUPROFEN
Pain Reliever/Fever Reducer/Nasal Decongestant

(See PDR For Nonprescription Drugs.)

VICKS® 44 OTC
COUGH RELIEF
Dextromethorphan Hydrobromide
Cough Suppressant

(See PDR For Nonprescription Drugs.)

VICKS® 44D OTC
COUGH & HEAD CONGESTION RELIEF
Cough Suppressant/Nasal Decongestant

(See PDR For Nonprescription Drugs.)

VICKS® 44E OTC
COUGH & CHEST CONGESTION RELIEF
Cough Suppressant/Expectorant

(See PDR For Nonprescription Drugs.)

VICKS® 44M OTC
COUGH, COLD & FLU RELIEF
Cough Suppressant/Nasal
Decongestant/Antihistamine/
Pain Reliever-Fever Reducer

(See PDR For Nonprescription Drugs.)

VICKS® NYQUIL® LIQUID OTC
VICKS® NYQUIL® LIQUICAPS®
[nī quĭl]
Multi-Symptom Cold/Flu Relief
Antihistamine/Cough Suppressant/
Pain Reliever/Nasal Decongestant/
Fever Reducer

(See PDR For Nonprescription Drugs.)

VICKS® SINEX® OTC
[sī ′nĕx]
NASAL SPRAY AND
ULTRA FINE MIST FOR SINUS RELIEF
Phenylephrine HCl Decongestant

(See PDR For Nonprescription Drugs.)

VICKS® SINEX® 12 HOUR OTC
[sī ′nĕx]
NASAL SPRAY AND ULTRA FINE MIST
FOR SINUS RELIEF
Oxymetazoline HCl Nasal Decongestant

(See PDR For Nonprescription Drugs.)

VICKS® VAPOR INHALER OTC
l-Dexoxyephedrine
Nasal Decongestant

(See PDR For Nonprescription Drugs.)

VICKS® VAPORUB® OTC
(cream) (ointment)
[vā ′pō-rub]
Nasal Decongestant/Cough
Suppresssant/Topical Analgesic

(See PDR For Nonprescription Drugs.)

VICKS® VAPOSTEAM® OTC
[vā ′pō ″stēm]
Liquid Medication for
Hot Steam Vaporizers.
Camphor/Cough
Suppressant

(See PDR For Nonprescription Drugs.)

Procter & Gamble Pharmaceuticals, Inc.

HEALTH CARE RESEARCH CENTER
8700 MASON MONTGOMERY RD
MASON, OH 45040

Direct Inquiries to:
Customer Service
(800) 448-4878

For Medical Information Contact:
Medical Communications
(800) 836-0658
Fax: (800) 438-0138
or write
Procter & Gamble Company
Medical Communications Department
Health Care Research Center
P.O. Box 8006
Mason, OH 45040-8006

In Emergencies:
Medical Communications
(800) 836-0658

Information on these Procter & Gamble Pharmaceuticals products is based on labeling in effect July, 2000. Further information on these and other Procter & Gamble Pharmaceuticals products may be obtained by direct inquiry to Procter & Gamble Pharmaceuticals, Medical Communications Department, Health Care Research Center P.O. Box 8006 Mason, OH 45040-8006, or phone 800-836-0658/FAX 800-438-0138.

ACTONEL® ℞
[ac′tŏn-ĕl]
(risedronate sodium tablets)

DESCRIPTION

ACTONEL (risedronate sodium tablets) is a pyridinyl bisphosphonate that inhibits osteoclast-mediated bone resorption and modulates bone metabolism. Each ACTONEL tablet for oral administration contains the equivalent of 5 or 30 mg of anhydrous risedronate sodium in the form of the hemi-pentahydrate with small amounts of monohydrate. The empirical formula for risedronate sodium hemi-pentahydrate is $C_7H_{10}NO_7P_2Na \cdot 2.5\ H_2O$. The chemical name of risedronate sodium is [1-hydroxy-2-(3-pyridinyl)ethylidene]bis[phosphonic acid] monosodium salt. The chemical structure of risedronate sodium hemi-pentahydrate is the following:

Molecular Weight:
Anhydrous: 305.10
Hemi-pentahydrate: 350.13

Risedronate sodium is a fine, white to off-white, odorless, crystalline powder. It is soluble in water and in aqueous solutions, and essentially insoluble in common organic solvents.

Inactive Ingredients: Crospovidone, ferric oxide yellow (5 mg tablets only), hydroxypropyl cellulose, hydroxypropyl methylcellulose, lactose monohydrate, magnesium stearate, microcrystalline cellulose, polyethylene glycol, silicon dioxide, titanium dioxide.

CLINICAL PHARMACOLOGY

Mechanism of Action: ACTONEL has an affinity for hydroxyapatite crystals in bone and acts as an antiresorptive agent. At the cellular level, ACTONEL inhibits osteoclasts. The osteoclasts adhere normally to the bone surface, but show evidence of reduced active resorption (e.g., lack of ruffled border). Histomorphometry in rats, dogs, and minipigs showed that ACTONEL treatment reduces bone turnover (activation frequency, i.e., the rate at which bone remodeling sites are activated) and bone resorption at remodeling sites.

Pharmacokinetics:

Absorption: Absorption after an oral dose is relatively rapid (t_{max} ~1 hour) and occurs throughout the upper gastrointestinal tract. The fraction of the dose absorbed is independent of dose over the range studied (single dose, 2.5 to 30 mg; multiple dose, 2.5 to 5 mg). Steady-state conditions in the serum are observed within 57 days of daily dosing. Mean absolute oral bioavailability of the 30 mg tablet is 0.63% (90% CI: 0.54% to 0.75%) and is comparable to a solution. The extent of absorption of a 30-mg dose (three, 10-mg tablets) when administered 0.5 hours before breakfast is reduced by 55% compared to dosing in the fasting state (no food or drink for 10 hours prior to or 4 hours after dosing). Dosing 1 hour prior to breakfast reduces the extent of absorption by 30% compared to dosing in the fasting state. Dosing either 0.5 hours prior to breakfast or 2 hours after dinner (evening meal) results in a similar extent of absorption. ACTONEL is effective when administered at least 30 minutes before breakfast.

Distribution: The mean steady-state volume of distribution is 6.3 L/kg in humans. Human plasma protein binding of drug is about 24%. Preclinical studies in rats and dogs dosed intravenously with single doses of [^{14}C] risedronate indicate that approximately 60% of the dose is distributed to bone. The remainder of the dose is excreted in the urine. After multiple oral dosing in rats, the uptake of risedronate in soft tissues was in the range of 0.001% to 0.01%.

Metabolism: There is no evidence of systemic metabolism of risedronate.

Elimination: Approximately half of the absorbed dose is excreted in urine within 24 hours, and 85% of an intravenous dose is recovered in the urine over 28 days. Mean renal clearance is 105 mL/min (CV = 34%) and mean total clearance is 122 mL/min (CV = 19%), with the difference primarily reflecting nonrenal clearance or clearance due to adsorption to bone. The renal clearance is not concentration dependent, and there is a linear relationship between renal clearance and creatinine clearance. Unabsorbed drug is eliminated unchanged in feces. Once risedronate is absorbed, the serum concentration-time profile is multi-phasic with an initial half-life of about 1.5 hours and a terminal exponential half-life of 480 hours. This terminal half-life is hypothesized to represent the dissociation of risedronate from the surface of bone.

Special Populations:

Pediatric: Risedronate pharmacokinetics have not been studied in patients < 18 years of age.

Gender: Bioavailability and pharmacokinetics following oral administration are similar in men and women.

Geriatric: Bioavailability and disposition are similar in elderly (> 60 years of age) and younger subjects. No dosage adjustment is necessary.

Race: Pharmacokinetic differences due to race have not been studied.

Renal Insufficiency: Risedronate is excreted unchanged primarily via the kidney. As compared to persons with normal renal function, the renal clearance of risedronate was decreased by about 70% in patients with creatinine clearance of approximately 30 mL/min. ACTONEL is not recommended for use in patients with severe renal impairment (creatinine clearance < 30 mL/min) because of lack of clinical experience. No dosage adjustment is necessary in patients with a creatinine clearance ≥ 30 mL/min.

Hepatic Insufficiency: No studies have been performed to assess risedronate's safety or efficacy in patients with hepatic impairment. Risedronate is not metabolized in rat, dog, and human liver preparations. Insignificant amounts (< 0.1% of intravenous dose) of drug are excreted in the bile in rats. Therefore, dosage adjustment is unlikely to be needed in patients with hepatic impairment.

Pharmacodynamics:

Treatment and Prevention of Osteoporosis in Postmenopausal Women: Osteoporosis is characterized by decreased bone mass and increased fracture risk, most commonly at the spine, hip, and wrist.

The diagnosis can be confirmed by the finding of low bone mass, evidence of fracture on x-ray, a history of osteoporotic fracture, or height loss or kyphosis indicative of vertebral fracture. Osteoporosis occurs in both men and women but is more common among women following menopause. In healthy humans, bone formation and resorption are closely linked; old bone is resorbed and replaced by newly-formed bone. In postmenopausal osteoporosis, bone resorption exceeds bone formation, leading to bone loss and increased risk of bone fracture. After menopause, the risk of fractures of the spine and hip increases; approximately 40% of 50-year-old women will experience an osteoporosis-related fracture during their remaining lifetimes. After experiencing one osteoporosis-related fracture, the risk of future fracture increases five-fold compared to the risk among a non-fractured population.

ACTONEL treatment decreases the elevated rate of bone turnover that is typically seen in postmenopausal osteoporosis. In clinical trials, administration of ACTONEL to postmenopausal women resulted in decreases in biochemical markers of bone turnover, including urinary deoxypyridinoline/creatinine (a marker of bone resorption) and bone specific alkaline phosphatase (a marker of bone formation). At the 5-mg dose, decreases in deoxypyridinoline/creatinine were evident within 14 days of treatment. Changes in bone formation markers were observed later than changes in resorption markers, as expected, due to the coupled nature of bone resorption and bone formation; decreases in bone specific alkaline phosphatase of about 20% were evident within 3 months of treatment. Bone turnover markers reached a nadir of about 40% below baseline values by the sixth month of treatment and remained stable with continued treatment for up to 3 years. Bone turnover is decreased as early as 14 days and maximally within about 6 months of treatment, with achievement of a new steady-state which more nearly approximates the rate of bone turnover seen in premenopausal women. ACTONEL is not an estrogen and does not have the benefits and risks of estrogen therapy.

As a result of the inhibition of bone resorption, asymptomatic and usually transient decreases from baseline in serum calcium (< 1%) and serum phosphate (< 3%) and compensatory increases in serum PTH levels (< 30%) were observed within 6 months in patients in osteoporosis clinical trials. There were no significant differences in serum calcium, phosphate, or PTH levels between the ACTONEL and placebo groups at 3 years.

Glucocorticoid-Induced Osteoporosis: Sustained use of glucocorticoids is commonly associated with development of osteoporosis and resulting fractures (especially vertebral, hip, and rib). It occurs both in males and females of all ages. The relative risk of a hip fracture in patients on > 7.5 mg/day prednisone is more than doubled (RR = 2.27); the relative risk of vertebral fracture is increased five-fold (RR = 5.18). Bone loss occurs most rapidly during the first 6 months of therapy with persistent but slowing bone loss for as long as glucocorticoid therapy continues. Osteoporosis occurs as a result of inhibited bone formation and increased bone resorption resulting in net bone loss. ACTONEL decreases bone resorption without directly inhibiting bone formation.

In two 1-year clinical trials in the treatment and prevention of glucocorticoid-induced osteoporosis, ACTONEL 5 mg decreased urinary collagen cross-linked N-Telopeptide (a marker of bone resorption) and serum bone specific alkaline phosphatase (a marker of bone formation) by 50% to 55% and 25% to 30%, respectively, within 3 to 6 months after initiation of therapy.

Paget's Disease: Paget's disease of bone is a chronic, focal skeletal disorder characterized by greatly increased and disordered bone remodeling. Excessive osteoclastic bone resorption is followed by osteoblastic new bone formation, leading to the replacement of the normal bone architecture by disorganized, enlarged, and weakened bone structure.

Clinical manifestations of Paget's disease range from no symptoms to severe bone pain, bone deformity, pathological fractures, and neurological disorders. Serum alkaline phosphatase, the most frequently used biochemical marker of disease activity, provides an objective measure of disease severity and response to therapy.

In pagetic patients treated with ACTONEL 30 mg/day for 2 months, bone turnover returned to normal in a majority of patients as evidenced by significant reductions in serum alkaline phosphatase, a marker of bone formation, and in urinary hydroxyproline/creatinine and deoxypyridinoline/creatinine, markers of bone resorption. Radiographic structural changes of bone lesions, especially improvement of a majority of lesions with an osteolytic front in weight-bearing bones, were also observed after ACTONEL treatment. In addition, histomorphometric data provide further support that ACTONEL can lead to a more normal bone structure in these patients.

Radiographs taken at baseline and after 6 months from patients treated with ACTONEL 30 mg daily demonstrate that ACTONEL decreases the extent of osteolysis in both the appendicular and axial skeleton. Osteolytic lesions in the lower extremities improved or were unchanged in 15/16 (94%) of assessed patients; 9/16 (56%) patients showed clear improvement in osteolytic lesions. No evidence of new fractures was observed.

CLINICAL STUDIES

Treatment of Osteoporosis in Postmenopausal Women: The fracture efficacy of ACTONEL 5 mg daily in the treatment of postmenopausal osteoporosis was demonstrated in two large, randomized, placebo-controlled, double-blind studies which enrolled a total of almost 4000 postmenopausal women under similar protocols. The Multinational study (VERT MN) (ACTONEL 5 mg, n = 408) was conducted primarily in Europe and Australia; a second study was conducted in North America (VERT NA) (ACTONEL 5 mg, n = 821). Patients were selected on the basis of radiographic evidence of previous vertebral fracture, and therefore, had established disease. The average number of prevalent vertebral fractures per patient at study entry was 4 in VERT MN, and 2.5 in VERT NA, with a broad range of baseline BMD levels. All patients in these studies received supplemental calcium 1000 mg/day. Patients with low vitamin D levels (approximately 40 nmol/L or less) also received supplemental vitamin D 500 IU/day.

Positive effects of ACTONEL treatment on BMD were also demonstrated in each of two large, randomized, placebo-controlled trials (BMD MN and BMD NA) in which almost 1200 postmenopausal women (ACTONEL 5 mg, n = 394) were recruited on the basis of low lumbar spine bone mass (more than 2 SD below the premenopausal-mean) rather than a history of vertebral fracture.

Effect on Vertebral Fractures: Fractures of previously undeformed vertebrae (new fractures) and worsening of pre-

Table 1
The Effect of ACTONEL on the Risk of Vertebral Fractures

	Proportion of Patients with Fracture (%)[a]			
VERT NA	Placebo n = 678	ACTONEL 5 mg n = 696	Absolute Risk Reduction (%)	Relative Risk Reduction (%)
New and Worsening				
0 – 1 Year	7.2	3.9	3.3	49
0 – 2 Years	12.8	8.0	4.8	42
0 – 3 Years	18.5	13.9	4.6	33
New				
0 – 1 Year	6.4	2.4	4.0	65
0 – 2 Years	11.7	5.8	5.9	55
0 – 3 Years	16.3	11.3	5.0	41
VERT MN	Placebo n = 346	ACTONEL 5 mg n = 344	Absolute Risk Reduction (%)	Relative Risk Reduction (%)
New and Worsening				
0 – 1 Year	15.3	8.2	7.1	50
0 – 2 Years	28.3	13.9	14.4	56
0 – 3 Years	34.0	21.8	12.2	46
New				
0 – 1 Year	13.3	5.6	7.7	61
0 – 2 Years	24.7	11.6	13.1	59
0 – 3 Years	29.0	18.1	10.9	49

[a] Calculated by Kaplan-Meier methodology.

Table 2
Mean Percent Increase in BMD from Baseline in Patients Taking ACTONEL 5 mg or Placebo at Endpoint[a]

	VERT MN[b]		VERT NA[b]		BMD MN[c]		BMD NA[c]	
	Placebo N = 323	5 mg N = 323	Placebo N = 599	5 mg N = 606	Placebo N = 161	5 mg N = 148	Placebo N = 191	5 mg N = 193
Lumbar Spine	1.0	6.6	0.8	5.0	0.0	4.0	0.2	4.8
Femoral Neck	−1.4	1.6	−1.0	1.4	−1.1	1.3	0.1	2.4
Femoral Trochanter	−1.9	3.9	−0.5	3.0	−0.6	2.5	1.3	4.0
Midshaft Radius	−1.5*	0.2*	−1.2*	0.1*	ND		ND	

[a] The endpoint value is the value at the study's last time point for all patients who had BMD measured at that time; otherwise the last postbaseline BMD value prior to the study's last time point is used.
[b] The duration of the studies was 3 years.
[c] The duration of the studies was 1.5 to 2 years.
* BMD of the midshaft radius was measured in a subset of centers in the VERT MN (placebo, n = 222; 5 mg, n = 214) and VERT NA (placebo, n = 310; 5 mg, n = 306)
ND = analysis not done

existing vertebral fractures were diagnosed radiographically; some of these fractures were also associated with symptoms (i.e., clinical fractures). Spinal radiographs were scheduled annually and prospectively planned analyses were based on the time to a patient's first diagnosed fracture. The primary endpoint for these studies was the incidence of new and worsening vertebral fractures across the period of 0 to 3 years. ACTONEL 5 mg daily significantly reduced the incidence of new and worsening vertebral fractures and of new vertebral fractures in both VERT NA and VERT MN at all time points (Table 1). The reduction in risk seen in the subgroup of patients who had two or more vertebral fractures at study entry was similar to that seen in the overall study population.

[See table 1 above]

Effect on Osteoporosis Related Nonvertebral Fractures: In VERT MN and VERT NA, a prospectively planned efficacy endpoint was defined consisting of all radiographically confirmed fractures of skeletal sites accepted as associated with osteoporosis. Fractures at these sites were collectively referred to as osteoporosis-related nonvertebral fractures. ACTONEL 5 mg daily significantly reduced the incidence of nonvertebral osteoporosis-related fractures over 3 years in VERT NA (8% vs. 5%; relative risk reduction 39%) and reduced the fracture incidence in VERT MN from 16% to 11%. There was a significant reduction from 11% to 7% when the studies were combined, with a corresponding 36% reduction in relative risk. Figure 1 shows the overall results as well as the results at the individual skeletal sites for the combined studies.

[See figure at top of next column]

Effect on Height: In the two 3-year osteoporosis treatment studies, standing height was measured yearly by stadiometer. Both ACTONEL and placebo-treated groups lost height during the studies. Patients who received ACTONEL had a statistically significant smaller loss of height than those who received placebo. In VERT MN, the median annual height change was - 1.3 mm/yr in the ACTONEL 5 mg daily group compared with - 2.4 mm/yr in the placebo group. In VERT NA , the median annual height change was - 0.7 mm/yr in the ACTONEL 5 mg daily group compared with - 1.1 mm/yr in the placebo group.

Effect on Bone Mineral Density: The results of four, randomized, placebo-controlled trials in women with postmenopausal osteoporosis (VERT MN, VERT NA, BMD MN, BMD NA) demonstrate that ACTONEL 5 mg daily increases BMD at the spine, hip, and wrist compared to the effects seen with placebo. Table 2 displays the significant increases

Figure 1
Nonvertebral Osteoporosis-Related Fractures Cumulative Incidence over 3 Years Combined VERT MN and VERT NA

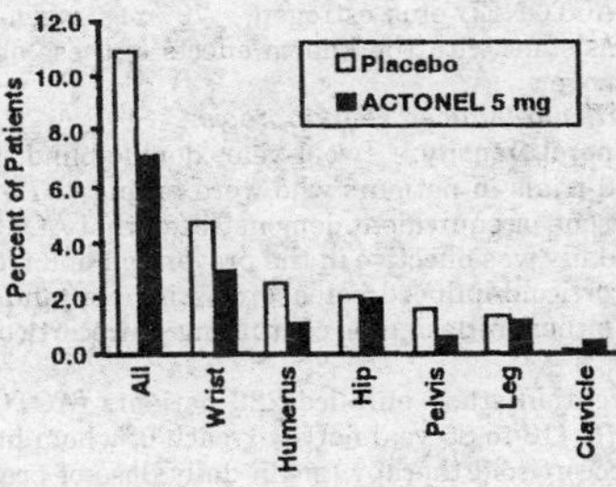

in BMD seen at the lumbar spine, femoral neck, femoral trochanter, and midshaft radius in these trials compared to placebo. Thus, overall ACTONEL reverses the loss of BMD, a central factor in the progression of osteoporosis. In both VERT studies (VERT MN and VERT NA), ACTONEL 5 mg daily produced increases in lumbar spine BMD which were progressive over the 3 years of treatment, and were statistically significant relative to baseline and to placebo at 6 months and at all later time points.

[See table 2 above]

Histology/Histomorphometry: Bone biopsies from 110 postmenopausal women were obtained at endpoint. Patients had received daily ACTONEL (2.5 mg or 5 mg) or placebo for 2 to 3 years. Histologic evaluation (n = 103) showed no osteomalacia, impaired bone mineralization, or other adverse effects on bone in ACTONEL-treated women. These findings demonstrate that bone formed during ACTONEL administration is of normal quality. The histomorphometric parameter mineralizing surface, an index of bone turnover, was assessed based upon baseline and post-treatment biopsy samples from 23 patients treated with ACTONEL 5 mg and 21 treated with placebo. Mineralizing surface decreased moderately in ACTONEL-treated patients (median percent

Continued on next page

Actonel—Cont.

change: ACTONEL 5 mg, - 74%; placebo, - 21%), consistent with the known effects of treatment on bone turnover.

Prevention of Osteoporosis in Postmenopausal Women: ACTONEL 5 mg daily prevented bone loss in a majority of postmenopausal women (age range 42 to 63 years) within 3 years of menopause in a 2-year, double-blind, placebo-controlled study in 383 patients (ACTONEL 5 mg, n = 129). All patients in this study received supplemental calcium 1000 mg/day. Increases in BMD were observed as early as 3 months following initiation of ACTONEL treatment. ACTONEL 5 mg produced significant mean increases in BMD at the lumbar spine, femoral neck, and trochanter compared to placebo at the end of the study (Figure 2). ACTONEL 5 mg daily was also effective in patients with lower baseline lumbar spine BMD (more than 1 SD below the premenopausal mean) and in those with normal baseline lumbar spine BMD. Bone mineral density at the distal radius decreased in both ACTONEL and placebo-treated women following 1 year of treatment.

Figure 2
Change in BMD from Baseline
2-Year Prevention Study

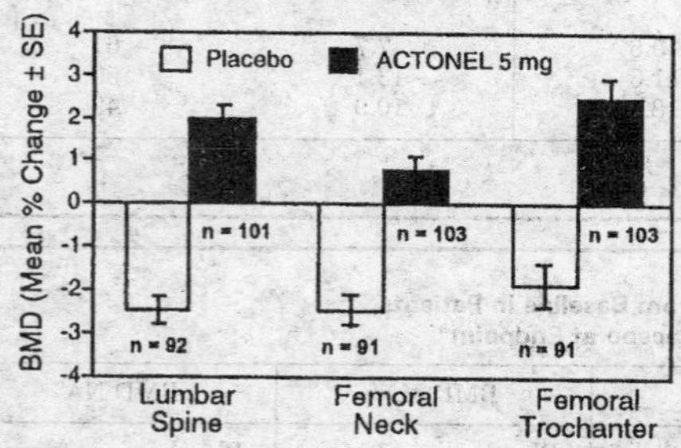

Combined Administration with Hormone Replacement Therapy: The effects of combining ACTONEL 5 mg daily with conjugated estrogen 0.625 mg daily (n = 263) were compared to the effects of conjugated estrogen alone (n = 261) in a 1-year, randomized, double-blind study of women ages 37 to 82 years, who were on average 14 years postmenopausal. The BMD results for this study are presented in Table 3.

[See table 3 above]

Table 3
Percent Change from Baseline in BMD after 1 Year of Treatment

	Estrogen 0.625 mg N = 261	ACTONEL 5 mg + Estrogen 0.625 mg N = 263
Lumbar Spine	4.6 ± 0.20	5.2 ± 0.23
Femoral Neck	1.8 ± 0.25	2.7 ± 0.25
Femoral Trochanter	3.2 ± 0.28	3.7 ± 0.25
Midshaft Radius	0.4 ± 0.14	0.7 ± 0.17
Distal Radius	1.7 ± 0.24	1.6 ± 0.28

Values shown are mean (± SEM) percent change from baseline

Histology/Histomorphometry: Bone biopsies from 53 postmenopausal women were obtained at endpoint. Patients had received ACTONEL 5 mg plus estrogen or estrogen alone once daily for 1 year. Histologic evaluation (n = 47) demonstrated that the bone of patients treated with ACTONEL plus estrogen was of normal lamellar structure and normal mineralization. The histomorphometric parameter mineralizing surface, a measure of bone turnover, was assessed based upon baseline and post-treatment biopsy samples from 12 patients treated with ACTONEL plus estrogen and 12 treated with estrogen alone. Mineralizing surface decreased in both treatment groups (median percent change: ACTONEL plus estrogen, - 79%; estrogen alone, - 50%), consistent with the known effects of these agents on bone turnover.

Glucocorticoid-Induced Osteoporosis:

Bone Mineral Density: Two 1-year, double-blind, placebo-controlled trials in patients who were taking ≥ 7.5 mg/day of prednisone or equivalent demonstrated that ACTONEL 5 mg once daily was effective in the prevention and treatment of glucocorticoid-induced osteoporosis in men and women who are either initiating or continuing glucocorticoid therapy.

The prevention study enrolled 228 patients (ACTONEL 5 mg, n = 76) (18 to 85 years of age), each of whom had initiated glucocorticoid therapy (mean daily dose of prednisone 21 mg) within the previous 3 months (mean duration of use prior to study 1.8 months) for rheumatic, skin, and pulmonary diseases. The mean lumbar spine BMD was normal at baseline (average T score 0.684). All patients in this study received supplemental calcium 500 mg/day. By the third month of treatment, and continuing through the year-long treatment, the placebo group experienced losses in BMD at the lumbar spine, femoral neck, and trochanter, while BMD was maintained or increased in the ACTONEL 5 mg group. At each skeletal site there were statistically significant differences between the ACTONEL 5 mg group and the placebo group at all timepoints (Months 3, 6, 9, and 12). The treatment differences increased with continued treatment. Although BMD increased at the distal radius in the ACTONEL 5 mg group compared with the placebo group, the difference was not statistically significant. The differences between placebo and ACTONEL 5 mg after 1 year were 3.8% at the lumbar spine, 4.1% at the femoral neck, and 4.6% at the trochanter, as shown in Figure 3. The results at these skeletal sites were similar to the overall results when the subgroups of men and postmenopausal women, but not premenopausal women, were analyzed separately. ACTONEL was effective at the lumbar spine, femoral neck, and trochanter regardless of age (< 65 vs. ≥ 65), gender, prior and concomitant glucocorticoid dose, or baseline BMD. Positive treatment effects were also observed in patients taking glucocorticoids for a broad range of rheumatologic disorders, the most common of which were rheumatoid arthritis, temporal arteritis, and polymyalgia rheumatica.

The treatment study of similar design enrolled 290 patients (ACTONEL 5 mg, n = 100) (19 to 85 years of age) with continuing, long-term (≥ 6 months) use of glucocorticoids (mean duration of use prior to study 60 months; mean daily dose of prednisone 15 mg) for rheumatic, skin, and pulmonary diseases. The baseline mean lumbar spine BMD was low (1.63 SD below the young healthy population mean), with 28% of the patients more than 2.5 SD below the mean. All patients in this study received supplemental calcium 1000 mg/day and vitamin D 400 IU/day.

After 1 year of treatment, the BMD of the placebo group was within ± 1% of baseline levels at the lumbar spine, femoral neck, and trochanter. ACTONEL 5 mg increased BMD at the lumbar spine (2.9%), femoral neck (1.8%), and trochanter (2.4%). The differences between ACTONEL and placebo were 2.7% at the lumbar spine, 1.9% at the femoral neck, and 1.6% at the trochanter as shown in Figure 4. The differences were statistically significant for the lumbar spine and femoral neck, but not at the femoral trochanter. ACTONEL was similarly effective on lumbar spine BMD regardless of age (< 65 vs. ≥ 65), gender, or pre-study glucocorticoid dose. Positive treatment effects were also observed in patients taking glucocorticoids for a broad range of rheumatologic disorders, the most common of which were rheumatoid arthritis, temporal arteritis, and polymyalgia rheumatica.

Figure 3
Change in BMD from Baseline
Patients Recently Initiating
Glucocorticoid Therapy

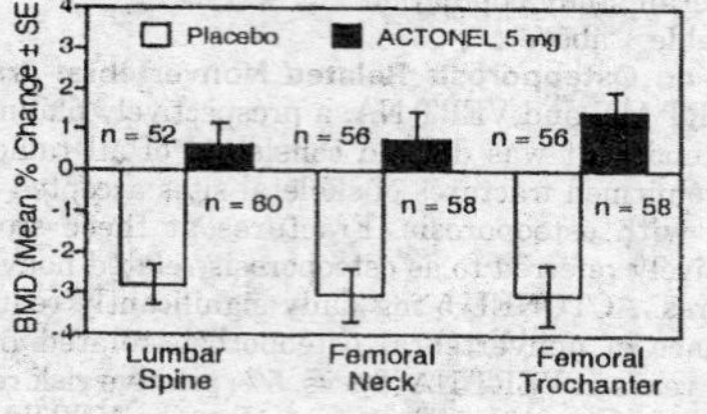

Figure 4
Change in BMD from Baseline
Patients on Long-Term
Glucocorticoid Therapy

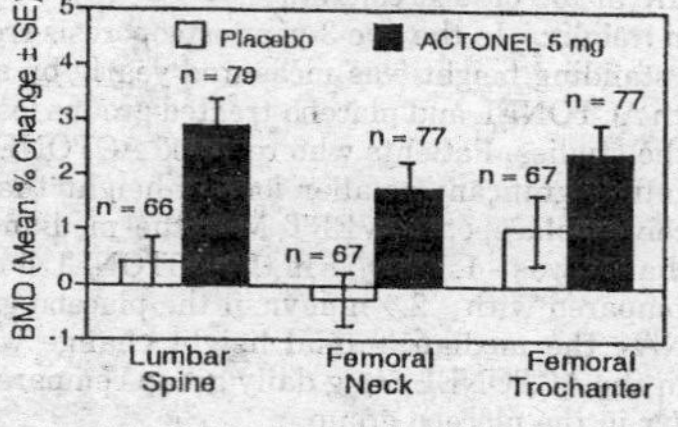

Vertebral Fractures: In the prevention study of patients initiating glucocorticoids, the incidence of vertebral fractures at 1 year was reduced from 17% in the placebo group to 6% in the ACTONEL group. In the treatment study of patients continuing glucocorticoids, the incidence of vertebral fractures was reduced from 15% in the placebo group to 5% in the ACTONEL group (Figure 5). The statistically significant reduction in vertebral fracture incidence in the analysis of the combined studies corresponded to an absolute risk reduction of 11% and a relative risk reduction of 70%. All vertebral fractures were diagnosed radiographically; some of these fractures also were associated with symptoms (i.e., clinical fractures).

Figure 5
Incidence of Vertebral Fractures in Patients Initiating or Continuing Glucocorticoid Therapy

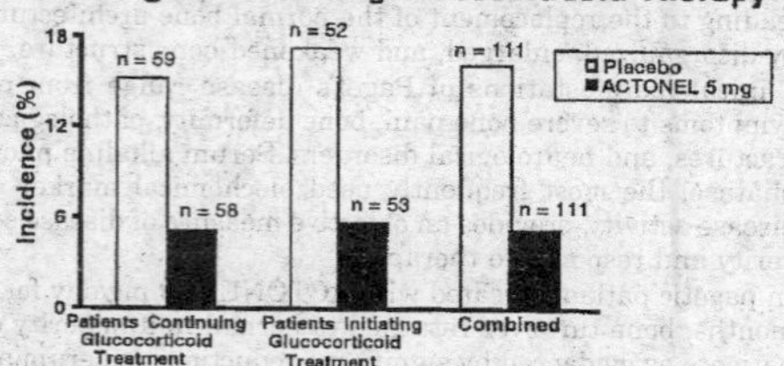

Histology/Histomorphometry: Bone biopsies from 40 patients on glucocorticoid therapy were obtained at endpoint. Patients had received daily ACTONEL (2.5 mg or 5 mg) or placebo for 1 year. Histologic evaluation (n = 33) showed that bone formed during treatment with ACTONEL was of normal lamellar structure and normal mineralization, with no bone or marrow abnormalities observed. The histomorphometric parameter mineralizing surface, a measure of bone turnover, was assessed based upon baseline and post-treatment biopsy samples from 10 patients treated with ACTONEL 5 mg. Mineralizing surface decreased 24% (median percent change) in these patients. Only a small number of placebo-treated patients had both baseline and post-treatment biopsy samples, precluding a meaningful quantitative assessment.

Treatment of Paget's Disease: The efficacy of ACTONEL was demonstrated in two clinical studies involving 120 men and 65 women. In a double-blind, active-controlled study of patients with moderate-to-severe Paget's disease (serum alkaline phosphatase levels of at least two times the upper limit of normal), patients were treated with ACTONEL 30 mg daily for 2 months or Didronel® (etidronate disodium) 400 mg/day for 6 months. At Day 180, 77% (43/56) of ACTONEL-treated patients achieved normalization of serum alkaline phosphatase levels compared to 10.5% (6/57) of patients treated with Didronel ($p < 0.001$). At Day 540, 16 months after discontinuation of therapy, 53% (17/32) of ACTONEL-treated patients and 14% (4/29) of Didronel-treated patients with available data remained in biochemical remission.

During the first 180 days of the active-controlled study, 85% (51/60) of ACTONEL-treated patients demonstrated a ≥ 75% reduction from baseline in serum alkaline phosphatase excess (difference between measured level and mid-point of the normal range) with 2 months of treatment compared to 20% (12/60) in the Didronel-treated group with 6 months of treatment ($p < 0.001$). Changes in serum alkaline phosphatase excess over time (shown in Figure 6) are significant following only 30 days of treatment, with a 36% reduction in serum alkaline phosphatase excess at that time compared to only a 6% reduction seen with Didronel treatment at the same time point ($p < 0.01$).

[See figure at top of next column]

Response to ACTONEL therapy was similar in patients with mild to very severe Paget's disease. Table 4 shows the

Table 4
Mean Percent Reduction From Baseline at Day 180 in Total Serum Alkaline Phosphatase Excess by Disease Severity

	30mg ACTONEL			400 mg DIDRONEL		
Subgroup: Baseline Disease Severity (AP)	N	Baseline Serum AP (U/L)*	Mean % Reduction	N	Baseline Serum AP (U/L)*	Mean % Reduction
> 2, <3× ULN	32	271.6 ± 5.3	−88.1	22	277.9 ± 7.45	−44.6
≥ 3, <7× ULN	14	475.3 ± 28.8	−87.5	25	480.5 ± 26.44	−35.0
≥ 7× ULN	8	1336.5 ± 134.19	−81.8	6	1331.5 ± 167.58	−47.2

* Values shown are mean ± SEM; ULN = upper limit of normal

Figure 6
Mean Percent Change from Baseline in Serum Alkaline Phosphatase Excess by Visit

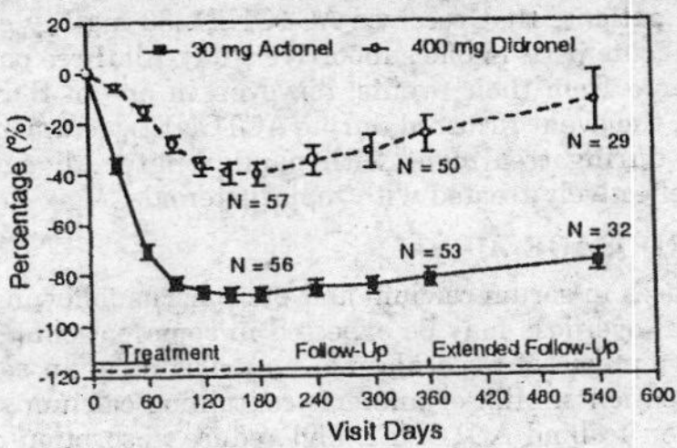

mean percent reduction from baseline at Day 180 in excess serum alkaline phosphatase in patients with mild, moderate, or severe disease.

[See table 4 at top of previous page]

Response to ACTONEL therapy was similar between patients who had previously received anti-pagetic therapy and those who had not. In the active-controlled study, four patients previously non-responsive to one or more courses of anti-pagetic therapy (calcitonin, Didronel) responded to treatment with ACTONEL 30 mg daily (defined by at least a 30% change from baseline). Each of these patients achieved at least 90% reduction from baseline in serum alkaline phosphatase excess with three patients achieving normalization of serum alkaline phosphatase levels.

Histomorphometry of the bone was studied in 14 patients with bone biopsies: nine patients had biopsies from pagetic bone lesions and five patients from non-pagetic bone. Bone biopsy results in non-pagetic bone did not reveal osteomalacia, impairment of bone remodeling, or induction of a significant decline in bone turnover in patients treated with ACTONEL.

ANIMAL PHARMACOLOGY AND/OR TOXICOLOGY:

Risedronate demonstrated potent anti-osteoclast, antiresorptive activity in ovariectomized rats and minipigs. Bone mass and biomechanical strength were increased dose-dependently at oral doses up to 4 and 25 times the human recommended oral dose of 5 mg based on surface area, (mg/m^2) for rats and mini-pigs, respectively. Risedronate treatment maintained the positive correlation between BMD and bone strength and did not have a negative effect on bone structure or mineralization. In intact dogs, risedronate induced positive bone balance at the level of the bone remodeling unit at oral doses ranging from 0.35 to 1.4 times the human 5-mg dose based on surface area (mg/m^2).

In dogs treated with an oral dose of 1 mg/kg/day (approximately 5 times the human 5-mg dose based on surface area, mg/m^2), risedronate caused a delay in fracture healing of the radius. The observed delay in fracture healing is similar to other bisphosphonates. This effect did not occur at a dose of 0.1 mg/kg/day (approximately 0.5 times the human 5-mg dose based on surface area, mg/m^2).

The Schenk rat assay, based on histologic examination of the epiphyses of growing rats after drug treatment, demonstrated that risedronate did not interfere with bone mineralization even at the highest dose tested (5 mg/kg/day, subcutaneously), which was approximately 3500 times the lowest antiresorptive dose (1.5 mcg/kg/day in this model) and approximately 8 times the human 5-mg dose based on surface area (mg/m^2). This indicates that ACTONEL administered at the therapeutic dose is unlikely to induce osteomalacia.

INDICATIONS AND USAGE

Postmenopausal Osteoporosis: ACTONEL is indicated for the treatment and prevention of osteoporosis in postmenopausal women.

Treatment of Osteoporosis: In postmenopausal women with osteoporosis, ACTONEL increases BMD and reduces the incidence of vertebral fractures and a composite endpoint of nonvertebral osteoporosis-related fractures (see CLINICAL STUDIES). Osteoporosis may be confirmed by the presence or history of osteoporotic fracture, or by the finding of low bone mass (for example, at least 2 SD below the premenopausal mean).

Prevention of Osteoporosis: ACTONEL may be considered in postmenopausal women who are at risk of developing osteoporosis and for whom the desired clinical outcome is to maintain bone mass and to reduce the risk of fracture.

Factors such as family history of osteoporosis, previous fracture, smoking, BMD (at least 1 SD below the premenopausal mean), high bone turnover, thin body frame, Caucasian or Asian race, and early menopause are associated with an increased risk of developing osteoporosis and fractures. The presence of these risk factors may be important when considering the use of ACTONEL for prevention of osteoporosis.

Glucocorticoid-Induced Osteoporosis: ACTONEL is indicated for the prevention and treatment of glucocorticoid-induced osteoporosis in men and women who are either initiating or continuing systemic glucocorticoid treatment (daily dosage equivalent to 7.5 mg or greater of prednisone) for chronic diseases. Patients treated with glucocorticoids should receive adequate amounts of calcium and vitamin D.

Paget's Disease: ACTONEL is indicated for treatment of Paget's disease of bone (osteitis deformans).

Treatment is indicated in patients with Paget's disease of bone (1) who have a level of serum alkaline phosphatase (SAP) at least two times the upper limit of normal, or (2) who are symptomatic, or (3) who are at risk for future complications from their disease, to induce remission (normalization of serum alkaline phosphatase).

CONTRAINDICATIONS

- Hypocalcemia (See PRECAUTIONS, General)
- Known hypersensitivity to any component of this product
- Inability to stand or sit upright for at least 30 minutes

WARNINGS: Bisphosphonates may cause upper gastrointestinal disorders such as dysphagia, esophagitis, and esophageal or gastric ulcer (see PRECAUTIONS).

PRECAUTIONS

General: Hypocalcemia and other disturbances of bone and mineral metabolism should be effectively treated before starting ACTONEL therapy. Adequate intake of calcium and vitamin D is important in all patients, especially in patients with Paget's disease in whom bone turnover is significantly elevated. ACTONEL is not recommended for use in patients with severe renal impairment (creatinine clearance < 30 mL/min).

Bisphosphonates have been associated with gastrointestinal disorders such as dysphagia, esophagitis, and esophageal or gastric ulcers. This association has been reported for bisphosphonates in postmarketing experience, but has not been found in most pre-approval clinical trials, including those conducted with ACTONEL. Patients should be advised that taking the medication according to the instructions is important to minimize the risk of these events. They should take ACTONEL with sufficient plain water (6 to 8 oz) to facilitate delivery to the stomach, and should not lie down for 30 minutes after taking the drug.

Glucocorticoid-Induced Osteoporosis: The risk versus benefit of ACTONEL for the prevention and treatment of glucocorticoid-induced osteoporosis at daily doses of glucocorticoids < 7.5 mg of prednisone or equivalent has not been established. Before initiating treatment, the hormonal status of both men and women should be ascertained and appropriate replacement considered.

The efficacy of ACTONEL has been established in studies of 1-year's duration. The efficacy of ACTONEL beyond 1 year has not been studied.

Information for Patients: The patient should be informed to pay particular attention to the dosing instructions as clinical benefits may be compromised by failure to take the drug according to instructions. Specifically, ACTONEL should be taken at least 30 minutes before the first food or drink of the day other than water.

To facilitate delivery to the stomach, and thus reduce the potential for esophageal irritation, patients should take ACTONEL while in an upright position (sitting or standing) with a full glass of plain water (6 to 8 oz). Patients should not lie down for 30 minutes after taking the medication (see PRECAUTIONS, General). Patients should not chew or suck on the tablet because of a potential for oropharyngeal irritation.

Patients should be instructed that if they develop symptoms of esophageal disease (such as difficulty or pain upon swallowing, retrosternal pain or severe persistent or worsening heartburn) they should consult their physician before continuing ACTONEL.

Patients should receive supplemental calcium and vitamin D if dietary intake is inadequate (see PRECAUTIONS, General). Calcium supplements or calcium-, aluminum-, and magnesium-containing medications may interfere with the absorption of ACTONEL and should be taken at a different time of the day, as with food.

Weight-bearing exercise should be considered along with the modification of certain behavioral factors, such as excessive cigarette smoking, and/or alcohol consumption, if these factors exist.

Drug Interactions: No specific drug-drug interaction studies were performed. Risedronate is not metabolized and does not induce or inhibit hepatic microsomal drug-metabolizing enzymes (Cytochrome P450).

Calcium Supplements/Antacids: Co-administration of ACTONEL and calcium, antacids, or oral medications containing divalent cations will interfere with the absorption of ACTONEL.

Hormone Replacement Therapy: One study of about 500 early postmenopausal women has been conducted to date in which treatment with ACTONEL (5 mg/day) plus estrogen replacement therapy was compared with estrogen replacement therapy alone. Exposure to study drugs was approximately 12 to 18 months and the primary endpoint was change in BMD. If considered appropriate, ACTONEL may be used concomitantly with hormone replacement therapy.

Aspirin/Nonsteroidal Anti-Inflammatory Drugs (NSAIDs): Of over 5700 patients enrolled in the ACTONEL Phase 3 osteoporosis studies, aspirin use was reported by 31% of patients, 24% of whom were regular users (3 or more days per week). Forty-eight percent of patients reported NSAID use, 21% of whom were regular users. Among regular aspirin or NSAID users, the incidence of upper gastrointestinal adverse experiences in ACTONEL-treated patients (24.5%) was similar to that in placebo-treated patients (24.8%).

H_2 Blockers and Proton Pump Inhibitors (PPIs): Of over 5700 patients enrolled in the ACTONEL Phase 3 osteoporosis studies, 21% used H_2 blockers and/or PPIs. Among these patients, the incidence of upper gastrointestinal adverse experiences in the ACTONEL-treated patients was similar to that in placebo-treated patients.

Drug/Laboratory Test Interactions: Bisphosphonates are known to interfere with the use of bone-imaging agents. Specific studies with ACTONEL have not been performed.

Carcinogenesis, Mutagenesis, Impairment of Fertility:

Carcinogenesis: In a 104-week carcinogenicity study, rats were administered daily oral doses up to 24 mg/kg/day (approximately 7.7 times the maximum recommended human daily dose of 30 mg based on surface area, mg/m^2). There were no significant drug-induced tumor findings in male or female rats. The high dose male group of 24 mg/kg/day was terminated early in the study (Week 93) due to excessive toxicity, and data from this group were not included in the statistical evaluation of the study results. In an 80-week carcinogenicity study, mice were administered daily oral doses up to 32 mg/kg/day (approximately 6.4 times the 30 mg/day human dose based on surface area, mg/m^2). There were no significant drug-induced tumor findings in male or female mice.

Mutagenesis: Risedronate did not exhibit genetic toxicity in the following assays: *In vitro* bacterial mutagenesis in *Salmonella* and *E. coli* (Ames assay), mammalian cell mutagenesis in CHO/HGPRT assay, unscheduled DNA synthesis in rat hepatocytes and an assessment of chromosomal aberrations *in vivo* in rat bone marrow. Risedronate was positive in a chromosomal aberration assay in CHO cells at highly cytotoxic concentrations (> 675 mcg/mL, survival of 6% to 7%). When the assay was repeated at doses exhibiting appropriate cell survival (29%), there was no evidence of chromosomal damage.

Impairment of Fertility: In female rats, ovulation was inhibited at an oral dose of 16 mg/kg/day (approximately 5.2 times the 30 mg/day human dose based on surface area, mg/m^2). Decreased implantation was noted in female rats treated with doses ≥ 7 mg/kg/day (approximately 2.3 times the 30 mg/day human dose based on surface area, mg/m^2). In male rats, testicular and epididymal atrophy and inflammation were noted at 40 mg/kg/day (approximately 13 times the 30 mg/day human dose based on surface area, mg/m^2). Testicular atrophy was also noted in male rats after 13 weeks of treatment at oral doses of 16 mg/kg/day (approximately 5.2 times the 30 mg/day human dose based on surface area, mg/m^2). There was moderate-to-severe spermatid maturation block after 13 weeks in male dogs at an oral dose of 8 mg/kg/day (approximately 8 times the 30 mg/day human dose based on surface area, mg/m^2). These findings tended to increase in severity with increased dose and exposure time.

Pregnancy: Pregnancy Category C: Survival of neonates was decreased in rats treated during gestation with oral doses ≥ 16 mg/kg/day (approximately 5.2 times the 30 mg/day human dose based on surface area, mg/m^2). Body weight was decreased in neonates from dams treated with 80 mg/kg (approximately 26 times the 30 mg/day human dose based on surface area, mg/m^2). In rats treated during gestation, the number of fetuses exhibiting incomplete ossification of sternebrae or skull was statistically significantly increased at 7.1 mg/kg/day (approximately 2.3 times the 30 mg/day human dose based on surface area, mg/m^2). Both incomplete ossification and unossified sternebrae were increased in rats treated with oral doses ≥ 16 mg/kg/day (approximately 5.2 times the 30 mg/day human dose based on surface area, mg/m^2). A low incidence of cleft palate was observed in fetuses from female rats treated with oral doses ≥ 3.2 mg/kg/day (approximately 1 time the 30 mg/day human dose based on surface area, mg/m^2). The relevance of this finding to human use of ACTONEL is unclear. No significant fetal ossification effects were seen in rabbits treated with oral doses up to 10 mg/kg/day during gestation (approximately 6.7 times the 30 mg/day human dose based on surface area, mg/m^2). However, in rabbits treated with 10 mg/kg/day, 1 of 14 litters were aborted and 1 of 14 litters were delivered prematurely.

Similar to other bisphosphonates, treatment during mating and gestation with doses as low as 3.2 mg/kg/day (approximately 1 time the 30 mg/day human dose based on surface area, mg/m^2) has resulted in periparturient hypocalcemia and mortality in pregnant rats allowed to deliver.

There are no adequate and well-controlled studies of ACTONEL in pregnant women. ACTONEL should be used during pregnancy only if the potential benefit justifies the potential risk to the mother and fetus.

Nursing Women: Risedronate was detected in feeding pups exposed to lactating rats for a 24-hour period postdosing, indicating a small degree of lacteal transfer. It is not known whether risedronate is excreted in human milk. Because many drugs are excreted in human milk and because of the potential for serious adverse reactions in nursing infants from bisphosphonates, a decision should be made whether to discontinue nursing or to discontinue the drug, taking into account the importance of the drug to the mother.

Pediatric Use: Safety and effectiveness in pediatric patients have not been established.

Geriatric Use: Of the patients receiving ACTONEL in postmenopausal osteoporosis studies (see CLINICAL STUDIES), 43% were between 65 and 75 years of age, and 20% were over 75. The corresponding proportions were 26% and 11% in glucocorticoid-induced osteoporosis trials, and 40% and 26% in Paget's disease trials. No overall differences in efficacy or safety were observed between these patients and younger patients.

Use in Men: Safety and effectiveness have been demonstrated in clinical studies in men receiving ACTONEL both

Continued on next page

Actonel—Cont.

for Paget's disease and for treatment and prevention of glucocorticoid-induced osteoporosis. However, the safety and effectiveness in men for osteoporosis due to other causes have not been established.

ADVERSE REACTIONS

Osteoporosis: ACTONEL has been studied in over 5700 patients enrolled in the Phase 3 glucocorticoid-induced osteoporosis clinical trials and in postmenopausal osteoporosis trials of up to 3 years duration. The overall adverse event profile of ACTONEL 5 mg in these studies was similar to that of placebo. Most adverse events were either mild or moderate and did not lead to discontinuation from the study. The incidence of serious adverse events in the placebo group was 24.9% and in the ACTONEL 5 mg group was 26.3%. The percentage of patients who withdrew from the study due to adverse events was 14.4% and 13.5% for the placebo and ACTONEL 5 mg groups, respectively. Table 5 lists adverse events from the Phase 3 osteoporosis trials reported in ≥ 2% of patients and in more ACTONEL-treated patients than placebo-treated patients. Adverse events are shown without attribution of causality.

[See table 5 below]

Duodenitis and glossitis have been reported uncommonly (0.1% to 1%). There have been rare reports (< 0.1%) of abnormal liver function tests.

Laboratory Test Findings: Asymptomatic and small decreases were observed in serum calcium and phosphorus levels. Overall, mean decreases of 0.8% in serum calcium and of 2.7% in phosphorus were observed at 6 months in patients receiving ACTONEL. Throughout the Phase 3 studies, serum calcium levels below 8 mg/dL were observed in 18 patients, 9 (0.5%) in each treatment arm (ACTONEL and placebo). Serum phosphorus levels below 2 mg/dL were observed in 14 patients, 11 (0.6%) treated with ACTONEL and 3 (0.2%) treated with placebo.

Endoscopic Findings: ACTONEL clinical studies enrolled over 5700 patients, many with pre-existing gastrointestinal disease and concomitant use of NSAIDs or aspirin. Investigators were encouraged to perform endoscopies in any patients with moderate-to-severe gastrointestinal complaints while maintaining the blind. These endoscopies were ultimately performed on equal numbers of patients between the treated and placebo groups [75 (14.5%) placebo; 75 (11.9%) ACTONEL]. Across treatment groups, the percentage of patients with normal esophageal, gastric, and duodenal mucosa on endoscopy was similar (20% placebo, 21% ACTONEL). The number of patients who withdrew from the studies due to the event prompting endoscopy was similar across treatment groups. Positive findings on endoscopy were also generally comparable across treatment groups. There was a higher number of reports of mild duodenitis in the ACTONEL group, however there were more duodenal ulcers in the placebo group. Clinically important findings (perforations, ulcers, or bleeding) among this symptomatic population were similar between groups (51% placebo; 39% ACTONEL).

Paget's Disease: ACTONEL has been studied in 392 patients with Paget's disease of bone. As in trials of ACTONEL for other indications, the adverse experiences reported in the Paget's disease trials have generally been mild or moderate, have not required discontinuation of treatment, and have not appeared to be related to patient age, gender, or race.

In a double-blind, active-controlled study, the adverse event profile was similar for ACTONEL and Didronel: 6.6% (4/61) of patients treated with ACTONEL 30 mg/day for 2 months discontinued treatment due to adverse events, compared with 8.2% (5/61) of patients treated with Didronel 400 mg/day for 6 months.

[See table at bottom of next page]

Three patients that received ACTONEL 30 mg/day experienced acute iritis in one supportive study. All three patients recovered from their events; however, in one of these patients, the event recurred during ACTONEL treatment and again during treatment with pamidronate. All patients were effectively treated with topical steroids.

Table 5
Adverse Events Occurring at a Frequency ≥ 2% and in More ACTONEL-Treated Patients than Placebo-Treated Patients
Combined Phase 3 Osteoporosis Trials

Body System	Placebo % (N = 1914)	ACTONEL 5 mg % (N = 1916)
Body as a Whole		
Infection	29.7	29.9
Back Pain	23.6	26.1
Pain	13.1	13.6
Abdominal Pain	9.4	11.6
Neck Pain	4.5	5.3
Asthenia	4.3	5.1
Chest Pain	4.9	5.0
Neoplasm	3.0	3.3
Hernia	2.5	2.9
Cardiovascular		
Hypertension	9.0	10.0
Cardiovascular Disorder	1.7	2.5
Angina Pectoris	2.4	2.5
Digestive		
Nausea	10.7	10.9
Diarrhea	9.6	10.6
Flatulence	4.2	4.6
Gastritis	2.3	2.5
Gastrointestinal Disorder	2.1	2.3
Rectal Disorder	1.9	2.2
Tooth Disorder	2.0	2.1
Hemic and Lymphatic		
Ecchymosis	4.0	4.3
Anemia	1.9	2.4
Musculoskeletal		
Arthralgia	21.1	23.7
Joint Disorder	5.4	6.8
Myalgia	6.3	6.6
Bone Pain	4.3	4.6
Bone Disorder	3.2	4.0
Leg Cramps	2.6	3.5
Bursitis	2.9	3.0
Tendon Disorder	2.5	3.0
Nervous		
Depression	6.2	6.8
Dizziness	5.4	6.4
Insomnia	4.5	4.7
Anxiety	3.0	4.3
Neuralgia	3.5	3.8
Vertigo	3.2	3.3
Hypertonia	2.1	2.2
Paresthesia	1.8	2.1
Respiratory		
Pharyngitis	5.0	5.8
Rhinitis	5.0	5.7
Dyspnea	3.2	3.8
Pneumonia	2.6	3.1
Skin and Appendages		
Rash	7.2	7.7
Pruritus	2.2	3.0
Skin Carcinoma	1.8	2.0
Special Senses		
Cataract	5.4	5.9
Conjunctivitis	2.8	3.1
Otitis Media	2.4	2.5
Urogenital		
Urinary Tract Infection	9.7	10.9
Cystitis	3.5	4.1

OVERDOSAGE

Decreases in serum calcium and phosphorus following substantial overdose may be expected in some patients. Signs and symptoms of hypocalcemia may also occur in some of these patients. Milk or antacids containing calcium should be given to bind ACTONEL and reduce absorption of the drug.

In cases of substantial overdose, gastric lavage may be considered to remove unabsorbed drug. Standard procedures that are effective for treating hypocalcemia, including the administration of calcium intravenously, would be expected to restore physiologic amounts of ionized calcium and to relieve signs and symptoms of hypocalcemia.

Lethality after single oral doses was seen in female rats at 903 mg/kg and male rats at 1703 mg/kg. The minimum lethal dose in mice and rabbits was 4000 mg/kg and 1000 mg/kg. These values represent 320 to 620 times the 30-mg human dose based on surface area (mg/m^2).

DOSAGE AND ADMINISTRATION

ACTONEL should be taken once per day at least 30 minutes before the first food or drink of the day other than water.

To facilitate delivery to the stomach, ACTONEL should be swallowed while the patient is in an upright position and with a full glass of plain water (6 to 8 oz). Patients should not lie down for 30 minutes after taking the medication (see PRECAUTIONS, General).

Patients should receive supplemental calcium and vitamin D if dietary intake is inadequate (see PRECAUTIONS, General). Calcium supplements and calcium-, aluminum-, and magnesium-containing medications may interfere with the absorption of ACTONEL and should be taken at a different time of the day. ACTONEL is not recommended for use in patients with severe renal impairment (creatinine clearance < 30 mL/min). No dosage adjustment is necessary in patients with a creatinine clearance ≥ 30 mL/min or in the elderly.

Treatment and Prevention of Postmenopausal Osteoporosis/Glucocorticoid-Induced Osteoporosis (see INDICATIONS AND USAGE): The recommended regimen is 5 mg orally daily.

Paget's Disease (see INDICATIONS AND USAGE): The recommended treatment regimen is 30 mg once daily for 2 months. Retreatment may be considered (following post-treatment observation of at least 2 months) if relapse occurs, or if treatment fails to normalize serum alkaline phosphatase. For retreatment, the dose and duration of therapy are the same as for initial treatment. No data are available on more than one course of retreatment.

HOW SUPPLIED

ACTONEL is available as follows:

5-mg film-coated, oval, yellow tablets with RSN on one face and 5 mg on the other.

NDC 0149-0471-01 bottle of 30

30-mg film-coated, oval, white tablets with RSN on one face and 30 mg on the other.

NDC 0149-0470-01 bottle of 30

Store at controlled room temperature 20°–25°C (68°–77°F) [See USP].

Sold Under U.S. Patent No. 5,583,122

Mfg. and Dist. by:
Procter & Gamble Pharmaceuticals, TM Owner
Cincinnati, Ohio 45202
Mkt. with:
Aventis Pharmaceuticals Inc. (formerly Hoechst Marion Roussel, Inc.)
Kansas City, Missouri 64137
APRIL 2000

ACTONEL® (AK-toh-nel) Tablets
Patient Information
generic name: risedronate sodium

This leaflet tells you about ACTONEL and how to take it. Read this information carefully before you begin taking ACTONEL. It is important to take ACTONEL exactly as recommended. Read this information each time your prescription is refilled in case new information is available. This leaflet does not take the place of discussions with your health care provider because it does not describe all the risks and benefits of ACTONEL. ACTONEL can be prescribed and dispensed only by licensed health care professionals; they have information about your medical condition and more information about ACTONEL. Talk with your health care provider about ACTONEL before you start taking the medicine and during your regular checkups.

What is the most important information I should know about ACTONEL?

Take ACTONEL once a day or as directed by your health care provider. You must take ACTONEL exactly as recommended so that it will work and to reduce the risk of harmful side effects (see **How should I take ACTONEL?**).

What is ACTONEL?
ACTONEL is a drug to treat and prevent osteoporosis. ACTONEL can reverse bone loss and help reduce the risk of breaking bones (fractures) by stopping further loss of bone and increasing bone mass. ACTONEL is not a hormone like estrogen (hormone replacement therapy used in postmenopausal women). Therefore, it does not have all the benefits and risks of estrogen.

What is osteoporosis?
Osteoporosis is a disease that causes bones to become thinner. Thin bones can break easily. Most people think of their bones as being solid like a rock. Actually, bone is tissue, just like other parts of the body—your heart, brain, or skin, for example. Bone just happens to be a harder type of tissue. Bone is always changing. Your body keeps your bones strong and healthy by replacing old bone with new bone.
When someone has osteoporosis, the body removes more bone than it replaces. This means that bones get weaker and more likely to break. Osteoporosis is a bone disease that is quite common, especially in older women. However, young people and men can develop osteoporosis, too.
Osteoporosis can be prevented, and with proper therapy it can be effectively managed.

How can osteoporosis affect me?
In the early stages of osteporosis, people often have no pain or other symptoms. As bones become weaker, they are more likely to break when someone falls—or even without a fall. While osteoporosis can affect any bone, the spine, wrist, and hip are the bones most likely to break. People with osteoporosis may "shrink" (lost height), develop a curved back, or have severe back pain that forces them to limit their activities.

Who is at risk for osteoporosis?
Many things put people at risk for osteoporosis. Some are just part of who you are, like being a woman, going through menopause or already being postmenopausal, being Caucasian or Asian, being thin, or having a family history of osteoporosis. Other factors include not getting enough calcium or vitamin D, having an inactive lifestyle, smoking cigarettes, or drinking too much alcohol. Long-term use of cortisone-type medicines (such as prednisone) can also cause osteoporosis in both men and women of all ages.

Who should not take ACTONEL?
Do not take ACTONEL if you have:
- low blood calcium (hypocalcemia)
- the inability to sit or stand upright for 30 minutes
- an allergy to ACTONEL
- severe kidney disease

If you are pregnant or nursing (breast-feeding), or have severe kidney disease, talk to your health care provider before taking ACTONEL.

How should I take ACTONEL?
Take ACTONEL once daily or as directed by your health care provider. It is important to take ACTONEL as recommended so that you can benefit from the medicine. Following these recommendations also helps ACTONEL work correctly and helps you avoid possible irritation of the esophagus, the tube connecting the mouth and the stomach.
Take one ACTONEL tablet first thing in the morning while in an upright position (sitting or standing) before you have anything to eat or drink (other than plain water). Do not eat or drink anything except plain water for 30 minutes after taking ACTONEL.

Remember:
- Take one ACTONEL tablet with 6 to 8 ounces (about 1 cup) of plain water (not coffee, tea, or juice, and **especially not milk or other dairy products**).
- After taking ACTONEL, wait at least 30 minutes before lying down. You may sit, stand, or do normal activities like read the newspaper, take a walk, etc.
- Swallow ACTONEL whole rather than chewing it or waiting for it to dissolve.
- If you take vitamins, calcium, and antacids, take them at a different time of the day from when you take ACTONEL, at least 30 minutes after you take ACTONEL.
- If you forget to take ACTONEL, do not double your next dose. Simply take ACTONEL as you normally would for your next dose.
- You should continue to take ACTONEL for as long as your health care provider receommends. ACTONEL can treat your osteoporosis or help keep you from getting osteoporosis only if you continue to take it.

What should I avoid while taking ACTONEL?
Foods and some supplements and medicines can stop your body from absorbing ACTONEL. Therefore, do not take these products at or near the time you take ACTONEL: food, milk, calcium supplements, or calcium-, aluminum-, or magnesium-containing medicines, such as antacids (see How should I take ACTONEL?). Ask your health care provider if there is anything else you should avoid while taking this medicine.

What are the possible side effects of ACTONEL?
Most people have no problems with ACTONEL. However, ACTONEL may cause side effects. Side effects from ACTONEL are usually mild. They generally do not cause patients to stop taking ACTONEL.
In studies of ACTONEL in patients with osteoporosis, the most common side effects were reported about as often with ACTONEL as with placebo (sugar pill). They include upset stomach, abdominal (stomach area) pain, constipation, diarrhea, gas, and headache.
This summary does not include all the possible side effects of ACTONEL. Talk to your health care provider about possible side effects. Tell your health care provider if you feel discomfort in your stomach or esophagus (the tube connecting the mouth and the stomach). Stop taking ACTONEL and tell your health care provider right away if swallowing is difficult or painful, if you have chest pain or if you have severe or continuing heartburn.

Other important information

How can I tell if ACTONEL is working?
ACTONEL can build bone mass in most people who take it, even though they won't be able to see or feel a difference. Your health care provider may measure the thickness (density) of your bones to check your progress. This is called a bone mineral density measurement.

What if I have other questions about ACTONEL?
If you have questions about ACTONEL, ask your health care provider or pharmacist. If you want to read more about ACTONEL, ask your health care provider or pharmacist for the labeling written for health care professionals. For more information, call 1-877-ACTONEL (toll-free) or visit our web site at www.actonel.com

Table 6
Adverse Events Reported in ≥ 2% of ACTONEL-Treated Patients*
in Phase 3 Paget's Disease Trials

Body System	30 mg/day × 2 months ACTONEL % (N = 61)	400 mg/day × 6 months Didronel % (N = 61)
Body as a Whole		
Flu Syndrome	9.8	1.6
Chest Pain	6.6	3.3
Asthenia	4.9	0
Neoplasm	3.3	1.6
Gastrointestinal		
Diarrhea	19.7	14.8
Abdominal Pain	11.5	8.2
Nausea	9.8	9.8
Constipation	6.6	8.2
Belching	3.3	1.6
Colitis	3.3	3.3
Metabolic & Nutritional		
Peripheral Edema	8.2	6.6
Musculoskeletal		
Arthralgia	32.8	29.5
Bone Pain	4.9	4.9
Leg Cramps	3.3	3.3
Myasthenia	3.3	0
Nervous		
Headache	18.0	16.4
Dizziness	6.6	4.9
Respiratory		
Bronchitis	3.3	4.9
Sinusitis	4.9	1.6
Skin		
Rash	11.5	8.2
Special Senses		
Amblyopia	3.3	3.3
Tinnitus	3.3	3.3
Dry Eye	3.3	0

* Considered to be possibly or probably causally related in at least one patient

ACTONEL® is marketed by:
Procter & Gamble Pharmaceuticals
Cincinnati, Ohio 45202
and
Aventis Pharmaceuticals Inc. (formerly Hoechst Marion Roussel, Inc.)
Kansas City, Missouri 64137

APRIL 2000
Shown in Product Identification Guide, page 331

ASACOL® ℞
[*āce 'ah-kol*]
(mesalamine)
Delayed-Release Tablets

DESCRIPTION
Each **Asacol** delayed-release tablet for oral administration contains 400 mg of mesalamine, an anti-inflammatory drug. The **Asacol** delayed-release tablets are coated with acrylic based resin, Eudragit S (methacrylic acid copolymer B, NF), which dissolves at pH 7 or greater, releasing mesalamine in the terminal ileum and beyond for topical anti-inflammatory action in the colon. Mesalamine has the chemical name 5-amino-2-hydroxybenzoic acid; its structural formula is:

COOH
OH
H_2N
Molecular Weight: 153.1
Molecular Formula: $C_7H_7NO_3$

Inactive Ingredients: Each tablet contains colloidal silicon dioxide, dibutyl phthalate, edible black ink, iron oxide red, iron oxide yellow, lactose, magnesium stearate, methacrylic acid copolymer B (Eudragit S), polyethylene glycol, povidone, sodium starch glycolate, and talc.

CLINICAL PHARMACOLOGY
Mesalamine is thought to be the major therapeutically active part of the sulfasalazine molecule in the treatment of ulcerative colitis. Sulfasalazine is converted to equimolar amounts of sulfapyridine and mesalamine by bacterial action in the colon. The usual oral dose of sulfasalazine for active ulcerative colitis is 3 to 4 grams daily in divided doses, which provides 1.2 to 1.6 grams of mesalamine to the colon.
The mechanism of action of mesalamine (and sulfasalazine) is unknown, but appears to be topical rather than systemic. Mucosal production of arachidonic acid (AA) metabolites, both through the cyclooxygenase pathways, i.e., prostanoids, and through the lipoxygenase pathways, i.e., leukotrienes (LTs) and hydroxyeicosatetraenoic acids (HETEs), is increased in patients with chronic inflammatory bowel disease, and it is possible that mesalamine diminishes inflammation by blocking cyclooxygenase and inhibiting prostaglandin (PG) production in the colon.

Pharmacokinetics: **Asacol** tablets are coated with an acrylic-based resin that delays release of mesalamine until it reaches the terminal ileum and beyond. This has been demonstrated in human studies conducted with radiological and serum markers. Approximately 28% of the mesalamine in **Asacol** tablets is absorbed after oral ingestion, leaving the remainder available for topical action and excretion in the feces. Absorption of mesalamine is similar in fasted and fed subjects. The absorbed mesalamine is rapidly acetylated in the gut mucosal wall and by the liver. It is excreted mainly by the kidney as N-acetyl-5-aminosalicylic acid.
Mesalamine from orally administered **Asacol** tablets appears to be more extensively absorbed than the mesalamine released from sulfasalazine. Maximum plasma levels of mesalamine and N-acetyl-5-aminosalicylic acid following multiple **Asacol** doses are about 1.5 to 2 times higher than those following an equivalent dose of mesalamine in the form of sulfasalazine. Combined mesalamine and N-acetyl-5-aminosalicylic acid AUC's and urine drug dose recoveries following multiple doses of **Asacol** tablets are about 1.3 to 1.5 times higher than those following an equivalent dose of mesalamine in the form of sulfasalazine.
The t_{max} for mesalamine and its metabolite, N-acetyl-5-aminosalicylic acid, is usually delayed, reflecting the delayed release, and ranges from 4 to 12 hours. The half-lives of elimination ($t1/2_{elm}$) for mesalamine and N-acetyl-5-aminosalicylic acid are usually about 12 hours, but are variable, ranging from 2 to 15 hours. There is a large intersubject variability in the plasma concentrations of mesalamine and N-acetyl-5-aminosalicylic acid and in their elimination half-lives following administration of **Asacol** tablets.

Clinical Studies:
Mildly to moderately active ulcerative colitis: Two placebo-controlled studies have demonstrated the efficacy of **Asacol** tablets in patients with mildly to moderately active ulcerative colitis. In one randomized, double-blind, multi-center trial of 158 patients, **Asacol** doses of 1.6 g/day and 2.4

Continued on next page

Asacol—Cont.

g/day were compared to placebo. At the dose of 2.4 g/day, **Asacol** tablets reduced the disease activity, with 21 of 43 (49%) **Asacol** patients showing improvement in sigmoidoscopic appearance of the bowel compared to 12 of 44 (27%) placebo patients (p = 0.048). In addition, significantly more patients in the **Asacol** 2.4 g/day group showed improvement in rectal bleeding and stool frequency. The 1.6 g/day dose did not produce consistent evidence of effectiveness.

In a second randomized, double-blind, placebo-controlled clinical trial of 6 weeks duration in 87 ulcerative colitis patients, **Asacol** tablets, at a dose of 4.8 g/day, gave sigmoidoscopic improvement in 28 of 38 (74%) patients compared to 10 of 38 (26%) placebo patients ($p < 0.001$). Also, more patients in the **Asacol** 4.8 g/day group showed improvement in overall symptoms.

Maintenance of remission of ulcerative colitis: A 6-month, randomized, double-blind, placebo-controlled, multi-center study involved 264 patients treated with **Asacol** 0.8 g/day (n = 90), 1.6 g/day (n = 87), or placebo (n = 87). The proportion of patients treated with 0.8 g/day who maintained endoscopic remission was not statistically significant compared to placebo. In the intention to treat (ITT) analysis of all 174 patients treated with **Asacol** 1.6 g/day or placebo, **Asacol** maintained endoscopic remission of ulcerative colitis in 61 of 87 (70.1%) of patients, compared to 42 of 87 (48.3%) of placebo recipients (p = 0.005).

A pooled efficacy analysis of 4 maintenance trials compared **Asacol**, at doses of 0.8 g/day to 2.8 g/day, with sulfasalazine, at doses of 2 g/day to 4 g/day (n = 200). Treatment success was 59 of 98 (59%) for **Asacol** and 70 of 102 (69%) for sulfasalazine, a non-significant difference.

Study to assess the effect on male fertility: The effect of **Asacol** (mesalamine) on sulfasalazine-induced impairment of male fertility was examined in an open-label study. Nine patients (age < 40 years) with chronic ulcerative colitis in clinical remission on sulfasalazine 2 g/day to 3 g/day were crossed over to an equivalent **Asacol** dose (0.8 g/day to 1.2 g/day) for 3 months. Improvement in sperm count ($p < 0.02$) and morphology ($p < 0.02$) occurred in all cases. Improvement in sperm motility ($p < 0.001$) occurred in 8 of the 9 patients.

INDICATIONS AND USAGE

Asacol tablets are indicated for the treatment of mildly to moderately active ulcerative colitis and for the maintenance of remission of ulcerative colitis.

CONTRAINDICATIONS

Asacol tablets are contraindicated in patients with hypersensitivity to salicylates or to any of the components of the **Asacol** tablet.

PRECAUTIONS

General: Patients with pyloric stenosis may have prolonged gastric retention of **Asacol** tablets which could delay release of mesalamine in the colon.

Exacerbation of the symptoms of colitis has been reported in 3% of **Asacol**-treated patients in controlled clinical trials. This acute reaction, characterized by cramping, abdominal pain, bloody diarrhea, and occasionally by fever, headache, malaise, pruritus, rash, and conjunctivitis, has been reported after the initiation of **Asacol** tablets as well as other mesalamine products. Symptoms usually abate when **Asacol** tablets are discontinued.

Some patients who have experienced a hypersensitivity reaction to sulfasalazine may have a similar reaction to **Asacol** tablets or to other compounds which contain or are converted to mesalamine.

Renal: Renal impairment, including minimal change nephropathy, and acute and chronic interstitial nephritis, has been reported in patients taking **Asacol** tablets as well as other compounds which contain or are converted to mesalamine. In animal studies (rats, dogs), the kidney is the principal target organ for toxicity. At doses of approximately 750 mg/kg to 1000 mg/kg [15 to 20 times the administered recommended human dose (based on a 50 kg person) on a mg/kg basis and 3 to 4 times on a mg/m^2 basis], mesalamine causes renal papillary necrosis. **Therefore, caution should be exercised when using Asacol (or other compounds which contain or are converted to mesalamine or its metabolites) in patients with known renal dysfunction or history of renal disease. It is recommended that all patients have an evaluation of renal function prior to initiation of Asacol tablets and periodically while on Asacol therapy.**

Information for Patients: Patients should be instructed to swallow the **Asacol** tablets whole, taking care not to break the outer coating. The outer coating is designed to remain intact to protect the active ingredient and thus ensure mesalamine availability for action in the colon. In 2% to 3% of patients in clinical studies, intact or partially intact tablets have been reported in the stool. If this occurs repeatedly, patients should contact their physician.

Patients with ulcerative colitis should be made aware that ulcerative colitis rarely remits completely, and that the risk of relapse can be substantially reduced by continued administration of **Asacol** at a maintenance dosage.

Drug Interactions: There are no known drug interactions.

Carcinogenesis, Mutagenesis, Impairment of Fertility: Dietary mesalamine was not carcinogenic in rats at doses as high as 480 mg/kg/day, or in mice at 2000 mg/kg/day. These doses are 2.4 and 5.1 times the maximum recommended human maintenance dose of **Asacol** of 1.6 g/day (32 mg/kg/day if 50 kg body weight assumed or 1184 mg/m^2), respectively, based on body surface area. Mesalamine was negative in the Ames assay for mutagenesis, negative for induction of sister chromatid exchanges (SCE) and chromosomal aberrations in Chinese hamster ovary cells *in vitro*, and negative for induction of micronuclei (MN) in mouse bone marrow polychromatic erythrocytes. Mesalamine, at oral doses up to 480 mg/kg/day, had no adverse effect on fertility or reproductive performance of male and female rats.

Pregnancy: Teratogenic Effects: Pregnancy Category B: Reproduction studies in rats and rabbits at oral doses up to 480 mg/kg/day have revealed no evidence of teratogenic effects or fetal toxicity due to mesalamine. There are, however, no adequate and well-controlled studies in pregnant women. Because animal reproduction studies are not always predictive of human response, this drug should be used during pregnancy only if clearly needed.

Nursing Mothers: Low concentrations of mesalamine and higher concentrations of its N-acetyl metabolite have been detected in human breast milk. While the clinical significance of this has not been determined, caution should be exercised when mesalamine is administered to a nursing woman.

Pediatric Use: Safety and effectiveness of **Asacol** tablets in pediatric patients have not been established.

Geriatric Use: Clinical studies of **Asacol** did not include sufficient numbers of subjects aged 65 and over to determine whether they respond differently from younger subjects. Other reported clinical experience has not identified differences in responses between the elderly and younger patients. In general, the greater frequency of decreased hepatic, renal, or cardiac function, and of concomitant disease or other drug therapy in elderly patients should be considered when prescribing **Asacol**.

This drug is known to be substantially excreted by the kidney, and the risk of toxic reactions to this drug may be greater in patients with impaired renal function. Because elderly patients are more likely to have decreased renal function, care should be taken when prescribing this drug therapy. As stated in the PRECAUTIONS section, it is recommended that all patients have an evaluation of renal function prior to initiation of **Asacol** tablets and periodically while on **Asacol** therapy.

ADVERSE REACTIONS

Asacol tablets have been evaluated in 3685 inflammatory bowel disease patients (most patients with ulcerative colitis) in controlled and open-label studies. Adverse events seen in clinical trials with **Asacol** tablets have generally been mild and reversible. Adverse events presented in the following sections may occur regardless of length of therapy and similar events have been reported in short- and long-term studies and in the post-marketing setting.

In two short-term (6 weeks) placebo-controlled clinical studies involving 245 patients, 155 of whom were randomized to **Asacol** tablets, five (3.2%) of the **Asacol** patients discontinued **Asacol** therapy because of adverse events as compared to two (2.2%) of the placebo patients. Adverse reactions leading to withdrawal from **Asacol** tablets included (each in one patient): diarrhea and colitis flare; dizziness, nausea, joint pain, and headache; rash, lethargy and constipation; dry mouth, malaise, lower back discomfort, mild disorientation, mild indigestion and cramping; headache, nausea, malaise, aching, vomiting, muscle cramps, a stuffy head, plugged ears, and fever.

Adverse events occurring in **Asacol**-treated patients at a frequency of 2% or greater in the two short-term, double-blind, placebo-controlled trials mentioned above are listed in Table 1 below. Overall, the incidence of adverse events seen with **Asacol** tablets was similar to placebo.

Table 1
Frequency (%) of Common Adverse Events Reported in Ulcerative Colitis Patients Treated with **Asacol** Tablets or Placebo in Short-Term (6-Week) Double-Blind Controlled Studies

	Percent of Patients with Adverse Events	
Event	Placebo (n = 87)	Asacol tablets (n = 152)
Headache	36	35
Abdominal pain	14	18
Eructation	15	16
Pain	8	14
Nausea	15	13
Pharyngitis	9	11
Dizziness	8	8
Asthenia	15	7
Diarrhea	9	7
Back pain	5	7
Fever	8	6
Rash	3	6
Dyspepsia	1	6
Rhinitis	5	5
Arthralgia	3	5
Hypertonia	3	5
Vomiting	2	5
Constipation	1	5
Flatulence	7	3
Dysmenorrhea	3	3
Chest pain	2	3
Chills	2	3
Flu syndrome	2	3
Peripheral edema	2	3
Myalgia	1	3
Sweating	1	3
Colitis exacerbation	0	3
Pruritus	0	3
Acne	1	2
Increased cough	1	2
Malaise	1	2
Arthritis	0	2
Conjunctivitis	0	2
Insomnia	0	2

Of these adverse events, only rash showed a consistently higher frequency with increasing **Asacol** dose in these studies.

In a 6-month placebo-controlled maintenance trial involving 264 patients, 177 of whom were randomized to **Asacol** tablets, six (3.4%) of the **Asacol** patients discontinued **Asacol** therapy because of adverse events, as compared to four (4.6%) of the placebo patients. Adverse reactions leading to withdrawal from **Asacol** tablets included (each in one patient): anxiety; headache; pruritus; decreased libido; rheumatoid arthritis; and stomatitis and asthenia.

In the 6-month placebo-controlled maintenance trial, the incidence of adverse events seen with **Asacol** tablets was similar to that seen with placebo. In addition to events listed in Table 1, the following adverse events occurred in **Asacol**-treated patients at a frequency of 2% or greater in this study: abdominal enlargement, anxiety, bronchitis, ear disorder, ear pain, gastroenteritis, gastrointestinal hemorrhage, infection, joint disorder, migraine, nervousness, paresthesia, rectal disorder, rectal hemorrhage, sinusitis, stool abnormalities, tenesmus, urinary frequency, vasodilation, and vision abnormalities.

In 3342 patients in uncontrolled clinical studies, the following adverse events occurred at a frequency of 5% or greater and appeared to increase in frequency with increasing dose: asthenia, fever, flu syndrome, pain, abdominal pain, back pain, flatulence, gastrointestinal bleeding, arthralgia, and rhinitis.

In addition to the adverse events listed above, the following events have been reported in clinical studies, literature reports, and postmarketing use of products which contain (or have been metabolized to) mesalamine. Because many of these events were reported voluntarily from a population of unknown size, estimates of frequency cannot be made. These events have been chosen for inclusion due to their seriousness of potential causal connection to mesalamine:

Body as a Whole: Neck pain, facial edema, edema, lupus-like syndrome.

Cardiovascular: Pericarditis (rare), myocarditis (rare).

Gastrointestinal: Anorexia, pancreatitis, gastritis, increased appetite, cholecystitis, dry mouth, oral ulcers, perforated peptic ulcer (rare), bloody diarrhea. There have been rare reports of hepatotoxicity including, jaundice, cholestatic jaundice, hepatitis, and possible hepatocellular damage including liver necrosis and liver failure. Some of these cases were fatal. Asymptomatic elevations of liver enzymes which usually resolve during continued use or with discontinuation of the drug have also been reported. One case of Kawasaki-like syndrome which included changes in liver enzymes was also reported.

Hematologic: Agranulocytosis (rare), aplastic anemia (rare), thrombocytopenia, eosinophilia, leukopenia, anemia, lymphadenopathy.

Musculoskeletal: Gout.

Nervous: Depression, somnolence, emotional lability, hyperesthesia, vertigo, confusion, tremor, peripheral neuropathy (rare), transverse myelitis (rare), Guillain-Barré syndrome (rare).

Respiratory/Pulmonary: Eosinophilic pneumonia, interstitial pneumonitis, asthma exacerbation, pleuritis.

Skin: Alopecia, psoriasis (rare), pyoderma gangrenosum (rare), dry skin, erythema nodosum, urticaria.

Special Senses: Eye pain, taste perversion, blurred vision, tinnitus.

Urogenital: Interstitial nephritis (See also Renal subsection in PRECAUTIONS), minimal change nephropathy (See also Renal subsection in PRECAUTIONS), dysuria, urinary urgency, hematuria, epididymitis, menorrhagia.

Laboratory Abnormalities: Elevated AST (SGOT) or ALT (SGPT), elevated alkaline phosphatase, elevated GGT, elevated LDH, elevated bilirubin, elevated serum creatinine and BUN.

DRUG ABUSE AND DEPENDENCY

Abuse: None reported.

Dependency: Drug dependence has not been reported with chronic administration of mesalamine.

OVERDOSAGE

Two cases of pediatric overdosage have been reported. A 3-year-old male who ingested 2 grams of **Asacol** tablets was treated with ipecac and activated charcoal; no adverse events occurred. Another 3-year-old male, approximately 16 kg, ingested an unknown amount of a maximum of 24 grams of **Asacol** crushed in solution (i.e., uncoated mesalamine); he was treated with orange juice and activated charcoal, and experienced no adverse events. In dogs, single doses of 6 grams of delayed-release **Asacol** tablets resulted in renal papillary necrosis but were not fatal. This was approximately 12.5 times the recommended human dose (based on a dose of 2.4 g/day in a 50 kg person). Single oral doses of uncoated mesalamine in mice and rats of 5000 mg/kg and 4595 mg/kg, respectively, or of 3000 mg/kg in cynomolgus monkeys, caused significant lethality.

DOSAGE AND ADMINISTRATION

For the treatment of mildly to moderately active ulcerative colitis: The usual dosage in adults is two 400-mg tablets to be taken three times a day for a total daily dose of 2.4 grams for a duration of 6 weeks.

For the maintenance of remission of ulcerative colitis: The recommended dosage in adults is 1.6 grams daily, in divided doses. Treatment duration in the prospective, well-controlled trial was 6 months.

HOW SUPPLIED

Asacol tablets are available as red-brown, capsule-shaped tablets containing 400 mg mesalamine and imprinted "Asacol NE" in black.

NDC 0149-0752-02 Bottle of 100

Store at controlled room temperature 20°–25°C (68°–77°F) [See USP].

CAUTION: Federal law prohibits dispensing without prescription.

Procter & Gamble Pharmaceuticals
Cincinnati, Ohio 45202
under license from Tillotts Pharma AG,
the registered trademark owner, and Medeva PLC
Made in Germany, D-64331 Weiterstadt
U.S. Patent Nos. 5,541,170 and 5,541,171
REVISED OCTOBER 1999

Shown in Product Identification Guide, page 331

DANTRIUM® capsules ℞

[dan 'trē-um]
(dantrolene sodium)

Dantrium (dantrolene sodium) has a potential for hepatotoxicity, and should not be used in conditions other than those recommended. Symptomatic hepatitis (fatal and non-fatal) has been reported at various dose levels of the drug. The incidence reported in patients taking up to 400 mg/day is much lower than in those taking doses of 800 mg or more per day. Even sporadic short courses of these higher dose levels within a treatment regimen markedly increased the risk of serious hepatic injury. Liver dysfunction as evidenced by blood chemical abnormalities alone (liver enzyme elevations) has been observed in patients exposed to **Dantrium** for varying periods of time. Overt hepatitis has occurred at varying intervals after initiation of therapy, but has been most frequently observed between the third and twelfth month of therapy. The risk of hepatic injury appears to be greater in females, in patients over 35 years of age, and in patients taking other medication(s) in addition to **Dantrium** (dantrolene sodium). **Dantrium** should be used only in conjunction with appropriate monitoring of hepatic function including frequent determination of SGOT or SGPT. If no observable benefit is derived from the administration of **Dantrium** after a total of 45 days, therapy should be discontinued. The lowest possible effective dose for the individual patient should be prescribed.

DESCRIPTION

The chemical formula of Dantrium (dantrolene sodium) is hydrated 1-[[[5-(4-nitrophenyl)-2-furanyl]methylene]amino]-2, 4-imidazolidinedione sodium salt. It is an orange powder, slightly soluble in water, but due to its slightly acidic nature the solubility increases somewhat in alkaline solution. The anhydrous salt has a molecular weight of 336. The hydrated salt contains approximately 15% water (3-1/2 moles) and has a molecular weight of 399. The structural formula for the hydrated salt is:

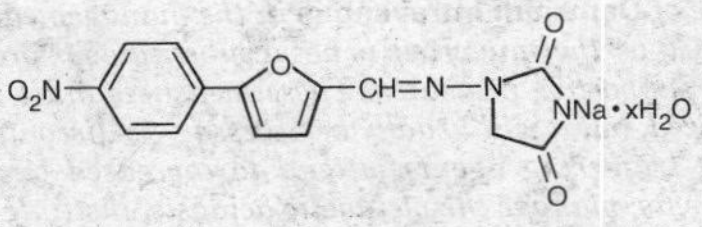

Dantrium is supplied in capsules of 25 mg, 50 mg, and 100 mg.

Inactive Ingredients: Each capsule contains edible black ink, FD&C Yellow No. 6, gelatin, lactose, magnesium stearate, starch, synthetic iron oxide red, synthetic iron oxide yellow, talc, and titanium dioxide.

CLINICAL PHARMACOLOGY

In isolated nerve-muscle preparation, **Dantrium** has been shown to produce relaxation by affecting the contractile response of the skeletal muscle at a site beyond the myoneural junction, directly on the muscle itself. In skeletal muscle, Dantrium dissociates the excitation-contraction coupling, probably by interfering with the release of Ca++ from the sarcoplasmic reticulum. This effect appears to be more pronounced in fast muscle fibers as compared to slow ones, but generally affects both. A central nervous system effect occurs, with drowsiness, dizziness, and generalized weakness occasionally present. Although **Dantrium** does not appear to directly affect the CNS, the extent of its indirect effect is unknown. The absorption of **Dantrium** after oral administration in humans is incomplete and slow but consistent, and dose-related blood levels are obtained. The duration and intensity of skeletal muscle relaxation is related to the dosage and blood levels. The mean biologic half-life of **Dantrium** in adults is 8.7 hours after a 100-mg dose. Specific metabolic pathways in the degradation and elimination of **Dantrium** in human subjects have been established. Metabolic patterns are similar in adults and pediatric patients. In addition to the parent compound, dantrolene, which is found in measurable amounts in blood and urine, the major metabolites noted in body fluids are the 5-hydroxy analog and the acetamido analog. Since **Dantrium** is probably metabolized by hepatic microsomal enzymes, enhancement of its metabolism by other drugs is possible. However, neither phenobarbital nor diazepam appears to affect **Dantrium** metabolism.

Clinical experience in the management of fulminant human malignant hyperthermia, as well as experiments conducted in malignant hyperthermia susceptible swine, have revealed that the administration of intravenous dantrolene, combined with indicated supportive measures, is effective in reversing the hypermetabolic process of malignant hyperthermia. Known differences between human and swine malignant hyperthermia are minor. The prophylactic administration of oral or intravenous dantrolene to malignant hyperthermia susceptible swine will attenuate or prevent the development of signs of malignant hyperthermia in a manner dependent upon the dosage of dantrolene administered and the intensity of the malignant hyperthermia triggering stimulus. Limited clinical experience with the administration of oral dantrolene to patients judged malignant hyperthermia susceptible, when combined with clinical experience in the use of intravenous dantrolene for the treatment of malignant hyperthermia and data derived from the above cited animal model experiments, suggests that oral dantrolene will also attenuate or prevent the development of signs of human malignant hyperthermia, provided that currently accepted practices in the management of such patients are adhered to (see INDICATIONS AND USAGE); intravenous dantrolene should also be available for use should the signs of malignant hyperthermia appear.

INDICATIONS AND USAGE

In Chronic Spasticity:
Dantrium is indicated in controlling the manifestations of clinical spasticity resulting from upper motor neuron disorders (e.g., spinal cord injury, stroke, cerebral palsy, or multiple sclerosis). It is of particular benefit to the patient whose functional rehabilitation has been retarded by the sequelae of spasticity. Such patients must have presumably reversible spasticity where relief of spasticity will aid in restoring residual function. **Dantrium** is not indicated in the treatment of skeletal muscle spasm resulting from rheumatic disorders.

If improvement occurs, it will ordinarily occur within the dosage titration (see DOSAGE AND ADMINISTRATION), and will be manifested by a decrease in the severity of spasticity and the ability to resume a daily function not quite attainable without **Dantrium**.

Occasionally, subtle but meaningful improvement in spasticity may occur with **Dantrium** therapy. In such instances, information regarding improvement should be solicited from the patient and those who are in constant daily contact and attendance with him. Brief withdrawal of **Dantrium** for a period of 2 to 4 days will frequently demonstrate exacerbation of the manifestations of spasticity and may serve to confirm a clinical impression.

A decision to continue the administration of **Dantrium** on a long-term basis is justified if introduction of the drug into the patient's regimen:

produces a significant reduction in painful and/or disabling spasticity such as clonus, or
permits a significant reduction in the intensity and/or degree of nursing care required, or
rids the patient of any annoying manifestation of spasticity considered important by the patient himself.

In Malignant Hyperthermia:
Oral **Dantrium** is also indicated preoperatively to prevent or attenuate the development of signs of malignant hyperthermia in known, or strongly suspect, malignant hyperthermia susceptible patients who require anesthesia and/or surgery. Currently accepted clinical practices in the management of such patients must still be adhered to (careful monitoring for early signs of malignant hyperthermia, minimizing exposure to triggering mechanisms and prompt use of intravenous dantrolene sodium and indicated supportive measures should signs of malignant hyperthermia appear); see also the package insert for **Dantrium®** (dantrolene sodium) **Intravenous**.

Oral **Dantrium** should be administered following a malignant hyperthermic crisis to prevent recurrence of the signs of malignant hyperthermia.

CONTRAINDICATIONS

Active hepatic disease, such as hepatitis and cirrhosis, is a contraindication for use of **Dantrium**. **Dantrium** is contraindicated where spasticity is utilized to sustain upright posture and balance in locomotion or whenever spasticity is utilized to obtain or maintain increased function.

WARNINGS

It is important to recognize that fatal and non-fatal liver disorders of an idiosyncratic or hypersensitivity type may occur with **Dantrium** therapy.

At the start of **Dantrium** therapy, it is desirable to do liver function studies (SGOT, SGPT, alkaline phosphatase, total bilirubin) for a baseline or to establish whether there is preexisting liver disease. If baseline liver abnormalities exist and are confirmed, there is a clear possibility that the potential for **Dantrium** hepatotoxicity could be enhanced, although such a possibility has not yet been established.

Liver function studies (e.g., SGOT or SGPT) should be performed at appropriate intervals during **Dantrium** therapy. If such studies reveal abnormal values, therapy should generally be discontinued. Only where benefits of the drug have been of major importance to the patient, should reinitiation or continuation of therapy be considered. Some patients have revealed a return to normal laboratory values in the face of continued therapy while others have not.

If symptoms compatible with hepatitis, accompanied by abnormalities in liver function tests or jaundice appear, **Dantrium** should be discontinued. If caused by Dantrium and detected early, the abnormalities in liver function characteristically have reverted to normal when the drug was discontinued.

Dantrium therapy has been reinstituted in a few patients who have developed clinical and/or laboratory evidence of hepatocellular injury. If such reinstitution of therapy is done, it should be attempted only in patients who clearly need **Dantrium** and only after previous symptoms and laboratory abnormalities have cleared. The patient should be hospitalized and the drug should be restarted in very small and gradually increasing doses. Laboratory monitoring should be frequent and the drug should be withdrawn immediately if there is any indication of recurrent liver involvement. Some patients have reacted with unmistakable signs of liver abnormality upon administration of a challenge dose, while others have not.

Dantrium should be used with particular caution in females and in patients over 35 years of age in view of apparent greater likelihood of drug-induced, potentially fatal, hepatocellular disease in these groups.

Long-term safety of **Dantrium** in humans has not been established. Chronic studies in rats, dogs, and monkeys at dosages greater than 30 mg/kg/day showed growth or weight depression and signs of hepatopathy and possible occlusion nephropathy, all of which were reversible upon cessation of treatment. Sprague-Dawley female rats fed dantrolene sodium for 18 months at dosage levels of 15, 30, and 60 mg/kg/day showed an increased incidence of benign and malignant mammary tumors compared with concurrent controls. At the highest dose level, there was an increase in the incidence of benign hepatic lymphatic neoplasms. In a 30-month study at the same dose levels also in Sprague-Dawley rats, dantrolene sodium produced a decrease in the time of onset of mammary neoplasms. Female rats at the highest dose level showed an increased incidence of hepatic lymphangiomas and hepatic angiosarcomas.

The only drug-related effect seen in a 30-month study in Fischer-344 rats was a dose-related reduction in the time of onset of mammary and testicular tumors. A 24-month study in HaM/ICR mice revealed no evidence of carcinogenic activity. Carcinogenicity in humans cannot be fully excluded, so that this possible risk of chronic administration must be weighed against the benefits of the drug (i.e., after a brief trial) for the individual patient.

USAGE IN PREGNANCY

The safety of Dantrium for use in women who are or who may become pregnant has not been established. **Dantrium** should not be used in nursing mothers.

Usage in Pediatric Patients: The long-term safety of **Dantrium** in pediatric patients under the age of 5 years has not been established. Because of the possibility that adverse effects of the drug could become apparent only after many years, a benefit-risk consideration of the long-term use of **Dantrium** is particularly important in pediatric patients.

Drug Interactions:
Drowsiness may occur with Dantrium therapy, and the concomitant administration of CNS depressants such as sedatives and tranquilizing agents may result in further drowsiness.

While a definite drug interaction with estrogen therapy has not yet been established, caution should be observed if the two drugs are to be given concomitantly. Hepatotoxicity has occurred more often in women over 35 years of age receiving concomitant estrogen therapy.

Cardiovascular collapse in patients treated simultaneously with verapamil and dantrolene sodium is rare. The combination of therapeutic doses of intravenous dantrolene sodium and verapamil in halothane/α-chloralose anesthetized swine has resulted in ventricular fibrillation and cardiovascular collapse in association with marked hyperkalemia. Until the relevance of these findings to humans is established, the combination of dantrolene sodium and calcium channel blockers is not recommended during the management of malignant hyperthermia.

Administration of **Dantrium** may potentiate vecuronium-induced neuromuscular block.

PRECAUTIONS

Dantrium should be used with caution in patients with impaired pulmonary function, particularly those with obstructive pulmonary disease, and in patients with severely impaired cardiac function due to myocardial disease. It should be used with caution in patients with a history of previous liver disease or dysfunction (see WARNINGS).

Continued on next page

Dantrium Capsules—Cont.

Patients should be cautioned against driving a motor vehicle or participating in hazardous occupations while taking **Dantrium**. Caution should be exercised in the concomitant administration of tranquilizing agents.

Dantrium might possibly evoke a photosensitivity reaction; patients should be cautioned about exposure to sunlight while taking it.

ADVERSE REACTIONS

The most frequently occurring side effects of **Dantrium** have been drowsiness, dizziness, weakness, general malaise, fatigue, and diarrhea. These are generally transient, occurring early in treatment, and can often be obviated by beginning with a low dose and increasing dosage gradually until an optimal regimen is established. Diarrhea may be severe and may necessitate temporary withdrawal of **Dantrium** therapy. If diarrhea recurs upon readministration of **Dantrium**, therapy should probably be withdrawn permanently.

Other less frequent side effects, listed according to system, are:

Gastrointestinal: Constipation, rarely progressing to signs of intestinal obstruction, GI bleeding, anorexia, swallowing difficulty, gastric irritation, abdominal cramps, nausea and/or vomiting.

Hepatobiliary: Hepatitis (see WARNINGS).

Neurologic: Speech disturbance, seizure, headache, lightheadedness, visual disturbance, diplopia, alteration of taste, insomnia, drooling.

Cardiovascular: Tachycardia, erratic blood pressure, phlebitis, heart failure.

Hematologic: Aplastic anemia, leukopenia, lymphocytic lymphoma, thrombocytopenia.

Psychiatric: Mental depression, mental confusion, increased nervousness.

Urogenital: Increased urinary frequency, crystalluria, hematuria, difficult erection, urinary incontinence and/or nocturia, difficult urination and/or urinary retention.

Integumentary: Abnormal hair growth, acne-like rash, pruritus, urticaria, eczematoid eruption, sweating.

Musculoskeletal: Myalgia, backache.

Respiratory: Feeling of suffocation, respiratory depression.

Special Senses: Excessive tearing.

Hypersensitivity: Pleural effusion with pericarditis, anaphylaxis.

Other: Chills and fever.

The published literature has included some reports of **Dantrium** use in patients with Neuroleptic Malignant Syndrome (NMS). **Dantrium** capsules are not indicated for the treatment of NMS and patients may expire despite treatment with **Dantrium** capsules.

DOSAGE AND ADMINISTRATION

For Use in Chronic Spasticity:

Prior to the administration of **Dantrium**, consideration should be given to the potential response to treatment. A decrease in spasticity sufficient to allow a daily function not otherwise attainable should be the therapeutic goal of treatment with **Dantrium**. Refer to INDICATIONS AND USAGE section for description of response to be anticipated.

It is important to establish a therapeutic goal (regain and maintain a specific function such as therapeutic exercise program, utilization of braces, transfer maneuvers, etc.) before beginning **Dantrium** therapy. Dosage should be increased until the maximum performance compatible with the dysfunction due to underlying disease is achieved. No further increase in dosage is then indicated.

Usual Dosage: It is important that the dosage be titrated and individualized for maximum effect. The lowest dose compatible with optimal response is recommended.

In view of the potential for liver damage in long-term **Dantrium** *use, therapy should be stopped if benefits are not evident within 45 days.*

Adults: The following gradual titration schedule is suggested. Some patients will not respond until higher daily dosage is achieved. Each dosage level should be maintained for seven days to determine the patient's response. If no further benefit is observed at the next higher dose, dosage should be decreased to the previous lower dose.

25 mg once daily for seven days, then
25 mg t.i.d. for seven days
50 mg t.i.d. for seven days
100 mg t.i.d.

Therapy with a dose four times daily may be necessary for some individuals. Doses higher than 100 mg four times daily should not be used. (See Box Warning.)

Pediatric Patients: The following gradual titration schedule is suggested. Some patients will not respond until higher daily dosage is achieved. Each dosage level should be maintained for seven days to determine the patient's response. If no further benefit is observed at the next higher dose, dosage should be decreased to the previous lower dose.

0.5 mg/kg once daily for seven days, then
0.5 mg/kg t.i.d. for seven days
1 mg/kg t.i.d. for seven days
2 mg/kg t.i.d.

Therapy with a dose four times daily may be necessary for some individuals. Doses higher than 100 mg four times daily should not be used. (See Box Warning.)

For Malignant Hyperthermia:

Preoperatively: Administer 4 to 8 mg/kg/day of oral **Dantrium** in 3 or 4 divided doses for one or two days prior to surgery, with the last dose being given approximately 3 to 4 hours before scheduled surgery with a minimum of water. This dosage will usually be associated with skeletal muscle weakness and sedation (sleepiness or drowsiness); adjustment can usually be made within the recommended dosage range to avoid incapacitation or excessive gastrointestinal irritation (including nausea and/or vomiting).

Post Crisis Follow-up:

Oral **Dantrium** should also be administered following a malignant hyperthermia crisis, in doses of 4 to 8 mg/kg per day in four divided doses, for a one to three day period to prevent recurrence of the manifestations of malignant hyperthermia.

OVERDOSAGE

Symptoms which may occur in case of overdose include, but are not limited to, muscular weakness and alterations in the state of consciousness (e.g. lethargy, coma), vomiting, diarrhea, and crystalluria. For acute overdosage, general supportive measures should be employed along with immediate gastric lavage.

Intravenous fluids should be administered in fairly large quantities to avert the possibility of crystalluria. An adequate airway should be maintained and artificial resuscitation equipment should be at hand. Electrocardiographic monitoring should be instituted, and the patient carefully observed. To date, no experience has been reported with dialysis and its value in Dantrium overdosage is not known.

HOW SUPPLIED

Dantrium (dantrolene sodium) is available in

25-mg opaque, orange and tan capsules:
NDC 0149-0030-05 bottle of 100
NDC 0149-0030-66 bottle of 500
NDC 0149-0030-77 hospital unit-dose strips in boxes of 100

50-mg opaque, orange and tan capsules:
NDC 0149-0031-05 bottle of 100

100-mg opaque, orange and tan capsules:
NDC 0149-0033-05 bottle of 100
NDC 0149-0033-77 hospital unit-dose strips in boxes of 100

Avoid excessive heat (over 104°F or 40°C).

Address medical inquiries to Procter & Gamble Pharmaceuticals, Medical Communications Department, 11450 Grooms Rd, Cincinnati, Ohio 45242.

CAUTION: Federal law prohibits dispensing without prescription.

Procter & Gamble Pharmaceuticals
Cincinnati, Ohio 45202
REVISED FEBRUARY 1997

DANTRIUM® INTRAVENOUS ℞
(dantrolene sodium for injection)

DESCRIPTION

Dantrium Intravenous is a sterile, non-pyrogenic, lyophilized formulation of dantrolene sodium for injection. **Dantrium Intravenous** is supplied in 70 mL vials containing 20 mg dantrolene sodium, 3000 mg mannitol, and sufficient sodium hydroxide to yield a pH of approximately 9.5 when reconstituted with 60 mL sterile water for injection USP (without a bacteriostatic agent).

Dantrium is classified as a direct-acting skeletal muscle relaxant. Chemically, **Dantrium** is hydrated 1-[[[5-(4-nitrophenyl)-2-furanyl]methylene]amino]-2,4-imidazolidinedione sodium salt. The structural formula for the hydrated salt is:

O_2N— —CH = N – N NNa ·xH_2O

The hydrated salt contains approximately 15% water (3-1/2 moles) and has a molecular weight of 399. The anhydrous salt (dantrolene) has a molecular weight of 336.

CLINICAL PHARMACOLOGY

In isolated nerve-muscle preparation, **Dantrium** has been shown to produce relaxation by affecting the contractile response of the muscle at a site beyond the myoneural junction. In skeletal muscle, **Dantrium** dissociates excitation-contraction coupling, probably by interfering with the release of Ca^{++} from the sarcoplasmic reticulum. The administration of intravenous **Dantrium** to human volunteers is associated with loss of grip strength and weakness in the legs, as well as subjective CNS complaints (see also PRECAUTIONS, Information for Patients). Information concerning the passage of **Dantrium** across the blood-brain barrier is not available.

In the anesthetic-induced malignant hyperthermia syndrome, evidence points to an intrinsic abnormality of skeletal muscle tissue. In affected humans, it has been postulated that "triggering agents" (e.g., general anesthetics and depolarizing neuromuscular blocking agents) produce a change within the cell which results in an elevated myoplasmic calcium. This elevated myoplasmic calcium activates acute cellular catabolic processes that cascade to the malignant hyperthermia crisis.

It is hypothesized that addition of **Dantrium** to the "triggered" malignant hyperthermic muscle cell reestablishes a normal level of ionized calcium in the myoplasm. Inhibition of calcium release from the sarcoplasmic reticulum by **Dantrium** reestablishes the myoplasmic calcium equilibrium, increasing the percentage of bound calcium. In this way, physiologic, metabolic, and biochemical changes associated with the malignant hyperthermia crisis may be reversed or attenuated. Experimental results in malignant hyperthermia susceptible swine show that prophylactic administration of intravenous or oral dantrolene prevents or attenuates the development of vital sign and blood gas changes characteristic of malignant hyperthermia in a dose related manner. The efficacy of intravenous dantrolene in the treatment of human and porcine malignant hyperthermia crisis, when considered along with prophylactic experiments in malignant hyperthermia susceptible swine, lends support to prophylactic use of oral or intravenous dantrolene in malignant hyperthermia susceptible humans. When prophylactic intravenous dantrolene is administered as directed, whole blood concentrations remain at a near steady state level for 3 or more hours after the infusion is completed. Clinical experience has shown that early vital sign and/or blood gas changes characteristic of malignant hyperthermia may appear during or after anesthesia and surgery despite the prophylactic use of dantrolene and adherence to currently accepted patient management practices. These signs are compatible with attenuated malignant hyperthermia and respond to the administration of additional i.v. dantrolene (see DOSAGE AND ADMINISTRATION). The administration of the recommended prophylactic dose of intravenous dantrolene to healthy volunteers was not associated with clinically significant cardiorespiratory changes.

Specific metabolic pathways for the degradation and elimination of **Dantrium** in humans have been established. Dantrolene is found in measurable amounts in blood and urine. Its major metabolites in body fluids are 5-hydroxy dantrolene and an acetylamino metabolite of dantrolene. Another metabolite with an unknown structure appears related to the latter. **Dantrium** may also undergo hydrolysis and subsequent oxidation forming nitrophenylfuroic acid.

The mean biologic half-life of **Dantrium** after intravenous administration is variable, between 4 to 8 hours under most experimental conditions. Based on assays of whole blood and plasma, slightly greater amounts of dantrolene are associated with red blood cells than with the plasma fraction of blood. Significant amounts of dantrolene are bound to plasma proteins, mostly albumin, and this binding is readily reversible.

Cardiopulmonary depression has not been observed in malignant hyperthermia susceptible swine following the administration of up to 7.5 mg/kg i.v. dantrolene. This is twice the amount needed to maximally diminish twitch response to single supramaximal peripheral nerve stimulation (95% inhibition). A transient, inconsistent, depressant effect on gastrointestinal smooth muscles has been observed at high doses.

INDICATIONS AND USAGE

Dantrium Intravenous is indicated, along with appropriate supportive measures, for the management of the fulminant hypermetabolism of skeletal muscle characteristic of malignant hyperthermia crises in patients of all ages. **Dantrium Intravenous** should be administered by continuous rapid intravenous push as soon as the malignant hyperthermia reaction is recognized (i.e., tachycardia, tachypnea, central venous desaturation, hypercarbia, metabolic acidosis, skeletal muscle rigidity, increased utilization of anesthesia circuit carbon dioxide absorber, cyanosis and mottling of the skin, and, in many cases, fever).

Dantrium Intravenous is also indicated preoperatively, and sometimes postoperatively, to prevent or attenuate the development of clinical and laboratory signs of malignant hyperthermia in individuals judged to be malignant hyperthermia susceptible.

CONTRAINDICATIONS

None.

WARNINGS

The use of **Dantrium Intravenous** *in the management of malignant hyperthermia crisis is not a substitute for previously known supportive measures. These measures must be individualized, but it will usually be necessary to discontinue the suspect triggering agents, attend to increased oxygen requirements, manage the metabolic acidosis, institute cooling when necessary, monitor urinary output, and monitor for electrolyte imbalance.*

Since the effect of disease state and other drugs on **Dantrium** related skeletal muscle weakness, including possible respiratory depression, cannot be predicted, patients who receive i.v. **Dantrium** preoperatively should have vital signs monitored.

If patients judged malignant hyperthermia susceptible are administered intravenous or oral **Dantrium** preoperatively, anesthetic preparation must still follow a standard malignant hyperthermia susceptible regimen, including the avoidance of known triggering agents. Monitoring for early clinical and metabolic signs of malignant hyperthermia is indicated because attenuation of malignant hyperthermia, rather than prevention, is possible. These signs usually call for the administration of additional i.v. dantrolene.

PRECAUTIONS

General: Care must be taken to prevent extravasation of **Dantrium** solution into the surrounding tissues due to the high pH of the intravenous formulation.

When mannitol is used for prevention or treatment of late renal complications of malignant hyperthermia, the 3 g of mannitol needed to dissolve each 20 mg vial of i.v. **Dantrium** should be taken into consideration.

Information for Patients: Based upon data in human volunteers, it will sometimes be appropriate to tell patients who receive **Dantrium Intravenous** that decrease in grip strength and weakness of leg muscles, especially walking down stairs, can be expected postoperatively. In addition, symptoms such as "lightheadedness" may be noted. Since some of these symptoms may persist for up to 48 hours, patients must not operate an automobile or engage in other hazardous activity during this time. Caution is also indicated at meals on the day of administration because difficulty swallowing and choking has been reported. Caution should be exercised in the concomitant administration of tranquilizing agents.

Hepatotoxicity seen with **Dantrium Capsules: Dantrium** (dantrolene sodium) has a potential for hepatotoxicity, and should not be used in conditions other than those recommended. Symptomatic hepatitis (fatal and non-fatal) has been reported at various dose levels of the drug. The incidence reported in patients taking up to 400 mg/day is much lower than in those taking doses of 800 mg or more per day. Even sporadic short courses of these higher dose levels within a treatment regimen markedly increased the risk of serious hepatic injury. Liver dysfunction as evidenced by blood chemical abnormalities alone (liver enzyme elevations) has been observed in patients exposed to **Dantrium** for varying periods of time. Overt hepatitis has occurred at varying intervals after initiation of therapy, but has been most frequently observed between the third and twelfth month of therapy. The risk of hepatic injury appears to be greater in females, in patients over 35 years of age, and in patients taking other medication(s) in addition to **Dantrium** (dantrolene sodium). **Dantrium** should be used only in conjunction with appropriate monitoring of hepatic function including frequent determination of SGOT or SGPT.

Fatal and non-fatal liver disorders of an idiosyncratic or hypersensitivity type may occur with **Dantrium** therapy.

Drug Interactions: Dantrium is metabolized by the liver, and it is theoretically possible that its metabolism may be enhanced by drugs known to induce hepatic microsomal enzymes. However, neither phenobarbital nor diazepam appears to affect **Dantrium** metabolism. Binding to plasma protein is not significantly altered by diazepam, diphenylhydantoin, or phenylbutazone. Binding to plasma proteins is reduced by warfarin and clofibrate and increased by tolbutamide.

Cardiovascular collapse in patients treated simultaneously with verapamil and dantrolene sodium is rare. The combination of therapeutic doses of intravenous dantrolene sodium and verapamil in halothane/alpha-chloralose anesthetized swine has resulted in ventricular fibrillation and cardiovascular collapse in association with marked hyperkalemia. It is recommended that the combination of intravenous dantrolene sodium and calcium channel blockers, such as verapamil, not be used together during the management of malignant hyperthermia crisis until the relevance of these findings to humans is established.

Administration of dantrolene may potentiate vecuronium-induced neuromuscular block.

Carcinogenesis, Mutagenesis, and Impairment of Fertility: Sprague-Dawley female rats fed **Dantrium** for 18 months at dosage levels of 15, 30, and 60 mg/kg/day showed an increased incidence of benign and malignant mammary tumors compared with concurrent controls. At the highest dose levels, there was an increase in the incidence of benign hepatic lymphatic neoplasms. In a 30-month study at the same dose levels also in Sprague-Dawley rats, dantrolene sodium produced a decrease in the time of onset of mammary neoplasms. Female rats at the highest dose level showed an increased incidence of hepatic lymphangiomas and hepatic angiosarcomas.

The only drug-related effect seen in a 30-month study in Fischer-344 rats was a dose-related reduction in the time of onset of mammary and testicular tumors. A 24-month study in HaM/ICR mice revealed no evidence of carcinogenic activity.

The significance of carcinogenicity data relative to use of **Dantrium** in humans is unknown.

Dantrolene sodium has produced positive results in the Ames *S. Typhimurium* bacterial mutagenesis assay in the presence and absence of a liver activating system.

Dantrolene sodium administered to male and female rats at dose levels up to 45 mg/kg/day showed no adverse effects on fertility or general reproductive performance.

Pregnancy: Pregnancy Category C: **Dantrium** has been shown to be embryocidal in the rabbit and has been shown to decrease pup survival in the rat when given at doses seven times the human oral dose. There are no adequate and well-controlled studies in pregnant women. **Dantrium Intravenous** should be used during pregnancy only if the potential benefit justifies the potential risk to the fetus.

Labor and Delivery: In one uncontrolled study, 100 mg per day of prophylactic oral **Dantrium** was administered to term pregnant patients awaiting labor and delivery. Dantrolene readily crossed the placenta, with maternal and fetal whole blood levels approximately equal at delivery; neonatal levels then fell approximately 50% per day for 2 days before declining sharply. No neonatal respiratory and neuromuscular side effects were detected at low dose. More data, at higher doses, are needed before more definitive conclusions can be made.

ADVERSE REACTIONS

There have been occasional reports of death following malignant hyperthermia crisis even when treated with intravenous dantrolene; incidence figures are not available (the pre-dantrolene mortality of malignant hyperthermia crisis was approximately 50%). Most of these deaths can be accounted for by late recognition, delayed treatment, inadequate dosage, lack of supportive therapy, intercurrent disease and/or the development of delayed complications such as renal failure or disseminated intravascular coagulopathy. In some cases there are insufficient data to completely rule out therapeutic failure of dantrolene.

There are rare reports of fatality in malignant hyperthermia crisis, despite initial satisfactory response to i.v. dantrolene, which involve patients who could not be weaned from dantrolene after initial treatment.

The administration of intravenous **Dantrium** to human volunteers is associated with loss of grip strength and weakness in the legs, as well as drowsiness and dizziness.

The following adverse reactions are in approximate order of severity:

There are rare reports of pulmonary edema developing during the treatment of malignant hyperthermia crisis in which the diluent volume and mannitol needed to deliver i.v. dantrolene possibly contributed.

There have been reports of thrombophlebitis following administration of intravenous dantrolene; actual incidence figures are not available.

There have been rare reports of urticaria and erythema possibly associated with the administration of i.v. **Dantrium**. There has been one case of anaphylaxis.

None of the serious reactions occasionally reported with long-term oral **Dantrium** use, such as hepatitis, seizures, and pleural effusion with pericarditis, have been reasonably associated with short-term **Dantrium Intravenous** therapy.

The following events have been reported in patients receiving oral dantrolene: aplastic anemia, leukopenia, lymphocytic lymphoma, and heart failure. (See package insert for **Dantrium** (dantrolene sodium) **Capsules** for a complete listing of adverse reactions.)

The published literature has included some reports of **Dantrium** use in patients with Neuroleptic Malignant Syndrome (NMS). **Dantrium Intravenous** is not indicated for the treatment of NMS and patients may expire despite treatment with **Dantrium Intravenous.**

OVERDOSAGE

Because **Dantrium Intravenous** must be administered at a low concentration in a large volume of fluid, acute toxicity of **Dantrium** could not be assessed in animals. In 14-day (subacute) studies, the intravenous formulation of **Dantrium** was relatively non-toxic to rats at doses of 10 mg/kg/day and 20 mg/kg/day. While 10 mg/kg/day in dogs for 14 days evoked little toxicity, 20 mg/kg/day for 14 days caused hepatic changes of questionable biologic significance.

Symptoms which may occur in case of overdose include, but are not limited to, muscular weakness and alterations in the state of consciousness (e.g. lethargy, coma), vomiting, diarrhea, and crystalluria.

For acute overdosage, general supportive measures should be employed.

Intravenous fluids should be administered in fairly large quantities to avert the possibility of crystalluria. An adequate airway should be maintained and artificial resuscitation equipment should be at hand. Electrocardiographic monitoring should be instituted, and the patient carefully observed. The value of dialysis in **Dantrium** overdose is not known.

DOSAGE AND ADMINISTRATION

As soon as the malignant hyperthermia reaction is recognized, all anesthetic agents should be discontinued; the administration of 100% oxygen is recommended. **Dantrium Intravenous** should be administered by continuous rapid intravenous push beginning at a minimum dose of 1 mg/kg, and continuing until symptoms subside or the maximum cumulative dose of 10 mg/kg has been reached.

If the physiologic and metabolic abnormalities reappear, the regimen may be repeated. It is important to note that administration of **Dantrium Intravenous** should be continuous until symptoms subside. The effective dose to reverse the crisis is directly dependent upon the individual's degree of susceptibility to malignant hyperthermia, the amount and time of exposure to the triggering agent, and the time elapsed between onset of the crisis and initiation of treatment.

Pediatric Dose: Experience to date indicates that the dose of **Dantrium Intravenous** for pediatric patients is the same as for adults.

Preoperatively: Dantrium Intravenous and/or **Dantrium Capsules** may be administered preoperatively to patients judged malignant hyperthermia susceptible as part of the overall patient management to prevent or attenuate the development of clinical and laboratory signs of malignant hyperthermia.

Dantrium Intravenous: The recommended prophylactic dose of **Dantrium Intravenous** is 2.5 mg/kg, starting approximately 1-1/4 hours before anticipated anesthesia and infused over approximately 1 hour. This dose should prevent or attenuate the development of clinical and laboratory signs of malignant hyperthermia provided that the usual precautions, such as avoidance of established malignant hyperthermia triggering agents, are followed.

Additional **Dantrium Intravenous** may be indicated during anesthesia and surgery because of the appearance of early clinical and/or blood gas signs of malignant hyperthermia or because of prolonged surgery (see also CLINICAL PHARMACOLOGY, WARNINGS, and PRECAUTIONS). Additional doses must be individualized.

Oral Administration of Dantrium Capsules: Administer 4 to 8 mg/kg/day of oral **Dantrium** in three or four divided doses for 1 or 2 days prior to surgery, with the last dose being given with a minimum of water approximately 3 to 4 hours before scheduled surgery. Adjustment can usually be made within the recommended dosage range to avoid incapacitation (weakness, drowsiness, etc.) or excessive gastrointestinal irritation (nausea and/or vomiting). See also the package insert for **Dantrium Capsules.**

Post Crisis Follow-Up: Dantrium Capsules, 4 to 8 mg/kg/day, in four divided doses should be administered for 1 to 3 days following a malignant hyperthermia crisis to prevent recurrence of the manifestations of malignant hyperthermia.

Intravenous **Dantrium** may be used postoperatively to prevent or attenuate the recurrence of signs of malignant hyperthermia when oral **Dantrium** administration is not practical. The i.v. dose of **Dantrium** in the postoperative period must be individualized, starting with 1 mg/kg or more as the clinical situation dictates.

PREPARATION:

Each vial of **Dantrium Intravenous** should be reconstituted by adding 60 mL of *sterile water for injection USP (without a bacteriostatic agent), and the vial shaken until the solution is clear.* 5% Dextrose Injection USP, 0.9% Sodium Chloride Injection USP, and other acidic solutions are not compatible with **Dantrium Intravenous** and should not be used. The contents of the vial must be *protected from direct light* and *used within 6 hours* after reconstitution. Store reconstituted solutions at controlled room temperature (59°F to 86°F or 15°C to 30°C).

Reconstituted **Dantrium Intravenous** should *not* be transferred to large glass bottles for prophylactic infusion due to precipitate formation observed with the use of some glass bottles as reservoirs.

For prophylactic infusion, the required number of individual vials of **Dantrium Intravenous** should be reconstituted as outlined above. The contents of individual vials are then transferred to a larger volume sterile intravenous plastic bag. Stability data on file at Procter & Gamble Pharmaceuticals indicate commercially available sterile plastic bags are acceptable drug delivery devices. However, it is recommended that the prepared infusion be inspected carefully for cloudiness and/or precipitation prior to dispensing and administration. Such solutions should not be used. While stable for 6 hours, it is recommended that the infusion be prepared immediately prior to the anticipated dosage administration time.

Parenteral drug products should be inspected visually for particulate matter and discoloration prior to administration.

HOW SUPPLIED

Dantrium Intravenous (NDC 0149-0734-02) is available in vials containing a sterile lyophilized mixture of 20 mg dantrolene sodium, 3000 mg mannitol, and sufficient sodium hydroxide to yield a pH of approximately 9.5 when reconstituted with 60 mL sterile water for injection USP (without a bacteriostatic agent).

Store unreconstituted product at controlled room temperature (59°F to 86°F or 15°C to 30°C) and avoid prolonged exposure to light.

Address medical inquiries to Procter & Gamble Pharmaceuticals, Medical Communications Department, PO Box 8006, Mason, Ohio 45040-8006

To place an order, call Procter & Gamble Pharmaceuticals Customer Service 800-448-4878.

CAUTION: Rx only

Procter & Gamble Pharmaceuticals
Cincinnati, Ohio 45202
REVISED OCTOBER 1999

DIDRONEL® ℞

[dī 'drō-nel]
(etidronate disodium)

DESCRIPTION

Didronel tablets contain either 200 mg or 400 mg of etidronate disodium, the disodium salt of (1-hydroxyethylidene) diphosphonic acid, for oral administration. This compound, also known as EHDP, regulates bone metabolism. It is a white powder, highly soluble in water, with a molecular weight of 250 and the following structural formula:

$$HO-\overset{\overset{\large ONa}{|}}{\underset{\underset{\large O}{\downarrow}}{P}}-\overset{\overset{\large OH}{|}}{\underset{\underset{\large CH_3}{|}}{C}}-\overset{\overset{\large ONa}{|}}{\underset{\underset{\large O}{\downarrow}}{P}}-OH$$

Inactive Ingredients: Each tablet contains magnesium stearate, microcrystalline cellulose, and starch.

CLINICAL PHARMACOLOGY

Didronel acts primarily on bone. It can inhibit the formation, growth, and dissolution of hydroxyapatite crystals and

Continued on next page

Didronel—Cont.

their amorphous precursors by chemisorption to calcium phosphate surfaces. Inhibition of crystal resorption occurs at lower doses than are required to inhibit crystal growth. Both effects increase as the dose increases.

Didronel is not metabolized. The amount of drug absorbed after an oral dose is approximately 3%. In normal subjects, plasma half-life ($t_{1/2}$) of etidronate, based on non-compartmental pharmacokinetics is 1 to 6 hours. Within 24 hours, approximately half the absorbed dose is excreted in urine; the remainder is distributed to bone compartments from which it is slowly eliminated. Animal studies have yielded bone clearance estimates up to 165 days. In humans, the residence time on bone may vary due to such factors as specific metabolic condition and bone type. Unabsorbed drug is excreted intact in the feces. Preclinical studies indicate etidronate disodium does not cross the blood-brain barrier.

Didronel therapy does not adversely affect serum levels of parathyroid hormone or calcium.

Paget's Disease: Paget's disease of bone (osteitis deformans) is an idiopathic, progressive disease characterized by abnormal and accelerated bone metabolism in one or more bones. Signs and symptoms may include bone pain and/or deformity, neurologic disorders, elevated cardiac output and other vascular disorders, and increased serum alkaline phosphatase and/or urinary hydroxyproline levels. Bone fractures are common in patients with Paget's disease.

Didronel slows accelerated bone turnover (resorption and accretion) in pagetic lesions and, to a lesser extent, in normal bone. This has been demonstrated histologically, scintigraphically, biochemically, and through calcium kinetic and balance studies. Reduced bone turnover is often accompanied by symptomatic improvement, including reduced bone pain. Also, the incidence of pagetic fractures may be reduced, and elevated cardiac output and other vascular disorders may be improved by **Didronel** therapy.

Heterotopic Ossification: Heterotopic ossification, also referred to as myositis ossificans (circumscripta, progressiva or traumatica), ectopic calcification, periarticular ossification, or paraosteoarthropathy, is characterized by metaplastic osteogenesis. It usually presents with signs of localized inflammation or pain, elevated skin temperature, and redness. When tissues near joints are involved, functional loss may also be present.

Heterotopic ossification may occur for no known reason as in myositis ossificans progressiva or may follow a wide variety of surgical, occupational, and sports trauma (e.g., hip arthroplasty, spinal cord injury, head injury, burns, and severe thigh bruises). Heterotopic ossification has also been observed in non-traumatic conditions (e.g., infections of the central nervous system, peripheral neuropathy, tetanus, biliary cirrhosis, Peyronie's disease, as well as in association with a variety of benign and malignant neoplasms).

Clinical trials have demonstrated the efficacy of **Didronel** in heterotopic ossification following total hip replacement, or due to spinal cord injury.

— *Heterotopic ossification complicating total hip replacement* typically develops radiographically 3 to 8 weeks postoperatively in the pericapsular area of the affected hip joint. The overall incidence is about 50%; about one-third of these cases are clinically significant.

— *Heterotopic ossification due to spinal cord injury* typically develops radiographically 1 to 4 months after injury. It occurs below the level of injury, usually at major joints. The overall incidence is about 40%; about one-half of these cases are clinically significant.

Didronel chemisorbs to calcium hydroxyapatite crystals and their amorphous precursors, blocking the aggregation, growth, and mineralization of these crystals. This is thought to be the mechanism by which **Didronel** prevents or retards heterotopic ossification. There is no evidence **Didronel** affects mature heterotopic bone.

INDICATIONS AND USAGE

Didronel is indicated for the treatment of symptomatic Paget's disease of bone and in the prevention and treatment of heterotopic ossification following total hip replacement or due to spinal cord injury. **Didronel** is not approved for the treatment of osteoporosis.

Paget's Disease: **Didronel** is indicated for the treatment of symptomatic Paget's disease of bone. **Didronel** therapy usually arrests or significantly impedes the disease process as evidenced by:

— Symptomatic relief, including decreased pain and/or increased mobility (experienced by 3 out of 5 patients).

— Reductions in serum alkaline phosphatase and urinary hydroxyproline levels (30% or more in 4 out of 5 patients).

— Histomorphometry showing reduced numbers of osteoclasts and osteoblasts, and more lamellar bone formation.

— Bone scans showing reduced radionuclide uptake at pagetic lesions.

In addition, reductions in pagetically elevated cardiac output and skin temperature have been observed in some patients.

In many patients, the disease process will be suppressed for a period of at least 1 year following cessation of therapy. The upper limit of this period has not been determined.

The effects of the **Didronel** treatment in patients with asymptomatic Paget's disease have not been studied. However, **Didronel** treatment of such patients may be warranted if extensive involvement threatens irreversible neurologic damage, major joints, or major weight-bearing bones.

Heterotopic Ossification: **Didronel** is indicated in the prevention and treatment of heterotopic ossification following total hip replacement or due to spinal cord injury.

Didronel reduces the incidence of clinically important heterotopic bone by about two-thirds. Among those patients who form heterotopic bone, **Didronel** retards the progression of immature lesions and reduces the severity by at least half. Follow-up data (at least 9 months posttherapy) suggest these benefits persist.

In total hip replacement patients, **Didronel** does not promote loosening of the prosthesis or impede trochanteric reattachment.

In spinal cord injury patients, **Didronel** does not inhibit fracture healing or stabilization of the spine.

CONTRAINDICATIONS

Didronel tablets are contraindicated in patients with known hypersensitivity to etidronate disodium or in patients with clinically overt osteomalacia.

WARNINGS

Paget's Disease: In Paget's patients the response to therapy may be of slow onset and continue for months after **Didronel** therapy is discontinued. Dosage should not be increased prematurely. A 90-day drug-free interval should be provided between courses of therapy.

Heterotopic Ossification: No specific warnings.

PRECAUTIONS

General: Patients should maintain an adequate nutritional status, particularly an adequate intake of calcium and vitamin D.

Therapy has been withheld from some patients with enterocolitis since diarrhea may be experienced, particularly at higher doses.

Didronel is not metabolized and is excreted intact via the kidney. Hyperphosphatemia may occur at doses of 10 to 20 mg/kg/day, apparently as a result of drug-related increases in tubular reabsorption of phosphate. Serum phosphate levels generally return to normal 2 to 4 weeks post-therapy. There is no experience to specifically guide treatment in patients with impaired renal function. **Didronel** dosage should be reduced when reductions in glomerular filtration rates are present. Patients with renal impairment should be closely monitored. In approximately 10% of patients in clinical trials of **Didronel® I. V. Infusion** (etidronate disodium) for hypercalcemia of malignancy, occasional, mild-to-moderate abnormalities in renal function (increases of > 0.5 mg/dl serum creatinine) were observed during or immediately after treatment.

Didronel suppresses bone turnover, and may retard mineralization of osteoid laid down during the bone accretion process. These effects are dose and time dependent. Osteoid, which may accumulate noticeably at doses of 10 to 20 mg/kg/day, mineralizes normally posttherapy. In patients with fractures, especially of long bones, it may be advisable to delay or interrupt treatment until callus is evident.

Paget's Disease: In Paget's patients, treatment regimens exceeding the recommended (see DOSAGE AND ADMINISTRATION) daily maximum dose of 20 mg/kg or continuous administration of medication for periods greater than 6 months may be associated with osteomalacia and an increased risk of fracture.

Long bones predominantly affected by lytic lesions, particularly in those patients unresponsive to **Didronel** therapy, may be especially prone to fracture.

Patients with predominantly lytic lesions should be monitored radiographically and biochemically to permit termination of **Didronel** in those patients unresponsive to treatment.

Drug Interactions: There have been isolated reports of patients experiencing increases in their prothrombin times when etidronate was added to warfarin therapy. The majority of these reports concerned variable elevations in prothrombin times without clinically significant sequelae. Although the relevance of these reports and any mechanism of coagulation alterations is unclear, patients on warfarin should have their prothrombin time monitored.

Carcinogenesis: Long-term studies in rats have indicated that **Didronel** is not carcinogenic.

Pregnancy: Teratogenic Effects: Pregnancy Category C. In teratology and developmental toxicity studies conducted in rats and rabbits treated with dosages of up to 100 mg/kg (5 to 20 times the clinical dose), no adverse or teratogenic effects have been observed in the offspring. Etidronate disodium has been shown to cause skeletal abnormalities in rats when given at oral dose levels of 300 mg/kg (15 to 60 times the human dose). Other effects on the offspring (including decreased live births) are at dosages that cause significant toxicity in the parent generation and are 25 to 200 times the human dose. The skeletal effects are thought to be the result of the pharmacological effects of the drug on bone. There are no adequate and well-controlled studies in pregnant women. **Didronel** (etidronate disodium) should be used during pregnancy only if the potential benefit justifies the potential risk to the fetus.

Nursing Mothers: It is not known whether this drug is excreted in human milk. Because many drugs are excreted in human milk, caution should be exercised when **Didronel** is administered to a nursing woman.

Pediatric Use: Safety and effectiveness in pediatric patients have not been established. Pediatric patients have been treated with **Didronel**, at doses recommended for adults, to prevent heterotopic ossifications or soft tissue calcifications. A rachitic syndrome has been reported infrequently at doses of 10 mg/kg/day and more for prolonged periods approaching or exceeding a year. The epiphyseal radiologic changes associated with retarded mineralization of new osteoid and cartilage, and occasional symptoms reported, have been reversible when medication is discontinued.

ADVERSE REACTIONS

The incidence of gastrointestinal complaints (diarrhea, nausea) is the same for **Didronel** at 5 mg/kg/day as for placebo, about 1 patient in 15. At 10 to 20 mg/kg/day the incidence may increase to 2 or 3 in 10. These complaints are often alleviated by dividing the total daily dose.

Paget's Disease: In Paget's patients, increased or recurrent bone pain at pagetic sites, and/or the onset of pain at previously asymptomatic sites has been reported. At 5 mg/kg/day about 1 patient in 10 (versus 1 in 15 in the placebo group) report these phenomena. At higher doses the incidence rises to about 2 in 10. When therapy continues, pain resolves in some patients but persists in others.

Heterotopic Ossification: No specific adverse reactions.

Worldwide Postmarketing Experience: The worldwide postmarketing experience for etidronate disodium reflects its use in the following approved indications: Paget's disease, heterotopic ossification, and hypercalcemia of malignancy. It also reflects the use of etidronate disodium for osteoporosis where approved in countries outside the US. Other adverse events that have been reported and were thought to be possibly related to etidronate disodium include the following: alopecia; arthropathies, including arthralgia and arthritis; bone fracture; esophagitis; glossitis; hypersensitivity reactions, including angioedema, follicular eruption, macular rash, maculopapular rash, pruritus, a single case of Stevens-Johnson syndrome, and urticaria; osteomalacia; neuropsychiatric events, including amnesia, confusion, depression, and hallucination; and paresthesias. In patients receiving etidronate disodium, there have been rare reports of agranulocytosis, pancytopenia, and a report of leukopenia with recurrence on rechallenge. In addition, there have been rare reports of exacerbation of asthma. Exacerbation of existing peptic ulcer disease has been reported in a few patients. In one patient, perforation also occurred. In osteoporosis clinical trials, headache, gastritis, leg cramps, and arthralgia occurred at a significantly greater incidence in patients who received etidronate as compared with those who received placebo.

OVERDOSAGE

Clinical experience with acute **Didronel** overdosage is extremely limited. Decreases in serum calcium following substantial overdosage may be expected in some patients. Signs and symptoms of hypocalcemia also may occur in some of these patients. Some patients may develop vomiting. In one event, an 18-year-old female who ingested an estimated single dose of 4000 to 6000 mg (67 to 100 mg/kg) of **Didronel** was reported to be mildly hypocalcemic (7.52 mg/dl) and experienced paresthesia of the fingers. Hypocalcemia resolved 6 hours after lavage and treatment with intravenous calcium gluconate. A 92-year-old female who accidentally received 1600 mg of etidronate disodium per day for 3.5 days experienced marked diarrhea and required treatment for electrolyte imbalance. Orally administered etidronate disodium may cause hematologic abnormalities in some patients (see ADVERSE REACTIONS).

Etidronate disodium suppresses bone turnover and may retard mineralization of osteoid laid down during the bone accretion process. These effects are dose and time dependent. Osteoid which may accumulate noticeably at doses of 10 to 20 mg/kg/day of chronic, continuous dosing mineralizes normally posttherapy.

Prolonged continuous treatment (chronic overdosage) has been reported to cause nephrotic syndrome and fracture.

Gastric lavage may remove unabsorbed drug. Standard procedures for treating hypocalcemia, including the administration of Ca++ intravenously, would be expected to restore physiologic amounts of ionized calcium and relieve signs and symptoms of hypocalcemia. Such treatment has been effective.

DOSAGE AND ADMINISTRATION

Didronel should be taken as a single, oral dose. However, should gastrointestinal discomfort occur, the dose may be divided. To maximize absorption, patients should avoid taking the following items within two hours of dosing:

— Food, especially food high in calcium, such as milk or milk products.

— Vitamins with mineral supplements or antacids which are high in metals such as calcium, iron, magnesium, or aluminum.

***Paget's Disease:* Initial Treatment Regimens:** 5 to 10 mg/kg/day, not to exceed 6 months, or 11 to 20 mg/kg/day, not to exceed 3 months.

The recommended initial dose is 5 mg/kg/day for a period not to exceed 6 months. Doses above 10 mg/kg/day should be reserved for when 1) lower doses are ineffective or 2) there is an overriding need to suppress rapid bone turnover (especially when irreversible neurologic damage is possible) or reduce elevated cardiac output. Doses in excess of 20 mg/kg/day are not recommended.

Retreatment Guidelines: Retreatment should be initiated only after 1) a **Didronel**-free period of at least 90 days and 2) there is biochemical, symptomatic or other evidence of active disease process. It is advisable to monitor patients every 3 to 6 months although some patients may go drug free for extended periods. Retreatment regimens are the same as for initial treatment. For most patients the original dose will be adequate for retreatment. If not, consideration should be given to increasing the dose within the recommended guidelines.

Heterotopic Ossification: The following treatment regimens have been shown to be effective:

— Total Hip Replacement Patients: 20 mg/kg/day for 1 month before and 3 months after surgery (4 months total).

— Spinal Cord Injured Patients: 20 mg/kg/day for 2 weeks followed by 10 mg/kg/day for 10 weeks (12 weeks total). **Didronel** therapy should begin as soon as medically feasible following the injury, preferably prior to evidence of heterotopic ossification.

Retreatment has not been studied.

HOW SUPPLIED

Didronel is available as 200-mg, white, rectangular tablets with "P & G" on one face and "402" on the other.

NDC 0149-0405-60 bottle of 60

400-mg, white, scored, capsule-shaped tablets with "N E" on one face and "406" on the other.

NDC 0149-0406-60 bottle of 60

Avoid excessive heat (over 104°F or 40°C).

Procter & Gamble Pharmaceuticals
Cincinnati, Ohio 45202
REVISED AUGUST 1998

Shown in Product Identification Guide, page 331

MACROBID® ℞

[*mak 'rō bid*]
(nitrofurantoin monohydrate/macrocrystals)
Capsules

DESCRIPTION

Nitrofurantoin is an antibacterial agent specific for urinary tract infections. The **Macrobid®** brand of nitrofurantoin is a hard gelatin capsule shell containing the equivalent of 100 mg of nitrofurantoin in the form of 25 mg of nitrofurantoin macrocrystals and 75 mg of nitrofurantoin monohydrate. The chemical name of nitrofurantoin macrocrystals is 1-[[[5-nitro-2-furanyl]methylene]amino]-2,4- imidazolidinedione. The chemical structure is the following:

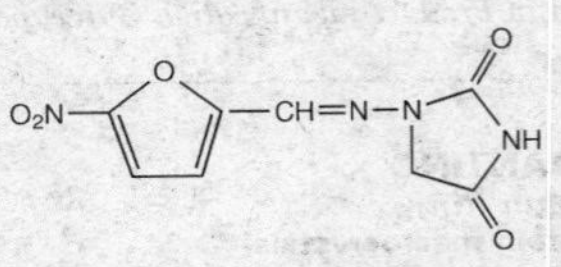

Molecular Weight: 238.16

The chemical name of nitrofurantoin monohydrate is 1-[[[5-nitro-2-furanyl]methylene]amino]-2,4- imidazolidinedione monohydrate. The chemical structure is the following:

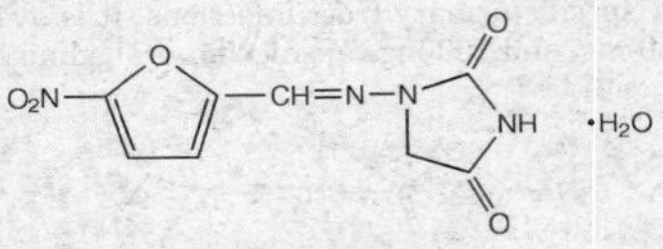

Molecular Weight: 256.17

Inactive Ingredients: Each capsule contains carbomer 934P, corn starch, compressible sugar, D&C Yellow No. 10, edible gray ink, FD&C Blue No. 1, FD&C Red No. 40, gelatin, lactose, magnesium stearate, povidone, talc, and titanium dioxide.

CLINICAL PHARMACOLOGY

Each **Macrobid** capsule contains two forms of nitrofurantoin. Twenty-five percent is macrocrystalline nitrofurantoin, which has slower dissolution and absorption than nitrofurantoin monohydrate. The remaining 75% is nitrofurantoin monohydrate contained in a powder blend which, upon exposure to gastric and intestinal fluids, forms a gel matrix that releases nitrofurantoin over time. Based on urinary pharmacokinetic data, the extent and rate of urinary excretion of nitrofurantoin from the 100-mg **Macrobid** capsule are similar to those of the 50-mg or 100-mg **Macrodantin®** (nitrofurantoin macrocrystals) capsule. Approximately 20–25% of a single dose of nitrofurantoin is recovered from the urine unchanged over 24 hours.

Plasma nitrofurantoin concentrations after a single oral dose of the 100-mg **Macrobid** capsule are low, with peak levels usually less than 1 mcg/mL. Nitrofurantoin is highly soluble in urine, to which it may impart a brown color. When **Macrobid** is administered with food, the bioavailability of nitrofurantoin is increased by approximately 40%.

Microbiology: Nitrofurantoin is bactericidal in urine at therapeutic doses. The mechanism of the antimicrobial action of nitrofurantoin is unusual among antibacterials. Nitrofurantoin is reduced by bacterial flavoproteins to reactive intermediates which inactivate or alter bacterial ribosomal proteins and other macromolecules. As a result of such inactivations, the vital biochemical processes of protein synthesis, aerobic energy metabolism, DNA synthesis, RNA synthesis, and cell wall synthesis are inhibited. The broad-based nature of this mode of action may explain the lack of acquired bacterial resistance to nitrofurantoin, as the necessary multiple and simultaneous mutations of the target macromolecules would likely be lethal to the bacteria. Development of resistance to nitrofurantoin has not been a significant problem since its introduction in 1953. Cross-resistance with antibiotics and sulfonamides has not been observed, and transferable resistance is, at most, a very rare phenomenon. Nitrofurantoin, in the form of **Macrobid**, has been shown to be active against most strains of the following bacteria both *in vitro* and in clinical infections: (See **INDICATIONS AND USAGE.**)

Gram-Positive Aerobes
Staphylococcus saprophyticus

Gram-Negative Aerobes
Escherichia coli

Nitrofurantoin also demonstrates *in vitro* activity against the following microorganisms, although the clinical significance of these data with respect to treatment with **Macrobid** is unknown:

Gram-Positive Aerobes
Coagulase-negative staphylococci
(including *Staphylococcus epidermidis*)
Enterococcus faecalis
Staphylococcus aureus
Streptococcus agalactiae
Group D streptococci
Viridans group streptococci

Gram-Negative Aerobes
Citrobacter amalonaticus
Citrobacter diversus
Citrobacter freundii
Klebsiella oxytoca
Klebsiella ozaenae

Nitrofurantoin is not active against most strains of *Proteus* species or *Serratia* species. It has no activity against *Pseudomonas* species.

Antagonism has been demonstrated *in vitro* between nitrofurantoin and quinolone antimicrobials. The clinical significance of this finding is unknown.

Susceptibility Tests:

Dilution techniques:

Quantitative methods are used to determine antimicrobial minimal inhibitory concentrations (MIC's). These MIC's provide estimates of the susceptibility of bacteria to antimicrobial compounds. The MIC's should be determined using a standardized procedure. Standardized procedures are based on a dilution method[1] (broth or agar) or equivalent with standardized inoculum concentrations and standardized concentrations of nitrofurantoin powder. The MIC values should be interpreted according to the following criteria:

MIC (µg/mL)	Interpretation
≤ 32	Susceptible (S)
64	Intermediate (I)
≥ 128	Resistant (R)

A report of "Susceptible" indicates that the pathogen is likely to be inhibited if the antimicrobial compound in the urine reaches the concentrations usually achievable. A report of "Intermediate" indicates that the result should be considered equivocal, and, if the microorganism is not fully susceptible to alternative, clinically feasible drugs, the test should be repeated. This category implies possible clinical applicability in body sites where the drug is physiologically concentrated or in situations where high dosage of drug can be used. This category also provides a buffer zone which prevents small uncontrolled technical factors from causing major discrepancies in interpretation. A report of "Resistant" indicates that the pathogen is not likely to be inhibited if the antimicrobial compound in the urine reaches the concentrations usually achievable; other therapy should be selected.

Standardized susceptibility test procedures require the use of laboratory control microorganisms to control the technical aspects of the laboratory procedures. Standard nitrofurantoin powder should provide the following MIC values:

Microorganism	MIC (µg/mL)
E. coli ATCC 25922	4–16
S. aureus ATCC 29213	8–32
E. faecalis ATCC 29212	4–16

Diffusion techniques:

Quantitative methods that require measurement of zone diameters also provide reproducible estimates of the susceptibility of bacteria to antimicrobial compounds. One such standardized procedure[2] requires the use of standardized inoculum concentrations. This procedure uses paper disks impregnated with 300-µg nitrofurantoin to test the susceptibility of microorganisms to nitrofurantoin.

Reports from the laboratory providing results of the standard single-disk susceptibility test with a 300-µg nitrofurantoin disk should be interpreted according to the following criteria:

Zone Diameter (mm)	Interpretation
≥ 17	Susceptible (S)
15–16	Intermediate (I)
≤ 14	Resistant (R)

Interpretation should be as stated above for results using dilution techniques. Interpretation involves correlation of the diameter obtained in the disk test with the MIC for nitrofurantoin.

As with standardized dilution techniques, diffusion methods require the use of laboratory control microorganisms that are used to control the technical aspects of the laboratory procedures. For the diffusion technique, the 300-µg nitrofurantoin disk should provide the following zone diameters in these laboratory test quality control strains:

Microorganism	Zone Diameter (mm)
E. coli ATCC 25922	20–25
S. aureus ATCC 25923	18–22

INDICATIONS AND USAGE

Macrobid is indicated only for the treatment of acute uncomplicated urinary tract infections (acute cystitis) caused by susceptible strains of *Escherichia coli* or *Staphylococcus saprophyticus*.

Nitrofurantoin is not indicated for the treatment of pyelonephritis or perinephric abscesses. Nitrofurantoins lack the broader tissue distribution of other therapeutic agents approved for urinary tract infections. Consequently, many patients who are treated with **Macrobid** are predisposed to persistence or reappearance of bacteriuria. (See **CLINICAL STUDIES.**) Urine specimens for culture and susceptibility testing should be obtained before and after completion of therapy. If persistence or reappearance of bacteriuria occurs after treatment with **Macrobid**, other therapeutic agents with broader tissue distribution should be selected. In considering the use of **Macrobid**, lower eradication rates should be balanced against the increased potential for systemic toxicity and for the development of antimicrobial resistance when agents with broader tissue distribution are utilized.

CONTRAINDICATIONS

Anuria, oliguria, or significant impairment of renal function (creatinine clearance under 60 mL per minute or clinically significant elevated serum creatinine) are contraindications. Treatment of this type of patient carries an increased risk of toxicity because of impaired excretion of the drug.

Because of the possibility of hemolytic anemia due to immature erythrocyte enzyme systems (glutathione instability), the drug is contraindicated in pregnant patients at term (38–42 weeks gestation), during labor and delivery, or when the onset of labor is imminent. For the same reason, the drug is contraindicated in neonates under one month of age. **Macrobid** is also contraindicated in those patients with known hypersensitivity to nitrofurantoin.

WARNINGS

ACUTE, SUBACUTE, OR CHRONIC PULMONARY REACTIONS HAVE BEEN OBSERVED IN PATIENTS TREATED WITH NITROFURANTOIN. IF THESE REACTIONS OCCUR, MACROBID SHOULD BE DISCONTINUED AND APPROPRIATE MEASURES TAKEN. REPORTS HAVE CITED PULMONARY REACTIONS AS A CONTRIBUTING CAUSE OF DEATH.

CHRONIC PULMONARY REACTIONS (DIFFUSE INTERSTITIAL PNEUMONITIS OR PULMONARY FIBROSIS, OR BOTH) CAN DEVELOP INSIDIOUSLY. THESE REACTIONS OCCUR RARELY AND GENERALLY IN PATIENTS RECEIVING THERAPY FOR SIX MONTHS OR LONGER. CLOSE MONITORING OF THE PULMONARY CONDITION OF PATIENTS RECEIVING LONG-TERM THERAPY IS WARRANTED AND REQUIRES THAT THE BENEFITS OF THERAPY BE WEIGHED AGAINST POTENTIAL RISKS. (SEE RESPIRATORY REACTIONS.)

Hepatic reactions, including hepatitis, cholestatic jaundice, chronic active hepatitis, and hepatic necrosis, occur rarely. Fatalities have been reported. The onset of chronic active hepatitis may be insidious, and patients should be monitored periodically for changes in biochemical tests that would indicate liver injury. If hepatitis occurs, the drug should be withdrawn immediately and appropriate measures should be taken.

Peripheral neuropathy, which may become severe or irreversible, has occurred. Fatalities have been reported. Conditions such as renal impairment (creatinine clearance under 60 mL per minute or clinically significant elevated serum creatinine), anemia, diabetes mellitus, electrolyte imbalance, vitamin B deficiency, and debilitating disease may enhance the occurrence of peripheral neuropathy. Patients receiving long-term therapy should be monitored periodically for changes in renal function.

Optic neuritis has been reported rarely in postmarketing experience with nitrofurantoin formulations.

Cases of hemolytic anemia of the primaquine-sensitivity type have been induced by nitrofurantoin. Hemolysis appears to be linked to a glucose-6-phosphate dehydrogenase deficiency in the red blood cells of the affected patients. This deficiency is found in 10 percent of Blacks and a small percentage of ethnic groups of Mediterranean and Near-Eastern origin. Hemolysis is an indication for discontinuing **Macrobid**; hemolysis ceases when the drug is withdrawn.

Pseudomembranous colitis has been reported with nearly all antibacterial agents, including nitrofurantoin, and may range from mild to life threatening. Therefore, it is important to consider this diagnosis in patients with diarrhea subsequent to the administration of antibacterial agents.

Treatment with antibacterial agents alters the normal flora of the colon and may permit overgrowth of clostridia. Studies indicate that a toxin produced by *Clostridium difficile* is one primary cause of antibiotic-associated colitis.

Continued on next page

Macrobid—Cont.

After the diagnosis of pseudomembranous colitis has been established, appropriate therapeutic measures should be initiated. Mild cases of pseudomembranous colitis usually respond to drug discontinuation alone. In moderate to severe cases, consideration should be given to management with fluids and electrolytes, protein supplementation, and treatment with an antibacterial drug clinically effective against *Clostridium difficile* colitis.

PRECAUTIONS

Information for Patients: Patients should be advised to take **Macrobid** with food (ideally breakfast and dinner) to further enhance tolerance and improve drug absorption. Patients should be instructed to complete the full course of therapy; however, they should be advised to contact their physician if any unusual symptoms occur during therapy.

Patients should be advised not to use antacid preparations containing magnesium trisilicate while taking **Macrobid**.

Drug Interactions: Antacids containing magnesium trisilicate, when administered concomitantly with nitrofurantoin, reduce both the rate and extent of absorption. The mechanism for this interaction probably is adsorption of nitrofurantoin onto the surface of magnesium trisilicate.

Uricosuric drugs, such as probenecid and sulfinpyrazone, can inhibit renal tubular secretion of nitrofurantoin. The resulting increase in nitrofurantoin serum levels may increase toxicity, and the decreased urinary levels could lessen its efficacy as a urinary tract antibacterial.

Drug/Laboratory Test Interactions: As a result of the presence of nitrofurantoin, a false-positive reaction for glucose in the urine may occur. This has been observed with Benedict's and Fehling's solutions but not with the glucose enzymatic test.

Carcinogenesis, Mutagenesis, Impairment of Fertility: Nitrofurantoin was not carcinogenic when fed to female Holtzman rats for 44.5 weeks or to female Sprague-Dawley rats for 75 weeks. Two chronic rodent bioassays utilizing male and female Sprague-Dawley rats and two chronic bioassays in Swiss mice and in BDF_1 mice revealed no evidence of carcinogenicity. Nitrofurantoin presented evidence of carcinogenic activity in female $B6C3F_1$ mice as shown by increased incidences of tubular adenomas, benign mixed tumors, and granulosa cell tumors of the ovary. In male F344/N rats, there were increased incidences of uncommon kidney tubular cell neoplasms, osteosarcomas of the bone, and neoplasms of the subcutaneous tissue. In one study involving subcutaneous administration of 75 mg/kg nitrofurantoin to pregnant female mice, lung papillary adenomas of unknown significance were observed in the F1 generation. Nitrofurantoin has been shown to induce point mutations in certain strains of *Salmonella typhimurium* and forward mutations in L5178Y mouse lymphoma cells. Nitrofurantoin induced increased numbers of sister chromatid exchanges and chromosomal aberrations in Chinese hamster ovary cells but not in human cells in culture. Results of the sex-linked recessive lethal assay in Drosophila were negative after administration of nitrofurantoin by feeding or by injection. Nitrofurantoin did not induce heritable mutation in the rodent models examined.

The significance of the carcinogenicity and mutagenicity findings relative to the therapeutic use of nitrofurantoin in humans is unknown. The administration of high doses of nitrofurantoin to rats causes temporary spermatogenic arrest; this is reversible on discontinuing the drug. Doses of 10 mg/kg/day or greater in healthy human males may, in certain unpredictable instances, produce a slight to moderate spermatogenic arrest with a decrease in sperm count.

Pregnancy:

Teratogenic effects: Pregnancy Category B. Several reproduction studies have been performed in rabbits and rats at doses up to six times the human dose and have revealed no evidence of impaired fertility or harm to the fetus due to nitrofurantoin. In a single published study conducted in mice at 68 times the human dose (based on mg/kg administered to the dam), growth retardation and a low incidence of minor and common malformations were observed. However, at 25 times the human dose, fetal malformations were not observed; the relevance of these findings to humans is uncertain. There are, however, no adequate and well-controlled studies in pregnant women. Because animal reproduction studies are not always predictive of human response, this drug should be used during pregnancy only if clearly needed.

Non-teratogenic effects: Nitrofurantoin has been shown in one published transplacental carcinogenicity study to induce lung papillary adenomas in the F1 generation mice at doses 19 times the human dose on a mg/kg basis. The relationship of this finding to potential human carcinogenesis is presently unknown. Because of the uncertainty regarding the human implications of these animal data, this drug should be used during pregnancy only if clearly needed.

Labor and Delivery: See **CONTRAINDICATIONS**.

Nursing Mothers: Nitrofurantoin has been detected in human breast milk in trace amounts. Because of the potential for serious adverse reactions from nitrofurantoin in nursing infants under one month of age, a decision should be made whether to discontinue nursing or to discontinue the drug, taking into account the importance of the drug to the mother. (See **CONTRAINDICATIONS**.)

Pediatric Use: **Macrobid** is contraindicated in infants below the age of one month. (See **CONTRAINDICATIONS**.) Safety and effectiveness in pediatric patients below the age of twelve years have not been established.

ADVERSE REACTIONS

In clinical trials of **Macrobid**, the most frequent clinical adverse events that were reported as possibly or probably drug-related were nausea (8%), headache (6%), and flatulence (1.5%). Additional clinical adverse events reported as possibly or probably drug-related occurred in less than 1% of patients studied and are listed below within each body system in order of decreasing frequency:

Gastrointestinal: Diarrhea, dyspepsia, abdominal pain, constipation, emesis

Neurologic: Dizziness, drowsiness, amblyopia

Respiratory: Acute pulmonary hypersensitivity reaction (see **WARNINGS**)

Allergic: Pruritus, urticaria

Dermatologic: Alopecia

Miscellaneous: Fever, chills, malaise

The following additional clinical adverse events have been reported with the use of nitrofurantoin:

Gastrointestinal: Sialadenitis, pancreatitis. There have been sporadic reports of pseudomembranous colitis with the use of nitrofurantoin. The onset of pseudomembranous colitis symptoms may occur during or after antimicrobial treatment. (See **WARNINGS**.)

Neurologic: Peripheral neuropathy, which may become severe or irreversible, has occurred. Fatalities have been reported. Conditions such as renal impairment (creatinine clearance under 60 mL per minute or clinically significant elevated serum creatinine), anemia, diabetes mellitus, electrolyte imbalance, vitamin B deficiency, and debilitating diseases may increase the possibility of peripheral neuropathy. (See **WARNINGS**.)

Asthenia, vertigo, and nystagmus also have been reported with the use of nitrofurantoin. Benign intracranial hypertension (pseudotumor cerebri), confusion, depression, optic neuritis, and psychotic reactions have been reported rarely. Bulging fontanels, as a sign of benign intracranial hypertension in infants, have been reported rarely.

Respiratory:

CHRONIC, SUBACUTE, OR ACUTE PULMONARY HYPERSENSITIVITY REACTIONS MAY OCCUR WITH THE USE OF NITROFURANTOIN.

CHRONIC PULMONARY REACTIONS GENERALLY OCCUR IN PATIENTS WHO HAVE RECEIVED CONTINUOUS TREATMENT FOR SIX MONTHS OR LONGER. MALAISE, DYSPNEA ON EXERTION, COUGH, AND ALTERED PULMONARY FUNCTION ARE COMMON MANIFESTATIONS WHICH CAN OCCUR INSIDIOUSLY. RADIOLOGIC AND HISTOLOGIC FINDINGS OF DIFFUSE INTERSTITIAL PNEUMONITIS OR FIBROSIS, OR BOTH, ARE ALSO COMMON MANIFESTATIONS OF THE CHRONIC PULMONARY REACTION. FEVER IS RARELY PROMINENT.

THE SEVERITY OF CHRONIC PULMONARY REACTIONS AND THEIR DEGREE OF RESOLUTION APPEAR TO BE RELATED TO THE DURATION OF THERAPY AFTER THE FIRST CLINICAL SIGNS APPEAR. PULMONARY FUNCTION MAY BE IMPAIRED PERMANENTLY, EVEN AFTER CESSATION OF THERAPY. THE RISK IS GREATER WHEN CHRONIC PULMONARY REACTIONS ARE NOT RECOGNIZED EARLY.

In subacute pulmonary reactions, fever and eosinophilia occur less often than in the acute form. Upon cessation of therapy, recovery may require several months. If the symptoms are not recognized as being drug-related and nitrofurantoin therapy is not stopped, the symptoms may become more severe.

Acute pulmonary reactions are commonly manifested by fever, chills, cough, chest pain, dyspnea, pulmonary infiltration with consolidation or pleural effusion on x-ray, and eosinophilia. Acute reactions usually occur within the first week of treatment and are reversible with cessation of therapy. Resolution often is dramatic. (See **WARNINGS**.)

Changes in EKG (e.g., non-specific ST/T wave changes, bundle branch block) have been reported in association with pulmonary reactions. Cyanosis has been reported rarely.

Hepatic: Hepatic reactions, including hepatitis, cholestatic jaundice, chronic active hepatitis, and hepatic necrosis, occur rarely. (See **WARNINGS**.)

Allergic: Lupus-like syndrome associated with pulmonary reaction to nitrofurantoin has been reported. Also, angioedema; maculopapular, erythematous, or eczematous eruptions; anaphylaxis; arthralgia; myalgia; drug fever; and chills have been reported. Hypersensitivity reactions represent the most frequent spontaneously-reported adverse events in worldwide postmarketing experience with nitrofurantoin formulations.

Dermatologic: Exfoliative dermatitis and erythema multiforme (including Stevens-Johnson syndrome) have been reported rarely.

Hematologic: Cyanosis secondary to methemoglobinemia has been reported rarely.

Miscellaneous: As with other antimicrobial agents, superinfections caused by resistant organisms, e.g., *Pseudomonas* species or *Candida* species, can occur.

In clinical trials of **Macrobid**, the most frequent laboratory adverse events (1–5%), without regard to drug relationship, were as follows: eosinophilia, increased AST (SGOT), increased ALT (SGPT), decreased hemoglobin, increased serum phosphorus. The following laboratory adverse events also have been reported with the use of nitrofurantoin: glucose-6-phosphate dehydrogenase deficiency anemia (see **WARNINGS**), agranulocytosis, leukopenia, granulocytopenia, hemolytic anemia, thrombocytopenia, megaloblastic anemia. In most cases, these hematologic abnormalities resolved following cessation of therapy. Aplastic anemia has been reported rarely.

OVERDOSAGE

Occasional incidents of acute overdosage of nitrofurantoin have not resulted in any specific symptoms other than vomiting. Induction of emesis is recommended. There is no specific antidote, but a high fluid intake should be maintained to promote urinary excretion of the drug. Nitrofurantoin is dialyzable.

DOSAGE AND ADMINISTRATION

Macrobid capsules should be taken with food.

Adults and Pediatric Patients Over 12 Years: One 100-mg capsule every 12 hours for seven days.

HOW SUPPLIED

Macrobid is available as 100-mg opaque black and yellow capsules imprinted "Macrobid" on one half and "Norwich Eaton" on the other.

NDC 0149-0710-01 bottle of 100

Store at controlled room temperature (59° to 86°F or 15° to 30°C).

Rx Only

REFERENCES

1. National Committee for Clinical Laboratory Standards. Methods for Dilution Antimicrobial Susceptibility Tests for Bacteria that Grow Aerobically—Third Edition. Approved Standard NCCLS Document M7-A3, Vol. 13, No. 25, NCCLS, Villanova, PA, December 1993.
2. National Committee for Clinical Laboratory Standards. Performance Standards for Antimicrobial Disk Susceptibility Tests—Fifth Edition. Approved Standard NCCLS Document M2-A5, Vol. 13, No. 24, NCCLS, Villanova, PA, December 1993.

CLINICAL STUDIES

Controlled clinical trials comparing **Macrobid** 100 mg p.o. q12h and **Macrodantin** 50 mg p.o. q6h in the treatment of acute uncomplicated urinary tract infections demonstrated approximately 75% microbiologic eradication of susceptible pathogens in each treatment group.

Procter & Gamble Pharmaceuticals
Cincinnati, Ohio 45202
REVISED FEBRUARY 1998

Shown in Product Identification Guide, page 331

MACRODANTIN® ℞

[mak" rō-dan' tin]

(nitrofurantoin macrocrystals)

DESCRIPTION

Macrodantin (nitrofurantoin macrocrystals) is a synthetic chemical of controlled crystal size. It is a stable, yellow, crystalline compound. **Macrodantin** is an antibacterial agent for specific urinary tract infections. It is available in 25-mg, 50-mg, and 100-mg capsules for oral administration.

1-[[(5-NITRO-2-FURANYL)METHYLENE]AMINO]-2,4-IMIDAZOLIDINEDIONE

Inactive Ingredients: Each capsule contains edible black ink, gelatin, lactose, starch, talc, titanium dioxide, and may contain FD&C Yellow No. 6 and D&C Yellow No. 10.

CLINICAL PHARMACOLOGY

Macrodantin is a larger crystal form of **Furadantin®** (nitrofurantoin). The absorption of **Macrodantin** is slower and its excretion somewhat less when compared to **Furadantin**. Blood concentrations at therapeutic dosage are usually low. It is highly soluble in urine, to which it may impart a brown color.

Following a dose regimen of 100 mg q.i.d. for 7 days, average urinary drug recoveries (0-24 hours) on day 1 and day 7 were 37.9% and 35.0%.

Unlike many drugs, the presence of food or agents delaying gastric emptying can increase the bioavailability of **Macrodantin**, presumably by allowing better dissolution in gastric juices.

Microbiology: Nitrofurantoin is bactericidal in urine at therapeutic doses. The mechanism of the antimicrobial action of nitrofurantoin is unusual among antibacterials. Nitrofurantoin is reduced by bacterial flavoproteins to reactive intermediates which inactivate or alter bacterial ribosomal proteins and other macromolecules. As a result of such inactivations, the vital biochemical processes of protein synthesis, aerobic energy metabolism, DNA synthesis, RNA synthesis, and cell wall synthesis are inhibited. The broad-based nature of this mode of action may explain the lack of acquired bacterial resistance to nitrofurantoin, as the necessary multiple and simultaneous mutations of the target macromolecules would likely be lethal to the bacteria. Development of resistance to nitrofurantoin has not been a significant problem since its introduction in 1953. Cross-resistance with antibiotics and sulfonamides has not been observed, and transferable resistance is, at most, a very rare phenomenon.

Nitrofurantoin, in the form of **Macrodantin**, has been shown to be active against most strains of the following bacteria both *in vitro* and in clinical infections: (See **INDICATIONS AND USAGE**.)

Gram-Positive Aerobes

Staphylococcus aureus

Enterococci (e.g., *Enterococcus faecalis*)

Gram-Negative Aerobes

Escherichia coli

NOTE: Some strains of *Enterobacter* species and *Klebsiella* species are resistant to nitrofurantoin.

Nitrofurantoin also demonstrates in vitro activity against the following microorganisms, although the clinical significance of these data with respect to treatment with **Macrodantin** is unknown:

Gram-Positive Aerobes

Coagulase-negative staphylococci (including *Staphylococcus epidermidis* and *Staphylococcus saprophyticus*)

Streptococcus agalactiae

Group D streptococci

Viridans group streptococci

Gram-Negative Aerobes

Citrobacter amalonaticus

Citrobacter diversus

Citrobacter freundii

Klebsiella oxytoca

Klebsiella ozaenae

Nitrofurantoin is not active against most strains of *Proteus* species or *Serratia* species. It has no activity against *Pseudomonas species.*

Antagonism has been demonstrated *in vitro* between nitrofurantoin and quinolone antimicrobial agents. The clinical significance of this finding is unknown.

Susceptibility Tests:

Dilution techniques:

Quantitative methods are used to determine antimicrobial minimal inhibitory concentrations (MIC's). These MIC's provide estimates of the susceptibility of bacteria to antimicrobial compounds. The MIC's should be determined using a standardized procedure. Standardized procedures are based on a dilution method[1] (broth or agar) or equivalent with standardized inoculum concentrations and standardized concentrations of nitrofurantoin powder. The MIC values should be interpreted according to the following criteria:

MIC (µg/mL)	Interpretation
≤ 32	Susceptible (S)
64	Intermediate (I)
≥ 128	Resistant (R)

A report of "Susceptible" indicates that the pathogen is likely to be inhibited if the antimicrobial compound in the urine reaches the concentrations usually achievable. A report of "Intermediate" indicates that the result should be considered equivocal, and, if the microorganism is not fully susceptible to alternative, clinically feasible drugs, the test should be repeated. This category implies possible clinical applicability in body sites where the drug is physiologically concentrated or in situations where high dosage of drug can be used. This category also provides a buffer zone which prevents small uncontrolled technical factors from causing major discrepancies in interpretation. A report of "Resistant" indicates that the pathogen is not likely to be inhibited if the antimicrobial compound in the urine reaches the concentrations usually achievable; other therapy should be selected.

Standardized susceptibility test procedures require the use of laboratory control microorganisms to control the technical aspects of the laboratory procedures. Standard nitrofurantoin powder should provide the following MIC values:

Microorganism	MIC (µg/mL)
E. coli ATCC 25922	4–16
S. aureus ATCC 29213	8–32
E. faecalis ATCC 29212	4–16

Diffusion techniques:

Quantitative methods that require measurement of zone diameters also provide reproducible estimates of the susceptibility of bacteria to antimicrobial compounds. One such standardized procedure[2] requires the use of standardized inoculum concentrations. This procedure uses paper disks impregnated with 300-µg nitrofurantoin to test the susceptibility of microorganisms to nitrofurantoin.

Reports from the laboratory providing results of the standard single-disk susceptibility test with a 300-µg nitrofurantoin disk should be interpreted according to the following criteria:

Zone Diameter (mm)	Interpretation
≥ 17	Susceptible (S)
15-16	Intermediate (I)
≤ 14	Resistant (R)

Interpretation should be as stated above for results using dilution techniques. Interpretation involves correlation of the diameter obtained in the disk test with the MIC for nitrofurantoin.

As with standardized dilution techniques, diffusion methods require the use of laboratory control microorganisms that are used to control the technical aspects of the laboratory procedures. For the diffusion technique, the 300-æg nitrofurantoin disk should provide the following zone diameters in these laboratory test quality control strains:

Microorganism	Zone Diameter (mm)
E. coli ATCC 25922	20–25
S. aureus ATCC 25923	18–22

INDICATIONS AND USAGE

Macrodantin is specifically indicated for the treatment of urinary tract infections when due to susceptible strains of *Escherichia coli*, enterococci, *Staphylococcus aureus*, and certain susceptible strains of *Klebsiella* and *Enterobacter* species.

Nitrofurantoin is not indicated for the treatment of pyelonephritis or perinephric abscesses.

Nitrofurantoins lack the broader tissue distribution of other therapeutic agents approved for urinary tract infections. Consequently, many patients who are treated with **Macrodantin** are predisposed to persistence or reappearance of bacteriuria. Urine specimens for culture and susceptibility testing should be obtained before and after completion of therapy. If persistence or reappearance of bacteriuria occurs after treatment with **Macrodantin**, other therapeutic agents with broader tissue distribution should be selected. In considering the use of **Macrodantin**, lower eradication rates should be balanced against the increased potential for systemic toxicity and for the development of antimicrobial resistance when agents with broader tissue distribution are utilized.

CONTRAINDICATIONS

Anuria, oliguria, or significant impairment of renal function (creatinine clearance under 60 mL per minute or clinically significant elevated serum creatinine) are contraindications. Treatment of this type of patient carries an increased risk of toxicity because of impaired excretion of the drug.

Because of the possibility of hemolytic anemia due to immature erythrocyte enzyme systems (glutathione instability), the drug is contraindicated in pregnant patients at term (38-42 weeks gestation), during labor and delivery, or when the onset of labor is imminent. For the same reason, the drug is contraindicated in neonates under one month of age.

Macrodantin is also contraindicated in those patients with known hypersensitivity to nitrofurantoin.

WARNINGS

ACUTE, SUBACUTE, OR CHRONIC PULMONARY REACTIONS HAVE BEEN OBSERVED IN PATIENTS TREATED WITH NITROFURANTOIN. IF THESE REACTIONS OCCUR, MACRODANTIN SHOULD BE DISCONTINUED AND APPROPRIATE MEASURES TAKEN. REPORTS HAVE CITED PULMONARY REACTIONS AS A CONTRIBUTING CAUSE OF DEATH.

CHRONIC PULMONARY REACTIONS (DIFFUSE INTERSTITIAL PNEUMONITIS OR PULMONARY FIBROSIS, OR BOTH) CAN DEVELOP INSIDIOUSLY. THESE REACTIONS OCCUR RARELY AND GENERALLY IN PATIENTS RECEIVING THERAPY FOR SIX MONTHS OR LONGER. CLOSE MONITORING OF THE PULMONARY CONDITION OF PATIENTS RECEIVING LONG-TERM THERAPY IS WARRANTED AND REQUIRES THAT THE BENEFITS OF THERAPY BE WEIGHED AGAINST POTENTIAL RISKS. (SEE RESPIRATORY REACTIONS.)

Hepatic reactions, including hepatitis, cholestatic jaundice, chronic active hepatitis, and hepatic necrosis, occur rarely. Fatalities have been reported. The onset of chronic active hepatitis may be insidious, and patients should be monitored periodically for changes in biochemical tests that would indicate liver injury. If hepatitis occurs, the drug should be withdrawn immediately and appropriate measures should be taken.

Peripheral neuropathy, which may become severe or irreversible, has occurred. Fatalities have been reported. Conditions such as renal impairment (creatinine clearance under 60 mL per minute or clinically significant elevated serum creatinine), anemia, diabetes mellitus, electrolyte imbalance, vitamin B deficiency, and debilitating disease may enhance the occurrence of peripheral neuropathy. Patients receiving long-term therapy should be monitored periodically for changes in renal function.

Optic neuritis has been reported rarely in postmarketing experience with nitrofurantoin formulations.

Cases of hemolytic anemia of the primaquine-sensitivity type have been induced by nitrofurantoin. Hemolysis appears to be linked to a glucose-6-phosphate dehydrogenase deficiency in the red blood cells of the affected patients. This deficiency is found in 10 percent of Blacks and a small percentage of ethnic groups of Mediterranean and Near-Eastern origin. Hemolysis is an indication for discontinuing **Macrodantin**; hemolysis ceases when the drug is withdrawn.

Pseudomembranous colitis has been reported with nearly all antibacterial agents, including nitrofurantoin, and may range from mild to life threatening. Therefore, it is important to consider this diagnosis in patients with diarrhea subsequent to the administration of antibacterial agents.

Treatment with antibacterial agents alters the normal flora of the colon and may permit overgrowth of clostridia. Studies indicate that a toxin produced by *Clostridium difficile* is one primary cause of antibiotic-associated colitis.

After the diagnosis of pseudomembranous colitis has been established, appropriate therapeutic measures should be initiated. Mild cases of pseudomembranous colitis usually respond to drug discontinuation alone. In moderate to severe cases, consideration should be given to management with fluids and electrolytes, protein supplementation, and treatment with an antibacterial drug clinically effective against *Clostridium difficile* colitis.

PRECAUTIONS

Information for Patients: Patients should be advised to take **Macrodantin** with food to further enhance tolerance and improve drug absorption. Patients should be instructed to complete the full course of therapy; however, they should be advised to contact their physician if any unusual symptoms occur during therapy.

Many patients who cannot tolerate microcrystalline nitrofurantoin are able to take **Macrodantin** without nausea.

Patients should be advised not to use antacid preparations containing magnesium trisilicate while taking **Macrodantin.**

Drug Interactions: Antacids containing magnesium trisilicate, when administered concomitantly with nitrofurantoin, reduce both the rate and extent of absorption. The mechanism for this interaction probably is adsorption of nitrofurantoin onto the surface of magnesium trisilicate.

Uricosuric drugs, such as probenecid and sulfinpyrazone, can inhibit renal tubular secretion of nitrofurantoin. The resulting increase in nitrofurantoin serum levels may increase toxicity, and the decreased urinary levels could lessen its efficacy as a urinary tract antibacterial.

Drug/Laboratory Test Interactions: As a result of the presence of nitrofurantoin, a false-positive reaction for glucose in the urine may occur. This has been observed with Benedict's and Fehling's solutions but not with the glucose enzymatic test.

Carcinogenesis, Mutagenesis, Impairment of Fertility: Nitrofurantoin was not carcinogenic when fed to female Holtzman rats for 44.5 weeks or to female Sprague-Dawley rats for 75 weeks. Two chronic rodent bioassays utilizing male and female Sprague-Dawley rats and two chronic bioassays in Swiss mice and in BDF_1 mice revealed no evidence of carcinogenicity.

Nitrofurantoin presented evidence of carcinogenic activity in female $B6C3F_1$ mice as shown by increased incidences of tubular adenomas, benign mixed tumors, and granulosa cell tumors of the ovary. In male F344/N rats, there were increased incidences of uncommon kidney tubular cell neoplasms, osteosarcomas of the bone, and neoplasms of the subcutaneous tissue. In one study involving subcutaneous administration of 75 mg/kg nitrofurantoin to pregnant female mice, lung papillary adenomas of unknown significance were observed in the F1 generation.

Nitrofurantoin has been shown to induce point mutations in certain strains of *Salmonella typhimurium* and forward mutations in L5178Y mouse lymphoma cells. Nitrofurantoin induced increased numbers of sister chromatid exchanges and chromosomal aberrations in Chinese hamster ovary cells but not in human cells in culture. Results of the sex-linked recessive lethal assay in Drosophila were negative after administration of nitrofurantoin by feeding or by injection. Nitrofurantoin did not induce heritable mutation in the rodent models examined.

The significance of the carcinogenicity and mutagenicity findings relative to the therapeutic use of nitrofurantoin in humans is unknown.

The administration of high doses of nitrofurantoin to rats causes temporary spermatogenic arrest; this is reversible on discontinuing the drug. Doses of 10 mg/kg/day or greater in healthy human males may, in certain unpredictable instances, produce a slight to moderate spermatogenic arrest with a decrease in sperm count.

Pregnancy:

Teratogenic effects: Pregnancy Category B. Several reproduction studies have been performed in rabbits and rats at doses up to six times the human dose and have revealed no evidence of impaired fertility or harm to the fetus due to nitrofurantoin. In a single published study conducted in mice at 68 times the human dose (based on mg/kg administered to the dam), growth retardation and a low incidence of minor and common malformations were observed. However, at 25 times the human dose, fetal malformations were not observed; the relevance of these findings to humans is uncertain. There are, however, no adequate and well-controlled studies in pregnant women. Because animal reproduction studies are not always predictive of human response, this drug should be used during pregnancy only if clearly needed.

Non-teratogenic effects: Nitrofurantoin has been shown in one published transplacental carcino-genicity study to induce lung papillary adenomas in the F1 generation mice at doses 19 times the human dose on a mg/kg basis. The relationship of this finding to potential human carcinogenesis is presently unknown. Because of the uncertainty regarding the human implications of these animal data, this drug should be used during pregnancy only if clearly needed.

Labor and Delivery: See **CONTRAINDICATIONS.**

Nursing Mothers: Nitrofurantoin has been detected in human breast milk in trace amounts. Because of the potential for serious adverse reactions from nitrofurantoin in nursing infants under one month of age, a decision should be made whether to discontinue nursing or to discontinue the drug, taking into account the importance of the drug to the mother. (See **CONTRAINDICATIONS.**)

Pediatric Use: **Macrodantin** is contraindicated in infants below the age of one month. (See **CONTRAINDICATIONS.**)

Continued on next page

Macrodantin—Cont.

ADVERSE REACTIONS

Respiratory:

CHRONIC, SUBACUTE, OR ACUTE PULMONARY HYPERSENSITIVITY REACTIONS MAY OCCUR.

CHRONIC PULMONARY REACTIONS OCCUR GENERALLY IN PATIENTS WHO HAVE RECEIVED CONTINUOUS TREATMENT FOR SIX MONTHS OR LONGER. MALAISE, DYSPNEA ON EXERTION, COUGH, AND ALTERED PULMONARY FUNCTION ARE COMMON MANIFESTATIONS WHICH CAN OCCUR INSIDIOUSLY. RADIOLOGIC AND HISTOLOGIC FINDINGS OF DIFFUSE INTERSTITIAL PNEUMONITIS OR FIBROSIS, OR BOTH, ARE ALSO COMMON MANIFESTATIONS OF THE CHRONIC PULMONARY REACTION. FEVER IS RARELY PROMINENT.

THE SEVERITY OF CHRONIC PULMONARY REACTIONS AND THEIR DEGREE OF RESOLUTION APPEAR TO BE RELATED TO THE DURATION OF THERAPY AFTER THE FIRST CLINICAL SIGNS APPEAR. PULMONARY FUNCTION MAY BE IMPAIRED PERMANENTLY, EVEN AFTER CESSATION OF THERAPY. THE RISK IS GREATER WHEN CHRONIC PULMONARY REACTIONS ARE NOT RECOGNIZED EARLY.

In subacute pulmonary reactions, fever and eosinophilia occur less often than in the acute form. Upon cessation of therapy, recovery may require several months. If the symptoms are not recog-nized as being drug-related and nitrofurantoin therapy is not stopped, the symptoms may become more severe.

Acute pulmonary reactions are commonly manifested by fever, chills, cough, chest pain, dyspnea, pulmonary infiltration with consolidation or pleural effusion on x-ray, and eosinophilia. Acute reactions usually occur within the first week of treatment and are reversible with cessation of therapy. Resolution often is dramatic. (See **WARNINGS**.)

Changes in EKG (e.g., non-specific ST/T wave changes, bundle branch block) have been reported in association with pulmonary reactions.

Cyanosis has been reported rarely.

Hepatic: Hepatic reactions, including hepatitis, cholestatic jaundice, chronic active hepatitis, and hepatic necrosis, occur rarely. (See **WARNINGS**.)

Neurologic: Peripheral neuropathy, which may become severe or irreversible, has occurred. Fatalities have been reported. Conditions such as renal impairment (creatinine clearance under 60 mL per minute or clinically significant elevated serum creatinine), anemia, diabetes mellitus, electrolyte imbalance, vitamin B deficiency, and debilitating diseases may increase the possibility of peripheral neuropathy. (See **WARNINGS**.)

Asthenia, vertigo, nystagmus, dizziness, headache, and drowsiness also have been reported with the use of nitrofurantoin.

Benign intracranial hypertension (pseudotumor cerebri), confusion, depression, optic neuritis, and psychotic reactions have been reported rarely. Bulging fontanels, as a sign of benign intracranial hypertension in infants, have been reported rarely.

Dermatologic: Exfoliative dermatitis and erythema multiforme (including Stevens-Johnson syndrome) have been reported rarely. Transient alopecia also has been reported.

Allergic: A lupus-like syndrome associated with pulmonary reactions to nitrofurantoin has been reported. Also, angioedema; maculopapular, erythematous, or eczematous eruptions; pruritus; urticaria; anaphylaxis; arthralgia; myalgia; drug fever; and chills have been reported. Hyper sensitivity reactions represent the most frequent spontaneously-reported adverse events in worldwide postmarketing experience with nitrofurantoin formulations.

Gastrointestinal: Nausea, emesis, and anorexia occur most often. Abdominal pain and diarrhea are less common gastrointestinal reactions. These dose-related reactions can be minimized by reduction of dosage. Sialadenitis and pancreatitis have been reported. There have been sporadic reports of pseudomembranous colitis with the use of nitrofurantoin. The onset of pseudomembranous colitis symptoms may occur during or after antimicrobial treatment. (See **WARNINGS**.)

Hematologic: Cyanosis secondary to methemoglobinemia has been reported rarely.

Miscellaneous: As with other antimicrobial agents, superinfections caused by resistant organisms, e.g., *Pseudomonas* species or *Candida* species, can occur.

Laboratory Adverse Events: The following laboratory adverse events have been reported with the use of nitrofurantoin: increased AST (SGOT), increased ALT (SGPT), decreased hemoglobin, increased serum phosphorus, eosinophilia, glucose-6-phosphate dehydrogenase deficiency anemia (see **WARNINGS**), agranulocytosis, leukopenia, granulo-cytopenia, hemolytic anemia, thrombocytopenia, megaloblastic anemia. In most cases, these hematologic abnormalities resolved following cessation of therapy. Aplastic anemia has been reported rarely.

OVERDOSAGE

Occasional incidents of acute overdosage of **Macrodantin** have not resulted in any specific symptoms other than vomiting. Induction of emesis is recommended. There is no specific antidote, but a high fluid intake should be maintained to promote urinary excretion of the drug. It is dialyzable.

DOSAGE AND ADMINISTRATION

Macrodantin should be given with food to improve drug absorption and, in some patients, tolerance.

Adults: 50–100 mg four times a day — the lower dosage level is recommended for uncomplicated urinary tract infections.

Pediatric Patients: 5–7 mg/kg of body weight per 24 hours, given in four divided doses (contraindicated under one month of age).

Therapy should be continued for one week or for at least 3 days after sterility of the urine is obtained. Continued infection indicates the need for reevaluation.

For long-term suppressive therapy in adults, a reduction of dosage to 50-100 mg at bedtime may be adequate. For long-term suppressive therapy in pediatric patients, doses as low as 1 mg/kg per 24 hours, given in a single dose or in two divided doses, may be adequate. **SEE WARNINGS SECTION REGARDING RISKS ASSOCIATED WITH LONG-TERM THERAPY.**

HOW SUPPLIED

Macrodantin is available as follows:

25-mg opaque, white capsule imprinted with one black line encircling the capsule and coded "MACRODANTIN 25 mg" and "0149-0007".*

NDC 0149-0007-05 bottle of 100

50-mg opaque, yellow and white capsule imprinted with two black lines encircling the capsule and coded "MACRODANTIN 50 mg" and "0149-0008".*

NDC 0149-0008-05 bottle of 100
NDC 0149-0008-66 bottle of 500
NDC 0149-0008-67 bottle of 1000
NDC 0149-0008-77 hospital unit-dose strips in box of 100

100-mg opaque, yellow capsule imprinted with three black lines encircling the capsule and coded "MACRODANTIN 100 mg" and "0149-0009".*

NDC 0149-0009-05 bottle of 100
NDC 0149-0009-66 bottle of 500
NDC 0149-0009-67 bottle of 1000
NDC 0149-0009-77 hospital unit-dose strips in box of 100

*Capsule design, registered trademark of Procter & Gamble Pharmaceuticals.

Rx Only

REFERENCES

1. National Committee for Clinical Laboratory Standards. Methods for Dilution Antimicrobial Susceptibility Tests for Bacteria that Grow Aerobically -- Third Edition. Approved Standard NCCLS Document M7-A3, Vol. 13, No. 25, NCCLS, Villanova, PA, December 1993.
2. National Committee for Clinical Laboratory Standards. Performance Standards for Antimicrobial Disk Susceptibility Tests -- Fifth Edition. Approved Standard NCCLS Document M2-A5, Vol. 13, No. 24, NCCLS, Villanova, PA, December 1993.

Procter & Gamble Pharmaceuticals
Cincinnati, Ohio 45202
REVISED FEBRUARY 1998

Shown in Product Identification Guide, page 331

The Purdue Frederick Company

ONE STAMFORD FORUM
STAMFORD, CT 06901-3431

For Medical Information Contact:
888-726-7535
Adverse Drug Experiences:
888-726-7535
Customer Service:
800-877-5666
FAX 800-877-3210

OxyContin® 10 mg Tablets
OxyContin® 20 mg Tablets
OxyContin® 40 mg Tablets
OxyContin® 80 mg Tablets
OxyContin® 160 mg Tablets
see listing under Purdue Pharma L.P., page 2697

OxyIR® Capsules—see listing under Purdue Pharma L.P., page 2701

BETADINE® BRAND PLUS OTC
First Aid Antibiotics + Pain Reliever Ointment
[*bā 'tăh-dīn"*]

Each gram contains: Polymyxin B Sulfate (10,000 IU), Bacitracin Zinc (500 IU), and Pramoxine HCl 10 mg in a cholesterolized ointment base.

ACTIONS

Topical broad-spectrum antibiotics plus topical anesthetic in a cholesterolized ointment* (moisturizer) base to help prevent infection and temporarily relieve pain; active ingredients per gram: polymyxin B sulfate (10,000 IU), bacitracin zinc (500 IU), and pramoxine HCl 10 mg.

INDICATIONS

Help prevent infection and provide temporary pain relief in minor cuts, scrapes and burns.

ADMINISTRATION

Clean affected area. Apply small amount of this product (an amount equal to the surface area of the tip of the finger) on the area 1 to 3 times daily. May be covered with a sterile bandage. **Children under 2 years of age: Consult a doctor.**

WARNINGS

For External Use Only. Do not use in the eyes or apply over large areas of the body. In case of deep or puncture wounds, animal bites, or serious burns, consult a physician. Stop use and consult a physician if the condition persists or gets worse. Do not use longer than 1 week unless directed by a physician. Keep this and all medications out of the reach of children. In case of accidental ingestion, seek professional assistance or contact a Poison Control Center immediately.

HOW SUPPLIED

1/2 oz. plastic tube with an applicator tip, and 1/32 oz. packettes.

*Formulated with Aquaphor®—a registered trademark of Beiersdorf AG.

Stamford, CT 06901-3431

BETADINE® OTC
BRAND First Aid Antibiotics + Moisturizer Ointment
[*Bā 'tăh-dīn"*]

Each gram contains: Polymyxin B Sulfate (10,000 IU) and Bacitracin Zinc (500 IU) in a cholesterolized ointment base.

ACTION AND USES

BETADINE Brand First Aid Antibiotics + Moisturizer Ointment is a topical antibiotic in a cholesterolized ointment* base. It is formulated to help prevent infection in minor cuts, scrapes and burns.

ADVANTAGES

Its unique nonprescription formula of two broad-spectrum antibiotics plus moisturizer helps prevent infection while helping to heal damaged skin.

ADMINISTRATION

Clean affected area. Apply small amount (an amount equal to the surface area of the tip of the finger) on the area 1 to 3 times daily. May be covered with a sterile bandage.

WARNINGS

For External Use Only. Do not use in the eyes or apply over large areas of the body. In case of deep or puncture wounds, animal bites, or serious burns, consult a physician. Stop use and consult a physician if the condition persists or gets worse or if a rash or other allergic reaction develops. Do not use this product if you are allergic to any of the ingredients. Do not use longer than 1 week unless directed by a physician. Keep this and all medications out of the reach of children. In case of accidental ingestion, seek professional assistance or contact a Poison Control Center immediately.

SUPPLIED

$^1/_2$ oz. plastic tubes, with an applicator-tip for easy and economical application, and $^1/_{32}$ oz. packettes. Store at room temperature.

*Formulated with Aquaphor®—a registered trademark of Beiersdorf AG.

Stamford, CT 06901-3431

BETADINE® MEDICATED DOUCHE CONCENTRATE OTC
[*bā 'tăh-dīn"*]
(povidone-iodine, 10%)

A pleasantly scented solution, BETADINE Medicated Douche is indicated for the prompt symptomatic relief of minor vaginal irritation, itching and soreness. May be used as a cleansing douche.

ADVANTAGES

Low surface tension, with uniform wetting action to assist penetration into vaginal crypts and crevices. Microbicidal activity is retained in the presence of moderate quantities of blood, pus, mucosal secretions and soap and water. Virtually nonirritating to vaginal mucosa. Will not stain skin or natural fabrics.

DIRECTIONS FOR USE

Directions for prompt symptomatic relief of minor vaginal irritation and itching: Fill 2 capfuls (2 tablespoonfuls) with douche. Mix with a quart of lukewarm water. Repeat procedure each day and use once daily for five days. Continue use for the full five days, even if symptoms are relieved earlier.

Directions For Deodorizing and Cleansing Douche: Two (2) tablespoonfuls of BETADINE Douche Concentrate to a quart of lukewarm water once or twice per week. Do not use more often than twice weekly.

When Not to Douche: Douching does not prevent pregnancy, nor should it be used for self-treatment or prevention of a sexually transmitted disease (STD). Do not use during pregnancy, while breast-feeding, or when symptoms of Pelvic Inflammatory Disease (PID) or an STD are present, except with the approval of your physician. Women with iodine sensitivity should not use this product.
When to Stop Use: If symptoms persist after five days of use, or redness, swelling or pain develops, discontinue use and consult a physician.

WARNINGS
Douching is reported to be associated with Pelvic Inflammatory Disease, a serious infection of the reproductive system which can lead to infertility and/or tubal (ectopic) pregnancy. Symptoms of PID and STD pain or tenderness in the lower part of the abdomen and pelvis; vaginal discharge and/or bleeding; nausea or fever; frequent urination; genital sores, and genital ulcers. If you suspect you have a STD or PID, stop using this product and see a physician immediately. Read and save the leaflet, *Important Information for Women*, which accompanies each package.

HOW SUPPLIED
8 oz. plastic bottles. Disposable $^1/_2$ oz. (1 tablespoonful) packets. Also available: BETADINE Medicated Disposable Douche (twin-pack) and BETADINE Pre-Mixed Medicated Disposable Douche, which requires no measuring or mixing (twin-pack).

Stamford, CT 06901-3431

BETADINE® OINTMENT — OTC
[*bā 'tăh-dīn"*]
(povidone-iodine, 10%)

ACTION
Betadine Ointment, in a water-soluble base, is a topical microbicide active against organisms commonly encountered in skin and wound infections.

INDICATIONS
Therapeutically, It may be used as an adjunct to systemic therapy where indicated; for primary or secondary topical infections, infected surgical incisions, infected decubitus or stasis ulcers, pyodermas, secondarily infected dermatoses, and infected traumatic lesions.
Prophylactically: It may be used to prevent microbial contamination in burns, incisions and other topical lesions; for degerming skin in hyperalimentation and catheter care. Its use for abrasions, minor cuts and wounds may prevent the development of infections and permit wound healing.

ADMINISTRATION
Apply directly to affected area as needed. Nonocclusion allows air to reach the wound. May be bandaged.

WARNINGS
For External Use Only. In case of deep or puncture wounds or serious burns, consult physician. If redness, irritation, swelling or pain persists or increases, or if infection occurs, discontinue use and consult physician. Keep out of reach of children.

SUPPLIED
$^1/_{32}$ oz. and $^1/_8$ oz. packettes; 1 oz. tubes.

Stamford, CT 06901-3431

BETADINE® PREPSTICK® APPLICATOR — OTC
[*bā' tăh-dīn''*]
[povidone-iodine, 10%]
Topical Antiseptic Bactericide/Virucide

Individually wrapped applicators are packaged dry with approximately 2.6 grams of microbicidal Betadine® Solution stored in the handle of the applicator. Antiseptic solution is released into the $1^{3/8}$-inch-long, soft foam swab head by gently squeezing the 4-inch-long plastic handle.

ACTIONS
Reduces bacterial load and the risk of infection.

INDICATIONS
For degerming skin and mucous membranes. Provides sufficient antiseptic solution for most kinds of site prepping—including prior to IM injections, venous punctures, and minor surgical procedures.

ADMINISTRATION
Gently squeeze plastic handle. This allows the release of the antiseptic solution into the foam swab head. Apply to prep site with the moistened foam tip, working in a circular motion from inside to the outside. Apply as often as needed.

WARNINGS
For External Use Only. Do not use in the eyes. Discontinue use if irritation and redness develop. **Do not heat prior to application.**

HOW SUPPLIED
150 individually packaged applicators per dispensing unit. Each applicator contains approximately 2.6 grams of solution.

Stamford, CT 06901-3431

BETADINE® PREPSTICK PLUS™ APPLICATOR — OTC
[*bā 'tăh-dīn"*]
povidone-iodine, 10%
with alcohol for faster drying
Topical Antiseptic Bactericide/Virucide

Povidone-iodine with alcohol is stored in the 4-inch-long plastic handle of these individually wrapped applicators which are packaged dry. Antiseptic solution is released into the soft foam swab head by gently squeezing the handle.

ACTIONS
Reduces bacterial load and the risk of infection.

INDICATIONS
For degerming skin and mucous membranes. Provides sufficient antiseptic solution for most types of site prepping—including prior to IM injections, venous punctures, and minor surgical procedures.

ADMINISTRATION
Gently squeeze plastic handle. This allows the release of the antiseptic solution into the foam swab head. Apply to prep site with the moistened foam tip, working in a circular motion from inside to outside. Apply as often as needed.

WARNINGS
For External Use Only. Do not use in the eyes. Discontinue use if irritation and redness develop. **Do not heat prior to application. FLAMMABLE. KEEP AWAY FROM FIRE, FLAME OR ELECTRICAL SPARK.**

HOW SUPPLIED
150 individually packaged applicators per dispensing unit. Each applicator contains approximately 2.6 grams of solution.

Stamford, CT 06901-3431

BETADINE® SKIN CLEANSER — OTC
[*bā 'tăh-dīn"*]
(povidone-iodine, 7.5%)

BETADINE Skin Cleanser, a sudsing, antiseptic bactericidal, virucidal liquid cleanser, forms a rich, golden lather.

INDICATIONS
Helps prevent infection in cuts, scrapes and minor burns; used routinely for general hygiene; virtually nonirritating, nonstaining to skin.

DIRECTIONS FOR USE
Wet the skin, apply a sufficient amount to work up a rich golden lather. Allow lather to remain about 3 minutes and rinse off. Repeat 2–3 times a day or as directed by physician.

WARNINGS
For External Use Only. In case of deep or puncture wounds or serious burns, consult physician. If redness, irritation, swelling or pain persists or increases, or if infection occurs, discontinue use and consult physician. Keep out of reach of children. Avoid storing at excessive heat.

HOW SUPPLIED
4 fl. oz. plastic bottles.

NOTE
Blue stains on starched linen will wash off with soap and water.

Stamford, CT 06901-3431

BETADINE® SOLUTION — OTC
[*bā 'tăh-dīn"*]
(povidone-iodine,10%)
Topical Antiseptic Bactericide/Virucide

INDICATIONS
For preoperative prepping of operative site, including the vagina, and as a general topical bactericide/virucide for: disinfection of wounds; emergency treatment of lacerations and abrasions; second- and third-degree burns; as a prophylactic anti-infective agent in hospital and office procedures, including postoperative application to incisions to help prevent infection; bacterial and mycotic skin infections; decubitus and stasis ulcers; as a preoperative swab in the mouth and throat.

ADMINISTRATION
Apply full strength as often as needed as a paint, spray, or wet soak. May be bandaged.

WARNINGS
For External Use Only. In preoperative prepping, avoid "pooling" beneath the patient. Prolonged exposure to wet solution may cause irritation or rarely, severe skin reactions. In rare instance of local irritation or sensitivity, discontinue use. Do not heat prior to application.

HOW SUPPLIED
$^1/_2$ oz., 4 oz., 8 oz., 16 oz. (1 pt.), 32 oz. (1 qt.) and 1 gal. plastic bottles.

ALSO AVAILABLE
BETADINE® Solution Swab Aid® Pads for degerming small areas of skin or mucous membranes prior to injections, aspirations, catheterization and surgery; boxes of 100 packettes. Also: disposable BETADINE® Solution Swabsticks, in packettes of 1's and 3's. BETADINE® Aerosol Spray povidone-iodine, 5% in 3 oz. bottles.

Stamford, CT 06901-3431

BETADINE® SURGICAL SCRUB — OTC
[*bā 'tăh-dīn "*]
(povidone-iodine, 7.5%)
Topical Antiseptic Bactericide/Virucide

INDICATIONS
A broad-spectrum antiseptic, bactericidal, virucidal sudsing skin cleanser for pre- and postoperative scrubbing or washing by hospital operating room personnel; for preoperative use on patients; and general use as an antiseptic microbicide in physician's office. Forms rich, golden lather.

DIRECTIONS FOR USE
A. **For Preoperative Washing by Operating Personnel**
1. Wet hands and forearms with water. Pour about 5 cc. (1 teaspoonful) of BETADINE Surgical Scrub on the palm of the hand and spread over both hands and forearms. Without adding more water, rub the Scrub thoroughly over all areas for about five minutes. Use a brush if desired. Clean thoroughly under fingernails. Add a little water and develop copious suds. Rinse thoroughly under running water.
2. Complete the wash by scrubbing with another 5 cc. of BETADINE Surgical Scrub in the same way.

B. **For Preoperative Use on Patients**
After the skin area is shaved, wet it with water. Apply BETADINE Surgical Scrub (1 cc. is sufficient to cover an area of 20-30 square inches), develop lather and scrub thoroughly for about five minutes. Rinse off by aid of sterile gauze saturated with water. The area may then be painted with BETADINE Solution or sprayed with BETADINE Aerosol Spray and allowed to dry.

C. **For Use in the Physician's Office**
Use for washing whenever a germicidal soap is required. For maximum degerming of the hands proceed as under (A). To prepare the patient's skin proceed as under (B).
Note: Blue stains on starched linen will wash off with soap and water.

WARNINGS
For External Use Only. Do not heat prior to application. In rare instances of local irritation or sensitivity, discontinue use. Keep out of reach of children.

SUPPLIED
4 oz. plastic bottle, 16 oz. (1 pint) plastic bottle with and without pump, 32 oz. (1 quart) and 1 gal. plastic bottles.

Stamford, CT 06901-3431

BETASEPT® Surgical Scrub 4% — OTC
[*bā 'tăh-sĕp-t "*]
(chlorhexidine gluconate)

ACTION AND USES
BETASEPT Surgical Scrub (chlorhexidine gluconate) is an antiseptic/antimicrobial skin cleanser for hand scrubbing or washing by operating room personnel, for hand-washing by medical personnel, for pre-operative skin preparation, and for skin wound and general skin cleansing.
BETASEPT Surgical Scrub provides rapid bactericidal action and has a persistent antimicrobial effect against a wide range of microorganisms.

ADVANTAGES
BETASEPT Surgical Scrub is uniquely kind to hands—a feature that encourages hospital personnel to follow correct hand-washing procedures.
BETASEPT Surgical Scrub is formulated in a highly viscous base which can help reduce waste and per-use cost during prepping and hand-washing. No unnecessary pink tint has been added.

DIRECTIONS FOR USE
Surgical Hand Scrub:
Wet hands and forearms with water. Scrub for 3 minutes with about 5 mL of BETASEPT Surgical Scrub and a wet brush, paying particular attention to the nails, cuticles and interdigital spaces. A separate nail cleaner may be used. Rinse thoroughly. Wash for an additional 3 minutes with 5 mL of BETASEPT Surgical Scrub and rinse under running water. Dry thoroughly.
Personnel Hand Wash:
Wet hands with water. Dispense about 5 mL of BETASEPT Surgical Scrub into cupped hands and wash in a vigorous manner for 15 seconds. Rinse and dry thoroughly.

Continued on next page

Betasept—Cont.

Pre-Operative Skin Preparation:
Apply BETASEPT Surgical Scrub liberally to surgical site and swab for at least 2 minutes. Dry with a sterile towel. Repeat procedure for an additional 2 minutes and again dry with a sterile towel.

Skin Wound and General Skin Cleansing:
Wounds which involve more than the superficial layers of the skin should not be routinely treated with BETASEPT Surgical Scrub. BETASEPT Surgical Scrub should not be used for repeated general skin cleansing of large body areas except in those patients whose underlying condition makes it necessary to reduce the bacterial population of the skin. To use, thoroughly rinse the area to be cleansed with water. Apply the minimum amount of BETASEPT Surgical Scrub necessary to cover the skin or wound area and wash gently. Rinse again thoroughly.

WARNINGS

FOR EXTERNAL USE ONLY. KEEP OUT OF EYES, EARS AND MOUTH, BETASEPT SURGICAL SCRUB SHOULD NOT BE USED AS A PRE-OPERATIVE SKIN PREPARATION OF THE FACE OR HEAD, MISUSE OF PRODUCTS CONTAINING CHLORHEXIDINE GLUCONATE HAS BEEN REPORTED TO CAUSE SERIOUS AND PERMANENT EYE INJURY WHEN IT HAS BEEN PERMITTED TO ENTER AND REMAIN IN THE EYE DURING SURGICAL PROCEDURES. IF BETASEPT SURGICAL SCRUB SHOULD CONTACT THESE AREAS, RINSE OUT PROMPTLY AND THOROUGHLY WITH WATER.

Avoid contact with meninges. Betasept Surgical Scrub should not be used by persons who have sensitivity to it or its components. Chlorhexidine gluconate has been reported to cause deafness when instilled in the middle ear through perforated ear drums. Irritation, sensitization and generalized allergic reactions have been reported with chlorhexidine-containing products, especially in the genital areas. If adverse reactions occur, discontinue use immediately and if severe, contact a physician. Keep this and all drugs out of the reach of children. In case of accidental ingestion, seek professional assistance or contact a Poison Control Center immediately.

Avoid excessive heat (above 104°F).

HOW SUPPLIED

BETASEPT Surgical Scrub 4% is packaged in 1 gallon, 32 oz., 32 oz. with pump, 16 oz., 8 oz., and 4 oz. plastic bottles.

Stamford, CT 06901-3431

CERUMENEX® EARDROPS ℞

[*sĕ-rū 'mĕn-ĕx"*]

(triethanolamine polypeptide oleate-condensate)

DESCRIPTION

CERUMENEX Eardrops contain Triethanolamine Polypeptide Oleate-Condensate (10%). Inactive Ingredients: Chlorobutanol 0.5%, Propylene Glycol and Water. Triethanolamine Polypeptide Oleate is a hygroscopic-miscible solution with low surface tension and optimal viscosity of 50–90 cps. It also has a slightly acid pH range (5.0–6.0) to approximate the surface of a normal ear canal.

CLINICAL PHARMACOLOGY

CERUMENEX Eardrops emulsify and disperse excess or impacted earwax. The triethanolamine polypeptide oleate, a surfactant, in a hygroscopic vehicle lyses cerumen to facilitate removal by subsequent water irrigation.

INDICATIONS AND USAGE

For removal of impacted cerumen prior to ear examination, otologic therapy and/or audiometry.

CONTRAINDICATIONS

Perforated tympanic membrane or otitis media is considered a contraindication to the use of this medication in the external ear canal.

A history of hypersensitivity to CERUMENEX Eardrops or to any of its components is also a contraindication to the use of this medication.

WARNINGS

Discontinue promptly if sensitization or irritation occurs.

PRECAUTIONS

General

It is recommended that the following precautions be observed in prescribing and administration of this agent:

1. Extreme caution is indicated in patients with demonstrable dermatologic idiosyncrasies or with history of allergic reactions in general.
2. Exposure of the ear canal to the CERUMENEX Eardrops should be limited to 15–30 minutes.
3. When administering CERUMENEX Eardrops, care must be taken to avoid undue exposure of the skin outside the ear during the instillation and the flushing out of the medication. If the medication comes in contact with the skin, the area should be washed with soap and water. Use of proper technique (see **DOSAGE AND ADMINISTRATION**) will help avoid such undue exposure.
4. CERUMENEX Eardrops should be used only with caution in external otitis.

Information for Patients

1. Patients should be cautioned to avoid placing the applicator tip into the ear canal.
2. Patients should be cautioned to gently flush the ear with lukewarm water.
3. Patients should be warned to use CERUMENEX Eardrops in ears only. Surrounding skin should be promptly rinsed of any excess drops.
4. Patients should be instructed not to leave CERUMENEX Eardrops in the ear for longer than 30 minutes. A second application may be made, if needed, but more frequent use must be indicated by the physician.
5. Patients must be instructed not to exceed the time of exposure, nor to use the medication more frequently than directed by the physician.
6. Patients should be advised to discontinue the use of the medication in case of a possible reaction and to consult their physician promptly.

Carcinogenesis, Mutagenesis, Impairment of Fertility

Long-term animal studies have not been performed to evaluate the carcinogenic potential or the effect on fertility of CERUMENEX Eardrops.

Pregnancy

Teratogenic Effects: Pregnancy Category C. Animal reproduction studies have not yet been conducted with CERUMENEX Eardrops. It is also not known whether CERUMENEX Eardrops can cause fetal harm when administered to a pregnant woman or can affect reproduction capacity. CERUMENEX Eardrops should be given to a pregnant woman only if clearly needed.

Nursing Mothers

It is not known whether this drug is excreted in human milk. Because many drugs are excreted in human milk, caution should be exercised when CERUMENEX Eardrops are administered to a nursing mother.

Pediatric Use

Safety and effectiveness in children have not been established.

ADVERSE REACTIONS

Clinical Reactions of Possible Allergic Origin

Localized dermatitis reactions were reported in about 1% of 2,700 patients treated, ranging from a very mild erythema and pruritus of the external canal to a severe eczematoid reaction involving the external ear and periauricular tissue, generally with duration of 2–10 days. Other reactions which have been reported in connection with the use of CERUMENEX Eardrops include allergic contact dermatitis, skin ulcerations, burning and pain at the application site and skin rash.

DOSAGE AND ADMINISTRATION

1. Fill ear canal with CERUMENEX Eardrops with the patient's head tilted at a 45° angle.
2. Insert cotton plug and allow to remain 15–30 minutes.
3. Then gently flush with lukewarm water, using a soft rubber syringe (avoid excessive pressure). Exposure of skin outside the ear to the drug should be avoided. The procedure may be repeated if the first application fails to clear the impaction.

CAUTION: Federal Law Prohibits Dispensing Without a Prescription.

FOR EXTERNAL USE IN THE EAR ONLY

HOW SUPPLIED

CERUMENEX Eardrops (triethanolamine polypeptide oleate-condensate) are supplied in 6 ml (NDC 0034-5490-06) and 12 ml (NDC 0034-5490-12) bottles with a cellophane wrapped dropper.

Store at Controlled Room Temperature 15–30°C (59–86°F).

Stamford, CT 06901-3431

June 9, 2000 L8037

MS CONTIN® 15 mg Tablets Ⓒ ℞
MS CONTIN® 30 mg Tablets Ⓒ ℞
MS CONTIN® 60 mg Tablets Ⓒ ℞
MS CONTIN® 100 mg Tablets Ⓒ ℞

MS CONTIN® 200 mg Tablets* Ⓒ ℞
(For use in opioid tolerant patients only.)

[*em es "kŏn "tĕn*]

Morphine Sulfate Controlled-Release

I3220

DESCRIPTION

Chemically, morphine sulfate is 7,8-didehydro-4,5α-epoxy-17-methylmorphinan-3,6 α-diol sulfate (2:1) (salt) pentahydrate and has the following structural formula:

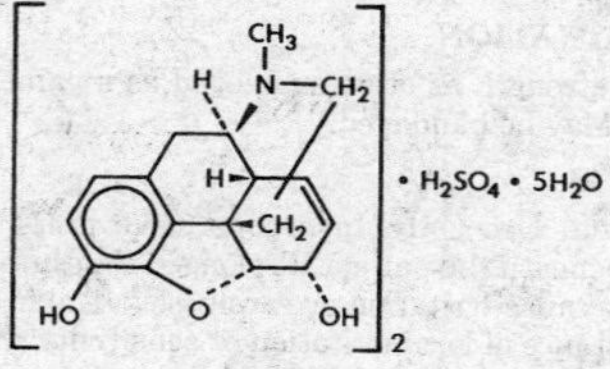

Each MS CONTIN 15 mg Controlled-Release Tablet contains: 15 mg Morphine sulfate U.S.P. Inactive ingredients: Cetostearyl alcohol, FD&C Blue No. 2, Hydroxyethyl cellulose, Hydroxypropyl methylcellulose, Lactose, Magnesium stearate, Talc, Titanium dioxide and other ingredients.

Each MS CONTIN 30 mg Controlled-Release Tablet contains: 30 mg Morphine sulfate U.S.P. Inactive ingredients: Cetostearyl alcohol, D&C Red No. 7, FD&C Blue No. 1, Hydroxyethyl cellulose, Hydroxypropyl methylcellulose, Lactose, Magnesium stearate, Talc, Titanium dioxide and other ingredients.

Each MS CONTIN 60 mg Controlled-Release Tablet contains: 60 mg Morphine sulfate U.S.P. Inactive ingredients: Cetostearyl alcohol, D&C Red No. 30, D&C Yellow No. 10, Hydroxyethyl cellulose, Hydroxypropyl methylcellulose, Lactose, Magnesium stearate, Talc, Titanium dioxide and other ingredients.

Each MS CONTIN 100 mg Controlled-Release Tablet contains: 100 mg Morphine sulfate U.S.P. Inactive ingredients: Cetostearyl alcohol, Hydroxyethyl cellulose, Hydroxypropyl methylcellulose, Magnesium stearate, Synthetic black iron oxide, Talc, Titanium dioxide and other ingredients.

MS CONTIN 200 mg Tablets*

(For use in opioid tolerant patients only.)

Each MS CONTIN 200 mg Controlled-Release Tablet* contains: 200 mg Morphine sulfate U.S.P. Inactive ingredients: Cetostearyl alcohol, D&C Yellow No. 10, FD&C Blue No. 1, Hydroxyethyl cellulose, Hydroxypropyl cellulose, Hydroxypropyl methylcellulose, Magnesium stearate, Polyethylene glycol, Talc, Titanium dioxide.

***FOR USE IN OPIOID TOLERANT PATIENTS ONLY.**

CLINICAL PHARMACOLOGY

Metabolism and Pharmacokinetics

MS CONTIN is a controlled-release tablet containing morphine sulfate. Following oral administration of a given dose of morphine, the amount ultimately absorbed is essentially the same whether the source is MS CONTIN or a conventional formulation. Morphine is released from MS CONTIN somewhat more slowly than from conventional oral preparations. Because of pre-systemic elimination (i.e., metabolism in the gut wall and liver) only about 40% of the administered dose reaches the central compartment.

Once absorbed, morphine is distributed to skeletal muscle, kidneys, liver, intestinal tract, lungs, spleen and brain. Morphine also crosses the placental membranes and has been found in breast milk.

Although a small fraction (less than 5%) of morphine is demethylated, for all practical purposes, virtually all morphine is converted to glucuronide metabolites; among these, morphine-3-glucuronide is present in the highest plasma concentration following oral administration.

The glucuronide system has a very high capacity and is not easily saturated even in disease. Therefore, rate of delivery of morphine to the gut and liver should not influence the total and, probably, the relative quantities of the various metabolites formed. Moreover, even if rate affected the relative amounts of each metabolite formed, it should be unimportant clinically because morphine's metabolites are ordinarily inactive.

The following pharmacokinetic parameters show considerable inter-subject variation but are representative of average values reported in the literature. The volume of distribution (Vd) for morphine is 4 liters per kilogram, and its terminal elimination half-life is normally 2 to 4 hours.

Following the administration of conventional oral morphine products, approximately fifty percent of the morphine that will reach the central compartment intact reaches it within 30 minutes. Following the administration of an equal amount of MS CONTIN to normal volunteers, however, this extent of absorption occurs, on average, after 1.5 hours.

The possible effect of food upon the systemic bioavailability of MS CONTIN has not been systematically evaluated for all strengths. Data from at least one study suggests that concurrent administration of MS CONTIN with a fatty meal may cause a slight decrease in peak plasma concentration.

Variation in the physical/mechanical properties of a formulation of an oral morphine drug product can affect both its absolute bioavailability and its absorption rate constant (k_a). The formulation employed in MS CONTIN has not been shown to affect morphine's oral bioavailability, but does decrease its apparent k_a. Other basic pharmacokinetic parameters (e.g., volume of distribution [Vd], elimination rate constant [k_e], clearance [Cl]), are unchanged as they are fundamental properties of morphine in the organism. However, in chronic use, the possibility that shifts in metabolite to parent drug ratios may occur cannot be excluded.

When immediate-release oral morphine or MS CONTIN is given on a fixed dosing regimen, steady state is achieved in about a day.

For a given dose and dosing interval, the AUC and average blood concentration of morphine at steady state (Css) will be independent of the specific type of oral formulation administered so long as the formulations have the same absolute bioavailability. The absorption rate of a formulation will, however, affect the maximum (Cmax) and minimum (Cmin) blood levels and the times of their occurrence.

PHARMACODYNAMICS

The effects described below are common to all morphine-containing products.

Central Nervous System

The principal actions of therapeutic value of morphine are analgesia and sedation (i.e., sleepiness and anxiolysis).

The precise mechanism of the analgesic action is unknown. However, specific CNS opiate receptors and endogenous compounds with morphine-like activity have been identified throughout the brain and spinal cord and are likely to play a role in the expression of analgesic effects.
Morphine produces respiratory depression by direct action on brain stem respiratory centers. The mechanism of respiratory depression involves a reduction in the responsiveness of the brain stem respiratory centers to increases in carbon dioxide tension, and to electrical stimulation.
Morphine depresses the cough reflex by direct effect on the cough center in the medulla. Antitussive effects may occur with doses lower than those usually required for analgesia.
Morphine causes miosis, even in total darkness. Pinpoint pupils are a sign of narcotic overdose but are not pathognomonic (e.g., pontine lesions of hemorrhagic or ischemic origins may produce similar findings). Marked mydriasis rather than miosis may be seen with worsening hypoxia.

Gastrointestinal Tract and Other Smooth Muscle

Gastric, biliary and pancreatic secretions are decreased by morphine. Morphine causes a reduction in motility associated with an increase in tone in the antrum of the stomach and duodenum. Digestion of food in the small intestine is delayed and propulsive contractions are decreased. Propulsive peristaltic waves in the colon are decreased, while tone is increased to the point of spasm. The end result is constipation. Morphine can cause a marked increase in biliary tract pressure as a result of spasm of sphincter of Oddi.

Cardiovascular System

Morphine produces peripheral vasodilation which may result in orthostatic hypotension. Release of histamine can occur and may contribute to narcotic-induced hypotension. Manifestations of histamine release and/or peripheral vasodilation may include pruritus, flushing, red eyes and sweating.

Plasma Level- Analgesia Relationships

In any particular patient, both analgesic effects and plasma morphine concentrations are related to the morphine dose. In non-tolerant individuals, plasma morphine concentration-efficacy relationships have been demonstrated and suggest that opiate receptors occupy effector compartments, leading to a lag-time, or hysteresis, between rapid changes in plasma morphine concentrations and effects of such changes. The most direct and predictable concentration-effect relationships can, therefore, be expected at distribution equilibrium and/or steady state conditions. In general, the minimum effective analgesic concentration in the plasma of non tolerant patients ranges from approximately 5 to 20ng/ml.
While plasma morphine-efficacy relationships can be demonstrated in non-tolerant individuals, they are influenced by a wide variety of factors and are not generally useful as a guide to the clinical use of morphine. The effective dose in opioid-tolerant patients may be 10–50 times as great (or greater) than the appropriate dose for opioid-naive individuals. Dosages of morphine should be chosen and must be titrated on the bases of clinical evaluation of the patient and the balance between therapeutic and adverse effects.
For any fixed dose and dosing interval, MS CONTIN will have at steady state, a lower Cmax and a higher Cmin than conventional morphine. This is a potential advantage; a reduced fluctuation in morphine concentration during the dosing interval should keep morphine blood levels more centered within the theoretical "therapeutic window." (Fluctuation for a dosing interval is defined as [Cmax-Cmin]/[Css-average].) On the other hand, the degree of fluctuation in serum morphine concentration might conceivably affect other phenomena. For example, reduced fluctuations in blood morphine concentrations might influence the rate of tolerance induction.
The elimination of morphine occurs primarily as renal excretion of 3-morphine glucuronide. A small amount of the glucuronide conjugate is excreted in the bile, and there is some minor enterohepatic recycling. Because morphine is primarily metabolized to inactive metabolites, the effects of renal disease on morphine's elimination are not likely to be pronounced. However, as with any drug, caution should be taken to guard against unanticipated accumulation if renal and/or hepatic function is seriously impaired.

INDICATIONS AND USAGE

MS CONTIN is a controlled-release oral morphine formulation indicated for the relief of moderate to severe pain. It is intended for use in patients who require repeated dosing with potent opioid analgesics over periods of more than a few days.
The MS CONTIN 200 mg Tablet strength is a high dose, controlled-release, oral morphine formulation indicated for the relief of pain in opioid tolerant patients only.

CONTRAINDICATIONS

MS CONTIN is contraindicated in patients with known hypersensitivity to the drug, in patients with respiratory depression in the absence of resuscitative equipment, and in patients with acute or severe bronchial asthma.
MS CONTIN is contraindicated in any patient who has or is suspected of having a paralytic ileus.

WARNINGS

(See also: CLINICAL PHARMACOLOGY)

Impaired Respiration

Respiratory depression is the chief hazard of all morphine preparations. Respiratory depression occurs most frequently in the elderly and debilitated patients, as well as in those suffering from conditions accompanied by hypoxia or hypercapnia when even moderate therapeutic doses may dangerously decrease pulmonary ventilation.
Morphine should be used with extreme caution in patients with chronic obstructive pulmonary disease or cor pulmonale, and in patients having a substantially decreased respiratory reserve, hypoxia, hypercapnia, or preexisting respiratory depression. In such patients, even usual therapeutic doses of morphine may decrease respiratory drive while simultaneously increasing airway resistance to the point of apnea.

Head Injury and Increased Intracranial Pressure

The respiratory depressant effects of morphine with carbon dioxide retention and secondary elevation of cerebrospinal fluid pressure may be markedly exaggerated in the presence of head injury, other intracranial lesions, or preexisting increase in intracranial pressure. Morphine produces effects which may obscure neurologic signs of further increases in pressure in patients with head injuries.

Hypotensive Effect

MS CONTIN, like all opioid analgesics, may cause severe hypotension in an individual whose ability to maintain his blood pressure has already been compromised by a depleted blood volume, or a concurrent administration of drugs such as phenothiazines or general anesthetics. (See also: PRECAUTIONS: Drug Interactions.) MS CONTIN may produce orthostatic hypotension in ambulatory patients.
MS CONTIN, like all opioid analgesics, should be administered with caution to patients in circulatory shock, since vasodilation produced by the drug may further reduce cardiac output and blood pressure.

Interactions with other CNS Depressants

MS CONTIN, like all opioid analgesics, should be used with great caution and in reduced dosage in patients who are concurrently receiving other central nervous system depressants including sedatives or hypnotics, general anesthetics, phenothiazines, other tranquilizers and alcohol because respiratory depression, hypotension and profound sedation or coma may result.

Interactions with Mixed Agonist/Antagonist Opioid Analgesics

From a theoretical perspective, agonist/antagonist analgesics (i.e., pentazocine, nalbuphine, butorphanol and buprenorphine) should NOT be administered to a patient who has received or is receiving a course of therapy with a pure opioid agonist analgesic. In these patients, mixed agonist/antagonist analgesics may reduce the analgesic effect or may precipitate withdrawal symptoms.

Drug Dependence

Morphine can produce drug dependence and has a potential for being abused. Tolerance as well as psychological and physical dependence may develop upon repeated administration. Physical dependence, however, is not of paramount importance in the management of terminally ill patients or any patients in severe pain. Abrupt cessation or a sudden reduction in dose after prolonged use may result in withdrawal symptoms. After prolonged exposure to opioid analgesics, if withdrawal is necessary, it must be undertaken gradually. (See DRUG ABUSE AND DEPENDENCE.)
Infants born to mothers physically dependent on opioid analgesics may also be physically dependent and exhibit respiratory depression and withdrawal symptoms. (See DRUG ABUSE AND DEPENDENCE.)

PRECAUTIONS

(See also: CLINICAL PHARMACOLOGY)

Special precautions regarding MS CONTIN 200 mg Tablets

MS CONTIN 200 mg Tablets are for use only in opioid tolerant patients requiring daily morphine equivalent dosages of 400 mg or more. Care should be taken in its prescription and patients should be instructed against use by individuals other than the patient for whom it was prescribed, as this may have severe medical consequences for that individual.

General

MS CONTIN is intended for use in patients who require more than several days continuous treatment with a potent opioid analgesic. The controlled-release nature of the formulation allows it to be administered on a more convenient schedule than conventional immediate-release oral morphine products. (See CLINICAL PHARMACOLOGY: "Metabolism and Pharmacokinetics".) However, MS CONTIN does not release morphine continuously over the course of a dosing interval. The administration of single doses of MS CONTIN on a q12 hour dosing schedule will result in higher peak and lower trough plasma levels than those that occur when an identical daily dose of morphine is administered using conventional oral formulations on a q4h regimen. The clinical significance of greater fluctuations in morphine plasma level has not been systematically evaluated. (See DOSAGE AND ADMINISTRATION)
As with any potent opioid, it is critical to adjust the dosing regimen for each patient individually, taking into account the patient's prior analgesic treatment experience. Although it is clearly impossible to enumerate every consideration that is important to the selection of the initial dose and dosing interval of MS CONTIN, attention should be given to 1) the daily dose, potency, and characteristics of the opioid the patient has been taking previously (e.g., whether it is a pure agonist or mixed agonist-antagonist), 2) the reliability of the relative potency estimate used to calculate the dose of morphine needed [N.B. potency estimates may vary with the route of administration], 3) the degree of opioid tolerance, if any, and 4) the general condition and medical status of the patient.
Selection of patients for treatment with MS CONTIN should be governed by the same principles that apply to the use of morphine or other potent opioid analgesics. Specifically, the increased risks associated with its use in the following populations should be considered: the elderly or debilitated and those with severe impairment of hepatic, pulmonary or renal function; myxedema or hypothyroidism; adrenocortical insufficiency (e.g., Addison's Disease); CNS depression or coma; toxic psychosis; prostatic hypertrophy or urethral stricture; acute alcoholism; delirium tremens; kyphoscoliosis, or inability to swallow.
The administration of morphine, like all opioid analgesics, may obscure the diagnosis or clinical course in patients with acute abdominal conditions.
Morphine may aggravate preexisting convulsions in patients with convulsive disorders. Morphine should be used with caution in patients about to undergo surgery of the biliary tract since it may cause spasm of the sphincter of Oddi. Similarly, morphine should be used with caution in patients with acute pancreatitis secondary to biliary tract disease.

Information for Patients

If clinically advisable, patients receiving MS CONTIN should be given the following instructions by the physician:

1. Appropriate pain management requires changes in the dose to maintain best pain control. Patients should be advised of the need to contact their physician if pain control is inadequate, but not to change the dose of MS CONTIN without consulting their physician.
2. Morphine may impair mental and/or physical ability required for the performance of potentially hazardous tasks (e.g., driving, operating machinery). Patients started on MS CONTIN or whose dose has been changed should refrain from dangerous activity until it is established that they are not adversely affected.
3. Morphine should not be taken with alcohol or other CNS depressants (sleep aids, tranquilizers) because additive effects including CNS depression may occur. A physician should be consulted if other prescription medications are currently being used or are prescribed for future use.
4. For women of childbearing potential who become or are planning to become pregnant, a physician should be consulted regarding analgesics and other drug use.
5. Upon completion of therapy, it may be appropriate to taper the morphine dose, rather than abruptly discontinue it.
6. While psychological dependence ("addiction") to morphine used in the treatment of pain is very rare, morphine is one of a class of drugs known to be abused and should be handled accordingly.
7. The MS CONTIN 200 mg Tablet is for use only in opioid tolerant patients requiring daily morphine equivalent dosages of 400 mg or more. Special care must be taken to avoid accidental ingestion or the use by individuals (including children) other than the patient for whom it was originally prescribed, as such unsupervised use may have severe, even fatal, consequences.

Drug Interactions (See WARNINGS)

The concomitant use of other central nervous system depressants including sedatives or hypnotics, general anesthetics, phenothiazines, tranquilizers and alcohol may produce additive depressant effects. Respiratory depression, hypotension and profound sedation or coma may occur. When such combined therapy is contemplated, the dose of one or both agents should be reduced. Opioid analgesics, including MS CONTIN, may enhance the neuromuscular blocking action of skeletal muscle relaxants and produce an increased degree of respiratory depression.

Carcinogenicity/Mutagenicity/Impairment of Fertility

Studies of morphine sulfate in animals to evaluate the drug's carcinogenic and mutagenic potential or the effect on fertility have not been conducted.

Pregnancy

Teratogenic effects—CATEGORY C: Adequate animal studies on reproduction have not been performed to determine whether morphine affects fertility in males or females. There are no well-controlled studies in women, but marketing experience does not include any evidence of adverse effects on the fetus following routine (short-term) clinical use of morphine sulfate products. Although there is no clearly defined risk, such experience cannot exclude the possibility of infrequent or subtle damage to the human fetus.
MS CONTIN should be used in pregnant women only when clearly needed. (See also: PRECAUTIONS: Labor and Delivery, and DRUG ABUSE AND DEPENDENCE.)
Nonteratogenic effects: Infants born from mothers who have been taking morphine chronically may exhibit withdrawal symptoms.

Labor and Delivery

MS CONTIN is not recommended for use in women during and immediately prior to labor. Occasionally, opioid analgesics may prolong labor through actions which temporarily reduce the strength, duration and frequency of uterine contractions. However, this effect is not consistent and may be offset by an increased rate of cervical dilatation which tends to shorten labor.
Neonates whose mothers received opioid analgesics during labor should be observed closely for signs of respiratory de-

Continued on next page

MS Contin—Cont.

pression. A specific narcotic antagonist, naloxone, should be available for reversal of narcotic-induced respiratory depression in the neonate.

Nursing Mothers

Low levels of *morphine* have been detected in the breast milk. Withdrawal symptoms can occur in breast-feeding infants when maternal administration of morphine sulfate is stopped. Ordinarily, nursing should not be undertaken while a patient is receiving MS CONTIN since morphine may be excreted in the milk.

Pediatric Use

Use of MS CONTIN has not been evaluated systematically in children.

ADVERSE REACTIONS

The adverse reactions caused by morphine are essentially those observed with other opioid analgesics. They include the following major hazards: respiratory depression, apnea, and to a lesser degree, circulatory depression; respiratory arrest, shock and cardiac arrest.

Most Frequently Observed

Constipation, lightheadedness, dizziness, sedation, nausea, vomiting, sweating, dysphoria and euphoria.

Some of these effects seem to be more prominent in ambulatory patients and in those not experiencing severe pain. Some adverse reactions in ambulatory patients may be alleviated if the patient lies down.

Less Frequently Observed Reactions

Central Nervous System: Weakness, headache, agitation, tremor, uncoordinated muscle movements, seizure, alterations of mood (nervousness, apprehension, depression, floating feelings), dreams, muscle rigidity, transient hallucinations and disorientation, visual disturbances, insomnia and increased intracranial pressure.

Gastrointestinal: Dry mouth, constipation, biliary tract spasm, laryngospasm, anorexia, diarrhea, cramps and taste alterations.

Cardiovascular: Flushing of the face, chills, tachycardia, bradycardia, palpitation, faintness, syncope, hypotension and hypertension.

Genitourinary: Urine retention or hesitance, reduced libido and/or potency.

Dermatologic: Pruritus, urticaria, other skin rashes, edema and diaphoresis.

Other: Antidiuretic effect, paresthesia, muscle tremor, blurred vision, nystagmus, diplopia and miosis.

DRUG ABUSE AND DEPENDENCE

Opioid analgesics may cause psychological and physical dependence (see WARNINGS). Physical dependence results in withdrawal symptoms in patients who abruptly discontinue the drug or may be precipitated through the administration of drugs with narcotic antagonist activity, e.g., naloxone or mixed agonist/antagonist analgesics (pentazocine, etc.; See also OVERDOSAGE). Physical dependence usually does not occur to a clinically significant degree until after several weeks of continued narcotic usage. Tolerance, in which increasingly large doses are required in order to produce the same degree of analgesia, is initially manifested by a shortened duration of analgesic effect, and, subsequently, by decreases in the intensity of analgesia.

In chronic-pain patients, and in narcotic-tolerant cancer patients, the administration of MS CONTIN should be guided by the degree of tolerance manifested. Physical dependence, per se, is not ordinarily a concern when one is dealing with opioid-tolerant patients whose pain and suffering is associated with an irreversible illness.

If MS CONTIN is abruptly discontinued, a moderate to severe abstinence syndrome may occur. The opioid agonist abstinence syndrome is characterized by some or all of the following: restlessness, lacrimation, rhinorrhea, yawning, perspiration, gooseflesh, restless sleep or "yen" and mydriasis during the first 24 hours. These symptoms often increase in severity and over the next 72 hours may be accompanied by increasing irritability, anxiety, weakness, twitching and spasms of muscles; kicking movements; severe backache, abdominal and leg pains; abdominal and muscle cramps; hot and cold flashes, insomnia; nausea, anorexia, vomiting, intestinal spasm, diarrhea; coryza and repetitive sneezing; increase in body temperature, blood pressure, respiratory rate and heart rate. Because of excessive loss of fluids through sweating, vomiting and diarrhea, there is usually marked weight loss, dehydration, ketosis, and disturbances in acid-base balance. Cardiovascular collapse can occur. Without treatment most observable symptoms disappear in 5–14 days; however, there appears to be a phase of secondary or chronic abstinence which may last for 2–6 months characterized by insomnia, irritability, and muscular aches.

If treatment of physical dependence of patients on MS CONTIN is necessary, the patient may be detoxified by gradual reduction of the dosage. Gastrointestinal disturbances or dehydration should be treated accordingly.

OVERDOSAGE

Acute overdosage with morphine is manifested by respiratory depression, somnolence progressing to stupor or coma, skeletal muscle flaccidity, cold and clammy skin, constricted pupils, and, sometimes, bradycardia and hypotension.

In the treatment of overdosage, primary attention should be given to the re-establishment of a patent airway and institution of assisted or controlled ventilation. The pure opioid antagonist, naloxone, is a specific antidote against respiratory depression which results from opioid overdose. Naloxone (usually 0.4 to 2.0 mg) should be administered intravenously; however, because its duration of action is relatively short, the patient must be carefully monitored until spontaneous respiration is reliably re-established. If the response to naloxone is suboptimal or not sustained, additional naloxone may be re-administered, as needed, or given by continuous infusion to maintain alertness and respiratory function; however, there is no information available about the cumulative dose of naloxone that may be safely administered.

Naloxone should not be administered in the absence of clinically significant respiratory or circulatory depression secondary to morphine overdose. Naloxone should be administered cautiously to persons who are known, or suspected to be physically dependent on MS CONTIN. In such cases, an abrupt or complete reversal of narcotic effects may precipitate an acute abstinence syndrome.

Note: In an individual physically dependent on opioids, administration of the usual dose of the antagonist will precipitate an acute withdrawal syndrome. The severity of the withdrawal syndrome produced will depend on the degree of physical dependence and the dose of the antagonist administered. Use of a narcotic antagonist in such a person should be avoided. If necessary to treat serious respiratory depression in the physically dependent patient, the antagonist should be administered with care and by titration with smaller than usual doses of the antagonist.

Supportive measures (including oxygen, vasopressors) should be employed in the management of circulatory shock and pulmonary edema accompanying overdose as indicated. Cardiac arrest or arrhythmias may require cardiac massage or defibrillation.

DOSAGE AND ADMINISTRATION

(See also: CLINICAL PHARMACOLOGY, WARNINGS AND PRECAUTIONS sections)

MS CONTIN TABLETS ARE TO BE TAKEN WHOLE, AND ARE NOT TO BE BROKEN, CHEWED OR CRUSHED. TAKING BROKEN, CHEWED OR CRUSHED MS CONTIN TABLETS COULD LEAD TO THE RAPID RELEASE AND ABSORPTION OF A POTENTIALLY TOXIC DOSE OF MORPHINE.

MS CONTIN is intended for use in patients who require more than several days continuous treatment with a potent opioid analgesic. The controlled-release nature of the formulation allows it to be administered on a more convenient schedule than conventional immediate-release oral morphine products. (See CLINICAL PHARMACOLOGY: "Metabolism and Pharmacokinetics".) However, MS CONTIN does not release morphine continuously over the course of a dosing interval. The administration of single doses of MS CONTIN on a q12h dosing schedule will result in higher peak and lower trough plasma levels than those that occur when an identical daily dose of morphine is administered using conventional oral formulations on a q4h regimen. The clinical significance of greater fluctuations in morphine plasma level has not been systematically evaluated.

As with any potent opioid drug product, it is critical to adjust the dosing regimen for each patient individually, taking into account the patient's prior analgesic treatment experience. Although it is clearly impossible to enumerate every consideration that is important to the selection of initial dose and dosing interval of MS CONTIN, attention should be given to 1) the daily dose, potency and precise characteristics of the opioid the patient has been taking previously (e.g., whether it is a pure agonist or mixed agonist/antagonist), 2) the reliability of the relative potency estimate used to calculate the dose of morphine needed [N.B. potency estimates may vary with the route of administration], 3) the degree of opioid tolerance, if any, and 4) the general condition and medical status of the patient.

The following dosing recommendations, therefore, can only be considered suggested approaches to what is actually a series of clinical decisions in the management of the pain of an individual patient.

Conversion from Conventional Oral Morphine to MS CONTIN

A patient's daily morphine requirement is established using immediate-release oral morphine (dosing every 4 to 6 hours). The patient is then converted to MS CONTIN in either of two ways: 1) by administering one-half of the patient's 24-hour requirement as MS CONTIN on an every 12-hour schedule; or, 2) by administering one-third of the patient's daily requirement as MS CONTIN on an every eight hour schedule. With either method, dose and dosing interval is then adjusted as needed (see discussion below). The 15 mg tablet should be used for initial conversion for patients whose total daily requirement is expected to be less than 60 mg. The 30 mg tablet strength is recommended for patients with a daily morphine requirement of 60 to 120 mg. When the total daily dose is expected to be greater than 120 mg, the appropriate combination of tablet strengths should be employed.

Conversion from Parenteral Morphine or Other Opioids (Parenteral or Oral) to MS CONTIN

MS CONTIN can be administered as the initial oral morphine drug product; in this case, however, particular care must be exercised in the conversion process. Because of uncertainty about, and intersubject variation in, relative estimates of opioid potency and cross tolerance, initial dosing regimens should be conservative; that is, an underestimation of the 24-hour oral morphine requirement is preferred to an overestimate. To this end, initial individual doses of MS CONTIN should be estimated conservatively. In patients whose daily morphine requirements are expected to be less than or equal to 120 mg per day, the 30 mg tablet strength is recommended for the initial titration period. Once a stable dose regimen is reached, the patient can be converted to the 60 mg or 100 mg tablet strength, or appropriate combination of tablet strengths, if desired.

Estimates of the relative potency of opioids are only approximate and are influenced by route of administration, individual patient differences, and possibly, by an individual's medical condition. Consequently, it is difficult to recommend any fixed rule for converting a patient to MS CONTIN directly. The following general points should be considered, however.

1. *Parenteral to oral morphine ratio:* Estimates of the oral to parenteral potency of morphine vary. Some authorities suggest that a dose of oral morphine only three times the daily parenteral morphine requirement may be sufficient in chronic use settings.
2. *Other parenteral or oral opioids to oral morphine:* Because there is lack of systemic evidence bearing on these types of analgesic substitutions, specific recommendations are not possible.

Physicians are advised to refer to published relative potency data, keeping in mind that such ratios are only approximate. In general, it is safer to underestimate the daily dose of MS CONTIN required and rely upon ad hoc supplementation to deal with inadequate analgesia. (See discussion which follows.)

Use of MS CONTIN as the first opioid analgesic

There has been no systematic evaluation of MS CONTIN as an initial opioid analgesic in the management of pain. Because it may be more difficult to titrate a patient using a controlled-release morphine, it is ordinarily advisable to begin treatment using an immediate-release formulation.

Considerations in the Adjustment of Dosing Regimens

Whatever the approach, if signs of excessive opioid effects are observed early in a dosing interval, the next dose should be reduced. If this adjustment leads to inadequate analgesia, that is, "breakthrough" pain occurs late in the dosing interval, the dosing interval may be shortened. Alternatively, a supplemental dose of a short-acting analgesic may be given. As experience is gained, adjustments can be made to obtain an appropriate balance between pain relief, opioid side effects, and the convenience of the dosing schedule.

In adjusting dosing requirements, it is recommended that the dosing interval never be extended beyond 12 hours because the administration of very large single doses may lead to acute overdose. (N.B. MS CONTIN is a controlled-release formulation; it does not release morphine continuously over the dosing interval.)

For patients with low daily morphine requirements, the 15 mg tablet should be used.

Special Instructions for MS CONTIN 200 mg Tablets (For use in opioid tolerant patients only.)

The MS CONTIN 200 mg tablet is for use only in opioid tolerant patients requiring daily morphine equivalent dosages of 400 mg or more. It is recommended that this strength be reserved for patients that have already been titrated to a stable analgesic regimen using lower strengths of MS CONTIN or other opioid.

Conversion from MS CONTIN to parenteral opioids:

When converting a patient from MS CONTIN to parenteral opioids, it is best to assume that the parenteral to oral potency is high. NOTE THAT THIS IS THE CONVERSE OF THE STRATEGY USED WHEN THE DIRECTION OF CONVERSION IS FROM THE PARENTERAL TO ORAL FORMULATIONS. IN BOTH CASES, HOWEVER, THE AIM IS TO ESTIMATE THE NEW DOSE CONSERVATIVELY. For example, to estimate the required 24-hour dose of morphine for IM use, one could employ a conversion of 1 mg of morphine IM for every 6 mg of morphine as MS CONTIN. Of course, the IM 24-hour dose would have to be divided by six and administered on a q4h regimen. This approach is recommended because it is least likely to cause overdose.

Safety and Handling

MS CONTIN TABLETS ARE TO BE TAKEN WHOLE, AND ARE NOT TO BE BROKEN, CHEWED, OR CRUSHED. TAKING BROKEN, CHEWED, OR CRUSHED MS CONTIN TABLETS COULD LEAD TO THE RAPID RELEASE AND ABSORPTION OF A POTENTIALLY TOXIC DOSE OF MORPHINE.

The MS CONTIN 200 mg Tablet strength is for use only in opioid tolerant patients requiring daily morphine equivalent dosages of 400 mg or more. This strength is potentially toxic if accidentally ingested and patients and their families should be instructed to take special care to avoid accidental or intentional ingestion by individuals other than those for whom the medication was originally prescribed.

HOW SUPPLIED

NDC 0034-0514-10: MS CONTIN (morphine sulfate controlled-release tablets) 15 mg are supplied in opaque plastic bottles containing 100 tablets.

NDC 0034-0514-90: MS CONTIN (morphine sulfate controlled-release tablets) 15 mg are supplied in opaque plastic bottles containing 500 tablets.

NDC 0034-0514-25: MS CONTIN (morphine sulfate controlled-release tablets) 15 mg are supplied in unit dose packaging with 25 individually numbered tablets per card; one card per glue end carton.

NDC 0034-0515-50: MS CONTIN (morphine sulfate controlled-release tablets) 30 mg are supplied in opaque plastic bottles containing 50 tablets.
NDC 0034-0515-10: MS CONTIN (morphine sulfate controlled-release tablets) 30 mg are supplied in opaque plastic bottles containing 100 tablets.
NDC 0034-0515-45: MS CONTIN (morphine sulfate controlled-release tablets) 30 mg are supplied in opaque plastic bottles containing 250 tablets.
NDC 0034-0515-90: MS CONTIN (morphine sulfate controlled-release tablets) 30 mg are supplied in opaque plastic bottles containing 500 tablets.
NDC 0034-0515-25: MS CONTIN (morphine sulfate controlled-release tablets) 30 mg are supplied in unit dose packaging with 25 individually numbered tablets per card; one card per glue end carton.
NDC 0034-0516-10: MS CONTIN (morphine sulfate controlled-release tablets) 60 mg are supplied in opaque plastic bottles containing 100 tablets.
NDC 0034-0516-90: MS CONTIN (morphine sulfate controlled-release tablets) 60 mg are supplied in opaque plastic bottles containing 500 tablets.
NDC 0034-0516-25: MS CONTIN (morphine sulfate controlled-release tablets) 60 mg are supplied in unit dose packaging with 25 individually numbered tablets per card; one card per glue end carton.
NDC 0034-0517-10: MS CONTIN (morphine sulfate controlled-release tablets) 100 mg are supplied in opaque plastic bottles containing 100 tablets.
NDC 0034-0517-90: MS CONTIN (morphine sulfate controlled-release tablets) 100 mg are supplied in opaque plastic bottles containing 500 tablets.
NDC 0034-0517-25: MS CONTIN (morphine sulfate controlled-release tablets) 100 mg are supplied in unit dose packaging with 25 individually numbered tablets per card; one card per glue end carton.
NDC 0034-0513-10: MS CONTIN (morphine sulfate controlled-release tablets) 200 mg are supplied in opaque plastic bottles containing 100 tablets.
NDC 0034-0513-25: MS CONTIN (morphine sulfate controlled-release tablets) 200 mg are supplied in unit dose packaging with 25 individually numbered tablets per card; one card per glue end carton.
15 mg: Each round, blue-colored tablet bears the symbol PF on one side and M15 on the other side.
30 mg: Each round, lavender-colored tablet bears the symbol PF on one side and M30 on the other side.
60 mg: Each round, orange-colored tablet bears the symbol PF on one side and M60 on the other side.
100 mg: Each round, gray-colored tablet bears the symbol PF on one side and 100 on the other side.
200 mg: Each capsule-shaped, green-colored tablet bears the symbol PF on one side and 200 on the other side.
Store tablets at controlled room temperature 15°–30°C (59°–86°F).
Dispense in tight, light-resistant container.

CAUTION

DEA Order Form Required.
THE PURDUE FREDERICK COMPANY
Stamford, CT 06901-3431

U.S. Patent Number 4366310
June 9, 2000 **I3220**
Shown in Product Identification Guide, page 331

MSIR® Ⓒ℞
[em 'es ī "ahr]
Oral Solution
(morphine sulfate)

MSIR® Ⓒ℞
Oral Solution Concentrate*
(morphine sulfate)

MSIR® Ⓒ℞
Immediate-Release Oral Tablets
(morphine sulfate)

MSIR® Ⓒ℞
Immediate-Release Oral Capsules
(morphine sulfate)

***This product contains dry natural rubber**

DESCRIPTION

Chemically, morphine sulfate is 7,8 didehydro-4,5 α-epoxy-17-methylmorphinan-3,6 α-diol sulfate (2:1) (salt) pentahydrate and has the following structural formula:

MSIR Oral Solution
Each 5 mL of MSIR Oral Solution contains:
Morphine Sulfate .... 10 or 20 mg
Inactive Ingredients: Edetate disodium, FD&C Red. No. 40, Glycerin, Invert Sugar, Sodium benzoate, Sodium chloride, Sucrose, Artificial & Natural Flavors, and other ingredients.

MSIR Oral Solution Concentrate
Each 1 mL of MSIR Oral Solution Concentrate contains:
Morphine Sulfate .... 20 mg
Inactive Ingredients: Edetate disodium, Sodium benzoate, and other ingredients.

MSIR Tablets
Each MSIR Tablet for oral administration contains:
Morphine Sulfate .... 15 or 30 mg
Inactive Ingredients: Croscarmellose sodium, Lactose, Magnesium stearate, Microcrystalline cellulose, and Talc.

MSIR Capsules
Each MSIR Capsule for oral administration contains:
Morphine Sulfate .... 15 or 30 mg
Inactive Ingredients: FD&C Blue No. 1, FD&C Blue No. 2, FD&C Red No. 40, FD&C Yellow No. 6, Gelatin, Hydroxypropyl methylcellulose, Lactose, Polyethylene glycol, Polysorbate 80, Polyvinylpyrrolidone, Starch, Sucrose, Titanium dioxide, and other ingredients. In addition, the 30 mg capsule contains Black iron oxide and D&C Red No. 28.

CLINICAL PHARMACOLOGY

Metabolism and Pharmacokinetics

MSIR Solutions, Tablets and Capsules containing morphine sulfate are for oral administration and are conventional immediate release products. Only about 40% of the administered dose reaches the central compartment because of presystemic elimination (i.e., metabolism in the gut wall and liver).

Once absorbed, morphine is distributed to skeletal muscle, kidneys, liver, intestinal tract, lungs, spleen and brain. Morphine also crosses the placental membranes and has been found in breast milk.

Although a small fraction (less than 5%) of morphine is demethylated, for all practical purposes, virtually all morphine is converted to glucuronide metabolites; among these, morphine-3-glucuronide is present in the highest plasma concentration following oral administration.

The glucuronide system has a very high capacity and is not easily saturated even in disease. Therefore, rate of delivery of morphine to the gut and liver should not influence the total and, probably, the relative quantities of the various metabolites formed. Moreover, even if rate affected the relative amounts of each metabolite formed, it should be unimportant clinically because morphine's metabolites are ordinarily inactive.

The following pharmacokinetic parameters show considerable intersubject variation but are representative of average values reported in the literature. The volume of distribution (Vd) for morphine is 4 liters per kilogram, and its terminal elimination half-life is approximately 2 to 4 hours. Following the administration of conventional oral morphine products, approximately fifty percent of the morphine that will reach the central compartment intact, reaches it within 30 minutes.

Variation in the physical/mechanical properties of a formulation of an oral morphine drug product can affect both its absolute bioavailability and its absorption rate constant (k_a). The basic pharmacokinetic parameters (e.g., volume of distribution [Vd], elimination rate constant [k_e], clearance [Cl]) are fundamental properties of morphine in the organism. However, in chronic use, the possibility that shifts in metabolite to parent drug ratios may occur cannot be excluded.

When immediate-release oral morphine is given on a fixed dosing regimen, steady state is achieved in about a day.

For a given dose and dosing interval, the AUC and average blood concentration of morphine at steady state (Css) will be independent of the specific type of oral formulation administered so long as the formulations have the same absolute bioavailability. The absorption rate of a formulation will, however, affect the maximum (Cmax) and minimum (Cmin) blood levels and the times of their occurrence.

While there is no predictable relationship between morphine blood levels and analgesic response, effective analgesia will not occur below some minimum blood level in a given patient. The minimum effective blood level for analgesia will vary among patients, especially among patients who have been previously treated with potent mu (μ) agonist opioids. Similarly, there is no predictable relationship between blood morphine concentration and untoward clinical responses; again, however, higher concentrations are more likely to be toxic than lower ones.

The elimination of morphine occurs primarily as renal excretion of 3-morphine glucuronide. A small amount of the glucuronide conjugate is excreted in the bile, and there is some minor enterohepatic recycling.

The elimination half-life of morphine is reported to vary between 2 and 4 hours. Thus, steady-state is probably achieved on most regimens within a day. Because morphine is primarily metabolized to inactive metabolites, the effects of renal disease on morphine's elimination are not likely to be pronounced. However, as with any drug, caution should be taken to guard against unanticipated accumulation if renal and/or hepatic function is seriously impaired.

Individual differences in the metabolism of morphine suggest that MSIR Oral Solutions, Tablets and Capsules be dosed conservatively according to the dosing initiation and titration recommendations in the Dosage and Administration section.

PHARMACODYNAMICS

The effects described below are common to all morphine-containing products.

Central Nervous System

The principal actions of therapeutic value of morphine are analgesia and sedation (i.e., sleepiness and anxiolysis).

The precise mechanism of analgesic action is unknown. However, specific CNS opiate receptors and endogenous compounds with morphine-like activity have been identified throughout the brain and spinal cord and are likely to play a role in the expression of analgesic effects.

Morphine produces respiratory depression by direct action on brain stem respiratory centers. The mechanism of respiratory depression involves a reduction in the responsiveness of the brain stem respiratory centers to increases in carbon dioxide tension, and to electrical stimulation.

Morphine depresses the cough reflex by direct effect on the cough center in the medulla. Antitussive effects may occur with doses lower than those usually required for analgesia.

Morphine causes miosis, even in total darkness. Pinpoint pupils are a sign of narcotic overdose but are not pathognomonic (e.g., pontine lesions of hemorrhagic or ischemic origins may produce similar findings). Marked mydriasis rather than miosis may be seen with worsening hypoxia.

Gastrointestinal Tract and Other Smooth Muscle

Gastric, biliary and pancreatic secretions are decreased by morphine. Morphine causes a reduction in motility associated with an increase in tone in the antrum of the stomach and duodenum. Digestion of food in the small intestine is delayed and propulsive contractions are decreased. In addition, propulsive peristaltic waves in the colon are decreased, while tone is increased to the point of spasm. The end result is constipation. Morphine can cause a marked increase in biliary tract pressure as a result of spasm of the sphincter of Oddi.

Cardiovascular System

Morphine produces peripheral vasodilation which may result in orthostatic hypotension. Release of histamine can occur and may contribute to narcotic-induced hypotension. Manifestations of histamine release and/or peripheral vasodilation may include pruritus, flushing, red eyes and sweating.

INDICATIONS AND USAGE

MSIR Oral Solutions, Tablets and Capsules are indicated for the relief of moderate to severe pain.

CONTRAINDICATIONS

MSIR Oral Solutions, Tablets and Capsules are contraindicated in patients with known hypersensitivity to the drug, in patients with respiratory depression in the absence of resuscitative equipment, and in patients with acute or severe bronchial asthma.

MSIR Oral Solutions, Tablets and Capsules are contraindicated in any patient who has or is suspected of having a paralytic ileus.

WARNINGS (See also: CLINICAL PHARMACOLOGY)

Impaired Respiration

Respiratory depression is the chief hazard of all morphine preparations. Respiratory depression occurs most frequently in elderly and debilitated patients, and those suffering from conditions accompanied by hypoxia or hypercapnia when even moderate therapeutic doses may dangerously decrease pulmonary ventilation.

Morphine should be used with extreme caution in patients with chronic obstructive pulmonary disease or cor pulmonale, and in patients having a substantially decreased respiratory reserve, hypoxia, hypercapnia, or preexisting respiratory depression. In such patients, even usual therapeutic doses of morphine may decrease respiratory drive while simultaneously increasing airway resistance to the point of apnea.

Head Injury and Increased Intracranial Pressure

The respiratory depressant effects of morphine with carbon dioxide retention and secondary elevation of cerebrospinal fluid pressure may be markedly exaggerated in the presence of head injury, other intracranial lesions, or preexisting increase in intracranial pressure. Morphine produces effects which may obscure neurologic signs of further increase in pressure in patients with head injuries.

Hypotensive Effects

MSIR Oral Solutions, Tablets and Capsules, like all opioid analgesics, may cause severe hypotension in an individual whose ability to maintain his blood pressure has already been compromised by a depleted blood volume, or a concurrent administration of drugs such as phenothiazines, or general anesthetics. (See also: PRECAUTIONS: Drug Interactions.) MSIR Oral Solutions, Tablets and Capsules may produce orthostatic hypotension in ambulatory patients.

MSIR Oral Solutions, Tablets and Capsules, like all opioid analgesics, should be administered with caution to patients in circulatory shock, since vasodilation produced by the drug may further reduce cardiac output and blood pressure.

Interactions with Other CNS Depressants

MSIR Oral Solutions, Tablets and Capsules, like all opioid analgesics, should be used with great caution and in reduced dosage in patients who are concurrently receiving other central nervous system depressants including sedatives or hypnotics, general anesthetics, phenothiazines,

Continued on next page

MSIR—Cont.

other tranquilizers and alcohol, because respiratory depression, hypotension and profound sedation or coma may result.

Interactions with Mixed Agonist/Antagonist Opioid Analgesics

From a theoretical perspective, agonist/antagonist analgesics (i.e., pentazocine, nalbuphine, butorphanol and buprenorphine) should NOT be administered to a patient who has received or is receiving a course of therapy with a pure agonist opioid analgesic. In these patients, mixed agonist-antagonist analgesics may reduce the analgesic effect or may precipitate withdrawal symptoms.

Drug Dependence

Morphine can produce drug dependence and has a potential for being abused. Tolerance and psychological and physical dependence may develop upon repeated administration. Physical dependence, however, is not of paramount importance in the management of terminally ill patients or any patient in severe pain. Abrupt cessation or a sudden reduction in dose after prolonged use may result in withdrawal symptoms. After prolonged exposure to opioid analgesics, if withdrawal is necessary, it must be undertaken gradually. (See DRUG ABUSE AND DEPENDENCE.)

Infants born to mothers physically dependent on opioid analgesics may also be physically dependent and exhibit respiratory depression and withdrawal symptoms. (See DRUG ABUSE AND DEPENDENCE.)

PRECAUTIONS (See also: CLINICAL PHARMACOLOGY)

General

MSIR Oral Solutions, Tablets and Capsules are intended for use in patients who require a potent opioid analgesic for relief of moderate to severe pain.

Selection of patients for treatment with MSIR Oral Solutions, Tablets and Capsules should be governed by the same principles that apply to the use of morphine and other potent opioid analgesics. Specifically, the increased risks associated with its use in the following populations should be considered: the elderly or debilitated and those with severe impairment of hepatic, pulmonary or renal function; myxedema or hypothyroidism; adrenocortical insufficiency (e.g., Addison's Disease); CNS depression or coma; toxic psychoses; prostatic hypertrophy or urethral stricture; acute alcoholism; delirium tremens; kyphoscoliosis or inability to swallow.

The administration of morphine, like all opioid analgesics, may obscure the diagnosis or clinical course in patients with acute abdominal conditions.

Morphine may aggravate preexisting convulsions in patients with convulsive disorders.

Morphine should be used with caution in patients about to undergo surgery of the biliary tract, since it may cause spasm of the sphincter of Oddi. Similarly, morphine should be used with caution in patients with acute pancreatitis secondary to biliary tract disease.

Information for Patients

If clinically advisable, patients receiving MSIR Oral Solutions, Tablets and Capsules should be given the following instructions by the physician.

1. Morphine may produce physical and/or psychological dependence. For this reason, the dose of the drug should not be adjusted without consulting a physician.
2. Morphine may impair mental and/or physical ability required for the performance of potentially hazardous tasks (e.g., driving, operating machinery).
3. Morphine should not be taken with alcohol or other CNS depressants (sleep aids, tranquilizers) because additive effects including CNS depression may occur. A physician should be consulted if other prescription medications are currently being used or are prescribed for future use.
4. For women of childbearing potential who become or are planning to become pregnant, a physician should be consulted regarding analgesics and other drug use.

Drug Interactions (See also WARNINGS)

The concomitant use of other central nervous system depressants including sedatives or hypnotics, general anesthetics, phenothiazines, tranquilizers and alcohol may produce additive depressant effects. Respiratory depression, hypotension and profound sedation or coma may occur. When such combined therapy is contemplated, the dose of one or both agents should be reduced. Opioid analgesics, including MSIR Oral Solutions, Tablets and Capsules, may enhance the neuromuscular blocking action of skeletal muscle relaxants and produce an increased degree of respiratory depression.

Carcinogenicity/Mutagenicity/Impairment of Fertility

Studies of morphine sulfate in animals to evaluate the drug's carcinogenic and mutagenic potential or the effect on fertility have not been conducted.

Pregnancy

Teratogenic effects—CATEGORY C: Adequate animal studies on reproduction have not been performed to determine whether morphine affects fertility in males or females. There are no well-controlled studies in women, but marketing experience does not include any evidence of adverse effects on the fetus following routine (short-term) clinical use of morphine sulfate products. Although there is no clearly defined risk, such experience cannot exclude the possibility of infrequent or subtle damage to the human fetus. MSIR Oral Solutions, Tablets and Capsules should be used in pregnant women only when clearly needed. (See also: PRECAUTIONS: Labor and Delivery, and DRUG ABUSE AND DEPENDENCE.)

Nonteratogenic effects: Infants born from mothers who have been taking morphine chronically may exhibit withdrawal symptoms.

Labor and Delivery

MSIR Oral Solutions, Tablets and Capsules are not recommended for use in women during and immediately prior to labor. Occasionally, opioid analgesics may prolong labor through actions which temporarily reduce the strength, duration and frequency of uterine contractions. However, this effect is not consistent and may be offset by an increased rate of cervical dilatation which tends to shorten labor.

Neonates whose mothers received opioid analgesics during labor should be observed closely for signs of respiratory depression. A specific narcotic antagonist, naloxone, should be available for reversal of narcotic-induced respiratory depression in the neonate.

Nursing Mothers

Low levels of morphine have been detected in human milk. Withdrawal symptoms can occur in breast-feeding infants when maternal administration of morphine sulfate is stopped. Nursing should not be undertaken while a patient is receiving MSIR Oral Solutions, Tablets and Capsules since morphine may be excreted in the milk.

Pediatric Use

MSIR Oral Solutions, Tablets and Capsules have not been evaluated systematically in children.

ADVERSE REACTIONS

The adverse reactions caused by morphine are essentially the same as those observed with other opioid analgesics. They include the following major hazards: respiratory depression, apnea, and to a lesser degree, circulatory depression; respiratory arrest, shock, and cardiac arrest.

Most Frequently Observed

Constipation, lightheadedness, dizziness, sedation, nausea, vomiting, sweating, dysphoria and euphoria.

Some of these effects seem to be more prominent in ambulatory patients and in those not experiencing severe pain. Some adverse reactions in ambulatory patients may be alleviated if the patient lies down.

Less Frequently Observed Reactions

Central Nervous System: Weakness, headache, agitation, tremor, uncoordinated muscle movements, seizure, alterations of mood (nervousness, apprehension, depression, floating feelings), dreams, muscle rigidity, transient hallucinations and disorientation, visual disturbances, insomnia and increased intracranial pressure.

Gastrointestinal: Dry mouth, biliary tract spasm, laryngospasm, anorexia, diarrhea, cramps and taste alterations.

Cardiovascular: Flushing of the face, chills, tachycardia, bradycardia, palpitation, faintness, syncope, hypotension and hypertension.

Genitourinary: Urinary retention or hesitance, reduced libido, and/or potency.

Dermatologic: Pruritus, urticaria, other skin rashes, edema and diaphoresis.

Other: Antidiuretic effect, paresthesia, muscle tremor, blurred vision, nystagmus, diplopia and miosis.

DRUG ABUSE AND DEPENDENCE

Opioid analgesics may cause psychological and physical dependence. (See WARNINGS.) Physical dependence results in withdrawal symptoms in patients who abruptly discontinue the drug or may be precipitated through the administration of drugs with narcotic antagonist activity, e.g., naloxone or mixed agonist/antagonist analgesics (pentazocine, etc.: see also OVERDOSE). Physical dependence usually does not occur to a clinically significant degree until after several weeks of continued narcotic usage. Tolerance, in which increasingly large doses are required in order to produce the same degree of analgesia, is initially manifested by a shortened duration of analgesic effect, and, subsequently, by decreases in the intensity of analgesia.

In chronic-pain patients and in narcotic-tolerant cancer patients, the administration of MSIR Oral Solutions, Tablets and Capsules should be guided by the degree of tolerance manifested. Physical dependence, per se, is not ordinarily a concern when one is dealing with opioid-tolerant patients whose pain and suffering is associated with an irreversible illness.

If MSIR Oral Solutions, Tablets and Capsules are abruptly discontinued, a moderate to severe abstinence syndrome may occur. The opioid agonist abstinence syndrome is characterized by some or all of the following: restlessness, lacrimation, rhinorrhea, yawning, perspiration, cutis anserina, restless sleep known as the "yen" and mydriasis during the first 24 hours. These symptoms often increase in severity and over the next 72 hours may be accompanied by increasing irritability, anxiety, weakness, twitching and spasms of muscles; kicking movements; severe backache, abdominal and leg pains; abdominal and muscle cramps; hot and cold flashes; insomnia; nausea, anorexia, vomiting, intestinal spasm, diarrhea; coryza and repetitive sneezing; and increase in body temperature, blood pressure, respiratory rate and heart rate. Because of excessive loss of fluids through sweating, vomiting and diarrhea, there is usually marked weight loss, dehydration, ketosis, and disturbances in acid-base balance. Cardiovascular collapse can occur. Without treatment, most observable symptoms disappear in 5–14 days; however, there appears to be a phase of secondary or chronic abstinence which may last for 2–6 months, characterized by insomnia, irritability, and muscular aches.

If treatment of physical dependence on MSIR Oral Solutions, Tablets and Capsules is necessary, the patient may be detoxified by gradual reduction of the dosage. Gastrointestinal disturbances or dehydration should be treated accordingly.

OVERDOSE

Acute overdosage with morphine is manifested by respiratory depression, somnolence progressing to stupor or coma, skeletal muscle flaccidity, cold and clammy skin, constricted pupils, and, sometimes, bradycardia and hypotension.

In the treatment of overdosage, primary attention should be given to the re-establishment of a patent airway and institution of assisted or controlled ventilation. The pure opioid antagonist, naloxone, is a specific antidote against respiratory depression which results from opioid overdose. Naloxone (usually 0.4 to 2.0 mg) should be administered intravenously; however, because its duration of action is relatively short, the patient must be carefully monitored until spontaneous respiration is reliably reestablished. If the response to naloxone is suboptimal or not sustained, additional naloxone may be re-administered, as needed, or given by continuous infusion to maintain alertness and respiratory function; however, there is no information available about the cumulative dose of naloxone that may be safely administered.

Naloxone should not be administered in the absence of clinically significant respiratory or circulatory depression secondary to morphine overdose. Naloxone should be administered cautiously to persons who are known or suspected to be physically dependent on morphine. In such cases, an abrupt or complete reversal of narcotic effects may precipitate an acute abstinence syndrome.

Note: In an individual physically dependent on opioids, administration of the usual dose of the antagonist will precipitate an acute withdrawal syndrome. The severity of the withdrawal syndrome produced will depend on the degree of physical dependence and the dose of the antagonist administered. Use of a narcotic antagonist in such a person should be avoided. If necessary to treat serious respiratory depression in the physically dependent patient the antagonist should be administered with extreme care and by titration with smaller than usual doses of the antagonist.

Supportive measures (including oxygen, vasopressors) should be employed in the management of circulatory shock and pulmonary edema accompanying overdose as indicated. Cardiac arrest or arrhythmias may require cardiac massage or defibrillation.

DOSAGE AND ADMINISTRATION

(See also: CLINICAL PHARMACOLOGY, WARNINGS AND PRECAUTIONS sections)

Dosage of morphine is a patient-dependent variable, which must be individualized according to patient metabolism, age and disease state and also response to morphine. Each patient should be maintained at the lowest dosage level that will produce acceptable analgesia. As the patient's well-being improves after successful relief of moderate to severe pain, periodic reduction of dosage and/or extension of dosing interval should be attempted to minimize exposure to morphine.

Usual Adult Oral Dose: 5 to 30 mg every four (4) hours or as directed by physician, administered either as MSIR Oral Solutions, MSIR Oral Tablets or MSIR Oral Capsules. For control of pain in terminal illness, it is recommended that the appropriate dose of MSIR Oral Solutions, MSIR Oral Tablets or MSIR Oral Capsules be given on a regularly scheduled basis every four hours at the minimum dose to achieve acceptable analgesia. If converting a patient from another narcotic to morphine sulfate on the basis of standard equivalence tables, a 1 to 3 ratio of parenteral to oral morphine equivalence is suggested. This ratio is conservative and may underestimate the amount of morphine required. If this is the case, the dose of MSIR Oral Solutions, MSIR Oral Tablets or MSIR Oral Capsules should be gradually increased to achieve acceptable analgesia and tolerable side effects.

Sprinkling Contents of Capsule on Food or Liquids: MSIR Oral Capsules may be carefully opened and the entire beaded contents added to a small amount of cool, soft food, such as applesauce or pudding, or a liquid, such as water or orange juice. The bead-food mixture should be swallowed immediately and not stored for future use.

HOW SUPPLIED

MSIR (morphine sulfate) Oral Solution: (pleasantly flavored)

10 mg per 5 mL.

NDC 0034-0521-02: high density polyethylene plastic bottle of 120 mL with child-resistant closure.

20 mg per 5 mL.

NDC 0034-0522-02: high density polyethylene plastic bottle of 120 mL with child-resistant closure.

MSIR (morphine sulfate) Oral Solution Concentrate: (unflavored)

20 mg per 1 mL.

NDC 0034-0523-01: high density polyethylene plastic, child-resistant closure bottle with child-resistant dropper in 30 mL size.

NDC 0034-0523-02: high density polyethylene plastic, child-resistant closure bottle with child-resistant dropper in 120 mL size.

Discard opened bottle of Oral Solution after 90 days. Protect from light.

MSIR (morphine sulfate) Tablets:

15 mg round, white scored tablets

NDC 0034-0518-10: opaque plastic bottle containing 100 tablets. Each tablet bears the symbol *PF* on the scored side and *MI 15* on the other side.

30 mg capsule-shaped, white scored tablets

NDC 0034-0519-10: opaque plastic bottle containing 100 tablets. Each tablet bears the symbol *PF* on the scored side and *MI 30* on the other side.

MSIR (morphine sulfate) Capsules:

15 mg capsules, white opaque capsule body with blue cap

NDC 0034-1025-10: opaque plastic bottle containing 100 capsules. Each capsule bears the symbols *"PF MSIR 15"* and *"THIS END UP."*

30 mg capsules, gray opaque capsule body with lavender cap

NDC 0034-1026-10: opaque plastic bottle containing 100 capsules. Each capsule bears the symbols *"PF MSIR 30"* and *"THIS END UP."*

Store MSIR Oral Solutions, Tablets and Capsules at controlled room temperature 15°to 30°C (59°– 86°F).

CAUTION: DEA Order Form Required.

Rx Only

THE PURDUE FREDERICK COMPANY
Stamford, CT 06901-3431

June 9, 2000 I3154

Shown in Product Identification Guide, page 331 and 332

Senna

X-PREP® BOWEL EVACUANT LIQUID **OTC**

[*ĕx 'prep*]

(extract of senna concentrate)

INDICATIONS

An easy-to-administer, palatable, highly effective bowel evacuant for cleansing the colon prior to x-ray, endoscopic examination or surgery. Permits excellent visualization without residual oil droplets. X-PREP Liquid is fully prepared in a single dose container—all the patient has to do is drink the contents of one small bottle (2$^1/_2$ fl. oz.). Good patient cooperation is ensured because of highly pleasant taste. Predictable effectiveness helps reduce or eliminate the need for enemas prior to radiography.

DESCRIPTION

Each bottle contains 130 mg sennosides. Active Ingredient: Extract of Senna Concentrate. Inactive Ingredients: Methylparaben, Potassium sorbate, Propylparaben, Sucrose, Water, Natural and Artificial Flavors, and other ingredients.

CONTRAINDICATIONS

Acute surgical abdomen.

WARNINGS

Do not use this product unless directed by a physician. Do not use when abdominal pain, nausea or vomiting is present, unless directed by a physician. As with any drug, if you are pregnant or nursing a baby, seek the advice of a health professional before using this product. In case of accidental overdose, seek professional assistance or contact a Poison Control Center immediately. Keep out of children's reach.

CAUTION

In diabetic patients, the physician should be aware of the sugar content of X-PREP Liquid (50 grams per 2$^1/_2$ fl. oz. dose).

ADMINISTRATION AND DOSAGE

Recommended Dosage (or as directed by physician):

Adults and children 12 years of age and older: Take one bottle between 2 and 4 p.m. on day prior to x-ray or other diagnostic procedures. Drink entire contents. For children under 12 years of age, consult a doctor. A strong bowel action can be expected approximately 6 hours after drinking. After X-PREP Liquid is taken, diet should be confined to clear fluids.

HOW SUPPLIED

2$^1/_2$ fl. oz. bottles, each providing a single, complete adult dose.

Also Available—Two X-PREP® Bowel Evacuant Kits.

Kit #1 contains: Two SENOKOT-S® Tablets (standardized senna concentrate and docusate sodium), one bottle of X-PREP Liquid 2$^1/_2$ fl. oz., and one RECTOLAX® Suppository (bisacodyl 10 mg), plus easy-to-follow patient instructions for hydration, clear liquid diet, and the correct time sequence for administering the above laxatives.

Kit #2 contains: One dose CITRALAX® Granules 1.06 oz. (effervescent citrate/sulfate of magnesia), one bottle of X-PREP Liquid 2$^1/_2$ fl. oz., and one RECTOLAX Suppository (bisacodyl 10 mg), plus easy-to-follow patient instructions.

SENOKOT® CHILDREN'S SYRUP **OTC**

[*sĕn 'ō-kŏt*]

(extract of senna concentrate)

ACTION AND USES

To relieve functional constipation in children from two to under 12 years of age, Senokot Children's Syrup generally produces bowel movement in 6 to 12 hours. Taken at bedtime, it works gently overnight.

DESCRIPTION

Each teaspoon of Senokot Children's Syrup contains 8.8 mg sennosides. Active Ingredient: Extract of Senna Concentrate. Inactive Ingredients: Methylparaben, Potassium sorbate, Propylparaben, Sucrose, Water, Natural and artificial chocolate flavor, and other ingredients.

ADMINISTRATION AND DOSAGE

Recommended Dosage (or as directed by a doctor):

Take preferably at bedtime.

AGE	STARTING	MAXIMUM
6 to under 12 years of age	1-1$^1/_2$ tsp. once/day	1$^1/_2$ tsp. twice/day
2 to under 6 years of age	$^1/_2$–$^3/_4$ tsp. once/day	$^3/_4$ tsp. twice/day
Under 2 years	Consult a physician	

SENOKOT Children's Syrup is packaged with a free measuring cup to help assure accurate dosing. Formulated without alcohol, Senokot Children's Syrup has an appealing chocolaty flavor. It may be given with ice cream or stirred into milk. Its natural active ingredient is concentrated, making it effective with smaller doses than other children's laxatives.

WARNINGS

Do not use laxative products when abdominal pain, nausea, or vomiting are present unless directed by a doctor. If there has been a sudden change in the child's bowel movements that persists over a period of 2 weeks, consult a doctor before using a laxative. Laxative products should not be used for a period longer than 1 week unless directed by a doctor. Rectal bleeding or failure to have a bowel movement after use of a laxative may indicate a serious condition. Discontinue use and consult a doctor. As with any drug, if the user is pregnant or nursing a baby, seek the advice of a health professional before taking this product. In case of accidental overdose, seek professional assistance or contact a Poison Control Center immediately. Keep out of children's reach.

HOW SUPPLIED

2.5 fl. oz. plastic bottles; packaged with measuring cup.

SENOKOT® TABLETS/GRANULES **OTC**

[*sen 'o-kot*]

SenokotXTRA® Tablets **OTC**

(standardized senna concentrate)

SENOKOT-S® Tablets **OTC**

(standardized senna concentrate and docusate sodium)
Natural Vegetable Laxative/Stool Softener Combination

INDICATIONS

SENOKOT Tablets/Granules and Double-Strength SenokotXTRA Tablets contain a natural vegetable derivative, standardized for uniform action. Each Double-Strength SenokotXTRA Tablet contains twice the active ingredient in one SENOKOT Tablet; patients may take one Double-Strength SenokotXTRA Tablet instead of two SENOKOT Tablets.

Senokot Laxatives provide a virtually colon-specific action which is gentle, effective and predictable, generally producing bowel movement in 6 to 12 hours. SENOKOT has been found to be effective even in many previously intractable cases of functional constipation. SENOKOT preparations may aid in rehabilitation of the constipated patient by facilitating regular elimination. At proper dosage levels, SENOKOT preparations are virtually free of adverse reactions (such as loose stools or abdominal discomfort) and enjoy high patient acceptance. Numerous and extensive clinical studies show their high degree of effectiveness in several types of functional constipation: geriatric and postpartum, drug-induced, pediatric, as well as in functional constipation concurrent with heart disease or anorectal surgery.

SENOKOT-S Tablets are designed to relieve both aspects of functional constipation—bowel inertia and hard, dry stools. They provide a natural neuroperistaltic stimulant combined with a classic stool softener, standardized senna concentrate gently stimulates the colon while docusate sodium softens the stool for smoother and easier evacuation. This coordinated dual action of the two ingredients results in colon-specific, predictable laxative effect, generally producing bowel movement in 6 to 12 hours. Flexibility of dosage permits fine adjustment to individual requirements. SENOKOT-S Tablets are highly suitable for relief of postsurgical and postpartum constipation, and effectively counter-act drug-induced constipation.

DESCRIPTION

SENOKOT Tablets: Each tablet contains 8.6 mg sennosides.

Active Ingredient: Standardized Senna Concentrate.

Inactive Ingredients: Corn starch, Glycerin, Lactose, Magnesium Stearate, Talc and other ingredients.

SENOKOT Granules: (cocoa-flavored): Each teaspoonful contains 15 mg sennosides.

Active Ingredient: Standardized Senna Concentrate.

Inactive Ingredients: Cocoa, Malt extract, Sodium lauryl sulfate, Sucrose, Vanillin and other ingredients.

SenokotXTRA Tablets: Each tablet contains 17 mg sennosides.

Active Ingredient: Standardized Senna Concentrate.

Inactive Ingredients: Corn Starch, Glycerin, Lactose, Magnesium stearate, Talc and other ingredients.

SENOKOT-S Tablets: Each tablet contains 8.6 mg sennosides and 50 mg of docusate sodium. Active Ingredients: Docusate Sodium and Standardized Senna Concentrate. Inactive Ingredients: Cellulosic polymers, Corn starch, FD&C Yellow No. 10, FD&C Yellow No. 6 (Sunset Yellow), Guar Gum, Lactose, Polyethylene glycol, Talc, Titanium dioxide, and other ingredients.

RECOMMENDED DOSAGE

(or as directed by a doctor): Take preferably at bedtime.

For older, debilitated patients, the physician may consider prescribing $^1/_2$ the initial dose.

Senokot Tablets and Granules are available for children under 6 years of age. For children under 2 years of age, consult a physician.

SENOKOT Tablets and SENOKOT-S Tablets:
Recommended Dosage (or as directed by a doctor):
Take preferably at bedtime.

AGE	STARTING	MAXIMUM
Adults and children 12 years of age and over	2 tablets once a day	4 tablets twice a day
6 to under 12 years of age	1 tablet once a day	2 tablets twice a day
2 to under 6 years of age	$^1/_2$ tablet once a day	1 tablet twice a day
Under 2 years	Consult a physician.	

Double-Strength SenokotXTRA Tablets:
Recommended Dosage (or as directed by a doctor): Take preferably at bedtime.

AGE	STARTING	MAXIMUM
Adults and children 12 years of age and over	1 tablet once a day	2 tablets twice a day
6 to under 12 years of age	$^1/_2$ tablet once a day	1 tablet twice a day

SENOKOT Granules (May be eaten plain, mixed with liquids such as milk to make a delicious drink, or sprinkled on foods.):

AGE	STARTING	MAXIMUM
Adults and children 12 years of age and over	1 teaspoon once a day	2 teaspoons twice a day
6 to under 12 years of age	$^1/_2$ teaspoon once a day	1 teaspoon twice a day
2 to under 6 years of age	$^1/_4$ teaspoon once a day	$^1/_2$ teaspoon twice a day
Under 2 years	Consult a physician.	

WARNINGS

Do not use laxative products when abdominal pain, nausea or vomiting are present unless directed by a doctor. If you have noticed a sudden change in bowel movements that persists over a period of 2 weeks, consult a doctor before using a laxative. Laxative products should not be used for a period longer than 1 week unless directed by a doctor. Rectal bleeding or failure to have a bowel movement after use of a laxative may indicate a serious condition. Discontinue use and consult your doctor. As with any drug, if you are pregnant or nursing a baby, seek the advice of a health professional before using this product. In case of accidental overdose, seek professional assistance or contact a Poison Control Center immediately. Keep out of children's reach.

HOW SUPPLIED

Tablets: Boxes of 20; bottles of 50, 100 and 1000. Unit Strip Packs in boxes of 100 tablets: each tablet individually sealed. Double-Strength SenokotXTRA Tablets: Boxes of 12 and 36.

Continued on next page

Senokot Tablets/Granules—Cont.

Senokot-S Tablets are supplied in packages of 10, bottles of 30, 60, and 1000 tablets, and Unit Strip Boxes of 100 tablets.
Granules: 2, 6, and 12 oz. plastic containers.
ALSO AVAILABLE
SENOKOT Syrup (extract of senna concentrate) in bottles of 2 and 8 fl. oz. Each teaspoon of SENOKOT Syrup contains 8.8 mg sennosides.
Active Ingredient: Extract of Senna Concentrate.
Inactive Ingredients: Methylparaben, Potassium sorbate, Propylparaben, Sucrose, Water, Natural and artificial chocolate flavor and other ingredients.

TRILISATE® TABLETS/LIQUID ℞
[*trĭl 'ĭ-sāt "*]
(choline magnesium trisalicylate)
500 mg, 750 mg, or 1000 mg
salicylate content

DESCRIPTION

TRILISATE Tablets/Liquid are nonsteroidal, anti-inflammatory preparations containing choline magnesium trisalicylate which is freely soluble in water. The absolute structure of choline magnesium trisalicylate is not known at this time. Choline magnesium trisalicylate has a molecular formula of $C_{26}H_{29}O_{10}NMg$, a molecular weight of 539.8, and it may be represented in the solid form as:

$$HO-CH_2-CH_2-N(CH_3)_3 \left[O_2C-C_6H_4(HO) \right]_3 Mg$$

This substance when dissolved in water would appear to form 5 ions (1 choline ion, 1 magnesium ion and 3 salicylate ions) which may be represented as:

$$\left[HO\ CH_2\ CH_2\ N(CH_3)_3\right]^+ \left[Mg^{+2}\right] \text{ and } 3\left[O_2C-C_6H_4(HO)\right]^-$$

TRILISATE Tablets/Liquid are available in scored, salmon-colored, film-coated 500 mg tablets; in scored, white, film-coated 750 mg tablets, and in scored, red, film-coated 1000 mg tablets. TRILISATE Liquid is a cherry cordial-flavored liquid providing 500 mg salicylate content per teaspoonful (5 ml) for oral administration.
Each 500 mg tablet contains 293 mg of choline salicylate combined with 362 mg of magnesium salicylate to provide 500 mg salicylate content. Each 750 mg tablet contains 440 mg of choline salicylate combined with 544 mg of magnesium salicylate to provide 750 mg salicylate content. Each 1000 mg tablet contains 587 mg of choline salicylate combined with 725 mg magnesium salicylate to provide 1000 mg salicylate content. TRILISATE Liquid contains 293 mg of choline salicylate combined with 362 mg of magnesium salicylate to provide 500 mg salicylate per teaspoonful (5 ml) in a clear amber, cherry cordial-flavored vehicle.
Inactive Ingredients: Each 500 mg tablet contains Carboxymethylcellulose sodium, Edetate disodium, FD&C Yellow No. 6, Polyethylene glycol, Polysorbate 20, Polysorbate 80, Stearic acid, Talc, and other ingredients.
Each 750 mg tablet contains Carboxymethylcellulose sodium, Edetate disodium, Hydroxypropyl methylcellulose, Polyethylene glycol, Polysorbate 20, Stearic acid, Talc, Titanium dioxide, and other ingredients.
Each 1000 mg tablet contains Carboxymethylcellulose sodium, Edetate disodium, FD&C Red No. 40, FD&C Yellow No. 6, FD&C Blue No. 2, Hydroxypropyl methylcellulose, Polyethylene glycol, Polysorbate 20, Polysorbate 80, Stearic acid, Talc, Titanium dioxide and other ingredients.
Each teaspoonful (5 ml) of Liquid contains: Caramel, Carboxymethylcellulose sodium, Edetate disodium, FD&C Yellow No. 6, Glycerin, High fructose corn syrup, Potassium sorbate, Water, and Artificial flavors.

CLINICAL PHARMACOLOGY

TRILISATE Tablets/Liquid contain salicylate with anti-inflammatory, analgesic and antipyretic action. On ingestion of TRILISATE Tablets/Liquid, the salicylate moiety is absorbed rapidly and reaches peak blood levels within an average of one to two hours after single doses of the tablets or liquid. The primary route of excretion is renal: the excretion products are chiefly the glycine and glucuronide conjugates. At higher serum salicylate concentrations, the glycine conjugation pathway becomes rapidly saturated. Thus, the slower glucuronide conjugation pathway becomes the rate limiting step for salicylate excretion. In addition, salicylate excreted in the bile as glucuronide conjugate may be reabsorbed. These factors account for the prolongation of salicylate half-life and the nonlinear increase in plasma salicylate level as the salicylate dose is increased. The serum concentration of salicylate is increased by conditions that decrease glomerular filtration rate or proximal tubular secretion.
The bioequivalence of TRILISATE Liquid and Tablets 500 mg/750 mg/1000 mg has been established. With the tablets, a steady-state condition is usually reached after 4 to 5 doses, and the half-life of elimination, on repeated administration of tablets, is 9 to 17 hours. This permits a maintenance dosage schedule of once or twice daily. Unlike aspirin and certain other non-steroidal anti-inflammatory agents, such as arylpropionic acid derivatives and arylacetic acid derivatives, choline magnesium trisalicylate, at therapeutic dosage levels, does not affect platelet aggregation, as shown by in-vitro and in-vivo studies.

INDICATIONS AND USAGE

Osteoarthritis, Rheumatoid Arthritis and Acute Painful Shoulder: Salicylates are considered the base therapy of choice in the arthritides; and TRILISATE preparations are indicated for the relief of the signs and symptoms of rheumatoid arthritis, osteoarthritis and other arthritides. TRILISATE Tablets or Liquid are indicated in the long-term management of these diseases and especially in the acute flare of rheumatoid arthritis. TRILISATE Tablets or Liquid are also indicated for the treatment of acute painful shoulder.
TRILISATE preparations are effective and generally well tolerated, and are logical choices whenever salicylate treatment is indicated. They are particularly suitable when a once-a-day or b.i.d. dosage regimen is important to patient compliance; when gastrointestinal intolerance to aspirin is encountered; when gastrointestinal microbleeding or hematologic effects of aspirin are considered a patient hazard; and when interference (or the risk of interference) with normal platelet function by aspirin or by propionic acid derivatives is considered to be clinically undesirable. Use of TRILISATE Liquid is appropriate when a liquid dosage form is preferred, as in the elderly patient.
The efficacy of TRILISATE preparations has not been studied in those patients who are designated by the American Rheumatism Association as belonging in Functional Class IV (incapacitated, largely or wholly bedridden or confined to a wheelchair, with little or no self-care). Analgesic and Antipyretic Action: TRILISATE Tablets/Liquid are also indicated for the relief of mild to moderate pain and for antipyresis.
Pediatric Use: **In children**, TRILISATE preparations are indicated for conditions requiring anti-inflammatory or analgesic action—such as juvenile rheumatoid arthritis and other appropriate conditions. In a four-week open label pilot study of patients with juvenile rheumatoid arthritis, children from 6 to 16 years of age previously on aspirin received weight adjusted doses (50–60 mg/kg) of TRILISATE 500 mg tablets on a divided b.i.d. schedule with subsequent dose titration to achieve therapeutic serum salicylate levels. Eighty-three percent (83%) of the patients rated the therapeutic effect of TRILISATE as good or excellent. Tinnitus was reported by one patient and elevated SGOT levels at Week 1, which decreased during the trial, were detected in two patients. (See WARNINGS section).

CONTRAINDICATIONS

Patients who are hypersensitive to non-acetylated salicylates should not take TRILISATE Tablets or Liquid.

WARNINGS

Reye Syndrome is a rare but serious disease which may develop in children and teenagers who have chicken pox, influenza, or flu symptoms. While the cause of Reye Syndrome is unknown, some studies suggest a possible association between the development of Reye Syndrome and the use of medicines containing acetylated salicylates or aspirin. TRILISATE Tablets and Liquid are a combination of choline salicylate and magnesium salicylate which are nonacetylated salicylates, and there have been no reported cases associating TRILISATE with Reye Syndrome. Nevertheless, TRILISATE, as a salicylate-containing product, is not recommended for use in children and teenagers with chicken pox, influenza or flu symptoms.
The FDA has determined that routine heavy alcohol use (three or more alcoholic drinks every day), in combination with analgesic/antipyretic drug products containing NSAID ingredients (including choline and magnesium salicylates), increases the risk of adverse GI events, including stomach bleeding.

PRECAUTIONS

General Precautions: As with other salicylates and nonsteroidal anti-inflammatory drugs, TRILISATE preparations should be used with caution in patients with acute or chronic renal insufficiency, with acute or chronic hepatic dysfunction, or with gastritis or peptic ulcer disease.
Although reports exist of cross reactivity, including bronchospasm, with the use of non-acetylated salicylate products in aspirin-sensitive patients, TRILISATE preparations were found to be well tolerated with regard to pulmonary function and respiratory symptoms when these parameters were monitored in a group of documented aspirin-sensitive asthmatics dosed with TRILISATE in both controlled and open label studies.[1]
Concurrent use of other salicylate-containing products and TRILISATE preparations can lead to an increase in plasma salicylate concentration and may result in potentially toxic salicylate levels.
Laboratory Tests: Plasma salicylate levels can be periodically assessed during treatment with TRILISATE preparations to determine whether a therapeutically effective anti-inflammatory concentration of 15 to 30 mg/100 ml (150–300 micrograms/ml) is being maintained. Manifestations of systemic salicylate intoxication are usually not seen until the concentration exceeds 30 mg/100 ml. However, such tests rarely differentiate between the active free and inactive protein bound salicylate components. Since protein binding of salicylate is affected by age, nutritional status, competitive binding of other drugs, and underlying disease (e.g. rheumatoid arthritis), plasma salicylate level determinations may not always accurately reflect efficacious or toxic levels of active free salicylate. Acidification of the urine can significantly diminish the renal clearance of salicylate and increase plasma salicylate concentrations.
Drug Interactions: Foods and drugs that alter urine pH may affect renal clearance of salicylate and plasma salicylate concentrations. Raising urine pH, as with chronic antacid use, can enhance renal salicylate clearance and diminish plasma salicylate concentration; urine acidification can decrease urinary salicylate excretion and increase plasma levels.
When salicylate drug products are concurrently dosed with other plasma protein bound drug products, adverse effects may result. Although TRILISATE preparations are a rational choice for anti-inflammatory and analgesic therapy in patients on oral anticoagulants due to their demonstrated lack of effect in vivo and in vitro on platelet aggregation, bleeding time, platelet count, prothrombin time, and serum thromboxane B2 generation[1–7], the potential exists for increased levels of unbound warfarin with their concurrent use. Prothrombin time should be closely monitored and warfarin dose appropriately adjusted when therapy with TRILISATE preparations is initiated. The effect of TRILISATE on blood prothrombin levels has not been established. Salicylates may increase the therapeutic as well as toxic effects of methotrexate, particularly when administered in chemotherapeutic doses, by inhibition of renal methotrexate excretion and by displacement of plasma protein bound methotrexate. Caution should be exercised in administering TRILISATE to rheumatoid arthritis patients on methotrexate. When sulfonylurea oral hypoglycemic agents are co-administered with salicylates, the hypoglycemic effect may be enhanced via increased insulin secretion or by displacement of sulfonylurea agents from binding sites. Insulin-treated diabetics on high doses of salicylates should also be closely monitored for a similar hypoglycemic response. Other drugs with which salicylate competes for protein binding sites, and whose plasma concentration or free fraction may be altered by concurrent salicylate administration, include the following: phenytoin, valproic acid, and carbonic anhydrase inhibitors.
The efficacy of uricosuric agents may be decreased when administered with salicylate products. Although low doses of salicylate (1 to 2 grams per day) have been reported to decrease urate excretion and elevate plasma urate concentrations, intermediate doses (2 to 3 grams per day) usually do not alter urate excretion. Larger salicylate doses (over 5 grams per day) can induce uricosuria and lower plasma urate levels.
Corticosteroids can reduce plasma salicylate levels by increasing renal elimination and perhaps by also stimulating hepatic metabolism of salicylates. By monitoring plasma salicylate levels, salicylate dosage may be titrated to accommodate changes in corticosteroid dose or to avoid salicylate toxicity during corticosteroid taper.
Drug/Laboratory Test Interactions: Free T4 values may be increased in patients on salicylate drug products due to competitive plasma protein binding; a concurrent decrease in total plasma T4 may be observed. Thyroid function is not affected.
Carcinogenesis: No long-term animal studies have been performed with TRILISATE to evaluate its carcinogenic potential.
Use in Pregnancy: Pregnancy Category C. Animal reproduction studies have not been conducted with TRILISATE preparations. It is also not known whether TRILISATE can cause fetal harm when administered to a pregnant woman or can affect reproduction capacity. TRILISATE should be given to a pregnant woman only if clearly needed. Because of the known effects of other salicylate drug products on the fetal cardiovascular system (closure of ductus arteriosus), use during late pregnancy should be avoided.
Labor and Delivery: The effects of TRILISATE on labor and delivery in pregnant women are unknown. Since prolonged gestation and prolonged labor due to prostaglandin inhibition have been reported with the use of other salicylate products, the use of TRILISATE preparations near term is not recommended. Other salicylate products have also been associated with alterations in maternal and neonatal hemostasis mechanisms and with perinatal mortality.
Nursing Mothers: Salicylate is excreted in human milk. Peak milk salicylate levels are delayed, occurring as long as 9 to 12 hours post dose, and the milk:plasma ratio has been reported to be as high as 0.34. Because of the potential for significant salicylate absorption by the nursing infant, caution should be exercised when TRILISATE is administered to a nursing woman.
Geriatric Use: The elderly may be prone to more side effects from salicylates than younger patients due to an age-related decline in renal clearance and/or increased use of concomitant medication. The elderly are more likely than younger patients to be taking a number of medications, some of which may affect the plasma protein binding of salicylate and thus increase the amount of free salicylate.

ADVERSE REACTIONS

The most frequent adverse reactions observed with TRILISATE preparations in clinical trials[7–12] are tinnitus and gastrointestinal complaints (including nausea, vomiting, gastric upset, indigestion, heartburn, diarrhea, constipation and epigastric pain). These occur in less than twenty percent (20%) of patients. Should tinnitus develop, reduction of daily dosage is recommended until the tinnitus is resolved. Less frequent adverse reactions, occurring in less than two percent (2%) of patients, are: hearing impairment, headache, lightheadedness, dizziness, drowsiness, and lethargy. Adverse reactions occurring in less than one percent (1%) of patients are: gastric ulceration, positive fecal occult blood, elevation in serum BUN and creatinine, rash, pruritus, anorexia, weight gain, edema, epistaxis and dysgeusia.

Spontaneous reporting has yielded isolated or rare reports of the following adverse experiences: duodenal ulceration, elevated hepatic transaminases, hepatitis, esophagitis, asthma, erythema multiforme, urticaria, ecchymoses, irreversible hearing loss and/or tinnitus, mental confusion, hallucinations.

DRUG ABUSE AND DEPENDENCE

Drug abuse and dependence have not been reported with TRILISATE preparations.

OVERDOSAGE

Death in adults has been reported following ingestion of doses from 10 to 30 grams of salicylate; however, larger doses have been taken without resulting fatality.

Symptoms: Salicylate intoxication, known as salicylism, may occur with large doses or extended therapy. Common symptoms of salicylism include headache, dizziness, tinnitus, hearing impairment, confusion, drowsiness, sweating, vomiting, diarrhea, and hyperventilation. A more severe degree of salicylate intoxication can lead to CNS disturbances, alteration in electrolyte balance, respiratory and metabolic acidosis, hyperthermia, and dehydration.

Treatment: Reduction of further absorption of salicylate from the gastrointestinal tract can be achieved via emesis, gastric lavage, use of activated charcoal, or a combination of the above. Appropriate I.V. fluids should be administered to correct dehydration, electrolyte imbalance, and acidosis and to maintain adequate renal function. To accelerate salicylate excretion, forced diuresis with alkalinizing solution is recommended. In extreme cases, peritoneal dialysis or hemodialysis should be considered for effective salicylate removal.

DOSAGE AND ADMINISTRATION

ADULTS: In rheumatoid arthritis, osteoarthritis, the more severe arthritides, and acute painful shoulder, the recommended starting dosage is 1500 mg given b.i.d. Some patients may be treated with 3000 mg given once per day (h.s.). Dosage should be adjusted in accordance with the patient's response. In patients with renal dysfunction, monitor salicylate levels and adjust dose accordingly.

ELDERLY: In the elderly patient, a daily dosage of 2250 mg given as 750 mg t.i.d. may be efficacious and well tolerated. Dosage should be adjusted in accordance with the patient's response. In patients with renal dysfunction, monitor salicylate levels and adjust dose accordingly.

For mild to moderate pain or for antipyresis, the usual dosage is 2000 mg to 3000 mg daily in divided doses (b.i.d.). Based on patient response or salicylate blood levels, dosage may be adjusted to achieve optimum therapeutic effect. Salicylate blood levels should be in the range of 15 to 30 mg/100 ml for anti-inflammatory effect and 5 to 15 mg/100 ml for analgesia and antipyresis.

Each 500 mg tablet or teaspoonful is equivalent in salicylate content to 10 gr of aspirin; each 750 mg tablet, to 15 gr of aspirin; and each 1000 mg tablet, to 20 gr of aspirin.

If the physician prefers, the recommended daily dosage may be administered on a t.i.d. schedule.

As with other therapeutic agents, individual dosage adjustment is advisable, and a number of patients may require higher or lower dosages than those recommended. Certain patients require 2 to 3 weeks of therapy for optimal effect.

CHILDREN: Usual daily dose for children for anti-inflammatory or analgesic action:

TRILISATE 500 mg Tablets/Liquid and TRILISATE 750 mg and 1000 mg Tablets, 50 mg/kg/day.

Weight (kg)	Total daily dose
12–13	500 mg
14–17	750 mg
18–22	1000 mg
23–27	1250 mg
28–32	1500 mg
33–37	1750 mg

Total daily doses should be administered in divided doses (b.i.d.). Doses of TRILISATE preparations are calculated as the total daily dose of 50 mg/kg/day for children of 37 kg body weight or less and 2250 mg/day for heavier children. TRILISATE Liquid is available for greater convenience in treating younger patients and those adult patients unable to swallow a solid dosage form.

Rx Only

HOW SUPPLIED

NDC 0034-0500-80: TRILISATE 500 mg Tablets (scored, salmon-colored, film-coated) supplied in bottles of 100 tablets.

NDC 0034-0500-50: TRILISATE 500 mg Tablets (scored, salmon-colored, film-coated) supplied in bottles of 500 tablets.

NDC 0034-0505-80: TRILISATE 750 mg Tablets (scored, white, film-coated) in bottles of 100 tablets.

NDC 0034-0505-50: TRILISATE 750 mg Tablets (scored, white, film-coated) in bottles of 500 tablets.

NDC 0034-0510-80: TRILISATE 1000 mg Tablets (scored, red, film-coated) in bottles of 100 tablets.

NDC 0034-0520-80: TRILISATE Liquid in bottles of 8 fl. oz. (237 ml).

Store at controlled room temperature 59° to 86°F (15° to 30°C).

REFERENCES

1. Szczeklik, A et al; Choline magnesium trisalicylate in patients with aspirin-induced asthma; *Eur Respir J*; 3:535–539, 1990.
2. Zucker, MB and Rothwell KB; Differential influences of salicylate compounds on platelet aggregation and serotonin release; *Current Therapeutic Research*; 23(2), Feb 1987.
3. Stuart, JJ and Pisko, EJ; Choline magnesium trisalicylate does not impair platelet aggregation; *Pharmatherapeutica*; 2(8):547, 1981.
4. Danesh, BJZ, Saniabadi, AR, Russell, RI et al; Therapeutic potential of choline magnesium trisalicylate as an alternative to aspirin for patients with bleeding tendencies; *Scottish Medical Journal*; 32:167–168, 1987.
5. Danesh, BJZ, McLaren, M. Russell, RI et al; Does nonacetylated salicylate inhibit thromboxane biosynthesis in human platelets? *Scottish Medical Journal*; 33: 315–316, 1988.
6. Danesh, BJZ, McLaren, M, Russell, RI et al; Comparison of the effect of aspirin and choline magnesium trisalicylate on thromboxane biosynthesis in human platelets: role of the acetyl moiety; *Haemostasis*; 19: 169–173, 1989.
7. Data on file. Medical Department. The Purdue Frederick Company, 1989.
8. Blechman, WJ, and Lechner, BL; Clinical comparative evaluation of choline magnesium trisalicylate and acetylsalicylic acid in rheumatoid arthritis; *Rheumatology and Rehabilitation*; 18:119–124, 1979.
9. McLaughlin, G; Choline magnesium trisalicylate vs. naproxen in rheumatoid arthritis; *Current Therapeutic Research*; 32(4):579–585, 1982.
10. Ehrlich, GE; Miller, SB; and Zeiders, RS; Choline magnesium trisalicylate vs. ibuprofen in rheumatoid arthritis; *Rheumatology and Rehabilitation*; 19:30–41, 1980.
11. Goldenberg, A; Rudnicki, RD, and Koonce, ML; Clinical comparison of efficacy and safety of choline magnesium trisalicylate and indomethacin in treating osteoarthritis; *Current Therapeutic Research*; 24(3):245–260, 1978.
12. Guerin, BK and Burnstein, SL; Conservative therapy of acute painful shoulder; *Orthopedic Review*; XI(7):29–37, 1982.

The Purdue Frederick Company, Stamford, CT 06901-3431

June 9, 2000 S145-BL

Shown in Product Identification Guide, page 332

UNIPHYL® ℞

[*ū 'nĭ-fĭl*]

400 mg and 600 mg Tablets
(theophylline)

UNICONTIN® Controlled-Release System

DESCRIPTION

Uniphyl® (theophylline, anhydrous) Tablets in a controlled-release system allows a 24-hour dosing interval for appropriate patients.

Theophylline is structurally classified as a methylxanthine. It occurs as a white, odorless, crystalline powder with a bitter taste. Anhydrous theophylline has the chemical name 1H-Purine-2,6-dione,3,7-dihydro-1,3-dimethyl-, and is represented by the following structural formula:

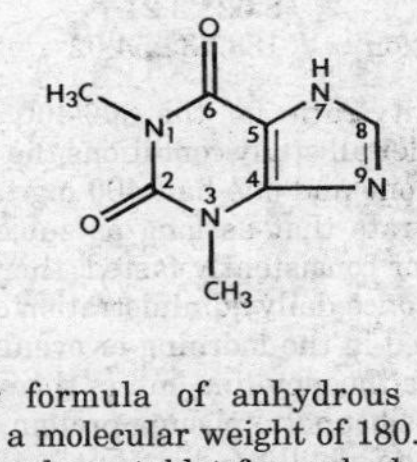

The molecular formula of anhydrous theophylline is $C_7H_8N_4O_2$ with a molecular weight of 180.17.

Each controlled-release tablet for oral administration, contains 400 or 600 mg of anhydrous theophylline per tablet.

Inactive Ingredients: Cetostearyl alcohol, Hydroxyethyl cellulose, Magnesium stearate, Povidone and Talc.

CLINICAL PHARMACOLOGY

Mechanism of Action: Theophylline has two distinct actions in the airways of patients with reversible obstruction; smooth muscle relaxation (i.e., bronchodilation) and suppression of the response of the airways to stimuli (i.e., non-bronchodilator prophylactic effects). While the mechanisms of action of theophylline are not known with certainty, studies in animals suggest that bronchodilatation is mediated by the inhibition of two isozymes of phosphodiesterase (PDE III and, to a lesser extent, PDE IV) while non-bronchodilator prophylactic actions are probably mediated through one or more different molecular mechanisms, that do not involve inhibition of PDE III or antagonism of adenosine receptors. Some of the adverse effects associated with theophylline appear to be mediated by inhibition of PDE III (e.g., hypotension, tachycardia, headache, and emesis) and adenosine receptor antagonism (e.g., alterations in cerebral blood flow). Theophylline increases the force of contraction of diaphragmatic muscles. This action appears to be due to enhancement of calcium uptake through an adenosine-mediated channel.

Serum Concentration-Effect Relationship: Bronchodilation occurs over the serum theophylline concentration range of 5–20 mcg/mL. Clinically important improvement in symptom control has been found in most studies to require peak serum theophylline concentrations >10 mcg/mL, but patients with mild disease may benefit from lower concentrations. At serum theophylline concentrations >20 mcg/mL, both the frequency and severity of adverse reactions increase. In general, maintaining peak serum theophylline concentrations between 10 and 15 mcg/mL will achieve most of the drug's potential therapeutic benefit while minimizing the risk of serious adverse events.

Pharmacokinetics:

Overview Theophylline is rapidly and completely absorbed after oral administration in solution or immediate-release solid oral dosage form. Theophylline does not undergo any appreciable pre-systemic elimination, distributes freely into fat-free tissues and is extensively metabolized in the liver. The pharmacokinetics of theophylline vary widely among similar patients and cannot be predicted by age, sex, body weight or other demographic characteristics. In addition, certain concurrent illnesses and alterations in normal physiology (see Table I) and co-administration of other drugs (see Table II) can significantly alter the pharmacokinetic characteristics of theophylline. Within-subject variability in metabolism has also been reported in some studies, especially in acutely ill patients. It is, therefore, recommended that serum theophylline concentrations be measured frequently in acutely ill patients (e.g., at 24-hr intervals) and periodically in patients receiving long-term therapy, e.g., at 6–12 month intervals. More frequent measurements should be made in the presence of any condition that may significantly alter theophylline clearance (see PRECAUTIONS, Laboratory tests).

[See table at top of next page]

Absorption Uniphyl® administered in the fed state is completely absorbed after oral administration.

In a single-dose crossover study, two 400 mg Uniphyl® Tablets were administered to 19 normal volunteers in the morning or evening immediately following the same standardized meal (769 calories consisting of 97 grams carbohydrates, 33 grams protein and 27 grams fat). There was no evidence of dose dumping nor were there any significant differences in pharmacokinetic parameters attributable to time of drug administration. On the morning arm, the pharmacokinetic parameters were AUC=241.9±83.0 mcg hr/mL, Cmax=9.3±2.0 mcg/mL, Tmax=12.8±4.2 hours. On the evening arm, the pharmacokinetic parameters were AUC=219.7±83.0 mcg hr/mL, Cmax=9.2±2.0 mcg/mL, Tmax=12.5±4.2 hours.

A study in which Uniphyl® 400 mg tablets were administered to 17 fed adult asthmatics produced similar theophylline level-time curves when administered in the morning or evening. Serum levels were generally higher in the evening regimen but there were no statistically significant differences between the two regimens.

	MORNING	EVENING
AUC (0–24 hrs) (mcg hr/mL)	236.0±76.7	256.0±80.4
Cmax (mcg/mL)	14.5±4.1	16.3±4.5
Cmin (mcg/mL)	5.5±2.9	5.0±2.5
Tmax (hours)	8.1±3.7	10.1±4.1

A single-dose study in 15 normal fasting male volunteers whose theophylline inherent mean elimination half-life was verified by a liquid theophylline product to be 6.9±2.5 (S.D.) hours were administered two or three 400 mg Uniphyl® Tablets. The relative bioavailability of Uniphyl® given in the fasting state in comparison to an immediate-release product was 59%. Peak serum theophylline levels occurred at 6.9±5.2 (S.D.) hours, with a normalized (to 800 mg) peak level being 6.2±2.1 (S.D.). The apparent elimination half-life for the 400 mg Uniphyl® Tablets was 17.2±5.8 (S.D.) hours.

Steady-state pharmacokinetics were determined in a study in 12 fasted patients with chronic reversible obstructive pulmonary disease. All were dosed with two 400 mg Uniphyl® Tablets given once daily in the morning and a reference controlled-release BID product administered as two 200 mg tablets given 12 hours apart. The pharmacokinetic parameters obtained for Uniphyl® Tablets given at doses of 800 mg once daily in the morning were virtually identical to the corresponding parameters for the reference drug when given as 400 mg BID. In particular, the AUC, Cmax and Cmin values obtained in this study were as follows:

	Uniphyl® Tablets 800 mg Q24h±S.D.	Reference Drug 400 mg Q12h±S.D.
AUC, (0–24 hours), mcg hr/mL	288.9±21.5	283.5±38.4

Continued on next page

Uniphyl—Cont.

Cmax, mcg/mL	15.7±2.8	15.2±2.1
Cmin, mcg/mL	7.9±1.6	7.8±1.7
Cmax-Cmin diff.	7.7±1.5	7.4±1.5

Single-dose studies in which subjects were fasted for twelve (12) hours prior to and an additional four (4) hours following dosing, demonstrated reduced bioavailability as compared to dosing with food. One single-dose study in 20 normal volunteers dosed with two (2) 400 mg tablets in the morning, compared dosing under these fasting conditions with dosing immediately prior to a standardized breakfast (769 calories, consisting of 97 grams carbohydrates, 33 grams protein and 27 grams fat). Under fed conditions, the pharmacokinetic parameters were: AUC=231.7±92.4 mcg hr/mL, Cmax=8.4±2.6 mcg/mL, Tmax=17.3±6.7 hours. Under fasting conditions, these parameters were AUC=141.2±6.53 mcg hr/mL, Cmax=5.5±1.5 mcg/mL, Tmax=6.5±2.1 hours. Another single-dose study in 21 normal male volunteers, dosed in the evening, compared fasting to a standardized high calorie, high fat meal (870–1,020 calories, consisting of 33 grams protein, 55–75 grams fat, 58 grams carbohydrates). In the fasting arm subjects received one Uniphyl® 400 mg Tablet at 8 p.m. after an eight hour fast followed by a further four hour fast. In the fed arm, subjects were again dosed with one 400 mg Uniphyl® Tablet, but at 8 p.m. immediately after the high fat content standardized meal cited above. The pharmacokinetic parameters (normalized to 800 mg) fed were AUC=221.8±40.9 mcg hr/mL, Cmax=10.9±1.7 mcg/mL, Tmax=11.8±2.2 hours. In the fasting arm, the pharmacokinetic parameters (normalized to 800 mg) were AUC=146.4±40.9 mcg hr/mL, Cmax=6.7±1.7 mcg/mL, Tmax=7.3±2.2 hours.

Thus, administration of single Uniphyl® doses to healthy normal volunteers, under prolonged fasted conditions (at least 10 hour overnight fast before dosing followed by an additional four (4) hour fast after dosing) results in decreased bioavailability. However, there was no failure of this delivery system leading to a sudden and unexpected release of a large quantity of theophylline with Uniphyl® Tablets even when they are administered with a high fat, high calorie meal.

Similar studies were conducted with the 600 mg Uniphyl® Tablet. A single-dose study in 24 subjects with an established theophylline clearance of ≤ 4 L/hr, compared the pharmacokinetic evaluation of one 600 mg Uniphyl® Tablet and one and one-half 400 mg Uniphyl® Tablets under fed (using a standard high fat diet) and fasted conditions. The results of this 4-way randomized crossover study demonstrate the bioequivalence of the 400 mg and 600 mg Uniphyl® Tablets. Under fed conditions, the pharmacokinetic results for the one and one-half 400 mg Tablets were AUC=214.64±55.88 mcg hr/mL, Cmax=10.58±2.21 mcg/mL and Tmax=9.00±2.64 hours, and for the 600 mg Tablet were AUC=207.85±48.9 mcg hr/mL, Cmax=10.39±1.91 mcg/mL and Tmax=9.58 ±1.86 hours. Under fasted conditions the pharmacokinetic results for the one and one-half 400 mg Tablets were AUC=191.85±51.1 mcg hr/mL, Cmax=7.37±1.83 mcg/mL and Tmax=8.08±4.39 hours, and for the 600 mg Tablet were AUC=199.39±70.27 mcg hr/mL, Cmax=7.66±2.09 mcg/mL and Tmax=9.67±4.89 hours.

In this study the mean fed/fasted ratios for the one and one-half 400 mg Tablets and the 600 mg Tablet were about 112% and 104%, respectively.

In another study, the bioavailability of the 600 mg Uniphyl® Tablet was examined with morning and evening administration. This single-dose, crossover study in 22 healthy males was conducted under fed (standard high fat diet) conditions. The results demonstrated no clinically significant difference in the bioavailability of the 600 mg Uniphyl® Tablet administered in the morning or in the evening. The results were: AUC=233.6±45.1 mcg hr/mL, Cmax=10.6±1.3 mcg/mL and Tmax=12.5±3.2 hours with morning dosing; AUC=209.8±46.2 mcg hr/mL, Cmax=9.7±1.4 mcg/mL and Tmax=13.7±3.3 hours with evening dosing. The PM/AM ratio was 89.3%.

The absorption characteristics of Uniphyl® Tablets (theophylline, anhydrous) have been extensively studied. A steady-state crossover bioavailability study in 22 normal males compared two Uniphyl® 400 mg Tablets administered q24h at 8 a.m. immediately after breakfast with a reference controlled-release theophylline product administered BID in fed subjects at 8 a.m. immediately after breakfast and 8 p.m. immediately after dinner (769 calories, consisting of 97 grams carbohydrates, 33 grams protein and 27 grams fat).

The pharmacokinetic parameters for Uniphyl® 400 mg Tablets under these steady-state conditions were AUC=203.3±87.1 mcg hr/mL, Cmax=12.1±3.8 mcg/mL, Cmin=4.50±3.6, Tmax=8.8±4.6 hours. For the reference BID product, the pharmacokinetic parameters were AUC=219.2±88.4 mcg hr/mL, Cmax=11.0±4.1 mcg/mL, Cmin=7.28±3.5, Tmax=6.9±3.4 hours. The mean percent fluctuation [(Cmax-Cmin/Cmin) × 100] = 169% for the once-daily regimen and 51% for the reference product BID regimen.

The bioavailability of the 600 mg Uniphyl® tablet was further evaluated in a multiple dose, steady-state study in 26 healthy males comparing the 600 mg Tablet to one and one-half 400 mg Uniphyl® tablets. All subjects had previously established theophylline clearances of ≤ 4L/hr and were dosed once-daily for 6 days under fed conditions. The results

Table I. Mean and range of total body clearance and half-life of theophylline related to age and altered physiological states.¶

Population Characteristics	Total body clearance* mean (range)‡ (mL/kg/min)	Half-life mean (range)‡ (hr)
Age		
Premature neonates		
postnatal age 3–15 days	0.29 (0.09–0.49)	30 (17–43)
postnatal age 25–57 days	0.64 (0.04–1.2)	20 (9.4–30.6)
Term infants		
postnatal age 1–2 days	NR†	25.7 (25–26.5)
postnatal age 3–30 weeks	NR†	11 (6–29)
Children		
1–4 years	1.7 (0.5–2.9)	3.4 (1.2–5.6)
4–12 years	1.6 (0.8–2.4)	NR†
13–15 years	0.9 (0.48–1.3)	NR†
6–17 years	1.4 (0.2–2.6)	3.7 (1.5–5.9)
Adults (16–60 years)		
otherwise healthy		
non-smoking asthmatics	0.65 (0.27–1.03)	8.7 (6.1–12.8)
Elderly (>60 years)		
non-smokers with normal cardiac,		
liver, and renal function	0.41 (0.21–0.61)	9.8 (1.6–18)
Concurrent illness or altered physiological state		
Acute pulmonary edema	0.33** (0.07–2.45)	19** (3.1–82)
COPD->60 years, stable		
non-smoker >1 year	0.54 (0.44–0.64)	11 (9.4–12.6)
COPD with cor pulmonale	0.48 (0.08–0.88)	NR†
Cystic fibrosis (14–28 years)	1.25 (0.31–2.2)	6.0 (1.8–10.2)
Fever associated with		
acute viral respiratory illness		
(children 9–15 years)	NR†	7.0 (1.0–13)
Liver disease		
cirrhosis	0.31 ** (0.1–0.7)	32** (10–56)
acute hepatitis	0.35 (0.25–0.45)	19.2 (16.6–21.8)
cholestasis	0.65 (0.25–1.45)	14.4 (5.7–31.8)
Pregnancy		
1st trimester	NR†	8.5 (3.1–13.9)
2nd trimester	NR†	8.8 (3.8–13.8)
3rd trimester	NR†	13.0 (8.4–17.6)
Sepsis with multi-organ failure	0.47 (0.19–1.9)	18.8 (6.3–24.1)
Thyroid disease		
hypothyroid	0.38 (0.13–0.57)	11.6 (8.2–25)
hyperthyroid	0.8 (0.68–0.97)	4.5 (3.7–5.6)

¶ For various North American patient populations from literature reports. Different rates of elimination and consequent dosage requirements have been observed among other peoples.
* Clearance represents the volume of blood completely cleared of theophylline by the liver in one minute. Values listed were generally determined at serum theophylline concentrations <20 mcg/mL; clearance may decrease and half-life may increase at higher serum concentrations due to non-linear pharmacokinetics.
‡ Reported range or estimated range (mean ± 2 SD) where actual range not reported.
† NR = not reported or not reported in a comparable format.
** Median

Note: In addition to the factors listed above, theophylline clearance is increased and half-life decreased by low carbohydrate/high protein diets, parenteral nutrition, and daily consumption of charcoal-broiled beef. A high carbohydrate/low protein diet can decrease the clearance and prolong the half-life of theophylline.

showed no clinically significant difference between the 600 mg and one and one-half 400 mg Uniphyl® tablet regimens. Steady-state results were:

	600 MG TABLET FED	600 MG (ONE + ONE-HALF 400 MG TABLETS) FED
AUC 0–24hrs (mcg hr/mL)	209.77±51.04	212.32±56.29
Cmax (mcg/mL)	12.91±2.46	13.17±3.11
Cmin (mcg/mL)	5.52±1.79	5.39±1.95
Tmax (hours)	8.62±3.21	7.23±2.35
Percent Fluctuation	183.73±54.02	179.72±28.86

The bioavailability ratio for the 600/400 mg tablets was 98.8%. Thus, under all study conditions the 600 mg tablet is bioequivalent to one and one-half 400 mg tablets.

Studies demonstrate that as long as subjects were either consistently fed or consistently fasted, there is similar bioavailability with once-daily administration of Uniphyl® tablets whether dosed in the morning or evening.

Distribution Once theophylline enters the systemic circulation, about 40% is bound to plasma protein, primarily albumin. Unbound theophylline distributes throughout body water, but distributes poorly into body fat. The apparent volume of distribution of theophylline is approximately 0.45 L/kg (range 0.3–0.7 L/kg) based on ideal body weight. Theophylline passes freely across the placenta, into breast milk and into the cerebrospinal fluid (CSF). Saliva theophylline concentrations approximate unbound serum concentrations, but are not reliable for routine or therapeutic monitoring unless special techniques are used. An increase in the volume of distribution of theophylline, primarily due to reduction in plasma protein binding, occurs in premature neonates, patients with hepatic cirrhosis, uncorrected acidemia, the elderly and in women during the third trimester of pregnancy. In such cases, the patient may show signs of toxicity at total (bound + unbound) serum concentrations of theophylline in the therapeutic range (10–20 mcg/mL) due to elevated concentrations of the pharmacologically active unbound drug. Similarly, a patient with decreased theophylline binding may have a sub-therapeutic total drug concentration while the pharmacologically active unbound concentration is in the therapeutic range. If only total serum theophylline concentration is measured, this may lead to an unnecessary and potentially dangerous dose increase. In patients with reduced protein binding, measurement of unbound serum theophylline concentration provides a more reliable means of dosage adjustment than measurement of total serum theophylline concentration. Generally, concentrations of unbound theophylline should be maintained in the range of 6–12 mcg/mL.

Metabolism Following oral dosing, theophylline does not undergo any measurable first-pass elimination. In adults and children beyond one year of age, approximately 90% of the dose is metabolized in the liver. Biotransformation takes place through demethylation to 1-methylxanthine and 3-methylxanthine and hydroxylation to 1,3-dimethyluric acid. 1-methylxanthine is further hydroxylated, by xanthine oxidase, to 1-methyluric acid. About 6% of a theophylline dose is N-methylated to caffeine. Theophylline demethylation to 3-methylxanthine is catalyzed by cytochrome P-450 1A2, while cytochromes P-450 2E1 and P-450 3A3 catalyze the hydroxylation to 1,3-dimethyluric acid. Demethylation to 1-methylxanthine appears to be catalyzed either by cytochrome P-450 1A2 or a closely related cytochrome. In neonates, the N-demethylation pathway is absent while the function of the hydroxylation pathway is markedly deficient. The activity of these pathways slowly increases to maximal levels by one year of age.

Caffeine and 3-methylxanthine are the only theophylline metabolites with pharmacologic activity. 3-methylxanthine has approximately one tenth the pharmacologic activity of theophylline and serum concentrations in adults with normal renal function are <1 mcg/mL. In patients with end-stage renal disease, 3-methylxanthine may accumulate to concentrations that approximate the unmetabolized theophylline concentration. Caffeine concentrations are usually undetectable in adults regardless of renal function. In neonates, caffeine may accumulate to concentrations that approximate the unmetabolized theophylline concentration and thus, exert a pharmacologic effect.

Both the N-demethylation and hydroxylation pathways of theophylline biotransformation are capacity-limited. Due to the wide intersubject variability of the rate of theophylline metabolism, non-linearity of elimination may begin in some patients at serum theophylline concentrations <10 mcg/mL. Since this non-linearity results in more than proportional changes in serum theophylline concentrations with changes in dose, it is advisable to make increases or decreases in dose in small increments in order to achieve desired changes in serum theophylline concentrations (see DOSAGE AND ADMINISTRATION, Table VI). Accurate prediction of dose-dependency of theophylline metabolism in patients *a priori* is not possible, but patients with very high initial clearance rates (i.e., low steady-state serum theophylline concentrations at above average doses) have the greatest likelihood of experiencing large changes in serum theophylline concentration in response to dosage changes.

Excretion In neonates, approximately 50% of the theophylline dose is excreted unchanged in the urine. Beyond the first three months of life, approximately 10% of the theophylline dose is excreted unchanged in the urine. The remainder is excreted in the urine mainly as 1,3-dimethyluric acid (35–40%), 1-methyluric acid (20–25%) and 3-methylxanthine (15–20%). Since little theophylline is excreted unchanged in the urine and since active metabolites of theophylline (i.e., caffeine, 3-methylxanthine) do not accumulate to clinically significant levels even in the face of end-stage renal disease, no dosage adjustment for renal insufficiency is necessary in adults and children >3 months of age. In contrast, the large fraction of the theophylline dose excreted in the urine as unchanged theophylline and caffeine in neonates requires careful attention to dose reduction and frequent monitoring of serum theophylline concentrations in neonates with reduced renal function (See WARNINGS).

Serum Concentrations at Steady State After multiple doses of theophylline, steady state is reached in 30–65 hours (average 40 hours) in adults. At steady state, on a dosage regimen with 24-hour intervals, the expected mean trough concentration is approximately 50% of the mean peak concentration, assuming a mean theophylline half-life of 8 hours. The difference between peak and trough concentrations is larger in patients with more rapid theophylline clearance. In these patients administration of Uniphyl® may be required more frequently (every 12 hours).

Special Populations (See Table I for mean clearance and half-life values)

Geriatric The clearance of theophylline is decreased by an average of 30% in healthy elderly adults (>60 yrs) compared to healthy young adults. Careful attention to dose reduction and frequent monitoring of serum theophylline concentrations are required in elderly patients (see WARNINGS).

Pediatrics The clearance of theophylline is very low in neonates (see WARNINGS). Theophylline clearance reaches maximal values by one year of age, remains relatively constant until about 9 years of age and then slowly decreases by approximately 50% to adult values at about age 16. Renal excretion of unchanged theophylline in neonates amounts to about 50% of the dose, compared to about 10% in children older than three months and in adults. Careful attention to dosage selection and monitoring of serum theophylline concentrations are required in pediatric patients (see WARNINGS and DOSAGE AND ADMINISTRATION).

Gender Gender differences in theophylline clearance are relatively small and unlikely to be of clinical significance. Significant reduction in theophylline clearance, however, has been reported in women on the 20th day of the menstrual cycle and during the third trimester of pregnancy.

Race Pharmacokinetic differences in theophylline clearance due to race have not been studied.

Renal insufficiency Only a small fraction, e.g., about 10%, of the administered theophylline dose is excreted unchanged in the urine of children greater than three months of age and adults. Since little theophylline is excreted unchanged in the urine and since active metabolites of theophylline (i.e., caffeine, 3-methylxanthine) do not accumulate to clinically significant levels even in the face of end-stage renal disease, no dosage adjustment for renal insufficiency is necessary in adults and children >3 months of age. In contrast, approximately 50% of the administered theophylline dose is excreted unchanged in the urine in neonates. Careful attention to dose reduction and frequent monitoring of serum theophylline concentrations are required in neonates with decreased renal function (see WARNINGS).

Hepatic Insufficiency Theophylline clearance is decreased by 50% or more in patients with hepatic insufficiency (e.g., cirrhosis, acute hepatitis, cholestasis). Careful attention to dose reduction and frequent monitoring of serum theophylline concentrations are required in patients with reduced hepatic function (see WARNINGS).

Congestive Heart Failure (CHF) Theophylline clearance is decreased by 50% or more in patients with CHF. The extent of reduction in theophylline clearance in patients with CHF appears to be directly correlated to the severity of the cardiac disease. Since theophylline clearance is independent of liver blood flow, the reduction in clearance appears to be due to impaired hepatocyte function rather than reduced perfusion. Careful attention to dose reduction and frequent monitoring of serum theophylline concentrations are required in patients with CHF (see WARNINGS).

Smokers Tobacco and marijuana smoking appears to increase the clearance of theophylline by induction of metabolic pathways. Theophylline clearance has been shown to increase by approximately 50% in young adult tobacco smokers and by approximately 80% in elderly tobacco smokers compared to non-smoking subjects. Passive smoke exposure has also been shown to increase theophylline clearance by up to 50%. Abstinence from tobacco smoking for one week causes a reduction of approximately 40% in theophylline clearance. Careful attention to dose reduction and frequent monitoring of serum theophylline concentrations are required in patients who stop smoking (see WARNINGS). Use of nicotine gum has been shown to have no effect on theophylline clearance.

Fever Fever, regardless of its underlying cause, can decrease the clearance of theophylline. The magnitude and duration of the fever appear to be directly correlated to the degree of decrease of theophylline clearance. Precise data are lacking, but a temperature of 39°C (102°F) for at least 24 hours is probably required to produce a clinically significant increase in serum theophylline concentrations. Children with rapid rates of theophylline clearance (i.e., those who require a dose that is substantially larger than average [e.g., >22 mg/kg/day] to achieve a therapeutic peak serum theophylline concentration when afebrile) may be at greater risk of toxic effects from decreased clearance during sustained fever. Careful attention to dose reduction and frequent monitoring of serum theophylline concentrations are required in patients with sustained fever (see WARNINGS).

Miscellaneous Other factors associated with decreased theophylline clearance include the third trimester of pregnancy, sepsis with multiple organ failure, and hypothyroidism. Careful attention to dose reduction and frequent monitoring of serum theophylline concentrations are required in patients with any of these conditions (see WARNINGS). Other factors associated with increased theophylline clearance include hyperthyroidism and cystic fibrosis.

Clinical Studies: In patients with chronic asthma, including patients with severe asthma requiring inhaled corticosteroids or alternate-day oral corticosteroids, many clinical studies have shown that theophylline decreases the frequency and severity of symptoms, including nocturnal exacerbations, and decreases the "as needed" use of inhaled beta-2 agonists. Theophylline has also been shown to reduce the need for short courses of daily oral prednisone to relieve exacerbations of airway obstruction that are unresponsive to bronchodilators in asthmatics.

In patients with chronic obstructive pulmonary disease (COPD), clinical studies have shown that theophylline decreases dyspnea, air trapping, the work of breathing, and improves contractility of diaphragmatic muscles with little or no improvement in pulmonary function measurements.

INDICATIONS AND USAGE

Theophylline is indicated for the treatment of the symptoms and reversible airflow obstruction associated with chronic asthma and other chronic lung diseases, e.g., emphysema and chronic bronchitis.

CONTRAINDICATIONS

Uniphyl® is contraindicated in patients with a history of hypersensitivity to theophylline or other components in the product.

WARNINGS

Concurrent Illness: Theophylline should be used with extreme caution in patients with the following clinical conditions due to the increased risk of exacerbation of the concurrent condition.

Active peptic ulcer disease
Seizure disorders
Cardiac arrhythmias (not including bradyarrhythmias)

Conditions That Reduce Theophylline Clearance: There are several readily identifiable causes of reduced theophylline clearance. ***If the total daily dose is not appropriately reduced in the presence of these risk factors, severe and potentially fatal theophylline toxicity can occur.*** Careful consideration must be given to the benefits and risks of theophylline use and the need for more intensive monitoring of serum theophylline concentrations in patients with the following risk factors:

Age

Neonates (term and premature)
Children <1 year
Elderly (>60 years)

Concurrent Diseases

Acute pulmonary edema
Congestive heart failure
Cor-pulmonale
Fever; ≥102° for 24 hours or more; or lesser temperature elevations for longer periods
Hypothyroidism
Liver disease, cirrhosis, acute hepatitis
Reduced renal function in infants <3 months of age
Sepsis with multi-organ failure
Shock

Cessation of Smoking

Drug Interactions

Adding a drug that inhibits theophylline metabolism (e.g., cimetidine, erythromycin, tacrine) or stopping a concurrently administered drug that enhances theophylline metabolism (e.g., carbamazepine, rifampin). (See PRECAUTIONS, Drug Interactions, Table II).

When Signs or Symptoms of Theophylline Toxicity Are Present:

Whenever a patient receiving theophylline develops nausea or vomiting, particularly repetitive vomiting, or other signs or symptoms consistent with theophylline toxicity (even if another cause may be suspected), additional doses of theophylline should be withheld and a serum theophylline concentration measured immediately. Patients should be instructed not to continue any dosage that causes adverse effects and to withhold subsequent doses until the symptoms have resolved, at which time the clinician may instruct the patient to resume the drug at a lower dosage (see DOSAGE AND ADMINISTRATION, Dosing Guidelines, Table VI).

Dosage Increases: Increases in the dose of theophylline should not be made in response to an acute exacerbation of symptoms of chronic lung disease since theophylline provides little added benefit to inhaled $beta_2$-selective agonists and systemically administered corticosteroids in this circumstance and increases the risk of adverse effects. A peak steady-state serum theophylline concentration should be measured before increasing the dose in response to persistent chronic symptoms to ascertain whether an increase in dose is safe. Before increasing the theophylline dose on the basis of a low serum concentration, the clinician should consider whether the blood sample was obtained at an appropriate time in relationship to the dose and whether the patient has adhered to the prescribed regimen (see PRECAUTIONS, Laboratory Tests).

As the rate of theophylline clearance may be dose-dependent (i.e., steady-state serum concentrations may increase disproportionately to the increase in dose), an increase in dose based upon a sub-therapeutic serum concentration measurement should be conservative. In general, limiting dose increases to about 25% of the previous total daily dose will reduce the risk of unintended excessive increases in serum theophylline concentration (see DOSAGE AND ADMINISTRATION, Table VI).

PRECAUTIONS

General: Careful consideration of the various interacting drugs and physiologic conditions that can alter theophylline clearance and require dosage adjustment should occur prior to initiation of theophylline therapy, prior to increases in theophylline dose, and during follow up (see WARNINGS). The dose of theophylline selected for initiation of therapy should be low and, ***if tolerated,*** increased slowly over a period of a week or longer with the final dose guided by monitoring serum theophylline concentrations and the patient's clinical response (see DOSAGE AND ADMINISTRATION, Table V).

Monitoring Serum Theophylline Concentrations: Serum theophylline concentration measurements are readily available and should be used to determine whether the dosage is appropriate. Specifically, the serum theophylline concentration should be measured as follows:

1. When initiating therapy to guide final dosage adjustment after titration.
2. Before making a dose increase to determine whether the serum concentration is sub-therapeutic in a patient who continues to be symptomatic.
3. Whenever signs or symptoms of theophylline toxicity are present.
4. Whenever there is a new illness, worsening of a chronic illness or a change in the patient's treatment regimen that may alter theophylline clearance (e.g., fever >102°F sustained for ≥24 hours, hepatitis, or drugs listed in Table II are added or discontinued).

To guide a dose increase, the blood sample should be obtained at the time of the expected peak serum theophylline concentration; 12 hours after an evening dose or 9 hours after a morning dose at steady-state. For most patients, steady-state will be reached after 3 days of dosing when no doses have been missed, no extra doses have been added, and none of the doses have been taken at unequal intervals. A trough concentration (i.e., at the end of the dosing interval) provides no additional useful information and may lead to an inappropriate dose increase since the peak serum theophylline concentration can be two or more times greater than the trough concentration with an immediate-release formulation. If the serum sample is drawn more than 12 hours after the evening dose, or more than 9 hours after a morning dose, the results must be interpreted with caution since the concentration may not be reflective of the peak concentration. In contrast, when signs or symptoms of theophylline toxicity are present, a serum sample should be obtained as soon as possible, analyzed immediately, and the result reported to the clinician without delay. In patients in whom decreased serum protein binding is suspected (e.g., cirrhosis, women during the third trimester of pregnancy), the concentration of unbound theophylline should be measured and the dosage adjusted to achieve an unbound concentration of 6–12 mcg/mL.

Saliva concentrations of theophylline cannot be used reliably to adjust dosage without special techniques.

Effects on Laboratory Tests: As a result of its pharmacological effects, theophylline at serum concentrations within the 10–20 mcg/mL range modestly increases plasma glucose (from a mean of 88 mg% to 98 mg%), uric acid (from a mean of 4 mg/dl to 6 mg/dl), free fatty acids (from a mean of 451 µEq/l to 800 µEq/l, total cholesterol (from a mean of 140 vs 160 mg/dl), HDL (from a mean of 36 to 50 mg/dl), HDL/LDL ratio (from a mean of 0.5 to 0.7), and urinary free cortisol excretion (from a mean of 44 to 63 mcg/24 hr). Theophylline at serum concentrations within the 10–20 mcg/mL range may also transiently decrease serum concentrations of triiodothyronine (144 before, 131 after one week and 142 ng/dL after 4 weeks of theophylline). The clinical importance of these changes should be weighed against the potential therapeutic benefit of theophylline in individual patients.

Continued on next page

Uniphyl—Cont.

Information for Patients: The patient (or parent/care giver) should be instructed to seek medical advice whenever nausea, vomiting, persistent headache, insomnia or rapid heart beat occurs during treatment with theophylline, even if another cause is suspected. The patient should be instructed to contact their clinician if they develop a new illness, especially if accompanied by a persistent fever, if they experience worsening of a chronic illness, if they start or stop smoking cigarettes or marijuana, or if another clinician adds a new medication or discontinues a previously prescribed medication. Patients should be instructed to inform all clinicians involved in their care that they are taking theophylline, especially when a medication is being added or deleted from their treatment. Patients should be instructed to not alter the dose, timing of the dose, or frequency of administration without first consulting their clinician. If a dose is missed, the patient should be instructed to take the next dose at the usually scheduled time and to not attempt to make up for the missed dose.

Uniphyl® tablets can be taken once a day in the morning or evening. It is recommended that Uniphyl® be taken with meals. Patients should be advised that if they choose to take Uniphyl® with food it should be taken consistently with food and if they take it in a fasted condition it should routinely be taken fasted. It is important that the product whenever dosed be dosed consistently with or without food. Uniphyl® tablets are not to be chewed or crushed. The scored tablet may be split. Patients receiving Uniphyl® tablets may pass an intact matrix tablet in the stool or via colostomy. These matrix tablets usually contain little or no residual theophylline.

Table II. Clinically significant drug interactions with theophylline*

Drug	Type of Interaction	Effect**
Adenosine	Theophylline blocks adenosine receptors.	Higher doses of adenosine may be required to achieve desired effect.
Alcohol	A single large dose of alcohol (3 mL/kg of whiskey) decreases theophylline clearance for up to 24 hours.	30% increase
Allopurinol	Decreases theophylline clearance at allopurinol doses ≥600 mg/day.	25% increase
Aminoglutethimide	Increases theophylline clearance by induction of microsomal enzyme activity.	25% decrease
Carbamazepine	Similar to aminoglutethimide.	30% decrease
Cimetidine	Decreases theophylline clearance by inhibiting cytochrome P450 1A2.	70% increase
Ciprofloxacin	Similar to cimetidine.	40% increase
Clarithromycin	Similar to erythromycin.	25% increase
Diazepam	Benzodiazepines increase CNS concentrations of adenosine, a potent CNS depressant, while theophylline blocks adenosine receptors.	Larger diazepam doses may be required to produce desired level of sedation. Discontinuation of theophylline without reduction of diazepam dose may result in respiratory depression.
Disulfiram	Decreases theophylline clearance by inhibiting hydroxylation and demethylation.	50% increase
Enoxacin	Similar to cimetidine.	300% increase
Ephedrine	Synergistic CNS effects	Increased frequency of nausea, nervousness, and insomnia.
Erythromycin	Erythromycin metabolite decreases theophylline clearance by inhibiting cytochrome P450 3A3.	35% increase. Erythromycin steady-state serum concentrations decrease by a similar amount.
Estrogen	Estrogen containing oral contraceptives decrease theophylline clearance in a dose-dependent fashion. The effect of progesterone on theophylline clearance is unknown.	30% increase
Flurazepam	Similar to diazepam.	Similar to diazepam
Fluvoxamine	Similar to cimetidine	Similar to cimetidine
Halothane	Halothane sensitizes the myocardium to catecholamines, theophylline increases release of endogenous catecholamines.	Increased risk of ventricular arrhythmias.
Interferon, human recombinant alpha-A	Decreases theophylline clearance.	100% increase
Isoproterenol (IV)	Increases theophylline clearance.	20% decrease
Ketamine	Pharmacologic	May lower theophylline seizure threshold.
Lithium	Theophylline increases renal lithium clearance.	Lithium dose required to achieve a therapeutic serum concentration increased an average of 60%.
Lorazepam	Similar to diazepam.	Similar to diazepam.
Methotrexate (MTX)	Decreases theophylline clearance.	20% increase after low dose MTX, higher dose MTX may have a greater effect.
Mexiletine	Similar to disulfiram.	80% increase
Midazolam	Similar to diazepam.	Similar to diazepam.
Moricizine	Increases theophylline clearance.	25% decrease
Pancuronium	Theophylline may antagonize non-depolarizing neuromuscular blocking effects; possibly due to phosphodiesterase inhibition.	Larger dose of pancuronium may be required to achieve neuromuscular blockade.
Pentoxifylline	Decreases theophylline clearance.	30% increase
Phenobarbital (PB)	Similar to aminoglutethimide.	25% decrease after two weeks of concurrent PB.
Phenytoin	Phenytoin increases theophylline clearance by increasing microsomal enzyme activity. Theophylline decreases phenytoin absorption.	Serum theophylline and phenytoin concentrations decrease about 40%.
Propafenone	Decreases theophylline clearance and pharmacologic interaction.	40% increase. Beta-2 blocking effect may decrease efficacy of theophylline.
Propranolol	Similar to cimetidine and pharmacologic interaction.	100% increase. Beta-2 blocking effect may decrease efficacy of theophylline.
Rifampin	Increases theophylline clearance by increasing cytochrome P450 1A2 and 3A3 activity.	20–40% decrease
Sulfinpyrazone	Increases theophylline clearance by increasing demethylation and hydroxylation. Decreases renal clearance of theophylline.	20% decrease
Tacrine	Similar to cimetidine, also increases renal clearance of theophylline.	90% increase
Thiabendazole	Decreases theophylline clearance.	190% increase
Ticlopidine	Decreases theophylline clearance.	60% increase
Troleandomycin	Similar to erythromycin.	33–100% increase depending on troleandomycin dose.
Verapamil	Similar to disulfiram.	20% increase

*** Refer to PRECAUTIONS, Drug Interactions for further information regarding table.**

**** Average effect on steady-state theophylline concentration or other clinical effect for pharmacologic interactions. Individual patients may experience larger changes in serum theophylline concentration than the value listed.**

Drug Interactions: Theophylline interacts with a wide variety of drugs. The interaction may be pharmacodynamic, i.e., alterations in the therapeutic response to theophylline or another drug or occurrence of adverse effects without a change in serum theophylline concentration. More frequently, however, the interaction is pharmacokinetic, i.e., the rate of theophylline clearance is altered by another drug resulting in increased or decreased serum theophylline concentrations. Theophylline only rarely alters the pharmacokinetics of other drugs.

The drugs listed in Table II have the potential to produce clinically significant pharmacodynamic or pharmacokinetic interactions with theophylline. The information in the "Effect" column of Table II assumes that the interacting drug is being added to a steady-state theophylline regimen. If theophylline is being initiated in a patient who is already taking a drug that inhibits theophylline clearance (e.g., cimetidine, erythromycin), the dose of theophylline required to achieve a therapeutic serum theophylline concentration will be smaller. Conversely, if theophylline is being initiated in a patient who is already taking a drug that enhances theophylline clearance (e.g., rifampin), the dose of theophylline required to achieve a therapeutic serum theophylline concentration will be larger. Discontinuation of a concomitant drug that increases theophylline clearance will result in accumulation of theophylline to potentially toxic levels, unless the theophylline dose is appropriately reduced. Discontinuation of a concomitant drug that inhibits theophylline clearance will result in decreased serum theophylline concentrations, unless the theophylline dose is appropriately increased.

The drugs listed in Table III have either been documented not to interact with theophylline or do not produce a clinically significant interaction (i.e., <15% change in theophylline clearance).

The listing of drugs in Tables II and III are current as of February 9, 1995. New interactions are continuously being reported for theophylline, especially with new chemical entities. **The clinician should not assume that a drug does not interact with theophylline if it is not listed in Table II.** Before addition of a newly available drug in a patient receiving theophylline, the package insert of the new drug and/or the medical literature should be consulted to determine if an interaction between the new drug and theophylline has been reported.

[See table above]

Table III. Drugs that have been documented not to interact with theophylline or drugs that produce no clinically significant interaction with theophylline.*

albuterol, systemic and inhaled
amoxicillin
ampicillin, with or without sulbactam
atenolol
azithromycin
caffeine, dietary ingestion
cefaclor
co-trimoxazole (trimethoprim and sulfamethoxazole)
diltiazem
dirithromycin
enflurane
famotidine
felodipine
finasteride
hydrocortisone
isoflurane
isoniazid
isradipine
influenza vaccine
ketoconazole
lomefloxacin
mebendazole
medroxyprogesterone
methylprednisolone
metronidazole
metoprolol
nadolol
nifedipine
nizatidine
norfloxacin
ofloxacin
omeprazole
prednisone, prednisolone
ranitidine
rifabutin
roxithromycin
sorbitol (purgative doses do not inhibit theophylline absorption)
sucralfate
terbutaline, systemic
terfenadine
tetracycline
tocainide

*** Refer to PRECAUTIONS, Drug Interactions for information regarding table.**

Drug-Food Interactions: The bioavailability of Uniphyl® tablets (theophylline, anhydrous) has been studied with coadministration of food. In three single-dose studies, subjects given Uniphyl® 400 mg or 600 mg tablets with a standardized high-fat meal were compared to fasted conditions. Under fed conditions, the peak plasma concentration and bioavailability were increased; however, a precipitous increase in the rate and extent of absorption was not evident (**See Pharmacokinetics-Absorption**). The increased peak and extent of absorption under fed conditions suggests that dosing should be ideally administered consistently either with or without food.

The Effect of Other Drugs on Theophylline Serum Concentration Measurements: Most serum theophylline assays in clinical use are immunoassays which are specific for theophylline. Other xanthines such as caffeine, dyphylline, and pentoxifylline are not detected by these assays. Some drugs (e.g., cefazolin, cephalothin), however, may interfere with certain HPLC techniques. Caffeine and xanthine metabolites in neonates or patients with renal dysfunction may cause the reading from some dry reagent office methods to be higher than the actual serum theophylline concentration.

Carcinogenesis, Mutagenesis, and Impairment of Fertility: Long term carcinogenicity studies have been carried out in mice (oral doses 30–150 mg/kg) and rats (oral doses 5–75 mg/kg). Results are pending.

Theophylline has been studied in Ames salmonella, *in vivo* and *in vitro* cytogenetics, micronucleus and Chinese hamster ovary test systems and has not been shown to be genotoxic.

In a 14 week continuous breeding study, theophylline, administered to mating pairs of $B6C3F_1$ mice at oral doses of 120, 270 and 500 mg/kg (approximately 1.0–3.0 times the human dose on a mg/m^2 basis) impaired fertility, as evidenced by decreases in the number of live pups per litter, decreases in the mean number of litters per fertile pair, and increases in the gestation period at the high dose as well as decreases in the proportion of pups born alive at the mid and high dose. In 13 week toxicity studies, theophylline was administered to F344 rats and $B6C3F_1$ mice at oral doses of 40–300 mg/kg (approximately 2.0 times the human dose on a mg/m^2 basis). At the high dose, systemic toxicity was observed in both species including decreases in testicular weight.

Pregnancy: CATEGORY C: There are no adequate and well controlled studies in pregnant women. Additionally, there are no teratogenicity studies in non-rodents (e.g., rabbits). Theophylline was not shown to be teratogenic in CD-1 mice at oral doses up to 400 mg/kg, approximately 2.0 times the human dose on a mg/m^2 basis or in CD-1 rats at oral doses up to 260 mg/kg, approximately 3.0 times the recommended human dose on a mg/m^2 basis. At a dose of 220 mg/kg, embryotoxicity was observed in rats in the absence of maternal toxicity.

Nursing Mothers: Theophylline is excreted into breast milk and may cause irritability or other signs of mild toxicity in nursing human infants. The concentration of theophylline in breast milk is about equivalent to the maternal serum concentration. An infant ingesting a liter of breast milk containing 10–20 mcg/mL of theophylline per day is likely to receive 10–20 mg of theophylline per day. Serious adverse effects in the infant are unlikely unless the mother has toxic serum theophylline concentrations.

Pediatric Use: Theophylline is safe and effective for the approved indications in pediatric patients. The maintenance dose of theophylline must be selected with caution in pediatric patients since the rate of theophylline clearance is highly variable across the pediatric age range (see CLINICAL PHARMACOLOGY, Table I, WARNINGS, and DOSAGE AND ADMINISTRATION, Table V).

Geriatric Use: Elderly patients are at significantly greater risk of experiencing serious toxicity from theophylline than younger patients due to pharmacokinetic and pharmacodynamic changes associated with aging. Theophylline clearance is reduced in patients greater than 60 years of age, resulting in increased serum theophylline concentrations in response to a given theophylline dose. Protein binding may be decreased in the elderly resulting in a larger proportion of the total serum theophylline concentration in the pharmacologically active unbound form. For these reasons, the maximum daily dose of theophylline in patients greater than 60 years of age ordinarily should not exceed 400 mg/day unless the patient continues to be symptomatic and the peak steady-state serum theophylline concentration is <10 mcg/mL (see DOSAGE AND ADMINISTRATION). Theophylline doses greater than 400 mg/d should be prescribed with caution in elderly patients.

ADVERSE REACTIONS

Adverse reactions associated with theophylline are generally mild when peak serum theophylline concentrations are <20 mcg/mL and mainly consist of transient caffeine-like adverse effects such as nausea, vomiting, headache, and insomnia. When peak serum theophylline concentrations exceed 20 mcg/mL, however, theophylline produces a wide range of adverse reactions including persistent vomiting, cardiac arrhythmias, and intractable seizures which can be lethal (see OVERDOSAGE). The transient caffeine-like adverse reactions occur in about 50% of patients when theophylline therapy is initiated at doses higher than recommended initial doses (e.g., >300 mg/day in adults and >12 mg/kg/day in children beyond >1 year of age). During the initiation of theophylline therapy, caffeine-like adverse effects may transiently alter patient behavior, especially in school age children, but this response rarely persists. Initiation of theophylline therapy at a low dose with subsequent slow titration to a predetermined age-related maximum dose will significantly reduce the frequency of these transient adverse effects (see DOSAGE AND ADMINISTRATION, Table V). In a small percentage of patients (<3% of children and <10% of adults) the caffeine-like adverse effects persist during maintenance therapy, even at peak serum theophylline concentrations within the therapeutic range (i.e., 10–20 mcg/mL). Dosage reduction may alleviate the caffeine-like adverse effects in these patients, however, persistent adverse effects should result in a reevaluation of the need for continued theophylline therapy and the potential therapeutic benefit of alternative treatment.

Other adverse reactions that have been reported at serum theophylline concentrations <20 mcg/mL include diarrhea, irritability, restlessness, fine skeletal muscle tremors, and transient diuresis. In patients with hypoxia secondary to COPD, multifocal atrial tachycardia and flutter have been reported at serum theophylline concentrations ≥15 mcg/mL. There have been a few isolated reports of seizures at serum theophylline concentrations <20 mcg/mL in patients with an underlying neurological disease or in elderly patients. The occurrence of seizures in elderly patients with serum theophylline concentrations <20 mcg/mL may be secondary to decreased protein binding resulting in a larger proportion of the total serum theophylline concentration in the pharmacologically active unbound form. The clinical characteristics of the seizures reported in patients with serum theophylline concentrations <20 mcg/mL have generally been milder than seizures associated with excessive serum theophylline concentrations resulting from an overdose (i.e. they have generally been transient, often stopped without anticonvulsant therapy, and did not result in neurological residua).

Table IV. Manifestations of theophylline toxicity.*

	Percentage of patients reported with sign or symptom			
	Acute Overdose (Large Single Ingestion)		Chronic Overdosage (Multiple Excessive Doses)	
Sign/Symptom	Study 1 (n=157)	Study 2 (n=14)	Study 1 (n=92)	Study 2 (n=102)
Asymptomatic	NR**	0	NR**	6
Gastrointestinal				
Vomiting	73	93	30	61
Abdominal Pain	NR**	21	NR**	12
Diarrhea	NR**	0	NR**	14
Hematemesis	NR**	0	NR**	2
Metabolic/Other				
Hypokalemia	85	79	44	43
Hyperglycemia	98	NR**	18	NR**
Acid/base disturbance	34	21	9	5
Rhabdomyolysis	NR**	7	NR**	0
Cardiovascular				
Sinus tachycardia	100	86	100	62
Other supraventricular tachycardias	2	21	12	14
Ventricular premature beats	3	21	10	19
Atrial fibrillation or flutter	1	NR**	12	NR**
Multifocal atrial tachycardia	0	NR**	2	NR**
Ventricular arrhythmias with hemodynamic instability	7	14	40	0
Hypotension/shock	NR**	21	NR**	8
Neurologic				
Nervousness	NR**	64	NR**	21
Tremors	38	29	16	14
Disorientation	NR**	7	NR**	11
Seizures	5	14	14	5
Death	3	21	10	4

* These data are derived from two studies in patients with serum theophylline concentrations >30 mcg/mL. In the first study (Study #1—Shanon, *Ann Intern Med* 1993; 119:1161–67), data were prospectively collected from 249 consecutive cases of theophylline toxicity referred to a regional poison center for consultation. In the second study (Study #2—Sessler, *Am J Med* 1990;88:567–76), data were retrospectively collected from 116 cases with serum theophylline concentrations >30 mcg/mL among 6000 blood samples obtained for measurement of serum theophylline concentrations in three emergency departments. Differences in the incidence of manifestations of theophylline toxicity between the two studies may reflect sample selection as a result of study design (e.g., in Study #1, 48% of the patients had acute intoxications versus only 10% in Study #2) and different methods of reporting results.

**NR=Not reported in a comparable manner.

OVERDOSAGE

General: The chronicity and pattern of theophylline overdosage significantly influences clinical manifestations of toxicity, management and outcome. There are two common presentations: (1) *acute overdose,* i.e., ingestion of a single large excessive dose (>10 mg/kg), as occurs in the context of an attempted suicide or isolated medication error, and (2) *chronic overdosage,* i.e., ingestion of repeated doses that are excessive for the patient's rate of theophylline clearance. The most common causes of chronic theophylline overdosage include patient or care giver error in dosing, clinician prescribing of an excessive dose or a normal dose in the presence of factors known to decrease the rate of theophylline clearance, and increasing the dose in response to an exacerbation of symptoms without first measuring the serum theophylline concentration to determine whether a dose increase is safe.

Severe toxicity from theophylline overdose is a relatively rare event. In one health maintenance organization, the frequency of hospital admissions for chronic overdosage of theophylline was about 1 per 1000 person-years exposure. In another study, among 6000 blood samples obtained for measurement of serum theophylline concentration, for any reason, from patients treated in an emergency department, 7% were in the 20–30 mcg/mL range and 3% were >30 mcg/mL. Approximately two-thirds of the patients with serum theophylline concentrations in the 20–30 mcg/mL range had one or more manifestations of toxicity while >90% of patients with serum theophylline concentrations >30 mcg/mL were clinically intoxicated. Similarly, in other reports, serious toxicity from theophylline is seen principally at serum concentrations >30 mcg/mL.

Several studies have described the clinical manifestations of theophylline overdose and attempted to determine the factors that predict life-threatening toxicity. In general, patients who experience an acute overdose are less likely to experience seizures than patients who have experienced a chronic overdosage, unless the peak serum theophylline concentration is >100 mcg/mL. After a chronic overdosage, generalized seizures, life-threatening cardiac arrhythmias, and death may occur at serum theophylline concentrations >30 mcg/mL. The severity of toxicity after chronic overdosage is more strongly correlated with the patient's age than the peak serum theophylline concentration; patients >60 years are at the greatest risk for severe toxicity and mortality after a chronic overdosage. Pre-existing or concurrent disease may also significantly increase the susceptibility of a patient to a particular toxic manifestation, e.g., patients with neurologic disorders have an increased risk of seizures and patients with cardiac disease have an increased risk of cardiac arrhythmias for a given serum theophylline concentration compared to patients without the underlying disease.

The frequency of various reported manifestations of theophylline overdose according to the mode of overdose are listed in Table IV.

Other manifestations of theophylline toxicity include increases in serum calcium, creatine kinase, myoglobin and leukocyte count, decreases in serum phosphate and magnesium, acute myocardial infarction, and urinary retention in men with obstructive uropathy.

Seizures associated with serum theophylline concentrations >30 mcg/mL are often resistant to anticonvulsant therapy and may result in irreversible brain injury if not rapidly controlled. Death from theophylline toxicity is most often secondary to cardiorespiratory arrest and/or hypoxic encephalopathy following prolonged generalized seizures or intractable cardiac arrhythmias causing hemodynamic compromise.

Overdose Management: General Recommendations for Patients with Symptoms of Theophylline Overdose or Serum Theophylline Concentrations >30 mcg/mL (Note: Serum theophylline concentrations may continue to increase after presentation of the patient for medical care.)

1. While simultaneously instituting treatment, contact a regional poison center to obtain updated information and advice on individualizing the recommendations that follow.
2. Institute supportive care, including establishment of intravenous access, maintenance of the airway, and electrocardiographic monitoring.
3. Treatment of seizures Because of the high morbidity and mortality associated with theophylline-induced seizures, treatment should be rapid and aggressive. Anticonvulsant therapy should be initiated with an intravenous benzodiazepine, e.g., diazepam, in increments of 0.1–0.2 mg/kg every 1–3 minutes until seizures are terminated. Repetitive seizures should be treated with a loading dose of phenobarbital (20 mg/kg infused over 30–60 minutes). Case reports of theophylline overdose in humans and animal studies suggest that phenytoin is ineffective in terminating theophylline-induced seizures. The doses of benzodiazepines and phenobarbital required to terminate theophylline-induced seizures are close to the doses that may cause severe respiratory depression or respiratory arrest; the clinician should therefore be prepared to provide assisted ventilation. Elderly patients and patients with COPD may be more susceptible to the respiratory depressant effects of anticonvulsants. Barbiturate-induced coma or administration of general anesthesia may be required to terminate repetitive seizures or status epilepticus. General anesthesia should be used with caution in patients with theophylline overdose because fluorinated volatile anesthetics may sensitize the myocardium to endogenous catecholamines released by theophylline.

Continued on next page

Uniphyl—Cont.

Enflurane appears less likely to be associated with this effect than halothane and may, therefore, be safer. Neuromuscular blocking agents alone should not be used to terminate seizures since they abolish the musculoskeletal manifestations without terminating seizure activity in the brain.

4. Anticipate Need for Anticonvulsants in patients with theophylline overdose who are at high risk for theophylline-induced seizures, e.g., patients with acute overdoses and serum theophylline concentrations >100 mcg/mL or chronic overdosage in patients >60 years of age with serum theophylline concentrations >30 mcg/mL, the need for anticonvulsant therapy should be anticipated. A benzodiazepine such as diazepam should be drawn into a syringe and kept at the patient's bedside and medical personnel qualified to treat seizures should be immediately available. In selected patients at high risk for theophylline-induced seizures, consideration should be given to the administration of prophylactic anticonvulsant therapy. Situations where prophylactic anticonvulsant therapy should be considered in high risk patients include anticipated delays in instituting methods for extracorporeal removal of theophylline (e.g., transfer of a high risk patient from one health care facility to another for extracorporeal removal) and clinical circumstances that significantly interfere with efforts to enhance theophylline clearance (e.g., a neonate where dialysis may not be technically feasible or a patient with vomiting unresponsive to antiemetics who is unable to tolerate multiple-dose oral activated charcoal). In animal studies, prophylactic administration of phenobarbital, but not phenytoin, has been shown to delay the onset of theophylline-induced generalized seizures and to increase the dose of theophylline required to induce seizures (i.e., markedly increases the LD_{50}). Although there are no controlled studies in humans, a loading dose of intravenous phenobarbital (20 mg/kg infused over 60 minutes) may delay or prevent life-threatening seizures in high risk patients while efforts to enhance theophylline clearance are continued. Phenobarbital may cause respiratory depression, particularly in elderly patients and patients with COPD.
5. Treatment of cardiac arrhythmias Sinus tachycardia and simple ventricular premature beats are not harbingers of life-threatening arrhythmias, they do not require treatment in the absence of hemodynamic compromise, and they resolve with declining serum theophylline concentrations. Other arrhythmias, especially those associated with hemodynamic compromise, should be treated with antiarrhythmic therapy appropriate for the type of arrhythmia.
6. Gastrointestinal decontamination Oral activated charcoal (0.5 g/kg up to 20 g and repeat at least once 1–2 hours after the first dose) is extremely effective in blocking the absorption of theophylline throughout the gastrointestinal tract, even when administered several hours after ingestion. If the patient is vomiting, the charcoal should be administered through a nasogastric tube or after administration of an antiemetic. Phenothiazine antiemetics such as prochlorperazine or perphenazine should be avoided since they can lower the seizure threshold and frequently cause dystonic reactions. A single dose of sorbitol may be used to promote stooling to facilitate removal of theophylline bound to charcoal from the gastrointestinal tract. Sorbitol, however, should be dosed with caution since it is a potent purgative which can cause profound fluid and electrolyte abnormalities, particularly after multiple doses. Commercially available fixed combinations of liquid charcoal and sorbitol should be avoided in young children and after the first dose in adolescents and adults since they do not allow for individualization of charcoal and sorbitol dosing. Ipecac syrup should be avoided in theophylline overdoses. Although ipecac induces emesis, it does not reduce the absorption of theophylline unless administered within 5 minutes of ingestion and even then is less effective than oral activated charcoal. Moreover, ipecac induced emesis may persist for several hours after a single dose and significantly decrease the retention and the effectiveness of oral activated charcoal.
7. Serum Theophylline Concentration Monitoring The serum theophylline concentration should be measured immediately upon presentation, 2–4 hours later, and then at sufficient intervals, e.g., every 4 hours, to guide treatment decisions and to assess the effectiveness of therapy. Serum theophylline concentrations may continue to increase after presentation of the patient for medical care as a result of continued absorption of theophylline from the gastrointestinal tract. Serial monitoring of serum theophylline serum concentrations should be continued until it is clear that the concentration is no longer rising and has returned to non-toxic levels.
8. General Monitoring Procedures Electrocardiographic monitoring should be initiated on presentation and continued until the serum theophylline level has returned to a non-toxic level. Serum electrolytes and glucose should be measured on presentation and at appropriate intervals indicated by clinical circumstances. Fluid and electrolyte abnormalities should be promptly corrected. **Monitoring and treatment should be continued until the serum concentration decreases below 20 mcg/mL.**
9. Enhance clearance of theophylline Multiple-dose oral activated charcoal (e.g., 0.5 mg/kg up to 20 g, every two hours) increases the clearance of theophylline at least twofold by adsorption of theophylline secreted into gastrointestinal fluids. Charcoal must be retained in, and pass through, the gastrointestinal tract to be effective; emesis should therefore be controlled by administration of appropriate antiemetics. Alternatively, the charcoal can be administered continuously through a nasogastric tube in conjunction with appropriate antiemetics. A single dose of sorbitol may be administered with the activated charcoal to promote stooling to facilitate clearance of the adsorbed theophylline from the gastrointestinal tract. Sorbitol alone does not enhance clearance of theophylline and should be dosed with caution to prevent excessive stooling which can result in severe fluid and electrolyte imbalances. Commercially available fixed combinations of liquid charcoal and sorbitol should be avoided in young children and after the first dose in adolescents and adults since they do not allow for individualization of charcoal and sorbitol dosing. In patients with intractable vomiting, extracorporeal methods of theophylline removal should be instituted (see OVERDOSAGE, Extracorporeal Removal).

Specific Recommendations:

Acute Overdose

A. Serum Concentration >20 <30 mcg/mL
   1. Administer a single dose of oral activated charcoal.
   2. Monitor the patient and obtain a serum theophylline concentration in 2–4 hours to insure that the concentration is not increasing.

B. Serum Concentration >30 <100 mcg/mL
   1. Administer multiple dose oral activated charcoal and measures to control emesis.
   2. Monitor the patient and obtain serial theophylline concentrations every 2–4 hours to gauge the effectiveness of therapy and to guide further treatment decisions.
   3. Institute extracorporeal removal if emesis, seizures, or cardiac arrhythmias cannot be adequately controlled (see OVERDOSAGE, Extracorporeal Removal).

C. Serum Concentration >100 mcg/mL
   1. Consider prophylactic anticonvulsant therapy.
   2. Administer multiple-dose oral activated charcoal and measures to control emesis.
   3. Consider extracorporeal removal, even if the patient has not experienced a seizure (see OVERDOSAGE, Extracorporeal Removal).
   4. Monitor the patient and obtain serial theophylline concentrations every 2–4 hours to gauge the effectiveness of therapy and to guide further treatment decisions.

Chronic Overdosage

A. Serum Concentration >20 <30 mcg/mL (with manifestations of theophylline toxicity)
   1. Administer a single dose of oral activated charcoal.
   2. Monitor the patient and obtain a serum theophylline concentration in 2–4 hours to insure that the concentration is not increasing.

B. Serum Concentration >30 mcg/mL in patients <60 years of age
   1. Administer multiple-dose oral activated charcoal and measures to control emesis.
   2. Monitor the patient and obtain serial theophylline concentrations every 2–4 hours to gauge the effectiveness of therapy and to guide further treatment decisions.
   3. Institute extracorporeal removal if emesis, seizures, or cardiac arrhythmias cannot be adequately controlled (see OVERDOSAGE, Extracorporeal Removal).

C. Serum Concentration >30 mcg/mL in patients ≥60 years of age
   1. Consider prophylactic anticonvulsant therapy.
   2. Administer multiple-dose oral activated charcoal and measures to control emesis.
   3. Consider extracorporeal removal even if the patient has not experienced a seizure (see OVERDOSAGE, Extracorporeal Removal).
   4. Monitor the patient and obtain serial theophylline concentrations every 2–4 hours to gauge the effectiveness of therapy and to guide further treatment decisions.

Extracorporeal Removal: Increasing the rate of theophylline clearance by extracorporeal methods may rapidly decrease serum concentrations, but the risks of the procedure must be weighed against the potential benefit. Charcoal hemoperfusion is the most effective method of extracorporeal removal, increasing theophylline clearance up to six fold, but serious complications, including hypotension, hypocalcemia, platelet consumption and bleeding diatheses may occur. Hemodialysis is about as efficient as multiple-dose oral activated charcoal and has a lower risk of serious complications than charcoal hemoperfusion. Hemodialysis should be considered as an alternative when charcoal hemoperfusion is not feasible and multiple-dose oral charcoal is ineffective because of intractable emesis. Serum theophylline concentrations may rebound 5–10 mcg/mL after discontinuation of charcoal hemoperfusion or hemodialysis due to redistribution of theophylline from the tissue compartment. Peritoneal dialysis is ineffective for theophylline removal; exchange transfusions in neonates have been minimally effective.

DOSAGE AND ADMINISTRATION

Uniphyl® 400 or 600 mg Tablets can be taken once a day in the morning or evening. It is recommended that Uniphyl be taken with meals. Patients should be advised that if they choose to take Uniphyl® with food it should be taken consistently with food and if they take it in a fasted condition it should routinely be taken fasted. It is important that the product whenever dosed be dosed consistently with or without food.

Uniphyl® Tablets are not to be chewed or crushed. The scored tablet may be split. Infrequently, patients receiving Uniphyl® 400 or 600 mg Tablets may pass an intact matrix tablet in the stool or via colostomy. These matrix tablets usually contain little or no residual theophylline.

Stabilized patients, 12 years of age or older, who are taking an immediate-release or controlled-release theophylline product may be transferred to once-daily administration of 400 mg or 600 mg Uniphyl® Tablets on a mg-for-mg basis. It must be recognized that the peak and trough serum theophylline levels produced by the once-daily dosing may vary from those produced by the previous product and/or regimen.

General Considerations: The steady-state peak serum theophylline concentration is a function of the dose, the dosing interval, and the rate of theophylline absorption and clearance in the individual patient. Because of marked individual differences in the rate of theophylline clearance, the dose required to achieve a peak serum theophylline concentration in the 10–20 mcg/mL range varies fourfold among otherwise similar patients in the absence of factors known to alter theophylline clearance (e.g., 400–1600 mg/day in adults <60 years old and 10–36 mg/kg/day in children 1–9 years old). For a given population there is no single theophylline dose that will provide both safe and effective serum concentrations for all patients. Administration of the median theophylline dose required to achieve a therapeutic serum theophylline concentration in a given population may result in either sub-therapeutic or potentially toxic serum theophylline concentrations in individual patients. For example, at a dose of 900 mg/d in adults <60 years or 22 mg/kg/d in children 1–9 years, the steady-state peak serum theophylline concentration will be <10 mcg/mL in about 30% of patients, 10–20 mcg/mL in about 50% and 20–30 mcg/mL in about 20% of patients. **The dose of theophylline must be individualized on the basis of peak serum theophylline concentration measurements in order to achieve a dose that will provide maximum potential benefit with minimal risk of adverse effects.**

Transient caffeine-like adverse effects and excessive serum concentrations in slow metabolizers can be avoided in most patients by starting with a sufficiently low dose and slowly increasing the dose, if judged to be clinically indicated, in small increments (See Table V). Dose increases should only be made if the previous dosage is well tolerated and at intervals of no less than 3 days to allow serum theophylline concentrations to reach the new steady-state. Dosage adjustment should be guided by serum theophylline concentration measurement (see PRECAUTIONS, Laboratory Tests and DOSAGE AND ADMINISTRATION, Table VI). Health care providers should instruct patients and care givers to discontinue any dosage that causes adverse effects, to withhold the medication until these symptoms are gone and to then resume therapy at a lower, previously tolerated dosage (see WARNINGS).

If the patient's symptoms are well controlled, there are no apparent adverse effects, and no intervening factors that might alter dosage requirements (see WARNINGS and PRECAUTIONS), serum theophylline concentrations should be monitored at 6 month intervals for rapidly growing children and at yearly intervals for all others. In acutely ill patients, serum theophylline concentrations should be monitored at frequent intervals, e.g., every 24 hours.

Theophylline distributes poorly into body fat, therefore, mg/kg dose should be calculated on the basis of ideal body weight.

Table V contains theophylline dosing titration schema recommended for patients in various age groups and clinical circumstances. Table VI contains recommendations for theophylline dosage adjustment based upon serum theophylline concentrations. **Application of these general dosing recommendations to individual patients must take into account the unique clinical characteristics of each patient. In general, these recommendations should serve as the upper limit for dosage adjustments in order to decrease the risk of potentially serious adverse events associated with unexpected large increases in serum theophylline concentration.**

Table V. Dosing initiation and titration (as anhydrous theophylline).*

A. Children (12–15 years) and adults (16–60 years) without risk factors for impaired clearance.

Titration Step	*Children < 45 kg*	*Children > 45 kg and adults*
1. Starting Dosage	12–14 mg/kg/day up to a maximum of 300 mg/day admin. QD*	300–400 mg/day† admin. QD*
2. After 3 days, if tolerated, increase dose to:	16 mg/kg/day up to a maximum of 400 mg/day admin. QD*	400–600 mg/day† admin. QD*

3. After 3 more days, if tolerated and if needed increase dose to:	20 mg/kg/day up to a maximum of 600 mg/day admin. QD*	As with all theophylline products, doses greater than 600 mg should be titrated according to blood level (See Table VI)

†If caffeine-like adverse effects occur, then consideration should be given to a lower dose and titrating the dose more slowly (see ADVERSE REACTIONS).

B. **Patients With Risk Factors For Impaired Clearance, The Elderly (>60 Years), And Those In Whom It Is Not Feasible To Monitor Serum Theophylline Concentrations:**
In children 12–15 years of age, the theophylline dose should not exceed 16 mg/kg/day up to a maximum of 400 mg/day in the presence of risk factors for reduced theophylline clearance (see WARNINGS) or if it is not feasible to monitor serum theophylline concentrations.
In adolescents ≥16 years and adults, including the elderly, the theophylline dose should not exceed 400 mg/day in the presence of risk factors for reduced theophylline clearance (see WARNINGS) or if it is not feasible to monitor serum theophylline concentrations.
*Patients with more rapid metabolism clinically identified by higher than average dose requirements, should receive a smaller dose more frequently (every 12 hours) to prevent breakthrough symptoms resulting from low trough concentrations before the next dose.

Table VI. Dosage adjustment guided by serum theophylline concentration.

Peak Serum Concentration	Dosage Adjustment
<9.9 mcg/mL	If symptoms are not controlled and current dosage is tolerated, increase dose about 25%. Recheck serum concentration after three days for further dosage adjustment.
10–14.9 mcg/mL	If symptoms are controlled and current dosage is tolerated, maintain dose and recheck serum concentration at 6–12 month intervals.¶ If symptoms are not controlled and current dosage is tolerated consider adding additional medication(s) to treatment regimen.
15–19.9 mcg/mL	Consider 10% decrease in dose to provide greater margin of safety even if current dosage is tolerated.¶
20–24.9 mcg/mL	Decrease dose by 25% even if no adverse effects are present. Recheck serum concentration after 3 days to guide further dosage adjustment.
25–30 mcg/mL	Skip next dose and decrease subsequent doses at least 25% even if no adverse effects are present. Recheck serum concentration after 3 days to guide further dosage adjustment. If symptomatic, consider whether overdose treatment is indicated (see recommendations for chronic overdosage).
>30 mcg/mL	Treat overdose as indicated (see recommendations for chronic overdosage). If theophylline is subsequently resumed, decrease dose by at least 50% and recheck serum concentration after 3 days to guide further dosage adjustment.

¶ Dose reduction and/or serum theophylline concentration measurement is indicated whenever adverse effects are present, physiologic abnormalities that can reduce theophylline clearance occur (e.g., sustained fever), or a drug that interacts with theophylline is added or discontinued (see WARNINGS).

HOW SUPPLIED

Uniphyl® (theophylline, anhydrous) 400 mg Controlled-Release Tablets are supplied in white-opaque plastic bottles containing 100 tablets (NDC 0034-7004-80) or 500 tablets (NDC 0034-7004-70).
Each round, white, scored 400 mg tablet bears the symbol PF on one side and is marked U400 on the other side.
Uniphyl® (theophylline, anhydrous) 600 mg Controlled-Release Tablets are supplied in white-opaque plastic bottles containing 100 tablets (NDC 0034-7006-80).
Each rectangular, concave, white 600 mg scored tablet bears the symbol PF on one side and is marked U600 on the other side.
Store at controlled room temperature 15°–30°C (59°–86°F).
Dispense in tight, light-resistant container.
The Purdue Frederick Company
Stamford, CT 06901-3431

U.S. Patent Number 4,366,310
June 9, 2000 S1374
Shown in Product Identification Guide, page 332

EDUCATIONAL MATERIAL

www.senokot.com provides dosing information for the Senokot® products family of laxatives, as well as patient education about constipation and its causes. A special section on toilet training, written by a pediatrician, describes the popular child-centered approach.

Medication-Induced Constipation continuing education program for pharmacists. Available at www.powerpak.com

Website containing pain management information for healthcare professionals and patients. Available at www.partnersagainstpain.com

EDUCATIONAL MATERIAL

Laxative Protocol Sheets (00PS77) 1 page (pad of 25)
Available to physicians, nurses and pharmacists

Purdue Pharma L.P.

ONE STAMFORD FORUM
STAMFORD, CT 06901-3431

For Medical Inquiries:
888-726-7535
Adverse Drug Experiences:
888-726-7535
Customer Service:
800-877-5666
FAX 800-877-3210

MS Contin® Tablets—see listing under The Purdue Frederick Company, page 2680

MSIR® Capsules—see listing under The Purdue Frederick Company, page 2683

MSIR® Tablets—see listing under The Purdue Frederick Company, page 2683

MSIR® Liquid—see listing under The Purdue Frederick Company, page 2683

CHIROCAINE® ℞
[*kī′-rō-kān*]
Levobupivacaine Injection

DESCRIPTION

Chirocaine (levobupivacaine injection) contains a single enantiomer of bupivacaine hydrochloride which is chemically described as (S)-1-butyl-2-piperidylformo-2′, 6′-xylidide hydrochloride and it is related chemically and pharmacologically to the amino amide class of local anesthetics.
Levobupivacaine hydrochloride, the S-enantiomer of bupivacaine, is a white crystalline powder with a molecular formula of $C_{18}H_{28}N_2O \cdot HCl$, a molecular weight of 324.9, and with the following structural formula:

* -indicates the chiral center

The solubility of levobupivacaine hydrochloride in water is about 100 mg per mL at 20°C, the partition coefficient (oleyl alcohol/water) is 1624 and the pKa is 8.09. The pKa of levobupivacaine hydrochloride is the same as that of bupivacaine hydrochloride and the partition coefficient is very similar to that of bupivacaine hydrochloride (1565).

Chirocaine is a sterile, non-pyrogenic, colorless solution (pH 4.0–6.5) containing levobupivacaine hydrochloride equivalent to 2.5 mg/mL, 5.0 mg/mL, and 7.5 mg/mL of levobupivacaine, sodium chloride for isotonicity, and Water for Injection. Sodium hydroxide and/or hydrochloric acid may have been added to adjust pH. Chirocaine is preservative free and is available in 10 mL and 30 mL single dose vials.

CLINICAL PHARMACOLOGY

Mechanism of Action

Chirocaine® is a member of the amino amide class of local anesthetics. Local anesthetics block the generation and the conduction of nerve impulses by increasing the threshold for electrical excitation in the nerve, by slowing propagation of the nerve impulse, and by reducing the rate of rise of the action potential. In general, the progression of anesthesia is related to the diameter, myelination, and conduction velocity of affected nerve fibers. Clinically, the order of loss of nerve function is as follows: 1) pain, 2) temperature, 3) touch, 4) proprioception, and 5) skeletal muscle tone.

Pharmacokinetics

[See table 1 below]
After IV infusion of equivalent doses of levobupivacaine and bupivacaine, the mean clearance, volume of distribution, and terminal half-life values of levobupivacaine and bupivacaine were similar. No detectable levels of R (+)-bupivacaine were found after the administration of levobupivacaine.
A comparison of the estimates for plasma AUC and C_{max} between Chirocaine and bupivacaine in two Phase III clinical trials involving short duration administration of either agent found that neither total plasma exposure or C_{max} differed between the two drugs when compared within studies. Between study values differed somewhat, likely due to differences in the injection sites, volume, and total dose administered in each of the studies. These data suggest that Chirocaine and bupivacaine have a similar pharmacokinetic profile. Pharmacokinetic data from two Phase III studies are presented below:
[See table 2 at top of next page]
Between 0.5% and 0.75% levobupivacaine given epidurally at doses of 75 mg and 112.5 mg respectively, the mean C_{max} and AUC_{0-24} of levobupivacaine were approximately dose-proportional. Similarly, between 0.25% and 0.5% levobupivacaine used for brachial plexus block at doses of 1 mg/kg and 2 mg/kg respectively, the mean C_{max} and AUC_{0-24} of levobupivacaine were approximately dose-proportional.

Absorption

The plasma concentration of levobupivacaine following therapeutic administration depends on dose and also on route of administration, because absorption from the site of administration is affected by the vascularity of the tissue. Peak levels in blood were reached approximately 30 minutes after epidural administration, and doses up to 150 mg resulted in mean C_{max} levels of up to 1.2 µg/mL.

Distribution

Plasma protein binding of levobupivacaine evaluated *in vitro* was found to be >97% at concentrations between 0.1 and 1 µg/mL. The association of levobupivacaine with human blood cells was very low (0–2%) over the concentration range 0.01–1 µg/mL and increased to 32% at 10 µg/mL. The volume of distribution of levobupivacaine after intravenous administration was 67 liters.

Metabolism

Levobupivacaine is extensively metabolized with no unchanged levobupivacaine detected in urine or feces. *In vitro* studies using [^{14}C]levobupivacaine showed that CYP3A4 isoform and CYP1A2 isoform mediate the metabolism of levobupivacaine to desbutyl levobupivacaine and 3-hydroxy levobupivacaine, respectively. *In vivo*, the 3-hydroxy levobupivacaine appears to undergo further transformation to glucuronide and sulfate conjugates. Metabolic inversion of levobupivacaine to R(+)-bupivacaine was not evident both *in vitro* and *in vivo*.

Elimination

Following intravenous administration, recovery of the radiolabelled dose of levobupivacaine was essentially quantitative with a mean total of about 95% being recovered in urine and feces in 48 hours. Of this 95%, about 71% was in urine while 24% was in feces. The mean elimination half-life of total radioactivity in plasma was 3.3 hours. The mean clearance and terminal half-life of levobupivacaine after intravenous infusion were 39 liters/hour and 1.3 hours, respectively.

Continued on next page

Table 1. Pharmacokinetic parameter values of levobupivacaine after the administration of 40 mg levobupivacaine, and those of racemic bupivacaine, R(+)- and S(-)- enantiomers after the administration of 40 mg of bupivacaine intravenously in healthy volunteers (mean ± SD).

Parameter	Levobupivacaine	Bupivacaine Racemate	R(+)-bupivacaine	S(-)-bupivacaine
C_{max}, µg/mL	1.445 ± 0.237	1.421 ± 0.224	0.629 ± 0.100	0.794 ± 0.131
$AUC_{0-\infty}$, µg hour/mL	1.153 ± 0.447	1.166 ± 0.400	0.478 ± 0.166	0.715 ± 0.261
$t_{1/2}$, hour	1.27 ± 0.37	1.15 ± 0.41	1.08 ± 0.17	1.34 ± 0.44
V_d, Liter	66.91 ± 18.23	59.97 ± 17.65	68.58 ± 21.02	56.73 ± 15.14
Cl, Liter/hour	39.06 ± 13.29	38.12 ± 12.64	46.72 ± 16.07	46.72 ± 16.07

Chirocaine—Cont.

Special Populations

Elderly: The limited data available indicate that while there are some differences in T_{max}, C_{max} and AUC with regards to age (between age groups of <65, 65–75, and >75 years), these differences are small and vary depending on the site of administration.

Gender: The small number of subjects in either of the male and female groups and the different routes of administration (data could not be pooled) in the different studies did not permit the assessment of gender differences in the pharmacokinetics of levobupivacaine.

Pediatrics: No pharmacokinetic data of levobupivacaine are available in the pediatric population.

Maternal/Fetal Ratio: The ratio of umbilical venous and maternal concentration of levobupivacaine ranged from 0.252–0.303 after the epidural administration of levobupivacaine for cesarean section. These are within the range normally seen for bupivacaine.

Nursing Mothers: It is known that some local anesthetic drugs are excreted in human milk and caution should be exercised when they are administered to a nursing woman. The excretion of levobupivacaine or its metabolites in human milk has not been studied (see PRECAUTIONS).

Renal Failure: No special studies were conducted in renal failure patients. Unchanged levobupivacaine is not excreted in the urine. Although there is no evidence that levobupivacaine accumulates in patients with renal failure, some of its metabolites may accumulate because they are primarily excreted by the kidney.

Hepatic Failure: No special studies were conducted in hepatic failure patients. Levobupivacaine is eliminated primarily by hepatic metabolism and changes in hepatic function may have significant consequences. Levobupivacaine should be used with caution in patients with severe hepatic disease, and repeated doses may need to be reduced due to delayed elimination.

Drug-Drug Interactions: In vitro studies showed that morphine, fentanyl, clonidine, and sufentanil are not likely to have an inhibitory effect on the oxidative metabolism of levobupivacaine. However, none of these tested compounds was an inhibitor of the CYP3A4 or CYP1A2 isoforms. Although no clinical studies have been conducted, it is likely that the metabolism of levobupivacaine may be affected by the known CYP3A4 inducers (such as phenytoin, phenobarbital, rifampin), CYP3A4 inhibitors (azole antimycotics e.g., ketoconazole; certain protease inhibitors e.g., ritonavir; macrolide antibiotics e.g., erythromycin; and calcium channel antagonists e.g., verapamil), CYP1A2 inducers (omeprazole) and CYP1A2 inhibitors (furafylline and clarithromycin).

Relative Potency

The relative potency of Chirocaine compared to bupivacaine has not been established.

Pharmacodynamics

Chirocaine® can be expected to share the pharmacodynamic properties of other local anesthetics. Systemic absorption of local anesthetics can produce effects on the central nervous and cardiovascular systems. At blood concentrations achieved with therapeutic doses, changes in cardiac conduction, excitability, refractoriness, contractility, and peripheral vascular resistance have been reported. Toxic blood concentrations depress cardiac conduction and excitability, which may lead to atrioventricular block, ventricular arrhythmias, and cardiac arrest, sometimes resulting in death. In addition, myocardial contractility is depressed and peripheral vasodilation occurs, leading to decreased cardiac output and arterial blood pressure.

Following systemic absorption, local anesthetics can produce central nervous system stimulation, depression, or both. Apparent central nervous system stimulation is usually manifested as restlessness, tremors, and shivering, progressing to convulsions. Ultimately central nervous system depression may progress to coma and cardio-respiratory arrest. However, the local anesthetics have a primary depressant effect on the medulla and on higher centers. The depressed stage may occur without a prior excited stage.

In nonclinical pharmacology studies comparing Chirocaine and bupivacaine in animal species, both the CNS and the cardiac toxicity of Chirocaine were less than that of bupivacaine. Arrhythmogenic effects were seen in animals at higher doses of Chirocaine than bupivacaine. Animal data comparing the difficulty of resuscitation from levobupivacaine- and bupivacaine-induced arrhythmia are not available. Central nervous system toxicity occurred with both drugs at lower doses and at lower plasma concentrations than those doses and plasma concentrations associated with cardiotoxicity.

In two intravenous infusion studies in conscious sheep, the convulsive doses of levobupivacaine were found to be significantly higher than for bupivacaine. Following repeated intravenous bolus administration mean (± SD) convulsive doses for levobupivacaine and bupivacaine were 9.7 (7.9) mg/kg and 6.1 (3.4) mg/kg respectively. The associated median total serum concentrations were 3.2 µg/mL and 1.6 µg/mL. In a second study following a 3 minute intravenous infusion the mean convulsant dose (95% CI) for levobupivacaine was 101 mg (87–116 mg) and for bupivacaine 79 mg (72–87 mg).

A study in human volunteers was designed to assess the effects of Chirocaine and bupivacaine on the EEG following an intravenous dose (40 mg) that was predicted to be below the threshold to cause CNS symptoms. In this study, levobupivacaine decreased high alpha power in the parietal, temporal and occipital regions, but to a lesser extent than bupivacaine. Levobupivacaine had no effect on high alpha power in the frontal and central regions, nor did it produce the increase in theta power observed at some electrodes following bupivacaine.

Table 2. Pharmacokinetic parameter values of levobupivacaine and bupivacaine in patients administered the respective drugs epidurally and for brachial plexus block.

Route	Epidural			Brachial Plexus Block		
	Levobupivacaine		Bupivacaine	Levobupivacaine		Bupivacaine
Concentration (%)	**0.50**	**0.75**	**0.50**	**0.25**	**0.50**	**0.50**
Dose received	**75mg**	**112.5mg**	**75mg**	**1 mg/kg**	**2 mg/kg**	**2 mg/kg**
n	9	9	8	10	10	9
C_{max} (µ/mL)	0.582	0.811	0.414	0.474	0.961	1.029
T_{max} (h)	0.52	0.44	0.36	0.50	0.71	0.68
$AUC_{(0\text{-}t)}$ (µg.h/mL)	3.561	4.930	2.044	2.999	5.311	6.832

In another study, 14 subjects received Chirocaine or bupivacaine infusions intravenously until significant CNS symptoms occurred (occurrence of numbness of the tongue, lightheadedness, tinnitus, dizziness, blurred vision, or muscle (twitching). The mean dose at which CNS symptoms occurred was 56 mg (range 17.5–150 mg) for Chirocaine and 48 mg (range 22.5–110 mg) for bupivacaine; this difference did not reach statistical significance. The primary endpoints of the study were cardiac contractility and standard electrocardiograph parameters. Although some differences were seen between treatments, the clinical relevance of these is unknown.

CLINICAL TRIALS

The clinical trial program included 1220 patients and subjects who received Chirocaine in 31 clinical trials. Chirocaine has been studied as a local anesthetic in adults administered as an epidural block for surgical cases, including cesarean section; in peripheral neural blockade; and for post-operative pain control. Although relative potency has not been established, clinical trials have demonstrated that Chirocaine and bupivacaine exhibit similar anesthetic effects (see CLINICAL PHARMACOLOGY; Relative Potency).

Central Administration

Epidural Administration in Cesarean Section

In one study, Chirocaine and bupivacaine, 0.50%, were evaluated as an epidural block in 62 patients undergoing cesarean section in a randomized, double-blind comparative trial. The mean (± S.D.) time to sensory block measured at T4 to T6 was 10 ± 8 minutes for Chirocaine and 6 ± 4 minutes for bupivacaine. The mean duration of sensory and motor block was 8 ± 1 and 4 ± 1 hours for Chirocaine and 7 ±1 and 4 ± 1 hours for bupivacaine, respectively. Ninety-four percent of patients receiving Chirocaine and 100% of patients receiving bupivacaine achieved a block adequate for surgery. In a second bupivacaine-controlled cesarean section study involving 62 patients, the mean time to onset of T4 to T6 sensory block for Chirocaine and bupivacaine was 10 ± 7 minutes and 9 ± 7 minutes, respectively, with 94% of Chirocaine patients and 91% of bupivacaine patients achieving a bilateral block adequate for surgery. The mean time to complete regression of sensory block was 8 ± 2 hours for both treatments.

Epidural Administration During Labor and Delivery

Chirocaine 0.25% was evaluated as intermittent injections via an epidural catheter in 68 patients during labor in a randomized double-blind comparative trial to bupivacaine 0.25%. The median duration of pain relief in the subset of patients receiving 0.25% Chirocaine who had relief was 49 minutes; for bupivacaine patients the median duration was 51 minutes. Following the first top-up injections, 91% of patients receiving Chirocaine and 90% of patients receiving bupivacaine achieved pain relief.

Epidural Administration for Surgery

Chirocaine® concentrations of 0.50% and 0.75% administered by epidural injection were evaluated in 85 patients undergoing lower limb or major abdominal surgery in randomized, double-blind comparisons to bupivacaine. Anesthesia sufficient for surgery was achieved in almost all patients on either treatment. In patients having abdominal surgery, the mean (± S.D.) time to onset of sensory block was 14 ± 6 minutes for Chirocaine and 14 ± 10 minutes for bupivacaine. With respect to the duration of block, the time to complete regression was 551 ± 88 minutes for Chirocaine and 506 ± 71 minutes for bupivacaine.

Post-operative Pain Management

Post-operative pain control was evaluated in 258 patients in three studies including one dose-ranging study and two studies assessing Chirocaine in combination with epidural fentanyl or clonidine. The dose ranging study evaluated Chirocaine in patients undergoing orthopedic surgery; the highest concentration, 0.25%, was significantly more effective than lower concentrations. The Chirocaine combination studies in post-operative pain management tested 0.125% Chirocaine in combination with 4 µg/mL fentanyl and 0.125% Chirocaine in combination with clonidine 50 µg/hour in orthopedic surgery. In these studies, the efficacy variable was time to first request for rescue analgesia during the 24 hour epidural infusion period. In both studies, the combination treatment provided better pain control than clonidine, opioid or local anesthetic alone.

Peripheral Nerve Administration

Chirocaine has been evaluated for its anesthetic efficacy when used as a peripheral nerve block. These clinical trials included brachial plexus (by supraclavicular approach) block study, infiltration anesthesia studies (for inguinal hernia repair), peribulbar block studies.

Brachial Plexus Block

Chirocaine 0.25% and 0.5% were compared with 0.5% bupivacaine in 74 patients receiving a brachial plexus (supraclavicular) block for elective surgery. In the Chirocaine 0.25% treated group 68% of patients achieved satisfactory block and in the Chirocaine 0.5% treated group, 81% of patients achieved satisfactory block for surgery. In the bupivacaine 0.5% treated group, 74% of patients achieved satisfactory block for surgery.

Infiltration Anesthesia

Chirocaine 0.25% was evaluated in 68 patients in two randomized, double-blind, bupivacaine-controlled clinical trials for infiltration anesthesia during surgery and for post-operative pain management in patients undergoing inguinal hernia repair. No clear differences between the treatments were seen.

Peribulbar Block Anesthesia

Two clinical trials were conducted to evaluate 0.75% Chirocaine and bupivacaine in 110 patients for peribulbar block for anterior segment ophthalmic surgery, including cataract, glaucoma, and graft surgery, and for post-operative pain management. In one study, a 10 mL injection of 0.75% Chirocaine or bupivacaine produced a block adequate for surgery at a median time of 10 minutes. In the second study, a 5 mL dose of 0.75% Chirocaine or bupivacaine injected in a technique more closely resembling a retrobulbar block resulted in a median time to adequate block of 2 minutes for both treatments. Post-operative pain was reported in fewer than 10% of patients overall.

INDICATIONS AND USAGE

Chirocaine is indicated for the production of local or regional anesthesia for surgery and obstetrics, and for post-operative pain management.

Surgical Anesthesia: Epidural, peripheral neural blockade; and local infiltration.

Pain Mangement: continuous epidural infusion or intermittent epidural neural blockade; continuous or intermittent peripheral neural blockade or local infiltration.

For continuous epidural analgesia, Chirocaine may be administered in combination with epidural fentanyl or clonidine.

CONTRAINDICATIONS

Chirocaine is contraindicated in patients with a known hypersensitivity to Chirocaine or to any local anesthetic agent of the amide type.

WARNINGS

IN PERFORMING CHIROCAINE® BLOCKS, UNINTENDED INTRAVENOUS INJECTION IS POSSIBLE AND MAY RESULT IN CARDIAC ARREST. DESPITE RAPID DETECTION AND APPROPRIATE TREATMENT, PROLONGED RESUSCITATION MAY BE REQUIRED. THE RESUSCITABILITY RELATIVE TO BUPIVACAINE IS UNKNOWN AT THIS POINT IN TIME AS IT HAS NOT BEEN STUDIED. AS WITH ALL LOCAL ANESTHETICS OF THE AMIDE TYPE, CHIROCAINE SHOULD BE ADMINISTERED IN INCREMENTAL DOSES. SINCE CHIROCAINE SHOULD NOT BE INJECTED RAPIDLY IN LARGE DOSES, IT IS NOT RECOMMENDED FOR EMERGENCY SITUATIONS, WHERE A FAST ONSET OF SURGICAL ANESTHESIA IS NECESSARY.

HISTORICALLY, PREGNANT PATIENTS WERE REPORTED TO HAVE A HIGH RISK FOR CARDIAC ARRHYTHMIAS, CARDIAC/CIRCULATORY ARREST AND DEATH WHEN BUPIVACAINE WAS INADVERTENTLY RAPIDLY INJECTED INTRAVENOUSLY. AVOID 0.75% CHIROCAINE IN OBSTETRICAL PATIENTS. THIS CONCENTRATION IS INDICATED ONLY FOR NON-OBSTETRICAL SURGERY REQUIRING PROFOUND MUSCLE RELAXATION AND LONG DURATION. FOR CESAREAN SECTION, THE 5 MG/ML (0.5%) CHIROCAINE SOLUTION IN DOSES UP TO 150 MG IS RECOMMENDED.

LOCAL ANESTHETICS SHOULD ONLY BE ADMINISTERED BY CLINICIANS WHO ARE WELL VERSED IN THE DIAGNOSIS AND MANAGEMENT OF DRUG-RELATED TOXICITY AND OTHER ACUTE EMERGENCIES WHICH MIGHT ARISE FROM THE BLOCK BEING ADMINISTERED. THE IMMEDIATE AVAILABILITY OF OXYGEN, OTHER RESUSCITATIVE DRUGS, CARDIOPULMONARY RESUSCITATIVE EQUIPMENT, AND THE PERSONNEL RESOURCES NEEDED FOR PROPER MANAGEMENT OF TOXIC REACTIONS AND RELATED EMERGENCIES MUST BE ENSURED. (see also **ADVERSE REACTIONS** and **PRECAUTIONS**). DELAY IN PROPER MANAGEMENT OF DRUG-RELATED TOXICITY, UNDERVENTILATION FROM ANY CAUSE, AND/OR

ALTERED SENSITIVITY MAY LEAD TO THE DEVELOPMENT OF ACIDOSIS, CARDIAC ARREST, AND POSSIBLY DEATH.

SOLUTIONS OF CHIROCAINE SHOULD NOT BE USED FOR THE PRODUCTION OF OBSTETRICAL PARACERVICAL BLOCK ANESTHESIA. THERE ARE NO DATA TO SUPPORT SUCH USE AND THERE IS THE ADDITIONAL RISK OF FETAL BRADYCARDIA AND DEATH.

INTRAVENOUS REGIONAL ANESTHESIA (BIER BLOCK) SHOULD NOT BE PERFORMED USING CHIROCAINE BECAUSE OF THE LACK OF CLINICAL EXPERIENCE AND THE RISK OF ATTAINING TOXIC BLOOD LEVELS OF LEVOBUPIVACAINE.

It is essential that aspiration for blood or cerebrospinal fluid (where applicable), be done prior to injecting ay local anesthetic, both before the original dose and all subsequent doses, to avoid intravascular or intrathecal injection. However, a negative aspiration does *not* ensure against intravascular or intrathecal injection. Chirocaine should be used with caution in patients receiving other local anesthetics or agents structurally related to amide-type local anesthetics, since the toxic effects of these drugs are additive.

When contemplating a peripheral nerve block, where large volumes of local anesthetic are needed, caution should be exercised when using the higher mg/mL concentrations of Chirocaine. Animal studies demonstrate CNS and cardiac toxicity that is dose related, thus equal volumes of higher concentration will be more likely to produce cardiac toxicity.

PRECAUTIONS

General

The safe and effective use of local anesthetics depends on proper dosage, correct technique, adequate precautions, and readiness for emergencies.

Resuscitative equipment, oxygen, and resuscitative drugs should be available for immediate use (see **WARNINGS** and **ADVERSE REACTIONS**). The lowest dosage that results in effective anesthesia should be used to avoid high plasma or dermatomal levels and serious adverse effects. Injections should be made slowly and incrementally, with frequent aspirations before and during the injection to avoid intravascular injection. When a continuous catheter technique is used, syringe aspirations should also be performed before and during each supplemental injection. During the administration of epidural anesthesia, it is recommended that a test dose of a local anesthetic with a fast onset be administered initially and that the patint be monitored for central nervous system and cardiovascular toxicity, as well as for signs of unintended intrathecal administration before proceeding. When clinical conditions permit, consideration should be given to employing local anesthetic solutions that contain epinephrine for the test dose because circulatory changes compatible with epinephrine may also serve as a warning sign of unintended intravascular injection. An intravascular injection is still possible even if aspirations for blood are negative.

Injection of repeated doses of local anesthetics may cause significant increases in plasma levels with each repeated dose due to slow accumulation of the drug or its metabolites or to slow metabolic degradation. Tolerance to elevated blood levels varies with the physical condition of the patient. Local anesthetics should also be used with caution in patients with hypotension, hypovolemia, or impaired cardiovascular function, especially heart block.

Careful and constant monitoring of cardiovascular and respiratory vital signs (adequacy of ventilation) and the patient's state of consciousness should be performed after each local anesthetic injection. The clinician must be aware that restlessness, anxiety, incoherent speech, lightheadedness, numbness and tingling of the mouth and lips, metallic taste, tinnitus, dizziness, blurred vision, tremors, twitching, depression, or drowsiness may be early warning signs of central nervous system toxicity.

Amide-type local anesthetics such as Chirocaine are metabolized by the liver, therefore these drugs, especially repeat doses, should be used cautiously in patients with hepatic disease. Patients with severe hepatic disease, because of their inability to metabolize local anesthetics normally, are at a greater risk for developing toxic plasma concentrations. Local anesthetics should also be used with caution in patients with impaired cardiovascular function as they may be less able to compensate for functional changes associated with prolonged A-V conduction caused by these drugs.

Many drugs used during the conduct of anesthesia are considered potential triggering agents for malignant hyperthermia. Amide-type local anesthetics are not known to trigger this reaction.

Epidural Anesthesia

During epidural administration, Chirocaine should be administered in incremental volumes of 3 to 5 mL with sufficient time between doses to detect toxic manifestations of unintentional intravascular or intrathecal injection. Syringe aspirations should also be performed before and during each supplemental injection in continuous catheter techniques. An intravascular injection is still possible even if aspirations for blood are negative. During the administration of epidural anesthesia, it is recommended that a test dose is administered initially and the effects monitored before the full dose is given. A test dose of a short-acting amide anesthetic, such as 3 mL of lidocaine, is recommended to detect unintentional intrathecal administration. This will be manifested within a few minutes by signs of a subarachnoid block (e.g., decreased sensation of the buttocks, paresis of the legs or, in the sedated patient, absent knee jerk). Unintentional intrathecal injection of local anesthetics can lead to very high spinal anesthesia, possibly apnea, severe hypotension and loss of consciousness. An intravascular or intrathecal injection is still possible even if the results of the test dose are negative. The test dose itself may produce a systemic toxic reaction, extensive subarachnoid block, or cardiovascular effects.

ADVERSE EVENTS REPORTED WITH AN INCIDENCE OF ≥ 1% IN THE PHASE II/III BUPIVACAINE-CONTROLLED STUDIES

Event	Levobupivacaine N=509		Bupivacaine N=453	
	N	(%)	N	(%)
Hypotension	100	(19.6)	93	(20.5)
Nausea	59	(11.6)	66	(14.6)
Anemia	49	(9.6)	37	(8.2)
Post-operative Pain	37	(7.3)	37	(8.2)
Vomiting	42	(8.3)	30	(6.6)
Back Pain	29	(5.7)	19	(4.2)
Fever	33	(6.5)	35	(7.7)
Dizziness	26	(5.1)	22	(4.9)
Fetal Distress	49	(9.6)	41	(9.1)
Headache	23	(4.5)	18	(4.0)
Delivery Delayed	32	(6.3)	31	(6.8)
Pruritus	19	(3.7)	26	(5.7)
Pain	18	(3.5)	17	(3.8)
ECG Abnormal	16	(3.1)	17	(3.8)
Abdomen Enlarged	15	(2.9)	12	(2.6)
Albuminuria	15	(2.9)	6	(1.3)
Rigors	15	(2.9)	12	(2.6)
Constipation	14	(2.8)	20	(4.4)
Diplopia	13	(2.6)	14	(3.1)
Hypoesthesia	13	(2.6)	15	(3.3)
Flatulence	12	(2.4)	11	(2.4)
Abdominal Pain	11	(2.2)	6	(1.3)
Hypothermia	11	(2.2)	6	(1.3)
Bradycardia	11	(2.2)	10	(2.2)
Dyspepsia	10	(2.0)	11	(2.4)
Hematuria	10	(2.0)	5	(1.1)
Hemorrhage in Pregnancy	9	(1.8)	12	(2.6)
Paresthesia	9	(1.8)	2	(0.4)
Tachycardia	9	(1.8)	7	(1.5)
Urine Abnormal	9	(1.8)	6	(1.3)
Purpura	7	(1.4)	4	(0.9)
Wound Drainage Increased	7	(1.4)	13	(2.9)
Coughing	6	(1.2)	3	(0.7)
Leukocytosis	6	(1.2)	3	(0.7)
Somnolence	6	(1.2)	4	(0.9)
Urinary Incontinence	6	(1.2)	1	(0.2)
Anesthesia Local	5	(1.0)	5	(1.1)
Anxiety	5	(1.0)	6	(1.3)
Breast Pain (Female)	5	(1.0)	4	(0.9)
Hypertension	5	(1.0)	8	(1.8)
Urine Flow Decreased	5	(1.0)	3	(0.7)
Urinary Tract Infection	5	(1.0)	3	(0.7)
Diarrhea	5	(1.0)	6	(1.3)

Use in Head and Neck Area

Small doses of local anesthetics injected into the head and neck area may produce adverse reactions similar to systemic toxicity seen with unintentional intravascular injections of larger doses. The injection procedures require the utmost care. Confusion, convulsions, respiratory depression, and/or respiratory arrest and cardiovascular stimulation or depression have been reported. These reactions may be due to intraarterial injection of the local anesthetic with retrograde flow to the cerebral circulation. Patients receiving these blocks should have their respirations and circulation monitored and be constantly observed. Resuscitative equipment and personnel for treating adverse reactions should be immediately available. Dosage recommendations should not be exceeded (see **DOSAGE AND ADMINISTRATION**).

Information for Patients

When appropriate, patients should be informed in advance that they may experience temporary loss of sensation and

Continued on next page

Chirocaine—Cont.

motor activity in the anesthetized part of the body following correct administration of regional anesthesia. Also, when appropriate, the physician should discuss other information including adverse reactions in the Chirocaine package insert.

Clinically Significant Drug-Drug Interactions
Chirocaine® should be used with caution in patients receiving other local anesthetics or agents structurally related to amide-type local anesthetics since the toxic effects of these drugs could be additive. *In vitro* studies indicate CYP3A4 isoform and CYP1A2 isoform mediate the metabolism of levobupivacaine to desbutyl levobupivacaine and 3-hydroxy levobupivacaine, respectively. Thus agents likely to be concomitantly administered with Chirocaine that are metabolized by this isoenzyme family may potentially interact with Chirocaine. Although no clinical studies have been conducted, it is likely that the metabolism of levobupivacaine may be affected by the known CYP3A4 inducers (such as phenytoin, phenobarbital, rifampin), CYP3A4 inhibitors (azole antimycotics e.g., ketoconazole; certain protease inhibitors e.g., ritanovir; macrolide antibiotics e.g., erythromycin; and calcium channel antagonists e.g., verapamil), CYP1A2 inducers (omeprazole) and CYP1A2 inhibitors (furafylline and clarithromycin). Dosage adjustment may be warranted when levobupivacaine is concurrently administered with CYP3A4 inhibitors and CYP1A2 inhibitors as systemic levobupivacaine levels may rise resulting in toxicity.

Carcinogenesis, Mutagenesis, Impairment of Fertility
Long-term studies in animals of most local anesthetics, including Chirocaine, to evaluate the carcinogenic potential have not been conducted. Mutagenicity was not observed in bacterial mutation assay, mouse lymphoma cells mutation assay, chromosome aberrations in human blood lymphocytes, and micronuclei in the bone marrow of treated mice. Studies performed with Chirocaine in rats at 30 mg/kg/day (180 mg/m^2/day) did not demonstrate an effect on fertility or general reproductive performance over two generations. This dose is approximately one-half the maximum recommended human dose (570 mg/person) based on body surface area (352 mg/m^2).

Pregnancy Category B
Teratogenicity studies in rats (180 mg/m^2/day) and rabbits (220 mg/m^2/day) did not show evidence of any adverse effects on organogenesis or early fetal development. The doses used were approximately one-half the maximum recommended human dose (570 mg/person or 352 mg/m^2) based on body surface area. There were no treatment-related effects on late fetal development, parturition, lactation, neonatal viability, or growth of the offspring in a perinatal and postnatal study in rats at dose levels up to approximately one-half the maximum recommended human dose based on body surface area. There were no adequate and well-controlled studies in pregnant women of the effects of Chirocaine on the developing fetus. Chirocaine should only be used during pregnancy if the benefits outweigh the risks.

Labor and Delivery
Local anesthetics, including Chirocaine, rapidly cross the placenta, and, when used for epidural block, can cause varying degrees of maternal, fetal, and neonatal toxicity. The incidence and degree of toxicity depend upon the procedure performed, the type and amount of drug used, and the technique of drug administration. Adverse reactions in the parturient, fetus, and neonate involve alterations of the central nervous system, peripheral vascular tone, and cardiac function. Maternal hypotension, fetal bradycardia and fetal decelerations have resulted from regional anesthesia with Chirocaine for obstetrical pain relief. Local anesthetics produce vasodilation by blocking sympathetic nerves. Administration of intravenous fluids, elevation of the patient's legs and left uterine displacement will help prevent decreases in blood pressure. The fetal heart rate should also be monitored continuously and electronic fetal monitoring is highly advisable.

Nursing Mothers
Some local anesthetic drugs are excreted in human milk and caution should be exercised when Chirocaine is administered to a nursing woman. The excretion of Chirocaine or its metabolites in human milk has not been studied. Studies in rats demonstrated that small amounts of Chirocaine can be detected in the pups after administration of Chirocaine to the nursing mothers.

Pediatric Use
The safety and effectiveness of Chirocaine in pediatric patients have not been established.

Geriatric Use
Of the total number of subjects in clinical studies of Chirocaine, 16% were 65 and over, while 8% were 75 and over. No overall differences in safety or effectiveness were observed between these subjects and younger subjects, and other reported clinical experience has not identified differences in responses between the elderly and younger patients, but greater sensitivity of some older individuals cannot be ruled out.

ADVERSE REACTIONS

Reactions to Chirocaine are characteristic of those associated with other amide-type local anesthetics. A major cause of the adverse reactions to this group of drugs is associated with excessive plasma levels, or high dermatol levels, which may be due to overdose, unintentional intravascular injection, or slow metabolic degradation. The reported adverse events are derived from studies conducted in the United States and Europe. The reference drug was primarily bupivacaine. While the adverse event profile from clinical trials in patients was similar between the two drugs, their relative potency has not been established. The studies were conducted using a variety of premedications, sedatives, and surgical procedures of varying length. A total of 1220 patients were exposed to Chirocaine. Each patient was counted once for each type of adverse event.

In the Phase II/III studies, 78% of patients who received Chirocaine® reported at least one adverse event. Of those patients who received the 0.75% levobupivacaine concentration, 85% reported at least one adverse event.

Adverse events that occurred in >5% of all Chirocaine-treated patients in Phase II/III studies (N=1141) were hypotension (31%), nausea (21%), post-operative pain (18%), fever (17%), vomiting (14%), anemia (12%), pruritus (9%), pain (8%), headache (7%), constipation (7%), dizziness (6%), and fetal distress (5%).

[See table at top of previous page]

Dosage Recommendations

	% Concentration	Dose mL	Dose mg	Motor Block
Surgical Anesthesia				
Epidural for surgery	0.5-0.75	10-20	50-150	Moderate to complete
Epidural for Cesarean Section	0.5	20-30	100-150	Moderate to complete
Peripheral Nerve	0.25-0.5	30 0.4 mL/kg	75-150 1-2 mg/kg	Moderate to complete
Ophthalmic	0.75	5-15	37.5-112.5	Moderate to complete
Local Infiltration	0.25	60	150	Not applicable
Pain Management[a]				
Labor Analgesia (epidural bolus)	0.25	10-20	25-50	Minimal to moderate
Post-operative pain (epidural infusion)	0.125[b]-0.25[c]	4-10 mL/h	5-25 mg/h	Minimal to moderate

[a] In pain management Chirocaine® can be used epidurally with fentanyl or clonidine.
[b] 0.125% is to be used only as adjunct therapy in combination with fentanyl or clonidine.
[c] Dilutions of Chirocaine standard solutions should be made with preservative free 0.9% saline according to standard hospital procedures for sterility.

The following adverse events were reported during the Chirocaine clinical program in more than one patient, occurred at an overall incidence of <1%, and were considered clinically relevant:

Body as a Whole: asthenia, edema.
Cardiovascular Disorders, General: postural hypotension.
Central and Peripheral Nervous System Disorders: hypokinesia, involuntary muscle contraction, spasm (generalized), tremor, syncope.
Heart Rate and Rhythm Disorders: arrhythmia, extrasystoles, fibrillation (atrial), cardiac arrest.
Gastrointestinal System Disorders: ileus.
Liver and Biliary System Disorders: elevated bilirubin.
Psychiatric Disorders: confusion.
Respiratory System Disorders: apnea, bronchospasm, dyspnea, pulmonary edema, respiratory insufficiency.
Skin and Appendage Disorders: increased sweating, skin discoloration.

OVERDOSAGE

Acute emergencies from local anesthetics are generally related to high plasma levels or high dermatomal levels ("high spinal") encountered during therapeutic use of local anesthetics or to unintended intrathecal or intravascular injection of local anesthetic solution (see **ADVERSE REACTIONS, WARNINGS**, and **PRECAUTIONS**). There was one case of suspected unintentional intravascular injection which occurred during the clinical trial program. That patient received 19 mL of 0.75% levobupivacaine (142.5 mg) and experienced CNS excitation which was treated with thiopental. No abnormal cardiovascular changes were observed and the patient recovered without sequelae.

Management of Local Anesthetic Emergencies
The first consideration is prevention, best accomplished by incremental injection of Chirocaine, careful and constant monitoring of cardiovascular and respiratory vital signs and the patient's state of consciousness after each local anesthetic injection and during continuous infusion. At the first sign of change, oxygen should be administered.

The first step in the management of systemic toxic reactions, as well as under-ventilation or apnea due to unintentional subarachnoid injection of drug solution, consists of immediate attention to the establishment and maintenance of a patent airway and effective assisted or controlled ventilation with 100% oxygen with a delivery system capable of permitting immediate positive airway pressure by mask. This may prevent convulsions if they have not already occurred.

If necessary, use drugs to control convulsions. Intravenous barbiturates, anti-convulsant agents, or muscle relaxants should only be administered by those familiar with their use. Immediately after the institution of these ventilatory measures, the adequacy of the circulation should be evaluated. Supportive treatment of circulatory depression may require administration of intravenous fluids, and, when appropriate, a vasopressor dictated by the clinical situation (such as ephedrine or epinephrine to enhance myocardial contractile force).

If difficulty is encountered in the maintenance of a patent airway or if prolonged ventilatory support (assisted or controlled) is indicated, endotracheal intubation, employing drugs and techniques familiar to the clinician, may be indicated after initial administration of oxygen by mask.

The supine position is dangerous in pregnant women at term because of aortocaval compression by the gravid uterus. Therefore, during treatment of systemic toxicity, maternal hypotension or fetal bradycardia following regional block, the parturient should be maintained in the left lateral decubitus position if possible, or manual displacement of the uterus off the great vessels should be accomplished. Resuscitation of obstetrical patients may take longer than resuscitation of non-pregnant patients and closed-chest cardiac compression may be ineffective. Rapid delivery of the fetus may improve the response to resuscitation efforts.

DOSAGE AND ADMINISTRATION

The rapid injection of a large volume of local anesthetic solution should be avoided and fractional (incremental) doses should always be used. The smallest dose and concentration required to produce the desired result should be administered. The dose of any local anesthetic differs with the anesthetic procedure, the area to be anesthetized, the vascularity of the tissues, the number of neuronal segments to be blocked, the intensity of the block, the degree of muscle relaxation required, the duration of the anesthesia desired, individual tolerance, and the physical condition of the patient. Patients in poor general condition due to aging or other compromising factors such as impaired cardiovascular function, advanced liver disease, or severe renal dysfunction, require special attention.

To reduce the risk of potentially serious adverse reactions, attempts should be made to optimize the patient's condition before major blocks are performed, and the dosage should be adjusted accordingly. Use an adequate test dose (3–5 mL) of a short-acting local anesthetic solution containing epinephrine prior to induction of complete nerve block. This test dose should be repeated if the patient is moved in such a fashion as to have displaced the epidural catheter. It is recommended that adequate time be allowed for the onset of anesthesia following administration of each test dose.

Disinfecting agents containing heavy metals, which cause release of ions (mercury, zinc, copper, etc.), should not be used for skin or mucous membrane disinfection since they have been related to incidents of swelling and edema.

When chemical disinfection of the container surface is desired, either isopropyl alcohol (91%) or ethyl alcohol (70%) is recommended. It is recommended that chemical disinfection be accomplished by wiping the vial stopper thoroughly with cotton or gauze that has been moistened with the recommended alcohol just prior to use.

When a container is required to have a sterile outside, glass containers may be autoclaved once. Stability has been demonstrated following an autoclave cycle at 121°C for 15 minutes.

These products are intended for single use and do not contain preservatives; any solution remaining from an open container should be discarded.

For specific techniques and procedures, refer to standard contemporary textbooks.

Chirocaine Compatibility and Admixtures
Chirocaine may not be compatible with alkaline solutions having a pH greater than 8.5. Studies have shown that Chi-

rocaine is compatible with 0.9% Sodium Chloride Injection USP and with saline solutions containing fentanyl and clonidine. Compatibility studies with other parenteral products have not been studied.

Dilution Stability

Chirocaine® diluted in 0.9% Sodium Chloride Injection is physically and chemically stable when stored in PVC (polyvinyl chloride) bags at ambient room temperature for up to 24 hours. Aseptic techniques should be used to prepare the diluted product. Admixtures of Chirocaine should be prepared for single patient use only and used within 24 hours of preparation. The unused portion of diluted Chirocaine should be discarded after each use.

NOTE: Parenteral products should be inspected visually for particulate matter and discoloration prior to administration whenever solution and container permit. Solutions that are not clear and colorless should not be used.

[See table at top of previous page]

The doses in the table are those considered to be necessary to produce a successful block and should be regarded as guidelines for use in adults. Individual variations in onset and duration occur.

Epidural doses of up to 375 mg have been administered incrementally to patients during a surgical procedure.

The maximum dose in 24 hours for intraoperative block and post-operative pain management was 695 mg.

The maximum dose administered as a post-operative epidural infusion over 24 hours was 570 mg.

The maximum dose administered to patients as a single fractionated injection was 300 mg for brachial plexus block.

HOW SUPPLIED

Chirocaine, 2.5 mg levobupivacaine in each mL.
10 mL Single Use Vials. (NDC 59011-997-10)
30 mL Single Use Vials. (NDC 59011-997-30)
Chirocaine, 5.0 mg levobupivacaine in each mL.
10 mL Single Use Vials. (NDC 59011-998-10)
30 mL Single Use Vials. (NDC 59011-998-30)
Chirocaine, 7.5 mg levobupivacaine in each mL.
10 mL Single Use Vials. (NDC 59011-999-10)
30 mL Single Use Vials. (NDC 59011-999-30)

STORAGE

Store Chirocaine at controlled room temperature, 20–25°C (68–77°F), excursions permitted to 15–30°C (59–86°F).

Rx ONLY

Manufactured by
Ben Venue Laboratories, Inc.
Bedford, OH 44146
For
Purdue Pharma L.P.
Stamford, CT 06901-3431

Licensed under U.S. Patent Numbers:
5,708,011; 5,777,124; 5,786,484; 5,849,763; 5,919,804
June 9, 2000 C6246

Shown in Product Identification Guide, page 332

OXYCONTIN® Ⓒ℞

(OXYCODONE HCl CONTROLLED-RELEASE) TABLETS
10 mg 20 mg 40 mg 80 mg* 160 mg*

***80 mg and 160 mg For use in opioid tolerant patients only.**

DESCRIPTION

OxyContin® (oxycodone hydrochloride controlled-release) tablets are an opioid analgesic supplied in 10 mg, 20 mg, 40 mg, 80 mg, and 160 mg tablet strengths for oral administration. The tablet strengths describe the amount of oxycodone per tablet as the hydrochloride salt. The structural formula for oxycodone hydrochloride is as follows:

$C_{18}H_{21}NO_4 \cdot HCl$ MW 351.83

The chemical formula is 4, 5-epoxy-14-hydroxy-3-methoxy-17-methylmorphinan-6-one hydrochloride.

Oxycodone is a white, odorless crystalline powder derived from the opium alkaloid, thebaine. Oxycodone hydrochloride dissolves in water (1 g in 6 to 7 mL). It is slightly soluble in alcohol (octanol water partition coefficient 0.7). The tablets contain the following inactive ingredients: ammonio methacrylate copolymer, hydroxypropyl methylcellulose, lactose, magnesium stearate, povidone, red iron oxide (20 mg strength tablet only), stearyl alcohol, talc, titanium dioxide, triacetin, yellow iron oxide (40 mg strength tablet only), yellow iron oxide with FD&C blue No. 2 (80 mg strength tablet only), FD&C blue No. 2 (160 mg strength tablet only) and other ingredients.

OxyContin® 80 mg and 160 mg Tablets ARE FOR USE IN OPIOID TOLERANT PATIENTS ONLY.

CLINICAL PHARMACOLOGY

Central Nervous System

Oxycodone is a pure agonist opioid whose principal therapeutic action is analgesia. Other therapeutic effects of oxycodone include anxiolysis, euphoria and feelings of relaxation. Like all pure opioid agonists, there is no ceiling effect to analgesia, such as is seen with partial agonists or non-opioid analgesics.

The precise mechanism of the analgesic action is unknown. However, specific CNS opioid receptors for endogenous compounds with opioid-like activity have been identified throughout the brain and spinal cord and play a role in the analgesic effects of this drug.

Oxycodone produces respiratory depression by direct action on brain stem respiratory centers. The respiratory depression involves both a reduction in the responsiveness of the brain stem respiratory centers to increases in carbon dioxide tension and to electrical stimulation.

Oxycodone depresses the cough reflex by direct effect on the cough center in the medulla. Antitussive effects may occur with doses lower than those usually required for analgesia. Oxycodone causes miosis, even in total darkness. Pinpoint pupils are a sign of opioid overdose but are not pathognomonic. Marked mydriasis rather than miosis may be seen due to hypoxia in overdose situations.

Gastrointestinal Tract and Other Smooth Muscle

Oxycodone causes a reduction in motility associated with an increase in smooth muscle tone in the antrum of the stomach and duodenum. Digestion of food in the small intestine is delayed and propulsive contractions are decreased. Propulsive peristaltic waves in the colon are decreased, while tone may be increased to the point of spasm resulting in constipation. Other opioid-induced effects may include a reduction in gastric, biliary and pancreatic secretions, spasm of sphincter of Oddi, and transient elevations in serum amylase.

Cardiovascular System

Oxycodone may produce release of histamine with or without associated peripheral vasodilation. Manifestations of histamine release and/or peripheral vasodilation may include pruritus, flushing, red eyes, sweating, and/or orthostatic hypotension.

Concentration—Efficacy Relationships (Pharmacodynamics)

Studies in normal volunteers and patients reveal predictable relationships between oxycodone dosage and plasma oxycodone concentrations, as well as between concentration and certain expected opioid effects. In normal volunteers these include pupillary constriction, sedation and overall "drug effect" and in patients, analgesia and feelings of "relaxation." In non-tolerant patients, analgesia is not usually seen at a plasma oxycodone concentration of less than 5–10 ng/mL.

As with all opioids, the minimum effective plasma concentration for analgesia will vary widely among patients, especially among patients who have been previously treated with potent agonist opioids. As a result, patients need to be treated with individualized titration of dosage to the desired effect. The minimum effective analgesic concentration of oxycodone for any individual patient may increase with repeated dosing due to an increase in pain and/or the development of tolerance.

Concentration—Adverse Experience Relationships

OxyContin tablets are associated with typical opioid-related adverse experiences similar to those seen with immediate-release oxycodone and all opioids. There is a general relationship between increasing oxycodone plasma concentration and increasing frequency of dose-related opioid adverse experiences such as nausea, vomiting, CNS effects, and respiratory depression. In opioid-tolerant patients, the situation is altered by the development of tolerance to opioid-related side effects, and the relationship is poorly understood.

As with all opioids, the dose must be individualized (see **DOSAGE AND ADMINISTRATION**), because the effective analgesic dose for some patients will be too high to be tolerated by other patients.

PHARMACOKINETICS AND METABOLISM

The activity of OxyContin® (oxycodone hydrochloride controlled-release) tablets is primarily due to the parent drug oxycodone. OxyContin tablets are designed to provide controlled delivery of oxycodone over 12 hours. Oxycodone release from OxyContin tablets is pH independent. Oxycodone is well absorbed from OxyContin tablets with an oral bioavailability of from 60% to 87%. The relative oral bioavailability of OxyContin to immediate-release oral dosage forms is 100%. Upon repeated dosing in normal volunteers, steady-state levels were achieved within 24–36 hours. Dose proportionality and/or bioavailability has been established for the 10 mg, 20 mg, 40 mg, 80 mg, and 160 mg tablet strengths for both peak plasma levels (C_{max}) and extent of absorption (AUC). Oxycodone is extensively metabolized and eliminated primarily in the urine as both conjugated and unconjugated metabolites. The apparent elimination half-life of oxycodone following the administration of OxyContin was 4.5 hours compared to 3.2 hours for immediate-release oxycodone.

Absorption

About 60% to 87% of an oral dose of oxycodone reaches the central compartment in comparison to a parenteral dose. This high oral bioavailability is due to low pre-systemic and/or first-pass metabolism. In normal volunteers the t½ of absorption is 0.4 hours for immediate-release oral oxycodone. In contrast, OxyContin tablets exhibit a biphasic absorption pattern with two apparent absorption half-times of 0.6 and 6.9 hours, which describes the initial release of oxycodone from the tablet followed by a prolonged release.

Plasma Oxycodone By Time

Dose proportionality has been established for the 10 mg, 20 mg, 40 mg, and 80 mg tablet strengths for both peak plasma concentrations (C_{max}) and extent of absorption (AUC) (see Table 1 below). Another study established that the 160 mg tablet is bioequivalent to 2 × 80 mg tablets as well as to 4 × 40 mg for both peak plasma concentrations (C_{max}) and extent of absorption (AUC) (see Table 2 below). Given the short half-life of elimination of oxycodone from OxyContin, steady-state plasma concentrations of oxycodone are

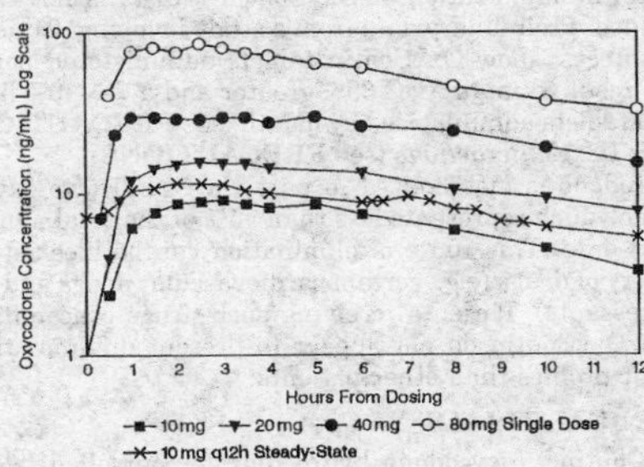

achieved within 24–36 hours of initiation of dosing with OxyContin tablets. In a study comparing 10 mg of OxyContin every 12 hours to 5 mg of immediate-release oxycodone every 6 hours, the two treatments were found to be equivalent for AUC and C_{max}, and similar for C_{min} (trough) concentrations. There was less fluctuation in plasma concentrations for the OxyContin tablets than for the immediate-release formulation.

[See table 1 at top of next page]
[See table 2 at top of next page]

Food Effects

Food has no significant effect on the extent of absorption of oxycodone from OxyContin. However, the peak plasma concentration of oxycodone increased by 25% when OxyContin 160 mg tablet was administered with a high fat meal.

Distribution

Following intravenous administration, the volume of distribution (Vss) for oxycodone was 2.6 L/kg. Oxycodone binding to plasma protein at 37°C and a pH of 7.4 was about 45%. Once absorbed, oxycodone is distributed to skeletal muscle, liver, intestinal tract, lungs, spleen, and brain. Oxycodone has been found in breast milk (see **PRECAUTIONS**).

Metabolism

Oxycodone hydrochloride is extensively metabolized to noroxycodone, oxymorphone, and their glucuronides. The major circulating metabolite is noroxycodone with an AUC ratio of 0.6 relative to that of oxycodone. Noroxycodone is reported to be a considerably weaker analgesic than oxycodone. Oxymorphone, although possessing analgesic activity, is present in the plasma only in low concentrations. The correlation between oxymorphone concentrations and opioid effects was much less than that seen with oxycodone plasma concentrations. The analgesic activity profile of other metabolites is not known at present.

The formation of oxymorphone, but not noroxycodone, is mediated by CYP2D6 and as such its formation can, in theory, be affected by other drugs (see *Drug-Drug Interactions*).

Excretion

Oxycodone and its metabolites are excreted primarily via the kidney. The amounts measured in the urine have been reported as follows: free oxycodone up to 19%; conjugated oxycodone up to 50%; free oxymorphone 0%; conjugated oxymorphone ≤14%; both free and conjugated noroxycodone have been found in the urine but not quantified. The total plasma clearance was 0.8 L/min for adults.

Special Populations

Elderly

The plasma concentrations of oxycodone are only nominally affected by age, being 15% greater in elderly as compared to young subjects. There were no differences in adverse event reporting between young and elderly subjects.

Gender

Female subjects have, on average, plasma oxycodone concentrations up to 25% higher than males on a body weight adjusted basis. The reason for this difference is unknown.

Renal Impairment

Preliminary data from a study involving patients with mild to severe renal dysfunction (creatinine clearance <60 mL/min) show peak plasma oxycodone and noroxycodone concentrations 50% and 20% higher, respectively and AUC values for oxycodone, noroxycodone, and oxymorphone 60%, 50%, and 40% higher than normal subjects, respectively. This is accompanied by an increase in sedation but not by

Continued on next page

OxyContin—Cont.

differences in respiratory rate, pupillary constriction, or several other measures of drug effect. There was an increase in t½ of elimination for oxycodone of only 1 hour (see **PRECAUTIONS**).

Hepatic Impairment

Preliminary data from a study involving patients with mild to moderate hepatic dysfunction show peak plasma oxycodone and noroxycodone concentrations 50% and 20% higher, respectively, than normal subjects. AUC values are 95% and 65% higher, respectively. Oxymorphone peak plasma concentrations and AUC values are lower by 30% and 40%. These differences are accompanied by increases in some, but not other, drug effects. The t½ elimination for oxycodone increased by 2.3 hours (see **PRECAUTIONS**).

Rectal Administration

Rectal administration of OxyContin tablets is not recommended. Preliminary data from a study involving 21 normal volunteers, show OxyContin tablets administered per rectum resulted in an AUC 39% greater and a C_{max} 9% higher than tablets administered by mouth (see **PRECAUTIONS**).

Drug-Drug Interactions (see **PRECAUTIONS**)

Oxycodone is metabolized in part via CYP2D6 to oxymorphone which represents less than 15% of the total administered dose. This route of elimination can be blocked by a variety of drugs (e.g., certain cardiovascular drugs and antidepressants). Patients receiving such drugs concomitantly with OxyContin do not appear to present different therapeutic profiles than other patients.

Table 1
Mean [% coefficient variation]

Regimen/ Dosage Form	AUC (ng•hr/mL)†	C_{max} (ng/mL)	T_{max} (hrs)	Trough Conc. (ng/mL)
Single Dose 10 mg OxyContin	100.7 [26.6]	10.6 [20.1]	2.7 [44.1]	n.a.
20 mg OxyContin	207.5 [35.9]	21.4 [36.6]	3.2 [57.9]	n.a.
40 mg OxyContin	423.1 [33.3]	39.3 [34.0]	3.1 [77.4]	n.a.
80 mg OxyContin*	1085.5 [32.3]	98.5 [32.1]	2.1 [52.3]	n.a.
Multiple Dose 10 mg OxyContin Tablets q12h	103.6 [38.6]	15.1 [31.0]	3.2 [69.5]	7.2 [48.1]
5 mg immediate-release q6h	99.0 [36.2]	15.5 [28.8]	1.6 [49.7]	7.4 [50.9]

Table 2
Mean [% coefficient variation]

Regimen/ Dosage Form	AUC_∞ (ng•hr/mL)†	C_{max} (ng/mL)	T_{max} (hrs)	Trough Conc. (ng/mL)
Single Dose* 4×40 mg OxyContin	1935.3 [34.7]	152.0 [28.9]	2.56 [42.3]	n.a.
2×80 mg OxyContin	1859.3 [30.1]	153.4 [25.1]	2.78 [69.3]	n.a.
1×160 mg OxyContin*	1856.4 [30.5]	156.4 [24.8]	2.54 [36.4]	n.a.

†for single-dose AUC=$AUC_{0\text{-}inf}$; for multiple-dose AUC=$AUC_{0\text{-}T}$
*data obtained while volunteers received naltrexone which can enhance absorption.

CLINICAL TRIALS

OxyContin® (oxycodone hydrochloride controlled-release) tablets were evaluated in studies involving 713 patients with either cancer or non-cancer pain. All patients receiving OxyContin were dosed q12h. Efficacy comparable to other forms of oral oxycodone was demonstrated in clinical studies using pharmacokinetic, pharmacodynamic, and efficacy outcomes. The outcome of these trials indicated: (1) a positive relationship between dose and plasma oxycodone concentration, (2) a positive relationship between plasma oxycodone concentration and analgesia, and (3) an observed peak to trough variation in plasma concentration with OxyContin lying within the observed range established with qid dosing of immediate-release oxycodone in clinical populations at the same total daily dose.

In clinical trials, OxyContin tablets were substituted for a wide variety of analgesics, including acetaminophen (APAP), aspirin (ASA), other non-steroidal anti-inflammatory drugs (NSAIDs), opioid combination products and single-entity opioids, primarily morphine. In cancer patients receiving adequate opioid therapy at baseline, pain intensity scores and acceptability of therapy remained unchanged by transfer to OxyContin. For non-cancer pain patients who had moderate to severe pain at baseline on prn opioid therapy, pain control and acceptability of therapy improved with the introduction of fixed-interval therapy with OxyContin.

Use in Cancer Pain

OxyContin was studied in three double-blind, controlled clinical trials involving 341 cancer patients and several open-label trials with therapy durations of over 10 months. Two, double-blind, controlled clinical studies indicated that OxyContin dosed q12h produced analgesic efficacy equivalent to immediate-release oxycodone dosed qid at the same total daily dose. Peak and trough plasma concentrations attained were similar to those attained with immediate-release oxycodone at equivalent total daily doses. With titration to analgesic effect and proper use of rescue medication, nearly every patient achieved adequate pain control with OxyContin.

In the third study, a double-blind, active-controlled, crossover trial, OxyContin dosed q12h was shown to be equivalent in efficacy and safety to immediate-release oxycodone dosed qid at the same total daily dose. Patients were able to be titrated to an acceptable analgesic effect with either OxyContin or immediate-release oxycodone with both treatments providing stable pain control within 2 days in most patients.

In patients with cancer pain, the total daily OxyContin doses tested ranged from 20 mg to 640 mg per day. The average total daily dose was approximately 105 mg per day.

Studies in Non-Cancer Pain

A double-blind, placebo-controlled, fixed-dose, parallel group study was conducted in 133 patients with moderate to severe osteoarthritis pain, who were judged as having inadequate pain control with prn opioids and maximal non-steroidal anti-inflammatory therapy. In this study, 20 mg OxyContin q12h significantly decreased pain and improved quality of life, mood, and sleep, relative to placebo. Both dose-concentration and concentration-effect relationships were noted with a minimum effective plasma oxycodone concentration of approximately 5–10 ng/mL.

In a double-blind, active-controlled, crossover study involving 57 patients with low-back pain inadequately controlled with prn opioids and non-opioid therapy, OxyContin administered q12h provided analgesia equivalent to immediate-release oxycodone administered qid. Patients could be titrated to an acceptable analgesic effect with either OxyContin or immediate-release forms of oxycodone.

Single-Dose Comparison with Standard Therapy

A single-dose, double-blind, placebo-controlled, post-operative study of 182 patients was conducted utilizing graded doses of OxyContin (10, 20, and 30 mg). Twenty and 30 mg of OxyContin gave equivalent peak analgesic effect compared to two oxycodone 5 mg/acetaminophen 325 mg tablets and to 15 mg immediate-release oxycodone, while the 10 mg dose of OxyContin was intermediate between both the immediate-release and combination products and placebo. The onset of analgesic action with OxyContin occurred within 1 hour in most patients following oral administration.

OxyContin is not recommended pre-operatively (preemptive analgesia) or for the management of pain in the immediate post-operative period (the first 12 to 24 hours following surgery) because the safety or appropriateness of fixed-dose, long-acting opioids in this setting has not been established.

Other Clinical Trials

In open-label trials involving approximately 200 patients with cancer-related and non-cancer pain, dosed according to the package insert recommendations, appropriate analgesic effectiveness was noted without regard to age, gender, race, or disease state. There were no unusual drug interactions observed in patients receiving a wide range of medications common in these populations.

For opioid-naive patients, the average total daily dose of OxyContin was approximately 40 mg per day. There was no evidence of oxycodone and metabolite accumulation during 8 months of therapy. For cancer pain patients the average total daily dose was 105 mg (range 20 to 720 mg) per day. There was a significant decrease in acute opioid-related side effects, except for constipation, during the first several weeks of therapy. Development of significant tolerance to analgesia was uncommon.

A cohort of patients have been treated with OxyContin 80 mg tablets. There were no differences in the efficacy or safety profiles than seen with the other tablet strengths.

INDICATIONS AND USAGE

OxyContin® tablets are a controlled-release oral formulation of oxycodone hydrochloride indicated for the management of moderate to severe pain where use of an opioid analgesic is appropriate for more than a few days (see **CLINICAL PHARMACOLOGY; CLINICAL TRIALS**).

CONTRAINDICATIONS

OxyContin® is contraindicated in patients with known hypersensitivity to oxycodone, or in any situation where opioids are contraindicated. This includes patients with significant respiratory depression (in unmonitored settings or the absence of resuscitative equipment), and patients with acute or severe bronchial asthma or hypercarbia. OxyContin is contraindicated in any patient who has or is suspected of having paralytic ileus.

WARNINGS

OxyContin® (oxycodone hydrochloride controlled-release) TABLETS ARE TO BE SWALLOWED WHOLE, AND ARE NOT TO BE BROKEN, CHEWED OR CRUSHED. TAKING BROKEN, CHEWED OR CRUSHED OxyContin TABLETS COULD LEAD TO THE RAPID RELEASE AND ABSORPTION OF A POTENTIALLY TOXIC DOSE OF OXYCODONE.

Respiratory Depression

Respiratory depression is the chief hazard from all opioid agonist preparations. Respiratory depression occurs most frequently in elderly or debilitated patients, usually following large initial doses in non-tolerant patients, or when opioids are given in conjunction with other agents that depress respiration.

Oxycodone should be used with extreme caution in patients with significant chronic obstructive pulmonary disease or cor pulmonale, and in patients having a substantially decreased respiratory reserve, hypoxia, hypercapnia, or preexisting respiratory depression. In such patients, even usual therapeutic doses of oxycodone may decrease respiratory drive to the point of apnea. In these patients alternative non-opioid analgesics should be considered, and opioids should be employed only under careful medical supervision at the lowest effective dose.

Head Injury

The respiratory depressant effects of opioids include carbon dioxide retention and secondary elevation of cerebrospinal fluid pressure, and may be markedly exaggerated in the presence of head injury, intracranial lesions, or other sources of preexisting increased intracranial pressure. Oxycodone produces effects on pupillary response and consciousness which may obscure neurologic signs of further increases in intracranial pressure in patients with head injuries.

Hypotensive Effect

OxyContin®, like all opioid analgesics, may cause severe hypotension in an individual whose ability to maintain blood pressure has been compromised by a depleted blood volume, or after concurrent administration with drugs such as phenothiazines or other agents which compromise vasomotor tone. OxyContin may produce orthostatic hypotension in ambulatory patients. OxyContin, like all opioid analgesics, should be administered with caution to patients in circulatory shock, since vasodilation produced by the drug may further reduce cardiac output and blood pressure.

PRECAUTIONS

Special precautions regarding OxyContin® 80 mg and 160 mg Tablets

OxyContin® 80 mg and 160 mg Tablets are for use only in opioid tolerant patients requiring daily oxycodone equivalent dosages of 160 mg or more for the 80 mg tablet and 320 mg or more for the 160 mg tablet. Care should be taken in the prescription of this tablet strength. Patients should be instructed against use by individuals other than the patient for whom it was prescribed, as such inappropriate use may have severe medical consequences.

One OxyContin® 160 mg tablet is comparable to two 80 mg tablets when taken on an empty stomach. With a high fat meal, however, there is a 25% greater peak plasma concentration following one 160 mg tablet. Dietary caution should be taken when patients are initially titrated to 160 mg tablets (see DOSAGE AND ADMINISTRATION).

General

OxyContin® (oxycodone hydrochloride controlled-release) tablets are intended for use in patients who require oral pain therapy with an opioid agonist of more than a few days duration. As with any opioid analgesic, it is critical to adjust the dosing regimen individually for each patient (see **DOSAGE AND ADMINISTRATION**).

Selection of patients for treatment with OxyContin should be governed by the same principles that apply to the use of similar controlled-release opioid analgesics (see **INDICATIONS AND USAGE**). Opioid analgesics given on a fixed-dosage schedule have a narrow therapeutic index in certain patient populations, especially when combined with other drugs, and should be reserved for cases where the benefits of opioid analgesia outweigh the known risks of respiratory depression, altered mental state, and postural hypotension. Physicians should individualize treatment in every case, using non-opioid analgesics, prn opioids and/or combination products, and chronic opioid therapy with drugs such as

OxyContin in a progressive plan of pain management such as outlined by the World Health Organization, the Agency for Health Care Policy and Research, and the American Pain Society.

Use of OxyContin is associated with increased potential risks and should be used only with caution in the following conditions: acute alcoholism; adrenocortical insufficiency (e.g., Addison's disease); CNS depression or coma; delirium tremens; debilitated patients; kyphoscoliosis associated with respiratory depression; myxedema or hypothyroidism; prostatic hypertrophy or urethral stricture; severe impairment of hepatic, pulmonary or renal function; and toxic psychosis.

The administration of oxycodone, like all opioid analgesics, may obscure the diagnosis or clinical course in patients with acute abdominal conditions. Oxycodone may aggravate convulsions in patients with convulsive disorders, and all opioids may induce or aggravate seizures in some clinical settings.

Interactions with other CNS Depressants

OxyContin, like all opioid analgesics, should be used with caution and started in a reduced dosage ($^1/_3$ to $^1/_2$ of the usual dosage) in patients who are concurrently receiving other central nervous system depressants including sedatives or hypnotics, general anesthetics, phenothiazines, other tranquilizers, and alcohol. Interactive effects resulting in respiratory depression, hypotension, profound sedation, or coma may result if these drugs are taken in combination with the usual doses of OxyContin.

Interactions with Mixed Agonist/Antagonist Opioid Analgesics

Agonist/antagonist analgesics (i.e., pentazocine, nalbuphine, butorphanol, and buprenorphine) should be administered with caution to a patient who has received or is receiving a course of therapy with a pure opioid agonist analgesic such as oxycodone. In this situation, mixed agonist/antagonist analgesics may reduce the analgesic effect of oxycodone and/or may precipitate withdrawal symptoms in these patients.

Ambulatory Surgery

OxyContin is not recommended pre-operatively (preemptive analgesia) or for the management of pain in the immediate post-operative period (the first 12 to 24 hours following surgery) for patients not previously taking the drug, because its safety in this setting has not been established.

Patients who are already receiving OxyContin tablets as part of ongoing analgesic therapy may be safely continued on the drug if appropriate dosage adjustments are made considering the procedure, other drugs given and the temporary changes in physiology caused by the surgical intervention (see **PRECAUTIONS**: *Drug-Drug Interactions*, and **DOSAGE AND ADMINISTRATION**).

Post-Operative Use

Morphine and other opioids have been shown to decrease bowel motility. Ileus is a common post-operative complication, especially after intra-abdominal surgery with opioid analgesia. Caution should be taken to monitor for decreased bowel motility in post-operative patients receiving opioids. Standard supportive therapy should be implemented.

Use in Pancreatic/Biliary Tract Disease

Oxycodone may cause spasm of the sphincter of Oddi and should be used with caution in patients with biliary tract disease, including acute pancreatitis. Opioids like oxycodone may cause increases in the serum amylase level.

Tolerance and Physical Dependence

Tolerance is the need for increasing doses of opioids to maintain a defined effect such as analgesia (in the absence of disease progression or other external factors). Physical dependence is the occurrence of withdrawal symptoms after abrupt discontinuation of a drug or upon administration of an antagonist. Physical dependence and tolerance are not unusual during chronic opioid therapy.

Significant tolerance should not occur in most of the patients treated with the lowest doses of oxycodone. It should be expected, however, that a fraction of cancer patients will develop some degree of tolerance and require progressively higher dosages of OxyContin to maintain pain control during chronic treatment. Regardless of whether this occurs as a result of increased pain secondary to disease progression or pharmacological tolerance, dosages can usually be increased safely by adjusting the patient's dose to maintain an acceptable balance between pain relief and side effects. The dosage should be selected according to the patient's individual analgesic response and ability to tolerate side effects. Tolerance to the analgesic effect of opioids is usually paralleled by tolerance to side effects, except for constipation.

Physical dependence results in withdrawal symptoms in patients who abruptly discontinue the drug or may be precipitated through the administration of drugs with opioid antagonist activity (see **OVERDOSAGE**). If OxyContin is abruptly discontinued in a physically dependent patient, an abstinence syndrome may occur. This is characterized by some or all of the following: restlessness, lacrimation, rhinorrhea, yawning, perspiration, chills, myalgia, and mydriasis. Other symptoms also may develop, including: irritability, anxiety, backache, joint pain, weakness, abdominal cramps, insomnia, nausea, anorexia, vomiting, diarrhea, or increased blood pressure, respiratory rate, or heart rate.

If signs and symptoms of withdrawal occur, patients should be treated by reinstitution of opioid therapy followed by a gradual, tapered dose reduction of OxyContin combined with symptomatic support (see **DOSAGE AND ADMINISTRATION**: *Cessation of Therapy*).

Information for Patients/Caregivers

If clinically advisable, patients receiving OxyContin (oxycodone hydrochloride controlled-release) tablets or their caregivers should be given the following information by the physician, nurse, pharmacist, or caregiver:

1. Patients should be advised that OxyContin tablets were designed to work properly only if swallowed whole. They may release all their contents at once if broken, chewed or crushed, resulting in a risk of overdose.
2. Patients should be advised to report episodes of breakthrough pain and adverse experiences occurring during therapy. Individualization of dosage is essential to make optimal use of this medication.
3. Patients should be advised not to adjust the dose of OxyContin without consulting the prescribing professional.
4. Patients should be advised that OxyContin may impair mental and/or physical ability required for the performance of potentially hazardous tasks (e.g., driving, operating heavy machinery).
5. Patients should not combine OxyContin with alcohol or other central nervous system depressants (sleep aids, tranquilizers) except by the orders of the prescribing physician, because additive effects may occur.
6. Women of childbearing potential who become, or are planning to become, pregnant should be advised to consult their physician regarding the effects of analgesics and other drug use during pregnancy on themselves and their unborn child.
7. Patients should be advised that OxyContin is a potential drug of abuse. They should protect it from theft, and it should never be given to anyone other than the individual for whom it was prescribed.
8. Patients should be advised that they may pass empty matrix "ghosts" (tablets) via colostomy or in the stool, and that this is of no concern since the active medication has already been absorbed.
9. Patients should be advised that if they have been receiving treatment with OxyContin for more than a few weeks and cessation of therapy is indicated, it may be appropriate to taper the OxyContin dose, rather than abruptly discontinue it, due to the risk of precipitating withdrawal symptoms. Their physician can provide a dose schedule to accomplish a gradual discontinuation of the medication.

Laboratory Monitoring

Due to the broad range of plasma concentrations seen in clinical populations, the varying degrees of pain, and the development of tolerance, plasma oxycodone measurements are usually not helpful in clinical management. Plasma concentrations of the active drug substance may be of value in selected, unusual or complex cases.

Interactions with Alcohol and Drugs of Abuse

Oxycodone may be expected to have additive effects when used in conjunction with alcohol, other opioids or illicit drugs which cause central nervous system depression.

Use in Drug and Alcohol Addiction

OxyContin is an opioid with no approved use in the management of addictive disorders. Its proper usage in individuals with drug or alcohol dependence, either active or in remission, is for the management of pain requiring opioid analgesia.

Drug-Drug Interactions

Opioid analgesics, including OxyContin, may enhance the neuromuscular blocking action of skeletal muscle relaxants and produce an increased degree of respiratory depression.

Oxycodone is metabolized in part to oxymorphone via CYP2D6. While this pathway may be blocked by a variety of drugs (e.g., certain cardiovascular drugs and antidepressants), such blockade has not yet been shown to be of clinical significance with this agent. Clinicians should be aware of this possible interaction, however.

Use with CNS Depressants

OxyContin, like all opioid analgesics, should be started at $^1/_3$ to $^1/_2$ of the usual dosage in patients who are concurrently receiving other central nervous system depressants including sedatives or hypnotics, general anesthetics, phenothiazines, centrally acting anti-emetics, tranquilizers, and alcohol because respiratory depression, hypotension, and profound sedation or coma may result. No specific interaction between oxycodone and monoamine oxidase inhibitors has been observed, but caution in the use of any opioid in patients taking this class of drugs is appropriate.

Mutagenicity/Carcinogenicity

Oxycodone was not mutagenic in the following assays: Ames Salmonella and E. Coli test with and without metabolic activation at doses of up to 5000 μg, chromosomal aberration test in human lymphocytes in the absence of metabolic activation at doses of up to 1500 μg/ml and with activation 48 hours after exposure at doses of up to 5000 μg/ml, and in the in vivo bone marrow micronucleus test in mice (at plasma levels of up to 48 μg/ml). Mutagenic results occurred in the presence of metabolic activation in the human chromosomal aberration test (at greater than or equal to 1250 μg/ml) at 24 but not 48 hours of exposure and in the mouse lymphoma assay at doses of 50 μg/ml or greater with metabolic activation and at 400 μg/ml or greater without metabolic activation. The data from these tests indicate that the genotoxic risk to humans may be considered low.

Studies of oxycodone in animals to evaluate its carcinogenic potential have not been conducted owing to the length of clinical experience with the drug substance.

Pregnancy

Teratogenic Effects—Category B: Reproduction studies have been performed in rats and rabbits by oral administration at doses up to 8 mg/kg (48 mg/m^2) and 125 mg/kg (1375 mg/m^2), respectively. These doses are 3 and 47 times a human dose of 160 mg/day (90 mg/m^2), based on mg/kg of a 60 kg adult (0.5 and 15 times this human dose based upon mg/m^2). The results did not reveal evidence of harm to the fetus due to oxycodone. There are, however, no adequate and well-controlled studies in pregnant women. Because animal reproduction studies are not always predictive of human response, this drug should be used during pregnancy only if clearly needed.

Nonteratogenic Effects—Neonates whose mothers have been taking oxycodone chronically may exhibit respiratory depression and/or withdrawal symptoms, either at birth and/or in the nursery.

Labor and Delivery

OxyContin is not recommended for use in women during and immediately prior to labor and delivery because oral opioids may cause respiratory depression in the newborn.

Nursing Mothers

Low concentrations of oxycodone have been detected in breast milk. Withdrawal symptoms can occur in breast-feeding infants when maternal administration of an opioid analgesic is stopped. Ordinarily, nursing should not be undertaken while a patient is receiving OxyContin since oxycodone may be excreted in the milk.

Pediatric Use

Safety and effectiveness in pediatric patients below the age of 18 have not been established with this dosage form of oxycodone. However, oxycodone has been used extensively in the pediatric population in other dosage forms, as have the excipients used in this formulation. No specific increased risk is expected from the use of this form of oxycodone in pediatric patients old enough to safely take tablets if dosing is adjusted for the patient's weight (see **DOSAGE AND ADMINISTRATION**). **It must be remembered that OxyContin tablets cannot be crushed or divided for administration.**

Geriatric Use

In controlled pharmacokinetic studies in elderly subjects (greater than 65 years) the clearance of oxycodone appeared to be slightly reduced. Compared to young adults, the plasma concentrations of oxycodone were increased approximately 15%. In clinical trials with appropriate initiation of therapy and dose titration, no untoward or unexpected side effects were seen based on age, and the usual doses and dosing intervals are appropriate for the geriatric patient. As with all opioids, the starting dose should be reduced to $^1/_3$ to $^1/_2$ of the usual dosage in debilitated, non-tolerant patients.

Hepatic Impairment

A study of OxyContin in patients with hepatic impairment indicates greater plasma concentrations than those with normal function. The initiation of therapy at $^1/_3$ to $^1/_2$ the usual doses and careful dose titration is warranted.

Renal Impairment

In patients with renal impairment, as evidenced by decreased creatinine clearance (<60 mL/min.), the concentrations of oxycodone in the plasma are approximately 50% higher than in subjects with normal renal function. Dose initiation should follow a conservative approach. Dosages should be adjusted according to the clinical situation.

Gender Differences

In pharmacokinetic studies, opioid-naive females demonstrate up to 25% higher average plasma concentrations and greater frequency of typical opioid adverse events than males, even after adjustment for body weight. The clinical relevance of a difference of this magnitude is low for a drug intended for chronic usage at individualized dosages, and there was no male/female difference detected for efficacy or adverse events in clinical trials.

Rectal Administration

OxyContin® Tablets are not recommended for administration per rectum. A study in normal volunteers showed a significantly greater AUC and higher C_{max} during this route of administration (see **PHARMACOKINETICS AND METABOLISM**).

ADVERSE REACTIONS

Serious adverse reactions which may be associated with OxyContin® (oxycodone hydrochloride controlled-release) tablet therapy in clinical use are those observed with other opioid analgesics, including: respiratory depression, apnea, respiratory arrest, and (to an even lesser degree) circulatory depression, hypotension, or shock (see **OVERDOSAGE**).

The non-serious adverse events seen on initiation of therapy with OxyContin are typical opioid side effects. These events are dose-dependent, and their frequency depends upon the dose, the clinical setting, the patient's level of opioid tolerance, and host factors specific to the individual. They should be expected and managed as a part of opioid analgesia. The most frequent (>5%) include constipation, nausea, somnolence, dizziness, vomiting, pruritus, headache, dry mouth, sweating, and asthenia.

In many cases the frequency of these events during initiation of therapy may be minimized by careful individualization of starting dosage, slow titration, and the avoidance of large swings in the plasma concentrations of the opioid. Many of these adverse events will cease or decrease in intensity as OxyContin therapy is continued and some degree of tolerance is developed.

In clinical trials comparing OxyContin with immediate-release oxycodone and placebo, the most common adverse events (>5%) reported by patients (pts) at least once during therapy were:

Continued on next page

OxyContin—Cont.

Table 3

	OxyContin (n=227) # Pts	(%)	Immediate-Release (n=225) # Pts	(%)	Placebo (n=45) # Pts	(%)
Constipation	52	(23)	58	(26)	3	(7)
Nausea	52	(23)	60	(27)	5	(11)
Somnolence	52	(23)	55	(24)	2	(4)
Dizziness	29	(13)	35	(16)	4	(9)
Pruritus	29	(13)	28	(12)	1	(2)
Vomiting	27	(12)	31	(14)	3	(7)
Headache	17	(7)	19	(8)	3	(7)
Dry Mouth	13	(6)	15	(7)	1	(2)
Asthenia	13	(6)	16	(7)	—	—
Sweating	12	(5)	13	(6)	1	(2)

The following adverse experiences were reported in OxyContin treated patients with an incidence between 1% and 5%. In descending order of frequency they were anorexia, nervousness, insomnia, fever, confusion, diarrhea, abdominal pain, dyspepsia, rash, anxiety, euphoria, dyspnea, postural hypotension, chills, twitching, gastritis, abnormal dreams, thought abnormalities, and hiccups.

The following adverse reactions occurred in less than 1% of patients involved in clinical trials:

General: accidental injury, chest pain, facial edema, malaise, neck pain, pain

Cardiovascular: migraine, syncope, vasodilation, ST depression

Digestive: dysphagia, eructation, flatulence, gastrointestinal disorder, increased appetite, nausea and vomiting, stomatitis, ileus

Hemic and Lymphatic: lymphadenopathy

Metabolic and Nutritional: dehydration, edema, hyponatremia, peripheral edema, syndrome of inappropriate antidiuretic hormone secretion, thirst

Nervous: abnormal gait, agitation, amnesia, depersonalization, depression, emotional lability, hallucination, hyperkinesia, hypesthesia, hypotonia, malaise, paresthesia, seizures, speech disorder, stupor, tinnitus, tremor, vertigo, withdrawal syndrome with or without seizures

Respiratory: cough increased, pharyngitis, voice alteration

Skin: dry skin, exfoliative dermatitis, urticaria

Special Senses: abnormal vision, taste perversion

Urogenital: dysuria, hematuria, impotence, polyuria, urinary retention, urination impaired

DRUG ABUSE AND DEPENDENCE (Addiction)

OxyContin® is a mu-agonist opioid with an abuse liability similar to morphine and is a Schedule II controlled substance. Oxycodone products are common targets for both drug abusers and drug addicts. Delayed absorption, as provided by OxyContin tablets, is believed to reduce the abuse liability of a drug.

Drug addiction (drug dependence, psychological dependence) is characterized by a preoccupation with the procurement, hoarding, and abuse of drugs for non-medicinal purposes. Drug dependence is treatable, utilizing a multi-disciplinary approach, but relapse is common. Iatrogenic "addiction" to opioids legitimately used in the management of pain is very rare. "Drug seeking" behavior is very common to addicts. Tolerance and physical dependence in pain patients are not signs of psychological dependence. Preoccupation with achieving adequate pain relief can be appropriate behavior in a patient with poor pain control. Most chronic pain patients limit their intake of opioids to achieve a balance between the benefits of the drug and dose-limiting side effects.

Physicians should be aware that psychological dependence may not be accompanied by concurrent tolerance and symptoms of physical dependence in all addicts. In addition, abuse of opioids can occur in the absence of true psychological dependence and is characterized by misuse for non-medical purposes, often in combination with other psychoactive substances.

OxyContin consists of a dual-polymer matrix, intended for oral use only. Parenteral venous injection of the tablet constituents, especially talc, can be expected to result in local tissue necrosis and pulmonary granulomas.

OVERDOSAGE

Acute overdosage with oxycodone can be manifested by respiratory depression, somnolence progressing to stupor or coma, skeletal muscle flaccidity, cold and clammy skin, constricted pupils, bradycardia, hypotension, and death.

In the treatment of oxycodone overdosage, primary attention should be given to the re-establishment of a patent airway and institution of assisted or controlled ventilation. Supportive measures (including oxygen and vasopressors) should be employed in the management of circulatory shock and pulmonary edema accompanying overdose as indicated. Cardiac arrest or arrhythmias may require cardiac massage or defibrillation.

The pure opioid antagonists such as naloxone or nalmefene are specific antidotes against respiratory depression from opioid overdose. Opioid antagonists should not be administered in the absence of clinically significant respiratory or circulatory depression secondary to oxycodone overdose. They should be administered cautiously to persons who are known, or suspected to be, physically dependent on any opioid agonist including OxyContin®. In such cases, an abrupt or complete reversal of opioid effects may precipitate an acute abstinence syndrome. The severity of the withdrawal syndrome produced will depend on the degree of physical dependence and the dose of the antagonist administered. Please see the prescribing information for the specific opioid antagonist for details of their proper use.

DOSAGE AND ADMINISTRATION

General Principles

OxyContin® (oxycodone hydrochloride controlled-release) TABLETS ARE TO BE SWALLOWED WHOLE, AND ARE NOT TO BE BROKEN, CHEWED OR CRUSHED. TAKING BROKEN, CHEWED OR CRUSHED OxyContin TABLETS COULD LEAD TO THE RAPID RELEASE AND ABSORPTION OF A POTENTIALLY TOXIC DOSE OF OXYCODONE.

ONE OXYCONTIN® 160 MG TABLET IS COMPARABLE TO TWO 80 MG TABLETS WHEN TAKEN ON AN EMPTY STOMACH. WITH A HIGH FAT MEAL, HOWEVER, THERE IS A 25% GREATER PEAK PLASMA CONCENTRATION FOLLOWING ONE 160 MG TABLET. DIETARY CAUTION SHOULD BE TAKEN WHEN PATIENTS ARE INITIALLY TITRATED TO 160 MG TABLETS.

In treating pain it is vital to assess the patient regularly and systematically. Therapy should also be regularly reviewed and adjusted based upon the patient's own reports of pain and side effects and the health professional's clinical judgment.

OxyContin is intended for the management of moderate to severe pain in patients who require treatment with an oral opioid analgesic for more than a few days. The controlled-release nature of the formulation allows it to be effectively administered every 12 hours (see **CLINICAL PHARMACOLOGY; PHARMACOKINETICS AND METABOLISM**). While symmetric (same dose AM and PM), around-the-clock, q12h dosing is appropriate for the majority of patients, some patients may benefit from asymmetric (different dose given in AM than in PM) dosing, tailored to their pain pattern. It is usually appropriate to treat a patient with only one opioid for around-the-clock therapy.

Initiation of Therapy

It is critical to initiate the dosing regimen for each patient individually, taking into account the patient's prior opioid and non-opioid analgesic treatment. Attention should be given to:

(1) the general condition and medical status of the patient
(2) the daily dose, potency and kind of the analgesic(s) the patient has been taking
(3) the reliability of the conversion estimate used to calculate the dose of oxycodone
(4) the patient's opioid exposure and opioid tolerance (if any)
(5) special safety issues associated with conversion to OxyContin doses at or exceeding 160 mg q12h (see **Special instructions for OxyContin 80 mg and 160 mg Tablets**)
(6) the balance between pain control and adverse experiences

Care should be taken to use low initial doses of OxyContin in patients who are not already opioid tolerant, especially those who are receiving concurrent treatment with muscle relaxants, sedatives, or other CNS active medications (see **PRECAUTIONS**: *Drug-Drug Interactions*).

Patients Not Already Taking Opioids (opioid naive)

Clinical trials have shown that patients may initiate analgesic therapy with OxyContin. A reasonable starting dose for most patients who are opioid naive is 10 mg q12h. If a non-opioid analgesic [aspirin (ASA), acetaminophen (APAP) or a non-steroidal anti-inflammatory (NSAID)] is being provided, it may be continued. If the current non-opioid is discontinued, early upward dose titration may be necessary.

Conversion from Fixed-Ratio Opioid/APAP, ASA, or NSAID Combination Drugs

Patients who are taking 1 to 5 tablets/capsules/caplets per day of a regular strength fixed-combination opioid/non-opioid should be started on 10 to 20 mg OxyContin q12h. For patients taking 6 to 9 tablets/capsules/caplets, a starting dose of 20 to 30 mg q12h is suggested. For those taking 10 to 12 tablets/capsules/caplets a day, 30 to 40 mg q12h should be considered. The non-opioid may be continued as a separate drug. Alternatively, a different non-opioid analgesic may be selected. If the decision is made to discontinue the non-opioid analgesic, consideration should be given to early upward titration.

Patients Currently on Opioid Therapy

If a patient has been receiving opioid-containing medications prior to OxyContin therapy, the total daily (24-hour) dose of the other opioids should be determined.

1. Using standard conversion ratio estimates (see Table 4 below), multiply the mg/day of the previous opioids by the appropriate multiplication factors to obtain the equivalent total daily dose of oral oxycodone.
2. Divide this 24-hour oxycodone dose in half to obtain the twice a day (q12h) dose of OxyContin.
3. Round down to a dose which is appropriate for the tablet strengths available (10 mg, 20 mg, 40 mg, 80 mg, and 160 mg tablets).
4. Discontinue all other around-the-clock opioid drugs when OxyContin therapy is initiated.

No fixed conversion ratio is likely to be satisfactory in all patients, especially patients receiving large opioid doses. The recommended doses shown in Table 4 are only a starting point, and close observation and frequent titration are indicated until patients are stable on the new therapy.

Table 4

*Multiplication Factors for Converting the Daily Dose of Prior Opioids to the Daily Dose of Oral Oxycodone**

(Mg/Day Prior Opioid × Factor=Mg/Day Oral Oxycodone)

	Oral Prior Opioid	Parenteral Prior Opioid
Oxycodone	1	—
Codeine	0.15	—
Fentanyl TTS	SEE BELOW	SEE BELOW
Hydrocodone	0.9	—
Hydromorphone	4	20
Levorphanol	7.5	15
Meperidine	0.1	0.4
Methadone	1.5	3
Morphine	0.5	3

***To be used only for conversion to oral oxycodone.** For patients receiving high-dose parenteral opioids, a more conservative conversion is warranted. For example, for high-dose parenteral morphine, use 1.5 instead of 3 as a multiplication factor.

In all cases, supplemental analgesia (see below) should be made available in the form of immediate-release oral oxycodone or another suitable short-acting analgesic.

OxyContin can be safely used concomitantly with usual doses of non-opioid analgesics and analgesic adjuvants, provided care is taken to select a proper initial dose (see **PRECAUTIONS**).

Conversion from Transdermal Fentanyl to OxyContin

Eighteen hours following the removal of the transdermal fentanyl patch, OxyContin treatment can be initiated. Although there has been no systematic assessment of such conversion, a conservative oxycodone dose, approximately 10 mg q12h of OxyContin, should be initially substituted for each 25 μg/hr fentanyl transdermal patch. The patient should be followed closely for early titration as there is very limited clinical experience with this conversion.

Managing Expected Opioid Adverse Experiences

Most patients receiving opioids, especially those who are opioid naive, will experience side effects. Frequently the side effects from OxyContin are transient, but may require evaluation and management. Adverse events such as constipation should be anticipated and treated aggressively and prophylactically with a stimulant laxative and/or stool softener. Patients do not usually become tolerant to the constipating effects of opioids.

Other opioid-related side effects such as sedation and nausea are usually self-limited and often do not persist beyond the first few days. If nausea persists and is unacceptable to the patient, treatment with anti-emetics or other modalities may relieve these symptoms and should be considered.

Patients receiving OxyContin may pass an intact matrix "ghost" in the stool or via colostomy. These ghosts contain little or no residual oxycodone and are of no clinical consequence.

Individualization of Dosage

Once therapy is initiated, pain relief and other opioid effects should be frequently assessed. Patients should be titrated to adequate effect (generally mild or no pain with the regular use of no more than two doses of supplemental analgesia per 24 hours). Rescue medication should be available (see *Supplemental Analgesia*). Because steady-state plasma concentrations are approximated within 24 to 36 hours, dosage adjustment may be carried out every 1 to 2 days. It is most appropriate to increase the q12h dose, not the dosing frequency. There is no clinical information on dosing intervals shorter than q12h. As a guideline, except for the increase from 10 mg to 20 mg q12h, the total daily oxycodone dose usually can be increased by 25% to 50% of the current dose at each increase.

If signs of excessive opioid-related adverse experiences are observed, the next dose may be reduced. If this adjustment leads to inadequate analgesia, a supplemental dose of immediate-release oxycodone may be given. Alternatively, non-opioid analgesic adjuvants may be employed. Dose adjustments should be made to obtain an appropriate balance between pain relief and opioid-related adverse experiences.

If significant adverse events occur before the therapeutic goal of mild or no pain is achieved, the events should be treated aggressively. Once adverse events are under control, upward titration should continue to an acceptable level of pain control.

During periods of changing analgesic requirements, including initial titration, frequent contact is recommended between physician, other members of the health-care team, the patient and the caregiver/family.

Special instructions for OxyContin® 80 mg and 160 mg Tablets

(For use in opioid tolerant patients only.)

OxyContin® 80 mg and 160 mg Tablets are for use only in opioid tolerant patients requiring daily oxycodone equivalent dosages of 160 mg or more for the 80 mg tablet and 320 mg or more for the 160 mg tablet. Care should be taken in the prescription of this tablet strength. Patients should be instructed against use by individuals other than the patient for whom it was prescribed, as such inappropriate use may have severe medical consequences.

One OxyContin® 160 mg tablet is comparable to two 80 mg tablets when taken on an empty stomach. With a high fat meal, however, there is a 25% greater peak plasma con-

centration following one 160 mg tablet. Dietary caution should be taken when patients are initially titrated to 160 mg tablets.

Supplemental Analgesia

Most cancer patients given around-the-clock therapy with controlled-release opioids will need to have immediate-release medication available for "rescue" from breakthrough pain or to prevent pain that occurs predictably during certain patient activities (incident pain).

Rescue medication can be immediate-release oxycodone, either alone or in combination with acetaminophen, aspirin or other NSAIDs as a supplemental analgesic. The supplemental analgesic should be prescribed at $^1/_4$ to $^1/_3$ of the 12-hour OxyContin dose as shown in Table 5. The rescue medication is dosed as needed for breakthrough pain and administered one hour before anticipated incident pain. If more than two doses of rescue medication are needed within 24 hours, the dose of OxyContin should be titrated upward. Caregivers and patients using prn rescue analgesia in combination with around-the-clock opioids should be advised to report incidents of breakthrough pain to the physician managing the patient's analgesia (see *Information for Patients/Caregivers*).

Table 5

Table of Appropriate Supplemental Analgesia

OxyContin q12h Dose (mg)	Rescue Dose (immediate-release oxycodone) (mg) dosed PRN
10 (1×10 mg)	5
20 (2×10 mg)	5
30 (3×10 mg)	10
40 (2×20 mg)	10
60 (3×20 mg)	15
80 (2×40 mg)	20
120 (3×40 mg)	30
160 (2×80 mg)	40
240 (3×80 mg)	60
320 (2×160 mg)	80
480 (3×160 mg)	120

Maintenance of Therapy

The intent of the titration period is to establish a patient-specific q12h dose that will maintain adequate analgesia with acceptable side effects for as long as pain relief is necessary. Should pain recur then the dose can be incrementally increased to re-establish pain control. The method of therapy adjustment outlined above should be employed to re-establish pain control.

During chronic therapy, especially for non-cancer pain syndromes, the continued need for around-the-clock opioid therapy should be reassessed periodically (e.g., every 6 to 12 months) as appropriate.

Cessation of Therapy

When the patient no longer requires therapy with OxyContin tablets, patients receiving doses of 20–60 mg/day can usually have the therapy stopped abruptly without incident. However, higher doses should be tapered over several days to prevent signs and symptoms of withdrawal in the physically dependent patient. The daily dose should be reduced by approximately 50% for the first two days and then reduced by 25% every two days thereafter until the total dose reaches the dose recommended for opioid naive patients (10 or 20 mg q12h). Therapy can then be discontinued.

If signs of withdrawal appear, tapering should be stopped. The dose should be slightly increased until the signs and symptoms of opioid withdrawal disappear. Tapering should then begin again but with longer periods of time between each dose reduction.

Conversion from OxyContin to Parenteral Opioids

To avoid overdose, conservative dose conversion ratios should be followed. Initiate treatment with about 50% of the estimated equianalgesic daily dose of parenteral opioid divided into suitable individual doses based on the appropriate dosing interval, and titrate based upon the patient's response.

SAFETY AND HANDLING

OxyContin® (oxycodone hydrochloride controlled-release) tablets are solid dosage forms that pose no known health risk to health-care providers beyond that of any controlled substance. As with all such drugs, care should be taken to prevent diversion or abuse by proper handling.

HOW SUPPLIED

OxyContin® (oxycodone hydrochloride controlled-release) 10 mg tablets are round, unscored, white-colored, convex tablets bearing the symbol OC on one side and 10 on the other. They are supplied as follows:

NDC 59011-100-10: child-resistant closure, opaque plastic bottles of 100

NDC 59011-100-25: unit dose packaging with 25 individually numbered tablets per card; one card per glue end carton

OxyContin® (oxycodone hydrochloride controlled-release) 20 mg tablets are round, unscored, pink-colored, convex tablets bearing the symbol OC on one side and 20 on the other. They are supplied as follows:

NDC 59011-103-10: child-resistant closure, opaque plastic bottles of 100

NDC 59011-103-25: unit dose packaging with 25 individually numbered tablets per card; one card per glue end carton

OxyContin® (oxycodone hydrochloride controlled-release) 40 mg tablets are round, unscored, yellow-colored, convex tablets bearing the symbol OC on one side and 40 on the other. They are supplied as follows:

NDC 59011-105-10: child-resistant closure, opaque plastic bottles of 100

NDC 59011-105-25: unit dose packaging with 25 individually numbered tablets per card; one card per glue end carton

OxyContin® (oxycodone hydrochloride controlled-release) 80 mg tablets are round, unscored, green-colored, convex tablets bearing the symbol OC on one side and 80 on the other. They are supplied as follows:

NDC 59011-107-10: child-resistant closure, opaque plastic bottles of 100

NDC 59011-107-25: unit dose packaging with 25 individually numbered tablets per card; one card per glue end carton

OxyContin® (oxycodone hydrochloride controlled-release) 160 mg tablets are modified caplet-shaped, unscored, blue-colored, convex tablets bearing the symbol OC on one side and 160 on the other. They are supplied as follows:

NDC 59011-109-10: child-resistant closure, opaque plastic bottles of 100

NDC 59011-109-25: unit dose packaging with 25 individually numbered tablets per card; one card per glue end carton

Store at 25°C (77°F); excursions permitted between 15°–30°C (59°–86°F).

Dispense in tight, light-resistant container.

CAUTION

DEA Order Form Required.

Manufactured by The PF Laboratories, Inc.
Totowa, N.J. 07512

Distributed by Purdue Pharma L.P.
Stamford, CT 06901-3431

U.S. Patent Numbers 4,861,598; 4,970,075; 5,266,331; 5,508,042; 5,549,912; and 5,656,295

June 6, 2000 M4909 00PO10

Shown in Product Identification Guide, page 332

OXYIR® Ⓒ℞

(oxycodone hydrochloride)
Immediate-Release Oral Capsules
5 mg

OXYFAST® Ⓒ℞

(oxycodone hydrochloride)
Immediate-Release
Oral CONCENTRATE Solution*
20 mg/1mL
***This product contains dry natural rubber**

DESCRIPTION

Oxycodone is 14-hydroxydihydrocodeinone, a white odorless crystalline powder which is derived from the opium alkaloid, thebaine, and may be represented by the following structural formula:

OxyIR Oral Capsules

Each 5 mg of OxyIR Capsules contains:

Oxycodone hydrochloride .... 5 mg

Inactive ingredients: Hydroxypropyl methylcellulose, Maize starch, Polyethylene glycol, Polysorbate 80, Sucrose, Synthetic red iron oxide E172, Synthetic yellow iron oxide E172, Titanium dioxide E171.

OxyFast Oral CONCENTRATE Solution

Each 1 mL of OxyFast **Concentrate** Solution contains:

Oxycodone hydrochloride .... 20 mg

Inactive ingredients: Citric acid, FD&C Yellow #10, Sodium benzoate, Sodium citrate, Sodium saccharine and water.

ACTIONS

The analgesic ingredient, oxycodone, is a semisynthetic narcotic with multiple actions qualitatively similar to those of morphine; the most prominent of these involve the central nervous system and organs composed of smooth muscle. The principal actions of therapeutic value of oxycodone are analgesia and sedation.

CLINICAL PHARMACOLOGY

Central Nervous System: Oxycodone is a pure agonist opioid whose principal therapeutic action is analgesia. Other therapeutic effects of oxycodone include anxiolysis, euphoria and feelings of relaxation. Like all pure opioid agonists, there is no ceiling effect to analgesia, such as is seen with partial agonists or non-opioid analgesics.

The precise mechanism of the analgesic action is unknown. However, specific CNS opioid receptors for endogenous compounds with opioid-like activity have been identified throughout the brain and spinal cord and play a role in the analgesic effects of this drug.

Oxycodone produces respiratory depression by direct action on brain stem respiratory centers. The respiratory depression involves both a reduction in the responsiveness of the brain stem respiratory centers to increases in carbon dioxide tension and to electrical stimulation.

Oxycodone depresses the cough reflex by direct effect on the cough center in the medulla. Antitussive effects may occur with doses lower than those usually required for analgesia.

Oxycodone causes miosis, even in total darkness. Pinpoint pupils are a sign of opioid overdose but are not pathognomonic. Marked mydriasis rather than miosis may be seen due to hypoxia in overdose situations.

Gastrointestinal Tract and Other Smooth Muscle: Oxycodone causes a reduction in motility associated with an increase in smooth muscle tone in the antrum of the stomach and duodenum. Digestion of food in the small intestine is delayed and propulsive contractions are decreased. Propulsive peristaltic waves in the colon are decreased, while tone may be increased to the point of spasm resulting in constipation. Other opioid-induced effects may include a reduction in gastric, biliary and pancreatic secretions, spasm of sphincter of Oddi, and transient elevations in serum amylase.

Cardiovascular System: Oxycodone may produce release of histamine with or without associated peripheral vasodilation. Manifestations of histamine release and/or peripheral vasodilation may include pruritus, flushing, red eyes, sweating, and/or orthostatic hypotension.

Concentration—Effect Relationships (Pharmacodynamics): Studies in normal volunteers and patients reveal predictable relationships between oxycodone dosage and plasma oxycodone concentrations, as well as between concentration and certain expected opioid effects. In normal volunteers these include pupillary constriction, sedation and overall "drug effect" and in patients, analgesia and feelings of "relaxation." In non-tolerant patients, analgesia is not usually seen at a plasma oxycodone concentration of less than 5–10 ng/mL.

As with all opioids, the minimum effective plasma concentration for analgesia will vary widely among patients, especially among patients who have been previously treated with potent agonist opioids. As a result, patients need to be treated with individualized titration of dosage to the desired effect. The minimum effective analgesic concentration of oxycodone for any individual patient may increase with repeated dosing due to an increase in pain and/or the development of tolerance.

Concentration—Adverse Experience Relationships: OxyIR Capsules and OxyFast **CONCENTRATE** Solution are associated with typical opioid-related adverse experiences similar to those seen with all opioids. There is a general relationship between increasing oxycodone plasma concentration and increasing frequency of dose-related opioid adverse experiences such as nausea, vomiting, CNS effects and respiratory depression. In opioid-tolerant patients, the situation is altered by the development of tolerance to opioid-related side effects, and the relationship is poorly understood.

As with all opioids, the dose must be individualized (see DOSAGE AND ADMINISTRATION), because the effective analgesic dose for some patients will be too high to be tolerated by other patients.

INDICATIONS AND USAGE

For the relief of moderate to moderately severe pain.

CONTRAINDICATIONS

OxyIR and OxyFast are contraindicated in patients with known hypersensitivity to oxycodone, or in any situation where opioids are contraindicated. This includes patients with significant respiratory depression (in unmonitored settings or the absence of resuscitative equipment), and patients with acute or severe bronchial asthma or hypercarbia. OxyIR and OxyFast are contraindicated in any patient who has or is suspected of having paralytic ileus.

WARNINGS

Respiratory Depression: Respiratory depression is the chief hazard from all opioid agonist preparations. Respiratory depression occurs most frequently in elderly or debilitated patients, usually following large initial doses in non-tolerant patients, or when opioids are given in conjunction with other agents that depress respiration.

Oxycodone should be used with extreme caution in patients with significant chronic obstructive pulmonary disease or cor pulmonale, and in patients having a substantially decreased respiratory reserve, hypoxia, hypercapnia, or preexisting respiratory depression. In such patients, even usual therapeutic doses of oxycodone may decrease respiratory drive to the point of apnea. In these patients alternative non-opioid analgesics should be considered, and opioids should be employed only under careful medical supervision at the lowest effective dose.

Hypotensive Effect: OxyIR® Capsules and OxyFast® **CONCENTRATE** Solution, like all opioid analgesics, may cause severe hypotension in an individual whose ability to maintain blood pressure has been compromised by a depleted blood volume, or after concurrent administration with drugs such as phenothiazines or other agents which compromise vasomotor tone. OxyIR and OxyFast may produce orthostatic hypotension in ambulatory patients. OxyIR and OxyFast, like all opioid analgesics, should be administered with caution to patients in circulatory shock, since va-

Continued on next page

OxyIR/OxyFAST—Cont.

sodilation produced by the drug may further reduce cardiac output and blood pressure.

Drug Dependence: Oxycodone can produce drug dependence of the morphine type, and therefore, has the potential for being abused. Psychic dependence, physical dependence and tolerance may develop upon repeated administration of this drug, and it should be prescribed and administered with the same degree of caution appropriate to the use of other oral narcotic-containing medications. Like other narcotic-containing medications, this drug is subject to the Federal Controlled Substances Act.

Usage in Ambulatory Patients: Oxycodone may impair the mental and/or physical abilities required for the performance of potential hazardous tasks such as driving a car or operating machinery. The patient using this drug should be cautioned accordingly.

Interaction with Other Central Nervous System Depressants: Patients receiving other narcotic analgesics, general anesthetics, phenothiazines, other tranquilizers, sedative-hypnotics or other CNS depressants (including alcohol) concomitantly with oxycodone hydrochloride may exhibit an additive CNS depression. When such combined therapy is contemplated, the dose of one or both agents should be reduced.

Usage in Pregnancy: Safe use in pregnancy has not been established relative to possible adverse effects on fetal development. Therefore, this drug should not be used in pregnant women unless, in the judgment of the physician, the potential benefits outweigh the possible hazards.

Usage in Children: This drug should not be administered to children.

PRECAUTIONS

Special Precautions Regarding OxyFast Oral CONCENTRATE 20 mg/1mL Solution

OxyFast 20 mg/1 mL solution is a highly concentrated solution. Care should be taken in the prescription and dispensing of this solution strength. Patients should be instructed against use by individuals other than the patient, as inappropriate use may cause acute overdosage.

General

Opioid analgesics given on a fixed-dosage schedule have a narrow therapeutic index in certain patient populations, especially when combined with other drugs, and should be reserved for cases where the benefits of opioid analgesia outweigh the known risks of respiratory depression, altered mental state, and postural hypotension.

Use of OxyIR® and OxyFast® is associated with increased potential risks and should be used only with caution in the following conditions: acute alcoholism; adrenocortical insufficiency (e.g., Addison's disease); CNS depression or coma; delirium tremens; debilitated patients; kyphoscoliosis associated with respiratory depression; myxedema or hypothyroidism; prostatic hypertrophy or urethral stricture; severe impairment of hepatic, pulmonary or renal function; and toxic psychosis.

The administration of oxycodone, like all opioid analgesics, may obscure the diagnosis or clinical course in patients with acute abdominal conditions. Oxycodone may aggravate convulsions in patients with convulsive disorders, and all opioids may induce or aggravate seizures in some clinical settings.

Interactions with Mixed Agonist/Antagonist Opioid Analgesics: Agonist/antagonist and partial agonist analgesics (i.e., pentazocine, nalbuphine, butorphanol and buprenorphine) should be administered with caution to a patient who has received or is receiving a course of therapy with a pure opioid agonist analgesic such as oxycodone. In this situation, mixed agonist/antagonist and partial agonist analgesics may reduce the analgesic effect of oxycodone and/or may precipitate withdrawal symptoms in these patients.

Use in Pancreatic/Biliary Tract Disease: Oxycodone may cause spasm of the sphincter of Oddi and should be used with caution in patients with biliary tract disease, including acute pancreatitis. Opioids like oxycodone may cause increases in the serum amylase level.

Head Injury and Increased Intracranial Pressure: The respiratory depressant effects of opioids and their capacity to elevate cerebrospinal fluid pressure may be markedly exaggerated in the presence of head injury, other intracranial lesions or a pre-existing increase in intracranial pressure. Furthermore, opioids produce adverse reactions which may obscure the clinical course of patients with head injuries.

Acute Abdominal Conditions: The administration of this drug or other opioids may obscure the diagnosis or clinical course in patients with acute abdominal conditions.

Information for Patients/Caregivers: If clinically advisable, patients receiving OxyIR (immediate-release) Capsules or OxyFast **CONCENTRATE** Solution or their caregivers should be given the following information by the physician, nurse, pharmacist or caregiver:

1. Patients should be advised not to adjust the dose of this drug without consulting the prescribing professional.
2. Patients should be advised that this drug may impair mental and/or physical ability required for the performance of potentially hazardous tasks (e.g., driving, operating heavy machinery).
3. Patients should not combine this drug with alcohol or other central nervous system depressants (sleep aids, tranquilizers) except by the orders of the prescribing physician, because additive effects may occur.
4. Women of childbearing potential who become, or are planning to become, pregnant should be advised to consult their physician regarding the effects of analgesics and other drug use during pregnancy on themselves and their unborn child.
5. Patients should be advised that this drug is a potential drug of abuse. They should protect it from theft, and it should never be given to anyone other than the individual for whom it was prescribed.
6. Patients should be advised that if they have been receiving treatment with this drug for more than a few weeks and cessation of therapy is indicated, it may be appropriate to taper this drug dose, rather than abruptly discontinue it, due to the risk of precipitating withdrawal symptoms. Their physician can provide a dose schedule to accomplish a gradual discontinuation of the medication.

Laboratory Monitoring: Due to the broad range of plasma concentrations seen in clinical populations, the varying degrees of pain, and the development of tolerance, plasma oxycodone measurements are usually not helpful in clinical management. Plasma concentrations of the active drug substance may be of value in selected, unusual or complex cases.

Use in Drug and Alcohol Addiction: OxyIR and OxyFast are opioids with no approved use in the management of addictive disorders. Their proper usage in individuals with drug or alcohol dependence, either active or in remission, is for the management of pain requiring opioid analgesia.

Drug-Drug Interactions: The CNS depressant effects of oxycodone hydrochloride may be additive with that of other CNS depressants. See WARNINGS.

Opioid analgesics, including OxyIR and OxyFast, may enhance the neuromuscular blocking action of skeletal muscle relaxants and produce an increased degree of respiratory depression.

Oxycodone is metabolized in part to oxymorphone via CYP2D6. While this pathway may be blocked by a variety of drugs (e.g., certain cardiovascular drugs and antidepressants), such blockade has not yet been shown to be of clinical significance with this agent. Clinicians should be aware of this possible interaction, however.

Mutagenicity/Carcinogenicity: Oxycodone was not mutagenic in the following assays: Ames Salmonella and E. Coli test with and without metabolic activation at doses of up to 5000 μg, chromosomal aberration test in human lymphocytes (in the absence of metabolic activation at doses of up to 1500 μg/ml and with activation 48 hours after exposure) at doses of up to 5000 μg/ml, and in the in vivo bone marrow micronucleus test in mice (at plasma levels of up to 48 μg/ml). Mutagenic results occurred in the presence of metabolic activation in the human chromosomal aberration test (at greater than or equal to 1250 μg/ml) at 24 but not 48 hours of exposure and in the mouse lymphoma assay at doses of 50 μg/ml or greater with metabolic activation and at 400 μg/ml or greater without metabolic activation. The data from these tests indicate that the genotoxic risk to humans may be considered low.

Studies of oxycodone in animals to evaluate its carcinogenic potential have not been conducted owing to the length of clinical experience with the drug substance.

Pregnancy: Teratogenic Effects—Category B: Reproduction studies have been performed in rats and rabbits by oral administration at doses up to 8 mg/kg (48 mg/m^2) and 125 mg/kg (1375 mg/m^2), respectively. These doses are 3 and 47 times a human dose of 160 mg/day (90 mg/m^2), based on mg/kg of a 60 kg adult (0.5 and 15 times this human dose based upon mg/m^2). The results did not reveal evidence of harm to the fetus due to oxycodone. There are, however, no adequate and well-controlled studies in pregnant women. Because animal reproduction studies are not always predictive of human response, this drug should be used during pregnancy only if clearly needed.

Nonteratogenic Effects—Neonates whose mothers have been taking oxycodone chronically may exhibit respiratory depression and/or withdrawal symptoms, either at birth and/or in the nursery.

Labor and Delivery: OxyIR® and OxyFast® are not recommended for use in women during and immediately prior to labor and delivery because oral opioids may cause respiratory depression in the newborn.

Nursing Mothers: Low concentrations of oxycodone have been detected in breast milk. Withdrawal symptoms can occur in breast-feeding infants when maternal administration of an opioid analgesic is stopped. Ordinarily, nursing should not be undertaken while a patient is receiving OxyIR or OxyFast since oxycodone may be excreted in the milk.

Pediatric Use: Safety and effectiveness in pediatric patients have not been established.

Special Risk Patients: This drug should be given with caution to certain patients such as the elderly, or debilitated, and those with severe impairment of hepatic or renal function, hypothyroidism, Addison's disease and prostatic hypertrophy or urethral stricture.

ADVERSE REACTIONS

The most frequently observed reactions include light-headedness, dizziness, sedation, nausea and vomiting. These effects seem to be more prominent in ambulatory than in nonambulatory patients, and some of these adverse reactions may be alleviated if the patient lies down. Many of these adverse events will cease or decrease in intensity as oxycodone therapy is continued and some degree of tolerance is developed.

Other adverse reactions include euphoria, dysphoria, constipation, skin rash and pruritus.

DRUG ABUSE AND DEPENDENCE (Addiction)

Oxycodone products are common targets for both drug abusers and drug addicts.

Drug addiction (drug dependence, psychological dependence) is characterized by a preoccupation with the procurement, hoarding, and abuse of drugs for non-medicinal purposes. Drug dependence is treatable, utilizing a multi-disciplinary approach, but relapse is common. Iatrogenic "addiction" to opioids legitimately used in the management of pain is very rare. "Drug seeking" behavior is very common to addicts. Tolerance and physical dependence in pain patients are not signs of psychological dependence. Preoccupation with achieving adequate pain relief can be appropriate behavior in a patient with poor pain control. Most chronic pain patients limit their intake of opioids to achieve a balance between the benefits of the drug and dose-limiting side effects. Physicians should be aware that psychological dependence may not be accompanied by concurrent tolerance and symptoms of physical dependence in all addicts. In addition, abuse of opioids can occur in the absence of true psychological dependence and is characterized by misuse for non-medical purposes, often in combination with other psychoactive substances.

MANAGEMENT OF OVERDOSAGE

Signs and Symptoms: Serious overdose of oxycodone hydrochloride is characterized by respiratory depression (a decrease in respiratory rate and/or tidal volume, Cheyne-Stokes respiration, cyanosis), extreme somnolence progressing to stupor or coma, skeletal muscle flaccidity, cold and clammy skin, and sometimes bradycardia and hypotension. In severe overdosage, apnea, circulatory collapse, cardiac arrest and death may occur.

Treatment: Primary attention should be given to the reestablishment of adequate respiratory exchange through provision of a patent airway and the institution of assisted or controlled ventilation. The narcotic antagonist naloxone is a specific antidote against respiratory depression which may result from overdosage or unusual sensitivity to narcotics, including oxycodone. Therefore, an appropriate dose of naloxone (usual initial adult dose: 0.4 mg) should be administered, preferably by the intravenous route, simultaneously with efforts at respiratory resuscitation. Since the duration of action of oxycodone may exceed that of the antagonist, the patient should be kept under continued surveillance and repeated doses of the antagonist should be administered as needed to maintain adequate respiration. An antagonist should not be administered in the absence of clinically significant respiratory or cardiovascular depression.

Oxygen, intravenous fluids, vasopressors and other supportive measures should be employed as indicated.

Gastric emptying may be useful in removing unabsorbed drug.

DOSAGE AND ADMINISTRATION

Special Precautions Regarding OxyFast Oral CONCENTRATE 20 mg/1 mL Solution

OxyFast 20 mg/1 mL solution is a highly concentrated solution. Care should be taken in the prescription and dispensing of this solution strength. Patients should be instructed against use by individuals other than the patient, as inappropriate use may cause acute overdosage.

Dosage should be adjusted to the severity of the pain and the response of the patient. It may occasionally be necessary to exceed the usual dosage recommended below in cases of more severe pain or in those patients who have become tolerant to the analgesic effects of opioids. This drug is given orally. The usual adult dosage is 5 mg every 6 hours as needed for pain.

Nurse/Patient Instructions: Fill dropper to the level of the prescribed dose (1.0 mL=20 mg; 0.75 mL=15 mg; 0.5 mL=10 mg and 0.25 mL=5 mg). For ease of administration, add dose to approximately 30 mL (1 fl. oz.) or more of juice or other liquid. May also be added to applesauce, pudding or other semi-solid foods. The drug-food mixture should be used immediately and not stored for future use.

HOW SUPPLIED

OxyIR (oxycodone hydrochloride) Capsules:

5 mg capsules, Cap: Beige Imprinted with O-IR; Body: Orange Imprinted with PF5mg.

NDC 59011-201-10: Opaque plastic bottle containing 100 Capsules

OxyFast (oxycodone hydrochloride) Oral CONCENTRATE Solution:

20 mg per 1 mL.

NDC 59011-225-20: High density polyethylene plastic, with child-resistant closure bottle with child-resistant dropper in 30 mL size.

Discard opened bottle of oral solution after 90 days. Protect from light.

Store OxyFast oral CONCENTRATE solutions and capsules at controlled room temperature 15° to 30°C (59°–86°F).

Caution

DEA Order Form Required.

Printed in U.S.A.

Purdue Pharma L.P., Stamford, CT 06901-3431

June 9, 2000

F4597-811 00PO11
Shown in Product Identification Guide, page 332

EDUCATIONAL MATERIAL

Website containing pain management information for healthcare professionals and patients. Available at www.partnersagainstpain.com

Questcor Pharmaceuticals, Inc.

26118 RESEARCH ROAD
HAYWARD, CA 94545

Direct Inquiries to:
(510) 732-5551
FAX: (510) 732-7741

ETHAMOLIN® ℞

[*ē-tham-ō-lin*]
(ethanolamine oleate)
Injection, 5%
For Local Intravenous Use Only

DESCRIPTION

ETHAMOLIN® (ethanolamine oleate) Injection is a mild sclerosing agent.
Chemically it is $C_{17}H_{33}COOH.\ NH_2CH_2CH_2OH$. It has the following structure:

$$\left[\begin{matrix} CH_2CH_2-OH \\ \overset{|}{N}H_2^{+} \\ H \end{matrix}\right] \quad CH_3-(CH_2)_7-CH{=}CH-(CH_2)_7-\overset{O}{\overset{\|}{C}}-O^-$$

The empirical formula is $C_{20}H_{41}NO_3$, representing a molecular weight of 343.55.
ETHAMOLIN Injection consists of ethanolamine, a basic substance, which when combined with oleic acids forms a clear, straw to pale yellow colored, deliquescent oleate. The pH ranges from 8.0 to 9.0.
ETHAMOLIN Injection is a sterile, apyrogenic, aqueous solution containing in each mL approximately 50 mg of ethanolamine oleate with benzyl alcohol 2% by volume as preservative.

HOW SUPPLIED

ETHAMOLIN® (ethanolamine oleate) Injection, 5% is available in 2 mL ampules in boxes of 10 (NDC 63004-4790-6).
Store at Controlled Room Temperature, 15°–30°C (59°–86°F). Protect from light.

GLOFIL™-125 ℞

[*glōw-fill*]
Sodium Iothalamate I-125
Injection, USP

INULIN AND SODIUM CHLORIDE INJECTION USP ℞

[*in-ū-lynn*]
For Intravenous Injection

R&D Laboratories, Inc.

4640 ADMIRALTY WAY, SUITE 710
MARINA DEL REY, CA 90292

Direct Inquiries to:
Gregory Little,
(310) 305-8053, extension 227
(800) 338-9066
FAX (310) 305-8103

For Medical Emergencies:
Jur Strobos, MD
(310) 345-6370

CALCI–CHEW®
Medical Food

1.25 gm USP grade calcium carbonate chewable tablets—500 mg elemental calcium. Packaged as three separate flavors—cherry, lemon, orange.

DESCRIPTION

Tablets supplying 1.25 gm USP grade calcium carbonate. Contains no dyes and no sodium.

INDICATIONS

For the distinctive nutritional needs of renal patients as calcium supplementation, in the treatment of hypocalcemia, and the binding of phosphorous in the G.I. tract.

DOSAGE

For hypocalcemia, use as necessary to restore calcium to normal levels. For patients with impaired calcium absorption or on a calcium restricted diet, give under a physician's guidance.

HOW SUPPLIED

Plastic bottles of 100 tablets.

FLAVOR	NDC No.
CHERRY	54391-0025-2
LEMON	54391-0225-2
ORANGE	54391-0325-2

CALCI–MIX®
Medical Food

1.25 gm USP grade calcium carbonate powdered in pull apart capsules. Contains 500 mg of elemental calcium. Can be swallowed or pulled apart and sprinkled on food or in drink.

DESCRIPTION

Gelatin capsules containing 1.25 gm USP grade calcium carbonate. Contains no sodium and no dyes.

INDICATIONS

For the distinctive nutritional needs of renal patients as calcium supplementation, in the treatment of hypocalcemia, and the binding of phosphorous in the G.I. tract.

DOSAGE

For hypocalcemia, use as necessary to restore calcium to normal levels. For patients with impaired calcium absorption or on a calcium restricted diet, give under a physician's guidance.

SUPPLIED

Plastic bottles of 100 capsules. NDC 54391-0027-3.

L-CARNITINE
Medical Food

250 mg capsules.
Plastic bottles of 60 capsules
NDC 54391-0050-9

MAG-CARB®
[*măg-kărb*]
Medical Food

DESCRIPTION

A 250 mg magnesium carbonate medical food packaged in a gel capsule, delivering 70 mg of elemental magnesium. Used as a general supplement and especially suitable for the transplant recipient on cyclosporin therapy who is at risk for magnesium deficiency, and in the binding of phosphorous in the G.I. tract.

INGREDIENTS

Magnesium carbonate, magnesium stearate, cellulose, and gelatin.

DOSAGE

As needed or prescribed.

HOW SUPPLIED

Clear gelatin capsules in plastic bottles of 100. Store tightly in a cool, dry place.
NDC #54391-0031-3

NEPHRO–CALCI®
Medical Food

1.5 gm USP grade calcium carbonate tablets—600 mg elemental calcium.

DESCRIPTION

Tablets supplying 1.5 gm of (USP grade) calcium carbonate. Contains no dyes.

INDICATIONS

For the distinctive nutritional needs of renal patients as calcium supplementation, in the treatment of hypocalcemia, and the binding of phosphorous in the G.I. tract.

DOSAGE

For hypocalcemia, use as necessary to restore calcium to normal levels. For patients with impaired calcium absorption and patients on a calcium restricted diet, give under a physician's guidance.

SUPPLIED

Plastic bottles of 100 tablets. NDC 54391-0026-3.

NEPHRO–FER®
Medical Food

High-potency iron for the distinctive nutritional needs of renal patients.

DESCRIPTION

Each tablet supplies 350 mg of ferrous fumarate—115 mg of elemental iron.

INDICATIONS

Patients taking EPO requiring oral iron supplementation—particularly patients who experience gastric problems with ferrous sulfate. Appropriate for any iron supplementation. (See Nephro-Fer® Rx for side effects.)

DOSAGE

One tablet daily or as directed by a physician.

SUPPLIED

Brown oval tablets marked RD13.
Tablets in unit dose blister packs of 30. NDC 54391-0013-8.

NEPHRO-FER® Rx ℞
Iron Supplement With Folic Acid

Oral iron supplement. For any patient needing iron supplementation for documented iron deficiency. Suitable for certain patients undergoing therapy with erythropoietin.

DESCRIPTION

Each tablet contains 324 mg ferrous fumarate—106.9 mg elemental iron—and 1 mg folic acid. Ferrous fumarate may be better tolerated than ferrous sulfate in some patients.

INDICATIONS

Renal failure patients and patients who have documented iron deficiency. Patients undergoing erythropoietin therapy who risk iron deficiency.

DOSAGE

One to three tablets daily between meals as required to correct iron deficiency, or as prescribed by physician.

SIDE EFFECTS

Transient bloating, flatulence, constipation, and diarrhea. Ingestion of greater than 400 mg per day of elemental iron can result in nausea and vomiting.

PRECAUTION

See folic acid precaution under NEPHRO-VITE® + FE

SUPPLIED

Brown, oval tablets marked RD33.
Tablets in unit dose blister packs of 30. NDC 54391-1313-8.
For use under medical supervision.

NEPHRAMINE® ℞
5.4% Essential Amino Acid Injection

DESCRIPTION

5.4% NephrAmine® (Essential Amino Acid Injection) is a sterile, nonpyrogenic solution containing crystalline essential amino acids plus histidine. Each 250 mL unit provides Rose's recommended daily intake of essential amino acids[1] plus 625 mg of histidine, considered essential for uremics. The total nitrogen content of a 250 mL unit is approximately 1.6 grams (10 g of protein equivalent) in 14 grams of amino acids. All amino acids designated USP are the "L" isomer.

Each 100 mL contains:

Histidine USP*	0.25 g
Isoleucine USP	0.56 g
Leucine USP	0.88 g
Lysine	0.64 g
(added as Lysine Acetate USP	0.90 g)
Methionine USP	0.88 g
Phenylalanine USP	0.88 g
Threonine USP	0.40 g
Tryptophan USP	0.20 g
Valine USP	0.64 g
Cysteine	<0.014 g
(as Cysteine HCl·H_2O USP	<0.020 g)
Sodium Bisulfite (as an antioxidant)	<0.05 g
Water for Injection USP	qs

pH adjusted with Sodium Hydroxide NF as required
pH: 6.5 (6.0–7.0); Calculated Osmolarity: 435 mOsmol/liter
Total Nitrogen: Approx. 0.65 g/100 mL
Concentration of Electrolytes (mEq/liter): Sodium 5
Chloride <3; Acetate Approx. 44

*Histidine is considered an essential amino acid in uremic patients
[1] Rose WC: The sequence of events leading to the establishment of the amino acid needs of man. **Am J Public Health; 1968: 58(11): 2020–2027**

CLINICAL PHARMACOLOGY

NephrAmine® provides an intravenously compatible mixture of essential amino acids which, when infused with hypertonic dextrose as a source of calories, plus electrolytes, minerals, and vitamins, provides in a small volume of fluid all ingredients (with the exception of essential fatty acids) needed for total parenteral nutrition in patients with renal disease.
Infusion of NephrAmine® and hypertonic dextrose provides essential amino acids and calories for protein synthesis to

Continued on next page

Nephramine—Cont.

promote improved cellular metabolic balance. Infusion of these components can decrease the rate of rise of blood urea nitrogen (bun) and minimize deterioration of serum potassium, magnesium and phosphorus balance in patients with impaired renal function. The extent to which essential amino acids and calories promote incorporation of waste urea nitrogen into newly synthesized amino acids in man, as it does in experimental animals, is, so far, not established.

The accelerated decrease in serum creatinine levels seen in patients with limited extra-renal complications suggests that treatment with NephrAmine® and hypertonic dextrose leads to earlier return of renal function in patients with potentially reversible acute renal failure. By providing nutritional support and promoting biochemical improvement as well as earlier return of renal function, NephrAmine® and hypertonic dextrose decrease morbidity associated with acute renal failure.

It is thought that acetate from lysine acetate, under the condition of parenteral nutrition, does not impact net acid-base balance when renal and respiratory functions are normal. Clinical evidence seems to support this thinking; however, confirmatory experimental evidence is not available.

The amounts of sodium and chloride present are not of clinical significance.

INDICATIONS AND USAGE

5.4% NephrAmine® (Essential Amino Acid Injection) is indicated for adult and pediatric use, in conjunction with other measures, to provide nutritional support for uremic patients, particularly when oral nutrition is infeasible or impractical. See ***Special Precautions in Pediatric Patients*** for additional information.

CONTRAINDICATIONS

NephrAmine® is contraindicated in patients with severe, uncorrected electrolyte and acid-base imbalance, hyperammonemia, decreased (subcritical) circulating blood volume, inborn errors of amino acid metabolism, or hypersensitivity to one or more amino acids present in the solution.

WARNINGS

This product contains sodium bisulfite, a sulfite that may cause allergic-type reactions including anaphylactic symptoms and life-threatening or less severe asthmatic episodes in certain susceptible people. The overall prevalence of sulfite sensitivity in the general population is unknown and probably low. Sulfite sensitivity is seen more frequently in asthmatic than in nonasthmatic people.

Safe and effective use of central venous nutrition requires a knowledge of nutrition as well as clinical expertise in recognition and treatment of the complications which can occur. **Frequent clinical evaluation and laboratory determinations are necessary for proper monitoring of central venous nutrition.** Studies should include blood sugar, serum proteins, kidney and liver function tests, electrolytes, hemogram, carbon dioxide combining power, serum osmolarity, blood cultures, blood ammonia levels, and circulating blood volume.

NephrAmine® does not replace dialysis and conventional supportive therapy in patients with renal failure.

Administration of NephrAmine® to children or low birth-weight infants, especially in high doses, may result in hyperammonemia.

Clinically significant hypokalemia, hypophosphatemia, or hypomagnesemia may occur as a result of therapy with NephrAmine® and hypertonic dextrose and replacement therapy may become necessary.

Administration of nitrogen in any form to patients with marked hepatic insufficiency or hepatic coma may result in plasma amino acid imbalances, hyperammonemia, or central nervous system deterioration. NephrAmine® should, therefore, be used with caution in such patients.

The intravenous administration of these solutions can cause fluid and/or solute overload resulting in dilution of serum electrolyte concentrations, overhydration, congested states or pulmonary edema. The risk of dilutional states is inversely proportional to the solute concentration of the solution infused. The risk of solute overload causing congested states with peripheral and pulmonary edema is directly proportional to the concentration of the solution.

Conservative doses of amino acids should be given, dictated by the nutritional status of the patient.

PRECAUTIONS

General

Clinical evaluation and periodic laboratory determinations are necessary to monitor changes in fluid balance, electrolyte concentrations, and acid-base balance during prolonged parenteral therapy or whenever the condition of the patient warrants such evaluation. Significant deviations from normal concentrations may require the use of additional electrolyte supplements.

In order to promote urea nitrogen reutilization in patients with renal failure, it is essential to provide adequate calories with minimal amounts of the essential amino acids, and to severely restrict the intake of nonessential nitrogen. Hypertonic dextrose solutions are a convenient and metabolically effective source of concentrated calories.

Fluid balance must be carefully monitored in patients with renal failure and care should be taken to avoid circulatory overload, particularly in association with cardiac insufficiency.

In patients with myocardial infarct, infusion of amino acids should always be accompanied by dextrose, since in anoxia, free fatty acids cannot be utilized by the myocardium, and energy must be produced anaerobically from glycogen or glucose.

Strongly hypertonic nutrient solutions should be administered through an indwelling intravenous catheter with the tip located in the superior vena cava.

Special care must be taken when giving hypertonic dextrose to glucose-intolerant patients such as diabetic or prediabetic and uremic patients; especially when the latter are receiving peritoneal dialysis. To prevent severe hyperglycemia in such patients, insulin may be required.

Administration of glucose at a rate exceeding the patient's utilization may lead to hyperglycemia, coma, and death.

Administration of amino acids without carbohydrates may result in the accumulation of ketone bodies in the blood. Correction of this ketonemia may be achieved by the administration of carbohydrates. Abrupt cessation of hypertonic dextrose infusion may result in rebound hypoglycemia.

When 5.4% NephrAmine® (Essential Amino Acid Injection) is subjected to changes in temperature, there is a chance that some transient crystallization of amino acids may occur. Thorough shaking of the bottle for about one minute should redissolve the amino acids. If the amino acids do not completely redissolve, the bottle must be rejected.

To minimize the risk of possible incompatibilities arising from mixing this solution with other additives that may be prescribed, the final infusate should be inspected for cloudiness or precipitation immediately after mixing, prior to administration, and periodically during administration.

Use only if solution is clear and vacuum is present.

Usage in Pregnancy

Pregnancy Category C. Animal reproduction studies have not been conducted with 5.4% NephrAmine® (Essential Amino Acid Injection). It is also not known whether NephrAmine® can cause fetal harm when administered to a pregnant woman or can affect reproduction capacity. NephrAmine® should be given to a pregnant woman only if clearly needed.

Special Precautions for Central Venous Nutrition

Administration by central venous catheter should be used only by those familiar with this technique and its complications.

Central venous nutrition may be associated with complications which can be prevented or minimized by careful attention to all aspects of the procedure including solution preparation, administration, and patient monitoring. **It is essential that a carefully prepared protocol, based on current medical practices, be followed, preferably by an experienced team.**

SEE PACKAGE INSERT FOR ADDITIONAL INFORMATION ON CENTRAL VENOUS ADMINISTRATION.

Special Precautions in Patients with Renal Insufficiency

Frequent laboratory studies are necessary in patients with renal insufficiency due to underlying metabolic abnormalities. Hyperglycemia, a frequent complication, may not be reflected by glycosuria in renal failure. Blood glucose, therefore, must be determined frequently, often every six hours to guide dosage of dextrose and insulin if required.

Serum concentrations of potassium, phosphorus, and magnesium may dramatically decline with successful treatment, individually or together; these substances should be supplemented as required. Special care must be taken to avoid hypokalemia in digitalized patients, or those with cardiac arrhythmias.

Special Precautions in Pediatric Patients

5.4% NephrAmine® (Essential Amino Acid Injection) should be used with special caution in pediatric patients, especially low birth-weight infants, due to limited clinical experience.

Laboratory and clinical monitoring of pediatric patients, especially when nutritionally depleted, must be extensive and frequent. Initial total daily dose should be low, and increased slowly. Dosage of NephrAmine® above one gram of essential amino acids per kilogram body weight per day is not recommended.

Frequent monitoring of blood glucose is required in low birth-weight or septic infants as infusion of hypertonic dextrose carries a greater risk of hyperglycemia in such patients.

The absence of arginine in NephrAmine® may accentuate the risk of hyperammonemia in infants.

ADVERSE REACTIONS

See **WARNINGS** and ***Special Precautions for Central Venous Nutrition.***

Reactions which may occur because of the solution or the technique of administration include febrile response, infection at the site of injection, venous thrombosis, and hypervolemia.

Symptoms may result from an excess or deficit of one or more of the ions present in the solution infused, therefore, frequent monitoring of electrolyte levels is essential.

Infrequent instances of hyperammonemia have been reported following administration of essential amino acid solutions to patients with massive gastrointestinal hemorrhage, nonuremic infants and children or following administration of higher than recommended doses to adult or pediatric patients. Serum ammonia levels and clinical symptoms may subside when the infusions are discontinued.

Phosphorus deficiency may lead to impaired tissue oxygenation and acute hemolytic anemia. Relative to calcium, excessive phosphorus intake can precipitate hypocalcemia with cramps, tetany and muscular hyperexcitability.

If an adverse reaction does occur, discontinue the infusion, evaluate the patient, institute appropriate therapeutic countermeasures and save the remainder of the fluid for examination if deemed necessary.

OVERDOSAGE

In the event of a fluid or solute overload during parenteral therapy, reevaluate the patient's condition, and institute appropriate corrective treatment.

DOSAGE AND ADMINISTRATION

The objective of nutritional management of renal decompensation is the provision of sufficient amino acid and caloric support for protein synthesis without greatly exceeding the renal capacity to excrete metabolic wastes.

Three grams of nitrogen per day provided as essential amino acids with adequate calories produce nitrogen equilibrium in many stable patients with chronic uremia. Although nitrogen requirements may be higher in stressed or acutely uremic patients, or those on dialysis, provision of additional nitrogen may not be possible due to fluid intake limits or glucose intolerance.

The usual methods of determining individual patient requirements for amino acids such as nitrogen balance or daily body weight are difficult to perform or interpret in the uremic patient. Therefore, dosage is guided by the patient's fluid intake limits and glucose and nitrogen tolerances, as well as metabolic and clinical response. Rate of rise of blood urea nitrogen generally diminishes with infusion of essential amino acids. However, excessive intake of dietary protein or increased protein catabolism may alter this response.

Adults: Generally, 250 to 500 mL of 5.4% NephrAmine® (Essential Amino Acid Injection), containing approximately 1.6 to 3.2 grams of nitrogen (in 13.4 to 26.8 grams of essential amino acids), are given daily. Adequate calories should be provided simultaneously. Each 250 mL of NephrAmine® is typically mixed aseptically with 500 mL of 70% dextrose to yield a solution of 1.8% NephrAmine® in 47% dextrose. This mixture provides a calorie-to-nitrogen ratio of 744:1.

Children: Initial total daily dose should be low and increased slowly. Dosage of NephrAmine® above one gram of essential amino acids per kg of body weight per day is not recommended. See ***Special Precautions in Pediatric Patients*** for additional information.

Fat emulsion coadministration should be considered when prolonged (more than 5 days) parenteral nutrition is required in order to prevent essential fatty acid deficiency (E.F.A.D.). Serum lipids should be monitored for evidence of E.F.A.D. in patients maintained on fat free TPN.

Electrolyte supplementation may be required. Undiluted NephrAmine® contains 5 mEq/liter of sodium. Elevated serum potassium, phosphorus, and magnesium levels generally decrease during treatment with NephrAmine®. Although these effects are beneficial, especially in acute renal failure, in some instances the reduction may be so great that supplementation of these electrolytes is required, especially in the presence of cardiac arrhythmias or digitalis toxicity. During periods of anuria or oliguria, electrolyte supplementation should be done with caution, even if serum levels are in the low normal range.

Compatibility of electrolyte additives to the 5.4% NephrAmine® (Essential Amino Acid Injection)/hypertonic dextrose mixture must be considered, and potentially incompatible ions such as calcium and phosphate may be added to alternate infusion bottles to avoid precipitation. In patients with hyperchloremic or other metabolic acidosis, sodium and potassium may be added as acetate or lactate salts to provide bicarbonate precursor. The electrolyte content of NephrAmine® must be considered when calculating daily electrolyte intake. Serum electrolytes, including magnesium and phosphorus, should be monitored frequently.

If a patient's nutritional intake is primarily parenteral, vitamins, especially the water soluble vitamins, should also be provided.

Hypertonic mixtures of essential amino acids and dextrose may be safely administered by continuous infusion through a central venous catheter with the tip located in the superior vena cava. Initial infusion rates should be slow, generally 20–30 mL/hour. Increases by increments of 10 mL/hour each 24 hours are recommended to a maximum of 60–100 mL/hour. If administration rate should fall behind schedule, no attempt to "catch up" to planned intake should be made. Administration rate is governed by the patient's nitrogen, fluid, and glucose tolerance. Uremic patients are frequently glucose intolerant, especially in association with peritoneal dialysis, and may require the administration of exogenous insulin to prevent hyperglycemia. Blood glucose levels must be determined frequently. To prevent rebound hypoglycemia, a solution containing 5% dextrose should be administered when hypertonic dextrose infusions are abruptly discontinued.

Parenteral drug products should be inspected visually for particulate matter and discoloration prior to administration, whenever solution and container permit.

Care must be taken to avoid incompatible admixtures. Consult with pharmacist.

HOW SUPPLIED

5.4% NephrAmine® (Essential Amino Acid Injection) is supplied sterile and nonpyrogenic in glass containers packaged 12 per case.

NDC No.: 54391-1909-5 **Size:** 250 mL
Exposure of pharmaceutical products to heat should be minimized. Avoid excessive heat. Protect from freezing. It is recommended that the product be stored at room temperature (25°C); however, brief exposure up to 40°C does not adversely affect the product. Protect from light until use.

Manufactured By B. Braun Medical, Inc. For R&D Laboratories, Inc.
For Medical Emergencies:
McGaw Stat Line
(800) 854-6851

NEPHRO–VITE®Rx ℞

Vitamin Formulation For Renal Patients

DESCRIPTION

Kidney failure and the process of dialysis causes vitamin losses necessitating the regular replacement of the water soluble vitamins. It is important not to over supplement some vitamins. Vitamin A should not be supplemented and vitamin C supplementation should be limited to 60 mg per day to avoid the risk of increased oxalate formation.

Each tablet provides:

	Nephro-Vite®Rx	Nephro-Vite®
Vitamin C	60mg	60mg
Vitamin B_1	1.5mg	1.5mg
Vitamin B_2	1.7mg	1.7mg
Niacinamide	20mg	20mg
Vitamin B_6	10mg	10mg
Vitamin B_{12}	6mcg	6mcg
Folic Acid	1mg	.8mg
Pantothenic Acid	10mg	10mg
Biotin	300mcg	300mcg

INDICATIONS

Dialysis patients; Azotemic patients not on dialysis who eat poorly.

PRECAUTION

See Folic Acid Precaution under Nephro-Vite® +Fe

DOSAGE

One tablet daily, or as prescribed by physician.

SUPPLIED

Film coated, round yellow tablets, marked RD 12.
Plastic bottles of 100. NDC 54391-1002-1.
For use under medical supervision.

NEPHRO–VITE®

Vitamin Formulation For Renal Patients
Medical Food

Renal vitamin replacement formulation—see table under Nephro-Vite® Rx for description. Same dosage as Nephro-Vite® Rx.
Film coated, round yellow tablets marked RD 02.
Supplied in plastic bottles of 100. NDC 54391-0002-1.

NEPHRO-VITE® +Fe ℞

Vitamin Formulation For Renal Patients
With Iron

COMPOSITION

Same as Nephro-Vite® Rx with the addition of 304 mg of ferrous fumarate—100 mg of elemental iron.

INDICATIONS

For any patient needing vitamin and iron supplementation for documented iron deficiency. Suitable for pre-dialysis and end stage renal disease patients.

PRECAUTION

Folic acid may partially correct the hematological damage due to vitamin B_{12} deficiency of pernicious anemia while the associated neurological damage progresses.

ADVERSE REACTIONS

Allergic sensitization has been reported following administration of folic acid. Sensitivity to low doses of iron has been reported. High doses of iron may result in iron toxicity, which may be characterized by: transient bloating, flatulence, constipation and diarrhea. Ingestion of greater than 400 mg/day of elemental iron can result in nausea and vomiting.

DOSAGE

One tablet daily between meals or as prescribed by a physician.

HOW SUPPLIED

Film coated, oval tablets marked RD23. Tablets in unit dose blister packs of 30.
NDC 54391-2213-8
For use under medical supervision.

Reckitt Benckiser Pharmaceuticals Inc.

1909 HUGUENOT ROAD
RICHMOND, VA 23235

Direct Inquiries to:
Professional Services
(804) 379-1090
FAX: (804) 379-1215

For Medical Information Contact:
In Emergencies
Medical Department
(804) 379-1090
FAX: (804) 379-1215

BUPRENEX® ℂ ℞

[*būp ′rĕn-ex*]
(buprenorphine hydrochloride)
INJECTABLE

DESCRIPTION

Buprenex (buprenorphine hydrochloride) is a narcotic under the Controlled Substances Act due to its chemical derivation from thebaine. Chemically, it is 17-(cyclopropylmethyl)-α-(1,1-dimethylethyl)-4, 5-epoxy-18, 19-dihydro-3-hydroxy-6-methoxy-α-methyl-6, 14-ethenomorphinan-7-methanol, hydrochloride [5α, 7α(S)]. Buprenorphine hydrochloride is a white powder, weakly acidic and with limited solubility in water. Buprenex is a clear, sterile, injectable agonist-antagonist analgesic intended for intravenous or intramuscular administration. Each ml of Buprenex contains 0.324 mg buprenorphine hydrochloride (equivalent to 0.3 mg buprenorphine), 50 mg anhydrous dextrose, water for injection and HCl to adjust pH. Buprenorphine hydrochloride has the molecular formula, $C_{29}H_{41}NO_4$-HCl, and the following structure:

Molecular weight: 504.09

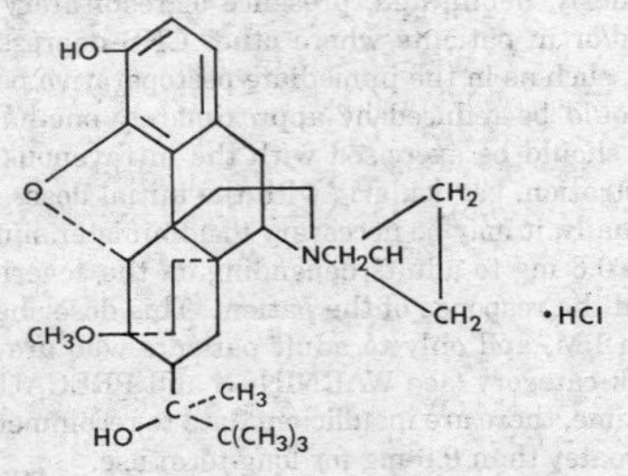

CLINICAL PHARMACOLOGY

Buprenex is a parenteral opioid analgesic with 0.3 mg Buprenex being approximately equivalent to 10 mg morphine sulfate in analgesic and respiratory depressant effects in adults. Pharmacological effects occur as soon as 15 minutes after intramuscular injection and persist for 6 hours or longer. Peak pharmacologic effects usually are observed at 1 hour. When used intravenously, the times to onset and peak effect are shortened.

The limits of sensitivity of available analytical methodology precluded demonstration of bioequivalence between intramuscular and intravenous routes of administration. In postoperative adults, pharmacokinetic studies have shown elimination half-lives ranging from 1.2–7.2 hours (mean 2.2 hours) after intravenous administration of 0.3 mg of buprenorphine. A single, ten-patient, pharmacokinetic study of doses of 3 μg/kg in children (age 5-7 years) showed a high inter-patient variability, but suggests that the clearance of the drug may be higher in children than in adults. This is supported by at least one repeat-dose study in postoperative pain that showed an optimal inter-dose interval of 4–5 hours in pediatric patients as opposed to the recommended 6–8 hours in adults.

Buprenorphine, in common with morphine and other phenolic opioid analgesics, is metabolized by the liver and its clearance is related to hepatic blood flow. Studies in patients anesthetized with 0.5% halothane have shown that this anesthetic decreases hepatic blood flow by about 30%.

Mechanism of Analgesic Action: Buprenex exerts its analgesic effect via high affinity binding to μ subclass opiate receptors in the central nervous system. Although Buprenex may be classified as a partial agonist, under the conditions of recommended use it behaves very much like classical μ agonists such as morphine. One unusual property of Buprenex observed in *in vitro* studies is its very slow rate of dissociation from its receptor. This could account for its longer duration of action than morphine, the unpredictability of its reversal by opioid antagonists, and its low level of manifest physical dependence.

Narcotic Antagonist Activity: Buprenorphine demonstrates narcotic antagonist activity and has been shown to be equipotent with naloxone as an antagonist of morphine in the mouse tail flick test.

Cardiovascular Effects: Buprenex may cause a decrease or, rarely, an increase in pulse rate and blood pressure in some patients.

Effects on Respiration: Under usual conditions of use in adults, both Buprenex and morphine show similar dose-related respiratory depressant effects. At adult therapeutic doses, Buprenex (0.3 mg buprenorphine) can decrease respiratory rate in an equivalent manner to an equianalgesic dose of morphine (10 mg). (See WARNINGS.)

INDICATIONS AND USAGE

Buprenex is indicated for the relief of moderate to severe pain.

CONTRAINDICATIONS

Buprenex should not be administered to patients who have been shown to be hypersensitive to the drug.

WARNINGS

Impaired Respiration: As with other potent opioids, clinically significant respiratory depression may occur within the recommended dose range in patients receiving therapeutic doses of buprenorphine. Buprenex should be used with caution in patients with compromised respiratory function (e.g., chronic obstructive pulmonary disease, cor pulmonale, decreased respiratory reserve, hypoxia, hypercapnia, or preexisting respiratory depression). Particular caution is advised if Buprenex is administered to patients taking or recently receiving drugs with CNS/respiratory depressant effects. In patients with the physical and/or pharmacological risk factors above, the dose should be reduced by approximately one-half.

NALOXONE MAY NOT BE EFFECTIVE IN REVERSING THE RESPIRATORY DEPRESSION PRODUCED BY BUPRENEX. THEREFORE, AS WITH OTHER POTENT OPIOIDS, THE PRIMARY MANAGEMENT OF OVERDOSE SHOULD BE THE REESTABLISHMENT OF ADEQUATE VENTILATION WITH MECHANICAL ASSISTANCE OF RESPIRATION, IF REQUIRED.

Interaction with Other Central Nervous System Depressants: Patients receiving Buprenex in the presence of other narcotic analgesics, general anesthetics, antihistamines, benzodiazepines, phenothiazines, other tranquilizers, sedative/hypnotics or other CNS depressants (including alcohol) may exhibit increased CNS depression. When such combined therapy is contemplated, it is particularly important that the dose of one or both agents be reduced.

Head Injury and Increased Intracranial Pressure: Buprenex, like other potent analgesics, may itself elevate cerebrospinal fluid pressure and should be used with caution in head injury, intracranial lesions and other circumstances where cerebrospinal pressure may be increased. Buprenex can produce miosis and changes in the level of consciousness which may interfere with patient evaluation.

Use in Ambulatory Patients: Buprenex may impair the mental or physical abilities required for the performance of potentially dangerous tasks such as driving a car or operating machinery. Therefore, Buprenex should be administered with caution to ambulatory patients who should be warned to avoid such hazards.

Use in Narcotic-Dependent Patients: Because of the narcotic antagonist activity of Buprenex, use in the physically dependent individual may result in withdrawal effects.

PRECAUTIONS

General: Buprenex should be administered with caution in the elderly, debilitated patients, in children and those with severe impairment of hepatic, pulmonary, or renal function; myxedema or hypothyroidism; adrenal cortical insufficiency (e.g., Addison's disease); CNS depression or coma; toxic psychoses; prostatic hypertrophy or urethral stricture; acute alcoholism, delirium tremens; or kyphoscoliosis.

Because Buprenex is metabolized by the liver, the activity of Buprenex may be increased and/or extended in those individuals with impaired hepatic function or those receiving other agents known to decrease hepatic clearance.

Buprenex has been shown to increase intracholedochal pressure to a similar degree as other opioid analgesics, and thus should be administered with caution to patients with dysfunction of the biliary tract.

Information for Patients: The effects of Buprenex, particularly drowsiness, may be potentiated by other centrally acting agents such as alcohol or benzodiazepines. It is particularly important that in these circumstances patients must not drive or operate machinery. Buprenex has some pharmacologic effects similar to morphine which in susceptible patients may lead to self-administration of the drug when pain no longer exists. Patients must not exceed the dosage of Buprenex prescribed by their physician. Patients should be urged to consult their physician if other prescription medications are currently being used or are prescribed for future use.

Drug Interactions: Drug interactions common to other potent opioid analgesics also may occur with Buprenex. Particular care should be taken when Buprenex is used in combination with central nervous system depressant drugs (see WARNINGS). Although specific information is not presently available, caution should be exercised when Buprenex is used in combination with MAO inhibitors. There have been reports of respiratory and cardiovascular collapse in patients who received therapeutic doses of diazepam and Buprenex. A suspected interaction between Buprenex and phenprocoumon resulting in purpura has been reported.

Continued on next page

Buprenex—Cont.

Carcinogenesis, Mutagenesis, Impairment of Fertility: The effects of Buprenex on fertility and gestation indices were investigated in rats by the subcutaneous and intramuscular routes at doses 10 to 1,000 times the proposed human doses. Dystocia was noted in dams treated with 1,000 times the human dose. No effects on fertility or gestation were noted in these Segment 1 studies.

Pregnancy: Pregnancy Category C. Reproduction studies have been performed in the rat at doses which ranged from 10 to 1,000 times the proposed human dose by the subcutaneous and intramuscular routes and 160 times the proposed human dose by the intravenous route. By the intramuscular route, Buprenex produced mild but statistically significant ($p < 0.05$) post-implantation losses and early fetal deaths at 10 and 100 but not 1,000 times the proposed human dose. No fetal malformations were noted in rats at any dose when Buprenex was administered by subcutaneous, intramuscular, or intravenous routes. In rabbits, intramuscularly administered Buprenex produced a dose-related trend for extra rib formation which attained statistical significance ($p < 0.01$) at 1,000 times the proposed human dose. By the intravenous route, doses in rats of 40 and 160 times the proposed human dose of Buprenex caused a slight increase in post-implantation losses that may have been treatment-related. No major fetal malformations were noted in drug treated groups when administered by intramuscular or intravenous routes.

There are no adequate and well-controlled studies in pregnant women. Buprenex should be used during pregnancy only if the potential benefit justifies the potential risk to the fetus.

Labor and Delivery: The safety of Buprenex given during labor and delivery has not been established.

Nursing Mothers: An apparent lack of milk production during general reproduction studies with Buprenex in rats caused decreased viability and lactation indices. It is unknown at this time whether or not Buprenex is excreted in human milk. Despite the lack of specific knowledge on this issue, it is reasonable to assume that Buprenex will enter human milk and caution should be exercised in the use of Buprenex when it is administered to nursing mothers.

Pediatric Use: The safety and effectiveness of Buprenex have been established for children between 2 and 12 years of age. Use of Buprenex in children is supported by evidence from adequate and well controlled trials of Buprenex in adults, with additional data from studies of 960 children ranging in age from 9 months to 18 years of age. Data is available from a pharmacokinetic study, several controlled clinical trials, and several large post-marketing studies and case series. The available information provides reasonable evidence that Buprenex may be used safely in children ranging from 2–12 years of age, and that it is of similar effectiveness in children as in adults.

ADVERSE REACTIONS

The most frequent side effect in clinical studies involving 1,133 patients was sedation which occurred in approximately two-thirds of the patients. Although sedated, these patients could easily be aroused to an alert state.

Other less frequent adverse reactions occurring in 5–10% of the patients were:

Nausea
Dizziness/Vertigo

Occurring in 1–5% of the patients:

Sweating
Hypotension
Vomiting
Miosis
Headache
Nausea/Vomiting
Hypoventilation

The following adverse reactions were reported to have occurred in less than 1% of the patients:

CNS Effect: confusion, blurred vision, euphoria, weakness/fatigue, dry mouth, nervousness, depression, slurred speech, paresthesia.

Cardiovascular: hypertension, tachycardia, bradycardia.

Gastrointestinal: constipation.

Respiratory: dyspnea, cyanosis.

Dermatological: pruritus.

Ophthalmological: diplopia, visual abnormalities.

Miscellaneous: injection site reaction, urinary retention, dreaming, flushing/warmth, chills/cold, tinnitus, conjunctivitis, Wenckebach block, and psychosis.

Other effects observed infrequently include malaise, hallucinations, depersonalization, coma, dyspepsia, flatulence, apnea, rash, amblyopia, tremor, and pallor.

The following reactions have been reported to occur rarely: loss of appetite, dysphoria/agitation, diarrhea, urticaria, and convulsions/lack of muscle coordination.

In the United Kingdom, buprenorphine hydrochloride was made available under monitored release regulation during the first year of sale, and yielded data from 1,736 physicians on 9,123 patients (17,120 administrations). Data on 240 children under the age of 18 years were included in this monitored release program. No important new adverse effects attributable to buprenorphine hydrochloride were observed.

DRUG ABUSE AND DEPENDENCE

Buprenorphine hydrochloride is a partial agonist of the morphine type: *i.e.,* it has certain opioid properties which may lead to psychic dependence of the morphine type due to an opiate-like euphoric component of the drug. Direct dependence studies have shown little physical dependence upon withdrawal of the drug. However, caution should be used in prescribing to individuals who are known to be drug abusers or ex-narcotic addicts. The drug may not substitute in acutely dependent narcotic addicts due to its antagonist component and may induce withdrawal symptoms.

OVERDOSAGE

Manifestations: Clinical experience with Buprenex overdosage has been insufficient to define the signs of this condition at this time. Although the antagonist activity of buprenorphine may become manifest at doses somewhat above the recommended therapeutic range, doses in the recommended therapeutic range may produce clinically significant respiratory depression in certain circumstances. (See WARNINGS.)

Treatment: The respiratory and cardiac status of the patients should be monitored carefully. Primary attention should be given to the reestablishment of adequate respiratory exchange through provision of a patent airway and institution of assisted or controlled ventilation. Oxygen, intravenous fluids, vasopressors, and other supportive measures should be employed as indicated. Doxapram, a respiratory stimulant, may be used. **NALOXONE MAY NOT BE EFFECTIVE IN REVERSING THE RESPIRATORY DEPRESSION PRODUCED BY BUPRENEX. THEREFORE, AS WITH OTHER POTENT OPIOIDS, THE PRIMARY MANAGEMENT OF OVERDOSE SHOULD BE THE REESTABLISHMENT OF ADEQUATE VENTILATION WITH MECHANICAL ASSISTANCE OF RESPIRATION, IF REQUIRED.**

DOSAGE AND ADMINISTRATION

Adults: The usual dosage for persons 13 years of age and over is 1 ml Buprenex (0.3 mg buprenorphine) given by deep intramuscular or slow (over at least 2 minutes) intravenous injection at up to 6-hour intervals, as needed. Repeat once (up to 0.3 mg) if required, 30 to 60 minutes after initial dosage, giving consideration to previous dose pharmacokinetics, and thereafter only as needed. In high-risk patients (e.g., elderly, debilitated, presence of respiratory disease, etc.) and/or in patients where other CNS depressants are present, such as in the immediate postoperative period, the dose should be reduced by approximately one-half. Extra caution should be exercised with the intravenous route of administration, particularly with the initial dose.

Occasionally, it may be necessary to administer single doses of up to 0.6 mg to adults depending on the severity of the pain and the response of the patient. This dose should only be given I.M. and only to adult patients who are not in a high risk category (see WARNINGS and PRECAUTIONS). At this time, there are insufficient data to recommend single doses greater than 0.6 mg for long-term use.

Children: Buprenex has been used in children 2–12 years of age at doses between 2–6 micrograms/kg of body weight given every 4–6 hours. There is insufficient experience to recommend a dose in infants below the age of two years, single doses greater than 6 micrograms/kg of body weight, or the use of a repeat or second dose at 30–60 minutes (such as is used in adults). Since there is some evidence that not all children clear buprenorphine faster than adults, fixed interval or "round-the-clock" dosing should not be undertaken until the proper inter-dose interval has been established by clinical observation of the child. Physicians should recognize that, as with adults, some pediatric patients may not need to be remedicated for 6–8 hours.

Safety and Handling: Buprenex is supplied in sealed ampuls and poses no known environmental risk to health care providers. Accidental dermal exposure should be treated by removal of any contaminated clothing and rinsing the affected area with water.

Buprenex is a potent narcotic, and like all drugs of this class has been associated with abuse and dependence among health care providers. To control the risk of diversion, it is recommended that measures appropriate to the health care setting be taken to provide rigid accounting, control of wastage, and restriction of access.

Parenteral drug products should be inspected visually for particulate matter and discoloration prior to administration, whenever solution and container permit.

HOW SUPPLIED

Buprenex (buprenorphine hydrochloride) is supplied in clear glass snap-ampuls of 1 ml (0.3 mg buprenorphine).
NDC 12496-0757-1

Avoid excessive heat (over 104°F or 40°C). Protect from prolonged exposure to light.

Manufactured by:
Reckitt Benckiser
Hull, England HU8 7DS.

Distributed by:
Reckitt Benckiser Pharmaceuticals Inc.,
Richmond, VA 23235.
Buprenex® is a trademark of Reckitt Benckiser (Overseas) Limited.
REVISED July 1998

912801

Shown in Product Identification Guide, page 332

Respa® Pharmaceuticals, Inc.

P.O. BOX 88222 , CAROL STREAM, IL 60188

Direct Inquiries to:
(630) 462-9986
FAX: (630) 462-9934

RESPA®-DM TABLETS / Dye & Sugar Free ℞

Each tablet contain 28 mg Dextromethorphan and 600 mg Guaifenesin

DOSAGE

12 yr. and older 1 or 2 tab. B.I.D. 6 to 12 1 tab. B.I.D.

RESPA-GF® TABLETS / Dye & Sugar Free ℞

Each tablet contain 600 mg Guaifenesin

DOSAGE

12 yr. and older 1 or 2 tab. B.I.D. 6 to 12 1 tab. B.I.D.

RESPA-1ST® TABLETS / Dye & Sugar Free ℞

Each tab. contain 58 mg Pseudoephedrine and 600 mg Guaifenesin

DOSAGE

12 yr. and older 1 or 2 tab. B.I.D. 6 to 12 1 tab. B.I.D.

RESPAHIST® CAPSULES / Dye Free ℞

Each capsule contain 6 mg Brompheniramine and 60 mg Pseudoephedrine

DOSAGE

12 yr. and older 1 or 2 capsules B.I.D. 6 to 12 1 Capsule B.I.D.

RESPA-A.R.M.® TABLETS / Dye & Sugar Free ℞

Each tablet contains: 25 mg Phenylephrine HCL, 50 mg Phenylpropanolamine HCL, 8 mg Chlorpheniramine MAL, Belladonna Alkaloids (Hyoscyamine Sulfate, Atropine Sulfate and Scopolamine Hydrobromide)

DOSAGE

Adults and Children over 12 years of age 1 tab B.I.D.

TRIKOF-D® TABLETS / Dye & Sugar Free ℞

Each tablet contain 600mg Guaifenesin, 30mg Dextromethorphan, 37.5mg Phenylpropanolamine

DOSAGE

12yr. and older 1 or 2 tab. B.I.D. 6 to 12 1 tab. B.I.D.

Rhône-Poulenc Rorer Pharmaceuticals Inc.

Due to the merger of Hoechst Marion Roussel and Rhône-Poulenc Rorer, please refer to Aventis Pharmaceuticals for product information.

Richwood Pharmaceutical Company Inc.

7900 TANNER'S GATE DRIVE, SUITE 200
FLORENCE, KENTUCKY 41042
(For product information see Shire US Inc.)

Roberts Pharmaceutical Corp.

4 INDUSTRIAL WAY WEST
EATONTOWN, NJ 07724
(For product information see Shire US Inc.)

A. H. Robins Company

1407 CUMMINGS DRIVE
RICHMOND, VA 23220

Direct General Inquiries to:
(610) 688-4400

For Emergency Medical Information Contact:
Day: (800) 934-5556 8:30 AM to 4:30 PM (Eastern Standard Time), Weekdays only
Night: (610) 688-4400 (Emergencies only; non-emergencies should wait until the next day)

For Medical/Pharmacy Inquiries on Marketed Products Call:
Medical Affairs, (800) 934-5556 8:30 AM to 4:30 PM (Eastern Standard Time), Weekdays only

A.H. Robins Products

The following is a list of products listed under A.H. Robins. All oral solid dosage forms are listed with their corresponding National Drug Code (NDC) numbers. All numbers are preceded by 0031.
[See table above]

NDC Number	Product
–	DIMETANE®-DX Cough Syrup (each teaspoonful [5 mL] contains 2 mg brompheniramine maleate, 30 mg pseudoephedrine HCl and 10 mg dextromethorphan hydrobromide)
1535	MITROLAN® (calcium polycarbophil) Tablets
4207	DONNATAL® Capsules (each capsule contains 16.2 mg phenobarbital, 0.1037 mg hyoscyamine sulfate, 0.0194 mg atropine sulfate and 0.0065 mg scopolamine hydrobromide)
–	DONNATAL® Elixir (each teaspoonful [5 mL] contains 16.2 mg phenobarbital, 0.1037 mg hyoscyamine sulfate, 0.0194 mg atropine sulfate and 0.0065 mg scopolamine hydrobromide)
4235	DONNATAL® EXTENTABS® (each Extentabs tablet contains 48.6 mg phenobarbital, 0.3111 mg hyoscyamine sulfate, 0.0582 mg atropine sulfate and 0.0195 mg scopolamine hydrobromide)
4250	DONNATAL® Tablets (each tablet contains 16.2 mg phenobarbital, 0.1037 mg hyoscyamine sulfate, 0.0194 mg atropine sulfate and 0.0065 mg scopolamine hydrobromide)
4650	DONNAZYME® Tablets (each tablet contains 500 mg pancreatin)
6257	PHENAPHEN® with Codeine C-III (acetaminophen and codeine phosphate) No. 3 Capsules, (325 mg/30 mg)
6274	PHENAPHEN® with Codeine C-III (acetaminophen and codeine phosphate) No. 4 Capsules, (325 mg/60 mg)
6649	QUINIDEX EXTENTABS® (quinidine sulfate extended-release tablets, USP), 300 mg
–	REGLAN® (metoclopramide HCl) Syrup, 5 mg/5 mL
6701	REGLAN® (metoclopramide HCl) Tablets, 10 mg
6705	REGLAN® (metoclopramide HCl) Tablets, 5 mg
7429	ROBAXIN® (methocarbamol tablets, USP) Tablets, 500 mg
7449	ROBAXIN®-750 (methocarbamol tablets, USP) Tablets, 750 mg
7469	ROBAXISAL® Tablets (each tablet contains 400 mg methocarbamol and 325 mg aspirin)
–	ROBITUSSIN A-C® Syrup C-V (each teaspoonful [5 mL] contains 100 mg guaifenesin and 10 mg codeine phosphate)
–	ROBITUSSIN®-DAC Syrup C-V (each teaspoonful [5 mL] contains 100 mg guaifenesin, 30 mg pseudoephedrine hydrochloride, and 10 mg codeine phosphate)
8901	TENEX® (guanfacine HCl) Tablets, 1 mg
8903	TENEX® (guanfacine HCl) Tablets, 2 mg

DIMETANE®–DX ℞

[dī ′mĕ-tān]
COUGH SYRUP
SUGAR-FREE

DESCRIPTION

Dimetane-DX Cough Syrup is a light-red syrup with a butterscotch flavor.
Each 5 mL (1 teaspoonful) contains:

Brompheniramine Maleate, USP	2 mg
Pseudoephedrine Hydrochloride, USP	30 mg
Dextromethorphan Hydrobromide, USP	10 mg

Alcohol 0.95 percent
In a palatable, aromatic vehicle.
Inactive Ingredients: Citric Acid, FD&C Red 40, FD&C Yellow 6, Flavors, Glycerin, Saccharin Sodium, Sodium Benzoate, Sorbitol, Water.
Antihistamine/Nasal Decongestant/Antitussive syrup for oral administration.

CLINICAL PHARMACOLOGY

Brompheniramine maleate is a histamine antagonist, specifically an H_1-receptor-blocking agent belonging to the alkylamine class of antihistamines. Antihistamines appear to compete with histamine for receptor sites on effector cells. Brompheniramine also has anticholinergic (drying) and sedative effects. Among the antihistaminic effects, it antagonizes the allergic response (vasodilatation, increased vascular permeability, increased mucus secretion) of nasal tissue. Brompheniramine is well absorbed from the gastrointestinal tract, with peak plasma concentration after single, oral dose of 4 mg reached in 5 hours; urinary excretion is the major route of elimination, mostly as products of biodegradation; the liver is assumed to be the main site of metabolic transformation.
Pseudoephedrine acts on sympathetic nerve endings and also on smooth muscle, making it useful as a nasal decongestant. The nasal decongestant effect is mediated by the action of pseudoephedrine on α-sympathetic receptors, producing vasoconstriction of the dilated nasal arterioles. Following oral administration, effects are noted within 30 minutes with peak activity occurring at approximately one hour.
Dextromethorphan acts centrally to elevate the threshold for coughing. It has no analgesic or addictive properties. The onset of antitussive action occurs in 15 to 30 minutes after administration and is of long duration.

INDICATIONS AND USAGE

For relief of coughs and upper respiratory symptoms, including nasal congestion, associated with allergy or the common cold.

CONTRAINDICATIONS

Hypersensitivity to any of the ingredients. Do not use in the newborn, in premature infants, in nursing mothers, in patients with severe hypertension or severe coronary artery disease. Do not use dextromethorphan in patients receiving monoamine oxidase (MAO) inhibitors (see "DRUG INTERACTIONS").
Antihistamines should not be used to treat lower respiratory tract conditions including asthma.

WARNINGS

Especially in infants and small children, antihistamines in overdosage may cause hallucinations, convulsions, and death.
Antihistamines may diminish mental alertness. In the young child, they may produce excitation.

PRECAUTIONS

General
Because of its antihistamine component, Dimetane-DX Cough Syrup should be used with caution in patients with a history of bronchial asthma, narrow angle glaucoma, gastrointestinal obstruction, or urinary bladder neck obstruction. Because of its sympathomimetic component, Dimetane-DX Cough Syrup should be used with caution in patients with diabetes, hypertension, heart disease, or thyroid disease.

Information for Patients
Patients should be warned about engaging in activities requiring mental alertness, such as driving a car or operating dangerous machinery.

Drug Interactions
Monoamine oxidase (MAO) inhibitors—Hyperpyrexia, hypotension, and death have been reported coincident with the co-administration of MAO inhibitors and products containing dextromethorphan. In addition, MAO inhibitors prolong and intensify the anticholinergic (drying) effects of antihistamines and may enhance the effect of pseudoephedrine. Concomitant administration of Dimetane-DX and MAO inhibitors should be avoided (see **"Contraindications"**).
Central nervous system (CNS) depressants—Antihistamines have additive effects with alcohol and other CNS depressants (hypnotics, sedatives, tranquilizers, antianxiety agents, etc).
Antihypertensive drugs—Sympathomimetics may reduce the effects of antihypertensive drugs.

Carcinogenesis, Mutagenesis, Impairment of Fertility
Animal studies of Dimetane-DX Cough Syrup to assess the carcinogenic and mutagenic potential or the effect on fertility have not been performed.

Pregnancy
Teratogenic Effects —Pregnancy Category C
Animal reproduction studies have not been conducted with Dimetane-DX Cough Syrup. It is also not known whether Dimetane-DX Cough Syrup can cause fetal harm when administered to a pregnant woman or can affect reproduction capacity. Dimetane-DX Cough Syrup should be given to a pregnant woman only if clearly needed.
Reproduction studies of brompheniramine maleate (a component of Dimetane-DX Cough Syrup) in rats and mice at doses up to 16 times the maximum human dose have revealed no evidence of impaired fertility or harm to the fetus.

Nursing Mothers
Because of the higher risk of intolerance of antihistamines in small infants generally, and in newborns and prematures in particular, Dimetane-DX Cough Syrup is contraindicated in nursing mothers.

Pediatric Use
Safety and effectiveness in pediatric patients below the age of 6 months have not been established (see **"DOSAGE AND ADMINISTRATION"**).

ADVERSE REACTIONS

The most frequent adverse reactions to Dimetane-DX Cough Syrup are: sedation; dryness of mouth, nose and throat; thickening of bronchial secretions; dizziness. Other adverse reactions may include:
Dermatologic: Urticaria, drug rash, photosensitivity, pruritus.
Cardiovascular System: Hypotension, hypertension, cardiac arrhythmias, palpitation.
CNS: Disturbed coordination, tremor, irritability, insomnia, visual disturbances, weakness, nervousness, convulsions, headache, euphoria, and dysphoria.
G. U. System: Urinary frequency, difficult urination.
G. I. System: Epigastric discomfort, anorexia, nausea, vomiting, diarrhea, constipation.
Respiratory System: Tightness of chest and wheezing, shortness of breath.
Hematologic System: Hemolytic anemia, thrombocytopenia, agranulocytosis.

OVERDOSAGE

Signs and Symptoms
Central nervous system effects from overdosage of brompheniramine may vary from depression to stimulation, especially in children. Anticholinergic effects may be noted. Toxic doses of pseudoephedrine may result in CNS stimulation, tachycardia, hypertension, and cardiac arrhythmias; signs of CNS depression may occasionally be seen. Dextromethorphan in toxic doses will cause drowsiness, ataxia, nystagmus, opisthotonos, and convulsive seizures.

Toxic Doses
Data suggest that individuals may respond in an unexpected manner to apparently small amounts of a particular drug. A $2\frac{1}{2}$-year-old child survived the ingestion of 21 mg/kg of dextromethorphan exhibiting only ataxia, drowsiness, and fever, but seizures have been reported in 2 children following the ingestion of 13–17 mg/kg. Another $2\frac{1}{2}$-year-old child survived a dose of 300–900 mg of brompheniramine.

Continued on next page

Dimetane-Dx—Cont.

iramine. The toxic dose of pseudoephedrine should be less than that of ephedrine, which is estimated to be 50 mg/kg.

Treatment

Induce emesis if patient is alert and is seen prior to 6 hours following ingestion. Precautions against aspiration must be taken, especially in infants and small children. Gastric lavage may be carried out, although in some instances tracheostomy may be necessary prior to lavage. Naloxone hydrochloride 0.005 mg/kg intravenously may be of value in reversing the CNS depression that may occur from an overdose of dextromethorphan. CNS stimulants may counter CNS depression. Should CNS hyperactivity or convulsive seizures occur, intravenous short-acting barbiturates may be indicated. Hypertensive responses and/or tachycardia should be treated appropriately. Oxygen, intravenous fluids, and other supportive measures should be employed as indicated.

DOSAGE AND ADMINISTRATION

Adults and pediatric patients 12 years of age and over: 2 teaspoonfuls every 4 hours. Children 6 to under 12 years: 1 teaspoonful every 4 hours. Children 2 to under 6 years: $^1/_2$ teaspoonful every 4 hours. Infants 6 months to under 2 years: Dosage to be established by physician.
Do not exceed 6 doses during a 24-hour period.

HOW SUPPLIED

Dimetane®-DX Cough Syrup is a light-red syrup containing in each 5 mL (1 teaspoonful) brompheniramine maleate 2 mg, pseudoephedrine hydrochloride 30 mg and dextromethorphan hydrobromide 10 mg, available in pints (NDC 0031-1836-25).

Store at controlled room temperature, between 20°C and 25°C (68°F and 77°F).

Dispense in tight, light-resistant container.

Manufactured by:
Pharmaceutical Division
A.H. Robins Company
Richmond, VA 23220
CI 4691-1 Issued June 4, 1997

DONNATAL® TABLETS ℞
DONNATAL® CAPSULES ℞
DONNATAL® ELIXIR ℞

[don 'nă-tal]

DESCRIPTION

Each Donnatal tablet, capsule or 5 mL (teaspoonful) of elixir (23% alcohol) contains:

Phenobarbital, USP	16.2 mg
(Warning: May be habit forming)	
Hyoscyamine Sulfate, USP	0.1037 mg
Atropine Sulfate, USP	0.0194 mg
Scopolamine Hydrobromide, USP	0.0065 mg

INACTIVE INGREDIENTS:

Tablets: Dibasic Calcium Phosphate, Magnesium Stearate, Microcrystalline Cellulose, Silicon Dioxide, Sodium Starch Glycolate, Stearic Acid, Sucrose. May contain Corn Starch, Dextrose, or Invert Sugar.

Capsules: Corn Starch, Edible Ink, D&C Yellow 10 and FD&C Green 3 or FD&C Blue 1 and FD&C Yellow 6, FD&C Blue 2 Aluminum Lake, Gelatin, Lactose, Sucrose. May contain FD&C Red 40 and Yellow 6 Aluminum Lakes.

Elixir: D&C Yellow 10, FD&C Blue 1, FD&C Yellow 6, Flavors, Glucose, Saccharin Sodium, Water.

ACTIONS

This drug combination provides natural belladonna alkaloids in a specific, fixed ratio combined with phenobarbital to provide peripheral anticholinergic/antispasmodic action and mild sedation.

INDICATIONS

Based on a review of this drug by the National Academy of Sciences—National Research Council and/or other information, FDA has classified the following indications as "possibly" effective:
For use as adjunctive therapy in the treatment of irritable bowel syndrome (irritable colon, spastic colon, mucous colitis) and acute enterocolitis.
May also be useful as adjunctive therapy in the treatment of duodenal ulcer. IT HAS NOT BEEN SHOWN CONCLUSIVELY WHETHER ANTICHOLINERGIC/ ANTISPASMODIC DRUGS AID IN THE HEALING OF A DUODENAL ULCER, DECREASE THE RATE OF RECURRENCES OR PREVENT COMPLICATIONS.

CONTRAINDICATIONS

Glaucoma, obstructive uropathy (for example, bladder neck obstruction due to prostatic hypertrophy); obstructive disease of the gastrointestinal tract (as in achalasia, pyloroduodenal stenosis, etc.); paralytic ileus, intestinal atony of the elderly or debilitated patient; unstable cardiovascular status in acute hemorrhage; severe ulcerative colitis especially if complicated by toxic megacolon; myasthenia gravis; hiatal hernia associated with reflux esophagitis.
Donnatal is contraindicated in patients with known hypersensitivity to any of the ingredients. Phenobarbital is contraindicated in acute intermittent porphyria and in those patients in whom phenobarbital produces restlessness and/or excitement.

WARNINGS

In the presence of a high environmental temperature, heat prostration can occur with belladonna alkaloids (fever and heatstroke due to decreased sweating).
Diarrhea may be an early symptom of incomplete intestinal obstruction, especially in patients with ileostomy or colostomy. In this instance treatment with this drug would be inappropriate and possibly harmful.
Donnatal may produce drowsiness or blurred vision. The patient should be warned, should these occur, not to engage in activities requiring mental alertness, such as operating a motor vehicle or other machinery, and not to perform hazardous work.
Phenobarbital may decrease the effect of anticoagulants and necessitate larger doses of the anticoagulant for optimal effect. When the phenobarbital is discontinued, the dose of the anticoagulant may have to be decreased.
Phenobarbital may be habit forming and should not be administered to individuals known to be addiction prone or to those with a history of physical and/or psychological dependence upon drugs.
Since barbiturates are metabolized in the liver, they should be used with caution and initial doses should be small in patients with hepatic dysfunction.

PRECAUTIONS

Use with caution in patients with: autonomic neuropathy, hepatic or renal disease, hyperthyroidism, coronary heart disease, congestive heart failure, cardiac arrhythmias, tachycardia, and hypertension.
Belladonna alkaloids may produce a delay in gastric emptying (antral stasis) which would complicate the management of gastric ulcer.
Theoretically, with overdosage, a curare-like action may occur.
CARCINOGENESIS, MUTAGENESIS. Long-term studies in animals have not been performed to evaluate carcinogenic potential.
PREGNANCY CATEGORY C. Animal reproduction studies have not been conducted with Donnatal. It is not known whether Donnatal can cause fetal harm when administered to a pregnant woman or can affect reproduction capacity. Donnatal should be given to a pregnant woman only if clearly needed.
NURSING MOTHERS. It is not known whether this drug is excreted in human milk. Because many drugs are excreted in human milk, caution should be exercised when Donnatal is administered to a nursing mother.

ADVERSE REACTIONS

Adverse reactions may include xerostomia; urinary hesitancy and retention; blurred vision; tachycardia; palpitation; mydriasis; cycloplegia; increased ocular tension; loss of taste sense; headache; nervousness; drowsiness; weakness; dizziness; insomnia; nausea; vomiting; impotence; suppression of lactation; constipation; bloated feeling; musculoskeletal pain; severe allergic reaction or drug idiosyncrasies, including anaphylaxis, urticaria and other dermal manifestations; and decreased sweating. Elderly patients may react with symptoms of excitement, agitation, drowsiness, and other untoward manifestations to even small doses of the drug.
Phenobarbital may produce excitement in some patients, rather than a sedative effect. In patients habituated to barbiturates, abrupt withdrawal may produce delirium or convulsions.

DOSAGE AND ADMINISTRATION

The dosage of Donnatal should be adjusted to the needs of the individual patient to assure symptomatic control with a minimum of adverse effects.
Donnatal Tablets or Capsules. Adults: One or two Donnatal tablets or capsules three or four times a day according to condition and severity of symptoms.
Donnatal Elixir. Adults: One or two teaspoonfuls of elixir three or four times a day according to conditions and severity of symptoms.
Children (Elixir)—may be dosed every 4 or 6 hours.:

Body Weight	Starting Dosage q4h	q6h
10 lb (4.5 kg)	0.5 mL	0.75 mL
20 lb (9.1 kg)	1.0 mL	1.5 mL
30 lb (13.6 kg)	1.5 mL	2.0 mL
50 lb (22.7 kg)	$^1/_2$ tsp	$^3/_4$ tsp
75 lb (34.0 kg)	$^3/_4$ tsp	1 tsp
100 lb (45.4 kg)	1 tsp	$1^1/_2$ tsp

OVERDOSAGE

The signs and symptoms of overdose are headache, nausea, vomiting, blurred vision, dilated pupils, hot and dry skin, dizziness, dryness of the mouth, difficulty in swallowing, CNS stimulation. Treatment should consist of gastric lavage, emetics, and activated charcoal. If indicated, parenteral cholinergic agents such as physostigmine or bethanechol chloride should be added.

HOW SUPPLIED

Donnatal® Tablets. White, compressed, scored and embossed "R"; in bottles of 100 (NDC 0031-4250-63), 1000 (NDC 0031-4250-74) and Dis-Co® Unit Dose Packs of 100 (NDC 0031-4250-64).
Donnatal® Capsules. Green and white, monogrammed "AHR" and "4207"; in bottles of 100 (NDC 0031-4207-63).
Donnatal® Elixir. Green, citrus flavored, in 4 fl. oz. (NDC 0031-4221-12), pints (NDC 0031-4221-25), gallons (NDC 0031-4221-29) and 5 mL Dis-Co® Unit Dose Packs (4 × 25s) (NDC 0031-4221-13).
Store at controlled room temperature, between 20°C and 25°C (68°F and 77°F).
Dispense in tight, light-resistant container.

Manufactured by:
Pharmaceutical Division
A.H. Robins Company
Richmond, VA 23220
CI 4692-2 Revised June 6, 1996

Shown in Product Identification Guide, page 332

DONNATAL EXTENTABS® ℞

[don 'nă-tal ĕks"tĕn 'tabs]

DESCRIPTION

Each Donnatal Extentabs tablet contains:

Phenobarbital, USP ($^3/_4$ gr)	48.6 mg
(Warning: May be habit forming)	
Hyoscyamine Sulfate, USP	0.3111 mg
Atropine Sulfate, USP	0.0582 mg
Scopolamine Hydrobromide, USP	0.0195 mg

Each Donnatal Extentabs tablet contains the equivalent of three Donnatal tablets. Extentabs are designed to release the ingredients gradually to provide effects for up to twelve (12) hours.

Inactive Ingredients: Acacia, Acetylated Monoglycerides, Calcium Sulfate, Carnauba Wax, D&C Yellow 10, Edible Ink, FD&C Blue 1, FD&C Blue 2 Aluminum Lake, FD&C Yellow 6, Gelatin, Guar Gum, Magnesium Stearate, Polysorbates, Shellac, Sodium Phosphate, Sucrose, Titanium Dioxide, Wheat Flour, White Wax and other ingredients, one of which is a corn derivative. May include FD&C Red 40 and Yellow 6 Aluminum Lakes.

ACTIONS

This drug combination provides natural belladonna alkaloids in a specific, fixed ratio combined with phenobarbital to provide peripheral anticholinergic/antispasmodic action and mild sedation.

INDICATIONS

Based on a review of this drug by the National Academy of Sciences—National Research Council and/or other information, FDA has classified the following indications as "possibly" effective:
For use as adjunctive therapy in the treatment of irritable bowel syndrome (irritable colon, spastic colon, mucous colitis) and acute enterocolitis.
May also be useful as adjunctive therapy in the treatment of duodenal ulcer. IT HAS NOT BEEN SHOWN CONCLUSIVELY WHETHER ANTICHOLINERGIC/ ANTISPASMODIC DRUGS AID IN THE HEALING OF A DUODENAL ULCER, DECREASE THE RATE OF RECURRENCES OR PREVENT COMPLICATIONS.

CONTRAINDICATIONS

Glaucoma, obstructive uropathy (for example, bladder neck obstruction due to prostatic hypertrophy); obstructive disease of the gastrointestinal tract (as in achalasia, pyloroduodenal stenosis, etc.); paralytic ileus, intestinal atony of the elderly or debilitated patient; unstable cardiovascular status in acute hemorrhage; severe ulcerative colitis especially if complicated by toxic megacolon; myasthenia gravis; hiatal hernia associated with reflux esophagitis.
Donnatal is contraindicated in patients with known hypersensitivity to any of the ingredients. Phenobarbital is contraindicated in acute intermittent porphyria and in those patients in whom phenobarbital produces restlessness and/or excitement.

WARNINGS

In the presence of a high environmental temperature, heat prostration can occur with belladonna alkaloids (fever and heatstroke due to decreased sweating).
Diarrhea may be an early symptom of incomplete intestinal obstruction, especially in patients with ileostomy or colostomy. In this instance treatment with this drug would be inappropriate and possibly harmful.
Donnatal may produce drowsiness or blurred vision. The patient should be warned, should these occur, not to engage in activities requiring mental alertness, such as operating a motor vehicle or other machinery, and not to perform hazardous work.
Phenobarbital may decrease the effect of anticoagulants and necessitate larger doses of the anticoagulant for optimal effect. When the phenobarbital is discontinued, the dose of the anticoagulant may have to be decreased.
Phenobarbital may be habit forming and should not be administered to individuals known to be addiction prone or to those with a history of physical and/or psychological dependence upon drugs.
Since barbiturates are metabolized in the liver, they should be used with caution and initial doses should be small in patients with hepatic dysfunction.

PRECAUTIONS

Use with caution in patients with: autonomic neuropathy, hepatic or renal disease, hyperthyroidism, coronary heart disease, congestive heart failure, cardiac arrhythmias, tachycardia, and hypertension.

Belladonna alkaloids may produce a delay in gastric emptying (antral stasis) which would complicate the management of gastric ulcer.

Theoretically, with overdosage, a curare-like action may occur.

Carcinogenesis, mutagenesis. Long-term studies in animals have not been performed to evaluate carcinogenic potential.

Pregnancy Category C. Animal reproduction studies have not been conducted with Donnatal. It is not known whether Donnatal can cause fetal harm when administered to a pregnant woman or can affect reproduction capacity. Donnatal should be given to a pregnant woman only if clearly needed.

Nursing mothers. It is not known whether this drug is excreted in human milk. Because many drugs are excreted in human milk, caution should be exercised when Donnatal is administered to a nursing mother.

ADVERSE REACTIONS

Adverse reactions may include xerostomia; urinary hesitancy and retention; blurred vision; tachycardia; palpitation; mydriasis; cycloplegia; increased ocular tension; loss of taste sense; headache; nervousness; drowsiness; weakness; dizziness; insomnia; nausea; vomiting; impotence; suppression of lactation; constipation; bloated feeling; musculoskeletal pain; severe allergic reaction or drug idiosyncrasies, including anaphylaxis, urticaria and other dermal manifestations; and decreased sweating. Elderly patients may react with symptoms of excitement, agitation, drowsiness, and other untoward manifestations to even small doses of the drug.

Phenobarbital may produce excitement in some patients, rather than a sedative effect. In patients habituated to barbiturates, abrupt withdrawal may produce delirium or convulsions.

DOSAGE AND ADMINISTRATION

The dosage of Donnatal Extentabs should be adjusted to the needs of the individual patient to assure symptomatic control with a minimum of adverse reactions. The usual dose is one tablet every twelve (12) hours. If indicated, one tablet every eight (8) hours may be given.

OVERDOSAGE

The signs and symptoms of overdose are headache, nausea, vomiting, blurred vision, dilated pupils; hot and dry skin, dizziness, dryness of the mouth, difficulty in swallowing, CNS stimulation. Treatment should consist of gastric lavage, emetics, and activated charcoal. If indicated, parenteral cholinergic agents such as physostigmine or bethanechol chloride should be added.

HOW SUPPLIED

Pale green, coated tablets, monogrammed AHR and Donnatal Extentab in bottles of 100 (NDC 0031-4235-63) and 500 (NDC 0031-4235-70); and Dis-Co® Unit Dose Packs of 100 (NDC 0031-4235-64).

Store at controlled room temperature, between 20°C and 25°C (68°F and 77°F).

Dispense in well-closed, light-resistant container.

Manufactured by:
Pharmaceutical Division
A.H. Robins Company
Richmond, VA 23220
CI 4693-1 Issued November 1994

Shown in Product Identification Guide, page 332

DONNAZYME® Tablets ℞

[don 'nă " zīm]

Pancreatic Enzyme Replacement

DESCRIPTION

Donnazyme tablets are available for oral administration. Each tablet contains:

Pancreatin, USP equivalent .... 500 mg

which provides not less than the following enzymatic activity—

Lipase .... 1,000 USP Units
Protease .... 12,500 USP Units
Amylase .... 12,500 USP Units

Inactive Ingredients: Acacia, Acetylated Monoglycerides, Calcium Sulfate, Carnauba Wax, Cellulose Acetate Phthalate, Corn Starch, D&C Yellow 10 Aluminum Lake, Diethyl Phthalate, Edible Ink, FD&C Blue 1 Aluminum Lake, FD&C Yellow 6 Aluminum Lake, Gelatin, Methylparaben, Microcrystalline Cellulose, Polysorbates, Povidone, Propylparaben, Shellac, Sodium Benzoate, Stearic Acid, Sucrose, Titanium Dioxide, Wheat Flour, White Wax. May contain Docusate Sodium.

CLINICAL PHARMACOLOGY

The outer layer of Donnazyme tablets is gastric-soluble. The core of the tablet contains pancreatin. It is designed to disintegrate in the alkaline medium of the duodenum where it releases the active enzyme components of pancreatin (trypsin, amylase and lipase). Trypsin breaks down larger protein fractions into peptides; amylase converts starch into maltose; lipase splits fat into fatty acids and glycerin.

INDICATIONS AND USAGE

Donnazyme is indicated for the treatment of exocrine pancreatic insufficiency.

CONTRAINDICATIONS

Donnazyme is contraindicated in patients with known hypersensitivity to the drug.

WARNINGS

Do not take this product if you are allergic to pork.
Do not take this product unless directed by a physician.
Do not exceed the labeled dose unless directed by a physician.
Do not chew tablets.
Swallow tablets quickly to lessen potential for mouth irritation.

PRECAUTIONS

Carcinogenesis, mutagenesis: Long-term studies in animals have not been performed to evaluate carcinogenic potential.

Pregnancy Category C. Animal reproduction studies have not been conducted with Donnazyme. It is not known whether Donnazyme can cause fetal harm when administered to a pregnant woman or can affect reproduction capacity. Donnazyme should be given to a pregnant woman only if clearly needed.

Nursing mothers: It is not known whether this drug is excreted in human milk. Because many drugs are excreted in human milk, caution should be exercised when Donnazyme is administered to a nursing mother.

Pediatric Use: Safety and effectiveness in children have not been established.

ADVERSE REACTIONS

Skin rash is the most frequently reported adverse reaction to Donnazyme and appears to be associated with hypersensitivity to pork protein in the pancreatin. At high doses, a laxative effect may occur.

OVERDOSAGE

Excessive dosage may produce a laxative effect. Systemic toxicity does not occur.

DOSAGE AND ADMINISTRATION

Two tablets with each meal and 2 tablets taken with food eaten between meals or as directed by a physician. Donnazyme tablets should be swallowed whole and not crushed or chewed.

HOW SUPPLIED

Kelly green tablets in bottles of 100 (NDC 0031-4650-63). Store at controlled room temperature, between 20°C and 25°C (68°F and 77°F). Dispense in tight container.

Manufactured by:
Pharamaceutical Division
A.H. Robins Company
Richmond, VA 23220
rev. 2/95

Shown in Product Identification Guide, page 332

DOPRAM® INJECTABLE ℞

[do 'pram]

brand of Doxapram Hydrochloride Injection, USP

DESCRIPTION

Dopram Injectable (Doxapram Hydrochloride Injection, USP) is a clear, colorless, sterile, non-pyrogenic, aqueous solution with pH 3.5—5.0, for intravenous administration.

Each 1 mL contains:

Doxapram Hydrochloride, USP .... 20 mg
Benzyl Alcohol, NF (as preservative) 0.9%
Water for Injection, USP .... q.s.

Due to its benzyl alcohol content, Dopram Injectable should not be used in newborns.

Dopram Injectable is a respiratory stimulant.

Doxapram hydrochloride is a white to off-white, crystalline powder, sparingly soluble in water, alcohol and chloroform. It has the following chemical name:

1-ethyl-4-[2-(4-morpholinyl)ethyl]-3,3-diphenyl-2-pyrrolidinone monohydrochloride, monohydrate.

CLINICAL PHARMACOLOGY

Doxapram hydrochloride produces respiratory stimulation mediated through the peripheral carotid chemoreceptors. As the dosage level is increased, the central respiratory centers in the medulla are stimulated with progressive stimulation of other parts of the brain and spinal cord.

The onset of respiratory stimulation following the recommended single intravenous injection of doxapram hydrochloride usually occurs in 20–40 seconds with peak effect at 1–2 minutes. The duration of effect may vary from 5–12 minutes.

The respiratory stimulant action is manifested by an increase in tidal volume associated with a slight increase in respiratory rate.

A pressor response may result following doxapram administration. Provided there is no impairment of cardiac function, the pressor effect is more marked in hypovolemic than in normovolemic states. The pressor response is due to the improved cardiac output rather than peripheral vasoconstriction. Following doxapram administration, an increased release of catecholamines has been noted.

Although opiate induced respiratory depression is antagonized by doxapram, the analgesic effect is not affected.

INDICATIONS

1. ***Postanesthesia.***
   a. When the possibility of airway obstruction and/or hypoxia have been eliminated, doxapram may be used to stimulate respiration in patients with drug-induced postanesthesia respiratory depression or apnea other than that due to muscle relaxant drugs.
   b. To pharmacologically stimulate deep breathing in the so-called "stir-up" regimen in the postoperative patient. (Simultaneous administration of oxygen is desirable.)
2. ***Drug-induced central nervous system depression.***
   Exercising care to prevent vomiting and aspiration, doxapram may be used to stimulate respiration, hasten arousal, and to encourage the return of laryngopharyngeal reflexes in patients with mild to moderate respiratory and CNS depression due to drug overdosage.
3. ***Chronic pulmonary disease associated with acute hypercapnia.***
   Doxapram is indicated as a temporary measure in hospitalized patients with acute respiratory insufficiency superimposed on chronic obstructive pulmonary disease. Its use should be for a short period of time (approximately 2 hours) as an aid in the prevention of elevation of arterial CO_2 tension during the administration of oxygen. It should not be used in conjuction with mechanical ventilation.

CONTRAINDICATIONS

Due to its benzyl alcohol content, Dopram Injectable should not be used in newborns.

Doxapram should not be used in patients with epilepsy or other convulsive disorders.

Doxapram is contraindicated in patients with mechanical disorders of ventilation such as mechanical obstruction, muscle paresis, flail chest, pneumothorax, acute bronchial asthma, pulmonary fibrosis or other conditions resulting in restriction of chest wall, muscles of respiration or alveolar expansion.

Doxapram is contraindicated in patients with evidence of head injury or cerebral vascular accident and in those with significant cardiovascular impairment, severe hypertension, or known hypersensitivity to the drug.

WARNINGS

1. ***In postanesthetic use.***
   a. Doxapram is neither an antagonist to muscle relaxant drugs nor a specific narcotic antagonist. Adequacy of airway and oxygenation must be assured prior to doxapram administration.
   b. Doxapram should be administered with great care and only under careful supervision to patients with hypermetabolic states such as hyperthyroidism or pheochromocytoma.
   c. Since narcosis may recur after stimulation with doxapram, care should be taken to maintain close observation until the patient has been fully alert for $^1/_2$ to 1 hour.
2. ***In drug-induced CNS and respiratory depression.***
   Doxapram alone may not stimulate adequate spontaneous breathing or provide sufficient arousal in patients who are ***severely*** depressed either due to respiratory failure or to CNS depressant drugs, but should be used as an adjunct to established supportive measures and resuscitative techniques.
3. ***In chronic obstructive pulmonary disease.***
   a. Because of the associated increased work of breathing, do not increase the rate of infusion of doxapram in severely ill patients in an attempt to lower pCO_2.
   b. Doxapram should not be used in conjunction with mechanical ventilation.

PRECAUTIONS

1. ***General.***
   a. An adequate airway is essential.
   b. Recommended dosages of doxapram should be employed and maximum total dosages should not be exceeded. In order to avoid side effects, it is advisable to use the minimum effective dosage.
   c. Monitoring of the blood pressure and deep tendon reflexes is recommended to prevent overdosage.
   d. Vascular extravasation or use of a single injection site over an extended period should be avoided since either may lead to thrombophlebitis or local skin irritation.
   e. Rapid infusion may result in hemolysis.
   f. Lowered pCO_2 induced by hyperventilation produces cerebral vasoconstriction and slowing of the cerebral circulation. This should be taken into consideration on an individual basis.
   g. Intravenous short-acting barbiturates, oxygen and resuscitative equipment should be readily available to manage overdosage manifested by excessive central nervous system stimulation. Slow administration of the drug, and careful observation of the patient during administration and for some time subsequently are ad-

Continued on next page

Dopram—Cont.

visable. These precautions are to assure that the protective reflexes have been restored and to prevent possible post-hyperventilation hypoventilation.

h. Doxapram should be administered cautiously to patients receiving sympathomimetic or monoamine oxidase inhibiting drugs, since an additive pressor effect may occur.

i. Blood pressure increases are generally modest but significant increases have been noted in some patients. Because of this doxapram is not recommended for use in severe hypertension (see Contraindications).

j. If sudden hypotension or dyspnea develops, doxapram should be stopped.

2. ***In postanesthetic use.***

a. The same consideration to pre-existing disease states should be exercised as in non-anesthetized individuals. See Contraindications and Warnings covering use in hypertension, asthma, disturbances of respiratory mechanics including airway obstruction, CNS disorders including increased cerebrospinal fluid pressure, convulsive disorders, acute agitation, and profound metabolic disorders.

b. See Drug Interactions.

3. ***In chronic obstructive pulmonary disease.***

a. Arrhythmias seen in some patients in acute respiratory failure secondary to chronic obstructive pulmonary disease are probably the result of hypoxia. Doxapram should be used with caution in these patients.

b. Arterial blood gases should be drawn prior to the initiation of doxapram infusion and oxygen administration, then at least every 1/2 hour. Doxapram administration does not diminish the need for careful monitoring of the patient or the need for supplemental oxygen in patients with acute respiratory failure. Doxapram should be stopped if the arterial blood gases deteriorate, and mechanical ventilation initiated.

Drug Interactions: Administration of doxapram to patients who are receiving sympathomimetic or monoamine oxidase inhibiting drugs may result in an additive pressor effect. (See Precautions).

In patients who have received muscle relaxants, doxapram may temporarily mask the residual effects of muscle relaxant drugs.

In patients who have received anesthetics known to sensitize the myocardium to catecholamines, such as halothane, cyclopropane and enflurane, initiation of doxapram therapy should be delayed for at least 10 minutes following discontinuance of anesthesia, since an increase in epinephrine release has been noted with doxapram.

Carcinogenesis, mutagenesis, impairment of fertility. No carcinogenic or mutagenic studies have been performed using doxapram. Doxapram did not adversely affect the breeding performance of rats.

Pregnancy Category B. Reproduction studies have been performed in rats at doses up to 1.6 times the human dose and have revealed no evidence of impaired fertility or harm to the fetus due to doxapram. There are, however, no adequate and well-controlled studies in pregnant women. Since the animals in the reproduction studies were dosed by the IM and oral routes and animal reproduction studies, in general, are not always predictive of human response, this drug should be used during pregnancy only if clearly needed.

Nursing mothers. It is not known whether this drug is excreted in human milk. Because many drugs are excreted in human milk, caution should be exercised when doxapram hydrochloride is administered to a nursing mother.

Pediatric use. The use of the preservative benzyl alcohol in the newborn has been associated with metabolic, CNS, respiratory, circulatory, and renal dysfunction. Safety and effectiveness in children below the age of 12 years have not been established.

ADVERSE REACTIONS

The following adverse reactions have been reported:

1. ***Central and autonomic nervous systems.***
Pyrexia, flushing, sweating; pruritus and paresthesia, such as a feeling of warmth, burning, or hot sensation, especially in the area of genitalia and perineum; apprehension, disorientation, pupillary dilatation, headache, dizziness, hyperactivity, involuntary movements, muscle spasticity, increased deep tendon reflexes, clonus, bilateral Babinski, and convulsions.
2. ***Respiratory.***
Dyspnea, cough, tachypnea, laryngospasm, bronchospasm, hiccough, and rebound hypoventilation.
3. ***Cardiovascular.***
Phlebitis, variations in heart rate, lowered T-waves, arrhythmias, chest pain, tightness in chest. A mild to moderate increase in blood pressure is commonly noted and may be of concern in patients with severe cardiovascular diseases.
4. ***Gastrointestinal.***
Nausea, vomiting, diarrhea, desire to defecate.
5. ***Genitourinary.***
Stimulation of urinary bladder with spontaneous voiding; urinary retention.
6. ***Laboratory determinations.***
A decrease in hemoglobin, hematocrit, or red blood cell count has been observed in postoperative patients. In the presence of pre-existing leukopenia, a further decrease in WBC has been observed following anesthesia and treatment with doxapram hydrochloride. Elevation of BUN and albuminuria have also been observed. As some of the patients cited above had received multiple drugs concomitantly, a cause and effect relationship could not be determined.

Table I. Dosage for postanesthetic use—I.V.

I.V. Administration	Recommended dosage mg/kg	Recommended dosage mg/lb	Maximum dose per single injection mg/kg	Maximum dose per single injection mg/lb	Maximum total dose mg/kg	Maximum total dose mg/lb
Single Injection	0.5–1.0	0.25–0.5	1.5	0.70	1.5	0.70
Repeat Injections (5 min. intervals)	0.5–1.0	0.25–0.5	1.5	0.70	2.0	1.0
Infusion	0.5–1.0	0.25–0.5	—	—	4.0	2.0

Table II. Dosage for drug-induced CNS depression.

Level of Depression	METHOD ONE Priming dose single/repeat i.v. injection mg/kg	METHOD ONE mg/lb	METHOD TWO Rate of intermittent i.v. infusion mg/kg/hr	METHOD TWO mg/lb/hr
Mild*	1.0	0.5	1.0–2.0	0.5–1.0
Moderate†	2.0	1.0	2.0–3.0	1.0–1.5

*Mild Depression
Class 0: Asleep, but can be aroused and can answer questions.
Class 1: Comatose, will withdraw from painful stimuli, reflexes intact.
†Moderate Depression
Class 2: Comatose, will not withdraw from painful stimuli, reflexes intact.
Class 3: Comatose, reflexes absent, no depression of circulation or respiration.

OVERDOSAGE

Signs and Symptoms. Symptoms of overdosage are extensions of the pharmacologic effects of the drug. Excessive pressor effect, tachycardia, skeletal muscle hyperactivity, and enhanced deep tendon reflexes may be early signs of overdosage. Therefore, the blood pressure, pulse rate and deep tendon reflexes should be evaluated periodically and the dosage or infusion rate adjusted accordingly.

Convulsive seizures are unlikely at recommended dosages. In unanesthetized animals, the convulsant dose is 70 times greater than the respiratory stimulant dose. Intravenous LD_{50} values in the mouse and rat were approximately 75 mg/kg and in the cat and dog were 40–80 mg/kg.

Except for management of chronic obstructive pulmonary disease associated with acute hypercapnia, the maximum recommended dosage is 3 GRAMS/24 HOURS. (See Dosage and Administration.)

Management. There is no specific antidote for doxapram. Management should be symptomatic. Short-acting intravenous barbiturates, oxygen and resuscitative equipment should be used as needed for supportive treatment.

There is no evidence that doxapram is dialyzable; further, the half-life of doxapram makes it unlikely that dialysis would be appropriate in managing overdose with this drug.

DOSAGE AND ADMINISTRATION

1. Doxapram hydrochloride is compatible with 5% and 10% dextrose in water or normal saline. ADMIXTURE OF DOXAPRAM WITH ALKALINE SOLUTIONS SUCH AS 2.5% THIOPENTAL SODIUM, BICARBONATE, OR AMINOPHYLLINE WILL RESULT IN PRECIPITATION OR GAS FORMATION.
2. ***In postanesthetic use.***

a. By i.v. injection (see Table I. Dosage for postanesthetic use—I.V.) Slow administration of the drug and careful observation of the patient during administration and for some time subsequently are advisable.

[See table I above]

b. By infusion. The solution is prepared by adding 250 mg of doxapram (12.5 mL) to 250 mL of dextrose or saline solution. The infusion is initiated at a rate of approximately 5 mg/minute until a satisfactory respiratory response is observed, and maintained at a rate of 1–3 mg/minute. The rate of infusion should be adjusted to sustain the desired level of respiratory stimulation with a minimum of side effects. The recommended total dosage by infusion is 4 mg/kg (2.0 mg/lb), or approximately 300 mg for the average adult.

3. ***In the management of drug-induced CNS depression.***
(See Table II. Dosage for drug-induced CNS depression.)

[See table II above]

METHOD ONE

Using Single and/or Repeat Single I.V. ***Injections.***

a. Give priming dose of 1.0 mg/lb (2.0 mg/kg) body weight and repeat in 5 minutes.

b. Repeat same dose q1–2h until patient wakens. Watch for relapse into unconsciousness or development of respiratory depression, since Dopram does not affect the metabolism of CNS-depressant drugs.

c. If relapse occurs, resume injections q1–2h until arousal is sustained, or total maximum daily dose (3 grams) is given. Allow patients to sleep until 24 hours have elapsed from first injection of Dopram, using assisted or automatic respiration if necessary.

d. Repeat procedure the following day until patient breathes spontaneously and sustains desired level of consciousness, or until maximum dosage (3 grams) is given.

e. Repetitive doses should be administered only to patients who have shown response to the initial dose.

f. Failure to respond appropriately indicates the need for neurologic evaluation for a possible central nervous system source of sustained coma.

METHOD TWO

By Intermittent I.V. ***Infusion.***

a. Give priming dose as in Method One.

b. If patient wakens, watch for relapse; if no response, continue general supportive treatment for 1–2 hours and repeat Dopram. If some respiratory stimulation occurs, prepare I.V. infusion by adding 250 mg of Dopram (12.5 mL) to 250 mL of saline or dextrose solution. Deliver at rate of 1–3 mg/min (60–180 mL/hr) according to size of patient and depth of coma. Discontinue Dopram if patient begins to waken or at end of 2 hours.

c. Continue supportive treatment for 1/2 to 2 hours and repeat Step b.

d. Do not exceed 3 grams/day.

4. ***Chronic obstructive pulmonary disease associated with acute hypercapnia.***

a. One vial of doxapram (400 mg) should be mixed with 180 mL of dextrose or saline solution (concentration of 2.0 mg/mL). The infusion should be started at 1–2 mg/minute (1/2–1 mL/minute); if indicated, increase to a maximum of 3 mg/minute. Arterial blood gases should be determined prior to the onset of doxapram's administration and at least every half hour during the two hours of infusion to insure against the insidious development of CO_2-RETENTION AND ACIDOSIS. Alteration of oxygen concentration or flow rate may necessitate adjustment in the rate of doxapram infusion.

b. Predictable blood gas patterns are more readily established with a continuous infusion of doxapram. If the blood gases show evidence of deterioration, the infusion of doxapram should be discontinued.

c. ADDITIONAL INFUSIONS BEYOND THE SINGLE MAXIMUM TWO HOUR ADMINISTRATION PERIOD ARE NOT RECOMMENDED.

Parenteral drug products should be inspected visually for particulate matter and discoloration prior to administration, whenever solution and container permit.

HOW SUPPLIED

Dopram Injectable (Doxapram Hydrochloride Injection) is available in 20 mL multiple dose vials containing 20 mg of doxapram hydrochloride per mL. with benzyl alcohol 0.9% as the preservative (NDC 0031-4849-83).

Store at Controlled Room Temperature, Between 15°C and 30°C (59°F and 86°F).

Manufactured for Pharmaceutical Division
A. H. Robins Co.
Richmond, Virginia 23220
by Elkins-Sinn, Inc., Cherry Hill, New Jersey 08003-4099.
J-9702 rev. 4/86

PHENAPHEN® WITH CODEINE

Ⓒ ℞

[fen 'ah-fen"]

(Acetaminophen and Codeine Phosphate Capsules)

DESCRIPTION

Each Phenaphen® with Codeine No. 3 capsule contains:
Acetaminophen, USP .... 325 mg
Codeine Phosphate, USP .... 30 mg
(Warning: May be habit forming)

Inactive Ingredients: D&C Yellow 10, Edible Ink, FD&C Blue 1, (FD&C Green 3 and Red 40), FD&C Yellow 6, Gelatin, Magnesium Stearate, Sodium Starch Glycolate, Stearic Acid.

Each Phenaphen® with Codeine No. 4 capsule contains:

Acetaminophen, USP	325 mg
Codeine Phosphate, USP	60 mg

(Warning: May be habit forming)

Inactive Ingredients: Corn Starch, D&C Yellow 10, Edible Ink, FD&C Green 3 or Blue 1, FD&C Yellow 6, Gelatin, Lactose, Magnesium Stearate, Sodium Starch Glycolate, Stearic Acid.

Acetaminophen, 4′-hydroxyacetanilide, is a non-opiate, non-salicylate analgesic and antipyretic which occurs as a white, odorless, crystalline powder, possessing a slightly bitter taste.

Codeine is an alkaloid, obtained from opium or prepared from morphine by methylation. Codeine phosphate occurs as fine, white, needle-shaped crystals, or white, crystalline powder. It is affected by light. Its chemical name is: 7,8-didehydro-4, 5α-epoxy-3-methoxy-17-methylmorphinan-6α-ol phosphate (1:1) (salt) hemihydrate.

HOW SUPPLIED

Phenaphen with Codeine No. 3, black and green capsules in bottles of 100 (NDC 0031-6257-63) and 500 (NDC 0031-6257-70).

Phenaphen with Codeine No. 4, green and white capsules in bottles of 100 (NDC 0031-6274-63).

Store at controlled room temperature, between 20°– 25°C (68°–77°F).

Dispense capsules in tight, light-resistant container.

Manufactured by:
Pharmaceutical Division
A.H. Robins Company
Richmond, VA 23220
CI 4695-1 Issued February 28, 1997

For prescribing information write to Professional Service, Wyeth-Ayerst Pharmaceuticals, P.O. Box 8299, Philadelphia, PA 19101, or contact your local Wyeth-Ayerst representative.

QUINIDEX EXTENTABS® Tablets ℞

[*kwĭn ′ĭ ″deks ĕks ″tĕn ′tabs*]
(quinidine sulfate extended-release tablets, USP)

DESCRIPTION

Quinidine is an antimalarial schizonticide and an antiarrhythmic agent with Class la activity; it is the d-isomer of quinine, and its molecular weight is 324.43. Quinidine sulfate is the sulfate salt of quinidine; its chemical name is cinchonan-9-ol, 6′-methoxy-, (9S)-, sulfate(2:1) dihydrate; its structural formula is

its empirical formula is $(C_{20}H_{24}N_2O_2)_2 \cdot H_2SO_4 \cdot 2H_2O$; and its molecular weight is 782.95, of which 82.9% is quinidine base.

Each Quinidex Extentabs® tablet contains 300 mg of quinidine sulfate (249 mg of quinidine base) in a formulation to provide extended release; the inactive ingredients are acacia, acetylated monoglycerides, calcium sulfate, carnauba wax, edible ink, FD&C Blue 2, gelatin, guar gum, magnesium oxide, magnesium stearate, polysorbates, shellac, sucrose, titanium dioxide, white wax, and other ingredients, one of which is a corn derivative. Tablets may also contain FD&C Red 40 and FD&C Yellow 6 Aluminum Lakes. These tablets comply with USP Drug Release Test 1.

CLINICAL PHARMACOLOGY

Pharmacokinetics

The absolute bioavailability of quinidine from Quinidex is about 70%, but this varies widely (45–100%) between patients. The less-than-complete bioavailability is the result of first-pass metabolism in the liver. Peak serum levels generally appear about 6 hours after dosing.

Although the effect of food upon Quinidex absorption has not been studied, peak serum quinidine levels obtained from immediate-release quinidine sulfate are known to be delayed by nearly an hour (without change in total absorption) when these products are taken with food.

The **volume of distribution** of quinidine is 2 to 3 L/kg in healthy young adults, but this may be reduced to as little as 0.5 L/kg in patients with congestive heart failure, or increased to 3 to 5 L/kg in patients with cirrhosis of the liver. At concentrations of 2 to 5 mg/L (6.5 to 16.2 μmol/L), the fraction of quinidine bound to plasma proteins (mainly to α_1-acid glycoprotein and to albumin) is 80 to 88% in adults and older children, but it is lower in pregnant women, and in infants and neonates it may be as low as 50 to 70%. Because α_1-acid glycoprotein levels are increased in response to stress, serum levels of total quinidine may be greatly increased in settings such as acute myocardial infarction, even though the serum content of unbound (active) drug may remain normal. Protein binding is also increased in chronic renal failure, but binding abruptly descends toward or below normal when heparin is administered for hemodialysis.

Quinidine **clearance** typically proceeds at 3 to 5 mL/min/kg in adults, but clearance in children may be twice or three times as rapid. The elimination half-life is 6 to 8 hours in adults and 3 to 4 hours in children. Quinidine clearance is unaffected by hepatic cirrhosis, so the increased volume of distribution seen in cirrhosis leads to a proportionate increase in the elimination half-life.

Most quinidine is eliminated hepatically via the action of cytochrome $P_{450}IIIA_4$; there are several different hydroxylated metabolites, and some of these have antiarrhythmic activity.

The most important of quinidine's metabolites is 3-hydroxyquinidine (3HQ), serum levels of which can approach those of quinidine in patients receiving conventional doses of Quinidex. The volume of distribution of 3HQ appears to be larger than that of quinidine, and the elimination half-life of 3HQ is about 12 hours.

As measured by antiarrhythmic effects in animals, by QT_c prolongation in human volunteers, or by various *in vitro* techniques, 3HQ has at least half the antiarrhythmic activity of the parent compound, so it may be responsible for a substantial fraction of the effect of Quinidex in chronic use.

When the urine pH is less than 7, about 20% of administered quinidine appears unchanged in the urine, but this fraction drops to as little as 5% when the urine is more alkaline. Renal clearance involves both glomerular filtration and active tubular secretion, moderated by (pH-dependent) tubular reabsorption. The new renal clearance is about 1 mL/min/kg in healthy adults.

When renal function is taken into account, quinidine clearance is apparently independent of patient age.

Assays of serum quinidine levels are widely available, but the results of modern assays may not be consistent with results cited in the older medical literature. The serum levels of quinidine cited in this package insert are those derived from specific assays, using either benzene extraction or (preferably) reverse-phase high-pressure liquid chromatography. In matched samples, older assays might unpredictably have given results that were as much as two or three times higher. A typical "therapeutic" concentration range is 2 to 6 mg/L (6.2 to 18.5 μmol/L).

Mechanisms of Action

In patients with malaria, quinidine acts primarily as an intra-erythrocytic schizonticide, with little effect upon sporozites or upon pre-erythrocytic parasites. Quinidine is gametocidal to *Plasmodium vivax* and *P. malariae,* but not to *P. falciparum.*

In cardiac muscle and in Purkinje fibers, quinidine depresses the rapid inward depolarizing sodium current, thereby slowing phase-0 depolarization and reducing the amplitude of the action potential without affecting the resting potential. In normal Purkinje fibers, it reduces the slope of phase-4 depolarization, shifting the threshold voltage upward toward zero. The result is slowed conduction and reduced automaticity in all parts of the heart, with increase of the effective refractory period relative to the duration of the action potential in the atria, ventricles, and Purkinje tissues. Quinidine also raises the fibrillation thresholds of the atria and ventricles, and it raises the ventricular *de*fibrillation threshold as well. Quinidine's actions fall into Class Ia in the Vaughan-Williams classification.

By slowing conduction and prolonging the effective refractory period, quinidine can interrupt or prevent reentrant arrhythmias and arrhythmias due to increased automaticity, including atrial flutter, atrial fibrillation, and paroxysmal supraventricular tachycardia.

In patients with the sick sinus syndrome, quinidine can cause marked sinus node depression and bradycardia. In most patients, however, use of quinidine is associated with an increase in the sinus rate.

Quinidine prolongs the QT interval in a dose-related fashion. This may lead to increased ventricular automaticity and polymorphic ventricular tachycardias, including *torsades de pointes* (see **WARNINGS**).

In addition, quinidine has anticholinergic activity, it has negative inotropic activity, and it acts peripherally as an α-adrenergic antagonist (that is, as a vasodilator).

Clinical Effects

Maintenance of sinus rhythm after conversion from atrial fibrillation: In six clinical trials (published between 1970 and 1984) with a total of 808 patients, quinidine (418 patients) was compared to nontreatment (258 patients) or placebo (132 patients) for the maintenance of sinus rhythm after cardioversion from chronic atrial fibrillation. Quinidine was consistently more efficacious in maintaining sinus rhythm, but a meta-analysis found that mortality in the quinidine-exposed patients (2.9%) was significantly greater than mortality in the patients who had not been treated with active drug (0.8%). Suppression of atrial fibrillation with quinidine has theoretical patient benefits (e.g., improved exercise tolerance; reduction in hospitalization for cadioversion; lack of arrhythmia-related palpitations, dyspnea, and chest pain; reduced incidence of systemic embolism and/or stroke), but these benefits have never been demonstrated in clinical trials. Some of these benefits (e.g., reduction in stroke incidence) may be achievable by other means (anticoagulation).

By slowing the rate of atrial flutter/fibrillation, quinidine can decrease the degree of atrioventricular block and cause an increase, sometimes marked, in the rate at which supraventricular impulses are successfully conducted by the atrioventricular node, with a resultant paradoxical increase in ventricular rate (see **WARNINGS**).

Non-life-threatening ventricular arrhythmias: In studies of patients with a variety of ventricular arrhythmias (mainly frequent ventricular premature beats and non-sustained ventricular tachycardia), quinidine (total N=502) has been compared to flecainide (N=141), mexiletine (N=246), propafenone (N=53), and tocainide (N=67). In each of these studies, the mortality in the quinidine group was numerically greater than the mortality in the comparator group. When the studies were combined in a meta-analysis, quinidine was associated with a statistically significant threefold relative risk of death.

At therapeutic doses, quinidine's only consistent effect upon the surface electrocardiogram is an increase in the QT interval. This prolongation can be monitored as a guide to safety, and it may provide better guidance than serum drug levels (see **WARNINGS**).

INDICATIONS AND USAGE

Conversion of Atrial Fibrillation/Flutter

In patients with symptomatic atrial fibrillation/flutter whose symptoms are not adequately controlled by measures that reduce the rate of ventricular response, Quinidex is indicated as a means of restoring normal sinus rhythm. If this use of Quinidex does not restore sinus rhythm within a reasonable time (see **DOSAGE AND ADMINISTRATION**), then Quinidex should be discontinued.

Reduction of Frequency of Relapse into Atrial Fibrillation/Flutter

Chronic therapy with Quinidex is indicated for some patients at high risk of symptomatic atrial fibrillation/flutter; generally patients who have had previous episodes of atrial fibrillation/flutter that were so frequent and poorly tolerated as to outweigh, in the judgment of the physician and the patient, the risks of prophylactic therapy with Quinidex. The increased risk of death should specifically be considered. Quinidex should be used only after alternative measures (e.g., use of other drugs to control ventricular rate) have been found to be inadequate.

In patients with histories of frequent symptomatic episodes of atrial fibrillation/flutter, the goal of therapy should be an increase in the average time between episodes. In most patients, the tachyarrhythmia *will recur* during therapy, and a single recurrence should not be interpreted as therapeutic failure.

Suppression of Ventricular Arrhythmias

Quinidex is also indicated for the suppression of recurrent documented ventricular arrhythmias, such as sustained ventricular tachycardia, that in the judgment of the physician are life-threatening. Because of the proarrhythmic effects of quinidine, its use with ventricular arrhythmias of lesser severity is generally not recommended, and treatment of patients with asymptomatic ventricular premature contractions should be avoided. Where possible, therapy should be guided by the results of programmed electrical stimulation and/or Holter monitoring with exercise.

Antiarrhythmic drugs (including Quinidex) have not been shown to enhance survival in patients with ventricular arrhythmias.

CONTRAINDICATIONS

Quinidine is contraindicated in patients who are known to be allergic to it, or who have developed thrombocytopenic purpura during prior therapy with quinidine or quinine.

In the absence of a functioning artificial pacemaker, quinidine is also contraindicated in any patient whose cardiac rhythm is dependent upon a junctional or idioventricular pacemaker, including patients in complete atrioventricular block.

Quinidine is also contraindicated in patients who, like those will myasthenia gravis, might be adversely affected by an anticholinergic agent.

WARNINGS

Mortality

In many trials of antiarrhythmic therapy for non-life-threatening arrhythmias, active antiarrhythmic therapy has resulted in increased mortality; the risk of active therapy is probably greatest in patients with structural heart disease.

In the case of quinidine used to prevent or defer recurrence of atrial flutter/fibrillation, the best available data come from a meta-analysis described under CLINICAL PHARMACOLOGY—Clinical Effects above. In the patients studied in the trials there analyzed, the mortality associated with the use of quinidine was more than three times as great as the mortality associated with the use of placebo.

Another meta-analysis, also described under CLINICAL PHARMACOLOGY—Clinical Effects, showed that in patients with various non-life-threatening ventricular arrhythmias, the mortality associated with the use of quinidine was consistently greater than that associated with the use of any of a variety of alternative antiarrhythmics.

Proarrhythmic Effects

Like many other drugs (including all other Class la antiarrhythmics), quinidine prolongs the QT_c interval, and this

Continued on next page

Quinidex—Cont.

can lead to *torsades de pointes*, a life-threatening ventricular arrhythmia (see **OVERDOSAGE**). The risk of *torsades* is increased by bradycardia, hypokalemia, hypomagnesemia, or high serum levels of quinidine, but it may appear in the absence of any of these risk factors. The best predictor of this arrhythmia appears to be the length of the QT_c interval, and quinidine should be used with extreme care in patients who have preexisting long-QT syndromes, who have histories of *torsades de pointes* of any cause, or who have previously responded to quinidine (or other drugs that prolong ventricular repolarization) with marked lengthening of the QT_c interval. Estimation of the incidence of *torsades* in patients with therapeutic levels of quinidine is not possible from the available data.

Other ventricular arrhythmias that have been reported with quinidine include frequent extrasystoles, ventricular tachycardia, ventricular flutter, and ventricular fibrillation.

Paradoxical Increase in Ventricular Rate in Atrial Flutter/Fibrillation

When quinidine is administered to patients with atrial flutter/fibrillation the desired pharmacologic reversion to sinus rhythm may (rarely) be preceded by a showing of the atrial rate with a consequent increase in the rate of beats conducted to the ventricles. The resulting ventricular rate may be very high (greater than 200 beats per minute) and poorly tolerated. This hazard may be decreased if partial atrioventricular block is achieved prior to initiation of quinidine therapy, using conduction-reducing drugs such as digitalis, verapamil, diltiazem, or a β-receptor blocking agent.

Exacerbated Bradycardia in Sick Sinus Syndrome

In patients with the sick sinus syndrome, quinidine has been associated with marked sinus node depression and bradycardia.

Pharmacokinetic Considerations

Renal or hepatic dysfunction causes the elimination of quinidine to be slowed, while congestive heart failure causes a reduction in quinidine's apparent volume of distribution. Any of these conditions can lead to quinidine toxicity if dosage is not appropriately reduced. In addition, interactions with coadministered drugs can alter the serum concentration and activity of quinidine, leading either to toxicity or to lack of efficacy if the dose of quinidine is not appropriately modified. (See **PRECAUTIONS—Drug Interactions.**)

Vagolysis

Because quinidine opposes the atrial and A-V nodal effects of vagal stimulation, physical or pharmacological vagal maneuvers undertaken to terminate paroxysmal supraventricular tachycardia may be ineffective in patients receiving quinidine.

PRECAUTIONS

General

All the precautions applying to regular quinidine therapy apply to this product. Hypersensitivity or anaphylactoid reactions to quinidine, although rare, should be considered, especially during the first weeks of therapy. Hospitalization for close clinical observation, electrocardiographic monitoring, and determination of serum quinidine levels are indicated when large doses of quinidine are used or with patients who present an increased risk.

Laboratory Tests

Periodic blood counts and liver and kidney function tests should be performed during long-term therapy; the drug should be discontinued if blood dyscrasias or evidence of hepatic or renal dysfunction occurs.

Heart Block

In patients without implanted pacemakers who are at high risk of complete atrioventricular block (e.g., those with digitalis intoxication, second-degree atrioventricular block, or severe intraventricular conduction defects), quinidine should be used only with caution.

Drug Interactions

Altered pharmacokinetics of quinidine: Drugs that alkalinize the urine (**carbonic-anhydrase inhibitors, sodium bicarbonate, thiazide diuretics**) reduce renal elimination of quinidine.

By pharmacokinetic mechanisms that are not well understood, quinidine levels are increased by coadministration of **amiodarone** or **cimetidine**. Very rarely, and again by mechanisms not understood, quinidine levels are decreased by coadministration of **nifedipine**.

Hepatic elimination of quinidine may be accelerated by coadministration of drugs (**phenobarbital, phenytoin, rifampin**) that induce production of cytochrome $P_{450}IIIA_4$.

Perhaps because of competition for the $P_{450}IIIA_4$ metabolic pathway, quinidine levels rise when **ketoconazole** is coadministered.

Coadministration of **propranolol** usually does not affect quinidine pharmacokinetics, but in some studies the β-blocker appeared to cause increases in the peak serum levels of quinidine, decreases in quinidine's volume of distribution, and decreases in total quinidine clearance. The effects (if any) of coadministration of **other β-blockers** on quinidine pharmacokinetics have not been adequately studied.

Diltiazem significantly decreases the clearance and increases the $t_{½}$ of quinidine, but quinidine does not alter the kinetics of diltiazem.

Hepatic clearance of quinidine is significantly reduced during coadministration of **verapamil**, with corresponding increases in serum levels and half-life.

Altered pharmacokinetics of other drugs: Quinidine slows the elimination of **digoxin** and simultaneously reduces digoxin's apparent volume of distribution. As a result, serum digoxin levels may be as much as doubled. When quinidine and digoxin are coadministered, digoxin doses usually need to be reduced. Serum levels of **digitoxin** are also raised when quinidine is coadministered, although the effect appears to be smaller.

By a mechanism that is not understood, quinidine potentiates the anticoagulatory action of **warfarin**, and the anticoagulant dosage may need to be reduced.

Cytochrome $P_{450}IID_6$ is an enzyme critical to the metabolism of many drugs, notably including **mexiletine**, some **phenothiazines**, and most **polycyclic antidepressants**. Constitutional deficiency of cytochrome $P_{450}IID_6$ is found in less than 1% of Orientals, in about 2% of American blacks, and in about 8% of American whites. Testing with debrisoquine is sometimes used to distinguish the $P_{450}IID_6$-deficient "poor metabolizers" from the majority-phenotype "extensive metabolizers."

When drugs whose metabolism is $P_{450}IID_6$-dependent are given to poor metabolizers, the serum levels achieved are higher, sometimes much higher, than the serum levels achieved when identical doses are given to extensive metabolizers. To obtain similar clinical benefit without toxicity, doses given to poor metabolizers may need to be greatly reduced. In the cases of prodrugs whose actions are actually mediated by $P_{450}IID_6$-produced metabolites (for example, **codeine** and **hydrocodone**, whose analgesic and antitussive effects appear to be mediated by morphine and hydromorphone, respectively), it may not be possible to achieve the desired clinical benefits in poor metabolizers.

Quinidine is not metabolized by cytochrome $P_{450}IID_6$, but therapeutic serum levels of quinidine inhibit the action of cytochrome $P_{450}IID_6$, effectively converting extensive metabolizers into poor metabolizers. Caution must be exercised whenever quinidine is prescribed together with drugs metabolized by cytochrome $P_{450}IID_6$.

Perhaps by competing for pathways of renal clearance, coadministration of quinidine causes an increase in serum levels of **procainamide**.

Serum levels of **haloperidol** are increased when quinidine is coadministered.

Presumably because both drugs are metabolized by cytochrome $P_{450}IIIA_4$, coadministration of quinidine causes variable slowing of the metabolism of **nifedipine**. Interactions with other dihydropyridine calcium-channel blockers have not been reported, but these agents (including **felodipine, nicardipine,** and **nimodipine**) are all dependent upon $P_{450}IIIA_4$ for metabolism, so similar interactions with quinidine should be anticipated.

Altered pharmacodynamics of other drugs: Quinidine's anticholinergic, vasodilating, and negative inotropic actions may be additive to those of other drugs with these effects, and antagonistic to those of drugs with cholinergic, vasoconstricting, and positive inotropic effects. For example, when quinidine and **verapamil** are coadministered in doses that are each well tolerated as monotherapy, hypotension attributable to additive peripheral α-blockade is sometimes reported.

Quinidine potentiates the actions of depolarizing (succinylcholine, decamethonium) and nondepolarizing (d-tubocurarine, pancuronium) **neuromuscular blocking agents**. These phenomena are not well understood, but they are observed in animals models as well as in humans. In addition, *in vitro* addition of quinidine to the serum of pregnant women reduces the activity of pseudocholinesterase, an enzyme that is essential to the metabolism of succinylcholine.

Non-interactions of quinidine with other drugs: Quinidine has no clinically significant effect on the pharmacokinetics of **diltiazem, flecainide, mephenytoin, metoprolol, propafenone, propranolol, quinine, timolol,** or **tocainide**.

Conversely, the pharmacokinetics of quinidine are not significantly affected by **caffeine, ciprofloxacin, digoxin, diltiazem, felodipine, omeprazole,** or **quinine**. Quinidine's pharmacokinetics are also unaffected by cigarette smoking.

Information for Patients

Before prescribing Quinidex Extentabs® as prophylaxis against recurrence of atrial fibrillation, the physician should inform the patient of the risks and benefits to be expected (see **CLINICAL PHARMACOLOGY**).

Discussion should include the facts

- that the goal of therapy will be a reduction (probably not to zero) in the frequency of episodes of atrial fibrillation; and
- that reduced frequency of fibrillatory episodes may be expected, if achieved, to bring symptomatic benefit; but
- that no data are available to show that reduced frequency of fibrillatory episodes will reduce the risks of irreversible harm through stroke or death; and in fact
- that such data as are available suggest that treatment with Quinidex is likely to increase the patient's risk of death.

Carcinogenesis, Mutagenesis, Impairment of Fertility

Animal studies to evaluate quinidine's carcinogenic or mutagenic potential have not been performed. Similarly, there are no animal data as to quinidine's potential to impair fertility.

Pregnancy

Pregnancy Category C: Animal reproductive studies have not been conducted with quinidine. There are no adequate and well-controlled studies in pregnant women. Quinidine should be given to a pregnant woman only if clearly needed.

In one neonate whose mother had received quinidine throughout her pregnancy, the serum level of quinidine was equal to that of the mother, with no apparent ill effect. The level of quinidine in amniotic fluid was about three times higher than that found in serum.

Labor and Delivery

Quinine is said to be oxytocic in humans, but there are no adequate data as to quinidine's effects (if any) on human labor and delivery.

Nursing Mothers

Quinidine is present in human milk at levels slightly lower than those in maternal serum; a human infant ingesting such milk should (scaling directly by weight) be expected to develop serum quinidine levels at least an order of magnitude lower than those of the mother. On the other hand, the pharmacokinetics and pharmacodynamics of quinidine in human infants have not been adequately studied, and neonates' reduced protein binding of quinidine may increase their risk of toxicity at low total serum levels. Administration of quinidine should (if possible) be avoided in lactating women who continue to nurse.

Geriatric Use

Safety and efficacy of quinidine in elderly patients have not been systematically studied.

Pediatric Use

In antimalarial trials, quinidine was as safe and effective in pediatric patients as in adults. Notwithstanding the known pharmacokinetic differences between the pediatric population and adults (see **CLINICAL PHARMACOLOGY—Pharmacokinetics**), pediatric patients in these trials received the same doses (on a mg/kg basis) as adults.

Safety and effectiveness of the antiarrhythmic use of quinidine in pediatric patients have not been established in well-controlled clinical trials.

ADVERSE REACTIONS

Quinidine preparations have been used for many years, but there are only sparse data from which to estimate the incidence of various adverse reactions. The adverse reactions most frequently reported have consistently been gastrointestinal, including diarrhea, nausea, vomiting, and heartburn/esophagitis. In one study of 245 adult outpatients who received quinidine to suppress premature ventricular contractions, the incidences of reported adverse experiences were as shown in the table below. The most serious quinidine-associated adverse reactions are described above under **WARNINGS**.

Adverse Experiences in a 245-Patient PVC Trial

	Incidence (%)
diarrhea	85 (35)
"upper gastrointestinal distress"	55 (22)
light-headedness	37 (15)
headache	18 (7)
fatigue	17 (7)
palpitations	16 (7)
angina-like pain	14 (6)
weakness	13 (5)
rash	11 (5)
visual problems	8 (3)
change in sleep habits	7 (3)
tremor	6 (2)
nervousness	5 (2)
discoordination	3 (1)

Vomiting and diarrhea can occur as isolated reactions to therapeutic levels of quinidine, but they also may be the first signs of **cinchonism**, a syndrome that also may include tinnitus, reversible high-frequency hearing loss, deafness, vertigo, blurred vision, diplopia, photophobia, headache, confusion, and delirium. Cinchonism is most often a sign of chronic quinidine toxicity, but it may appear in sensitive patients after a single moderate dose.

A few cases of **hepatotoxicity**, including granulomatous hepatitis, have been reported in patients receiving quinidine. All of these have appeared during the first few weeks of therapy, and most (not all) have remitted once quinidine was withdrawn.

Autoimmune and inflammatory syndromes associated with quinidine therapy have included pneumonitis, fever, urticaria, flushing, exfoliative rash, bronchospasm, psoriasiform rash, pruritus and lymphadenopathy, hemolytic anemia, vasculitis, thrombocytopenic purpura, uveitis, angioedema, agranulocytosis, the sicca syndrome, arthralgia, myalgia, elevation in serum levels of skeletal-muscle enzymes, and a disorder resembling systemic lupus erythematosus.

Convulsions, apprehension, and ataxia have been reported, but it is not clear that these were not simply the results of hypotension and consequent cerebral hypoperfusion. There are many reports of syncope. Acute psychotic reactions have been reported to follow the first dose of quinidine, but these reactions appear to be extremely rare.

Other adverse reactions occasionally reported include depression, mydriasis, disturbed color perception, night blindness, scotomata, optic neuritis, visual field loss, photosensitivity, and abnormalities of pigmentation.

OVERDOSAGE

Overdoses with various oral formulations of quinidine have been well described. Death has been described after a 5-gram ingestion by a toddler, while an adolescent was reported to survive after ingesting 8 grams of quinidine.

The most important ill effects of acute quinidine overdoses are ventricular arrhythmias and hypotension. Other signs and symptoms of overdose may include vomiting, diarrhea, tinnitus, high-frequency hearing loss, vertigo, blurred vision, diplopia, photophobia, headache, confusion, and delirium.

Arrhythmias

Serum quinidine levels can be conveniently assayed and monitored, but the electrocardiographic QT_c interval is a better predictor of quinidine-induced ventricular arrhythmias.

The necessary treatment of hemodynamically unstable polymorphic ventricular tachycardia (including *torsades de pointes*) is withdrawal of treatment with quinidine and either immediate cardioversion or, if a cardiac pacemaker is in place or immediately available, immediate overdrive pacing. After pacing or cardioversion, further management must be guided by the length of the QT_c interval.

Quinidine-associated ventricular tachyarrhythmias with normal underlying QT_c intervals have not been adequately studied. Because of the theoretical possibility of QT-prolonging effects that might be additive to those of quinidine, other antiarrhythmics with Class I (disopyramide, procainamide) or Class III activities should (if possible) be avoided. Similarly, although the use of bretylium in quinidine overdose has not been reported, it is reasonable to expect that the α-blocking properties of bretylium might be additive to those of quinidine, resulting in problematic hypotension.

If the post-cardioversion QT_c interval is prolonged, then the pre-cardioversion polymorphic ventricular tachyarrhythmia was (by definition) *torsades de pointes*. In this case, lidocaine and bretylium are unlikely to be of value, and other Class I antiarrhythmics (disopyramide, procainamide) are likely to exacerbate the situation. Factors contributing to QT_c prolongation (especially hypokalemia and hypomagnesemia) should be sought out and (if possible) aggressively corrected. Prevention of recurrent *torsades* may require sustained overdrive pacing or the cautious administration of isoproterenol (30 to 150 ng/kg/min).

Hypotension

Quinidine-induced hypotension that is not due to an arrhythmia is likely to be a consequence of quinidine-related α-blockade and vasorelaxation. Simple repletion of central volume (Trendelenburg positioning, saline infusion) may be sufficient therapy; other interventions reported to have been beneficial in this setting are those that increase peripheral vascular resistance, including α-agonist catecholamines (norepinephrine, metaraminol) and the Military Anti-Shock Trousers.

Treatment

Adequate studies of orally-administered activated charcoal in human overdoses of quinidine have not been reported, but there are animal data showing significant enhancement of systemic elimination following this intervention, and there is at least one human case report in which the elimination half-life of quinidine in the serum was apparently shortened by repeated gastric lavage. Activated charcoal should be avoided if an ileus is present; the conventional dose is 1 gram/kg, administered every 2 to 6 hours as a slurry with 8 mL/kg of tap water. Although renal elimination of quinidine might theoretically be accelerated by maneuvers to acidify the urine, such maneuvers are potentially hazardous and of no demonstrated benefit.

Quinidine is not usefully removed from the circulation by dialysis. Following quinidine overdose, drugs that delay elimination of quinidine (cimetidine, carbonic-anhydrase inhibitors, thiazide diuretics) should be withdrawn unless absolutely required.

In managing overdose, consider the possibilities of multiple-drug overdoses, drug-drug interactions, and unusual drug kinetics in your patient.

DOSAGE AND ADMINISTRATION

Conversion of Atrial Fibrillation/Flutter to Sinus Rhythm

Especially in patients with known structural heart disease or other risk factors for toxicity, initiation or dose-adjustment of treatment with Quinidex should generally be performed in a setting where facilities and personnel for monitoring and resuscitation are continuously available.

Patients with symptomatic atrial fibrillation/flutter should be treated with Quinidex only after ventricular rate control (e.g., with digitalis or β-blockers) has failed to provide satisfactory control of symptoms. Adequate trials have not identified an optimal regimen of Quinidex for conversion of atrial fibrillation/flutter to sinus rhythm. Therapy with Quinidex should begin with one tablet (300 mg; 249 mg of quinidine base) every 8 to 12 hours. If this regimen is well tolerated, if the serum quinidine level is still well within the laboratory's therapeutic range, and if this regimen has not resulted in conversion, then the dose may be cautiously raised. If, at any point during administration, the QRS complex widens to 130% of its pre-treatment duration; the QT_c interval widens to 130% of its pre-treatment duration and is then longer than 500 ms; P waves disappear; or the patient develops significant tachycardia, symptomatic bradycardia, or hypotension, then Quinidex is discontinued, and other means of conversion (e.g., direct-current cardioversion) are considered.

Reduction of Frequency of Relapse into Atrial Fibrillation/Flutter

In a patient with a history of frequent symptomatic episodes of atrial fibrillation/flutter, the goal of therapy with Quinidex should be an increase in the average time between episodes. In most patients, the tachyarrhythmia *will recur* during therapy with Quinidex, and a single recurrence should not be interpreted as therapeutic failure.

Especially in patients with known structural heart disease or other risk factors for toxicity, initiation or dose-adjustment of treatment with Quinidex should generally be performed in a setting where facilities and personnel for monitoring and resuscitation are continously available.

Monitoring should be continued for two or three days after initiation of the regimen on which the patient will be discharged.

Therapy with Quinidex should begin with one tablet (300 mg; 249 mg of quinidine base) every eight to twelve hours. If this regimen is well tolerated, if the serum quinidine level is still well within the laboratory's therapeutic range, and if the average time between arrhythmic episodes has not been satisfactorily increased, then the dose may be cautiously raised. The total daily dosage should be reduced if the QRS complex widens to 130% of its pre-treatment duration; the QT_c interval widens to 130% of its pre-treatment duration and is then longer than 500 ms; P waves disappear; or the patient develops significant tachycardia, symptomatic bradycardia, or hypotension.

Suppression of Ventricular Arrhythmias

Dosing regimens for the use of quinidine sulfate in suppressing life-threatening ventricular arrhythmias have not been adequately studied.

Described regimens have generally been similar to the regimen described just above for the prophylaxis of symptomatic atrial fibrillation/flutter. Where possible, therapy should be guided by the results of programmed electrical stimulation and/or Holter monitoring with exercise.

HOW SUPPLIED

Quinidex Extentabs® Tablets (quinidine sulfate extended-release tablets, USP) are 300 mg, white, sugar-coated, round tablets marked with "QUINIDEX" and "AHR". The tablets are available in bottles and in DIS-CO® unit-dose packages as follows:

bottle of 100	NDC 0031-6649-63
bottle of 250	NDC 0031-6649-67
unit-dose pack of 100	NDC 0031-6649-64

Store at controlled room temperature, 20°–25°C (68°–77°F).

Dispense in well-closed, light-resistant container.

Caution: Federal law prohibits dispensing without prescription.

Manufactured by:
Pharmaceutical Division
A.H. Robins Company
Richmond, VA 23220
CI 4675-2 Revised January 20, 1998

Shown in Product Identification Guide, page 332

REGLAN® Tablets ℞
[*rĕg 'lăn*]
(Metoclopramide Tablets, USP)
REGLAN® Syrup
(Metoclopramide Oral Solution, USP)
REGLAN® Injectable
(Metoclopramide Injection, USP)

DESCRIPTION

For oral administration, Reglan Tablets (Metoclopramide Tablets, USP) 10 mg are white. scored, capsule-shaped tablets engraved Reglan on one side and AHR 10 on the opposite side.

Each tablet contains:
Metoclopramide base 10 mg
(as the monohydrochloride monohydrate)

Inactive Ingredients

Magnesium Stearate, Mannitol, Microcrystalline Cellulose, Stearic Acid.

Reglan Tablets (Metoclopramide Tablets, USP) 5 mg are green, elliptical-shaped tablets engraved Reglan 5 on one side and AHR on the opposite side.

Each tablet contains:
Metoclopramide base 5 mg
(as the monohydrochloride monohydrate)

Inactive Ingredients

Corn Starch, D&C Yellow 10 Lake, FD&C Blue 1 Aluminum Lake, Lactose, Microcrystalline Cellulose, Silicon Dioxide, Stearic Acid.

Reglan Syrup (Metoclopramide Oral Solution, USP) is an orange-colored, palatable, aromatic, sugar-free liquid.

Each 5 mL (1 teaspoonful) contains:
Metoclopramide base 5 mg
(as the monohydrochloride monohydrate)

Inactive Ingredients

Citric Acid, FD&C Yellow 6, Flavors, Glycerin, Methylparaben, Propylparaben, Sorbitol, Water.

For parenteral administration, Reglan Injectable (Metoclopramide Injection, USP) is a clear, colorless, sterile solution with a pH of 4.5–6.5 for intravenous or intramuscular administration.

CONTAINS NO PRESERVATIVE.

2 mL single dose vials/ampuls; 10 mL and 30 mL single dose vials

Each 1 mL contains:
Metoclopramide base 5 mg
(as the monohydrochloride monohydrate)
Sodium Chloride, USP 8.5 mg, Water for Injection, USP q.s. pH adjusted, when necessary, with hydrochloric acid and/or sodium hydroxide.

Metoclopramide hydrochloride is a white crystalline, odorless substance, freely soluble in water. Chemically, it is 4-amino-5-chloro-N-[2-(diethylamino)ethyl]-2-methoxy benzamide monohydrochloride monohydrate. Molecular weight: 354.3.

Cl, $CONHCH_2CH_2N(C_2H_5)_2$, H_2N, OCH_3 · HCl · H_2O

CLINICAL PHARMACOLOGY

Metoclopramide stimulates motility of the upper gastrointestinal tract without stimulating gastric, biliary, or pancreatic secretions. Its mode of action is unclear. It seems to sensitize tissues to the action of acetylcholine. The effect of metoclopramide on motility is not dependent on intact vagal innervation, but it can be abolished by anticholinergic drugs.

Metoclopramide increases the tone and amplitude of gastric (especially antral) contractions, relaxes the pyloric sphincter and the duodenal bulb, and increases peristalsis of the duodenum and jejunum resulting in accelerated gastric emptying and intestinal transit. It increases the resting tone of the lower esophageal sphincter. It has little, if any, effect on the motility of the colon or gallbladder.

In patients with gastroesophageal reflux and low LESP (lower esophageal sphincter pressure), single oral doses of metoclopramide produce dose-related increases in LESP. Effects begin at about 5 mg and increase through 20 mg (the largest dose tested). The increase in LESP from a 5 mg dose lasts about 45 minutes and that of 20 mg lasts between 2 and 3 hours. Increased rate of stomach emptying has been observed with single oral doses of 10 mg.

The antiemetic properties of metoclopramide appear to be a result of its antagonism of central and peripheral dopamine receptors. Dopamine produces nausea and vomiting by stimulation of the medullary chemoreceptor trigger zone (CTZ), and metoclopramide blocks stimulation of the CTZ by agents like l-dopa or apomorphine which are known to increase dopamine levels or to possess dopamine-like effects. Metoclopramide also abolishes the slowing of gastric emptying caused by apomorphine.

Like the phenothiazines and related drugs, which are also dopamine antagonists, metoclopramide produces sedation and may produce extrapyramidal reactions, although these are comparatively rare (see **WARNINGS**).

Metoclopramide inhibits the central and peripheral effects of apomorphine, induces release of prolactin and causes a transient increase in circulating aldosterone levels, which may be associated with transient fluid retention.

The onset of pharmacological action of metoclopramide is 1 to 3 minutes following an intravenous dose, 10 to 15 minutes following intramuscular administration, and 30 to 60 minutes following an oral dose; pharmacological effects persist for 1 to 2 hours.

Pharmacokinetics

Metoclopramide is rapidly and well absorbed. Relative to an intravenous dose of 20 mg, the absolute oral bioavailability of metoclopramide is 80% ± 15.5% as demonstrated in a crossover study of 18 subjects. Peak plasma concentrations occur at about 1–2 hr after a single oral dose. Similar time to peak is observed after individual doses at steady state.

In a single dose study of 12 subjects, the area under the drug concentration-time curve increases linearly with doses from 20 to 100 mg. Peak concentrations increase linearly with dose; time to peak concentrations remains the same; whole body clearance is unchanged; and the elimination rate remains the same. The average elimination half-life in individuals with normal renal function is 5–6 hr. Linear kinetic processes adequately describe the absorption and elimination of metoclopramide.

Approximately 85% of the radioactivity of an orally administered dose appears in the urine within 72 hr. Of the 85% eliminated in the urine, about half is present as free or conjugated metoclopramide.

The drug is not extensively bound to plasma proteins (about 30%). The whole body volume of distribution is high (about 3.5 L/kg) which suggests extensive distribution of drug to the tissues.

Renal impairment affects the clearance of metoclopramide. In a study with patients with varying degrees of renal impairment, a reduction in creatinine clearance was correlated with a reduction in plasma clearance, renal clearance, non-renal clearance, and increase in elimination half-life. The kinetics of metoclopramide in the presence of renal impairment remained linear however. The reduction in clearance as a result of renal impairment suggests that adjustment downward of maintenance dosage should be done to avoid drug cumulation.

Adult Pharmacokinetic Data

Parameter	Value
Vd (L/kg)	~ 3.5
Plasma Protein Binding	~ 30%
$t_{1/2}$ (hr)	5—6
Oral Bioavailability	80%±15.5%

Continued on next page

Reglan—Cont.

In pediatric patients, the pharmacodynamics of metoclopramide following oral and intravenous administration are highly variable and a concentration-effect relationship has not been established.
There are insufficient reliable data to conclude whether the pharmacokinetics of metoclopramide in adults and the pediatric population are similar.
Although there are insufficient data to support the efficacy of metoclopramide in pediatric patients with symptomatic gastroesophageal reflux (GER) or cancer chemotherapy-related nausea and vomiting, its pharmacokinetics have been studied in these patient populations.
In an open-label study, six pediatric patients (age range, 3.5 weeks to 5.4 months) with GER received metoclopramide 0.15 mg/kg oral solution every 6 hours for 10 doses. The mean peak plasma concentration of metoclopramide after the tenth dose was 2-fold (56.8 μg/L) higher compared to that observed after the first dose (29 μg/L) indicating drug accumulation with repeated dosing. After the tenth dose, the mean time to reach peak concentrations (2.2 hr), half-life (4.1 hr), clearance (0.67 L/h/kg), and volume of distribution (4.4 L/kg) of metoclopramide were similar to those observed after the first dose. In the youngest patient (age, 3.5 weeks), metoclopramide half-life after the first and the tenth dose (23.1 and 10.3 hr, respectively) was significantly longer compared to other infants due to reduced clearance. This may be attributed to immature hepatic and renal systems at birth.
Single intravenous doses of metoclopramide 0.22 to 0.46 mg/kg (mean, 0.35 mg/kg) were administered over 5 minutes to 9 pediatric cancer patients receiving chemotherapy (mean age, 11.7 years; range, 7 to 14 yr) for prophylaxis of cytotoxic-induced vomiting. The metoclopramide plasma concentrations extrapolated to time zero ranged from 65 to 395 μg/L (mean, 152 μg/L). The mean elimination half-life, clearance, and volume of distribution of metoclopramide were 4.4 hr (range, 1.7 to 8.3 hr), 0.56 L/h/kg (range, 0.12 to 1.20 L/h/kg), and 3.0 L/kg (range, 1.0 to 4.8 L/kg), respectively.
In another study, nine pediatric cancer patients (age range, 1 to 9 yr) received 4 to 5 intravenous infusions (over 30 minutes) of metoclopramide at a dose of 2 mg/kg to control emesis. After the last dose, the peak serum concentrations of metoclopramide ranged from 1060 to 5680 μg/L. The mean elimination half-life, clearance, and volume of distribution of metoclopramide were 4.5 hr (range, 2.0 to 12.5 hr), 0.37 L/h/kg (range, 0.10 to 1.24 L/h/kg), and 1.93 L/kg (range, 0.95 to 5.50 L/kg), respectively.
[See table above]

Pediatric Pharmacokinetic Studies

Reference	Dose, Route	$t_{1/2}$ (hr)	Cl (L/hr/kg)	Vd (L/kg)	Cmax (μg/L)
1.	0.15 mg/kg oral soln, multiple dose	4.1[a,b]	0.67±0.14	4.4±0.65 (Vd_{area})	1st dose = 29±2.3 10th dose = 56.8±10.5
2.	0.35 mg/kg, IV over 5 min	4.4±0.56	0.56±0.10	3.0±0.38 (Dose/Cp^0)	152±31
3.	2 mg/kg 30 min IV infusion 4–5 times within 9.5 hours	4.5[b]	0.37[b]	1.93[b]	1060 to 5680[b]

a. Data presented as means ± SEM.
b. SEM not available.
1. Kearns, GL, et al. *J Pediatric Gastroenterol Nutr* 7(6):823–829, 1988.
2. Bateman, DN, et al. *Br J Clin Pharmac* 15:557–559, 1983.
3. Ford, C. *Clin Pharmac Ther* 43:196, 1988.

INDICATIONS AND USAGE

Symptomatic Gastroesophageal Reflux

Reglan Tablets and Syrup are indicated as short-term (4 to 12 weeks) therapy for adults with symptomatic, documented gastroesophageal reflux who fail to respond to conventional therapy.
The principal effect of metoclopramide is on symptoms of postprandial and daytime heartburn with less observed effect on nocturnal symptoms. If symptoms are confined to particular situations, such as following the evening meal, use of metoclopramide as single doses prior to the provocative situation should be considered, rather than using the drug throughout the day. Healing of esophageal ulcers and erosions has been endoscopically demonstrated at the end of a 12-week trial using doses of 15 mg q.i.d. As there is no documented correlation between symptoms and healing of esophageal lesions, patients with documented lesions should be monitored endoscopically.

Diabetic Gastroparesis (Diabetic Gastric Stasis)

Reglan (Metoclopramide Hydrochloride, USP) is indicated for the relief of symptoms associated with acute and recurrent diabetic gastric stasis. The usual manifestations of delayed gastric emptying (e.g., nausea, vomiting, heartburn, persistent fullness after meals, and anorexia) appear to respond to Reglan within different time intervals. Significant relief of nausea occurs early and continues to improve over a three-week period. Relief of vomiting and anorexia may precede the relief of abdominal fullness by one week or more.

The Prevention of Nausea and Vomiting Associated with Emetogenic Cancer Chemotherapy

Reglan Injectable is indicated for the prophylaxis of vomiting associated with emetogenic cancer chemotherapy.

The Prevention of Postoperative Nausea and Vomiting

Reglan Injectable is indicated for the prophylaxis of postoperative nausea and vomiting in those circumstances where nasogastric suction is undesirable.

Small Bowel Intubation

Reglan Injectable may be used to facilitate small bowel intubation in adults and pediatric patients in whom the tube does not pass the pylorus with conventional maneuvers.

Radiological Examination

Reglan Injectable may be used to stimulate gastric emptying and intestinal transit of barium in cases where delayed emptying interferes with radiological examination of the stomach and/or small intestine.

CONTRAINDICATIONS

Metoclopramide should not be used whenever stimulation of gastrointestinal motility might be dangerous, e.g., in the presence of gastrointestinal hemorrhage, mechanical obstruction, or perforation.
Metoclopramide is contraindicated in patients with pheochromocytoma because the drug may cause a hypertensive crisis, probably due to release of catecholamines from the tumor. Such hypertensive crises may be controlled by phentolamine.
Metoclopramide is contraindicated in patients with known sensitivity or intolerance to the drug.
Metoclopramide should not be used in epileptics or patients receiving other drugs which are likely to cause extrapyramidal reactions, since the frequency and severity of seizures or extrapyramidal reactions may be increased.

WARNINGS

Mental depression has occurred in patients with and without prior history of depression. Symptoms have ranged from mild to severe and have included suicidal ideation and suicide. Metoclopramide should be given to patients with a prior history of depression only if the expected benefits outweigh the potential risks.
Extrapyramidal symptoms, manifested primarily as acute dystonic reactions, occur in approximately 1 in 500 patients treated with the usual adult dosages of 30–40 mg/day of metoclopramide. These usually are seen during the first 24–48 hours of treatment with metoclopramide, occur more frequently in pediatric patients and young patients less than 30 years of age and are even more frequent at the higher doses used in prophylaxis of vomiting due to cancer chemotherapy. These symptoms may include involuntary movements of limbs and facial grimacing, torticollis, oculogyric crisis, rhythmic protrusion of tongue, bulbar type of speech, trismus, or dystonic reactions resembling tetanus. Rarely, dystonic reactions may present as stridor and dyspnea, possibly due to laryngospasm. If these symptoms should occur, inject 50 mg Benadryl® (diphenhydramine hydrochloride) intramuscularly, and they usually will subside. Cogentin® (benztropine mesylate), 1 to 2 mg intramuscularly, may also be used to reverse these reactions.
Parkinsonian-like symptoms have occurred, more commonly within the first 6 months after beginning treatment with metoclopramide, but occasionally after longer periods. These symptoms generally subside within 2–3 months following discontinuance of metoclopramide. Patients with preexisting Parkinson's disease should be given metoclopramide cautiously, if at all, since such patients may experience exacerbation of parkinsonian symptoms when taking metoclopramide.

Tardive Dyskinesia

Tardive dyskinesia, a syndrome consisting of potentially irreversible, involuntary, dyskinetic movements may develop in patients treated with metoclopramide. Although the prevalence of the syndrome appears to be highest among the elderly, especially elderly women, it is impossible to predict which patients are likely to develop the syndrome. Both the risk of developing the syndrome and the likelihood that it will become irreversible are believed to increase with the duration of treatment and the total cumulative dose.
Less commonly, the syndrome can develop after relatively brief treatment periods at low doses; in these cases, symptoms appear more likely to be reversible.
There is no known treatment for established cases of tardive dyskinesia although the syndrome may remit, partially or completely, within several weeks-to-months after metoclopramide is withdrawn. Metoclopramide itself, however, may suppress (or partially suppress) the signs of tardive dyskinesia, thereby masking the underlying disease process. The effect of this symptomatic suppression upon the long-term course of the syndrome is unknown. Therefore, the use of metoclopramide for the symptomatic control of tardive dyskenesia is not recommended.

PRECAUTIONS

General

In one study in hypertensive patients, intravenously administered metoclopramide was shown to release catecholamines; hence, caution should be exercised when metoclopramide is used in patients with hypertension.
Intravenous injections of undiluted metoclopramide should be made slowly allowing 1 to 2 minutes for 10 mg since a transient but intense feeling of anxiety and restlessness, followed by drowsiness, may occur with rapid administration.
Intravenous administration of Reglan Injectable diluted in a parenteral solution should be made slowly over a period of not less than 15 minutes.
Giving a promotility drug such as metoclopramide theoretically could put increased pressure on suture lines following a gut anastomosis or closure. Although adverse events related to this possibility have not been reported to date, the possibility should be considered and weighed when deciding whether to use metoclopramide or nasogastric suction in the prevention of postoperative nausea and vomiting.

Information for Patients

Metoclopramide may impair the mental and/or physical abilities required for the performance of hazardous tasks such as operating machinery or driving a motor vehicle. The ambulatory patient should be cautioned accordingly.

Drug Interactions

The effects of metoclopramide on gastrointestinal motility are antagonized by anticholinergic drugs and narcotic analgesics. Additive sedative effects can occur when metoclopramide is given with alcohol, sedatives, hypnotics, narcotics or tranquilizers.
The finding that metoclopramide releases catecholamines in patients with essential hypertension suggests that it should be used cautiously, if at all, in patients receiving monoamine oxidase inhibitors.
Absorption of drugs from the stomach may be diminished (e.g., digoxin) by metoclopramide, whereas the rate and/or extent of absorption of drugs from the small bowel may be increased (e.g., acetaminophen, tetracycline, levodopa, ethanol, cyclosporine).
Gastroparesis (gastric stasis) may be responsible for poor diabetic control in some patients. Exogenously administered insulin may begin to act before food has left the stomach and lead to hypoglycemia. Because the action of metoclopramide will influence the delivery of food to the intestines and thus the rate of absorption, insulin dosage or timing of dosage may require adjustment.

Carcinogenesis, Mutagenesis, Impairment of Fertility

A 77-week study was conducted in rats with oral doses up to about 40 times the maximum recommended human daily dose. Metoclopramide elevates prolactin levels and the elevation persists during chronic administration. Tissue culture experiments indicate that approximately one-third of human breast cancers are prolactin-dependent *in vitro*, a factor of potential importance if the prescription of metoclopramide is contemplated in a patient with previously detected breast cancer. Although disturbances such as galactorrhea, amenorrhea, gynecomastia, and impotence have been reported with prolactin-elevating drugs, the clinical significance of elevated serum prolactin levels is unknown for most patients. An increase in mammary neoplasms has been found in rodents after chronic administration of prolactin-stimulating neuroleptic drugs and metoclopramide. Neither clinical studies nor epidemiologic studies conducted to date, however, have shown an association between chronic administration of these drugs and mammary tumorigenesis; the available evidence is too limited to be conclusive at this time.
An Ames mutagenicity test performed on metoclopramide was negative.

Pregnancy Category B

Reproduction studies performed in rats, mice, and rabbits by the I.V., I.M., S.C., and oral routes at maximum levels ranging from 12 to 250 times the human dose have demonstrated no impairment of fertility or significant harm to the fetus due to metoclopramide. There are, however, no adequate and well-controlled studies in pregnant women. Because animal reproduction studies are not always predictive of human response, this drug should be used during pregnancy only if clearly needed.

Nursing Mothers

Metoclopramide is excreted in human milk. Caution should be exercised when metoclopramide is administered to a nursing mother.

Pediatric Use

Safety and effectiveness in pediatric patients have not been established except as stated to facilitate small bowel intubation (see **OVERDOSAGE** and **DOSAGE AND ADMINISTRATION**).
Care should be exercised in administering metoclopramide to neonates since prolonged clearance may produce exces-

sive serum concentrations (see **CLINICAL PHARMACOLOGY—Pharmacokinetics**). In addition, neonates have reduced levels of nicotinamide adenine dinucleotide-methemoglobin reductase which, in combination with the aforementioned pharmacokinetic factors, make neonates more susceptible to methemoglobinemia (see **OVERDOSAGE**).

The safety profile of metoclopramide in adults cannot be extrapolated to pediatric patients. Dystonias and other extrapyramidal reactions associated with metoclopramide are more common in the pediatric population than in adults. (See **WARNINGS** and **ADVERSE REACTIONS—Extrapyramidal Reactions.**)

ADVERSE REACTIONS

In general, the incidence of adverse reactions correlates with the dose and duration of metoclopramide administration. The following reactions have been reported, although in most instances, data do not permit an estimate of frequency:

CNS Effects

Restlessness, drowsiness, fatigue and lassitude occur in approximately 10% of patients receiving the most commonly prescribed dosage of 10 mg q.i.d. (see **PRECAUTIONS**). Insomnia, headache, confusion, dizziness, or mental depression with suicidal ideation (see **WARNINGS**) occur less frequently. In cancer chemotherapy patients being treated with 1–2 mg/kg per dose, incidence of drowsiness is about 70%. There are isolated reports of convulsive seizures without clearcut relationship to metoclopramide. Rarely, hallucinations have been reported.

Extrapyramidal Reactions (EPS)

Acute dystonic reactions, the most common type of EPS associated with metoclopramide, occur in approximately 0.2% of patients (1 in 500) treated with 30 to 40 mg of metoclopramide per day. In cancer chemotherapy patients receiving 1–2 mg/kg per dose, the incidence is 2% in patients over the ages of 30–35, and 25% or higher in pediatric patients and adult patients less than 30 years of age who have not had prophylactic administration of diphenhydramine. Symptoms include involuntary movements of limbs, facial grimacing, torticollis, oculogyric crisis, rhythmic protrusion of tongue, bulbar type of speech, trismus, opisthotonus (tetanus-like reactions) and, rarely, stridor and dyspnea possibly due to laryngospasm; ordinarily these symptoms are readily reversed by diphenhydramine (see **WARNINGS**).

Parkinsonian-like symptoms may include bradykinesia, tremor, cogwheel rigidity, mask-like facies (see **WARNINGS**).

Tardive dyskinesia most frequently is characterized by involuntary movements of the tongue, face, mouth, or jaw, and sometimes by involuntary movements of the trunk and/or extremities; movements may be choreoathetotic in appearance (see **WARNINGS**).

Motor restlessness (akathisia) may consist of feelings of anxiety, agitation, jitteriness, and insomnia, as well as inability to sit still, pacing, foot tapping. These symptoms may disappear spontaneously or respond to a reduction in dosage.

Endocrine Disturbances

Galactorrhea, amenorrhea, gynecomastia, impotence secondary to hyperprolactinemia (see **PRECAUTIONS**). Fluid retention secondary to transient elevation of aldosterone (see **CLINICAL PHARMACOLOGY**).

Cardiovascular

Hypotension, hypertension, supraventricular tachycardia, bradycardia and possible AV block (see **CONTRAINDICATIONS** and **PRECAUTIONS**).

Gastrointestinal

Nausea and bowel disturbances, primarily diarrhea.

Hepatic

Rarely, cases of hepatotoxicity, characterized by such findings as jaundice and altered liver function tests, when metoclopramide was administered with other drugs with known hepatotoxic potential.

Renal

Urinary frequency and incontinence.

Hematologic

A few cases of neutropenia, leukopenia, or agranulocytosis, generally without clearcut relationship to metoclopramide. Methemoglobinemia, especially with overdosage in neonates (see **OVERDOSAGE**). Sulfhemoglobinemia in adults.

Allergic Reactions

A few cases of rash, urticaria, or bronchospasm, especially in patients with a history of asthma. Rarely, angioneurotic edema, including glossal or laryngeal edema.

Miscellaneous

Visual disturbances. Porphyria. Rare occurrences of neuroleptic malignant syndrome (NMS) have been reported. This potentially fatal syndrome is comprised of the symptom complex of hyperthermia, altered consciousness, muscular rigidity, and autonomic dysfunction.

Transient flushing of the face and upper body, without alterations in vital signs, following high doses intravenously.

OVERDOSAGE

Symptoms of overdosage may include drowsiness, disorientation and extrapyramidal reactions. Anticholinergic or antiparkinson drugs or antihistamines with anticholinergic properties may be helpful in controlling the extrapyramidal reactions. Symptoms are self-limiting and usually disappear within 24 hours.

Hemodialysis removes relatively little metoclopramide, probably because of the small amount of the drug in blood relative to tissues. Similarly, continuous ambulatory peritoneal dialysis does not remove significant amounts of drug. It is unlikely that dosage would need to be adjusted to compensate for losses through dialysis. Dialysis is not likely to be an effective method of drug removal in overdose situations.

Unintentional overdose due to misadministration has been reported in infants and children with the use of Reglan syrup. While there was no consistent pattern to the reports associated with these overdoses, events included seizures, extrapyramidal reactions, and lethargy.

Methemoglobinemia has occurred in premature and full-term neonates who were given overdoses of metoclopramide (1–4 mg/kg/day orally, intramuscularly or intravenously for 1–3 or more days). Methemoglobinemia has not been reported in neonates treated with 0.5 mg/kg/day in divided doses. Methemoglobinemia can be reversed by the intravenous administration of methylene blue.

DOSAGE AND ADMINISTRATION

For the Relief of Symptomatic Gastroesophageal Reflux

Administer from 10 mg to 15 mg Reglan (Metoclopramide Hydrochloride, USP) orally up to q.i.d. 30 minutes before each meal and at bedtime, depending upon symptoms being treated and clinical response (see **CLINICAL PHARMACOLOGY** and **INDICATIONS AND USAGE**). If symptoms occur only intermittently or at specific times of the day, use of metoclopramide in single doses up to 20 mg prior to the provoking situation may be preferred rather than continuous treatment. Occasionally, patients (such as elderly patients) who are more sensitive to the therapeutic or adverse effects of metoclopramide will require only 5 mg per dose.

Experience with esophageal erosions and ulcerations is limited, but healing has thus far been documented in one controlled trial using q.i.d. therapy at 15 mg/dose, and this regimen should be used when lesions are present, so long as it is tolerated (see **ADVERSE REACTIONS**). Because of the poor correlation between symptoms and endoscopic appearance of the esophagus, therapy directed at esophageal lesions is best guided by endoscopic evaluation.

Therapy longer than 12 weeks has not been evaluated and cannot be recommended.

For the Relief of Symptoms Associated with Diabetic Gastroparesis (Diabetic Gastric Stasis)

Administer 10 mg of metoclopramide 30 minutes before each meal and at bedtime for two to eight weeks, depending upon response and the likelihood of continued well-being upon drug discontinuation.

The initial route of administration should be determined by the severity of the presenting symptoms. If only the earliest manifestations of diabetic gastric stasis are present, oral administration of Reglan may be initiated. However, if severe symptoms are present, therapy should begin with Reglan Injectable (I.M. or I.V.). Doses of 10 mg may be administered slowly by the intravenous route over a 1- to 2-minute period.

Administration of Reglan Injectable (Metoclopramide Injection, USP) up to 10 days may be required before symptoms subside, at which time oral administration may be instituted. Since diabetic gastric stasis is frequently recurrent, Reglan therapy should be reinstituted at the earliest manifestation.

For the Prevention of Nausea and Vomiting Associated with Emetogenic Cancer Chemotherapy

For doses in excess of 10 mg, Reglan Injectable should be diluted in 50 mL of a parenteral solution.

The preferred parenteral solution is Sodium Chloride Injection (normal saline), which when combined with Reglan Injectable, can be stored frozen for up to 4 weeks. Reglan Injectable is degraded when admixed and frozen with Dextrose-5% in Water. Reglan Injectable diluted in Sodium Chloride Injection, Dextrose-5% in Water, Dextrose-5% in 0.45% Sodium Chloride, Ringer's Injection or Lactated Ringer's Injection may be stored up to 48 hours (without freezing) after preparation if protected from light. All dilutions may be stored unprotected from light under normal light conditions up to 24 hours after preparation.

Intravenous infusions should be made slowly over a period of not less than 15 minutes, 30 minutes before beginning cancer chemotherapy and repeated every 2 hours for two doses, then every 3 hours for three doses.

The initial two doses should be 2 mg/kg if highly emetogenic drugs such as cisplatin or dacarbazine are used alone or in combination. For less emetogenic regimens, 1 mg/kg per dose may be adequate.

If extrapyramidal symptoms should occur, inject 50 mg Benadryl® (diphenhydramine hydrochloride) intramuscularly, and EPS usually will subside.

For the Prevention of Postoperative Nausea and Vomiting

Reglan Injectable should be given intramuscularly near the end of surgery. The usual adult dose is 10 mg; however, doses of 20 mg may be used.

To Facilitate Small Bowel Intubation

If the tube has not passed the pylorus with conventional maneuvers in 10 minutes, a single dose (undiluted) may be administered slowly by the intravenous route over a 1- to 2-minute period.

The recommended single dose is: Pediatric patients above 14 years of age and adults—10 mg metoclopramide base. Pediatric patients (6–14 years of age)—2.5 to 5 mg metoclopramide base; (under 6 years of age)—0.1 mg/kg metoclopramide base.

To Aid in Radiological Examinations

In patients where delayed gastric emptying interferes with radiological examination of the stomach and/or small intestine, a single dose may be administered slowly by the intravenous route over a 1- to 2-minute period.

For dosage, see intubation above.

USE IN PATIENTS WITH RENAL OR HEPATIC IMPAIRMENT

Since metoclopramide is excreted principally through the kidneys, in those patients whose creatinine clearance is below 40 mL/min, therapy should be initiated at approximately one-half the recommended dosage. Depending upon clinical efficacy and safety considerations, the dosage may be increased or decreased as appropriate.

See **OVERDOSAGE** section for information regarding dialysis.

Metoclopramide undergoes minimal hepatic metabolism, except for simple conjugation. Its safe use has been described in patients with advanced liver disease whose renal function was normal.

NOTE: Parenteral drug products should be inspected visually for particulate matter and discoloration prior to administration, whenever solution and container permit.

ADMIXTURE COMPATIBILITIES

Reglan Injectable (Metoclopramide Injection, USP) is compatible for mixing and injection with the following dosage forms to the extent indicated below:

Physically and Chemically Compatible Up to 48 Hours

Cimetidine Hydrochloride (SK&F), Mannitol, USP (Abbott), Potassium Acetate, USP (Invenex), Potassium Chloride, USP (ESI), Potassium Phosphate, USP (Invenex).

Physically Compatible up to 48 Hours

Ascorbic Acid, USP (Abbott), Benztropine Mesylate, USP (MS&D), Cytarabine, USP (Upjohn), Dexamethasone Sodium Phosphate, USP (ESI, MS&D), Diphenhydramine Hydrochloride, USP (Parke-Davis), Doxorubicin Hydrochloride, USP (Adria), Heparin Sodium, USP (ESI), Hydrocortisone Sodium Phosphate (MS&D), Lidocaine Hydrochloride, USP (ESI), Magnesium Sulfate, USP (ESI), Multi-Vitamin Infusion (must be refrigerated-USV), Vitamin B Complex with Ascorbic Acid (Roche).

Physically Compatible Up to 24 Hours (*Do not use if precipitation occurs*)

Aminophylline, USP (ESI), Clindamycin Phosphate, USP (Upjohn), Cyclophosphamide, USP (Mead-Johnson), Insulin, USP (Lilly), Methylprednisolone Sodium Succinate, USP (ESI).

Conditionally Compatible (*Use within one hour after mixing or may be infused directly into the same running IV line*)

Ampicillin Sodium, USP (Bristol), Calcium Gluconate, USP (ESI), Cisplatin (Bristol), Erythromycin Lactobionate, USP (Abbott), Methotrexate Sodium, USP (Lederle), Penicillin G Potassium, USP (Squibb), Tetracycline Hydrochloride, USP (Lederle).

Incompatible (*Do Not Mix*)

Cephalothin Sodium, USP (Lilly), Chloramphenicol Sodium, USP (Parke-Davis), Sodium Bicarbonate, USP (Abbott).

HOW SUPPLIED

Each white, capsule-shaped, scored Reglan® Tablet contains 10 mg metoclopramide base (as the monohydrochloride monohydrate). Available in bottles of 100 (NDC 0031-6701-63), and 500 tablets (NDC 0031-6701-70) and Dis-Co® Unit Dose Packs of 100 tablets (NDC 0031-6701-64).

Each green, elliptical-shaped Reglan® Tablet contains 5 mg metoclopramide base (as the monohydrochloride monohydrate). Available in bottles of 100 (NDC 0031-6705-63) and Dis-Co® Unit Dose Packs of 100 tablets (NDC 0031-6705-64). **Dispense tablets in tight, light-resistant container.**

Reglan® Syrup, 5 mg metoclopramide base (as the monohydrochloride monohydrate) per 5 mL, available in pints (NDC 0031-6706-25). **Dispense syrup in tight, light-resistant container.**

PRESERVATIVE-FREE

Reglan® Injectable 5 mg metoclopramide base (as the monohydrochloride monohydrate) per mL; available in 2 mL single dose vials in cartons of 25 (NDC 0031-6709-72), 10 mL single dose vials in cartons of 25 (NDC 0031-6709-78), 30 mL single dose vials in cartons of 25 (NDC 0031-6709-24), 2 mL ampuls in cartons of 25 (NDC 0031-6709-95). [See table above]

Container	Contents #	Total Concentration #	Administration
2 mL single dose vial/ampul	10 mg	5 mg/mL	FOR IV or IM ADMINISTRATION
10 mL single dose vial	50 mg	5 mg/mL	FOR IV INFUSION ONLY; DILUTE BEFORE USING
30 mL single dose vial	150 mg	5 mg/mL	FOR IV INFUSION ONLY; DILUTE BEFORE USING

Metoclopramide base (as the monohydrochloride monohydrate)

Continued on next page

Reglan—Cont.

Store vials and ampuls in carton until used. Do not store open single dose vials or ampuls for later use, as they contain no preservative.

Dilutions may be stored unprotected from light under normal light conditions up to 24 hours after preparation.

Tablets, Syrup and Injectable should be stored at controlled room temperature, between 20°C and 25°C (68°F and 77°F).

Reglan Injectable is manufactured for Pharmaceutical Division, A. H. Robins Company, Richmond, Virginia 23220 by Elkins-Sinn, Cherry Hill, NJ 08003, a subsidiary of A.H. Robins

CI 6015-1 Issued December 15, 1999

Shown in Product Identification Guide, page 332

ROBAXIN® INJECTABLE ℞

[ro "baks 'in]

brand of Methocarbamol Injection, USP

DESCRIPTION

Methocarbamol has the following structural formula:

$O{-}CH_2{-}CH(OH){-}CH_2O{-}C(=O){-}NH_2$ (on a benzene ring with OCH_3)

3-(2-methoxyphenoxy)-1,2-propanediol
1-carbamate, or methocarbamol

Robaxin Injectable is a parenteral dosage form.

Each mL contains:

Methocarbamol, USP **100 mg**; Polyethylene Glycol 300, NF 0.5 mL; Water for Injection, USP q.s. pH adjusted, when necessary, with hydrochloric acid and/or sodium hydroxide. AFTER MIXING WITH I.V. INFUSION FLUIDS, **DO NOT REFRIGERATE.**

ACTIONS

The mechanism of action of methocarbamol in humans has not been established, but may be due to general central nervous system depression. It has no direct action on the contractile mechanism of striated muscle, the motor end plate or the nerve fiber.

INDICATIONS

The injectable form of methocarbamol is indicated as an adjunct to rest, physical therapy, and other measures for the relief of discomfort associated with acute, painful musculoskeletal conditions. The mode of action of this drug has not been clearly identified, but may be related to its sedative properties. Methocarbamol does not directly relax tense skeletal muscles in man.

CONTRAINDICATIONS

Robaxin Injectable should not be administered to patients with known or suspected renal pathology. This caution is necessary because of the presence of polyethylene glycol 300 in the vehicle.

A much larger amount of polyethylene glycol 300 than is present in recommended doses of Robaxin Injectable is known to have increased pre-existing acidosis and urea retention in patients with renal impairment. Although the amount present in this preparation is well within the limits of safety, caution dictates this contraindication.

Robaxin Injectable is contraindicated in patients hypersensitive to any of the ingredients.

WARNINGS

Since methocarbamol may possess a general central nervous system depressant effect, patients receiving Robaxin Injectable (methocarbamol injection) should be cautioned about combined effects with alcohol and other CNS depressants.

Safe use of Robaxin Injectable has not been established with regard to possible adverse effects upon fetal development. Therefore, Robaxin Injectable should not be used in women who are or may become pregnant and particularly during early pregnancy unless in the judgment of the physician the potential benefits outweigh the possible hazards.

PRECAUTIONS

As with other agents administered either intravenously or intramuscularly, careful supervision of dose and rate of injection should be observed. Rate of injection should not exceed 3 mL per minute—i.e., one 10 mL vial in approximately three minutes. Since Robaxin Injectable is hypertonic, vascular extravasation must be avoided. A recumbent position will reduce the likelihood of side reactions.

Blood aspirated into the syringe does not mix with the hypertonic solution. This phenomenon occurs with many other intravenous preparations. The blood may be safely injected with the methocarbamol, or the injection may be stopped when the plunger reaches the blood, whichever the physician prefers.

The total dosage should not exceed 30 mL (three vials) a day for more than three consecutive days except in the treatment of tetanus.

Caution should be observed in using the injectable form in suspected or known epileptic patients.

Safety and effectiveness in children below the age of 12 years have not been established except in tetanus. See special directions for use in tetanus.

It is not known whether this drug is secreted in human milk. As a general rule, nursing should not be undertaken while a patient is on a drug since many drugs are excreted in human milk.

Methocarbamol may cause a color interference in certain screening tests for 5-hydroxyindoleacetic acid (5-HIAA) and vanillylmandelic acid (VMA).

ADVERSE REACTIONS

Dizziness, lightheadedness, drowsiness, vertigo, fainting, syncope, hypotension, gastrointestinal upset, metallic taste, thrombophlebitis, sloughing at the site of injection, pain at the site of injection, anaphylactic reaction, urticaria, pruritus, rash, conjunctivitis with nasal congestion, flushing, nystagmus, diplopia, mild muscular incoordination, bradycardia, blurred vision, headache, fever. In most cases of syncope there was spontaneous recovery. In others, epinephrine, injectable steroids and/or injectable antihistamines were employed to hasten recovery. Certain of these complaints may have been due to any overly rapid rate of intravenous injection.

The onset of convulsive seizures during intravenous administration has been reported, including instances in known epileptics. The psychic trauma of the procedure may have been a contributing factor. Although several observers have reported success in terminating epileptiform seizures with Robaxin Injectable, its administration to patients with epilepsy is not recommended.

DOSAGE AND ADMINISTRATION

For Intravenous and Intramuscular Use Only. Total adult dosage should not exceed 30 mL (3 vials) a day for more than 3 consecutive days except in the treatment of tetanus. A like course may be repeated after a lapse of 48 hours if the condition persists. Dosage and frequency of injection should be based on the severity of the condition being treated and therapeutic response noted.

For the relief of symptoms of moderate degree, 10 mL (one vial) may be adequate. Ordinarily this injection need not be repeated, as the administration of the oral form will usually sustain the relief initiated by the injection. For the severest cases or in postoperative conditions in which oral administration is not feasible, 20 to 30 mL (two to three vials) may be required.

Directions for Intravenous Use. Robaxin Injectable may be administered undiluted directly into the vein at a ***maximum rate of three mL per minute.*** It may also be added to an intravenous drip of Sodium Chloride Injection (Sterile Isotonic Sodium Chloride Solution for Parenteral Use) or five per cent Dextrose Injection (Sterile 5 percent Dextrose Solution); one vial given as a single dose should not be diluted to more than 250 mL for I. V. infusion. Care should be exercised to avoid vascular extravasation of this hypertonic solution which may result in thrombophlebitis. It is preferable that the patient be in a recumbent position during and for at least 10 to 15 minutes following the injection.

Directions for Intramuscular Use. When the intramuscular route is indicated, not more than five mL (one-half vial) should be injected into each gluteal region. The injections may be repeated at eight hour intervals, if necessary. When satisfactory relief of symptoms is achieved, it can usually be maintained with tablets.

Not Recommended for Subcutaneous Administration.

Special Directions for Use in Tetanus: There is clinical evidence which suggests that methocarbamol may have a beneficial effect in the control of the neuromuscular manifestations of tetanus. It does not, however, replace the usual procedure of debridement, tetanus antitoxin, penicillin, tracheotomy, attention to fluid balance, and supportive care. Robaxin Injectable should be added to the regimen as soon as possible.

For adults: Inject one or two vials directly into the tubing of a previously inserted indwelling needle. An additional 10 mL or 20 mL may be added to the infusion bottle so that a total of up to 30 mL (three vials) is given as the initial dose (note Precautions). This procedure should be repeated every six hours until conditions allow for the insertion of a nasogastric tube. Crushed Robaxin (methocarbamol) tablets suspended in water or saline may then be given through this tube. Total daily oral doses up to 24 grams may be required as judged by patient response.

For children: A minimum initial dose of 15 mg/kg is recommended. This dosage may be repeated every six hours as indicated. The maintenance dosage may be given by injection into the tubing or by I.V. infusion with an appropriate quantity of fluid. See directions for I.V. use.

HOW SUPPLIED

Robaxin Injectable—10 mL single dose vials in packages of 5 (NDC 0031-7409-87) and 25 (NDC 0031-7409-94).

Manufactured for Pharmaceutical Division, A. H. ROBINS CO., Richmond, VA 23220, by ELKINS-SINN, INC., Cherry Hill, NJ 08034, a subsidiary of A.H. Robins.

J-9667 rev. 12/81

Shown in Product Identification Guide, page 332

ROBAXIN® ℞

[ro "baks 'in]

brand of Methocarbamol Tablets, USP
500 mg per tablet

ROBAXIN®–750 ℞

brand of Methocarbamol Tablets, USP
750 mg per tablet

DESCRIPTION

Inactive Ingredients: ROBAXIN—Corn Starch, FD&C Yellow 6 Aluminum Lake, Hydroxypropyl Cellulose, Hydroxypropyl Methylcellulose, Magnesium Stearate, Polysorbate 20, Povidone, Propylene Glycol, Saccharin Sodium, Sodium Lauryl Sulfate, Sodium Starch Glycolate, Stearic Acid, Titanium Dioxide.

ROBAXIN-750—Corn Starch, D&C Yellow 10 Aluminum Lake, FD&C Yellow 6 Aluminum Lake, Hydroxypropyl Cellulose, Hydroxypropyl Methylcellulose, Magnesium Stearate, Polysorbate 20, Povidone, Propylene Glycol, Saccharin Sodium, Sodium Lauryl Sulfate, Sodium Starch Glycolate, Stearic Acid, Titanium Dioxide.

Methocarbamol has the following structural formula:

$O{-}CH_2{-}CH(OH){-}CH_2O{-}C(=O){-}NH_2$ (on a benzene ring with OCH_3)

1,2-Propanediol, 3-(2-methoxyphenoxy)-,
1-carbamate, (±)-.

ACTIONS

The mechanism of action of methocarbamol in humans has not been established, but may be due to general central nervous system depression. It has no direct action on the contractile mechanism of striated muscle, the motor end plate or the nerve fiber.

INDICATIONS

Robaxin (methocarbamol) is indicated as an adjunct to rest, physical therapy, and other measures for the relief of discomforts associated with acute, painful musculoskeletal conditions. The mode of action of this drug has not been clearly identified, but may be related to its sedative properties. Methocarbamol does not directly relax tense skeletal muscles in man.

CONTRAINDICATIONS

Robaxin is contraindicated in patients hypersensitive to any of the ingredients.

WARNINGS

Since methocarbamol may possess a general central nervous system depressant effect, patients receiving Robaxin/Robaxin-750 (methocarbamol tablets) should be cautioned about combined effects with alcohol and other CNS depressants.

Safe use of methocarbamol has not been established with regard to possible adverse effects upon fetal development. Therefore, methocarbamol tablets should not be used in women who are or may become pregnant and particularly during early pregnancy unless in the judgment of the physician the potential benefits outweigh the possible hazards.

PRECAUTIONS

Safety and effectiveness in children below the age of 12 years have not been established.

It is not known whether this drug is secreted in human milk. As a general rule, nursing should not be undertaken while a patient is on a drug since many drugs are excreted in human milk.

Methocarbamol may cause a color interference in certain screening tests for 5-hydroxyindoleacetic acid (5-HIAA) and vanillylmandelic acid (VMA).

ADVERSE REACTIONS

Lightheadedness, dizziness, drowsiness, nausea, allergic manifestations such as urticaria, pruritus, rash, conjunctivitis with nasal congestion, blurred vision, headache, fever.

DOSAGE AND ADMINISTRATION

Robaxin (methocarbamol), 500 mg—Adults: initial dosage, 3 tablets q.i.d.; maintenance dosage, 2 tablets q.i.d.

Robaxin-750 (methocarbamol), 750 mg — Adults: initial dosage, 2 tablets q.i.d.; maintenance dosage, 1 tablet q.4h. or 2 tablets t.i.d.

Six grams a day are recommended for the first 48 to 72 hours of treatment. (For severe conditions 8 grams a day may be administered.) Thereafter, the dosage can usually be reduced to approximately 4 grams a day.

HOW SUPPLIED

Robaxin—light orange, round, film-coated tablets monogrammed Robaxin and AHR in bottles of 100 (NDC 0031-7429-63), and 500 (NDC 0031-7429-70).

Robaxin-750—orange, capsule-shaped, film-coated tablets monogrammed Robaxin-750 and AHR in bottles of 100 (NDC 0031-7449-63), 500 (NDC 0031-7449-70), and Dis-Co® unit dose packs of 100 (NDC 0031-7449-64).

Store at Controlled Room Temperature, between 20°C and 25°C (68°F and 77°F).

Dispense in tight container.

Also available in the injectable form, 1 g methocarbamol in each 10 ml vial (NDC 0031-7409).

Manufactured by:
Pharmaceutical Division
A.H. Robins Company
Richmond, VA 23220
CI 4696-1 Issued December 17, 1996

Shown in Product Identification Guide, page 332

ROBAXISAL® TABLETS ℞

[*ro "baks 'ĭ-sal "*]

DESCRIPTION

For oral administration, Robaxisal is available as a pink and white laminated tablet containing:

Methocarbamol, USP .... 400 mg
Aspirin, USP .... 325 mg

Inactive Ingredients: Corn Starch, FD&C Red 3, Magnesium Stearate, Povidone, Sodium Lauryl Sulfate, Sodium Starch Glycolate, Stearic Acid.

Methocarbamol has the following structural formula and chemical name:

O–CH₂–CH(OH)–CH₂O–C(=O)–NH₂ (benzene ring with OCH₃)

3-(2-Methoxyphenoxy)-1,2-propanediol 1-Carbamate

ACTIONS

Robaxisal provides a double approach to the management of discomforts associated with musculoskeletal disorders.

METHOCARBAMOL

The mechanism of action of methocarbamol in humans has not been established, but may be due to general central nervous system depression. It has no direct action on the contractile mechanism of striated muscle, the motor end plate or the nerve fiber.

ASPIRIN

Aspirin is a mild analgesic with anti-inflammatory and antipyretic activity.

INDICATIONS

Robaxisal is indicated as an adjunct to rest, physical therapy, and other measures for the relief of discomfort associated with acute, painful musculoskeletal conditions. The mode of action of methocarbamol has not been clearly identified but may be related to its sedative properties. Methocarbamol does not directly relax tense skeletal muscles in man.

CONTRAINDICATIONS

Hypersensitivity to methocarbamol or aspirin.

WARNINGS

Since methocarbamol may possess a general central nervous system depressant effect, patients receiving Robaxisal should be cautioned about combined effects with alcohol and other CNS depressants.

PRECAUTIONS

Products containing aspirin should be administered with caution to patients with gastritis or peptic ulceration, or those receiving hypoprothrombinemic anticoagulants.

Methocarbamol may cause a color interference in certain screening tests for 5-hydroxyindoleacetic acid (5-HIAA) and vanillylmandelic acid (VMA).

PREGNANCY

Safe use of Robaxisal has not been established with regard to possible adverse effects upon fetal development. Therefore, Robaxisal should not be used in women who are or may become pregnant and particularly during early pregnancy unless in the judgment of the physician the potential benefits outweigh the possible hazards.

NURSING MOTHERS

It is not known whether methocarbamol is secreted in human milk; however, aspirin does appear in human milk in moderate amounts. It can produce a bleeding tendency either by interfering with the function of the infant's platelets or by decreasing the amount of prothrombin in the blood. The risk is minimal if the mother takes the aspirin just after nursing and if the infant has an adequate store of vitamin K. As a general rule, nursing should not be undertaken while a patient is on a drug.

PEDIATRIC USE

Safety and effectiveness in children 12 years of age and below have not been established.

USE IN ACTIVITIES REQUIRING MENTAL ALERTNESS

Robaxisal may rarely cause drowsiness. Until the patient's response has been determined, he should be cautioned against the operation of motor vehicles or dangerous machinery.

ADVERSE REACTIONS

The most frequent adverse reaction to methocarbamol is dizziness or lightheadedness and nausea. This occurs in about one in 20–25 patients. Less frequent reactions are drowsiness, blurred vision, headache, fever, allergic manifestations such as urticaria, pruritus, and rash.

Adverse reactions that have been associated with the use of aspirin include: nausea and other gastrointestinal discomfort, gastritis, gastric erosion, vomiting, constipation, diarrhea, angio-edema, asthma, rash, pruritus, urticaria.

Gastrointestinal discomfort may be minimized by taking Robaxisal with food.

DOSAGE AND ADMINISTRATION

Adults and children over 12 years of age: Two tablets four times daily. Three tablets four times daily may be used in severe conditions for one to three days in patients who are able to tolerate salicylates. These dosage recommendations provide respectively 3.2 and 4.8 grams of methocarbamol per day.

OVERDOSAGE

Toxicity due to overdosage of methocarbamol is unlikely; however, acute overdosage of aspirin may cause symptoms of salicylate intoxication.

TREATMENT OF OVERDOSAGE

Supportive therapy for 24 hours, as methocarbamol is excreted within that time. If salicylate intoxication occurs, especially in children, the hyperpnea may be controlled with sodium bicarbonate. Judicious use of 5% CO_2 with 95% O_2 may be of benefit. Abnormal electrolyte patterns should be corrected with appropriate fluid therapy.

HOW SUPPLIED

Robaxisal® is supplied as pink and white laminated, compressed tablets in bottles of 100 (NDC 0031-7469-63) and 500 (NDC 0031-7469-70).

Store at controlled room temperature, between 20° and 25°C (68° and 77°F).

Dispense in well-closed container.

Manufactured by:
Pharmaceutical Division
A.H. Robins Company
Richmond, VA 23220
CI 4697-1 Issued February 6, 1997

Shown in Product Identification Guide, page 332

ROBINUL® INJECTABLE ℞

[*ro 'bĭ-nul*]

(Glycopyrrolate Injection, USP)

DESCRIPTION

Robinul (glycopyrrolate) is a synthetic anticholinergic agent. Each 1 mL contains:

Glycopyrrolate, USP .... 0.2 mg
Water for Injection, USP .... q.s.
Benzyl Alcohol, NF (preservative) 0.9%

pH adjusted, when necessary, with hydrochloric acid and/or sodium hydroxide.

For Intramuscular or Intravenous administration.

Glycopyrrolate is a quaternary ammonium compound with the following chemical name:

3[(cyclopentylhydroxyphenylacetyl)oxy]-1,1-dimethyl pyrrolidinium bromide.

Unlike atropine, glycopyrrolate is completely ionized at physiological pH values.

Robinul Injectable is a clear, colorless, sterile liquid; pH 2.0–3.0.

CLINICAL PHARMACOLOGY

Glycopyrrolate, like other anticholinergic (antimuscarinic) agents, inhibits the action of acetylcholine on structures innervated by postganglionic cholinergic nerves and on smooth muscles that respond to acetylcholine but lack cholinergic innervation. These peripheral cholinergic receptors are present in the autonomic effector cells of smooth muscle, cardiac muscle, the sinoatrial node, the atrioventricular node, exocrine glands, and, to a limited degree, in the autonomic ganglia. Thus, it diminishes the volume and free acidity of gastric secretions and controls excessive pharyngeal, tracheal, and bronchial secretions.

Glycopyrrolate antagonizes muscarinic symptoms (e.g., bronchorrhea, bronchospasm, bradycardia, and intestinal hypermotility) induced by cholinergic drugs such as the anticholinesterases.

The highly polar quaternary ammonium group of glycopyrrolate limits its passage across lipid membranes, such as the blood-brain barrier, in contrast to atropine sulfate and scopolamine hydrobromide, which are non-polar tertiary amines which penetrate lipid barriers easily.

Peak effects occur approximately 30 to 45 minutes after intramuscular administration. The vagal blocking effects persist for 2 to 3 hours and the antisialagogue effects persist up to 7 hours, periods longer than for atropine. With intravenous injection, the onset of action is generally evident within one minute.

INDICATIONS AND USAGE

In Anesthesia: Robinul (glycopyrrolate) Injectable is indicated for use as a preoperative antimuscarinic to reduce salivary, tracheobronchial, and pharyngeal secretions; to reduce the volume and free acidity of gastric secretions; and, to block cardiac vagal inhibitory reflexes during induction of anesthesia and intubation. When indicated, Robinul Injectable may be used intraoperatively to counteract drug-induced or vagal traction reflexes with the associated arrhythmias. Glycopyrrolate protects against the peripheral muscarinic effects (e.g., bradycardia and excessive secretions) of cholinergic agents such as neostigmine and pyridostigmine given to reverse the neuromuscular blockade due to nondepolarizing muscle relaxants.

In Peptic Ulcer: For use in adults as adjunctive therapy for the treatment of peptic ulcer when rapid anticholinergic effect is desired or when oral medication is not tolerated.

CONTRAINDICATIONS

Known hypersensitivity to glycopyrrolate.

Due to its benzyl alcohol content, Robinul Injectable should not be used in newborns (children less than 1 month of age).

In addition, in the management of *peptic ulcer* patients, because of the longer duration of therapy, Robinul Injectable may be contraindicated in patients with concurrent glaucoma; obstructive uropathy (for example, bladder neck obstruction due to prostatic hypertrophy); obstructive disease of the gastrointestinal tract (as in achalasia, pyloroduodenal stenosis, etc.); paralytic ileus, intestinal atony of the elderly or debilitated patient; unstable cardiovascular status in acute hemorrhage; severe ulcerative colitis; toxic megacolon complicating ulcerative colitis; myasthenia gravis.

WARNINGS

This drug should be used with great caution, if at all, in patients with glaucoma or asthma.

In the ambulatory patient. Robinul (glycopyrrolate) may produce drowsiness or blurred vision. The patient should be cautioned regarding activities requiring mental alertness such as operating a motor vehicle or other machinery or performing hazardous work while taking this drug.

In addition, in the presence of a high environmental temperature, heat prostration (fever and heat stroke due to decreased sweating) can occur with use of Robinul (glycopyrrolate).

Diarrhea may be an early symptom of incomplete intestinal obstruction, especially in patients with ileostomy or colostomy. In this instance treatment with Robinul (glycopyrrolate) would be inappropriate and possibly harmful.

PRECAUTIONS

General

Investigate any tachycardia before giving glycopyrrolate since an increase in the heart rate may occur.

Use with caution in patients with: coronary artery disease; congestive heart failure; cardiac arrhythmias; hypertension; hyperthyroidism.

In managing ulcer patients, use Robinul with caution in the elderly and in all patients with autonomic neuropathy, hepatic or renal disease, ulcerative colitis or hiatal hernia, since anticholinergic drugs may aggravate these conditions.

With overdosage, a curare-like action may occur.

Drug Interactions

The intravenous administration of any anticholinergic in the presence of cyclopropane anesthesia can result in ventricular arrhythmias; therefore, caution should be observed if Robinul (glycopyrrolate) Injectable is used during cyclopropane anesthesia. If the drug is given in small incremental doses of 0.1 mg or less, the likelihood of producing ventricular arrhythmias is reduced.

Carcinogenesis, Mutagenesis, Impairment of Fertility

Long-term studies in animals have not been performed to evaluate carcinogenic potential. In the teratology studies, diminished rates of conception and of survival at weaning were observed in rats, in a dose-related manner. Studies in dogs suggest that this may be due to diminished seminal secretion which is evident at high doses of glycopyrrolate.

Pregnancy Category B

Reproduction studies have been performed in rats and rabbits up to 1000 times the human dose and have revealed no teratogenic effects from glycopyrrolate. There are, however, no adequate and well-controlled studies in pregnant women. Because animal reproduction studies are not always predictive of human response, this drug should be used during pregnancy only if clearly needed.

Nursing Mothers

It is not known whether this drug is excreted in human milk. Because many drugs are excreted in human milk, caution should be exercised when Robinul is administered to a nursing woman.

Pediatric Use

Safety and effectiveness in children below the age of 12 years have not been established for the management of peptic ulcer.

ADVERSE REACTIONS

Anticholinergics produce certain effects, most of which are extensions of their pharmacologic actions. Adverse reactions to anticholinergics in general may include dry mouth; urinary hesitancy and retention; blurred vision due to mydriasis; increased ocular tension; tachycardia; palpitation; decreased sweating; loss of taste; headache; nervousness; drowsiness; weakness; dizziness; insomnia; nausea; vomiting; impotence; suppression of lactation; constipation; bloated feeling; severe allergic reaction or drug idiosyncrasies including anaphylaxis; urticaria and other dermal manifestations; some degree of mental confusion and/or excitement, especially in elderly persons.

Robinul is chemically a quaternary ammonium compound; hence, its passage across lipid membranes, such as the blood-brain barrier is limited in contrast to atropine sulfate and scopolamine hydrobromide. For this reason the occurrence of CNS related side effects is lower, in comparison to their incidence following administration of anticholinergics which are chemically tertiary amines that can cross this barrier readily.

Continued on next page

Robinul—Cont.

OVERDOSAGE

To combat peripheral anticholinergic effects, a quaternary ammonium anticholinesterase such as neostigmine methylsulfate (which does not cross the blood-brain barrier) may be given intravenously in increments of 0.25 mg in adults. This dosage may be repeated every five to ten minutes until anticholinergic overactivity is reversed or up to a maximum of 2.5 mg. Proportionately smaller doses should be used in children. Indication for repetitive doses of neostigmine should be based on close monitoring of the decrease in heart rate and the return of bowel sounds.

In the unlikely event that CNS symptoms (excitement, restlessness, convulsions, psychotic behavior) occur, physostigmine (which does cross the blood-brain barrier) should be used. Physostigmine 0.5 to 2 mg should be slowly administered intravenously and repeated as necessary up to a total of 5 mg in adults. Proportionately smaller doses should be used in children.

Fever should be treated symptomatically. In the event of a curare-like effect on respiratory muscles, artificial respiration should be instituted and maintained until effective respiratory action returns.

DOSAGE AND ADMINISTRATION

Robinul (glycopyrrolate) Injectable may be administered intramuscularly, or intravenously, without dilution, in the following indications.

Adults: *Preanesthetic Medication.* The recommended dose of Robinul (glycopyrrolate) Injectable is 0.002 mg (0.01 mL) per pound of body weight by intramuscular injection, given 30 to 60 minutes prior to the anticipated time of induction of anesthesia or at the time the preanesthetic narcotic and/or sedative are administered.

Intraoperative Medication. Robinul (glycopyrrolate) Injectable may be used during surgery to counteract drug induced or vagal traction reflexes with the associated arrhythmias (e.g., bradycardia). It should be administered intravenously as single doses of 0.1 mg (0.5 mL) and repeated, as needed, at intervals of 2–3 minutes. The usual attempts should be made to determine the etiology of the arrhythmia, and the surgical or anesthetic manipulations necessary to correct parasympathetic imbalance should be performed.

Reversal of Neuromuscular Blockade. The recommended dose of Robinul (glycopyrrolate) Injectable is 0.2 mg (1.0 mL) for each 1.0 mg of neostigmine or 5.0 mg of pyridostigmine. In order to minimize the appearance of cardiac side effects, the drugs may be administered simultaneously by intravenous injection and may be mixed in the same syringe.

Children: (Read Contraindications). *Preanesthetic Medication.* The recommended dose of Robinul (glycopyrrolate) Injectable in children 1 month to 12 years of age is 0.002 mg (0.01 mL) per pound of body weight intramuscularly, given 30 to 60 minutes prior to the anticipated time of induction of anesthesia or at the time the preanesthetic narcotic and/or sedative are administered.

Children 1 month to 2 years of age may require up to 0.004 mg (0.02 mL) per pound of body weight.

Intraoperative Medication. Because of the long duration of action of Robinul (glycopyrrolate) if used as preanesthetic medication, additional Robinul (glycopyrrolate) Injectable for anticholinergic effect intraoperatively is rarely needed; in the event it is required the recommended pediatric dose is 0.002 mg (0.01 mL) per pound of body weight intravenously, not to exceed 0.1 mg (0.5 mL) in a single dose which may be repeated, as needed, at intervals of 2–3 minutes. The usual attempts should be made to determine the etiology of the arrhythmia, and the surgical or anesthetic manipulations necessary to correct parasympathetic imbalance should be performed.

Reversal of Neuromuscular Blockade. The recommended pediatric dose of Robinul (glycopyrrolate) Injectable is 0.2 mg (1.0 mL) for each 1.0 mg of neostigmine or 5.0 mg of pyridostigmine. In order to minimize the appearance of cardiac side effects, the drugs may be administered simultaneously by intravenous injection and may be mixed in the same syringe.

Adults: *Peptic Ulcer.* The usual recommended dose of Robinul Injectable is 0.1 mg (0.5 mL) administered at 4-hour intervals, 3 or 4 times daily intravenously or intramuscularly. Where more profound effect is required, 0.2 mg (1.0 mL) may be given. Some patients may need only a single dose, and frequency of administration should be dictated by patient response up to a maximum of four times daily.

Robinul Injectable is not recommended for peptic ulcers in children under 12 years of age. (See Precautions.)

NOTE: Parenteral drug products should be inspected visually for particulate matter and discoloration prior to administration whenever solution and container permit.

Admixture Compatibilities. Robinul (glycopyrrolate) Injectable is compatible for mixing and injection with the following injectable dosage forms: 5% and 10% glucose in water or saline; atropine sulfate, USP; Antilirium® (physostigmine salicylate); Benadryl® (diphenhydramine HCl); codeine phosphate, USP; Emete-Con® (benzquinamide HCl); hydromorphone HCl, USP; Inapsine® (droperidol); Innovar® (droperidol and fentanyl citrate); Largon® (propiomazine HCl); Levo-Dromoran® (levorphanol tartrate); lidocaine, USP; Mepergan® (meperidine and promethazine HCls); meperidine HCl, USP; Mestinon®/Regonol® (pyridostigmine bromide); morphine sulfate, USP; Nisentil® (alphaprodine HCl); Nubain® (nalbuphine HCl); Numorphan® (oxymorphone HCl); Pantopon® (opium alkaloids HCls); procaine HCl, USP; promethazine HCl, USP; Prostigmin® (neostigmine methylsulfate, USP); scopolamine HBr, USP; Sparine® (promazine HCl); Stadol® (butorphanol tartrate); Sublimaze® (fentanyl citrate); Talwin® (pentazocine lactate); Tigan® (trimethobenzamide HCl); Vesprin® (triflupromazine HCl); and Vistaril® (hydroxyzine HCl). Robinul Injectable may be administered via the tubing of a running infusion of physiological saline or lactated Ringer's solution. Since the stability of glycopyrrolate is questionable above a pH of 6.0, do *not* combine Robinul Injectable in the same syringe with Brevital® (methohexital Na); Chloromycetin® (chloramphenicol Na succinate); Dramamine® (dimenhydrinate); Nembutal® (pentobarbital Na); Pentothal® (thiopental Na); Seconal® (secobarbital Na); sodium bicarbonate (Abbott); or Valium® (diazepam). A gas will evolve or a precipitate may form. Mixing with Decadron® (dexamethasone Na phosphate) or a buffered solution of lactated Ringer's solution will result in a pH higher than 6.0. Mixing chlorpromazine HCl, USP, or Compazine® (prochlorperazine) with other agents in a syringe is not recommended by the manufacturer, although the mixture with Robinul Injectable is physically compatible.

HOW SUPPLIED

Robinul (glycopyrrolate) Injectable, 0.2 mg/mL, is available in 1 mL single dose vials packaged in 25's (NDC 0031-7890-11), 2 mL single dose vials packaged in 25's (NDC 0031-7890-95), 5 mL multiple dose vials packaged in 25's (NDC 0031-7890-06), and 20 mL (NDC 0031-7890-83) multiple dose vials.

Store at controlled room temperature, between 20°C and 25°C (68°F and 77°F).

Manufactured by:
Pharmaceutical Division
A. H. Robins Company
Richmond, VA 23220
CI 4932-1 Issued April 25, 1997

Shown in Product Identification Guide, page 332

ROBITUSSIN A–C® Ⓒ

[*ro "bī-tuss 'in*]
Expectorant
Cough Suppressant
Sugar-Free

Robitussin and Codeine
Each 5 mL (1 teaspoonful) contains:

Guaifenesin, USP	100 mg
Codeine Phosphate, USP	10 mg

(Warning: May be habit forming)
Alcohol 3.5 percent
In a palatable, aromatic syrup

Inactive Ingredients: Caramel, Citric Acid, FD&C Red 40, Flavors, Glycerin, Saccharin Sodium, Sodium Benzoate, Sorbitol, Water.

ACTIONS

Robitussin A-C combines the expectorant, guaifenesin, with the cough suppressant, codeine. Guaifenesin enhances the output of lower respiratory tract fluid. The enhanced flow of less viscid secretions promotes and facilitates the removal of mucus. Codeine is a centrally acting agent which elevates the threshold for cough.

As a result, dry, unproductive coughs become more productive and less frequent.

Under Federal law, Robitussin A-C is available without a prescription. Certain state laws may differ. The container label contains the following indications, warnings and drug interaction precaution statements and directions:

INDICATIONS

Temporarily controls cough due to minor throat and bronchial irritation as may occur with the common cold or inhaled irritants. Helps loosen phlegm (mucus) and thin bronchial secretions to make coughs more productive.

WARNINGS

A persistent cough may be a sign of a serious condition. If cough persists for more than 1 week, tends to recur, or is accompanied by fever, rash, or persistent headache, consult a doctor. Do not take this product for persistent or chronic cough such as occurs with smoking, asthma, chronic bronchitis, emphysema, or if cough is accompanied by excessive phlegm (mucus) unless directed by a doctor. Adults and children who have a chronic pulmonary disease or shortness of breath, or children who are taking other drugs, should not take this product unless directed by a doctor. May cause or aggravate constipation. As with any drug, if you are pregnant or nursing a baby, seek the advice of a health professional before using this product.

PROFESSIONAL NOTE: Guaifenesin has been shown to produce a color interference with certain clinical laboratory determinations of 5-hydroxyindoleacetic acid (5-HIAA) and vanillylmandelic acid (VMA).

DRUG INTERACTION PRECAUTION

Caution should be used when taking this product with sedatives, tranquilizers and drugs used for depression, especially monoamine oxidase inhibitors (MAOIs). These combinations may cause greater sedation (drowsiness) than is caused by the products used alone.

DIRECTIONS

Take orally as stated below or use as directed by a doctor. Adults and children 12 years of age and over: 2 teaspoonfuls every 4 hours, not to exceed 12 teaspoonfuls in a 24-hour period; children 6 to under 12 years: 1 teaspoonful every 4 hours, not to exceed 6 teaspoonfuls in a 24-hour period; children under 6 years: consult a doctor. A special measuring device should be used to give an accurate dose of this product to children under 6 years of age. Giving a higher dose than recommended by a doctor could result in serious side effects for a child. Use of codeine-containing preparations is not recommended for children under 2 years of age. Do not exceed recommended dosage.

HOW SUPPLIED

Bottles of 4 fl. oz. (NDC 0031-8674-12), pints (NDC 0031-8674-25), and gallons (NDC 0031-8674-29).

Manufactured by:
Pharmaceutical Division
A.H. Robins Company
Richmond, VA 23220
rev. 6/89

ROBITUSSIN® -DAC Ⓒ

[*ro "bī-tuss 'in*]
Expectorant
Nasal Decongestant
Cough-Suppressant
Sugar-Free

Each 5 mL (1 teaspoonful) contains:

Guaifenesin, USP	100 mg
Pseudoephedrine Hydrochloride, USP	30 mg
Codeine Phosphate, USP	10 mg

(Warning: May be habit forming)
In a palatable, aromatic syrup
Alcohol 1.9 percent

Inactive Ingredients: Caramel, Citric Acid, FD&C Red 40, Flavors, Glycerin, Saccharin Sodium, Sodium Benzoate, Sorbitol, Water.

ACTIONS

Robitussin-DAC combines the expectorant, guaifenesin, the nasal decongestant, pseudoephedrine, and the cough suppressant, codeine. Guaifenesin enhances the output of lower respiratory tract fluid. The enhanced flow of less viscid secretions promotes and facilitates the removal of mucus. Codeine is a centrally acting agent which elevates the threshold for cough. As a result, dry, unproductive coughs become more productive and less frequent. The nasal decongestant, pseudoephedrine, reduces the swelling of nasal passages.

Under Federal law, Robitussin-DAC is available without a prescription. Certain state laws may differ. The container label contains the following indications, warnings and drug interaction precaution statements and directions:

INDICATIONS

Temporarily relieves nasal congestion and controls cough due to minor throat and bronchial irritation as may occur with the common cold or inhaled irritants. Temporarily restores freer breathing through the nose. Helps loosen phlegm (mucus) and thin bronchial secretions to make coughs more productive.

WARNINGS

A persistent cough may be a sign of a serious condition. If cough persists for more than 1 week, tends to recur, or is accompanied by fever, rash, or persistent headache, consult a doctor. Do not take this product for persistent or chronic cough such as occurs with smoking, asthma, chronic bronchitis, emphysema, or if cough is accompanied by excessive phlegm (mucus) unless directed by a doctor. Adults and children who have a chronic pulmonary disease or shortness of breath, or children who are taking other drugs, should not take this product unless directed by a doctor. Do not take this product if you have high blood pressure, heart disease, diabetes or thyroid disease, except under the advice and supervision of a doctor. Do not exceed recommended dosage because at higher doses nervousness, dizziness or sleeplessness may occur. May cause or aggravate constipation. As with any drug, if you are pregnant or nursing a baby, seek the advice of a health professional before using this product.

PROFESSIONAL NOTE: Guaifenesin has been shown to produce a color interference with certain clinical laboratory determinations of 5-hydroxyindoleacetic acid (5-HIAA) and vanillylmandelic acid (VMA).

DRUG INTERACTION PRECAUTION

Do not take this product if you are presently taking a prescription drug for high blood pressure or depression, especially monoamine oxidase inhibitors (MAOIs), without first consulting your doctor.

DIRECTIONS

Take orally as stated below or use as directed by a doctor. Adults and children 12 years of age and over: 2 teaspoonfuls every 4 hours, not to exceed 8 teaspoonfuls in a 24-hour period; children 6 to under 12 years: 1 teaspoonful every 4 hours, not to exceed 4 teaspoonfuls in a 24-hour period; children under 6 years: consult a doctor. A special measuring device should be used to give an accurate dose of this product to children under 6 years of age. Giving a higher dose than recommended by a doctor could result in serious side effects for a child. Use of codeine-containing preparations is not recommended for children under 2 years of age. Do not exceed recommended dosage.

HOW SUPPLIED

Bottles of 4 fl. oz. (NDC 0031-8680-12) and one pint (NDC 0031-8680-25).
Manufactured by:
Pharmaceutical Division
A.H. Robins Company
Richmond, VA 23220
rev. 6/89

TENEX® ℞

[těn' ěks]
(Guanfacine Hydrochloride)
Tablets

DESCRIPTION

Tenex (guanfacine hydrochloride) is a centrally acting antihypertensive with α_2-adrenoceptor agonist properties in tablet form for oral administration.
The chemical name of Tenex (guanfacine hydrochloride) is N-amidino-2-(2,6-dichlorophenyl) acetamide hydrochloride and its molecular weight is 282.56.
Guanfacine hydrochloride is a white to off-white powder; sparingly soluble in water and alcohol and slightly soluble in acetone. The tablets contain the following inactive ingredients:
1 mg—FD&C Red 40 aluminum lake, lactose, microcrystalline cellulose, povidone, stearic acid.
2 mg—D&C Yellow 10 aluminum lake, lactose, microcrystalline cellulose, povidone, stearic acid.

CLINICAL PHARMACOLOGY

Tenex (guanfacine hydrochloride) is an orally active antihypertensive agent whose principal mechanism of action appears to be stimulation of central α_2-adrenergic receptors. By stimulating these receptors, guanfacine reduces sympathetic nerve impulses from the vasomotor center to the heart and blood vessels. This results in a decrease in peripheral vascular resistance and a reduction in heart rate.
The dose-response relationship for blood pressure and adverse effects of guanfacine given once a day as monotherapy has been evaluated in patients with mild to moderate hypertension. In this study patients were randomized to placebo or to 0.5 mg, 1 mg, 2 mg, 3 mg, or 5 mg of Tenex. Results are shown in the following table. A useful effect was not observed overall until doses of 2 mg were reached, although responses in white patients were seen at 1 mg; 24 hour effectiveness of 1 mg to 3 mg doses was documented using 24 hour ambulatory monitoring. While the 5 mg dose added an increment of effectiveness, it caused an unacceptable increase in adverse reactions.
[See first table above]
Controlled clinical trials in patients with mild to moderate hypertension who were receiving a thiazide-type diuretic have defined the dose-response relationship for blood pressure response and adverse reactions of guanfacine given at bedtime and have shown that the blood pressure response to guanfacine can persist for 24 hours after a single dose. In the 12-week, placebo-controlled dose-response study, patients were randomized to placebo or to doses of 0.5, 1, 2, and 3 mg of guanfacine, in addition to 25 mg chlorthalidone, each given at bedtime. The observed mean changes from baseline, tabulated below, indicate the similarity of response for placebo and the 0.5 mg dose. Doses of 1, 2, and 3 mg resulted in decreased blood pressure in the sitting position with no real differences among the three doses. In the standing position there was some increase in response with dose.
[See second table above]
While most of the effectiveness of guanfacine in combination (and as monotherapy in white patients) was present at 1 mg, adverse reactions at this dose were not clearly distinguishable from those associated with placebo. Adverse reactions were clearly present at 2 and 3 mg (see **ADVERSE REACTIONS**).
In a second 12-week, placebo-controlled study of 1, 2 or 3 mg of Tenex (guanfacine hydrochloride) administered with 25 mg of chlorthalidone once daily, a significant decrease in blood pressure was maintained for a full 24 hours after dosing. While there was no significant difference between the 12 and 24 hour blood pressure readings, the fall in blood pressure at 24 hours was numerically smaller, suggesting possible escape of blood pressure in some patients and the need for individualization of therapy.
In a double-blind, randomized trial, either guanfacine or clonidine was given at recommended doses with 25 mg chlorthalidone for 24 weeks and then abruptly discontinued. Results showed equal degrees of blood pressure reduction with the two drugs and there was no tendency for blood pressures to increase despite maintenance of the same daily dose of the two drugs. Signs and symptoms of rebound phenomena were infrequent upon discontinuation of either drug. Abrupt withdrawal of clonidine produced a rapid return of diastolic and especially, systolic blood pressure to approximately pretreatment levels, with occasional values significantly greater than baseline, whereas guanfacine withdrawal produced a more gradual increase to pretreatment levels, but also with occasional values significantly greater than baseline.

Mean Changes (mm Hg) from Baseline in Seated Systolic and Diastolic Blood Pressure for Patients Completing 4 to 8 Weeks of Treatment with Guanfacine Monotherapy

Mean Change S/D* Seated	n = (range)	Placebo	0.5 mg	1 mg	2 mg	3 mg	5 mg
White Patients	11–30	–1/–5	–6/–8	–8/–9	–12/–11	–15/–12	–18/–16
Black Patients	8–28	–3/–5	0/–2	–3/–5	–7/–7	–8/–9	–19/–15

* S/D = Systolic/diastolic blood pressure.

Mean Decreases (mm Hg) in Seated and Standing Blood Pressure for Patients Treated with Guanfacine in Combination with Chlorthalidone

Mean Change	n =	Placebo 63	0.5 mg 63	1 mg 64	2 mg 58	3 mg 59
S/D* Seated		–5/–7	–5/–6	–14/–13	–12/–13	–16/–13
S/D* Standing		–3/–5	–5/–4	–11/–9	–9/–10	–15/–12

* S/D = Systolic/diastolic blood pressure

Adverse Reaction	Placebo n=59	0.5 mg n=60	1 mg n=61	2 mg n=60	3 mg n=59
Dry Mouth	0%	10%	10%	42%	54%
Somnolence	8%	5%	10%	13%	39%
Asthenia	0%	2%	3%	7%	3%
Dizziness	8%	12%	2%	8%	15%
Headache	8%	13%	7%	5%	3%
Impotence	0%	0%	0%	7%	3%
Constipation	0%	2%	0%	5%	15%
Fatigue	2%	2%	5%	8%	10%

Adverse Reaction	Placebo n=73	0.5 mg n=72	1 mg n=72	2 mg n=72	3 mg n=72
Dry Mouth	5 (7%)	4 (5%)	6 (8%)	8 (11%)	20 (28%)
Somnolence	1 (1%)	3 (4%)	0 (0%)	1 (1%)	10 (14%)
Asthenia	0 (0%)	2 (3%)	0 (0%)	2 (2%)	7 (10%)
Dizziness	2 (2%)	1 (1%)	3 (4%)	6 (8%)	3 (4%)
Headache	3 (4%)	4 (3%)	3 (4%)	1 (1%)	2 (2%)
Impotence	1 (1%)	1 (0%)	0 (0%)	1 (1%)	3 (4%)
Constipation	0 (0%)	0 (0%)	0 (0%)	1 (1%)	1 (1%)
Fatigue	3 (3%)	2 (3%)	2 (3%)	5 (6%)	3 (4%)

Pharmacodynamics

Hemodynamic studies in man showed that the decrease in blood pressure observed after single-dose or long-term oral treatment with guanfacine was accompanied by a significant decrease in peripheral resistance and a slight reduction in heart rate (5 beats/min). Cardiac output under conditions of rest or exercise was not altered by guanfacine.
Tenex (guanfacine hydrochloride) lowered elevated plasma renin activity and plasma catecholamine levels in hypertensive patients, but this does not correlate with individual blood-pressure responses.
Growth hormone secretion was stimulated with single oral doses of 2 and 4 mg of guanfacine. Long-term use of Tenex had no effect on growth hormone levels.
Guanfacine had no effect on plasma aldosterone. A slight but insignificant decrease in plasma volume occurred after one month of guanfacine therapy. There were no changes in mean body weight or electrolytes.

Pharmacokinetics

Relative to an intravenous dose of 3 mg, the absolute oral bioavailability of guanfacine is about 80%. Peak plasma concentrations occur from 1 to 4 hours with an average of 2.6 hours after single oral doses or at steady state.
The area under the concentration-time curve (AUC) increases linearly with the dose.
In individuals with normal renal function, the average elimination half-life is approximately 17 hr (range 10–30 hr). Younger patients tend to have shorter elimination half-lives (13–14 hr) while older patients tend to have half-lives at the upper end of the range. Steady state blood levels were attained within 4 days in most subjects.
In individuals with normal renal function, guanfacine and its metabolites are excreted primarily in the urine. Approximately 50% (40–75%) of the dose is eliminated in the urine as unchanged drug; the remainder is eliminated mostly as conjugates of metabolites produced by oxidative metabolism of the aromatic ring.
The guanfacine-to-creatinine clearance ratio is greater than 1.0, which would suggest that tubular secretion of drug occurs.
The drug is approximately 70% bound to plasma proteins, independent of drug concentration.
The whole body volume of distribution is high (a mean of 6.3 L/kg), which suggests a high distribution of drug to the tissues.
The clearance of guanfacine in patients with varying degrees of renal insufficiency is reduced, but plasma levels of drug are only slightly increased compared to patients with normal renal function. When prescribing for patients with renal impairment, the low end of the dosing range should be used. Patients on dialysis also can be given usual doses of guanfacine hydrochloride as the drug is poorly dialyzed.

INDICATIONS AND USAGE

Tenex (guanfacine hydrochloride) is indicated in the management of hypertension. Tenex may be given alone or in combination with other antihypertensive agents, especially thiazide-type diuretics.

CONTRAINDICATIONS

Tenex is contraindicated in patients with known hypersensitivity to guanfacine hydrochloride.

PRECAUTIONS

General

Like other antihypertensive agents, Tenex (guanfacine hydrochloride) should be used with caution in patients with severe coronary insufficiency, recent myocardial infarction, cerebrovascular disease or chronic renal or hepatic failure.

Sedation

Tenex, like other orally active central α-2-adrenergic agonists, causes sedation or drowsiness, especially when beginning therapy. These symptoms are dose-related (see **ADVERSE REACTIONS**). When Tenex is used with other centrally active depressants (such as phenothiazines, barbiturates, or benzodiazepines), the potential for additive sedative effects should be considered.

Rebound

Abrupt cessation of therapy with orally active central α-2 adrenergic agonists may be associated with increases (from depressed on-therapy levels) in plasma and urinary catecholamines, symptoms of "nervousness and anxiety" and, less commonly, increases in blood pressure to levels significantly greater than those prior to therapy.

Information for Patients

Patients who receive Tenex should be advised to exercise caution when operating dangerous machinery or driving motor vehicles until it is determined that they do not become drowsy or dizzy from the medication. Patients should be warned that their tolerance for alcohol and other CNS depressants may be diminished. Patients should be advised not to discontinue therapy abruptly.

Laboratory Tests

In clinical trials, no clinically relevant laboratory test abnormalities were identified as causally related to drug during short-term treatment with Tenex (guanfacine hydrochloride).

Drug Interactions

The potential for increased sedation when Tenex is given with other CNS-depressant drugs should be appreciated.
The administration of guanfacine concomitantly with a known microsomal enzyme inducer (phenobarbital or phenytoin) to two patients with renal impairment reportedly resulted in significant reductions in elimination half-life and

Continued on next page

Tenex—Cont.

plasma concentration. In such cases, therefore, more frequent dosing may be required to achieve or maintain the desired hypotensive response. Further, if guanfacine is to be discontinued in such patients, careful tapering of the dosage may be necessary in order to avoid rebound phenomena (see **Rebound** above).

Anticoagulants

Ten patients who were stabilized on oral anticoagulants were given guanfacine, 1–2 mg/day, for 4 weeks. No changes were observed in the degree of anticoagulation.

In several well-controlled studies, guanfacine was administered together with diuretics with no drug interactions reported. In the long-term safety studies, Tenex was given concomitantly with many drugs without evidence of any interactions. The principal drugs given (number of patients in parentheses) were: cardiac glycosides (115), sedatives and hypnotics (103), coronary vasodilators (52), oral hypoglycemics (45), cough and cold preparations (45), NSAIDs (38), antihyperlipidemics (29), antigout drugs (24), oral contraceptives (18), bronchodilators (13), insulin (10), and beta blockers (10).

Drug/Laboratory Test Interactions

No laboratory test abnormalities related to the use of Tenex (guanfacine hydrochloride) have been identified.

Carcinogenesis, Mutagenesis, Impairment of Fertility

No carcinogenic effect was observed in studies of 78 weeks in mice at doses more than 150 times the maximum recommended human dose and 102 weeks in rats at doses more than 100 times the maximum recommended human dose. In a variety of test models, guanfacine was not mutagenic.

No adverse effects were observed in fertility studies in male and female rats.

Pregnancy Category B

Administration of guanfacine to rats at 70 times the maximum recommended human dose and to rabbits at 20 times the maximum recommended human dose resulted in no evidence of harm to the fetus. Higher doses (100 and 200 times the maximum recommended human dose in rabbits and rats respectively) were associated with reduced fetal survival and maternal toxicity. Rat experiments have shown that guanfacine crosses the placenta.

There are, however, no adequate and well-controlled studies in pregnant women. Because animal reproduction studies are not always predictive of human response, this drug should be used during pregnancy only if clearly needed.

Labor and Delivery

Tenex (guanfacine hydrochloride) is not recommended in the treatment of acute hypertension associated with toxemia of pregnancy. There is no information available on the effects of guanfacine on the course of labor and delivery.

Nursing Mothers

It is not known whether Tenex (guanfacine hydrochloride) is excreted in human milk. Because many drugs are excreted in human milk, caution should be exercised when Tenex is administered to a nursing woman. Experiments with rats have shown that guanfacine is excreted in the milk.

Pediatric Use

Safety and effectiveness in children under 12 years of age have not been demonstrated. Therefore, the use of Tenex in this age group is not recommended.

ADVERSE REACTIONS

Adverse reactions noted with Tenex (guanfacine hydrochloride) are similar to those of other drugs of the central α–2 adrenoreceptor agonist class: dry mouth, sedation (somnolence), weakness (asthenia), dizziness, constipation, and impotence. While the reactions are common, most are mild and tend to disappear on continued dosing.

Skin rash with exfoliation has been reported in a few cases; although clear cause and effect relationships to Tenex could not be established, should a rash occur, Tenex should be discontinued and the patient monitored appropriately.

In the dose-response monotherapy study described under **CLINICAL PHARMACOLOGY**, the frequency of the most commonly observed adverse reactions showed a dose relationship from 0.5 to 3 mg as follows:

[See third table at top of previous page]

The percent of patients who dropped out because of adverse reactions are shown below for each dosage group.

	Placebo	0.5 mg	1 mg	2 mg	3 mg
Percent dropouts	0%	2.0%	5.0%	13%	32%

The most common reasons for dropouts among patients who received guanfacine were dry mouth, somnolence, dizziness, fatigue, weakness, and constipation.

In the 12-week, placebo-controlled, dose-response study of guanfacine administered with 25 mg chlorthalidone at bedtime, the frequency of the most commonly observed adverse reactions showed a clear dose relationship from 0.5 to 3 mg as follows:

[See fourth table at top of previous page]

There were 41 premature terminations because of adverse reactions in this study. The percent of patients who dropped out and the dose at which the dropout occurred were as follows:

Dose:	Placebo	0.5 mg	1 mg	2 mg	3 mg
Percent dropouts	6.9%	4.2%	3.2%	6.9%	8.3%

Reasons for dropouts among patients who received guanfacine were: somnolence, headache, weakness, dry mouth, dizziness, impotence, insomnia, constipation, syncope, urinary incontinence, conjunctivitis, paresthesia, and dermatitis.

In a second 12-week placebo-controlled combination therapy study in which the dose could be adjusted upward to 3 mg per day in 1-mg increments at 3-week intervals, i.e., a setting more similar to ordinary clinical use, the most commonly recorded reactions were: dry mouth, 47%; constipation, 16%; fatigue, 12%; somnolence, 10%; asthenia, 6%; dizziness, 6%; headache, 4%; and insomnia, 4%.

Reasons for dropouts among patients who received guanfacine were: somnolence, dry mouth, dizziness, impotence, constipation, confusion, depression, and palpitations.

In the clonidine/guanfacine comparison described in **CLINICAL PHARMACOLOGY**, the most common adverse reactions noted were as follows:

Adverse Reactions	Guanfacine (n = 279)	Clonidine (n = 278)
Dry mouth	30%	37%
Somnolence	21%	35%
Dizziness	11%	8%
Constipation	10%	5%
Fatigue	9%	8%
Headache	4%	4%
Insomnia	4%	3%

Adverse reactions occurring in 3% or less of patients in the three controlled trials of Tenex with a diuretic were:

Cardiovascular—	bradycardia, palpitations, substernal pain
Gastrointestinal—	abdominal pain, diarrhea, dyspepsia, dysphagia, nausea
CNS—	amnesia, confusion, depression, insomnia, libido decrease
ENT disorders—	rhinitis, taste perversion, tinnitus
Eye disorders—	conjunctivitis, iritis, vision disturbance
Musculoskeletal—	leg cramps, hypokinesia
Respiratory—	dyspnea
Dermatologic—	dermatitis, pruritus, purpura, sweating
Urogenital—	testicular disorder, urinary incontinence
Other—	malaise, paresthesia, paresis

Adverse reaction reports tend to decrease over time. In an open-label trial of one year's duration, 580 hypertensive subjects were given guanfacine, titrated to achieve goal blood pressure, alone (51%), with diuretic (38%), with beta blocker (3%), with diuretic plus beta blocker (6%), or with diuretic plus vasodilator (2%). The mean daily dose of guanfacine reached was 4.7 mg.

Adverse Reaction	Incidence of adverse reactions at any time during the study	Incidence of adverse reactions at the end of one year
	n=580	n=580
Dry mouth	60%	15%
Drowsiness	33%	6%
Dizziness	15%	1%
Constipation	14%	3%
Weakness	5%	1%
Headache	4%	0.2%
Insomnia	5%	0%

There were 52 (8.9%) dropouts due to adverse effects in this 1-year trial. The causes were: dry mouth (n = 20), weakness (n = 12), constipation (n = 7), somnolence (n = 3), nausea (n = 3), orthostatic hypotension (n = 2), insomnia (n = 1), rash (n = 1), nightmares (n = 1), headache (n = 1), and depression (n = 1).

Postmarketing Experience

An open-label postmarketing study involving 21,718 patients was conducted to assess the safety of Tenex (guanfacine hydrochloride) 1 mg/day given at bedtime for 28 days. Tenex was administered with or without other antihypertensive agents. Adverse events reported in the postmarketing study at an incidence greater than 1% included dry mouth, dizziness, somnolence, fatigue, headache and nausea. The most commonly reported adverse events in this study were the same as those observed in controlled clinical trials.

Less frequent, possibly Tenex-related events observed in the postmarketing study and/or reported spontaneously include:

BODY AS A WHOLE	asthenia, chest pain, edema, malaise, tremor
CARDIOVASCULAR	bradycardia, palpitations, syncope, tachycardia
CENTRAL NERVOUS SYSTEM	paresthesias, vertigo
EYE DISORDERS	blurred vision
GASTROINTESTINAL SYSTEM	abdominal pain, constipation, diarrhea, dyspepsia
LIVER AND BILIARY SYSTEM	abnormal liver function tests
MUSCULO-SKELETAL SYSTEM	arthralgia, leg cramps, leg pain, myalgia
PSYCHIATRIC	agitation, anxiety, confusion, depression, insomnia, nervousness
REPRODUCTIVE SYSTEM, MALE	impotence
RESPIRATORY SYSTEM	dyspnea
SKIN AND APPENDAGES	alopecia, dermatitis, exfoliative dermatitis, pruritus, rash
SPECIAL SENSES	alterations in taste
URINARY SYSTEM	nocturia, urinary frequency

Rare, serious disorders with no definitive cause and effect relationship to Tenex have been reported spontaneously and/or in the postmarketing study. These events include acute renal failure, cardiac fibrillation, cerebrovascular accident, congestive heart failure, heart block, and myocardial infarction.

DRUG ABUSE AND DEPENDENCE

No reported abuse or dependence has been associated with the administration of Tenex (guanfacine hydrochloride).

OVERDOSAGE

Signs and Symptoms

Drowsiness, lethargy, bradycardia and hypotension have been observed following overdose with guanfacine.

A 25-year-old female intentionally ingested 60 mg. She presented with severe drowsiness and bradycardia of 45 beats/minute. Gastric lavage was performed and an infusion of isoproterenol (0.8 mg in 12 hours) was administered. She recovered quickly and without sequelae.

A 28-year-old female who ingested 30–40 mg developed only lethargy, was treated with activated charcoal and a cathartic, was monitored for 24 hours, and was discharged in good health.

A 2-year-old male weighing 12 kg, who ingested up to 4 mg of guanfacine, developed lethargy. Gastric lavage (followed by activated charcoal and sorbitol slurry via NG tube) removed some tablet fragments within 2 hours after ingestion, and vital signs were normal.

During 24-hour observation in ICU, systolic pressure was 58 and heart rate 70 at 16 hours post-ingestion. No intervention was required, and the child was discharged fully recovered the next day.

Treatment of Overdosage

Gastric lavage and supportive therapy as appropriate. Guanfacine is not dialyzable in clinically significant amounts (2.4%).

DOSAGE AND ADMINISTRATION

The recommended initial dose of Tenex (guanfacine hydrochloride) when given alone or in combination with another antihypertensive drug is 1 mg daily given at bedtime to minimize somnolence. If after 3 to 4 weeks of therapy, 1 mg does not give a satisfactory result, a dose of 2 mg may be given, although most of the effect of Tenex is seen at 1 mg (see **CLINICAL PHARMACOLOGY**). Higher daily doses have been used, but adverse reactions increase significantly with doses above 3 mg/day.

The frequency of rebound hypertension is low, but it can occur. When rebound occurs, it does so after 2–4 days, which is delayed compared with clonidine hydrochloride. This is consistent with the longer half-life of guanfacine. In most cases, after abrupt withdrawal of guanfacine, blood pressure returns to pretreatment levels slowly (within 2–4 days) without ill effects.

HOW SUPPLIED

Tenex® (guanfacine hydrochloride) Tablets are available in the following dosing strengths (expressed in equivalent amounts of guanfacine):

1 mg—light pink, diamond-shaped tablet embossed with a 1 and engraved AHR on one side and engraved TENEX on the other side in bottles of 100 (NDC 0031-8901-63) and 500 (NDC 0031-8901-70) and Dis-Co® Unit Dose Packs of 100 (NDC 0031-8901-64).

2 mg—yellow, diamond-shaped tablet, one side engraved TENEX, other side engraved 2 with AHR below it in bottles of 100 (NDC 0031-8903-63).

Store at controlled room temperature, between 20°C and 25°C (68°F and 77°F).

Dispense in tight, light-resistant container.

Manufactured by:
Pharmaceutical Division
A.H. Robins Company
Richmond, VA 23220
CI 4688-3 Revised August 13, 1998

Shown in Product Identification Guide, page 332

Roche Pharmaceuticals
Roche Laboratories Inc.
340 Kingsland Street
Nutley, NJ 07110-1199

For Medical Information:
(Including routine inquiries, adverse drug events and product complaints)
Call: (800) 526-6367
In Emergencies: 24-hour service
For the Medical Needs Program:
Call: (800) 285-4487
Write: Professional Product Information

ACCUTANE® ℞

[*acc 'u-tane*]
(isotretinoin)
CAPSULES

The following text is complete prescribing information based on official labeling in effect June 2000.

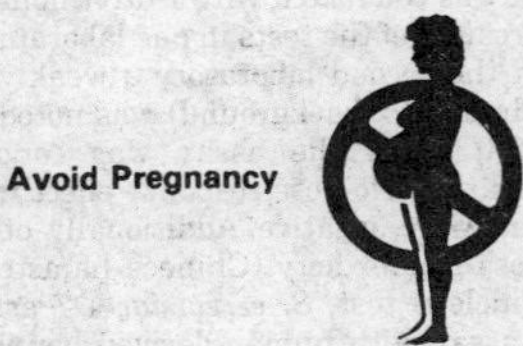

Avoid Pregnancy

CONTRAINDICATIONS AND WARNINGS: Accutane must not be used by females who are pregnant or who may become pregnant while undergoing treatment. Although not every fetus exposed to Accutane has resulted in a deformed child, there is an extremely high risk that a deformed infant can result if pregnancy occurs while taking Accutane in any amount even for short periods of time. Potentially any fetus exposed during pregnancy can be affected. Presently, there are no accurate means of determining after Accutane exposure which fetus has been affected and which fetus has not been affected.

Accutane is contraindicated in females of childbearing potential unless the patient meets all of the following conditions:

- **must have severe disfiguring nodular acne that is recalcitrant to standard therapies (see INDICATIONS AND USAGE for definition)**
- **must be reliable in understanding and carrying out instructions**
- **must be capable of complying with the mandatory contraceptive measures required for Accutane therapy and understand behaviors associated with an increased risk of pregnancy**
- **must have received both oral and written warnings of the hazards of taking Accutane during pregnancy and exposing a fetus to the drug**
- **must have received both oral and written information on the types of contraceptive methods and warnings about the rates of possible contraceptive failure, and of the need to use two separate, effective forms of contraception simultaneously, unless abstinence is the chosen method, or the patient has undergone a hysterectomy and has acknowledged in writing her understanding of the information and warnings and of the need for using two contraceptive methods simultaneously**
- **must have had a negative urine or serum pregnancy test with a sensitivity of at least 50 mIU/mL when the patient is qualified for Accutane therapy by the prescriber, and must have had a second negative urine or serum pregnancy test on the second day of the next normal menstrual period or at least 11 days after the last unprotected act of sexual intercourse, whichever is later**
- **must understand and agree that her prescriber will issue her a prescription for Accutane only after she has contacted the prescriber to confirm that she has obtained a negative result for the second urine pregnancy test which is to be conducted on the second day of the next normal menstrual period or at least 11 days after the last unprotected act of sexual intercourse, whichever is later**
- **must have received instruction to join the Accutane Survey and have watched a videotape, provided by Roche to her prescriber, that provides information about contraceptive methods, possible reasons for contraceptive failure, and importance of using effective contraception when taking teratogenic drugs.**

Major human fetal abnormalities related to Accutane administration have been documented: CNS abnormalities (including cerebral abnormalities, cerebellar malformation, hydrocephalus, microcephaly, cranial nerve deficit); skull abnormality; external ear abnormalities (including anotia, micropinna, small or absent external auditory canals); eye abnormalities (including microphthalmia); cardiovascular abnormalities; facial dysmorphia; cleft palate; thymus gland abnormality; parathyroid hormone deficiency. In some cases death has occurred with certain of the abnormalities previously noted. Cases of IQ scores less than 85 with or without obvious CNS abnormalities have also been reported. There is an increased risk of spontaneous abortion. In addition, premature births have been reported.

It is strongly recommended that a prescription for Accutane should not be issued by the prescriber until a female patient has had negative results from two urine or serum pregnancy tests, one of which is performed in the prescriber's office when the patient is qualified for Accutane therapy, the second of which is performed on the second day of the next normal menstrual period or 11 days after the last unprotected act of sexual intercourse, whichever is later. It is also recommended that pregnancy testing and counseling about contraception and behaviors associated with an increased risk of pregnancy be repeated on a monthly basis. To assure compliance, the prescriber should not issue a prescription for a female patient, until after the second negative pregnancy test result is obtained. In addition, the prescriber should prescribe no more than a 1-month supply of the drug for all Accutane patients and no automatic refills should be permitted. Roche will supply urine pregnancy test kits for female Accutane patients for the initial, second, and monthly testing during therapy.

Effective contraception must be used for at least 1 month before beginning Accutane therapy, during therapy, and for 1 month following discontinuation of therapy even where there has been a history of infertility, unless due to hysterectomy. The patient must be counseled about and understand the limitations of any chosen contraceptive method. The patient must also understand the risks associated with not using two contraceptive methods, even when one of the chosen methods is a hormonal contraceptive method.

Any birth control method can fail. Therefore, it is critically important that women of childbearing potential use two effective forms of contraception simultaneously, unless absolute abstinence is the chosen method, even when one of the forms is a hormonal contraceptive method. Although hormonal contraceptives are highly effective, there have been reports of pregnancy from women who have used oral contraceptives, as well as injectable/implantable contraceptive products. These reports are more frequent for women who use only a single method of contraception. It is not known if hormonal contraceptives differ in their effectiveness when used with Accutane.

If a pregnancy does occur during treatment, the prescriber and patient should discuss the desirability of continuing the pregnancy. Prescribers are encouraged to report all cases of pregnancy with specific information about the contraceptive forms used during Accutane therapy and for 1 month following therapy, either to the Roche Medical Services @ 1-800-526-6367 or to the Food and Drug Administration MedWatch Program @ 1-800-FDA-1088.

Accutane should be prescribed only by prescribers who have special competence in the diagnosis and treatment of severe recalcitrant nodular acne, are experienced in the use of systemic retinoids, and understand the risk of teratogenicity if Accutane is used during pregnancy.

Prescribers who prescribe Accutane should use the Pregnancy Prevention Program℠ kit provided by Roche for the counseling of patients, should instruct the patient to participate in the Accutane Survey, and should receive medical education sponsored by Roche about effective contraception, the limitations of contraceptive methods and behaviors associated with an increased risk of contraceptive failure and pregnancy.

DESCRIPTION

Isotretinoin, a retinoid, is available as Accutane in 10-mg, 20-mg and 40-mg soft gelatin capsules for oral administration. Each capsule also contains beeswax, butylated hydroxyanisole, edetate disodium, hydrogenated soybean oil flakes, hydrogenated vegetable oil, and soybean oil. Gelatin capsules contain glycerin and parabens (methyl and propyl), with the following dye systems: 10 mg — iron oxide (red) and titanium dioxide; 20 mg — C Red No. 3, FD&C Blue No. 1, and titanium dioxide; 40 mg — FD&C Yellow No. 6, D&C Yellow No. 10, and titanium dioxide.

Chemically, isotretinoin is 13-*cis*-retinoic acid and is related to both retinoic acid and retinol (vitamin A). It is a yellow-orange to orange crystalline powder with a molecular weight of 300.44. The structural formula is:

COOH

CLINICAL PHARMACOLOGY

Isotretinoin is a retinoid, which when administered in pharmacologic dosages of 0.5 to 2.0 mg/kg/day, inhibits sebaceous gland function and keratinization. The exact mechanism of action of Accutane is unknown.

Nodular Acne: Clinical improvement in nodular acne patients occurs in association with a reduction in sebum secretion. The decrease in sebum secretion is temporary and is related to the dose and duration of treatment with Accutane, and reflects a reduction in sebaceous gland size and an inhibition of sebaceous gland differentiation.[1]

Pharmacokinetics: *Absorption:* Oral absorption of isotretinoin is optimal when taken with food or milk. After administration of a single 80-mg oral dose (two 40-mg capsules) of isotretinoin to 15 healthy male subjects, maximum blood concentrations ranged from 167 to 459 ng/mL (mean 256 ng/mL) and were achieved in 1 to 6 hours (mean 3.2 hours). The oral absorption of isotretinoin is consistent with first-order kinetics and can be described with a linear two-compartment model. Nodular acne does not alter the absorption of the drug: In a 27-day study of isotretinoin in 10 male patients with nodular acne treated with an oral dose of 40 mg bid, the mean peak concentration ranged from 98 ng/mL to 535 ng/mL (mean 262 ng/mL) and occurred at 2 to 4 hours after administration (mean 2.9 hours). In these patients, the mean ± SD minimum steady-state blood concentration of isotretinoin was 160 ± 19 ng/mL. The terminal elimination half-life was consistent with that observed in normal subjects.

Distribution: Isotretinoin is more than 99.9% bound to plasma proteins, primarily albumin.

Metabolism: After oral administration of isotretinoin, 4-*oxo*-isotretinoin is the major metabolite identified in the blood. Maximum concentrations of 4-*oxo*-isotretinoin (87 to 399 ng/mL) were achieved at 6 to 20 hours after oral administration of two 40-mg capsules; the blood concentration of the major metabolite generally exceeded that of isotretinoin after 6 hours. Isotretinoin also undergoes isomerization to the all-trans-isomer, tretinoin, which is then metabolized to its corresponding 4-*oxo*-metabolite; both have been detected. Both parent compound and metabolites are further metabolized into conjugates which are excreted.

Elimination: Following administration of an 80-mg liquid suspension oral dose of ^{14}C-isotretinoin, ^{14}C-activity in blood declined with a half-life of 90 hours. The metabolites of isotretinoin and any conjugates are ultimately excreted in the feces and urine in relatively equal amounts (total of 65% to 83%). The terminal elimination half-life of isotretinoin ranges from 10 to 20 hours. The mean elimination half-life of 4-*oxo*-isotretinoin is 25 hours (range 17 to 50 hours). After both single and multiple doses, the accumulation ratio of 4-*oxo*-isotretinoin to parent compound is 3 to 3.5.

INDICATIONS AND USAGE

Severe recalcitrant nodular acne: Accutane is indicated for the treatment of severe recalcitrant nodular acne. Nodules are inflammatory lesions with a diameter of 5 mm or greater. The nodules may become suppurative or hemorrhagic. "Severe," by definition,[2] means "many" as opposed to "few or several" nodules. Because of significant adverse effects associated with its use, Accutane should be reserved for patients with severe nodular acne who are unresponsive to conventional therapy, including systemic antibiotics. In addition, for female patients of childbearing potential, Accutane is indicated only for those females who are not pregnant (see boxed CONTRAINDICATIONS AND WARNINGS).

A single course of therapy for 15 to 20 weeks has been shown to result in complete and prolonged remission of disease in many patients.[1,3,4] If a second course of therapy is needed, it should not be initiated until at least 8 weeks after completion of the first course, because experience has shown that patients may continue to improve while off Accutane. The optimal interval before retreatment has not been defined for patients who have not completed skeletal growth (see WARNINGS: *Skeletal: Hyperostosis* and *Premature Epiphyseal Closure*).

CONTRAINDICATIONS

Pregnancy: Category X. See boxed CONTRAINDICATIONS AND WARNINGS.

Allergic Reactions: Accutane is contraindicated in patients who are hypersensitive to this medication or to any of its components. Accutane should not be given to patients who are sensitive to parabens, which are used as preservatives in the gelatin capsule (see PRECAUTIONS: *Hypersensitivity*).

WARNINGS

Psychiatric Disorders: **Accutane may cause depression, psychosis and, rarely, suicidal ideation, suicide attempts and suicide. Discontinuation of Accutane therapy may be insufficient; further evaluation may be necessary. No mechanism of action has been established for these events (see ADVERSE REACTIONS: *Psychiatric*).**

Pseudotumor Cerebri: **Accutane use has been associated with a number of cases of pseudotumor cerebri (benign intracranial hypertension), some of which involved concomitant use of tetracyclines. Concomitant treatment with tetracyclines should therefore be avoided. Early signs and symptoms of pseudotumor cerebri include papilledema, headache, nausea and vomiting, and visual disturbances. Patients with these symptoms should be screened for papilledema and, if present, they should be told to discontinue Accutane immediately and be referred to a neurologist for further diagnosis and care (see ADVERSE REACTIONS: *Neurological*).**

Pancreatitis: Acute pancreatitis has been reported in patients with either elevated or normal serum triglyceride levels. **In rare instances, fatal hemorrhagic pancreatitis has been reported.** Accutane should be stopped if hypertriglyc-

Continued on next page

Accutane—Cont.

eridemia cannot be controlled at an acceptable level or if symptoms of pancreatitis occur.

Lipids: Elevations of serum triglycerides have been reported in patients treated with Accutane. Marked elevations of serum triglycerides in excess of 800 mg/dL were reported in approximately 25% of patients receiving Accutane in clinical trials. In addition, approximately 15% developed a decrease in high-density lipoproteins and about 7% showed an increase in cholesterol levels. In clinical trials, the effects on triglycerides, HDL, and cholesterol were reversible upon cessation of Accutane therapy. Some patients have been able to reverse triglyceride elevation by reduction in weight, restriction of dietary fat and alcohol, and reduction in dose while continuing Accutane.[5]

Blood lipid determinations should be performed before Accutane is given and then at intervals until the lipid response to Accutane is established, which usually occurs within 4 weeks. Especially careful consideration must be given to risk/benefit for patients who may be at high risk during Accutane therapy (patients with diabetes, obesity, increased alcohol intake, lipid metabolism disorder or familial history of lipid metabolism disorder). If Accutane therapy is instituted, more frequent checks of serum values for lipids and/or blood sugar are recommended (see PRECAUTIONS: *Laboratory Tests*).

The cardiovascular consequences of hypertriglyceridemia associated with Accutane are unknown. *Animal Studies:* In rats given 8 or 32 mg/kg/day of isotretinoin (0.7 or 2.7 times the maximum clinical dose after normalization for total body surface area) for 18 months or longer, the incidences of focal calcification, fibrosis and inflammation of the myocardium, calcification of coronary, pulmonary and mesenteric arteries, and metastatic calcification of the gastric mucosa were greater than in control rats of similar age. Focal endocardial and myocardial calcifications associated with calcification of the coronary arteries were observed in two dogs after approximately 6 to 7 months of treatment with isotretinoin at a dosage of 60 to 120 mg/kg/day (15 to 30 times the maximum clinical dose, respectively, after normalization for total body surface area).

Hearing Impairment: Impaired hearing has been reported in patients taking Accutane; in some cases, the hearing impairment has been reported to persist after therapy has been discontinued. Mechanism(s) and causality for this event have not been established. Patients who experience tinnitus or hearing impairment should discontinue Accutane treatment and be referred to specialized care for further evaluation (see ADVERSE REACTIONS: *Special Senses*).

Hepatotoxicity: Clinical hepatitis considered to be possibly or probably related to Accutane therapy has been reported. Additionally, mild to moderate elevations of liver enzymes have been observed in approximately 15% of individuals treated during clinical trials, some of which normalized with dosage reduction or continued administration of the drug. If normalization does not readily occur or if hepatitis is suspected during treatment with Accutane, the drug should be discontinued and the etiology further investigated.

Inflammatory Bowel Disease: Accutane has been associated with inflammatory bowel disease (including regional ileitis) in patients without a prior history of intestinal disorders. In some instances, symptoms have been reported to persist after Accutane treatment has been stopped. Patients experiencing abdominal pain, rectal bleeding or severe diarrhea should discontinue Accutane immediately (see ADVERSE REACTIONS: *Gastrointestinal*).

Skeletal: *Hyperostosis:* A high prevalence of skeletal hyperostosis was noted in clinical trials for disorders of keratinization with a mean dose of 2.24 mg/kg/day. Additionally, skeletal hyperostosis was noted in 6 of 8 patients in a prospective study of disorders of keratinization.[6] Minimal skeletal hyperostosis and calcification of ligaments and tendons have also been observed by x-ray in prospective studies of nodular acne patients treated with a single course of therapy at recommended doses. The skeletal effects of multiple Accutane treatment courses for acne are unknown.

Premature Epiphyseal Closure: There are spontaneous reports of premature epiphyseal closure in acne patients receiving recommended doses, but it is not known if there is a causal relationship with Accutane. In clinical trials for disorders of keratinization with a mean dose of 2.24 mg/kg/day, two children showed x-ray findings suggestive of premature epiphyseal closure. The skeletal effects of multiple Accutane treatment courses for acne are unknown.

Vision Impairment: Visual problems should be carefully monitored. All Accutane patients experiencing visual difficulties should discontinue Accutane treatment and have an ophthalmological examination (see ADVERSE REACTIONS: *Special Senses*).

Corneal Opacities: Corneal opacities have occurred in patients receiving Accutane for acne and more frequently when higher drug dosages were used in patients with disorders of keratinization. The corneal opacities that have been observed in clinical trial patients treated with Accutane have either completely resolved or were resolving at follow-up 6 to 7 weeks after discontinuation of the drug (see ADVERSE REACTIONS: *Special Senses*).

Decreased Night Vision: Decreased night vision has been reported during Accutane therapy and in some instances the event has persisted after therapy was discontinued. Because the onset in some patients was sudden, patients should be advised of this potential problem and warned to be cautious when driving or operating any vehicle at night.

PRECAUTIONS

***Information for Patients and Prescribers:* Females of childbearing potential should be instructed that they must not be pregnant when Accutane therapy is initiated, and that they should use effective contraception while taking Accutane and for 1 month after Accutane has been stopped. They should also sign a consent form prior to beginning Accutane therapy. They should be instructed to join the Accutane Survey and to review the patient videotape provided by Roche to the prescriber that provides information about contraception, the most common reasons that contraception fails, and the importance of using effective contraception when taking teratogenic drugs. Female patients should also be seen monthly and have a urine or serum pregnancy test performed each month during treatment to confirm negative pregnancy status (see boxed CONTRAINDICATIONS AND WARNINGS).**

- Patients should be informed that they must not share Accutane with anyone else because of the risk of birth defects and other serious adverse events.
- Patients should not donate blood during therapy and for 1 month following discontinuance of the drug because the blood might be given to a pregnant woman whose fetus must not be exposed to Accutane.
- Patients should be informed that transient exacerbation (flare) of acne has been seen, generally during the initial period of therapy.
- Wax epilation and skin resurfacing procedures (such as dermabrasion, laser) should be avoided during Accutane therapy and for at least 6 months thereafter due to the possibility of scarring (see ADVERSE REACTIONS: *Skin and Appendages*).
- Patients should be advised to avoid prolonged exposure to UV rays or sunlight.
- Patients should be informed that they may experience decreased tolerance to contact lenses during and after therapy.
- Patients should be informed that approximately 16% of patients treated with Accutane in a clinical trial developed musculoskeletal symptoms (including arthralgia) during treatment. In general, these symptoms were mild to moderate, but occasionally required discontinuation of the drug. Transient pain in the chest has been reported less frequently. In the clinical trial, these symptoms generally cleared rapidly after discontinuation of Accutane, but in some cases persisted (see ADVERSE REACTIONS: *Musculoskeletal*).
- Neutropenia and rare cases of agranulocytosis have been reported. Accutane should be discontinued if clinically significant decreases in white cell counts occur.

Hypersensitivity: Anaphylactic reactions and other allergic reactions have been reported. Cutaneous allergic reactions and serious cases of allergic vasculitis, often with purpura (bruises and red patches) of the extremities and extracutaneous involvement (including renal) have been reported. Severe allergic reaction necessitates discontinuation of therapy and appropriate medical management.

Drug Interactions:

- Because of the relationship of Accutane to vitamin A, patients should be advised against taking vitamin supplements containing vitamin A to avoid additive toxic effects.
- Concomitant treatment with Accutane and tetracyclines should be avoided because Accutane use has been associated with a number of cases of pseudotumor cerebri (benign intracranial hypertension), some of which involved concomitant use of tetracyclines.
- Microdosed progesterone preparations (minipills) may be an inadequate method of contraception during Accutane therapy. Although other hormonal contraceptives are highly effective, there have been reports of pregnancy from women who have used oral contraceptives, as well as injectable/implantable contraceptive products. These reports are more frequent for women who use only a single method of contraception. It is not known if hormonal contraceptives differ in their effectiveness when used with Accutane. Therefore, it is critically important that women of childbearing potential use two effective forms of contraception simultaneously, unless absolute abstinence is the chosen method, even when one of the forms is a hormonal contraceptive method (see boxed CONTRAINDICATIONS AND WARNINGS).

Laboratory Tests:

- *Pregnancy Test:* Female patients of childbearing potential must have negative results from two urine or serum pregnancy tests with a sensitivity of at least 50 mIU/mL before a prescription is given. The first test is to be performed at the office visit when the patient is qualified for Accutane therapy by her prescriber. The second test is to be performed on the second day of her next menstrual cycle or 11 days after her last unprotected act of sexual intercourse, whichever is later. Additional pregnancy tests are to be conducted monthly during treatment.
- *Lipids:* Pretreatment and follow-up blood lipids should be obtained under fasting conditions. After consumption of alcohol, at least 36 hours should elapse before these determinations are made. It is recommended that these tests be performed at weekly or biweekly intervals until the lipid response to Accutane is established. The incidence of hypertriglyceridemia is 1 patient in 4 on Accutane therapy (see WARNINGS: *Lipids*).
- *Liver Function Tests:* Since elevations of liver enzymes have been observed during clinical trials, and hepatitis has been reported, pretreatment and follow-up liver function tests should be performed at weekly or biweekly intervals until the response to Accutane has been established (see WARNINGS: *Hepatotoxicity*).
- *Glucose:* Some patients receiving Accutane have experienced problems in the control of their blood sugar. In addition, new cases of diabetes have been diagnosed during Accutane therapy, although no causal relationship has been established.
- *CPK:* Some patients undergoing vigorous physical activity while on Accutane therapy have experienced elevated CPK levels; however, the clinical significance is unknown.

Carcinogenesis, Mutagenesis and Impairment of Fertility: In male and female Fischer 344 rats given oral isotretinoin at dosages of 8 or 32 mg/kg/day (0.7 or 2.7 times the maximum clinical dose, respectively, after normalization for total body surface area) for greater than 18 months, there was a dose-related increased incidence of pheochromocytoma relative to controls. The incidence of adrenal medullary hyperplasia was also increased at the higher dosage in both sexes. The relatively high level of spontaneous pheochromocytomas occurring in the male Fischer 344 rat makes it an equivocal model for study of this tumor; therefore, the relevance of this tumor to the human population is uncertain.

The Ames test was conducted with isotretinoin in two laboratories. The results of the tests in one laboratory were negative while in the second laboratory a weakly positive response (less than 1.6 x background) was noted in *S. typhimurium* TA100 when the assay was conducted with metabolic activation. No dose-response effect was seen and all other strains were negative. Additionally, other tests designed to assess genotoxicity (Chinese hamster cell assay, mouse micronucleus test, *S. cerevisiae* D7 assay, in vitro clastogenesis assay with human-derived lymphocytes, and unscheduled DNA synthesis assay) were all negative.

In rats, no adverse effects on gonadal function, fertility, conception rate, gestation or parturition were observed at oral dosages of isotretinoin of 2, 8, or 32 mg/kg/day (0.2, 0.7, or 2.7 times the maximum clinical dose, respectively, after normalization for total body surface area).

In dogs, testicular atrophy was noted after treatment with oral isotretinoin for approximately 30 weeks at dosages of 20 or 60 mg/kg/day (5 or 15 times the maximum clinical dose, respectively, after normalization for total body surface area). In general, there was microscopic evidence for appreciable depression of spermatogenesis but some sperm were observed in all testes examined and in no instance were completely atrophic tubules seen. In studies of 66 men, 30 of whom were patients with nodular acne under treatment with oral isotretinoin, no significant changes were noted in the count or motility of spermatozoa in the ejaculate. In a study of 50 men (ages 17 to 32 years) receiving Accutane (isotretinoin) therapy for nodular acne, no significant effects were seen on ejaculate volume, sperm count, total sperm motility, morphology or seminal plasma fructose.

***Pregnancy:* Category X. See boxed CONTRAINDICATIONS AND WARNINGS.**

Nursing Mothers: It is not known whether this drug is excreted in human milk. Because of the potential for adverse effects, nursing mothers should not receive Accutane.

ADVERSE REACTIONS

Clinical Trials and Postmarketing Surveillance: The adverse reactions listed below reflect the experience from investigational studies of Accutane, and the postmarketing experience. The relationship of some of these events to Accutane therapy is unknown. Many of the side effects and adverse reactions seen in patients receiving Accutane are similar to those described in patients taking very high doses of vitamin A (dryness of the skin and mucous membranes, eg, of the lips, nasal passage, and eyes).

Dose Relationship: Cheilitis and hypertriglyceridemia are usually dose related. Most adverse reactions reported in clinical trials were reversible when therapy was discontinued; however, some persisted after cessation of therapy (see WARNINGS and ADVERSE REACTIONS).

Body as a Whole: allergic reactions, including vasculitis, systemic hypersensitivity (see PRECAUTIONS: *Hypersensitivity*), edema, fatigue, lymphadenopathy, weight loss

Cardiovascular: palpitation, tachycardia, vascular thrombotic disease, stroke

Endocrine/Metabolic: hypertriglyceridemia (see WARNINGS: *Lipids*), alterations in blood sugar levels (see PRECAUTIONS: *Laboratory Tests*)

Gastrointestinal: inflammatory bowel disease (see WARNINGS: *Inflammatory Bowel Disease*), hepatitis (see WARNINGS: *Hepatotoxicity*), pancreatitis (see WARNINGS: *Lipids*), bleeding and inflammation of the gums, colitis, ileitis, nausea, other nonspecific gastrointestinal symptoms

Hematologic: allergic reactions (see PRECAUTIONS: *Hypersensitivity*), anemia, thrombocytopenia, neutropenia, rare reports of agranulocytosis (see PRECAUTIONS: *Information for Patients and Prescribers*). See PRECAUTIONS: *Laboratory* for other hematological parameters.

Musculoskeletal: skeletal hyperostosis, calcification of tendons and ligaments, premature epiphyseal closure (see WARNINGS: *Skeletal*), mild to moderate musculoskeletal symptoms including arthralgia (see PRECAUTIONS: *Information for Patients and Prescribers*), transient pain in the chest (see PRECAUTIONS: *Information for Patients and Prescribers*), elevations of CPK (see PRECAUTIONS: *Labo-*

ratory Tests), arthritis, tendonitis, other types of bone abnormalities
Neurological: pseudotumor cerebri (see WARNINGS: *Pseudotumor Cerebri*), dizziness, drowsiness, headache, insomnia, lethargy, malaise, nervousness, paresthesias, seizures, stroke, syncope, weakness
Psychiatric: suicidal ideation, suicide attempts, suicide, depression, psychosis (see WARNINGS: *Psychiatric Disorders*), emotional instability
Of the patients reporting depression, some reported that the depression subsided with discontinuation of therapy and recurred with reinstitution of therapy.
Reproductive System: abnormal menses
Respiratory: bronchospasms (with or without a history of asthma), respiratory infection, voice alteration
Skin and Appendages: acne fulminans, alopecia (which in some cases persists), bruising, cheilitis (dry lips), dry mouth, dry nose, dry skin, epistaxis, eruptive xanthomas,[7] flushing, fragility of skin, hair abnormalities, hirsutism, hyperpigmentation and hypopigmentation, infections (including disseminated herpes simplex), nail dystrophy, paronychia, peeling of palms and soles, photoallergic/photosensitizing reactions, pruritus, pyogenic granuloma, rash (including facial erythema, seborrhea, and eczema), sunburn susceptibility increased, sweating, urticaria, vasculitis (including Wegener's granulomastosis; see PRECAUTIONS: *Hypersensitivity*), abnormal wound healing (delayed healing or exuberant granulation tissue with crusting; see PRECAUTIONS: *Information for Patients and Prescribers*)
Special Senses: Hearing: hearing impairment (see WARNINGS: *Hearing Impairment*), tinnitus. *Vision:* corneal opacities (see WARNINGS: *Corneal Opacities*), decreased night vision which may persist (see WARNINGS: *Decreased Night Vision*), cataracts, color vision disorder, conjunctivitis, dry eyes, eyelid inflammation, keratitis, optic neuritis, photophobia, visual disturbances
Urinary System: glomerulonephritis (see PRECAUTIONS: *Hypersensitivity*), nonspecific urogenital findings (see PRECAUTIONS: *Laboratory* for other urological parameters)
Laboratory: Elevation of plasma triglycerides (see WARNINGS: *Lipids*), decrease in serum high-density lipoprotein (HDL) levels, elevations of serum cholesterol during treatment
Increased alkaline phosphatase, SGOT (AST), SGPT (ALT), GGTP or LDH (see WARNINGS: *Hepatotoxicity*)
Elevation of fasting blood sugar, elevations of CPK (see PRECAUTIONS: *Laboratory Tests*), hyperuricemia
Decreases in red blood cell parameters, decreases in white blood cell counts (including severe neutropenia and rare reports of agranulocytosis; see PRECAUTIONS: *Information for Patients and Prescribers*), elevated sedimentation rates, elevated platelet counts, thrombocytopenia
White cells in the urine, proteinuria, microscopic or gross hematuria

OVERDOSAGE

The oral LD_{50} of isotretinoin is greater than 4000 mg/kg in rats and mice (>300 times the maximum clinical dose after normalization of the rat dose for total body surface area and >150 times the maximum clinical dose after normalization of the mouse dose for total body surface area) and is approximately 1960 mg/kg in rabbits (327 times the maximum clinical dose after normalization for total body surface area). In humans, overdosage has been associated with vomiting, facial flushing, cheilosis, abdominal pain, headache, dizziness, and ataxia. All symptoms quickly resolved without apparent residual effects.

DOSAGE AND ADMINISTRATION

The recommended dosage range for Accutane is 0.5 to 2 mg/kg given in 2 divided doses daily for 15 to 20 weeks. In studies comparing 0.1, 0.5, and 1 mg/kg/day,[8] it was found that all dosages provided initial clearing of disease, but there was a greater need for retreatment with the lower dosages.
It is recommended that for most patients the initial dosage of Accutane be 0.5 to 1 mg/kg/day. Patients whose disease is very severe or is primarily manifested on the trunk may require up to the maximum recommended dosage, 2 mg/kg/day. During treatment, the dose may be adjusted according to response of the disease and/or the appearance of clinical side effects — some of which may be dose related.
If the total nodule count has been reduced by more than 70% prior to completing 15 to 20 weeks of treatment, the drug may be discontinued. After a period of 2 months or more off therapy, and if warranted by persistent or recurring severe nodular acne, a second course of therapy may be initiated. The optimal interval before retreatment has not been defined for patients who have not completed skeletal growth (see WARNINGS: *Skeletal: Hyperostosis* and *Premature Epiphyseal Closure*).
Contraceptive measures must be followed for any subsequent course of therapy (see boxed CONTRAINDICATIONS AND WARNINGS).
Accutane should be administered with food.
[See table above]

ACCUTANE DOSING BY BODY WEIGHT

Body Weight kilograms	Body Weight pounds	Total Mg/Day 0.5 mg/kg	Total Mg/Day 1 mg/kg	Total Mg/Day 2 mg/kg
40	88	20	40	80
50	110	25	50	100
60	132	30	60	120
70	154	35	70	140
80	176	40	80	160
90	198	45	90	180
100	220	50	100	200

HOW SUPPLIED

Soft gelatin capsules, 10 mg (light pink), imprinted ACCUTANE 10 ROCHE. Boxes of 100 containing 10 Prescription Paks of 10 capsules (NDC 0004-0155-49).
Soft gelatin capsules, 20 mg (maroon), imprinted ACCUTANE 20 ROCHE. Boxes of 100 containing 10 Prescription Paks of 10 capsules (NDC 0004-0169-49).
Soft gelatin capsules, 40 mg (yellow), imprinted ACCUTANE 40 ROCHE. Boxes of 100 containing 10 Prescription Paks of 10 capsules (NDC 0004-0156-49).
Store at controlled room temperature (59° to 86°F, 15° to 30°C). Protect from light.

REFERENCES

1. Peck GL, Olsen TG, Yoder FW, et al. Prolonged remissions of cystic and conglobate acne with 13-*cis*-retinoic acid. *N Engl J Med* 300:329–333, 1979. 2. Pochi PE, Shalita AR, Strauss JS, Webster SB. Report of the consensus conference on acne classification. *J Am Acad Dermatol* 24:495–500, 1991. 3. Farrell LN, Strauss JS, Stranieri AM. The treatment of severe cystic acne with 13-*cis*-retinoic acid: evaluation of sebum production and the clinical response in a multiple-dose trial. *J Am Acad Dermatol* 3:602–611, 1980. 4. Jones H, Blanc D, Cunliffe WJ. 13-*cis*-retinoic acid and acne. *Lancet* 2:1048–1049, 1980. 5. Katz RA, Jorgensen H, Nigra TP. Elevation of serum triglyceride levels from oral isotretinoin in disorders of keratinization. *Arch Dermatol* 116:1369–1372, 1980. 6. Ellis CN, Madison KC, Pennes DR, Martel W, Voorhees JJ. Isotretinoin therapy is associated with early skeletal radiographic changes. *J Am Acad Dermatol* 10:1024–1029, 1984. 7. Dicken CH, Connolly SM. Eruptive xanthomas associated with isotretinoin (13-*cis*-retinoic acid). *Arch Dermatol* 116:951–952, 1980. 8. Strauss JS, Rapini RP, Shalita AR, et al. Isotretinoin therapy for acne: results of a multicenter dose-response study. *J Am Acad Dermatol* 10:490–496, 1984.

PATIENT CONSENT FORM:

To be completed by the patient, her parent/guardian* and signed by her prescriber.
Please read each item below and initial in the space provided to indicate that you understand each item and agree to follow your prescriber's instructions. **DO NOT SIGN THIS CONSENT AND DO NOT TAKE ACCUTANE IF THERE IS ANYTHING THAT YOU DO NOT UNDERSTAND.** A parent or guardian of a minor patient must also read and understand each item before signing the consent.

1. I, ______________________________________,
(Patient's Name)
understand that Accutane is a very powerful medicine with the potential for serious Adverse Effects that is used to treat severe nodular acne that did not get better with other treatments including oral antibiotics.
INITIALS: ____________
2. I understand that I must not take Accutane (isotretinoin) if I am pregnant. I understand that I must not take Accutane if I am able to become pregnant and I am not using the required two separate forms of effective methods of birth control.
INITIALS: ____________
3. I understand from my prescriber that although not every fetus exposed to Accutane has resulted in a deformed child, there is an extremely high risk that my unborn baby could have severe birth defects if I am pregnant or become pregnant while taking Accutane in any amount even for short periods of time. Potentially any fetus exposed during pregnancy can be affected.
INITIALS: ____________
4. I understand that I must avoid pregnancy during the entire time of my treatment and for 1 month after the end of my treatment with Accutane.
INITIALS: ____________
5. I understand that if I am able to become pregnant and unless I absolutely and consistently abstain from sexual intercourse, I must use two separate, effective forms of birth control (contraception) **AT THE SAME TIME.**
INITIALS: ____________
6. I understand from discussions with my prescriber that birth control pills and injectable/implantable birth control products are the most effective forms of birth control. I understand that there have been reports of pregnancy from women who have used birth control pills, as well as women who have used injectable/implantable birth control products and I understand that pregnancies occur more often when only a single method of birth control is used. Therefore, I understand that it is essential that I use two different methods, even if one of the methods I choose is birth control pills or injectable/implantable birth control products.
INITIALS: ____________
7. I understand that the following are considered effective forms of contraception:
Primary: Tubal ligation, partner's vasectomy, birth control pills, injectable/implantable birth control products, and an IUD
Secondary: Diaphragms, latex condoms, and cervical caps; each must be used with a spermicide.
I understand that at least one of my two chosen methods of birth control must be a primary method, and that any birth control method can fail, even when two forms are used at the same time.
INITIALS: ____________
8. I understand that I may receive free initial contraceptive counseling and pregnancy testing from a consulting physician or family planning center. I understand that my Accutane prescriber can provide me with an Accutane Patient Referral Form for this consultation.
INITIALS: ____________
9. I understand that I must begin actively avoiding pregnancy as described above at least 1 month before taking the first dose of Accutane, throughout treatment with Accutane and for 1 month after I have completed Accutane treatment.
INITIALS: ____________
10. I understand that I cannot receive a prescription for Accutane unless I have 2 negative pregnancy test results. The first pregnancy test should be during the office visit when my prescriber decides to prescribe Accutane. The second test should be on the second day of my next menstrual cycle or 11 days after the last time I had unprotected sexual intercourse, whichever is later. I understand that I will have additional pregnancy testing, monthly, throughout my Accutane therapy.
INITIALS: ____________
11. I understand that I should not start Accutane until I am sure that I am not pregnant and have negative results from 2 pregnancy tests.
INITIALS: ____________
12. I have read and understand the materials my prescriber has given to me, including the brochure *Important Information Concerning Your Treatment with Accutane® (isotretinoin)*. I have watched and understand the Roche video provided to me by my prescriber about contraception. I have also been told about a confidential counseling line that I may call for additional information about birth control and I have received information on emergency contraception.
INITIALS: ____________
13. I understand that I must not share my medication with anyone else and that I should not give blood until 1 month after taking my last dose of Accutane, because if I do, someone else's unborn baby may be exposed to Accutane.
INITIALS: ____________
14. I understand that I must immediately stop taking Accutane and inform my prescriber if I become pregnant, miss my menstrual period, or stop using birth control.
INITIALS: ____________
15. I have been given information about the confidential Accutane Survey by my prescriber and he/she has explained to me how important it is to join the Accutane Survey.

My prescriber has answered all my questions about Accutane and the Accutane information provided to me. I understand all the information I have received and that avoiding pregnancy during Accutane treatment is my responsibility.
INITIALS: ____________
I now authorize my prescriber ________________ to begin my treatment with Accutane.

____
Patient signature Date

____
Parent/guardian signature Date

____
Please print: Patient name and address

____
Telephone (area code)

I have fully explained to the patient, ________________________, the nature and purpose of the treatment described above and the risks to females of childbearing potential. I have asked the patient if she has any questions regarding her treatment with Accutane and have answered those questions to the best of my ability.

____
Prescriber signature Date

*if patient is a minor under the age of 18.

Roche Pharmaceuticals
Roche Laboratories Inc., 340 Kingsland Street, Nutley, New Jersey 07110-1199

Revised: May 2000

Shown in Product Identification Guide, page 332

Continued on next page

BACTRIM™ ℞

[*bac 'trim*]

brand of trimethoprim and sulfamethoxazole

IV INFUSION

The following text is complete prescribing information based on official labeling in effect June 2000.

DESCRIPTION

Bactrim (trimethoprim and sulfamethoxazole) IV Infusion, a sterile solution for intravenous infusion only, is a synthetic antibacterial combination product. Each 5 mL contains 80 mg trimethoprim (16 mg/mL) and 400 mg sulfamethoxazole (80 mg/mL) compounded with 40% propylene glycol, 10% ethyl alcohol and 0.3% diethanolamine; 1% benzyl alcohol and 0.1% sodium metabisulfite added as preservatives, water for injection, and pH adjusted to approximately 10 with sodium hydroxide.

Trimethoprim is 2,4-diamino-5-(3,4,5-trimethoxybenzyl)pyrimidine. It is a white to light yellow, odorless, bitter compound with a molecular weight of 290.3.

Sulfamethoxazole is N^1-(5-methyl-3-isoxazolyl)sulfanilamide. It is an almost white, odorless, tasteless compound with a molecular weight of 253.28.

CLINICAL PHARMACOLOGY

Following a 1-hour intravenous infusion of a single dose of 160 mg trimethoprim and 800 mg sulfamethoxazole to 11 patients whose weight ranged from 105 lbs to 165 lbs (mean, 143 lbs), the peak plasma concentrations of trimethoprim and sulfamethoxazole were 3.4 ± 0.3 µg/mL and 46.3 ± 2.7 µg/mL, respectively. Following repeated intravenous administration of the same dose at 8-hour intervals, the mean plasma concentrations just prior to and immediately after each infusion at steady state were 5.6 ± 0.6 µg/mL and 8.8 ± 0.9 µg/mL for trimethoprim and 70.6 ± 7.3 µg/mL and 105.6 ± 10.9 µg/mL for sulfamethoxazole. The mean plasma half-life was 11.3 ± 0.7 hours for trimethoprim and 12.8 ± 1.8 hours for sulfamethoxazole. All of these 11 patients had normal renal function, and their ages ranged from 17 to 78 years (median, 60 years).[1]

Pharmacokinetic studies in children and adults suggest an age-dependent half-life of trimethoprim, as indicated in the following table.[2]

Age (years)	No. of Patients	Mean TMP Half-life (hours)
<1	2	7.67
1–10	9	5.49
10–20	5	8.19
20–63	6	12.82

Patients with severely impaired renal function exhibit an increase in the half-lives of both components, requiring dosage regimen adjustment (See DOSAGE AND ADMINISTRATION section).

Both trimethoprim and sulfamethoxazole exist in the blood as unbound, protein-bound and metabolized forms; sulfamethaxazole also exists as the conjugated form. The metabolism of sulfamethoxazole occurs predominately by N_4-acetylation, although the glucuronide conjugate has been identified. The principal metabolites of trimethoprim are the 1- and 3-oxides and the 3′- and 4′-hydroxy derivatives. The free forms of trimethoprim and sulfamethoxazole are considered to be the therapeutically active forms. Approximately 44% of trimethoprim and 70% of sulfamethoxazole are bound to plasma proteins. The presence of 10 mg percent sulfamethoxazole in plasma decreases the protein binding of trimethoprim by an insignificant degree; trimethoprim does not influence the protein binding of sulfamethoxazole.

Excretion of trimethoprim and sulfamethoxazole is primarily by the kidneys through both glomerular filtration and tubular secretion. Urine concentrations of both trimethoprim and sulfamethoxazole are considerably higher than are the concentrations in the blood. The percent of dose excreted in urine over a 12-hour period following the intravenous administration of the first dose of 240 mg of trimethoprim and 1200 mg of sulfamethoxazole on day 1 ranged from 17% to 42.4% as free trimethoprim; 7% to 12.7% as free sulfamethoxazole; and 36.7% to 56% as total (free plus the N_4-acetylated metabolite) sulfamethoxazole. When administered together as Bactrim, neither trimethoprim nor sulfamethoxazole affects the urinary excretion pattern of the other. Both trimethoprim and sulfamethoxazole distribute to sputum and vaginal fluid; trimethoprim also distributes to bronchial secretions, and both pass the placental barrier and are excreted in breast milk.

Microbiology: Sulfamethoxazole inhibits bacterial synthesis of dihydrofolic acid by competing with *para* -aminobenzoic acid (PABA). Trimethoprim blocks the production of tetrahydrofolic acid from dihydrofolic acid by binding to and reversibly inhibiting the required enzyme, dihydrofolate reductase. Thus, Bactrim blocks two consecutive steps in the biosynthesis of nucleic acids and proteins essential to many bacteria.

In vitro studies have shown that bacterial resistance develops more slowly with Bactrim than with either trimethoprim or sulfamethoxazole alone.

In vitro serial dilution tests have shown that the spectrum of antibacterial activity of Bactrim includes common bacterial pathogens with the exception of *Pseudomonas aeruginosa.* The following organisms are usually susceptible: *Escherichia coli, Klebsiella* species, *Enterobacter* species, *Morganella morganii, Proteus mirabilis,* indole-positive *Proteus* species including *Proteus vulgaris, Haemophilus influenzae* (including ampicillin-resistant strains), *Streptococcus pneumoniae, Shigella flexneri* and *Shigella sonnei.* It should be noted, however, that there are little clinical data on the use of Bactrim IV Infusion in serious systemic infections due to *Haemophilus influenzae* and *Streptococcus pneumoniae.*

[See table below]

The recommended quantitative disc susceptibility method may be used for estimating the susceptibility of bacteria to Bactrim.[3,4] With this procedure, a report from the laboratory of "Susceptible to trimethoprim and sulfamethoxazole" indicates that the infection is likely to respond to therapy with Bactrim. If the infection is confined to the urine, a report of "Intermediate susceptibility to trimethoprim and sulfamethoxazole" also indicates that the infection is likely to respond. A report of "Resistant to trimethoprim and sulfamethoxazole" indicates that the infection is unlikely to respond to therapy with Bactrim.

INDICATIONS AND USAGE

Pneumocystis Carinii Pneumonia: Bactrim IV Infusion is indicated in the treatment of *Pneumocystis carinii* pneumonia in children and adults.

Shigellosis: Bactrim IV Infusion is indicated in the treatment of enteritis caused by susceptible strains of *Shigella flexneri* and *Shigella sonnei* in children and adults.

Urinary Tract Infections: Bactrim IV Infusion is indicated in the treatment of severe or complicated urinary tract infections due to susceptible strains of *Escherichia coli, Klebsiella* species, *Enterobacter* species, *Morganella morganii* and *Proteus* species when oral administration of Bactrim is not feasible and when the organism is not susceptible to single-agent antibacterials effective in the urinary tract.

Although appropriate culture and susceptibility studies should be performed, therapy may be started while awaiting the results of these studies.

CONTRAINDICATIONS

Bactrim is contraindicated in patients with a known hypersensitivity to trimethoprim or sulfonamides and in patients with documented megaloblastic anemia due to folate deficiency. Bactrim is also contraindicated in pregnant patients and nursing mothers, because sulfonamides pass the placenta and are excreted in the milk and may cause kernicterus. Bactrim is contraindicated in infants less than 2 months of age.

WARNINGS

FATALITIES ASSOCIATED WITH THE ADMINISTRATION OF SULFONAMIDES, ALTHOUGH RARE, HAVE OCCURRED DUE TO SEVERE REACTIONS, INCLUDING STEVENS-JOHNSON SYNDROME, TOXIC EPIDERMAL NECROLYSIS, FULMINANT HEPATIC NECROSIS, AGRANULOCYTOSIS, APLASTIC ANEMIA AND OTHER BLOOD DYSCRASIAS. BACTRIM SHOULD BE DISCONTINUED AT THE FIRST APPEARANCE OF SKIN RASH OR ANY SIGN OF ADVERSE REACTION. Clinical signs, such as rash, sore throat, fever, arthralgia, cough, shortness of breath, pallor, purpura or jaundice may be early indications of serious reactions. In rare instances a skin rash may be followed by more severe reactions, such as Stevens-Johnson syndrome, toxic epidermal necrolysis, hepatic necrosis or serious blood disorder. Complete blood counts should be done frequently in patients receiving sulfonamides.

BACTRIM SHOULD NOT BE USED IN THE TREATMENT OF STREPTOCOCCAL PHARYNGITIS. Clinical studies have documented that patients with group A β-hemolytic streptococcal tonsillopharyngitis have a greater incidence of bacteriologic failure when treated with Bactrim than do those patients treated with penicillin, as evidenced by failure to eradicate this organism from the tonsillopharyngeal area.

Bactrim IV Infusion contains sodium metabisulfite, a sulfite that may cause allergic-type reactions, including anaphylactic symptoms and life-threatening or less severe asthmatic episodes in certain susceptible people. The overall prevalence of sulfite sensitivity in the general population is unknown and probably low. Sulfite sensitivity is seen more frequently in asthmatic than in nonasthmatic people.

PRECAUTIONS

General: Bactrim should be given with caution to patients with impaired renal or hepatic function, to those with possible folate deficiency (eg, the elderly, chronic alcoholics, patients receiving anticonvulsant therapy, patients with malabsorption syndrome, and patients in malnutrition states) and to those with severe allergies or bronchial asthma. In glucose-6-phosphate dehydrogenase deficient individuals, hemolysis may occur. This reaction is frequently dose-related.

Local irritation and inflammation due to extravascular infiltration of the infusion have been observed with Bactrim IV Infusion. If these occur the infusion should be discontinued and restarted at another site.

Use in the Elderly: There may be an increased risk of severe adverse reactions in elderly patients, particularly when complicating conditions exist, eg, impaired kidney and/or liver function, or concomitant use of other drugs. Severe skin reactions, generalized bone marrow suppression (see WARNINGS and ADVERSE REACTIONS sections) or a specific decrease in platelets (with or without purpura) are the most frequently reported severe adverse reactions in elderly patients. In those concurrently receiving certain diuretics, primarily thiazides, an increased incidence of thrombocytopenia with purpura has been reported. Appropriate dosage adjustments should be made for patients with impaired kidney function (see DOSAGE AND ADMINISTRATION section).

Use in the Treatment of Pneumocystis Carinii Pneumonia in Patients with Acquired Immunodeficiency Syndrome (AIDS): AIDS patients may not tolerate or respond to Bactrim in the same manner as non-AIDS patients. The incidence of side effects, particularly rash, fever, leukopenia, and elevated aminotransferase (transaminase) values, with Bactrim therapy in AIDS patients who are being treated for *Pneumocystis carinii* pneumonia has been reported to be greatly increased compared with the incidence normally associated with the use of Bactrim in non-AIDS patients.

Laboratory Tests: Appropriate culture and susceptibility studies should be performed before and throughout treatment. Complete blood counts should be done frequently in patients receiving Bactrim; if a significant reduction in the count of any formed blood element is noted, Bactrim should be discontinued. Urinalyses with careful microscopic examination and renal function tests should be performed during therapy, particularly for those patients with impaired renal function.

Drug Interactions: In elderly patients concurrently receiving certain diuretics, primarily thiazides, an increased incidence of thrombocytopenia with purpura has been reported. It has been reported that Bactrim may prolong the prothrombin time in patients who are receiving the anticoagulant warfarin. This interaction should be kept in mind when Bactrim is given to patients already on anticoagulant therapy, and the coagulation time should be reassessed.

Bactrim may inhibit the hepatic metabolism of phenytoin. Bactrim, given at a common clinical dosage, increased the phenytoin half-life by 39% and decreased the phenytoin metabolic clearance rate by 27%. When administering these drugs concurrently, one should be alert for possible excessive phenytoin effect.

Sulfonamides can also displace methotrexate from plasma protein binding sites, thus increasing free methotrexate concentrations.

Drug/Laboratory Test Interactions: Bactrim, specifically the trimethoprim component, can interfere with a serum methotrexate assay as determined by the competitive binding protein technique (CBPA) when a bacterial dihydrofolate reductase is used as the binding protein. No interference occurs, however, if methotrexate is measured by a radioimmunoassay (RIA).

The presence of trimethoprim and sulfamethoxazole may also interfere with the Jaffé alkaline picrate reaction assay for creatinine, resulting in overestimations of about 10% in the range of normal values.

Carcinogenesis, Mutagenesis, Impairment of Fertility:

Carcinogenesis: Long-term studies in animals to evaluate carcinogenic potential have not been conducted with Bactrim IV Infusion.

REPRESENTATIVE MINIMUM INHIBITORY CONCENTRATION VALUES FOR BACTRIM-SUSCEPTIBLE ORGANISMS (MIC—µg/mL)

Bacteria	TMP alone	SMX alone	TMP/SMX(1:20) TMP	SMX
Escherichia coli	0.05–1.5	1.0–245	0.05–0.5	0.95–9.5
Proteus species (indole positive)	0.5–5.0	7.35–300	0.05–1.5	0.95–28.5
Morganella morganii	0.5–5.0	7.35–300	0.05–1.5	0.95–28.5
Proteus mirabilis	0.5–1.5	7.35–30	0.05–0.15	0.95–2.85
Klebsiella species	0.15–5.0	2.45–245	0.05–1.5	0.95–28.5
Enterobacter species	0.15–5.0	2.45–245	0.05–1.5	0.95–28.5
Haemophilus influenzae	0.15–1.5	2.85–95	0.015–0.15	0.285–2.85
Streptococcus pneumoniae	0.15–1.5	7.35–24.5	0.05–0.15	0.95–2.85
*Shigella flexneri**	<0.01–0.04	<0.16–>320	<0.002–0.03	0.04–0.625
*Shigella sonnei**	0.02–0.08	0.625–>320	0.004–0.06	0.08–1.25

TMP = trimethoprim

SMX = sulfamethoxazole

* Rudoy RC, Nelson JD, Haltalin KC. *Antimicrob Agents Chemother.* May 1974;5:439–443.

Mutagenesis: Bacterial mutagenic studies have not been performed with sulfamethoxazole and trimethoprim in combination. Trimethoprim was demonstrated to be nonmutagenic in the Ames assay. No chromosomal damage was observed in human leukocytes cultured in vitro with sulfamethoxazole and trimethoprim alone or in combination; the concentrations used exceeded blood levels of these compounds following therapy with Bactrim. Observations of leukocytes obtained from patients treated with Bactrim revealed no chromosomal abnormalities.

Impairment of Fertility: Bactrim IV Infusion has not been studied in animals for evidence of impairment of fertility. However, studies in rats at oral dosages as high as 70 mg/kg trimethoprim plus 350 mg/kg sulfamethoxazole daily showed no adverse effects on fertility or general reproductive performance.

Pregnancy: Teratogenic Effects: Pregnancy Category C. In rats, oral doses of 533 mg/kg sulfamethoxazole or 200 mg/kg trimethoprim produced teratological effects manifested mainly as cleft palates.

The highest dose which did not cause cleft palates in rats was 512 mg/kg sulfamethoxazole or 192 mg/kg trimethoprim when administered separately. In two studies in rats, no teratology was observed when 512 mg/kg of sulfamethoxazole was used in combination with 128 mg/kg of trimethoprim. In one study, however, cleft palates were observed in one litter out of 9 when 355 mg/kg of sulfamethoxazole was used in combination with 88 mg/kg of trimethoprim.

In some rabbit studies, an overall increase in fetal loss (dead and resorbed and malformed conceptuses) was associated with doses of trimethoprim six times the human therapeutic dose.

While there are no large, well-controlled studies on the use of trimethoprim and sulfamethoxazole in pregnant women, Brumfitt and Pursell,[5] in a retrospective study, reported the outcome of 186 pregnancies during which the mother received either placebo or oral trimethoprim and sulfamethoxazole. The incidence of congenital abnormalities was 4.5% (3 of 66) in those who received placebo and 3.3% (4 of 120) in those receiving trimethoprim and sulfamethoxazole. There were no abnormalities in the 10 children whose mothers received the drug during the first trimester. In a separate survey, Brumfitt and Pursell also found no congenital abnormalities in 35 children whose mothers had received oral trimethoprim and sulfamethoxazole at the time of conception or shortly thereafter.

Because trimethoprim and sulfamethoxazole may interfere with folic acid metabolism, Bactrim IV Infusion should be used during pregnancy only if the potential benefit justifies the potential risk to the fetus.

Nonteratogenic Effects: See CONTRAINDICATIONS section.

Nursing Mothers: See CONTRAINDICATIONS section.

Pediatric Use: Bactrim IV Infusion is not recommended for infants younger than two months of age (see CONTRAINDICATIONS section).

ADVERSE REACTIONS

The most common adverse effects are gastrointestinal disturbances (nausea, vomiting, anorexia) and allergic skin reactions (such as rash and urticaria). **FATALITIES ASSOCIATED WITH THE ADMINISTRATION OF SULFONAMIDES, ALTHOUGH RARE, HAVE OCCURRED DUE TO SEVERE REACTIONS, INCLUDING STEVENS-JOHNSON SYNDROME, TOXIC EPIDERMAL NECROLYSIS, FULMINANT HEPATIC NECROSIS, AGRANULOCYTOSIS, APLASTIC ANEMIA AND OTHER BLOOD DYSCRASIAS (SEE WARNINGS SECTION).** Local reaction, pain and slight irritation on IV administration are infrequent. Thrombophlebitis has rarely been observed.

Hematologic: Agranulocytosis, aplastic anemia, thrombocytopenia, leukopenia, neutropenia, hemolytic anemia, megaloblastic anemia, hypoprothrombinemia, methemoglobinemia, eosinophilia.

Allergic Reactions: Stevens-Johnson syndrome, toxic epidermal necrolysis, anaphylaxis, allergic myocarditis, erythema multiforme, exfoliative dermatitis, angioedema, drug fever, chills, Henoch-Schoenlein purpura, serum sickness-like syndrome, generalized allergic reactions, generalized skin eruptions, conjunctival and scleral injection, photosensitivity, pruritus, urticaria and rash. In addition, periarteritis nodosa and systemic lupus erythematosus have been reported.

Gastrointestinal: Hepatitis (including cholestatic jaundice and hepatic necrosis), elevation of serum transaminase and bilirubin, pseudomembraneous enterocolitis, pancreatitis, stomatitis, glossitis, nausea, emesis, abdominal pain, diarrhea, anorexia.

Genitourinary: Renal failure, interstitial nephritis, BUN and serum creatinine elevation, toxic nephrosis with oliguria and anuria, and crystalluria.

Neurologic: Aseptic meningitis, convulsions, peripheral neuritis, ataxia, vertigo, tinnitus, headache.

Psychiatric: Hallucinations, depression, apathy, nervousness.

Endocrine: The sulfonamides bear certain chemical similarities to some goitrogens, diuretics (acetazolamide and the thiazides) and oral hypoglycemic agents. Cross-sensitivity may exist with these agents. Diuresis and hypoglycemia have occurred rarely in patients receiving sulfonamides.

Musculoskeletal: Arthralgia and myalgia.

Respiratory: Pulmonary infiltrates.

Miscellaneous: Weakness, fatigue, insomnia.

OVERDOSAGE

Acute: Since there has been no extensive experience in humans with single doses of Bactrim IV Infusion in excess of 25 mL (400 mg trimethoprim and 2000 mg sulfamethoxazole), the maximum tolerated dose in humans is unknown. Signs and symptoms of overdosage reported with sulfonamides include anorexia, colic, nausea, vomiting, dizziness, headache, drowsiness and unconsciousness. Pyrexia, hematuria and crystalluria may be noted. Blood dyscrasias and jaundice are potential late manifestations of overdosage.

Signs of acute overdosage with trimethoprim include nausea, vomiting, dizziness, headache, mental depression, confusion and bone marrow depression.

General principles of treatment include the administration of intraveneous fluids if urine output is low and renal function is normal. Acidification of the urine will increase renal elimination of trimethoprim. The patient should be monitored with blood counts and appropriate blood chemistries, including electrolytes. If a significant blood dyscrasia or jaundice occurs, specific therapy should be instituted for these complications. Peritoneal dialysis is not effective and hemodialysis is only moderately effective in eliminating trimethoprim and sulfamethoxazole.

Chronic: Use of Bactrim IV Infusion at high doses and/or for extended periods of time may cause bone marrow depression manifested as thrombocytopenia, leukopenia and/or megaloblastic anemia. If signs of bone marrow depression occur, the patient should be given leucovorin 5 to 15 mg daily until normal hematopoiesis is restored.

Animal Toxicity: The LD_{50} of Bactrim IV Infusion in mice is 700 mg/kg or 7.3 mL/kg; in rats and rabbits the LD_{50} is >500 mg/kg or >5.2 mL/kg. The vehicle produced the same LD_{50} in each of these species as the active drug.

The signs and symptoms noted in mice, rats and rabbits with Bactrim IV Infusion or its vehicle at the high IV doses used in acute toxicity studies included ataxia, decreased motor activity, loss of righting reflex, tremors or convulsions, and/or respiratory depression.

DOSAGE AND ADMINISTRATION

CONTRAINDICATED IN INFANTS LESS THAN 2 MONTHS OF AGE. CAUTION—BACTRIM IV INFUSION MUST BE DILUTED IN 5% DEXTROSE IN WATER SOLUTION PRIOR TO ADMINISTRATION. DO NOT MIX BACTRIM IV INFUSION WITH OTHER DRUGS OR SOLUTIONS. RAPID INFUSION OR BOLUS INJECTION MUST BE AVOIDED.

Dosage:

CHILDREN AND ADULTS:

Pneumocystis Carinii Pneumonia: Total daily dose is 15 to 20 mg/kg (based on the trimethoprim component) given in 3 or 4 equally divided doses every 6 to 8 hours for up to 14 days. One investigator noted that a total daily dose of 10 to 15 mg/kg was sufficient in 10 adult patients with normal renal function.[6]

Severe Urinary Tract Infections and Shigellosis: Total daily dose is 8 to 10 mg/kg (based on the trimethoprim component) given in 2 or 4 equally divided doses every 6, 8 or 12 hours for up to 14 days for severe urinary tract infections and 5 days for shigellosis. The maximum recommended daily dose is 60 mL per day.

For Patients with Impaired Renal Function: When renal function is impaired, a reduced dosage should be employed using the following table:

Creatinine Clearance (mL/min)	Recommended Dosage Regimen
Above 30	Usual standard regimen
15–30	1/2 the usual regimen
Below 15	Use not recommended

Method of Preparation: Bactrim IV Infusion must be diluted. EACH 5 ML SHOULD BE ADDED TO 125 ML OF 5% DEXTROSE IN WATER. After diluting with 5% dextrose in water the solution should not be refrigerated and should be used within 6 hours. If a dilution of 5 mL per 100 mL of 5% dextrose in water is desired, it should be used within 4 hours. If upon visual inspection there is cloudiness or evidence of crystallization after mixing, the solution should be discarded and a fresh solution prepared.

Multidose Vials: After initial entry into the vial, the remaining contents must be used within 48 hours.

The following infusion systems have been tested and found satisfactory: unit-dose glass containers; unit-dose polyvinyl chloride and polyolefin containers. No other systems have been tested and therefore no others can be recommended.

Dilution: EACH 5 ML OF BACTRIM IV INFUSION SHOULD BE ADDED TO 125 ML OF 5% DEXTROSE IN WATER.

Note: In those instances where fluid restriction is desirable, each 5 mL may be added to 75 mL of 5% dextrose in water. Under these circumstances the solution should be mixed just prior to use and should be administered within 2 hours. If upon visual inspection there is cloudiness or evidence of crystallization after mixing, the solution should be discarded and a fresh solution prepared.

DO NOT MIX BACTRIM IV INFUSION–5% DEXTROSE IN WATER WITH DRUGS OR SOLUTIONS IN THE SAME CONTAINER.

Administration: The solution should be given by intravenous infusion over a period of 60 to 90 minutes. Rapid infusion or bolus injection must be avoided. Bactrim IV Infusion should not be given intramuscularly.

HOW SUPPLIED

10-mL *Vials,* containing 160 mg trimethoprim (16 mg/mL) and 800 mg sulfamethoxazole (80 mg/mL) for infusion with 5% dextrose in water. Boxes of 10 (NDC 0004-1955-01).

30-mL *Multidose Vials,* each 5 mL containing 80 mg trimethoprim (16 mg/mL) and 400 mg sulfamethoxazole (80 mg/mL) for infusion with 5% dextrose in water. Boxes of 1 (NDC 0004-1958-01).

STORE AT ROOM TEMPERATURE (15°–30°C or 59°–86°F). DO NOT REFRIGERATE.

Bactrim is also available as *DS (double strength) Tablets* (white, notched, capsule shaped), containing 160 mg trimethoprim and 800 mg sulfamethoxazole—bottles of 100 (NDC 0004-0117-01), 250 (NDC 0004-0117-04) and 500 (NDC 0004-0117-14). Imprint on tablets: (front) BACTRIM-DS; (back) ROCHE.

Tablets (light green, scored, capsule shaped), containing 80 mg trimethoprim and 400 mg sulfamethoxazole—bottles of 100 (NDC 0004-0050-01). Imprint on tablets: (front) BACTRIM; (back) ROCHE.

Pediatric Suspension (pink, cherry flavored), containing 40 mg trimethoprim and 200 mg sulfamethoxazole per teaspoonful (5 mL)—bottles of 16 oz (1 pint) (NDC 0004-1033-28).

REFERENCES

1. Grose WE, Bodey GP, Loo TL. Clinical Pharmacology of Intravenously Administered Trimethoprim-Sulfamethoxazole. *Antimicrob Agents Chemother.* Mar 1979;15:447-451. 2. Siber GR, Gorham C, Durbin W, Lesko L, Levin MJ. Pharmacology of Intravenous Trimethoprim-Sulfamethoxazole in Children and Adults. *Current Chemotherapy and Infectious Diseases.* American Society for Microbiology, Washington, D.C., 1980, Vol. 1, pp. 691-692. 3. Bauer AW, Kirby WMM, Sherris JC, Turck M. Antibiotic Susceptibility Testing by a Standardized Single Disk Method. *Am J Clin Pathol.* Apr 1966;45:493-496.4. National Committee for Clinical Laboratory Standards. *Performance Standards for Antimicrobial Disc Susceptibility Test.* 771 East Lancaster Avenue, Villanova, Pennsylvania 19085: Approved Standard ASM-2. 5. Brumfitt W, Pursell R. Trimethoprim/Sulfamethoxazole in the Treatment of Bacteriuria in Women. *J Infect Dis.* Nov 1973;128 (Suppl):S657-S663. 6. Winston DJ, Lau WK, Gale RP, Young LS. Trimethoprim-Sulfamethoxazole for the Treatment of *Pneumocystis carinii* pneumonia. *Ann Intern Med.* June 1980;92:762-769.

Revised: March 1994

BACTRIM™ ℞

[*băc ' trĭm*]

brand of trimethoprim and sulfamethoxazole
DS (double strength) TABLETS,
TABLETS and PEDIATRIC SUSPENSION

The following text is complete prescribing information based on official labeling in effect June 2000.

DESCRIPTION

Bactrim (trimethoprim and sulfamethoxazole) is a synthetic antibacterial combination product available in DS (double strength) tablets, tablets and pediatric suspension for oral administration. Each DS tablet contains 160 mg trimethoprim and 800 mg sulfamethoxazole plus magnesium stearate, pregelatinized starch and sodium starch glycolate. Each tablet contains 80 mg trimethoprim and 400 mg sulfamethoxazole plus magnesium stearate, pregelatinized starch, sodium starch glycolate, FD&C Blue No. 1 lake, FD&C Yellow No. 6 lake and D&C Yellow No. 10 lake. Each teaspoonful (5 mL) of the pediatric suspension contains 40 mg trimethoprim and 200 mg sulfamethoxazole in a vehicle containing 0.3 percent alcohol, edetate disodium, glycerin, microcrystalline cellulose, parabens (methyl and propyl), polysorbate 80, saccharin sodium, simethicone, sorbitol, sucrose, FD&C Yellow No. 6, FD&C Red No. 40, flavors and water.

Trimethoprim is 2, 4-diamino-5-(3,4,5 trimethoxybenzyl)pyrimidine; the molecular formula is $C_{14}H_{18}N_4O_3$. It is a white to light yellow, odorless, bitter compound with a molecular weight of 290.3 and the following structural formula:

Sulfamethoxazole is N^1-(5-methyl-3-isoxazolyl)sulfanilamide; the molecular formula is $C_{10}H_{11}N_3O_3S$. It is almost white, odorless, tasteless compound with a molecular weight of 253.28 and the following structural formula:

Continued on next page

Bactrim—Cont.

CLINICAL PHARMACOLOGY

Bactrim is rapidly absorbed following oral administration. Both sulfamethoxazole and trimethoprim exist in the blood as unbound, protein-bound and metabolized forms; sulfamethoxazole also exists as the conjugated form. The metabolism of sulfamethoxazole occurs predominately by N_4-acetylation, although the glucuronide conjugate has been identified. The principal metabolites of trimethoprim are the 1- and 3-oxides and the 3'- and 4'- hydroxy derivatives. The free forms of sulfamethoxazole and trimethoprim are considered to be the therapeutically active forms. Approximately 44% of trimethoprim and 70% of sulfamethoxazole are bound to plasma proteins. The presence of 10 mg percent sulfamethoxazole in plasma decreases the protein binding of trimethoprim by an insignificant degree; trimethoprim does not influence the protein binding of sulfamethoxazole.

Peak blood levels for the individual components occur 1 to 4 hours after oral administration. The mean serum half-lives of sulfamethoxazole and trimethoprim are 10 and 8 to 10 hours, respectively. However, patients with severely impaired renal function exhibit an increase in the half-lives of both components, requiring dosage regimen adjustment (see DOSAGE AND ADMINISTRATION section). Detectable amounts of trimethoprim and sulfamethoxazole are present in the blood 24 hours after drug administration. During administration of 160 mg trimethoprim and 800 mg sulfamethoxazole bid, the mean steady-state plasma concentration of trimethoprim was 1.72 µg/mL. The steady-state mean plasma levels of free and total sulfamethoxazole were 57.4 µg/mL and 68.0 µg/mL, respectively. These steady-state levels were achieved after three days of drug administration.[1]

Excretion of sulfamethoxazole and trimethoprim is primarily by the kidneys through both glomerular filtration and tubular secretion. Urine concentrations of both sulfamethoxazole and trimethoprim are considerably higher than are the concentrations in the blood. The average percentage of the dose recovered in urine from 0 to 72 hours after a single oral dose of Bactrim is 84.5% for total sulfonamide and 66.8% for free trimethoprim. Thirty percent of the total sulfonamide is excreted as free sulfamethoxazole, with the remaining as N_4-acetylated metabolite.[2] When administered together as Bactrim, neither sulfamethoxazole nor trimethoprim affects the urinary excretion pattern of the other.

Both trimethoprim and sulfamethoxazole distribute to sputum, vaginal fluid and middle ear fluid; trimethoprim also distributes to bronchial secretion, and both pass the placental barrier and are excreted in human milk.

Microbiology: Trimethoprim blocks the production of tetrahydrofolic acid from dihydrofolic acid by binding to and reversibly inhibiting the required enzyme, dihydrofolate reductase. Sulfamethoxazole inhibits bacterial synthesis of dihydrofolic acid by competing with *para*-aminobenzoic acid (PABA). Thus, trimethoprim and sulfamethoxazole block two consecutive steps in the biosynthesis of nucleic acids and proteins essential to many bacteria.

In vitro studies have shown that bacterial resistance develops more slowly with both trimethoprim and sulfamethoxazole in combination than with either trimethoprim or sulfamethoxazole alone.

Trimethoprim and sulfamethoxazole have been shown to be active against most strains of the following microorganisms, both in vitro and in clinical infections as described in the INDICATIONS and USAGE section.

Aerobic gram-positive microorganisms:
Streptococcus pneumoniae

Aerobic gram-negative microorganisms:
Escherichia coli (including susceptible enterotoxigenic strains implicated in traveler's diarrhea)
Klebsiella species
Enterobacter species
Haemophilus influenzae
Morganella morganii
Proteus mirabilis
Proteus vulgaris
Shigella flexneri[3]
Shigella sonnei[3]

Other Organisms:
Pneumocystis carinii

Susceptibility Testing Methods:

Dilution Techniques: Quantitative methods are used to determine antimicrobial minimum inhibitory concentrations (MICs). These MICs provide estimates of the susceptibility of bacteria to antimicrobial compounds. The MICs should be determined using a standardized procedure. Standardized procedures are based on a dilution method[4] (broth or agar) or equivalent with standardized inoculum concentrations and standardized concentrations of trimethoprim/sulfamethoxazole powder. The MIC values should be interpreted according to the following criteria:

For testing *Enterobacteriaceae*:

MIC (µg/mL)	Interpretation
≤ 2/38	Susceptible (S)
≥ 4/76	Resistant (R)

When testing either *Haemophilus influenzae*[a] or *Streptococcus pneumoniae*[b]:

Microorganism		MIC (µg/mL)
Escherichia coli	ATCC 25922	≤ 0.5/9.5
Haemophilus influenzae[c]	ATCC 49247	0.03/0.59 – 0.25/4.75
Streptococcus pneumoniae[d]	ATCC 49619	0.12/2.4 – 1/19

c. This quality control range is applicable only to *Haemophilus influenzae* ATCC 49247 tested by broth microdilution procedure using *Haemophilus* Test Medium (HTM)[4].

d. This quality control range is applicable to tests performed by the broth microdilution method only using cation-adjusted Mueller-Hinton broth with 2% to 5% lysed horse blood[4].

Microorganism		Zone Diameter Ranges (mm)
Escherichia coli	ATCC 25922	24 – 32
Haemophilus influenzae[g]	ATCC 49247	24 – 32
Streptococcus pneumoniae[h]	ATCC 49619	20 – 28

* Mueller-Hinton agar should be checked for excessive levels of thymidine or thymine. To determine whether Mueller-Hinton medium has sufficiently low levels of thymidine and thymine, an *Enterococcus faecalis* (ATCC 29212 or ATCC 33186) may be tested with trimethoprim/sulfamethoxazole disks. A zone of inhibition ≥ 20 mm that is essentially free of fine colonies indicates a sufficiently low level of thymidine and thymine.

g. This quality control range is applicable only to *Haemophilus influenzae* ATCC 49247 tested by a disk diffusion procedure using *Haemophilus* Test Medium (HTM)[5].

h. This quality control range is applicable only to tests performed by disk diffusion using Mueller-Hinton agar supplemented with 5% defibrinated sheep blood when incubated in 5% CO_2[5].

MIC (µg/mL)	Interpretation[b]
≤ 0.5/9.5	Susceptible (S)
1/19–2/38	Intermediate (I)
≥ 4/76	Resistant (R)

a. These interpretative standards are applicable only to broth microdilution susceptibility tests with *Haemophilus influenzae* using *Haemophilus* Test Medium (HTM)[4].

b. These interpretative standards are applicable only to broth microdilution susceptibility tests using cation-adjusted Mueller-Hinton broth with 2% to 5% lysed horse blood[4].

A report of "Susceptible" indicates that the pathogen is likely to be inhibited if the antimicrobial compound in the blood reaches the concentrations usually achievable. A report of "Intermediate" indicates that the result should be considered equivocal, and, if the microorganism is not fully susceptible to alternative, clinically feasible drugs, the test should be repeated. This category implies possible clinical applicability in body sites where the drug is physiologically concentrated or in situations where high dosage of drug can be used. This category also provides a buffer zone which prevents small uncontrolled technical factors from causing major discrepancies in interpretation. A report of "Resistant" indicates that the pathogen is not likely to be inhibited if the antimicrobial compound in the blood reaches the concentrations usually achievable; other therapy should be selected.

Quality Control

Standardized susceptibility test procedures require the use of laboratory control microorganisms to control the technical aspects of the laboratory procedures. Standard trimethoprim/sulfamethoxazole powder should provide the following range of values:

[See table above]

Diffusion Techniques:

Quantitative methods that require measurement of zone diameters also provide reproducible estimates of the susceptibility of bacteria to antimicrobial compounds. One such standardized procedure[5] requires the use of standardized inoculum concentrations. This procedure uses paper disks impregnated with 1.25/23.75 µg of trimethoprim/sulfamethoxazole to test the susceptibility of microorganisms to trimethoprim/sulfamethoxazole.

Reports from the laboratory providing results of the standard single-disk susceptibility test with a 1.25/23.75 µg of trimethoprim/sulfamethoxazole disk should be interpreted according to the following criteria:

For testing either *Enterobacteriaceae* or *Haemophilus influenzae*[e]:

Zone Diameter (mm)	Interpretation
16	Susceptible (S)
11 – 15	Intermediate (I)
10	Resistant (R)

e. These zone diameter standards are applicable only for disk diffusion testing with *Haemophilus influenzae* and *Haemophilus* Test Medium (HTM)[5].

When testing *Streptococcus pneumoniae*[f]:

Zone Diameter (mm)	Interpretation
19	Susceptible (S)
16 – 18	Intermediate (I)
15	Resistant (R)

f. These zone diameter interpretative standards are applicable only to tests performed using Mueller-Hinton agar supplemented with 5% defibrinated sheep blood when incubated in 5% CO_2[5].

Interpretation should be as stated above for results using dilution techniques. Interpretation involves correlation of the diameter obtained in the disk test with the MIC for trimethoprim/sulfamethoxazole.

Quality Control

As with standardized dilution techniques, diffusion methods require the use of laboratory control microorganisms that are used to control the technical aspects of the laboratory procedures. For the diffusion technique, the 1.25/23.75 µg trimethoprim/sulfamethoxazole disk* should provide the following zone diameters in these laboratory test quality control strains:

[See table above]

INDICATIONS AND USAGE

Urinary Tract Infections: For the treatment of urinary tract infections due to susceptible strains of the following organisms: *Escherichia coli, Klebsiella* species, *Enterobacter* species, *Morganella morganii, Proteus mirabilis* and *Proteus vulgaris*. It is recommended that initial episodes of uncomplicated urinary tract infections be treated with a single effective antibacterial agent rather than the combination.

Acute Otitis Media: For the treatment of acute otitis media in pediatric patients due to susceptible strains of *Streptococcus pneumoniae* or *Haemophilus influenzae* when in the judgment of the physician Bactrim offers some advantage over the use of other antimicrobial agents. To date, there are limited data on the safety of repeated use of Bactrim in pediatric patients under two years of age. Bactrim is not indicated for prophylactic or prolonged administration in otitis media at any age.

Acute Exacerbations of Chronic Bronchitis in Adults: For the treatment of acute exacerbations of chronic bronchitis due to susceptible strains of *Streptococcus pneumoniae* or *Haemophilus influenzae* when in the judgment of the physician Bactrim offers some advantage over the use of a single antimicrobial agent.

Shigellosis: For the treatment of enteritis caused by susceptible strains of *Shigella flexneri* and *Shigella sonnei* when antibacterial therapy is indicated.

Pneumocystis Carinii Pneumonia: For the treatment of documented *Pneumocystis carinii* pneumonia and for prophylaxis against *Pneumocystis carinii* pneumonia in individuals who are immunosuppressed and considered to be at an increased risk of developing *Pneumocystis carinii* pneumonia.

Traveler's Diarrhea in Adults: For the treatment of traveler's diarrhea due to susceptible strains of enterotoxigenic *E. coli*.

CONTRAINDICATIONS

Bactrim is contraindicated in patients with a known hypersensitivity to trimethoprim or sulfonamides and in patients with documented megaloblastic anemia due to folate deficiency. Bactrim is also contraindicated in pregnant patients and nursing mothers, because sulfonamides pass the placenta and are excreted in the milk and may cause kernicterus. Bactrim is contraindicated in pediatric patients less than 2 months of age. Bactrim is also contraindicated in patients with marked hepatic damage or with severe renal insufficiency when renal function status cannot be monitored.

WARNINGS: FATALITIES ASSOCIATED WITH THE ADMINISTRATION OF SULFONAMIDES, ALTHOUGH RARE, HAVE OCCURRED DUE TO SEVERE REACTIONS INCLUDING STEVENS-JOHNSON SYNDROME, TOXIC EPIDERMAL NECROLYSIS, FULMINANT HEPATIC NECROSIS, AGRANULOCYTOSIS, APLASTIC ANEMIA AND OTHER BLOOD DYSCRASIAS.

SULFONAMIDES, INCLUDING SULFONAMIDE-CONTAINING PRODUCTS SUCH AS TRIMETHOPRIM/SULFAMETHOXAZOLE, SHOULD BE DISCONTINUED AT THE FIRST APPEARANCE OF SKIN RASH OR ANY SIGN OF ADVERSE REACTION. In rare instances, a skin rash may be followed by a more severe reaction, such as Stevens-Johnson syndrome, toxic epidermal necrolysis, hepatic necrosis, and serious blood disorders (see PRECAUTIONS). Clinical signs such as rash, sore throat, fever, arthralgia, pallor, purpura, or jaundice may be early indications of serious reactions.

Cough, shortness of breath, and pulmonary infiltrates are hypersensitivity reactions of the respiratory tract that have been reported in association with sulfonamide treatment.

The sulfonamides should not be used for the treatment of group A β-hemolytic streptococcal infections. In an established infection, they will not eradicate the streptococcus and, therefore, will not prevent sequelae such as rheumatic fever.

Pseudomembranous colitis has been reported with nearly all antibacterial agents, including trimethoprim/sulfamethoxazole, and may range in severity from mild to life-threatening. Therefore, it is important to consider this diagnosis in patients who present with diarrhea subsequent to the administration of antibacterial agents.

Treatment with antibacterial agents alters the normal flora of the colon and may permit overgrowth of clostridia. Studies indicate that a toxin produced by *Clostridium difficile* is one primary cause of "antibiotic-associated colitis."
After the diagnosis of pseudomembranous colitis has been established, therapeutic measures should be initiated. Mild cases of pseudomembranous colitis usually respond to drug discontinuation alone. In moderate to severe cases, consideration should be given to management with fluids and electrolytes, protein supplementation, and treatment with an antibacterial drug effective against *C. difficile*.

PRECAUTIONS

General: Bactrim should be given with caution to patients with impaired renal or hepatic function, to those with possible folate deficiency (eg, the elderly, chronic alcoholics, patients receiving anticonvulsant therapy, patients with malabsorption syndrome, and patients in malnutrition states) and to those with severe allergies or bronchial asthma. In glucose-6-phosphate dehydrogenase deficient individuals, hemolysis may occur. This reaction is frequently dose-related (see CLINICAL PHARMACOLOGY and DOSAGE AND ADMINISTRATION).
Cases of hypoglycemia in non-diabetic patients treated with Bactrim are seen rarely, usually occurring after a few days of therapy. Patients with renal dysfunction, liver disease, malnutrition or those receiving high doses of Bactrim are particularly at risk.
Hematological changes indicative of folic acid deficiency may occur in elderly patients or in patients with preexisting folic acid deficiency or kidney failure. These effects are reversible by folinic acid therapy.
Trimethoprim has been noted to impair phenylalanine metabolism, but this is of no significance in phenylketonuric patients on appropriate dietary restriction.
As with all drugs containing sulfonamides, caution is advisable in patients with porphyria or thyroid dysfunction.
Use in the Elderly: There may be an increased risk of severe adverse reactions in elderly patients, particularly when complicating conditions exist, eg, impaired kidney and/or liver function, or concomitant use of other drugs. Severe skin reactions, generalized bone marrow suppression (see WARNINGS and ADVERSE REACTIONS sections) or a specific decrease in platelets (with or without purpura) are the most frequently reported severe adverse reactions in elderly patients. In those concurrently receiving certain diuretics, primarily thiazides, an increased incidence of thrombocytopenia with purpura has been reported. Appropriate dosage adjustments should be made for patients with impaired kidney function and duration of use should be as short as possible to minimize risks of undesired reactions (see DOSAGE AND ADMINISTRATION section). The trimethoprim component of Bactrim may cause hyperkalemia when administered to patients with underlying disorders of potassium metabolism, with renal insufficiency, or when given concomitantly with drugs known to induce hyperkalemia. Close monitoring of serum potassium is warranted in these patients. Discontinuation of Bactrim treatment is recommended to help lower potassium serum levels.
Use in the Treatment of and Prophylaxis for Pneumocystis Carinii Pneumonia in Patients with Acquired Immunodeficiency Syndrome (AIDS): AIDS patients may not tolerate or respond to Bactrim in the same manner as non-AIDS patients. The incidence of side effects, particularly rash, fever, leukopenia and elevated aminotransferase (transaminase) values, with Bactrim therapy in AIDS patients who are being treated for *Pneumocystis carinii* pneumonia has been reported to be greatly increased compared with the incidence normally associated with the use of Bactrim in non-AIDS patients. The incidence of hyperkalemia appears to be increased in AIDS patients receiving Bactrim. Adverse effects are generally less severe in patients receiving Bactrim for prophylaxis. A history of mild intolerance to Bactrim in AIDS patients does not appear to predict intolerance of subsequent secondary prophylaxis.[6] However, if a patient develops skin rash or any sign of adverse reaction, therapy with Bactrim should be reevaluated (see WARNINGS).
High dosage of trimethoprim, as used in patients with *Pneumocystis carinii* pneumonia, induces a progressive but reversible increase of serum potassium concentrations in a substantial number of patients. Even treatment with recommended doses may cause hyperkalemia when trimethoprim is administered to patients with underlying disorders of potassium metabolism, with renal insufficiency, or if drugs known to induce hyperkalemia are given concomitantly. Close monitoring of serum potassium is warranted in these patients.
During treatment, adequate fluid intake and urinary output should be ensured to prevent crystalluria. Patients who are "slow acetylators" may be more prone to idiosyncratic reactions to sulfonamides.
Information for Patients: Patients should be instructed to maintain an adequate fluid intake in order to prevent crystalluria and stone formation.
Laboratory Tests: Complete blood counts should be done frequently in patients receiving Bactrim; if a significant reduction in the count of any formed blood element is noted, Bactrim should be discontinued. Urinalyses with careful microscopic examination and renal function tests should be performed during therapy, particularly for those patients with impaired renal function.
Drug Interactions: In elderly patients concurrently receiving certain diuretics, primarily thiazides, an increased incidence of thrombocytopenia with purpura has been reported.

Weight		Dose–every 12 hours	
lb	kg	Teaspoonfuls	Tablets
22	10	1 (5 mL)	—
44	20	2 (10 mL)	1
66	30	3 (15 mL)	$1^1/_2$
88	40	4 (20 mL)	2 or 1 DS tablet

Weight		Dose–every 6 hours	
lb	kg	Teaspoonfuls	Tablets
18	8	1 (5 mL)	—
35	16	2 (10 mL)	1
53	24	3 (15 mL)	$1^1/_2$
70	32	4 (20 mL)	2 or 1 DS tablet
88	40	5 (25 mL)	$2^1/_2$
106	48	6 (30 mL)	3 or $1^1/_2$DS tablets
141	64	8 (40 mL)	4 or 2 DS tablets
176	80	10 (50 mL)	5 or $2^1/_2$ DS Tablets

Body Surface Area	Dose–every 12 hours	
(m^2)	Teaspoonfuls	Tablets
0.26	$^1/_2$ (2.5 mL) (2.5 mL)	—
0.53	1 (5 mL)	$^1/_2$
1.06	2 (10 mL)	1

It has been reported that Bactrim may prolong the prothrombin time in patients who are receiving the anticoagulant warfarin. This interaction should be kept in mind when Bactrim is given to patients already on anticoagulant therapy, and the coagulation time should be reassessed.
Bactrim may inhibit the hepatic metabolism of phenytoin. Bactrim, given at a common clinical dosage, increased the phenytoin half-life by 39% and decreased the phenytoin metabolic clearance rate by 27%. When administering these drugs concurrently, one should be alert for possible excessive phenytoin effect.
Sulfonamides can also displace methotrexate from plasma protein binding sites and can compete with the renal transport of methotrexate, thus increasing free methotrexate concentrations.
There have been reports of marked but reversible nephrotoxicity with coadministration of Bactrim and cyclosporine in renal transplant recipients.
Increased digoxin blood levels can occur with concomitant Bactrim therapy, especially in elderly patients. Serum digoxin levels should be monitored.
Increased sulfamethoxazole blood levels may occur in patients who are also receiving indomethacin.
Occasional reports suggest that patients receiving pyrimethamine as malaria prophylaxis in doses exceeding 25 mg weekly may develop megaloblastic anemia if Bactrim is prescribed.
The efficacy of tricyclic antidepressants can decrease when coadministered with Bactrim.
Like other sulfonamide-containing drugs, Bactrim potentiates the effect of oral hypoglycemics.
In the literature, a single case of toxic delirium has been reported after concomitant intake of trimethoprim/sulfamethoxazole and amantadine.
Drug/Laboratory Test Interactions: Bactrim, specifically the trimethoprim component, can interfere with a serum methotrexate assay as determined by the competitive binding protein technique (CBPA) when a bacterial dihydrofolate reductase is used as the binding protein. No interference occurs, however, if methotrexate is measured by a radioimmunoassay (RIA).
The presence of trimethoprim and sulfamethoxazole may also interfere with the Jaffé alkaline picrate reaction assay for creatinine, resulting in overestimations of about 10% in the range of normal values.
Carcinogenesis, Mutagenesis, Impairment of Fertility:
Carcinogenesis: Long-term studies in animals to evaluate carcinogenic potential have not been conducted with Bactrim.
Mutagenesis: Bacterial mutagenic studies have not been performed with sulfamethoxazole and trimethoprim in combination. Trimethoprim was demonstrated to be nonmutagenic in the Ames assay. No chromosomal damage was observed in human leukocytes cultured in vitro with sulfamethoxazole and trimethoprim alone or in combination; the concentrations used exceeded blood levels of these compounds following therapy with Bactrim. Observations of leukocytes obtained from patients treated with Bactrim revealed no chromosomal abnormalities.
Impairment of Fertility: No adverse effects on fertility or general reproductive performance were observed in rats given oral dosages as high as 70 mg/kg/day trimethoprim plus 350 mg/kg/day sulfamethoxazole. These doses are 10.9-fold higher than the recommended human dose for trimethoprim and sulfamethoxazole.
Pregnancy: Teratogenic Effects: Pregnancy Category C. In rats, oral doses of 533 mg/kg sulfamethoxazole (16.7-fold higher than the recommended human dose) or 200 mg/kg trimethoprim (31.3-fold higher than the recommended human dose) produced teratologic effects manifested mainly as cleft palates.
The highest dose which did not cause cleft palates in rats was 512 mg/kg sulfamethoxazole (16-fold higher than the recommended human dose) or 192 mg/kg trimethoprim (30-fold higher than the recommended human dose) when administered separately. In two studies in rats, no teratology was observed when 512 mg/kg of sulfamethoxazole (16-fold higher than the recommended human dose) was used in combination with 128 mg/kg of trimethoprim (20-fold higher than the recommended human dose). In one study, however, cleft palates were observed in one litter out of 9 when 355 mg/kg of sulfamethoxazole (11.1-fold higher than the recommended human dose) was used in combination with 88 mg/kg of trimethoprim (13.8-fold higher than the recommended human dose).
In some rabbit studies, an overall increase in fetal loss (dead and resorbed and malformed conceptuses) was associated with doses of trimethoprim 6 times the human therapeutic dose.
While there are no large, well-controlled studies on the use of trimethoprim and sulfamethoxazole in pregnant women, Brumfitt and Pursell,[7] in a retrospective study, reported the outcome of 186 pregnancies during which the mother received either placebo or trimethoprim and sulfamethoxazole. The incidence of congenital abnormalities was 4.5% (3 of 66) in those who received placebo and 3.3% (4 of 120) in those receiving trimethoprim and sulfamethoxazole. There were no abnormalities in the 10 children whose mothers received the drug during the first trimester. In a separate survey, Brumfitt and Pursell also found no congenital abnormalities in 35 children whose mothers had received oral trimethoprim and sulfamethoxazole at the time of conception or shortly thereafter.
Because trimethoprim and sulfamethoxazole may interfere with folic acid metabolism, Bactrim should be used during pregnancy only if the potential benefit justifies the potential risk to the fetus.
Nonteratogenic Effects: See CONTRAINDICATIONS section.
Nursing Mothers: See CONTRAINDICATIONS section.
Pediatric Use: Bactrim is not recommended for pediatric patients younger than 2 months of age (see INDICATIONS and CONTRAINDICATIONS sections).

ADVERSE REACTIONS: The most common adverse effects are gastrointestinal disturbances (nausea, vomiting, anorexia) and allergic skin reactions (such as rash and urticaria). **FATALITIES ASSOCIATED WITH THE ADMINISTRATION OF SULFONAMIDES, ALTHOUGH RARE, HAVE OCCURRED DUE TO SEVERE REACTIONS, INCLUDING STEVENS-JOHNSON SYNDROME, TOXIC EPIDERMAL NECROLYSIS, FULMINANT HEPATIC NECROSIS, AGRANULOCYTOSIS, APLASTIC ANEMIA AND OTHER BLOOD DYSCRASIAS (SEE WARNINGS SECTION).**
Hematologic: Agranulocytosis, aplastic anemia, thrombocytopenia, leukopenia, neutropenia, hemolytic anemia, megaloblastic anemia, hypoprothrombinemia, methemoglobinemia, eosinophilia, pancytopenia, purpura.
Allergic Reactions: Stevens-Johnson syndrome, toxic epidermal necrolysis, anaphylaxis, allergic myocarditis, erythema multiforme, exfoliative dermatitis, angioedema, drug fever, chills, Henoch-Schoenlein purpura, serum sickness-like syndrome, generalized allergic reactions, generalized skin eruptions, photosensitivity, conjunctival and scleral injection, pruritus, urticaria and rash. In addition, periarteritis nodosa and systemic lupus erythematosus have been reported.
Gastrointestinal: Hepatitis (including cholestatic jaundice and hepatic necrosis), elevation of serum transaminase and bilirubin, pseudomembranous enterocolitis, pancreatitis, stomatitis, glossitis, nausea, emesis, abdominal pain, diarrhea, anorexia.
Genitourinary: Renal failure, interstitial nephritis, BUN and serum creatinine elevation, toxic nephrosis with oligu-

Continued on next page

Bactrim—Cont.

ria and anuria, crystalluria and nephrotoxicity in association with cyclosporine.

Metabolic and Nutritional: Hyperkalemia (see PRECAUTIONS: *Use in the Elderly* and *Use in the Treatment of and Prophylaxis for Pneumocystis Carinii Pneumonia in Patients with Acquired Immunodeficiency Syndrome [AIDS]*).
Neurologic: Aseptic meningitis, convulsions, peripheral neuritis, ataxia, vertigo, tinnitus, headache.
Psychiatric: Hallucinations, depression, apathy, nervousness.
Endocrine: The sulfonamides bear certain chemical similarities to some goitrogens, diuretics (acetazolamide and the thiazides) and oral hypoglycemic agents. Cross-sensitivity may exist with these agents. Diuresis and hypoglycemia have occurred rarely in patients receiving sulfonamides.
Musculoskeletal: Arthralgia and myalgia. Isolated cases of rhabdomyolysis have been reported with Bactrim, mainly in AIDS patients.
Respiratory: Cough, shortness of breath, and pulmonary infiltrates (see WARNINGS).
Miscellaneous: Weakness, fatigue, insomnia.

OVERDOSAGE

Acute: The amount of a single dose of Bactrim that is either associated with symptoms of overdosage or is likely to be life-threatening has not been reported. Signs and symptoms of overdosage reported with sulfonamides include anorexia, colic, nausea, vomiting, dizziness, headache, drowsiness and unconsciousness. Pyrexia, hematuria and crystalluria may be noted. Blood dyscrasias and jaundice are potential late manifestations of overdosage.
Signs of acute overdosage with trimethoprim include nausea, vomiting, dizziness, headache, mental depression, confusion and bone marrow depression.
General principles of treatment include the institution of gastric lavage or emesis, forcing oral fluids, and the administration of intravenous fluids if urine output is low and renal function is normal. Acidification of the urine will increase renal elimination of trimethoprim. The patient should be monitored with blood counts and appropriate blood chemistries, including electrolytes. If a significant blood dyscrasia or jaundice occurs, specific therapy should be instituted for these complications. Peritoneal dialysis is not effective and hemodialysis is only moderately effective in eliminating trimethoprim and sulfamethoxazole.
Chronic: Use of Bactrim at high doses and/or for extended periods of time may cause bone marrow depression manifested as thrombocytopenia, leukopenia and/or megaloblastic anemia. If signs of bone marrow depression occur, the patient should be given leucovorin 5 to 15 mg daily until normal hematopoiesis is restored.

DOSAGE AND ADMINISTRATION

Not recommended for use in pediatric patients less than 2 months of age.
Urinary Tract Infections and Shigellosis in Adults and Pediatric Patients, and Acute Otitis Media in Pediatric Patients:
Adults: The usual adult dosage in the treatment of urinary tract infections is 1 Bactrim DS (double strength) tablet, 2 Bactrim tablets or 4 teaspoonfuls (20 mL) of Bactrim Pediatric Suspension every 12 hours for 10 to 14 days. An identical daily dosage is used for 5 days in the treatment of shigellosis.
Pediatric Patients: The recommended dose for pediatric patients with urinary tract infections or acute otitis media is 8 mg/kg trimethoprim and 40 mg/kg sulfamethoxazole per 24 hours, given in two divided doses every 12 hours for 10 days. An identical daily dosage is used for 5 days in the treatment of shigellosis. The following table is a guideline for the attainment of this dosage:
Pediatric Patients 2 months of age or older:
[See table at top of previous page]
For Patients with Impaired Renal Function: When renal function is impaired, a reduced dosage should be employed using the following table:

Creatinine Clearance (mL/min)	Recommended Dosage Regimen
Above 30	Usual standard regimen
15–30	$\frac{1}{2}$ the usual regimen
Below 15	Use not recommended

Acute Exacerbations of Chronic Bronchitis in Adults:
The usual adult dosage in the treatment of acute exacerbations of chronic bronchitis is 1 Bactrim DS (double strength) tablet, 2 Bactrim tablets or 4 teaspoonfuls (20 mL) of Bactrim Pediatric Suspension every 12 hours for 14 days.
Pneumocystis Carinii Pneumonia:
Treatment: Adults and Pediatric Patients:
The recommended dosage for treatment of patients with documented *Pneumocystis carinii* pneumonia is 15 to 20 mg/kg trimethoprim and 75 to 100 mg/kg sulfamethoxazole per 24 hours given in equally divided doses every 6 hours for 14 to 21 days.8 The following table is a guideline for the upper limit of this dosage.
[See table at top of previous page]
For the lower limit dose (15 mg/kg trimethoprim and 75 mg/kg sulfamethoxazole per 24 hours) administer 75% of the dose in the above table.

Prophylaxis:
Adults:
The recommended dosage for prophylaxis in adults is 1 Bactrim DS (double strength) tablet daily.[9]
Pediatric Patients:
For pediatric patients, the recommended dose is 150 mg/m^2/day trimethoprim with 750 mg/m^2/day sulfamethoxazole given orally in equally divided doses twice a day, on 3 consecutive days per week. The total daily dose should not exceed 320 mg trimethoprim and 1600 mg sulfamethoxazole.[10]
The following table is a guideline for the attainment of this dosage in pediatric patients:
[See table at top of previous page]
Traveler's Diarrhea in Adults:
For the treatment of traveler's diarrhea, the usual adult dosage is 1 Bactrim DS (double strength) tablet; 2 Bactrim tablets or 4 teaspoonfuls (20 mL) of Pediatric Suspension every 12 hours for 5 days.

HOW SUPPLIED

DS (double strength) Tablets (white, notched, capsule shaped), containing 160 mg trimethoprim and 800 mg sulfamethoxazole—bottles of 100 (NDC 0004-0117-01), 250 (NDC 0004-0117-04) and 500 (NDC 0004-0117-14). Imprint on tablets: (front) BACTRIM-DS; (back) ROCHE.
Tablets (light green, scored, capsule shaped), containing 80 mg trimethoprim and 400 mg sulfamethoxazole—bottles of 100 (NDC 0004-0050-01). Imprint on tablets: (front) BACTRIM; (back) ROCHE.
Pediatric Suspension (pink, cherry flavored), containing 40 mg trimethoprim and 200 mg sulfamethoxazole per teaspoonful (5 mL)—bottles of 16 oz (1 pint) (NDC 0004-1033-28).
TABLETS SHOULD BE STORED AT 15° to 30°C (59° to 86°F) IN A DRY PLACE AND PROTECTED FROM LIGHT. SUSPENSION SHOULD BE STORED AT 15° to 30°C (59° to 86°F) AND PROTECTED FROM LIGHT.

REFERENCES

1. Kremers P, Duvivier J, Heusghem C. Pharmacokinetic Studies of Co-Trimoxazole in Man after Single and Repeated Doses. *J Clin Pharmacol*. Feb-Mar 1974; 14:112–117.
2. Kaplan SA, et al. Pharmacokinetic Profile of Trimethoprim-Sulfamethoxazole in Man. *J Infect Dis*. Nov 1973; 128 (Suppl): S547–S555.
3. Rudoy RC, Nelson JD, Haltalin KC. *Antimicrobial Agents Chemother*. May 1974;5:439–443.
4. National Committee for Clinical Laboratory Standards. *Methods for Dilution Antimicrobial Susceptibility Tests for Bacteria that Grow Aerobically*; Approved Standard—Fourth Edition. NCCLS Document M7-A4, Vol.17, No. 2, NCCLS, Wayne, PA, January, 1997.
5. National Committee for Clinical Laboratory Standards. *Performance Standards for Antimicrobial Disk Susceptibility Tests*. Approved Standard—Sixth Edition. NCCLS Document M2–A6, Vol. 17, No. 1, NCCLS, Wayne, PA, January, 1997.
6. Hardy DW, et al. A controlled trial of trimethoprim-sulfamethoxazole or aerosolized pentamidine for secondary prophylaxis of *Pneumocystis carinii* pneumonia in patients with the acquired immuno-deficiency syndrome. *N Engl J Med*. 1992; 327: 1842–1848.
7. Brumfitt W, Pursell R. Trimethoprim/Sulfamethoxazole in the Treatment of Bacteriuria in Women. *J Infect Dis*. Nov 1973; 128 (Suppl):S657–S663.
8. Masur H. Prevention and treatment of *Pneumocystis* pneumonia. *N Engl J Med*. 1992; 327: 1853–1880.
9. Recommendations for prophylaxis against *Pneumocystis carinii* pneumonia for adults and adolescents infected with human immunodefficiency virus. *MMWR*. 1992; 41(RR-4):1–11.
10. CDC Guidelines for prophylaxis against *Pneumocystis carinii* pneumonia for children infected with human immunodeficiency virus. *MMWR*. 1991; 40(RR-2):1–13.

℞ only
Revised: July 2000
Shown in Product Identification Guide, page 332

CELLCEPT® ℞

[cĕll-cĕpt]
(mycophenolate mofetil capsules)
(mycophenolate mofetil tablets)
CELLCEPT® ORAL SUSPENSION
(mycophenolate mofetil for oral suspension)
CELLCEPT® INTRAVENOUS
(mycophenolate mofetil hydrochloride for injection)

The following text is complete prescribing information based on official labeling in effect June 2000.

WARNING: **Increased susceptibility to infection and the possible development of lymphoma may result from immunosuppression. Only physicians experienced in immunosuppressive therapy and management of renal, cardiac or hepatic transplant patients should use CellCept. Patients receiving the drug should be managed in facilities equipped and staffed with adequate laboratory and supportive medical resources. The physician responsible for maintenance therapy should have complete information requisite for the follow-up of the patient.**

DESCRIPTION

CellCept (mycophenolate mofetil) is the 2-morpholinoethyl ester of mycophenolic acid (MPA), an immunosuppressive agent; inosine monophosphate dehydrogenase (IMPDH) inhibitor.
The chemical name for mycophenolate mofetil (MMF) is 2-morpholinoethyl (E)-6-(1,3-dihydro-4-hydroxy-6-methoxy-7-methyl-3-oxo-5-isobenzofuranyl)-4-methyl-4-hexenoate. It has an empirical formula of $C_{23}H_{31}NO_7$, a molecular weight of 433.50, and the following structural formula:

Mycophenolate mofetil is a white to off-white crystalline powder. It is slightly soluble in water (43 µg/mL at pH 7.4); the solubility increases in acidic medium (4.27 mg/mL at pH 3.6). It is freely soluble in acetone, soluble in methanol, and sparingly soluble in ethanol. The apparent partition coefficient in 1-octanol/water (pH 7.4) buffer solution is 238. The pKa values for mycophenolate mofetil are 5.6 for the morpholino group and 8.5 for the phenolic group.
Mycophenolate mofetil hydrochloride has a solubility of 65.8 mg/mL in 5% Dextrose Injection USP (D5W). The pH of the reconstituted solution is 2.4 to 4.1.
CellCept is available for oral administration as capsules containing 250 mg of mycophenolate mofetil, tablets containing 500 mg of mycophenolate mofetil, and as a powder for oral suspension, which when constituted contains 200 mg/mL mycophenolate mofetil.
Inactive ingredients in CellCept 250 mg capsules include croscarmellose sodium, magnesium stearate, povidone (K-90) and pregelatinized starch. The capsule shells contain black iron oxide, FD&C blue #2, gelatin, red iron oxide, silicon dioxide, sodium lauryl sulfate, titanium dioxide, and yellow iron oxide.
Inactive ingredients in CellCept 500 mg tablets include black iron oxide, croscarmellose sodium, FD&C blue #2 aluminum lake, hydroxypropyl cellulose, hydroxypropyl methylcellulose, magnesium stearate, microcrystalline cellulose, polyethylene glycol 400, povidone (K-90), red iron oxide, talc, and titanium dioxide; may also contain ammonium hydroxide, ethyl alcohol, methyl alcohol, n-butyl alcohol, propylene glycol, and shellac.
Inactive ingredients in CellCept Oral Suspension include aspartame, citric acid anhydrous, colloidal silicon dioxide, methylparaben, mixed fruit flavor, sodium citrate dihydrate, sorbitol, soybean lecithin, and xanthan gum.
CellCept Intravenous is the hydrochloride salt of mycophenolate mofetil. The chemical name for the hydrochloride salt of mycophenolate mofetil is 2-morpholinoethyl (E)-6-(1,3-dihydro-4-hydroxy-6-methoxy-7-methyl-3-oxo-5-isobenzofuranyl)-4-methyl-4-hexenoate hydrochloride. It has an empirical formula of $C_{23}H_{31}NO_7$ HCl and a molecular weight of 469.96.
CellCept Intravenous is available as a sterile white to off-white lyophilized powder in vials containing mycophenolate mofetil hydrochloride for administration by intravenous infusion only. Each vial of CellCept Intravenous contains the equivalent of 500 mg mycophenolate mofetil as the hydrochloride salt. The inactive ingredients are polysorbate 80, 25 mg, and citric acid, 5 mg. Sodium hydroxide may have been used in the manufacture of CellCept Intravenous to adjust the pH. Reconstitution and dilution with 5% Dextrose Injection USP yields a slightly yellow solution of mycophenolate mofetil, 6 mg/mL. (For detailed method of preparation, see DOSAGE AND ADMINISTRATION.)

CLINICAL PHARMACOLOGY

Mechanism of Action: Mycophenolate mofetil has been demonstrated in experimental animal models to prolong the survival of allogeneic transplants (kidney, heart, liver, intestine, limb, small bowel, pancreatic islets, and bone marrow).
Mycophenolate mofetil has also been shown to reverse ongoing acute rejection in the canine renal and rat cardiac allograft models. Mycophenolate mofetil also inhibited proliferative arteriopathy in experimental models of aortic and heart allografts in rats, as well as in primate cardiac xenografts. Mycophenolate mofetil was used alone or in combination with other immunosuppressive agents in these studies. Mycophenolate mofetil has been demonstrated to inhibit immunologically mediated inflammatory responses in animal models and to inhibit tumor development and prolong survival in murine tumor transplant models.
Mycophenolate mofetil is rapidly absorbed following oral administration and hydrolyzed to form MPA, which is the active metabolite. MPA is a potent, selective, uncompetitive, and reversible inhibitor of inosine monophosphate dehydrogenase (IMPDH), and therefore inhibits the de novo pathway of guanosine nucleotide synthesis without incorporation into DNA. Because T- and B-lymphocytes are critically dependent for their proliferation on de novo synthesis of purines, whereas other cell types can utilize salvage pathways, MPA has potent cytostatic effects on lymphocytes. MPA inhibits proliferative responses of T- and B-lymphocytes to both mitogenic and allospecific stimulation. Addition of guanosine or deoxyguanosine reverses the cytostatic effects of MPA on lymphocytes. MPA also suppresses antibody formation by B-lymphocytes. MPA prevents the glycosylation of lymphocyte and monocyte glycoproteins that are involved in intercellular adhesion to endothelial cells and

may inhibit recruitment of leukocytes into sites of inflammation and graft rejection. Mycophenolate mofetil did not inhibit early events in the activation of human peripheral blood mononuclear cells, such as the production of interleukin-1 (IL-1) and interleukin-2 (IL-2), but did block the coupling of these events to DNA synthesis and proliferation.

Pharmacokinetics: Following oral and intravenous administration, mycophenolate mofetil undergoes rapid and complete metabolism to MPA, the active metabolite. Oral absorption of the drug is rapid and essentially complete. MPA is metabolized to form the phenolic glucuronide of MPA (MPAG) which is not pharmacologically active. The parent drug, mycophenolate mofetil, can be measured systemically during the intravenous infusion; however, shortly (about 5 minutes) after the infusion is stopped or after oral administration, MMF concentration is below the limit of quantitation (0.4 µg/mL).

Absorption: In 12 healthy volunteers, the mean absolute bioavailability of oral mycophenolate mofetil relative to intravenous mycophenolate mofetil (based on MPA AUC) was 94%. The area under the plasma-concentration time curve (AUC) for MPA appears to increase in a dose-proportional fashion in renal transplant patients receiving multiple doses of mycophenolate mofetil up to a daily dose of 3 g (see table below on pharmacokinetic parameters).

Food (27 g fat, 650 calories) had no effect on the extent of absorption (MPA AUC) of mycophenolate mofetil when administered at doses of 1.5 g bid to renal transplant patients. However, MPA C_{max} was decreased by 40% in the presence of food (see DOSAGE AND ADMINISTRATION).

Distribution: The mean (±SD) apparent volume of distribution of MPA in 12 healthy volunteers is approximately 3.6 (±1.5) and 4.0 (±1.2) L/kg following intravenous and oral administration, respectively. MPA, at clinically relevant concentrations, is 97% bound to plasma albumin. MPAG is 82% bound to plasma albumin at MPAG concentration ranges that are normally seen in stable renal transplant patients; however, at higher MPAG concentrations (observed in patients with renal impairment or delayed graft function), the binding of MPA may be reduced as a result of competition between MPAG and MPA for protein binding. Mean blood to plasma ratio of radioactivity concentrations was approximately 0.6 indicating that MPA and MPAG do not extensively distribute into the cellular fractions of blood.

In vitro studies to evaluate the effect of other agents on the binding of MPA to human serum albumin (HSA) or plasma proteins showed that salicylate (at 25 mg/dL with HSA) and MPAG (at ≥460 µg/mL with plasma proteins) increased the free fraction of MPA. At concentrations that exceeded what is encountered clinically, cyclosporine, digoxin, naproxen, prednisone, propranolol, tacrolimus, theophylline, tolbutamide, and warfarin did not increase the free fraction of MPA. MPA at concentrations as high as 100 µg/mL had little effect on the binding of warfarin, digoxin or propranolol, but decreased the binding of theophylline from 53% to 45% and phenytoin from 90% to 87%.

Metabolism: Following oral and intravenous dosing, mycophenolate mofetil undergoes complete metabolism to MPA, the active metabolite. Metabolism to MPA occurs presystemically after oral dosing. MPA is metabolized principally by glucuronyl transferase to form the phenolic glucuronide of MPA (MPAG) which is not pharmacologically active. In vivo, MPAG is converted to MPA via enterohepatic recirculation. The following metabolites of the 2-hydroxyethyl-morpholino moiety are also recovered in the urine following oral administration of mycophenolate mofetil to healthy subjects: N-(2-carboxymethyl)-morpholine, N-(2-hydroxyethyl)-morpholine, and the N-oxide of N-(2-hydroxyethyl)-morpholine.

Secondary peaks in the plasma MPA concentration-time profile are usually observed 6 to 12 hours postdose. The coadministration of cholestyramine (4 g tid) resulted in approximately a 40% decrease in the MPA AUC (largely as a consequence of lower concentrations in the terminal portion of the profile). These observations suggest that enterohepatic recirculation contributes to MPA plasma concentrations.

Increased plasma concentrations of mycophenolate mofetil metabolites (MPA 50% increase and MPAG about a 3-fold to 6-fold increase) are observed in patients with renal insufficiency (see CLINICAL PHARMACOLOGY: *Special Populations*).

Excretion: Negligible amount of drug is excreted as MPA (<1% of dose) in the urine. Orally administered radiolabeled mycophenolate mofetil resulted in complete recovery of the administered dose, with 93% of the administered dose recovered in the urine and 6% recovered in feces. Most (about 87%) of the administered dose is excreted in the urine as MPAG. At clinically encountered concentrations, MPA and MPAG are usually not removed by hemodialysis. However, at high MPAG plasma concentrations (>100 µg/mL), small amounts of MPAG are removed. Bile acid sequestrants, such as cholestyramine, reduce MPA AUC by interfering with enterohepatic circulation of the drug (see OVERDOSAGE).

Mean (±SD) apparent half-life and plasma clearance of MPA are 17.9 (±6.5) hours and 193 (±48) mL/min following oral administration and 16.6 (±5.8) hours and 177 (±31) mL/min following intravenous administration, respectively.

Pharmacokinetics in Healthy Volunteers, Renal, Cardiac, and Hepatic Transplant Patients: Shown below are the mean (±SD) pharmacokinetic parameters for MPA following the administration of mycophenolate mofetil given as single doses to healthy volunteers and multiple doses to renal, cardiac, and hepatic transplant patients. In the early posttransplant period (<40 days posttransplant), renal, cardiac, and hepatic transplant patients had mean MPA AUCs approximately 20% to 41% lower and mean C_{max} approximately 32% to 44% lower compared to the late transplant period (3 to 6 months posttransplant).

Mean MPA AUC values following administration of 1 g bid intravenous mycophenolate mofetil over 2 hours to renal transplant patients for 5 days were about 24% higher than those observed after oral administration of a similar dose in the immediate posttransplant phase. In hepatic transplant patients, administration of 1 g bid intravenous CellCept followed by 1.5 g bid oral CellCept resulted in mean MPA AUC values similar to those found in renal transplant patients administered 1 g CellCept bid.

[See table above]

Pharmacokinetic Parameters for MPA [mean (±SD)] Following Administration of Mycophenolate Mofetil to Healthy Volunteers (Single Dose), Renal, Cardiac, and Hepatic Transplant Patients (Multiple Doses)

	Dose/Route	T_{max} (h)	C_{max} (µg/mL)	Total AUC (µg•h/mL)
Healthy Volunteers (single dose)	1 g/oral	0.80 (±0.36) (n=129)	24.5 (±9.5) (n=129)	63.9 (±16.2) (n=117)
Renal Transplant Patients (bid dosing) Time After Transplantation	**Dose/Route**	**T_{max} (h)**	**C_{max} (µg/mL)**	**Interdosing Interval AUC(0–12h) (µg•h/mL)**
5 days	1 g/iv	1.58 (±0.46) (n=31)	12.0 (±3.82) (n=31)	40.8 (±11.4) (n=31)
6 days	1 g/oral	1.33 (±1.05) (n=31)	10.7 (±4.83) (n=31)	32.9 (±15.0) (n=31)
Early (<40 days)	1 g/oral	1.31 (±0.76) (n=25)	8.16 (±4.50) (n=25)	27.3 (±10.9) (n=25)
Early (<40 days)	1.5 g/oral	1.21 (±0.81) (n=27)	13.5 (±8.18) (n=27)	38.4 (±15.4) (n=27)
Late (>3 months)	1.5 g/oral	0.90 (±0.24) (n=23)	24.1 (±12.1) (n=23)	65.3 (±35.4) (n=23)
Cardiac Transplant Patients (bid dosing) Time After Transplantation	**Dose/Route**	**T_{max} (h)**	**C_{max} (µg/mL)**	**Interdosing Interval AUC(0–12h) (µg•h/mL)**
Early (Day before discharge)	1.5 g/oral	1.8 (±1.3) (n=11)	11.5 (±6.8) (n=11)	43.3 (±20.8) (n=9)
Late (>6 months)	1.5 g/oral	1.1 (±0.7) (n=52)	20.0 (±9.4) (n=52)	54.1* (±20.4) (n=49)
Hepatic Transplant Patients (bid dosing) Time After Transplantation	**Dose/Route**	**T_{max} (h)**	**C_{max} (µg/mL)**	**Interdosing Interval AUC(0–12h) (µg•h/mL)**
4 to 9 days	1 g/iv	1.50 (±0.517) (n=22)	17.0 (±12.7) (n=22)	34.0 (±17.4) (n=22)
Early (5 to 8 days)	1.5 g/oral	1.15 (±0.432) (n=20)	13.1 (±6.76) (n=20)	29.2 (±11.9) (n=20)
Late (>6 months)	1.5 g/oral	1.54 (±0.51) (n=6)	19.3 (±11.7) (n=6)	49.3 (±14.8) (n=6)

**AUC(0–12h) values quoted are extrapolated from data from samples collected over 4 hours.*

Two 500 mg tablets have been shown to be bioequivalent to four 250 mg capsules. Five mL of the 200 mg/mL constituted oral suspension have been shown to be bioequivalent to four 250 mg capsules.

Special Populations: Shown below are the mean (±SD) pharmacokinetic parameters for MPA following the administration of oral mycophenolate mofetil given as single doses to non-transplant subjects with renal or hepatic impairment.

[See first table at top of next page]

Renal Insufficiency: In a single-dose study, MMF was administered as capsule or intravenous infusion over 40 minutes. Plasma MPA AUC observed after oral dosing to volunteers with severe chronic renal impairment [glomerular filtration rate (GFR) <25 mL/min/1.73 m²] was about 75% higher relative to that observed in healthy volunteers (GFR >80 mL/min/1.73 m²). In addition, the single-dose plasma MPAG AUC was 3-fold to 6-fold higher in volunteers with severe renal impairment than in volunteers with mild renal impairment or healthy volunteers, consistent with the known renal elimination of MPAG. No data are available on the safety of long-term exposure to this level of MPAG.

Plasma MPA AUC observed after single-dose (1 g) intravenous dosing to volunteers (n=4) with severe chronic renal impairment (GFR <25 mL/min/1.73 m²) was 62.4 µg•h/mL (±19.3). Multiple dosing of mycophenolate mofetil in patients with severe chronic renal impairment has not been studied (see PRECAUTIONS: *General* and DOSAGE AND ADMINISTRATION).

In patients with delayed renal graft function posttransplant, mean MPA AUC(0–12h) was comparable to that seen in posttransplant patients without delayed graft function. There is a potential for a transient increase in the free fraction and concentration of plasma MPA in patients with delayed graft function. However, dose adjustment does not appear to be necessary in patients with delayed graft function. Mean plasma MPAG AUC(0–12h) was 2-fold to 3-fold higher than in posttransplant patients without delayed graft function (see PRECAUTIONS: *General* and DOSAGE AND ADMINISTRATION).

In 8 patients with primary non-function of the organ following renal transplantation, plasma concentrations of MPAG accumulated about 6-fold to 8-fold after multiple dosing for 28 days. Accumulation of MPA was about 1-fold to 2-fold.

The pharmacokinetics of mycophenolate mofetil are not altered by hemodialysis. Hemodialysis usually does not remove MPA or MPAG. At high concentrations of MPAG (>100 µg/mL), hemodialysis removes only small amounts of MPAG.

Hepatic Insufficiency: In a single-dose (1 g oral) study of 18 volunteers with alcoholic cirrhosis and 6 healthy volunteers, hepatic MPA glucuronidation processes appeared to be relatively unaffected by hepatic parenchymal disease when pharmacokinetic parameters of healthy volunteers and alcoholic cirrhosis patients within this study were compared. However, it should be noted that for unexplained reasons, the healthy volunteers in this study had about a 50% lower AUC as compared to healthy volunteers in other studies,

Continued on next page

CellCept—Cont.

thus making comparisons between volunteers with alcoholic cirrhosis and healthy volunteers difficult. Effects of hepatic disease on this process probably depend on the particular disease. Hepatic disease with other etiologies, such as primary biliary cirrhosis, may show a different effect. In a single-dose (1 g intravenous) study of 6 volunteers with severe hepatic impairment (aminopyrine breath test less than 0.2% of dose) due to alcoholic cirrhosis, MMF was rapidly converted to MPA. MPA AUC was 44.1 µg•h/mL (±15.5).

Pediatrics: Very limited pharmacokinetic data are available for pediatric renal transplant recipients. Data on these patients are presented in the table below:

[See second table at right]

Gender: Data obtained from several studies were pooled to look at any gender-related differences in the pharmacokinetics of MPA (data were adjusted to 1 g oral dose). Mean (±SD) MPA AUC(0–12h) for males (n=79) was 32.0 (±14.5) and for females (n=41) was 36.5 (±18.8) µg•h/mL while mean (±SD) MPA C_{max} was 9.96 (±6.19) in the males and 10.6 (±5.64) µg/mL in the females. These differences are not of clinical significance.

Geriatric Use: Pharmacokinetics in the elderly have not been studied.

Pharmacokinetic Parameters for MPA [mean (±SD)] Following Single Doses of Mycophenolate Mofetil Capsules in Chronic Renal and Hepatic Impairment

Renal Impairment (no. of patients)	Dose	T_{max} (h)	C_{max} (µg/mL)	AUC(0–96h) (µg·h/mL)
Healthy Volunteers GFR >80 mL/min/1.73 m^2 (n=6)	1 g	0.75 (±0.27)	25.3 (±7.99)	45.0 (±22.6)
Mild Renal Impairment GFR 50 to 80 mL/min/1.73 m^2 (n=6)	1 g	0.75 (±0.27)	26.0 (±3.82)	59.9 (±12.9)
Moderate Renal Impairment GFR 25 to 49 mL/min/1.73 m^2 (n=6)	1 g	0.75 (±0.27)	19.0 (±13.2)	52.9 (±25.5)
Severe Renal Impairment GFR <25 mL/min/1.73 m^2 (n=7)	1 g	1.00 (±0.41)	16.3 (±10.8)	78.6 (±46.4)
Hepatic Impairment (no. of patients)	**Dose**	**T_{max} (h)**	**C_{max} (µg/mL)**	**AUC(0–48h) (µg·h/mL)**
Healthy Volunteers (n=6)	1 g	0.63 (±0.14)	24.3 (±5.73)	29.0 (±5.78)
Alcoholic Cirrhosis (n=18)	1 g	0.85 (±0.58)	22.4 (±10.1)	29.8 (±10.7)

Pharmacokinetic Parameters for MPA [mean ± (SD)] Following Multiple Oral Doses of Mycophenolate Mofetil in Pediatric Renal Transplant Patients 21 Days Posttransplant

Age Range	Dose	T_{max} (h)	C_{max} (µg/mL)	AUC(0–12h) (µg·h/mL)
≥3 mo to <6 yr (Mean = 2.75) (n=4)	15 mg/kg bid	1.25 (±0.87)	3.70 (±2.08)	13.6 (±8.69)
≥6 yr to <12 yr (Mean = 9.0) (n=4)	15 mg/kg bid	0.50 (±0.00)	13.5 (±4.48)	23.4 (±2.84)
≥12 yr to 18 yr (Mean = 15.6) (n=5)	15 mg/kg bid	0.50 (±0.00)	13.2 (±6.86)	30.0 (±8.34)
≥6 yr to <12 yr (Mean = 9.8) (n=5)	23 mg/kg bid	1.46 (±0.79)	17.0 (±20.0)	40.1 (±17.6)
≥12 yr to 18 yr (Mean = 14.6) (n=6)	23 mg/kg bid	1.32 (±0.76)	11.5 (±10.2)	31.1 (±11.4)

CLINICAL STUDIES

The safety and efficacy of CellCept in combination with corticosteroids and cyclosporine for the prevention of organ rejection were assessed in randomized, double-blind, multicenter trials in renal (3 trials), in cardiac (1 trial), and in hepatic (1 trial) transplant patients.

Renal Transplant: The three renal studies compared two dose levels of oral CellCept (1 g bid and 1.5 g bid) with azathioprine (2 studies) or placebo (1 study) when administered in combination with cyclosporine (Sandimmune®*) and corticosteroids to prevent acute rejection episodes. One study also included antithymocyte globulin (ATGAM®†) induction therapy. These studies are described by geographic location of the investigational sites. One study was conducted in the USA at 14 sites, one study was conducted in Europe at 20 sites, and one study was conducted in Europe, Canada, and Australia at a total of 21 sites.

The primary efficacy endpoint was the proportion of patients in each treatment group who experienced treatment failure within the first 6 months after transplantation (defined as biopsy-proven acute rejection on treatment or the occurrence of death, graft loss or early termination from the study for any reason without prior biopsy-proven rejection). CellCept, when administered with antithymocyte globulin (ATGAM®) induction (one study) and with cyclosporine and corticosteroids (all three studies), was compared to the following three therapeutic regimens: (1) antithymocyte globulin (ATGAM®) induction/azathioprine/cyclosporine/corticosteroids, (2) azathioprine/cyclosporine/corticosteroids, and (3) cyclosporine/corticosteroids.

CellCept, in combination with corticosteroids and cyclosporine reduced (statistically significant at 0.05 level) the incidence of treatment failure within the first 6 months following transplantation. The following tables summarize the results of these studies. These tables show (1) the proportion of patients experiencing treatment failure, (2) the proportion of patients who experienced biopsy-proven acute rejection on treatment, and (3) early termination, for any reason other than graft loss or death, without a prior biopsy-proven acute rejection episode. Patients who prematurely discontinued treatment were followed for the occurrence of death or graft loss, and the cumulative incidence of graft loss and patient death are summarized separately. Patients who prematurely discontinued treatment were not followed for the occurrence of acute rejection after termination. More patients discontinued receiving CellCept (without prior biopsy-proven rejection, death or graft loss) than discontinued in the control groups, with the highest rate in the CellCept 3 g/day group. Therefore, the acute rejection rates may be underestimates, particularly in the CellCept 3 g/day group.

* Sandimmune is a registered trademark of Novartis Pharmaceuticals Corporation.

† ATGAM is a registered trademark of Pharmacia and Upjohn Company.

[See first table at bottom of next page]

The cumulative incidence of 12-month graft loss or patient death is presented below. No advantage of CellCept with respect to graft loss or patient death was established. Numerically, patients receiving CellCept 2 g/day and 3 g/day experienced a better outcome than controls in all three studies; patients receiving CellCept 2 g/day experienced a better outcome than CellCept 3 g/day in two of the three studies. Patients in all treatment groups who terminated treatment early were found to have a poor outcome with respect to graft loss or patient death at 1 year.

[See second table at bottom of next page]

Cardiac Transplant: A double-blind, randomized, comparative, parallel-group, multicenter study in primary cardiac transplant recipients was performed at 20 centers in the United States, 1 in Canada, 5 in Europe and 2 in Australia. The total number of patients enrolled was 650; 72 never received study drug and 578 received study drug. Patients received CellCept 1.5 g bid (n=289) or azathioprine 1.5 to 3 mg/kg/day (n=289), in combination with cyclosporine (Sandimmune® or Neoral®*) and corticosteroids as maintenance immunosuppressive therapy. The two primary efficacy endpoints were: (1) the proportion of patients who, after transplantation, had at least one endomyocardial biopsy-proven rejection with hemodynamic compromise, or were retransplanted or died, within the first 6 months, and (2) the proportion of patients who died or were retransplanted during the first 12 months following transplantation. Patients who prematurely discontinued treatment were followed for the occurrence of allograft rejection for up to 6 months and for the occurrence of death for 1 year.

(1) Rejection: No difference was established between CellCept and azathioprine (AZA) with respect to biopsy-proven rejection with hemodynamic compromise.

(2) Survival: CellCept was shown to be at least as effective as AZA in preventing death or retransplantation at 1 year (see table next page).

* Neoral is a registered trademark of Novarits Pharmaceuticals Corporation.

[See third table at bottom of next page]

Hepatic Transplant: A double-blind, randomized, comparative, parallel-group, multicenter study in primary hepatic transplant recipients was performed at 16 centers in the United States, 2 in Canada, 4 in Europe and 1 in Australia. The total number of patients enrolled was 565. Per protocol, patients received CellCept 1g bid intravenously for up to 14 days followed by CellCept 1.5 g bid orally or azathioprine 1 to 2 mg/kg/day intravenously followed by azathioprine 1 to 2 mg/kg/day orally, in combination with cyclosporine (Neoral®) and corticosteroids as maintenance immunosuppressive therapy. The actual median oral dose of azathioprine on study was 1.5 mg/kg/day (range of 0.3 to 3.8 mg/kg/day) initially and 1.26 mg/kg/day (range of 0.3 to 3.8 mg/kg/day) at 12 months. The two primary endpoints were: (1) the proportion of patients who experienced, in the first 6 months posttransplantation, one or more episodes of biopsy-proven and treated rejection or death or retransplantation, and (2) the proportion of patients who experienced graft loss (death or retransplantation) during the first 12 months posttransplantation. Patients who prematurely discontinued treatment were followed for the occurrence of allograft rejection and for the occurrence of graft loss (death or retransplantation) for 1 year.

Results: In combination with corticosteroids and cyclosporine, CellCept obtained a lower rate of acute rejection at 6 months and a similar rate of death or retransplantation at 1 year compared to azathioprine.

[See fourth table at bottom of next page]

INDICATIONS AND USAGE

Renal, Cardiac, and Hepatic Transplant: CellCept is indicated for the prophylaxis of organ rejection in patients receiving allogeneic renal, cardiac or hepatic transplants. CellCept should be used concomitantly with cyclosporine and corticosteroids.

CellCept Intravenous is an alternative dosage form to CellCept capsules, tablets and oral suspension. CellCept Intravenous should be administered within 24 hours following transplantation. CellCept Intravenous can be administered for up to 14 days; patients should be switched to oral CellCept as soon as they can tolerate oral medication.

CONTRAINDICATIONS

Allergic reactions to CellCept have been observed; therefore, CellCept is contraindicated in patients with a hypersensitivity to mycophenolate mofetil, mycophenolic acid or any component of the drug product. CellCept Intravenous is contraindicated in patients who are allergic to Polysorbate 80 (TWEEN).

WARNINGS (see boxed WARNING)

Patients receiving immunosuppressive regimens involving combinations of drugs, including CellCept, as part of an immunosuppressive regimen are at increased risk of developing lymphomas and other malignancies, particularly of the skin. The risk appears to be related to the intensity and duration of immunosuppression rather than to the use of any specific agent. Oversuppression of the immune system can also increase susceptibility to infection, including opportunistic infections, fatal infections, and sepsis.

As usual for patients with increased risk for skin cancer, exposure to sunlight and UV light should be limited by wearing protective clothing and using a sunscreen with a high protection factor.

CellCept has been administered in combination with the following agents in clinical trials: antithymocyte globulin (ATGAM®), OKT3 (Orthoclone OKT® 3*), cyclosporine (Sandimmune®, Neoral®) and corticosteroids. The efficacy and safety of the use of CellCept in combination with other immunosuppressive agents have not been determined.

* Orthoclone OKT is a registered trademark of Ortho Biotech Inc.

Lymphoproliferative disease or lymphoma developed in 0.4% to 1% of patients receiving CellCept (2 g or 3 g) with other immunosuppressive agents in controlled clinical trials of renal, cardiac, and hepatic transplant patients (see ADVERSE REACTIONS).

Adverse effects on fetal development (including malformations) occurred when pregnant rats and rabbits were dosed during organogenesis. These responses occurred at doses lower than those associated with maternal toxicity, and at doses below the recommended clinical dose for renal or cardiac transplantation. There are no adequate and well-controlled studies in pregnant women. However, as CellCept has been shown to have teratogenic effects in animals, it may cause fetal harm when administered to a pregnant woman. Therefore, CellCept should not be used in pregnant women unless the potential benefit justifies the potential risk to the fetus.

Women of childbearing potential should have a negative serum or urine pregnancy test with a sensitivity of at least 50 mIU/mL within 1 week prior to beginning therapy. It is recommended that CellCept therapy should not be initiated by the physician until a report of a negative pregnancy test has been obtained.

Effective contraception must be used before beginning CellCept therapy, during therapy, and for 6 weeks following discontinuation of therapy, even where there has been a history of infertility, unless due to hysterectomy. Two reliable forms of contraception must be used simultaneously unless abstinence is the chosen method. If pregnancy does occur during treatment, the physician and patient should discuss the desirability of continuing the pregnancy (see PRECAUTIONS: *Pregnancy* and *Information for Patients*).

In patients receiving CellCept (2 g or 3 g) in controlled studies for prevention of renal, cardiac or hepatic rejection, fatal infection/sepsis occurred in approximately 2% of renal and cardiac patients and in 5% of hepatic patients (see ADVERSE REACTIONS).

Severe neutropenia [absolute neutrophil count (ANC) <0.5 × 10^3/μL] developed in up to 2.0% of renal, up to 2.8% of cardiac, and up to 3.6% of hepatic transplant patients receiving CellCept 3 g daily (see ADVERSE REACTIONS).

Patients receiving CellCept should be monitored for neutropenia (see PRECAUTIONS: *Laboratory Tests*). The development of neutropenia may be related to CellCept itself, concomitant medications, viral infections, or some combination of these causes. If neutropenia develops (ANC <1.3 × 10^3/μL), dosing with CellCept should be interrupted or the dose reduced, appropriate diagnostic tests performed, and the patient managed appropriately (see DOSAGE AND ADMINISTRATION). Neutropenia has been observed most frequently in the period from 31 to 180 days posttransplant in patients treated for prevention of renal, cardiac, and hepatic rejection.

Patients receiving CellCept should be instructed to report immediately any evidence of infection, unexpected bruising, bleeding or any other manifestation of bone marrow depression.

Renal Transplant Studies
Incidence of Treatment Failure
(Biopsy-proven Rejection or Early Termination for Any Reason)

USA Study (N=499 patients)	CellCept 2 g/day (n=167 patients)	CellCept 3 g/day (n=166 patients)	Azathioprine 1 to 2 mg/kg/day (n=166 patients)
All treatment failures	31.1%	31.3%	47.6%
Early termination without prior acute rejection*	9.6%	12.7%	6.0%
Biopsy-proven rejection episode on treatment	19.8%	17.5%	38.0%
Europe/Canada/ Australia Study (N=503 patients)	**CellCept 2 g/day (n=173 patients)**	**CellCept 3 g/day (n=164 patients)**	**Azathioprine 100 to 150 mg/day (n=166 patients)**
All treatment failures	38.2%	34.8%	50.0%
Early termination without prior acute rejection*	13.9%	15.2%	10.2%
Biopsy-proven rejection episode on treatment	19.7%	15.9%	35.5%
Europe Study (N=491 patients)	**CellCept 2 g/day (n=165 patients)**	**CellCept 3 g/day (n=160 patients)**	**Placebo (n=166 patients)**
All treatment failures	30.3%	38.8%	56.0%
Early termination without prior acute rejection*	11.5%	22.5%	7.2%
Biopsy-proven rejection episode on treatment	17.0%	13.8%	46.4%

*Does not include death and graft loss as reason for early termination.

Renal Transplant Studies
Cumulative Incidence of Combined Graft Loss or Patient Death at 12 Months

Study	CellCept 2 g/day	CellCept 3 g/day	Control (Azathioprine or Placebo)
USA	8.5%	11.5%	12.2%
Europe/Canada/Australia	11.7%	11.0%	13.6%
Europe	8.5%	10.0%	11.5%

Rejection at 6 Months/
Death or Retransplantation at 1 Year

	All Patients		Treated Patients	
	AZA N = 323	CellCept N = 327	AZA N = 289	CellCept N = 289
Biopsy-proven rejection with hemodynamic compromise at 6 months*	121 (38%)	120 (37%)	100 (35%)	92 (32%)
Death or retransplantation at 1 year	49 (15.2%)	42 (12.8%)	33 (11.4%)	18 (6.2%)

* Hemodynamic compromise occurred if any of the following criteria were met: pulmonary capillary wedge pressure ≥20 mm or a 25% increase; cardiac index <2.0 L/min/m^2 or a 25% decrease; ejection fraction ≤30%; pulmonary artery oxygen saturation ≤60% or a 25% decrease; presence of new S_3 gallop; fractional shortening was ≤20% or a 25% decrease; inotropic support required to manage the clinical condition.

Rejection at 6 Months/
Death or Retransplantation at 1 Year

	AZA N = 287	CellCept N = 278
Biopsy proven, treated rejection at 6 months (including death or retransplantation)	137 (47.7%)	107 (38.5%)
Death or retransplantation at 1 year	42 (14.6%)	41 (14.7%)

PRECAUTIONS

General: Gastrointestinal bleeding (requiring hospitalization) has been observed in approximately 3% of renal, in 1.7% of cardiac, and in 5.4% of hepatic transplant patients treated with CellCept 3 g daily. Gastrointestinal perforations have rarely been observed. Most patients receiving CellCept were also receiving other drugs known to be associated with these complications. Patients with active peptic ulcer disease were excluded from enrollment in studies with mycophenolate mofetil. Because CellCept has been associated with an increased incidence of digestive system adverse events, including infrequent cases of gastrointestinal tract ulceration, hemorrhage, and perforation, CellCept should be administered with caution in patients with active serious digestive system disease.

Subjects with severe chronic renal impairment (GFR <25 mL/min/1.73 m^2) who have received single doses of CellCept showed higher plasma MPA and MPAG AUCs relative to subjects with lesser degrees of renal impairment or normal healthy volunteers. No data are available on the safety of long-term exposure to these levels of MPAG. Doses of CellCept greater than 1 g administered twice a day to renal transplant patients should be avoided and they should be carefully observed (see CLINICAL PHARMACOLOGY: *Pharmacokinetics* and DOSAGE AND ADMINISTRATION). No data are available for cardiac or hepatic transplant patients with severe chronic renal impairment. CellCept may be used for cardiac or hepatic transplant patients with severe chronic renal impairment if the potential benefits outweigh the potential risks.

In patients with delayed renal graft function posttransplant, mean MPA AUC(0–12h) was comparable, but MPAG AUC(0–12h) was 2-fold to 3-fold higher, compared to that seen in posttransplant patients without delayed renal graft function. In the three controlled studies of prevention of renal rejection, there were 298 of 1483 patients (20%) with delayed graft function. Although patients with delayed graft function have a higher incidence of certain adverse events (anemia, thrombocytopenia, hyperkalemia) than patients without delayed graft function, these events were not more frequent in patients receiving CellCept than azathioprine or placebo. No dose adjustment is recommended for these patients; however, they should be carefully observed (see CLINICAL PHARMACOLOGY: *Pharmacokinetics* and DOSAGE AND ADMINISTRATION).

In cardiac transplant patients, the overall incidence of opportunistic infections was approximately 10% higher in patients treated with CellCept than in those receiving azathioprine therapy, but this difference was not associated with excess mortality due to infection/sepsis among patients treated with CellCept (see ADVERSE REACTIONS).

There were more herpes virus (H. simplex, H. zoster, and cytomegalovirus) infections in cardiac transplant patients treated with CellCept compared to those treated with azathioprine (see ADVERSE REACTIONS).

It is recommended that CellCept not be administered concomitantly with azathioprine because both have the potential to cause bone marrow suppression and such concomitant administration has not been studied clinically.

In view of the significant reduction in the AUC of MPA by cholestyramine, caution should be used in the concomitant administration of CellCept with drugs that interfere with enterohepatic recirculation because of the potential to reduce the efficacy of CellCept (see PRECAUTIONS: *Drug Interactions*).

On theoretical grounds, because CellCept is an IMPDH (inosine monophosphate dehydrogenase) inhibitor, it should be avoided in patients with rare hereditary deficiency of hypoxanthine-guanine phosphoribosyl-transferase (HGPRT) such as Lesch-Nyhan and Kelley-Seegmiller syndrome.

During treatment with CellCept, the use of live attenuated vaccines should be avoided and patients should be advised that vaccinations may be less effective (see PRECAUTIONS: *Drug Interactions: Live Vaccines*).

Phenylketonurics: CellCept Oral Suspension contains aspartame, a source of phenylalanine (0.56 mg phenylalanine/mL suspension). Therefore, care should be taken if CellCept Oral Suspension is administered to patients with phenylketonuria.

CAUTION: CELLCEPT INTRAVENOUS SOLUTION SHOULD NEVER BE ADMINISTERED BY RAPID OR BOLUS INTRAVENOUS INJECTION.

Continued on next page

CellCept—Cont.

Information for Patients: Patients should be informed of the need for repeated appropriate laboratory tests while they are receiving CellCept. Patients should be given complete dosage instructions and informed of the increased risk of lymphoproliferative disease and certain other malignancies. Women of childbearing potential should be instructed of the potential risks during pregnancy, and that they should use effective contraception before beginning CellCept therapy, during therapy, and for 6 weeks after CellCept has been stopped (see WARNINGS and PRECAUTIONS: *Pregnancy*).

Laboratory Tests: Complete blood counts should be performed weekly during the first month, twice monthly for the second and third months of treatment, then monthly through the first year (see WARNINGS, ADVERSE REACTIONS and DOSAGE AND ADMINISTRATION).

Drug Interactions: Drug interaction studies with mycophenolate mofetil have been conducted with acyclovir, antacids, cholestyramine, cyclosporine, ganciclovir, oral contraceptives, and trimethoprim/sulfamethoxazole. Drug interaction studies have not been conducted with other drugs that may be commonly administered to renal, cardiac or hepatic transplant patients. CellCept has not been administered concomitantly with azathioprine.

Acyclovir: Coadministration of mycophenolate mofetil (1 g) and acyclovir (800 mg) to 12 healthy volunteers resulted in no significant change in MPA AUC and C_{max}. However, MPAG and acyclovir plasma AUCs were increased 10.6% and 21.9%, respectively. Because MPAG plasma concentrations are increased in the presence of renal impairment, as are acyclovir concentrations, the potential exists for the two drugs to compete for tubular secretion, further increasing the concentrations of both drugs.

Antacids With Magnesium and Aluminum Hydroxides: Absorption of a single dose of mycophenolate mofetil (2 g) was decreased when administered to ten rheumatoid arthritis patients also taking Maalox®* TC (10 mL qid). The C_{max} and AUC(0-24h) for MPA were 33% and 17% lower, respectively, than when mycophenolate mofetil was administered alone under fasting conditions. CellCept may be administered to patients who are also taking antacids containing magnesium and aluminum hydroxides; however, it is recommended that CellCept and the antacid not be administered simultaneously.

* Maalox is a registered trademark of Novartis Consumer Health, Inc.

Cholestyramine: Following single-dose administration of 1.5 g mycophenolate mofetil to 12 healthy volunteers pretreated with 4 g tid of cholestyramine for 4 days, MPA AUC decreased approximately 40%. This decrease is consistent with interruption of enterohepatic recirculation which may be due to binding of recirculating MPAG with cholestyramine in the intestine. Some degree of enterohepatic recirculation is also anticipated following intravenous administration of CellCept. Therefore, CellCept is not recommended to be given with cholestyramine or other agents that may interfere with enterohepatic recirculation.

Cyclosporine: Cyclosporine (Sandimmune®) pharmacokinetics (at doses of 275 to 415 mg/day) were unaffected by single and multiple doses of 1.5 g bid of mycophenolate mofetil in 10 stable renal transplant patients. The mean (±SD) AUC(0–12h) and C_{max} of cyclosporine after 14 days of multiple doses of mycophenolate mofetil were 3290 (±822) ng•h/mL and 753 (±161) ng/mL, respectively, compared to 3245 (±1088) ng•h/mL and 700 (±246) ng/mL, respectively, 1 week before administration of mycophenolate mofetil. The effect of cyclosporine on mycophenolate mofetil pharmacokinetics could not be evaluated in this study; however, plasma concentrations of MPA were similar to that for healthy volunteers.

Ganciclovir: Following single-dose administration to 12 stable renal transplant patients, no pharmacokinetic interaction was observed between mycophenolate mofetil (1.5 g) and intravenous ganciclovir (5 mg/kg). Mean (±SD) ganciclovir AUC and C_{max} (n=10) were 54.3 (±19.0) μg•h/mL and 11.5 (±1.8) μg/mL, respectively, after coadministration of the two drugs, compared to 51.0 (±17.0) μg•h/mL and 10.6 (±2.0) μg/mL, respectively, after administration of intravenous ganciclovir alone. The mean (±SD) AUC and C_{max} of MPA (n=12) after coadministration were 80.9 (±21.6) μg•h/mL and 27.8 (±13.9) μg/mL, respectively, compared to values of 80.3 (±16.4) μg•h/mL and 30.9 (±11.2) μg/mL, respectively, after administration of mycophenolate mofetil alone. Because MPAG plasma concentrations are increased in the presence of renal impairment, as are ganciclovir concentrations, the two drugs will compete for tubular secretion and thus further increases in concentrations of both drugs may occur. In patients with renal impairment in which MMF and ganciclovir are coadministered, patients should be monitored carefully.

Oral Contraceptives: A study of coadministration of CellCept (1 g bid) and combined oral contraceptives containing ethinylestradiol (0.02 mg to 0.04 mg) and levonorgestrel (0.05 mg to 0.20 mg), desogestrel (0.15 mg) or gestodene (0.05 mg to 0.10 mg) was conducted in 18 women with psoriasis over 3 consecutive menstrual cycles. Mean AUC(0–24h) was similar for ethinylestradiol and 3-keto desogestrel; however, mean levonorgestrel AUC(0–24h) significantly decreased by about 15%. There was large inter-patient variability (%CV in the range of 60% to 70%) in the data, especially for ethinylestradiol. Mean serum levels of LH, FSH and progesterone were not significantly affected. CellCept may not have any influence on the ovulation-suppressing action of the studied oral contraceptives. However, it is recommended that oral contraceptives are coadministered with CellCept with caution and additional birth control methods be considered (see PRECAUTIONS: *Pregnancy*).

Trimethoprim/sulfamethoxazole: Following single-dose administration of mycophenolate mofetil (1.5 g) to 12 healthy male volunteers on day 8 of a 10 day course of Bactrim™* DS (trimethoprim 160 mg/sulfamethoxazole 800 mg) administered bid, no effect on the bioavailability of MPA was observed. The mean (±SD) AUC and C_{max} of MPA after concomitant administration were 75.2 (±19.8) μg•h/mL and 34.0 (±6.6) μg/mL, respectively, compared to 79.2 (±27.9) μg•h/mL and 34.2 (±10.7) μg/mL, respectively, after administration of mycophenolate mofetil alone.

* Bactrim is a trademark of Hoffmann-La Roche Inc.

Other Interactions: The measured value for renal clearance of MPAG indicates removal occurs by renal tubular secretion as well as glomerular filtration. Consistent with this, coadministration of probenecid, a known inhibitor of tubular secretion, with mycophenolate mofetil in monkeys results in a 3-fold increase in plasma MPAG AUC and a 2-fold increase in plasma MPA AUC. Thus, other drugs known to undergo renal tubular secretion may compete with MPAG and thereby raise plasma concentrations of

Adverse Events in Controlled Studies in Prevention of Renal, Cardiac or Hepatic Allograft Rejection (Reported in ≥10% of Patients in the CellCept Group)

	Renal Studies			Cardiac Study		Hepatic Study	
	CellCept 2 g/day	CellCept 3 g/day	Azathioprine 1 to 2 mg/kg/day or 100 to 150 mg/day	CellCept 3 g/day	Azathioprine 1.5 to 3 mg/kg/day	CellCept 3 g/day	Azathioprine 1 to 2 mg/kg/day
	(n=336)	(n=330)	(n=326)	(n=289)	(n=289)	(n=277)	(n=287)
	%	%	%	%	%	%	%
Body as a Whole							
Pain	33.0	31.2	32.2	75.8	74.7	74.0	77.7
Abdominal pain	24.7	27.6	23.0	33.9	33.2	62.5	51.2
Fever	21.4	23.3	23.3	47.4	46.4	52.3	56.1
Headache	21.1	16.1	21.2	54.3	51.9	53.8	49.1
Infection	18.2	20.9	19.9	25.6	19.4	27.1	25.1
Sepsis	17.6	19.7	15.6	18.7	18.7	27.4	26.5
Asthenia	13.7	16.1	19.9	43.3	36.3	35.4	33.8
Chest pain	13.4	13.3	14.7	26.3	26.0	15.9	13.2
Back pain	11.6	12.1	14.1	34.6	28.4	46.6	47.4
Accidental injury	—	—	—	19.0	14.9	11.2	15.0
Chills	—	—	—	11.4	11.4	10.8	10.1
Ascites	—	—	—	—	—	24.2	22.6
Abdomen enlarged	—	—	—	—	—	18.8	17.8
Hernia	—	—	—	—	—	11.6	8.7
Peritonitis	—	—	—	—	—	10.1	12.5
Hemic and Lymphatic							
Anemia	25.6	25.8	23.6	42.9	43.9	43.0	53.0
Leukopenia	23.2	34.5	24.8	30.4	39.1	45.8	39.0
Thrombocytopenia	10.1	8.2	13.2	23.5	27.0	38.3	42.2
Hypochromic anemia	7.4	11.5	9.2	24.6	23.5	13.7	10.8
Leukocytosis	7.1	10.9	7.4	40.5	35.6	22.4	21.3
Ecchymosis	—	—	—	16.6	8.0	—	—
Urogenital							
Urinary tract infection	37.2	37.0	33.7	13.1	11.8	18.1	17.8
Hematuria	14.0	12.1	11.3	—	—	—	—
Kidney tubular necrosis	6.3	10.0	5.8	—	—	—	—
Kidney function abnormal	—	—	—	21.8	26.3	25.6	28.9
Oliguria	—	—	—	14.2	12.8	17.0	20.6
Cardiovascular							
Hypertension	32.4	28.2	32.2	77.5	72.3	62.1	59.6
Hypotension	—	—	—	32.5	36.0	18.4	20.9
Cardiovascular disorder	—	—	—	25.6	24.2	—	—
Tachycardia	—	—	—	20.1	18.0	22.0	15.7
Arrhythmia	—	—	—	19.0	18.7	—	—
Bradycardia	—	—	—	17.3	17.3	—	—
Pericardial effusion	—	—	—	15.9	13.5	—	—
Heart failure	—	—	—	11.8	8.7	—	—

(continued on next page)

MPAG or the other drug undergoing tubular secretion. Drugs that alter the gastrointestinal flora may interact with mycophenolate mofetil by disrupting enterohepatic recirculation. Interference of MPAG hydrolysis may lead to less MPA available for absorption.

Live Vaccines: During treatment with CellCept, the use of live attenuated vaccines should be avoided and patients should be advised that vaccinations may be less effective (see PRECAUTIONS: *General*).

Carcinogenesis, Mutagenesis, Impairment of Fertility: In a 104-week oral carcinogenicity study in mice, mycophenolate mofetil in daily doses up to 180 mg/kg was not tumorigenic. The highest dose tested was 0.5 times the recommended clinical dose (2 g/day) in renal transplant patients and 0.3 times the recommended clinical dose (3 g/day) in cardiac transplant patients when corrected for differences in body surface area (BSA). In a 104-week oral carcinogenicity study in rats, mycophenolate mofetil in daily doses up to 15 mg/kg was not tumorigenic. The highest dose was 0.08 times the recommended clinical dose in renal transplant patients and 0.05 times the recommended clinical dose in cardiac transplant patients when corrected for BSA. While these animal doses were lower than those given to patients, they were maximal in those species and were considered adequate to evaluate the potential for human risk (see WARNINGS).

The genotoxic potential of mycophenolate mofetil was determined in five assays. Mycophenolate mofetil was genotoxic in the mouse lymphoma/thymidine kinase assay and the in vivo mouse micronucleus assay. Mycophenolate mofetil was not genotoxic in the bacterial mutation assay, the yeast mitotic gene conversion assay or the Chinese hamster ovary cell chromosomal aberration assay.

Mycophenolate mofetil had no effect on fertility of male rats at oral doses up to 20 mg/kg/day. This dose represents 0.1 times the recommended clinical dose in renal transplant patients and 0.07 times the recommended clinical dose in cardiac transplant patients when corrected for BSA. In a female fertility and reproduction study conducted in rats, oral doses of 4.5 mg/kg/day caused malformations (principally of the head and eyes) in the first generation offspring in the absence of maternal toxicity. This dose was 0.02 times the recommended clinical dose in renal transplant patients and 0.01 times the recommended clinical dose in cardiac transplant patients when corrected for BSA. No effects on fertility or reproductive parameters were evident in the dams or in the subsequent generation.

Pregnancy: *Category C.* In teratology studies in rats and rabbits, fetal resorptions and malformations occurred in rats at 6 mg/kg/day and in rabbits at 90 mg/kg/day, in the absence of maternal toxicity. These levels are equivalent to 0.03 to 0.92 times the recommended clinical dose in renal transplant patients and 0.02 to 0.61 times the recommended clinical dose in cardiac transplant patients on a BSA basis. In a female fertility and reproduction study conducted in rats, oral doses of 4.5 mg/kg/day caused malformations (principally of the head and eyes) in the first generation offspring in the absence of maternal toxicity. This dose was 0.02 times the recommended clinical dose in renal transplant patients and 0.01 times the recommended clinical dose in cardiac transplant patients when corrected for BSA.

There are no adequate and well-controlled studies in pregnant women. CellCept should not be used in pregnant women unless the potential benefit justifies the potential risk to the fetus. Effective contraception must be used before beginning CellCept therapy, during therapy and for 6 weeks after CellCept has been stopped (see WARNINGS and PRECAUTIONS: *Information for Patients*).

Nursing Mothers: Studies in rats treated with mycophenolate mofetil have shown mycophenolic acid to be excreted in milk. It is not known whether this drug is excreted in human milk. Because many drugs are excreted in human milk, and because of the potential for serious adverse reactions in nursing infants from mycophenolate mofetil, a decision should be made whether to discontinue nursing or to discontinue the drug, taking into account the importance of the drug to the mother.

Pediatric Patients: Safety and effectiveness in pediatric patients have not been established. Very limited pharmacokinetic data are available in pediatric patients (see CLINICAL PHARMACOLOGY: *Pharmacokinetics*).

Geriatric Use: Clinical studies of CellCept did not include sufficient numbers of subjects aged 65 and over to determine whether they respond differently from younger subjects. Other reported clinical experience has not identified differences in responses between the elderly and younger patients. In general dose selection for an elderly patient should be cautious, reflecting the greater frequency of decreased hepatic, renal or cardiac function and of concomitant or other drug therapy. Elderly patients may be at an increased risk of adverse reactions compared with younger individuals (see ADVERSE REACTIONS).

ADVERSE REACTIONS

The principal adverse reactions associated with the administration of CellCept include diarrhea, leukopenia, sepsis, vomiting, and there is evidence of a higher frequency of certain types of infections. The adverse event profile associated with the administration of CellCept Intravenous has been shown to be similar to that observed after administration of oral dosage forms of CellCept.

Adverse Events in Controlled Studies in Prevention of Renal, Cardiac or Hepatic Allograft Rejection (Reported in ≥10% of Patients in the CellCept Group)

	Renal Studies			Cardiac Study		Hepatic Study	
	CellCept 2 g/day	CellCept 3 g/day	Azathioprine 1 to 2 mg/kg/day or 100 to 150 mg/day	CellCept 3 g/day	Azathioprine 1.5 to 3 mg/kg/day	CellCept 3 g/day	Azathioprine 1 to 2 mg/kg/day
	(n=336)	(n=330)	(n=326)	(n=289)	(n=289)	(n=277)	(n=287)
	%	%	%	%	%	%	%
Metabolic and Nutritional							
Peripheral edema	28.6	27.0	28.2	64.0	53.3	48.4	47.7
Hypercholesteremia	12.8	8.5	11.3	41.2	38.4	—	—
Hypophosphatemia	12.5	15.8	11.7	—	—	14.4	9.1
Edema	12.2	11.8	13.5	26.6	25.6	28.2	28.2
Hypokalemia	10.1	10.0	8.3	31.8	25.6	37.2	41.1
Hyperkalemia	8.9	10.3	16.9	14.5	19.7	22.0	23.7
Hyperglycemia	8.6	12.4	15.0	46.7	52.6	43.7	48.8
Creatinine increased	—	—	—	39.4	36.0	19.9	21.6
BUN increased	—	—	—	34.6	32.5	10.1	12.9
Lactic dehydrogenase increased	—	—	—	23.2	17.0	—	—
Bilirubinemia	—	—	—	18.0	21.8	14.4	18.8
Hypervolemia	—	—	—	16.6	22.8	—	—
Generalized edema	—	—	—	18.0	20.1	14.8	16.0
Hyperuricemia	—	—	—	16.3	17.6	—	—
SGOT increased	—	—	—	17.3	15.6	—	—
Hypomagnesemia	—	—	—	18.3	12.8	39.0	37.6
Acidosis	—	—	—	14.2	16.6	—	—
Weight gain	—	—	—	15.6	15.2	—	—
SGPT increased	—	—	—	15.6	12.5	—	—
Hyponatremia	—	—	—	11.4	11.8	—	—
Hyperlipemia	—	—	—	10.7	9.3	—	—
Hypocalcemia	—	—	—	—	—	30.0	30.0
Hypoproteinemia	—	—	—	—	—	13.4	13.9
Hypoglycemia	—	—	—	—	—	10.5	9.1
Healing abnormal	—	—	—	—	—	10.5	8.7
Digestive							
Diarrhea	31.0	36.1	20.9	45.3	34.3	51.3	49.8
Constipation	22.9	18.5	22.4	41.2	37.7	37.9	38.3
Nausea	19.9	23.6	24.5	54.0	54.3	54.5	51.2
Dyspepsia	17.6	13.6	13.8	18.7	19.4	22.4	20.9
Vomiting	12.5	13.6	9.2	33.9	28.4	32.9	33.4
Nausea and vomiting	10.4	9.7	10.7	11.1	7.6	—	—
Oral moniliasis	10.1	12.1	11.3	11.4	11.8	10.1	10.1
Flatulence	—	—	—	13.8	15.6	12.6	9.8
Anorexia	—	—	—	—	—	25.3	17.1
Liver function tests abnormal	—	—	—	—	—	24.9	19.2
Cholangitis	—	—	—	—	—	14.1	13.6
Hepatitis	—	—	—	—	—	13.0	16.0
Cholestatic jaundice	—	—	—	—	—	11.9	10.8

(continued on next page)

CellCept Oral: The incidence of adverse events for CellCept was determined in randomized, comparative, double-blind trials in prevention of rejection in renal (2 active, 1 placebo-controlled trials), cardiac (1 active-controlled trial), and hepatic (1 active-controlled trial) transplant patients.

Elderly patients, particularly those who are receiving CellCept as part of a combination immunosuppressive regimen, may be at increased risk of certain infections (including CMV tissue invasive disease) and possibly gastrointestinal hemorrhage and pulmonary edema, compared to younger individuals (see PRECAUTIONS).

Safety data are summarized below for all active-controlled trials in renal (2 trials), cardiac (1 trial), and hepatic (1 trial) transplant patients. Approximately 53% of the renal

Continued on next page

CellCept—Cont.

patients, 65% of the cardiac patients, and 48% of the hepatic patients have been treated for more than 1 year. Adverse events reported in ≥10% of patients in the CellCept treatment groups are presented below.

[See table beginning on page 2732]

The placebo-controlled renal transplant study generally showed fewer adverse events occurring in ≥10% of patients. In addition, those that occurred were not only qualitatively similar to the azathioprine-controlled renal transplant studies, but also occurred at lower rates, particularly for infection, leukopenia, hypertension, diarrhea and respiratory infection. However, the following adverse events were reported in the placebo-controlled renal transplant study but not reported in the azathioprine-controlled renal transplant studies with an incidence of ≥10%: urinary tract disorder, bronchitis, and pneumonia.

The above data demonstrate that in three controlled trials for prevention of renal rejection, patients receiving 2 g/day of CellCept had an overall better safety profile than did patients receiving 3 g/day of CellCept.

The above data demonstrate that the types of adverse events observed in multicenter controlled trials in renal, cardiac, and hepatic transplant patients are qualitatively similar except for those that are unique to the specific organ involved.

Sepsis, which was generally CMV viremia, was slightly more common in renal transplant patients treated with CellCept compared to patients treated with azathioprine.

Adverse Events in Controlled Studies in Prevention of Renal, Cardiac or Hepatic Allograft Rejection (Reported in ≥10% of Patients in the CellCept Group)

	Renal Studies			Cardiac Study		Hepatic Study	
	CellCept 2 g/day	CellCept 3 g/day	Azathioprine 1 to 2 mg/kg/day or 100 to 150 mg/day	CellCept 3 g/day	Azathioprine 1.5 to 3 mg/kg/day	CellCept 3 g/day	Azathioprine 1 to 2 mg/kg/day
	(n=336)	(n=330)	(n=326)	(n=289)	(n=289)	(n=277)	(n=287)
	%	%	%	%	%	%	%
Respiratory							
Infection	22.0	23.9	19.6	37.0	35.3	15.9	19.9
Dyspnea	15.5	17.3	16.6	36.7	36.3	31.0	30.3
Cough increased	15.5	13.3	15.0	31.1	25.6	15.9	12.5
Pharyngitis	9.5	11.2	8.0	18.3	13.5	14.1	12.5
Lung disorder	—	—	—	30.1	29.1	22.0	18.8
Sinusitis	—	—	—	26.0	19.0	11.2	9.8
Rhinitis	—	—	—	19.0	15.6	—	—
Pleural effusion	—	—	—	17.0	13.8	34.3	35.9
Asthma	—	—	—	11.1	11.4	—	—
Pneumonia	—	—	—	10.7	10.4	13.7	11.5
Atelectasis	—	—	—	—	—	13.0	12.9
Skin and Appendages							
Acne	10.1	9.7	6.4	12.1	9.3	—	—
Rash	—	—	—	22.1	18.0	17.7	18.5
Skin disorder	—	—	—	12.5	8.7	—	—
Pruritus	—	—	—	—	—	14.1	10.5
Sweating	—	—	—	—	—	10.8	10.1
Nervous System							
Tremor	11.0	11.8	12.3	24.2	23.9	33.9	35.5
Insomnia	8.9	11.8	10.4	40.8	37.7	52.3	47.0
Dizziness	5.7	11.2	11.0	28.7	27.7	16.2	14.3
Anxiety	—	—	—	28.4	23.9	19.5	17.8
Paresthesia	—	—	—	20.8	18.0	15.2	15.3
Hypertonia	—	—	—	15.6	14.5	—	—
Depression	—	—	—	15.6	12.5	17.3	16.7
Agitation	—	—	—	13.1	12.8	—	—
Somnolence	—	—	—	11.1	10.4	—	—
Confusion	—	—	—	13.5	7.6	17.3	18.8
Nervousness	—	—	—	11.4	9.0	10.1	10.5
Musculoskeletal System							
Leg cramps	—	—	—	16.6	15.6	—	—
Myasthenia	—	—	—	12.5	9.7	—	—
Myalgia	—	—	—	12.5	9.3	—	—
Special Senses							
Amblyopia	—	—	—	14.9	6.6	—	—

The incidence of sepsis was comparable in CellCept and in azathioprine-treated patients in cardiac and hepatic studies.

In the digestive system, diarrhea was increased in renal and cardiac transplant patients receiving CellCept compared to patients receiving azathioprine, but was comparable in hepatic transplant patients treated with CellCept or azathioprine.

The incidence of malignancies among the 1483 patients treated in controlled trials for the prevention of renal allograft rejection who were followed for ≥1 year was similar to the incidence reported in the literature for renal allograft recipients.

Lymphoproliferative disease or lymphoma developed in 0.4% to 1% of patients receiving CellCept (2 g or 3 g daily) with other immunosuppressive agents in controlled clinical trials of renal, cardiac, and hepatic transplant patients followed for at least 1 year (see WARNINGS). Non-melanoma skin carcinomas occurred in 1.6% to 4.2% of patients, other types of malignancy in 0.7% to 2.1% of patients. Three-year safety data in renal and cardiac transplant patients did not reveal any unexpected changes in incidence of malignancy compared to the 1-year data.

Severe neutropenia (ANC $<0.5 \times 10^3/\mu L$) developed in up to 2.0% of renal transplant patients, up to 2.8% of cardiac transplant patients and up to 3.6% of hepatic transplant patients receiving CellCept 3 g daily (see WARNINGS, PRECAUTIONS: *Laboratory Tests* and DOSAGE AND ADMINISTRATION).

The following table shows the incidence of opportunistic infections that occurred in the renal, cardiac, and hepatic transplant populations in the azathioprine-controlled prevention trials:

[See table at bottom of next page]

The following other opportunistic infections occurred with an incidence of less than 4% in CellCept patients in the above azathioprine-controlled studies: Herpes zoster, visceral disease; Candida, urinary tract infection, fungemia/disseminated disease, tissue invasive disease; Cryptococcosis; Aspergillus/Mucor; Pneumocystis carinii.

In the placebo-controlled renal transplant study, the same pattern of opportunistic infection was observed compared to the azathioprine-controlled renal studies, with a notably lower incidence of the following: Herpes simplex and CMV tissue-invasive disease.

In patients receiving CellCept (2 g or 3 g) in controlled studies for prevention of renal, cardiac or hepatic rejection, fatal infection/sepsis occurred in approximately 2% of renal and cardiac patients and in 5% of hepatic patients (see WARNINGS).

In cardiac transplant patients, the overall incidence of opportunistic infections was approximately 10% higher in patients treated with CellCept than in those receiving azathioprine, but this difference was not associated with excess mortality due to infection/sepsis among patients treated with CellCept.

The following adverse events were reported with 3% to <10% incidence in renal, cardiac, and hepatic transplant patients treated with CellCept, in combination with cyclosporine and corticosteroids.

[See table at top of page 2736]

CellCept Intravenous: The adverse event profile of CellCept Intravenous was determined from a single, double-blind, controlled comparative study of the safety of 2 g/day of intravenous and oral CellCept in renal transplant patients in the immediate posttransplant period (administered for the first 5 days). The potential venous irritation of CellCept Intravenous was evaluated by comparing the adverse events attributable to peripheral venous infusion of CellCept Intravenous with those observed in the intravenous placebo group; patients in this group received active medication by the oral route.

Adverse events attributable to peripheral venous infusion were phlebitis and thrombosis, both observed at 4% in patients treated with CellCept Intravenous.

In the active controlled study in hepatic transplant patients, 2 g/day of CellCept Intravenous were administered in the immediate posttransplant period (up to 14 days). The safety profile of intravenous CellCept was similar to that of intravenous azathioprine.

Postmarketing Experience

Digestive: colitis (sometimes caused by cytomegalovirus), pancreatitis.

Resistance Mechanism Disorders: Serious life-threatening infections such as meningitis and infectious endocarditis have been reported occasionally and there is evidence of a higher frequency of certain types of serious infections such as tuberculosis and atypical mycobacterial infection.

Respiratory: Interstitial lung disorders, including fatal pulmonary fibrosis, have been reported rarely and should be considered in the differential diagnosis of pulmonary symptoms ranging from dyspnea to respiratory failure in posttransplant patients receiving CellCept.

OVERDOSAGE

There has been no reported experience of overdosage of mycophenolate mofetil in humans. The highest dose administered to renal transplant patients in clinical trials has been 4 g/day. In limited experience with cardiac and hepatic transplant patients in clinical trials, the highest doses used were 4 g/day or 5 g/day. At doses of 4 g/day or 5 g/day, there appears to be a higher rate, compared to the use of 3 g/day or less, of gastrointestinal intolerance (nausea, vomiting, and/or diarrhea), and occasional hematologic abnormalities,

principally neutropenia, leading to a need to reduce or discontinue dosing.
In acute oral toxicity studies, no deaths occurred in adult mice at doses up to 4000 mg/kg or in adult monkeys at doses up to 1000 mg/kg; these were the highest doses of mycophenolate mofetil tested in these species. These doses represent 11 times the recommended clinical dose in renal transplant patients and approximately 7 times the recommended clinical dose in cardiac transplant patients when corrected for BSA. In adult rats, deaths occurred after single-oral doses of 500 mg/kg of mycophenolate mofetil. The dose represents approximately 3 times the recommended clinical dose in cardiac transplant patients when corrected for BSA.
MPA and MPAG are usually not removed by hemodialysis. However, at high MPAG plasma concentrations (>100 µg/mL), small amounts of MPAG are removed. By increasing excretion of the drug, MPA can be removed by bile acid sequestrants, such as cholestyramine (see CLINICAL PHARMACOLOGY: *Pharmacokinetics*).

DOSAGE AND ADMINISTRATION

RENAL TRANSPLANTATION: A dose of 1 g administered orally or intravenously (over 2 hours) twice a day (daily dose of 2 g) is recommended for use in renal transplant patients. Although a dose of 1.5 g administered twice daily (daily dose of 3 g) was used in clinical trials and was shown to be safe and effective, no efficacy advantage could be established for renal transplant patients. Patients receiving 2 g/day of CellCept demonstrated an overall better safety profile than did patients receiving 3 g/day of CellCept.
CARDIAC TRANSPLANTATION: A dose of 1.5 g bid administered intravenously (over NO LESS THAN 2 HOURS) or 1.5 g bid oral (daily dose of 3 g) is recommended for use in cardiac transplant patients.
HEPATIC TRANSPLANTATION: A dose of 1 g bid administered intravenously (over NO LESS THAN 2 HOURS) or 1.5 g bid oral (daily dose of 3 g) is recommended for use in hepatic transplant patients.
CellCept Capsules, Tablets, and Oral Suspension: The initial oral dose of CellCept should be given as soon as possible following renal, cardiac or hepatic transplantation. Food had no effect on MPA AUC, but has been shown to decrease MPA C_{max} by 40%. Therefore, it is recommended that CellCept be administered on an empty stomach. However, in stable renal transplant patients, CellCept may be administered with food if necessary.
Note:
If required, CellCept Oral Suspension can be administered via a nasogastric tube with a minimum size of 8 French (minimum 1.7 mm interior diameter).
Patients With Hepatic Impairment: No dose adjustments are recommended for renal patients with severe hepatic parenchymal disease. However, it is not known whether dose adjustments are needed for hepatic disease with other etiologies (see CLINICAL PHARMACOLOGY: *Pharmacokinetics*).
No data are available for cardiac transplant patients with severe hepatic parenchymal disease.
Geriatric Use: The recommended dose of 1 g bid for renal transplant patients, 1.5 g bid for cardiac transplant patients, and 1 g bid administered intravenously or 1.5 g bid administered orally in hepatic transplant patients is appropriate for elderly patients (see PRECAUTIONS: *Geriatric Use*).

Preparation of Oral Suspension
It is recommended that CellCept Oral Suspension be constituted by the pharmacist prior to dispensing to the patient. CellCept Oral Suspension should not be mixed with any other medication.
Mycophenolate mofetil has demonstrated teratogenic effects in rats and rabbits. There are no adequate and well-controlled studies in pregnant women. (See WARNINGS, PRECAUTIONS, ADVERSE REACTIONS, and HANDLING AND DISPOSAL.) Care should be taken to avoid inhalation or direct contact with skin or mucous membranes of the dry powder or the constituted suspension. If such contact occurs, wash thoroughly with soap and water; rinse eyes with water.
1. Tap the closed bottle several times to loosen the powder.
2. Measure 94 mL of water in a graduated cylinder.
3. Add approximately half the total amount of water for constitution to the bottle and shake the closed bottle well for about 1 minute.
4. Add the remainder of water and shake the closed bottle well for about 1 minute.
5. Remove the child-resistant cap and push bottle adapter into neck of bottle.
6. Close bottle with child-resistant cap tightly. This will assure the proper seating of the bottle adapter in the bottle and child-resistant status of the cap.

Dispense with patient instruction sheet and oral dispensers. It is recommended to write the date of expiration of the constituted suspension on the bottle label. (The shelf-life of the constituted suspension is 60 days.)
After constitution the oral suspension contains 200 mg/mL mycophenolate mofetil. Store constituted suspension at 25°C (77°F); excursions permitted to 15° to 30°C (59° to 86°F). Storage in a refrigerator at 2° to 8°C (36° to 46°F) is acceptable. Do not freeze. Discard any unused portion 60 days after constitution.
CellCept Intravenous: CellCept Intravenous is an alternative dosage form to CellCept capsules, tablets and oral suspension recommended for patients unable to take oral CellCept. CellCept Intravenous should be administered within 24 hours following transplantation. CellCept Intravenous can be administered for up to 14 days; patients should be switched to oral CellCept as soon as they can tolerate oral medication.
CellCept Intravenous must be reconstituted and diluted to a concentration of 6 mg/mL using 5% Dextrose Injection USP. CellCept Intravenous is incompatible with other intravenous infusion solutions. Following reconstitution, CellCept Intravenous must be administered by slow intravenous infusion over a period of NO LESS THAN 2 HOURS by either peripheral or central vein.
CAUTION: CELLCEPT INTRAVENOUS SOLUTION SHOULD NEVER BE ADMINISTERED BY RAPID OR BOLUS INTRAVENOUS INJECTION.

Preparation of Infusion Solution (6 mg/mL)
Caution should be exercised in the handling and preparation of solutions of CellCept Intravenous. Avoid direct contact of the prepared solution of CellCept Intravenous with skin or mucous membranes. If such contact occurs, wash thoroughly with soap and water; rinse eyes with plain water. (See WARNINGS, PRECAUTIONS, ADVERSE REACTIONS, and HANDLING AND DISPOSAL.
CellCept Intravenous does not contain an antibacterial preservative; therefore, reconstitution and dilution of the product must be performed under aseptic conditions.
CellCept Intravenous infusion solution must be prepared in two steps: the first step is a reconstitution step with 5% Dextrose Injection USP, and the second step is a dilution step with 5% Dextrose Injection USP. A detailed description of the preparation is given below:
Step 1
a. Two (2) vials of CellCept Intravenous are used for preparing each 1 g dose, whereas three (3) vials are needed for each 1.5 g dose. Reconstitute the contents of each vial by injecting 14 mL of 5% Dextrose Injection USP.
b. Gently shake the vial to dissolve the drug.
c. Inspect the resulting slightly yellow solution for particulate matter and discoloration prior to further dilution. Discard the vial if particulate matter or discoloration is observed.

Step 2
a. To prepare a 1 g dose, further dilute the contents of the two reconstituted vials (approx. 2 × 15 mL) into 140 mL of 5% Dextrose Injection USP. To prepare a 1.5 g dose, further dilute the contents of the three reconstituted vials (approx. 3 × 15 mL) into 210 mL of 5% Dextrose Injection USP. The final concentration of both solutions is 6 mg mycophenolate mofetil per mL.
b. Inspect the infusion solution for particulate matter or discoloration. Discard the infusion solution if particulate matter or discoloration is observed.

If the infusion solution is not prepared immediately prior to administration, the commencement of administration of the infusion solution should be within 4 hours from reconstitution and dilution of the drug product. Keep solutions at 25°C (77°F); excursions permitted to 15° to 30°C (59° to 86°F).
CellCept Intravenous should not be mixed or administered concurrently via the same infusion catheter with other intravenous drugs or infusion admixtures.
Dosage Adjustments: In renal transplant patients with severe chronic renal impairment (GFR <25 mL/min/1.73 m^2) outside the immediate posttransplant period, doses of CellCept greater than 1 g administered twice a day should be avoided. These patients should also be carefully observed. No dose adjustments are needed in renal transplant patients experiencing delayed graft function postoperatively (see CLINICAL PHARMACOLOGY: *Pharmacokinetics* and PRECAUTIONS: *General*).
No data are available for cardiac or hepatic transplant patients with severe chronic renal impairment. CellCept may be used for cardiac or hepatic transplant patients with severe chronic renal impairment if the potential benefits outweigh the potential risks.
If neutropenia develops (ANC <1.3 x 10^3/µL), dosing with CellCept should be interrupted or the dose reduced, appropriate diagnostic tests performed, and the patient managed appropriately (see WARNINGS, ADVERSE REACTIONS, and PRECAUTIONS: *Laboratory Tests*).

HANDLING AND DISPOSAL

Mycophenolate mofetil has demonstrated teratogenic effects in rats and rabbits. CellCept tablets should not be crushed and CellCept capsules should not be opened or crushed. Avoid inhalation or direct contact with skin or mucous membranes of the powder contained in CellCept capsules and CellCept Oral Suspension (before or after constitution). If such contact occurs, wash thoroughly with soap and water; rinse eyes with plain water. Should a spill occur, wipe up using paper towels wetted with water to remove spilled powder or suspension. Caution should be exercised in the handling and preparation of solutions of CellCept Intravenous. Avoid direct contact of the prepared solution of CellCept Intravenous with skin or mucous membranes. If such contact occurs, wash thoroughly with soap and water; rinse eyes with plain water.

HOW SUPPLIED

CellCept (mycophenolate mofetil capsules)
250 mg
Blue-brown, two-piece hard gelatin capsules, printed in black with "CellCept 250" on the blue cap and "Roche" on the brown body. Supplied in the following presentations:

NDC Number	Size
NDC 0004-0259-01	Bottle of 100
NDC 0004-0259-05	Package containing 12 bottles of 120
NDC 0004-0259-43	Bottle of 500

Storage: Store at 25°C (77°F); excursions permitted to 15° to 30°C (59° to 86°F).

CellCept (mycophenolate mofetil tablets)
500 mg
Lavender-colored, caplet-shaped, film-coated tablets printed in black with "CellCept 500" on one side and "Roche" on the other. Supplied in the following presentations:

NDC Number	Size
NDC 0004-0260-01	Bottle of 100
NDC 0004-0260-43	Bottle of 500

Storage and Dispensing Information: Store at 25°C (77°F); excursions permitted to 15° to 30°C (59° to 86°F). Dispense in light-resistant containers, such as the manufacturer's original containers.

CellCept Oral Suspension (mycophenolate mofetil for oral suspension)
Supplied as a white to off-white powder blend for constitution to a white to off-white mixed-fruit flavor suspension. Supplied in the following presentation:

NDC Number	Size
NDC 0004-0261-29	225 mL bottle with bottle adapter and 2 oral dispensers

Storage: Store dry powder at 25°C (77°F); excursions permitted to 15° to 30°C (59° to 86°F). Store constituted suspension at 25°C (77°F); excursions permitted to 15° to 30°C (59° to 86°F) for up to 60 days. Storage in a refrigerator at 2° to 8°C (36° to 46°F) is acceptable. Do not freeze.

CellCept Intravenous (mycophenolate mofetil hydrochloride for injection)

Continued on next page

Viral and Fungal Infections in Controlled Studies in Prevention of Renal, Cardiac or Hepatic Transplant Rejection

	Renal Studies			Cardiac Study		Hepatic Study	
	CellCept 2 g/day	CellCept 3 g/day	Azathioprine 1 to 2 mg/kg/day or 100 to 150 mg/day	CellCept 3 g/day	Azathioprine 1.5 to 3 mg/kg/day	CellCept 3 g/day	Azathioprine 1 to 2 mg/kg/day
	(n=336)	(n=330)	(n=326)	(n=289)	(n=289)	(n=277)	(n=287)
	%	%	%	%	%	%	%
Herpes simplex	16.7	20.0	19.0	20.8	14.5	10.1	5.9
CMV							
–Viremia/syndrome	13.4	12.4	13.8	12.1	10.0	14.1	12.2
–Tissue invasive disease	8.3	11.5	6.1	11.4	8.7	5.8	8.0
Herpes zoster	6.0	7.6	5.8	10.7	5.9	4.3	4.9
–Cutaneous disease	6.0	7.3	5.5	10.0	5.5	4.3	4.9
Candida	17.0	17.3	18.1	18.7	17.6	22.4	24.4
–Mucocutaneous	15.5	16.4	15.3	18.0	17.3	18.4	17.4

Adverse Events Reported in 3% to <10% of Patients Treated With CellCept in Combination With Cyclosporine and Corticosteroids

Body System	Renal	Cardiac	Hepatic
Body as a Whole	abdomen enlarged, accidental injury, chills occurring with fever, cyst, face edema, flu syndrome, hemorrhage, hernia, malaise, plevic pain	abdomen enlarged, cellulitis, chills occurring with fever, cyst, face edema, flu syndrome, hemorrhage, hernia, malaise, neck pain, pelvic pain	abscess, cellulitis, chills occurring with fever, cyst, flu syndrome, hemorrhage, lab test abnormal, malaise, neck pain
Hemic and Lymphatic	ecchymosis, polycythemia	petechia, prothrombin time increased, thromboplastin time increased	coagulation disorder, ecchymosis, pancytopenia, prothrombin time increased
Urogenital	albuminuria, dysuria, hydronephrosis, impotence, pain, pyelonephritis, urinary frequency, urinary tract disorder	dysuria, hematuria, impotence, kidney failure, nocturia, prostatic disorder, urine abnormality, urinary frequency, urinary incontinence, urinary retention	acute kidney failure, dysuria, hematuria, kidney failure, scrotal edema, urinary frequency, urinary incontinence
Cardiovascular	angina pectoris, atrial fibrillation, cardiovascular disorder, hypotension, palpitation, peripheral vascular disorder, postural hypotension, tachycardia thrombosis, vasodilatation	angina pectoris, atrial fibrillation, atrial flutter, congestive heart failure, extrasystole, heart arrest, palpitation, pallor, peripheral vascular disorder, postural hypotension, pulmonary hypertension, supraventricular tachycardia, supraventricular extrasystoles, syncope, vasospasm, ventricular extrasystole, ventricular tachycardia, venous pressure increased	arrhythmia, arterial thrombosis, atrial fibrillation, bradycardia, palpitation, syncope, vasodilatation
Metabolic and Nutritional	acidosis, alkaline phosphatase increased, creatinine increased, dehydration, gamma glutamyl transpeptidase increased, hypercalcemia, hyperlipemia, hyperuricemia, hypervolemia, hypocalcemia, hypoglycemia, hypoproteinemia, lactic dehydrogenase increased, SGOT increased, SGPT increased, weight gain	abnormal healing, alkaline phosphatase increased, alkalosis, dehydration, gout, hypocalcemia, hypochloremia, hypoglycemia, hypophosphatemia, hypoproteinemia, hypovolemia, hypoxia, respiratory acidosis, thirst, weight loss	acidosis, alkaline phosphatase increased, dehydration, hypercholesteremia, hyperlipemia, hyperphosphatemia, hypervolemia, hyponatremia, hypoxia, hypovolemia, SGOT increased, SGPT increased, weight gain, weight loss
Digestive	anorexia, esophagitis, flatulence, gastritis, gastroenteritis, gastrointestinal hemorrhage, gastrointestinal moniliasis, gingivitis, gum hyperplasia, hepatitis, ileus, infection, liver function tests abnormal, mouth ulceration, rectal disorder	anorexia, dysphagia, esophagitis, gastritis, gastroenteritis, gastrointestinal disorder, gingivitis, gum hyperplasia, infection, jaundice, liver damage, liver function tests abnormal, melena, rectal disorder, stomatitis	dysphagia, esophagitis, gastritis, gastrointestinal disorder, gastrointestinal hemorrhage, ileus, infection, jaundice, melena, mouth ulceration, nausea and vomiting, rectal disorder, stomach ulcer
Respiratory	asthma, bronchitis, lung edema, lung disorder, pleural effusion, pneumonia, rhinitis, sinusitis	apnea, atelectasis, bronchitis, epistaxis, hemoptysis, hiccup, lung edema, neoplasm, pain, pneumothorax, respiratory disorder, sputum increased, voice alteration	asthma, bronchitis, epistaxis, hyperventilation, lung edema, pneumothorax, respiratory disorder, respiratory moniliasis, rhinitis
Skin and Appendages	alopecia, fungal dermatitis, hirsutism, pruritus, rash, skin benign neoplasm, skin carcinoma, skin disorder, skin hypertrophy, skin ulcer, sweating	fungal dermatitis, hemorrhage, pruritus, skin benign neoplasm, skin carcinoma, skin hypertrophy, skin ulcer, sweating	acne, fungal dermatitis hemorrhage, hirsutism, skin benign neoplasm, skin disorder, skin ulcer, vesiculobullous rash
Nervous	anxiety, depression, hypertonia, paresthesia, somnolence	convulsion, emotional lability, hallucinations, neuropathy, thinking abnormal, vertigo	agitation, convulsion, delirium, dry mouth, hypertonia, hypesthesia, neuropathy, psychosis, thinking anormal, somnolence
Endocrine	diabetes mellitus, parathroid disorder	Cushing's syndrome, diabetes mellitus, hypothyroidism	diabetes mellitus
Musculoskeletal	arthralgia, joint disorder, leg cramps, myalgia, myasthenia	arthralgia, joint disorder	arthralgia, leg cramps, myalgia, myasthenia, osteoporosis
Special Senses	amblyopia, cataract (not specified), conjunctivitis	abnormal vision, conjunctivitis, deafness, ear disorder, ear pain, eye hemorrhage, tinnitus, lacrimation disorder	abnormal vision, amblyopia, conjunctivitis, deafness

CellCept—Cont.

Supplied in a 20 mL, sterile vial containing the equivalent of 500 mg mycophenolate mofetil as the hydrochloride salt in cartons of 4 vials:

NDC Number

NDC 0004-0298-09

Storage: Store powder and reconstituted/infusion solutions at 25°C (77°F); excursions permitted to 15° to 30°C (59° to 86°F).

Rx only

Revised: July 2000

Shown in Product Identification Guide, page 332

CYTOVENE®-IV ℞

(ganciclovir sodium for injection)
FOR INTRAVENOUS INFUSION ONLY
CYTOVENE®
(ganciclovir capsules)
FOR ORAL ADMINISTRATION

The following text is complete prescribing information based on official labeling in effect June 2000.

WARNING: THE CLINICAL TOXICITY OF CYTOVENE AND CYTOVENE-IV INCLUDES GRANULOCYTOPENIA, ANEMIA AND THROMBOCYTOPENIA. IN ANIMAL STUDIES GANCICLOVIR WAS CARCINOGENIC, TERATOGENIC AND CAUSED ASPERMATOGENESIS.

CYTOVENE-IV IS INDICATED FOR USE *ONLY* IN THE TREATMENT OF CYTOMEGALOVIRUS (CMV) RETINITIS IN IMMUNOCOMPROMISED PATIENTS AND FOR THE PREVENTION OF CMV DISEASE IN TRANSPLANT PATIENTS AT RISK FOR CMV DISEASE.

CYTOVENE CAPSULES ARE INDICATED *ONLY* FOR PREVENTION OF CMV DISEASE IN PATIENTS WITH ADVANCED HIV INFECTION AT RISK FOR CMV DISEASE, FOR MAINTENANCE TREATMENT OF CMV RETINITIS IN IMMUNOCOMPROMISED PATIENTS, AND FOR PREVENTION OF CMV DISEASE IN SOLID ORGAN TRANSPLANT RECIPIENTS (see INDICATIONS AND USAGE).

BECAUSE CYTOVENE CAPSULES ARE ASSOCIATED WITH A RISK OF MORE RAPID RATE OF CMV RETINITIS PROGRESSION, THEY SHOULD BE USED AS MAINTENANCE TREATMENT ONLY IN THOSE PATIENTS FOR WHOM THIS RISK IS BALANCED BY THE BENEFIT ASSOCIATED WITH AVOIDING DAILY INTRAVENOUS INFUSIONS.

DESCRIPTION

Ganciclovir is a synthetic guanine derivative active against cytomegalovirus (CMV). CYTOVENE-IV and CYTOVENE are the brand names for ganciclovir sodium for injection and ganciclovir capsules, respectively.

CYTOVENE-IV is available as sterile lyophilized powder in strength of 500 mg per vial for intravenous administration only. Each vial of CYTOVENE-IV contains the equivalent of 500 mg ganciclovir as the sodium salt (46 mg sodium). Reconstitution with 10 mL of Sterile Water for Injection, USP, yields a solution with pH 11 and a ganciclovir concentration of approximately 50 mg/mL. Further dilution in an appropriate intravenous solution must be performed before infusion (see DOSAGE AND ADMINISTRATION).

CYTOVENE is available as 250 mg and 500 mg capsules. Each capsule contains 250 mg or 500 mg ganciclovir, respectively, and inactive ingredients croscarmellose sodium, magnesium stearate and povidone. Both hard gelatin shells consist of gelatin, titanium dioxide, yellow iron oxide and FD&C Blue No. 2.

Ganciclovir is a white to off-white crystalline powder with a molecular formula of $C_9H_{13}N_5O_4$ and a molecular weight of 255.23. The chemical name for ganciclovir is 9-[[2-hydroxy-1-(hydroxymethyl)ethoxy]methyl]guanine. Ganciclovir is a polar hydrophilic compound with a solubility of 2.6 mg/mL in water at 25°C and an n-octanol/water partition coefficient of 0.022. The pK_as for ganciclovir are 2.2 and 9.4.

Ganciclovir, when formulated as monosodium salt in the IV dosage form, is a white to off-white lyophilized powder with a molecular formula of $C_9H_{12}N_5NaO_4$, and a molecular weight of 277.22. The chemical name for ganciclovir sodium is 9-[[2-hydroxy-1-(hydroxymethyl) ethoxy]methyl]guanine, monosodium salt. The lyophilized powder has an aqueous solubility of greater than 50 mg/mL at 25°C. At physiological pH, ganciclovir sodium exists as the un-ionized form with a solubility of approximately 6 mg/mL at 37°C.

All doses in this insert are specified in terms of ganciclovir.

VIROLOGY

Mechanism of Action: Ganciclovir is an acyclic nucleoside analogue of 2′-deoxyguanosine that inhibits replication of herpes viruses. Ganciclovir has been shown to be active against cytomegalovirus (CMV) and herpes simplex virus (HSV) in human clinical studies.

To achieve anti-CMV activity, ganciclovir is phosphorylated first to the monophosphate form by a CMV-encoded (UL97 gene) protein kinase homologue, then to the di- and triphosphate forms by cellular kinases. Ganciclovir triphosphate concentrations may be 100-fold greater in CMV-infected than in uninfected cells, indicating preferential phosphorylation in infected cells. Ganciclovir triphosphate, once formed, persists for days in the CMV-infected cell. Ganciclovir triphosphate is believed to inhibit viral DNA synthesis by (1) competitive inhibition of viral DNA polymerases; and (2) incorporation into viral DNA, resulting in eventual termination of viral DNA elongation.

Antiviral Activity: The median concentration of ganciclovir that inhibits CMV replication (IC_{50}) in vitro (laboratory strains or clinical isolates) has ranged from 0.02 to 3.48 µg/mL. Ganciclovir inhibits mammalian cell proliferation (CIC_{50}) in vitro at higher concentrations ranging from 30 to 725 µg/mL. Bone marrow-derived colony-forming cells are more sensitive (CIC_{50} 0.028 to 0.7 µg/mL). The relationship of in vitro sensitivity of CMV to ganciclovir and clinical response has not been established.

Clinical Antiviral Effect of CYTOVENE-IV and CYTOVENE Capsules: *CYTOVENE-IV:* In a study of CYTOVENE-IV treatment of life- or sight-threatening CMV disease in immunocompromised patients, 121 of 314 patients had CMV cultured within 7 days prior to treatment and sequential posttreatment viral cultures of urine, blood, throat and/or semen. As judged by conversion to culture negativity, or a greater than 100-fold decrease in in vitro CMV titer, at least 83% of patients had a virologic response with a median response time of 7 to 15 days.

Antiviral activity of CYTOVENE-IV was demonstrated in two randomized studies for the prevention of CMV disease in transplant recipients (see table below).

[See first table at top of next page]

CYTOVENE Capsules: In trials comparing CYTOVENE-IV with CYTOVENE capsules for the maintenance treatment of CMV retinitis in patients with AIDS, serial urine cultures and other available cultures (semen, biopsy specimens, blood and others) showed that a small proportion of patients remained culture-positive during maintenance therapy with no statistically significant differences in CMV isolation rates between treatment groups.

A study of CYTOVENE capsules (1000 mg q8h) for prevention of CMV disease in individuals with advanced HIV infection (ICM 1654) evaluated antiviral activity as measured by CMV isolation in culture; most cultures were from urine. At baseline, 40% (176/436) and 44% (92/210) of ganciclovir and placebo recipients, respectively, had positive cultures (urine or blood). After 2 months on treatment, 10% vs 44% of ganciclovir vs placebo recipients had positive cultures.

Viral Resistance: The current working definition of CMV resistance to ganciclovir in in vitro assays is IC_{50} >3.0 µg/mL (12.0 µM). CMV resistance to ganciclovir has been observed in individuals with AIDS and CMV retinitis who have never received ganciclovir therapy. Viral resistance has also been observed in patients receiving prolonged treatment for CMV retinitis with CYTOVENE-IV. In a controlled study of oral ganciclovir for prevention of AIDS-associated CMV disease, 364 individuals had one or more cultures performed after at least 90 days of ganciclovir treatment. Of these, 113 had at least one positive culture. The last available isolate from each subject was tested for reduced sensitivity, and 2 of 40 were found to be resistant to ganciclovir. These resistant isolates were associated with subsequent treatment failure for retinitis.

The possibility of viral resistance should be considered in patients who show poor clinical response or experience persistent viral excretion during therapy. The principal mechanism of resistance to ganciclovir in CMV is the decreased ability to form the active triphosphate moiety; resistant viruses have been described that contain mutations in the UL97 gene of CMV that controls phosphorylation of ganciclovir. Mutations in the viral DNA polymerase have also been reported to confer viral resistance to ganciclovir.

CLINICAL PHARMACOLOGY

Pharmacokinetics:

BECAUSE THE MAJOR ELIMINATION PATHWAY FOR GANCICLOVIR IS RENAL, DOSAGE REDUCTIONS ACCORDING TO CREATININE CLEARANCE ARE REQUIRED FOR CYTOVENE-IV AND SHOULD BE CONSIDERED FOR CYTOVENE CAPSULES. FOR DOSING INSTRUCTIONS IN PATIENTS WITH RENAL IMPAIRMENT, REFER TO DOSAGE AND ADMINISTRATION.

Absorption: The absolute bioavailability of oral ganciclovir under fasting conditions was approximately 5% (n=6) and following food was 6% to 9% (n=32). When ganciclovir was administered orally with food at a total daily dosage of 3 g/day (500 mg q3h, 6 times daily and 1000 mg tid), the steady-state absorption as measured by area under the serum concentration vs time curve (AUC) over 24 hours and maximum serum concentrations (C_{max}) were similar following both regimens with an AUC_{0-24} of 15.9 ± 4.2 (mean ± SD) and 15.4 ± 4.3 µg·hr/mL and C_{max} of 1.02 ± 0.24 and 1.18 ± 0.36 µg/mL, respectively (n=16).

At the end of a 1-hour intravenous infusion of 5 mg/kg ganciclovir, total AUC ranged between 22.1 ± 3.2 (n=16) and 26.8 ± 6.1 µg·hr/mL (n=16) and C_{max} ranged between 8.27 ± 1.02 (n=16) and 9.0 ± 1.4 µg/mL (n=16).

Food Effects: When CYTOVENE capsules were given with a meal containing 602 calories and 46.5% fat at a dosage of 1000 mg every 8 hours to 20 HIV-positive subjects, the steady-state AUC increased by 22 ± 22% (range: -6% to 68%) and there was a significant prolongation of time to peak serum concentrations (T_{max}) from 1.8 ± 0.8 to 3.0 ± 0.6 hours and a higher C_{max} (0.85 ± 0.25 vs 0.96 ± 0.27 µg/mL) (n=20).

Distribution: The steady-state volume of distribution of ganciclovir after intravenous administration was 0.74 ± 0.15 L/kg (n=98). For CYTOVENE capsules, no correlation was observed between AUC and reciprocal weight (range: 55 to 128 kg); oral dosing according to weight is not required. Cerebrospinal fluid concentrations obtained 0.25 to 5.67 hours postdose in 3 patients who received 2.5 mg/kg ganciclovir intravenously q8h or q12h ranged from 0.31 to 0.68 µg/mL representing 24% to 70% of the respective plasma concentrations. Binding to plasma proteins was 1% to 2% over ganciclovir concentrations of 0.5 and 51 µg/mL.

Metabolism: Following oral administration of a single 1000 mg dose of ^{14}C-labeled ganciclovir, 86 ± 3% of the administered dose was recovered in the feces and 5 ± 1% was recovered in the urine (n=4). No metabolite accounted for more than 1% to 2% of the radioactivity recovered in urine or feces.

Elimination: When administered intravenously, ganciclovir exhibits linear pharmacokinetics over the range of 1.6 to 5.0 mg/kg and when administered orally, it exhibits linear kinetics up to a total daily dose of 4 g/day. Renal excretion of unchanged drug by glomerular filtration and active tubular secretion is the major route of elimination of ganciclovir. In patients with normal renal function, 91.3 ± 5.0% (n=4) of intravenously administered ganciclovir was recovered unmetabolized in the urine. Systemic clearance of intravenously administered ganciclovir was 3.52 ± 0.80 mL/min/kg (n=98) while renal clearance was 3.20 ± 0.80 mL/min/kg (n=47), accounting for 91 ± 11% of the systemic clearance (n=47). After oral administration of ganciclovir, steady-state is achieved within 24 hours. Renal clearance following oral administration was 3.1 ± 1.2 mL/min/kg (n=22). Half-life was 3.5 ± 0.9 hours (n=98) following IV administration and 4.8 ± 0.9 hours (n=39) following oral administration.

Patients With Positive CMV Cultures

Time	Heart Allograft* (n=147) CYTOVENE-IV†	Heart Allograft* (n=147) Placebo	Bone Marrow Allograft (n=72) CYTOVENE-IV‡	Bone Marrow Allograft (n=72) Placebo
Pretreatment	1/67 (2%)	5/64 (8%)	37/37 (100%)	35/35 (100%)
Week 2	2/75 (3%)	11/67 (16%)	2/31 (6%)	19/28 (68%)
Week 4	3/66 (5%)	28/66 (43%)	0/24 (0%)	16/20 (80%)

* CMV seropositive or receiving graft from seropositive donor
† 5 mg/kg bid for 14 days followed by 6 mg/kg qd for 5 days/week for 14 days
‡ 5 mg/kg bid for 7 days followed by 5 mg/kg qd until day 100 posttransplant

Estimated Creatinine Clearance (mL/min)	n	Dose	Clearance (mL/min) Mean ± SD	Half-life (hours) Mean ± SD
50–79	4	3.2 – 5 mg/kg	128 ± 63	4.6 ± 1.4
25–49	3	3 – 5 mg/kg	57 ± 8	4.4 ± 0.4
<25	3	1.25 – 5 mg/kg	30 ± 13	10.7 ± 5.7

Special Populations: *Renal Impairment:* The pharmacokinetics following intravenous administration of CYTOVENE-IV solution were evaluated in 10 immunocompromised patients with renal impairment who received doses ranging from 1.25 to 5.0 mg/kg.

[See second table above]

The pharmacokinetics of ganciclovir following oral administration of CYTOVENE capsules were evaluated in 44 patients, who were either solid organ transplant recipients or HIV positive. Apparent oral clearance of ganciclovir decreased and AUC_{0-24h} increased with diminishing renal function (as expressed by creatinine clearance). Based on these observations, it is necessary to modify the dosage of ganciclovir in patients with renal impairment (see DOSAGE AND ADMINISTRATION).

Hemodialysis reduces plasma concentrations of ganciclovir by about 50% after both intravenous and oral administration.

Race/Ethnicity and Gender: The effects of race/ethnicity and gender were studied in subjects receiving a dose regimen of 1000 mg every 8 hours. Although the numbers of blacks (16%) and Hispanics (20%) were small, there appeared to be a trend towards a lower steady-state C_{max} and AUC_{0-8} in these subpopulations as compared to Caucasians. No definitive conclusions regarding gender differences could be made because of the small number of females (12%); however, no differences between males and females were observed.

Pediatrics: Ganciclovir pharmacokinetics were studied in 27 neonates, aged 2 to 49 days. At an intravenous dose of 4 mg/kg (n=14) or 6 mg/kg (n=13), the pharmacokinetic parameters were, respectively, C_{max} of 5.5 ± 1.6 and 7.0 ± 1.6 µg/mL, systemic clearance of 3.14 ± 1.75 and 3.56 ± 1.27 mL/min/kg, and $t_{1/2}$ of 2.4 hours (harmonic mean) for both. Ganciclovir phrmacokinetics were also studied in 10 pediatric patients, aged 9 months to 12 years. The pharmacokinetic characteristics of ganciclovir were the same after single and multiple (q12h) intravenous doses (5 mg/kg). The steady-state volume of distribution was 0.64 ± 0.22 L/kg, C_{max} was 7.9 ± 3.9 µg/mL, systemic clearance was 4.7 ± 2.2 mL/min/kg, and $t_{1/2}$ was 2.4 ± 0.7 hours. The pharmacokinetics of intravenous ganciclovir in pediatric patients are similar to those observed in adults.

Elderly: No studies have been conducted in adults older than 65 years of age.

INDICATIONS AND USAGE

CYTOVENE-IV is indicated for the treatment of CMV retinitis in immunocompromised patients, including patients with acquired immunodeficiency syndrome (AIDS). CYTOVENE-IV is also indicated for the prevention of CMV disease in transplant recipients at risk for CMV disease (see CLINICAL TRIALS).

CYTOVENE capsules are indicated for the prevention of CMV disease in solid organ transplant recipients and in individuals with advanced HIV infection at risk for developing CMV disease. CYTOVENE capsules are also indicated as an alternative to the intravenous formulation for maintenance treatment of CMV retinitis in immunocompromised patients, including patients with AIDS, in whom retinitis is stable following appropriate induction therapy and for whom the risk of more rapid progression is balanced by the benefit associated with avoiding daily IV infusions (see CLINICAL TRIALS).

SAFETY AND EFFICACY OF **CYTOVENE-IV** AND **CYTOVENE** HAVE NOT BEEN ESTABLISHED FOR CONGENITAL OR NEONATAL CMV DISEASE; NOR FOR THE TREATMENT OF ESTABLISHED CMV DISEASE OTHER THAN RETINITIS; NOR FOR USE IN NON-IMMUNOCOMPROMISED INDIVIDUALS. THE SAFETY AND EFFICACY OF **CYTOVENE** CAPSULES HAVE NOT BEEN ESTABLISHED FOR TREATING ANY MANIFESTATION OF CMV DISEASE OTHER THAN MAINTENANCE TREATMENT OF CMV RETINITIS.

CLINICAL TRIALS

1. Treatment of CMV Retinitis

The diagnosis of CMV retinitis should be made by indirect ophthalmoscopy. Other conditions in the differential diagnosis of CMV retinitis include candidiasis, toxoplasmosis, histoplasmosis, retinal scars and cotton wool spots, any of which may produce a retinal appearance similar to CMV. For this reason it is essential that the diagnosis of CMV be established by an ophthalmologist familiar with the retinal presentation of these conditions. The diagnosis of CMV retinitis may be supported by culture of CMV from urine, blood, throat or other sites, but a negative CMV culture does not rule out CMV retinitis.

Studies With CYTOVENE-IV: In a retrospective, non-randomized, single-center analysis of 41 patients with AIDS and CMV retinitis diagnosed by ophthalmologic examination between August 1983 and April 1988, treatment with CYTOVENE-IV solution resulted in a significant delay in mean (median) time to first retinitis progression compared to untreated controls [105 (71) days from diagnosis vs 35 (29) days from diagnosis]. Patients in this series received induction treatment of CYTOVENE-IV 5 mg/kg bid for 14 to 21 days followed by maintenance treatment with either 5 mg/kg once daily, 7 days per week or 6 mg/kg once daily, 5 days per week (see DOSAGE AND ADMINISTRATION).

In a controlled, randomized study conducted between February 1989 and December 1990,[1] immediate treatment with CYTOVENE-IV was compared to delayed treatment in 42 patients with AIDS and peripheral CMV retinitis; 35 of 42 patients (13 in the immediate-treatment group and 22 in the delayed-treatment group) were included in the analysis of time to retinitis progression. Based on masked assessment of fundus photographs, the mean [95% CI] and median [95% CI] times to progression of retinitis were 66 days [39, 94] and 50 days [40, 84], respectively, in the immediate-treatment group compared to 19 days [11, 27] and 13.5 days [8, 18], respectively, in the delayed-treatment group.

Studies Comparing CYTOVENE Capsules to CYTOVENE-IV:

[See first table at top of next page]

ICM 1653: In this randomized, open-label, parallel group trial, conducted between March 1991 and November 1992, patients with AIDS and newly diagnosed CMV retinitis received a 3-week induction course of CYTOVENE-IV solution, 5 mg/kg bid for 14 days followed by 5 mg/kg once daily for 1 additional week.[2] Following the 21-day intravenous induction course, patients with stable CMV retinitis were randomized to receive 20 weeks of maintenance treatment with either CYTOVENE-IV solution, 5 mg/kg once daily, or CYTOVENE capsules, 500 mg 6 times daily (3000 mg/day). The study showed that the mean [95% CI] and median [95% CI] times to progression of CMV retinitis, as assessed by masked reading of fundus photographs, were 57 days [44, 70] and 29 days [28, 43], respectively, for patients on oral therapy compared to 62 days [50, 73] and 49 days [29, 61], respectively, for patients on intravenous therapy. The difference [95% CI] in the mean time to progression between the oral and intravenous therapies (oral - IV) was -5 days [-22, 12]. See Figure 1 for comparison of the proportion of patients remaining free of progression over time.

ICM 1774: In this three-arm, randomized, open-label, parallel group trial, conducted between June 1991 and August 1993, patients with AIDS and stable CMV retinitis following from 4 weeks to 4 months of treatment with CYTOVENE-IV solution were randomized to receive maintenance treatment with CYTOVENE-IV solution, 5 mg/kg once daily, CYTOVENE capsules, 500 mg 6 times daily, or CYTOVENE capsules, 1000 mg tid for 20 weeks. The study showed that the mean [95% CI] and median [95% CI] times to progression of CMV retinitis, as assessed by masked reading of fundus photographs, were 54 days [48, 60] and 42 days [31, 54], respectively, for patients on oral therapy compared to 66 days [56, 76] and 54 days [41, 69], respectively, for patients on intravenous therapy. The difference [95% CI] in the mean time to progression between the oral and intravenous therapies (oral - IV) was -12 days [-24, 0]. See Figure 2 for comparison of the proportion of patients remaining free of progression over time.

AVI 034: In this randomized, open-label, parallel group trial, conducted between June 1991 and February 1993, patients with AIDS and newly diagnosed (81%) or previously treated (19%) CMV retinitis who had tolerated 10 to 21 days of induction treatment with CYTOVENE-IV, 5 mg/kg twice daily, were randomized to receive 20 weeks of maintenance treatment with either CYTOVENE capsules, 500 mg 6 times daily or CYTOVENE-IV solution, 5 mg/kg/day.[3] The mean [95% CI] and median [95% CI] times to progression of CMV retinitis, as assessed by masked reading of fundus photographs, were 51 days [44, 57] and 41 days [31, 45], respectively, for patients on oral therapy compared to 62 days [52, 72] and 60 days [42, 83], respectively, for patients on

Continued on next page

Cytovene—Cont.

intravenous therapy. The difference [95% CI] in the mean time to progression between the oral and intravenous therapies (oral - IV) was -11 days [-24, 1]. See Figure 3 for comparison of the proportion of patients remaining free of progression over time.
Comparison of other CMV retinitis outcomes between oral and IV formulations (development of bilateral retinitis, progression into Zone 1, and deterioration of visual acuity), while not definitive, showed no marked differences between treatment groups in these studies. Because of low event rates among these endpoints, these studies are underpowered to rule out significant differences in these endpoints.

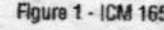
Figure 1 - ICM 1653

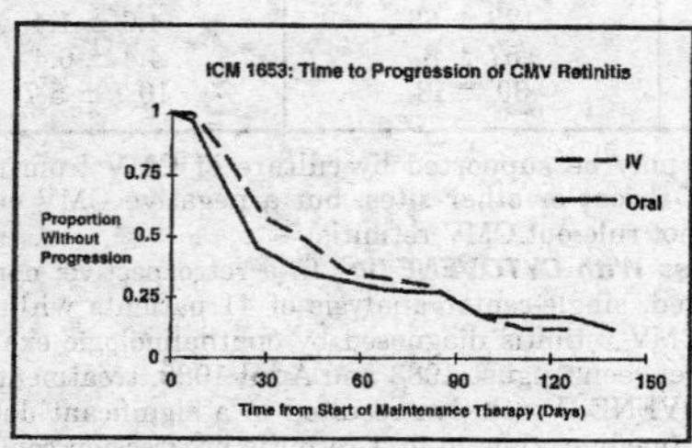

Figure 2 - ICM 1774

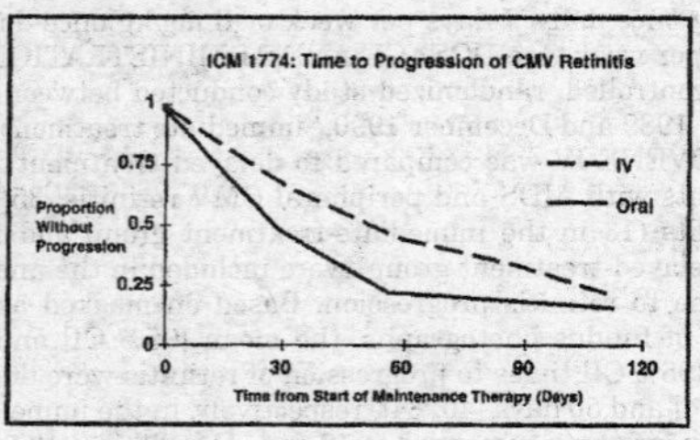

Figure 3 - AVI 034

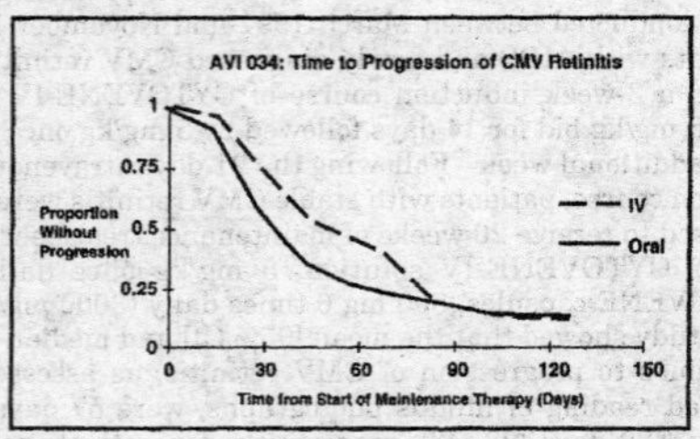

2. *Prevention of CMV Disease in Subjects With AIDS*
ICM 1654: In a double-blind study conducted between November 1992 and July 1994, 725 subjects with AIDS, who were CMV seropositive and/or culture positive, were randomized to receive CYTOVENE capsules, 1000 mg, every 8 hours, or placebo.[4] The study population had a median age of 38 years (range: 21 to 69); were 99% male; were 82% Caucasian, 10% Hispanic, 7% African-American and 1% Asian; and had a median CD_4 count of 21 (range: 0 to 100). The mean observation time was 351 days (range: 5 to 621). As shown in the following table, significantly more placebo recipients developed CMV disease.

Incidence of CMV Disease at 6, 12 and 18 Months After Enrollment (Kaplan-Meier Estimates)

	Incidence (Number Still At Risk) CMV Disease	
	Ganciclovir	Placebo
6 months	8% (397)	11% (190)
12 months	14% (225)	26% (92)
18 months	20% (27)	39% (9)

3. *Prevention of CMV Disease In Transplant Recipients*
CYTOVENE-IV: CYTOVENE-IV was evaluated in three randomized, controlled trials of prevention of CMV disease in organ transplant recipients.
ICM 1496: In a randomized, double-blind, placebo-controlled study of 149 heart transplant recipients[5] at risk for CMV infection (CMV seropositive or a seronegative recipient of an organ from a CMV seropositive donor), there was a statistically significant reduction in the overall incidence of CMV disease in patients treated with CYTOVENE-IV. Immediately posttransplant, patients received CYTOVENE-IV solution 5 mg/kg bid for 14 days followed by 6 mg/kg qd for 5 days/week for an additional 14 days. Twelve of the 76 (16%) patients treated with CYTOVENE-IV vs 31 of the 73 (43%) placebo-treated patients developed CMV disease during the 120-day posttransplant observation period. No significant differences in hematologic toxicities were seen between the two treatment groups (refer to table in ADVERSE EVENTS).

Population Characteristics in Studies ICM 1653, ICM 1774 and AVI 034

		ICM 1653 (n=121)	ICM 1774 (n=225)	AVI 034 (n=159)
Median age (years) Range		38 24–62	37 22–56	39 23–62
Sex	Males	116 (96%)	222 (99%)	148 (93%)
	Females	5 (4%)	3 (1%)	10 (6%)
Ethnicity	Asian	3 (3%)	5 (2%)	7 (4%)
	Black	11 (9%)	9 (4%)	3 (2%)
	Caucasian	98 (81%)	186 (83%)	140 (88%)
	Other	9 (7%)	25 (11%)	8 (5%)
Median CD_4 Count Range		9.5 0 – 141	7.0 0 – 80	10.0 0 – 320
Mean (SD) Observation Time (days)		107.9 (43.0)	97.6 (42.5)	80.9 (47.0)

Incidence of CMV Disease at 6 Months (Kaplan-Meier Estimates)

CMV Disease at 6 months	Ganciclovir (n=150)	Placebo (n=154)	Relative Risk (95% CI)
CMV Disease,* N (%)	7 (4.8%)	29 (18.9%)	0.22 (0.10, 0.51)
CMV syndrome†	6 (4.1%)	19 (12.4%)	
CMV hepatitis	1 (0.7%)	9 (5.9%)	
CMV GI disease	0 (0.0%)	3 (2.0%)	
CMV lung disease	0 (0.0%)	4 (2.6%)	

* One or more CMV endpoints
† CMV syndrome: CMV viremia and unexplained fever, accompanied by malaise and/or neutropenia.

ICM 1689: In a randomized, double-blind, placebo-controlled study of 72 bone marrow transplant recipients[6] with asymptomatic CMV infection (CMV positive culture of urine, throat or blood) there was a statistically significant reduction in the incidence of CMV disease in patients treated with CYTOVENE-IV following successful hematopoietic engraftment. Patients with virologic evidence of CMV infection received CYTOVENE-IV solution 5 mg/kg bid for 7 days followed by 5 mg/kg qd through day 100 posttransplant. One of the 37 (3%) patients treated with CYTOVENE-IV vs 15 of the 35 (43%) placebo-treated patients developed CMV disease during the study. At 6 months posttransplant, there continued to be a statistically significant reduction in the incidence of CMV disease in patients treated with CYTOVENE-IV. Six of 37 (16%) patients treated with CYTOVENE-IV vs 15 of the 35 (43%) placebo-treated patients developed disease through 6 months posttransplant. The overall rate of survival was statistically significantly higher in the group treated with CYTOVENE-IV, both at day 100 and day 180 posttransplant. Although the differences in hematologic toxicities were not statistically significant, the incidence of neutropenia was higher in the group treated with CYTOVENE-IV (refer to table in ADVERSE EVENTS).
ICM 1570: A second, randomized, unblinded study evaluated 40 allogeneic bone marrow transplant recipients at risk for CMV disease.[7] Patients underwent bronchoscopy and bronchoalveolar lavage (BAL) on day 35 posttransplant. Patients with histologic, immunologic or virologic evidence of CMV infection in the lung were then randomized to observation or treatment with CYTOVENE-IV solution (5 mg/kg bid for 14 days followed by 5 mg/kg qd 5 days/week until day 120). Four of 20 (20%) patients treated with CYTOVENE-IV and 14 of 20 (70%) control patients developed interstitial pneumonia. The incidence of CMV disease was significantly lower in the group treated with CYTOVENE-IV, consistent with the results observed in ICM 1689.
CYTOVENE Capsules: *GAN040:* CYTOVENE capsules were evaluated in a randomized, double-blind, placebo-controlled study of 304 orthotopic liver transplant recipients who were CMV seropositive or recipients of an organ from a seropositive donor. Administration of CYTOVENE capsules (1000 mg three times daily) or matching placebo commenced as soon as patients were able to take medication by mouth, but no later than 10 days following transplantation, and continued through 14 weeks after transplantation. Dosing was adjusted for patients with an estimated creatinine clearance <50 mL/min. The incidence of CMV disease at 6 months is summarized in the table below.
[See second table above]
CYTOVENE capsules significantly reduced the 6-month incidence of CMV disease in patients at increased risk of CMV disease, including seronegative recipients of organs from seropositive donors (15% [3/21] with CYTOVENE capsules vs 44% [11/25] with placebo), and patients receiving antilymphocyte antibodies (5% [2/44] with CYTOVENE capsules vs 33% [12/37] with placebo). The incidence of HSV infection at 6 months was 4% (5/150) in ganciclovir vs 24% (36/154) in placebo recipients (relative risk: 0.13; 95% CI: 0.05, 0.32).

CONTRAINDICATIONS

CYTOVENE-IV and CYTOVENE are contraindicated in patients with hypersensitivity to ganciclovir or acyclovir.

WARNINGS

Hematologic: **CYTOVENE-IV and CYTOVENE should not be administered if the absolute neutrophil count is less than 500 cells/μL or the platelet count is less than 25,000 cells/μL.** Granulocytopenia (neutropenia), anemia and thrombocytopenia have been observed in patients treated with CYTOVENE-IV and CYTOVENE. The frequency and severity of these events vary widely in different patient populations (see ADVERSE EVENTS).
CYTOVENE-IV and CYTOVENE should, therefore, be used with caution in patients with pre-existing cytopenias or with a history of cytopenic reactions to other drugs, chemicals or irradiation. Granulocytopenia usually occurs during the first or second week of treatment but may occur at any time during treatment. Cell counts usually begin to recover within 3 to 7 days of discontinuing drug. Colony-stimulating factors have been shown to increase neutrophil and white blood cell counts in patients receiving CYTOVENE-IV solution for treatment of CMV retinitis.
Impairment of Fertility: Animal data indicate that administration of ganciclovir causes inhibition of spermatogenesis and subsequent infertility. These effects were reversible at lower doses and irreversible at higher doses (see PRECAUTIONS: *Carcinogenesis, Mutagenesis* and *Impairment of Fertility*). Although data in humans have not been obtained regarding this effect, it is considered probable that ganciclovir at the recommended doses causes temporary or permanent inhibition of spermatogenesis. Animal data also indicate that suppression of fertility in females may occur.
Teratogenesis: Because of the mutagenic and teratogenic potential of ganciclovir, women of childbearing potential should be advised to use effective contraception during treatment. Similarly, men should be advised to practice barrier contraception during and for at least 90 days following treatment with CYTOVENE-IV or CYTOVENE (see *Pregnancy:* Category C).

PRECAUTIONS

General: In clinical studies with CYTOVENE-IV, the maximum single dose administered was 6 mg/kg by intravenous infusion over 1 hour. Larger doses have resulted in increased toxicity. It is likely that more rapid infusions would also result in increased toxicity (see OVERDOSAGE). Administration of CYTOVENE-IV solution should be accompanied by adequate hydration.
Initially reconstituted solutions of CYTOVENE-IV have a high pH (pH 11). Despite further dilution in intravenous flu-

Laboratory Data:

Selected Laboratory Abnormalities in Trials for Treatment of CMV Retinitis and Prevention of CMV Diseases

	CMV Retinitis Treatment*		CMV Disease Prevention§	
Treatment	CYTOVENE Capsules† 3000 mg/day	CYTOVENE-IV‡ 5 mg/kg/day	CYTOVENE Capsules[ll] 3000 mg/day	Placebo¶
Subjects, number	320	175	478	234
Neutropenia:				
<500 ANC/µL	18%	25%	10%	6%
500 – <749	17%	14%	16%	7%
750 – <1000	19%	26%	22%	16%
Anemia: Hemoglobin:				
<6.5 g/dL	2%	5%	1%	<1%
6.5 – <8.0	10%	16%	5%	3%
8.0 – <9.5	25%	26%	15%	16%
Maximum Serum Creatinine:				
≥2.5 mg/dL	1%	2%	1%	2%
≥1.5 – <2.5	12%	14%	19%	11%

* Pooled data from Treatment Studies, ICM 1653. Study ICM 1774 and Study AVI 034
† Mean time on therapy = 91 days, including allowed reinduction treatment periods
‡ Mean time on therapy = 103 days, including allowed reinduction treatment periods
§ Data from Prevention Study, ICM 1654
ll Mean time on ganciclovir = 269 days
¶ Mean time on placebo = 240 days
(See discussion of clinical trials under INDICATIONS AND USAGE.)

Selected Adverse Events Reported ≥5% of Subjects in Three Randomized Phase 3 Studies Comparing CYTOVENE Capsules to CYTOVENE-IV Solution for Maintenance Treatment of CMV Retinitis and in One Phase 3 Randomized Study Comparing Cytovene Capsules to Placebo for Prevention of CMV Disease

		Maintenance Treatment Studies		Prevention Study	
Body System	Adverse Event	Capsules (n=326)	IV (n=179)	Capsules (n=478)	Placebo (n=234)
Body as a Whole	Fever	38%	48%	35%	33%
	Infection	9%	13%	8%	4%
	Chills	7%	10%	7%	4%
	Sepsis	4%	15%	3%	2%
Digestive System	Diarrhea	41%	44%	48%	42%
	Anorexia	15%	14%	19%	16%
	Vomiting	13%	13%	14%	11%
Hemic and Lymphatic System	Leukopenia	29%	41%	17%	9%
	Anemia	19%	25%	9%	7%
	Thrombocytopenia	6%	6%	3%	1%
Nervous System	Neuropathy	8%	9%	21%	15%
Other	Sweating	11%	12%	14%	12%
	Pruritus	6%	5%	10%	9%
Catheter Related*	Total Catheter Events	6%	22%	–	–
	Catheter Infection	4%	9%	–	–
	Catheter Sepsis	1%	8%	–	–

* Some of these events also appear under other body systems.

ids, phlebitis and/or pain may occur at the site of intravenous infusion. Care must be taken to infuse solutions containing CYTOVENE-IV only into veins with adequate blood flow to permit rapid dilution and distribution (see DOSAGE AND ADMINISTRATION).

Since ganciclovir is excreted by the kidneys, normal clearance depends on adequate renal function. IF RENAL FUNCTION IS IMPAIRED, DOSAGE ADJUSTMENTS ARE REQUIRED FOR CYTOVENE-IV AND SHOULD BE CONSIDERED FOR CYTOVENE CAPSULES. Such adjustments should be based on measured or estimated creatinine clearance values (see DOSAGE AND ADMINISTRATION).

Information for Patients: All patients should be informed that the major toxicities of ganciclovir are granulocytopenia (neutropenia), anemia and thrombocytopenia and that dose modifications may be required, including discontinuation. The importance of close monitoring of blood counts while on therapy should be emphasized. Patients should be informed that ganciclovir has been associated with elevations in serum creatinine.

Patients should be instructed to take CYTOVENE capsules with food to maximize bioavailability.

Patients should be advised that ganciclovir has caused decreased sperm production in animals and may cause infertility in humans. Women of childbearing potential should be advised that ganciclovir causes birth defects in animals and should not be used during pregnancy. Women of childbearing potential should be advised to use effective contraception during treatment with CYTOVENE-IV or CYTOVENE. Similarly, men should be advised to practice barrier contraception during and for at least 90 days following treatment with CYTOVENE-IV or CYTOVENE.

Patients should be advised that ganciclovir causes tumors in animals. Although there is no information from human studies, ganciclovir should be considered a potential carcinogen.

All HIV+ Patients: These patients may be receiving zidovudine (Retrovir®*). Patients should be counseled that treatment with both ganciclovir and zidovudine simultaneously may not be tolerated by some patients and may result in severe granulocytopenia (neutropenia). Patients with AIDS may be receiving didanosine (Videx®†). Patients should be counseled that concomitant treatment with both ganciclovir and didanosine can cause didanosine serum concentrations to be significantly increased.

HIV+ Patients With CMV Retinitis: Ganciclovir is not a cure for CMV retinitis, and immunocompromised patients may continue to experience progression of retinitis during or following treatment. Patients should be advised to have ophthalmologic follow-up examinations at a minimum of every 4 to 6 weeks while being treated with CYTOVENE-IV or CYTOVENE. Some patients will require more frequent follow-up.

Transplant Recipients: Transplant recipients should be counseled regarding the high frequency of impaired renal function in transplant recipients who received CYTOVENE-IV solution in controlled clinical trials, particularly in patients receiving concomitant administration of nephrotoxic agents such as cyclosporine and amphotericin B. Although the specific mechanism of this toxicity, which in most cases was reversible, has not been determined, the higher rate of renal impairment in patients receiving CYTOVENE-IV solution compared with those who received placebo in the same trials may indicate that CYTOVENE-IV played a significant role.

Laboratory Testing: Due to the frequency of neutropenia, anemia and thrombocytopenia in patients receiving CYTOVENE-IV and CYTOVENE (see ADVERSE EVENTS), it is recommended that complete blood counts and platelet counts be performed frequently, especially in patients in whom ganciclovir or other nucleoside analogues have previously resulted in leukopenia or in whom neutrophil counts are less than 1000 cells/µL at the beginning of treatment. Increased serum creatinine levels have been observed in trials evaluating both CYTOVENE-IV and CYTOVENE. Patients should have serum creatinine or creatinine clearance values monitored carefully to allow for dosage adjustments in renally impaired patients (see DOSAGE AND ADMINISTRATION).

Drug Interactions: *Didanosine:* At an oral dose of 1000 mg of CYTOVENE every 8 hours and didanosine, 200 mg every 12 hours, the steady-state didanosine AUC_{0-12} increased 111 ± 114% (range: 10% to 493%) when didanosine was administered either 2 hours prior to or concurrent with administration of CYTOVENE (n=12 patients, 23 observations). A decrease in steady-state ganciclovir AUC of 21 ± 17% (range: -44% to 5%) was observed when didanosine was administered 2 hours prior to administration of CYTOVENE, but ganciclovir AUC was not affected by the presence of didanosine when the two drugs were administered simultaneously (n=12). There were no significant changes in renal clearance for either drug.

When the standard intravenous ganciclovir induction dose (5 mg/kg infused over 1 hour every 12 hours) was coadministered with didanosine at a dose of 200 mg orally every 12 hours, the steady-state didanosine AUC_{0-12} increased 70 ± 40% (range: 3% to 121%, n=11) and C_{max} increased 49 ± 48% (range: -28% to 125%). In a separate study, when the standard intravenous ganciclovir maintenance dose (5 mg/kg infused over 1 hour every 24 hours) was coadministered with didanosine at a dose of 200 mg orally every 12 hours, didanosine AUC_{0-12} increased 50 ± 26% (range: 22% to 110%, n=11) and C_{max} increased 36 ± 36% (range: -27% to 94%) over the first didanosine dosing interval. Didanosine plasma concentrations (AUC_{12-24}) were unchanged during the dosing intervals when ganciclovir was not coadministered. Ganciclovir pharmacokinetics were not affected by didanosine. In neither study were there significant changes in the renal clearance of either drug.

Zidovudine: At an oral dose of 1000 mg of CYTOVENE every 8 hours, mean steady-state ganciclovir AUC_{0-8} decreased 17 ± 25% (range: -52% to 23%) in the presence of zidovudine, 100 mg every 4 hours (n=12). Steady-state zidovudine AUC_{0-4} increased 19 ± 27% (range: -11% to 74%) in the presence of ganciclovir.

Since both zidovudine and ganciclovir have the potential to cause neutropenia and anemia, some patients may not tolerate concomitant therapy with these drugs at full dosage.

Probenecid: At an oral dose of 1000 mg of CYTOVENE every 8 hours (n=10), ganciclovir AUC_{0-8} increased 53 ± 91% (range: -14% to 299%) in the presence of probenecid, 500 mg every 6 hours. Renal clearance of ganciclovir decreased 22 ± 20% (range: -54% to -4%), which is consistent with an interaction involving competition for renal tubular secretion.

Imipenem-cilastatin: Generalized seizures have been reported in patients who received ganciclovir and imipenem-cilastatin. These drugs should not be used concomitantly unless the potential benefits outweigh the risks.

Other Medications: It is possible that drugs that inhibit replication of rapidly dividing cell populations such as bone marrow, spermatogonia and germinal layers of skin and gastrointestinal mucosa may have additive toxicity when administered concomitantly with ganciclovir. Therefore, drugs such as dapsone, pentamidine, flucytosine, vincristine, vinblastine, adriamycin, amphotericin B, trimethoprim/sulfamethoxazole combinations or other nucleoside analogues, should be considered for concomitant use with ganciclovir only if the potential benefits are judged to outweigh the risks.

No formal drug interaction studies of CYTOVENE-IV or CYTOVENE and drugs commonly used in transplant recipients have been conducted. Increases in serum creatinine were observed in patients treated with CYTOVENE-IV plus either cyclosporine or amphotericin B, drugs with known potential for nephrotoxicity (see ADVERSE EVENTS). In a retrospective analysis of 93 liver allograft recipients receiving ganciclovir (5 mg/kg infused over 1 hour every 12 hours) and oral cyclosporine (at therapeutic doses), there was no evidence of an effect on cyclosporine whole blood concentrations.

Carcinogenesis, Mutagenesis‡: Ganciclovir was carcinogenic in the mouse at oral doses of 20 and 1000 mg/kg/day (approximately 0.1× and 1.4×, respectively, the mean drug exposure in humans following the recommended intravenous dose of 5 mg/kg, based on area under the plasma concentration curve [AUC] comparisons). At the dose of 1000 mg/kg/day there was a significant increase in the incidence of tumors of the preputial gland in males, forestomach (nonglandular mucosa) in males and females, and reproductive tissues (ovaries, uterus, mammary gland, clitoral gland and vagina) and liver in females. At the dose of 20 mg/kg/day, a slightly increased incidence of tumors was noted in the preputial and harderian glands in males, forestomach in males and females, and liver in females. No carcinogenic effect was observed in mice administered ganciclovir at 1 mg/kg/day (estimated as 0.01× the human dose based on AUC comparison). Except for histiocytic sarcoma of the liver, ganciclovir-induced tumors were generally of epithelial or vascular origin. Although the preputial and clitoral glands, forestomach and harderian glands of mice do not have human counterparts, ganciclovir should be considered a potential carcinogen in humans.

Ganciclovir increased mutations in mouse lymphoma cells and DNA damage in human lymphocytes in vitro at concen-

Continued on next page

Cytovene—Cont.

trations between 50 to 500 and 250 to 2000 μg/mL, respectively. In the mouse micronucleus assay, ganciclovir was clastogenic at doses of 150 and 500 mg/kg (IV) (2.8 to 10× human exposure based on AUC) but not 50 mg/kg (exposure approximately comparable to the human based on AUC). Ganciclovir was not mutagenic in the Ames Salmonella assay at concentrations of 500 to 5000 μg/mL.

Impairment of Fertility‡: Ganciclovir caused decreased mating behavior, decreased fertility, and an increased incidence of embryolethality in female mice following intravenous doses of 90 mg/kg/day (approximately 1.7× the mean drug exposure in humans following the dose of 5 mg/kg, based on AUC comparisons). Ganciclovir caused decreased fertility in male mice and hypospermatogenesis in mice and dogs following daily oral or intravenous administration of doses ranging from 0.2 to 10 mg/kg. Systemic drug exposure (AUC) at the lowest dose showing toxicity in each species ranged from 0.03 to 0.1× the AUC of the recommended human intravenous dose.

***Pregnancy:* Category C‡:** Ganciclovir has been shown to be embryotoxic in rabbits and mice following intravenous administration and teratogenic in rabbits. Fetal resorptions were present in at least 85% of rabbits and mice administered 60 mg/kg/day and 108 mg/kg/day (2× the human exposure based on AUC comparisons), respectively. Effects observed in rabbits included: fetal growth retardation, embryolethality, teratogenicity and/or maternal toxicity. Teratogenic changes included cleft palate, anophthalmia/microphthalmia, aplastic organs (kidney and pancreas), hydrocephaly and brachygnathia. In mice, effects observed were maternal/fetal toxicity and embryolethality.

Daily intravenous doses of 90 mg/kg administered to female mice prior to mating, during gestation, and during lactation caused hypoplasia of the testes and seminal vesicles in the month-old male offspring, as well as pathologic changes in the nonglandular region of the stomach (see *Carcinogenesis, Mutagenesis*). The drug exposure in mice as estimated by the AUC was approximately 1.7× the human AUC.

Ganciclovir may be teratogenic or embryotoxic at dose levels recommended for human use. There are no adequate and well-controlled studies in pregnant women. CYTOVENE-IV or CYTOVENE should be used during pregnancy only if the potential benefits justify the potential risk to the fetus.

‡Footnote: All dose comparisons presented in the *Carcinogenesis, Mutagenesis, Impairment of Fertility* and *Pregnancy* subsections are based on the human AUC following administration of a single 5 mg/kg intravenous infusion of CYTOVENE-IV as used during the maintenance phase of treatment. Compared with the single 5 mg/kg intravenous infusion, human exposure is doubled during the intravenous induction phase (5 mg/kg bid) and approximately halved during maintenance treatment with CYTOVENE capsules (1000 mg tid). The cross-species dose comparisons should be divided by 2 for intravenous induction treatment with CYTOVENE-IV and multiplied by 2 for CYTOVENE capsules.

Nursing Mothers: It is not known whether ganciclovir is excreted in human milk. However, many drugs are excreted in human milk and, because carcinogenic and teratogenic effects occurred in animals treated with ganciclovir, the possibility of serious adverse reactions from ganciclovir in nursing infants is considered likely (see *Pregnancy:* Category C). Mothers should be instructed to discontinue nursing if they are receiving CYTOVENE-IV or CYTOVENE. The minimum interval before nursing can safely be resumed after the last dose of CYTOVENE-IV or CYTOVENE is unknown.

Pediatric Use: **SAFETY AND EFFICACY OF CYTOVENE-IV AND CYTOVENE IN PEDIATRIC PATIENTS HAVE NOT BEEN ESTABLISHED. THE USE OF CYTOVENE-IV OR CYTOVENE IN THE PEDIATRIC POPULATION WARRANTS EXTREME CAUTION DUE TO THE PROBABILITY OF LONG-TERM CARCINOGENICITY AND REPRODUCTIVE TOXICITY. ADMINISTRATION TO PEDIATRIC PATIENTS SHOULD BE UNDERTAKEN ONLY AFTER CAREFUL EVALUATION AND ONLY IF THE POTENTIAL BENEFITS OF TREATMENT OUTWEIGH THE RISKS.**

The spectrum of adverse events reported in 120 immunocompromised pediatric clinical trial participants with serious CMV infections receiving CYTOVENE-IV solution were similar to those reported in adults. Granulocytopenia (17%) and thrombocytopenia (10%) were the most common adverse events reported.

Sixteen pediatric patients (8 months to 15 years of age) with life- or sight-threatening CMV infections were evaluated in an open-label, CYTOVENE-IV solution, pharmacokinetics study. Adverse events reported for more than one pediatric patient were as follows: hypokalemia (4/16, 25%), abnormal kidney function (3/16, 19%), sepsis (3/16, 19%), thrombocytopenia (3/16, 19%), leukopenia (2/16, 13%), coagulation disorder (2/16, 13%), hypertension (2/16, 13%), pneumonia (2/16, 13%) and immune system disorder (2/16, 13%).

There has been very limited clinical experience using CYTOVENE-IV for the treatment of CMV retinitis in patients under the age of 12 years. Two pediatric patients (ages 9 and 5 years) showed improvement or stabilization of retinitis for 23 and 9 months, respectively. These pediatric patients received induction treatment with 2.5 mg/kg tid followed by maintenance therapy with 6 to 6.5 mg/kg once per day, 5 to 7 days per week. When retinitis progressed during once-daily maintenance therapy, both pediatric patients were treated with the 5 mg/kg bid regimen. Two other pediatric patients (ages 2.5 and 4 years) who received similar induction regimens showed only partial or no response to treatment. Another pediatric patient, a 6-year-old with T-cell dysfunction, showed stabilization of retinitis for 3 months while receiving continuous infusions of CYTOVENE-IV at doses of 2 to 5 mg/kg/24 hours. Continuous infusion treatment was discontinued due to granulocytopenia.

Eleven of the 72 patients in the placebo-controlled trial in bone marrow transplant recipients were pediatric patients, ranging in age from 3 to 10 years (5 treated with CYTOVENE-IV and 6 with placebo). Five of the pediatric patients treated with CYTOVENE-IV received 5 mg/kg intravenously bid for up to 7 days; 4 patients went on to receive 5 mg/kg qd up to day 100 posttransplant. Results were similar to those observed in adult transplant recipients treated with CYTOVENE-IV. Two of the 6 placebo-treated pediatric patients developed CMV pneumonia vs none of the 5 patients treated with CYTOVENE-IV. The spectrum of adverse events in the pediatric group was similar to that observed in the adult patients.

CYTOVENE capsules have not been studied in pediatric patients under age 13.

Use in Patients With Renal Impairment: CYTOVENE-IV and CYTOVENE should be used with caution in patients with impaired renal function because the half-life and plasma/serum concentrations of ganciclovir will be increased due to reduced renal clearance (see DOSAGE AND ADMINISTRATION and ADVERSE EVENTS: *Renal Toxicity*). Hemodialysis has been shown to reduce plasma levels of ganciclovir by approximately 50%.

Geriatric Use: The pharmacokinetic profiles of CYTOVENE-IV and CYTOVENE in elderly patients have not been established. Since elderly individuals frequently have a reduced glomerular filtration rate, particular attention should be paid to assessing renal function before and during administration of CYTOVENE-IV or CYTOVENE (see DOSAGE AND ADMINISTRATION).

Clinical studies of CYTOVENE-IV and CYTOVENE did not include sufficient numbers of subjects aged 65 and over to determine whether they respond differently from younger subjects. Other reported clinical experience has not identified differences in responses between the elderly and younger patients. In general, dose selection for an elderly patient should be cautious, usually starting at the low end of the dosing range, reflecting the greater frequency of decreased hepatic, renal, or cardiac function, and of concomitant disease or other drug therapy.

ADVERSE EVENTS

Adverse events that occurred during clinical trials of CYTOVENE-IV solution and CYTOVENE capsules are summarized below, according to the participating study subject population.

Subjects With AIDS: Three controlled, randomized, phase 3 trials comparing CYTOVENE-IV and CYTOVENE capsules for maintenance treatment of CMV retinitis have been completed. During these trials, CYTOVENE-IV or CYTOVENE capsules were prematurely discontinued in 9% of subjects because of adverse events. In a placebo-controlled, randomized, phase 3 trial of CYTOVENE capsules for prevention of CMV disease in AIDS, treatment was prematurely discontinued because of adverse events, new or worsening intercurrent illness, or laboratory abnormalities in 19.5% of subjects treated with CYTOVENE capsules and 16% of subjects receiving placebo. Laboratory data and adverse events reported during the conduct of these controlled trials are summarized below.

[See first table at top of previous page]

Adverse Events: The following table shows selected adverse events reported in 5% or more of the subjects in three controlled clinical trials during treatment with either CYTOVENE-IV solution (5 mg/kg/day) or CYTOVENE capsules (3000 mg/day), and in one controlled clinical trial in which CYTOVENE capsules (3000 mg/day) were compared to placebo for the prevention of CMV disease.

[See second table at top of previous page]

Controlled Trials – Transplant Recipients

	CYTOVENE-IV				CYTOVENE Capsules	
	Heart Allograft*		Bone Marrow Allograft†		Liver Allograft‡	
	CYTOVENE-IV (n=76)	Placebo (n=73)	CYTOVENE-IV (n=57)	Control (n=55)	CYTOVENE Capsules (n=150)	Placebo (n=154)
Neutropenia						
Minimum ANC <500/μL	4%	3%	12%	6%	3%	1%
Minimum ANC 500–1000/μL	3%	8%	29%	17%	3%	2%
TOTAL ANC ≤1000/μL	7%	11%	41%	23%	6%	3%
Thrombocytopenia						
Platelet count <25,000/μL	3%	1%	32%	28%	0%	3%
Platelet count 25,000–50,000/μL	5%	3%	25%	37%	5%	3%
TOTAL Platelet ≤50,000/μL	8%	4%	57%	65%	5%	6%

* Study ICM 1496. Mean duration of treatment = 28 days
† Study ICM 1570 and ICM 1689. Mean duration of treatment = 45 days
‡ Study GAN040. Mean duration of ganciclovir treatment = 82 days
(See discussion of clinical trials under INDICATIONS AND USAGE.)

Controlled Trials – Transplant Recipients

	CYTOVENE-IV						CYTOVENE Capsules	
	Heart Allograft ICM 1496		Bone Marrow Allograft ICM 1570		Bone Marrow Allograft ICM 1689		Liver Allograft Study 040	
Maximum Serum Creatinine Levels	CYTOVENE-IV (n=76)	Placebo (n=73)	CYTOVENE-IV (n=20)	Control (n=20)	CYTOVENE-IV (n=37)	Placebo (n=35)	CYTOVENE Capsules (n=150)	Placebo (n=154)
Serum Creatinine ≥2.5 mg/dL	18%	4%	20%	0%	0%	0%	16%	10%
Serum Creatinine ≥1.5–<2.5 mg/dL	58%	69%	50%	35%	43%	44%	39%	42%

The following events were frequently observed in clinical trials but occurred with equal or greater frequency in placebo-treated subjects: abdominal pain, nausea, flatulence, pneumonia, paresthesia, rash.

Retinal Detachment: Retinal detachment has been observed in subjects with CMV retinitis both before and after initiation of therapy with ganciclovir. Its relationship to therapy with ganciclovir is unknown. Retinal detachment occurred in 11% of patients treated with CYTOVENE-IV solution and in 8% of patients treated with CYTOVENE capsules. Patients with CMV retinitis should have frequent ophthalmologic evaluations to monitor the status of their retinitis and to detect any other retinal pathology.

Transplant Recipients: There have been three controlled clinical trials of CYTOVENE-IV solution and one controlled clinical trial of CYTOVENE capsules for the prevention of CMV disease in transplant recipients. Laboratory data and adverse events reported during these trials are summarized below.

Laboratory Data: The following table shows the frequency of granulocytopenia (neutropenia) and thrombocytopenia observed:

[See table at top of previous page]

The following table shows the frequency of elevated serum creatinine values in these controlled clinical trials:

[See table at bottom of previous page]

In 3 out of 4 trials, patients receiving either CYTOVENE-IV solution or CYTOVENE capsules had elevated serum creatinine levels when compared to those receiving placebo. Most patients in these studies also received cyclosporine. The mechanism of impairment of renal function is not known. However, careful monitoring of renal function during therapy with CYTOVENE-IV solution or CYTOVENE capsules is essential, especially for those patients receiving concomitant agents that may cause nephrotoxicity.

General: Other adverse events that were thought to be "probably" or "possibly" related to CYTOVENE-IV solution or CYTOVENE capsules in controlled clinical studies in either subjects with AIDS or transplant recipients are listed below. These events all occurred in at least 3 subjects.

Body as a Whole: abdomen enlarged, asthenia, chest pain, edema, headache, injection site inflammation, malaise, pain

Digestive System: abnormal liver function test, aphthous stomatitis, constipation, dyspepsia, eructation

Hemic and Lymphatic System: pancytopenia

Respiratory System: cough increased, dyspnea

Nervous System: abnormal dreams, anxiety, confusion, depression, dizziness, dry mouth, insomnia, seizures, somnolence, thinking abnormal, tremor

Skin and Appendages: alopecia, dry skin

Special Senses: abnormal vision, taste perversion, tinnitus, vitreous disorder

Metabolic and Nutritional Disorders: creatinine increased, SGOT increased, SGPT increased, weight loss

Cardiovascular System: hypertension, phlebitis, vasodilatation

Urogenital System: creatinine clearance decreased, kidney failure, kidney function abnormal, urinary frequency

Musculoskeletal System: arthralgia, leg cramps, myalgia, myasthenia

The following adverse events reported in patients receiving ganciclovir may be potentially fatal: gastrointestinal perforation, multiple organ failure, pancreatitis and sepsis.

Adverse Events Reported During Postmarketing Experience With CYTOVENE-IV and CYTOVENE Capsules: The following events have been identified during post-approval use of the drug. Because they are reported voluntarily from a population of unknown size, estimates of frequency cannot be made. These events have been chosen for inclusion due to either the seriousness, frequency of reporting, the apparent causal connection or a combination of these factors:

acidosis, allergic reaction, anaphylactic reaction, arthritis, bronchospasm, cardiac arrest, cardiac conduction abnormality, cataracts, cholelithiasis, cholestasis, congenital anomaly, dry eyes, dysesthesia, dysphasia, elevated triglyceride levels, encephalopathy, exfoliative dermatitis, extrapyramidal reaction, facial palsy, hallucinations, hemolytic anemia, hemolytic uremic syndrome, hepatic failure, hepatitis, hypercalcemia, hyponatremia, inappropriate serum ADH, infertility, intestinal ulceration, intracranial hypertension, irritability, loss of memory, loss of sense of smell, myelopathy, oculomotor nerve paralysis, peripheral ischemia, pulmonary fibrosis, renal tubular disorder, rhabdomyolysis, Stevens-Johnson syndrome, stroke, testicular hypotrophy, Torsades de Pointes, vasculitis, ventricular tachycardia

OVERDOSAGE

CYTOVENE-IV: Overdosage with CYTOVENE-IV has been reported in 17 patients (13 adults and 4 children under 2 years of age). Five patients experienced no adverse events following overdosage at the following doses: 7 doses of 11 mg/kg over a 3-day period (adult), single dose of 3500 mg (adult), single dose of 500 mg (72.5 mg/kg) followed by 48 hours of peritoneal dialysis (4-month-old), single dose of approximately 60 mg/kg followed by exchange transfusion (18-month-old), 2 doses of 500 mg instead of 31 mg (21-month-old).

Irreversible pancytopenia developed in 1 adult with AIDS and CMV colitis after receiving 3000 mg of CYTOVENE-IV solution on each of 2 consecutive days. He experienced worsening GI symptoms and acute renal failure that required short-term dialysis. Pancytopenia developed and persisted until his death from a malignancy several months later.

Creatinine Clearance* (mL/min)	CYTOVENE-IV Induction Dose (mg/kg)	Dosing Interval (hours)	CYTOVENE-IV Maintenance Dose (mg/kg)	Dosing Interval (hours)
≥70	5.0	12	5.0	24
50 – 69	2.5	12	2.5	24
25 – 49	2.5	24	1.25	24
10 – 24	1.25	24	0.625	24
<10	1.25	3 times per week, following hemodialysis	0.625	3 times per week, following hemodialysis

*Creatinine clearance can be related to serum creatinine by the formulas given below.

Creatinine Clearance* mL/min	CYTOVENE Capsule Dosages
≥70	1000 mg tid or 500 mg q3h, 6x/day
50 – 69	1500 mg qd or 500 mg tid
25 – 49	1000 mg qd or 500 mg bid
10 – 24	500 mg qd
<10	500 mg 3 times per week, following hemodialysis

* Creatinine clearance can be related to serum creatinine by the following formulas:

$$\text{Creatinine clearance for males} = \frac{(140 - \text{age [yrs]})\ (\text{body wt [kg]})}{(72)\ (\text{serum creatinine [mg/dL]})}$$

Creatinine clearance for females = $0.85 \times$ male value

Other adverse events reported following overdosage included: persistent bone marrow suppression (1 adult with neutropenia and thrombocytopenia after a single dose of 6000 mg), reversible neutropenia or granulocytopenia (4 adults, overdoses ranging from 8 mg/kg daily for 4 days to a single dose of 25 mg/kg), hepatitis (1 adult receiving 10 mg/kg daily, and one 2 kg infant after a single 40 mg dose), renal toxicity (1 adult with transient worsening of hematuria after a single 500 mg dose, and 1 adult with elevated creatinine (5.2 mg/dL) after a single 5000 to 7000 mg dose), and seizure (1 adult with known seizure disorder after 3 days of 9 mg/kg). In addition, 1 adult received 0.4 mL (instead of 0.1 mL) CYTOVENE-IV solution by intravitreal injection, and experienced temporary loss of vision and central retinal artery occlusion secondary to increased intraocular pressure related to the injected fluid volume.

CYTOVENE Capsules: There have been no reports of overdosage with CYTOVENE capsules. Doses as high as 6000 mg/day, given either as 1000 mg 6 times daily or as 2000 mg tid, did not result in overt toxicity other than transient neutropenia. Daily doses of more than 6000 mg have not been studied.

Since ganciclovir is dialyzable, dialysis may be useful in reducing serum concentrations. Adequate hydration should be maintained. The use of hematopoietic growth factors should be considered.

DOSAGE AND ADMINISTRATION

CAUTION—DO NOT ADMINISTER CYTOVENE-IV SOLUTION BY RAPID OR BOLUS INTRAVENOUS INJECTION. THE TOXICITY OF CYTOVENE-IV MAY BE INCREASED AS A RESULT OF EXCESSIVE PLASMA LEVELS.

CAUTION—INTRAMUSCULAR OR SUBCUTANEOUS INJECTION OF RECONSTITUTED CYTOVENE-IV SOLUTION MAY RESULT IN SEVERE TISSUE IRRITATION DUE TO HIGH pH (11).

Dosage: THE RECOMMENDED DOSE FOR CYTOVENE-IV SOLUTION AND CYTOVENE CAPSULES SHOULD NOT BE EXCEEDED. THE RECOMMENDED INFUSION RATE FOR CYTOVENE-IV SOLUTION SHOULD NOT BE EXCEEDED.

For Treatment of CMV Retinitis in Patients With Normal Renal Function:

1. Induction Treatment

The recommended initial dosage for patients with normal renal function is 5 mg/kg (given intravenously at a constant rate over 1 hour) every 12 hours for 14 to 21 days. CYTOVENE capsules should not be used for induction treatment.

2. Maintenance Treatment

CYTOVENE-IV: Following induction treatment, the recommended maintenance dosage of CYTOVENE-IV solution is 5 mg/kg given as a constant-rate intravenous infusion over 1 hour once daily, 7 days per week or 6 mg/kg once daily, 5 days per week.

CYTOVENE Capsules: Following induction treatment, the recommended maintenance dosage of CYTOVENE capsules is 1000 mg tid with food. Alternatively, the dosing regimen of 500 mg 6 times daily every 3 hours with food, during waking hours, may be used.

For patients who experience progression of CMV retinitis while receiving maintenance treatment with either formulation of ganciclovir, reinduction treatment is recommended.

For the Prevention of CMV Disease in Patients With Advanced HIV Infection and Normal Renal Function:

CYTOVENE Capsules: The recommended prophylactic dose of CYTOVENE capsules is 1000 mg tid with food.

For the Prevention of CMV Disease in Transplant Recipients With Normal Renal Function:

CYTOVENE-IV: The recommended initial dosage of CYTOVENE-IV solution for patients with normal renal function is 5 mg/kg (given intravenously at a constant rate over 1 hour) every 12 hours for 7 to 14 days, followed by 5 mg/kg once daily, 7 days per week or 6 mg/kg once daily, 5 days per week.

CYTOVENE Capsules: The recommended prophylactic dosage of CYTOVENE capsules is 1000 mg tid with food.

The duration of treatment with CYTOVENE-IV solution and CYTOVENE capsules in transplant recipients is dependent upon the duration and degree of immunosuppression. In controlled clinical trials in bone marrow allograft recipients, treatment with CYTOVENE-IV was continued until day 100 to 120 posttransplantation. CMV disease occurred in several patients who discontinued treatment with CYTOVENE-IV solution prematurely. In heart allograft recipients, the onset of newly diagnosed CMV disease occurred after treatment with CYTOVENE-IV was stopped at day 28 posttransplant, suggesting that continued dosing may be necessary to prevent late occurrence of CMV disease in this patient population. In a controlled clinical trial of liver allograft recipients, treatment with CYTOVENE capsules was continued through week 14 posttransplantation (see INDICATIONS AND USAGE section for a more detailed discussion).

Renal Impairment:

CYTOVENE-IV: For patients with impairment of renal function, refer to the table below for recommended doses of CYTOVENE-IV solution and adjust the dosing interval as indicated:

[See first table above]

Dosing for patients undergoing hemodialysis should not exceed 1.25 mg/kg 3 times per week, following each hemodialysis session. CYTOVENE-IV should be given shortly after completion of the hemodialysis session, since hemodialysis has been shown to reduce plasma levels by approximately 50%.

CYTOVENE Capsules: In patients with renal impairment, the dose of CYTOVENE capsules should be modified as shown below:

[See second table above]

Patient Monitoring: Due to the frequency of granulocytopenia, anemia and thrombocytopenia in patients receiving ganciclovir (see ADVERSE EVENTS), it is recommended that complete blood counts and platelet counts be performed frequently, especially in patients in whom ganciclovir or other nucleoside analogues have previously resulted in cytopenia, or in whom neutrophil counts are less than 1000 cells/µL at the beginning of treatment. Patients should have serum creatinine or creatinine clearance values followed carefully to allow for dosage adjustments in renally impaired patients (see DOSAGE AND ADMINISTRATION).

Reduction of Dose: Dosage reductions in renally impaired patients are required for CYTOVENE-IV and should be considered for CYTOVENE capsules (see *Renal Impairment*). Dosage reductions should also be considered for those with neutropenia, anemia and/or thrombocytopenia (see ADVERSE EVENTS). Ganciclovir should not be administered in patients with severe neutropenia (ANC less than 500/µL) or severe thrombocytopenia (platelets less than 25,000/µL).

Method of Preparation of CYTOVENE IV Solution: Each 10 mL clear glass vial contains ganciclovir sodium equivalent to 500 mg of ganciclovir and 46 mg of sodium. The contents of the vial should be prepared for administration in the following manner:

1. *Reconstituted Solution:*
   a. Reconstitute lyophilized CYTOVENE-IV by injecting 10 mL of Sterile Water for Injection, USP, into the vial. DO NOT USE BACTERIOSTATIC WATER FOR INJECTION CONTAINING PARABENS. IT IS INCOMPATIBLE WITH CYTOVENE-IV AND MAY CAUSE PRECIPITATION.
   b. Shake the vial to dissolve the drug.
   c. Visually inspect the reconstituted solution for particulate matter and discoloration prior to proceeding with infusion solution. Discard the vial if particulate matter or discoloration is observed.

Continued on next page

Cytovene—Cont.

d. Reconstituted solution in the vial is stable at room temperature for 12 hours. It should not be refrigerated.

2. *Infusion Solution:*
Based on patient weight, the appropriate volume of the reconstituted solution (ganciclovir concentration 50 mg/mL) should be removed from the vial and added to an acceptable (see below) infusion fluid (typically 100 mL) for delivery over the course of 1 hour. Infusion concentrations greater than 10 mg/mL are not recommended. The following infusion fluids have been determined to be chemically and physically compatible with CYTOVENE-IV solution: 0.9% Sodium Chloride, 5% Dextrose, Ringer's Injection and Lactated Ringer's Injection, USP.
CYTOVENE-IV, when reconstituted with sterile water for injection, further diluted with 0.9% sodium chloride injection, and stored refrigerated at 5°C in polyvinyl chloride (PVC) bags, remains physically and chemically stable for 14 days.
However, because CYTOVENE-IV is reconstituted with nonbacteriostatic sterile water, it is recommended that the infusion solution be used within 24 hours of dilution to reduce the risk of bacterial contamination. The infusion should be refrigerated. Freezing is not recommended.

Handling and Disposal: Caution should be exercised in the handling and preparation of solutions of CYTOVENE-IV and in the handling of CYTOVENE capsules. Solutions of CYTOVENE-IV are alkaline (pH 11). Avoid direct contact with the skin or mucous membranes of the powder contained in CYTOVENE capsules or of CYTOVENE-IV solutions. If such contact occurs, wash thoroughly with soap and water; rinse eyes thoroughly with plain water. CYTOVENE capsules should not be opened or crushed.
Because ganciclovir shares some of the properties of antitumor agents (ie, carcinogenicity and mutagenicity), consideration should be given to handling and disposal according to guidelines issued for antineoplastic drugs. Several guidelines on this subject have been published.[8–10]
There is no general agreement that all of the procedures recommended in the guidelines are necessary or appropriate.

HOW SUPPLIED

CYTOVENE®-IV (ganciclovir sodium for injection) is supplied in 10 mL sterile vials, each containing ganciclovir sodium equivalent to 500 mg of ganciclovir, in cartons of 25 (NDC 0004-6940-03).
Store vials at temperatures below 40°C (104°F).
CYTOVENE® (ganciclovir capsules) 250 mg are two-pieced, size No. 1, opaque green hard gelatin capsules with ROCHE and CYTOVENE 250 mg imprinted on the capsules in dark blue ink and with two blue lines partially encircling the capsule body. Each capsule contains 250 mg of ganciclovir as a white to off-white powder. CYTOVENE capsules are supplied as follows: Bottles of 180 capsules (NDC 0004-0269-48).
CYTOVENE® (ganciclovir capsules) 500 mg are two-pieced, size No. 0 elongated, opaque yellow/opaque green hard gelatin capsules with ROCHE and CYTOVENE 500 mg imprinted on the capsules in dark blue ink and with two blue lines partially encircling the capsule body. Each capsule contains 500 mg of ganciclovir as a white to off-white powder. CYTOVENE capsules are supplied as follows:
Bottles of 180 capsules (NDC 0004-0278-48).
Store between 5° and 25°C (41° and 77°F).
*Retrovir is a registered trademark of Glaxo Wellcome.
†Videx is a registered trademark of Bristol-Meyers Squibb.

REFERENCES

1. Spector SA, Weingeis T, Pollard R, et al. A randomized, controlled study of intravenous ganciclovir therapy for cytomegalovirus peripheral retinitis in patients with AIDS. *J Inf Dis.* 1993; 168:557–563. **2.** Drew WL, Ives D, Lalezari JP, et al. Oral ganciclovir as maintenance treatment for cytomegalovirus retinitis in patients with AIDS. *New Engl J Med.* 1995; 333:615–620. **3.** The Oral Ganciclovir European and Australian Cooperative Study Group. Intravenous vs oral ganciclovir: European/Australian comparative study of efficacy and safety in the prevention of cytomegalovirus retinitis recurrence in patients with AIDS. *AIDS.* 1995; 9:471–477. **4.** Spector SA, McKinley GF, Lalezari JP, Samo T, et al. Oral ganciclovir for the prevention of cytomegalovirus disease in persons with AIDS. *New Engl J Med.* 1996; 334: 1491–1497. **5.** Merigan TC, Renlund DG, Keay S, et al. A controlled trial of ganciclovir to prevent cytomegalovirus disease after heart transplantation. *New Engl J Med.* 1992; 326:1182–1186. **6.** Goodrich JM, Mori M, Gleaves CA, et al. Early treatment with ganciclovir to prevent cytomegalovirus disease after allogeneic bone marrow transplantation. *New Engl J Med.* 1991; 325:1601–1607. **7.** Schmidt GM, Horak DA, Niland JC, et al. The City of Hope-Stanford-Syntex CMV Study Group. A randomized, controlled trial of prophylactic ganciclovir for cytomegalovirus pulmonary infection in recipients of allogeneic bone marrow transplants. *New Engl J Med.* 1991; 15:1005–1011. **8.** Recommendations for the Safe Handling of Cytotoxic Drugs. US Department of Health and Human Services, National Institutes of Health, Bethesda, MD, September, 1992. NIH Publication No. 92–2621. **9.** American Society of Hospital Pharmacists technical assistance bulletin on handling cytotoxic and hazardous drugs. *Am J Hosp Pharm.* 1990; 47:1033–1049. **10.** Controlling Occupational Exposures to Hazardous Drugs. US Department of Labor. Occupational Health and Safety Administration. OSHA Technical Manual. Section V - Chapter 3, September 22, 1995.

CYTOVENE-IV for intravenous infusion manufactured by Parkedale Pharmaceuticals, Inc., Rochester, MI 48307 or Abbott Laboratories, North Chicago, IL 60064 and CYTOVENE Capsules for oral administration manufactured by Syntex Puerto Rico, Inc., Humacao, Puerto Rico 00791 for:
Roche Pharmaceuticals
Roche Laboratories Inc.
340 Kingsland Street
Nutley, New Jersey 07110-1199

Revised: September 1999

Shown in Product Identification Guide, page 332

DEMADEX® ℞

[dē'-mă-dex]
(torsemide)
TABLETS
INJECTION

The following text is complete prescribing information based on official labeling in effect June 2000.

DESCRIPTION

DEMADEX® (torsemide) is a diuretic of the pyridine-sulfonylurea class. Its chemical name is 1-isopropyl-3-[(4-*m*-toluidino-3-pyridyl) sulfonyl]urea.
Its empirical formula is $C_{16}H_{20}N_4O_3S$, its pKa is 7.1, and its molecular weight is 348.43.
Torsemide is a white to off-white crystalline powder. The tablets for oral administration also contain lactose NF, crospovidone NF, povidone USP, microcrystalline cellulose NF, and magnesium stearate NF. Torsemide ampuls for intravenous injection contain a sterile solution of torsemide (10 mg/mL), polyethylene glycol-400 NF, tromethamine USP, and sodium hydroxide NF (as needed to adjust pH) in water for injection USP.

CLINICAL PHARMACOLOGY

Mechanism of Action: Micropuncture studies in animals have shown that torsemide acts from within the lumen of the thick ascending portion of the loop of Henle, where it inhibits the $Na^+/K^+/2Cl^-$-carrier system. Clinical pharmacology studies have confirmed this site of action in humans, and effects in other segments of the nephron have not been demonstrated. Diuretic activity thus correlates better with the rate of drug excretion in the urine than with the concentration in the blood.
Torsemide increases the urinary excretion of sodium, chloride, and water, but it does not significantly alter glomerular filtration rate, renal plasma flow, or acid-base balance.

Pharmacokinetics and Metabolism: The bioavailability of DEMADEX tablets is approximately 80%, with little intersubject variation; the 90% confidence interval is 75% to 89%. The drug is absorbed with little first-pass metabolism, and the serum concentration reaches its peak (C_{max}) within 1 hour after oral administration. C_{max} and area under the serum concentration-time curve (AUC) after oral administration are proportional to dose over the range of 2.5 mg to 200 mg. Simultaneous food intake delays the time to C_{max} by about 30 minutes, but overall bioavailability (AUC) and diuretic activity are unchanged. Absorption is essentially unaffected by renal or hepatic dysfunction.
The volume of distribution of torsemide is 12 liters to 15 liters in normal adults or in patients with mild to moderate renal failure or congestive heart failure. In patients with hepatic cirrhosis, the volume of distribution is approximately doubled.
In normal subjects the elimination half-life of torsemide is approximately 3.5 hours. Torsemide is cleared from the circulation by both hepatic metabolism (approximately 80% of total clearance) and excretion into the urine (approximately 20% of total clearance in patients with normal renal function). The major metabolite in humans is the carboxylic acid derivative, which is biologically inactive. Two of the lesser metabolites possess some diuretic activity, but for practical purposes metabolism terminates the action of the drug.
Because torsemide is extensively bound to plasma protein (>99%), very little enters tubular urine via glomerular filtration. Most renal clearance of torsemide occurs via active secretion of the drug by the proximal tubules into tubular urine.
In patients with decompensated congestive heart failure, hepatic and renal clearance are both reduced, probably because of hepatic congestion and decreased renal plasma flow, respectively. The total clearance of torsemide is approximately 50% of that seen in healthy volunteers, and the plasma half-life and AUC are correspondingly increased. Because of reduced renal clearance, a smaller fraction of any given dose is delivered to the intraluminal site of action, so at any given dose there is less natriuresis in patients with congestive heart failure than in normal subjects.
In patients with renal failure, renal clearance of torsemide is markedly decreased but total plasma clearance is not significantly altered. A smaller fraction of the administered dose is delivered to the intraluminal site of action, and the natriuretic action of any given dose of diuretic is reduced. A diuretic response in renal failure may still be achieved if patients are given higher doses. The total plasma clearance and elimination half-life of torsemide remain normal under the conditions of impaired renal function because metabolic elimination by the liver remains intact.
In patients with hepatic cirrhosis, the volume of distribution, plasma half-life, and renal clearance are all increased, but total clearance is unchanged.
The pharmacokinetic profile of torsemide in healthy elderly subjects is similar to that in young subjects except for a decrease in renal clearance related to the decline in renal function that commonly occurs with aging. However, total plasma clearance and elimination half-life remain unchanged.

Clinical Effects: The diuretic effects of DEMADEX begin within 10 minutes of intravenous dosing and peak within the first hour. With oral dosing, the onset of diuresis occurs within 1 hour and the peak effect occurs during the first or second hour. Independent of the route of administration, diuresis lasts about 6 to 8 hours. In healthy subjects given single doses, the dose-response relationship for sodium excretion is linear over the dose range of 2.5 mg to 20 mg. The increase in potassium excretion is negligible after a single dose of up to 10 mg and only slight (5 mEq to 15 mEq) after a single dose of 20 mg.

Congestive Heart Failure: DEMADEX has been studied in controlled trials in patients with New York Heart Association Class II to Class IV congestive heart failure. Patients who received 10 mg to 20 mg of daily DEMADEX in these studies achieved significantly greater reductions in weight and edema than did patients who received placebo.

Nonanuric Renal Failure: In single-dose studies in patients with nonanuric renal failure, high doses of DEMADEX (20 mg to 200 mg) caused marked increases in water and sodium excretion. In patients with nonanuric renal failure, severe enough to require hemodialysis, chronic treatment with up to 200 mg of daily DEMADEX has not been shown to change steady-state fluid retention. When patients in a study of acute renal failure received total daily doses of 520 mg to 1200 mg of DEMADEX, 19% experienced seizures. Ninety-six patients were treated in this study; 6/32 treated with torsemide experienced seizures, 6/32 treated with comparably high doses of furosemide experienced seizures, and 1/32 treated with placebo experienced a seizure.

Hepatic Cirrhosis: When given with aldosterone antagonists, DEMADEX also caused increases in sodium and fluid excretion in patients with edema or ascites due to hepatic cirrhosis. Urinary sodium excretion rate relative to the urinary excretion rate of DEMADEX is less in cirrhotic patients than in healthy subjects (possibly because of the hyperaldosteronism and resultant sodium retention that are characteristic of portal hypertension and ascites). However, because of the increased renal clearance of DEMADEX in patients with hepatic cirrhosis, these factors tend to balance each other, and the result is an overall natriuretic response that is similar to that seen in healthy subjects. Chronic use of any diuretic in hepatic disease has not been studied in adequate and well-controlled trials.

Essential Hypertension: In patients with essential hypertension, DEMADEX has been shown in controlled studies to lower blood pressure when administered once a day at doses of 5 mg to 10 mg. The antihypertensive effect is near maximal after 4 to 6 weeks of treatment, but it may continue to increase for up to 12 weeks. Systolic and diastolic supine and standing blood pressures are all reduced. There is no significant orthostatic effect, and there is only a minimal peak-trough difference in blood pressure reduction.
The antihypertensive effects of DEMADEX are, like those of other diuretics, on the average greater in black patients (a low-renin population) than in nonblack patients.
When DEMADEX is first administered, daily urinary sodium excretion increases for at least a week. With chronic administration, however, daily sodium loss comes into balance with dietary sodium intake. If the administration of DEMADEX is suddenly stopped, blood pressure returns to pretreatment levels over several days, without overshoot.
DEMADEX has been administered together with β-adrenergic blocking agents, ACE inhibitors, and calcium-channel blockers. Adverse drug interactions have not been observed, and special dosage adjustment has not been necessary.

INDICATIONS AND USAGE

DEMADEX is indicated for the treatment of edema associated with congestive heart failure, renal disease, or hepatic disease. Use of torsemide has been found to be effective for the treatment of edema associated with chronic renal failure. Chronic use of any diuretic in hepatic disease has not been studied in adequate and well-controlled trials.
DEMADEX intravenous injection is indicated when a rapid onset of diuresis is desired or when oral administration is impractical.
DEMADEX is indicated for the treatment of hypertension alone or in combination with other antihypertensive agents.

CONTRAINDICATIONS

DEMADEX is contraindicated in patients with known hypersensitivity to DEMADEX or to sulfonylureas.
DEMADEX is contraindicated in patients who are anuric.

WARNINGS

Hepatic Disease With Cirrhosis and Ascites: DEMADEX should be used with caution in patients with hepatic disease with cirrhosis and ascites, since sudden alterations of fluid and electrolyte balance may precipitate hepatic coma. In these patients, diuresis with DEMADEX (or any other diuretic) is best initiated in the hospital. To prevent hypokalemia and metabolic alkalosis, an aldosterone antagonist or potassium-sparing drug should be used concomitantly with DEMADEX.

Ototoxicity: Tinnitus and hearing loss (usually reversible) have been observed after rapid intravenous injection of other loop diuretics and have also been observed after oral DEMADEX. It is not certain that these events were attributable to DEMADEX. Ototoxicity has also been seen in animal studies when very high plasma levels of torsemide were induced. Administered intravenously, DEMADEX should be injected slowly over 2 minutes, and single doses should not exceed 200 mg.

Volume and Electrolyte Depletion: Patients receiving diuretics should be observed for clinical evidence of electrolyte imbalance, hypovolemia, or prerenal azotemia. Symptoms of these disturbances may include one or more of the following: dryness of the mouth, thirst, weakness, lethargy, drowsiness, restlessness, muscle pains or cramps, muscular fatigue, hypotension, oliguria, tachycardia, nausea, and vomiting. Excessive diuresis may cause dehydration, blood-volume reduction, and possibly thrombosis and embolism, especially in elderly patients. In patients who develop fluid and electrolyte imbalances, hypovolemia, or prerenal azotemia, the observed laboratory changes may include hyper- or hyponatremia, hyper- or hypochloremia, hyper- or hypokalemia, acid-base abnormalities, and increased blood urea nitrogen (BUN). If any of these occur, DEMADEX should be discontinued until the situation is corrected; DEMADEX may be restarted at a lower dose.

In controlled studies in the United States, DEMADEX was administered to hypertensive patients at doses of 5 mg or 10 mg daily. After 6 weeks at these doses, the mean decrease in serum potassium was approximately 0.1 mEq/L. The percentage of patients who had a serum potassium level below 3.5 mEq/L at any time during the studies was essentially the same in patients who received DEMADEX (1.5%) as in those who received placebo (3%). In patients followed for 1 year, there was no further change in mean serum potassium levels. In patients with congestive heart failure, hepatic cirrhosis, or renal disease treated with DEMADEX at doses higher than those studied in United States antihypertensive trials, hypokalemia was observed with greater frequency, in a dose-related manner.

In patients with cardiovascular disease, especially those receiving digitalis glycosides, diuretic-induced hypokalemia may be a risk factor for the development of arrhythmias. The risk of hypokalemia is greatest in patients with cirrhosis of the liver, in patients experiencing a brisk diuresis, in patients who are receiving inadequate oral intake of electrolytes, and in patients receiving concomitant therapy with corticosteroids or ACTH.

Periodic monitoring of serum potassium and other electrolytes is advised in patients treated with DEMADEX.

PRECAUTIONS

Laboratory Values: *Potassium:* See WARNINGS.

Calcium: Single doses of DEMADEX increased the urinary excretion of calcium by normal subjects, but serum calcium levels were slightly increased in 4- to 6-week hypertension trials. In a long-term study of patients with congestive heart failure, the average 1-year change in serum calcium was a decrease of 0.10 mg/dL (0.02 mmol/L). Among 426 patients treated with DEMADEX for an average of 11 months, hypocalcemia was not reported as an adverse event.

Magnesium: Single doses of DEMADEX caused healthy volunteers to increase their urinary excretion of magnesium, but serum magnesium levels were slightly increased in 4- to 6-week hypertension trials. In long-term hypertension studies, the average 1-year change in serum magnesium was an increase of 0.03 mg/dL (0.01 mmol/L). Among 426 patients treated with DEMADEX for an average of 11 months, one case of hypomagnesemia (1.3 mg/dL (0.53 mmol/L)) was reported as an adverse event.

In a long-term clinical study of DEMADEX in patients with congestive heart failure, the estimated annual change in serum magnesium was an increase of 0.2 mg/dL (0.08 mmol/L), but these data are confounded by the fact that many of these patients received magnesium supplements. In a 4-week study in which magnesium supplementation was not given, the rate of occurrence of serum magnesium levels below 1.7 mg/dL (0.70 mmol/L) was 6% and 9% in the groups receiving 5 mg and 10 mg of DEMADEX, respectively.

Blood Urea Nitrogen (BUN), Creatinine and Uric Acid: DEMADEX produces small dose-related increases in each of these laboratory values. In hypertensive patients who received 10 mg of DEMADEX daily for 6 weeks, the mean increase in blood urea nitrogen was 1.8 mg/dL (0.6 mmol/L), the mean increase in serum creatinine was 0.05 mg/dL (4 mmol/L), and the mean increase in serum uric acid was 1.2 mg/dL (70 mmol/L). Little further change occurred with long-term treatment, and all changes reversed when treatment was discontinued.

Symptomatic gout has been reported in patients receiving DEMADEX, but its incidence has been similar to that seen in patients receiving placebo.

Glucose: Hypertensive patients who received 10 mg of daily DEMADEX experienced a mean increase in serum glucose concentration of 5.5 mg/dL (0.3 mmol/L) after 6 weeks of therapy, with a further increase of 1.8 mg/dL (0.1 mmol/L) during the subsequent year. In long-term studies in diabetics, mean fasting glucose values were not significantly changed from baseline. Cases of hyperglycemia have been reported but are uncommon.

Dose	*Shape*	*Bottle*	*Tel-E-Dose*
5 mg	oval	NDC 0004-0262-01	NDC 0004-0262-49
10 mg	oval	NDC 0004-0263-01	NDC 0004-0263-49
20 mg	oval	NDC 0004-0264-01	NDC 0004-0264-49
100 mg	capsule-shaped	NDC 0004-0265-01	NDC 0004-0265-49

Serum Lipids: In the controlled short-term hypertension studies in the United States, daily doses of 5 mg, 10 mg, and 20 mg of DEMADEX were associated with increases in total plasma cholesterol of 4, 4, and 8 mg/dL (0.10 to 0.20 mmol/L), respectively. The changes subsided during chronic therapy.

In the same short-term hypertension studies, daily doses of 5 mg, 10 mg and 20 mg of DEMADEX were associated with mean increases in plasma triglycerides of 16, 13 and 71 mg/dL (0.15 to 0.80 mmol/L), respectively.

In long-term studies of 5 mg to 20 mg of DEMADEX daily, no clinically significant differences from baseline lipid values were observed after 1 year of therapy.

Other: In long-term studies in hypertensive patients, DEMADEX has been associated with small mean decreases in hemoglobin, hematocrit, and erythrocyte count and small mean increases in white blood cell count, platelet count, and serum alkaline phosphatase. Although statistically significant, all of these changes were medically inconsequential. No significant trends have been observed in any liver enzyme tests other than alkaline phosphatase.

Drug Interactions: In patients with essential hypertension, DEMADEX has been administered together with beta-blockers, ACE inhibitors, and calcium-channel blockers. In patients with congestive heart failure, DEMADEX has been administered together with digitalis glycosides, ACE inhibitors, and organic nitrates. None of these combined uses was associated with new or unexpected adverse events.

Torsemide does not affect the protein binding of glyburide or of warfarin, the anticoagulant effect of phenprocoumon (a related coumarin derivative), or the pharmacokinetics of digoxin or carvedilol (a vasodilator/beta-blocker). In healthy subjects, coadministration of DEMADEX was associated with significant reduction in the renal clearance of spironolactone, with corresponding increases in the AUC. However, clinical experience indicates that dosage adjustment of either agent is not required.

Because DEMADEX and salicylates compete for secretion by renal tubules, patients receiving high doses of salicylates may experience salicylate toxicity when DEMADEX is concomitantly administered. Also, although possible interactions between torsemide and nonsteroidal anti-inflammatory agents (including aspirin) have not been studied, coadministration of these agents with another loop diuretic (furosemide) has occasionally been associated with renal dysfunction.

The natriuretic effect of DEMADEX (like that of many other diuretics) is partially inhibited by the concomitant administration of indomethacin. This effect has been demonstrated for DEMADEX under conditions of dietary sodium restriction (50 mEq/day) but not in the presence of normal sodium intake (150 mEq/day).

The pharmacokinetic profile and diuretic activity of torsemide are not altered by cimetidine or spironolactone. Coadministration of digoxin is reported to increase the area under the curve for torsemide by 50%, but dose adjustment of DEMADEX is not necessary.

Concomitant use of torsemide and cholestyramine has not been studied in humans but, in a study in animals, coadministration of cholestyramine decreased the absorption of orally administered torsemide. If DEMADEX and cholestyramine are used concomitantly, simultaneous administration is not recommended.

Coadministration of probenecid reduces secretion of DEMADEX into the proximal tubule and thereby decreases the diuretic activity of DEMADEX.

Other diuretics are known to reduce the renal clearance of lithium, inducing a high risk of lithium toxicity, so coadministration of lithium and diuretics should be undertaken with great caution, if at all. Coadministration of lithium and DEMADEX has not been studied.

Other diuretics have been reported to increase the ototoxic potential of aminoglycoside antibiotics and of ethacrynic acid, especially in the presence of impaired renal function. These potential interactions with DEMADEX have not been studied.

Carcinogenesis, Mutagenesis and Impairment of Fertility: No overall increase in tumor incidence was found when torsemide was given to rats and mice throughout their lives at doses up to 9 mg/kg/day (rats) and 32 mg/kg/day (mice). On a body-weight basis, these doses are 27 to 96 times a human dose of 20 mg; on a body-surface-area basis, they are 5 to 8 times this dose. In the rat study, the high-dose female group demonstrated renal tubular injury, interstitial inflammation, and a statistically significant increase in renal adenomas and carcinomas. The tumor incidence in this group was, however, not much higher than the incidence sometimes seen in historical controls. Similar signs of chronic non-neoplastic renal injury have been reported in high-dose animal studies of other diuretics such as furosemide and hydrochlorothiazide.

No mutagenic activity was detected in any of a variety of in vivo and in vitro tests of torsemide and its major human metabolite. The tests included the Ames test in bacteria (with and without metabolic activation), tests for chromosome aberrations and sister-chromatid exchanges in human lymphocytes, tests for various nuclear anomalies in cells found in hamster and murine bone marrow, tests for unscheduled DNA synthesis in mice and rats, and others.

In doses up to 25 mg/kg/day (75 times a human dose of 20 mg on a body-weight basis; 13 times this dose on a body-surface-area basis), torsemide had no adverse effect on the reproductive performance of male or female rats.

Pregnancy: Pregnancy Category B. There was no fetotoxicity or teratogenicity in rats treated with up to 5 mg/kg/day of torsemide (on a mg/kg basis, this is 15 times a human dose of 20 mg/day; on a mg/m^2 basis, the animal dose is 10 times the human dose), or in rabbits, treated with 1.6 mg/kg/day (on a mg/kg basis, 5 times the human dose of 20 mg/kg/day; on a mg/m^2 basis, 1.7 times this dose). Fetal and maternal toxicity (decrease in average body weight, increase in fetal resorption and delayed fetal ossification) occurred in rabbits and rats given doses 4 (rabbits) and 5 (rats) times larger. Adequate and well-controlled studies have not been carried out in pregnant women. Because animal reproduction studies are not always predictive of human response, this drug should be used during pregnancy only if clearly needed.

Labor and Delivery: The effect of DEMADEX on labor and delivery is unknown.

Nursing Mothers: It is not known whether DEMADEX is excreted in human milk. Because many drugs are excreted in human milk, caution should be exercised when DEMADEX is administered to a nursing woman.

Pediatric Use: Safety and effectiveness in pediatric patients have not been established.

Administration of another loop diuretic to severely premature infants with edema due to patent ductus arteriosus and hyaline membrane disease has occasionally been associated with renal calcifications, sometimes barely visible on X-ray but sometimes in staghorn form, filling the renal pelves. Some of these calculi have been dissolved, and hypercalciuria has been reported to have decreased, when chlorothiazide has been coadministered along with the loop diuretic. In other premature neonates with hyaline membrane disease, another loop diuretic has been reported to increase the risk of persistent patent ductus arteriosus, possibly through a prostaglandin-E-mediated process. The use of DEMADEX in such patients has not been studied.

Geriatric Use: Of the total number of patients who received DEMADEX in United States clinical studies, 24% were 65 or older while about 4% were 75 or older. No specific age-related differences in effectiveness or safety were observed between younger patients and elderly patients.

ADVERSE REACTIONS

At the time of approval, DEMADEX had been evaluated for safety in approximately 4000 subjects: over 800 of these subjects received DEMADEX for at least 6 months, and over 380 were treated for more than 1 year. Among these subjects were 564 who received DEMADEX during United States-based trials in which 274 other subjects received placebo.

The reported side effects of DEMADEX were generally transient, and there was no relationship between side effects and age, sex, race, or duration of therapy. Discontinuation of therapy due to side effects occurred in 3.5% of United States patients treated with DEMADEX and in 4.4% of patients treated with placebo. In studies conducted in the United States and Europe, discontinuation rates due to side effects were 3.0% (38/1250) with DEMADEX and 3.4% (13/380) with furosemide in patients with congestive heart failure, 2.0% (8/409) with DEMADEX and 4.8% (11/230) with furosemide in patients with renal insufficiency, and 7.6% (13/170) with DEMADEX and 0% (0/33) with furosemide in patients with cirrhosis.

The most common reasons for discontinuation of therapy with DEMADEX were (in descending order of frequency) dizziness, headache, nausea, weakness, vomiting, hyperglycemia, excessive urination, hyperuricemia, hypokalemia, excessive thirst, hypovolemia, impotence, esophageal hemorrhage, and dyspepsia. Dropout rates for these adverse events ranged from 0.1% to 0.5%.

The side effects considered possibly or probably related to study drug that occurred in United States placebo-controlled trials in more than 1% of patients treated with DEMADEX are shown in the table below.

Reactions Possibly or Probably Drug-Related United States Placebo-Controlled Studies Incidence (Percentages of Patients)

	DEMADEX (N=564)	Placebo (N=274)
Headache	7.3	9.1
Excessive Urination	6.7	2.2
Dizziness	3.2	4.0
Rhinitis	2.8	2.2
Asthenia	2.0	1.5
Diarrhea	2.0	1.1
ECG Abnormality	2.0	0.4
Cough Increase	2.0	1.5

Continued on next page

Demadex—Cont.

Constipation	1.8	0.7
Nausea	1.8	0.4
Arthralgia	1.8	0.7
Dyspepsia	1.6	0.7
Sore Throat	1.6	0.7
Myalgia	1.6	1.5
Chest Pain	1.2	0.4
Insomnia	1.2	1.8
Edema	1.1	1.1
Nervousness	1.1	0.4

The daily doses of DEMADEX used in these trials ranged from 1.25 mg to 20 mg, with most patients receiving 5 mg to 10 mg; the duration of treatment ranged from 1 to 52 days, with a median of 41 days. Of the side effects listed in the table, only "excessive urination" occurred significantly more frequently in patients treated with DEMADEX than in patients treated with placebo. In the placebo-controlled hypertension studies whose design allowed side-effect rates to be attributed to dose, excessive urination was reported by 1% of patients receiving placebo, 4% of those treated with 5 mg of daily DEMADEX, and 15% of those treated with 10 mg. The complaint of excessive urination was generally not reported as an adverse event among patients who received DEMADEX for cardiac, renal, or hepatic failure.

Serious adverse events reported in the clinical studies for which a drug relationship could not be excluded were atrial fibrillation, chest pain, diarrhea, digitalis intoxication, gastrointestinal hemorrhage, hyperglycemia, hyperuricemia, hypokalemia, hypotension, hypovolemia, shunt thrombosis, rash, rectal bleeding, syncope, and ventricular tachycardia.

Angioedema has been reported in a patient exposed to DEMADEX who was later found to be allergic to sulfa drugs.

Of the adverse reactions during placebo-controlled trials listed without taking into account assessment of relatedness to drug therapy, arthritis and various other nonspecific musculoskeletal problems were more frequently reported in association with DEMADEX than with placebo, even though gout was somewhat more frequently associated with placebo. These reactions did not increase in frequency or severity with the dose of DEMADEX. One patient in the group treated with DEMADEX withdrew due to myalgia, and one in the placebo group withdrew due to gout.

Hypokalemia: See WARNINGS.

OVERDOSAGE

There is no human experience with overdoses of DEMADEX, but the signs and symptoms of overdosage can be anticipated to be those of excessive pharmacologic effect: dehydration, hypovolemia, hypotension, hyponatremia, hypokalemia, hypochloremic alkalosis, and hemoconcentration. Treatment of overdosage should consist of fluid and electrolyte replacement.

Laboratory determinations of serum levels of torsemide and its metabolites are not widely available.

No data are available to suggest physiological maneuvers (eg, maneuvers to change the pH of the urine) that might accelerate elimination of torsemide and its metabolites. Torsemide is not dialyzable, so hemodialysis will not accelerate elimination.

DOSAGE AND ADMINISTRATION

General: DEMADEX tablets may be given at any time in relation to a meal, as convenient. Special dosage adjustment in the elderly is not necessary.

Because of the high bioavailability of DEMADEX, oral and intravenous doses are therapeutically equivalent, so patients may be switched to and from the intravenous form with no change in dose. DEMADEX intravenous injection should be administered either slowly as a bolus over a period of 2 minutes or administered as a continuous infusion.

If DEMADEX is administered through an IV line, it is recommended that, as with other IV injections, the IV line be flushed with Normal Saline (Sodium Chloride Injection, USP) before and after administration. DEMADEX injection is formulated above pH 8.3. Flushing the line is recommended to avoid the potential for incompatibilities caused by differences in pH which could be indicated by color change, haziness or the formation of a precipitate in the solution.

If DEMADEX is administered as a continuous infusion, stability has been demonstrated through 24 hours at room temperature in plastic containers for the following fluids and concentrations:

200 mg DEMADEX (10 mg/mL) added to:
- 250 mL Dextrose 5% in water
- 250 mL 0.9% Sodium Chloride
- 500 mL 0.45% Sodium Chloride

50 mg DEMADEX (10 mg/mL) added to:
- 500 mL Dextrose 5% in water
- 500 mL 0.9% Sodium Chloride
- 500 mL 0.45% Sodium Chloride

Before administration, the solution of DEMADEX should be visually inspected for discoloration and particulate matter. If either is found, the ampul should not be used.

Congestive Heart Failure: The usual initial dose is 10 mg or 20 mg of once-daily oral or intravenous DEMADEX. If the diuretic response is inadequate, the dose should be titrated upward by approximately doubling until the desired diuretic response is obtained. Single doses higher than 200 mg have not been adequately studied.

Chronic Renal Failure: The usual initial dose of DEMADEX is 20 mg of once-daily oral or intravenous DEMADEX. If the diuretic response is inadequate, the dose should be titrated upward by approximately doubling until the desired diuretic response is obtained. Single doses higher than 200 mg have not been adequately studied.

Hepatic Cirrhosis: The usual initial dose is 5 mg or 10 mg of once-daily oral or intravenous DEMADEX, administered together with an aldosterone antagonist or a potassium-sparing diuretic. If the diuretic response is inadequate, the dose should be titrated upward by approximately doubling until the desired diuretic response is obtained. Single doses higher than 40 mg have not been adequately studied.

Chronic use of any diuretic in hepatic disease has not been studied in adequate and well-controlled trials.

Hypertension: The usual initial dose is 5 mg once daily. If the 5 mg dose does not provide adequate reduction in blood pressure within 4 to 6 weeks, the dose may be increased to 10 mg once daily. If the response to 10 mg is insufficient, an additional antihypertensive agent should be added to the treatment regimen.

HOW SUPPLIED

DEMADEX for oral administration is available as white, scored tablets containing 5 mg, 10 mg, 20 mg, or 100 mg of torsemide. The tablets are supplied in bottles and Tel-E-Dose®* packages of 100 as follows:

[See table at top of previous page]

Each tablet is debossed on the scored side with the Boehringer Mannheim logo and 102, 103, 104, or 105 (for 5 mg, 10 mg, 20 mg, or 100 mg, respectively). On the opposite side, the tablet is debossed with 5, 10, 20, or 100 to indicate the dose.

DEMADEX for intravenous injection is supplied in clear ampuls containing 2 mL (20 mg, NDC 0004-0267-06) or 5 mL (50 mg, NDC 0004-0268-06) of a 10 mg/mL sterile solution.

Storage: Store all dosage forms at 15° to 30°C (59° to 86°F). Do not freeze.

*Tel-E-Dose is a registered trademark of Hoffmann-La Roche Inc.

Tablets manufactured by:
Boehringer Mannheim, GmbH, Mannheim, Germany
Ampuls manufactured by:
Abbott Laboratories, North Chicago, IL 60064

Revised: April 1998

Shown in Product Identification Guide, page 332

EC-NAPROSYN® ℞
(naproxen)
Delayed-Release Tablets

NAPROSYN® ℞
(naproxen)
Tablets

ANAPROX®/ANAPROX® DS ℞
[an' ă-prox]
(naproxen sodium)
Tablets

NAPROSYN® ℞
(naproxen)
Suspension

The following text is complete prescribing information based on official labeling in effect June 2000.

DESCRIPTION

Naproxen is a member of the arylacetic acid group of nonsteroidal anti-inflammatory drugs.

The chemical names for naproxen and naproxen sodium are (S)-6-methoxy-α-methyl-2-naphthaleneacetic acid and (S)-6-methoxy-α-methyl-2-naphthaleneacetic acid, sodium salt, respectively. Naproxen and naproxen sodium have the following structures, respectively:

R
H
CH_3
CH_3O

naproxen (R=-COOH) $C_{14}H_{14}O_3$ mol wt 230.26

naproxen sodium (R=-COONa) $C_{14}H_{13}NaO_3$ mol wt 252.23

Naproxen is an odorless, white to off-white crystalline substance. It is lipid-soluble, practically insoluble in water at low pH and freely soluble in water at high pH. The octanol/water partition coefficient of naproxen at pH 7.4 is 1.6 to 1.8. Naproxen sodium is a white to creamy white, crystalline solid, freely soluble in water at neutral pH.

NAPROSYN (naproxen) Tablets contain 250 mg, 375 mg or 500 mg of naproxen and croscarmellose sodium, iron oxides, povidone and magnesium stearate.

EC-NAPROSYN (naproxen) Delayed-Release Tablets are enteric-coated tablets containing 375 mg or 500 mg of naproxen and croscarmellose sodium, povidone and magnesium stearate. The enteric coating dispersion contains methacrylic acid copolymer, talc, triethyl citrate, sodium hydroxide and purified water. The dispersion may also contain simethicone emulsion. The dissolution of this enteric-coated naproxen tablet is pH dependent with rapid dissolution above pH 6. There is no dissolution below pH 4.

Each ANAPROX 275 mg and ANAPROX DS 550 mg tablet contains naproxen sodium, the active ingredient, with magnesium stearate, microcrystalline cellulose, povidone and talc. The coating suspension for the ANAPROX 275 mg tablet may contain hydroxypropyl methylcellulose 2910, Opaspray K-1-4210A, polyethylene glycol 8000 or Opadry YS-1-4215. The coating suspension for the ANAPROX DS 550 mg tablet may contain hydroxypropyl methylcellulose 2910, Opaspray K-1-4227, polyethylene glycol 8000 or Opadry YS-1-4216.

NAPROSYN (naproxen) Suspension for oral administration contains 125 mg/5 mL of naproxen in a vehicle containing sucrose, magnesium aluminum silicate, sorbitol solution and sodium chloride (30 mg/5 mL, 1.5 mEq), methylparaben, fumaric acid, FD&C Yellow No. 6, imitation pineapple flavor, imitation orange flavor and purified water. The pH of the suspension ranges from 2.2 to 3.7.

CLINICAL PHARMACOLOGY

Naproxen is a nonsteroidal anti-inflammatory drug (NSAID) with analgesic and antipyretic properties. The sodium salt of naproxen has been developed as a more rapidly absorbed formulation of naproxen for use as an analgesic. The naproxen anion inhibits prostaglandin synthesis but beyond this its mode of action is unknown.

Pharmacokinetics: Naproxen itself is rapidly and completely absorbed from the gastrointestinal tract with an in vivo bioavailability of 95%. The different dosage forms of NAPROSYN are bioequivalent in terms of extent of absorption (AUC) and peak concentration (C_{max}); however, the products do differ in their pattern of absorption. These differences between naproxen products are related to both the chemical form of naproxen used and its formulation. Even with the observed differences in pattern of absorption, the elimination half-life of naproxen is unchanged across products ranging from 12 to 17 hours. Steady-state levels of naproxen are reached in 4 to 5 days, and the degree of naproxen accumulation is consistent with this half-life. This suggests that the differences in pattern of release play only a negligible role in the attainment of steady-state plasma levels.

Absorption:

Immediate Release: After administration of NAPROSYN tablets, peak plasma levels are attained in 2 to 4 hours. After oral administration of ANAPROX, peak plasma levels are attained in 1 to 2 hours. The difference in rates between the two products is due to the increased aqueous solubility of the sodium salt of naproxen used in ANAPROX. Peak plasma levels of naproxen given as NAPROSYN Suspension are attained in 1 to 4 hours.

Delayed Release: EC-NAPROSYN is designed with a pH-sensitive coating to provide a barrier to disintegration in the acidic environment of the stomach and to lose integrity in the more neutral environment of the small intestine. The enteric polymer coating selected for EC-NAPROSYN dissolves above pH 6. When EC-NAPROSYN was given to fasted subjects, peak plasma levels were attained about 4 to 6 hours following the first dose (range: 2 to 12 hours). An in vivo study in man using radiolabeled EC-NAPROSYN tablets demonstrated that EC-NAPROSYN dissolves primarily in the small intestine rather than the stomach, so the absorption of the drug is delayed until the stomach is emptied.

When EC-NAPROSYN and NAPROSYN were given to fasted subjects (n=24) in a crossover study following 1 week of dosing, differences in time to peak plasma levels (T_{max}) were observed, but there were no differences in total absorption as measured by C_{max} and AUC:

[See table at bottom of next page]

Antacid Effects: When EC-NAPROSYN was given as a single dose with antacid (54 mEq buffering capacity), the peak plasma levels of naproxen were unchanged, but the time to peak was reduced (mean T_{max} fasted 5.6 hours, mean T_{max} with antacid 5 hours), although not significantly.

Food Effects: When EC-NAPROSYN was given as a single dose with food, peak plasma levels in most subjects were achieved in about 12 hours (range: 4 to 24 hours). Residence time in the small intestine until disintegration was independent of food intake. The presence of food prolonged the time the tablets remained in the stomach, time to first detectable serum naproxen levels, and time to maximal naproxen levels (T_{max}), but did not affect peak naproxen levels (C_{max}).

Distribution:

Naproxen has a volume of distribution of 0.16 L/kg. At therapeutic levels naproxen is greater than 99% albumin-bound. At doses of naproxen greater than 500 mg/day there is less than proportional increase in plasma levels due to an increase in clearance cause by saturation of plasma protein binding at higher doses (average trough C_{ss} 36.5, 49.2 and 56.4 mg/L with 500, 1000 and 1500 mg daily doses of naproxen). However, the concentration of unbound naproxen continues to increase proportionally to dose.

Metabolism:

Naproxen is extensively metabolized to 6-0-desmethyl naproxen, and both parent and metabolites do not induce metabolizing enzymes.

Elimination:
The clearance of naproxen is 0.13 mL/min/kg. Approximately 95% of the naproxen from any dose is excreted in the urine, primarily as naproxen (less than 1%), 6-0-desmethyl naproxen (less than 1%) or their conjugates (66% to 92%). The plasma half-life of the naproxen anion in humans ranges from 12 to 17 hours. The corresponding half-lives of both naproxen's metabolites and conjugates are shorter than 12 hours, and their rates of excretion have been found to coincide closely with the rate of naproxen disappearance from the plasma. In patients with renal failure metabolites may accumulate.

Special Populations:
Pediatric Patients: In pediatric patients aged 5 to 16 years with arthritis, plasma naproxen levels following a 5 mg/kg single dose of naproxen suspension (see DOSAGE AND ADMINISTRATION) were found to be similar to those found in normal adults following a 500 mg dose. The terminal half-life appears to be similar in pediatric and adult patients. Pharmacokinetic studies of naproxen were not performed in pediatric patients younger than 5 years of age. Pharmacokinetic parameters appear to be similar following administration of naproxen suspension or tablets in pediatric patients. EC-NAPROXYN has not been studied in subjects under the age of 18.

Renal Insufficiency: Naproxen pharmacokinetics has not been determined in subjects with renal insufficiency. Given that naproxen, its metabolites and conjugates are primarily excreted by the kidney, the potential exists for naproxen metabolites to accumulate in the presence of renal insufficiency.

CLINICAL STUDIES

General Information: Naproxen has been studied in patients with rheumatoid arthritis, osteoarthritis, juvenile arthritis, ankylosing spondylitis, tendonitis and bursitis, and acute gout. Improvement in patients treated for rheumatoid arthritis was demonstrated by a reduction in joint swelling, a reduction in duration of morning stiffness, a reduction in disease activity as assessed by both the investigator and patient, and by increased mobility as demonstrated by a reduction in walking time. Generally, response to naproxen has not been found to be dependent on age, sex, severity or duration of rheumatoid arthritis.

In patients with osteoarthritis, the therapeutic action of naproxen has been shown by a reduction in joint pain or tenderness, an increase in range of motion in knee joints, increased mobility as demonstrated by a reduction in walking time, and improvement in capacity to perform activities of daily living impaired by the disease.

In a clinical trial comparing standard formulations of naproxen 375 mg bid (750 mg a day) vs 750 mg bid (1500 mg/day), 9 patients in the 750 mg group terminated prematurely because of adverse events. Nineteen patients in the 1500 mg group terminated prematurely because of adverse events. Most of these adverse events were gastrointestinal events.

In clinical studies in patients with rheumatoid arthritis, osteoarthritis, and juvenile arthritis, naproxen has been shown to be comparable to aspirin and indomethacin in controlling the aforementioned measures of disease activity, but the frequency and severity of the milder gastrointestinal adverse effects (nausea, dyspepsia, heartburn) and nervous system adverse effects (tinnitus, dizziness, lightheadedness) were less in naproxen-treated patients than in those treated with aspirin or indomethacin.

In patients with ankylosing spondylitis, naproxen has been shown to decrease night pain, morning stiffness and pain at rest. In double-blind studies the drug was shown to be as effective as aspirin, but with fewer side effects.

In patients with acute gout, a favorable response to naproxen was shown by significant clearing of inflammatory changes (eg, decrese in swelling, heat) within 24 to 48 hours, as well as by relief of pain and tenderness.

Naproxen has been studied in patients with mild to moderate pain secondary to postoperative, orthopedic, postpartum episiotomy and uterine contraction pain and dysmenorrhea. Onset of pain relief can begin within 1 hour in patients taking naproxen and within 30 minutes in patients taking naproxen sodium. Analgesic effect was shown by such measures as reduction of pain intensity scores, increase in pain relief scores, decrease in numbers of patients requiring additional analgesic medication, and delay in time to remedication. The analgesic effect has been found to last for up to 12 hours.

Naproxen may be used safely in combination with gold salts and/or corticosteroids; however, in controlled clinical trials, when added to the regimen of patients receiving corticosteroids, it did not appear to cause greater improvement over that seen with corticosteroids alone. Whether naproxen has a "steroid-sparing" effect has not been adequately studied. When added to the regimen of patients receiving gold salts, naproxen did result in greater improvement. Its use in combination with salicylates is not recommended because there is evidence that aspirin increases the rate of excretion of naproxen and data are inadequate to demonstrate that naproxen and aspirin produce greater improvement over that achieved with aspirin alone. In addition, as with other NSAIDs, the combination may result in higher frequency of adverse events than demonstrated for either product alone.

In ^{51}Cr blood loss and gastroscopy studies with normal volunteers, daily administration of 1000 mg of naproxen as 1000 mg of NAPROSYN (naproxen) or 1100 mg of ANAPROX (naproxen sodium) has been demonstrated to cause statistically significantly less gastric bleeding and erosion than 3250 mg of aspirin.

Three 6-week, double-blind, multicenter studies with EC-NAPROSYN (naproxen) (375 or 500 mg bid, n=385) and NAPROSYN (375 or 500 mg bid, n=279) were conducted comparing EC-NAPROSYN with NAPROSYN, including 355 rheumatoid arthritis and osteoarthritis patients who had a recent history of NSAID-related GI symptoms. These studies indicated that EC-NAPROSYN and NAPROSYN showed no significant differences in efficacy or safety and had similar prevalence of minor GI complaints. Individual patients, however, may find one formulation preferable to the other.

Five hundred and fifty-three patients received EC-NAPROSYN during long-term open label trials (mean length of treatment was 159 days). The rates for clinically-diagnosed peptic ulcers and GI bleeds were similar to what has been historically reported for long-term NSAID use.

INDIVIDUALIZATION OF DOSAGE

Although NAPROSYN, NAPROSYN Suspension, EC-NAPROSYN, ANAPROX and ANAPROX DS all circulate in the plasma as naproxen, they have pharmacokinetic differences that may affect onset of action. Onset of pain relief can begin within 30 minutes in patients taking naproxen sodium and within 1 hour in patients taking naproxen. Because EC-NAPROSYN dissolves in the small intestine rather than in the stomach, the absorption of the drug is delayed compared to the other naproxen formulations (see CLINICAL PHARMACOLOGY).

The recommended strategy for initiating therapy is to choose a formulation and a starting dose likely to be effective for the patient and then adjust the dosage based on observation of benefit and/or adverse events. A lower dose should be considered in patients with renal or hepatic impairment or in elderly patients (see PRECAUTIONS).

Analgesia/Dysmenorrhea/Bursitis and Tendonitis: Because the sodium salt of naproxen is more rapidly absorbed, ANAPROX/ANAPROX DS is recommended for the management of acute painful conditions when prompt onset of pain relief is desired. The recommended starting dose is 550 mg followed by 550 mg every 12 hours or 275 mg every 6 to 8 hours, as required. The initial total daily dose should not exceed 1375 mg of naproxen sodium. Thereafter, the total daily dose should not exceed 1100 mg of naproxen sodium. NAPROSYN may also be used for treatment of acute pain and dysmenorrhea. EC-NAPROSYN is not recommended for initial treatment of acute pain because absorption of naproxen is delayed compared to other naproxen-containing products (see CLINICAL PHARMACOLOGY and INDICATIONS AND USAGE).

Acute Gout: The recommended starting dose is 750 mg of NAPROSYN followed by 250 mg every 8 hours until the attack has subsided. ANAPROX may also be used at a starting dose of 825 mg followed by 275 mg every 8 hours as needed EC-NAPROSYN is not recommended because of the delay in absorption (see CLINICAL PHARMACOLOGY).

Osteoarthritis/Rheumatoid Arthritis/Ankylosing Spondylitis: The recommended dose of naproxen is NAPROSYN or NAPROSYN Suspension 250 mg, 375 mg or 500 mg taken twice daily (morning and evening) or EC-NAPROSYN 375 mg or 500 mg taken twice daily. Naproxen sodium may also be used (see DOSAGE AND ADMINISTRATION).

During long-term administration the dose of naproxen may be adjusted up or down depending on the clinical response of the patient. A lower daily dose may suffice for long-term administration. In patients who tolerate lower doses well, the dose may be increased to 1500 mg per day when a higher level of anti-inflammatory/analgesic activity is required. When treating patients with naproxen 1500 mg/day (as NAPROSYN or 1650 mg of ANAPROX), the physician should observe sufficient increased clinical benefit to offset the potential increased risk. The morning and evening doses do not have to be equal in size and administration of the drug more frequently than twice daily does not generally make a difference in response (see CLINICAL PHARMACOLOGY).

Juvenile Arthritis: The use of NAPROSYN Suspension allows for more flexible dose titration. In pediatric patients, doses of 5 mg/kg/day produced plasma levels of naproxen similar to those seen in adults taking 500 mg of naproxen (see CLINICAL PHARMACOLOGY).

The recommended total daily dose is approximately 10 mg/kg given in two divided doses (ie, 5 mg/kg given twice a day) (see DOSAGE AND ADMINISTRATION).

INDICATIONS AND USAGE

Naproxen as NAPROSYN, EC-NAPROSYN, ANAPROX, ANAPROX DS or NAPROSYN Suspension are indicated for the treatment of rheumatoid arthritis, osteoarthritis, ankylosing spondylitis and juvenile arthritis.

Naproxen as NAPROSYN Suspension is recommended for juvenile rheumatoid arthritis in order to obtain the maximum dosage flexibility based on the patient's weight.

Naproxen as NAPROSYN, ANAPROX, ANAPROX DS and NAPROSYN Suspension are also indicated for the treatment of tendonitis, bursitis, acute gout, and for the management of pain and primary dysmenorrhea. EC-NAPROSYN is not recommended for initial treatment of acute pain because the absorption of naproxen is delayed compared to absorption from other naproxen-containing products (see CLINICAL PHARMACOLOGY and DOSAGE AND ADMINISTRATION).

CONTRAINDICATIONS

All naproxen products are contraindicated in patients who have had allergic reactions to prescription as well as to over-the-counter products containing naproxen. It is also contraindicated in patients in whom aspirin or other nonsteroidal anti-inflammatory/analgesic drugs induce the syndrome of asthma, rhinitis, and nasal polyps. Both types of reactions have the potential of being fatal. Anaphylactoid reactions to naproxen, whether of the true allergic type or the pharmacologic idiosyncratic (eg, aspirin hypersensitivity syndrome) type, usually but not always occur in patients with a known history of such reactions. Therefore, careful questioning of patients for such things as asthma, nasal polyps, urticaria, and hypotension associated with nonsteroidal antinflammatory drugs before starting therapy is important. In addition, if such symptoms occur during therapy, treatment should be discontinued.

WARNINGS

Risk of GI Ulceration, Bleeding and Perforation with NSAID Therapy: Serious gastrointestinal toxicity such as bleeding, ulceration and perforation can occur at any time, with or without warning symptoms, in patients treated chronically with NSAID therapy. Although minor upper gastrointestinal problems, such as dyspepsia, are common, usually developing early in therapy, physicians should remain alert for ulceration and bleeding in patients treated chronically with NSAIDs even in the absence of previous GI tract symptoms. In patients observed in clinical trials of several months to 2 years' duration, symptomatic upper GI ulcers, gross bleeding or perforation appear to occur in approximately 1% of patients treated for 3 to 6 months and in about 2% to 4% of patients treated for 1 year.

Physicians should inform patients about the signs and/or symptoms of serious GI toxicity and what steps to take if they occur.

Studies to date with all naproxen products have not identified any subset of patients not at risk of developing peptic ulceration and bleeding or any differences between different naproxen products in their propensity to cause peptic ulceration and bleeding. Except for a prior history of serious GI events and other risk factors known to be associated with peptic ulcer disease, such as alcoholism, smoking, etc., no risk factors (eg, age, sex) have been associated with increased risk. Elderly or debilitated patients seem to tolerate ulceration or bleeding less well than other individuals and most spontaneous reports of fatal GI events are in this population. Studies to date are inconclusive concerning the relative risk of various NSAIDs in causing such reactions. High doses of any NSAID probably carry a greater risk of these reactions, although controlled clinical trials showing this do not exist in most cases. In considering the use of relatively large doses (within the recommended dosage range), sufficient benefit should be anticipated to offset the potential increased risk of GI toxicity.

PRECAUTIONS

General: **NAPROXEN-CONTAINING PRODUCTS SUCH AS NAPROSYN, EC-NAPROSYN, ANAPROX, ANAPROX DS, NAPROSYN SUSPENSION, ALEVE®*, AND OTHER NAPROXEN PRODUCTS SHOULD NOT BE USED CONCOMITANTLY SINCE THEY ALL CIRCULATE IN THE PLASMA AS THE NAPROXEN ANION.**

If the steroid dose is reduced or eliminated during therapy, the steroid dosage should be reduced slowly and the patient should be observed closely for any evidence of adverse effects, including adrenal insufficiency and exacerbation of symptoms of arthritis.

Patients with initial hemoglobin values of 10 grams or less who are to receive long-term therapy should have hemoglobin values determined periodically.

The antipyretic and anti-inflammatory activities of the drug may reduce fever and inflammation, thus diminishing their utility as diagnostic signs in detecting complications of presumed noninfectious, noninflammatory painful conditions.

Because of adverse eye findings in animal studies with drugs of this class, it is recommended that ophthalmic studies be carried out if any change or disturbance in vision occurs.

Renal Effects: As with other nonsteroidal anti-inflammatory drugs, long-term administration of naproxen to animals has resulted in renal papillary necrosis and other abnormal renal pathology. In humans, there have been reports of acute interstitial nephritis, hematuria, proteinuria and occasionally nephrotic syndrome associated with naproxen-

Continued on next page

	EC-NAPROSYN* 500 mg bid	NAPROSYN* 500 mg bid
C_{max} (μg/mL)	94.9 (18%)	97.4 (13%)
T_{max} (hours)	4 (39%)	1.9 (61%)
$AUC_{0-12\ hr}$ (μg•hr/mL)	845 (20%)	767 (15%)

* Mean value (coefficient of variation)

EC-Naprosyn/Anaprox—Cont.

containing products and other NSAIDs since they have been marketed.

A second form of renal toxicity has been seen in patients taking naproxen as well as other nonsteroidal anti-inflammatory drugs. In patients with prerenal conditions leading to a reduction in renal blood flow or blood volume, where the renal prostaglandins have a supportive role in the maintenance of renal perfusion, administration of a nonsteroidal anti-inflammatory drug may cause a dose-dependent reduction in prostaglandin formation and precipitate overt renal decompensation. Patients at greatest risk of this reaction are those with impaired renal function, heart failure, liver dysfunction, those taking diuretics and the elderly. Discontinuation of nonsteroidal anti-inflammatory therapy is typically followed by recovery to the pretreatment state.

Naproxen and its metabolites are eliminated primarily by the kidneys; therefore, the drug should be used with caution in patients with significantly impaired renal function, and the monitoring of serum creatinine and/or creatinine clearance is advised in these patients. Caution should be used if the drug is given to patients with creatinine clearance of less than 20 mL/minute because accumulation of naproxen metabolites has been seen in such patients.

Chronic alcoholic liver disease and probably other diseases with decreased or abnormal plasma proteins (albumin) reduce the total plasma concentration of naproxen, but the plasma concentration of unbound naproxen is increased. Caution is advised when high doses are required and some adjustment of dosage may be required in these patients. It is prudent to use the lowest effective dose.

Studies indicate that although total plasma concentration of naproxen is unchanged, the unbound plasma fraction of naproxen is increased in the elderly. Caution is advised when high doses are required and some adjustment of dosage may be required in elderly patients. As with other drugs used in the elderly, it is prudent to use the lowest effective dose.

Hepatic Function: As with other nonsteroidal anti-inflammatory drugs, borderline elevations of one or more liver tests may occur in up to 15% of patients. These abnormalities may progress, may remain essentially unchanged, or may be transient with continued therapy. The SGPT (ALT) test is probably the most sensitive indicator of liver dysfunction. Meaningful (3 times the upper limit of normal) elevations of SGPT or SGOT (AST) occurred in controlled clinical trials in less than 1% of patients. A patient with symptoms and/or signs suggesting liver dysfunction or in whom an abnormal liver test has occurred, should be evaluated for evidence of the development of more severe hepatic reaction while on therapy with naproxen. Severe hepatic reactions, including jaundice and cases of fatal hepatitis, have been reported with naproxen as with other nonsteroidal anti-inflammatory drugs. Although such reactions are rare, if abnormal liver tests persist or worsen, if clinical signs and symptoms consistent with liver disease develop, or if systemic manifestations occur (eg, eosinophilia, rash, etc.), naproxen should be discontinued.

Fluid Retention and Edema: Peripheral edema has been observed in some patients receiving naproxen. Since each ANAPROX or ANAPROX DS tablet contains 25 mg or 50 mg of sodium (about 1 mEq per each 250 mg of naproxen), and each teaspoonful of NAPROSYN Suspension contains 39 mg (about 1.5 mEq per each 125 mg of naproxen) of sodium, this should be considered in patients whose overall intake of sodium must be severely restricted. For these reasons, ANAPROX, ANAPROX DS and NAPROSYN Suspension should be used with caution in patients with fluid retention, hypertension or heart failure.

Information for Patients: Naproxen, in NAPROSYN, EC-NAPROSYN, ANAPROX, ANAPROX DS and NAPROSYN Suspension, like other drugs of this class, is not free of side effects. The side effects of these formulations of naproxen can cause discomfort and, rarely, there are more serious side effects, such as gastrointestinal bleeding, which may result in hospitalization and even fatal outcomes.

NSAIDs (Nonsteroidal Anti-Inflammatory Drugs) are often essential agents in the management of arthritis and have a major role in the treatment of pain, but they also may be commonly employed for conditions that are less serious. Physicians may wish to discuss with their patients the potential risks (see WARNINGS, PRECAUTIONS and ADVERSE REACTIONS) and likely benefits of naproxen treatment, particularly when it is used for less serious conditions where treatment without NSAIDs may represent an acceptable alternative to both the patient and physician.

Caution should be exercised by patients whose activities require alertness if they experience drowsiness, dizziness, vertigo or depression during therapy with naproxen.

Laboratory Tests: Because serious GI tract ulceration and bleeding can occur without warning symptoms, physicians should follow patients chronically treated with naproxen for signs and symptoms of ulceration and bleeding and should inform them of the importance of this follow-up and what they should do if certain signs and symptoms do appear (see WARNINGS: *Risk of GI Ulcerations, Bleeding and Perforation with NSAID Therapy*).

Drug Interactions: The use of NSAIDs in patients who are receiving ACE inhibitors may potentiate renal disease states (see PRECAUTIONS: *Renal Effects*).

In vitro studies have shown that naproxen anion, because of its affinity for protein, may displace from their binding sites other drugs that are also albumin-bound (see CLINICAL PHARMACOLOGY: *Pharmacokinetics*).

Theoretically, the naproxen anion itself could likewise be displaced. Short-term controlled studies failed to show that taking the drug significantly affects prothrombin times when administered to individuals on coumarin-type anticoagulants. Caution is advised nonetheless, since interactions have been seen with other nonsteroidal agents of this class. Similarly, patients receiving the drug and a hydantoin, sulfonamide or sulfonylurea should be observed for signs of toxicity to these drugs (see CLINICAL STUDIES: *General Information*).

Concomitant administration of naproxen and aspirin is not recommended because naproxen is displaced from its binding sites during the concomitant administration of aspirin, resulting in lower plasma concentrations and peak plasma levels.

The natriuretic effect of furosemide has been reported to be inhibited by some drugs of this class. Inhibition of renal lithium clearance leading to increases in plasma lithium concentrations has also been reported. Naproxen and other nonsteroidal anti-inflammatory drugs can reduce the antihypertensive effect of propranolol and other beta-blockers. Probenecid given concurrently increases naproxen anion plasma levels and extends its plasma half-life significantly. Caution should be used if naproxen is administered concomitantly with methotrexate. Naproxen, naproxen sodium and other nonsteroidal anti-inflammatory drugs have been reported to reduce the tubular secretion of methotrexate in an animal model, possibly increasing the toxicity of methotrexate.

Due to the gastric pH elevating effects of H_2-blockers, sucralfate and intensive antacid therapy, concomitant administration of EC-NAPROSYN is not recommended.

Drug/Laboratory Test Interactions: Naproxen may decrease platelet aggregation and prolong bleeding time. This effect should be kept in mind when bleeding times are determined.

The administration of naproxen may result in increased urinary values for 17-ketogenic steroids because of an interaction between the drug and/or its metabolites with m-dinitrobenzene used in this assay. Although 17-hydroxy-corticosteroid measurements (Porter-Silber test) do not appear to be artifactually altered, it is suggested that therapy with naproxen be temporarily discontinued 72 hours before adrenal function tests are performed if the Porter-Silber test is to be used.

Naproxen may interfere with some urinary assays of 5-hydroxy indoleacetic acid (5HIAA).

Carcinogenesis: A 2-year study was performed in rats to evaluate the carcinogenic potential of naproxen at rat doses of 8, 16, and 24 mg/kg/day (50, 100, and 150 mg/m^2). The maximum dose used was 0.28 times the systemic exposure to humans at the recommended dose. No evidence of tumorigenicity was found.

Pregnancy: *Teratogenic Effects:* **Pregnancy Category B.** Reproduction studies have been performed in rats at 20 mg/kg/day (125 mg/m^2/day, 0.23 times the human systemic exposure), rabbits at 20 mg/kg/day (220 mg/m^2/day, 0.27 times the human systemic exposure), and mice at 170 mg/kg/day (510 mg/m^2/day, 0.28 times the human systemic exposure) with no evidence of impaired fertility or harm to the fetus due to the drug. There are no adequate and well-controlled studies in pregnant women. Because animal reproduction studies are not always predictive of human response, naproxen should not be used during pregnancy unless clearly needed.

Nonteratogenic Effects: There is some evidence to suggest that when inhibitors of prostaglandin synthesis are used to delay preterm labor there is an increased risk of neonatal complications such as necrotizing enterocolitis, patent ductus areteriosus and intracranial hemorrhage. Naproxen treatment given in late pregnancy to delay parturition has been associated with persistent pulmonary hypertension, renal dysfunction and abnormal prostaglandin E levels in preterm infants. Because of the known effect of drugs of this class on the human fetal cardiovascular system (closure of ductus arteriosus), use during third trimester should be avoided.

Nursing Mothers: The naproxen anion has been found in the milk of lactating women at a concentration of approximately 1% of that found in plasma. Because of the possible adverse effects of prostaglandin-inhibiting drugs on neonates, use in nursing mothers should be avoided.

Pediatric Use: Safety and effectiveness in pediatric patients below the age of 2 years have not been established. Pediatric dosing recommendations for juvenile arthritis are based on well-controlled studies (see DOSAGE AND ADMINISTRATION). There are no adequate effectiveness or dose-response data for other pediatric conditions, but the experience in juvenile arthritis and other use experience have established that single doses of 2.5 to 5 mg/kg (as naproxen suspension, see DOSAGE AND ADMINISTRATION), with total daily dose not exceeding 15 mg/kg/day, are well tolerated in pediatric patients over 2 years of age.

ADVERSE REACTIONS

The following adverse reactions are divided into three parts based on frequency and whether or not the possibility exists of a causal relationship between naproxen and these adverse events. In those reactions listed as "Probable Causal Relationship" there is at least 1 case for each adverse reaction where there is evidence to suggest that there is a causal relationship between drug usage and the reported event.

Adverse reactions reported in controlled clinical trials in 960 patients treated for rheumatoid arthritis or osteoarthritis are listed below. In general, reactions in patients treated chronically were reported 2 to 10 times more frequently than they were in short-term studies in the 962 patients treated for mild to moderate pain or for dysmenorrhea. The most frequent complaints reported related to the gastrointestinal tract.

A clinical study found gastrointestinal reactions to be more frequent and more severe in rheumatoid arthritis patients taking daily doses of 1500 mg naproxen compared to those taking 750 mg naproxen (see CLINICAL PHARMACOLOGY).

In controlled clinical trials with about 80 pediatric patients and in well-monitored, open-label studies with about 400 pediatric patients with juvenile arthritis treated with naproxen, the incidence of rash and prolonged bleeding times were increased, the incidence of gastrointestinal and central nervous system reactions were about the same, and the incidence of other reactions were lower in pediatric patients than in adults.

The following adverse reactions are divided into three parts based on frequency and causal relationship.

Incidence greater than 1% (Probable Causal Relationship):

Gastrointestinal: constipation*, heartburn*, abdominal pain*, nausea*, dyspepsia, diarrhea, stomatitis

Central Nervous System: headache*, dizziness*, drowsiness*, lightheadedness, vertigo

Dermatologic: itching (pruritus)*, skin eruptions*, ecchymoses*, sweating, purpura

Special Senses: tinnitus*, hearing disturbances, visual disturbances

Cardiovascular: edema*, dyspnea*, palpitations

General: thirst

*Incidence of reported reaction between 3% and 9%. Those reactions occurring in less than 3% of the patients are unmarked.

Incidence less than 1% (Probable Causal Relationship):

The following adverse reactions were reported less frequently than 1% during controlled clinical trials and through voluntary reports since marketing. Those reactions observed through voluntary reporting since marketing are italicized.

Gastrointestinal: *abnormal liver function tests, colitis,* gastrointestinal bleeding and/or *perforation, hematemesis,* jaundice, pancreatitis, melena, vomiting

Renal: *glomerular nephritis, hematuria, hyperkalemia, interstitial nephritis, nephrotic syndrome, renal disease, renal failure, renal papillary necrosis*

Hematologic: agranulocytosis, *eosinophilia, granulocytopenia, leukopenia,* thrombocytopenia

Central Nervous System: *depression, dream abnormalities,* inability to concentrate, *insomnia, malaise, myalgia, muscle weakness*

Dermatologic: *alopecia, photosensitive dermatitis, urticaria,* skin rashes, *photosensitivity reactions resembling porphyria cutanea tarda, epidermolysis bullosa*

Special Senses: *hearing impairment*

Cardiovascular: *congestive heart failure*

Respiratory: *eosinophilic pneumonitis*

General: *anaphylactoid reactions, angioneurotic edema, menstrual disorders, pyrexia (chills and fever)*

Incidence less than 1% (Causal Relationship Unknown):

These observations are being listed to serve as alerting information to the physician.

Hematologic: *aplastic anemia, hemolytic anemia*

Central Nervous System: *aseptic meningitis, cognitive dysfunction*

Dermatologic: *epidermal necrolysis, erythema multiforme, Stevens-Johnson syndrome*

Gastrointestinal: *nonpeptic gastrointestinal ulceration, ulcerative stomatitis*

Cardiovascular: *vasculitis*

General: *hyperglycemia, hypoglycemia*

OVERDOSAGE

Significant naproxen overdosage may be characterized by drowsiness, heartburn, indigestion, nausea or vomiting. Because naproxen sodium may be rapidly absorbed, high and early blood levels should be anticipated. A few patients have experienced seizures, but is is not clear whether or not these were drug-related. It is not known what dose of the drug would be life-threatening. The oral LD_{50} of the drug is 543 mg/kg in rats, 1234 mg/kg in mice, 4110 mg/kg in hamsters, and greater than 1000 mg/kg in dogs.

Should a patient ingest a large number of tablets or a large volume of suspension, accidentally or purposefully, the stomach may be emptied and usual supportive measures employed. In animals 0.5 g/kg of activated charcoal was effective in reducing plasma levels of naproxen. Hemodialysis does not decrease the plasma concentration of naproxen because of the high degree of its protein binding.

DOSAGE AND ADMINISTRATION

Rheumatoid Arthritis, Osteoarthritis, and Ankylosing Spondylitis

[See table at top of next page]

To maintain the integrity of the enteric coating, the EC-NAPROSYN tablet should not be broken, crushed or chewed during ingestion.

During long-term administration, the dose of naproxen may be adjusted up or down depending on the clinical response of the patient. A lower daily dose may suffice for long-term administration. The morning and evening doses do not have to be equal in size and the administration of the drug more frequently than twice daily is not necessary.

NAPROSYN	250 mg or 375 mg or 500 mg	twice daily twice daily twice daily
ANAPROX	275 mg (naproxen 250 mg with 25 mg sodium)	twice daily
ANAPROX DS	550 mg (naproxen 500 mg with 50 mg sodium)	twice daily
NAPROSYN Suspension	250 mg (10 mL/2 tsp) or 375 mg (15 mL/3 tsp) or 500 mg (20 mL/4 tsp)	twice daily twice daily twice daily
EC-NAPROSYN	375 mg or 500 mg	twice daily twice daily

In patients who tolerate lower doses well, the dose may be increased to naproxen 1500 mg per day for limited periods when a higher level of anti-inflammatory/analgesic activity is required. When treating such patients with naproxen 1500 mg/day, the physician should observe sufficient increased clinical benefits to offset the potential increased risk (see CLINICAL PHARMACOLOGY and INDIVIDUALIZATION OF DOSAGE).

Juvenile Arthritis: The recommended total daily dose of naproxen is approximately 10 mg/kg given in 2 divided doses (ie, 5 mg/kg given twice a day). A measuring cup marked in 1/2 teaspoon and 2.5 milliliter increments is provided with the NAPROSYN Suspension. The following table may be used as a guide for dosing of NAPROSYN Suspension:

Patient's Weight	Dose	Administered as
13 kg (29 lb)	62.5 mg bid	2.5 mL (1/2 tsp) twice daily
25 kg (55 lb)	125 mg bid	5.0 mL (1 tsp) twice daily
38 kg (84 lb)	187.5 mg bid	7.5 mL (1 1/2 tsp) twice daily

Management of Pain, Primary Dysmenorrhea and Acute Tendonitis and Bursitis: The recommended starting dose is 550 mg of naproxen sodium as ANAPROX/ANAPROX DS followed by 550 mg every 12 hours or 275 mg every 6 to 8 hours as required. The initial total daily dose should not exceed 1375 mg of naproxen sodium. Thereafter, the total daily dose should not exceed 1100 mg of naproxen sodium. NAPROSYN may also be used but EC-NAPROSYN is not recommended for initial treatment of acute pain because absorption of naproxen is delayed compared to other naproxen-containing products (see CLINICAL PHARMACOLOGY, INDICATIONS AND USAGE and INDIVIDUALIZATION OF DOSAGE).

Acute Gout: The recommended starting dose is 750 mg of NAPROSYN followed by 250 mg every 8 hours until the attack has subsided. ANAPROX may also be used at a starting dose of 825 mg followed by 275 mg every 8 hours. EC-NAPROSYN is not recommended because of the delay in absorption (see CLINICAL PHARMACOLOGY).

HOW SUPPLIED

NAPROSYN Tablets: 250 mg: round, yellow, biconvex, debossed with ROCHE on one side and NAPROSYN 250 on the other. Packaged in light-resistant bottles of 100.

100's (bottle): NDC 0004-6312-01.

375 mg: peach, capsule-shaped, debossed with NAPROSYN on one side and 375 on the other. Packaged in light-resistant bottles of 100 and 500.

100's (bottle): NDC 0004-6311-01; 500's (bottle): NDC 0004-6311-14.

500 mg: yellow, capsule-shaped, debossed with NAPROSYN on one side and 500 on the other. Packaged in light-resistant bottles of 100 and 500.

100's (bottle): NDC 0004-6310-01; 500's (bottle): NDC 0004-6310-14.

Store at 15° to 30°C (59° to 86°F) in well-closed containers; dispense in light-resistant containers.

NAPROSYN Suspension: 125 mg/5mL (contains 39 mg sodium, about 1.5 mEq/teaspoon): Available in 1 pint (473 mL) light-resistant bottles (NDC 0004-0028-28).

Store at 15° to 30°C (59° to 86°F); avoid excessive heat, above 40°C (104°F). Dispense in light-resistant containers.

EC-NAPROSYN Delayed-Release Tablets: 375 mg: white, capsule-shaped, imprinted with EC-NAPROSYN on one side and 375 on the other. Packaged in light-resistant bottles of 100.

100's (bottle): NDC 0004-6415-01.

500 mg: white, capsule-shaped, imprinted with EC-NAPROSYN on one side and 500 on the other. Packaged in light-resistant bottles of 100.

100's (bottle): NDC 0004-6416-01.

Store at 15° to 30°C (59° to 86°F) in well-closed containers; dispense in light-resistant containers.

ANAPROX Tablets: Naproxen sodium 275 mg: blue, biconvex oval-shaped, debossed with ROCHE on one side and 274 on the other. Packaged in bottles of 100.

100's (bottle): NDC 0004-6201-01.

Store at 15° to 30°C (59° to 86°F) in well-closed containers.

ANAPROX DS Tablets: Naproxen sodium 550 mg: dark blue, capsule-shaped, film-coated, debossed with ROCHE on one side and ANAPROX DS on the other. Packaged in bottles of 100 and 500.

100's (bottle): NDC 0004-6200-01; 500's (bottle): NDC 0004-6200-14.

Store at 15° to 30°C (59° to 86°F) in well-closed containers.

*ALEVE is a registered trademark of Bayer-Roche L.L.C.

Naprosyn Suspension manufactured by Patheon Inc., Mississauga, Ontario, Canada L5N 7K9

Distributed by:
Roche Pharmaceuticals
Roche Laboratories Inc.
340 Kingsland Street
Nutley, New Jersey 07110-1199

25768605-0999 Revised: September 1999

Shown in Product Identification Guide, page 332 & 333

FORTOVASE™ ℞
(saquinavir)
SOFT GELATIN CAPSULES

The following text is complete prescribing information based on official labeling in effect June 2000.

DESCRIPTION

FORTOVASE brand of saquinavir is an inhibitor of the human immunodeficiency virus (HIV) protease. FORTOVASE is available as beige, opaque, soft gelatin capsules for oral administration in a 200-mg strength (as saquinavir free base). Each capsule also contains the inactive ingredients medium chain mono- and diglycerides, povidone and dl-alpha tocopherol. Each capsule shell contains gelatin and glycerol 85% with the following colorants: red iron oxide, yellow iron oxide and titanium dioxide. The chemical name for saquinavir is N-tert-butyl-decahydro-2-[2(R)-hydroxy-4-phenyl-3(S)- [[N- (2-quinolylcarbonyl) -L-asparaginyl] amino]butyl]-(4aS,8aS)-isoquinoline-3(S)-carboxamide which has a molecular formula $C_{38}H_{50}N_6O_5$ and a molecular weight of 670.86.

Saquinavir is a white to off-white powder and is insoluble in aqueous medium at 25°C.

MICROBIOLOGY

Mechanism of Action: Saquinavir is an inhibitor of HIV protease. HIV protease is an enzyme required for the proteolytic cleavage of viral polyprotein precursors into individual functional proteins found in infectious HIV. Saquinavir is a peptide-like substrate analogue that binds to the protease active site and inhibits the activity of the enzyme. Saquinavir inhibition prevents cleavage of the viral polyproteins resulting in the formation of immature noninfectious virus particles.

Antiviral Activity In Vitro: In vitro antiviral activity of saquinavir was assessed in lymphoblastoid and monocytic cell lines and in peripheral blood lymphocytes. Saquinavir inhibited HIV activity in both acutely and chronically infected cells. IC_{50} and IC_{90} values (50% and 90% inhibitory concentrations) were in the range of 1 to 30 nM and 5 to 80 nM, respectively; however, these concentrations may be altered in the presence of human plasma due to protein binding of saquinavir. In cell culture saquinavir demonstrated additive to synergistic effects against HIV in double- and triple-combination regimens with reverse transcriptase inhibitors zidovudine, zalcitabine, didanosine, lamivudine, stavudine and nevirapine, without enhanced cytotoxicity. The relationship between in vitro susceptibility of HIV to saquinavir and inhibition of HIV replication in humans has not been established.

Drug Resistance: HIV isolates with reduced susceptibility to saquinavir (4-fold or greater increase in IC_{50} from baseline; ie, phenotypic resistance) have been selected in vitro. Genotypic analyses of these HIV isolates showed several mutations in the HIV-protease gene but only those at codons 48 (Gly→Val) and/or 90 (Leu→Met) were consistently associated with saquinavir resistance.

Isolates from selected patients with loss of antiviral activity and prolonged (range: 24 to 147 weeks) therapy with INVIRASE® (saquinavir mesylate) (alone or in combination with nucleoside analogues) showed reduced susceptibility to saquinavir. Genotypic analysis of these isolates showed that mutations at amino acid positions 48 and/or 90 of the HIV-protease gene were most consistently associated with saquinavir resistance. Other mutations in the protease gene were also observed. Mutations at codons 48 and 90 have not been detected in isolates from protease inhibitor naive patients.

In a study (NV15107) of treatment-experienced patients receiving FORTOVASE monotherapy (1200 mg tid) for 8 weeks followed by antiretroviral combination therapy for a period of 4 to 48 weeks (median 32 weeks), 10 of 32 patients showed genotypic changes associated with reduced susceptibility to saquinavir. However, for resistance evaluation virus could not be recovered from 11 of 32 patients.

In a study (NV15355) of treatment-naive patients receiving FORTOVASE in combination with two nucleoside analogues for a period of 16 weeks, 1 of 28 patient isolates showed genotypic changes at codon 71 and 90 in the HIV-protease gene.

Cross-resistance: Among protease inhibitors variable cross-resistance has been recognized. Analysis of saquinavir-resistant isolates from patients following prolonged (24 to 147 weeks) therapy with INVIRASE showed that a majority of patients had resistance to at least one of four other protease inhibitors (indinavir, nelfinavir, ritonavir, 141W94).

CLINICAL PHARMACOLOGY

Pharmacokinetics: The pharmacokinetic properties of saquinavir when administered as FORTOVASE have been evaluated in healthy volunteers (n=207) and HIV-infected patients (n=91) after single-oral doses (range: 300 mg to 1200 mg) and multiple-oral doses (range: 400 mg to 1200 mg tid). The disposition properties of saquinavir have been studied in healthy volunteers after intravenous doses of 6, 12, 36 or 72 mg (n=21).

ABSORPTION AND BIOAVAILABILITY IN ADULTS: Following multiple dosing of FORTOVASE (1200 mg tid) in HIV-infected patients in study NV15107, the mean steady-state area under the plasma concentration versus time curve (AUC) at week 3 was 7249 ng·h/mL (n=31) compared to 866 ng·h/mL (n=10) following multiple dosing with 600 mg tid of INVIRASE (Table 1). Preliminary results from a pharmacokinetic substudy of NV15182 showed a mean saquinavir AUC of 3485 (CV 66%) ng·h/mL (n=11) in patients sampled between weeks 61 to 69 of therapy (see PRECAUTIONS: *General*). While this mean AUC value was lower than that of the week 3 steady-state value for FORTOVASE (1200 mg tid) from study NV15107, it remained higher than the mean AUC value for INVIRASE in study NV15107.

Table 1. Mean AUC_8 in Patients Treated With FORTOVASE and INVIRASE (Week 3)

Treatment	n	AUC_8 ng·h/mL	± SD
FORTOVASE 1200 mg tid	31	7249	± 6174
INVIRASE 600 mg tid	10	866	± 533

The absolute bioavailability of saquinavir administered as FORTOVASE has not been assessed. However, following single 600-mg doses, the relative bioavailability of saquinavir as FORTOVASE compared to saquinavir administered as INVIRASE was estimated as 331% (95% CI 207% to 530%). The absolute bioavailability of saquinavir administered as INVIRASE average 4% (CV 73%, range: 1% to 9%) in 8 healthy volunteers who received a single 600-mg dose of INVIRASE following a high-fat breakfast (48 g protein, 60 g carbohydrate, 57 g fat; 1006 kcal). In healthy volunteers receiving single doses of FORTOVASE (300 mg to 1200 mg) and in HIV-infected patients receiving multiple doses of FORTOVASE (400 mg to 1200 mg tid), a greater than dose-proportional increase in saquinavir plasma concentrations has been observed.

Comparison of pharmacokinetic parameters between single- and multiple-dose studies shows that following multiple dosing of FORTOVASE (1200 mg tid) in healthy male volunteers (n=18), the steady-state AUC was 80% (95% CI 22% to 176%) higher than that observed after a single 1200-mg dose (n=30).

HIV-infected patients administered FORTOVASE (1200 mg tid) had AUC and maximum plasma concentration (C_{max}) values approximately twice those observed in healthy volunteers receiving the same treatment regimen. The mean AUC values at week 1 were 4159 (CV 88%) and 8839 (CV 82%) ng·h/mL, and C_{max} values were 1420 (CV 81%) and 2477 (CV 76%) ng/mL for healthy volunteers and HIV-infected patients, respectively.

FOOD EFFECT: The mean 12-hour AUC after a single 800-mg oral dose of saquinavir in healthy volunteers (n=12) was increased from 167 ng·h/mL (CV 45%), under fasting conditions, to 1120 ng·h/mL (CV 54%) when FORTOVASE was given with breakfast (48 g protein, 60 g carbohydrate, 57 g fat; 1006 kcal).

DISTRIBUTION IN ADULTS: The mean steady-state volume of distribution following intravenous administration of a 12-mg dose of saquinavir (n=8) was 700 L (CV 39%), suggesting saquinavir partitions into tissues. It has been shown that saquinavir, up to 30 µg/mL is approximately 97% bound to plasma proteins.

METABOLISM AND ELIMINATION IN ADULTS: In vitro studies using human liver microsomes have shown that the metabolism of saquinavir is cytochrome P450 mediated with the specific isoenzyme, CYP3A4, responsible for more than 90% of the hepatic metabolism. Based on in vitro studies, saquinavir is rapidly metabolized to a range of mono- and di-hydroxylated inactive compounds. In a mass balance study using 600 mg ^{14}C-saquinavir mesylate (n=8), 88% and 1% of the orally administered radioactivity was recovered in feces and urine, respectively, within 5 days of dosing. In an

Continued on next page

Fortovase—Cont.

additional 4 subjects administered 10.5 mg ^{14}C-saquinavir intravenously, 81% and 3% of the intravenously administered radioactivity was recovered in feces and urine, respectively, within 5 days of dosing. In mass balance studies, 13% of circulating radioactivity in plasma was attributed to unchanged drug after oral administration and the remainder attributed to saquinavir metabolites. Following intravenous administration, 66% of circulating radioactivity was attributed to unchanged drug and the remainder attributed to saquinavir metabolites, suggesting that saquinavir undergoes extensive first-pass metabolism.

Systemic clearance of saquinavir was rapid, 1.14 L/h/kg (CV 12%) after intravenous doses of 6, 36 and 72 mg. The mean residence time of saquinavir was 7 hours (n=8).

SPECIAL POPULATIONS: Hepatic or Renal Impairment: Saquinavir pharmacokinetics in patients with hepatic or renal insufficiency has not been investigated (see PRECAUTIONS). Only 1% of saquinavir is excreted in the urine, so the impact of renal impairment on saquinavir elimination should be minimal.

Gender, Race and Age: The effect of gender was investigated in healthy volunteers receiving single 1200-mg doses of FORTOVASE (n=12 females, 18 males). No effect of gender was apparent on the pharmacokinetics of saquinavir in this study.

The effect of race on the pharmacokinetics of saquinavir when administered as FORTOVASE is unknown.

The pharmacokinetics of saquinavir when administered as FORTOVASE has not been investigated in patients >65 years of age or in pediatric patients (<16 years of age).

DRUG INTERACTIONS (see PRECAUTIONS: *Drug Interactions*): Several drug interaction studies have been completed with both INVIRASE and FORTOVASE. Results from studies conducted with INVIRASE may not be applicable to FORTOVASE. Table 2 summarizes the effect of FORTOVASE on the geometric mean AUC and C_{max} of coadministered drugs. Table 3 summarizes the effect of coadministered drugs on the geometric mean AUC and C_{max} of saquinavir.

For information regarding clinical recommendations, see PRECAUTIONS: *Drug Interactions*.

[See table 2 below]

[See table 3 below]

INDICATIONS AND USAGE

FORTOVASE is indicated for use in combination with other antiretroviral agents for the treatment of HIV infection. This indication is based on a study that showed a reduction in both mortality and AIDS-defining clinical events for patients who received INVIRASE in combination with HIVID® (zalcitabine) compared to patients who received either HIVID or INVIRASE alone. This indication is also based on studies that showed increased saquinavir concentrations and improved antiviral activity for FORTOVASE 1200 mg tid compared to INVIRASE 600 mg tid.

Description of Clinical Studies: *STUDIES WITH FORTOVASE (saquinavir):*

Study NV15355: Efficacy Study

Study NV15355 is an ongoing, open-label, randomized, parallel study comparing FORTOVASE (n=90) and INVIRASE (n=81) in combination with two nucleoside reverse transcriptase inhibitors of choice in treatment-naive patients. The median age was 35 (range: 18 to 63), 92% of patients were male, and 68% were Caucasian. Mean baseline CD_4 cell count was 429 cells/mm^3, and mean baseline plasma HIV-RNA was 4.8 log_{10} copies/mL.

At week 16, 60 patients on the FORTOVASE arm compared to 30 patients on the INVIRASE arm had plasma HIV RNA levels below the limit of assay quantification (<400 copies/mL, Amplicor HIV-1 Monitor™ Test).

At week 16, mean changes from baseline in CD_4 cell counts and plasma HIV-RNA levels between the two treatment arms were statistically indistinguishable. The mean change in CD_4 cell count was 97 cells/mm^3 for the FORTOVASE arm and 115 cells/mm^3 for the INVIRASE arm. The mean changes in plasma HIV-RNA levels are summarized in Figure 1.

[See figure 1 at top of next column]

Study NV15182: Safety Study

Study NV15182 was an open-label safety study of FORTOVASE in combination with other antiretroviral agents in 442 patients (median age 39 [range: 15 to 71], 90% male and 73% Caucasian). The mean baseline CD_4 cell count was 227 cells/mm^3 and mean baseline HIV-RNA was 4.14 log_{10} copies/mL. The safety results from this study are displayed in the ADVERSE REACTIONS section.

Table 2. Effect of FORTOVASE on the Pharmacokinetics of Coadministered Drugs

Coadministered Drug	FORTOVASE Dose	N	% Change for Coadminstered Drug AUC (95%CI)	C_{max} (95%CI)
Clarithromycin 500 mg bid × 7 days	1200 mg tid × 7 days	12V		
Clarithromycin			↑45% (17-81%)	↑39% (10-76%)
14-OH clarithromycin metabolite			↓24% (5-40%)	↓34% (14-50%)
Nelfinavir 750-mg single dose	1200 mg tid × 4 days	14P	↑18% (5-33%)	↔
Ritonavir 400 mg bid × 14 days	400 mg bid × 14 days	8V	↔	↔
Terfenadine 60 mg bid × 11 days*	1200 mg tid × 4 days	12V		
Terfenadine			↑368% (257-514%)	↑253% (164-373%)
Terfenadine acid metabolite			↑120% (89-156%)	↑93% (59-133%)

↑ Denotes an average increase in exposure by the percentage indicated.
↓ Denotes an average decrease in exposure by the percentage indicated.
↔Denotes no statistically significant change in exposure was observed.
* FORTOVASE should not be coadministered with terfenadine (see PRECAUTIONS: *Drug Interactions*).
P Patient
V Healthy Volunteers.

Table 3. Effect of Coadministered Drugs on FORTOVASE and INVIRASE Pharmacokinetics

Coadministered Drug	FORTOVASE Dose	N	% Change for Saquinavir AUC (95%CI)	C_{max} (95%CI)
Clarithromycin 500 mg bid × 7 days	1200 mg tid × 7 days	12V	↑177% (108-269%)	↑187% (105-300%)
Indinavir 800 mg q8h × 2 days	800-mg single dose	6V	↑620% (273-1288%)	↑551% (320-908%)
	1200-mg single dose	6V	↑364% (190-644%)	↑299% (138-568%)
Nelfinavir 750 mg × 4 days	1200-mg single dose	14P	↑392% (271-553%)	↑179% (105-280%)
Ritonavir 400 mg bid × 14 days*	400 mg bid × 14 days†	8V	↑121% (7-359%)	↑64%§

Coadministered Drug	INVIRASE Dose	N	% Change for Saquinavir AUC (95%CI)	C_{max} (95%CI)
Delavirdine 400 mg tid × 14 days	600 mg tid × 21 days	13V	↑5-fold	Not available
Ketoconazole 200 mg qd × 6 days	600 mg tid × 6 days	12V	↑130% (58-235%)	↑147% (53-298%)
Nevirapine 200 mg bid × 21 days	600 mg tid × 7 days	23P	↓24% (1-42%)	↓28% (1-47%)
Ranitidine 150 mg × 2 doses	600-mg single dose	12V	↑67%§	↑74% (16-161%)
Rifabutin 300 mg qd × 14 days	600 mg tid × 14 days	12P	↓43% (29-53%)	↓30%§
Rifampin 600 mg qd × 7 days	600 mg tid × 14 days	12V	↓84% (79-88%)	↓79% (68-86%)
Ritonavir 400 mg bid steady state*	400 mg bid steady state‡	7P	↑1587% (808-3034%)	↑1277% (577-2702%)
Zalcitabine (ddC) 0.75 mg tid × 7 days	600 mg tid × 7 days	27P	↔	↔
Zidovudine (ZDV) 200 mg tid × > 7 days	600 mg tid × > 7 days	20P	↔	↔

↑ Denotes an average increase in exposure by the percentage indicated.
↓ Denotes an average decrease in exposure by the percentage indicated.
↔Denotes no statistically significant change in exposure was observed.
* When ritonavir was combined with the same dose of either INVIRASE or FORTOVASE, actual mean plasma exposures (AUC_{12}, 18.2 µg·h/mL, 20.0 µg·h/mL, respectively) were not significantly different.
† Compared to standard FORTOVASE 1200 mg tid regimen (n=33).
‡ Compared to standard INVIRASE 600 mg tid regimen (n=114).
§ Did not reach statistical significance.
P Patient
V Healthy Volunteers.

Figure 1. Mean Change from Baseline in Plasma HIV-RNA Levels in Study NV15355*

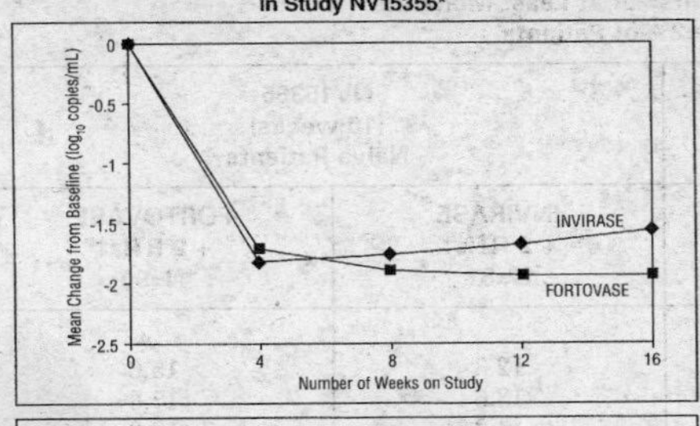

Number of Patients					
Week	0	4	8	12	16
INVIRASE	81	74	71	75	69†
FORTOVASE	90	83	79	78	75†

* Amplicor HIV-1 Monitor™ Test. Limit of quantification = 400 copies/mL.
† By 16 weeks of therapy, 15 patients receiving FORTOVASE and 7 receiving INVIRASE had discontinued study treatment; 5 patients on INVIRASE had missing data at week 16.

STUDIES WITH INVIRASE (saquinavir mesylate):

Study NV14256: INVIRASE + HIVID Versus Either Monotherapy

Study NV14256 (North America) was a randomized, double-blind study comparing the combination of INVIRASE 600 mg tid + HIVID to HIVID monotherapy and INVIRASE monotherapy. The study accrued 970 patients, with median baseline CD_4 cell count at study entry of 170 cells/mm^3. Median duration of prior ZDV treatment was 17 months. Median duration of follow-up was 17 months. There were 88 first AIDS-defining events or deaths in the HIVID monotherapy group, 84 in the INVIRASE monotherapy group and 51 in the combination group. For survival there were 30 deaths in the HIVID group, 40 in the INVIRASE group and 11 deaths in the combination group.

The analysis of clinical endpoints from this study showed that the 18-month cumulative incidence of clinical disease progression to AIDS-defining event or death was 17.7% for patients randomized to INVIRASE + HIVID compared to 30.7% for patients randomized to HIVID monotherapy and 28.3% for patients randomized to INVIRASE monotherapy. The reduction in the number of clinical events for the combination regimen relative to both monotherapy regimens was statistically significant (see Figure 2 for Kaplan-Meier estimates of time to disease progression).

Figure 2. Time to First AIDS-Defining Event (or Death) (days) NV14256

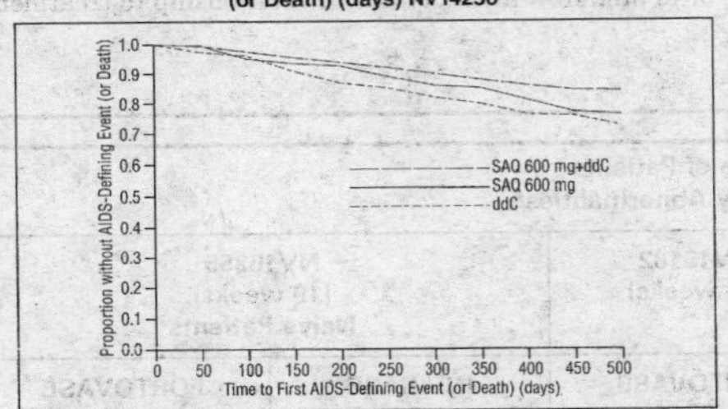

The 18-month cumulative mortality was 4% for patients randomized to INVIRASE + HIVID, 8.9% for patients randomized to HIVID monotherapy and 12.6% for patients randomized to INVIRASE monotherapy. The reduction in the number of deaths for the combination regimen relative to both monotherapy regimens was statistically significant (see Figure 3 for Kaplan-Meier estimates of time to death).

Figure 3. Time to Death (days) NV14256

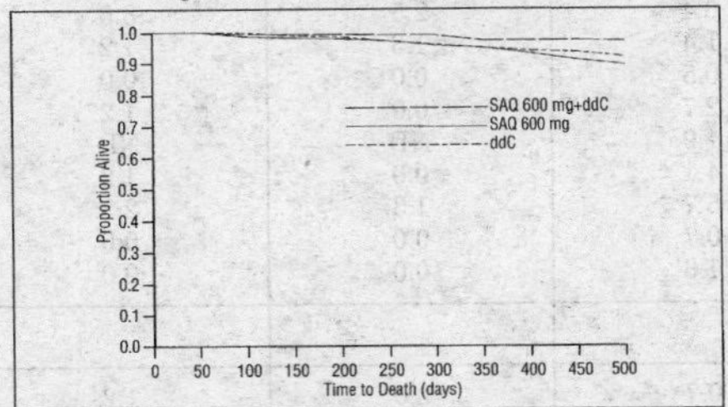

CONTRAINDICATIONS

FORTOVASE is contraindicated in patients with clinically significant hypersensitivity to saquinavir or to any of the components contained in the capsule.

FORTOVASE should not be administered concurrently with terfenadine, cisapride, astemizole, triazolam, midazolam or ergot derivatives, because competition for CYP3A by saquinavir could result in inhibition of the metabolism of these drugs and create the potential for serious and/or life-threatening reactions such as cardiac arrhythmias or prolonged sedation (see PRECAUTIONS: *Drug Interactions*).

WARNINGS

New onset diabetes mellitus, exacerbation of pre-existing diabetes mellitus and hyperglycemia have been reported during post-marketing surveillance in HIV-infected patients receiving protease-inhibitor therapy. Some patients required either initiation or dose adjustments of insulin or oral hypoglycemic agents for the treatment of these events. In some cases diabetic ketoacidosis has occurred. In those patients who discontinued protease-inhibitor therapy, hyperglycemia persisted in some cases. Because these events have been reported voluntarily during clinical practice, estimates of frequency cannot be made and a causal relationship between protease-inhibitor therapy and these events has not been established.

Drugs That Should Not Be Coadministered With FORTOVASE

Antihistamines	Astemizole, Terfenadine
Antimigraine	Ergot Derivatives
GI Motility Agents	Cisapride
Sedatives/Hypnotics	Midazolam, Triazolam

Clinically Significant Drug Interactions Which Decrease Saquinavir Plasma Concentrations

HIV Non-nucleoside Reverse Transcriptase Inhibitors	Nevirapine*
Antimycobacterial Agents	Rifabutin*, Rifampin*

Clinically Significant Drug Interactions Which Increase Saquinavir Plasma Concentrations

Antibiotics	Clarithromycin†
HIV Protease Inhibitors	Indinavir†, Ritonavir*† Nelfinavir†
HIV Non-nucleoside Reverse Transcriptase Inhibitors	Delavirdine*
Antifungal Agents	Ketoconazole*

Other Potential Drug Interactions‡

Anticonvulsants: Carbamazepine, Phenobarbital, Phenytoin	May decrease saquinavir plasma concentrations
Corticosteroids: Dexamethasone	May decrease saquinavir plasma concentrations

*Studied with INVIRASE.
†Studied with FORTOVASE.
‡This table is not all inclusive.

PRECAUTIONS

General: If a serious or severe toxicity occurs during treatment with FORTOVASE, FORTOVASE should be interrupted until the etiology of the event is identified or the toxicity resolves. At that time, resumption of treatment with full-dose FORTOVASE may be considered.

Preliminary results from a pharmacokinetic substudy of NV15182 from patients sampled between weeks 61 to 69 of treatment showed that the mean saquinavir AUC was lower than the week 3 mean AUC from study NV15107. However, the mean AUC of saquinavir at week 61 to 69 remained higher than the mean AUC of INVIRASE in study NV15107 (see CLINICAL PHARMACOLOGY: *Pharmacokinetics*). The clinical significance of this finding is unknown.

Hepatic Insufficiency: Saquinavir is principally metabolized by the liver. Therefore, caution should be exercised when administering FORTOVASE to patients with hepatic insufficiency since patients with baseline liver function tests >5 times the upper limit of normal were not included in clinical studies. Although a causal relationship has not been established, there have been reports of exacerbation of chronic liver dysfunction, including portal hypertension, in patients with underlying hepatitis B or C, cirrhosis or other underlying liver abnormalities.

Hemophilia: There have been reports of spontaneous bleeding in patients with hemophilia A and B treated with protease inhibitors. In some patients additional factor VIII was required. In the majority of reported cases treatment with protease inhibitors was continued or restarted. A causal relationship between protease-inhibitor therapy and these episodes has not been established.

Resistance/Cross-resistance: Varying degrees of cross-resistance among protease inhibitors have been observed. Continued administration of saquinavir therapy following loss of viral suppression may increase the likelihood of cross-resistance to other protease inhibitors (see MICROBIOLOGY).

Information for Patients: Patients should be informed that any change from INVIRASE to FORTOVASE should be made only under the supervision of a physician.

Patients should be informed that FORTOVASE is not a cure for HIV infection and that they may continue to contract illnesses associated with advanced HIV infection, including opportunistic infections. They should be informed that FORTOVASE therapy has not been shown to reduce the risk of transmitting HIV to others through sexual contact or blood contamination.

FORTOVASE may interact with some drugs; therefore, patients should be advised to report to their physician the use of any other prescription or nonprescription medication.

Patients should be advised that FORTOVASE should be taken within 2 hours after a full meal (see CLINICAL PHARMACOLOGY: *Pharmacokinetics*). Patients should be advised of the importance of taking their medication every day, as prescribed, to achieve maximum benefit. Patients should not alter the dose or discontinue therapy without consulting their physician. If a dose is missed, patients should take the next dose as soon as possible. However, the patient should not double the next dose.

Patients should be told that the long-term effects of FORTOVASE are unknown at this time.

Patients should be informed that refrigerated (36° to 46°F, 2° to 8°C) capsules of FORTOVASE remain stable until the expiration date printed on the label. Once brought to room temperature [at or below 77°F (25°C)], capsules should be used within 3 months.

Laboratory Tests: Clinical chemistry tests should be performed prior to initiating FORTOVASE therapy and at appropriate intervals thereafter. Elevated nonfasting triglyceride levels have been observed in patients in saquinavir trials. Triglyceride levels should be periodically monitored during therapy. For comprehensive information concerning laboratory test alterations associated with use of other antiretroviral therapies, physicians should refer to the complete product information for these drugs.

Drug Interactions: **Several drug interaction studies have been completed with both INVIRASE and FORTOVASE. Observations from drug interaction studies with INVIRASE may not be predictive for FORTOVASE.**

[See table above]

ANTIBIOTICS:

Clarithromycin: Coadministration of clarithromycin with FORTOVASE resulted in a 177% increase in saquinavir plasma AUC, a 45% increase in clarithromycin AUC and a 24% decrease in clarithromycin 14-OH metabolite AUC.

ANTIHISTAMINES:

Terfenadine: Coadministration of terfenadine with FORTOVASE resulted in increased terfenadine plasma levels; therefore, FORTOVASE should not be administered concurrently with terfenadine because of the potential for serious and/or life-threatening cardiac arrhythmias.

Astemizole: Because a similar interaction to that seen with terfenadine is likely from the coadministration of FORTOVASE and astemizole, FORTOVASE should not be administered concurrently with astemizole.

HIV PROTEASE INHIBITORS:

Indinavir: Coadministration of indinavir with FORTOVASE (1200-mg single dose) resulted in a 364% in-

Continued on next page

Fortovase—Cont.

crease in saquinavir plasma AUC. Currently, there are no safety and efficacy data available from the use of this combination.

Nelfinavir: Coadministration of nelfinavir with FORTOVASE resulted in an 18% increase in nelfinavir plasma AUC and a 392% increase in saquinavir plasma AUC. Currently, there are no safety and efficacy data available from the use of this combination.

Ritonavir: Following approximately 4 weeks of a combination regimen of saquinavir (400 mg or 600 mg bid) and ritonavir (400 mg or 600 mg bid) in HIV-infected patients, saquinavir AUC values were at least 17-fold greater than historical AUC values from patients who received saquinavir 600 mg tid without ritonavir. When used in combination therapy for up to 24 weeks, doses greater than 400 mg bid of either ritonavir or saquinavir were associated with an increase in adverse events. Plasma exposures achieved with INVIRASE (400 mg bid) and ritonavir (400 mg bid) are similar to those achieved with FORTOVASE (400 mg bid) and ritonavir (400 mg bid).

HIV REVERSE TRANSCRIPTASE INHIBITORS:

Based on known metabolic pathways and routes of elimination for nucleoside reverse transcriptase inhibitors, no interaction with saquinavir is expected.

HIV NON-NUCLEOSIDE REVERSE TRANSCRIPTASE INHIBITORS:

Delavirdine: Coadministration of delaviridine with INVIRASE resulted in a 5-fold increase in saquinavir plasma AUC. Currently there are limited safety and no efficacy data available from the use of this combination. In a small, preliminary study, hepatocellular enzyme elevations occurred in 13% of subjects during the first several weeks of the delaviridine and saquinavir combination (6% Grade 3 or 4). Hepatocellular changes should be monitored frequently if this combination is prescribed.

Nevirapine: Coadministration of nevirapine with INVIRASE resulted in a 24% decrease in saquinavir plasma AUC. Currently, there are no safety and efficacy data available from the use of this combination.

ANTIFUNGAL AGENTS:

Ketoconazole: Coadministration of ketoconazole with INVIRASE resulted in a 130% increase in saquinavir plasma AUC.

ANTIMYCOBACTERIAL AGENTS:

Rifabutin: Coadministration of rifabutin with INVIRASE resulted in a 43% decrease in saquinavir plasma AUC. Physicians should consider using an alternative to rifabutin when a patient is taking FORTOVASE.

Rifampin: Coadministration of rifampin with INVIRASE resulted in an 84% decrease in saquinavir plasma AUC. Physicians should consider using an alternative to rifampin when a patient is taking FORTOVASE.

H_2 ANTAGONISTS:

Ranitidine: Little or no change in the pharmacokinetics of INVIRASE was observed when coadministered with ranitidine. No significant interaction would be expected between FORTOVASE and ranitidine.

GI MOTILITY AGENTS:

Cisapride: Although no interaction study has been conducted, cisapride should not be administered concurrently with FORTOVASE because of the potential for serious and/or life-threatening cardiac arrhythmias.

Carcinogenesis, Mutagenesis and Impairment of Fertility:

Carcinogenesis: Carcinogenicity studies in rats and mice have not yet been completed.

Mutagenesis: Mutagenicity and genotoxicity studies, with and without metabolic activation where appropriate, have shown that saquinavir has no mutagenic activity in vitro in either bacterial (Ames test) or mammalian cells (Chinese hamster lung V79/HPRT test). Saquinavir does not induce chromosomal damage in vivo in the mouse micronucleus assay or in vitro in human peripheral blood lymphocytes and does not induce primary DNA damage in vitro in the unscheduled DNA synthesis test.

Impairment of Fertility: Fertility and reproductive performance were not affected in rats at plasma exposures (AUC values) approximately 50% of those achieved in humans at the recommended dose.

Pregnancy: *Teratogenic Effects:* Category B. Reproduction studies conducted with saquinavir in rats have shown no embryotoxicity or teratogenicity at plasma exposures (AUC values) approximately 50% of those achieved in humans at the recommended dose or in rabbits at plasma exposures approximately 40% of those achieved at the recommended clinical dose of FORTOVASE. Distribution studies in these species showed that placental transfer of saquinavir is low (less than 5% of maternal plasma concentrations).

Studies in rats indicated that exposure to saquinavir from late pregnancy through lactation at plasma concentrations (AUC values) approximately 50% of those achieved in humans at the recommended dose of FORTOVASE had no effect on the survival, growth and development of offspring to weaning. Because animal reproduction studies are not always predictive of human response, FORTOVASE should only be used during pregnancy after taking into account the importance of the drug to the mother. Presently, there are no reports of women receiving FORTOVASE in clinical trials who became pregnant.

Table 4. Percentage of Patients With Treatment-Emergent Adverse Events* of at Least Moderate Intensity, Occurring in ≥2% of Patients

	NV15182 (48 weeks)	NV15355 (16 weeks) Naiva Patients	
ADVERSE EVENT	**FORTOVASE + TOC† N=442**	**INVIRASE + 2 RTIs‡ N=81**	**FORTOVASE + 2 RTIs‡ N=90**
GASTROINTESTINAL			
Diarrhea	19.9	12.3	15.6
Nausea	10.6	13.6	17.8
Abdominal Discomfort	8.6	4.9	13.3
Dyspepsia	8.4	—	8.9
Flatulence	5.7	7.4	12.2
Vomiting	2.9	1.2	4.4
Abdominal Pain	2.3	1.2	7.8
Constipation	—	—	3.3
BODY AS A WHOLE			
Fatigue	4.8	6.2	6.7
CENTRAL AND PERIPHERAL NERVOUS SYSTEM			
Headaches	5.0	4.9	8.9
PSYCHIATRIC DISORDERS			
Depression	2.7	—	—
Insomnia	—	1.2	5.6
Anxiety	—	2.5	2.2
Libido Disorder	—	—	2.2
SPECIAL SENSES DISORDERS			
Taste Alteration		1.2	4.4
MUSCULOSKELETAL DISORDERS			
Pain	—	3.7	3.3
DERMATOLOGICAL DISORDERS			
Eczema	—	2.5	—
Rash	—	2.5	—
Verruca	—	—	2.2

* Includes adverse events at least possibly related to study drug or of unknown intensity and/or relationship to treatment (corresponding to ACTG Grade 3 and 4).
† Antiretroviral Treatment of Choice.
‡ Reverse Transcriptase Inhibitor.

Table 5. Percentage of Patients With Marked Laboratory Abnormalities*

		NV15182 (48 weeks)	NV15355 (16 weeks) Naive Patients	
BIOCHEMISTRY	**Limit**	**FORTOVASE + TOC† N=442**	**INVIRASE + 2 RTIs‡ N=81**	**FORTOVASE + 2 RTIs‡ N=90**
Alkaline Phosphatase	>5 × ULN§	0.5	0.0	0.0
Calcium (high)	>12.5 mg/dL	0.2	0.0	0.0
Creatine Kinase	>4 × ULN§	7.8	0.0	4.8
Gamma GT	>5 × ULN§	5.7	2.6	7.1
Glucose (low)	<40 mg/dL	6.4	2.5	3.5
Glucose (high)	>250 mg/dL	1.4	1.3	1.2
Phosphate	<1.5 mg/dL	0.5	0.0	0.0
Potassium (high)	>6.5 mEq/L	2.7	0.0	1.2
Serum Amylase	>2 × ULN§	1.9	ND	ND
SGOT (AST)	>5 × ULN§	4.1	0.0	1.2
SGPT (ALT)	>5 × ULN§	5.7	1.3	2.3
Sodium (high)	>157 mEq/L	0.7	0.0	0.0
Total Bilirubin	>2.5 × ULN§	1.6	0.0	0.0
HEMATOLOGY				
Hemoglobin	<7.0 gm/dL	0.7	0.0	1.2
Absolute Neutrophil Count	<750 mm^3	2.9	2.9	1.2
Platelets	<50,000 mm^3	0.9	2.5	0.0

* ACTG Grade 3 or above.
† Antiretroviral Treatment of Choice.
‡ Reverse Transcriptase Inhibitor.
§ ULN = Upper limit of normal range.
ND Not done.

Nursing Mothers: The US Public Health Service Centers for Disease Control and Prevention advises HIV-infected women not to breastfeed to avoid postnatal transmission of HIV to a child who may not be infected. It is not known whether saquinavir is excreted in human milk.

Pediatric Use: Safety and effectiveness of FORTOVASE in HIV-infected pediatric patients younger than 16 years of age have not been established.

Geriatric Use: Safety and effectiveness of FORTOVASE in HIV-infected geriatric patients older than 65 years of age have not been established.

ADVERSE REACTIONS (see PRECAUTIONS)

The safety of FORTOVASE was studied in more than 500 patients who received the drug either alone or in combination with other antiretroviral agents. The majority of treatment-related adverse events were of mild intensity. The

most frequently reported treatment-emergent adverse events among patients receiving FORTOVASE in combination with other antiretroviral agents were diarrhea, nausea, abdominal discomfort and dyspepsia.
Clinical adverse events of at least moderate intensity which occurred in ≥2% of patients in studies NV15182 and NV15355 are summarized in Table 4. The median duration of treatment in studies NV15182 and NV15355 were 52 and 18 weeks, respectively. In NV15182, more than 300 patients were on treatment for approximately 1 year.
[See table 4 at top of previous page]
FORTOVASE did not appear to alter the pattern, frequency or severity of known major toxicities associated with the use of nucleoside analogues. Physicians should refer to the complete product information for other antiretroviral agents as appropriate for drug-associated adverse reactions to these other agents.
Rare occurrences of the following serious adverse experiences have been reported during clinical trials of FORTOVASE and/or INVIRASE and were considered at least possibly related to use of study drugs: confusion, ataxia and weakness; seizures; headache; acute myeloblastic leukemia; hemolytic anemia; thrombocytopenia; thrombocytopenia and intracranial hemorrhage leading to death; attempted suicide; Stevens-Johnson syndrome; bullous skin eruption and polyarthritis; severe cutaneous reaction associated with increased liver function tests; isolated elevation of transaminases, exacerbation of chronic liver disease with Grade 4 elevated liver function tests, jaundice, ascites, and right and left upper quadrant abdominal pain; pancreatitis leading to death; intestinal obstruction; portal hypertension; thrombophlebitis; peripheral vasoconstriction; drug fever; nephrolithiasis; and acute renal insufficiency.
Table 5 summarizes the percentage of patients with marked laboratory abnormalities in study NV15182 and NV15355 (median duration of treatment was 52 and 18 weeks, respectively). In study NV15182, by 48 weeks <1% of patients discontinued treatment due to laboratory abnormalities.
[See table 5 at top of previous page]
Additional marked lab abnormalities have been observed with INVIRASE. These include: calcium (low), phosphate (low), potassium (low), sodium (low).
Monotherapy and Combination Studies: Other clinical adverse experiences of any intensity, at least remotely related to FORTOVASE and INVIRASE, including those in <2% of patients, are listed below by body system.
Autonomic Nervous System: Mouth dry, night sweats, sweating increased
Body as a Whole: Allergic reaction, anorexia, appetite decreased, appetite disturbances, asthenia, chest pain, edema, fever, intoxication, malaise, olfactory disorder, pain body, pain pelvic, retrosternal pain, shivering, trauma, wasting syndrome, weakness generalized, weight decrease
Cardiovascular/Cerebrovascular: Cyanosis, heart murmur, heart rate disorder, heart valve disorder, hypertension, hypotension, stroke, syncope, vein distended
Central and Peripheral Nervous System: Ataxia, cerebral hemorrhage, confusion, convulsions, dizziness, dysarthria, dysesthesia, hyperesthesia, hyperreflexia, hyporeflexia, light-headed feeling, myelopolyradiculoneuritis, neuropathy, numbness extremities, numbness face, paresis, paresthesia, peripheral neuropathy, poliomyelitis, prickly sensation, progressive multifocal leukoencephalopathy, spasms, tremor, unconsciousness
Dermatological: Acne, alopecia, chalazion, dermatitis, dermatitis seborrheic, erythema, folliculitis, furunculosis, hair changes, hot flushes, nail disorder, papillomatosis, papular rash, photosensitivity reaction, pigment changes skin, parasites external, pruritus, psoriasis, rash maculopapular, rash pruritic, red face, skin disorder, skin nodule, skin syndrome, skin ulceration, urticaria, verruca, xeroderma
Endocrine/Metabolic: Dehydration, diabetes mellitus, hyperglycemia, hypoglycemia, hypothyroidism, thirst, triglyceride increase, weight increase
Gastrointestinal: Abdominal distention, bowel movements frequent, buccal mucosa ulceration, canker sores oral, cheilitis, colic abdominal, dysphagia, esophageal ulceration, esophagitis, eructation, fecal incontinence, feces bloodstained, feces discolored, gastralgia, gastritis, gastroesophageal reflux, gastrointestinal inflammation, gingivitis, glossitis, hemorrhage rectum, hemorrhoids, infectious diarrhea, melena, painful defecation, parotid disorder, pruritus ani, pyrosis, salivary glands disorder, stomach upset, stomatitis, taste unpleasant, toothache, tooth disorder, ulcer gastrointestinal
Hematologic: Anemia, neutropenia, pancytopenia, splenomegaly
Liver and Biliary: Cholangitis sclerosing, cholelithiasis, hepatitis, hepatomegaly, hepatosplenomegaly, jaundice, liver enzyme disorder, pancreatitis
Musculoskeletal: Arthralgia, arthritis, back pain, cramps leg, cramps muscle, lumbago, musculoskeletal disorders, myalgia, myopathy, pain facial, pain jaw, pain leg, pain musculoskeletal, stiffness, tissue changes
Neoplasm: Kaposi's sarcoma, tumor
Platelet, Bleeding, Clotting: Bleeding dermal, hemorrhage, microhemorrhages, thrombocytopenia
Psychiatric: Agitation, amnesia, anxiety attack, behavior disturbances, dreaming excessive, euphoria, hallucination, intellectual ability reduced, irritability, lethargy, overdose effect, psychic disorder, psychosis, somnolence, speech disorder
Reproductive System: Epididymitis, erectile impotence, impotence, menstrual disorder, menstrual irregularity, penis disorder, prostate enlarged, vaginal discharge
Resistance Mechanism: Abscess, angina tonsillaris, candidiasis, cellulitis, herpes simplex, herpes zoster, infection bacterial, infection mycotic, infection staphylococcal, infestation parasitic, influenza, lymphadenopathy, molluscum contagiosum, moniliasis
Respiratory: Asthma bronchial, bronchitis, cough, dyspnea, epistaxis, hemoptysis, laryngitis, pharyngitis, pneumonia, pulmonary disease, respiratory disorder, rhinitis, rhinitis allergic atopic, sinusitis, upper respiratory tract infection
Special Senses: Blepharitis, conjunctivitis, cytomegalovirus retinitis, dry eye syndrome, earache, ear pressure, eye irritation, hearing decreased, otitis, taste unpleasant, tinnitus, visual disturbance, xerophthalmia
Urinary System: Micturition disorder, nocturia, renal calculus, renal colic, urinary tract bleeding, urinary tract infection

OVERDOSAGE

Overdosage with FORTOVASE has not been reported. There were 2 patients who had overdoses with INVIRASE. No sequelae were noted in the first patient after ingesting 8 grams of INVIRASE as a single dose. The patient was treated with induction of emesis within 2 to 4 hours after ingestion. The second patient ingested 2.4 grams of INVIRASE in combination with 600 mg of ritonavir and experienced pain in the throat that lasted for 6 hours and then resolved.

DOSAGE AND ADMINISTRATION

The recommended dose of FORTOVASE is six 200-mg capsules orally, three times a day (1200 mg tid). FORTOVASE should be taken with a meal or up to 2 hours after a meal. When used in combination with nucleoside analogues, the dosage of FORTOVASE should not be reduced as this will lead to greater than dose proportional decreases in saquinavir plasma levels.
Patients should be advised that FORTOVASE, like other protease inhibitors, is recommended for use in combination with active antiretroviral therapy. Greater activity has been observed when new antiretroviral therapies are begun at the same time as FORTOVASE. As with all protease inhibitors, adherence to the prescribed regimen is strongly recommended. Concomitant therapy should be based on a patient's prior drug exposure.
Monitoring of Patients: Clinical chemistry tests should be performed prior to initiating FORTOVASE therapy and at appropriate intervals thereafter. For comprehensive patient monitoring recommendations for other antiretroviral therapies, physicians should refer to the complete product information for these drugs.
Dose Adjustment for Combination Therapy With FORTOVASE: For toxicities that may be associated with FORTOVASE, the drug should be interrupted. For recipients of combination therapy with FORTOVASE and other antiretroviral agents, dose adjustment of the other antiretroviral agents should be based on the known toxicity profile of the individual drug. Physicians should refer to the complete product information for these drugs for comprehensive dose adjustment recommendations and drug-associated adverse reactions.

HOW SUPPLIED

FORTOVASE 200-mg capsules are beige, opaque, soft gelatin capsules with ROCHE and 0246 imprinted on the capsule shell — bottles of 180 (NDC 0004-0246-48).
The capsules should be refrigerated at 36° to 46°F (2° to 8°C) in tightly closed bottles until dispensed.
For patient use, refrigerated (36° to 46°F, 2° to 8°C) capsules of FORTOVASE remain stable until the expiration date printed on the label. Once brought to room temperature [at or below 77°F (25°C)], capsules should be used within 3 months.
Active ingredient manufactured by:
F. Hoffmann-La Roche Ltd., Basel, Switzerland

Issued: November 1997

Shown in Product Identification Guide, page 332

STERILE
FUDR ℞
[ef-u-dee-are]
brand of floxuridine

The following text is complete prescribing information based on official labeling in effect June 2000.

> **WARNING**
> It is recommended that FUDR be given only by or under the supervision of a qualified physician who is experienced in cancer chemotherapy and intra-arterial drug therapy and is well versed in the use of potent antimetabolites.
> Because of the possibility of severe toxic reactions, all patients should be hospitalized for initiation of the first course of therapy.

DESCRIPTION

Sterile FUDR (floxuridine), an antineoplastic antimetabolite, is available as a sterile, nonpyrogenic, lyophilized powder for reconstitution. Each vial contains 500 mg of floxuridine which is to be reconstituted with 5 mL of sterile water for injection. An appropriate amount of reconstituted solution is then diluted with a parenteral solution for intra-arterial infusion (see DOSAGE AND ADMINISTRATION).
Floxuridine is a fluorinated pyrimidine. Chemically, floxuridine is 2′-deoxy-5-fluorouridine with an empirical formula of $C_9H_{11}FN_2O_5$. It is a white to off-white odorless solid which is freely soluble in water.
The 2% aqueous solution has a pH of between 4.0 to 5.5. The molecular weight of floxuridine is 246.19.

CLINICAL PHARMACOLOGY

When FUDR is given by rapid intra-arterial injection it is apparently rapidly catabolized to 5-fluorouracil. Thus, rapid injection of FUDR produces the same toxic and antimetabolic effects as does 5-fluorouracil. The primary effect is to interfere with the synthesis of deoxyribonucleic acid (DNA) and to a lesser extent inhibit the formation of ribonucleic acid (RNA). However, when FUDR is given by continuous intra-arterial infusion its direct anabolism to FUDR-monophosphate is enhanced, thus increasing the inhibition of DNA.
Floxuridine is metabolized in the liver. The drug is excreted intact and as urea, fluorouracil, α-fluoro-β-ureidopropionic acid, dihydrofluorouracil, α-fluoro-β-guanidopropionic acid and α-fluoro-β-alanine in the urine; it is also expired as respiratory carbon dioxide. Pharmacokinetic data on intra-arterial infusion of FUDR are not available.

INDICATIONS AND USAGE

FUDR is effective in the palliative management of gastrointestinal adenocarcinoma metastatic to the liver, when given by continuous regional intra-arterial infusion in carefully selected patients who are considered incurable by surgery or other means. Patients with known disease extending beyond an area capable of infusion via a single artery should, except in unusual circumstances, be considered for systemic therapy with other chemotherapeutic agents.

CONTRAINDICATIONS

FUDR therapy is contraindicated for patients in a poor nutritional state, those with depressed bone marrow function or those with potentially serious infections.

WARNINGS

BECAUSE OF THE POSSIBILITY OF SEVERE TOXIC REACTIONS, ALL PATIENTS SHOULD BE HOSPITALIZED FOR THE FIRST COURSE OF THERAPY.
FUDR should be used with extreme caution in poor risk patients with impaired hepatic or renal function or a history of high-dose pelvic irradiation or previous use of alkylating agents. The drug is not intended as an adjuvant to surgery.
FUDR may cause fetal harm when administered to a pregnant woman. It has been shown to be teratogenic in the chick embryo, mouse (at doses of 2.5 to 100 mg/kg) and rat (at doses of 75 to 150 mg/kg). Malformations included cleft palates; skeletal defects; and deformed appendages, paws and tails. The dosages which were teratogenic in animals are 4.2 to 125 times the recommended human therapeutic dose.
There are no adequate and well-controlled studies with FUDR in pregnant women. If this drug is used during pregnancy or if the patient becomes pregnant while taking (receiving) this drug, the patient should be apprised of the potential hazard to the fetus. Women of childbearing potential should be advised to avoid becoming pregnant.
Combination Therapy: Any form of therapy which adds to the stress of the patient, interferes with nutrition or depresses bone marrow function will increase the toxicity of FUDR.

PRECAUTIONS

General: Sterile FUDR is a highly toxic drug with a narrow margin of safety. Therefore, patients should be carefully supervised since therapeutic response is unlikely to occur without some evidence of toxicity. Severe hematological toxicity, gastrointestinal hemorrhage and even death may result from the use of FUDR despite meticulous selection of patients and careful adjustment of dosage. Although severe toxicity is more likely in poor risk patients, fatalities may be encountered occasionally even in patients in relatively good condition.
Therapy is to be discontinued promptly whenever one of the following signs of toxicity appears:
Myocardial ischemia
Stomatitis or esophagopharyngitis, at the first visible sign
Leukopenia (WBC under 3500) or a rapidly falling white blood count
Vomiting, intractable
Diarrhea, frequent bowel movements or watery stools
Gastrointestinal ulceration and bleeding
Thrombocytopenia (platelets under 100,000)
Hemorrhage from any site
Information For Patients: Patients should be informed of expected toxic effects, particularly oral manifestations. Patients should be alerted to the possibility of alopecia as a result of therapy and should be informed that it is usually a transient effect.
Laboratory Tests: Careful monitoring of the white blood count and platelet count is recommended.
Drug Interactions: See WARNINGS section.

Continued on next page

FUDR—Cont.

Carcinogenesis, Mutagenesis, Impairment Of Fertility:
Carcinogenesis: Long-term studies in animals to evaluate the carcinogenic potential of floxuridine have not been conducted. On the basis of the available data, no evaluation can be made of the carcinogenic risk of FUDR to humans.
Mutagenesis: Oncogenic transformation of fibroblasts from mouse embryo has been induced in vitro by FUDR, but the relationship between oncogenicity and mutagenicity is not clear. Floxuridine has also been shown to be mutagenic in human leukocytes in vitro and in the *Drosophila* test system. In addition, 5-fluorouracil, to which floxuridine is catabolized when given by intra-arterial injection, has been shown to be mutagenic in in vitro tests.
Impairment Of Fertility: The effects of floxuridine on fertility and general reproductive performance have not been studied in animals. However, because floxuridine is catabolized to 5-fluorouracil, it should be noted that 5-fluorouracil has been shown to induce chromosomal aberrations and changes in chromosome organization of spermatogonia in rats at doses of 125 or 250 mg/kg, administered intraperitoneally.
Spermatogonial differentiation was also inhibited by fluorouracil, resulting in transient infertility. In female rats, fluorouracil, administered intraperitoneally at doses of 25 or 50 mg/kg during the preovulatory phase of oogenesis, significantly reduced the incidence of fertile matings, delayed the development of pre- and post-implantation embryos, increased the incidence of preimplantation lethality and induced chromosomal anomalies in these embryos. Compounds such as FUDR, which interfere with DNA, RNA and protein synthesis, might be expected to have adverse effects on gametogenesis.
Pregnancy: *Teratogenic Effects:* Pregnancy Category D (see WARNINGS). Floxuridine has been shown to be teratogenic in the chick embryo, mouse (at doses of 2.5 to 100 mg/kg) and rat (at doses of 75 to 150 mg/kg). Malformations included cleft palates, skeletal defects and deformed appendages, paws and tails. The dosages which were teratogenic in animals are 4.2 to 125 times the recommended human therapeutic dose.
There are no adequate and well-controlled studies with FUDR in pregnant women. While there is no evidence of teratogenicity in humans due to FUDR, it should be kept in mind that other drugs which inhibit DNA synthesis (eg, methotrexate and aminopterin) have been reported to be teratogenic in humans. FUDR should be used during pregnancy only if the potential benefit justifies the potential risk to the fetus.
Nonteratogenic Effects: Floxuridine has not been studied in animals for its effects on peri- and postnatal development. However, compounds which inhibit DNA, RNA and protein synthesis might be expected to have adverse effects on peri- and postnatal development.
Nursing Mothers: It is not known whether FUDR is excreted in human milk. Because FUDR inhibits DNA and RNA synthesis, mothers should not nurse while receiving this drug.
Pediatric Use: Safety and effectiveness in pediatric patients have not been established.

ADVERSE REACTIONS

Adverse reactions to the arterial infusion of FUDR are generally related to the procedural complications of regional arterial infusion.
The more common adverse reactions to the drug are nausea, vomiting, diarrhea, enteritis, stomatitis and localized erythema. The more common laboratory abnormalities are anemia, leukopenia, thrombocytopenia and elevations of alkaline phosphatase, serum transaminase, serum bilirubin and lactic dehydrogenase.
Other adverse reactions are:
Gastrointestinal: duodenal ulcer, duodenitis, gastritis, bleeding, gastroenteritis, glossitis, pharyngitis, anorexia, cramps, abdominal pain; possible intra- and extrahepatic biliary sclerosis, as well as acalculous cholecystitis.
Dermatologic: alopecia, dermatitis, nonspecific skin toxicity, rash.
Cardiovascular: myocardial ischemia.
Miscellaneous Clinical Reactions: fever, lethargy, malaise, weakness.
Laboratory Abnormalities: BSP, prothrombin, total proteins, sedimentation rate and thrombopenia.
Procedural Complications of Regional Arterial Infusion: arterial aneurysm; arterial ischemia; arterial thrombosis; embolism; fibromyositis; thrombophlebitis; hepatic necrosis; abscesses; infection at catheter site; bleeding at catheter site; catheter blocked, displaced or leaking.
The following adverse reactions have not been reported with FUDR but have been noted following the administration of 5-fluorouracil. While the possibility of these occurring following FUDR therapy is remote because of its regional administration, one should be alert for these reactions following the administration of FUDR because of the pharmacological similarity of these two drugs: pancytopenia, agranulocytosis, myocardial ischemia, angina, anaphylaxis, generalized allergic reactions, acute cerebellar syndrome, nystagmus, headache, dry skin, fissuring, photosensitivity, pruritic maculopapular rash, increased pigmentation of the skin, vein pigmentation, lacrimal duct stenosis, visual changes, lacrimation, photophobia, disorientation, confusion, euphoria, epistaxis and nail changes, including loss of nails.

OVERDOSAGE

The possibility of overdosage with FUDR is unlikely in view of the mode of administration. Nevertheless, the anticipated manifestations would be nausea, vomiting, diarrhea, gastrointestinal ulceration and bleeding, bone marrow depression (including thrombocytopenia, leukopenia and agranulocytosis). No specific antidotal therapy exists. Patients who have been exposed to an overdosage of FUDR should be monitored hematologically for at least 4 weeks. Should abnormalities appear, appropriate therapy should be utilized.
The acute intravenous toxicity of floxuridine is as follows:

Species	LD_{50} (mg/kg ± S.E.)
Mouse	880 ± 51
Rat	670 ± 73
Rabbit	94 ± 19 .6
Dog	157 ± 46

DOSAGE AND ADMINISTRATION

Each vial must be reconstituted with 5 mL of sterile water for injection to yield a solution containing approximately 100 mg of floxuridine/mL. The calculated daily dose(s) of the drug is then diluted with 5% dextrose or 0.9% sodium chloride injection to a volume appropriate for the infusion apparatus to be used. The administration of FUDR is best achieved with the use of an appropriate pump to overcome pressure in large arteries and to ensure a uniform rate of infusion.
Parenteral drug products should be inspected visually for particulate matter and discoloration prior to administration whenever solution and container permit.
The recommended therapeutic dosage schedule of FUDR by continuous arterial infusion is 0.1 to 0.6 mg/kg/day. The higher dosage ranges (0.4 mg to 0.6 mg) are usually employed for hepatic artery infusion because the liver metabolizes the drug, thus reducing the potential for systemic toxicity. Therapy can be given until adverse reactions appear. (See PRECAUTIONS section.) When these side effects have subsided, therapy may be resumed. The patient should be maintained on therapy as long as response to FUDR continues.
Procedures for proper handling and disposal of anticancer drugs should be considered. Several guidelines on this subject have been published.[1–6] There is no general agreement that all of the procedures recommended in the guidelines are necessary or appropriate.

HOW SUPPLIED

500 mg Sterile FUDR (floxuridine) powder in a 5-mL vial (NDC 0004-1935-08). This is to be reconstituted with 5 mL sterile water for injection.
The sterile powder should be stored at 59° to 86°F (15° to 30°C). Reconstituted vials should be stored under refrigeration (36° to 46°F, 2° to 8°C) for not more than 2 weeks.

REFERENCES

1. Recommendations for the safe handling of parenteral antineoplastic drugs. Washington, DC, US Government Printing Office NIH publication 83-2621.
2. AMA Council Report. Guidelines for handling parenteral antineoplastics. *JAMA.* Mar 15, 1985, 253:1590–1592.
3. National Study Commission on Cytotoxic Exposure: Recommendations for handling cytotoxic agents. Available from Louis P. Jeffrey, ScD, Director of Pharmacy Services, Rhode Island Hospital, 593 Eddy Street, Providence, Rhode Island 02902.
4. Clinical Oncological Society of Australia: Guidelines and recommendations for safe handling of antineoplastic agents. *Med J Aust.* Apr 30, 1983, 1:426–428.
5. Jones RB, Frank R, Mass T: Safe handling of chemotherapeutic agents: a report from the Mount Sinai Medical Center. *CA* Sept–Oct, 1983, 33:258–263.
6. ASHP technical assistance bulletin on handling cytotoxic drugs in hospitals. *Am J Hosp Pharm.* Jan, 1985, 42:131–137.

Revised: September 1997

HIVID® ℞
[hiv' 'id]
(zalcitabine)
TABLETS

The following text is complete prescribing information based on official labeling in effect June 2000.

WARNING:
THE USE OF HIVID HAS BEEN ASSOCIATED WITH SIGNIFICANT CLINICAL ADVERSE REACTIONS, SOME OF WHICH ARE POTENTIALLY FATAL. HIVID CAN CAUSE SEVERE PERIPHERAL NEUROPATHY AND BECAUSE OF THIS SHOULD BE USED WITH EXTREME CAUTION IN PATIENTS WITH PREEXISTING NEUROPATHY. HIVID MAY ALSO RARELY CAUSE PANCREATITIS AND PATIENTS WHO DEVELOP ANY SYMPTOMS SUGGESTIVE OF PANCREATITIS WHILE USING HIVID SHOULD HAVE THERAPY SUSPENDED IMMEDIATELY UNTIL THIS DIAGNOSIS IS EXCLUDED.
LACTIC ACIDOSIS AND SEVERE HEPATOMEGALY WITH STEATOSIS, INCLUDING FATAL CASES, HAVE BEEN REPORTED WITH THE USE OF ANTIRETROVIRAL NUCLEOSIDE ANALOGUES ALONE OR IN COMBINATION, INCLUDING HIVID (SEE WARNINGS).
IN ADDITION, RARE CASES OF HEPATIC FAILURE AND DEATH CONSIDERED POSSIBLY RELATED TO UNDERLYING HEPATITIS B AND HIVID HAVE BEEN REPORTED (SEE WARNINGS AND PRECAUTIONS).

DESCRIPTION

HIVID is the Hoffman-La Roche brand of zalcitabine [formerly called 2',3'-dideoxycytidine (ddC)], a synthetic pyrimidine nucleoside analogue active against the human immunodeficiency virus (HIV). HIVID is available as film-coated tablets for oral administration in strengths of 0.375 mg and 0.750 mg. Each tablet also contains the inactive ingredients lactose, microcrystalline cellulose, croscarmellose sodium, magnesium stearate, hydroxypropyl methylcellulose, polyethylene glycol, and polysorbate 80 along with the following colorant system: 0.375 mg tablet—synthetic brown, black, red and yellow iron oxides, and titanium dioxide; 0.750 mg tablet—synthetic black iron oxide and titanium dioxide. The chemical name for zalcitabine is 4-amino-1-beta-D-2', 3'-dideoxyribofuranosyl-2-(1H)-pyrimidone for 2',3'-dideoxycytidine with the molecular formula $C_9H_{13}N_3O_3$ and a molecular weight of 211.22. Zalcitabine has the following structural formula:

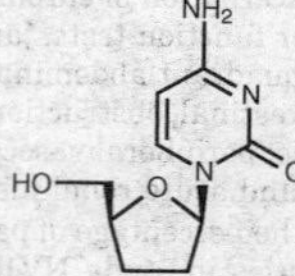

Zalcitabine is a white to off-white crystalline powder with an aqueous solubility of 76.4 mg/mL at 25°C.

MICROBIOLOGY

Mechanism of Action: Zalcitabine is a synthetic nucleoside analogue of the naturally occurring nucleoside deoxycytidine, in which the 3'-hydroxyl group is replaced by hydrogen. Within cells, zalcitabine is converted to the active metabolites, dideoxycytidine 5'-triphosphate (ddCTP), by the sequential action of cellular enzymes. Dideoxycytidine 5'-triphosphate inhibits the activity of the HIV-reverse transcriptase both by competing for utilization of the natural substrate, deoxycytidine 5'-triphosphate (dCTP), and by its incorporation into viral DNA. The lack of a 3'-OH group in the incorporated nucleoside analogue prevents the formation of the 5' to 3' phosphodiester linkage essential for DNA chain elongation and, therefore, the viral DNA growth is terminated. The active metabolite, ddCTP, is also an inhibitor of cellular DNA polymerase-beta and mitochondrial DNA polymerase-gamma and has been reported to be incorporated into the DNA of cells in culture.
In Vitro HIV Susceptibility: The in vitro anti-HIV activity of zalcitabine was assessed by infecting cell lines of lymphoblastic and monocytic origin and peripheral blood lymphocytes with laboratory and clinical isolates of HIV. The IC_{50} and IC_{95} values (50% and 95% inhibitory concentration) were in the range of 30 to 500 nM and 100 to 1000 nM, respectively (1 nM = 0.21 ng/mL). Zalcitabine showed antiviral activity in all acute infections; however, activity was substantially less in chronically infected cells. In drug combination studies with zidovudine (ZDV) or saquinavir, zalcitabine showed additive to synergistic activity in cell culture. The relationship between the in vitro susceptibility of HIV to reverse-transcriptase inhibitors and the inhibition of HIV replication in humans has not been established.
Drug Resistance: HIV isolates with a reduction in sensitivity to zalcitabine (ddC) have been isolated from a small number of patients treated with HIVID by 1 year of therapy. Genetic analysis of these isolates showed point mutations (Lys 65 Arg or Asn, Thr 69 Asp, Leu 74 Val, Val 75 Thr or Ala, Met 184 Val or Tyr 215 Cys) in the pol gene that encodes for the reverse transcriptase. Combination therapy with HIVID and ZDV does not appear to prevent the emergency of zidovudine-resistant isolates.
Cross-resistance: The potential for cross-resistance between HIV-reverse transcriptase inhibitors and HIV-protease inhibitors is low because of the different enzyme targets involved. The point mutation at position 69 appears to be specific to ddC in its selection and effect. Additionally, the point mutations at positions 65, 74, 75, and 184 are associated with resistance to didanosine (ddl), that at position 75 with resistance to stavudine (d4T), and those at positions 65 (Lys to Arg), and 184 (Met to Val) with resistance to lamivudine (3TC). HIV isolates with multidrug resistance to ZDV, ddl, ddC, d4T, and 3TC were recovered from a small number of patients treated for 1 year with the combination of ZDV, ddl or ddC. The pattern of resistance mutations in the combination therapy was different (Ala 62 Val, Val 75 lle, Phe 77 Leu, Phe 116 Tyr and Gin 151 Met) from monotherapy with mutation 151 being most significant for multidrug resistance.

CLINICAL PHARMACOLOGY

Pharmacokinetics: The pharmacokinetics of zalcitabine has been evaluated in studies in HIV-infected patients following 0.01 mg/kg, 0.03 mg/kg, and 1.5 mg oral doses, and a 1.5 mg intravenous dose administered as a 1-hour infusion.
Absorption and Bioavailability in Adults: Following oral administration to HIV-infected patients, the mean absolute

bioavailability of zalcitabine was >80% (30% CV, range 23% to 124%, n = 19). The absorption rate of a 1.5 mg oral dose of zalcitabine (n=20) was reduced when administered with food. This resulted in a 39% decrease in mean maximum plasma concentrations (C_{max}) from 25.2 ng/mL (35% CV, range 11.6 to 37.5 ng/mL) to 15.5 ng/mL (24% CV, range 9.1 to 23.7 ng/mL), and a twofold increase in time to achieve maximum plasma concentrations from a mean of 0.8 hours under fasting conditions to 1.6 hours when the drug was given with food. The extent of absorption (as reflected by AUC) was decreased by 14%, from 72 ng•hr/mL (28% CV, range 43 to 119 ng•hr/mL) to 62 ng•hr/mL (23% CV, range 42 to 91 ng•hr/mL). The clinical relevance of these decreases is unknown. Absorption of zalcitabine does not appear to be reduced in patients with diarrhea not caused by an identified pathogen.

Distribution in Adults: The steady-state volume of distribution following intravenous administration of a 1.5 mg dose of zalcitabine averaged 0.534 (± 0.127) L/kg (24% CV, range 0.304 to 0.734 L/kg, n=20). Cerebrospinal fluid obtained from 9 patients at 2 to 3.5 hours following 0.06 mg/kg or 0.09 mg/kg intravenous infusion showed measurable concentrations of zalcitabine. The CSF plasma concentration ratio ranged from 9% to 37% (mean 20%), demonstrating penetration of the drug through the blood-brain barrier. The clinical relevance of these ratios has not been evaluated.

Metabolism and Elimination in Adults: Zalcitabine is phosphorylated intracellularly to zalcitabine triphosphate, the active substrate for HIV-reverse transcriptase. Concentrations of zalcitabine triphosphate are too low for quantitation following administration of therapeutic doses to humans.

Zalcitabine does not undergo a significant degree of metabolism by the liver. The primary metabolite of zalcitabine that has been identified is dideoxyuridine (ddU), which accounts for less than 15% of an oral dose in both urine and feces (n=4). Approximately 10% of an orally administered radiolabeled dose of zalcitabine appears in the feces (n=10), comprised primarily of unchanged drug and ddU. Renal excretion of unchanged drug appears to be the primary route of elimination, accounting for approximately 80% of an intravenous dose and 60% of an orally administered dose within 24 hours after dosing (n=19). The mean elimination half-life is 2 hours and generally ranges from 1 to 3 hours in individual patients. Total clearance following an intravenous dose averaged 285 mL/min (29% CV, range 165 to 447 mL/min, n=20). Renal clearance averaged approximately 235 mL/min or about 80% of total clearance (30% CV, range 129 to 348 mL/min, n=20). Renal clearance exceeds glomerular filtration rate suggesting renal tubular secretion contributes to the elimination of zalcitabine by the kidneys.

In patients with impaired kidney function, prolonged elimination of zalcitabine may be expected. Preliminary results from 7 patients with renal impairment (estimated creatinine clearance <55 mL/min) indicate that the half-life was prolonged (up to 8.5 hours) in these patients compared to those with normal renal function. Maximum plasma concentrations were higher in some patients after a single dose (see PRECAUTIONS).

In patients with normal renal function, the pharmacokinetics of zalcitabine was not altered during 3 times daily multiple dosing (n=9). Accumulation of drug in plasma during this regimen was negligible. The drug was <4% bound to plasma proteins, indicating that drug interactions involving binding-site displacement are unlikely (see *Drug Interactions*).

Drug Interactions: *Zidovudine:* There was no significant pharmacokinetic interaction between zidovudine and zalcitabine when single doses of zalcitabine (1.5 mg) and zidovudine (200 mg) were coadministered to 12 HIV-positive patients.

Probenecid: Following administration of a single oral 1.5 mg dose of zalcitabine alone during probenecid treatment (500 mg at 8 and 2 hours before and 4 hours after zalcitabine dosing) to 12 HIV-positive patients, mean renal clearance decreased from 310 mL/min (28% CV) to 180 mL/min (22% CV) and AUC increased from 59 ng•hr/mL (27% CV) to 91 ng•hr/mL (22% CV), indicating an increase in exposure of approximately 50% to zalcitabine. Mean half-life of zalcitabine increased from 1.7 to 2.5 hours (see PRECAUTIONS).

Cimetidine: Administration of a single dose of 1.5 mg zalcitabine with a single dose of 800 mg cimetidine to 12 HIV-positive patients resulted in a decrease in renal clearance from 224 mL/min (27% CV) to 171 mL/min (39% CV) and an increase in AUC from 75 ng•hr/mL (29% CV) to 102 ng•hr/mL (35% CV) (see PRECAUTIONS) indicating an increase in exposure of approximately 36% to zalcitabine.

Maalox: Concomitant administration of Maalox®* TC (30 mL) with single dose of 1.5 mg zalcitabine to 12 HIV-positive patients resulted in a decrease in mean C_{max} from 25.2 ng/mL (28% CV) to 18.4 ng/mL (34% CV) and AUC from 75 ng•hr/mL (29% CV, n=10) to 58 ng•hr/mL (36% CV, n=10) indicating a decrease in bioavailability of approximately 25% to zalcitabine (see PRECAUTIONS).

Metoclopramide: Administration of a single dose of 1.5 mg zalcitabine with 20 mg metoclopramide (10 mg 1 hour before and 10 mg 4 hours after zalcitabine dose) to 12 HIV-positive patients resulted in a decrease in AUC from 69 ng•hr/mL (16% CV) to 62 ng•hr/mL (21% CV) indicating a decrease in bioavailability of approximately 10% (see PRECAUTIONS).

Loperamide: Administration of a single dose of 1.5 mg zalcitabine during loperamide treatment (4 mg 16 hours before zalcitabine, 2 mg at 10 hours and 4 hours before zalcitabine, and 2 mg 2 hours after the zalcitabine dose) to 12 HIV-positive patients with diarrhea resulted in no significant pharmacokinetic interaction between zalcitabine and loperamide.

Pharmacokinetics in Pediatric Patients: For pharmacokinetic properties in pediatric patients, see PRECAUTIONS: *Pediatric Use.* Limited pharmacokinetic data have been reported for 5 HIV-positive pediatric patients using doses of 0.03 and 0.04 mg/kg HIVID administered orally every 6 hours.[1] The mean bioavailability of zalcitabine in these pediatric patients was 54% and mean apparent systemic clearance was 150 mL/min/m^2. Due to the small number of subjects and different analytical techniques, it is difficult to make comparisons between pediatric and adult data.

Table 1. First AIDS-defining Event or Death and Death Only by Study Arm and Antiretroviral Experience in ACTG 175

Antiretroviral Experience	Event	Treatment			
		zidovudine	zidovudine + didanosine	zidovudine + HIVID	didanosine
Overall	n	619	613	615	620
	AIDS/Death	96 (16%)	65 (11%)	76 (12%)	71 (11%)
	Death Only	54 (9%)	31 (5%)	40 (7%)	29 (5%)
Naive	n	269	263	267	268
	AIDS/Death	32 (12%)	20 (8%)	16 (6%)	23 (9%)
	Death Only	18 (7%)	11 (4%)	9 (3%)	11 (4%)
Experienced	n	350	350	348	352
	AIDS/Death	64 (18%)	45 (13%)	60 (17%)	48 (14%)
	Death Only	36 (10%)	20 (6%)	31 (9%)	18 (5%)

INDICATIONS AND USAGE

HIVID is indicated in combination with antiretroviral agents for the treatment of HIV infection. This indication is based on study results showing a reduction in the rate of disease progression (AIDS-defining events or death) in patients with limited prior antiretroviral therapy who were treated with the combination of HIVID and zidovudine (see *Description of Clinical Studies*). This indication is also based on a study showing a reduction in both mortality and AIDS-defining clinical events for patients who received INVIRASE®† (saquinavir mesylate) in combination with HIVID compared to patients who received either HIVID or INVIRASE alone.

Description of Clinical Studies: The use of HIVID in combination with zidovudine is based on the clinical results from study ACTG 175. ACTG 175 was a randomized, double-blind, controlled trial that compared zidovudine 200 mg three times daily; didanosine 200 mg twice daily; zidovudine+didanosine; and zidovudine+HIVID 0.750 mg three times daily. A total of 2467 HIV-infected adults (mean baseline CD_4 count = 352 cells/mm^3) with no prior AIDS-defining event enrolled with the following demographics: male (82%), Caucasian (70%), mean age of 35 years, asymptomatic HIV infection (81%) and prior antiretroviral use (57%, mean duration = 89.5 weeks). The overall mean duration of study treatment was 99 weeks. The incidence of AIDS-defining events or death is shown in the table below. Although no antiretroviral agent should be used as monotherapy, a description of CPCRA 002 is included here as it provides a comparison of the safety and efficacy of HIVID compared to ddI.

CPCRA 002 was a randomized, multicenter, open-label study in which HIVID was compared to ddI as treatment for patients with advanced HIV infection (median CD_4 cell count = 37 cells/mm^3) who were clinically intolerant to ZDV, or who had met criteria for having disease progression while receiving ZDV.[2] Patients in this study had a mean of 17.5 months of prior ZDV use. The median duration of treatment for both HIVID and ddI was 34 weeks. The results demonstrate that HIVID was at least as efficacious as ddI in terms of time to an AIDS-defining event or death, while for survival alone the results favored HIVID. However, most of the patients (66%) in either group had disease progression over the median 16 months of follow-up. Overall rates of study drug intolerance, discontinuation and adverse events were similar for the two groups, although the types of events were different.

A clinical study (N3300/ACTG 114) has demonstrated ZDV to be superior to HIVID as monotherapy for advanced HIV disease (CD_4 cell count ≤200 cells/mm^3) in previously untreated patients.[3,4] The final analysis of this study indicated that 134 patients (42%) in the HIVID group with a median follow-up of 85 weeks and 120 patients (38%) in the ZDV group with a median follow-up of 96 weeks died with a relative risk for mortality of ZDV to HIVID of 0.54.

CONTRAINDICATIONS

HIVID is contraindicated in patients with clinically significant hypersensitivity to zalcitabine or to any of the excipients contained in the tablets.

WARNINGS

SIGNIFICANT CLINICAL ADVERSE REACTIONS, SOME OF WHICH ARE POTENTIALLY FATAL, HAVE BEEN REPORTED WITH HIVID. PATIENTS WITH DECREASED CD_4 CELL COUNTS APPEAR TO HAVE AN INCREASED INCIDENCE OF ADVERSE EVENTS.

1. Peripheral Neuropathy:

THE MAJOR CLINICAL TOXICITY OF HIVID IS PERIPHERAL NEUROPATHY, WHICH MAY OCCUR IN UP TO 1/3 OF PATIENTS WITH ADVANCED DISEASE TREATED WITH HIVID. The incidence in patients with less-advanced disease is lower.

HIVID-related peripheral neuropathy is a sensorimotor neuropathy characterized initially by numbness and burning dysesthesia involving the distal extremities. These symptoms may be followed by sharp shooting pains or severe continuous burning pain if the drug is not withdrawn. The neuropathy may progress to severe pain requiring narcotic analgesics and is potentially irreversible. In some patients, symptoms of neuropathy may initially progress despite discontinuation of HIVID. With prompt discontinuation of HIVID, the neuropathy is usually slowly reversible. There are no data regarding the use of HIVID in patients with preexisting peripheral neuropathy since these patients were excluded from clinical trials; therefore, HIVID should be used with extreme caution in these patients. Individuals with moderate or severe peripheral neuropathy, as evidenced by symptoms accompanied by objective findings, are advised to avoid HIVID.

HIVID should be used with caution in patients with a risk of developing peripheral neuropathy: patients with low CD_4 cell counts (CD_4 <50 cells/mm3), diabetes, weight loss and/or patients receiving HIVID concomitantly with drugs that have the potential to cause peripheral neuropathy (see PRECAUTIONS: *Drug Interactions*). Careful monitoring is strongly recommended for these individuals.

[See table above]

HIVID should be stopped promptly if signs or symptoms of peripheral neuropathy occurs, such as when moderate discomfort from numbness, tingling, burning or pain of the extremities progresses, or any related symptoms occur that are accompanied by an objective finding (see DOSAGE AND ADMINISTRATION).

2. Pancreatitis:

PANCREATITIS, WHICH HAS BEEN FATAL IN SOME CASES, HAS BEEN OBSERVED WITH THE ADMINISTRATION OF HIVID. Pancreatitis is an uncommon complication of HIVID occurring in up to 1.1% of patients.

Patients with a history of pancreatitis or known risk factors for the development of pancreatitis should be followed more closely while on HIVID therapy. Of 528 HIVID-treated patients enrolled in an expanded-access safety study (N3544), who had a history of prior pancreatitis or increased amylase, 28 (5.3%) developed pancreatitis and an additional 23 (4.4%) developed asymptomatic elevated serum amylase.

Treatment with HIVID should be stopped immediately if clinical signs or symptoms (nausea, vomiting, abdominal pain) or if abnormalities in laboratory values (hyperamylasemia associated with dysglycemia, rising triglyceride level, decreasing serum calcium) suggestive of pancreatitis should occur. If clinical pancreatitis develops during HIVID administration, it is recommended that HIVID be permanently discontinued. Treatment with HIVID should also be interrupted if treatment with another drug known to cause pancreatitis (eg, intravenous pentamidine) is required (see *Drug Interactions*).

3. Lactic Acidosis/Severe Hepatomegaly With Steatosis and Hepatic Toxicity:

Lactic acidosis and severe hepatomegaly with steatosis, including fatal cases, have been reported with the use of nucleoside analogues alone or in combination, including HIVID and other antiretrovirals.[5,6] A majority of these cases have been in women. Obesity and prolonged nucleoside exposure may be risk factors. Particular caution should be exercised when administering HIVID to any patient with known risk factors for liver disease; however, cases have also been reported in patients with no known risk factors. Treatment with HIVID should be suspended in any patient who develops clinical or laboratory findings suggestive of lactic acidosis or pronounced hepatotoxicity (which may include hepatomegaly and steatosis even in the absence of marked transaminase elevations).

IN ADDITION, RARE CASES OF HEPATIC FAILURE AND DEATH CONSIDERED POSSIBLY RELATED TO UNDERLYING HEPATITIS B AND HIVID HAVE BEEN REPORTED. Treatment with HIVID in patients with preexisting liver disease, liver enzyme abnormalities, a history of ethanol abuse or hepatitis should be approached with caution. Treatment with HIVID should be suspended in any patient who develops clinical or laboratory findings suggestive of pronounced hepatotoxicity. In clinical trials, drug interruption was recommended if liver function tests exceeded >5 times the upper limit of normal.

4. Other Serious Toxicities:

a) *Oral Ulcers:* Severe oral ulcers occurred in up to 3% of patients receiving HIVID in CPCRA 002 and ACTG 175;

Continued on next page

Hivid—Cont.

less severe oral ulcerations have occurred at higher frequencies in other clinical trials.

b) *Esophageal Ulcers:* Infrequent cases of esophageal ulcers have also been attributed to HIVID therapy. Interruption of HIVID should be considered in patients who develop esophageal ulcers that do not respond to specific treatment for opportunistic pathogens in order to assess a possible relationship to HIVID.

c) *Cardiomyopathy/Congestive Heart Failure:* Cardiomyopathy and congestive heart failure in patients with AIDS have been associated with the use of nucleoside analogues. Infrequent cases have been reported in patients receiving HIVID. Treatment with HIVID in patients with baseline cardiomyopathy or history of congestive heart failure should be approached with caution.

d) *Anaphylactoid Reaction:* An anaphylactoid reaction was reported in a patient receiving both HIVID and zidovudine. In addition, there have been several reports of hypersensitivity reactions (including anaphylactic reaction or urticaria without other signs of anaphylaxis).

PRECAUTIONS

General:

1. *Renal Impairment:* Patients with renal impairment (estimated creatinine clearance <55 mL/min) may be at a greater risk of toxicity from HIVID due to decreased drug clearance. Dosage adjustment is recommended in these patients (see DOSAGE AND ADMINISTRATION).
2. *Lymphoma:* High doses of zalcitabine, administered for 3 months to $B_6C_3F_1$ mice (resulting in plasma concentrations over 1000 times those seen in patients taking the recommended doses of HIVID) induced an increased incidence of thymic lymphoma.[7] Although the pathogenesis of the effect is uncertain, a predisposition to chemically induced thymic lymphoma and high rates of spontaneous lymphoreticular neoplasms have previously been noted in this strain of mice.[8]

The incidence of lymphomas was reviewed in 13 comparative studies conducted by Roche, the NIAID and the NCI, as well as 7 Roche expanded-access studies that included HIVID. In one study, ACTG 155, a statistically significant increased rate of lymphomas was seen in patients receiving HIVID or combination HIVID and zidovudine compared to zidovudine alone (rates of 0, 1.3, and 2.3 per 100 person years for zidovudine, HIVID, and combination HIVID and zidovudine, respectively; log rank p-value=0.001, pooling HIVID, and combination HIVID and zidovudine vs zidovudine, p-value=0.003). Based on review of the literature, the incidence of lymphomas in HIV-infected patients with advanced disese on zidovudine monotherapy would be expected to be approximately 1 to 2 per 100 person years of follow-up.

None of the other comparative studies evaluated showed a statistically significant difference in rates of lymphomas in patients receiving HIVID. In a large, controlled clinical trial (ACTG 175) HIVID in combination with zidovudine was not associated with an increase in the incidence of lymphoma over that seen with zidovudine monotherapy (6 of 615 and 9 of 619, respectively).

Lymphoma has been identified as a consequence of HIV infection. This most likely represents a consequence of prolonged immunosuppression; however, an association between the occurrrence of lymphoma and antiviral therapy cannot be excluded.

Patients receiving HIVID or any other antiretroviral therapy may continue to develop opportunistic infections and other complications of HIV infections, and therefore should remain under close clinical observation by physicians experienced in the treatment of patients with associated HIV diseases.

The duration of clinical benefit from antiretroviral therapy may be limited. Alterations in antiretroviral therapy should be considered in cases of disease progression, either clinical or as demonstrated by viral rebound (increase in HIV RNA after initial decline).

Information for Patients: Patients should be informed that HIVID is not a cure for HIV infection and that they may continue to acquire illnesses associated with advanced HIV infection, including opportunistic infections.

Patients should be told that there is currently no data demonstrating that HIVID therapy can reduce the risk of transmitting HIV to others through sexual contact or blood contamination.

Patients should be advised to take HIVID every day as prescribed. Patients should not alter the dose or discontinue therapy without consulting with their physician. If a dose is missed, patients should take the dose as soon as possible and then return to their normal schedule. However, if a dose is skipped, the patient should not double the next dose.

Patients should be instructed that the major toxicity of HIVID is peripheral neuropathy. Pancreatitis and hepatic toxicity are other serious potentially life-threatening toxicities that have been reported in patients treated with HIVID. Patients should be advised of the early symptoms of these conditions and instructed to promptly report them to their physician. Since the development of peripheral neuropathy appears to be dose-related to HIVID, patients should be advised to follow their physicians' instructions regarding the prescribed dose.

Laboratory Tests: Complete blood counts and clinical chemistry tests should be performed prior to initiating HIVID therapy and at appropriate intervals thereafter. Baseline testing of serum amylase and triglyceride levels should be performed in individuals with a prior history of pancreatitis, increased amylase, those on parenteral nutrition or with a history of ethanol abuse.

Drug Interactions: *Zidovudine:* There is no significant pharmacokinetic interaction between ZDV and zalcitabine which has been confirmed clinically. Zalcitabine also has no significant effect on the intracellular phosphorylation of ZDV, as shown in vitro in peripheral blood mononuclear cells or in the lymphoblastoid cell line h1A2v2. No information is available on pharmacokinetic interactions of zalcitabine with didanosine, lamivudine, and stravudine.

Saquinavir: The combination of HIVID, saquinavir, and ZDV has been studied (as triple combination) in adults. Pharmacokinetic data suggest that absorption, metabolism, and elimination of each of these drugs are unchanged when they are used together.

Drugs Associated With Peripheral Neuropathy: The concomitant use of HIVID with drugs that have the potential to cause peripheral neuropathy should be avoided where possible. Drugs that have been associated with peripheral neuropathy include antiretroviral nucleoside analogues, chloramphenicol, cisplatin, dapsone, disulfiram, ethionamide, glutethimide, gold, hydralazine, iodoquinol, isoniazid, metronidazole, nitrofurantoin, phenytoin, ribavirin, and vincristine. Concomitant use of HIVID with didanosine is not recommended.

Intravenous Pentamidine: Treatment with HIVID should be interrupted when the use of a drug that has the potential to cause pancreatitis is required. Death due to fulminant pancreatitis possibly related to intravenous pentamidine and HIVID has been reported. If intravenous pentamidine is required to treat *Pneumocystis carinii* pneumonia, treatment with HIVID should be interrupted (see WARNINGS).

Amphotericin, Foscarnet, and Aminoglycosides: Drugs such as amphotericin, foscarnet, and aminoglycosides may increase the risk of developing peripheral neuropathy (see WARNINGS: *Peripheral Neuropathy*) or other HIVID-associated adverse events by interfering with the renal clearance of zalcitabine (thereby raising systemic exposure). Patients who require the use of one of these drugs with HIVID should have frequent clinical and laboratory monitoring with dosage adjustment for any significant change in renal function.

Probenecid or Cimetidine: Concomitant administration of probenecid or cimetidine decreases the elimination of zalcitabine, most likely by inhibition of renal tubular secretion of zalcitabine. Patients receiving these drugs in combination with zalcitabine should be monitored for signs of toxicity and the dose of zalcitabine reduced if warranted.

Magnesium/Aluminum-containing Antacid Products: Absorption of zalcitabine is moderately reduced (approximately 25%) when coadministered with magnesium/aluminum-containing antacid products. The clinical significance of this reduction is not known, hence zalcitabine is not recommended to be ingested simultaneously with magnesium/aluminum-containing antacids.

Metoclopramide: Bioavailability is mildly reduced (approximately 10%) when zalcitabine and metoclopramide are coadministered (see CLINICAL PHARMACOLOGY: *Drug Interactions*).

Doxorubicin: Doxorubicin caused a decrease in zalcitabine phosphorylation (>50% inhibition of total phosphate formation) in U937/Molt 4 cells. Although there may be decreased zalcitabine activity because of lessened active metabolite formation, the clinical relevance of these in vitro results are not known.

Carcinogenesis, Mutagenesis, and Impairment of Fertility:

Carcinogensis: Zalcitabine was administered orally by dietary admixture to CRL:CD-1® (ICR) Br mice at dosages of 3, 83, or 250 mg/kg/day for 2 years. Plasma exposures (as measured by AUC) at these doses were 6-fold to 704-fold greater than the systemic exposure in humans with the therapeutic dose. Zalcitabine was administered orally by dietary admixture to CDF® (F-344)/CrIBR/CdBR rats at dosages of 3, 28, 83, or 250 mg/kg/day. At the highest dose tested, the systemic exposure to zalcitabine was 833 times the systemic exposure in humans with the therapeutic dose. A significant increase in thymic lymphoma in all zalcitabine dose groups and Harderian gland (a gland of the eye of rodents) adenoma in the two highest dose groups was observed in female CD1 mice after 2 years of dosing. No increase in tumor incidence was observed in rats or male mice treated with zalcitabine. In an independent study, administration of zalcitabine to $B_6C_3F_1$ mice at a dose of 1000 mg/kg/day for 3 months induced an increased incidence of thymic lymphoma. A high rate of spontaneous lymphoreticular neoplasms have previously been noted in this strain of mice.

Mutagenesis: Zalcitabine was positive in a cell transformation assay and induced chromosomal aberrations in vitro in human peripheral blood lymphocytes. Oral doses of zalcitabine at 2500 and 4500 mg/kg were clastogenic in the mouse micronucleus assay. Zalcitabine showed no evidence of mutagenicity in Ames tests, Chinese hamster lung cell assays and the mouse lymphoma assay. An unscheduled DNA synthesis assay in rat hepatocytes showed that zalcitabine had no effect on DNA repair.

Impairment of Fertility: Fertility and reproductive performance were assessed in rats at plasma concentrations up to 2142 times those achieved with the maximum recommended human dose (MRHD) based on AUC measurements. No adverse effects on rate of conception or general reproductive performance were observed. The highest dose was associated with embryolethality and evidence of teratogenicity. The next lower dose studied (plasma concentrations equivalent to 485 times the MHRD) was associated with a lower frequency of embryotoxicity but no teratogenicity. The fertility of F_1 males was significantly reduced at a calculated dose of 2142 (but not 485) times the MRHD (based on AUC measurements) in a teratology study in which rat mothers were dosed on gestation days 7 to 15. No adverse effects were observed on the fertility of parents or F_1 generation in the study of fertility and general reproductive performance or in the perinatal and postnatal reproduction study.

Pregnancy: *Teratogenic Effects:* Pregnancy Category C. Zalcitabine has been shown to be teratogenic in mice at calculated exposure levels of 1365 and 2730 times that of the MRHD (based on AUC measurements). In rats, zalcitabine was teratogenic at a calculated exposure level of 2142 times the MRHD but not at an exposure level of 485 times the MRHD. In a perinatal and postnatal study in the rat, a high incidence of hydrocephalus was observed in the F_1 offspring derived from litters of dams treated with 1071 (but not 485) times the MRHD (based on AUC measurements). There are no adequate and well-controlled studies of zalcitabine in pregnant women. HIVID should be used during pregnancy only if the potential benefit justifies the potential risk to the fetus. Fertile women should not receive HIVID unless they are using effective contraception during therapy. If pregnancy occurs, physicians are encouraged to report such cases by calling (800) 526-6367.

Nonteratogenic Effects: Increased embryolethality was observed in pregnant mice at doses 2730 times the MRHD and in pregnant rats above 485 (but not 98) times the MRHD (based on AUC measurements). Average fetal body weight was significantly decreased in mice at doses of 1365 times the MRHD and in rats at 2142 times the MRHD (based on AUC measurements). In a perinatal and postnatal study, the learning and memory of a significant number of F_1 offspring were impaired, and they tended to stay hyperactive for a longer period of time. These effects, observed at a calculated exposure level of 1071 (but not 485) times the MRHD (based on AUC measurements), were considered to result from extensive damage to or gross underdevelopment of the brain of these F_1 offspring consistent with the finding of hydrocephalus.

Nursing Mothers: The US Public Health Service Centers for Disease Control and Prevention advises HIV-infected women not to breastfeed to avoid postnatal transmission of HIV to a child who may not yet be infected. It is not known whether zalcitabine is excreted in human milk.

Pediatric Use: *Pharmacokinetics in Pediatric Patients:* Limited pharmacokinetic data have been reported for 5 HIV-positive pediatric patients using doses of 0.03 and 0.04 mg/kg HIVID administered orally every 6 hours.[1] The mean bioavailability of zalcitabine in these pediatric patients was 54% and mean apparent systemic clearance was 150 mL/min/m^2. Due to the small number of subjects and different analytical techniques, it is difficult to make comparisons between pediatric and adult data.

Safety and effectiveness of HIVID and HIV-infected pediatric patients younger than 13 years of age have not been established.

Geriatric Use: Clinical studies of HIVID did not include sufficient numbers of subjects aged 65 and over to determine whether they respond differently from younger subjects. In general, dose selection for an elderly patient should be cautious, reflecting the greater frequency of decreased hepatic, renal, or cardiac function, and of concomitant disease or other drug therapy. HIVID is known to be substantially excreted by the kidney, and the risk of toxic reactions to this drug may be greater in patients with impaired renal function. Because elderly patients are more likely to have decreased renal function, care should be taken in dose selection. In addition, renal function should be monitored and dosage adjustments should be made accordingly (see PRECAUTIONS: *General: Renal Impairment* and DOSAGE AND ADMINISTRATION).

ADVERSE REACTONS

(See WARNINGS.) Tables 2 and 3 summarize the clinical adverse events and laboratory abnormalities, respectively that occurred in ≥1% of patients in the comparative monotherapy trial (CPCRA 002) of HIVID vs didanosine (ddI), and the comparative combination trial (ACTG 175) of zidovudine (ZDV) monotherapy vs HIVID and zidovudine combination therapy, respectively. Other studies have found a higher or lower incidence of adverse experiences depending upon disease status, generally being lower in patients with less advanced disease.

[See table 2 at top of next page]

[See table 3 at top of next page]

Additional clinical adverse experiences associated with HIVID that occurred in <1% of patients in CPCRA 002 (at least possibly related, Grade 3 or higher), ACTG 175 (any relationship, Grade 3/4) or in other clinical studies are listed below by body system. Several of these events occurred in slightly higher rates in other studies. The incidence of adverse experiences varied in different studies, generally being lower in patients with less-advanced disease.

Body as a Whole: abnormal weight loss, asthenia, cachexia, chest tightness or pain, chills, cutaneous/allergic reaction, debilitation, difficulty moving, dry eyes/mouth, edema, facial pain or swelling, flank pain, flushing, increased sweating, lymphadenopathy, hypersensitivity reactions (see WARNINGS), malaise, night sweats, pain, pelvic/groin pain, rigors.
Cardiovascular: abnormal cardiac movement, arrhythmia, atrial fibrillation, cardiac failure, cardiac dysrhythmias, cardiomyopathy, heart racing, hypertension, palpitation, subarachnoid hemorrhage, syncope, tachycardia, ventricular ectopy.
Endocrine/Metabolic: abnormal triglycerides, abnormal lipase, altered serum glucose, decreased bicarbonate, diabetes mellitus, glycosuria, gout, hot flushes, hypercalcemia, hyperkalemia, hyperlipemia, hypernatremia, hyperuricemia, hypocalcemia, hypoglycemia, hypokalemia, hypomagnesemia, hyponatremia, hypophosphatemia, increased nonprotein nitrogen, lactic acidosis.
Gastrointestinal: abdominal bloating or cramps, acute pancreatitis, anal/rectal pain, anorexia, bleeding gums, bloody or black stools, colitis, dental abscess, dry mouth, dyspepsia, dysphagia, enlarged abdomen, epigastric pain, eructation, esophageal pain, esophageal ulcers, esophagitis, flatulence, gagging with pills, gastritis, gastrointestinal hemorrhage, gingivitis, glossitis, gum disorder, heartburn, hemorrhagic pancreatitis, hemorrhoids, increased saliva, left quadrant pain, melena, mouth lesion, odynophagia, painful sore gums, painful swallowing, pancreatitis, rectal hemorrhage, rectal mass, rectal ulcers, salivary gland enlargement, sore tongue, sore throat, tongue disorder, tongue ulcer, toothache, unformed/loose stools, vomiting.
Hematologic: absolute neutrophil count alteration, anemia, epistaxis, decreased hematocrit, granulocytosis, hemoglobinemia, leukopenia, neutrophilia, platelet alteration, purpura, thrombus, unspecified hematologic toxicity, white blood cell alteration.
Hepatic: abnormal lactate dehydrogenase, bilirubinemia, cholecystitis, decreased alkaline phosphatase, hepatitis, hepatocellular damage, hepatomegaly, increased alkaline phosphatase, jaundice.
Musculoskeletal: arthralgia, arthritis, arthropathy, arthrosis, back pain, backache, bone pains/aches, bursitis, cold extremities, extremity pain, joint inflammation, leg cramps, muscle aches, muscle weakness, muscle disorder, muscle stiffness, muscle cramps, myalgia, myopathy, myositis, neck pain, rib pain, stiff neck.
Neurological: abnormal coordination, aphasia, ataxia, Bell's palsy, confusion, decreased concentration, decreased neurological function, disequilibrium, dizziness, dysphonia, facial nerve palsy, focal motor seizure, grand mal seizure, hyperkinesia, hypertonia, hypokinesia, memory loss, migraine, neuralgia, neuritis, paralysis, seizures, speech disorder, status epilepticus, stupor, tremor, twitch, vertigo.
Psychological: acute psychotic disorder, acute stress reaction, agitation, amnesia, anxiety, confusion, decreased motivation, decreased sexual desire, depersonalization, emotional lability, euphoria, hallucination, impaired concentration, insomnia, manic reaction, mood swings, nervousness, paranoid state, somnolence, suicide attempt, dementia.
Respiratory: acute nasopharyngitis, chest congestion, coughing, cyanosis, difficulty breathing, dry nasal mucosa, dyspnea, flu-like symptoms, hemoptysis, nasal discharge, pharyngitis, rales/rhonchi, respiratory distress, sinus congestion, sinus pain, sinusitis, wheezing.
Skin: acne, alopecia, bullous eruptions, carbuncle/furuncle, cellulitis, cold sore, dermatitis, dry skin, dry rash desquamation, erythematous rash, exfoliative dermatitis, finger inflammation, follicular rash, impetigo, infection, itchy rash, lip blisters/lesions, macular/papular rash, maculopapular rash, moniliasis, mucocutaneous/skin disorder, nail disorder, photosensitivity reaction, pruritic disorder, pruritus, skin disorder, skin lesions, skin fissure, skin ulcer, urticaria.
Special Senses: abnormal vision, blurred vision, burning eyes, decreased taste, decreased vision, ear pain/problem, ear blockage, eye abnormality, eye inflammation, eye itching, eye pain, eye irritation, eye redness, eye hemorrhage, fluid in ears, hearing loss, increased tears, loss of taste, mucopurulent conjunctivitis, parosmia, photophobia, smell dysfunction, taste perversion, tinnitus, unequal-sized pupils, xerophthalmia, yellow sclera.
Urogenital: abnormal renal function, acute renal failure, albuminuria, bladder pain, dysuria, frequent urination, genital lesion/ulcer, increased blood urea nitrogen, increased creatinine, micturition frequency, nocturia, painful penis sore, pain on urination, penile edema, polyuria, renal cyst, renal calculus, testicular swelling, toxic nephropathy, urinary retention, vaginal itch, vaginal ulcer, vaginal pain, vaginal/cervix disorder, vaginal discharge.

Table 2. Percentage of Patients With Clinical Adverse Experience ≥ Grade 3*† in ≥1% of Patients Receiving HIVID

	CPCRA 002* ZDV Intolerant or Failure		ACTG 175‡ ZDV Naive/Experienced	
	HIVID 0.750 mg q8h n=237	ddI 250 mg q12h n=230	ZDV 200 mg q8h n=619	HIVID+ZDV 0.750 mg q8h+200 mg q8h n=615
Body System/Adverse Event				
Systemic				
Fatigue	3.8	2.6	2.7	2.3
Headache	2.1	1.3	2.4	2.6
Fever	1.7	0.4	2.7	2.9
Gastrointestinal				
Abdominal pain	3.0	7.0	2.3	1.8
Oral Lesions/Stomatitis§	3.0	0.0	0.6	1.5
Vomiting/Nausea§	3.4	7.0	4.9	2.1
Diarrhea/Constipation§	2.5	17.4	2.9	1.0
Hepatic				
Abnormal Hepatic Function	8.9	7.0	‖	‖
Neurological				
Convulsions	1.3	2.2		
Peripheral Neuropathy¶	28.3	13.0	3.1	3.3
Skin				
Rash/Pruritus/Urticaria	3.4	3.9	1.8	1.6
Metabolic and Nutrition				
Pancreatitis	0.0	1.7	0.2	0.5
Psychological				
Depression	0.4	0.0	1.1	1.8
Musculoskeletal				
Painful/Swollen Joints	0.4	0.0	0.3	1.0

* Grade 2 Adverse Events possibly or related to treatment or unassessable were included if study drug dosage was changed or interrupted.
† Grade 3 severity: event causing marked limitation in activity, requiring medical care and possible hospitalization.
Grade 4 severity: completely disabling, unable to care for self, requiring active medical intervention, probable hospitalization or hospice care.
‡ All relationships.
§ Adverse experiences were combined to form this category.
‖ See Table 3.
¶CPCRA 002 included patients who were dose-adjusted for Grade 2 events; ACTG 175 required dose adjustment for Grade 2 peripheral neuropathy but recorded only Grade 3 events.

Table 3. Percentage of Patients With Laboratory Abnormalities—Protocol Grade 3/4

	CPCRA 002* ZDV Intolerant or Failure		ACTG 175 ZDV Naive/Experienced	
	HIVID 0.750 mg q8h n=237	ddI 250 mg q12h n=230	ZDV 200 mg q8h n=619	HIVID+ZDV 0.750 mg q8h+200 mg q8h n=615
Laboratory Abnormality				
Anemia (<7.5 gm/dL)	8.4	7.4	1.8	3.1
Leukopenia (<1500 cells/mm^3)	13.1	9.6	N/A	N/A
Eosinophilia (>1000 cells/mm^3 or 25%)	2.5	1.7	N/A	N/A
Neutropenia (<750 cells/mm^3)	16.9	11.7	1.9	4.2
Thrombocytopenia (<50,000 cells/mm^3)	1.3	4.8	1.1	1.8
CPK Elevation* (>4 × ULN)	0.8	0.0	5.8	5.7
ALT (SGPT) (>5 × ULN)	N/A	N/A	3.6	5.0
AST (SGOT) (>5 × ULN)	7.6	5.7	2.9	4.1
Bilirubin (>2.5 × ULN)	0.8	0.9	0.5	1.0
GGT (>5 × ULN)	N/A	N/A	0.5	1.0
Amylase (>2 × ULN)	5.1	3.9	1.0	1.5
Hyperglycemia* (>250 mg/dL)	0.0	1.7	0 8	2.0

*Grade 3 or higher reported for CPCRA 002.
N/A Not available.

OVERDOSAGE

Acute Overdosage: Inadvertent pediatric overdoses have occurred with doses up to 1.5 mg/kg HIVID. Pediatric patients had prompt gastric lavage and treatment with activated charcoal and had no sequelae. Mixed overdoses including HIVID and other drugs have led to drowsiness and vomiting (with HIVID or placebo, zidovudine and trimethoprim/sulfamethoxazole [TMP/SMX]), or increased GGT (with 18.75 mg HIVID with zidovudine and lormetazepam) or increased creatine phosphokinase (with HIVID or placebo, zidovudine, fluconazole, dapsone and wine). There is no experience with acute HIVID overdosage at higher doses and sequelae are unknown. There is no known antidote for HIVID overdosage. It is not known whether zalcitabine is dialyzable by peritoneal dialysis or hemodialysis.
Chronic Overdosage: In an initial dose-finding study in which zalcitabine was administered at doses 25 times (0.25 mg/kg every 8 hours) the currently recommended dose, one patient discontinued HIVID after 1½ weeks of treatment subsequent to the development of a rash and fever. In the early Phase 1 studies, all patients receiving zalcitabine at approximately 6 times the current total daily recommended dose experienced peripheral neuropathy by week 10. Eighty percent of patients who received approximately 2 times the current total daily recommended dose experienced peripheral neuropathy by week 12.

DOSAGE AND ADMINISTRATION

Patients should be advised that HIVID is recommended for use in combination with active antiretroviral therapy. Greater activity has been observed when new antiretroviral therapies are begun at the same time as HIVID. Concomitant therapy should be based on a patient's prior drug exposure. The recommended regimen is one 0.750 mg tablet of HIVID orally every 8 hours (2.25 mg HIVID total daily dose) in combination with other antiretroviral agents. Please refer to the complete product information for each of the other antiretroviral agents for the recommended doses of these agents. Based on preliminary data, the recommended HIVID dosage reduction for patients with impaired renal function is: creatinine clearance 10 to 40 mL/min: 0.750 mg of HIVID every 12 hours; creatinine clearance <10 mL/min: 0.750 mg of HIVID every 24 hours.
Monitoring of Patients: Complete blood counts and clinical chemistry tests should be performed prior to initiating HIVID therapy and at appropriate intervals thereafter. For comprehensive patient monitoring recommendations for other antiretroviral therapies, physicians should refer to the complete product information for these drugs. Serum amylase levels should be monitored in those individuals who have a history of elevated amylase, pancreatitis, ethanol abuse, who are on parenteral nutrition or who are otherwise at high risk of pancreatitis. Careful monitoring for signs or symptoms suggestive of peripheral neuropathy is recommended, particularly in individuals with a low CD_4 cell count or who are at a greater risk of developing peripheral neuropathy while on therapy (see WARNINGS).
Dose Adjustment for HIVID: For toxicities that are likely to be associated with HIVID (eg, peripheral neuropathy, severe oral ulcers, pancreatitis, elevated liver function tests especially in patients with chronic Hepatitis B), HIVID

Continued on next page

Hivid—Cont.

should be interrupted or dose reduced. FOR SEVERE TOXICITIES OR THOSE PERSISTING AFTER DOSE REDUCTION, HIVID SHOULD BE INTERRUPTED. For recipients of combination therapy with HIVID and other antiretroviral agents, dose adjustments or interruption for each drug should be based on the known toxicity profile of the individual drugs. SEE INFORMATION FOR EACH DRUG USED IN COMBINATION FOR A DESCRIPTION OF KNOWN DRUG-ASSOCIATED ADVERSE REACTIONS.

Patients developing moderate discomfort with signs or symptoms of peripheral neuropathy should stop HIVID. HIVID-associated peripheral neuropathy may continue to worsen despite interruption of HIVID. HIVID should be reintroduced at 50% dose—0.375 mg every 8 hours only if all findings related to peripheral neuropathy have improved to mild symptoms. HIVID should be permanently discontinued if patients experience severe discomfort related to peripheral neuropathy or moderate discomfort that progresses. If other moderate to severe clinical adverse reactions or laboratory abnormalities (such as increased liver function tests) occur, then HIVID and/or other potential causative agent(s) should be interrupted until the adverse reaction abates. HIVID and/or the other potential causative agent(s) should then be carefully reintroduced at lower doses if appropriate. If adverse reactions recur at the reduced dose, therapy should be discontinued. The minimum effective dose of HIVID in combination with zidovudine for the treatment of adult patients with advanced HIV infection has not been established.

In patients with poor bone marrow reserve, particularly those patients with advanced symptomatic HIV disease, frequent monitoring of hematologic indices is recommended to detect serious anemia or granulocytopenia. Significant toxicities, such as anemia (hemoglobin of <7.5 gm/dL or reduction of >25% of baseline) and/or granulocytopenia (granulocyte count of <750 cells/mm^3 or reduction of >50% from baseline), may require a treatment interruption of HIVID and zidovudine until evidence of marrow recovery is observed. For less severe anemia or granulocytopenia, a reduction in daily dose of zidovudine in those patients receiving combination therapy may be adequate. In patients who experience hematologic toxicity, reduction in hemoglobin may occur as early as 2 to 4 weeks after initiation of therapy, and granulocytopenia usually occurs after 6 to 8 weeks of therapy. In patients who develop significant anemia, dose modification does not necessarily eliminate the need for transfusion. If marrow recovery occurs following dose modification, gradual increases in dose may be appropriate depending on hematologic indices and patient tolerance. For more details, refer to the complete product information for zidovudine.

HOW SUPPLIED

HIVID 0.375 mg tablets are oval, beige, film-coated tablets with "HIVID 0.375" imprinted on one side and "ROCHE" on the other side—bottles of 100 (NDC 0004-0220-01). HIVID 0.750 mg tablets are oval, gray, film-coated tablets with "HIVID 0.750" imprinted on one side and "ROCHE" on the other side—bottles of 100 (NDC 0004-0221-01).

The tablets should be stored in tightly closed bottles at 59° to 86°F (15° to 30°C).

REFERENCES

1. Pizzo PA, Butler K, Balis F, et al. Dideoxycytidine alone and in an alternating schedule with zidovudine in children with symptomatic human immunodeficiency virus infection. *J Pediatr.* 1990;117(5): 799–808.
2. Abrams DI, Goldman AI, Launer C, et al. A comparative trial of didanosine or zalcitabine after treatment with zidovudine in patients with human immunodeficiency virus infection. *N Engl J Med.* 1994;330(10): 657–662.
3. Follansbee S, Drew L, Olson R, et al. The efficacy of zalcitabine (ddC, HIVID) versus zidovudine (ZDV) as monotherapy in ZDV-naive patients with advanced HIV disease; a randomized, double-blind, comparative trial (ACTG 114; N3300). IXth International Conference on AIDS/IV STD World Congress, Berlin, Germany, June 7–11, 1993. Poster PO-B26-2113.
4. Remick S, Follansbee S, Olson R, et al. Safety and tolerance of zalcitabine (ddC, HIVID) in a double-blind comparative trial (ACTG 114; N3300). IXth International Conference on AIDS/IV STD World Congress, Berlin, Germany, June 7–11, 1993. Poster PO-B26-2115.
5. "Dear Doctor" letter, Burroughs Wellcome Co., June 1, 1993.
6. Food and Drug Administration Antiviral Drugs Advisory Committee Meeting, "Mitochondrial Damage Associated with Nucleoside Analogues," Rockville, MD, September 21, 1993.
7. Sanders VM, Elwell MR, Heath JE, et al. Induction of Thymic Lymphoma in Mice Administered the Dideoxynucleoside ddC. *Fundamental and Applied Toxicology.* 1995;27:263–269.
8. Irons RD, Le AT, Som DB, et al. 2'3'-Dideoxycytidine-induced Thymic Lymphoma Correlates with Species-specific Suppression of a Subpopulation of Primitive Hematopoietic Progenitor Cells in Mouse but Not Rat or Human Bone Marrow. *J Clin Invest.* 1995;95: 2777–2782.

*Maalox is a registered trademark of Novartis.

†INVIRASE is a registered trademark of Hoffmann-La Roche Inc.

Roche Pharmaceuticals
Roche Laboratories Inc.
340 Kingsland Street
Nutley, New Jersey 07110-1199

Revised: May 2000

27897190-0500

Shown in Product Identification Guide, page 332

INVIRASE®
(saquinavir mesylate)
CAPSULES ℞

The following text is complete prescribing information based on official labeling in effect June 2000.

DESCRIPTION

INVIRASE brand of saquinavir mesylate is an inhibitor of the human immunodeficiency virus (HIV) protease. INVIRASE is available as light brown and green, opaque hard gelatin capsules for oral administration in a 200-mg strength (as saquinavir free base). Each capsule also contains the inactive ingredients lactose, microcrystalline cellulose, povidone K30, sodium starch glycolate, talc and magnesium stearate. Each capsule shell contains gelatin and water with the following dye systems: red iron oxide, yellow iron oxide, black iron oxide, FD&C Blue #2 and titanium dioxide. The chemical name for saquinavir mesylate is N-tert-butyl-decahydro-2- [2(R)-hydroxy-4-phenyl-3(S)-[[N-(2-quinolylcarbonyl)-L-asparaginyl]amino]butyl]-(4aS,8aS) -isoquinoline-3(S)-carboxamide methanesulfonate with a molecular formula $C_{38}H_{50}N_6O_5 \cdot CH_4O_3S$ and a molecular weight of 766.96. The molecular weight of the free base is 670.86.

Saquinavir mesylate is a white to off-white, very fine powder with an aqueous solubility of 2.22 mg/mL at 25°C.

CLINICAL PHARMACOLOGY

Mechanism of Action: HIV protease cleaves viral polyprotein precursors to generate functional proteins in HIV-infected cells. The cleavage of viral polyprotein precursors is essential for maturation of infectious virus. Saquinavir mesylate, henceforth referred to as saquinavir, is a synthetic peptide-like substrate analogue that inhibits the activity of HIV protease and prevents the cleavage of viral polyproteins.

Microbiology: *Antiviral Activity In Vitro:* The in vitro antiviral activity of saquinavir was assessed in lymphoblastoid and monocytic cell lines and in peripheral blood lymphocytes. Saquinavir inhibited HIV activity in both acutely and chronically infected cells. IC50 values (50% inhibitory concentration) were in the range of 1 to 30 nM. In cell culture saquinavir demonstrated additive to synergistic effects against HIV in double- and triple-combination regimens with reverse transcriptase inhibitors zidovudine (ZDV), zalcitabine (ddC) and didanosine (ddI), without enhanced cytotoxicity.

Resistance: HIV isolates with reduced susceptibility to saquinavir have been selected in vitro. Genotypic analyses of these isolates showed substitution mutations in the HIV protease at amino acid positions 48 (Glycine to Valine) and 90 (Leucine to Methionine).

Phenotypic and genotypic changes in HIV isolates from patients treated with saquinavir were also monitored in Phase 1/2 clinical trials. Phenotypic changes were defined as a 10-fold decrease in sensitivity from baseline. Two viral protease mutations (L90M and/or G48V, the former predominating) were found in virus from treated, but not untreated, patients. The incidence across studies of phenotypic and genotypic changes in the subsets of patients studied for a period of 16 to 74 weeks (median observation time approximately 1 year) is shown in Table 1. However, the clinical relevance of phenotypic and genotypic changes associated with saquinavir therapy has not been established.

[See table below]

Cross-resistance to Other Antiretrovirals: The potential for HIV cross-resistance between protease inhibitors has not been fully explored. Therefore, it is unknown what effect saquinavir therapy will have on the activity of subsequent protease inhibitors. Cross-resistance between saquinavir and reverse transcriptase inhibitors is unlikely because of the different enzyme targets involved. ZDV-resistant HIV isolates have been shown to be sensitive to saquinavir in vitro.

Pharmacokinetics: The pharmacokinetic properties of saquinavir have been evaluated in healthy volunteers (n=351) and HIV-infected patients (n=270) after single- and multiple-oral doses of 25, 75, 200 and 600 mg tid and in healthy volunteers after intravenous doses of 6, 12, 36 or 72 mg (n=21).

ABSORPTION AND BIOAVAILABILITY IN ADULTS: Following multiple dosing (600 mg tid) in HIV-infected patients (n=30), the steady-state area under the plasma concentration versus time curve (AUC) was 2.5 times (95% CI 1.6 to 3.8) higher than that observed after a single dose. HIV-infected patients administered saquinavir 600 mg tid, with the instructions to take saquinavir after a meal or substantial snack, had AUC and maximum plasma concentration (C_{max}) values which were about twice those observed in healthy volunteers receiving the same treatment regimen (Table 2).

Table 2. Mean (%CV) AUC and C_{max} in Patients and Healthy Volunteers

	AUC_8 (dose interval) (ng·h/mL)	C_{max} (ng/mL)
Healthy Volunteers (n=6)	359.0 (46)	90.39 (49)
Patients (n=113)	757.2 (84)	253.3 (99)

Absolute bioavailability averaged 4% (CV 73%, range: 1% to 9%) in 8 healthy volunteers who received a single 600-mg dose (3 × 200 mg) of saquinavir following a high fat breakfast (48 g protein, 60 g carbohydrate, 57 g fat; 1006 kcal). The low bioavailability is thought to be due to a combination of incomplete absorption and extensive first-pass metabolism.

FOOD EFFECT: The mean 24-hour AUC after a single 600-mg oral dose (6 × 100 mg) in healthy volunteers (n=6) was increased from 24 ng·h/mL (CV 33%), under fasting conditions, to 161 ng·h/mL (CV 35%) when saquinavir was given following a high fat breakfast (48 g protein, 60 g carbohydrate, 57 g fat; 1006 kcal). Saquinavir 24-hour AUC and C_{max} (n=6) following the administration of a higher calorie meal (943 kcal, 54 g fat) were on average two times higher than after a lower calorie, lower fat meal (355 kcal, 8 g fat). The effect of food has been shown to persist for up to 2 hours.

DISTRIBUTION IN ADULTS: The mean steady-state volume of distribution following intravenous administration of a 12-mg dose of saquinavir (n=8) was 700 L (CV 39%), suggesting saquinavir partitions into tissues. Saquinavir was approximately 98% bound to plasma proteins over a concentration range of 15 to 700 ng/mL. In 2 patients receiving saquinavir 600 mg tid, cerebrospinal fluid concentrations were negligible when compared to concentrations from matching plasma samples.

METABOLISM AND ELIMINATION IN ADULTS: In vitro studies using human liver microsomes have shown that the metabolism of saquinavir is cytochrome P450 mediated with the specific isoenzyme, CYP3A4, responsible for more than 90% of the hepatic metabolism. Based on in vitro studies, saquinavir is rapidly metabolized to a range of mono- and di-hydroxylated inactive compounds. In a mass balance study using 600 mg ^{14}C-saquinavir (n=8), 88% and 1% of the orally administered radioactivity, was recovered in feces and urine, respectively, within 5 days of dosing. In an additional 4 subjects administered 10.5 mg ^{14}C-saquinavir intravenously, 81% and 3% of the intravenously administered radioactivity was recovered in feces and urine, respectively, within 5 days of dosing. In mass balance studies, 13% of circulating radioactivity in plasma was attributed to unchanged drug after oral administration and the remainder attributed to saquinavir metabolites. Following intravenous administration, 66% of circulating radioactivity was attributed to unchanged drug and the remainder attributed to saquinavir metabolites, suggesting that saquinavir undergoes extensive first-pass metabolism.

Systemic clearance of saquinavir was rapid, 1.14 L/h/kg (CV 12%) after intravenous doses of 6, 36 and 72 mg. The mean residence time of saquinavir was 7 hours (n=8).

SPECIAL POPULATIONS: Hepatic or Renal Impairment: Saquinavir pharmacokinetics in patients with hepatic or renal insufficiency has not been investigated (see PRECAUTIONS).

Gender, Race and Age: Pharmacokinetic data were available for 17 women in the Phase 1/2 studies. Pooled data did not reveal an apparent effect of gender on the pharmacokinetics of saquinavir.

The effect of race on the pharmacokinetics of saquinavir has not been evaluated, due to the small numbers of minorities for whom pharmacokinetic data were available.

Saquinavir pharmacokinetics has not been investigated in patients >65 years of age or in pediatric patients (<16 years).

DRUG INTERACTIONS: HIVID and ZDV: Concomitant use of INVIRASE with HIVID® (zalcitabine, ddC) and ZDV has been studied (as triple combination) in adults. Pharmacokinetic data suggest that the absorption, metabolism and elimination of each of these drugs are unchanged when they are used together.

Table 1. Frequency of Genotypic and Phenotypic Changes in Selected Patients Treated With Saquinavir

	Genotypic*		Phenotypic†	
	24 Week	1 Year	24 Week	1 Year
Monotherapy	3/8 (38%)	15/33 (45%)	2/22 (9%)	5/11 (45%)
Combination Therapy	5/30 (17%)	16/52 (31%)	0/23 (0%)	11/29 (38%)

*Double mutation (G48V and L90M) has occurred in 2 of 33 patients receiving monotherapy. The double mutation has not occurred with combination therapy.

†Phenotypic changes have been defined as at least a 10-fold change in sensitivity relative to baseline. In a few patients genotypic and phenotypic changes were unrelated.

Table 3. Summary of Mean Log 10 Plasma RNA Results From Major INVIRASE Clinical Studies

	V13330 (Italy) Naive patients			NV14255/ACTG229 (USA) ZDV-experienced			NV14256 (North America) ZDV-experienced		
	ZDV	SAQ*	ZDV+SAQ	ZDV+ddC	ZDV+SAQ	ZDV+ddC+SAQ	ddC	SAQ	SAQ+ddC
n Enrolled	17	19	20	100	99	98	314	318	308
Prior ZDV									
n	—	—	—	99	98	97	305	315	304
Median Duration (days)	—	—	—	659	713	647	521	523	477
Log_{10} Plasma RNA by PCR (copies/mL)									
n	17	19	20	100	97	96	300	307	294
Mean Baseline (n)	5.2 (17)	5.2 (19)	5.3 (20)	4.7 (100)	4.8 (97)	4.8 (96)	5.0 (300)	5.1 (307)	5.0 (294)
Mean Change from Baseline Week 16 (n)	−0.5 (15)	−0.2 (17)	−1.0 (17)	−0.3 (93)	0.0 (81)	−0.5 (86)	−0.4 (253)	−0.1 (262)	−0.6 (258)
Mean Change from Baseline Week 24 (n)	—	—	—	−0.2 (86)	0.0 (83)	−0.6 (84)	−0.3 (228)	−0.1 (244)	−0.6 (232)
Mean Change from Baseline Week 48 (n)	—	—	—	—	—	—	−0.3 (147)	−0.1 (167)	−0.6 (169)

*Saquinavir (SAQ) at 600 mg tid –Indicates not applicable

Nelfinavir: In 14 HIV-positive patients, coadministration of nelfinavir (750 mg) with saquinavir (given as FORTOVASE, 1200 mg) resulted in an 18% (95% CI 5–33%) increase in nelfinavir plasma AUC and a 392% (95% CI 271–553%) increase in saquinavir plasma AUC (see PRECAUTIONS: *Drug Interactions*).

Ritonavir: Following approximately 4 weeks of a combination regimen of saquinavir (400 or 600 mg bid) and ritonavir (400 or 600 mg bid) in HIV-positive patients, saquinavir AUC and C_{max} values increased at least 17-fold (95% CI 9–31-fold) and 14-fold, respectively (see PRECAUTIONS: *Drug Interactions*).

Delavirdine: In 13 healthy volunteers, coadministration of saquinavir (600 mg tid) with delavirdine (400 mg tid) resulted in a 5-fold increase in saquinavir AUC. In 7 healthy volunteers, coadministration of saquinavir (600 mg tid) with delavirdine (400 mg tid) resulted in a 15 ± 16% decrease in delavirdine AUC (see PRECAUTIONS: *Drug Interactions*).

Nevirapine: In 23 HIV-positive patients, coadministration of saquinavir (600 mg tid) with nevirapine (200 mg bid) resulted in a 24% (95% CI 1–42%) and 28% (95% CI 1–47%) decrease in saquinavir plasma AUC and C_{max}, respectively (see PRECAUTIONS: *Drug Interactions*).

Ketoconazole: Concomitant administration of ketoconazole (200 mg qd) and saquinavir (600 mg tid) to 12 healthy volunteers resulted in steady-state saquinavir AUC and C_{max} values which were three times those seen with saquinavir alone. No dose adjustment is required when the two drugs are coadministered at the doses studied. Ketoconazole pharmacokinetics was unaffected by coadministration with saquinavir.

Rifampin: Coadministration of rifampin (600 mg qd) and saquinavir (600 mg tid) to 12 healthy volunteers decreased the steady-state AUC and C_{max} of saquinavir by approximately 80%.

Rifabutin: Preliminary data from 12 HIV-infected patients indicate that the steady-state AUC of saquinavir (600 mg tid) was decreased by 40% when saquinavir was coadministered with rifabutin (300 mg qd).

INDICATIONS AND USAGE

INVIRASE in combination with other antiretroviral agents is indicated for the treatment of HIV infection. This indication is based on results from studies of surrogate marker responses and from a clinical study that showed a reduction in both mortality and AIDS-defining clinical events for patients who received INVIRASE in combination with HIVID compared to patients who received either HIVID or INVIRASE alone.

Description of Clinical Studies: *Patients With Advanced HIV Infection and Prior ZDV Therapy:* Study NV14256 (North America) was a randomized, double-blind study comparing the combination of INVIRASE 600 mg tid + HIVID to HIVID monotherapy and INVIRASE monotherapy. The study accrued 970 patients, with median baseline CD_4 cell count at study entry of 170 cells/mm^3. Median duration of prior ZDV treatment was 17 months. Median duration of follow-up was 17 months. There were 88 first AIDS-defining events or deaths in the HIVID monotherapy group, 84 in the INVIRASE monotherapy group and 51 in the combination group. For survival there were 30 deaths in the HIVID group, 40 in the INVIRASE group and 11 deaths in the combination group.

The analysis of clinical endpoints from this study showed that the 18-month cumulative incidence of clinical disease progression to AIDS-defining event or death was 17.7% for patients randomized to INVIRASE + HIVID compared to 30.7% for patients randomized to HIVID monotherapy and 28.3% for patients randomized to INVIRASE monotherapy. The reduction in the number of clinical events for the combination regimen relative to both monotherapy regimens was statistically significant (see Figure 1 for Kaplan-Meier estimates of time to disease progression).

[See figure 1 at top of next column]

The 18-month cumulative mortality was 4% for patients randomized to INVIRASE + HIVID, 8.9% for patients randomized to HIVID monotherapy and 12.6% for patients randomized to INVIRASE monotherapy. The reduction in the number of deaths for the combination regimen relative to both monotherapy regimens was statistically significant (see Figure 2 for Kaplan-Meier estimates of time to death).

Fig. 1. Time to First AIDS-Defining Event (or Death) (days) NV14256

Fig. 2. Time to Death (days) NV14256

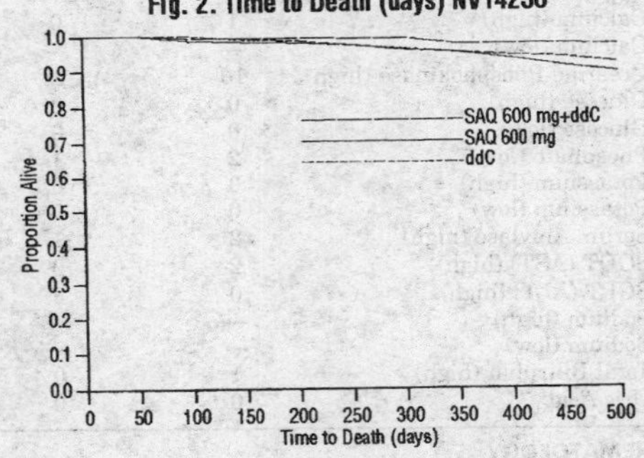

Figure 5 shows mean CD_4 changes over 48 weeks for the three treatment arms in study NV14256. Table 3 displays log RNA reductions at 16, 24 and 48 weeks among INVIRASE combination treatment arms in three clinical trials, including NV14256. Monotherapy arms are included for reference.

Fig. 5. Mean CD_4 Changes (cells/mm^3) from Baseline in Study NV14256

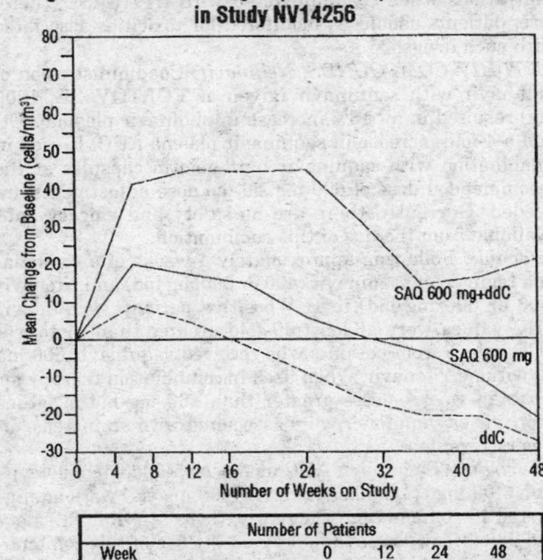

Number of Patients				
Week	0	12	24	48
ddC	313	258	235	154
SAQ+ddC	307	271	255	179
SAQ	317	263	242	175

[See table 3 above]

In ACTG229/NV14255, 295 patients (mean baseline CD_4=165) with prolonged ZDV treatment (median 713 days) were randomized to receive either INVIRASE 600 mg tid + HIVID + ZDV (triple combination), INVIRASE 600 mg tid + ZDV or HIVID + ZDV. In analyses of average CD_4 changes over 24 weeks, the triple combination produced greater increases in CD_4 cell counts (see Figure 4) compared to that of HIVID + ZDV. There were no significant differences in CD_4 changes among patients receiving INVIRASE + ZDV and HIVID + ZDV.

Fig. 4. Mean CD_4 Changes (cells/mm^3) from Baseline in Study ACTG229/NV14255

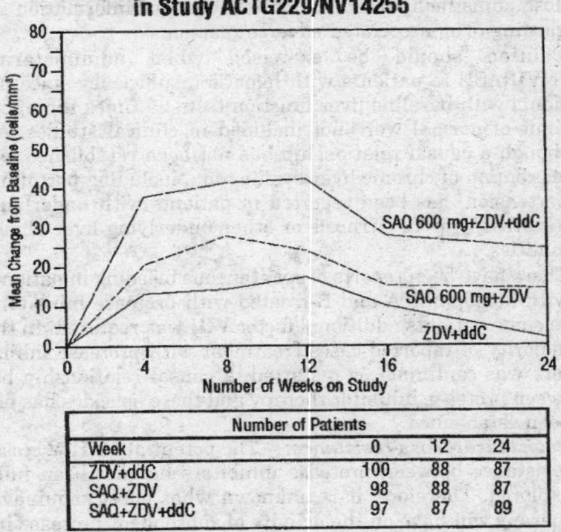

Number of Patients			
Week	0	12	24
ZDV+ddC	100	88	87
SAQ+ZDV	98	88	87
SAQ+ZDV+ddC	97	87	89

Comparisons of data across studies (NV14256 compared to ACTG229/NV14255) suggest that when INVIRASE was added to a regimen of prolonged prior zidovudine, there was little activity contributed by continuing ZDV.

Advanced Patients Without Prior ZDV Therapy: A dose-ranging study (Italy, V13330) conducted in 92 ZDV-naive patients (mean baseline CD_4=179) studied INVIRASE at doses of 75 mg, 200 mg and 600 mg tid in combination with ZDV 200 mg tid compared to INVIRASE 600 mg tid alone and ZDV alone.

In analyses of average CD_4 changes over 16 weeks, treatment with the combination of INVIRASE 600 mg tid + ZDV produced greater CD_4 cell increases than ZDV monotherapy (see Figure 3). The CD_4 changes of ZDV in combination with doses of INVIRASE lower than 600 mg tid were no greater than that of ZDV alone.

Fig. 3. Mean CD_4 Changes (cells/mm^3) from Baseline in Study V13330 (Italy)

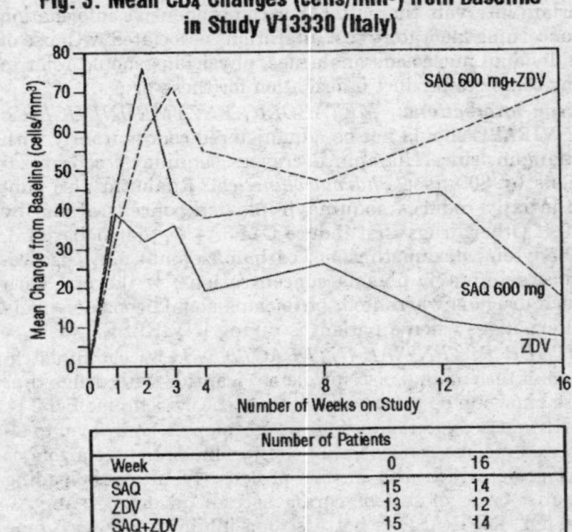

Number of Patients		
Week	0	16
SAQ	15	14
ZDV	13	12
SAQ+ZDV	15	14

Continued on next page

Invirase—Cont.

CONTRAINDICATIONS

INVIRASE is contraindicated in patients with clinically significant hypersensitivity to saquinavir or to any of the components contained in the capsule.

INVIRASE should not be administered concurrently with terfenadine, cisapride, astemizole, triazolam, midazolam or ergot derivatives. Inhibition of CYP3A4 by saquinavir could result in elevated plasma concentrations of these drugs, potentially causing serious or life-threatening reactions.

WARNING: New onset diabetes mellitus, exacerbation of pre-existing diabetes mellitus and hyperglycemia have been reported during postmarketing surveillance in HIV-infected patients receiving protease inhibitor therapy. Some patients required either initiation or dose adjustments of insulin or oral hypoglycemic agents for treatment of these events. In some cases diabetic ketoacidosis has occurred. In those patients who discontinued protease inhibitor therapy, hyperglycemia persisted in some cases. Because these events have been reported voluntarily during clinical practice, estimates of frequency cannot be made and a causal relationship between protease inhibitor therapy and these events has not been established.

PRECAUTIONS

General: The safety profile of INVIRASE in pediatric patients younger than 16 years has not been established.

If a serious or severe toxicity occurs during treatment with INVIRASE, INVIRASE should be interrupted until the etiology of the event is identified or the toxicity resolves. At that time, resumption of treatment with full-dose INVIRASE may be considered. For nucleoside analogues used in combination with INVIRASE, physicians should refer to the complete product information for these drugs for dose adjustment recommendations and for information regarding drug-associated adverse reactions.

Caution should be exercised when administering INVIRASE to patients with hepatic insufficiency since patients with baseline liver function tests >5 times the upper limit of normal were not included in clinical studies. Although a causal relationship has not been established, exacerbation of chronic liver dysfunction, including portal hypertension, has been reported in patients with underlying hepatitis B or C, cirrhosis or other underlying liver abnormalities.

There have been reports of spontaneous bleeding in patients with hemophilia A and B treated with protease inhibitors. In some patients additional factor VIII was required. In the majority of reported cases treatment with protease inhibitors was continued or restarted. A causal relationship between protease inhibitor therapy and these episodes has not been established.

Resistance/Cross-resistance: The potential for HIV cross-resistance between protease inhibitors has not been fully explored. Therefore, it is unknown what effect saquinavir therapy will have on the activity of subsequent protease inhibitors (see *Microbiology*).

Information for Patients: Patients should be informed that INVIRASE is not a cure for HIV infection and that they may continue to acquire illnesses associated with advanced HIV infection, including opportunistic infections. Patients should be advised that INVIRASE should be used only in combination with an active nucleoside analogue regimen.

Patients should be told that the long-term effects of INVIRASE are unknown at this time. They should be informed that INVIRASE therapy has not been shown to reduce the risk of transmitting HIV to others through sexual contact or blood contamination.

Patients should be advised that INVIRASE should be taken within 2 hours after a full meal (see *Pharmacokinetics*). When INVIRASE is taken without food, concentrations of saquinavir in the blood are substantially reduced and may result in no antiviral activity.

Laboratory Tests: Clinical chemistry tests should be performed prior to initiating INVIRASE therapy and at appropriate intervals thereafter. For comprehensive information concerning laboratory test alterations associated with use of individual nucleoside analogues, physicians should refer to the complete product information for these drugs.

Drug Interactions: *METABOLIC ENZYME INDUCERS:* INVIRASE should not be administered concomitantly with rifampin, since rifampin decreases saquinavir concentrations by 80% (see *Pharmacokinetics*). Rifabutin also substantially reduces saquinavir plasma concentrations by 40%. Other drugs that induce CYP3A4 (eg, phenobarbital, phenytoin, dexamethasone, carbamazepine) may also reduce saquinavir plasma concentrations. If therapy with such drugs is warranted, physicians should consider using alternatives when a patient is taking INVIRASE.

OTHER POTENTIAL INTERACTIONS: Coadministration of terfenadine, astemizole or cisapride with drugs that are known to be potent inhibitors of the cytochrome P4503A pathway (ie, ketoconazole, itraconazole, etc.) may lead to elevated plasma concentrations of terfenadine, astemizole or cisapride, which may in turn prolong QT intervals leading to rare cases of serious cardiovascular adverse events. Although INVIRASE is not a strong inhibitor of cytochrome P4503A, pharmacokinetic interaction studies with INVIRASE and terfenadine, astemizole or cisapride have not been conducted. Physicians should use alternatives to terfenadine, astemizole or cisapride when a patient is taking INVIRASE. Other compounds that are substrates of CYP3A4 (eg, calcium channel blockers, clindamycin, dapsone, quinidine, triazolam) may have elevated plasma concentrations when coadministered with INVIRASE; therefore, patients should be monitored for toxicities associated with such drugs.

Table 4. Percentage of Patients, by Study Arm, With Clinical Adverse Experiences Considered at Least Possibly Related to Study Drug or of Unknown Relationship and of Moderate, Severe or Life-threatening Intensity, Occurring in ≥2% of Patients in NV14255/ACTG229 and NV14256

	NV14255/ACTG229			NV14256		
ADVERSE EVENT	SAQ+ZDV n=99	SAQ+ddC+ZDV n=98	ddC+ZDV n=100	ddC n=325	SAQ n=327	SAQ+ddC n=318
GASTROINTESTINAL						
Diarrhea	3.0	1.0	—	0.9	4.9	4.4
Abdominal Discomfort	2.0	3.1	4.0	0.9	0.9	0.9
Nausea	—	3.1	3.0	1.5	2.4	0.9
Dyspepsia	1.0	1.0	2.0	0.6	0.9	0.9
Abdominal Pain	2.0	1.0	2.0	0.6	1.2	0.3
Mucosa Damage	—	—	4.0	—	—	0.3
Buccal Mucosa Ulceration	—	2.0	2.0	6.2	2.1	3.8
CENTRAL AND PERIPHERAL NERVOUS SYSTEM						
Headache	2.0	2.0	2.0	3.4	2.4	0.9
Paresthesia	2.0	3.1	4.0	1.2	0.3	0.3
Extremity Numbness	2.0	1.0	4.0	1.5	0.6	0.9
Dizziness	—	2.0	1.0	—	0.3	—
Peripheral Neuropathy	—	1.0	2.0	11.4	3.1	11.3
BODY AS A WHOLE						
Asthenia	6.1	9.2	10.0	—	0.3	—
Appetite Disturbances	—	1.0	2.0	—	—	—
SKIN AND APPENDAGES						
Rash	—	—	3.0	1.5	2.1	1.3
Pruritus	—	—	2.0	—	0.6	—
MUSCULOSKELETAL DISORDERS						
Musculoskeletal Pain	2.0	2.0	4.0	0.6	0.6	0.6
Myalgia	1.0	—	3.0	0.6	0.3	0.3

—Indicates no events reported

Table 5. Percentage of Patients, by Treatment Group, With Marked Laboratory Abnormalities* in NV14255/ACTG229 and NV14256

	NV14255/ACTG229			NV14256		
	SAQ+ZDV n=99	SAQ+ddC+ZDV n=98	ddC+ZDV n=100	ddC n=325	SAQ n=327	SAQ+ddC n=318
BIOCHEMISTRY						
Calcium (high)	1	0	0	<1	0	0
Calcium (low)	—	—	—	<1	<1	0
Creatine Phosphokinase (high)	10	12	7	6	3	7
Glucose (high)	0	0	0	<1	1	1
Glucose (low)	0	0	0	5	5	5
Phosphate (low)	2	1	0	0	<1	<1
Potassium (high)	0	0	0	2	2	3
Potassium (low)	0	0	0	0	1	0
Serum Amylase (high)	2	1	1	2	1	1
SGOT (AST) (high)	2	2	0	2	2	3
SGPT (ALT) (high)	0	3	1	2	2	2
Sodium (high)	—	—	—	0	0	<1
Sodium (low)	—	—	—	0	<1	0
Total Bilirubin (high)	1	0	0	0	<1	1
Uric Acid	0	0	1	Not assessed	Not assessed	Not assessed
HEMATOLOGY						
Neutrophils (low)	2	2	8	1	1	1
Hemoglobin (low)	0	0	1	<1	<1	0
Platelets (low)	0	0	2	1	1	<1

*Marked Laboratory Abnormality defined as a shift from Grade 0 to at least Grade 3 or from Grade 1 to Grade 4 (ACTG Grading System)

ANTI-HIV COMPOUNDS: Nelfinavir: Coadministration of nelfinavir with saquinavir (given as FORTOVASE, 1200 mg) resulted in an 18% increase in nelfinavir plasma AUC and a 4-fold increase in saquinavir plasma AUC. If used in combination with saquinavir hard-gelatin capsules at the recommended dose of 600 mg tid, no dose adjustments are needed. Currently, there are no safety and efficacy data available from the use of this combination.

Ritonavir: Following approximately 4 weeks of a combination regimen of saquinavir (400 or 600 mg bid) and ritonavir (400 or 600 mg bid) in HIV-positive patients, saquinavir AUC values were at least 17-fold greater than historical AUC values from patients who received saquinavir 600 mg tid without ritonavir. When used in combination therapy for up to 24 weeks, doses greater than 400 mg bid of either ritonavir or saquinavir were associated with an increase in adverse events.

Delavirdine: Saquinavir AUC increased 5-fold when delavirdine (400 mg tid) and saquinavir (600 mg tid) were administered in combination. Currently, there are limited safety and no efficacy data available from the use of this combination. In a small, preliminary study, hepatocellular enzyme elevations occurred in 15% of subjects during the first several weeks of the delavirdine and saquinavir combination (6% Grade 3 or 4). Hepatocellular enzymes (ALT/AST) should be monitored frequently if this combination is prescribed.

Nevirapine: Coadministration of nevirapine with INVIRASE resulted in a 24% decrease in saquinavir plasma AUC. Currently, there are no safety and efficacy data available from the use of this combination.

Carcinogenesis, Mutagenesis and Impairment of Fertility:

Carcinogenesis: Carcinogenicity studies in rats and mice have not yet been completed.

Mutagenesis: Mutagenicity and genotoxicity studies, with and without metabolic activation where appropriate, have shown that saquinavir has no mutagenic activity in vitro in either bacterial (Ames test) or mammalian cells (Chinese hamster lung V79/HPRT test). Saquinavir does not induce chromosomal damage in vivo in the mouse micronucleus assay or in vitro in human peripheral blood lymphocytes, and does not induce primary DNA damage in vitro in the unscheduled DNA synthesis test.

Impairment of Fertility: Fertility and reproductive performance were not affected in rats at plasma exposures (AUC values) up to five times those achieved in humans at the recommended dose.

Pregnancy: *Teratogenic Effects:* Category B. Reproduction studies conducted with saquinavir in rats have shown no embryotoxicity or teratogenicity at plasma exposures (AUC values) up to five times those achieved in humans at the recommended dose or in rabbits at plasma exposures four times those achieved at the recommended clinical dose. Studies in rats indicated that exposure to saquinavir from late pregnancy through lactation at plasma concentrations (AUC values) up to five times those achieved in humans at the recommended dose had no effect on the survival, growth and development of offspring to weaning. Because animal reproduction studies are not always predictive of human response, INVIRASE should be used during pregnancy after taking into account the importance of the drug to the mother. Presently, there are no reports of infants being born after women receiving INVIRASE in clinical trials became pregnant.

Nursing Mothers: The US Public Health Service Centers for Disease Control and Prevention advises HIV-infected women not to breastfeed to avoid postnatal transmission of HIV to a child who may not yet be infected. It is not known whether INVIRASE is excreted in human milk.

Pediatric Use: Safety and effectiveness of INVIRASE in HIV-infected pediatric patients younger than 16 years of age have not been established.

ADVERSE REACTIONS (see PRECAUTIONS)

The safety of INVIRASE was studied in patients who received the drug either alone or in combination with ZDV and/or HIVID (zalcitabine, ddC). The majority of adverse events were of mild intensity. The most frequently reported adverse events among patients receiving INVIRASE (excluding those toxicities known to be associated with ZDV and HIVID when used in combinations) were diarrhea, abdominal discomfort and nausea.

INVIRASE did not alter the pattern, frequency or severity of known major toxicities associated with the use of HIVID and/or ZDV. Physicians should refer to the complete product information for these drugs (or other antiretroviral agents as appropriate) for drug-associated adverse reactions to other nucleoside analogues.

In an open-label protocol, NV15114, in which 33 patients received treatment with INVIRASE, ZDV and lamivudine for 4 to 16 weeks, no unexpected toxicities were reported.

Table 4 lists clinical adverse events that occurred in ≥2% of patients receiving INVIRASE 600 mg tid alone or in combination with ZDV and/or HIVID in two trials. Median duration of treatment in NV14255/ACTG229 (triple-combination study) was 48 weeks; median duration of treatment in NV14256 (double-combination study) was approximately 1 year.

[See table 4 at top of previous page]

Rare occurrences of the following serious adverse experiences have been reported during clinical trials of INVIRASE and were considered at least possibly related to use of study drugs: confusion, ataxia and weakness; acute myeloblastic leukemia; hemolytic anemia; attempted suicide; Stevens-Johnson syndrome; seizures; severe cutaneous reaction associated with increased liver function tests; isolated elevation of transaminases; thrombophlebitis; headache; thrombocytopenia; exacerbation of chronic liver disease with Grade 4 elevated liver function tests, jaundice, ascites, and right and left upper quadrant abdominal pain; drug fever; bullous skin eruption and polyarthritis; pancreatitis leading to death; nephrolithiasis; thrombocytopenia and intracranial hemorrhage leading to death; peripheral vasoconstriction; portal hypertension; intestinal obstruction. These events were reported from a database of >6000 patients. Over 100 patients on saquinavir therapy have been followed for >2 years.

Table 5 shows the percentage of patients with marked laboratory abnormalities in studies NV14255/ACTG229 and NV14256. Marked laboratory abnormalities are defined as a Grade 3 or 4 abnormality in a patient with a normal baseline value or a Grade 4 abnormality in a patient with a Grade 1 abnormality at baseline (ACTG Grading System).

[See table 5 at top of previous page]

Monotherapy and Combination Studies: Other clinical adverse experiences of any intensity, at least remotely related to INVIRASE, including those in <2% of patients on arms containing INVIRASE in studies NV14255/ACTG229 and NV14256, and those in smaller clinical trials, are listed below by body system.

Body as a Whole: Allergic reaction, anorexia, chest pain, edema, fatigue, fever, intoxication, parasites external, retrosternal pain, shivering, wasting syndrome, weakness generalized, weight decrease

Cardiovascular: Cyanosis, heart murmur, heart valve disorder, hypertension, hypotension, syncope, vein distended

Endocrine/Metabolic: Dehydration, diabetes mellitus, dry eye syndrome, hyperglycemia, weight increase, xerophthalmia

Gastrointestinal: Cheilitis, colic abdominal, constipation, dyspepsia, dysphagia, esophagitis, eructation, feces bloodstained, feces discolored, flatulence, gastralgia, gastritis, gastrointestinal inflammation, gingivitis, glossitis, hemorrhage rectum, hemorrhoids, hepatitis, hepatomegaly, hepatosplenomegaly, infectious diarrhea, jaundice, liver enzyme disorder, melena, pain pelvic, painful defecation, pancreatitis, parotid disorder, salivary glands disorder, stomach upset, stomatitis, toothache, tooth disorder, vomiting

Hematologic: Anemia, bleeding dermal, microhemorrhages, neutropenia, pancytopenia, splenomegaly, thrombocytopenia

Musculoskeletal: Arthralgia, arthritis, back pain, cramps leg, cramps muscle, creatine phosphokinase increased, musculoskeletal disorders, stiffness, tissue changes, trauma

Neurological: Ataxia, bowel movements frequent, confusion, convulsions, dysarthria, dysesthesia, heart rate disorder, hyperesthesia, hyperreflexia, hyporeflexia, light-headed feeling, mouth dry, myelopolyradiculoneuritis, numbness face, pain facial, paresis, poliomyelitis, prickly sensation, progressive multifocal leukoencephalopathy, spasms, tremor, unconsciousness

Psychological: Agitation, amnesia, anxiety, anxiety attack, depression, dreaming excessive, euphoria, hallucination, insomnia, intellectual ability reduced, irritability, lethargy, libido disorder, overdose effect, psychic disorder, psychosis, somnolence, speech disorder, suicide attempt

Reproductive System: Impotence, prostate enlarged, vaginal discharge

Resistance Mechanism: Abscess, angina tonsillaris, candidiasis, cellulitis, herpes simplex, herpes zoster, infection bacterial, infection mycotic, infection staphylococcal, influenza, lymphadenopathy, moniliasis, tumor

Respiratory: Bronchitis, cough, dyspnea, epistaxis, hemoptysis, laryngitis, pharyngitis, pneumonia, pulmonary disease, respiratory disorder, rhinitis, sinusitis, upper respiratory tract infection

Skin and Appendages: Acne, alopecia, chalazion, dermatitis, dermatitis seborrheic, eczema, erythema, folliculitis, furunculosis, hair changes, hot flushes, nail disorder, night sweats, papillomatosis, photosensitivity reaction, pigment changes skin, rash maculopapular, skin disorder, skin nodule, skin ulceration, sweating increased, urticaria, verruca, xeroderma

Special Senses: Blepharitis, earache, ear pressure, eye irritation, hearing decreased, otitis, taste alteration, tinnitus, visual disturbance

Urinary System: Micturition disorder, renal calculus, urinary tract bleeding, urinary tract infection

OVERDOSAGE

No acute toxicities or sequelae were noted in 1 patient who ingested 8 grams of INVIRASE as a single dose. The patient was treated with induction of emesis within 2 to 4 hours after ingestion. In an exploratory Phase 2 study of oral dosing with INVIRASE at 7200 mg/day (1200 mg q4h), there were no serious toxicities reported through the first 25 weeks of treatment.

DOSAGE AND ADMINISTRATION

The recommended dose for INVIRASE in combination with a nucleoside analogue is three 200-mg capsules three times daily taken within 2 hours after a full meal. Please refer to the complete product information for each of the nucleoside analogues for the recommended doses of these agents.

INVIRASE should be used only in combination with an active antiretroviral nucleoside analogue regimen. Concomitant therapy should be based on a patient's prior drug exposure.

Monitoring of Patients: Clinical chemistry tests should be performed prior to initiating INVIRASE therapy and at appropriate intervals thereafter. For comprehensive patient monitoring recommendations for other nucleoside analogues, physicians should refer to the complete product information for these drugs.

Dose Adjustment for Combination Therapy With INVIRASE: For toxicities that may be associated with INVIRASE, the drug should be interrupted. INVIRASE at doses less than 600 mg tid are not recommended since lower doses have not shown antiviral activity. For recipients of combination therapy with INVIRASE and nucleoside analogues, dose adjustment of the nucleoside analogue should be based on the known toxicity profile of the individual drug. Physicians should refer to the complete product information for these drugs for comprehensive dose adjustment recommendations and drug-associated adverse reactions of nucleoside analogues.

HOW SUPPLIED

INVIRASE 200-mg capsules are light brown and green opaque capsules with ROCHE and 0245 imprinted on the capsule shell – bottles of 270 (NDC 0004-0245-15).

The capsules should be stored at 59° to 86°F (15° to 30°C) in tightly closed bottles.

Manufactured by F. Hoffmann-La Roche Ltd., Basel, Switzerland or Hoffmann-La Roche Laboratories Inc., Nutley, New Jersey

Revised: January 1998

Shown in Product Identification Guide, page 333

KLONOPIN® C-IV

[*klon 'o-pin*]

(clonazepam)

TABLETS

The following text is complete prescribing information based on official labeling in effect June 2000.

DESCRIPTION

Klonopin, a benzodiazepine, is available as scored tablets with a K-shaped perforation containing 0.5 mg of clonazepam, and unscored tablets with a K-shaped perforation containing 1 mg or 2 mg of clonazepam. Each tablet also contains lactose, magnesium stearate, microcrystalline cellulose and corn starch, with the following colorants: 0.5 mg—FD&C Yellow No. 6 Lake; 1 mg—FD&C Blue No. 1 Lake and FD&C Blue No. 2 Lake.

Chemically, clonazepam is 5-(2-chlorophenyl)-1,3-dihydro-7-nitro-2*H*-1,4-benzodiazepin-2-one. It is a light yellow crystalline powder. It has a molecular weight of 315.72.

CLINICAL PHARMACOLOGY

Pharmacodynamics: The precise mechanism by which clonazepam exerts its antiseizure and antipanic effects is unknown, although it is believed to be related to its ability to enhance the activity of gamma aminobutyric acid (GABA), the major inhibitory neurotransmitter in the central nervous system. Convulsions produced in rodents by pentylenetetrazol or, to a lesser extent, electrical stimulation are antagonized, as are convulsions produced by photic stimulation in susceptible baboons. A taming effect in aggressive primates, muscle weakness and hypnosis are also produced. In humans, clonazepam is capable of suppressing the spike and wave discharge in absence seizures (petit mal) and decreasing the frequency, amplitude, duration and spread of discharge in minor motor seizures.

Pharmacokinetics: Clonazepam is rapidly and completely absorbed after oral administration. The absolute bioavailability of clonazepam is about 90%. Maximum plasma concentrations of clonazepam are reached within 1 to 4 hours after oral administration. Clonazepam is approximately 85% bound to plasma proteins. Clonazepam is highly metabolized, with less than 2% unchanged clonazepam being excreted in the urine. Biotransformation occurs mainly by reduction of the 7-nitro group to the 4-amino derivative. This derivative can be acetylated, hydroxylated and glucuronidated. Cytochrome P-450 including CYP3A, may play an important role in clonazepam reduction and oxidation. The elimination half-life of clonazepam is typically 30 to 40 hours. Clonazepam pharmacokinetics are dose-independent throughout the dosing range. There is no evidence that clonazepam induces its own metabolism or that of other drugs in humans.

Pharmacokinetics in Demographic Subpopulations and in Disease States: Controlled studies examining the influence of gender and age on clonazepam pharmacokinetics have not been conducted, nor have the effects of renal or liver disease on clonazepam pharmacokinetics been studied. Because clonazepam undergoes hepatic metabolism, it is possible that liver disease will impair clonazepam elimination. Thus, caution should be exercised when administering clonazepam to these patients.

Clinical Trials: *Panic Disorder:* The effectiveness of Klonopin in the treatment of panic disorder was demonstrated in two double-blind, placebo-controlled studies of adult outpatients who had a primary diagnosis of panic disorder (DSM-IIIR) with or without agoraphobia. In these studies, Klonopin was shown to be significantly more effective than placebo in treating panic disorder on change from baseline in panic attack frequency, the Clinician's Global Impression Severity of Illness Score and the Clinician's Global Impression Improvement Score.

Study 1 was a 9-week, fixed-dose study involving Klonopin doses of 0.5, 1.0, 2.0, 3.0 or 4.0 mg/day or placebo. This study was conducted in four phases: a 1-week placebo lead-in, a 3-week upward titration, a 6-week fixed dose and a 7-week discontinuance phase. A significant difference from placebo was observed consistently only for the 1.0 mg/day group. The difference between the 1.0 mg dose group and placebo in reduction from baseline in the number of full panic attacks was approximately 1 panic attack per week. At endpoint, 74% of patients receiving clonazepam 1.0 mg/day were free of full panic attacks, compared to 56% of placebo-treated patients.

Study 2 was a 6-week, flexible-dose study involving Klonopin in a dose range of 0.5 to 4 mg/day or placebo. This study was conducted in three phases: a 1-week placebo lead-in, a 6-week optimal-dose and a 6-week discontinuance phase. The mean clonazepam dose during the optimal dosing period was 2.3 mg/day. The difference between Klonopin and placebo in reduction from baseline in the number of full panic attacks was approximately 1 panic attack per week. At endpoint, 62% of patients receiving clonazepam were free of full panic attacks, compared to 37% of placebo-treated patients.

Subgroup analyses did not indicate that there were any differences in treatment outcomes as a function of race or gender.

INDICATIONS AND USAGE

Seizure Disorders: Klonopin is useful alone or as an adjunct in the treatment of the Lennox-Gastaut syndrome (petit mal variant), akinetic and myoclonic seizures. In patients with absence seizures (petit mal) who have failed to respond to succinimides, Klonopin may be useful.

In some studies, up to 30% of patients have shown a loss of anticonvulsant activity, often within 3 months of administration. In some cases, dosage adjustment may reestablish efficacy.

Panic Disorder: Klonopin is indicated for the treatment of panic disorder, with or without agoraphobia, as defined in DSM-IV. Panic disorder is characterized by the occurrence of unexpected panic attacks and associated concern about having additional attacks, worry about the implications or consequences of the attacks, and/or a significant change in behavior related to the attacks.

The efficacy of Klonopin was established in two 6- to 9-week trials in panic disorder patients whose diagnoses corresponded to the DSM-IIIR category of panic disorder (see CLINICAL PHARMACOLOGY: *Clinical Trials*).

Panic disorder (DSM-IV) is characterized by recurrent unexpected panic attacks, ie, a discrete period of intense fear or discomfort in which four (or more) of the following symptoms develop abruptly and reach a peak within 10 minutes: (1) palpitations, pounding heart or accelerated heart rate; (2) sweating; (3) trembling or shaking; (4) sensations of shortness of breath or smothering; (5) feeling of choking; (6) chest pain or discomfort; (7) nausea or abdominal distress; (8) feeling dizzy, unsteady, lightheaded or faint; (9) dereal-

Continued on next page

Klonopin—Cont.

ization (feelings of unreality) or depersonalization (being detached from oneself); (10) fear of losing control; (11) fear of dying; (12) paresthesias (numbness or tingling sensations); (13) chills or hot flushes.

The effectiveness of Klonopin in long-term use, that is, for more than 9 weeks, has not been systematically studied in controlled clinical trials. The physician who elects to use Klonopin for extended periods should periodically reevaluate the long-term usefulness of the drug for the individual patient (see DOSAGE AND ADMINISTRATION).

CONTRAINDICATIONS

Klonopin should not be used in patients with a history of sensitivity to benzodiazepines, nor in patients with clinical or biochemical evidence of significant liver disease. It may be used in patients with open angle glaucoma who are receiving appropriate therapy but is contraindicated in acute narrow angle glaucoma.

WARNINGS

Interference with Cognitive and Motor Performance: Since Klonopin produces CNS depression, patients receiving this drug should be cautioned against engaging in hazardous occupations requiring mental alertness, such as operating machinery or driving a motor vehicle. They should also be warned about the concomitant use of alcohol or other CNS-depressant drugs during Klonopin therapy (see *Drug Interactions* and *Information for Patients* under PRECAUTIONS).

Pregnancy Risks: Data from several sources raise concerns about the use of Klonopin during pregnancy.

Animal Findings: In three studies in which Klonopin was administered orally to pregnant rabbits at doses of 0.2, 1.0, 5.0 or 10.0 mg/kg/day (low dose approximately 0.2 times the maximum recommended human dose of 20 mg/day for seizure disorders and equivalent to the maximum dose of 4 mg/day for panic disorder, on a mg/m^2 basis) during the period of organogenesis, a similar pattern of malformations (cleft palate, open eyelid, fused sternebrae and limb defects) was observed in a low, non-dose-related incidence in exposed litters from all dosage groups. Reductions in maternal weight gain occurred at dosages of 5 mg/kg/day or greater and reduction in embryo-fetal growth occurred in one study at a dosage of 10 mg/kg/day. No adverse maternal or embryo-fetal effects were observed in mice and rats following administration during organogenesis of oral doses up to 15 mg/kg/day or 40 mg/kg/day, respectively (4 and 20 times the maximum recommended human dose of 20 mg/day for seizure disorders and 20 and 100 times the maximum dose of 4 mg/day for panic disorder, respectively, on a mg/m^2 basis).

General Concerns and Considerations About Anticonvulsants: Recent reports suggest an association between the use of anticonvulsant drugs by women with epilepsy and an elevated incidence of birth defects in children born to these women. Data are more extensive with respect to diphenylhydantoin and phenobarbital, but these are also the most commonly prescribed anticonvulsants; less systematic or anecdotal reports suggest a possible similar association with the use of all known anticonvulsant drugs.

In children of women treated with drugs for epilepsy, reports suggesting an elevated incidence of birth defects cannot be regarded as adequate to prove a definite cause and effect relationship. There are intrinsic methodologic problems in obtaining adequate data on drug teratogenicity in humans; the possibility also exists that other factors (eg, genetic factors or the epileptic condition itself) may be more important than drug therapy in leading to birth defects. The great majority of mothers on anticonvulsant medication deliver normal infants. It is important to note that anticonvulsant drugs should not be discontinued in patients in whom the drug is administered to prevent seizures because of the strong possibility of precipitating status epilepticus with attendant hypoxia and threat to life. In individual cases where the severity and frequency of the seizure disorder are such that the removal of medication does not pose a serious threat to the patient, discontinuation of the drug may be considered prior to and during pregnancy; however, it cannot be said with any confidence that even mild seizures do not pose some hazards to the developing embryo or fetus.

General Concerns About Benzodiazepines: An increased risk of congenital malformations associated with the use of benzodiazepine drugs has been suggested in several studies. There may also be non-teratogenic risks associated with the use of benzodiazepines during pregnancy. There have been reports of neonatal flaccidity, respiratory and feeding difficulties, and hypothermia in children born to mothers who have been receiving benzodiazepines late in pregnancy. In addition, children born to mothers receiving benzodiazepines late in pregnancy may be at some risk of experiencing withdrawal symptoms during the postnatal period.

Advice Regarding the Use of Klonopin in Women of Childbearing Potential: In general, the use of Klonopin in women of childbearing potential, and more specifically during known pregnancy, should be considered only when the clinical situation warrants the risk to the fetus.

The specific considerations addressed above regarding the use of anticonvulsants for epilepsy in women of childbearing potential should be weighed in treating or counseling these women.

Because of experience with other members of the benzodiazepine class, Klonopin is assumed to be capable of causing an increased risk of congenital abnormalities when administered to a pregnant woman during the first trimester. Because use of these drugs is rarely a matter of urgency in the treatment of panic disorder, their use during the first trimester should almost always be avoided. The possibility that a woman of childbearing potential may be pregnant at the time of institution of therapy should be considered. If this drug is used during pregnancy, or if the patient becomes pregnant while taking this drug, the patient should be apprised of the potential hazard to the fetus. Patients should also be advised that if they become pregnant during therapy or intend to become pregnant, they should communicate with their physician about the desirability of discontinuing the drug.

Withdrawal Symptoms: Withdrawal symptoms of the barbiturate type have occurred after the discontinuation of benzodiazepines (see DRUG ABUSE AND DEPENDENCE section).

PRECAUTIONS

General: *Worsening of Seizures:* When used in patients in whom several different types of seizure disorders coexist, Klonopin may increase the incidence or precipitate the onset of generalized tonic-clonic seizures (grand mal). This may require the addition of appropriate anticonvulsants or an increase in their dosages. The concomitant use of valproic acid and Klonopin may produce absence status.

Laboratory Testing During Long-Term Therapy: Periodic blood counts and liver function tests are advisable during long-term therapy with Klonopin.

Risks of Abrupt Withdrawal: The abrupt withdrawal of Klonopin, particularly in those patients on long-term, high-dose therapy, may precipitate status epilepticus. Therefore, when discontinuing Klonopin, gradual withdrawal is essential. While Klonopin is being gradually withdrawn, the simultaneous substitution of another anticonvulsant may be indicated.

Caution in Renally Impaired Patients: Metabolites of Klonopin are excreted by the kidneys; to avoid their excess accumulation, caution should be exercised in the administration of the drug to patients with impaired renal function.

Hypersalivation: Klonopin may produce an increase in salivation. This should be considered before giving the drug to patients who have difficulty handling secretions. Because of this and the possibility of respiratory depression, Klonopin should be used with caution in patients with chronic respiratory diseases.

Information for Patients: Physicians are advised to discuss the following issues with patients for whom they prescribe Klonopin:

Dose Changes: To assure the safe and effective use of benzodiazepines, patients should be informed that, since benzodiazepines may produce psychological and physical dependence, it is advisable that they consult with their physician before either increasing the dose or abruptly discontinuing this drug.

Interference with Cognitive and Motor Performance: Because benzodiazepines have the potential to impair judgment, thinking or motor skills, patients should be cautioned about operating hazardous machinery, including automobiles, until they are reasonably certain that Klonopin therapy does not affect them adversely.

Pregnancy: Patients should be advised to notify their physician if they become pregnant or intend to become pregnant during therapy with Klonopin (see WARNINGS).

Nursing: Patients should be advised not to breastfeed an infant if they are taking Klonopin.

Concomitant Medication: Patients should be advised to inform their physicians if they are taking, or plan to take, any prescription or over-the-counter drugs, since there is a potential for interactions.

Alcohol: Patients should be advised to avoid alcohol while taking Klonopin.

Drug Interactions: *Effect of Clonazepam on the Pharmacokinetics of Other Drugs:* Clonazepam does not appear to alter the pharmacokinetics of phenytoin, carbamazepine or phenobarbital. The effect of clonazepam on the metabolism of other drugs has not been investigated.

Effect of Other Drugs on the Pharmacokinetics of Clonazepam: Ranitidine and propantheline, agents that decrease stomach acidity, do not greatly alter clonazepam pharmacokinetics. Fluoxetine does not affect the pharmacokinetics of clonazepam. Cytochrome P-450 inducers, such as phenytoin, carbamazepine and phenobarbital, induce clonazepam metabolism, causing an approximately 30% decrease in plasma clonazepam levels. Although clinical studies have not been performed, based on the involvement of the cytochrome P-450 3A family in clonazepam metabolism, inhibitors of this enzyme system, notably oral antifungal agents, should be used cautiously in patients receiving clonazepam.

Pharmacodynamic Interactions: The CNS-depressant action of the benzodiazepine class of drugs may be potentiated by alcohol, narcotics, barbiturates, nonbarbiturate hypnotics, antianxiety agents, the phenothiazines, thioxanthene and butyrophenone classes of antipsychotic agents, monoamine oxidase inhibitors and the tricyclic antidepressants, and by other anticonvulsant drugs.

Carcinogenesis, Mutagenesis, Impairment of Fertility: Carcinogenicity studies have not been conducted with clonazepam.

The data currently available are not sufficient to determine the genotoxic potential of clonazepam.

In a two-generation fertility study in which clonazepam was given orally to rats at 10 and 100 mg/kg/day (low dose approximately 5 times and 24 times the maximum recommended human dose of 20 mg/day for seizure disorder and 4 mg/day for panic disorder, respectively, on a mg/m^2 basis), there was a decrease in the number of pregnancies and in the number of offspring surviving until weaning.

Pregnancy: Teratogenic Effects: Pregnancy Category D (see WARNINGS).

Labor and Delivery: The effect of Klonopin on labor and delivery in humans has not been specifically studied; however, perinatal complications have been reported in children born to mothers who have been receiving benzodiazepines late in pregnancy, including findings suggestive of either excess benzodiazepine exposure or of withdrawal phenomena (see *Pregnancy Risks* under WARNINGS).

Nursing Mothers: Mothers receiving Klonopin should not breastfeed their infants.

Pediatric Use: Because of the possibility that adverse effects on physical or mental development could become apparent only after many years, a benefit-risk consideration of the long-term use of Klonopin is important in pediatric patients being treated for seizure disorder (see INDICATIONS and DOSAGE AND ADMINISTRATION sections).

Safety and effectiveness in pediatric patients with panic disorder below the age of 18 have not been established.

ADVERSE REACTIONS

The adverse experiences for Klonopin are provided separately for patients with seizure disorders and with panic disorder.

Seizure Disorders: The most frequently occurring side effects of Klonopin are referable to CNS depression. Experience in treatment of seizures has shown that drowsiness has occurred in approximately 50% of patients and ataxia in approximately 30%. In some cases, these may diminish with time; behavior problems have been noted in approximately 25% of patients. Others, listed by system, are:

Neurologic: Abnormal eye movements, aphonia, choreiform movements, coma, diplopia, dysarthria, dysdiadochokinesis, "glassy-eyed" appearance, headache, hemiparesis, hypotonia, nystagmus, respiratory depression, slurred speech, tremor, vertigo.

Psychiatric: Confusion, depression, amnesia, hallucinations, hysteria, increased libido, insomnia, psychosis, suicidal attempt (the behavior effects are more likely to occur in patients with a history of psychiatric disturbances). The following paradoxical reactions have been observed: excitability, irritability, aggressive behavior, agitation, nervousness, hostility, anxiety, sleep disturbances, nightmares and vivid dreams.

Respiratory: Chest congestion, rhinorrhea, shortness of breath, hypersecretion in upper respiratory passages.

Cardiovascular: Palpitations.

Dermatologic: Hair loss, hirsutism, skin rash, ankle and facial edema.

Gastrointestinal: Anorexia, coated tongue, constipation, diarrhea, dry mouth, encopresis, gastritis, increased appetite, nausea, sore gums.

Genitourinary: Dysuria, enuresis, nocturia, urinary retention.

Musculoskeletal: Muscle weakness, pains.

Miscellaneous: Dehydration, general deterioration, fever, lymphadenopathy, weight loss or gain.

Hematopoietic: Anemia, leukopenia, thrombocytopenia, eosinophilia.

Hepatic: Hepatomegaly, transient elevations of serum transaminases and alkaline phosphatase.

Panic Disorder: Adverse events during exposure to Klonopin were obtained by spontaneous report and recorded by clinical investigators using terminology of their own choosing. Consequently, it is not possible to provide a meaningful estimate of the proportion of individuals experiencing adverse events without first grouping similar types of events into a smaller number of standardized event categories. In the tables and tabulations that follow, CIGY dictionary terminology has been used to classify reported adverse events, except in certain cases in which redundant terms were collapsed into more meaningful terms, as noted below.

The stated frequencies of adverse events represent the proportion of individuals who experienced, at least once, a treatment-emergent adverse event of the type listed. An event was considered treatment-emergent if it occurred for the first time or worsened while receiving therapy following baseline evaluation.

Adverse Findings Observed in Short-Term, Placebo-Controlled Trials: *Adverse Events Associated with Discontinuation of Treatment:*

Overall, the incidence of discontinuation due to adverse events was 17% in Klonopin compared to 9% for placebo in the combined data of two 6- to 9-week trials. The most common events (≥1%) associated with discontinuation and a dropout rate twice or greater for Klonopin than that of placebo included the following:

Adverse Event	Klonopin (N=574)	Placebo (N=294)
Somnolence	7%	1%
Depression	4%	1%
Dizziness	1%	<1%
Nervousness	1%	0%

Ataxia	1%	0%
Intellectual Ability Reduced	1%	0%

Adverse Events Occurring at an Incidence of 1% or More Among Klonopin-Treated Patients:
Table 1 enumerates the incidence, rounded to the nearest percent, of treatment-emergent adverse events that occurred during acute therapy of panic disorder from a pool of two 6- to 9-week trials. Events reported in 1% or more of patients treated with Klonopin (doses ranging from 0.5 to 4 mg/day) and for which the incidence was greater than that in placebo-treated patients are included.
The prescriber should be aware that the figures in Table 1 cannot be used to predict the incidence of side effects in the course of usual medical practice where patient characteristics and other factors differ from those that prevailed in the clinical trials. Similarly, the cited frequencies cannot be compared with figures obtained from other clinical investigations involving different treatments, uses and investigators. The cited figures, however, do provide the prescribing physician with some basis for estimating the relative contribution of drug and nondrug factors to the side effect incidence in the population studied.
[See table above]
Commonly Observed Adverse Events:

Table 2. Incidence of Most Commonly Observed Adverse Events* in Acute Therapy in Pool of 6- to 9-Week Trials

Adverse Event (Roche Preferred Term)	Clonazepam (N=574)	Placebo (N=294)
Somnolence	37%	10%
Depression	7%	1%
Coordination Abnormal	6%	0%
Ataxia	5%	0%

*Treatment-emergent events for which the incidence in the clonazepam patients was ≥5% and at least twice that in the placebo patients.

Treatment-Emergent Depressive Symptoms: In the pool of two short-term placebo-controlled trials, adverse events classified under the preferred term "depression" were reported in 7% of Klonopin-treated patients compared to 1% of placebo-treated patients, without any clear pattern of dose relatedness. In these same trials, adverse events classified under the preferred term "depression" were reported as leading to discontinuation in 4% of Klonopin-treated patients compared to 1% of placebo-treated patients. While these findings are noteworthy, Hamilton Depression Rating Scale (HAM-D) data collected in these trials revealed a larger decline in HAM-D scores in the clonazepam group than the placebo group suggesting that clonazepam-treated patients were not experiencing a worsening or emergence of clinical depression.
Other Adverse Events Observed During the Premarketing Evaluation of Klonopin in Panic Disorder:
Following is a list of modified CIGY terms that reflect treatment-emergent adverse events reported by patients treated with Klonopin at multiple doses during clinical trials. All reported events are included except those already listed in Table 1 or elsewhere in labeling, those events for which a drug cause was remote, those event terms which were so general as to be uninformative, and events reported only once and which did not have a substantial probability of being acutely life-threatening. It is important to emphasize that, although the events occurred during treatment with Klonopin, they were not necessarily caused by it.
Events are further categorized by body system and listed in order of decreasing frequency. These adverse events were reported infrequently, which is defined as occurring in 1/100 to 1/1000 patients.
Body as a Whole: weight increase, accident, weight decrease, wound, edema, fever, shivering, abrasions, ankle edema, edema foot, edema periorbital, injury, malaise, pain, cellulitis, inflammation localized
Cardiovascular Disorders: chest pain, hypotension postural
Central and Peripheral Nervous System Disorders: migraine, paresthesia, drunkenness, feeling of enuresis, paresis, tremor, burning skin, falling, head fullness, hoarseness, hyperactivity, hypoesthesia, tongue thick, twitching
Gastrointestinal System Disorders: abdominal discomfort, gastrointestinal inflammation, stomach upset, toothache, flatulence, pyrosis, saliva increased, tooth disorder, bowel movements frequent, pain pelvic, dyspepsia, hemorrhoids
Hearing and Vestibular Disorders: vertigo, otitis, earache, motion sickness
Heart Rate and Rhythm Disorders: palpitation
Metabolic and Nutritional Disorders: thirst, gout
Musculoskeletal System Disorders: back pain, fracture traumatic, sprains and strains, pain leg, pain nape, cramps muscle, cramps leg, pain ankle, pain shoulder, tendinitis, arthralgia, hypertonia, lumbago, pain feet, pain jaw, pain knee, swelling knee
Platelet, Bleeding and Clotting Disorders: bleeding dermal
Psychiatric Disorders: insomnia, organic disinhibition, anxiety, depersonalization, dreaming excessive, libido loss, appetite increased, libido increased, reactions decreased, aggressive reaction, apathy, attention lack, excitement, feeling mad, hunger abnormal, illusion, nightmares, sleep disorder, suicide ideation, yawning

Table 1. Treatment-Emergent Adverse Event Incidence in 6- to 9-Week Placebo-Controlled Clinical Trials*
Clonazepam Maximum Daily Dose

Adverse Event by Body System	<1 mg n=96 %	1-<2 mg n=129 %	2-<3 mg n=113 %	≥3 mg n=235 %	All Klonopin Groups N=574 %	Placebo N=294 %
Central & Peripheral Nervous System						
Somnolence†	26	35	50	36	37	10
Dizziness	5	5	12	8	8	4
Coordination Abnormal†	1	2	7	9	6	0
Ataxia†	2	1	8	8	5	0
Dysarthria†	0	0	4	3	2	0
Psychiatric						
Depression	7	6	8	8	7	1
Memory Disturbance	2	5	2	5	4	2
Nervousness	1	4	3	4	3	2
Intellectual Ability Reduced	0	2	4	3	2	0
Emotional Lability	0	1	2	2	1	1
Libido Decreased	0	1	3	1	1	0
Confusion	0	2	2	1	1	0
Respiratory System						
Upper Respiratory Tract Infection†	10	10	7	6	8	4
Sinusitis	4	2	8	4	4	3
Rhinitis	3	2	4	2	2	1
Coughing	2	2	4	0	2	0
Pharyngitis	1	1	3	2	2	1
Bronchitis	1	0	2	2	1	1
Gastrointestinal System						
Constipation†	0	1	5	3	2	2
Appetite Decreased	1	1	0	3	1	1
Abdominal Pain†	2	2	2	0	1	1
Body as a Whole						
Fatigue	9	6	7	7	7	4
Allergic Reaction	3	1	4	2	2	1
Musculoskeletal						
Myalgia	2	1	4	0	1	1
Resistance Mechanism Disorders						
Influenza	3	2	5	5	4	3
Urinary System						
Micturition Frequency	1	2	2	1	1	0
Urinary Tract Infection†	0	0	2	2	1	0
Vision Disorders						
Blurred Vision	1	2	3	0	1	1
Reproductive Disorders‡						
Female						
Dysmenorrhea	0	6	5	2	3	2
Colpitis	4	0	2	1	1	1
Male						
Ejaculation Delayed	0	0	2	2	1	0
Impotence	3	0	2	1	1	0

* Events reported by at least 1% of patients treated with Klonopin and for which the incidence was greater than that for placebo.
† Indicates that the p-value for the dose-trend test (Cochran-Mantel-Haenszel) for adverse event incidence was ≤0.10.
‡ Denominators for events in gender-specific systems are n=240 (clonazepam), 102 (placebo) for male, and 334 (clonazepam), 192 (placebo) for female.

Reproductive Disorders, Female: breast pain, menstrual irregularity
Reproductive Disorders, Male: ejaculation decreased
Resistance Mechanism Disorders: infection mycotic, infection viral, infection streptococcal, herpes simplex infection, infectious mononucleosis, moniliasis
Respiratory System Disorders: sneezing excessive, asthmatic attack, dyspnea, nosebleed, pneumonia, pleurisy
Skin and Appendages Disorders: acne flare, alopecia, xeroderma, dermatitis contact, flushing, pruritus, pustular reaction, skin burns, skin disorder
Special Senses Other, Disorders: taste loss
Urinary System Disorders: dysuria, cystitis, polyuria, urinary incontinence, bladder dysfunction, urinary retention, urinary tract bleeding, urine discoloration
Vascular (Extracardiac) Disorders: thrombophlebitis leg
Vision Disorders: eye irritation, visual disturbance, diplopia, eye twitching, styes, visual field defect, xerophthalmia

DRUG ABUSE AND DEPENDENCE

Controlled Substance Class: Clonazepam is a Schedule IV controlled substance.
Physical and Psychological Dependence: Withdrawal symptoms, similar in character to those noted with barbiturates and alcohol (eg, convulsions, psychosis, hallucinations, behavioral disorder, tremor, abdominal and muscle cramps) have occurred following abrupt discontinuance of clonazepam. The more severe withdrawal symptoms have usually been limited to those patients who received excessive doses over an extended period of time. Generally milder withdrawal symptoms (eg, dysphoria and insomnia) have been reported following abrupt discontinuance of benzodiazepines taken continuously at therapeutic levels for several months. Consequently, after extended therapy, abrupt discontinuation should generally be avoided and a gradual dosage tapering schedule followed (see DOSAGE AND ADMINISTRATION section). Addiction-prone individuals (such as drug addicts or alcoholics) should be under careful surveillance when receiving clonazepam or other psychotropic agents because of the predisposition of such patients to habituation and dependence.
Following the short-term treatment of patients with panic disorder in Studies 1 and 2 (see CLINICAL PHARMACOLOGY: *Clinical Trials*), patients were gradually withdrawn during a 7-week downward-titration (discontinuance) period. Overall, the discontinuance period was associated with good tolerability and a very modest clinical deterioration, without evidence of a significant rebound phenomenon. However, there are not sufficient data from adequate and well-controlled long-term clonazepam studies in patients with panic disorder to accurately estimate the risks of withdrawal symptoms and dependence that may be associated with such use.

OVERDOSAGE

Human Experience: Symptoms of clonazepam overdosage, like those produced by other CNS depressants, include somnolence, confusion, coma and diminished reflexes.
Overdose Management: Treatment includes monitoring of respiration, pulse and blood pressure, general supportive measures and immediate gastric lavage. Intravenous fluids should be administered and an adequate airway maintained. Hypotension may be combated by the use of levarterenol or metaraminol. Dialysis is of no known value.
Flumazenil, a specific benzodiazepine-receptor antagonist, is indicated for the complete or partial reversal of the sedative effects of benzodiazepines and may be used in situations when an overdose with a benzodiazepine is known or suspected. Prior to the administration of flumazenil, necessary measures should be instituted to secure airway, ventilation and intravenous access. Flumazenil is intended as an adjunct to, not as a substitute for, proper management of benzodiazepine overdose. Patients treated with flumazenil should be monitored for resedation, respiratory depression

Continued on next page

Klonopin—Cont.

and other residual benzodiazepine effects for an appropriate period after treatment. **The prescriber should be aware of a risk of seizure in association with flumazenil treatment, particularly in long-term benzodiazepine users and in cyclic antidepressant overdose.** The complete flumazenil package insert, including CONTRAINDICATIONS, WARNINGS and PRECAUTIONS, should be consulted prior to use.
Flumazenil is not indicated in patients with epilepsy who have been treated with benzodiazepines. Antagonism of the benzodiazepine effect in such patients may provoke seizures.
Serious sequelae are rare unless other drugs or alcohol have been taken concomitantly.

DOSAGE AND ADMINISTRATION

Seizure Disorders: *Adults*: The initial dose for adults with seizure disorders should not exceed 1.5 mg/day divided into three doses. Dosage may be increased in increments of 0.5 to 1 mg every 3 days until seizures are adequately controlled or until side effects preclude any further increase. Maintenance dosage must be individualized for each patient depending upon response. Maximum recommended daily dose is 20 mg.
The use of multiple anticonvulsants may result in an increase of depressant adverse effects. This should be considered before adding Klonopin to an existing anticonvulsant regimen.
Pediatric Patients: Klonopin is administered orally. In order to minimize drowsiness, the initial dose for infants and children (up to 10 years of age or 30 kg of body weight) should be between 0.01 and 0.03 mg/kg/day but not to exceed 0.05 mg/kg/day given in two or three divided doses. Dosage should be increased by no more than 0.25 to 0.5 mg every third day until a daily maintenance dose of 0.1 to 0.2 mg/kg of body weight has been reached, unless seizures are controlled or side effects preclude further increase. Whenever possible, the daily dose should be divided into three equal doses. If doses are not equally divided, the largest dose should be given before retiring.
Panic Disorder: *Adults*: The initial dose for adults with panic disorder is 0.25 mg bid. An increase to the target dose for most patients of 1 mg/day may be made after 3 days. The recommended dose of 1 mg/day is based on the results from a fixed dose study in which the optimal effect was seen at 1 mg/day. Higher doses of 2, 3 and 4 mg/day in that study were less effective than the 1 mg/day dose and were associated with more adverse effects. Nevertheless, it is possible that some individual patients may benefit from doses of up to a maximum dose of 4 mg/day, and in those instances, the dose may be increased in increments of 0.125 to 0.25 mg bid every 3 days until panic disorder is controlled or until side effects make further increases undesired. To reduce the inconvenience of somnolence, administration of one dose at bedtime may be desirable.
Treatment should be discontinued gradually, with a decrease of 0.125 mg bid every 3 days, until the drug is completely withdrawn.
There is no body of evidence available to answer the question of how long the patient treated with clonazepam should remain on it. Therefore, the physician who elects to use Klonopin for extended periods should periodically reevaluate the long-term usefulness of the drug for the individual patient.
Pediatric Patients: There is no clinical trial experience with Klonopin in panic disorder patients under 18 years of age.

HOW SUPPLIED

Scored tablets with a K-shaped perforation—0.5 mg, orange (NDC 0004-0068-01); and unscored tablets with a K-shaped perforation—1 mg, blue (NDC 0004-0058-01); 2 mg, white (NDC 0004-0098-01)—bottles of 100. Imprint on tablets:

0.5 mg—1/2 KLONOPIN (front)
ROCHE (scored side)

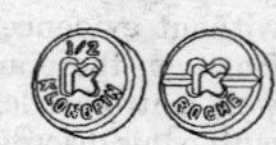

1 mg—1 KLONOPIN (front)
ROCHE (reverse side)

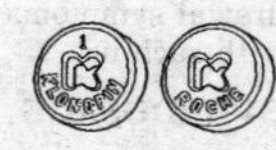

2 mg—2 KLONOPIN (front)
ROCHE (reverse side)

Store at 59° to 86°F (15° to 30°C).

Revised: April 1999

Shown in Product Identification Guide, page 333

LARIAM® ℞

[lar-é-um]
brand of mefloquine hydrochloride
TABLETS

DESCRIPTION

Lariam (mefloquine hydrochloride) is an antimalarial agent available as 250-mg tablets of mefloquine hydrochloride (equivalent to 228.0 mg of the free base) for oral administration.
Mefloquine hydrochloride is a 4-quinolinemethanol derivative with the specific chemical name of (R*, S*)-(±)-α-2-piperidinyl-2,8-bis (trifluoromethyl)-4-quinolinemethanol hydrochloride. It is a 2-aryl substituted chemical structural analog of quinine. The drug is a white to almost white crystalline compound, slightly soluble in water.
Mefloquine hydrochloride has a calculated molecular weight of 414.78 and the following structural formula:

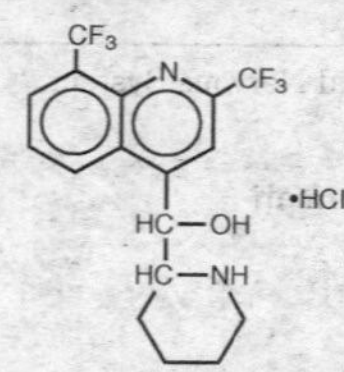

The inactive ingredients are ammonium-calcium alginate, corn starch, crospovidone, lactose, magnesium stearate, microcrystalline cellulose, poloxamer #331, and talc.

CLINICAL PHARMACOLOGY

Mefloquine is an antimalarial agent which acts as a blood schizonticide. Its exact mechanism of action is not known.
Pharmacokinetic studies of mefloquine in healthy male subjects showed that a significant lagtime occurred after drug administration, and the terminal elimination half-life varied widely (13 to 24 days) with a mean of about 3 weeks. Mefloquine is a mixture of enantiomeric molecules whose rates of release, absorption, transport, action, degradation and elimination may differ. A valid pharmacokinetic model may not exist in such a case.
Additional studies in European subjects showed slightly greater concentrations of drug for longer periods of time. The absorption half-life was 0.36 to 2 hours, and the terminal elimination half-life was 15 to 33 days. The primary metabolite was identified and its concentrations were found to surpass the concentrations of mefloquine.
Multiple-dose kinetic studies confirmed the long elimination half-lives previously observed. The mean metabolite to mefloquine ratio measured at steady-state was found to range between 2.3 and 8.6.
The total clearance of the drug, which is essentially all hepatic, is approximately 30 mL/min. The volume of distribution, approximately 20 L/kg, indicates extensive distribution. The drug is highly bound (98%) to plasma proteins and concentrated in blood erythrocytes, the target cells in malaria, at a relatively constant erythrocyte-to-plasma concentration ratio of about 2.
The pharmacokinetics of mefloquine in patients with compromised renal function and compromised hepatic function have not been studied.
In vitro and in vivo studies showed no hemolysis associated with glucose-6-phosphate dehydrogenase deficiency (see **ANIMAL TOXICOLOGY**).
Microbiology: Strains of *Plasmodium falciparum* resistant to mefloquine have been reported.

INDICATIONS AND USAGE

Treatment of Acute Malaria Infections: Lariam is indicated for the treatment of mild to moderate acute malaria caused by mefloquine-susceptible strains of *P. falciparum* (both chloroquine-susceptible and resistant strains) or by *Plasmodium vivax*. There are insufficient clinical data to document the effect of mefloquine in malaria caused by *P. ovale* or *P. malariae*.
Note: Patients with acute *P. vivax* malaria, treated with Lariam, are at high risk of relapse because Lariam does not eliminate exoerythrocytic (hepatic phase) parasites. To avoid relapse, after initial treatment of the acute infection with Lariam, patients should subsequently be treated with an 8-aminoquinoline (eg, primaquine).
Prevention of Malaria: Lariam is indicated for the prophylaxis of *P. falciparum* and *P. vivax* malaria infections, including prophylaxis of chloroquine-resistant strains of *P. falciparum*.

CONTRAINDICATIONS

Use of Lariam is contraindicated in patients with a known hypersensitivity to mefloquine or related compounds (eg, quinine and quinidine). Lariam should not be prescribed for prophylaxis in patients with active depression or with a history of psychosis or convulsions.

WARNINGS

In case of life-threatening, serious or overwhelming malaria infections due to *P. falciparum*, patients should be treated with an intravenous antimalarial drug. Following completion of intravenous treatment, Lariam may be given to complete the course of therapy.
Data on the use of halofantrine subsequent to administration of Lariam suggests a significant, potentially fatal prolongation of the QTc interval of the ECG. Therefore, halofantrine must not be given simultaneously with or subsequent to Lariam. No data are available on the use of Lariam after halofantrine (see PRECAUTIONS: *Drug Interactions*).
Concomitant administration of Lariam and quinine or quinidine may produce electrocardiographic abnormalities.
Concomitant administration of Lariam and quinine or chloroquine may increase the risk of convulsions.

PRECAUTIONS

General: In patients with epilepsy, Lariam may increase the risk of convulsions. The drug should therefore be prescribed only for curative treatment in such patients and only if there are compelling medical reasons for its use (see **PRECAUTIONS: *Drug Interactions***).
Caution should be exercised with regard to activities requiring alertness and fine motor coordination such as driving, piloting aircraft and operating machinery, as dizziness, a loss of balance, or other disorders of the central or peripheral nervous system have been reported during and following the use of Lariam. These effects may occur after therapy is discontinued due to the long half-life of the drug. During prophylactic use, if signs of acute anxiety, depression, restlessness or confusion occur, these may be considered prodromal to a more serious event. In these cases, the drug must be discontinued. Lariam should be used with caution in patients with psychiatric disturbances because mefloquine use has been associated with emotional disturbances (see **ADVERSE REACTIONS**).
In patients with impaired liver function the elimination of mefloquine may be prolonged, leading to higher plasma levels.
This drug has been administered for longer than 1 year. If the drug is to be administered for a prolonged period, periodic evaluations including liver function tests should be performed. Although retinal abnormalities seen in humans with long-term chloroquine use have not been observed with mefloquine use, long-term feeding of mefloquine to rats resulted in dose-related ocular lesions (retinal degeneration, retinal edema and lenticular opacity at 12.5 mg/kg/day and higher) (see **ANIMAL TOXICOLOGY**). Therefore, periodic ophthalmic examinations are recommended.
Parenteral studies in animals show that mefloquine, a myocardial depressant, possesses 20% of the antifibrillatory action of quinidine and produces 50% of the increase in the PR interval reported with quinine. The effect of mefloquine on the compromised cardiovascular system has not been evaluated. However, transitory and clinically silent ECG alterations have been reported during the use of mefloquine. Alterations included sinus bradycardia, sinus arrhythmia, first degree AV-block, prolongation of the QTc interval and abnormal T waves (see also cardiovascular effects under **PRECAUTIONS: *Drug Interactions*** and **ADVERSE REACTIONS**). The benefits of Lariam therapy should be weighed against the possibility of adverse effects in patients with cardiac disease.
Laboratory Tests: Periodic evaluation of hepatic function should be performed during prolonged prophylaxis.
Information for Patients: Patients should be advised:

- that malaria can be a life-threatening infection in the traveler;
- that Lariam is being prescribed to help prevent or treat this serious infection;
- that in a small percentage of cases, patients are unable to take this medication because of side effects, and it may be necessary to change medications;
- that when used as prophylaxis, the first dose of Lariam should be taken one week prior to departure;
- that if the patient experiences any symptom that may affect the patient's ability to take this drug as prescribed, the physician should be contacted and alternative antimalarial medication should be considered;
- that no chemoprophylactic regimen is 100% effective, and protective clothing, insect repellents, and bednets are important components of malaria prophylaxis;
- to seek medical attention for any febrile illness that occurs after return from a malarious area and inform their physician that they may have been exposed to malaria.

Drug Interactions: Drug-drug interactions with Lariam have not been explored in detail. There is one report of cardiopulmonary arrest, with full recovery, in a patient who was taking a beta blocker (propranolol) (see **PRECAUTIONS: *General***). The effects of mefloquine on the compromised cardiovascular system have not been evaluated. The benefits of Lariam therapy should be weighed against the possibility of adverse effects in patients with cardiac disease.
Because of the danger of a potentially fatal prolongation of the QTc interval, halofantrine should not be given simultaneously with or subsequent to Lariam (see **WARNINGS**).
Concomitant administration of Lariam and other related compounds (eg, quinine, quinidine and chloroquine) may produce electrocardiographic abnormalities and increase the risk of convulsions (see **CONTRAINDICATIONS**). If these drugs are to be used in the initial treatment of severe malaria, Lariam administration should be delayed at least 12 hours after the last dose. There is evidence that the use of halofantrine after mefloquine causes a significant lengthening of the QTc interval. Clinically significant QTc prolongation has not been found with mefloquine alone.
This appears to be the only clinically relevant interaction of this kind with Lariam, although theoretically, coadministration of other drugs known to alter cardiac conduction (eg, anti-arrhythmic or beta-adrenergic blocking agents, calcium channel blockers, antihistamines or H1-blocking agents, tricyclic antidepressants and phenothiazines) might also contribute to a prolongation of the QTc interval. There are no data that conclusively establish whether the concomitant administration of mefloquine and the above listed agents has an effect on cardiac function.
In patients taking an anticonvulsant (eg, valproic acid, carbamazepine, phenobarbital or phenytoin), the concomitant use of Lariam may reduce seizure control by lowering the plasma levels of the anticonvulsant. Therefore, patients concurrently taking antiseizure medication and Lariam

should have the blood level of their antiseizure medication monitored and the dosage adjusted appropriately (see **PRECAUTIONS:** ***General***).

When Lariam is taken concurrently with oral live typhoid vaccines, attenuation of immunization cannot be excluded. Vaccinations with attenuated live bacteria should therefore be completed at least 3 days before the first dose of Lariam. No other drug interactions are known. Nevertheless, the effects of Lariam on travelers receiving comedication, particularly those on anticoagulants or antidiabetics, should be checked before departure.

In clinical trials, the concomitant administration of sulfadoxine and pyrimethamine did not alter the adverse reaction profile.

Carcinogenesis, Mutagenesis, Impairment of Fertility: *Carcinogenesis:* The carcinogenic potential of mefloquine was studied in rats and mice in 2-year feeding studies at doses of up to 30 mg/kg/day. No treatment-related increases in tumors of any type were noted.

Mutagenesis: The mutagenic potential of mefloquine was studied in a variety of assay systems including: Ames test, a host-mediated assay in mice, fluctuation tests and a mouse micronucleus assay. Several of these assays were performed with and without prior metabolic activation. In no instance was evidence obtained for the mutagenicity of mefloquine.

Impairment of Fertility: Fertility studies in rats at doses of 5, 20, and 50 mg/kg/day of mefloquine have demonstrated adverse effects on fertility in the male at the high dose of 50 mg/kg/day, and in the female at doses of 20 and 50 mg/kg/day. Histopathological lesions were noted in the epididymides from male rats at doses of 20 and 50 mg/kg/day. Administration of 250 mg/week of mefloquine (base) in adult males for 22 weeks failed to reveal any deleterious effects on human spermatozoa.

Pregnancy: Teratogenic Effects. Pregnancy Category C. Mefloquine has been demonstrated to be teratogenic in rats and mice at a dose of 100 mg/kg/day. In rabbits, a high dose of 160 mg/kg/day was embryotoxic and teratogenic, and a dose of 80 mg/kg/day was teratogenic but not embryotoxic. There are no adequate and well-controlled studies in pregnant women. However, clinical experience with Lariam has not revealed an embryotoxic or teratogenic effect. Mefloquine should be used during pregnancy only if the potential benefit justifies the potential risk to the fetus. Women of childbearing potential who are traveling to areas where malaria is endemic should be warned against becoming pregnant. Women of childbearing potential should also be advised to practice contraception during malaria prophylaxis with Lariam.

Nursing Mothers: Mefloquine is excreted in human milk. Based on a study in a few subjects, low concentrations (3% to 4%) of mefloquine were excreted in human milk following a dose equivalent to 250 mg of the free base. Because of the potential for serious adverse reactions in nursing infants from mefloquine, a decision should be made whether to discontinue the drug, taking into account the importance of the drug to the mother.

Pediatric Use: Use of Lariam to treat acute, uncomplicated *P. falciparum* malaria in pediatric patients is supported by evidence from adequate and well-controlled studies of Lariam in adults with additional data from published open-label and comparative trials using Lariam to treat malaria caused by *P. falciparum* in patients younger than 16 years of age. The safety and effectiveness of Lariam for the treatment of malaria in pediatric patients below the age of 6 months have not been established.

In several studies, the administration of Lariam for the treatment of malaria was associated with early vomiting in pediatric patients. Early vomiting was cited in some reports as a possible cause of treatment failure. If a second dose is not tolerated, the patient should be monitored closely and alternative malaria treatment considered if improvement is not observed within a reasonable period of time (see **DOSAGE AND ADMINISTRATION**).

ADVERSE REACTIONS

Clinical: At the doses used for treatment of acute malaria infections, the symptoms possibly attributable to drug administration cannot be distinguished from those symptoms usually attributable to the disease itself.

Among subjects who received mefloquine for prophylaxis of malaria, the most frequently observed adverse experience was vomiting (3%). Dizziness, syncope, extrasystoles and other complaints affecting less than 1% were also reported.

Among subjects who received mefloquine for treatment, the most frequently observed adverse experiences included: dizziness, myalgia, nausea, fever, headache, vomiting, chills, diarrhea, skin rash, abdominal pain, fatigue, loss of appetite, and tinnitus. Those side effects occurring in less than 1% included bradycardia, hair loss, emotional problems, pruritus, asthenia, transient emotional disturbances and telogen effluvium (loss of resting hair). Seizures have also been reported.

Two serious adverse reactions were cardiopulmonary arrest in one patient shortly after ingesting a single prophylactic dose of mefloquine while concomitantly using propranolol (see **PRECAUTIONS**), and encephalopathy of unknown etiology during prophylactic mefloquine administration. The relationship of encephalopathy to drug administration could not be clearly established.

Postmarketing: Postmarketing surveillance indicates that the same adverse experiences are reported during prophylaxis, as well as acute treatment.

The most common adverse reactions to Lariam prophylaxis, namely nausea, vomiting, and dizziness, are generally mild and may decrease with prolonged use, in spite of increasing plasma drug levels. In a large study of tourists receiving various prophylactic antimalarials, the rate of subjects reporting adverse events on Lariam was similar to that of tourists on chloroquine.

The most frequently reported adverse events are nausea, vomiting, dizziness or vertigo, loss of balance, headache, somnolence, sleep disorders (insomnia, abnormal dreams), loose stools or diarrhea, and abdominal pain.

Less frequently reported adverse events:

Central and peripheral nervous system: convulsions, depression, hallucinations, psychotic or paranoid reactions, anxiety, agitation, aggression, confusion, forgetfulness, hearing impairment, restlessness, sensory and motor neuropathies (including paresthesia), tinnitus and vestibular disorders, visual disturbances. Suicidal ideation has also rarely been reported, but no relationship to drug administration has been established.

Cardiovascular system: circulatory disturbances (hypotension, hypertension, flushing, syncope), tachycardia or palpitations, bradycardia, irregular pulse, extrasystoles and other transient cardiac conduction alterations.

Skin: rash, exanthema, erythema, urticaria, pruritus, hair loss, sweating.

Musculoskeletal system: muscle weakness, muscle cramps, myalgia, arthralgia.

General symptoms: asthenia, malaise, fatigue, fever, chills, loss of appetite.

Isolated cases of erythema multiforme, Stevens-Johnson syndrome, AV-block, and encephalopathy, have been reported.

Laboratory: The most frequently observed laboratory alterations which could be possibly attributable to drug administration were decreased hematocrit, transient elevation of transaminases, leukopenia and thrombocytopenia. These alterations were observed in patients with acute malaria who received treatment doses of the drug and were attributed to the disease itself.

During prophylactic administration of mefloquine to indigenous populations in malaria-endemic areas, the following occasional alterations in laboratory values were observed: transient elevation of transaminases, leukocytosis or thrombocytopenia.

Because of the long half-life of mefloquine, adverse reactions to Lariam may occur or persist up to several weeks after the last dose.

OVERDOSAGE

In cases of overdosage with Lariam, the symptoms mentioned under **ADVERSE REACTIONS** may be more pronounced. The following procedure is recommended in case of overdosage: Induce vomiting or perform gastric lavage, as appropriate. Monitor cardiac function (if possible by ECG) and neurologic and psychiatric status for at least 24 hours. Provide symptomatic and intensive supportive treatment as required, particularly for cardiovascular disturbances. Treat vomiting or diarrhea with standard fluid therapy.

DOSAGE AND ADMINISTRATION (see INDICATIONS AND USAGE)

Adult Patients: *Treatment of mild to moderate malaria in adults caused by P. vivax or mefloquine-susceptible strains of P. falciparum:* Five tablets (1250 mg) mefloquine hydrochloride to be given as a single oral dose. The drug should not be taken on an empty stomach and should be administered with at least 8 oz (240 mL) of water.

If a full treatment course has been administered without clinical cure, alternative treatment should be given. Similarly, if previous prophylaxis with mefloquine has failed, Lariam should not be used for curative treatment.

Note: Patients with acute *P. vivax* malaria, treated with Lariam, are at high risk of relapse because Lariam does not eliminate exoerythrocytic (hepatic phase) parasites. To avoid relapse after initial treatment of the acute infection with Lariam, patients should subsequently be treated with an 8-aminoquinoline (eg, primaquine).

Malaria prophylaxis: One 250 mg Lariam tablet once weekly.

Prophylactic drug administration should begin 1 week before departure to an endemic area. Subsequent weekly doses should always be taken on the same day of the week. To reduce the risk of malaria after leaving an endemic area, prophylaxis should be continued for 4 additional weeks. Tablets should not be taken on an empty stomach and should be administered with at least 8 oz (240 mL) of water.

In certain cases, eg, when a traveler is taking other medication, it may be desirable to start prophylaxis 2 to 3 weeks prior to departure, in order to ensure that the combination of drugs is well tolerated.

Pediatric Patients: *Treatment of mild to moderate malaria in pediatric patients caused by mefloquine-susceptible strains of P. falciparum:* 20 to 25 mg/kg for non-immune patients. Splitting the total curative dose into 2 doses taken 6 to 8 hours apart may reduce the occurrence or severity of adverse effects. Experience with Lariam in infants less than 3 months old or weighing less than 5 kg is limited. The drug should not be taken on an empty stomach and should be administered with ample water. For very young patients, the dose may be crushed, mixed with water or sugar water and may be administered via an oral syringe.

If a full-treatment course has been administered without clinical cure, alternative treatment should be given. Similarly, if previous prophylaxis with mefloquine has failed, Lariam should not be used for curative treatment.

In pediatric patients, the administration of Lariam for the treatment of malaria has been associated with early vomiting. In some cases, early vomiting has been cited as a possible cause of treatment failure (see **PRECAUTIONS**). If a significant loss of drug product is observed or suspected because of vomiting, a second full dose of Lariam should be administered to patients who vomit less than 30 minutes after receiving the drug. If vomiting occurs 30 to 60 minutes after a dose, an additional half-dose should be given. If vomiting recurs, the patient should be monitored closely and alternative malaria treatment considered if improvement is not observed within a reasonable period of time.

The safety and effectiveness of Lariam to treat malaria in pediatric patients below the age of 6 months have not been established.

Malaria Prophylaxis: The following doses have been extrapolated from the recommended adult dose. Neither the pharmacokinetics, nor the clinical efficacy of these doses have been determined in children owing to the difficulty of acquiring this information in pediatric subjects. The recommended prophylactic dose of Lariam is 3 to 5 mg/kg once weekly. One 250 mg Lariam tablet should be taken once weekly in pediatric patients weighing over 45 kg. In pediatric patients weighing less than 45 kg, the weekly dose decreases in proportion to body weight:

>30 to 45 kg: ¾ tablet
>20 to 30 kg: ½ tablet
up to 20 kg: ¼ tablet

Experience with Lariam in infants less than 3 months old or weighing less than 5 kg is limited.

HOW SUPPLIED

Lariam is available as scored, white, round tablets, containing 250 mg of mefloquine hydrochloride in unit-dose packages of 25 (NDC 0004-0172-02). Imprint on tablets: LARIAM 250 ROCHE

Tablets should be stored at 15° to 30°C (59° to 86°F).

ANIMAL TOXICOLOGY

Ocular lesions were observed in rats fed mefloquine daily for 2 years. All surviving rats given 30 mg/kg/day had ocular lesions in both eyes characterized by retinal degeneration, opacity of the lens, and retinal edema. Similar but less severe lesions were observed in 80% of female and 22% of male rats fed 12.5 mg/kg/day for 2 years. At doses of 5 mg/kg/day, only corneal lesions were observed. They occurred in 9% of rats studied.

Manufactured by
F. HOFFMANN-LA ROCHE LTD
Basel, Switzerland
Distributed by
Roche Pharmaceuticals
Revised: August 1999

Shown in Product Identification Guide, page 333

ROCALTROL® ℞

[ro-cal 'trol]
brand of calcitriol
CAPSULES and ORAL SOLUTION

The following text is complete prescribing information based on official labeling in effect June 2000.

DESCRIPTION

Rocaltrol (calcitriol) is a synthetic vitamin D analog which is active in the regulation of the absorption of calcium from the gastrointestinal tract and its utilization in the body. Rocaltrol is available as capsules containing 0.25 mcg or 0.5 mcg calcitriol and as an oral solution containing 1 mcg/mL of calcitriol. All dosage forms contain butylated hydroxyanisole (BHA) and butylated hydroxytoluene (BHT) as antioxidants. The capsules contain a fractionated triglyceride of coconut oil, and the oral solution contains a fractionated triglyceride of palm seed oil. Gelatin capsule shells contain glycerin, parabens (methyl and propyl) and sorbitol, with the following dye systems: 0.25 mcg—FD&C Yellow No. 6 and titanium dioxide; 0.5 mcg—FD&C Red No. 3, FD&C Yellow No. 6 and titanium dioxide. The oral solution contains no additional adjuvants or coloring principles.

Calcitriol is a white, crystalline compound which occurs naturally in humans. It has a calculated molecular weight of 416.65 and is soluble in organic solvents but relatively insoluble in water. Chemically, calcitriol is 9,10-seco(5Z,7E)-5,7,10(19)-cholestatriene-1α, 3β, 25-triol.

The other names frequently used for calcitriol are 1α,25-dihydroxycholecalciferol, 1,25-dihydroxyvitamin D_3, 1,25-DHCC, 1,25$(OH)_2D_3$ and 1,25-diOHC.

CLINICAL PHARMACOLOGY

Man's natural supply of vitamin D depends mainly on exposure to the ultraviolet rays of the sun for conversion of 7-dehydrocholesterol in the skin to vitamin D_3 (cholecalciferol). Vitamin D_3 must be metabolically activated in the liver and the kidney before it is fully active as a regulator of calcium and phosphorus metabolism at target tissues. The initial transformation of vitamin D_3 is catalyzed by a vitamin D_3-25-hydroxylase enzyme (25-OHase) present in the liver, and

Continued on next page

Rocaltrol—Cont.

the product of this reaction is 25-hydroxyvitamin D_3 [25-$(OH)D_3$]. Hydroxylation of 25-$(OH)D_3$ occurs in the mitochondria of kidney tissue, activated by the renal 25-hydroxyvitamin D_3-1 alpha-hydroxylase (alpha-OHase), to produce 1,25-$(OH)_2D_3$ (calcitriol), the active form of vitamin D_3. Endogenous synthesis and catabolism of calcitriol, as well as physiological control mechanisms affecting these processes, play a critical role regulating the serum level of calcitriol.

Pharmacodynamics: The two known sites of action of calcitriol are intestine and bone. A calcitriol receptor-binding protein appears to exist in the mucosa of human intestine. Additional evidence suggests that calcitriol may also act on the kidney and the parathyroid glands. Calcitriol is the most active known form of vitamin D_3 in stimulating intestinal calcium transport. In acutely uremic rats calcitriol has been shown to stimulate intestinal calcium absorption. The kidneys of uremic patients cannot adequately synthesize calcitriol, the active hormone formed from precursor vitamin D. Resultant hypocalcemia and secondary hyperparathyroidism are a major cause of the metabolic bone disease of renal failure. However, other bone-toxic substances which accumulate in uremia (eg, aluminum) may also contribute. The beneficial effect of Rocaltrol in renal osteodystrophy appears to result from correction of hypocalcemia and secondary hyperparathyroidism. It is uncertain whether Rocaltrol produces other independent beneficial effects. Rocaltrol treatment is not associated with an accelerated rate of renal function deterioration. No radiographic evidence of extraskeletal calcification has been found in predialysis patients following treatment. The duration of pharmacologic activity of a single dose of calcitriol is about 3 to 5 days.

Pharmacokinetics: *Absorption:* Calcitriol is rapidly absorbed from the intestine. Peak serum concentrations (above basal values) were reached within 3 to 6 hours following oral administration of single doses of 0.25 to 1.0 mcg of Rocaltrol. Following a single oral dose of 0.5 mcg, mean serum concentrations of calcitriol rose from a baseline value of 40.0±4.4 (S.D.) pg/mL to 60.0±4.4 pg/mL at 2 hours, and declined to 53.0±6.9 at 4 hours, 50±7.0 at 8 hours, 44±4.6 at 12 hours and 41.5±5.1 at 24 hours.

Distribution: Calcitriol is approximately 99.9% bound in blood. Calcitriol and other vitamin D metabolites are transported in blood, by an alpha-globulin vitamin D binding protein. There is evidence that maternal calcitriol may enter the fetal circulation. Calcitriol is transferred into human milk at low levels (ie, 2.2±0.1 pg/mL).

Metabolism: In vivo and in vitro studies indicate the presence of two pathways of metabolism for calcitriol. The first pathway involves the 24-hydroxylase as the first step in catabolism of calcitriol. There is definite evidence of 24-hydroxylase activity in the kidney; this enzyme is also present in many target tissues which possess the vitamin D receptor such as the intestine. The end product of this pathway is a side chain shortened metabolite, calcitroic acid. The second pathway involves the conversion of calcitriol via the stepwise hydroxylation of carbon-26 and carbon-23, and cyclization to yield ultimately 1α, 25R$(OH)_2$-26, 23S-lactone D_3. The lactone appears to be the major metabolite circulating in humans, with mean serum concentrations of 131±17 pg/mL. In addition, several other metabolites of calcitriol have been identified: 1α, 25$(OH)_2$-24-oxo-D_3; 1α, 23,25$(OH)_3$-24-oxo-D_3; 1α, 24R,25$(OH)_3D_3$; 1α, 25S,26$(OH)_3D_3$; 1α, 25$(OH)_2$-23-oxo-D_3; 1α, 25R,26$(OH)_3$-23-oxo-D_3; 1α, (OH)24,25,26,27-tetranor-COOH-D_3.

Excretion: Enterohepatic recycling and biliary excretion of calcitriol occur. The metabolites of calcitriol are excreted primarily in feces. Following intravenous administration of radiolabeled calcitriol in normal subjects, approximately 27% and 7% of the radioactivity appeared in the feces and urine, respectively, within 24 hours. When a 1-mcg oral dose of radiolabeled calcitriol was administered to normal subjects, approximately 10% of the total radioactivity appeared in urine within 24 hours. Cumulative excretion of radioactivity on the sixth day following intravenous administration of radiolabeled calcitriol averaged 16% in urine and 49% in feces. The elimination half-life of calcitriol in serum after single oral doses is about 5 to 8 hours in normal subjects.

Special Populations: *Pediatric Pharmacokinetics:* The steady-state pharmacokinetics of oral Rocaltrol were determined in a small group of pediatric patients (age range: 1.8 to 16 years) undergoing peritoneal dialysis. Rocaltrol was administered for 2 months at an average dose of 10.2 ng/kg (SD 5.5 ng/kg). In this pediatric population, mean C_{max} was 116 pmol/L, mean serum half-life was 27.4 hours, and mean clearance was 15.3 mL/hr/kg.[1]

Geriatric: No studies have examined the pharmacokinetics of calcitriol in geriatric patients.

Gender: Controlled studies examining the influence of gender on calcitriol have not been conducted.

Hepatic Insufficiency: Controlled studies examining the influence of hepatic disease on calcitriol have not been conducted.

Renal Insufficiency: Lower predose and peak calcitriol levels in serum were observed in patients with nephrotic syndrome and patients undergoing hemodialysis compared with healthy subjects. The elimination half-life of calcitriol increased by at least twofold in chronic renal failure and hemodialysis patients compared with healthy subjects. Peak serum levels in patients with nephrotic syndrome were reached in 4 hours. For patients requiring hemodialysis peak serum levels were reached in 8 to 12 hours; half-lives were estimated to be 16.2 and 21.9 hours, respectively.

INDICATIONS AND USAGE

Predialysis Patients: Rocaltrol is indicated in the management of secondary hyperparathyroidism and resultant metabolic bone disease in patients with moderate to severe chronic renal failure (Ccr 15 to 55 mL/min) not yet on dialysis. In children, the creatinine clearance value must be corrected for a surface area of 1.73 square meters. A serum iPTH level of ≥ 100 pg/mL is strongly suggestive of secondary hyperparathyroidism.

Dialysis Patients: Rocaltrol is indicated in the management of hypocalcemia and the resultant metabolic bone disease in patients undergoing chronic renal dialysis. In these patients, Rocaltrol administration enhances calcium absorption, reduces serum alkaline phosphatase levels and may reduce elevated parathyroid hormone levels and the histological manifestations of osteitis fibrosa cystica and defective mineralization.

Hypoparathyroidism Patients: Rocaltrol is also indicated in the management of hypocalcemia and its clinical manifestations in patients with postsurgical hypoparathyroidism, idiopathic hypoparathyroidism, and pseudohypoparathyroidism.

CONTRAINDICATIONS

Rocaltrol should not be given to patients with hypercalcemia or evidence of vitamin D toxicity.

WARNINGS

Overdosage of any form of vitamin D is dangerous (see OVERDOSAGE). Progressive hypercalcemia due to overdosage of vitamin D and its metabolites may be so severe as to require emergency attention. Chronic hypercalcemia can lead to generalized vascular calcification, nephrocalcinosis and other soft-tissue calcification. **The serum calcium times phospate (Ca × P) product should not be allowed to exceed 70.** Radiographic evaluation of suspect anatomical regions may be useful in the early detection of this condition. Rocaltrol is the most potent metabolite of vitamin D available. The administration of Rocaltrol to patients in excess of their daily requirements can cause hypercalcemia, hypercalciuria and hyperphosphatemia. Therefore, pharmacologic doses of vitamin D and its derivatives should be withheld during Rocaltrol treatment to avoid possible additive effects and hypercalcemia.

A non-aluminum phosphate-binding compound and a low-phosphate diet should be used to control serum phosphorus levels in patients undergoing dialysis.

Magnesium-containing antacids and Rocaltrol should not be used concomitantly in patients on chronic renal dialysis because such use may lead to the development of hypermagnesemia.

Studies in dogs and rats given calcitriol for up to 26 weeks have shown that small increases of calcitriol above endogenous levels can lead to abnormalities of calcium metabolism with the potential for calcification of many tissues in the body.

PRECAUTIONS

General: Excessive dosage of Rocaltrol induces hypercalcemia and in some instances hypercalciuria; therefore, early in treatment during dosage adjustment, serum calcium should be determined twice weekly. In dialysis patients, a fall in serum alkaline phosphatase levels usually antedates the appearance of hypercalcemia and may be an indication of impending hypercalcemia. Should hypercalcemia develop, the drug should be discontinued immediately. Rocaltrol should be given cautiously to patients on digitalis, because hypercalcemia in such patients may precipitate cardiac arrhythmias.

In patients with normal renal function, chronic hypercalcemia may be associated with an increase in serum creatinine. While this is usually reversible, it is important in such patients to pay careful attention to those factors which may lead to hypercalcemia. Rocaltrol therapy should always be started at the lowest possible dose and should not be increased without careful monitoring of the serum calcium. An estimate of daily dietary calcium intake should be made and the intake adjusted when indicated.

Patients with normal renal function taking Rocaltrol should avoid dehydration. Adequate fluid intake should be maintained.

Information for Patients: The patient and his or her parents or spouse should be informed about compliance with dosage instructions, adherence to instructions about diet and calcium supplementation and avoidance of the use of unapproved nonprescription drugs. Patients should also be carefully informed about the symptoms of hypercalcemia (see ADVERSE REACTIONS).

The effectiveness of Rocaltrol therapy is predicated on the assumption that each patient is receiving an adequate daily intake of calcium. Patients are advised to have a dietary intake of calcium at a minimum of 600 mg daily. The U.S. RDA for calcium in adults is 800 mg to 1200 mg.

Laboratory Tests: For dialysis patients, serum calcium, phosphorus, magnesium and alkaline phosphatase should be determined periodically. For hypoparathyroid patients, serum calcium, phosphorus and 24-hour urinary calcium should be determined periodically. For predialysis patients, serum calcium, phosphorus, alkaline phosphatase, creatinine and intact PTH (iPTH) should be determined initially. Thereafter, serum calcium, phosphorus, alkaline phosphatase and creatine should be determined monthly for a 6-month period and then determined periodically. Intact PTH (iPTH) should be determined periodically every 3 to 4 months at the time of visits.

Drug Interactions: Cholestyramine has been reported to reduce intestinal absorption of fat-soluble vitamins; as such it may impair intestinal absorption of Rocaltrol. (see WARNINGS and PRECAUTIONS: *General*).

The coadministration of phenytoin or phenobarbital will not affect plasma concentrations of calcitriol, but may reduce endogenous plasma levels of 25(OH)D3 by inhibiting 25-hydroxylase in liver. Since endogenous synthesis of calcitriol will be inhibited, higher doses of Rocaltrol may be necessary if these drugs are administered simultaneously.

Thiazides are known to induce hypercalcemia by the reduction of calcium excretion in urine. Some reports have shown that the concomitant administration of thiazides with Rocaltrol causes hypercalcemia. Therefore, precaution should be taken when coadministration is necessary.

Ketoconazole may inhibit both synthetic and catabolic enzymes of calcitriol. Reductions in serum endogenous calcitriol concentrations have been observed following the administration of 300 mg/day to 1200 mg/day ketoconazole for a week to healthy men. However, in vivo drug interaction studies of ketoconazole with Rocaltrol have not been investigated.

Carcinogenesis, Mutagenesis and Impairment of Fertility: Long-term studies in animals have not been conducted to evaluate the carcinogenic potential of Rocaltrol. Rocaltrol is not mutagenic in vitro in the Ames Test, nor is it genotoxic in vivo in the Mouse Micronucleus Test. No significant effects of Rocaltrol on fertility and/or general reproductive performances were observed in a Segment I study in rats at doses of up to 0.3 µg/kg (approximately 3 times the maximum recommended dose based on body surface area).

Pregnancy: *Teratogenic Effects:* Pregnancy Category C. Rocaltrol has been found to be teratogenic in rabbits when given at doses of 0.08 and 0.3 µg/kg (approximately 2 and 6 times the maximum recommended dose based on mg/m^2). All 15 fetuses in 3 litters at these doses showed external and skeletal abnormalities. However, none of the other 23 litters (156 fetuses) showed external and skeletal abnormalities compared with controls.

Teratogenicity studies in rats at doses up to 0.45 µg/kg (approximately 5 times maximum recommended dose based on mg/m^2) showed no evidence of teratogenic potential. There are no adequate and well-controlled studies in pregnant women. Rocaltrol should be used during pregnancy only if the potential benefit justifies the potential risk to the fetus.

Nonteratogenic Effects: In the rabbit, dosages of 0.3 mcg/kg/day (approximately 6 times maximum recommended dose based on surface area) administered on days 7 to 18 of gestation resulted in 19% maternal mortality, a decrease in mean fetal body weight and a reduced number of newborn surviving to 24 hours. A study of perinatal and postnatal development in rats resulted in hypercalcemia in the offspring of dams given Rocaltrol at doses of 0.08 or 0.3 mcg/kg/day (approximately 1 and 3 times the maximum recommended dose based on mg/m^2), hypercalcemia and hypophosphatemia in dams given Rocaltrol at a dose of 0.08 or 0.3 mcg/kg/day, and increased serum urea nitrogen in dams given Rocaltrol at a dose of 0.3 mcg/kg/day. In another study in rats, maternal weight gain was slightly reduced at a dose of 0.3 mcg/kg/day (approximately 3 times the maximum recommended dose based on mg/m^2) administered on days 7 to 15 of gestation.

The offspring of a woman administered 17 mcg/day to 36 mcg/day of Rocaltrol (approximately 17 to 36 times the maximum recommended dose), during pregnancy manifested mild hypercalcemia in the first 2 days of life which returned to normal at day 3.

Nursing Mothers: Calcitriol from ingested Rocaltrol may be excreted in human milk. Because many drugs are excreted in human milk and because of the potential for serious adverse reactions from Rocaltrol in nursing infants, a mother should not nurse while taking Rocaltrol.

Pediatric Use: Safety and effectiveness of Rocaltrol in pediatric patients undergoing dialysis have not been established. The safety and effectiveness of Rocaltrol in pediatric predialysis patients is based on evidence from adequate and well-controlled studies of Rocaltrol in adults with predialysis chronic renal failure and additional supportive data from non-placebo controlled studies in pediatric patients. Dosing guidelines have not been established for pediatric patients under 1 year of age with hypoparathyroidism or for pediatric patients less than 6 years of age with pseudohypoparathyroidism (see DOSAGE AND ADMINISTRATION: *Hypoparathyroidism*).

Oral doses of Rocaltrol ranging from 10 to 55 ng/kg/day have been shown to improve calcium homeostasis and bone disease in pediatric patients with chronic renal failure for whom hemodialysis is not yet required (predialysis). Long-term calcitriol therapy is well-tolerated by pediatric patients. The most common safety issues are mild, transient episodes of hypercalcemia, hyperphosphatemia, and increases in the serum calcium times phosphate (Ca × P) product which are managed effectively by dosage adjustment or temporary discontinuation of the vitamin D derivative.

Geriatric Use: Safety and effectiveness of Rocaltrol in geriatric patients undergoing dialysis have not been established.

ADVERSE REACTIONS

Since Rocaltrol is believed to be the active hormone which exerts vitamin D activity in the body, adverse effects are, in general, similar to those encountered with excessive vitamin D intake. The early and late signs and symptoms of vitamin D intoxication associated with hypercalcemia include:

Early: weakness, headache, somnolence, nausea, vomiting, dry mouth, constipation, muscle pain, bone pain and metallic taste.

Late: polyuria, polydipsia, anorexia, weight loss, nocturia, conjunctivitis (calcific), pancreatitis, photophobia, rhinorrhea, pruritus, hyperthermia, decreased libido, elevated BUN, albuminuria, hypercholesterolemia, elevated SGOT and SGPT, ectopic calcification, nephrocalcinosis, hypertension, cardiac arrhythmias and, rarely, overt psychosis.

In clinical studies on hypoparathyroidism and pseudohypoparathyroidism, hypercalcemia was noted on at least one occasion in about 1 in 3 patients and hypercalciuria in about 1 in 7 patients. Elevated serum creatinine levels were observed in about 1 in 6 patients (approximately one half of whom had normal levels at baseline).

One case of erythema multiforme and one case of allergic reaction (swelling of lips and hives all over the body) were confirmed by rechallenge.

OVERDOSAGE

Administration of Rocaltrol to patients in excess of their daily requirements can cause hypercalcemia, hypercalciuria and hyperphosphatemia. High intake of calcium and phosphate concomitant with Rocaltrol may lead to similar abnormalities. High levels of calcium in the dialysate bath may contribute to the hypercalcemia (see WARNINGS).

Treatment of Hypercalcemia and Overdosage in Dialysis Patients and Hypoparathyroidism Patients: General treatment of hypercalcemia (greater than 1 mg/dL above the upper limit of the normal range) consists of immediate discontinuation of Rocaltrol therapy, institution of a low-calcium diet and withdrawal of calcium supplements. Serum calcium levels should be determined daily until normocalcemia ensues. Hypercalcemia frequently resolves in 2 to 7 days. When serum calcium levels have returned to within normal limits, Rocaltrol therapy may be reinstituted at a dose of 0.25 mcg/day less than prior therapy. Serum calcium levels should be obtained at least twice weekly after all dosage changes and subsequent dosage titration. In dialysis patients, persistent or markedly elevated serum calcium levels may be corrected by dialysis against a calcium-free dialysate.

Treatment of Hypercalcemia and Overdosage in Predialysis Patients: If hypercalcemia ensues (greater than 1 mg/dL above the upper limit of the normal range), adjust dosage to achieve normocalcemia by reducing Rocaltrol therapy from 0.5 mcg to 0.25 mcg daily. If the patient is receiving a therapy of 0.25 mcg daily, discontinue Rocaltrol until patient becomes normocalcemic. Calcium supplements should also be reduced or discontinued. Serum calcium levels should be determined 1 week after withdrawal of calcium supplements. If serum calcium levels have returned to normal, Rocaltrol therapy may be reinstituted at a dosage of 0.25 mcg/day if previous therapy was at a dosage of 0.5 mcg/day. If Rocaltrol therapy was previously administered at a dosage of 0.25 mcg/day, Rocaltrol therapy may be reinstituted at a dosage of 0.25 mcg every other day. If hypercalcemia is persistent at the reduced dosage, serum PTH should be measured. If serum PTH is normal, discontinue Rocaltrol therapy and monitor patient in 3 months' time.

Treatment of Hyperphospatemia in Predialysis Patients: If serum phosphorus levels exceed 5.0 mg/dL to 5.5 mg/dL, a calcium-containing phosphate binding agent (ie, calcium carbonate or calcium acetate) should be taken with meals. Serum phosphorus levels should be determined as described earlier (see PRECAUTIONS: *Laboratory Tests*). Aluminum-containing gels should be used with caution as phosphate binding agents because of the risk of slow aluminum accumulation.

Treatment of Accidental Overdosage of Rocaltrol: The treatment of acute accidental overdosage of Rocaltrol should consist of general supportive measures. If drug ingestion is discovered within a relatively short time, induction of emesis or gastric lavage may be of benefit in preventing further absorption. If the drug has passed through the stomach, the administration of mineral oil may promote its fecal elimination. Serial serum electrolyte determinations (especially calcium), rate of urinary calcium excretion and assessment of electrocardiographic abnormalities due to hypercalcemia should be obtained. Such monitoring is critical in patients receiving digitalis. Discontinuation of supplemental calcium and a low-calcium diet are also indicated in accidental overdosage. Due to the relatively short duration of the pharmacological action of calcitriol, further measures are probably unnecessary. Should, however, persistent and markedly elevated serum calcium levels occur, there are a variety of therapeutic alternatives which may be considered, depending on the patient's underlying condition. These include the use of drugs such as phosphates and corticosteroids as well as measures to induce an appropriate forced diuresis. The use of peritoneal dialysis against a calcium-free dialysate has also been reported.

DOSAGE AND ADMINISTRATION

The optimal daily dose of Rocaltrol must be carefully determined for each patient. Rocaltrol can be administered orally either as a capsule (0.25 mcg or 0.50 mcg) or an an oral solution (1 mcg/mL).

The effectiveness of Rocaltrol therapy is predicated on the assumption that each patient is receiving an adequate daily intake of calcium. Patients are advised to have a dietary intake of calcium at a minimum of 600 mg daily. The U.S. RDA for calcium in adults is 800 mg to 1200 mg. To ensure that each patient receives an adequate daily intake of calcium, the physician should either prescribe a calcium supplement or instruct the patient in proper dietary measures.

Dialysis Patients: The recommended initial dose of Rocaltrol is 0.25 mcg/day. If a satisfactory response in the biochemical parameters and clinical manifestations of the disease state is not observed, dosage may be increased by 0.25 mcg/day at 4- to 8-week intervals. During this titration period, serum calcium levels should be obtained at least twice weekly, and if hypercalcemia is noted, the drug should be immediately discontinued until normocalcemia ensues.

Patients with normal or only slightly reduced serum calcium levels may respond to Rocaltrol doses of 0.25 mcg every other day. Most patients undergoing hemodialysis respond to doses between 0.5 and 1 mcg/day.

Oral Rocaltrol may normalize plasma ionized calcium in some uremic patients, yet fail to suppress parathyroid hyperfunction. In these individuals with autonomous parathyroid hyperfunction, oral Rocaltrol may be useful to maintain normocalcemia, but has not been shown to be adequate treatment for hyperparathyroidism.

Hypoparathyroidism: The recommended initial dosage of Rocaltrol is 0.25 mcg/day given in the morning. If a satisfactory response in the biochemical parameters and clinical manifestations of the disease is not observed, the dose may be increased at 2- to 4-week intervals. During the dosage titration period, serum calcium levels should be obtained at least twice weekly and, if hypercalcemia is noted, Rocaltrol should be immediately discontinued until normocalcemia ensues. Careful consideration should also be given to lowering the dietary calcium intake.

Most adult patients and pediatric patients age 6 years and older have responded to dosages in the range of 0.5 mcg to 2 mcg daily. Pediatric patients in the 1 to 5 year age group with hypoparathyroidism have usually been given 0.25 mcg to 0.75 mcg daily. The number of treated patients with pseudohypoparathyroidism less than 6 years of age is too small to make dosage recommendations.

Predialysis Patients: The recommended initial dosage of Rocaltrol is 0.25 mcg/day in adults and pediatric patients 3 years of age and older. This dosage may be increased if necessary to 0.5 mcg/day.

For pediatric patients less than 3 years of age, the recommended initial dosage of Rocaltrol is 10 to 15 ng/kg/day.

HOW SUPPLIED

Capsules: 0.25 mcg calcitriol in soft gelatin, light orange, oval capsules, imprinted with ROCALTROL 0.25 ROCHE; bottles of 30 (NDC 0004-0143-23), and bottles of 100, (NDC 0004-0143-01).

Capsules: 0.5 mcg calcitriol in soft gelatin, dark orange, oblong capsules, imprinted with ROCALTROL 0.5 ROCHE; bottles of 100 (NDC 0004-0144-01).

Oral Solution: a clear, colorless to pale yellow oral solution containing 1 mcg/mL of calcitriol; each amber glass bottle of 15 mL of oral solution supplied with 20 single-use, graduated oral dispensers (NDC 0004-9115-00).

Rocaltrol Capsules and Oral Solution should be protected from light.

Store at 59° to 86°F (15° to 30°C).

REFERENCE

1. Jones CL, et al. Comparisons between oral and intraperitoneal 1,25–dihydroxyvitamin D_3, therapy in children treated with peritoneal dialysis. *Clin Nephrol.* 1994; 42:44–49.

Revised: November 1998

Shown in Product Identification Guide, page 333

ROCEPHIN® ℞

[ro-sef ' in]

(ceftriaxone sodium)

FOR INJECTION

The following text is complete prescribing information based on official labeling in effect June 2000.

DESCRIPTION

Rocephin is a sterile, semisynthetic, broad-spectrum cephalosporin antibiotic for intravenous or intramuscular administration. Ceftriaxone sodium is (6*R*,7*R*)-7-[2-(2-Amino-4-thiazolyl) glyoxylamido] - 8 - oxo - 3 - [[(1,2,5,6 - tetrahydro - 2 - methyl-5,6-dioxo-*as*-triazin-3-yl) thio] methyl] -5-thia-1-azabicyclo[4.2.0]oct-2-ene-2-carboxylic acid, 7^2-(*Z*)-(*O*-methyloxime), disodium salt, sesquaterhydrate.

The chemical formula of ceftriaxone sodium is $C_{18}\ H_{16}\ N_8\ Na_2\ O_7\ S_3\ 3.5\ H_2O$. It has a calculated molecular weight of 661.59.

Rocephin is a white to yellowish-orange crystalline powder which is readily soluble in water, sparingly soluble in methanol and very slightly soluble in ethanol. The pH of a 1% aqueous solution is approximately 6.7. The color of Rocephin solutions ranges from light yellow to amber, depending on the length of storage, concentration and diluent used.

Rocephin contains approximately 83 mg (3.6 mEq) of sodium per gram of ceftriaxone activity.

CLINICAL PHARMACOLOGY

Average plasma concentrations of ceftriaxone following a single 30-minute intravenous (IV) infusion of a 0.5, 1 or 2 gm dose and intramuscular (IM) administration of a single 0.5 (250 mg/mL or 350 mg/mL concentrations) or 1 gm dose in healthy subjects are presented in Table 1.

[See table 1 below]

Ceftriaxone was completely absorbed following IM administration with mean maximum plasma concentrations occurring between 2 and 3 hours postdosing. Multiple IV or IM doses ranging from 0.5 to 2 gm at 12- to 24-hour intervals resulted in 15% to 36% accumulation of ceftriaxone above single dose values.

Ceftriaxone concentrations in urine are high, as shown in Table 2.

[See table 2 at top of next page]

Thirty-three percent to 67% of a ceftriaxone dose was excreted in the urine as unchanged drug and the remainder was secreted in the bile and ultimately found in the feces as microbiologically inactive compounds. After a 1 gm IV dose, average concentrations of ceftriaxone, determined from 1 to 3 hours after dosing, were 581 mcg/mL in the gallbladder bile, 788 mcg/mL in the common duct bile, 898 mcg/mL in the cystic duct bile, 78.2 mcg/gm in the gallbladder wall and 62.1 mcg/mL in the concurrent plasma.

Over a 0.15 to 3 gm dose range in healthy adult subjects, the values of elimination half-life ranged from 5.8 to 8.7 hours; apparent volume of distribution from 5.78 to 13.5 L; plasma clearance from 0.58 to 1.45 L/hour; and renal clearance from 0.32 to 0.73 L/hour. Ceftriaxone is reversibly bound to human plasma proteins, and the binding decreased from a value of 95% bound at plasma concentrations of <25 mcg/mL to a value of 85% bound at 300 mcg/mL.

The average values of maximum plasma concentration, elimination half-life, plasma clearance and volume of distribution after a 50 mg/kg IV dose and after a 75 mg/kg IV dose in pediatric patients suffering from bacterial meningitis are shown in Table 3. Ceftriaxone penetrated the inflamed meninges of infants and children; CSF concentrations after a 50 mg/kg IV dose and after a 75 mg/kg IV dose are also shown in Table 3.

[See table 3 at top of next page]

Compared to that in healthy adult subjects, the pharmacokinetics of ceftriaxone were only minimally altered in elderly subjects and in patients with renal impairment or hepatic dysfunction (Table 4); therefore, dosage adjustments are not necessary for these patients with ceftriaxone dosages up to 2 gm per day. Ceftriaxone was not removed to any significant extent from the plasma by hemodialysis. In 6 of 26 dialysis patients, the elimination rate of ceftriaxone was markedly reduced, suggesting that plasma concentrations of ceftriaxone should be monitored in these patients to determine if dosage adjustments are necessary.

[See table 4 at top of next page]

Pharmacokinetics in the Middle Ear Fluid: In one study, total ceftriaxone concentrations (bound and unbound) were measured in middle ear fluid obtained during the insertion of tympanostomy tubes in 42 pediatric patients with otitis media. Sampling times were from 1 to 50 hours after a single intramuscular injection of 50 mg/kg of ceftriaxone. Mean (± SD) ceftriaxone levels in the middle ear reached a peak of 35 (± 12) μg/mL at 24 hours, and remained at 19 (± 7) μg/mL at 48 hours. Based on middle ear fluid ceftriaxone concentrations in the 23 to 25 hour and the 46 to 50 hour sampling time intervals, a half-life of 25 hours was calculated. Ceftriaxone is highly bound to plasma proteins. The extent of binding to proteins in the middle ear fluid is unknown.

Continued on next page

TABLE 1 Ceftriaxone Plasma Concentrations After Single Dose Administration

Dose/Route	Average Plasma Concentrations (mcg/mL)								
	0.5 hr	1 hr	2 hr	4 hr	6 hr	8 hr	12 hr	16 hr	24 hr
0.5 gm IV*	82	59	48	37	29	23	15	10	5
0.5 gm IM 250 mg/mL	22	33	38	35	30	26	16	ND	5
0.5 gm IM 350 mg/mL	20	32	38	34	31	24	16	ND	5
1 gm IV*	151	111	88	67	53	43	28	18	9
1 gm IM	40	68	76	68	56	44	29	ND	ND
2 gm IV*	257	192	154	117	89	74	46	31	15

*IV doses were infused at a constant rate over 30 minutes.
ND = Not determined.

Rocephin—Cont.

Microbiology: The bactericidal activity of ceftriaxone results from inhibition of cell wall synthesis. Ceftriaxone has a high degree of stability in the presence of beta-lactamases, both penicillinases and cephalosporinases, of gram-negative and gram-positive bacteria. Ceftriaxone is usually active against the following microorganisms in vitro and in clinical infections (see INDICATIONS AND USAGE):

GRAM-NEGATIVE AEROBES:
Acinetobacter calcoaceticus
Enterobacter aerogenes
Enterobacter cloacae
Escherichia coli
Haemophilus influenzae (including ampicillin-resistant and beta-lactamase producing strains)
Haemophilus parainfluenzae
Klebsiella oxytoca
Klebsiella pneumoniae
Moraxella catarrhalis (including beta-lactamase producing strains)
Morganella morganii
Neisseria gonorrhoeae (including penicillinase- and nonpenicillinase-producing strains)
Neisseria meningitidis
Proteus mirabilis
Proteus vulgaris
Serratia marcescens
Ceftriaxone is also active against many strains of *Pseudomonas aeruginosa.*
NOTE: Many strains of the above organisms that are multiply resistant to other antibiotics, eg, penicillins, cephalosporins and aminoglycosides, are susceptible to ceftriaxone.
GRAM-POSITIVE AEROBES:
Staphylococcus aureus (including penicillinase-producing strains)
Staphylococcus epidermidis
Streptococcus pneumoniae
Streptococcus pyogenes
Viridans group streptococci
NOTE: Methicillin-resistant staphylococci are resistant to cephalosporins, including ceftriaxone. Most strains of Group D streptococci and enterococci, eg, *Enterococcus (Streptococcus) faecalis,* are resistant.
ANAEROBES:
Bacteroides fragilis
Clostridium species
Peptostreptococcus species
NOTE: Most strains of *C. difficile* are resistant.
Ceftriaxone also demonstrates in vitro activity against most strains of the following microorganisms, although the clinical significance is unknown:
GRAM-NEGATIVE AEROBES:
Citrobacter diversus
Citrobacter freundii
Providencia species (including *Providencia rettgeri*)
Salmonella species (including *S. typhi*)
Shigella species
GRAM-POSITIVE AEROBES:
Streptococcus agalactiae
ANAEROBES:
Bacteroides bivius
Bacteroides melaninogenicus

Susceptibility Tests: *Diffusion Techniques:* Quantitative methods that require the measurement of zone diameters give the most precise estimate of the susceptibility of bacteria to antimicrobial agents. One such standard procedure[1] which has been recommended for use with disks to test susceptibility of organisms to ceftriaxone uses a 30-mcg ceftriaxone disk. Interpretation involves the correlation of the diameters obtained in the disk test with the minimum inhibitory concentration (MIC) for ceftriaxone.
Reports from the laboratory giving results of the standardized single disk susceptibility test using a 30-mcg ceftriaxone disk should be interpreted for ceftriaxone according to the following criteria:

Zone Diameter (mm)		Interpretation
≥18	(S)	Susceptible
14–17	(MS)	Moderately Susceptible
≤13	(R)	Resistant

A report of "Susceptible" indicates that the pathogen is likely to be inhibited by generally achievable levels. A report of "Moderately Susceptible" suggests that the organism would be susceptible if high dosage (not to exceed 4 gm per day) is used or if the infection is confined to tissues and fluids in which high antimicrobial levels are attained. A report of "Resistant" indicates that achievable concentrations are unlikely to be inhibitory, and other therapy should be selected.
Standardized procedures require the use of laboratory control organisms. The 30-mcg ceftriaxone disk should give the following zone diameters:

Organism	Zone Diameter (mm)
Staphylococcus aureus ATCC® 25923	22–28
Escherichia coli ATCC® 25922	29–35
Pseudomonas aeruginosa ATCC® 27853	17–23

Dilution Techniques:
Use a standardized dilution method[2] (broth, agar, microdilution) or equivalent with ceftriaxone powder. The MIC values obtained should be interpreted according to the following criteria:

MIC (mcg/mL)	Interpretation
≤16	Susceptible
>16–<64	Moderately Susceptible
≥64	Resistant

As with standard diffusion techniques, dilution methods require the use of laboratory control organisms. Standard ceftriaxone powder should provide the following MIC values:

Organism	MIC (mcg/mL)
Staphylococcus aureus ATCC® 29213	1–8
Escherichia coli ATCC® 25922	0.03–0.12
Pseudomonas aeruginosa ATCC® 27853	8–32

TABLE 2 Urinary Concentrations of Ceftriaxone After Single Dose Administration

Dose/Route	Average Urinary Concentrations (mcg/mL)					
	0–2 hr	2–4 hr	4–8 hr	8–12 hr	12–24 hr	24–48 hr
0.5 gm IV	526	366	142	87	70	15
0.5 gm IM	115	425	308	127	96	28
1 gm IV	995	855	293	147	132	32
1 gm IM	504	628	418	237	ND*	ND
2 gm IV	2692	1976	757	274	198	40

*ND = Not determined.

TABLE 3 Average Pharmacokinetic Parameters of Ceftriaxone in Pediatric Patients With Meningitis

	50 mg/kg IV	75 mg/kg IV
Maximum Plasma Concentrations (mcg/mL)	216	275
Elimination Half-life (hr)	4.6	4.3
Plasma Clearance (mL/hr/kg)	49	60
Volume of Distribution (mL/kg)	338	373
CSF Concentration—inflamed meninges (mcg/mL)	5.6	6.4
Range (mcg/mL)	1.3–18.5	1.3–44
Time after dose (hr)	3.7 (± 1.6)	3.3 (± 1.4)

TABLE 4 Average Pharmacokinetic Parameters of Ceftriaxone in Humans

Subject Group	Elimination Half-Life (hr)	Plasma Clearance (L/hr)	Volume of Distribution (L)
Healthy Subjects	5.8–8.7	0.58–1.45	5.8–13.5
Elderly Subjects (mean age, 70.5 yr)	8.9	0.83	10.7
Patients with renal impairment			
Hemodialysis patients (0–5 mL/min)*	14.7	0.65	13.7
Severe (5–15 mL/min)	15.7	0.56	12.5
Moderate (16–30 mL/min)	11.4	0.72	11.8
Mild (31–60 mL/min)	12.4	0.70	13.3
Patients with liver disease	8.8	1.1	13.6

*Creatinine clearance.

INDICATIONS AND USAGE

Rocephin is indicated for the treatment of the following infections when caused by susceptible organisms:
LOWER RESPIRATORY TRACT INFECTIONS caused by *Streptococcus pneumoniae, Staphylococcus aureus, Haemophilus influenzae, Haemophilus parainfluenzae, Klebsiella pneumoniae, Escherichia coli, Enterobacter aerogenes, Proteus mirabilis* or *Serratia marcescens.*
ACUTE BACTERIAL OTITIS MEDIA caused by *Streptococcus pneumoniae, Haemophilus influenzae* (including beta-lactamase producing strains) or *Moraxella catarrhalis* (including beta-lactamase producing strains).
NOTE: In one study lower clinical cure rates were observed with a single dose of Rocephin compared to 10 days of oral therapy. In a second study comparable cure rates were observed between single dose Rocephin and the comparator. The potentially lower clinical cure rate of Rocephin should be balanced against the potential advantages of parenteral therapy (see CLINICAL STUDIES).
SKIN AND SKIN STRUCTURE INFECTIONS caused by *Staphylococcus aureus, Staphylococcus epidermidis, Streptococcus pyogenes, Viridans* group streptococci, *Escherichia coli, Enterobacter cloacae, Klebsiella oxytoca, Klebsiella pneumoniae, Proteus mirabilis, Morganella morganii*, Pseudomonas aeruginosa, Serratia marcescens, Acinetobacter calcoaceticus, Bacteroides fragilis** or *Peptostreptococcus* species.
URINARY TRACT INFECTIONS (complicated and uncomplicated) caused by *Escherichia coli, Proteus mirabilis, Proteus vulgaris, Morganella morganii* or *Klebsiella pneumoniae.*
UNCOMPLICATED GONORRHEA (cervical/urethral and rectal) caused by *Neisseria gonorrhoeae,* including both penicillinase- and nonpenicillinase-producing strains, and pharyngeal gonorrhea caused by nonpenicillinase-producing strains of *Neisseria gonorrhoeae.*
PELVIC INFLAMMATORY DISEASE caused by *Neisseria gonorrhoeae.* Rocephin, like other cephalosporins, has no activity against *Chlamydia trachomatis.* Therefore, when cephalosporins are used in the treatment of patients with pelvic inflammatory disease and *C. trachomatis* is one of the suspected pathogens, appropriate antichlamydial coverage should be added.
BACTERIAL SEPTICEMIA caused by *Staphylococcus aureus, Streptococcus pneumoniae, Escherichia coli, Haemophilus influenzae* or *Klebsiella pneumoniae.*
BONE AND JOINT INFECTIONS caused by *Staphylococcus aureus, Streptococcus pneumoniae, Escherichia coli, Proteus mirabilis, Klebsiella pneumoniae* or *Enterobacter* species.
INTRA-ABDOMINAL INFECTIONS caused by *Escherichia coli, Klebsiella pneumoniae, Bacteroides fragilis, Clostridium* species (Note: most strains of *C. difficile* are resistant) or *Peptostreptococcus* species.
MENINGITIS caused by *Haemophilus influenzae, Neisseria meningitidis* or *Streptococcus pneumoniae.* Rocephin has also been used successfully in a limited number of cases of meningitis and shunt infection caused by *Staphylococcus epidermidis** and *Escherichia coli.**
*Efficacy for this organism in this organ system was studied in fewer than ten infections.
SURGICAL PROPHYLAXIS: The preoperative administration of a single 1 gm dose of Rocephin may reduce the incidence of postoperative infections in patients undergoing surgical procedures classified as contaminated or potentially contaminated (eg, vaginal or abdominal hysterectomy or cholecystectomy for chronic calculous cholecystitis in high-risk patients, such as those over 70 years of age, with acute cholecystitis not requiring therapeutic antimicrobials, obstructive jaundice or common duct bile stones) and in surgical patients for whom infection at the operative site would present serious risk (eg, during coronary artery bypass surgery). Although Rocephin has been shown to have been as effective as cefazolin in the prevention of infection following coronary artery bypass surgery, no placebo-controlled trials have been conducted to evaluate any cephalosporin antibiotic in the prevention of infection following coronary artery bypass surgery.
When administered prior to surgical procedures for which it is indicated, a single 1 gm dose of Rocephin provides protection from most infections due to susceptible organisms throughout the course of the procedure.
Before instituting treatment with Rocephin, appropriate specimens should be obtained for isolation of the causative organism and for determination of its susceptibility to the drug. Therapy may be instituted prior to obtaining results of susceptibility testing.

CONTRAINDICATIONS

Rocephin is contraindicated in patients with known allergy to the cephalosporin class of antibiotics.

WARNINGS

BEFORE THERAPY WITH ROCEPHIN IS INSTITUTED, CAREFUL INQUIRY SHOULD BE MADE TO DETERMINE WHETHER THE PATIENT HAS HAD PREVIOUS HYPERSENSITIVITY REACTIONS TO CEPHALOSPORINS, PENICILLINS OR OTHER DRUGS. THIS PRODUCT SHOULD BE GIVEN CAUTIOUSLY TO PENICILLIN-SENSITIVE PATIENTS. ANTIBIOTICS SHOULD BE ADMINISTERED WITH CAUTION TO ANY PATIENT WHO HAS DEMONSTRATED SOME FORM OF ALLERGY, PARTICULARLY TO DRUGS. SERIOUS ACUTE HYPER-

SENSITIVITY REACTIONS MAY REQUIRE THE USE OF SUBCUTANEOUS EPINEPHRINE AND OTHER EMERGENCY MEASURES.

Pseudomembranous colitis has been reported with nearly all antibacterial agents, including ceftriaxone, and may range in severity from mild to life-threatening. Therefore, it is important to consider this diagnosis in patients who present with diarrhea subsequent to the administration of antibacterial agents.

Treatment with antibacterial agents alters the normal flora of the colon and may permit overgrowth of clostridia. Studies indicate that a toxin produced by *Clostridium difficile* is one primary cause of "antibiotic-associated colitis."

After the diagnosis of pseudomembranous colitis has been established, appropriate therapeutic measures should be initiated. Mild cases of pseudomembranous colitis usually respond to drug discontinuation alone. In moderate to severe cases, consideration should be given to management with fluids and electrolytes, protein supplementation and treatment with an antibacterial drug clinically effective against *C. difficile* colitis.

PRECAUTIONS

General: Although transient elevations of BUN and serum creatinine have been observed, at the recommended dosages, the nephrotoxic potential of Rocephin is similar to that of other cephalosporins.

Ceftriaxone is excreted via both biliary and renal excretion (see CLINICAL PHARMACOLOGY). Therefore, patients with renal failure normally require no adjustment in dosage when usual doses of Rocephin are administered, but concentrations of drug in the serum should be monitored periodically. If evidence of accumulation exists, dosage should be decreased accordingly.

Dosage adjustments should not be necessary in patients with hepatic dysfunction; however, in patients with both hepatic dysfunction and significant renal disease, Rocephin dosage should not exceed 2 gm daily without close monitoring of serum concentrations.

Alterations in prothrombin times have occurred rarely in patients treated with Rocephin. Patients with impaired vitamin K synthesis or low vitamin K stores (eg, chronic hepatic disease and malnutrition) may require monitoring of prothrombin time during Rocephin treatment. Vitamin K administration (10 mg weekly) may be necessary if the prothrombin time is prolonged before or during therapy.

Prolonged use of Rocephin may result in overgrowth of nonsusceptible organisms. Careful observation of the patient is essential. If superinfection occurs during therapy, appropriate measures should be taken.

Rocephin should be prescribed with caution in individuals with a history of gastrointestinal disease, especially colitis.

There have been reports of sonographic abnormalities in the gallbladder of patients treated with Rocephin; some of these patients also had symptoms of gallbladder disease. These abnormalities appear on sonography as an echo without acoustical shadowing suggesting sludge or as an echo with acoustical shadowing which may be misinterpreted as gallstones. The chemical nature of the sonographically detected material has been determined to be predominantly a ceftriaxone-calcium salt. **The condition appears to be transient and reversible upon discontinuation of Rocephin and institution of conservative management.** Therefore, Rocephin should be discontinued in patients who develop signs and symptoms suggestive of gallbladder disease and/or the sonographic findings described above.

Carcinogenesis, Mutagenesis, Impairment of Fertility: *Carcinogenesis:* Considering the maximum duration of treatment and the class of the compound, carcinogenicity studies with ceftriaxone in animals have not been performed. The maximum duration of animal toxicity studies was 6 months.

Mutagenesis: Genetic toxicology tests included the Ames test, a micronucleus test and a test for chromosomal aberrations in human lymphocytes cultured in vitro with ceftriaxone. Ceftriaxone showed no potential for mutagenic activity in these studies.

Impairment of Fertility: Ceftriaxone produced no impairment of fertility when given intravenously to rats at daily doses up to 586 mg/kg/day, approximately 20 times the recommended clinical dose of 2 gm/day.

Pregnancy: Teratogenic Effects: Pregnancy Category B. Reproductive studies have been performed in mice and rats at doses up to 20 times the usual human dose and have no evidence of embryotoxicity, fetotoxicity or teratogenicity. In primates, no embryotoxicity or teratogenicity was demonstrated at a dose approximately 3 times the human dose.

There are, however, no adequate and well-controlled studies in pregnant women. Because animal reproductive studies are not always predictive of human response, this drug should be used during pregnancy only if clearly needed.

Nonteratogenic Effects: In rats, in the Segment I (fertility and general reproduction) and Segment III (perinatal and postnatal) studies with intravenously administered ceftriaxone, no adverse effects were noted on various reproductive parameters during gestation and lactation, including postnatal growth, functional behavior and reproductive ability of the offspring, at doses of 586 mg/kg/day or less.

Nursing Mothers: Low concentrations of ceftriaxone are excreted in human milk. Caution should be exercised when Rocephin is administered to a nursing woman.

Pediatric Use: Safety and effectiveness of Rocephin in neonates, infants and children have been established for the dosages described in the DOSAGE AND ADMINISTRATION section. In vitro studies have shown that ceftriaxone, like some other cephalosporins, can displace bilirubin from serum albumin. Rocephin should not be administered to hyperbilirubinemic neonates, especially prematures.

Diluent	Concentration mg/mL	Storage Room Temp. (25°C)	Storage Refrigerated (4°C)
Sterile Water for	100	3 days	10 days
Injection	250, 350	24 hours	3 days
0.9% Sodium	100	3 days	10 days
Chloride Solution	250, 350	24 hours	3 days
5% Dextrose	100	3 days	10 days
Solution	250, 350	24 hours	3 days
Bacteriostatic Water + 0.9%	100	24 hours	10 days
Benzyl Alcohol	250, 350	24 hours	3 days
1% Lidocaine Solution	100	24 hours	10 days
(without epinephrine)	250, 350	24 hours	3 days

Diluent	Storage Room Temp. (25°C)	Storage Refrigerated (4°C)
Sterile Water	3 days	10 days
0.9% Sodium Chloride Solution	3 days	10 days
5% Dextrose Solution	3 days	10 days
10% Dextrose Solution	3 days	10 days
5% Dextrose + 0.9% Sodium Chloride Solution*	3 days	Incompatible
5% Dextrose + 0.45% Sodium Chloride Solution	3 days	Incompatible

*Data available for 10 to 40 mg/mL concentrations in this diluent in PVC containers only.

Clinical Efficacy in Evaluable Population

Study Day	Ceftriaxone Single Dose	Comparator – 10 days of Oral Therapy	95% Confidence Interval	Statistical Outcome
Study 1—US		amoxicillin/clavulanate		
14	74% (220/296)	82% (247/302)	(-14.4%, -0.5%)	Ceftriaxone is lower than control at study day 14 and 28.
28	58% (167/288)	67% (200/297)	(-17.5%, -1.2%)	
Study 2—US[3]		TMP-SMZ		
14	54% (113/210)	60% (124/206)	(-16.4%, 3.6%)	Ceftriaxone is equivalent to control at study day 14 and 28.
28	35% (73/206)	45% (93/205)	(-19.9%, 0.0%)	

Organism	Study Day 13–15 No. Analyzed	Study Day 13–15 No. Erad. (%)	Study Day 30+2 No. Analyzed	Study Day 30+2 No. Erad. (%)
S. pneumoniae	38	32 (84)	35	25 (71)
H. influenzae	33	28 (85)	31	22 (71)
M. catarrhalis	15	12 (80)	15	9 (60)

ADVERSE REACTIONS

Rocephin is generally well tolerated. In clinical trials, the following adverse reactions, which were considered to be related to Rocephin therapy or of uncertain etiology, were observed:

LOCAL REACTIONS—pain, induration and tenderness was 1% overall. Phlebitis was reported in <1% after IV administration. The incidence of injection site reaction was 17% (3/17) after IM administration of 350 mg/mL and 5% (1/20) after IM administration of 250 mg/mL.

HYPERSENSITIVITY—rash (1.7%). Less frequently reported (<1%) were pruritus, fever or chills.

HEMATOLOGIC—eosinophilia (6%), thrombocytosis (5.1%) and leukopenia (2.1%). Less frequently reported (<1%) were anemia, hemolytic anemia, neutropenia, lymphopenia, thrombocytopenia and prolongation of the prothrombin time.

GASTROINTESTINAL—diarrhea (2.7%). Less frequently reported (<1%) were nausea or vomiting, and dysgeusia. The onset of pseudomembranous colitis symptoms may occur during or after antibacterial treatment (see WARNINGS).

HEPATIC—elevations of SGOT (3.1%) or SGPT (3.3%). Less frequently reported (<1%) were elevations of alkaline phosphatase and bilirubin.

RENAL—elevations of the BUN (1.2%). Less frequently reported (<1%) were elevations of creatinine and the presence of casts in the urine.

CENTRAL NERVOUS SYSTEM—headache or dizziness were reported occasionally (<1%).

GENITOURINARY—moniliasis or vaginitis were reported occasionally (<1%).

MISCELLANEOUS—diaphoresis and flushing were reported occasionally (<1%).

Other rarely observed adverse reactions (<0.1%) include leukocytosis, lymphocytosis, monocytosis, basophilia, a decrease in the prothrombin time, jaundice, gallbladder sludge, glycosuria, hematuria, anaphylaxis, bronchospasm, serum sickness, abdominal pain, colitis, flatulence, dyspepsia, palpitations and epistaxis.

DOSAGE AND ADMINISTRATION

Rocephin may be administered intravenously or intramuscularly.

ADULTS: The usual adult daily dose is 1 to 2 grams given once a day (or in equally divided doses twice a day) depending on the type and severity of infection. The total daily dose should not exceed 4 grams.

If *C. trachomatis* is a suspected pathogen, appropriate antichlamydial coverage should be added, because ceftriaxone sodium has no activity against this organism.

For the treatment of uncomplicated gonococcal infections, a single intramuscular dose of 250 mg is recommended.

For preoperative use (surgical prophylaxis), a single dose of 1 gram administered intravenously ½ to 2 hours before surgery is recommended.

PEDIATRIC PATIENTS: For the treatment of skin and skin structure infections, the recommended total daily dose is 50 to 75 mg/kg given once a day (or in equally divided doses twice a day). The total daily dose should not exceed 2 grams.

For the treatment of acute bacterial otitis media, a single intramuscular dose of 50 mg/kg (not to exceed 1 gram) is recommended (see INDICATIONS AND USAGE).

For the treatment of serious miscellaneous infections other than meningitis, the recommended total daily dose is 50 to 75 mg/kg, given in divided doses every 12 hours. The total daily dose should not exceed 2 grams.

In the treatment of meningitis, it is recommended that the initial therapeutic dose be 100 mg/kg (not to exceed 4 grams). Thereafter, a total daily dose of 100 mg/kg/day (not to exceed 4 grams daily) is recommended. The daily dose may be administered once a day (or in equally divided doses every 12 hours). The usual duration of therapy is 7 to 14 days.

Generally, Rocephin therapy should be continued for at least 2 days after the signs and symptoms of infection have disappeared. The usual duration of therapy is 4 to 14 days; in complicated infections, longer therapy may be required. When treating infections caused by *Streptococcus pyogenes*, therapy should be continued for at least 10 days.

No dosage adjustment is necessary for patients with impairment of renal or hepatic function; however, blood levels should be monitored in patients with severe renal impairment (eg, dialysis patients) and in patients with both renal and hepatic dysfunctions.

DIRECTIONS FOR USE: Intramuscular Administration: Reconstitute Rocephin powder with the appropriate diluent (see COMPATIBILITY AND STABILITY section).

After reconstitution, each 1 mL of solution contains approximately 250 mg or 350 mg equivalent of ceftriaxone according to the amount of diluent indicated below. If required, more dilute solutions could be utilized. **A 350 mg/mL concentration is not recommended for the 250 mg vial since it may not be possible to withdraw the entire contents.** As with all intramuscular preparations, Rocephin should be in-

Continued on next page

Rocephin—Cont.

jected well within the body of a relatively large muscle; aspiration helps to avoid unintentional injection into a blood vessel.

Vial Dosage Size	Amount of Diluent to be Added	
	250 mg/mL	350 mg/mL
250 mg	0.9 mL	—
500 mg	1.8 mL	1.0 mL
1 gm	3.6 mL	2.1 mL
2 gm	7.2 mL	4.2 mL

Intramuscular Convenience Kit: For the 500 mg vial, withdraw 1 mL of diluent, discard the remainder. Inject diluent into vial, shake vial thoroughly to form solution. Withdraw entire contents of vial into syringe to equal approximately 1.4 mL.
For 1 gm vial, withdraw entire contents of diluent (2.1 mL). Inject diluent into vial, shake vial thoroughly to form solution. Withdraw entire contents of vial into syringe to equal approximately 2.8 mL.
Intravenous Administration: Rocephin should be administered intravenously by infusion over a period of 30 minutes. Concentrations between 10 mg/mL and 40 mg/mL are recommended; however, lower concentrations may be used if desired. Reconstitute vials or "piggyback" bottles with an appropriate IV diluent (see COMPATIBILITY AND STABILITY section).

Vial Dosage Size	Amount of Diluent to be Added
250 mg	2.4 mL
500 mg	4.8 mL
1 gm	9.6 mL
2 gm	19.2 mL

After reconstitution, each 1 mL of solution contains approximately 100 mg equivalent of ceftriaxone. Withdraw entire contents and dilute to the desired concentration with the appropriate IV diluent.

Piggyback Bottle Dosage Size	Amount of Diluent to be Added
1 gm	10 mL
2 gm	20 mL

After reconstitution, further dilute to 50 mL or 100 mL volumes with the appropriate IV diluent.
COMPATIBILITY AND STABILITY: Rocephin sterile powder should be stored at room temperature—77°F (25°C)—or below and protected from light. After reconstitution, protection from normal light is not necessary. The color of solutions ranges from light yellow to amber, depending on the length of storage, concentration and diluent used.
Rocephin *intramuscular* solutions remain stable (loss of potency less than 10%) for the following time periods:
[See first table at top of previous page]
Rocephin *intravenous* solutions, at concentrations of 10, 20 and 40 mg/mL, remain stable (loss of potency less than 10%) for the following time periods stored in glass or PVC containers:
[See second table at top of previous page]
Similarly, Rocephin *intravenous* solutions, at concentrations of 100 mg/mL, remain stable in the IV piggyback glass containers for the above specified time periods.
The following *intravenous* Rocephin solutions are stable at room temperature (25°C) for 24 hours, at concentrations between 10 mg/mL and 40 mg/mL: Sodium Lactate (PVC container), 10% Invert Sugar (glass container), 5% Sodium Bicarbonate (glass container), Freamine III (glass container), Normosol-M in 5% Dextrose (glass and PVC containers), Ionosol-B in 5% Dextrose (glass container), 5% Mannitol (glass container), 10% Mannitol (glass container).
After the indicated stability time periods, unused portions of solutions should be discarded.
Rocephin reconstituted with 5% Dextrose or 0.9% Sodium Chloride solution at concentrations between 10 mg/mL and 40 mg/mL, and then stored in frozen state (−20°C) in PVC or polyolefin containers, remains stable for 26 weeks.
Frozen solutions should be thawed at room temperature before use. After thawing, unused portions should be discarded. **DO NOT REFREEZE.**
Rocephin solutions should *not* be physically mixed with or piggybacked into solutions containing other antimicrobial drugs or into diluent solutions other than those listed above, due to possible incompatibility.

ANIMAL PHARMACOLOGY

Concretions consisting of the precipitated calcium salt of ceftriaxone have been found in the gallbladder bile of dogs and baboons treated with ceftriaxone.
These appeared as a gritty sediment in dogs that received 100 mg/kg/day for 4 weeks. A similar phenomenon has been observed in baboons but only after a protracted dosing period (6 months) at higher dose levels (335 mg/kg/day or more). The likelihood of this occurrence in humans is considered to be low, since ceftriaxone has a greater plasma half-life in humans, the calcium salt of ceftriaxone is more soluble in human gallbladder bile and the calcium content of human gallbladder bile is relatively low.

HOW SUPPLIED

Rocephin is supplied as a sterile crystalline powder in glass vials and piggyback bottles. The following packages are available:
Vials containing 250 mg equivalent of ceftriaxone. Box of 1 (NDC 0004-1962-02) and box of 10 (NDC 0004-1962-01).
Vials containing 500 mg equivalent of ceftriaxone. Box of 1 (NDC 0004-1963-02) and box of 10 (NDC 0004-1963-01).
Vials containing 1 gm equivalent of ceftriaxone. Box of 1 (NDC 0004-1964-04) and box of 10 (NDC 0004-1964-01).
Piggyback bottles containing 1 gm equivalent of ceftriaxone. Box of 1 (NDC 0004-1964-02).
Vials containing 2 gm equivalent of ceftriaxone. Box of 10 (NDC 0004-1965-01).
Piggyback bottles containing 2 gm equivalent of ceftriaxone. Box of 1 (NDC 0004-1965-02).
Bulk pharmacy containers, containing 10 gm equivalent of ceftriaxone. Box of 1 (NDC 0004-1971-01). NOT FOR DIRECT ADMINISTRATION.
Rocephin is also supplied in an Intramuscular Convenience Kit, available in two strengths, consisting of a vial of ceftriaxone sodium as a sterile crystalline powder and a vial of Xylocaine®-MPF 1% (lidocaine HCl Injection, USP).
The following strengths are available:
Kit containing 1 vial of 500 mg equivalent of ceftriaxone, plus 1 vial of 2.1 mL Xylocaine (NDC 0004-2014-92).
Kit containing 1 vial of 1 gm equivalent of ceftriaxone, plus 1 vial of 2.1 mL Xylocaine (NDC 0004-2013-92).
Xylocaine®-MPF 1% (lidocaine HCl Injection, USP) is manufactured for Roche Laboratories Inc. by Astra USA, Inc., Westborough, MA 01581.
Rocephin is also supplied as a sterile crystalline powder in ADD-Vantage®* Vials as follows:
ADD-Vantage Vials containing 1 gm equivalent of ceftriaxone. Box of 10 (NDC 0004-1964-05).
ADD-Vantage Vials containing 2 gm equivalent of ceftriaxone. Box of 10 (NDC 0004-1965-05).
Rocephin (ceftriaxone sodium injection), also supplied premixed as a frozen, iso-osmotic, sterile, nonpyrogenic solution of ceftriaxone sodium in 50 mL single dose Galaxy®† containers (PL 2040 plastic), is manufactured for Roche Laboratories Inc., by Baxter Healthcare Corporation, Deerfield, Illinois 60015. The following strengths are available:
1 gm equivalent of ceftriaxone, iso-osmotic with approximately 1.9 gm Dextrose Hydrous, USP, added (NDC 0004-2002-78).
2 gm equivalent of ceftriaxone, iso-osmotic with approximately 1.2 gm Dextrose Hydrous, USP, added (NDC 0004-2003-78).
NOTE: Store Rocephin in the frozen state at or below -20°C/-4°F.

*Registered trademark of Abbott Laboratories, Inc.
†Registered trademark of Baxter International Inc.

CLINICAL STUDIES

Clinical Trials in Pediatric Patients With Acute Bacterial Otitis Media: In two adequate and well controlled US clinical trials a single IM dose of ceftriaxone was compared with a 10 day course of oral antibiotic in pediatric patients between the ages of 3 months and 6 years. The clinical cure rates and statistical outcome appear in the table below:
[See third table at top of previous page]
An open-label bacteriologic study of ceftriaxone without a comparator enrolled 108 pediatric patients, 79 of whom had positive baseline cultures for one or more of the common pathogens. The results of this study are tabulated as follows:
Week 2 and 4 Bacteriologic Eradication Rates in the Per Protocol Analysis in the Roche Bacteriologic Study by pathogen:
[See fourth table at top of previous page]

REFERENCES

1. National Committee for Clinical Laboratory Standards, *Performance Standards for Antimicrobial Disk Susceptibility Tests.* 5th ed. Villanova, PA: 1993. Approved Standard NCCLS Document M2-A5, Vol. 13, No. 24. NCCLS.
2. National Committee for Clinical Laboratory Standards, *Methods for Dilution Antimicrobial Susceptibility Tests for Bacteria That Grow Aerobically.* 3rd ed. Villanova, PA: 1993. Approved Standard NCCLS Document M7-A3, Vol. 13, No. 25. NCCLS.
3. Barnett ED, Teele DW, Klein JO, et al. *Comparison of Ceftriaxone and Trimethoprim-Sulfamethoxazole for Acute Otitis Media.* Pediatrics. Vol. 99, No. 1, January 1997.

Revised: January 1998

ROFERON®-A ℞

[ro-fear 'on]
(Interferon alfa-2a, recombinant)

DESCRIPTION

Roferon-A (Interferon alfa-2a, recombinant) is a sterile protein product for use by injection. Roferon-A is manufactured by recombinant DNA technology that employs a genetically engineered *Escherichia coli* bacterium containing DNA that codes for the human protein. Interferon alfa-2a, recombinant is a highly purified protein containing 165 amino acids, and it has an approximate molecular weight of 19,000 daltons. Fermentation is carried out in a defined nutrient medium containing the antibiotic tetracycline hydrochloride, 5 mg/L. However, the presence of the antibiotic is not detectable in the final product. Roferon-A is supplied as an injectable solution in a vial or a prefilled syringe. Each glass syringe barrel contains 0.5 mL of product. In addition, there is a needle which is ½ inch in length.
Single Use Injectable Solution:
3 million IU (11.1 mcg/mL) Roferon-A per vial—The solution is colorless and each mL contains 3 MIU of Interferon alfa-2a, recombinant, 7.21 mg sodium chloride, 0.2 mg polysorbate 80, 10 mg benzyl alcohol as a preservative and 0.77 mg ammonium acetate.
6 million IU (22.2 mcg/mL) Roferon-A per vial—The solution is colorless and each mL contains 6 MIU of Interferon alfa-2a, recombinant, 7.21 mg sodium chloride, 0.2 mg polysorbate 80, 10 mg benzyl alcohol as a preservative and 0.77 mg ammonium acetate.
9 million IU (33.3 mcg/0.9 mL) Roferon-A per vial—The solution is colorless and each 0.9 mL contains 9 MIU of Interferon alfa-2a, recombinant, 6.49 mg sodium chloride, 0.18 mg polysorbate 80, 9 mg benzyl alcohol as a preservative and 0.69 mg ammonium acetate. For single dose administration, withdraw 0.9 mL using a 1 mL syringe. Also can be used as a multidose vial.
36 million IU (133.3 mcg/mL) Roferon-A per vial—The solution is colorless and each mL contains 36 MIU of Interferon alfa-2a, recombinant, 7.21 mg sodium chloride, 0.2 mg polysorbate 80, 10 mg benzyl alcohol as a preservative and 0.77 mg ammonium acetate.
Single Use Prefilled Syringes:
3 million IU (11.1 mcg/0.5 mL) Roferon-A per syringe—The solution is colorless and each 0.5 mL contains 3 MIU of Interferon alfa-2a, recombinant, 3.605 mg sodium chloride, 0.1 mg polysorbate 80, 5 mg benzyl alcohol as a preservative and 0.385 mg ammonium acetate.
6 million IU (22.2 mcg/0.5 mL) Roferon-A per syringe—The solution is colorless and each 0.5 mL contains 6 MIU of Interferon alfa-2a, recombinant, 3.605 mg sodium chloride, 0.1 mg polysorbate 80, 5 mg benzyl alcohol as a preservative and 0.385 mg ammonium acetate.
9 million IU (33.3 mcg/0.5 mL) Roferon-A per syringe—The solution is colorless and each 0.5 mL contains 9 MIU of Interferon alfa-2a, recombinant, 3.605 mg sodium chloride, 0.1 mg polysorbate 80, 5 mg benzyl alcohol as a preservative and 0.385 mg ammonium acetate.
Multidose Injectable Solution:
9 million IU (33.3 mcg/0.9 mL) Roferon-A per vial—The solution is colorless and each 0.9 mL contains 9 MIU of Interferon alfa-2a, recombinant, 6.49 mg sodium chloride, 0.18 mg polysorbate 80, 9 mg benzyl alcohol as a preservative and 0.69 mg ammonium acetate. Also can be used as a single use vial.
18 million IU (66.7 mcg/3 mL) Roferon-A per vial—The solution is colorless and each mL contains 6 MIU of Interferon alfa-2a, recombinant, 7.21 mg sodium chloride, 0.2 mg polysorbate 80, 10 mg benzyl alcohol as a preservative and 0.77 mg ammonium acetate. Each 0.5 mL contains 3 MIU of Interferon alfa-2a, recombinant.
Based on the specific activity of 2.7×10^8IU/mg protein, the corresponding quantities of Interferon alfa-2a, recombinant in the vials described above are approximately 3 MIU (11.1 mcg/mL), 6 MIU (22.2 mcg/mL), 9 MIU (33.3 mcg/0.9 mL), 18 MIU (66.7 mcg/3 mL) and 36 MIU (133.3 mcg/mL).
The route of administration for the vial is subcutaneous or intramuscular; the route of administration for the prefilled syringe is subcutaneous only.

CLINICAL PHARMACOLOGY

The mechanism by which Interferon alfa-2a, recombinant, or any other interferon, exerts antitumor or antiviral activity is not clearly understood. However, it is believed that direct antiproliferative action against tumor cells, inhibition of virus replication and modulation of the host immune response play important roles in antitumor and antiviral activity.
The biological activities of Interferon alfa-2a, recombinant are species-restricted, ie, they are expressed in a very limited number of species other than humans. As a consequence, preclinical evaluation of Interferon alfa-2a, recombinant has involved in vitro experiments with human cells and some in vivo experiments.[1] Using human cells in culture, Interferon alfa-2a, recombinant has been shown to have antiproliferative and immunomodulatory activities that are very similar to those of the mixture of interferon alfa subtypes produced by human leukocytes. In vivo, Interferon alfa-2a, recombinant has been shown to inhibit the growth of several human tumors growing in immunocompromised (nude) mice. Because of its species-restricted activity, it has not been possible to demonstrate antitumor activity in immunologically intact syngeneic tumor model systems, where effects on the host immune system would be observable. However, such antitumor activity has been repeatedly demonstrated with, for example, mouse interferon-alfa in transplantable mouse tumor systems. The clinical significance of these findings is unknown.
The metabolism of Interferon alfa-2a, recombinant is consistent with that of alfa interferons in general. Alfa interferons are totally filtered through the glomeruli and undergo rapid proteolytic degradation during tubular reabsorption, rendering a negligible reappearance of intact alfa interferon in the systemic circulation. Small amounts of radiolabeled Interferon alfa-2a, recombinant appear in the urine of isolated rat kidneys, suggesting near complete reabsorption of Interferon alfa-2a, recombinant catabolites. Liver metabolism and subsequent biliary excretion are considered minor pathways of elimination for alfa interferons.

The serum concentrations of Interferon alfa-2a, recombinant reflected a large intersubject variation in both healthy volunteers and patients with disseminated cancer.
In healthy people, Interferon alfa-2a, recombinant exhibited an elimination half-life of 3.7 to 8.5 hours (mean 5.1 hours), volume of distribution at steady-state of 0.223 to 0.748 L/kg (mean 0.400 L/kg) and a total body clearance of 2.14 to 3.62 mL/min/kg (mean 2.79 mL/min/kg) after a 36 MIU (2.2×10^8pg) intravenous infusion. After intramuscular and subcutaneous administrations of 36 MIU, peak serum concentrations ranged from 1500 to 2580 pg/mL (mean 2020 pg/mL) at a mean time to peak of 3.8 hours and from 1250 to 2320 pg/mL (mean 1730 pg/mL) at a mean time to peak of 7.3 hours, respectively. The apparent fraction of the dose absorbed after intramuscular injection was greater than 80%.
The pharmacokinetics of Interferon alfa-2a, recombinant after single intramuscular doses to patients with disseminated cancer were similar to those found in healthy volunteers. Dose proportional increases in serum concentrations were observed after single doses up to 198 MIU. There were no changes in the distribution or elimination of Interferon alfa-2a, recombinant during twice daily (0.5 to 36 MIU), once daily (1 to 54 MIU), or three times weekly (1 to 136 MIU) dosing regimens up to 28 days of dosing. Multiple intramuscular doses of Interferon alfa-2a, recombinant resulted in an accumulation of two to four times the single dose serum concentrations. There is no pharmacokinetic information in patients with chronic hepatitis C, hairy cell leukemia, AIDS-related Kaposi's sarcoma and chronic myelogenous leukemia.
Serum neutralizing activity, determined by a highly sensitive enzyme immunoassay, and a neutralization bioassay, was detected in approximately 25% of all patients who received Roferon-A.[2] Antibodies to human leukocyte interferon may occur spontaneously in certain clinical conditions (cancer, systemic lupus erythematosus, herpes zoster) in patients who have never received exogenous interferon.[3] The significance of the appearance of serum neutralizing activity is not known.

CLINICAL STUDIES: Studies have shown that Roferon-A can normalize serum ALT, improve liver histology and reduce viral load in patients with chronic hepatitis C. Other studies have shown that Roferon-A can produce clinically meaningful tumor regression or disease stabilization in patients with hairy cell leukemia or in patients with AIDS-related Kaposi's sarcoma.[4–6] In Ph-positive Chronic Myelogenous Leukemia, Roferon-A supplemented with intermittent chemotherapy has been shown to prolong overall survival and to delay disease progression compared to patients treated with chemotherapy alone.[7] In addition, Roferon-A has been shown to produce sustained complete cytogenetic responses in a small subset of patients with CML in chronic phase. The activity of Roferon-A in Ph-negative CML has not been determined.
EFFECTS ON CHRONIC HEPATITIS C: The safety and efficacy of Roferon-A was evaluated in multiple clinical trials involving over 2000 patients 18 years of age or older with hepatitis, with or without cirrhosis, who had elevated serum alanine aminotransferase (ALT) levels and tested positive for antibody to hepatitis C. Roferon-A was given three times a week (tiw) by subcutaneous (SC) or intramuscular (IM) injection in a variety of dosing regimens, including dose escalation and de-escalation regimens. Normalization of serum ALT was defined in all studies as two consecutive normal serum ALT values at least 21 days apart. A sustained response (SR) was defined as normalization of ALT both at the end of treatment and at the end of at least 6 months of treatment-free follow-up.
In trials in which Roferon-A was administered for 6 months, 6 MIU, 3 MIU, and 1 MIU were directly compared. Six MIU was associated with higher SR rates but greater toxicity (see ADVERSE REACTIONS). In studies in which the same dose of Roferon-A was administered for 6 or 12 months, the longer duration was associated with higher SR rates and adverse events were no more severe or frequent in the second 6 months than in the first 6 months. Based on these data, the recommended regimens are 3 MIU for 12 months or 6 MIU for the first 3 months followed by 3 MIU for the next 9 months (see Table 1 and DOSAGE AND ADMINISTRATION). There are no direct comparisons of these two regimens.
Younger patients (eg, less than 35 years of age) and patients without cirrhosis on liver biopsy were more likely to respond completely to Roferon-A than those patients greater than 35 years of age or patients with cirrhosis on liver biopsy.
In the two studies in which Roferon-A was administered subcutaneously three times weekly for 12 months, 20/173 (12%) patients experienced a sustained response to therapy (see Table 1). Of these patients, 15/173 (9%) maintained this sustained response during continuous follow-up for up to four years. Patients who have ALT normalization but who fail to have a sustained response following an initial course of therapy may benefit from retreatment with higher doses of Roferon-A (see DOSAGE AND ADMINISTRATION).
A subset of patients had liver biopsies performed both before and after treatment with Roferon-A. An improvement in liver histology as assessed by Knodell Histology Activity Index was generally observed.
A retrospective subgroup analysis of 317 patients from two studies suggested a correlation between improvement in liver histology, durable serum ALT response rates, and decreased viral load as measured by the polymerase chain reaction (PCR).
[See table above]

Table 1.—ALT Normalization in Patients Receiving Therapy With Roferon-A for 12 Months

Study No.	Dose (MIU)	N	End of Treatment [% (95% CI)]	End of Observation (Sustained Response SR) [% (95% CI)]*
1**	3	56	23	11
2	3	117	23	12
1 and 2 Combined	3	173	23 (17–30)	12 (7–17)
3	6–3	210	25 (19–31)	19 (14–25)

* All patients were followed for 6 months after end of treatment.
**EOT and SR rates for Placebo (study 1) were 0.

EFFECTS ON Ph-POSITIVE CHRONIC MYELOGENOUS LEUKEMIA (CML): Roferon-A was evaluated in two trials of patients with chronic phase CML. Study DM84-38 was a single center phase II study conducted at the MD Anderson Cancer Center, which enrolled 91 patients, 81% were previously treated, 82% were Ph positive, and 63% received Roferon-A within 1 year of diagnosis. Study MI400 was a multicenter randomized phase III study conducted in Italy by the Italian Cooperative Study Group on CML in 335 patients; 226 Roferon-A and 109 chemotherapy. Patients with Ph-positive, newly diagnosed or minimally treated CML were randomized (ratio 2:1) to either Roferon-A or conventional chemotherapy with either hydroxyurea or busulfan. In study DM84-38, patients started Roferon-A at 9 MIU/day, whereas in study MI400, it was progressively escalated from 3 to 9 MIU/day over the first month. In both trials, dose escalation for insufficient hematologic response, and dose attenuation or interruption for toxicity was permitted. No formal guidelines for dose attenuation were given in the chemotherapy arm of study MI400. In addition, in the Roferon-A arm, the MI400 protocol allowed the addition of intermittent single agent chemotherapy for insufficient hematologic response to Roferon-A alone. In this trial, 44% of the Roferon-A treated patients also received intermittent single agent chemotherapy at some time during the study. The two studies were analyzed according to uniform response criteria. For hematologic response: complete response (WBC $<9 \times 10^9$/L, normalization of the differential with no immature forms in the peripheral blood, disappearance of splenomegaly), partial response (>50% decrease from baseline of WBC to $<20\% \times 10^9$/L). For cytogenetic response: complete response (0% Ph-positive metaphases), partial response (1% to 34% Ph-positive metaphases).
In study DM84-38, the median survival from initiation of Roferon-A was 47 months. In study MI400, the median survival for the patients on the interferon arm was 69 months, which was significantly better than the 55 months seen in the chemotherapy control group (48 patients in study MI400 proceeded to BMT and in study DM84-38, 15 patients proceeded to BMT).
Roferon-A treatment significantly delayed disease progression to blastic phase as evidenced by a median time to disease progression of 69 months to 46 months with chemotherapy.
By multivariate analysis of prognostic factors associated with all 335 patients entered into the randomized study, treatment with Roferon-A (with or without intermittent additional chemotherapy; p=0.006), Sokal index[8] (p=0.006) and WBC (p=0.023) were the three variables associated with an improved survival, independent of other baseline characteristics (Karnofsky performance status and hemoglobin being the other factors entered into the model).
In study MI400, overall hematologic responses, [complete responses (CR) and partial responses (PR)], were observed in approximately 60% of patients treated with Roferon-A (40% CR, 20% PR), compared to 70% with chemotherapy (30% CR, 40% PR). The median time to reach a complete hematologic response was 5 months in the Roferon-A arm and 4 months in the chemotherapy arm. The overall cytogenetic response rate (CR+PR), in patients receiving Roferon-A, was 10% and 12% in studies MI400 and DM84-38, respectively, according to the intent-to-treat principle. In contrast, only 2% of the patients in the chemotherapy arm of study MI400 achieved a cytogenetic response (with no complete responses). Cytogenetic responses were observed only in patients who had complete hematologic responses.
In study DM84-38, hematologic and cytogenetic response rates were higher in the subset of patients treated with Roferon-A within 1 year of diagnosis (76% and 17%, respectively) compared to the subset initiating Roferon-A therapy more than 1 year from diagnosis (29% and 4%, respectively). In an exploratory analysis, patients who achieved a cytogenetic response lived longer than those who did not.
Severe adverse events were observed in 66% and 31% of patients on study DM84-38 and MI400, respectively. Dose reduction and temporary cessation of therapy was required frequently. Permanent cessation of Roferon-A, due to intolerable side effects, was required in 15% and 23% of patients on studies DM84-38 and MI400, respectively (see ADVERSE REACTIONS).
Limited data are available on the use of Roferon-A in children with Ph-positive, adult-type CML. A published report on 15 children with CML suggests a safety profile similar to that seen in adult CML; clinical responses were also observed[9] (see DOSAGE AND ADMINISTRATION).
EFFECTS ON HAIRY CELL LEUKEMIA: A multicenter US phase II study (N2752) enrolled 218 patients; 75 were evaluable for efficacy in a preliminary analysis; 218 patients were evaluable for safety. Patients were to receive a starting dose of Roferon-A up to 6 MIU/m^2/day, for an induction period of 4 to 6 months. Responding patients were to receive 12 months maintenance therapy.
During the first 1 to 2 months of treatment of patients with hairy cell leukemia, significant depression of hematopoiesis was likely to occur. Subsequently, there was improvement in circulating blood cell counts. Of the 75 patients who were evaluable for efficacy following at least 16 weeks of therapy, 46 (61%) achieved complete or partial response. Twenty-one patients (28%) had a minor remission, 8 (11%) remained stable, and none had worsening of disease. All patients who achieved either a complete or partial response had complete or partial normalization of all peripheral blood elements including hemoglobin level, white blood cell, neutrophil, monocyte and platelet counts with a concomitant decrease in peripheral blood and bone marrow hairy cells. Responding patients also exhibited a marked reduction in red blood cell and platelet transfusion requirements, a decrease in infectious episodes and improvement in performance status. The probability of survival for 2 years in patients receiving Roferon-A (94%) was statistically increased compared to a historical control group (75%).
EFFECTS ON AIDS-RELATED KAPOSI'S SARCOMA: In six studies with Roferon-A, doses of 3 to 54 MIU daily were evaluated for the treatment of AIDS-related Kaposi's sarcoma in more than 350 patients. Four dosage regimens of Roferon-A were evaluated for initial induction. Thirty-nine patients received 3 MIU daily; 99 patients received an escalating regimen of 3 MIU, 9 MIU and 18 MIU each daily for 3 days, followed by 36 MIU daily; 119 patients received 36 MIU daily; and 16 patients received doses greater than 36 MIU to a maximum of 54 MIU daily. An additional 91 patients received Roferon-A in combination with vinblastine. The best response rate associated with acceptable toxicity was observed when Roferon-A was administered as a single agent at a dose of 36 MIU daily. The escalating regimen of 3 to 36 MIU daily provided equivalent therapeutic benefit with some amelioration of acute toxicity in some patients. In AIDS-related Kaposi's sarcoma, lower doses were less effective in inducing tumor regression and doses higher than 36 MIU daily were associated with unacceptable toxicity.
As summarized in Table 2, the likelihood of response to Roferon-A varied with the clinical manifestations of human immunodeficiency virus (HIV) infection. Patients with prior opportunistic infection or B symptoms are unlikely to respond to treatment with Roferon-A.
[See table at top of next page]
Patients who were otherwise asymptomatic, with no prior opportunistic infection and near-normal levels of CD_4 lymphocytes, experienced higher response rates. Responding patients with a baseline CD_4 lymphocyte count greater than 200 cells/mm^3 had a distinct survival advantage over both responding patients with a baseline CD_4 lymphocyte count of 200 cells/mm^3 or less and nonresponding patients regardless of their baseline CD_4 lymphocyte count. Median survival for responding patients with CD_4 lymphocyte counts of greater than 200 to 400 cells/mm^3 had not been reached but was greater than 32.7 months from the initiation of therapy. For responding patients with CD_4 lymphocyte counts of greater than 400 cells/mm^3, the median survival had not been reached but was greater than 29.5 months.
A classification system for staging AIDS-related Kaposi's sarcoma has been described based on location and extent of disease. In studies of Roferon-A, no difference was noted in response rates for patients with different stages of Kaposi's sarcoma. Likelihood of response was related to manifestations of HIV infection (baseline CD_4 lymphocyte count, prior opportunistic infection or B symptoms) and not to extent of tumor involvement. The median time to response was 2.7 months. The median duration of response for patients achieving a partial or complete response was 6.3 and 20.7 months, respectively. Complete and partial responses lasting in excess of 3 years have been observed. Therapy was discontinued because of progression of Kaposi's sarcoma, development of severe opportunistic infection or severe adverse effects. The median time to discontinuation of treatment was 12.5 months for responding patients and 2.3 months for patients who did not respond.

INDICATIONS AND USAGE

Roferon-A is indicated for the treatment of chronic hepatitis C, hairy cell leukemia and AIDS-related Kaposi's sarcoma in patients 18 years of age or older. In addition, it is indicated for chronic phase, Philadelphia chromosome (Ph) positive chronic myelogenous leukemia (CML) patients who are minimally pretreated (within 1 year of diagnosis).
FOR PATIENTS WITH CHRONIC HEPATITIS C: Roferon-A is indicated for use in patients with chronic hepatitis C diagnosed by HCV antibody and/or a history of ex-

Continued on next page

Roferon-A—Cont.

posure to hepatitis C who have compensated liver disease and are 18 years of age or older. A liver biopsy and a serum test for the presence of antibody to HCV should be performed to establish the diagnosis of chronic hepatitis C. Other causes of hepatitis, including hepatitis B, should be excluded prior to therapy with Roferon-A.

FOR PATIENTS WITH AIDS-RELATED KAPOSI'S SARCOMA: Roferon-A is indicated for the treatment of AIDS-related Kaposi's sarcoma in a select group of patients. In determining whether a patient should be treated, the physician should assess the likelihood of response based on the clinical manifestations of HIV infection, including prior opportunistic infections, presence of B symptoms, and CD_4 count, and the manifestations of Kaposi's sarcoma requiring treatment (see CLINICAL PHARMACOLOGY).

CONTRAINDICATIONS

Roferon-A is contraindicated in patients with known hypersensitivity to alfa interferon or any component of the product. The injectable solutions contain benzyl alcohol and are contraindicated in any individual with a known allergy to that preservative.

WARNINGS

Roferon-A should be administered under the guidance of a qualified physician (see DOSAGE AND ADMINISTRATION). Appropriate management of the therapy and its complications is possible only when adequate facilities are readily available.

DEPRESSION AND SUICIDAL BEHAVIOR INCLUDING SUICIDAL IDEATION, SUICIDAL ATTEMPTS AND SUICIDES HAVE BEEN REPORTED IN ASSOCIATION WITH TREATMENT WITH ALFA INTERFERONS, INCLUDING ROFERON-A. Patients to be treated with Roferon-A should be informed that depression and suicidal ideation may be side effects of treatment and should be advised to report these side effects immediately to the prescribing physician. Patients receiving Roferon-A therapy should receive close monitoring for the occurrence of depressive symptomatology. Cessation of treatment should be considered for patients experiencing depression. Although dose reduction or treatment cessation may lead to resolution of the depressive symptomatology, depression may persist and suicides have occurred after withdrawing therapy (see PRECAUTIONS and ADVERSE REACTIONS).

Central nervous system adverse reactions have been reported in a number of patients. These reactions included decreased mental status, dizziness, impaired memory, agitation, manic behavior and psychotic reactions. More severe obtundation and coma have been rarely observed. Most of these abnormalities were mild and reversible within a few days to 3 weeks upon dose reduction or discontinuation of Roferon-A therapy. Careful periodic neuropsychiatric monitoring of all patients is recommended.

Roferon-A should be used with caution in patients with severe preexisting cardiac disease, severe renal or hepatic disease, seizure disorders and/or compromised central nervous system function.

Roferon-A should be administered with caution to patients with cardiac disease or with any history of cardiac illness. Acute, self-limited toxicities (ie, fever, chills) frequently associated with Roferon-A administration may exacerbate preexisting cardiac conditions. Rarely, myocardial infarction has occurred in patients receiving Roferon-A. Cases of cardiomyopathy have been observed on rare occasions in patients treated with alfa interferons.

Patients with a history of autoimmune hepatitis or a history of autoimmune disease and patients who are immunosuppressed transplant recipients should not be treated with Roferon-A. Controlled studies of Roferon-A therapy in patients with advanced cirrhosis and/or decompensated liver disease have not been performed. In chronic hepatitis C, initiation of alfa-interferon therapy, including Roferon-A, has been reported to cause transient liver abnormalities, which in patients with poorly compensated liver disease can result in increased ascites, hepatic failure or death.

Leukopenia and elevation of hepatic enzymes occurred frequently but were rarely dose-limiting. Thrombocytopenia occurred less frequently. Proteinuria and increased cells in urinary sediment were also seen infrequently. Dose-limiting hepatic or renal toxicities were unusual. Infrequently, severe renal toxicities, sometimes requiring renal dialysis, have been reported with alfa-interferon therapy alone or in combination with IL-2 (see PRECAUTIONS).

Infrequently, severe or fatal gastrointestinal hemorrhage has been reported in association with alfa-interferon therapy.

Caution should be exercised when administering Roferon-A to patients with myelosuppression or when Roferon-A is used in combination with other agents that are known to cause myelosuppression. Synergistic toxicity has been observed when Roferon-A is administered in combination with zidovudine (AZT).[10] The effects of Roferon-A when combined with other drugs used in the treatment of AIDS-related disease are not known.

Hyperglycemia has been observed rarely in patients treated with Roferon-A. Symptomatic patients should have their blood glucose measured and followed-up accordingly. Patients with diabetes mellitus may require adjustment of their anti-diabetic regimen.

Table 2.—Likelihood of Response to Roferon-A in Patients With AIDS-Related Kaposi's Sarcoma

No. Pts.*	$CD_4(T_4)$ Lymphocyte Count(cells/mm^3)	Objective Response Rate (%) CR	PR	Total
83	0–200	3.6	3.6	7.2
51	201–400	15.7	11.8	27.5
33	>400	24.2	21.2	45.4

In the 28 patients evaluated who had prior opportunistic infection or B symptoms, the response rate was 3.6%.
*Patients had no prior opportunistic infection or B symptoms. B symptoms include night sweats, weight loss of greater than 10% of body weight or 15 lbs, or fever greater than 100°F without an identifiable source of infection.

Roferon-A should not be used for the treatment of visceral AIDS-related Kaposi's sarcoma associated with rapidly progressive or life-threatening disease.

The injectable solutions contain benzyl alcohol and should not be used by patients with a known allergy to benzyl alcohol. This product is not indicated for use in neonates or infants and should not be used by patients in that age group. There have been rare reports of death in neonates and infants associated with excessive exposure to benzyl alcohol. There have been reports of permanent neuropsychiatric deficits and multiple system organ failure associated with benzyl alcohol in neonates and infants. The amount of benzyl alcohol at which toxicity or adverse effects may occur in neonates or infants is not known (see CONTRAINDICATIONS).

PRECAUTIONS

General: In all instances where the use of Roferon-A is considered for chemotherapy, the physician must evaluate the need and usefulness of the drug against the risk of adverse reactions. Most adverse reactions are reversible if detected early. If severe reactions occur, the drug should be reduced in dosage or discontinued and appropriate corrective measures should be taken according to the clinical judgment of the physician. Reinstitution of Roferon-A therapy should be carried out with caution and with adequate consideration of the further need for the drug and, alertness to possible recurrence of toxicity. The minimum effective doses of Roferon-A for treatment of hairy cell leukemia, AIDS-related Kaposi's sarcoma and chronic myelogenous leukemia have not been established.

Variations in dosage and adverse reactions exist among different brands of Interferon. Therefore, do not use different brands of Interferon in a single treatment regimen.

Rare cases of autoimmune diseases including thrombocytopenia, vasculitis, Raynaud's phenomenon, rheumatoid arthritis, lupus erythematosus, and rhabdomyolysis have been observed in patients treated with alpha interferons. Any patient developing an autoimmune disorder during treatment should be closely monitored and, if appropriate, treatment should be discontinued.

Information for Patient: Patients should be cautioned not to change brands of Interferon without medical consultation, as a change in dosage may result. Patients should be informed regarding the potential benefits and risks attendant to the use of Roferon-A. If home use is determined to be desirable by the physician, instructions on appropriate use should be given, including review of the contents of the enclosed Patient Information Sheet. Patients should be well hydrated, especially during the initial stages of treatment. Patients should be thoroughly instructed in the importance of proper disposal procedures and cautioned against reusing syringes and needles. If home use is prescribed, a puncture-resistant container for the disposal of used syringes and needles should be supplied to the patient. The full container should be disposed of according to directions provided by the physician.

Patients receiving high-dose alfa interferon should be cautioned against performing tasks that require complete mental alertness such as operating machinery or driving a motor vehicle. Patients to be treated with Roferon-A should be informed that depression and suicidal ideation may be side effects of treatment and should be advised to report these side effects immediately to the prescribing physician.

Laboratory Tests: Complete blood with differential platelet counts and clinical chemistry tests should be performed before initiation of Roferon-A therapy and at appropriate periods during therapy. Since responses of hairy cell leukemia, AIDS-related Kaposi's sarcoma, chronic hepatitis C and chronic myelogenous leukemia are not generally observed for 1 to 3 months after initiation of treatment, very careful monitoring for severe depression of blood cell counts is warranted during the initial phase of treatment.

Those patients who have preexisting cardiac abnormalities and/or are in advanced stages of cancer should have electrocardiograms taken before and during the course of treatment.

For patients being treated for chronic hepatitis C, serum ALT should be evaluated before therapy to establish baselines and repeated at week 2 and monthly thereafter following initiation of therapy for monitoring clinical response. Patients with neutrophil count $<1500/mm^3$, platelet count $<75{,}000/mm^3$, hemoglobin <10 g/dL and creatinine >1.5 mg/dL were excluded from several major chronic hepatitis C studies; patients with these laboratory abnormalities should be carefully monitored if treated with Roferon-A.

Patients with preexisting thyroid abnormalities may be treated if normal thyroid stimulating hormone (TSH) levels can be maintained by medication. Testing of TSH levels in these patients is recommended at baseline and every 3 months following initiation of therapy.

Drug Interactions: Roferon-A has been reported to reduce the clearance of theophylline.[11,12] The clinical relevance of this interaction is presently unknown. Interactions between Roferon-A and other drugs have not been fully evaluated. Caution should be exercised when administering Roferon-A in combination with other potentially myelosuppressive agents (see WARNINGS).

Other Drug Interactions: Alfa interferons may affect the oxidative metabolic process by reducing the activity of hepatic microsomal cytochrome enzymes in the P450 group. Although the clinical relevance is still unclear, this should be taken into account when prescribing concomitant therapy with drugs metabolized by this route.

The neurotoxic, hematotoxic or cardiotoxic effects of previously or concurrently administered drugs may be increased by interferons. Interactions could occur following concurrent administration of centrally acting drugs. Use of Roferon-A in conjunction with interleukin-2 may potentiate risks of renal failure.

Carcinogenesis, Mutagenesis, Impairment of Fertility:

Carcinogenesis: Roferon-A has not been tested for its carcinogenic potential.

Mutagenesis: A. Internal Studies—Ames tests using six different tester strains, with and without metabolic activation, were performed with Roferon-A up to a concentration of 1920 µg/plate. There was no evidence of mutagenicity. Human lymphocyte cultures were treated in vitro with Roferon-A at noncytotoxic concentrations. No increase in the incidence of chromosomal damage was noted.

B. Published Studies—There are no published studies on the mutagenic potential of Roferon-A. However, a number of studies on the genotoxicity of human leukocyte interferon have been reported.

A chromosomal defect following the addition of human leukocyte interferon to lymphocyte cultures from a patient suffering from a lymphoproliferative disorder has been reported.

In contrast, other studies have failed to detect chromosomal abnormalities following treatment of lymphocyte cultures from healthy volunteers with human leukocyte interferon. It has also been shown that human leukocyte interferon protects primary chick embryo fibroblasts from chromosomal aberrations produced by gamma rays.

Impairment of Fertility: Roferon-A has been studied for its effect on fertility in Macaca mulatta (rhesus monkeys). Nonpregnant rhesus females treated with Roferon-A at doses of 5 and 25 MIU/kg/day have shown menstrual cycle irregularities, including prolonged or shortened menstrual periods and erratic bleeding; these cycles were considered to be anovulatory on the basis that reduced progesterone levels were noted and that expected increases in preovulatory estrogen and luteinizing hormones were not observed. These monkeys returned to a normal menstrual rhythm following discontinuation of treatment.

Pregnancy: Teratogenic Effects: Pregnancy Category C. Roferon-A has been shown to demonstrate a statistically significant increase in abortifacient activity in rhesus monkeys when given at approximately 20 to 500 times the human dose. A study in pregnant rhesus monkeys treated with 1, 5 or 25 MIU/kg/day of Roferon-A in their early to midfetal period (days 22 to 70 of gestation) has failed to demonstrate teratogenic activity for Roferon-A.

There are no adequate and well-controlled studies in pregnant women.

Nonteratogenic Effects: Dose-related abortifacient activity was observed in pregnant rhesus monkeys treated with 1, 5 or 25 MIU/kg/day of Roferon-A in their early to midfetal period (days 22 to 70 of gestation). A late fetal period study (days 79 to 100 of gestation) is in progress and as yet there have been no reports of any increased rate of abortion.

Usage in Pregnancy: Safe use in human pregnancy has not been established. Therefore, Roferon-A should be used during pregnancy only if the potential benefit justifies the potential risk to the fetus. Information from primate studies showed dose-related menstrual irregularities and an increased incidence of spontaneous abortions. Decreases in serum estradiol and progesterone concentrations have been reported in women treated with human leukocyte interferon.[13] Therefore, fertile women should not receive Roferon-A unless they are using effective contraception during the therapy period.

The injectable solution contains benzyl alcohol. The excipient benzyl alcohol can be transmitted via the placenta. The possibility of toxicity should be taken into account in premature infants after the administration of Roferon-A solution for injection immediately prior to birth or Cesarean section.

Male fertility and teratologic evaluations have yielded no significant adverse effects to date.

Nursing Mothers: It is not known whether this drug is excreted in human milk. Because many drugs are excreted in human milk and because of the potential for serious adverse reactions in nursing infants from Roferon-A, a decision should be made whether to discontinue nursing or to discontinue the drug, taking into account the importance of the drug to the mother.

Pediatric Use: Use of Roferon-A in children with Ph-positive adult-type CML is supported by evidence from adequate and well-controlled studies of Roferon-A in adults with additional data from the literature on the use of alfa interferon in children with CML. A published report on 15 children with Ph-positive adult-type CML suggests a safety profile similar to that seen in adult CML; clinical responses were also observed[9] (see DOSAGE AND ADMINISTRATION).

For all other indications, safety and effectiveness have not been established in patients below the age of 18 years.

The injectable solutions are not indicated for use in neonates or infants and should not be used by patients in that age group. There have been rare reports of death in neonates and infants associated with excessive exposure to benzyl alcohol (see WARNINGS).

ADVERSE REACTIONS

Depressive illness and suicidal behavior, including suicidal ideation and suicides, have been reported in association with the use of alfa-interferon products. The incidence of reported depression has varied substantially among trials, possibly related to the underlying disease, dose, duration of therapy and degree of monitoring, but has been reported to be 15% or higher (see WARNINGS).

FOR PATIENTS WITH CHRONIC HEPATITIS C: The most frequent adverse experiences were reported to be possibly or probably related to therapy with 3 MIU tiw Roferon-A, were mostly mild to moderate in severity and manageable without the need for discontinuation of therapy. A relative increase in the incidence, severity and seriousness of adverse events was observed in patients receiving doses above 3 MIU tiw.

Adverse reactions associated with the 3 MIU dose include:

Flu-like Symptoms: Fatigue (58%), myalgia/arthralgia (51%), flu-like symptoms (33%), fever (28%), chills (23%), asthenia (6%), sweating (5%), leg cramps (3%) and malaise (1%).

Central and Peripheral Nervous System: Headache (52%), dizziness (13%), paresthesia (7%), confusion (7%), concentration impaired (4%) and change in taste or smell (3%).

Gastrointestinal: Nausea/vomiting (33%), diarrhea (20%), anorexia (14%), abdominal pain (12%), flatulence (3%), liver pain (3%), digestion impaired (2%) and gingival bleeding (2%).

Psychiatric: Depression (16%), irritability (15%), insomnia (14%), anxiety (5%) and behavior disturbances (3%).

Pulmonary and Cardiovascular: Dryness or inflammation of oropharynx (6%), epistaxis (4%), rhinitis (3%), arrhythmia (1%) and sinusitis (<1%).

Skin: Injection site reaction (29%), partial alopecia (19%), rash (8%), dry skin or pruritus (7%), hematoma (1%), psoriasis (<1%), cutaneous eruptions (<1%), eczema (<1%) and seborrhea (<1%).

Other: Conjunctivitis (4%), menstrual irregularity (2%) and visual acuity decreased (<1%).

Patients receiving 6 MIU tiw experienced a higher incidence of severe psychiatric events (9%) than those receiving 3 MIU tiw (6%) in two large US studies. In addition, more patients withdrew from these studies when receiving 6 MIU tiw (11%) than when receiving 3 MIU tiw (7%). Up to half of patients receiving 3 MIU or 6 MIU tiw withdrawing from the study experienced depression or other psychiatric adverse events. At higher doses anxiety, sleep disorders, and irritability were observed more frequently. An increased incidence of fatigue, myalgia/arthralgia, headache, fever, chills, alopecia, sleep disturbances and dry skin or pruritus was also generally observed during treatment with higher doses of Roferon-A.

Generally there were fewer adverse events reported in the second 6 months of treatment than in the first 6 months for patients treated with 3 MIU tiw. Patients tolerant of initial therapy with Roferon-A generally tolerate re-treatment at the same dose, but tend to experience more adverse reactions at higher doses.

Infrequent adverse events (>1% but <3% incidence) included: cold feeling, cough, muscle cramps, diaphoresis, dyspnea, eye pain, reactivation of herpes simplex, lethargy, edema, sexual dysfunction, shaking, skin lesions, stomatitis, tooth disorder, urinary tract infection, weakness in extremities.

FOR PATIENTS WITH CHRONIC MYELOGENOUS LEUKEMIA:

For patients with chronic myelogenous leukemia, the percentage of adverse events, whether related to drug therapy or not, experienced by patients treated with rIFNα-2a is given below. Severe adverse events were observed in 66% and 31% of patients on study DM84-38 and MI400, respectively. Dose reduction and temporary cessation of therapy were required frequently. Permanent cessation of Roferon-A, due to intolerable side effects, was required in 15% and 23% of patients on studies DM84-38 and MI400, respectively.

Flu-like Symptoms: Fever (92%), asthenia or fatigue (88%), myalgia (68%), chills (63%), arthralgia/bone pain (47%) and headache (44%).

Table 3.—Significant Abnormal Laboratory Test Values

	Chronic Hepatitis C (n=203) 3 MIU tiw	Chronic Myelogenous Leukemia‡ US Study (n=91)	Chronic Myelogenous Leukemia‡ Non-US Study (n=219)	Hairy Cell Leukemia (n=218)	AIDS-related Kaposi's Sarcoma (n=241)
Leukopenia	1.5%	20%	3%	45%*	49%
Neutropenia	10%	22%	0%	68%*	52%
Thrombocytopenia	4.5%	27%	5%	62%*	35%
Anemia (Hb)	0%	15%	4%	31%*	27%
SGOT	NAP	5%	1%	9%	46%
Alk. Phosphatase	0%	3%	1%	3%	11%
LDH	NAP	NA	NA	<1%	10%
Proteinuria	0%	NA	NA	10%†	<1%

* In the majority of patients, initial hematologic laboratory test values were abnormal due to their underlying disease.
† Ten percent of the patients experienced a proteinuria >1+ at least once.
‡ Patients enrolled in the two clinical studies receiving at least one dose of Roferon-A.
NAP = Not applicable.
NA = Not assessed.

Gastrointestinal: Anorexia (48%), nausea/vomiting (37%) and diarrhea (37%).

Central and Peripheral Nervous System: Headache (44%), depression (28%), decreased mental status (16%), dizziness (11%), sleep disturbances (11%), paresthesia (8%), involuntary movements (7%) and visual disturbance (6%).

Pulmonary and Cardiovascular: Coughing (19%), dyspnea (8%) and dysrhythmia (7%).

Skin: Hair changes (including alopecia) (18%), skin rash (18%), sweating (15%), dry skin (7%) and pruritus (7%).

Uncommon adverse events (< 4%) reported in clinical studies included chest pain, syncope, hypotension, impotence, alterations in taste or hearing, confusion, seizures, memory loss, disturbances of libido, bruising and coagulopathy. Miscellaneous adverse events that were rarely observed included Coombs' positive hemolytic anemia, aplastic anemia, hypothyroidism, cardiomyopathy, hypertriglyceridemia and bronchospasm.

FOR PATIENTS WITH HAIRY CELL LEUKEMIA:

Constitutional (100%): Fever (92%), fatigue (86%), headache (64%), chills (64%), weight loss (33%), dizziness (21%) and flu-like symptoms (16%).

Integumentary (79%): Skin rash (44%), diaphoresis (22%), partial alopecia (17%), dry skin (17%) and pruritus (13%).

Musculoskeletal (73%): Myalgia (71%), joint or bone pain (25%) and arthritis or polyarthritis (5%).

Gastrointestinal (69%): Anorexia (43%), nausea/vomiting (39%) and diarrhea (34%).

Head and Neck (45%): Throat irritation (21%), rhinorrhea (12%) and sinusitis (11%).

Pulmonary (40%): Coughing (16%), dyspnea (12%) and pneumonia (11%).

Central Nervous System (39%): Dizziness (21%), depression (16%), sleep disturbance (10%), decreased mental status (10%), anxiety (6%), lethargy (6%), visual disturbance (6%) and confusion (5%).

Cardiovascular (39%): Chest pain (11%), edema (11%) and hypertension (11%).

Pain (34%): Pain (24%) and pain in back (16%).

Peripheral Nervous System (23%): Paresthesia (12%) and numbness (12%).

Rarely (<5%), central nervous system effects including gait disturbance, nervousness, syncope and vertigo, as well as cardiac adverse events including murmur, thrombophlebitis and hypotension were reported. Adverse experiences that occurred rarely, and may have been related to underlying disease, included ecchymosis, epistaxis, bleeding gums and petechiae. Urticaria and inflammation at the site of injection were also rarely observed.

FOR PATIENTS WITH AIDS-RELATED KAPOSI'S SARCOMA:

Flu-like Symptoms: Fatigue (95%), fever (74%), myalgia (69%), headache (66%), chills (41%) and arthralgia (24%).

Gastrointestinal: Anorexia (65%), nausea (51%), diarrhea (42%), emesis (17%) and abdominal pain (15%).

Central and Peripheral Nervous System: Dizziness (40%), decreased mental status (17%), depression (16%), paresthesia (8%), confusion (8%), diaphoresis (7%), visual disturbances (5%), sleep disturbances (5%) and numbness (3%).

Pulmonary and Cardiovascular: Coughing (27%), dyspnea (11%), edema (9%), chest pain (4%) and hypotension (4%).

Skin: Partial alopecia (22%), rash (11%) and dry skin or pruritus (5%).

Other: Weight loss (25%), change in taste (25%), dryness or inflammation of the oropharynx (14%), night sweats (8%) and rhinorrhea (4%).

Occasionally (<3%) nervous system effects including anxiety, nervousness, emotional lability, vertigo and forgetfulness, as well as cardiac adverse events, including palpitations and arrhythmia, were reported. Other adverse experiences that occurred occasionally (<3%) and may have been related to underlying disease, included sinusitis, constipation, chest congestion, pneumonia, urticaria and flatulence. Adverse experiences which occurred rarely (<1%) included ataxia, seizures, cyanosis, gastric distress, bronchospasm, pain at injection site, earache, eye irritation and rhinitis. Miscellaneous adverse experiences such as poor coordination, lethargy, muscle contractions, neuropathy, tremor, involuntary movement, syncope, aphasia, aphonia, dysarthria, amnesia, weakness and flushing of skin were observed in less than 0.5% of patients. Cases of cardiomyopathy have been observed on rare occasions in patients treated with alfa interferons.

IN OTHER INVESTIGATIONAL STUDIES OF ROFERON-A:

The following infrequent adverse events have been reported in one or more of the approved clinical indications as well as with the investigational use of Roferon-A (<5%): pancreatitis, colitis, gastrointestinal hemorrhage, stomatitis, thyroid dysfunction (including hypothyroidism and hyperthyroidism), diabetes (in some patients requiring insulin therapy), and pneumonitis (some cases responding to interferon cessation and corticosteroid therapy). In addition to the adverse experiences noted above, other adverse experiences that occurred included: abdominal fullness, hypermotility, hepatitis, gait disturbance, hallucinations, encephalopathy, psychomotor retardation, coma, stroke, transient ischemic attacks, dysphasia, sedation, apathy, irritability, hyperactivity, claustrophobia, loss of libido, congestive heart failure, myocardial infarction, Raynaud's phenomenon, hot flashes, tachypnea, ischemic retinopathy, excessive salivation and anaphylactic reactions. These adverse experiences occurred rarely (<1%).

The following events have been rarely observed (<3%) in some patients receiving Roferon-A: autoimmune diseases, ie, vasculitis, arthritis, hemolytic anemia and lupus erythematosus syndrome. The mechanism by which these events develop and their relationship to Roferon-A therapy are unclear. Similar events have been reported for other types of interferon.

ABNORMAL LABORATORY TEST VALUES: The percentage of patients with chronic hepatitis C, hairy cell leukemia, with AIDS-related Kaposi's sarcoma, and with chronic myelogenous leukemia who experienced a significant abnormal laboratory test value *(NCI or WHO grades III or IV)* at least once during their treatment with Roferon-A is shown in the following table:

[See table above]

CHRONIC HEPATITIS C: The incidence of neutropenia *(WHO grades III or IV)* was over twice as high in those treated with 6 MIU tiw (21%) as those treated with 3 MIU tiw (10%).

CHRONIC MYELOGENOUS LEUKEMIA: In the two clinical studies, a severe or life-threatening anemia was seen in up to 15% of patients. A severe or life-threatening leukopenia and thrombocytopenia were observed in up to 20% and 27% of patients, respectively. Changes were usually reversible when therapy was discontinued. One case of aplastic anemia and one case of Coombs' positive hemolytic anemia were seen in 310 patients treated with rIFNα-2a in clinical studies. Severe cytopenias led to discontinuation of therapy in 4% of all Roferon-A treated patients.

Transient increases in liver transaminases or alkaline phosphatase of any intensity were seen in up to 50% of patients during treatment with Roferon-A. Only 5% of patients had a severe or life-threatening increase in SGOT. In the clinical studies, such abnormalities required termination of therapy in less than 1% of patients.

HAIRY CELL LEUKEMIA: Increases in serum phosphorus (≥1.6 mmol/L) and serum uric acid (≥9.1 mg/dL) were observed in 9% and 10% of patients, respectively. The increase in serum uric acid is likely to be related to the underlying disease. Decreases in serum calcium (≤1.9 mmol/L) and serum phosphorus (≤0.9 mmol/L) were seen in 28% and 22% of patients, respectively.

OVERDOSAGE

There are no reports of overdosage, but repeated large doses of interferon can be associated with profound lethargy, fatigue, prostration, and coma. Such patients should be hospitalized for observation and appropriate supportive treatment given.

DOSAGE AND ADMINISTRATION

Roferon-A recommended dosing regimens are different for each of the following indications as described below.

Note: Parenteral drug products should be inspected visually for particulate matter and discoloration before administration, whenever solution and container permit.

Continued on next page

Roferon-A—Cont.

Roferon-A vials are administered either subcutaneously or intramuscularly. The Roferon-A prefilled syringe is administered subcutaneously only, due to the length of the syringe needle (1/2 inch) provided in the packaging.

CHRONIC HEPATITIS C: The recommended dosage of Roferon-A for the treatment of chronic hepatitis C is 3 MIU three times a week (tiw) administered subcutaneously or intramuscularly for 12 months (48 to 52 weeks). As an alternative, patients may be treated with an induction dose of 6 MIU tiw for the first 3 months (12 weeks) followed by 3 MIU tiw for 9 months (36 weeks). Normalization of serum ALT generally occurs within a few weeks after initiation of treatment in responders. Approximately 90% of patients who respond to Roferon-A do so within the first 3 months of treatment; however, patients responding to Roferon-A with a reduction in ALT should complete 12 months of treatment. Patients who have no response to Roferon-A within the first 3 months of therapy are not likely to respond with continued treatment; treatment discontinuation should be considered in these patients.

Patients who tolerate and partially or completely respond to therapy with Roferon-A but relapse following its discontinuation may be re-treated. Re-treatment with either 3 MIU tiw or with 6 MIU tiw for 6 to 12 months may be considered. Please see ADVERSE REACTIONS regarding the increased frequency of adverse reactions associated with treatment with higher doses.

Temporary dose reduction by 50% is recommended in patients who do not tolerate the prescribed dose. If adverse events resolve, treatment with the original prescribed dose can be re-initiated. In patients who cannot tolerate the reduced dose, cessation of therapy, at least temporarily, is recommended.

CHRONIC MYELOGENOUS LEUKEMIA: For patients with Ph-positive CML in chronic phase: Prior to initiation of therapy, a diagnosis of Philadelphia chromosome positive CML in chronic phase by the appropriate peripheral blood, bone marrow and other diagnostic testing should be made. Monitoring of hematologic parameters should be done regularly (eg, monthly). Since significant cytogenetic changes are not readily apparent until after hematologic response has occurred, and usually not until several months of therapy have elapsed, cytogenetic monitoring may be performed at less frequent intervals. Achievement of complete cytogenetic response has been observed up to 2 years following the start of Roferon-A treatment.

The recommended initial dose of Roferon-A is 9 MIU daily administered as a subcutaneous or intramuscular injection. Based on clinical experience,[3] short-term tolerance may be improved by gradually increasing the dose of Roferon-A over the first week of administration from 3 MIU daily for 3 days to 6 MIU daily for 3 days to the target dose of 9 MIU daily for the duration of the treatment period.

The optimal dose and duration of therapy have not yet been determined. Even though the median time to achieve a complete hematologic response was 5 months in study MI400, hematologic responses have been observed up to 18 months after treatment start. Treatment should be continued until disease progression. If severe side effects occur, a treatment interruption or a reduction in either the dose or the frequency of injections may be necessary to achieve the individual maximally tolerated dose (see PRECAUTIONS).

Limited data are available on the use of Roferon-A in children with CML. In one report of 15 children with Ph-positive, adult-type CML doses between 2.5 to 5 MIU/m^2/day given intramuscularly were tolerated.[9] In another study, severe adverse effects including deaths were noted in children with previously untreated, Ph-negative, juvenile CML, who received interferon doses of 30 MIU/m^2/day.[14]

HAIRY CELL LEUKEMIA: Prior to initiation of therapy, tests should be performed to quantitate peripheral blood hemoglobin, platelets, granulocytes and hairy cells and bone marrow hairy cells. These parameters should be monitored periodically (eg, monthly) during treatment to determine whether response to treatment has occurred. If a patient does not respond within 6 months, treatment should be discontinued. If a response to treatment does occur, treatment should be continued until no further improvement is observed and these laboratory parameters have been stable for about 3 months. Patients with hairy cell leukemia have been treated for up to 24 consecutive months. The optimal duration of treatment for this disease has not been determined.

The induction dose of Roferon-A is 3 MIU daily for 16 to 24 weeks, administered as a subcutaneous or intramuscular injection. Subcutaneous administration is particularly suggested for, but not limited to, thrombocytopenic patients (platelet count <50,000) or for patients at risk for bleeding. The recommended maintenance dose is 3 MIU, three times a week (tiw). Dose reduction by one-half or withholding of individual doses may be needed when severe adverse reactions occur. The use of doses higher than 3 MIU is not recommended in hairy cell leukemia.

AIDS-RELATED KAPOSI'S SARCOMA: Roferon-A is useful for the treatment of AIDS-related Kaposi's sarcoma in a select group of patients. In determining whether a patient should be treated, the physician should assess the likelihood of response based on the clinical manifestations of HIV infection and the manifestations of Kaposi's sarcoma requiring treatment (see CLINICAL PHARMACOLOGY).

Indicator lesion measurements and total lesion count should be performed before initiation of therapy. These parameters should be monitored periodically (eg, monthly) during treatment to determine whether response to treatment or disease stabilization has occurred. When disease stabilization or a response to treatment occurs, treatment should continue until there is no further evidence of tumor or until discontinuation is required because of a severe opportunistic infection or adverse effects. The optimal duration of treatment for this disease has not been determined.

The recommended induction dose of Roferon-A is 36 MIU daily for 10 to 12 weeks, administered as an intramuscular or subcutaneous injection. Subcutaneous administration is particularly suggested for, but not limited to, patients who are thrombocytopenic (platelet count <50,000) or who are at risk for bleeding. The recommended maintenance dose is 36 MIU, three times a week (tiw). If severe reactions occur, the dose should be modified (50% reduction) or therapy should be temporarily discontinued until the adverse reactions abate. An escalating schedule of 3 MIU, 9 MIU and 18 MIU each daily for 3 days followed by 36 MIU daily for the remainder of the 10- to 12-week induction period has also produced equivalent therapeutic benefit with some amelioration of the acute toxicity in some patients.

HOW SUPPLIED

Single Use Injectable Solution: (for subcutaneous or intramuscular administration)

3 million IU Roferon-A per vial —Each 1 mL contains 3 MIU of Interferon alfa-2a, recombinant, 7.21 mg sodium chloride, 0.2 mg polysorbate 80, 10 mg benzyl alcohol as a preservative and 0.77 mg ammonium acetate. Boxes of 1 (NDC 0004-2009-09).

6 million IU Roferon-A per vial —Each 1 mL contains 6 MIU of Interferon alfa-2a, recombinant, 7.21 mg sodium chloride, 0.2 mg polysorbate 80, 10 mg benzyl alcohol as a preservative and 0.77 mg ammonium acetate. Boxes of 1 (NDC 0004-2007-09).

9 million IU Roferon-A per vial —Each 0.9 mL contains 9 MIU of Interferon alfa-2a, recombinant, 6.49 mg sodium chloride, 0.18 mg polysorbate 80, 9 mg benzyl alcohol as a preservative and 0.69 mg ammonium acetate. For single dose administration, withdraw 0.9 mL using a 1 mL syringe. Also can be used as a multidose vial. Boxes of 1 (NDC 0004-2010-09).

36 million IU Roferon-A per vial —Each 1 mL contains 36 MIU of Interferon alfa-2a, recombinant, 7.21 mg sodium chloride, 0.2 mg polysorbate 80, 10 mg benzyl alcohol as a preservative and 0.77 mg ammonium acetate. Boxes of 1 (NDC 0004-2012-09).

Single Use Prefilled Syringes: (for subcutaneous administration only)

3 million IU Roferon-A per syringe —Each 0.5 mL contains 3 MIU of Interferon alfa-2a, recombinant, 3.605 mg sodium chloride, 0.1 mg polysorbate 80, 5 mg benzyl alcohol as a preservative and 0.385 mg ammonium acetate. Boxes of 1 (NDC 0004-2015-09); Boxes of 6 (NDC 0004-2015-07).

6 million IU Roferon-A per syringe —Each 0.5 mL contains 6 MIU of Interferon alfa-2a, recombinant, 3.605 mg sodium chloride, 0.1 mg polysorbate 80, 5 mg benzyl alcohol as a preservative and 0.385 mg ammonium acetate. Boxes of 1 (NDC 0004-2016-09); Boxes of 6 (NDC 0004-2016-07).

9 million IU Roferon-A per syringe —Each 0.5 mL contains 9 MIU of Interferon alfa-2a, recombinant, 3.605 mg sodium chloride, 0.1 mg polysorbate 80, 5 mg benzyl alcohol as a preservative and 0.385 mg ammonium acetate. Boxes of 1 (NDC 0004-2017-09); Boxes of 6 (NDC 0004-2017-07).

Multidose Injectable Solution: (for subcutaneous or intramuscular administration)

9 million IU Roferon-A per vial —Each 0.3 mL contains 3 MIU of Interferon alfa-2a, recombinant, 2.16 mg sodium chloride, 0.06 mg polysorbate 80, 3 mg benzyl alcohol as a preservative and 0.23 mg ammonium acetate. Also can be used as a single use vial. Once the vial is entered, it must be used within 30 days. The 9 MIU multidose vial contains an average of 13 MIU of Interferon alfa-2a, recombinant in order to provide the delivery of three 0.3 mL doses, each containing 3 MIU of Roferon-A Interferon alfa-2a, recombinant for injection. Boxes of 1 (NDC 0004-2010-09).

18 million IU Roferon-A per vial —Each 1 mL contains 6 MIU of Interferon alfa-2a, recombinant, 7.21 mg sodium chloride, 0.2 mg polysorbate 80, 10 mg benzyl alcohol as a preservative and 0.77 mg ammonium acetate. Each 0.5 mL contains 3 MIU of Interferon alfa-2a, recombinant. Once the vial is entered, it must be used within 30 days. The 18 MIU multidose vial contains an average of 22.8 MIU of Interferon alfa-2a, recombinant in order to provide the delivery of six 0.5 mL doses, each containing 3 MIU of Roferon-A Interferon alfa-2a, recombinant for injection. Boxes of 1 (NDC 0004-2011-09).

Storage: The injectable solution and the prefilled syringe should be stored in the refrigerator at 36° to 46°F (2° to 8°C). Do *not* freeze or shake.

REFERENCES

1. Trown PW, et al. *Cancer.* 1986; 57(suppl):1648–1656. 2. Itri LM, et al. *Cancer.* 1987; 59:668–674. 3. Jones GJ, Itri LM. *Cancer.* 1986; 57(suppl):1709–1715. 4. Foon KA, et al. *Blood.* 1984; 64(suppl 1):164a. 5. Quesada Jr, et al. *Cancer.* 1986; 57(suppl):1678–1680. 6. Krown SE, et al. *N Eng J Med.* 1984; 308:1071–1076. 7. The Italian Cooperative Study Group on CML. *N Engl J Med.* 1994; 330:820–825. 8. Sokal JE, et al. *Blood.* 1984; 63(4):789–799. 9. Dow LW, et al. *Cancer.* 1991; 68:1678–1684. 10. Krown SE, et al. *Proc Am Soc Clin Oncol.* 1988; 7:1. 11. Williams SJ, et al. *Lancet.* 1987; 2:939–941. 12. Jonkman JHG, et al. *Br J Clin Pharmacol.* 1989; 2(27):795–802. 13. Kauppila A, et al. *Int J Cancer.* 1982; 29:291–294. 14. Maybee D, et al. *Proc Annu Meet Am Soc Clin Oncol.* 1992; 11:A950.

Revised: November 1999

ROMAZICON® ℞

[*ro-măs 'ĕ-kŏn*]
(flumazenil)
INJECTION

The following text is complete prescribing information based on official labeling in effect June 2000.

DESCRIPTION

ROMAZICON® (flumazenil) is a benzodiazepine receptor antagonist. Chemically, flumazenil is ethyl 8-fluoro-5,6-dihydro-5-methyl-6-oxo-4H-imidazo [1,5-a](1,4) benzodiazepine-3-carboxylate. Flumazenil has an imidazobenzodiazepine structure and a calculated molecular weight of 303.3.

Flumazenil is a white to off-white crystalline compound with an octanol:buffer partition coefficient of 14 to 1 at pH 7.4. It is insoluble in water but slightly soluble in acidic aqueous solutions. ROMAZICON is available as a sterile parenteral dosage form for intravenous administration. Each mL contains 0.1 mg of flumazenil compounded with 1.8 mg of methylparaben, 0.2 mg of propylparaben, 0.9% sodium chloride, 0.01% edetate disodium, and 0.01% acetic acid; the pH is adjusted to approximately 4 with hydrochloric acid and/or, if necessary, sodium hydroxide.

CLINICAL PHARMACOLOGY

Flumazenil, an imidazobenzodiazepine derivative, antagonizes the actions of benzodiazepines on the central nervous system. Flumazenil competitively inhibits the activity at the benzodiazepine recognition site on the GABA/benzodiazepine receptor complex. Flumazenil is a weak partial agonist in some animal models of activity, but has little or no agonist activity in man.

Flumazenil does not antagonize the central nervous system effects of drugs affecting GABA-ergic neurons by means other than the benzodiazepine receptor (including ethanol, barbiturates, or general anesthetics) and does not reverse the effects of opioids.

Pharmacodynamics: Intravenous ROMAZICON has been shown to antagonize sedation, impairment of recall, psychomotor impairment and ventilatory depression produced by benzodiazepines in healthy human volunteers.

The duration and degree of reversal of benzodiazepine effects are related to the dose and plasma concentrations of flumazenil as shown in the following data from a study in normal volunteers.

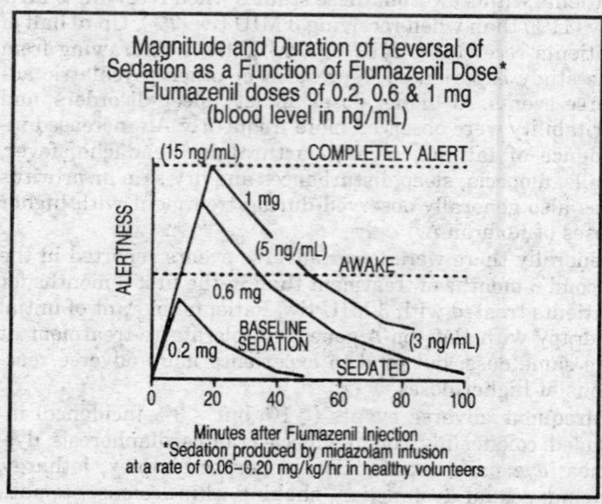

Generally, doses of approximately 0.1 mg to 0.2 mg (corresponding to peak plasma levels of 3 to 6 ng/mL) produce partial antagonism, whereas higher doses of 0.4 to 1 mg (peak plasma levels of 12 to 28 ng/mL) usually produce complete antagonism in patients who have received the usual sedating doses of benzodiazepines. The onset of reversal is usually evident within 1 to 2 minutes after the injection is completed. Eighty percent response will be reached within 3 minutes, with the peak effect occurring at 6 to 10 minutes. The duration and degree of reversal are related to the plasma concentration of the sedating benzodiazepine as well as the dose of ROMAZICON given.

In healthy volunteers, ROMAZICON did not alter intraocular pressure when given alone and reversed the decrease in intraocular pressure seen after administration of midazolam.

Pharmacokinetics in Adult Patients: After IV administration, plasma concentrations of flumazenil follow a two-compartment, open pharmacokinetic model with an initial distribution half-life of 7 to 15 minutes and a terminal half-life of 41 to 79 minutes. Peak concentrations of flumazenil are proportional to dose, with an apparent initial volume of distribution of 0.5 L/kg. After redistribution the apparent volume of distribution (V_{ss}) ranges from 0.77 to 1.60 L/kg. Protein binding is approximately 50% and the drug shows no preferential partitioning into red blood cells.

Flumazenil is a highly extracted drug. Clearance of flumazenil occurs primarily by hepatic metabolism and is dependent on hepatic blood flow. In pharmacokinetic studies of normal volunteers, total clearance ranges from 0.7 to 1.3 L/hr/kg, with less than 1% of the administered dose eliminated unchanged in the urine. The major metabolites of flumazenil identified in urine are the de-ethylated free acid and its glucuronide conjugate. In preclinical studies there was no evidence of pharmacologic activity exhibited by the de-ethylated free acid. Elimination of radiolabelled drug is essentially complete within 72 hours, with 90% to 95% of the radioactivity appearing in urine and 5% to 10% in the feces.

Pharmacokinetic parameters following a 5-minute infusion of a total of 1 mg of ROMAZICON mean (coefficient of variation, range):

C_{max}(ng/mL)	24 (38%, 11–43)
AUC (ng·hr/mL)	15 (22%, 10–22)
V_{ss}(L/kg)	1 (24%, 0.8–1.6)
Cl (L/hr/kg)	1 (20%, 0.7–1.4)
Half-life (min)	54 (21%, 41–79)

The pharmacokinetics of flumazenil are not significantly affected by gender, age, renal failure (creatinine clearance <10 mL/min), or hemodialysis beginning 1 hour after drug administration. Mean total clearance is decreased to 40% to 60% of normal in patients with moderate liver dysfunction and to 25% of normal in patients with severe liver dysfunction, compared with age-matched healthy subjects. This results in a prolongation of the half-life from 0.8 hours in healthy subjects to 1.3 hours in patients with moderate hepatic impairment and 2.4 hours in severely impaired patients. Ingestion of food during an intravenous infusion of the drug results in a 50% increase in clearance, most likely due to the increased hepatic blood flow that accompanies a meal. The pharmacokinetic profile of flumazenil is unaltered in the presence of benzodiazepine agonists and the kinetic profiles of those benzodiazepines are unaltered by flumazenil.

Pharmacokinetics in Pediatric Patients: The pharmacokinetics of flumazenil have been evaluated in 29 pediatric patients ranging in age from 1 to 17 years who had undergone minor surgical procedures. The average doses administered were 0.53 mg (0.044 mg/kg) in patients aged 1 to 5 years, 0.63 mg (0.020 mg/kg) in patients aged 6 to 12 years, and 0.8 mg (0.014 mg/kg) in patients aged 13 to 17 years. Compared to adults, the half-life was somewhat shorter and more variable in these patients, averaging 40 minutes and generally ranging from 20 to 75 minutes. Clearance and volume of distribution, normalized for body weight, were in the same range as those seen in adults, although more variability was seen in the pediatric patients.

CLINICAL TRIALS

ROMAZICON has been administered in adults to reverse the effects of benzodiazepines in conscious sedation, general anesthesia, and the management of suspected benzodiazepine overdose. Limited information from uncontrolled studies in pediatric patients is available regarding the use of ROMAZICON to reverse the effects of benzodiazepines in conscious sedation only.

Conscious Sedation in Adults: ROMAZICON was studied in four trials in 970 patients who received an average of 30 mg diazepam or 10 mg midazolam for sedation (with or without a narcotic) in conjunction with both inpatient and outpatient diagnostic or surgical procedures. ROMAZICON was effective in reversing the sedating and psychomotor effects of the benzodiazepine; however, amnesia was less completely and less consistently reversed. In these studies, ROMAZICON was administered as an initial dose of 0.4 mg IV (two doses of 0.2 mg) with additional 0.2 mg doses as needed to achieve complete awakening, up to a maximum total dose of 1 mg.

Seventy-eight percent of patients receiving flumazenil responded by becoming completely alert. Of those patients, approximately half responded to doses of 0.4 mg to 0.6 mg, while the other half responded to doses of 0.8 mg to 1 mg. Adverse effects were infrequent in patients who received 1 mg of ROMAZICON or less, although injection site pain, agitation and anxiety did occur. Reversal of sedation was not associated with any increase in the frequency of inadequate analgesia or increase in narcotic demand in these studies. While most patients remained alert throughout the 3-hour postprocedure observation period, resedation was observed to occur in 3% to 9% of the patients, and was most common in patients who had received high doses of benzodiazepines (see PRECAUTIONS).

General Anesthesia in Adults: ROMAZICON was studied in four trials in 644 patients who received midazolam as an induction and/or maintenance agent in both balanced and inhalational anesthesia. Midazolam was generally administered in doses ranging from 5 mg to 80 mg, alone and/or in conjunction with muscle relaxants, nitrous oxide, regional or local anesthetics, narcotics and/or inhalational anesthetics. Flumazenil was given as an initial dose of 0.2 mg IV, with additional 0.2 mg doses as needed to reach a complete response, up to a maximum total dose of 1 mg. These doses were effective in reversing sedation and restoring psychomotor function, but did not completely restore memory as tested by picture recall. ROMAZICON was not as effective in the reversal of sedation in patients who had received multiple anesthetic agents in addition to benzodiazepines.

Eighty-one percent of patients sedated with midazolam responded to flumazenil by becoming completely alert or just slightly drowsy. Of those patients, 36% responded to doses of 0.4 mg to 0.6 mg, while 64% responded to doses of 0.8 mg to 1 mg.

Resedation in patients who responded to ROMAZICON occurred in 10% to 15% of patients studied and was more common with larger doses of midazolam (>20 mg), long procedures (>60 minutes) and use of neuromuscular blocking agents (see PRECAUTIONS).

Management of Suspected Benzodiazepine Overdose in Adults: ROMAZICON was studied in two trials in 497 patients who were presumed to have taken an overdose of a benzodiazepine, either alone or in combination with a variety of other agents. In these trials, 299 patients were proven to have taken a benzodiazepine as part of the overdose, and 80% of the 148 who received ROMAZICON responded by an improvement in level of consciousness. Of the patients who responded to flumazenil, 75% responded to a total dose of 1 mg to 3 mg.

Reversal of sedation was associated with an increased frequency of symptoms of CNS excitation. Of the patients treated with flumazenil, 1% to 3% were treated for agitation or anxiety. Serious side effects were uncommon, but six seizures were observed in 446 patients treated with flumazenil in these studies. Four of these 6 patients had ingested a large dose of cyclic antidepressants, which increased the risk of seizures (see WARNINGS).

INDIVIDUALIZATION OF DOSAGE

General Principles: The serious adverse effects of ROMAZICON are related to the reversal of benzodiazepine effects. Using more than the minimally effective dose of ROMAZICON is tolerated by most patients but may complicate the management of patients who are physically dependent on benzodiazepines or patients who are depending on benzodiazepines for therapeutic effect (such as suppression of seizures in cyclic antidepressant overdose).

In high-risk patients, it is important to administer the smallest amount of ROMAZICON that is effective. The 1-minute wait between individual doses in the dose-titration recommended for general clinical populations may be too short for high-risk patients. This is because it takes 6 to 10 minutes for any single dose of flumazenil to reach full effects. Practitioners should slow the rate of administration of ROMAZICON administered to high-risk patients as recommended below.

Anesthesia and Conscious Sedation in Adult Patients: ROMAZICON is well tolerated at the recommended doses in individuals who have no tolerance to (or dependence on) benzodiazepines. The recommended doses and titration rates in anesthesia and conscious sedation (0.2 mg to 1 mg given at 0.2 mg/min) are well tolerated in patients receiving the drug for reversal of a single benzodiazepine exposure in most clinical settings (see ADVERSE EVENTS). The major risk will be resedation because the duration of effect of a long-acting (or large dose of a short-acting) benzodiazepine may exceed that of ROMAZICON. Resedation may be treated by giving a repeat dose at no less than 20-minute intervals. For repeat treatment, no more than 1 mg (at 0.2 mg/min doses) should be given at any one time and no more than 3 mg should be given in any one hour.

Overdose in Adult Patients: The risk of confusion, agitation, emotional lability and perceptual distortion with the doses recommended in patients with benzodiazepine overdose (3 mg to 5 mg administered as 0.5 mg/min) may be greater than that expected with lower doses and slower administration. The recommended doses represent a compromise between a desirable slow awakening and the need for prompt response and a persistent effect in the overdose situation. If circumstances permit, the physician may elect to use the 0.2 mg/minute titration rate to slowly awaken the patient over 5 to 10 minutes, which may help to reduce signs and symptoms on emergence.

ROMAZICON has no effect in cases where benzodiazepines are not responsible for sedation. Once doses of 3 mg to 5 mg have been reached without clinical response, additional ROMAZICON is likely to have no effect.

Patients Tolerant To Benzodiazepines: ROMAZICON may cause benzodiazepine withdrawal symptoms in individuals who have been taking benzodiazepines long enough to have some degree of tolerance. Patients who had been taking benzodiazepines prior to entry into the ROMAZICON trials, who were given flumazenil in doses over 1 mg, experienced withdrawal-like events 2 to 5 times more frequently than patients who received less than 1 mg.

In patients who may have tolerance to benzodiazepines, as indicated by clinical history or by the need for larger than usual doses of benzodiazepines, slower titration rates of 0.1 mg/min and lower total doses may help reduce the frequency of emergent confusion and agitation. In such cases, special care must be taken to monitor the patients for resedation because of the lower doses of ROMAZICON used.

Patients Physically Dependent on Benzodiazepines: ROMAZICON is known to precipitate withdrawal seizures in patients who are physically dependent on benzodiazepines, even if such dependence was established in a relatively few days of high dose sedation in Intensive Care Unit (ICU) environments. The risk of either seizures or resedation in such cases is high and patients have experienced seizures before regaining consciousness. ROMAZICON should be used in such settings with extreme caution, since the use of flumazenil in this situation has not been studied and no information as to dose and rate of titration is available. ROMAZICON should be used in such patients only if the potential benefits of using the drug outweigh the risks of precipitated seizures. Physicians are directed to the scientific literature for the most current information in this area.

INDICATIONS AND USAGE

Adult Patients: ROMAZICON is indicated for the complete or partial reversal of the sedative effects of benzodiazepines in cases where general anesthesia has been induced and/or maintained with benzodiazepines, where sedation has been produced with benzodiazepines for diagnostic and therapeutic procedures, and for the management of benzodiazepine overdose.

Pediatric Patients (aged 1 to 17): ROMAZICON is indicated for the reversal of conscious sedation induced with benzodiazepines (see PRECAUTIONS: *Pediatric Use*).

CONTRAINDICATIONS

ROMAZICON is contraindicated:

- in patients with a known hypersensitivity to flumazenil or benzodiazepines.
- in patients who have been given a benzodiazepine for control of a potentially life-threatening condition (eg, control of intracranial pressure or status epilepticus).
- in patients who are showing signs of serious cyclic antidepressant overdose (see WARNINGS).

WARNINGS

THE USE OF ROMAZICON HAS BEEN ASSOCIATED WITH THE OCCURRENCE OF SEIZURES.
THESE ARE MOST FREQUENT IN PATIENTS WHO HAVE BEEN ON BENZODIAZEPINES FOR LONG-TERM SEDATION OR IN OVERDOSE CASES WHERE PATIENTS ARE SHOWING SIGNS OF SERIOUS CYCLIC ANTIDEPRESSANT OVERDOSE.
PRACTITIONERS SHOULD INDIVIDUALIZE THE DOSAGE OF ROMAZICON AND BE PREPARED TO MANAGE SEIZURES.

Risk of Seizures: **The reversal of benzodiazepine effects may be associated with the onset of seizures in certain high-risk populations. Possible risk factors for seizures include: concurrent major sedative-hypnotic drug withdrawal, recent therapy with repeated doses of parenteral benzodiazepines, myoclonic jerking or seizure activity prior to flumazenil administration in overdose cases, or concurrent cyclic anti-depressant poisoning.**

ROMAZICON is not recommended in cases of serious cyclic antidepressant poisoning, as manifested by motor abnormalities (twitching, rigidity, focal seizure), dysrhythmia (wide QRS, ventricular dysrhythmia, heart block), anticholinergic signs (mydriasis, dry mucosa, hypoperistalsis), and cardiovascular collapse at presentation. In such cases ROMAZICON should be withheld and the patient should be allowed to remain sedated (with ventilatory and circulatory support as needed) until the signs of antidepressant toxicity have subsided. Treatment with ROMAZICON has no known benefit to the seriously ill mixed-overdose patient other than reversing sedation and should not be used in cases where seizures (from any cause) are likely.

Most convulsions associated with flumazenil administration require treatment and have been successfully managed with benzodiazepines, phenytoin or barbiturates. Because of the presence of flumazenil, higher than usual doses of benzodiazepines may be required.

Hypoventilation: **Patients who have received ROMAZICON for the reversal of benzodiazepine effects (after conscious sedation or general anesthesia) should be monitored for resedation, respiratory depression, or other residual benzodiazepine effects for an appropriate period (up to 120 minutes) based on the dose and duration of effect of the benzodiazepine employed.**

This is because ROMAZICON has not been established in patients as an effective treatment for hypoventilation due to benzodiazepine administration. In healthy male volunteers, ROMAZICON is capable of reversing benzodiazepine-induced depression of the ventilatory responses to hypercapnia and hypoxia after a benzodiazepine alone. However, such depression may recur because the ventilatory effects of typical doses of ROMAZICON (1 mg or less) may wear off before the effects of many benzodiazepines. The effects of ROMAZICON on ventilatory response following sedation with a benzodiazepine in combination with an opioid are inconsistent and have not been adequately studied. The availability of flumazenil does not diminish the need for prompt detection of hypoventilation and the ability to effectively intervene by establishing an airway and assisting ventilation.

Overdose cases should always be monitored for resedation until the patients are stable and resedation is unlikely.

PRECAUTIONS

Return of Sedation: ROMAZICON may be expected to improve the alertness of patients recovering from a procedure involving sedation or anesthesia with benzodiazepines, but

Continued on next page

Romazicon—Cont.

should not be substituted for an adequate period of post-procedure monitoring. The availability of ROMAZICON does not reduce the risks associated with the use of large doses of benzodiazepines for sedation.
Patients should be monitored for resedation, respiratory depression (see WARNINGS), or other persistent or recurrent agonist effects for an adequate period of time after administration of ROMAZICON.
Resedation is least likely in cases where ROMAZICON is administered to reverse a low dose of a short-acting benzodiazepine (<10 mg midazolam). It is most likely in cases where a large single or cumulative dose of a benzodiazepine has been given in the course of a long procedure along with neuromuscular blocking agents and multiple anesthetic agents.
Profound resedation was observed in 1% to 3% of adult patients in the clinical studies. In clinical situations where resedation must be prevented in adult patients, physicians may wish to repeat the initial dose (up to 1 mg of ROMAZICON given at 0.2 mg/min) at 30 minutes and possibly again at 60 minutes. This dosage schedule, although not studied in clinical trials, was effective in preventing resedation in a pharmacologic study in normal volunteers.
The use of ROMAZICON to reverse the effects of benzodiazepines used for conscious sedation has been evaluated in one open-label clinical trial involving 107 pediatric patients between the ages of 1 and 17 years. This study suggested that pediatric patients who have become fully awake following treatment with flumazenil may experience a recurrence of sedation, especially younger patients (ages 1 to 5). Resedation was experienced in 7 of 60 patients who were fully alert 10 minutes after the start of ROMAZICON administration. No patient experienced a return to the baseline level of sedation. Mean time to resedation was 25 minutes (range: 19 to 50 minutes) (see PRECAUTIONS: *Pediatric Use*). The safety and effectiveness of repeated flumazenil administration in pediatric patients experiencing resedation have not been established.
Use in the ICU: ROMAZICON should be used with caution in the ICU because of the increased risk of unrecognized benzodiazepine dependence in such settings. ROMAZICON may produce convulsions in patients physically dependent on benzodiazepines (see INDIVIDUALIZATION OF DOSAGE and WARNINGS).
Administration of ROMAZICON to diagnose benzodiazepine-induced sedation in the ICU is not recommended due to the risk of adverse events as described above. In addition, the prognostic significance of a patient's failure to respond to flumazenil in cases confounded by metabolic disorder, traumatic injury, drugs other than benzodiazepines, or any other reasons not associated with benzodiazepine receptor occupancy is unknown.
Use in Overdose: ROMAZICON is intended as an adjunct to, not as a substitute for, proper management of airway, assisted breathing, circulatory access and support, internal decontamination by lavage and charcoal, and adequate clinical evaluation.
Necessary measures should be instituted to secure airway, ventilation and intravenous access prior to administering flumazenil. Upon arousal, patients may attempt to withdraw endotracheal tubes and/or intravenous lines as the result of confusion and agitation following awakening.
Head Injury: ROMAZICON should be used with caution in patients with head injury as it may be capable of precipitating convulsions or altering cerebral blood flow in patients receiving benzodiazepines. It should be used only by practitioners prepared to manage such complications should they occur.
Use With Neuromuscular Blocking Agents: ROMAZICON should not be used until the effects of neuromuscular blockade have been fully reversed.
Use in Psychiatric Patients: ROMAZICON has been reported to provoke panic attacks in patients with a history of panic disorder.
Pain on Injection: To minimize the likelihood of pain or inflammation at the injection site, ROMAZICON should be administered through a freely flowing intravenous infusion into a large vein. Local irritation may occur following extravasation into perivascular tissues.
Use in Respiratory Disease: The primary treatment of patients with serious lung disease who experience serious respiratory depression due to benzodiazepines should be appropriate ventilatory support (see PRECAUTIONS) rather than the administration of ROMAZICON. Flumazenil is capable of partially reversing benzodiazepine-induced alterations in ventilatory drive in healthy volunteers, but has not been shown to be clinically effective.
Use in Cardiovascular Disease: ROMAZICON did not increase the work of the heart when used to reverse benzodiazepines in cardiac patients when given at a rate of 0.1 mg/min in total doses of less than 0.5 mg in studies reported in the clinical literature. Flumazenil alone had no significant effects on cardiovascular parameters when administered to patients with stable ischemic heart disease.
Use in Liver Disease: The clearance of ROMAZICON is reduced to 40% to 60% of normal in patients with mild to moderate hepatic disease and to 25% of normal in patients with severe hepatic dysfunction (see PHARMACOKINETICS). While the dose of flumazenil used for initial reversal of benzodiazepine effects is not affected, repeat doses of the drug in liver disease should be reduced in size or frequency.
Use in Drug and Alcohol Dependent Patients: ROMAZICON should be used with caution in patients with alcoholism and other drug dependencies due to the increased frequency of benzodiazepine tolerance and dependence observed in these patient populations.
ROMAZICON is not recommended either as a treatment for benzodiazepine dependence or for the management of protracted benzodiazepine abstinence syndromes, as such use has not been studied.
The administration of flumazenil can precipitate benzodiazepine withdrawal in animals and man. This has been seen in healthy volunteers treated with therapeutic doses of oral lorazepam for up to 2 weeks who exhibited effects such as hot flushes, agitation and tremor when treated with cumulative doses of up to 3 mg doses of flumazenil.
Similar adverse experiences suggestive of flumazenil precipitation of benzodiazepine withdrawal have occurred in some adult patients in clinical trials. Such patients had a short-lived syndrome characterized by dizziness, mild confusion, emotional lability, agitation (with signs and symptoms of anxiety), and mild sensory distortions. This response was dose-related, most common at doses above 1 mg, rarely required treatment other than reassurance and was usually short lived. When required (5 to 10 cases), these patients were successfully treated with usual doses of a barbiturate, a benzodiazepine, or other sedative drug.
Practitioners should assume that flumazenil administration may trigger dose-dependent withdrawal syndromes in patients with established physical dependence on benzodiazepines and may complicate the management of withdrawal syndromes for alcohol, barbiturates and cross-tolerant sedatives.
Drug Interactions: Interaction with central nervous system depressants other than benzodiazepines has not been specifically studied; however, no deleterious interactions were seen when ROMAZICON was administered after narcotics, inhalational anesthetics, muscle relaxants and muscle relaxant antagonists administered in conjunction with sedation or anesthesia.
Particular caution is necessary when using ROMAZICON in cases of mixed drug overdosage since the toxic effects (such as convulsions and cardiac dysrhythmias) of other drugs taken in overdose (especially cyclic antidepressants) may emerge with the reversal of the benzodiazepine effect by flumazenil. (see WARNINGS).
The pharmacokinetics of benzodiazepines are unaltered in the presence of flumazenil.
Use in Ambulatory Patients: The effects of ROMAZICON may wear off before a long-acting benzodiazepine is completely cleared from the body. In general, if a patient shows no signs of sedation within 2 hours after a 1-mg dose of flumazenil, serious resedation at a later time is unlikely. An adequate period of observation must be provided for any patient in whom either long-acting benzodiazepines (such as diazepam) or large doses of short-acting benzodiazepines (such as >10 mg of midazolam) have been used (see INDIVIDUALIZATION OF DOSAGE).
Because of the increased risk of adverse reactions in patients who have been taking benzodiazepines on a regular basis, it is particularly important that physicians query patients or their guardians carefully about benzodiazepine, alcohol and sedative use as part of the history prior to any procedure in which the use of ROMAZICON is planned (see PRECAUTIONS: *Use in Drug and Alcohol Dependent Patients*).
Information for Patients: ROMAZICON does not consistently reverse amnesia. Patients cannot be expected to remember information told to them in the post-procedure period and instructions given to patients should be reinforced in writing or given to a responsible family member. Physicians are advised to discuss with patients or their guardians, both before surgery and at discharge, that although the patient may feel alert at the time of discharge, the effects of the benzodiazepine may recur. As a result, the patient should be instructed, preferably in writing, that their memory and judgment may be impaired and specifically advised:

1. Not to engage in any activities requiring complete alertness, and not to operate hazardous machinery or a motor vehicle until at least 18 to 24 hours after discharge, and it is certain no residual sedative effects of the benzodiazepine remain.
2. Not to take any alcohol or non-prescription drugs for 18 to 24 hours after flumazenil administration or if the effects of the benzodiazepine persist.

Laboratory Tests: No specific laboratory tests are recommended to follow the patient's response or to identify possible adverse reactions.
Drug/Laboratory Test Interactions: The possible interaction of flumazenil with commonly used laboratory tests has not been evaluated.
Carcinogenesis, Mutagenesis, Impairment of Fertility: *Carcinogenesis:* No studies in animals to evaluate the carcinogenic potential of flumazenil have been conducted.
Mutagenesis: No evidence for mutagenicity was noted in the Ames test using five different tester strains. Assays for mutagenic potential in *S. cerevisiae* D7 and in Chinese hamster cells were considered to be negative as were blastogenesis assays in vitro in peripheral human lymphocytes and in vivo in a mouse micronucleus assay. Flumazenil caused a slight increase in unscheduled DNA synthesis in rat hepatocyte culture at concentrations which were also cytotoxic; no increase in DNA repair was observed in male mouse germ cells in an in vivo DNA repair assay.
Impairment of Fertility: A reproduction study in male and female rats did not show any impairment of fertility at oral dosages of 125 mg/kg/day. From the available data on the area under the curve (AUC) in animals and man the dose represented 120× the human exposure from a maximum recommended intravenous dose of 5 mg.
Pregnancy: *Pregnancy Category C:* There are no adequate and well-controlled studies of the use of flumazenil in pregnant women. Flumazenil should be used during pregnancy only if the potential benefit justifies the potential risk to the fetus.
Teratogenic Effects: Flumazenil has been studied for teratogenicity in rats and rabbits following oral treatments of up to 150 mg/kg/day. The treatments during the major organogenesis were on days 6 to 15 of gestation in the rat and days 6 to 18 of gestation in the rabbit. No teratogenic effects were observed in rats or rabbits at 150 mg/kg; the dose, based on the available data on the area under the plasma concentration-time curve (AUC) represented 120× to 600× the human exposure from a maximum recommended intravenous dose of 5 mg in humans. In rabbits, embryocidal effects (as evidenced by increased preimplantation and postimplantation losses) were observed at 50 mg/kg or 200× the human exposure from a maximum recommended intravenous dose of 5 mg. The no-effect dose of 15 mg/kg in rabbits represents 60× the human exposure.
Nonteratogenic Effects: An animal reproduction study was conducted in rats at oral dosages of 5, 25 and 125 mg/kg/day of flumazenil. Pup survival was decreased during the lactating period, pup liver weight at weaning was increased for the high-dose group (125 mg/kg/day) and incisor eruption and ear opening in the offspring were delayed; the delay in ear opening was associated with a delay in the appearance of the auditory startle response. No treatment-related adverse effects were noted for the other dose groups. Based on the available data from AUC, the effect level (125 mg/kg), represents 120× the human exposure from 5 mg, the maximum recommended intravenous dose in humans. The no-effect level represents 24× the human exposure from an intravenous dose of 5 mg.
Labor and Delivery: The use of ROMAZICON to reverse the effects of benzodiazepines used during labor and delivery is not recommended because the effects of the drug in the newborn are unknown.
Nursing Mothers: Caution should be exercised when deciding to administer ROMAZICON to a nursing woman because it is not known whether flumazenil is excreted in human milk.
Pediatric Use: The safety and effectiveness of ROMAZICON have been established in pediatric patients 1 year of age and older. Use of ROMAZICON in this age group is supported by evidence from adequate and well-controlled studies of ROMAZICON in adults with additional data from uncontrolled pediatric studies including one open-label trial.
The use of ROMAZICON to reverse the effects of benzodiazepines used for conscious sedation was evaluated in one uncontrolled clinical trial involving 107 pediatric patients between the ages of 1 and 17 years. At the doses used, ROMAZICON's safety was established in this population. Patients received up to 5 injections of 0.01 mg/kg flumazenil up to a maximum total dose of 1.0 mg at a rate not exceeding 0.2 mg/min.
Of 60 patients who were fully alert at 10 minutes, 7 experienced resedation. Resedation occurred between 19 and 50 minutes after the start of ROMAZICON administration. None of the patients experienced a return to the baseline level of sedation. All 7 patients were between the ages of 1 and 5 years. The types and frequency of adverse events noted in these pediatric patients were similar to those previously documented in clinical trials with ROMAZICON to reverse conscious sedation in adults. No patient experienced a serious adverse event attributable to flumazenil. The safety and efficacy of ROMAZICON in the reversal of conscious sedation in pediatric patients below the age of 1 year have not been established.
Pharmacokinetics In Pediatric Patients: The pharmacokinetics of flumazenil have been evaluated in 29 pediatric patients ranging in age from 1 to 17 years who had undergone minor surgical procedures. The average doses administered were 0.53 mg (0.044 mg/kg) in patients aged 1 to 5 years, 0.63 mg (0.020 mg/kg) in patients aged 6 to 12 years, and 0.8 mg (0.014 mg/kg) in patients aged 13 to 17 years. Compared to adults, the half-life was somewhat shorter and more variable in these patients, averaging 40 minutes and generally ranging from 20 to 75 minutes. Clearance and volume of distribution, normalized for body weight, were in the same range as those seen in adults, although more variability was seen in the pediatric patients.
The safety and efficacy of ROMAZICON have not been established in pediatric patients for reversal of the sedative effects of benzodiazepines used for induction of general anesthesia, for the management of overdose, or for the resuscitation of the newborn, as no well-controlled clinical studies have been performed to determine the risks, benefits and dosages to be used. However, published anecdotal reports discussing the use of ROMAZICON in pediatric patients for these indications have reported similar safety profiles and dosing guidelines to those described for the reversal of conscious sedation.
The risks identified in the adult population with ROMAZICON use also apply to pediatric patients. Therefore, consult the CONTRAINDICATIONS, WARNINGS, PRECAUTIONS, and ADVERSE REACTIONS sections when using ROMAZICON in pediatric patients.

Geriatric Use: Of the total number of subjects in clinical studies of flumazenil, 248 were 65 and over. No overall differences in safety or effectiveness were observed between these subjects and younger subjects. Other reported clinical experience has not identified differences in responses between the elderly and younger patients, but greater sensitivity of some older individuals cannot be ruled out.
The pharmacokinetics of flumazenil have been studied in the elderly and are not significantly different from younger patients. Several studies of ROMAZICON in subjects over the age of 65 and one study in subjects over the age of 80 suggest that while the doses of benzodiazepine used to induce sedation should be reduced, ordinary doses of ROMAZICON may be used for reversal.

ADVERSE REACTIONS

Serious Adverse Reactions: Deaths have occurred in patients who received ROMAZICON in a variety of clinical settings. The majority of deaths occurred in patients with serious underlying disease or in patients who had ingested large amounts of non-benzodiazepine drugs, (usually cyclic antidepressants), as part of an overdose.
Serious adverse events have occurred in all clinical settings, and convulsions are the most common serious adverse events reported. ROMAZICON administration has been associated with the onset of convulsions in patients who are relying on benzodiazepine effects to control seizures, are physically dependent on benzodiazepines, or who have ingested large doses of other drugs (see WARNINGS).
Two of the 446 patients who received ROMAZICON in controlled clinical trials for the management of a benzodiazepine overdose had cardiac dysrhythmias (1 ventricular tachycardia, 1 junctional tachycardia).

Adverse Events in Clinical Studies: The following adverse reactions were considered to be related to ROMAZICON administration (both alone and for the reversal of benzodiazepine effects) and were reported in studies involving 1875 individuals who received flumazenil in controlled trials. Adverse events most frequently associated with flumazenil alone were limited to dizziness, injection site pain, increased sweating, headache, and abnormal or blurred vision (3% to 9%).
Body as a Whole: fatigue (asthenia, malaise), headache, injection site pain* and injection site reaction (thrombophlebitis, skin abnormality, rash)
Cardiovascular System: cutaneous vasodilation (sweating, flushing, hot flushes)
Digestive System: nausea and vomiting (11%)
Nervous System: agitation (anxiety, nervousness, dry mouth, tremor, palpitations, insomnia, dyspnea, hyperventilation)*, dizziness (vertigo, ataxia) (10%) and emotional lability (crying abnormal, depersonalization, euphoria, increased tears, depression, dysphoria, paranoia)
Special Senses: abnormal vision (visual field defect, diplopia) and paresthesia (sensation abnormal, hypoesthesia)

All adverse reactions occurred in 1% to 3% of cases unless otherwise marked.
*indicates reaction in 3% to 9% of cases.
Observed percentage reported if greater than 9%.

The following adverse events were observed infrequently (less than 1%) in the clinical studies, but were judged as probably related to ROMAZICON administration and/or reversal of benzodiazepine effects:
Nervous System: confusion (difficulty concentrating, delirium), convulsions (see WARNINGS) and somnolence (stupor)
Special Senses: abnormal hearing (transient hearing impairment, hyperacusis, tinnitus)
The following adverse events occurred with frequencies less than 1% in the clinical trials. Their relationship to ROMAZICON administration is unknown, but they are included as alerting information for the physician.
Body as a Whole: rigors, shivering
Cardiovascular System: arrhythmia (atrial, nodal, ventricular extrasystoles), bradycardia, tachycardia, hypertension and chest pain
Digestive System: hiccup
Nervous System: speech disorder (dysphonia, thick tongue)
Not included in this list is operative site pain that occurred with the same frequency in patients receiving placebo as in patients receiving flumazenil for reversal of sedation following a surgical procedure.

DRUG ABUSE AND DEPENDENCE

ROMAZICON acts as a benzodiazepine antagonist, blocks the effects of benzodiazepines in animals and man, antagonizes benzodiazepine reinforcement in animal models, produces dysphoria in normal subjects, and has had no reported abuse in foreign marketing. Although ROMAZICON has a benzodiazepine-like structure it does not act as a benzodiazepine agonist in man and is not a controlled substance.

OVERDOSAGE

Large intravenous doses of ROMAZICON, when administered to healthy normal volunteers in the absence of a benzodiazepine agonist, produced no serious adverse reactions, severe signs or symptoms, or clinically significant laboratory test abnormalities. In clinical studies, most adverse reactions to flumazenil were an extension of the pharmacologic effects of the drug in reversing benzodiazepine effects.
Reversal with an excessively high dose of ROMAZICON may produce anxiety, agitation, increased muscle tone, hyperesthesia and possibly convulsions. Convulsions have been treated with barbiturates, benzodiazepines and phenytoin, generally with prompt resolution of the seizures (see WARNINGS).

DOSAGE AND ADMINISTRATION

ROMAZICON is recommended for intravenous use only. It is compatible with 5% dextrose in water, lactated Ringer's and normal saline solutions. If ROMAZICON is drawn into a syringe or mixed with any of these solutions, it should be discarded after 24 hours. For optimum sterility, ROMAZICON should remain in the vial until just before use. As with all parenteral drug products, ROMAZICON should be inspected visually for particulate matter and discoloration prior to administration, whenever solution and container permit.
To minimize the likelihood of pain at the injection site, ROMAZICON should be administered through a freely running intravenous infusion into a large vein.
Reversal of Conscious Sedation:
Adult Patients: For the reversal of the sedative effects of benzodiazepines administered for conscious sedation, the recommended initial dose of ROMAZICON is 0.2 mg (2 mL) administered intravenously over 15 seconds. If the desired level of consciousness is not obtained after waiting an additional 45 seconds, a further dose of 0.2 mg (2 mL) can be injected and repeated at 60-second intervals where necessary (up to a maximum of 4 additional times) to a maximum total dose of 1 mg (10 mL). The dosage should be individualized based on the patient's response, with most patients responding to doses of 0.6 mg to 1 mg (see INDIVIDUALIZATION OF DOSAGE).
In the event of resedation, repeated doses may be administered at 20-minute intervals as needed. For repeat treatment, no more than 1 mg (given as 0.2 mg/min) should be administered at any one time, and no more than 3 mg should be given in any one hour.
It is recommended that ROMAZICON be administered as the series of small injections described (not as a single bolus injection) to allow the practitioner to control the reversal of sedation to the approximate endpoint desired and to minimize the possibility of adverse effects (see INDIVIDUALIZATION OF DOSAGE).
Pediatric Patients: For the reversal of the sedative effects of benzodiazepines administered for conscious sedation in pediatric patients, the recommended initial dose is 0.01 mg/kg (up to 0.2 mg) administered intravenously over 15 seconds. If the desired level of consciousness is not obtained after waiting an additional 45 seconds, further injections of 0.01 mg/kg (up to 0.2 mg) can be administered and repeated at 60-second intervals where necessary (up to a maximum of 4 additional times) to a maximum total dose of 0.05 mg/kg or 1 mg, whichever is lower. The dose should be individualized based on the patient's response. The mean total dose administered in the pediatric clinical trial of flumazenil was 0.65 mg (range: 0.08 mg to 1.00 mg). Approximately one-half of patients required the maximum of five injections.
Resedation occurred in 7 of 60 pediatric patients who were fully alert 10 minutes after the start of ROMAZICON administration (see PRECAUTIONS: *Pediatric Use*). The safety and efficacy of repeated flumazenil administration in pediatric patients experiencing resedation have not been established.
It is recommended that ROMAZICON be administered as the series of small injections described (not as a single bolus injection) to allow the practitioner to control the reversal of sedation to the approximate endpoint desired and to minimize the possibility of adverse effects (see INDIVIDUALIZATION OF DOSAGE).
The safety and efficacy of ROMAZICON in the reversal of conscious sedation in pediatric patients below the age of 1 year have not been established.
Reversal of General Anesthesia in Adult Patients: For the reversal of the sedative effects of benzodiazepines administered for general anesthesia, the recommended initial dose of ROMAZICON is 0.2 mg (2 mL) administered intravenously over 15 seconds. If the desired level of consciousness is not obtained after waiting an additional 45 seconds, a further dose of 0.2 mg (2 mL) can be injected and repeated at 60-second intervals where necessary (up to a maximum of 4 additional times) to a maximum total dose of 1 mg (10 mL). The dosage should be individualized based on the patient's response, with most patients responding to doses of 0.6 mg to 1 mg (see INDIVIDUALIZATION OF DOSAGE).
In the event of resedation, repeated doses may be administered at 20-minute intervals as needed. For repeat treatment, no more than 1 mg (given as 0.2 mg/min) should be administered at any one time, and no more than 3 mg should be given in any one hour.
It is recommended that ROMAZICON be administered as the series of small injections described (not as a single bolus injection) to allow the practitioner to control the reversal of sedation to the approximate endpoint desired and to minimize the possibility of adverse effects (see INDIVIDUALIZATION OF DOSAGE).
Management of Suspected Benzodiazepine Overdose in Adult Patients: For initial management of a known or suspected benzodiazepine overdose, the recommended initial dose of ROMAZICON is 0.2 mg (2 mL) administered intravenously over 30 seconds. If the desired level of consciousness is not obtained after waiting 30 seconds, a further dose of 0.3 mg (3 mL) can be administered over another 30 seconds. Further doses of 0.5 mg (5 mL) can be administered over 30 seconds at 1-minute intervals up to a cumulative dose of 3 mg.
Do not rush the administration of ROMAZICON. Patients should have a secure airway and intravenous access before administration of the drug and be awakened gradually (see PRECAUTIONS).
Most patients with a benzodiazepine overdose will respond to a cumulative dose of 1 mg to 3 mg of ROMAZICON, and doses beyond 3 mg do not reliably produce additional effects. On rare occasions, patients with a partial response at 3 mg may require additional titration up to a total dose of 5 mg (administered slowly in the same manner).
If a patient has not responded 5 minutes after receiving a cumulative dose of 5 mg of ROMAZICON, the major cause of sedation is likely not to be due to benzodiazepines, and additional ROMAZICON is likely to have no effect.
In the event of resedation, repeated doses may be given at 20-minute intervals if needed. For repeat treatment, no more than 1 mg (given as 0.5 mg/min) should be given at any one time and no more than 3 mg should be given in any one hour.
Safety and Handling: ROMAZICON is supplied in sealed dosage forms and poses no known risk to the health care provider. Routine care should be taken to avoid aerosol generation when preparing syringes for injection, and spilled medication should be rinsed from the skin with cool water.

HOW SUPPLIED

5 mL multiple-use vials containing 0.1 mg/mL flumazenil—boxes of 10 (NDC 0004-6911-06); 10 mL multiple-use vials containing 0.1 mg/mL flumazenil—boxes of 10 (NDC 0004-6912-06).
Store at 59° to 86° F (15° to 30° C).
Revised: May 2000

SORIATANE® ℞
[*sŏr 'ĭa tane*]
(acitretin)
CAPSULES

The following text is complete prescribing information based on official labeling in effect June 2000.

CONTRAINDICATIONS AND WARNINGS: Soriatane must not be used by females who are pregnant, or who intend to become pregnant during therapy or at any time for at least 3 years following discontinuation of therapy. Soriatane also must not be used by females who may not use reliable contraception while undergoing treatment or for at least 3 years following discontinuation of treatment. Acitretin is a metabolite of etretinate (Tegison®), and major human fetal abnormalities have been reported with the administration of etretinate and acitretin. Potentially, any fetus exposed can be affected.
Clinical evidence has shown that concurrent ingestion of acitretin and ethanol has been associated with the formation of etretinate, which has a longer elimination half-life than acitretin. Because the longer elimination half-life of etretinate would increase the duration of teratogenic potential for female patients, ethanol must not be ingested by female patients either during treatment with Soriatane or for 2 months after cessation of therapy. This allows for elimination of acitretin, thus removing the substrate for transesterification to etretinate. The mechanism of the metabolic process for conversion of acitretin to etretinate has not been fully defined. It is not known whether substances other than ethanol are associated with transesterification.
Acitretin has been shown to be embryotoxic and/or teratogenic in rabbits, mice, and rats at doses approximately 0.6, 3 and 15 times the maximum recommended therapeutic dose, respectively.
Major human fetal abnormalities associated with etretinate and/or acitretin administration have been reported including meningomyelocele, meningoencephalocele, multiple synostoses, facial dysmorphia, syndactylies, absence of terminal phalanges, malformations of hip, ankle and forearm, low set ears, high palate, decreased cranial volume, cardiovascular malformation and alterations of the skull and cervical vertebrae on x-ray.
Females of reproductive potential must not be given Soriatane until pregnancy is excluded. It is contraindicated in females of reproductive potential unless the patient meets ALL of the following conditions:

- **has severe psoriasis and is unresponsive to other therapies or whose clinical condition contraindicates the use of other treatments;**
- **has received both oral and written warnings of the hazards of taking Soriatane during pregnancy;**
- **has received both oral and written warnings of the risk of possible contraception failure and of the need to use two reliable forms of contraception simultaneously both during therapy and for at least 3 years *after* discontinuation of therapy and has acknowledged in writing her understanding of these warnings and of the need for using dual contraceptive methods (unless the patient has undergone a hysterectomy or practices abstinence);**
- **has had a negative serum or urine pregnancy test with a sensitivity of at least 50 mIU/mL within 1 week prior to beginning therapy;**

Continued on next page

Soriatane—Cont.

- **will begin therapy only on the second or third day of the next normal menstrual period;**
- **is capable of complying with the mandatory contraceptive measures; and**
- **is reliable in understanding and carrying out instructions.**

A prescription for Soriatane should not be issued by the physician until a report of a negative pregnancy test has been obtained and the patient has begun her menstrual period. Pregnancy testing and contraception counseling should be repeated on a regular basis. To encourage compliance with this recommendation, the physician should prescribe a limited supply of the drug. Effective contraception must be used for at least 1 month before beginning Soriatane therapy, during therapy and for at least 3 years following discontinuation of therapy even where there has been a history of infertility, unless due to hysterectomy. It is recommended that two reliable forms of contraception be used simultaneously unless abstinence is the chosen method. Patients who have undergone tubal ligation should use a second form of contraception.

It is not known whether residual acitretin in seminal fluid poses risk to a fetus while a male patient is taking the drug or after it is discontinued. There have been five pregnancies reported in which the male partner was undergoing Soriatane treatment. One pregnancy resulted in a normal infant. Two pregnancies ended in spontaneous abortions. In another case, the fetus had bilateral cystic hygromas and multiple cardiopulmonary malformations. The relationship of these malformations to the drug is unknown. The outcome of the fifth case is unknown.

Samples of seminal fluid from 3 male patients treated with acitretin and 6 male patients treated with etretinate have been assayed for the presence of acitretin. The maximum concentration of acitretin observed in the seminal fluid of these men was 12.5 ng/mL. Assuming an ejaculate volume of 10 mL, the amount of drug transferred in semen would be 125 ng, which is 1/200,000 of a single 25 mg capsule.

Females who have taken Tegison (etretinate) must continue to follow the contraceptive recommendations for Tegison.

Acitretin, the active metabolite of etretinate, is teratogenic and is contraindicated during pregnancy. The risk of severe fetal malformations is well established when systemic retinoids are taken during pregnancy. Pregnancy must also be prevented after stopping acitretin therapy, while the drug is being eliminated to below a threshold blood concentration that would be associated with an increased incidence of birth defects. Because this threshold has not been established for acitretin in humans and because elimination rates vary among patients, the duration of posttherapy contraception to achieve adequate elimination cannot be calculated precisely. It is strongly recommended that contraception be continued for at least 3 years after stopping treatment with acitretin, based on the following considerations:

- **In the absence of transesterification to form etretinate, greater than 98% of the acitretin would be eliminated within 2 months, assuming a mean elimination half-life of 49 hours.**
- **In cases where etretinate is formed, as has been demonstrated with concomitant administration of acitretin and ethanol,**
  - **greater than 98% of the etretinate formed would be eliminated in 2 years, assuming a mean elimination half-life of 120 days.**
  - **greater than 98% of the etretinate formed would be eliminated in 3 years, based on the longest demonstrated elimination half-life of 168 days. However, etretinate was found in plasma and subcutaneous fat in one patient reported to have had sporadic alcohol intake, 52 months after she stopped acitretin therapy.[1]**
- **An increased incidence of birth defects was estimated based on a limited number of cases which have been reported to Roche, which were identified before the outcome was known, and where pregnancy occurred during the time interval when the patient was being treated with acitretin or etretinate. For cases identified after the outcome was known, severe birth defects have been reported where pregnancy occurred during the time interval when the patient was being treated with acitretin or etretinate.**
- **There have been 202 cases reported before the outcome was known where pregnancy occurred after the last dose of etretinate or acitretin. Fetal outcome remained unknown in approximately one-half of these cases, of which 62 were terminated and 11 were spontaneous abortions. Fetal outcome is known for 103 of these prospectively reported cases. Fifteen of the outcomes were abnormal: hernia, hypocalcemia, hypotonia, undescended testicle, laparoschisis, absent hand/wrist, clubfoot, ichthyosis, apnea/anemia, placental disorder/death and premature birth (5). Birth defects have also been reported retrospectively (ie, after the outcome was known). Among the retrospectively reported cases where pregnancy occurred more than 2 years after the last dose of etretinate or acitretin, there are 2 normal outcomes, 3 unknown outcomes and 7 abnormal outcomes. The 7 abnormal outcomes reported are: malformation unspecified, aplasia of the forearm, stillbirth, right ventricular/aortic duct defect, heart malformation unspecified, and chromosomal disorder (2). For these listed reports, the relationship of the birth defects to the drug is unknown.**

If pregnancy does occur during Soriatane therapy or at any time for at least 3 years following discontinuation of Soriatane therapy, the physician and patient should discuss the possible effects on the pregnancy.

Soriatane should be prescribed only by physicians who have special competence in the diagnosis and treatment of severe psoriasis, are experienced in the use of systemic retinoids, and understand the risk of teratogenicity.

DESCRIPTION

Soriatane (acitretin), a retinoid, is available in 10 mg and 25 mg gelatin capsules for oral administration. Chemically, acitretin is all-*trans*-9-(4-methoxy-2,3,6-trimethylphenyl)-3,7-dimethyl-2,4,6,8-nonatetraenoic acid. It is a metabolite of etretinate and is related to both retinoic acid and retinol (vitamin A). It is a yellow to greenish-yellow powder with a molecular weight of 326.44.

Each capsule contains acitretin, microcrystalline cellulose, sodium ascorbate, gelatin, black monogramming ink and maltodextrin (a mixture of polysaccharides).

Gelatin capsule shells contain gelatin, parabens (methyl and propyl), iron oxide (yellow, black, and red), and titanium dioxide. They may also contain benzyl alcohol, butyl paraben, carboxymethylcellulose sodium, edetate calcium disodium, potassium sorbate and/or sodium propionate.

CLINICAL PHARMACOLOGY

The mechanism of action of Soriatane is unknown.

Pharmacokinetics: *Absorption:* Oral absorption of acitretin is optimal when given with food. For this reason, acitretin was given with food in all of the following studies. After administration of a single 50 mg oral dose of acitretin to 18 healthy subjects, maximum plasma concentrations ranged from 196 to 728 ng/mL (mean 416 ng/mL) and were achieved in 2 to 5 hours (mean 2.7 hours). The oral absorption of acitretin is linear and proportional with increasing doses from 25 to 100 mg. Approximately 72% (range 47% to 109%) of the administered dose was absorbed after a single 50 mg dose of acitretin was given to 12 healthy subjects.

Distribution: Acitretin is more than 99.9% bound to plasma proteins, primarily albumin.

Metabolism (see Pharmacokinetic Drug Interactions: Ethanol): Following oral absorption, acitretin undergoes extensive metabolism and interconversion by simple isomerization to its 13-*cis* form (*cis*-acitretin). The formation of *cis*-acitretin relative to parent compound is not altered by dose or fed/fast conditions of oral administration of acitretin. Both parent compound and isomer are further metabolized into chain-shortened breakdown products and conjugates which are excreted.

Following multiple-dose administration of acitretin, steady-state concentrations of acitretin and *cis*-acitretin in plasma are achieved within approximately 3 weeks.

Elimination: The chain-shortened metabolites and conjugates of acitretin and *cis*-acitretin are ultimately excreted in the feces (34% to 54%) and urine (16% to 53%). The terminal elimination half-life of acitretin following multiple-dose administration is 49 hours (range 33 to 96 hours), and that of *cis*-acitretin under the same conditions is 63 hours (range 28 to 157 hours). The accumulation ratio of the parent compound is 1.2; that of *cis*-acitretin is 6.6.

Special Populations: *Psoriasis:* In an 8-week study of acitretin pharmacokinetics in patients with psoriasis, mean steady-state trough concentrations of acitretin increased in a dose proportional manner with dosages ranging from 10 to 50 mg daily. Acitretin plasma concentrations were nonmeasurable (<4 ng/mL) in all patients 3 weeks after cessation of therapy.

Elderly: In a multiple-dose study in healthy young (n=6) and elderly (n=8) subjects, a two-fold increase in acitretin plasma concentrations were seen in elderly subjects, although the elimination half-life did not change.

Renal Failure: Plasma concentrations of acitretin were significantly (59.3%) lower in end-stage renal failure subjects (n=6) when compared to age-matched controls, following single 50 mg oral doses. Acitretin was not removed by hemodialysis in these subjects.

Pharmacokinetic Drug Interactions (see also boxed CONTRAINDICATIONS AND WARNINGS and PRECAUTIONS: *Drug Interactions*): In studies of in vivo pharmacokinetic drug interactions, no interaction was seen between acitretin and cimetidine, digoxin, phenprocoumon or glyburide.

Ethanol: Clinical evidence has shown that etretinate (a retinoid with a much longer half-life, see below) can be formed with concurrent ingestion of acitretin and ethanol. In a two-way crossover study, all 10 subjects formed etretinate with concurrent ingestion of a single 100 mg oral dose of acitretin during a 3-hour period of ethanol ingestion (total ethanol, approximately 1.4 g/kg body weight). A mean peak etretinate concentration of 59 ng/mL (range 22 to 105 ng/mL) was observed, and extrapolation of AUC values indicated that the formation of etretinate in this study was comparable to a single 5 mg oral dose of etretinate. There was no detectable formation of etretinate when a single 100 mg oral dose of acitretin was administered without concurrent ethanol ingestion, although the formation of etretinate without concurrent ethanol ingestion cannot be excluded (see boxed CONTRAINDICATIONS AND WARNINGS). Of 93 evaluable psoriatic patients on acitretin therapy in several foreign studies (10 to 80 mg/day), 16% had measurable etretinate levels (>5 ng/mL).

Etretinate has a much longer elimination half-life compared to that of acitretin. In one study the apparent mean terminal half-life after 6 months of therapy was approximately 120 days (range 84 to 168 days). In another study of 47 patients treated chronically with etretinate, 5 had detectable serum drug levels (in the range of 0.5 to 12 ng/mL) 2.1 to 2.9 years after therapy was discontinued. The long half-life appears to be due to storage of etretinate in adipose tissue.

Progestin-only Contraceptives: It has not been established if there is a pharmacokinetic interaction between acitretin and combined oral contraceptives. However, it *has been* established that acitretin interferes with the contraceptive effect of microdosed progestin preparations.[2] *It is not known whether other progestational contraceptives, such as implants and injectables, are inadequate methods of contraception during acitretin therapy.*

INDICATIONS AND USAGE

Soriatane is indicated for the treatment of severe psoriasis, including the erythrodermic and generalized pustular types, in adults. Because of significant adverse effects associated with its use, Soriatane should be prescribed only by physicians knowledgeable in the systemic use of retinoids. In females of reproductive potential, Soriatane should be reserved for patients who are unresponsive to other therapies or whose clinical condition contraindicates the use of other treatments.

Most patients experience relapse of psoriasis after discontinuing therapy. Subsequent courses, when clinically indicated, have produced results similar to the initial course of therapy.

CONTRAINDICATIONS

Pregnancy Category X (see boxed CONTRAINDICATIONS AND WARNINGS)

WARNINGS

(See also boxed CONTRAINDICATIONS AND WARNINGS)

Hepatotoxicity: **Of the 525 patients treated in US clinical trials, 2 had clinical jaundice with elevated serum bilirubin and transaminases considered related to Soriatane treatment. Liver function test results in these patients returned to normal after Soriatane was discontinued. Two of the 1289 patients treated in European clinical trials developed biopsy-confirmed toxic hepatitis. A second biopsy in one of these patients revealed nodule formation suggestive of cirrhosis. One patient in a Canadian clinical trial of 63 patients developed a three-fold increase of transaminases. A liver biopsy of this patient showed mild lobular disarray, multifocal hepatocyte loss and mild triaditis of the portal tracts compatible with acute reversible hepatic injury. The patient's transaminase levels returned to normal 2 months after Soriatane was discontinued.**

The potential of acitretin therapy to induce hepatotoxicity was prospectively evaluated using liver biopsies in an open-label study of 128 patients. Pretreatment and posttreatment biopsies were available for 87 patients. A comparison of liver biopsy findings before and after therapy revealed 49 (58%) patients showed no change, 21 (25%) improved and 14 (17%) patients had a worsening of their liver biopsy status. For 6 patients, the classification changed from class 0 (no pathology) to class I (normal fatty infiltration; nuclear variability and portal inflammation; both mild); for 7 patients, the change was from class I to class II (fatty infiltration, nuclear variability, portal inflammation and focal necrosis; all moderate to severe); and for 1 patient, the change was from class II to class IIIb (fibrosis, moderate to severe). No correlation could be found between liver function test result abnormalities and the change in liver biopsy status, and no cumulative dose relationship was found.

Elevations of AST (SGOT), ALT (SGPT), GGT (GGTP) or LDH have occurred in approximately 1 in 3 patients treated with Soriatane. Of the 525 patients treated in clinical trials in the US, treatment was discontinued in 20 (3.8%) due to elevated liver function test results. If hepatotoxicity is suspected during treatment with Soriatane, the drug should be discontinued and the etiology further investigated.

Ten of 652 patients treated in US clinical trials of etretinate, of which acitretin is the active metabolite, had clinical or histologic hepatitis considered to be possibly or probably related to etretinate treatment. There have been reports of hepatitis-related deaths worldwide; a few of these patients had received etretinate for a month or less before presenting with hepatic symptoms or signs.

Pancreatitis: **Lipid elevations occur in 25% to 50% of patients treated with acitretin. Triglyceride increases sufficient to be associated with pancreatitis are much less common, although fatal fulminant pancreatitis has been reported for one patient.**

Pseudotumor cerebri: Soriatane and other retinoids administered orally have been associated with cases of pseudotumor cerebri (benign intracranial hypertension). Some of these events involved concomitant use of isotretinoin and tetracyclines. However, the event seen in a single Soriatane patient was not associated with tetracyline use. Early signs and symptoms include papilledema, headache, nausea and vomiting and visual disturbances. Patients with these signs and symptoms should be examined for papilledema and, if present, should discontinue Soriatane immediately and be referred for neurological evaluation and care.

Ophthalmologic Effects: The eyes and vision of 329 patients treated with Soriatane were examined by ophthalmologists. The findings included dry eyes (23%), irritation of eyes (9%) and brow and lash loss (5%). The following were reported in less than 5% of patients: Bell's Palsy, blepharitis and/or crusting of lids, blurred vision, conjunctivitis, corneal epithelial abnormality, cortical cataract, decreased night vision, diplopia, itchy eyes or eyelids, nuclear cataract, pannus, papilledema, photophobia, posterior subcapsular cataract, recurrent sties and subepithelial corneal lesions.
Any patient treated with Soriatane who is experiencing visual difficulties should discontinue the drug and undergo ophthalmologic evaluation.

Hyperostosis: In clinical trials with Soriatane, patients were prospectively evaluated for evidence of development or change in bony abnormalities of the vertebral column, knees and ankles.

Vertebral Results: Of 380 patients treated with Soriatane, 15% had preexisting abnormalities of the spine which showed new changes or progression of preexisting findings. Changes included degenerative spurs, anterior bridging of spinal vertebrae, diffuse idiopathic skeletal hyperostosis, ligament calcification and narrowing and destruction of a cervical disc space.
De novo changes (formation of small spurs) were seen in 3 patients after 1 1/2 to 2 1/2 years.

Skeletal Appendicular Results: Six of 128 patients treated with Soriatane showed abnormalities in the knees and ankles before treatment that progressed during treatment. In 5, these changes involved the formation of additional spurs or enlargement of existing spurs. The sixth patient had degenerative joint disease which worsened. No patients developed spurs de novo. Clinical complaints did not predict radiographic changes.

Lipids: Blood lipid determinations should be performed before Soriatane is administered and again at intervals of 1 to 2 weeks until the lipid response to the drug is established, usually within 4 to 8 weeks. In patients receiving Soriatane during clinical trials, 66% and 33% experienced elevation in triglycerides and cholesterol, respectively. Decreased high density lipoproteins (HDL) occurred in 40%. These effects of Soriatane were generally reversible upon cessation of therapy.
Patients with an increased tendency to develop hypertriglyceridemia included those with diabetes mellitus, obesity, increased alcohol intake or a familial history of these conditions.
Hypertriglyceridemia and lowered HDL may increase a patient's cardiovascular risk status. In addition, elevation of serum triglycerides to greater than 800 mg/dL has been associated with fatal fulminant pancreatitis. Therefore, dietary modifications, reduction in Soriatane dose, or drug therapy should be employed to control significant elevations of triglycerides.

Animal Studies: Subchronic and chronic toxicity studies in rats and dogs revealed dose-related, reversible signs of intolerance typical of retinoids. In rats, decreased body weight gain and increases in serum cholesterol, triglycerides, lipoproteins and alkaline phosphatase were observed; fractures and evidence of healed fractures were also noted. In dogs, signs of intolerance included erythema, skin hypertrophy/hyperplasia and testicular changes. In dogs, the dosages studied were as much as ten times the recommended human dosage; in rats, one to two times. Most of the side effects were readily reversible after cessation of treatment, except for epiphyseal ossification.
Acitretin shares with vitamin A and other retinoids the potential to cause malformations in the offspring of various species, including mouse, rat and rabbit, even at dosage levels recommended for humans. Since acitretin is teratogenic in animals at human dosage levels, females of reproductive potential must not be treated if pregnancy cannot be excluded.

PRECAUTIONS

General: Caution is advised in patients with severely impaired liver or kidney function (see CLINICAL PHARMACOLOGY). Soriatane should not be given to patients who are sensitive to parabens, which are used as preservatives in the gelatin capsule.

Information for Patients: Females of reproductive potential should be advised that they must not be pregnant when Soriatane therapy is initiated and that they should use effective contraception for at least 1 month prior to Soriatane therapy, and while taking Soriatane. Acitretin, the active metabolite of etretinate, is teratogenic and is contraindicated during pregnancy. The risk of severe fetal malformation is well established when systemic retinoids are taken during pregnancy. Pregnancy must also be prevented after stopping acitretin therapy, while the drug is being eliminated to below a threshold blood concentration that would be associated with an increased incidence of birth defects. Because this threshold has not been established for acitretin in humans and because elimination rates vary among patients, the duration of posttherapy contraception to achieve adequate elimination cannot be calculated precisely. It is strongly recommended that contraception be continued for at least 3 years after stopping treatment with acitretin, based on the following considerations:

- In the absence of transesterification to form etretinate, greater than 98% of the acitretin would be eliminated within 2 months, assuming a mean elimination half-life of 49 hours.
- In cases where etretinate is formed, as has been demonstrated with concomitant administration of acitretin and ethanol,
  - greater than 98% of the etretinate formed would be eliminated in 2 years, assuming a mean elimination half-life of 120 days.
  - greater than 98% of the etretinate formed would be eliminated in 3 years, based on the longest demonstrated elimination half-life of 168 days. However, etretinate was found in plasma and subcutaneous fat in one patient reported to have had sporadic alcohol intake, 52 months after she stopped acitretin therapy.[1]
- An increased incidence of birth defects was estimated based on a limited number of cases which have been reported to Roche, which were identified before the outcome was known, and where pregnancy occurred during the time interval when the patient was being treated with acitretin or etretinate. For cases identified after the outcome was known, severe birth defects have been reported where pregnancy occurred during the time interval when the patient was being treated with acitretin or etretinate.
- There have been 202 cases reported before the outcome was known where pregnancy occurred after the last dose of etretinate or acitretin. Fetal outcome remained unknown in approximately one-half of these cases, of which 62 were terminated and 11 were spontaneous abortions. Fetal outcome is known for 103 of these prospectively reported cases. Fifteen of the outcomes were abnormal: hernia, hypocalcemia, hypotonia, undescended testicle, laparoschisis, absent hand/wrist, clubfoot, ichthyosis, apnea/anemia, placental disorder/death and premature birth (5). Birth defects have also been reported retrospectively (ie, after the outcome was known). Among the retrospectively reported cases where pregnancy occurred more than 2 years after the last dose of etretinate or acitretin, there are 2 normal outcomes, 3 unknown outcomes and 7 abnormal outcomes. The 7 abnormal outcomes reported are: malformation unspecified, aplasia of the forearm, stillbirth, right ventricular/aortic duct defect, heart malformation unspecified, and chromosomal disorder (2). For these listed reports, the relationship of the birth defects to the drug is unknown.

Females of reproductive potential should also be advised that they must not ingest beverages or products containing ethanol while taking Soriatane and for 2 months after Soriatane treatment has been discontinued. This allows for elimination of the acitretin which can be converted to etretinate in the presence of alcohol. They should be advised that certain methods of birth control can fail, including tubal ligation and microdosed progestin "minipill" preparations. Data from one patient who received a very low-dosed progestin contraceptive (levonorgestrel 0.03 mg) had a significant increase of the progesterone level after three menstrual cycles during acitretin treatment.[2] Female patients should sign a consent form prior to beginning Soriatane therapy (see boxed CONTRAINDICATIONS AND WARNINGS).
Because of the relationship of Soriatane to vitamin A, patients should be advised against taking vitamin A supplements in excess of minimum recommended daily allowances to avoid possible additive toxic effects.
Patients should be advised that a transient worsening of psoriasis is sometimes seen during the initial treatment period.
Patients should be advised that they may have to wait 2 or 3 months before they get the full benefit of Soriatane.

Table 1. Adverse Events Frequently Reported During Clinical Trials Percent of Patients Reporting (N=525)

BODY SYSTEM	>75%	50% to 75%	25% to 50%	10% to 25%
Mucous Membranes	Cheilitis		Rhinitis	Dry mouth Epistaxis
Skin and Appendages		Alopecia Skin peeling	Dry skin Nail disorder Pruritus	Erythematous rash Hyperesthesia Paresthesia Paronychia Skin atrophy Sticky skin
Eye Disorders				Xerophthalmia
Musculoskeletal				Arthralgia Spinal hyperostosis (progression of existing lesions)
CNS				Rigors

Patients should be advised that they may experience decreased tolerance to contact lenses during the treatment period.
It is recommended that patients not donate blood during and for 3 years following therapy.
Patients should avoid the use of sun lamps and excessive exposure to sunlight because the effects of UV light are enhanced by retinoid therapy.
Patients should be advised that they must not give their Soriatane capsules to any other person.

Laboratory Tests: In clinical studies, the incidence of hypertriglyceridemia was 66%, hypercholesterolemia was 33% and that of decreased HDL was 40%. Pretreatment and follow-up measurements should be obtained under fasting conditions. It is recommended that these tests be performed weekly or every other week until the lipid response to Soriatane has stabilized (see WARNINGS).
Elevations of AST (SGOT), ALT (SGPT) or LDH were experienced by approximately 1 in 3 patients treated with Soriatane. It is recommended that these tests be performed prior to initiation of Soriatane therapy, at 1- to 2-week intervals until stable and thereafter at intervals as clinically indicated.
Certain patients receiving retinoids have experienced problems in the control of their blood sugar. In addition, new cases of diabetes have been diagnosed during retinoid therapy, although no causal relationship has been established.

Drug Interactions: Clinical evidence has shown that etretinate can be formed with concurrent ingestion of acitretin and ethanol (see boxed CONTRAINDICATIONS AND WARNINGS and CLINICAL PHARMACOLOGY: *Pharmacokinetics*).
In a study of 7 healthy male volunteers, acitretin treatment enhanced clearance of blood glucose in the presence of glibenclamide (a sulfonylurea similar to chlorpropamide) in 3 of the 7 subjects. Repeating the study with 6 healthy male volunteers in the absence of glibenclamide did not detect an effect of acitretin on glucose tolerance. Careful supervision of diabetic patients under treatment with Soriatane is recommended (see CLINICAL PHARMACOLOGY: *Pharmacokinetics* and DOSAGE AND ADMINISTRATION).
There may be the possibility of an increased risk of hepatotoxicity in patients treated with etretinate and methotrexate concomitantly. Consequently, the concomitant use of Soriatane and methotrexate should be avoided.
There appears to be no pharmacokinetic interaction between acitretin and cimetidine, digoxin, phenprocoumon or glyburide.
It has not been established if there is a pharmacokinetic interaction between acitretin and combined oral contraceptives. However, it *has been* established that acitretin interferes with the contraceptive effect of microdosed progestin "minipill" preparations. *It is not known whether other progestational contraceptives, such as implants and injectables, may be inadequate methods of contraception during acitretin therapy.*

Carcinogenesis, Mutagenesis and Impairment of Fertility: *Carcinogenesis:* A carcinogenesis study of acitretin in Wistar rats, at doses up to 2 mg/kg/day administered 7 days/week for 104 weeks, has been completed. There were no neoplastic lesions observed that were considered to have been related to treatment with acitretin. A carcinogenesis study in mice has been completed with etretinate, the ethyl ester of acitretin. Blood level data obtained during this study demonstrated that etretinate was metabolized to acitretin and that blood levels of acitretin exceeded those of etretinate at all times studied. In the etretinate study, an increased incidence of blood vessel tumors (hemangiomas and hemangiosarcomas at several different sites) was noted in male, but not female, mice at doses approximately 5.7 to 7.1 times the maximum recommended human therapeutic dose.
Mutagenesis: Acitretin was evaluated for mutagenic potential in the Ames test, in the Chinese hamster (V79/HGPRT) assay, in unscheduled DNA synthesis assays using rat hepatocytes and human fibroblasts and in an in vivo mouse micronucleus assay. No evidence of mutagenicity of acitretin was demonstrated in any of these assays.

Continued on next page

Soriatane—Cont.

Impairment of Fertility: In a fertility study in rats, the fertility of treated animals was not impaired at the highest dosage of acitretin tested, 3 mg/kg/day (approximately three times the maximum recommended therapeutic dose). Chronic toxicity studies in dogs revealed testicular changes (reversible mild to moderate spermatogenic arrest and appearance of multinucleated giant cells) in the highest dosage group (50 then 30 mg/kg/day).

No decreases in sperm count or concentration and no changes in sperm motility or morphology were noted in 31 men (17 psoriatic patients, 8 patients with disorders of keratinization and 6 healthy volunteers) given 30 to 50 mg/day of acitretin for at least 12 weeks. In these studies, no deleterious effects were seen on either testosterone production, LH or FSH in any of the 31 men.[3-5] No deleterious effects were seen on the hypothalamic-pituitary axis in any of the 18 men where it was measured.[3,4]

Pregnancy: *Teratogenic Effects:* **Pregnancy Category X (see boxed CONTRAINDICATIONS AND WARNINGS).**

Effective contraception must be used by female patients of reproductive potential for at least 1 month before beginning Soriatane therapy, during therapy and for at least 3 years following discontinuation of therapy. This warning applies even where there has been a history of infertility, unless due to hysterectomy.

In a study in which acitretin was administered to male rats only at a dosage of 5 mg/kg/day for 10 weeks (approximate duration of one spermatogenic cycle) prior to and during mating with untreated female rats, no teratogenic effects were observed in the progeny.

Samples of seminal fluid from 3 male patients treated with acitretin and 6 male patients treated with etretinate have been assayed for the presence of acitretin. The maximum concentration of acitretin observed in the seminal fluid of these men was 12.5 ng/mL. Assuming an ejaculate volume of 10 mL, the amount of drug transferred in semen would be 125 ng, which is 1/200,000 of a single 25 mg capsule.

It is not known whether residual acitretin in seminal fluid poses risk to a fetus while a male patient is taking the drug or after it is discontinued. There have been five pregnancies reported in which the male partner was undergoing Soriatane treatment. One pregnancy resulted in a normal infant. Two pregnancies ended in spontaneous abortions. In one case the fetus had bilateral cystic hygromas and multiple cardiopulmonary malformations: the relationship of these malformations to the drug is unknown. The outcome of the fifth case is unknown.

Nonteratogenic Effects: In rats dosed at 3 mg/kg/day (approximately three times the maximum recommended therapeutic dose), slightly decreased pup survival and delayed incisor eruption were noted. At the next lowest dose tested, 1 mg/kg/day, no treatment-related adverse effects were observed.

Nursing Mothers: Studies on lactating rats have shown that etretinate is excreted in the milk. However, it is not known whether either etretinate or acitretin is excreted in human milk. However, nursing mothers should not receive Soriatane because of the potential for excretion in milk and serious adverse reactions in nursing infants.

Pediatric Use: No clinical studies have been conducted in pediatric patients. Therefore, safety and effectiveness in pediatric patients have not been established. Ossification of interosseous ligaments and tendons of the extremities, skeletal hyperostoses and premature epiphyseal closure have been reported with other systemic retinoids. While it is not known that these occurrences are more severe or more frequent in children, there is concern in pediatric patients because of the implications for growth potential.

ADVERSE EVENTS

During clinical trials with acitretin, 513/525 (98%) of patients reported a total of 3545 adverse events. One-hundred sixteen patients left studies prematurely, primarily because of adverse experiences involving the mucous membranes and skin. Three patients died. Two of the deaths were not drug related (pancreatic adenocarcinoma and lung cancer); the other patient died of an acute myocardial infarction, considered remotely related to drug therapy.

In clinical trials, Soriatane has been associated with elevations in liver function test results or triglyceride levels and hepatitis. A case of fatal fulminant pancreatitis has been reported during Soriatane therapy.

Soriatane has also been associated with a case of pseudotumor cerebri (see WARNINGS). One case of myopathy with peripheral neuropathy has been reported during Soriatane therapy. Both conditions improved with discontinuation of the drug.

Hypervitaminosis A produces a wide spectrum of signs and symptoms primarily of the mucocutaneous, musculoskeletal, hepatic, and central nervous systems. Many of the clinical adverse reactions reported to date with Soriatane administration resemble those of the hypervitaminosis A syndrome. The tables below list by body system and frequency the adverse events reported during clinical trials of 525 patients with psoriasis.

[See table 1 at top of previous page]

[See table 2 above and at top of next page]

Laboratory: Soriatane therapy induces changes in liver function tests in a significant number of patients. Elevations of AST (SGOT), ALT (SGPT) or LDH were experienced by approximately 1 in 3 patients treated with Soriatane. In most patients, elevations were slight to moderate and returned to normal either during continuation of therapy or after cessation of treatment. In patients receiving Soriatane during clinical trials, 66% and 33% experienced elevation in triglycerides and cholesterol, respectively. Decreased high density lipoproteins (HDL) occurred in 40% (see WARNINGS).

Table 3 lists the laboratory abnormalities reported during clinical trials.

[See table 3 at bottom of next page]

Table 2. Adverse Events Less Frequently Reported During Clinical Trials (Some of Which May Bear No Relationship to Therapy) Percent of Patients Reporting (N=525)

BODY SYSTEM	1% to 10%	<1%
Mucous Membranes	Gingival bleeding Gingivitis Increased saliva Stomatitis Thirst Ulcerative stomatitis	Altered saliva Anal disorder Gum hyperplasia Hemorrhage Pharyngitis
Skin and Appendages	Abnormal skin odor Abnormal hair texture Bullous eruption Cold/clammy skin Dermatitis Increased sweating Infection Psoriasiform rash Purpura Pyogenic granuloma Rash Seborrhea Skin fissures Skin ulceration Sunburn	Acne Breast pain Cyst Eczema Fungal infection Furunculosis Hair discoloration Herpes simplex Hyperkeratosis Hypertrichosis Hypoesthesia Impaired healing Otitis media Otitis externa Photosensitivity reaction Psoriasis aggravated Scleroderma Skin nodule Skin hypertrophy Skin disorder Skin irritation Sweat gland disorder Urticaria Verrucae
Eye Disorders	Abnormal/blurred vision Blepharitis Conjunctivitis/irritation Corneal epithelial abnormality Decreased night vision/ night blindness Eye abnormality Eye pain Photophobia	Abnormal lacrimation Chalazion Conjunctival hemorrhage Corneal ulceration Diplopia Ectropion Itchy eyes and lids Papilledema Recurrent sties Subepithelial corneal lesions
Musculoskeletal	Arthritis Arthrosis Back pain Hypertonia Myalgia Osteodynia Peripheral joint hyperostosis (progression of existing lesions)	Bone disorder Olecranon bursitis Spinal hyperostosis (new lesions) Tendinitis
CNS	Headache Pain	Abnormal gait Migraine Neuritis Pseudotumor cerebri (intracranial hypertension)
Gastrointestinal	Abdominal pain Diarrhea Nausea Tongue disorder	Constipation Dyspepsia Esophagitis Gastritis Gastroenteritis Glossitis Hemorrhoids Melena Tenesmus Tongue ulceration

OVERDOSAGE

One overdose case has been reported. A 32-year-old mentally handicapped male with Darier's disease took 21 × 25 mg capsules (525 mg single dose). He vomited several hours later but experienced no other ill effects. His therapeutic treatment was continued. The acute oral toxicity (LD_{50}) of acitretin in both mice and rats was greater than 4000 mg/kg.

DOSAGE AND ADMINISTRATION

There is intersubject variation in the pharmacokinetics, clinical efficacy and incidence of side effects with Soriatane. A number of the more common side effects are dose related. Individualization of dosage is required to achieve maximum therapeutic response while minimizing side effects. Soriatane therapy should be initiated at 25 or 50 mg per day, given as a single dose with the main meal. Maintenance doses of 25 to 50 mg per day may be given after initial response to treatment; although, in general, therapy should be terminated when lesions have resolved sufficiently. Relapses may be treated as outlined for initial therapy.

Females who have taken Tegison (etretinate) must continue to follow the contraceptive recommendations for Tegison.

HOW SUPPLIED

Brown and white capsules, 10 mg, imprinted SORIATANE 10 ROCHE; Prescription Paks of 30 (NDC 0004-0213-57).

Brown and yellow capsules, 25 mg, imprinted SORIATANE 25 ROCHE; Prescription Paks of 30 (NDC 0004-0214-57).

Store between 15° and 25°C (59° and 77°F). Protect from light. Avoid exposure to high temperatures and humidity after the bottle is opened.

REFERENCES:

1. Maier H, Honigsmann H: Concentration of etretinate in plasma and subcutaneous fat after long-term acitretin. *Lancet* 348:1107, 1996.
2. Berbis Ph, et al.: *Arch Dermatol Res*(1988) 280:388-389.
3. Sigg C, et al.: Andrological investigations in patients treated with etretin. *Dermatologica* 175:48-49, 1987.
4. Parsch EM, et al.: Andrological investigation in men treated with acitretin (Ro 10-1670). *Andrologia* 22:479-482, 1990.
5. Kadar L, et al.: Spermatological investigations in psoriatic patients treated with acitretin. In: Pharmacology of

Table 2. Adverse Events Less Frequently Reported During Clinical Trials (Some of Which May Bear No Relationship to Therapy) Percent of Patients Reporting (N=525)

BODY SYSTEM	1% to 10%	<1%
Special Senses/Other	Earache Taste perversion Tinnitus	Ceruminosis Deafness Taste loss
Psychiatric	Depression Insomnia Somnolence	Anxiety Dysphonia Libido decreased Nervousness
Respiratory	Sinusitis	Coughing Increased sputum Laryngitis
Urinary		Abnormal urine Dysuria Penis disorder
Reproductive		Atrophic vaginitis Leukorrhea
Cardiovascular	Flushing	Chest pain Cyanosis Increased bleeding time Intermittent claudication Peripheral ischemia
Body as a Whole	Anorexia Edema Fatigue Hot flashes Increased appetite	Alcohol tolerance Dizziness Fever Influenza-like symptoms Malaise Moniliasis Muscle weakness Weight increase
Liver and Biliary		Hepatic function abnormal Hepatitis Jaundice

Table 3. Abnormal Laboratory Test Results Reported During Clinical Trials Percent of Patients Reporting

BODY SYSTEM	50% to 75%	25% to 50%	10% to 25%	1% to 10%
Hematologic		Increased reticulocytes	Decreased: – Hematocrit – Hemoglobin – WBC Increased: – Haptoglobin – Neutrophils – WBC	Increased: – Bands – Basophils – Eosinophils – Hematocrit – Hemoglobin – Lymphocytes – Monocytes Decreased: – Haptoglobin – Lymphocytes – Neutrophils – Reticulocytes Increased or decreased: – Platelets – RBC
Electrolytes			Increased: – Phosphorus – Potassium – Sodium Increased and decreased magnesium	Decreased: – Phosphorus – Potassium – Sodium Increased and decreased: – Calcium – Chloride
Renal			Increased uric acid	Increased: – BUN – Creatinine
Hepatic		Increased: – Cholesterol – LDH – SGOT – SGPT Decreased HDL cholesterol	Increased: – Alkaline phosphatase – Direct bilirubin – GGTP	Increased: – Globulin – Total bilirubin – Total protein Increased and decreased Serum albumin
Urinary		WBC in urine	Acetonuria Hematuria RBC in urine	Glycosuria Proteinuria
Miscellaneous	Increased triglycerides	Increased: – CPK – Fasting blood sugar	Decreased: fasting blood sugar High occult blood	Increased and decreased iron

Retinoids in the Skin; Reichert U. et al., ed, KARGER, Basel, vol. 3, pp 253-254, 1988.

PATIENT INFORMATION/CONSENT:

IMPORTANT INFORMATION AND WARNINGS FOR *ALL* PATIENTS:

Small amounts of Soriatane have been detected in the ejaculate of males taking Soriatane. The amount of Soriatane detected corresponds to less than 1/200,000 of a 25 mg dose. You should discuss any questions you have about this information with your physician.

Alcohol intake can cause Soriatane to be changed into a related drug, etretinate, which may not leave the body for many years.

In addition, you must not donate blood during your treatment with Soriatane and for 3 years after you stop taking Soriatane.

It is recommended that you and your doctor schedule appointments regularly to check your body's response to Soriatane. For your health and well-being, be sure to keep your appointments as scheduled.

Do not give your Soriatane capsules to any other person.

IMPORTANT INFORMATION AND WARNINGS FOR *FEMALE* PATIENTS:

Soriatane must not be used by females who are pregnant or who may become pregnant while undergoing treatment or at any time for at least 3 years after treatment is discontinued.

If you do become pregnant during Soriatane therapy, or at any time for at least 3 years after you stop taking Soriatane, you should discuss with your physician the possible effects on the pregnancy.

Soriatane can cause severe birth defects if it is taken when a female is pregnant. In addition, birth defects have occurred in babies of females who became pregnant after stopping Soriatane treatment. Therefore:

- you must not be pregnant when you start taking Soriatane,
- you must not become pregnant while you are taking Soriatane,
- you must wait at least 3 years after you stop taking Soriatane before becoming pregnant.

Alcohol must be avoided during the entire Soriatane treatment course and for 2 months after you stop taking Soriatane. This is because alcohol intake can cause Soriatane to be changed into a related drug, etretinate. Etretinate may not leave the body for many years and, like Soriatane, can cause severe birth defects. It is recommended that you and your doctor schedule appointments regularly to repeat the pregnancy test and check your body's response to Soriatane. For your health and well-being, be sure to keep your appointments as scheduled.

In addition, you must not donate blood during your treatment with Soriatane and for 3 years after you stop taking Soriatane.

Do not give your Soriatane capsules to any other person.

THE CONSENT FOR *FEMALE* PATIENTS:

My treatment with Soriatane has been personally explained to me by Dr. ______________. The following points of information, among others, have been specifically discussed and made clear:

1. I, ______________________________________,
(Patient's Name)
understand that Soriatane is used to treat severe psoriasis that is unresponsive to other therapies.
INITIALS: ______________
2. I understand that severe birth defects related to treatment with Soriatane have occurred in babies of women who have taken Soriatane during pregnancy. In addition, birth defects have occurred in babies of women who became pregnant after stopping Soriatane treatment.
INITIALS: ______________
3. I understand that I must not be pregnant when I start taking Soriatane.
INITIALS: ______________
4. I understand that I must not become pregnant while I am taking Soriatane.
INITIALS: ______________
5. I understand that I must wait at least 3 years after I stop taking Soriatane before becoming pregnant.
INITIALS: ______________
6. I have been told by my doctor that effective birth control (contraception) must be used for at least 1 month before starting Soriatane, for the entire duration of Soriatane therapy and for at least 3 years after Soriatane treatment has stopped. My doctor has told me that I must either abstain from sexual intercourse or use two reliable kinds of birth control at the same time. I have also been told that any method of birth control can fail, including tubal ligation or microdosed progestin "minipill" preparations. I must use two forms of reliable birth control simultaneously, even if I think I cannot become pregnant, unless I abstain from sexual intercourse or have had a hysterectomy.
INITIALS: ______________
7. I understand that if I have taken Tegison (etretinate), I must continue to follow the birth control (contraception) recommendations for Tegison.
INITIALS: ______________
8. I know that I must have a blood or urine test done by my doctor that shows I am not pregnant within 1 week be-

Continued on next page

Soriatane—Cont.

fore starting Soriatane. I understand that I must wait until the second or third day of my next normal menstrual period before starting Soriatane.

INITIALS: __________

9. My doctor has told me that I can participate in the "Patient Referral" program for an initial free pregnancy test and birth control counseling session by a consulting physician.

INITIALS: __________

10. I know that I must immediately stop taking Soriatane if I become pregnant and immediately contact my doctor to discuss possible effects on the pregnancy. I also know that I must immediately contact my doctor if I become pregnant at any time for at least 3 years after stopping Soriatane.

INITIALS: __________

11. I have carefully read the Soriatane patient brochure, "Important information concerning your treatment with Soriatane," given to me by my doctor. I understand all of its contents and have talked over any questions I have with my doctor.

INITIALS: __________

12. I am not now pregnant, nor do I plan to become pregnant while taking Soriatane and for at least 3 years after I have completely finished taking Soriatane.

INITIALS: __________

13. I know that I must avoid ingesting any beverage or product that contains alcohol during the entire Soriatane treatment course and for 2 months after I have completely finished taking Soriatane.

INITIALS: __________

14. I understand that if I consume any beverage or product that contains alcohol during my treatment with Soriatane or during the 2 months after I stop taking Soriatane, the risk of birth defects will persist for a longer period of time.

INITIALS: __________

15. I have been told not to donate blood during my treatment with Soriatane and for 3 years after I have completely finished taking Soriatane.

INITIALS: __________

I now authorize Dr. ____________________
to begin my treatment with Soriatane.

____
Patient signature, Parent or Guardian signature if patient is a minor Date

____
Address

____

____
Telephone Number

I have fully explained to the patient, ________________, the nature and purpose of the treatment described above and the teratogenic risk. I have asked the patient if there are any questions regarding treatment with Soriatane and have answered those questions to the best of my ability.

____
Physician signature Date

Issued: August 1997

Shown in Product Identification Guide, page 333

TAMIFLU™ ℞
(oseltamivir phosphate)
CAPSULES

The following text is complete prescribing information based on official labeling in effect June 2000.

DESCRIPTION

TAMIFLU (oseltamivir phosphate) is available as a capsule containing 75-mg oseltamivir for oral use, in the form of oseltamivir phosphate. In addition to the active ingredient, each capsule contains pregelatinized starch, talc, povidone K 30, croscarmellose sodium, sodium stearyl fumarate, ethanol, and purified water. The capsule shell contains gelatin, titanium dioxide, yellow iron oxide, black iron oxide, and red iron oxide. Each capsule is printed with blue ink, which includes FD&C Blue #2 as the colorant. Oseltamivir phosphate is a white crystalline solid with the chemical name (3R,4R,5S)-4-acetylamino-5-amino-3(1-ethylpropoxy)-1-cyclohexene-1-carboxylic acid, ethyl ester, phosphate (1:1). The chemical formula is $C_{16}H_{28}N_2O_4$ (free base). The molecular weight is 312.4 for oseltamivir free base and 410.4 for oseltamivir phosphate salt. The structural formula is as follows:

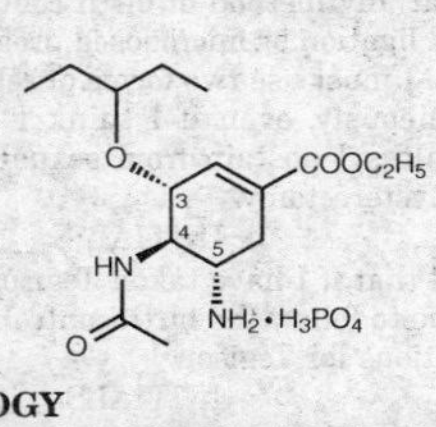

MICROBIOLOGY

Mechanism of Action: Oseltamivir is an ethyl ester prodrug requiring ester hydrolysis for conversion to the active form, oseltamivir carboxylate. The proposed mechanism of action of oseltamivir is via inhibition of influenza virus neuraminidase with the possibility of alteration of virus particle aggregation and release.

Table 1. Mean (% CV) Pharmacokinetic Parameters of Oseltamivir and Oseltamivir Carboxylate After a Multiple 75-mg Twice Daily Oral Dose (n=20)

Parameter	Oseltamivir	Oseltamivir Carboxylate
Cmax (ng/mL)	65.2 (26)	348 (18)
$AUC_{0\text{-}12h}$ (ng·h/mL)	112 (25)	2719 (20)

Antiviral Activity In Vitro: The antiviral activity of oseltamivir carboxylate against laboratory strains and clinical isolates of influenza virus was determined in cell culture assays. The concentrations of oseltamivir carboxylate required for inhibition of influenza virus were highly variable depending on the assay method used and the virus tested. The 50% and 90% inhibitory concentrations (IC50 and IC90) were in the range of 0.0008 μM to >35 μM and 0.004 μM to >100 μM, respectively (1 μM=0.284 μg/mL). The relationship between the in vitro antiviral activity in cell culture and the inhibition of influenza virus replication in humans has not been established.

Drug Resistance: Influenza A virus with reduced susceptibility to oseltamivir carboxylate have been recovered in vitro by passage of virus in the presence of increasing concentrations of oseltamivir carboxylate. Genetic analysis of these isolates showed that reduced susceptibility to oseltamivir carboxylate is associated with mutations that result in amino acid changes in the viral neuraminidase or viral hemagglutinin or both.

In challenge studies of human subjects infected with influenza virus; 3% (3/102) of the post-treatment isolates showed emergence of influenza variants with decreased neuraminidase susceptibility to oseltamivir carboxylate. Genotypic analysis of these variants showed a specific mutation in the active site of neuraminidase compared to challenge virus.

In clinical studies of naturally acquired infection with influenza virus, 1.3% (4/301) of post-treatment isolates showed emergence of influenza variants with decreased neuraminidase susceptiblity to oseltamivir carboxylate.

Genotypic analysis of these variants showed a specific mutation in the active site of neuraminidase compared to pretreatment isolates. The contribution of resistance due to alterations in the viral hemagglutinin has not been fully evaluated.

Cross-resistance: Cross-resistance between zanamivir-resistant influenza mutants and oseltamivir-resistant influenza mutants has been observed in vitro.

Due to limitations in the assays available to detect drug-induced shifts in virus susceptibility, an estimate of the incidence of oseltamivir resistance and possible cross-resistance to zanamivir in clinical isolates cannot be made. However, one of the three oseltamivir-induced mutations in the viral neuraminidase from clinical isolates is the same as one of the three mutations observed in zanamivir-resistant virus.

Insufficient information is available to fully characterize the risk of emergence of TAMIFLU resistance in clinical use.

Immune Response: No influenza vaccine interaction study has been conducted. In studies of naturally acquired and experimental influenza, treatment with TAMIFLU did not impair normal humoral antibody response to infection.

Influenza Challenge Studies: Antiviral activity of TAMIFLU was supported for influenza A and B by experimental challenge studies in volunteers who received intranasal inoculations of challenge strains of influenza virus. These subjects received TAMIFLU or placebo shortly after viral inoculation.

CLINICAL PHARMACOLOGY: ***Pharmacokinetics: Absorption and Bioavailability:*** Oseltamivir is readily absorbed from the gastrointestinal tract after oral administration of oseltamivir phosphate and is extensively converted predominantly by hepatic esterases to oseltamivir carboxylate. At least 75% of an oral dose reaches the systemic circulation as oseltamivir carboxylate. Exposure to oseltamivir is less than 5% of the total exposure after oral dosing (Table 1).

[See table above]

Plasma concentrations of oseltamivir carboxylate are proportional to doses up to 500 mg given twice daily (see DOSAGE AND ADMINISTRATION).

Coadministration with food has no significant effect on the peak plasma concentration (551 ng/mL under fasted conditions and 441 ng/mL under fed conditions) and the area under the plasma concentration time curve (6218 ng·h/mL under fasted conditions and 6069 ng·h/mL under fed conditions) of oseltamivir carboxylate.

Distribution: The volume of distribution (Vss) of oseltamivir carboxylate, following intravenous administration in 24 subjects, ranged between 23 and 26 liters.

The binding of oseltamivir carboxylate to human plasma protein is low (3%). The binding of oseltamivir to human plasma protein is 42%, which is insufficient to cause significant displacement-based drug interactions.

Metabolism: Oseltamivir is extensively converted to oseltamivir carboxylate by esterases located predominantly in the liver. Neither oseltamivir nor oseltamivir carboxylate is a substrate for, or inhibitor of, cytochrome P450 isoforms.

Elimination: Absorbed oseltamivir is primarily (>90%) eliminated by conversion to oseltamivir carboxylate. Plasma concentrations of oseltamivir declined with a half-life of 1 to 3 hours in most subjects after oral administration. Oseltamivir carboxylate is not further metabolized and is eliminated in the urine. Plasma concentrations of oseltamivir carboxylate declined with a half-life of 6 to 10 hours in most subjects after oral administration. Oseltamivir carboxylate is eliminated entirely (>99%) by renal excretion. Renal clearance (18.8 L/h) exceeds glomerular filtration rate (7.5 L/h) indicating that tubular secretion occurs, in addition to glomerular filtration. Less than 20% of an oral radiolabeled dose is eliminated in feces.

Special Populations: *Renal Impairment:* Administration of 100 mg of oseltamivir phosphate twice daily for 5 days to patients with various degrees of renal impairment showed that exposure to oseltamivir carboxylate is inversely proportional to declining renal function. Dose adjustment is recommended for patients with creatinine clearance below 30 mL/min. There are no data available in patients with renal failure (creatinine clearance <10 mL/min); therefore, caution is advised when administering the drug to those patients (see DOSAGE AND ADMINISTRATION: *Special Dosage Instructions*).

Geriatric Patients: Exposure to oseltamivir carboxylate at steady-state was 25% to 35% higher in geriatric patients (age range 65 to 78 years) compared to young adults given comparable doses of oseltamivir. Half-lives observed in the geriatric patients were similar to those seen in young adults. Based on drug exposure and tolerability, dose adjustments are not required for geriatric patients (see DOSAGE AND ADMINISTRATION: *Special Dosage Instructions*).

INDICATIONS AND USAGE

TAMIFLU is indicated for the treatment of uncomplicated acute illness due to influenza infection in adults who have been symptomatic for no more than 2 days. This indication is based on studies of naturally occurring influenza in which the predominant infection was influenza A, and influenza challenge studies in which antiviral activity of TAMIFLU was supported for influenza A and B (see *Description of Clinical Studies* and PRECAUTIONS).

Description of Clinical Studies:

Naturally Occurring Influenza Trials: Two phase 3 placebo-controlled and double-blind clinical trials were conducted: one in the USA and one outside the USA. Patients were eligible for these trials if they had fever >100°F, accompanied by at least one respiratory symptom (cough, nasal symptoms or sore throat) and at least one systemic symptom (myalgia, chills/sweats, malaise, fatigue or headache) and influenza virus was known to be circulating in the community. In addition, all patients enrolled in the trials were allowed to take fever-reducing medications.

Of 1355 patients enrolled in these two trials, 849 (63%) patients were influenza-infected (age range 18 to 65 years; median age 34 years; 52% male; 90% Caucasian; 31% smokers). Of these 849 patients, 95% were infected with influenza A, 3% with influenza B, and 2% with influenza of unknown type.

TAMIFLU was started within 40 hours of onset of symptoms. Subjects participating in the trials were required to self-assess the influenza-associated symptoms as "none," "mild," "moderate" or "severe." Time to improvement was calculated from the time of treatment initiation to the time when all symptoms (nasal congestion, sore throat, cough, aches, fatigue, headaches, and chills/sweats) were assessed as "none" or "mild." In both studies, at the recommended dose of TAMIFLU 75 mg twice daily for 5 days, there was a 1.3 day reduction in the median time to improvement in influenza-infected subjects receiving TAMIFLU compared to subjects receiving placebo. Subgroup analyses of these studies by gender showed no differences in the treatment effect of TAMIFLU in men and women.

No increased efficacy was demonstrated in subjects receiving treatment of 150-mg TAMIFLU twice daily for 5 days.

CONTRAINDICATIONS

TAMIFLU is contraindicated in patients with known hypersensitivity to any of the components of the product.

PRECAUTIONS

General: There is no evidence for efficacy of TAMIFLU in any illness caused by agents other than influenza viruses Types A and B. Data on treatment of influenza B are limited (see INDICATIONS AND USAGE: *Description of Clinical Studies*).

Efficacy of TAMIFLU in patients who begin treatment after 40 hours of symptoms has not been established.

Efficacy of TAMIFLU in subjects with chronic cardiac disease and/or respiratory disease has not been established. No difference in the incidence of complications was observed between the treatment and placebo groups in this population.

No information is available regarding treatment of influenza in patients with any medical condition sufficiently severe or unstable to be considered at imminent risk of requiring hospitalization.

Use of TAMIFLU should not affect the evaluation of individuals for annual influenza vaccination in accordance with guidelines of the Center for Disease Controls and Preven-

Table 2. Adverse Events ≥1% in the Treatment of Naturally Acquired Influenza With Dose of TAMIFLU 75 mg Twice Daily

	TAMIFLU 75 mg twice daily N=724		Placebo N=716	
Nausea (without vomiting)	72	(9.9%)	40	(5.6%)
Vomiting	68	(9.4%)	21	(2.9%)
Diarrhea	48	(6.6%)	70	(9.8%)
Bronchitis	17	(2.3%)	15	(2.1%)
Abdominal pain	16	(2.2%)	16	(2.2%)
Dizziness	15	(2.1%)	25	(3.5%)
Headache	13	(1.8%)	14	(2.0%)
Cough	9	(1.2%)	12	(1.7%)
Insomnia	8	(1.1%)	6	(0.8%)
Vertigo	7	(1.0%)	3	(0.4%)
Fatigue	7	(1.0%)	7	(1.0%)

tion Advisory Committee on Immunization Practices. Efficacy of TAMIFLU has not been established for prophylactic use to prevent influenza.

Safety and efficacy of repeated treatment courses have not been studied.

Information for Patients: Patients should be instructed to begin treatment with TAMIFLU as soon as possible from the first appearance of flu symptoms.

Patients should be instructed to take any missed doses as soon as they remember, except if it is near the next scheduled dose (within 2 hours), and then continue to take TAMIFLU at the usual times.

TAMIFLU is not a substitute for a flu shot. Patients should continue receiving an annual flu shot according to guidelines on immunization practices.

Drug Interactions: Information derived from pharmacology and pharmacokinetic studies of oseltamivir suggests that clinically significant drug interactions are unlikely.

Oseltamivir is extensively converted to oseltamivir carboxylate by esterases, located predominantly in the liver. Drug interactions involving competition for esterases have not been extensively reported in literature. Low protein binding of oseltamivir and oseltamivir carboxylate suggests that the probability of drug displacement interactions is low.

In vitro studies demonstrate that neither oseltamivir nor oseltamivir carboxylate is a good substrate for P450 mixed-function oxidases or for glucuronyl transferases.

Cimetidine, a non-specific inhibitor of cytochrome P450 isoforms and competitor for renal tubular secretion of basic or cationic drugs, has no effect on plasma levels of oseltamivir or oseltamivir carboxylate.

Clinically important drug interactions involving competition for renal tubular secretion are unlikely due to the known safety margin for most of these drugs, the elimination characteristics of oseltamivir carboyxlate (glomerular filtration and anionic tubular secretion) and the excretion capacity of these pathways. Coadministration of probenecid results in an approximate twofold increase in exposure to oseltamivir carboxylate due to a decrease in active anionic tubular secretion in the kidney. However, due to the safety margin of oseltamivir carboxylate, no dose adjustments are required when coadministering with probenecid.

Preliminary information shows that coadministration with amoxicillin does not alter plasma levels of either compound, indicating that competition for the anionic secretion pathway is weak.

In six subjects, multiple doses of oseltamivir did not affect the single-dose pharmacokinetics of acetaminophen.

Carcinogenesis, Mutagenesis, and Impairment of Fertility: Oseltamivir was found to be non-mutagenic in the Ames, human lymphocyte chromosome and mouse micronucleus tests. Oseltamivir carboxylate was also found to be non-mutagenic in the Ames and mouse lymphoma cell mutation tests.

In a fertility and early embryonic development study in rats, doses of oseltamivir at 50, 250 and 1500 mg/kg/day were administered to females for 2 weeks before mating, during mating and until Day 6 of pregnancy. Males were dosed for 4 weeks before mating, during and for 2 weeks after mating. There were no effects on fertility, mating performance or early embryonic development at any dose level. The highest dose was approximately 100 times the human systemic exposure (AUC 0 to 24 h) of oseltamivir carboxylate.

Long-term carcinogenicity tests with oseltamivir have not been completed.

Pregnancy: Pregnancy Category C: There are insufficient human data upon which to base an evaluation of risk of TAMIFLU to the pregnant woman or developing fetus. Studies for effects on embryo-fetal development were conducted in rats (50, 250, and 1500 mg/kg/day) and rabbits (50, 150, and 500 mg/kg/day) by the oral route. Relative exposures at these doses were, respectively, 2, 13, and 100 times human exposure in the rat and 4, 8, and 50 times human exposure in the rabbit. Pharmacokinetic studies indicated that fetal exposure was seen in both species. In the rat study, minimal maternal toxicity was reported in the 1500 mg/kg/day group. In the rabbit study, slight and marked maternal toxicities were observed, respectively, in the 150 and 500 mg/kg/day groups. There was a dose-dependent increase in the incidence rates of a variety of minor skeleton adnormalities and variants in the exposed offspring in these studies. However, the individual incidence rate of each skeletal abnormality or variant remained within the background rates of occurrence in the species studied.

Because animal reproductive studies may not be predictive of human response and there are no adequate and well-controlled studies in pregnant women, TAMIFLU should be used during pregnancy only if the potential benefit justifies the potential risk to the fetus.

Nursing Mothers: In lactating rats, oseltamivir and oseltamivir carboxylate are excreted in the milk. It is not known whether oseltamivir or oseltamivir carboxylate is excreted in human milk. TAMIFLU should, therefore, be used only if the potential benefit for the lactating mother justifies the potential risk to the breast-fed infant.

Pediatric Use: The safety and efficacy of TAMIFLU in children (<18 years) have not been established.

Geriatric Use: In an ongoing study of otherwise healthy elderly patients, >65 years (n=168), given the recommended dosing regimen of TAMIFLU, there was a reduction in the median time to improvement in the subjects receiving TAMIFLU similar to that seen in younger adults. No overall difference in safety was observed between these subjects and younger adults.

ADVERSE REACTIONS

A total of 1171 patients who participated in adult phase 3 controlled clinical trials for the treatment of influenza were treated with TAMIFLU. The most frequently reported adverse events in these studies were nausea and vomiting. These events were generally of mild to moderate degree and usually occurred on the first 2 days of administration. Less than 1% of subjects discontinued prematurely from clinical trials due to nausea and vomiting.

Adverse events that occurred with an incidence of ≥1% in 1440 patients taking placebo or TAMIFLU 75 mg twice daily in adult phase 3 treatment studies are shown in Table 2. This summary includes 945 healthy young adults and 495 "at risk" patients (elderly patients and patients with chronic cardiac or respiratory disease). Those events reported numerically more frequently in patients taking TAMIFLU compared with placebo were nausea, vomiting, bronchitis, insomnia, and vertigo.

[See table above]

Additional adverse events occurring in <1% of patients receiving TAMIFLU included unstable angina, anemia, pseudomembranous colitis, humerus fracture, pneumonia, pyrexia, and peritonsillar abscess.

OVERDOSAGE

At present, there has been no experience with overdose. Single doses of up to 1000 mg of TAMIFLU have been associated with nausea and/or vomiting. A complete pack of ten capsules of TAMIFLU contains a total of 750 mg of oseltamivir.

DOSAGE AND ADMINISTRATION

Standard Dosage: The recommended oral dose of TAMIFLU is 75 mg twice daily for 5 days. Treatment should begin within 2 days of onset of symptoms of influenza. TAMIFLU may be taken with or without food (see *PHARMACOKINETICS*). However, when taken with food, tolerability may be enhanced in some patients.

Special Dosage Instructions: *Hepatic Impairment:* The safety and pharmacokinetics in patients with hepatic impairment have not been evaluated.

Renal Impairment: No dose adjustment is necessary for patients with creatinine clearance above 30 mL/min. In patients with a creatinine clearance of less than 30 mL/min, it is recommended that the dose be reduced to 75 mg of TAMIFLU once daily for 5 days. The drug has not been studied in patients with renal failure (creatinine clearance below 10 mL/min); therefore, caution is advised when administering the drug to those patient populations (see *PHARMACOKINETICS*: *Special Populations*).

Pediatric Patients: The safety and efficacy of TAMIFLU in children have not been established.

Geriatric Patients: No dose adjustment is required for geriatric patients (see *PHARMACOKINETICS*: *Special Populations* and PRECAUTIONS).

HOW SUPPLIED

TAMIFLU is supplied as 75-mg (75 mg free base equivalent of the phosphate salt) grey/light yellow hard gelatin capsules. "ROCHE" is printed in blue ink on the grey body and "75 mg" is printed in blue ink on the light yellow cap. Available in blister packages of 10 (NDC 0004-0800-85).

Storage: Store at 25°C (77°F); excursions permitted to 15° to 30°C (59° to 86°F). [See USP Controlled Room Temperature]

Manufactured by:
F. Hoffmann-La Roche Ltd.
Basel, Switzerland
Distributed by:
Roche Laboratories Inc.
340 Kingsland Street
Nutley, New Jersey 07110-1199
Licensor:
Gilead Sciences, Inc.
Foster City, California 94404
Issued: October 1999
Printed in USA

Patient Information About:
TAMIFLU™
(oseltamivir phosphate)
75 mg CAPSULES

This leaftlet contains important patient information about TAMIFLU (oseltamivir phosphate), and should be read completely before beginning treatment. It does not, however, take the place of discussions with your doctor or health care professional about your medical condition or your treatment. This summary does not list all benefits and risks of TAMIFLU. The medication described here can only be prescribed and dispensed by a licensed health care professional, who has information about your medical condition and more information about the drug, including how to take it, what to expect, and potential side effects. If you have any questions about TAMIFLU talk with your doctor. Only your health care professional can determine if TAMIFLU is right for you.

What is TAMIFLU?

TAMIFLU (TAM-ih-floo) is a medicine to treat flu (infection caused by influenza virus). It belongs to a group of medicines called neuraminidase inhibitors. These medications attack the influenza virus and prevent it from spreading inside your body. TAMIFLU treats the cause of flu at its source, rather than simply masking symptoms. Each TAMIFLU capsule (grey/light-yellow) contains 75 mg of active drug and should be taken by mouth.

Who should not take TAMIFLU?

You should not take TAMIFLU if you are allergic to oseltamivir phosphate or any other ingredients of TAMIFLU. Before starting treatment, make sure your doctor knows if you are taking any other medication or have any type of kidney disease.

Who should consider taking TAMIFLU?

Adult patients who have flu symptoms that appeared within the previous day or two. Typical symptoms of flu include sudden onset of fever, cough, headache, fatigue, muscular weakness, and sore throat.

What can I expect if I take TAMIFLU?

In two large clinical trials, one conducted in the USA and one conducted outside the USA, flu patients who took TAMIFLU recovered 1.3 days (30%) faster than flu patients who did not take TAMIFLU.

Can I take other medications with TAMIFLU?

TAMIFLU has been shown to have a good safety profile, with minimal risk of drug interactions. Your doctor or health care professional may recommend taking over-the-counter medications to reduce fever or other symptoms while the antiviral action of TAMIFLU takes effect. Before starting treatment make sure that your health care professional knows if you are taking any other medication.

How and when should I take TAMIFLU?

TAMIFLU should be taken twice daily (once in the morning and once in the evening) for five days. TAMIFLU can be taken with food. As with many medicines, if taken with a light snack, milk, or a meal, the potential for stomach upset may be reduced. You should complete the entire treatment of ten capsules, even if you are feeling better. Never share TAMIFLU with anyone, even if they have the same symptoms.

It is important that you begin your treatment with TAMIFLU as soon as possible from the first appearance of your flu symptoms.

What if I miss a dose?

If you forget to take your medicine at any time, take the missed dose as soon as you remember, except if it is near the next dose (within 2 hours). Then continue to take TAMIFLU at the usual times. You do not need to take a double-dose. If you have missed several doses, inform your doctor and follow the advice given to you.

What are common possible side effects of TAMIFLU treatment?

TAMIFLU is generally well tolerated. The most common side effects are nausea and vomiting. Taking TAMIFLU with food may reduce the potential of these side effects. If you notice any side effects not mentioned in this leaflet or if you have any concerns about the side effects you are experiencing, please inform your health care professional.

Should I get a flu shot?

TAMIFLU is not a substitute for a flu shot. You should continue receiving an annual flu shot according to guidelines on immunization practices that your physician can discuss with you.

What if I am pregnant or nursing?

If you are pregnant or planning to become pregnant while taking TAMIFLU, talk to your doctor before taking this

Continued on next page

Tamiflu—Cont.

medication. TAMIFLU is normally not recommended for use during pregnancy or nursing, as the effects on the unborn child or nursing infant are unknown.

How and where should I store TAMIFLU?
TAMIFLU capsules should be stored at room temperature before 77°F (25°C) and kept in a dry place. Keep this medication out of the reach of children.
Manufactured by:
F. Hoffmann-La Roche Ltd.
Basel, Switzerland
Distributed by:
Roche Laboratories Inc.
340 Kingsland Street
Nutley, New Jersey 07110-1199
Licensor:
Gilead Sciences, Inc.
Foster City, California 94404
Issued: October 1999

Shown in Product Identification Guide, page 333

TASMAR® ℞
(tolcapone)
TABLETS

The following text is complete prescribing information based on official labeling in effect June 2000.

Before prescribing TASMAR, the physician should be thoroughly familiar with the details of this prescribing information.

TASMAR SHOULD NOT BE USED BY PATIENTS UNTIL THERE HAS BEEN A COMPLETE DISCUSSION OF THE RISKS AND THE PATIENT HAS PROVIDED WRITTEN INFORMED CONSENT (SEE PATIENT CONSENT SECTION).

WARNING:

Because of the risk of potentially fatal, acute fulminant liver failure, TASMAR (tolcapone) should ordinarily be used in patients with Parkinson's disease on l-dopa/carbidopa who are experiencing symptom fluctuations and are not responding satisfactorily to or are not appropriate candidates for other adjunctive therapies (see INDICATIONS and DOSAGE AND ADMINISTRATION sections).

Because of the risk of liver injury and because TASMAR, when it is effective, provides an observable symptomatic benefit, the patient who fails to show substantial clinical benefit within 3 weeks of initiation of treatment, should be withdrawn from TASMAR.

TASMAR therapy should not be initiated if the patient exhibits clinical evidence of liver disease or two SGPT/ALT or SGOT/AST values greater than the upper limit of normal. Patients with severe dyskinesia or dystonia should be treated with caution (see PRECAUTIONS: *Rhabdomyolysis*).

Patients who develop evidence of hepatocellular injury while on TASMAR and are withdrawn from the drug for any reason may be at increased risk for liver injury if TASMAR is reintroduced. Accordingly, such patients should not ordinarily be considered for retreatment.

Cases of severe hepatocellular injury, including fulminant liver failure resulting in death, have been reported in postmarketing use. As of October 1998, 3 cases of fatal fulminant hepatic failure have been reported from approximately 60,000 patients providing about 40,000 patient years of worldwide use. This incidence may be 10- to 100-fold higher than the background incidence in the general population. Underreporting of cases may lead to significant underestimation of the increased risk associated with the use of TASMAR.

A prescriber who elects to use TASMAR in face of the increased risk of liver injury is strongly advised to monitor patients for evidence of emergent liver injury. Patients should be advised of the need for self-monitoring for both the classical signs of liver disease (eg, clay colored stools, jaundice) and the nonspecific ones (eg, fatigue, loss of appetite, lethargy).

Although a program of frequent laboratory monitoring for evidence of hepatocellular injury is deemed essential, it is not clear that baseline and periodic monitoring of liver enzymes will prevent the occurrence of fulminant liver failure. However, it is generally believed that early detection of drug-induced hepatic injury along with immediate withdrawal of the suspect drug enhances the likelihood for recovery. It is also widely held, without a robust body of evidence, that patients with preexisting hepatic disease are more vulnerable to hepatotoxins. Accordingly, the following liver monitoring program is recommended.

Before starting treatment with TASMAR, the physician should conduct appropriate tests to exclude the presence of liver disease. In patients determined to be appropriate candidates for treatment with TASMAR, serum glutamic-pyruvic transaminase (SGPT/ALT) and serum glutamic-oxaloacetic transaminase (SGOT/AST) levels should be determined at baseline and then every 2 weeks for the first year of therapy, every 4 weeks for the next 6 months, and then every 8 weeks thereafter. If the dose is increased to 200 mg tid (see DOSAGE AND ADMINISTRATION section), liver enzyme monitoring should take place before increasing the dose and then be reinitiated at the frequency above.

TASMAR should be discontinued if SGPT/ALT or SGOT/AST exceeds the upper limit of normal or if clinical signs and symptoms suggest the onset of hepatic failure (persistent nausea, fatigue, lethargy, anorexia, jaundice, dark urine, pruritus, and right upper quadrant tenderness).

DESCRIPTION

TASMAR® is available as tablets containing 100 mg or 200 mg tolcapone.

Tolcapone, an inhibitor of catechol-*O*-methyltransferase (COMT), is used in the treatment of Parkinson's disease as an adjunct to levodopa/carbidopa therapy. It is a yellow, odorless, non-hygroscopic, crystalline compound with a relative molecular mass of 273.25. The chemical name of tolcapone is 3,4-dihydroxy-4'-methyl-5-nitrobenzophenone. Its empirical formula is $C_{14}H_{11}NO_5$.

Inactive ingredients: Core: lactose monohydrate, microcrystalline cellulose, dibasic calcium phosphate anhydrous, povidone K-30, sodium starch glycolate, talc and magnesium stearate. Film coating: hydroxypropyl methyl-cellulose, titanium dioxide, talc, ethylcellulose, triacetin and sodium lauryl sulfate, with the following dye systems: 100 mg—yellow and red iron oxide; 200 mg—red iron oxide.

CLINICAL PHARMACOLOGY

Mechanism of Action: Tolcapone is a selective and reversible inhibitor of catechol-*O*-methyltransferase (COMT).

In mammals, COMT is distributed throughout various organs. The highest activities are in the liver and kidney. COMT also occurs in the heart, lung, smooth and skeletal muscles, intestinal tract, reproductive organs, various glands, adipose tissue, skin, blood cells and neuronal tissues, especially in glial cells. COMT catalyzes the transfer of the methyl group of S-adenosyl-L-methionine to the phenolic group of substrates that contain a catechol structure. Physiological substrates of COMT include dopa, catecholamines (dopamine, norepinephrine, epinephrine) and their hydroxylated metabolites. The function of COMT is the elimination of biologically active catechols and some other hydroxylated metabolites. In the presence of a decarboxylase inhibitor, COMT becomes the major metabolizing enzyme for levodopa catalyzing the metabolism to 3-methoxy-4-hydroxy-L-phenylalanine (3-OMD) in the brain and periphery.

The precise mechanism of action of tolcapone is unknown, but it is believed to be related to its ability to inhibit COMT and alter the plasma pharmacokinetics of levodopa. When tolcapone is given in conjunction with levodopa and an aromatic amino acid decarboxylase inhibitor, such as carbidopa, plasma levels of levodopa are more sustained than after administration of levodopa and an aromatic amino acid decarboxylase inhibitor alone. It is believed that these sustained plasma levels of levodopa result in more constant dopaminergic stimulation in the brain, leading to greater effects on the signs and symptoms of Parkinson's disease in patients as well as increased levodopa adverse effects, sometimes requiring a decrease in the dose of levodopa. Tolcapone enters the CNS to a minimal extent, but has been shown to inhibit central COMT activity in animals.

Pharmacodynamics: *COMT Activity in Erythrocytes:* Studies in healthy volunteers have shown that tolcapone reversibly inhibits human erythrocyte catechol-*O*-methyltransferase (COMT) activity after oral administration. The inhibition is closely related to plasma tolcapone concentrations. With a 200-mg single dose of tolcapone, maximum inhibition of erythrocyte COMT activity is on average greater than 80%. During multiple dosing with tolcapone (200 mg tid), erythrocyte COMT inhibition at trough tolcapone blood concentrations is 30% to 45%.

Effect on the Pharmacokinetics of Levodopa and its Metabolites: When tolcapone is administered together with levodopa/carbidopa, it increases the relative bioavailability (AUC) of levodopa by approximately twofold. This is due to a decrease in levodopa clearance resulting in a prolongation of the terminal elimination half-life of levodopa (from approximately 2 hours to 3.5 hours). In general, the average peak levodopa plasma concentration (C_{max}) and the time of its occurrence (T_{max}) are unaffected. The onset of effect occurs after the first administration and is maintained during long-term treatment. Studies in healthy volunteers and Parkinson's disease patients have confirmed that the maximal effect occurs with 100 mg to 200 mg tolcapone. Plasma levels of 3-OMD are markedly and dose-dependently decreased by tolcapone when given with levodopa/carbidopa. Population pharmacokinetic analyses in patients with Parkinson's disease have shown the same effects of tolcapone on levodopa plasma concentrations that occur in healthy volunteers.

Pharmacokinetics of Tolcapone: Tolcapone pharmacokinetics are linear over the dose range of 50 mg to 400 mg, independent of levodopa/carbidopa coadministration. The elimination half-life of tolcapone is 2 to 3 hours and there is no significant accumulation. With tid dosing of 100 mg or 200 mg, C_{max} is approximately 3 µg/mL and 6 µg/mL, respectively.

Absorption: Tolcapone is rapidly absorbed, with a T_{max} of approximately 2 hours. The absolute bioavailability following oral administration is about 65%. Food given within 1 hour before and 2 hours after dosing of tolcapone decreases the relative bioavailability by 10% to 20% (see DOSAGE AND ADMINISTRATION).

Distribution: The steady-state volume of distribution of tolcapone is small (9 L). Tolcapone does not distribute widely into tissues due to its high plasma protein binding. The plasma protein binding of tolcapone is >99.9% over the concentration range of 0.32 to 210 µg/mL. In vitro experiments have shown that tolcapone binds mainly to serum albumin.

Metabolism and Elimination: Tolcapone is almost completely metabolized prior to excretion, with only a very small amount (0.5% of dose) found unchanged in urine. The main metabolic pathway of tolcapone is glucuronidation; the glucuronide conjugate is inactive. In addition, the compound is methylated by COMT to 3-*O*-methyl-tolcapone. Tolcapone is metabolized to a primary alcohol (hydroxylation of the methyl group), which is subsequently oxidized to the carboxylic acid. In vitro experiments suggest that the oxidation may be catalyzed by cytochrome P450 3A4 and P450 2A6. The reduction to an amine and subsequent *N*-acetylation occur to a minor extent. After oral administration of a ^{14}C-labeled dose of tolcapone, 60% of labeled material is excreted in urine and 40% in feces.

Tolcapone is a low-extraction-ratio drug (extraction ratio = 0.15) with a moderate systemic clearance of about 7 L/h.

Special Populations: Tolcapone pharmacokinetics are independent of sex, age, body weight, and race (Japanese, Black and Caucasian). Polymorphic metabolism is unlikely based on the metabolic pathways involved.

Hepatic Impairment: A study in patients with hepatic impairment has shown that moderate non-cirrhotic liver disease had no impact on the pharmacokinetics of tolcapone. In patients with moderate cirrhotic liver disease (Child-Pugh Class B), however, clearance and volume of distribution of unbound tolcapone was reduced by almost 50%. This reduction may increase the average concentration of unbound drug by twofold (see DOSAGE AND ADMINISTRATION). TASMAR therapy should not be initiated if the patient exhibits clinical evidence of active liver disease or two SGPT/ALT or SGOT/AST values greater than the upper limit of normal (see BOXED WARNING).

Renal Impairment: The pharmacokinetics of tolcapone have not been investigated in a specific renal impairment study. However, the relationship of renal function and tolcapone pharmacokinetics has been investigated using population pharmacokinetics during clinical trials. The data of more than 400 patients have confirmed that over a wide range of creatinine clearance values (30 mL/min to 130 mL/min) the pharmacokinetics of tolcapone are unaffected by renal function. This could be explained by the fact that only a negligible amount of unchanged tolcapone (0.5%) is excreted in the urine. The glucuronide conjugate of tolcapone is mainly excreted in the urine but is also excreted in the bile. Accumulation of this stable and inactive metabolite should not present a risk in renally impaired patients with creatinine clearance above 25 mL/min (see DOSAGE AND ADMINISTRATION). Given the very high protein binding of tolcapone, no significant removal of the drug by hemodialysis would be expected.

Drug Interactions: See PRECAUTIONS: *Drug Interactions.*

Clinical Studies: The effectiveness of TASMAR as an adjunct to levodopa in the treatment of Parkinson's disease was established in three multicenter randomized controlled trials of 13 to 26 weeks' duration, supported by four 6-week trials whose results were consistent with those of the longer trials. In two of the longer trials, tolcapone was evaluated in patients whose Parkinson's disease was characterized by deterioration in their response to levodopa at the end of a dosing interval (so-called fluctuating patients with wearing-off phenomena). In the remaining trial, tolcapone was evaluated in patients whose response to levodopa was relatively stable (so-called non-fluctuators).

Fluctuating Patients: In two 3-month trials, patients with documented episodes of wearing-off phenomena, despite optimum levodopa therapy, were randomized to receive placebo, tolcapone 100 mg tid or 200 mg tid. The formal double-blind portion of the trial was 3 months long, and the primary outcome was a comparison between treatments in the change from baseline in the amount of time spent "On" (a period of relatively good functioning) and "Off" (a period of relatively poor functioning). Patients recorded periodically, throughout the duration of the trial, the time spent in each of these states.

In addition to the primary outcome, patients were also assessed using sub-parts of the Unified Parkinson's Disease Rating Scale (UPDRS), a frequently used multi-item rating scale intended to evaluate mentation (Part I), activities of daily living (Part II), motor function (Part III), complications of therapy (Part IV), and disease staging (Parts V and VI); an Investigator's Global Assessment of Change (IGA), a subjective scale designed to assess global functioning in 5 areas of Parkinson's disease; the Sickness Impact Profile (SIP), a multi-item scale in 12 domains designed to assess the patient's functioning in multiple areas; and the change in daily levodopa/carbidopa dose.

In one of the studies, 202 patients were randomized in 11 centers in the United States and Canada. In this trial, all patients were receiving concomitant levodopa and carbidopa. In the second trial, 177 patients were randomized in 24 centers in Europe. In this trial, all patients were receiving concomitant levodopa and benserazide.

The following tables display the results of these 2 trials:

[See table 1 at bottom of next page]

[See table 2 at bottom of next page]

Effects on "Off" time and levodopa dose did not differ by age or sex.

Non-fluctuating Patients: In this study, 298 patients with idiopathic Parkinson's disease on stable doses of levodopa/carbidopa who were not experiencing wearing-off phenomena were randomized to placebo, tolcapone 100 mg tid, or tolcapone 200 mg tid for 6 months at 20 centers in the United States and Canada. The primary measure of effectiveness was the Activities of Daily Living portion (Subscale II) of the UPDRS. In addition, the change in daily levodopa dose, other subscales of the UPDRS, and the SIP were assessed as secondary measures. The results are displayed in the following table:

[See table 3 at top of next page]

Effects on Activities of Daily Living did not differ by age or sex.

Table 1.
US/Canadian Fluctuator Study

Primary Measure

	Baseline (hrs)	Change from Baseline at Month 3 (hrs)	p-value*
*Hours of Wake Time "Off"***			
Placebo	6.2	−1.2	—
100 mg tid	6.4	−2.0	0.169
200 mg tid	5.9	−3.0	<0.001
*Hours of Wake Time "On"***			
Placebo	8.7	1.4	—
100 mg tid	8.1	2.0	0.267
200 mg tid	9.1	2.9	0.008

Secondary Measures

	Baseline	Change from Baseline at Month 3	p-value*
Levodopa Total Daily Dose (mg)			
Placebo	948	16	
100 mg tid	788	−166	<0.001
200 mg tid	865	−207	<0.001
Global (overall) % Improved			
Placebo	—	42	—
100 mg tid	—	71	<0.001
200 mg tid	—	91	<0.001
UPDRS Motor			
Placebo	19.5	−0.4	—
100 mg tid	17.6	−1.9	0.217
200 mg tid	20.6	−2.0	0.210
UPDRS ADL			
Placebo	7.5	−0.3	—
100 mg tid	7.7	−0.8	0.487
200 mg tid	8.3	0.2	0.412
SIP (total)			
Placebo	14.7	−2.2	—
100 mg tid	14.9	−0.4	0.210
200 mg tid	17.6	−0.3	0.216

*Compared to placebo.
**Hours "Off" or "On" are based on the percent of waking day "Off" or "On", assuming a 16-hour waking day.

Table 2.
European Fluctuator Study

Primary Measure

	Baseline (hrs)	Change from Baseline at Month 3 (hrs)	p-value*
*Hours of Wake Time "Off"***			
Placebo	6.1	−0.7	—
100 mg tid	6.5	−2.0	0.008
200 mg tid	6.0	−1.6	0.081
*Hours of Wake Time "On"***			
Placebo	8.5	−0.1	—
100 mg tid	8.1	1.7	0.003
200 mg tid	8.4	1.7	0.003

Secondary Measures

	Baseline	Change from Baseline at Month 3	p-value*
Levodopa Total Daily Dose (mg)			
Placebo	660	−29	—
100 mg tid	667	−109	0.025
200 mg tid	675	−122	0.010
Global (overall) % Improved			
Placebo	—	37	—
100 mg tid	—	70	0.003
200 mg tid	—	78	<0.001
UPDRS Motor			
Placebo	24.0	−2.1	—
100 mg tid	22.4	−4.2	0.163
200 mg tid	22.4	−6.5	0.004
UPDRS ADL			
Placebo	7.9	−0.5	—
100 mg tid	7.5	−0.9	0.408
200 mg tid	7.7	−1.3	0.097
SIP (total)			
Placebo	21.6	−0.9	—
100 mg tid	16.6	−1.9	0.419
200 mg tid	18.4	−4.2	0.011

*Compared to placebo.
**Hours "Off" or "On" are based on the percent of waking day "Off" or "On", assuming a 16-hour waking day.

INDICATIONS

TASMAR is indicated as an adjunct to levodopa and carbidopa for the treatment of the signs and symptoms of idiopathic Parkinson's disease. Because of the risk of potentially fatal, acute fulminant liver failure, TASMAR (tolcapone) should ordinarily be used in patients with Parkinson's disease on l-dopa/carbidopa who are experiencing symptom fluctuations and are not responding satisfactorily to or are not appropriate candidates for other adjunctive therapies. Because of the risk of liver injury and because TASMAR, when it is effective, provides an observable symptomatic benefit, the patient who fails to show substantial clinical benefit within 3 weeks of initiation of treatment, should be withdrawn from TASMAR.

The effectiveness of TASMAR was demonstrated in randomized controlled trials in patients receiving concomitant levodopa therapy with carbidopa or another aromatic amino acid decarboxylase inhibitor who experienced end of dose wearing-off phenomena as well as in patients who did not experience such phenomena (see CLINICAL PHARMACOLOGY: *Clinical Studies*).

CONTRAINDICATIONS

TASMAR tablets are contraindicated in patients with liver disease, in patients who were withdrawn from TASMAR because of evidence of TASMAR-induced hepatocellular injury or who have demonstrated hypersensitivity to the drug or its ingredients.

TASMAR is also contraindicated in patients with a history of non-traumatic rhabdomyolysis or hyperpyrexia and confusion possibly related to medication (see PRECAUTIONS: *Events Reported With Dopaminergic Therapy*).

WARNINGS

(SEE BOXED WARNING) Because of the risk of potentially fatal, acute fulminant liver failure, TASMAR (tolcapone) should ordinarily be used in patients with Parkinson's disease on l-dopa/carbidopa who are experiencing symptom fluctuations and are not responding satisfactorily to or are not appropriate candidates for other adjunctive therapies (see INDICATIONS and DOSAGE AND ADMINISTRATION sections).

Because of the risk of liver injury and because TASMAR, when it is effective, provides an observable symptomatic benefit, the patient who fails to show substantial clinical benefit within 3 weeks of initiation of treatment, should be withdrawn from TASMAR.

TASMAR therapy should not be initiated if the patient exhibits clinical evidence of liver disease or two SGPT/ALT or SGOT/AST values greater than the upper limit of normal. Patients with severe dyskinesia or dystonia should be treated with caution (see PRECAUTIONS: *Rhabdomyolysis*).

Patients who develop evidence of hepatocellular injury while on TASMAR and are withdrawn from the drug for any reason may be at increased risk for liver injury if TASMAR is reintroduced. Accordingly, such patients should not ordinarily be considered for retreatment.

In controlled Phase 3 trials, increases to more than 3 times the upper limit of normal in ALT or AST occurred in approximately 1% of patients at 100 mg tid and 3% of patients at 200 mg tid. Females were more likely than males to have an increase in liver enzymes (approximately 5% vs 2%). Approximately one third of patients with elevated enzymes had diarrhea. Increases to more than 8 times the upper limit of normal in liver enzymes occurred in 0.3% at 100 mg tid and 0.7% at 200 mg tid. Elevated enzymes led to discontinuation in 0.3% and 1.7% of patients treated with 100 mg tid and 200 mg tid, respectively. Elevations usually occurred within 6 weeks to 6 months of starting treatment. In about half the cases with elevated liver enzymes, enzyme levels returned to baseline values within 1 to 3 months while patients continued TASMAR treatment. When treatment was discontinued, enzymes generally declined within 2 to 3 weeks but in some cases took as long as 1 to 2 months to return to normal.

Monoamine oxidase (MAO) and COMT are the two major enzyme systems involved in the metabolism of catecholamines. It is theoretically possible, therefore, that the combination of TASMAR and a non-selective MAO inhibitor (eg, phenelzine and tranylcypromine) would result in inhibition of the majority of the pathways responsible for normal catecholamine metabolism. For this reason, patients should ordinarily not be treated concomitantly with TASMAR and a non-selective MAO inhibitor.

Tolcapone can be taken concomitantly with a selective MAO-B inhibitor (eg, selegiline).

PRECAUTIONS

Hypotension/Syncope: Dopaminergic therapy in Parkinson's disease patients has been associated with orthostatic hypotension. Tolcapone enhances levodopa bioavailability and, therefore, may increase the occurrence of orthostatic hypotension. In TASMAR clinical trials, orthostatic hypotension was documented at least once in 8%, 14% and 13% of the patients treated with placebo, 100 mg and 200 mg TASMAR tid, respectively. A total of 2%, 5% and 4% of the patients treated with placebo, 100 mg and 200 mg TASMAR tid, respectively, reported orthostatic symptoms at some time during their treatment and also had at least one episode of orthostatic hypotension documented (however, the episode of orthostatic symptoms itself was invariably not accompanied by vital sign measurements). Patients with

Continued on next page

Tasmar—Cont.

orthostasis at baseline were more likely than patients without symptoms to have orthostatic hypotension during the study, irrespective of treatment group. In addition, the effect was greater in tolcapone-treated patients than in placebo-treated patients. Baseline treatment with dopamine agonists or selegiline did not appear to increase the likelihood of experiencing orthostatic hypotension when treated with TASMAR. Approximately 0.7% of the patients treated with TASMAR (5% of patients who were documented to have had at least one episode of orthostatic hypotension) eventually withdrew from treatment due to adverse events presumably related to hypotension.

In controlled Phase 3 trials, approximately 5%, 4% and 3% of tolcapone 200 mg tid, 100 mg tid and placebo patients, respectively, reported at least one episode of syncope. Reports of syncope were generally more frequent in patients in all three treatment groups who had an episode of documented hypotension (although the episodes of syncope, obtained by history, were themselves not documented with vital sign measurement) compared to patients who did not have any episodes of documented hypotension.

Diarrhea: In clinical trials, diarrhea developed in approximately 8%, 16% and 18% of patients treated with placebo, 100 mg and 200 mg TASMAR tid, respectively. While diarrhea was generally regarded as mild to moderate in severity, approximately 3% to 4% of patients on tolcapone had diarrhea which was regarded as severe. Diarrhea was the adverse event which most commonly led to discontinuation, with approximately 1%, 5% and 6% of patients treated with placebo, 100 mg and 200 mg TASMAR tid, respectively, withdrawing from the trials prematurely. Discontinuing TASMAR for diarrhea was related to the severity of the symptom. Diarrhea resulted in withdrawal in approximately 8%, 40% and 70% of patients with mild, moderate and severe diarrhea, respectively. Although diarrhea generally resolved after discontinuation of TASMAR, it led to hospitalization in 0.3%, 0.7% and 1.7% of patients in the placebo, 100 mg and 200 mg TASMAR tid groups.

Typically, diarrhea presents 6 to 12 weeks after tolcapone is started, but it may appear as early as 2 weeks and as late as many months after the initiation of treatment. Clinical trial data suggested that diarrhea associated with tolcapone use may sometimes be associated with anorexia (decreased appetite).

No consistent description of tolcapone-induced diarrhea has been derived from clinical trial data, and the mechanism of action is currently unknown.

It is recommended that all cases of persistent diarrhea should be followed up with an appropriate work-up (including occult blood samples).

Hallucinations: In clinical trials, hallucinations developed in approximately 5%, 8% and 10% of patients treated with placebo, 100 mg and 200 mg TASMAR tid, respectively. Hallucinations led to drug discontinuation and premature withdrawal from clinical trials in 0.3%, 1.4% and 1.0% of patients treated with placebo, 100 mg and 200 mg TASMAR tid, respectively. Hallucinations led to hospitalization in 0.0%, 1.7% and 0.0% of patients in the placebo, 100 mg and 200 mg TASMAR tid groups, respectively.

In general, hallucinations present shortly after the initiation of therapy with tolcapone (typically within the first 2 weeks). Clinical trial data suggest that hallucinations associated with tolcapone use may be responsive to levodopa dose reduction. Patients whose hallucinations resolved had a mean levodopa dose reduction of 175 mg to 200 mg (20% to 25%) after the onset of the hallucinations. Hallucinations were commonly accompanied by confusion and to a lesser extent sleep disorder (insomnia) and excessive dreaming.

Dyskinesia: TASMAR may potentiate the dopaminergic side effects of levodopa and may cause and/or exacerbate preexisting dyskinesia. Although decreasing the dose of levodopa may ameliorate this side effect, many patients in controlled trials continued to experience frequent dyskinesias despite a reduction in their dose of levodopa. The rates of withdrawal for dyskinesia were 0.0%, 0.3% and 1.0% for placebo, 100 mg and 200 mg TASMAR tid, respectively.

Rhabdomyolysis: Cases of severe rhadbomyolysis, with one case of multiorgan system failure rapidly progressing to death, have been reported. The complicated nature of these cases makes it impossible to determine what role, if any, TASMAR played in their pathogenesis. Severe prolonged motor activity including dyskinesia may account for rhabdomyolysis. Some cases, however, included fever, alteration of consciousness and muscular rigidity. It is possible, therefore, that the rhabdomyolysis may be a result of the syndrome described in *Hyperpyrexia and Confusion* (see PRECAUTIONS: *Events Reported With Dopaminergic Therapy*).

Renal Impairment: No dosage adjustment is needed in patients with mild to moderate renal impairment, however, patients with severe renal impairment should be treated with caution (see CLINICAL PHARMACOLOGY: *Pharmacokinetics of Tolcapone* and DOSAGE AND ADMINISTRATION).

Renal Toxicity: When rats were dosed daily for 1 or 2 years (exposures 6 times the human exposure or greater) there was a high incidence of proximal tubule cell damage consisting of degeneration, single cell necrosis, hyperplasia, karyocytomegaly and atypical nuclei. These effects were not associated with changes in clinical chemistry parameters, and there is no established method for monitoring for the possible occurrence of these lesions in humans. Although it has

Table 3.
US/Canadian Non-fluctuator Study

	Baseline	Change from Baseline at Month 6	p-value*
Primary Measure			
UPDRS ADL			
Placebo	8.5	0.1	—
100 mg tid	7.5	-1.4	<0.001
200 mg tid	7.9	-1.6	<0.001
Secondary Measures			
Levodopa Total Daily Dose (mg)			
Placebo	364	47	—
100 mg tid	370	-21	<0.001
200 mg tid	381	-32	<0.001
UPDRS Motor			
Placebo	19.7	0.1	—
100 mg tid	17.3	-2.0	0.018
200 mg tid	16.0	-2.3	0.008
SIP (total)			
Placebo	6.9	0.4	—
100 mg tid	7.3	-0.9	0.044
200 mg tid	7.3	-0.7	0.078
Percent of Patients who Developed Fluctuations			
Placebo	—	26	—
100 mg tid	—	19	0.297
200 mg tid	—	14	0.047

* Compared to placebo.

been speculated that these toxicities may occur as the result of a species-specific mechanism, experiments which would confirm that theory have not been conducted.

Hepatic Impairment: Because of the risk of liver injury, TASMAR therapy should not be initiated in any patient with liver disease. For similar reasons, treatment should not be initiated in patients who have two SGPT/ALT or SGOT/AST values greater than the upper limit of normal (see BOXED WARNING) or any other evidence of hepatocellular dysfunction.

Hematuria: The rates of hematuria in placebo-controlled trials were approximately 2%, 4% and 5% in placebo, 100 mg and 200 mg TASMAR tid, respectively. The etiology of the increase with TASMAR has not always been explained (for example, by urinary tract infection or coumadin therapy). In placebo-controlled trials in the United States (N=593) rates of microscopically confirmed hematuria were approximately 3%, 2% and 2% in placebo, 100 mg and 200 mg TASMAR tid, respectively.

Events Reported With Dopaminergic Therapy: The events listed below are known to be associated with the use of drugs that increase dopaminergic activity, although they are most often associated with the use of direct dopamine agonists. While cases of Hyperpyrexia and Confusion have been reported in association with tolcapone withdrawal (see paragraph below), the expected incidence of fibrotic complications is so low that even if tolcapone caused these complications at rates similar to those attributable to other dopaminergic therapies, it is unlikely that even a single example would have been detected in a cohort of the size exposed to tolcapone.

Hyperpyrexia and Confusion: In clinical trials, four cases of a symptom complex resembling the neuroleptic malignant syndrome (characterized by elevated temperature, muscular rigidity, and altered consciousness), similar to that reported in association with the rapid dose reduction or withdrawal of other dopaminergic drugs, have been reported in association with the abrupt withdrawal or lowering of the dose of tolcapone. In 3 of these cases, CPK was elevated as well. One patient died, and the other 3 patients recovered over periods of approximately 2, 4 and 6 weeks. Rare cases of this symptom complex have been reported during marketed use. These cases are of a complicated nature including the concomitant administration of several medications affecting brain monoaminergic (ie, MAO-I, tricyclic and selective serotonin reuptake inhibitors) and anticholinergic systems. It is difficult, therefore, to determine what role, if any, TASMAR played in the pathogenesis. It may, therefore, be prudent to be particularly cautious if several concomitant medications of these types are used.

Fibrotic Complications: Cases of retroperitoneal fibrosis, pulmonary infiltrates, pleural effusion, and pleural thickening have been reported in some patients treated with ergot derived dopaminergic agents. While these complications may resolve when the drug is discontinued, complete resolution does not always occur. Although these adverse events are believed to be related to the ergoline structure of these compounds, whether other, nonergot derived drugs (eg, tolcapone) that increase dopaminergic activity can cause them is unknown.

Three cases of pleural effusion, one with pulmonary fibrosis, occurred during clinical trials. These patients were also on concomitant dopamine agonists (pergolide or bromocriptine) and had a prior history of cardiac disease or pulmonary pathology (nonmalignant lung lesion).

Information for Patients: Patients should be instructed to take TASMAR only as prescribed.

TASMAR should not be used by patients until there has been a complete discussion of the risks and the patient has provided written informed consent (see PATIENT CONSENT section).

Patients should be informed of the clinical signs and symptoms that suggest the onset of hepatic injury (persistent nausea, fatigue, lethargy, anorexia, jaundice, dark urine, pruritus, and right upper quadrant tenderness) (**see WARNINGS**). If symptoms of hepatic failure occur, patients should be advised to contact their physician immediately.

Patients should be informed that hallucinations can occur.

Patients should be informed of the need to have regular blood tests to monitor liver enzymes.

Patients should be advised that they may develop postural (orthostatic) hypotension with or without symptoms such as dizziness, nausea, syncope, and sometimes sweating. Hypotension may occur more frequently during initial therapy. Accordingly, patients should be cautioned against rising rapidly after sitting or lying down, especially if they have been doing so for prolonged periods, and especially at the initiation of treatment with TASMAR.

Patients should be advised that they should neither drive a car nor operate other complex machinery until they have gained sufficient experience on TASMAR to gauge whether or not it affects their mental and/or motor performance adversely. Because of the possible additive sedative effects, caution should be used when patients are taking other CNS depressants in combination with TASMAR.

Patients should be informed that nausea may occur, especially at the initiation of treatment with TASMAR.

Patients should be advised of the possibility of an increase in dyskinesia and/or dystonia.

Although TASMAR has not been shown to be teratogenic in animals, it is always given in conjunction with levodopa/carbidopa, which is known to cause visceral and skeletal malformations in the rabbit. Accordingly, patients should be advised to notify their physicians if they become pregnant or intend to become pregnant during therapy (see PRECAUTIONS: *Pregnancy*).

Tolcapone is excreted into maternal milk in rats. Because of the possibility that tolcapone may be excreted into human maternal milk, patients should be advised to notify their physicians if they intend to breastfeed or are breastfeeding an infant.

Laboratory Tests: **Although a program of frequent laboratory monitoring for evidence of hepatocellular injury is deemed essential, it is not clear that baseline and periodic monitoring of liver enzymes will prevent the occurrence of fulminant liver failure. However, it is generally believed that early detection of drug-induced hepatic injury along with immediate withdrawal of the suspect drug enhances the likelihood for recovery. It is also widely held, without a robust body of evidence, that patients with preexisting hepatic disease are more vulnerable to hepatotoxins. Accordingly, the following liver monitoring program is recommended.**

Before starting treatment with TASMAR, the physician should conduct appropriate tests to exclude the presence of liver disease. In patients determined to be appropriate candidates for treatment with TASMAR, serum glutamic-pyruvic transaminase (SGPT/ALT) and serum glutamic-oxaloacetic transaminase (SGOT/AST) levels should be determined at baseline and then every 2 weeks for the first year of therapy, every 4 weeks for the next 6 months and then every 8 weeks thereafter.

If the dose is increased to 200 mg tid (see DOSAGE AND ADMINISTRATION section), liver enzyme monitoring should take place before increasing the dose and then be reinitiated at the frequency above.

TASMAR should be discontinued if SGPT/ALT or SGOT/AST exceeds the upper limit of normal or if clinical signs and symptoms suggest the onset of hepatic failure (persistent nausea, fatigue, lethargy, anorexia, jaundice, dark urine, pruritus, and right upper quadrant tenderness).

Special Populations: TASMAR therapy should not be initiated if the patient exhibits clinical evidence of active liver disease or two SGPT/ALT or SGOT/AST values greater than the upper limit of normal. Patients with severe dyskinesia or dystonia should be treated with caution (see PRECAUTIONS: *Rhabdomyolysis*). Patients with severe renal impairment should be treated with caution (see INDICATIONS, DOSAGE AND ADMINISTRATION, BOXED WARNING and WARNINGS).

Drug Interactions: *Protein Binding:* Although tolcapone is highly protein bound, in vitro studies have shown that tolcapone at a concentration of 50 µg/mL did not displace other highly protein-bound drugs from their binding sites at therapeutic concentrations. The experiments included warfarin (0.5 to 7.2 µg/mL), phenytoin (4.0 to 38.7 µg/mL), tolbutamide (24.5 to 96.1 µg/mL) and digitoxin (9.0 to 27.0 µg/mL).

Drugs Metabolized by Catechol-O-Methyltransferase (COMT): Tolcapone may influence the pharmacokinetics of drugs metabolized by COMT. However, no effects were seen on the pharmacokinetics of the COMT substrate carbidopa. The effect of tolcapone on the pharmacokinetics of other drugs of this class such as α-methyldopa, dobutamine, apomorphine, and isoproterenol has not been evaluated. A dose reduction of such compounds should be considered when they are coadministered with tolcapone.

Effect of Tolcapone on the Metabolism of Other Drugs: In vitro experiments have been performed to assess the potential of tolcapone to interact with isoenzymes of cytochrome P450 (CYP). No relevant interactions with substrates for CYP 2A6 (coumadin), CYP 1A2 (caffeine), CYP 3A4 (midazolam, terfenadine, cyclosporine), CYP 2C19 (S-mephenytoin) and CYP 2D6 (desipramine) were observed in vitro. The absence of an interaction with desipramine, a drug metabolized by cytochrome P450 2D6, was also confirmed in an in vivo study where tolcapone did not change the pharmacokinetics of desipramine.

Due to its affinity to cytochrome P450 2C9 in vitro, tolcapone may interfere with drugs, whose clearance is dependent on this metabolic pathway, such as tolbutamide and warfarin. However, in an in vivo interaction study, tolcapone did not change the pharmacokinetics of tolbutamide. Therefore, clinically relevant interactions involving cytochrome P450 2C9 appear unlikely. Similarly, tolcapone did not affect the pharmacokinetics of desipramine, a drug metabolized by cytochrome P450 2D6, indicating that interactions with drugs metabolized by that enzyme are unlikely. Since clinical information is limited regarding the combination of warfarin and tolcapone, coagulation parameters should be monitored when these two drugs are coadministered.

Drugs That Increase Catecholamines: Tolcapone did not influence the effect of ephedrine, an indirect sympathomimetic, on hemodynamic parameters or plasma catecholamine levels, either at rest or during exercise. Since tolcapone did not alter the tolerability of ephedrine, these drugs can be coadministered.

When TASMAR was given together with levodopa/carbidopa and desipramine, there was no significant change in blood pressure, pulse rate and plasma concentrations of desipramine. Overall, the frequency of adverse events increased slightly. These adverse events were predictable based on the known adverse reactions to each of the three drugs individually. Therefore, caution should be exercised when desipramine is administered to Parkinson's disease patients being treated with TASMAR and levodopa/carbidopa.

In clinical trials, patients receiving TASMAR/levodopa preparations reported a similar adverse event profile independent of whether or not they were also concomitantly administered selegiline (a selective MAO-B inhibitor).

Carcinogenesis, Mutagenesis and Impairment of Fertility:

Carcinogenesis: Carcinogenicity studies in which tolcapone was administered in the diet were conducted in mice and rats. Mice were treated for 80 (female) or 95 (male) weeks with doses of 100, 300 and 800 mg/kg/day, equivalent to 0.8, 1.6 and 4 times human exposure (AUC = 80 µg·hr/mL) at the recommended daily clinical dose of 600 mg.

Rats were treated for 104 weeks with doses of 50, 250 and 450 mg/kg/day. Tolcapone exposures were 1, 6.3 and 13 times the human exposure in male rats and 1.7, 11.8 and 26.4 times the human exposure in female rats. There was an increased incidence of uterine adenocarcinomas in female rats at exposure equivalent to 26.4 times the human exposure. There was evidence of renal tubular injury and renal tubular tumor formation in rats. A low incidence of renal tubular cell adenomas occurred in middle- and high-dose female rats; tubular cell carcinomas occurred in middle- and high-dose male and high-dose female rats, with a statistically significant increase in high-dose males. Exposures were equivalent to 6.3 (males) or 11.8 (females) times the human exposure or greater; no renal tumors were observed at exposures of 1 (males) or 1.7 (females) times the human exposure. Minimal-to-marked damage to the renal tubules, consisting of proximal tubule cell degeneration, single cell necrosis, hyperplasia and karyocytomegaly, occurred at the doses associated with renal tumors. Renal tubule damage, characterized by proximal tubule cell degeneration and the presence of atypical nuclei, as well as one adenocarcinoma in a high-dose male, were observed in a 1-year study in rats receiving doses of tolcapone of 150 and 450 mg/kg/day. These histopathological changes suggest the possibility that renal tumor formation might be secondary to chronic cell damage and sustained repair, but this relationship has not been established, and the relevance of these findings to humans is not known. There was no evidence of carcinogenic effects in the long-term mouse study. The carcinogenic potential of tolcapone in combination with levodopa/carbidopa has not been examined.

Mutagenesis: Tolcapone was clastogenic in the in vitro mouse lymphoma/thymidine kinase assay in the presence of metabolic activation. Tolcapone was not mutagenic in the Ames test, the in vitro V79/HPRT gene mutation assay, or the unscheduled DNA synthesis assay. It was not clastogenic in an in vitro chromosomal aberration assay in cultured human lymphocytes, or in an in vivo micronucleus assay in mice.

Impairment of Fertility: Tolcapone did not affect fertility and general reproductive performance in rats at doses up to 300 mg/kg/day (5.7 times the human dose on a mg/m^2 basis).

Pregnancy: Pregnancy Category C. Tolcapone, when administered alone during organogenesis, was not teratogenic at doses of up to 300 mg/kg/day in rats or up to 400 mg/kg/day in rabbits (5.7 times and 15 times the recommended daily clinical dose of 600 mg, on a mg/m^2 basis, respectively). In rabbits, however, an increased rate of abortion occurred at a dose of 100 mg/kg/day (3.7 times the daily clinical dose on a mg/m^2 basis) or greater. Evidence of maternal toxicity (decreased weight gain, death) was observed at 300 mg/kg in rats and 400 mg/kg in rabbits. When tolcapone was administered to female rats during the last part of gestation and throughout lactation, decreased litter size and impaired growth and learning performance in female pups were observed at a dose of 250/150 mg/kg/day (dose reduced from 250 to 150 mg/kg/day during late gestation due to high rate of maternal mortality; equivalent to 4.8/2.9 times the clinical dose on a mg/m^2 basis).

Tolcapone is always given concomitantly with levodopa/carbidopa, which is known to cause visceral and skeletal malformations in rabbits. The combination of tolcapone (100 mg/kg/day) with levodopa/carbidopa (80/20 mg/kg/day) produced an increased incidence of fetal malformations (primarily external and skeletal digit defects) compared to levodopa/carbidopa alone when pregnant rabbits were treated throughout organogenesis. Plasma exposures to tolcapone (based on AUC) were 0.5 times the expected human exposure, and plasma exposures to levodopa were 6 times higher than those in humans under therapeutic conditions. In a combination embryo-fetal development study in rats, fetal body weights were reduced by the combination of tolcapone (10, 30 and 50 mg/kg/day) and levodopa/carbidopa (120/30 mg/kg/day) and by levodopa/carbidopa alone. Tolcapone exposures were 0.5 times expected human exposure or greater; levodopa exposures were 21 times the expected human exposure or greater. The high dose of 50 mg/kg/day of tolcapone given alone was not associated with reduced fetal body weight (plasma exposures of 1.4 times the expected human exposure).

There is no experience from clinical studies regarding the use of TASMAR in pregnant women. Therefore, TASMAR should be used during pregnancy only if the potential benefit justifies the potential risk to the fetus.

Nursing Women: In animal studies, tolcapone was excreted into maternal rat milk.

It is not known whether tolcapone is excreted in human milk. Because many drugs are excreted in human milk, caution should be exercised when tolcapone is administered to a nursing woman.

Pediatric Use: There is no identified potential use of tolcapone in pediatric patients.

ADVERSE REACTIONS

Cases of severe hepatocellular injury, including fulminant liver failure resulting in death, have been reported in postmarketing use. As of October 1998, 3 cases of fatal fulminant hepatic failure have been reported from approximately 60,000 patients providing about 40,000 patient years of worldwide use. This incidence may be 10- to 100-fold higher than the background incidence in the general population.

The imprecision of the estimated increase is due to uncertainties about the base rate and the actual number of cases occurring in association with TASMAR. The incidence of idiopathic potentially fatal fulminant hepatic failure (ie, not due to viral hepatitis or alcohol) is low. One estimate, based upon transplant registry data, is approximately 3/1,000,000 patients per year in the United States. Whether this estimate is an appropriate basis for estimating the increased risk of liver failure among TASMAR users is uncertain. TASMAR users, for example, differ in age and general health status from candidates for liver transplantation. Similarly, underreporting of cases may lead to significant underestimation of the increased risk associated with the use of TASMAR.

During the premarketing development of tolcapone, two distinct patient populations were studied, patients with end-of-dose wearing-off phenomena and patients with stable responses to levodopa therapy. All patients received concomitant treatment with levodopa preparations, however, and were similar in other clinical aspects. Adverse events are, therefore, shown for these two populations combined.

The most commonly observed adverse events (>5%) in the double-blind, placebo-controlled trials (N=892) associated with the use of TASMAR not seen at an equivalent frequency among the placebo-treated patients were dyskinesia, nausea, sleep disorder, dystonia, dreaming excessive, anorexia, cramps muscle, orthostatic complaints, somnolence, diarrhea, confusion, dizziness, headache, hallucination, vomiting, constipation, fatigue, upper respiratory tract infection, falling, sweating increased, urinary tract infection, xerostomia, abdominal pain, urine discoloration.

Approximately 16% of the 592 patients who participated in the double-blind, placebo-controlled trials discontinued treatment due to adverse events compared to 10% of the 298 patients who received placebo. Diarrhea was by far the most frequent cause of discontinuation (approximately 6% in tolcapone patients vs 1% on placebo).

Adverse Event Incidence in Controlled Clinical Studies: Table 4 lists treatment emergent adverse events that occurred in at least 1% of patients treated with tolcapone participating in the double-blind, placebo-controlled studies and were numerically more common in at least one of the tolcapone groups. In these studies, either tolcapone or placebo were added to levodopa/carbidopa (or benserazide).

The prescriber should be aware that these figures cannot be used to predict the incidence of adverse events in the course of usual medical practice where patient characteristics and other factors differ from those that prevailed in the clinical studies. Similarly, the cited frequencies cannot be compared with figures obtained from other clinical investigations involving different treatments, uses, and investigators. However, the cited figures do provide the prescriber with some basis for estimating the relative contribution of drug and nondrug factors to the adverse events incidence rate in the population studied.

Table 4.
Summary of Patients With Adverse Events After Start of Trial Drug Administration
(At Least 1% in TASMAR Group and at Least One TASMAR Dose Group > Placebo)

	Placebo	Tolcapone tid	
		100 mg	200 mg
	N = 298	N = 296	N = 298
Adverse Events	(%)	(%)	(%)
Dyskinesia	20	42	51
Nausea	18	30	35
Sleep Disorder	18	24	25
Dystonia	17	19	22
Dreaming Excessive	17	21	16
Anorexia	13	19	23
Cramps Muscle	17	17	18
Orthostatic Complaints	14	17	17
Somnolence	13	18	14
Diarrhea	8	16	18
Confusion	9	11	10
Dizziness	10	13	6
Headache	7	10	11
Hallucination	5	8	10
Vomiting	4	8	10
Constipation	5	6	8
Fatigue	6	7	3
Upper Respiratory Tract Infection	3	5	7
Falling	4	4	6
Sweating Increased	2	4	7
Urinary Tract Infection	4	5	5
Xerostomia	2	5	6
Abdominal Pain	3	5	6
Syncope	3	4	5
Urine Discoloration	1	2	7
Dyspepsia	2	4	3
Influenza	2	3	4
Dyspnea	2	3	3
Balance Loss	2	3	2
Flatulence	2	2	4
Hyperkinesia	1	3	2
Chest Pain	1	3	1
Hypotension	1	2	2
Paresthesia	2	3	1
Stiffness	1	2	2
Arthritis	1	2	1
Chest Discomfort	1	1	2
Hypokinesia	1	1	3
Micturition Disorder	1	2	1
Pain Neck	1	2	2
Burning	0	2	1
Sinus Congestion	0	2	1
Agitation	0	1	1
Bleeding Dermal	0	1	1
Irritability	0	1	1
Mental Deficiency	0	1	1
Hyperactivity	0	1	1
Malaise	0	1	0
Panic Reaction	0	1	0
Tumor Skin	0	1	0
Cataract	0	1	0
Euphoria	0	1	0

Continued on next page

Tasmar—Cont.

Fever	0	0	1
Alopecia	0	1	0
Eye Inflamed	0	1	0
Hypertonia	0	0	1
Tumor Uterus	0	1	0

Other events reported by 1% or more of patients treated with TASMAR but that were equally or more frequent in the placebo group were arthralgia, pain limbs, anxiety, micturition frequency, fractures, vision blurred, pneumonia, paresis, lethargy, asthenia, edema peripheral, gait abnormal, taste alteration, weight decrease and sinusitis.

Effects of Gender and Age on Adverse Reactions: Experience in clinical trials have suggested that patients greater than 75 years of age may be more likely to develop hallucinations than patients less than 75 years of age, while patients over 75 may be less likely to develop dystonia. Females may be more likely to develop somnolence than males.

Other Adverse Events Observed During All Trials in Patients With Parkinson's Disease: TASMAR has been administered in 1536 patients with Parkinson's disease in clinical trials. During these trials, all adverse events were recorded by the clinical investigators using terminology of their own choosing. To provide a meaningful estimate of the proportion of individuals having adverse events, similar types of adverse events were grouped into a smaller number of standardized categories using COSTART dictionary terminology. These categories are used in the listing below.

All reported events that occurred at least twice (or once for serious or potentially serious events), except those already listed above, trivial events and terms too vague to be meaningful are included, without regard to determination of a causal relationship to TASMAR.

Events are further classified within body system categories and enumerated in order of decreasing frequency using the following definitions: frequent adverse events are defined as those occurring in at least 1/100 patients; infrequent adverse events are defined as those occurring in between 1/100 and 1/1000 patients; and rare adverse events are defined as those occurring in fewer than 1/1000 patients.

Nervous System—frequent: depression, hypesthesia, tremor, speech disorder, vertigo, emotional lability; *infrequent:* neuralgia, amnesia, extrapyramidal syndrome, hostility, libido increased, manic reaction, nervousness, paranoid reaction, cerebral ischemia, cerebrovascular accident, delusions, libido decreased, neuropathy, apathy, choreoathetosis, myoclonus, psychosis, thinking abnormal, twitching; *rare:* antisocial reaction, delirium, encephalopathy, hemiplegia, meningitis.

Digestive System—frequent: tooth disorder; *infrequent:* dysphagia, gastrointestinal hemorrhage, gastroenteritis, mouth ulceration, increased salivation, abnormal stools, esophagitis, cholelithiasis, colitis, tongue disorder, rectal disorder; *rare:* cholecystitis, duodenal ulcer, gastrointestinal carcinoma, stomach atony.

Body as a Whole—frequent: flank pain, accidental injury, abdominal pain, infection; *infrequent:* hernia, pain, allergic reaction, cellulitis, infection fungal, viral infection, carcinoma, chills, infection bacterial, neoplasm, abscess, face edema; *rare:* death.

Cardiovascular System—frequent: palpitation; *infrequent:* hypertension, vasodilation, angina pectoris, heart failure, atrial fibrillation, tachycardia, migraine, aortic stenosis, arrhythmia, arteriospasm, bradycardia, cerebral hemorrhage, coronary artery disorder, heart arrest, myocardial infarct, myocardial ischemia, pulmonary embolus; *rare:* arteriosclerosis, cardiovascular disorder, pericardial effusion, thrombosis.

Musculoskeletal System—frequent: myalgia; *infrequent:* tenosynovitis, arthrosis, joint disorder.

Urogenital System—frequent: urinary incontinence, impotence; *infrequent:* prostatic disorder, dysuria, nocturia, polyuria, urinary retention, urinary tract disorder, hematuria, kidney calculus, prostatic carcinoma, breast neoplasm, oliguria, uterine atony, uterine disorder, vaginitis; *rare:* bladder calculus, ovarian carcinoma, uterine hemorrhage.

Respiratory System—frequent: bronchitis, pharyngitis; *infrequent:* cough increased, rhinitis, asthma, epistaxis, hyperventilation, laryngitis, hiccup; *rare:* apnea, hypoxia, lung edema.

Skin and Appendages—frequent: rash; *infrequent:* herpes zoster, pruritus, seborrhea, skin discoloration, eczema, erythema multiforme, skin disorder, furunculosis, herpes simplex, urticaria.

Special Senses—frequent: tinnitus; *infrequent:* diplopia, ear pain, eye hemorrhage, eye pain, lacrimation disorder, otitis media, parosmia; *rare:* glaucoma.

Metabolic and Nutritional—infrequent: edema, hypercholesteremia, thirst, dehydration.

Hemic and Lymphatic System—infrequent: anemia; *rare:* leukemia, thrombocytopenia.

Endocrine System—infrequent: diabetes mellitus.

Unclassified—infrequent: surgical procedure.

DRUG ABUSE AND DEPENDENCE

Tolcapone is not a controlled substance.

Studies conducted in rats and monkeys did not reveal any potential for physical or psychological dependence. Although clinical trials have not revealed any evidence of the potential for abuse, tolerance or physical dependence, systematic studies in humans designed to evaluate these effects have not been performed.

OVERDOSAGE

The highest dose of tolcapone administered to humans was 800 mg tid, with and without levodopa/carbidopa coadministration. This was in a 1-week study in elderly, healthy volunteers. The peak plasma concentrations of tolcapone at this dose were on average 30 µg/mL (compared to 3 µg/mL and 6 µg/mL with 100 mg and 200 mg tolcapone, respectively). Nausea, vomiting and dizziness were observed, particularly in combination with levodopa/carbidopa.

The threshold for the lethal plasma concentration for tolcapone based on animal data is >100 µg/mL. Respiratory difficulties were observed in rats at high oral (gavage) and intravenous doses and in dogs with rapidly injected intravenous doses.

Management of Overdose: Hospitalization is advised. General supportive care is indicated. Based on the physicochemical properties of the compound, hemodialysis is unlikely to be of benefit.

DOSAGE AND ADMINISTRATION

Because of the risk of potentially fatal, acute fulminant liver failure, TASMAR (tolcapone) should ordinarily be used in patients with Parkinson's disease on l-dopa/carbidopa who are experiencing symptom fluctuations and are not responding satisfactorily to or are not appropriate candidates for other adjunctive therapies (see INDICATIONS and DOSAGE AND ADMINISTRATION sections).

Because of the risk of liver injury and because TASMAR when it is effective provides an observable symptomatic benefit, the patient who fails to show substantial clinical benefit within 3 weeks of initiation of treatment, should be withdrawn from TASMAR.

TASMAR therapy should not be initiated if the patient exhibits clinical evidence of liver disease or two SGPT/ALT or SGOT/AST values greater than the upper limit of normal. Patients with severe dyskinesia or dystonia should be treated with caution (see PRECAUTIONS: *Rhabdomyolysis*).

Patients who develop evidence of hepatocellular injury while on TASMAR and are withdrawn from the drug for any reason may be at increased risk for liver injury if TASMAR is reintroduced. Accordingly, such patients should not ordinarily be considered for retreatment.

Treatment with TASMAR should always be initiated at a dose of 100 mg tid, always as an adjunct to levodopa/carbidopa therapy. The recommended daily dose of TASMAR is also 100 mg tid. In clinical trials, elevations in ALT occurred more frequently at the dose of 200 mg tid. While it is unknown whether the risk of acute fulminant liver failure is increased at the 200-mg dose, it would be prudent to use 200 mg only if the anticipated incremental clinical benefit is justified (see BOXED WARNING, WARNINGS, PRECAUTIONS: *Laboratory Tests*). If a patient fails to show the expected incremental benefit on the 200-mg dose after a total of 3 weeks of treatment (regardless of dose), TASMAR should be discontinued.

In clinical trials, the first dose of the day of TASMAR was always taken together with the first dose of the day of levodopa/carbidopa, and the subsequent doses of TASMAR were given approximately 6 and 12 hours later.

In clinical trials, the majority of patients required a decrease in their daily levodopa dose if their daily dose of levodopa was >600 mg or if patients had moderate or severe dyskinesias before beginning treatment.

To optimize an individual patient's response, reductions in daily levodopa dose may be necessary. In clinical trials, the average reduction in daily levodopa dose was about 30% in those patients requiring a levodopa dose reduction. (Greater than 70% of patients with levodopa doses above 600 mg daily required such a reduction.)

TASMAR can be combined with both the immediate and sustained release formulations of levodopa/carbidopa.

TASMAR may be taken with or without food (see CLINICAL PHARMACOLOGY).

Patients With Impaired Hepatic Function: TASMAR therapy should not be initiated if any patient with liver disease or two SGPT/ALT or SGOT/AST values greater than the upper limit of normal. (See BOXED WARNING, WARNINGS, and CLINICAL PHARMACOLOGY).

Patients With Impaired Renal Function: No dose adjustment of TASMAR is recommended for patients with mild to moderate renal impairment. However, patients with severe renal impairment should be treated with caution. The safety of tolcapone has not been examined in subjects who had creatinine clearance less than 25 mL/min (see CLINICAL PHARMACOLOGY).

Withdrawing Patients From TASMAR: As with any dopaminergic drug, withdrawal or abrupt reduction in the TASMAR dose may lead to emergence of signs and symptoms of Parkinson's disease or Hyperpyrexia and Confusion, a syndrome complex resembling the neuroleptic malignant syndrome (see PRECAUTIONS: *Events Reported With Dopaminergic Therapy*). If a decision is made to discontinue treatment with TASMAR, then it is recommended to closely monitor the patient and adjust other dopaminergic treatments as needed. This syndrome should be considered in the differential diagnosis for any patient who develops a high fever or severe rigidity. Tapering TASMAR has not been systematically evaluated. As the duration of COMT inhibition with TASMAR is generally 5 to 6 hours on average, decreasing the frequency of dosage to twice or once a day may not in itself prevent withdrawal effects.

HOW SUPPLIED

TASMAR is supplied as film-coated tablets containing 100 mg or 200 mg tolcapone. The 100 mg beige tablet and the 200 mg reddish-brown tablet are hexagonal and biconvex. Imprinted with black ink on one side of the tablet is TASMAR and the tablet strength (100 or 200), on the other side is ROCHE.

TASMAR 100 mg Tablets: bottles of 90 (NDC 0004-5920-01).

TASMAR 200 mg Tablets: bottles of 90 (NDC 0004-5921-01).

Storage: Store at controlled room temperature 20° to 25°C (68° to 77°F) in tight containers as defined in USP/NF.

PATIENT CONSENT

TASMAR SHOULD NOT BE USED BY PATIENTS UNTIL THERE HAS BEEN A COMPLETE DISCUSSION OF THE RISKS AND WRITTEN INFORMED CONSENT HAS BEEN OBTAINED.

IMPORTANT INFORMATION AND WARNING

Reports of potentially life threatening cases of severe hepatocellular injury, including fulminant liver failure resulting in death, have been reported in association with use of TASMAR.

PATIENT CONSENT

My, ____________________, treatment with TASMAR has been personally described to me by Dr.________________.

The following points of information, among others, have been specifically discussed and made clear and I have had the opportunity to ask any questions concerning this information:

1. I. ____________________ (patient's name) understand that TASMAR is used to treat certain types of patients with Parkinson's disease and my physician has told me that I am this type of patient.
   Initials: ______________
2. I understand that there is a serious risk that I could develop severe liver failure, which may be potentially fatal, by using TASMAR.
   Initials: ______________
3. I understand that there are no laboratory tests that will predict if I am at an increased risk for fatal liver failure.
   Initials: ______________
4. I understand that I should have the recommended blood work before my treatment with TASMAR is begun or continued and every 2 weeks for the first year, then every 4 weeks for the next 6 months, and then every 8 weeks thereafter while taking TASMAR. I understand that although this blood work may help detect if I develop liver failure it may do so only after significant, irreversible and potentially fatal damage has already occurred.
   Initials: ______________
5. I understand that I must immediately report any unusual symptoms to Dr. ______________ and be especially aware of persistent nausea, fatigue, lethargy, decreased appetite, jaundice (yellowing of skin or the whites of the eyes), dark urine, itchiness or right-sided abdominal pain.
   Initials: ______________

I now authorize Dr. ______________ to begin my treatment with TASMAR; OR, if my treatment has already begun with TASMAR, to continue such treatment.

Patient/Caretaker______________________________

Address______________________________

____

Telephone______________________________

PHYSICIAN STATEMENT:

I have fully explained to the patient, ____________________, the nature and purpose of the treatment with TASMAR (tolcapone) and the potential risks associated with that treatment. I have asked the patient if he/she has any questions regarding this treatment or the risks and have answered those questions to the best of my ability. I also acknowledge that I have read and understand the prescribing information listed above.

____

Physician Date

NOTE TO PHYSICIAN: It is strongly recommended that you retain a signed copy of the informed consent with the patient's medical records.

SUPPLY OF PATIENT CONSENT FORMS:

A supply of "Patient Consent" forms as printed above, is available, free of charge, from your local Roche representative, or may be obtained by calling 1-800-526-6367. Permission to use the above Patient Consent by photocopy reproduction is also hereby granted by Roche Laboratories Inc.

Revised November 1998

Shown in Product Identification Guide, page 333

TICLID® ℞

[tye'klid]

(ticlopidine hydrochloride)

Tablets

The following text is complete prescribing information based on official labeling in effect June 2000.

WARNING: TICLID can cause life-threatening hematological adverse reactions, including neutropenia/

agranulocytosis and thrombotic thrombocytopenic purpura (TTP).

Neutropenia/Agranulocytosis: **Among 2048 patients in clinical trials, there were 50 cases (2.4%) of neutropenia (less than 1200 neutrophils/mm^3), and the neutrophil count was below 450/mm^3 in 17 of these patients (0.8% of the total population).**

TTP: **One case of thrombotic thrombocytopenic purpura was reported during clinical trials. Based on postmarketing data, US physicians reported about 100 cases between 1992 and 1997. Based on an estimated patient exposure of 2 million to 4 million, and assuming an event reporting rate of 10% (the true rate is not known), the incidence of ticlopidine-associated TTP may be as high as one case in every 2000 to 4000 patients exposed.**

Monitoring of Clinical and Hematologic Status: **Severe hematological adverse reactions may occur within a few days of the start of therapy. The incidence of TTP peaks after about 3 to 4 weeks of therapy and neutropenia peaks at approximately 4 to 6 weeks with both declining thereafter. Only a few cases have arisen after more than 3 months of treatment.**

Hematological adverse reactions cannot be reliably predicted by any identified demographic or clinical characteristics. During the first 3 months of treatment, patients receiving TICLID must, therefore, be hematologically and clinically monitored for evidence of neutropenia or TTP. If any such evidence is seen, TICLID should be immediately discontinued.

The detection and treatment of ticlopidine-associated hematological adverse reactions are further described under WARNINGS.

DESCRIPTION

TICLID (ticlopidine hydrochloride) is a platelet aggregation inhibitor. Chemically it is 5-[(2-chlorophenyl)methyl]-4,5,6,7-tetrahydrothieno [3,2-c] pyridine hydrochloride.

Ticlopidine hydrochloride is a white crystalline solid. It is freely soluble in water and self-buffers to a pH of 3.6. It also dissolves freely in methanol, is sparingly soluble in methylene chloride and ethanol, slightly soluble in acetone and insoluble in a buffer solution of pH 6.3. It has a molecular weight of 300.25.

TICLID tablets for oral administration are provided as white, oval, film-coated, blue-imprinted tablets containing 250 mg of ticlopidine hydrochloride. Each tablet also contains citric acid, magnesium stearate, microcrystalline cellulose, povidone, starch and stearic acid as inactive ingredients. The white film-coating contains hydroxypropylmethyl cellulose, polyethylene glycol and titanium dioxide. Each tablet is printed with blue ink, which includes FD&C Blue #1 aluminum lake as the colorant. The tablets are identified with Ticlid on one side and 250 on the reverse side.

CLINICAL PHARMACOLOGY

Mechanism of Action: When taken orally, ticlopidine hydrochloride causes a time- and dose-dependent inhibition of both platelet aggregation and release of platelet granule constituents, as well as a prolongation of bleeding time. The intact drug has no significant in vitro activity at the concentrations attained in vivo; and, although analysis of urine and plasma indicates at least 20 metabolites, no metabolite which accounts for the activity of ticlopidine has been isolated.

Ticlopidine hydrochloride, after oral ingestion, interferes with platelet membrane function by inhibiting ADP-induced platelet-fibrinogen binding and subsequent platelet-platelet interactions. The effect on platelet function is irreversible for the life of the platelet, as shown both by persistent inhibition of fibrinogen binding after washing platelets ex vivo and by inhibition of platelet aggregation after resuspension of platelets in buffered medium.

Pharmacokinetics and Metabolism: After oral administration of a single 250-mg dose, ticlopidine hydrochloride is rapidly absorbed with peak plasma levels occurring at approximately 2 hours after dosing and is extensively metabolized. Absorption is greater than 80%. Administration after meals results in a 20% increase in the AUC of ticlopidine.

Ticlopidine hydrochloride displays nonlinear pharmacokinetics and clearance decreases markedly on repeated dosing. In older volunteers the apparent half-life of ticlopidine after a single 250-mg dose is about 12.6 hours; with repeat dosing at 250 mg bid, the terminal elimination half-life rises to 4 to 5 days and steady-state levels of ticlopidine hydrochloride in plasma are obtained after approximately 14 to 21 days.

Ticlopidine hydrochloride binds reversibly (98%) to plasma proteins, mainly to serum albumin and lipoproteins. The binding to albumin and lipoproteins is nonsaturable over a wide concentration range. Ticlopidine also binds to alpha-1 acid glycoprotein. At concentrations attained with the recommended dose, only 15% or less ticlopidine in plasma is bound to this protein.

Ticlopidine hydrochloride is metabolized extensively by the liver; only trace amounts of intact drug are detected in the urine. Following an oral dose of radioactive ticlopidine hydrochloride administered in solution, 60% of the radioactivity is recovered in the urine and 23% in the feces. Approximately 1/3 of the dose excreted in the feces is intact ticlopidine hydrochloride, possibly excreted in the bile. Ticlopidine hydrochloride is a minor component in plasma (5%) after a single dose, but at steady-state is the major component (15%). Approximately 40% to 50% of the radioactive metabolites circulating in plasma are covalently bound to plasma proteins, probably by acylation.

Clearance of ticlopidine decreases with age. Steady-state trough values in elderly patients (mean age 70 years) are about twice those in younger volunteer populations.

Hepatically Impaired Patients: The effect of decreased hepatic function on the pharmacokinetics of TICLID was studied in 17 patients with advanced cirrhosis. The average plasma concentration of ticlopidine in these subjects was slightly higher than that seen in older subjects in a separate trial (see CONTRAINDICATIONS).

Renally Impaired Patients: Patients with mildly (Ccr 50 to 80 mL/min) or moderately (Ccr 20 to 50 mL/min) impaired renal function were compared to normal subjects (Ccr 80 to 150 mL/min) in a study of the pharmacokinetic and platelet pharmacodynamic effects of TICLID (250 mg bid) for 11 days. Concentrations of unchanged TICLID were measured after a single 250-mg dose and after the final 250-mg dose on Day 11.

AUC values of ticlopidine increased by 28% and 60% in mild and moderately impaired patients, respectively, and plasma clearance decreased by 37% and 52%, respectively, but there were no statistically significant differences in ADP-induced platelet aggregation. In this small study (26 patients), bleeding times showed significant prolongation only in the moderately impaired patients.

Pharmacodynamics: In healthy volunteers over the age of 50, substantial inhibition (over 50%) of ADP-induced platelet aggregation is detected within 4 days after administration of ticlopidine hydrochloride 250 mg bid, and maximum platelet aggregation inhibition (60% to 70%) is achieved after 8 to 11 days. Lower doses cause less, and more delayed, platelet aggregation inhibition, while doses above 250 mg bid give little additional effect on platelet aggregation but an increased rate of adverse effects. The dose of 250 mg bid is the only dose that has been evaluated in controlled clinical trials.

After discontinuation of ticlopidine hydrochloride, bleeding time and other platelet function tests return to normal within 2 weeks, in the majority of patients.

At the recommended therapeutic dose (250 mg bid), ticlopidine hydrochloride has no known significant pharmacological actions in man other than inhibition of platelet function and prolongation of the bleeding time.

CLINICAL TRIALS

The effect of ticlopidine on the risk of stroke and cardiovascular events was studied in two multicenter, randomized, double-blind trials.

1. Study in Patients Experiencing Stroke Precursors: In a trial comparing ticlopidine and aspirin (The Ticlopidine Aspirin Stroke Study or TASS), 3069 patients (1987 men, 1082 women) who had experienced such stroke precursors as transient ischemic attack (TIA), transient monocular blindness (amaurosis fugax), reversible ischemic neurological deficit or minor stroke, were randomized to ticlopidine 250 mg bid or aspirin 650 mg bid. The study was designed to follow patients for at least 2 years and up to 5 years.

Over the duration of the study, TICLID significantly reduced the risk of fatal and nonfatal stroke by 24% (p = .011) from 18.1 to 13.8 per 100 patients followed for 5 years, compared to aspirin. During the first year, when the risk of stroke is greatest, the reduction in risk of stroke (fatal and nonfatal) compared to aspirin was 48%; the reduction was similar in men and women.

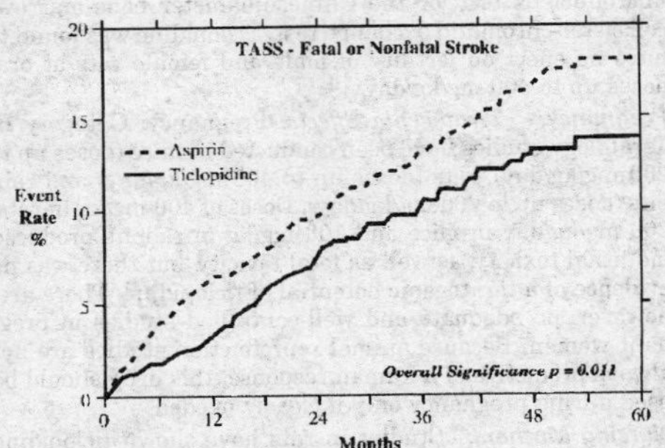

2. Study in Patients Who Had a Completed Atherothrombotic Stroke: In a trial comparing ticlopidine with placebo (The Canadian American Ticlopidine Study or CATS) 1073 patients who had experienced a previous atherothrombotic stroke were treated with TICLID 250 mg bid or placebo for up to 3 years.

TICLID significantly reduced the overall risk of stroke by 24% (p = .017) from 24.6 to 18.6 per 100 patients followed for 3 years, compared to placebo. During the first year the reduction in risk of fatal and nonfatal stroke over placebo was 33%.

[See figure at top of next column]

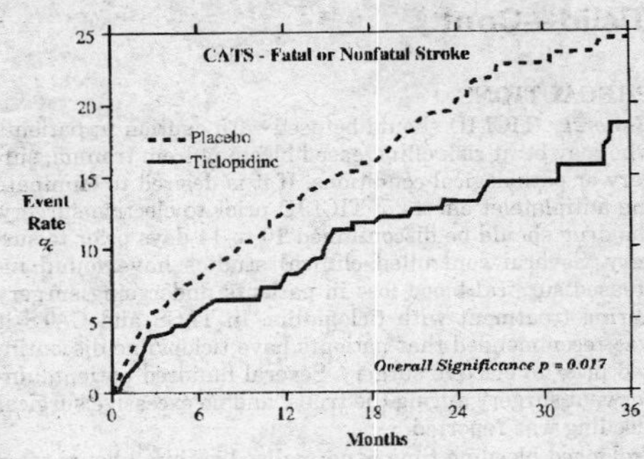

INDICATIONS AND USAGE

TICLID is indicated to reduce the risk of thrombotic stroke (fatal or nonfatal) in patients who have experienced stroke precursors, and in patients who have had a completed thrombotic stroke.

Because TICLID is associated with a risk of life-threatening blood dyscrasias including thrombotic thrombocytopenic purpura (TTP) and neutropenia/agranulocytosis (see BOXED WARNING and WARNINGS), TICLID should be reserved for patients who are intolerant or allergic to aspirin therapy or who have failed aspirin therapy.

CONTRAINDICATIONS

The use of TICLID is contraindicated in the following conditions:

- Hypersensitivity to the drug
- Presence of hematopoietic disorders such as neutropenia and thrombocytopenia or a past history of TTP
- Presence of a hemostatic disorder or active pathological bleeding (such as bleeding peptic ulcer or intracranial bleeding)
- Patients with severe liver impairment

WARNINGS

Hematological Adverse Reactions: *Neutropenia:* Neutropenia may occur suddenly. Bone-marrow examination typically shows a reduction in myeloid precursors. After withdrawal of ticlopidine, the neutrophil count usually rises to >1200/mm^3 within 1 to 3 weeks.

Thrombocytopenia: Rarely, thrombocytopenia may occur in isolation or together with neutropenia.

Thrombotic Thrombocytopenic Purpura (TTP): TTP is characterized by thrombocytopenia, microangiopathic hemolytic anemia (schistocytes [fragmented RBCs] seen on peripheral smear), neurological findings, renal dysfunction, and fever. The signs and symptoms can occur in any order, in particular, clinical symptoms may precede laboratory findings by hours or days. With **prompt** treatment (often including plasmapheresis), 70% to 80% of patients will survive with minimal or no sequelae. Because platelet transfusions may accelerate thrombosis in patients with TTP on ticlopidine, they should, if possible, be avoided.

Monitoring for Hematologic Adverse Reactions: Starting just before initiating treatment and continuing through the third month of therapy, patients receiving TICLID must be monitored every 2 weeks. Because of ticlopidine's long plasma half-life, patients who discontinue ticlopidine during this 3-month period should continue to be monitored for 2 weeks after discontinuation. More frequent monitoring, and monitoring after the first 3 months of therapy, is necessary only in patients with clinical signs (eg, signs or symptoms suggestive of infection) or laboratory signs (eg, neutrophil count less than 70% of the baseline count, decrease in hematocrit or platelet count) that suggest incipient hematological adverse reactions.

Clinically, fever might suggest either neutropenia or TTP; TTP might also be suggested by weakness, pallor, petechiae or purpura, dark urine (due to blood, bile pigments, or hemoglobin) or jaundice, or neurological changes. Patients should be told to discontinue TICLID and to contact the physician immediately upon the occurrence of any of these findings.

Laboratory monitoring should include a complete blood count, with special attention to the absolute neutrophil count (WBC × % neutrophils), platelet count, and the appearance of the peripheral smear. Ticlopidine is occasionally associated with thrombocytopenia unrelated to TTP. Any acute, unexplained reduction in **hemoglobin** or platelet count should prompt further investigation for a diagnosis of TTP, and the appearance of **schistocytes** (fragmented RBCs) on the smear should be treated as presumptive evidence of TTP. If there are laboratory signs of TTP, or if the neutrophil count is confirmed to be <1200/mm^3, then the drug should be discontinued.

Other Hematological Effects: Rare cases of agranulocytosis, pancytopenia or aplastic anemia have been reported in postmarketing experience, some of which have been fatal. All forms of hematological adverse reactions are potentially fatal.

Cholesterol Elevation: TICLID therapy causes increased serum cholesterol and triglycerides. Serum total cholesterol levels are increased 8% to 10% within 1 month of therapy and persist at that level. The ratios of the lipoprotein subfractions are unchanged.

Anticoagulant Drugs: The tolerance and safety of coadministration of TICLID with heparin, oral anticoagulants or fibrinolytic agents have not been established. If a patient is switched from an anticoagulant or fibrinolytic drug to TICLID, the former drug should be discontinued prior to TICLID administration.

Continued on next page

Ticlid—Cont.

PRECAUTIONS

General: TICLID should be used with caution in patients who may be at risk of increased bleeding from trauma, surgery or pathological conditions. If it is desired to eliminate the antiplatelet effects of TICLID prior to elective surgery, the drug should be discontinued 10 to 14 days prior to surgery. Several controlled clinical studies have found increased surgical blood loss in patients undergoing surgery during treatment with ticlopidine. In TASS and CATS it was recommended that patients have ticlopidine discontinued prior to elective surgery. Several hundred patients underwent surgery during the trials, and no excessive surgical bleeding was reported.

Prolonged bleeding time is normalized within 2 hours after administration of 20 mg methylprednisolone IV. Platelet transfusions may also be used to reverse the effect of TICLID on bleeding. Because platelet transfusions may accelerate thrombosis in patients with TTP on ticlopidine, they should, if possible, be avoided.

GI Bleeding: TICLID prolongs template bleeding time. The drug should be used with caution in patients who have lesions with a propensity to bleed (such as ulcers). Drugs that might induce such lesions should be used with caution in patients on TICLID (see CONTRAINDICATIONS).

Use in Hepatically Impaired Patients: Since ticlopidine is metabolized by the liver, dosing of TICLID or other drugs metabolized in the liver may require adjustment upon starting or stopping concomitant therapy. Because of limited experience in patients with severe hepatic disease, who may have bleeding diatheses, the use of TICLID is not recommended in this population (see CLINICAL PHARMACOLOGY and CONTRAINDICATIONS).

Use in Renally Impaired Patients: There is limited experience in patients with renal impairment. Decreased plasma clearance, increased AUC values and prolonged bleeding times can occur in renally impaired patients. In controlled clinical trials no unexpected problems have been encountered in patients having mild renal impairment, and there is no experience with dosage adjustment in patients with greater degrees of renal impairment. Nevertheless, for renally impaired patients, it may be necessary to reduce the dosage of ticlopidine or discontinue it altogether if hemorrhagic or hematopoietic problems are encountered (see CLINICAL PHARMACOLOGY).

***Information for the Patient* (see PPI):** Patients should be told that a decrease in the number of white blood cells (neutropenia) or platelets (thrombocytopenia) can occur with TICLID, especially during the first 3 months of treatment and that neutropenia, if it is severe, can result in an increased risk of infection. They should be told it is critically important to obtain the scheduled blood tests to detect neutropenia or thrombocytopenia. Patients should also be reminded to contact their physicians if they experience any indication of infection such as fever, chills, or sore throat, any of which might be a consequence of neutropenia. Thrombocytopenia may be part of a syndrome called TTP. Symptoms and signs of TTP, such as fever, weakness, difficulty speaking, seizures, yellowing of skin or eyes, dark or bloody urine, pallor or petechiae (pinpoint hemorrhagic spots on the skin), should be reported immediately.

All patients should be told that it may take them longer than usual to stop bleeding when they take TICLID and that they should report any unusual bleeding to their physician. Patients should tell physicians and dentists that they are taking TICLID before any surgery is scheduled and before any new drug is prescribed.

Patients should be told to promptly report side effects of TICLID such as severe or persistent diarrhea, skin rashes or subcutaneous bleeding or any signs of cholestasis, such as yellow skin or sclera, dark urine, or light-colored stools. Patients should be told to take TICLID with food or just after eating in order to minimize gastrointestinal discomfort.

Laboratory Tests: *Liver Function:* TICLID therapy has been associated with elevations of alkaline phosphatase and transaminases, which generally occurred within 1 to 4 months of therapy initiation. In controlled clinical trials the incidence of elevated alkaline phosphatase (greater than two times upper limit of normal) was 7.6% in ticlopidine patients, 6% in placebo patients and 2.5% in aspirin patients. The incidence of elevated AST (SGOT) (greater than two times upper limit of normal) was 3.1% in ticlopidine patients, 4% in placebo patients and 2.1% in aspirin patients. No progressive increases were observed in closely monitored clinical trials (eg, no transaminase greater than 10 times the upper limit of normal was seen), but most patients with these abnormalities had therapy discontinued. Occasionally patients had developed minor elevations in bilirubin.

Based on postmarketing and clinical trial experience, liver function testing, including SGPT and GGTP, should be considered whenever liver dysfunction is suspected, particularly during the first 4 months of treatment.

Drug Interactions: Therapeutic doses of TICLID caused a 30% increase in the plasma half-life of antipyrine and may cause analogous effects on similarly metabolized drugs. Therefore, the dose of drugs metabolized by hepatic microsomal enzymes with low therapeutic ratios or being given to patients with hepatic impairment may require adjustment to maintain optimal therapeutic blood levels when starting or stopping concomitant therapy with ticlopidine. Studies of specific drug interactions yielded the following results:

Aspirin and Other NSAIDs: Ticlopidine potentiates the effect of aspirin or other NSAIDs on platelet aggregation. The safety of concomitant use of ticlopidine with aspirin or other NSAIDs has not been established. Aspirin did not modify the ticlopidine-mediated inhibition of ADP-induced platelet aggregation, but ticlopidine potentiated the effect of aspirin on collagen-induced platelet aggregation. Concomitant use of aspirin and ticlopidine is not recommended (see PRECAUTIONS: *GI Bleeding*).

Antacids: Administration of TICLID after antacids resulted in an 18% decrease in plasma levels of ticlopidine.

Cimetidine: Chronic administration of cimetidine reduced the clearance of a single dose of TICLID by 50%.

Digoxin: Coadministration of TICLID with digoxin resulted in a slight decrease (approximately 15%) in digoxin plasma levels. Little or no change in therapeutic efficacy of digoxin would be expected.

Theophylline: In normal volunteers, concomitant administration of TICLID resulted in a significant increase in the theophylline elimination half-life from 8.6 to 12.2 hours and a comparable reduction in total plasma clearance of theophylline.

Phenobarbital: In 6 normal volunteers, the inhibitory effects of TICLID on platelet aggregation were not altered by chronic administration of phenobarbital.

Phenytoin: In vitro studies demonstrated that ticlopidine does not alter the plasma protein binding of phenytoin. However, the protein binding interactions of ticlopidine and its metabolites have not been studied in vivo. Several cases of elevated phenytoin plasma levels with associated somnolence and lethargy have been reported following coadministration with TICLID. Caution should be exercised in coadministering this drug with TICLID, and it may be useful to remeasure phenytoin blood concentrations.

Propranolol: In vitro studies demonstrated that ticlopidine does not alter the plasma protein binding of propranolol. However, the protein binding interactions of ticlopidine and its metabolites have not been studied in vivo. Caution should be exercised in coadministering this drug with TICLID.

Other Concomitant Therapy: Although specific interaction studies were not performed, in clinical studies TICLID was used concomitantly with beta blockers, calcium channel blockers and diuretics without evidence of clinically significant adverse interactions (see PRECAUTIONS).

Food Interaction: The oral bioavailability of ticlopidine is increased by 20% when taken after a meal. Administration of TICLID with food is recommended to maximize gastrointestinal tolerance. In controlled trials TICLID was taken with meals.

Carcinogenesis, Mutagenesis, Impairment of Fertility: In a 2-year oral carcinogenicity study in rats, ticlopidine at daily doses of up to 100 mg/kg (610 mg/m^2) was not tumorigenic. For a 70-kg person (1.73m^2 body surface area) the dose represents 14 times the recommended clinical dose on a mg/kg basis and two times the clinical dose on body surface area basis. In a 78-week oral carcinogenicity study in mice, ticlopidine at daily doses up to 275 mg/kg (1180 mg/m^2) was not tumorigenic. The dose represents 40 times the recommended clinical dose on a mg/kg basis and four times the clinical dose on body surface area basis.

Ticlopidine was not mutagenic in vitro in the Ames test, the rat hepatocyte DNA-repair assay, or the Chinese-hamster fibroblast chromosomal aberration test; or in vivo in the mouse spermatozoid morphology test, the Chinese-hamster micronucleus test, or the Chinese-hamster bone-marrow-cell sister-chromatid exchange test. Ticlopidine was found to have no effect on fertility of male and female rats at oral doses up to 400 mg/kg/day.

Pregnancy: *Teratogenic Effects:* Pregnancy: Category B. Teratology studies have been conducted in mice (doses up to 200 mg/kg/day), rats (doses up to 400 mg/kg/day) and rabbits (doses up to 200 mg/kg/day). Doses of 400 mg/kg in rats, 200 mg/kg/day in mice and 100 mg/kg in rabbits produced maternal toxicity, as well as fetal toxicity, but there was no evidence of a teratogenic potential of ticlopidine. There are, however, no adequate and well-controlled studies in pregnant women. Because animal reproduction studies are not always predictive of a human response, this drug should be used during pregnancy only if clearly needed.

Nursing Mothers: Studies in rats have shown ticlopidine is excreted in the milk. It is not known whether this drug is excreted in human milk. Because many drugs are excreted in human milk and because of the potential for serious adverse reactions in nursing infants from ticlopidine, a decision should be made whether to discontinue nursing or to discontinue the drug, taking into account the importance of the drug to the mother.

Pediatric Use: Safety and effectiveness in pediatric patients have not been established.

Geriatric Use: Clearance of ticlopidine is somewhat lower in elderly patients and trough levels are increased. The major clinical trials with TICLID were conducted in an elderly population with an average age of 64 years. Of the total number of patients in the therapeutic trials, 45% of patients were over 65 years old and 12% were over 75 years old. No overall differences in effectiveness or safety were observed between these patients and younger patients, and other reported clinical experience has not identified differences in responses between the elderly and younger patients, but greater sensitivity of some older individuals cannot be ruled out.

ADVERSE REACTIONS

Adverse reactions were relatively frequent with over 50% of patients reporting at least one. Most (30% to 40%) involved the gastrointestinal tract. Most adverse effects are mild, but 21% of patients discontinued therapy because of an adverse event, principally diarrhea, rash, nausea, vomiting, GI pain and neutropenia. Most adverse effects occur early in the course of treatment, but a new onset of adverse effects can occur after several months.

The incidence rates of adverse events listed in the following table were derived from multicenter, controlled clinical trials described above comparing TICLID, placebo and aspirin over study periods of up to 5.8 years. Adverse events considered by the investigator to be probably drug-related that occurred in at least 1% of patients treated with TICLID are shown in the following table:

Percent of Patients With Adverse Events in Controlled Studies

Event	TICLID (n = 2048) Incidence		Aspirin (n = 1527) Incidence		Placebo (n = 536) Incidence	
Any Events	*60.0*	*(20.9)*	*53.2*	*(14.5)*	*34.3*	*(6.1)*
Diarrhea	12.5	(6.3)	5.2	(1.8)	4.5	(1.7)
Nausea	7.0	(2.6)	6.2	(1.9)	1.7	(0.9)
Dyspepsia	7.0	(1.1)	9.0	(2.0)	0.9	(0.2)
Rash	5.1	(3.4)	1.5	(0.8)	0.6	(0.9)
GI Pain	3.7	(1.9)	5.6	(2.7)	1.3	(0.4)
Neutropenia	2.4	(1.3)	0.8	(0.1)	1.1	(0.4)
Purpura	2.2	(0.2)	1.6	(0.1)	0.0	(0.0)
Vomiting	1.9	(1.4)	1.4	(0.9)	0.9	(0.4)
Flatulence	1.5	(0.1)	1.4	(0.3)	0.0	(0.0)
Pruritus	1.3	(0.8)	0.3	(0.1)	0.0	(0.0)
Dizziness	1.1	(0.4)	0.5	(0.4)	0.0	(0.0)
Anorexia	1.0	(0.4)	0.5	(0.3)	0.0	(0.0)
Abnormal Liver Function Test	1.0	(0.7)	0.3	(0.3)	0.0	(0.0)

Incidence of discontinuation, regardless of relationship to therapy, is shown in parentheses.

Hematological: Neutropenia/thrombocytopenia, TTP (see BOXED WARNING and WARNINGS), agranulocytosis, eosinophilia, pancytopenia, thrombocytosis and bone-marrow depression have been reported.

Gastrointestinal: TICLID therapy has been associated with a variety of gastrointestinal complaints including diarrhea and nausea. The majority of cases are mild, but about 13% of patients discontinued therapy because of these. They usually occur within 3 months of initiation of therapy and typically are resolved within 1 to 2 weeks without discontinuation of therapy. If the effect is severe or persistent, therapy should be discontinued. In some cases of severe or bloody diarrhea, colitis was later diagnosed.

Hemorrhagic: TICLID has been associated with increased bleeding, spontaneous posttraumatic bleeding and perioperative bleeding including, but not limited to, gastrointestinal bleeding. It has also been associated with a number of bleeding complications such as ecchymosis, epistaxis, hematuria and conjunctival hemorrhage.

Intracerebral bleeding was rare in clinical trials with TICLID, with an incidence no greater than that seen with comparator agents (ticlopidine 0.5%, aspirin 0.6%, placebo 0.75%). It has also been reported postmarketing.

Rash: Ticlopidine has been associated with a maculopapular or urticarial rash (often with pruritus). Rash usually occurs within 3 months of initiation of therapy with a mean onset time of 11 days. If drug is discontinued, recovery occurs within several days. Many rashes do not recur on drug rechallenge. There have been rare reports of severe rashes, including Stevens-Johnson syndrome, erythema multiforme and exfoliative dermatitis.

Less Frequent Adverse Reactions (Probably Related): Clinical adverse experiences occurring in 0.5% to 1% of patients in the controlled trials include:

Digestive System: GI fullness
Skin and Appendages: urticaria
Nervous System: headache
Body as a Whole: asthenia, pain
Hemostatic System: epistaxis
Special Senses: tinnitus

In addition, rarer, relatively serious events have also been reported from postmarketing experience: Hemolytic anemia with reticulocytosis, aplastic anemia, immune thrombocytopenia, hepatitis, hepatocellular jaundice, cholestatic jaundice, hepatic necrosis, peptic ulcer, renal failure, nephrotic syndrome, hyponatremia, vasculitis, sepsis, angioedema, allergic pneumonitis, systemic lupus (positive ANA), peripheral neuropathy, serum sickness, arthropathy and myositis.

OVERDOSAGE

One case of deliberate overdosage with TICLID has been reported by a foreign postmarketing surveillance program. A 38-year-old male took a single 6000-mg dose of TICLID (equivalent to 24 standard 250-mg tablets). The only abnormalities reported were increased bleeding time and increased SGPT. No special therapy was instituted and the patient recovered without sequelae.

Single oral doses of ticlopidine at 1600 mg/kg and 500 mg/kg were lethal to rats and mice, respectively. Symptoms of acute toxicity were GI hemorrhage, convulsions, hypothermia, dyspnea, loss of equilibrium and abnormal gait.

DOSAGE AND ADMINISTRATION

The recommended dose of TICLID is 250 mg bid taken with food. Other doses have not been studied in controlled trials for these indications.

HOW SUPPLIED

TICLID is available in white, oval, film-coated 250-mg tablets, printed in blue with Ticlid on one side and 250 on the other. They are provided in unit of use bottles of 30 tablets (NDC 0004-0018-23) and 60 tablets (NDC 0004-0018-22) and 500 tablets (NDC 0004-0018-14).

Store at 15° to 30°C (59° to 86°F).

IMPORTANT INFORMATION ABOUT TICLID (ticlopidine HCl) TABLETS

The information in this leaflet is intended to help you use TICLID safely. Please read the leaflet carefully. Although it does not contain all the detailed medical information that is provided to your doctor, it provides facts about TICLID that are important for you to know. If you still have questions after reading this leaflet or if you have questions at any time during your treatment with TICLID, check with your doctor.

Special Warning for Users of TICLID/Necessary Blood Tests: TICLID is recommended to help reduce your risk of having a stroke, but only for patients who have had a stroke or early stroke warning symptoms while on aspirin, or for those who have these symptoms but are intolerant or allergic to aspirin.

TICLID is not prescribed for those who can take aspirin to prevent a stroke because TICLID can cause life-threatening blood problems. **Getting your blood tests done and reporting symptoms to your doctor as soon as possible can avoid serious complications.**

The white cells of the blood that fight infection may drop to dangerous levels (a condition called neutropenia). This occurs in about 2.4% (1 in 40) of people on ticlopidine. You should be on the lookout for signs of infection such as fever, chills or sore throat. If this problem is caught early, it can almost always be reversed, but if undetected it can be fatal. Another problem that has occurred in some patients taking ticlopidine is a decrease in cells called platelets (a condition called thrombocytopenia). This may occur as part of a syndrome that includes injury to red blood cells, causing anemia, kidney abnormalities, neurologic changes and fever. This condition is called TTP and can be fatal.

Things you should watch for as possible early signs of TTP are yellow skin or eye color, pinpoint dots (rash) on the skin, pale color, fever, weakness on a side of the body, or dark urine. **If any of these occur, contact your doctor immediately.**

Both complications occur most frequently in the first 90 days after TICLID is started. To make sure you don't develop either of these problems, your doctor will arrange for you to have your blood tested before you start taking TICLID and then every 2 weeks for the first 3 months you are on TICLID. If detected, neutropenia and thrombocytopenia can almost always be reversed. It is essential that you keep your appointments for the blood tests and that you call your doctor immediately if you have any indication that you may have TTP or neutropenia. If you stop taking TICLID for any reason within the first 3 months, you will still need to have your blood tested for an additional 2 weeks after you have stopped taking TICLID.

Other Warnings and Precautions: A few people may develop jaundice while being treated with TICLID. The signs of jaundice are yellowing of the skin or the whites of the eyes or consistent darkening of the urine or lightening in the color of the stools. These symptoms should be reported to your physician promptly.

If any of the symptoms described above for neutropenia, TTP or jaundice occur, contact your doctor immediately.

TICLID should be used only as directed by your doctor. Do not give TICLID to anyone else. **Keep TICLID out of reach of children!**

Some people may have such side effects as diarrhea, skin rash, stomach or intestinal discomfort. If any of these problems are persistent, or if you are concerned about them, bring them to your doctor's attention.

It may take longer than usual to stop bleeding when taking TICLID. Tell your doctor if you have any more bleeding or bruising than usual, and, if you have emergency surgery, be sure to let your doctor or dentist know that you are taking TICLID. Also, tell your doctor well in advance of any planned surgery (including tooth extraction), because he or she may recommend that you stop taking TICLID temporarily.

How TICLID Works: A stroke occurs when a clot (or thrombus) forms in a blood vessel in the brain or forms in another part of the body and breaks off, then travels to the brain (an embolus). In both cases the blood supply to part of the brain is blocked and that part of the brain is damaged. TICLID works by making the blood less likely to clot, although not so much less that it causes you to become likely to bleed, unless you have a bleeding disorder or some injury (such as a bleeding ulcer of the stomach or intestine) that is especially likely to bleed.

Who Should Not Take TICLID? Contact your doctor immediately and do not take TICLID if:

- you have an allergic reaction to TICLID
- you have a blood disorder or a serious bleeding problem, such as a bleeding stomach ulcer
- you have previously been told you had TTP
- you have severe liver disease or other liver problems
- you are pregnant or you are planning to become pregnant
- you are breastfeeding

Distributed by:
Roche Pharmaceuticals
Roche Laboratories Inc
340 Kingsland Street
Nutley, New Jersey 07110-1199

Revised: June 1999

Shown in Product Identification Guide, page 333

TORADOL® IV/IM ℞
[tō rah-dol]
(ketorolac tromethamine injection)
TORADOL® ORAL
(ketorolac tromethamine tablets)

The following text is complete prescribing information based on official labeling in effect June 2000.

WARNING

TORADOL, a nonsteroidal anti-inflammatory drug (NSAID), is indicated for the short-term (up to 5 days) management of moderately severe acute pain that requires analgesia at the opioid level. It is NOT indicated for minor or chronic painful conditions. TORADOL is a potent NSAID analgesic, and its administration carries many risks. The resulting NSAID-related adverse events can be serious in certain patients for whom TORADOL is indicated, especially when the drug is used inappropriately. Increasing the dose of TORADOL beyond the label recommendations will not provide better efficacy but will result in increasing the risk of developing serious adverse events.

GASTROINTESTINAL EFFECTS

- TORADOL can cause peptic ulcers, gastrointestinal bleeding and/or perforation. Therefore, TORADOL is CONTRAINDICATED in patients with active peptic ulcer disease, in patients with recent gastrointestinal bleeding or perforation, and in patients with a history of peptic ulcer disease or gastrointestinal bleeding.

RENAL EFFECTS

- TORADOL is CONTRAINDICATED in patients with advanced renal impairment and in patients at risk for renal failure due to volume depletion (see WARNINGS).

RISK OF BLEEDING

- TORADOL inhibits platelet function and is, therefore, CONTRAINDICATED in patients with suspected or confirmed cerebrovascular bleeding, patients with hemorrhagic diathesis, incomplete hemostasis and those at high risk of bleeding (see WARNINGS and PRECAUTIONS).
- TORADOL is CONTRAINDICATED as prophylactic analgesic before any major surgery and is CONTRAINDICATED intraoperatively when hemostasis is critical because of the increased risk of bleeding.

HYPERSENSITIVITY

- Hypersensitivity reactions, ranging from bronchospasm to anaphylactic shock, have occurred and appropriate counteractive measures must be available when administering the first dose of TORADOL IV/IM (see CONTRAINDICATIONS and WARNINGS). TORADOL is CONTRAINDICATED in patients with previously demonstrated hypersensitivity to ketorolac tromethamine or allergic manifestations to aspirin or other nonsteroidal anti-inflammatory drugs (NSAIDs).

INTRATHECAL OR EPIDURAL ADMINISTRATION

- TORADOL is CONTRAINDICATED for intrathecal or epidural administration due to its alcohol content.

LABOR, DELIVERY AND NURSING

- The use of TORADOL in labor and delivery is CONTRAINDICATED because it may adversely affect fetal circulation and inhibit uterine contractions.
- The use of TORADOL is CONTRAINDICATED in nursing mothers because of the potential adverse effects of prostaglandin-inhibiting drugs on neonates.

CONCOMITANT USE WITH NSAIDs

- TORADOL is CONTRAINDICATED in patients currently receiving ASA or NSAIDs because of the cumulative risk of inducing serious NSAID-related side effects.

DOSAGE AND ADMINISTRATION

TORADOL ORAL

- TORADOL ORAL is indicated only as continuation therapy to TORADOL IV/IM, and the combined duration of use of TORADOL IV/IM and TORADOL ORAL is not to exceed 5 days because of the increased risk of serious adverse events.
- The recommended total daily dose of TORADOL ORAL (maximum 40 mg) is significantly lower than for TORADOL IV/IM (maximum 120 mg) (see DOSAGE AND ADMINISTRATION and *Transition from TORADOL IV/IM to TORADOL ORAL*).

SPECIAL POPULATIONS

- Dosage should be adjusted for patients 65 years or older, for patients under 50 kg (110 lbs) of body weight (see DOSAGE AND ADMINISTRATION) and for patients with moderately elevated serum creatinine (see WARNINGS). Doses of TORADOL IV/IM are not to exceed 60 mg (total dose per day) in these patients.

DESCRIPTION

TORADOL (ketorolac tromethamine) is a member of the pyrrolo-pyrrole group of nonsteroidal anti-inflammatory drugs (NSAIDs). The chemical name for ketorolac tromethamine is (±)-5-benzoyl-2,3-dihydro-1H-pyrrolizine-1-carboxylic acid, compound with 2-amino-2-(hydroxymethyl)-1,3-propanediol.

TORADOL is a racemic mixture of [−]S and [+]R ketorolac tromethamine. Ketorolac tromethamine may exist in three crystal forms. All forms are equally soluble in water. Ketorolac tromethamine has a pKa of 3.5 and an n-octanol/water partition coefficient of 0.26. The molecular weight of ketorolac tromethamine is 376.41.

TORADOL is available for intravenous (IV) or intramuscular (IM) administration as: 15 mg in 1 mL (1.5%) and 30 mg in 1 mL (3%) in sterile solution; 60 mg in 2 mL (3%) of ketorolac tromethamine in sterile solution is available for IM administration only. For the TUBEX syringe units, the solutions contain 10% (w/v) alcohol, USP, and 6.68 mg, 4.35 mg and 8.70 mg, respectively, of sodium chloride in sterile water. For the vials, the solutions contain 0.1% citric acid, 10% (w/v) alcohol, USP, and 6.68 mg, 4.35 mg and 8.70 mg, respectively, of sodium chloride in sterile water. The pH is adjusted with sodium hydroxide or hydrochloric acid, and the solutions are packaged with nitrogen. The sterile solutions are clear and slightly yellow in color.

TORADOL ORAL is available as round, white, film-coated, red-printed tablets. Each tablet contains 10 mg ketorolac tromethamine, the active ingredient, with added lactose, magnesium stearate and microcrystalline cellulose. The white film-coating contains hydroxypropyl methylcellulose, polyethylene glycol and titanium dioxide.

The tablets are printed with red ink that includes FD&C Red #40 Aluminum lake as the colorant. There is a large T printed on both sides of the tablet, as well as the word TORADOL on one side, and the word ROCHE on the other.

CLINICAL PHARMACOLOGY

Pharmacodynamics: Ketorolac tromethamine is a nonsteroidal anti-inflammatory drug (NSAID). Ketorolac tromethamine inhibits synthesis of prostaglandins and may be considered a peripherally acting analgesic. The biological activity of ketorolac tromethamine is associated with the S-form. Ketorolac tromethamine possesses no sedative or anxiolytic properties.

Pain relief was statistically different after TORADOL dosing from that of placebo at $^1/_2$ hour (the first time point at which it was measured) following the largest recommended doses of TORADOL and by 1 hour following the smallest recommended doses. The peak analgesic effect occurred within 2 to 3 hours and was not statistically significantly different over the recommended dosage range of TORADOL. The greatest difference between large and small doses of TORADOL by either route was in the duration of analgesia.

Pharmacokinetics: Ketorolac tromethamine is a racemic mixture of [−]S- and [+]R-enantiomeric forms, with the S-form having analgesic activity.

Comparison of IV, IM and Oral Pharmacokinetics: The pharmacokinetics of ketorolac tromethamine, following IV, IM and oral doses of TORADOL, are compared in Table 1. The extent of bioavailability following administration of the oral and IM forms of TORADOL was equal to that following an IV bolus.

Linear Kinetics: Following administration of single ORAL, IM or IV doses of TORADOL in the recommended dosage ranges, the clearance of the racemate does not change. This implies that the pharmacokinetics of ketorolac tromethamine in humans, following single or multiple IM, IV or recommended oral doses of TORADOL, are linear. At the higher recommended doses, there is a proportional increase in the concentrations of free and bound racemate.

Binding and Distribution: The ketorolac tromethamine racemate has been shown to be highly protein bound (99%). Nevertheless, even plasma concentrations as high as 10 μg/mL will only occupy approximately 5% of the albumin binding sites. Thus, the unbound fraction for each enantiomer will be constant over the therapeutic range. A decrease in serum albumin, however, will result in increased free drug concentrations.

The mean apparent volume (Vβ) of ketorolac tromethamine following complete distribution was approximately 13 liters. This parameter was determined from single-dose data.

Metabolism: Ketorolac tromethamine is largely metabolized in the liver. The metabolic products are hydroxylated and conjugated forms of the parent drug. The products of metabolism, and some unchanged drug, are excreted in the urine.

Clearance and Excretion: A single-dose study with 10 mg TORADOL (n=9) demonstrated that the S-enantiomer is cleared approximately two times faster than the R-enantiomer and that the clearance was independent of the route of administration. This means that the ratio of S/R plasma concentrations decreases with time after each dose. There is little or no inversion of the R- to S- form in humans. The clearance of the racemate in normal subjects, elderly individuals and in hepatically and renally impaired patients is outlined in Table 2.

The half-life of the ketorolac tromethamine S-enantiomer was approximately 2.5 hours (SD ± 0.4) compared with 5 hours (SD ± 1.7) for the R-enantiomer. In other studies, the half-life for the racemate has been reported to lie within the range of 5 to 6 hours.

Continued on next page

Toradol—Cont.

Accumulation: TORADOL administered as an IV bolus every 6 hours for 5 days to healthy subjects (n=13), showed no significant difference in C_{max} on Day 1 and Day 5. Trough levels averaged 0.29 µg/mL (SD ± 0.13) on Day 1 and 0.55 µg/mL (SD ± 0.23) on Day 6. Steady state was approached after the fourth dose.

Accumulation of ketorolac tromethamine has not been studied in special populations (elderly patients, renal failure patients or hepatic disease patients).

Effect of Food: Oral administration of TORADOL after a high-fat meal resulted in decreased peak and delayed time-to-peak concentrations of ketorolac tromethamine by about 1 hour. Antacids did not affect the extent of absorption.

Kinetics in Special Populations: Elderly Patients: Based on single-dose data only, the half-life of the ketorolac tromethamine racemate increased from 5 to 7 hours in the elderly (65 to 78 years) compared with young healthy volunteers (24 to 35 years) (see Table 2). There was little difference in the C_{max} for the two groups (elderly, 2.52 µg/mL ± 0.77; young, 2.99 µg/mL ± 1.03) (see PRECAUTIONS—*Use in the Elderly*).

Renally Impaired Patients: Based on single-dose data only, the mean half-life of ketorolac tromethamine in renally impaired patients is between 6 and 19 hours and is dependent on the extent of the impairment. There is poor correlation between creatinine clearance and total ketorolac tromethamine clearance in the elderly and populations with renal impairment (r=0.5).

In patients with renal disease, the AUC_∞ of each enantiomer increased by approximately 100% compared with healthy volunteers. The volume of distribution doubles for the S-enantiomer and increases by 1/5th for the R-enantiomer. The increase in volume of distribution of ketorolac tromethamine implies an increase in unbound fraction.

The AUC_∞-ratio of the ketorolac tromethamine enantiomers in healthy subjects and patients remained similar, indicating there was no selective excretion of either enantiomer in patients compared to healthy subjects (see WARNINGS—*Renal Effects*).

Hepatic Effects: There was no significant difference in estimates of half-life, AUC_∞ and C_{max} in 7 patients with liver disease compared to healthy volunteers (see PRECAUTIONS—*Hepatic Effects*).

Clinical Studies: The analgesic efficacy of intramuscularly, intravenously and orally administered TORADOL was investigated in two postoperative pain models: general surgery (orthopedic, gynecologic and abdominal) and oral surgery (removal of impacted third molars). The studies were double-blind, single- and multiple-dose, parallel trial designs in patients with moderate to severe pain at baseline. TORADOL$^{\underline{IV/IM}}$ was compared as follows: IM to meperidine or morphine administered intramuscularly and IV to morphine administered either directly IV or through a PCA (Patient-Controlled Analgesia) pump.

Short-Term Use (up to 5 days) Studies: In the comparisons of intramuscular administration during the first hour, the onset of analgesic action was similar for TORADOL and the narcotics, but the duration of analgesia was longer with TORADOL than with the opioid comparators meperidine or morphine.

[See table 1 above]
[See table 2 at right]

Table 1
Table of Approximate Average Pharmacokinetic Parameters (Mean ± SD) Following Oral, Intramuscular and Intravenous Doses of TORADOL

Pharmacokinetic Parameters (units)	Oral*	Intramuscular†			Intravenous Bolus‡	
	10 mg	15 mg	30 mg	60 mg	15 mg	30 mg
Bioavailability (extent)	100%					
T_{max}[1] (min)	44 ± 34	33 ± 21§	44 ± 29	33 ± 21§	1.1 ± 0.7§	2.9 ± 1.8
C_{max}[2] (µg/mL) [single-dose]	0.87 ± 0.22	1.14 ± 0.32§	2.42 ± 0.68	4.55 ± 1.27§	2.47 ± 0.51§	4.65 ± 0.96
C_{max} (µg/mL) [steady state qid]	1.05 ± 0.26§	1.56 ± 0.44§	3.11 ± 0.87§	N/A″	3.09 ± 1.17§	6.85 ± 2.61
C_{min}[3] (µg/mL) [steady state qid]	0.29 ± 0.07§	0.47 ± 0.13§	0.93 ± 0.26§	N/A	0.61 ± 0.21§	1.04 ± 0.35
C_{avg}[4] (µg/mL) [steady state qid]	0.59 ± 0.20§	0.94 ± 0.29§	1.88 ± 0.59§	N/A	1.09 ± 0.30§	2.17 ± 0.59
$V\beta$[5] (L/kg)	—0.175 ± 0.039—				0.210 ± 0.044	

% Dose metabolized = <50 — % Dose excreted in feces = 6
% Dose excreted in urine = 91 — % Plasma protein binding = 99

[1]Time-to-peak plasma concentration
[2]Peak plasma concentration
[3]Trough plasma concentration
[4]Average plasma concentration
[5]Volume of distribution

* Derived from PO pharmacokinetic studies in 77 normal fasted volunteers
† Derived from IM pharmacokinetic studies in 54 normal volunteers
‡ Derived from IV pharmacokinetic studies in 24 normal volunteers
§ Mean value was simulated from observed plasma concentration data and standard deviation was simulated from percent coefficient of variation for observed C_{max} and T_{max} data
″ Not applicable because 60 mg is only recommended as a single dose

Table 2
The Influence of Age, Liver and Kidney Function, on the Clearance and Terminal Half-life of TORADOL (IM[1] and ORAL[2])

Type of Subjects	Total Clearance [In L/h/kg][3] IM Mean (range)	Total Clearance ORAL Mean (range)	Terminal Half-life [In hours] IM Mean (range)	Terminal Half-life ORAL Mean (range)
Normal Subjects IM (n=54) mean age=32, range=18–60 Oral (n=77) mean age=32, range=20–60	0.023 (0.010–0.046)	0.025 (0.013–0.050)	5.3 (3.5–9.2)	5.3 (2.4–9.0)
Healthy Elderly Subjects IM (n=13), Oral (n=12) mean age=72, range=65–78	0.019 (0.013–0.034)	0.024 (0.018–0.034)	7.0 (4.7–8.6)	6.1 (4.3–7.6)
Patients with Hepatic Dysfunction IM and Oral (n=7) mean age=51, range 43–64	0.029 (0.013–0.066)	0.033 (0.019–0.051)	5.4 (2.2–6.9)	4.5 (1.6–7.6)
Patients with Renal Impairment IM (n=25), Oral (n=9) serum creatinine=1.9–5.0 mg/dL, mean age (IM)=54, range=35–71 mean age (Oral)=57, range=39–70	0.015 (0.005–0.043)	0.016 (0.007–0.052)	10.3 (5.9–19.2)	10.8 (3.4–18.9)
Renal Dialysis Patients IM and Oral (n=9) mean age=40, range =27–63	0.016 (0.003–0.036)		13.6 (8.0–39.1)	—

[1]Estimated from 30 mg single IM doses of ketorolac tromethamine
[2]Estimated from 10 mg single oral doses of ketorolac tromethamine
[3]Liters/hour/kilogram

IV Administration: In normal subjects (n=37), the total clearance of 30 mg IV-administered TORADOL was 0.030 (0.017–0.051) L/h/kg. The terminal half-life was 5.6 (4.0–7.9) hours.

In a multidose, postoperative (general surgery) double-blind trial of TORADOL^{IM} 30 mg versus morphine 6 and 12 mg IM, each drug given on an as needed basis for up to 5 days, the overall analgesic effect of TORADOL^{IM} 30 mg was between that of morphine 6 and 12 mg. The majority of patients treated with either TORADOL or morphine were dosed for up to 3 days; a small percentage of patients received 5 days of dosing.

In clinical settings where perioperative morphine was allowed, TORADOL$^{\underline{IV}}$ 30 mg, given once or twice as needed, provided analgesia comparable to morphine 4 mg IV once or twice as needed.

There was relatively limited experience with 5 consecutive days of TORADOL$^{\underline{IV}}$ use in controlled clinical trials, as most patients were given the drug for 3 days or less. The adverse events seen with IV-administered TORADOL were similar to those observed with IM-administered TORADOL, as would be expected based on the similar pharmacokinetics and bioequivalence (AUC, clearance, plasma half-life) of IV and IM routes of TORADOL administration.

Clinical Studies with Concomitant Use of Opioids: Clinical studies in postoperative pain management have demonstrated that TORADOL$^{\underline{IV/IM}}$, when used in combination with opioids, significantly reduced opioid consumption. This combination may be useful in the subpopulation of patients especially prone to opioid-related complications. TORADOL and narcotics should not be administered in the same syringe.

In a postoperative study, where all patients received morphine by a PCA device, patients treated with TORADOL$^{\underline{IV}}$ as fixed intermittent boluses (eg, 30 mg initial dose followed by 15 mg q3h), required significantly less morphine (26%) than the placebo group. Analgesia was significantly superior, at various postdosing pain assessment times, in the patients receiving TORADOL^{IV} plus PCA morphine as compared to patients receiving PCA-administered morphine alone.

Postmarketing Surveillance Study: A large postmarketing observational, nonrandomized study, involving approximately 10,000 patients receiving TORADOL, demonstrated that the risk of clinically serious gastrointestinal (GI) bleeding was dose-dependent (see Tables 3A and 3B). This was particularly true in elderly patients who received an average daily dose greater than 60 mg/day of TORADOL (Table 3A).

Table 3
Incidence of Clinically Serious GI Bleeding as Related to Age, Total Daily Dose, and History of GI Perforation, Ulcer, Bleeding (PUB) after up to 5 Days of Treatment with TORADOL$^{\underline{IV/IM}}$

A. Patients without History of PUB

Age of Patients	Total Daily Dose of TORADOL$^{IV/IM}$ ≤60 mg	>60 to 90 mg	>90 to 120 mg	>120 mg
<65 years of age	0.4%	0.4%	0.9%	4.6%
≥65 years of age	1.2%	2.8%	2.2%	7.7%

B. Patients with History of PUB

Age of Patients	Total Daily Dose of TORADOL$^{IV/IM}$ ≤60 mg	>60 to 90 mg	>90 to 120 mg	>120 mg
<65 years of age	2.1%	4.6%	7.8%	15.4%
≥65 years of age	4.7%	3.7%	2.8%	25.0%

INDICATIONS AND USAGE

TORADOL is indicated for the short-term (≤5 days) management of moderately severe acute pain that requires analgesia at the opioid level, usually in a postoperative setting. Therapy should always be initiated with TORADOL$^{\underline{IV/IM}}$, and TORADOL$^{\underline{ORAL}}$ is to be used only as continuation treatment, if necessary. Combined use of TORADOL$^{\underline{IV/IM}}$ and TORADOL$^{\underline{ORAL}}$ is not to exceed 5 days of use because of the potential of increasing the frequency and severity of adverse reactions associated with the recommended doses (see WARNINGS, PRECAUTIONS, DOSAGE AND ADMINISTRATION and ADVERSE REACTIONS). Patients should be switched to alternative analgesics as soon as possible, but TORADOL therapy is not to exceed 5 days.

TORADOL$^{IV/IM}$ has been used concomitantly with morphine and meperidine and has shown an opioid-sparing effect. For breakthrough pain, it is recommended to supplement the lower end of the TORADOL$^{IV/IM}$ dosage range with low doses of narcotics prn, unless otherwise contraindicated. TORADOL$^{IV/IM}$ and narcotics should not be administered in the same syringe (see DOSAGE AND ADMINISTRATION: *Pharmaceutical Information for TORADOL$^{IV/IM}$*).

CONTRAINDICATIONS

(see also Boxed WARNING):

- TORADOL is CONTRAINDICATED in patients with active peptic ulcer disease, in patients with recent gastrointestinal bleeding or perforation and in patients with a history of peptic ulcer disease or gastrointestinal bleeding.
- TORADOL is CONTRAINDICATED in patients with advanced renal impairment or in patients at risk for renal failure due to volume depletion (see WARNINGS for correction of volume depletion).
- TORADOL is CONTRAINDICATED in labor and delivery because, through its prostaglandin synthesis inhibitory effect, it may adversely affect fetal circulation and inhibit uterine contractions, thus increasing the risk of uterine hemorrhage.
- The use of TORADOL is CONTRAINDICATED in nursing mothers because of the potential adverse effects of prostaglandin-inhibiting drugs on neonates.
- TORADOL is CONTRAINDICATED in patients with previously demonstrated hypersensitivity to ketorolac tromethamine, allergic manifestations to aspirin or other nonsteroidal anti-inflammatory drugs (NSAIDs).
- TORADOL is CONTRAINDICATED as prophylactic analgesic before any major surgery and is CONTRAINDICATED intraoperatively when hemostasis is critical because of the increased risk of bleeding.
- TORADOL inhibits platelet function and is, therefore, CONTRAINDICATED in patients with suspected or confirmed cerebrovascular bleeding, hemorrhagic diathesis, incomplete hemostasis and those at high risk of bleeding (see WARNINGS and PRECAUTIONS).
- TORADOL is CONTRAINDICATED in patients currently receiving ASA or NSAIDs because of the cumulative risks of inducing serious NSAID-related adverse events.
- TORADOL$^{IV/IM}$ is CONTRAINDICATED for neuraxial (epidural or intrathecal) administration due to its alcohol content.
- The concomitant use of TORADOL and probenecid is CONTRAINDICATED.

WARNINGS

(see also Boxed WARNING):

The combined use of TORADOL$^{IV/IM}$ and TORADOL^{ORAL} is not to exceed 5 days.

The most serious risks associated with TORADOL are:

- ***Gastrointestinal Ulcerations, Bleeding and Perforation:*** TORADOL is CONTRAINDICATED in patients with previously documented peptic ulcers and/or GI bleeding. Serious gastrointestinal toxicity, such as bleeding, ulceration and perforation, can occur at any time, with or without warning symptoms, in patients treated with TORADOL. Studies to date with NSAIDs have not identified any subset of patients not at risk of developing peptic ulceration and bleeding. Elderly or debilitated patients seem to tolerate ulceration or bleeding less well than other individuals, and most spontaneous reports of fatal GI events are in this population. Postmarketing experience with parenterally administered TORADOL suggests that there may be a greater risk of gastrointestinal ulcerations, bleeding and perforation in the elderly.

  The incidence and severity of gastrointestinal complications increases with increasing dose of, and duration of treatment with, TORADOL. In a nonrandomized, in-hospital postmarketing surveillance study comparing parenteral TORADOL to parenteral opioids, higher rates of clinically serious GI bleeding were seen in patients <65 years of age who received an average total daily dose of more than 90 mg of TORADOL$^{IV/IM}$ per day (see CLINICAL PHARMACOLOGY: *Postmarketing Surveillance Study*).

  The same study showed that elderly (≥65 years of age) and debilitated patients are more susceptible to gastrointestinal complications. A history of peptic ulcer disease was revealed as another risk factor that increases the possibility of developing serious gastrointestinal complications during TORADOL therapy (see Tables 3A and 3B).
- ***Impaired Renal Function: TORADOL should be used with caution in patients with impaired renal function or a history of kidney disease because it is a potent inhibitor of prostaglandin synthesis.*** Renal toxicity with TORADOL has been seen in patients with conditions leading to a reduction in blood volume and/or renal blood flow where renal prostaglandins have a supportive role in the maintenance of renal perfusion. In these patients administration of TORADOL may cause a dose-dependent reduction in renal prostaglandin formation and may precipitate acute renal failure. Patients at greatest risk of this reaction are those with impaired renal function, dehydration, heart failure, liver dysfunction, those taking diuretics and the elderly. Discontinuation of TORADOL therapy is usually followed by recovery to the pretreatment state.

  Renal Effects: TORADOL and its metabolites are eliminated primarily by the kidneys, which, in patients with reduced creatinine clearance, will result in diminished clearance of the drug (see CLINICAL PHARMACOLOGY). Therefore, TORADOL should be used with caution in patients with impaired renal function (see DOSAGE AND ADMINISTRATION) and such patients should be followed closely. With the use of TORADOL, there have been reports of acute renal failure, nephritis and nephrotic syndrome.

  Because patients with underlying renal insufficiency are at increased risk of developing acute renal failure, the risks and benefits should be assessed prior to giving TORADOL to these patients. Hence, in patients with moderately elevated serum creatinine, it is recommended that the daily dose of TORADOL$^{IV/IM}$ be reduced by half, not to exceed 60 mg/day. **TORADOL IS CONTRAINDICATED IN PATIENTS WITH SERUM CREATININE CONCENTRATIONS INDICATING ADVANCED RENAL IMPAIRMENT** (see CONTRAINDICATIONS).

  Hypovolemia should be corrected before treatment with TORADOL is initiated.
- ***Fluid Retention and Edema:*** Fluid retention, edema, retention of NaCl, oliguria, elevations of serum urea nitrogen and creatinine have been reported in clinical trials with TORADOL. Therefore, TORADOL should be used only very cautiously in patients with cardiac decompensation, hypertension or similar conditions.
- ***Hemorrhage:*** Because prostaglandins play an important role in hemostasis and NSAIDs affect platelet aggregation as well, use of TORADOL in patients who have coagulation disorders should be undertaken very cautiously, and those patients should be carefully monitored. Patients on therapeutic doses of anticoagulants (eg, heparin or dicumarol derivatives) have an increased risk of bleeding complications if given TORADOL concurrently; therefore, physicians should administer such concomitant therapy only extremely cautiously. The concurrent use of TORADOL and prophylactic low-dose heparin (2500 to 5000 units q12h), warfarin and dextrans have not been studied extensively, but may also be associated with an increased risk of bleeding. Until data from such studies are available, physicians should carefully weigh the benefits against the risks and use such concomitant therapy in these patients only extremely cautiously. In patients who receive anticoagulants for any reason, there is an increased risk of intramuscular hematoma formation from administered TORADOL^{IM} (see PRECAUTIONS: *Drug Interactions*). Patients receiving therapy that affects hemostasis should be monitored closely.

  In postmarketing experience, postoperative hematomas and other signs of wound bleeding have been reported in association with the perioperative use of TORADOL$^{IV/IM}$. Therefore, perioperative use of TORADOL should be avoided and postoperative use be undertaken with caution when hemostasis is critical (see WARNINGS and PRECAUTIONS).
- ***Anaphylactoid Reactions:*** Anaphylactoid reactions may occur in patients without a known previous exposure or hypersensitivity to aspirin, TORADOL or other NSAIDs, or in individuals with a history of angioedema, bronchospastic reactivity (eg, asthma) and nasal polyps. Anaphylactoid reactions, like anaphylaxis, may have a fatal outcome.

PRECAUTIONS

General:

- *Hepatic Effects: TORADOL should be used with caution in patients with impaired hepatic function or a history of liver disease.* Treatment with TORADOL may cause elevations of liver enzymes, and, in patients with preexisting liver dysfunction, it may lead to the development of a more severe hepatic reaction. The administration of TORADOL should be discontinued in patients in whom an abnormal liver test has occurred as a result of TORADOL therapy.
- *Hematologic Effects:* TORADOL inhibits platelet aggregation and may prolong bleeding time; therefore, it is contraindicated as a preoperative medication, and caution should be used when hemostasis is critical. Unlike aspirin, the inhibition of platelet function by TORADOL disappears within 24 to 48 hours after the drug is discontinued. TORADOL does not appear to affect platelet count, prothrombin time (PT) or partial thromboplastin time (PTT). In controlled clinical studies, where TORADOL was administered intramuscularly or intravenously postoperatively, the incidence of clinically significant postoperative bleeding was 0.4% for TORADOL compared to 0.2% in the control groups receiving narcotic analgesics.

Information for Patients: TORADOL is a potent NSAID and may cause serious side effects such as gastrointestinal bleeding or kidney failure, which may result in hospitalization and even fatal outcome.

Physicians, when prescribing TORADOL, should inform their patients of the potential risks of TORADOL treatment (see Boxed WARNING, WARNINGS, PRECAUTIONS and ADVERSE REACTIONS sections). *Advise patients not to give TORADOL^{ORAL} to other family members and to discard any unused drug.*

Remember that the total duration of TORADOL therapy is not to exceed 5 days.

Drug Interactions: Ketorolac is highly bound to human plasma protein (mean 99.2%).

The in vitro binding of ***warfarin*** to plasma proteins is only slightly reduced by ketorolac tromethamine (99.5% control vs 99.3%) when ketorolac plasma concentrations reach 5 to 10 µg/mL. Ketorolac does not alter ***digoxin*** protein binding. In vitro studies indicate that, at therapeutic concentrations of ***salicylate*** (300 µg/mL), the binding of ketorolac was reduced from approximately 99.2% to 97.5%, representing a potential twofold increase in unbound ketorolac plasma levels. Therapeutic concentrations of ***digoxin, warfarin, ibuprofen, naproxen, piroxicam, acetaminophen, phenytoin*** and ***tolbutamide*** did not alter ketorolac tromethamine protein binding.

In a study involving 12 volunteers, TORADOL^{ORAL} was coadministered with a single dose of 25 mg ***warfarin***, causing no significant changes in pharmacokinetics or pharmacodynamics of warfarin. In another study, TORADOL$^{IV/IM}$ was given with two doses of 5000 U of ***heparin*** to 11 healthy volunteers, resulting in a mean template bleeding time of 6.4 minutes (3.2 to 11.4 min) compared to a mean of 6.0 minutes (3.4 to 7.5 min) for heparin alone and 5.1 minutes (3.5 to 8.5 min) for placebo. Although these results do not indicate a significant interaction between TORADOL and warfarin or heparin, the administration of TORADOL to patients taking anticoagulants should be done extremely cautiously, and patients should be closely monitored (see WARNINGS and PRECAUTIONS).

TORADOL$^{IV/IM}$ reduced the diuretic response to ***furosemide*** in normovolemic healthy subjects by approximately 20% (mean sodium and urinary output decreased 17%).

Concomitant administration of TORADOL^{ORAL} and ***probenecid*** resulted in decreased clearance of ketorolac and significant increases in ketorolac plasma levels (total AUC increased approximately threefold from 5.4 to 17.8 µg/h/mL) and terminal half-life increased approximately twofold from 6.6 to 15.1 hours. Therefore, concomitant use of TORADOL and probenecid is contraindicated.

Inhibition of renal ***lithium*** clearance, leading to an increase in plasma lithium concentration, has been reported with some prostaglandin synthesis-inhibiting drugs. The effect of TORADOL on plasma lithium has not been studied, but cases of increased lithium plasma levels during TORADOL therapy have been reported.

Concomitant administration of ***methotrexate*** and some NSAIDs has been reported to reduce the clearance of methotrexate, enhancing the toxicity of methotrexate. The effect of TORADOL on methotrexate clearance has not been studied.

In postmarketing experience there have been reports of a possible interaction between TORADOL$^{IV/IM}$ and ***nondepolarizing muscle relaxants*** that resulted in apnea. The concurrent use of TORADOL with muscle relaxants has not been formally studied.

Concomitant use of ***ACE inhibitors*** may increase the risk of renal impairment, particularly in volume-depleted patients.

Sporadic cases of seizures have been reported during concomitant use of TORADOL and ***antiepileptic drugs*** (phenytoin, carbamazepine).

Hallucinations have been reported when TORADOL was used in patients taking ***psychoactive drugs*** (fluoxetine, thiothixene, alprazolam).

TORADOL$^{IV/IM}$ has been administered concurrently with ***morphine*** in several clinical trials of postoperative pain without evidence of adverse interactions. Do not mix TORADOL and morphine in the same syringe.

There is no evidence in animal or human studies that TORADOL induces or inhibits hepatic enzymes capable of metabolizing itself or other drugs.

Carcinogenesis, Mutagenesis and Impairment of Fertility: An 18-month study in mice with oral doses of ketorolac tromethamine at 2 mg/kg/day (0.9 times the human systemic exposure at the recommended IM or IV dose of 30 mg qid, based on area-under-the-plasma-concentration curve [AUC]), and a 24-month study in rats at 5 mg/kg/day (0.5 times the human AUC) showed no evidence of tumorigenicity.

Ketorolac tromethamine was not mutagenic in the Ames test, unscheduled DNA synthesis and repair, and in forward mutation assays. Ketorolac tromethamine did not cause chromosome breakage in the in vivo mouse micronucleus assay. At 1590 µg/mL and at higher concentrations, ketorolac tromethamine increased the incidence of chromosomal aberrations in Chinese hamster ovarian cells.

Impairment of fertility did not occur in male or female rats at oral doses of 9 mg/kg (0.9 times the human AUC) and 16 mg/kg (1.6 times the human AUC) of ketorolac tromethamine, respectively.

Pregnancy: Pregnancy Category C. Reproduction studies have been performed during organogenesis using daily oral doses of ketorolac tromethamine at 3.6 mg/kg (0.37 times the human AUC) in rabbits and at 10 mg/kg (1.0 times the human AUC) in rats. Results of these studies did not reveal evidence of teratogenicity to the fetus. Oral doses of ketorolac tromethamine at 1.5 mg/kg (0.14 times the human AUC), administered after gestation Day 17, caused dystocia and higher pup mortality in rats. There are no adequate and well-controlled studies of TORADOL in pregnant women. TORADOL should be used during pregnancy only if the potential benefit justifies the potential risk to the fetus.

Labor and Delivery: The use of TORADOL is contraindicated in labor and delivery because, through its prostaglandin synthesis inhibitory effect, it may adversely affect fetal circulation and inhibit uterine contractions, thus increasing the risk of uterine hemorrhage (see CONTRAINDICATIONS).

Continued on next page

Toradol—Cont.

Lactation and Nursing: After a single administration of 10 mg of TORADOL^{ORAL} to humans, the maximum milk concentration observed was 7.3 ng/mL, and the maximum milk-to-plasma ratio was 0.037. After 1 day of dosing (qid), the maximum milk concentration was 7.9 ng/mL, and the maximum milk-to-plasma ratio was 0.025. Because of the possible adverse effects of prostaglandin-inhibiting drugs on neonates, use in nursing mothers is contraindicated.

Pediatric Use: Safety and efficacy in children (less than 16 years of age) have not been established. Therefore, use of TORADOL in children is not recommended.

Use in the Elderly (≥65 years of age): Because ketorolac tromethamine may be cleared more slowly by the elderly (see CLINICAL PHARMACOLOGY) who are also more sensitive to the adverse effects of NSAIDs (see WARNINGS: *Renal Effects*), extra caution and reduced dosages (see DOSAGE AND ADMINISTRATION) must be used when treating the elderly with TORADOL$^{IV/IM}$. The lower end of the TORADOL$^{IV/IM}$ dosage range is recommended for patients over 65 years of age, and total daily dose is not to exceed 60 mg. The incidence and severity of gastrointestinal complications increases with increasing dose of, and duration of treatment with, TORADOL.

ADVERSE REACTIONS

Adverse reaction rates increase with higher doses of TORADOL. Practitioners should be alert for the severe complications of treatment with TORADOL, such as GI ulceration, bleeding and perforation, postoperative bleeding, acute renal failure, anaphylactic and anaphylactoid reactions and liver failure (see Boxed WARNING, WARNINGS, PRECAUTIONS and DOSAGE AND ADMINISTRATION). These NSAID-related complications can be serious in certain patients for whom TORADOL is indicated, especially when the drug is used inappropriately.

The Adverse Reactions Listed Below Were Reported In Clinical Trials As Probably Related To TORADOL:

- ***Incidence Greater Than 1%***

Percentage of incidence in parentheses for those events reported in 3% or more patients.

Body as a Whole: edema (4%)
Cardiovascular: hypertension
Dermatologic: pruritus, rash
Gastrointestinal: nausea (12%), dyspepsia (12%), gastrointestinal pain (13%), diarrhea (7%), constipation, flatulence, gastrointestinal fullness, vomiting, stomatitis
Hemic and Lymphatic: purpura
Nervous System: headache (17%), drowsiness (6%), dizziness (7%), sweating
Injection-site pain was reported by 2% of patients in multidose studies.

- ***Incidence 1% or Less***

Body as a Whole: weight gain, fever, infections, asthenia
Cardiovascular: palpitation, pallor, syncope
Dermatologic: urticaria
Gastrointestinal: gastritis, rectal bleeding, eructation, anorexia, increased appetite
Hemic and Lymphatic: epistaxis, anemia, eosinophilia
Nervous System: tremors, abnormal dreams, hallucinations, euphoria, extrapyramidal symptoms, vertigo, paresthesia, depression, insomnia, nervousness, excessive thirst, dry mouth, abnormal thinking, inability to concentrate, hyperkinesis, stupor
Respiratory: dyspnea, pulmonary edema, rhinitis, cough
Special Senses: abnormal taste, abnormal vision, blurred vision, tinnitus, hearing loss
Urogenital: hematuria, proteinuria, oliguria, urinary retention, polyuria, increased urinary frequency

The Following Adverse Events Were Reported From Postmarketing Experience:

Body as a Whole: hypersensitivity reactions such as anaphylaxis, anaphylactoid reaction, laryngeal edema, tongue edema (see Boxed WARNING, WARNINGS), myalgia
Cardiovascular: hypotension, flushing
Dermatologic: Lyell's syndrome, Stevens-Johnson syndrome, exfoliative dermatitis, maculopapular rash, urticaria
Gastrointestinal: peptic ulceration, GI hemorrhage, GI perforation (see Boxed WARNING, WARNINGS), melena, acute pancreatitis
Hemic and Lymphatic: postoperative wound hemorrhage (rarely requiring blood transfusion—see Boxed WARNING, WARNINGS and PRECAUTIONS), thrombocytopenia, leukopenia
Hepatic: hepatitis, liver failure, cholestatic jaundice
Nervous System: convulsions, psychosis, aseptic meningitis
Respiratory: asthma, bronchospasm
Urogenital: acute renal failure (see Boxed WARNING, WARNINGS), flank pain with or without hematuria and/or azotemia, nephritis, hyponatremia, hyperkalemia, hemolytic uremic syndrome

OVERDOSAGE

In controlled overdosage, daily doses of 360 mg of TORADOL$^{IV/IM}$ given for 5 days (three times the highest recommended dose), caused abdominal pain and peptic ulcers which healed after discontinuation of dosing. Metabolic acidosis has been reported following intentional overdosage. Dialysis does not significantly clear ketorolac tromethamine from the blood stream.

DOSAGE AND ADMINISTRATION

THE COMBINED DURATION OF USE OF TORADOL$^{IV/IM}$ AND TORADOL^{ORAL} IS NOT TO EXCEED 5 DAYS.

THE USE OF TORADOL^{ORAL} IS ONLY INDICATED AS CONTINUATION THERAPY TO TORADOL$^{IV/IM}$.

TORADOL$^{IV/IM}$

TORADOL$^{IV/IM}$ may be used as a single or multiple dose on a regular or prn schedule for the management of moderately severe acute pain that requires analgesia at the opioid level, usually in a postoperative setting. Hypovolemia should be corrected prior to the administration of TORADOL (see WARNINGS: *Renal Effects*). Patients should be switched to alternative analgesics as soon as possible, but TORADOL therapy is not to exceed 5 days.

When administering TORADOL$^{IV/IM}$, the IV bolus must be given over no less than 15 seconds. The IM administration should be given slowly and deeply into the muscle. The analgesic effect begins in 30 minutes with maximum effect in 1 to 2 hours after dosing IV or IM. Duration of analgesic effect is usually 4 to 6 hours.

Single-Dose Treatment: The Following Regimen Should Be Limited To Single Administration Use Only

IM Dosing:

- *Patients <65 years of age:* One dose of 60 mg.
- *Patients ≥65 years of age, renally impaired and/or less than 50 kg (110 lbs) of body weight:* One dose of 30 mg.

IV Dosing:

- *Patients <65 years of age:* One dose of 30 mg.
- *Patients ≥65 years of age, renally impaired and/or less than 50 kg (110 lbs) of body weight:* One dose of 15 mg.

Multiple-Dose Treatment (IV or IM)

- *Patients <65 years of age:* The recommended dose is 30 mg TORADOL$^{IV/IM}$ every 6 hours. The maximum daily dose should not exceed 120 mg.
- *For Patients ≥65 years of age, renally impaired patients (see WARNINGS) and patients less than 50 kg (110 lbs):* The recommended dose is 15 mg TORADOL$^{IV/IM}$ every 6 hours. The maximum daily dose for these populations should not exceed 60 mg.

For breakthrough pain do not increase the dose or the frequency of TORADOL. Consideration should be given to supplementing these regimens with low doses of opioids prn unless otherwise contraindicated.

Pharmaceutical Information for TORADOL$^{IV/IM}$: Parenteral drug products should be inspected visually for particulate matter and discoloration prior to administration whenever solution and container permit.

TORADOL$^{IV/IM}$ should not be mixed in a small volume (eg, in a syringe) with morphine sulfate, meperidine hydrochloride, promethazine hydrochloride or hydroxyzine hydrochloride; this will result in precipitation of ketorolac from solution.

TORADOL^{ORAL} is indicated ONLY as continuation therapy to TORADOL$^{IV/IM}$ for the management of moderately severe acute pain that requires analgesia at the opioid level (see also PRECAUTIONS: *Information for Patients*).

Transition from TORADOL$^{IV/IM}$ to TORADOL^{ORAL}: The recommended TORADOL^{ORAL} dose is as follows:

- *Patients <65 years of age:* 2 tablets as a first oral dose for patients who received **60 mg IM single dose, 30 mg IV single dose or 30 mg multiple dose.** TORADOL$^{IV/IM}$ followed by 1 tablet TORADOL^{ORAL} every 4 to 6 hours, not to exceed 40 mg/24 h of TORADOL^{ORAL}
- *Patients ≥65 years of age, renally impaired and/or less than 50 kg (110 lbs) of body weight:* 1 tablet as a first oral dose for patients who received **30 mg IM single dose, 15 mg IV single dose or 15 mg multiple dose.** TORADOL$^{IV/IM}$ followed by 1 tablet TORADOL^{ORAL} every 4 to 6 hours, not to exceed 40 mg/24 h of TORADOL^{ORAL}.

Shortening the recommended dosing intervals may result in increased frequency and severity of adverse reactions.

The maximum combined duration of use (parenteral and oral TORADOL) is limited to 5 days.

The TUBEX® BLUNT POINTE™ Sterile Cartridge Unit is suitable for substances to be administered intravenously only. It is intended for use with injection sets specifically manufactured as "needle-less" injection systems. TUBEX® BLUNT POINTE™ is compatible with Abbott's LifeShield® prepierced reseal injection site, Baxter's InterLink® Injection Site, and B. Braun Medical's SafSite® Reflux Valve. Consult manufacturer's recommendations regarding "Directions for Use" of the "needle-less" system. It is also intended for admixture with, and convenient administration of, various medicaments when using Drug Vial Adapters for "needle-less" injection systems.

The TUBEX® Sterile Cartridge-Needle Unit and sterile vial are suitable for substances to be administered intravenously and intramuscularly.

HOW SUPPLIED

TORADOL$^{IV/IM}$ for intramuscular or intravenous use is available in a TUBEX® Cartridge-Needle Unit or a sterial vial:

15 mg: 15 mg/mL, 1 mL TUBEX® Sterile Cartridge-Needle Unit (22 gauge × 1-1/4 inch needle) box of 10 (NDC 0004-6921-06) or 1 mL fill per 2 mL single use vial, box of 10 (NDC 0004-6925-06).

30 mg: 30 mg/mL, 1 mL TUBEX® Sterile Cartridge-Needle Unit (22 gauge × 1-1/4 inch needle) box of 10 (NDC 0004-6923-06) or 1 mL fill per 2 mL single use vial, box of 10 (NDC 0004-6926-06).

For IM Single-Dose Use Only Not Intended for IV Use—60 mg: 30 mg/mL, 2 mL TUBEX® Sterile Cartridge-Needle Unit (22 gauge × 1-1/4 inch needle) box of 1 (NDC 0004-6924-09 or 2 mL fill per 2 mL single use vial, box of 1 (NDC 0004-6927-09).

TORADOL^{IV} for intravenous use is available in a TUBEX® BLUNT POINTE™ Sterile Cartridge Unit:

15 mg: 15 mg/mL, 1 mL TUBEX® BLUNT POINTE™ Sterile Cartridge Unit, box of 10 (NDC 0004-6920-06).

30 mg: 30 mg/mL, 1 mL TUBEX® BLUNT POINTE™ Sterile Cartridge Unit, box of 10 (NDC 0004-6922-06).

Syringes manufactured by Wyeth Laboratories, Inc., Philadelphia, PA 19101 for Roche Laboratories Inc., Nutley, NJ 07110.

Vials manufactured by Hoffmann-La Roche Inc., Nutley, NJ 07110.

Store at 15° to 30°C (59° to 86°F) with protection from light.

TORADOL^{ORAL} 10 mg tablets are available in bottles of 100 tablets (NDC 0004-0273-01).

Store bottles at 15° to 30°C (59° to 86°F).

Manufactured by Syntex Puerto Rico, Inc., Humacao, PR 00791

TUBEX® Injector

NOTE: The TUBEX® Injector is reusable: do not discard.

TUBEX® Sterile Cartridge-Needle Unit
DIRECTIONS FOR USE

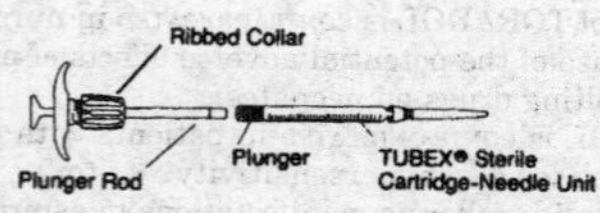

TUBEX® BLUNT POINTE™ Sterile Cartridge Unit
DIRECTIONS FOR USE:

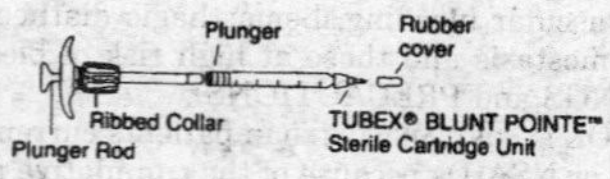

TUBEX® BLUNT POINTE™ Sterile Cartridge Unit is intended for use with injection sets specifically manufactured as "needle-less" injection systems.

TUBEX® BLUNT POINTE™ Sterile Cartridge Unit is compatible with Abbott's LifeShield® prepierced reseal injection site, Baxter's InterLink® Injection Site and B. Braun Medical's SafSite® Reflux Valve. Consult manufacturer's recommendations regarding "Directions for Use" of the "needle-less" injection system.

To load a TUBEX® Sterile Cartridge Unit into the TUBEX® Injector

1. Turn the ribbed collar to the "OPEN" position until it stops.

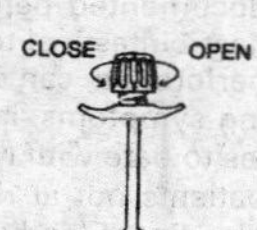

2. Hold the Injector with the open end

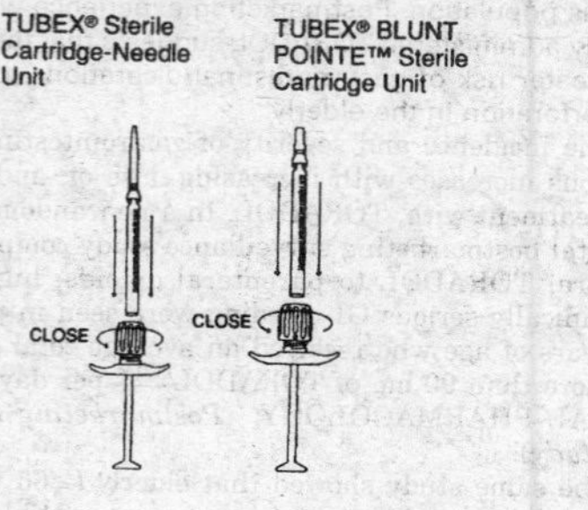

up and fully insert the TUBEX® Sterile Cartridge Unit. Firmly tighten the ribbed collar in the direction of the "CLOSE" arrow.

3. Thread the plunger rod into the plunger of the TUBEX® Sterile Cartridge Unit until slight resistance is felt. The Injector is now ready for use in the usual manner.

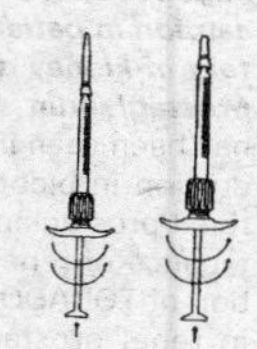

To administer TUBEX® Sterile Cartridge-Needle Units

Method of administration is the same as with conventional syringe. Remove needle cover by grasping it securely; twist and pull. Introduce needle into patient, aspirate by pulling back slightly on the plunger, and inject.

To administer TUBEX® BLUNT POINTE™ Sterile Cartridge Units

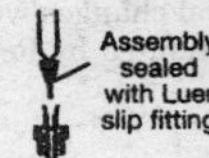

"Needle-less" IV set administration is similar to administration with conventional syringes. Remove rubber cover by grasping it securely; twist and pull. For B. Braun Medical's SafSite® Reflux Valves, aseptically swab the luer slip fitting of the BLUNT POINTE™ sterile cartridge tip assembly with a sterile, individually wrapped, saturated 70% Isopropyl Alcohol swab. This action will remove the lubricant coating from the tip to facilitate a tight seal. Introduce TUBEX® BLUNT POINTE™ Sterile Cartridge Unit into the "needle-less" IV set as per manufacturer's "Directions for Use."

To remove the empty TUBEX® Cartridge Unit and dispose into a vertical disposal container

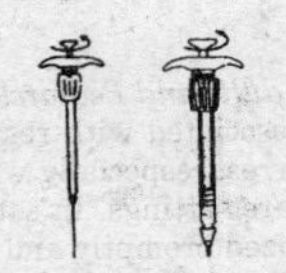

1. Do not recap the needle/point. Disengage the plunger rod.

2. Hold the Injector, needle/point down, over a vertical disposal container and loosen the ribbed collar. TUBEX® Cartridge Unit will drop into the container.

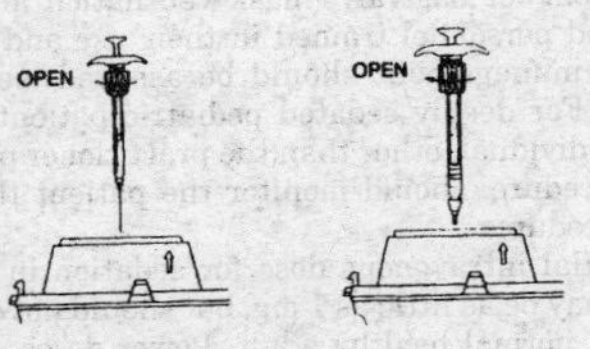

3. Discard the cover.

To remove the empty TUBEX® Cartridge Unit and dispose into a horizontal (mailbox) disposal container

1. Do not recap the needle/point. Disengage the plunger rod.
2. Open the horizontal (mailbox) disposal container. Insert TUBEX® Cartridge Unit, needle/point pointing down, halfway into container. Close the container lid on cartridge. Loosen ribbed collar; TUBEX® Cartridge Unit will drop into the container.

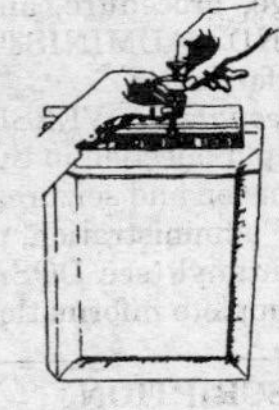

3. Discard the cover.

The TUBEX® Injector is reusable and should not be discarded.

Used TUBEX® Cartridge Units should not be employed for successive injections or as multiple-dose containers. They are intended to be used only once and discarded.

NOTE: Any graduated markings on TUBEX® Sterile Cartridge Units are to be used only as a guide in mixing, withdrawing, or administering measured doses.

Wyeth-Ayerst does not recommend and will not accept responsibility for the use of any cartridge-needle units or needle-less units other than TUBEX® Cartridge Units in the TUBEX® Injector.

Revised August 1997

Shown in Product Identification Guide, page 333

VALIUM® Ⓒ

[val 'ee-um]

brand of diazepam

INJECTION

The following text is complete prescribing information based on official labeling in effect June 2000.

DESCRIPTION

Each mL contains 5 mg diazepam compounded with 40% propylene glycol, 10% ethyl alcohol, 5% sodium benzoate and benzoic acid as buffers, and 1.5% benzyl alcohol as preservative.

Diazepam is a benzodiazepine derivative developed through original Roche research. Chemically, diazepam is 7-chloro-1, 3-dihydro-1-methyl-5-phenyl-2H-1,4-benzodiazepin-2-one. It is a colorless crystalline compound, insoluble in water and has a molecular weight of 284.74.

ACTIONS

In animals, diazepam appears to act on parts of the limbic system, the thalamus and hypothalamus, and induces calming effects. Diazepam, unlike chlorpromazine and reserpine, has no demonstrable peripheral autonomic blocking action, nor does it produce extrapyramidal side effects; however, animals treated with diazepam do have a transient ataxia at higher doses. Diazepam was found to have transient cardiovascular depressor effects in dogs. Long-term experiments in rats revealed no disturbances of endocrine function. Injections into animals have produced localized irritation of tissue surrounding injection sites and some thickening of veins after intravenous use.

INDICATIONS

Valium is indicated for the management of anxiety disorders or for the short-term relief of the symptoms of anxiety. Anxiety or tension associated with the stress of everyday life usually does not require treatment with an anxiolytic.

In acute alcohol withdrawal, Valium may be useful in the symptomatic relief of acute agitation, tremor, impending or acute delirium tremens and hallucinosis.

As an adjunct prior to endoscopic procedures if apprehension, anxiety or acute stress reactions are present, and to diminish the patient's recall of the procedures. (See WARNINGS.)

Valium is a useful adjunct for the relief of skeletal muscle spasm due to reflex spasm to local pathology (such as inflammation of the muscles or joints, or secondary to trauma); spasticity caused by upper motor neuron disorders (such as cerebral palsy and paraplegia); athetosis; stiff-man syndrome; and tetanus.

Valium Injection is a useful adjunct in status epilepticus and severe recurrent convulsive seizures.

Valium is a useful premedication (the IM route is preferred) for relief of anxiety and tension in patients who are to undergo surgical procedures. Intravenously, prior to cardioversion for the relief of anxiety and tension and to diminish the patient's recall of the procedure.

CONTRAINDICATIONS

Valium Injection is contraindicated in patients with a known hypersensitivity to this drug; acute narrow angle glaucoma; and open angle glaucoma unless patients are receiving appropriate therapy.

WARNINGS

When used intravenously, the following procedures should be undertaken to reduce the possibility of venous thrombosis, phlebitis, local irritation, swelling, and, rarely, vascular impairment: the solution should be injected slowly, taking at least 1 minute for each 5 mg (1 mL) given; do not use small veins, such as those on the dorsum of the hand or wrist; extreme care should be taken to avoid intra-arterial administration or extravasation.

Do not mix or dilute Valium with other solutions or drugs in syringe or infusion flask. If it is not feasible to administer Valium directly IV, it may be injected slowly through the infusion tubing as close as possible to the vein insertion.

Extreme care must be used in administering Valium Injection, particularly by the IV route, to the elderly, to very ill patients and to those with limited pulmonary reserve because of the possibility that apnea and/or cardiac arrest may occur. Concomitant use of barbiturates, alcohol or other central nervous system depressants increases depression with increased risk of apnea. Resuscitative equipment including that necessary to support respiration should be readily available.

When Valium is used with a narcotic analgesic, the dosage of the narcotic should be reduced by at least one-third and administered in small increments. In some cases the use of a narcotic may not be necessary.

Valium Injection should not be administered to patients in shock, coma or in acute alcoholic intoxication with depression of vital signs. As is true of most CNS-acting drugs, patients receiving Valium should be cautioned against engaging in hazardous occupations requiring complete mental alertness, such as operating machinery or driving a motor vehicle.

Tonic status epilepticus has been precipitated in patients treated with IV Valium for petit mal status or petit mal variant status.

***Usage in Pregnancy:* An increased risk of congenital malformations associated with the use of minor tranquilizers (diazepam, meprobamate and chlordiazepoxide) during the first trimester of pregnancy has been suggested in several studies. Because use of these drugs is rarely a matter of urgency, their use during this period should almost always be avoided. The possibility that a woman of childbearing potential may be pregnant at the time of institution of therapy should be considered. Patients should be advised that if they become pregnant during therapy or intend to become pregnant they should communicate with their physicians about the desirability of discontinuing the drug.**

In humans, measurable amounts of diazepam were found in maternal and cord blood, indicating placental transfer of the drug. Until additional information is available, Valium Injection is not recommended for obstetrical use.

Withdrawal symptoms of the barbiturate type have occurred after the discontinuation of benzodiazepines (see DRUG ABUSE AND DEPENDENCE section).

PRECAUTIONS

Although seizures may be brought under control promptly, a significant proportion of patients experience a return to seizure activity, presumably due to the short-lived effect of Valium after IV administration. The physician should be prepared to readminister the drug. However, Valium is not recommended for maintenance, and once seizures are brought under control, consideration should be given to the administration of agents useful in longer term control of seizures.

If Valium is to be combined with other psychotropic agents or anticonvulsant drugs, careful consideration should be given to the pharmacology of the agents to be employed—particularly with known compounds which may potentiate the action of Valium, such as phenothiazines, narcotics, barbiturates, MAO inhibitors and other antidepressants. In highly anxious patients with evidence of accompanying depression, particularly those who may have suicidal tendencies, protective measures may be necessary. The usual precautions in treating patients with impaired hepatic function should be observed. Metabolites of Valium are excreted by the kidney; to avoid their excess accumulation, caution should be exercised in the administration to patients with compromised kidney function.

Since an increase in cough reflex and laryngospasm may occur with peroral endoscopic procedures, the use of a topical anesthetic agent and the availability of necessary countermeasures are recommended.

Until additional information is available, diazepam injection is not recommended for obstetrical use.

Valium Injection has produced hypotension or muscular weakness in some patients particularly when used with narcotics, barbiturates or alcohol.

Lower doses (usually 2 mg to 5 mg) should be used for elderly and debilitated patients.

The clearance of Valium and certain other benzodiazepines can be delayed in association with Tagamet (cimetidine) administration. The clinical significance of this is unclear.

Pediatric Use: Safety and effectiveness in pediatric patients below the age of 30 days have not been established. Prolonged central nervous system depression has been observed in neonates, apparently due to inability to biotransform Valium into inactive metabolites.

In pediatric use, in order to obtain maximal clinical effect with the minimum amount of drug and thus to reduce the risk of hazardous side effects, such as apnea or prolonged periods of somnolence, it is recommended that the drug be given slowly over a 3-minute period in a dosage not to exceed 0.25 mg/kg. After an interval of 15 to 30 minutes the initial dosage can be safely repeated. If, however, relief of symptoms is not obtained after a third administration, adjunctive therapy appropriate to the condition being treated is recommended.

ADVERSE REACTIONS

Side effects most commonly reported were drowsiness, fatigue and ataxia; venous thrombosis and phlebitis at the site of injection. Other adverse reactions less frequently reported include: *CNS:* confusion, depression, dysarthria, headache, hypoactivity, slurred speech, syncope, tremor, vertigo. *GI:* constipation, nausea. *GU:* incontinence, changes in libido, urinary retention. *Cardiovascular:* bradycardia, cardiovascular collapse, hypotension. *EENT:* blurred vision, diplopia, nystagmus. *Skin:* urticaria, skin rash. *Other:* hiccups, changes in salivation, neutropenia, jaundice. Paradoxical reactions such as acute hyperexcited states, anxiety, hallucinations, increased muscle spasticity, insomnia, rage, sleep disturbances and stimulation have been reported; should these occur, use of the drug should be discontinued. Minor changes in EEG patterns, usually low-voltage fast activity, have been observed in patients during and after Valium therapy and are of no known significance.

In peroral endoscopic procedures, coughing, depressed respiration, dyspnea, hyperventilation, laryngospasm and pain in throat or chest have been reported.

Because of isolated reports of neutropenia and jaundice, periodic blood counts and liver function tests are advisable during long-term therapy.

DRUG ABUSE AND DEPENDENCE

Withdrawal symptoms, similar in character to those noted with barbiturates and alcohol (convulsions, tremor, abdominal and muscle cramps, vomiting and sweating), have occurred following abrupt discontinuance of diazepam. The more severe withdrawal symptoms have usually been limited to those patients who had received excessive doses over an extended period of time. Generally milder withdrawal symptoms (eg, dysphoria and insomnia) have been reported following abrupt discontinuance of benzodiazepines taken continuously at therapeutic levels for several months. Consequently, after extended therapy, abrupt discontinuation should generally be avoided and a gradual dosage tapering schedule followed. Addiction-prone individuals (such as drug addicts or alcoholics) should be under careful surveillance when receiving diazepam or other psychotropic agents because of the predisposition of such patients to habituation and dependence.

DOSAGE AND ADMINISTRATION

Dosage should be individualized for maximum beneficial effect. The usual recommended dose in adults ranges from 2 mg to 20 mg IM or IV, depending on the indication and its severity. In some conditions, eg, tetanus, larger doses may be required. (See dosage for specific indications.) In acute conditions the injection may be repeated within 1 hour although an interval of 3 to 4 hours is usually satisfactory. Lower doses (usually 2 mg to 5 mg) and slow increase in dosage should be used for elderly or debilitated patients and when other sedative drugs are administered (see WARNINGS and ADVERSE REACTIONS).

Continued on next page

Valium Injectable—Cont.

For dosage in pediatric patients above the age of 30 days, see the specific indications below. When intravenous use is indicated, facilities for respiratory assistance should be readily available.

Intramuscular: Valium Injection should be injected deeply into the muscle.

Intravenous Use: (See WARNINGS and PRECAUTIONS: *Pediatric Use.*) The solution should be injected slowly, taking at least 1 minute for each 5 mg (1 mL) given. Do not use small veins, such as those on the dorsum of the hand or wrist. Extreme care should be taken to avoid intra-arterial administration or extravasation.

Do not mix or dilute Valium with other solutions or drugs in syringe or infusion flask. If it is not feasible to administer Valium directly IV, it may be injected slowly through the infusion tubing as close as possible to the vein insertion.

[See table below]

Once the acute symptomatology has been properly controlled with Valium Injection, the patient may be placed on oral therapy with Valium if further treatment is required.

Management of Overdosage:

Manifestations of Valium overdosage include somnolence, confusion, coma and diminished reflexes. Respiration, pulse and blood pressure should be monitored, as in all cases of drug overdosage, although, in general, these effects have been minimal. General supportive measures should be employed, along with intravenous fluids, and an adequate airway maintained. Hypotension may be combated by the use of Levophed® (levarterenol) or Aramine (metaraminol). Dialysis is of limited value.

Flumazenil, a specific benzodiazepine-receptor antagonist, is indicated for the complete or partial reversal of the sedative effects of benzodiazepines and may be used in situations when an overdose with a benzodiazepine is known or suspected. Prior to the administration of flumazenil, necessary measures should be instituted to secure airway, ventilation and intravenous access. Flumazenil is intended as an adjunct to, not as a substitute for, proper management of benzodiazepine overdose. Patients treated with flumazenil should be monitored for resedation, respiratory depression and other residual benzodiazepine effects for an appropriate period after treatment. **The prescriber should be aware of a risk of seizure in association with flumazenil treatment, particularly in long-term benzodiazepine users and in cyclic antidepressant overdose.** The complete flumazenil package insert, including CONTRAINDICATIONS, WARNINGS and PRECAUTIONS, should be consulted prior to use.

HOW SUPPLIED

Vials, 10 mL, boxes of 1 (NDC 0004-1932-09). *Tel-E-Ject* ® (disposable syringes), 2 mL, boxes of 10 (NDC 0004-1933-06).

ANIMAL PHARMACOLOGY

Oral LD_{50} of diazepam is 720 mg/kg in mice and 1240 mg/kg in rats. Intraperitoneal administration of 400 mg/kg to a monkey resulted in death on the sixth day.

Reproduction Studies: A series of rat reproduction studies was performed with diazepam in oral doses of 1, 10, 80 and 100 mg/kg given for periods ranging from 60 to 228 days prior to mating. At 100 mg/kg there was a decrease in the number of pregnancies and surviving offspring in these rats. These effects may be attributable to prolonged sedative activity, resulting in lack of interest in mating and lessened maternal nursing and care of the young. Neonatal survival of rats at doses lower than 100 mg/kg was within normal limits. Several neonates, both controls and experimentals, in these rat reproduction studies showed skeletal or other defects. Further studies in rats at doses up to and including 80 mg/kg/day did not reveal significant teratological effects on the offspring. Rabbits were maintained on doses of 1, 2, 5 and 8 mg/kg from day 6 through day 18 of gestation. No adverse effects on reproduction and no teratological changes were noted.

Distributed by Roche Laboratories Inc, Nutley, NJ 07110

Revised: March 1999

	USUAL ADULT DOSAGE	*DOSAGE RANGE IN PEDIATRIC PATIENTS* **(IV administration should be made slowly)**
Moderate Anxiety Disorders and Symptoms of Anxiety.	2 mg to 5 mg, IM or IV. Repeat in 3 to 4 hours, if necessary.	
Severe Anxiety Disorders and Symptoms of Anxiety.	5 mg to 10 mg, IM or IV. Repeat in 3 to 4 hours, if necessary.	
Acute Alcohol Withdrawal: As an aid in symptomatic relief of acute agitation, tremor, impending or acute delirium tremens and hallucinosis.	10 mg, IM or IV initially, then 5 mg to 10 mg in 3 to 4 hours, if necessary.	
Endoscopic Procedures: Adjunctively, if apprehension, anxiety or acute stress reactions are present prior to endoscopic procedures. Dosage of narcotics should be reduced by at least a third and in some cases may be omitted. See *Precautions* for peroral procedures.	Titrate IV dosage to desired sedative response, such as slurring of speech, with slow administration immediately prior to the procedure. Generally 10 mg or less is adequate, but up to 20 mg IV may be given, particularly when concomitant narcotics are omitted. If IV cannot be used, 5 mg to 10 mg IM approximately 30 minutes prior to the procedure.	
Muscle Spasm: Associated with local pathology, cerebral palsy, athetosis, stiff-man syndrome or tetanus.	5 mg to 10 mg, IM or IV initially, then 5 mg to 10 mg in 3 to 4 hours, if necessary. For tetanus, larger doses may be required.	For tetanus in pediatric patients between 30 days and 5 years of age, 1 mg to 2 mg IM or IV, slowly, repeated every 3 to 4 hours as necessary. In pediatric patients 5 years or older, 5 mg to 10 mg repeated every 3 to 4 hours may be required to control tetanus spasms. Respiratory assistance should be available.
Status Epilepticus and Severe Recurrent Convulsive Seizures: In the convulsing patient, the IV route is by far preferred. This injection should be administered slowly. However, if IV administration is impossible, the IM route may be used.	5 mg to 10 mg initially (IV preferred). This injection may be repeated if necessary at 10 to 15 minute intervals up to a maximum dose of 30 mg. If necessary, therapy with Valium may be repeated in 2 to 4 hours; however, residual active metabolites may persist, and readministration should be made with this consideration. Extreme caution must be exercised with individuals with chronic lung disease or unstable cardiovascular status.	Pediatric patients between the ages of 30 days and 5 years, 0.2 mg to 0.5 mg slowly every 2 to 5 minutes up to a maximum of 5 mg (IV preferred). Pediatric patients 5 years or older, 1 mg every 2 to 5 minutes up to a maximum of 10 mg (slow IV administration preferred). Repeat in 2 to 4 hours if necessary. EEG monitoring of the seizure may be helpful.
Preoperative Medication: To relieve anxiety and tension. (If atropine, scopolamine or other premedications are desired, they must be administered in separate syringes.)	10 mg, IM (preferred route), before surgery.	
Cardioversion: To relieve anxiety and tension and to reduce recall of procedure.	5 mg to 15 mg, IV, within 5 to 10 minutes prior to the procedure.	

VERSED® Ⓒ IV

[ver-sed ']

(midazolam HCl)

INJECTION

The following text is complete prescribing information based on official labeling in effect June 2000.

WARNING

Adults and Pediatrics: Intravenous VERSED has been associated with respiratory depression and respiratory arrest, especially when used for sedation in noncritical care settings. In some cases, where this was not recognized promptly and treated effectively, death or hypoxic encephalopathy has resulted. Intravenous VERSED should be used only in hospital or ambulatory care settings, including physicians' and dental offices, that provide for continuous monitoring of respiratory and cardiac function, ie, pulse oximetry. Immediate availability of resuscitative drugs and age- and size-appropriate equipment for bag/valve/mask ventilation and intubation, and personnel trained in their use and skilled in airway management should be assured (see WARNINGS). For deeply sedated pediatric patients, a dedicated individual, other than the practitioner performing the procedure, should monitor the patient throughout the procedure.

The initial intravenous dose for sedation in adult patients may be as little as 1 mg, but should not exceed 2.5 mg in a normal healthy adult. Lower doses are necessary for older (over 60 years) or debilitated patients and in patients receiving concomitant narcotics or other central nervous system (CNS) depressants. The initial dose and all subsequent doses should always be titrated slowly; administer over at least 2 minutes and allow an additional 2 or more minutes to fully evaluate the sedative effect. The use of the 1 mg/mL formulation or dilution of the 1 mg/mL or 5 mg/mL formulation is recommended to facilitate slower injection. Doses of sedative medications in pediatric patients must be calculated on a mg/kg basis, and initial doses and all subsequent doses should always be titrated slowly. The initial pediatric dose of VERSED for sedation/anxiolysis/amnesia is age, procedure, and route dependent (see DOSAGE AND ADMINISTRATION for complete dosing information).

Neonates: VERSED should not be administered by rapid injection in the neonatal population. Severe hypotension and seizures have been reported following rapid IV administration, particularly with concomitant use of fentanyl (see DOSAGE AND ADMINISTRATION for complete information).

DESCRIPTION

VERSED is a water-soluble benzodiazepine available as a sterile, nonpyrogenic parenteral dosage form for intravenous or intramuscular injection. Each mL contains midazolam hydrochloride equivalent to 1 mg or 5 mg midazolam compounded with 0.8% sodium chloride and 0.01% edetate disodium, with 1% benzyl alcohol as preservative; the pH is adjusted to approximately 3 with hydrochloric acid and, if necessary, sodium hydroxide.

Midazolam is a white to light yellow crystalline compound, insoluble in water. The hydrochloride salt of midazolam, which is formed *in situ*, is soluble in aqueous solutions. Chemically, midazolam HCl is 8-chloro-6-(2-fluorophenyl)-1-methyl-4*H*-imidazo[1,5-a][1,4]benzodiazepine hydrochloride. Midazolam hydrochloride has the empirical formula $C_{18}H_{13}ClFN_3 \cdot HCl$, a calculated molecular weight of 362.25 and the following structural formula:

Under the acidic conditions required to solubilize midazolam in the product, midazolam is present as an equilibrium mixture (shown below) of the closed ring form shown above and an open-ring structure formed by the acid-catalyzed ring opening of the 4,5-double bond of the diazepine ring. The amount of open-ring form is dependent upon the pH of the solution. At the specified pH of the product, the solution may contain up to about 25% of the open-ring compound. At the physiologic conditions under which the product is absorbed (pH of 5 to 8) into the systemic circulation, any open-ring form present reverts to the physiologically active, lipophilic, closed-ring form (midazolam) and is absorbed as such.

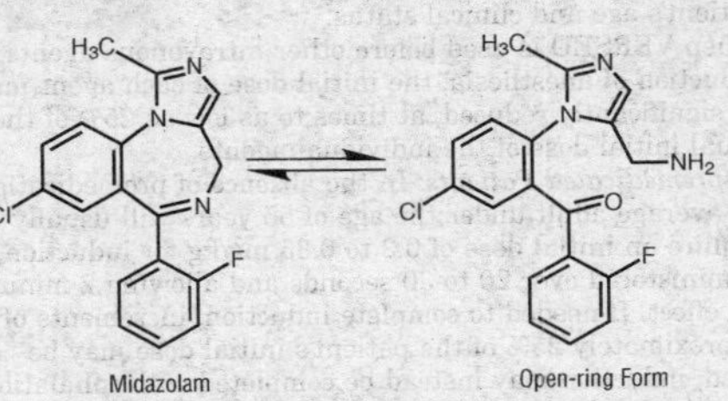

Midazolam Open-ring Form

The following chart plots the percentage of midazolam present as the open-ring form as a function of pH in aqueous solutions. As indicated in the graph, the amount of open-ring compound present in solution is sensitive to changes in pH over the pH range specified for the product: 3.0 to 4.0 for the 1 mg/mL concentration and 3.0 to 3.6 for the 5 mg/mL concentration. Above pH 5, at least 99% of the mixture is present in the closed-ring form.

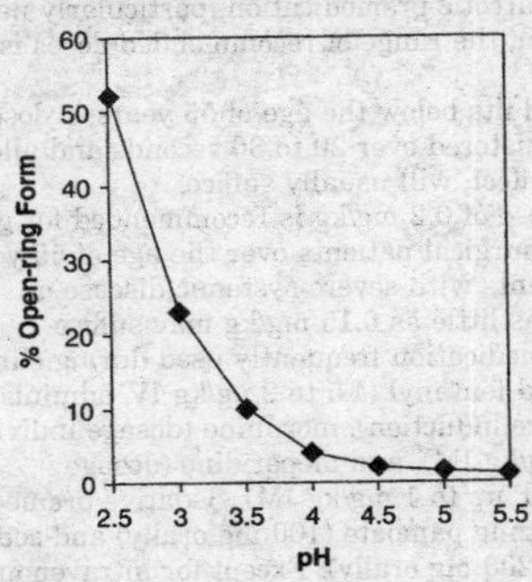

CLINICAL PHARMACOLOGY

VERSED is a short-acting benzodiazepine central nervous system (CNS) depressant.

The effects of VERSED on the CNS are dependent on the dose administered, the route of administration, and the presence or absence of other medications. Onset time of sedative effects after IM administration in adults is 15 minutes, with peak sedation occurring 30 to 60 minutes following injection. In one adult study, when tested the following day, 73% of the patients who received VERSED intramuscularly had no recall of memory cards shown 30 minutes following drug administration; 40% had no recall of the memory cards shown 60 minutes following drug administration. Onset time of sedative effects in the pediatric population begins within 5 minutes and peaks at 15 to 30 minutes depending upon the dose administered. In pediatric patients, up to 85% had no recall of pictures shown after receiving intramuscular VERSED compared with 5% of the placebo controls.

Sedation in adult and pediatric patients is achieved within 3 to 5 minutes after intravenous (IV) injection; the time of onset is affected by total dose administered and the concurrent administration of narcotic premedication. Seventy-one percent of the adult patients in endoscopy studies had no recall of introduction of the endoscope; 82% of the patients had no recall of withdrawal of the endoscope. In one study of pediatric patients undergoing lumbar puncture or bone marrow aspiration, 88% of patients had impaired recall vs 9% of the placebo controls. In another pediatric oncology study, 91% of VERSED treated patients were amnestic compared with 35% of patients who had received fentanyl alone.

When VERSED is given IV as an anesthetic induction agent, induction of anesthesia occurs in approximately 1.5 minutes when narcotic premedication has been administered and in 2 to 2.5 minutes without narcotic premedication or other sedative premedication. Some impairment in a test of memory was noted in 90% of the patients studied. A dose response study of pediatric patients premedicated with 1.0 mg/kg intramuscular (IM) meperidine found that only 4 out of 6 pediatric patients who received 600 µg/kg IV VERSED lost consciousness, with eye closing at 108 ± 140 seconds. This group was compared with pediatric patients who were given thiopental 5 mg/kg IV; 6 out of 6 closed their eyes at 20 ± 3.2 seconds. VERSED did not dependably induce anesthesia at this dose despite concomitant opioid administration in pediatric patients.

VERSED, used as directed, does not delay awakening from general anesthesia in adults. Gross tests of recovery after awakening (orientation, ability to stand and walk, suitability for discharge from the recovery room, return to baseline Trieger competency) usually indicate recovery within 2 hours but recovery may take up to 6 hours in some cases. When compared with patients who received thiopental, patients who received midazolam generally recovered at a slightly slower rate. Recovery from anesthesia or sedation for procedures in pediatric patients depends on the dose of VERSED administered, coadministration of other medications causing CNS depression and duration of the procedure.

In patients without intracranial lesions, induction of general anesthesia with IV VERSED is associated with a moderate decrease in cerebrospinal fluid pressure (lumbar puncture measurements), similar to that observed following IV thiopental. Preliminary data in neurosurgical patients with normal intracranial pressure but decreased compliance (subarachnoid screw measurements) show comparable elevations of intracranial pressure with VERSED and with thiopental during intubation. No similar studies have been reported in pediatric patients.

The usual recommended intramuscular premedicating doses of VERSED do not depress the ventilatory response to carbon dioxide stimulation to a clinically significant extent in adults. Intravenous induction doses of VERSED depress the ventilatory response to carbon dioxide stimulation for 15 minutes or more beyond the duration of ventilatory depression following administration of thiopental in adults. Impairment of ventilatory response to carbon dioxide is more marked in adult patients with chronic obstructive pulmonary disease (COPD). Sedation with IV VERSED does not adversely affect the mechanics of respiration (resistance, static recoil, most lung volume measurements); total lung capacity and peak expiratory flow decrease significantly but static compliance and maximum expiratory flow at 50% of awake total lung capacity (V_{max}) increase. In one study of pediatric patients under general anesthesia, intramuscular VERSED (100 or 200 µg/kg) was shown to depress the response to carbon dioxide in a dose-related manner.

In cardiac hemodynamic studies in adults, IV induction of general anesthesia with VERSED was associated with a slight to moderate decrease in mean arterial pressure, cardiac output, stroke volume and systemic vascular resistance. Slow heart rates (less than 65/minute), particularly in patients taking propranolol for angina, tended to rise slightly; faster heart rates (eg, 85/minute) tended to slow slightly. In pediatric patients, a comparison of IV VERSED (500 µg/kg) with propofol (2.5 mg/kg) revealed a mean 15% decrease in systolic blood pressure in patients who had received IV VERSED vs a mean 25% decrease in systolic blood pressure following propofol.

Pharmacokinetics: Midazolam's activity is primarily due to the parent drug. Elimination of the parent drug takes place via hepatic metabolism of midazolam to hydroxylated metabolites that are conjugated and excreted in the urine. Six single-dose pharmacokinetic studies involving healthy adults yield pharmacokinetic parameters for midazolam in the following ranges: volume of distribution (Vd), 1.0 to 3.1 L/kg; elimination half-life, 1.8 to 6.4 hours (mean approximately 3 hours); total clearance (Cl), 0.25 to 0.54 L/hr/kg. In a parallel group study, there was no difference in the clearance, in subjects administered 0.15 mg/kg (n=4) and 0.30 mg/kg (n=4) IV doses indicating linear kinetics. The clearance was successively reduced by approximately 30% at doses of 0.45 mg/kg (n=4) and 0.6 mg/kg (n=5) indicating non-linear kinetics in this dose range.

Continued on next page

USUAL ADULT DOSE

INTRAMUSCULARLY

For preoperative sedation/anxiolysis/amnesia (induction of sleepiness or drowsiness and relief of apprehension and to impair memory of perioperative events).

For intramuscular use, VERSED should be injected deep in a large muscle mass.

The recommended premedication dose of VERSED for good risk (ASA Physical Status I & II) adult patients below the age of 60 years is 0.07 to 0.08 mg/kg IM (approximately 5 mg IM) administered up to 1 hour before surgery.

The dose must be individualized and reduced when IM VERSED is administered to patients with chronic obstructive pulmonary disease, other higher risk surgical patients, patients 60 or more years of age, and patients who have received concomitant narcotics or other CNS depressants (see ADVERSE REACTIONS). In a study of patients 60 years or older, who did not receive concomitant administration of narcotics, 2 to 3 mg (0.02 to 0.05 mg/kg) of VERSED produced adequate sedation during the preoperative period. The dose of 1 mg IM VERSED may suffice for some older patients if the anticipated intensity and duration of sedation is less critical. As with any potential respiratory depressant, these patients require observation for signs of cardiorespiratory depression after receiving IM VERSED.

Onset is within 15 minutes, peaking at 30 to 60 minutes. It can be administered concomitantly with atropine sulfate or scopolamine hydrochloride and reduced doses of narcotics.

INTRAVENOUSLY

Sedation/anxiolysis/amnesia for procedures (see INDICATIONS): Narcotic premedication results in less variability in patient response and a reduction in dosage of VERSED. For peroral procedures, the use of an appropriate topical anesthetic is recommended. For bronchoscopic procedures, the use of narcotic premedication is recommended.

VERSED 1 mg/mL formulation is recommended for sedation/anxiolysis/amnesia for procedures to facilitate slower injection. Both the 1 mg/mL and the 5 mg/mL formulations may be diluted with 0.9% sodium chloride or 5% dextrose in water.

When used for sedation/anxiolysis/amnesia for a procedure, dosage must be individualized and titrated. VERSED should always be titrated slowly; administer over at least 2 minutes and allow an additional 2 or more minutes to fully evaluate the sedative effect. Individual response will vary with age, physical status and concomitant medications, but may also vary independent of these factors. (see WARNINGS concerning cardiac/respiratory arrest/airway obstruction/hypoventilation.)

1. *Healthy Adults Below the Age of 60:* Titrate slowly to the desired effect (eg, the initiation of slurred speech). Some patients may respond to as little as 1 mg. No more than 2.5 mg should be given over a period of at least 2 minutes. Wait an additional 2 or more minutes to fully evaluate the sedative effect. If further titration is necessary, continue to titrate, using small increments, to the appropriate level of sedation. Wait an additional 2 or more minutes after each increment to fully evaluate the sedative effect. A total dose greater than 5 mg is not usually necessary to reach the desired endpoint.

If narcotic premedication or other CNS depressants are used, patients will require approximately 30% less VERSED than unpremedicated patients.

2. *Patients Age 60 or Older, and Debilitated or Chronically Ill Patients:* Because the danger of hypoventilation, airway obstruction, or apnea is greater in elderly patients and those with chronic disease states or decreased pulmonary reserve, and because the peak effect may take longer in these patients, increments should be smaller and the rate of injection slower.

Titrate slowly to the desired effect (eg, the initiation of slurred speech). Some patients may respond to as little as 1 mg. No more than 1.5 mg should be given over a period of no less than 2 minutes. Wait an additional 2 or more minutes to fully evaluate the sedative effect. If additional titration is necessary, it should be given at a rate of no more than 1 mg over a period of 2 minutes, waiting an additional 2 or more minutes each time to fully evaluate the sedative effect. Total doses greater than 3.5 mg are not usually necessary.

If concomitant CNS depressant premedications are used in these patients, they will require at least 50% less VERSED than healthy young unpremedicated patients.

3. *Maintenance Dose:* Additional doses to maintain the desired level of sedation may be given in increments of 25% of the dose used to first reach the sedative endpoint, but again only by slow titration, especially in the elderly and chronically ill or debilitated patient. These additional doses should be given only after a thorough clinical evaluation clearly indicates the need for additional sedation.

Versed—Cont.

Absorption: The absolute bioavailability of the intramuscular route was greater than 90% in a crossover study in which healthy subjects (n=17) were administered a 7.5 mg IV or IM dose. The mean peak concentration (C_{max}) and time to peak (T_{max}) following the IM dose was 90 ng/mL (20% CV) and 0.5 hour (50% CV). C_{max} for the 1-hydroxy metabolite following the IM dose was 8 ng/mL (T_{max}=1.0 hour).

Following IM administration, C_{max} for midazolam and its 1-hydroxy metabolite were approximately one-half of those achieved after intravenous injection.

Distribution: The volume of distribution (Vd) determined from six single-dose pharmacokinetic studies involving healthy adults ranged from 1.0 to 3.1 L/kg. Female gender, old age, and obesity are associated with increased values of midazolam Vd. In humans, midazolam has been shown to cross the placenta and enter into fetal circulation and has been detected in human milk and CSF (see *Special Populations*).

In adults and pediatric patients older than 1 year, midazolam is approximately 97% bound to plasma protein, principally albumin.

Metabolism: In vitro studies with human liver microsomes indicate that the biotransformation of midazolam is mediated by cytochrome P450 3A4. This cytochrome also appears to be present in gastrointestinal tract mucosa as well as liver. Sixty to seventy percent of the biotransformation products is 1-hydroxy-midazolam (also termed alpha-hydroxy-midazolam) while 4-hydroxy-midazolam constitutes 5% or less. Small amounts of a dihydroxy derivative have also been detected but not quantified. The principal urinary excretion products are glucuronide conjugates of the hydroxylated derivatives.

Drugs that inhibit the activity of cytochrome P450 3A4 may inhibit midazolam clearance and elevate steady-state midazolam concentrations.

Studies of the intravenous administration of 1-hydroxy-midazolam in humans suggest that 1-hydroxy-midazolam is at least as potent as the parent compound and may contribute to the net pharmacologic activity of midazolam. In vitro studies have demonstrated that the affinities of 1- and 4-hydroxy-midazolam for the benzodiazepine receptor are approximately 20% and 7%, respectively, relative to midazolam.

Excretion: Clearance of midazolam is reduced in association with old age, congestive heart failure, liver disease (cirrhosis) or conditions which diminish cardiac output and hepatic blood flow.

The principal urinary excretion product is 1-hydroxy-midazolam in the form of a glucuronide conjugate; smaller amounts of the glucuronide conjugates of 4-hydroxy- and dihydroxy-midazolam are detected as well. The amount of midazolam excreted unchanged in the urine after a single IV dose is less than 0.5% (n=5). Following a single IV infusion in 5 healthy volunteers, 45% to 57% of the dose was excreted in the urine as 1-hydroxymethyl midazolam conjugate.

Pharmacokinetics-Continuous Infusion: The pharmacokinetic profile of midazolam following continuous infusion, based on 282 adult subjects, has been shown to be similar to that following single-dose administration for subjects of comparable age, gender, body habitus and health status. However, midazolam can accumulate in peripheral tissues with continuous infusion. The effects of accumulation are greater after long-term infusions than after short-term infusions. The effects of accumulation can be reduced by maintaining the lowest midazolam infusion rate that produces satisfactory sedation.

Infrequent hypotensive episodes have occurred during continuous infusion; however, neither the time to onset nor the duration of the episode appeared to be related to plasma concentrations of midazolam or alpha-hydroxy-midazolam. Further, there does not appear to be an increased chance of occurrence of a hypotensive episode with increased loading doses.

Patients with renal impairment may have longer elimination half-lives for midazolam (see *Special Populations: Renal Failure*).

Special Populations: Changes in the pharmacokinetic profile of midazolam due to drug interactions, physiological variables, etc., may result in changes in the plasma concentration-time profile and pharmacological response to midazolam in these patients. For example, patients with acute renal failure appear to have a longer elimination half-life for midazolam and may experience delayed recovery (see *Special Populations: Renal Failure*). In other groups, the relationship between prolonged half-life and duration of effect has not been established.

Pediatrics and Neonates: In pediatric patients aged 1 year and older, the pharmacokinetic properties following a single dose of VERSED reported in 10 separate studies of midazolam are similar to those in adults. Weight-normalized clearance is similar or higher (0.19 to 0.80 L/hr/kg) than in adults and the terminal elimination half-life (0.78 to 3.3 hours) is similar to or shorter than in adults. The pharmacokinetic properties during and following continuous intravenous infusion in pediatric patients in the operating room as an adjunct to general anesthesia and in the intensive care environment are similar to those in adults.

In seriously ill neonates, however, the terminal elimination half-life of midazolam is substantially prolonged (6.5 to 12.0

USUAL ADULT DOSE Induction of Anesthesia: For induction of general anesthesia, before administration of other anesthetic agents.	Individual response to the drug is variable, particularly when a narcotic premedication is not used. The dosage should be titrated to the desired effect according to the patient's age and clinical status. When VERSED is used before other intravenous agents for induction of anesthesia, the initial dose of each agent may be significantly reduced, at times to as low as 25% of the usual initial dose of the individual agents. *Unpremedicated Patients:* In the absence of premedication, an average adult under the age of 55 years will usually require an initial dose of 0.3 to 0.35 mg/kg for induction, administered over 20 to 30 seconds and allowing 2 minutes for effect. If needed to complete induction, increments of approximately 25% of the patient's initial dose may be used; induction may instead be completed with inhalational anesthetics. In resistant cases, up to 0.6 mg/kg total dose may be used for induction, but such larger doses may prolong recovery. Unpremedicated patients over the age of 55 years usually require less VERSED for induction; an initial dose of 0.3 mg/kg is recommended. Unpremedicated patients with severe systemic disease or other debilitation usually require less VERSED for induction. An initial dose of 0.2 to 0.25 mg/kg will usually suffice; in some cases, as little as 0.15 mg/kg may suffice. *Premedicated Patients:* When the patient has received sedative or narcotic premedication, particularly narcotic premedication, the range of recommended doses is 0.15 to 0.35 mg/kg. In average adults below the age of 55 years, a dose of 0.25 mg/kg, administered over 20 to 30 seconds and allowing 2 minutes for effect, will usually suffice. The initial dose of 0.2 mg/kg is recommended for good risk (ASA I & II) surgical patients over the age of 55 years. In some patients with severe systemic disease or debilitation, as little as 0.15 mg/kg may suffice. Narcotic premedication frequently used during clinical trials included fentanyl (1.5 to 2 μg/kg IV, administered 5 minutes before induction), morphine (dosage individualized, up to 0.15 mg/kg IM), and meperidine (dosage individualized, up to 1 mg/kg IM). Sedative premedications were hydroxyzine pamoate (100 mg orally) and sodium secobarbital (200 mg orally). Except for intravenous fentanyl, administered 5 minutes before induction, all other premedications should be administered approximately 1 hour prior to the time anticipated for VERSED induction.
Injectable VERSED can also be used during maintenance of anesthesia, for surgical procedures, as a component of balanced anesthesia. Effective narcotic premedication is especially recommended in such cases.	Incremental injections of approximately 25% of the induction dose should be given in response to signs of lightening of anesthesia and repeated as necessary.
CONTINUOUS INFUSION For continuous infusion, VERSED 5 mg/mL formulation is recommended diluted to a concentration of 0.5 mg/mL with 0.9% sodium chloride or 5% dextrose in water.	*Usual Adult Dose:* If a loading dose is necessary to rapidly initiate sedation, 0.01 to 0.05 mg/kg (approximately 0.5 to 4.0 mg for a typical adult) may be given slowly or infused over several minutes. This dose may be repeated at 10 to 15 minute intervals until adequate sedation is achieved. For maintenance of sedation, the usual initial infusion rate is 0.02 to 0.10 mg/kg/hr (1 to 7 mg/hr). Higher loading or maintenance infusion rates may occasionally be required in some patients. The lowest recommended doses should be used in patients with residual effects from anesthetic drugs, or in those concurrently receiving other sedatives or opioids. Individual response to VERSED is variable. The infusion rate should be titrated to the desired level of sedation, taking into account the patient's age, clinical status and current medications. In general, VERSED should be infused at the lowest rate that produces the desired level of sedation. Assessment of sedation should be performed at regular intervals and the VERSED infusion rate adjusted up or down by 25% to 50% of the initial infusion rate so as to assure adequate titration of sedation level. Larger adjustments or even a small incremental dose may be necessary if rapid changes in the level of sedation are indicated. In addition, the infusion rate should be decreased by 10% to 25% every few hours to find the minimum effective infusion rate. Finding the minimum effective infusion rate decreases the potential accumulation of midazolam and provides for the most rapid recovery once the infusion is terminated. Patients who exhibit agitation, hypertension, or tachycardia in response to noxious stimulation, but who are otherwise adequately sedated, may benefit from concurrent administration of an opioid analgesic. Addition of an opioid will generally reduce the minimum effective VERSED infusion rate.
PEDIATRIC PATIENTS	**UNLIKE ADULT PATIENTS, PEDIATRIC PATIENTS GENERALLY RECEIVE INCREMENTS OF VERSED ON A MG/KG BASIS.** As a group, pediatric patients generally require higher dosages of VERSED (mg/kg) than do adults. Younger (less than six years) pediatric patients may require higher dosages (mg/kg) than older pediatric patients, and may require close monitoring (see tables below). In obese PEDIATRIC PATIENTS, the dose should be calculated based on ideal body weight. When VERSED is given in conjunction with opioids or other sedatives, the potential for respiratory depression, airway obstruction, or hypoventilation is increased. For appropriate patient monitoring (see Boxed WARNING, WARNINGS, *MONITORING* subsection of DOSAGE AND ADMINISTRATION). The health care practitioner who uses this medication in pediatric patients should be aware of and follow accepted professional guidelines for pediatric sedation appropriate to their situation.

hours) and the clearance reduced (0.07 to 0.12 L/hr/kg) compared to healthy adults or other groups of pediatric patients. It cannot be determined if these differences are due to age, immature organ function or metabolic pathways, underlying illness or debility.

Obese: In a study comparing normals (n=20) and obese patients (n=20) the mean half-life was greater in the obese group (5.9 vs 2.3 hours). This was due to an increase of approximately 50% in the Vd corrected for total body weight. The clearance was not significantly different between groups.

Geriatric: In three parallel group studies, the pharmacokinetics of midazolam administered IV or IM were compared in young (mean age 29, n=52) and healthy elderly subjects (mean age 73, n=53). Plasma half-life was approximately two-fold higher in the elderly. The mean Vd based on total body weight increased consistently between 15% to 100% in the elderly. The mean Cl decreased approximately 25% in the elderly in two studies and was similar to that of the younger patients in the other.

Congestive Heart Failure: In patients suffering from congestive heart failure, there appeared to be a two-fold increase in the elimination half-life, a 25% decrease in the plasma clearance and a 40% increase in the volume of distribution of midazolam.

Hepatic Insufficiency: Midazolam pharmacokinetics were studied after an IV single dose (0.075 mg/kg) was administered to 7 patients with biopsy proven alcoholic cirrhosis and 8 control patients. The mean half-life of midazolam increased 2.5-fold in the alcoholic patients. Clearance was reduced by 50% and the Vd increased by 20%. In another study in 21 male patients with cirrhosis, without ascites and with normal kidney function as determined by creatinine clearance, no changes in the pharmacokinetics of midazolam or 1-hydroxy-midazolam were observed when compared to healthy individuals.

Renal Failure: Patients with renal impairment may have longer elimination half-lives for midazolam and its metabolites which may result in slower recovery.

Midazolam and 1-hydroxy-midazolam pharmacokinetics in 6 ICU patients who developed acute renal failure (ARF) were compared with a normal renal function control group. Midazolam was administered as an infusion (5 to 15 mg/hr). Midazolam clearance was reduced (1.9 vs 2.8 mL/min/kg) and the half-life was prolonged (7.6 vs 13 hours) in the ARF patients. The renal clearance of the 1-hydroxy-midazolam glucuronide was prolonged in the ARF group (4 vs 136 mL/min) and the half-life was prolonged (12 vs >25 hours). Plasma levels accumulated in all ARF patients to about ten times that of the parent drug. The relationship between accumulating metabolite levels and prolonged sedation is unclear.

In a study of chronic renal failure patients (n=15) receiving a single IV dose, there was a two-fold increase in the clearance and volume of distribution but the half-life remained unchanged. Metabolite levels were not studied.

Plasma Concentration-Effect Relationship: Concentration-effect relationships (after an IV dose) have been demonstrated for a variety of pharmacodynamic measures (eg, reaction time, eye movement, sedation) and are associated with extensive intersubject variability. Logistic regression analysis of sedation scores and steady-state plasma concentration indicated that at plasma concentrations greater than 100 ng/mL there was at least a 50% probability that patients would be sedated, but respond to verbal commands (sedation score = 3). At 200 ng/mL there was at least a 50% probability that patients would be asleep, but respond to glabellar tap (sedation score = 4).

Drug Interactions: For information concerning pharmacokinetic drug interactions with VERSED (see PRECAUTIONS).

INDICATIONS

Injectable VERSED is indicated:

- intramuscularly or intravenously for preoperative sedation/anxiolysis/amnesia;
- intravenously as an agent for sedation/anxiolysis/amnesia prior to or during diagnostic, therapeutic or endoscopic procedures, such as bronchoscopy, gastroscopy, cystoscopy, coronary angiography, cardiac catheterization, oncology procedures, radiologic procedures, suture of lacerations and other procedures either alone or in combination with other CNS depressants;
- intravenously for induction of general anesthesia, before administration of other anesthetic agents. With the use of narcotic premedication, induction of anesthesia can be attained within a relatively narrow dose range and in a short period of time. Intravenous VERSED can also be used as a component of intravenous supplementation of nitrous oxide and oxygen (balanced anesthesia);
- continuous intravenous infusion for sedation of intubated and mechanically ventilated patients as a component of anesthesia or during treatment in a critical care setting.

VERSED is associated with a high incidence of partial or complete impairment of recall for the next several hours (see CLINICAL PHARMACOLOGY).

CONTRAINDICATIONS

Injectable VERSED is contraindicated in patients with a known hypersensitivity to the drug. Benzodiazepines are contraindicated in patients with acute narrow-angle glaucoma. Benzodiazepines may be used in patients with open-angle glaucoma only if they are receiving appropriate therapy. Measurements of intraocular pressure in patients without eye disease show a moderate lowering following induction with VERSED; patients with glaucoma have not been studied.

VERSED is not intended for intrathecal or epidural administration due to the presence of the preservative benzyl alcohol in the dosage form.

OBSERVER'S ASSESSMENT OF ALERTNESS/SEDATION (OAA/S)

Assessment Categories				
Responsiveness	Speech	Facial Expression	Eyes	Composite Score
Responds readily to name spoken in normal tone	normal	normal	clear, no ptosis	5 (alert)
Lethargic response to name spoken in normal tone	mild slowing or thickening	mild relaxation	glazed or mild ptosis (less than half the eye)	4
Responds only after name is called loudly and/or repeatedly	slurring or prominent slowing	marked relaxation (slack jaw)	glazed and marked ptosis (half the eye or more)	3
Responds only after mild prodding or shaking	few recognizable words	—	—	2
Does not respond to mild prodding or shaking	—	—	—	1 (deep sleep)

FREQUENCY OF OBSERVER'S ASSESSMENT OF ALERTNESS/SEDATION COMPOSITE SCORES IN ONE STUDY OF PEDIATRIC PATIENTS UNDERGOING PROCEDURES WITH INTRAVENOUS MIDAZOLAM FOR SEDATION

Age Range (years)	n	OAA/S Score				
		1 (deep sleep)	2	3	4	5 (alert)
1–2	16	6 (38%)	4 (25%)	3 (19%)	3 (19%)	0
>2–5	22	9 (41%)	5 (23%)	8 (36%)	0	0
>5–12	34	1 (3%)	6 (18%)	22 (65%)	5 (15%)	0
>12–17	18	0	4 (22%)	14 (78%)	0	0
Total (1–17)	90	16 (18%)	19 (21%)	47 (52%)	8 (9%)	0

WARNINGS

VERSED must never be used without individualization of dosage particularly when used with other medications capable of producing central nervous system depression. Prior to the intravenous administration of VERSED in any dose, the immediate availability of oxygen, resuscitative drugs, age- and size-appropriate equipment for bag/valve/mask ventilation and intubation, and skilled personnel for the maintenance of a patent airway and support of ventilation should be ensured. Patients should be continuously monitored with some means of detection for early signs of hypoventilation, airway obstruction, or apnea, ie, pulse oximetry. Hypoventilation, airway obstruction, and apnea can lead to hypoxia and/or cardiac arrest unless effective countermeasures are taken immediately. The immediate availability of specific reversal agents (flumazenil) is highly recommended. Vital signs should continue to be monitored during the recovery period. Because intravenous VERSED depresses respiration (see CLINICAL PHARMACOLOGY) and because opioid agonists and other sedatives can add to this depression, VERSED should be administered as an induction agent only by a person trained in general anesthesia and should be used for sedation/anxiolysis/amnesia only in the presence of personnel skilled in early detection of hypoventilation, maintaining a patent airway and supporting ventilation. **When used for sedation/anxiolysis/amnesia, VERSED should always be titrated slowly in adult or pediatric patients.** Adverse hemodynamic events have been reported in pediatric patients with cardiovascular instability; rapid intravenous administration should also be avoided in this population (see DOSAGE AND ADMINISTRATION for complete information).

Serious cardiorespiratory adverse events have occurred after administration of VERSED. These have included respiratory depression, airway obstruction, oxygen desaturation, apnea, respiratory arrest and/or cardiac arrest, sometimes resulting in death or permanent neurologic injury. There have also been rare reports of hypotensive episodes requiring treatment during or after diagnostic or surgical manipulations particularly in adult or pediatric patients with hemodynamic instability. Hypotension occurred more frequently in the sedation studies in patients premedicated with a narcotic.

Reactions such as agitation, involuntary movements (including tonic/clonic movements and muscle tremor), hyperactivity and combativeness have been reported in both adult and pediatric patients. These reactions may be due to inadequate or excessive dosing or improper administration of VERSED; however, consideration should be given to the possibility of cerebral hypoxia or true paradoxical reactions. Should such reactions occur, the response to each dose of VERSED and all other drugs, including local anesthetics, should be evaluated before proceeding. Reversal of such responses with flumazenil has been reported in pediatric patients.

Concomitant use of barbiturates, alcohol or other central nervous system depressants may increase the risk of hypoventilation, airway obstruction, desaturation, or apnea and may contribute to profound and/or prolonged drug effect. Narcotic premedication also depresses the ventilatory response to carbon dioxide stimulation.

Higher risk adult and pediatric surgical patients, elderly patients and debilitated adult and pediatric patients require lower dosages, whether or not concomitant sedating medications have been administered. Adult or pediatric patients with COPD are unusually sensitive to the respiratory depressant effect of VERSED. Pediatric and adult patients undergoing procedures involving the upper airway such as upper endoscopy or dental care, are particularly vulnerable to episodes of desaturation and hypoventilation due to partial airway obstruction. Adult and pediatric patients with chronic renal failure and patients with congestive heart failure eliminate midazolam more slowly (see CLINICAL PHARMACOLOGY). Because elderly patients frequently have inefficient function of one or more organ systems and because dosage requirements have been shown to decrease with age, reduced initial dosage of VERSED is recommended, and the possibility of profound and/or prolonged effect should be considered.

Injectable VERSED should not be administered to adult or pediatric patients in shock or coma, or in acute alcohol intoxication with depression of vital signs. Particular care should be exercised in the use of intravenous VERSED in adult or pediatric patients with uncompensated acute illnesses, such as severe fluid or electrolyte disturbances.

There have been limited reports of intra-arterial injection of VERSED. Adverse events have included local reactions, as well as isolated reports of seizure activity in which no clear causal relationship was established. Precautions against unintended intra-arterial injection should be taken. Extravasation should also be avoided.

The safety and efficacy of VERSED following nonintravenous and nonintramuscular routes of administration have not been established. VERSED should only be administered intramuscularly or intravenously.

The decision as to when patients who have received injectable VERSED, particularly on an outpatient basis, may again engage in activities requiring complete mental alertness, operate hazardous machinery or drive a motor vehicle must be individualized. Gross tests of recovery from the effects of VERSED (see CLINICAL PHARMACOLOGY) cannot be relied upon to predict reaction time under stress. It is recommended that no patient operate hazardous machinery or a motor vehicle until the effects of the drug, such as drowsiness, have subsided or until 1 full day after anesthesia and surgery, whichever is longer. For pediatric patients, particular care should be taken to assure safe ambulation.

Usage in Pregnancy: **An increased risk of congenital malformations associated with the use of benzodiazepine drugs (diazepam and chlordiazepoxide) has been suggested in several studies. If this drug is used during pregnancy, the patient should be apprised of the potential hazard to the fetus.**

Withdrawal symptoms of the barbiturate type have occurred after the discontinuation of benzodiazepines (see DRUG ABUSE AND DEPENDENCE).

Usage in Preterm Infants and Neonates: Rapid injection should be avoided in the neonatal population. VERSED administered rapidly as an intravenous injection (less than 2 minutes) has been associated with severe hypotension in

Continued on next page

Versed—Cont.

neonates, particularly when the patient has also received fentanyl. Likewise, severe hypotension has been observed in neonates receiving a continuous infusion of midazolam who then receive a rapid intravenous injection of fentanyl. Seizures have been reported in several neonates following rapid intravenous administration.

The neonate also has reduced and/or immature organ function and is also vulnerable to profound and/or prolonged respiratory effects of VERSED.

Exposure to excessive amounts of benzyl alcohol has been associated with toxicity (hypotension, metabolic acidosis), particularly in neonates, and an increased incidence of kernicterus, particularly in small preterm infants. There have been rare reports of deaths, primarily in preterm infants, associated with exposure to excessive amounts of benzyl alcohol. The amount of benzyl alcohol from medications is usually considered negligible compared to that received in flush solutions containing benzyl alcohol. Administration of high dosages of medications (including VERSED) containing this preservative must take into account the total amount of benzyl alcohol administered. The recommended dosage range of VERSED for preterm and term infants includes amounts of benzyl alcohol well below that associated with toxicity; however, the amount of benzyl alcohol at which toxicity may occur is not known. If the patient requires more than the recommended dosages or other medications containing this preservative, the practitioner must consider the daily metabolic load of benzyl alcohol from these combined sources.

PRECAUTIONS

General: Intravenous doses of VERSED should be decreased for elderly and for debilitated patients (see WARNINGS and DOSAGE AND ADMINISTRATION). These patients will also probably take longer to recover completely after VERSED administration for the induction of anesthesia.

VERSED does not protect against the increase in intracranial pressure or against the heart rate rise and/or blood pressure rise associated with endotracheal intubation under light general anesthesia.

Use With Other CNS Depressants: The efficacy and safety of VERSED in clinical use are functions of the dose administered, the clinical status of the individual patient, and the use of concomitant medications capable of depressing the CNS. Anticipated effects range from mild sedation to deep levels of sedation virtually equivalent to a state of general anesthesia where the patient may require external support of vital functions. Care must be taken to individualize and carefully titrate the dose of VERSED to the patient's underlying medical/surgical conditions, administer to the desired effect being certain to wait an adequate time for peak CNS effects of both VERSED and concomitant medications, and have the personnel and size-appropriate equipment and facilities available for monitoring and intervention (see Boxed WARNING, WARNINGS and DOSAGE AND ADMINISTRATION). Practitioners administering VERSED must have the skills necessary to manage reasonably foreseeable adverse effects, particularly skills in airway management. For information regarding withdrawal (see DRUG ABUSE AND DEPENDENCE).

Information for Patients: To assure safe and effective use of benzodiazepines, the following information and instructions should be communicated to the patient when appropriate:

1. Inform your physician about any alcohol consumption and medicine you are now taking, especially blood pressure medication and antibiotics, including drugs you buy without a prescription. Alcohol has an increased effect when consumed with benzodiazepines; therefore, caution should be exercised regarding simultaneous ingestion of alcohol during benzodiazepine treatment.
2. Inform your physician if you are pregnant or are planning to become pregnant.
3. Inform your physician if you are nursing.
4. Patients should be informed of the pharmacological effects of VERSED, such as sedation and amnesia, which in some patients may be profound. The decision as to when patients who have received injectable VERSED, particularly on an outpatient basis, may again engage in activities requiring complete mental alertness, operate hazardous machinery or drive a motor vehicle must be individualized.
5. Patients receiving continuous infusion of midazolam in critical care settings over an extended period of time, may experience symptoms of withdrawal following abrupt discontinuation.

Drug Interactions: The sedative effect of intravenous VERSED is accentuated by any concomitantly administered medication, which depresses the central nervous system, particularly narcotics (eg, morphine, meperidine and fentanyl) and also secobarbital and droperidol. Consequently, the dosage of VERSED should be adjusted according to the type and amount of concomitant medications administered and the desired clinical response (see DOSAGE AND ADMINISTRATION).

Caution is advised when midazolam is administered concomitantly with drugs that are known to inhibit the P450 3A4 enzyme system such as cimetidine (not ranitidine), erythromycin, diltiazem, verapamil, ketoconazole and itraconazole. These drug interactions may result in prolonged sedation due to a decrease in plasma clearance of midazolam.

The effect of single oral doses of 800 mg cimetidine and 300 mg ranitidine on steady-state concentrations of midazolam was examined in a randomized crossover study (n=8). Cimetidine increased the mean midazolam steady-state concentration from 57 to 71 ng/mL. Ranitidine increased the mean steady-state concentration to 62 ng/mL. No change in choice reaction time or sedation index was detected after dosing with the H2 receptor antagonists.

In a placebo-controlled study, erythromycin administered as a 500 mg dose, tid, for 1 week (n=6), reduced the clearance of midazolam following a single 0.5 mg/kg IV dose. The half-life was approximately doubled.

Caution is advised when midazolam is administered to patients receiving erythromycin since this may result in a decrease in the plasma clearance of midazolam.

The effects of diltiazem (60 mg tid) and verapamil (80 mg tid) on the pharmacokinetics and pharmacodynamics of midazolam were investigated in a three-way crossover study (n=9). The half-life of midazolam increased from 5 to 7 hours when midazolam was taken in conjunction with verapamil or diltiazem. No interaction was observed in healthy subjects between midazolam and nifedipine.

In a placebo-controlled study, saquinvair administered as a 1200 mg dose, tid, for 5 days (n=12), a 56% reduction in the clearance of midazolam following a single 0.05 mg/kg IV dose was observed. The half-life was approximately doubled.

A moderate reduction in induction dosage requirements of thiopental (about 15%) has been noted following use of intramuscular VERSED for premedication in adults.

The intravenous administration of VERSED decreases the minimum alveolar concentration (MAC) of halothane required for general anesthesia. This decrease correlates with the dose of VERSED administered; no similar studies have been carried out in pediatric patients but there is no scientific reason to expect that pediatric patients would respond differently than adults.

Although the possibility of minor interactive effects has not been fully studied, VERSED and pancuronium have been used together in patients without noting clinically significant changes in dosage, onset or duration in adults. VERSED does not protect against the characteristic circulatory changes noted after administration of succinylcholine or pancuronium and does not protect against the increased intracranial pressure noted following administration of succinylcholine. VERSED does not cause a clinically significant change in dosage, onset or duration of a single intubating dose of succinylcholine; no similar studies have been carried out in pediatric patients but there is no scientific reason to expect that pediatric patients would respond differently than adults.

No significant adverse interactions with commonly used premedications or drugs used during anesthesia and surgery (including atropine, scopolamine, glycopyrrolate, diazepam, hydroxyzine, d-tubocurarine, succinylcholine and other nondepolarizing muscle relaxants) or topical local anesthetics (including lidocaine, dyclonine HCl and Cetacaine) have been observed in adults or pediatric patients. In neonates, however, severe hypotension has been reported with concomitant administration of fentanyl. This effect has been observed in neonates on an infusion of midazolam who received a rapid injection of fentanyl and in patients on an infusion of fentanyl who have received a rapid injection of midazolam.

Drug/Laboratory Test Interactions: Midazolam has not been shown to interfere with results obtained in clinical laboratory tests.

Carcinogenesis, Mutagenesis and Impairment of Fertility:
Carcinogenesis: Midazolam maleate was administered with

INTRAMUSCULARLY For sedation/anxiolysis/amnesia prior to anesthesia or for procedures, intramuscular VERSED can be used to sedate pediatric patients to facilitate less traumatic insertion of an intravenous catheter for titration of additional medication.	USUAL PEDIATRIC DOSE (NON-NEONATAL) Sedation after intramuscular VERSED is age and dose dependent: higher doses may result in deeper and more prolonged sedation. Doses of 0.1 to 0.15 mg/kg are usually effective and do not prolong emergence from general anesthesia. For more anxious patients, doses up to 0.5 mg/kg have been used. Although not systematically studied, the total dose usually does not exceed 10 mg. If VERSED is given with an opioid, the initial dose of each must be reduced.
INTRAVENOUSLY BY INTERMITTENT INJECTION For sedation/anxiolysis/amnesia prior to and during procedures or prior to anesthesia.	USUAL PEDIATRIC DOSE (NON-NEONATAL) It should be recognized that the depth of sedation/anxiolysis needed for pediatric patients depends on the type of procedure to be performed. For example, simple light sedation/anxiolysis in the preoperative period is quite different from the deep sedation and analgesia required for an endoscopic procedure in a child. For this reason, there is a broad range of dosage. For all pediatric patients, regardless of the indications for sedation/anxiolysis, it is vital to titrate VERSED and other concomitant medications slowly to the desired clinical effect. The initial dose of VERSED should be administered over 2 to 3 minutes. Since VERSED is water soluble, it takes approximately three times longer than diazepam to achieve peak EEG effects, therefore one must wait an additional 2 to 3 minutes to fully evaluate the sedative effect before initiating a procedure or repeating a dose. If further sedation is necessary, continue to titrate with small increments until the appropriate level of sedation is achieved. If other medications capable of depressing the CNS are coadministered, the peak effect of those concomitant medications must be considered and the dose of VERSED adjusted. The importance of drug titration to effect is vital to the safe sedation/anxiolysis of the pediatric patient. The total dose of VERSED will depend on patient response, the type and duration of the procedure, as well as the type and dose of concomitant medications. 1. *Pediatric Patients Less Than 6 Months of Age:* Limited information is available in non-intubated pediatric patients less than 6 months of age. It is uncertain when the patient transfers from neonatal physiology to pediatric physiology, therefore the dosing recommendations are unclear. Pediatric patients less than 6 months of age are particularly vulnerable to airway obstruction and hypoventilation, therefore titration with small increments to clinical effect and careful monitoring are essential. 2. *Pediatric Patients 6 Months to 5 Years of Age:* Initial dose 0.05 to 0.1 mg/kg; total dose up to 0.6 mg/kg may be necessary to reach the desired endpoint but usually does not exceed 6 mg. Prolonged sedation and risk of hypoventilation may be associated with the higher doses. 3. *Pediatric Patients 6 to 12 Years of Age:* Initial dose 0.025 to 0.05 mg/kg; total dose up to 0.4 mg/kg may be needed to reach the desired endpoint but usually does not exceed 10 mg. Prolonged sedation and risk of hypoventilation may be associated with the higher doses. 4. *Pediatric Patients 12 to 16 Years of Age:* Should be dosed as adults. Prolonged sedation may be associated with higher doses; some patients in this age range will require higher than recommended adult doses but the total dose usually does not exceed 10 mg. The dose of VERSED must be reduced in patients premedicated with opioid or other sedative agents including VERSED. Higher risk or debilitated patients may require lower dosages whether or not concomitant sedating medications have been administered (see WARNINGS).

CONTINUOUS INTRAVENOUS INFUSION For sedation/anxiolysis/amnesia in critical care settings.	USUAL PEDIATRIC DOSE (NON-NEONATAL) To initiate sedation, an intravenous loading dose of 0.05 to 0.2 mg/kg administered over at least 2 to 3 minutes can be used to establish the desired clinical effect IN PATIENTS WHOSE TRACHEA IS INTUBATED. (VERSED should not be administered as a rapid intravenous dose.) This loading dose may be followed by a continuous intravenous infusion to maintain the effect. An infusion of VERSED has been used in patients whose trachea was intubated but who were allowed to breathe spontaneously. Assisted ventilation is recommended for pediatric patients who are receiving other central nervous system depressant medications such as opioids. Based on pharmacokinetic parameters and reported clinical experience, continuous intravenous infusions of VERSED should be initiated at a rate of 0.06 to 0.12 mg/kg/hr (1 to 2 µg/kg/min). The rate of infusion can be increased or decreased (generally by 25% of the initial or subsequent infusion rate) as required, or supplemental intravenous doses of VERSED can be administered to increase or maintain the desired effect. Frequent assessment at regular intervals using standard pain/sedation scales is recommended. Drug elimination may be delayed in patients receiving erythromycin and/or other P450 3A4 enzyme inhibitors (see PRECAUTIONS: *Drug Interactions*) and in patients with liver dysfunction, low cardiac output (especially those requiring inotropic support), and in neonates. Hypotension may be observed in patients who are critically ill, particularly those receiving opioids and/or when VERSED is rapidly administered. When initiating an infusion with VERSED in hemodynamically compromised patients, the usual loading dose of VERSED should be titrated in small increments and the patient monitored for hemodynamic instability (eg, hypotension). These patients are also vulnerable to the respiratory depressant effects of VERSED and require careful monitoring of respiratory rate and oxygen saturation.
CONTINUOUS INTRAVENOUS INFUSION For sedation in critical care settings.	USUAL NEONATAL DOSE Based on pharmacokinetic parameters and reported clinical experience in preterm and term neonates WHOSE TRACHEA WAS INTUBATED, continuous intravenous infusions of VERSED should be initiated at a rate of 0.03 mg/kg/hr (0.5 µg/kg/min) in neonates <32 weeks and 0.06 mg/kg/hr (1 µg/kg/min) in neonates >32 weeks. Intravenous loading doses should not be used in neonates, rather the infusion may be run more rapidly for the first several hours to establish therapeutic plasma levels. The rate of infusion should be carefully and frequently reassessed, particularly after the first 24 hours so as to administer the lowest possible effective dose and reduce the potential for drug accumulation. This is particularly important because of the potential for adverse effects related to metabolism of the benzyl alcohol (see WARNINGS: *Usage in Preterm Infants and Neonates*). Hypotension may be observed in patients who are critically ill and in preterm and term infants, particularly those receiving fentanyl and/or when VERSED is administered rapidly. Due to an increased risk of apnea, extreme caution is advised when sedating preterm and former preterm patients whose trachea is not intubated.

diet in mice and rats for 2 years at dosages of 1, 9 and 80 mg/kg/day. In female mice in the highest dose group there was a marked increase in the incidence of hepatic tumors. In high-dose male rats there was a small but statistically significant increase in benign thyroid follicular cell tumors. Dosages of 9 mg/kg/day of midazolam maleate (25 times a human dose of 0.35 mg/kg) do not increase the incidence of tumors. The pathogenesis of induction of these tumors is not known. These tumors were found after chronic administration, whereas human use will ordinarily be of single or several doses.

Mutagenesis: Midazolam did not have mutagenic activity in *Salmonella typhimurium* (5 bacterial strains), Chinese hamster lung cells (V79), human lymphocytes or in the micronucleus test in mice.

Impairment of Fertility: A reproduction study in male and female rats did not show any impairment of fertility at dosages up to 10 times the human IV dose of 0.35 mg/kg.

Pregnancy: *Teratogenic Effects:* Pregnancy Category D (see WARNINGS).

Segment II teratology studies, performed with midazolam maleate injectable in rabbits and rats at 5 and 10 times the human dose of 0.35 mg/kg, did not show evidence of teratogenicity.

Nonteratogenic Effects: Studies in rats showed no adverse effects on reproductive parameters during gestation and lactation. Dosages tested were approximately 10 times the human dose of 0.35 mg/kg.

Labor and Delivery: In humans, measurable levels of midazolam were found in maternal venous serum, umbilical venous and arterial serum and amniotic fluid, indicating placental transfer of the drug. Following intramuscular administration of 0.05 mg/kg of midazolam, both the venous and the umbilical arterial serum concentrations were lower than maternal concentrations.

The use of injectable VERSED in obstetrics has not been evaluated in clinical studies. Because midazolam is transferred transplacentally and because other benzodiazepines given in the last weeks of pregnancy have resulted in neonatal CNS depression, VERSED is not recommended for obstetrical use.

Nursing Mothers: Midazolam is excreted in human milk. Caution should be exercised when VERSED is administered to a nursing woman.

Pediatric Use: The safety and efficacy of VERSED for sedation/anxiolysis/amnesia following single dose intramuscular administration, intravenously by intermittent injections and continuous infusion have been established in pediatric and neonatal patients. For specific safety monitoring and dosage guidelines (see Boxed WARNING, CLINICAL PHARMACOLOGY, INDICATIONS, WARNINGS, PRECAUTIONS, ADVERSE REACTIONS, OVERDOSAGE and DOSAGE AND ADMINISTRATION). UNLIKE ADULT PATIENTS, PEDIATRIC PATIENTS GENERALLY RECEIVE INCREMENTS OF VERSED ON A MG/KG BASIS. As a group, pediatric patients generally require higher dosages of VERSED (mg/kg) than do adults. Younger (less than six years) pediatric patients may require higher dosages (mg/kg) than older pediatric patients, and may require closer monitoring. In obese PEDIATRIC PATIENTS, the dose should be calculated based on ideal body weight. When VERSED is given in conjunction with opioids or other sedatives, the potential for respiratory depression, airway obstruction, or hypoventilation is increased. The health care practitioner who uses this medication in pediatric patients should be aware of and follow accepted professional guidelines for pediatric sedation appropriate to their situation.

VERSED should not be administered by rapid injection in the neonatal population. Severe hypotension and seizures have been reported following rapid IV administration, particularly, with concomitant use of fentanyl.

Geriatric Use: Because geriatric patients may have altered drug distribution and diminished hepatic and/or renal function, reduced doses of VERSED are recommended: Intravenous and intramuscular doses of VERSED should be decreased for elderly and for debilitated patients (see WARNINGS and DOSAGE AND ADMINISTRATION) and subjects over 70 years of age may be particularly sensitive. These patients will also probably take longer to recover completely after VERSED administration for the induction of anesthesia. Administration of IM and IV VERSED to elderly and/or high-risk surgical patients has been associated with rare reports of death under circumstances compatible with cardiorespiratory depression. In mose of these cases, the patients also received other central nervous system depressants capable of depressing respiration, especially narcotics (see DOSAGE AND ADMINISTRATION).

Specific dosing and monitoring guidelines for geriatric patients are provided in the DOSAGE AND ADMINISTRATION section for premedicated patients for sedation/anxiolysis/amnesia following IV and IM administration, for induction of anesthesia following IV administration and for continuous infusion.

ADVERSE REACTIONS

See WARNINGS concerning serious cardiorespiratory events and possible paradoxical reactions. Fluctuations in vital signs were the most frequently seen findings following parenteral administration of VERSED in adults and included decreased tidal volume and/or respiratory rate decrease (23.3% of patients following IV and 10.8% of patients following IM administration) and apnea (15.4% of patients following IV administration), as well as variations in blood pressure and pulse rate. The majority of serious adverse effects, particularly those associated with oxygenation and ventilation, have been reported when VERSED is administered with other medications capable of depressing the central nervous system. **The incidence of such events is higher in patients undergoing procedures involving the airway without the protective effect of an endotracheal tube (eg, upper endoscopy and dental procedures).**

Adults: The following additional adverse reactions were reported after intramuscular administration:

headache (1.3%)

Local effects at IM Injection site

pain (3.7%)
induration (0.5%)
redness (0.5%)
muscle stiffness (0.3%)

Administration of IM VERSED to elderly and/or higher risk surgical patients has been associated with rare reports of death under circumstances compatible with cardiorespiratory depression. In most of these cases, the patients also received other central nervous system depressants capable of depressing respiration, especially narcotics (see DOSAGE AND ADMINISTRATION).

The following additional adverse reactions were reported subsequent to intravenous administration as a single sedative/anxiolytic/amnestic agent in adult patients:

hiccoughs (3.9%)
nausea (2.8%)
vomiting (2.6%)
coughing (1.3%)
"oversedation" (1.6%)
headache (1.5%)
drowsiness (1.2%)

Local effects at the IV site

tenderness (5.6%)
pain during injection (5.0%)
redness (2.6%)
induration (1.7%)
phlebitis (0.4%)

Pediatric Patients: The following adverse events related to the use of IV VERSED in pediatric patients were reported in the medical literature: desaturation 4.6%, apnea 2.8%, hypotension 2.7%, paradoxical reactions 2.0%, hiccough 1.2%, seizure-like activity 1.1% and nystagmus 1.1%. The majority of airway-related events occurred in patients receiving other CNS depressing medications and in patients where VERSED was not used as a single sedating agent.

Neonates: For information concerning hypotensive episodes and seizures following the administration of VERSED to neonates (see Boxed WARNING, CONTRAINDICATIONS, WARNINGS and PRECAUTIONS).

Other adverse experiences, observed mainly following IV injection as a single sedative/anxiolytic/amnesia agent and occurring at an incidence of <1.0% in adult and pediatric patients, are as follows:

Respiratory: Laryngospasm, bronchospasm, dyspnea, hyperventilation, wheezing, shallow respirations, airway obstruction, tachypnea

Cardiovascular: Bigeminy, premature ventricular contractions, vasovagal episode, bradycardia, tachycardia, nodal rhythm

Gastrointestinal: Acid taste, excessive salivation, retching

CNS/Neuromuscular: Retrograde amnesia, euphoria, hallucination, confusion, argumentativeness, nervousness, anxiety, grogginess, restlessness, emergence delirium or agitation, prolonged emergence from anesthesia, dreaming during emergence, sleep disturbance, insomnia, nightmares, athetoid movements, seizure-like activity, ataxia, dizziness, dysphoria, slurred speech, dysphonia, paresthesia

Special Senses: Blurred vision, diplopia, nystagmus, pinpoint pupils, cyclic movements of eyelids, visual disturbance, difficulty focusing eyes, ears blocked, loss of balance, light-headedness

Integumentary: Hive-like elevation at injection site, swelling or feeling of burning, warmth or coldness at injection site

Hypersensitivity: Allergic reactions including anaphylactoid reactions, hives, rash, pruritus

Miscellaneous: Yawning, lethargy, chills, weakness, toothache, faint feeling, hematoma

Continued on next page

Versed—Cont.

DRUG ABUSE AND DEPENDENCE

Midazolam is subject to Schedule IV control under the Controlled Substances Act of 1970.

Midazolam was actively self-administered in primate models used to assess the positive reinforcing effects of psychoactive drugs.

Midazolam produced physical dependence of a mild to moderate intensity in cynomolgus monkeys after 5 to 10 weeks of administration. Available data concerning the drug abuse and dependence potential of midazolam suggest that its abuse potential is at least equivalent to that of diazepam.

Withdrawal symptoms, similar in character to those noted with barbiturates and alcohol (convulsions, hallucinations, tremor, abdominal and muscle cramps, vomiting and sweating), have occurred following abrupt discontinuation of benzodiazepines, including midazolam. Abdominal distention, nausea, vomiting, and tachycardia are prominent symptoms of withdrawal in infants. The more severe withdrawal symptoms have usually been limited to those patients who had received excessive doses over an extended period of time. Generally milder withdrawal symptoms (eg, dysphoria and insomnia) have been reported following abrupt discontinuance of benzodiazepines taken continuously at therapeutic levels for several months. Consequently, after extended therapy, abrupt discontinuation should generally be avoided and a gradual dosage tapering schedule followed. There is no consensus in the medical literature regarding tapering schedules; therefore, practitioners are advised to individualize therapy to meet patient's needs. In some case reports, patients who have had severe withdrawal reactions due to abrupt discontinuation of high-dose long-term midazolam, have been successfully weaned off of midazolam over a period of several days.

OVERDOSAGE

The manifestations of VERSED overdosage reported are similar to those observed with other benzodiazepines, including sedation, somnolence, confusion, impaired coordination, diminished reflexes, coma and untoward effects on vital signs. No evidence of specific organ toxicity from VERSED overdosage has been reported.

Treatment of Overdosage: Treatment of injectable VERSED overdosage is the same as that followed for overdosage with other benzodiazepines. Respiration, pulse rate and blood pressure should be monitored and general supportive measures should be employed. Attention should be given to the maintenance of a patent airway and support of ventilation, including administration of oxygen. An intravenous infusion should be started. Should hypotension develop, treatment may include intravenous fluid therapy, repositioning, judicious use of vasopressors appropriate to the clinical situation, if indicated, and other appropriate countermeasures. There is no information as to whether peritoneal dialysis, forced diuresis or hemodialysis are of any value in the treatment of midazolam overdosage.

Flumazenil, a specific benzodiazepine-receptor antagonist, is indicated for the complete or partial reversal of the sedative effects of benzodiazepines and may be used in situations when an overdose with a benzodiazepine is known or suspected. There are anecdotal reports of reversal of adverse hemodynamic responses associated with VERSED following administration of flumazenil to pediatric patients. Prior to the administration of flumazenil, necessary measures should be instituted to secure the airway, assure adequate ventilation, and establish adequate intravenous access. Flumazenil is intended as an adjunct to, not as a substitute for, proper management of benzodiazepine overdose. Patients treated with flumazenil should be monitored for resedation, respiratory depression and other residual benzodiazepine effects for an appropriate period after treatment. **Flumazenil will only reverse benzodiazepine-induced effects but will not reverse the effects of other concomitant medications.** The reversal of benzodiazepine effects may be associated with the onset of seizures in certain high-risk patients. **The prescriber should be aware of a risk of seizure in association with flumazenil treatment, particularly in long-term benzodiazepine users and in cyclic antidepressant overdose.** The complete flumazenil package insert, including CONTRAINDICATIONS, WARNINGS and PRECAUTIONS, should be consulted prior to use.

DOSAGE AND ADMINISTRATION

VERSED is a potent sedative agent that requires slow administration and individualization of dosage. Clinical experience has shown VERSED to be 3 to 4 times as potent per mg as diazepam. BECAUSE SERIOUS AND LIFE-THREATENING CARDIORESPIRATORY ADVERSE EVENTS HAVE BEEN REPORTED, PROVISION FOR MONITORING, DETECTION AND CORRECTION OF THESE REACTIONS MUST BE MADE FOR EVERY PATIENT TO WHOM VERSED INJECTION IS ADMINISTERED, REGARDLESS OF AGE OR HEALTH STATUS. Excessive single doses or rapid intravenous administration may result in respiratory depression, airway obstruction and/or arrest. The potential for these latter effects is increased in debilitated patients, those receiving concomitant medications capable of depressing the CNS, and patients without an endotracheal tube but undergoing a procedure involving the upper airway such as endoscopy or dental (see Boxed WARNING and WARNINGS).

Reactions such as agitation, involuntary movements, hyperactivity and combativeness have been reported in adult and pediatric patients. Should such reactions occur, caution should be exercised before continuing administration of VERSED (see WARNINGS).

VERSED should only be administered IM or IV (see WARNINGS).

Care should be taken to avoid intra-arterial injection or extravasation (see WARNINGS).

VERSED Injection may be mixed in the same syringe with the following frequently used premedications: morphine sulfate, meperidine, atropine sulfate or scopolamine. VERSED, at a concentration of 0.5 mg/mL, is compatible with 5% dextrose in water and 0.9% sodium chloride for up to 24 hours and with lactated Ringer's solution for up to 4 hours. Both the 1 mg/mL and 5 mg/mL formulations of VERSED may be diluted with 0.9% sodium chloride or 5% dextrose in water.

MONITORING: Patient response to sedative agents, and resultant respiratory status, is variable. Regardless of the intended level of sedation or route of administration, sedation is a continuum; a patient may move easily from light to deep sedation, with potential loss of protective reflexes. This is especially true in pediatric patients. Sedative doses should be individually titrated, taking into account patient age, clinical status and concomitant use of other CNS depressants. Continuous monitoring of respiratory and cardiac function is required (ie, pulse oximetry).

Adults and Pediatrics: Sedation guidelines recommend a careful presedation history to determine how a patient's underlying medical conditions or concomitant medications might affect their response to sedation/analgesia as well as a physical examination including a focused examination of the airway for abnormalities. Further recommendations include appropriate presedation fasting.

Titration to effect with multiple small doses is essential for safe administration. It should be noted that adequate time to achieve peak central nervous system effect (3 to 5 minutes) for midazolam should be allowed between doses to minimize the potential for oversedation. Sufficient time must elapse between doses of concomitant sedative medications to allow the effect of each dose to be assessed before subsequent drug administration. This is an important consideration for all patients who receive intravenous VERSED.

Immediate availability of resuscitative drugs and *age- and size-appropriate* equipment and personnel trained in their use and skilled in airway management should be assured (see WARNINGS).

Pediatrics: For deeply sedated pediatric patients a dedicated individual, other than the practitioner performing the procedure, should monitor the patient throughout the procedure.

Intravenous access is not thought to be necessary for all pediatric patients sedated for a diagnostic or therapeutic procedure because in some cases the difficulty of gaining IV access would defeat the purpose of sedating the child; rather, emphasis should be placed upon having the intravenous equipment available and a practitioner skilled in establishing vascular access in pediatric patients immediately available.

[See table on pages 2795 and 2796]
[See first table at top of page 2797]
[See second table at top of page 2797]
[See table on page 2798 and previous page]

Note: Parenteral drug products should be inspected visually for particulate matter and discoloration prior to administration, whenever solution and container permit.

HOW SUPPLIED

Package configurations containing midazolam hydrochloride equivalent to **5 mg** midazolam/**mL:**
1-mL vials (5 mg) — boxes of 10 (NDC 0004-1974-01); 2-mL vials (10 mg) — boxes of 10 (NDC 0004-1973-01); 5-mL vials (25 mg) — boxes of 10 (NDC 0004-1975-01); 10-mL vials (50 mg) — boxes of 10 (NDC 0004-1946-01); 2-mL Tel-E-Ject® disposable syringes (10 mg) box of 1 (NDC 0004-1947-09); — package of 10 boxes (NDC 0004-1947-01).

Package configurations containing midazolam hydrochloride equivalent to **1 mg** midazolam/**mL:**
2-mL vials (2 mg) — boxes of 10 (NDC 0004-1998-06); 5-mL vials (5 mg) — boxes of 10 (NDC 0004-1999-01); 10-mL vials (10 mg) — boxes of 10 (NDC 0004-2000-06).

Store at 59° to 86°F (15° to 30°C).

Distributed by:
Roche Pharmaceuticals
Roche Laboratories Inc.
340 Kingsland Street
Nutley, New Jersey 07110-1199

27897253-0600 Revised: June 2000

VERSED® (midazolam HCl) SYRUP ℞

The following text is complete prescribing information based on official labeling in effect June 1999.

VERSED Syrup has been associated with respiratory depression and respiratory arrest, especially when used for sedation in noncritical care settings. VERSED Syrup has been associated with reports of respiratory depression, airway obstruction, desaturation, hypoxia, and apnea, most often when used concomitantly with other central nervous system depressants (eg, opioids). VERSED Syrup should be used only in hospital or ambulatory care settings, including physicians' and dentists' offices, THAT CAN PROVIDE FOR CONTINUOUS MONITORING OF RESPIRATORY AND CARDIAC FUNCTION. IMMEDIATE AVAILABILITY OF RESUSCITATIVE DRUGS AND AGE- AND SIZE-APPROPRIATE EQUIPMENT FOR VENTILATION AND INTUBATION, AND PERSONNEL TRAINED IN THEIR USE AND SKILLED IN AIRWAY MANAGEMENT SHOULD BE ASSURED (see WARNINGS). For deeply sedated patients, a dedicated individual, other than the practitioner performing the procedure, should monitor the patient throughout the procedure.

DESCRIPTION

Midazolam is a benzodiazepine available as VERSED Syrup for oral administration. Midazolam, a white to light yellow crystalline compound, is insoluble in water, but can be solubilized in aqueous solutions by formation of the hydrochloride salt *in situ* under acidic conditions. Chemically, midazolam HCl is 8-chloro-6-(2-fluorophenyl)-1-methyl-4*H*-imidazo[1,5-a][1,4]benzodiazepine hydrochloride. Midazolam hydrochloride has the empirical formula $C_{18}H_{13}ClFN_3 \cdot HCl$, and a calculated molecular weight of 362.25.

Each mL of the syrup contains midazolam hydrochloride equivalent to 2 mg midazolam compounded with sorbitol, glycerin, citric acid anhydrous, sodium citrate, sodium benzoate, sodium saccharin, edetate disodium, FD&C Red #33, artificial cough syrup flavor, artificial bitterness modifier and water; the pH is adjusted to approximately 3 with hydrochloric acid.

Under the acidic conditions required to solubilize midazolam in the syrup, midazolam is present as an equilibrium mixture (shown below) of the closed ring form shown above and an open-ring structure formed by the acid-catalyzed ring opening of the 4,5-double bond of the diazepine ring. The amount of open-ring form is dependent upon the pH of the solution. At the specified pH of the syrup, the solution may contain up to about 40% of the open-ring compound. At the physiologic conditions under which the product is absorbed (pH of 5 to 8) into the systemic circulation, any open-ring form present reverts to the physiologically active, lipophilic, closed-ring form (midazolam) and is absorbed as such.

The following chart plots the percentage of midazolam present as the open-ring form as a function of pH in aqueous solutions. As indicated in the graph, the amount of open-ring compound present in solution is sensitive to changes in pH over the pH range specified for the product: 2.8 to 3.6. Above pH 5, at least 99% of the mixture is present in the closed-ring form.

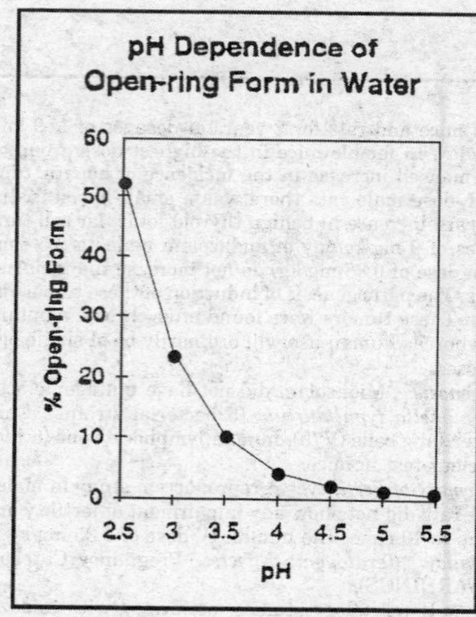

CLINICAL PHARMACOLOGY

Midazolam is a short-acting benzodiazepine central nervous system (CNS) depressant.

Pharmacodynamics: Pharmacodynamic properties of midazolam and its metabolites, which are similar to those of other benzodiazepines, include sedative, anxiolytic, amnesic and hypnotic activities. Benzodiazepine pharmacologic effects appear to result from reversible interactions with the γ-amino butyric acid (GABA) benzodiazepine receptor in the CNS, the major inhibitory neurotransmitter in the central nervous system. The action of midazolam is readily reversed by the benzodiazepine receptor antagonist, flumazenil.

Data from published reports of studies in pediatric patients clearly demonstrate that oral midazolam provides safe and effective sedation and anxiolysis prior to surgical procedures that require anesthesia as well as before other procedures that require sedation but may not require anesthesia.

Table 1. Pharmacokinetics of Midazolam Following Single Dose Administration of VERSED Syrup

Number of subjects/age	Dose (mg/kg)	T_{max} (h)	C_{max} (ng/mL)	$t_{1/2}$ (h)	$AUC_{0-\infty}$ (ng•h/mL)
6 months to <2 years old					
1	0.25	0.17	28.0	5.82	67.6
1	0.50	0.35	66.0	2.22	152
1	1.00	0.17	61.2	2.97	224
2 to <12 years old					
18	0.25	0.72 ± 0.44	63.0 ± 30.0	3.16 ± 1.50	138 ± 89.5
18	0.50	0.95 ± 0.53	126 ± 75.8	2.71 ± 1.09	306 ± 196
18	1.00	0.88 ± 0.99	201 ± 101	2.37 ± 0.96	743 ± 642
12 to <16 years old					
4	0.25	2.09 ± 1.35	29.1 ± 8.2	6.83 ± 3.84	155 ± 84.6
4	0.50	2.65 ± 1.58	118 ± 81.2	4.35 ± 3.31	821 ± 568
2	1.00	0.55 ± 0.28	191 ± 47.4	2.51 ± 0.18	566 ± 15.7

Table 2.

Interacting Drug	Adult Doses Studied	% Increase in C_{max} of Oral Midazolam	% Increase in AUC of Oral Midazolam
Erythromycin	500 mg tid	170–171	281–341
Cimetidine	800–1200 mg up to qid in divided doses	6–138	10–102
Diltiazem	60 mg tid	105	275
Fluconazole	200 mg qd	150	250
Grapefruit Juice	200 mL	56	52
Itraconazole	100–200 mg qd	80–240	240–980
Ketoconazole	400 mg qd	309	1490
Ranitidine	150 mg bid or tid; 300 mg qd	15–67	9–66
Roxithromycin	300 mg qd	37	47
Verapamil	80 mg tid	97	192

Table 3.

Interacting Drug	Adult Doses Studied	% Decrease in C_{max} of Oral Midazolam	% Decrease in AUC of Oral Midazolam
Carbamazepine	Therapeutic Doses	93	94
Phenytoin	Therapeutic Doses	93	94
Rifampin	600 mg/day	94	96

The most commonly reported effective doses range from 0.25 to 1.0 mg/kg in children (6 months to <16 years). The single most commonly reported effective dose is 0.5 mg/kg. Time to onset of effect is most frequently reported as 10 to 20 minutes.

The effects of midazolam on the CNS are dependent on the dose administered, the route of administration, and the presence or absence of other medications.

Following premedication with oral midazolam, time to recovery has been assessed in pediatric patients using various measures, such as time to eye opening, time to extubation, time in the recovery room, and time to discharge from the hospital. Most placebo-controlled trials (8 total) have shown little effect of oral midazolam on recovery time from general anesthesia; however, a number of other placebo-controlled studies (5 total) have demonstrated some prolongation in recovery time following premedication with oral midazolam. Prolonged recovery may be related to duration of the surgical procedure and/or use of other medications with central nervous system depressant properties.

Partial or complete impairment of recall following oral midazolam has been demonstrated in several studies. Amnesia for the surgical experience was greater after oral midazolam when used as a premedicant than after placebo and was generally considered a benefit. In one study, 69% of midazolam patients did not remember mask application versus 6% of placebo patients.

Episodes of oxygen desaturation, respiratory depression, apnea, and airway obstruction have been reported in <1% of pediatric patients following premedication (eg, sedation prior to induction of anesthesia) with VERSED Syrup; the potential for such adverse events are markedly increased when oral midazolam is combined with other central nervous system depressing agents and in patients with abnormal airway anatomy, patients with cyanotic congenital heart disease, or patients with sepsis or severe pulmonary disease (see WARNINGS).

Concomitant use of barbiturates or other central nervous system depressants may increase the risk of hypoventilation, airway obstruction, desaturation or apnea, and may contribute to profound and/or prolonged drug effect. In one study of pediatric patients undergoing elective repair of congenital cardiac defects, premedication regimens (oral dose of 0.75 mg/kg midazolam or IM morphine plus scopolamine) increased transcutaneous carbon dioxide ($PtcCO_2$), decreased SpO_2 (as measured by pulse oximetry), and decreased respiratory rates preferentially in patients with pulmonary hypertension. This suggests that hypercarbia or hypoxia following premedication might pose a risk to children with congenital heart disease and pulmonary hypertension. In a study of an adult population 65 years and older, the preinduction administration of oral midazolam 7.5 mg resulted in a 60% incidence of hypoxemia (paO_2<90% for over 30 seconds) at some time during the operative procedure versus 15% for the nonpremedicated group.

Pharmacokinetics: *Absorption:* Midazolam is rapidly absorbed after oral administration and is subject to substantial intestinal and hepatic first-pass metabolism. The pharmacokinetics of midazolam and its major metabolite, α-hydroxymidazolam, and the absolute bioavailability of VERSED Syrup were studied in pediatric patients of different ages (6 months to <16 years old) over a 0.25 to 1.0 mg/kg dose range. Pharmacokinetic parameters from this study are presented in Table 1. The mean T_{max} values across dose groups (0.25, 0.5, and 1.0 mg/kg) range from 0.17 to 2.65 hours. Midazolam exhibits linear pharmacokinetics between oral doses of 0.25 to 1.0 mg/kg (up to a maximum dose of 40 mg) across the age groups ranging from 6 months to <16 years. Linearity was also demonstrated across the doses within the age group of 2 years to <12 years having 18 patients at each of the three doses. The absolute bioavailability of the midazolam syrup in pediatric patients is about 36%, which is not affected by pediatric age or weight. The $AUC_{0-\infty}$ ratio of α-hydroxymidazolam to midazolam for the oral dose in pediatric patients is higher than for an IV dose (0.38 to 0.75 versus 0.21 to 0.39 across the age group of 6 months to <16 years), and the $AUC_{0-\infty}$ ratio of α-hydroxymidazolam to midazolam for the oral dose is higher in pediatric patients than in adults (0.38 to 0.75 versus 0.40 to 0.56). Food effect has not been tested using VERSED Syrup. When a 15 mg oral tablet of midazolam was administered with food to adults, the absorption and disposition of midazolam was not affected. Feeding is generally contraindicated prior to sedation of pediatric patients for procedures.

[See table 1 above]

Distribution: The extent of plasma protein binding of midazolam is moderately high and concentration independent. In adults and pediatric patients older than 1 year, midazolam is approximately 97% bound to plasma protein, principally albumin. In healthy volunteers, α-hydroxymidazolam is bound to the extent of 89%. In pediatric patients (6 months to <16 years) receiving 0.15 mg/kg IV midazolam, the mean steady-state volume of distribution ranged from 1.24 to 2.02 L/kg.

Metabolism: Midazolam is primarily metabolized in the liver and gut by human cytochrome P450 IIIA4 (CYP3A4) to its pharmacologic active metabolite, α-hydroxymidazolam, followed by glucuronidation of the α-hydroxyl metabolite which is present in unconjugated and conjugated forms in human plasma. The α-hydroxymidazolam glucuronide is then excreted in urine. In a study in which adult volunteers were administered intravenous midazolam (0.1 mg/kg) and α-hydroxymidazolam (0.15 mg/kg), the pharmacodynamic parameter values of the maximum effect (E_{max}) and concentration eliciting half-maximal effect (EC_{50}) were similar for both compounds. The effects studied were reaction time and errors in tracing tests. The results indicate that α-hydroxymidazolam is equipotent and equally effective as unchanged midazolam on a total plasma concentration basis. After oral or intravenous administration, 63% to 80% of midazolam is recovered in urine as α-hydroxymidazolam glucuronide. No significant amount of parent drug or metabolites is extractable from urine before beta-glucuronidase and sulfatase deconjugation, indicating that the urinary metabolites are excreted mainly as conjugates.

Midazolam is also metabolized to two other minor metabolites: 4-hydroxy metabolite (about 3% of the dose) and 1,4-dihydroxy metabolite (about 1% of the dose) are excreted in small amounts in the urine as conjugates.

Elimination: The mean elimination half-life of midazolam ranged from 2.2 to 6.8 hours following single, oral doses of 0.25, 0.5, and 1.0 mg/kg of midazolam (VERSED Syrup). Similar results (ranged from 2.9 to 4.5 hours) for the mean elimination half-life were observed following IV administration of 0.15 mg/kg of midazolam to pediatric patients (6 months to <16 years old). In the same group of patients receiving the 0.15 mg/kg IV dose, the mean total clearance ranged from 9.3 to 11.0 mL/min/kg.

Pharmacokinetic-Pharmacodynamic Relationships: The relationship between plasma concentration and sedation and anxiolysis scores of oral midazolam syrup (single oral doses of 0.25, 0.5, or 1.0 mg/kg) was investigated in three age groups of pediatric patients (6 months to <2 years, 2 to <12 years, and 12 to <16 years old). In this study, the patient's sedation scores were recorded at baseline and at 10-minute intervals up to 30 minutes after oral dosing until satisfactory sedation ("drowsy" or "asleep but responsive to mild shaking" or "asleep and not responsive to mild shaking") was achieved. Anxiolysis scores were measured at the time when the patient was separated from his/her parents and at mask induction. The results of the analyses showed that the mean midazolam plasma concentration as well as the mean of midazolam plus α-hydroxymidazolam for those patients with a sedation score of 4 (asleep but responsive to mild shaking) is significantly different than the mean concentrations for those patients with a sedation score of 3 (drowsy), which is significantly different than the mean concentrations for patients with a sedation score of 2 (awake/calm). The statistical analysis indicates that the greater the midazolam, or midazolam plus α-hydroxymidazolam concentration, the greater the maximum sedation score for pediatric patients. No such trend was observed between anxiolysis scores and the mean midazolam concentration or mean of midazolam plus α-hydroxymidazolam concentration; however, anxiolysis is a more variable surrogate measurement of clinical response.

Special Populations:

Renal Impairment: Although the pharmacokinetics of intravenous midazolam in adult patients with chronic renal failure differed from those of subjects with normal renal function, there were no alterations in the distribution, elimination, or clearance of unbound drug in the renal failure patients. However, the effects of renal impairment on the active metabolite α-hydroxymidazolam are unknown.

Hepatic Dysfunction: Chronic hepatic disease alters the pharmacokinetics of midazolam. Following oral administration of 15 mg of midazolam, C_{max} and bioavailability values were 43% and 100% higher, respectively, in adult patients with hepatic cirrhosis than adult subjects with normal liver function. In the same patients with hepatic cirrhosis, following IV administration of 7.5 mg of midazolam, the clearance of midazolam was reduced by about 40% and the elimination half-life was increased by about 90% compared with subjects with normal liver function. Midazolam should be titrated for the desired effect in patients with chronic hepatic disease.

Continued on next page

Versed Syrup—Cont.

Congestive Heart Failure: Following oral administration of 7.5 mg of midazolam, elimination half-life values were 43% higher in adult patients with congestive heart failure than in control subjects.
Neonates: VERSED Syrup has not been studied in pediatric patients less than 6 months of age.
Drug-Drug Interactions: See PRECAUTIONS: *Drug Interactions.*
INHIBITORS OF CYP3A4 ISOZYMES:
Table 2 summarizes the changes in the C_{max} and AUC of midazolam when drugs known to inhibit CYP3A4 were concurrently administered with oral midazolam in adult subjects.
[See table 2 at top of previous page]
Other drugs known to inhibit the effects of CYP3A4 would be expected to have similar effects on these midazolam pharmacokinetic parameters.
INDUCERS OF CYP3A4 ISOZYMES:
Table 3 summarizes the changes in the C_{max} and AUC of midazolam when drugs known to induce CYP3A4 were concurrently administered with oral midazolam in adult subjects. The clinical significance of these changes is unclear.
[See table 3 at top of previous page]
Although not tested, phenobarbital, rifabutin and other drugs known to induce the effects of CYP3A4 would be expected to have similar effects on these midazolam pharmacokinetic parameters.
Drugs that did not affect midazolam pharmacokinetics are presented in Table 4.

Table 4.

Interacting Drug	Adult Doses Studied
Azithromycin	500 mg/day
Magnesium	Not available
Nitrendipine	20 mg
Terbinafine	200 mg/day

Clinical Trials: Dose Ranging, Safety and Efficacy Study With VERSED Syrup in Pediatric Patients: The effectiveness of VERSED Syrup as a premedicant to sedate and calm pediatric patients prior to induction of general anesthesia was compared among three different doses in a randomized, double-blind, parallel-group study. Patients of ASA physical status I, II or III were stratified to 1 of 3 age groups (6 months to <2 years, 2 to <6 years, and 6 to <16 years), and within each age group randomized to 1 of 3 dosing groups (0.25, 0.5, and 1.0 mg/kg up to a maximum dose of 20 mg). Greater than 90% of treated patients achieved satisfactory sedation and anxiolysis at at least one timepoint within 30 minutes posttreatment. Similarly high proportions of patients exhibited satisfactory ease of separation from parent or guardian and were cooperative at the time of mask induction with nitrous oxide and halothane administration. Onset time of satisfactory sedation or anxiolysis occurred within 10 minutes after treatment for >70% of patients who started with an unsatisfactory baseline rating. Whereas pairwise comparisons (0.25 mg/kg versus 0.5 mg/kg groups, and 0.5 mg/kg versus 1.0 mg/kg groups) on satisfactory sedation did not yield significant p-values (p=0.08 in both cases), comparative analysis of the clinical response between the high and low doses demonstrated that a higher proportion of patients in the 1.0 mg/kg dose group exhibited satisfactory sedation and anxiolysis as compared to the 0.25 mg/kg group ($p<0.05$).

INDICATIONS AND USAGE

VERSED Syrup is indicated for use in pediatric patients for sedation, anxiolysis and amnesia prior to diagnostic, therapeutic or endoscopic procedures or before induction of anesthesia.
VERSED Syrup is intended for use in monitored settings only and not for chronic or home use (see WARNINGS).
VERSED SYRUP MUST BE USED AS SPECIFIED IN THE LABEL.
Midazolam is associated with a high incidence of partial or complete impairment of recall for the next several hours (see CLINICAL PHARMACOLOGY).

CONTRAINDICATIONS

VERSED is contraindicated in patients with a known hypersensitivity to the drug or allergies to cherries or formulation excipients. Benzodiazepines are contraindicated in patients with acute narrow-angle glaucoma. Benzodiazepines may be used in patients with open-angle glaucoma only if they are receiving appropriate therapy. Measurements of intraocular pressure in patients without eye disease show a moderate lowering following induction of general anesthesia with injectable VERSED; patients with glaucoma have not been studied.

WARNINGS

Serious respiratory adverse events have occurred after administration of oral VERSED, most often when VERSED was used in combination with other central nervous system depressants. These adverse events have included respiratory depression, airway obstruction, oxygen desaturation, apnea, and rarely, respiratory and/or cardiac arrest (see box WARNING). When oral midazolam is administered as the sole agent at recommended doses respiratory depression, airway obstruction, oxygen desaturation, and apnea occur infrequently (see DOSAGE AND ADMINISTRATION).
Prior to the administration of VERSED in any dose, the immediate availability of oxygen, resuscitative drugs, age- and size-appropriate equipment for bag/valve/mask ventilation and intubation, and skilled personnel for the maintenance of a patent airway and support of ventilation should be ensured. VERSED Syrup must never be used without individualization of dosage, particularly when used with other medications capable of producing central nervous system depression.
VERSED Syrup should be used only in hospital or ambulatory care settings, including physicians' and dentists' offices, that are equipped to provide continuous monitoring of respiratory and cardiac function. VERSED Syrup must only be administered to patients if they will be monitored by direct visual observation by a health care professional. If VERSED Syrup will be administered in combination with other anesthetic drugs or drugs which depress the central nervous system, patients must be monitored by persons specifically trained in the use of these drugs and, in particular, in the management of respiratory effects of these drugs, including respiratory and cardiac resuscitation of patients in the age group being treated.
For deeply sedated patients, a dedicated individual whose sole responsibility is to observe the patient, other than the practitioner performing the procedure, should monitor the patient throughout the procedure.
Patients should be continuously monitored for early signs of hypoventilation, airway obstruction, or apnea with means for detection readily available (eg, pulse oximetry). Hypoventilation, airway obstruction, and apnea can lead to hypoxia and/or cardiac arrest unless effective countermeasures are taken immediately. The immediate availability of specific reversal agents (flumazenil) is highly recommended. Vital signs should continue to be monitored during the recovery period. Because VERSED can depress respiration (see CLINICAL PHARMACOLOGY), especially when used concomitantly with opioid agonists and other sedatives (see DOSAGE AND ADMINISTRATION), it should be used for sedation/anxiolysis/amnesia only in the presence of personnel skilled in early detection of hypoventilation, maintaining a patent airway, and supporting ventilation.
Episodes of oxygen desaturation, respiratory depression, apnea, and airway obstruction have been occasionally reported following premedication (sedation prior to induction of anesthesia) with oral midazolam; such events are markedly increased when oral midazolam is combined with other central nervous system depressing agents and in patients with abnormal airway anatomy, patients with cyanotic congenital heart disease, or patients with sepsis or severe pulmonary disease.
Reactions such as agitation, involuntary movements (including tonic/clonic movements and muscle tremor), hyperactivity and combativeness have been reported in both adult and pediatric patients. Consideration should be given to the possibility of paradoxical reaction. Should such reactions occur, the response to each dose of VERSED and all other drugs, including local anesthetics, should be evaluated before proceeding. Reversal of such responses with flumazenil has been reported in pediatric and adult patients.
Concomitant use of barbiturates, alcohol or other central nervous system depressants may increase the risk of hypoventilation, airway obstruction, desaturation, or apnea and may contribute to profound and/or prolonged drug effect. Narcotic premedication also depresses the ventilatory response to carbon dioxide stimulation.
Coadministration of oral midazolam in patients who are taking ketoconazole and itraconazole has been shown to result in large increases in C_{max} and AUC of midazolam due to a decrease in plasma clearance of midazolam (see PHARMACOKINETICS: *Drug-Drug Interactions* and PRECAUTIONS). Due to the potential for intense and prolonged sedation and respiratory depression, VERSED Syrup should only be coadministered with these medications if absolutely necessary and with appropriate equipment and personnel available to respond to respiratory insufficiency.
Higher risk pediatric surgical patients may require lower doses, whether or not concomitant sedating medications have been administered. Pediatric patients with cardiac or respiratory compromise may be unusually sensitive to the respiratory depressant effect of VERSED. Pediatric patients undergoing procedures involving the upper airway such as upper endoscopy or dental care, are particularly vulnerable to episodes of desaturation and hypoventilation due to partial airway obstruction. Patients with chronic renal failure and patients with congestive heart failure eliminate midazolam more slowly (see CLINICAL PHARMACOLOGY).
The decision as to when patients who have received VERSED Syrup, particularly on an outpatient basis, may again engage in activities requiring complete mental alertness, operate hazardous machinery or drive a motor vehicle must be indivdualized. Gross tests of recovery from the effects of VERSED Syrup (see CLINICAL PHARMACOLOGY) cannot be relied upon to predict reaction time under stress. It is recommended that no patient operate hazardous machinery or a motor vehicle until the effects of the drug, such as drowsiness, have subsided or until one full day after anesthesia and surgery, whichever is longer. Particular care should be taken to assure safe ambulation.
Usage in Pregnancy: Although VERSED Syrup has not been studied in pregnant patients, an increased risk of congenital malformations associated with the use of benzodiazepine drugs (diazepam and chlordiazepoxide) have been suggested in several studies. If this drug is used during pregnancy, the patient should be apprised of the potential hazard to the fetus.
Usage in Preterm Infants and Neonates: VERSED Syrup has not been studied in patients less than 6 months of age.

PRECAUTIONS

Use With Other CNS Depressants: The efficacy and safety of VERSED in clinical use are functions of the dose administered, the clinical status of the individual patient, and the use of concomitant medications capable of depressing the CNS. Anticipated effects may range from mild sedation to deep levels of sedation with a potential loss of protective reflexes, particularly when coadministered with anesthetic agents or other CNS depressants. Care must be taken to individualize the dose of VERSED based on the patient's age, underlying medical/surgical conditions, concomitant medications, and to have the personnel, age- and size-appropriate equipment and facilities available for monitoring and intervention. Practitioners administering VERSED must have the skills necessary to manage reasonably foreseeable adverse effects, particularly skills in airway management.
Use With Inhibitors of CYP3A4 Isozymes: Oral midazolam should be used with caution in patients treated with drugs known to inhibit CYP3A4 because inhibition of metabolism may lead to more intense and prolonged sedation (see PHARMACOKINETICS: *Drug-Drug Interactions*). Patients being treated with medications known to inhibit CYP3A4 isozymes should be treated with lower than recommended doses of VERSED Syrup and the clinician should expect a more intense and prolonged effect.
Information for Patients: To assure safe and effective use of VERSED Syrup, the following information and instructions should be communicated to the patient when appropriate:

1. Inform your physician about any alcohol consumption and medicine you are now taking, especially blood pressure medication and antibiotics, including drugs you buy without a prescription. Alcohol has an increased effect when consumed with benzodiazepines; therefore, caution should be exercised regarding simultaneous ingestion of alcohol during benzodiazepine treatment.
2. Inform your physician if you are pregnant or are planning to become pregnant.
3. Inform your physician if you are nursing.
4. Patients should be informed of the pharmacological effects of VERSED Syrup, such as sedation and amnesia, which in some patients may be profound. The decision as to when patients who have received VERSED Syrup, particularly on an outpatient basis, may again engage in activities requiring complete mental alertness, operate hazardous machinery or drive a motor vehicle must be individualized.
5. VERSED Syrup should not be taken in conjunction with grapefruit juice.
6. For pediatric patients, particular care should be taken to assure safe ambulation.

Drug Interactions: *Inhibitors of CYP3A4 Isozymes:* Caution is advised when midazolam is administered concomitantly with drugs that are known to inhibit the cytochrome P450 3A4 enzyme system (ie, some drugs in the drug classes of azole antimycotics, protease inhibitors, calcium channel antagonists, and macrolide antibiotics). Drugs such as erythromycin, diltiazem, verapamil, ketoconazole, fluconazole and itraconazole were shown to significantly increase the C_{max} and AUC of orally administered midazolam. These drug interactions may result in increased and prolonged sedation due to a decrease in plasma clearance of midazolam. Although not studied, the potent cytochrome P450 3A4 inhibitors ritonavir and nelfinavir may cause intense and prolonged sedation and respiratory depression due to a decrease in plasma clearance of midazolam. Caution is advised when VERSED Syrup is used concomitantly with these drugs. Dose adjustments should be considered and possible prolongation and intensity of effect should be anticipated (see PHARMACOKINETICS: *Drug-Drug Interactions*).
Inducers of CYP3A4 Isozymes: Cytochrome P450 inducers, such as rifampin, carbamazepine, and phenytoin, induce metabolism and caused a markedly decreased C_{max} and AUC of oral midazolam in adult studies. Although clinical studies have not been performed, phenobarbital is expected to have the same effect. Caution is advised when administering VERSED Syrup to patients receiving these medications and if necessary dose adjustments should be considered.
CNS Depressants: One case was reported of inadequate sedation with chloral hydrate and later with oral midazolam due to a possible interaction with methylphenidate administered chronically in a 2-year-old boy with a history of William's syndrome. The difficulty in achieving adequate sedation may have been the result of decreased absorption of the sedatives due to both the gastrointestinal effects and stimulant effects of methylphenidate.
The sedative effect of VERSED Syrup is accentuated by any concomitantly administered medication which depresses

the central nervous system, particularly narcotics (eg, morphine, meperidine and fentanyl), propofol, ketamine, nitrous oxide, secobarbital and droperidol. Consequently, the dose of VERSED Syrup should be adjusted according to the type and amount of concomitant medications administered and the desired clinical response (see DOSAGE AND ADMINISTRATION).
No significant adverse interactions with common premedications (such as atropine, scopolamine, glycopyrrolate, diazepam, hydroxyzine, and other muscle relaxants) or local anesthetics have been observed.
Drug/Laboratory Test Interactions: Midazolam has not been shown to interfere with results obtained in clinical laboratory tests.
Carcinogenesis, Mutagenesis and Impairment of Fertility:
Carcinogenesis: Midazolam maleate was administered with diet in mice and rats for 2 years at dosages of 1, 9, and 80 mg/kg/day. In female mice in the highest dose (10 times the highest oral dose of 1.0 mg/kg for a pediatric patient, on a mg/m^2 basis) group there was a marked increase in the incidence of hepatic tumors. In high-dose (19 times the pediatric dose) male rats there was a small but statistically significant increase in benign thyroid follicular cell tumors. Dosages of 9 mg/kg/day of midazolam maleate (1 to 2 times the pediatric dose) did not increase the incidence of tumors in mice or rats. The pathogenesis of induction of these tumors is not known. These tumors were found after chronic administration, whereas human use will ordinarily be single or intermittent doses.
Mutagenesis: Midazolam did not have mutagenic activity in *Salmonella typhimurium* (5 bacterial strains), Chinese hamster lung cells (V79), human lymphocytes or in the micronucleus test in mice.
Impairment of Fertility: A reproduction study in male and female rats did not show any impairment of fertility at dosages up to 16 mg/kg/day PO (3 times the human dose of 1.0 mg/kg, on a mg/m^2 basis).
Pregnancy: *Teratogenic Effects:* Pregnancy Category D (see WARNINGS).
Embryo-fetal development studies, performed with midazolam maleate in mice (at up to 120 mg/kg/day PO, 10 times the human dose of 1.0 mg/kg on a mg/m^2 basis), rats (at up to 4 mg/kg/day IV, 8 times the human IV dose of 5 mg) and rabbits (at up to 100 mg/kg/day PO, 32 times the human oral dose of 1.0 mg/kg on a mg/m^2 basis), did not show evidence of teratogenicity.
Nonteratogenic Effects: Studies in rats showed no adverse effects on reproductive parameters during gestation and lactation. Dosages tested (4 mg/kg IV and 50 mg/kg PO) were approximately 8 times each of the human doses on a mg/m^2 basis.
Labor and Delivery: In humans, measurable levels of midazolam were found in maternal venous serum, umbilical venous and arterial serum and amniotic fluid, indicating placental transfer of the drug.
The use of VERSED Syrup in obstetrics has not been evaluated in clinical studies. Because midazolam is transferred transplacentally and because other benzodiazepines given in the last weeks of pregnancy have resulted in neonatal CNS depression, VERSED Syrup is not recommended for obstetrical use.
Nursing Mothers: Midazolam is excreted in human milk. Caution should be exercised when VERSED Syrup is administered to a nursing woman.
Geriatric Use: The safety and efficacy of this product have not been fully studied in geriatric patients. Therefore, there are no available data on a safe dosing regimen. One study in geratric subjects, using midazolam 7.5 mg as a premedicant prior to general anesthesia, noted a 60% incidence of hypoxemia (pO_2<90% for over 30 seconds) at sometime during the operative procedure versus 15% for the nonpremedicated group. Until further information is available it is recommended that this product should not be used in geriatric patients.
Use in Patients With Heart Disease: Following oral administration of 7.5 mg of midazolam to adult patients with congestive heart failure, the half-life of midazolam was 43% higher than in control subjects. One study suggests that hypercarbia or hypoxia following premedication with oral midazolam might pose a risk to children with congenital heart disease and pulmonary hypertension, although there are no known reports of pulmonary hypertensive crises that had been triggered by premedication. In the study, 22 children were premedicated with oral midazolam (0.75 mg/kg) or IM morphine plus scopolamine prior to elective repair of congenital cardiac defects. Both premedication regimens increased $PtcCO_2$ and decreased SpO_2 and respiratory rates preferentially in patients with pulmonary hypertension.

ADVERSE REACTIONS

The distribution of adverse events occurring in patients evaluated in a randomized, double-blind, parallel-group trial are presented in Tables 5 and 6 by body system in order of decreasing frequency: for the premedication period (eg, sedation period prior to induction of anesthesia) alone, see Table 5; for over the entire monitoring period including premedication, anesthesia and recovery, see Table 6.
The distribution of adverse events occurring during the premedication period, before induction of anesthesia, is presented in Table 5. Emesis, which occurred in 31/397 (8%) patients over the entire monitoring period, occurred in 3/397 (0.8%) of patients during the premedication period (from midazolam administration to mask induction). Nausea, which occurred in 14/397 (4%) patients over the entire monitoring period (premedication, anesthesia and recovery), occurred in 2/397 (0.5%) patients during the premedication period.

Table 5. Adverse Events Occurring During the Premedication Period Before Mask Induction in the Randomized, Double-Blind, Parallel-Group Trial

Body System	**Treatment Regimen**						**Overall**	
No. Patients with Adverse Events	0.25 mg/kg (n=132)		0.50 mg/kg (n=132)		1.0 mg/kg (n=133)		(n=397)	
	No.	(%)	No.	(%)	No.	(%)	No.	(%)
Gastrointestinal System Disorders								
Emesis	1	(0.76%)	1	(0.76%)	1	(0.75%)	3	(0.76%)
Nausea					2	(1.5%)	2	(0.50%)
Respiratory System Disorders								
Laryngospasm					1*	(0.75%)	1	(0.25%)
Sneezing/Rhinorrhea					1	(0.75%)	1	(0.25%)
ALL BODY SYSTEMS	1	(0.76%)	1	(0.76%)	5	(3.8%)	7	(1.8%)

*This adverse event occurred precisely at the time of induction.

Table 6. Adverse Events (≥1 %) From the Randomized, Double-Blind, Parallel-Group Trial on Entire Monitoring Period (premedication, anesthesia, recovery)

Body System	**Treatment Regimen**						**Overall**	
No. Patients with Adverse Events	0.25 mg/kg (n=132)		0.50 mg/kg (n=132)		1.0 mg/kg (n=133)		(n=397)	
	No.	(%)	No.	(%)	No.	(%)	No.	(%)
Gastrointestinal System Disorders								
Emesis	11	(8%)	5	(4%)	15	(11%)	31	(8%)
Nausea	6	(5%)	2	(2%)	6	(5%)	14	(4%)
Overall	16	(12%)	8	(6%)	16	(12%)	40	(10%)
Respiratory System Disorders								
Hypoxia	0		5	(4%)	4	(3%)	9	(2%)
Laryngospasm	0		1	(<1%)	5	(4%)	6	(2%)
Respiratory Depression	2	(2%)	1	(<1%)	2	(2%)	5	(1%)
Rhonchi	2	(2%)	1	(<1%)	2	(2%)	5	(1%)
Airway Obstruction	2	(2%)	2	(2%)	0		4	(1%)
Upper Airway Congestion	2	(2%)	0		2	(2%)	4	(1%)
Overall	7	(5%)	9	(7%)	15	(11%)	31	(8%)
Psychiatric Disorders								
Agitated	1	(<1%)	2	(2%)	3	(2%)	6	(2%)
Overall	1	(<1%)	3	(2%)	4	(3%)	8	(2%)
Heart Rate Rhythm Disorders								
Bradycardia	1	(<1%)	3	(2%)	0		4	(1%)
Bigeminy	2	(2%)	0		0		2	(<1%)
Overall	3	(2%)	3	(2%)	1	(<1%)	7	(2%)
Central & Peripheral Nervous System Disorders								
Prolonged Sedation	0		0		2	(2%)	2	(<1%)
Overall	2	(2%)	0		3	(2%)	5	(1%)
Skin and Appendages Disorders								
Rash	2	(2%)	0		0		2	(<1%)
Overall	2	(2%)	2	(2%)	0		4	(1%)
ALL BODY SYSTEMS	26	(20%)	23	(17%)	33	(25%)	82	(21%)

The distribution of all adverse events occurring in ≥1% of patients over the entire monitoring period are presented in Table 6. For the entire monitoring period (premedication, anesthesia and recovery), adverse events were reported by 82/397 (21%) patients who received midazolam overall. The most frequently reported adverse events were emesis occurring in 31/397 (8%) patients and nausea occurring in 14/397 (4%) patients. Most of these gastrointestinal events occurred after the administration of other anesthetic agents. For the respiratory system overall, adverse events (hypoxia, laryngospasm, rhonchi, coughing, respiratory depression, airway obstruction, upper-airway congestion, shallow respirations), occurred during the entire monitoring period in 31/397 (8%) patients and increased in frequency as dosage was increased: 71/132 (5%) patients in the 0.25 mg/kg dose group, 9/132 (7%) patients in the 0.5 mg/kg dose group, and 15/133 (11%) patients in the 1.0 mg/kg dose group.
Most of the respiratory adverse events occurred during induction, general anesthesia or recovery. One patient (0.25%) experienced a respiratory system adverse event (laryngospasm) during the premedication period. This adverse event occurred precisely at the time of induction. Although many of the respiratory complications occurred in settings of upper airway procedures or concurrently administered opioids, a number of these events occurred outside of these settings as well. In this study, administration of VERSED Syrup was generally accompanied by a slight decrease in both systolic and diastolic blood pressures, as well as a slight increase in heart rate.
[See table 5 above]
[See table 6 above]
There were no deaths during the study and no patient withdrew from the study due to adverse events. Serious adverse events (both respiratory disorders) were experienced postoperatively by two patients: one case of airway obstruction and desaturation (SpO_2 of 33%) in a patient given VERSED Syrup 0.25 mg/kg, and one case of upper airway obstruction and respiratory depression following 0.5 mg/kg. Both patients had received intravenous morphine sulfate (1.5 mg total for both patients).
Other adverse events that have been reported in the literature with the oral administration of midazolam (not necessarily VERSED Syrup), are listed below. The incidence rate for these events was generally <1%.
Respiratory: apnea, hypercarbia, desaturation, stridor.
Cardiovascular: decreased systolic and diastolic blood pressure, increased heart rate.
Gastrointestinal: nausea, vomiting, hiccoughs, gagging, salivation, drooling.
Central Nervous System: dysphoria, disinhibition, excitation, aggression, mood swings, hallucinations, adverse behavior, agitation, dizziness, confusion, ataxia, vertigo, dysarthria.
Special Senses: diplopia, strabismus, loss of balance, blurred vision.

DRUG ABUSE AND DEPENDENCE

VERSED Syrup is a benzodiazepine and is a Schedule IV controlled substance that can produce drug dependence of the diazepam-type. Therefore, VERSED Syrup may be subject to misuse, abuse and addiction. Benzodiazepines can cause physical dependence. Physical dependence results in withdrawal symptoms in patients who abruptly discontinue the drug. Withdrawal symptoms (ie, convulsions, hallucinations, tremors, abdominal and muscle cramps, vomiting and sweating), similar in characteristics to those noted with barbiturates and alcohol have occurred following abrupt discontinuation of midazolam following chronic administration. Abdominal distention, nausea, vomiting, and tachycardia are prominent symptoms of withdrawal in infants.
The handling of VERSED Syrup should be managed to minimize the risk of diversion, including restriction of access and accounting procedures as appropriate to the clinical setting and as required by law.

OVERDOSAGE

The manifestations of VERSED overdosage reported are similar to those observed with other benzodiazepines, including sedation, somnolence, confusion, impaired coordination, diminished reflexes, coma, and deleterious effects on vital signs. No evidence of specific organ toxicity from VERSED overdosage has been reported.
Treatment of Overdosage: Treatment of VERSED overdosage is the same as that followed for overdosage with other benzodiazepines. Respiration, pulse rate and blood pressure should be monitored and general supportive measures should be employed. Attention should be given to the maintenance of a patent airway and support of ventilation, including administration of oxygen. Should hypotension develop, treatment may include intravenous fluid therapy, repositioning, judicious use of vasopressors appropriate to the clinical situation, if indicated, and other appropriate countermeasures. There is no information as to whether peritoneal dialysis, forced diuresis or hemodialysis are of any value in the treatment of midazolam overdosage.

Continued on next page

Versed Syrup—Cont.

Gastrointestinal decontamination with lavage and/or activated charcoal once the patient's airway is secure is also recommended.

Flumazenil, a specific benzodiazepine-receptor antagonist, is indicated for the complete or partial reversal of the sedative effects of VERSED and may be used in situations when an overdose with a benzodiazepine is known or suspected. There are anecdotal reports of adverse hemodynamic responses associated with VERSED following administration of flumazenil to pediatric patients. Prior to the administration of flumazenil, necessary measures should be instituted to secure the airway, assure adequate ventilation, and establish adequate intravenous access. Flumazenil is intended as an adjunct to, not as a substitute for, proper management of benzodiazepine overdose. Patients treated with flumazenil should be monitored for resedation, respiratory depression and other residual benzodiazepine effects for an appropriate period after treatment. The prescriber should be aware of a risk of seizure in association with flumazenil treatment, particularly in long-term benzodiazepine users and in cyclic antidepressant overdose. The complete flumazenil package insert, including CONTRAINDICATIONS, WARNINGS and PRECAUTIONS, should be consulted prior to use.

DOSAGE AND ADMINISTRATION

VERSED Syrup is indicated for use as a single dose (0.25 to 1.0 mg/kg with a maximum dose of 20 mg) for preprocedural sedation and anxiolysis in pediatric patients. VERSED Syrup is not intended for chronic administration.

Monitoring: VERSED Syrup should only be used in hospital or ambulatory care settings, including physicians' and dentists' offices, that can provide for continuous monitoring of respiratory and cardiac function. Immediate availability of resuscitative drugs and age- and size-appropriate equipment for bag/valve/mask ventilation and intubation, and personnel trained in their use and skilled in airway management should be assured (see WARNINGS). For deeply sedated patients, a dedicated individual whose sole responsibility it is to observe the patient, other than the practitioner performing the procedure, should monitor the patient throughout the procedure. Continuous monitoring of respiratory and cardiac function is required.

VERSED Syrup must be given only to patients if they will be monitored by direct visual observation by a health care professional. VERSED Syrup should only be administered by persons specifically trained in the use of anesthetic drugs and the management of respiratory effects of anesthetic drugs, including respiratory and cardiac resuscitation of patients in the age group being treated.

Patient response to sedative agents, and resultant respiratory status, is variable. Regardless of the intended level of sedation or route of administration, sedation is a continuum; a patient may move easily from light to deep sedation, with potential loss of protective reflexes, particularly when coadministered with anesthetic agents and other CNS depressants. This is especially true in pediatric patients. The health care practitioner who uses this medication in pediatric patients should be aware of and follow accepted professional guidelines for pediatric sedation appropriate to their situation.

Sedation guidelines recommend a careful presedation history to determine how a patient's underlying medical conditions or concomitant medications might affect their response to sedation/analgesia as well as a physical examination including a focused examination of the airway for abnormalities. Further recommendations include appropriate presedation fasting.

Intravenous access is not thought to be necessary for all pediatric patients sedated for a diagnostic or therapeutic procedure because in some cases the difficulty of gaining IV access would defeat the purpose of sedating the child; rather, emphasis should be placed upon having the intravenous equipment available and a practitioner skilled in establishing vascular access in pediatric patients immediately available.

VERSED Syrup must never be used without individualization of dosage, particularly when used with other medications capable of producing CNS depression. Younger (<6 years of age) pediatric patients may require higher dosages (mg/kg) than older pediatric patients, and may require close monitoring.

When VERSED Syrup is given in conjunction with opioids or other sedatives, the potential for respiratory depression, airway obstruction, or hypoventilation is increased. For appropriate patient monitoring, see WARNINGS and *Monitoring* subsection of DOSAGE AND ADMINISTRATION. The health care practitioner who uses this medication in pediatric patients should be aware of and follow accepted professional guidelines for pediatric sedation appropriate to their situation.

The recommended dose for pediatric patients is a single dose of 0.25 to 0.5 mg/kg, depending on the status of the patient and desired effect, up to a maximum dose of 20 mg. In general, it is recommended that the dose be individualized and modified based on patient age, level of anxiety, and medical need. The younger (6 months to <6 years of age) and less cooperative patients may require a higher than usual dose up to 1.0 mg/kg. A dose of 0.25 mg/kg may suffice for older (6 to <16 years of age) or cooperative patients, especially if the anticipated intensity and duration of sedation is less critical. For all pediatric patients, a dose of 0.25 mg/kg should be considered when VERSED Syrup is administered to patients with cardiac or respiratory compromise, other higher risk surgical patients, and patients who have received concomitant narcotics or other CNS depressants. As with any potential respiratory depressant, these patients must be monitored for signs of cardiorespiratory depression after receiving VERSED Syrup. In obese pediatric patients, the dose should be calculated based on ideal body weight. VERSED Syrup has not been studied, nor is it intended for chronic use.

INSERTION OF PRESS-IN BOTTLE ADAPTER (PIBA)

1. Remove the cap and push bottle adapter into neck of bottle.
2. Close the bottle tightly with cap. This will assure the proper seating of the bottle adapter in the bottle.

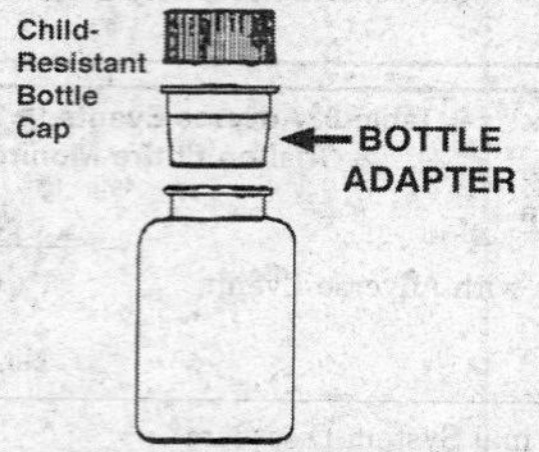

USE OF ORAL DISPENSERS AND PIBA

1. Remove the cap.
2. Before inserting the tip of the oral dispenser into bottle adapter, push the plunger completely down toward the tip of the oral dispenser. Insert tip firmly into opening of the bottle adapter.
3. Turn the entire unit (bottle and oral dispenser) upside down.
4. Pull the plunger out slowly until the desired amount of medication is withdrawn into the oral dispenser.

ORAL DISPENSER

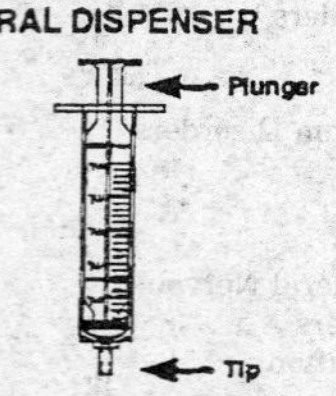

5. Turn the entire unit right side up and remove the oral dispenser slowly from the bottle.
6. The tip of the dispenser may be covered with a tip cap, until time of use.

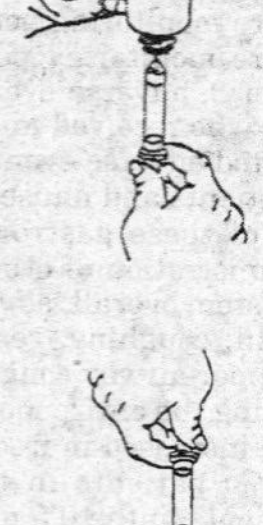

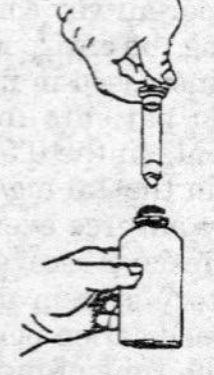

7. Close bottle with cap after each use.
8. Dispense directly into mouth. Do not mix with any liquid (such as grapefruit juice) prior to dispensing.

DISPOSAL OF VERSED SYRUP

The disposal of Schedule IV controlled substances must be consistent with State and Federal Regulations.

HOW SUPPLIED

VERSED Syrup is supplied as a clear, red to purplish-red, cherry-flavored syrup containing midazolam hydrochloride equivalent to 2 mg of midazolam/mL; each amber glass bottle of 118 mL of syrup is supplied with 1 press-in bottle adapter, 4 single-use, graduated, oral dispensers and 4 tip caps (NDC 0004-0168-51).

Storage: Store at 25°C (77°F); excursions permitted to 15° to 30°C (59° to 86°F). [See USP Controlled Room Temperature]

Revised: December 1998

VESANOID® ℞

[*ves' ă noid*]
(tretinoin)
CAPSULES

The following text is complete prescribing information based on official labeling in effect June 2000.

WARNINGS:

1. ***Experienced Physician and Institution:*** Patients with acute promyelocytic leukemia (APL) are at high risk in general and can have severe adverse reactions to VESANOID (tretinoin). VESANOID should therefore be administered under the supervision of a physician who is experienced in the management of patients with acute leukemia and in a facility with laboratory and supportive services sufficient to monitor drug tolerance and protect and maintain a patient compromised by drug toxicity, including respiratory compromise. Use of VESANOID requires that the physician concludes that the possible benefit to the patient outweighs the following known adverse effects of the therapy.
2. ***Retinoic Acid-APL Syndrome:*** About 25% of patients with APL treated with VESANOID have experienced a syndrome called the retinoic-acid-APL (RA-APL) syndrome characterized by fever, dyspnea, weight gain, radiographic pulmonary infiltrates and pleural or pericardial effusions. This syndrome has occasionally been accompanied by impaired myocardial contractility and episodic hypotension. It has been observed with or without concomitant leukocytosis. Endotracheal intubation and mechanical ventilation have been required in some cases due to progressive hypoxemia, and several patients have expired with multiorgan failure. The syndrome generally occurs during the first month of treatment, with some cases reported following the first dose of VESANOID.
   The management of the syndrome has not been defined rigorously, but high-dose steroids given at the first suspicion of the RA-APL syndrome appear to reduce morbidity and mortality. At the first signs suggestive of the syndrome (unexplained fever, dyspnea and/or weight gain, abnormal chest auscultatory findings or radiographic abnormalities), high-dose steroids (dexamethasone 10 mg intravenously administered every 12 hours for 3 days or until the resolution of symptoms) should be immediately initiated, irrespective of the leukocyte count. The majority of patients do not require termination of VESANOID therapy during treatment of the RA-APL syndrome.
3. ***Leukocytosis at Presentation and Rapidly Evolving Leukocytosis During VESANOID Treatment:*** During VESANOID treatment about 40% of patients will develop rapidly evolving leukocytosis. Patients who present with high WBC at diagnosis ($>5\times10^9$/L) have an increased risk of a further rapid increase in WBC counts. Rapidly evolving leukocytosis is associated with a higher risk of life-threatening complications. If signs and symptoms of the RA-APL syndrome are present together with leukocytosis, treatment with high-dose steroids should be initiated immediately. Some investigators routinely add chemotherapy to VESANOID treatment in the case of patients presenting with a WBC count of $>5\times10^9$/L or in the case of a rapid increase in WBC count for patients leukopenic at start of treatment, and have reported a lower incidence of the RA-APL syndrome. Consideration could be given to adding full-dose chemotherapy (including an anthracycline if not contraindicated) to the VESANOID therapy on day 1 or 2 for patients presenting with a WBC count of $>5\times10^9$/L, or immediately, for patients presenting with a WBC count of $<5\times10^9$/L, if the WBC count reaches $\geq6\times10^9$/L by day 5, or $\geq10\times10^9$/L by day 10, or $\geq15\times10^9$/L by day 28.
4. ***Teratogenic Effects. Pregnancy Category D—see WARNINGS:*** There is a high risk that a severely deformed infant will result if VESANOID is administered durign pregnancy. If, nonetheless, it is determined that VESANOID represents the best available treatment for a pregnant woman or a woman of childbearing potential, it must be assured that the patient has received full information and warnings of the risk to the fetus if she were to be pregnant and of the risk of possible contraception failure and has been instructed in the need to use two reliable forms of contraception simultaneously during therapy and for 1 month following discontinuation of therapy, and has acknowledged her understanding of the need for using dual contraception, unless abstinence is the chosen method.
   Within 1 week prior to the institution of VESANOID therapy, the patient should have blood or urine collected for a serum or urine pregnancy test with a sensitivity of at least 50 mIU/L. When possible, VESANOID therapy should be delayed until a negative result from this test is obtained. When a delay is not possible, the patient should be placed on two reliable forms of contraception. Pregnancy testing and contraception counseling should be repeated monthly throughout the period of VESANOID treatment.

DESCRIPTION

VESANOID (tretinoin) is a retinoid that induces maturation of acute promyelocytic leukemia (APL) cells in culture. It is available in a 10 mg soft gelatin capsule for oral administration. Each capsule also contains beeswax, butyl-

ated hydroxyanisole, edetate disodium, hydrogenated soybean oil flakes, hydrogenated vegetable oils and soybean oil. The gelatin capsule shell contains glycerin, yellow iron oxide, red iron oxide, titanium dioxide, methylparaben and propylparaben.
Chemically, tretinoin is all-*trans* retinoic acid and is related to retinol (Vitamin A). It is a yellow to light orange crystalline powder with a molecular weight of 300.44.
The structural formula is as follows:

CLINICAL PHARMACOLOGY

Mechanism of Action: Tretinoin is not a cytolytic agent but instead induces cytodifferentiation and decreased proliferation of APL cells in culture and in vivo. In APL patients, tretinoin treatment produces an initial maturation of the primitive promyelocytes derived from the leukemic clone, followed by a repopulation of the bone marrow and peripheral blood by normal, polyclonal hematopoietic cells in patients achieving complete remission (CR). The exact mechanism of action of tretinoin in APL is unknown.
Pharmacokinetics: Tretinoin activity is primarily due to the parent drug. In human pharmacokinetics studies, orally administered drug was well absorbed into the systemic circulation, with approximately two-thirds of the administered radiolabel recovered in the urine. The terminal elimination half-life of tretinoin following initial dosing is 0.5 to 2 hours in patients with APL. There is evidence that tretinoin induces its own metabolism. Plasma tretinoin concentrations decrease on average to one-third of their day 1 values during 1 week of continuous therapy. Mean ± SD peak tretinoin concentrations decreased from 394 ± 89 to 138 ± 139 ng/mL, while area under the curve (AUC) values decreased from 537 ± 191 ng·h/mL to 249 ± 185 ng·h/mL during 45 mg/m^2 daily dosing in 7 APL patients. Increasing the dose to "correct" for this change has not increased response.
Absorption: A single 45 mg/m^2 (~ 80 mg) oral dose to APL patients resulted in a mean ± SD peak tretinoin concentration of 347 ± 266 ng/mL. Time to reach peak concentration was between 1 and 2 hours.
Distribution: The apparent volume of distribution of tretinoin has not been determined. Tretinoin is greater than 95% bound in plasma, predominately to albumin. Plasma protein binding remains constant over the concentration range of 10 to 500 ng/mL.
Metabolism: Tretinoin metabolites have been identified in plasma and urine. Cytochrome P450 enzymes have been implicated in the oxidative metabolism of tretinoin. Metabolites include 13-*cis* retinoic acid, 4-oxo *trans* retinoic acid, 4-oxo *cis* retinoic acid, and 4-oxo *trans* retinoic acid glucuronide. In APL patients, daily administration of a 45 mg/m^2 dose of tretinoin resulted in an approximately tenfold increase in the urinary excretion of a 4-oxo *trans* retinoic acid glucuronide after 2 to 6 weeks of continuous dosing, when compared to baseline values.
Excretion: Studies with radiolabeled drug have demonstrated that after the oral administration of 2.75 and 50 mg doses of tretinoin, greater than 90% of the radioactivity was recovered in the urine and feces. Based upon data from 3 subjects, approximately 63% of radioactivity was recovered in the urine within 72 hours and 31% appeared in the feces within 6 days.
Special Populations: The pharmacokinetics of tretinoin have not been separately evaluated in women, in members of different ethnic groups, or in individuals with renal or hepatic insufficiency.
Drug-Drug Interactions: In 13 patients who had received daily doses of tretinoin for 4 consecutive weeks, administration of ketoconazole (400 to 1200 mg oral dose) 1 hour prior to the administration of the tretinoin dose on day 29 led to a 72% increase (218 ± 224 vs 375 ± 285 ng·h/mL) in tretinoin mean plasma AUC. The precise cytochrome P450 enzymes involved in these interactions have not been specified; *CYP, 3A4, 2C8* and 2E have been implicated in various preliminary reports.

Clinical Studies: VESANOID has been investigated in 114 previously treated APL patients and in 67 previously untreated ("de novo") patients in one open-label, uncontrolled single investigator clinical study (Memorial Sloan-Kettering Cancer Center [MSKCC]) and in two cohorts of compassionate cases treated by multiple investigators under the auspices of the National Cancer Institute (NCI). All patients received 45 mg/m^2/day as a divided oral dose for up to 90 days or 30 days beyond the day that CR was reached. Results are shown in the following table:
[See table above]

	MSKCC		NCI Cohort 1		NCI Cohort 2	
	Relapsed n=20	De Novo n=15	Relapsed* n=48	De Novo n=14	Relapsed n=46	De Novo† n=38
Complete Remission	16 (80%)	11 (73%)	24 (50%)	5 (36%)	24 (52%)	26 (68%)
Median Survival (Mo)	10.8	NR	5.8	0.5	8.8	NR
Median Follow-up (Mo)	9.9	42.9	5.6	1.2	8.0	13.1
RA-APL Syndrome	4 (20%)	5 (33%)	10 (21%)	6 (43%)	NA	NA

NR = Not Reached
NA = Not Available
* Including 9 chemorefractory patients
† Including 8 patients who received chemotherapy but failed to enter remission

The median time to CR was between 40 and 50 days (range: 2 to 120 days). Most patients in these studies received cytotoxic chemotherapy during the remission phase. These results compare to the 30% to 50% CR rate and ≤6 month median survival reported for cytotoxic chemotherapy of APL in the treatment of relapse.
Ten of 15 pediatric cases achieved CR (8 of 10 males and 2 of 5 females). There were insufficient patients of black, Hispanic or Asian derivation to estimate relative response rates in these groups, but responses were seen in each category. Responses were seen in 3 of 4 patients for whom cytogenic analysis failed to detect the t(15;17) translocation typically seen in APL. The t(15;17) translocation results in the PML/RARα gene, which appears necessary for this disease. Molecular genetic studies were not conducted in these cases, but it is likely they represent cases with a masked translocation giving rise to PML/RARα. Responses to tretinoin have not been observed in cases in which PML/RARα fusion has been shown to be absent.

INDICATIONS AND USAGE

VESANOID (tretinoin) capsules are indicated for the induction of remission in patients with acute promyelocytic leukemia (APL), French-American-British (FAB) classification M3 (including the M3 variant), characterized by the presence of the t(15;17) translocation and/or the presence of the PML/RARα gene who are refractory to, or who have relapsed from, anthracycline chemotherapy, or for whom anthracycline-based chemotherapy is contraindicated. VESANOID is for the induction of remission only. The optimal consolidation or maintenance regimens have not been defined, but all patients should receive an accepted form of remission consolidation and/or maintenance therapy for APL after completion of induction therapy with VESANOID.

CONTRAINDICATIONS

VESANOID is contraindicated in patients with a known hypersensitivity to retinoids. VESANOID should not be given to patients who are sensitive to parabens, which are used as preservatives in the gelatin capsule.

WARNINGS

Pregnancy Category D—see boxed WARNINGS: Tretinoin has teratogenic and embryotoxic effects in mice, rats, hamsters, rabbits and pigtail monkeys, and may be expected to cause fetal harm when administered to a pregnant woman. Tretinoin causes fetal resorptions and a decrease in live fetuses in all animals studied. Gross external, soft tissue and skeletal alterations occurred at doses higher than 0.7 mg/kg/day in mice, 2 mg/kg/day in rats, 7 mg/kg/day in hamsters, and at a dose of 10 mg/kg/day, the only dose tested, in pigtail monkeys (about 1/20, 1/4, and 1/2 and 4 times the human dose, respectively, on a mg/m^2 basis).
There are no adequate and well-controlled studies in pregnant women. Although experience with humans administered VESANOID is extremely limited, increased spontaneous abortions and major human fetal abnormalities related to the use of other retinoids have been documented in humans. Reported defects include abnormalities of the CNS, musculoskeletal system, external ear, eye, thymus and great vessels; and facial dysmorphia, cleft palate, and parathyroid hormone deficiency. Some of these abnormalities were fatal. Cases of IQ scores less than 85, with or without obvious CNS abnormalities, have also been reported. All fetuses exposed during pregnancy can be affected and at the present time there is no antepartum means of determining which fetuses are and are not affected.
Effective contraception must be used by all females during VESANOID therapy and for 1 month following discontinuation of therapy. Contraception must be used even when there is a history of infertility or menopause, unless a hysterectomy has been performed. Whenever contraception is required, it is recommended that two reliable forms of contraception be used simultaneously, unless abstinence is the chosen method. If pregnancy does occur during treatment, the physician and patient should discuss the desirability of continuing or terminating the pregnancy.
Patients Without the t(15;17) Translocation: Initiation of therapy with VESANOID may be based on the morphological diagnosis of acute promyelocytic leukemia. Confirmation of the diagnosis of APL should be sought by detection or the t(15;17) genetic marker by cytogenic studies. If these are negative, PML/RARα fusion should be sought using molecular diagnostic techniques. The response rate of other AML subtypes to VESANOID has not been demonstrated; therefore, patients who lack the genetic marker should be considered for alternative treatment.
Retinoic Acid-APL (RA-APL) Syndrome: In up to 25% of patients with APL treated with VESANOID, a syndrome occurs which can be fatal (see boxed WARNINGS and ADVERSE REACTIONS).
Leukocytosis at Presentation and Rapidly Evolving Leukocytosis During VESANOID Treatment: (see boxed WARNINGS).
Pseudotumor Cerebri: Retinoids, including VESANOID, have been associated with pseudomotor cerebri (benign intracranial hypertension), especially in pediatric patients. Early signs and symptoms of pseudotumor cerebri include papilledema, headache, nausea and vomiting, and visual disturbances. Patients with these symptoms should be evaluated for pseudotumor cerebri, and, if present, appropriate care should be instituted in concert with neurological assessment.
Lipids: Up to 60% of patients experienced hypercholesterolemia and/or hypertriglyceridemia, which were reversible upon completion of treatment. The clinical consequences of temporary elevation of triglycerides and cholesterol are unknown, but venous thrombosis and myocardial infarction have been reported in patients who ordinarily are at low risk for such complications.
Elevated Liver Function Test Results: Elevated liver function test results occur in 50% to 60% of patients during treatment. Liver function test results should be carefully monitored during treatment and consideration be given to a temporary withdrawal of VESANOID if test results reach >5 times the upper limit of normal values. However, the majority of these abnormalities resolve without interruption of VESANOID or after completion of treatment.

PRECAUTIONS

General: VESANOID has potentially significant toxic side effects in APL patients. Patients undergoind therapy should be closely observed for signs of respiratory compromise and/or leukocytosis (see boxed WARNINGS). Supportive care appropriate for APL patients; eg, prophylaxis for bleeding, prompt therapy for infeciton, should be maintained during therapy with VESANOID.
Laboratory Tests: The patient's hematologic profile, coagulation profile, liver function test results, and triglyceride and cholesterol levels should be monitored frequently.
Drug Interactions: Limited clinical data on potential drug interactions are available. As VESANOID is metabolized by the hepatic P450 system, there is a potential for alteration of pharmacokinetics parameters in patients administered concomitant medications that are also inducers or inhibitors of this system. Medications that generally induce hepatic P450 enzymes include rifampicin, glucocorticoids, phenobarbital and pentobarbital. Medications that generally inhibit hepatic P450 enzymes include ketoconazole, cimetidine, erythromycin, verapamil, diltiazem and cyclosporin. To date there are no data to suggest that co-use with these medications increases or decreases either efficacy or toxicity of VESANOID.
Effect of Food: No data on the effect of food on the absorption of VESANOID are available. The absorption of retinoids as a class has been shown to be enhanced when taken together with food.
Carcinogenesis, Mutagenesis and Impairment of Fertility: No long-term carcinogenicity studies with tretinoin have been conducted. In short-term carcinogenicity studies, tretinoin at a dose of 30 mg/kg/day (about 2 times the human dose on a mg/m^2 basis) was shown to increase the rate of diethylnitrosamine (DEN)-induced mouse liver adenomas and carcinomas. Tretinoin was negative when tested in the Ames and Chinese hamster V79 cell HGPRT assays for mutagenicity. A twofold increase in the sister chromatid exchange (SCE) has been demonstrated in human diploid fibroblasts, but other chromosome aberration assays, including an in vitro assay in human peripheral lymphocytes and an in vivo mouse micronucleus assay, did not show a clastogenic or aneuploidogenic effect. Adverse effects on fertility and reproductive performance were not observed in studies conducted in rats at doses up to 5 mg/kg/day (about 2/3 the human dose on a mg/m^2 basis). In a 6-week toxicology study in dogs, minimal to marked testicular degeneration, with increased numbers of immature spermatozoa, were observed at 10 mg/kg/day (about 4 times the equivalent human dose in mg/m^2).
Nursing Mothers: It is not known whether this drug is excreted in human milk. Because many drugs are excreted in human milk, and because of the potential for serious adverse reactions from VESANOID in nursing infants, mothers should discontinue nursing prior to taking this drug.
Pediatric Use: There are limited clinical data on the pediatric use of VESANOID. Of 15 pediatric patients (age range: 1 to 16 years) treated with VESANOID, the incidence of complete remission was 67%. Safety and effectiveness in pediatric patients below the age of 1 year have not been established. Some pediatric patients experience severe headache and pseudotumor cerebri, requiring analgesic treatment and lumbar puncture for relief. Increased caution is recommended in the treatment of pediatric patients. Dose reduction may be considered for pediatric patients experiencing serious and/or intolerable toxicity; however, the efficacy and safety of VESANOID at doses lower than 45 mg/m^2/day have not been evaluated in the pediatric population.
Geriatric Use: Of the total number of subjects in clinical studies of VESANOID, 21.4% were 60 and over. No overall differences in safety or effectiveness were observed between these subjects and younger subjects, and other reported clinical experience has not identified differences in re-

Continued on next page

Vesanoid—Cont.

sponses between the elderly and younger patients, but greater sensitivity of some older individuals cannot be ruled out.

ADVERSE REACTIONS

Virtually all patients experience some drug related toxicity, especially headache, fever, weakness, and fatigue. These adverse effects are seldom permanent or irreversible nor do they usually require interruption of therapy. Some of the adverse events are common in patients with APL, including hemorrhage, infections, gastrointestinal hemorrhage, disseminated intravascular coagulation, pneumonia, septicemia, and cerebral hemorrhage. The following describes the adverse events, regardless of drug relationship, that were observed in patients treated with VESANOID.

Typical Retinoid Toxicity: The most frequently reported adverse events were similar to those described in patients taking high doses of vitamin A and included headache (86%), fever (83%), skin/mucous membrane dryness (77%), bone pain (77%), nausea/vomiting (57%), rash (54%), mucositis (26%), pruritus (20%), increased sweating (20%), visual disturbances (17%), ocular disorders (17%), alopecia (14%), skin changes (14%), changed visual acuity (6%), bone inflammation (3%), visual field defects (3%).

RA-APL Syndrome: APL patients treated with VESANOID have experienced a syndrome characterized by fever, dyspnea, weight gain, radiographic pulmonary infiltrates and pleural or pericardial effusions. This syndrome has occasionally been accompanied by impaired myocardial contractility and episodic hypotension and has been observed with or without concomitant leukocytosis. Some patients have expired due to progressive hypoxemia and multiorgan failure. The syndrome generally occurs during the first month of treatment, with some cases reported following the first dose of VESANOID. The management of the syndrome has not been defined rigorously, but high-dose steroids given at the first signs of the syndrome appear to reduce morbidity and mortality. Treatment with dexamethasone, 10 mg intravenously administered every 12 hours for 3 days or until resolution of symptoms, should be initiated without delay at the first suspicion of symptoms (one or more of the following: fever, dyspnea, weight gain, abnormal chest ausculatory findings or radiographic abnormalities). Sixty percent or more of patients treated with VESANOID may require high-dose steroids because of these symptoms. The majority of patients do not require termination of VESANOID therapy during treatment of the syndrome.

Body as a Whole: General disorders related to VESANOID administration and/or associated with APL included malaise (66%), shivering (63%), hemorrhage (60%), infections (58%), peripheral edema (52%), pain (37%), chest discomfort (32%), edema (29%), disseminated intravascular coagulation (26%), weight increase (23%), injection site reactions (17%), anorexia (17%), weight decrease (17%), myalgia (14%), flank pain (9%), cellulitis (8%), face edema (6%), fluid imbalance (6%), pallor (6%), lymph disorders (6%), acidosis (3%), hypothermia (3%), ascites (3%).

Respiratory System Disorders: Respiratory system disorders were commonly reported in APL patients administered VESANOID. The majority of these events are symptoms of the RA-APL syndrome (see boxed WARNINGS). Respiratory system adverse events included upper respiratory tract disorders (63%), dyspnea (60%), respiratory insufficiency (26%), pleural effusion (20%), pneumonia (14%), rales (14%), expiratory wheezing (14%), lower respiratory tract disorders (9%), pulmonary infiltration (6%), bronchial asthma (3%), pulmonary edema (3%), larynx edema (3%), unspecified pulmonary disease (3%).

Ear Disorders: Ear disorders were consistently reported, with earache or feeling of fullness in the ears reported by 23% of the patients. Hearing loss and other unspecified auricular disorders were observed in 6% of patients, with infrequent (<1%) reports of irreversible hearing loss.

Gastrointestinal Disorders: GI disorders included GI hemorrhage (34%), abdominal pain (31%), other gastrointestinal disorders (26%), diarrhea (23%), constipation (17%), dyspepsia (14%), abdominal distention (11%), hepatosplenomegaly (9%), hepatitis (3%), ulcer (3%), unspecified liver disorder (3%).

Cardiovascular and Heart Rate and Rhythm Disorders: Arrhythmias (23%), flushing (23%), hypotension (14%), hypertension (11%), phlebitis (11%), cardiac failure (6%) and for 3% of patients: cardiac arrest, myocardial infarction, enlarged heart, heart murmur, ischemia, stroke, myocarditis, pericarditis, pulmonary hypertension, secondary cardiomyopathy.

Central and Peripheral Nervous System Disorders and Psychiatric: Dizziness (20%), paresthesias (17%), anxiety (17%), insomnia (14%), depression (14%), confusion (11%), cerebral hemorrhage (9%), intracranial hypertension (9%), agitation (9%), hallucination (6%) and for 3% of patients: abnormal gait, agnosia, aphasia, asterixis, cerebellar edema, cerebellar disorders, convulsions, coma, CNS depression, dysarthria, encephalopathy, facial paralysis, hemiplegia, hyporeflexia, hypotaxia, no light reflex, neurologic reaction, spinal cord disorder, tremor, leg weakness, unconsciousness, dementia, forgetfulness, somnolence, slow speech.

Urinary System Disorders: Renal insufficiency (11%), dysuria (9%), acute renal failure (3%), micturition frequency (3%), renal tubular necrosis (3%), enlarged prostate (3%).

Miscellaneous Adverse Events: Isolated cases of erythema nodosum, basophilia and hyperhistaminemia, Sweet's syndrome, organomegaly, hypercalcemia, pancreatitis and myositis have been reported.

OVERDOSAGE

There has been no experience with acute overdosage in humans. The maximal tolerated dose in patients with myelodysplastic syndrome or solid tumors was 195 mg/m^2/day. The maximal tolerated dose in pediatric patients was lower at 60 mg/m^2/day. Overdosage with other retinoids has been associated with transient headache, facial flushing, cheilosis, abdominal pain, dizziness and ataxia. These symptoms have quickly resolved without apparent residual effects.

DOSAGE AND ADMINISTRATION

The recommended dose is 45 mg/m^2/day administered as two evenly divided doses until complete remission is documented. Therapy should be discontinued 30 days after achievement of complete remission or after 90 days of treatment, whichever occurs first.

If after initiation of treatment of VESANOID the presence of the t(15;17) translocation is not confirmed by cytogenetics and/or by polymerase chain reaction studies and the patient has not responded to VESANOID, alternative therapy appropriate for acute myelogenous leukemia should be considered.

VESANOID is for the induction of remission only. Optimal consolidation or maintenance regimens have not been determined. All patients should, therefore, receive a standard consolidation and/or maintenance chemotherapy regimen for APL after induction therapy with VESANOID, unless otherwise contraindicated.

HOW SUPPLIED

VESANOID is supplied as 10 mg capsules, two-tone (lengthwise), orange-yellow and reddish-brown and imprinted VESANOID 10 ROCHE. Supplied in high-density polyethylene, opaque Prescription Pak Bottles of 100 capsules with child-resistant closure (NDC 0004-0250-01).

Store at 15° to 30°C (59° to 86°F). Protect from light.

Roche Pharmaceuticals
Roche Laboratories Inc.
340 Kingsland Street
Nutley, New Jersey 07110-1199

27897174-0500 Revised: May 2000

Shown in Product Identification Guide, page 333

XELODA® ℞

[zĕl-ōda]
(capecitabine)
TABLETS

The following text is complete prescribing information based on official labeling in effect June 2000.

DESCRIPTION

XELODA (capecitabine) is a fluoropyrimidine carbamate with antineoplastic activity. It is an orally administered systemic prodrug of 5′-deoxy-5-fluorouridine (5′-DFUR) which is converted to 5-fluorouracil.

The chemical name for capecitabine is 5′-deoxy-5-fluoro-N-[(pentyloxy)carbonyl]-cytidine and has a molecular weight of 359.35. Capecitabine has the following structural formula:

Capecitabine is a white to off-white crystalline powder with an aqueous solubility of 26 mg/mL at 20°C.

XELODA is supplied as biconvex, oblong film-coated tablets for oral administration. Each light peach-colored tablet contains 150 mg capecitabine and each peach-colored tablet contains 500 mg capecitabine. The inactive ingredients in XELODA include: anhydrous lactose, croscarmellose sodium, hydroxypropyl methylcellulose, microcrystalline cellulose, magnesium stearate and purified water. The peach or light peach film coating contains hydroxypropyl methylcellulose, talc, titanium dioxide, and synthetic yellow and red iron oxides.

CLINICAL PHARMACOLOGY

Capecitabine is relatively non-cytotoxic in vitro. This drug is enzymatically converted to 5-fluorouracil (5-FU) in vivo.

Bioactivation: Capecitabine is readily absorbed from the gastrointestinal tract. In the liver, a 60 kDa carboxyesterase hydrolyzes much of the compound to 5′-deoxy-5-fluorocytidine (5′-DFCR). Cytidine deaminase, an enzyme found in most tissues, including tumors, subsequently converts 5′-DFCR to 5′-deoxy-5-fluorouridine (5′-DFUR). The enzyme, thymidine phosphorylase (dThdPase), then hydrolyzes 5′-DFUR to the active drug 5-FU. Many tissues throughout the body express thymidine phosphorylase. Some human carcinomas express this enzyme in higher concentrations than surrounding normal tissues.

Metabolic Pathway of capecitabine to 5-FU
[See chemical structure at top of next column]

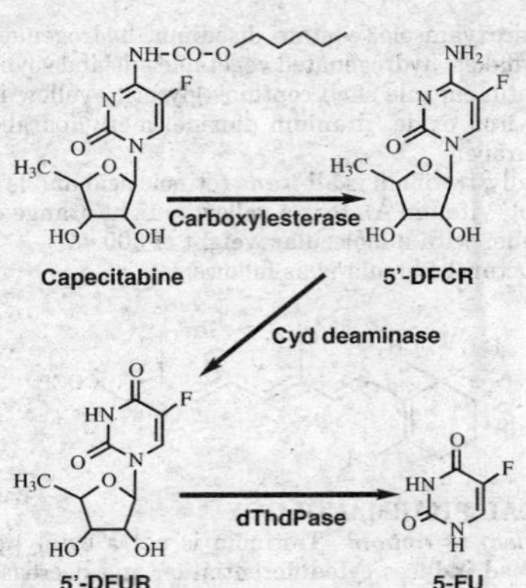

Mechanism of Action: Both normal and tumor cells metabolize 5-FU to 5-fluoro-2-deoxyuridine monophosphate (FdUMP) and 5-fluorouridine triphosphate (FUTP). These metabolites cause cell injury by two different mechanisms. First, FdUMP and the folate cofactor, N^{5-10}-methylenetetrahydrofolate, bind to thymidylate synthase (TS) to form a covalently bound ternary complex. This binding inhibits the formation of thymidylate from uracil. Thymidylate is the necessary precursor of thymidine triphosphate, which is essential for the synthesis of DNA, so that a deficiency of this compound can inhibit cell division. Second, nuclear transcriptional enzymes can mistakenly incorporate FUTP in place of uridine triphosphate (UTP) during the synthesis of RNA. This metabolic error can interfere with RNA processing and protein synthesis.

Pharmacokinetics in Colorectal Tumors and Adjacent Healthy Tissue: Following oral administration of capecitabine 7 days before surgery in patients with colorectal cancer, the median ratio of 5-FU concentration in colorectal tumors to adjacent tissues was 2.9 (range from 0.9 to 8.0). These ratios have not been evaluated in breast cancer patients or compared to 5-FU infusion.

Human Pharmacokinetics: The pharmacokinetics of XELODA and its metabolites have been evaluated in about 200 cancer patients over a dosage range of 500 to 3500 mg/m^2/day. Over this range, the pharmacokinetics of capecitabine and its metabolite, 5′-DFCR were dose proportional and did not change over time. The increases in the AUCs of 5′-DFUR and 5-FU, however, were greater than proportional to the increase in dose and the AUC of 5-FU was 34% higher on day 14 than on day 1. The elimination half-life of both parent capecitabine and 5-FU was about ¾ of an hour. The inter-patient variability in the C_{max} and AUC of 5-FU was greater than 85%.

Absorption, Distribution, Metabolism and Excretion: Capecitabine reached peak blood levels in about 1.5 hours (T_{max}) with peak 5-FU levels occurring slightly later, at 2 hours. Food reduced both the rate and extent of absorption of capecitabine with mean C_{max} and $AUC_{0-\infty}$ decreased by 60% and 35%, respectively. The C_{max} and $AUC_{0-\infty}$ of 5-FU were also reduced by food by 43% and 21%, respectively. Food delayed T_{max} of both parent and 5-FU by 1.5 hours (see PRECAUTIONS and DOSAGE AND ADMINISTRATION).

Plasma protein binding of capecitabine and its metabolites is less than 60% and is not concentration-dependent. Capecitabine was primarily bound to human albumin (approximately 35%).

Capecitabine is extensively metabolized enzymatically to 5-FU. The enzyme dihydropyrimidine dehydrogenase hydrogenates 5-FU, the product of capecitabine metabolism, to the much less toxic 5-fluoro-5,6-dihydro-fluorouracil (FUH_2). Dihydropyrimidinase cleaves the pyrimidine ring to yield 5-fluoro-ureido-propionic acid (FUPA). Finally, β-ureido-propionase cleaves FUPA to α-fluoro-β-alanine (FBAL) which is cleared in the urine.

Capecitabine and its metabolites are predominantly excreted in urine; 95.5% of administered capecitabine dose is recovered in urine. Fecal excretion is minimal (2.6%). The major metabolite excreted in urine is FBAL which represents 57% of the administered dose. About 3% of the administered dose is excreted in urine as unchanged drug.

Special Populations:

Age, Gender and Ethnicity: No formal studies were conducted to examine the effect of age or gender or ethnicity on the pharmacokinetics of capecitabine and its metabolites.

Hepatic Insufficiency: XELODA has been evaluated in 13 patients with mild to moderate hepatic dysfunction due to liver metastases defined by a composite score including bilirubin, AST/ALT and alkaline phosphatase following a single 1255 mg/m^2 dose of capecitabine. Both $AUC_{0-\infty}$ and C_{max} of capecitabine increased by 60% in patients with hepatic dysfunction compared to patients with normal hepatic function (n=14). The $AUC_{0-\infty}$ and C_{max} of 5-FU was not affected. In patients with mild to moderate hepatic dysfunction due to liver metastases, caution should be exercised when XELODA is administered. The effect of severe hepatic dysfunction on XELODA is not known (see PRECAUTIONS and DOSAGE AND ADMINISTRATION).

Renal Insufficiency: No formal pharmacokinetic study was conducted in patients with renal impairment (see PRECAUTIONS).

Drug-Drug Interactions:

Drugs Metabolized by Cytochrome P450 Enzymes: In vitro enzymatic studies with human liver microsomes indicated that capecitabine and 5′-DFUR had no inhibitory effects on substrates of cytochrome P450 for the major isoenzymes such as 1A2, 2A6, 3A4, 2C9, 2C19, 2D6, and 2E1, suggesting a low likelihood of interactions with drugs metabolized by cytochrome P450 enzymes.

Antacid: When Maalox®* (20 mL), an aluminum hydroxide- and magnesium hydroxide-containing antacid, was administered immediately after capecitabine (1250 mg/m^2, n=12 cancer patients), AUC and C_{max} increased by 16% and 35%, respectively, for capecitabine and by 18% and 22%, respectively, for 5′-DFCR. No effect was observed on the other three major metabolites (5′-DFUR, 5-FU, FBAL) of capecitabine.

XELODA has a low potential for pharmacokinetic interactions related to plasma protein binding.

CLINICAL STUDIES

In a phase 1 study with XELODA in patients with solid tumors, the maximum tolerated dose as a single agent was 3000 mg/m^2 when administered daily for 2 weeks, followed by a 1-week rest period. The dose-limiting toxicities were diarrhea and leukopenia.

Breast Carcinoma: The antitumor activity of XELODA was evaluated in an open-label single-arm trial conducted in 24 centers in the US and Canada. A total of 162 patients with stage IV breast cancer were enrolled. The primary endpoint was tumor response rate in patients with measurable disease, with response defined as a ≥50% decrease in sum of the products of the perpendicular diameters of bidimensionally measurable disease for at least 1 month. XELODA was administered at a daily dose of 2510 mg/m^2 for 2 weeks followed by a 1-week rest period and given as 3-week cycles. The baseline demographics and clinical characteristics for all patients (n=162) and those with measurable disease (n=135) are shown in the table below. Resistance was defined as progressive disease while on treatment, with or without an initial response, or relapse within 6 months of completing treatment with an anthracycline-containing adjuvant chemotherapy regimen.

[See table 1 above]

Antitumor responses for patients with disease resistant to both paclitaxel and an anthracycline are shown in the table below.

Table 2. Response Rates in Doubly-Resistant Patients

	Resistance to Both Paclitaxel and an Anthracycline (n=43)
CR	0
PR[1]	11
CR + PR[1]	11
Response Rate[1]	25.6%
(95% C.I.)	(13.5, 41.2)
Duration of Response,[1]	
Median in days[2]	154
(Range)	(63 to 233)

[1]Includes 2 patients treated with an anthracenedione
[2]From date of first response

For the subgroup of 43 patients who were doubly resistant, the median time to progression was 102 days and the median survival was 255 days. The objective response rate in this population was supported by a response rate of 18.5% (1 CR, 24 PRs) in the overall population of 135 patients with measurable disease, who were less resistant to chemotherapy (see Table 1). The median time to progression was 90 days and the median survival was 306 days.

INDICATIONS AND USAGE

XELODA is indicated for the treatment of patients with metastatic breast cancer resistant to both paclitaxel and an anthracycline-containing chemotherapy regimen or resistant to paclitaxel and for whom further anthracycline therapy is not indicated, eg, patients who have received cumulative doses of 400 mg/m^2 of doxorubicin or doxorubicin equivalents. Resistance is defined as progressive disease while on treatment, with or without an initial response, or relapse within 6 months of completing treatment with an anthracycline-containing adjuvant regimen.

This indication is based on demonstration of a response rate. No results are available from controlled trials that demonstrate a clinical benefit resulting from treatment, such as improvement in disease-related symptoms, disease progression, or survival.

CONTRAINDICATIONS

XELODA is contraindicated in patients who have a known hypersensitivity to 5-fluorouracil.

WARNINGS

Coagulopathy: Altered coagulation parameters and/or bleeding have been reported in patients taking XELODA concomitantly with coumarin-derivative anticoagulants such as warfarin and phenprocoumon. These events occurred within several days and up to several months after initiating XELODA therapy and, in a few cases, within one month after stopping XELODA. These events occurred in patients with and without liver metastases. Patients taking coumarin-derivative anticoagulants concomitantly with XELODA should be monitored regularly for alterations in their coagulation parameters (PT or INR) (see PRECAUTIONS: *Drug-Drug Interactions*).

Table 1. Baseline Demographics and Clinical Characteristics

	Patients with Measurable Disease (n=135)	All Patients (n=162)
Age (median, years)	55	56
Karnofsky PS	90	90
No. Disease Sites		
1–2	43 (32%)	60 (37%)
3–4	63 (46%)	69 (43%)
>5	29 (22%)	34 (21%)
Dominant Site of Disease		
Visceral[1]	101 (75%)	110 (68%)
Soft Tissue	30 (22%)	35 (22%)
Bone	4 (3%)	17 (10%)
Prior Chemotherapy		
Paclitaxel	135 (100%)	162 (100%)
Anthracycline[2]	122 (90%)	147 (91%)
5-FU	110 (81%)	133 (82%)
Resistance to Paclitaxel	103 (76%)	124 (77%)
Resistance to an Anthracycline[2]	55 (41%)	67 (41%)
Resistance to both Paclitaxel and an Anthracycline[2]	43 (32%)	51 (31%)

[1]Lung, pleura, liver, peritoneum
[2]Includes 2 patients treated with an anthracenedione

Table 3. Percent of Adverse Events Considered Remotely, Possibly, or Probably Related to Treatment in ≥5% of Patients

Adverse Event	Phase 2 Trial in Stage IV Breast Cancer (n=162)			Overall Safety Database (n=570)		
Body System/Adverse Event	Total	Grade 3	Grade 4	Total	Grade 3	Grade 4
GI						
Diarrhea	57	12	3	50	11	2
Nausea	53	4	—	44	4	—
Vomiting	37	4	—	26	3	—
Stomatitis	24	7	—	23	4	—
Abdominal pain	20	4	—	17	4	—
Constipation	15	1	—	9	1	—
Dyspepsia	8	—	—	6	—	—
Skin and Subcutaneous						
Hand-and-Foot Syndrome	57	11	—	45	13	—
Dermatitis	37	1	—	31	1	—
Nail disorder	7	—	—	4	—	—
General						
Fatigue	41	8	—	34	5	—
Pyrexia	12	1	—	10	—	—
Pain in limb	6	1	—	4	—	—
Neurological						
Paraesthesia	21	1	—	12	—	—
Headache	9	1	—	7	1	—
Dizziness	8	—	—	5	—	—
Insomnia	8	—	—	3	—	—
Metabolism						
Anorexia	23	3	—	20	2	—
Dehydration	7	4	1	5	2	1
Eye						
Eye irritation	15	—	—	10	—	—
Musculoskeletal						
Myalgia	9	—	—	4	—	—
Cardiac						
Edema	9	1	—	6	—	—
Blood						
Neutropenia	26	2	2	22	3	2
Thrombocytopenia	24	3	1	21	1	1
Anemia	72	3	1	74	2	1
Lymphopenia	94	44	15	94	36	10
Hepatobiliary						
Hyperbilirubinemia	22	9	2	34	14	3

—Not observed or applicable.

Diarrhea: XELODA can induce diarrhea, sometimes severe. Patients with severe diarrhea should be carefully monitored and given fluid and electrolyte replacement if they become dehydrated. The median time to first occurrence of grade 2–4 diarrhea was 31 days (range from 1 to 322 days). National Cancer Institute of Canada (NCIC) grade 2 diarrhea is defined as an increase of 4 to 6 stools/day or nocturnal stools, grade 3 diarrhea as an increase of 7 to 9 stools/day or incontinence and malabsorption, and grade 4 diarrhea as an increase of ≥10 stools/day or grossly bloody diarrhea or the need for parenteral support. If grade 2, 3 or 4 diarrhea occurs, administration of XELODA should be immediately interrupted until the diarrhea resolves or decreases in intensity to grade 1. Following grade 3 or 4 diarrhea, subsequent doses of XELODA should be decreased (see DOSAGE AND ADMINISTRATION). Standard antidiarrheal treatments (eg, loperamide) are recommended.

Necrotizing enterocolitis (typhlitis) has been reported.

Geriatric Patients (gastrointestinal toxicity): Patients ≥80 years old may experience a greater incidence of gastrointestinal grade 3 or 4 adverse events (see PRECAUTIONS: *Geriatric Use*). Among the 14 patients 80 years of age and greater treated with capecitabine, three (21.4%), three (21.4%) and one (7.1%) patients experienced reversible grade 3 or 4 diarrhea, nausea and vomiting, respectively. Among the 313 patients age 60 to 79 years old, the incidence of gastrointestinal toxicity was similar to that in the overall population.

Pregnancy: XELODA may cause fetal harm when given to a pregnant woman. Capecitabine at doses of 198 mg/kg/day during organogenesis caused teratogenic malformations and embryo death in mice. In separate pharmacokinetic

Continued on next page

Xeloda—Cont.

studies, this dose in mice produced 5′-DFUR AUC values about 0.2 times the corresponding values in patients administered the recommended daily dose. Teratogenic malformations in mice included cleft palate, anophthalmia, microphthalmia, oligodactyly, polydactyly, syndactyly, kinky tail and dilation of cerebral ventricles. At doses of 90 mg/kg/day, capecitabine given to pregnant monkeys during organogenesis caused fetal death. This dose produced 5′-DFUR AUC values about 0.6 times the corresponding values in patients administered the recommended daily dose. There are no adequate and well-controlled studies in pregnant women using XELODA. If the drug is used during pregnancy, or if the patient becomes pregnant while receiving this drug, the patient should be apprised of the potential hazard to the fetus. Women of childbearing potential should be advised to avoid becoming pregnant while receiving treatment with XELODA.

PRECAUTIONS

General: Patients receiving therapy with XELODA should be monitored by a physician experienced in the use of cancer chemotherapeutic agents. Most adverse events are reversible and do not need to result in discontinuation, although doses may need to be withheld or reduced (see DOSAGE AND ADMINISTRATION).

Hand-and-Foot Syndrome: Hand-and-foot syndrome (palmar-plantar erythrodysesthesia or chemotherapy induced acral erythema) is characterized by the following: numbness, dysesthesia/paresthesia, tingling, painless or painful swelling, erythema, desquamation, blistering and severe pain. Grade 2 hand-and-foot syndrome is defined as painful erythema and swelling of the hands and/or feet and/or discomfort affecting the patient's activities of daily living. Grade 3 hand-and-foot syndrome is defined as moist desquamation, ulceration, blistering and severe pain of the hands and/or feet and/or severe discomfort that causes the patient to be unable to work or perform activities of daily living. If grade 2 or 3 hand-and-foot syndrome occurs, administration of XELODA should be interrupted until the event resolves or decreases in intensity to grade 1. Following grade 3 hand-and-foot syndrome, subsequent doses of XELODA should be decreased (see DOSAGE AND ADMINISTRATION).

Cardiac: There has been cardiotoxicity associated with fluorinated pyrimidine therapy, including myocardial infarction, angina, dysrhythmias, cardiogenic shock, sudden death and electrocardiograph changes. These adverse events may be more common in patients with a prior history of coronary artery disease.

Hepatic Insufficiency: Patients with mild to moderate hepatic dysfunction due to liver metastases should be carefully monitored when XELODA is administered. The effect of severe hepatic dysfunction on the disposition of XELODA is not known (see CLINICAL PHARMACOLOGY and DOSAGE AND ADMINISTRATION).

Hyperbilirubinemia: Grade 3 or 4 hyperbilirubinemia occurred in 17% (n=97) of 570 patients with either metastatic breast or colorectal cancer who received a dose of 2510 mg/m^2 daily for 2 weeks followed by a 1-week rest period. Of 339 patients who had hepatic metastases at baseline and 231 patients without hepatic metastases at baseline, grade 3 or 4 hyperbilirubinemia occurred in 21.2% and 10.4%, respectively. Seventy-four (76%) of the 97 patients with grade 3 or 4 hyperbilirubinemia also had concurrent elevations in alkaline phosphatase and/or hepatic transaminases; 6% of these were grade 3 or 4. Only 4 patients (4%) had elevated hepatic transaminases without a concurrent elevation in alkaline phosphatase. If drug related grade 2–4 elevations in bilirubin occur, administration of XELODA should be immediately interrupted until the hyperbilirubinemia resolves or decreases in intensity to grade 1. NCIC grade 2 hyperbilirubinemia is defined as 1.5 × normal, grade 3 hyperbilirubinemia as 1.5–3 × normal and grade 4 hyperbilirubinemia as >3 × normal. (See recommended dose modifications under DOSAGE AND ADMINISTRATION.)

Renal Insufficiency: There is little experience in patients with renal impairment. Physicians should exercise caution when XELODA is administered (see DOSAGE AND ADMINISTRATION).

Hematologic: In 570 patients with either metastatic breast or colorectal cancer who received a dose of 2510 mg/m^2 administered daily for 2 weeks followed by a 1-week rest period, 4%, 2%, and 3% of patients had grade 3 or 4 neutropenia, thrombocytopenia and decreases in hemoglobin, respectively.

Carcinogenesis, Mutagenesis and Impairment of Fertility: Long-term studies in animals to evaluate the carcinogenic potential of capecitabine have not been conducted. Capecitabine was not mutagenic in vitro to bacteria (Ames test) or mammalian cells (Chinese hamster V79/HPRT gene mutation assay). Capecitabine was clastogenic in vitro to human peripheral blood lymphocytes but not clastogenic in vivo to mouse bone marrow (micronucleus test). Fluorouracil causes mutations in bacteria and yeast. Fluorouracil also causes chromosomal abnormalities in the mouse micronucleus test in vivo.

Impairment of Fertility: In studies of fertility and general reproductive performance in mice, oral capecitabine doses of 760 mg/kg/day disturbed estrus and consequently caused a decrease in fertility. In mice that became pregnant, no fetuses survived this dose. The disturbance in estrus was reversible. In males, this dose caused degenerative changes in the testes, including decreases in the number of spermatocytes and spermatids. In separate pharmacokinetic studies, this dose in mice produced 5′-DFUR AUC values about 0.7 times the corresponding values in patients administered the recommended daily dose.

Information for Patients (see Patient Package Insert): Patients and patients' caregivers should be informed of the expected adverse effects of XELODA, particularly nausea, vomiting, diarrhea, and hand-and-foot syndrome, and should be made aware that patient-specific dose adaptations during therapy are expected and necessary (see DOSAGE AND ADMINISTRATION). Patients should be encouraged to recognize the common grade 2 toxicities associated with XELODA treatment.

Diarrhea: Patients experiencing grade 2 diarrhea (an increase of 4 to 6 stools/day or nocturnal stools) or greater should be instructed to stop taking XELODA immediately. Standard antidiarrheal treatments (eg, loperamide) are recommended.

Nausea: Patients experiencing grade 2 nausea (food intake significantly decreased but able to eat intermittently) or greater should be instructed to stop taking XELODA immediately. Initiation of symptomatic treatment is recommended.

Vomiting: Patients experiencing grade 2 vomiting (2 to 5 episodes in a 24-hour period) or greater should be instructed to stop taking XELODA immediately. Initiation of symptomatic treatment is recommended.

Hand-and-Foot Syndrome: Patients experiencing grade 2 hand-and-foot syndrome (painful erythema and swelling of the hands and/or feet and/or discomfort affecting the patients' activities of daily living) or greater should be instructed to stop taking XELODA immediately.

Stomatitis: Patients experiencing grade 2 stomatitis (painful erythema, edema or ulcers of the mouth or tongue, but able to eat) or greater should be instructed to stop taking XELODA immediately. Initiation of symptomatic treatment is recommended (see DOSAGE AND ADMINISTRATION).

Fever and Neutropenia: Patients who develop a fever of 100.5°F or greater or other evidence of potential infection should be instructed to call their physician.

Drug-Food Interaction: In all clinical trials, patients were instructed to administer XELODA within 30 minutes after a meal. Since current safety and efficacy data are based upon administration with food, it is recommended that XELODA be administered with food (see DOSAGE AND ADMINISTRATION).

Drug-Drug Interactions:

Antacid: The effect of an aluminum hydroxide- and magnesium hydroxide-containing antacid (Maalox)* on the pharmacokinetics of capecitabine was investigated in 12 cancer patients. There was a small increase in plasma concentrations of capecitabine and one metabolite (5′-DFCR); there was no effect on the 3 major metabolites (5′-DFUR, 5-FU and FBAL).

Coumarin Anticoagulants: Altered coagulation parameters and/or bleeding have been reported in patients taking capecitabine concomitantly with coumarin-derivative anticoagulants such as warfarin and phenprocoumon. Patients taking coumarin-derivative anticoagulants concomitantly with capecitabine should be monitored regularly for alterations in their coagulation parameters (PT or INR) (see WARNINGS: *Coagulopathy*).

Phenytoin: Postmarketing reports indicate that some patients receiving capecitabine and phenytoin had toxicity associated with elevated phenytoin levels. The level of phenytoin should be carefully monitored in patients taking XELODA and phenytoin dose may need to be reduced (see DOSAGE AND ADMINISTRATION: *Dose Modification Guidelines*).

Leucovorin: The concentration of 5-fluorouracil is increased and its toxicity may be enhanced by leucovorin. Deaths from severe enterocolitis, diarrhea, and dehydration have been reported in elderly patients receiving weekly leucovorin and fluorouracil.

Pregnancy: *Teratogenic Effects:* Category D (see WARNINGS). Women of childbearing potential should be advised to avoid becoming pregnant while receiving treatment with XELODA.

Nursing Women: It is not known whether the drug is excreted in human milk. Because many drugs are excreted in human milk and because of the potential for serious adverse reactions in nursing infants, it is recommended that nursing be discontinued when receiving XELODA therapy.

Pediatric Use: The safety and effectiveness of XELODA in persons <18 years of age have not been established.

Geriatric Use: No separate studies have been conducted to examine the effect of age on the pharmacokinetics of capecitabine and its metabolites. Patients ≥80 years old may experience a greater incidence of gastrointestinal grade 3 or 4 adverse events (see WARNINGS). Among the 14 patients 80 years of age and greater treated with capecitabine, 21.4%, 21.4% and 7.1% experienced grade 3 or 4 diarrhea, nausea and vomiting, respectively. Among the 313 patients 60 to 79 years old, the incidence was similar to the overall population.

The elderly may be pharmacodynamically more sensitive to the toxic effects of 5-FU. Physicians should pay particular attention to monitoring the adverse effects of XELODA in the elderly.

ADVERSE REACTIONS

The following table shows the adverse events occurring in ≥5% of patients reported as at least remotely related to the administration of XELODA. Rates are rounded to the nearest whole number. The data are shown both for the study in stage IV breast cancer and for a group of 570 patients with breast and colorectal cancer who received a dose of 2510 mg/m^2 administered daily for 2 weeks followed by a 1-week rest period. The 570 patients were enrolled in 6 clinical trials (162 from the breast cancer trial described under CLINICAL STUDIES, 83 other patients with breast cancer and 325 patients with colorectal cancer). The mean duration of treatment was 121 days. A total of 71 patients (13%) discontinued treatment because of adverse events/intercurrent illness.

[See table 3 at top of previous page]

Shown below by body system are the adverse events in <5% of patients reported as related to the administration of XELODA and that were clinically at least remotely relevant. In parentheses is the incidence of grade 3 or 4 occurrences of each adverse event.

Gastrointestinal: intestinal obstruction (1.1), rectal bleeding (0.4), GI hemorrhage (0.2), esophagitis (0.4), gastritis, colitis, duodenitis, haematemesis, necrotizing enterocolitis

Skin: increased sweating (0.2), photosensitivity (0.2), radiation recall syndrome (0.2)

General: chest pain (0.2)

Neurological: ataxia (0.4), encephalopathy (0.2), depressed level of consciousness (0.2), loss of consciousness (0.2)

Metabolism: cachexia (0.4), hypertriglyceridemia (0.2)

Respiratory: dyspnea (0.5), epistaxis (0.2), bronchospasm (0.2), respiratory distress (0.2)

Infections: oral candidiasis (0.2), upper respiratory tract infection (0.2), urinary tract infection (0.2), bronchitis (0.2), pneumonia (0.2), sepsis (0.4), bronchopneumonia (0.2), gastroenteritis (0.2), gastrointestinal candidiasis (0.2), laryngitis (0.2), esophageal candidiasis (0.2)

Musculoskeletal: bone pain (0.2), joint stiffness (0.2)

Cardiac: angina pectoris (0.2), cardiomyopathy

Vascular: hypotension (0.2), hypertension (0.2), venous phlebitis and thrombophlebitis (0.2), deep venous thrombosis (0.7), lymphoedema (0.2), pulmonary embolism (0.4), cerebrovascular accident (0.2)

Blood: coagulation disorder (0.2), idiopathic thrombocytopenic purpura (0.2), pancytopenia (0.2)

Psychiatric: confusion (0.2)

Renal and Urinary: nocturia (0.2)

Hepatobiliary: hepatic fibrosis (0.2), cholestatic hepatitis (0.2), hepatitis (0.2)

Immune System: drug hypersensitivity (0.2)

OVERDOSAGE

Acute: Based on experience in animals and in humans treated up to doses of 3514 mg/m^2/day, the anticipated manifestations of acute overdose would be nausea, vomiting, diarrhea, gastrointestinal irritation and bleeding, and bone marrow depression. Medical management of overdose should include customary supportive medical interventions aimed at correcting the presenting clinical manifestations. Although no clinical experience has been reported, dialysis may be of benefit in reducing circulating concentrations of 5′-DFUR, a low-molecular weight metabolite of the parent compound.

Single doses of XELODA were not lethal to mice, rats, and monkeys at doses up to 2000 mg/kg (2.4, 4.8, and 9.6 times the recommended human daily dose on a mg/m^2 basis).

DOSAGE AND ADMINISTRATION

The recommended dose of XELODA is 2500 mg/m^2 administered orally daily with food for 2 weeks followed by a 1-week rest period given as 3 week cycles. The XELODA daily dose is given orally in two divided doses (approximately 12 hours apart) at the end of a meal. XELODA tablets should be swallowed with water. The following table displays the total daily dose by body surface area and the number of tablets to be taken at each dose.

Table 4. XELODA Dose Calculation According to Body Surface Area

Dose level 2500 mg/m^2/day		Number of tablets to be taken at each dose (morning and evening)	
Surface Area (m^2)	Total Daily* Dose (mg)	150 mg	500 mg
≤ 1.24	3000	0	3
1.25–1.36	3300	1	3
1.37–1.51	3600	2	3
1.52–1.64	4000	0	4
1.65–1.76	4300	1	4
1.77–1.91	4600	2	4
1.92–2.04	5000	0	5
2.05–2.17	5300	1	5
≥ 2.18	5600	2	5

*Total Daily Dose divided by 2 to allow equal morning and evening doses.

Table 5. Recommended Dose Modifications

Toxicity NCIC Grades*	During a Course of Therapy	Dose Adjustment for Next Cycle (% of starting dose)
• *Grade 1*	Maintain dose level	Maintain dose level
• *Grade 2*		
-1st appearance	Interrupt until resolved to grade 0–1	100%
-2nd appearance	Interrupt until resolved to grade 0–1	75%
-3rd appearance	Interrupt until resolved to grade 0–1	50%
-4th appearance	Discontinue treatment permanently	
• *Grade 3*		
-1st appearance	Interrupt until resolved to grade 0–1	75%
-2nd appearance	Interrupt until resolved to grade 0–1	50%
-3rd appearance	Discontinue treatment permanently	
• *Grade 4*		
-1st appearance	Discontinue permanently *or* If physician deems it to be in the patient's best interest to continue, interrupt until resolved to grade 0–1	50%

*National Cancer Institute of Canada Common Toxicity Criteria were used except for the Hand-and-Foot Syndrome (see PRECAUTIONS).

Dose Modification Guidelines: Patients should be carefully monitored for toxicity. Toxicity due to XELODA administration may be managed by symptomatic treatment, dose interruptions and adjustment of XELODA dose. Once the dose has been reduced it should not be increased at a later time.

The phenytoin dose may need to be reduced when phenytoin is concomitantly administered with XELODA (see PRECAUTIONS: *Drug-Drug Interactions*).

[See table 5 above]

Dosage modifications are not recommended for grade 1 events. Therapy with XELODA should be interrupted upon the occurrence of a grade 2 or 3 adverse experience. Once the adverse event has resolved or decreased in intensity to grade 1, then XELODA therapy may be restarted at full dose or as adjusted according to the above table. If a grade 4 experience occurs, therapy should be discontinued or interrupted until resolved or decreased to grade 1, and therapy should be restarted at 50% of the original dose. Doses of capecitabine omitted for toxicity are not replaced or restored; instead the patient should resume the planned treatment cycles.

Adjustment of Starting Dose in Special Populations:

Hepatic Impairment: In patients with mild to moderate hepatic dysfunction due to liver metastases, no starting dose adjustment is necessary; however, patients should be carefully monitored. Patients with severe hepatic dysfunction have not been studied.

Renal Impairment: Insufficient data are available in patients with renal impairment to provide a dosage recommendation.

Geriatrics: The elderly may be pharmacodynamically more sensitive to the toxic effects of 5-FU and therefore, physicians should exercise caution in monitoring the effects of XELODA in the elderly. Insufficient data are available to provide a dosage recommendation.

HOW SUPPLIED

XELODA is supplied as biconvex, oblong film-coated tablets, available in bottles as follows:

150 mg

color: light peach

engraving: XELODA on one side, 150 on the other

150 mg tablets packaged in bottles of 120

(NDC 0004-1100-51)

500 mg

color: peach

engraving: XELODA on one side, 500 on the other

500 mg tablets packaged in bottles of 240

(NDC 0004-1101-16)

Storage Conditions: **Store at 25°C (77°F); excursions permitted to 15° to 30°C (59° to 86°F), keep tightly closed.** [See USP Controlled Room Temperature]

*Maalox is a registered trademark of Novartis.

Revised: July 2000

PATIENT PACKAGE INSERT (text only):

Patient Information About XELODA® (capecitabine) Tablets

This information will help you learn more about XELODA® (capecitabine) Tablets. It cannot, however, cover all possible precautions or side effects associated with XELODA nor does it list all the benefits and risks of XELODA. Your doctor should always be your first choice for detailed information about your medical condition and your treatment. Be sure to ask your doctor about any questions you may have.

What is XELODA?

- XELODA [zeh-LOE-duh] is an oral medication for the treatment of advanced breast cancer resistant to treatment with paclitaxel [pak-lih-TAK-sil] and an anthracycline [ann-thruh-SYE-kleen]-containing chemotherapy regimen. Paclitaxel is also known as Taxol®*. Anthracyclines include Adriamycin®† or doxorubicin.
- XELODA tablets come in two strengths: 150 mg (light peach) and 500 mg (peach).

How does XELODA work?

XELODA is converted in the body to the substance 5-fluorouracil. In some patients, this substance kills cancer cells and decreases the size of the tumor.

Who should not take XELODA?

- Patients allergic to 5-fluorouracil.
- Studies in animals suggest that XELODA may cause serious harm to an unborn child. No studies have been done with pregnant women. If you are pregnant, be sure to discuss with your doctor whether XELODA is right for you. Also, tell your doctor if you are nursing.

How should I take XELODA?

Your doctor will prescribe a dose and treatment regimen that is right for *you*. Your doctor may want you to take a combination of *150 mg* and *500 mg* tablets for each dose. If a combination of tablets is prescribed, it is very important that you correctly identify the tablets. Taking the wrong tablets could result in an overdose (too much medication) or underdose (too little medication). The 150 mg tablets are light peach in color and have 150 engraved on one side. The 500 mg tablets are peach in color and have 500 engraved on one side.

- Take the tablets in the combination prescribed by your doctor for your **morning and evening** doses.
- Take the tablets within **30 minutes after the end of a meal** (breakfast and dinner).
- XELODA tablets should be **swallowed with water.**
- It is important that you take all your medication as prescribed by your doctor.
- If you are taking the vitamin folic acid, please inform your doctor.
- If you are taking phenytoin (also known as Dilantin®‡), please inform your doctor. Your doctor may need to more frequently test the levels of phenytoin in your blood and/or change the dose of phenytoin that you are taking.
- If you are taking warfarin (also known as Coumadin®§), please inform your doctor. Your doctor may need to more frequently check how quickly your blood is clotting.

How long will I have to take XELODA?

It is recommended that XELODA be taken for 14 days followed by a 7-day rest period (no drug) given as a 21-day cycle. Your doctor will determine how many cycles of treatment you will need.

What if I miss a dose?

If you miss a dose of XELODA, do not take the missed dose at all and do not double the next one. Instead, continue your regular dosing schedule and check with your doctor.

What are the most common side effects of XELODA?

The most common side effects of XELODA are:

- diarrhea, nausea, vomiting, stomatitis (sores in mouth and throat), abdominal pain, constipation, loss of appetite or decreased appetite, and dehydration (excessive water loss from the body).
- hand-and-foot syndrome (palms of the hands or soles of the feet tingle, become numb, painful, swollen or red), rash, dry or itchy skin.
- tiredness, weakness, dizziness, headache, and fever.

When should I call my doctor?

It is important that you **CONTACT YOUR DOCTOR IMMEDIATELY** if you experience the following side effects. This will help reduce the likelihood that the side effect will continue or become serious. Your doctor may instruct you to decrease the dose and/or temporarily discontinue treatment with XELODA.

STOP taking XELODA immediately and contact your doctor if any of these symptoms occur:

- ***Diarrhea:*** if you have more than 4 bowel movements each day or any diarrhea at night.
- ***Vomiting:*** if you vomit more than once in a 24-hour time period.
- ***Nausea:*** if you lose your appetite, and the amount of food you eat each day is much less than usual.
- ***Stomatitis:*** if you have pain, redness, swelling, or sores in your mouth.
- ***Hand-and-foot syndrome:*** if you have pain, swelling or redness of hands and/or feet.
- ***Fever or Infection:*** if you have a temperature of 100.5°F or greater, or other evidence of infection.

If caught early, most of these side effects usually improve within 2 to 3 days after you stop taking XELODA. If they don't improve within 2 to 3 days, call your doctor again. After side effects have improved, your doctor will tell you whether to start taking XELODA again or what dose to use.

How should I store and use XELODA?

- Never share XELODA with anyone.
- XELODA should be stored at normal room temperature (about 65° to 85°F).
- Keep this and all other medications out of the reach of children.
- In case of accidental ingestion or if you suspect that more than the prescribed dose of this medication has been taken, contact your doctor or local poison control center or emergency room IMMEDIATELY.
- Medicines are sometimes prescribed for uses other than those listed in this leaflet. If you have any questions or concerns, or want more information about XELODA, contact your doctor or pharmacist.

*Taxol is a registered trademark of Bristol-Myers Squibb Company.

†Adriamycin is a registered trademark of Pharmacia & Upjohn Company.

‡Dilantin is a registered trademark of Parke-Davis.

§Coumadin is a registered trademark of DuPont Pharma.

Shown in Product Identification Guide, page 333

XENICAL® ℞
(orlistat)
CAPSULES

DESCRIPTION

XENICAL (orlistat) is a lipase inhibitor for obesity management that acts by inhibiting the absorption of dietary fats. Orlistat is (S)-2-formylamino-4-methyl-pentanoic acid (S)-1-[[(2S, 3S)-3-hexyl-4-oxo-2-oxetanyl] methyl]-dodecyl ester. Its empirical formula is $C_{29}H_{53}NO_5$, and its molecular weight is 495.7. It is a single diastereomeric molecule that contains four chiral centers, with a negative optical rotation in ethanol at 529 nm.

Orlistat is a white to off-white crystalline powder. Orlistat is practically insoluble in water, freely soluble in chloroform, and very soluble in methanol and ethanol. Orlistat has no pK_a within the physiological pH range.

XENICAL is available for oral administration in dark-blue, hard-gelatin capsules, with light-blue imprinting. Each capsule contains 120 mg of the active ingredient, orlistat. The capsules also contain the inactive ingredients microcrystalline cellulose, sodium starch glycolate, sodium lauryl sulfate, povidone, and talc. Each capsule shell contains gelatin, titanium dioxide, and FD&C Blue No. 1, with printing of pharmaceutical glaze NF, titanium dioxide, and FD&C Blue No. 1 aluminum lake.

CLINICAL PHARMACOLOGY

Mechanism of Action: Orlistat is a reversible inhibitor of lipases. It exerts its therapeutic activity in the lumen of the stomach and small intestine by forming a covalent bond with the active serine residue site of gastric and pancreatic lipases. The inactivated enzymes are thus unavailable to hydrolyze dietary fat in the form of triglycerides into absorbable free fatty acids and monoglycerides. As undigested triglycerides are not absorbed, the resulting caloric deficit may have a positive effect on weight control. Systemic absorption of the drug is therefore not needed for activity. At the recommended therapeutic dose of 120 mg three times a day, orlistat inhibits dietary fat absorption by approximately 30%.

Pharmacokinetics: *Absorption:* Systemic exposure to orlistat is minimal. Following oral dosing with 360 mg ^{14}C-orlistat, plasma radioactivity peaked at approximately 8 hours; plasma concentrations of intact orlistat were near the limits of detection (<5 ng/mL). In therapeutic studies involving monitoring of plasma samples, detection of intact orlistat in plasma was sporadic and concentrations were low (<10 ng/mL or 0.02 μM), without evidence of accumulation, and consistent with minimal absorption.

The average absolute bioavailability of intact orlistat was assessed in studies with male rats at oral doses of 150 and

Continued on next page

Xenical—Cont.

1000 mg/kg/day and in male dogs at oral doses of 100 and 1000 mg/kg/day and found to be 0.12%, 0.59% in rats and 0.7%, 1.9% in dogs, respectively.

Distribution: In vitro orlistat was >99% bound to plasma proteins (lipoproteins and albumin were major binding proteins). Orlistat minimally partitioned into erythrocytes.

Metabolism: Based on animal data, it is likely that the metabolism of orlistat occurs mainly within the gastrointestinal wall. Based on an oral ^{14}C-orlistat mass balance study in obese patients, two metabolites, M1 (4-member lactone ring hydrolyzed) and M3 (M1 with N-formyl leucine moiety cleaved), accounted for approximately 42% of total radioactivity in plasma. M1 and M3 have an open β-lactone ring and extremely weak lipase inhibitory activity (1000- and 2500-fold less than orlistat, respectively). In view of this low inhibitory activity and the low plasma levels at the therapeutic dose (average of 26 ng/mL and 108 ng/mL for M1 and M3, respectively, 2 to 4 hours after a dose), these metabolites are considered pharmacologically inconsequential. The primary metabolite M1 had a short half-life (approximately 3 hours) whereas the secondary metabolite M3 disappeared at a slower rate (half-life approximately 13.5 hours). In obese patients, steady-state plasma levels of M1, but not M3, increased in proportion to orlistat doses.

Elimination: Following a single oral dose of 360 mg ^{14}C-orlistat in both normal weight and obese subjects, fecal excretion of the unabsorbed drug was found to be the major route of elimination. Orlistat and its M1 and M3 metabolites were also subject to biliary excretion. Approximately 97% of the administered radioactivity was excreted in feces; 83% of that was found to be unchanged orlistat. The cumulative renal excretion of total radioactivity was <2% of the given dose of 360 mg ^{14}C-orlistat. The time to reach complete excretion (fecal plus urinary) was 3 to 5 days. The disposition of orlistat appeared to be similar between normal weight and obese subjects. Based on limited data, the half-life of the absorbed orlistat is in the range of 1 to 2 hours.

Special Populations: Because the drug is minimally absorbed, studies in special populations (geriatric, pediatric, different races, patients with renal and hepatic insufficiency) were not conducted.

Drug-Drug Interactions: Drug-drug interaction studies indicate that XENICAL had no effect on pharmacokinetics and/or pharmacodynamics of alcohol, digoxin, glyburide, nifedipine (extended-release tablets), oral contraceptives, phenytoin, or warfarin. XENICAL induced a modest increase of the bioavailability and lipid-lowering effect of pravastatin (see CLINICAL STUDIES and PRECAUTIONS). Alcohol did not affect the pharmacodynamics of orlistat.

Other Short-term Studies: In several studies of up to 6-weeks duration, the effects of therapeutic doses of XENICAL on gastrointestinal and systemic physiological processes were assessed in normal-weight and obese subjects. Postprandial cholecystokinin plasma concentrations were lowered after multiple doses of XENICAL in two studies but not significantly different from placebo in two other experiments. There were no clinically significant changes observed in gallbladder motility, bile composition or lithogenicity, or colonic cell proliferation rate, and no clinically significant reduction of gastric emptying time or gastric acidity. In addition, no effects on plasma triglyceride levels or systemic lipases were observed with the administration of XENICAL in these studies. In a 3-week study of 28 healthy male volunteers, XENICAL (120 mg three times a day) did not significantly affect the balance of calcium, magnesium, phosphorus, zinc, copper, and iron.

Dose-response Relationship: A simple maximum effect (E_{max}) model was used to define the dose-response curve of the relationship between XENICAL daily dose and fecal fat excretion as representative of gastrointestinal lipase inhibition. The dose-response curve demonstrated a steep portion for doses up to approximately 400 mg daily, followed by a plateau for higher doses. At doses greater than 120 mg three times a day, the percentage increase in effect was minimal.

CLINICAL STUDIES

Observational epidemiologic studies have established a relationship between obesity and visceral fat and the risks for cardiovascular disease, type 2 diabetes, certain forms of cancer, gallstones, certain respiratory disorders, and an increase in overall mortality. These studies suggest that weight loss, if maintained, may produce health benefits for obese patients who have or are at risk of developing weight-related comorbidities. The long-term effects of orlistat on morbidity and mortality associated with obesity have not been established.

The effects of XENICAL on weight loss, weight maintenance, and weight regain and on a number of comorbidities (eg, type 2 diabetes, lipids, blood pressure) were assessed in seven long-term (1- to 2-years duration) multicenter, double-blind, placebo-controlled clinical trials. During the first year of therapy, weight loss and weight maintenance were assessed. During the second year of therapy, some studies assessed continued weight loss and weight maintenance and others assessed the effect of orlistat on weight regain. These studies included over 2800 patients treated with XENICAL and 1400 patients treated with placebo. The majority of these patients had obesity-related risk factors and comorbidities. In these 7 studies, treatment with XENICAL and placebo designates treatment with XENICAL plus diet and placebo plus diet, respectively.

Table 1. Percentage of Patients Losing ≥5% and ≥10% of Body Weight From Randomization After 1-Year Treatment*

Intent-to-Treat Population†

	≥5% Weight Loss			≥10% Weight Loss		
Study No.	XENICAL n	Placebo n	p-value	XENICAL n	Placebo n	p-value
14119B	35.5% 110	21.3% 108	0.021	16.4% 110	6.5% 108	0.022
14119C	54.8% 343	27.4% 340	<0.001	24.8% 343	8.2% 340	<0.001
14149	50.6% 241	26.3% 236	<0.001	22.8% 241	11.9% 236	0.02
14161‡	37.1% 210	16.0% 212	<0.001	19.5% 210	3.8% 212	<0.001
14185	42.6% 657	22.4% 223	<0.001	17.7% 657	9.9% 223	0.006

The diet utilized during year 1 was a reduced-calorie diet.
*Treatment designates XENICAL 120 mg three times a day plus diet or placebo plus diet
†Last observation carried forward
‡All studies, with the exception of 14161, were conducted at centers specialized in treating obesity and complications of obesity. Study 14161 was conducted with primary care physicians.

Table 3. Percentage of Patients Losing ≥5% and ≥10% of Body Weight From Randomization After 2-Year Treatment*

Intent-to-Treat Population†

	≥5% Weight Loss			≥10% Weight Loss		
Study No.	XENICAL n	Placebo n	p-value	XENICAL n	Placebo n	p-value
14119C	45.1% 133	23.6% 123	<0.001	24.8% 133	6.5% 123	<0.001
14149	43.3% 178	27.2% 158	0.002	18.0% 178	9.5% 158	0.025
14161‡	25.0% 148	15.0% 113	0.049	16.9% 148	3.5% 113	0.001
14185	34.0% 147	27.9% 122	0.279	17.7% 147	11.5% 122	0.154

The diet utilized during year 2 was designed for weight maintenance and not weight loss.
*Treatment designates XENICAL 120 mg three times a day plus diet or placebo plus diet
†Last observation carried forward
‡All studies, with the exception of 14161 were conducted at centers specializing in treating obesity or complications of obesity. Study 14161 was conducted with primary care physicians.

During the weight loss and weight maintenance period, a well-balanced, reduced-calorie diet that was intended to result in an approximate 20% decrease in caloric intake and provide 30% of calories from fat was recommended to all patients. In addition, all patients were offered nutritional counseling.

One-year Results: Weight Loss, Weight Maintenance, and Risk Factors: Weight loss was observed within 2 weeks of initiation of therapy and continued for 6 to 12 months.

Pooled data from five clinical trials indicated that the overall mean weight loss from randomization to the end of 6 months and 1 year of treatment in the intent-to-treat population were 12.4 lbs and 13.4 lbs in the patients treated with XENICAL and 6.2 lbs and 5.8 lbs in the placebo-treated patients, respectively. During the 4-week placebo lead-in period of the studies, an additional 5 to 6 lb weight loss was also observed in the same patients. Of the patients who completed 1 year of treatment, 57% of the patients treated with XENICAL (120 mg three times a day) and 31% of the placebo-treated patients lost at least 5% of their baseline body weight.

The percentages of patients achieving ≥5% and ≥10% weight loss after 1 year in five large multicenter studies for the intent-to-treat populations are presented in Table 1.

[See table 1 above]

The relative changes in risk factors associated with obesity following 1 year of therapy with XENICAL and placebo are presented for the population as a whole and for the population with abnormal values at randomization.

Population as a Whole: The changes in metabolic, cardiovascular and anthropometric risk factors associated with obesity based on pooled data for five clinical studies, regardless of the patient's risk factor status at randomization, are presented in Table 2. One year of therapy with XENICAL resulted in relative improvement in several risk factors.

Table 2. Mean Change in Risk Factors From Randomization Following 1-Year Treatment* – Population as a Whole

Risk Factor	XENICAL 120 mg†	Placebo†
Metabolic:		
Total Cholesterol	−2.0%	+5.0%
LDL-Cholesterol	−4.0%	+5.0%
HDL-Cholesterol	+9.3%	+12.8%
LDL/HDL	−0.37%	−0.20
Triglycerides	+1.34%	+2.9%
Fasting Glucose, mmol/L	−0.04	+0.0
Fasting Insulin, pmol/L	−6.7	+5.2
Cardiovascular:		
Systolic Blood Pressure, mm Hg	−1.01	+0.58
Diastolic Blood Pressure, mm Hg	−1.19	+0.46
Anthropometric:		
Waist Circumference, cm	−6.45	−4.04
Hip Circumference, cm	−5.31	−2.96

*Treatment designates XENICAL 120 mg three times a day plus diet or placebo plus diet
†Intent-to-treat population at week 52, observed data based on pooled data from 5 studies

Population With Abnormal Risk Factors at Randomization: The changes from randomization following 1-year treatment in the population with abnormal lipid levels (LDL ≥130 mg/dL, LDL/HDL ≥3.5, HDL <35 mg/dL) were greater for XENICAL compared to placebo with respect to LDL-cholesterol (−7.83% vs +1.14%) and the LDL/HDL ratio (−0.64 vs −0.46). HDL increased in the placebo group by 20.1% and in the XENICAL group by 18.8%. In the population with abnormal blood pressure at baseline (systolic BP ≥140 mm Hg), the change in SBP from randomization to 1 year was greater for XENICAL (−10.89 mm Hg) than placebo (−5.07 mm Hg). For patients with a diastolic blood pressure ≥90 mm Hg, XENICAL patients decreased by −7.9 mm Hg while the placebo patients decreased by −5.5 mm Hg. Fasting insulin decreased more for XENICAL than placebo (−39 vs −16 pmol/L) from randomization to 1 year in the population with abnormal baseline values (≥120 pmol/L). A greater reduction in waist circumference for XENICAL vs placebo (−7.29 vs −4.53 cm) was observed in the population with abnormal baseline values (≥100 cm).

Effect on Weight Regain: Three studies were designed to evaluate the effects of XENICAL compared to placebo in reducing weight regain after a previous weight loss achieved following either diet alone (one study, 14302) or prior treatment with XENICAL (two studies, 14119C and 14185). The diet utilized during the 1-year weight regain portion of the studies was a weight-maintenance diet, rather than a weight-loss diet, and patients received less nutritional counseling than patients in weight-loss studies. For studies 14119C and 14185, patients' previous weight loss was due to 1 year of treatment with XENICAL in conjunction with a mildly hypocaloric diet. Study 14302 was conducted to evaluate the effects of 1 year of treatment with XENICAL on weight regain in patients who had lost 8% or more of their body weight in the previous 6 months on diet alone.

In study 14119C, patients treated with placebo regained 52% of the weight they had previously lost while the patients treated with XENICAL regained 26% of the weight they had previously lost (p<0.001). In study 14185, patients treated with placebo regained 63% of the weight they had previously lost while the patients treated with XENICAL regained 35% of the weight they had lost (p<0.001). In study 14302, patients treated with placebo regained 53% of the weight they had previously lost while the patients treated with XENICAL regained 32% of the weight that they had lost (p<0.001).

Two-year Results: Long-term Weight Control and Risk Factors: The treatment effects of XENICAL were examined for 2 years in four of the five 1-year weight management clinical studies previously discussed (see Table 1). At the end of year 1, the patients' diets were reviewed and changed where necessary. The diet prescribed in the second year was designed to maintain patient's current weight. XENICAL was shown to be more effective than placebo in long-term weight control in four large, multicenter, 2-year double-blind, placebo-controlled studies.

Pooled data from four clinical studies indicate that 40% of all patients treated with 120 mg three times a day of XENICAL and 24% of patients treated with placebo who completed 2 years of the same therapy had ≥5% loss of body weight from randomization. Pooled data from four clinical studies indicate that the relative weight loss advantage between XENICAL 120 mg three times a day and placebo treatment groups was the same after 2 years as for 1 year, indicating that the pharmacologic advantage of XENICAL was maintained over 2 years. In the same studies cited in the *One-year Results* (see Table 1), the percentages of patients achieving a ≥5% and ≥10% weight loss after 2 years are shown in Table 3.

[See table 3 at top of previous page]

The relative changes in risk factors associated with obesity following 2 years of therapy were also assessed in the population as a whole and the population with abnormal risk factors at randomization.

Population as a Whole: The relative differences in risk factors between treatment with XENICAL and placebo were similar to the results following 1 year of therapy for total cholesterol, LDL-cholesterol, LDL/HDL ratio, triglycerides, fasting glucose, fasting insulin, diastolic blood pressure, waist circumference, and hip circumference. The relative differences between treatment groups for HDL cholesterol and systolic blood pressure were less than that observed in the year one results.

Population With Abnormal Risk Factors at Randomization: The relative differences in risk factors between treatment with XENICAL and placebo were similar to the results following 1 year of therapy for LDL- and HDL-cholesterol, triglycerides, fasting insulin, diastolic blood pressure, and waist circumference. The relative differences between treatment groups for LDL/HDL ratio and isolated systolic blood pressure were less than that observed in the year one results.

Study of Patients With Type 2 Diabetes: A 1-year double-blind, placebo-controlled study in type 2 diabetics (N=321) stabilized on sulfonylureas was conducted. Thirty percent of patients treated with XENICAL achieved at least a 5% or greater reduction in body weight from randomization compared to 13% of the placebo-treated patients (p<0.001). Table 4 describes the changes over 1 year of treatment with XENICAL compared to placebo, in sulfonylurea usage and dose reduction as well as in hemoglobin HbA1c, fasting glucose, and insulin.

Table 4. Mean Changes in Body Weight and Glycemic Control From Randomization Following 1-Year Treatment in Patients With Type 2 Diabetes

	XENICAL 120 mg* (n=162)	Placebo* (n=159)	Statistical Significance
% patients who discontinued dose of oral sulfonylurea	11.7%	7.5%	†
% patients who decreased dose of oral sulfonylurea	31.5%	21.4%	
Average reduction in sulfonylurea medication dose	−22.8%	−9.1%	†
Body weight change (lbs)	−8.9	−4.2	†
HbA1c	−0.18%	+0.28%	†
Fasting glucose, mmol/L	−0.02	+0.54	†
Fasting insulin, pmol/L	−19.68	−18.02	ns

Statistical significance based on intent-to-treat population, last observation carried forward.
* Treatment designates XENICAL 120 mg three times a day plus diet or placebo plus diet
† Statistically significant (p≤0.05) based on intent-to-treat, last observation carried forward
ns nonsignificant, p>0.05

In addition, XENICAL (n=162) compared to placebo (n=159) was associated with significant lowering for total cholesterol (−1.0% vs +9.0%, p≤0.05), LDL-cholesterol (−3.0% vs +10.0%, p≤0.05), LDL/HDL ratio (−0.26 vs −0.02, p≤0.05) and triglycerides (+2.54% vs +16.2%, p≤0.05), respectively. For HDL cholesterol, there was a +6.49% increase on XENICAL and +8.6% increase on placebo, p>0.05. Systolic blood pressure increased by +0.61 mm Hg on XENICAL and increased by +4.33 mm Hg on placebo, p>0.05. Diastolic blood pressure decreased by −0.47 mm Hg for XENICAL and by −0.5 mm Hg for placebo, p>0.05.

Glucose Tolerance in Obese Patients: Two-year studies that included oral glucose tolerance tests were conducted in obese patients not previously diagnosed or treated for type 2 diabetes and whose baseline oral glucose tolerance test (OGTT) status at randomization was either normal, impaired, or diabetic.

The progression from a normal OGTT at randomization to a diabetic or impaired OGTT following 2 years of treatment with XENICAL (n=251) or placebo (n=207) were compared. Following treatment with XENICAL, 0.0% and 7.2% of the patients progressed from normal to diabetic and normal to impaired, respectively, compared to 1.9% and 12.6% of the placebo treatment group, respectively.

In patients found to have an impaired OGTT at randomization, the percent of patients improving to normal or deteriorating to diabetic status following 1 and 2 years of treatment with XENICAL compared to placebo are presented. After 1 year of treatment, 45.8% of the placebo patients and 73% of the XENICAL patients had a normal oral glucose tolerance test while 10.4% of the placebo patients and 2.6% of the XENICAL patients became diabetic. After 2 years of treatment, 50% of the placebo patients and 71.7% of the XENICAL patients had a normal oral glucose tolerance test while 7.5% of placebo patients were found to be diabetic and 1.7% of XENICAL patients were found to be diabetic after treatment.

INDICATIONS AND USAGE

XENICAL is indicated for obesity management including weight loss and weight maintenance when used in conjunction with a reduced-calorie diet. XENICAL is also indicated to reduce the risk for weight regain after prior weight loss. XENICAL is indicated for obese patients with an initial body mass index (BMI) ≥30 kg/m^2 or ≥27 kg/m^2 in the presence of other risk factors (e.g., hypertension, diabetes, dyslipidemia).

Table 5 illustrates body mass index (BMI) according to a variety of weights and heights. The BMI is calculated by dividing weight in kilograms by height in meters squared. For example, a person who weighs 180 lbs and is 5′5″ would have a BMI of 30.

[See graphic above]

Table 5. Body Mass Index (BMI), kg/m^2*

HEIGHT (ft/in) \ WEIGHT (lb)	120	130	140	150	160	170	180	190	200	210	220	230	240	250	260	270	280	290	300	310	320
4'10"	25	27	29	31	34	36	38	40	42	44	46	48	50	52	54	57	59	61	63	65	67
4'11"	24	26	28	30	32	34	36	38	40	43	45	47	49	51	53	55	57	59	61	63	65
5'0"	23	25	27	29	31	33	35	37	39	41	43	45	47	48	51	53	55	57	59	61	63
5'1"	23	25	27	28	30	32	34	36	38	40	42	44	45	47	49	51	53	55	57	59	61
5'2"	22	24	26	27	29	31	33	35	37	38	40	42	44	46	48	49	51	53	55	57	59
5'3"	21	23	25	27	28	30	32	34	36	37	39	41	43	44	46	48	50	51	53	55	57
5'4"	21	22	24	26	28	29	31	33	34	36	38	40	41	43	45	46	48	50	52	53	55
5'5"	20	22	23	25	27	28	30	32	33	35	37	38	40	42	43	45	47	48	50	52	53
5'6"	19	21	23	24	26	27	29	31	32	34	36	37	39	40	42	44	45	47	49	50	52
5'7"	19	20	22	24	25	27	28	30	31	33	35	36	38	39	41	42	44	46	47	49	50
5'8"	18	20	21	23	24	26	27	29	30	32	34	35	37	38	40	41	43	44	46	47	49
5'9"	18	19	21	22	24	25	27	28	30	31	33	34	36	37	38	40	41	43	44	46	47
5'10"	17	19	20	22	23	24	26	27	29	30	32	33	35	36	37	39	40	42	43	45	46
5'11"	17	18	20	21	22	24	25	27	28	29	31	32	34	35	36	38	39	41	42	43	45
6'0"	16	18	19	20	22	23	24	26	27	29	30	31	33	34	35	37	38	39	41	42	43
6'1"	16	17	19	20	21	22	24	25	26	28	29	30	32	33	34	36	37	38	40	41	42
6'2"	15	17	18	19	21	22	23	24	26	27	28	30	31	32	33	35	36	37	39	40	41

*Conversion Factors:
Weight in lbs ÷ 2.2 = weight in kilograms (kg)
Height in inches x 0.0254 = height in meters (m)
1 foot = 12 inches

Table 7. Commonly Observed Adverse Events

	Year 1		Year 2	
Adverse Event	XENICAL* % Patients (N=1913)	Placebo* % Patients (N=1466)	XENICAL* % Patients (N=613)	Placebo* % Patients (N=524)
Oily Spotting	26.6	1.3	4.4	0.2
Flatus with Discharge	23.9	1.4	2.1	0.2
Fecal Urgency	22.1	6.7	2.8	1.7
Fatty/Oily Stool	20.0	2.9	5.5	0.6
Oily Evacuation	11.9	0.8	2.3	0.2
Increased Defecation	10.8	4.1	2.6	0.8
Fecal Incontinence	7.7	0.9	1.8	0.2

*Treatment designates XENICAL three times a day plus diet or placebo plus diet

CONTRAINDICATIONS

XENICAL is contraindicated in patients with chronic malabsorption syndrome or cholestasis, and in patients with known hypersensitivity to XENICAL or to any component of this product.

WARNINGS

Miscellaneous: Organic causes of obesity (e.g., hypothyroidism) should be excluded before prescribing XENICAL. Preliminary data from a XENICAL and cyclosporine drug interaction study indicate a reduction in cyclosporine plasma levels when XENICAL was coadministered with cyclosporine. Therefore, XENICAL and cyclosporine should not be coadministered. To reduce the chance of a drug-drug interaction, cyclosporine should be taken at least 2 hours before or after XENICAL in patients taking both drugs. In addition, in those patients whose cyclosporine levels are being measured, more frequent monitoring should be considered.

PRECAUTIONS

General: Patients should be advised to adhere to dietary guidelines (see DOSAGE AND ADMINISTRATION). Gastrointestinal events (see ADVERSE REACTIONS) may increase when XENICAL is taken with a diet high in fat (>30% total daily calories from fat). The daily intake of fat should be distributed over three main meals. If XENICAL is taken with any one meal very high in fat, the possibility of gastrointestinal effects increases.

Patients should be counseled to take a multivitamin supplement that contains fat-soluble vitamins to ensure adequate nutrition because XENICAL has been shown to reduce the absorption of some fat-soluble vitamins and beta-carotene. In addition, the levels of vitamin D and beta-carotene may be low in obese patients compared with non-obese subjects. The supplement should be taken once a day at least 2 hours before or after the administration of XENICAL, such as at bedtime.

Table 6 illustrates the percentage of patients on XENICAL and placebo who developed a low vitamin level on two or more consecutive visits during 1 and 2 years of therapy in studies in which patients were not previously receiving vitamin supplementation.

Table 6. Incidence of Low Vitamin Values on Two or More Consecutive Visits (Nonsupplemented Patients With Normal Baseline Values – First and Second Year)

	Placebo*	XENICAL*
Vitamin A	1.0%	2.2%
Vitamin D	6.6%	12.0%

Continued on next page

Xenical—Cont.

Vitamin E	1.0%	5.8%
Beta-carotene	1.7%	6.1%

*Treatment designates placebo plus diet or XENICAL plus diet

Some patients may develop increased levels of urinary oxalate following treatment with XENICAL. Caution should be exercised when prescribing XENICAL to patients with a history of hyperoxaluria or calcium oxalate nephrolithiasis. Weight-loss induction by XENICAL may be accompanied by improved metabolic control in diabetics, which might require a reduction in dose of oral hypoglycemic medication (e.g., sulfonylureas, metformin) or insulin (see CLINICAL STUDIES).

Misuse Potential: As with any weight-loss agent, the potential exists for misuse of XENICAL in inappropriate patient populations (eg, patients with anorexia nervosa or bulimia). See INDICATIONS AND USAGE for recommended prescribing guidelines.

Information for Patients: Patients should read the Patient Information before starting treatment with XENICAL and each time their prescription is renewed.

Drug Interactions: *Alcohol:* In a multiple-dose study in 30 normal weight subjects, coadministration of XENICAL and 40 grams of alcohol (e.g., approximately 3 glasses of wine) did not result in alteration of alcohol pharmacokinetics, orlistat pharmacodynamics (fecal fat excretion), or systemic exposure to orlistat.

Cyclosporine: Preliminary data from XENICAL and cyclosporine drug interaction study indicate a reduction in cyclosporine plasma levels when XENICAL was coadministered with cyclosporine (see WARNINGS).

Digoxin: In 12 normal-weight subjects receiving XENICAL 120 mg three times a day for 6 days, XENICAL did not alter the pharmacokinetics of a single dose of digoxin.

Fat-soluble Vitamin Supplements and Analogues: A pharmacokinetic interaction study showed a 30% reduction in beta-carotene supplement absorption when concomitantly administered with XENICAL. XENICAL inhibited absorption of a vitamin E acetate supplement by approximately 60%. The effect of orlistat on the absorption of supplemental vitamin D, vitamin A, and nutritionally-derived vitamin K is not known at this time.

Glyburide: In 12 normal-weight subjects receiving orlistat 80 mg three times a day for 5 days, orlistat did not alter the pharmacokinetics or pharmacodynamics (blood glucose-lowering) of glyburide.

Nifedipine (extended-release tablets): In 17 normal-weight subjects receiving XENICAL 120 mg three times a day for 6 days, XENICAL did not alter the bioavailability of nifedipine (extended-release tablets).

Oral Contraceptives: In 20 normal-weight female subjects, the treatment of XENICAL 120 mg three times a day for 23 days resulted in no changes in the ovulation-suppressing action of oral contraceptives.

Phenytoin: In 12 normal-weight subjects receiving XENICAL 120 mg three times a day for 7 days, XENICAL did not alter the pharmacokinetics of a single 300-mg dose of phenytoin.

Pravastatin: In a parallel study of 24 normal-weight, mildly hypercholesterolemic subjects receiving XENICAL 120 mg three times a day for 10 days, the effect of XENICAL was additive to the lipid-lowering effect of pravastatin. Modest increases (approximately 30%) in pravastatin plasma concentrations were observed during coadministration with XENICAL.

Warfarin: In 12 normal-weight subjects, administration of XENICAL 120 mg three times a day for 16 days did not result in any change in either warfarin pharmacokinetics (both R- and S-enantiomers) or pharmacodynamics (prothrombin time and serum Factor VII). Although undercarboxylated osteocalcin, a marker of vitamin K nutritional status, was unaltered with XENICAL administration, vitamin K levels tended to decline in subjects taking XENICAL. Therefore, as vitamin K absorption may be decreased with XENICAL, patients on chronic stable doses of warfarin who are prescribed XENICAL should be monitored closely for changes in coagulation parameters.

Carcinogenesis, Mutagenesis, Impairment of Fertility: Carcinogenicity studies in rats and mice did not show a carcinogenic potential for orlistat at doses up to 1000 mg/kg/day and 1500 mg/kg/day, respectively. For mice and rats, these doses are 38 and 46 times the daily human dose calculated on an area under concentration vs times curve basis of total drug-related material.

Orlistat had no detectable mutagenic or genotoxic activity as determined by the Ames test, a mammalian forward mutation assay (V79/HPRT), an in vitro clastogenesis assay in peripheral human lymphocytes, an unscheduled DNA synthesis assay (UDS) in rat hepatocytes in culture, and an in vivo mouse micronucleus test.

When given to rats at a dose of 400 mg/kg/day in a fertility and reproduction study, orlistat had no observable adverse effects. This dose is 12 times the daily human dose calculated on a body surface area (mg/m^2) basis.

Pregnancy: Teratogenic Effects: Pregnancy Category B. Teratogenicity studies were conducted in rats and rabbits at doses up to 800 mg/kg/day. Neither study showed embryotoxicity or teratogenicity. This dose is 23 and 47 times the daily human dose calculated on a body surface area (mg/m^2) basis for rats and rabbits, respectively.

The incidence of dilated cerebral ventricles was increased in the mid- and high-dose groups of the rat teratology study. These doses were 6 and 23 times the daily human dose calculated on a body surface area (mg/m^2) basis for the mid- and high-dose levels, respectively. This finding was not reproduced in two additional rat teratology studies at similar doses.

There are no adequate and well-controlled studies of XENICAL in pregnant women. Because animal reproductive studies are not always predictive of human response, XENICAL is not recommended for use during pregnancy.

Nursing Mothers: It is not known if orlistat is secreted in human milk. Therefore, XENICAL should not be taken by nursing women.

Pediatric Use: The safety and efficacy of XENICAL in pediatric patients have not been established.

Geriatric Use: Clinical studies of XENICAL did not include sufficient numbers of patients aged 65 years and older to determine whether they respond differently from younger patients.

ADVERSE REACTIONS

Commonly Observed (based on first year and second year data — XENICAL 120 mg three times a day versus placebo): Gastrointestinal (GI) symptoms were the most commonly observed treatment-emergent adverse events associated with the use of XENICAL in double-blind, placebo-controlled clinical trials and are primarily a manifestation of the mechanism of action. (Commonly observed is defined as an incidence of ≥5% and an incidence in the XENICAL 120 mg group that is at least twice that of placebo.)

[See table 7 at top of previous page]

These and other commonly observed adverse reactions were generally mild and transient, and they decreased during the second year of treatment. In general, the first occurrence of these events was within 3 months of starting therapy. Overall, approximately 50% of all episodes of GI adverse events associated with orlistat treatment lasted for less than 1 week, and a majority lasted for no more than 4 weeks. However, GI adverse events may occur in some individuals over a period of 6 months or longer.

Discontinuation of Treatment: In controlled clinical trials, 8.8% of patients treated with XENICAL discontinued treatment due to adverse events, compared with 5.0% of placebo-treated patients. For XENICAL, the most common adverse events resulting in discontinuation of treatment were gastrointestinal.

Incidence in Controlled Clinical Trials: The following table lists other treatment-emergent adverse events from seven multicenter, double-blind, placebo-controlled clinical trials that occurred at a frequency of ≥2% among patients treated with XENICAL 120 mg three times a day and with an incidence that was greater than placebo during year 1 and year 2, regardless of relationship to study medication.

[See table 8 below]

Table 8. Other Treatment-Emergent Adverse Events From Seven Placebo-Controlled Clinical Trials

Body System/ Adverse Events	Year 1		Year 2	
	XENICAL* % Patients (N=1913)	Placebo* % Patients (N=1466)	XENICAL* % Patients (N=613)	Placebo* % Patients (N=524)
Gastrointestinal System				
Abdominal Pain/Discomfort	25.5	21.4	—	—
Nausea	8.1	7.3	3.6	2.7
Infectious Diarrhea	5.3	4.4	—	—
Rectal Pain/Discomfort	5.2	4.0	3.3	1.9
Tooth Disorder	4.3	3.1	2.9	2.3
Gingival Disorder	4.1	2.9	2.0	1.5
Vomiting	3.8	3.5	—	—
Respiratory System				
Influenza	39.7	36.2	—	—
Upper Respiratory Infection	38.1	32.8	26.1	25.8
Lower Respiratory Infection	7.8	6.6	—	—
Ear, Nose & Throat Symptoms	2.0	1.6	—	—
Musculoskeletal System				
Back Pain	13.9	12.1	—	—
Pain Lower Extremities	—	—	10.8	10.3
Arthritis	5.4	4.8	—	—
Myalgia	4.2	3.3	—	—
Joint Disorder	2.3	2.2	—	—
Tendonitis	—	—	2.0	1.9
Central Nervous System				
Headache	30.6	27.6	—	—
Dizziness	5.2	5.0	—	—
Body as a Whole				
Fatigue	7.2	6.4	3.1	1.7
Sleep Disorder	3.9	3.3	—	—
Skin & Appendages				
Rash	4.3	4.0	—	—
Dry Skin	2.1	1.4	—	—
Reproductive, Female				
Menstrual Irregularity	9.8	7.5	—	—
Vaginitis	3.8	3.6	2.6	1.9
Urinary System				
Urinary Tract Infection	7.5	7.3	5.9	4.8
Psychiatric Disorder				
Psychiatric Anxiety	4.7	2.9	2.8	2.1
Depression	—	—	3.4	2.5
Hearing & Vestibular Disorders				
Otitis	4.3	3.4	2.9	2.5
Cardiovascular Disorders				
Pedal Edema	—	—	2.8	1.9

* Treatment designates XENICAL 120 mg three times a day plus diet or placebo plus diet
—None reported at a frequency ≥2% and greater than placebo

Other Clinical Studies or Postmarketing Surveillance: Rare cases of hypersensitivity have been reported with the use of XENICAL. Signs and symptoms have included pruritus, rash, urticaria, angioedema, and anaphylaxis.

Preliminary data from XENICAL and cyclosporine drug interaction study indicate a reduction in cyclosporine plasma levels when XENICAL was coadministered with cyclosporine (see WARNINGS).

OVERDOSAGE

Single doses of 800 mg XENICAL and multiple doses of up to 400 mg three times a day for 15 days have been studied in normal weight and obese subjects without significant adverse findings.

Should a significant overdose of XENICAL occur, it is recommended that the patient be observed for 24 hours. Based on human and animal studies, systemic effects attributable to the lipase-inhibiting properties of orlistat should be rapidly reversible.

DOSAGE AND ADMINISTRATION

The recommended dose of XENICAL is one 120 mg capsule three times a day with each main meal containing fat (during or up to 1 hour after the meal).

The patient should be on a nutritionally balanced, reduced-calorie diet that contains approximately 30% of calories from fat. The daily intake of fat, carbohydrate, and protein should be distributed over three main meals. If a meal is occasionally missed or contains no fat, the dose of XENICAL can be omitted.

Because XENICAL has been shown to reduce the absorption of some fat-soluble vitamins and beta-carotene, patients should be counseled to take a multivitamin containing fat-soluble vitamins to ensure adequate nutrition. The supplement should be taken at least 2 hours before or after the administration of XENICAL, such as at bedtime.

Doses above 120 mg three times a day have not been shown to provide additional benefit.

Based on fecal fat measurements, the effect of XENICAL is seen as soon as 24 to 48 hours after dosing. Upon discontinuation of therapy, fecal fat content usually returns to pretreatment levels within 48 to 72 hours.

The safety and effectiveness of XENICAL beyond 2 years have not been determined at this time.

HOW SUPPLIED

XENICAL is a dark-blue, hard-gelatin capsule containing pellets of powder.

XENICAL 120 mg Capsules: Dark-blue, two-piece, No. 1 opaque hard-gelatin capsule imprinted with Roche and XENICAL 120 in light-blue ink — bottle of 90 (NDC 0004-0256-52).

Storage Conditions: **Store at 25°C (77°F); excursions permitted to 15° to 30°C (59° to 86°F)** [see USP Controlled Room Temperature]. **Keep bottle tightly closed.**

XENICAL should not be used after the given expiration date.

Roche Pharmaceuticals
Roche Laboratories Inc.
340 Kingsland Street
Nutley, New Jersey 07110-1199

Revised: September 1999

Shown in Product Identification Guide, page 333

ZENAPAX® ℞
(Daclizumab)
STERILE CONCENTRATE
FOR INJECTION

The following text is complete prescribing information based on official labeling in effect June 2000.

WARNING:

Only physicians experienced in immunosuppressive therapy and management of organ transplant patients should prescribe ZENAPAX® (Daclizumab). The physician responsible for ZENAPAX administration should have complete information requisite for the follow-up of the patient. ZENAPAX should only be administered by healthcare personnel trained in the administration of the drug who have available adequate laboratory and supportive medical resources.

DESCRIPTION

ZENAPAX® (Daclizumab) is an immunosuppressive, humanized IgG1 monoclonal antibody produced by recombinant DNA technology that binds specifically to the alpha subunit (p55 alpha, CD25, or Tac subunit) of the human high-affinity interleukin-2 (IL-2) receptor that is expressed on the surface of activated lymphocytes.

Daclizumab is a composite of human (90%) and murine (10%) antibody sequences. The human sequences were derived from the constant domains of human IgG1 and the variable framework regions of the Eu myeloma antibody. The murine sequences were derived from the complementarity-determining regions of a murine anti-Tac antibody. The molecular weight predicted from DNA sequencing is 144 kilodaltons.

ZENAPAX 25 mg/5mL is supplied as a clear, sterile, colorless concentrate for further dilution and intravenous administration. Each milliliter of ZENAPAX contains 5 mg of Daclizumab and 3.6 mg sodium phosphate monobasic monohydrate, 11 mg sodium phosphate dibasic heptahydrate, 4.6 mg sodium chloride, 0.2 mg polysorbate 80 and may contain hydrochloric acid or sodium hydroxide to adjust the pH to 6.9. No preservatives are added.

CLINICAL PHARMACOLOGY

Mechanism of Action: Daclizumab functions as an IL-2 receptor antagonist that binds with high-affinity to the Tac subunit of the high-affinity IL-2 receptor complex and inhibits IL-2 binding. Daclizumab binding is highly specific for Tac, which is expressed on activated but not resting lymphocytes. Administration of ZENAPAX inhibits IL-2–mediated activation of lymphocytes, a critical pathway in the cellular immune response involved in allograft rejection.

While in the circulation, ZENAPAX impairs the response of the immune system to antigenic challenges. Whether the ability to respond to repeated or ongoing challenges with those antigens returns to normal after ZENAPAX is cleared is unknown (see PRECAUTIONS).

Pharmacokinetics: In clinical trials involving renal allograft patients treated with a 1 mg/kg IV dose of ZENAPAX every 14 days for a total of five doses, peak serum concentration (mean ± SD) rose between the first dose (21 ± 14 µg/mL) and fifth dose (32 ± 22 µg/mL). The mean trough serum concentration before the fifth dose was 7.6 ± 4.0 µg/mL. In vitro and in vivo data suggest that serum levels of 5 to 10 µg/mL are necessary for saturation of the Tac subunit of the IL-2 receptors to block the responses of activated T lymphocytes.

Population pharmacokinetic analysis of the data using a two-compartment open model gave the following values for a reference patient (45-year-old male Caucasian patient with a body weight of 80 kg and no proteinuria): systemic clearance = 15 mL/hour, volume of central compartment = 2.5 liter, volume of peripheral compartment = 3.4 liter. The estimated terminal elimination half-life for the reference patient was 20 days (480 hours), which is similar to the terminal elimination half-life for human IgG (18 to 23 days). Bayesian estimates of terminal elimination half-life ranged from 11 to 38 days for the 123 patients included in the population analysis.

The influence of body weight on systemic clearance supports the dosing of ZENAPAX on a milligram per kilogram (mg/kg) basis. For patients studied, this dosing maintained drug exposure within 30% of the reference exposure. Covariate analyses showed that no dosage adjustments based on age, race, gender or degree of proteinuria, are required for renal allograft patients. The estimated interpatient variability (percent coefficient of variation) in systemic clearance and central volume of distribution were 15% and 27%, respectively.

Pharmacodynamics: At the recommended dosage regimen, Daclizumab saturates the Tac subunit of the IL-2 receptor for approximately 120 days post-transplant. The duration of clinically significant IL-2 receptor blockade after the recommended course of ZENAPAX is not known. No significant changes to circulating lymphocyte numbers or cell phenotypes were observed by flow cytometry. Cytokine release syndrome has not been observed after ZENAPAX administration.

CLINICAL STUDIES

The safety and efficacy of ZENAPAX for the prophylaxis of acute organ rejection in adult patients receiving their first cadaveric kidney transplant were assessed in two randomized, double-blind, placebo-controlled, multicenter trials. These trials compared a dose of 1.0 mg/kg of ZENAPAX with placebo when each was administered as part of standard immunosuppressive regimens containing either cyclosporine and corticosteroids (double-therapy trial, no US sites) or cyclosporine, corticosteroids, and azathioprine (triple-therapy trial, predominantly US sites) to prevent acute renal allograft rejection. ZENAPAX dosing was initiated within 24 hours pretransplant, with subsequent doses given every 14 days for a total of five doses.

The primary efficacy endpoint of both trials was the proportion of patients who developed a biopsy-proven acute rejection episode within the first 6 months following transplantation. As shown in Table 1, this incidence was significantly lower in the ZENAPAX-treated group in both the double-therapy and triple-therapy trials.

[See table above]

Table 1. Efficacy Parameters

	Triple-therapy Regimen (cyclosporine, corticosteroids, and azathioprine)			Double-therapy Regimen (cyclosporine and corticosteroids)		
	Placebo (N=134)	**ZENAPAX (N=126)**	**p-value**	**Placebo (N=134)**	**ZENAPAX (N=141)**	**p-value**
Primary Endpoint						
Incidence of biopsy-proven acute rejection at 6 months						
No. of patients	47 (35%)	28 (22%)	0.03	63 (47%)	39 (28%)	0.001
Secondary Endpoints						
Incidence of biopsy-proven acute rejection at 1 year						
No. of patients	51 (38%)	35 (28%)	0.09	65 (49%)	39 (28%)	<0.001
Patient survival at 1 year post-transplant						
No. of patients	129 (96%)	123 (98%)	0.51	126 (94%)	140 (99%)	0.01
Graft survival at 1 year post-transplant						
No. of patients with functioning graft	121 (90%)	120 (95%)	0.08	111 (83%)	124 (88%)	0.30

No difference in patient survival was observed in the triple-therapy study between ZENAPAX- and placebo-treated patients. Treatment with ZENAPAX was associated with better patient survival at 1 year post-transplant in the double-therapy study.

The incidence of delayed graft function was no different between placebo-treated and ZENAPAX-treated patients in either study. No difference in graft function was observed 1 year post-transplant in either study between placebo-treated and ZENAPAX-treated patients.

In a randomized, double-blind study, ZENAPAX (50 patients) or placebo (25 patients) was added to an immunosuppressive regimen of cyclosporine, mycophenolate mofetil, and steroids to assess tolerability, pharmacokinetics, and drug interactions. The addition of ZENAPAX to an immunosuppressive regimen of cyclosporine, mycophenolate mofetil, and steroids did not result in an increased incidence of adverse events or a change in the types of adverse events reported. The incidence of the combined endpoint of biopsy-proven or clinically presumptive acute rejection was 20% (5 of 25 patients) in the placebo group and 12% (6 of 50 patients) in the ZENAPAX group. Although numerically lower, the difference in acute rejection was not significant.

INDICATION AND USAGE

ZENAPAX is indicated for the prophylaxis of acute organ rejection in patients receiving renal transplants. It is used as part of an immunosuppressive regimen that includes cyclosporine and corticosteroids.

CONTRAINDICATION

ZENAPAX is contraindicated in patients with known hypersensitivity to Daclizumab or to any components of this product.

WARNINGS

See Boxed WARNING.

ZENAPAX should be administered under qualified medical supervision. Patients should be informed of the potential benefits of therapy and the risks associated with administration of immunosuppressive therapy.

While the incidence of lymphoproliferative disorders and opportunistic infections, in the limited clinical trial experience, was no higher in ZENAPAX-treated patients compared with placebo-treated patients, patients on immunosuppressive therapy are at increased risk for developing lymphoproliferative disorders and opportunistic infections and should be monitored accordingly.

Anaphylactic reactions following administration of proteins can occur. Severe hypersensitivity reactions following administration of ZENAPAX have been reported rarely. Therefore, medications for the treatment of severe hypersensitivity reactions should be available for immediate use.

PRECAUTIONS

General: It is not known whether ZENAPAX use will have a long-term effect on the ability of the immune system to respond to antigens first encountered during ZENAPAX-induced immunosuppression.

Re-administration of ZENAPAX after an initial course of therapy has not been studied in humans. The potential risks of such re-administration, specifically those associated with immunosuppression and/or the occurrence of anaphylaxis/anaphylactoid reactions, are not known.

Immunogenicity: Low titers of anti-idiotype antibodies to Daclizumab were detected in the ZENAPAX-treated patients with an overall incidence of 8.4%. No antibodies that affected efficacy, safety, serum Daclizumab levels or any other clinically relevant parameter examined were detected.

Drug Interactions: The following medications have been administered in clinical trials with ZENAPAX with no incremental increase in adverse reactions: cyclosporine, mycophenolate mofetil, ganciclovir, acyclovir, azathioprine, and corticosteroids. Very limited experience exists with the use of ZENAPAX concomitantly with tacrolimus, muromonab-CD3, antithymocyte globulin, and antilymphocyte globulin. In renal allograft recipients treated with ZENAPAX and mycophenolate mofetil, no pharmacokinetic interaction between Daclizumab and mycophenolic acid, the active metabolite of mycophenolate mofetil, was observed.

Carcinogenesis, Mutagenesis and Impairment of Fertility: Long-term studies to evaluate the carcinogenic potential of ZENAPAX have not been performed. ZENAPAX was not genotoxic in the Ames or the V79 chromosomal aberration assays, with or without metabolic activation. The effect of ZENAPAX on fertility is not known, because animal reproduction studies have not been conducted with ZENAPAX (see WARNINGS and ADVERSE REACTIONS).

Pregnancy: Pregnancy Category C: Animal reproduction studies have not been conducted with ZENAPAX. Therefore, it is not known whether ZENAPAX can cause fetal harm when administered to pregnant women or can affect reproductive capacity. In general, IgG molecules are known to cross the placental barrier. ZENAPAX should not be used in pregnant women unless the potential benefit justifies the potential risk to the fetus. Women of childbearing potential should use effective contraception before beginning ZENAPAX therapy, during therapy, and for 4 months after completion of ZENAPAX therapy.

Nursing Mothers: It is not known whether ZENAPAX is excreted in human milk. Because many drugs are excreted

Continued on next page

Zenapax—Cont.

in human milk, including human antibodies, and because of the potential for adverse reactions, a decision should be made to discontinue nursing or to discontinue the drug, taking into account the importance of the drug to the mother.
Pediatric Use: No adequate and well-controlled studies have been completed in pediatric patients. The preliminary results of an ongoing safety and pharmacokinetic study (N=25) in pediatric patients (median age: 12 years of age, range: 11 months to 17 years of age; 11 months to 5 years = 7 patients; 6 years to 12 years = 6 patients; 13 years to 17 years = 12 patients) treated with ZENAPAX in addition to standard immunosuppressive agents including mycophenolate mofetil, cyclosporine, tacrolimus, azathioprine, and corticosteroids indicate that the most frequently reported adverse events were hypertension (48%), post-operative (post-traumatic) pain (44%), diarrhea (36%), and vomiting (32%). The reported rates of hypertension and dehydration were higher for pediatric patients than for adult patients. It is not known whether the immune response to vaccines, infection, and other antigenic stimuli administered or encountered during ZENAPAX therapy is impaired or whether such response will remain impaired after ZENAPAX therapy.
The preliminary pharmacokinetic results from this ongoing study in pediatric patients indicate Daclizumab serum levels (N=6) appear to be somewhat lower in pediatric renal transplant patients than in adult transplant patients administered the same dosing regimen. However, Daclizumab levels in these pediatric patients were sufficient to saturate the Tac subunit of the IL-2 receptor on lymphocytes as measured by flow cytometry (N=24). The Tac subunit of the IL-2 receptor was saturated immediately after the first dose of 1.0 mg/kg of Daclizumab and remained saturated for at least the first 3 months post-transplant. Saturation of the Tac subunit of the IL-2 receptor was similar to that observed in adult patients receiving the same dose regimen.
Geriatric Use: Clinical studies of ZENAPAX did not include sufficient numbers of subjects age 65 and older to determine whether they respond differently from younger subjects. Caution must be used in giving immunosuppressive drugs to elderly patients.

ADVERSE REACTIONS

The safety of ZENAPAX was determined in four clinical studies, three of which were randomized controlled clinical trials, in 629 patients receiving renal allografts of whom 336 received ZENAPAX and 293 received placebo. All patients received concomitant cyclosporine and corticosteroids.
ZENAPAX did not appear to alter the pattern, frequency or severity of known major toxicities associated with the use of immunosuppressive drugs.
Adverse events were reported by 95% of the patients in the placebo-treated group and 96% of the patients in the ZENAPAX-treated group. The proportion of patients prematurely withdrawn from the combined studies because of adverse events was 8.5% in the placebo-treated group and 8.6% in the ZENAPAX-treated group.
ZENAPAX did not increase the number of serious adverse events observed compared with placebo. The most frequently reported adverse events were gastrointestinal disorders, which were reported with equal frequency in ZENAPAX- (67%) and placebo-treated (68%) patient groups.
The incidence and types of adverse events were similar in both placebo-treated and ZENAPAX-treated patients. The following adverse events occurred in ≥5% of ZENAPAX-treated patients. These events included: *Gastrointestinal System:* constipation, nausea, diarrhea, vomiting, abdominal pain, pyrosis, dyspepsia, abdominal distention, epigastric pain not food-related; *Metabolic and Nutritional:* edema extremities, edema; *Central and Peripheral Nervous System:* tremor, headache, dizziness; *Urinary System:* oliguria, dysuria, renal tubular necrosis; *Body as a Whole—General:* post-traumatic pain, chest pain, fever, pain, fatigue; *Autonomic Nervous System:* hypertension, hypotension, aggravated hypertension; *Respiratory System:* dyspnea, pulmonary edema, coughing; *Skin and Appendages:* impaired wound healing without infection, acne; *Psychiatric:* insomnia; *Musculoskeletal System:* musculoskeletal pain, back pain; *Heart Rate and Rhythm:* tachycardia; *Vascular Extracardiac:* thrombosis; *Platelet, Bleeding and Clotting Disorders:* bleeding; *Hemic and Lymphatic:* lymphocele.
The following adverse events occurred in <5% and ≥2% of ZENAPAX-treated patients. These included: *Gastrointestinal System:* flatulence, gastritis, hemorrhoids; *Metabolic and Nutritional:* fluid overload, diabetes mellitus, dehydration; *Urinary System:* renal damage, hydronephrosis, urinary tract bleeding, urinary tract disorder, renal insufficiency; *Body as a Whole—General:* shivering, generalized weakness; *Central and Peripheral Nervous System:* urinary retention, leg cramps, prickly sensation; *Respiratory System:* atelectasis, congestion, pharyngitis, rhinitis, hypoxia, rales, abnormal breath sounds, pleural effusion; *Skin and Appendages:* pruritus, hirsutism, rash, night sweats, increased sweating; *Psychiatric:* depression, anxiety; *Musculoskeletal System:* arthralgia, myalgia; *Vision:* vision blurred; *Application Site:* application site reaction.
Incidence of Malignancies: One year after treatment, the incidence of malignancies was 2.7% in the placebo group compared with 1.5% in the ZENAPAX group. Addition of ZENAPAX did not increase the number of post-transplant lymphomas, which occurred with a frequency of <1% in both placebo-treated and ZENAPAX-treated groups.
Hyperglycemia: No differences in abnormal hematologic or chemical laboratory test results were seen between placebo-treated and ZENAPAX-treated groups with the exception of fasting blood glucose. Fasting blood glucose was measured in a small number of placebo- and ZENAPAX-treated patients. A total of 16% (10 of 64 patients) of placebo-treated and 32% (28 of 88 patients) of ZENAPAX-treated patients had high fasting blood glucose values. Most of these high values occurred either on the first day post-transplant when patients received high doses of corticosteroids or in patients with diabetes.
Incidence of Infectious Episodes: The overall incidence of infectious episodes, including viral infections, fungal infections, bacteremia and septicemia, and pneumonia, was not higher in ZENAPAX-treated patients than in placebo-treated patients. The types of infections reported were similar in both the ZENAPAX-treated and the placebo-treated groups. Cytomegalovirus infection was reported in 16% of the patients in the placebo group and 13% of the patients in the ZENAPAX group. One exception was cellulitis and wound infections, which occurred in 4.1% of placebo-treated and 8.4% of ZENAPAX-treated patients. At 1 year post-transplant, 7 placebo patients and only 1 ZENAPAX-treated patient had died of an infection.

OVERDOSAGE

There have not been any reports of overdoses with ZENAPAX. A maximum tolerated dose has not been determined in patients. A dose of 1.5 mg/kg has been administered to bone marrow transplant recipients without any associated adverse events.

DOSAGE AND ADMINISTRATION

ZENAPAX is used as part of an immunosuppressive regimen that includes cyclosporine and corticosteroids. The recommended dose for ZENAPAX is 1.0 mg/kg. The calculated volume of ZENAPAX should be mixed with 50 mL of sterile 0.9% sodium chloride solution and administered via a peripheral or central vein over a 15-minute period.
Based on the clinical trials, the standard course of ZENAPAX therapy is five doses. The first dose should be given no more than 24 hours before transplantation. The four remaining doses should be given at intervals of 14 days.
No dosage adjustment is necessary for patients with severe renal impairment. No dosage adjustments based on other identified covariates (age, gender, proteinuria, race) are required for renal allograft patients. No data are available for administration in patients with severe hepatic impairment.
Instructions for Administration:

- ZENAPAX IS NOT FOR DIRECT INJECTION. The calculated volume should be diluted in 50 mL of sterile 0.9% sodium chloride solution before intravenous administration to patients. When mixing the solution, gently invert the bag in order to avoid foaming; DO NOT SHAKE.
- Parenteral drug products should be inspected visually for particulate matter and discoloration before administration. If particulate matter is present or the solution colored, do not use.
- Care must be taken to assure sterility of the prepared solution, since the drug product does not contain any antimicrobial preservative or bacteriostatic agents.
- ZENAPAX is a colorless solution provided as a single-use vial; any unused portion of the drug should be discarded.
- Once the infusion is prepared, it should be administered intravenously within 4 hours. If it must be held longer, it should be refrigerated between 2° to 8°C (36° to 46°F) for up to 24 hours. After 24 hours, the prepared solution should be discarded.
- No incompatibility between ZENAPAX and polyvinyl chloride or polyethylene bags or infusion sets has been observed. No data are available concerning the incompatibility of ZENAPAX with other drug substances. However, other drug substances should not be added or infused simultaneously through the same intravenous line.
- ZENAPAX may be administered by healthcare personnel trained in the administration of the drug who have available adequate laboratory and supportive medical resources.

HOW SUPPLIED

ZENAPAX is supplied in single-use glass vials. Each vial contains 25 mg of Daclizumab in 5 mL of solution (NDC 0004-0501-09). Vials should be stored between the temperatures of 2° to 8°C (36° to 46°F); do not shake or freeze. Protect undiluted solution against direct light. Diluted medication is stable for 24 hours at 4°C or for 4 hours at room temperature.

Revised: July 1999

EDUCATIONAL MATERIAL

Please contact your Roche representative concerning availability of educational programs and material.

Roche Pharmaceuticals

Roche Products Inc.
Manati, Puerto Rico 00674

Direct Medical Inquiries to:
Roche Laboratories Inc
(800) 526-6367
Direct Customer Service (Distribution) Inquiries to:
Roche Laboratories Inc
(800) 526-0625

VALIUM® Ⓒ

[val 'ee-um]
brand of diazepam
TABLETS

The following text is complete prescribing information based on official labeling in effect June 2000.

DESCRIPTION

Valium (diazepam) is a benzodiazepine derivative developed through original Roche research. Chemically, diazepam is 7-chloro-1,3-dihydro-1-methyl -5- phenyl-2H-1,4-benzodiazepin-2-one. It is a colorless crystalline compound, insoluble in water and has a molecular weight of 284.74.
Valium 5-mg tablets contain FD&C Yellow No. 6 and D&C Yellow No. 10 dyes. Valium 10-mg tablets contain FD&C Blue No. 1 dye. Valium 2-mg tablets contain no dye.

PHARMACOLOGY

In animals, Valium appears to act on parts of the limbic system, the thalamus and hypothalamus, and induces calming effects. Valium, unlike chlorpromazine and reserpine, has no demonstrable peripheral autonomic blocking action, nor does it produce extrapyramidal side effects; however, animals treated with Valium do have a transient ataxia at higher doses. Valium was found to have transient cardiovascular depressor effects in dogs. Long-term experiments in rats revealed no disturbances of endocrine function.
Oral LD_{50} of diazepam is 720 mg/kg in mice and 1240 mg/kg in rats. Intraperitoneal administration of 400 mg/kg to a monkey resulted in death on the sixth day.
Reproduction Studies: A series of rat reproduction studies was performed with diazepam in oral doses of 1, 10, 80 and 100 mg/kg. At 100 mg/kg there was a decrease in the number of pregnancies and surviving offspring in these rats. Neonatal survival of rats at doses lower than 100 mg/kg was within normal limits. Several neonates in these rat reproduction studies showed skeletal or other defects. Further studies in rats at doses up to and including 80 mg/kg/day did not reveal teratological effects on the offspring.
In humans, measurable blood levels of Valium were obtained in maternal and cord blood, indicating placental transfer of the drug.

INDICATIONS

Valium is indicated for the management of anxiety disorders or for the short-term relief of the symptoms of anxiety. Anxiety or tension associated with the stress of everyday life usually does not require treatment with an anxiolytic.
In acute alcohol withdrawal, Valium may be useful in the symptomatic relief of acute agitation, tremor, impending or acute delirium tremens and hallucinosis.
Valium is a useful adjunct for the relief of skeletal muscle spasm due to reflex spasm to local pathology (such as inflammation of the muscles or joints, or secondary to trauma); spasticity caused by upper motor neuron disorders (such as cerebral palsy and paraplegia); athetosis; and stiff-man syndrome.
Oral Valium may be used adjunctively in convulsive disorders, although it has not proved useful as the sole therapy.
The effectiveness of Valium in long-term use, that is, more than 4 months, has not been assessed by systematic clinical studies. The physician should periodically reassess the usefulness of the drug for the individual patient.

CONTRAINDICATIONS

Valium is contraindicated in patients with a known hypersensitivity to this drug and, because of lack of sufficient clinical experience, in pediatric patients under 6 months of age. It may be used in patients with open angle glaucoma who are receiving appropriate therapy, but is contraindicated in acute narrow angle glaucoma.

WARNINGS

Valium is not of value in the treatment of psychotic patients and should not be employed in lieu of appropriate treatment. As is true of most preparations containing CNS-acting drugs, patients receiving Valium should be cautioned against engaging in hazardous occupations requiring complete mental alertness such as operating machinery or driving a motor vehicle.
As with other agents which have anticonvulsant activity, when Valium is used as an adjunct in treating convulsive disorders, the possibility of an increase in the frequency and/or severity of grand mal seizures may require an increase in the dosage of standard anticonvulsant medication. Abrupt withdrawal of Valium in such cases may also be associated with a temporary increase in the frequency and/or severity of seizures.

Since Valium has a central nervous system depressant effect, patients should be advised against the simultaneous ingestion of alcohol and other CNS-depressant drugs during Valium therapy.

Usage in Pregnancy: **An increased risk of congenital malformations associated with the use of minor tranquilizers (diazepam, meprobamate and chlordiazepoxide) during the first trimester of pregnancy has been suggested in several studies. Because use of these drugs is rarely a matter of urgency, their use during this period should almost always be avoided. The possibility that a woman of childbearing potential may be pregnant at the time of institution of therapy should be considered. Patients should be advised that if they become pregnant during therapy or intend to become pregnant they should communicate with their physicians about the desirability of discontinuing the drug.**

Management of Overdosage: Manifestations of Valium overdosage include somnolence, confusion, coma and diminished reflexes. Respiration, pulse and blood pressure should be monitored, as in all cases of drug overdosage, although, in general, these effects have been minimal following overdosage. General supportive measures should be employed, along with immediate gastric lavage. Intravenous fluids should be administered and an adequate airway maintained. Hypotension may be combated by the use of Levophed® (levarterenol) or Aramine (metaraminol). Dialysis is of limited value. As with the management of intentional overdosage with any drug, it should be borne in mind that multiple agents may have been ingested.

Flumazenil, a specific benzodiazepine-receptor antagonist, is indicated for the complete or partial reversal of the sedative effects of benzodiazepines and may be used in situations when an overdose with a benzodiazepine is known or suspected. Prior to the administration of flumazenil, necessary measures should be instituted to secure airway, ventilation, and intravenous access. Flumazenil is intended as an adjunct to, not as a substitute for, proper management of benzodiazepine overdose. Patients treated with flumazenil should be monitored for resedation, respiratory depression and other residual benzodiazepine effects for an appropriate period after treatment. **The prescriber should be aware of a risk of seizure in association with flumazenil treatment, particularly in long-term benzodiazepine users and in cyclic antidepressant overdose.** The complete flumazenil package insert, including CONTRAINDICATIONS, WARNINGS and PRECAUTIONS, should be consulted prior to use.

Withdrawal symptoms of the barbiturate type have occurred after the discontinuation of benzodiazepines. (See DRUG ABUSE AND DEPENDENCE section.)

PRECAUTIONS

If Valium is to be combined with other psychotropic agents or anticonvulsant drugs, careful consideration should be given to the pharmacology of the agents to be employed—particularly with known compounds which may potentiate the action of Valium, such as phenothiazines, narcotics, barbiturates, MAO inhibitors and other antidepressants. The usual precautions are indicated for severely depressed patients or those in whom there is any evidence of latent depression; particularly the recognition that suicidal tendencies may be present and protective measures may be necessary. The usual precautions in treating patients with impaired renal or hepatic function should be observed.

In elderly and debilitated patients, it is recommended that the dosage be limited to the smallest effective amount to preclude the development of ataxia or oversedation (2 mg to $2^1/_2$ mg once or twice daily, initially, to be increased gradually as needed and tolerated).

The clearance of Valium and certain other benzodiazepines can be delayed in association with Tagamet (cimetidine) administration. The clinical significance of this is unclear.

Information for Patients: To assure the safe and effective use of benzodiazepines, patients should be informed that, since benzodiazepines may produce psychological and physical dependence, it is advisable that they consult with their physician before either increasing the dose or abruptly discontinuing this drug.

Pediatric Use: Safety and effectiveness in pediatric patients below the age of 6 months have not been established.

ADVERSE REACTIONS

Side effects most commonly reported were drowsiness, fatigue and ataxia. Infrequently encountered were confusion, constipation, depression, diplopia, dysarthria, headache, hypotension, incontinence, jaundice, changes in libido, nausea, changes in salivation, skin rash, slurred speech, tremor, urinary retention, vertigo and blurred vision. Paradoxical reactions such as acute hyperexcited states, anxiety, hallucinations, increased muscle spasticity, insomnia, rage, sleep disturbances and stimulation have been reported; should these occur, use of the drug should be discontinued. Because of isolated reports of neutropenia and jaundice, periodic blood counts and liver function tests are advisable during long-term therapy. Minor changes in EEG patterns, usually low-voltage fast activity, have been observed in patients during and after Valium therapy and are of no known significance.

DRUG ABUSE AND DEPENDENCE

Withdrawal symptoms, similar in character to those noted with barbiturates and alcohol (convulsions, tremor, abdominal and muscle cramps, vomiting and sweating), have occurred following abrupt discontinuance of diazepam. The more severe withdrawal symptoms have usually been limited to those patients who had received excessive doses over an extended period of time. Generally milder withdrawal symptoms (eg, dysphoria and insomnia) have been reported following abrupt discontinuance of benzodiazepines taken continuously at therapeutic levels for several months. Consequently, after extended therapy, abrupt discontinuation should generally be avoided and a gradual dosage tapering schedule followed. Addiction-prone individuals (such as drug addicts or alcoholics) should be under careful surveillance when receiving diazepam or other psychotropic agents because of the predisposition of such patients to habituation and dependence.

DOSAGE AND ADMINISTRATION

Dosage should be individualized for maximum beneficial effect. While the usual daily dosages given below will meet the needs of most patients, there will be some who may require higher doses. In such cases dosage should be increased cautiously to avoid adverse effects.

ADULTS:	*USUAL DAILY DOSE*
Management of Anxiety Disorders and Relief of Symptoms of Anxiety.	Depending upon severity of symptoms—2 mg to 10 mg, 2 to 4 times daily
Symptomatic Relief in Acute Alcohol Withdrawal.	10 mg, 3 or 4 times during the first 24 hours, reducing to 5 mg, 3 or 4 times daily as needed
Adjunctively for Relief of Skeletal Muscle Spasm.	2 mg to 10 mg, 3 or 4 times daily
Adjunctively in Convulsive Disorders.	2 mg to 10 mg, 2 to 4 times daily
Geriatric Patients, or in the presence of debilitating disease.	2 mg to $2^1/_2$ mg, 1 or 2 times daily initially; increase gradually as needed and tolerated
PEDIATRIC PATIENTS: Because of varied responses to CNS-acting drugs, initiate therapy with lowest dose and increase as required. Not for use in pediatric patients under 6 months.	1 mg to $2^1/_2$ mg, 3 or 4 times daily initially; increase gradually as needed and tolerated

HOW SUPPLIED

For oral administration, round, scored tablets with a cut out "V" design—2 mg, white—bottles of 100 (NDC 0140-0004-01) and 500 (NDC 0140-0004-14); 5 mg, yellow—bottles of 100 (NDC 0140-0005-01) and 500 (NDC 0140-0005-14); 10 mg, blue—bottles of 100 (NDC 0140-0006-01) and 500 (NDC 0140-0006-14).

Imprint on tablets:

2 mg:
2 VALIUM® (front)
ROCHE (scored side)

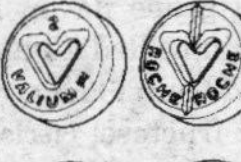

5 mg:
5 VALIUM® (front)
ROCHE (scored side)

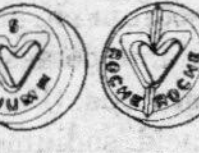

10 mg:
10 VALIUM® (front)
ROCHE (scored side)

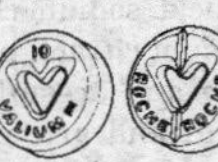

Revised: April 1997

Shown in Product Identification Guide, page 333

Roerig Division

235 EAST 42ND STREET
NEW YORK, NY 10017-5755

For Medical Information Contact:
24 hours a day, seven days a week:
(800) 438-1985

Distribution:
1855 Shelby Oaks Drive North
Memphis, TN 38134
(901) 387-5200
Customer Service:
(800) 533-4535

EXPORT INQUIRIES:
Pfizer International Inc.
(212) 573-2323
(See Pfizer Inc.)

Ross Products Division

ABBOTT LABORATORIES
COLUMBUS, OH 43215-1724 USA

Direct Inquiries to:
1-800-227-5767

CLEAR EYES® OTC

[*klēr īz*]
Lubricant Eye Redness Reliever Drops

(See PDR For Ophthalmology.)

CLEAR EYES® ACR OTC

[*klēr īz*]
Astringent/Lubricant Redness Reliever Eye Drops

(See PDR For Ophthalmology.)

CLEAR EYES® CLR OTC

[*klēr īz*]
Soothing Drops
Contact Lens Relief

(See PDR For Opthalmic Medicines.)

EAR DROPS BY MURINE® OTC

See Murine Ear Wax Removal System/Murine Ear Drops

ELECARE® OTC

[*el' e-cāre*]
Nutritionally Complete Amino Acid-Based Medical Food

USAGE

For meeting the nutritional needs of children 1 year of age and older who need an amino acid-based medical food or who cannot tolerate intact protein; for the dietary management of maldigestion, malabsorption, severe food allergies, GI tract impairment, or other conditions in which an elemental (amino acid-based) diet is required.

Features:

- Useful in such conditions as short-bowel syndrome.
- The only free amino acid-based medical food specifically indicated for children 1 year of age and older that has been clinically documented to be hypoallergenic.
- Well tolerated.
- Clinically shown to support growth when used as a primary source of nutrition.
- One third of fat as medium-chain triglycerides, an easily digested and well-absorbed fat source.
- Stringent manufacturing standards to reduce risk of whole-protein contamination.
- Milk-protein-free; fructose-free; galactose-free; lactose-free; gluten-free; soy-protein-free.

AVAILABILITY

Powder:
14.1-oz (400-g) cans; 6 per case; No. 54665.

INGREDIENTS

(Pareve, ⓤ) 53% Corn Syrup Solids, 8.9% High-Oleic Safflower Oil, 7.5% Fractionated Coconut Oil (Medium-Chain Triglycerides), 6.4% Soy Oil; less than 2% of: L-Glutamine, L-Asparagine Monohydrate, L-Leucine, DATEM (an Emulsifier), L-Lysine Acetate, Calcium Phosphate Tribasic, Potassium Phosphate Dibasic, L-Valine, L-Isoleucine, L-Arginine, L-Phenylalanine, L-Tyrosine, Sodium Citrate, L-Thre-

Continued on next page

Elecare—Cont.

onine, Potassium Citrate, L-Proline, L-Serine, L-Alanine, Ascorbic Acid, Glycine, L-Histidine, L-Methionine, Magnesium Chloride, L-Cystine Dihydrochloride, L-Tryptophan, Calcium Carbonate, Choline Chloride, Taurine, m-Inositol, Ferrous Sulfate, Sodium Chloride, Ascorbyl Palmitate, L-Carnitine, Zinc Sulfate, Alpha-Tocopheryl Acetate, Niacinamide, Calcium Pantothenate, Cupric Sulfate, Thiamine Chloride Hydrochloride, Manganese Sulfate, Vitamin A Palmitate, Beta-Carotene, Riboflavin, Pyridoxine Hydrochloride, Folic Acid, Biotin, Phylloquinone, Chromium Chloride, Potassium Iodide, Sodium Selenate, Sodium Molybdate, Vitamin D_3 and Cyanocobalamin.

[See first table above]

PHENYLKETONURICS: Contains phenylalanine

PREPARATION

Use as directed by physician. To prepare standard dilution of 30 Cal/fl oz (1 Cal/mL) in a 1-Liter container, add 210 grams of Powder to container and add water to yield 1 Liter.

WARNINGS

Do not heat EleCare mixture as it may damage some nutrients as well as affect the taste. Never use a microwave oven to prepare or warm mixture. Serious burns can result.

(FAN 3584-01)

MURINE TEARS® OTC

[*mur 'ēn*]

Lubricant Eye Drops

(See PDR For Ophthalmology.)

MURINE TEARS® PLUS OTC

[*mur 'ēn*]

Lubricant Redness Reliever Eye Drops

(See PDR For Ophthalmology.)

MURINE® EAR WAX REMOVAL SYSTEM/MURINE® EAR DROPS OTC

[*mur 'ēn*]

Carbamide Peroxide Ear Wax Removal Aid

PEDIALYTE® OTC

[*pē 'dē-ah-līt "*]

Oral Electrolyte Maintenance Solution

USAGE

To quickly replace fluids and electrolytes lost during diarrhea and vomiting to help prevent dehydration in infants and children; for maintenance of water and electrolytes following corrective parenteral therapy for severe diarrhea. Pedialyte is designed to promote fluid absorption more effectively than common household beverages.

Features:

- Ready To Use—no mixing or dilution necessary.
- Balanced electrolytes to replace diarrheal stool losses and provide maintenance requirements.
- Provides glucose to promote sodium and water absorption.
- Unflavored liquid form available for young infants; fruit-flavored, bubble gum-flavored and grape-flavored liquids formulated with improved taste to enhance compliance in older infants and children.
- Plastic liter bottles are resealable and allow easy measuring and pouring.
- 8-oz, single-serving size; cherry flavor is easy for children to hold and drink.
- Freezer Pops (2.1 fl oz Pedialyte per sleeve) are available in multiple flavors to encourage compliance with fluid intake recommendations for children 1 year of age and older.
- Widely available in grocery, drug and discount stores.

AVAILABILITY

Ready To Use:

1-liter (33.8-fl-oz) plastic bottles; 8 per case; Unflavored, No. 00336; Fruit Flavor, No. 00365; Bubble Gum Flavor, No. 51752; Grape Flavor, No. 00240.

8-fl-oz glass bottles; 4 six-packs per case; Unflavored, No. 00160.

2.1-fl-oz sleeve Freezer Pops; 8 sixteen-sleeve boxes per case; Grape, Cherry, Orange and Blue Raspberry, No. 00245.

8-fl-oz plastic bottles; 8 four-packs per case; Cherry, No. 54981.

DOSAGE

Refer to Administration Guide to restore fluid and minerals lost in diarrhea and vomiting.

Pedialyte should be offered frequently in amounts tolerated. Total daily intake should be adjusted to meet individual needs, based on thirst and response to therapy. The suggested intakes for maintenance are based on water requirements for ordinary energy expenditure.[1]

[See second table above]

NUTRIENTS:	PER 100 g POWDER	PER 1000 Cal
Protein Equivalent, g	14.3	30.1
Fat, g	22.6	47.6
Carbohydrate, g	51	107
Water, g	1.0	2.1
Calories	475	1000
VITAMINS:		
Vitamin A, IU	1300	2737
(mcg RE)	(390)	(821)
Vitamin D, IU	200	421
(mcg)	(5.00)	(10.5)
Vitamin E, IU	10.0	21.1
(mg α-TE)	(6.7)	(14.2)
Vitamin K, mcg	30	63.2
Thiamin (Vit. B_1), mg	1.0	2.1
Riboflavin (Vit. B_2), mg	0.50	1.05
Vitamin B_6, mg	0.48	1.01
Vitamin B_{12}, mcg	2.0	4.21
Niacin, mg	8	16.8
(mg NE)	(12.3)	(25.9)
Folic Acid (Folacin), mcg	140	295
Pantothenic Acid, mg	2.0	4.21
Biotin, mcg	20	42.1
Vitamin C (Ascorbic Acid), mg	43	90.5
Choline, mg	38	80
Inositol, mg	24	50.5
MINERALS:		
Calcium, mg	515	1084
Phosphorus, mg	385	811
Magnesium, mg	40	84
Iron, mg	8.4	17.7
Zinc, mg	5.3	11.2
Manganese, mg	0.50	1.05
Copper, mg	0.60	1.26
Iodine, mcg	34	71.6
Selenium, mcg	11	23.2
Chromium, mcg	11	23.2
Molybdenum, mcg	12	25.3
Sodium, mg	215	453
(mEq)	(9.35)	(19.7)
Potassium, mg	715	1505
(mEq)	(18.29)	(38.5)
Chloride, mg	285	600
(mEq)	(8.04)	(16.9)

Osmolality, prepared at standard dilution = 596 mosm/kg water.

Pedialyte Administration Guide for Infants and Young Children*

Age	2 Weeks	3 Months	6 Months	9 Months	1 Year	1½ Years	2 Years	2½ Years	3 Years	3½ Years	4 Years
Approximate Weight† (lb)	9	14	18	21	23	26	28	30	32	34	36
(kg)	4.0	6.4	8.2	9.5	10.5	11.8	12.7	13.6	14.4	15.3	16.3
PEDIALYTE fl oz/day for maintenance**	16 to 20	30 to 34	36 to 42	39 to 45	42 to 47	47 to 52	48 to 53	51 to 56	53 to 57	54 to 57	55 to 59

* Administration Guide does not apply to infants less than 1 week of age. For children over 4 years, maintenance intakes may exceed 2 liters daily. If there is vomiting or fever, or if diarrhea continues beyond 24 hours, consult the child's physician.

** Fluid intake is total fluid requirement from oral electrolyte solution, formula or other fluids, but does not take into account ongoing stool losses. Fluid loss in the stool should be replaced by consumption of an extra amount of Pedialyte equal to stool losses, in addition to fluid maintenance requirement in this Administration Guide. Pedialyte Freezer Pops are to be used with Pedialyte Oral Electrolyte Maintenance Solution or other appropriate fluids to help prevent dehydration.

† Weight based on the 50th percentile of weight for age for boys from the National Center for Health Statistics (NCHS) Centers for Disease Control and Prevention (CDC) growth charts. Kuczmarski RJ, Ogden CL, Grummer-Strawn LM, et al: CDC Growth Charts: United States. Advance data from vital and health statistics; no. 314. Hyattsville, Md: National Center for Health Statistics, June 8, 2000.

1. Extrapolated from Barness L: Nutrition and nutritional disorders, in Behrman RE, Kliegman RM, Nelson WE, Vaughan VC III: *Nelson Textbook of Pediatrics*, ed 14. Philadelphia: WB Saunders Co, 1992, pp 105-107.

INGREDIENTS:

Unflavored: (Pareve, Ⓤ) Water, dextrose, potassium citrate, sodium chloride and sodium citrate.

Fruit Flavor: (Pareve, Ⓤ) Water, dextrose; Less than 2% of: fructose, citric acid, natural and artificial fruit flavors, potassium citrate, sodium chloride, sodium citrate, sucralose, acesulfame potassium and Yellow 6.

Grape Flavor: (Pareve, Ⓤ) Water, dextrose; Less than 2% of: fructose, citric acid, potassium citrate, sodium chloride, artificial grape flavor, sodium citrate, sucralose, acesulfame potassium, Red 40 and Blue 1.

Bubble Gum Flavor: (Pareve, Ⓤ) Water, dextrose; Less than 2% of: fructose, citric acid, potassium citrate, sodium chloride, sodium citrate, artificial bubble gum flavor, sucralose, acesulfame potassium and Red 40.

Freezer Pops: (Pareve,Ⓤ) Water, dextrose; Less than 2% of: citric acid, sodium chloride, sodium carboxymethylcellulose, potassium citrate, potassium sorbate, sodium benzoate, sucralose and acesulfame potassium; **Grape** also contains: Natural and artificial grape flavor, Red 40 and Blue 1; **Cherry** also contains: Natural and artificial cherry flavor and Red 40; **Orange** also contains: Natural and artificial orange flavor, Yellow 6 and Red 40; **Blue Raspberry** also contains: Natural and artificial blue raspberry flavor and Blue 1.

Singles: (Pareve, Ⓤ) Water, dextrose; Less than 2% of: fructose, citric acid, sodium chloride, potassium citrate, sodium citrate, artificial cherry flavor, potassium sorbate, sodium benzoate, sucralose, acesulfame potassium and Red 40.

UNFLAVORED PEDIALYTE LIQUID PROVIDES (per liter):

Sodium, 45 mEq; potassium, 20 mEq; chloride, 35 mEq; citrate, 30 mEq; dextrose, 25 g; Calories, 100.

(FAN 3536)

PEDIALYTE LIQUID PROVIDES (per liter):

Sodium, 45 mEq; potassium, 20 mEq; chloride, 35 mEq; citrate, 30 mEq; dextrose, 20 g; fructose, 5 g; Calories, 100.

PEDIALYTE FREEZER POPS PROVIDE (per liter):

Sodium, 45 mEq; potassium, 20 mEq; chloride, 35 mEq; citrate, 30 mEq; dextrose, 25 g; Calories, 100.

PEDIALYTE SINGLES PROVIDE (8 fl oz):

Sodium, 10.6 mEq; potassium, 4.7 mEq; chloride, 8.3 mEq; citrate, 7.1 mEq; dextrose, 4.7 g; fructose, 1.2 g; Calories 24.

(FAN 3691)

PEDIAZOLE® ℞

(8030)

erythromycin ethylsuccinate and sulfisoxazole acetyl for oral suspension

DESCRIPTION

Pediazole is a combination of erythromycin ethylsuccinate, USP, and sulfisoxazole acetyl, USP. When reconstituted with water as directed on the label, the granules form a white, strawberry-banana flavor suspension that provides the equivalent of 200 mg erythromycin activity and the equivalent of 600 mg of sulfisoxazole activity per teaspoonful (5 mL).

Erythromycin is produced by a strain of *Saccaropolyspora erythraea* and belongs to the macrolide group of antibiotics. It is basic and readily forms salts and esters. Erythromycin ethylsuccinate is the 2′-ethylsuccinyl ester of erythromycin. It is essentially a tasteless form of the antibiotic suitable for oral administration, particularly in suspension dosage forms. The chemical name is erythromycin 2′-(ethyl succinate). Erythromycin ethylsuccinate has the following structural formula:

Sulfisoxazole acetyl or N^1-acetyl sulfisoxazole is an ester of sulfisoxazole. Chemically, sulfisoxazole is N-(3,4-Dimethyl-5-isoxazolyl)-N-sulfanilylacetamide. Sulfisoxazole acetyl has the following structural formula:

Inactive Ingredients: Citric acid, magnesium aluminum silicate, poloxamer, sodium carboxymethylcellulose, sodium citrate, sucrose and artificial flavoring.

CLINICAL PHARMACOLOGY

Orally administered erythromycin ethylsuccinate suspensions are readily and reliably absorbed. Erythromycin ethylsuccinate products have demonstrated rapid and consistent absorption in both fasting and nonfasting conditions. However, higher serum concentrations are obtained when these products are given with food. Bioavailability data are available from Ross Products Division. Erythromycin is largely bound to plasma proteins. After absorption, erythromycin diffuses readily into most body fluids. In the absence of meningeal inflammation, low concentrations are normally achieved in the spinal fluid, but the passage of the drug across the blood-brain barrier increases in meningitis. Erythromycin crosses the placental barrier and is excreted in human milk. Erythromycin is not removed by peritoneal dialysis or hemodialysis.

In the presence of normal hepatic function, erythromycin is concentrated in the liver and is excreted in the bile; the effect of hepatic dysfunction on biliary excretion of erythromycin is not known. After oral administration, less than 5% of the administered dose can be recovered in the active form in the urine.

Wide variation in blood levels may result following identical doses of a sulfonamide. Blood levels should be measured in patients receiving these drugs for serious infections. Free sulfonamide blood levels of 50 to 150 mcg/mL may be considered therapeutically effective for most infections, with blood levels of 120 to 150 mcg/mL being optimal for serious infections. The maximum sulfonamide level should be 200 mcg/mL, because adverse reactions occur more frequently above this concentration.

Following oral administration, sulfisoxazole is rapidly and completely absorbed; the small intestine is the major site of absorption, but some of the drug is absorbed from the stomach. Sulfonamides are present in the blood as free, conjugated (acetylated and possibly other forms), and protein-bound forms. The amount present as "free" drug is considered to be the therapeutically active form. Approximately 85% of a dose of sulfisoxazole is bound to plasma proteins, primarily to albumin; 65% to 72% of the unbound portion is in the nonacetylated form.

Maximum plasma concentrations of intact sulfisoxazole following a single 2-g oral dose of sulfisoxazole to healthy adult volunteers ranged from 127 to 211 mcg/mL (mean, 169 mcg/mL), and the time of peak plasma concentration ranged from 1 to 4 hours (mean, 2.5 hours). The elimination half-life of sulfisoxazole ranged from 4.6 to 7.8 hours after oral administration. The elimination of sulfisoxazole has been shown to be slower in elderly subjects (63 to 75 years) with diminished renal function (creatine clearance 37 to 68 mL/min).[1] After multiple-dose oral administration of 500 mg q.i.d. to healthy volunteers, the average steady-state plasma concentrations of intact sulfisoxazole ranged from 49.9 to 88.8 mcg/mL (mean, 63.4 mcg/mL).[2]

Sulfisoxazole and its acetylated metabolites are excreted primarily by the kidneys through glomerular filtration. Concentrations of sulfisoxazole are considerably higher in the urine than in the blood. The mean urinary recovery following oral administration of sulfisoxazole is 97% within 48 hours; 52% of this is intact drug, and the remainder is the N^4-acetylated metabolite.

Sulfisoxazole is distributed only in extracellular body fluids. It is excreted in human milk. It readily crosses the placental barrier. In healthy subjects, cerebrospinal fluid concentrations of sulfisoxazole vary; in patients with meningitis, however, concentrations of free drug in cerebrospinal fluid as high as 94 mcg/mL have been reported.

Microbiology:

Pediazole has been formulated to contain sulfisoxazole for concomitant use with erythromycin.

Erythromycin acts by inhibition of protein synthesis by binding 50 S ribosomal subunits of susceptible organisms. It does not affect nucleic acid synthesis. Antagonism has been demonstrated *in vitro* between erythromycin and clindamycin, lincomycin, and chloramphenicol.

The sulfonamides are bacteriostatic agents, and the spectrum of activity is similar for all. Sulfonamides inhibit bacterial synthesis of dihydrofolic acid by preventing the condensation of the pteridine with *para*-aminobenzoic acid through competitive inhibition of the enzyme dihydropteroate synthetase. Resistant strains have altered dihydropteroate synthetase with reduced affinity for sulfonamides or produce increased quantities of *para*-aminobenzoic acid.

Susceptibility Testing:

Quantitative methods that require measurement of zone diameter give the most precise estimates of the susceptibility of bacteria to antimicrobial agents. One such standardized single-disc procedure[3] has been recommended for use with discs to test susceptibility to erythromycin and sulfisoxazole. Interpretation involves correlation of the zone diameters obtained in the disc test with minimal inhibitory concentration (MIC) values for erythromycin and sulfisoxazole.

If the standardized procedure of disc susceptibility is used, a 15-mcg erythromycin disc should give a zone diameter of at least 18 mm when tested against an erythromycin-susceptible bacterial strain, and a 250-300 mcg sulfisoxazole disc should give a zone diameter of at least 17 mm when tested against a sulfisoxazole-susceptible bacterial strain.

In vitro sulfonamide susceptibility tests are not always reliable because media containing excessive amounts of thymidine are capable of reversing the inhibitory effect of sulfonamides, which may result in false resistant reports. The tests must be carefully coordinated with bacteriological and clinical responses. When the patient is already taking sulfonamides, follow-up cultures should have aminobenzoic acid added to the isolation media but not to subsequent susceptibility test media.

INDICATIONS AND USAGE

For treatment of ACUTE OTITIS MEDIA in children that is caused by susceptible strains of *Haemophilus influenzae.*

CONTRAINDICATIONS

Pediazole is contraindicated in the following patient populations:

Patients with a known hypersensitivity to either of its components, children younger than 2 months, pregnant women *at term,* and mothers nursing infants less than 2 months of age.

Use in pregnant women at term, in children less than 2 months of age, and in mothers nursing infants less than 2 months of age is contraindicated because sulfonamides may promote kernicterus in the newborn by displacing bilirubin from plasma proteins.

Erythromycin is contraindicated in patients taking terfenadine. **(See PRECAUTIONS—Drug Interactions.)**

WARNINGS

FATALITIES ASSOCIATED WITH THE ADMINISTRATION OF SULFONAMIDES, ALTHOUGH RARE, HAVE OCCURRED DUE TO SEVERE REACTIONS INCLUDING STEVENS-JOHNSON SYNDROME, TOXIC EPIDERMAL NECROLYSIS, FULMINANT HEPATIC NECROSIS, AGRANULOCYTOSIS, APLASTIC ANEMIA, AND OTHER BLOOD DYSCRASIAS.

SULFONAMIDES, INCLUDING SULFONAMIDE-CONTAINING PRODUCTS SUCH AS PEDIAZOLE, SHOULD BE DISCONTINUED AT THE FIRST APPEARANCE OF SKIN RASH OR ANY SIGN OF ADVERSE REACTION. In rare instances, a skin rash may be followed by a more severe reaction, such as Stevens-Johnson syndrome, toxic epidermal necrolysis, hepatic necrosis, and serious blood disorders. **(See PRECAUTIONS.)**

Clinical signs such as sore throat, fever, pallor, rash, purpura, or jaundice may be early indications of serious reactions.

There have been reports of hepatic dysfunction with or without jaundice, occurring in patients receiving oral erythromycin products.

Cough, shortness of breath, and pulmonary infiltrates are hypersensitivity reactions of the respiratory tract that have been reported in association with sulfonamide treatment.

The sulfonamides should not be used for the treatment of group A beta-hemolytic streptococcal infections. In an established infection, they will not eradicate the streptococcus and, therefore, will not prevent sequelae such as rheumatic fever.

Pseudomembranous colitis has been reported with nearly all antibacterial agents, including Pediazole, and may range in severity from mild to life-threatening. Therefore, it is important to consider this diagnosis in patients who present with diarrhea subsequent to the administration of antibacterial agents.

Treatment with antibacterial agents alters the normal flora of the colon and may permit overgrowth of clostridia. Studies indicate that a toxin produced by *Clostridium difficile* is one primary cause of "antibiotic-associated colitis."

After diagnosis of pseudomembranous colitis has been established, therapeutic measures should be initiated. Mild cases of pseudomembranous colitis usually respond to drug discontinuation alone. In moderate to severe cases, consideration should be given to management with fluids and electrolytes, protein supplementation, and treatment with an antibacterial drug clinically effective against *Clostridium difficile* colitis.

There have been reports suggesting that erythromycin does not reach the fetus in adequate concentration to prevent congenital syphilis. Infants born to women treated during pregnancy with erythromycin for early syphilis should be treated with an appropriate penicillin regimen.

Rhabdomyolysis with or without renal impairment has been reported in seriously ill patients receiving erythromycin concomitantly with lovastatin. Therefore, patients receiving concomitant lovastatin and erythromycin should be carefully monitored for creatine kinase (CK) and serum transaminase levels. (See package insert for lovastatin.)

PRECAUTIONS

General: Erythromycin is principally excreted by the liver. Caution should be exercised when erythromycin is administered to patients with impaired hepatic function. **(See CLINICAL PHARMACOLOGY and WARNING sections.)**

Prolonged or repeated use of erythromycin may result in an overgrowth of nonsusceptible bacteria or fungi. If superinfection occurs, erythromycin should be discontinued and appropriate therapy instituted.

There have been reports that erythromycin may aggravate the weakness of patients with myasthenia gravis.

When indicated, incision and drainage or other surgical procedures should be performed in conjunction with antibiotic therapy.

Sulfonamides should be given with caution to patients with impaired renal or hepatic function and to those with severe allergy or bronchial asthma. In glucose-6-phosphate dehydrogenase-deficient individuals, hemolysis may occur; this reaction is frequently dose-related.

Information for Patients: Patients should maintain an adequate fluid intake to prevent crystalluria and stone formation.

Laboratory Tests: Complete blood counts should be done frequently in patients receiving sulfonamides. If a significant reduction in the count of any formed blood element is noted, Pediazole should be discontinued. Urinalysis with careful microscopic examination and renal function tests should be performed during therapy, particularly for those patients with impaired renal function. Blood levels should be measured in patients receiving a sulfonamide for serious infections. **(See INDICATIONS AND USAGE.)**

Drug/laboratory Test Interactions: Erythromycin interferes with the fluorometric determination of urinary catecholamines.

Drug Interactions: Erythromycin use in patients who are receiving high doses of theophylline may be associated with an increase in serum theophylline levels and potential theophylline toxicity. In case of theophylline toxicity and/or elevated serum theophylline levels, the dose of theophylline should be reduced while the patient is receiving concomitant erythromycin therapy.

Concomitant administration of erythromycin and digoxin has been reported to result in elevated digoxin serum levels. There have been reports of increased anticoagulant effects when erythromycin and oral anticoagulants were used concomitantly. Increased anticoagulation effects due to this drug may be more pronounced in the elderly.

Concurrent use of erythromycin and ergotamine or dihydroergotamine has been associated in some patients with acute ergot toxicity characterized by severe peripheral vasospasm and dysesthesia.

Erythromycin has been reported to decrease the clearance of triazolam and midazolam and thus may increase the pharmacologic effect of these benzodiazepines.

The use of erythromycin in patients concurrently taking drugs metabolized by the cytochrome P450 system may be associated with elevations in serum levels of these other drugs. There have been reports of interactions of erythromycin with carbamazepine, cyclosporine, hexobarbital, phenytoin, alfentanil, diisopyramide, lovastatin, and bromocriptine. Serum concentrations of drugs metabolized by the cytochrome P450 system should be monitored closely in patients concurrently receiving erythromycin.

Erythromycin significantly alters the metabolism of terfenadine when taken concomitantly. Rare cases of serious cardiovascular adverse events, including death, cardiac arrest, torsades de pointes, and other ventricular arrhythmias, have been observed. **(See CONTRAINDICATIONS.)**

It has been reported that sulfisoxazole may prolong the prothrombin time in patients who are receiving the anticoagulant warfarin. This interaction should be kept in mind when Pediazole is given to patients already on anticoagulant therapy, and the coagulation time should be reassessed.

It has been proposed that sulfisoxazole competes with thiopental for plasma protein binding. In one study involving 48 patients, intravenous sulfisoxazole resulted in a decrease in the amount of thiopental required for anesthesia and in a shortening of the awakening time. It is not known whether chronic oral doses of sulfisoxazole have a similar effect. Until more is known about this interaction, physicians should be aware that patients receiving sulfisoxazole might require less thiopental for anesthesia.

Sulfonamides can displace methotrexate from plasma protein binding sites, thus increasing free methotrexate concentrations. Studies in man have shown sulfisoxazole infusions to decrease plasma protein-bound methotrexate by one fourth.

Sulfisoxazole can also potentiate the blood-sugar-lowering activity of sulfonylureas.

Carcinogenesis, Mutagenesis, Impairment of Fertility:

Carcinogenesis: Pediazole has not undergone adequate trials relating to carcinogenicity; each component, however, has been evaluated separately. Long-term (21 month) oral studies conducted in rats with erythromycin ethylsuccinate did not provide evidence of tumorigenicity. Sulfisoxazole was not carcinogenic in either sex when administered to mice by gavage for 103 weeks at dosages up to approximately 18 times the recommended human dose or to rats at 4 times the human dose. Rats appear to be especially susceptible to the goitrogenic effects of sulfonamides, and long-term administration of sulfonamides has resulted in thyroid malignancies in this species.

Mutagenesis: There are no studies available that adequately evaluate the mutagenic potential of Pediazole or either of its components. However, sulfisoxazole was not observed to be mutagenic in *E. coli* Sd-4-73 when tested in the absence of a metabolic activating system. There was no apparent effect on male or female fertility in rats fed erythromycin (base) at levels up to 0.25% of diet.

Impairment of Fertility: Pediazole has not undergone adequate trials relating to impairment of fertility. In a reproduction study in rats given 7 times the human dose per day of sulfisoxazole, no effects were observed regarding mating behavior, conception rate or fertility index (percent pregnant).

Continued on next page

Pediazole—Cont.

Pregnancy: Teratogenic Effects. Pregnancy Category C. At dosages 7 times the human daily dose, sulfisoxazole was not teratogenic in either rats or rabbits. However, in two other teratogenicity studies, cleft palates developed in both rats and mice after administration of 5 to 9 times the human therapeutic dose of sulfisoxazole.

There is no evidence of teratogenicity or any other adverse effect on reproduction in female rats fed erythromycin base (up to 0.25% of diet) prior to and during mating, during gestation, and through weaning of two successive litters. There are, however, no adequate and well-controlled studies in pregnant women. Because animal reproduction studies are not always predictive of human response, this drug should be used during pregnancy only if clearly needed. Erythromycin has been reported to cross the placental barrier in humans, but fetal plasma levels are generally low.

There are no adequate or well-controlled studies of Pediazole in either laboratory animals or in pregnant women. It is not known whether Pediazole can cause fetal harm when administered to a pregnant woman prior to term or can affect reproduction capacity. Pediazole should be used during pregnancy only if the potential benefit justifies the potential risk to the fetus.

Nonteratogenic Effects: Kernicterus may occur in the newborn as a result of treatment of a pregnant woman *at term* with sulfonamides. **(See CONTRAINDICATIONS.)**

Labor and Delivery: The effects of erythromycin and sulfisoxazole on labor and delivery are unknown.

Nursing Mothers: Both erythromycin and sulfisoxazole are excreted in human milk. **Because of the potential for the development of kernicterus in neonates due to the displacement of bilirubin from plasma proteins by sulfisoxazole, a decision should be made whether to discontinue nursing or discontinue the drug, taking into account the importance of the drug to the mother. (See CONTRAINDICATIONS.)**

Pediatric Use: **See INDICATIONS AND USAGE** and **DOSAGE AND ADMINISTRATION** sections. Not for use in children under 2 months of age. **(See CONTRAINDICATIONS.)**

ADVERSE REACTIONS

Erythromycin ethylsuccinate: The most frequent side effects of oral erythromycin preparations are gastrointestinal and are dose-related. They include nausea, vomiting, abdominal pain, diarrhea and anorexia. Symptoms of hepatic dysfunction and/or abnormal liver-function test results may occur **(see WARNINGS section).** Pseudomembranous colitis has been rarely reported in association with erythromycin therapy.

Allergic reactions ranging from urticaria and mild skin eruptions to anaphylaxis have occurred.

There have been isolated reports of reversible hearing loss occurring chiefly in patients with renal insufficiency and in patients receiving high doses of erythromycin.

Onset of pseudomembranous colitis symptoms may occur during or after antibiotic treatment. **(See WARNINGS.)**

Sulfisoxazole acetyl: Included in the listing that follows are adverse reactions that have been reported with other sulfonamide products: pharmacologic similarities require that each of the reactions be considered with Pediazole administration.

Allergic/Dermatologic: Anaphylaxis, erythema multiforme (Stevens-Johnson syndrome), toxic epidermal necrolysis (Lyell's syndrome), exfoliative dermatitis, angioedema, arteritis, vasculitis, allergic myocarditis, serum sickness, rash, urticaria, pruritus, photosensitivity, and conjunctival and scleral injection. In addition, periarteritis nodosa and systemic lupus erythematosus have been reported. **(See WARNINGS.)**

Cardiovascular: Tachycardia, palpitations, syncope, and cyanosis.

Rarely, erythromycin has been associated with the production of ventricular arrhythmias, including ventricular tachycardia and torsade de pointes, in individuals with prolonged QT intervals.

Endocrine: The sulfonamides bear certain chemical similarities to some goitrogens, diuretics (acetazolamide and the thiazides) and oral hypoglycemic agents. Cross-sensitivity may exist with these agents. Developments of goiter, diuresis, and hypoglycemia have occurred rarely in patients receiving sulfonamides.

Gastrointestinal: Hepatitis, hepatocellular necrosis, jaundice, pseudomembranous colitis, nausea, emesis, anorexia, abdominal pain, diarrhea, gastrointestinal hemorrhage, melena, flatulence, glossitis, stomatitis, salivary gland enlargement, and pancreatitis. Onset of pseudomembranous colitis symptoms may occur during or after treatment with sulfisoxazole, a component of Pediazole. **(See WARNINGS.)**

The sulfisoxazole acetyl component of Pediazole has been reported to cause increased elevation of liver-associated enzymes in patients with hepatitis.

Genitourinary: Crystalluria, hematuria, BUN and creatinine elevations, nephritis, and toxic nephrosis with oliguria and anuria. Acute renal failure and urinary retention have also been reported.

The frequency of renal complications, commonly associated with some sulfonamides, is lower in patients receiving the more soluble sulfonamides such as sulfisoxazole.

Hematologic: Leukopenia, agranulocytosis, aplastic anemia, thrombocytopenia, purpura, hemolytic anemia, anemia, eosinophilia, clotting disorders including hypoprothrombinemia and hypofibrinogenemia, sulfhemoglobinemia, and methemoglobinemia.

Neurologic: Headache, dizziness, peripheral neuritis, paresthesia, convulsions, tinnitus, vertigo, ataxia, and intracranial hypertension.

Psychiatric: Psychosis, hallucinations, disorientation, depression, and anxiety.

Respiratory: Cough, shortness of breath, and pulmonary infiltrates. **(See WARNINGS.)**

Vascular: Angioedema, arteritis, and vasculitis.

Miscellaneous: Edema (including periorbital), pyrexia, drowsiness, weakness, fatigue, lassitude, rigors, flushing, hearing loss, insomnia, and pneumonitis.

OVERDOSAGE

No information is available on a specific result of overdose with Pediazole. Overdosage of erythromycin should be handled with the prompt elimination of unabsorbed drug and all other appropriate measures. Erythromycin is not removed by peritoneal dialysis or hemodialysis.

The amount of a single dose of sulfisoxazole that is either associated with symptoms of overdosage or is likely to be life-threatening has not been reported. Signs and symptoms of overdosage reported with sulfonamides include anorexia, colic, nausea, vomiting, dizziness, headache, drowsiness and unconsciousness. Pyrexia, hematuria and crystalluria may be noted. Blood dyscrasias and jaundice are potential late manifestations of overdosage.

General principles of treatment include the immediate discontinuation of the drug, instituting gastric lavage or emesis, forcing oral fluids, and administering intravenous fluids if urine output is low and renal function is normal. The patient should be monitored with blood counts and appropriate blood chemistries, including electrolytes. If the patient becomes cyanotic, the possibility of methemoglobinemia should be considered and, if present, the condition should be treated appropriately with intravenous 1% methylene blue. If a significant blood dyscrasia or jaundice occurs, specific therapy should be instituted for these complications. Peritoneal dialysis is not effective, and hemodialysis is only moderately effective in removing sulfonamides.

The acute toxicity of sulfisoxazole in animals is as follows:

Species	LD_{50} ± S.E. (mg/kg)
mouse	5700 ± 235
rats	>10,000
rabbits	>2000

DOSAGE AND ADMINISTRATION

PEDIAZOLE SHOULD NOT BE ADMINISTERED TO INFANTS UNDER 2 MONTHS OF AGE BECAUSE OF CONTRAINDICATIONS OF SYSTEMIC SULFONAMIDES IN THIS AGE GROUP.

For Acute Otitis Media in Children: The dose of Pediazole can be calculated based on the erythromycin component (50 mg/kg/day) or the sulfisoxazole component (150 mg/kg/day to a maximum of 6 g/day). The total daily dose of Pediazole should be administered in equally divided doses three or four times a day for 10 days. Pediazole may be administered without regard to meals.

The following approximate dosage schedules are recommended for using Pediazole:

Children: Two months of age or older

FOUR-TIMES-A-DAY SCHEDULE

Weight	Dose—every 6 hours
Less than 8 kg (<18 lbs)	Adjust dosage by body weight
8 kg (18 lbs)	1/2 teaspoonful (2.5 mL)
16 kg (35 lbs)	1 teaspoonful (5 mL)
24 kg (53 lbs)	1 1/2 teaspoonfuls (7.5 mL)
Over 32 kg (over 70 lbs)	2 teaspoonfuls (10 mL)

THREE-TIMES-A-DAY SCHEDULE

Weight	Dose—every 8 hours
Less than 6 kg (<13 lbs)	Adjust dosage by body weight
6 kg (13 lbs)	1/2 teaspoonful (2.5 mL)
12 kg (26 lbs)	1 teaspoonful (5 mL)
18 kg (40 lbs)	1 1/2 teaspoonfuls (7.5 mL)
24 kg (53 lbs)	2 teaspoonfuls (10 mL)
Over 30 kg (over 66 lbs)	2 1/2 teaspoonfuls (12.5 mL)

TO PATIENT: Shake before using. Oversize bottle provides shake space. Keep tightly closed. Store in the refrigerator. Use within 14 days. Unused portion should be discarded after 14 days.

HOW SUPPLIED

Pediazole Suspension is available for teaspoon dosage in 100-mL (**NDC** 0074-8030-13), 150-mL (**NDC** 0074-8030-43), 200-mL (**NDC** 0074-8030-53) and 250-mL (**NDC** 0074-8030-73) bottles, in the form of granules to be reconstituted with water. The suspension provides erythromycin ethylsuccinate equivalent to 200 mg erythromycin activity and sulfisoxazole acetyl equivalent to 600 mg sulfisoxazole per teaspoonful (5 mL).

Before mixing, store below 86°F (30°C).

REFERENCES

1. Biovert A, Barbeau G, Belanger PM: Pharmacokinetics of sulfisoxazole in young and elderly subjects. *Gerontology* 1984;30:125-131.
2. Oie S, Gambertoglio JG, Fleckenstein L: Comparison of the disposition of total and unbound sulfisoxazole after single and multiple dosing. *J Pharmacokinet Biopharm* 1982;10:157-172.
3. National Committee for Clinical Laboratory Standards: *Performance Standards for Antimicrobial Disk Susceptibility Tests,* ed. 4. Approved Standard NCCLS Document M2-A4, Vol 10, No. 7. Villanova, Pa: NCCLS, 1990.

July, 1994

PEDIASURE® OTC

[*pē 'dē-ah-shur"*]

Complete, Balanced Nutrition®

USAGE

As a nutritionally complete, balanced, enteral formula especially designed for tube or oral feeding of children 1 to 10 years of age. Also available with fiber. The fiber level in PediaSure With Fiber helps maintain normal bowel function. May be used as the sole source of nutrition or as a supplement. PediaSure meets or exceeds 100% of the NAS-NRC RDAs for protein, vitamins and minerals for children 1 to 6 years of age in 1000 mL (approx. 34 fl oz), and for children 7 to 10 years of age in 1300 mL (approx. 44 fl oz). Calcium: phosphorus ratio of 1.2:1 meets recommendations by the American Academy of Pediatrics Committee on Nutrition (AAP-CON) for growing children. Contains selenium, chromium, molybdenum, inositol, taurine and carnitine.

Not for parenteral use.

Not intended for infants under 1 year of age unless specified by a doctor.

AVAILABILITY

Ready To Use:

8-fl-oz (237 mL) cans: 24 per case; Vanilla, No. 00373 (retail), Vanilla, No. 51804 (institution); Chocolate, No. 51812 (retail), Chocolate, No. 51882 (institution); Strawberry, No. 51810 (retail), Strawberry, No. 51880 (institution); Banana Cream, No. 51808 (retail), Banana Cream, No. 51884 (institution); PediaSure With Fiber, Vanilla, No. 50652 (retail), Vanilla No. 51806 (institution).

COMPOSITION

Ready To Use PediaSure Vanilla. (Other flavors have similar composition and nutrient values. For specific information, see product labels.)

INGREDIENTS (institution)

Ⓤ-D Water, Maltodextrin (Corn), Sugar (Sucrose), Sodium Caseinate, High-Oleic Safflower Oil, Soy Oil, Fractionated Coconut Oil (Medium-Chain Triglycerides), Whey Protein Concentrate, Less than 0.5% of: Calcium Phosphate Tribasic, Natural and Artificial Flavor, Potassium Citrate, Magnesium Chloride, Cellulose Gel, Potassium Phosphate Dibasic, Potassium Chloride, Soy Lecithin, Mono- and Diglycerides, Choline Chloride, Carrageenan, Ascorbic Acid, Cellulose Gum, m-Inositol, Taurine, Ferrous Sulfate, Zinc Sulfate, Niacinamide, Alpha-Tocopheryl Acetate, L-Carnitine, Calcium Pantothenate, Thiamine Chloride Hydrochloride, Pyridoxine Hydrochloride, Riboflavin, Manganese Sulfate, Cupric Sulfate, Vitamin A Palmitate, Folic Acid, Biotin, Potassium Iodide, Sodium Selenate, Sodium Molybdate, Phylloquinone, Vitamin D_3 and Cyanocobalamin.

(FAN 7403-01)

INGREDIENTS (retail)

Ⓤ-D Water, Sugar (Sucrose), Maltodextrin (Corn), Sodium Caseinate, High-Oleic Safflower Oil, Soy Oil, Fractionated Coconut Oil (Medium-Chain Triglycerides), Whey Protein Concentrate; Less than 0.5% of: Calcium Phosphate Tribasic, Natural and Artificial Flavor, Potassium Citrate, Magnesium Chloride, Cellulose Gel, Potassium Phosphate Dibasic, Potassium Chloride, Soy Lecithin, Mono- and Diglycerides, Choline Chloride, Carrageenan, Ascorbic Acid, Cellulose Gum, m-Inositol, Taurine, Ferrous Sulfate, Zinc Sulfate, Sodium Chloride, Niacinamide, Alpha-Tocopheryl Acetate, L-Carnitine, Calcium Pantothenate, Thiamine Chloride Hydrochloride, Pyridoxine Hydrochloride, Riboflavin, Manganese Sulfate, Cupric Sulfate, Vitamin A Palmitate, Folic Acid, Biotin, Potassium Iodide, Sodium Selenate, Sodium Molybdate, Phylloquinone, Vitamin D_3 and Cyanocobalamin. PediaSure With Fiber also contains soy fiber.

NUTRIENTS (PER 8 FL OZ):

Energy	237	Cal
Protein	7.1	g
Fat	11.8	g
Carbohydrate	26 (26.9)*	g
L-Carnitine	4	mg
Taurine	17	mg
Water	200	g

VITAMINS/MINERALS PER 8 FL OZ:

Vitamin A	610	IU
Vitamin D	120	IU
Vitamin E	5.4	IU
Vitamin K	9.0	mcg
Vitamin C	24	mg
Folic Acid	88	mcg
Thiamin (Vit B_1)	0.64	mg
Riboflavin (Vit B_2)	0.50	mg
Vitamin B_6	0.62	mg
Vitamin B_{12}	1.4	mcg
Niacin	4.0	mg
Choline	71	mg
Biotin	76	mcg
Pantothenic Acid	2.4	mg
Inositol	19	mg
Sodium	90	mg
Potassium	310	mg
Chloride	240	mg
Calcium	230	mg
Phosphorus	190	mg
Magnesium	47	mg
Iodine	23	mcg
Manganese	0.24	mg
Copper	0.24	mg
Zinc	2.8	mg
Iron	3.3	mg
Chromium	7.1	mcg
Molybdenum	8.5	mcg
Selenium	5.4	mcg

*PediaSure With Fiber includes soy fiber (a source of dietary fiber that provides 1.2 calories and 1.2 g of total dietary fiber).

(FAN 3705-02)

REHYDRALYTE® OTC

[rē-hy' drah-līt"]

Oral Electrolyte Rehydration Solution

USAGE

To restore fluid and minerals lost during moderate to severe diarrhea.

Features:

- Ready To Use—No mixing or dilution necessary.
- Safe, economical alternative to IV therapy.
- 75 mEq of sodium per liter for effective replacement of fluid deficits.
- 2.5% glucose solution to promote sodium and water absorption and provide energy.
- Available in pharmacies.

AVAILABILITY

Ready To Use:

8-fl-oz bottles; 4 six-packs per case; No. 00162.

DOSAGE

Refer to Administration Guide for management of mild to moderate dehydration secondary to moderate to severe diarrhea. Rehydralyte should be offered frequently in amounts tolerated. Total daily intake should be adjusted to meet individual needs, based on thirst and response to therapy. The suggested intakes for replacement are based on fluid losses of 5% to 10% of body weight, including maintenance requirement, which is based on water requirements for ordinary energy expenditure.[1]

[See table above]

INGREDIENTS

(Pareve,Ⓤ) Water, dextrose, sodium chloride, potassium citrate and sodium citrate.

Provides:	Per 8 Fl Oz	Per Liter
Sodium (mEq)	17.7	75
Potassium (mEq)	4.7	20
Chloride (mEq)	15.4	65
Citrate (mEq)	7.1	30
Dextrose (g)	5.9	25
Energy (Cal)	24	100

(FAN 3518-01)

Rehydralyte Administration Guide for Infants and Young Children*

Age	2 Weeks	3	6 Months	9	1	$1^1/_2$	2	$2^1/_2$ Years	3	$3^1/_2$	4
Approximate Weight** (lb)	9	14	18	21	23	26	28	30	32	34	36
(kg)	4.0	6.4	8.2	9.5	10.5	11.8	12.7	13.6	14.4	15.3	16.3
REHYDRALYTE fl oz/day for Replacement for 5% Dehydration (including maintenance)¶	23 to 26	41 to 45	49 to 56	55 to 61	60 to 65	66 to 71	69 to 74	74 to 79	77 to 81	79 to 83	82 to 86
REHYDRALYTE fl oz/day for Replacement for 10% Dehydration (including maintenance)¶	29 to 33	51 to 55	63 to 69	70 to 76	77 to 82	86 to 91	90 to 95	97 to 102	101 to 105	105 to 109	108 to 113

* Administration Guide does not apply to infants less than 1 week of age. For children over 4 years, maintenance intakes alone may exceed 2 liters daily. If there is vomiting or fever, or if diarrhea continues beyond 24 hours, consult the child's physician.

** Weight based on the 50th percentile of weight for age for boys from the National Center for Health Statistics (NCHS) Centers for Disease Control and Prevention (CDC) growth charts. Kuczmarski RJ, Ogden CL, Grummer-Strawn LM, et al: CDC Growth Charts: United States. Advance data from vital and health statistics; no. 314. Hyattsville, Md: National Center for Health Statistics, June 8, 2000.

¶ Fluid intake is total fluid requirement from oral electrolyte solution, formula or other fluids, but does not take into account ongoing stool losses. Fluid loss in the stool should be replaced by consumption of an extra amount of Rehydralyte equal to stool losses, in addition to the fluid maintenance requirements in this Administration Guide.

1. Extrapolated from Barness L: Nutrition and nutritional disorders, in Behrman RE, Kliegman RM, Nelson WE, Vaughan VC III: *Nelson Textbook of Pediatrics*, ed 14. Philadelphia: WB Saunders Co, 1992, pp 105–107.

ROSS METABOLIC FORMULA SYSTEM

CALCILO XD®

Low-Calcium/Vitamin D-Free Infant Formula With Iron

USAGE:

For use in the nutrition support of infants with hypercalcemia, as may occur in infants with Williams syndrome, or in management of infants with osteopetrosis and when a low-calcium/vitamin D-free formula is needed.

Powder: 14.1-oz (400-g) cans; measuring scoop enclosed; 6 per case; No. 00378.

CYCLINEX®-1

Amino Acid-Modified Medical Food With Iron

USAGE:

When a nonessential amino acid-free medical food is needed for nutrition support of infants and toddlers with a defect in a urea cycle enzyme or with gyrate atrophy of the choroid and retina.

Powder: 12.3-oz (350-g) cans; 6 per case; No. 51144.

CYCLINEX®-2

Amino Acid-Modified Medical Food

USAGE:

When a nonessential amino acid-free medical food is needed for nutrition support of children and adults with a defect in a urea cycle enzyme or with gyrate atrophy of the choroid and retina.

Powder: 11.4-oz (325-g) cans; 6 per case; No. 51146.

FLAVONEX® Flavored Energy Supplement

USAGE:

With amino acid-modified medical foods for children and adults.

Powder: Red Punch, 21.1-oz (600-g) cans; 6 per case; No. 51530. Grapefruit, 21.1-oz (600-g) cans; 6 per case; No. 51280.

GLUTAREX®-1

Amino Acid-Modified Medical Food With Iron

USAGE:

When a lysine- and tryptophan-free medical food is needed for nutrition support of infants and toddlers with glutaric aciduria type I.

Powder: 12.3-oz (350-g) cans; 6 per case; No. 51140.

GLUTAREX®-2

Amino Acid-Modified Medical Food

USAGE:

When a lysine- and tryptophan-free medical food is needed for nutrition support of children and adults with glutaric aciduria type I.

Powder: 11.4-oz (325-g) cans; 6 per case; No. 51142.

HOMINEX®-1

Amino Acid-Modified Medical Food With Iron

USAGE:

When a methionine-free medical food is needed for nutrition support of infants and toddlers with vitamin B_6-nonresponsive homocystinuria or hypermethioninemia.

Powder: 12.3-oz (350-g) cans; 6 per case; No. 51116.

HOMINEX®-2

Amino Acid-Modified Medical Food

USAGE:

When a methionine-free medical food is needed for nutrition support of children and adults with vitamin B_6-nonresponsive homocystinuria or hypermethioninemia.

Powder: 11.4-oz (325-g) cans; 6 per case; No. 51118.

I-VALEX®-1

Amino Acid-Modified Medical Food With Iron

USAGE:

When a leucine-free medical food is needed for nutrition support of infants and toddlers with isovaleric acidemia or other disorders of leucine catabolism.

Powder: 12.3-oz (350-g) cans; 6 per case; No. 51136.

I-VALEX®-2

Amino Acid-Modified Medical Food

USAGE:

When a leucine-free medical food is needed for nutrition support of children and adults with isovaleric acidemia or other disorders of leucine catabolism.

Powder: 11.4-oz (325-g) cans; 6 per case; No. 51138.

KETONEX®-1

Amino Acid-Modified Medical Food With Iron

USAGE:

When a branched-chain amino acid-free medical food is needed for nutrition support of infants and toddlers with branched-chain ketoaciduria (maple syrup urine disease—MSUD).

Powder: 12.3-oz (350-g) cans; 6 per case; No. 51112.

KETONEX®-2

Amino Acid-Modified Medical Food

USAGE:

When a branched-chain amino acid-free medical food is needed for nutrition support of children and adults with branched-chain ketoaciduria (maple syrup urine disease—MSUD).

Powder: 11.4-oz (325-g) cans; 6 per case; No. 51114.

PHENEX™-1

Amino Acid-Modified Medical Food With Iron

USAGE:

When a phenylalanine-free medical food is needed for nutrition support of infants and toddlers with phenylketonuria (PKU) or hyperphenylalaninemia.

Powder: 12.3-oz (350-g) cans; 6 per case; No. 51120.

PHENEX™-2

Amino Acid-Modified Medical Food

USAGE:

When a phenylalanine-free medical food is needed for nutrition support of children and adults with phenylketonuria (PKU) or hyperphenylalaninemia.

Powder: 11.4-oz (325-g) cans; 6 per case; No. 51122.

PRO-PHREE®

Protein-Free Energy Module With Iron, Vitamins & Minerals

USAGE:

When a protein-free medical food is indicated for nutrition support of infants and toddlers requiring reduced protein intake, specific mixtures of L-amino acids or increased energy, minerals and vitamins.

Powder: 12.3-oz (350-g) cans; 6 per case; No. 51148.

PROPIMEX®-1

Amino Acid-Modified Medical Food With Iron

USAGE:

When a methionine- and valine-free, low-isoleucine and low-threonine medical food is needed for nutrition support of infants and toddlers with propionic or methylmalonic acidemia.

Powder: 12.3-oz (350-g) cans; 6 per case; No. 51132.

PROPIMEX®-2

Amino Acid-Modified Medical Food

USAGE:

When a methionine- and valine-free, low-isoleucine and low-threonine medical food is needed for nutrition support

Continued on next page

Ross Metabolic Formula—Cont.

of children and adults with propionic or methylmalonic acidemia.
Powder: 11.4-oz (325-g) cans; 6 per case; No. 51134.

PROVIMIN®
Protein-Vitamin-Mineral Formula Component With Iron
USAGE:
For use in management of patients who require a formula modified in carbohydrate and fat.
Powder: 5.3-oz (150-g) cans; 6 per case; No. 50260.

RCF®
Ross Carbohydrate Free Soy Formula Base With Iron
USAGE:
For use in the dietary management of patients unable to tolerate the type or amount of carbohydrate in milk or conventional infant formulas; or with seizure disorders requiring a ketogenic diet.
Concentrated Liquid: 13-fl-oz (384-mL) cans; 12 per case; No. 00108.

SIMILAC® PM 60/40
Low-Iron Infant Formula
USAGE:
For infants predisposed to or being treated for hypocalcemia with hyperphosphatemia, or those with impaired renal function who would benefit from lowered mineral intake.
Powder: 1-lb (454-g) cans, measuring scoop enclosed; 6 per case; No. 00850.
For hospital/institutional use, Similac PM 60/40 in 4-oz cans is available in the Ross Hospital Formula System.

TYROMEX®-1
Amino Acid-Modified Medical Food With Iron
USAGE:
When a phenylalanine-, tyrosine- and methionine-free medical food is needed for nutrition support of infants and toddlers with tyrosinemia type I.
Powder: 12.3-oz (350-g) cans; 6 per case; No. 51128.

TYREX®-2
Amino Acid-Modified Medical Food
USAGE:
When a phenylalanine- and tyrosine-free medical food is needed for nutrition support of children and adults with tyrosinemia type II.
Powder: 11.4-oz (325-g) cans; 6 per case; No. 51126.

SELSUN® Rx ℞
[sel 'sun]
(2.5% selenium sulfide lotion, USP)

DESCRIPTION
A liquid antiseborrheic, antifungal preparation for topical application. Contains: Selenium sulfide 2 $^1/_2$% w/v in aqueous suspension; also contains: bentonite, lauric diethanolamide, ethylene glycol monostearate, titanium dioxide, amphoteric-2, sodium lauryl sulfate, sodium phosphate (monobasic), glyceryl monoricinoleate, citric acid, captan and perfume.

CLINICAL PHARMACOLOGY
Selenium sulfide appears to have a cytostatic effect on cells of the epidermis and follicular epithelium, reducing corneocyte production.

INDICATIONS AND USAGE
Treatment of tinea versicolor, seborrheic dermatitis of scalp and treatment of dandruff.

CONTRAINDICATIONS
Not to be used by patients allergic to ingredients.

PRECAUTIONS
General: Not to be used when inflammation or exudation is present as increased absorption may occur.
Information for Patients: See Warnings and Precautions section under Application Instructions.
Carcinogenesis: Dermal application of 25% and 50% solutions of 2.5% selenium sulfide lotion on mice over an 88-week period indicated no carcinogenic effects.
Pregnancy: WHEN USED FOR THE TREATMENT OF TINEA VERSICOLOR, SELSUN IS CLASSIFIED AS PREGNANCY CATEGORY C. Animal reproduction studies have not been conducted with SELSUN. It is also not known whether SELSUN can cause fetal harm when applied to body surfaces of a pregnant woman or can affect reproduction capacity. Under ordinary circumstances SELSUN should not be used for the treatment of tinea versicolor in pregnant women.
Pediatric Use: Safety and effectiveness in infants have not been established.

ADVERSE REACTIONS
In decreasing order of severity: skin irritation; occasional reports of increase in normal hair loss; discoloration of hair (can be avoided or minimized by thorough rinsing of hair after treatment). As with other shampoos, oiliness or dryness of hair and scalp may occur.

OVERDOSAGE
Accidental Oral Ingestion:
No documented reports of serious toxicity in humans resulting from acute ingestion of SELSUN, however, acute toxicity studies in animals suggest that ingestion of large amounts could result in potential human toxicity. Evacuation of the stomach contents should be considered in cases of acute oral ingestion.

DOSAGE AND ADMINISTRATION
See application instructions.
Treatment of tinea versicolor: Apply to affected areas and lather with a small amount of water. Allow product to remain on skin for 10 minutes, then rinse thoroughly. Repeat procedure once a day for 7 days.
Treatment of seborrheic dermatitis and dandruff: Usually two applications each week for two weeks will afford control. After this, may be used at less frequent intervals—weekly, every two weeks, or every 3 or 4 weeks in some cases. Should not be applied more frequently than required to maintain control.
APPLICATION INSTRUCTIONS: Keep tightly capped.
Shake well before using. Product may damage jewelry; remove jewelry before use.
For treatment of tinea versicolor:
1. Apply to affected areas and lather with a small amount of water.
2. Allow to remain on skin for 10 minutes.
3. Rinse body thoroughly.
4. Repeat this procedure once a day for 7 days.

For treatment of dandruff and seborrheic dermatitis of the scalp:
1. Massage about 1 or 2 teaspoonfuls of shampoo into wet scalp.
2. Allow to remain on scalp for 2 to 3 minutes.
3. Rinse scalp thoroughly.
4. Repeat application and rinse thoroughly.
5. After treatment, wash hands well.
6. Repeat treatments as directed by physician.

WARNINGS AND PRECAUTIONS:
For External Use Only. Do not use on broken skin or inflamed areas. If allergic reactions occur, discontinue use. Avoid getting shampoo in eyes or in contact with genital area and skin folds as it may cause irritation and burning. These areas should be thoroughly rinsed after application. Keep this and all medicines out of reach of children.
Store below 86°F (30°C).

HOW SUPPLIED
4-fl-oz bottles (NDC 0074-2660-04).
(.2960)
December, 1998

SELSUN BLUE® OTC
[sel 'sun]
Dandruff Shampoo
(selenium sulfide lotion, 1%)

SURVANTA® ℞
(beractant)
intratracheal suspension

Sterile Suspension
For Intratracheal Administration Only

DESCRIPTION
SURVANTA® (beractant) Intratracheal Suspension is a sterile, non-pyrogenic pulmonary surfactant intended for intratracheal use only. It is a natural bovine lung extract containing phospholipids, neutral lipids, fatty acids, and surfactant-associated proteins to which colfosceril palmitate (dipalmitoylphosphatidylcholine), palmitic acid, and tripalmitin are added to standardize the composition and to mimic surface-tension lowering properties of natural lung surfactant. The resulting composition provides 25 mg/mL phospholipids (including 11.0-15.5 mg/mL disaturated phosphatidylcholine), 0.5-1.75 mg/mL triglycerides, 1.4-3.5 mg/mL free fatty acids, and less than 1.0 mg/mL protein. It is suspended in 0.9% sodium chloride solution, and heat-sterilized. SURVANTA contains no preservatives. Its protein content consists of two hydrophobic, low molecular weight, surfactant-associated proteins commonly known as SP-B and SP-C. It does not contain the hydrophilic, large molecular weight surfactant-associated protein known as SP-A.
Each mL of SURVANTA contains 25 mg of phospholipids. It is an off-white to light brown liquid supplied in single-use glass vials containing 4 mL (100 mg phospholipids) or 8 mL (200 mg phospholipids).

CLINICAL PHARMACOLOGY
Endogenous pulmonary surfactant lowers surface tension on alveolar surfaces during respiration and stabilizes the alveoli against collapse at resting transpulmonary pressures. Deficiency of pulmonary surfactant causes Respiratory Distress Syndrome (RDS) in premature infants. SURVANTA replenishes surfactant and restores surface activity to the lungs of these infants.

Activity
In vitro, SURVANTA reproducibly lowers minimum surface tension to less than 8 dynes/cm as measured by the pulsating bubble surfactometer and Wilhelmy Surface Balance. *In situ,* SURVANTA restores pulmonary compliance to excised rat lungs artificially made surfactant-deficient. *In vivo,* single SURVANTA doses improve lung pressure-volume measurements, lung compliance, and oxygenation in premature rabbits and sheep.

Animal Metabolism
SURVANTA is administered directly to the target organ, the lungs, where biophysical effects occur at the alveolar surface. In surfactant-deficient premature rabbits and lambs, alveolar clearance of radio-labelled lipid components of SURVANTA is rapid. Most of the dose becomes lung-associated within hours of administration, and the lipids enter endogenous surfactant pathways of reutilization and recycling. In surfactant-sufficient adult animals, SURVANTA clearance is more rapid than in premature and young animals. There is less reutilization and recycling of surfactant in adult animals.
Limited animal experiments have not found effects of SURVANTA on endogenous surfactant metabolism. Precursor incorporation and subsequent secretion of saturated phosphatidylcholine in premature sheep are not changed by SURVANTA treatments.
No information is available about the metabolic fate of the surfactant-associated proteins in SURVANTA. The metabolic disposition in humans has not been studied.

Clinical Studies
Clinical effects of SURVANTA were demonstrated in six single-dose and four multiple-dose randomized, multicenter, controlled clinical trials involving approximately 1700 infants. Three open trials, including a Treatment IND, involved more than 8500 infants. Each dose of SURVANTA in all studies was 100 mg phospholipids/kg birth weight and was based on published experience with Surfactant TA, a lyophilized powder dosage form of SURVANTA having the same composition.

Prevention Studies
Infants of 600-1250 g birth weight and 23 to 29 weeks estimated gestational age were enrolled in two *multiple-dose* studies. A dose of SURVANTA was given within 15 minutes of birth to prevent the development of RDS. Up to three additional doses in the first 48 hours, as often as every 6 hours, were given if RDS subsequently developed and infants required mechanical ventilation with an $FiO_2 \geq 0.30$. Results of the studies at 28 days of age are shown in Table 1.

TABLE 1

Study 1

	SURVANTA	Control	*P*-Value
Number infants studied	119	124	
Incidence of RDS (%)	27.6	63.5	<0.001
Death due to RDS (%)	2.5	19.5	<0.001
Death or BPD due to RDS (%)	48.7	52.8	0.536
Death due to any cause (%)	7.6	22.8	0.001
Air Leaks[a](%)	5.9	21.7	0.001
Pulmonary interstitial emphysema (%)	20.8	40.0	0.001

Study 2[b]

	SURVANTA	Control	*P*-Value
Number infants studied	91	96	
Incidence of RDS (%)	28.6	48.3	0.007
Death due to RDS (%)	1.1	10.5	0.006
Death or BPD due to RDS (%)	27.5	44.2	0.018
Death due to any cause[c](%)	16.5	13.7	0.633
Air Leaks[a](%)	14.5	19.6	0.374
Pulmonary interstitial emphysema (%)	26.5	33.2	0.298

[a] Pneumothorax or pneumopericardium
[b] Study discontinued when Treatment IND initiated
[c] No cause of death in the SURVANTA group was significantly increased; the higher number of deaths in this group was due to the sum of all causes.

Rescue Studies
Infants of 600-1750 g birth weight with RDS requiring mechanical ventilation and an $FiO_2 \geq 0.40$ were enrolled in two *multiple-dose* rescue studies. The initial dose of SURVANTA was given after RDS developed and before 8 hours of age. Infants could receive up to three additional doses in the first 48 hours, as often as every 6 hours, if they required mechanical ventilation and an $FiO_2 \geq 0.30$. Results of the studies at 28 days of age are shown in Table 2.

TABLE 2

Study 3[a]

	SURVANTA	Control	P-Value
Number infants studied	198	193	
Death due to RDS (%)	11.6	18.1	0.071
Death or BPD due to RDS (%)	59.1	66.8	0.102
Death due to any cause (%)	21.7	26.4	0.285
Air Leaks[b](%)	11.8	29.5	<0.001
Pulmonary interstitial emphysema (%)	16.3	34.0	<0.001

Study 4

	SURVANTA	Control	P-Value
Number infants studied	204	203	
Death due to RDS (%)	6.4	22.3	<0.001
Death or BPD due to RDS (%)	43.6	63.4	<0.001
Death due to any cause (%)	15.2	28.2	0.001
Air Leaks[b] (%)	11.2	22.2	0.005
Pulmonary interstitial emphysema (%)	20.8	44.4	<0.001

[a] Study discontinued when Treatment IND initiated
[b] Pneumothorax or pneumopericardium

Acute Clinical Effects
Marked improvements in oxygenation may occur within minutes of administration of SURVANTA.
All controlled clinical studies with SURVANTA provided information regarding the acute effects of SURVANTA on the arterial-alveolar oxygen ratio (a/APO$_2$), FiO$_2$, and mean airway pressure (MAP) during the first 48 to 72 hours of life. Significant improvements in these variables were sustained for 48-72 hours in SURVANTA-treated infants in four single-dose and two multiple-dose rescue studies and in two multiple-dose prevention studies. In the single-dose prevention studies, FiO$_2$ improved significantly.

INDICATIONS AND USAGE

SURVANTA is indicated for prevention and treatment ("rescue") of Respiratory Distress Syndrome (RDS) (hyaline membrane disease) in premature infants. SURVANTA significantly reduces the incidence of RDS, mortality due to RDS and air leak complications.

Prevention
In premature infants less than 1250 g birth weight or with evidence of surfactant deficiency, give SURVANTA as soon as possible, preferably within 15 minutes of birth.

Rescue
To treat infants with RDS confirmed by x-ray and requiring mechanical ventilation, give SURVANTA as soon as possible, preferably by 8 hours of age.

CONTRAINDICATIONS

None known.

WARNINGS

SURVANTA is intended for intratracheal use only.
SURVANTA CAN RAPIDLY AFFECT OXYGENATION AND LUNG COMPLIANCE. Therefore, its use should be restricted to a highly supervised clinical setting with immediate availability of clinicians experienced with intubation, ventilator management, and general care of premature infants. Infants receiving SURVANTA should be frequently monitored with arterial or transcutaneous measurement of systemic oxygen and carbon dioxide.
DURING THE DOSING PROCEDURE, TRANSIENT EPISODES OF BRADYCARDIA AND DECREASED OXYGEN SATURATION HAVE BEEN REPORTED. If these occur, stop the dosing procedure and initiate appropriate measures to alleviate the condition. After stabilization, resume the dosing procedure.

PRECAUTIONS

General
Rales and moist breath sounds can occur transiently after administration. Endotracheal suctioning or other remedial action is not necessary unless clear-cut signs of airway obstruction are present.
Increased probability of post-treatment nosocomial sepsis in SURVANTA-treated infants was observed in the controlled clinical trials (Table 3). The increased risk for sepsis among SURVANTA-treated infants was not associated with increased mortality among these infants. The causative organisms were similar in treated and control infants. There was no significant difference between groups in the rate of post-treatment infections other than sepsis.
Use of SURVANTA in infants less than 600 g birth weight or greater than 1750 g birth weight has not been evaluated in controlled trials. There is no controlled experience with use of SURVANTA in conjunction with experimental therapies for RDS (eg, high-frequency ventilation or extracorporeal membrane oxygenation).
No information is available on the effects of doses other than 100 mg phospholipids/kg, more than four doses, dosing more frequently than every 6 hours, or administration after 48 hours of age.

Carcinogenesis, Mutagenesis, Impairment of Fertility
Carcinogenicity studies have not been performed with SURVANTA. SURVANTA was negative when tested in the Ames test for mutagenicity. Using the maximum feasible dose volume, SURVANTA up to 500 mg phospholipids/kg/day (approximately one-third the premature infant dose based on mg/m^2/day) was administered subcutaneously to newborn rats for 5 days. The rats reproduced normally and there were no observable adverse effects in their offspring.

ADVERSE REACTIONS

The most commonly reported adverse experiences were associated with the dosing procedure. In the multiple-dose controlled clinical trials, each dose of SURVANTA was divided into four quarter-doses which were instilled through a catheter inserted into the endotracheal tube by briefly disconnecting the endotracheal tube from the ventilator. Transient bradycardia occurred with 11.9% of *doses.* Oxygen desaturation occurred with 9.8% of *doses.*
Other reactions during the dosing procedure occurred with fewer than 1% of doses and included endotracheal tube reflux, pallor, vasoconstriction, hypotension, endotracheal tube blockage, hypertension, hypocarbia, hypercarbia, and apnea. No deaths occurred during the dosing procedure, and all reactions resolved with symptomatic treatment.
The occurrence of concurrent illnesses common in premature infants was evaluated in the controlled trials. The rates in all controlled studies are in Table 3.

TABLE 3

	All Controlled Studies		
Concurrent Event	**SURVANTA (%)**	**Control (%)**	**P-Value[a]**
Patent ductus arteriosus	46.9	47.1	0.814
Intracranial hemorrhage	48.1	45.2	0.241
Severe intracranial hemorrhage	24.1	23.3	0.693
Pulmonary air leaks	10.9	24.7	<0.001
Pulmonary interstitial emphysema	20.2	38.4	<0.001
Necrotizing enterocolitis	6.1	5.3	0.427
Apnea	65.4	59.6	0.283
Severe apnea	46.1	42.5	0.114
Post-treatment sepsis	20.7	16.1	0.019
Post-treatment infection	10.2	9.1	0.345
Pulmonary hemorrhage	7.2	5.3	0.166

[a]*P*-value comparing groups in controlled studies

When all controlled studies were pooled, there was no difference in intracranial hemorrhage. However, in one of the single-dose rescue studies and one of the multiple-dose prevention studies, the rate of intracranial hemorrhage was significantly higher in SURVANTA patients than control patients (63.3% *v* 30.8%, *P*=0.001; and 48.8% *v* 34.2%, *P*=0.047, respectively). The rate in a Treatment IND involving approximately 8100 infants was lower than in the controlled trials.
In the controlled clinical trials, there was no effect of SURVANTA on results of common laboratory tests: white blood cell count and serum sodium, potassium, bilirubin, creatinine.
More than 4300 pretreatment and posttreatment serum samples from approximately 1500 patients were tested by Western Blot Immunoassay for antibodies to surfactant-associated proteins SP-B and SP-C. No IgG or IgM antibodies were detected.
Several other complications are known to occur in premature infants. The following conditions were reported in the controlled clinical studies. The rates of the complications were not different in treated and control infants, and none of the complications were attributed to SURVANTA.
Respiratory: lung consolidation, blood from the endotracheal tube, deterioration after weaning, respiratory decompensation, subglottic stenosis, paralyzed diaphragm, respiratory failure.
Cardiovascular: hypotension, hypertension, tachycardia, ventricular tachycardia, aortic thrombosis, cardiac failure, cardio-respiratory arrest, increased apical pulse, persistent fetal circulation, air embolism, total anomalous pulmonary venous return.
Gastrointestinal: abdominal distention, hemorrhage, intestinal perforations, volvulus, bowel infarct, feeding intolerance, hepatic failure, stress ulcer.
Renal: renal failure, hematuria.
Hematologic: coagulopathy, thrombocytopenia, disseminated intravascular coagulation.
Central Nervous System: seizures.
Endocrine/Metabolic: adrenal hemorrhage, inappropriate ADH secretion, hyperphosphatemia.
Musculoskeletal: inguinal hernia.
Systemic: fever, deterioration.

Follow-Up Evaluations
To date, no long-term complications or sequelae of SURVANTA therapy have been found.

Single-Dose Studies
Six-month adjusted-age follow-up evaluations of 232 infants (115 treated) demonstrated no clinically important differences between treatment groups in pulmonary and neurologic sequelae, incidence or severity of retinopathy of prematurity, rehospitalizations, growth, or allergic manifestations.

Multiple-Dose Studies
Six-month adjusted-age follow-up evaluations have been completed in 631 (345 treated) of 916 surviving infants. There were significantly less cerebral palsy and need for supplemental oxygen in SURVANTA infants than controls. Wheezing at the time of examination was significantly more frequent among SURVANTA infants, although there was no difference in bronchodilator therapy.
Final twelve-month follow-up data from the multiple-dose studies are available from 521 (272 treated) of 909 surviving infants. There was significantly less wheezing in SURVANTA infants than controls, in contrast to the six-month results. There was no difference in the incidence of cerebral palsy at twelve months.
Twenty-four month adjusted-age evaluations were completed in 429 (226 treated) of 906 surviving infants. There were significantly fewer SURVANTA infants with rhonchi, wheezing, and tachypnea at the time of examination. No other differences were found.

OVERDOSAGE

Overdosage with SURVANTA has not been reported. Based on animal data, overdosage might result in acute airway obstruction. Treatment should be symptomatic and supportive.
Rales and moist breath sounds can transiently occur after SURVANTA is given, and do not indicate overdosage. Endotracheal suctioning or other remedial action is not required unless clear-cut signs of airway obstruction are present.

DOSAGE AND ADMINISTRATION

FOR INTRATRACHEAL ADMINISTRATION ONLY.
SURVANTA should be administered by or under the supervision of clinicians experienced in intubation, ventilator management, and general care of premature infants.
Marked improvements in oxygenation may occur within minutes of administration of SURVANTA. Therefore, frequent and careful clinical observation and monitoring of systemic oxygenation are essential to avoid hyperoxia.
Review of audiovisual instructional materials describing dosage and administration procedures is recommended before using SURVANTA. Materials are available upon request from Ross Products Division, Abbott Laboratories Inc.

Dosage
Each dose of SURVANTA is 100 mg of phospholipids/kg birth weight (4 mL/kg). The SURVANTA DOSING CHART shows the total dosage for a range of birth weights.

SURVANTA DOSING CHART

WEIGHT (grams)	TOTAL DOSE (mL)	WEIGHT (grams)	TOTAL DOSE (mL)
600- 650	2.6	1301-1350	5.4
651- 700	2.8	1351-1400	5.6
701- 750	3.0	1401-1450	5.8
751- 800	3.2	1451-1500	6.0
801- 850	3.4	1501-1550	6.2
851- 900	3.6	1551-1600	6.4
901- 950	3.8	1601-1650	6.6
951-1000	4.0	1651-1700	6.8
1001-1050	4.2	1701-1750	7.0
1051-1100	4.4	1751-1800	7.2
1101-1150	4.6	1801-1850	7.4
1151-1200	4.8	1851-1900	7.6
1201-1250	5.0	1901-1950	7.8
1251-1300	5.2	1951-2000	8.0

Four doses of SURVANTA can be administered in the first 48 hours of life. Doses should be given no more frequently than every 6 hours.

Directions for Use
SURVANTA should be inspected visually for discoloration prior to administration. The color of SURVANTA is off-white to light brown. If settling occurs during storage, swirl the vial gently (DO NOT SHAKE) to redisperse. Some foaming at the surface may occur during handling and is inherent in the nature of the product.
SURVANTA is stored refrigerated (2–8°C). Date and time need to be recorded in the box on front of the carton or vial, whenever SURVANTA is removed from the refrigerator. Before administration, SURVANTA should be warmed by standing at room temperature for at least 20 minutes or warmed in the hand for at least 8 minutes. ARTIFICIAL WARMING METHODS SHOULD NOT BE USED. If a prevention dose is to be given, preparation of SURVANTA should begin before the infant's birth.
Unopened, unused vials of SURVANTA that have been warmed to room temperature may be returned to the refrigerator within 24 hours of warming, and stored for future use. SURVANTA SHOULD NOT BE REMOVED FROM THE REFRIGERATOR FOR MORE THAN 24 HOURS. SURVANTA SHOULD NOT BE WARMED AND RETURNED TO THE REFRIGERATOR MORE THAN ONCE.
Each single-use vial of SURVANTA should be entered only once. Used vials with residual drug should be discarded.
SURVANTA DOES NOT REQUIRE RECONSTITUTION OR SONICATION BEFORE USE.

Dosing Procedures

General
SURVANTA is administered intratracheally by instillation through a 5 French end-hole catheter. The catheter can be inserted into the infant's endotracheal tube without interrupting ventilation by passing the catheter through a neonatal suction valve attached to the endotracheal tube. Alter-

Continued on next page

Survanta—Cont.

natively, SURVANTA can be instilled through the catheter by briefly disconnecting the endotracheal tube from the ventilator.
The neonatal suction valve used for administering SURVANTA should be a type that allows entry of the catheter into the endotracheal tube without interrupting ventilation and also maintains a closed airway circuit system by sealing the valve around the catheter.
If the neonatal suction valve is used, the catheter should be rigid enough to pass easily into the endotracheal tube. A very soft and pliable catheter may twist or curl within the neonatal suction valve. The length of the catheter should be shortened so that the tip of the catheter protrudes just beyond the end of the endotracheal tube above the infant's carina. SURVANTA should not be instilled into a mainstem bronchus.
To ensure homogenous distribution of SURVANTA throughout the lungs, each dose is divided into *four quarter-doses.* Each quarter-dose is administered with the infant in a different position. The recommended positions are:

- Head and body inclined 5–10° down, head turned to the right
- Head and body inclined 5–10° down, head turned to the left
- Head and body inclined 5–10° up, head turned to the right
- Head and body inclined 5–10° up, head turned to the left

The dosing procedure is facilitated if one person administers the dose while another person positions and monitors the infant.

First Dose

Determine the total dose of SURVANTA from the SURVANTA DOSING CHART based on the infant's birth weight. Slowly withdraw the entire contents of the vial into a plastic syringe through a large-gauge needle (eg, at least 20 gauge). DO NOT FILTER SURVANTA AND AVOID SHAKING.
Attach the premeasured 5 French end-hole catheter to the syringe. Fill the catheter with SURVANTA. Discard excess SURVANTA through the catheter so that only the total dose to be given remains in the syringe.
BEFORE ADMINISTERING SURVANTA, assure proper placement and patency of the endotracheal tube. At the discretion of the clinician, the endotracheal tube may be suctioned before administering SURVANTA. The infant should be allowed to stabilize before proceeding with dosing.
In the prevention strategy, weigh, intubate and stabilize the infant. Administer the dose as soon as possible after birth, preferably within 15 minutes. Position the infant appropriately and gently inject the first quarter-dose through the catheter over 2-3 seconds.
After administration of the first quarter-dose, remove the catheter from the endotracheal tube. Manually ventilate with a hand-bag with sufficient oxygen to prevent cyanosis, at a rate of 60 breaths/minute, and sufficient positive pressure to provide adequate air exchange and chest wall excursion.
In the rescue strategy, the first dose should be given as soon as possible after the infant is placed on a ventilator for management of RDS. In the clinical trials, immediately before instilling the first quarter-dose, the infant's ventilator settings were changed to rate 60/minute, inspiratory time 0.5 second, and FiO_2 1.0.
Position the infant appropriately and gently inject the first quarter-dose through the catheter over 2–3 seconds. After administration of the first quarter-dose, remove the catheter from the endotracheal tube and continue mechanical ventilation.
In both strategies, ventilate the infant for at least 30 seconds or until stable. Reposition the infant for instillation of the next quarter-dose.
Instill the remaining quarter-doses using the same procedures. After instillation of each quarter-dose, remove the catheter and ventilate for at least 30 seconds or until the infant is stabilized. After instillation of the final quarter-dose, remove the catheter without flushing it. Do not suction the infant for 1 hour after dosing unless signs of significant airway obstruction occur.
AFTER COMPLETION OF THE DOSING PROCEDURE, RESUME USUAL VENTILATOR MANAGEMENT AND CLINICAL CARE.

Repeat Doses

The dosage of SURVANTA for repeat doses is also 100 mg phospholipids/kg and is based on the infant's birth weight. The infant should not be reweighed for determination of the SURVANTA dosage. Use the SURVANTA DOSING CHART to determine the total dosage.
The need for additional doses of SURVANTA is determined by evidence of continuing respiratory distress. Using the following criteria for redosing, significant reductions in mortality due to RDS were observed in the multiple-dose clinical trials with SURVANTA.

Dose no sooner than 6 hours after the preceding dose if the infant remains intubated and requires at least 30% inspired oxygen to maintain a PaO_2 less than or equal to 80 torr.

Radiographic confirmation of RDS should be obtained before administering additional doses to those who received a prevention dose.

Prepare SURVANTA and position the infant for administration of each quarter-dose as previously described. After instillation of each quarter-dose, remove the dosing catheter from the endotracheal tube and ventilate the infant for at least 30 seconds or until stable.
In the clinical studies, ventilator settings used to administer repeat doses were different than those used for the first dose. For repeat doses, the FiO_2 was increased by 0.20 or an amount sufficient to prevent cyanosis. The ventilator delivered a rate of 30/minute with an inspiratory time less than 1.0 second. If the infant's pretreatment rate was 30 or greater, it was left unchanged during SURVANTA instillation.
Manual hand-bag ventilation should not be used to administer repeat doses. DURING THE DOSING PROCEDURE, VENTILATOR SETTINGS MAY BE ADJUSTED AT THE DISCRETION OF THE CLINICIAN TO MAINTAIN APPROPRIATE OXYGENATION AND VENTILATION.
AFTER COMPLETION OF THE DOSING PROCEDURE, RESUME USUAL VENTILATOR MANAGEMENT AND CLINICAL CARE.

Dosing Precautions

If an infant experiences bradycardia or oxygen desaturation during the dosing procedure, stop the dosing procedure and initiate appropriate measures to alleviate the condition. After the infant has stabilized, resume the dosing procedure. Rales and moist breath sounds can occur transiently after administration of SURVANTA. Endotracheal suctioning or other remedial action is unnecessary unless clear-cut signs of airway obstruction are present.

HOW SUPPLIED

SURVANTA (beractant) Intratracheal Suspension is supplied in single-use glass vials containing 4 mL (NDC 0074-1040-04) or 8 mL (NDC 0074-1040-08) of SURVANTA. Each milliliter contains 25 mg of phospholipids suspended in 0.9% sodium chloride solution. The color is off-white to light brown.
Store unopened vials at refrigeration temperature (2-8°C). Protect from light. Store vials in carton until ready for use. Vials are for single use only. Upon opening, discard unused drug.

October, 1999

TRONOLANE® OTC
[tron 'e-lān]
Anesthetic Cream for Hemorrhoids
Hemorrhoidal Suppositories

PEDIAFLOR® Drops ℞
Sodium Fluoride Oral Solution, USP
1.7 fl oz (50 mL) bottles, calibrated dropper

VI-DAYLIN® ADC VITAMINS Drops OTC
Dietary Supplement of Vitamins A,D, and C
50 mL Spil-gard® bottles, calibrated dropper

VI-DAYLIN® ADC VITAMINS + IRON Drops OTC
Dietary Supplement of Vitamins A,D, and C with Iron
50 mL Spil-gard® bottles, calibrated dropper

VI-DAYLIN® MULTIVITAMIN DROPS OTC
Multivitamin Supplement
50 mL Spil-gard® bottles, calibrated dropper

VI-DAYLIN® MULTIVITAMIN + IRON Drops OTC
Multivitamin/Iron Supplement
50 mL Spil-gard® bottles, calibrated dropper

VI-DAYLIN®/F ADC VITAMINS Drops With Fluoride ℞
ADC Vitamins/Fluoride
50 mL Spil-gard® bottles, calibrated dropper

VI-DAYLIN®/F ADC VITAMINS + IRON Drops With Fluoride ℞
ADC Vitamins/Fluoride/Iron Supplement
50 mL Spil-gard® bottles, calibrated dropper

VI-DAYLIN®/F MULTIVITAMIN Drops With Fluoride ℞
Multivitamins/Fluoride
50 mL Spil-gard® bottles, calibrated dropper

VI-DAYLIN®/F MULTIVITAMIN + IRON Drops With Fluoride ℞
Multivitamins/Fluoride/Iron Supplement
50 mL Spil-gard® bottles, calibrated dropper

VI-DAYLIN® MULTIVITAMIN Chewable Tablets OTC
Multivitamin Supplement
100 tablet bottles

VI-DAYLIN® MULTIVITAMIN + IRON Chewable Tablets OTC
Multivitamin/Iron Supplement
100 tablet bottles

VI-DAYLIN®/F MULTIVITAMIN Chewable Tablets With Fluoride ℞
Multivitamins/Fluoride
100 tablet bottles

VI-DAYLIN®/F MULTIVITAMIN + IRON Chewable Tablets With Fluoride ℞
Multivitamins/Fluoride/Iron
100 tablet bottles

VI-DAYLIN® MULTIVITAMIN Liquid OTC
Multivitamin Supplement
16-fl-oz (473 mL) bottles
8-fl-oz (237 mL) bottles

VI-DAYLIN® MULTIVITAMIN + IRON Liquid OTC
Multivitamin/Iron Supplement
16-fl-oz (473 mL) bottles
8-fl-oz (237 mL) bottles

EDUCATIONAL MATERIAL

A complete program of educational services for health care professionals and patients is available.
Contact your local Ross representative.

Roxane Laboratories, Inc.

P.O. 16532
COLUMBUS, OH 43216-6532

Direct Inquiries to:
Technical Product Information
P.O. 16532
Columbus, OH 43216-6532
1-800-962-8364

ROXANE LABORATORIES, INC PRODUCT LIST

Acetaminophen 120mg and Codeine Phosphate Oral Solution USP 120mg/12mL per 5mL
Acetaminophen and Codeine Phosphate Tablets USP 300mg/30mg
Acetylcysteine Solution USP 10%, 20%
Alprazolam Intensol™ Oral Solution (Concentrate) 1mg/mL
Aminophylline Oral Solution USP 105mg/5mL
Aromatic Cascara Fluidextract USP
Azathioprine Tablets USP 50mg
Cafcit® (Caffeine Citrate) Oral Solution 20mg/mL
Calcium Carbonate Tablets USP 1250mg
Calcium Carbonate Oral Suspension (not USP) 1250mg/5mL
Calcium Gluconate Tablets USP 500mg
Chlorpromazine Hydrochloride Intensol™ (oral concentrate USP) 30 mg per mL, 100 mg per mL
Cocaine Hydrochloride Topical Solution 4%,10%
Codeine Phosphate Oral Solution 15mg/5mL
Codeine Sulfate Tablets USP 15mg, 30mg, 60mg
Cromolyn Sodium Inhalation Solution USP 20mg/mL
Cyclophosphamide Tablets USP 25mg, 50mg
Dexamethasone Intensol™ Oral Solution (concentrate) 1 mg per mL
Dexamethasone Oral Solution 0.5mg/5mL
Dexamethasone Tablets USP 0.5 mg, 0.75mg, 1mg, 1.5mg, 2mg, 4mg, 6mg
Diazepam Intensol™ Oral Solution (Concentrate) 5 mg/mL
Diazepam Oral Solution 5 mg/5 mL, 10 mg/10 mL
Diclofenac Sodium Delayed-Release Tablets USP 25mg, 50mg, 75mg
Digoxin Elixir USP 0.05mg/mL, 0.125mg/2.5mL, 0.25mg/5mL
DHT™ Dihydrotachysterol Tablets USP 0.125mg, 0.2mg, 0.4mg
DHT™ Intensol™ 0.2 mg/mL
Diluent (Flavored) for Oral Use
Diphenoxylate Hydrochloride and Atropine Sulfate Oral Solution USP
Docusate Sodium Syrup USP 50mg/15mL, 100mg/30mL
Duraclon™ Clonidine HCl Injection 100mcg/mL
Furosemide Oral Solution 10mg/mL, 40mg/5mL
Furosemide Tablets USP 20mg, 40mg, 80mg
Guaifenesin Syrup USP 100mg/5mL, 200mg/10mL
Hydrochlorothiazide Oral Solution 50mg/5mL
Hydromorphone Hydrochloride Tablets USP 2mg, 4mg, 8 mg
Hydromorphone Hydrochloride Oral Solution 1 mg per mL
Hydroxyurea Capsules USP 500mg
Ipratropium Bromide Inhalation Solution 0.02%
Isoetharine Inhalation Solution USP 1%
Kaolin-Pectin Suspension
Lactulose Solution USP 10g/15mL
Leucovorin Calcium Tablets USP 5mg, 10mg, 15mg, 25mg
Levorphanol Tartrate Tablets USP 2 mg
Lidocaine Viscous 2%
Lidocaine Hydrochloride Oral Topical Solution USP
Lidocaine Hydrochloride Topical Solution USP 4%
Lithium Carbonate Capsules USP 150mg, 300mg, 600mg
Lithium Carbonate Tablets USP 300mg
Lithium Citrate Syrup USP 8mEq per 5mL, 16mEq per 10mL
Loperamide Hydrochloride Oral Solution 1mg/5mL, 2mg/10mL
Lorazepam Intensol™ Oral Concentrate USP 2mg/mL
Marinol® (Dronabinol) Capsules 2.5 mg, 5 mg, 10 mg
Megestrol Acetate Tablets USP 20mg, 40mg
Meperidine Hydrochloride Tablets USP 50mg, 100mg

Meperidine Hydrochloride Syrup USP 50mg/5mL
Methadone Hydrochloride Intensol™ Oral Concentrate USP 10mg/mL
Methadone Hydrochloride Tablets USP 5mg, 10mg
Methadone Hydrochloride Oral Solution USP 5mg/5mL, 10mg/5mL
Methadone Hydrochloride USP Powder 50 g/100 g
Methotrexate Tablets USP 2.5mg
Metoclopramide Intensol™ (Metoclopramide Hydrochloride Oral Solution, Concentrate) 10mg/mL
Metoclopramide Oral Solution USP 5mg/5mL, 10mg/10mL
Mexiletine Hydrochloride Capsules USP 150mg, 200mg, 250mg
Milk of Magnesia Concentrated (Flavored) 100mL, 400mL
Milk of Magnesia—Cascara Suspension Concentrated 15mL
Mineral Oil, Topical Light USP (Sterile) 10mL, 30mL
Morphine Sulfate Immediate Release Tablets 15mg, 30mg
Morphine Sulfate (Immediate Release) Oral Solution 10mg/5mL, 20mg/10mL, 20mg/5mL
Naproxen Oral Suspension USP 125mg/5mL, 375mg/15mL, 500mg/20mL
Nystatin Oral Suspension USP 100,000 USP units per mL, 500,000 USP units per mL
Oramorph® SR Tablets (Morphine Sulfate Sustained Release Tablets) 15mg, 30mg, 60mg, 100mg
Potassium Chloride Oral Solution USP 10%, 20%
Prednisone Intensol™ Oral Solution (Concentrate) 5mg/mL
Prednisone Oral Solution USP 5mg/5mL
Prednisone Tablets USP 1mg, 2.5mg, 5mg, 10mg, 20mg, 50mg
Prelu-2® Timed Release Capsules (Phendimetrazine Tartrate) 105mg
Propantheline Bromide Tablets USP 15mg
Propranolol Hydrochloride Intensol™ Oral Solution (Concentrate) 80mg/mL
Propranolol Hydrochloride Oral Solution 20mg/5mL and 40mg/5 mL
Pseudoephedrine Hydrochloride Tablets USP 30mg, 60mg
Roxanol™ Morphine Sulfate (Immediate Release) Oral Solution (Concentrated) 20mg/mL
Roxanol 100™ Morphine Sulfate Oral Solution (Concentrate) 100mg/5mL
Roxanol™-T Morphine Sulfate (Immediate Release) Oral Solution (Concentrated) tinted flavored 20mg/mL
Roxicet™ Oral Solution Oxycodone Hydrochloride and Acetaminophen 5mg/325mg per 5mL
Roxicet™ Oxycodone and Acetaminophen Tablets USP 5mg/325mg
Roxicet™ 5/500 Caplets (Oxycodone and Acetaminophen Tablets USP)
Roxicodone™ (Oxycodone Hydrochloride Oral Solution USP) 5mg/5mL
Roxicodone™ (Oxycodone Hydrochloride Tablets USP) (Immediate Release) 15mg, 30mg
Roxicodone™ Oxycodone Hydrochloride Intensol™ Oral Solution (Concentrate) 20mg per mL
Roxilox™ (Oxycodone and Acetaminophen Capsules USP) 5mg/500mg
Saliva Substitute
Sodium Chloride Inhalation Solution USP (Normal Saline) Sterile 0.9% 3mL, 5mL
Sodium Polystyrene Sulfonate Suspension USP 15g/60mL; 30g/120mL and 50g/200mL
Theophylline Oral Solution 80mg/15mL, 100mg/18.75mL
Thioridazine Hydrochloride Intensol™ Oral Solution USP (Concentrate) 30mg per mL, 100mg per mL
Torecan® Injection (Thiethylperazine Malate) USP 10mg
Torecan® Tablets (Thiethylperazine Maleate Tablets USP) 10mg
Triazolam Tablets USP 0.125mg, 0.25mg
Viramune (Nevirapine)Tablets 200mg
Viramune (Nevirapine) Oral Suspension, 50 mg/5mL

CAFCIT® ℞

(caffeine citrate) 20 mg/mL
Injection/Oral Solution
℞only

DESCRIPTION

CAFCIT® (caffeine citrate) Injection for intravenous administration and CAFCIT® (caffeine citrate) Oral Solution are clear, colorless, sterile non-pyrogenic, preservative-free, aqueous solutions adjusted to pH 4.7. Each mL contains 20 mg caffeine citrate (equivalent to 10 mg of caffeine base) prepared in solution by the addition of 10 mg caffeine anhydrous to 5.0 mg citric acid monohydrate, 8.3 mg sodium citrate dihydrate and Water for Injection.

Caffeine, a central nervous system stimulant, is an odorless white crystalline powder or granule, with a bitter taste. It is sparingly soluble in water and ethanol at room temperature. The chemical name of caffeine is 3,7-dihydro-1,3,7-trimethyl-1*H*-purine-2,6-dione. In the presence of citric acid it forms caffeine citrate salt in solution. The structural formula and molecular weight of caffeine citrate follows:
[See chemical structure at top of next column]

CLINICAL PHARMACOLOGY

Mechanism of Action

Caffeine is structurally related to other methylxanthines, theophylline and theobromine. It is a bronchial smooth muscle relaxant, a CNS stimulant, a cardiac muscle stimulant and a diuretic.

	CAFCIT®	Placebo	p-value
Number of patients evaluated[1]	45	37	
% of patients with zero apnea events on day 2	26.7	8.1	0.03
Apnea rate on day 2 (per 24 hrs.)	4.9	7.2	0.134
% of patients with 50% reduction in apnea events from baseline on day 2	76	57	0.07

[1]Of 85 patients who received drug, 3 were not included in the efficacy analysis because they had < 6 apnea episodes/24 hours at baseline.

Caffeine citrate
$C_{14}H_{18}N_4O_9$ Mol. Wt. 386.31

Although the mechanism of action of caffeine in apnea of prematurity is not known, several mechanisms have been hypothesized. These include: (1) stimulation of the respiratory center, (2) increased minute ventilation, (3) decreased threshold to hypercapnia, (4) increased response to hypercapnia, (5) increased skeletal muscle tone, (6) decreased diaphragmatic fatigue, (7) increased metabolic rate, and (8) increased oxygen consumption.

Most of these effects have been attributed to antagonism of adenosine receptors, both A_1 and A_2 subtypes, by caffeine, which has been demonstrated in receptor binding assays and observed at concentrations approximating those achieved therapeutically.

Pharmacokinetics

Absorption: After oral administration of 10 mg caffeine base/kg to preterm neonates, the peak plasma level (C_{max}) for caffeine ranged from 6–10 mg/L and the mean time to reach peak concentration (T_{max}) ranged from 30 minutes to 2 hours. The T_{max} was not affected by formula feeding. The absolute bioavailability; however, was not fully examined in preterm neonates.

Distribution: Caffeine is rapidly distributed into the brain. Caffeine levels in the cerebrospinal fluid of preterm neonates approximate their plasma levels. The mean volume of distribution of caffeine in infants (0.8–0.9 L/kg) is slightly higher than that in adults (0.6 L/kg). Plasma protein binding data are not available for neonates or infants. In adults, the mean plasma protein binding *in vitro* is reported to be approximately 36%.

Metabolism: Hepatic cytochrome P450 1A2 (CYP1A2) is involved in caffeine biotransformation. Caffeine metabolism in preterm neonates is limited due to their immature hepatic enzyme systems.

Interconversion between caffeine and theophylline has been reported in preterm neonates; caffeine levels are approximately 25% of theophylline levels after theophylline administration and approximately 3–8% of caffeine administered would be expected to convert to theophylline.

Elimination: In young infants, the elimination of caffeine is much slower than that in adults due to immature hepatic and/or renal function. Mean half-life ($T_{1/2}$) and fraction excreted unchanged in urine (A_e) of caffeine in infants have been shown to be inversely related to gestational/postconceptual age. In neonates, the $T_{1/2}$ is approximately 3–4 days and the A_e is approximately 86% (within 6 days). By 9 months of age, the metabolism of caffeine approximates that seen in adults ($T_{1/2}$ = 5 hours and A_e = 1%).

Special Populations: Studies examining the pharmacokinetics of caffeine in neonates with hepatic or renal insufficiency have not been conducted. CAFCIT® (caffeine citrate) should be administered with caution in preterm neonates with impaired renal or hepatic function.

Clinical Studies

One multicenter, randomized, double-blind trial compared CAFCIT® (caffeine citrate) to placebo in eighty-five (85) preterm infants (gestational age 28 to < 33 weeks) with apnea of prematurity. Apnea of prematurity was defined as having at least 6 apnea episodes of greater than 20 seconds duration in a 24-hour period with no other identifiable cause of apnea. A 1 mL/kg (20 mg/kg caffeine citrate providing 10 mg/kg as caffeine base) loading dose of CAFCIT® was administered intravenously, followed by a 0.25 mL/kg (5 mg/kg caffeine citrate providing 2.5 mg/kg of caffeine base) daily maintenance dose administered either intravenously or orally (generally through a feeding tube). The duration of treatment in this study was limited to 10 to 12 days. The protocol allowed infants to be "rescued" with open-label caffeine citrate treatment if their apnea remained uncontrolled during the double-blind phase of the trial.

The percentage of patients without apnea on day 2 of treatment (24–48 hours after the loading dose) was significantly greater with CAFCIT® than placebo. The following table summarizes the clinically relevant endpoints evaluated in this study:
[See table above]

In this 10–12 day trial, the mean number of days with zero apnea events was 3.0 in the CAFCIT® group and 1.2 in the placebo group. The mean number of days with a 50% reduction from baseline in apnea events was 6.8 in the CAFCIT® group and 4.6 in the placebo group.

INDICATIONS AND USAGE

CAFCIT® (caffeine citrate) is indicated for the short term treatment of apnea of prematurity in infants between 28 and <33 weeks gestational age.

CONTRAINDICATIONS

CAFCIT® (caffeine citrate) is contraindicated in patients who have demonstrated hypersensitivity to any of its components.

WARNINGS

During the double-blind, placebo-controlled clinical trial, six cases of necrotizing enterocolitis developed among the 85 infants studied (caffeine=46, placebo=39), with three cases resulting in death. Five of the six patients with necrotizing enterocolitis were randomized to or had been exposed to CAFCIT® (caffeine citrate).

Reports in the published literature have raised a question regarding the possible association between the use of methylxanthines and development of necrotizing enterocolitis, although a causal relationship between methylxanthine use and necrotizing enterocolitis has not been established. Therefore, as with all preterm infants, patients being treated with CAFCIT® should be carefully monitored for the development of necrotizing enterocolitis.

PRECAUTIONS

General

Apnea of prematurity is a diagnosis of exclusion. Other causes of apnea (e.g., central nervous system disorders, primary lung disease, anemia, sepsis, metabolic disturbances, cardiovascular abnormalities, or obstructive apnea) should be ruled out or properly treated prior to initiation of CAFCIT® (caffeine citrate).

Caffeine is a central nervous system stimulant and in cases of caffeine overdose, seizures have been reported. CAFCIT® should be used with caution in infants with seizure disorders.

The duration of treatment of apnea of prematurity in the placebo-controlled trial was limited to 10 to 12 days. The safety and efficacy of CAFCIT® for longer periods of treatment have not been established. Safety and efficacy of CAFCIT® for use in the prophylaxis treatment of sudden infant death syndrome (SIDS) or prior to extubation in mechanically ventilated infants have also not been established.

Cardiovascular

Although no cases of cardiac toxicity were reported in the placebo-controlled trial, caffeine has been shown to increase heart rate, left ventricular output, and stroke volume in published studies. Therefore, CAFCIT® should be used with caution in infants with cardiovascular disease.

Renal and Hepatic Systems

CAFCIT® should be administered with caution in infants with impaired renal or hepatic function. (See **CLINICAL PHARMACOLOGY**, *Elimination, Special Populations.*)

Information for Patients

Parents/caregivers of patients receiving CAFCIT® (caffeine citrate) Oral Solution should receive the following instructions:

1. CAFCIT® does not contain any preservatives and each vial is for single use only. Any unused portion of the medication should be discarded.
2. It is important that the dose of CAFCIT® be measured accurately, i.e., with a 1cc or other appropriate syringe.
3. Consult your physician if the baby continues to have apnea events; do not increase the dose of CAFCIT® without medical consultation.
4. Consult your physician if the baby begins to demonstrate signs of gastrointestinal intolerance, such as abdominal distention, vomiting, or bloody stools, or seems lethargic.
5. CAFCIT® should be inspected visually for particulate matter and discoloration prior to its administration. Vials containing discolored solution or visible particulate matter should be discarded.

Laboratory Tests

Prior to initiation of CAFCIT® (caffeine citrate), baseline serum levels of caffeine should be measured in infants previously treated with theophylline, since preterm infants metabolize theophylline to caffeine. Likewise, baseline serum levels of caffeine should be measured in infants born to mothers who consumed caffeine prior to delivery, since caffeine readily crosses the placenta.

In the placebo-controlled clinical trial, caffeine levels ranged from 8 to 40 mg/mL. A therapeutic plasma concentration range of caffeine could not be determined from the placebo-controlled clinical trial. Serious toxicity has been reported in the literature when serum caffeine levels exceed 50 mg/L. In clinical studies reported in the literature, cases of hypoglycemia and hyperglycemia have been observed. Therefore, serum glucose may need to be periodically monitored in infants receiving CAFCIT®.

Drug Interactions

Cytochrome P450 1A2 (CYP1A2) is known to be the major enzyme involved in the metabolism of caffeine. Therefore, caffeine has the potential to interact with drugs that are substrates for CYP1A2, inhibit CYP1A2, or induce CYP1A2.

Continued on next page

Cafcit—Cont.

Few data exist on drug interactions with caffeine in preterm neonates. Based on adult data, lower doses of caffeine may be needed following coadministration of drugs which are reported to decrease caffeine elimination (e.g., cimetidine and ketoconazole) and higher caffeine doses may be needed following coadministration of drugs that increase caffeine elimination (e.g., phenobarbital and phenytoin).

Caffeine administered concurrently with ketoprofen reduced the urine volume of 4 healthy volunteers. The clinical significance of this interaction in preterm neonates is not known.

Interconversion between caffeine and theophylline has been reported in preterm neonates. The concurrent use of these drugs is not recommended.

Carcinogenesis, Mutagenesis, Impairment of Fertility

In a 2-year study in Sprague-Dawley rats, caffeine (as caffeine base) administered in drinking water was not carcinogenic in male rats at doses up to 102 mg/kg or in female rats at doses up to 170 mg/kg (approximately 2 and 4 times, respectively, the maximum recommended intravenous loading dose for infants on a mg/m^2 basis). In an 18-month study in C57BL/6 mice, no evidence of tumorigenicity was seen at dietary doses up to 55 mg/kg (less than the maximum recommended intravenous loading dose for infants on a mg/m^2 basis).

Caffeine (as caffeine base) increased the sister chromatid exchange (SCE) SCE/cell metaphase (exposure time dependent) in an *in vivo* mouse metaphase analysis. Caffeine also potentiated genotoxicity of known mutagens and enhanced the micronuclei formation (5-fold) in folate-deficient mice. However, caffeine did not increase chromosomal aberrations in *in vitro* Chinese hamster ovary cell (CHO) and human lymphocyte assays and was not mutagenic in an *in vitro* CHO/hypoxanthine guanine phosphoribosyltransferease (HGPRT) gene mutation assay, except at cytotoxic concentrations In addition, caffeine was not clastogenic in an *in vivo* mouse micronucleus assay.

Caffeine (as caffeine base) administered to male rats at 50 mg/kg/day subcutaneously (approximately equal to the maximum recommended intravenous loading dose for infants on a mg/m^2 basis) for four days prior to mating with untreated females, caused decreased male reproductive performance in addition to causing embryotoxicity. In addition, long-term exposure to high oral doses of caffeine (3.0 g over 7 weeks) was toxic to rat testes as manifested by spermatogenic cell degeneration.

Pregnancy: Pregnancy Category C

Concern for the teratogenicity of caffeine is not relevant when administered to infants. In studies performed in adult animals, caffeine (as caffeine base) administered to pregnant mice as sustained-release pellets at 50 mg/kg (less than the maximum recommended intravenous loading dose for infants on a mg/m^2 basis), during the period of organogenesis, caused a low incidence of cleft palate and exencephaly in the fetuses. There are no adequate and well-controlled studies in pregnant women.

ADVERSE REACTIONS

Overall, the reported number of adverse events in the double-blind period of the controlled trial was similar for CAFCIT® (caffeine citrate) and placebo groups. The following table shows adverse events that occurred in the double-blind period of the controlled trial and that were more frequent in CAFCIT® treated patients than placebo.

[See first table above]

ADVERSE EVENTS THAT OCCURRED MORE FREQUENTLY IN CAFCIT® TREATED PATIENTS THAN PLACEBO DURING DOUBLE-BLIND THERAPY

Adverse Event (AE)	CAFCIT® N=46 n (%)	Placebo N=39 n (%)
BODY AS A WHOLE		
Accidental Injury	1 (2.2)	0 (0.0)
Feeding Intolerance	4 (8.7)	2 (5.1)
Sepsis	2 (4.3)	0 (0.0)
CARDIOVASCULAR SYSTEM		
Hemorrhage	1 (2.2)	0 (0.0)
DIGESTIVE SYSTEM		
Necrotizing Enterocolitis	2 (4.3)	1 (2.6)
Gastritis	1 (2.2)	0 (0.0)
Gastrointestinal Hemorrhage	1 (2.2)	0 (0.0)
HEMIC AND LYMPHATIC SYSTEM		
Disseminated Intravascular Coagulation	1 (2.2)	0 (0.0)
METABOLIC AND NUTRITIVE DISORDERS		
Acidosis	1 (2.2)	0 (0.0)
Healing Abnormal	1 (2.2)	0 (0.0)
NERVOUS SYSTEM		
Cerebral Hemorrhage	1 (2.2)	0 (0.0)
RESPIRATORY SYSTEM		
Dyspnea	1 (2.2)	0 (0.0)
Lung Edema	1 (2.2)	0 (0.0)
SKIN AND APPENDAGES		
Dry Skin	1 (2.2)	0 (0.0)
Rash	4 (8.7)	3 (7.7)
Skin Breakdown	1 (2.2)	0 (0.0)
SPECIAL SENSES		
Retinopathy of Prematurity	1 (2.2)	0 (0.0)
UROGENITAL SYSTEM		
Kidney Failure	1 (2.2)	0 (0.0)

In addition to the cases above, three cases of necrotizing enterocolitis were diagnosed in patients receiving CAFCIT® (caffeine citrate) during the open-label phase of the study.

Three of the infants who developed necrotizing enterocolitis during the trial died. All had been exposed to caffeine. Two were randomized to caffeine, and one placebo patient was "rescued" with open-label caffeine for uncontrolled apnea.

Adverse events described in the published literature include: central nervous system stimulation (i.e., irritability, restlessness, jitteriness), cardiovascular effects (i.e., tachycardia, increased left ventricular output, and increased stroke volume), gastrointestinal effects (i.e., increased gastric aspirate, gastrointestinal intolerance), alterations in serum glucose (hypoglycemia and hyperglycemia) and renal effects (increased urine flow rate, increased creatinine clearance, and increased sodium and calcium excretion). Published long-term follow-up studies have not shown caffeine to adversely affect neurological development of growth parameters.

OVERDOSAGE

Following overdose, serum caffeine levels have ranged from approximately 50 mg/L to 350 mg/L. Signs and symptoms reported in the literature after caffeine overdose in preterm infants include fever, tachypnea, jitteriness, fine tremor of the extremities, hypertonia, opisthotonos, tonic-clonic movements, nonpurposeful jaw and lip movements, vomiting, hyperglycemia, elevated blood urea nitrogen, and elevated total leukocyte concentration. Seizures have also been reported in cases of overdose. One case of caffeine overdose complicated by development of intraventricular hemorrhage and long-term neurological sequelae has been reported. No deaths associated with caffeine overdose have been reported in preterm infants.

Treatment of caffeine overdose is primarily symptomatic and supportive. Caffeine levels have been shown to decrease after exchange transfusions. Convulsions may be treated with intravenous administration of diazepam or a barbiturate such as pentobarbital sodium.

DOSAGE AND ADMINISTRATION

Prior to initiation of CAFCIT® (caffeine citrate), baseline serum levels of caffeine should be measured in infants previously treated with theophylline, since preterm infants metabolize theophylline to caffeine. Likewise, baseline serum levels of caffeine should be measured in infants born to mothers who consumed caffeine prior to delivery, since caffeine readily crosses the placenta.

The recommended loading dose and maintenance doses of CAFCIT® follow.

[See second table above]

	Dose of CAFCIT® (caffeine citrate) Volume	Dose of CAFCIT® (caffeine citrate) mg/kg	Route	Frequency
Loading Dose	1 mL/kg	20 mg/kg	Intravenous* (over 30 minutes)	One Time
Maintenance Dose	0.25 mL/kg	5 mg/kg	Intravenous* (over 10 minutes) or Orally	Every 24 hours†

* using a syringe infusion pump
† beginning 24 hours after the loading dose

NOTE THAT THE DOSE OF CAFFEINE BASE IS ONE-HALF THE DOSE WHEN EXPRESSED AS CAFFEINE CITRATE (e.g., 20 mg of caffeine citrate is equivalent to 10 mg of caffeine base).

Serum concentrations of caffeine may need to be monitored periodically throughout treatment to avoid toxicity. Serious toxicity has been associated with serum levels greater than 50 mg/L.

CAFCIT® should be inspected visually for particulate matter and discoloration prior to administration. Vials containing discolored solution or visible particulate matter should be discarded.

Drug Compatibility

To test for drug compatibility with common intravenous solutions or medications, twenty (20) mL of CAFCIT® (caffeine citrate) Injection were combined with 20 mL of a solution or medication, with the exception of an Intralipid® admixture, which was combined as 80 mL/80 mL. The physical appearance of the combined solutions was evaluated for precipitation. The admixtures were mixed for 10 minutes and then assayed for caffeine. The admixtures were then continually mixed for 24 hours, with further sampling for caffeine assays at 2, 4, 8, and 24 hours.

Based on this testing, CAFCIT® (caffeine citrate) Injection, 60 mg/3 mL is chemically stable for 24 hours at room temperature when combined with the following test products.

- Dextrose Injection, USP 5%
- 50% Dextrose Injection USP
- Intralipid® 20% IV Fat Emulsion
- Aminosyn® 8.5% Crystalline Amino Acid Solution
- Dopamine HCl Injection, USP 40 mg/mL diluted to 0.6 mg/mL with Dextrose Injection, USP 5%
- Calcium Gluconate Injection, USP 10% (0.465 mEq/Ca^{+2}/mL)
- Heparin Sodium Injection, USP 1000 units/mL diluted to 1 unit/mL with Dextrose Injection, USP 5%
- Fentanyl Citrate Injection, USP 50 μg/mL diluted to 10 μg/mL with Dextrose Injection, USP 5%

HOW SUPPLIED

Both CAFCIT® (caffeine citrate) Injection and CAFCIT® Oral Solution are available as clear, colorless, sterile, non-pyrogenic, preservative-free, aqueous solutions in 3 mL colorless glass vials. The vials of CAFCIT® Injection are sealed with a teflon-faced gray rubber stopper and an aluminum overseal with a white flip-off polypropylene disk inset. The vials of CAFCIT® Oral Solution are sealed with a teflon-faced gray rubber stopper and a peel-off aluminum overseal with a blue flip-off polypropylene disk inset.

Both the injection and oral solution vials contain 3 mL solution at a concentration of 20 mg/mL caffeine citrate (60 mg/vial) equivalent to 10 mg/mL caffeine base (30 mg/vial).

CAFCIT® (caffeine citrate) Injection
NDC 0054-8219-01: 3 mL vial, individually packaged in a carton.

CAFCIT® (caffeine citrate) Oral Solution
NDC 0054-8069-06: 3 mL vial (NOT CHILD RESISTANT), 10 vials per white polypropylene child-resistant container.

Store at 15°–30°C (59°–86°F).

Preservative Free. For single use only. Discard unused portion.

ATTENTION PHARMACIST: Detach "Instructions for Use" from the package insert and dispense with CAFCIT® (caffeine citrate) Oral Solution prescription.

Manufactured by:
Ben Venue Laboratories, Inc., Bedford, Ohio 44146.
Distributed by:
Roxane Laboratories, Inc., Columbus, Ohio 43216
4043450
040
 Revised April 2000

DOLOPHINE® HYDROCHLORIDE ℂ ℞

(Methadone Hydrochloride Tablets USP) 5 mg, 10 mg
Methadone Hydrochloride Injection USP 10 mg per mL

Rx only.

CONDITIONS FOR DISTRIBUTION AND USE OF METHADONE PRODUCTS:
Code of Federal Regulations,
Title 21, Sec. 291.505

METHADONE PRODUCTS, WHEN USED FOR TREATMENT OF NARCOTIC ADDICTION IN DETOXIFICATION OR MAINTENANCE PROGRAMS, SHALL BE DISPENSED ONLY BY APPROVED HOSPITAL PHARMACIES, APPROVED COMMUNITY PHARMACIES, AND MAINTENANCE PROGRAMS APPROVED BY THE FOOD AND DRUG ADMINISTRATION AND THE DESIGNATED STATE AUTHORITY.

APPROVED MAINTENANCE PROGRAMS SHALL DISPENSE AND USE METHADONE IN ORAL FORM ONLY AND ACCORDING TO THE TREATMENT REQUIREMENTS STIPULATED IN THE FEDERAL METHADONE REGULATIONS (21 CFR 291.505).

FAILURE TO ABIDE BY THE REQUIREMENTS IN THESE REGULATIONS MAY RESULT IN CRIMINAL PROSECUTION, SEIZURE OF THE DRUG SUPPLY, REVOCATION OF THE PROGRAM APPROVAL, AND INJUNCTION PRECLUDING OPERATION OF THE PROGRAM.

A METHADONE PRODUCT, WHEN USED AS AN ANALGESIC, MAY BE DISPENSED IN ANY LICENSED PHARMACY.

DESCRIPTION

Dolophine® Hydrochloride (Methadone Hydrochloride Tablets USP) (3-heptanone, 6-(dimethyl-amino)-4,4-diphenyl-,hydrochloride), is a white, essentially odorless, bitter-tasting powder. It is very soluble in water, soluble in isopropanol and in chloroform, and practically insoluble in ether and in glycerine. Methadone hydrochloride has a pKa of 8.25 in water at 20°C. Its molecular weight is 345.91 and it has the following structural formula.

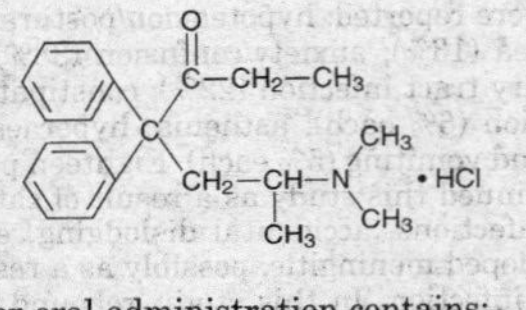

Each tablet for oral administration contains:
Methadone Hydrochloride .... 5 mg, 10 mg

Inactive Ingredients:
The tablets also contain magnesium stearate, microcrystalline cellulose and starch.
Each mL of the injection contains methadone hydrochloride 10 mg (0.029 mmol) and sodium chloride 0.9%. Sodium hydroxide and/or hydrochloric acid may have been added during manufacture to adjust the pH. The 20 mL vials also contain chlorobutanol (chloroform derivative), 0.5%, as a preservative.

HOW SUPPLIED

DOLOPHINE HYDROCHLORIDE®
(Methadone Hydrochloride Tablets USP)
5 mg white scored tablets (Identified 54 162).
NDC 0054-4218-25: Bottles of 100 tablets.
NDC 0054-8218-24: Unit dose, 25 tablets per card (reverse numbered), 4 cards per shipper
10 mg white scored tablets (Identified 54 549).
NDC 0054-4219-25: Bottles of 100 tablets.
NDC 0054-8219-24: Unit dose, 25 tablets per card (reverse numbered), 4 cards per shipper
DOLOPHINE HYDROCHLORIDE®
(Methadone Hydrochloride Injection USP)
10 mg per mL, Multiple-Dose Vials.
NDC 0054-1218-42: Single 20 mL multiple-dose vials.
Store at 25°C (77°F); excursions permitted to 15°–30°C (59°–86°F) [see USP Controlled Room Temperature].
Dispense in a tight, light-resistant container as defined in the USP/NF.

DURACLON™ ℞

[dūră clŏn]
clonidine hydrochloride injection

The 500 µg/mL strength product should be diluted prior to use in an appropriate solution.

NOTE: Duraclon™ (epidural clonidine) is not recommended for obstetrical, post-partum, or peri-operative pain management. The risk of hemodynamic instability, especially hypotension and bradycardia, from epidural clonidine may be unacceptable in these patients. However, in a rare obstetrical, post-partum or peri-operative patient, potential benefits may outweigh the possible risks.

DESCRIPTION

Duraclon (clonidine hydrochloride injection) is a centrally-acting analgesic for use in continuous epidural infusion devices.
Clonidine Hydrochloride, USP, is an imidazoline derivative and exists as a mesomeric compound. The chemical names are Benzenamine, 2,6-dichloro-N-2-imidazolindinylidene-monohydrochloride and 2-[(2, 6-dichlorophenyl)imino]imidazolidine monohydrochloride. The following is the structural formula:

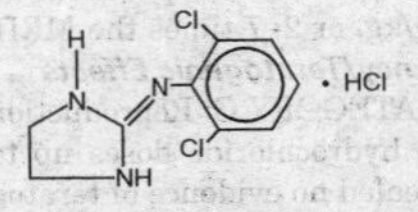

$C_9H_9Cl_2N_3 \cdot HCl$ Mol. Wt. 266.56

Duraclon (clonidine hydrochloride injection) is supplied as a clear, colorless, preservative-free, pyrogen-free, aqueous sterile solution (pH 5 to 7) in a single-dose, 10 mL vial. Each mL of the 100 µg/mL (0.1 mg/mL) concentration contains 100 µg of Clonidine Hydrochloride, USP and 9 mg Sodium Chloride, USP in Water for Injection, USP. Hydrochloric Acid and/or Sodium Hydroxide may have been added for pH adjustment. Each 10 mL vial contains 1 mg (1000 µg) of clonidine hydrochloride. Each mL of the 500 µg/mL (0.5 mg/mL) concentration contains 500 µg of Clonidine Hydrochloride, USP and 9 mg Sodium Chloride, USP in Water for injection, USP. Hydrochloric Acid and/or Sodium Hydroxide may have been added for pH adjustment. Each 10 mL vial contains 5 mg (5000 µg) of clonidine hydrochloride.

CLINICAL PHARMACOLOGY

Mechanism of Action

Epidurally administered clonidine produces dose-dependent analgesia not antagonized by opiate antagonists. The analgesia is limited to the body regions innervated by the spinal segments where analgesic concentrations of clonidine are present. Clonidine is thought to produce analgesia at presynaptic and postjunctional alpha-2-adrenoceptors in the spinal cord by preventing pain signal transmission to the brain.

Pharmacokinetics

Following a 10 minute intravenous infusion of 300 mcg clonidine HCl to five male volunteers, plasma clonidine levels showed an initial rapid distribution phase (mean±SD $t_{1/2}$=11±9 minutes) followed by a slower elimination phase ($t_{1/2}$=9±2 hours) over 24 hours. Clonidine's total body clearance (CL) was 219±92 mL/min.
Following a 700 mcg clonidine HCl epidural dose given over five minutes to four male and five female volunteers, peak clonidine plasma levels (4.4±1.4 ng/mL) were obtained in 19±27 minutes. The plasma elimination half-life was determined to be 22±15 hours following sample collection for 24 hours. CL was 190±70 mL/min. In cerebral spinal fluid (CSF), peak clonidine levels (418±255 ng/mL) were achieved in 26±11 minutes. The clonidine CSF elimination half-life was 1.3±0.5 hours when samples were collected for 6 hours. Compared to men, women had a lower mean plasma clearance, longer mean plasma half-life, and higher mean peak level of clonidine in both plasma and CSF.
In cancer patients who received 14 days of clonidine HCl epidural infusion (rate=30 mcg/hr) plus morphine by patient-controlled analgesia (PCA), steady state clonidine plasma concentrations of 2.2±1.1 and 2.4±1.4 ng/mL were obtained on dosing days 7 and 14, respectively. CL was 279±184 and 272±163 mL/min on these days. CSF concentrations were not determined in these patients.

Distribution

Clonidine is highly lipid soluble and readily distributes into extravascular sites including the central nervous system. Clonidine's volume of distribution is 2.1±0.4 L/kg. The binding of clonidine to plasma protein is primarily to albumin and varies between 20 and 40% *in vitro*. Epidurally administered clonidine readily partitions into plasma via the epidural veins and attains systemic concentrations (0.5–2.0 ng/mL) that are associated with a hypotensive effect mediated by the central nervous system.

Excretion

Following an intravenous dose of ^{14}C-clonidine, 72% of the administered dose was excreted in urine in 96 hours of which 40–50% was unchanged clonidine. Renal clearance for clonidine was determined to be 133±66 mL/min. In a study where ^{14}C-clonidine was given to subjects with varying degrees of kidney function, elimination half-lives varied (17.5 to 41 hours) as a function of creatinine clearance. In subjects undergoing hemodialysis only 5% of body clonidine stores was removed.

Metabolism

In humans, clonidine metabolism follows minor pathways with the major metabolite, p-hydroxyclonidine, being present at less than 10% of the concentration of unchanged drug in urine.

Special Populations

The pharmacokinetics of epidurally administered clonidine has not been studied in the pediatric population or in patients with renal or hepatic disease.

Clinical Trials

In a double-blind, randomized study of cancer patients with severe intractable pain below the C4 dermatome not controlled by morphine, 38 patients were randomized to an epidural infusion of Duraclon plus epidural morphine, whereas 47 subjects received epidural placebo plus epidural morphine. Both groups were allowed rescue doses of epidural morphine. Successful analgesia, defined as a decrease in either morphine use or Visual Analog Score (VAS) pain, was significantly more common with epidural clonidine than placebo (45% vs 21%, p=0.016). Only the subgroup of 36 patients with "neuropathic" pain, characterized by the investigator as well-localized, burning, shooting, or electric-like pain in a dermatomal or peripheral nerve distribution had significant analgesic effects relative to placebo in this study. The most frequent adverse events with clonidine were hypotension (45% vs 11% for placebo, p< 0.001), postural hypotension (32% vs 0%, p< 0.001), dizziness (13% vs 4%, p=0.234), anxiety (11% vs 2%, p=0.168) and dry mouth (13% vs 9%, p=0.505). Both mean blood pressure and heart rate were reduced in the clonidine group. At the conclusion of the two week study period in the clinical trial, all patients were abruptly withdrawn from study drug or placebo. Four patients of the clonidine group suffered rebound hypertension upon withdrawal of clonidine; one of these patients suffered a cerebrovascular accident. Asymptomatic bradycardia was noted in one clonidine patient.

INDICATIONS AND USAGE

Duraclon is indicated in combination with opiates for the treatment of severe pain in cancer patients that is not adequately relieved by opioid analgesics alone. Epidural clonidine is more likely to be effective in patients with neuropathic pain than somatic or visceral pain (see ***Clinical Trials***).
The safety of this drug product has only been established in a highly selected group of cancer patients, and only after an adequate trial of opioid analgesia. Other use is of unproven safety and is not recommended. In a rare patient, the potential benefits may outweigh the known risks (see **WARNINGS**).

CONTRAINDICATIONS

Duraclon is contraindicated in patients with a history of sensitization or allergic reactions to clonidine. Epidural administration is contraindicated in the presence of an injection site infection, in patients on anticoagulant therapy, and in those with a bleeding diathesis. Administration of Duraclon above the C4 dermatome is contraindicated since there are no adequate safety data to support such use. (See **WARNINGS**).

WARNINGS

Use in Postoperative or Obstetrical Analgesia

Duraclon (epidural clonidine) is not recommended for obstetrical, post-partum, or perioperative pain management. The risk of hemodynamic instability, especially hypotension and bradycardia, from epidural clonidine may be unacceptable in these patients.

Hypotension

Because severe hypotension may follow the administration of clonidine, it should be used with caution in all patients. It is not recommended in most patients with severe cardiovascular disease or in those who are otherwise hemodynamically unstable. The benefit of its administration in these patients should be carefully balanced against the potential risks resulting from hypotension.
Vital signs should be monitored frequently, especially during the first few days of epidural clonidine therapy. When clonidine is infused into the upper thoracic spinal segments, more pronounced decreases in the blood pressure may be seen.
Clonidine decreases sympathetic outflow from the central nervous system resulting in decreases in peripheral resistance, renal vascular resistance, heart rate, and blood pressure. However, in the absence of profound hypotension, renal blood flow and glomerular filtration rate remain essentially unchanged.
In the pivotal double-blind, randomized study of cancer patients, where 38 subjects were administered epidural Duraclon at 30 mcg/hr in addition to epidural morphine, hypotension occurred in 45% of subjects. Most episodes of hypotension occurred within the first four days after beginning epidural clonidine. However, hypotensive episodes occurred throughout the duration of the trial. There was a tendency for these episodes to occur more commonly in women, and in those with higher serum clonidine levels. Patients experiencing hypotension also tended to weigh less than those who did not experience hypotension. The hypotension usually responded to intravenous fluids and, if necessary, parenteral ephedrine.
Published reports on the use of epidural clonidine for intraoperative or postoperative analgesia also show a consistent and marked hypotensive response to clonidine. Severe hypotension may occur even if intravenous fluid pretreatment is given.

Withdrawal

Sudden cessation of clonidine treatment, regardless of the route of administration, has, in some cases, resulted in symptoms such as nervousness, agitation, headache, and tremor, accompanied or followed by a rapid rise in blood

Continued on next page

Duraclon—Cont.

pressure. The likelihood of such reactions appears to be greater after administration of higher doses or with concomitant beta-blocker treatment. Special caution is therefore advised in these situations. Rare instances of hypertensive encephalopathy, cerebrovascular accidents and death have been reported after abrupt clonidine withdrawal. Patients with a history of hypertension and/or other underlying cardiovascular conditions may be at particular risk of the consequences of abrupt discontinuation of clonidine. In the pivotal double-blind, randomized cancer pain study, four of 38 subjects receiving 720 mcg of clonidine per day experienced rebound hypertension following abrupt withdrawal. One of these patients with rebound hypertension subsequently experienced a cerebrovascular accident.
Careful monitoring of infusion pump function and inspection of catheter tubing for obstruction or dislodgment can help reduce the risk of inadvertent abrupt withdrawal of epidural clonidine. Patients should notify their physician immediately if clonidine administration is inadvertently interrupted for any reason. Patients should also be instructed not to discontinue therapy without consulting their physician.
When discontinuing therapy with epidural clonidine, the physician should reduce the dose gradually over 2 to 4 days to avoid withdrawal symptoms.
An excessive rise in blood pressure following discontinuation of epidural clonidine can be treated by administration of clonidine or by intravenous phentolamine. If therapy is to be discontinued in patients receiving a beta-blocker and clonidine concurrently, the beta-blocker should be withdrawn several days before the gradual discontinuation of epidural clonidine.

Infections

Infections related to implantable epidural catheters pose a serious risk. Evaluation of fever in a patient receiving epidural clonidine should include the possibility of a catheter-related infection such as meningitis or epidural abscess.

PRECAUTIONS

General

Cardiac Effects: Epidural clonidine frequently causes decreases in heart rate. Symptomatic bradycardia can be treated with atropine. Rarely, atrioventricular block greater than first degree has been reported. Clonidine does not alter the hemodynamic response to exercise, but may mask the increase in heart rate associated with hypovolemia.
Respiratory Depression and Sedation: Clonidine administration may result in sedation through the activation of alpha-adrenoceptors in the brainstem. High doses of clonidine cause sedation and ventilatory abnormalities that are usually mild. Tolerance to these effects can develop with chronic administration. These effects have been reported with bolus doses that are significantly larger than the infusion rate recommended for treating cancer patients.
Depression: Depression has been seen in a small percentage of patients treated with oral or transdermal clonidine. Depression commonly occurs in cancer patients and may be exacerbated by treatment with clonidine. Patients, especially those with a known history of affective disorders, should be monitored for the signs and symptoms of depression.
Pain of Visceral or Somatic Origin: In the clinical investigations, at doses tested, Duraclon was most effective in well-localized, "neuropathic" pain that was characterized as electrical, burning, or shooting in nature, and which was localized to a dermatomal or peripheral nerve distribution. Duraclon may be less effective, or possibly ineffective in the treatment of pain that is diffuse, poorly localized, or visceral in origin.

Information for Patients

Patients should be instructed about the risks of rebound hypertension and warned not to discontinue clonidine except under the supervision of a physician. Patients should notify their physician immediately if clonidine administration is inadvertently interrupted for any reason. Patients who engage in potentially hazardous activities, such as operating machinery or driving, should be advised of the potential sedative and hypotensive effects of epidural clonidine. They should also be informed that sedative effects may be increased by CNS-depressing drugs such as alcohol and barbiturates, and that hypotensive effects may be increased by opiates.

Drug Interactions

Clonidine may potentiate the CNS-depressive effect of alcohol, barbiturates or other sedating drugs. Narcotic analgesics may potentiate the hypotensive effects of clonidine. Tricyclic antidepressants may antagonize the hypotensive effects of clonidine. The effects of tricyclic antidepressants on clonidine's analgesic actions are not known.
Beta blockers may exacerbate the hypertensive response seen with clonidine withdrawal. Also, due to the potential for additive effects such as bradycardia and AV block, caution is warranted in patients receiving clonidine with agents known to affect sinus node function or AV nodal conduction, e.g., digitalis, calcium channel blockers, and beta-blockers.
There is one reported case of a patient with acute delirium associated with the simultaneous use of fluphenazine and oral clonidine. Symptoms resolved when clonidine was withdrawn and recurred when the patient was rechallenged with clonidine.

Epidural clonidine may prolong the duration of pharmacologic effects of epidural local anesthetics, including both sensory and motor blockade.

Carcinogenesis, Mutagenesism, Impairment of Fertility

In a 132-week study in rats, clonidine hydrochloride administered as a dietary admixture at 5–8 times (based on body surface area) the 50 mcg/kg maximum recommended daily human dose (MRDHD) for hypertension did not show any carcinogenic potential. Clonidine was inactive in the Ames test of mutagenicity.
Fertility of male or female rats was unaffected by oral clonidine hydrochloride doses as high as 150 mcg/kg, or about 0.5 times the MRDHD. Fertility of female rats did, however, appear to be affected in another experiment at oral dose levels of 500–2000 mcg/kg, or 2–7 times the MRDHD.

Usage in Pregnancy/Teratogenic Effects

PREGNANCY CATEGORY C: Reproduction studies in rabbits at clonidine hydrochloride doses up to approximately the MRDHD revealed no evidence of teratogenic or embryotoxic potential. In rats, however, doses as low as one-third the MRDHD were associated with increased resorptions in a study in which dams were treated continuously from 2 months prior to mating. Increased resorptions were not associated with treatment with the same or higher doses up to 0.5 times the MRDHD when dams were treated on days 6–15 of gestation. Increased resorptions were observed at higher levels (7-times the MRDHD) in rats and mice treated on days 1–14 of gestation.
Clonidine readily crosses the placenta and its concentrations are equal in maternal and umbilical cord plasma; amniotic fluid concentrations can be 4-times those found in serum. There are no adequate and well-controlled studies in pregnant women during early gestation when organ formation takes place. Studies using epidural clonidine during labor have demonstrated no apparent adverse effects on the infant at the time of delivery. However, these studies did not monitor the infants for hemodynamic effects in the days following delivery. Clonidine hydrochloride injection should be used during pregnancy only if the potential benefits justify the potential risk to the fetus.

Labor and Delivery

There are no adequate controlled clinical trials evaluating the safety, efficacy, and dosing of Duraclon in obstetrical settings. Because maternal perfusion of the placenta is critically dependent on blood pressure, use of Duraclon as an analgesic during labor and delivery is not indicated (see **WARNINGS**).

Nursing Mothers

Concentrations of clonidine in human breast milk are approximately twice those found in maternal plasma. Caution should be exercised when clonidine is administered to a nursing women. Because of the potential for severe adverse reactions in nursing infants, a decision should be made to either discontinue nursing or to discontinue clonidine.

Pediatric Use

The safety and effectiveness of Duraclon in this limited indication and clinical population have been established in patients old enough to tolerate placement and management of an epidural catheter, based on evidence from adequate and well controlled studies in adults and experience with the use of clonidine in the pediatric age group for other indications. The use of Duraclon should be restricted to pediatric patients with severe intractable pain from malignancy that is unresponsive to epidural or spinal opiates or other more conventional analgesic techniques. The starting dose of Duraclon should be selected on per kilogram basis (0.5 mcg per kg per hour) and cautiously adjusted based on the clinical response.

ADVERSE REACTIONS

Adverse reactions seen during continuous epidural clonidine infusion are dose-dependent and typical for a compound of this pharmacologic class. The adverse events most frequently reported in the pivotal controlled clinical trial of continuous epidural clonidine administration consisted of hypotension, postural hypotension, decreased heart rate, rebound hypertension, dry mouth, nausea, confusion, dizziness, somnolence, and fever. Hypotension is the adverse event that most frequently requires treatment. The hypotension is usually responsive to intravenous fluids and, if necessary, parenterally-administered ephedrine. Hypotension was observed more frequently in women and in lower weight patients, but no dose-related response was established.
Implantable epidural catheters are associated with a risk of catheter-related infections, including meningitis and/or epidural abscess. The risk depends on the clinical situation and the type of catheter used, but catheter related infections occur in 5%–20% of patients, depending on the kind of catheter used, catheter placement techniques, quality of catheter care, and length of catheter placement.
The inadvertent intrathecal administration of clonidine has not been associated with a significantly increased risk of adverse events, but there are inadequate safety and efficacy data to support the use of intrathecal clonidine.
Epidural clonidine was compared to placebo in a two week double-blind study of 85 terminal cancer patients with intractable pain receiving epidural morphine. The following adverse events were reported in two or more patients and may be related to administration of either Duraclon or morphine.

Incidence of Adverse Events in the Two-Week Trial

Adverse Events	Clonidine N = 38 n (%)	Placebo N = 47 n (%)
Total Number of Patients Who Experienced At Least One Adverse Event	37 (97.4)	38 (80.5)
Hypotension	17 (44.8)	5 (10.6)
Postural Hypotension	12 (31.6)	0 (0)
Dry Mouth	5 (13.2)	4 (8.5)
Nausea	5 (13.2)	10 (21.3)
Somnolence	5 (13.2)	10 (21.3)
Dizziness	5 (13.2)	2 (4.3)
Confusion	5 (13.2)	5 (10.6)
Vomiting	4 (10.5)	7 (14.9)
Nausea/Vomiting	3 (7.9)	1 (2.1)
Sweating	2 (5.3)	0 (0)
Chest Pain	2 (5.3)	0 (0)
Hallucination	2 (5.3)	1 (2.1)
Tinnitus	2 (5.3)	0 (0)
Constipation	1 (2.6)	2 (4.3)
Tachycardia	1 (2.6)	2 (4.3)
Hypoventilation	1 (2.6)	2 (4.3)

An open label long-term extension of the above trial was performed. Thirty-two subjects received epidural clonidine and morphine for up to 94 weeks with a median dosing period of 10 weeks. The following adverse events (and percent incidence) were reported: hypotension/postural hypotension (47%); nausea (13%); anxiety/confusion (38%); somnolence (25%); urinary tract infection (22%); constipation, dyspnea, fever, infection (6% each); asthenia, hyperaesthesia, pain, skin ulcer, and vomiting (5% each). Eighteen percent of subjects discontinued this study as a result of catheter-related problems (infections, accidental dislodging, etc.), and one subject developed meningitis, possibly as a result of a catheter-related infection. In this study, rebound hypertension was not assessed, and ECG and laboratory data were not systematically sought.
The following adverse reactions have also been reported with the use of any dosage form of clonidine. In many cases patients were receiving concomitant medication and a causal relationship has not been established:
Body as a Whole: Weakness, 10%; fatigue, 4%; headache and withdrawal syndrome, each 1%. Also reported were pallor, a weakly positive Coomb's test, and increased sensitivity to alcohol.
Cardiovascular: Palpitations and tachycardia, and bradycardia, each 0.5%. Syncope, Raynaud's phenomenon, congestive heart failure, and electrocardiographic abnormalities (i.e., sinus node arrest, functional bradycardia, high degree AV block) have been reported rarely. Rare cases of sinus bradycardia and atrioventricular block have been reported, both with and without the use of concomitant digitalis.
Central Nervous System: Nervousness and agitation, 3%; mental depression, 1%; insomnia, 0.5%. Cerebrovascular accidents, other behavioral changes, vivid dreams or nightmares, restlessness, and delirium have been reported rarely.
Dermatological: Rash, 1%; pruritus, 0.7%; hives, angioneurotic edema and urticaria, 0.5%; alopecia, 0.2%.
Gastrointestinal: Anorexia and malaise, each 1%; mild transient abnormalities in liver function tests, 1%; hepatitis, parotitis, ileus and pseudoobstruction, and abdominal pain, rarely.
Genitourinary: Decreased sexual activity, impotence, and libido, 3%; nocturia, about 1%; difficulty in micturition, about 0.2%; urinary retention, about 0.1%.
Hematologic: Thrombocytopenia, rarely.
Metabolic: Weight gain, 0.1%; gynecomastia, 1%; transient elevation of glucose or serum phosphatase, rarely.
Musculoskeletal: Muscle or joint pain, about 0.6%; leg cramps, 0.3%.
Oro-otolaryngeal: Dryness of the nasal mucosa was rarely reported.
Ophthalmological: Dryness of the eyes, burning of the eyes and blurred vision were rarely reported.

OVERDOSAGE

Hypertension may develop early and may be followed by hypotension, bradycardia, respiratory depression, hypothermia, drowsiness, decreased or absent reflexes, irritability, and miosis. With large oral overdoses, reversible cardiac conduction defects or arrhythmias, apnea, coma, and seizures have been reported. As little as 100 mcg of oral clonidine has produced signs of toxicity in pediatric patients.

There is no specific antidote for clonidine overdosage. Supportive care may include atropine sulfate for bradycardia, intravenous fluids and/or vasopressor agents for hypotension. Hypertension associated with overdosage has been treated with intravenous furosemide, diazoxide, or alpha-blocking agents such as phentolamine.
Naloxone may be a useful adjunct in the treatment of clonidine-induced respiratory depression, hypotension, and/or coma; blood pressure should be monitored since the administration of naloxone has occasionally resulted in paradoxical hypertension. Tolazoline administration has yielded inconsistent results and is not recommended as first-line therapy. Dialysis is not likely to significantly enhance the elimination of clonidine.
The largest overdose reported to date involved a 28-year old white male who ingested 100 mg of clonidine hydrochloride powder. This patient developed hypertension followed by hypotension, bradycardia, apnea, hallucinations, semicoma, and premature ventricular contractions. The patient fully recovered after intensive treatment. Plasma clonidine levels were 60 ng/mL after 1 hour, 190 ng/mL after 1.5 hours, 370 ng/mL after 2 hours, and 120 ng/mL after 5.5 and 6.5 hours. In mice and rats, the oral LD50 of clonidine is 206 and 465 mg/kg, respectively.

DOSAGE AND ADMINISTRATION

The recommended starting dose of Duraclon for continuous epidural infusion is 30 mcg/hr. Although dosage may be titrated up or down depending on pain relief and occurrence of adverse events, experience with dosage rates above 40 mcg/hr is limited.
Familiarization with the continuous epidural infusion device is essential. Patients receiving epidural clonidine from a continuous infusion device should be closely monitored for the first few days to assess their response.
The 500μg/mL (0.5 mg/mL) strength product must be diluted prior to use in 0.9% Sodium Chloride for Injection, U.S.P., to a final concentration of 100 μg/mL:

Volume of Duraction 500 μg/mL	Volume of 0.9% Sodium Chloride for injection, U.S.P.	Resulting Final Duraclon Concentration (100 μg/mL)
1 mL	4 mL	500 μg/5 mL
2 mL	8 mL	1000 μg/10 mL
3 mL	12 mL	1500 μg/15 mL
4 mL	16 mL	2000 μg/20 mL
5 mL	20 mL	2500 μg/25 mL
6 mL	24 mL	3000 μg/30 mL
7 mL	28 mL	3500 μg/35 mL
8 mL	32 mL	4000 μg/40 mL
9mL	36 mL	4500 μg/45 mL
10 mL	40 mL	5000 μg/50 mL

Renal Impairment: Dosage should be adjusted according to the degree of renal impairment, and patients should be carefully monitored. Since only a minimal amount of clonidine is removed during routine hemodialysis, there is no need to give supplemental clonidine following dialysis.

Duraclon must *not* be used with a preservative.
Parenteral drug products should be inspected visually for particulate matter and discoloration prior to administration, whenever solution and container permit.

HOW SUPPLIED

NDC 0054-8233-01 100 mcg/mL solution in 10 mL vials, packaged individually.
NDC 0054-8234-01 500 μg/mL solution in 10 mL vials, packaged individually.
Store at 25°C controlled room temperature, see USP.
Preservative Free. Discard unused portion.
Manufactured for:
Roxane Laboratories, Inc.
By: American Pharmaceutical Partners, Inc.
Los Angeles, CA 90024
456320/Revised: May 2000
010
Roxane Laboratories, Inc.
Columbus, Ohio 43216

LITHIUM CARBONATE ℞

CAPSULES USP 150 mg, 300 mg, and 600 mg
TABLETS USP 300 mg
Rx only

WARNING

Lithium toxicity is closely related to serum lithium levels, and can occur at doses close to therapeutic levels. Facilities for prompt and accurate serum lithium determinations should be available before initiating therapy.

DESCRIPTION

Each tablet for oral administration contains:
Lithium Carbonate .... 300 mg
Each capsule for oral administration contains:
Lithium Carbonate .... 150 mg, 300 mg, or 600 mg

Inactive Ingredients:
The capsules contain talc, gelatin, FD&C Red No. 40, titanium dioxide, and the imprinting ink contains FD&C Blue No. 2, FD&C Yellow No. 6, FD&C Red No. 40, synthetic black iron oxide, and pharmaceutical glaze. The tablets contain calcium stearate, microcrystalline cellulose, povidone, sodium lauryl sulfate, and sodium starch glycolate.
Lithium is an element of the alkali-metal group with atomic number 3, atomic weight 6.94 and an emission line at 671 nm on the flame photometer.
Lithium Carbonate is a white, light alkaline powder with molecular formula Li_2CO_3 and molecular weight 73.89. Lithium acts as an antimanic.

CLINICAL PHARMACOLOGY

Preclinical studies have shown that lithium alters sodium transport in nerve and muscle cells and effects a shift toward intraneuronal metabolism of catecholamines, but the specific biochemical mechanism of lithium action in mania is unknown.

INDICATIONS AND USAGE

Lithium carbonate is indicated in the treatment of manic episodes of Bipolar Disorder. Bipolar Disorder, Manic (DSM-III) is equivalent to Manic Depressive illness, Manic, in the older DSM-II terminology.
Lithium is also indicated as a maintenance treatment for individuals with a diagnosis of Bipolar Disorder. Maintenance therapy reduces the frequency of manic episodes and diminishes the intensity of those episodes which may occur. Typical symptoms of mania include pressure of speech, motor hyperactivity, reduced need for sleep, flight of ideas, grandiosity elation, or poor judgment, aggressiveness, and possibly hostility. When given to a patient experiencing a manic episode, lithium may produce a normalization of symptomatology within 1 to 3 weeks.

CONTRAINDICATIONS

Lithium should generally not be given to patients with significant renal or cardiovascular disease, severe debilitation or dehydration, or sodium depletion, and to patients receiving diuretics, since the risk of lithium toxicity is very high in such patients. If the psychiatric indication is life-threatening, and if such a patient fails to respond to other measures, lithium treatment may be undertaken with extreme caution, including daily serum lithium determinations and adjustment to the usually low doses ordinarily tolerated by these individuals. In such instances, hospitalization is a necessity.

WARNINGS

Lithium may cause fetal harm when administered to a pregnant woman. There have been reports of lithium having adverse effects on nidations in rats, embryo viability in mice, and metabolism in-vitro of rat testis and human spermatozoa have been attributed to lithium, as have teratogenicity in submammalian species and cleft palates in mice. Studies in rats, rabbits and monkeys have shown no evidence of lithium-induced teratology. Data from lithium birth registries suggest an increase in cardiac and other anomalies, especially Ebstein's anomaly. If the patient becomes pregnant while taking lithium, she should be apprised of the potential risk to the fetus. If possible, lithium should be withdrawn for at least the first trimester unless it is determined that this would seriously endanger the mother.
Chronic lithium therapy may be associated with diminution of renal concentrating ability, occasionally presenting as nephrogenic diabetes insipidus, with polyuria and polydipsia. Such patients should be carefully managed to avoid dehydration with resulting lithium retention and toxicity. This condition is usually reversible when lithium is discontinued. Morphologic changes with glomerular and interstitial fibrosis and nephron-atrophy have been reported in patients on chronic lithium therapy. Morphologic changes have also been seen in bipolar patients never exposed to lithium. The relationship between renal functional and morphologic changes and their association with lithium therapy has not been established. To date, lithium in therapeutic doses has not been reported to cause end-stage renal disease.
When kidney function is assessed, for baseline data prior to starting lithium therapy or thereafter, routine urinalysis and other tests may be used to evaluate tubular function (e.g., urine specific gravity or osmolality following a period of water deprivation, or 24-hour urine volume) and glomerular function (e.g., serum creatinine or creatinine clearance). During lithium therapy, progressive or sudden changes in renal function, even within the normal range, indicate the need for reevaluation of treatment.
Lithium toxicity is closely related to serum lithium levels, and can occur at doses close to therapeutic levels (see DOSAGE AND ADMINISTRATION).

PRECAUTIONS

General: The ability to tolerate lithium is greater during the acute manic phase and decreases when manic symptoms subside (See DOSAGE AND ADMINISTRATION).
The distribution space of lithium approximates that of total body water. Lithium is primarily excreted in urine with insignificant excretion in feces. Renal excretion of lithium is proportional to its plasma concentration. The half-life of elimination of lithium is approximately 24 hours. Lithium decreases sodium reabsorption by the renal tubules which could lead to sodium depletion. Therefore, it is essential for the patient to maintain a normal diet, including salt, and an adequate fluid intake (2500-3000 mL) at least during the initial stabilization period. Decreased tolerance to lithium has been reported to ensue from protracted sweating or diarrhea and, if such occur, supplemental fluid and salt should be administered.
In addition to sweating and diarrhea, concomitant infection with elevated temperatures may also necessitate a temporary reduction or cessation of medication.
Previously existing underlying thyroid disorders do not necessarily constitute a contraindication to lithium treatment; where hypothyroidism exists, careful monitoring of thyroid function during lithium stabilization and maintenance allows for correction of changing thyroid parameters, if any. Where hypothyroidism occurs during lithium stabilization and maintenance, supplemental thyroid treatment may be used.
Information for the patients: Outpatients and their families should be warned that the patient must discontinue lithium therapy and contact his physician if such clinical signs of lithium toxicity as diarrhea, vomiting, tremor, mild ataxia, drowsiness, or muscular weakness occur.
Lithium may impair mental and/or physical abilities. Caution patients about activities requiring alertness (e.g., operating vehicles or machinery).
Drug interactions: Combined use of haloperidol and lithium: An encephalopathic syndrome (characterized by weakness, lethargy, fever, tremulousness and confusion, extrapyramidal symptoms, leucocytosis, elevated serum enzymes, BUN and FBS) followed by irreversible brain damage has occurred in a few patients treated with lithium plus haloperidol. A causal relationship between these events and the concomitant administration of lithium and haloperidol has not been established; however, patients receiving such combined therapy should be monitored closely for early evidence of neurological toxicity and treatment discontinued promptly if such signs appear.
The possibility of similar adverse interactions with other antipsychotic medication exists.
Lithium may prolong the effects of neuromuscular blocking agents. Therefore, neuromuscular blocking agents should be given with caution to patients receiving lithium.
Indomethacin and piroxicam have been reported to increase significantly steady state plasma lithium levels. In some cases lithium toxicity has resulted from such interactions. There is also evidence that other non-steroidal, anti-inflammatory agents may have a similar effect. When such combinations are used, increased plasma lithium level monitoring is recommended.
Caution should be used when lithium and diuretics or angiotensin converting enzyme (ACE) inhibitors are used concomitantly because sodium loss may reduce the renal clearance of lithium and increase serum lithium levels with risk of lithium toxicity. When such combinations are used, the lithium dosage may need to be decreased, and more frequent monitoring of lithium plasma levels is recommended.
Pregnancy: Teratogenic effects—Pregnancy Category D, See WARNINGS section.
Nursing mothers: Lithium is excreted in human milk. Nursing should not be undertaken during lithium therapy except in rare and unusual circumstances where, in the view of the physician, the potential benefits to the mother outweigh possible hazards to the child.
Usage in Children: Since information regarding the safety and effectiveness of lithium in children under 12 years of age is not available, its use in such patients is not recommended at this time. There has been a report of a transient syndrome of acute dystonia and hyperreflexia occurring in a 15 kg child who ingested 300 mg lithium carbonate.

ADVERSE REACTIONS

Lithium toxicity: The likelihood of toxicity increases with increasing serum lithium levels. Serum lithium levels greater than 1.5 mEq/l carry a greater risk than lower levels. However, patients sensitive to lithium may exhibit toxic signs at serum levels below 1.5 mEq/l.
Diarrhea, vomiting, drowsiness, muscular weakness and lack of coordination may be early signs of lithium toxicity, and can occur at lithium levels below 2.0 mEq/l. At higher levels, giddiness, ataxia, blurred vision, tinnitus and a large output of dilute urine may be seen. Serum lithium levels above 3.0 mEq/l may produce a complex clinical picture involving multiple organs and organ systems. Serum lithium levels should not be permitted to exceed 2.0 mEq/l during the acute treatment phase.
Fine hand tremor, polyuria and mild thirst may occur during initial therapy for the acute manic phase, and may persist throughout treatment. Transient and mild nausea and general discomfort may also appear during the first few days of lithium administration.
These side effects are an inconvenience rather than a disabling condition, and usually subside with continued treatment or a temporary reduction or cessation of dosage. If persistent, a cessation of dosage is indicated.
The following adverse reactions have been reported and do not appear to be directly related to serum lithium levels.
Neuromuscular: tremor, muscle hyperirritability (fasciculations, twitching, clonic movements of whole limbs), ataxia, choreo-athetotic movements, hyperactive deep tendon reflexes.

Continued on next page

Lithium Carbonate—Cont.

Central Nervous System: Blackout spells, epileptiform seizures, slurred speech, dizziness, vertigo, incontinence of urine or feces, somnolence, psychomotor retardation, restlessness, confusion, stupor, coma, acute dystonia, downbeat nystagmus.
Cardiovascular: cardiac arrhythmia, hypotension, peripheral circulatory collapse, sinus node dysfunction with severe bradycardia (which may result in syncope).
Neurological: Cases of pseudotumor cerebri (increased intracranial pressure and papilledema) have been reported with lithium use. If undetected, this condition may result in enlargement of the blind spot, constriction of visual fields and eventual blindness due to optic atrophy. Lithium should be discontinued, if clinically possible, if this syndrome occurs.
Gastrointestinal: anorexia, nausea, vomiting, diarrhea.
Genitourinary: albuminuria, oliguria, polyuria, glycosuria.
Dermatologic: drying and thinning of hair, anesthesia of skin, chronic folliculitis, xerosis cutis, alopecia and exacerbation of psoriasis.
Autonomic Nervous System: blurred vision, dry mouth.
Thyroid Abnormalities: euthyroid goiter and/or hypothyroidism (including myxedema) accompanied by lower T_3 and T_4. Iodine 131 uptake may be elevated. (See PRECAUTIONS). Paradoxically, rare cases of hyperthyroidism have been reported.
EEG Changes: diffuse slowing, widening of frequency spectrum, potentiation and disorganization of background rhythm.
EKG Changes: reversible flattening, isoelectricity or inversion of T-waves.
Miscellaneous: fatigue, lethargy, transient scotomata, dehydration, weight loss, tendency to sleep.
Miscellaneous reactions unrelated to dosage are: transient electroencephalographic and electrocardiographic changes, leucocytosis, headache, diffuse nontoxic goiter with or without hypothyroidism, transient hyperglycemia, generalized pruritis with or without rash, cutaneous ulcers, albuminuria, worsening of organic brain syndromes, excessive weight gain, edematous swelling of ankles or wrists, and thirst or polyuria, sometimes resembling diabetes insipidus, and metallic taste.
A single report has been received of the development of painful discoloration of fingers and toes and coldness of the extremities within one day of the starting of treatment of lithium. The mechanism through which these symptoms (resembling Raynaud's Syndrome) developed is not known. Recovery followed discontinuance.

OVERDOSAGE

The toxic levels for lithium are close to the therapeutic levels. It is therefore important that patients and their families be cautioned to watch for early symptoms and to discontinue the drug and inform the physician should they occur. Toxic symptoms are listed in detail under ADVERSE REACTIONS.
Treatment: No specific antidote for lithium poisoning is known. Early symptoms of lithium toxicity can usually be treated by reduction or cessation of dosage of the drug and resumption of the treatment at a lower dose after 24 to 48 hours. In severe cases of lithium poisoning, the first and foremost goal of treatment consists of elimination of this ion from the patient.
Treatment is essentially the same as that used in barbiturate poisoning: 1) gastric lavage, 2) correction of fluid and electrolyte imbalance and 3) regulation of kidney functioning. Urea, mannitol, and aminophylline all produce significant increases in lithium excretion. Hemodialysis is an effective and rapid means of removing the ion from the severely toxic patient. Infection prophylaxis, regular chest X-rays, and preservation of adequate respiration are essential.

DOSAGE AND ADMINISTRATION

Acute Mania: Optimal patient response to Lithium Carbonate usually can be established and maintained with 600 mg t.i.d. Such doses will normally produce an effective serum lithium level ranging between 1.0 and 1.5 mEq/l. Dosage must be individualized according to serum levels and clinical response. Regular monitoring of the patient's clinical state and of serum lithium levels is necessary. Serum levels should be determined twice per week during the acute phase, and until the serum level and clinical condition of the patient have been stabilized.
Long-term Control: The desirable serum lithium levels are 0.6 to 1.2 mEq/l. Dosage will vary from one individual to another, but usually 300 mg of lithium carbonate t.i.d. or q.i.d. will maintain this level. Serum lithium levels in uncomplicated cases receiving maintenance therapy during remission should be monitored at least every two months.
Patients abnormally sensitive to lithium may exhibit toxic signs at serum levels of 1.0 to 1.5 mEq/l. Elderly patients often respond to reduced dosage, and may exhibit signs of toxicity at serum levels ordinarily tolerated by other patients.
N.B.: Blood samples for serum lithium determination should be drawn immediately prior to the next dose when lithium concentrations are relatively stable (i.e., 8–12 hours after the previous dose.) Total reliance must not be placed on serum levels alone. Accurate patient evaluation requires both clinical and laboratory analysis.

HOW SUPPLIED

Lithium Carbonate Tablets USP
300 mg white, scored tablets (Identified 54 452)
NDC 0054-8528-25: Unit dose, 10 tablets per strip, 10 strips per shelf pack, 10 shelf packs per shipper.
(For Institutional Use Only).
NDC 0054-4527-25: Bottles of 100 tablets.
NDC 0054-4527-31: Bottles of 1000 tablets.
Lithium Carbonate Capsules USP
150 mg white opaque colored capsules (size 4) (Identified 54 213).
NDC 0054-8526-25: Unit dose, 10 capsules per strip, 10 strips per shelf pack, 10 shelf packs per shipper.
(For Institutional Use Only).
NDC 0054-2526-25: Bottles of 100 capsules.
300 mg flesh-colored capsules (size 2) (Identified 54 463).
NDC 0054-8527-25: Unit dose, 10 capsules per strip, 10 strips per shelf pack, 10 shelf packs per shipper.
(For Institutional Use Only).
NDC 0054-2527-25: Bottles of 100 capsules.
NDC 0054-2527-31: Bottles of 1000 capsules.
600 mg white opaque/flesh colored capsules (size 0) (Identified 54 702).
NDC 0054-8531-25: Unit dose, 10 capsules per strip, 10 strips per shelf pack, 10 shelf packs per shipper.
(For Institutional Use Only.)
NDC 0054-2531-25: Bottles of 100 capsules.
4055501 Revised May 1999
059 ©RLI, 1999
Roxane Laboratories, Inc.
Columbus, OH 43216

LITHIUM CITRATE SYRUP USP ℞

8 mEq of Lithium per 5 mL
SUGAR FREE
FOR ORAL ADMINISTRATION ONLY

DESCRIPTION

Lithium Citrate Syrup is a palatable oral dosage form of lithium ion. Lithium citrate is prepared in solution from lithium hydroxide and citric acid in a ratio approximating di-lithium citrate:
Each 5 mL of Lithium Citrate Syrup contains 8 mEq of lithium ion (Li+), equivalent to the amount of lithium in 300 mg of lithium carbonate, and alcohol 0.3% v/v.
Inactive ingredients:
The syrup contains alcohol, sorbitol, flavoring, water, and other ingredients.
Lithium is an element of the alkali-metal group with atomic number 3, atomic weight 6.94, and an emission line at 671 nm on the flame photometer.

HOW SUPPLIED

Lithium Citrate Syrup, 8 mEq per 5 mL
NDC 0054-8529-04: Unit dose Patient Cup™ filled to deliver 5 mL, ten 5 mL Patient Cups™ per shelf pack, ten shelf packs per shipper. (For Institutional Use Only).
NDC 0054-3527-63: Bottles of 500 mL.
NDC 0054-8530-04: Unit dose Patient Cup™ filled to deliver 10 mL, ten 10 mL Patient Cups™ per shelf pack, ten shelf packs per shipper. (For Institutional Use Only).
Refer to Lithium Carbonate Capsules and Tablets heading for complete text.

MARINOL® CIII ℞

(dronabinol)
Capsules
Rx only.

DESCRIPTION

Dronabinol is a cannabinoid designated chemically as (6a*R-trans*)-6a,7,8,10a-tetrahydro-6,6,9-trimethyl-3-phentyl-6*H*-dibenzo[*b,d*]pyran-1-ol. Dronabinol has the following empirical and structural formulas:

$C_{21}H_{30}O_2$ (molecular weight = 314.47)

Dronabinol, the active ingredient in Marinol, is synthetic delta-9-tetrahydrocannabinol (delta-9-THC). Delta-9-tetrahydrocannabinol is also a naturally occurring component of *Cannabis sativa L.* (Marijuana).
Dronabinol is a light yellow resinous oil that is sticky at room temperature and hardens upon refrigeration. Dronabinol is insoluble in water and is formulated in sesame oil. It has a pK_a of 10.6 and an octanol-water partition coefficient: 6,0000:1 at pH 7.
Capsules for oral administration: Marinol is supplied as round, soft gelatin capsules containing either 2.5 mg, 5 mg, or 10 mg dronabinol. Each Marinol capsule is formulated with the following inactive ingredients: FD&C Blue No. 1 (5 mg), FD&C Red No. 40 (5 mg), FD&C Yellow No. 6 (5 mg and 10 mg), gelatin, glycerin, methylparaben, propylparaben, sesame oil, and titanium dioxide.

CLINICAL PHARMACOLOGY

Dronabinol is an orally active cannabinoid which, like other cannabinoids, has complex effects on the central nervous system (CNS), including central sympathomimetic activity. Cannabinoid receptors have been discovered in neural tissues. These receptors may play a role in mediating the effects of dronabinol and other cannabinoids.
Pharmacodynamics: Dronabinol-induced sympathomimetic activity may result in tachycardia and/or conjunctival injection. Its effects on blood pressure are inconsistent, but occasional subjects have experienced orthostatic hypotension and/or syncope upon abrupt standing.
Dronabinol also demonstrates reversible effects on appetite, mood, cognition, memory, and perception. These phenomena appear to be dose-related, increasing in frequency with higher dosages, and subject to great interpatient variability.
After oral administration, dronabinol has an onset of action of approximately 0.5 to 1 hours and peak effect at 2 to 4 hours. Duration of action for psychoactive effects is 4 to 6 hours, but the appetite stimulant effect of dronabinol may continue for 24 hours or longer after administration.
Tachyphylaxis and tolerance develop to some of the pharmacologic effects of dronabinol and other cannabinoids with chronic use, suggesting an indirect effect on sympathetic neurons. In a study of the pharmacodynamics of chronic dronabinol exposure, healthy male volunteers (N = 12) received 210 mg/day dronabinol, administered orally in divided doses, for 16 days. An initial tachycardia induced by dronabinol was replaced successively by normal sinus rhythm and then bradycardia. A decrease in supine blood pressure, made worse by standing, was also observed initially. These volunteers developed tolerance to the cardiovascular and subjective adverse CNS effects of dronabinol within 12 days of treatment initiation.
Tachyphylaxis and tolerance do not, however, appear to develop to the appetite stimulant effect of Marinol. In studies involving patients with Acquired Immune Deficiency Syndrome (AIDS), the appetite stimulant effect of Marinol has been sustained for up to five months in clinical trials, at dosages ranging from 2.5 mg/day to 20 mg/day.
Pharmacokinetics:
Absorption and Distribution: Marinol (dronabinol) is almost completely absorbed (90 to 95%) after single oral doses. Due to the combined effects of first pass hepatic metabolism and high lipid solubility, only 10% to 20% of the administered dose reaches the systemic circulation. Dronabinol has a large apparent volume of distribution, approximately 10 L/kg, because of its liquid solubility. The plasma protein binding of dronabinol and its metabolites is approximately 97%.
The elimination phase of dronabinol can be described using a two compartment model with an initial (alpha) half-life of about 4 hours and a terminal (beta) half-life of 25 to 36 hours. Because of its large volume of distribution, dronabinol and its metabolites may be excreted at low levels for prolonged periods of time.
Metabolism: Dronabinol undergoes extensive first-pass hepatic metabolism, primarily by microsomal hydroxylation, yielding both active and inactive metabolites. Dronabinol and its principal active metabolite, 11-OH-delta-9-THC, are present in approximately equal concentrations in plasma. Concentrations of both parent drug and metabolite peak at approximately 2 to 4 hours after oral dosing and decline over several days. Values for clearance average about 0.2 L/kg-hr, but are highly variable due to the complexity of cannabinoid distribution.
Elimination: Dronabinol and its biotransformation products are excreted in both feces and urine. Biliary excretion is the major route of elimination with about half of a radiolabeled oral dose being recovered from the feces within 72 hours as contrasted with 10 to 15% recovered from urine. Less than 5% of an oral dose is recovered unchanged in the feces.
Following single dose administration, low levels of dronabinol metabolites have been detected for more than 5 weeks in the urine and feces.
In a study of Marinol involving AIDS patients, urinary cannabinoid/creatinine concentration ratios were studied biweekly over a six week period. The urinary cannabinoid/creatinine ratio was closely correlated with dose. No increase in the cannabinoid/creatinine ratio was observed after the first two weeks of treatment, indicating that steady-state cannabinoid levels had been reached. This conclusion is consistent with predictions based on the observed terminal half-life of dronabinol.
Special Populations: The pharmacokinetic profile of Marinol has not been investigated in either pediatric or geriatric patients.

CLINICAL TRIALS

Appetite Stimulation: The appetite stimulant effect of Marinol (dronabinol) in the treatment of AIDS-related anorexia associated with weight loss was studied in a randomized, double-blind, placebo-controlled study involving 139 patients. The initial dosage of Marinol in all patients was 5 mg/day, administered in doses of 2.5 mg one hour before lunch and one hour before supper. In pilot studies, early morning administration of Marinol appeared to have been associated with an increased frequency of adverse experiences, as compared to dosing later in the day. The effect of Marinol on appetite, weight, mood, and nausea was measured at scheduled intervals during the six-week treatment period. Side effects (feeling high, dizziness, confusion, somnolence) occurred in 13 of 72 patients (18%) at this dosage

level and the dosage was reduced to 2.5 mg/day, administered at a single dose at supper or bedtime.
As compared to placebo, Marinol treatment resulted in a statistically significant improvement in appetite as measured by visual analog scale (see figure). Trends toward improved body weight and mood, and decreases in nausea were also seen.
After completing the 6-week study, patients were allowed to continue treatment with Marinol in an open-label study, in which there was a sustained improvement in appetite.

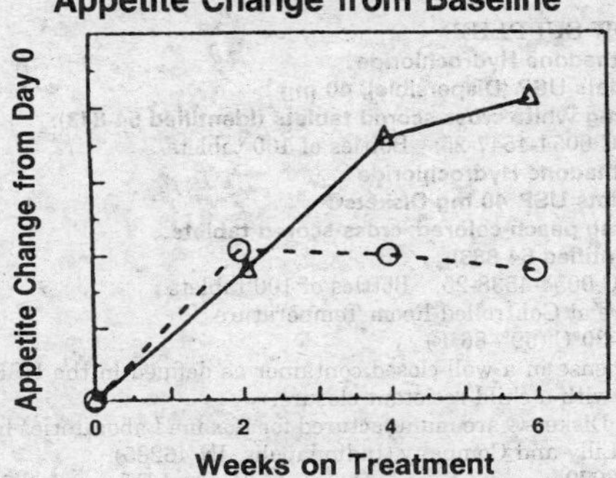

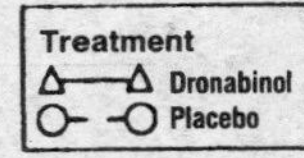

Antiemetic: Marinol (dronabinol) treatment of chemotherapy-induced emesis was evaluated in 454 patients with cancer, who received a total of 750 courses of treatment of various malignancies. The antiemetic efficacy of Marinol was greatest in patients receiving cytotoxic therapy with MOPP for Hodgkin's and non-Hodgkin's lymphomas. Marinol dosages ranged from 2.5 mg/day to 40 mg/day, administered in equally divided doses every four to six hours (four times daily). As indicated in the following table, escalating the Marinol dose above 7 mg/m² increased the frequency of adverse experiences, with no additional antiemetic benefit.
[See table above]
Combination antiemetic therapy with Marinol and a phenothiazine (prochlorperazine) may result in synergistic or additive antiemetic effects and attenuate the toxicities associated with each of the agents.

Marinol Dose: Response Frequency and Adverse Experiences*
(N = 750 treatment courses)

Marinol Dose	Response Frequency (%)			Adverse Events Frequency (%)		
	Complete	Partial	Poor	None	Nondysphoric	Dysphoric
< 7 mg/m²	36	32	32	23	65	12
> 7 mg/m²	33	31	36	13	58	28

*Nondysphoric events consisted of drowsiness, tachycardia, etc.

INDIVIDUALIZATION OF DOSAGES

The pharmacologic effects of Marinol (dronabinol) are dose-related and subject to considerable interpatient variability. Therefore, dosage individualization is critical in achieving the maximum benefit of Marinol treatment.
Appetite Stimulation: In the clinical trials, the majority of patients were treated with 5 mg/day Marinol, although the dosages ranged from 2.5 to 20 mg/day. For an adult:

1. Begin with 2.5 mg before lunch and 2.5 mg before supper. If CNS symptoms (feeling high, dizziness, confusion, somnolence) do occur, they usually resolve in 1 to 3 days with continued dosage.
2. If CNS symptoms are severe or persistent, reduce the dose to 2.5 mg before supper. If symptoms continue to be a problem, taking the single dose in the evening or at bedtime may reduce their severity.
3. When adverse effects are absent or minimal and further therapeutic effect is desired, increase the dose to 2.5 mg before lunch and 5 mg before supper or 5 and 5 mg. Although most patients respond to 2.5 mg twice daily, 10 mg twice daily has been tolerated in about half of the patients in appetite stimulation studies.

The pharmacologic effects of Marinol are reversible upon treatment cessation.
Antiemetic: Most patients respond to 5 mg three or four times daily. Dosage may be escalated during a chemotherapy cycle or at subsequent cycles, based upon initial results. Therapy should be initiated at the lowest recommended dosage and titrated to clinical response. Administration of Marinol with phenothiazines, such as prochlorperazine, has resulted in improved efficacy as compared to either drug alone, without additional toxicity.
Pediatrics: Marinol is not recommended for AIDS-related anorexia in pediatric patients because it has not been studied in this population. The pediatric dosage for the treatment of chemotherapy-induced emesis is the same as in adults. Caution is recommended in prescribing Marinol for children because of the psychoactive effects.
Geriatrics: Caution is advised in prescribing Marinol in elderly patients because they are generally more sensitive to the psychoactive effects of drugs. In antiemetic studies, no difference in tolerance or efficacy was apparent in patients > 55 years old.

INDICATIONS AND USAGE

Marinol (dronabinol) is indicated for the treatment of:

1. anorexia associated with weight loss in patients with AIDS; and
2. nausea and vomiting associated with cancer chemotherapy in patients who have failed to respond adequately to conventional antiemetic treatments.

CONTRAINDICATIONS

Marinol (dronabinol) is contraindicated in any patient who has a history of hypersensitivity to any cannabinoid or sesame oil.

WARNINGS

Patients receiving treatment with Marinol should be specifically warned not to drive, operate machinery, or engage in any hazardous activity until it is established that they are able to tolerate the drug and to perform such tasks safely.

PRECAUTIONS

General: The risk/benefit ratio of Marinol (dronabinol) use should be carefully evaluated in patients with the following medical conditions because of individual variation in response and tolerance to the effects of Marinol.
Marinol should be used with caution in patients with cardiac disorders because of occasional hypotension, possible hypertension, syncope, or tachycardia (see CLINICAL PHARMACOLOGY).
Marinol should be used with caution in patients with a history of substance abuse, including alcohol abuse or dependence, because they may be more prone to abuse Marinol as well. Multiple substance abuse is common and marijuana, which contains the same active compound, is a frequently abused substance.
Marinol should be used with caution and careful psychiatric monitoring in patients with mania, depression, or schizophrenia because Marinol may exacerbate these illnesses.
Marinol should be used with caution in patients receiving concomitant therapy with sedatives, hypnotics or other psychoactive drugs because of the potential for additive or synergistic CNS effects.
Marinol should be used with caution in pregnant patients, nursing mothers, or pediatric patients because it has not been studied in these patient populations.
Marinol should be used with caution for treatment of anorexia and weight loss in elderly patients with AIDS because they may be more sensitive to the psychoactive effects and because its use in these patients has not been studied.
Information for Patients: Patients receiving treatment with Marinol (dronabinol) should be altered to the potential for additive central nervous system depression if Marinol is used concomitantly with alcohol or other CNS depressants such as benzodiazepines and barbiturates.
Patients receiving treatment with Marinol should be specifically warned not to drive, operate machinery, or engage in any hazardous activity until it is established that they are able to tolerate the drug and to perform such tasks safely.
Patients using Marinol should be advised of possible changes in mood and other adverse behavioral effects of the drug so as to avoid panic in the event of such manifestations. Patients should remain under the supervision of a responsible adult during initial use of Marinol and following dosage adjustments.
Drug Interactions: In studies involving patients with AIDS and/or cancer, Marinol (dronabinol) has been co-administered with a variety of medications (e.g., cytotoxic agents, anti-infective agents, sedatives, or opioid analgesics) without resulting in any clinically significant drug/drug interactions. Although no drug/drug interactions were discovered during the clinical trials of Marinol, cannabinoids may interact with other medications through both metabolic and pharmacodynamic mechanisms. Dronabinol is highly protein bound to plasma proteins, and therefore, might displace other protein-bound drugs. Although this displacement has not been confirmed *in vivo*, practitioners should monitor patients for a change in dosage requirements when administering dronabinol to patients receiving other highly protein-bound drugs. Published reports of drug/drug interactions involving cannabinoids are summarized in the following table.

CONCOMITANT DRUG	CLINICAL EFFECT(S)
Amphetamines, cocaine, other sympathomimetic agents	Additive hypertension, tachycardia, possibly cardiotoxicity
Atropine, scopolamine, antihistamines, other anticoholinergic agents	Additive or super-additive tachycardia, drowsiness
Amitriptyline, amoxapine, desipramine, other tricyclic antidepressants	Additive tachycardia, hypertension drowsiness
Barbiturates, benzodiazepines, ethanol, lithium, opioids, buspirone, antihistamines, muscle relaxants, other CNS depressants	Additive drownsiness and CNS depression
Disulfiram	A reversible hypomanic reaction was reported in a 28 y/o man who smoked marijuana; confirmed by dechallenge and rechallenge
Fluoxetine	A 21 y/o female with depression and bulimia receiving 20 mg/day fluoxetine X 4 wks became hypomanic after smoking marijuana; symptoms resolved after 4 days
Antipyrine, barbiturates	Decreased clearance of these agents, presumably via competitive inhibition of metabolism
Theophylline	Increased theophylline metabolism reported with smoking of marijuana; effect similar to that following smoking tobacco

Carcinogenesis, Mutagenesis, Impairment of Fertility: Carcinogenicity studies have not been performed with dronabinol. Mutagenicity testing of dronabinol was negative in an Ames test. In a long-term study (77 days) in rats, oral administration of dronabinol at doses of 30 to 150 mg/m², equivalent to 0.3 to 1.5 times maximum recommended human dose (MRHD) of 90 mg/m²/day in cancer patients or 2 to 10 times MRHD of 15 mg/m²/day in AIDS patients, reduced ventral prostate, seminal vesicle and epididymal weights and caused a decrease in seminal fluid volume. Decreases in spermatogenesis, number of developing germ cells, and number of Leydig cells in the testis were also observed. However, sperm count, mating success and testosterone levels were not affected. The significance of these animal findings in humans is not known.
Pregnancy: Pregnancy Category C. Reproduction studies with dronabinol have been performed in mice at 15 to 450 mg/m², equivalent to 0.2 to 5 times maximum recommended human dose (MRHD) of 90 mg/m²/day in cancer patients or 1 to 30 times MRHD of 15 mg/m²/day in AIDS patients, and in rats at 74 to 295 mg/m² (equivalent to 0.8 to 3 times MRHD of 90 mg/m² in cancer patients or 5 to 20 times MRHD of 15 mg/m²/day in AIDS patients). These studies have revealed no evidence of teratogenicity due to dronabinol. At these dosages in mice and rats, dronabinol decreased maternal weight gain and number of viable pups and increased fetal mortality and early resorptions. Such effects were dose dependent and less apparent at lower doses which produced less maternal toxicity. There are no adequate and well-controlled studies in pregnant women. Dronabinol should be used only if the potential benefit justifies the potential risk to the fetus.
Nursing Mothers: Use of Marinol is not recommended in nursing mothers since, in addition to the secretion of HIV virus in breast milk, dronabinol is concentrated in and secreted in human breast milk and is absorbed by the nursing baby.

ADVERSE REACTIONS

Adverse experiences information summarized in the tables below was derived from well-controlled clinical trials conducted in the US and US territories involving 474 patients exposed to Marinol (dronabinol). Studies of AIDS-related weight loss included 157 patients receiving dronabinol at a dose of 2.5 mg twice daily and 67 receiving placebo. Studies of different durations were combined by considering the first occurrence of events during the first 28 days. Studies of nausea and vomiting related to cancer chemotherapy included 317 patients receiving dronabinol and 68 receiving placebo.
A cannabinoid dose-related "high" (easy laughing, elation and heightened awareness) has been reported by patients receiving Marinol in both the antiemetic (24%) and the lower dose appetite stimulant clinical trials (8%) (see CLINICAL TRIALS).
The most frequently reported adverse experiences in patients with AIDS during placebo-controlled clinical trials involved the CNS and were reported by 33% of patients receiving Marinol. About 25% of patients reported a minor CNS adverse event during the first 2 weeks and about 4% reported such an event each week for the next 6 weeks thereafter.
PROBABLY CAUSALLY RELATED: Incidence greater than 1%.
Rates derived from clinical trials in AIDS-related anorexia (N=157) and chemotherapy-related nausea (N=317). Rates were generally higher in the anti-emetic use (given in parentheses).

Continued on next page

Marinol—Cont.

Body as a whole: Asthenia.
Cardiovascular: Palpitations, tachycardia, vasodilation/facial flush.
Digestive: Abdominal pain*, nausea*, vomiting*.
Nervous system: (Amnesia), anxiety/nervousness, (ataxia), confusion, depersonalization, dizziness*, euphoria*, (hallucination), paranoid reaction*, somnolence*, thinking abnormal*.

*Incidence of events 3% to 10%

PROBABLY CAUSALLY RELATED: Incidence less than 1%.
Event rates derived from clinical trials in AIDS-related anorexia (N=157) and chemotherapy-related nausea (N=317).

Cardiovascular: Conjunctivitis*, hypotension*.
Digestive: Diarrhea*, fecal incontinence.
Musculoskeletal: Myalgias.
Nervous system: Depression, nightmares, speech difficulties, tinnitus.
Skin and Appendages: Flushing*.
Special senses: Vision difficulties.

*Incidence of events 0.3% to 1%.

CAUSAL RELATIONSHIP UNKNOWN: Incidence less than 1%.
The clinical significance of the association of these events with Marinol treatment is unknown, but they are reported as alerting information for the clinician.

Body as a whole: Chills, headache, malaise.
Digestive: Anorexia, hepatic enzyme elevation.
Respiratory: Cough, rhinitis, sinusitis.
Skin and Appendages: Sweating.

DRUG ABUSE AND DEPENDENCE

Marinol (dronabinol) is one of the psychoactive compounds present in cannabis, and is abusable and controlled [Schedule III (CIII)] under the Controlled Substances Act. Both psychological and physiological dependence have been noted in healthy individuals receiving dronabinol, but addiction is uncommon and has only been seen after prolonged high dose administration.

Chronic abuse of cannabis has been associated with decrements in motivation, cognition, judgement, and perception. The etiology of these impairments is unknown, but may be associated with the complex process of addiction rather than an isolated effect of the drug. No such decrements in psychological, social or neurological status have been associated with the administration of Marinol for therapeutic purposes.

In an open-label study in patients with AIDS who received Marinol for up to five months, no abuse, diversion or systematic change in personality or social functioning were observed despite the inclusion of a substantial number of patients with a past history of drug abuse.

An abstinence syndrome has been reported after the abrupt discontinuation of dronabinol in volunteers receiving dosages of 210 mg/day for 12 to 16 consecutive days. Within 12 hours after discontinuation, these volunteers manifested symptoms such as irritability, insomnia, and restlessness. By approximately 24 hours post-dronabinol discontinuation, withdrawal symptoms intensified to include "hot flashes", sweating, rhinorrhea, loose stools, hiccoughs and anorexia. These withdrawal symptoms gradually dissipated over the next 48 hours. Electroencephalographic changes consistent with the effects of drug withdrawal (hyperexcitation) were recorded in patients after abrupt dechallenge. Patients also complained of disturbed sleep for several weeks after discontinuing therapy with high dosages of dronabinol.

OVERDOSAGE

Signs and symptoms following MILD Marinol (dronabinol) intoxication include drowsiness, euphoria, heightened sensory awareness, altered time perception, reddened conjunctiva, dry mouth and tachycardia; following MODERATE intoxication include memory impairment, depersonalization, mood alteration, urinary retention, and reduced bowel motility; and following SEVERE intoxication include decreased motor coordination, lethargy, slurred speech, and postural hypotension. Apprehensive patients may experience panic reactions and seizures may occur in patients with existing seizure disorders.

The estimated lethal human dose of intravenous dronabinol is 30 mg/kg (2100 mg/70kg). Significant CNS symptoms in antiemetic studies followed oral doses of 0.4 mg/kg (28 mg/70 kg) of Marinol.

Management: A potentially serious oral ingestion, if recent, should be managed with gut decontamination. In unconscious patients with a secure airway, instill activated charcoal (30 to 100 g in adults, 1 to 2 g/kg infants) via a nasogastric tube. A saline cathartic or sorbitol may be added to the first dose of activated charcoal. Patients experiencing depressive, hallucinatory or psychotic reactions should be placed in a quiet area and offered reassurance. Benzodiazepines (5 to 10 mg diazepam *po*) may be used for treatment of extreme agitation. Hypotension usually responds to Trendelenburg position and IV fluids. Pressors are rarely required.

DOSAGE AND ADMINISTRATION

Appetite stimulation: Initially, 2.5 mg Marinol (dronabinol) should be administered orally twice daily (b.i.d.), before lunch and supper. For patients unable to tolerate this 5 mg/day dosage of Marinol, the dosage can be reduced to 2.5 mg/day, administered as a single dose in the evening or at bedtime. If clinically indicated and in the absence of significant adverse effects, the dosage may be gradually increased to a maximum of 20 mg/day Marinol, administered in divided oral doses. Caution should be exercised in escalating the dosage of Marinol because of the increased frequency of dose-related adverse experiences at higher dosages (see PRECAUTIONS).

Antiemetic: Marinol is best administered at an initial dose of 5 mg/m^2, given 1 to 3 hours prior to the administration of chemotherapy, then every 2 to 4 hours after chemotherapy is given, for a total of 4 to 6 doses/day. Should the 5 mg/m^2 dose prove to be ineffective, and in the absence of significant side effects, the dose may be escalated by 2.5 mg/m^2 increments to a maximum of 15 mg/m^2 per dose. Caution should be exercised in dose escalation, however, as the incidence of disturbing psychiatric symptoms increases significantly at maximum dose (see PRECAUTIONS).

STORAGE CONDITIONS
Marinol (dronabinol) should be packaged in a well-closed container and stored in a cool environment between 8° and 15°C (46° and 59°F) and alternatively could be stored in a refrigerator. Protect from freezing.

HOW SUPPLIED

MARINOL® CAPSULES (dronabinol solution in sesame oil in soft gelatin capsules)
2.5 mg white capsules (Identified RL).
NDC 0054-2601-11: Bottles of 25 capsules.
NDC 0054-2601-21: Bottles of 60 capsules.
NDC 0054-2601-25: Bottles of 100 capsules.
5 mg dark brown capsules (Identified RL).
NDC 0054-2602-11: Bottles of 25 capsules.
NDC 0054-2602-25: Bottles of 100 capsules.
10 mg orange capsules (Identified RL).
NDC 0054-2603-11: Bottles of 25 capsules.
NDC 0054-2603-21: Bottles of 60 capsules.
MARINOL® is a registered trademark of Unimed Pharmaceuticals, Inc. and is marketed by Roxane Laboratories, Inc. under license from Unimed Pharmaceuticals, Inc.
Manufactured by Banner Pharmacaps, Inc.
Chatsworth CA 91311
4056020 **Revised October 1999**
109 ® RLI, 1999
Shown in Product Identification Guide, page 333

METHADONE HYDROCHLORIDE ℂ ℞

[*mĕth 'ă-dōn hī-drō- klō-rīd*]
DISKETS® (dispersible tablets)
Tablets, USP
(See also **Dolophine® Hydrochloride)**

Rx only

CONDITIONS FOR DISTRIBUTION AND USE OF METHADONE PRODUCTS:
Code of Federal Regulations,
Title 21, Sec. 291.505

METHADONE PRODUCTS, WHEN USED FOR TREATMENT OF NARCOTIC ADDICTION IN DETOXIFICATION OR MAINTENANCE PROGRAMS, SHALL BE DISPENSED ONLY BY APPROVED HOSPITAL PHARMACIES, APPROVED COMMUNITY PHARMACIES, AND MAINTENANCE PROGRAMS APPROVED BY THE FOOD AND DRUG ADMINISTRATION AND THE DESIGNATED STATE AUTHORITY.

APPROVED MAINTENANCE PROGRAMS SHALL DISPENSE AND USE METHADONE IN ORAL FORM ONLY AND ACCORDING TO THE TREATMENT REQUIREMENTS STIPULATED IN THE FEDERAL METHADONE REGULATIONS (21 CFR 291.505).

FAILURE TO ABIDE BY THE REQUIREMENTS IN THESE REGULATIONS MAY RESULT IN CRIMINAL PROSECUTION, SEIZURE OF THE DRUG SUPPLY, REVOCATION OF THE PROGRAM APPROVAL, AND INJUNCTION PRECLUDING OPERATION OF THE PROGRAM.

DESCRIPTION

Each tablet for oral administration contains:
Methadone Hydrochloride .... 40 mg
Inactive Ingredients:
The dispersible tablets contain magnesium stearate, microcrystalline cellulose, and starch (corn). The Diskets® contain cellulose, FD&C Yellow No. 6, flavors, magnesium stearate, potassium phosphate, silicon dioxide, cornstarch, and stearic acid.

Methadone hydrochloride is a white crystalline material which is water soluble. However, the methadone hydrochloride dispersible tablets have been specially formulated with insoluble excipients to deter the use of this drug by injection.

Chemically, Methadone Hydrochloride is 6-(Dimethylamino)-4,4-diphenyl-3-heptanone hydrochloride, which can be represented by the following structural formula:
[See chemical structure at top of next column]

CH2CH3
CO CH3
C—CH2CHN(CH3)2 • HCl

$C_{21}H_{27}NO \cdot HCl$ M.W. 345.91

HOW SUPPLIED

Methadone Hydrochloride
Tablets USP (Dispersible), 40 mg
40 mg white cross-scored tablets (Identified 54 843).
NDC 0054-4547-25: Bottles of 100 tablets.
Methadone Hydrochloride
Tablets USP, 40 mg Diskets®
40 mg peach-colored, cross-scored tablets (Identified 54 883).
NDC 0054-4538-25: Bottles of 100 tablets.
Store at Controlled Room Temperature
15°–30°C (59°–86°F)
Dispense in a well-closed container as defined in the USP/NF, with a child-resistant closure.
The Diskets® are manufactured for Roxane Laboratories by Eli Lilly and Company (Indianapolis, IN 46285).
4056070 Revised February 1999
029 © RLI. 1999.

METHADONE HYDROCHLORIDE ℂ ℞

Oral Concentrate USP
10 mg per mL
For Methadone Treatment Programs Only

Rx only.

CONDITIONS FOR DISTRIBUTION AND USE OF METHADONE PRODUCTS:
Code of Federal Regulations,
Title 21, Sec. 291.505

METHADONE PRODUCTS, WHEN USED FOR TREATMENT OF NARCOTIC ADDICTION IN DETOXIFICATION OR MAINTENANCE PROGRAMS, SHALL BE DISPENSED ONLY BY APPROVED HOSPITAL PHARMACIES, APPROVED COMMUNITY PHARMACIES, AND MAINTENANCE PROGRAMS APPROVED BY THE FOOD AND DRUG ADMINISTRATION AND THE DESIGNATED STATE AUTHORITY.
APPROVED MAINTENANCE PROGRAMS SHALL DISPENSE AND USE METHADONE IN ORAL FORM ONLY AND ACCORDING TO THE TREATMENT REQUIREMENTS STIPULATED IN THE FEDERAL METHADONE REGULATIONS (21 CFR 291.505).
FAILURE TO ABIDE BY THE REQUIREMENTS IN THESE REGULATIONS MAY RESULT IN CRIMINAL PROSECUTION, SEIZURE OF THE DRUG SUPPLY, REVOCATION OF THE PROGRAM APPROVAL, AND INJUNCTION PRECLUDING OPERATION OF THE PROGRAM.

DESCRIPTION

Each mL for oral administration contains:
Methadone Hydrochloride .... 10 mg
Chemically, Methadone Hydrochloride is 3-Heptan-one, 6-(dimethylamino)-4,4-diphenyl-, hydrochloride, which can be represented by the following structural formula:

CH2CH3
CO CH3
C—CH2CHN(CH3)2 • HCl

$C_{21}H_{27}NO \cdot HCl$ M.W. 345.91

Each mL, for oral administration, contains 10 mg of methadone hydrochloride.
Inactive ingredients: sodium benzoate, citric acid, and water.

HOW SUPPLIED

Methadone Hydrochloride Oral Concentrate USP
10 mg per mL
Clear, flavorless solution.
NDC 0054-3553-67: Bottles of 1 quart (946 mL).
Store at Controlled Room Temperature
15°–30°C (59°–86°F)
Protect from light.
Dispense in a tight, light-resistant container as defined in the USP/NF.
4056322 Revised August 1999
089 © RLI, 1999.
Roxane Laboratories, Inc.
Columbus, Ohio 43216

ORAMORPH® SR ℂ

(morphine sulfate)
Sustained Release Tablets
15 mg, 30 mg, 60 mg, 100 mg
Rx only.

> **NOTE**
> THIS IS A SUSTAINED RELEASE DOSAGE FORM. PATIENT SHOULD BE INSTRUCTED TO SWALLOW THE TABLET AS A WHOLE; THE TABLET SHOULD NOT BE BROKEN IN HALF, NOR SHOULD IT BE CRUSHED OR CHEWED.
> THE SUSTAINED RELEASE OF MORPHINE FROM **ORAMORPH SR** SHOULD BE TAKEN INTO CONSIDERATION IN EVENT OF ADVERSE REACTIONS OR OVERDOSAGE.

DESCRIPTION

Each tablet for oral administration contains:
Morphine sulfate .... 15 mg, 30 mg, 60 mg, or 100 mg in a tablet that provides for sustained release of the medication.
Morphine sulfate occurs as white, feathery, silky crystals, cubical masses of crystals, or white crystalline powder; it is soluble in water and slightly soluble in alcohol. Morphine has a pKa of 7.9, with an octanol/water partition coefficient of 1.42 at pH 7.4. At this pH, the tertiary amino group is mostly ionized, making the molecule water-soluble. Morphine is significantly more water-soluble than any other opioid in clinical use.
Chemically, morphine sulfate is 7,8-didehydro-4,5α-epoxy-17-methyl-morphinian-3,6α-diol sulfate (2:1)(salt) pentahydrate, and has the following structural formula:

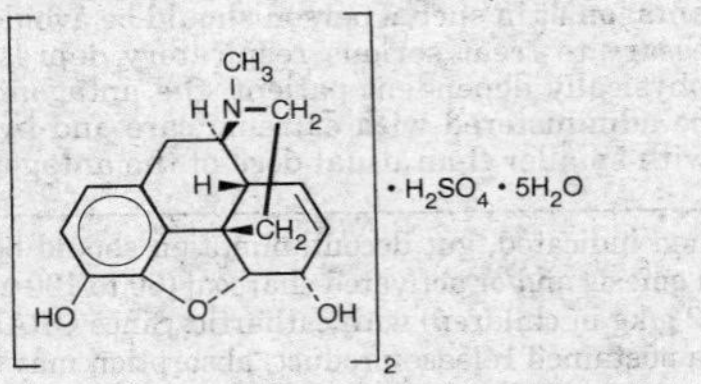

$$[C_{17}H_{19}NO_3]_2 \cdot H_2SO_4 \cdot 5H_2O$$

Each ORAMORPH SR Tablet contains 15 mg, 30 mg, 60 mg, or 100 mg Morphine Sulfate USP. Inactive ingredients: Lactose, Hydroxypropyl Methylcellulose, Colloidal Silicon Dioxide, and Stearic Acid.

CLINICAL PHARMACOLOGY

Morphine is the prototype of many narcotic drugs that interact predominantly with the opioid μ-receptor. These μ-binding sites are discretely distributed in the human brain, with high densities in the posterior amygdala, hypothalamus, thalamus, nucleus caudatus, putamen, and certain cortical areas. They are also found on the terminal axons of primary afferents with laminae I and II (substantia gelatinosa) of the spinal cord and in the spinal nucleus of the trigeminal nerve.
In clinical settings, morphine exerts its principal pharmacological effect on the central nervous system and gastrointestinal tract. Its primary actions of therapeutic value are analgesia and sedation. Morphine appears to increase the patient's tolerance for pain and to decrease discomfort, although the presence of the pain itself may still be recognized. In addition to analgesia, alterations in mood, euphoria and dysphoria, and drowsiness commonly occur.
Morphine depresses various respiratory centers, depresses the cough reflex, and constricts the pupils. Analgesically effective blood levels of morphine may cause nausea and vomiting directly by stimulating the chemoreceptor trigger zone, but nausea and vomiting are significantly more common in ambulatory than in recumbent patients, as is postural syncope.
Morphine increases the tone and decreases the propulsive contractions of the smooth muscle of the gastrointestinal tract. The resultant prolongation in gastrointestinal transit time is responsible for the constipating effect of morphine. Because morphine may increase biliary-tract pressure, some patients with biliary colic may experience worsening rather than relief of pain.
While morphine generally increases the tone of urinary-tract smooth muscle, the net effect tends to be variable, in some cases producing urinary urgency, in others, difficulty in urination.
In therapeutic doses, morphine does not usually exert major effects on the cardiovascular system. Some patients, however, exhibit a propensity to develop orthostatic hypotension and fainting. Rapid intravenous injection is more likely to precipitate a fall in blood pressure than oral dosing.
Morphine can cause histamine release, which appears to be responsible for dilation of cutaneous blood vessels, with resulting flushing of the face and neck, pruritus, and sweating.

PHARMACOKINETICS

ORAMORPH SR Tablets are a sustained release oral dosage form of morphine sulfate. Only about 40% of the administered dose reaches the central compartment because of first-pass effect (i.e., metabolism in the gut wall and liver). Once absorbed, morphine is distributed to skeletal muscle, kidneys, liver, intestinal tract, lungs, spleen and brain. Morphine also crosses the placental membrane and has been found in breast milk.
For all practical purposes, virtually all morphine is converted to glucuronide metabolites; only a small fraction (less than 5%) of absorbed morphine is demethylated. Among these glucuronide metabolites, morphine-3-glucuronide is present in the highest plasma concentration following oral administration; a smaller fraction is converted to morphine-6-glucuronide, which has the greater analgesic activity of these two metabolites.
The glucuronide system has a high capacity and is not easily saturated, even in disease. Therefore, the rate of delivery of morphine to the gut and liver does not influence the total and/or the relative quantities of the various metabolites formed.
The pharmacokinetic parameters following oral administration of ORAMORPH SR, presented in the table below, show considerable inter-subject variation, but are representative of average values reported in the literature. The volume of distribution (Vd) for morphine is 4 liters per kilogram (L/kg), and the terminal elimination half-life is approximately 2 to 4 hours.
[See table above]

TABLE OF APPROXIMATE[1] AVERAGE PHARMACOKINETIC PARAMETERS FOLLOWING ORAL DOSING OF ORAMORPH SR

Pharmacokinetic Parameter (scientific notation) (unit)		Dose of ORAMORPH SR			
		Dose of 2 × 15 mg	30 mg	60 mg	100 mg
Bioavailability (oral compared to injectable)		approximately 40%			
Time-to-peak plasma concentration $\{T_{max}\}$(h)	mean (range)	3.7 (1–6)	3.8 (1–7)	3.8 (2–7)	3.6 (1.5–12)
Peak plasma concentration $\{C_{max}\}$ (ng/mL) [single dose]	mean (range)	11.1 (6.5–16.2)	9.9 (5.0–18.6)	16.1 (10.0–25.3)	27.4 (14.1–46.1)
Volume of distribution (calculated from mean clearance and terminal half-life) **{Vd(β)}** (L/kg)	mean	4 L/kg			

Dose metabolized = approximately 90%
Morphine metabolites (%) = morphine-3-glucuronide (55–75%), morphine-6-glucuronide (1–5%)

[1]Derived from pharmacokinetic studies in 24 normal volunteers

Following the administration of conventional, immediate-release, oral morphine products, approximately 50% of the morphine, that will ever reach the central compartment, reaches it within 30 minutes. Following the administration of an equal amount of ORAMORPH SR to normal volunteers, however, 50% of absorption occurs, on average, after 1.5 hours.
The possible effect of food upon the systemic bioavailability of ORAMORPH SR has not been evaluated.
Although variation in the physico-mechanical properties of a formulation of an oral morphine drug product can affect both its absolute bioavailability and its absorption rate constant (k_a), morphine distribution and clearance are unchanged, as they are fundamental properties of morphine in the organism. However, in chronic use, the possibility of shifts in metabolite-to-parent drug ratios cannot be excluded.
When immediate-release oral morphine or ORAMORPH SR is given on a fixed dosing regimen, steady-state is achieved in about one or two days.
For a given dose and dosing interval, the Area-Under-the-Curve (AUC) and average blood concentration of morphine at steady-state (C_{SS}) will be independent of the type of oral formulation administered, as long as the formulations have the same absolute bioavailability. The absorption rate of a formulation will, however, affect the maximum (C_{max}) and minimum (C_{min}) plasma concentrations and the time between administration and their occurrence. For any fixed dose and dosing interval, ORAMORPH SR will have, at steady-state, a lower C_{max} and a higher C_{min} than conventional immediate-release morphine, which might be a therapeutic advantage in chronic pain control (see also PHARMACODYNAMICS).
The clearance of morphine occurs primarily as renal excretion of morphine-3-glucuronide. A small amount of the glucuronide conjugate is excreted in the bile, and there is some minor enterohepatic recycling; about 10% of the glucuronide conjugate is excreted in the feces. Because morphine is essentially metabolized in the liver, the effects of renal disease on morphine's clearance are not likely to be pronounced. As with any drug, however, caution should be taken to guard against unanticipated accumulation if renal and/or hepatic function is seriously impaired.

PHARMACODYNAMICS

In clinical settings, morphine's primary actions of therapeutic value are analgesia and sedation. Opiate analgesia involves at least three anatomical areas of the central nervous system: the periaqueductal-periventricular gray matter, the ventromedial medulla, and the spinal cord. Morphine appears to increase the patient's tolerance for pain, and to decrease the discomfort, although the presence of pain itself may still be recognized.
While there is considerable variability in the relationship between morphine blood concentration and analgesic response, effective analgesia probably will not occur below some minimum blood level in a given patient. The minimum effective blood level for analgesia will vary among patients, especially among patients who have been previously treated with potent μ-agonist opioids. Similarly, there is a considerable variability in the relationship between morphine plasma concentration and untoward clinical responses, but higher concentrations are more likely to be toxic.
In contrast to immediate-release morphine, after dosing with ORAMORPH SR, the morphine blood levels show reduced fluctuation between peak and trough plasma levels; that means that they are more centered within the theoretical 'therapeutic window'. On the other hand, the reduced fluctuation in morphine plasma concentration might conceivably affect other phenomena, as for example, the rate of tolerance induction.
ORAMORPH SR is an analgesic intended for patients who require chronic morphine analgesia and who will have, in consequence, markedly different degrees of pharmacodynamic tolerance for opioid drugs. Morphine and similar opioids induce tolerance to their effects, so that a shortening of the duration of satisfactory analgesia may be the first sign of an increase in tolerance.
Once patients are started on morphine, the dose required for satisfactory analgesia will rise, with the rate of development of tolerance varying, depending on the patient's prior narcotic use, level of pain, degree of anxiety, use of other CNS-active drugs, circulatory status, total daily dose, and the dosing interval.

INDICATIONS AND USAGE

ORAMORPH SR is indicated for the relief of pain in patients who require opioid analgesics for more than a few days.

CONTRAINDICATIONS

ORAMORPH SR is contraindicated in patients with respiratory depression in the absence of resuscitative equipment, in patients with acute or severe bronchial asthma and in patients with known hypersensitivity to morphine.
ORAMORPH SR is contraindicated in any patient who has or is suspected of having a paralytic ileus.

WARNINGS

IMPAIRED RESPIRATION:
Respiratory depression is the chief hazard of all morphine preparations. Respiratory depression occurs more frequently in the elderly and debilitated patients, as well as in those suffering from conditions accompanied by hypoxia or hypercapnia when even moderate therapeutic doses may dangerously decrease pulmonary ventilation.
Morphine should be used with extreme caution in patients who have a decreased respiratory reserve (e.g., emphysema, severe obesity, kyphoscoliosis, or paralysis of the phrenic nerve). ORAMORPH SR should not be given in cases of chronic asthma, upper airway obstruction, or in any other chronic pulmonary disorder without due consideration of the known risk of acute respiratory failure following morphine administration in such patients.
DRUG ABUSE AND DEPENDENCE - CONTROLLED SUBSTANCE:
Morphine sulfate is a Schedule II narcotic under the United States Controlled Substance Act (21 U.S.C. 801–886).
Morphine is the most commonly cited prototype for narcotic substances that possess an addiction-forming or addiction-sustaining liability. A patient may be at risk for developing a dependence to morphine if used improperly or for overly long periods of time. As with all potent opioids which are

Continued on next page

Oramorph SR—Cont.

μ-agonists, tolerance as well as psychological and physical dependence to morphine may develop irrespective of the route of administration (oral, intravenous, intramuscular, intrathecal, epidural). Individuals with a prior history of opioid or other substance abuse or dependence, being more apt to respond to eurphorogenic and reinforcing properties of morphine, would be considered to be at greater risk.

Care must be taken to avert withdrawal symptoms when morphine is discontinued abruptly or upon administration of a narcotic antagonist.

PRECAUTIONS

General Precautions: Selection of patients for treatment with ORAMORPH SR should be governed by the same principles that apply to the use of morphine or other potent opioid analgesics. Narcotic analgesics are drugs that have a narrow therapeutic index in the old, the sick, and the infirm, i.e., the very population in which their use is indicated. Physicians should individualize treatment with ORAMORPH SR in every case, weighing the need for analgesia against the risks of serious or fatal reactions to the drug.

Use in Patients with Increased Intracranial Pressure or with Head Injury: ORAMORPH SR should be used with extreme caution in patients with increased intracranial pressure or with head injury. The respiratory depressant effects of morphine (increased pCO_2) may result in elevation of cerebrospinal fluid pressure and may thus be markedly exaggerated in the presence of head injury, other intracranial lesions, or a pre-existing increased intracranial pressure. Morphine produces effects which may obscure neurologic signs of further increases in pressure in patients with head injuries. Pupillary changes (miosis), associated with morphine, may conceal the existence, extent, and course of intracranial pathology.

Use in Hepatic or Renal Disease: The clearance of morphine may be reduced in patients with hepatic dysfunction, while the clearance of its metabolites may be decreased in renal dysfunction. This will be manifested by both a prolonged elimination half-life and the accumulation of levels of either morphine or its metabolites in excess of those produced in normals, with the potential for an increase of adverse effects (see WARNINGS and ADVERSE REACTIONS). These changes in morphine pharmacodynamics, in patients with hepatic or renal dysfunctions, should be considered when adjusting the dose and dosage intervals, taking also into account the slow-release character of ORAMORPH SR.

Drug Interactions

Use with Other Central Nervous System Depressants: The depressant effects of morphine are potentiated by the presence of other CNS depressants such as alcohol, sedatives, antihistaminics, or psychotropic drugs. Use of neuroleptics in conjunction with oral morphine may increase the risk of respiratory depression, hypotension and profound sedation or coma.

Interaction with Mixed Agonist/Antagonist Opioid Analgesics: Agonist/antagonist analgesics (i.e., pentazocine, nalbuphine, butorphanol, or buprenorphine) should NOT be administered to patients who have received or are receiving a course of therapy with a pure opioid agonist analgesic. In these patients, the mixed agonist/antagonist may alter the analgesic effect or may precipitate withdrawal symptoms.

Carcinogenesis, Mutagenesis, Impairment of Fertility: Studies of morphine sulfate in animals to evaluate the drug's carcinogenic and mutagenic potential or the effect on fertility have not been conducted.

Pregnancy:

Teratogenic Effects—Category C: There are no well-controlled studies in women, but marketing experience does not include any evidence of adverse effects on the fetus following routine (short-term) clinical use of morphine sulfate products. Although there is no clearly defined risk, such experience cannot exclude the possibility of infrequent or subtle damage to the human fetus.

ORAMORPH SR should be used in pregnant women only when clearly needed. (See also: PRECAUTIONS: Labor and Delivery, and DRUG ABUSE AND DEPENDENCE CONTROLLED SUBSTANCE.)

Nonteratogenic Effects: Infants born from mothers who have been taking morphine chronically may exhibit withdrawal symptoms.

Labor and Delivery: ORAMORPH SR is not recommended for use in women during and immediately prior to labor. Occasionally, opioid analgesics may prolong labor through actions which temporarily reduce the strength, duration and frequency of uterine contractions.

Neonates, whose mothers received opioid analgesics during labor, should be observed closely for signs of respiratory depression. A specific narcotic antagonist, naloxone, should be available for reversal of narcotic-induced respiratory depression in the neonate.

Nursing Mothers: ORAMORPH SR should not be given to nursing mothers because morphine is excreted in maternal milk. Effects on the nursing infant are not known, but withdrawal symptoms can occur in breast-fed infants when maternal administration of morphine sulfate is stopped.

Pediatric Use: ORAMORPH SR has not been evaluated in children. Its use in the pediatric population is, therefore, not recommended.

Use in the Aged: The pharmacodynamic effects of morphine in the aged are more variable than in the younger population. Patients will vary widely in the effective initial dose, rate of development of tolerance, and the frequency and magnitude of associated adverse effects as the dose is increased. Individualization of doses must receive careful attention in elderly patients.

Information for Patients: If clinically advisable, patients receiving ORAMORPH SR brand or morphine sulfate sustained release tablets, should be given the following instructions by the physician:

1. Morphine may produce psychological and/or physical dependence. For this reason, the dose of the drug should not be increased without consulting a physician.
2. Morphine may impair mental and/or physical ability required for the performance of potentially hazardous tasks (e.g., driving, operating machinery).
3. Morphine should not be taken with alcohol or other CNS depressants (sleep aids, tranquilizers) because additive effects, including CNS depression, may occur. A physician should be consulted if other prescription and/or over-the-counter medications are currently being used or are prescribed for future use.
4. For women of childbearing potential, who become or are planning to become pregnant, a physician should be consulted regarding analgesics and other drug use.

ADVERSE REACTIONS

NOTE: THE SUSTAINED RELEASE OF MORPHINE FROM ORAMORPH SR SHOULD BE TAKEN INTO CONSIDERATION IN THE EVENT OF OCCURRING ADVERSE REACTIONS.

Adverse reactions caused by morphine are essentially those observed with other opioid analgesics. They include the following *major hazards:* **respiratory depression,** and less frequently, **circulatory depression, apnea, shock** and **cardiac arrest** secondary to respiratory and/or circulatory depression.

Most Frequently Observed Reactions:
Constipation, nausea, vomiting, lightheadedness, dizziness, sedation, dysphoria, euphoria, and sweating. Some of these effects seem to be more prominent in ambulatory patients and in those not experiencing severe pain. Some adverse reactions in ambulatory patients may be alleviated if the patient is in a supine position.

Less Frequently Observed Reactions:

Body as a Whole: Edema, antidiuretic effect, chills, muscle tremor, muscle rigidity.

Cardiovascular: Flushing of the face, tachycardia, bradycardia, palpitation, faintness, syncope, hypotension, hypertension.

Gastrointestinal: Dry mouth, biliary tract spasm, laryngospasm, anorexia, diarrhea, cramps, taste alterations.

Genitourinary: Urine retention or hesitance, reduced libido and/or potency.

Nervous System: Weakness, headache, agitation, tremor, uncoordinated muscle movements, seizure, paresthesia, alterations of mood (nervousness, apprehension, depression, floating feelings), dreams, transient hallucination and disorientation, visual disturbances, insomnia, increased intracranial pressure.

Skin: Pruritus, urticaria and other skin rashes.

Special Senses: Blurred vision, nystagmus, diplopia, miosis.

DRUG ABUSE AND DEPENDENCE

Opioid analgesics may cause psychological and physical dependence (see WARNINGS). Physical dependence results in withdrawal symptoms in patients who abruptly discontinue the drug, or these symptoms may be precipitated through the administration of drugs with antagonistic activity, e.g., naloxone or mixed agonist/antagonist analgesics (pentazocine, etc.; see also OVERDOSAGE). Physical dependence usually does not occur, to a clinically significant degree, until several weeks of continued opioid usage. Tolerance, in which increasingly larger doses are required to produce the same degree of analgesia, is initially manifested by a shortened duration of a analgesic effect and, subsequently, by decreases in the intensity of analgesia. In patients with chronic pain, as well as in opioid-tolerant cancer patients, the administration of ORAMORPH SR (morphine sulfate) should be guided by the degree of tolerance manifested. Physical dependence, *per se,* is not ordinarily a concern when one is dealing with opioid-tolerant patients whose pain and suffering is associated with an irreversible illness. If ORAMORPH SR is abruptly discontinued, an abstinence syndrome may occur. Withdrawal symptoms, in patients dependent on morphine, begin shortly before the time of the next scheduled dose, reaching a peak at 36 to 72 hours after the last dose, and then slowly subside over a period of 7 to 10 days. Symptoms include yawning, sweating, lacrimation, rhinorrhea, restless sleep, dilated pupils, gooseflesh, irritability, tremor, nausea, vomiting, and diarrhea.

Treatment of the abstinence syndrome is primarily symptomatic and supportive, including maintenance of proper fluid and electrolyte balance. If withdrawal has inadvertently been precipitated in a patient who requires narcotics for pain management, the withdrawal syndrome can be terminated rapidly by the administration of an appropriate dose of a pure agonist opioid, such as morphine. The degree of physical dependence of a patient on ORAMORPH SR can be intentionally reduced by a gradual reduction of dosage and symptomatic treatment of withdrawal symptomatology.

OVERDOSAGE

NOTE: THE SUSTAINED RELEASE OF MORPHINE FROM **ORAMORPH SR** SHOULD BE TAKEN INTO CONSIDERATION IN THE EVENT OF AN OVERDOSAGE.

Overdosage of morphine is characterized by respiratory depression, with or without concomitant CNS depression. Since respiratory arrest may result either through direct depression of the respiratory center, or as the result of hypoxia, primary attention should be given to the establishment of adequate respiratory exchange through provision of a patent airway and institution of assisted, or controlled, ventilation. The narcotic antagonist, naloxone, is a specific antidote. An initial dose of 0.4 to 2 mg of naloxone should be administered intravenously, simultaneously with respiratory resuscitation. If the desired degree of counteraction and improvement in respiratory function is not obtained, naloxone may be repeated at 2 to 3 minute intervals. If no response is observed after 10 mg of naloxone has been administered, the diagnosis of narcotic-induced, or partial narcotic-induced, toxicity should be questioned. Intramuscular or subcutaneous administration may be used if the intravenous route is not available.

As the duration of effect of naloxone is considerably shorter than that of ORAMORPH SR, repeated administration may be necessary. Patients should be closely observed for evidence of renarcotization.

NOTE: In a individual physically dependent on opioids, administration of the usual doses of the antagonist will precipitate an acute withdrawal syndrome. The severity of the withdrawal syndrome produced will depend on the degree of physical dependence and the dose of the antagonist administered. Use of a narcotic antagonist in such a person should be avoided. If necessary to treat serious respiratory depression in a physically dependent patient, the antagonist should be administered with extreme care and by titration with smaller than usual dose of the antagonist.

When indicated, gut decontamination should be performed via emesis and/or activated charcoal (60 to 100 g in adults, 1 to 2 g/kg in children) with cathartic. Since ORAMORPH SR is a sustained release product, absorption may be expected to continue for many hours, particularly following an overdose, combined with decreased peristaltic activity of the gastrointestinal tract.

Supportive measures (including oxygen, vasopressors) should be employed in the management of circulatory shock and pulmonary edema accompanying overdose as indicated. Cardiac arrest or arrhythmias may require cardiac massage or defibrillation.

DOSAGE AND ADMINISTRATION

(See also: CLINICAL PHARMACOLOGY, WARNINGS and PRECAUTIONS sections.)

NOTE: ORAMORPH SR TABLET MUST BE SWALLOWED WHOLE. DO NOT BREAK THE TABLET IN HALF. DO NOT CRUSH OR CHEW. TAKING BROKEN, CHEWED OR CRUSHED TABLETS COULD LEAD TO THE RAPID RELEASE AND ABSORPTION OF A POTENTIALLY TOXIC DOSE OF MORPHINE.

ORAMORPH SR is intended for use in patients who require more than several days of continuous treatment with a potent opioid analgesic. The sustained release nature of the formulation allows it to be administered on a more convenient schedule than conventional immediate-release oral morphine products (see CLINICAL PHARMACOLOGY—PHARMACOKINETICS). However, ORAMORPH SR does not release morphine continuously over the course of a dosing interval. The administration of single doses of ORAMORPH SR on a q12h dosing schedule will result in peak and trough plasma levels similar to those following an identical daily dose of morphine administered using conventional oral formulations on a q4h regimen. If pain is not controlled for a full 12 hours, then the dosing interval should be shortened, but to no less than 8 hours.

As with any potent opioid, it is critical to adjust the dosing regimen for each patient individually, taking into account the patient's prior analgesic treatment experience. Although it is not possible to enumerate every condition that is important to the selection of the initial dose and dosing interval of ORAMORPH SR, attention should be given to (1) the daily dose, potency and characteristics of a pure agonist, or mixed agonist-antagonist, the patient has been taking previously, (2) the reliability of the relative potency estimate to calculate the dose of morphine needed [N.B.: potency estimates may vary with the route of administration], (3) the fact that roughly only 40% of the morphine sulfate in ORAMORPH SR becomes available after pre-systemic metabolization in the intestinal wall and liver, (4) the degree of opioid tolerance, and (5) the general condition and medical status of the patient.

The following dosing recommendation for ORAMORPH SR therefore, can only be considered suggested approaches to the series of clinical decisions in the management of pain of an individual patient.

Conversion from Conventional Immediate-Release Oral Morphine to ORAMORPH SR: A patient's daily morphine requirement is established by using the Daily Oral Morphine Requirement of the immediate-release formulation which gives the Daily Oral Morphine Requirement for

ORAMORPH SR. Since ORAMORPH SR is given on an 'every 12 hour' schedule, the single dose of ORAMORPH SR is half of the Daily Oral Morphine Requirement. Dose and dosing interval is adjusted as needed (see discussion below). For initial conversion, the 30 mg tablet strength is recommended for patients with a daily morphine requirement of 120 mg or less.

Conversion from Parental Morphine or Other Opioid Analgesics (parental or oral) to ORAMORPH SR:

Because of uncertainty about relative estimates of opioid potency and cross tolerance, as well as intersubject variation, initial dosing regimens should be conservative, i.e., an underestimation of the 24-hour oral morphine requirement is preferred to an overestimate. To this end, initial individual doses of ORAMORPH SR should be estimated conservatively. In patients whose daily morphine requirements are expected to be less than or equal to 120 mg per day, the 30 mg tablet strength is recommended for the initial titration period. Once a stable dose regimen is reached, the patient can be converted to the 60 mg or 100 mg tablet strength, as appropriate.

Estimates of the relative potency of opioids are only approximate, and are influenced by route of administration, individual patient differences, and possibly, by the patient's medical condition. Consequently, it is difficult to recommend any precise rule for converting a patient to ORAMORPH SR directly. However, the following general points should be considered:

1. *Parenteral to oral morphine ratio:* Estimates of the oral-to-parenteral potency of morphine vary. Some authorities suggest that a dose of morphine only 3 times the daily parenteral morphine requirement may be sufficient in chronic use settings. (3 times the Daily **Parenteral** Morphine Requirement = the Daily **Oral** Morphine Requirement)
2. *Other parenteral or oral opioids to oral morphine:* Because of a lack of reliable relative potency assays, specific recommendations are not possible. In general, it is safer to underestimate the Total Daily Dose of ORAMORPH SR required and rely upon *ad hoc* supplementation to deal with inadequate analgesia (see discussion which follows).

Use of ORAMORPH SR as the First Opioid Analgesic:

There has been no systematic evaluation of ORAMORPH SR as an initial opioid analgesic in the management of pain. Because it may be more difficult to titrate a patient using a sustained release morphine, it is ordinarily advisable to begin treatment using an immediate release formulation.

Considerations in the Adjustment of Dosing Regimens:

Whatever the approach, if signs of excessive opioid effects are observed early in a dosing interval, the next dose should be reduced. If this adjustment leads to inadequate analgesia, i.e., 'breakthrough' pain occurs late in the dosing interval, the dosing interval may be shortened. Alternatively, a supplemental dose of a short-acting analgesic may be given. As experience is gained, adjustments can be made to obtain an appropriate balance between pain relief, opioid side effects and the convenience of the dosing schedule.

In adjusting dose requirements, it is recommended that the dosing interval never be extended beyond 12 hours, because the administration of very large single doses of ORAMORPH SR may lead to acute overdosage.

For patients with low daily morphine requirements, the 15 mg tablet should be used. In this regard, adjustment in dose should NOT be attempted by breaking or crushing the tablets. ORAMORPH SR tablets are intended to be swallowed whole.

Conversion from ORAMORPH SR to Parenteral Opioids:

When converting a patient from ORAMORPH SR to parenteral opioids, it is best to assume that the parenteral to oral potency relationship is high. NOTE THAT THIS IS THE CONVERSE OF THE STRATEGY USED WHEN THE DIRECTION OF CONVERSION IS FROM THE PARENTERAL TO ORAL FORMULATIONS. IN BOTH CASES, HOWEVER, THE AIM IS TO ESTIMATE THE NEW DOSE CONSERVATIVELY. For example, to estimate the required 24-hour dose of morphine for IM use, one could employ a conversion of 1 mg of morphine IM for every 6 mg of morphine as ORAMORPH SR. Of course, the IM 24-hour dose would have to be divided by six and administered on a q4h regimen. This approach is recommended because it is least likely to cause overdosage.

HOW SUPPLIED

ORAMORPH SR® (Morphine Sulfate)
Sustained Release Tablets
15 mg white tablets (Identified 54 782)
[Embossed with 15]

NDC 0054-8790-24: Unit dose, 25 tablets per card (reverse numbered), 4 cards per shipper.
NDC 0054-4790-25: Bottles of 100 tablets.
NDC 0054-4790-29: Bottles of 500 tablets.

30 mg white tablets (Identified 54 409)
[Embossed with 30]

NDC 0054-8805-24: Unit dose, 25 tablets per card (reverse numbered), 4 cards per shipper.
NDC 0054-4805-19: Bottles of 50 tablets.
NDC 0054-4805-25: Bottles of 100 tablets.
NDC 0054-4805-27: Bottles of 250 tablets.

60 mg white tablets (Identified 54 933)
[Embossed with 60]

NDC 0054-8792-11: Unit dose, 25 tablets per card (reverse numbered), 1 card per shipper.
NDC 0054-4792-25: Bottles of 100 tablets.

100 mg white tablets (Identified 54 862)
[Embossed with 100]

NDC 0054-8793-11: Unit dose, 25 tablets per card (reverse numbered), 1 card per shipper.
NDC 0054-4793-25: Bottles of 100 tablets.

DEA Order Form Required.

Dispense in a tight, light-resistant container.

Storage: ORAMORPH SR Tablets should be stored in unopened containers at or below room temperature.

Federal law prohibits the transfer of this drug to any person other than the patient for whom it was prescribed.

Safety and Handling Instructions:

ORAMORPH SR is supplied as tablets that pose little risk of direct exposure to health care personnel and should be handled and disposed of in accordance with hospital policy. Patients and their families should be instructed to dispose of ORAMORPH SR tablets, that are no longer needed, down the toilet.

4073305 Revised February 1999
029 © RLI, 1999

Roxane Laboratories, Inc.
Columbus, Ohio 43216

Shown in Product Identification Guide, page 333

ORLAAM® Ⓒ℞

Levomethadyl Acetate Hydrochloride
Oral Solution
Rx only.

> CONDITIONS FOR DISTRIBUTION AND USE OF ORLAAM (21 CFR 291.505)
>
> ORLAAM, used for the treatment of narcotic addiction, shall be dispensed only by treatment programs approved by FDA, DEA and the designated state authority. Approved treatment programs shall dispense and use ORLAAM in oral form only and according to the treatment requirements stipulated in Federal regulations. Failure to abide by these requirements may result in injunction precluding operation of the program, seizure of the drug supply, revocation of the program approval, and possible criminal prosecution.
>
> ORLAAM has no recommended uses outside of the treatment of opiate addiction.

DESCRIPTION

ORLAAM (brand of levomethadyl acetate hydrochloride) is a synthetic opiate agonist. Chemically, it is levo-alpha-6-dimethylamino-4, 4-diphenyl-3-heptyl acetate hydrochloride, $C_{23}H_{31}NO_2$ • HCl. It is also known as levo-alpha-acetylmethadol hydrochloride (LAAM). The structural formula is:

$(CH_3)_2N$ — CH_3CHCH_2 — C — $CHCH_2CH_3$ •HCl, with $OCCH_3$ (C=O)

The compound is a white crystalline powder, soluble in water (>15 mg/mL), ethanol, and methyl ethyl ketone. The octanol:water partition coefficient of LAAM is 405:1 at physiologic pH. Doses of ORLAAM (LAAM) are always expressed as the weight of the hydrochloride salt (molecular weight 389.95).

ORLAAM is an aqueous solution which is diluted for oral administration. Each one mL of ORLAAM contains: Levomethadyl acetate hydrochloride (LAAM) 10 mg. Inactive ingredients: Methylparaben, propylparaben, hydrochloric acid and water.

CLINICAL PHARMACOLOGY

LAAM is a synthetic opioid agonist with actions qualitatively similar to morphine (a prototypic mu agonist) and affecting the central nervous system (CNS) and smooth muscle. Principal actions include analgesia and sedation. Tolerance to these effects develops with repeated use. An abstinence syndrome generally occurs upon cessation of chronic administration similar to that observed with other opiates, but with slower onset, more prolonged course, and less severe symptoms.

LAAM exerts its clinical effects in the treatment of opiate abuse through two mechanisms. First, LAAM cross-substitutes for opiates of the morphine-type, suppressing symptoms of withdrawal in opiate-dependent individuals. Second, chronic oral administration of LAAM can produce sufficient tolerance to block the subjective "high" of usual doses of parenterally administered opiates.

LAAM is metabolized by N-demethylation to nor-LAAM and dinor-LAAM, which are also opioid agonists. These metabolites are more potent than the parent drug. The opioid effect which occurs when LAAM is administered is slower in onset and longer in duration (72 hours) than that of methadone (24 hours). This extended duration of action allows three-times-weekly administration (see CLINICAL TRIALS).

PHARMACODYNAMICS

The duration of action of a single dose of LAAM is due to the sum of the opioid activity of the parent drug and its metabolites. A single dose of orally administered LAAM has an onset of opioid effects averaging 2 to 4 hours after ingestion and a duration of action of 48 to 72 hours (as measured by pupillary constriction and suppression of abstinence signs). LAAM cross-substitutes for opiates like morphine in opiate-dependent individuals, suppressing symptoms of withdrawal from these compounds. Single oral doses of 30 to 60 mg of LAAM eliminate signs of abstinence for 24 to 48 hours in individuals maintained on high doses of morphine who are abruptly withdrawn. At higher doses (80 mg and above), suppression of withdrawal can increase to 48 to 72 hours in most individuals.

Repeated oral administration of LAAM can produce sufficient tolerance to block the effects of parenterally administered opiates. Chronic oral administration of 70 to 100 mg of LAAM three times weekly produces tolerance which blocks the "high" of a 25 mg dose of intravenously administered heroin for up to 72 hours; maintenance on lower doses (50 mg) of LAAM produces only partial blockage for the same period.

PHARMACOKINETICS

Absorption

LAAM is rapidly absorbed from an oral solution. Plasma levels are detectable within 15 to 30 minutes after ingestion and reach their peak within 1.5 to 2 hours at steady-state. LAAM undergoes first-pass metabolism to its demethylated metabolite nor-LAAM, which is sequentially N-demethylated to dinor-LAAM. Both metabolites are active and contribute to the extent and duration of ORLAAM's clinical activity (see PHARMACODYNAMICS).

Pharmacokinetic Model

The steady-state pharmacokinetics of LAAM were modeled from a study in 25 healthy adult addicts using three-times-a-week dosing over a 15-day observation period. LAAM and its metabolites were found to follow a multi-compartment model with extensive tissue distribution (Vd ~ 20 L/kg). LAAM had a clearance of about 0.22 L/kg/hr, mostly by conversion to nor-LAAM. Kinetic studies of the pure metabolites in man have not yet provided accurate estimates of their clearance in the absence of the precursor, but the half-lives observed in this study were 2.6 days for LAAM, approximately 2 days for nor-LAAM, and approximately 4 days for dinor-LAAM.

The pharmacokinetic model used to estimate steady-state plasma levels for each subject in this study assumed a common 3 mg/kg/wk dosage regimen (0.94 mg/kg on Mon. and Wed., 1.125 mg/kg on Fri.). The estimates (which fit the observed data with a correlation of better than 0.95) revealed a large inter-patient variability. There was at least a 5-fold range in peak plasma concentrations for LAAM and its metabolites across the 25 subjects over the 72-hour interval from Friday to Monday on a 3-times-a-week dosage regimen. Table 1 contains these estimates of peak and trough plasma concentrations of LAAM, nor-LAAM, and dinor-LAAM.

Table 1: Peak and Trough Estimated Steady-State Plasma Concentrations During the 72 Hour Interval (Friday to Monday) for a 65-kg Patient Given 3 mg/kg/Week on Mon./Wed./Fri.

	LAAM Mean (CV)	Nor-LAAM Mean (CV)	Dinor-LAAM Mean (CV)
Cmax(ng/mL)*	204 (34%)	173 (34%)	114 (28%)
Cmin(ng/mL)**	36 (62%)	85 (58%)	96 (34%)

*Following Friday Morning Dose
**Prior to Monday Morning Dose

Figure 1: Simulated Steady-State Plasma Concentrations of LAAM, Nor-LAAM and Dinor-LAAM following Thrice Weekly Dosing with ORLAAM

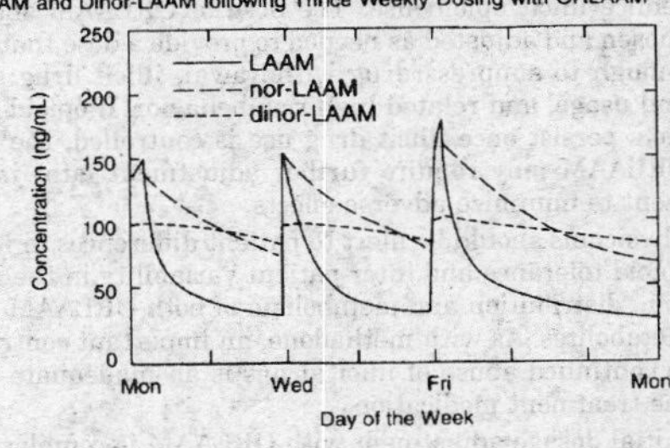

Metabolism and Elimination

ORLAAM is metabolized by the cytochrome P450 isoform, CYP3A4. As noted above, the formation of nor-LAAM and dinor-LAAM is by sequential demethylation, such that dinor-LAAM is formed from nor-LAAM, not directly from LAAM. While N-demethylation is the primary route of me-

Continued on next page

Orlaam—Cont.

tabolism, minor pathways of elimination include direct excretion and deacetylation to methadol, nor-methadol, and dinor-methadol.

Special Populations

Gender—An analysis of the data from the above study showed some difference in the plasma clearance of LAAM in 8 females versus 17 males. Males showed a trend toward a slower conversion of LAAM to nor-LAAM, which may alter the plasma concentration profile of LAAM and its active opioid metabolites. Although this effect was much smaller than the observed inter-individual differences, physicians should be alert to a possible gender difference (see INDIVIDUALIZATION OF DOSAGE).

Hepatic and Renal Disease—At the present time no pharmacokinetics studies have been carried out in subjects with clinically significant hepatic insufficiency or serious renal impairment. Since both the pharmacokinetics and pharmacodynamics of opiate agonists may be altered in these subjects, and any additional risks of ORLAAM therapy are not well understood in such patients, physicians may choose to manage such patients with methadone due to its simpler metabolic profile.

CLINICAL TRIALS

ORLAAM has been studied in 2666 street addicts and 3319 methadone maintenance patients, including 5697 males and 288 females. During the course of 27 studies, 4610 patients received orally administered ORLAAM for up to three years in thrice-weekly doses ranging from 10 to 140 mg. Twenty-one studies provide the primary evidence upon which the dosing recommendations for ORLAAM are based. The vast majority of patients who received ORLAAM were treated on a thrice-weekly basis, typically on Mondays, Wednesdays and Fridays (Mon./Wed./Fri.), although every-other-day dosing schedules were used in some settings. Most of the sites dosing patients with LAAM on a 3-times-a-week (Mon./Wed./Fri. or Tues./Thurs./Sat.) schedule increased the dose prior to the 72-hour inter-dose interval by 20 to 40% to obtain coverage for the full 72 hours.

In controlled clinical trials, treatment with ORLAAM was found to be comparable to treatment with methadone with respect to reduction in use of illicit opioids. ORLAAM doses in the range of 60 to 100 mg 3-times-a-week reduced the average frequency of urine samples positive for opiates to 15–20%, as did therapy with 50 to 100 mg a day of methadone. There was a trend for more patients to drop out of ORLAAM therapy than methadone therapy in the first 4 weeks of treatment (16% dropouts for ORLAAM v. 12% for methadone), but the dropout rates for both treatments rapidly declined and both were in the range of 1 to 2% per week for the remaining patients by the third month of the studies. Global ratings of patient acceptability and response to treatment were similar for both LAAM and methadone.

In the Phase III studies, ORLAAM tended to be more effective in patients perceived by staff to benefit from a reduced frequency of clinic visits and less effective in patients perceived as needing the added support of daily clinic visits.

Four independent studies were concerned with other research objectives, including induction regimens, methadone-to-ORLAAM (and ORLAAM-to-methadone) crossover ratios, and detoxification. This research involved 800 adults (including 11 females), approximately 440 of whom were methadone maintenance patients. The results of these studies, as well as the results of a nationwide Phase III usage study of 623 patients (including 204 females) in 25 representative clinics across the country, are reflected in the dosing recommendations.

INDIVIDUALIZATION OF DOSAGE

ORLAAM is intended for use as part of a comprehensive treatment plan for narcotic dependence of the opioid type. Supplying narcotic drugs to narcotic addicts for the treatment of addiction without appropriate medical evaluation, treatment planning, and counseling has not been shown to be effective, and is a violation of the law except in special circumstances.

The therapeutic goal early in treatment with ORLAAM is to reduce illicit opioid use. The dose of ORLAAM should be chosen and adjusted as needed to provide a dose that is high enough to suppress drug withdrawal, illicit drug seeking and usage, and related high-risk behavior. If opioid side effects persist once illicit drug use is controlled, the dose of ORLAAM may require further adjustment later in treatment to minimize adverse effects.

Physicians should be alert to patient differences in levels of opioid tolerance and inter-patient variability in the absorption, distribution and metabolism of both ORLAAM and its metabolites. As with methadone, an important contribution to continued abuse of illicit drugs is an inadequate dose of the treatment medication.

Initial dosage adjustment with ORLAAM is complex due to its delayed onset of action. If the starting dose is too high or if the dose is escalated too rapidly for the patient's level of tolerance, symptoms characteristic of excessive opioid effect may occur, i.e., poor concentration, sedation, and orthostatic hypotension. Patients should be watched for such symptoms, and the dose should be lowered if they appear. In rare instances, serious symptoms of narcotic overdosage may occur, leading to profound CNS and respiratory depression.

ORLAAM and its metabolites quickly accumulate to toxic levels if the doses intended for 3-times-a-week dosing are given too frequently. The recommended doses are intended for every-other-day or 3-times-a-week dosing and **should not be given daily.**

The recommended initial dose for patients with low or unknown tolerance to opioids is 20 to 40 mg **three-times-a-week** or **every-other-day.** Successive doses may be increased by 5 to 10 mg. At least two weeks are needed to achieve a clinical plateau after a dosage adjustment. Adjustment to a dosing schedule is dependent upon the rate at which an individual develops tolerance to the increasing level of ORLAAM (and its metabolites) as well as the time required for ORLAAM and its metabolites to accumulate to steady-state levels.

The goal of dosage titration is to suppress narcotic withdrawal while avoiding excessive opioid effects due to the build-up of long-acting metabolites. It may be safer to provide extra counseling and support rather than to attempt to completely suppress a patient's withdrawal or narcotic hunger during the first week or two of therapy. On the other hand, there is the ever-present danger that patients who receive sub-therapeutic starting doses will supplement with street drugs, resulting in overdose. Patients should be strongly warned against this practice. Later in the titration process, dosage adjustments are better made on a weekly basis whenever possible.

For patients on methadone maintenance whose level of tolerance is known, the recommended initial dose of ORLAAM is 1.2 to 1.3 times the patient's daily dose of methadone, not to exceed 120 mg. Care should be taken not to adjust the dose too frequently thereafter (usually 5 to 10 mg changes every second or third dose) since increasing the dose too rapidly may result in oversedation.

One major advantage of ORLAAM therapy is reduction in need for daily clinic visits and for take-home medication. In some patients, ORLAAM may not provide adequate suppression of withdrawal for a full 72 hours. For such individuals, several therapeutic options are available: (1) extra support and an explanation of reasons for the effect, (2) increasing the dose given prior to the 72-hour interval, (3) switching to an every-other-day dosing schedule, (4) dispensing a supplemental methadone dose.

Most patients do not experience withdrawal during the 72-hour inter-dose interval after reaching pharmacological steady-state **with or without** adjustment of the Friday dose. If additional opioids are required, small doses of supplemental methadone should be given rather than giving ORLAAM on two consecutive days. Take-home doses of methadone always pose a risk in this setting and physicians should carefully weigh the potential therapeutic benefit against the risk of diversion (see DOSAGE AND ADMINISTRATION).

Patients should receive extra support and counseling and be warned against supplementing with street drugs as they make the switch from methadone to ORLAAM. The variability in the clearance of LAAM, nor-LAAM, and dinor-LAAM and clinical experience suggest that there will be a small number of patients who require either lower or higher doses than those recommended.

DURATION OF ORLAAM THERAPY

There is no information from controlled clinical trials as to the appropriate duration of ORLAAM therapy. There are reports from investigators that some patients on ORLAAM may experience less variation in opioid effects and have less drug craving than with methadone, so ORLAAM should be considered for patients who need long-term maintenance during social and vocational rehabilitation.

When a patient has eliminated illicit drug use, achieved social and occupational stability, and made lifestyle changes to reduce the risk of relapse, consideration may be given to discontinuation of ORLAAM therapy. Such a decision should be carefully considered as part of an individualized treatment plan. Stable long-term ORLAAM therapy is preferable to repeated cycles of premature discontinuation of medication followed by relapse to uncontrolled addiction.

A patient is most likely to remain abstinent if discontinuation of medication is attempted after the achievement of behavioral objectives and is accompanied by appropriate non-pharmacological support. The rate of dose reduction should vary according to patient's response. Discontinuation of ORLAAM therapy for administrative reasons or because of adverse reactions to the drug should be managed as described below under DOSAGE AND ADMINISTRATION.

INDICATIONS

ORLAAM is indicated for the management of opiate dependence.

CONTRAINDICATIONS

ORLAAM is contraindicated in patients with known or suspected QT prolongation (QTc interval greater than 440 or 450 ms). This would include patients with congenital long QT syndrome, or conditions which may lead to QT prolongation (see WARNINGS, Effects on Cardiac Conduction) such as: 1) clinically significant bradycardia (less than 50 bpm), 2) any clinically significant cardiac disease, 3) treatment with Class I and Class III antiarrhythmics, 4) treatment with monoamine oxidase inhibitors (MAOI's), 5) concomitant treatement with other drug products known to prolong the QT interval (see PRECAUTIONS, Drug Interactions), and 6) electrolyte imbalance, in particular hypokalemia and hypomagnesemia.

ORLAAM is contraindicated in patients with known hypersensitivity to LAAM.

ORLAAM is not recommended for any use other than for the treatment of opioid dependence (see WARNINGS).

WARNINGS

Administration of ORLAAM on a daily basis has led to excessive drug accumulation and risk of fatal overdose. ORLAAM has only been studied on a thrice-weekly or every-other-day dosing regimen. Routine daily dosing after a patient has been inducted onto ORLAAM treatment is not allowed by current treatment regulations.

Any decision to administer ORLAAM more frequently than every other day for any reason should be approached with extreme caution. Even then only very small doses (5 to 10 mg) should be considered.

Risk of Overdose

Analysis of some of the deaths from overdose observed in the development of ORLAAM has shown that when ORLAAM is diverted into channels of abuse, the uninformed addict can become impatient with the slow onset of ORLAAM (2 to 4 hours) and take illicit drugs, resulting in a potentially lethal combined overdose when the peak ORLAAM effect develops. Due to these risks of diversion and accidental death, ORLAAM has been approved for use only when **dispensed** by a licensed facility and is not given in take-home doses.

Effects on Cardiac Conduction

ORLAAM has been shown to prolong the ST segment of the electrocardiogram in beagle dogs dosed five days a week. Serial EKGs performed in a pharmacokinetics study showed a prolongation of the QTc interval in some patients which was not associated with dose. Such a prolongation of the QTc interval has been seen with other opioids, and it is not known if this is an effect specific to LAAM or if it is also seen with methadone. In either case, careful monitoring is recommended when using ORLAAM in patients with a history of known cardiac conduction defects, those taking medications affecting cardiac conduction, and in other cases where an unusual risk of dysrhythmia is suggested by history or physical examination. This information is provided to alert the prescribing physician, and is not intended to deter the appropriate use of opioid agonists in patients with a history of cardiac disease.

Cases of QT prolongation and severe arrhythmia (torsade de pointes) have been observed during post-marketing treatment with ORLAAM. Based on these reports, all patients should undergo a 12-lead ECG prior to administration of ORLAAM to determine if a prolonged QT interval (QTc greater than 440 or 450 ms) is present. If there is a prolonged QT interval, ORLAAM should NOT be administered. For patients in whom the potential benefit of ORLAAM treatment is felt to outweigh the risks of potentially severe arrhythmias, an ECG should be performed prior to treatment and 12–14 days after initiating treatement to rule out any alterations in the QT interval.

ORLAAM should be administered with extreme caution to patients who may be at risk for development of prolonged QT syndrome (e.g., congestive heart failure, bradycardia, use of a diuretic, cardiac hypertrophy, hypokalemia, or hypomagnesemia).

ORLAAM is metabolized to active metabolites by the cytochrome P450 isoform, CYP3A4. Therefore, the addition of drugs that induce this enzyme could increase the levels of active metabolites in a patient that was previously at steady-state, and this could potentially precipitate severe arrhythmias, including torsade de pointes (see PRECAUTIONS, Drug Interactions).

Use of Narcotic Antagonists

In an individual receiving ORLAAM, the administration of the usual dose of a narcotic antagonist may precipitate an acute withdrawal syndrome. The severity of this syndrome depends on the dose of the antagonist administered and the patient's level of physical dependence. Narcotic antagonists should be used in patients receiving ORLAAM only if needed. If a narcotic antagonist is used to treat respiratory depression in the physically dependent patient, it should be administered with care and titration should begin with much smaller-than-usual doses (0.1 to 0.2 mg recommended). If the desired effect is not achieved, escalating doses may be administered every 2 to 3 minutes. If a cumulative dose of 10 mg of naloxone has been given without effect, further administration is unlikely to be of benefit (see OVERDOSAGE).

If the patient does respond to narcotic antagonists, physicians should remember that naloxone has a much shorter duration of action than ORLAAM. Such patients should remain under prolonged observation rather than being allowed to leave emergency treatment, since ORLAAM's action will outlast naloxone-induced reversal, putting the unsupervised patient at risk of relapse, a return of respiratory depression and possible death if continuing medical attention is not available. Use of other parenteral opioid antagonists may be appropriate in some cases, but only if the dosage of such drugs can be readily titrated. Oral naltrexone would not be appropriate for the treatment of ORLAAM overdose, as it has been associated with the precipitation of prolonged opioid withdrawal symptoms when used in overdose settings.

Warnings to Patients

Patients must be warned that the peak activity of ORLAAM is not immediate, and that use or abuse of other psychoactive drugs, including alcohol, may result in **fatal** overdose, especially with the first few doses of ORLAAM, either during initiation of treatment or after a lapse in treatment.

Use in High Risk Patients
Suicide attempts with opiates, especially in combination with tricyclic antidepressants, alcohol, and other CNS active agents, are part of the clinical pattern of addiction. Although outpatient therapy with ORLAAM and other drugs of this class is usually associated with a reduction in the risk of suicide, such risk is not eliminated. Individualized evaluation and treatment planning, including hospitalization, should be considered for patients who continue to exhibit uncontrolled drug use and persistent high-risk behavior despite adequate pharmacotherapy.

PRECAUTIONS

Initial Administration and Dosage Adjustment
Due to the long half-lives of ORLAAM and its metabolites, patients will not feel the full effects of the medication for at least several days. Consequently, extra care is needed when starting patients on ORLAAM and when making initial dosage adjustments (see INDIVIDUALIZATION OF DOSAGE and DOSAGE AND ADMINISTRATION).

Use in Ambulatory Patients
Initiation of therapy or excessive doses of ORLAAM may impair the mental and/or physical abilities required for performance of potentially hazardous tasks, such as driving a car or operating machinery. Patients should be warned not to engage in such activities if their alertness and behavior are affected. Most patients show no detectable impairment of ordinary tasks on ORLAAM therapy.

Head Injury and Increased Intracranial Pressure
The respiratory depressant effects of narcotics and their capacity to elevate cerebrospinal fluid pressure may be markedly exaggerated in the presence of increased intracranial pressure. Furthermore, narcotics produce side effects that may make it difficult to evaluate the clinical course of patients with head injuries. In view of LAAM's profile as a mu agonist, it should be used with extreme caution and only if deemed essential in such patients.

Asthma and Other Respiratory Conditions
ORLAAM, as with other opioids, should be used with caution in patients with asthma, in those with chronic obstructive pulmonary disease or cor pulmonale, and in individuals with a substantially decreased respiratory reserve, preexisting respiratory depression, hypoxia, or hypercapnea. In such patients, even usual therapeutic doses of narcotics may decrease respiratory drive while simultaneously increasing airway resistance to the point of apnea.

Special Risk Patients
Opioids should be given with caution and at reduced initial dose in certain patients, such as the elderly or debilitated and those with significant hepatic or renal dysfunction, hypothyroidism, Addison's Disease, prostatic hypertrophy, or urethral stricture.

Acute Abdominal Conditions
As with other mu agonists, treatment with ORLAAM may obscure the diagnosis or clinical course in patients with acute abdominal conditions.

Drug Interactions
No interaction studies have been performed in humans. ORLAAM is metabolized by the cytochrome P450 isoform, CYP3A4. The addition of drugs that induce this enzyme could increase the levels of active metabolites in a patient that was previously at steady-state.

Potentially Arrhythmogenic Agents—Any drug known to have the potential to prolong the QT interval should not be used together with ORLAAM. Possible pharmacodynamic interactions can occur between ORLAAM and potentially arrhythmogenic agents such as class I or III antiarrhythmics, antihistamines that prolong the QT interval, antimalarials, calcium channel blockers, neuroleptics that prolong the QT interval, and antidepressants

Caution should be used when prescribing concomitant drugs known to induce hypokalemia or hypomagnesemia as they may precipitate QT prolongation and interact with ORLAAM. These would include diuretics, laxatives and supraphysiological use of steroid hormones with mineralocorticoid potential.

Polydrug and Alcohol Abusers—Patients who are known to abuse sedatives, tranquilizers, propoxyphene, antidepressants, benzodiazepines, and alcohol should be warned of the risk of serious overdose if these substances are taken while on ORLAAM maintenance.

Interaction with Narcotic Antagonists, Mixed Agonists/Antagonists, Partial Agonists, and Pure Agonists—As with other mu agonists, patients maintained on ORLAAM may experience withdrawal symptoms when administered pure narcotic antagonists, mixed agonists/antagonists or partial agonists such as naloxone, naltrexone, pentazocine, nalbuphine, butorphanol, and buprenorphine.

In addition, agonists such as meperidine and propoxyphene, which are N-demethylated to long-acting, excitatory metabolites, should not be used by patients taking ORLAAM because they would be ineffective unless given in such high doses that the risk of toxic effects of the metabolites becomes unacceptable.

Anesthesia and Analgesia—Patients receiving ORLAAM will develop a similar level of tolerance for opioids as patients receiving methadone. Anesthetists and other practitioners should be prepared to adjust their management of these patients accordingly.

Other Drug Interactions—The anti-tuberculosis drug rifampin has been found to produce a marked (50%) reduction in serum methadone levels, leading to the appearance of symptoms of withdrawal in well-stabilized methadone maintenance patients. Similar effects on serum methadone levels have been observed for carbamazepine, phenobarbital, and phenytoin. The presumed mechanism for this effect is the induction of methadone metabolizing enzymes. Since ORLAAM is metabolized into a **more** active metabolite, nor-LAAM, administration of these drugs may **increase** ORLAAM's peak activity and/or **shorten** its duration of action. Conversely, drugs like erythromycin, cimetidine, and antifungal drugs like ketoconazole that inhibit hepatic metabolism, may **slow** the onset, **lower** the activity, and/or **increase** the duration of action of ORLAAM. Caution and close observation of patients receiving these drugs are advised to allow early detection of any need to adjust the dose or dosing interval.

Information for Patients
Patients should be provided the patient package insert for ORLAAM if they are new to the drug, and in addition should be advised that:

ORLAAM, unlike methadone, is not to be taken daily, and daily use of the usual doses will lead to serious overdose.

If a patient taking ORLAAM experiences symptoms suggestive of an arrhythmia (such as palpitations, dizziness, lightheadedness, syncope, or seizures), that patient should seek medical attention immediately.

ORLAAM is slow acting and patients should be alerted to the risk of abusing any psychoactive drug, including alcohol, while on ORLAAM therapy. This is particularly important during the first 7 to 10 days of treatment, before ORLAAM has had time to exert its full pharmacologic effect.

In addition to being warned of the delay in onset of ORLAAM, patients who are transferring from ORLAAM to methadone should be informed that they should wait 48 hours after the last dose of ORLAAM before ingesting their first dose of methadone or other narcotic (see DOSAGE AND ADMINISTRATION).

Patients should inform their adult family members that, in the event of overdose, the treating physician or emergency room staff should be told that the patient is being treated with ORLAAM, a long-acting opioid which is likely to outlast naloxone-induced reversal and which requires prolonged observation and careful monitoring. In addition, the treating physician or emergency room staff should be informed that the patient is physically dependent on narcotics and that naloxone should be administered with care so as to minimize any precipitated abstinence syndrome.

As with most mu agonists, ORLAAM may interact with other CNS depressants and should be used with caution, and in reduced dosage, in patients concurrently receiving other narcotic analgesics, antihistamines, benzodiazepines, phenothiazines or other major tranquilizers, anxiolytics, sedative-hypnotics, tricyclic antidepressants, and other CNS depressants, including alcohol. Patients should be warned of the importance of reporting the use of any of these compounds to their physicians, as serious side effects could result, including respiratory depression, hypotension, profound sedation or coma.

Carcinogenesis, Mutagenesis and Impairment of Fertility
Two-year carcinogenicity studies with LAAM in rats at 13 mg/kg (77 mg/m^2) and in mice at 30 mg/kg (90 mg/m^2) given orally in the diet did not show carcinogenic changes. LAAM is not mutagenic in the Ames test, the unscheduled DNA synthesis and repair test, mouse lymphoma cells in vitro, or chromosomal aberration tests in rats in vivo. LAAM tested positive in the forward mutation assay in N. crassa at 150 μg/mL in vitro and in the heritable translocation assay in mice at 21 mg/kg (63 mg/m^2). The clinical significance of these findings is not known.

Chronic treatment with LAAM at 80 mg three times a week did not produce chromosomal aberrations in peripheral human lymphocytes. Effects of LAAM on fertility in animals has not been fully evaluated.

Use in Pregnancy: Pregnancy Category C
Animal reproduction studies are not complete and there are no clinical data on the safety of ORLAAM in pregnancy. For these reasons, ORLAAM is not recommended for use in pregnancy. Women who may become pregnant should be advised of the risks of ORLAAM therapy and of the desirability of discontinuing ORLAAM prior to a planned pregnancy. Current regulations mandate monthly pregnancy tests in female patients of childbearing potential who are using ORLAAM.

If a female patient becomes pregnant on ORLAAM despite these precautions, it is recommended she be transferred to methadone for the remainder of the pregnancy (see TRANSFER FROM ORLAAM TO METHADONE, in DOSAGE AND ADMINISTRATION). If it appears wiser to continue a specific patient on ORLAAM, the physician should be alert to possible respiratory depression of the newborn and other perinatal complications (see Labor and Delivery).

Labor and Delivery
The effects of ORLAAM on labor and delivery are not known. Like other mu agonist opioids, however, ORLAAM is expected to produce respiratory depression and a possible neonatal dependence syndrome with a delayed emergence of withdrawal symptoms. Use of ORLAAM in labor and delivery is not recommended unless, in the opinion of the treating physician, the potential benefits outweigh the possible hazards.

Nursing Mothers
The effects of LAAM on infants of nursing mothers have not been studied. It is not known if LAAM is excreted in human milk in sufficient concentration to affect an infant. Use of ORLAAM in nursing mothers is not recommended unless, in the opinion of the treating physician, the potential benefits outweigh the possible hazards.

Pediatric Use
The use of ORLAAM in addicts under 18 years of age has not been studied. Its use is not recommended and is contrary to current regulations.

ADVERSE REACTIONS

Physicians should be alert to palpitations, syncope, or other symptoms suggestive of episodes of irregular cardiac rhythm in patients taking ORLAAM and promptly evaluate such cases (see WARNINGS, Effects on Cardiac Conduction).

Heroin or Methadone Withdrawal Reactions
Patients presenting for ORLAAM treatment are frequently in withdrawal from heroin or other opiates. They may display typical withdrawal symptoms which should be differentiated from ORLAAM's side effects. Patients may exhibit some or all of the following signs and symptoms associated with withdrawal from opiates: lacrimation, rhinorrhea, sneezing, yawning, perspiration, gooseflesh, fever, chilliness alternating with flushing, restlessness, irritability, insomnia, weakness, anxiety, depression, dilated pupils, tremors, tachycardia, abdominal cramps, body aches, anorexia, nausea, vomiting, diarrhea, and weight loss. Control of such symptoms is a primary goal of therapy. However, because of the slow onset and long half-lives of ORLAAM, nor-LAAM and dinor-LAAM, overly aggressive increases in dosage to control these withdrawal symptoms with ORLAAM may result in overdose (see INDIVIDUALIZATION OF DOSAGE).

Signs and Symptoms of ORLAAM Excess
The interaction between the development and maintenance of opioid tolerance and ORLAAM dose can be complex. Dose reduction is recommended in cases where patients develop signs and symptoms of excessive ORLAAM effect, characterized by complaints of "feeling wired", poor concentration, drowsiness, and possibly dizziness on standing.

ORLAAM Withdrawal
Patients may experience withdrawal symptoms (nasal congestion, abdominal symptoms, diarrhea, muscle aches, anxiety) over the 72-hour dosing interval if the dose of ORLAAM is too low. This may be managed as described under INDIVIDUALIZATION OF DOSAGE, but physicians should be alert to the possible need for dose or dose schedule adjustments if patients complain of weekend withdrawal symptoms in the last day of the 72-hour dosing interval.

Adverse Reactions on Stable Therapy
The following adverse events were observed in the 25-site, 623-patient usage study in male and female opiate addicts (see CLINICAL TRIALS). These signs and symptoms were reported during the second and third months of treatment with ORLAAM, and were considered severe enough to require medical evaluation. In this study, both questionnaires and spontaneous reports were used to gather information. Questionnaire-elicited symptom frequencies were about five times as frequent as the spontaneous reporting frequencies given below.

Incidence greater than 1%, Probably Causally Related

Body as a Whole—	Asthenia*, back pain, chills, edema, hot flashes (males 2:1), flu syndrome and malaise (11%).
Gastrointestinal—	Abdominal pain*, constipation*, diarrhea, dry mouth, nausea and vomiting.
Musculoskeletal—	Arthralgia*
Nervous System—	Abnormal dreams, anxiety, decreased sex drive, depression, euphoria, headache, hypesthesia, insomnia (9.1%), nervousness*, somnolence.
Respiratory—	Cough, rhinitis, and yawning.
Skin/appendages—	Rash, sweating*.
Special Senses—	Blurred vision.
Urogenital—	Difficult ejaculation*, impotence*.

*Reactions in 3–9% of patients; reactions in 1–3% are unmarked.

Incidence less than 1%, Probably Causally Related

Cardiovascular—	Postural hypotension.
Musculoskeletal—	Myalgia.
Special Senses—	Tearing.

Causal Relationship Unknown
These reactions were reported with low frequency in controlled and uncontrolled studies of LAAM, are not known to be causally related to the administration of the drug, and are provided as alerting information for physicians.

Cardiovascular—	Hypertension
Hepatic—	Hepatitis and abnormal liver function tests.
Urogenital—	Amenorrhea, pyuria.

The following adverse reactions have been reported in the post-marketing setting (all reactions in less than 1% of patients).

Body as a Whole—	Altered hormone level, chest pain.
Cardiovascular—	QT interval prolongation, torsade de pointes, cardiac arrest, ST segment elevation, ventricular tachycardia, myocardial infarction, angina pectoris, syncope, migraine.
Nervous System—	Convulsions, confusion, hallucination, incoordination, amnesia.
Respiratory—	Apnea, dyspnea.
Urogenital—	Breast enlargement.

Continued on next page

Orlaam—Cont.

DRUG DEPENDENCE

ORLAAM is a Schedule II controlled substance under the Federal Controlled Substances Act. ORLAAM produces dependence of the morphine-type and has potential for abuse. Tolerance and physical dependence will develop upon repeated administration. As with methadone and any other narcotic administered to narcotic addicts, ORLAAM is at risk for diversion and illicit use, and should be handled accordingly (see WARNINGS).

OVERDOSE

Signs and Symptoms

All but a few cases of ORLAAM overdose have involved multiple drugs. Overdose on ORLAAM alone is rare and has always been the result of too frequent (daily) dosing. Overdose is primarily of concern in persons not tolerant to opiates, since in such individuals a dose of 20 to 40 mg of ORLAAM may cause somnolence, and a larger initial dose may cause serious overdose. Tolerant individuals will generally not show symptoms unless higher doses are administered.

In ORLAAM overdose, as with other mu agonist opioids, the following signs and symptoms should be anticipated: respiratory depression (decrease in respiratory rate and/or tidal volume, Cheyenne-Stokes respiration, cyanosis), extreme somnolence progressing to stupor or coma, maximally constricted pupils, skeletal muscle flaccidity, cold and clammy skin, bradycardia, and hypotension. In severe overdose, apnea, circulatory collapse, pulmonary edema, cardiac arrest and death may occur.

Treatment

In the case of ORLAAM overdose, protect the patient's airway and support ventilation and circulation. Absorption of ORLAAM from the gastrointestinal tract may be decreased by gastric emptying and/or administration of activated charcoal. (Safeguard the patient's airway when employing gastric emptying or administering charcoal in any patient with diminished consciousness). Forced diuresis, peritoneal dialysis, hemodialysis, or charcoal hemoperfusion are unlikely to be beneficial for ORLAAM overdose due to its high lipid solubility and large volume of distribution.

In managing ORLAAM overdose, the physician should consider the possibility of multiple drugs, the interaction between drugs, and any unusual drug kinetics in the patient. Naloxone may be given to antagonize opiate effects, but the airway must be secured as vomiting may ensue. If possible, naloxone should be titrated to clinical effect rather than given as a large single bolus, since rapid reversal of opioid effects by large naloxone doses can cause severe precipitated withdrawal effects that may include cardiac instability. If a patient has received a total of 10 mg of naloxone without clinical response, the diagnosis of opioid overdose is unlikely.

If the patient does respond to naloxone, the physician should remember that the duration of ORLAAM activity is much longer (days) than that of naloxone (minutes) and repeated dosing with or continuous intravenous infusion of naloxone is likely to be required. Use of oral naltrexone in this setting is not recommended because it may precipitate prolonged opioid withdrawal symptoms (see Use of Narcotic Antagonists).

DOSAGE AND ADMINISTRATION

ORLAAM produces opioid effects and a high degree of opioid tolerance that inhibits drug-seeking behavior and blocks the euphoria produced by the usual doses of heroin. The dose of ORLAAM in each patient should be adjusted to achieve the optimal therapeutic benefit with acceptable adverse opioid effects (see INDIVIDUALIZATION OF DOSAGE).

ORLAAM must always be diluted before administration, and should be mixed with diluent prior to dispensing. To avoid confusion between prepared doses of ORLAAM and methadone, the liquid used to dilute ORLAAM should be a different color from that used to dilute methadone in any specific clinic setting.

ORLAAM DOSING

Dosing Schedules

ORLAAM is usually administered three times a week, either on Monday, Wednesday and Friday, or on Tuesday, Thursday and Saturday. If withdrawal is a problem during the 72-hour inter-dose interval, the preceding dose may be increased. In some cases, an every-other-day schedule may be appropriate (see INDIVIDUALIZATION OF DOSAGE).

The usual doses of ORLAAM must not be given on consecutive days because of the risk of fatal overdose. No dose mentioned in this label is **ever** meant to be given as a daily dose (see WARNINGS).

INDUCTION

The initial dose of ORLAAM for street addicts should be 20 to 40 mg. Each subsequent dose, administered at 48- or 72-hour intervals, may be adjusted in increments of 5 to 10 mg until a pharmacokinetic and pharmacodynamic steady-state is reached, usually within 1 or 2 weeks (see INDIVIDUALIZATION OF DOSAGE).

Patients dependent on methadone may require higher initial doses of ORLAAM. The suggested initial 3-times-a-week dose of ORLAAM for such patients is 1.2 to 1.3 times the daily methadone maintenance dose being replaced. This initial dose should not exceed 120 mg and subsequent doses, administered at 48- or 72-hour intervals, should be adjusted according to clinical response.

Most patients can tolerate the 72-hour inter-dose interval during the induction period. Some patients may require additional intervention (see INDIVIDUALIZATION OF DOSAGE). If additional opioids are required, supplemental methadone in small doses should be given rather than giving ORLAAM on two consecutive days. Take-home doses of methadone always pose a risk in this setting and physicians should carefully weigh the potential therapeutic benefit against the risk of diversion.

In some cases, where the degree of tolerance is unknown, patients can be started on methadone to facilitate more rapid titration to an effective dose, then converted to ORLAAM after a few weeks of methadone therapy.

The crossover from methadone to ORLAAM should be accomplished in a single dose; complete transfer to ORLAAM is simpler and preferable to more complex regimens involving escalating doses of ORLAAM and decreasing doses of methadone.

Dosage should be carefully titrated to the individual; induction too rapid for the patient's level of tolerance may result in overdose. Serious hazards, as seen in association with all narcotic analgesics, are respiratory depression and, to a lesser extent, circulatory depression.

MAINTENANCE

Most patients will be stabilized on doses in the range of 60 to 90 mg, 3-times-a-week. Doses as low as 10 mg and as high as 140 mg three times a week have been given in clinical studies.

Supplemental dosing over the 72-hour inter-dose interval (weekend) is rarely needed. For example, if a patient on a Mon./Wed./Fri. schedule complains of withdrawal on Sundays, the recommended dosage adjustment is to increase the Friday dose in 5 to 10 mg increments up to 40% over the Mon./Wed. dose or to a maximum of 140 mg.

If withdrawal symptoms persist after adjustment of dose, consideration may be given to every-other-day dosing if clinic hours permit. If the clinic is not open seven days a week and every-other day dosing is not practical, the patient's schedule may be adjusted so the 72-hour interval occurs during the week and the patient can come to the clinic to receive a supplemental dose of methadone (see INDIVIDUALIZATION OF DOSAGE).

The maximum **total** amount of ORLAAM recommended for any patient is 140-140-140 mg or 130-130-180 mg on a thrice-weekly schedule or 140 mg every other day.

PLANNED TEMPORARY INTERRUPTION OF ORLAAM MAINTENANCE

ORLAAM take-home doses are not permitted by regulation. Thus, several circumstances may cause the planned temporary discontinuation of treatment with ORLAAM. Patients eligible for one or more take-home doses of methadone, who are unable to attend the clinic for their next regularly scheduled ORLAAM dose because of illness, personal or family crisis, other hardships, travel and/or state/federal holidays, may be temporarily transferred directly to methadone.

Patients meeting these criteria may receive one or more methadone doses. Methadone doses should be 80% of the patient's Monday/Wednesday ORLAAM dose (e.g., patients receiving 80-80-100 mg of ORLAAM on a Monday/Wednesday/Friday regimen would be transferred to a daily methadone dose of 64 mg). The first dose of methadone should be ingested no sooner than 48 hours after the last ORLAAM dose. The number of take-home methadone doses should be **two less** than the number of days of expected absence and should not exceed, in any case, the number of take-homes allowed in the methadone regulations.

Upon return to clinic, patients should resume ORLAAM maintenance following the same dosage regimen used prior to the temporary interruption (see above). If more than 48 hours has elapsed since their last methadone dose, patients should be reinducted on ORLAAM at a dose determined by clinical and/or toxicological evaluation of the patient by the physician.

REINDUCTION AFTER AN UNPLANNED LAPSE IN DOSING

Following a lapse of one ORLAAM dose:

1) If a patient comes to the clinic to be dosed **on the day following a missed scheduled dose** (misses Monday, arrives Tuesday), the regular Monday dose should be administered on Tuesday, with the scheduled Wednesday dose administered on Thursday and the Friday dose given on Saturday. The patient's regular schedule may be resumed the following Monday (misses Wednesday, receives the regular dose on Thursday and Saturday, and returns to the regular Monday/Wednesday/Friday dosing schedule the next week).
2) If a patient misses one dose and comes to the clinic **on the day of the next scheduled dose** (misses Monday, arrives Wednesday), the usual dose will be well tolerated in most instances, although a reduced dose may be appropriate in selected cases.

Following a lapse of more than one ORLAAM dose:

Patients should be reinducted at an initial dose of 1/2 or 3/4 their previous ORLAAM dose, followed by increases of 5 to 10 mg every dosing day (48- or 72-hours intervals) until their previous maintenance dose is achieved. Patients who have been off of ORLAAM treatment for more than a week should be reinducted.

TRANSFER FROM ORLAAM TO METHADONE

Patients maintained on ORLAAM may be transferred directly to methadone. Because of the difference between the two compounds' metabolites and their pharmacological half-lives, it is recommended that methadone be started on a daily dose at 80% of the ORLAAM dose being replaced; the initial methadone dose must be given no sooner than 48 hours after the last ORLAAM dose. Subsequent increases or decreases of 5 to 10 mg in the daily methadone dose may be given to control symptoms of withdrawal or, less likely, symptoms of excessive sedation, in accordance with clinical observations.

DETOXIFICATION FROM ORLAAM

There is a limited experience with detoxifying patients from ORLAAM in a systematic manner, and both gradual reduction (5 to 10% a week) and abrupt withdrawal schedules have been used successfully. The decision to discontinue ORLAAM therapy should be made as part of a comprehensive treatment plan (see INDIVIDUALIZATION OF DOSAGE).

SAFETY AND HANDLING

ORLAAM is a solution of a potent narcotic (LAAM). There are no known specific hazards associated with dermal and aerosol exposure to ORLAAM. In case of accidental dermal exposure, promptly remove contaminated clothing and rinse the affected skin with cool water.

For the first six to twelve months, sales of ORLAAM will be restricted to clinics that have received training in its use, until there is general knowledge about how to use the drug safely. Since ORLAAM can be potentially dangerous if diverted, appropriate security measures should be taken to safeguard stock of ORLAAM as required by 21 CFR 1301.74 & 1304.28.

HOW SUPPLIED

ORLAAM Oral Solution (10 mg/mL) is a clear, colorless liquid supplied in plastic bottles as follows:
NDC 0054-3649-63: **500 mL per bottle**
Store at controlled room temperature 15°–30°C (59°–86°F). Protect from direct sunlight.
ORLAAM is compatible with the materials used in most dispensing systems. Information about obtaining appropriate dispensing systems suitable for use with ORLAAM is available from the manufacturer upon request.

4065000 **Revised June 2000**
060
Roxane Laboratories, Inc.
Columbus, Ohio 43216

ROXANOL™ ROXANOL™–T ROXANOL 100™ Ⓒ

MORPHINE SULFATE (IMMEDIATE RELEASE) ORAL SOLUTION (CONCENTRATE)

Rx only.

DESCRIPTION

Each mL of Roxanol™ contains:
Morphine Sulfate .... 20 mg
Each mL of Roxanol™–T contains:
Morphine Sulfate .... 20 mg
Solution is also tinted/flavored
Each 5 mL of Roxanol 100™ contains:
Morphine Sulfate .... 100 mg

Chemically, Morphine Sulfate is, Morphinan-3,6-diol, 7,8-didehydro-4,5-epoxy-17-methyl-,(5α,6α)-, sulfate(2:1)(salt), pentahydrate, which can be represented by the following structural formula:

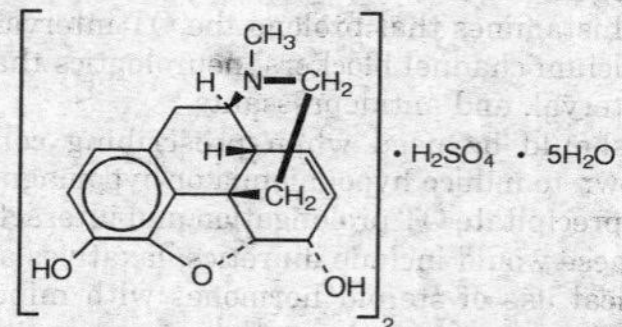

Morphine Sulfate acts as a narcotic analgesic.

CLINICAL PHARMACOLOGY

The major effects of morphine are on the central nervous system and the bowel. Opioids act as agonists, interacting with stereospecific and saturable binding sites or receptors in the brain and other tissues.

Morphine is about two-thirds absorbed from the gastrointestinal tract with the maximum analgesic effect occurring 60 minutes post administration.

INDICATIONS AND USAGE

Morphine is indicated for the relief of severe acute and severe chronic pain.

CONTRAINDICATIONS

Hypersensitivity to morphine; respiratory insufficiency or depression; severe CNS depression; attack of bronchial asthma; heart failure secondary to chronic lung disease; cardiac arrhythmias; increased intracranial or cerebrospinal pressure; head injuries; brain tumor; acute alcoholism; delirium tremens; convulsive disorders; after biliary tract surgery; suspected surgical abdomen; surgical anastomosis; concomitantly with MAO inhibitors or within 14 days of such treatment.

WARNINGS

Morphine can cause tolerance, psychological and physical dependence. Withdrawal will occur on abrupt discontinuation or administration of a narcotic antagonist.

Interaction with Other Central-Nervous-System Depressants —Morphine should be used with caution and in reduced dosage in patients who are concurrently receiving other narcotic analgesics, general anesthetics, phenothiazines, other tranquilizers, sedative-hypnotics, tricyclic antidepressants, and other CNS depressants (including alcohol). Respiratory depression, hypotension, and profound sedation or coma may result.

PRECAUTIONS

General

Head Injury and Increased Intracranial Pressure: The respiratory depressant effects of morphine and its capacity to elevate cerebrospinal-fluid pressure may be markedly exaggerated in the presence of increased intracranial pressure. Furthermore, narcotics produce side effects that may obscure the clinical course of patients with head injuries. In such patients, morphine must be used with caution and only if it is deemed essential.

Asthma and Other Respiratory Conditions: Morphine should be used with caution in patients having an acute asthmatic attack, in those with chronic obstructive pulmonary disease or cor pulmonale, and in individuals with a substantially decreased respiratory reserve, preexisting respiratory depression, hypoxia, or hypercapnia. In such patients, even usual therapeutic doses of narcotics may decrease respiratory drive while simultaneously increasing airway resistance to the point of apnea.

Hypotensive Effect: The administration of morphine may result in severe hypotension in an individual whose ability to maintain his blood pressure has already been compromised by a depleted blood volume or concurrent administration of such drugs as the phenothiazines or certain anesthetics.

Special-Risk Patients: Morphine should be given with caution and the initial dose should be reduced in certain patients, such as the elderly or debilitated and those with severe impairment of hepatic or renal function, hypothyroidism, Addison's disease, prostatic hypertrophy, or urethral stricture.

Acute Abdominal Conditions: The administration of morphine or other narcotics may obscure the diagnosis or clinical course in patients with acute abdominal conditions.

Information for Patients

Use in Ambulatory Patients —Morphine may impair the mental and/or physical abilities required for the performance of potentially hazardous tasks, such as driving a car or operating machinery. The patient should be cautioned accordingly.

Morphine, like other narcotics, may produce orthostatic hypotension in ambulatory patients.

Patients should be cautioned about the combined effects of alcohol or other central nervous system depressants with morphine.

Drug Interactions

Generally, effects of morphine may be potentiated by alkalizing agents and antagonized by acidifying agents. Analgesic effect of morphine is potentiated by chlorpromazine and methocarbamol. CNS depressants such as anaesthetics, hypnotics, barbiturates, phenothiazines, chloral hydrate, glutethimide, sedatives, MAO inhibitors (including procarbazine hydrochloride), antihistamines, β-blockers (propranolol), alcohol, furazolidone and other narcotics may enhance the depressant effects of morphine.

Morphine may increase anticoagulant activity of coumarin and other anticoagulants.

Carcinogenicity/Mutagenicity

Long-term studies to determine the carcinogenic and mutagenic potential of morphine are not available.

Pregnancy:

Teratogenic Effects: Pregnancy Category C. Animal production studies have not been conducted with morphine. It is also not known whether morphine can cause fetal harm when administered to a pregnant woman or can affect reproduction capacity. Morphine should be given to a pregnant woman only if clearly needed.

Labor and Delivery

Morphine readily crosses the placental barrier and, if administered during labor, may lead to respiratory depression in the neonate.

Nursing Mothers

Morphine has been detected in human milk. For this reason, caution should be exercised when morphine is administered to a nursing woman.

Pediatric Usage

Safety and effectiveness in children have not been established.

ADVERSE REACTIONS

THE MAJOR HAZARDS OF MORPHINE, AS OF OTHER NARCOTIC ANALGESICS, ARE RESPIRATORY DEPRESSION AND, TO A LESSER DEGREE, CIRCULATORY DEPRESSION, RESPIRATORY ARREST, SHOCK, AND CARDIAC ARREST HAVE OCCURRED.

The most frequently observed adverse reactions include lightheadedness, dizziness, sedation, nausea, vomiting, and sweating. These effects seem to be more prominent in ambulatory patients and in those who are not suffering severe pain. In such individuals, lower doses are available. Some adverse reactions may be alleviated in the ambulatory patient if he lies down.

Other adverse reactions include the following:

Central Nervous System: Euphoria, dysphoria, weakness, headache, insomnia, agitation, disorientation, and visual disturbances.

Gastrointestinal: Dry mouth, anorexia, constipation, and biliary tract spasm.

Cardiovascular: Flushing of the face, bradycardia, palpitation, faintness, and syncope.

Allergic: Pruritus, urticaria, other skin rashes, edema, and, rarely hemorrhagic urticaria.

Treatment of the most frequent adverse reactions

Constipation: Ample intake of water or other liquids should be encouraged. Concomitant administration of a stool softener and a peristaltic stimulant with the narcotic analgesic can be an effective preventive measure for those patients in need of therapeutics. If elimination does not occur for two days, an enema should be administered to prevent impaction.

In the event diarrhea occurs, seepage around a fecal impaction is a possible cause to consider before antidiarrheal measures are employed.

Nausea and Vomiting: Phenothiazines and antihistamines can be effective treatments for nausea of the medullary and vestibular sources respectively. However, these drugs may potentiate the side effects of the narcotics or the antinauseant.

Drowsiness (sedation): Once pain control is achieved, undesirable sedation can be minimized by titrating the dosage to a level that just maintains a tolerable pain or pain free state.

DRUG ABUSE AND DEPENDENCE

Morphine Sulfate, a narcotic, is a Schedule II controlled substance under the Federal Controlled Substance Act. As with other narcotics, some patients may develop a physical and psychological dependence on morphine. They may increase dosage without consulting a physician and subsequently may develop a physical dependence on the drug. In such cases, abrupt discontinuance may precipitate typical withdrawal symptoms, including convulsions. Therefore the drug should be withdrawn gradually from any patient known to be taking excessive dosages over a long period of time.

In treating the terminally ill patient the benefit of pain relief may outweigh the possibility of drug dependence. The chance of drug dependence is substantially reduced when the patient is placed on scheduled narcotic programs instead of a "pain to relief-of-pain" cycle typical of a PRN regimen.

OVERDOSAGE

Signs and Symptoms: Serious overdose with morphine is characterized by respiratory depression (a decrease in respiratory rate and/or tidal volume, Cheyne-Stokes respiration, cyanosis), extreme somnolence progressing to stupor or coma, skeletal muscle flaccidity, cold or clammy skin, and sometimes bradycardia and hypotension. In severe overdosage, apnea, circulatory collapse, cardiac arrest and death may occur.

Treatment: Primary attention should be given to the reestablishment of adequate respiratory exchange through provision of a patent airway and the institution of assisted or controlled ventilation. The narcotic antagonist naloxone is a specific antidote against respiratory depression which may result from overdosage or unusual sensitivity to narcotics, including morphine. Therefore, an appropriate dose of naloxone (usual initial adult dose: 0.4 mg) should be administered, preferably by the intravenous route and simultaneously with efforts at respiratory resuscitation. Since the duration of action of morphine may exceed that of the antagonist, the patient should be kept under continued surveillance and repeated doses of the antagonist should be administered as needed to maintain adequate respiration.

An antagonist should not be administered in the absence of clinically significant respiratory or cardiovascular depression.

Oxygen, intravenous fluids, vasopressors and other supportive measures should be employed as indicated.

Gastric emptying may be useful in removing unabsorbed drug.

DOSAGE AND ADMINISTRATION

Usual Adult Oral Dose: 10 to 30 mg every 4 hours or as directed by physician. Dosage is a patient dependent variable, therefore increased dosage may be required to achieve adequate analgesia.

For control of severe, chronic pain in patients with certain terminal disease, this drug should be administered on a regularly scheduled basis, every 4 hours, at the lowest dosage level that will achieve adequate analgesia.

Note: Medication may suppress respiration in the elderly, the very ill, and those patients with respiratory problems, therefore lower doses may be required.

Morphine Dosage Reduction: During the first two to three days of effective pain relief, the patient may sleep for many hours. This can be misinterpreted as the effect of excessive analgesic dosing rather than the first sign of relief in a pain exhausted patient. The dose, therefore, should be maintained for at least three days before reduction, if respiratory activity and other vital signs are adequate.

Following successful relief of severe pain, periodic attempts to reduce the narcotic dose should be made. Smaller doses or complete discontinuation of the narcotic analgesic may become feasible due to a physiologic change or the improved mental state of the patient.

HOW SUPPLIED

Roxanol™
Morphine Sulfate (Immediate Release)
Oral Solution (Concentrate)
20 mg per mL

NDC 0054-3751-44: Bottles of 30 mL with calibrated dropper.

NDC 0054-3751-50: Bottles of 120 mL with calibrated dropper.

Roxanol™–T
Morphine Sulfate (Immediate Release)
Oral Solution (Concentrate)
20 mg per mL (tinted/flavored)

NDC 0054-3774-44: Bottles of 30 mL with calibrated dropper.

NDC 0054-3774-50: Bottles of 120 mL with calibrated dropper.

Roxanol 100™
Morphine Sulfate (Immediate Release)
Oral Solution (Concentrate)
100 mg per 5 mL

NDC 0054-3751-58: Bottles of 240 mL with calibrated patient spoon.

DEA Order Form Required

4073001 Revised February 1999
029 ©RLI, 1999
Roxane Laboratories, Inc.
Columbus, OH 43216

Shown in Product Identification Guide, page 333

ROXICODONE™ C℞

[*rox-ē-cō-dōne*]
(oxycodone hydrochloride)
Tablets USP, Oral Solution USP, and Intensol™

DESCRIPTION

Each tablet contains:
Oxycodone Hydrochloride .... 5 mg
Each 5 mL Oral Solution contains:
Oxycodone Hydrochloride .... 5 mg
Each mL Intensol™ contains:
Oxycodone Hydrochloride .... 20 mg

Inactive Ingredients:

The tablets contain microcrystalline cellulose and stearic acid.

The oral solution contains alcohol, FD&C Red No. 40, flavoring, glycol, sorbitol, water, and other ingredients.

The Intensol™ contains citric acid, sodium benzoate, and water.

Oxycodone is 14-hydroxydihydrocodeinone, a white odorless crystalline powder which is derived from the opium alkaloid, thebaine, and may be represented by the following structural formula:

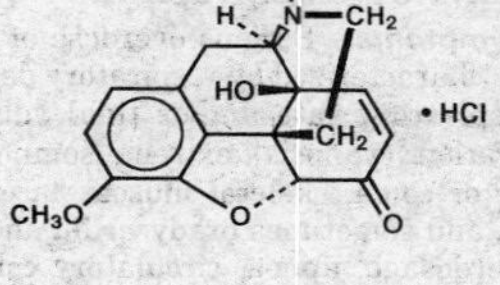

ACTIONS

The analgesic ingredient, oxycodone, is a semisynthetic narcotic with multiple actions qualitatively similar to those of morphine; the most prominent of these involve the central nervous system and organs composed of smooth muscle. The principal actions of therapeutic value of oxycodone are analgesia and sedation.

Oxycodone is similar to codeine and methadone in that it retains at least one half of its analgesic activity when administered orally.

INDICATIONS

For the relief of moderate to moderately severe pain.

CONTRAINDICATIONS

Hypersensitivity to oxycodone.

WARNINGS

Drug Dependence: Oxycodone can produce drug dependence of the morphine type, and therefore, has the potential for being abused. Psychic dependence, physical dependence and tolerance may develop upon repeated administration of this drug, and it should be prescribed and administered with the same degree of caution appropriate to the use of other oral narcotic-containing medications. Like other narcotic-containing medications, this drug is subject to the Federal Controlled Substances Act.

Usage in Ambulatory Patients: Oxycodone may impair the mental and/or physical abilities required for the performance of potentially hazardous tasks such as driving a car or operating machinery. The patient using this drug should be cautioned accordingly.

Interaction with Other Central Nervous System Depressants: Patients receiving other narcotic analgesics, general anesthetics, phenothiazines, other tranquilizers, sedative-hypnotics or other CNS depressants (including alcohol) concomitantly with oxycodone hydrochloride may exhibit an additive CNS depression. When such combined therapy is contemplated, the dose of one or both agents should be reduced.

Usage In Pregnancy: Safe use in pregnancy has not been established relative to possible adverse effects on fetal de-

Continued on next page

Roxicodone—Cont.

velopment. Therefore, this drug should not be used in pregnant women unless, in the judgment of the physician, the potential benefits outweigh the possible hazards.

Usage In Children: This drug should not be administered to children.

PRECAUTIONS

Head Injury and Increased Intracranial Pressure: The respiratory depressant effects of narcotics and their capacity to elevate cerebrospinal fluid pressure may be markedly exaggerated in the presence of head injury, other intracranial lesions or a pre-existing increase in intracranial pressure. Furthermore, narcotics produce adverse reactions which may obscure the clinical course of patients with head injuries.

Acute Abdominal Conditions: The administration of this drug or other narcotics may obscure the diagnosis or clinical course in patients with acute abdominal conditions.

Special Risk Patients: This drug should be given with caution to certain patients such as the elderly, or debilitated, and those with severe impairment of hepatic or renal function, hypothyroidism, Addison's disease and prostatic hypertrophy or urethral stricture.

ADVERSE REACTIONS

The most frequently observed adverse reactions include light headedness, dizziness, sedation, nausea and vomiting. These effects seem to be more prominent in ambulatory than in nonambulatory patients, and some of these adverse reactions may be alleviated if the patient lies down.

Other adverse reactions include euphoria, dysphoria, constipation, skin rash and pruritus.

DOSAGE AND ADMINISTRATION

The usual adult oral dose is 10 to 30 mg every 4 hours as needed for pain or as directed by physician. The dose must be individually adjusted according to severity of pain, patient response and patient size. More severe pain may require 30 mg or more every 4 hours. If the pain increases in severity, analgesia is not adequate or tolerance occurs, a gradual increase in dosage may be required.

For control of severe, chronic pain in patients with certain terminal diseases, this drug should be administered on a regularly scheduled basis, every 4 hours, at the lowest dosage level that will achieve adequate analgesia.

DRUG INTERACTIONS

The CNS depressant effects of oxycodone hydrochloride may be additive with that of other CNS depressants. See WARNINGS.

MANAGEMENT OF OVERDOSAGE

Signs and Symptoms: Serious overdose of oxycodone hydrochloride is characterized by respiratory depression (a decrease in respiratory rate and/or tidal volume, Cheyne-Stokes respiration, cyanosis), extreme somnolence progressing to stupor or coma, skeletal muscle flaccidity, cold and clammy skin, and sometimes bradycardia and hypotension. In severe overdosage, apnea, circulatory collapse, cardiac arrest and death may occur.

Treatment: Primary attention should be given to the reestablishment of adequate respiratory exchange through provision of a patent airway and the institution of assisted or controlled ventilation. The narcotic antagonist naloxone is a specific antidote against respiratory depression which may result from overdosage or unusual sensitivity to narcotics, including oxycodone. Therefore, an appropriate dose of naloxone (usual initial adult dose: 0.4 mg) should be administered, preferably by the intravenous route, simultaneously with efforts at respiratory resuscitation. Since the duration of action of oxycodone may exceed that of the antagonist, the patient should be kept under continued surveillance and repeated doses of the antagonist should be administered as needed to maintain adequate respiration.

An antagonist should not be administered in the absence of clinically significant respiratory or cardiovascular depression.

Oxygen, intravenous fluids, vasopressors and other supportive measures should be employed as indicated.

Gastric emptying may be useful in removing unabsorbed drug.

HOW SUPPLIED

5 mg white scored tablets. (Identified 54 582).

NDC 0054-8657-24: Unit dose, 25 tablets per card (reverse numbered), 4 cards per shipper.

NDC 0054-4657-25: Bottles of 100 tablets.

5 mg per 5 mL Oral Solution.

NDC 0054-8782-16: Unit dose Patient Cups™ filled to deliver 5 mL (oxycodone hydrochloride 5 mg), ten 5 mL Patient Cups™ per shelf pack, 4 shelf packs per shipper.

NDC 0054-3682-63: Bottles of 500 mL.

20 mg per mL Intensol™ (Concentrated Oral Solution)

NDC 0054-3683-44: Bottles of 30 mL with calibrated dropper [graduations of 0.25 mL (5 mg), 0.5 mL (10 mg), 0.75 mL (15 mg), and 1 mL (20 mg) on the dropper].

DEA Order Form Required

Rx only.

4064401 Revised June 1998
068

Roxane Laboratories, Inc.
Columbus, OH 43216

VIRAMUNE® ℞
[*vī'ră-mūne*]
(nevirapine) Tablets

VIRAMUNE ℞
(nevirapine) Oral Suspension

> WARNING:
> SEVERE, LIFE-THREATENING SKIN REACTIONS, INCLUDING FATAL CASES, HAVE OCCURRED IN PATIENTS TREATED WITH VIRAMINE®. THESE HAVE INCLUDED CASES OF STEVENS-JOHNSON SYNDROME, TOXIC EPIDERMAL NECROLYSIS, AND HYPERSENSITIVITY REACTIONS CHARACTERIZED BY RASH, CONSTITUTIONAL FINDINGS, AND ORGAN DYSFUNCTION. PATIENTS DEVELOPING SIGNS OR SYMPTOMS OF SEVERE SKIN REACTIONS OR HYPERSENSITIVITY REACTIONS MUST DISCONTINUE VIRAMUNE® AS SOON AS POSSIBLE. (See WARNINGS)
> SEVERE AND LIFE-THREATENING HEPATOTOXICITY, INCLUDING FATAL HEPATIC NECROSIS, HAS OCCURRED IN PATIENTS TREATED WITH VIRAMUNE®. (See WARNINGS)
> RESISTANT VIRUS EMERGES RAPIDLY AND UNIFORMLY WHEN VIRAMUNE® IS ADMINISTERED AS MONOTHERAPY. THEREFORE, VIRAMUNE® SHOULD ALWAYS BE ADMINISTERED IN COMBINATION WITH ANTIRETROVIRAL AGENTS.

DESCRIPTION

VIRAMUNE® is the brand name for nevirapine (NVP), a non-nucleoside reverse transcriptase inhibitor with activity against Human Immunodeficiency Virus Type 1 (HIV-1). Nevirapine is structurally a member of the dipyridodiazepinone chemical class of compounds.

VIRAMUNE® Tablets are for oral administration. Each tablet contains 200 mg of nevirapine and the inactive ingredients microcrystalline cellulose, lactose monohydrate, povidone, sodium starch glycolate, colloidal silicon dioxide and magnesium stearate.

VIRAMUNE® Oral Suspension is for oral administration. Each 5 mL of VIRAMUNE® suspension contains 50 mg of nevirapine (as nevirapine hemihydrate). The suspension also contains the following excipients: carbomer 934P, methylparaben, propylparaben, sorbitol, sucrose, polysorbate 80, sodium hydroxide and water.

The chemical name of nevirapine is 11-cyclopropyl-5,11-dihydro-4-methyl-6H-dipyrido [3,2-b:2',3'-][1,4] diazepin-6-one. Nevirapine is a white to off-white crystalline powder with the molecular weight of 266.3 and the molecular formula $C_{15}H_{14}N_4O$. Nevirapine has the following structural formula:

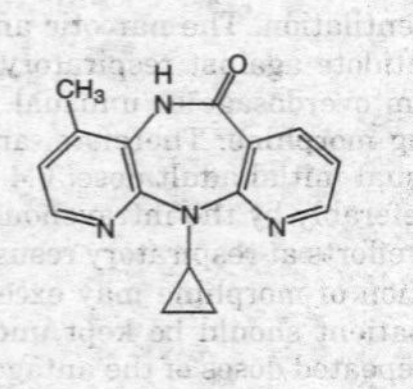

MICROBIOLOGY

Mechanism of Action: Nevirapine is a non-nucleoside reverse transcriptase inhibitor (NNRTI) of HIV-1. Nevirapine binds directly to reverse transcriptase (RT) and blocks the RNA-dependent and DNA-dependent DNA polymerase activities by causing a disruption of the enzyme's catalytic site. The activity of nevirapine does not compete with template or nucleoside triphosphates. HIV-2 RT and eukaryotic DNA polymerases (such as human DNA polymerases α, β, γ, or δ) are not inhibited by nevirapine.

In Vitro HIV Susceptibility: The relationship between *in vitro* susceptibility of HIV-1 to nevirapine and the inhibition of HIV-1 replication in humans has not been established. The *in vitro* antiviral activity of nevirapine was measured in peripheral blood mononuclear cells, monocyte derived macrophages, and lymphoblastoid cell lines. IC_{50} values (50% inhibitory concentration) ranged from 10 – 100 nM against laboratory and clinical isolates of HIV-1. In cell culture, nevirapine demonstrated additive to synergistic activity against HIV in drug combination regimens with zidovudine (ZDV), didanosine (ddI), stavudine (d4T), lamivudine (3TC), saquinavir, and indinavir.

Resistance: HIV isolates with reduced susceptibility (100 – 250-fold) to nevirapine emerge *in vitro*. Genotypic analysis showed mutations in the HIV RT gene at amino acid positions 181 and/or 106 depending upon the virus strain and cell line employed. Time to emergence of nevirapine resistance *in vitro* was not altered when selection included nevirapine in combination with several other NNRTIs.

Phenotypic and genotypic changes in HIV-1 isolates from patients treated with either nevirapine (n=24) or nevirapine and ZDV (n=14) were monitored in Phase I/II trials over 1 to ≥12 weeks. After 1 week of nevirapine monotherapy, isolates from 3/3 patients had decreased susceptibility to nevirapine *in vitro*; one or more of the RT mutations at amino acid positions 103, 106, 108, 181, 188 and 190 were detected in some patients as early as 2 weeks after therapy initiation. By week eight of nevirapine monotherapy, 100% of the patients tested (n=24) had HIV isolates with a >100-fold decrease in susceptibility to nevirapine *in vitro* compared to baseline, and had one or more of the nevirapine-associated RT resistance mutations; 19 of 24 patients (80%) had isolates with a position 181 mutation regardless of dose. Nevirapine+ZDV combination therapy did not alter the emergence rate of nevirapine-resistant virus or the magnitude of nevirapine resistance *in vitro*; however, a different RT mutation pattern, predominantly distributed amongst amino acid positions 103, 106, 188, and 190, was observed. In patients (6 of 14) whose baseline isolates possessed a wild type RT gene, nevirapine+ZDV combination therapy did not appear to delay emergence of ZDV-resistant RT mutations. The clinical relevance of phenotypic and genotypic changes associated with nevirapine therapy has not been established.

Cross-resistance: Rapid emergence of HIV strains which are cross-resistant to NNRTIs has been observed *in vitro*. Data on cross-resistance between the NNRTI nevirapine and nucleoside analogue RT inhibitors are very limited. In four patients, ZDV-resistant isolates tested *in vitro* retained susceptibility to nevirapine and in six patients, nevirapine-resistant isolates were susceptible to ZDV and ddI. Cross-resistance between nevirapine and HIV protease inhibitors is unlikely because the enzyme targets involved are different.

ANIMAL PHARMACOLOGY

Animal studies have shown that nevirapine is widely distributed to nearly all tissues and readily crosses the blood-brain barrier.

CLINICAL PHARMACOLOGY

Pharmacokinetics in Adults: **Absorption and Bioavailability:** Nevirapine is readily absorbed (>90%) after oral administration in healthy volunteers and in adults with HIV-1 infection. Absolute bioavailability in 12 healthy adults following single-dose administration was 93 ± 9% (mean ± SD) for a 50 mg tablet and 91 ± 8% for an oral solution. Peak plasma nevirapine concentrations of 2 ± 0.4 µg/mL (7.5 µM) were attained by 4 hours following a single 200 mg dose. Following multiple doses, nevirapine peak concentrations appear to increase linearly in the dose range of 200 to 400 mg/day. Steady state trough nevirapine concentrations of 4.5 ± 1.9 µg/mL (17 ± 7 µM), (n = 242) were attained at 400 mg/day. Nevirapine tablets and suspension have been shown to be comparably bioavailable and interchangeable at doses up to 200 mg. When VIRAMUNE® (200 mg) was administered to 24 healthy adults (12 female, 12 male), with either a high fat breakfast (857 kcal, 50 g fat, 53% of calories from fat) or antacid (Maalox® 30 mL), the extent of nevirapine absorption (AUC) was comparable to that observed under fasting conditions. In a separate study in HIV-1-infected patients (n=6), nevirapine steady-state systemic exposure (AUCτ) was not significantly altered by ddI, which is formulated with an alkaline buffering agent. VIRAMUNE® may be administered with or without food, antacid or ddI.

Distribution: Nevirapine is highly lipophilic and is essentially nonionized at physiologic pH. Following intravenous administration to healthy adults, the apparent volume of distribution (Vdss) of nevirapine was 1.21 ± 0.09 L/kg, suggesting that nevirapine is widely distributed in humans. Nevirapine readily crosses the placenta and is found in breast milk. (See PRECAUTIONS, *Nursing Mothers*) Nevirapine is about 60% bound to plasma proteins in the plasma concentration range of 1–10 µg/mL. Nevirapine concentrations in human cerebrospinal fluid (n=6) were 45% (± 5%) of the concentrations in plasma; this ratio is approximately equal to the fraction not bound to plasma protein.

Metabolism/Elimination: *In vivo* studies in humans and *in vitro* studies with human liver microsomes have shown that nevirapine is extensively biotransformed via cytochrome P450 (oxidative) metabolism to several hydroxylated metabolites. *In vitro* studies with human liver microsomes suggest that oxidative metabolism of nevirapine is mediated primarily by cytochrome P450 isozymes from the CYP3A family, although other isozymes may have a secondary role. In a mass balance/excretion study in eight healthy male volunteers dosed to steady state with nevirapine 200 mg given twice daily followed by a single 50 mg dose of ^{14}C-nevirapine, approximately 91.4 ± 10.5% of the radiolabeled dose was recovered, with urine (81.3 ± 11.1%) representing the primary route of excretion compared to feces (10.1 ± 1.5%). Greater than 80% of the radioactivity in urine was made up of glucuronide conjugates of hydroxylated metabolites. Thus cytochrome P450 metabolism, glucuronide conjugation, and urinary excretion of glucuronidated metabolites represent the primary route of nevirapine biotransformation and elimination in humans. Only a small fraction (<5%) of the radioactivity in urine (representing <3% of the total dose) was made up of parent compound; therefore, renal excretion plays a minor role in elimination of the parent compound.

Nevirapine has been shown to be an inducer of hepatic cytochrome P450 metabolic enzymes. The pharmacokinetics of autoinduction are characterized by an approximately 1.5 to 2 fold increase in the apparent oral clearance of nevirapine as treatment continues from a single dose to two-to-four weeks of dosing with 200 – 400 mg/day. Autoinduction also results in a corresponding decrease in the terminal phase half-life of nevirapine in plasma from approximately 45 hours (single dose) to approximately 25 – 30 hours following multiple dosing with 200 – 400 mg/day.

Pharmacokinetics in Special Populations: **Renal/Hepatic Dysfunction:** The pharmacokinetics of nevirapine have not been evaluated in patients with either renal or hepatic dysfunction.

Gender: In one Phase I study in healthy volunteers (15 females, 15 males), the weight-adjusted apparent volume of distribution (Vdss/F) of nevirapine was higher in the female subjects (1.54 L/kg) compared to the males (1.38 L/kg), suggesting that nevirapine was distributed more extensively in the female subjects. However, this difference was offset by a slightly shorter terminal-phase half-life in the females resulting in no significant gender difference in nevirapine oral clearance or plasma concentrations following either single- or multiple-dose administration(s).

Race: An evaluation of nevirapine plasma concentrations (pooled data from several clinical trials) from HIV-1-infected patients (27 Black, 24 Hispanic, 189 Caucasian) revealed no marked difference in nevirapine steady-state trough concentrations (median Cminss = 4.7 µg/mL Black, 3.8 µg/mL Hispanic, 4.3 µg/mL Caucasian) with long-term nevirapine treatment at 400 mg/day. However, the pharmacokinetics of nevirapine have not been evaluated specifically for the effects of ethnicity.

Geriatric Patients: Nevirapine pharmacokinetics in HIV-1 infected adults do not appear to change with age (range 18 – 68 years); however, nevirapine has not been extensively evaluated in patients beyond the age of 55 years.

Pediatric Patients: See PRECAUTIONS, *Pediatric Use*.

Drug Interactions: *Nucleoside Analogues:* No dosage adjustments are required when VIRAMUNE® is taken in combination with ZDV, ddI, or zalcitabine (ddC). Results from studies in HIV-1 infected patients who were administered VIRAMUNE® with different combinations of ddI or ddC, on a background of ZDV therapy, indicated that no clinically significant pharmacokinetic interactions occurred when the nucleoside analogues were administered in combination with VIRAMUNE®.

Protease Inhibitors: In the following three studies, VIRAMUNE® was given 200 mg once daily for two weeks followed by 200mg twice daily for 28 days:

Ritonavir: No dosage adjustments are required when VIRAMUNE® is taken in combination with ritonavir. Results from a 49-day study in HIV-infected patients (n=14) administered VIRAMUNE® and ritonavir (600 mg b.i.d. [using a gradual dose escalation regimen]) indicated that their coadministration did not affect ritonavir AUC or Cmax. Comparison of nevirapine pharmacokinetics from this study to historical data suggested that coadministration did not affect the pharmacokinetics of nevirapine.

Indinavir: Results from a 36-day study in HIV-infected patients (n=19) administered VIRAMUNE® and indinavir (800 mg q8h) indicated that their coadministration led to a 28% mean decrease (95% CI −39, −16) in indinavir AUC and an 11% mean decrease (95% CI −49, +59) in indinavir Cmax. The clinical significance of this interaction is not known. Comparison of nevirapine pharmacokinetics from this study to historical data suggested that coadministration did not affect the pharmacokinetics of nevirapine.

Saquinavir: Results from a 42-day study in HIV-infected patients (n=23) administered VIRAMUNE® and saquinavir (hard gelatin capsules, 600 mg t.i.d.) indicated that their coadministration led to a 24% mean decrease (95% CI −42, −1) in saquinavir AUC and a 28% mean decrease (95% CI −47, −1) in saquinavir Cmax. The clinical significance of this interaction is not known. Coadministration did not affect the pharmacokinetics of nevirapine.

In vitro: Studies using human liver microsomes indicated that the formation of nevirapine hydroxylated metabolites was not affected by the presence of dapsone, rifabutin, rifampin, and trimethoprim/sulfamethoxazole. Ketoconazole significantly inhibited the formation of nevirapine hydroxylated metabolites.

In vivo: ketoconazole: VIRAMUNE® and ketoconazole should not be administered concomitantly. Ketoconazole AUC and Cmax decreased by a median 63% (95% CI −95, +33) and 40% (95% CI −52, +11), respectively, in HIV-infected patients (n=22) who were given VIRAMUNE® 200 mg once daily for two weeks followed by 200 mg twice daily for two weeks along with ketoconazole 400 mg daily. (See PRECAUTIONS, *Drug Interactions*) Comparison of the pharmacokinetics from this study to historical data suggested that coadministration with ketoconazole may result in a 15 – 30% increase in nevirapine plasma concentrations. The clinical significance of this observation is not known.

Monitoring of nevirapine plasma concentrations in patients who received long-term VIRAMUNE® treatment indicate that steady-state nevirapine trough plasma concentrations were elevated in patients who received cimetidine (+21%, n=11) and macrolides (+12%, n=24), known inhibitors of CYP3A.

Steady-state nevirapine trough concentrations were reduced in patients who received rifabutin (−16%, n=19) and rifampin (−37%, n=3), known inducers of CYP3A. Nevirapine is an inducer of CYP3A, with maximal induction occurring within 2 – 4 weeks of initiating multiple-dose therapy. Other compounds that are substrates of CYP3A may have decreased plasma concentrations when co-administered with VIRAMUNE®. Therefore, careful monitoring of the therapeutic effectiveness of CYP3A-metabolized drugs is recommended when taken in combination with VIRAMUNE®. (See PRECAUTIONS, *Drug Interactions*, for recommendations regarding rifampin, rifabutin and oral contraceptives and methadone)

INDICATIONS AND USAGE

VIRAMUNE® (nevirapine) is indicated for use in combination with other antiretroviral agents for the treatment of HIV-1 infection. This indication is based on analyses of changes in surrogate endpoints. At present, there are no results from controlled clinical trials evaluating the effect of VIRAMUNE® in combination with other antiretroviral agents on the clinical progression of HIV-1 infection, such as the incidence of opportunistic infections or survival.

Resistant virus emerges rapidly and uniformly when VIRAMUNE® is administered as monotherapy. Therefore, VIRAMUNE® should always be administered in combination with at least one additional antiretroviral agent.

Description of Clinical Studies: **Patients with a prior history of nucleoside therapy:** ACTG 241 compared treatment with VIRAMUNE®+ZDV+ddI versus ZDV+ddI in 398 HIV-1-infected patients (median age 38 years, 74% Caucasian, 80% male) with CD4+ cell counts ≤350 cells/mm^3 (mean 153 cells/mm^3) and a mean baseline plasma HIV-1 RNA concentration of 4.59 $\log_{10}$ copies/mL (38,905 copies/mL), who had received at least 6 months of nucleoside therapy prior to enrollment (median 115 weeks). Treatment doses were VIRAMUNE®, 200 mg daily for two weeks, followed by 200 mg twice daily, or placebo; ZDV, 200 mg three times daily; ddI, 200 mg twice daily. Mean changes in CD4+ cell counts are shown in Figure 1. For 198 patients in the virology substudy, mean HIV-1 RNA concentration changes from baseline are shown in Figure 2.

Figure 1: Mean Change From Baseline for CD4+ Cell Count (absolute number of CD4+ cells/mm^3), Trial ACTG 241

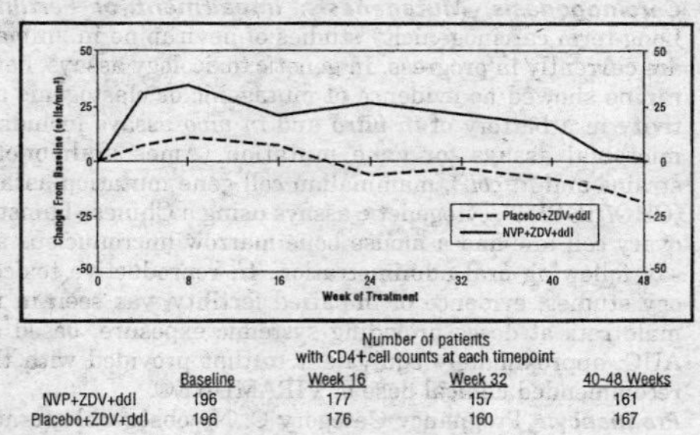

Number of patients with CD4+cell counts at each timepoint

	Baseline	Week 16	Week 32	40-48 Weeks
NVP+ZDV+ddI	196	177	157	161
Placebo+ZDV+ddI	196	176	160	167

Figure 2: Mean Change From Baseline in HIV-1 RNA* Concentrations ($\log_{10}$ copies/mL), Virology Sub-study of Trial ACTG 241

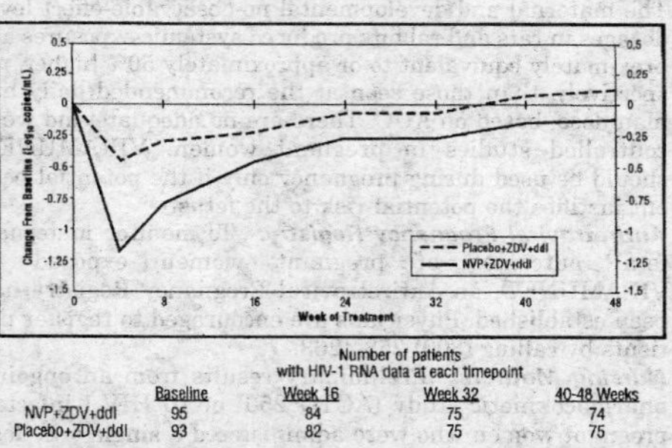

Number of patients with HIV-1 RNA data at each timepoint

	Baseline	Week 16	Week 32	40-48 Weeks
NVP+ZDV+ddI	95	84	75	74
Placebo+ZDV+ddI	93	82	75	75

* the clinical significance of changes in serum viral RNA measurements during treatment with VIRAMUNE® has not been established

Trial BI 1037 compared treatment with VIRAMUNE®+ZDV versus ZDV in 60 HIV-1-infected patients (median age 33 years, 70% Caucasian, 93% male) with CD4+ cell counts between 200 and 500 cells/mm^3 (mean 373 cells/mm^3) and a mean baseline plasma HIV-1 RNA concentration of 4.24 $\log_{10}$ copies/mL (17,378 copies/mL), who had received between 3 and 24 months of prior ZDV therapy (median 35 weeks). Treatment doses were VIRAMUNE® 200 mg daily for 2 weeks, followed by 200 mg twice daily, or placebo; ZDV, 500 – 600 mg/day. Mean changes in CD4+ cell counts are shown in Figure 3. Mean HIV-1 RNA concentration changes from baseline are shown in Figure 4.

Figure 3: Mean Change From Baseline for CD4+ Cell Count (absolute number of CD4+ cells/mm^3), Trial BI 1037

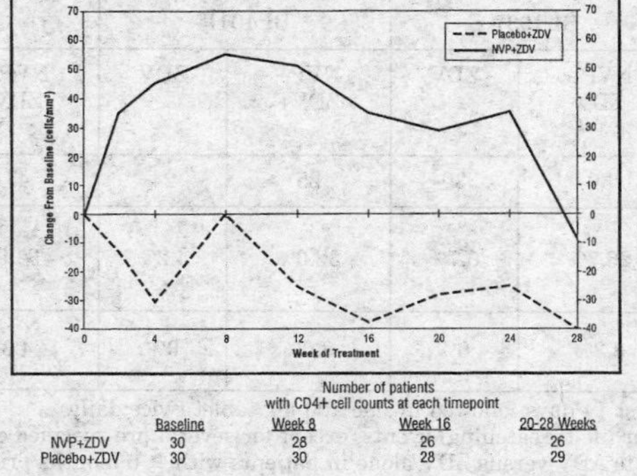

Number of patients with CD4+ cell counts at each timepoint

	Baseline	Week 8	Week 16	20-28 Weeks
NVP+ZDV	30	28	26	26
Placebo+ZDV	30	30	28	29

Figure 4: Mean Change From Baseline in HIV-1 RNA Concentrations ($\log_{10}$ copies/mL), Trial BI 1037

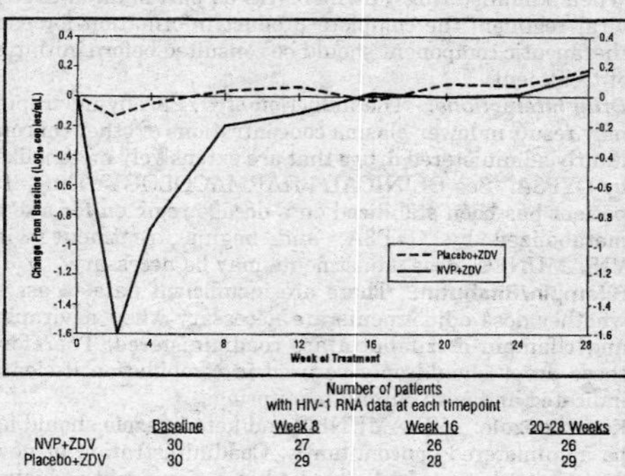

Number of patients with HIV-1 RNA data at each timepoint

	Baseline	Week 8	Week 16	20-28 Weeks
NVP+ZDV	30	27	26	26
Placebo+ZDV	30	29	28	29

Patients without a history of prior antiretroviral therapy: BI Trial 1046 compared treatment with VIRAMUNE® +ZDV+ddI versus VIRAMUNE®+ZDV versus ZDV+ddI in 151 HIV-1-infected patients (median age 36 years, 94% Caucasian, 93% male) with CD4+ cell counts of 200 – 600 cells/mm^3 (mean 376 cells/mm^3) and a mean baseline plasma HIV-1 RNA concentration of 4.41 $\log_{10}$ copies/mL (25,704 copies/mL). Treatment doses were VIRAMUNE®, 200 mg daily for two weeks, followed by 200 mg twice daily, or placebo; ZDV, 200 mg three times daily; ddI, 125 or 200 mg twice daily. Changes in CD4+ cell counts at 24 weeks: mean levels of CD4+ cell counts in those randomized to VIRAMUNE®+ZDV+ddI and ZDV+ddI remained significantly above baseline; however there was no significant difference between these arms. Changes in HIV-1 viral RNA at 24 weeks: there was no significant difference as measured by mean changes in plasma viral RNA between those randomized to VIRAMUNE®+ZDV+ddI and ZDV+ddI. However, the proportion of patients whose HIV-1 RNA decreased below the limit of detection (400 copies/mL) was significantly greater for the VIRAMUNE®+ZDV+ddI group (27/36 or 75%), when compared to the ZDV+ddI group (18/39 or 46%) or the VIRAMUNE®+ZDV group (0/28 or 0%); the clinical significance of this finding is unknown.

CONTRAINDICATIONS

VIRAMUNE® is contraindicated in patients with clinically significant hypersensitivity to any of the components contained in the tablet or the oral suspension.

WARNINGS

Severe, life-threatening skin reactions, including fatal cases, have occurred in patients treated with VIRAMUNE®. These have included cases of Stevens-Johnson syndrome, toxic epidermal necrolysis, and hypersensitivity reactions characterized by rash, constitutional findings, and organ dysfunction. Patients developing signs or symptoms of severe skin reactions or hypersensitivity reactions (including, but not limited to, severe rash or rash accompanied by fever, blisters, oral lesions, conjunctivitis, facial edema, muscle or joint aches, general malaise and/or significant hepatic abnormalities) must discontinue VIRAMUNE® as soon as possible. (See PRECAUTIONS, *Information for Patients;* ADVERSE REACTIONS) VIRAMUNE® therapy must be initiated with a 14-day lead-in period of 200 mg/day (4 mg/kg/day in pediatric patients), which has been shown to reduce the frequency of rash. If rash is observed during this lead-in period, dose escalation should not occur until the rash has resolved. (See DOSAGE AND ADMINISTRATION)

Severe or life-threatening hepatotoxicity, including fatal fulminant hepatitis (transaminase elevations, with or without hyperbilirubinemia, prolonged partial thromboplastin time, or eosinophilia), has occurred in patients treated with VIRAMUNE®. Some of these cases began in the first few weeks of therapy and some were accompanied by rash. VIRAMUNE® administration should be interrupted in patients experiencing moderate or severe ALT or AST abnormalities until these return to baseline values. VIRAMUNE® should be permanently discontinued if liver function abnormalities recur upon readministration. Monitoring of ALT and AST is strongly recommended, especially during the first six months of VIRAMUNE® treatment. (See PRECAUTIONS, *Information for Patients;* ADVERSE REACTIONS; DOSAGE AND ADMINISTRATION)

PRECAUTIONS

General: Nevirapine is extensively metabolized by the liver and nevirapine metabolites are extensively eliminated by the kidney. However, the pharmacokinetics of nevirapine have not been evaluated in patients with either hepatic or renal dysfunction. Therefore, VIRAMUNE® should be used with caution in these patient populations.

The duration of clinical benefit from antiretroviral therapy may be limited. Patients receiving VIRAMUNE® or any other antiretroviral therapy may continue to develop opportunistic infections and other complications of HIV infection, and therefore should remain under close clinical observation by physicians experienced in the treatment of patients with associated HIV diseases.

Continued on next page

Viramune—Cont.

When administering VIRAMUNE® as part of an antiretroviral regimen, the complete product information for each therapeutic component should be consulted before initiation of treatment.

Drug Interactions: The induction of CYP3A by nevirapine may result in lower plasma concentrations of other concomitantly administered drugs that are extensively metabolized by CYP3A. (See CLINICAL PHARMACOLOGY) Thus, if a patient has been stabilized on a dosage regimen for a drug metabolized by CYP3A, and begins treatment with VIRAMUNE®, dose adjustments may be necessary.

Rifampin/Rifabutin: There are insufficient data to assess whether dose adjustments are necessary when nevirapine and rifampin or rifabutin are coadministered. Therefore, these drugs should only be used in combination if clearly indicated and with careful monitoring.

Ketoconazole: VIRAMUNE® and ketoconazole should not be administered concomitantly. Coadministration of nevirapine and ketoconazole resulted in a significant reduction in ketoconazole plasma concentrations. (See CLINICAL PHARMACOLOGY, Drug Interactions)

Oral Contraceptives: There are no clinical data on the effects of nevirapine on the pharmacokinetics of oral contraceptives. Nevirapine may decrease plasma concentrations of oral contraceptives (also other hormonal contraceptives); therefore, these drugs should not be administered concomitantly with VIRAMUNE®.

Methadone: Based on the known metabolism of methadone, nevirapine may decrease plasma concentrations of methadone by increasing its hepatic metabolism. Narcotic withdrawal syndrome has been reported in patients treated with VIRAMUNE® and methadone concomitanly. Methadone-maintained patients beginning nevirapine therapy should be monitored for evidence of withdrawal and methadone dose should be adjusted accordingly.

Information for Patients: **Patients should be instructed that the major toxicity of VIRAMUNE® is rash and should be advised to promptly notify their physician of any rash.** Fatal skin reactions have been reported. The majority of rashes associated with VIRAMUNE® occur within the first 6 weeks of initiation of therapy. Patients should be instructed that if any rash occurs during the two-week lead-in period, the VIRAMUNE® dose should not be escalated until the rash resolves. Any patient experiencing severe rash or hypersensitivity reactions (rash accompanied by constitutional findings such as fever, blistering, oral lesions, conjunctivitis, facial edema, muscle or joint aches, general malaise, or significant hepatic abnormalities) should immediately discontinue medication and consult a physician.

Patients should be instructed that abnormal liver function tests and cases of clinical hepatitis, including fatal fulminant hepatitis, have been reported with VIRAMUNE®. Liver function tests should be monitored, especially during the first six months of therapy. VIRAMUNE® administration should be interrupted in patients experiencing moderate or severe liver function test abnormalities, until liver function tests return to baseline values; VIRAMUNE® should be permanently discontinued if liver function abnormalities recur upon readministration. Patients should be instructed to consult their physicians immediately should symptoms of hepatitis occur.

Oral contraceptives and other hormonal methods of birth control should not be used as a method of contraception in women taking VIRAMUNE®. (See PRECAUTIONS, *Drug Interactions*)

Patients should be informed that VIRAMUNE® therapy has not been shown to reduce the risk of transmission of HIV-1 to others through sexual contact or blood contamination. The long term effects of VIRAMUNE® are unknown at this time.

VIRAMUNE® is not a cure for HIV-1 infection; patients may continue to experience illnesses associated with advanced HIV-1 infection, including opportunistic infections. Treatment with VIRAMUNE® has not been shown to reduce the incidence or frequency of such illnesses; patients should be advised to remain under the care of a physician when using VIRAMUNE®.

Patients should be informed to take VIRAMUNE® every day as prescribed. Patients should not alter the dose without consulting their doctor. If a dose is missed, patients should take the next dose as soon as possible. However, if a dose is skipped, the patient should not double the next dose. Patients should be advised to report to their doctor the use of any other medications. Based on the known metabolism of methadone, nevirapine may decrease plasma concentrations of methadone by increasing its hepatic metabolism. Narcotic withdrawal syndrome has been reported in patients treated with VIRAMUNE® and methadone concomitantly. Methadone-maintained patients beginning nevirapine therapy should be monitored for evidence of withdrawal and methadone dose should be adjusted accordingly.

Table 1: Number of Pediatric Patients (%) with Marked Laboratory Abnormalities in Trials BI 882 and BI 892 Combined.

	No. (%) of Patients n=37
Hematology	
Decreased Hg (<8.0 g/dL)	7 (19)
Decreased platelets (<50,000/mm³)	4 (11)
Decreased neutrophils (<750/mm³)	14 (38)
Increased MCV (>100 F/L)	13 (35)
Blood Chemistry	
Increased ALT (>250 U/L)	4 (11)
Increased AST (>250 U/L)	5 (14)
Increased GGT (>450 U/L)	4 (11)
Increased total bilirubin (>2.5 mg/dL)	1 (3)
Increased alkaline phosphatase (>2x ULN)	19 (51)
Increased amylase (>2x ULN)	6 (16)

Carcinogenesis, Mutagenesis, Impairment of Fertility: Long-term carcinogenicity studies of nevirapine in animals are currently in progress. In genetic toxicology assays, nevirapine showed no evidence of mutagenic or clastogenic activity in a battery of *in vitro* and *in vivo* assays including microbial assays for gene mutation (Ames: Salmonella strains and *E. coli*), mammalian cell gene mutation assays (CHO/HGPRT), cytogenetic assays using a Chinese hamster ovary cell line and a mouse bone marrow micronucleus assay following oral administration. In reproductive toxicology studies, evidence of impaired fertility was seen in female rats at doses providing systemic exposure, based on AUC, approximately equivalent to that provided with the recommended clinical dose of VIRAMUNE®.

Pregnancy: Pregnancy Category C: No observable teratogenicity was detected in reproductive studies performed in pregnant rats and rabbits. In rats, a significant decrease in fetal body weight occurred at doses providing systemic exposure approximately 50% higher, based on AUC, than that seen at the recommended human clinical dose.

The maternal and developmental no-observable-effect level dosages in rats and rabbits produced systemic exposures approximately equivalent to or approximately 50% higher, respectively, than those seen at the recommended daily human dose, based on AUC. There are no adequate and well-controlled studies in pregnant women. VIRAMUNE® should be used during pregnancy only if the potential benefit justifies the potential risk to the fetus.

Antiretroviral Pregnancy Registry: To monitor maternal-fetal outcomes of pregnant women exposed to VIRAMUNE®, an Antiretroviral Pregnancy Registry has been established. Physicians are encouraged to register patients by calling (800) 258-4263.

Nursing Mothers: Preliminary results from an ongoing pharmacokinetic study (ACTG 250) of 10 HIV-1-infected pregnant women who were administered a single oral dose of 100 or 200 mg VIRAMUNE® at a median of 5.8 hours before delivery, indicate that nevirapine readily crosses the placenta and is found in breast milk.

Consistent with the recommendation by the U.S. Public Health Service Centers for Disease Control and Prevention that HIV-infected mothers not breast-feed their infants to avoid risking postnatal transmission of HIV, mothers should discontinue nursing if they are receiving VIRAMUNE®.

Pediatric Use: The pharmacokinetics of nevirapine have been studied in two open-label studies in children with HIV-1 infection. In one study (BI 853; ACTG 165), nine HIV-1-infected children ranging in age from 9 months to 14 years were administered a single dose (7.5 mg, 30 mg, or 120 mg per m²; n=3 per dose) of nevirapine suspension after an overnight fast. The mean nevirapine apparent clearance adjusted for body weight was greater in children compared to adults.

In a multiple dose study (BI 882; ACTG 180), nevirapine suspension or tablets (240 or 400 mg/m²/day) were administered as monotherapy or in combination with ZDV or ZDV+ddI to 37 HIV-1-infected pediatric patients with the following demographics: male (54%), racial minority groups (73%), median age of 11 months (range: 2 months- 15 years). The majority of these patients received 120 mg/m²/day of nevirapine for approximately 4 weeks followed by 120 mg/m²/b.i.d. (patients > 9 years of age) or 200 mg/m²/b.i.d. (patients ≤ 9 years of age). Nevirapine apparent clearance adjusted for body weight reached maximum values by age 1 to 2 years and then decreased with increasing age. Nevirapine apparent clearance adjusted for body weight was at least two-fold greater in children younger than 8 years compared to adults. The relationship between nevirapine clearance with long term drug administration and age is shown in Figure 5. The pediatric dosing regimens were selected in order to achieve steady-state plasma concentrations in pediatric patients that approximate those in adults. (See DOSAGE AND ADMINISTRATION, *Pediatric Patients*)

Figure 5: Nevirapine Apparent Clearance (mL/kg/hr) in Pediatric Patients

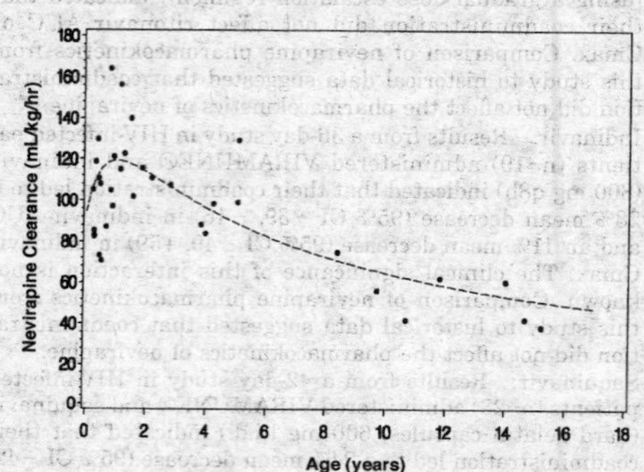

Evaluation of the pharmacokinetics of nevirapine in neonates is ongoing.

Safety was assessed in trial BI 882 in which patients were followed for a mean duration of 33.9 months (range: 6.8 months to 5.3 years, including long-term follow-up in 29 of these patients in trial BI 892). The most frequently reported adverse events related to VIRAMUNE® in pediatric patients were similar to those observed in adults, with the exception of granulocytopenia which was more commonly observed in children. Serious adverse events were assessed in ACTG 245, a double-blind, placebo controlled trial of VIRAMUNE® (n = 305) in which pediatric patients received combination treatment with VIRAMUNE®. In this trial two patients were reported to experience Stevens-Johnson syndrome or Stevens-Johnson/toxic epidermal necrolysis transition syndrome. Cases of allergic reaction, including one case of anaphylaxis, were also reported. The evaluation of the antiviral activity of VIRAMUNE® in pediatric patients is ongoing.

Table 2: Percentage of Patients with Rashes in Adult Controlled Trials[a]

	ACTG 241[b]		BI 1037		BI 1011[c]			BI 1046		COMBINED DATA	
	NVP+ ZDV+ ddI	ZDV+ ddI	NVP+ ZDV	ZDV	NVP+ ZDV+	ZDV	NVP+ ZDV	NVP+ ZDV+ ddI	ZDV+ ddI	NVP	Control
n	197	201	30	30	25	24	47	51	53	350	308
Rash events of all Grades and all causality	39.6%	23.9%	26.7%	6.7%	32.0%	4.2%	31.9	29.4%	13.2%	35.4%	18.8%
Grade 3 or 4 rash events; all causality	8.1%	1.5%	3.3%	0%	8.0%	0%	4.3	3.9%	1.9%	6.6%	1.3%

a At recommended dose of one 200 mg tablet daily for the first 14 days followed by one 200 mg tablet twice daily
b Trial ACTG 241 was designed to report Grade 3/4 (severe or life-threatening) events; except for several pre-specified events including rash for which all grades are reported
c Trial BI 1011 was an open-label comparison of NVP added to ADV versus ZDV alone in patients with ≥ 6 months prior antiretroviral therapy.

Table 3: Comparative Incidence of Selected Drug-Related Events in Adult Controlled Trials

	ACTG 241 Grade 3/4 Events		Trials BI 1037 and BI 1011[a] All Severities		Trial BI 1046 All Severities			COMBINED DATA	
	NVP+ ZDV+ ddI	ZDV+ ddI	NVP+ ZDV	ZDV Alone	NVP+ ZDV	NVP+ ZDV+ ddI	ZDV+ ddI	NVP	Control
Number of patients	197	201	55	30	47	51	53	350	284
Overall incidence of related adverse events	31%	23%	42%	33%	87%	71%	57%	46%	30%
Rash	8	2	20	3	24	24	6	14	2
Nausea	4	3	9	3	43	41	30	15	8
Headache	2	2	11	0	23	12	11	8	3
Abnormal LFT	5	3	2	3	17	10	4	7	3
Fatigue	1	0	10	0	19	16	23	7	4
Fever	3	1	11	3	6	4	6	5	2
Vomiting	2	1	4	0	15	6	8	5	2
Myalgia	1	0	2	3	13	8	8	4	1
Somnolence	0	0	6	0	4	8	8	3	1
Abdominal pain	1	1	2	0	13	2	2	3	1
Arthralgia	0	0	2	0	4	6	0	2	0
Hepatitis	1	0	4	0	2	0	0	1	0
Paraesthesia	1	0	2	0	2	2	0	1	0
Ulcerative Stomatitis	0	0	4	0	2	0	0	1	0
Diarrhea	2	2	0	0	11	12	13	4	4
Peripheral Neuropathy	0	2	0	0	0	0	0	0	1

a Total does not include patients who received ZDV alone in open label trial BI 1011.

Table 1 summarizes the marked laboratory abnormalities occurring in pediatric patients in Trial BI 882 and in follow-up Trial BI 892.

[See table 1 at top of previous page]

ADVERSE REACTIONS

Adults: The safety of VIRAMUNE® has been assessed in 2861 patients in clinical trials. The most clinically important adverse events associated with VIRAMUNE® therapy are rash and increases in liver function tests. Cases of hypersensitivity reactions have been observed.

The major clinical toxicity of VIRAMUNE® is rash, with VIRAMUNE®-attributable rash occurring in 16% of patients in combination regimens in Phase II/III controlled studies. Thirty-five percent of patients treated with VIRAMUNE® experienced rash compared with 19% of patients treated in control groups of either ZDV+ddI or ZDV alone (Table 2). Severe or life-threatening rash occurred in 6.6% of VIRAMUNE®-treated patients compared with 1.3% of patients treated in the control groups.

Rashes are usually mild to moderate, maculopapular erythematous cutaneous eruptions, with or without pruritus, located on the trunk, face and extremities. The majority of severe rashes occurred within the first 28 days of treatment; 25% of the patients with severe rashes required hospitalization; and one patient required surgical intervention. Overall, 7% of patients discontinued VIRAMUNE® due to rash.

[See table 2 at bottom of previous page]

[See table 3 above]

Laboratory Abnormalities: Table 4 summarizes marked laboratory abnormalities occurring in three controlled studies.

[See table 4 below]

Asymptomatic elevations in GGT levels are more frequent in VIRAMUNE® recipients than in controls. Because clinical hepatitis has been reported in VIRAMUNE®-treated patients, monitoring of ALT (SGPT) and AST (SGOT) is strongly recommended, especially during the first six months of VIRAMUNE® treatment. (See WARNINGS)

Post Marketing Surveillance: In addition to the adverse events identified during clinical trials, the following events have been reported with the use of VIRAMUNE® in clinical practice. Body as a whole: drug withdrawal (See PRECAUTIONS: *drug interactions*

Liver and Biliary: jaundice

Hematology: eosinophilia

Skin and Appendages: allergic reactions including anaphylaxis, angioedema, bullous eruptions, and urticaria have all been reported. In addition, hypersensitivity reactions with rash associated with constitutional findings such as fever, blistering, oral lesions, conjunctivitis, facial edema, muscle or joint aches, general malaise or significant hepatic abnormalities (See WARNINGS) plus one or more of the following: hepatitis, eosinophilia, granulocytopenia and/or renal dysfunction have been reported with the use of VIRAMUNE®.

Pediatric Patients: The most frequently reported adverse events related to VIRAMUNE® in pediatric patients were similar to those observed in adults, with the exception of granulocytopenia which was more commonly observed in children (See PRECAUTIONS: *Pediatric Use.*) The safety profile of VIRAMUNE® in neonates has not been established.

OVERDOSAGE

There is no known antidote for VIRAMUNE® overdosage. Cases of VIRAMUNE® overdose at doses ranging from 800 to 1800 mg per day for up to 15 days have been reported. Patients have experienced events including edema, erythema nodosum, fatigue, fever, headache, insomnia, nausea, pulmonary infiltrates, rash, vertigo, vomiting and weight decrease. All events subsided following discontinuation of VIRAMUNE®.

DOSAGE AND ADMINISTRATION

Adults: The recommended dose for VIRAMUNE® is one 200 mg tablet daily for the first 14 days **(this lead-in period should be used because it has been found to lessen the frequency of rash)**, followed by one 200 mg tablet twice daily, in combination with antiretroviral agents. For concomitantly administered antiretroviral therapy, the manufacturer's recommended dosage and monitoring should be followed.

Pediatric Patients: The recommended oral dose of VIRAMUNE® for pediatric patients 2 months up to 8 years of age is 4 mg/kg once daily for the first 14 days followed by 7 mg/kg twice daily thereafter. For patients 8 years and older the recommended dose is 4 mg/kg once daily for two weeks followed by 4 mg/kg twice daily thereafter. The total daily dose should not exceed 400 mg for any patient.

VIRAMUNE® suspension should be shaken gently prior to administration. It is important to administer the entire measured dose of suspension by using an oral dosing syringe or dosing cup. An oral dosing syringe is recommended, particularly for volumes of 5 mL or less. If a dosing cup is used, it should be thoroughly rinsed with water and the rinse should also be administered to the patient.

Monitoring of Patients: Clinical chemistry tests, which include liver function tests, should be performed prior to initiating VIRAMUNE® therapy and at appropriate intervals during therapy. (See WARNINGS)

Dosage Adjustment: **VIRAMUNE® should be discontinued if patients experience severe rash or a rash accompanied by constitutional findings. (See WARNINGS) Patients experiencing rash during the 14-day lead-in period of 200 mg/day (4 mg/kg/day in pediatric patients) should not have their VIRAMUNE® dose increased until the rash has resolved. (See PRECAUTIONS, *Information for Patients*)**

VIRAMUNE® administration should be interrupted in patients experiencing moderate or severe liver function test abnormalities (excluding GGT), until the liver function test elevations have returned to baseline. VIRAMUNE® may then be restarted at 200 mg per day (or 4 mg/kg/day in pediatric patients). Increasing the daily dose to 200 mg twice daily (4 or 7 mg/kg twice daily, according to age, for pediatric patients) should be done with caution, after extended observation. VIRAMUNE® should be permanently discontinued if moderate or severe liver function test abnormalities recur. (See WARNINGS)

Patients who interrupt VIRAMUNE® dosing for more than 7 days should restart the recommended dosing, using one 200 mg tablet daily (4 mg/kg/day in pediatric patients) for the first 14 days (lead-in) followed by one 200 mg tablet twice daily (4 or 7 mg/kg twice daily, according to age, for pediatric patients).

No data are available to recommend a dosage of VIRAMUNE® in patients with hepatic dysfunction, renal insufficiency, or undergoing dialysis.

HOW SUPPLIED

VIRAMUNE® (nevirapine) Tablets, 200 mg, are white, oval, biconvex tablets, 9.3 mm × 19.1 mm. One side is embossed with "54 193", with a single bisect separating the "54" and "193". The opposite side has a single bisect.

Table 4: Percentage of Adult Patients with Marked Laboratory Abnormalities

	Data combined for controlled trials ACTG 241, BI 1037, BI 1011 & BI 1046	
	VIRAMUNE® n=350	Control n=308
Hematology		
Decreased Hg (<8.0 g/dL)	1.1%	1.6%
Decreased platelets (<50,000/mm^3)	0.9	0.6
Decreased neutrophils (<750/mm^3)	9.1	9.4
Blood chemistry		
Increased ALT (>250 U/L)	5.1	3.9
Increased AST (>250 U/L)	3.4	2.3
Increased GGT (>450 U/L)	3.1	1.3
Increased total bilirubin (>2.5 mg/dL)	0.6	1.6

Continued on next page

Viramune—Cont.

VIRAMUNE® Tablets are supplied in bottles of 100 (NDC 0054-4647-25), bottles of 60 (NDC 0054-4647-21), and individually blister-sealed unit-dose cartons of 100 tablets as 10 × 10 cards (NDC 0054-8647-25).

VIRAMUNE® (nevirapine) Oral Suspension, is a white to off-white preserved suspension containing 50 mg nevirapine (as nevirapine hemihydrate) in each 5 mL. VIRAMUNE® suspension is supplied in plastic bottles with child-resistant closures containing 240 mL of suspension (NDC 0054-3905-58).

VIRAMUNE® Tablets and Oral Suspension should be stored at 15°C – 30°C (59°F – 86°F).

Roxane Laboratories, Inc
Columbus, OH 43216
Rx only
Revised 7/8/99

Shown in Product Identification Guide, page 333

Salix Pharmaceuticals, Inc.

4101 LAKE BOONE TRAIL, SUITE 418
RALEIGH, NORTH CAROLINA 27607

Direct Inquiries to:
phone: (919) 788-8550
fax (919) 788-8611

COLAZAL™ ℞

[*kōl a zal*]
(balsalazide disodium)
Capsules

DESCRIPTION

Each *COLAZAL™* capsule contains 750 mg of balsalazide disodium, a prodrug that is enzymatically cleaved in the colon to produce mesalamine (5–aminosalicylic acid), an anti inflammatory drug. Each daily dose of *COLAZAL™* (6.75 grams) is equivalent to 2.4 grams of mesalamine. Balsalazide disodium has the chemical name (E)-5-[[-4-[[(2-carboxyethyl) amino]carbonyl] phenyl]azo]-2-hydroxybenzoic acid, disodium salt, dihydrate. Its structural formula is:

[Structural formula: NaOOC, HO–C6H3–N=N–C6H4–C(=O)–NH–CH2–CH2–COONa • 2 H2O]

Molecular Weight: 437.32
Molecular Formula: $C_{17}H_{13}N_3O_6Na_2 \cdot 2H_2O$

Balsalazide disodium is a stable, odorless orange to yellow microcrystalline powder. It is freely soluble in water and isotonic saline, sparingly soluble in methanol and ethanol, and practically insoluble in all other organic solvents.

Inactive Ingredients: Each hard gelatin capsule contains colloidal silicon dioxide and magnesium stearate. The sodium content of each capsule is approximately 86 mg.

CLINICAL PHARMACOLOGY

Balsalazide disodium is delivered intact to the colon where it is cleaved by bacterial azoreduction to release equimolar quantities of mesalamine, which is the therapeutically active portion of the molecule, and 4-aminobenzoyl-β-alanine. The recommended dose of 6.75 grams/day, for the treatment of active disease, provides 2.4 grams of free 5-aminosalicylic acid to the colon.

The 4-aminobenzoyl-β-alanine carrier moiety released when balsalazide disodium is cleaved is only minimally absorbed and largely inert. The mechanism of action of 5-aminosalicylic acid is unknown, but appears to be topical rather than systemic. Mucosal production of arachidonic acid metabolites, both through the cyclooxygenase pathways, i.e., prostanoids, and through the lipoxygenase pathways, i.e., leukotrienes and hydroxyeicosatetraenoic acids, is increased in patients with chronic inflammatory bowel disease, and it is possible that 5-aminosalicylic acid diminishes inflammation by blocking production of arachidonic acid metabolites in the colon.

Pharmacokinetics: *COLAZAL™* capsules contain granules of balsalazide disodium which are insoluble in acid and designed to be delivered to the colon intact. Upon reaching the colon, bacterial azoreductases cleave the compound to release 5-aminosalicylic acid the therapeutically active portion of the molecule, and 4-aminobenzoyl-β-alanine.

Absorption: In healthy individuals, the systemic absorption of intact balsalazide was very low and variable. The mean C_{max} occurs approximately 1–2 hours after single oral doses of 1.5 grams or 2.25 grams. The absolute bioavailability of this compound was not determined. In a study of ulcerative colitis patients receiving balsalazide, 1.5 grams twice daily, for over one year, systemic drug exposure, based on mean AUC values, was up to 60 times greater (8 ng*hr/mL to 480 ng*hr/mL) after equivalent multiple doses of 1.5 grams twice daily when compared to healthy subjects who received the same dose. There was a large intersubject variability in the plasma concentration of balsalazide versus time profiles in all studies, thus its half-life could not be determined. The effect of food intake on the absorption of this compound was not studied.

Distribution: The binding of balsalazide to human plasma proteins was ≥ 99%.

Metabolism: The products of the azoreduction of this compound, 5-aminosalicylic acid and 4-aminobenzoyl-β-alanine, and their N-acetylated metabolites have been identified in plasma, urine and feces.

Elimination: Less than 1% of an oral dose was recovered as parent compound, 5-aminosalicylic acid or 4-aminobenzoyl-β-alanine in the urine of healthy subjects after single and multiple doses of *COLAZAL™*, while up to 25% of the dose was recovered as the N-acetylated metabolites. In a study with 10 healthy volunteers, 65% of a single 2.25 grams dose of *COLAZAL™* was recovered as 5-aminosalicylic acid, 4–aminobenzoyl-β-alanine, and the N-acetylated metabolites in feces, while <1% of the dose was recovered as parent compound.

In a study that examined the disposition of balsalazide in patients who were taking 3–6 grams of *COLAZAL™* daily for more than one year and who were in remission from ulcerative colitis, less than 1% of an oral dose was recovered as intact balsalazide in the urine. Less than 4% of the dose was recovered as 5-aminosalicylic acid, while virtually no 4-aminobenzoyl-β-alanine was detected in urine. The urinary recovery of the N-acetylated metabolites comprised 20–25% of the balsalazide dose. No fecal recovery studies were performed in this population.

Special Populations

Geriatric: No information is available for the geriatric population.

Pediatric: The safety and effectiveness of balsalazide in the pediatric population have not been established.

Gender: No adequate and well-controlled studies which examine balsalazide in males versus females are available.

Renal Insufficiency: No adequate and well-controlled studies which examine balsalazide disposition in patients with mild, moderate, and severe renal impairment are available.

Hepatic Insufficiency: No information is available for patients with hepatic impairment.

Race: No information is available which examines balsalazide in different races.

Pharmacodynamic/Pharmacokinetic Relationship: No information is available.

Drug-Drug Interactions: Neither in vitro nor in vivo drug-drug interaction studies have been performed with balsalazide.

Figure 1 :Percentage of Patients Improved at 8 Weeks

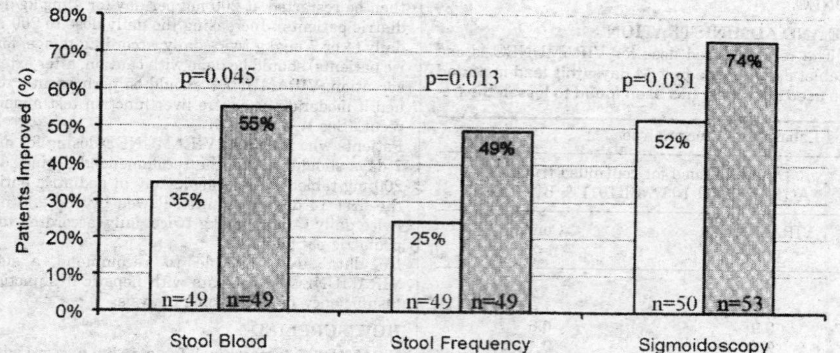

CLINICAL TRIALS

Two randomized, double blind studies were conducted.

In the first trial, 103 patients with active mild to moderate ulcerative colitis with sigmoidoscopy findings of friable or spontaneously bleeding mucosa were randomized and treated with balsalazide 6.75 grams/day or balsalazide 2.25 grams/day. The primary efficacy endpoint was reduction of rectal bleeding and improvement of at least one of the other assessed symptoms (stool frequency, patient functional assessment, abdominal pain, sigmoidoscopic grade, and physician's global assessment (PGA)). Outcome assessment for rectal bleeding at each interim period (week 2, 4, and 8) encompassed a 4 day period (96 hours). Results demonstrated a statistically significant difference between high and low doses of *COLAZAL™* (Figure 1).

[See graphic below]

A second study, conducted in Europe, confirmed findings of symptomatic improvement.

INDICATIONS AND USAGE

COLAZAL™ is indicated for the treatment of mildly to moderately active ulcerative colitis. Safety and effectiveness of *COLAZAL™* beyond 12 weeks has not been established.

CONTRAINDICATIONS

COLAZAL™ is contraindicated in patients with hypersensitivity to salicylates or to any of the components of *COLAZAL™* capsules or balsalazide metabolites.

PRECAUTIONS

Of the 259 patients treated with *COLAZAL™* 6.75 grams/day in controlled clinical trials of active disease, exacerbation of the symptoms of colitis, possibly related to drug use, has been reported by 3 patients.

General: Patients with pyloric stenosis may have prolonged gastric retention of *COLAZAL™* Capsules.

Renal: There have been no reported incidents of renal impairment in patients taking *COLAZAL™*. At doses up to 2000 mg/kg (approximately 21 times the recommended 6.75 grams/day dose on a mg/kg basis for a 70 kg person), *COLAZAL™* had no nephrotoxic effects in rats or dogs. Renal toxicity has been observed in animals and patients given other mesalamine products. Therefore, caution should be exercised when administering *COLAZAL™* to patients with known renal dysfunction or a history of renal disease.

Drug Interactions: No drug interaction studies have been conducted for *COLAZAL™*, however the use of orally administered antibiotics could, theoretically, interfere with the release of mesalamine in the colon.

Carcinogenesis, Mutagenesis, Impairment of Fertility: In a 24 month rat (Sprague Dawley) carcinogenicity study, oral (dietary) balsalazide disodium at doses up to 2 grams/kg/day was not tumorigenic. For a 50 kg person of average height this dose represents 2.4 times the recommended human dose on a body surface area basis.

Balsalazide disodium was not genotoxic in the following in vitro or in vivo tests: Ames test, human lymphocyte chromosomal aberration test, and mouse lymphoma cell (L5178Y/TK+/−) forward mutation test, or mouse micronucleus test. However, it was genotoxic in the in vitro Chinese hamster lung cell (CH V79/HGPRT) forward mutation test.

4-aminobenzoyl-β-alanine, a metabolite of balsalazide disodium, was not genotoxic in the Ames test and the mouse lymphoma cell (L5178Y/TK+/−) forward mutation test but was positive in the human lymphocyte chromosomal aberration test. N-acetyl-4-aminobenzoyl-β-alanine, a conjugated metabolite of balsalazide disodium, was not genotoxic in Ames test, the mouse lymphoma cell (L5178Y/TK+/−) forward mutation test, or the human lymphocyte chromosomal aberration test. Balsalazide disodium at oral doses up to 2 grams/kg/day, 2.4 times the recommended human dose based on body surface area, was found to have no effect on fertility and reproductive performance in rats.

Pregnancy—Teratogenic Effects: Pregnancy Category B. Reproduction studies were performed in rats and rabbits at oral doses up to 2 grams/kg/day, 2.4 and 4.7 times the recommended human dose based on body surface area for the rat and rabbit, respectively, and revealed no evidence of impaired fertility or harm to the fetus due to balsalazide disodium. There are, however, no adequate and well-controlled studies in pregnant women. Because animal reproduction studies are not always predictive of human response, this drug should be used during pregnancy only if clearly needed.

Nursing Mothers: It is not known whether balsalazide disodium is excreted in human milk. Because many drugs are excreted in human milk, caution should be exercised when *COLAZAL™* is administered to a nursing woman.

Pediatric Use: Safety and effectiveness of *COLAZAL™* in pediatric patients have not been established.

ADVERSE REACTIONS

Over 1000 patients received treatment with *COLAZAL™* in domestic and foreign clinical trials. In four controlled clinical trials patients receiving a *COLAZAL™* dose of 6.75 grams/day most frequently reported the following events (reporting frequency ≥3%), headache (8%), abdominal pain (6%), diarrhea (5%), nausea (5%), vomiting (4%), respiratory infection (4%), and arthralgia (4%). Withdrawal from therapy due to adverse events was comparable among patients on *COLAZAL™* and placebo.

Adverse events reported by 1% or more of patients who participated in the four well-controlled, Phase 3 trials are presented by treatment group (Table 1).

Table 1. Adverse Events Occurring in at Least 1% of *COLAZAL™* and Ulcerative Colitis Patients in Controlled Trials

Adverse Event	COLAZAL™ 6.75 grams/day [N = 259]	Placebo [N = 35]
Headache	22 (8%)	3 (9%)
Abdominal pain	16 (6%)	1 (3%)
Nausea	14 (5%)	2 (6%)
Diarrhea	14 (5%)	1 (3%)
Vomiting	11 (4%)	2 (6%)
Respiratory	9 (4%)	5 (14%)
Arthralgia	9 (4%)	–
Rhinitis	6 (2%)	–
Insomnia	6 (2%)	–
Fatigue	6 (2%)	–
Rectal bleeding	5 (2%)	1 (3%)
Flatulence	5 (2%)	–
Fever	5 (2%)	–
Dyspepsia	5 (2%)	–
Pharyngitis	4 (2%)	–
Pain	4 (2%)	1 (3%)
Coughing	4 (2%)	–
Back pain	4 (2%)	1 (3%)
Anorexia	4 (2%)	–
Urinary Tract	3 (1%)	–
Sinusitis	3 (1%)	1 (3%)
Myalgia	3 (1%)	–
Frequent stools	3 (1%)	1 (3%)
Flu-like Disorder	3 (1%)	–
Dry mouth	3 (1%)	–
Dizziness	3 (1%)	2 (6%)
Cramps	3 (1%)	–
Constipation	3 (1%)	

The number of placebo patients is too small for valid comparisons. Some adverse events, such as abdominal pain, fatigue, and nausea were reported more frequently in women subjects than in men. Abdominal pain, rectal bleeding, and anemia can be part of the clinical presentation of ulcerative colitis.

The following adverse events, presented by body system, have also been infrequently reported by patients taking *COLAZAL™* during clinical trials (n = 513) for the treatment of active acute ulcerative colitis or from foreign post-marketing reports. In most cases no relationship to *COLAZAL™* has been established.

Body as a Whole: abdomen enlarged, asthenia, chest pain, chills, edema, hot flushes, malaise

Cardiovascular and vascular: bradycardia, deep venous thrombosis, hypertension, leg ulcer, palpitations, pericarditis

Gastrointestinal: amylase increased, bowel irregularity, colitis ulcerative aggravated, diarrhea with blood, diverticulosis, epigastric pain, eructation, fecal incontinence, feces abnormal, gastroenteritis, giardiasis, glossitis, hemorrhoids, melena, neoplasm benign, pancreatitis, ulcerative stomatitis, stools frequent, tenesmus, tongue discoloration

Hematologic: anemia, epistaxis, fibrinogen plasma increase, hemorrhage, prothrombin decrease, prothrombin increase, thrombocythemia

Liver and biliary: bilirubin increase, hepatic function abnormal, SGOT increase, SGPT increase

Lymphatic: eosinophilia, granulocytopenia, leukocytosis, leukopenia, lymphadenopathy, lymphoma-like disorder, lymphopenia

Metabolic and nutritional: creatinine phosphokinase increased, hypocalcemia, hypokalemia, hypoproteinemia, LDH increase, weight decrease, weight increase

Musculoskeletal: arthritis, arthropathy, stiffness in legs

Nervous: aphasia, dysphonia, gait abnormal, hypertonia, hypoesthesia, paresis, spasm generalized, tremor

Psychiatric: anxiety, depression, nervousness, somnolence

Reproductive: menstrual disorder

Resistance Mechanism: abscess, immunoglobulins decrease, infection, moniliasis, viral infection

Respiratory: bronchospasm, dyspnea, hemoptysis

Skin: alopecia, angioedema, dermatitis, dry skin, erythema nodosum, erythematous rash, pruritus, pruritus ani, psoriasis, skin ulceration

Special Senses: conjunctivitis, earache, ear infection, iritis, parosmia, taste perversion, tinnitus, vision abnormal

Urinary: hematuria, interstitial nephritis, micturition frequency, polyuria, pyuria

Post Marketing Reports:

The following events have been identified during post-approval use in clinical practice, of products which contain (or are metabolized to) mesalamine. Because they are reported voluntarily from a population of unknown size estimates of frequency cannot be made. These events have been chosen for inclusion due to a combination of seriousness, frequency of reporting, or potential causal connection to mesalamine.

Gastrointestinal: Reports of hepatotoxicity, including elevated liver function tests (SGOT/AST, SGPT/ALT, GGT, LDH, alkaline phosphatase, bilirubin), jaundice, cholestatic jaundice, cirrhosis, hepatocellular damage including liver necrosis and liver failure. Some of these cases were fatal, however, no fatalities associated with these events were reported in *COLAZAL™* clinical trials. One case of Kawasaki-like syndrome which included hepatic function changes was also reported, however, this event was not reported in *COLAZAL™* clinical trials.

DRUG ABUSE AND DEPENDENCY

Abuse: None reported

Dependency: Drug dependence has not been reported with chronic administration of mesalamine.

OVERDOSAGE

No case of overdose has occurred with *COLAZAL™*. A 3–year-old boy is reported to have ingested 2 grams of another mesalamine product. He was treated with ipecac and activated charcoal with no adverse reactions.

If an overdose occurs with *COLAZAL™* use, treatment should be supportive, with particular attention to correction of electrolyte abnormalities.

A single oral dose of balsalazide disodium at 5 grams/kg or 4-aminobenzoyl-β-alanine, a metabolite of balsalazide disodium, at 1 gram/kg was non-lethal in mice and rats. No symptoms of acute toxicity were seen at these doses.

DOSAGE AND ADMINISTRATION

For Treatment of Active Ulcerative Colitis the usual dose in adults is three 750 mg *COLAZAL™* capsules to be taken three times a day for a total daily dose of 6.75 grams for a duration of 8 weeks. Some patients in the clinical trials required treatment for up to 12 weeks.

HOW SUPPLIED

COLAZAL™ is available as beige capsules containing 750 mg balsalazide and BZ imprinted in black.

NDC 65649-101-02 Bottles of 280 capsules

Store at 25°C (77°F); excursions permitted to 15–30°C (59–86°F). See USP Controlled Room Temperature.

Rx only

Manufactured for Salix Pharmaceuticals, Inc., Raleigh, N.C. 27607

by: Anabolic, Inc., Irvine, CA 92712

* *COLAZAL™* is a trademark of Salix Pharmaceuticals, Inc.

(07/00)

Shown in Product Identification Guide, page 333

Samra Health & Beauty, Inc.

3000 S. ROBERTSON BLVD.
SUITE 420
LOS ANGELES, CA 90034

For Direct Inquiries Contact:
1-888-417-2672

CALM COLON™ OTC
IBS FORMULA
HERBAL SUPPLEMENT

DESCRIPTION

Composition

Each Calm Colon capsule contains 500 mg of a 5:1 aqueous extract consisting of the following herbs:

Chinese Name	Common Name
Yin Chen	Capillary Artemisia Leaf
Bai Zhu	Atracylodes Root
Wu Wei Zi	Schisandra Fruit
Yi Yi Ren	Job's Tears Seed
Dang Shen	Codonopsis Root
Huo Xiang	Agastache Leaf
Chai Hu	Chinese Thouroughwax Root
Qin Pi	Fraxinus Chinensis Bark
Fu Ling	Wolfporia Cocos
Che Qian Zi	Asian Psyllium Seed
Huang Bai	Phellodendron Bark
Zhi Gan Cao	Licorice Root
Pao Jiang	Ginger Root
Huo Po	Magnolia Bark
Fang Feng	Fang Feng Root
Chen Pi	Tangerine Peel
Bai Shao	White Peony Root
Mu Xiang	Costus Root
Huang Lian	Chinese Goldthread Root
Bai Zhi	Fragrant Angelica Root

INDICATIONS AND USAGE

Calm Colon is indicated for irritable bowel syndrome.

DOSAGE

1 capsule 3 times daily one half hour before meals with water.

SUPPLIED

Bottle of 60 and 90 clear two piece gelatin capsules.

Sandoz Pharmaceuticals Corporation

PLEASE NOTE:

Due to the merger of CibaGeneva Pharmaceuticals and Sandoz Pharmaceuticals Corporation, please refer to **Novartis Pharmaceuticals Corporation** for branded product information and Geneva Pharmaceuticals, Inc. for branded generic product information.

Sankyo Pharma Inc.

TWO HILTON COURT
PARISPPANY, NJ 07054

Direct Inquiries to:
1-877-4SANKYO
www.welchol@sankyopharma.com

WELCHOL™ TABLETS ℞
(colesevelam hydrochloride)
[koe le sev' e lam]
Rx only

DESCRIPTION

WelChol™ contains colesevelam hydrochloride (hereafter referred to as colesevelam), a non-absorbed, polymeric, lipid-lowering agent intended for oral administration.

Colesevelam is a high capacity bile acid binding molecule.

Colesevelam is poly(allylamine hydrochloride) cross-linked with epichlorohydrin and alkylated with 1-bromodecane and (6-bromohexyl)-trimethylammonium bromide.

Colesevelam is hydrophilic, and insoluble in water.

WelChol™ is an off-white, film-coated, solid tablet containing 625 mg colesevelam. In addition, each tablet contains the following inactive ingredients: magnesium stearate, microcrystalline cellulose, and silicon dioxide. The tablets are imprinted using a water-soluble black ink.

CLINICAL PHARMACOLOGY

Mechanism of Action

The mechanism of action for the lipid-lowering activity of colesevelam, the active pharmaceutical ingredient in WelChol™, has been evaluated in various *in vitro* and *in vivo* studies. These studies have demonstrated that colesevelam binds bile acids, including glycocholic acid, the major bile acid in humans.

Cholesterol is the sole precursor of bile acids. During normal digestion, bile acids are secreted into the intestine. A major portion of bile acids are then absorbed from the intestinal tract and returned to the liver via the enterohepatic circulation.

Colesevelam is a non-absorbed, lipid-lowering polymer that binds bile acids in the intestine, impeding their reabsorption. As the bile acid pool becomes depleted, the hepatic enzyme, cholesterol 7-α-hydroxylase, is upregulated, which increases the conversion of cholesterol to bile acids. This causes an increased demand for cholesterol in the liver cells, resulting in the dual effect of increasing transcription and activity of the cholesterol biosynthetic enzyme, hydroxymethyl-glutaryl-coenzyme A (HMG-CoA) reductase, and increasing the number of hepatic low-density lipoprotein (LDL) receptors. These compensatory effects result in increased clearance of LDL cholesterol (LDL-C) from the blood, resulting in decreased serum LDL-C levels.[1, 2]

Clinical studies have demonstrated that elevated levels of total cholesterol (total-C), LDL-C, and apolipoprotein B (Apo B, a protein associated with LDL-C) are associated with an increased risk of atherosclerosis in humans. Similarly, decreased levels of high-density lipoprotein cholesterol (HDL-C) are associated with the development of atherosclerosis[1]. Epidemiological investigations have established that cardiovascular morbidity and mortality vary directly with the levels of total-C and LDL-C, and inversely with the level of HDL-C.

The combination of colesevelam and an HMG-CoA reductase inhibitor is effective in further lowering serum total-C and LDL-C levels beyond that achieved by either agent alone. The effects of colesevelam either alone or with an HMG-CoA reductase inhibitor on cardiovascular morbidity and mortality have not been determined.

Pharmacokinetics

Colesevelam is a hydrophilic, water-insoluble polymer that is not hydrolyzed by digestive enzymes and is not absorbed. In 16 healthy volunteers, an average of 0.05% of a single ^{14}C-labeled colesevelam dose was excreted in the urine when given following 28 days of chronic dosing of 1.9 grams of colesevelam twice per day.

Clinical Trials

WelChol™ reduces total-C, LDL-C, and Apo B, and increases HDL-C when administered either alone or in combination with an HMG-CoA reductase inhibitor in patients with primary hypercholesterolemia.

Continued on next page

Welchol—Cont.

Approximately 1400 patients were studied in eight clinical trials with treatment durations ranging from 4 to 50 weeks. With the exception of one long-term study, all studies were multicenter, randomized, double-blind, and placebo-controlled. A maximum therapeutic response to WelChol™ was achieved within 2 weeks and was maintained during long-term therapy.

In a study in patients with LDL-C between 130 and 200 mg/dL (mean 158 mg/dL), WelChol™ was given for 24 weeks in divided doses with the morning and evening meals. As shown in Table 1 below, the mean LDL-C reductions were 15% and 18% at the 3.8 g and 4.5 g doses. The respective mean total-C reductions were 7% and 10%. The mean Apo B reductions were 12% in both treatment groups. WelChol™ at both doses increased HDL-C by 3%. There were small increases in triglycerides (TG) at both WelChol™ doses that were not statistically different from placebo.

[See table 1 above]

In a study in 98 patients with LDL-C between 145 and 250 mg/dL (mean 169 mg/dL), WelChol™ 3.8 g was given for 6 weeks as a single dose with breakfast, a single dose with dinner, or as divided doses with breakfast and dinner. The mean LDL-C reductions were 18%, 15%, and 18% for the three dosing regimens, respectively. The reductions with these three regimens were not statistically different from one another.

Co-administration of WelChol™ and an HMG-CoA reductase inhibitor (atorvastatin, lovastatin, or simvastatin) demonstrated an additive reduction of LDL-C in three clinical studies. As demonstrated in Table 2 below, WelChol™ doses of 2.3 g to 3.8 g resulted in additional 8% to 16% reductions in LDL-C above that seen with the HMG-CoA reductase inhibitor alone.

[See table 2 above]

In all three studies, the LDL-C reduction achieved with the combination of WelChol™ and any given doses of HMG-CoA reductase inhibitor therapy was statistically superior to that achieved with WelChol™ or that dose of the HMG-CoA reductase inhibitor alone.

The LDL-C reduction with atorvastatin 80 mg was not statistically significantly different from the combination of WelChol™ 3.8 g and atorvastatin 10 mg.

Table 1: WelChol™ 24 Week Trial - Percentage Change in Lipid Parameters From Baseline

GRAMS/DAY	N	LDL-C	TOTAL-C	HDL-C	TG	APO B
Placebo	88	0	+1	−1	+5	0
3.8 g (6 tablets)	95	−15*	−7*	+3*	+10	−12*
4.5 g (7 tablets)	94	−18*	−10*	+3	+9	−12*

*$p<0.05$ for lipid parameters compared to placebo, for Apo B compared to baseline LDL-C, total-C, and Apo B are mean values; HDL-C and TG are median values.

Table 2: WelChol™ in Combination with Atorvastatin, Simvastatin, and Lovastatin - Percentage Change in Lipid Parameters

DOSE/DAY	N	LDL-C	TOTAL-C	HDL-C	TG	APO B
Atorvastatin Trial (4-week)						
Placebo	19	+3	+4	+4	+10	−2
Atorvastatin 10 mg	18	−38*	−27*	+8	−24*	−32*
WelChol™ 3.8 g/ Atorvastatin 10 mg	18	−48*	−31*	+11	−1	−38*
Atorvastatin 80 mg	20	−53*	−39*	+6	−33*	−46*
Simvastatin Trial (6-week)						
Placebo	33	−4	−2	−3	+6	−4*
Simvastatin 10 mg	35	−26*	−19*	+3*	−17*	−20*
WelChol™ 3.8 g/ Simvastatin 10 mg	34	−42*	−28*	+10*	−12*	−33*
Simvastatin 20 mg	39	−34*	−23*	+7*	−12*	−26*
WelChol™ 2.3 g/ Simvastatin 20 mg	37	−42*	−29*	+4*	−12*	−32*
Lovastatin Trial (4-week)						
Placebo	26	0	+1	+1	+1	0
Lovastatin 10 mg	26	−22*	−14*	+5	0	−16*
WelChol™ 2.3 g/ Lovastatin 10 mg together	27	−34*	−21*	+4	−1	−24*
WelChol™ 2.3 g/ Lovastatin 10 mg apart	23	−32*	−21*	+2	−2	−24*

*$p<0.05$ for lipid parameters compared to placebo, for Apo B compared to baseline LDL-C, total-C and Apo B are mean values; HDL-C and TG are median values.

INDICATIONS AND USAGE

WelChol™, administered alone or in combination with an HMG-CoA reductase inhibitor, is indicated as adjunctive therapy to diet and exercise for the reduction of elevated LDL cholesterol in patients with primary hypercholesterolemia (Fredrickson Type IIa).

Therapy with lipid lowering agents should be a component of multiple risk-factor intervention in patients at significant increased risk for atherosclerotic vascular disease due to hypercholesterolemia. Lipid altering agents should be used in addition to a diet restricted in saturated fat and cholesterol and when the response to diet and other non-pharmacological means has been inadequate.

Prior to initiating therapy with WelChol™, secondary causes of hypercholesterolemia (i.e., poorly controlled diabetes mellitus, hypothyroidism, nephrotic syndrome, dysproteinemias, obstructive liver disease, other drug therapy, alcoholism) should be excluded, and a lipid profile obtained to assess total-C, HDL-C, and TG. For individuals with TG less than 400 mg/dL, LDL-C can be estimated using the following equation.[3]

LDL-C = Total-C - [(TG/5) + HDL-C]

Periodic determination of serum cholesterol levels in patients as outlined in the National Cholesterol Education Program (NCEP) guidelines should be done to confirm a favorable initial and long-term response. The NCEP treatment guidelines are presented in Table 3.

Table 3: NCEP Guideline

PATIENT ASSESSMENT CRITERIA	LDL-C	
	INITIATION LEVEL	MINIMUM GOAL
Without CHD and with fewer than two risk factors	≥ 190 mg/dL	< 160 mg/dL
Without CHD and with two or more risk factors	≥ 160 mg/dL	< 130 mg/dL
With CHD	≥ 130 mg/dL	≤ 100 mg/dL

- CHD = Coronary Heart Disease
- 1. Other risk factors for CHD include the following: age (males >45 years, females >55 years or premature menopause without estrogen replacement therapy); family history of premature CHD; current cigarette smoking; hypertension; confirmed HDL-C, <35mg/dL (<0.01 mmol/L); and diabetes mellitus. Subtract risk factor if HDL-C >60 mg/dL (>1.6 mmol/L).
- 2. In CHD patients with LDL-C levels of 100–129 mg/dL, the physician should exercise clinical judgment in deciding whether to initiate drug treatment.

CONTRAINDICATIONS

WelChol™ is contraindicated in individuals with bowel obstruction and in individuals who have shown hypersensitivity to any of the components of WelChol™.

PRECAUTIONS

General

Patients with TG levels greater than 300 mg/dL were excluded from WelChol™ clinical trials. Caution should be exercised when treating patients with TG levels greater than 300 mg/dL.

In non-clinical safety studies, rats administered colesevelam at doses greater than 30-fold the projected human clinical dose experienced hemorrhage from Vitamin K deficiency. WelChol™ did not induce any clinically significant reduction in the absorption of vitamins A, D, E, or K during clinical trials of up to one year. However, caution should be exercised when treating patients with a susceptibility to vitamin K or fat soluble vitamin deficiencies.

The safety and efficacy of WelChol™ in patients with dysphagia, swallowing disorders, severe gastrointestinal motility disorders, or major gastrointestinal tract surgery have not been established. Consequently, caution should be exercised when WelChol™ is used in patients with these gastrointestinal disorders.

Information for the Patient

WelChol™ may be taken once per day with a meal, or taken twice per day in divided doses with meals. Patients should be directed to take WelChol™ with a liquid and a meal, and adhere to their NCEP-recommended diet. Patients should tell their physicians if they are pregnant, are intending to become pregnant, or are breastfeeding.

Laboratory Tests

Serum total-C, LDL-C and TG levels should be determined periodically based on NCEP guidelines to confirm favorable initial and adequate long-term responses.

Drug Interactions

WelChol™ has been studied in several human drug interaction studies in which it was administered with a meal and the test drug. WelChol™ was found to have no significant effect on the bioavailability of digoxin, lovastatin, metoprolol, quinidine, valproic acid, and warfarin. WelChol™ decreased the Cmax and AUC of sustained-release verapamil (Calan SR®) by approximately 31% and 11%, respectively. Since there is a high degree of variability in the bioavailability of verapamil, the clinical significance of this finding is unclear. In clinical studies, coadministration of WelChol™ with atorvastatin, lovastatin, or simvastatin did not interfere with the lipid-lowering activity of the HMG-CoA reductase inhibitor. Other drugs have not been studied. When administering other drugs for which alterations in blood levels could have a clinically significant effect on safety or efficacy, physicians should consider monitoring drug levels or effects.

Carcinogenesis, Mutagenesis, Impairment of Fertility

A 104-week carcinogenicity study with colesevelam (WelChol™) was conducted in CD-1 mice, at oral dietary doses up to 3 g/kg/day. This dose was approximately 50 times the maximum recommended human dose of 4.5 g/day, based on body weight, mg/kg. There were no significant drug-induced tumor findings in male or female mice. In a 104-week carcinogenicity study with colesevelam (WelChol™) in Harlan Sprague-Dawley rats, a statistically significant increase in the incidence of pancreatic acinar cell adenoma was seen in male rats at doses >1.2 g/kg/day (approximately 20 times the maximum human dose, based on body weight, mg/kg) (trend test only). A statistically significant increase in thyroid C-cell adenoma was seen in female rats at 2.4 g/kg/day (approximately 40 times the maximum human dose, based on body weight, mg/kg).

Colesevelam and four degradants present in the drug substance have been evaluated for mutagenicity in the Ames test and a mammalian chromosomal aberration test. The four degradants and an extract of the parent compound did not exhibit genetic toxicity in an *in vitro* bacterial mutagenesis assay in *S. typhimurium* and *E. coli* (Ames assay) with or without rat liver metabolic activation. An extract of the parent compound was positive in the Chinese Hamster Ovary (CHO) cell chromosomal aberration assay in the presence of metabolic activation and negative in the absence of metabolic activation. The results of the CHO cell chromosomal aberration assay with two of the four degradants, declyamine HCl and aminohexyltrimethyl ammonium chloride HCl, were equivocal in the absence of metabolic activation and negative in the presence of metabolic activation. The other two degradants, didecylamine HCl and 6-decylamino-hexyltrimethyl ammonium chloride HCl, were negative in the presence and absence of metabolic activation.

Colesevelam did not impair fertility in rats at doses of up to 3 g/kg/day (approximately 50 times the maximum human dose, based on body weight, mg/kg).

PREGNANCY

Pregnancy Category B

Reproduction studies have been performed in rats and rabbits at doses up to 3 g/kg/day and 1 g/kg/day, respectively (approximately 50 and 17 times the maximum human dose, based on body weight, mg/kg) and have revealed no evidence of harm to the fetus due to colesevelam. There are, however, no adequate and well-controlled studies in pregnant women. Because animal reproduction studies are not always predictive of human response, this drug should be used during pregnancy only if clearly needed.

Requirements for vitamins and other nutrients are increased in pregnancy. The effect of WelChol™ on the absorption of vitamins has not been studied in pregnant women.

Pediatric Use

The safety and efficacy of colesevelam (WelChol™) have not been established in pediatric patients.

Geriatric Use

There is no evidence for special considerations when colesevelam (WelChol™) is administered to elderly patients.

ADVERSE REACTIONS

WelChol™ treatment-emergent adverse events that occurred in greater than 2% of patients in an integrated safety analysis are presented in Table 4.

Table 4: Frequent (>2%) Treatment-Emergent Adverse Events By Treatment Category

BODY SYSTEM/ ADVERSE EVENT	PLACEBO (N=258) %	WELCHOL™ ONLY (N=807) %
Body as a Whole		
Infection	13	10
Headache	8	6
Pain	7	5
Back Pain	6	3
Abdominal Pain	5	5
Flu Syndrome	3	3
Accidental Injury	3	4
Asthenia	2	4
Digestive System		
Flatulence	14	12
Constipation	7	11
Diarrhea	7	5
Nausea	4	4
Dyspepsia	3	8
Respiratory System		
Sinusitis	4	2
Rhinitis	3	3
Cough Increased	2	2
Pharyngitis	2	3
Musculoskeletal System		
Myalgia	0	2

OVERDOSAGE

Because WelChol™ is not absorbed, the risk of systemic toxicity is low. Doses in excess of 4.5 g per day have not been tested.

DOSAGE AND ADMINISTRATION

Monotherapy

The recommended starting dose of WelChol™ is 3 tablets taken twice per day with meals or 6 tablets once per day with a meal. The WelChol™ dose can be increased to 7 tablets, depending upon the desired therapeutic effect. WelChol™ should be taken with a liquid.

Combination Therapy

Welchol™, at doses of 4 to 6 tablets per day, has been shown to be safe and effective when dosed at the same time (i.e., co-administered) as an HMG-CoA reductase inhibitor or when the two drugs are dosed apart. [**CLINICAL PHARMACOLOGY, Clinical Trials**]. WelChol™ should be taken with a liquid. For maximal therapeutic effect in combination with an HMG-CoA reductase inhibitor, the recommended dose of WelChol™ is 3 tablets taken twice per day with meals or 6 tablets taken once per day with a meal.

HOW SUPPLIED

WelChol™ is supplied as an off-white, solid tablet imprinted with the word "Sankyo" over "C01," containing 625 mg colesevelam, magnesium stearate, microcrystalline cellulose, silicon dioxide, HPMC (hydroxypropyl methylcellulose), and acetylated monoglyceride.

WelChol™ Tablets are available as follows:

Bottles of 180-NDC 65597-701-18

Storage

Store at room temperature (25 °C). Brief exposure to 40 °C does not adversely affect the product. [See USP controlled room temperature.] Protect from moisture.

REFERENCES

1. Grundy SM, Ahrens EH, Salen G. Interruption of the enterohepatic circulation of bile acids in man: comparative effects of cholestyramine and ileal exclusion on cholesterol metabolism. J Lab Clin Med 1971; 78: 94–121.
2. Shepherd J, Packard CJ, Bicker S, Veitch LTD, Gemmell MH. Cholestyramine promotes receptor-mediated low-density-lipoprotein catabolism. N Engl J Med 1980; 302: 1219–22.
3. Friedewald WT, Levy RI, Fredrickson DS: Estimation of the concentration of LDL cholesterol in plasma without use of a preparative ultracentifuge. Clin. Chem. 1972; 18(6): 499.

Marketed for:
Sankyo Pharma Inc.
New York, New York 10017
by:
Sankyo Parke Davis
Parsippany, New Jersey 07054
Licensed From: GelTex Pharmaceuticals, Inc.
Issued: June 2000
Version 3 (06/21/00)

Shown in Product Identification Guide, page 333

Sanofi-Synthelabo Inc.
90 PARK AVENUE
NEW YORK, NY 10016

Direct Inquiries to:
(212) 551-4000

For Medical Information Contact:
Product Information Services
(800) 446-6267

Sales and Ordering:
East Coast: (800) 223-1062
West Coast: (800) 223-5511

ARALEN® ℞
chloroquine hydrochloride injection, USP

For Malaria and Extraintestinal Amebiasis

WARNING: PHYSICIANS SHOULD COMPLETELY FAMILIARIZE THEMSELVES WITH THE COMPLETE CONTENTS OF THIS LEAFLET BEFORE PRESCRIBING ARALEN.

DESCRIPTION

Parenteral solution, each mL containing 50 mg of the dihydrochloride salt equivalent to 40 mg of chloroquine base. Chloroquine hydrochloride, a 4-aminoquinoline compound, is chemically 7-(Chloro-4-[[4-diethylamino)-1-methylbutyl] amino]-quinoline dihydrochloride, a white, crystalline substance, freely soluble in water.

ACTIONS

The compound is a highly active antimalarial and amebicidal agent.

ARALEN has been found to be highly active against the erythrocytic forms of *Plasmodium vivax* and *malariae* and most strains of *Plasmodium falciparum* (but not the gametocytes of *P. falciparum*). The precise mechanism of action of the drug is not known.

ARALEN does not prevent relapses in patients with vivax or malariae malaria because it is not effective against exoerythrocytic forms of the parasite, nor will it prevent vivax or malariae infection when administered as a prophylactic. It is highly effective as a suppressive agent in patients with vivax or malariae malaria, in terminating acute attacks, and significantly lengthening the interval between treatment and relapse. In patients with falciparum malaria it abolishes the acute attack and effects complete cure of the infection, unless due to a resistant strain of *P. falciparum.*

INDICATIONS

ARALEN is indicated for the treatment of extraintestinal amebiasis and for treatment of acute attacks of malaria due to *P. vivax, P. malariae, P. ovale,* and susceptible strains of *P. falciparum* when oral therapy is not feasible.

CONTRAINDICATIONS

Use of this drug is contraindicated in the presence of retinal or visual field changes either attributable to 4- aminoquinoline compounds or to any other etiology, and in patients with known hypersensitivity to 4-aminoquinoline compounds. However, in the treatment of acute attacks of malaria caused by susceptible strains of plasmodia, the physician may elect to use this drug after carefully weighing the possible benefits and risks to the patient.

WARNINGS

Children and infants are extremely susceptible to adverse effects from an overdose of parenteral ARALEN and sudden deaths have been recorded after such administration. In no instance should the single dose of parenteral ARALEN administered to infants or children exceed 5 mg base per kg.

In recent years it has been found that certain strains of *P. falciparum* have become resistant to 4-aminoquinoline compounds (including chloroquine and hydroxychloroquine) as shown by the fact that normally adequate doses have failed to prevent or cure clinical malaria or parasitemia. Treatment with quinine or other specific forms of therapy is therefore advised for patients infected with a resistant strain of parasites.

Use of ARALEN should be avoided in patients with psoriasis, for it may precipitate a severe attack of psoriasis. Some authors consider the use of 4-aminoquinoline compounds contraindicated in patients with porphyria since the condition may be exacerbated.

Irreversible retinal damage has been observed in some patients who had received long-term or high-dosage 4-aminoquinoline therapy. Retinopathy has been reported to be dose related.

If there is any indication (past or present) of abnormality in the visual acuity, visual field, or retinal macular areas (such as pigmentary changes, loss of foveal reflex), or any visual symptoms (such as light flashes and streaks) which are not fully explainable by difficulties of accommodation or corneal opacities, the drug should be discontinued immediately and the patient closely observed for possible progression. Retinal changes (and visual disturbances) may progress even after cessation of therapy.

Usage in Pregnancy. Usage of this drug during pregnancy should be avoided except in the suppression or treatment of malaria when in the judgment of the physician the benefit outweighs the possible hazard. It should be noted that radioactively tagged chloroquine administered intravenously to pregnant pigmented CBA mice passed rapidly across the placenta, accumulated selectively in the melanin structures of the fetal eyes and was retained in the ocular tissues for five months after the drug had been eliminated from the rest of the body.[1]

PRECAUTIONS

Since the drug is known to concentrate in the liver, it should be used with caution in patients with hepatic disease or alcoholism or in conjunction with known hepatotoxic drugs.

The drug should be administered with caution to patients having G-6-PD (glucose-6-phosphate dehydrogenase) deficiency.

ADVERSE REACTIONS

Respiratory depression, cardiovascular collapse, shock, convulsions, and death have been reported with overdoses of ARALEN, brand of chloroquine hydrochloride injection, especially in infants and children.

Any of the adverse reactions associated with short-term oral administration of chloroquine phosphate must be considered a possibility with chloroquine hydrochloride. Cardiovascular effects, such as hypotension and electrocardiographic changes (particularly inversion or depression of the T-wave, widening of the QRS complex), have rarely been noted in patients receiving usual antimalarial doses of the drug. Mild and transient headache, pruritus, psychic stimulation, visual disturbances (blurring of vision and difficulty of focusing or accommodation), pleomorphic skin eruptions, and gastrointestinal complaints (anorexia, nausea, vomiting, diarrhea, abdominal cramps) have been observed.

Instances of convulsive seizures associated with oral chloroquine therapy in patients with extraintestinal amebiasis have been reported.

A few cases of a nerve type of deafness have been reported after prolonged therapy, usually in high doses. Tinnitus and reduced hearing have been reported, in a patient with preexistent auditory damage, after administration of only 500 mg once a week for a few months. Since neuromyopathy, blood dyscrasias, lichen planus-like eruptions, and skin and mucosal pigmentary changes have been noted during prolonged oral therapy, their occurrence with this dosage form is possible.

Patients with retinal changes may be asymptomatic, especially in early cases, or may complain of nyctalopia and scotomatous vision with field defects of paracentral, pericentral

Continued on next page

This product information was prepared in September 2000. On these and other products of Sanofi-Synthelabo Inc., detailed information may be obtained on a current basis by direct inquiry to Product Information Services, 90 Park Avenue, New York, NY 10016 (toll free 1-800-446-6267).

Aralen—Cont.

ring types, and typically temporal scotomas, eg, difficulty in reading with words tending to disappear, seeing only half an object, misty vision, and fog before the eyes. Rarely scotomatous vision may occur without observable retinal changes.

DOSAGE AND ADMINISTRATION

Malaria — **Adult Dose.** An initial dose of 4 mL or 5 mL (160 mg to 200 mg chloroquine base) may be injected intramuscularly and repeated in 6 hours if necessary. The total parenteral dosage in the first 24 hours should not exceed 800 mg chloroquine base. Treatment by mouth should be started as soon as practicable and continued until a course of approximately 1.5 g of base in 3 days is completed.

Pediatric Dose. Infants and children are extremely susceptible to overdosage of parenteral ARALEN. Severe reactions and deaths have occurred. In the pediatric age range, parenteral ARALEN dosage should be calculated in proportion to the adult dose based upon body weight. The recommended single dose in infants and children is 5 mg base per kg. This dose may be repeated in 6 hours; however, the total dose in any 24 hour period should not exceed 10 mg base per kg of body weight. Parenteral administration should be terminated and oral therapy instituted as soon as possible.

Extraintestinal Amebiasis—In adult patients not able to tolerate oral therapy, from 4 mL to 5 mL (160 mg to 200 mg chloroquine base) may be injected daily for 10 to 12 days. Oral administration should be substituted or resumed as soon as possible.

OVERDOSAGE

Inadvertent toxic doses may produce respiratory depression or shock with hypotension. Respiratory depression is treated by artificial respiration and administration of oxygen. In shock with hypotension, a potent vasopressor, such as NEO-SYNEPHRINE® hydrochloride, brand of phenylephrine hydrochloride, USP, should be given intramuscularly in doses of 2 mg to 5 mg.

HOW SUPPLIED

Ampuls of 5 mL (250 mg/5 mL), box of 5 (NDC 0024-0074-01)

Store at room temperature up to 30°C (86°F).

REFERENCE

Ullberg S, Lindquist N G, Sjostrand S E: Accumulation of chorio-retinotoxic drugs in the foetal eye. *Nature* 1970; 227: 1257.

Revised September 1999

ASW-3B

ARALEN® ℞
chloroquine phosphate, USP

For Malaria and Extraintestinal Amebiasis

WARNING
PHYSICIANS SHOULD COMPLETELY FAMILIARIZE THEMSELVES WITH THE COMPLETE CONTENTS OF THIS LEAFLET BEFORE PRESCRIBING ARALEN.

DESCRIPTION

ARALEN, chloroquine phosphate, USP, is a 4-aminoquinoline compound for oral administration. It is a white, odorless, bitter tasting, crystalline substance, freely soluble in water.

ARALEN is an antimalarial and amebicidal drug.

Chemically, it is 7-chloro- 4-[[4- (diethylamino) -1-methylbutyl]amino] quinoline phosphate (1:2).

Inactive Ingredients: Carnauba Wax, Colloidal Silicon Dioxide, D&C Red No 27, Dibasic Calcium Phosphate, Hydroxypropyl Methylcellulose, Magnesium Stearate, Microcrystalline Cellulose, Polyethylene Glycol, Polysorbate 80, Pregelatinized Starch, Sodium Starch Glycolate, Stearic Acid, Titanium Dioxide.

CLINICAL PHARMACOLOGY

ARALEN has been found to be highly active against the erythrocytic forms of *Plasmodium vivax* and *Plasmodium malariae* and most strains of *Plasmodium falciparum* (but not the gametocytes of *P. falciparum*).

The mechanism of plasmodicidal action of chloroquine is not completely certain. While the drug can inhibit certain enzymes, its effect is believed to result, at least in part, from its interaction with DNA.

Chloroquine is rapidly and almost completely absorbed from the gastrointestinal tract, and only a small proportion of the administered dose is found in the stools. Approximately 55% of the drug in the plasma is bound to nondiffusible plasma constituents. Excretion of chloroquine is quite slow, but is increased by acidification of the urine. Chloroquine is deposited in the tissues in considerable amounts. In animals, from 200 to 700 times the plasma concentration may be found in the liver, spleen, kidney, and lung; leukocytes also concentrate the drug. The brain and spinal cord, in contrast, contain only 10 to 30 times the amount present in plasma.

Chloroquine undergoes appreciable degradation in the body. The main metabolite is desethylchloroquine, which accounts for one fourth of the total material appearing in the urine; bisdesethylchloroquine, a carboxylic acid derivative, and other metabolic products as yet uncharacterized are found in small amounts. Slightly more than half of the urinary drug products can be accounted for as unchanged chloroquine.

Microbiology

ARALEN has been found to be highly active against the erythrocytic forms of *Plasmodium vivax* and *malariae* and most strains of *Plasmodium falciparum* (but not the gametocytes of *P. falciparum*). The precise mechanism of action of the drug is not known.

In vitro studies with trophozoites of *Entamoeba histolytica* have demonstrated that ARALEN also possesses amebicidal activity comparable to that of emetine.

INDICATIONS AND USAGE

ARALEN is indicated for the suppressive treatment and for acute attacks of malaria due to *P. vivax, P. malariae, P. ovale,* and susceptible strains of *P. falciparum.* The drug is also indicated for the treatment of extraintestinal amebiasis.

ARALEN does not prevent relapses in patients with vivax or malariae malaria because it is not effective against exoerythrocytic forms of the parasite, nor will it prevent vivax or malariae infection when administered as a prophylactic. It is highly effective as a suppressive agent in patients with vivax or malariae malaria, in terminating acute attacks, and significantly lengthening the interval between treatment and relapse. In patients with falciparum malaria it abolishes the acute attack and effects complete cure of the infection, unless due to a resistant strain of *P. falciparum.*

CONTRAINDICATIONS

Use of this drug is contraindicated in the presence of retinal or visual field changes either attributable to 4-aminoquinoline compounds or to any other etiology, and in patients with known hypersensitivity to 4-aminoquinoline compounds. However, in the treatment of acute attacks of malaria caused by susceptible strains of plasmodia, the physician may elect to use this drug after carefully weighing the possible benefits and risks to the patient.

WARNINGS

In recent years it has been found that certain strains of *P. falciparum* have become resistant to 4-aminoquinoline compounds (including chloroquine and hydroxychloroquine) as shown by the fact that normally adequate doses have failed to prevent or cure clinical malaria or parasitemia. Treatment with quinine or other specific forms of therapy is therefore advised for patients infected with a resistant strain of parasites.

Irreversible retinal damage has been observed in some patients who had received long-term or high-dosage 4-aminoquinoline therapy. Retinopathy has been reported to be dose related.

When prolonged therapy with any antimalarial compound is contemplated, initial (base line) and periodic ophthalmologic examinations (including visual acuity, expert slit-lamp, funduscopic, and visual field tests) should be performed.

If there is any indication (past or present) of abnormality in the visual acuity, visual field, or retinal macular areas (such as pigmentary changes, loss of foveal reflex), or any visual symptoms (such as light flashes and streaks) which are not fully explainable by difficulties of accommodation or corneal opacities, the drug should be discontinued immediately and the patient closely observed for possible progression. Retinal changes (and visual disturbances) may progress even after cessation of therapy.

All patients on long-term therapy with this preparation should be questioned and examined periodically, including testing knee and ankle reflexes, to detect any evidence of muscular weakness. If weakness occurs, discontinue the drug.

A number of fatalities have been reported following the accidental ingestion of chloroquine, sometimes in relatively small doses (0.75 g or 1 g chloroquine phosphate in one 3-year-old child). Patients should be strongly warned to keep this drug out of the reach of children because they are especially sensitive to the 4-aminoquinoline compounds.

Use of ARALEN in patients with psoriasis may precipitate a severe attack of psoriasis. When used in patients with porphyria the condition may be exacerbated. The drug should not be used in these conditions unless in the judgment of the physician the benefit to the patient outweighs the possible hazard.

PRECAUTIONS

General

If any severe blood disorder appears which is not attributable to the disease under treatment, discontinuance of the drug should be considered.

Since this drug is known to concentrate in the liver, it should be used with caution in patients with hepatic disease or alcoholism or in conjunction with known hepatotoxic drugs.

The drug should be administered with caution to patients having G-6-PD (glucose-6-phosphate dehydrogenase) deficiency.

Laboratory Tests

Complete blood cell counts should be made periodically if patients are given prolonged therapy.

Nursing Mothers

Because of the potential for serious adverse reactions in nursing infants from chloroquine, a decision should be made whether to discontinue nursing or to discontinue the drug, taking into account the importance of the drug to the mother.

Pediatric Use

See WARNINGS and DOSAGE AND ADMINISTRATION.

ADVERSE REACTIONS

Ocular reactions: Irreversible retinal damage in patients receiving long-term or high-dosage 4-aminoquinoline therapy; visual disturbances (blurring of vision and difficulty of focusing or accommodation); nyctalopia; scotomatous vision with field defects of paracentral, pericentral ring types, and typically temporal scotomas, e.g., difficulty in reading with words tending to disappear, seeing half an object, misty vision, and fog before the eyes.

Neuromuscular reactions: Convulsive seizures.

Auditory reactions: Nerve type deafness; tinnitus, reduced hearing in patients with preexisting auditory damage.

Gastrointestinal reactions: Anorexia, nausea, vomiting, diarrhea, abdominal cramps.

Dermatologic reactions: Pleomorphic skin eruptions, skin and mucosal pigmentary changes; lichen planus-like eruptions, pruritus, and hair loss.

CNS reactions: Mild and transient headache, psychic stimulation.

Cardiovascular reactions: Rarely, hypotension, electrocardiographic change.

OVERDOSAGE

Symptoms: Chloroquine is very rapidly and completely absorbed after ingestion. Toxic doses of chloroquine can be fatal. As little as 1 g may be fatal in children. Toxic symptoms can occur within minutes. These consist of headache, drowsiness, visual disturbances, nausea and vomiting, cardiovascular collapse, and convulsions followed by sudden and early respiratory and cardiac arrest. The electrocardiogram may reveal atrial standstill, nodal rhythm, prolonged intraventricular conduction time, and progressive bradycardia leading to ventricular fibrillation and/or arrest.

Treatment: Treatment is symptomatic and must be prompt with immediate evacuation of the stomach by emesis (at home, before transportation to the hospital) or gastric lavage until the stomach is completely emptied. If finely powdered, activated charcoal is introduced by stomach tube, after lavage, and within 30 minutes after ingestion of the antimalarial, it may inhibit further intestinal absorption of the drug. To be effective, the dose of activated charcoal should be at least five times the estimated dose of chloroquine ingested.

Convulsions, if present, should be controlled before attempting gastric lavage. If due to cerebral stimulation, cautious administration of an ultra short-acting barbiturate may be tried but, if due to anoxia, it should be corrected by oxygen administration and artificial respiration. In shock with hypotension, a potent vasopressor should be administered. Because of the importance of supporting respiration, tracheal intubation or tracheostomy, followed by gastric lavage, may also be necessary. Peritoneal dialysis and exchange transfusions have also been suggested to reduce the level of the drug in the blood.

A patient who survives the acute phase and is asymptomatic should be closely observed for at least six hours. Fluids may be forced, and sufficient ammonium chloride (8 g daily in divided doses for adults) may be administered for a few days to acidify the urine to help promote urinary excretion in cases of both overdosage or sensitivity.

DOSAGE AND ADMINISTRATION

The dosage of chloroquine phosphate is often expressed in terms of equivalent chloroquine base. Each 500 mg tablet of ARALEN contains the equivalent of 300 mg chloroquine base. In infants and children the dosage is preferably calculated by body weight.

Malaria: Suppression—**Adult Dose:** 500 mg (= 300 mg base) on exactly the same day of each week.

Pediatric Dose: The weekly suppressive dosage is 5 mg calculated as base, per kg of body weight, but should not exceed the adult dose regardless of weight.

If circumstances permit, suppressive therapy should begin two weeks prior to exposure. However, failing this in adults, an initial double (loading) dose of 1 g (= 600 mg base), or in children 10 mg base/kg may be taken in two divided doses, six hours apart. The suppressive therapy should be continued for eight weeks after leaving the endemic area.

For Treatment of Acute Attack

Adults: An initial dose of 1 g (= 600 mg base) followed by an additional 500 mg (= 300 mg base) after six to eight hours and a single dose of 500 mg (= 300 mg base) on each of two consecutive days. This represents a total dose of 2.5 g chloroquine phosphate or 1.5 g base in three days.

The dosage for adults may also be calculated on the basis of body weight; this method is preferred for infants and children. A total dose representing 25 mg of base per kg of body weight is administered in three days, as follows:

First dose: 10 mg base per kg (but not exceeding a single dose of 600 mg base).

Second dose: 5 mg base per kg (but not exceeding a single dose of 300 mg base) 6 hours after first dose.

Third dose: 5 mg base per kg 18 hours after second dose.

Fourth dose: 5 mg base per kg 24 hours after third dose.

For radical cure of *vivax* and *malariae* malaria concomitant therapy with an 8-aminoquinoline compound is necessary.

Extraintestinal Amebiasis: Adults, 1 g (600 mg base) daily for two days, followed by 500 mg (300 mg base) daily for at least two to three weeks. Treatment is usually combined with an effective intestinal amebicide.

HOW SUPPLIED

Tablets of 500 mg (= 300 mg base), bottles of 25 (NDC 0024-0084-01).

Pink, film-coated convex tablets, $^1/_2$ inch in diameter with an uncoated core, containing 500 mg chloroquine phosphate, equivalent to 300 mg of chloroquine base.

Dispense in tight, light-resistant containers as defined in the USP/NF.

Store at 25°C (77°F); excursions permitted to 15°–30°C (59°–86°F) [see USP Controlled Room Temperature]

ASW-2B

Revised September 1999

Shown in Product Identification Guide, page 333

AVAPRO® ℞
(irbesartan) Tablets

USE IN PREGNANCY
When used in pregnancy during the second and third trimesters, drugs that act directly on the renin-angiotensin system can cause injury and even death to the developing fetus. When pregnancy is detected, AVAPRO should be discontinued as soon as possible. See **WARNINGS: Fetal/Neonatal Morbidity and Mortality.**

DESCRIPTION

AVAPRO* (irbesartan) is an angiotensin II receptor (AT_1 subtype) antagonist.

Irbesartan is a non-peptide compound, chemically described as a 2-butyl-3- [[2'- (1*H*-tetrazol-5-yl) [1, 1'-biphenyl]-4-yl] methyl]-1,3-diazaspiro [4,4] non-1-en-4-one.

Its empirical formula is $C_{25}H_{28}N_6O$, and the structural formula:

Irbesartan is a white to off-white crystalline powder with a molecular weight of 428.5. It is a nonpolar compound with a partition coefficient (octanol/water) of 10.1 at pH of 7.4. Irbesartan is slightly soluble in alcohol and methylene chloride and practically insoluble in water.

AVAPRO is available for oral administration in unscored tablets containing 75 mg, 150 mg, or 300 mg of irbesartan. Inactive ingredients include: lactose, microcrystalline cellulose, pregelatinized starch, croscarmellose sodium, poloxamer 188, silicon dioxide and magnesium stearate.

CLINICAL PHARMACOLOGY

Mechanism of Action

Angiotensin II is a potent vasoconstrictor formed from angiotensin I in a reaction catalyzed by angiotensin-converting enzyme (ACE, kininase II). Angiotensin II is the principal pressor agent of the renin-angiotensin system (RAS) and also stimulates aldosterone synthesis and secretion by adrenal cortex, cardiac contraction, renal resorption of sodium, activity of sympathetic nervous system, and smooth muscle cell growth. Irbesartan blocks the vasoconstrictor and aldosterone-secreting effects of angiotensin II by selectively binding to the AT_1 angiotensin II receptor. There is also an AT_2 receptor in many tissues, but it is not involved in cardiovascular homeostasis.

Irbesartan is a specific competitive antagonist of AT_1 receptors with a much greater affinity (more than 8500-fold) for the AT_1 receptor than for the AT_2 receptor and no agonist activity.

Blockade of the AT_1 receptor removes the negative feedback of angiotensin II on renin secretion, but the resulting increased plasma renin activity and circulating angiotensin II do not overcome the effects of irbesartan on blood pressure.

Irbesartan does not inhibit ACE or renin or affect other hormone receptors or ion channels known to be involved in the cardiovascular regulation of blood pressure and sodium homeostasis. Because irbesartan does not inhibit ACE, it does not affect the response to bradykinin; whether this has clinical relevance is not known.

Pharmacokinetics

Irbesartan is an orally active agent that does not require biotransformation into an active form. The oral absorption of irbesartan is rapid and complete with an average absolute bioavailability of 60–80%. Following oral administration of AVAPRO, peak plasma concentrations of irbesartan are attained at 1.5–2 hours after dosing. Food does not affect the bioavailability of AVAPRO.

Irbesartan exhibits linear pharmacokinetics over the therapeutic dose range.

The terminal elimination half-life of irbesartan averaged 11–15 hours. Steady-state concentrations are achieved within 3 days. Limited accumulation of irbesartan (<20%) is observed in plasma upon repeated once-daily dosing.

Metabolism and Elimination

Irbesartan is metabolized via glucuronide conjugation and oxidation. Following oral or intravenous administration of ^{14}C-labeled irbesartan, more than 80% of the circulating plasma radioactivity is attributable to unchanged irbesartan. The primary circulating metabolite is the inactive irbesartan glucuronide conjugate (approximately 6%). The remaining oxidative metabolites do not add appreciably to irbesartan's pharmacologic activity.

Irbesartan and its metabolites are excreted by both biliary and renal routes. Following either oral or intravenous administration of ^{14}C-labeled irbesartan, about 20% of radioactivity is recovered in the urine and the remainder in the feces, as irbesartan or irbesartan glucuronide.

In vitro studies of irbesartan oxidation by cytochrome P450 isoenzymes indicated irbesartan was oxidized primarily by 2C9; metabolism by 3A4 was negligible. Irbesartan was neither metabolized by, nor did it substantially induce or inhibit, isoenzymes commonly associated with drug metabolism (1A1, 1A2, 2A6, 2B6, 2D6, 2E1). There was no induction or inhibition of 3A4.

Distribution

Irbesartan is 90% bound to serum proteins (primarily albumin and α_1-acid glycoprotein) with negligible binding to cellular components of blood. The average volume of distribution is 53–93 liters. Total plasma and renal clearances are in the range of 157–176 and 3.0–3.5 mL/min, respectively. With repetitive dosing, irbesartan accumulates to no clinically relevant extent.

Studies in animals indicate that radiolabeled irbesartan weakly crosses the blood brain barrier and placenta. Irbesartan is excreted in the milk of lactating rats.

* Registered trademark of Sanofi

Special Populations

Pediatric: Irbesartan pharmacokinetics have not been investigated in patients <18 years of age.

Gender: No gender related differences in pharmacokinetics were observed in healthy elderly (age 65–80 years) or in healthy young (age 18–40 years) subjects. In studies of hypertensive patients, there was no gender difference in half-life or accumulation, but somewhat higher plasma concentrations of irbesartan were observed in females (11–44%). No gender-related dosage adjustment is necessary.

Geriatric: In elderly subjects (age 65–80 years), irbesartan elimination half-life was not significantly altered, but AUC and C_{max} values were about 20–50% greater than those of young subjects (age 18–40 years). No dosage adjustment is necessary in the elderly.

Race: In healthy black subjects, irbesartan AUC values were approximately 25% greater than whites; there was no difference in C_{max} values.

Renal Insufficiency: The pharmacokinetics of irbesartan were not altered in patients with renal impairment or in patients on hemodialysis. Irbesartan is not removed by hemodialysis. No dosage adjustment is necessary in patients with mild to severe renal impairment unless a patient with renal impairment is also volume depleted. (See **WARNINGS: Hypotension in Volume- or Salt-depleted Patients** and **DOSAGE AND ADMINISTRATION.)**

Hepatic Insufficiency: The pharmacokinetics of irbesartan following repeated oral administration were not significantly affected in patients with mild to moderate cirrhosis of the liver. No dosage adjustment is necessary in patients with hepatic insufficiency.

Drug Interactions: (See **PRECAUTIONS: Drug Interactions.)**

Pharmacodynamics

In healthy subjects, single oral irbesartan doses of up to 300 mg produced dose-dependent inhibition of the pressor effect of angiotensin II infusions. Inhibition was complete (100%) 4 hours following oral doses of 150 mg or 300 mg and partial inhibition was sustained for 24 hours (60% and 40% at 300 mg and 150 mg, respectively).

In hypertensive patients, angiotensin II receptor inhibition following chronic administration of irbesartan causes a 1.5–2 fold rise in angiotensin II plasma concentration and a 2–3 fold increase in plasma renin levels. Aldosterone plasma concentrations generally decline following irbesartan administration, but serum potassium levels are not significantly affected at recommended doses.

In hypertensive patients, chronic oral doses of irbesartan (up to 300 mg) had no effect on glomerular filtration rate, renal plasma flow or filtration rate, renal plasma flow or filtration fraction. In multiple dose studies in hypertensive patients, there were no clinically important effects on fasting triglycerides, total cholesterol, HDL-cholesterol, or fasting glucose concentrations. There was no effect on serum uric acid during chronic oral administration, and no uricosuric effect.

Clinical Studies

The antihypertensive effects of AVAPRO (irbesatan) were examined in seven (7) major placebo-controlled 8–12 week trials in patients with baseline diastolic blood pressures of 95–110 mmHg. Doses of 1–900 mg were included in these trials in order to fully explore the dose-range of irbesartan. These studies allowed comparison of once- or twice-daily regimens at 150 mg/day, comparisons of peak and trough effects, and comparisons of response by gender, age, and race. Two of the seven placebo-controlled trials identified above examined the antihypertensive effects of irbesartan and hydrochlorothiazide in combination.

The seven (7) studies of irbesartan monotherapy included a total of 1915 patients randomized to irbesartan (1–900 mg) and 611 patients randomized to placebo. Once-daily doses of 150 and 300 mg provided statistically and clinically significant decreases in systolic and diastolic blood pressure with trough (24 hours post-dose) effects after 6–12 weeks of treatment compared to placebo, of about 8–10/5–6 and 8–12/5–8 mmHg, respectively. No further increase in effect was seen at dosages greater than 300 mg. The dose-response relationships for effects on systolic and diastolic pressure are shown in Figures 1 and 2.

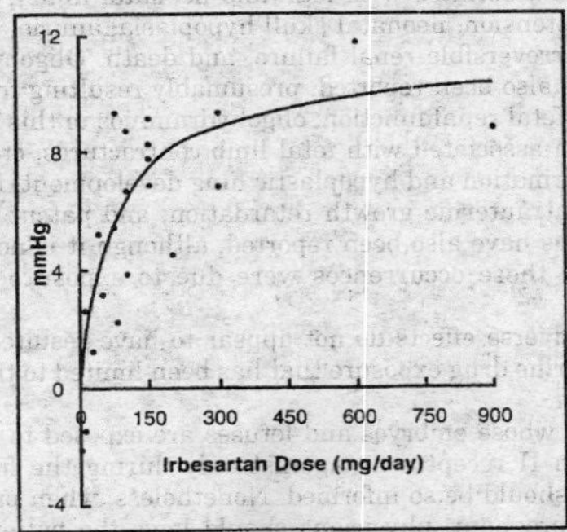

Figure 1. Placebo-subtracted reduction in trough SeSBP; integrated analysis

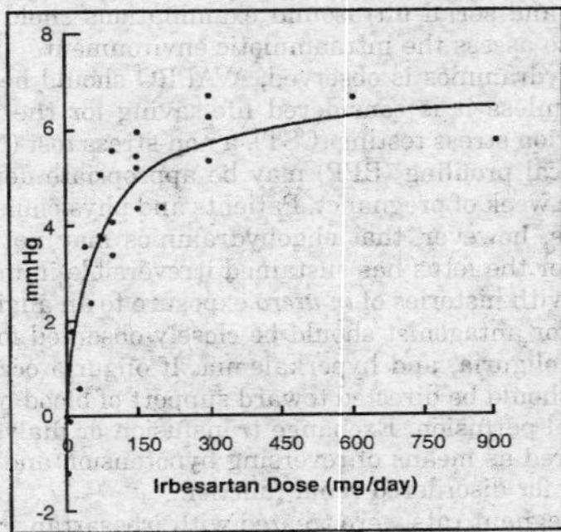

Figure 2. Placebo-subtracted reduction in trough SeDBP; integrated analysis

Once-daily administration of therapeutic doses of irbesartan gave peak effects at around 3–6 hours and, in one ambulatory blood pressure monitoring study, again around 14 hours. This was seen with both once-daily and twice-daily dosing. Trough-to-peak ratios by systolic and diastolic response were generally between 60–70%. In a continuous blood pressure monitoring study, once-daily dosing with 150 mg gave trough and mean 24-hour responses similar to those observed in patients receiving twice-daily dosing at the same total daily dose.

In controlled trials, the addition of irbesartan to hydrochlorothiazide doses of 6.25, 12.5, or 25 mg produced further dose-related reductions in blood pressure similar to those achieved with the same monotherapy dose of irbesartan. HCTZ aldo had an approximately additive effect.

Analysis of age, gender, and race subgroups of patients showed that men and women, and patients over and under 65 years of age, had generally similar responses. Irbesartan was effective in reducing blood pressure regardless of race, although the effect was somewhat less in blacks (usually a low-renin population).

The effect of irbesartan is apparent after the first dose and it is close to its full observed effect at 2 weeks. At the end of an 8-week exposure, about 2/3 of the antihypertensive effect was still present one week after the last dose. Rebound hypertension was not observed. There was essentially no change in average heart rate in irbesartan-treated patients in controlled trials.

INDICATIONS AND USAGE

AVAPRO (irbesartan) is indicated for the treatment of hypertension. It may be used alone or in combination with other antihypertensive agents.

Continued on next page

This product information was prepared in September 2000. On these and other products of Sanofi-Synthelabo Inc., detailed information may be obtained on a current basis by direct inquiry to Product Information Services, 90 Park Avenue, New York, NY 10016 (toll free 1-800-446-6267).

Avapro—Cont.

CONTRAINDICATIONS

AVAPRO is contraindicated in patients who are hypersensitive to any component of this product.

WARNINGS

Fetal/Neonatal Morbidity and Mortality

Drugs that act directly on the renin-angiotensin system can cause fetal and neonatal morbidity and death when administered to pregnant women. Several dozen cases have been reported in the world literature in patients who were taking angiotensin-converting-enzyme inhibitors. When pregnancy is detected, AVAPRO should be discontinued as soon as possible.

The use of drugs that act directly on the renin-angiotensin system during the second and third trimesters of pregnancy has been associated with fetal and neonatal injury, including hypotension, neonatal skull hypoplasia, anuria, reversible or irreversible renal failure, and death. Oligohydramnios has also been reported, presumably resulting from decreased fetal renal function; oligohydramnios in this setting has been associated with fetal limb contractures, craniofacial deformation and hypoplastic lung development. Prematurity, intrauterine growth retardation, and patent ductus arteriosus have also been reported, although it is not clear whether these occurrences were due to exposure to the drug.

These adverse effects do not appear to have resulted from intrauterine drug exposure that has been limited to the first trimester.

Mothers whose embryos and fetuses are exposed to an angiotensin II receptor antagonist only during the first trimester should be so informed. Nonetheless, when patients become pregnant, physicians should have the patient discontinue the use of AVAPRO as soon as possible.

Rarely (probably less often than once in every thousand pregnancies), no alternative to a drug acting on the renin-angiotensin system will be found. In these rare cases, the mothers should be apprised of the potential hazards to their fetuses, and serial ultrasound examinations shold be performed to assess the intraamniotic environment.

If oligohydramnios is observed, AVAPRO should be discontinued unless it is considered life-saving for the mother. Contraction stress testing (CST), a non-stress test (NST), or biophysical profiling (BPP) may be appropriate depending upon the week of pregnancy. Patients and physicians should be aware, however, that oligohydramnios may not appear until after the fetus has sustained irreversible injury.

Infants with histories of *in utero* exposure to an angiotensin II receptor antagonist should be closely observed for hypotension, oliguria, and hyperkalemia. If oliguria occurs, attention should be directed toward support of blood pressure and renal perfusion. Exchange transfusion or dialysis may be required as means of reversing hypotension and/or substituting for disordered renal function.

When pregnant rats were treated with irbesartan from day 0 to day 20 of gestation (oral doses of 50, 180, and 650 mg/kg/day), increased incidences of renal pelvic cavitation, hydroureter and/or absence of renal papilla were observed in fetuses at doses ≥50 mg/kg/day [approximately equivalent to the maximum recommended human dose (MRHD), 300 mg/day, on a body surface area basis]. Subcutaneous edema was observed in fetuses at doses ≥180 mg/kg/day (about 4 times the MRHD on a body surface area basis). As these anomalies were not observed in rats in which irbesartan exposure (oral doses of 50, 150 and 450 mg/kg/day) was limited to gestation days 6–15, they appear to reflect late gestational effects of the drug. In pregnant rabbits, oral doses of 30 mg irbesartan/kg/day were associated with maternal mortality and abortion. Surviving females receiving this dose (about 1.5 times the MRHD of a body surface area basis) had a slight increase in early resorptions and a corresponding decrease in live fetuses. Irbesartan was found to cross the placental barrier in rats and rabbits.

Radioactivity was present in the rat and rabbit fetus during late gestation and in rat milk following oral doses of radiolabeled irbesartan.

Hypotension in Volume- or Salt-depleted Patients

Excessive reduction of blood pressure was rarely seen (<0.1%) in patients with uncomplicated hypertension. Initiation of antihypertensive therapy may cause symptomatic hypotension in patients with intravascular volume- or sodium-depletion, e.g., in patients treated virgorously with diuretics or in patients on dialysis. Such volume depletion should be corrected prior to administration of AVAPRO (irbesartan), or a low starting dose should be used (see **DOSAGE AND ADMINISTRATION**).

If hypotension occurs, the patient should be placed in the supine position and, if necessary, given an intravenous infusion of normal saline. A transient hypotensive response is not a contraindication to further treatment, which usually can be continued without difficulty once the blood pressure has stabilized.

PRECAUTIONS

Impaired Renal Function

As a consequence of inhibiting the renin-angiotensin-aldosterone system, changes in renal function may be anticipated in susceptible individuals. In patients whose renal function may depend on the activity of the renin-angiotensin-aldosterone system (e.g., patients with severe congestive heart failure), treatment with angiotensin-converting-enzyme inhibitors has been associated with oliguria and/or progressive azotemia and (rarely) with acute renal failure and/or death. AVAPRO would be expected to behave similarly. In studies of ACE inhibitors in patients with unilateral or bilateral renal artery stenosis, increases in serum creatinine or BUN have been reported. There has been no known use of AVAPRO in patients with unilateral or bilateral renal artery stenosis, but a similar effect should be anticipated.

Information for Patients

Pregnancy: Female patients of childbearing age should be told about the consequences of second- and third-trimester exposure to drugs that act on the renin-angiotensin system, and they should also be told that these consequences do not appear to have resulted from intrauterine drug exposure that has been limited to the first trimester. These patients should be asked to report pregnancies to their physicians as soon as possible.

Drug Interactions

No significant drug-drug pharmacokinetic (or pharmacodynamic) interactions have been found in interaction studies with hydrochlorothiazide, digoxin, warfarin, and nifedipine. *In vitro* studies show significant inhibition of the formation of oxidized irbesartan metabolites with the known cytochrome CYP 2C9 substrates/inhibitors sulphenazole, tolbutamide and nifedipine. However, in clinical studies the consequences of concomitant irbesartan on the pharmacodynamics of warfarin were negligible. Based on *in vitro* data, no interaction would be expected with drugs whose metabolism is dependent upon cytochrome P450 isozymes 1A1, 1A2, 2A6, 2B6, 2D6, 2E1, or 3A4.

In separate studies of patients receiving maintenance doses of warfarin, hydrochlorothiazide, or digoxin, irbesartan administration for 7 days had no effect on the pharmacodynamics of warfarin (prothrombin time) or pharmacokinetics of digoxin. The pharmacokinetics of irbesartan were not affected by coadministration of nifedipine or hydrochlorothiazide.

Carcinogenesis, Mutagenesis, Impairment of Fertility

No evidence of carcinogenicity was observed when irbesartan was administered at doses of up to 500/1000 mg/kg/day (males/females, respectively) in rats and 1000 mg/kg/day in mice for up to two years. For male and female rats, 500 mg/kg/day provided an average systemic exposure to irbesartan (AUC_{0-24h}, bound plus unbound) about 3 and 11 times, respectively, the average systemic exposure in humans receiving the maximum recommended dose (MRD) of 300 mg irbesartan/day, whereas 1000 mg/kg/day (administered to females only) provided an average systemic exposure about 21 times that reported for humans at the MRD. For male and female mice, 1000 mg/kg/day provided an exposure to irbesartan about 3 and 5 times, respectively, the human exposure at 300 mg/day.

Irbesartan was not mutagenic in a battery of *in vitro* tests (Ames microbial test, rat hepatocyte DNA repair test, V79 mammalian-cell forward gene-mutation assay). Irbesartan was negative in several tests for induction of chromosomal aberrations (*in vitro*—human lymphocyte assay; *in vivo*—mouse micronucleus study).

Irbesartan had no adverse effects on fertility or mating of male or female rats at oral doses ≤650 mg/kg/day, the highest dose providing a systemic exposure to irbesartan (AUC_{0-24h}, bound plus unbound) about 5 times that found in humans receiving the maximum recommended dose of 300 mg/day.

Pregnancy

Pregnancy Categories C (first trimester) and D (second and third trimester).

See **WARNINGS: Fetal/Neonatal Morbidity and Mortality.**

Nursing Mothers

It is not known whether irbesartan is excreted in human milk, but irbesartan or some metabolite of irbesartan is secreted at low concentration in the milk of lactating rats. Because of the potential for adverse effects on the nursing infant, a decision should be made whether to discontinue nursing or discontinue the drug, taking into account the importance of the drug to the mother.

Pediatric Use

Safety and effectiveness in pediatric patients have not been established.

Geriatric Use

Of the total number of patients receiving AVAPRO (irbesartan) in controlled clinical studies, 911 patients (18.5%) were 65 years and over, while 150 patients (3.0%) were 75 years and over. No overall differences in effectiveness or safety were observed between these patients and younger patients, but greater sensitivity of some older individuals cannot be ruled out.

ADVERSE REACTIONS

AVAPRO has been evaluated for safety in more than 4300 patients with hypertension and about 5000 subjects overall. This experience includes 1303 patients treated for over 6 months and 407 patients for 1 year or more. Treatment with AVAPRO was well-tolerated, with an incidence of adverse events similar to placebo. These events generally were mild and transient with no relationship to the doses of AVAPRO.

In placebo-controlled clinical trials, discontinuation of therapy due to a clinical adverse event was required in 3.3 percent of patients treated with AVAPRO, versus 4.5 percent of patients given placebo.

In placebo-controlled clinical trials, the adverse event experiences that occurred in at least 1% of patients treated with AVAPRO (n=1965) and at a higher incidence versus placebo (n=641) included diarrhea (3% vs. 2%), dyspepsia/heartburn (2% vs. 1%), musculoskeletal trauma (2% vs. 1%), fatigue (4% vs. 3%), and upper respiratory infection (9% vs. 6%). None of these differences were significant.

The following adverse events occurred at an incidence of 1% or greater in patients treated with irbesartan, but were at least as frequent or more frequent in patients recieving placebo: abdominal pain, anxiety/nervousness, chest pain, dizziness, edema, headache, influenza, musculoskeletal pain, pharyngitis, nausea/vomiting, rash, rhinitis, sinus abnormailty, tachycardia and urinary tract infection.

Irbesartan use was not associated with an increased incidence of dry cough, as is typically associated with ACE inhibitor use. In placebo controlled studies, the incidence of cough in irbesartan treated patients was 2.8% versus 2.7% in patients receiving placebo.

The incidence of hypotension or orthostatic hypotension was low in irbesartan treated patients (0.4%), unrelated to dosage, and similar to the incidence among placebo treated patients (0.2%). Dizziness, syncope, and vertigo were reported with equal or less frequency in patients receiving irbesartan compared with placebo.

In addition, the following potentially important events occurred in less than 1% of the 1965 patients and at least 5 patients (0.3%) receiving irbesartan in clinical studies, and those less frequent, clinically significant events (listed by body system). It cannot be determined whether these events were causally related to irbesartan:

Body as a Whole: fever, chills, facial edema, upper extremity edema;

Cardiovascular: flushing, hypertension, cardiac murmur, myocardial infarction, angina pectoris, arrhythmic/conduction disorder, cardio-respiratory arrest, heart failure, hypertensive crisis;

Dermatologic: pruritus, dermatitis, ecchymosis, erythema face, urticaria;

Endocrine/Metabolic/Electrolyte Imbalances: sexual dysfunction, libido change, gout;

Gastrointestinal: constipation, oral lesion, gastroenteritis, flatulence, abdominal distention;

Musculoskeletal/Connective Tissue: extremity swelling, muscle cramp, arthritis, muscle ache, musculoskeletal chest pain, joint stiffness, bursitis, muscle weakness;

Nervous System: sleep disturbance, numbness, somnolence, emotional disturbance, depression, paresthesia, tremor, transient ischemic attack, cerebrovascular accident;

Renal/Genitourinary: abnormal urination, prostate disorder;

Respiratory: epistaxis, tracheobronchitis, congestion, pulmonary congestion, dyspnea, wheezing;

Special Senses: vision disturbance, hearing abnormality, ear infection, ear pain, conjunctivitis, other eye disturbance, eyelid abnormality, ear abnormality.

Post-Marketing Experience: The following adverse reactions have been reported in post-marketing experience: Rare cases of urticaria and angioedema (involving swelling of the face, lips, pharynx, and/or tongue); hyperkalemia.

Laboratory Test Findings

In controlled clinical trials, clincally important differences in laboratory tests were rarely associated with administration of AVAPRO.

Creatinine, Blood Urea Nitrogen: Minor increases in blood urea nitrogen (BUN) or serum creatinine were observed in less than 0.7% of patients with essential hypertension treated with AVAPRO alone versus 0.9% on placebo. (See **PRECAUTIONS: Impaired Renal Function.**)

Hematologic: Mean decreases in hemoglobin of 0.2 g/dL were observed in 0.2% of patients receiving AVAPRO compared to 0.3% of placebo treated patients. Neutropenia (<1000 cells/mm^3) occurred at similar frequencies among patients receiving AVAPRO (0.3%) and placebo treated patients (0.5%).

OVERDOSAGE

No data are available in regard to overdosage in humans. However, daily doses of 900 mg for 8 weeks were well-tolerated. The most likely manifestations of overdosage are expected to be hypotension and tachycardia; bradycardia might also occur from overdose. Irbesartan is not removed by hemodialysis.

To obtain up-to-date information about the treatment of overdosage, a good resource is a certified Regional Poison-Control Center. Telephone numbers of certified poison-con-

	75 mg	150 mg	300 mg
Debossing	2771	2772	2773
Bottle of 30	0087-2771-31	0087-2772-31	0087-2773-31
Bottle of 90	0087-2771-32	0087-2772-32	0087-2773-32
Bottle of 500	0087-2771-15	0087-2772-15	0087-2773-15
Blister of 100	0087-2771-35	0087-2772-35	0087-2773-35

trol centers are listed in the *Physicians' Desk Reference* (PDR). In managing overdose, consider the possibilities of multiple-drug interactions, drug-drug interactions, and unusual drug kinetics in the patient.

Laboratory determinations of serum levels of irbesartan are not widely available, and such determinations have, in any event, no known established role in the management of irbesartan overdose.

Acute oral toxicity studies with irbesartan in mice and rats indicated acute lethal doses were in excess of 2000 mg/kg, about 25- and 50-fold the maximum recommended human dose (300 mg) on a mg/m^2 basis, respectively.

DOSAGE AND ADMINISTRATION

The recommended initial dose of AVAPRO is 150 mg once daily. Patients requiring further reduction in blood pressure should be titrated to 300 mg once daily.

A low dose of a diuretic may be added, if blood pressure is not controlled by AVAPRO alone. Hydrochlorothiazide has been shown to have an additive effect (see **CLINICAL PHARMACOLOGY: Clinical Studies**). Patients not adequately treated by the maximum dose of 300 mg once daily are unlikely to derive additional benefit from a higher dose or twice-daily dosing.

No dosage adjustment is necessary in elderly patients, or in patients with hepatic impairment or mild to severe renal impairment.

AVAPRO may be administered with other antihypertensive agents.

AVAPRO may be administered with or without food.

Volume- and Salt-depleted Patients

A lower initial dose or AVAPRO (75 mg) is recommended in patients with depletion of intravascular volume or salt (e.g., patients treated vigorously with diuretics or on hemodialysis) (see **WARNINGS: Hypotension in Volume- of Salt-depleted Patients**).

HOW SUPPLIED

AVAPRO® (irbesartan) is available as white to off-white biconvex oval tablets, debossed with a heart shape on one side and a portion of the NDC code on the other. Unit-of-use bottles contain 30, 90, or 500 tablets and blister packs contain 100 tablets, as follows:

[See table at top of previous page]

Storage

Store at a temperature between 15° C and 30° C (59° F and 85° F) [USP].

Manufactured and Distributed by:
Bristol-Myers Squibb Company
Princeton, NJ 08543-4500
Comarketed by:
Sanofi-Synthelabo Inc.
New York, NY 10016
Revised November 1999 1092944A1 J4-641C

Shown in Product Identification Guide, page 333

BRONCHOLATE® SYRUP ℞

Each teaspoonful (5 ml) orange flavored syrup contains:

Ephedrine HCl	6.25 mg
Guaifenesin	100.00 mg

HOW SUPPLIED

Bottles of 16 oz.

CHEMET® ℞
SUCCIME

DESCRIPTION

CHEMET (succimer) is an orally active, heavy metal chelating agent. The chemical name for succimer is *meso* 2, 3-dimercaptosuccinic acid (DMSA). Its empirical formula is $C_4H_6O_4S_2$ and molecular weight is 182.2. The *meso*-structural formula is:

```
     COOH
      |
  H—C—SH
      |
  H—C—SH
      |
     COOH
```

Succimer is a white crystalline powder with an unpleasant, characteristic mercaptan odor and taste.

Each CHEMET opaque white capsule for oral administration, contains beads coated with 100 mg of succimer and is imprinted black with CHEMET 100. Inactive ingredients in medicated beads are: povidone, sodium starch glycolate, starch and sucrose. Inactive ingredients in capsule are: gelatin, iron oxide, titanium dioxide and other ingredients.

CLINICAL PHARMACOLOGY

Succimer is a lead chelator; it forms water soluble chelates and, consequently, increases the urinary excretion of lead.

Preclinical Toxicology: In an ongoing six month chronic oral toxicity study in dogs, thrombocytopenia was observed in animals receiving succimer at 80 or 140 mg/kg/day after three months of dosing. Preliminary gross pathology findings in the affected dogs included ecchymoses in a number of organs. No depressed platelet counts were observed in dogs receiving succimer at 10 mg/kg/day for three months. Platelets were not enumerated in previous oral toxicity studies up to 28 days. In those studies, daily doses of succimer up to 200 mg/kg/day did not produce any significant overt toxicity in rats and dogs. However, six and twenty-eight day oral toxicity studies in dogs have shown that doses of 300 mg/kg/ day or higher were toxic and lethal to some dogs. Kidney and gastrointestinal tract were the major target organs for succimer toxicity. Toxicity was manifested by anorexia, emesis, mucoid and/or bloody diarrhea, increased blood urea nitrogen concentration, increased SGPT, SGOT and alkaline phosphatase levels, renal tubular necrosis, purulent nephritis and severe gastrointestinal bleeding and ulceration. Deaths were due to renal failure.

Pharmacokinetics: In a study performed in healthy adult volunteers, after a single dose of ^{14}C-succimer at 16, 32, or 48 mg/kg, absorption was rapid but variable with peak blood radioactivity levels between one and two hours. On average, 49% of the radiolabeled dose was excreted: 39% in the feces, 9% in the urine and 1% as carbon dioxide from the lungs. Since fecal excretion probably represented non-absorbed drug, most of the absorbed drug was excreted by the kidneys. The apparent elimination half-life of the radiolabeled material in the blood was about two days.

In other studies of healthy adult volunteers receiving a single oral dose of 10 mg/kg, the chemical analysis of succimer and its metabolites in the urine showed that succimer was rapidly and extensively metabolized. Approximately 25% of the administered dose was excreted in the urine with the peak blood level and urinary excretion occurring between two and four hours. Of the total amount of drug eliminated in the urine, approximately 90% was eliminated in altered form as mixed succimer-cysteine disulfides; the remaining 10% was eliminated unchanged. The majority of mixed disulfides consisted of succimer in disulfide linkages with two molecules of L-cysteine, the remaining disulfides contained one L-cysteine per succimer molecule.

Pharmacodynamics: Dose ranging studies were performed in 18 men with blood lead levels of 44–96 µg/dL. Three groups of 6 patients received either 10.0, 6.7 or 3.3 mg/kg succimer orally every 8 hours for 5 days. After five days the mean blood levels of the three groups decreased 72.5%, 58.3% and 35.5% respectively. The mean urinary lead excretions in the initial 24 hours were 28.6, 18.6 and 12.3 times the pretreatment 24 hour urinary lead excretion. As the chelatable pool was reduced during therapy, urinary lead output decreased. A mean of 19 mg of lead was excreted during a five-day course of 30 mg/kg/day succimer. Clinical symptoms, such as headache and colic and biochemical indices of lead toxicity also improved. Decrease in urinary excretion of d-aminolevulinic acid (ALA) and coproporphyrin paralleled the improvement in erythrocyte d-aminolevulinic acid dehydratase (ALA-D). Three control patients with lead poisoning of similar severity received $CaNa_2$ EDTA intravenously at a dose of 50 mg/kg/day for five days. The mean blood lead level decreased 47.4% and the mean urinary lead excretion was 21 mg in the control patients.

Effect on Essential Minerals: In the above studies succimer had no significant effect on the urinary elimination of iron, calcium or magnesium. Zinc excretion doubled during treatment. The effect of succimer on the excretion of essential minerals was small compared to that of $CaNa_2$ EDTA, which can induce more than a ten-fold increase in urinary excretion of zinc and doubling of copper and iron excretion.

Efficacy: A dose ranging study was performed in 15 pediatric patients aged 2 to 7 years with blood lead levels of 30–49 µg/dL and positive $CaNa_2$ EDTA lead mobilization tests. Each group of five patients received 350, 233 or 116 mg/m^2 succimer every 8 hours for 5 days. These doses corresponded to 10, 6.7 and 3.3 mg/kg. Six control patients received 1000 mg/m^2/day $CaNa_2$ EDTA intravenously for 5 days. Following therapy, the mean blood lead levels decreased 78, 63 and 42% respectively in the three groups treated with succimer. The response of the 350 mg/m^2 every 8 hours (10 mg/kg q 8 hr) group was significantly better than that of the other succimer treated groups as well as that of the control group, whose mean blood lead level fell 48%. No adverse reactions or changes in essential mineral excretion were reported in the succimer treated groups. In the $CaNa_2$ EDTA treated group, the cumulative amount of urinary lead excreted was slightly but significantly greater than in the succimer group. After $CaNa_2$ EDTA, the urinary excretion of copper, zinc, iron and calcium were significantly increased.

As with other chelators, both adults and pediatric patients experienced a rebound in blood lead levels after discontinuation of CHEMET. In these studies, after treatment with a dose of 350 mg/m^2 (10 mg/kg) every 8 hours for five days, the mean lead level rebounded and plateaued at 60–85% of pretreatment levels two weeks after therapy. The rebound plateau was somewhat higher with lower doses of succimer and with intravenous $CaNa_2$ EDTA.

In an attempt to control rebound of blood lead levels, 19 pediatric patients, ages 1–7 years, with blood lead levels of 42–67 µg/dL, were treated with 350 mg/m^2 succimer every 8 hours for five days and then divided into three groups. One group was followed for two weeks with no further therapy, the second group was treated for two weeks with 350 mg/m^2 daily, and the third with 350 mg/m^2 every 12 hours. After the initial 5 days of therapy, the mean blood lead level in all subjects declined 61%. While the untreated group and the group treated with 350 mg/m^2 daily experienced rebound during the ensuing two weeks, the group who received the 350 mg/ m^2 every 12 hours experienced no such rebound during the treatment period and less rebound following cessation of therapy.

In another study, ten pediatric patients, ages 21 to 72 months, with blood lead levels of 30–57 µg/dL were treated with succimer 350 mg/m^2 every eight hours for five days followed by an additional 19–22 days of therapy at a dose of 350 mg/m^2 every 12 hours. The mean blood lead levels decreased and remained stable at under 15 µg/dL during the extended dosing period.

In addition to the controlled studies, approximately 250 patients with lead poisoning have been treated with succimer either orally or parenterally in open U.S. and foreign studies with similar results reported. Succimer has been used for the treatment of lead poisoning in one patient with sickle cell anemia and in five patients with glucose-6-phosphodehydrogenase (G6PD) deficiency without adverse reactions.

Lead Encephalopathy: Three adults with lead encephalopathy have been reported in the literature to have improved with succimer therapy. However, data are not available regarding the use of succimer for the treatment of this rare and sometimes fatal complication of lead poisoning in pediatric patients.

Other Heavy Metal Poisoning: No controlled clinical studies have been conducted with succimer in poisoning with other heavy metals. A limited number of patients have received succimer for mercury or arsenic poisoning. These patients showed increased urinary excretion of the heavy metal and varying degrees of symptomatic improvement.

INDICATIONS AND USAGE

CHEMET is indicated for the treatment of lead poisoning in pediatric patients with blood lead levels above 45 µg/dL. CHEMET is not indicated for prophylaxis of lead poisoning in a lead-containing environment; the use of CHEMET should always be accompanied by identification and removal of the source of the lead exposure.

CONTRAINDICATIONS

CHEMET should not be administered to patients with a history of allergy to the drug.

WARNINGS

Keep out of reach of pediatric patients. CHEMET is not a substitute for effective abatement of lead exposure.

Mild to moderate neutropenia has been observed in some patients receiving succimer. While a causal relationship to succimer has not been definitely established, neutropenia has been reported with other drugs in the same chemical class. A complete blood count with white blood cell differential and direct platelet counts should be obtained prior to and weekly during treatment with succimer. Therapy should either be withheld or discontinued if the absolute neutrophil count (ANC) is below 1200/µL and the patient followed closely to document recovery of the ANC to above 1500/µL or to the patient's baseline neutrophil count. There is limited experience with reexposure in patients who have developed neutropenia. Therefore, such patients should be rechallenged only if the benefit of succimer therapy clearly outweighs the potential risk of another episode of neutropenia and then only with careful patient monitoring.

Patients treated with succimer should be instructed to promptly report any signs of infection. If infection is suspected, the above laboratory tests should be conducted immediately.

PRECAUTIONS

The extent of clinical experience with CHEMET is limited. Therefore, patients should be carefully observed during treatment.

General: Elevated blood lead levels and associated symptoms may return rapidly after discontinuation of CHEMET because of redistribution of lead from bone stores to soft tissues and blood. After therapy, patients should be monitored for rebound of blood lead levels, by measuring blood lead levels at least once weekly until stable. However, the severity of lead intoxication (as measured by the initial blood lead level and the rate and degree of rebound of blood lead) should be used as a guide for more frequent blood lead monitoring.

All patients undergoing treatment should be adequately hydrated. Caution should be exercised in using CHEMET therapy in patients with compromised renal function. Limited data suggests that CHEMET is dialyzable, but that the lead chelates are not.

Transient mild elevations of serum transaminases have been observed in 6–10% of patients during the course of succimer therapy. Serum transaminases should be monitored before the start of therapy and at least weekly during therapy. Patients with a history of liver disease should be monitored closely. No data are available regarding the metabolism of succimer in patients with liver disease.

Clinical experience with repeated courses is limited. The safety of uninterrupted dosing longer than three weeks has not been established and it is not recommended.

The possibility of allergic or other mucocutaneous reactions to the drug must be borne in mind on readministration (as

Continued on next page

This product information was prepared in September 2000. On these and other products of Sanofi-Synthelabo Inc., detailed information may be obtained on a current basis by direct inquiry to Product Information Services, 90 Park Avenue, New York, NY 10016 (toll free 1-800-446-6267).

Chemet—Cont.

well as during initial courses). Patients requiring repeated courses of CHEMET should be monitored during each treatment course. One patient experienced recurrent mucocutaneous vesicular eruptions of increasing severity affecting the oral mucosa, the external urethral meatus and the perianal area on the third, fourth and fifth courses of the drug. The reaction resolved between courses and upon discontinuation of therapy.

Information for Patients: Patients should be instructed to maintain adequate fluid intake. If rash occurs, patients should consult their physician. Patients should be instructed to promptly report any indication of infection, which may be a sign of neutropenia (see WARNINGS and ADVERSE REACTIONS).

In young pediatric patients unable to swallow capsules, the contents of the capsule can be administered in a small amount of food (see DOSAGE AND ADMINISTRATION).

Drug Interaction: CHEMET is not known to interact with other drugs including iron supplements; interactions have not been systematically studied. Concomitant administration of CHEMET with other chelation therapy, such as $CaNa_2$ EDTA is not recommended.

Drug/Laboratory Tests Interaction: Succimer may interfere with serum and urinary laboratory tests. *In vitro* studies have shown succimer to cause false positive results for ketones in urine using nitroprusside reagents such as Ketostix® and falsely decreased measurements of serum uric acid and CPK.

Carcinogenesis, Mutagenesis and Impairment of Fertility: CHEMET has not been tested for carcinogenic potential in long-term animal studies. CHEMET has not been tested in animals for its effect on fertility and reproductive performance in males and females. It was not mutagenic in the Ames bacterial assay and in the mammalian cell forward gene mutation assay.

Pregnancy: *Teratogenic Effects —Pregnancy Category C.* CHEMET has been shown to be teratogenic and fetotoxic in pregnant mice when given subcutaneously in a dose range of 410 to 1640 mg/kg/day during the period of organogenesis. There are no adequate and well controlled studies in pregnant women. CHEMET should be used during pregnancy only if the potential benefit justifies the potential risk to the fetus.

Nursing Mothers: It is not known whether this drug is excreted in human milk. Because many drugs and heavy metals are excreted in human milk, nursing mothers requiring CHEMET therapy should be discouraged from nursing their infants.

Pediatric Use: Refer to the INDICATIONS and DOSAGE AND ADMINISTRATION sections. Safety and efficacy in pediatric patients less than 12 months of age have not been established.

ADVERSE REACTIONS

Clinical experience with CHEMET has been limited. Consequently, the full spectrum and incidence of adverse reactions including the possibility of hypersensitivity or idiosyncratic reactions have not been determined. The most common events attributable to succimer, i.e., gastrointestinal symptoms or increases in serum transaminases, have been observed in about 10% of patients (see PRECAUTIONS). Rashes, some necessitating discontinuation of therapy, have been reported in about 4% of patients. If rash occurs, other causes (e.g. measles) should be considered before ascribing the reaction to succimer. Rechallenge with succimer may be considered if lead levels are high enough to warrant retreatment. One allergic mucocutaneous reaction has been reported on repeated administration of the drug (See PRECAUTIONS). Mild to moderate neutropenia has been observed in some patients receiving succimer (see WARNINGS). Table I presents adverse events reported with the administration of succimer for the treatment of lead and other heavy metal intoxication.

TABLE I
INCIDENCE OF ADVERSE EVENTS IN DOMESTIC STUDIES REGARDLESS OF ATTRIBUTION OR SUCCIMER DOSAGE

	Pediatric Patients (191)		Adults (134)	
	%	(n)	%	(n)
Digestive:	12.0	23	20.9	28
Nausea, vomiting, diarrhea, appetite loss, hemorrhoidal symptoms, loose stools, metallic taste in mouth.				
Body as a Whole:	5.2	10	15.7	21
Back pain, abdominal cramps, stomach pains, head pain, rib pain, chills, flank pain, fever, flu-like symptoms, heavy head/tired, head cold, headache, moniliasis.				
Metabolic:	4.2	8	10.4	14
Elevated SGPT, SGOT, alkaline phosphatase, elevated serum cholesterol.				
Nervous:	1.0	2	12.7	17
Drowsiness, dizziness, sensorimotor neuropathy, sleepiness, paresthesia.				
Skin and Appendages:	2.6	5	11.2	15
Papular rash, herpetic rash, rash, mucocutaneous eruptions, pruritus.				
Special Senses:	1.0	2	3.7	5
Cloudy film in eye, ears plugged, otitis media, eyes watery.				
Respiratory:	3.7	7	0.7	1
Throat sore, rhinorrhea, nasal congestion, cough.				
Urogenital:	0.0	—	3.7	5
Decreased urination, voiding difficulty, proteinuria increased.				
Cardiovascular:	0.0	—	1.8	2
Arrhythmia				
Heme/Lymphatic:	0.5*	1	1.5*	2
Mild to moderate neutropenia				
Increased platelet count, intermittent eosinophilia.				
Musculoskeletal:	0.0	—	3.0	4
Kneecap pain, leg pains.				

* Does not include neutropenia - see WARNINGS

OVERDOSAGE

Doses of 2300 mg/kg in the rat and 2400 mg/kg in the mouse produced ataxia, convulsions, labored respiration and frequently death. No case of overdosage has been reported in humans. Limited data indicate that succimer is dialyzable. In case of acute overdosage, induction of vomiting or gastric lavage followed by administration of an activated charcoal slurry and appropriate supportive therapy are recommended.

DOSAGE AND ADMINISTRATION

Start dosage at 10 mg/kg or 350 mg/m^2 every eight hours for five days. Initiation of therapy at higher doses is not recommended. (See Table II for Dosing chart and number of capsules.) Reduce frequency of administration to 10 mg/kg or 350 mg/m^2 every 12 hours (two-thirds of initial daily dosage) for an additional two weeks of therapy. A course of treatment lasts 19 days. Repeated courses may be necessary if indicated by weekly monitoring of blood lead concentration. A minimum of two weeks between courses is recommended unless blood lead levels indicate the need for more prompt treatment.

TABLE II
CHEMET (SUCCIMER) PEDIATRIC DOSING CHART

LBS	KG	DOSE (MG)*	Number of CAPSULES*
18–35	8–15	100	1
36–55	16–23	200	2
56–75	24–34	300	3
76–100	35–44	400	4
>100	>45	500	5

* To be administered every 8 hours for 5 days, followed by dosing every 12 hours for 14 days.

In young pediatric patients who cannot swallow capsules, CHEMET can be administered by separating the capsule and sprinkling the medicated beads on a small amount of soft food or putting them in a spoon and following with fruit drink.

Identification of the source of lead in the pediatric patient's environment and its abatement are critical to a successful therapy outcome. Chelation therapy is not a substitute for preventing further exposure to lead and should not be used to permit continued exposure to lead.

Patients who have received $CaNa_2$ EDTA with or without BAL may use CHEMET for subsequent treatment after an interval of four weeks. Data on the concomitant use of CHEMET with $CaNa_2$ EDTA with or without BAL are not available, and such use is not recommended.

HOW SUPPLIED

100 mg capsules in bottle of 100 (NDC 0024-0333-01)

Storage

Store between 15°C and 25°C and avoid excessive heat.

Rev. 5/00

CSP-1C

Shown in Product Identification Guide, page 333

DANOCRINE® ℞
DANAZOL, USP

DESCRIPTION

DANOCRINE, brand of danazol, is a synthetic steroid derived from ethisterone. It is a white to pale yellow crystalline powder, practically insoluble or insoluble in water, and sparingly soluble in alcohol. Chemically, danazol is 17α-Pregna-2,4-dien-20-yno [2,3-*d*]-isoxazol-17-ol. The molecular formula is $C_{22}H_{27}NO_2$. It has a molecular weight of 337.46 and the following structural formula:

Danocrine capsules for oral administration contain 50 mg, 100 mg or 200 mg danazol.

Inactive Ingredients: Corn Starch, Lactose, Magnesium Stearate, Talc. Capsules 50 mg, 100 mg and 200 mg contain D&C Yellow #10, FD&C Red #40, Gelatin, Silicon Dioxide, Sodium Lauryl Sulfate, Titanium Dioxide. The 50 mg and 200 mg capsules also contain D&C Red #28.

CLINICAL PHARMACOLOGY

DANOCRINE suppresses the pituitary-ovarian axis. This suppression is probably a combination of depressed hypothalamic-pituitary response to lowered estrogen production, the alteration of sex steroid metabolism, and interaction of danazol with sex hormone receptors. The only other demonstrable hormonal effect is weak androgenic activity. DANOCRINE depresses the output of both follicle-stimulating hormone (FSH) and luteinizing hormone (LH).

Recent evidence suggests a direct inhibitory effect at gonadal sites and a binding of DANOCRINE to receptors of gonadal steroids at target organs. In addition, DANOCRINE has been shown to significantly decrease IgG, IgM and IgA levels, as well as phospholipid and IgG isotope autoantibodies in patients with endometriosis and associated elevations of autoantibodies, suggesting this could be another mechanism by which it facilitates regression of the disease.

Bioavailability studies indicate that blood levels do not increase proportionally with increases in the administered dose. When the dose of DANOCRINE is doubled the increase in plasma levels is only about 35% to 40%.

Separate single dosing of 100 mg and 200 mg capsules of DANOCRINE to female volunteers showed that both the extent of availability and the maximum plasma concentration increased by three-to-four fold, respectively, following a meal (> 30 grams of fat), when compared to the fasted state. Further, food also delayed mean time to peak concentration of DANOCRINE by about 30 minutes.

In the treatment of endometriosis, DANOCRINE alters the normal and ectopic endometrial tissue so that it becomes inactive and atrophic. Complete resolution of endometrial lesions occurs in the majority of cases.

Changes in vaginal cytology and cervical mucus reflect the suppressive effect of DANOCRINE on the pituitary-ovarian axis.

In the treatment of fibrocystic breast disease, DANOCRINE usually produces partial to complete disappearance of nodularity and complete relief of pain and tenderness. Changes in the menstrual pattern may occur.

Generally, the pituitary-suppressive action of DANOCRINE is reversible. Ovulation and cyclic bleeding usually return within 60 to 90 days when therapy with DANOCRINE is discontinued.

In the treatment of hereditary angioedema, DANOCRINE at effective doses prevents attacks of the disease characterized by episodic edema of the abdominal viscera, extremities, face, and airway which may be disabling and, if the airway is involved, fatal. In addition, DANOCRINE corrects partially or completely the primary biochemical abnormality of hereditary angioedema by increasing the levels of the deficient C1 esterase inhibitor (C1EI). As a result of this action the serum levels of the C4 component of the complement system are also increased.

INDICATIONS AND USAGE

Endometriosis. DANOCRINE is indicated for the treatment of endometriosis amenable to hormonal management.

Fibrocystic Breast Disease. Most cases of symptomatic fibrocystic breast disease may be treated by simple measures (e.g., padded brassieres and analgesics).

In infrequent patients, symptoms of pain and tenderness may be severe enough to warrant treatment by suppression of ovarian function. DANOCRINE is usually effective in decreasing nodularity, pain, and tenderness. It should be stressed to the patient that this treatment is not innocuous in that it involves considerable alterations of hormone levels and that recurrence of symptoms is very common after cessation of therapy.

Hereditary Angioedema. DANOCRINE is indicated for the prevention of attacks of angioedema of all types (cutaneous, abdominal, laryngeal) in males and females.

CONTRAINDICATIONS

DANOCRINE should not be administered to patients with:

1. Undiagnosed abnormal genital bleeding.
2. Markedly impaired hepatic, renal, or cardiac function.
3. Pregnancy. (See WARNINGS.)
4. Breast feeding.
5. Porphyria—DANOCRINE can induce ALA synthetase activity and hence porphyrin metabolism.

WARNINGS

Use of danazol in pregnancy is contraindicated. A sensitive test (e.g., beta subunit test if available) capable of determining early pregnancy is recommended immediately prior to start of therapy. Additionally a non-hormonal method of contraception should be used during therapy. If a patient becomes pregnant while taking danazol, administration of the drug should be discontinued and the patient should be apprised of the potential risk to the fetus. Exposure to danazol in utero may result in androgenic effects on the female fetus; reports of clitoral hypertrophy, labial fusion, urogenital sinus defect, vaginal atresia, and ambiguous genitalia have been received. (See PRECAUTIONS: Pregnancy, Teratogenic Effects.)

Thromboembolism, thrombotic and thrombophlebitic events including sagittal sinus thrombosis and life-threatening or fatal strokes have been reported.

Experience with long-term therapy with danazol is limited. Peliosis hepatis and benign hepatic adenoma have

been observed with long-term use. Peliosis hepatis and hepatic adenoma may be silent until complicated by acute, potentially life-threatening intra-abdominal hemorrhage. The physician therefore should be alert to this possibility. Attempts should be made to determine the lowest dose that will provide adequate protection. If the drug was begun at a time of exacerbation of hereditary angioneurotic edema due to trauma, stress or other cause, periodic attempts to decrease or withdraw therapy should be considered.
Danazol has been associated with several cases of benign intracranial hypertension also known as pseudotumor cerebri. Early signs and symptoms of benign intracranial hypertension include papilledema, headache, nausea and vomiting, and visual disturbances. Patients with these symptoms should be screened for papilledema and, if present, the patients should be advised to discontinue danazol immediately and be referred to a neurologist for further diagnosis and care.

A temporary alteration of lipoproteins in the form of decreased high density lipoproteins and possibly increased low density lipoproteins has been reported during danazol therapy. These alterations may be marked, and prescribers should consider the potential impact on the risk of atherosclerosis and coronary artery disease in accordance with the potential benefit of the therapy to the patient.
Before initiating therapy of fibrocystic breast disease with DANOCRINE, carcinoma of the breast should be excluded. However, nodularity, pain, tenderness due to fibrocystic breast disease may prevent recognition of underlying carcinoma before treatment is begun. Therefore, if any nodule persists or enlarges during treatment, carcinoma should be considered and ruled out.
Patients should be watched closely for signs of androgenic effects some of which may not be reversible even when drug administration is stopped.

PRECAUTIONS

Because DANOCRINE may cause some degree of fluid retention, conditions that might be influenced by this factor, such as epilepsy, migraine, or cardiac or renal dysfunction, require careful observation.
Since hepatic dysfunction manifested by modest increases in serum transaminase levels has been reported in patients treated with DANOCRINE, periodic liver function tests should be performed (see WARNINGS and ADVERSE REACTIONS).
Administration of danazol has been reported to cause exacerbation of the manifestations of acute intermittent porphyria. (See CONTRAINDICATIONS.)
Drug Interactions: Prolongation of prothrombin time occurs in patients stabilized on warfarin. Therapy with danazol may cause an increase in carbamazepine levels in patients taking both drugs.
Laboratory Tests: Danazol treatment may interfere with laboratory determinations of testosterone, androstenedione and dehydroepiandrosterone.
Carcinogenesis, Mutagenesis, Impairment of Fertility: No valid studies have been performed to assess the carcinogenicity of DANOCRINE.
Pregnancy, Teratogenic Effects: (See CONTRAINDICATIONS.) Pregnancy Category X. DANOCRINE administered orally to pregnant rats from the 6th through the 15th day of gestation at doses up to 250 mg/kg/day (7–15 times the human dose) did not result in drug-induced embryotoxicity or teratogenicity, nor difference in litter size, viability or weight of offspring compared to controls. In rabbits, the administration of DANOCRINE on days 6–18 of gestation at doses of 60 mg/kg/day and above (2–4 times the human dose) resulted in inhibition of fetal development.
Nursing Mothers: (See CONTRAINDICATIONS.)
Pediatric Use: Safety and effectiveness in pediatric patients have not been established.

ADVERSE REACTIONS

The following events have been reported in association with the use of DANOCRINE:
Androgen like effects include weight gain, acne and seborrhea. Mild hirsutism, edema, hair loss, voice change, which may take the form of hoarseness, sore throat or of instability or deepening of pitch, may occur and may persist after cessation of therapy. Hypertrophy of the clitoris is rare.
Other possible endocrine effects are menstrual disturbances including spotting, alteration of the timing of the cycle and amenorrhea. Although cyclical bleeding and ovulation usually return within 60–90 days after discontinuation of therapy with DANOCRINE, persistent amenorrhea has occasionally been reported.
Flushing, sweating, vaginal dryness and irritation and reduction in breast size, may reflect lowering of estrogen. Nervousness and emotional lability have been reported. In the male a modest reduction in spermatogenesis may be evident during treatment. Abnormalities in semen volume, viscosity, sperm count, and motility may occur in patients receiving long-term therapy.
Hepatic dysfunction, as evidenced by reversible elevated serum enzymes and/or jaundice, has been reported in patients receiving a daily dosage of DANOCRINE of 400 mg or more. It is recommended that patients receiving DANOCRINE be monitored for hepatic dysfunction by laboratory tests and clinical observation. Serious hepatic toxicity including cholestatic jaundice, peliosis hepatis, and hepatic adenoma have been reported. (See WARNINGS and PRECAUTIONS.)
Abnormalities in laboratory tests may occur during therapy with DANOCRINE including CPK, glucose tolerance, glucagon, thyroid binding globulin, sex hormone binding globulin, other plasma proteins, lipids and lipoproteins.
The following reactions have been reported, a causal relationship to the administration of DANOCRINE has neither been confirmed nor refuted; *allergic:* urticaria, pruritus and rarely, nasal congestion; *CNS effects:* headache, nervousness and emotional lability, dizziness and fainting, depression, fatigue, sleep disorders, tremor, paresthesias, weakness, visual disturbances, and rarely, benign intracranial hypertension, anxiety, changes in appetite, chills, and rarely convulsions, Guillain-Barre syndrome; *gastrointestinal:* gastroenteritis, nausea, vomiting, constipation, and rarely, pancreatitis; *musculoskeletal:* muscle cramps or spasms, or pains, joint pain, joint lockup, joint swelling, pain in back, neck, or extremities, and rarely, carpal tunnel syndrome which may be secondary to fluid retention; *genitourinary:* hematuria, prolonged posttherapy amenorrhea; *hematologic:* an increase in red cell and platelet count. Reversible erythrocytosis, leukocytosis or polycythemia may be provoked. Eosinophilia, leukopenia and thrombocytopenia have also been noted. *Skin:* rashes (maculopapular, vesicular, papular, purpuric, petechial), and rarely, sun sensitivity, Stevens-Johnson syndrome; *other:* increased insulin requirements in diabetic patients, change in libido, elevation in blood pressure, and rarely, cataracts, bleeding gums, fever, pelvic pain, nipple discharge. Malignant liver tumors have been reported in rare instances, after long-term use.

DOSAGE AND ADMINISTRATION

Endometriosis. In moderate to severe disease, or in patients infertile due to endometriosis, a starting dose of 800 mg given in two divided doses is recommended. Amenorrhea and rapid response to painful symptoms is best achieved at this dosage level. Gradual downward titration to a dose sufficient to maintain amenorrhea may be considered depending upon patient response. For mild cases, an initial daily dose of 200 mg to 400 mg given in two divided doses is recommended and may be adjusted depending on patient response. **Therapy should begin during menstruation. Otherwise, appropriate tests should be performed to ensure that the patient is not pregnant while on therapy with DANOCRINE. (See CONTRAINDICATIONS and WARNINGS.) It is essential that therapy continue uninterrupted for 3 to 6 months but may be extended to 9 months if necessary.** After termination of therapy, if symptoms recur, treatment can be reinstituted.
Fibrocystic Breast Disease. The total daily dosage of DANOCRINE for fibrocystic breast disease ranges from 100 mg to 400 mg given in two divided doses depending upon patient response. **Therapy should begin during menstruation. Otherwise, appropriate tests should be performed to ensure that the patient is not pregnant while on therapy with DANOCRINE.** A nonhormonal method of contraception is recommended when DANOCRINE is administered at this dose, since ovulation may not be suppressed.
In most instances, breast pain and tenderness are significantly relieved by the first month and eliminated in 2 to 3 months. Usually elimination of nodularity requires 4 to 6 months of uninterrupted therapy. Regular menstrual patterns, irregular menstrual patterns, and amenorrhea each occur in approximately one-third of patients treated with 100 mg of DANOCRINE. Irregular menstrual patterns and amenorrhea are observed more frequently with higher doses. Clinical studies have demonstrated that 50% of patients may show evidence of recurrence of symptoms within one year. In this event, treatment may be reinstated.
Hereditary Angioedema. The dosage requirements for continuous treatment of hereditary angioedema with DANOCRINE should be individualized on the basis of the clinical response of the patient. It is recommended that the patient be started on 200 mg, two or three times a day. After a favorable initial response is obtained in terms of prevention of episodes of edematous attacks, the proper continuing dosage should be determined by decreasing the dosage by 50% or less at intervals of one to three months or longer if frequency of attacks prior to treatment dictates. If an attack occurs, the daily dosage may be increased by up to 200 mg. During the dose adjusting phase, close monitoring of the patient's response is indicated, particularly if the patient has a history of airway involvement.

HOW SUPPLIED

Capsules of 200 mg (orange), bottles of 60 (NDC 0024-0305-60).
Capsules of 200 mg (orange), bottles of 100 (NDC 0024-0305-06).
Capsules of 100 mg (yellow), bottles of 100 (NDC 0024-0304-06).
Capsules of 50 mg (orange and white), bottles of 100 (NDC 0024-0303-06).
Store at controlled room temperature, 15° C to 30° C (59° F to 86° F).

DSW-5 I (O)

Revised September 1999

Shown in Product Identification Guide, page 333

DEMEROL® Ⓒ℞

MEPERIDINE HYDROCHLORIDE, USP
WARNING: May be habit forming

DESCRIPTION

Meperidine hydrochloride is ethyl 1-methyl-4-phenylisonipecotate hydrochloride, a white crystalline substance with a melting point of 186° C to 189° C. It is readily soluble in water and has a neutral reaction and a slightly bitter taste. The solution is not decomposed by a short period of boiling.
The syrup is a pleasant-tasting, nonalcoholic, banana-flavored solution containing 50 mg of DEMEROL, brand of meperidine hydrochloride, per 5 mL teaspoon (25 drops contain 13 mg of DEMEROL). The tablets contain 50 mg or 100 mg of the analgesic.
Inactive Ingredients—TABLETS: Calcium Sulfate, Dibasic Calcium Phosphate, Starch, Stearic Acid, Talc. SYRUP: Benzoic Acid, Flavor, Liquid Glucose, Purified Water, Saccharin Sodium.

CLINICAL PHARMACOLOGY

Meperidine hydrochloride is a narcotic analgesic with multiple actions qualitatively similar to those of morphine; the most prominent of these involve the central nervous system and organs composed of smooth muscle. The principal actions of therapeutic value are analgesia and sedation.
There is some evidence which suggests that meperidine may produce less smooth muscle spasm, constipation, and depression of the cough reflex than equianalgesic doses of morphine. Meperidine, in 60 mg to 80 mg parenteral doses, is approximately equivalent in analgesic effect to 10 mg of morphine. The onset of action is slightly more rapid than with morphine, and the duration of action is slightly shorter. Meperidine is significantly less effective by the oral than by the parenteral route, but the exact ratio of oral to parenteral effectiveness is unknown.

INDICATIONS AND USAGE

For the relief of moderate to severe pain

CONTRAINDICATIONS

Hypersensitivity to meperidine.
Meperidine is contraindicated in patients who are receiving monoamine oxidase (MAO) inhibitors or those who have recently received such agents. Therapeutic doses of meperdine have occasionally precipitated unpredictable, severe, and occasionally fatal reactions in patients who have received such agents within 14 days. The mechanism of these reactions is unclear, but may be related to a preexisting hyperphenylalaninemia. Some have been characterized by coma, severe respiratory depression, cyanosis, and hypotension, and have resembled the syndrome of acute narcotic overdose. In other reactions the predominant manifestations have been hyperexcitability, convulsions, tachycardia, hyperpyrexia, and hypertension. Although it is not known that other narcotics are free of the risk of such reactions, virtually all of the reported reactions have occurred with meperidine. If a narcotic is needed in such patients, a sensitivity test should be performed in which repeated, small, incremental doses of morphine are administered over the course of several hours while the patient's condition and vital signs are under careful observation. (Intravenous hydrocortisone or prednisolone have been used to treat severe reactions, with the addition of intravenous chlorpromazine in those cases exhibiting hypertension and hyperpyrexia. The usefulness and safety of narcotic antagonists in the treatment of these reactions is unknown.)

WARNINGS

Drug Dependence. Meperidine can produce drug dependence of the morphine type and therefore has the potential for being abused. Psychic dependence, physical dependence, and tolerance may develop upon repeated administration of meperidine, and it should be prescribed and administered with the same degree of caution appropriate to the use of morphine. Like other narcotics, meperidine is subject to the provisions of the Federal narcotic laws.
Interaction with Other Central Nervous System Depressants. MEPERIDINE SHOULD BE USED WITH GREAT CAUTION AND IN REDUCED DOSAGE IN PATIENTS WHO ARE CONCURRENTLY RECEIVING OTHER NARCOTIC ANALGESICS, GENERAL ANESTHETICS, PHENOTHIAZINES, OTHER TRANQUILIZERS (SEE DOSAGE AND ADMINISTRATION), SEDATIVE-HYPNOTICS (INCLUDING BARBITUATES), TRICYCLIC ANTIDEPRESSANTS AND OTHER CNS DEPRESSANTS (INCLUDING ALCOHOL). RESPIRATORY DEPRESSION, HYPOTENSION, AND PROFOUND SEDATION OR COMA MAY RESULT.
Head Injury and Increased Intracranial Pressure. The respiratory depressant effects of meperidine and its capacity to elevate cerebrospinal fluid pressure may be markedly exaggerated in the presence of head injury, other intracranial lesions, or a preexisting increase in intracranial pressure. Furthermore, narcotics produce adverse reactions which may obscure the clinical course of patients with head injuries. In such patients, meperidine must be used with extreme caution and only if its use is deemed essential.
Asthma and Other Respiratory Conditions. Meperidine should be used with extreme caution in patients having an acute asthmatic attack, patients with chronic obstructive pulmonary disease or cor pulmonale, patients having a sub-

Continued on next page

This product information was prepared in September 2000. On these and other products of Sanofi-Synthelabo Inc., detailed information may be obtained on a current basis by direct inquiry to Product Information Services, 90 Park Avenue, New York, NY 10016 (toll free 1-800-446-6267).

Demerol—Cont.

stantially decreased respiratory reserve, and patients with preexisting respiratory depression, hypoxia, or hypercapnia. In such patients, even usual therapeutic doses of narcotics may decrease respiratory drive while simultaneously increasing airway resistance to the point of apnea.
Hypotensive Effect. The administration of meperidine may result in severe hypotension in the postoperative patient or any individual whose ability to maintain blood pressure has been compromised by a depleted blood volume or the administration of drugs such as the phenothiazines or certain anesthetics.
Usage in Ambulatory Patients. Meperidine may impair the mental and/or physical abilities required for the performance of potentially hazardous tasks such as driving a car or operating machinery. The patient should be cautioned accordingly.
Meperidine, like other narcotics, may produce orthostatic hypotension in ambulatory patients.
Usage in Pregnancy and Lactation. Meperidine should not be used in pregnant women prior to the labor period, unless in the judgment of the physician the potential benefits outweigh the possible hazards, because safe use in pregnancy prior to labor has not been established relative to possible adverse effects on fetal development.
Meperidine crosses the placental barrier and can produce depression of respiration and psychophysiologic functions in the newborn. Resuscitation may be required (see section on OVERDOSAGE).
Meperidine appears in the milk of nursing mothers receiving the drug.

PRECAUTIONS

Supraventricular Tachycardias. Meperidine should be used with caution in patients with atrial flutter and other supraventricular tachycardias because of a possible vagolytic action which may produce a significant increase in the ventricular response rate.
Convulsions. Meperidine may aggravate preexisting convulsions in patients with convulsive disorders. If dosage is escalated substantially above recommended levels because of tolerance development, convulsions may occur in indivduals without a history of convulsive disorders.
Acute Abdominal Conditions. The administration of meperidine or other narcotics may obscure the diagnosis or clinical course in patients with acute abdominal conditions.
Special Risk Patients. Meperidine should be given with caution and the initial dose should be reduced in certain patients such as the elderly or debilitated, and those with severe impairment of hepatic or renal function, hypothyroidism, Addison's disease, and prostatic hypertrophy or urethral stricture.
Pregnancy. For usage during pregnancy see WARNINGS.
Nursing Mothers. See WARNINGS

ADVERSE REACTIONS

The major hazards of meperidine, as with other narcotic analgesics, are respiratory depression and, to a lesser degree, circulatory depression; respiratory arrest, shock, and cardiac arrest have occurred.
The most frequently observed adverse reactions include lightheadedness, dizziness, sedation, nausea, vomiting, and sweating. These effects seem to be more prominent in ambulatory patients and in those who are not experiencing severe pain. In such individuals, lower doses are advisable. Some adverse reactions in ambulatory patients may be alleviated if the patient lies down.
Other adverse reactions include:
Nervous System. Euphoria, dysphoria, weakness, headache, agitation, tremor, uncoordinated muscle movements, severe convulsions, transient hallucinations and disorientation, visual disturbances.
Gastrointestinal. Dry mouth, constipation, biliary tract spasm.
Cardiovascular. Flushing of the face, tachycardia, bradycardia, palpitation, hypotension (see WARNINGS), syncope, phlebitis following intravenous injection.
Genitourinary. Urinary retention.
Allergic. Pruritus, urticaria, other skin rashes, wheal and flare over the vein with intravenous injection.
Other. Pain at injection site; local tissue irritation and induration following subcutaneous injection, particularly when repeated; antidiuretic effect.

DOSAGE AND ADMINISTRATION

For Relief of Pain

Dosage should be adjusted according to the severity of the pain and the response of the patient. Meperidine is less effective orally than on parenteral administration. The dose of DEMEROL should be proportionately reduced (usually by 25 to 50 percent) when administered concomitantly with phenothiazines and many other tranquilizers since they potentiate the action of DEMEROL.
Adults. The usual dosage is 50 mg to 150 mg, orally, every 3 or 4 hours as necessary.
Pediatric Patients. The usual dosage is 0.5 mg/lb to 0.8 mg/lb, or orally, up to the adult dose, every 3 or 4 hours as necessary.
Each dose of the syrup should be taken in one-half glass of water, since if taken undiluted, it may exert a slight topical anesthetic effect on mucous membranes.

OVERDOSAGE

Symptoms. Serious overdosage with meperidine is characterized by respiratory depression (a decrease in respiratory rate and/or tidal volume, Cheyne-Stokes respiration, cyanosis), extreme somnolence progressing to stupor or coma, skeletal muscle flaccidity, cold and clammy skin, and sometimes bradycardia and hypotension. In severe overdosage, particularly by the intravenous route, apnea, circulatory collapse, cardiac arrest, and death may occur.
Treatment. Primary attention should be given to the reestablishment of adequate respiratory exchange through provision of a patent airway and institution of assisted or controlled ventilation. The narcotic antagonist, naloxone hydrochloride, is a specific antidote against respiratory depression which may result from overdosage or unusual sensitivity to narcotics, including meperidine. Therefore, an appropriate dose of this antagonist should be administered, preferably by the intravenous route, simultaneously with efforts at respiratory resuscitation.
An antagonist should not be administered in the absence of clinically significant respiratory or cardiovascular depression.
Oxygen, intravenous fluids, vasopressors, and other supportive measures should be employed as indicated.
In cases of overdosage with DEMEROL tablets, the stomach should be evacuated by emesis or gastric lavage.
NOTE: In an individual physically dependent on narcotics, the administration of the usual dose of a narcotic antagonist will precipitate an acute withdrawal syndrome. The severity of this syndrome will depend on the degree of physical dependence and the dose of antagonist administered. The use of narcotic antagonists in such individuals should be avoided if possible. If a narcotic antagonist must be used to treat serious respiratory depression in the physically dependent patient, the antagonist should be administered with extreme care and only one-fifth to one-tenth the usual initial dose administered.

HOW SUPPLIED

For Oral Use

Tablets are white, round and convex: the 50 mg tablet is scored.

Tablets of 50 mg.
bottles of 100 (NDC 0024-0335-04),
bottles of 500 (NDC 0024-0335-06),
Hospital Blister Pak of 25 (NDC 0024-0335-02).
100 mg: bottles of 100 (NDC 0024-0337-04),
bottles of 500 (NDC 0024-0337-06),

Syrup

Nonalcoholic, banana-flavored 50 mg per 5 mL teaspoon, bottles of 16 fl oz (NDC 0024-0332-06).
Store at room temperature up to 25° C (77° F), excursions permitted to 15°–30°C (59°–86°F) [See USP controlled Room Temperature].

DSW-3 I(0)
Revised September 1999

Shown in Product Identification Guide, page 333

HISTUSSIN® D ℂ ℞

Antihistamine Free

DESCRIPTION

Each 5 ml teaspoonful of HISTUSSIN D for oral use contains

Hydrocodone Bitartrate	5 mg
Pseudoephedrine Hydrochloride	60 mg

Antitussive-Decongestant Liquid

HOW SUPPLIED

HISTUSSIN D liquid is supplied as a deep red syrup with a wild cherry/black raspberry flavor Pints NDC 0024-0864-16

HISTUSSIN® HC ℂ ℞

Each 5 ml orange/pineapple flavored alcohol-free, sugar-free orange syrup contains:

Hydrocodone Bitartrate	2.5 mg
(Warning: May be habit forming.)	
Phenylephrine Hydrochloride	5.0 mg
Chlorpheniramine Maleate	2.0 mg

HOW SUPPLIED

Bottles of 16 oz.
NDC 0024-0860-16

HYALGAN® ℞

sodium hyaluronate

LABELING

CAUTION

Federal law restricts this device to sale by or on the order of a physician.

DESCRIPTION

Hyalgan® is a viscous solution consisting of a high molecular weight (500,000–730,000 daltons) fraction of purified natural sodium hyaluronate in buffered physiological sodium chloride, having a pH of 6.8–7.5. The sodium hyaluronate is extracted from rooster combs. Hyaluronic acid is a natural complex sugar of the glycosaminoglycan family and is a long-chain polymer containing repeating disaccharide units of Na-glucuronate-N-acetylglucosamine.

INDICATIONS

Hyalgan® is indicated for the treatment of pain in osteoarthritis (OA) of the knee in patients who have failed to respond adequately to conservative nonpharmacologic therapy, and to simple analgesics, e.g., acetaminophen.

CONTRAINDICATIONS

- Do not administer to patients with known hypersensitivity to hyaluronate preparations.
- Intra-articular injections are contraindicated in cases of past and present infections or skin diseases in the area of the injection site.

WARNINGS

- Do not concomitantly use disinfectants containing quaternary ammonium salts for skin preparation because hyaluronic acid can precipitate in their presence.
- Anaphylactoid and allergic reactions have been reported with this product. See Adverse Events Section for more detail.
- Transient increases in inflammation in the injected knee following Hyalgan® injection in some patients with inflammatory arthritis such as rheumatoid arthritis or gouty arthritis have been reported.

PRECAUTIONS

General

- The effectiveness of a single treatment cycle of less than 5 injections has not been established. Pain relief may not be seen until after the fifth injection.
- The safety and effectiveness of the use of Hyalgan® in joints other than the knee have not been established.
- The safety and effectiveness of the use of Hyalgan® concomitantly with other intra-articular injectables have not been established.
- Use caution when injecting Hyalgan® into patients who are allergic to avian proteins, feathers, and egg products.
- Strict aseptic administration technique must be followed.
- **STERILE CONTENTS.** The vial/syringe is intended for single use. The contents of the vial must be used immediately once the container has been opened. Discard any unused Hyalgan®.
- Do not use Hyalgan® if the package is opened or damaged. Store in the original packaging (protected from light) below 77° F (25° C). DO NOT FREEZE.
- Remove joint effusion, if present, before injecting Hyalgan®.

Information for Patients

- Provide patients with a copy of the Patient Information prior to use.
- Transient pain and/or swelling of the injected joint may occur after intra-articular injection of Hyalgan®.
- As with any invasive joint procedure, it is recommended that the patient avoid any strenuous activities or prolonged (i.e., more than 1 hour) weight-bearing activities such as jogging or tennis within 48 hours following the intra-articular injection.

Use in Specific Populations

- **Pregnancy:** *Teratogenic Effects*—Reproductive toxicity studies, including multigeneration studies, have been performed in rats and rabbits at doses up to 11 times the anticipated human dose (1.43 mg/kg per treatment cycle) and have revealed no evidence of impaired fertility or harm to the experimental animal fetus due to intra-articular injections of Hyalgan®. Animal reproduction studies are not always predictive of human response. The safety and effectiveness of Hyalgan® have not been established in pregnant women.
- **Nursing Mothers:** It is not known if Hyalgan® is excreted in human milk. The safety and effectiveness of Hyalgan® have not been established in lactating women.
- **Pediatrics:** The safety and effectiveness of Hyalgan® have not been demonstrated in children.

ADVERSE EVENTS

Hyalgan® was investigated in a pivotal clinical investigation conducted in the United States in which there were three arms (164 subjects treated with Hyalgan®; 168 with placebo; and 163 with naproxen) (refer to Table 1). Common adverse events reported for the Hyalgan®-treated subjects were gastrointestinal complaints, injection site pain, knee swelling/effusion, local skin reactions (rash, ecchymosis), pruritus, and headache. Swelling and effusion, local skin reactions (ecchymosis and rash), and headache occurred at equal frequency in the Hyalgan®- and placebo-treated groups. Hyalgan®-treated subjects had 48/164 (29%) incidents of gastrointestinal complaints that were not statistically different from the placebo-treated group. A statistically significant difference in the occurrence of pain at the injection site was noted in the Hyalgan®-treated subjects: 38/164 (23%) in comparison to 22/168 (13%) in the placebo-treated subjects ($p = 0.022$). There were 6/164 (4%) premature discontinuations in Hyalgan®-treated subjects due to injection site pain in comparison to 1/168 (<1%) in the placebo-treated subjects. These differences were not statistically significant.
Two (2/164, 1.2%) Hyalgan®-treated subjects and 3/168 (1.8%) placebo-treated subjects were reported to have positive bacterial cultures of effusion aspirated from the treated knee. The two Hyalgan®-treated subjects and two of the

TABLE 2. STUDY DESIGN

Routes of Administration	Hyalgan®	Placebo	Naproxen
s.c.	Lidocaine (1%)	Lidocaine (1%)	Lidocaine (1%)
i.a.*	Hyalgan® (20 mg/2 mL)	Phosphate-Buffered Saline (2 mL)	none
p.o./b.i.d.	Placebo for naproxen capsules	Placebo for naproxen capsules	Naproxen capsules (500 mg)
p.o./p.r.n. (not to exceed 4 grams/day)	Acetaminophen	Acetaminophen	Acetaminophen

Legend: s.c. = subcutaneous; i.a. = intra-articular; p.o. = by mouth; b.i.d. = twice a day; p.r.n. = as needed
* Synovial fluid was aspirated (when present) in the Hyalgan® and placebo groups.

TABLE 3
Demographic Characteristics of All Randomized Subjects

DEMOGRAPHIC VARIABLE	TREATMENT			
	Hyalgan® N = 164	Placebo N = 168	Naproxen N = 163	TOTAL N = 495
AGE (years):				
Mean	63.5	64.3	63.2	63.7
SD	10.1	10.0	9.2	9.8
Range	41–90	44–85	40–80	40–90
Gender [N (%)]:				
Female	99 (60.3)	91 (54.1)	99 (60.7)	289 (58.4)
Male	65 (39.6)	77 (45.8)	64 (39.3)	206 (41.6)
Race [N (%)]:				
Caucasian	137 (83.6)	135 (80.4)	133 (81.6)	405 (81.8)
Black	23 (14.0)	32 (19.0)	25 (15.3)	80 (16.2)
Other	4 (4.2)	1 (1.0)	5 (3.1)	10 (2.0)
Height (cm):				
Mean	167.8	168.6	167.6	168.0
SD	8.8	10.7	11.9	10.5
Range	145–190	142–193	102–198	102–198
Weight (kg):				
Mean	88.4	88.1	89.7	88.7
SD	18.0	18.2	18.4	18.2
Range	46–139	49–170	45–150	45–170
NSAIDs Use (N, %)	107 (65.2)	117 (69.6)	113 (69.3)	337 (68.1)
Use of Assistive Devices (N, %)	35 (21.3)	34 (20.2)	32 (19.6)	101 (20.4)
Physical Therapy (N, %)	20 (12.2)	17 (10.1)	25 (15.3)	62 (12.5)

Legend: cm = centimeters; kg = kilograms; SD = standard deviation

TABLE 4
Clinical Results

Evaluation	Success Criteria	Results
100 mm VAS for pain during 50- foot walk.	A statistically significant (alpha = 0.05) reduction on mean VAS for Hyalgan® when compared to placebo at Week 26. This difference was also to exceed one fourth of the Standard Deviation of the mean change from baseline.	At Week 26, the difference between the Hyalgan®-treated group and the placebo-treated group adjusted means was 8.85 mm (p = 0.0043), which is a difference of approximately one-third of a standard deviation (Table 5).
Masked Evaluator Categorical Assessment of subject pain (0=none to 5=disabled) during the 48 hours preceding visits.	The number of Hyalgan®-treated subjects showing improvement at Week 26 was to be concordant with the VAS results; however, not required to be independently statistically significant.	At Week 26 the masked evaluator's categorical assessment of pain indicated that the Hyalgan®-treated subjects experienced less pain than the placebo-treated subjects (Table 6).
Subjects' Categorical Assessment of pain (0=none to 5=disabled) during the 48 hours preceding visits.	The number of Hyalgan®-treated subjects showing improvement at Week 26 was to be concordant with the VAS results; however, not required to be independently statistically significant.	At Week 26 the subjects' categorical assessment of pain indicated that the Hyalgan®-treated subjects experienced less pain than the placebo-treated subjects (Table 7).
Magnitude of the observed effect for Hyalgan® versus placebo on both the VAS and the categorical pain assessments.	At Week 26 the magnitude of the observed effect for Hyalgan® versus placebo on both the VAS and the categorical pain assessments were to be at least 50% of those observed for the naproxen group.	The improvement in pain on the VAS exhibited by the Hyalgan®-treated group relative to the placebo-treated group were at least 50% of the benefits exhibited by the naproxen-treated group relative to the placebo-treated group. The results of the categorical assessments by the masked evaluator and the subject indicated that improvement of the Hyalgan®-treated group relative to the placebo-treated group was at least 50% of the benefits exhibited by the naproxen-treated group relative to the placebo-treated group (Table 8).

placebo-treated subjects did not exhibit evidence of infection clinically or subsequently and were not treated with antibiotics. One of the placebo-treated subjects was hospitalized and received presumptive treatment for septic arthritis.
Hyalgan® has been in clinical use in Europe since 1987. Analysis of the adverse events that have been reported with the use of Hyalgan® in Europe reveals that most of the events are related to local symptoms such as pain, swelling/effusion, and warmth or redness at the injection site. In the two events reported as anaphylactoid reactions, Hyalgan® treatment was discontinued and both had favorable outcomes. Three cases of allergic reactions were reported in which the patients were discontinued from Hyalgan® treatment and the incidents resolved. Seven cases of fever were reported in which three of the cases were reported to be associated with local reactions; pyogenic arthritis was reported to be ruled out in these three cases. All the fever patients were discontinued from Hyalgan® treatment and all incidents resolved. One incident of shock (which was described as a "hypotensive crisis") was reported. The incident resolved and Hyalgan® treatment was continued.
Adverse experience data from the literature contain no evidence of increased risk relating to retreatment with Hyalgan®. The frequency and severity of adverse events occurring during repeat treatment cycles did not increase over that reported for a single treatment cycle. (Carrabba et al., 1995; Carrabba et al., 1991; Kotz and Kolarz, 1999; Scali, 1995).

TABLE 1
Incidence[1] of Adverse Events Occurring in More Than 5% of All Subjects

Adverse Event	Hyalgan® N = 164	Placebo N = 168
Gastrointestinal Complaints[2]	48 (29%)	59 (36%)
Injection site pain[3]	38 (23%)[4]	22 (13%)
Headache	30 (18%)	29 (17%)
Local skin[5]	23 (14%)	17 (10%)
Local joint pain and swelling[6]	21 (13%)	22 (13%)
Pruritus (local)	12 (7%)	7 (4%)

Notes: [1] Number and % of subjects
[2] Severe in 4 Hyalgan®-treated subjects and 4 placebo-treated subjects
[3] Severe in 5 Hyalgan®-treated subjects and 2 placebo-treated subjects
[4] Statistically significant (p=0.02)
[5] Includes ecchymosis and rash
[6] Severe in 2 Hyalgan®-treated subjects (1.2%) and 1 placebo-treated subjects

CLINICAL STUDY

The use of Hyalgan® as a treatment for pain in OA of the knee was investigated in a multicenter clinical trial conducted in the United States.

Study Design

This study was a double-masked, placebo and naproxen-controlled, multicenter prospective clinical trial with three treatment arms, as summarized in Table 2. A total of 495 subjects with moderate to severe pain was randomized (at baseline evaluation) into three treatment groups in a ratio of 1:1:1 Hyalgan®, placebo, or naproxen.
[See table 2 above]

Patient Population and Demographics

The demographics of trial participants were comparable across treatment groups with regard to age, sex, race, height, weight, history of osteoarthritis, prior use of NSAIDs, prior physical therapy, and use of assistive devices (refer to Table 3).
[See table 3 above]

Evaluation Schedule

After meeting initial screening requirements NSAID therapy was discontinued. After 2 weeks, all subjects returned for baseline evaluations. The baseline evaluation included assessment of three primary effectiveness criteria; measurement of pain during a 50-foot walk test using a 100 mm Visual Analog Scale (VAS), a categorical assessment (0 = none to 5 = disabled) of pain, as assessed by a masked evaluator, during the 48 hours preceding the visit, and a categorical assessment (0 = none to 5 = disabled) of pain, as assessed by the subject, during the 48 hours preceding the visit.
All subjects who completed the NSAID washout period and met all entry requirements received their first injection after randomization. All subjects received subcutaneous lidocaine injections. Intra-articular injections (Hyalgan®, pla-

Continued on next page

This product information was prepared in September 2000. On these and other products of Sanofi-Synthelabo Inc., detailed information may be obtained on a current basis by direct inquiry to Product Information Services, 90 Park Avenue, New York, NY 10016 (toll free 1-800-446-6267).

Hyalgan—Cont.

cebo) were administered weekly for a total of 5 injections (Weeks 0–4). The naproxen group received 500 mg of naproxen to be taken b.i.d. for 26 weeks.
Subsequent visits and evaluations took place at Weeks 5, 9, 12, 16, 21, and 26. Safety and effectiveness criteria were assessed and recorded at these time periods.

Clinical Results
For this trial, overall success for effectiveness was defined as meeting all four of the success criteria listed in Table 4 using scores from week 26. The criteria were met (refer to Tables 4 through 8).
]See table 4 at bottom of previous page]
[See table 5 above]
[See table 6 at right]
[See table 7 below]
[See table 8 below]

Additional Analyses
a. An analysis of study completers was performed as follows: Success was defined as 1) achieving a 20 mm decrease in the VAS for the 50-foot walk test by Week 5, and 2) maintaining this improvement through Week 26. In this analysis greater proportions of Hyalgan®-treated subjects (59/105, 56%) than either placebo- (47/115, 41%) or naproxen-treated subjects (51/113, 45%) were successful under this definition. The Hyalgan®-placebo comparison was statistically significant (p = 0.031, Fisher's Exact Test).
Since patients were not followed beyond Week 26, it is unknown how long pain relief continued. There are reports in the literature of some patients experiencing benefit beyond 26 weeks.
b. *Categorical Assessment of Pain—Subjects:* A longitudinal analysis of categorical assessment of pain by the subject, which analyzed the percentage of subjects who attained success revealed that a significantly higher percentage of Hyalgan®-treated subjects as compared to the placebo-treated subjects (55/105, 52% vs 43/115, 37%, p = 0.030, Fisher's Exact Test) achieved success (an improvement of greater than or equal to one point on the five-point scale) and maintained this success from Week 5 until Week 26.

Safety
In order for the product to be considered safe, the incidence of severe swelling and pain consequent to intra-articular injection should be less than 5%. This criterion was met as indicated in Table 1. See the Adverse Events Section.

DETAILED DEVICE DESCRIPTION

Each vial or syringe contains:

Sodium Hyaluronate	20.0 mg
Sodium chloride	17.0 mg
Monobasic sodium phosphate • $2H_2O$	0.1 mg
Dibasic sodium phosphate • $12H_2O$	1.2 mg
Water for injection	q.s.* to 2.0 mL

*q.s. = up to

HOW SUPPLIED
Hyalgan® is supplied as a sterile, non-pyrogenic solution in 2 mL vials or 2 mL pre-filled syringes.

DIRECTIONS FOR USE
Hyalgan® is administered by intra-articular injection. A treatment cycle consists of a total of five injections given at weekly intervals.
Precaution: Do not use Hyalgan® if the package is opened or damaged. Store in the original packaging (protected from light) below 77° F (25° C). DO NOT FREEZE.
Precaution: Strict aseptic administration technique must be followed.
Warning: Do not concomitantly use disinfectants containing quaternary ammonium salts for skin preparation because hyaluronic acid can precipitate in their presence.
Inject subcutaneous lidocaine or similar local anesthetic prior to injection of Hyalgan®.
Precaution: Remove joint effusion, if present, before injection of Hyalgan®.
Do not use the same syringe for removing joint effusion and for injecting Hyalgan®.
Take care to remove the tip cap of the syringe and needle aseptically.
Inject Hyalgan® into the joint through a 20-gauge needle.
Precaution: The vial/syringe is intended for single use. The contents of the vial must be used immediately once the container has been opened. Discard any unused Hyalgan®. Inject the full 2 mL in one knee only. If treatment is bilateral, a separate vial should be used for each knee.

MANUFACTURED BY
FIDIA S.p.A.
Via Ponte della Fabbrica 3/A
35031 Abano Terme, Padua (PD), Italy

DISTRIBUTED BY
Sanofi-Synthelabo Inc.
90 Park Avenue
New York, NY 10016

TABLE 5
ANCOVA of 50-Foot Walk Test (mm) VAS by Week for All Completed Subjects

	Week							
	3	4	5	9	12	16	21	26
Adjusted Means Hyalgan®	27.23	21.54	19.29	20.04	20.26	20.83	18.44	17.88
Placebo	32.35	28.57	25.67	24.28	26.66	25.44	24.77	26.73
Hyalgan® versus Placebo	5.13	7.03	6.39	4.24	6.40	4.61	6.33	8.846
p-value	0.06	0.01	0.01	0.1	0.03	0.1	0.02	0.004

TABLE 6
Masked Evaluators' Categorical Assessments of Pain for Completed Subjects in Prior 48 Hours: Level of Pain by Treatment Group at Baseline and Week 26

	NUMBER (%) OF SUBJECTS IN CATEGORY					
	Hyalgan®		Placebo		Naproxen	
	Baseline	Week 26	Baseline	Week 26	Baseline	Week 26
None (0)	0 (0.0)	27 (25.7)	0 (0.0)	15 (13.0)	0 (0.0)	17 (15.0)
Slight (1)	1 (1.0)	23 (21.9)	0 (0.0)	27 (23.5)	0 (0.0)	32 (28.3)
Mild (2)	2 (1.9)	24 (22.9)	2 (1.7)	29 (25.2)	2 (1.8)	27 (23.9)
Moderate (3)	69 (65.7)	26 (24.8)	85 (73.9)	34 (29.6)	79 (70.5)	28 (24.8)
Marked (4)	33 (31.4)	5 (4.8)	28 (24.3)	10 (8.7)	31 (27.7)	9 (8.0)
TOTAL	105 (100)	105 (100)	115 (100)	115 (100)	112* (100)	113 (100)

*One Naproxen treated subject was missing a Baseline assessment.

TABLE 7
Subjects' Categorical Assessments of Pain for Completed Subjects in Prior 48 Hours: Level of Pain by Treatment Group at Baseline and Week 26

	NUMBER (%) OF SUBJECTS IN CATEGORY					
	Hyalgan®		Placebo		Naproxen	
	Baseline	Week 26	Baseline	Week 26	Baseline	Week 26
None (0)	1 (1.0)	23 (21.9)	0 (0.0)	14 (12.2)	0 (0.0)	13 (11.5)
Slight (1)	2 (1.9)	27 (25.7)	0 (0.0)	24 (20.9)	1 (0.9)	31 (27.4)
Mild (2)	6 (5.7)	19 (18.1)	8 (7.0)	24 (20.9)	7 (6.2)	26 (23.0)
Moderate (3)	62 (59.0)	26 (24.8)	78 (67.8)	40 (34.8)	72 (63.7)	31 (27.4)
Marked (4)	34 (32.4)	10 (9.5)	29 (25.2)	13 (11.3)	33 (29.2)	12 (10.6)
TOTAL	105 (100)	105 (100)	115 (100)	115 (100)	113 (100)	113 (100)

TABLE 8
Hyalgan® Effect as a Percentage of the Naproxen-Placebo Difference

Assessment	Hyalgan® (HYL)	Placebo (PLA)	Naproxen (NAP)	HYL-PLA	NAP-HYL	NAP-PLA	(HYL-PLA) % of (NAP-PLA)
VAS for 50 foot Walk Baseline Adjusted Mean Effect Sizes From ANCOVA				−8.85 mm on a 100 mm VAS	4.12 mm on a 100 mm VAS	−4.73* mm on a 100 mm VAS	187%
% of Subjects Improved by Masked Evaluators	78.1	69.6	73.2	8.5	−4.9	3.6	236%
% of Subjects Improved by Subjects	73.3	62.6	67.3	10.7	−6.0	4.7	228%

*Imputed as (NAP-HYL)+(HYL-PLA).
Note that Effectiveness Success Criterion D is satisfied since ((HYL-PLA) % of (NAP-PLA))>50% for all three of the above pain assessments.

REFERENCES

1. M. Carrabba et al., 1991 Hyaluronic acid sodium salt (Hyalgan®) in the treatment of patients with osteoarthritis of the knee: a controlled trial versus Orgotein, Final Report, April 1991. Data on file.
2. M. Carrabba et al., 1995. Effectiveness and safety of 1, 3 and 5 injections of 20 mg/2 ml Hyalgan® in comparison with a placebo and with arthrocentesis only, in the treatment of knee osteoarthritis. European Journal of Rheumatology and Inflammation 15:25–31.
3. M. Dougados et al., 1993. High molecular weight sodium hyaluronate (hyalectin) in osteoarthritis of the knee: a one-year placebo-controlled trial. Osteoarthritis and Cartilage 1:97–103.
4. R. Kotz and G. Kolarz, 1997 pulished as R. Kotz and G. Kolarz, 1999. Intra-articular hyaluronic acid: duration of effect and results of repeated treatment cycles. The American Journal of Orthopedics, 28:5–7.
5. G. Leardini et al., 1987. Intra-articular sodium hyaluronate (Hyalgan®) in gonarthrosis. Clinical Trials Journal 24(4):341–350.

6. J.J. Scali, 1995. Intra-articular hyaluronic acid in the treatment of osteoarthritis of the knee: a long term study 15(1):57–62.

0720131

Revised December 1999

Shown in Product Identification Guide, page 333

KAYEXALATE® ℞

brand of sodium polystyrene sulfonate, USP

Cation-Exchange Resin

DESCRIPTION

KAYEXALATE, brand of sodium polystyrene sulfonate, is a benzene, diethenyl- polymer, with ethenylbenzene, sulfonated, sodium salt and has the following structural formula:

$$\left[-CH-CH_2- \text{(benzene ring)}-SO_3^-Na^+ \right]$$

The drug is a light brown to brown, finely ground, powdered form of sodium polystyrene sulfonate, a cation-exchange resin prepared in the sodium phase with an *in vitro* exchange capacity of approximately 3.1 mEq (*in vivo* approximately 1 mEq) of potassium per gram. The sodium content is approximately 100 mg (4.1 mEq) per gram of the drug. It can be administered orally or in an enema.

CLINICAL PHARMACOLOGY

As the resin passes along the intestine or is retained in the colon after administration by enema, the sodium ions are partially released and are replaced by potassium ions. For the most part, this action occurs in the large intestine, which excretes potassium ions to a greater degree than does the small intestine. The efficiency of this process is limited and unpredictably variable. It commonly approximates the order of 33 percent but the range is so large that definitive indices of electrolyte balance must be clearly monitored. Metabolic data are unavailable.

INDICATION AND USAGE

KAYEXALATE is indicated for the treatment of hyperkalemia.

CONTRAINDICATIONS

KAYEXALATE is contraindicated in patients with hypokalemia or those patients who are hypersensitive to it.

WARNINGS

Alternative Therapy in Severe Hyperkalemia:
Since effective lowering of serum potassium with KAYEXALATE may take hours to days, treatment with this drug alone may be insufficient to rapidly correct severe hyperkalemia associated with states of rapid tissue breakdown (e.g., burns and renal failure) or hyperkalemia so marked as to constitute a medical emergency. Therefore, other definitive measures, including dialysis, should always be considered and may be imperative.

Hypokalemia: Serious potassium deficiency can occur from therapy with KAYEXALATE. The effect must be carefully controlled by frequent serum potassium determinations within each 24-hour period. Since intracellular potassium deficiency is not always reflected by serum potassium levels, the level at which treatment with KAYEXALATE should be discontinued must be determined individually for each patient. Important aids in making this determination are the patient's clinical condition and electrocardiogram. Early clinical signs of severe hypokalemia include a pattern of irritable confusion and delayed thought processes. Electrocardiographically, severe hypokalemia is often associated with a lengthened Q-T interval, widening, flattening, or inversion of the T wave, and prominent U waves. Also, cardiac arrhythmias may occur, such as premature atrial, nodal, and ventricular contractions, and supraventricular and ventricular tachycardias. The toxic effects of digitalis are likely to be exaggerated. Marked hypokalemia can also be manifested by severe muscle weakness, at times extending into frank paralysis.

Electrolyte Disturbances: Like all cation-exchange resins, KAYEXALATE is not totally selective (for potassium) in its actions, and small amounts of other cations such as magnesium and calcium can also be lost during treatment. Accordingly, patients receiving KAYEXALATE should be monitored for all applicable electrolyte disturbances.

Systemic Alkalosis: Systemic alkalosis has been reported after cation-exchange resins were administered orally in combination with nonabsorbable cation-donating antacids and laxatives such as magnesium hydroxide and aluminum carbonate. Magnesium hydroxide should not be administered with KAYEXALATE. One case of grand mal seizure has been reported in a patient with chronic hypocalcemia of renal failure who was given KAYEXALATE with magnesium hydroxide as laxative. (See PRECAUTIONS, Drug Interactions.)

PRECAUTIONS

Caution is advised when KAYEXALATE is administered to patients who cannot tolerate even a small increase in sodium loads (ie, severe congestive heart failure, severe hypertension, or marked edema). In such instances compensatory restriction of sodium intake from other sources may be indicated.

If constipation occurs, patients should be treated with sorbitol (from 10 mL to 20 mL of 70 percent syrup every two hours or as needed to produce one or two watery stools daily), a measure which also reduces any tendency to fecal impaction.

Drug Interactions

Antacids: The simultaneous oral administration of KAYEXALATE with nonabsorbable cation-donating antacids and laxatives may reduce the resin's potassium exchange capability.

Systemic alkalosis has been reported after cation-exchange resins were administered orally in combination with nonabsorbable cation-donating antacids and laxatives such as magnesium hydroxide and aluminum carbonate. Magnesium hydroxide should not be administered with KAYEXALATE. One case of grand mal seizure has been reported in a patient with chronic hypocalcemia of renal failure who was given KAYEXALATE with magnesium hydroxide as a laxative.

Intestinal obstruction due to concretions of aluminum hydroxide when used in combination with KAYEXALATE has been reported.

Digitalis: The toxic effects of digitalis on the heart, especially various ventricular arrhythmias and A-V nodal dissociation, are likely to be exaggerated by hypokalemia, even in the face of serum digoxin concentrations in the "normal range". (See WARNINGS.)

Carcinogenesis, Mutagenesis, Impairment of Fertility

Studies have not been performed.

Pregnancy Category C

Animal reproduction studies have not been conducted with KAYEXALATE. It is also not known whether KAYEXALATE can cause fetal harm when administered to a pregnant woman or can affect reproduction capacity. KAYEXALATE should be given to a pregnant woman only if clearly needed.

Nursing Mothers

It is not known whether this drug is excreted in human milk. Because many drugs are excreted in human milk, caution should be exercised when KAYEXALATE is administered to a nursing woman.

ADVERSE REACTIONS

KAYEXALATE may cause some degree of gastric irritation. Anorexia, nausea, vomiting, and constipation may occur especially if high doses are given. Also, hypokalemia, hypocalcemia, and significant sodium retention may occur. Occasionally diarrhea develops. Large doses in elderly individuals may cause fecal impaction (see PRECAUTIONS). This effect may be obviated through usage of the resin in enemas as described under DOSAGE AND ADMINISTRATION. Rare instances of colonic necrosis have been reported. Intestinal obstruction due to concretions of aluminum hydroxide, when used in combination with KAYEXALATE, has been reported.

DOSAGE AND ADMINISTRATION

Suspension of this drug should be freshly prepared and not stored beyond 24 hours.

The average daily adult dose of the resin is 15 g to 60 g. This is best provided by administering 15 g (approximately 4 *level* teaspoons) of KAYEXALATE one to four times daily. One gram of KAYEXALATE contains 4.1 mEq of sodium; one level teaspoon contains approximately 3.5 g of KAYEXALATE and 15 mEq of sodium. (A heaping teaspoon may contain as much as 10 g to 12 g of KAYEXALATE.) Since the *in vivo* efficiency of sodium-potassium exchange resins is approximately 33 percent, about one third of the resin's actual sodium content is being delivered to the body.

In smaller children and infants, lower doses should be employed by using as a guide a rate of 1 mEq of potassium per gram of resin as the basis for calculation.

Each dose should be given as a suspension in a small quantity of water or, for greater palatability, in syrup. The amount of fluid usually ranges from 20 mL to 100 mL, depending on the dose, or may be simply determined by allowing 3 mL to 4 mL per gram of resin. Sorbitol may be administered in order to combat constipation.

The resin may be introduced into the stomach through a plastic tube and, if desired, mixed with a diet appropriate for a patient in renal failure.

The resin may also be given, although with less effective results, in an enema consisting (for adults) of 30 g to 50 g every six hours. Each dose is administered as a warm emulsion (at body temperature) in 100 mL of aqueous vehicle, such as sorbitol. The emulsion should be agitated gently during administration. The enema should be retained as long as possible and followed by a cleansing enema.

After an initial cleansing enema, a soft, large size (French 28) rubber tube is inserted into the rectum for a distance of about 20 cm, with the tip well into the sigmoid colon, and taped in place. The resin is then suspended in the appropriate amount of aqueous vehicle at body temperature and introduced by gravity, while the particles are kept in suspension by stirring. The suspension is flushed with 50 mL or 100 mL of fluid, following which the tube is clamped and left in place. If back leakage occurs, the hips are elevated on pillows or a knee-chest position is taken temporarily. A somewhat thicker suspension may be used, but care should be taken that no paste is formed, because the latter has a greatly reduced exchange surface and will be particularly ineffective if deposited in the rectal ampulla. The suspension is kept in the sigmoid colon for several hours, if possible. Then, the colon is irrigated with nonsodium containing solution at body temperature in order to remove the resin. Two quarts of flushing solution may be necessary. The returns are drained constantly through a Y tube connection. Particular attention should be paid to this cleansing enema when sorbitol has been used.

The intensity and duration of therapy depend upon the severity and resistance of hyperkalemia.

KAYEXALATE should not be heated for to do so may alter the exchange properties of the resin.

HOW SUPPLIED

Store at room temperature.

KAYEXALATE is available as a cream to light brown, finely ground powder in jars of 1 pound (453.6g), NDC 0024-1075-01.

KSW-1C

Revised September 1999

MEBARAL® Ⓒ ℞

Brand of MEPHOBARBITAL TABLETS, USP

DESCRIPTION

Mephobarbital, 5-Ethyl-1-methyl-5-phenylbarbituric acid, is a barbiturate with sedative, hypnotic, and anticonvulsant properties. It occurs as a white, nearly odorless, tasteless powder and is slightly soluble in water and in alcohol.

MEBARAL is available as tablets for oral administration.

The structural formula is:

[Structural formula: CH_3, O, N, O, CH_3CH_2, NH, O, phenyl ring]

Inactive Ingredients: Lactose, Starch, Stearic Acid, Talc.

CLINICAL PHARMACOLOGY

Barbiturates are capable of producing all levels of CNS mood alteration from excitation to mild sedation, to hypnosis, and deep coma. Overdosage can produce death. In high enough therapeutic doses, barbiturates induce anesthesia.

Barbiturates depress the sensory cortex, decrease motor activity, alter cerebellar function, and produce drowsiness, sedation, and hypnosis.

Barbiturates are respiratory depressants. The degree of respiratory depression is dependent upon dose. With hypnotic doses, respiratory depression produced by barbiturates is similar to that which occurs during physiologic sleep with slight decrease in blood pressure and heart rate.

Studies in laboratory animals have shown that barbiturates cause reduction in the tone and contractility of the uterus, ureters, and urinary bladder. However, concentrations of the drugs required to produce this effect in humans are not reached with sedative-hypnotic doses.

Barbiturates do not impair normal hepatic function, but have been shown to induce liver microsomal enzymes, thus increasing and/or altering the metabolism of barbiturates and other drugs. (See PRECAUTIONS—Drug Interactions.)

MEBARAL exerts a strong sedative and anticonvulsant action but has a relatively mild hypnotic effect. It reduces the incidence of epileptic seizures in grand mal and petit mal. MEBARAL usually causes little or no drowsiness or lassitude. Hence, when it is used as a sedative or anticonvulsant, patients usually become more calm, more cheerful, and better adjusted to their surroundings without clouding of mental faculties. MEBARAL is reported to produce less sedation than does phenobarbital.

Barbiturates are weak acids that are absorbed and rapidly distributed to all tissues and fluids with high concentrations in the brain, liver, and kidneys. Lipid solubility of the barbiturates is the dominant factor in their distribution within the body. Barbiturates are bound to plasma and tissue proteins to a varying degree with the degree of binding increasing directly as a function of lipid solubility.

Approximately 50% of an oral dose of mephobarbital is absorbed from the gastrointestinal tract. Therapeutic plasma concentrations for mephobarbital have not been established nor has the half-life been determined. Following oral administration, the onset of action of the drug is 30 to 60 minutes and the duration of action is 10 to 16 hours. The primary route of mephobarbital metabolism is N-demethylation by the microsomal enzymes of the liver to form phenobarbital. Phenobarbital may be excreted in the urine unchanged or further metabolized to *p*-hydroxyphenobarbital and ex-

Continued on next page

This product information was prepared in September 2000. On these and other products of Sanofi-Synthelabo Inc., detailed information may be obtained on a current basis by direct inquiry to Product Information Services, 90 Park Avenue, New York, NY 10016 (toll free 1-800-446-6267).

Mebaral—Cont.

creted in the urine as glucuronide or sulfate conjugates. About 75% of a single oral dose of mephobarbital is converted to phenobarbital in 24 hours.
Therefore, chronic administration of mephobarbital may lead to an accumulation of phenobarbital (not mephobarbital) in plasma. It has not been determined whether mephobarbital or phenobarbital is the active agent during long-time mephobarbital therapy.

INDICATIONS AND USAGE

MEBARAL is indicated for use as a sedative for the relief of anxiety, tension, and apprehension, and as an anticonvulsant for the treatment of grand mal and petit mal epilepsy.

CONTRAINDICATIONS

Hypersensitivity to any barbiturate. Manifest or latent porphyria.

WARNINGS

Habit Forming

Barbiturates may be habit forming. Tolerance, psychological, and physical dependence may occur with continued use. (See DRUG ABUSE AND DEPENDENCE and CLINICAL PHARMACOLOGY.) Patients who have psychological dependence on barbiturates may increase the dosage or decrease the dosage interval without consulting a physician and may subsequently develop a physical dependence on barbiturates. To minimize the possibility of overdosage or the development of dependence, the prescribing and dispensing of sedative-hypnotic barbiturates should be limited to the amount required for the interval until the next appointment. Abrupt cessation after prolonged use in the dependent person may result in withdrawal symptoms, including delirium, convulsions, and possibly death. Barbiturates should be withdrawn gradually from any patient known to be taking excessive dosage over long periods of time. (See DRUG ABUSE AND DEPENDENCE.)

Acute or Chronic Pain

Caution should be exercised when barbiturates are administered to patients with acute or chronic pain, because paradoxical excitement could be induced or important symptoms could be masked. However, the use of barbiturates as sedatives in the postoperative surgical period and as adjuncts to cancer chemotherapy is well established.

Use in Pregnancy

Barbiturates can cause fetal damage when administered to a pregnant woman. Retrospective, case-controlled studies have suggested a connection between the maternal consumption of barbiturates and a higher than expected incidence of fetal abnormalities. Following oral or parenteral administration, barbiturates readily cross the placental barrier and are distributed throughout fetal tissues with highest concentrations found in the placenta, fetal liver, and brain. Fetal blood levels approach maternal blood levels following parenteral administration.
Withdrawal symptoms occur in infants born to mothers who receive barbiturates throughout the last trimester of pregnancy. (See DRUG ABUSE AND DEPENDENCE.) If this drug is used during pregnancy, or if the patient becomes pregnant while taking this drug, the patient should be apprised of the potential hazard to the fetus.

Synergistic Effects

The concomitant use of alcohol or other CNS depressants may produce additive CNS depressant effects.

PRECAUTIONS

General

Barbiturates may be habit forming. Tolerance and psychological and physical dependence may occur with continuing use. (See DRUG ABUSE AND DEPENDENCE.) Barbiturates should be administered with caution, if at all, to patients who are mentally depressed, have suicidal tendencies, or a history of drug abuse.
Elderly or debilitated patients may react to barbiturates with marked excitement, depression, and confusion. In some persons, barbiturates repeatedly produce excitement rather than depression.
In patients with hepatic damage, barbiturates should be administered with caution and initially in reduced doses. Barbiturates should not be administered to patients showing the premonitory signs of hepatic coma.
Status epilepticus may result from the abrupt discontinuation of MEBARAL, even when administered in small daily doses in the treatment of epilepsy.
Caution and careful adjustment of dosage are required when MEBARAL is used in patients with impaired renal, cardiac, or respiratory function and in patients with myasthenia gravis and myxedema. The least quantity feasible should be prescribed or dispensed at any one time in order to minimize the possibility of acute or chronic overdosage.
Vitamin D Deficiency: MEBARAL may increase vitamin D requirements, possibly by increasing vitamin D metabolism via enzyme induction. Rarely, rickets and osteomalacia have been reported following prolonged use of barbiturates.
Vitamin K: Bleeding in the early neonatal period due to coagulation defects may follow exposure to anticonvulsant drugs *in utero;* therefore, vitamin K should be given to the mother before delivery or to the child at birth.

Information for the Patient

Practitioners should give the following information and instructions to patients receiving barbiturates.

1. The use of barbiturates carries with it an associated risk of psychological and/or physical dependence. The patient should be warned against increasing the dose of the drug without consulting a physician.
2. Barbiturates may impair mental and/or physical abilities required for the performance of potentially hazardous tasks. (e.g., driving, operating machinery, etc.)
3. Alcohol should not be consumed while taking barbiturates. Concurrent use of the barbiturates with other CNS depressants (e.g., alcohol, narcotics, tranquilizers, and antihistamines) may result in additional CNS depressant effects.

Laboratory Tests

Prolonged therapy with barbiturates should be accompanied by periodic laboratory evaluation of organ systems, including hematopoietic, renal, and hepatic systems. (See PRECAUTIONS [General] and ADVERSE REACTIONS.)

Drug Interactions

Most reports of clinically significant drug interactions occurring with the barbiturates have involved phenobarbital. However, the application of these data to other barbiturates appears valid and warrants serial blood level determinations of the relevant drugs when there are multiple therapies.

1. *Anticoagulants.* Phenobarbital lowers the plasma levels of dicumarol (name previously used: bishydroxycoumarin) and causes a decrease in anticoagulant activity as measured by the prothrombin time. Barbiturates can induce hepatic microsomal enzymes resulting in increased metabolism and decreased anticoagulant response of oral anticoagulants (eg, warfarin, acenocoumarol, dicumarol, and phenprocoumon). Patients stabilized on anticoagulant therapy may require dosage adjustments if barbiturates are added to or withdrawn from their dosage regimen.
2. *Corticosteroids.* Barbiturates appear to enhance the metabolism of exogenous corticosteroids probably through the induction of hepatic microsomal enzymes. Patients stabilized on corticosteroid therapy may require dosage adjustments if barbiturates are added to or withdrawn from their dosage regimen.
3. *Griseofulvin.* Phenobarbital appears to interfere with the absorption of orally administered griseofulvin, thus decreasing its blood level. The effect of the resultant decreased blood levels of griseofulvin on therapeutic response has not been established. However, it would be preferable to avoid concomitant administration of these drugs.
4. *Doxycycline.* Phenobarbital has been shown to shorten the half-life of doxycycline for as long as 2 weeks after barbiturate therapy is discontinued.
This mechanism is probably through the induction of hepatic microsomal enzymes that metabolize the antibiotic. If phenobarbital and doxycycline are administered concurrently, the clinical response to doxycycline should be monitored closely.
5. *Phenytoin, Sodium Valproate, Valproic Acid.* The effect of barbiturates on the metabolism of phenytoin appears to be variable. Some investigators report an accelerating effect, while others report no effect. Because the effect of barbiturates on the metabolism of phenytoin is not predictable, phenytoin and barbiturate blood levels should be monitored more frequently if these drugs are given concurrently. Sodium valproate and valproic acid appear to decrease barbiturate metabolism; therefore, barbiturate blood levels should be monitored and appropriate dosage adjustments made as indicated.
6. *Central Nervous System Depressants.* The concomitant use of other central nervous system depressants, including other sedatives or hypnotics, antihistamines, tranquilizers, or alcohol, may produce additive depressant effects.
7. *Monoamine Oxidase Inhibitors (MAOI).* MAOI prolong the effects of barbiturates probably because metabolism of the barbiturate is inhibited.
8. *Estradiol, Estrone, Progesterone, and other Steroidal Hormones.* Pretreatment with or concurrent administration of phenobarbital may decrease the effect of estradiol by increasing its metabolism. There have been reports of patients treated with antiepileptic drugs (e.g. phenobarbital) who become pregnant while taking oral contraceptives. An alternant contraceptive method might be suggested to women taking phenobarbital.

Carcinogenesis

Animal Data. Phenobarbital sodium is carcinogenic in mice and rats after lifetime administration. In mice, it produced benign and malignant liver cell tumors. In rats, benign liver cell tumors were observed very late in life. Phenobarbital is the major metabolite of MEBARAL.
Human Data. In a 29-year epidemiological study of 9,136 patients who were treated on an anticonvulsant protocol which included phenobarbital, results indicated a higher than normal incidence of hepatic carcinoma. Previously, some of these patients were treated with thorotrast, a drug which is known to produce hepatic carcinomas. Thus, this study did not provide sufficient evidence that phenobarbital sodium is carcinogenic in humans. Phenobarbital is the major metabolite of MEBARAL.
A retrospective study of 84 children with brain tumors matched to 73 normal controls and 78 cancer controls (malignant disease other than brain tumors) suggested an association between exposure to barbiturates prenatally and an increased incidence of brain tumors.

Pregnancy

Teratogenic Effects. Pregnancy Category D—See WARNINGS—Use in Pregnancy.
Nonteratogenic Effects. Reports of infants suffering from long-term barbiturate exposure *in utero* included the acute withdrawal syndrome of seizures and hyperirritability from birth to a delayed onset of up to 14 days. (See DRUG ABUSE AND DEPENDENCE.)

Labor and Delivery.

Hypnotic doses of these barbiturates do not appear to significantly impair uterine activity during labor. Full anesthetic doses of barbiturates decrease the force and frequency of uterine contractions. Administration of sedative-hypnotic barbiturates to the mother during labor may result in respiratory depression in the newborn. Premature infants are particularly susceptible to the depressant effects of barbiturates. If barbiturates are used during labor and delivery, resuscitation equipment should be available.
Data are currently not available to evaluate the effect of these barbiturates when forceps delivery or other intervention is necessary. Also, data are not available to determine the effect of these barbiturates on the later growth, development, and functional maturation of the child.

Nursing Mothers.

Caution should be exercised when a barbiturate is administered to a nursing woman since small amounts of barbiturates are excreted in the milk.

ADVERSE REACTIONS

The following adverse reactions and their incidence were compiled from surveillance of thousands of hospitalized patients. Because such patients may be less aware of certain of the milder adverse effects of barbiturates, the incidence of these reactions may be somewhat higher in fully ambulatory patients.
More than 1 in 100 Patients. The most common adverse reaction estimated to occur at a rate of 1 to 3 patients per 100 is:
Nervous System: Somnolence.
Less than 1 in 100 Patients. Adverse reactions estimated to occur at a rate of less than 1 in 100 patients listed below, grouped by organ system, and by decreasing order of occurrence are:
Nervous System: Agitation, confusion, hyperkinesia, ataxia, CNS depression, nightmares, nervousness, psychiatric disturbance, hallucinations, insomnia, anxiety, dizziness, thinking abnormality.
Respiratory System: Hypoventilation, apnea.
Cardiovascular System: Bradycardia, hypotension, syncope.
Digestive System: Nausea, vomiting, constipation.
Other Reported Reactions: Headache, hypersensitivity reactions (angioedema, skin rashes, exfoliative dermatitis), fever, liver damage, megaloblastic anemia following chronic phenobarbital use.

DRUG ABUSE AND DEPENDENCE

Mephobarbital is a controlled substance in Narcotic Schedule IV. Barbiturates may be habit forming. Tolerance, psychological dependence, and physical dependence may occur especially following prolonged use of high doses of barbiturates. As tolerance to barbiturates develops, the amount needed to maintain the same level of intoxication increases; tolerance to a fatal dosage, however, does not increase more than two-fold. As this occurs, the margin between an intoxicating dosage and fatal dosage becomes smaller.
Symptoms of acute intoxication with barbiturates include unsteady gait, slurred speech, and sustained nystagmus. Mental signs of chronic intoxication include confusion, poor judgment, irritability, insomnia, and somatic complaints.
Symptoms of barbiturate dependence are similar to those of chronic alcoholism. If an individual appears to be intoxicated with alcohol to a degree that is radically disproportionate to the amount of alcohol in his or her blood the use of barbiturates should be suspected. The lethal dose of a barbiturate is far less if alcohol is also ingested.
The symptoms of barbiturate withdrawal can be severe and may cause death. Minor withdrawal symptoms may appear 8 to 12 hours after the last dose of a barbiturate. These symptoms usually appear in the following order: anxiety, muscle twitching, tremor of hands and fingers, progressive weakness, dizziness, distortion in visual perception, nausea, vomiting, insomnia, and orthostatic hypotension. Major withdrawal symptoms (convulsions and delirium) may occur within 16 hours and last up to 5 days after abrupt cessation of these drugs. Intensity of withdrawal symptoms gradually declines over a period of approximately 15 days. Individuals susceptible to a barbiturate abuse and dependence include alcoholics and opiate abusers, as well as other sedative-hypnotic and amphetamine abusers.
Drug dependence to barbiturates arises from repeated administration of a barbiturate or agent with barbiturate-like effect on a continuous basis, generally in amounts exceeding therapeutic dose levels. The characteristics of drug dependence to barbiturates include: (a) a strong desire or need to continue taking the drug; (b) a tendency to increase the dose; (c) a psychic dependence on the effects of the drug related to subjective and individual appreciation of those effects; and (d) a physical dependence on the effects of the drug requiring its presence for maintenance of homeostasis and resulting in a definite, characteristic, and self-limited abstinence syndrome when the drug is withdrawn.
Treatment of barbiturate dependence consists of cautious and gradual withdrawal of the drug. Barbiturate-dependent patients can be withdrawn by using a number of different withdrawal regimens. In all cases withdrawal takes an extended period of time. One method involves substituting a 30 mg dose of phenobarbital for each 100 mg to 200 mg dose of barbiturate that the patient has been taking. The total daily amount of phenobarbital is then administered in 3 to 4

divided doses, not to exceed 600 mg daily. Should signs of withdrawal occur on the first day of treatment, a loading dose of 100 mg to 200 mg of phenobarbital may be administered IM in addition to the oral dose. After stabilization on phenobarbital, the total daily dose is decreased by 30 mg a day as long as withdrawal is proceeding smoothly. A modification of this regimen involves initiating treatment at the patient's regular dosage level and decreasing the daily dosage by 10% if tolerated by the patient.
Infants physically dependent on barbiturates may be given phenobarbital 3 mg/kg/day to 10 mg/kg/day. After withdrawal symptoms (hyperactivity, disturbed sleep, tremors, hyperreflexia) are relieved, the dosage of phenobarbital should be gradually decreased and completely withdrawn over a 2-week period.

OVERDOSAGE

The toxic dose of barbiturates varies considerably. In general, an oral dose of 1 g of most barbiturates produces serious poisoning in an adult. Death commonly occurs after 2 g to 10 g of ingested barbiturate. Barbiturate intoxication may be confused with alcoholism, bromide intoxication, and with various neurological disorders.
Acute overdosage with barbiturates is manifested by CNS and respiratory depression which may progress to Cheyne-Stokes respiration, areflexia, constriction of the pupils to a slight degree (though in severe poisoning they may show paralytic dilation), oliguria, tachycardia, hypotension, lowered body temperature, and coma. Typical shock syndrome (apnea, circulatory collapse, respiratory arrest, and death) may occur.
In extreme overdose, all electrical activity in the brain may cease, in which case a "flat" EEG normally equated with clinical death cannot be accepted. This effect is fully reversible unless hypoxic damage occurs. Consideration should be given to the possibility of barbiturate intoxication even in situations that appear to involve trauma.
Complications such as pneumonia, pulmonary edema, cardiac arrhythmias, congestive heart failure, and renal failure may occur. Uremia may increase CNS sensitivity to barbiturates if renal function is impaired. Differential diagnosis should include hypoglycemia, head trauma, cerebrovascular accidents, convulsive states, and diabetic coma.
Treatment of overdosage is mainly supportive and consists of the following:

1. Maintenance of an adequate airway, with assisted respiration and oxygen administration as necessary.
2. Monitoring of vital signs and fluid balance.
3. If the patient is conscious and has not lost the gag reflex, emesis may be induced with ipecac. Care should be taken to prevent pulmonary aspiration of vomitus. After completion of vomiting, 30 g activated charcoal in a glass of water may be administered.
4. If emesis is contraindicated, gastric lavage may be performed with a cuffed endotracheal tube in place with the patient in the face down position. Activated charcoal may be left in the emptied stomach and a saline cathartic administered.
5. Fluid therapy and other standard treatment for shock, if needed.
6. If renal function is normal, forced diuresis may aid in the elimination of the barbiturate. Alkalinization of the urine increases renal excretion of some barbiturates, including mephobarbital (which is metabolized to phenobarbital).
7. Although not recommended as a routine procedure, hemodialysis may be used in severe barbiturate intoxications or if the patient is anuric or in shock.
8. Patient should be rolled from side to side every 30 minutes.
9. Antibiotics should be given if pneumonia is suspected.
10. Appropriate nursing care to prevent hypostatic pneumonia, decubiti aspiration, and other complications of patients with altered states of consciousness.

DOSAGE AND ADMINISTRATION

Epilepsy: Average dose for adults: 400 mg to 600 mg (6 grains to 9 grains) daily; children under 5 years: 16 mg to 32 mg ($^1/_4$ grain to $^1/_2$ grain) three or four times daily; children over 5 years: 32 mg to 64 mg ($^1/_2$ grain to 1 grain) three or four times daily. MEBARAL is best taken at bedtime if seizures generally occur at night, and during the day if attacks are diurnal.
Treatment should be started with a small dose which is gradually increased over four or five days until the optimum dosage is determined. If the patient has been taking some other antiepileptic drug, it should be tapered off as the doses of MEBARAL are increased, to guard against the temporary marked attacks that may occur when any treatment for epilepsy is changed abruptly. Similarly, when the dose is to be lowered to a maintenance level or to be discontinued, the amount should be reduced gradually over four or five days.
Special Patient Population. Dosage should be reduced in the elderly or debilitated because these patients may be more sensitive to barbiturates. Dosage should be reduced for patients with impaired renal function or hepatic disease.
Combination with Other Drugs: MEBARAL may be used in combination with phenobarbital, either in the form of alternating courses or concurrently. When the two drugs are used at the same time, the dose should be about one-half the amount of each used alone. The average daily dose for an adult is from 50 mg to 100 mg ($^3/_4$ grain to $1^1/_2$ grains) of phenobarbital and from 200 mg to 300 mg (3 grains to $4^1/_2$ grains) of MEBARAL.
MEBARAL may also be used with phenytoin sodium; in some cases, combined therapy appears to give better results than either agent used alone, since phenytoin sodium is particularly effective for the psychomotor types of seizure but relatively ineffective for petit mal. When the drugs are employed concurrently, a reduced dose of phenytoin sodium is advisable, but the full dose of MEBARAL may be given. Satisfactory results have been obtained with an average daily dose of 230 mg ($3^1/_2$ grains) of phenytoin sodium plus about 600 mg (9 grains) of MEBARAL.
Sedation: Adults: 32 mg to 100 mg ($^1/_2$ grain to $1^1/_2$ grains)—optimum dose, 50 mg ($^3/_4$ grain)—three to four times daily. Children: 16 mg to 32 mg ($^1/_4$ grain to $^1/_2$ grain) three to four times daily.

HOW SUPPLIED

Tablets—white, round, convex and the 32 mg and 50 mg tablets are scored.
32 mg ($^1/_2$ grain), bottles of 250
(NDC 0024-1231-05)
50 mg ($^3/_4$ grain), bottles of 250
(NDC 0024-1232-05)
100 mg ($1^1/_2$ grains), bottles of 250
(NDC 0024-1233-05)
Store at room temperature up to 25° C (77° F).

MSW-9D
Revised November 1999

NegGram® ℞
NALIDIXIC ACID, USP

DESCRIPTION

NegGram®, brand of nalidixic acid, is a quinolone antibacterial agent for oral administration. Nalidixic acid is 1-ethyl-1, 4-dihydro-7-methyl-4-oxo-1, 8-naphthyridine-3-carboxylic acid. It is a pale yellow, crystalline substance and a very weak organic acid.
Nalidixic acid has the following structural formula:

Inactive Ingredients—SUSPENSION: Carbomer 934P, FD&C Red #40, Flavor, Parabens, Purified Water, Saccharin Sodium, Sodium Chloride, Sorbitol Solution. CAPLETS: Hydrogenated Vegetable Oil, Methylcellulose, Microcrystalline Cellulose, Sodium Lauryl Sulfate, Yellow Ferric Oxide.

CLINICAL PHARMACOLOGY

Following oral administration, NegGram is rapidly absorbed from the gastrointestinal tract, partially metabolized in the liver, and rapidly excreted through the kidneys. Unchanged nalidixic acid appears in the urine along with an active metabolite, hydroxynalidixic acid, which has antibacterial activity similar to that of nalidixic acid. Other metabolites include glucuronic acid conjugates of nalidixic acid and hydroxy nalidixic acid, and the dicarboxylic acid derivative. The hydroxy metabolite represents 30 percent of the biologically active drug in the blood and 85 percent in the urine. Peak serum levels of active drug average approximately 20 mcg to 40 mcg per mL (90 percent protein bound), one to two hours after administration of a 1 g dose to a fasting normal individual, with a half-life of about 90 minutes. Peak urine levels of active drug average approximately 150 mcg to 200 mcg per mL, three to four hours after administration, with a half-life of about six hours. Approximately four percent of NegGram is excreted in the feces. Traces of nalidixic acid were found in blood and urine of an infant whose mother had received the drug during the last trimester of pregnancy. (See PRECAUTIONS—Drug Interactions.)

Microbiology
NegGram has marked antibacterial activity against gram-negative bacteria including *Enterobacter* species, *Escherichia coli, Morganella Morganii; Proteus Mirabilis, Proteus vulgaris,* and *Providencia rettgeri. Pseudomonas* species are generally resistant to the drug. NegGram is bactericidal and is effective over the entire urinary pH range. Conventional chromosomal resistance to NegGram taken in full dosage has been reported to emerge in approximately 2 to 14 percent of patients during treatment; however, bacterial resistance to NegGram has not been shown to be transferable via R factor.

Susceptibility Test
Diffusion Techniques: Quantitative methods that require measurement of zone diameters give the most precise estimates of antibacterial susceptibility. One such procedure recommended for use with a disc containing 30 mcg of nalidixic acid is the National Committee for Clinical Laboratory Standards (NCCLS) approved procedure. Only organisms from urinary tract infections should be tested. Results of laboratory tests using 30 mcg nalidixic acid discs should be interpreted using the following criteria:

Zone Diameter (mm)	Interpretation
≥ 19	(S) Susceptible
14–18	(I) Intermediate
≤ 13	(R) Resistant

Dilution Techniques: Broth and agar dilution methods, such as those recommended by the NCCLS, may be used to determine the minimum inhibitory concentration (MIC) of nalidixic acid. MIC test results should be interpreted according to the following criteria:

MIC (mcg/mL)	Interpretation
≤16	(S) Susceptible
≥32	(R) Resistant

For any susceptibility test, a report of "susceptible" indicates that the pathogen is likely to respond to nalidixic acid therapy. A report of "resistant" indicates that the pathogen is not likely to respond. A report of "intermediate" generally indicates that the test result is equivocal.
The Quality Control strains should have the following assigned daily ranges for nalidixic acid:

QC Strains
E. Coli
(ATCC 25922)
Disc Zone Diameter
22–28
MIC (mcg/mL)
1.0–4.0

INDICATIONS AND USAGE

NegGram is indicated for the treatment of urinary tract infections caused by susceptible gram-negative microorganisms, including the majority of *E. Coli, Enterobacter* species, *Klebsiella* species, and *Proteus* species. Disc susceptibility testing with the 30 mcg disc should be performed prior to administration of the drug, and during treatment if clinical response warrants.

CONTRAINDICATIONS

NegGram is contraindicated in patients with known hypersensitivity to nalidixic acid and in patients with a history of convulsive disorders.

WARNINGS

Central Nervous System (CNS) effects including convulsions, increased intracranial pressure, and toxic psychosis have been reported with nalidixic acid therapy. Convulsive seizures have been reported with other drugs in this class. Quinolones may also cause CNS stimulation which may lead to tremor, restlessness, lightheadedness, confusion, and hallucinations. Therefore, nalidixic acid should be used with caution in patients with known or suspected CNS disorders, such as, cerebral arteriosclerosis or epilepsy, or other factors which predispose seizures. (See ADVERSE REACTIONS.) If these reactions occur in patients receiving nalidixic acid, the drug should be discontinued and appropriate measures instituted.
Serious and occasionally fatal hypersensitivity (anaphylactoid) reactions, some following the first dose, have been reported in patients receiving quinolone therapy. Some reactions were accompanied by cardiovascular collapse, loss of consciousness, tingling, pharyngeal or facial edema, dyspnea, urticaria, and itching. Only a few patients had a history of hypersensitivity reactions. Serious anaphylactoid reactions required immediate emergency treatment with epinephrine. Oxygen, intravenous steroids, and airway management, including intubation, should be administered as indicated.
Nalidixic acid and other members of the quinolone drug class have been shown to cause arthropathy in juvenile animals. (See PRECAUTIONS and ANIMAL PHARMACOLOGY.)
Pseudomembranous colitis has been reported with nearly all antibacterial agents, including quinolones, and may range in severity from mild to life-threatening. Therefore, it is important to consider this diagnosis in patients who present with diarrhea subsequent to the administration of antibacterial agents.
Treatment with antibacterial agents alters the normal flora of the colon and may permit overgrowth of clostridia. Studies indicate that a toxin produced by *Clostridium difficile* is one primary cause of "antibiotic-associated colitis".
After the diagnosis of pseudomembranous colitis has been established, therapeutic measures should be initiated. Mild cases of pseudomembranous colitis usually respond to drug discontinuation alone. In moderate to severe cases, consideration should be given to management with fluids and electrolytes, protein supplementation, and treatment with an antibacterial drug clinically effective against *C. difficile* colitis.

PRECAUTIONS

General
Blood counts and renal and liver function tests should be performed periodically if treatment is continued for more

Continued on next page

This product information was prepared in September 2000. On these and other products of Sanofi-Synthelabo Inc., detailed information may be obtained on a current basis by direct inquiry to Product Information Services, 90 Park Avenue, New York, NY 10016 (toll free 1-800-446-6267).

NegGram—Cont.

than two weeks. NegGram should be used with caution in patients with liver disease, epilepsy, or severe cerebral arteriosclerosis. (See WARNINGS.) While caution should be used in patients with severe renal failure, therapeutic concentrations of NegGram in the urine, without increased toxicity due to drug accumulation in the blood, have been observed in patients on full dosage with creatinine clearances as low as 2 mL/minute to 8 mL/minute.

Moderate to severe phototoxicity reactions have been observed in patients who are exposed to direct sunlight while receiving NegGram or other members of this drug class. Excessive sunlight should be avoided. Therapy should be discontinued if phototoxicity occurs.

If bacterial resistance to NegGram emerges during treatment, it usually does so within 48 hours, permitting rapid change to another antimicrobial. Therefore, if the clinical response is unsatisfactory or if relapse occurs, cultures and sensitivity tests should be repeated. Underdosage with NegGram during initial treatment (with less than 4 g per day for adults) may predispose to emergence of bacterial resistance. (See DOSAGE AND ADMINISTRATION.)

Information for Patients

Patients should be advised NegGram may be taken with or without meals. Patients should be advised to drink fluids liberally and not take antacids.

Patients should be advised that quinolones may be associated with hypersensitivity reactions, even following a single dose, and to discontinue the drug at the first sign of a skin rash or other allergic reactions.

Quinolones may cause dizziness and lightheadedness, therefore, patients should know how they react to NegGram before they operate an automobile or machinery or engage in activities requiring mental alertness or coordination.

Patients should be advised that quinolones may increase the effects of theophylline and caffeine. There is a possibility of caffeine accumulation when products containing caffeine are consumed while taking quinolones. Patients should be advised to avoid excessive sunlight or artificial ultraviolet light while receiving nalidixic acid and to discontinue therapy if phototoxicity occurs.

Patients should be advised that convulsions have been reported in patients taking quinolones, including Nalidixic acid, and to notify their physician before taking this drug if there is a history of this condition. Patients should be advised that mineral supplements, vitamins with iron or minerals, calcium-, aluminum-, magnesium-based antacids, sucralfate or Videx®, (Didanosine), chewable/buffered tablets of the pediatric powder for oral solution should not be taken within the two-hour period before or within the two-hour period after taking nalidixic aid (see **Drug Interactions**).

Drug Interactions

Elevated plasma levels of theophylline have been reported with concomitant quinolone use. There have been reports of theophylline-related side effects in patients on concomitant therapy with quinolones and theophylline. Therefore, monitoring of theophylline plasma levels should be considered and dosage of theophylline adjusted, as required.

Quinolones have been shown to interfere with the metabolism of caffeine. This may lead to reduced clearance of caffeine and the prolongation of its plasma half-life.

Quinolones, including nalidixic acid, may enhance the effects of the oral anticoagulant warfarin or its derivatives. When these products are administered concomitantly, prothrombin time or other suitable coagulation test should be closely monitored.

Nitrofurantoin interferes with the therapeutic action of nalidixic acid.

Antacids containing magnesium, aluminum, or calcium; sucralfate or divalent or trivalent cations such as iron; multivitamins containing zinc; and Videx®, (Didanosine), chewable/buffered tablets or the pediatric powder for oral solution may substantially interfere with the absorption of quinolones, resulting in systemic levels considerably lower than desired. These agents should not be taken within the two hour period before or within the two-hour period after nalidixic acid administration.

Elevated serum levels of cyclosporine have been reported with the concomitant use of some quinolones and cyclosporine. Therefore, cyclosporine serum levels should be monitored and appropriate cyclosporine dosage adjustments made when these drugs are used concomitantly.

Drug Laboratory Test Interactions

When Benedict's or Fehling's solution or Clinitest® Reagent Tablets are used to test the urine of patients taking NegGram, a false-positive reaction for glucose may be obtained, due to the liberation of glucuronic acid from the metabolites excreted. However, a colorimetric test for glucose based on an enzyme reaction (e.g., with Clinistix® Reagent Strips or Tes-Tape®) does not give a false-positive reaction to the liberated glucuronic acid.

Incorrect values may be obtained for urinary 17-keto and ketogenic steroids in patients receiving NegGram, because of an interaction between the drug and the *m*-dinitrobenzene used in the usual assay method. In such cases, the Porter-Silber test for 17-hydroxycorticoids may be used.

Carcinogenesis, Mutagenesis, Impairment of Fertility

In lifetime studies in the rat given nalidixic acid in the diet, there was an increased incidence of preputial gland neoplasms in the treated males and clitoral gland neoplasms in the treated females. Studies in mice in which nalidixic acid was administered in the feed for two years, or was given in the feed for 76 weeks followed by no treatment for 9 weeks, gave equivocal evidence of carcinogenic activity.

Nalidixic acid was tested in the Ames bacterial mutagenicity test (maximum dose 33 mcg/plate) and the mouse lymphoma assay (L5178Y/TK; maximum dose 100 mcg/mL) with and without metabolic activation, and results were negative.

Pregnancy: Teratogenic Effects.

Pregnancy Category C.

NegGram has been shown to be teratogenic and embryocidal in rats when given in oral doses six times the human dose. NegGram also prolonged the duration of pregnancy especially at four times the clinical dose. There are no adequate and well-controlled studies in pregnant women. Since nalidixic acid, like other drugs in this class, causes arthropathy in immature animals, NegGram should be used during pregnancy only if the potential benefit justifies the potential risk to the fetus. (See WARNINGS and ANIMAL PHARMACOLOGY.)

Nursing Mothers

It is not known whether NegGram is excreted in human milk. Because other drugs are excreted in human milk and because of the potential for serious adverse reactions in nursing infants from NegGram, a decision should be made whether to discontinue nursing or to discontinue the drug taking into account the importance of the drug to the mother.

Pediatric Use

Safety and effectiveness in infants below the age of three months have not been established.

Usage in Patients Under 18 Years of Age

Toxicological studies have shown that nalidixic acid and related drugs can produce erosions of the cartilage in weight-bearing joints and other signs of arthropathy in immature animals of most species tested. No such joint lesions have been reported in humans to date. Nevertheless, until the significance of this finding is clarified, this drug should only be used in patients under 18 years of age when the potential benefit justifies the potential risk. (See WARNINGS and ANIMAL PHARMACOLOGY.)

Geriatric Use

Clinical studies of NegGram® did not include sufficient numbers of subjects aged 65 and over to determine whether they respond differently from younger subjects. Other reported clinical experience has not identified differences in responses between the elderly and younger patients. Caution should therefore be observed in using nalidixic acid in elderly patients. This drug is known to be substantially excreted by the kidney, and the risk of toxic reactions to this drug may be greater in patients with impaired renal function. Because elderly patients are more likely to have decreased renal function, care should be taken in dose selection, and it may be useful to monitor renal function. (See PRECAUTIONS, General.)

ADVERSE REACTIONS

Reactions reported after oral administration of NegGram include the following.

CNS effects: drowsiness, weakness, headache, and dizziness and vertigo. Reversible subjective visual disturbances without objective findings have occurred infrequently (generally with each dose during the first few days of treatment). These reactions include overbrightness of lights, change in color perception, difficulty in focusing, decrease in visual acuity, and double vision. They usually disappeared promptly when dosage was reduced or therapy was discontinued. Toxic psychosis or brief convulsions have been reported rarely, usually following excessive doses. In general, the convulsions have occurred in patients with predisposing factors such as epilepsy or cerebral arteriosclerosis. In infants and children receiving therapeutic doses of NegGram, increased intracranial pressure with bulging anterior fontanel, papilledema, and headache has occasionally been observed. A few cases of 6th cranial nerve palsy have been reported. Although the mechanisms of these reactions are unknown, the signs and symptoms usually disappeared rapidly with no sequelae when treatment was discontinued.

Gastrointestinal: abdominal pain, nausea, vomiting, and diarrhea.

Allergic: rash, pruritus, urticaria, angioedema, eosinophilia, arthralgia with joint stiffness and swelling, and anaphylactoid reaction. Erythema Multiforme and Stevens-Johnson syndrome have been reported with nalidixic acid and other drugs in this class. Rash was the most frequently reported adverse reaction. Photosensitivity reactions consisting of erythema and bullae on exposed skin surfaces usually resolve completely in 2 weeks to 2 months after NegGram is discontinued; however, bullae may continue to appear with successive exposures to sunlight or with mild skin trauma for up to 3 months after discontinuation of drug. (See PRECAUTIONS.)

Other: rarely, cholestasis, paresthesia, metabolic acidosis, thrombocytopenia, leukopenia, or hemolytic anemia, sometimes associated with glucose 6-phosphate dehydrogenase deficiency.

OVERDOSAGE

Manifestations: Toxic psychosis, convulsions, increased intracranial pressure, or metabolic acidosis may occur in patients taking more than the recommended dosage. Vomiting, nausea, and lethargy may also occur following overdosage.

Treatment: Reactions are short-lived (two or three hours) because the drug is rapidly excreted. If overdosage is noted early, gastric lavage is indicated. If absorption has occurred, increased fluid administration is advisable and supportive measures such as oxygen and means of artificial respiration should be available. Although anticonvulsant therapy has not been used in the few instances of overdosage reported, it may be indicated in a severe case.

DOSAGE AND ADMINISTRATION

Antacids containing calcium, magnesium, or aluminum; sucralfate; divalent or trivalent cations such as iron; multivitamins contaning zinc; or Videx® (didanosine), chewable/buffered tablets of the pediatric powder for oral solution should not be taken within the two-hour period before or within the two-hour period after taking nalidixic acid.

Adults. The recommended dosage for initial therapy in adults is 1 g administered four times daily for one or two weeks (total daily dose, 4 g). For prolonged therapy, the total daily dose may be reduced to 2 g after the initial treatment period. Underdosage during initial treatment may predispose to emergence of bacterial resistance.

Pediatric Patients. Until further experience is gained, NegGram should not be administered to infants younger than three months. Dosage in Pediatric Patients 12 years of age and under should be calculated on the basis of body weight. The recommended total daily dosage for initial therapy is 25 mg/lb/day (55 mg/kg/day), administered in four equally divided doses. For prolonged therapy, the total daily dose may be reduced to 15 mg/lb/day (33 mg/kg/day). NegGram Suspension or NegGram Caplets of 250 mg may be used. One 250 mg tablet is equivalent to one teaspoon (5 mL) of the suspension.

HOW SUPPLIED

Suspension (250 mg/5 mL tsp), raspberry flavored, bottles of 1 pint (NDC 0024-1318-06)

Caplets of 1 g, light buff-colored capsule-shaped tablets, bottles of 100 (NDC 0024-1323-04)

Caplets of 500 mg, light buff-colored capsule-shaped tablets, bottles of 56 (NDC 0024-1322-03) 500 (NDC 0024-1322-06)

Caplets of 250 mg, light buff-colored capsule-shaped tablets, bottles of 56 (NDC 0024-1321-03)

Store suspension at room temperature up to 25°C (77°F).

Store caplets at room temperature, up to 30°C (86°F).

ANIMAL PHARMACOLOGY

NegGram (nalidixic acid) and related drugs have been shown to cause arthropathy in juvenile animals of most species tested. (See WARNINGS.)

Long-term administration of nalidixic acid to rats resulted in retinal degeneration and cataracts.

Hydroxynalidixic acid, the principal metabolite of NegGram, did not produce any oculotoxic effects at any dosage level in seven species of animals including three primate species. However, oral administration of this metabolite in high doses has been shown to have oculotoxic potential, namely in dogs and cats where it produced retinal degeneration upon prolonged administration leading, in some cases, to blindness.

In experiments with NegGram itself, little if any such activity could be elicited in either dogs or cats. Sensitivity to CNS side effects in these species limited the doses of NegGram that could be used; this factor, together with a low conversion rate to the hydroxy metabolite in these species, may explain the absence of these effects.

NSW-6 F (0)

Revised January 2000

Shown in Product Identification Guide, page 333

NEO–SYNEPHRINE® Hydrochloride ℞

brand of phenylephrine hydrochloride ophthalmic solution, USP

Vasoconstrictor and Mydriatic

SOLUTIONS 2.5% AND 10%

VISCOUS SOLUTION 10%

For Use in Ophthalmology

WARNING: PHYSICIANS SHOULD COMPLETELY FAMILIARIZE THEMSELVES WITH THE COMPLETE CONTENTS OF THIS LEAFLET BEFORE PRESCRIBING NEO-SYNEPHRINE.

DESCRIPTION

NEO-SYNEPHRINE hydrochloride, brand of phenylephrine hydrochloride ophthalmic solution, is a sterile solution used as a vasoconstrictor and mydriatic for use in ophthalmology.

NEO-SYNEPHRINE hydrochloride is a synthetic sympathomimetic compound structurally similar to epinephrine and ephedrine.

Phenylephrine hydrochloride is (–)-*m* -Hydroxy-α-[(methylamino)methyl] benzyl alcohol hydrochloride, and has the following structural formula:

OH — C(H) — CH_2NHCH_3 · HCl (on benzene ring with OH)

CLINICAL PHARMACOLOGY

NEO-SYNEPHRINE possesses predominantly α-adrenergic effects. In the eye, phenylephrine acts locally as a potent vasoconstrictor and mydriatic, by constricting ophthalmic blood vessels and the radial muscle of the iris.

The ophthalmologic usefulness of NEO-SYNEPHRINE hydrochloride is due to its rapid effect and moderately prolonged action, as well as to the fact that it produces no compensatory vasodilatation.

The action of different concentrations of ophthalmic solutions of NEO-SYNEPHRINE hydrochloride is shown in the following table:

Strength of solution (%)	Mydriasis		Paralysis of accommodation
	Maximal (minutes)	Recovery time (hours)	
2.5	15–60	3	trace
10	10–60	6	slight

Although rare, systemic absorption of sufficient quantities of phenylephrine may lead to systemic α-adrenergic effects, such as rise in blood pressure which may be accompanied by a reflex atropine-sensitive bradycardia.

INDICATIONS AND USAGE

NEO-SYNEPHRINE hydrochloride is recommended for use as a decongestant and vasoconstrictor and for pupil dilatation in uveitis (posterior synechiae), wide angle glaucoma, prior to surgery, refraction, ophthalmoscopic examination, and diagnostic procedures.

CONTRAINDICATIONS

Ophthalmic solutions of NEO-SYNEPHRINE hydrochloride are contraindicated in persons with narrow angle glaucoma (and in those individuals who are hypersensitive to NEO-SYNEPHRINE). NEO-SYNEPHRINE hydrochloride 10 percent ophthalmic solutions are contraindicated in infants and in patients with aneurysms.

WARNINGS

There have been rare reports associating the use of NEO-SYNEPHRINE 10 percent ophthalmic solutions with the development of serious cardiovascular reactions, including ventricular arrhythmias and myocardial infarctions. These episodes, some ending fatally, have usually occurred in elderly patients with preexisting cardiovascular diseases.

PRECAUTIONS

Exceeding recommended dosages or applying NEO-SYNEPHRINE hydrochloride ophthalmic solutions to the instrumented, traumatized, diseased or postsurgical eye or adnexa, or to patients with suppressed lacrimation, as during anesthesia, may result in the absorption of sufficient quantities of phenylephrine to produce a systemic vasopressor response.

A significant elevation in blood pressure is rare but has been reported following conjunctival instillation of recommended doses of NEO-SYNEPHRINE 10 percent ophthalmic solutions. Caution, therefore, should be exercised in administering the 10 percent solutions to children of low body weight, the elderly, and patients with insulin-dependent diabetes, hypertension, hyperthyroidism, generalized arteriosclerosis, or cardiovascular disease. The posttreatment blood pressure of these patients, and any patients who develop symptoms, should be carefully monitored.

Ordinarily, any mydriatic, including NEO-SYNEPHRINE hydrochloride, solution, is contraindicated in patients with glaucoma, since it may occasionally raise intraocular pressure. However, when temporary dilatation of the pupil may free adhesions or when vasoconstriction of intrinsic vessels may lower intraocular tension, these advantages may temporarily outweigh the danger from coincident dilatation of the pupil.

Rebound miosis has been reported in older persons one day after receiving NEO-SYNEPHRINE hydrochloride ophthalmic solutions, and reinstillation of the drug produced a reduction in mydriasis. This may be of clinical importance in dilating the pupils of older subjects prior to retinal detachment or cataract surgery.

Due to a strong action of the drug on the dilator muscle, older individuals may also develop transient pigment floaters in the aqueous humor 30 to 45 minutes following the administration of NEO-SYNEPHRINE hydrochloride ophthalmic solutions. The appearance may be similar to anterior uveitis or to a microscopic hyphema.

To prevent pain, a drop of suitable topical anesthetic may be applied before using the 10 percent ophthalmic solution.

Drug Interaction: As with all other adrenergic drugs, when NEO-SYNEPHRINE 10 percent ophthalmic solutions or 2.5 percent ophthalmic solution is administered simultaneously with, or up to 21 days after, administration of monoamine oxidase (MAO) inhibitors, careful supervision and adjustment of dosages are required since exaggerated adrenergic effects may occur. The pressor response of adrenergic agents may also be potentiated by tricyclic antidepressants, propranolol, reserpine, guanethidine, methyldopa, and atropine-like drugs.

It has been reported that the concomitant use of NEO-SYNEPHRINE 10 percent ophthalmic solutions and systemic beta blockers has caused acute hypertension and, in one case, the rupture of a congenital cerebral aneurysm. NEO-SYNEPHRINE may potentiate the cardiovascular depressant effects of potent inhalation anesthetic agents.

Carcinogenesis, Mutagenesis, Impairment of Fertility: No long-term animal studies have been done to evaluate the potential of NEO-SYNEPHRINE in these areas.

Pregnancy Category C: Animal reproduction studies have not been conducted with NEO-SYNEPHRINE. It is also not known whether NEO-SYNEPHRINE can cause fetal harm when administered to a pregnant woman or can affect reproduction capacity. NEO-SYNEPHRINE should be given to a pregnant woman only if clearly needed.

Nursing Mothers: It is not known whether this drug is excreted in milk; many are. Caution should be exercised when NEO-SYNEPHRINE hydrochloride ophthalmic solution is administered to a nursing woman.

Pediatric Use: NEO-SYNEPHRINE hydrochloride 10 percent ophthalmic solutions are contraindicated in infants. (See CONTRAINDICATIONS.) For use in older children see DOSAGE AND ADMINISTRATION.

Exceeding recommended dosages or applying NEO-SYNEPHRINE hydrochloride ophthalmic solutions to the instrumented, traumatized, diseased or postsurgical eye or adnexa, or to patients with suppressed lacrimation, as during anesthesia, may result in the absorption of sufficient quantities of phenylephrine to produce a systemic vasopressor response.

The hypertensive effects of phenylephrine may be treated with an alpha-adrenergic blocking agent such as phentolamine mesylate, 5 mg to 10 mg intravenously, repeated as necessary.

The oral LD_{50} of phenylephrine in the rat: 350 mg/kg, in the mouse: 120 mg/kg.

DOSAGE AND ADMINISTRATION

Prolonged exposure to air or strong light may cause oxidation and discoloration. Do not use if solution is brown or contains a precipitate.

Vasoconstriction and Pupil Dilatation

NEO-SYNEPHRINE hydrochloride 10 percent ophthalmic solutions are especially useful when rapid and powerful dilatation of the pupil and reduction of congestion in the capillary bed are desired. A drop of a suitable topical anesthetic may be applied, followed in a few minutes by 1 drop of the NEO-SYNEPHRINE hydrochloride 10 percent ophthalmic solutions on the upper limbus. The anesthetic prevents stinging and consequent dilution of the solution by lacrimation. It may occasionally be necessary to repeat the instillation after one hour, again preceded by the use of the topical anesthetic.

Uveitis: Posterior Synechiae

NEO-SYNEPHRINE hydrochloride 10 percent ophthalmic solutions may be used in patients with uveitis when synechiae are present or may develop. The formation of synechiae may be prevented by the use of the 10 percent ophthalmic solutions and atropine to produce wide dilatation of the pupil. It should be emphasized, however, that the vasoconstrictor effect of NEO-SYNEPHRINE hydrochloride may be antagonistic to the increase of local blood flow in uveal infection.

To free recently formed posterior synechiae, 1 drop of the 10 percent ophthalmic solutions may be applied to the upper surface of the cornea. On the following day, treatment may be continued if necessary. In the interim, hot compresses should be applied for five or ten minutes three times a day, with 1 drop of a 1 or 2 percent solution of atropine sulfate before and after each series of compresses.

Glaucoma

In certain patients with glaucoma, temporary reduction of intraocular tension may be attained by producing vasoconstriction of the intraocular vessels; this may be accomplished by placing 1 drop of the 10 percent ophthalmic solutions on the upper surface of the cornea. This treatment may be repeated as often as necessary.

NEO-SYNEPHRINE hydrochloride, may be used with miotics in patients with wide angle glaucoma. It reduces the difficulties experienced by the patient because of the small field produced by miosis, and still it permits and often supports the effect of the miotic in lowering the intraocular pressure. Hence, there may be marked improvement in visual acuity after using NEO-SYNEPHRINE hydrochloride in conjunction with miotic drugs.

Surgery

When a short-acting mydriatic is needed for wide dilatation of the pupil before intraocular surgery, the 10 percent ophthalmic solutions or 2.5 percent ophthalmic solution may be applied topically from 30 to 60 minutes before the operation.

Refraction

Prior to determination of refractive errors, NEO-SYNEPHRINE hydrochloride 2.5 percent ophthalmic solution may be used effectively with homatropine hydrobromide, atropine sulfate, or a combination of homatropine and cocaine hydrochloride.

For *adults,* a drop of the preferred cycloplegic is placed in each eye, followed in five minutes by 1 drop of NEO-SYNEPHRINE hydrochloride 2.5 percent ophthalmic solution and in ten minutes by another drop of the cycloplegic. In 50 to 60 minutes, the eyes are ready for refraction.

For *children,* a drop of atropine sulfate 1 percent is placed in each eye, followed in 10 to 15 minutes by 1 drop of NEO-SYNEPHRINE hydrochloride 2.5 percent ophthalmic solution and in five to ten minutes by a second drop of atropine sulfate 1 percent. In one to two hours, the eyes are ready for refraction.

For a "one application method," NEO-SYNEPHRINE hydrochloride 2.5 percent ophthalmic solution may be combined with a cycloplegic to elicit synergistic action. The additive effect varies depending on the patient. Therefore, when using a "one application method," it may be desirable to increase the concentration of the cycloplegic.

Ophthalmoscopic Examination

One drop of NEO-SYNEPHRINE hydrochloride 2.5 percent ophthalmic solution is placed in each eye. Sufficient mydriasis to permit examination is produced in 15 to 30 minutes. Dilatation lasts from one to three hours.

Diagnostic Procedures

Provocative Test for Angle Block in Patients with Glaucoma: The 2.5 percent ophthalmic solution may be used as a provocative test when latent increased intraocular pressure is suspected. Tension is measured before application of NEO-SYNEPHRINE hydrochloride and again after dilatation. A 3 to 5 mm of mercury rise in pressure suggests the presence of angle block in patients with glaucoma; however, failure to obtain such a rise does not preclude the presence of glaucoma from other causes.

Shadow Test (Retinoscopy): When dilatation of the pupil without cycloplegic action is desired for the shadow test, the 2.5 percent ophthalmic solution may be used alone.

Blanching Test: One or 2 drops of the 2.5 percent ophthalmic solution should be applied to the injected eye. After five minutes, examine for perilimbal blanching. If blanching occurs, the congestion is superficial and probably does not indicate iritis.

HOW SUPPLIED

In Mono-Drop ® (plastic dropper) bottle:

Low surface tension solutions

2.5 percent ophthalmic solution —

NEO-SYNEPHRINE hydrochloride, 2.5 percent in a sterile, isotonic, buffered, low surface tension vehicle with sodium phosphate, sodium biphosphate, boric acid, and, as antiseptic preservative, benzalkonium chloride, NF, 1:7500. The pH is adjusted with phosphoric acid or sodium hydroxide.

Bottles of 15 mL (NDC 0024-1358-01)

10 percent ophthalmic solution —

NEO-SYNEPHRINE hydrochloride 10 percent in a sterile, buffered, low surface tension vehicle with sodium phosphate, sodium biphosphate, and, as antiseptic preservative, benzalkonium chloride 1:10,000. The pH is adjusted with phosphoric acid or sodium hydroxide.

Bottles of 5 mL (NDC 0024-1359-01)

Viscous solution

10 percent ophthalmic solution —

NEO-SYNEPHRINE hydrochloride 10 percent in a sterile, buffered, viscous vehicle with sodium phosphate, sodium biphosphate, methylcellulose, and, as antiseptic preservative, benzalkonium chloride 1:10,000. The pH is adjusted with phosphoric acid or sodium hydroxide.

Bottles of 5 mL (NDC 0024-1362-01)

Store at 25°C (77°F); excursions permitted to 15°C–30°C (59°F–86°F) [see USP Controlled Room Temperature]

Revised September 1999

NSW-5-E

PEDIACOF® Ⓒ ℞

DESCRIPTION

Each teaspoon (5 mL) contains:

Codeine phosphate, USP .... 5.0 mg

(Warning: May be habit forming.)

Phenylephrine hydrochloride, USP .... 2.5 mg

Chlorpheniramine maleate, USP .... 0.75 mg

Potassium iodide, USP .... 75.0 mg

with sodium benzoate 0.2% as preservative and alcohol 5%.

Inactive Ingredients: Alcohol, Citric Acid, FD&C Red #40, Flavor, Glycerin, Liquid Glucose, Purified Water, Saccharin Sodium, Sodium Benzoate.

HOW SUPPLIED

Raspberry flavored syrup

Bottle of 16 fl oz (**NDC** 0024-1509-06)

Store at room temperature up to 25° C (77° F)

Available on prescription only.

For complete prescribing information see package insert or contact Product Information Services.

Revised September 1999

PSW-10D

Continued on next page

This product information was prepared in September 2000. On these and other products of Sanofi-Synthelabo Inc., detailed information may be obtained on a current basis by direct inquiry to Product Information Services, 90 Park Avenue, New York, NY 10016 (toll free 1-800-446-6267).

pHisoHex® ℞
brand of hexachlorophene detergent cleanser
sudsing antibacterial soapless skin cleanser

DESCRIPTION

pHisoHex, brand of hexachlorophene detergent cleanser, is an antibacterial sudsing emulsion for topical administration. pHisoHex contains a colloidal dispersion of hexachlorophene 3% (w/w) in a stable emulsion consisting of entsufon sodium, petrolatum, lanolin cholesterols, methylcellulose, polyethylene glycol, polyethylene glycol monostearate, lauryl myristyl diethanolamide, sodium benzoate, and water. pH is adjusted with hydrochloric acid. Entsufon sodium is a synthetic detergent.

Chemically, hexachlorophene is Phenol, 2,2'-methylenebis[3,4,6-trichloro-].

CLINICAL PHARMACOLOGY

pHisoHex is a bacteriostatic cleansing agent. It cleanses the skin thoroughly and has bacteriostatic action against staphylococci and other gram-positive bacteria. Cumulative antibacterial action develops with repeated use. Cleansing with alcohol or soaps containing alcohol removes the antibacterial residue.

Detectable blood levels of hexachlorophene following absorption through intact skin have been found in subjects who regularly scrubbed with hexachlorophene emulsion 3%. (See **WARNINGS** for additional information.)

pHisoHex has the same slight acidity as normal skin (pH value 5.0 to 6.0).

INDICATIONS AND USAGE

pHisoHex is indicated for use as a surgical scrub and a bacteriostatic skin cleanser. It may also be used to control an outbreak of gram-positive infection where other infection control procedures have been unsuccessful. Use only as long as necessary for infection control.

CONTRAINDICATIONS

pHisoHex should not be used on burned or denuded skin.

It should not be used as an occlusive dressing, wet pack, or lotion.

It should not be used routinely for prophylactic total body bathing.

It should not be used as a vaginal pack or tampon, or on any mucous membranes.

pHisoHex should not be used on persons with sensitivity to any of its components. It should not be used on persons who have demonstrated primary light sensitivity to halogenated phenol derivatives because of the possibility of cross-sensitivity to hexachlorophene.

WARNINGS

RINSE THOROUGHLY AFTER EACH USE. Patients should be closely monitored and use should be immediately discontinued at the first sign of any of the symptoms described below. Rapid absorption of hexachlorophene may occur with resultant toxic blood levels when preparations containing hexachlorophene are applied to skin lesions such as ichthyosis congenita, the dermatitis of Letterer-Siwe's syndrome, or other generalized dermatological conditions. Application to burns has also produced neurotoxicity and death.

pHisoHex SHOULD BE DISCONTINUED PROMPTLY IF SIGNS OR SYMPTOMS OF CEREBRAL IRRITABILITY OCCUR.

Infants, especially premature infants or those with dermatoses, are particularly susceptible to hexachlorophene absorption. Systemic toxicity may be manifested by signs of stimulation (irritation) of the central nervous system, sometimes with convulsions.

Infants have developed dermatitis, irritability, generalized clonic muscular contractions and decerebrate rigidity following application of a 6 percent hexachlorophene powder. Examination of brainstems of those infants revealed vacuolization like that which can be produced in newborn experimental animals following repeated topical application of 3 percent hexachlorophene. Moreover, a study of histologic sections of premature infants who died of unrelated causes has shown a positive correlation between hexachlorophene baths and lesions in white matter of brains.

PRECAUTIONS

General

Avoid accidental contact of pHisoHex with the eyes.

If contact occurs, promptly rinse thoroughly with water. To assist in the detection of ocular irritation, applications to the head and periorbital skin areas should be performed only in responsive patients with unanesthetized eyes.

RINSE THOROUGHLY AFTER USE, especially from sensitive areas such as the scrotum and perineum.

pHisoHex is intended for external use only. If swallowed, pHisoHex is harmful, especially to infants and children. **pHisoHex should not be poured into measuring cups, medicine bottles, or similar containers since it may be mistaken for baby formula or other medications.**

Carcinogenesis, Mutagenesis, Impairment of Fertility

Carcinogenicity studies in animals: Hexachlorophene was tested in one experiment in rats by oral administration; it had no carcinogenic effect.

Hexachlorophene was not mutagenic in *Salmonella typhimurium* and was negative in a dominant lethal assay in male mice. Cytogenetic tests with cultured human lymphocytes were also negative.

Human data: No case reports or epidemiological studies were available.

Impairment of fertility: Topical exposure of neonatal rats to 3% hexachlorophene solution caused reduced fertility in 7-month-old males, due to inability to ejaculate.

Embryotoxicity and Teratogenicity

Placental transfer of hexachlorophene has been demonstrated in rats.

Hexachlorophene is embryotoxic and produces some teratogenic effects.

Pregnancy Category C

There are no adequate and well-controlled studies in pregnant women. Hexachlorophene should be used during pregnancy only if the potential benefit justifies potential risk to the fetus.

Hexachlorophene has been shown to be teratogenic and embryotoxic in rats when given by mouth or instilled into the vagina in large doses.

Administration of 500 mg/kg diet or 20 to 30 mg/kg bw/day by gavage to rats caused some malformations (angulated ribs, cleft palate, micro- and anophthalmia) and reduction in litter size.

Placental transfer and excretion in milk of hexachlorophene has been demonstrated in rats.

In another study, doses of up to 50 mg/kg diet failed to produce any effects in 3 generations of rats. Hexachlorophene did not interfere with reproduction in hamsters.

Nursing Mothers

It is not known whether this drug is excreted in human milk. Because many drugs are excreted in human milk and because of the potential for serious adverse reactions in nursing infants from hexachlorophene, a decision should be made whether to discontinue nursing or to discontinue the drug taking into account the importance of the drug to the mother.

Pediatric Use

pHisoHex, brand of hexachlorophene detergent cleanser, should not be used routinely for bathing infants. See **WARNINGS.** For premature infants: see **WARNINGS.**

ADVERSE REACTIONS

Adverse reactions to pHisoHex may include dermatitis and photosensitivity. Sensitivity to hexachlorophene is rare; however, persons who have developed photoallergy to similar compounds also may become sensitive to hexachlorophene.

In persons with highly sensitive skin the use of pHisoHex may at times produce a reaction characterized by redness and/or mild scaling or dryness, especially when it is combined with such mechanical factors as excessive rubbing or exposure to heat or cold.

OVERDOSAGE

The accidental ingestion of pHisoHex in amounts from 1 oz to 4 oz has caused anorexia, vomiting, abdominal cramps, diarrhea, dehydration, convulsions, hypotension, and shock, and in several reported instances, fatalities.

If patients are seen early, the stomach should be evacuated by emesis or gastric lavage. Olive oil or vegetable oil (60 mL or 2 fl oz) may then be given to delay absorption of hexachlorophene, followed by a saline cathartic to hasten removal. Treatment is symptomatic and supportive; intravenous fluids (5 percent dextrose in physiologic saline solution) may be given for dehydration. Any other electrolyte derangement should be corrected. If marked hypotension occurs, vasopressor therapy is indicated. Use of opiates may be considered if gastrointestinal symptoms (cramping, diarrhea) are severe. Scheduled medical or surgical procedures should be postponed until the patient's condition has been evaluated and stabilized.

DOSAGE AND ADMINISTRATION

Surgical Hand Scrub

1. Wet hands and forearms with water. Apply approximately 5 mL of pHisoHex over the hands and rub into a copious lather by adding small amounts of water. Spread suds over hands and forearms and scrub well with a wet brush for 3 minutes. Pay particular attention to the nails and interdigital spaces. A separate nail cleaner may be used. *Rinse thoroughly* under running water.
2. Apply 5 mL of pHisoHex to hands again and scrub as above for another 3 minutes. *Rinse thoroughly* with running water and dry.
3. For repeat surgical scrubs during the day, scrub thoroughly with the same amount of pHisoHex for 3 minutes only. *Rinse thoroughly* with water and dry.

Bacteriostatic Cleansing

Wet hands with water. Dispense approximately 5 mL of pHisoHex into the palm, work up a lather with water and apply to area to be cleansed.

Rinse thoroughly after each washing.

INFANT CARE: pHisoHex should not be used routinely for bathing infants. See **WARNINGS.**

PREMATURE INFANTS: See **WARNINGS.**

Use of baby skin products containing alcohol may decrease the antibacterial action of pHisoHex, brand of hexachlorophene detergent cleanser.

HOW SUPPLIED

5 oz plastic squeeze bottle
(NDC 0024-1535-02).
1 pint plastic squeeze bottle
(NDC 0024-1535-06).
1 gallon plastic bottle
(NDC 0024-1535-08).

Prolonged direct exposure of pHisoHex to strong light may cause brownish surface discoloration but does not affect its antibacterial or detergent properties. Shaking will disperse the color. If pHisoHex is spilled or splashed on porous surfaces, rinse off to avoid discoloration.

pHisoHex should not be dispensed from, or stored in, containers with ordinary metal parts. A special type of stainless steel must be used or undesirable discoloration of the product or oxidation of metal may occur.

Directions for Cleaning Dispensers: Before initial installation and use, run an antiseptic, such as an aqueous solution of benzalkonium chloride, NF, 1:500 to 1:750, or alcohol, through the working parts; rinse with sterile water. At weekly intervals thereafter, remove dispenser and pour off remainder of pHisoHex emulsion. Rinse empty dispenser with water. Run water through the working parts by operating the dispenser. Sanitize as described above. Rinse thoroughly with sterile water.

ANIMAL TOXICITY

The oral LD_{50} of hexachlorophene in male rats is 66 mg/kg bw, in females 56 mg/kg bw, and in weanling rats 120 mg/kg bw.

In suckling rats (10-days old), it is 9 mg/kg bw.

Store at room temperature up to 25°C (77°F)

Revised September 1999
PSW-9G

PLAQUENIL® ℞
HYDROXYCHLOROQUINE SULFATE, USP

WARNING
PHYSICIANS SHOULD COMPLETELY FAMILIARIZE THEMSELVES WITH THE COMPLETE CONTENTS OF THIS LEAFLET BEFORE PRESCRIBING HYDROXYCHLOROQUINE.

DESCRIPTION

Hydroxychloroquine sulfate is a colorless crystalline solid, soluble in water to at least 20 percent; chemically the drug is 2-[[4-[(7-Chloro-4- quinolyl) amino] pentyl] ethylamino] ethanol sulfate (1:1).

Plaquenil (hydroxychloroquine sulfate) tablets contain 200 mg hydroxychloroquine sulfate, equivalent to 155 mg base, and are for oral administration.

Inactive Ingredients: Dibasic Calcium Phosphate, Hydroxypropyl Methylcellulose, Magnesium Stearate, Polyethylene glycol 400, Polysorbate 80, Starch, Titanium Dioxide.

ACTIONS

The drug possesses antimalarial actions and also exerts a beneficial effect in lupus erythematosus (chronic discoid or systemic) and acute or chronic rheumatoid arthritis. The precise mechanism of action is not known.

INDICATIONS

PLAQUENIL is indicated for the suppressive treatment and treatment of acute attacks of malaria due to *Plasmodium vivax, P. malariae, P. ovale,* and susceptible strains of *P. falciparum.* It is also indicated for the treatment of discoid and systemic lupus erythematosus, and rheumatoid arthritis.

CONTRAINDICATIONS

Use of this drug is contraindicated (1) in the presence of retinal or visual field changes attributable to any 4-aminoquinoline compound, (2) in patients with known hypersensitivity to 4-aminoquinoline compounds, and (3) for long-term therapy in children.

WARNINGS, General

PLAQUENIL is not effective against chloroquine-resistant strains of *P. falciparum.*

Children are especially sensitive to the 4-aminoquinoline compounds. A number of fatalities have been reported following the accidental ingestion of chloroquine, sometimes in relatively small doses (0.75 g or 1 g in one 3- year-old child). Patients should be strongly warned to keep these drugs out of the reach of children.

Use of PLAQUENIL in patients with psoriasis may precipitate a severe attack of psoriasis. When used in patients with porphyria the condition may be exacerbated. The preparation should not be used in these conditions unless in the judgment of the physician the benefit to the patient outweighs the possible hazard.

Usage in Pregnancy—Usage of this drug during pregnancy should be avoided except in the suppression or treatment of malaria when in the judgment of the physician the benefit outweighs the possible hazard. It should be noted that radioactively-tagged chloroquine administered intravenously to pregnant, pigmented CBA mice passed rapidly across the placenta. It accumulated selectively in the melanin structures of the fetal eyes and was retained in the ocular tissues for five months after the drug had been eliminated from the rest of the body.

PRECAUTIONS, General

Antimalarial compounds should be used with caution in patients with hepatic disease or alcoholism or in conjunction with known hepatotoxic drugs.

Periodic blood cell counts should be made if patients are given prolonged therapy. If any severe blood disorder appears which is not attributable to the disease under treatment, discontinuation of the drug should be considered. The drug should be administered with caution in patients having G-6-PD (glucose-6-phosphate dehydrogenase) deficiency.

OVERDOSAGE

The 4-aminoquinoline compounds are very rapidly and completely absorbed after ingestion, and in accidental overdosage, or rarely with lower doses in hypersensitive patients, toxic symptoms may occur within 30 minutes. These consist of headache, drowsiness, visual disturbances, cardiovascular collapse, and convulsions, followed by sudden and early respiratory and cardiac arrest. The electrocardiogram may reveal atrial standstill, nodal rhythm, prolonged intraventricular conduction time, and progressive bradycardia leading to ventricular fibrillation and/or arrest. Treatment is symptomatic and must be prompt with immediate evacuation of the stomach by emesis (at home, before transportation to the hospital) or gastric lavage until the stomach is completely emptied. If finely powdered, activated charcoal is introduced by the stomach tube, after lavage, and within 30 minutes after ingestion of the tablets, it may inhibit further intestinal absorption of the drug. To be effective, the dose of activated charcoal should be at least five times the estimated dose of hydroxychloroquine ingested. Convulsions, if present, should be controlled before attempting gastric lavage. If due to cerebral stimulation, cautious administration of an ultrashort-acting barbiturate may be tried but, if due to anoxia, it should be corrected by oxygen administration, artificial respiration or, in shock with hypotension, by vasopressor therapy. Because of the importance of supporting respiration, tracheal intubation or tracheostomy, followed by gastric lavage, may also be necessary. Exchange transfusions have been used to reduce the level of 4-aminoquinoline drug in the blood.

A patient who survives the acute phase and is asymptomatic should be closely observed for at least six hours. Fluids may be forced, and sufficient ammonium chloride (8 g daily in divided doses for adults) may be administered for a few days to acidify the urine to help promote urinary excretion in cases of both overdosage and sensitivity.

MALARIA

ACTIONS

Like chloroquine phosphate, USP, PLAQUENIL is highly active against the erythrocytic forms of *P. vivax* and *malariae* and most strains of *P. falciparum* (but not the gametocytes of *P. falciparum*).

PLAQUENIL does not prevent relapses in patients with *vivax* or *malariae* malaria because it is not effective against exo-erythrocytic forms of the parasite, nor will it prevent *vivax* or *malariae* infection when administered as a prophylactic. It is highly effective as a suppressive agent in patients with *vivax* or *malariae* malaria, in terminating acute attacks, and significantly lengthening the interval between treatment and relapse. In patients with *falciparum* malaria, it abolishes the acute attack and effects complete cure of the infection, unless due to a resistant strain of *P. falciparum.*

INDICATIONS

PLAQUENIL is indicated for the treatment of acute attacks and suppression of malaria.

WARNING

In recent years, it has been found that certain strains of *P. falciparum* have become resistant to 4-aminoquinoline compounds (including hydroxychloroquine) as shown by the fact that normally adequate doses have failed to prevent or cure clinical malaria or parasitemia. Treatment with quinine or other specific forms of therapy is therefore advised for patients infected with a resistant strain of parasites.

ADVERSE REACTIONS

Following the administration in doses adequate for the treatment of an acute malarial attack, mild and transient headache, dizziness, and gastrointestinal complaints (diarrhea, anorexia, nausea, abdominal cramps and, on rare occasions, vomiting) may occur.

DOSAGE AND ADMINISTRATION

One tablet of 200 mg of hydroxychloroquine sulfate is equivalent to 155 mg base.

Malaria: Suppression—*In adults,* 400 mg (=310 mg base) on exactly the same day of each week. *In infants and children,* the weekly suppressive dosage is 5 mg, calculated as base, per kg of body weight, but should not exceed the adult dose regardless of weight.

If circumstances permit, suppressive therapy should begin two weeks prior to exposure. However, failing this, in adults an initial double (loading) dose of 800 mg (= 620 mg base), or in children 10 mg base/kg may be taken in two divided doses, six hours apart. The suppressive therapy should be continued for eight weeks after leaving the endemic area.

Treatment of the acute attack—*In adults,* an initial dose of 800 mg (= 620 mg base) followed by 400 mg (= 310 mg base) in six to eight hours and 400 mg (= 310 mg base) on each of two consecutive days (total 2 g hydroxychloroquine sulfate or 1.55 g base). An alternative method, employing a single dose of 800 mg (= 620 mg base), has also proved effective.

The dosage for adults may also be calculated on the basis of body weight; this method is preferred for infants and children. A total dose representing 25 mg of base per kg of body weight is administered in three days, as follows:

First dose: 10 mg base per kg (but not exceeding a single dose of 620 mg base).

Second dose: 5 mg base per kg (but not exceeding a single dose of 310 mg base) 6 hours after first dose.

Third dose: 5 mg base per kg 18 hours after second dose.

Fourth dose: 5 mg base per kg 24 hours after third dose.

For radical cure of *vivax* and *malariae* malaria concomitant therapy with an 8-aminoquinoline compound is necessary.

LUPUS ERYTHEMATOSUS AND RHEUMATOID ARTHRITIS

INDICATIONS

PLAQUENIL is useful in patients with the following disorders who have not responded satisfactorily to drugs with less potential for serious side effects: lupus erythematosus (chronic discoid and systemic) and acute or chronic rheumatoid arthritis.

WARNINGS

PHYSICIANS SHOULD COMPLETELY FAMILIARIZE THEMSELVES WITH THE COMPLETE CONTENTS OF THIS LEAFLET BEFORE PRESCRIBING PLAQUENIL.

Irreversible retinal damage has been observed in some patients who had received long-term or high-dosage 4-aminoquinoline therapy for discoid and systemic lupus erythematosus, or rheumatoid arthritis. Retinopathy has been reported to be dose related.

When prolonged therapy with any antimalarial compound is contemplated, initial (base line) and periodic (every three months) ophthalmologic examinations (including visual acuity, expert slit-lamp, funduscopic, and visual field tests) should be performed.

If there is any indication of abnormality in the visual acuity, visual field, or retinal macular areas (such as pigmentary changes, loss of foveal reflex), or any visual symptoms (such as light flashes and streaks) which are not fully explainable by difficulties of accommodation or corneal opacities, the drug should be discontinued immediately and the patient closely observed for possible progression. Retinal changes (and visual disturbances) may progress even after cessation of therapy.

All patients on long-term therapy with this preparation should be questioned and examined periodically, including the testing of knee and ankle reflexes, to detect any evidence of muscular weakness. If weakness occurs, discontinue the drug.

In the treatment of rheumatoid arthritis, if objective improvement (such as reduced joint swelling, increased mobility) does not occur within six months, the drug should be discontinued. Safe use of the drug in the treatment of juvenile arthritis has not been established.

PRECAUTIONS

Dermatologic reactions to PLAQUENIL may occur and, therefore, proper care should be exercised when it is administered to any patient receiving a drug with a significant tendency to produce dermatitis.

The methods recommended for early diagnosis of "chloroquine retinopathy" consist of (1) funduscopic examination of the macula for fine pigmentary disturbances or loss of the foveal reflex and (2) examination of the central visual field with a small red test object for pericentral or paracentral scotoma or determination of retinal thresholds to red. Any unexplained visual symptoms, such as light flashes or streaks should also be regarded with suspicion as possible manifestations of retinopathy.

If serious toxic symptoms occur from overdosage or sensitivity, it has been suggested that ammonium chloride (8 g daily in divided doses for adults) be administered orally three or four days a week for several months after therapy has been stopped, as acidification of the urine increases renal excretion of the 4-aminoquinoline compounds by 20 to 90 percent. However, caution must be exercised in patients with impaired renal function and/or metabolic acidosis.

ADVERSE REACTIONS

Not all of the following reactions have been observed with every 4-aminoquinoline compound during long-term therapy, but they have been reported with one or more and should be borne in mind when drugs of this class are administered. Adverse effects with different compounds vary in type and frequency.

CNS Reactions: Irritability, nervousness, emotional changes, nightmares, psychosis, headache, dizziness, vertigo, tinnitus, nystagmus, nerve deafness, convulsions, ataxia.

Neuromuscular Reactions: Extraocular muscle palsies, skeletal muscle weakness, absent or hypoactive deep tendon reflexes.

Ocular Reactions:

A. *Ciliary body:* Disturbance of accommodation with symptoms of blurred vision. This reaction is dose related and reversible with cessation of therapy.

B. *Cornea:* Transient edema, punctate to lineal opacities, decreased corneal sensitivity. The corneal changes, with or without accompanying symptoms (blurred vision, halos around lights, photophobia), are fairly common, but reversible. Corneal deposits may appear as early as three weeks following initiation of therapy.

The incidence of corneal changes and visual side effects appears to be considerably lower with hydroxychloroquine than with chloroquine.

C. *Retina:*

Macula: Edema, atrophy, abnormal pigmentation (mild pigment stippling to a "bull's-eye" appearance), loss of foveal reflex, increased macular recovery time following exposure to a bright light (photo-stress test), elevated retinal threshold to red light in macular, paramacular, and peripheral retinal areas.

Other fundus changes include optic disc pallor and atrophy, attenuation of retinal arterioles, fine granular pigmentary disturbances in the peripheral retina and prominent choroidal patterns in advanced stage.

D. *Visual field defects:* pericentral or paracentral scotoma, central scotoma with decreased visual acuity, rarely field constriction.

The most common visual symptoms attributed to the retinopathy are: reading and seeing difficulties (words, letters, or parts of objects missing), photophobia, blurred distance vision, missing or blacked out areas in the central or peripheral visual field, light flashes and streaks.

Retinopathy appears to be dose related and has occurred within several months (rarely) to several years of daily therapy; a small number of cases have been reported several years after antimalarial drug therapy was discontinued. It has not been noted during prolonged use of weekly doses of the 4-aminoquinoline compounds for suppression of malaria.

Patients with retinal changes may have visual symptoms or may be asymptomatic (with or without visual field changes). Rarely scotomatous vision or field defects may occur without obvious retinal change.

Retinopathy may progress even after the drug is discontinued. In a number of patients, early retinopathy (macular pigmentation sometimes with central field defects) diminished or regressed completely after therapy was discontinued. Paracentral scotoma to red targets (sometimes called "premaculopathy") is indicative of early retinal dysfunction which is usually reversible with cessation of therapy.

A small number of cases of retinal changes have been reported as occurring in patients who received only hydroxychloroquine. These usually consisted of alteration in retinal pigmentation which was detected on periodic ophthalmologic examination; visual field defects were also present in some instances. A case of delayed retinopathy has been reported with loss of vision starting one year after administration of hydroxychloroquine had been discontinued.

Dermatologic Reactions: Bleaching of hair, alopecia, pruritus, skin and mucosal pigmentation, skin eruptions (urticarial, morbilliform, lichenoid, maculopapular, purpuric, erythema annulare centrifugum and exfoliative dermatitis).

Hematologic Reactions: Various blood dyscrasias such as aplastic anemia, agranulocytosis, leukopenia, thrombocytopenia (hemolysis in individuals with glucose-6-phosphate dehydrogenase (G-6-PD) deficiency).

Gastrointestinal Reactions: Anorexia, nausea, vomiting, diarrhea, and abdominal cramps.

Miscellaneous Reactions: Weight loss, lassitude, exacerbation or precipitation of porphyria and nonlight-sensitive psoriasis.

Cardiomyopathy has been rarely reported and the relationship to hydroxychloroquine is unclear.

DOSAGE AND ADMINISTRATION

One tablet of hydroxychloroquine sulfate, 200 mg, is equivalent to 155 mg base.

Lupus erythematosus—Initially, the average *adult* dose is 400 mg (=310 mg base) once or twice daily. This may be continued for several weeks or months, depending on the response of the patient. For prolonged maintenance therapy, a smaller dose, from 200 mg to 400 mg (= 155 mg to 310 mg base) daily will frequently suffice.

The incidence of retinopathy has been reported to be higher when this maintenance dose is exceeded.

Rheumatoid arthritis—The compound is cumulative in action and will require several weeks to exert its beneficial therapeutic effects, whereas minor side effects may occur relatively early. Several months of therapy may be required before maximum effects can be obtained. If objective improvement (such as reduced joint swelling, increased mobility) does not occur within six months, the drug should be discontinued. Safe use of the drug in the treatment of juvenile rheumatoid arthritis has not been established.

Initial dosage—In **adults,** from 400 mg to 600 mg (=310 mg to 465 mg base) daily, each dose to be taken with a meal or a glass of milk. In a small percentage of patients, troublesome side effects may require temporary reduction of the initial dosage. Later (usually from five to ten days), the dose may gradually be increased to the optimum response level, often without return of side effects.

Maintenance dosage—When a good response is obtained (usually in four to twelve weeks), the dosage is reduced by 50 percent and continued at a usual maintenance level of

Continued on next page

This product information was prepared in September 2000. On these and other products of Sanofi-Synthelabo Inc., detailed information may be obtained on a current basis by direct inquiry to Product Information Services, 90 Park Avenue, New York, NY 10016 (toll free 1-800-446-6267).

Plaquenil—Cont.

200 mg to 400 mg (=155 mg to 310 mg base) daily, each dose to be taken with a meal or a glass of milk. The incidence of retinopathy has been reported to be higher when this maintenance dose is exceeded.

Should a relapse occur after medication is withdrawn, therapy may be resumed or continued on an intermittent schedule if there are no ocular contraindications.

Corticosteroids and salicylates may be used in conjunction with this compound, and they can generally be decreased gradually in dosage or eliminated after the drug has been used for several weeks. When gradual reduction of steroid dosage is indicated, it may be done by reducing every four to five days the dose of cortisone by no more than from 5 mg to 15 mg; of hydrocortisone from 5 mg to 10 mg; of prednisolone and prednisone from 1 mg to 2.5 mg; of methylprednisolone and triamcinolone from 1 mg to 2 mg; and of dexamethasone from 0.25 mg to 0.5 mg.

HOW SUPPLIED

Plaquenil tablets are white, to off-white, film coated tablets imprinted "PLAQUENIL" on one face in black ink. Each tablet contains 200 mg hydroxychloroquine sulfate (equivalent to 155 mg base). Bottles of 100 tablets (NDC 0024-1562-10).

Dispense in a tight, light-resistant container as defined in the USP/NF.

Store at room temperature up to 30°C (86°F).

PSW-5D

Shown in Product Identification Guide, page 333

Revised November 1998

PLAVIX®
clopidogrel bisulfate tablets ℞

DESCRIPTION

PLAVIX (clopidogrel bisulfate) is an inhibitor of ADP-induced platelet aggregation acting by direct inhibition of adenosine diphosphate (ADP) binding to its receptor and of the subsequent ADP-mediated activation of the glycoprotein GPIIb/IIIa complex. Chemically it is methyl (+)-(*S*)-α-(2-chlorophenyl)-6,7-dihydrothieno[3,2-c]pyridine-5(4*H*)-acetate sulfate (1:1). The empirical formula of clopidogrel bisulfate is $C_{16}H_{16}Cl\ NO_2S \bullet H_2SO_4$ and its molecular weight is 419.9.

The structural formula is as follows:

Clopidogrel bisulfate is a white to off-white powder. It is practically insoluble in water at neutral pH but freely soluble at pH 1. It also dissolves freely in methanol, dissolves sparingly in methylene chloride, and is practically insoluble in ethyl ether. It has a specific optical rotation of about +56°.

PLAVIX for oral administration is provided as pink, round, biconvex, debossed film-coated tablets containing 97.875 mg of clopidogrel bisulfate which is the molar equivalent of 75 mg of clopidogrel base.

Each tablet contains anhydrous lactose, hydrogenated castor oil, microcrystalline cellulose, polyethylene glycol 6000 and pregelatinized starch as inactive ingredients. The pink film coating contains ferric oxide (red), hydroxypropyl methylcellulose 2910, polyethylene glycol 6000 and titanium dioxide. The tablets are polished with Carnauba wax.

CLINICAL PHARMACOLOGY

Mechanism of Action

Clopidogrel is an inhibitor of platelet aggregation. A variety of drugs that inhibit platelet function have been shown to decrease morbid events in people with established atherosclerotic cardiovascular disease as evidenced by stroke or transient ischemic attacks, myocardial infarction, or need for bypass or angioplasty. This indicates that platelets participate in the initiation and/or evolution of these events and that inhibiting them can reduce the event rate.

Pharmacodynamic Properties

Clopidogrel selectively inhibits the binding of adenosine diphosphate (ADP) to its platelet receptor and the subsequent ADP-mediated activation of the glycoprotein GPIIb/IIIa complex, thereby inhibiting platelet aggregation. Biotransformation of clopidogrel is necessary to produce inhibition of platelet aggregation, but an active metabolite responsible for the activity of the drug has not been isolated. Clopidogrel also inhibits platelet aggregation induced by agonists other than ADP by blocking the amplification of platelet activation by released ADP. Clopidogrel does not inhibit phosphodiesterase activity.

Clopidogrel acts by irreversibly modifying the platelet ADP receptor. Consequently, platelets exposed to clopidogrel are affected for the remainder of their lifespan.

Dose dependent inhibition of platelet aggregation can be seen 2 hours after single oral doses of PLAVIX. Repeated doses of 75 mg PLAVIX per day inhibit ADP-induced platelet aggregation on the first day, and inhibition reaches steady state between Day 3 and Day 7. At steady state, the average inhibition level observed with a dose of 75 mg PLAVIX per day was between 40% and 60%. Platelet aggregation and bleeding time gradually return to baseline values after treatment is discontinued, generally in about 5 days.

Pharmacokinetics and Metabolism

After repeated 75–mg oral doses of clopidogrel (base), plasma concentrations of the parent compound, which has no platelet inhibiting effect, are very low and are generally below the quantification limit (0.00025 mg/L) beyond 2 hours after dosing. Clopidogrel is extensively metabolized by the liver. The main circulating metabolite is the carboxylic acid derivative, and it too has no effect on platelet aggregation. It represents about 85% of the circulating drug-related compounds in plasma.

Following an oral dose of ^{14}C-labeled clopidogrel in humans, approximately 50% was excreted in the urine and approximately 46% in the feces in the 5 days after dosing. The elimination half-life of the main circulating metabolite was 8 hours after single and repeated administration. Covalent binding to platelets accounted for 2% of radiolabel with a half-life of 11 days.

Effect of Food: Administration of PLAVIX (clopidogrel bisulfate) with meals did not significantly modify the bioavailability of clopidogrel as assessed by the pharmacokinetics of the main circulating metabolite.

Absorption and Distribution: Clopidogrel is rapidly absorbed after oral administration of repeated doses of 75 mg clopidogrel (base), with peak plasma levels (≅3 mg/L) of the main circulating metabolite occurring approximately 1 hour after dosing. The pharmacokinetics of the main circulating metabolite are linear (plasma concentrations increased in proportion to dose) in the dose range of 50 to 150 mg of clopidogrel. Absorption is at least 50% based on urinary excretion of clopidogrel-related metabolites.

Clopidogrel and the main circulating metabolite bind reversibly *in vitro* to human plasma proteins (98% and 94%, respectively). The binding is nonsaturable *in vitro* up to a concentration of 100 µg/mL.

Metabolism and Elimination: *In vitro* and *in vivo*, clopidogrel undergoes rapid hydrolysis into its carboxylic acid derivative. In plasma and urine, the glucuronide of the carboxylic acid derivative is also observed.

Special Populations

Geriatric Patients: Plasma concentrations of the main circulating metabolite are significantly higher in elderly (≥75 years) compared to young healthy volunteers but these higher plasma levels were not associated with differences in platelet aggregation and bleeding time. No dosage adjustment is needed for the elderly.

Renally Impaired Patients: After repeated doses of 75 mg PLAVIX per day, plasma levels of the main circulating metabolite were lower in patients with severe renal impairment (creatinine clearance from 5 to 15 mL/min) compared to subjects with moderate renal impairment (creatinine clearance 30 to 60 mL/min) or healthy subjects. Although inhibition of ADP-induced platelet aggregation was lower (25%) than that observed in healthy volunteers, the prolongation of bleeding time was similar to healthy volunteers receiving 75 mg of PLAVIX per day. No dosage adjustment is needed in renally impaired patients.

Gender: No significant difference was observed in the plasma levels of the main circulating metabolite between males and females. In a small study comparing men and women, less inhibition of ADP-induced platelet aggregation was observed in women, but there was no difference in prolongation of bleeding time. In the large, controlled clinical study (Clopidogrel vs. Aspirin in Patients at Risk of Ischemic Events; CAPRIE), the incidence of clinical outcome events, other adverse clinical events, and abnormal clinical laboratory parameters was similar in men and women.

Race: Pharmacokinetic differences due to race have not been studied.

CLINICAL STUDIES

The clinical evidence for the efficacy of PLAVIX is derived from the CAPRIE (Clopidogrel vs. Aspirin in Patients at Risk of Ischemic Events) trial. This was a 19,185-patient, 304-center, international, randomized, double-blind, parallel-group study comparing PLAVIX (75 mg daily) to aspirin (325 mg daily). The patients randomized had: 1) recent histories of myocardial infarction (within 35 days); 2) recent histories of ischemic stroke (within 6 months) with at least a week of residual neurological signs; or 3) objectively established peripheral arterial disease. Patients received randomized treatment for an average of 1.6 years (maximum of 3 years).

The trial's primary outcome was the time to first occurrence of new ischemic stroke (fatal or not), new myocardial infarction (fatal or not), or other vascular death. Deaths not easily attributable to nonvascular causes were all classified as vascular.

Outcome Events of the Primary Analysis

Patients	PLAVIX 9599	apririn 9586
IS (fatal or not)	438 (4.56%)	461 (4.81%)
MI (fatal or not)	275 (2.86%)	333 (3.47%)
Other vascular death	226 (2.35%)	226 (2.36%)
Total	939 (9.78%)	1020 (10.64%)

As shown in the table, PLAVIX (clopidogrel bisulfate) was associated with a lower incidence of outcome events of every kind. The overall risk reduction (9.78% vs. 10.64%) was 8.7%, P=0.045. Similar results were obtained when all-cause mortality and all-cause strokes were counted instead of vascular mortality and ischemic strokes (risk reduction 6.9%). In patients who survived an on-study stroke or myocardial infarction, the incidence of subsequent events was again lower in the PLAVIX group.

The curves showing the overall event rate are shown in the figure. The event curves separated early and continued to diverge over the 3-year follow-up period.

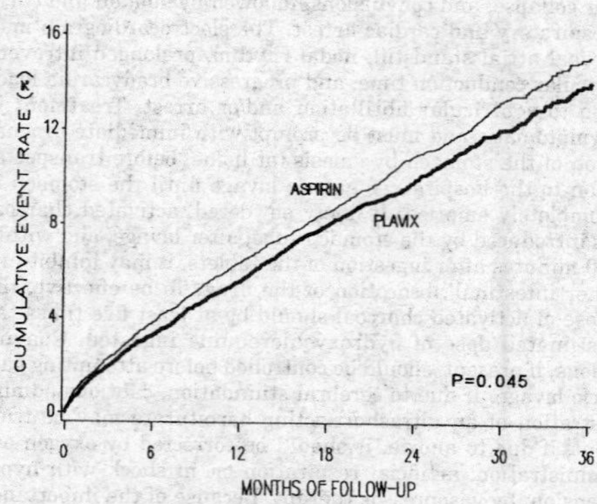

Although the statistical significance favoring PLAVIX over aspirin was marginal (P=0.045), and represents the result of a single trial that has not been replicated, the comparator drug, aspirin, is itself effective (vs. placebo) in reducing cardiovascular events in patients with recent myocardial infarction or stroke. Thus, the difference between PLAVIX and placebo, although not measured directly, is substantial.

The CAPRIE trial included a population that was randomized on the basis of 3 entry criteria. The efficacy of PLAVIX relative to aspirin was heterogeneous across these randomized subgroups (P=0.043). It is not clear whether this difference is real or a chance occurrence. Although the CAPRIE trial was not designed to evaluate the relative benefit of PLAVIX over aspirin in the individual patient subgroups, the benefit appeared to be strongest in patients who were enrolled because of peripheral vascular disease (especially those who also had a history of myocardial infarction) and weaker in stroke patients. In patients who were enrolled in the trial on the sole basis of a recent myocardial infarction, PLAVIX was not numerically superior to aspirin.

In the meta-analyses of studies of aspirin vs. placebo in patients similar to those in CAPRIE, aspirin was associated with a reduced incidence of atherothrombotic events. There was a suggestion of heterogeneity in these studies too, with the effect strongest in patients with a history of myocardial infarction, weaker in patients with a history of stroke, and not discernible in patients with a history of peripheral vascular disease. With respect to the inferred comparison of PLAVIX to placebo, there is no indication of heterogeneity.

INDICATIONS AND USAGE

PLAVIX (clopidogrel bisulfate) is indicated for the reduction of atherosclerotic events (myocardial infarction, stroke, and vascular death) in patients with atherosclerosis documented by recent stroke, recent myocardial infarction, or established peripheral arterial disease.

CONTRAINDICATIONS

The use of PLAVIX is contraindicated in the following conditions:

- Hypersensitivity to the drug substance or any component of the product.
- Active pathological bleeding such as peptic ulcer or intracranial hemorrhage.

WARNINGS

Thrombotic thrombocytopenic purpura (TTP): TTP has been reported rarely following use of PLAVIX, sometimes after a short exposure (<2 weeks). TTP is a serious condition requiring prompt treatment. It is characterized by thrombocytopenia, microangiopathic hemolytic anemia (schistocytes [fragmented RBCs] seen on peripheral smear), neurological findings, renal dysfunction, and fever. TTP was not seen during clopidogrel's clinical trials, which included over 11,300 clopidogrel-treated patients. In world-wide postmarketing experience, however, TTP has been reported at a rate of about four cases per million patients exposed, or about 11 cases per million patient-years. The background rate is thought to be about four cases per million person-years.

PRECAUTIONS

General

As with other anti-platelet agents, PLAVIX should be used with caution in patients who may be at risk of increased bleeding from trauma, surgery, or other pathological conditions. If a patient is to undergo elective surgery and an antiplatelet effect is not desired, PLAVIX should be discontinued 7 days prior to surgery.

GI Bleeding: PLAVIX prolongs the bleeding time. In CAPRIE, PLAVIX was associated with a rate of gastrointestinal bleeding of 2.0%, vs. 2.7% on aspirin. PLAVIX should be used with caution in patients who have lesions with a propensity to bleed (such as ulcers). Drugs that might induce such lesions (such as aspirin and other nonsteroidal anti-inflammatory drugs [NSAIDs]) should be used with caution in patients taking PLAVIX.

Use in Hepatically Impaired Patients: Experience is limited in patients with severe hepatic disease, who may have bleeding diatheses. PLAVIX should be used with caution in this population.

Information for Patients

Patients should be told that it may take them longer than usual to stop bleeding when they take PLAVIX, and that they should report any unusual bleeding to their physician. Patients should inform physicians and dentists that they are taking PLAVIX before any surgery is scheduled and before any new drug is taken.

Drug Interactions

Study of specific drug interactions yielded the following results:

Aspirin: Aspirin did not modify the clopidogrel-mediated inhibition of ADP-induced platelet aggregation. Concomitant administration of 500 mg of aspirin twice a day for 1 day did not significantly increase the prolongation of bleeding time induced by PLAVIX. PLAVIX potentiated the effect of aspirin on collagen-induced platelet aggregation. The safety of chronic concomitant administration of aspirin and PLAVIX has not been established.

Heparin: In a study in healthy volunteers, PLAVIX did not necessitate modification of the heparin dose or alter the effect of heparin on coagulation. Coadministration of heparin had no effect on inhibition of platelet aggregation induced by PLAVIX. The safety of this combination has not been established, however, and concomitant use should be undertaken with caution.

Nonsteroidal Anti-Inflammatory Drugs (NSAIDs): In healthy volunteers receiving naproxen, concomitant administration of PLAVIX was associated with increased occult gastrointestinal blood loss. NSAIDs and PLAVIX should be coadministered with caution.

Warfarin: The safety of the coadministration of PLAVIX with warfarin has not been established. Consequently, concomitant administration of these two agents should be undertaken with caution. (See **Precautions - General**).

Other Concomitant Therapy: No clinically significant pharmacodynamic interactions were observed when PLAVIX was coadministered with **atenolol, nifedipine**, or both atenolol and nifedipine. The pharmacodynamic activity of PLAVIX was also not significantly influenced by the coadministration of **phenobarbital, cimetidine** or **estrogen**.

The pharmacokinetics of **digoxin** or **theophylline** were not modified by the coadministration of PLAVIX (clopidogrel bisulfate).

At high concentrations *in vitro*, clopidogrel inhibits P_{450} (2C9). Accordingly, PLAVIX may interfere with the metabolism of **phenytoin, tamoxifen, tolbutamide, warfarin, torsemide, fluvastatin,** and many **nonsteroidal anti-inflammatory agents**, but there are no data with which to predict the magnitude of these interactions. Caution should be used when any of these drugs is coadministered with PLAVIX.

In addition to the above specific interaction studies, patients entered into CAPRIE received a variety of concomitant medications **including diuretics, beta-blocking agents, angiotensin converting enzyme inhibitors, calcium antagonists, cholesterol lowering agents, coronary vasodilators, antidiabetic agents, antiepileptic agents** and **hormone replacement therapy** without evidence of clinically significant adverse interactions.

Drug/Laboratory Test Interactions

None known.

Carcinogenesis, Mutagenesis, Impairment of Fertility

There was no evidence of tumorigenicity when clopidogrel was administered for 78 weeks to mice and 104 weeks to rats at dosages up to 77 mg/kg per day, which afforded plasma exposures >25 times that in humans at the recommended daily dose of 75 mg.

Clopidogrel was not genotoxic in four *in vitro* tests (Ames test, DNA-repair test in rat hepatocytes, gene mutation assay in Chinese hamster fibroblasts, and metaphase chromosome analysis of human lymphocytes) and in one *in vivo* test (micronucleus test by oral route in mice).

Clopidogrel was found to have no effect on fertility of male and female rats at oral doses up to 400 mg/kg per day (52 times the recommended human dose on a mg/m^2 basis).

Pregnancy

Pregnancy Category B. Reproduction studies performed in rats and rabbits at doses up to 500 and 300 mg/kg/day (respectively, 65 and 78 times the recommended daily human dose on a mg/m^2 basis), revealed no evidence of impaired fertility or fetotoxicity due to clopidogrel. There are, however, no adequate and well-controlled studies in pregnant women. Because animal reproduction studies are not always predictive of a human response, PLAVIX should be used during pregnancy only if clearly needed.

Nursing Mothers

Studies in rats have shown that clopidogrel and/or its metabolites are excreted in the milk. It is not known whether this drug is excreted in human milk. Because many drugs are excreted in human milk and because of the potential for serious adverse reactions in nursing infants, a decision should be made whether to discontinue nursing or to discontinue the drug, taking into account the importance of the drug to the nursing woman.

Pediatric Use

Safety and effectiveness in the pediatric population have not been established.

ADVERSE REACTIONS

PLAVIX has been evaluated for safety in more than 11,300 patients, including over 7,000 patients treated for 1 year or more. The overall tolerability of PLAVIX was similar to that of aspirin regardless of age, gender and race, with an approximately equal incidence (13%) of patients withdrawing from treatment because of adverse reactions. The clinically important adverse events observed in CAPRIE are discussed below.

Hemorrhagic: In patients receiving PLAVIX in CAPRIE, gastrointestinal hemorrhage occurred at a rate of 2.0%, and required hospitalization in 0.7%. In patients receiving aspirin, the corresponding rates were 2.7% and 1.1%, respectively. The incidence of intracranial hemorrhage was 0.4% for PLAVIX compared to 0.5% for aspirin.

Neutropenia/agranulocytosis: Ticlopidine, a drug chemically similar to PLAVIX, is associated with a 0.8% rate of severe neutropenia (less than 450 neutrophils/μL). Patients in CAPRIE (see Clinical Trials) were intensively monitored for neutropenia. Severe neutropenia was observed in six patients, four on PLAVIX and two on aspirin. Two of the 9599 patients who received PLAVIX and none of the 9586 patients who received aspirin had neutrophil counts of zero. One of the four PLAVIX patients was receiving cytotoxic chemotherapy, and another recovered and returned to the trial after only temporarily interrupting treatment with PLAVIX.

Although the risk of myelotoxicity with PLAVIX thus appears to be quite low, this possibility should be considerd when a patient receiving PLAVIX demonstrates fever or other sign of infection.

Gastrointestinal: Overall, the incidence of gastrointestinal events (e.g. abdominal pain, dyspepsia, gastritis and constipation) in patients receiving PLAVIX (clopidogrel bisulfate) was 27.1%, compared to 29.8% in those receiving aspirin.

The incidence of peptic, gastric or duodenal ulcers was 0.7% for PLAVIX and 1.2% for aspirin.

Cases of diarrhea were reported in 4.5% of patients in the PLAVIX group compared to 3.4% in the aspirin group. However, these were rarely severe (PLAVIX=0.2% and aspirin=0.1%).

The incidence of patients withdrawing from treatment because of gastrointestinal adverse reactions was 3.2% for PLAVIX and 4.0% for aspirin.

Rash and Other Skin Disorders: The incidence of skin and appendage disorders in patients receiving PLAVIX was 15.8% (0.7% serious); the corresponding rate in aspirin patients was 13.1% (0.5% serious).

The overall incidence of patients withdrawing from treatment because of skin and appendage disorders adverse reactions was 1.5% for PLAVIX and 0.8% for aspirin.

Adverse events occurring in ≥2.5% of patients on PLAVIX in the CAPRIE controlled clinical trial are shown below regardless of relationship to PLAVIX. The median duration of therapy was 20 months, with a maximum of 3 years.

Adverse Events Occurring in ≥2.5% of PLAVIX Patients

Body System Event	% Incidence (% Discontinuation) PLAVIX [n=9599]	 Aspirin [n=9586]
Body as a Whole - general disorders		
Chest Pain	8.3 (0.2)	8.3 (0.3)
Accidental Injury	7.9 (0.1)	7.3 (0.1)
Influenza-like symptoms	7.5 (<0.1)	7.0 (<0.1)
Pain	6.4 (0.1)	6.3 (0.1)
Fatigue	3.3 (0.1)	3.4 (0.1)
Cardiovascular disorders, general		
Edema	4.1 (<0.1)	4.5 (<0.1)
Hypertension	4.3 (<0.1)	5.1 (<0.1)
Central & peripheral nervous system disorders		
Headache	7.6 (0.3)	7.2 (0.2)
Dizziness	6.2 (0.2)	6.7 (0.3)
Gastrointestinal system disorders		
Abdominal pain	5.6 (0.7)	7.1 (1.0)
Dyspepsia	5.2 (0.6)	6.1 (0.7)
Diarrhea	4.5 (0.4)	3.4 (0.3)
Nausea	3.4 (0.5)	3.8 (0.4)
Metabolic & nutritional disorders		
Hypercholesterolemia	4.0 (0)	4.4 (<0.1)
Musculo-skeletal system disorders		
Arthralgia	6.3 (0.1)	6.2 (0.1)
Back Pain	5.8 (0.1)	5.3 (<0.1)
Platelet, bleeding, & clotting disorders		
Purpura	5.3 (0.3)	3.7 (0.1)
Epistaxis	2.9 (0.2)	2.5 (0.1)
Psychiatric disorders		
Depression	3.6 (0.1)	3.9 (0.2)
Respiratory system disorders		
Upper resp tract infection	8.7 (<0.1)	8.3 (<0.1)
Dyspnea	4.5 (0.1)	4.7 (0.1)
Rhinitis	4.2 (0.1)	4.2 (<0.1)
Bronchitis	3.7 (0.1)	3.7 (0)
Coughing	3.1 (<0.1)	2.7 (<0.1)
Skin & appendage disorders		
Rash	4.2 (0.5)	3.5 (0.2)
Pruritus	3.3 (0.3)	1.6 (0.1)
Urinary system disorders		
Urinary tract infection	3.1 (0)	3.5 (0.1)

Incidence of discontinuation, regardless of relationship to therapy, is shown in parentheses.

Other adverse experiences of potential importance occurring in 1% to 2.5% of patients receiving PLAVIX (clopidogrel bisulfate) in the CAPRIE controlled clinical trial are listed below regardless of relationship to PLAVIX. In general, the incidence of these events was similar in the aspirin-treated group.

Autonomic Nervous System Disorders: Syncope, Palpitation. *Body as a Whole - general disorders:* Asthenia, Hernia. *Cardiovascular disorders:* Cardiac failure. *Central and peripheral nervous system disorders:* Cramps legs, Hypoaesthesia, Neuralgia, Paraesthesia, Vertigo. *Gastrointestinal system disorders:* Constipation, Vomiting. *Heart rate and rhythm disorders:* Fibrillation atrial. *Liver and biliary system disorders:* Hepatic enzymes increased. *Metabolic and nutritional disorders:* Gout, hyperuricemia, non-protein nitrogen (NPN) increased. *Musculo-skeletal system disorders:* Arthritis, Arthrosis. *Platelet, bleeding & clotting disorders:* GI hemorrhage, hematoma, platelets decreased. *Psychiatric disorders:* Anxiety, Insomnia. *Red blood cell disorders:* Anemia. *Respiratory system disorders:* Pneumonia, Sinusitis. *Skin and appendage disorders:* Eczema, Skin ulceration. *Urinary system disorders:* Cystitis. *Vision disorders:* Cataract, Conjunctivitis.

Other potentially serious adverse events which may be of clinical interest but were rarely reported (<1%) in patients who received PLAVIX are listed below regardless of relationship to PLAVIX. In general, the incidence of these events was similar in the aspirin group.

Body as a whole: Allergic reaction, necrosis ischemic. *Cardiovascular disorders:* Edema generalized. *Gastrointestinal system disorders:* Gastric ulcer perforated, gastritis hemorrhagic, upper GI ulcer hemorrhagic. *Liver and Biliary system disorders:* Bilirubinemia, hepatitis infectious, liver fatty. *Platelet, bleeding and clotting disorders:* hemarthrosis, hematuria, hemoptysis, hemorrhage intracranial, hemorrhage retroperitoneal, hemorrhage of operative wound, ocular hemorrhage, pulmonary hemorrhage, purpura allergic, thrombocytopenia. *Red blood cell disorders:* Anemia aplastic, anemia hypochromic. *Reproductive disorders, female:* Menorrhagia. *Respiratory system disorders:* Hemothorax. *Skin and appendage disorders:* Bullous eruption, rash erythematous, rash maculopapular, urticaria. *White cell and reticuloendothelial system disorders:* Agranulocytosis, granulocytopenia, leukemia, leukopenia, neutrophils decreased.

Postmarketing Experience

The following events have been reported spontaneously from worldwide postmarketing experience: very rare cases of hypersensitivity reactions including angioedema, bronchospasms, and anaphylactoid reactions. Suspected thrombotic thrombocytopenic purpura (TTP) has been reported as part of the world-wide postmarketing experience, see **WARNINGS**.

OVERDOSAGE

One case of deliberate overdosage with PLAVIX was reported in the large, controlled clinical study. A 34-year-old woman took a single 1,050-mg dose of PLAVIX (equivalent to 14 standard 75-mg tablets). There were no associated adverse events. No special therapy was instituted, and she recovered without sequelae.

No adverse events were reported after single oral administration of 600 mg (equivalent to 8 standard 75-mg tablets) of PLAVIX in healthy volunteers. The bleeding time was prolonged by a factor of 1.7, which is similar to that typically observed with the therapeutic dose of 75 mg of PLAVIX per day.

A single oral dose or clopidogrel at 1500 or 2000 mg/kg was lethal to mice and to rats and at 3000 mg/kg to baboons. Symptoms of acute toxicity were vomiting (in baboons), prostration, difficult breathing, and gastrointestinal hemorrhage in all species.

Recommendations About Specific Treatment:

Based on biological plausibility, platelet transfusion may be appropriate to reverse the pharmacological effects of PLAVIX if quick reversal is required.

DOSAGE AND ADMINISTRATION

The recommended dose of PLAVIX is 75 mg once daily with or without food.

Continued on next page

This product information was prepared in September 2000. On these and other products of Sanofi-Synthelabo Inc., detailed information may be obtained on a current basis by direct inquiry to Product Information Services, 90 Park Avenue, New York, NY 10016 (toll free 1-800-446-6267).

Plavix—Cont.

No dosage adjustment is necessary for elderly patients or patients with renal disease. (See **Clinical Pharmacology: Special Populations.**)

HOW SUPPLIED

PLAVIX (clopidogrel bisulfate) is available as a pink, round, biconvex, film-coated tablet debossed with "75" on one side and "1171" on the other. Tablets are provided as follows:
NDC 63653-1171-6 bottles of 30
NDC 63653-1171-1 bottles of 90
NDC 63653-1171-5 bottles of 500
NDC 63653-1171-3 blisters of 100

Storage

Store at 25°C (77°F); excursions permitted to 15°-30°C (59°-86°F) [See USP Controlled Room Temperature]
Manufactured by:
Sanofi-Synthelabo Inc.
New York, NY 10016
Distributed by:
Bristol-Myers Squibb/Sanofi Pharmaceuticals Partnership
New York, NY 10016
PLAVIX® is a registered trademark of Sanofi-Synthelabo
Revised April 2000
1171 DIM-07 1081251AS
Shown in Product Identification Guide, page 333

POLY-HISTINE CS® ℂ ℞

Each 5 ml raspberry/strawberry flavored alcohol-free, red syrup contains:

Codeine Phosphate	10.0 mg
(Warning: May be habit forming.)	
Phenylpropanolamine HCl	12.5 mg
Brompheniramine Maleate	2.0 mg

HOW SUPPLIED

Bottles of 16 oz.
NDC 0024-1633-16

POLY-HISTINE ELIXIR® ℞

Each teaspoonful (5 ml) lemon-lime flavored green elixir contains:

Phenyltoloxamine Citrate	4.0 mg
Pyrilamine Maleate	4.0 mg
Pheniramine Maleate	4.0 mg
Alcohol	4%

HOW SUPPLIED

Bottles of 16 oz.
NDC 0024-1647-16

POLY-HISTINE-D® ELIXIR ℞

Each teaspoonful (5 ml) wild cherry flavored red elixir contains:

Phenylpropanolamine HCl	12.5 mg
Phenyltoloxamine Citrate	4.0 mg
Pyrilamine Maleate	4.0 mg
Pheniramine Maleate	4.0 mg
Alcohol	4%

HOW SUPPLIED

Bottles of 16 oz.
NDC 0024-1662-16

POLY-HISTINE DM® SYRUP ℞

Each 5 ml black-raspberry flavored alcohol-free, sugar free purple syrup contains:

Dextromethorphan HBr	10.0 mg
Phenylpropanolamine HCl	12.5 mg
Brompheniramine Maleate	2.0 mg

HOW SUPPLIED

Bottles of 16 oz.
NDC 0024-1686-16

PRENATE ADVANCE™ TABLETS ℞
PRENATAL VITAMINS

DESCRIPTION

PRENATE ADVANCE™ is a white oval oil-and water-soluble multivitamin/multimineral tablet which contains calcium carbonate and Microlron II® carbonyl iron. The tablet is imprinted with "PRENATE" on both sides.

Each tablet contains:

Elemental Iron (carbonyl iron)	90 mg
Calcium (calcium carbonate)	200 mg
Copper (cupric oxide)	2 mg
Zinc (zinc oxide)	25 mg
Folic Acid	1 mg
Vitamin A (beta carotene)	2700 IU
Vitamin D3 (cholecalciferol)	400 IU
Vitamin E (dl-alpha tocopheryl acetate)	30 IU
Vitamin C (ascorbic acid)	120 mg
Vitamin B1 (thiamine mononitrate)	3 mg
Vitamin B2 (riboflavin)	3.4 mg
Vitamin B6 (pyridoxine HCl)	20 mg
Vitamin B12 (cyanocobalamin)	12 mcg
Niacinamide	20 mg
Magnesium (magnesium oxide)	30 mcg
Docusate Sodium	50 mg

Other Ingredients: carnauba wax, crospovidone, hydroxypropyl methylcellulose, magnesium stearate, propylene glycol, silicon dioxide, stearic acid, titanium dioxide, and vanillin.

INDICATIONS

PRENATE ADVANCE is a multivitamin/multimineral nutritional supplement indicated for use in improving the nutritional status of women throughout pregnancy and in the postnatal period for both lactating and nonlactating mothers. PRENATE ADVANCE can also be beneficial in improving the nutritional status of women prior to conception.

CONTRAINDICATIONS

This product is contraindicated in patients with a known hypersensitivity to any of the ingredients.

WARNINGS

WARNING: Accidental overdose of iron-containing products is a leading cause of fatal poisoning in children under 6. Keep this product out of reach of children. In case of accidental overdose, call a doctor or poison control center immediately.

Folic acid alone is improper therapy in the treatment of pernicious anemia and other megaloblastic anemias where vitamin B12 is deficient.

PRECAUTIONS

Folic acid in doses above 0.1 mg daily may obscure pernicious anemia in that hematologic remission can occur while neurological manifestations progress.

ADVERSE REACTIONS

Allergic sensitization has been reported following both oral and parenteral administration of folic acid.

DOSAGE AND ADMINISTRATION

One tablet daily or as directed by a physician.

HOW SUPPLIED

Child-resistant unit-dose packs of 90 tablets—NDC 0024-1727-10

NOTICE: Contact with moisture may produce surface discoloration and/or erosion of the tablet.

KEEP THIS AND ALL DRUGS OUT OF THE REACH OF CHILDREN.

Store between 15° and 30°C (59° and 86°F).

Rx only

Manufactured for
Sanofi-Synthelabo Inc.
New York, NY 10016
by Patheon Inc.
Mississauga, ON L5N 7K9
For inquiries call 1-800-446-6267

HPM02920-01-0600SS
172711-0662
Shown in Product Identification Guide, page 333

PRIMACOR® ℞
MILRINONE LACTATE INJECTION

DESCRIPTION

PRIMACOR, brand of milrinone lactate injection, is a member of a new class of bipyridine inotropic/vasodilator agents with phosphodiesterase inhibitor activity, distinct from digitalis glycosides or catecholamines. PRIMACOR (milrinone lactate) is designated chemically as 1,6-dihydro-2-methyl-6-oxo-[3,4′-bipyridine]-5-carbonitrile lactate and has the following structure:

Milrinone is an off-white to tan crystalline compound with a molecular weight of 211.2 and an empirical formula of $C_{12}H_9N_3O$. It is slightly soluble in methanol, and very slightly soluble in chloroform and in water. As the lactate salt, it is stable and colorless to pale yellow in solution. PRIMACOR is available as sterile aqueous solutions of the lactate salt of milrinone for injection or infusion intravenously.

Sterile, single-dose vials: Single-dose vials of 10, 20 and 50 mL, contain in each mL milrinone lactate equivalent to 1 mg milrinone and 47 mg Dextrose, Anhydrous, USP, in Water for Injection, USP. The pH is adjusted to between 3.2 and 4.0 with lactic acid or sodium hydroxide. The total concentration of lactic acid can vary between 0.95 mg/mL and 1.29 mg/mL. These vials require preparation of dilutions prior to administration to patients intravenously.

Pre-Mix Flexible Container: The Flexible Container provide two ready-to-use dilutions of milrinone in volumes of 100 and 200 mL of 5% Dextrose Injection. Each mL contains milrinone lactate equivalent to 200 mcg milrinone. The nominal concentration of lactic acid is 0.282 mg/mL. Each mL also contains 49.4 mg Dextrose, Anhydrous, USP. The pH is adjusted to between 3.2 and 4.0 with lactic acid or sodium hydroxide. The flexible plastic container is comprised of polyvinyl chloride with a foil overwrap. Water can permeate the plastic into the overwrap, but the amount is insufficient to significantly affect the pre-mix solution.

CLINICAL PHARMACOLOGY

PRIMACOR is a positive inotrope and vasodilator, with little chronotropic activity different in structure and mode of action from either the digitalis glycosides or catecholamines.

PRIMACOR, at relevant inotropic and vasorelaxant concentrations, is a selective inhibitor of peak III cAMP phosphodiesterase isozyme in cardiac and vascular muscle. This inhibitory action is consistent with cAMP mediated increases in intracellular ionized calcium and contractile force in cardiac muscle, as well as with cAMP dependent contractile protein phosphorylation and relaxation in vascular muscle. Additional experimental evidence also indicates that PRIMACOR is not a beta-adrenergic agonist nor does it inhibit sodium-potassium adenosine triphosphatase activity as do the digitalis glycosides.

Clinical studies in patients with congestive heart failure have shown that PRIMACOR produces dose-related and plasma drug concentration-related increases in the maximum rate of increase of left ventricular pressure. Studies in normal subjects have shown that PRIMACOR produces increases in the slope of the left ventricular pressure-dimension relationship, indicating a direct inotropic effect of the drug. PRIMACOR also produces dose-related and plasma concentration-related increases in forearm blood flow in patients with congestive heart failure, indicating a direct arterial vasodilator activity of the drug.

Both the inotropic and vasodilatory effects have been observed over the therapeutic range of plasma milrinone concentrations of 100 ng/mL to 300 ng/mL.

In addition to increasing myocardial contractility, PRIMACOR improves diastolic function as evidenced by improvements in left ventricular diastolic relaxation.

The acute administration of intravenous milrinone has also been evaluated in clinical trials in excess of 1600 patients, with chronic heart failure, heart failure associated with cardiac surgery, and heart failure associated with myocardial infarction. The total number of deaths, either on therapy or shortly thereafter (24 hours) was 15, less than 0.9%, few of which were thought to be drug-related.

Pharmacokinetics

Following intravenous injections of 12.5 mcg/kg to 125 mcg/kg to congestive heart failure patients, PRIMACOR had a volume of distribution of 0.38 liters/kg, a mean terminal elimination half-life of 2.3 hours, and a clearance of 0.13 liters/kg/hr. Following intravenous infusions of 0.20 mcg/kg/min to 0.70 mcg/kg/min to congestive heart failure patients, the drug had a volume of distribution of about 0.45 liters/kg, a mean terminal elimination half-life of 2.4 hours, and a clearance of 0.14 liters/kg/hr. These pharmacokinetic parameters were not dose-dependent, and the area under the plasma concentration versus time curve following injections was significantly dose-dependent.

PRIMACOR has been shown (by equilibrium dialysis) to be approximately 70% bound to human plasma protein.

The primary route of excretion of PRIMACOR in man is via the urine. The major urinary excretions of orally administered PRIMACOR in man are milrinone (83%) and its 0-glucuronide metabolite (12%). Elimination in normal subjects via the urine is rapid, with approximately 60% recovered within the first two hours following dosing and approximately 90% recovered within the first eight hours following dosing. The mean renal clearance of PRIMACOR is approximately 0.3 liters/min, indicative of active secretion.

Pharmacodynamics

In patients with heart failure due to depressed myocardial function, PRIMACOR produced a prompt dose and plasma concentration related increase in cardiac output and decreases in pulmonary capillary wedge pressure and vascular resistance, which were accompanied by mild-to-moderate increases in heart rate. Additionally, there is no increased effect on myocardial oxygen consumption. In uncontrolled studies, hemodynamic improvement during intravenous therapy with PRIMACOR was accompanied by clinical symptomatic improvement, but the ability of PRIMACOR to relieve symptoms has not been evaluated in controlled clinical trials. The great majority of patients experience improvements in hemodynamic function within 5 to 15 minutes of the initiation of therapy.

In studies in congestive heart failure patients, PRIMACOR when administered as a loading injection followed by a maintenance infusion produced significant mean initial increases in cardiac index of 25 percent, 38 percent, and 42 percent at dose regimens of 37.5 mcg/kg/0.375 mcg/kg/min, 50 mcg/kg/0.50 mcg/kg/min, and 75 mcg/kg/0.75 mcg/kg/min, respectively. Over the same range of loading injections and maintenance infusions, pulmonary capillary wedge pressure significantly decreased by 20 percent, 23 percent, and 36 percent, respectively, while systemic vascular resistance significantly decreased by 17 percent, 21 percent, and 37 percent. Mean arterial pressure fell by up to 5 percent at the two lower dose regimens, but by 17 percent at the highest dose. Patients evaluated for 48 hours maintained improvements in hemodynamic function, with no evidence of diminished response (tachyphylaxis). A smaller number of patients have received infusions of PRIMACOR for periods up to 72 hours without evidence of tachyphylaxis.

The duration of therapy should depend upon patient responsiveness.

PRIMACOR has a favorable inotropic effect in fully digitalized patients without causing signs of glycoside toxicity. Theoretically, in cases of atrial flutter/fibrillation, it is possible that PRIMACOR may increase ventricular response rate because of its slight enhancement of AV node conduction. In these cases, digitalis should be considered prior to the institution of therapy with PRIMACOR.

Improvement in left ventricular function in patients with ischemic heart disease has been observed. The improvement has occurred without inducing symptoms or electrocardiographic signs of myocardial ischemia.

The steady-state plasma milrinone concentrations after approximately 6 to 12 hours of unchanging maintenance infusion of 0.50 mcg/kg/min are approximately 200 ng/mL. Near maximum favorable effects of PRIMACOR on cardiac output and pulmonary capillary wedge pressure are seen at plasma milrinone concentrations in the 150 ng/mL to 250 ng/mL range.

INDICATIONS AND USAGE

Primacor is indicated for the short-term intravenous treatment of patients with acute decompensated heart failure. Patients receiving PRIMACOR should be observed closely with appropriate electrocardiographic equipment. The facility for immediate treatment of potential cardiac events, which may include life threatening ventricular arrythmias, must be available. The majority of experience with intravenous PRIMACOR has been in patients receiving digoxin and diuretics. There is no experience in controlled trials with infusions of PRIMACOR for periods exceeding 48 hours.

CONTRAINDICATIONS

PRIMACOR is contraindicated in patients who are hypersensitive to it.

WARNINGS

Whether given orally or by continuous or intermittent intravenous infusion, PRIMACOR has not been shown to be safe or effective in the longer (greater than 48 hours) treatment of patients with heart failure. In a multicenter trial of 1088 patients with Class III and IV heart failure, long-term oral treatment with PRIMACOR was associated with no improvement in symptoms and an increased risk of hospitalization and death. In this study, patients with class IV symptoms appeared to be at particular risk of life-threatening cardiovascular reactions. There is no evidence that PRIMACOR given by long-term continuous or intermittent infusion does not carry a similar risk.

The use of PRIMACOR both intravenously and orally has been associated with increased frequency of ventricular arrhythmias, including nonsustained ventricular tachycardia. Long-term oral use has been associated with an increased risk of sudden death. Hence, patients receiving PRIMACOR should be observed closely with the use of continuous electrocardiographic monitoring to allow the prompt detection and management of ventricular arrhythmias.

PRECAUTIONS

General

PRIMACOR should not be used in patients with severe obstructive aortic or pulmonic valvular disease in lieu of surgical relief of the obstruction. Like other inotropic agents, it may aggravate outflow tract obstruction in hypertrophic subaortic stenosis.

Supraventricular and ventricular arrhythmias have been observed in the high-risk population treated. In some patients, injections of PRIMACOR and oral PRIMACOR have been shown to increase ventricular ectopy, including nonsustained ventricular tachycardia. The potential for arrhythmia, present in congestive heart failure itself, may be increased by many drugs or combinations of drugs. Patients receiving PRIMACOR should be closely monitored during infusion.

PRIMACOR produces a slight shortening of AV node conduction time, indicating a potential for an increased ventricular response rate in patients with atrial flutter/fibrillation which is not controlled with digitalis therapy.

During therapy with PRIMACOR, blood pressure and heart rate should be monitored and the rate of infusion slowed or stopped in patients showing excessive decreases in blood pressure.

If prior vigorous diuretic therapy is suspected to have caused significant decreases in cardiac filling pressure, PRIMACOR should be cautiously administered with monitoring of blood pressure, heart rate, and clinical symptomatology.

USE IN ACUTE MYOCARDIAL INFARCTION

No clinical studies have been conducted in patients in the acute phase of post myocardial infarction. Until further clinical experience with this class of drugs is gained, PRIMACOR is not recommended in these patients.

MAINTENANCE DOSE

	Infusion Rate	Total Daily Dose (24 Hours)	
Minimum	0. 375 mcg/kg/min	0.59 mg/kg	Administer as a
Standard	0. 50 mcg/kg/min	0.77 mg/kg	continuous
Maximum	0. 75 mcg/kg/min	1.13 mg/kg	intravenous infusion.

PRIMACOR Infusion Rate (mL/hr) Using 200 mcg/mL Concentration

Maintenance Dose	Patient Body Weight (kg)									
(mcg/kg/min)	-30	40	50	60	70	80	90	100	110	120
0.375	3.4	4.5	5.6	6.8	7.9	9.0	10.1	11.3	12.4	13.5
0.400	3.6	4.8	6.0	7.2	8.4	9.6	10.8	12.0	13.2	14.4
0.500	4.5	6.0	7.5	9.0	10.5	12.0	13.5	15.0	16.5	18.0
0.600	5.4	7.2	9.0	10.8	12.6	14.4	16.2	18.0	19.8	21.6
0.700	6.3	8.4	10.5	12.6	14.7	16.8	18.9	21.0	23.1	25.2
0.750	6.8	9.0	11.3	13.5	15.8	18.0	20.3	22.5	24.8	27.0

Laboratory Tests

Fluid and Electrolytes: Fluid and electrolyte changes and renal function should be carefully monitored during therapy with PRIMACOR. Improvement in cardiac output with resultant diuresis may necessitate a reduction in the dose of diuretic. Potassium loss due to excessive diuresis may predispose digitalized patients to arrhythmias. Therefore, hypokalemia should be corrected by potassium supplementation in advance of or during use of PRIMACOR.

Drug Interactions

No untoward clinical manifestations have been observed in limited experience with patients in whom PRIMACOR was used concurrently with the following drugs: digitalis glycosides; lidocaine, quinidine; hydralazine, prazosin; isosorbide dinitrate, nitroglycerin; chlorthalidone, furosemide, hydrochlorothiazide, spironolactone; captopril; heparin, warfarin, diazepam, insulin; and potassium supplements.

Chemical Interactions

There is an immediate chemical interaction which is evidenced by the formation of a precipitate when furosemide is injected into an intravenous line of an infusion of PRIMACOR. Therefore, furosemide should not be administered in intravenous lines containing PRIMACOR.

Carcinogenesis, Mutagenesis, Impairment of Fertility

Twenty-four months of oral administration of PRIMACOR to mice at doses up to 40 mg/kg/day (about 50 times the human oral therapeutic dose in a 50 kg patient) was unassociated with evidence of carcinogenic potential. Neither was there evidence of carcinogenic potential when PRIMACOR was orally administered to rats at doses up to 5 mg/kg/day (about 6 times the human oral therapeutic dose) for twenty-four months or at 25 mg/kg/day (about 30 times the human oral therapeutic dose) for up to 18 months in males and 20 months in females. Whereas the Chinese Hamster Ovary Chromosome Aberration Assay was positive in the presence of a metabolic activation system, results from the Ames Test, the Mouse Lymphoma Assay, the Micronucleus Test, and the in vivo Rat Bone Marrow Metaphase Analysis indicated an absence of mutagenic potential. In reproductive performance studies in rats, PRIMACOR had no effect on male or female fertility at oral doses up to 32 mg/kg/day.

Animal Toxicity

Oral and intravenous administration of toxic dosages of PRIMACOR to rats and dogs resulted in myocardial degeneration/fibrosis and endocardial hemorrhage, principally affecting the left ventricular papillary muscles. Coronary vascular lesions characterized by periarterial edema and inflammation have been observed in dogs only. The myocardial/endocardial changes are similar to those produced by beta-adrenergic receptor agonists such as isoproterenol, while the vascular changes are similar to those produced by minoxidil and hydralazine. Doses within the recommended clinical dose range (up to 1.13 mg/kg/day) for congestive heart failure patients have not produced significant adverse effects in animals.

Pregnancy Category C

Oral administration of PRIMACOR to pregnant rats and rabbits during organogenesis produced no evidence of teratogenicity at dose levels up to 40 mg/kg/day and 12 mg/kg/day, respectively. PRIMACOR did not appear to be teratogenic when administered intravenously to pregnant rats at doses up to 3 mg/kg/day (about 2.5 times the maximum recommended clinical intravenous dose) or pregnant rabbits at doses up to 12 mg/kg/day, although an increased resorption rate was apparent at both 8 mg/kg/day and 12 mg/kg/day (intravenous) in the latter species. There are no adequate and well-controlled studies in pregnant women. PRIMACOR should be used during pregnancy only if the potential benefit justifies the potential risk to the fetus.

Nursing Mothers

Caution should be exercised when PRIMACOR is administered to nursing women, since it is not known whether it is excreted in human milk.

Pediatric Use

Safety and effectiveness in pediatric patients have not been established.

Use in Elderly Patients

There are no special dosage recommendations for the elderly patient. Ninety percent of all patients administered PRIMACOR in clinical studies were within the age range of 45 to 70 years, with a mean age of 61 years. Patients in all age groups demonstrated clinically and statistically significant responses. No age-related effects on the incidence of adverse reactions have been observed. Controlled pharmacokinetic studies have not disclosed any age-related effects on the distribution and elimination of PRIMACOR.

ADVERSE REACTIONS

Cardiovascular Effects: In patients receiving PRIMACOR in Phase II and III clinical trials, ventricular arrhythmias were reported in 12.1%: Ventricular ectopic activity, 8.5%; nonsustained ventricular tachycardia, 2.8%; sustained ventricular tachycardia, 1% and ventricular fibrillation, 0.2%(2 patients experienced more than one type of arrhythmia). Holter recordings demonstrated that in some patients injection of PRIMACOR increased ventricular ectopy, including nonsustained ventricular tachycardia. Life-threatening arrhythmias were infrequent and when present have been associated with certain underlying factors such as preexisting arrhythmias, metabolic abnormalities (e.g. hypokalemia), abnormal digoxin levels and catheter insertion. PRIMACOR was not shown to be arrhythmogenic in an electrophysiology study. Supraventricular arrhythmias were reported in 3.8% of the patients receiving PRIMACOR. The incidence of both supraventricular and ventricular arrhythmias has not been related to the dose or plasma milrinone concentration.

Other cardiovascular adverse reactions include hypotension, 2.9% and angina/chest pain, 1.2%.

CNS Effects

Headaches, usually mild to moderate in severity, have been reported in 2.9% of patients receiving PRIMACOR.

Other Effects

Other adverse reactions reported, but not definitely related to the administration of PRIMACOR include hypokalemia, 0.6%; tremor, 0.4%; and thrombocytopenia, 0.4%.

Isolated spontaneous reports of bronchospasm have been received; and in the post-marketing experience, liver function test abnormalities have been reported.

OVERDOSAGE

Doses of PRIMACOR may produce hypotension because of its vasodilator effect. If this occurs, administration of PRIMACOR should be reduced or temporarily discontinued until the patient's condition stabilizes. No specific antidote is known, but general measures for circulatory support should be taken.

DOSAGE AND ADMINISTRATION

PRIMACOR should be administered with a loading dose followed by a continuous infusion (maintenance dose) according to the following guidelines:

LOADING DOSE

50 mcg/kg: Administer slowly over 10 minutes

The table below shows the loading dose in milliliters (mL) of PRIMACOR (1 mg/mL) by patient body weight (kg).

Loading Dose (mL) Using 1 mg/mL Concentration

	Patient Body Weight (kg)									
kg	30	40	50	60	70	80	90	100	110	120
mL	1.5	2.0	2.5	3.0	3.5	4.0	4.5	5.0	5.5	6.0

The loading dose may be given undiluted, but diluting to a rounded total volume of 10 or 20 mL (see Maintenance Dose for diluents) may simplify the visualization of the injection rate.

[See first table above]

PRIMACOR drawn from vials should be diluted prior to maintenance dose administration. The diluents that may be used are 0.45% Sodium Chloride Injection USP, 0.9% Sodium Chloride Injection USP, or 5% Dextrose Injection USP.

Continued on next page

This product information was prepared in September 2000. On these and other products of Sanofi-Synthelabo Inc., detailed information may be obtained on a current basis by direct inquiry to Product Information Services, 90 Park Avenue, New York, NY 10016 (toll free 1-800-446-6267).

Primacor—Cont.

The table below shows the volume of diluent in milliliters (mL) that must be used to achieve 200 mcg/mL concentration for infusion, and the resultant total volumes.

Desired Infusion Concentration mcg/mL	PRIMACOR 1 mg/mL (mL)	Diluent (mL)	Total Volume (mL)
200	10	40	50
200	20	80	100

The infusion rate should be adjusted according to hemodynamic and clinical response. Patients should be closely monitored. In controlled clinical studies, most patients showed an improvement in hemodynamic status as evidenced by increases in cardiac output and reductions in pulmonary capillary wedge pressure.

Note: See **"Dosage Adjustment in Renally Impaired Patients."** Dosage may be titrated to the maximum hemodynamic effect and should not exceed 1.13 mg/kg/day. Duration of therapy should depend upon patient responsiveness. The maintenance dose in mL/hr by patient body weight (kg) may be determined by reference to the following table.

Note: **PRIMACOR supplied in 100 mL and 200 mL Flexible Containers (200 mcg/mL in 5% Dextrose Injection) need not be diluted prior to use.**

[See second table at top of previous page]

When administering PRIMACOR (milrinone lactate) by continuous infusion, it is advisable to use a calibrated electronic infusion device.

The Flexible Container has a concentration of milrinone equivalent to 200 mcg/mL in 5% Dextrose Injection and is more convenient to use than dilutions prepared from the vials. To use the Flexible Container, tear the overwrap at the notch and remove the Pre-Mix solution container. Squeeze the container firmly to check for leaks. Discard the container if leaks are found since the sterility of the product could be affected. Do not add supplementary medication. To prepare the container for administration of PRIMACOR intravenously, use aseptic techniques.

1) The flow control clamp of the administration set is closed.
2) The cover of the outlet port at the bottom of the container is removed.
3) Noting the full directions on the administration set carton, the piercing pin of the set is inserted into the port with a twisting motion until it is firmly seated.
4) The container is suspended on the hanger.
5) The drip chamber is squeezed and released to establish the fill level.
6) The flow control clamp is opened to expel air from the set, and then closed.
7) The set is attached to the venipuncture device, primed, and if not indwelling, the venipuncture is performed.
8) The rate of administration is controlled with the flow control clamp. WARNING- DO NOT USE IN SERIES CONNECTIONS. Caution: Do not use plastic containers in series connections. Such use could result in air embolism due to residual air being drawn from the primary container before administration of the fluid from the secondary container is complete.

Intravenous drug products should be inspected visually and should not be used if particulate matter or discoloration is present.

Dosage Adjustment in Renally Impaired Patients

Data obtained from patients with severe renal impairment (creatinine clearance = 0 to 30 mL/min) but without congestive heart failure have demonstrated that the presence of renal impairment significantly increases the terminal elimination half-life of PRIMACOR. Reductions in infusion rate may be necessary in patients with renal impairment. For patients with clinical evidence of renal impairment, the recommended infusion rate can be obtained from the following table:

Creatinine Clearance (mL/min/1.73 m^2)	Infusion Rate (mcg/kg/min)
5	0.20
10	0.23
20	0.28
30	0.33
40	0.38
50	0.43

HOW SUPPLIED

PRIMACOR is supplied as 10 mL single-dose vials in a box of 10 NDC 0024-1200-10; as 20 mL single-dose vials box of 10 NDC 0024-1200-20 and in value packs of 50 units NDC 0024-1200-25; and as a 50 mL single-dose vial box of NDC 0024-1200-50, containing a sterile, clear, colorless to pale yellow solution. Each mL contains milrinone lactate equivalent to 1 mg milrinone.

PRIMACOR is also supplied as Carpuject® sterile cartridge unit with InterLink® System Cannula, 5 mL (1 mg/mL) NDC 0024-1200-06 in 5 mL cartridges, box of 10. Each mL contains milrinone lactate equivalent to 1 mg milrinone.

PRIMACOR is also supplied as Carpuject® sterile cartridge Unit (22-gauge, 1 1/4 Inch Needle) in 5 mL cartridges (1 mg/mL) box of 10 NDC 0024-1200-05. Each mL contains milrinone lactate equivalent to 1 mg milrinone.

Store at controlled room temperature 15° C to 30° C (59° F to 86° F). Avoid freezing.

The following PRIMACOR Flexible Containers are also supplied:

100 mL (200 mcg/mL) NDC 0024-1203-01 in 5% Dextrose Injection single units and in value packs of 50 units NDC 0024-1203-15.

200 mL (200 mcg/mL) NDC 0024-1203-02 in 5% Dextrose Injection single units and in value packs of 50 units NDC 0024-1203-25.

Exposure of pharmaceutical products to heat should be minimized. Avoid excessive heat. Protect from freezing. It is recommended that the Flexible Containers be stored at room temperature, 25° C (77° F), however, brief exposure up to 40° C (104° F) does not adversely affect the product.

InterLink® is a Trademark of Baxter International, Inc.

U.S. Pat. Nos. 5,158,554; 5,171,234; 5,188,620; Pat. Pending

Revised June 2000

PSW-1T(A)

Shown in Product Identification Guide, page 333

SKELID® ℞

[skel 'ĭd]

(tiludronate disodium)

DESCRIPTION

SKELID is a bisphosphonate characterized by a (4-chlorophenylthio) group on the carbon atom of the basic P-C-P structure common to all bisphosphonates. Its generic name is tiludronate disodium. Tiludronate disodium is the hydrated hemihydrate form of the disodium salt of tiludronic acid. Its chemical name is [[(4-Chlorophenyl) thio]methylene]bis [phosphonic acid], disodium salt, and its structural formula is as follows:

Cl–C6H4–S–CH[P(O)(OH)(ONa)]2 • 1/2 H_2O • 0.5 H_2O

tiludronate disodium
(molecular weight 380.6)

SKELID tablets for oral administration contain 240 mg tiludronate disodium, which is the molar equivalent of 200 mg tiludronic acid. SKELID tablets also contain sodium lauryl sulfate, hydroxypropyl methylcellulose 2910, crospovidone, magnesium stearate, and lactose monohydrate.

CLINICAL PHARMACOLOGY

Mechanism of Action

In vitro studies indicate that tiludronate disodium acts primarily on bone through a mechanism that involves inhibition of osteoclastic activity with a probable reduction in the enzymatic and transport processes that lead to resorption of the mineralized matrix.

Bone resorption occurs following recruitment, activation, and polarization of osteoclasts. Tiludronate disodium appears to inhibit osteoclasts through at least two mechanisms: disruption of the cytoskeletal ring structure, possibly by inhibition of protein-tyrosine-phosphatase, thus leading to detachment of osteoclasts from the bone surface and the inhibition of the osteoclastic proton pump.

Pharmacokinetics

Absorption

Relative to an intravenous (IV) reference dose, the mean oral bioavailability of tiludronate disodium in healthy male subjects was 6% after an oral dose equivalent to 400 mg tiludronic acid administered after an overnight fast and 4 hours before a standard breakfast. In single-dose studies, bioavailability was reduced by 90% when an oral dose equivalent to 400 mg tiludronic acid was administered with, or 2 hours after, a standard breakfast compared to the same dose administered after an overnight fast and 4 hours before a standard breakfast. However, in clinical studies, efficacy was seen when SKELID was dosed at least 2 hours before or after meals.

After administration of a single dose equivalent to 400 mg tiludronic acid to healthy male subjects, tiludronic acid was rapidly absorbed with peak plasma concentrations of approximately 3 mg/L occurring within 2 hours. In pagetic patients, after repeated administration of doses equivalent to 400 mg/day tiludronic acid (2 hours before or 2 hours after a meal) for durations of 12 days to 12 weeks, average plasma concentrations of tiludronic acid occurring between 1 and 2 hours after dosing ranged between 1 and 4.6 mg/L.

Distribution

Animal pharmacology studies in rats demonstrate that tiludronic acid is widely distributed to bone and soft tissues. Over a period of days, loss of drug occurs from most tissues with the exception of bone and cartilage. Tiludronate is then slowly released from bone with a half-life in rats of 30 days or longer depending on the status of bone turnover.

After oral administration of doses equivalent to 400 mg/day tiludronic acid to nonpagetic patients with osteoarthrosis, the steady state in bone was not reached after 30 days of dosing.

At plasma concentrations between 1 and 10 mg/L, tiludronic acid was approximately 90% bound to human serum protein (mainly albumin).

Metabolism

In laboratory animals, tiludronic acid undergoes little if any metabolism. *In vitro*, tiludronic acid is not metabolized in human liver microsomes and hepatocytes.

Elimination

The principal route of elimination of tiludronic acid is in the urine. After IV administration to healthy volunteers, approximately 60% of the dose was excreted in the urine as tiludronic acid within 13 days. Renal clearance is dose independent and is approximately 10 mL/min in healthy subjects. In pagetic patients treated with doses equivalent to 400 mg/day tiludronic acid for 12 days, the mean apparent plasma elimination half-life was approximately 150 hours. The elimination rate from human bone is unknown.

Special Populations

Geriatric: No dosage adjustment in elderly patients is necessary. Plasma concentrations of tiludronic acid were higher in elderly pagetic patients (≥65 years of age); however, this difference was not clinically significant.

Pediatric: SKELID pharmacokinetics have not been investigated in subjects under the age of 18 years.

Gender: There were no clinically significant differences in plasma concentrations after repeated administration of tiludronate disodium to male and female pagetic patients.

Race: Pharmacokinetic differences due to race have not been studied.

Renal Insufficiency: SKELID is not recommended for patients with severe renal failure (creatinine clearance <30 mL/min) due to lack of clinical experience. After a single oral dose equivalent to 400 mg tiludronic acid, subjects with creatinine clearance between 11 and 18 mL/min had C_{max} values (approximately 3 mg/L) in the range of healthy volunteers. However, the plasma elimination half-life was approximately 205 hours, which is longer than that observed in pagetic patients after repeated doses (150 hours) and healthy subjects after single doses (50 hours). These values were obtained in a cross-study comparison between healthy volunteers and pagetic patients.

Hepatic Insufficiency: No dosage adjustment is needed. Since tiludronate undergoes little or no metabolism, no studies were conducted in subjects with hepatic insufficiency.

Drug-Drug Interactions: (See also PRECAUTIONS, Drug Interactions.) The bioavailability of SKELID is decreased 80% by calcium, when calcium and SKELID are administered at the same time, and 60% by some aluminum- or magnesium-containing antacids, when administered 1 hour before SKELID. Aspirin may decrease bioavailability of SKELID by up to 50% when taken 2 hours after SKELID. The bioavailability of SKELID is increased 2–4 fold by indomethacin and is not significantly altered by coadministration of diclofenac. The pharmacokinetic parameters of digoxin are not significantly modified by SKELID coadministration. *In vitro* studies show that tiludronate disodium does not displace warfarin from its binding site on protein.

Summary of Pharmacokinetic Parameters in the Normal Population

Parameter	Mean (SD)
Absolute bioavailability of two 200-mg tablets taken 4 hrs before standard breakfast	6% (2%)*
Time to peak plasma concentration (taken 4 hrs before first meal of day, n=151)	1.5 (0.9) hr
Maximum plasma concentration after a single 400-mg dose (taken 4 hrs before first meal of day, n=151)	2.66 (1.22) mg/L
Renal Clearance after IV administration of 20-mg dose	0.54 (0.14) L/hr

*Bioavailability was reduced by 90% when this oral dose was administered with, or 2 hours after, a standard breakfast.

Pharmacodynamics

Paget's disease of bone is a chronic, focal skeletal disorder characterized by greatly increased and disorderly bone remodeling. Excessive osteoclastic bone resorption is followed by osteoblastic new bone formation, leading to the replacement of the normal bone architecture by disorganized, enlarged, and weakened bone structure.

Clinical manifestations of Paget's disease range from no symptoms to severe bone pain, bone deformity, pathological fractures, and neurological and other complications. Serum alkaline phosphatase, the most frequently used biochemical index of disease activity, provides an objective measure of disease severity and response to therapy.

In pagetic patients treated with SKELID 400 mg/day for 3 months, changes in urinary hydroxyproline, a biochemical marker of bone resorption, and in serum alkaline phosphatase, a marker of bone formation, indicate a reduction toward normal in the rate of bone turnover. In addition, reduced numbers of osteoclasts by histomorphometric analysis and radiological improvement of lytic lesions indicate that SKELID can suppress the pagetic disease process.

Clinical Studies

The efficacy of SKELID 400 mg/day treatment was demonstrated in two randomized, double-blind, placebo-controlled multicenter studies and one positive-controlled study. All three studies included male and female patients with Paget's disease of the bone (radiograph examination and level of serum alkaline phosphatase [SAP] at least twice the upper normal limit). In one placebo-controlled study, conducted in North America, patients were randomly assigned to receive a daily dose of placebo or 200 or 400 mg/day SKELID for 3 months followed by an additional 12 weeks without treatment. A second placebo-controlled study of similar design was conducted in the UK.

A positive-controlled study was conducted in Europe with treatment groups of 400 mg/day SKELID for 3 months with a 3-month treatment-free follow-up, 400 mg/day SKELID for 6 months, and 400 mg/day etidronate for 6 months. In all of these studies, the efficacy of SKELID was primarily assessed by SAP activity after 3 and 6 months.

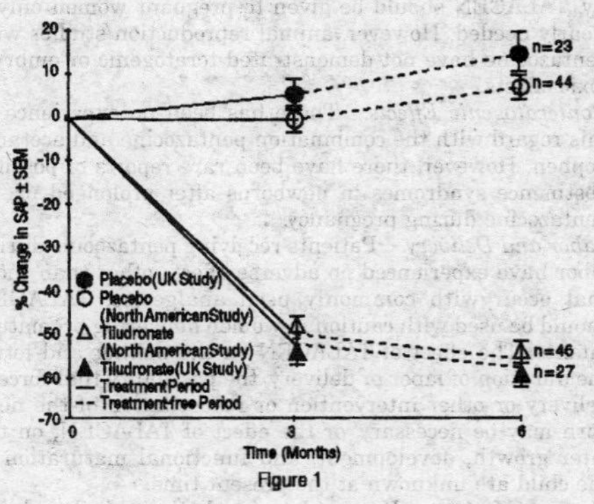

Figure 1

In the placebo-controlled trials, suppression of SAP levels was statistically significantly greater with 400 mg/day SKELID both at the end of treatment (3 months) and on follow-up (6 months) than with placebo (See Figure 1). The proportion of patients demonstrating at least a 50% reduction in SAP at 3 months with 400 mg/day SKELID was 61% in the North American study and 52% in the UK study.

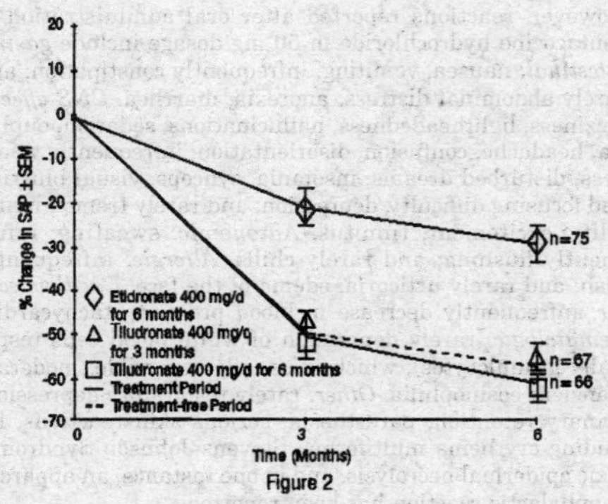

Figure 2

In the positive-controlled trial, six months after the start of dosing, the decrease in SAP levels in patients who ceased dosing after a 3-month course of SKELID was significantly greater than with 6 months of etidronate 400 mg/day, and was equivalent to levels in patients who completed a 6-month course of SKELID (See Figure 2).

Treatment effects of SKELID were similar, regardless of pagetic patients' baseline SAP level, gender or age in the population studied.

Histomorphometry of the bone was studied in 19 pagetic and 29 nonpagetic patients (34 biopsies in pagetic patients and 41 biopsies in nonpagetic patients). Bone biopsy results in nonpagetic bone confirmed that SKELID did not impair bone remodeling or induce a significant decline in bone turnover. Results obtained in pagetic and nonpagetic bone indicated no evidence of osteomalacia or accumulation of unmineralized osteoid, and there was no reduction in the mineralization rate.

INDICATIONS AND USAGE

SKELID is indicated for treatment of Paget's disease of bone (osteitis deformans).

Treatment is indicated in patients with Paget's disease of bone (1) who have a level of serum alkaline phosphatase (SAP) at least twice the upper limit of normal, or (2) who are symptomatic, or (3) who are at risk for future complications of their disease.

CONTRAINDICATION

SKELID is contraindicated in individuals with known hypersensitivity to any component of this product.

WARNINGS

Bisphosphonates may cause upper gastrointestinal disorders, such as dysphagia, esophagitis, esophageal ulcer, and gastric ulcer (See ADVERSE REACTIONS).

PRECAUTIONS

General

SKELID is not recommended for patients with severe renal failure, for example, those with creatinine clearance <30 mL/min (see CLINICAL PHARMACOLOGY, Renal Insufficiency).

Information for Patients

Patients receiving SKELID should be instructed to:

1. Take SKELID with 6 to 8 ounces of plain water.
2. SKELID should not be taken within 2 hours of food.
3. Maintain adequate vitamin D and calcium intake.
4. Calcium supplements, aspirin, and indomethacin should not be taken within 2 hours before or 2 hours after SKELID.
5. Aluminum- or magnesium-containing antacids, if needed, should be taken at least 2 hours after taking SKELID.

Drug Interactions

The bioavailability of SKELID is decreased 80% by calcium, when calcium and SKELID are administered at the same time, and 60% by some aluminum- or magnesium-containing antacids, when administered 1 hour before SKELID. Aspirin may decrease bioavailability of SKELID by up to 50% when taken 2 hours after SKELID. The bioavailability of SKELID is increased 2–4 fold by indomethacin but is not significantly altered by coadministration of diclofenac. The pharmacokinetic parameters of digoxin are not significantly modified by SKELID coadministration. *In vitro* studies show that tiludronate does not displace warfarin from its binding site on protein.

Carcinogenesis, Mutagenesis, Impairment of Fertility

Carcinogenicity studies have not yet been completed.

Tiludronate was not genotoxic in the following assays: an *in vitro* microbial mutagenesis assay with and without metabolic activation, a human lymphocyte assay, a yeast cell assay for forward mutation and mitotic crossing over, or the *in vivo* mouse micronucleus test.

Tiludronate had no effect on rat fertility (male or female) at exposures up to two times the 400 mg/day human dose, based on surface area, mg/m^2 (75 mg/kg/day tiludronic acid dose).

Pregnancy

Pregnancy Category C

In a teratology study in rabbits dosed during days 6-18 of gestation at 42 mg/kg/day and 130 mg/kg/day (2 and 5 times the 400 mg/day human dose based on body surface area), there was dose-related scoliosis likely attributable to the pharmacologic properties of the drug.

Mice receiving 375 mg/kg/day tiludronic acid (7 times the 400 mg/day human dose based on body surface area, mg/m^2) for days 6–15 of gestation showed slight maternal toxicity (decreased body weight gain), increased postimplantation loss, decreased number of fetuses/dam, and decreased fetus body weight. Uncommon malformations of the paw (shortened or missing digits, blood blisters between or in place of digits) were present in six fetuses at 375 mg/kg/day, all from the same litter.

Maternal toxicity (decreased body weight) was also observed in a teratology study in rats dosed during days 6–18 of gestation at 375 mg/kg/day tiludronic acid (10 times the 400 mg/day human dose based on body surface area, mg/m^2). There were reduced percent implantations, increased postimplantation loss, and increased intra-uterine deaths in the rats. There were no teratogenic effects on fetuses.

Protracted parturition and maternal death, presumably due to hypocalcemia, occurred at 75 mg/kg/day tiludronic acid (two times the 400 mg/day human dose based on body surface area, mg/m^2) when rats were treated from day 15 of gestation to day 25 postpartum.

There are no adequate and well-controlled studies in pregnant women. SKELID should be used during pregnancy only if the potential benefit justifies the potential risk to the fetus.

Nursing Mothers

It is not known whether tiludronate is excreted in human milk. Because many drugs are excreted in human milk, caution should be exercised when SKELID is administered to a nursing woman.

Pediatric Use

Safety and effectiveness of SKELID in pediatric patients have not been established.

ADVERSE REACTIONS

The safety of SKELID has been studied in more than 1100 patients, and the adverse experience profile is similar between controlled and uncontrolled clinical trials. Adverse events occurring in placebo-controlled trials of pagetic patients treated with SKELID 400 mg/day are presented in the table below.

The most frequently occurring adverse events in patients who received SKELID 400 mg/day were in the gastrointestinal body system: nausea (9.3%), diarrhea (9.3%), and dyspepsia (5.3%).

Adverse events associated with SKELID usually have been mild, and generally have not required discontinuation of therapy. In two placebo-controlled trials, 1.3% of patients receiving 400 mg SKELID and 5.4% of patients receiving placebo discontinued therapy due to any clinical adverse event.

Adverse Events[a] (%) Reported[b] in > 2% of Pagetic Patients from Placebo-Controlled Studies

	SKELID 400 mg/day (n=75)	Placebo (n=74)
Body as a Whole		
Pain	21.3	23.0
Back Pain	8.0	8.1
Accidental Injury	4.0	2.7
Influenza-like Symptoms	4.0	5.4
Chest Pain	2.7	0
Peripheral Edema	2.7	1.4
Cardiovascular, General		
Dependent Edema	2.7	0
Central and Peripheral Nervous System		
Headache	6.7	12.2
Dizziness	4.0	6.8
Paresthesia	4.0	0
Endocrine		
Hyperparathyroidism	2.7	0
Gastrointestinal		
Diarrhea	9.3	4.1
Nausea	9.3	5.4
Dyspepsia	5.3	8.1
Vomiting	4.0	0
Flatulence	2.7	0
Tooth Disorder	2.7	1.4
Metabolic and Nutritional		
Vitamin D Deficiency	2.7	2.7
Musculoskeletal System		
Arthralgia	2.7	5.4
Arthrosis	2.7	0
Resistance Mechanism		
Infection	2.7	0
Respiratory System		
Rhinitis	5.3	0
Sinusitis	5.3	1.4
Upper Respiratory Tract Infection	5.3	14.9
Coughing	2.7	2.7
Pharyngitis	2.7	1.4
Skin and Appendage		
Rash	2.7	1.4
Skin Disorder	2.7	1.4
Vision		
Cataract	2.7	0
Conjunctivitis	2.7	0
Glaucoma	2.7	0

[a] Reported using WHO terminology
[b] All events reported, irrespective of causality

Other adverse events not listed in the table above but reported in ≥ 1% of pagetic patients treated with SKELID in all clinical trials of at least one month duration, regardless of dose and causality assessment, are listed below. The adverse event terms within each body system are listed in the order of decreasing frequency occurring in the population.

Body as a Whole: Asthenia, syncope, fatigue
Cardiovascular: Hypertension
Central and Peripheral Nervous Systems: Vertigo, involuntary muscle contractions
Gastrointestinal: Abdominal pain, constipation, dry mouth, gastritis
Musculoskeletal: Fracture pathological
Psychiatric: Anorexia, somnolence, anxiety, nervousness, insomnia
Respiratory System: Bronchitis
Skin and Appendages: Pruritus, increased sweating
Urinary System: Urinary tract infection
Vascular (extracardiac): Flushing

Stevens-Johnson type syndrome has been observed rarely; the causality relationship of this to SKELID has not been established.

OVERDOSAGE

Based on the known action of tiludronate, hypocalcemia is a potential consequence of SKELID overdose. In one patient with hypercalcemia of malignancy, intravenous administration of high doses of SKELID (800 mg/day total dose, 6 mg/kg/day for 2 days) was associated with acute renal failure and death.

No specific information is available on the treatment of overdose with SKELID. Dialysis would not be beneficial. Standard medical practices may be used to manage renal insufficiency or hypocalcemia, if signs of these develop.

DOSAGE AND ADMINISTRATION

A single 400-mg daily oral dose of SKELID, taken with 6 to 8 ounces of plain water only, should be administered for a period of 3 months. Beverages other than plain water (in-

Continued on next page

This product information was prepared in September 2000. On these and other products of Sanofi-Synthelabo Inc., detailed information may be obtained on a current basis by direct inquiry to Product Information Services, 90 Park Avenue, New York, NY 10016 (toll free 1-800-446-6267).

Skelid—Cont.

cluding mineral water), food (see below), and some medications (see PRECAUTIONS, Drug Interactions) are likely to reduce the absorption of SKELID (see CLINICAL PHARMACOLOGY, Pharmacokinetics).
SKELID should not be taken within 2 hours of food.
Calcium or mineral supplements should be taken at least 2 hours before or two hours after SKELID. Aluminum- or magnesium-containing antacids, if needed, should be taken at least two hours after taking SKELID.
SKELID should not be taken within 2 hours of indomethacin.
Following therapy, allow an interval of 3 months to assess response. Specific data regarding retreatment are limited, although results from uncontrolled studies indicate favorable biochemical improvement similar to initial SKELID treatment.

HOW SUPPLIED

SKELID (NDC 0024-1800-02) is supplied as white to practically white, biconvex round tablets containing 240 mg tiludronate disodium, which is the molar equivalent of 200 mg tiludronic acid. SKELID tablets are engraved with "S.W" on one side and "200" on the other side and packaged, in foil strips in cartons of 56 tablets per carton.

Storage

SKELID should be stored at 25° C (77° F); excursions permitted to 15° C to 30° C (59° F to 86° F) [see USP Controlled Room Temperature]. Tablets should not be removed from the foil strips until they are to be used.
Distributed by *Sanofi Synthelabo Inc.*
NEW YORK, NY 10016
Manufactured by Sanofi Winthrop Industrie
1, Rue de la Vierge
33440 Ambarès, France
SSW-3C

Shown in Product Identification Guide, page 333

TALACEN® Ⓒ℞

Pentazocine hydrochloride, USP and acetaminophen, USP

DESCRIPTION

TALACEN is a combination of pentazocine hydrochloride, USP, equivalent to 25 mg base and acetaminophen, USP, 650 mg.
Pentazocine is a member of the benzazocine series (also known as the benzomorphan series). Chemically, pentazocine is 1,2,3,4,5,6-hexahydro-6,11-dimethyl-3-(3-methyl-2-butenyl)-2,6-methano-3-benzazocin-8-ol, a white, crystalline substance soluble in acidic aqueous solutions.
Chemically, acetaminophen is Acetamide, *N*- (4-hydroxyphenyl)-.
Pentazocine is an analgesic and acetaminophen is an analgesic and antipyretic.
TALACEN is a pale blue, scored caplet for oral administration.
Inactive Ingredients: Colloidal Silicon Dioxide, FD&C Blue #1, Gelatin, Microcrystalline Cellulose, Potassium Sorbate, Pregelatinized Starch, Sodium Lauryl Sulfate, Sodium Metabisulfite, Sodium Starch Glycolate, Stearic Acid.

CLINICAL PHARMACOLOGY

TALACEN is an analgesic possessing antipyretic actions.
Pentazocine is an analgesic with agonist/antagonist action which when administered orally is approximately equivalent on a mg for mg basis in analgesic effect to codeine.
Acetaminophen is an analgesic and antipyretic.
Onset of significant analgesia with pentazocine usually occurs between 15 and 30 minutes after oral administration, and duration of action is usually three hours or longer. Onset and duration of action and the degree of pain relief are related both to dose and the severity of pretreatment pain.
Pentazocine weakly antagonizes the analgesic effects of morphine, meperidine, and phenazocine; in addition, it produces incomplete reversal of cardiovascular, respiratory, and behavioral depression induced by morphine and meperidine. Pentazocine has about 1/50 the antagonistic activity of nalorphine. It also has sedative activity.
Pentazocine is well absorbed from the gastrointestinal tract. Plasma levels closely correspond to the onset, duration, and intensity of analgesia. The time to mean peak concentration in 24 normal volunteers was 1.7 hours (range 0.5 to 4 hours) after oral administration and the mean plasma elimination half-life was 3.6 hours (range 1.5 to 10 hours).
The action of pentazocine is terminated for the most part by biotransformation in the liver with some free pentazocine excreted in the urine. The products of the oxidation of the terminal methyl groups and glucuronide conjugates are excreted by the kidney. Elimination of approximately 60% of the total dose occurs within 24 hours. Pentazocine passes the placental barrier.
Onset of significant analgesic and antipyretic activity of acetaminophen when administered orally occurs within 30 minutes and is maximal at approximately $2^1/_2$ hours. The pharmacological mode of action of acetaminophen is unknown at this time.
Acetaminophen is rapidly and almost completely absorbed from the gastrointestinal tract. In 24 normal volunteers the time to mean peak plasma concentration was 1 hour (range 0.25 to 3 hours) after oral administration and the mean plasma elimination half-life was 2.8 hours (range 2 to 4 hours).
The effect of pentazocine on acetaminophen plasma protein binding or vice versa has not been established. For acetaminophen there is little or no plasma protein binding at normal therapeutic doses. When toxic doses of acetaminophen are ingested and drug plasma levels exceed 90 mcg/mL, plasma binding may vary from 8% to 43%.
Acetaminophen is conjugated in the liver with glucuronic acid and to a lesser extent with sulfuric acid. Approximately 80% of acetaminophen is excreted in the urine after conjugation and about 3% is excreted unchanged. The drug is also conjugated to a lesser extent with cysteine and additionally metabolized by hydroxylation.
If TALACEN is taken every 4 hours over an extended period of time, accumulation of pentazocine and to a lesser extent, acetaminophen, may occur.

INDICATIONS AND USAGE

TALACEN is indicated for the relief of mild to moderate pain.

CONTRAINDICATIONS

TALACEN should not be administered to patients who are hypersensitive to either pentazocine or acetaminophen.

WARNINGS

Contains sodium metabisulfite, a sulfite that may cause allergic-type reactions including anaphylactic symptoms and life-threatening or less severe asthmatic episodes in certain susceptible people. The overall prevalence of sulfite sensitivity in the general population is unknown and probably low. Sulfite sensitivity is seen more frequently in asthmatic than in nonasthmatic people.
Head Injury and Increased Intracranial Pressure. As in the case of other potent analgesics, the potential of pentazocine for elevating cerebrospinal fluid pressure may be attributed to CO_2 retention due to the respiratory depressant effects of the drug. These effects may be markedly exaggerated in the presence of head injury, other intracranial lesions, or a preexisting increase in intracranial pressure. Furthermore, pentazocine can produce effects which may obscure the clinical course of patients with head injuries. In such patients, TALACEN must be used with extreme caution and only if its use is deemed essential.
Acute CNS Manifestations. Patients receiving therapeutic doses of pentazocine have experienced hallucinations (usually visual), disorientation, and confusion which have cleared spontaneously within a period of hours. The mechanism of this reaction is not known. Such patients should be closely observed and vital signs checked. If the drug is reinstituted, it should be done with caution since these acute CNS manifestations may recur.
There have been instances of psychological and physical dependence on parenteral pentazocine in patients with a history of drug abuse, and rarely, in patients without such a history. (See DRUG ABUSE AND DEPENDENCE.)
Due to the potential for increased CNS depressant effects, alcohol should be used with caution in patients who are currently receiving pentazocine.
Pentazocine may precipitate opioid abstinence symptoms in patients receiving courses of opiates for pain relief.

PRECAUTIONS

In prescribing TALACEN for chronic use, the physician should take precautions to avoid increases in dose by the patient.
Myocardial Infarction. As with all drugs, TALACEN should be used with caution in patients with myocardial infarction who have nausea or vomiting.
Certain Respiratory Conditions. Although respiratory depression has rarely been reported after oral administration of pentazocine, the drug should be administered with caution to patients with respiratory depression from any cause, severely limited respiratory reserve, severe bronchial asthma and other obstructive respiratory conditions, or cyanosis.
Impaired Renal or Hepatic Function. Decreased metabolism of the drug by the liver in extensive liver disease may predispose to accentuation of side effects. Although laboratory tests have not indicated that pentazocine causes or increases renal or hepatic impairment, the drug should be administered with caution to patients with such impairment. Since acetaminophen is metabolized by the liver, the question of the safety of its use in the presence of liver disease should be considered.
Biliary Surgery. Narcotic drug products are generally considered to elevate biliary tract pressure for varying periods following their administration. Some evidence suggests that pentazocine may differ from other marketed narcotics in this respect (i.e., it causes little or no elevation in biliary tract pressures). The clinical significance of these findings, however, is not yet known.
CNS Effect. Caution should be used when TALACEN is administered to patients prone to seizures; seizures have occurred in a few such patients in association with the use of pentazocine although no cause and effect relationship has been established.
Information for Patients. Since sedation, dizziness, and occasional euphoria have been noted, ambulatory patients should be warned not to operate machinery, drive cars, or unnecessarily expose themselves to hazards. Pentazocine may cause physical and psychological dependence when taken alone and may have additive CNS depressant properties when taken in combination with alcohol or other CNS depressants.
Drug Interactions. Pentazocine is a mild narcotic antagonist. Some patients previously given narcotics, including methadone for the daily treatment of narcotic dependence, have experienced withdrawal symptoms after receiving pentazocine.
Carcinogenesis, Mutagenesis, Impairment of Fertility. Carcinogenesis, mutagenesis, and impairment of fertility studies have not been done with this combination product.
Pentazocine, when administered orally or parenterally, had no adverse effect on either the reproductive capabilities or the course of pregnancy in rabbits and rats. Embryotoxic effects on the fetuses were not shown.
The daily administration of 4 mg/kg to 20 mg/kg pentazocine subcutaneously to female rats during a 14 day premating period and until the 13th day of pregnancy did not have any adverse effects on the fertility rate.
There is no evidence in long-term animal studies to demonstrate that pentazocine is carcinogenic.
Pregnancy Category C. Animal reproduction studies have not been conducted with TALACEN. It is also not known whether TALACEN can cause fetal harm when administered to pregnant women or can affect reproduction capacity. TALACEN should be given to pregnant women only if clearly needed. However, animal reproduction studies with pentazocine have not demonstrated teratogenic or embryotoxic effects.
Nonteratogenic Effects. There has been no experience in this regard with the combination pentazocine and acetaminophen. However, there have been rare reports of possible abstinence syndromes in newborns after prolonged use of pentazocine during pregnancy.
Labor and Delivery. Patients receiving pentazocine during labor have experienced no adverse effects other than those that occur with commonly used analgesics. TALACEN should be used with caution in women delivering premature infants. The effect of TALACEN on the mother and fetus, the duration of labor or delivery, the possibility that forceps delivery or other intervention or resuscitation of the newborn may be necessary, or the effect of TALACEN, on the later growth, development, and functional maturation of the child are unknown at the present time.
Nursing Mothers. It is not known whether this drug is excreted in human milk. Because many drugs are excreted in human milk, caution should be exercised when TALACEN is administered to a nursing woman.
Pediatric Use. Safety and effectiveness in pediatric patients below the age of 12 have not been established.

ADVERSE REACTIONS

Clinical experience with TALACEN has been insufficient to define all possible adverse reactions with this combination. However, reactions reported after oral administration of pentazocine hydrochloride in 50 mg dosage include *gastrointestinal:* nausea, vomiting, infrequently constipation; and rarely abdominal distress, anorexia, diarrhea. *CNS effects:* dizziness, lightheadedness, hallucinations, sedation, euphoria, headache, confusion, disorientation; infrequently weakness, disturbed dreams, insomnia, syncope, visual blurring and focusing difficulty, depression; and rarely tremor, irritability, excitement, tinnitus. *Autonomic:* sweating; infrequently flushing; and rarely chills. *Allergic:* infrequently rash; and rarely urticaria, edema of the face. *Cardiovascular:* infrequently decrease in blood pressure, tachycardia. *Hematologic:* rarely depression of white blood cells (especially granulocytes), which is usually reversible, moderate transient eosinophilia. *Other:* rarely respiratory depression, urinary retention, paresthesia, serious skin reactions, including erythema multiforme, Stevens-Johnson Syndrome, toxic epidermal necrolysis, and in one instance, an apparent anaphylactic reaction has been reported.
Numerous clinical studies have shown that acetaminophen, when taken in recommended doses, is relatively free of adverse effects in most age groups, even in the presence of a variety of disease states.
A few cases of hypersensitivity to acetaminophen have been reported, as manifested by skin rashes, thrombocytopenic purpura, rarely hemolytic anemia and agranulocytosis. Occasional individuals respond to ordinary doses with nausea and vomiting and diarrhea.

DRUG ABUSE AND DEPENDENCE

Controlled Substance. TALACEN is a Schedule IV controlled substance.
Abuse and Dependence. There have been some reports of dependence and of withdrawal symptoms with orally administered pentazocine. There have been recorded instances of psychological and physical dependence in patients using parenteral pentazocine. Abrupt discontinuance following the extended use of parenteral pentazocine has resulted in withdrawal symptoms. Patients with a history of drug dependence should be under close supervision while receiving TALACEN. There have been rare reports of possible abstinence syndromes in newborns after prolonged use of pentazocine during pregnancy.
Some tolerance to the analgesic and subjective effects of pentazocine develops with frequent and repeated use.
Drug addicts who are given closely spaced doses of pentazocine (e.g., 60 mg to 90 mg every 4 hours) develop physical dependence which is demonstrated by abrupt withdrawal or by administration of naloxone. The withdrawal symptoms exhibited after chronic doses of more than 500 mg of pen-

tazocine per day have similar characteristics, but to a lesser degree, of opioid withdrawal and may be associated with drug seeking behavior.

OVERDOSAGE

Manifestations. Clinical experience with TALACEN has been insufficient to define the signs of overdosage with this product. It may be assumed that signs and symptoms of TALACEN overdose would be a combination of those observed with pentazocine overdose and acetaminophen overdose.

For pentazocine alone in single doses above 60 mg there have been reports of the occurrence of nalorphine-like psychotomimetic effects such as anxiety, nightmares, strange thoughts, and hallucinations. Marked respiratory depression associated with increased blood pressure and tachycardia have also resulted from excessive doses as have dizziness, nausea, vomiting, lethargy, and paresthesias. The respiratory depression is antagonized by naloxone (see *Treatment*).

In acute acetaminophen overdosage, dose-dependent, potentially fatal hepatic necrosis is the most serious adverse effect. Renal tubular necrosis, hypoglycemic coma, and thrombocytopenia may also occur.

In adults, a single dose of 10 g to 15 g (200 mg/kg to 250 mg/kg) of acetaminophen may cause hepatotoxicity. A dose of 25 g or more is potentially fatal. The potential seriousness of the intoxication may not be evident during the first two days of acute acetaminophen poisoning. During the first 24 hours, nausea, vomiting, anorexia, and abdominal pain occur. These may persist for a week or more. Liver injury may become evident the second day, initial signs being elevation of serum transaminase and lactic dehydrogenase activity, increased serum bilirubin concentration, and prolongation of prothrombin time. Serum albumin concentration and alkaline phosphatase activity may remain normal. The hepatotoxicity may lead to encephalopathy, coma, and death. Transient azotemia is evident in a majority of patients and acute renal failure occurs in some.

There have been reports of glycosuria and impaired glucose tolerance, but hypoglycemia may also occur. Metabolic acidosis and metabolic alkalosis have been reported. Cerebral edema and nonspecific myocardial depression have also been noted. Biopsy reveals centrolobular necrosis with sparing of the periportal area. The hepatic lesions are reversible over a period of weeks or months in nonfatal cases.

The severity of the liver injury can be determined by measurement of the plasma half-time of acetaminophen during the first day of acute poisoning. If the half-time exceeds 4 hours, hepatic necrosis is likely and if the half-time is greater than 12 hours, hepatic coma will probably occur. Only minimal liver damage has developed when the serum concentration was below 120 mcg/mL at 12 hours after ingestion of the drug. If serum bilirubin concentration is greater than 4 mg/100 mL during the first 5 days, encephalopathy may occur.

The seven day oral LD_{50} value for TALACEN in mice is 3570 mg/kg.

Treatment. Oxygen, intravenous fluids, vasopressors, and other supportive measures should be employed as indicated. Assisted or controlled ventilation should also be considered. For respiratory depression due to overdosage or unusual sensitivity to TALACEN, parenteral naloxone is a specific and effective antagonist.

The toxic effects of acetaminophen may be prevented or minimized by antidotal therapy with N-acetylcysteine. In order to obtain the best possible results, N-acetylcysteine should be administered within approximately 16 hours of ingestion of the overdose.

For complete prescribing information for the approved use of acetylcysteine in the treatment of acetaminophen overdose, see package insert for MUCOMYST® (acetylcysteine) Bristol-Myers Squibb.

Vigorous supportive therapy is required in severe intoxication. Procedures to limit the continuing absorption of the drug must be readily performed since the hepatic injury is dose dependent and occurs early in the course of intoxication. Induction of vomiting or gastric lavage, followed by oral administration of activated charcoal should be done in all cases.

If hemodialysis can be initiated within the first 12 hours, it is advocated for patients with a plasma acetaminophen concentration exceeding 120 mcg/mL at 4 hours after ingestion of the drug.

DOSAGE AND ADMINISTRATION

Adult. The usual adult dose is 1 caplet every 4 hours as needed for pain relief, up to a maximum of 6 caplets per day. The usual duration of therapy is dependent upon the condition being treated but in any case should be reviewed regularly by the physician. The effect of meals on the rate and extent of bioavailability of both pentazocine and acetaminophen has not been documented.

HOW SUPPLIED

Talacen is available as a pale blue, scored caplet embossed with "Winthrop" on one side and "T37" on the other side.

Bottles of 100 (NDC 0024-1937-04).

Unit Dose Dispenser Package of 250 (NDC 0024-1937-14), 10 sleeves of 25 caplets each.

Store at controlled room temperature 15° C to 30° C (59° F to 86° F).

Revised September 1999

TSW-6 D

Shown in Product Identification Guide, page 333

TALWIN® Compound pentazocine hydrochloride and aspirin, USP

Ⓒ℞

DESCRIPTION

TALWIN Compound is a combination of pentazocine hydrochloride, USP, equivalent to 12.5 mg base and aspirin, USP, 325 mg.

Pentazocine is a member of the benzazocine series (also known as the benzomorphan series). Chemically, pentazocine is 1, 2, 3, 4, 5, 6 -hexahydro - 6, 11-dimethyl-3-(3-methyl-2-butenyl)-2, 6-methano-3-benzazocin-8-ol, a white, crystalline substance soluble in acidic aqueous solutions and has the following structural formula:

H
N—$CH_2CH{=}C(CH_3)_2$
C--CH_3
H
HO
CH_3

Chemically, aspirin is Benzoic acid, 2-(acetyloxy)- and has the following structural formula:

COOH
$OCOCH_3$

Inactive Ingredients: Magnesium Stearate, Microcrystalline Cellulose, Sodium Lauryl Sulfate, Starch.

CLINICAL PHARMACOLOGY

Pentazocine is a potent analgesic which when administered orally is approximately equivalent, on a mg for mg basis, in analgesic effect to codeine. Two caplets of TALWIN Compound when administered orally have the additive analgesic effect equivalent to 25 mg of TALWIN plus 650 mg of aspirin. TALWIN Compound provides the analgesic effects of pentazocine and the analgesic, anti-inflammatory, and antipyretic actions of aspirin.

Onset of significant analgesia usually occurs between 15 and 30 minutes after oral administration, and duration of action is usually three hours or longer. Onset and duration of action and the degree of pain relief are related both to dose and the severity of pretreatment pain. Pentazocine weakly antagonizes the analgesic effects of morphine, meperidine, and phenazocine; in addition, it produces incomplete reversal of cardiovascular, respiratory, and behavioral depression induced by morphine and meperidine. Pentazocine has about $^1/_{50}$ the antagonistic activity of nalorphine. It also has sedative activity.

INDICATION AND USAGE

For the relief of moderate pain

CONTRAINDICATIONS

TALWIN Compound should not be administered to patients who are hypersensitive to either pentazocine or salicylates, or in any situation where aspirin is contraindicated.

WARNINGS

Drug Dependence. There have been instances of psychological and physical dependence on parenteral pentazocine in patients with a history of drug abuse, and rarely, in patients without such a history. Abrupt discontinuance following the extended use of parenteral pentazocine has resulted in withdrawal symptoms. There have been a few reports of dependence and of withdrawal symptoms with orally administered pentazocine. Patients with a history of drug dependence should be under close supervision while receiving TALWIN Compound orally. There have been rare reports of possible abstinence syndromes in newborns after prolonged use of pentazocine during pregnancy.

In prescribing TALWIN Compound for chronic use, the physician should take precautions to avoid increases in dose by the patient and to prevent the use of the drug in anticipation of pain rather than for the relief of pain.

Head Injury and Increased Intracranial Pressure. The respiratory depressant effects of pentazocine and its potential for elevating cerebrospinal fluid pressure may be markedly exaggerated in the presence of head injury, other intracranial lesions, or a preexisting increase in intracranial pressure. Furthermore, pentazocine can produce effects which may obscure the clinical course of patients with head injuries. In such patients, TALWIN Compound must be used with extreme caution and only if its use is deemed essential.

Usage in Pregnancy. Safe use of pentazocine during pregnancy (other than labor) has not been established. Animal reproduction studies have not demonstrated teratogenic or embryotoxic effects. However, TALWIN Compound should be administered to pregnant patients (other than labor) only when, in the judgment of the physician, the potential benefits outweigh the possible hazards. Patients receiving pentazocine during labor have experienced no adverse effects other than those that occur with commonly used analgesics. TALWIN Compound, should be used with caution in women delivering premature infants.

Acute CNS Manifestations. Patients receiving therapeutic doses of pentazocine have experienced hallucinations (usually visual), disorientation, and confusion which have cleared spontaneously within a period of hours. The mechanism of this reaction is not known. Such patients should be closely observed and vital signs checked. If the drug is reinstituted it should be done with caution since these acute CNS manifestations may recur.

Due to the potential for increased CNS depressant effects, alcohol should be used with caution in patients who are currently receiving pentazocine.

Usage in pediatric patients. Because clinical experience in children under 12 years of age is limited, administration of TALWIN Compound in this age group is not recommended.

Ambulatory Patients. Since sedation, dizziness, and occasional euphoria have been noted, ambulatory patients should be warned not to operate machinery, drive cars, or unnecessarily expose themselves to hazards.

Other. Because of its aspirin content, TALWIN Compound should be used with caution in the presence of peptic ulcer, in conjunction with anticoagulant therapy, or in any situation where the effects of aspirin may be deleterious.

PRECAUTIONS

Certain Respiratory Conditions. Although respiratory depression has rarely been reported after oral administration of pentazocine, TALWIN Compound, should be administered with caution to patients with respiratory depression from any cause, severely limited respiratory reserve, severe bronchial asthma and other obstructive respiratory conditions, or cyanosis.

Impaired Renal or Hepatic Function. Decreased metabolism of the drug by the liver in extensive liver disease may predispose to accentuation of side effects. Although laboratory tests have not indicated that pentazocine causes or increases renal or hepatic impairment, TALWIN Compound should be administered with caution to patients with such impairment.

Myocardial Infarction. As with all drugs, TALWIN Compound should be used with caution in patients with myocardial infarction who have nausea or vomiting.

Biliary Surgery. Narcotic drug products are generally considered to elevate biliary tract pressure for varying periods following administration. Some evidence suggests that pentazocine may differ in this respect (i.e., it causes little or no elevation in biliary tract pressures). The clinical significance of these findings, however, is not yet known.

Patients Receiving Narcotics. Pentazocine is a mild narcotic antagonist. Some patients previously given narcotics, including methadone for the daily treatment of narcotic dependence, have experienced withdrawal symptoms after receiving pentazocine.

CNS Effect. Caution should be used when pentazocine is administered to patients prone to seizures. Seizures have occurred in a few such patients in association with the use of pentazocine although no cause and effect relationship has been established.

Pediatric Use. For usage in pediatric patients see WARNINGS.

ADVERSE REACTIONS

Reactions reported after oral administration of pentazocine or TALWIN Compound include *Gastrointestinal:* nausea, vomiting; infrequently constipation; and rarely abdominal distress, anorexia, diarrhea. *CNS Effects:* dizziness, lightheadedness, hallucinations, sedation, euphoria, headache, confusion, disorientation; infrequently weakness, disturbed dreams, insomnia, syncope, visual blurring and focusing difficulty, depression; and rarely tremor, irritability, excitement, tinnitus. *Autonomic:* sweating; infrequently flushing; and rarely chills. *Allergic:* infrequently rash; and rarely urticaria, edema of the face, and angioneurotic edema. *Cardiovascular:* infrequently decrease in blood pressure, tachycardia. *Hematologic:* rarely depression of white blood cells (especially granulocytes), which is usually reversible, moderate transient eosinophilia. *Other:* rarely respiratory depression, urinary retention, paresthesia, angioneurotic edema, serious skin reactions, including erythema multiforme, Stevens-Johnson syndrome and toxic epidermal necrolysis.

DOSAGE AND ADMINISTRATION

Adults. The usual adult dose is 2 caplets three or four times a day.

Pediatric Patients. Since clinical experience in pediatric patients under 12 years of age is limited, administration of TALWIN Compound in this age group is not recommended.

Duration of Therapy. Patients with chronic pain who receive pentazocine orally for prolonged periods have only rarely been reported to experience withdrawal symptoms when administration was abruptly discontinued (see WARNINGS). Tolerance to the analgesic effect of pentazocine has also been reported only rarely. Significant abnormalities of liver and kidney function tests have not been reported, even after prolonged administration of pentazocine.

OVERDOSAGE

Manifestations: Clinical experience with pentazocine overdosage has been insufficient to define the signs of this condition. Signs of salicylate overdosage include headache, dizziness, confusion, tinnitus, diaphoresis, thirst, nausea, vomiting, diarrhea, tachycardia, tachypnea, Kussmaul breathing, convulsions, and coma. Death is usually from respiratory failure.

Continued on next page

This product information was prepared in September 2000. On these and other products of Sanofi-Synthelabo Inc., detailed information may be obtained on a current basis by direct inquiry to Product Information Services, 90 Park Avenue, New York, NY 10016 (toll free 1-800-446-6267).

Talwin Compound—Cont.

Treatment: Treatment for overdosage of TALWIN Compound, should include treatment for salicylate poisoning as outlined in standard references.
Oxygen, intravenous fluids, vasopressors, and other supportive measures should be employed as indicated. Assisted or controlled ventilation should also be considered. For respiratory depression due to overdosage or unusual sensitivity to pentazocine, parenteral naloxone is a specific and effective antagonist.

HOW SUPPLIED

Caplets, white, each containing pentazocine hydrochloride equivalent to 12.5 mg base and aspirin 325 mg. Bottles of 100 (NDC 0024-1927-04).
Store at room temperature up to 30° C (86° F).
Revised September 1999

TSW-5 O

TALWIN® Nx ℂ ℞
pentazocine and naloxone hydrochlorides USP

Analgesic for Oral Use Only

> TALWIN® Nx is intended for oral use only. Severe, potentially lethal, reactions may result from misuse of TALWIN® Nx by injection either alone or in combination with other substances. (See DRUG ABUSE AND DEPENDENCE section.)

DESCRIPTION

TALWIN Nx contains pentazocine hydrochloride, USP, equivalent to 50 mg base and is a member of the benzazocine series (also known as the benzomorphan series), and naloxone hydrochloride, USP, equivalent to 0.5 mg base.
TALWIN Nx is an analgesic for oral administration.
Chemically, pentazocine hydrochloride is 1,2,3,4,5,6-Hexahydro -6,11 -dimethyl -3-(3-methyl-2-butenyl)-2, 6-methano-3-benzazocin-8-ol hydrochloride, a white, crystalline substance soluble in acidic aqueous solutions.
Chemically, naloxone hydrochloride is Morphinan-6-one, 4, 5-epoxy-3, 14-dihydroxy-17-(2-propenyl)-, hydrochloride, (5α)-. It is a slightly off-white powder, and is soluble in water and dilute acids.
Inactive Ingredients: Colloidal Silicon Dioxide, Dibasic Calcium Phosphate, D&C Yellow #10, FD&C Yellow #6, Magnesium Stearate, Microcrystalline Cellulose, Sodium Lauryl Sulfate, Starch.

CLINICAL PHARMACOLOGY

Pentazocine is a potent analgesic which when administered orally in a 50 mg dose appears equivalent in analgesic effect to 60 mg (1 grain) of codeine. Onset of significant analgesia usually occurs between 15 and 30 minutes after oral administration, and duration of action is usually three hours or longer. Onset and duration of action and the degree of pain relief are related both to dose and the severity of pretreatment pain. Pentazocine weakly antagonizes the analgesic effects of morphine and meperidine; in addition, it produces incomplete reversal of cardiovascular, respiratory, and behavioral depression induced by morphine and meperidine. Pentazocine has about 1/50 the antagonistic activity of nalorphine. It also has sedative activity.
Pentazocine is well absorbed from the gastrointestinal tract. Concentrations in plasma coincide closely with the onset, duration, and intensity of analgesia; peak values occur 1 to 3 hours after oral administration. The half-life in plasma is 2 to 3 hours.
Pentazocine is metabolized in the liver and excreted primarily in the urine. Pentazocine passes into the fetal circulation.
Naloxone when administered orally at 0.5 mg has no pharmacologic activity. Naloxone hydrochloride administered parenterally at the same dose is an effective antagonist to pentazocine and a pure antagonist to narcotic analgesics.
TALWIN Nx is a potent analgesic when administered orally. However, the presence of naloxone in TALWIN Nx will prevent the effect of pentazocine if the product is misused by injection.
Studies in animals indicate that the presence of naloxone does not affect pentazocine analgesia when the combination is given orally. If the combination is given by injection the action of pentazocine is neutralized.

INDICATIONS AND USAGE

> TALWIN® Nx is intended for oral use only. Severe, potentially lethal, reactions may result from misuse of TALWIN® Nx by injection either alone or in combination with other substances. (See DRUG ABUSE AND DEPENDENCE section.)

TALWIN Nx is indicated for the relief of moderate to severe pain.
TALWIN Nx is indicated for oral use only.

CONTRAINDICATIONS

TALWIN Nx should not be administered to patients who are hypersensitive to either pentazocine or naloxone.

WARNINGS

> TALWIN® Nx is intended for oral use only. Severe, potentially lethal, reactions may result from misuse of TALWIN® Nx by injection either alone or in combination with other substances. (See DRUG ABUSE AND DEPENDENCE section.)

Drug Dependence. Pentazocine can cause a physical and psychological dependence. (See DRUG ABUSE AND DEPENDENCE.)
Head Injury and Increased Intracranial Pressure. As in the case of other potent analgesics, the potential of pentazocine for elevating cerebrospinal fluid pressure may be attributed to CO_2 retention due to the respiratory depressant effects of the drug. These effects may be markedly exaggerated in the presence of head injury, other intracranial lesions, or a preexisting increase in intracranial pressure. Furthermore, pentazocine can produce effects which may obscure the clinical course of patients with head injuries. In such patients, pentazocine must be used wth extreme caution and only if its use is deemed essential.
Usage with Alcohol. Due to the potential for increased CNS depressant effects, alcohol should be used with caution in patients who are currently receiving pentazocine.
Patients Receiving Narcotics. Pentazocine is a mild narcotic antagonist. Some patients previously given narcotics, including methadone for the daily treatment of narcotic dependence, have experienced withdrawal symptoms after receiving pentazocine.
Certain Respiratory Conditions. Although respiratory depression has rarely been reported after oral administration of pentazocine, the drug should be administered with caution to patients with respiratory depression from any cause, severely limited respiratory reserve, severe bronchial asthma, and other obstructive respiratory conditions, or cyanosis.
Acute CNS Manifestations. Patients receiving therapeutic doses of pentazocine have experienced hallucinations (usually visual), disorientation, and confusion which have cleared spontaneously within a period of hours. The mechanism of this reaction is not known. Such patients should be very closely observed and vital signs checked. If the drug is reinstituted, it should be done with caution since these acute CNS manifestations may recur.

PRECAUTIONS

CNS Effect. Caution should be used when pentazocine is administered to patients prone to seizures; seizures have occurred in a few such patients in association with the use of pentazocine though no cause and effect relationship has been established.
Impaired Renal or Hepatic Function. Decreased metabolism of pentazocine by the liver in extensive liver disease may predispose to accentuation of side effects. Although laboratory tests have not indicated that pentazocine causes or increases renal or hepatic impairment, the drug should be administered with caution to patients with such impairment.
In prescribing pentazocine for long-term use, the physician should take precautions to avoid increases in dose by the patient.
Biliary Surgery. Narcotic drug products are generally considered to elevate biliary tract pressure for varying periods following their administration. Some evidence suggests that pentazocine may differ from other marketed narcotics in this respect (i.e., it causes little or no elevation in biliary tract pressures). The clinical significance of these findings, however, is not yet known.
Information for Patients. Since sedation, dizziness, and occasional euphoria have been noted, ambulatory patients should be warned not to operate machinery, drive cars, or unnecessarily expose themselves to hazards. Pentazocine may cause physical and psychological dependence when taken alone and may have additive CNS depressant properties when taken in combination with alcohol or other CNS depressants.
Myocardial Infarction. As with all drugs, pentazocine should be used with caution in patients with myocardial infarction who have nausea or vomiting.
Drug Interactions. Usage with Alcohol: See WARNINGS.
Carcinogenesis, Mutagenesis, Impairment of Fertility. No long-term studies in animals to test for carcinogenesis have been performed with the components of TALWIN Nx.
Pregnancy Category C. Animal reproduction studies have not been conducted with TALWIN Nx. It is also not known whether TALWIN Nx can cause fetal harm when administered to pregnant women or can affect reproduction capacity. TALWIN Nx should be given to pregnant women only if clearly needed. However, animal reproduction studies with pentazocine have not demonstrated teratogenic or embryotoxic effects.
Labor and Delivery. Patients receiving pentazocine during labor have experienced no adverse effects other than those that occur with commonly used analgesics. TALWIN Nx should be used with caution in women delivering premature infants. The effect of TALWIN Nx on the mother and fetus, the duration of labor or delivery, the possibility that forceps delivery or other intervention or resuscitation of the newborn may be necessary, or the effect of TALWIN Nx on the later growth, development, and functional maturation of the child are unknown at the present time.
Nursing Mothers. It is not known whether this drug is excreted in human milk. Because many drugs are excreted in human milk, caution should be exercised when TALWIN Nx is administered to a nursing woman.
Pediatric Use. Safety and effectiveness in pediatric patients below the age of 12 years have not been established.

ADVERSE REACTIONS

Cardiovascular. Hypotension, tachycardia, syncope.
Respiratory. Rarely, respiratory depression.
Acute CNS Manifestations. Patients receiving therapeutic doses of pentazocine have experienced hallucinations (usually visual), disorientation, and confusion which have cleared spontaneously within a period of hours. The mechanism of this reaction is not known. Such patients should be closely observed and vital signs checked. If the drug is reinstituted it should be done with caution since these acute CNS manifestations may recur.
Other CNS Effects. Dizziness, lightheadedness, hallucinations, sedation, euphoria, headache, confusion, disorientation; infrequently weakness, disturbed dreams, insomnia, syncope, visual blurring and focusing difficulty, depression; and rarely tremor, irritability, excitement, tinnitus.
Autonomic. Sweating; infrequently flushing; and rarely chills.
Gastrointestinal. Nausea, vomiting, constipation, diarrhea, anorexia, rarely abdominal distress.
Allergic. Edema of the face; dermatitis, including pruritus; flushed skin, including plethora; infrequently rash, and rarely urticaria.
Ophthalmic. Visual blurring and focusing difficulty.
Hematologic. Depression of white blood cells (especially granulocytes), which is usually reversible, moderate transient eosinophilia.
Other. Headache, chills, insomnia, weakness, urinary retention, paresthesia, serious skin reactions, including erythema multiforme, Stevens-Johnson Syndrome and toxic epidermal necrolysis.

DRUG ABUSE AND DEPENDENCE

Controlled Substance. TALWIN Nx is a Schedule IV controlled substance.
There have been some reports of dependence and of withdrawal symptoms with orally administered pentazocine. Patients with a history of drug dependence should be under close supervision while receiving pentazocine orally. There have been rare reports of possible abstinence syndromes in newborns after prolonged use of pentazocine during pregnancy.
There have been instances of psychological and physical dependence on parenteral pentazocine in patients with a history of drug abuse and rarely, in patients without such a history. Abrupt discontinuance following the extended use of parenteral pentazocine has resulted in withdrawal symptoms.
In prescribing pentazocine for chronic use, the physician should take precautions to avoid increases in dose by the patient.
The amount of naloxone present in TALWIN Nx (0.5 mg per tablet) has no action when taken orally and will not interfere with the pharmacologic action of pentazocine. However, this amount of naloxone given by injection has profound antagonistic action to narcotic analgesics.
Severe, even lethal, consequences may result from misuse of tablets by injection either alone or in combination with other substances, such as pulmonary emboli, vascular occlusion, ulceration and abscesses, and withdrawal symptoms in narcotic dependent individuals.
TALWIN Nx contains an opioid antagonist, naloxone (0.5 mg). Naloxone is inactive when administered orally at this dose, and its inclusion in TALWIN Nx is intended to curb a form of misuse of oral pentazocine. Parenterally, naloxone is an active narcotic antagonist. Thus, TALWIN Nx has a lower potential for parenteral misuse than the previous oral pentazocine formulation TALWIN® 50, (pentazocine hydrochloride tablets, USP). However, it is still subject to patient misuse and abuse by the oral route.

OVERDOSAGE

Manifestations. Clinical experience of overdosage with this oral medication has been insufficient to define the signs of this condition.
Treatment. Oxygen, intravenous fluids, vasopressors, and other supportive measures should be employed as indicated. Assisted or controlled ventilation should also be considered. For respiratory depression due to overdosage or unusual sensitivity to pentazocine, parenteral naloxone is a specific and effective antagonist.

DOSAGE AND ADMINISTRATION

> TALWIN® Nx is intended for oral use only. Severe, potentially lethal, reactions may result from misuse of TALWIN® Nx by injection either alone or in combination with other substances. (See DRUG ABUSE AND DEPENDENCE section.)

Adults. The usual initial adult dose is 1 tablet every three or four hours. This may be increased to 2 tablets when needed. Total daily dosage should not exceed 12 tablets.
When anti-inflammatory or antipyretic effects are desired in addition to analgesia, aspirin can be administered concomitantly with this product.
Pediatric Patients. Since clinical experience in pediatric patients under 12 years of age is limited, administration of this product in this age group is not recommended.

Duration of Therapy. Patients with chronic pain who receive TALWIN Nx orally for prolonged periods have only rarely been reported to experience withdrawal symptoms when administration was abruptly discontinued (see WARNINGS). Tolerance to the analgesic effect of pentazocine has also been reported only rarely. However, there is no long-term experience with the oral administration of TALWIN Nx.

HOW SUPPLIED

Tablets (oblong), yellow, scored, each containing pentazocine hydrochloride equivalent to 50 mg base and naloxone hydrochloride equivalent to 0.5 mg base.
Bottles of 100 (NDC 0024-1951-04).
Store at controlled room temperature 15° C to 30° C (59° F to 80° F).
Revised September 1999

TSW-4 E

Shown in Product Identification Guide, page 334

WINSTROL® Ⓒ℞
stanozolol, USP

DESCRIPTION

WINSTROL, brand of stanozolol tablets, is an anabolic steroid, a synthetic derivative of testosterone. Each tablet for oral administration contains 2 mg of stanozolol. It is designated chemically as 17-methyl-2′*H*-5α-androst-2-eno[3,2-*c*]pyrazol-17β-ol, and has the following structural formula:

Inactive Ingredients: Dibasic Calcium Phosphate, D&C Red #28, FD&C Red #40, Lactose, Magnesium Stearate, Starch.

CLINICAL PHARMACOLOGY

Anabolic steroids are synthetic derivatives of testosterone. Certain clinical effects and adverse reactions demonstrate the androgenic properties of this class of drugs. Complete dissociation of anabolic and androgenic effects has not been achieved. The actions of anabolic steroids are therefore similar to those of male sex hormones with the possibility of causing serious disturbances of growth and sexual development if given to young children. They suppress the gonadotropic functions of the pituitary and may exert a direct effect upon the testes.
WINSTROL has been found to increase low-density lipoproteins and decrease high-density lipoproteins. These changes are not associated with any increase in total cholesterol or triglyceride levels and revert to normal on discontinuation of treatment.
Hereditary angioedema (HAE) is an autosomal dominant disorder caused by a deficient or nonfunctional C1 esterase inhibitor (C1 INH) and clinically characterized by episodes of swelling of the face, extremities, genitalia, bowel wall, and upper respiratory tract.
In small scale clinical studies, stanozolol was effective in controlling the frequency and severity of attacks of angioedema and in increasing serum levels of C1 INH and C4. WINSTROL is not effective in stopping HAE attacks while they are under way. The effect of WINSTROL on increasing serum levels of C1 INH and C4 may be related to an increase in protein anabolism.

INDICATIONS AND USAGE

Hereditary Angioedema. WINSTROL is indicated prophylactically to decrease the frequency and severity of attacks of angioedema.

CONTRAINDICATIONS

The use of WINSTROL is contraindicated in the following:
1. Male patients with carcinoma of the breast, or with known or suspected carcinoma of the prostate.
2. Carcinoma of the breast in females with hypercalcemia; androgenic anabolic steroids may stimulate osteolytic resorption of bone.
3. Nephrosis or the nephrotic phase of nephritis.
4. WINSTROL can cause fetal harm when administered to a pregnant woman.

WINSTROL is contraindicated in women who are or may become pregnant. If this drug is used during pregnancy, or if the patient becomes pregnant while taking this drug, the patient should be apprised of the potential hazard to the fetus.

WARNINGS

PELIOSIS HEPATIS, A CONDITION IN WHICH LIVER AND SOMETIMES SPLENIC TISSUE IS REPLACED WITH BLOOD-FILLED CYSTS, HAS BEEN REPORTED IN PATIENTS RECEIVING ANDROGENIC ANABOLIC STEROID THERAPY. THESE CYSTS ARE SOMETIMES PRESENT WITH MINIMAL HEPATIC DYSFUNCTION, BUT AT OTHER TIMES THEY HAVE BEEN ASSOCIATED WITH LIVER FAILURE. THEY ARE OFTEN NOT RECOGNIZED UNTIL LIFE-THREATENING LIVER FAILURE OR INTRA-ABDOMINAL HEMORRHAGE DEVELOPS. WITHDRAWAL OF DRUG USUALLY RESULTS IN COMPLETE DISAPPEARANCE OF LESIONS.
LIVER CELL TUMORS ARE ALSO REPORTED. MOST OFTEN THESE TUMORS ARE BENIGN AND ANDROGEN-DEPENDENT, BUT FATAL MALIGNANT TUMORS HAVE BEEN REPORTED. WITHDRAWAL OF DRUG OFTEN RESULTS IN REGRESSION OR CESSATION OF PROGRESSION OF THE TUMOR. HOWEVER, HEPATIC TUMORS ASSOCIATED WITH ANDROGENS OR ANABOLIC STEROIDS ARE MUCH MORE VASCULAR THAN OTHER HEPATIC TUMORS AND MAY BE SILENT UNTIL LIFE-THREATENING INTRA-ABDOMINAL HEMORRHAGE DEVELOPS.
BLOOD LIPID CHANGES THAT ARE KNOWN TO BE ASSOCIATED WITH INCREASED RISK OF ATHEROSCLEROSIS ARE SEEN IN PATIENTS TREATED WITH ANDROGENS AND ANABOLIC STEROIDS. THESE CHANGES INCLUDE DECREASED HIGH-DENSITY LIPOPROTEIN AND SOMETIMES INCREASED LOW-DENSITY LIPOPROTEIN. THE CHANGES MAY BE VERY MARKED AND COULD HAVE A SERIOUS IMPACT ON THE RISK OF ATHEROSCLEROSIS AND CORONARY ARTERY DISEASE.
Cholestatic hepatitis and jaundice occur with 17-alpha-alkylated androgens at relatively low doses. If cholestatic hepatitis with jaundice appears, the anabolic steroid should be discontinued. If liver function tests become abnormal, the patient should be monitored closely and the etiology determined. Generally, the anabolic steroid should be discontinued although in cases of mild abnormalities, the physician may elect to follow the patient carefully at a reduced drug dosage.
In patients with breast cancer, anabolic steroid therapy may cause hypercalcemia by stimulating osteolysis. In this case, the drug should be discontinued.
Edema with or without congestive heart failure may be a serious complication in patients with preexisting cardiac, renal, or hepatic disease. Concomitant administration of adrenal cortical steroids or ACTH may add to the edema.
Geriatric male patients treated with androgenic anabolic steroids may be at an increased risk for the development of prostatic hypertrophy and prostatic carcinoma.
In children, anabolic steroid treatment may accelerate bone maturation without producing compensatory gain in linear growth. This adverse effect may result in compromised adult stature. The younger the child, the greater the risk of compromising final mature height. The effect on bone maturation should be monitored by assessing bone age of the wrist and hand every six months.
Anabolic steroids have not been shown to enhance athletic ability.

PRECAUTIONS

General

Anabolic steroids may cause suppression of clotting factors II, V, VII, and X, and an increase in prothrombin time.
Women should be observed for signs of virilization (deepening of the voice, hirsutism, acne, and clitoromegaly). To prevent irreversible change, drug therapy must be discontinued, or the dosage significantly reduced when mild virilism is first detected. Such virilization is usual following androgenic anabolic steroid use at high doses. Some virilizing changes in women are irreversible even after prompt discontinuance of therapy and are not prevented by concomitant use of estrogens. Menstrual irregularities may also occur.
The insulin or oral hypoglycemic dosage may need adjustment in diabetic patients who receive anabolic steroids.
Information for the Patient. The physician should instruct patients to report any of the following side effects of androgens:
Adult or Adolescent Males. Too frequent or persistent erections of the penis, appearance or aggravation of acne.
Women. Hoarseness, acne, changes in menstrual periods, or more hair on the face.
All Patients. Any nausea, vomiting, changes in skin color, or ankle swelling.
Laboratory Tests. Women with disseminated breast carcinoma should have frequent determination of urine and serum calcium levels during the course of androgenic anabolic steroid therapy (see WARNINGS).
Because of the hepatotoxicity associated with the use of 17-alpha-alkylated androgens, liver function tests should be obtained periodically.
Periodic (every 6 months) x-ray examinations of bone age should be made during treatment of prepubertal patients to determine the rate of bone maturation and the effects of androgenic anabolic steroid therapy on the epiphyseal centers.
In common with other anabolic steroids, WINSTROL has been reported to lower the level of high-density lipoproteins and raise the level of low-density lipoproteins. These changes usually revert to normal on discontinuation of treatment. Increased low-density lipoproteins and decreased high-density lipoproteins are considered cardiovascular risk factors. Serum lipids and high-density lipoprotein cholesterol should be determined periodically.
Hemoglobin and hematocrit should be checked periodically for polycythemia in patients who are receiving high doses of anabolic steroids.
Drug Interaction. Anabolic steroids may increase sensitivity to anticoagulants; therefore, dosage of an anticoagulant may have to be decreased in order to maintain the prothrombin time at the desired therapeutic level.
Drug/Laboratory Test Interferences. Therapy with androgenic anabolic steroids may decrease levels of thyroxine-binding globulin resulting in decreased total T_4 serum levels and increase resin uptake of T_3 and T_4. Free thyroid hormone levels remain unchanged and there is no clinical evidence of thyroid dysfunction.
Carcinogenesis, Mutagenesis, Impairment of Fertility.
Animal data: Testosterone has been tested by subcutaneous injection and implantation in mice and rats. The implant induced cervical-uterine tumors in mice, which metastasized in some cases. There is suggestive evidence that injection of testosterone into some strains of female mice increases their susceptibility to hepatoma. Testosterone is also known to increase the number of tumors and decrease the degree of differentiation of chemically-induced carcinomas of the liver in rats.
Human data: There are rare reports of hepatocellular carcinoma in patients receiving long-term therapy with androgens in high doses. Withdrawal of the drugs did not lead to regression of the tumors in all cases.
Geriatric patients treated with androgens may be at an increased risk of developing prostatic hypertrophy and prostatic carcinoma although conclusive evidence to support this concept is lacking.
This compound has not been tested for mutagenic potential. However, as noted above, carcinogenic effects have been attributed to treatment with androgenic hormones. The potential carcinogenic effects likely occur through a hormonal mechanism rather than by a direct chemical interaction mechanism.
Impairment of fertility was not tested directly in animal species. However, as noted below under ADVERSE REACTIONS, oligospermia in males and amenorrhea in females are potential adverse effects of treatment with WINSTROL Tablets. Therefore, impairment of fertility is a possible outcome of treatment with WINSTROL.
Pregnancy Category X. See CONTRAINDICATIONS section.
Nursing Mothers. It is not known whether anabolic steroids are excreted in human milk. Many drugs are excreted in human milk and because of the potential for adverse reactions in nursing infants from WINSTROL, a decision should be made whether to discontinue nursing or discontinue the drug, taking into account the importance of the drug to the mother.
Pediatric Use. Anabolic agents may accelerate epiphyseal maturation more rapidly than linear growth in children, and the effect may continue for 6 months after the drug has been stopped. Therefore, therapy should be monitored by x-ray studies at 6 month intervals in order to avoid the risk of compromising the adult height. The safety and efficacy of WINSTROL in children with hereditary angioedema have not been established.

ADVERSE REACTIONS

Hepatic: Cholestatic jaundice with, rarely, hepatic necrosis and death. Hepatocellular neoplasms and peliosis hepatis have been reported in association with long-term androgenic-anabolic steroid therapy (see WARNINGS). Reversible changes in liver function tests also occur including increased bromsulphalein (BSP) retention and increases in serum bilirubin, glutamic oxaloacetic transaminase (SGOT), and alkaline phosphatase.
Genitourinary System: *In men. Prepubertal:* Phallic enlargement and increased frequency of erections.
Postpubertal: Inhibition of testicular function, testicular atrophy and oligospermia, impotence, chronic priapism, epididymitis and bladder irritability.
In women: Clitoral enlargement, menstrual irregularities.
In both sexes: Increased or decreased libido.
CNS: Habituation, excitation, insomnia, depression.
Gastrointestinal: Nausea, vomiting, diarrhea.
Hematologic: Bleeding in patients on concomitant anticoagulant therapy.
Breast: Gynecomastia.
Larynx: Deepening of the voice in women.
Hair: Hirsutism and male pattern baldness in women.
Skin: Acne (especially in women and prepubertal boys).
Skeletal: Premature closure of epiphyses in children (see PRECAUTIONS, **Pediatric Use**).
Fluid and Electrolytes: Edema, retention of serum electrolytes (sodium, chloride, potassium, phosphate, calcium).
Metabolic/Endocrine: Decreased glucose tolerance (see PRECAUTIONS), increased serum levels of low-density lipoproteins and decreased levels of high-density lipoproteins (see PRECAUTIONS, **Laboratory Tests**), increased creatine and creatinine excretion, increased serum levels of creatinine phosphokinase (CPK).

Some virilizing changes in women are irreversible even after prompt discontinuance of therapy and are not prevented by concomitant use of estrogens (see PRECAUTIONS).

DRUG ABUSE AND DEPENDENCE

Controlled Substance Class: WINSTROL is classified as a controlled substance under the Anabolic Steroids Control Act of 1990 and has been assigned to Schedule III.

Continued on next page

This product information was prepared in September 2000. On these and other products of Sanofi-Synthelabo Inc., detailed information may be obtained on a current basis by direct inquiry to Product Information Services, 90 Park Avenue, New York, NY 10016 (toll free 1-800-446-6267).

Winstrol—Cont.

DOSAGE AND ADMINISTRATION

The use of anabolic steroids may be associated with serious adverse reactions, many of which are dose related; therefore, patients should be placed on the lowest possible effective dose.

Hereditary Angioedema. The dosage requirements for continuous treatment of hereditary angioedema with WINSTROL should be individualized on the basis of the clinical response of the patient. It is recommended that the patient be started on 2 mg, three times a day. After a favorable initial response is obtained in terms of prevention of episodes of edematous attacks, the proper continuing dosage should be determined by decreasing the dosage at intervals of one to three months to a maintenance dosage of 2 mg a day. Some patients may be successfully managed on a 2 mg alternate day schedule. During the dose adjusting phase, close monitoring of the patient's response is indicated, particularly if the patient has a history of airway involvement.

The prophylactic dose of WINSTROL, to be used prior to dental extraction, or other traumatic or stressful situations has not been established and may be substantially larger.

Attacks of hereditary angioedema are generally infrequent in childhood and the risks from stanozolol administration are substantially increased. Therefore, long-term prophylactic therapy with this drug is generally not recommended in children, and should only be undertaken with due consideration of the benefits and risks involved (see PRECAUTIONS, **Pediatric Use**).

HOW SUPPLIED

WINSTROL tablets for oral administration are pink, round tablets scored on one side.

Bottles of 100—NDC 0024-2253-04

Store at controlled room temperature 15° to 30° C (59° to 86° F)

Revised September 1999

WSW-1-F(O)

Shown in Product Identification Guide, page 334

ZEPHREX® TABLETS ℞

DESCRIPTION

ZEPHREX® is a white film coated, oval-shaped tablet with a bisect on one side and SANOFI with 460 below the name on the other side.

Each tablet contains:

Pseudoephedrine HCl	60 mg
Guaifenesin	400 mg

HOW SUPPLIED

100's NDC 0024-2624-01

ZEPHREX LA® TABLETS ℞

Each timed release* orange, oval-shaped tablet embossed with bock on one side and a Z bisect LA on the other side contains:

Pseudoephedrine HCl	120.0 mg
Guaifenesin	600.0 mg

* In a special base to provide prolonged therapeutic action.

HOW SUPPLIED

Bottles of 100.

NDC 0024-2627-02

Santen Inc.

555 GATEWAY DRIVE
NAPA, CA 94558

For direct inquiries contact:

Customer Service Department
(877) 772-6836
(877) 473-5264 FAX

ALAMAST™ ℞

[ălā-măst]

(pemirolast potassium ophthalmic solution) 0.1%

Description: ALAMAST™ (pemirolast potassium ophthalmic solution) is a sterile, aqueous ophthalmic solution with a pH of approximately 8.0 containing 0.1% of the mast cell stabilizer, pemirolast potassium, for topical administration to the eyes. Pemirolast potassium is a slightly yellow, water-soluble powder with a molecular weight of 266.3

The chemical structure is presented below:

[See chemical structure at top of next column]

Chemical name:

9-methyl-3-(1H-tetrazol-5-yl)-4H-pyrido[1,2-α] pyrimidin-4-one potassium

Each mL contains: ACTIVE: pemirolast potassium 1 mg (0.1%); PRESERVATIVE: lauralkonium chloride 0.005%; INACTIVES: glycerin, dibasic sodium phosphate, monobasic sodium phosphate, phosphoric acid and/or sodium hydroxide to adjust pH, and purified water. The osmolality of ALAMAST™ ophthalmic solution is approximately 240 mOsmol/kg.

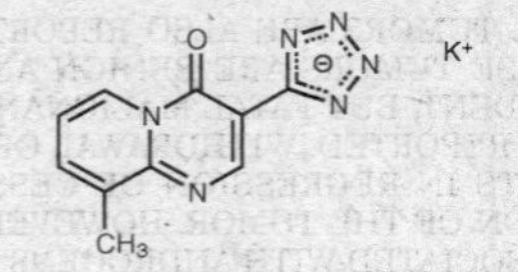

Clinical Pharmacology: Mechanism of Action: Pemirolast potassium is a mast cell stabilizer that inhibits the *in vivo* Type I immediate hypersensitivity reaction. *In vitro* and *in vivo* studies have demonstrated that pemirolast potassium inhibits the antigen-induced release of inflammatory mediators (e.g., histamine, leukotriene C_4, D_4, E_4) from human mast cells. In addition, pemirolast potassium inhibits the chemotaxis of eosinophils into ocular tissue and blocks the release of mediators from human eosinophils. Although the precise mechanism of action is unknown, the drug has been reported to prevent calcium influx into mast cells upon antigen stimulation.

Pharmacokinetics: Topical ocular administration of one to two drops of ALAMAST™ ophthalmic solution in each eye four times daily in 16 healthy volunteers for two weeks resulted in detectable concentrations in the plasma. The mean (±SE) peak plasma level of 4.7 ± 0.8 ng/mL occurred at 0.42 ± 0.05 hours and the mean $t_{½}$ was 4.5 ± 0.2 hours. When a single 10 mg pemirolast potassium dose was taken orally, a peak plasma concentration of 0.723 µg/mL was reached. Following topical administration, about 10–15% of the dose was excreted unchanged in the urine.

Clinical Studies: In clinical environmental studies, ALAMAST™ was significantly more effective than placebo after 28 days in preventing ocular itching associated with allergic conjunctivitis.

Indications And Usage: ALAMAST™ ophthalmic solution is indicated for the prevention of itching of the eye due to allergic conjunctivitis. Symptomatic response to therapy (decreased itching) may be evident within a few days, but frequently requires longer treatment (up to four weeks).

Contraindications: ALAMAST™ ophthalmic solution is contraindicated in patients with previously demonstrated hypersensitivity to any of the ingredients of this product.

Warnings: For topical ophthalmic use only. Not for injection or oral use.

Precautions: Information for patients: To prevent contaminating the dropper tip and solution, do not touch the eyelids or surrounding areas with the dropper tip. Keep the bottle tightly closed when not in use. Patients should be advised not to wear a contact lens if their eye is red. ALAMAST™ should not be used to treat contact lens related irritation. The preservative in ALAMAST™, lauralkonium chloride, may be absorbed by soft contact lenses. Patients who wear soft contact lenses and whose eyes are not red should be instructed to wait at least ten minutes after instilling ALAMAST™ before they insert their contact lenses.

Carcinogenesis, mutagenesis, impairment of fertility: Pemirolast potassium was not mutagenic or clastogenic when tested in a series of bacterial and mammalian tests for gene mutation and chromosomal injury *in vitro* nor was it clastogenic when tested *in vivo* in rats. Pemirolast potassium had no effect on mating and fertility in rats at oral doses up to 250 mg/kg (approximately 20,000 fold the human dose at 2 drops/eye, 40 µL/drop, QID for a 50 kg adult). A reduced fertility and pregnancy index occurred in the F_1 generation when F_0 dams were treated with 400 mg/kg pemirolast potassium during late pregnancy and lactation period (approximately 30,000 fold the human dose).

Pregnancy:

Teratogenic effects: **Pregnancy Category C.** Pemirolast potassium caused an increased incidence of thymic remnant in the neck, interventricular septal defect, fetuses with wavy rib, splitting of thoracic vertebral body, and reduced numbers of ossified sternebrae, sacral and caudal vertebrae, and metatarsi when rats were given oral doses ≥ 250 mg/kg (approximately 20,000 fold the human dose at 2 drops/eye, 40 µL/drop, QID for a 50 kg adult) during organogenesis. Increased incidence of dilation of renal pelvis/ureter in the fetuses and neonates was also noted when rats were given an oral dose of 400 mg/kg pemirolast potassium (approximately 30,000 fold the human dose). Pemirolast potassium was not teratogenic in rabbits given oral doses up to 150 mg/kg (approximately 12,000 fold the human dose) during the same time period. There are no adequate and well-controlled studies in pregnant women. Because animal reproductive studies are not always predictive of human response, ALAMAST™ ophthalmic solution should be used during pregnancy only if the benefit outweighs the risk.

Non-teratogenic effects: Pemirolast potassium produced increased pre- and post-implantation losses, reduced embryo/fetal and neonatal survival, decreased neonatal body weight, and delayed neonatal development in rats receiving an oral dose at 400 mg/kg (approximately 30,000 fold the human dose). Pemirolast potassium also caused a reduction in the number of corpus lutea, the number of implantations, and number of live fetuses in the F_1 generation in rats when F_0 dams were given oral doses ≥250 mg/kg (approximately 20,000 fold the human dose) during late gestation and the lactation period.

Nursing Mothers: Pemirolast potassium is excreted in the milk of lactating rats at concentrations higher than those in plasma. It is not known whether pemirolast potassium is excreted in human milk. Because many drugs are excreted in human milk, caution should be exercised when ALAMAST™ ophthalmic solution is administered to a nursing woman.

Pediatric Use: Safety and effectiveness in pediatric patients below the age of 3 years have not been established.

Adverse Reactions: In clinical studies lasting up to 17 weeks with ALAMAST™ ophthalmic solution, headache, rhinitis, and cold/flu symptoms were reported at an incidence of 10–25%. The occurrence of these side effects was generally mild. Some of these events were similar to the underlying ocular disease being studied.

The following ocular and non-ocular adverse reactions were reported at an incidence of less than 5%:

Ocular: burning, dry eye, foreign body sensation, and ocular discomfort.

Non-Ocular: allergy, back pain, bronchitis, cough, dysmenorrhea, fever, sinusitis, and sneezing/nasal congestion.

Overdosage: No accounts of ALAMAST™ ophthalmic solution overdose were reported following topical ocular application. Oral ingestion of the contents of a 10 mL bottle would be equivalent to 10 mg of pemirolast potassium.

Dosage And Administration: The recommended dose is one to two drops in each affected eye four times daily. Symptomatic response to therapy (decreased itching) may be evident within a few days, but frequently requires longer treatment (up to four weeks).

How Supplied: ALAMAST™ (pemirolast potassium ophthalmic solution) 0.1% is supplied as follows: 10 mL in a white, low density polyethylene bottle with a controlled dropper tip, and a white polypropylene screw cap.

10 mL bottle (NDC 65086-711-10)

Storage: Store at 15°–25°C (59°–77°F).

Rx only

Marketed by:

Santen Inc., Napa, CA 94558, USA

Manufactured by:

Parkedale Pharmaceuticals™, Inc.,
Rochester, MI 48307, USA

U.S. Patent No. 5,034,230

Shown in Product Identification Guide, page 334

BETIMOL® ℞

(timolol ophthalmic solution) 0.25%, 0.5%

DESCRIPTION

Betimol® (timolol ophthalmic) contains:

Active Ingredient: Each mL of Betimol® 0.25% contains 2.56 mg of timolol hemihydrate equivalent to 2.5 mg of timolol. Each mL of Betimol® 0.5% contains 5.12 mg of timolol hemihydrate equivalent to 5.0 mg of timolol.

Inactive Ingredients: monosodium and disodium phosphate dihydrate to adjust pH (6.5–7.5) and water for injection, benzalkonium chloride 0.01% added as a preservative.

HOW SUPPLIED

Betimol® (timolol ophthalmic solution) is a clear, colorless solution.

Betimol® 0.25% is supplied in a white, opaque, plastic ophthalmic dispenser bottle with a controlled drop tip as follows:

NDC 65086-522-99	2.5mL
NDC 65086-522-05	5mL
NDC 65086-522-10	10mL
NDC 65086-522-11	15mL

Betimol® 0.5% is supplied in a white, opaque, plastic, ophthalmic dispenser bottle with a controlled drop tip as follows:

NDC 65086-525-99	2.5mL
NDC 65086-525-05	5mL
NDC 65086-525-10	10mL
NDC 65086-525-15	15mL

MADE IN FINLAND

MANUFACTURED BY:

Santen Oy, P.O. Box 33
FIN-33721, Tampere, Finland

MARKETED BY:

Santen, Inc.
Napa, CA 94558

Revised: May 2000

Shown in Product Identification Guide, page 334

QUIXIN™ ℞

(levofloxacin ophthalmic solution) 0.5%

DESCRIPTION

QUIXIN™ (levofloxacin ophthalmic solution) 0.5% is a sterile topical ophthalmic solution. Levofloxacin is a fluoroquinolone antibacterial active against a broad spectrum of Gram-positive and Gram-negative ocular pathogens.

Levofloxacin is the pure (-)-(S)-enantiomer of the racemic drug substance, ofloxacin. It is more soluble in water at neutral pH than ofloxacin.

Structural formula

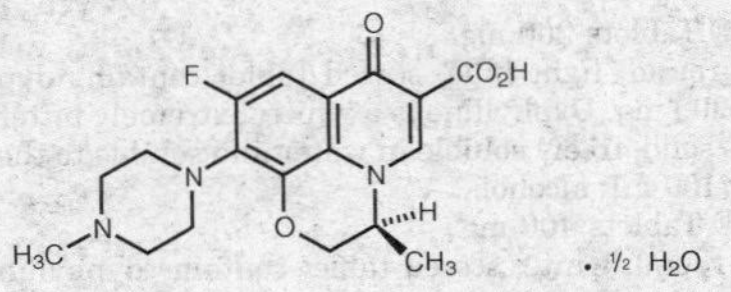

levofloxacin hemihydrate

$C_{18}H_{20}FN_3O_4 \cdot {}^1/_2\, H_2O$ Mol Wt 370.38

Chemical name: (-)-(S)-9-fluoro-2,3-dihydro-3-methyl-10-(4-methyl-1-piperazinyl)-7-oxo-7*H*-pyrido[1,2,3-*de*]-1,4 benzoxazine-6-carboxylic acid hemihydrate.

Levofloxacin (hemihydrate) is a yellowish-white crystalline powder.

Each mL of QUIXIN™ contains 5.12 mg of levofloxacin hemihydrate equivalent to 5 mg levofloxacin.

Contains: **Active**: Levofloxacin 0.5% (5 mg/mL); **Preservative:** benzalkonium chloride 0.005%; **Inactives:** sodium chloride and water. May also contain hydrochloric acid and/or sodium hydroxide to adjust pH.

QUIXIN™ solution is isotonic and formulated at pH 6.5 with an osmolality of approximately 300 mOsm/kg. Levofloxacin is a fluorinated 4-quinolone containing a six-member (pyridobenzoxazine) ring from positions 1 to 8 of the basic ring structure.

CLINICAL PHARMACOLOGY

Pharmacokinetics:

Levofloxacin concentration in plasma was measured in 15 healthy adult volunteers at various time points during a 15-day course of treatment with QUIXIN™ solution. The mean levofloxacin concentration in plasma 1 hour postdose, ranged from 0.86 ng/mL on Day 1 to 2.05 ng/mL on Day 15. The highest maximum mean levofloxacin concentration of 2.25 ng/mL was measured on Day 4 following 2 days of dosing every 2 hours for a total of 8 doses per day. Maximum mean levofloxacin concentrations increased from 0.94 ng/mL on Day 1 to 2.15 ng/mL on Day 15, which is more than 1,000 times lower than those reported after standard oral doses of levofloxacin.

Levofloxacin concentration in tears was measured in 30 healthy adult volunteers at various time points following instillation of a single drop of QUIXIN™ solution. Mean levofloxacin concentrations in tears ranged from 34.9 to 221.1 μg/mL during the 60-minute period following the single dose. The mean tear concentrations measured 4 and 6 hours postdose were 17.0 and 6.6 μg/mL. The clinical significance of these concentrations is unknown.

Microbiology:

Levofloxacin is the L-isomer of the racemate, ofloxacin, a quinolone antimicrobial agent. The antibacterial activity of ofloxacin resides primarily in the L-isomer. The mechanism of action of levofloxacin and other fluoroquinolone antimicrobials involves the inhibition of bacterial topoisomerase IV and DNA gyrase (both of which are type II topoisomerases), enzymes required for DNA replication, transcription, repair, and recombination.

Levofloxacin has *in vitro* activity against a wide range of Gram-negative and Gram-positive microorganisms and is often bactericidal at concentrations equal to or slightly greater than inhibitory concentrations.

Fluoroquinolones, including levofloxacin, differ in chemical structure and mode of action from β-lactam antibiotics and aminoglycosides, and therefore may be active against bacteria resistant to β-lactam antibiotics and aminoglycosides. Additionally, β-lactam antibiotics and aminoglycosides may be active against bacteria resistant to levofloxacin.

Resistance to levofloxacin due to spontaneous mutation *in vitro* is a rare occurrence (range: 10^{-9} to 10^{-10}).

Levofloxacin has been shown to be active against most strains of the following microorganisms, both *in vitro* and in clinical infections as described in the INDICATIONS AND USAGE section:

Aerobic Gram-positive microorganisms

Corynebacterium species*
Staphylococcus aureus (methicillin-susceptible strains only)
Staphylococcus epidermidis (methicillin-susceptible strains only)
Streptococcus pneumoniae
Streptococcus (Groups C/F)
Streptococcus (Group G)
Viridans group streptococci

Aerobic Gram-negative microorganisms

*Acinetobacter lwoffii**
Haemophilus influenzae
*Serratia marcescens**

*Efficacy for this organism was studied in fewer than 10 infections.

The following *in vitro* data are also available, but their clinical significance in ophthalmic infections is unknown. The safety and effectiveness of levofloxacin in treating ophthalmological infections due to these microorganisms have not been established in adequate and well-controlled trials.

These organisms are considered susceptible when evaluated using systemic breakpoints. However, a correlation between the *in vitro* systemic breakpoint and ophthalmological efficacy has not been established. The list of organisms is provided as guidance only in assessing the potential treatment of conjunctival infections. Levofloxacin exhibits *in vitro* minimal inhibitory concentrations (MICs) of 2 μg/mL or less (systemic susceptible breakpoint) against most (≥90%) strains of the following ocular pathogens.

Aerobic Gram-positive microorganisms

Enterococcus faecalis
Staphylococcus saprophyticus
Streptococcus agalactiae
Streptococcus pyogenes

Aerobic Gram-negative microorganisms

Acinetobacter anitratus
Acinetobacter baumannii
Citrobacter diversus
Citrobacter freundii
Enterobacter aerogenes
Enterobacter agglomerans
Enterobacter cloacae
Escherichia coli
Haemophilus parainfluenzae
Klebsiella oxytoca
Klebsiella pneumoniae
Legionella pneumophila
Moraxella catarrhalis
Morganella morganii
Neisseria gonorrhoeae
Proteus mirabilis
Proteus vulgaris
Providencia rettgeri
Providencia stuartii
Pseudomonas aeruginosa
Pseudomonas fluorescens

Clinical Studies:

In randomized, double-masked, multicenter controlled clinical trials where patients were dosed for 5 days, QUIXIN™ demonstrated clinical cures in 79% of patients treated for bacterial conjunctivitis on the final study visit day (day 6–10). Microbial outcomes for the same clinical trials demonstrated an eradication rate for presumed pathogens of 90%.

INDICATIONS AND USAGE

QUIXIN™ solution is indicated for the treatment of bacterial conjunctivitis caused by susceptible strains of the following organisms:

Aerobic Gram-positive microorganisms

Corynebacterium species*
Staphylococus aureus (methicillin-susceptible strains only)
Staphylococcus epidermidis (methicillin-susceptible strains only)
Streptococcus pneumoniae
Streptococcus (Groups C/F)
Streptococcus (Group G)
Viridans group streptococci

Aerobic Gram-negative microorganisms

*Acinetobacter lwoffii**
Haemophilus influenzae
*Serratia marcescens**

*Efficacy for this organism was studied in fewer than 10 infections.

CONTRAINDICATIONS

QUIXIN™ solution is contraindicated in patients with a history of hypersensitivity to levofloxacin, to other quinolones, or to any of the components in this medication.

WARNINGS

NOT FOR INJECTION.

QUIXIN™ solution should not be injected subconjunctivally, nor should it be introduced directly into the anterior chamber of the eye.

In patients receiving systemic quinolones, serious and occasionally fatal hypersensitivity (anaphylactic) reactions have been reported, some following the first dose. Some reactions were accompanied by cardiovascular collapse, loss of consciousness, angioedema (including laryngeal, pharyngeal or facial edema), airway obstruction, dyspnea, urticaria, and itching. If an allergic reaction to levofloxacin occurs, discontinue the drug. Serious acute hypersensitivity reactions may require immediate emergency treatment. Oxygen and airway management should be administered as clinically indicated.

PRECAUTIONS

General:

As with other anti-infectives, prolonged use may result in overgrowth of non-susceptible organisms, including fungi. If superinfection occurs, discontinue use and institute alternative therapy. Whenever clinical judgment dictates, the patient should be examined with the aid of magnification, such as slit-lamp biomicroscopy, and, where appropriate, fluorescein staining.

Patients should be advised not to wear contact lenses if they have signs and symptoms of bacterial conjunctivitis.

Information for Patients:

Avoid contaminating the applicator tip with material from the eye, fingers or other source.

Systemic quinolones have been associated with hypersensitivity reactions, even following a single dose. Discontinue use immediately and contact your physician at the first sign of a rash or allergic reaction.

Drug Interactions:

Specific drug interaction studies have not been conducted with QUIXIN™. However, the systemic administration of some quinolones has been shown to elevate plasma concentrations of theophylline, interfere with the metabolism of caffeine, and enhance the effects of the oral anticoagulant warfarin and its derivatives, and has been associated with transient elevations in serum creatinine in patients receiving systemic cyclosporine concomitantly.

Carcinogenesis, Mutagenesis, Impairment of Fertility:

In a long term carcinogenicity study in rats, levofloxacin exhibited no carcinogenic or tumorigenic potential following daily dietary administration for 2 years; the highest dose (100mg/kg/day) was 875 times the highest recommended human ophthalmic dose.

Levofloxacin was not mutagenic in the following assays: Ames bacterial mutation assay (*S. typhimurium* and *E. coli*), CHO/HGPRT forward mutation assay, mouse micronucleus test, mouse dominant lethal test, rat unscheduled DNA synthesis assay, and the *in vivo* mouse sister chromatid exchange assay. It was positive in the *in vitro* chromosomal aberration (CHL cell line) and *in vitro* sister chromatid exchange (CHL/IU cell line) assays.

Levofloxacin caused no impairment of fertility or reproduction in rats at oral doses as high as 360 mg/kg/day, corresponding to 3,150 times the highest recommended human ophthalmic dose.

Pregnancy: Teratogenic Effects. Pregnancy Category C:

Levofloxacin at oral doses of 810 mg/kg/day in rats, which corresponds to approximately 7,000 times the highest recommended human ophthalmic dose caused decreased fetal body weight and increased fetal mortality.

No teratogenic effect was observed when rabbits were dosed orally as high as 50 mg/kg/day, which corresponds to approximately 400 times the highest recommended maximum human ophthalmic dose, or when dosed intravenously as high as 25 mg/kg/day, corresponding to approximately 200 times the highest recommended human ophthalmic dose.

There are, however, no adequate and well-controlled studies in pregnant women. Levofloxacin should be used during pregnancy only if the potential benefit justifies the potential risk to the fetus.

Nursing Mothers:

Levofloxacin has not been measured in human milk. Based upon data from ofloxacin, it can be presumed that levofloxacin is excreted in human milk. Caution should be exercised when QUIXIN™ is administered to a nursing mother.

Pediatric Use:

Safety and effectiveness in infants below the age of one year have not been established. Oral administration of quinolones has been shown to cause arthropathy in immature animals. There is no evidence that the ophthalmic administration of levofloxacin has any effect on weight bearing joints.

Geriatric Use:

No overall differences in safety or effectiveness have been observed between elderly and other adult patients.

ADVERSE REACTIONS

The most frequently reported adverse events in the overall study population were transient decreased vision, fever, foreign body sensation, headache, transient ocular burning, ocular pain or discomfort, pharyngitis and photophobia. These events occurred in approximately 1–3% of patients. Other reported reactions occurring in less than 1% of patients included allergic reactions, lid edema, ocular dryness, and ocular itching.

DOSAGE AND ADMINISTRATION

Days 1 and 2: Instill one to two drops in the affected eye(s) every 2 hours while awake up to 8 times per day.

Days 3 through 7: Instill one to two drops in the affected eye(s) every 4 hours while awake up to 4 times per day.

HOW SUPPLIED

QUIXIN™ (levofloxacin ophthalmic solution) 0.5% is supplied in a white, low density polyethylene bottle with a controlled dropper tip and a tan, high density polyethylene cap in the following sizes:

2.5 mL NDC 65086-135-99 (Physician Sample)
2.5 mL NDC 65086-135-25
5 mL NDC 65086-135-05

Storage: Store at 15°–25°C (59°–77°F).

Rx Only.

Manufactured by:
Santen Oy, P. O. Box 33
FIN-33721 Tampere, Finland

Marketed by:
Santen Inc., Napa, CA 94558, U.S.A.

Licensed from Daiichi Pharmaceutical Co., Ltd., Tokyo, Japan

U.S. PAT. NOS. 4,382,892; 4,551,456; 5,503,407

Shown in Product Identification Guide, page 334

For information on over-the-counter drugs, consult **PDR For Nonprescription Drugs.**

Savage Laboratories®

a division of Altana Inc.
60 BAYLIS ROAD
MELVILLE, NY 11747

Direct Inquiries to:
Customer Service
(800) 231-0206
FAX: (631) 454-0732

AXOCET® ℞

(Butalbital and Acetaminophen capsules)
Rx only

DESCRIPTION

AXOCET® are opaque grey capsules imprinted with Savage logo and 0198. Each capsule contains Butalbital USP, 50 mg and Acetaminophen USP, 650 mg.

HOW SUPPLIED

AXOCET® Capsules are supplied as follows:
Bottle of 100, NDC 0281-0198-17

—NEW FORMULATION— CHROMAGEN® OB ℞

PRENATAL MULTI-VITAMIN/MINERAL SOFT GELATIN CAPSULES
Rx only

DESCRIPTION

CONTENTS: Each blue soft gelatin capsule, imprinted 0331 contains:

Calcium (as calcium carbonate)	200 mg
Vitamin C (ascorbic acid)	60 mg
Iron (as ferrous fumarate)	28 mg
Docusate Calcium	25 mg
Vitamin E (*d*-alpha tocopherol)	30 IU
Vitamin B_6 (pyridoxine hydrochloride)	20 mg
Vitamin B_2 (riboflavin)	1.8 mg
Vitamin B_1 (thiamine mononitrate)	1.6 mg
Folic Acid	1 mg
Vitamin B_{12} (cyanocobalamin)	12 mcg
Vitamin D (cholecalciferol)	400 IU

ACTIVE INGREDIENT: Each gelcap contains 1 mg folic acid.

DISCUSSION: The amount of elemental iron and the absorption of the iron components of commercial iron preparations vary widely. Certain accessory components enhance absorption and utilization of iron. Chromagen® OB gelcaps are formulated to provide the essential factors for a complete, versatile vitamin and mineral supplement.

ACTIONS

HIGH ELEMENTAL IRON CONTENT: Ferrous fumarate, used in Chromagen® OB gelcaps, is an organic iron complex which has the highest elemental iron content of any hematinic salt—33%. This compares with 20% for ferrous sulfate (heptahydrate) and 13% for ferrous gluconate.

MORE COMPLETE ABSORPTION: It has been shown that ascorbic acid, when given in sufficient amounts, can increase the absorption of ferrous iron from the gastrointestinal tract. The effect of ascorbic acid may be related both to its reducing effect, preventing the formation of insoluble ferric hydroxide, and to its ability to form soluble complexes with ferric iron, which preserve the iron solubility at the more alkaline duodenal pH. Studies indicate that 60 mg of ascorbic acid can increase iron absorption. Each Chromagen® OB gelcap contains 60 mg of ascorbic acid.

PROMOTES MOVEMENT OF PLASMA IRON: Ascorbic acid also plays a role in the movement of plasma iron to storage depots in the tissues. The action, which leads to the transport of plasma iron to ferritin, presumably involves its reducing effect, converting transferrin iron from the ferric to the ferrous state. There is also evidence that ascorbic acid improves iron utilization, presumably as a further result of its reducing action. It may also have a direct effect upon erythropoiesis. Ascorbic acid is further alleged to enhance the conversion of folic acid to a more physiologically active form, folinic acid, necessary for erythropoiesis.

EXCELLENT ORAL TOLERATION: Ferrous fumarate is used in Chromagen® OB gelcaps because it is less likely to cause gastric disturbances. Ferrous fumarate has a low ionization constant and high solubility in the entire pH range of the gastrointestinal tract. It does not precipitate proteins or have the astringency of ionizable forms of iron, and does not interfere with proteolytic or diastatic activities of the digestive system.

TOXICITY: Ferrous fumarate is the least toxic of three popular iron salts.

INDICATIONS

Chromagen® OB is a vitamin and mineral nutritional supplement indicated for use in women throughout pregnancy and in the postnatal period for both lactating and nonlactating mothers. It is also useful for improving the nutritional status of women prior to conception.

CONTRAINDICATIONS

This product is contraindicated in patients with a known hypersensitivity to any of the ingredients. Hemochromatosis and hemosiderosis are contraindications to iron therapy. Supplemental vitamins should also not be prescribed for patients with Wilson's disease.

WARNINGS

Folic acid alone is improper therapy in the treatment of pernicious anemia and other megaloblastic anemias where Vitamin B_{12} is deficient.

> **WARNING: Accidental overdose of iron-containing products is a leading cause of fatal poisoning in children under 6. Keep this product out of reach of children. In case of accidental overdose, call a doctor or poison control center immediately.**

Average gelcap doses in sensitive individuals or excessive dosage may cause nausea, skin rash, vomiting, diarrhea, precordial pain, or flushing of the face and extremities.

PRECAUTIONS

General:
Folic acid, in doses above 0.1 mg daily may obscure pernicious anemia, in that hematologic remission can occur while neurological manifestations remain progressive.
Information for Patients:
Patients should not exceed the recommended dosage unless directed by the physician. Patients should be informed that iron therapy can cause black or dark stools.

ADVERSE REACTIONS

The following adverse reactions, normally associated with iron products, such as Chromagen® OB, may include constipation, diarrhea, nausea, vomiting, dark stools and abdominal pain. Adverse reactions are usually transient.

USUAL ADULT DOSAGE

One soft gelatin capsule daily, to be taken with food and a full glass of water.

HOW SUPPLIED

NDC 0281-0331-53, bottle of 100 capsules.
Dispense in a tight, light resistant container with a child resistant closure.
Store at controlled room temperature 15°–30°C (59°–86°F). Avoid excessive heat 40°C (104°F). Avoid freezing.
Manufactured for:
SAVAGE LABORATORIES®
a division of Altana Inc.
MELVILLE, NEW YORK 11747 IF70331A
by: R.P. Scherer Corporation #242
St. Petersburg, Florida 33702 R6/00
Shown in Product Identification Guide, page 334

CHROMAGEN® FA ℞

SOFT GELATIN CAPSULES
Rx only

DESCRIPTION

Each maroon and brown soft gelatin capsule contains: ferrous fumarate USP, 200 mg (66 mg elemental iron), ascorbic acid USP, 250 mg, folic acid USP, 1 mg, cyanocobalamin USP, 10 mcg.

> **WARNING**
> **Accidental overdose of iron-containing products is a leading cause of fatal poisoning in children under 6. Keep this product out of reach of children. In case of accidental overdose, call a doctor or poison control center immediately.**

HOW SUPPLIED

Capsules: NDC 0281-0259-18, Unit Dose Box 100
Shown in Product Identification Guide, page 334

CHROMAGEN® FORTE ℞

SOFT GELATIN CAPSULES
Rx only

DESCRIPTION

Each brown soft gelatin capsule imprinted with and 0262 contains: ferrous fumarate USP, 460 mg (151 mg elemental iron), ascorbic acid USP, 60 mg, folic acid USP, 1 mg, cyanocobalamin USP, 10 mcg.

> **WARNING**
> **Accidental overdose of iron-containing products is a leading cause of fatal poisoning in children under 6. Keep this product out of reach of children. In case of accidental overdose, call a doctor or poison control center immediately.**

HOW SUPPLIED

Capsules: NDC 0281-0262-18, Unit Dose Box 100
Shown in Product Identification Guide, page 334

DILOR® ℞

(Dyphylline tablets, elixir, injection USP)
Rx only

DESCRIPTION

Dilor® Tablets 200 mg
Each round, light blue, scored tablet contains dyphylline USP, 200 mg. Dyphylline is a white, extremely bitter, amorphous solid, freely soluble in water and soluble to the extent of 2 g/100 mL alcohol.
Dilor® Tablets 400 mg
Each round, white, scored tablet contains dyphylline USP, 400 mg and the following inactive ingredients: colloidal silicon dioxide, corn starch, food starch, povidone, sodium lauryl sulfate, and stearic acid.
Dilor® Injection
Each 2 mL ampule contains dyphylline USP, 500 mg (250 mg/mL), in water for injection USP, Sodium hydroxide NF used to adjust pH.

HOW SUPPLIED

Dilor®-200 Tablets are supplied as follows:
NDC 0281-1115-53 Bottle of 100
NDC 0281-1115-63 Unit dose, Box of 100
Dilor®-400 Tablets are supplied as follows:
NDC 0281-1116-53 Bottle of 100
NDC 0281-1116-57 Bottle of 1000
NDC 0281-1116-63 Unit dose box of 100
Dilor® Injection (dyphylline injection USP) 250 mg/mL is supplied as follows:
NDC 0281-1112-31 Box of 6 × 2 mL ampules

DILOR-G® ℞

(dyphylline and guaifenesin tablets USP)
(dyphylline and guaifenesin Liquid USP)
Rx only

DESCRIPTION

Dilor-G® Tablets
Each round, pink scored tablet contains dyphylline USP 200 mg and guaifenesin USP 200 mg and the following inactive ingredients: colloidal silicon dioxide, corn starch, food starch, povidone, stearic acid and artificial coloring.
Dilor-G® Liquid
Each teaspoon (5 mL) contains dyphylline USP 100 mg and guaifenesin USP 100 mg in a pale-pink, mint flavored base containing: citric acid, glycerin, saccharin sodium, sorbitol, sucrose, artificial coloring and flavoring, purified water, and sodium hydroxide to adjust pH. Methylparaben and propylparaben added as preservatives.

HOW SUPPLIED

Dilor-G® Tablets are supplied as follows:
NDC 0281-1124-53, Bottle of 100.
NDC 0281-1124-57, Bottle of 1000.
NDC 0281-1124-63, Unit dose, Box of 100.
Dilor-G® Liquid
NDC 0281-1127-74, Pint.
1F71124C #84 R 5/99
1F71127C #79 R 3/99

ETHIODOL® ℞

BRAND OF ETHIODIZED OIL INJECTION
A Low Viscosity Radio-Opaque Diagnostic Agent
Rx only

> NOT FOR INTRAVASCULAR, INTRATHECAL OR INTRABRONCHIAL USE

DESCRIPTION

Ethiodol, brand of ethiodized oil, is a sterile injectable radio-opaque diagnostic agent for use in hysterosalpingography and lymphography. It contains 37% iodine (475 mg/mL) organically combined with ethyl esters of the fatty acids (primarily as ethyl monoiodostearate and ethyl diiodostearate) of poppyseed oil. Stabilized with poppyseed oil, 1%. The precise structure of Ethiodol is unknown at this time. Ethiodol is a straw to amber colored, oily fluid, which because of simplified molecular structure, possesses a greatly reduced viscosity (1.280 specific gravity at 15°C yields viscosity of 0.5–1.0 poise). This high fluidity provides a new flexibility for radiographic exploration.

CLINICAL PHARMACOLOGY

There has been little detailed investigation of the metabolic fate of Ethiodol in either man or animals. However, the fate of Ethiodol following lymphangiography in dogs has been reported.[1] Koehler et al. employed I^{131}-tagged Ethiodol for lymphangiography in dogs and analyses of individual organs at various time intervals were done. The investigators reported an average of only 25% of the injected medium was retained in the lymphatics at the end of three days. An average of 50% was recovered from the lungs. They found the remainder of injected activity was fairly uniformly distributed throughout the body. Urinary excretion in the form of inorganic iodine was revealed as the chief mode of iodine loss from the system.

INDICATIONS

Ethiodol is indicated for use as a radio-opaque medium for hysterosalpingography and lymphography.

IN HYSTEROSALPINGOGRAPHY

CONTRAINDICATIONS

Ethiodol is contraindicated in patients hypersensitive to it. Ethiodol should not be injected intrathecally or intravascularly, or used in bronchography. A history of sensitivity to iodine contraindicates the use of Ethiodol; iodine is split off from fatty compounds and becomes free iodine in the body. Hysterosalpingography is contraindicated in intrauterine pregnancy, acute pelvic inflammatory disease, marked cervical erosion, endocervicitis in the presence of intrauterine bleeding, in the immediate pre-or postmenstrual phase, or within 30 days of curettage or conization.

WARNINGS

Ethiodol is not intended for use in bronchography and, therefore, is not to be introduced into the bronchial tree. A history of sensitivity to iodine or to other contrast materials is not an absolute contraindication to Ethiodol, but calls for extreme caution. All procedures utilizing contrast media carry a definite risk of adverse reactions. While most reactions are minor, life threatening and fatal reactions may occur without warning. The risk/benefit factor should always be carefully evaluated. At all times a fully equipped emergency cart and resuscitation equipment should be readily available, and personnel competent in recognizing and treating reactions of all severity should be on hand.

PRECAUTIONS

General: Since iodine-containing contrast materials may alter the results of certain thyroid function tests, such tests, if indicated, should be performed prior to the administration of this drug. Pulmonary embolization of the contrast material may occur if hysterosalpingography is performed under conditions which may lead to intravasation of the contrast materials. These conditions include uterine bleeding, recent curettage or conization and injection of the contrast material under excessive pressure.

Carcinogenesis, Mutagenesis, and Impairment of Fertility: Long-term studies in animals have not been performed to evaluate carcinogenic potential, mutagenesis, or whether Ethiodol can affect fertility in males or females.

Pregnancy Category C: Animal reproduction studies have not been conducted with Ethiodol. It is also not known whether Ethiodol can cause fetal harm when administered to a pregnant woman or can affect reproduction capacity. Ethiodol should be administered to a pregnant woman only if clearly needed.

Nursing Mothers: It is not known whether this drug is excreted in human milk. Because many drugs are excreted in human milk and because of the potential for serious adverse reactions in nursing infants from Ethiodol, a decision should be made whether to discontinue nursing or to discontinue the drug, taking into account the importance of the drug to the mother.

ADVERSE REACTIONS

Hypersensitivity reactions, foreign body reactions and exacerbation of pelvic inflammatory disease, although infrequent, have been reported. In an occasional patient, abdominal pains may occur. Such pains may be the result of tubal torsion, or possibly due to too rapid a rate of instillation or excessive pressure, or both. The condition is usually only transitory, lasting one or two hours at most, and may be relieved by the administration of any of the commonly used analgesics.

DOSAGE AND ADMINISTRATION

The hysterosalpingogram is preferably taken during the patient's preovulatory phase (as determined from her basal body temperature record) and not less than two days after cessation of her menstrual flow. It has been frequently observed that some bleeding will occur during or after the onset of pregnancy which cannot be distinguished by the patient from a normal menstrual period. In such cases a basal body temperature record will reveal a sustained high temperature phase, and thus enable an operator to avoid hysterosalpingography when a pregnancy may exist. Salpingography should not be performed if the blood is exuding from the cervical os (which occasionally occurs without the patient being aware of it) or if any gross evidence of endocervicitis exists.

Careful aseptic technique should be employed as for any operative procedure in which the uterus is entered. A self-retaining cannula should be used thereby permitting removal of the vaginal speculum so that the outline of the cervical canal may be seen in the film. The use of a radio-opaque aluminum speculum may be employed in patients where a lacerated or patulous cervix does not permit the use of a retaining cannula.

The radio-opaque agent is introduced under pressure and preferably with fluoroscopic control. A preliminary film is exposed and a skiagram is made after the injection of 5 mL of the agent. The pressure is raised to 80–90 mm Hg. In cases of normal bilateral tubal patency, the pressure falls immediately to below 60 mm Hg. The wet film may be viewed immediately and if both tubes are seen to "fill", the apparatus is removed and the procedure is finished, except for the 24 hour follow-up to establish whether or not "spill" into the peritoneal cavity has occurred.

Increments of 2 mL of the agent are injected and successive films exposed until tubal patency is established or until the patient's limit of tolerance to discomfort is reached. Few patients will complain of discomfort at pressures under 200 mm Hg.

IN LYMPHOGRAPHY

CONTRAINDICATIONS

Ethiodol is contraindicated in patients hypersensitive to it. Ethiodol should not be injected intrathecally or intravascularly or introduced into the bronchial tree. Patients with known sensitivity to iodine should not have lymphography performed. Iodine is split off from fatty compounds and becomes free iodine in the body. Lymphography is contraindicated in patients with a right to left cardiac shunt, in patients with advanced pulmonary disease, especially those with alveolar-capillary block, and in patients who have had radiotherapy to the lungs.

WARNINGS

The use of intralymphatic Ethiodol presents a significant hazard in patients with pre-existing pulmonary disease characterized by a decrease in pulmonary diffusing capacity and/or pulmonary blood flow. A few fatalities have been noted in such patients. With reference to this potential complication, recent studies indicate a significant decrease in both pulmonary diffusing capacity and pulmonary capillary blood flow following Ethiodol lymphography without appreciable concomitant clinical manifestations. Also, care should be exercised in patients with other types of pulmonary disease in view of the more frequent incidence of overt pulmonary complications such as pulmonary infarction, in these groups. However, it is to be noted that pulmonary infarction, although rare, has occurred in patients without evidence of pre-existing pulmonary disease.

The safety of intralymphatic Ethiodol has not been established in pregnant women, and accordingly, its use should be restricted to such situations where it is deemed necessary.

PRECAUTIONS

General: Although subclinical pulmonary embolization occurs in a majority of patients following Ethiodol lymphography, clinical evidence of such embolization is infrequent and is usually of a transient nature. Such clinical manifestations are usually immediate, but may be delayed from a few hours to days. It would appear that it is advantageous to use the smallest volume of Ethiodol necessary for radiographic visualization. For this reason, and to prevent inadvertent venous administration, radiographic monitoring of patients is recommended during the injection of Ethiodol.

The timing and choice of anesthesia following Ethiodol injection may be influenced by consideration of the above noted decrease in pulmonary and capillary blood flow and diffusing capacity. It should be noted that although an average of 2 to 3 days was required for complete reversibility for such tests, an occasional patient required up to 12 days to return to baseline values.

PBI determination of thyroid uptake studies should be carried out prior to the lymphographic procedure because interference with these tests may be anticipated for as long as one year. In the presence of known iodine sensitivity, Ethiodol lymphography should be carried out with greatest precaution.

Carcinogenesis, Mutagenesis, and Impairment of Fertility: Long-term studies in animals have not been performed to evaluate carcinogenic potential, mutagenesis, or whether Ethiodol can affect fertility in males or females.

Pregnancy Category C: Animal reproduction studies have not been conducted with Ethiodol. It is also not known whether Ethiodol can cause fetal harm when administered to a pregnant woman or can affect reproduction capacity. Ethiodol should be administered to a pregnant woman only if clearly needed.

Nursing Mothers: It is not known whether this drug is excreted in human milk. Because many drugs are excreted in human milk and because of the potential for serious adverse reactions in nursing infants from Ethiodol, a decision should be made whether to discontinue nursing or to discontinue the drug, taking into account the importance of the drug to the mother.

ADVERSE REACTIONS

The occasional observation of pulmonary Ethiodol embolization (infarction) several hours after injection has been reported. This was noticed more frequently when excessive amounts of Ethiodol have been injected, in the presence of marked lymphatic obstruction or through accidental intravenous injection. Radiologic manifestations are fine, granular stippling throughout both lung fields. The clinical symptoms usually noted have been mild, consisting of moderate temperature elevation, dyspnea, and cough. However, severe acute symptoms developed in two patients both of whom were severely ill and required extensive care.[2] Fuchs[3] experienced 1 severe and 3 minor complications in a series of 20 bilateral procedures. Two are described by the author as cardiovascular collapse occurring at two hours respectively following the completion of the procedure. It was postulated that minute emboli may have been causative. Recovery was rapid and complete in both instances.

The occurrence of pulmonary invasion may be minimized if radiographic confirmation of intralymphatic (rather than venous) injection is secured, and the procedure discontinued when the medium becomes visible in the thoracic duct or the presence of lymphatic obstruction is noticed.

While rare, other side effects reported include transient fever, lymphangitis, iodism (headache, soreness of mouth and pharynx, coryza and skin rash), allergic dermatitis, and lipogranuloma formation. Delayed wound healing at the site of incision and secondary infection are occasionally seen, and can be prevented or minimized by adhering to a strict sterile technique.

Transient edema or temporary exacerbation of preexisting lymphedema, as well as thrombophlebitis have also been reported. In the extremely rare presence of concomitant lymphatic and inferior vena cava obstruction the contrast medium may be shunted partially to the liver, resulting in hepatic embolization. Also, when accidental intravenous administration of Ethiodol results in a considerable amount of this medium entering the circulation, embolization other than pulmonary may occur as reported in 2 cases.[4] Both cases developed a transient, psychotic-like manifestation, which in all probability stemmed from the entrance of fine oil droplets into the cerebral circulation. Recovery was uneventful and complete without evidence of neurological sequelae.

DOSAGE AND ADMINISTRATION

This method applies for both the upper and lower extremities. A lymphatic vessel is selected for cannulization.

The patient should be comfortably arranged in a supine position on a portable stretcher or an x-ray table. When available, a radiolucent pad will add to the patient's comfort during the one to two hours required for completion of the examination. It is important that the patient be in a cooperative state. Premedication might be advisable in the unusually apprehensive patient.

In the unusually restless patient, the extremities should be immobilized during the entire procedure to prevent displacement of the needle. Thomas splints have been satisfactorily employed for the legs and simple arm boards for the upper extremities. The cut-down and injection instruments and materials include the following:

- Sterile pediatric cut-down set
- Sterile towels for draping, sponges, etc.
- Local anesthetic, such as procaine hydrochloride, and a syringe
- Bactericidal painting solution
- 20 mL syringe containing 15 mL of Ethiodol with an 18 inch catheter to which is affixed a 27 or 30 gauge needle. (If bilateral lymphography is scheduled, two syringes should be prepared.)
- A manually driven or motorized unit (a pressure regulated pump) to provide for slow injection.

Under local infiltration anesthesia, a transverse, curvilinear or longitudinal small skin incision should be made near the ankle or wrist (just lateral and distal to the first metatarsal head on the dorsum of the foot, or just over the "snuff-box" in the dorsum of the hand).

Upon superficial dissection (but not penetrating the subcutaneous layer of tissue) lymph vessels will be noted in the immediate subcutaneous tissue, while larger lymph vessel trunks are found in the extrafascial plane. The deeper lymph trunks will be easier to cannulate.

One lymph vessel is then exposed, avoiding circumferential dissection. The less manipulation performed, the better the results that will be obtained. The lymphatic, thus isolated, is then cannulated with a 27 or 30 gauge 5/8 inch needle, depending upon the size of the lymphatic selected for injection. It is rarely possible to cannulate with a needle greater than 27 gauge. Insertion of the needle through the skin flap before cannulating the lymphatic serves to reduce the movement of the needle within the vessel. Additional security of the needle in the lymphatic is obtained by strapping, with sterile tape, the polyethylene tubing to the patient's foot.

The injection should be started at a slow rate, i.e., 0.1 mL to 0.2 mL per minute. Radiographic monitoring either by fluoroscopy or serial radiographs after 1 mL to 2 mL has been injected, will confirm the proper intralymphatic placement of the needle, rule out accidental intravenous injection or extravasation of the medium by perforation or rupture of the lymphatic. Monitoring will also permit prompt termination of the procedure in the event that lymphatic blockage is present. In such situations, continuation of the injection will result in unnecessary introduction of contrast material in the venous system via the lymphovenous communication channels. If the injection is satisfactory, approximately 6 to 8 mL, are then injected. However, as soon as it becomes radiographically evident that Ethiodol has entered the thoracic duct, the procedure should be terminated to minimize entry of the contrast material into the subclavian vein. Two to four mL of Ethiodol injected into the upper extremity will suffice to demonstrate the axillary and supraclavicular nodes. In penile lymphography approximately 2 to 3 mL of Ethiodol is required. In infants and children, a minimum of 1 mL to a maximum of 6 mL should be employed.

The rate of speed at which the contrast material may be introduced varies and is dependent upon receptivity of the lymphatics in the individual patient. If the injection is proceeding at too rapid a rate, extravasation will be noted and the patient may refer to pain in the foot, leg or arm.

At the completion of the injection, anteroposterior roentgenograms are obtained of the legs or arms, thighs, pelvis, abdomen and chest (dorsal spine technique). Lateral or oblique views as well as laminograms are obtained when in-

Continued on next page

Ethiodol—Cont.

dicated. Follow-up films at 24 or 48 hours provide better demonstration of lymph nodes and permit more concise evaluation of nodal architecture.

As a general rule, the smallest possible amount of Ethiodol should be employed according to the anatomical area to be visualized. Therefore, and to prevent inadvertent venous administration, fluoroscopic monitoring or serial radiographic guidance of patients is recommended during the injection of Ethiodol.

Average dose in the adult patient for unilateral lymphography of the upper extremities is 2 to 4 mL; of lower extremities, 6 to 8 mL; of penile lymphography, 2 to 3 mL; of cervical lymphography, 1 to 2 mL.

In the pediatric patient, a minimum of 1 mL to a maximum of 6 mL may be employed according to the anatomical area to be visualized.

SUMMARY OF STEPS TO AVOID COMPLICATIONS IN LYMPHOGRAPHY[5]

1. Contraindicate patients:
   A. With a known hypersensitivity to Ethiodol
   B. With a right to left cardiac shunt
   C. With advanced pulmonary disease, especially those with alveolar-capillary block. Pulmonary gas diffusion studies should be done if in doubt.
   D. Who have had radiation therapy to the lungs
2. Proceed with caution:
   A. Patients having markedly advanced neoplastic disease with expected lymphatic obstruction.
   B. Patients having undergone previous surgery interrupting the lymphatic system.
   C. Patients having had deep radiation therapy to the examined area.
   If in those cases in which extreme caution should be exercised, lymphography is still necessary, a smaller dose of oily contrast medium with protracted injection time with less pressure and careful monitoring is required.
3. Skin testing should be done on all patients before submitting them to lymphography. Be aware of possible hypersensitivity to local anesthetics and skin disinfectants. Careful history taking is important.
4. Technique of cannulation: extravasation is to be avoided and/or detected early. The injection site should be included on the "scout film" or observed under image amplification fluoroscopy. The needle tip must remain visible in the incision wound.
5. Oily contrast materials: once opened, ampules should be discarded. Ampules of Ethiodol should not be used if the color has darkened or if particulate matter is present. The average dose for each foot in an adult is 5 to 6 mL; one-half as much for the upper extremity. The amount for children should be determined by careful monitoring. It should stay below 0.25 mL/kg.
6. Injection pressure should be regulated to deliver the average dose in no less than 1 1/4 hours. Continuous monitoring helps to determine the speed most appropriate for each individual. Sensation of pain is a warning of too high pressure.
7. Scout roentgenograms: if scout roentgenograms are used for monitoring, they should be developed and viewed immediately in order to apply corrective measures when needed; e.g., discontinuation of the study when one sees intravenous injection or lymphatico-venous anastomosis. Reduction of injection speed is needed if evidence of collateral circulation occurs or if the higher abdomino-aortic nodes do not opacify in spite of the usual injection pressure. This is highly suggestive of lymphatic obstruction. Scout roentgenograms should be taken more frequently in such cases.
8. Surgical technique: strict aseptic surgical technique is followed including the wearing of a face mask. Before suturing the incision wound, the remnants of the lymphatic vessels and loose tissue are removed and the wound well washed with saline to remove any possible oil. In case of reflux type lymphedema, the cannulated large lymphatic vessel may have to be closed by catgut to avoid development of a lymphocyst.
   The patient is instructed to elevate the legs as often as possible to promote healing. The sutures are removed from the feet on the 10th day, and on the 5th or 6th from the hands.

HOW SUPPLIED

Ethiodol (ethiodized oil for injection) is supplied in a box of two 10 ml ampules, NDC 0281-7062-37.

Store at controlled room temperature 15°–30°C (59°–86°F). Protect from light. Remove from carton only upon use.

Parenteral drug products should be inspected visually for particulate matter and discoloration prior to administration, whenever solution and container permit. Ethiodol brand of ethiodized oil for injection is straw to amber color under normal conditions. (See **DESCRIPTION**).

A development of Guerbet Laboratories.

BIBLIOGRAPHY

1. P. Ruben Koehler, M.D. et al.: "Body Distribution of Ethiodol Following Lymphangiography", Radiology, 1964, 82, 5 866-871.
2. Bronk, et. al.: "Oil Embolism in Lymphography", Radiation, 80:194, February 1963.
3. Fuchs, S.A., "Complications in Lymphography With Oily Contrast Media", Acta Radiol., 57:247, November 1962.
4. Viamonte, M. Jr., University of Miami, Jackson Memorial Hospital, Miami, Florida, Private Communication.
5. Kuisk, H., "Techniques of Lymphography and Principles of Interpretation", 1971, Warren H. Green, Inc., St. Louis, Missouri, 63105.

SAVAGE LABORATORIES®
a division of Altana Inc.
MELVILLE, NEW YORK 11747

IF77062E
#45
R7/99

EVAC-Q-KWIK® OTC

DESCRIPTION

A bowel evacuant system comprised of three separate products that are intended to be administered sequentially at intervals intended to minimize the overlap of pharmacological activity.

EVAC-Q-MAG®

Active Ingredient: magnesium citrate.

Inactive Ingredients: citric acid, potassium citrate, sodium saccharin, in a lemon-flavored, carbonated water base.

EVAC-Q-TAB®

Active Ingredient: each tablet contains Bisacodyl 5 mg.

Inactive Ingredients: Lactose anhydrous, magnesium stearate, stearic acid, sodium starch glycolate, microcrystalline cellulose, silicone dioxide colloidal, acacia, gelatin, pharmaceutical glaze, polyvinyl acetate phthalate, D&C yellow #10, FD& C yellow #6, corn starch, calcium sulfate, sugar, talc, titanium dioxide, bees wax, carnauba wax, and other coating ingredients.

EVAC-Q-KWIK® SUPPOSITORY

Active Ingredient: bisacodyl 10 mg.

Inactive Ingredient: hydrogenated vegetable oil base.

HOW SUPPLIED

(NDC 0281-0297-76) Evac-Q-Kwik Kit

PANDEL® ℞
(hydrocortisone probutate cream)
Cream, 0.1%
Rx only.

For Dermatologic Use Only
Not for Ophthalmic Use

DESCRIPTION

Each gram of Pandel® (hydrocortisone probutate cream) Cream, 0.1% contains: 1 mg of hydrocortisone probutate in a cream base of propylene glycol, white petrolatum, light mineral oil, stearyl alcohol, polysorbate 60, sorbitan monostearate, glyceryl monostearate, PEG-20 stearate, glyceryl stearate SE, methylparaben, butylparaben, citric acid, sodium citrate anhydrous, and purified water.

HOW SUPPLIED

Pandel® (hydrocortisone probutate cream) Cream, 0.1%, a white to off-white opaque cream is supplied as follows:
15 g tubes (NDC 0281-0153-15)
45 g tubes (NDC 0281-0153-46)
80 g tubes (NDC 0281-0153-80)

—NEW FORMULATION—
CHROMAGEN® OB & ULTRAFORT™ Prenatal ComboPak ℞
Prenatal Multi-Vitamin/Mineral plus Iron Supplement Kit
Rx only

—NEW FORMULATION—
CHROMAGEN® OB

DESCRIPTION

CONTENTS: Each blue soft gelatin capsule, imprinted ▼0331 contains:

Calcium (as calcium carbonate)	200 mg
Vitamin C (ascorbic acid)	60 mg
Iron (as ferrous fumarate)	28 mg
Docusate Calcium	25 mg
Vitamin E (*d*-alpha tocopherol)	30 IU
Vitamin B_6 (pyridoxine hydrochloride)	20 mg
Vitamin B_2 (riboflavin)	1.8 mg
Vitamin B_1 (thiamine mononitrate)	1.6 mg
Folic Acid	1 mg
Vitamin B_{12} (cyanocobalamin)	12 mcg
Vitamin D (cholecalciferol)	400 IU

ACTIVE INGREDIENT: Each gelcap contains 1 mg folic acid.

DISCUSSION: The amount of elemental iron and the absorption of the iron components of commercial iron preparations vary widely. Certain accessory components enhance absorption and utilization of iron. Chromagen® OB gelcaps are formulated to provide the essential factors for a complete, versatile vitamin and mineral supplement.

ACTIONS

HIGH ELEMENTAL IRON CONTENT: Ferrous fumarate, used in Chromagen® OB gelcaps, is an organic iron complex which has the highest elemental iron content of any hematinic salt—33%. This compares with 20% for ferrous sulfate (heptahydrate) and 13% for ferrous gluconate.

MORE COMPLETE ABSORPTION: It has been shown that ascorbic acid, when given in sufficient amounts, can increase the absorption of ferrous iron from the gastrointestinal tract. The effect of ascorbic acid may be related both to its reducing effect, preventing the formation of insoluble ferric hydroxide, and to its ability to form soluble complexes with ferric iron, which preserve the iron solubility at the more alkaline duodenal pH. Studies indicate that 60 mg of ascorbic acid can increase iron absorption. Each Chromagen® OB gelcap contains 60 mg of ascorbic acid.

PROMOTES MOVEMENT OF PLASMA IRON: Ascorbic acid also plays a role in the movement of plasma iron to storage depots in the tissues. The action, which leads to the transport of plasma iron to ferritin, presumably involves its reducing effect, converting transferrin iron from the ferric to the ferrous state. There is also evidence that ascorbic acid improves iron utilization, presumably as a further result of its reducing action. It may also have a direct effect upon erythropoiesis. Ascorbic acid is further alleged to enhance the conversion of folic acid to a more physiologically active form, folinic acid, necesssary for erythropoiesis.

EXCELLENT ORAL TOLERATION: Ferrous fumarate is used in Chromagen® OB gelcaps because it is less likely to cause gastric disturbances. Ferrous fumarate has a low ionization constant and high solubility in the entire pH range of the gastrointestinal tract. It does not precipitate proteins or have the astringency of ionizable forms of iron, and does not interfere with proteolytic or diastatic activities of the digestive system.

TOXICITY: Ferrous fumarate is the least toxic of three popular iron salts.

INDICATIONS

Chromagen® OB is a vitamin and mineral nutritional supplement indicated for use in women prior to, throughout pregnancy and in the postnatal period for both lactating and non-lactating mothers. It is also useful for improving the nutritional status of women prior to conception.

CONTRAINDICATIONS

This product is contraindicated in patients with a known hypersensitivity to any of the ingredients. Hemochromatosis and hemosiderosis are contraindications to iron therapy. Supplemental vitamins should also not be prescribed for patients with Wilson's disease.

WARNINGS

Folic acid alone is improper therapy in the treatment of pernicious anemia and other megaloblastic anemias where Vitamin B_{12} is deficient.

WARNING: Accidental overdose of iron-containing products is a leading cause of fatal poisoning in children under 6. Keep this product out of reach of children. In case of accidental overdose, call a doctor or poison control center immediately.

Average gelcap doses in sensitive individuals or excessive dosage may cause nausea, skin rash, vomiting, diarrhea, precordial pain, or flushing of the face and extremities.

PRECAUTIONS

General:
Folic acid, in doses above 0.1 mg daily may obscure pernicious anemia, in that hematologic remission can occur while neurological manifestations remain progressive.

Information for Patients:
Patients should not exceed the recommended dosage unless directed by the physician. Patients should be informed that iron therapy can cause black or dark stools.

ADVERSE REACTIONS

The following adverse reactions, normally associated with iron products such as Chromagen® OB, may include constipation, diarrhea, nausea, vomiting, dark stools and abdominal pain. Adverse reactions are usually transient.

Dispense in a tight, light resistant container with a child resistant closure.

Store at controlled room temperature 15°–30°C (59°–86°F). Avoid excessive heat 40°C (104°F). Avoid freezing.

ULTRAFORT™

DESCRIPTION

CONTENTS: Each maroon soft gelatin capsule, imprinted ▼0260 contains: Vitamin C (ascorbic acid), 250 mg, Ferrous fumarate USP, 200 mg, Zinc (as Zinc Sulfate USP), 25 mg, Vitamin B_{12} (cyanocobalamin), 10 mcg.

DISCUSSION: The amount of elemental iron and the absorption of the iron components of commercial iron preparations vary widely. It is further established that certain "accessory components" may be included to enhance absorption and utilization of iron. UltraFort™ gelcaps are formulated to provide the essential factors for a complete, versatile hematinic.

ACTIONS

HIGH ELEMENTAL IRON CONTENT: Ferrous fumarate, used in UltraFort™ gelcaps, is an organic iron complex which has the highest elemental iron content of any hematinic salt—33%. This compares with 20% for ferrous sulfate (heptahydrate) and 13% for ferrous gluconate.[1,2]

MORE COMPLETE ABSORPTION: It has been repeatedly shown that ascorbic acid, when given in sufficient amounts, can increase the absorption of ferrous iron from the gastrointestinal tract.[3,4,5,6,7,8,9] The absorption-promoting effect is mainly due to the reducing action of ascorbic acid within the gastrointestinal lumen, which helps to prevent or delay the formation of insoluble or less dissociated ferric compounds.[3] Iron absorption has been shown to increase sharply with increasing amounts of ascorbic acid, showing a gain in absorption of approximately 40% at 250 mg. Above 250 mg, the gain becomes insignificant, with an additional gain of only approximately 8% at 500 mg.[3] Each UltraFort™ gelcap contains 250 mg of ascorbic acid, believed to be the optimal amount.

PROMOTES MOVEMENT OF PLASMA IRON: Ascorbic acid also plays an important role in the movement of plasma iron to storage depots in the tissues.[10] The action, which leads to the transport of plasma iron to ferritin, presumably involves its reducing effect, converting transferrin iron from the ferric to the ferrous state.[5] There is also evidence that ascorbic acid improves iron utilization, presumably as a further result of its reducing action,[6,9] and some evidence that it may have a direct effect upon erythropoiesis. Ascorbic acid is further alleged to enhance the conversion of folic acid to a more physiologically active form, folinic acid, which would make it even more important in the treatment of anemia since it would aid in the utilization of dietary folic acid.[11]

EXCELLENT ORAL TOLERATION: Ferrous fumarate is used in UltraFort™ gelcaps because it is less likely to cause the gastric disturbances so often associated with oral iron therapy. Ferrous fumarate has a low ionization constant and high solubility in the entire pH range of the gastrointestinal tract. It does not precipitate proteins or have the astringency of more ionizable forms of iron, and does not interfere with proteolytic or diastatic activities of the digestive system. Because of excellent oral toleration, UltraFort™ can usually be administered between meals when iron absorption is maximal.

ZINC SUPPLEMENTATION: Zinc is a necessary catalyst for over 200 enzymes functioning at the cellular level. Physiologic functions facilitated by zinc include wound healing, tissue repair, recovery from prolonged stress or trauma, and facilitation of host immunity, among others. These and other actions of zinc are beneficial in iron deficiency anemia.[12] Daily zinc supplementation, during pregnancy, is associated with improved infant birth weights and head circumference, in women with low zinc blood plasma levels.[13] During pregnancy low zinc plasma levels are also associated with an increased risk of low birth weight of infants, preterm labor, preterm delivery, placental ablation, perinatal death, abnormal labor, and other pregnancy complications.[14–17]

TOXICITY: Ferrous fumarate was found to be the least toxic of three popular oral iron salts, with an oral LD_{50} of 630 mg/kg. In the same report, the LD_{50} of ferrous gluconate was reported to be 320 mg/kg and ferrous sulfate 230 mg/kg.[1,18]

INDICATIONS

For the treatment of all anemias responsive to oral iron therapy, such as hypochromic anemia associated with pregnancy, chronic or acute blood loss, dietary restriction, metabolic disease and post-surgical convalescence.

CONTRAINDICATIONS

Hemochromatosis and hemosiderosis are contraindications to iron therapy.

WARNING
Accidental overdose of iron-containing products is a leading cause of fatal poisoning in children under 6. Keep this product out of reach of children. In case of accidental overdose, call a doctor or poison control center immediately.

SIDE EFFECTS

Average capsule doses in sensitive individuals or excessive dosage may cause nausea, skin rash, vomiting, diarrhea, precordial pain, or flushing of the face and extremities.

USUAL ADULT DOSAGE: Chromagen® OB—one soft gelatin capsule in the morning with food and a full glass of water. UltraFort™—one soft gelatin capsule at night.

HOW SUPPLIED

Prenatal ComboPak 30 Day Supply, NDC 0281-0338-30
Prenatal ComboPak 100 Day Supply, NDC 0281-0338-18
Store at controlled room temperature 15°–30°C (59°–86°F). Avoid excessive heat 40°C (104°F). Avoid freezing.

BIBLIOGRAPHY

1Berk, M.S. and Novich, M.A.: "Treatment of Iron Deficiency Anemia With Ferrous Fumarate," Am. J. Obst. & Gynec., 203–206, 1962. 2Shapleigh, J.B. and Montgomery, A.: Am. Pract. & Dig. Treat. 10–461, 1959. 3Brise, H. and Hallberg, L.: "Effect of Ascorbic Acid on Iron Absorption," Acta. Med. Scand., 171:376, 51–58, 1962. 4New Drugs, p. 309, AMA, Chicago, 1966. 5Mazur, A., Green, S. and Carleton, A.: "Mechanism of Plasma Iron Incorporation into Hepatic Ferritin," J. Bio. Chem., 3:595–603, 1960. 6Greenberg, S.M., Tucker, A.E., Mathues, H. and J.D.: "Iron Absorption and Metabolism I. Interrleationship of Ascorbic Acid and Vitamin E," J. Nutrition, 63:19–31, 1957. 7Moore, C.V. and Dubach, R.: "Observations on the Absorption of Iron from Foods Tagged with Radioiron," Trans. Assoc. Amer. Physic., 64:245, 1951. 8Steinkamp, R., Dubach, R. and Moore, C.V.: "Studies in Iron Transportation and Metabolism," Arch. Int. Med., 95:181, 1955. 9Gorten, M.K. and Bradley, J.E.: "The Treatment of Nutritional Anemia in Infancy and Childhood with Oral Iron and Ascorbic Acid," J. Pediatrics, 45:1, 1954. 10Mazur, A.: "Role of Ascorbic Acid in the Incorporation of Plasma Iron into Ferritin," Ann. N.Y. Acad. Sci., 92:223–229, 1961. 11Cox, E.V., et al: "The Anemia of Scurvy," Amer. J. Med., 42:220–227, 1967. 12"Drug Information for the Health Care Professional," U.S. Pharmacopeial Conven., Rockville, P. 2826–2828, 1995. 13Goldenberg, R.L., Tamura, T., Neggers, Y., Copper, R.L., Johston, K.E., DuBard, M.B., Hauth, J.C.: "The effect of zinc supplementation on pregnancy outcome," JAMA, 274:463–468, 1995. 14Jameson, S.: "Zinc status in pregnancy: The effects of zinc therapy on perinatal mortality, prematurity and placental ablation," Ann. N.Y. Acad. Sci., 678:178–192, 1993. 15Lazebnik, N., Kuhnert, B.R., Kuhnert, P.M. and Thompson, K.L.: "Zinc status, pregnancy complications, and labor abnormalities", Am. J. Obstet. Gynecol., 158:161–66, 1988. 16Sikorski, R., Juszkiewicz, T. and Paszkowski, P.: "Zinc status in women with premature rupture of the membranes at term." Obstet. Gynecol., 76:675–677, 1990. 17Cherry, F., Sandstead, H.H., Rojas, P., Johnson, L.K., Batson, H.K. and Wang, X.B., "Adolescent pregnancy: Associations among body weight, zinc nutriture, and pregnancy outcome", Am. J. Clin. Nutr., 50: 945–954, 1989. 18Berenbaum, M.C., et al.: Blood, 15:540, 1960.

Manufactured for:
SAVAGE LABORATORIES®
a division of Altana Inc. IF338A
Melville, New York 11747 R 6/00
by: R.P. Scherer Corporation, St. Petersburg, Florida 33702
Shown in Product Identification Guide, page 334

STRONGSTART™ CAPLETS ℞
Rx only

DESCRIPTION

CONTENTS: Each StrongStart™ Caplet, imprinted with Savage Laboratories logo 0343, contains:

Vitamin D (cholicalciferol)	400 IU
Vitamin E (alpha-tocopherol)	30 IU
Vitamin A (as betacarotene)	1,000 IU
Vitamin C (ascorbic acid)	100 mg
Vitamin B_1 (thiamine)	3 mg
Vitamin B_2 (riboflavin)	3 mg
Vitamin B_3 (niacinamide)	15 mg
Vitamin B_5 (pantothenic acid)	7 mg
Vitamin B_6 (pyridoxine)	20 mg
Vitamin B_9 (folic acid)	1 mg
Vitamin B_{12} (cyanocobalamin)	12 mcg
Calcium carbonate	200 mg
Docusate sodium	25 mg
Iron (as ferrous fumarate)	29 mg
Zinc oxide	20 mg

ACTIVE INGREDIENT: Each StrongStart™ Caplet contains 1 mg of folic acid (Vitamin B_9).

INDICATIONS

StrongStart™ Caplets are indicated for vitamin and mineral dietary supplementation in women throughout their pregnancy and in the postnatal period for both lactating and non-lactating mothers. StrongStart™ Caplets can also be administered to improve the nutritional status of women prior to conception.

WARNING

The administration of folic acid alone is inadequate for the treatment of pernicious anemia and other megablastic anemias caused by vitamin B_{12} deficiency.

WARNING
Accidental overdose of iron-containing products is a leading cause of fatal poisoning in children under 6 years old. Keep this product out of reach of children. In case of accidental overdose, call a physician or poison control center immediately.

PRECAUTIONS

General: Folic acid, in doses of 0.1 mg daily, may obscure pernicious anemia in that hematologic remission can occur while neurological manifestations remain progressive.

DOSAGE AND ADMINISTRATION

The usual dosage of StrongStart™ Caplets is one caplet daily, or as directed by a physician.

HOW SUPPLIED

NDC 0281-0343-53, bottle of 100 caplets.
NDC 0281-0343-30, bottle of 30 caplets.
Dispense StrongStart™ Caplets in a tight, light resistant container with a child resistant closure. Store StrongStart™ Caplets at controlled room temperature, 15°–30° C (59°–86° F). Avoid excessive heat 40° C (104° F).
Avoid freezing.
Manufactured for:
Savage Laboratories®
a Division of Altana, Inc.
Melville, NY 11747
Manufactured by:
Confab Laboratories, Inc
Quebec, Canada
J3Y 3X3.

STRONGSTART™ ℞
Chewable
Rx only

DESCRIPTION

CONTENTS: Each StrongStart™ Chewable, imprinted with Savage Laboratories logo 0344, contains:

Vitamin D (cholecalciferol)	400 IU
Vitamin E (dl-α-tocopherol)	30 IU
Vitamin A (as betacarotene)	1,000 IU
Vitamin C (ascorbic acid)	100 mg
Vitamin B_1 (thiamine)	3 mg
Vitamin B_2 (riboflavin)	3 mg
Vitamin B_3 (niacinamide)	15 mg
Vitamin B_5 (pantothenic acid)	7 mg
Vitamin B_6 (pyridoxine HCl)	20 mg
Vitamin B_9 (folic acid)	1 mg
Vitamin B_{12} (cyanocobalamin)	12 mcg
Calcium carbonate	200 mg
Iron (as ferrous fumarate)	29 mg
Zinc oxide	20 mg

ACTIVE INGREDIENT: Each StrongStart™ Chewable contains 1 mg of folic acid (vitamin B_9).

INDICATIONS

StrongStart™ Chewables are indicated for vitamin and mineral dietary supplementation in women throughout their pregnancy and in the postnatal period for both lactating and non-lactating mothers. StrongStart™ Chewable can also be administered to improve the nutritional status of women prior to conception.

WARNING

The administration of folic acid alone is inadequate for the treatment of pernicious anemia and other megablastic anemias caused by vitamin B_{12} deficiency.

WARNING: Accidental overdose of iron-containing products is a leading cause of fatal poisoning in children under 6. Keep this product out of reach of children. In case of accidental overdose, call a doctor or poison control center immediately.

Phenylketonurics: Contains Phenylaline 6 mg Per Tablet.

PRECAUTIONS

General: Folic acid, in doses of 0.1 mg daily, may obscure pernicious anemia in that hematologic remission can occur while neurological manifestations remain progressive.

DOSAGE AND ADMINISTRATION

The usual dosage of StrongStart™ Chewable is one chewable daily, or as directed by a physician.

HOW SUPPLIED

NDC 0281-0344-53, bottle of 100
NDC 0281-0344-30, bottle of 30
Dispense StrongStart™ Chewables in a tight, light resistant container with a child resistant closure. Store StrongStart™ Chewables at controlled room temperature, 15°–30° C (59°–86° F). Avoid excessive heat 40° C (104° F).
Avoid freezing.
Manufactured for
SAVAGE LABORATORIES®
a division of Altana Inc.
Melville, New York 11747
Manufactured by:
Confab Laboratories
St. Hubert, Quebec, Canada J3Y 3X3
IF70344
R8/00

TYMPAGESIC® ℞
(Analgesic-Decongestant Ear Drops)

DESCRIPTION

TYMPAGESIC® Otic Solution, analgesic-decongestant ear drops, contains phenylephrine hydrochloride USP 0.25%, antipyrine USP 5%, benzocaine USP 5%, sodium metabisulfite and edetate disodium USP in propylene glycol USP.

HOW SUPPLIED

TYMPAGESIC® Otic Solution is supplied as follows:
13 mL amber glass bottle with dropper
NDC 0281-7363-39

For information on over-the-counter drugs, consult **PDR For Nonprescription Drugs**.

Scandipharm, Inc.

22 INVERNESS CENTER PARKWAY
BIRMINGHAM, AL 35242

(For prescribing information, see listing under AXCAN SCANDIPHARM INC.)

Schein Pharmaceutical, Inc.

100 CAMPUS DRIVE
FLORHAM PARK, NJ 07932

Direct Inquiries to:
Customer Service
(800) 356-5790
FAX: 800-760-9224

For Medical Information Contact:
(800) 548-6236 (24 Hours)
(888) 397-4766 (24 Hours—Brand Products)

FERRLECIT® ℞
[fĕr "le'sit]
sodium ferric gluconate complex in sucrose injection
62.5 mg/5 mL

DESCRIPTION

Ferrlecit® (sodium ferric gluconate complex in sucrose injection) is a stable macromolecular complex with an apparent molecular weight on gel chromatography of 350,000±23,000 daltons. The macromolecular complex is negatively charged at alkaline pH and is present in solution with sodium cations. It is free of ferrous ion and dextran polysaccharides. The product has a deep red color indicative of ferric oxide linkages.
The structural formula is considered to be

$$[NaFe_2O_3(C_6H_{11}O_7)(C_{12}H_{22}O_{11})_5]_{\approx 200}$$

Each ampule of 5 mL of Ferrlecit® for intravenous injection contains 62.5 mg (12.5 mg/mL) of elemental iron as the sodium salt of a ferric ion carbohydrate complex in an alkaline aqueous solution with approximately 20% sucrose w/v (195 mg/mL) in water for injection, pH 7.7–9.7.
Each mL contains 9 mg of benzyl alcohol as an inactive ingredient.
Therapeutic Class: Hematinic

CLINICAL PHARMACOLOGY

Ferrlecit® is used to replete the total body content of iron. Iron is critical for normal hemoglobin synthesis to maintain oxygen transport. Additionally, iron is necessary for metabolism and synthesis of DNA and various enzymatic processes.
The total body iron content of an adult ranges from 2 to 4 grams. Approximately 2/3 is in hemoglobin and 1/3 in reticuloendothelial storage (bone marrow, spleen, liver) and ferritin. The body highly conserves iron (daily loss of 0.03%) requiring supplementation of about 1 mg/day to replenish losses in healthy, non-menstruating adults. The etiology of iron deficiency in hemodialysis patients is varied and can include increased iron utilization (e.g., from erythropoietin therapy), blood loss (e.g., from fistula, retention in dailyzer, hematologic testing, menses), decreased dietary intake or absorption, surgery, iron sequestration due to inflammatory process, and malignancy. The administration of exogenous erythropoietin increases red blood cell production and iron utilization. The increased iron utilization and blood losses in the hemodialysis patient may lead to absolute or functional iron deficiency. Iron deficiency is absolute when hematologic indicators of iron stores are low. Patients with functional iron deficiency do not meet laboratory criteria for absolute iron deficiency but demonstrate an increase in hemoglobin/hematocrit or a decrease in erythropoietin dosage with stable hemoglobin/hematocrit when parenteral iron is administered.

Pharmacokinetics

Human pharmacokinetic studies have not been performed with Ferrlecit®. *In vitro* experiments have shown that less than 1% of the iron species within Ferrlecit® can be dialyzed through membranes with pore sizes corresponding to 12,000 to 14,000 daltons over a period of up to 270 minutes. These studies were conducted with undiluted Ferrlecit®, and with Ferrlecit® diluted in 0.9% saline or double distilled water.

CLINICAL STUDIES

Two clinical studies were conducted to assess the safety and efficacy of Ferrlecit®.

Study A

Study A was a three-center, randomized, open-label study of the safety and efficacy of two doses of Ferrlecit® administered intravenously to iron-deficient hemodialysis patients. The study included both a dose-response concurrent control and an historical control. Enrolled patients received a test dose of Ferrlecit® (25 mg of elemental iron) and were then randomly assigned to receive Ferrlecit® at cumulative doses of either 500 mg (low dose) or 1000 mg (high dose) of elemental iron. Ferrlecit® was given to both dose groups in eight divided doses during sequential dialysis sessions (a period of 16 to 17 days). At each dialysis session, patients in the low-dose group received Ferrlecit® 62.5 mg of elemental iron over 30 minutes, and those in the high-dose group received Ferrlecit® 125 mg of elemental iron over 60 minutes. The primary endpoint was the change in hemoglobin from baseline to the last available observation through Day 40. Eligibility for this study included chronic hemodialysis patients with a hemoglobin below 10 g/dL (or hematocrit at or below 32%) and either serum ferritin below 100 ng/mL or iron saturation below 18%. Exclusion criteria included significant underlying disease or inflammatory conditions or an erythropoietin (EPO) requirement of greater than 10,000 units three times per week. Parenteral iron and red cell transfusion were not allowed for two months before the study. Oral iron and red cell transfusion were not allowed during the study for Ferrlecit® treated patients.
The historical control population consisted of 25 chronic hemodialysis patients who received only oral iron supplementation for 14 months and did not receive red cell transfusion. All patients had stable EPO doses and hematocrit values for at least two months before initiation of oral iron therapy.
The evaluated population consisted of 39 patients in the low-dose Ferrlecit® group, 44 patients in the high-dose Ferrlecit® group, and 25 historical control patients.
The mean baseline hemoglobin and hematocrit were similar between treatment and historical control patients: 9.8 g/dL and 29% and 9.6 g/dL and 29% in low- and high-dose Ferrlecit® treated patients, respectively, and 9.4 g/dL and 29% in historical control patients. Baseline serum iron saturation was 20% in the low-dose group, 16% in the high-dose group, and 14% in the historical control. Baseline serum ferritin was 106 ng/mL in the low-dose group, 88 ng/mL in the high-dose group, and 606 ng/mL in the historical control.
Patients in the high-dose Ferrlecit® group achieved significantly higher increases in hemoglobin and hematocrit than either patients in the low-dose Ferrlecit® group or patients in the historical control group (oral iron). Patients in the low-dose Ferrlecit® group did not achieve significantly higher increases in hemoglobin and hematocrit than patients receiving oral iron. See Table 1.
[See table 1 above]

TABLE 1
Hemoglobin, Hematocrit, and Iron Studies

Study A	Mean Change from Baseline to Two Weeks After Cessation of Therapy		
	Ferrlecit® 1000 mg IV (N=44)	Ferrlecit® 500 mg IV (N=39)	Historical Control-Oral Iron (N=25)
Hemoglobin	1.1 g/dL*	0.3 g/dL	0.4 g/dL
Hematocrit	3.6%*	1.4%	0.8%
Iron Saturation	8.5%	2.8%	6.1%
Serum Ferritin	199 ng/mL	132 ng/mL	NA

*p<0.01 verses both 500 mg group and the historical control group

Cumulative Ferrlecit® Dose (mg of elemental iron)	62.5	250	375	562.5	625	750	1000	1125	1187.5
Patients (#)	1	1	2	1	10	4	12	6	1

Study B

Study B was a single-center, non-randomized, open-label, historically-controlled study of the safety and efficacy of variable, cumulative doses of intravenous Ferrlecit® in iron-deficient hemodialysis patients. Ferrlecit® administration was identical to Study A. The primary efficacy variable was the change in hemoglobin from baseline to the last available observation through Day 50.
Inclusion and exclusion criteria were identical to those of Study A as was the historical control population. Sixty-three patients were evaluated in this study: 38 in the Ferrlecit®-treated group and 25 in the historical control group.
Ferrlecit®-treated patients were considered to have completed the study per protocol if they received at least eight Ferrlecit® doses of either 62.5 mg or 125 mg of elemental iron. A total of 14 patients (37%) completed the study per protocol. Twelve (32%) Ferrlecit®-treated patients received less than eight doses, and 12 (32%) patients had incomplete information on the sequence of dosing. Not all patients received Ferrlecit® at consecutive dialysis sessions and many received oral iron during the study.
[See second table above]
Baseline hemoglobin and hematocrit values were similar between the treatment and control groups, and were 9.1 g/dL and 27.3%, respectively, for Ferrlecit®-treated patients. Serum iron studies were also similar between treatment and control groups, with the exception of serum ferritin, which was 606 ng/mL for historical control patients, compared to 77 ng/mL for Ferrlecit®-treated patients.
In this patient population, only the Ferrlecit®-treated group achieved significant increase in hemoglobin and hematocrit from baseline. This increase was significantly greater than that seen in the historical oral iron treatment group. See Table 2.
[See table 2 above]

TABLE 2
Hemoglobin, Hematocrit, and Iron Studies

Study B	Mean Change from Baseline to One Month After Treatment	
	Ferrlecit® (N=38)	Oral Iron (N=25)
	change	change
Hemoglobin (g/dL)	1.3a,b	0.4
Hematocrit (%)	3.8a,b	0.2
Iron Saturation (%)	6.7b	1.7
Serum Ferritin (ng/mL)	73b	-145

a - p<0.05 on group comparison by the ANCOVA method
b - p<0.001 from baseline by the paired t-test method

INDICATIONS AND USAGE

Ferrlecit® is indicated for treatment of iron deficiency anemia in patients undergoing chronic hemodialysis who are receiving supplemental erythropoietin therapy.

CONTRAINDICATIONS

- All anemias not associated with iron deficiency.
- Hypersensitivity to Ferrlecit® or any of its inactive components.

WARNINGS

HYPERSENSITIVITY REACTIONS: **POTENTIALLY FATAL HYPERSENSITIVITY REACTIONS CHARACTERIZED BY CARDIOVASCULAR COLLAPSE, CARDIAC ARREST, BRONCHOSPASM, ORAL OR PHARYNGEAL EDEMA, DYSPNEA, ANGIOEDEMA, URTICARIA, OR PRURITUS SOMETIMES ASSOCIATED WITH PAIN AND MUSCLE SPASM OF THE CHEST OR BACK HAVE BEEN REPORTED RARELY IN PATIENTS RECEIVING FERRLECIT®. FATAL IMMEDIATE HYPERSENSITIVITY REACTIONS HAVE BEEN REPORTED IN PATIENTS RECEIVING THERAPY WITH MANY IRON CARBOHYDRATE COMPLEXES. SERIOUS ANAPHYLACTOID REACTIONS REQUIRE APPROPRIATE RESUSCITATIVE MEASURES. ALTHOUGH FATAL REACTIONS HAVE NOT BEEN OBSERVED IN FERRLECIT® CLINICAL STUDIES, INSUFFICIENT NUMBERS OF PATIENTS MAY HAVE BEEN ENROLLED TO OBSERVE THIS EVENT. See ADVERSE REACTIONS.**

FLUSHING AND HYPOTENSION: **HYPOTENSION ASSOCIATED WITH FLUSHING, LIGHT-HEADEDNESS, MALAISE, FATIGUE, WEAKNESS OR SEVERE PAIN IN THE CHEST, BACK, FLANKS, OR GROIN HAS BEEN ASSOCIATED WITH RAPID ADMINISTRATION OF INTRAVENOUS IRON. THESE HYPOTENSIVE REACTIONS ARE NOT ASSOCIATED WITH SIGNS OF HYPERSENSITIVITY AND HAVE USUALLY RESOLVED WITHIN ONE OR TWO HOURS. SUCCESSFUL TREATMENT MAY CONSIST OF OBSERVATION OR, IF THE HYPOTENSION CAUSES SYMPTOMS, VOLUME EXPANSION. IN NORTH AMERICAN TRIALS, FERRLECIT® DOSES OF 62.5 MG OF ELEMENTAL IRON WERE ADMINISTERED**

OVER 30 MINUTES, AND DOSES OF 125 MG OF ELEMENTAL IRON WERE ADMINISTERED OVER ONE HOUR. THIS RATE OF ADMINISTRATION (2.1 MG/MIN) SHOULD NOT BE EXCEEDED. See ADVERSE REACTIONS.

PRECAUTIONS

General: Iron is not easily eliminated from the body and accumulation can be toxic. Unnecessary therapy with parenteral iron will cause excess storage of iron with consequent possibility of iatrogenic hemosiderosis. Iron overload is particularly apt to occur in patients with hemoglobinopathies and other refractory anemias. Ferrlecit® should not be administered to patients with iron overload. See OVERDOSAGE.

Carcinogenesis, Mutagenesis, Impairment of Fertility: Long-term carcinogenicity studies in animals were not performed. Studies to assess the effects of Ferrlecit® on fertility were not conducted. Ferrlecit® was not mutagenic in the Ames test and the rat micronucleus test. It produced a clastogenic effect in an *in vitro* chromosomal aberration assay in Chinese hamster ovary cells.

Pregnancy Category B: Ferrlecit® was not teratogenic at doses of elemental iron up to 100 mg/kg/day (300 mg/m^2/day) in mice and 20 mg/kg/day (120 mg/m^2/day) in rats. On a body surface area basis, these doses were 1.3 and 3.24 times the recommended human dose (125 mg/day or 92.5 mg/m^2/day) for a person of 50 kg body weight, average height and body surface area of 1.46 m^2. There were no adequate and well-controlled studies in pregnant women. Ferrlecit® should be used during pregnancy only if the potential benefit justifies the potential risk to the fetus.

Nursing Mothers: It is not known whether this drug is excreted in human milk. Because many drugs are excreted in human milk, caution should be exercised when Ferrlecit® is administered to a nursing woman.

Pediatric Use: Safety and effectiveness of Ferrlecit® in pediatric patients has not been established. Ferrlecit® contains benzyl alcohol and therefore should not be used in neonates.

Geriatric Use: Clinical studies of Ferrlecit® did not include sufficient numbers of subjects aged 65 and over to determine whether they respond differently from younger subjects. Other reported clinical experience has not identified differences in responses between the elderly and younger patients. In particular, 51/159 hemodialysis patients in North American clinical studies were aged 65 years or older. Among these patients, no differences in safety or efficacy as a result of age were identified. In general, dose selection for an elderly patient should be cautious, usually starting at the low end of the dosing range, reflecting the greater frequency of decreased hepatic, renal, or cardiac function, and of concomitant disease or other drug therapy.

ADVERSE REACTIONS

Exposure to Ferrlecit® has been documented in 385 patients on hemodialysis. Of these, 159 were patients in North American studies and 226 were European patients described in the medical literature.

Flushing and Hypotension: See WARNINGS.

Flushing and hypotension have been reported following administration of Ferrlecit® in European case reports. Of the 226 renal dialysis patients exposed to Ferrlecit® and reported in the literature, 3 (1.3%) patients experienced serious hypotensive events which were accompanied by flushing in two. All completely reversed after one hour without sequelae.

In North American clinical studies the incidence of any hypotension in patients who received Ferrlecit® 62.5 mg of elemental iron over 30 minutes was similar to the incidence of hypotension in patients who received Ferrlecit® 125 mg of elemental iron over 60 minutes (34% vs. 36%).

Ferrlecit® is intended to be administered during dialysis during which many patients may experience transient hypotension. Administration of Ferrlecit® may augment hypotension caused by dialysis.

Among the 159 patients evaluated in North American clinical studies, one patient experienced a transient decreased level of consciousness without hypotension. Another patient discontinued treatment prematurely because of dizziness, lightheadedness, diplopia, malaise, and weakness without hypotension that resulted in a 3–4 hour hospitalization for observation following drug administration. The syndrome resolved spontaneously.

Hypersensitivity reactions: See WARNINGS.

Although fatal hypersensitivity reactions have not occurred in the 385 patients exposed to Ferrlecit®, insufficient numbers of patients may have been exposed to observe this event. The primary Ferrlecit®-associated hypersensitivity events in Study A were Type III reactions that occurred in three out of a total 88 (3.4%) Ferrlecit®-treated patients and which resulted in premature study discontinuation. The first patient withdrew after the development of pruritus and chest pain following the test dose of Ferrlecit®. The second patient, in the high-dose group, experienced nausea, abdominal and flank pain, fatigue and rash following the first dose of Ferrlecit®. The third patient, in the low-dose group, experienced a "red blotchy rash" following the first dose of Ferrlecit®. Of the 38 patients exposed to Ferrlecit® in Study B, none reported hypersensitivity reactions. Hypersensitivity reactions were not reported in 33 additional patients treated with maintenance Ferrlecit® in North American studies. This group includes five chronic hemodialysis patients with a history of anaphylaxis to iron dextran who received up to 1000 mg of Ferrlecit® without an allergic reaction.

Of the 226 renal dialysis patients exposed to Ferrlecit® and reported in the literature, 2 (0.9%) patients experienced adverse events that recurred on drug rechallenge and prohibited further drug use. These were: (1) malaise, heat, vomiting, and loin pain and (2) intense epigastric pain lasting 3–4 hours.

From a total of 387 Ferrlecit®-treated patients in medical reports and North American trials, six patients (1.6%) experienced serious reactions which precluded further therapy with Ferrlecit®.

Adverse Laboratory Changes: No differences in laboratory findings associated with Ferrlecit® were reported in North American clinical trials when normalized against a National Institute of Health database on laboratory findings in 1,100 hemodialysis patients.

Other Adverse Events Observed During Clinical Trials: Ferrlecit® has been administered to 159 patients in North American clinical trials. During these trials, all adverse events were recorded by clinical investigators using terminology of their own choosing. Adverse events, whether or not related to Ferrlecit® administration, reported in >1% of Ferrlecit®-treated patients from trials A and B are categorized below by body system using modified COSTART terminology and ranked in order of decreasing frequency within each system. Hemodialysis patients may have similar symptoms related to dialysis itself or to chronic renal failure.

Body as a Whole: injection site reaction, pain, chest pain, asthenia, headache, abdominal pain, fatigue, fever, malaise, infection, back pain, rigors, chills, arm pain, flu-like syndrome, sepsis, carcinoma.

Nervous System: cramps, dizziness, leg cramps, paresthesias, agitation, insomnia, somnolence.

Respiratory: dyspnea, coughing, upper respiratory infections, rhinitis, pneumonia.

Cardiovascular System: hypotension, hypertension, syncope, tachycardia, bradycardia, angina pectoris, myocardial infarction, pulmonary edema.

Gastrointestinal System: nausea, vomiting, diarrhea, rectal disorder, dyspepsia, eructation, flatulence, melena.

Musculoskeletal System: myalgia, arthralgia.

Skin and Appendages: pruritus, increased sweating, rash.

Genitourinary System: urinary tract infection.

Special Senses: conjunctivitis, abnormal vision.

Metabolic and Nutritional Disorders: hyperkalemia, generalized edema, leg edema, hypoglycemia, hypokalemia, edema, hypervolemia.

Hematologic System: abnormal erythrocytes, anemia, lymphadenopathy.

OVERDOSAGE

Dosages in excess of iron needs may lead to accumulation of iron in iron storage sites and hemosiderosis. Periodic monitoring of laboratory parameters of iron levels storage may assist in recognition of iron accumulation. Ferrlecit® should not be administered in patients with iron overload.

Serum iron levels greater than 300 µg/dL (combined with transferrin oversaturation) may indicate iron poisoning which is characterized by abdominal pain, diarrhea, or vomiting which progresses to pallor or cyanosis, lassitude, drowsiness, hyperventilation due to acidosis, and cardiovascular collapse. Symptoms attributed to oversaturation of transferrin following rapid IV infusions of Ferrlecit® have been reported in two patients.

The Ferrlecit® iron complex is not dialyzable.

Ferrlecit® at elemental iron doses of 125 mg/kg, 78.8 mg/kg, 62.5 mg/kg and 250 mg/kg caused deaths to mice, rats, rabbits, and dogs, respectively. The major symptoms of acute toxicity were decreased activity, staggering, ataxia, increases in the respiratory rate, tremor, and convulsions.

DOSAGE AND ADMINISTRATION

The dosage of Ferrlecit® is expressed in terms of mg of elemental iron. Each 5 mL ampule contains 62.5 mg of elemental iron (12.5 mg/mL).

Before initiating therapeutic doses of Ferrlecit®, administration of an intravenous test dose of 2 mL Ferrlecit® (25 mg of elemental iron) is recommended. This test dose should be diluted in 50 mL of 0.9% sodium chloride for injection and administered over sixty minutes.

The recommended dosage of Ferrlecit® for the repletion treatment of iron deficiency in hemodialysis patients is 10 mL of Ferrlecit® (125 mg of elemental iron) diluted in 100 mL of 0.9% sodium chloride for injection, administered by intravenous infusion over 1 hour. Most patients will require a minimum cumulative dose of 1.0 gram of elemental iron, administered over eight sessions at sequential dialysis treatment, to achieve a favorable hemoglobin or hematocrit response. Patients may continue to require therapy with Ferrlecit® or other intravenous iron preparations at the lowest dose necessary to maintain the target levels of hemoglobin, hematocrit, and laboratory parameters of iron storage within acceptable limits.

Ferrlecit® has been administered at sequential dialysis sessions by infusion during the dialysis session itself.

Note: Do not mix Ferrlecit® with other medications, or add to parenteral nutrition solutions for intravenous infusion. The compatibility of Ferrlecit® with intravenous infusion vehicles other than 0.9% sodium chloride for injection has not been evaluated. Parenteral drug products should be inspected visually for particulate matter and discoloration before administration, whenever the solution and container permit.

Use immediately after dilution in saline.

HOW SUPPLIED

Ferrlecit® is supplied in colorless glass ampules containing a viscous dark red solution with no visible particular matter. Each ampule contains 62.5 mg of elemental iron in 5 mL for intravenous use, packaged in cartons of 10 ampules.

Store at 20°C–25°C (68°F–77°F); excursions permitted to 15°C–30°C (59–86°F). See USP Controlled Room Temperature.

Caution: Rx Only

Shown in Product Identification Guide, page 334

INFeD®
(IRON DEXTRAN INJECTION, USP)

℞

WARNING
THE PARENTERAL USE OF COMPLEXES OF IRON AND CARBOHYDRATES HAS RESULTED IN ANAPHYLACTIC-TYPE REACTIONS. DEATHS ASSOCIATED WITH SUCH ADMINISTRATION HAVE BEEN REPORTED. THEREFORE, INFeD SHOULD BE USED ONLY IN THOSE PATIENTS IN WHOM THE INDICATIONS HAVE BEEN CLEARLY ESTABLISHED AND LABORATORY INVESTIGATIONS CONFIRM AN IRON DEFICIENT STATE NOT AMENABLE TO ORAL IRON THERAPY.

DESCRIPTION

INFeD (iron dextran injection,USP) is a dark brown, slightly viscous sterile liquid complex of ferric hydroxide and dextran for intravenous or intramuscular use.

Each mL contains the equivalent of 50 mg of elemental iron (as an iron dextran complex), approximately 0.9% sodium chloride, in water for injection. Sodium hydroxide and/or hydrochloric acid may have been used to adjust pH. The pH of the solution is between 5.2 and 6.5.

The iron dextran complex has an average apparent molecular weight of 165,000 g/mole with a range of approximately +/− 10%.

Therapeutic Class: Hematinic

CLINICAL PHARMACOLOGY

General: After intramuscular injection, iron dextran is absorbed from the injection site into the capillaries and the lymphatic system. Circulating iron dextran is removed from the plasma by cells of the reticuloendothelial system, which split the complex into its components of iron and dextran. The iron is immediately bound to the available protein moieties to form hemosiderin or ferritin, the physiological forms of iron, or to a lesser extent to transferrin. This iron which is subject to physiological control replenishes hemoglobin and depleted iron stores.

Dextran, a polyglucose, is either metabolized or excreted. Negligible amounts of iron are lost via the urinary or alimentary pathways after administration of iron dextran.

The major portion of intramuscular injections of iron dextran is absorbed within 72 hours; most of the remaining iron is absorbed over the ensuing 3 to 4 weeks.

Various studies involving intravenously administered ^{59}Fe iron dextran to iron deficient subjects, some of whom had coexisting diseases, have yielded half-life values ranging from 5 hours to more than 20 hours. The 5-hour value was determined for ^{59}Fe iron dextran from a study that used laboratory methods to separate the circulating ^{59}Fe iron dextran from the transferrin-bound ^{59}Fe. The 20-hour value reflects a half-life determined by measuring total ^{59}Fe, both circulating and bound. It should be understood that these half-life values do not represent clearance of iron from the body. Iron is not easily eliminated from the body and accumulation of iron can be toxic.

In vitro studies have shown that removal of iron dextran by dialysis is negligible.[1,2] Six different dialyzer membranes were investigated (polysulfone, cuprophane, cellulose acetate, cellulose triacetate, polymethylmethacrylate and polyacrylonitrile), including those considered high efficiency and high flux.

INDICATIONS AND USAGE

Intravenous or intramuscular injections of iron dextran are indicated for treatment of patients with documented iron deficiency in whom oral administration is unsatisfactory or impossible.

CONTRAINDICATIONS

Hypersensitivity to the product. All anemias not associated with iron deficiency.

WARNINGS

See BOXED WARNING.

A risk of carcinogenesis may attend the intramuscular injection of iron-carbohydrate complexes. Such complexes have been found under experimental conditions to produce sarcoma when large doses or small doses injected repeatedly at the same site were given to rats, mice, and rabbits, and possibly in hamsters.

The long latent period between the injection of a potential carcinogen and the appearance of a tumor makes it impossible to measure accurately the risk in man. There have, however, been several reports in the literature describing tumors at the injection site in humans who had previously

Continued on next page

INFeD—Cont.

received intramuscular injections of iron-carbohydrate complexes.
Large intravenous doses, such as used with total dose infusions (TDI), have been associated with an increased incidence of adverse effects. The adverse effects frequently are delayed (1–2 days) reactions typified by one or more of the following symptoms; arthralgia, backache, chills, dizziness, moderate to high fever, headache, malaise, myalgia, nausea, and vomiting. The onset is usually 24–48 hours after administration and symptoms generally subside within 3–4 days. These symptoms have also been reported following intramuscular injection and generally subside within 3–7 days. The etiology of these reactions is not known. The potential for a delayed reaction must be considered when estimating the risk/benefit of treatment.
The maximum daily dose should not exceed 2 mL undiluted iron dextran.
This preparation should be used with extreme care in patients with serious impairment of liver function.
It should not be used during the acute phase of infectious kidney disease.
Adverse reactions experienced following administration of INFeD may exacerbate cardiovascular complications in patients with pre-existing cardiovascular disease.

PRECAUTIONS

General: Unwarranted therapy with parenteral iron will cause excess storage of iron with the consequent possibility of exogenous hemosiderosis. Such iron overload is particularly apt to occur in patients with hemoglobinopathies and other refractory anemias that might be erroneously diagnosed as iron deficiency anemias.
INFeD should be used with caution in individuals with histories of significant allergies and/or asthma.
Anaphylaxis and other hypersensitivity reactions have been reported after uneventful test doses as well as therapeutic doses of iron dextran injection. Therefore, administration of subsequent test doses during therapy should be considered. (See DOSAGE AND ADMINISTRATION: Administration.)
Epinephrine should be immediately available in the event of acute hypersensitivity reactions. (Usual adult dose: 0.5 mL of a 1:1000 solution, by subcutaneous or intramuscular injection.)
Note: Patients using beta-blocking agents may not respond adequately to epinephrine. Isoproterenol or similar beta-agonist agents may be required in these patients.
Patients with rheumatoid arthritis may have an acute exacerbation of joint pain and swelling following the administration of INFeD.
Reports in the literature from countries outside the United States (in particular, New Zealand) have suggested that the use of intramuscular iron dextran in neonates has been associated with an increased incidence of gram-negative sepsis, primarily due to *E. Coli*.
Information For Patients: Patients should be advised of the potential adverse reactions associated with the use of INFeD.
Drug/Laboratory Test Interactions: Large doses of iron dextran (5 mL or more) have been reported to give a brown color to serum from a blood sample drawn 4 hours after administration.
The drug may cause falsely elevated values of serum bilirubin and falsely decreased values of serum calcium.
Serum iron determinations (especially by colorimetric assays) may not be meaningful for 3 weeks following the administration of iron dextran.
Serum ferritin peaks approximately 7 to 9 days after an intravenous dose of INFeD and slowly returns to baseline after about 3 weeks.
Examination of the bone marrow for iron stores may not be meaningful for prolonged periods following iron dextran therapy because residual iron dextran may remain in the reticuloendothelial cells.
Bone scans involving 99m Tc-diphosphonate have been reported to show a dense, crescentic area of activity in the buttocks, following the contour of the iliac crest, 1 to 6 days after intramuscular injections of iron dextran.
Bone scans with 99m Tc-labeled bone seeking agents, in the presence of high serum ferritin levels or following iron dextran infusions, have been reported to show reduction of bony uptake, marked renal activity, and excessive blood pool and soft tissue accumulation.
Carcinogenesis, Mutagenesis, Impairment Of Fertility: See WARNINGS.
Pregnancy: *Pregnancy Category C:* Iron dextran has been shown to be teratogenic and embryocidal in mice, rats, rabbits, dogs, and monkeys when given in doses of about 3 times the maximum human dose.
No consistent adverse fetal effects were observed in mice, rats, rabbits, dogs and monkeys at doses of 50 mg iron/kg or less. Fetal and maternal toxicity has been reported in monkeys at a total intravenous dose of 90 mg iron/kg over a 14 day period. Similar effects were observed in mice and rats on administration of a single dose of 125 mg iron/kg. Fetal abnormalities in rats and dogs were observed at doses of 250 mg iron/kg and higher. The animals used in these tests were not iron deficient. There are no adequate and well-controlled studies in pregnant women. INFeD should be used during pregnancy only if the potential benefit justifies the potential risk to the fetus.
Placental Transfer: Various animal studies and studies in pregnant humans have demonstrated inconclusive results with respect to the placental transfer of iron dextran as iron

$$\frac{\text{mg blood iron}}{\text{lb body weight}} = \frac{\text{mL blood}}{\text{lb body weight}} \times \frac{\text{g hemoglobin}}{\text{mL blood}} \times \frac{\text{mg iron}}{\text{g hemoglobin}}$$

a) Blood volume .... 65 mL/kg body weight
b) Normal hemoglobin (males and females)
  over 15 kg (33 lbs) .... 14.8 g/dl
  15 kg (33 lbs) or less .... 12.0 g/dl
c) Iron content of hemoglobin ... 0.34%
d) Hemoglobin deficit
e) Weight
Based on the above factors, individuals with normal hemoglobin levels will have approximately 33 mg of blood iron per kilogram of body weight (15 mg/lb).
Note: The table and accompanying formula are applicable for dosage determinations only in patients with iron deficiency anemia; they are not to be used for dosage determinations in patients requiring iron replacement for blood loss.

TOTAL INFeD® REQUIREMENT FOR HEMOGLOBIN RESTORATION AND IRON STORES REPLACEMENT*

PATIENT LEAN BODY WEIGHT		Milliliter Requirement of INFeD Based On Observed Hemoglobin of							
		3	4	5	6	7	8	9	10
kg	lb	(g/dl)	(g/dl)	(g/dl)	(g/dl)	(g/dl)	(g/dl)	(g/dl)	(g/dl)
5	11	3	3	3	3	2	2	2	2
10	22	7	6	6	5	5	4	4	3
15	33	10	9	9	8	7	7	6	5
20	44	16	15	14	13	12	11	10	9
25	55	20	18	17	16	15	14	13	12
30	66	23	22	21	19	18	17	15	14
35	77	27	26	24	23	21	20	18	17
40	88	31	29	28	26	24	22	21	19
45	99	35	33	31	29	27	25	23	21
50	110	39	37	35	32	30	28	26	24
55	121	43	41	38	36	33	31	28	26
60	132	47	44	42	39	36	34	31	28
65	143	51	48	45	42	39	36	34	31
70	154	55	52	49	45	42	39	36	33
75	165	59	55	52	49	45	42	39	35
80	176	63	59	55	52	48	45	41	38
85	187	66	63	59	55	51	48	44	40
90	198	70	66	62	58	54	50	46	42
95	209	74	70	66	62	57	53	49	45
100	220	78	74	69	65	60	56	52	47
105	231	82	77	73	68	63	59	54	50
110	242	86	81	76	71	67	62	57	52
115	253	90	85	80	75	70	64	59	54
120	264	94	88	83	78	73	67	62	57

* Table values were calculated based on a normal adult hemoglobin of 14.8 g/dl for weights greater than 15 kg (33 lbs) and a hemoglobin of 12.0 g/dl for weights less than or equal to 15 kg (33 lbs).

dextran. It appears that some iron does reach the fetus, but the form in which it crosses the placenta is not clear.
Nursing Mothers: Caution should be exercised when INFeD is administered to a nursing woman. Traces of unmetabolized iron dextran are excreted in human milk.
Pediatric Use: Not recommended for use in infants under 4 months of age (See DOSAGE AND ADMINISTRATION.)

ADVERSE REACTIONS

Severe/Fatal: Anaphylactic reactions have been reported with the use of iron dextran injection; on occasions these reactions have been fatal. Such reactions, which occur most often within the first several minutes of administration, have been generally characterized by sudden onset of respiratory difficulty and/or cardiovascular collapse. (See boxed WARNING and PRECAUTIONS: General, pertaining to immediate availability of epinephrine.)
Cardiovascular: Chest pain, chest tightness, shock, cardiac arrest, hypotension, hypertension, tachycardia, bradycardia, flushing, arrhythmias. (Flushing and hypotension may occur from too rapid injections by the intravenous route.)
Dermatologic: Urticaria, pruritus, purpura, rash, cyanosis.
Gastrointestinal: Abdominal pain, nausea, vomiting, diarrhea.
Hematologic/lymphatic: Leucocytosis, lymphadenopathy.
Musculoskeletal/soft tissue: Arthralgia, arthritis (may represent reactivation in patients with quiescent rheumatoid arthritis—See PRECAUTIONS: General), myalgia; backache; sterile abscess, atrophy/fibrosis (intramuscular injection site); brown skin and/or underlying tissue discoloration (staining), soreness or pain at or near intramuscular injection sites; cellulitis; swelling; inflammation; local phlebitis at or near intravenous injection site.
Neurologic: Convulsions, seizures, syncope, headache, weakness, unresponsiveness, paresthesia, febrile episodes, chills, dizziness, disorientation, numbness, unconsciousness.
Respiratory: Respiratory arrest, dyspnea, bronchospasm, wheezing.
Urologic: Hematuria.
Delayed reactions: Arthralgia, backache, chills, dizziness, fever, headache, malaise, myalgia, nausea, vomiting (See WARNINGS.).
Miscellaneous: Febrile episodes, sweating, shivering, chills, malaise, altered taste.

OVERDOSAGE

Overdosage with iron dextran is unlikely to be associated with any acute manifestations. Dosages of iron dextran in excess of the requirements for restoration of hemoglobin and replenishment of iron stores may lead to hemosiderosis. Periodic monitoring of serum ferritin levels may be helpful in recognizing a deleterious progressive accumulation of iron resulting from impaired uptake of iron from the reticuloendothelial system in concurrent medical conditions such as chronic renal failure, Hodgkin's disease, and rheumatoid arthritis. The LD_{50} of iron dextran is not less than 500 mg/kg in the mouse.

DOSAGE AND ADMINISTRATION

Oral iron should be discontinued prior to administration of INFeD.
Dosage:
I. *Iron Deficiency Anemia:* Periodic hematologic determination (hemoglobin and hematocrit) is a simple and accurate technique for monitoring hematological response, and should be used as a guide in therapy. It should be recognized that iron storage may lag behind the appearance of normal blood morphology. Serum iron, total iron binding capacity (TIBC) and percent saturation of transferrin are other important tests for detecting and monitoring the iron deficient state.
After administration of iron dextran complex, evidence of a therapeutic response can be seen in a few days as an increase in the reticulocyte count.
Although serum ferritin is usually a good guide to body iron stores, the correlation of body iron stores and serum ferritin may not be valid in patients on chronic renal dialysis who are also receiving iron dextran complex.
Although there are significant variations in body build and weight distribution among males and females, the accompanying table and formula represent a convenient means for estimating the total iron required. This total iron requirement reflects the amount of iron needed to restore hemoglobin concentration to normal or near normal levels plus an additional allowance to provide adequate replenishment of iron stores in most individuals with moderately or severely reduced levels of hemoglobin. It should be remembered that iron deficiency anemia will not appear until essentially all iron stores have been depleted. Therapy, thus, should aim at not only replenishment of hemoglobin iron but iron stores as well.
Factors contributing to the formula are shown below.
[See first table above]
[See second table above]

The total amount of INFeD in mL required to treat the anemia and replenish iron stores may be approximated as follows:

Adults and Children over 15 kg (33 lbs): See Dosage Table.

Alternatively the total dose may be calculated:

Dose (mL) = 0.0442 (Desired Hb−Observed Hb) × LBW + (0.26 × LBW)

Based on: Desired Hb = the target Hb in g/dl.

Observed Hb = the patient's current hemoglobin in g/dl.

LBW = Lean body weight in kg. A patient's lean body weight (or actual body weight if less than lean body weight) should be utilized when determining dosage.

For males: LBW = 50 kg + 2.3 kg for each inch of patient's height over 5 feet

For females: LBW = 45.5 kg + 2.3 kg for each inch of patient's height over 5 feet

To calculate a patient's weight in kg when lbs are known:

$$\frac{\text{patient's weight in pounds}}{2.2} = \text{weight in kilograms}$$

Children 5–15 kg (11–33 lbs): See Dosage Table.

INFeD should not normally be given in the first four months of life. (See PRECAUTIONS: Pediatric Use.)

Alternatively the total dose may be calculated:

Dose (mL) = 0.0442 (Desired Hb−Observed Hb) × W + (0.26 × W)

Based on: Desired Hb = the target Hb in g/dl. (Normal Hb for Children 15 kg or less is 12 g/dl.)

W = Weight in kg.

To calculate a patient's weight in kg when lbs are known:

$$\frac{\text{patient's weight in pounds}}{2.2} = \text{weight in kilograms}$$

II. *Iron Replacement for Blood Loss:* Some individuals sustain blood losses on an intermittent or repetitive basis. Such blood losses may occur periodically in patients with hemorrhagic diatheses (familial telangiectasia; hemophilia; gastrointestinal bleeding) and on a repetitive basis from procedures such as renal hemodialysis.

Iron therapy in these patients should be directed toward replacement of the equivalent amount of iron represented in the blood loss. The table and formula described under **I. *Iron Deficiency Anemia*** are ***not*** applicable for simple iron replacement values.

Quantitative estimates of the individual's periodic blood loss and hematocrit during the bleeding episode provide a convenient method for the calculation of the required iron dose.

The formula shown below is based on the approximation that 1 mL of normocytic, normochromic red cells contains 1 mg of elemental iron:

Replacement iron (in mg) = Blood loss (in mL) × hematocrit

Example: Blood loss of 500 mL with 20% hematocrit
Replacement Iron = 500 × 0.20 = 100 mg

$$\text{INFeD dose} = \frac{100 \text{ mg}}{50} = 2 \text{ mL}$$

Administration: The total amount of INFeD required for the treatment of iron deficiency anemia or iron replacement for blood loss is determined from the table or appropriate formula. (See Dosage.)

1. *Intravenous Injection*—PRIOR TO RECEIVING THEIR FIRST INFeD THERAPEUTIC DOSE, ALL PATIENTS SHOULD BE GIVEN AN INTRAVENOUS TEST DOSE OF 0.5 mL. (See PRECAUTIONS: General.) THE TEST DOSE SHOULD BE ADMINISTERED AT A GRADUAL RATE OVER AT LEAST 30 SECONDS. Although anaphylactic reactions known to occur following INFeD administration are usually evident within a few minutes, or sooner, it is recommended that a period of an hour or longer elapse before the remainder of the initial therapeutic dose is given.

Individual doses of 2 mL or less may be given on a daily basis until the calculated total amount required has been reached. INFeD is given undiluted at a **slow gradual rate** not to exceed 50 mg (1 mL) per minute.

2. *Intramuscular Injection*—PRIOR TO RECEIVING THEIR FIRST INFeD THERAPEUTIC DOSE, ALL PATIENTS SHOULD BE GIVEN AN INTRAMUSCULAR TEST DOSE OF 0.5 mL. (See PRECAUTIONS: General.) The test dose should be administered in the same recommended test site and by the same technique as described in the last paragraph of this section. Although anaphylactic reactions known to occur following INFeD administration are usually evident within a few minutes or sooner, it is recommended that at least an hour or longer elapse before the remainder of the initial therapeutic dose is given.

If no adverse reactions are observed, INFeD can be given according to the following schedule until the calculated total amount required has been reached. Each day's dose should ordinarily not exceed 0.5 mL (25 mg of iron) for infants under 5 kg (11 lbs); 1.0 mL (50 mg of iron) for children under 10 kg (22 lbs); and 2.0 mL (100 mg of iron) for other patients.

INFeD should be injected only into the muscle mass of the upper outer quadrant of the buttock—never into the arm or other exposed areas—and should be injected deeply, with a 2-inch or 3-inch 19 or 20 gauge needle. If the patient is standing, he/she should be bearing his/her weight on the leg opposite the injection site, or if in bed, he/she should be in the lateral position with injection site uppermost. To avoid injection or leakage into the subcutaneous tissue, a Z-track technique (displacement of the skin laterally prior to injection) is recommended.

NOTE: Do not mix INFeD with other medications or add to parenteral nutrition solutions for intravenous infusion.

Parenteral drug products should be inspected visually for particulate matter and discoloration prior to administration, whenever the solution and container permit.

HOW SUPPLIED

INFeD® (Iron Dextran Injection, USP) containing 50 mg of elemental iron per mL, is available in 2 mL single dose amber vials (for intramuscular or intravenous use) in cartons of 10 (NDC 0364-3012-47).

Store at controlled room temperature 15°–30°C (59°–86°F).

CAUTION: Federal law prohibits dispensing without prescription.

REFERENCES

1. Hatton RC, Portales IT, Finlay A, Ross EA. Removal of Iron Dextran by Hemodialysis: An In Vitro Study. Am J Kid Dis. 1995; 26(2):327–330.
2. Manuel MA, Stewart WK, St. Clair Neill GD, Hutchinson F. Loss of Iron - Dextran through Cuprophane Membrane of a Disposable Coil Dialyser. Nephron. 1972; 9:94–98.

Literature revised: September 1996
Product No.: 1001-02
SCHEIN PHARMACEUTICAL, INC.
Florham Park, NJ 07932 USA

Shown in Product Identification Guide, page 334

Schering Corporation

a wholly-owned subsidiary of Schering-Plough Corporation
GALLOPING HILL ROAD
KENILWORTH, NJ 07033

Direct Inquiries to:
(908) 298-4000
CUSTOMER SERVICE:
(800) 222-7579
FAX: (908) 820-6400

For Medical Information Contact:
Schering Laboratories
Drug Information Services
2000 Galloping Hill Road
Kenilworth, NJ 07033
(800) 526-4099
FAX: (908) 298-2188

Product Identification Codes

To provide quick and positive identification of Schering Products, we have imprinted the product identification number of the National Drug Code on most tablets and capsules. In some cases, identification letters also appear.

Additionally, the following telephone numbers are provided for inquiries:

Drug Information Services
9:00 AM to 5:00 PM EST
1-800-526-4099

After regular hours and on weekends: (908) 298-4000

CELESTONE® SOLUSPAN®* ℞

brand of betamethasone sodium phosphate and betamethasone acetate Injectable Suspension, USP
6 mg per mL

*brand of rapid and repository injectable

DESCRIPTION

Each mL of CELESTONE SOLUSPAN* Injectable Suspension contains: 3.0 mg betamethasone as betamethasone sodium phosphate; 3.0 mg betamethasone acetate; 7.1 mg dibasic sodium phosphate; 3.4 mg monobasic sodium phosphate; 0.1 mg edetate disodium; and 0.2 mg benzalkonium chloride. It is a sterile, aqueous suspension with a pH between 6.8 and 7.2.

The formula for betamethasone sodium phosphate is $C_{22}H_{28}FNa_2O_8P$ with a molecular weight of 516.41. Chemically, it is 9-Fluoro-11β,17,21-trihydroxy-16β-methylpregna-1,4-diene-3,20-dione 21-(disodium phosphate).

The formula for betamethasone acetate is $C_{24}H_{31}FO_6$ with a molecular weight of 434.50. Chemically, it is 9-Fluoro-11β, 17, 21-trihydroxy-16β-methylpregna-1,4-diene-3, 20-dione 21-acetate.

The chemical structures for betamethasone sodium phosphate and betamethasone acetate are as follows:

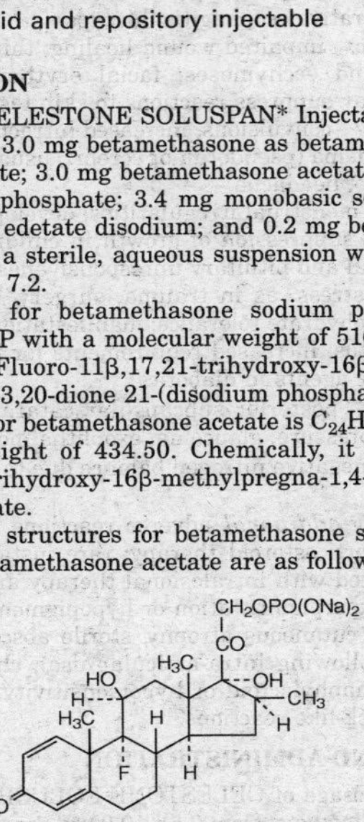

$CH_2OPO(ONa)_2$, CO, HO, H_3C, OH, CH_3, H, F

betamethasone sodium phosphate

[See chemical structure at top of next column]

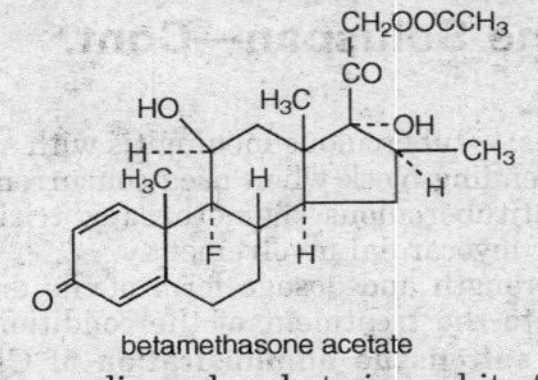

CH_2OOCCH_3, CO, HO, H_3C, OH, CH_3, H, F

betamethasone acetate

Betamethasone sodium phosphate is a white to practically white, odorless powder, and is hygroscopic. It is freely soluble in water and in methanol, but is practically insoluble in acetone and in chloroform.

Betamethasone acetate is a white to creamy white, odorless powder that sinters and resolidifies at about 165°C, and remelts at about 200°C to 220°C with decomposition. It is practically insoluble in water, but freely soluble in acetone, and is soluble in alcohol and in chloroform.

ACTIONS

Naturally occurring glucocorticoids (hydrocortisone), which also have salt-retaining properties, are used as replacement therapy in adrenocortical deficiency states. Their synthetic analogs are primarily used for their potent anti-inflammatory effects in disorders of many organ systems.

Betamethasone sodium phosphate, a soluble ester, provides prompt activity, while betamethasone acetate is only slightly soluble and affords sustained activity.

Glucocorticoids cause profound and varied metabolic effects. In addition, they modify the body's immune responses to diverse stimuli.

INDICATIONS

When oral therapy is not feasible and the strength, dosage form, and route of administration of the drug reasonably lend the preparation to the treatment of the condition, CELESTONE SOLUSPAN Injectable Suspension for intramuscular use is indicated as follows:

Endocrine disorders: primary or secondary adrenocortical insufficiency (hydrocortisone or cortisone is the drug of choice; synthetic analogs may be used in conjunction with mineralocorticoids where applicable; in infancy mineralocorticoid supplementation is of particular importance).

Acute adrenocortical insufficiency (hydrocortisone or cortisone is the drug of choice; mineralocorticoid supplementation may be necessary, particularly when synthetic analogs are used); preoperatively and in the event of serious trauma or illness, in patients with known adrenal insufficiency or when adrenocortical reserve is doubtful; shock unresponsive to conventional therapy if adrenocortical insufficiency exists or is suspected; congenital adrenal hyperplasia; nonsuppurative thyroiditis; hypercalcemia associated with cancer.

Rheumatic disorders: as adjunctive therapy for short-term administration (to tide the patient over an acute episode or exacerbation) in: post-traumatic osteoarthritis; synovitis of osteoarthritis; rheumatoid arthritis, including juvenile rheumatoid arthritis (selected cases may require low-dose maintenance therapy); acute and subacute bursitis; epicondylitis; acute nonspecific tenosynovitis; acute gouty arthritis; psoriatic arthritis; ankylosing spondylitis.

Collagen diseases: during an exacerbation or as maintenance therapy in selected cases of systemic lupus erythematosus, acute rheumatic carditis.

Dermatologic diseases: pemphigus, severe erythema multiforme (Stevens-Johnson syndrome), exfoliative dermatitis, bullous dermatitis herpetiformis, severe seborrheic dermatitis, severe psoriasis, mycosis fungoides.

Allergic states: control of severe or incapacitating allergic conditions intractable to adequate trials of conventional treatment in: bronchial asthma, contact dermatitis, atopic dermatitis, serum sickness, seasonal or perennial allergic rhinitis, drug hypersensitivity reactions, urticarial transfusion reactions, acute noninfectious laryngeal edema (epinephrine is the drug of first choice).

Ophthalmic diseases: severe acute and chronic allergic and inflammatory processes involving the eye, such as: herpes zoster ophthalmicus, iritis and iridocyclitis, chorioretinitis, diffuse posterior uveitis and choroiditis, optic neuritis, sympathetic ophthalmia, anterior segment inflammation, allergic conjunctivitis, allergic corneal marginal ulcers, keratitis.

Gastrointestinal diseases: to tide the patient over a critical period of disease in: ulcerative colitis (systemic therapy), regional enteritis (systemic therapy).

Respiratory diseases: symptomatic sarcoidosis, berylliosis, fulminating or disseminated pulmonary tuberculosis when used concurrently with appropriate antituberculous chemotherapy, Loeffler's syndrome not manageable by other means, aspiration pneumonitis.

Hematologic disorders: acquired (autoimmune) hemolytic anemia, secondary thrombocytopenia in adults, erythroblastopenia (RBC anemia), congenital (erythroid) hypoplastic anemia.

Neoplastic diseases: for palliative management of: leukemias and lymphomas in adults, acute leukemia of childhood.

Edematous states: to induce diuresis or remission of proteinuria in the nephrotic syndrome, without uremia, of the idiopathic type or that due to lupus erythematosus.

Continued on next page

Information on Schering products appearing on these pages is effective as of January 2000.

Celestone Soluspan—Cont.

Miscellaneous: tuberculous meningitis with subarachnoid block or impending block when used concurrently with appropriate antituberculous chemotherapy, trichinosis with neurologic or myocardial involvement.

When the strength and dosage form of the drug lend the preparation to the treatment of the condition, the **intra-articular or soft tissue administration** of CELESTONE SOLUSPAN Injectable Suspension is indicated as adjunctive therapy for short-term administration (to tide the patient over an acute episode or exacerbation) in: synovitis of osteoarthritis, rheumatoid arthritis, acute and subacute bursitis, acute gouty arthritis, epicondylitis, acute nonspecific tenosynovitis, post-traumatic osteoarthritis.

When the strength and dosage form of the drug lend the preparation to the treatment of the condition, the **intralesional administration** of CELESTONE SOLUSPAN Injectable Suspension is indicated for: keloids; localized hypertrophic, infiltrated, inflammatory lesions of: lichen planus, psoriatic plaques, granuloma annulare, and lichen simplex chronicus (neurodermatitis); discoid lupus erythematosus; necrobiosis lipoidica diabeticorum; alopecia areata.

CELESTONE SOLUSPAN Injectable Suspension may also be useful in cystic tumors of an aponeurosis or tendon (ganglia).

CONTRAINDICATIONS

CELESTONE SOLUSPAN Injectable Suspension is contraindicated in systemic fungal infections.

WARNINGS

CELESTONE SOLUSPAN Injectable Suspension should not be administered intravenously.

In patients on corticosteroid therapy subjected to any unusual stress, increased dosage of rapidly acting corticosteroids before, during, and after the stressful situation is indicated.

Corticosteroids may mask some signs of infection, and new infections may appear during their use. There may be decreased resistance and inability to localize infection when corticosteroids are used.

Prolonged use of corticosteroids may produce posterior subcapsular cataracts, glaucoma with possible damage to the optic nerves, and may enhance the establishment of secondary ocular infections due to fungi or viruses.

CELESTONE SOLUSPAN Injectable Suspension contains two betamethasone esters, one of which, betamethasone sodium phosphate, disappears rapidly from the injection site. The potential for systemic effect produced by the soluble portion of CELESTONE SOLUSPAN Injectable Suspension should therefore be taken into account by the physician when using the drug.

Average and large doses of cortisone or hydrocortisone can cause elevation of blood pressure, salt and water retention, and increased excretion of potassium. These effects are less likely to occur with the synthetic derivatives, except when used in large doses. Dietary salt restriction and potassium supplementation may be necessary. All corticosteroids increase calcium excretion.

While on corticosteroid therapy patients should not be vaccinated against smallpox. Other immunization procedures should not be undertaken in patients who are on corticosteroids, especially in high doses, because of possible hazards of neurological complications and lack of antibody response.

Persons who are on drugs which suppress the immune system are more susceptible to infections than healthy individuals. Chickenpox and measles, for example, can have a more serious or even fatal course in nonimmune children or adults on corticosteroids. In such children, or adults who have not had these diseases, particular care should be taken to avoid exposure. How the dose, route, and duration of corticosteroid administration affects the risk of developing a disseminated infection is not known. The contribution of the underlying disease and/or prior corticosteroid treatment to the risk is also not known. If exposed to chickenpox, prophylaxis with varicella-zoster immune globulin (VZIG) may be indicated. If exposed to measles, prophylaxis with pooled intramuscular immunoglobulin (IG) may be indicated. (See the respective package inserts for complete VZIG and IG prescribing information.) If chickenpox develops, treatment with antiviral agents may be considered.

Similarly, corticosteroids should be used with great care in patients with known or suspected *Strongyloides* (threadworm) infestation. In such patients, corticosteroid-induced immunosuppression may lead to *Strongyloides* hyperinfection and dissemination with widespread larval migration, often accompanied by severe enterocolitis and potentially fatal gram-negative septicemia.

The use of CELESTONE SOLUSPAN Injectable Suspension in active tuberculosis should be restricted to those cases of fulminating or disseminated tuberculosis in which the corticosteroid is used for the management of the disease in conjunction with appropriate antituberculous regimen.

If corticosteroids are indicated in patients with latent tuberculosis or tuberculin reactivity, close observation is necessary as reactivation of the disease may occur. During prolonged corticosteroid therapy, these patients should receive chemoprophylaxis.

Because rare instances of anaphylactoid reactions have occurred in patients receiving parenteral corticosteroid therapy, appropriate precautionary measures should be taken prior to administration, especially when the patient has a history of allergy to any drug.

Usage in pregnancy: Since adequate human reproduction studies have not been done with corticosteroids, the use of these drugs in pregnancy, nursing mothers, or women of childbearing potential requires that the possible benefits of the drug be weighed against the potential hazards to the mother and embryo or fetus. Infants born of mothers who have received substantial doses of corticosteroids during pregnancy should be carefully observed for signs of hypoadrenalism.

PRECAUTIONS

Information for Patients: Persons who are on immunosuppressant doses of corticosteroids should be warned to avoid exposure to chickenpox or measles. Patients should also be advised that if they are exposed, medical advice should be sought without delay.

General: Drug-induced secondary adrenocortical insufficiency may be minimized by gradual reduction of dosage. This type of relative insufficiency may persist for months after discontinuation of therapy; therefore, in any situation of stress occurring during that period, hormone therapy should be reinstituted. Since mineralocorticoid secretion may be impaired, salt and/or a mineralocorticoid should be administered concurrently.

There is an enhanced effect of corticosteroids in patients with hypothyroidism and in those with cirrhosis.

Corticosteroids should be used cautiously in patients with ocular herpes simplex for fear of corneal perforation.

The lowest possible dose of corticosteroid should be used to control the condition under treatment, and when reduction in dosage is possible, the reduction must be gradual.

Psychic derangements may appear when corticosteroids are used, ranging from euphoria, insomnia, mood swings, personality changes, and severe depression to frank psychotic manifestations. Also, existing emotional instability or psychotic tendencies may be aggravated by corticosteroids.

Aspirin should be used cautiously in conjunction with corticosteroids in hypoprothrombinemia.

Steroids should be used with caution in nonspecific ulcerative colitis, if there is a probability of impending perforation, abscess, or other pyogenic infection; diverticulitis; fresh intestinal anastomoses; active or latent peptic ulcer; renal insufficiency; hypertension; osteoporosis; and myasthenia gravis.

Growth and development of infants and children on prolonged corticosteroid therapy should be carefully followed.

The following additional precautions also apply for parenteral corticosteroids. **Intra-articular injection of a corticosteroid may produce systemic as well as local effects.**

Appropriate examination of any joint fluid present is necessary to exclude a septic process.

A marked increase in pain accompanied by local swelling, further restriction of joint motion, fever, and malaise are suggestive of septic arthritis. If this complication occurs and the diagnosis of sepsis is confirmed, appropriate antimicrobial therapy should be instituted.

Local injection of a steroid into a previously infected joint is to be avoided.

Corticosteroids should not be injected into unstable joints.

The slower rate of absorption by intramuscular administration should be recognized.

ADVERSE REACTIONS

Fluid and electrolyte disturbances: sodium retention, fluid retention, congestive heart failure in susceptible patients, potassium loss, hypokalemic alkalosis, hypertension.

Musculoskeletal: muscle weakness, steroid myopathy, loss of muscle mass, osteoporosis, vertebral compression fractures, aseptic necrosis of femoral and humeral heads, pathologic fracture of long bones.

Gastrointestinal: peptic ulcer with possible subsequent perforation and hemorrhage, pancreatitis, abdominal distention, ulcerative esophagitis, hiccups.

Dermatologic: impaired wound healing; thin, fragile skin; petechiae and ecchymoses; facial erythema; increased sweating; may suppress reactions to skin tests.

Neurological: convulsions, increased intracranial pressure with papilledema (pseudotumor cerebri) usually after treatment, vertigo, headache.

Endocrine: menstrual irregularities; development of cushingoid state; suppression of growth in children; secondary adrenocortical and pituitary unresponsiveness, particularly in times of stress, as in trauma, surgery, or illness; decreased carbohydrate tolerance; manifestations of latent diabetes mellitus; increased requirements for insulin or oral hypoglycemic agents in diabetics.

Ophthalmic: posterior subcapsular cataracts, increased intraocular pressure, glaucoma, exophthalmos.

Metabolic: negative nitrogen balance due to protein catabolism.

The following *additional* adverse reactions are related to parenteral corticosteroid therapy: rare instances of blindness associated with intralesional therapy around the face and head, hyperpigmentation or hypopigmentation, subcutaneous and cutaneous atrophy, sterile abscess, postinjection flare (following intra-articular use), charcot-like arthropathy, anaphylactoid or hypersensitivity and hypotensive and shock-like reactions.

DOSAGE AND ADMINISTRATION

The initial dosage of CELESTONE SOLUSPAN Injectable Suspension may vary from 0.5 to 9.0 mg per day depending on the specific disease entity being treated. In situations of less severity, lower doses will generally suffice while in selected patients higher initial doses may be required. Usually the parenteral dosage ranges are $^1/_3$ to $^1/_2$ the oral dose given every 12 hours. However, in certain overwhelming, acute, life-threatening situations, administration in dosages exceeding the usual dosages may be justified and may be in multiples of the oral dosages.

The initial dosage should be maintained or adjusted until a satisfactory response is noted. If after a reasonable period of time there is a lack of satisfactory clinical response, CELESTONE SOLUSPAN Injectable Suspension should be discontinued and the patient transferred to other appropriate therapy. *It Should Be Emphasized That Dosage Requirements Are Variable and Must Be Individualized on the Basis of the Disease Under Treatment and the Response of the Patient.* After a favorable response is noted, the proper maintenance dosage should be determined by decreasing the initial drug dosage in small decrements at appropriate time intervals until the lowest dosage which will maintain an adequate clinical response is reached. It should be kept in mind that constant monitoring is needed in regard to drug dosage. Included in the situations which may make dosage adjustments necessary are changes in clinical status secondary to remissions or exacerbations in the disease process, the patient's individual drug responsiveness, and the effect of patient exposure to stressful situations not directly related to the disease entity under treatment. In this latter situation it may be necessary to increase the dosage of CELESTONE SOLUSPAN Injectable Suspension for a period of time consistent with the patient's condition. If after long-term therapy the drug is to be stopped, it is recommended that it be withdrawn gradually rather than abruptly.

If coadministration of a local anesthetic is desired, CELESTONE SOLUSPAN Injectable Suspension may be mixed with 1% or 2% lidocaine hydrochloride, using the formulations which do not contain parabens. Similar local anesthetics may also be used. Diluents containing methylparaben, propylparaben, phenol, etc., should be avoided since these compounds may cause flocculation of the steroid. The required dose of CELESTONE SOLUSPAN Injectable Suspension is first withdrawn from the vial into the syringe. The local anesthetic is then drawn in, and the syringe shaken briefly. **Do not inject local anesthetics into the vial of CELESTONE SOLUSPAN Injectable Suspension.**

Bursitis, tenosynovitis, peritendinitis: In acute subdeltoid, subacromial, olecranon, and prepatellar bursitis, one intrabursal injection of 1.0 mL CELESTONE SOLUSPAN Injectable Suspension can relieve pain and restore full range of movement. Several intrabursal injections of corticosteroids are usually required in recurrent acute bursitis and in acute exacerbations of chronic bursitis. Partial relief of pain and some increase in mobility can be expected in both conditions after one or two injections. Chronic bursitis may be treated with reduced dosage once the acute condition is controlled. In tenosynovitis and tendinitis, three or four local injections at intervals of 1 to 2 weeks between injections are given in most cases. Injections should be made into the affected tendon sheaths rather than into the tendons themselves. In ganglions of joint capsules and tendon sheaths, injection of 0.5 mL directly into the ganglion cysts has produced marked reduction in the size of the lesions.

Rheumatoid arthritis and osteoarthritis: Following intra-articular administration of 0.5 to 2.0 mL of CELESTONE SOLUSPAN Injectable Suspension, relief of pain, soreness, and stiffness may be experienced. Duration of relief varies widely in both diseases. Intra-articular Injection—CELESTONE SOLUSPAN Injectable Suspension is well tolerated in joints and periarticular tissues. There is virtually no pain on injection, and the "secondary flare" that sometimes occurs a few hours after intra-articular injection of corticosteroids has not been reported with CELESTONE SOLUSPAN Injectable Suspension. Using sterile technique, a 20- to 24-gauge needle on an empty syringe is inserted into the synovial cavity and a few drops of synovial fluid are withdrawn to confirm that the needle is in the joint. The aspirating syringe is replaced by a syringe containing CELESTONE SOLUSPAN Injectable Suspension and injection is then made into the joint.

Recommended Doses for Intra-articular Injection

Size of joint	Location	Dose (mL)
Very Large	Hip	1.0–2.0
Large	Knee, Ankle, Shoulder	1.0
Medium	Elbow, Wrist	0.5–1.0
Small (Metacarpophalangeal, interphalangeal) (Sternoclavicular)	Hand Chest	0.25–0.5

A portion of the administered dose of CELESTONE SOLUSPAN Injectable Suspension is absorbed systemically following intra-articular injection. In patients being treated concomitantly with oral or parenteral corticosteroids, especially those receiving large doses, the systemic absorption of the drug should be considered in determining intra-articular dosage.

Dermatologic conditions: In intralesional treatment, 0.2 mL/sq cm of CELESTONE SOLUSPAN Injectable Suspension is injected intradermally (not subcutaneously) using a tuberculin syringe with a 25-gauge, $^1/_2$-inch needle. Care should be taken to deposit a uniform depot of medication intradermally. A total of no more than 1.0 mL at weekly intervals is recommended.

Disorders of the foot: A tuberculin syringe with a 25-gauge, 3/4-inch needle is suitable for most injections into the foot. The following doses are recommended at intervals of 3 days to a week.

Diagnosis	CELESTONE SOLUSPAN Injectable Suspension Dose (mL)
Bursitis	
under heloma durum or heloma molle	0.25–0.5
under calcaneal spur	0.5
over hallux rigidus or digiti quinti varus	0.5
Tenosynovitis, periostitis of cuboid	0.5
Acute gouty arthritis	0.5–1.0

HOW SUPPLIED

CELESTONE SOLUSPAN Injectable Suspension, 5-mL multiple-dose vial; box of one (NDC 0085-0566-05).

Shake well before using.

Store between 2° and 25°C (36° and 77°F).

Protect from light.

Schering Corporation
Kenilworth, NJ 07033 USA

Rev. 10/99 23504804

CELESTONE® ℞

brand of betamethasone
Syrup, USP

DESCRIPTION

Glucocorticoids are adrenocortical steroids, both naturally occurring and synthetic, that are readily absorbed from the gastrointestinal tract. A derivative of prednisolone, CELESTONE (betamethasone) has a 16β-methyl group that enhances the anti-inflammatory action of the molecule and reduces the sodium- and water-retaining properties of the fluorine atom bound at carbon 9.

The formula for betamethasone is $C_{22}H_{29}FO_5$ and has a molecular weight of 392.47. Chemically, it is 9-fluoro-11β,17,21-trihydroxy-16β-methylpregna-1,4-diene-3,20-dione and has the following structure:

Betamethasone is a white to practically white, odorless, crystalline powder. It melts at about 240°C with some decomposition. Betamethasone is sparingly soluble in acetone, alcohol, dioxane, and methanol; very slightly soluble in chloroform and ether; and is insoluble in water.

CELESTONE Syrup contains 0.6 mg betamethasone, USP, in each 5 mL.

The inactive ingredients for celestone Syrup include: alcohol, USP; cellulose powdered, NF; citric acid, USP anhydrous; FD&C Red No. 40; FD&C Yellow No. 6; Flavor Cherry Artificial 13506457 IFF; Flavor Orange Natural Terpeneless 73502530 IFF; propylene glycol, USP; sodium benzoate, NF; sodium chloride, USP; sorbitol solution, USP; sugar granulated; and water purified, USP.

ACTIONS

Naturally occurring glucocorticoids (hydrocortisone and cortisone), which also have salt-retaining properties, are used as replacement therapy in adrenocortical deficiency states. Their synthetic analogs, such as betamethasone, are primarily used for their potent anti-inflammatory effects in disorders of many organ systems.

Glucocorticoids, such as betamethasone, cause profound and varied metabolic effects. In addition, they modify the body's immune response to diverse stimuli.

INDICATIONS

Endocrine disorders: primary or secondary adrenocortical insufficiency (hydrocortisone or cortisone is the first choice; synthetic analogs may be used in conjunction with mineralocorticoids where applicable; in infancy mineralocorticoid supplementation is of particular importance); congenital adrenal hyperplasia; nonsuppurative thyroiditis; hypercalcemia associated with cancer.

Rheumatic disorders: as adjunctive therapy for short-term administration (to tide the patient over an acute episode or exacerbation) in: psoriatic arthritis; rheumatoid arthritis, including juvenile rheumatoid arthritis (selected cases may require low-dose maintenance therapy); ankylosing spondylitis; acute and subacute bursitis; acute nonspecific tenosynovitis; acute gouty arthritis; post-traumatic osteoarthritis; synovitis of osteoarthritis; epicondylitis.

Collagen diseases: during an exacerbation or as maintenance therapy in selected cases of: systemic lupus erythematosus, acute rheumatic carditis.

Dermatologic diseases: pemphigus, bullous dermatitis herpetiformis, severe erythema multiforme (Stevens-Johnson syndrome), exfoliative dermatitis, mycosis fungoides, severe psoriasis, severe seborrheic dermatitis.

Allergic states: control of severe or incapacitating allergic conditions intractable to adequate trials of conventional treatment: seasonal or perennial allergic rhinitis, serum sickness, bronchial asthma, contact dermatitis, atopic dermatitis, drug hypersensitivity reactions.

Ophthalmic diseases: severe acute and chronic allergic and inflammatory processes involving the eye and its adnexa, such as: allergic conjunctivitis, keratitis, allergic corneal marginal ulcers, herpes zoster ophthalmicus, iritis and iridocyclitis, chorioretinitis, anterior segment inflammation, diffuse posterior uveitis and choroiditis, optic neuritis, sympathetic ophthalmia.

Respiratory diseases: symptomatic sarcoidosis, Loeffler's syndrome not manageable by other means, berylliosis, fulminating or disseminated pulmonary tuberculosis when used concurrently with appropriate antituberculous chemotherapy, aspiration pneumonitis.

Hematologic disorders: idiopathic thrombocytopenic purpura in adults, secondary thrombocytopenia in adults, acquired (autoimmune) hemolytic anemia, erythroblastopenia (RBC anemia), congenital (erythroid) hypoplastic anemia.

Neoplastic diseases: for palliative management of: leukemias and lymphomas in adults, acute leukemia of childhood.

Edematous states: to induce a diuresis or remission of proteinuria in the nephrotic syndrome, without uremia, of the idiopathic type or that due to lupus erythematosus.

Gastrointestinal diseases: to tide the patient over a critical period of the disease in: ulcerative colitis, regional enteritis.

Miscellaneous: tuberculous meningitis with subarachnoid block or impending block when used concurrently with appropriate antituberculous chemotherapy, trichinosis with neurologic or myocardial involvement.

CONTRAINDICATIONS

CELESTONE Syrup is contraindicated in systemic fungal infections.

WARNINGS

In patients on corticosteroid therapy subjected to unusual stress, increased dosage of rapidly acting corticosteroids before, during, and after the stressful situation is indicated.

Corticosteroids may mask some signs of infection, and new infections may appear during their use. There may be decreased resistance and inability to localize infection when corticosteroids are used.

Prolonged use of corticosteroids may produce posterior subcapsular cataracts, glaucoma with possible damage to the optic nerves, and may enhance the establishment of secondary ocular infections due to fungi or viruses.

Average and large doses of hydrocortisone or cortisone can cause elevation of blood pressure, salt and water retention, and increased excretion of potassium. These effects are less likely to occur with the synthetic derivatives except when used in large doses. Dietary salt restrictions and potassium supplementation may be necessary. All corticosteroids increase calcium excretion.

While on corticosteroid therapy, patients should not be vaccinated against smallpox. Other immunization procedures should not be undertaken in patients who are on corticosteroids, especially on high doses, because of possible hazards of neurological complications and a lack of antibody response.

Persons who are on drugs which suppress the immune system are more susceptible to infections than healthy individuals. Chickenpox and measles, for example, can have a more serious or even fatal course in nonimmune children or adults on corticosteroids. In such children, or adults who have not had these diseases, particular care should be taken to avoid exposure. How the dose, route, and duration of corticosteroid administration affects the risk of developing a disseminated infection is not known. The contribution of the underlying disease and/or prior corticosteroid treatment to the risk is also not known. If exposed to chickenpox, prophylaxis with varicella-zoster immune globulin (VZIG) may be indicated. If exposed to measles, prophylaxis with pooled intramuscular immunoglobulin (IG) may be indicated. (See the respective package inserts for complete VZIG and IG prescribing information.) If chickenpox develops, treatment with antiviral agents may be considered.

Similarly, corticosteroids should be used with great care in patients with known or suspected *Strongyloides* (threadworm) infestation. In such patients, corticosteroid-induced immunosuppression may lead to *Strongyloides* hyper infection and dissemination with widespread larval migration, often accompanied by severe enterocolitis and potentially fatal gram-negative septicemia.

The use of CELESTONE Syrup in active tuberculosis should be restricted to those cases of fulminating or disseminated tuberculosis in which the corticosteroid is used for the management of the disease in conjunction with an appropriate antituberculous regimen.

If corticosteroids are indicated in patients with latent tuberculosis or tuberculin reactivity, close observation is necessary as reactivation of the disease may occur. During prolonged corticosteroid therapy, these patients should receive chemoprophylaxis.

Usage in pregnancy: Since adequate human reproduction studies have not been done with corticosteroids, the use of these drugs in pregnancy, nursing mothers, or women of childbearing potential requires that the possible benefits of the drug be weighed against the potential hazards to the mother and embryo or fetus. Infants born of mothers who have received substantial doses of corticosteroids during pregnancy should be carefully observed for signs of hypoadrenalism.

PRECAUTIONS

Information for Patients: Persons who are on immunosuppressant doses of corticosteroids should be warned to avoid exposure to chickenpox or measles. Patients should also be advised that if they are exposed, medical advice should be sought without delay.

General: Drug-induced secondary adrenocortical insufficiency may be minimized by gradual reduction of dosage. This type of relative insufficiency may persist for months after discontinuation of therapy; therefore, in any situation of stress occurring during that period, hormone therapy should be reinstituted. Since mineralocorticoid secretion may be impaired, salt and/or a mineralocorticoid should be administered concurrently.

There is an enhanced effect of corticosteroids on patients with hypothyroidism and in those with cirrhosis.

Corticosteroids should be used cautiously in patients with ocular herpes simplex because of possible corneal perforation.

The lowest possible dose of corticosteroid should be used to control the condition under treatment, and when reduction in dosage is possible, the reduction should be gradual.

Psychic derangements may appear when corticosteroids are used, ranging from euphoria, insomnia, mood swings, personality changes, and severe depression to frank psychotic manifestations. Also, existing emotional instability or psychotic tendencies may be aggravated by corticosteroids.

Aspirin should be used cautiously in conjunction with corticosteroids in hypoprothrombinemia.

Steroids should be used with caution in nonspecific ulcerative colitis, if there is a probability of impending perforation, abscess or other pyogenic infection; diverticulitis; fresh intestinal anastomoses; active or latent peptic ulcer; renal insufficiency; hypertension; osteoporosis; and myasthenia gravis.

Growth and development of infants and children on prolonged corticosteroid therapy should be carefully observed.

ADVERSE REACTIONS

Fluid and electrolyte disturbances: sodium retention, fluid retention, congestive heart failure in susceptible patients, potassium loss, hypokalemic alkalosis, hypertension.

Musculoskeletal: muscle weakness, steroid myopathy, loss of muscle mass, osteoporosis, vertebral compression fractures, aseptic necrosis of femoral and humeral heads, pathologic fracture of long bones.

Gastrointestinal: peptic ulcer with possible perforation and hemorrhage, pancreatitis, abdominal distention, ulcerative esophagitis, hiccups.

Dermatologic: impaired wound healing; thin, fragile skin; petechiae and ecchymoses; facial erythema; increased sweating; may suppress reactions to skin tests.

Neurological: convulsions, increased intra cranial pressure with papilledema (pseudotumor cerebri) usually after treatment, vertigo, headache.

Endocrine: menstrual irregularities; development of cushingoid state; suppression of growth in children; secondary adrenocortical and pituitary unresponsiveness, particularly in times of stress, as in trauma, surgery, or illness; decreased carbohydrate tolerance; manifestations of latent diabetes mellitus; increased requirements of insulin or oral hypoglycemic agents in diabetics.

Ophthalmic: posterior subcapsular cataracts, increased intraocular pressure, glaucoma, exophthalmos.

Metabolic: negative nitrogen balance due to protein catabolism.

Other: anaphylactoid or hypersensitivity and hypotensive or shock-like reactions.

DOSAGE AND ADMINISTRATION

The initial dosage of CELESTONE Syrup may vary from 0.6 mg to 7.2 mg per day depending on the specific disease entity being treated. In situations of less severity, lower doses will generally suffice, while in selected patients higher initial doses may be required. The initial dosage should be maintained or adjusted until a satisfactory response is noted. If after a reasonable period of time there is a lack of satisfactory clinical response, betamethasone should be discontinued and the patient transferred to other appropriate therapy. **IT SHOULD BE EMPHASIZED THAT DOSAGE REQUIREMENTS ARE VARIABLE AND MUST BE INDIVIDUALIZED ON THE BASIS OF THE DISEASE UNDER TREATMENT AND THE RESPONSE OF THE PATIENT.** After a favorable response is noted, the proper maintenance dosage should be determined by decreasing the initial drug dosage in small decrements at appropriate time intervals until the lowest dosage which will maintain an adequate clinical response is reached. It should be kept in mind that constant monitoring is needed in regard to drug dosage. Included in the situations which may make dosage adjustments necessary are changes in clinical status secondary to remissions or exacerbations in the disease process, the patient's individual

Continued on next page

Information on Schering products appearing on these pages is effective as of January 2000.

Celestone—Cont.

drug responsiveness, and the effect of patient exposure to stressful situations not directly related to the disease entity under treatment. In this latter situation, it may be necessary to increase the dosage of betamethasone for a period of time consistent with the patient's condition. If after long-term therapy the drug is to be stopped, it is recommended that it be withdrawn gradually rather than abruptly.

HOW SUPPLIED

CELESTONE Syrup, 0.6 mg per 5 mL, orange-red colored liquid, bottle of 4 fluid ounces (118 mL) (NDC 0085-0942-05). **Protect from light.**
Store between 2° and 30°C (36° and 86°F).
Schering Corporation
Kenilworth, NJ 07033 USA
Rev. 10/99 17979639

CLARITIN® ℞
brand of loratadine
TABLETS, SYRUP, and RAPIDLY-DISINTEGRATING TABLETS

DESCRIPTION

Loratadine is a white to off-white powder not soluble in water, but very soluble in acetone, alcohol, and chloroform. It has a molecular weight of 382.89, and empirical formula of $C_{22}H_{23}ClN_2O_2$; its chemical name is ethyl 4-(8-chloro-5, 6-dihydro-11*H*-benzo [5, 6] cyclohepta [1, 2-*b*] pyridin-11-ylidene)-1-piperidinecarboxylate and has the following structural formula:

CLARITIN Tablets contain 10 mg micronized loratadine, an antihistamine, to be administered orally. They also contain the following inactive ingredients: corn starch, lactose, and magnesium stearate.
CLARITIN Syrup contains 1 mg/mL micronized loratadine, an antihistamine, to be administered orally. It also contains the following inactive ingredients: citric acid, edetate disodium, artificial flavor, glycerin, propylene glycol, sodium benzoate, sugar, and water. The pH is between 2.5 and 3.1.
CLARITIN REDITABS (loratadine rapidly-disintegrating tablets) contain 10 mg micronized loratadine, an antihistamine, to be administered orally. It disintegrates in the mouth within seconds after placement on the tongue, allowing its contents to be subsequently swallowed with or without water. CLARITIN REDITABS (loratadine rapidly-disintegrating tablets) also contain the following inactive ingredients: citric acid, gelatin, mannitol, and mint flavor.

CLINICAL PHARMACOLOGY

Loratadine is a long-acting tricyclic antihistamine with selective peripheral histamine H_1-receptor antagonistic activity.
Human histamine skin wheal studies following single and repeated 10 mg oral doses of CLARITIN have shown that the drug exhibits an antihistaminic effect beginning within 1 to 3 hours, reaching a maximum at 8 to 12 hours, and lasting in excess of 24 hours. There was no evidence of tolerance to this effect after 28 days of dosing with CLARITIN.
Whole body autoradiographic studies in rats and monkeys, radiolabeled tissue distribution studies in mice and rats, and *in vivo* radioligand studies in mice have shown that neither loratadine nor its metabolites readily cross the blood-brain barrier. Radioligand binding studies with guinea pig pulmonary and brain H_1-receptors indicate that there was preferential binding to peripheral versus central nervous system H_1-receptors.
Repeated application of CLARITIN REDITABS (loratadine rapidly-disintegrating tablets) to the hamster cheek pouch did not cause local irritation.
Pharmacokinetics: Loratadine was rapidly absorbed following oral administration of 10 mg tablets, once daily for 10 days to healthy adult volunteers with times to maximum concentration (T_{max}) of 1.3 hours for loratadine and 2.5 hours for its major active metabolite, descarboethoxyloratadine. Based on a cross-study comparison of single doses of loratadine syrup and tablets given to healthy adult volunteers, the plasma concentration profile of descarboethoxyloratadine for the two formulations is comparable. The pharmacokinetics of loratadine and descarboethoxyloratadine are independent of dose over the dose range of 10 to 40 mg and are not altered by the duration of treatment. In a single-dose study, food increased the systemic bioavailability (AUC) of loratadine and descarboethoxyloratadine by approximately 40% and 15%, respectively. The time to peak plasma concentration (T_{max}) of loratadine and descarboethoxyloratadine was delayed by 1 hour. Peak plasma concentrations (C_{max}) were not affected by food.
Pharmacokinetic studies showed that CLARITIN REDITABS (loratadine rapidly-disintegrating tablets) provide plasma concentrations of loratadine and descarboethoxyloratadine similar to those achieved with CLARITIN Tablets. Following administration of 10 mg loratadine once daily for 10 days with each dosage form in a randomized crossover comparison in 24 normal adult subjects, similar mean exposures (AUC) and peak plasma concentrations (C_{max}) of loratadine were observed. CLARITIN REDITABS (loratadine rapidly-disintegrating tablets) mean AUC and C_{max} were 11% and 6% greater than that of the CLARITIN Tablet values, respectively. Descarboethoxyloratadine bioequivalence was demonstrated between the two formulations. After 10 days of dosing, mean peak plasma concentrations were attained at 1.3 hours and 2.3 hours (T_{max}) for parent and metabolite, respectively.
In a single-dose study with CLARITIN REDITABS (loratadine rapidly-disintegrating tablets), food increased the AUC of loratadine by approximately 48% and did not appreciably affect the AUC of descarboethoxyloratadine. The times to peak plasma concentration (T_{max}) of loratadine and descarboethoxyloratadine were delayed by approximately 2.4 and 3.7 hours, respectively, when food was consumed prior to CLARITIN REDITABS (loratadine rapidly-disintegrating tablets) administration. Parent and metabolite peak concentrations (C_{max}) were not affected by food.
In a single-dose study with CLARITIN REDITABS (loratadine rapidly-disintegrating tablets) in 24 subjects, the AUC of loratadine was increased by 26% when administered without water compared to administration with water, while C_{max} was not substantially affected. The bioavailability of descarboethoxyloratadine was not different when administered without water.
Approximately 80% of the total loratadine dose administered can be found equally distributed between urine and feces in the form of metabolic products within 10 days. In nearly all patients, exposure (AUC) to the metabolite is greater than to the parent loratadine. The mean elimination half-lives in normal adult subjects (n = 54) were 8.4 hours (range = 3 to 20 hours) for loratadine and 28 hours (range = 8.8 to 92 hours) for descarboethoxyloratadine. Loratadine and descarboethoxyloratadine reached steady-state in most patients by approximately the fifth dosing day. There was considerable variability in the pharmacokinetic data in all studies of CLARITIN Tablets and Syrup, probably due to the extensive first-pass metabolism.
In vitro studies with human liver microsomes indicate that loratadine is metabolized to descarboethoxyloratadine predominantly by cytochrome P450 3A4 (CYP3A4) and, to a lesser extent, by cytochrome P450 2D6 (CYP2D6). In the presence of a CYP3A4 inhibitor ketoconazole, loratadine is metabolized to descarboethoxyloratadine predominantly by CYP2D6. Concurrent administration of loratadine with either ketoconazole, erythromycin (both CYP3A4 inhibitors), or cimetidine (CYP2D6 and CYP3A4 inhibitor) to healthy volunteers was associated with substantially increased plasma concentrations of loratadine (see **Drug Interactions** section).
The pharmacokinetic profile of loratadine in children in the 6- to 12-year age group is similar to that of adults. In a single-dose pharmacokinetic study of 13 pediatric volunteers (aged 8–12 years) given 10 mL of CLARITIN Syrup containing 10 mg loratadine, the ranges of individual subject values of pharmacokinetic parameters (AUC and C_{max}) were comparable to those following administration of a 10 mg tablet or syrup to adult volunteers.
Special Populations: In a study involving twelve healthy geriatric subjects (66 to 78 years old), the AUC and peak plasma levels (C_{max}) of both loratadine and descarboethoxyloratadine were approximately 50% greater than those observed in studies of younger subjects. The mean elimination half-lives for the geriatric subjects were 18.2 hours (range = 6.7 to 37 hours) for loratadine and 17.5 hours (range = 11 to 38 hours) for descarboethoxyloratadine.
In a study involving 12 subjects with chronic renal impairment (creatinine clearance ≤ 30 mL/min) both AUC and C_{max} increased by approximately 73% for loratadine and by 120% for descarboethoxyloratadine, as compared to 6 subjects with normal renal function (creatinine clearance ≥ 80 mL/min). The mean elimination half-lives of loratadine (7.6 hours) and descarboethoxyloratadine (23.9 hours) were not substantially different from that observed in normal subjects. Hemodialysis does not have an effect on the pharmacokinetics of loratadine or descarboethoxyloratadine in subjects with chronic renal impairment.
In seven patients with chronic alcoholic liver disease, the AUC and C_{max} of loratadine were double while the pharmacokinetic profile of descarboethoxyloratadine was not substantially different from that observed in other trials enrolling normal subjects. The elimination half-lives for loratadine and descarboethoxyloratadine were 24 hours and 37 hours, respectively, and increased with increasing severity of liver disease.
Clinical Trials: Clinical trials of CLARITIN Tablets involved over 10,700 patients, 12 years of age and older, who received either CLARITIN Tablets or another antihistamine and/or placebo in double-blind randomized controlled studies. In placebo-controlled trials, 10 mg once daily of CLARITIN Tablets was superior to placebo and similar to clemastine (1 mg BID) or terfenadine (60 mg BID) in effects on nasal and non-nasal symptoms of allergic rhinitis. In these studies somnolence occurred less frequently with CLARITIN Tablets than with clemastine and at about the same frequency as terfenadine or placebo. In studies with CLARITIN Tablets at doses 2 to 4 times higher than the recommended dose of 10 mg, a dose-related increase in the incidence of somnolence was observed. Therefore, some patients, particularly those with hepatic or renal impairment and the elderly, or those on medications that impair clearance of loratadine and its metabolites may experience somnolence. In addition, three placebo-controlled, double-blind, 2-week trials in 188 pediatric patients with seasonal allergic rhinitis aged 6 to 12 years, were conducted at doses of CLARITIN Syrup up to 10 mg once daily.
Clinical trials of CLARITIN REDITABS (loratadine rapidly-disintegrating tablets) involved over 1300 patients who received either CLARITIN REDITABS (loratadine rapidly-disintegrating tablets), CLARITIN Tablets, or placebo. In placebo-controlled trials, one CLARITIN REDITABS (loratadine rapidly-disintegrating tablets) once daily was superior to placebo and similar to CLARITIN Tablets in effects on nasal and non-nasal symptoms of seasonal allergic rhinitis.
Among those patients involved in double-blind, randomized, controlled studies of CLARITIN Tablets, approximately 1000 patients (age 12 and older), were enrolled in studies of chronic idiopathic urticaria. In placebo-controlled clinical trials, CLARITIN Tablets 10 mg once daily were superior to placebo in the management of chronic idiopathic urticaria, as demonstrated by reduction of associated itching, erythema, and hives. In these studies, the incidence of somnolence seen with CLARITIN Tablets was similar to that seen with placebo.
In a study in which CLARITIN Tablets were administered to adults at 4 times the clinical dose for 90 days, no clinically significant increase in the QT_c was seen on ECGs.
In a single-rising dose study in which doses up to 160 mg (16 times the clinical dose) were studied, loratadine did not cause any clinically significant changes on the QTc interval in the ECGs.

INDICATIONS AND USAGE

CLARITIN is indicated for the relief of nasal and non-nasal symptoms of seasonal allergic rhinitis and for the treatment of chronic idiopathic urticaria in patients 6 years of age or older.

CONTRAINDICATIONS

CLARITIN is contraindicated in patients who are hypersensitive to this medication or to any of its ingredients.

PRECAUTIONS

General: Patients with liver impairment or renal insufficiency (GFR < 30 mL/min) should be given a lower initial dose (10 mg every other day). (See **CLINICAL PHARMACOLOGY: Special Populations.**)
Drug Interactions: Loratadine (10 mg once daily) has been coadministered with therapeutic doses of erythromycin, cimetidine, and ketoconazole in controlled clinical pharmacology studies in adult volunteers. Although increased plasma concentrations (AUC 0–24 hrs) of loratadine and/or descarboethoxyloratadine were observed following coadministration of loratadine with each of these drugs in normal volunteers (n = 24 in each study), there were no clinically relevant changes in the safety profile of loratadine, as assessed by electrocardiographic parameters, clinical laboratory tests, vital signs, and adverse events. There were no significant effects on QT_c intervals, and no reports of sedation or syncope. No effects on plasma concentrations of cimetidine or ketoconazole were observed. Plasma concentrations (AUC 0–24 hrs) of erythromycin decreased 15% with coadministration of loratadine relative to that observed with erythromycin alone. The clinical relevance of this difference is unknown. These above findings are summarized in the following table:
[See table below]
There does not appear to be an increase in adverse events in subjects who received oral contraceptives and loratadine.
Carcinogenesis, Mutagenesis, and Impairment of Fertility: In an 18-month carcinogenicity study in mice and a 2-year study in rats, loratadine was administered in the diet at doses up to 40 mg/kg (mice) and 25 mg/kg (rats). In the carcinogenicity studies, pharmacokinetic assessments were carried out to determine animal exposure to the drug. AUC data demonstrated that the exposure of mice given 40 mg/kg of loratadine was 3.6 (loratadine) and 18 (descarboethoxyloratadine) times higher than in humans given the maximum recommended daily oral dose. Exposure of rats given 25 mg/kg of loratadine was 28 (loratadine) and 67 (descarboethoxyloratadine) times higher than in humans given the maximum recommended daily oral dose. Male mice given 40 mg/kg had a significantly higher incidence of

Effects on Plasma Concentrations (AUC 0–24 hrs) of Loratadine and Descarboethoxyloratadine
After 10 Days of Coadministration (Loratadine 10 mg) in Normal Volunteers

	Loratadine	Descarboethoxyloratadine
Erythromycin (500 mg Q8h)	+ 40%	+46%
Cimetidine (300 mg QID)	+103%	+ 6%
Ketoconazole (200 mg Q12h)	+307%	+73%

hepatocellular tumors (combined adenomas and carcinomas) than concurrent controls. In rats, a significantly higher incidence of hepatocellular tumors (combined adenomas and carcinomas) was observed in males given 10 mg/kg and males and females given 25 mg/kg. The clinical significance of these findings during long-term use of CLARITIN is not known.

In mutagenicity studies, there was no evidence of mutagenic potential in reverse (Ames) or forward point mutation (CHO-HGPRT) assays, or in the assay for DNA damage (rat primary hepatocyte unscheduled DNA assay) or in two assays for chromosomal aberrations (human peripheral blood lymphocyte clastogenesis assay and the mouse bone marrow erythrocyte micronucleus assay). In the mouse lymphoma assay, a positive finding occurred in the nonactivated but not the activated phase of the study.

Decreased fertility in male rats, shown by lower female conception rates, occurred at an oral dose of 64 mg/kg (approximately 50 times the maximum recommended human daily oral dose on a mg/m^2 basis) and was reversible with cessation of dosing. Loratadine had no effect on male or female fertility or reproduction in the rat at an oral dose of approximately 24 mg/kg (approximately 20 times the maximum recommended human daily oral dose on a mg/m^2 basis).

Pregnancy Category B: There was no evidence of animal teratogenicity in studies performed in rats and rabbits at oral doses up to 96 mg/kg (approximately 75 times and 150 times, respectively, the maximum recommended human daily oral dose on a mg/m^2 basis). There are, however, no adequate and well-controlled studies in pregnant women. Because animal reproduction studies are not always predictive of human response, CLARITIN should be used during pregnancy only if clearly needed.

Nursing Mothers: Loratadine and its metabolite, descarboethoxyloratadine, pass easily into breast milk and achieve concentrations that are equivalent to plasma levels with an AUC_{milk}/AUC_{plasma} ratio of 1.17 and 0.85 for loratadine and descarboethoxyloratadine, respectively. Following a single oral dose of 40 mg, a small amount of loratadine and descarboethoxyloratadine was excreted into the breast milk (approximately 0.03% of 40 mg over 48 hours). A decision should be made whether to discontinue nursing or to discontinue the drug, taking into account the importance of the drug to the mother. Caution should be exercised when CLARITIN is administered to a nursing woman.

Pediatric Use: The safety of CLARITIN Syrup at a daily dose of 10 mg has been demonstrated in 188 pediatric patients 6–12 years of age in placebo-controlled 2-week trials. The effectiveness of CLARITIN for the treatment of seasonal allergic rhinitis and chronic idiopathic urticaria in this pediatric age group is based on an extrapolation of the demonstrated efficacy of CLARITIN in adults in these conditions and the likelihood that the disease course, pathophysiology, and the drug's effect are substantially similar to that of the adults. The recommended dose for the pediatric population is based on cross-study comparison of the pharmacokinetics of CLARITIN in adults and pediatric subjects and on the safety profile of loratadine in both adults and pediatric patients at doses equal to or higher than the recommended doses. The safety and effectiveness of CLARITIN in pediatric patients under 6 years of age have not been established.

ADVERSE REACTIONS

CLARITIN Tablets: Approximately 90,000 patients, aged 12 and older, received CLARITIN Tablets 10 mg once daily in controlled and uncontrolled studies. Placebo-controlled clinical trials at the recommended dose of 10 mg once a day varied from 2 weeks' to 6 months' duration. The rate of premature withdrawal from these trials was approximately 2% in both the treated and placebo groups.

[See first table above]

Adverse events reported in placebo-controlled chronic idiopathic urticaria trials were similar to those reported in allergic rhinitis studies.

Adverse event rates did not appear to differ significantly based on age, sex, or race, although the number of nonwhite subjects was relatively small.

CLARITIN REDITABS (loratadine rapidly-disintegrating tablets): Approximately 500 patients received CLARITIN REDITABS (loratadine rapidly-disintegrating tablets) in controlled clinical trials of 2 weeks' duration. In these studies, adverse events were similar in type and frequency to those seen with CLARITIN Tablets and placebo.

Administration of CLARITIN REDITABS (loratadine rapidly-disintegrating tablets) did not result in an increased reporting frequency of mouth or tongue irritation.

CLARITIN Syrup: Approximately 300 pediatric patients 6 to 12 years of age received 10 mg loratadine once daily in controlled clinical trials for a period of 8–15 days. Among these, 188 children were treated with 10 mg loratadine syrup once daily in placebo-controlled trials. Adverse events in these pediatric patients were observed to occur with type and frequency similar to those seen in the adult population. The rate of premature discontinuance due to adverse events among pediatric patients receiving loratadine 10 mg daily was less than 1%.

[See second table above]

In addition to those adverse events reported above (≥ 2%), the following adverse events have been reported in at least one patient in CLARITIN clinical trials in adult and pediatric patients:

Autonomic Nervous System: Altered lacrimation, altered salivation, flushing, hypoesthesia, impotence, increased sweating, thirst.

REPORTED ADVERSE EVENTS WITH AN INCIDENCE OF MORE THAN 2% IN PLACEBO-CONTROLLED ALLERGIC RHINITIS CLINICAL TRIALS IN PATIENTS 12 YEARS OF AGE AND OLDER

PERCENT OF PATIENTS REPORTING

	LORATADINE 10 mg QD n = 1926	PLACEBO n = 2545	CLEMASTINE 1 mg BID n = 536	TERFENADINE 60 mg BID n = 684
Headache	12	11	8	8
Somnolence	8	6	22	9
Fatigue	4	3	10	2
Dry Mouth	3	2	4	3

ADVERSE EVENTS OCCURRING WITH A FREQUENCY OF ≥2% IN LORATADINE SYRUP-TREATED PATIENTS (6–12 YEARS OLD) IN PLACEBO-CONTROLLED TRIALS, AND MORE FREQUENTLY THAN IN THE PLACEBO GROUP

PERCENT OF PATIENTS REPORTING

	LORATADINE 10 mg QD n = 188	PLACEBO n = 262	CHLORPHENIRAMINE 2-4 mg BID/TID n = 170
Nervousness	4	2	2
Wheezing	4	2	5
Fatigue	3	2	5
Hyperkinesia	3	1	1
Abdominal Pain	2	0	0
Conjunctivitis	2	<1	1
Dysphonia	2	<1	0
Malaise	2	0	1
Upper Respiratory Tract Infection	2	<1	0

Body As A Whole: Angioneurotic edema, asthenia, back pain, blurred vision, chest pain, earache, eye pain, fever, leg cramps, malaise, rigors, tinnitus, viral infection, weight gain.

Cardiovascular System: Hypertension, hypotension, palpitations, supraventricular tachyarrhythmias, syncope, tachycardia.

Central and Peripheral Nervous System: Blepharospasm, dizziness, dysphonia, hypertonia, migraine, paresthesia, tremor, vertigo.

Gastrointestinal System: Altered taste, anorexia, constipation, diarrhea, dyspepsia, flatulence, gastritis, hiccup, increased appetite, nausea, stomatitis, toothache, vomiting.

Musculoskeletal System: Arthralgia, myalgia.

Psychiatric: Agitation, amnesia, anxiety, confusion, decreased libido, depression, impaired concentration, insomnia, irritability, paroniria.

Reproductive System: Breast pain, dysmenorrhea, menorrhagia, vaginitis.

Respiratory System: Bronchitis, bronchospasm, coughing, dyspnea, epistaxis, hemoptysis, laryngitis, nasal dryness, pharyngitis, sinusitis, sneezing.

Skin and Appendages: Dermatitis, dry hair, dry skin, photosensitivity reaction, pruritus, purpura, rash, urticaria.

Urinary System: Altered micturition, urinary discoloration, urinary incontinence, urinary retention.

In addition, the following spontaneous adverse events have been reported rarely during the marketing of loratadine: abnormal hepatic function, including jaundice, hepatitis, and hepatic necrosis; alopecia; anaphylaxis; breast enlargement; erythema multiforme; peripheral edema; and seizures.

DRUG ABUSE AND DEPENDENCE

There is no information to indicate that abuse or dependency occurs with CLARITIN.

OVERDOSAGE

In adults, somnolence, tachycardia, and headache have been reported with overdoses greater than 10 mg with the Tablet formulation (40 to 180 mg). Extrapyramidal signs and palpitations have been reported in children with over doses of greater than 10 mg of CLARITIN Syrup. In the event of overdosage, general symptomatic and supportive measures should be instituted promptly and maintained for as long as necessary.

Treatment of overdosage would reasonably consist of emesis (ipecac syrup), except in patients with impaired consciousness, followed by the administration of activated charcoal to absorb any remaining drug. If vomiting is unsuccessful, or contraindicated, gastric lavage should be performed with normal saline. Saline cathartics may also be of value for rapid dilution of bowel contents. Loratadine is not eliminated by hemodialysis. It is not known if loratadine is eliminated by peritoneal dialysis.

No deaths occurred at oral doses up to 5000 mg/kg in rats and mice (greater than 2400 and 1200 times, respectively, the maximum recommended human daily oral dose on a mg/m^2 basis). Single oral doses of loratadine showed no effects in rats, mice, and monkeys at doses as high as 10 times the maximum recommended human daily oral dose on a mg/m^2 basis.

DOSAGE AND ADMINISTRATION

Adults and children 12 years of age and over: The recommended dose of CLARITIN is 10 mg once daily.

Children 6–11 years of age: The recommended dose of CLARITIN is 10 mg (2 teaspoonfuls) once daily.

In patients with liver failure or renal insufficiency (GFR < 30 mL/min), one tablet or two teaspoonfuls every other day should be the starting dose.

Administration of CLARITIN REDITABS (loratadine rapidly-disintegrating tablets): Place CLARITIN REDITABS (loratadine rapidly-disintegrating tablets) on the tongue. Tablet disintegration occurs rapidly. Administer with or without water.

HOW SUPPLIED

CLARITIN Tablets: 10 mg, white to off-white compressed tablets; impressed with the product identification number "458" on one side and "CLARITIN 10" on the other; high-density polyethylene plastic bottles of 100 (NDC 0085-0458-03) and 500 (NDC 0085-0458-06). Also available, CLARITIN Unit-of-Use packages of 14 tablets (7 tablets per blister card) (NDC 0085-0458-01) and 30 tablets (10 tablets per blister card) (NDC 0085-0458-05); and 10 × 10 tablet Unit Dose-Hospital Pack (NDC 0085-0458-04).

Protect Unit-of-Use packaging and Unit Dose-Hospital Pack from excessive moisture.

Store between 2° and 30°C (36° and 86°F).

CLARITIN Syrup: Clear, colorless to light-yellow liquid, containing 1 mg loratadine per mL; amber glass bottles of 16 fluid ounces (NDC 0085-1223-01).

Store between 2° and 25°C (36° and 77°F).

CLARITIN REDITABS (loratadine rapidly-disintegrating tablets): CLARITIN REDITABS (loratadine rapidly-disintegrating tablets), 10 mg, white to off-white blister-formed tablet; Unit-of-Use polyvinyl chloride blister packages of 30 tablets (3 laminated foil pouches, each containing one blister card of 10 tablets) supplied with Patient's Instructions for Use (NDC 0085-1128-02).

Keep CLARITIN REDITABS (loratadine rapidly-disintegrating tablets) in a dry place.

Store between 2° and 25°C (36° and 77°F). Use within 6 months of opening laminated foil pouch, and immediately upon opening individual tablet blister.

Schering Corporation
Kenilworth, NJ 07033 USA
Rev. 1/99 19649830
19628434T

CLARITIN REDITABS (loratadine rapidly-disintegrating tablets) are manufactured for Schering Corporation by Scherer DDS, England.

U.S. Patent Nos. 4,282,233 and 4,371,516.

Shown in Product Identification Guide, page 334

CLARITIN-D® 12 HOUR ℞

brand of loratadine and pseudoephedrine sulfate, USP Extended Release Tablets

CAUTION: Federal Law Prohibits Dispensing Without Prescription

DESCRIPTION

CLARITIN-D 12 HOUR Extended Release Tablets contain 5 mg loratadine in the tablet coating for immediate release and 120 mg pseudoephedrine sulfate, USP equally distributed between the tablet coating for immediate release and the barrier-coated extended release core.

Continued on next page

Information on Schering products appearing on these pages is effective as of January 2000.

Claritin-D 12 hr.—Cont.

Loratadine is a white to off-white powder, not soluble in water, but very soluble in acetone, alcohol, and chloroform. Loratadine has a molecular weight of 382.89 and empirical formula of $C_{22}H_{23}ClN_2O_2$; the chemical name, ethyl 4-(8-chloro-5,6-dihydro-11*H*-benzo[5,6]cyclohepta [1,2-*b*]pyridin-11-ylidene)-1-piperidinecarboxylate; and has the following chemical structure:

O OC₂H₅ N N Cl

Pseudoephedrine sulfate is the synthetic salt of one of the naturally occurring dextrorotatory diastereomers of ephedrine and is classified as an indirect sympathomimetic amine. The empirical formula for pseudoephedrine sulfate is $(C_{10}H_{15}NO)_2 \bullet H_2SO_4$; the chemical name is [S-(R*,R*)]-a-[1(methylamino)ethyl] benzenemethanol sulfate (2:1) (salt), and the following chemical structure:

$$\left[C_6H_5-\underset{OH}{\overset{H}{C}}-\underset{H}{\overset{NHCH_3}{C}}-CH_3 \right]_2 \bullet H_2SO_4$$

The molecular weight of pseudoephedrine sulfate is 428.54. It is a white powder, freely soluble in water and methanol and sparingly soluble in chloroform.

The inactive ingredients for CLARITIN-D 12 HOUR Extended Release Tablets are acacia, butylparaben, calcium sulfate, carnauba wax, corn starch, lactose, magnesium stearate, microcrystalline cellulose, neutral soap, oleic acid, povidone, rosin, sugar, talc, titanium dioxide, white wax, and zein.

CLINICAL PHARMACOLOGY

The following information is based upon studies of loratadine alone or pseudoephedrine alone, except as indicated.

Loratadine is a long-acting tricyclic antihistamine with selective peripheral histamine H_1-receptor antagonistic activity.

Human histamine skin wheal studies following single and repeated oral doses of loratadine have shown that the drug exhibits an antihistaminic effect beginning within 1 to 3 hours, reaching a maximum at 8 to 12 hours, and lasting in excess of 24 hours. There was no evidence of tolerance to this effect developing after 28 days of dosing with loratadine.

Pharmacokinetic studies following single and multiple oral doses of loratadine in 115 volunteers showed that loratadine is rapidly absorbed and extensively metabolized to an active metabolite (descarboethoxyloratadine). Approximately 80% of the total dose administered can be found equally distributed between urine and feces in the form of metabolic products after 10 days. The mean elimination half-lives found in studies in normal adult subjects (n = 54) were 8.4 hours (range = 3 to 20 hours) for loratadine and 28 hours (range = 8.8 to 92 hours) for the major active metabolite (descarboethoxyloratadine). In nearly all patients, exposure (AUC) to the metabolite is greater than exposure to parent loratadine. Loratadine and descarboethoxyloratadine reached steady-state in most patients by approximately the fifth dosing day. The pharmacokinetics of loratadine and descarboethoxyloratadine are dose independent over the dose range of 10 to 40 mg and are not significantly altered by the duration of treatment.

In vitro studies with human liver microsomes indicate that loratadine is metabolized to descarboethoxyloratadine predominantly by P450 CYP3A4 and, to a lesser extent, by P450 CYP2D6. In the presence of a CYP3A4 inhibitor ketoconazole, loratadine is metabolized to descarboethoxyloratadine predominantly by CYP2D6. Concurrent administration of loratadine with either ketoconazole, erythromycin (both CYP3A4 inhibitors), or cimetidine (CYP2D6 and CYP3A4 inhibitor) to healthy volunteers was associated with significantly increased plasma concentrations of loratadine (see **Drug Interactions** section).

In a study involving twelve healthy geriatric subjects (66 to 78 years old), the AUC and peak plasma levels (C_{max}) of both loratadine and descarboethoxyloratadine were significantly higher (approximately 50% increased) than in studies of younger subjects. The mean elimination half-lives for the elderly subjects were 18.2 hours (range = 6.7 to 37 hours) for loratadine and 17.5 hours (range = 11 to 38 hours) for the active metabolite.

In the clinical efficacy studies, loratadine was administered before meals. In a single-dose study, food increased the AUC of loratadine by approximately 40% and of descarboethoxyloratadine by approximately 15%. The time of peak plasma concentration (T_{max}) of loratadine and descarboethoxyloratadine was delayed by 1 hour with a meal.

In patients with chronic renal impairment (creatinine clearance ≤ 30 mL/min) both the AUC and peak plasma levels (C_{max}) increased on average by approximately 73% for loratadine; and approximately by 120% for descarboethoxyloratadine, compared to individuals with normal renal function. The mean elimination half-lives of loratadine (7.6 hours) and descarboethoxyloratadine (23.9 hours) were not significantly different from that observed in normal subjects. Hemodialysis does not have an effect on the pharmacokinetics of loratadine or its active metabolite (descarboethoxyloratadine) in subjects with chronic renal impairment.

In patients with chronic alcoholic liver disease the AUC and peak plasma levels (C_{max}) of loratadine were double while the pharmacokinetic profile of the active metabolite (descarboethoxyloratadine) was not significantly changed from that in normals. The elimination half-lives for loratadine and descarboethoxyloratadine were 24 hours and 37 hours, respectively, and increased with increasing severity of liver disease.

There was considerable variability in the pharmacokinetic data in all studies of loratadine, probably due to the extensive first-pass metabolism. Individual histograms of area under the curve, clearance, and volume of distribution showed a log normal distribution with a 25-fold range in distribution in healthy subjects.

Loratadine is about 97% bound to plasma proteins at the expected concentrations (2.5 to 100 ng/mL) after a therapeutic dose. Loratadine does not affect the plasma protein binding of warfarin and digoxin. The metabolite descarboethoxyloratadine is 73% to 77% bound to plasma proteins (at 0.5 to 100 ng/mL).

Whole body autoradiographic studies in rats and monkeys, radiolabeled tissue distribution studies in mice and rats, and *in vivo* radioligand studies in mice have shown that neither loratadine nor its metabolites readily cross the blood-brain barrier. Radioligand binding studies with guinea pig pulmonary and brain H_1-receptors indicate that there was preferential binding to peripheral versus central nervous system H_1-receptors.

In a study in which loratadine alone was administered at four times the clinical dose for 90 days, no clinically significant increase in the QT_c was seen on ECGs.

In a single-rising dose study of loratadine alone in which doses up to 160 mg (16 times the clinical dose) were administered, no clinically significant changes on the QT_c interval in the ECGs were observed.

Pseudoephedrine sulfate (d-isoephedrine sulfate) is an orally active sympathomimetic amine which exerts a decongestant action on the nasal mucosa. It is recognized as an effective agent for the relief of nasal congestion due to allergic rhinitis. Pseudoephedrine produces peripheral effects similar to those of ephedrine and central effects similar to, but less intense than, amphetamines. It has the potential for excitatory side effects.

The pseudoephedrine component of CLARITIN-D 12 HOUR Extended Release Tablets was absorbed at a similar rate and was equally available from the combination tablet as from a pseudoephedrine sulfate repetabs 120 mg tablet. Mean (%CV) steady-state peak plasma concentration of 464 ng/mL (22) was attained at 3.9 hours (50). The terminal half-life of pseudoephedrine from the combination tablet administered twice daily was 6.3 hours (23). The ingestion of food was found not to affect the absorption of pseudoephedrine from CLARITIN-D 12 HOUR Extended Release Tablets. Loratadine and pseudoephedrine sulfate do not influence the pharmacokinetics of each other when administered concomitantly.

CLINICAL STUDIES

Clinical trials of Claritin-D 12 HOUR Extended Release Tablets in seasonal allergic rhinitis involved approximately 3700 patients who received either the combination product, a comparative treatment, or placebo, in double-blind, randomized controlled studies. Four of the largest studies involved approximately 1600 patients in comparisons of the combination product, loratadine (5 mg bid), pseudoephedrine sulfate (120 mg bid), and placebo. Improvement in symptoms of seasonal allergic rhinitis for patients receiving CLARITIN-D 12 HOUR Extended Release Tablets was significantly greater than the improvement in those patients who received the individual components or placebo. The combination reduced the intensity of sneezing, rhinorrhea, nasal pruritus, and eye tearing more than pseudoephedrine and reduced the intensity of nasal congestion more than loratadine, demonstrating a contribution of each of the components. The onset of antihistamine and nasal decongestant actions occurred after the first dose of CLARITIN-D 12 HOUR Extended Release Tablets. CLARITIN-D 12 HOUR Extended Release Tablets were well tolerated, with a frequency of sedation similar to that seen with placebo, and an adverse event profile clinically similar to that of pseudoephedrine.

In a 6-week, placebo-controlled study of 193 patients with seasonal allergic rhinitis and concomitant mild to moderate asthma, CLARITIN-D 12 HOUR Extended Release Tablets twice daily improved seasonal allergic rhinitis signs and symptoms with no decrease in pulmonary function or adverse effect on asthma symptoms. This supports the safety of administering CLARITIN-D 12 Hour Extended Release Tablets to seasonal allergic rhinitis patients with asthma.

INDICATIONS AND USAGE

CLARITIN-D 12 HOUR Extended Release Tablets are indicated for the relief of symptoms of seasonal allergic rhinitis. CLARITIN-D 12 HOUR Extended Release Tablets should be administered when both the antihistaminic properties of CLARITIN (loratadine) and the nasal decongestant activity of pseudoephedrine are desired (see **CLINICAL PHARMACOLOGY**).

CONTRAINDICATIONS

CLARITIN-D 12 HOUR Extended Release Tablets are contraindicated in patients who are hypersensitive to this medication or to any of its ingredients.

This product, due to its pseudoephedrine component, is contraindicated in patients with narrow-angle glaucoma or urinary retention, and in patients receiving monoamine oxidase (MAO) inhibitor therapy or within fourteen (14) days of stopping such treatment (see **Drug Interactions** section). It is also contraindicated in patients with severe hypertension, severe coronary artery disease, and in those who have shown hypersensitivity or idiosyncrasy to its components, to adrenergic agents, or to other drugs of similar chemical structures. Manifestations of patient idiosyncrasy to adrenergic agents include: insomnia, dizziness, weakness, tremor, or arrhythmias.

WARNINGS

CLARITIN-D 12 HOUR Extended Release Tablets should be used with caution in patients with hypertension, diabetes mellitus, ischemic heart disease, increased intraocular pressure, hyperthyroidism, renal impairment, or prostatic hypertrophy. Central nervous system stimulation with convulsions or cardiovascular collapse with accompanying hypotension may be produced by sympathomimetic amines.

Use in Patients Approximately 60 Years and Older: The safety and efficacy of CLARITIN-D 12 HOUR Extended Release Tablets in patients greater than 60 years old have not been investigated in placebo-controlled clinical trials. The elderly are more likely to have adverse reactions to sympathomimetic amines.

PRECAUTIONS

General: Because the doses of this fixed combination product cannot be individually titrated and hepatic insufficiency results in a reduced clearance of loratadine to a much greater extent than pseudoephedrine, CLARITIN-D 12 HOUR Extended Release Tablets should generally be avoided in patients with hepatic insufficiency. Patients with renal insufficiency (GFR < 30 mL/min) should be given a lower initial dose (one tablet per day) because they have reduced clearance of loratadine and pseudoephedrine.

Information for Patients: Patients taking CLARITIN-D 12 HOUR Extended Release Tablets should receive the following information: CLARITIN-D 12 HOUR Extended Release Tablets are prescribed for the relief of symptoms of seasonal allergic rhinitis. Patients should be instructed to take CLARITIN-D 12 HOUR Extended Release Tablets only as prescribed and not to exceed the prescribed dose. Patients should also be advised against the concurrent use of CLARITIN-D 12 HOUR Extended Release Tablets with over-the-counter antihistamines and decongestants.

This product should not be used by patients who are hypersensitive to it or to any of its ingredients. Due to its pseudoephedrine component, this product should not be used by patients with narrow-angle glaucoma, urinary retention, or by patients receiving a monoamine oxidase (MAO) inhibitor or within 14 days of stopping use of an MAO inhibitor. It also should not be used by patients with severe hypertension or severe coronary artery disease.

Patients who are or may become pregnant should be told that this product should be used in pregnancy or during lactation only if the potential benefit justifies the potential risk to the fetus or nursing infant.

Patients should be instructed not to break or chew the tablet.

Drug Interactions: No specific interaction studies have been conducted with CLARITIN-D 12 HOUR Extended Release Tablets. However, loratadine (10 mg once daily) has been safely coadministered with therapeutic doses of erythromycin, cimetidine, and ketoconazole in controlled clinical pharmacology studies. Although increased plasma concentrations (AUC 0–24 hrs) of loratadine and/or descarboethoxyloratadine were observed following coadministration of loratadine with each of these drugs in normal volunteers (n = 24 in each study), there were no clinically relevant changes in the safety profile of loratadine, as assessed by electrocardiographic parameters, clinical laboratory tests, vital signs, and adverse events. There were no significant effects on QT_c intervals, and no reports of sedation or syncope. No effects on plasma concentrations of cimetidine or ketoconazole were observed. Plasma concentrations (AUC 0–24 hrs) of erythromycin decreased 15% with coadministration of loratadine relative to that observed with erythromycin alone. The clinical relevance of this difference is unknown. These above findings are summarized in the following table:

Effects on Plasma Concentrations (AUC 0-24 hrs) of Loratadine and Descarboethoxyloratadine After 10 Days of Coadministration (Loratadine 10 mg) in Normal Volunteers

	Loratadine	Descarboethoxyloratadine
Erythromycin (500 mg Q8h)	+ 40%	+46%
Cimetidine (300 mg QID)	+103%	+ 6%
Ketoconazole (200 mg Q12h)	+307%	+73%

There does not appear to be an increase in adverse events in subjects who received oral contraceptives and loratadine.

CLARITIN-D 12 HOUR Extended Release Tablets (pseudoephedrine component) are contraindicated in patients taking monoamine oxidase inhibitors and for 2 weeks after stopping use of an MAO inhibitor. The antihypertensive effects of beta-adrenergic blocking agents, methyldopa, mecamylamine, reserpine, and veratrum alkaloids may be reduced by sympathomimetics. Increased ectopic pacemaker activity can occur when pseudoephedrine is used concomitantly with digitalis.

Drug/Laboratory Test Interactions: The *in vitro* addition of pseudoephedrine to sera containing the cardiac isoenzyme MB of serum creatinine phosphokinase progressively inhibits the activity of the enzyme. The inhibition becomes complete over 6 hours.

Carcinogenesis, Mutagenesis, Impairment of Fertility: There are no animal or laboratory studies on the combination product loratadine and pseudoephedrine sulfate to evaluate carcinogenesis, mutagenesis, or impairment of fertility.

In an 18-month oncogenicity study in mice and a 2-year study in rats loratadine was administered in the diet at doses up to 40 mg/kg (mice) and 25 mg/kg (rats). In the carcinogenicity studies pharmacokinetic assessments were carried out to determine animal exposure to the drug. AUC data demonstrated that the exposure of mice given 40 mg/kg of loratadine was 3.6 (loratadine) and 18 (active metabolite) times higher than a human given 10 mg/day. Exposure of rats given 25 mg/kg of loratadine was 28 (loratadine) and 67 (active metabolite) times higher than a human given 10 mg/day. Male mice given 40 mg/kg had a significantly higher incidence of hepatocellular tumors (combined adenomas and carcinomas) than concurrent controls. In rats, a significantly higher incidence of hepatocellular tumors (combined adenomas and carcinomas) was observed in males given 10 mg/kg and males and females given 25 mg/kg. The clinical significance of these findings during long-term use of loratadine is not known.

In mutagenicity studies with loratadine alone, there was no evidence of mutagenic potential in reverse (Ames) or forward point mutation (CHO-HGPRT) assays, or in the assay for DNA damage (Rat Primary Hepatocyte Unscheduled DNA Assay) or in two assays for chromosomal aberrations (Human Peripheral Blood Lymphocyte Clastogenesis Assay and the Mouse Bone Marrow Erythrocyte Micronucleus Assay). In the Mouse Lymphoma Assay, a positive finding occurred in the nonactivated but not the activated phase of the study.

Loratadine administration produced hepatic microsomal enzyme induction in the mouse at 40 mg/kg and rat at 25 mg/kg, but not at lower doses.

Decreased fertility in male rats, shown by lower female conception rates, occurred at approximately 64 mg/kg of loratadine and was reversible with cessation of dosing. Loratadine had no effect on male or female fertility or reproduction in the rat at doses approximately 24 mg/kg.

Pregnancy Category B: There was no evidence of animal teratogenicity in reproduction studies performed on rats and rabbits with this combination at oral doses up to 150 mg/kg (885 mg/m^2 or 5 times the recommended daily human dosage of 250 mg or 185 mg/m^2), and 120 mg/kg (1416 mg/m^2 or 8 times the recommended daily human dosage), respectively. There are, however, no adequate and well-controlled studies in pregnant women. Because animal reproduction studies are not always predictive of human response, CLARITIN-D 12 HOUR Extended Release Tablets should be used during pregnancy only if clearly needed.

Nursing Mothers: It is not known if this combination product is excreted in human milk. However, loratadine when administered alone and its metabolite descarboethoxyloratadine pass easily into breast milk and achieve concentrations that are equivalent to plasma levels, with an AUC_{milk}/AUC_{plasma} ratio of 1.17 and 0.85 for the parent and active metabolite, respectively. Following a single oral dose of 40 mg, a small amount of loratadine and metabolite was excreted into the breast milk (approximately 0.03% of 40 mg after 48 hours). Pseudoephedrine administered alone also distributes into breast milk of the lactating human female. Pseudoephedrine concentrations in milk are consistently higher than those in plasma. The total amount of drug in milk as judged by the area under the curve (AUC) is 2 to 3 times greater than in plasma. The fraction of a pseudoephedrine dose excreted in milk is estimated to be 0.4% to 0.7%. A decision should be made whether to discontinue nursing or to discontinue the drug, taking into account the importance of the drug to the mother. Caution should be exercised when CLARITIN-D 12 HOUR Extended Release Tablets are administered to a nursing woman.

Pediatric Use: Safety and effectiveness in children below the age of 12 years have not been established.

ADVERSE REACTIONS

Experience from controlled and uncontrolled clinical studies involving approximately 10,000 patients who received the combination of loratadine and pseudoephedrine sulfate for a period of up to 1 month provides information on adverse reactions. The usual dose was one tablet every 12 hours for up to 28 days.

In controlled clinical trials using the recommended dose of one tablet every 12 hours, the incidence of reported adverse events was similar to those reported with placebo, with the exception of insomnia (16%) and dry mouth (14%).

[See table above]

Adverse event rates did not appear to differ significantly based on age, sex, or race, although the number of non-white subjects was relatively small.

In addition to those adverse events reported above (≥2%), the following less frequent adverse events have been reported in at least one patient treated with CLARITIN-D 12 HOUR Extended Release Tablets:

REPORTED ADVERSE EVENTS WITH AN INCIDENCE OF ≥2% ON CLARITIN-D 12 HOUR EXTENDED RELEASE TABLETS IN PLACEBO-CONTROLLED CLINICAL TRIALS PERCENT OF PATIENTS REPORTING

	CLARITIN-D® 12 HOUR n=1023	Loratadine n=543	Pseudo-ephedrine n=548	Placebo n=922
Headache	19	18	17	19
Insomnia	16	4	19	3
Dry Mouth	14	4	9	3
Somnolence	7	8	5	4
Nervousness	5	3	7	2
Dizziness	4	1	5	2
Fatigue	4	6	3	3
Dyspepsia	3	2	3	1
Nausea	3	2	3	2
Pharyngitis	3	3	2	3
Anorexia	2	1	2	1
Thirst	2	1	2	1

Autonomic Nervous System: Abnormal lacrimation, dehydration, flushing, hypoesthesia, increased sweating, mydriasis.

Body As A Whole: Asthenia, back pain, blurred vision, chest pain, conjunctivitis, earache, ear infection, eye pain, fever, flu-like symptoms, leg cramps, lymphadenopathy, malaise, photophobia, rigors, tinnitus, viral infection, weight gain.

Cardiovascular System: Hypertension, hypotension, palpitations, peripheral edema, syncope, tachycardia, ventricular extrasystoles.

Central and Peripheral Nervous System: Dysphonia, hyperkinesia, hypertonia, migraine, paresthesia, tremors, vertigo.

Gastrointestinal System: Abdominal distension, abdominal distress, abdominal pain, altered taste, constipation, diarrhea, eructation, flatulence, gastritis, gingival bleeding, hemorrhoids, increased appetite, stomatitis, taste loss, tongue discoloration, toothache, vomiting.

Liver and Biliary System: Hepatic function abnormal.

Musculoskeletal System: Arthralgia, myalgia, torticollis.

Psychiatric: Aggressive reaction, agitation, anxiety, apathy, confusion, decreased libido, depression, emotional lability, euphoria, impaired concentration, irritability, paroniria.

Reproductive System: Dysmenorrhea, impotence, intermenstrual bleeding, vaginitis.

Respiratory System: Bronchitis, bronchospasm, chest congestion, coughing, dry throat, dyspnea, epistaxis, halitosis, nasal congestion, nasal irritation, sinusitis, sneezing, sputum increased, upper respiratory infection, wheezing.

Skin and Appendages: Acne, bacterial skin infection, dry skin, eczema, edema, epidermal necrolysis, erythema, hematoma, pruritus, rash, urticaria.

Urinary System: Dysuria, micturition frequency, nocturia, polyuria, urinary retention.

The following additional adverse events have been reported with the use of CLARITIN Tablets: alopecia, altered salivation, amnesia, anaphylaxis, angioneurotic edema, blepharospasm, breast enlargement, breast pain, dermatitis, dry hair, erythema multiforme, hemoptysis, hepatic necrosis, hepatitis, jaundice, laryngitis, menorrhagia, nasal dryness, photosensitivity reaction, purpura, seizures, supraventricular tachyarrhythmias, and urinary discoloration.

Pseudoephedrine may cause mild CNS stimulation in hypersensitive patients. Nervousness, excitability, restlessness, dizziness, weakness, or insomnia may occur. Headache, drowsiness, tachycardia, palpitation, pressor activity, and cardiac arrhythmias have been reported. Sympathomimetic drugs have also been associated with other untoward effects, such as fear, anxiety, tenseness, tremor, hallucinations, seizures, pallor, respiratory difficulty, dysuria, and cardiovascular collapse.

DRUG ABUSE AND DEPENDENCE

There is no information to indicate that abuse or dependency occurs with loratadine or the combination of loratadine and pseudoephedrine. Pseudoephedrine, like other central nervous system stimulants, has been abused. At high doses, subjects commonly experience an elevation of mood, a sense of increased energy and alertness, and decreased appetite. Some individuals become anxious, irritable, and loquacious. In addition to the marked euphoria, the user experiences a sense of markedly enhanced physical strength and mental capacity. With continued use, tolerance develops, the user increases the dose, and toxic signs and symptoms appear. Depression may follow rapid withdrawal.

OVERDOSAGE

In the event of overdosage, general symptomatic and supportive measures should be instituted promptly and maintained for as long as necessary. Treatment of overdosage would reasonably consist of emesis (ipecac syrup), except in patients with impaired consciousness, followed by the administration of activated charcoal to absorb any remaining drug. If vomiting is unsuccessful, or contraindicated, gastric lavage should be performed with normal saline. Saline cathartics may also be of value for rapid dilution of bowel contents. Loratadine is not eliminated by hemodialysis. It is not known if loratadine is eliminated by peritoneal dialysis. Somnolence, tachycardia, and headache have been reported with doses of 40 to 180 mg of CLARITIN Tablets. In large doses, sympathomimetics may give rise to giddiness, headache, nausea, vomiting, sweating, thirst, tachycardia, precordial pain, palpitations, difficulty in micturition, muscular weakness and tenseness, anxiety, restlessness, and insomnia. Many patients can present a toxic psychosis with delusions and hallucinations. Some may develop cardiac arrhythmias, circulatory collapse, convulsions, coma, and respiratory failure.

The oral LD_{50} values for the mixture of the two drugs were greater than 525 and 1839 mg/kg in mice and rats, respectively. Oral LD_{50} values for loratadine were greater than 5000 mg/kg in rats and mice. Doses of loratadine as high as 10 times the recommended daily clinical dose showed no effect in rats, mice, and monkeys.

DOSAGE AND ADMINISTRATION

Adults and children 12 years of age and over: one tablet twice a day (every 12 hours). Because the doses of this fixed combination product cannot be individually titrated and hepatic insufficiency results in a reduced clearance of loratadine to a much greater extent than pseudoephedrine, CLARITIN-D 12 HOUR Extended Release Tablets should generally be avoided in patients with hepatic insufficiency. Patients with renal insufficiency (GFR < 30 mL/min) should be given a lower initial dose (one tablet per day) because they have reduced clearance of loratadine and pseudoephedrine.

HOW SUPPLIED

CLARITIN-D 12 HOUR Extended Release Tablets contain 5 mg loratadine and 120 mg pseudoephedrine sulfate. CLARITIN-D 12 HOUR Extended Release Tablets are white tablets branded in green with "CLARITIN-D", which are supplied in high-density polyethylene bottles of 100 (NDC 0085-0635-01). Also available are CLARITIN-D 12 HOUR Extended Release Tablets Unit-of-Use packages of 30 tablets (3 packs of 10 tablets each) (NDC 0085-0635-05); and 10 x 10 tablets Unit Dose-Hospital Pack (NDC 0085-0635-04).

Keep Unit-of-Use packaging and Unit Dose-Hospital Pack in a dry place.

Store between 2° and 25°C (36° and 77°F).

Schering Corporation
Kenilworth, NJ 07033 USA

Rev. 5/98 17798669

17762664T

Shown in Product Identification Guide, page 334

CLARITIN-D® 24 HOUR ℞

brand of loratadine and pseudoephedrine sulfate, USP Extended Release Tablets

DESCRIPTION

CLARITIN-D® 24 HOUR (loratadine and pseudoephedrine sulfate, USP) Extended Release Tablets contain 10 mg loratadine in the tablet coating for immediate release and 240 mg pseudoephedrine sulfate, USP in the tablet core which is released slowly allowing for once-daily administration.

Loratadine is a long-acting antihistamine having the empirical formula $C_{22}H_{23}ClN_2O_2$; the chemical name ethyl 4-(8-chloro-5,6-dihydro-11*H*-benzo[5,6]cyclohepta[1,2-*b*]pyridin-11-ylidene)-1-piperidinecarboxylate; and the following chemical structure:

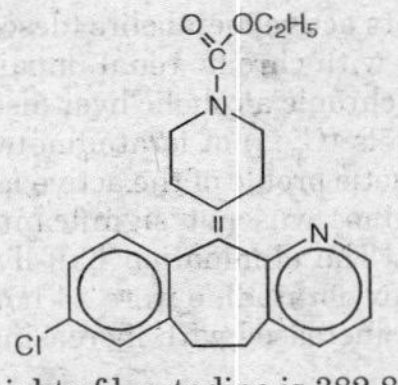

The molecular weight of loratadine is 382.89. It is a white to off-white powder, not soluble in water, but very soluble in acetone, alcohol, and chloroform.

Continued on next page

Information on Schering products appearing on these pages is effective as of January 2000.

Claritin-D 24 hr.—Cont.

Pseudoephedrine sulfate is the synthetic salt of one of the naturally occurring dextrorotatory diastereomers of ephedrine and is classified as an indirect sympathomimetic amine. The empirical formula for pseudoephedrine sulfate is $(C_{10}H_{15}NO)_2 \bullet H_2SO_4$; the chemical name is α-[1-(methylamino) ethyl]-[*S*-(*R**, *R**)]-benzenemethanol sulfate (2:1)(salt); and the chemical structure is:

$$\left[C_6H_5-\underset{OH}{\overset{H}{C}}-\underset{H}{\overset{NHCH_3}{C}}-CH_3 \right]_2 \bullet H_2SO_4$$

The molecular weight of pseudoephedrine sulfate is 428.54. It is a white powder, freely soluble in water and methanol and sparingly soluble in chloroform.

The inactive ingredients for oval, biconvex CLARITIN-D 24 HOUR Extended Release Tablets are calcium phosphate, carnauba wax, ethylcellulose, hydroxypropyl methylcellulose, magnesium stearate, polyethylene glycol, povidone, silicon dioxide, sugar, titanium dioxide, and white wax.

CLINICAL PHARMACOLOGY

The following information is based upon studies of loratadine alone or pseudoephedrine alone, except as indicated.

Loratadine is a long-acting tricyclic antihistamine with selective peripheral histamine H_1-receptor antagonistic activity.

Human histamine skin wheal studies following single and repeated oral doses of loratadine have shown that the drug exhibits an antihistaminic effect beginning within 1 to 3 hours, reaching a maximum at 8 to 12 hours, and lasting in excess of 24 hours. There was no evidence of tolerance to this effect developing after 28 days of dosing with loratadine.

Pharmacokinetic studies following single and multiple oral doses of loratadine in 115 volunteers showed that loratadine is rapidly absorbed and extensively metabolized to an active metabolite (descarboethoxyloratadine). Approximately 80% of the total dose administered can be found equally distributed between urine and feces in the form of metabolic products after 10 days. The mean elimination half-lives found in studies in normal adult subjects (n = 54) were 8.4 hours (range = 3 to 20 hours) for loratadine and 28 hours (range = 8.8 to 92 hours) for the major active metabolite (descarboethoxyloratadine). In nearly all patients, exposure (AUC) to the metabolite is greater than exposure to parent loratadine. Loratadine and descarboethoxyloratadine reached steady state in most patients by approximately the fifth dosing day. The pharmacokinetics of loratadine and descarboethoxyloratadine are dose independent over the dose range of 10 to 40 mg and are not significantly altered by the duration of treatment.

In vitro studies with human liver microsomes indicate that loratadine is metabolized to descarboethoxyloratadine predominantly by P450 CYP3A4 and, to a lesser extent, by P450 CYP2D6. In the presence of a CYP3A4 inhibitor ketoconazole, loratadine is metabolized to descarboethoxyloratadine predominantly by CYP2D6. Concurrent administration of loratadine with either ketoconazole, erythromycin (both CYP3A4 inhibitors), or cimetidine (CYP2D6 and CYP3A4 inhibitor) to healthy volunteers was associated with significantly increased plasma concentrations of loratadine (see **Drug Interactions** section).

In a study involving 12 healthy geriatric subjects (66 to 78 years old), the AUC and peak plasma levels (C_{max}) of both loratadine and descarboethoxyloratadine were significantly higher (approximately 50% increased) than in studies of younger subjects. The mean elimination half-lives for the elderly subjects were 18.2 hours (range = 6.7 to 37 hours) for loratadine and 17.5 hours (range = 11 to 38 hours) for the active metabolite.

In patients with chronic renal impairment (creatinine clearance ≤30 mL/min) both the AUC and peak plasma levels (C_{max}) increased on average by approximately 73% for loratadine; and approximately by 120% for descarboethoxyloratadine, compared to individuals with normal renal function. The mean elimination half-lives of loratadine (7.6 hours) and descarboethoxyloratadine (23.9 hours) were not significantly different from that observed in normal subjects. Hemodialysis does not have an effect on the pharmacokinetics of loratadine or its active metabolite (descarboethoxyloratadine) in subjects with chronic renal impairment.

In patients with chronic alcoholic liver disease the AUC and peak plasma levels (C_{max}) of loratadine were double while the pharmacokinetic profile of the active metabolite (descarboethoxyloratadine) was not significantly changed from that in normals. The elimination half-lives for loratadine and descarboethoxyloratadine were 24 hours and 37 hours, respectively, and increased with increasing severity of liver disease.

There was considerable variability in the pharmacokinetic data in all studies of loratadine, probably due to the extensive first-pass metabolism. Individual histograms of area under the curve, clearance, and volume of distribution showed a log normal distribution with a 25-fold range in distribution in healthy subjects.

Loratadine is about 97% bound to plasma proteins at the expected plasma concentrations (2.5 to 100 ng/mL) after a therapeutic dose. Loratadine does not affect the plasma protein binding of warfarin and digoxin. The metabolite descarboethoxyloratadine is 73% to 77% bound to plasma proteins (at 0.5 to 100 ng/mL).

Whole body autoradiographic studies in rats and monkeys, radio-labeled tissue distribution studies in mice and rats, and *in vivo* radioligand studies in mice have shown that neither loratadine nor its metabolites readily cross the blood-brain barrier. Radioligand binding studies with guinea pig pulmonary and brain H_1-receptors indicate that there was preferential binding to peripheral versus central nervous system H_1-receptors.

In a study in which loratadine alone was administered at four times the clinical dose for 90 days, no clinically significant increase in the QT_c was seen on ECGs.

In a single-rising dose study of loratadine alone in which doses up to 160 mg (16 times the clinical dose) were administered, no clinically significant changes on the QT_c interval in the ECGs were observed.

Pseudoephedrine sulfate (d-isoephedrine sulfate) is an orally active sympathomimetic amine which exerts a decongestant action on the nasal mucosa. It is recognized as an effective agent for the relief of nasal congestion due to allergic rhinitis. Pseudoephedrine produces peripheral effects similar to those of ephedrine and central effects similar to, but less intense than, amphetamines. It has the potential for excitatory side effects.

The bioavailability of loratadine and pseudoephedrine sulfate from CLARITIN-D 24 HOUR Extended Release Tablets is similar to that achieved with separate administration of the components. Coadministration of loratadine and pseudoephedrine does not significantly affect the bioavailability of either component.

In a single-dose study, food increased the AUC of loratadine by approximately 125% and C_{max} by approximately 80%. However, food did not significantly affect the pharmacokinetics of pseudoephedrine sulfate or descarboethoxyloratadine.

Clinical Studies: Clinical trials of CLARITIN-D 24 HOUR Extended Release Tablets involved a total of approximately 2000 patients with seasonal allergic rhinitis. One study involved 879 patients, who received either the combination product (loratadine 10 mg and pseudoephedrine sulfate 240 mg), loratadine (10 mg once daily) or pseudoephedrine sulfate (120 mg twice daily) alone, or placebo, in a double-blind randomized design. Improvement in nasal and non-nasal symptoms of seasonal allergic rhinitis including nasal congestion in patients receiving CLARITIN-D 24 HOUR Extended Release Tablets was significantly greater than in placebo recipients, and generally greater than that achieved with loratadine or pseudoephedrine sulfate alone. In this study, CLARITIN-D 24 HOUR Extended Release Tablets were well tolerated, with a frequency of sedation similar to that seen with placebo, and a frequency of nervousness and insomnia similar to that seen with pseudoephedrine sulfate given alone.

In another study of 469 patients, once-daily administration of CLARITIN-D 24 HOUR Extended Release Tablets provided effects similar to those achieved with twice-daily administration of CLARITIN-D 12 HOUR Extended Release Tablets, a combination product containing 5 mg loratadine plus 120 mg pseudoephedrine sulfate, USP, extended release.

The end of dosing interval efficacy of the pseudoephedrine component of CLARITIN-D 24 HOUR Extended Release Tablets on the symptom of nasal stuffiness was evaluated in a study of 695 patients who were randomized to receive CLARITIN-D 24 HOUR Extended Release Tablets, CLARITIN Tablets, or placebo. Patients who received CLARITIN-D 24 HOUR Extended Release Tablets had significantly more improvement in nasal stuffiness scores at the end of the dosing interval than those patients receiving CLARITIN Tablets or placebo throughout the course of the trial.

In a 6-week, placebo-controlled study of 193 patients with seasonal allergic rhinitis and concomitant mild to moderate asthma, CLARITIN-D 12 HOUR Extended Release Tablets twice daily improved seasonal allergic rhinitis signs and symptoms with no decrease in pulmonary function or adverse effect on asthma symptoms. This supports the safety of administering CLARITIN-D 24 HOUR Extended Release Tablets to seasonal allergic rhinitis patients with asthma.

INDICATIONS AND USAGE

CLARITIN-D 24 HOUR Extended Release Tablets are indicated for the relief of symptoms of seasonal allergic rhinitis. CLARITIN-D 24 HOUR Extended Release Tablets should be administered when both the antihistaminic properties of CLARITIN® (loratadine) and the nasal decongestant activity of pseudoephedrine sulfate are desired (see **CLINICAL PHARMACOLOGY** section).

CONTRAINDICATIONS

CLARITIN-D 24 HOUR Extended Release Tablets are contraindicated in patients who are hypersensitive to this medication or to any of its ingredients.

This product, due to its pseudoephedrine component, is contraindicated in patients with narrow-angle glaucoma or urinary retention, and in patients receiving monoamine oxidase (MAO) inhibitor therapy or within fourteen (14) days of stopping such treatment. (See **PRECAUTIONS: Drug Interactions** section.) It is also contraindicated in patients with severe hypertension, severe coronary artery disease, and in those who have shown hypersensitivity or idiosyncrasy to its components, to adrenergic agents, or to other drugs of similar chemical structures. Manifestations of patient idiosyncrasy to adrenergic agents include: insomnia, dizziness, weakness, tremor, or arrhythmias.

WARNINGS

CLARITIN-D 24 HOUR Extended Release Tablets should be used with caution in patients with hypertension, diabetes mellitus, ischemic heart disease, increased intraocular pressure, hyperthyroidism, renal impairment, or prostatic hypertrophy. Central nervous system stimulation with convulsions or cardiovascular collapse with accompanying hypotension may be produced by sympathomimetic amines.

Use in Patients Approximately 60 Years of Age and Older: The safety and efficacy of CLARITIN-D 24 HOUR Extended Release Tablets in patients greater than 60 years old have not been investigated in placebo-controlled clinical trials. The elderly are more likely to have adverse reactions to sympathomimetic amines.

PRECAUTIONS

General: Because there have been reports of esophageal obstruction and perforation in patients who have taken a previously marketed formulation of CLARITIN-D 24 HOUR Extended Release Tablets, it is recommended that patients who have a history of difficulty in swallowing tablets or who have known upper gastrointestinal narrowing or abnormal esophageal peristalsis not use this product. Furthermore, since it is not known whether this formulation of CLARITIN-D 24 HOUR Extended Release Tablets has the potential for this adverse event, it is reasonable to recommend that all patients take this product with a full glass of water (see **PRECAUTIONS: Information for Patients, ADVERSE REACTIONS, DOSAGE AND ADMINISTRATION**). Because the doses of this fixed combination product cannot be individually titrated and hepatic insufficiency results in a reduced clearance of loratadine to a much greater extent than pseudoephedrine, CLARITIN-D 24 HOUR Extended Release Tablets should generally be avoided in patients with hepatic insufficiency. Patients with renal insufficiency (GFR <30 mL/min) should be given a lower initial dose (one tablet every other day) because they have reduced clearance of loratadine and pseudoephedrine.

Information for Patients: Patients taking CLARITIN-D 24 HOUR Extended Release Tablets should receive the following information: CLARITIN-D 24 HOUR Extended Release Tablets are prescribed for the relief of symptoms of seasonal allergic rhinitis. Patients should be instructed to take CLARITIN-D 24 HOUR Extended Release Tablets only as prescribed and not to exceed the prescribed dose. Patients should also be advised against the concurrent use of CLARITIN-D 24 HOUR Extended Release Tablets with over-the-counter antihistamines and decongestants. Patients who have a history of difficulty in swallowing tablets or who have known upper gastrointestinal narrowing or abnormal esophageal peristalsis should not use this product. This product should not be used by patients who are hypersensitive to it or to any of its ingredients. Due to its pseudoephedrine component, this product should not be used by patients with narrow-angle glaucoma, urinary retention, or by patients receiving a monamine oxidase (MAO) inhibitor or within 14 days of stopping use of an MAO inhibitor. It also should not be used by patients with severe hypertension or severe coronary artery disease.

Patients who are or may become pregnant should be told that this product should be used in pregnancy or during lactation only if the potential benefit justifies the potential risk to the fetus or nursing infant.

Patients should be instructed not to break or chew the tablet and to take it with a full glass of water (see **PRECAUTIONS: General, ADVERSE REACTIONS, DOSAGE AND ADMINISTRATION**).

Drug Interactions: No specific interaction studies have been conducted with CLARITIN-D 24 HOUR Extended Release Tablets. However, loratadine (10 mg once daily) has been safely coadministered with therapeutic doses of erythromycin, cimetidine, and ketoconazole in controlled clinical pharmacology studies. Although increased plasma concentrations (AUC 0–24 hrs) of loratadine and/or descarboethoxyloratadine were observed following coadministration of loratadine with each of these drugs in normal volunteers (n = 24 in each study), there were no clinically relevant changes in the safety profile of loratadine, as assessed by electrocardiographic parameters, clinical laboratory tests, vital signs, and adverse events. There were no significant effects on QT_c intervals, and no reports of sedation or syncope. No effects on plasma concentrations of cimetidine or ketoconazole were observed. Plasma concentrations (AUC 0–24 hrs) of erythromycin decreased 15% with coadministration of loratadine relative to that observed with erythromycin alone. The clinical relevance of this difference is unknown. These above findings are summarized in the following table:

Effects on Plasma Concentrations (AUC 0-24 hrs) of Loratadine and Descarboethoxyloratadine After 10 Days of Coadministration (Loratadine 10 mg) in Normal Volunteers

	Loratadine	Descarboethoxy-loratadine
Erythromycin (500 mg Q8h)	+ 40%	+46%
Cimetidine (300 mg QID)	+103%	+ 6%
Ketoconazole (200 mg Q12h)	+307%	+73%

There does not appear to be an increase in adverse events in subjects who received oral contraceptives and loratadine. CLARITIN-D 24 HOUR Extended Release Tablets (pseudoephedrine component) are contraindicated in patients taking monoamine oxidase inhibitors and for 2 weeks after stopping use of an MAO inhibitor. The antihypertensive effects of beta-adrenergic blocking agents, methyldopa, mecamylamine, reserpine, and veratum alkaloids may be reduced by sympathomimetics. Increased ectopic pacemaker activity can occur when pseudoephedrine is used concomitantly with digitalis.

Drug/Laboratory Test Interactions: The *in vitro* addition of pseudoephedrine to sera containing the cardiac isoenzyme MB of serum creatinine phosphokinase progressively inhibits the activity of the enzyme. The inhibition becomes complete over 6 hours.

Carcinogenesis, Mutagenesis, Impairment of Fertility: There are no animal or laboratory studies on the combination product loratadine and pseudoephedrine sulfate to evaluate carcinogenesis, mutagenesis, or impairment of fertility.

In an 18-month carcinogenicity study in mice and a 2-year study in rats loratadine was administered in the diet at doses up to 40 mg/kg (mice) and 25 mg/kg (rats). In the carcinogenicity studies pharmacokinetic assessments were carried out to determine animal exposure to the drug. AUC data demonstrated that the exposure of mice given 40 mg/kg of loratadine was 3.6 (loratadine) and 18 (active metabolite) times higher than in humans given the maximum recommended daily oral dose. Exposure of rats given 25 mg/kg of loratadine was 28 (loratadine) and 67 (active metabolite) times higher than in humans given the maximum recommended daily oral dose. Male mice given 40 mg/kg had a significantly higher incidence of hepatocellular tumors (combined adenomas and carcinomas) than concurrent controls. In rats, a significantly higher incidence of hepatocellular tumors (combined adenomas and carcinomas) was observed in males given 10 mg/kg and in males and females given 25 mg/kg. The clinical significance of these findings during long-term use of loratadine is not known.

Two-year feeding studies in mice and rats conducted under the auspices of the National Toxicology Programs (NTP) uncovered no evidence of carcinogenic potential of ephedrine sulfate at doses up to 10 and 27 mg/kg, respectively (approximately 16% and 100% of the maximum recommended human daily oral dose of pseudoephedrine sulfate on a mg/m^2 basis).

In mutagenicity studies with loratadine alone, there was no evidence of mutagenic potential in reverse (Ames) or forward point mutation (CHO-HGPRT) assays, or in the assay for DNA damage (Rat Primary Hepatocyte Unscheduled DNA Assay) or in two assays for chromosomal aberrations (Human Peripheral Blood Lymphocyte Clastogenesis Assay and the Mouse Bone Marrow Erythrocyte Micronucleus Assay). In the Mouse Lymphoma Assay, a positive finding occurred in the nonactivated but not the activated phase of the study.

Decreased fertility in male rats, shown by lower female conception rates, occurred at 64 mg/kg of loratadine (approximately 50 times the maximum recommended human daily oral dose based on mg/m^2) and was reversible with cessation of dosing. Loratadine had no effect on male or female fertility or reproduction in the rat at 24 mg/kg (approximately 20 times the maximum recommended daily oral dose on a mg/m^2 basis).

Pregnancy Category B: The combination product loratadine and pseudoephedrine sulfate was evaluated for teratogenicity in rats and rabbits. There was no evidence of teratogenicity in reproduction studies with this combination of the same clinical ratio (1:24) at oral doses up to 150 mg/kg (approximately 5 times the maximum recommended human daily oral dose on a mg/m^2 basis) in rats, and 120 mg/kg (8 times the maximum recommended human daily oral dose on a mg/m^2 basis) in rabbits. Similarly, no evidence of animal teratogenicity in rats and rabbits was reported at oral doses up to 96 mg/kg of loratadine alone (approximately 75 and 150 times, respectively, the maximum human daily oral dose on a mg/m^2 basis). There are, however, no adequate and well-controlled studies in pregnant women. Because animal reproduction studies are not always predictive of human response, CLARITIN-D 24 HOUR Extended Release Tablets should be used during pregnancy only if clearly needed.

Nursing Mothers: It is not known if this combination product is excreted in human milk. However, loratadine when administered alone and its metabolite descarboethoxyloratadine pass easily into breast milk and achieve concentrations that are equivalent to plasma levels, with an AUC_{milk}/AUC_{plasma} ratio of 1.17 and 0.85 for the parent and active metabolite, respectively. Following a single oral dose of 40 mg, a small amount of loratadine and metabolite was excreted into the breast milk (approximately 0.03% of 40 mg over 48 hours). Pseudoephedrine administered alone also distributes into breast milk of the lactating human female. Pseudoephedrine concentrations in milk are consistently higher than those in plasma. The total amount of drug in milk as judged by the area under the curve (AUC) is 2 to 3 times greater than in plasma. The fraction of a pseudoephedrine dose excreted in milk is estimated to be 0.4% to 0.7%. A decision should be made whether to discontinue nursing or to discontinue the drug, taking into account the importance of the drug to the mother. Caution should be exercised when CLARITIN-D 24 HOUR Extended Release Tablets are administered to a nursing woman.

REPORTED ADVERSE EVENTS WITH AN INCIDENCE OF ≥2% IN CLARITIN-D 24 HOUR EXTENDED RELEASE TABLETS TREATMENT GROUP IN DOUBLE-BLIND, RANDOMIZED, PLACEBO-CONTROLLED CLINICAL TRIALS

PERCENT OF PATIENTS REPORTING

	CLARITIN-D® 24 HOUR (n = 605)	Loratadine 10 mg (n = 449)	Pseudo-ephedrine 120 mg q12h (n = 220)	Placebo (n = 605)
Dry Mouth	8	2	7	2
Somnolence	6	4	5	4
Insomnia	5	1	9	1
Pharyngitis	5	5	5	5
Dizziness	4	2	3	2
Coughing	3	2	3	1
Fatigue	3	4	1	2
Nausea	3	2	4	2
Nervousness	3	1	4	1
Anorexia	2	<1	2	0
Dysmenorrhea	2	2	2	1

Pediatric Use: Safety and effectiveness in children below the age of 12 years have not been established.

ADVERSE REACTIONS

Information on adverse reactions is provided from placebo-controlled studies involving over 2000 patients, 605 of whom received CLARITIN-D 24 HOUR Extended Release Tablets once daily for up to 2 weeks. In these studies, the incidence of adverse events reported with CLARITIN-D 24 HOUR Extended Release Tablets was similar to those reported with twice-daily (q12h) 120 mg sustained-release pseudoephedrine alone.

[See table above]

Adverse events occurring in greater than or equal to 2% of CLARITIN-D 24 HOUR Extended Release Tablets-treated patients, but that were more common in the placebo-treated group, include headache.

Adverse events did not appear to significantly differ based on age, sex, or race, although the number of non-whites was relatively small.

In addition to those adverse events reported above, the following adverse events have been reported in fewer than 2% of patients who received CLARITIN-D 24 HOUR Extended Release Tablets:

Autonomic Nervous System: Altered lacrimation, flushing, increased sweating, mydriasis, thirst.

Body As A Whole: Abnormal vision, asthenia, back pain, chest pain, conjunctivitis, earache, eye pain, facial edema, fever, flu-like symptoms, leg cramps, lymphadenopathy, malaise, rigors, tinnitus.

Cardiovascular System: Hypertension, palpitation, tachycardia.

Central and Peripheral Nervous System: Convulsions, dysphonia, hyperkinesis, hypertonia, migraine, paresthesia, tremor.

Gastrointestinal System: Abdominal distension, altered taste, constipation, diarrhea, dyspepsia, flatulence, gastritis, stomatitis, tongue ulceration, toothache, vomiting.

Liver and Biliary System: Cholelithiasis.

Musculoskeletal System: Arthralgia, musculoskeletal pain, myalgia, tendinitis.

Psychiatric: Agitation, depression, emotional lability, irritability.

Reproductive System: Vaginitis.

Resistance Mechanism: Abscess, viral infection.

Respiratory System: Bronchospasm, dyspnea, epistaxis, hemoptysis, nasal congestion, nasal irritation, pleurisy, pneumonia, sinusitis, sputum increased, wheezing.

Skin and Appendages: Acne, pruritus.

Urinary System: Oliguria, micturition frequency, urinary retention, urinary tract infection.

Additional adverse events reported with the combination of loratadine and pseudoephedrine include abnormal hepatic function, aggressive reaction, anxiety, apathy, confusion, euphoria, paroniria, postural hypotension, syncope, urticaria, vertigo, weight gain.

The following additional adverse events have been reported with CLARITIN Tablets: abdominal distress, alopecia, altered micturition, altered salivation, amnesia, anaphylaxis, angioneurotic edema, blepharospasm, breast enlargement, breast pain, bronchitis, decreased libido, dermatitis, dry hair, dry skin, erythema multiforme, hypoesthesia, impaired concentration, impotence, increased appetite, laryngitis, menorrhagia, nasal dryness, peripheral edema, photosensitivity reaction, purpura, rash, seizures, sneezing, supraventricular tachyarrhythmias, upper respiratory infection, urinary discoloration.

Pseudoephedrine may cause mild CNS stimulation in hypersensitive patients. Nervousness, excitability, restlessness, dizziness, weakness, or insomnia may occur. Headache, drowsiness, tachycardia, palpitation, pressor activity, and cardiac arrhythmias have been reported. Sympathomimetic drugs have also been associated with other untoward effects, such as fear, anxiety, tenseness, tremor, hallucinations, seizures, pallor, respiratory difficulty, dysuria, and cardiovascular collapse.

There have been postmarketing reports of mechanical upper gastrointestinal tract obstruction and esophageal perforation in patients taking a previously marketed formulation of CLARITIN-D 24 HOUR Extended Release Tablets. In some, but not all, of these cases, patients have had known upper gastrointestinal narrowing or abnormal esophageal peristalsis. It is not known whether this reformulation of CLARITIN-D 24 HOUR Extended Release Tablets has the potential for this adverse event (see **PRECAUTIONS, DOSAGE AND ADMINISTRATION**).

DRUG ABUSE AND DEPENDENCE

There is no information to indicate that abuse or dependency occurs with loratadine. Pseudoephedrine, like other central nervous system stimulants, has been abused. At high doses, subjects commonly experience an elevation of mood, a sense of increased energy and alertness, and decreased appetite. Some individuals become anxious, irritable, and loquacious. In addition to the marked euphoria, the user experiences a sense of markedly enhanced physical strength and mental capacity. With continued use, tolerance develops, the user increases the dose, and toxic signs and symptoms appear. Depression may follow rapid withdrawal.

OVERDOSAGE

In the event of overdosage, general symptomatic and supportive measures should be instituted promptly and maintained for as long as necessary. Treatment of overdosage would reasonably consist of emesis (ipecac syrup), except in patients with impaired consciousness, followed by the administration of activated charcoal to absorb any remaining drug. If vomiting is unsuccessful, or contraindicated, gastric lavage should be performed with normal saline. Saline cathartics may also be of value for rapid dilution of bowel contents. Loratadine is not eliminated by hemodialysis. It is not known if loratadine is eliminated by peritoneal dialysis. Somnolence, tachycardia, and headache have been reported with doses of 40 to 180 mg of loratadine. In large doses, sympathomimetics may give rise to giddiness, headache, nausea, vomiting, sweating, thirst, tachycardia, precordial pain, palpitations, difficulty in micturition, muscular weakness and tenseness, anxiety, restlessness, and insomnia. Many patients can present a toxic psychosis with delusions and hallucinations. Some may develop cardiac arrhythmias, circulatory collapse, convulsions, coma, and respiratory failure.

The oral median lethal dose for the mixture of the two drugs was greater than 525 and 1839 mg/kg in mice and rats, respectively (approximately 10 and 58 times the maximum recommended human daily oral dose on a mg/m^2 basis). The oral median lethal dose for loratadine was greater than 5000 mg/kg in rats and mice (greater than 2000 times the maximum recommended human daily oral dose on a mg/m^2 basis). Single oral doses of loratadine showed no effects in rats, mice, and monkeys at doses as high as 10 times the maximum recommended human daily oral dose on a mg/m^2 basis.

DOSAGE AND ADMINISTRATION

Adults and children 12 years of age and over: one tablet daily taken with a full glass of water (see **PRECAUTIONS, ADVERSE REACTIONS**). Because the doses of this fixed combination product cannot be individually titrated and hepatic insufficiency results in a reduced clearance of loratadine to a much greater extent than pseudoephedrine, CLARITIN-D 24 HOUR Extended Release Tablets should generally be avoided in patients with hepatic insufficiency. Patients with renal insufficiency (GFR <30 mL/min) should be given a lower initial dose (one tablet every other day) because they have reduced clearance of loratadine and pseudoephedrine. Patients who have a history of difficulty in swallowing tablets or who have known upper gastrointestinal narrowing or abnormal esophageal peristalsis should not use this product (see **PRECAUTIONS: Information for Patients,** and **ADVERSE REACTIONS**).

HOW SUPPLIED

CLARITIN-D 24 HOUR Extended Release Tablets contain 10 mg loratadine in the tablet coating for immediate release and 240 mg pseudoephedrine sulfate, USP in an extended-release core. CLARITIN-D 24 HOUR Extended Release Tablets are white to off-white oval, biconvex, coated tablets

Continued on next page

Information on Schering products appearing on these pages is effective as of January 2000.

Claritin-D 24 hr.—Cont.

branded in black with "CLARITIN-D 24 HOUR"; high-density polyethylene bottles of 100 (NDC 0085-1233-01) and blister packages of 10 x 10 tablet Unit Dose-Hospital Pack (NDC 0085-1233-02).

Protect Unit Dose-Hospital Pack from light and store in a dry place. Store between 15° and 25°C (59° and 77°F).
U.S. Patent Nos. 5,314,697; 4,731,447; and 4,282,233.
CLARITIN-D® 24 HOUR
brand of loratadine and
pseudoephedrine sulfate, USP
Extended Release Tablets
Rev. 4/98 21678406
21861804T

Shown in Product Identification Guide, page 334

DIPROLENE® AF ℞

brand of augmented
betamethasone dipropionate*
CREAM 0.05%
(potency expressed as betamethasone)
*Vehicle augments the penetration of the steroid.
For Dermatologic Use Only—Not for Ophthalmic Use

DESCRIPTION

DIPROLENE® AF Cream contains betamethasone dipropionate, USP, a synthetic adrenocorticosteroid, for dermatologic use in an emollient base. Betamethasone, an analog of prednisolone, has a high degree of corticosteroid activity and a slight degree of mineralocorticoid activity. Betamethasone dipropionate is the 17, 21-dipropionate ester of betamethasone.
Chemically, betamethasone dipropionate is 9-fluoro-11β, 17,21-trihydroxy-16β-methylpregna-1,4-diene-3,20-dione 17,21-dipropionate, with the empirical formula $C_{28}H_{37}FO_7$, a molecular weight of 504.6, and the following structural formula:

Betamethasone dipropionate is a white to creamy white, odorless crystalline powder, insoluble in water.
Each gram of DIPROLENE AF Cream 0.05% contains: 0.643 mg betamethasone dipropionate, USP (equivalent to 0.5 mg betamethasone) in an emollient cream base of purified water, USP; chlorocresol NF; propylene glycol, USP; white petrolatum, USP; white wax NF; cyclomethicone; sorbitol solution, USP; glyceryl oleate/propylene glycol; ceteareth-30; carbomer 940 NF; and sodium hydroxide R.

CLINICAL PHARMACOLOGY

The corticosteroids are a class of compounds comprising steroid hormones secreted by the adrenal cortex and their synthetic analogs. In pharmacologic doses, corticosteroids are used primarily for their anti-inflammatory and/or immunosuppressive effects.
Topical corticosteroids, such as betamethasone dipropionate, are effective in the treatment of corticosteroid-responsive dermatoses primarily because of their anti-inflammatory, anti-pruritic, and vasoconstrictive actions. However, while the physiologic, pharmacologic, and clinical effects of the corticosteroids are well-known, the exact mechanisms of their actions in each disease are uncertain. Betamethasone dipropionate, a corticosteroid, has been shown to have topical (dermatologic) and systemic pharmacologic and metabolic effects characteristic of this class of drugs.
Pharmacokinetics: The extent of percutaneous absorption of topical corticosteroids is determined by many factors including the vehicle, the integrity of the epidermal barrier, and the use of occlusive dressings. (See **DOSAGE AND ADMINISTRATION** section.)
Topical corticosteroids can be absorbed through normal intact skin. Inflammation and/or other disease processes in the skin may increase percutaneous absorption. Occlusive dressings substantially increase the percutaneous absorption of topical corticosteroids. (See **DOSAGE AND ADMINISTRATION** section.)
Once absorbed through the skin, topical corticosteroids enter pharmacokinetic pathways similar to systemically administered corticosteroids. Corticosteroids are bound to plasma proteins in varying degrees, are metabolized primarily in the liver and excreted by the kidneys. Some of the topical corticosteroids and their metabolites are also excreted into the bile.
DIPROLENE AF Cream was applied once daily at 7 grams per day for one week to diseased skin, in patients with psoriasis or atopic dermatitis, to study its effects on the hypothalamic-pituitary-adrenal (HPA) axis. The results suggested that the drug caused a slight lowering of adrenal corticosteroid secretion, although in no case did plasma cortisol levels go below the lower limit of the normal range.

INDICATIONS AND USAGE

DIPROLENE AF Cream is indicated for relief of the inflammatory and pruritic manifestations of corticosteroid-responsive dermatoses.

CONTRAINDICATIONS

DIPROLENE AF Cream is contraindicated in patients who are hypersensitive to betamethasone dipropionate, to other corticosteroids, or to any ingredient in this preparation.

PRECAUTIONS

General: Systemic absorption of topical corticosteroids has produced reversible HPA axis suppression, manifestations of Cushing's syndrome, hyperglycemia, and glucosuria in some patients.
Conditions which augment systemic absorption include the application of the more potent corticosteroids, use over large surface areas, prolonged use, and the addition of occlusive dressings. (See **DOSAGE AND ADMINISTRATION** section.)
Therefore, patients receiving a large dose of a potent topical steroid applied to a large surface area should be evaluated periodically for evidence of HPA axis suppression by using the urinary free cortisol and ACTH stimulation tests. If HPA axis suppression is noted, an attempt should be made to withdraw the drug, to reduce the frequency of application, or to substitute a less potent steroid.
Recovery of HPA axis function is generally prompt and complete upon discontinuation of the drug. Infrequently, signs and symptoms of steroid withdrawal may occur, requiring supplemental systemic corticosteroids.
Children may absorb proportionally larger amounts of topical corticosteroids and thus be more susceptible to systemic toxicity. (See **PRECAUTIONS—Pediatric Use.**)
If irritation develops, topical corticosteroids should be discontinued and appropriate therapy instituted.
In the presence of dermatological infections, the use of an appropriate antifungal or antibacterial agent should be instituted. If a favorable response does not occur promptly, the corticosteroid should be discontinued until the infection has been adequately controlled.
Information for Patients: Patients using topical corticosteroids should receive the following information and instructions. This information is intended to aid in the safe and effective use of this medication. It is not a disclosure of all possible adverse or intended effects.

1. This medication is to be used as directed by the physician and should not be used longer than the prescribed time period. It is for external use only. Avoid contact with the eyes.
2. Patients should be advised not to use this medication for any disorder other than that for which it was prescribed.
3. The treated skin area should not be bandaged or otherwise covered or wrapped as to be occlusive. (See **DOSAGE AND ADMINISTRATION** section.)
4. Patients should report any signs of local adverse reactions.

Laboratory Tests: The following tests may be helpful in evaluating HPA axis suppression:
Urinary free cortisol test
ACTH stimulation test
Carcinogenesis, Mutagenesis, and Impairment of Fertility: Long-term animal studies have not been performed to evaluate the carcinogenic potential or the effect on fertility of topically applied corticosteroids.
Studies to determine mutagenicity with prednisolone and hydrocortisone have revealed negative results.
Pregnancy Category C: Corticosteroids are generally teratogenic in laboratory animals when administered systemically at relatively low dosage levels. The more potent corticosteroids have been shown to be teratogenic after dermal application in laboratory animals. There are no adequate and well-controlled studies of the teratogenic effects of topically applied corticosteroids in pregnant women. Therefore, topical corticosteroids should be used during pregnancy only if the potential benefit justifies the potential risk to the fetus. Drugs of this class should not be used extensively on pregnant patients, in large amounts, or for prolonged periods of time.
Nursing Mothers: It is not known whether topical administration of corticosteroids can result in sufficient systemic absorption to produce detectable quantities in breast milk. Systemically administered corticosteroids are secreted into breast milk in quantities not likely to have a deleterious effect on the infant. Nevertheless, a decision should be made whether to discontinue nursing or to discontinue the drug, taking into account the importance of the drug to the mother.
Pediatric Use: Use of DIPROLENE AF Cream in children under 12 years is not recommended.
Pediatric patients may demonstrate greater susceptibility to topical corticosteroid-induced HPA axis suppression and Cushing's syndrome than mature patients because of a larger skin surface area to body weight ratio.
Hypothalamic-pituitary-adrenal (HPA) axis suppression, Cushing's syndrome, and intracranial hypertension have been reported in children receiving topical corticosteroids. Manifestations of adrenal suppression in children include linear growth retardation, delayed weight gain, low plasma cortisol levels, and absence of response to ACTH stimulation. Manifestations of intracranial hypertension include bulging fontanelles, headaches, and bilateral papilledema.
Chronic corticosteroid therapy may interfere with the growth and development of children.

ADVERSE REACTIONS

The only local adverse reaction reported to be possibly or probably related to treatment with DIPROLENE AF Cream during controlled clinical studies was stinging. It occurred in 0.4% of the 242 patients or subjects involved in the studies.
The following local adverse reactions are reported infrequently when topical corticosteroids are used as recommended. These reactions are listed in an approximate decreasing order of occurrence: burning, itching, irritation, dryness, folliculitis, hypertrichosis, acneiform eruptions, hypopigmentation, perioral dermatitis, allergic contact dermatitis, maceration of the skin, secondary infection, skin atrophy, striae, miliaria.

OVERDOSAGE

Topically applied corticosteroids can be absorbed in sufficient amounts to produce systemic effects. (See **PRECAUTIONS.**)

DOSAGE AND ADMINISTRATION

Apply a thin film of DIPROLENE AF Cream to the affected skin areas once or twice daily. Treatment with DIPROLENE AF Cream should be limited to 45 g per week.
DIPROLENE AF Cream is not to be used with occlusive dressings.

HOW SUPPLIED

DIPROLENE AF Cream 0.05% is supplied in 15 g (NDC 0085-0517-01), and 50 g (NDC 0085-0517-04) tubes; boxes of one.
Store between 2° and 30°C (36° and 86°F).
DIPROLENE® AF
brand of augmented
betamethasone dipropionate*
Cream, 0.05*
(potency expressed as betamethasone)
*Vehicle augments the penetration of the steroid.
For Dermatologic Use Only—
Not for Ophthalmic Use
Schering Corporation
Kenilworth, NJ 07033 USA
Rev. 1/99 17968629
18670313T

Shown in Product Identification Guide, page 334

DIPROLENE® ℞

brand of augmented
betamethasone dipropionate*
Gel 0.05%
(potency expressed as betamethasone)
*Vehicle augments the penetration of the steroid.
For Dermatologic Use Only —
Not for Ophthalmic Use

DESCRIPTION

DIPROLENE® Gel contains betamethasone dipropionate, USP, a synthetic fluorinated corticosteroid for topical dermatologic use. Betamethasone dipropionate is included in a class of compounds consisting primarily of synthetic corticosteroids for use topically as anti-inflammatory and antipruritic agents.
Chemically, betamethasone dipropionate is 9-fluoro-11β,17,21-trihydroxy-16β-methylpregna-1,4-diene-3,20-dione 17,21-dipropionate, with the empirical formula $C_{28}H_{37}FO_7$, a molecular weight of 504.6, and the following structural formula:

Betamethasone dipropionate is a white to creamy white, odorless crystalline powder, insoluble in water.
Each gram of DIPROLENE Gel contains: 0.643 mg betamethasone dipropionate, USP (equivalent to 0.5 mg betamethasone) in an augmented gel base of purified water, USP; propylene glycol, USP; carbomer 940, NF; and sodium hydroxide, NF or R. May also contain phosphoric acid, NF to adjust the pH to approximately 4.5.

CLINICAL PHARMACOLOGY

Like other topical corticosteroids, betamethasone dipropionate has anti-inflammatory, antipruritic, and vasoconstrictive properties. The mechanism of the anti-inflammatory activity of the topical steroids, in general, is unclear. However, corticosteroids are thought to act by the induction of phospholipase A_2 inhibitory proteins, collectively called lipocortins. It is postulated that these proteins control the biosynthesis of potent mediators of inflammation, such as prostaglandins and leukotrienes, by inhibiting the release of their common precursor, arachidonic acid. Arachidonic acid is released from membrane phospholipids by phospholipase A_2.

Pharmacokinetics: The extent of percutaneous absorption of topical corticosteroids is determined by many factors including the vehicle and the integrity of the epidermal barrier. Occlusive dressings with hydrocortisone for up to 24 hours have not been demonstrated to increase penetration; however, occlusion of hydrocortisone for 96 hours markedly enhances penetration. Topical corticosteroids can be absorbed from normal intact skin. In addition, inflammation and/or other disease processes in the skin may increase percutaneous absorption. Studies performed with DIPROLENE (augmented betamethasone dipropionate) Gel indicate that it is in the super-high range of potency as compared with other topical corticosteroids.

INDICATIONS AND USAGE

DIPROLENE Gel is a super-high potency corticosteroid indicated for the relief of the inflammatory and pruritic manifestations of corticosteroid-responsive dermatoses. Treatment beyond two consecutive weeks is not recommended, and the total dose should not exceed 50 g per week because of potential for the drug to suppress the hypothalamic-pituitary-adrenal (HPA) axis.

CONTRAINDICATIONS

DIPROLENE Gel is contraindicated in those patients with a history of hypersensitivity to any of the components of the preparation.

PRECAUTIONS

General: DIPROLENE Gel should not be used in the treatment of rosacea or perioral dermatitis, and it should not be used on the face, groin, or in the axillae.

Systemic absorption of topical corticosteroids can produce reversible hypothalamic-pituitary-adrenal (HPA) axis suppression with the potential for glucocorticosteroid insufficiency after withdrawal of treatment. Manifestations of Cushing's syndrome, hyperglycemia, and glucosuria can also be produced in some patients by systemic absorption of topical corticosteroids while on treatment.

At 7 g per day (applied once daily or as 3.5 g twice daily), DIPROLENE Gel was shown to cause inhibition of the HPA axis following application for 1, 2 or 3 weeks to diseased skin in some patients with psoriasis or atopic dermatitis. These effects were reversible upon discontinuation of treatment.

Patients receiving DIPROLENE Gel applied to large areas should be evaluated periodically for evidence of HPA axis suppression. This may be done by using the ACTH-stimulation, morning plasma cortisol and urinary free-cortisol tests. Patients should not be treated with DIPROLENE Gel for more than 2 weeks at a time, and amounts greater than 50 g per week should not be used because of the potential for the drug to suppress the HPA axis.

If HPA axis suppression is noted, an attempt should be made to withdraw the drug, to reduce the frequency of application, or to substitute a less potent corticosteroid. Recovery of HPA axis function is generally prompt and complete upon discontinuation of topical corticosteroids. Infrequently, signs and symptoms of glucocorticosteroid insufficiency may occur, requiring supplemental systemic corticosteroids. For information on systemic supplementation, see prescribing information for systemic corticosteroids.

Pediatric patients may be more susceptible to systemic toxicity from equivalent doses due to their larger skin surface to body mass ratios (see **PRECAUTIONS—Pediatric Use**).

If irritation develops, DIPROLENE Gel should be discontinued and appropriate therapy instituted. Allergic contact dermatitis with corticosteroids is usually diagnosed by observing failure to heal rather than noting clinical exacerbation as with most topical products not containing corticosteroids. Such an observation should be corroborated with appropriate diagnostic patch testing.

If concomitant fungal and/or bacterial skin infections are present or develop, an appropriate antifungal or antibacterial agent should be used. If a favorable response does not occur promptly, use of DIPROLENE Gel should be discontinued until the infection has been adequately controlled.

Information for Patients: Patients using topical corticosteroids should receive the following information and instructions:

1. The medication is to be used as directed by the physician. It is for external use only. Avoid contact with the eyes.
2. The medication should not be used for any disorder other than that for which it was prescribed.
3. The treated skin area should not be bandaged or otherwise covered or wrapped so as to be occlusive.
4. Patients should report to their physician any signs of local adverse reactions.

Laboratory Tests: The following tests may be helpful in evaluating patients for HPA axis suppression:

ACTH-stimulation test
Morning plasma-cortisol test
Urinary free-cortisol test

Carcinogenesis, Mutagenesis, and Impairment of Fertility: Long-term animal studies have not been performed to evaluate the carcinogenic potential of betamethasone dipropionate.

Studies in rabbits, mice, and rats using intramuscular doses up to 1.0, 33, and 2.0 mg/kg, respectively, resulted in dose-related increases in fetal resorptions in the rabbits and mice.

Pregnancy: Teratogenic Effects: Pregnancy Category C: Corticosteroids have been shown to be teratogenic in laboratory animals when administered systemically at relatively low dosage levels. Some corticosteroids have been shown to be teratogenic after dermal application to laboratory animals.

Betamethasone dipropionate has been shown to be teratogenic in rabbits when given by the intramuscular route at doses of 0.05 mg/kg. This dose is approximately 26 times the human topical dose of DIPROLENE Gel assuming human percutaneous absorption of approximately 3% and the use in a 70-kg person of 7 g per day. The abnormalities observed included umbilical hernias, cephalocele, and cleft palate. There are no adequate and well-controlled studies of the teratogenic potential of betamethasone dipropionate in pregnant women. Therefore, DIPROLENE Gel should be used during pregnancy only if the potential benefit justifies the potential risk to the fetus.

Nursing Mothers: Systemically administered corticosteroids appear in human milk and could suppress growth, interfere with endogenous corticosteroid production, or cause other untoward effects. It is not known whether topical administration of corticosteroids could result in sufficient systemic absorption to produce detectable quantities in human milk. Because many drugs are excreted in human milk, caution should be exercised when DIPROLENE Gel is administered to a nursing woman.

Pediatric Use: Data regarding use of Diprolene Gel in pediatric patients are not available, so use of this product in patients under the age of 12 is not recommended. *Because of a higher ratio of skin surface area to body mass, pediatric patients are at a greater risk than adults of HPA axis suppression when they are treated with topical corticosteroids. They are, therefore, also at greater risk of glucocorticosteroid insufficiency after withdrawal of treatment and of Cushing's syndrome while on treatment.* Adverse effects, including striae, have been reported with inappropriate use of topical corticosteroids in infants and children.

HPA axis suppression, Cushing's syndrome, and intracranial hypertension have been reported in pediatric patients receiving topical corticosteroids. Manifestations of adrenal suppression in pediatric patients include linear growth retardation, delayed weight gain, low plasma cortisol levels, and absence of response to ACTH stimulation. Manifestations of intracranial hypertension include bulging fontanelles, headaches, and bilateral papilledema.

ADVERSE REACTIONS

In controlled clinical trials, the total incidence of adverse events associated with the use of DIPROLENE (augmented betamethasone dipropionate) Gel was 10%. These included stinging or burning in 6% of patients, dry skin in 4% of patients, and pruritus in 2% of patients. Less frequently reported adverse reactions were irritation, skin atrophy, telangiectasia, erythema, cracking/ tightening of the skin, follicular rash, and allergic contact dermatitis.

The following additional local adverse reactions are reported infrequently with topical corticosteroids, but may occur more frequently with super-high potency corticosteroids, such as DIPROLENE Gel. These reactions are listed in approximate decreasing order of occurrence: acneiform eruptions, hypopigmentation, perioral dermatitis, secondary infection, striae, and miliaria.

OVERDOSAGE

Topically applied DIPROLENE Gel can be absorbed in sufficient amounts to produce systemic effects (see **PRECAUTIONS**).

DOSAGE AND ADMINISTRATION

Apply a thin layer of DIPROLENE Gel to the affected skin once or twice daily and rub in gently and completely.

DIPROLENE Gel is a super-high potency topical corticosteroid; therefore, treatment should be limited to 2 weeks, and amounts greater than 50 g per week should not be used. **DIPROLENE Gel should not be used with occlusive dressings.**

HOW SUPPLIED

DIPROLENE Gel 0.05% is supplied in 15-g (NDC 0085-0634-01) and 50-g (NDC 0085-0634-03) tubes; boxes of one.

Store between 2° and 25°C (36° and 77°F).

Schering Corporation
Kenilworth, NJ 07033 USA
Rev. 1/00 17969137
18671425T

Shown in Product Identification Guide, page 334

DIPROLENE® ℞

brand of augmented betamethasone dipropionate*
Lotion 0.05%
(potency expressed as betamethasone)
*Vehicle augments the penetration of the steroid.
For Dermatologic Use Only—Not for Ophthalmic Use

DESCRIPTION

DIPROLENE® Lotion contains betamethasone dipropionate, USP, a synthetic adrenocorticosteroid, for dermatologic use. Betamethasone, an analog of prednisolone, has a high degree of corticosteroid activity and a slight degree of mineralocorticoid activity. Betamethasone dipropionate is the 17, 21-dipropionate ester of betamethasone.

Chemically, betamethasone dipropionate is 9-fluoro-11β,17,21-trihydroxy-16β-methylpregna-1,4-diene-3,20-dione 17,21-dipropionate, with the empirical formula $C_{28}H_{37}FO_7$, a molecular weight of 504.6, and the following structural formula:

Betamethasone dipropionate is a white to creamy white, odorless crystalline powder, insoluble in water.

Each gram of DIPROLENE Lotion 0.05% contains: 0.643 mg betamethasone dipropionate, USP (equivalent to 0.5 mg betamethasone), in a lotion base of purified water, USP; isopropyl alcohol, USP (30%); hydroxypropyl cellulose, NF; propylene glycol, USP; sodium phosphate monobasic monohydrate R; phosphoric acid, NF used to adjust the pH to 4.5.

CLINICAL PHARMACOLOGY

The corticosteroids are a class of compounds comprising steroid hormones secreted by the adrenal cortex and their synthetic analogs. In pharmacologic doses, corticosteroids are used primarily for their anti-inflammatory and/or immunosuppressive effects.

Topical corticosteroids, such as betamethasone dipropionate, are effective in the treatment of corticosteroid-responsive dermatoses primarily because of their anti-inflammatory, antipruritic, and vasoconstrictive actions. However, while the physiologic, pharmacologic, and clinical effects of the corticosteroids are well known, the exact mechanisms of their actions in each disease are uncertain. Betamethasone dipropionate, a corticosteroid, has been shown to have topical (dermatologic) and systemic pharmacologic and metabolic effects characteristic of this class of drugs.

Pharmacokinetics: The extent of percutaneous absorption of topical corticosteroids is determined by many factors including the vehicle, the integrity of the epidermal barrier, and the use of occlusive dressings. (See **DOSAGE AND ADMINISTRATION** section.)

Topical corticosteroids can be absorbed through normal intact skin. Inflammation and/or other disease processes in the skin may increase percutaneous absorption. Occlusive dressings substantially increase the percutaneous absorption of topical corticosteroids. (See **DOSAGE AND ADMINISTRATION** section.)

Once absorbed through the skin, topical corticosteroids enter pharmacokinetic pathways similar to systemically administered corticosteroids. Corticosteroids are bound to plasma proteins in varying degrees, are metabolized primarily in the liver and excreted by the kidneys. Some of the topical corticosteroids and their metabolites are also excreted into the bile.

DIPROLENE Lotion was applied once daily at 7 mL per day for 21 days to diseased skin (in patients with scalp psoriasis) to study its effects on the hypothalamic-pituitary-adrenal (HPA) axis. In 2 out of 11 patients, the drug lowered plasma cortisol levels below normal limits. Adrenal depression in these patients was transient and returned to normal within a week. In one of these patients, plasma cortisol levels returned to normal while treatment continued.

INDICATIONS AND USAGE

DIPROLENE Lotion is indicated for treatment of the inflammatory and pruritic manifestations of moderate to severe corticosteroid-responsive dermatoses.

Treatment beyond 2 weeks is not recommended, and the total dosage should not exceed 50 mL per week because of potential for the drug to suppress the hypothalamic-pituitary-adrenal axis.

CONTRAINDICATIONS

DIPROLENE Lotion is contraindicated in patients who are hypersensitive to betamethasone dipropionate, to other corticosteroids, or to any ingredient in this preparation.

PRECAUTIONS

General: DIPROLENE Lotion is a highly potent topical corticosteroid that has been shown to suppress the HPA axis at 7 mL per day.

Systemic absorption of topical corticosteroids has produced reversible HPA axis suppression, manifestations of Cushing's syndrome, hyperglycemia, and glucosuria in some patients.

Conditions which augment systemic absorption include the application of the more potent corticosteroids such as

Continued on next page

Diprolene Lotion—Cont.

DIPROLENE, use over large surface areas, prolonged use, and the addition of occlusive dressings. (See **DOSAGE AND ADMINISTRATION** section.)

Therefore, patients receiving large doses of a potent topical steroid applied to a large surface area should be evaluated periodically for evidence of HPA axis suppression by using the urinary free cortisol and ACTH stimulation tests. If HPA axis suppression is noted, an attempt should be made to withdraw the drug, to reduce the frequency of application, or to substitute a less potent steroid.

Recovery of HPA axis function is generally prompt and complete upon discontinuation of the drug. Infrequently, signs and symptoms of steroid withdrawal may occur, requiring supplemental systemic corticosteroids.

Children may absorb proportionally larger amounts of topical corticosteroids and thus be more susceptible to systemic toxicity. (See **PRECAUTIONS—Pediatric Use.**)

If irritation develops, topical corticosteroids should be discontinued and appropriate therapy instituted.

In the presence of dermatological infections, the use of an appropriate antifungal or antibacterial agent should be instituted. If a favorable response does not occur promptly, the corticosteroid should be discontinued until the infection has been adequately controlled.

Information for Patients: Patients using topical corticosteroids should receive the following information and instructions. This information is intended to aid in the safe and effective use of this medication. It is not a disclosure of all possible adverse or intended effects.

1. This medication is to be used as directed by the physician and should not be used longer than the prescribed time period. It is for external use only. Avoid contact with the eyes.
2. Patients should be advised not to use this medication for any disorder other than that for which it was prescribed.
3. The treated skin areas should not be bandaged or otherwise covered or wrapped so as to be occlusive. (See **DOSAGE AND ADMINISTRATION** section.)
4. Patients should report any signs of local adverse reactions.

Laboratory Tests: The following tests may be helpful in evaluating HPA axis suppression:
Urinary free cortisol test
ACTH stimulation test

Carcinogenesis, Mutagenesis, and Impairment of Fertility: Long-term animal studies have not been performed to evaluate the carcinogenic potential or the effect on fertility of topically applied corticosteroids.

Studies to determine mutagenicity with prednisolone and hydrocortisone have revealed negative results.

Pregnancy Category C: Corticosteroids are generally teratogenic in laboratory animals when administered systemically at relatively low dosage levels. The more potent corticosteroids have been shown to be teratogenic after dermal application in laboratory animals. Betamethasone dipropionate has not been tested for teratogenicity by this route; however, it appears to be fairly well absorbed percutaneously. There are no adequate and well-controlled studies of the teratogenic effects of topically applied corticosteroids in pregnant women. Therefore, topical corticosteroids should be used during pregnancy only if the potential benefit justifies the potential risk to the fetus. Drugs of this class should not be used extensively on pregnant patients, in large amounts, or for prolonged periods of time.

Nursing Mothers: It is not known whether topical administration of corticosteroids can result in sufficient systemic absorption to produce detectable quantities in breast milk. Systemically administered corticosteroids are secreted into breast milk in quantities not likely to have a deleterious effect on the infant. Nevertheless, a decision should be made whether to discontinue nursing or to discontinue the drug, taking into account the importance of the drug to the mother.

Pediatric Use: Data regarding use of Diprolene Lotion in pediatric patients are not available, so use of this product in pediatric patients under the age of 12 is not recommended.

Pediatric patients may demonstrate greater susceptibility to topical corticosteroid-induced HPA axis suppression and Cushing's syndrome than mature patients because of a larger skin surface area to body weight ratio.

Hypothalamic-pituitary-adrenal (HPA) axis suppression, Cushing's syndrome, and intracranial hypertension have been reported in children receiving topical corticosteroids. Manifestations of adrenal suppression in children include linear growth retardation, delayed weight gain, low plasma cortisol levels, and absence of response to ACTH stimulation. Manifestations of intra-cranial hypertension include bulging fontanelles, headaches, and bilateral papilledema. Chronic corticosteroid therapy may interfere with the growth and development of children.

ADVERSE REACTIONS

The overall incidence of drug-related adverse reactions in the DIPROLENE Lotion clinical studies was 5%. The adverse reactions that were reported to be possibly or probably related to treatment with DIPROLENE Lotion during controlled clinical studies involving 327 patients or normal volunteers were as follows: folliculitis occurred in 2%, burning and acneiform papules each occurred in 1%, and hyperesthesia and irritation each occurred in less than 1% of patients.

The following adverse reactions are also reported infrequently when topical corticosteroids are used as recommended. These reactions are listed in approximate decreasing order of occurrence: itching, dryness, hypertrichosis, hypopigmentation, perioral dermatitis, allergic contact dermatitis, maceration of the skin, secondary infection, skin atrophy, striae, miliaria.

OVERDOSAGE

Topically applied corticosteroids can be absorbed in sufficient amounts to produce systemic effects. (See **PRECAUTIONS.**)

DOSAGE AND ADMINISTRATION

Apply a few drops of DIPROLENE Lotion to the affected area once or twice daily and massage lightly until the lotion disappears. Treatment must be limited to 14 days, and amounts greater than 50 mL per week should not be used. **DIPROLENE Lotion is not to be used with occlusive dressings.**

HOW SUPPLIED

DIPROLENE Lotion 0.05% is supplied in 30-mL (29 g) (NDC 0085-0962-01) and 60-mL (58 g) (NDC 0085-0962-02) plastic squeeze bottles; boxes of one.

Store between 2° and 25°C (36° and 77°F).

Schering Corporation
Kenilworth, NJ 07033 USA
Rev. 12/99 23409810
23816407T

DIPROLENE® ℞

brand of augmented
betamethasone dipropionate*
Ointment 0.05%
(potency expressed as betamethasone)
*Vehicle augments the penetration of the steroid.
For Dermatologic Use Only—Not for Ophthalmic Use

DESCRIPTION

DIPROLENE Ointment contains betamethasone dipropionate, USP, a synthetic adrenocorticosteroid, for dermatologic use. Betamethasone, an analog of prednisolone, has a high degree of corticosteroid activity and a slight degree of mineralocorticoid activity. Betamethasone dipropionate is the 17,21-dipropionate ester of betamethasone.

Chemically, betamethasone dipropionate is 9-fluoro-11β, 17,21-trihydroxy-16β-methylpregna-1,4-diene-3,20-dione 17,21-dipropionate, with the empirical formula $C_{28}H_{37}FO_7$, a molecular weight of 504.6, and the following structural formula:

Betamethasone dipropionate is a white to creamy white, odorless crystalline powder, insoluble in water.

Each gram of DIPROLENE Ointment 0.05% contains: 0.643 mg betamethasone dipropionate, USP (equivalent to 0.5 mg betamethasone), in ACTIBASE®, an optimized vehicle of propylene glycol, USP; propylene glycol stearate (55% monoester); white wax, NF; and white petrolatum, USP.

CLINICAL PHARMACOLOGY

The corticosteroids are a class of compounds comprising steroid hormones secreted by the adrenal cortex and their synthetic analogs. In pharmacologic doses, corticosteroids are used primarily for their anti-inflammatory and/or immunosuppressive effects.

Topical corticosteroids, such as betamethasone dipropionate, are effective in the treatment of corticosteroid-responsive dermatoses primarily because of their anti-inflammatory, antipruritic, and vasoconstrictive actions. However, while the physiologic, pharmacologic, and clinical effects of the corticosteroids are well known, the exact mechanisms of their actions in each disease are uncertain. Betamethasone dipropionate, a corticosteroid, has been shown to have topical (dermatologic) and systemic pharmacologic and metabolic effects characteristic of this class of drugs.

Pharmacokinetics: The extent of percutaneous absorption of topical corticosteroids is determined by many factors including the vehicle, the integrity of the epidermal barrier, and the use of occlusive dressings. (See **DOSAGE AND ADMINISTRATION** section.)

Topical corticosteroids can be absorbed from normal intact skin. Inflammation and/or other disease processes in the skin may increase percutaneous absorption. Occlusive dressings substantially increase the percutaneous absorption of topical corticosteroids. (See **DOSAGE AND ADMINISTRATION** section.)

Once absorbed through the skin, topical corticosteroids enter pharmacokinetic pathways similar to systemically administered corticosteroids. Corticosteroids are bound to plasma proteins in varying degrees. Corticosteroids are metabolized primarily in the liver and are then excreted by the kidneys. Some of the topical corticosteroids and their metabolites are also excreted into the bile.

At 14 g per day, DIPROLENE Ointment was shown to depress the plasma levels of adrenal cortical hormones following repeated application to diseased skin in patients with psoriasis. Adrenal depression in these patients was transient, and rapidly returned to normal upon cessation of treatment. At 7 g per day (3.5 g b.i.d.), DIPROLENE Ointment was shown to cause minimal inhibition of the hypothalamic-pituitary-adrenal (HPA) axis when applied two times daily for 2 to 3 weeks, in normal patients and in patients with psoriasis and eczematous disorders.

With 6 g to 7 g of DIPROLENE Ointment applied once daily for 3 weeks, no significant inhibition of the HPA axis was observed in patients with psoriasis and atopic dermatitis, as measured by plasma cortisol and 24-hour urinary 17-hydroxy-corticosteroid levels.

INDICATIONS AND USAGE

DIPROLENE Ointment is indicated for relief of the inflammatory and pruritic manifestations of corticosteroid-responsive dermatoses.

CONTRAINDICATIONS

DIPROLENE Ointment is contraindicated in patients who are hypersensitive to betamethasone dipropionate, to other corticosteroids, or to any ingredient in this preparation.

PRECAUTIONS

General: Systemic absorption of topical corticosteroids has produced reversible HPA axis suppression, manifestations of Cushing's syndrome, hyperglycemia, and glucosuria in some patients.

Conditions which augment systemic absorption include the application of the more potent corticosteroids, use over large surface areas, prolonged use, and the addition of occlusive dressings. (See **DOSAGE AND ADMINISTRATION** section.)

Therefore, patients receiving a large dose of a potent topical steroid applied to a large surface area should be evaluated periodically for evidence of HPA axis suppression by using the urinary free cortisol and ACTH stimulation tests. If HPA axis suppression is noted, an attempt should be made to withdraw the drug, reduce the frequency of application, or substitute a less potent steroid.

Recovery of HPA axis function is generally prompt and complete upon discontinuation of the drug. Infrequently, signs and symptoms of steroid withdrawal may occur, requiring supplemental systemic corticosteroids.

Children may absorb proportionally larger amounts of topical corticosteroids and thus be more susceptible to systemic toxicity. (See **PRECAUTIONS—Pediatric Use.**)

If irritation develops, topical corticosteroids should be discontinued and appropriate therapy instituted.

In the presence of dermatological infections, the use of an appropriate antifungal or antibacterial agent should be instituted. If a favorable response does not occur promptly, the corticosteroid should be discontinued until the infection has been adequately controlled.

Information for Patients: Patients using topical corticosteroids should receive the following information and instructions:

1. This medication is to be used as directed by the physician and should not be used longer than the prescribed time period. It is for external use only. Avoid contact with the eyes.
2. Patients should be advised not to use this medication for any disorder other than that for which it was prescribed.
3. The treated skin area should not be bandaged or otherwise covered or wrapped as to be occlusive. (See **DOSAGE AND ADMINISTRATION** section.)
4. Patients should report any signs of local adverse reactions.

Laboratory Tests: The following tests may be helpful in evaluating HPA axis suppression:
Urinary free cortisol test
ACTH stimulation test

Carcinogenesis, Mutagenesis, and Impairment of Fertility: Long-term animal studies have not been performed to evaluate the carcinogenic potential or the effect on fertility of topically applied corticosteroids.

Studies to determine mutagenicity with prednisolone have revealed negative results.

Pregnancy Category C: Corticosteroids are generally teratogenic in laboratory animals when administered systemically at relatively low dosage levels. The more potent corticosteroids have been shown to be teratogenic after dermal application in laboratory animals. There are no adequate and well-controlled studies of the teratogenic effects of topically applied corticosteroids in pregnant women. Therefore, topical corticosteroids should be used during pregnancy only if the potential benefit justifies the potential risk to the fetus. Drugs of this class should not be used extensively on pregnant patients, in large amounts, or for prolonged periods of time.

Nursing Mothers: It is not known whether topical administration of corticosteroids could result in sufficient systemic absorption to produce detectable quantities in breast milk. Systemically administered corticosteroids are secreted into breast milk in quantities not likely to have a deleterious effect on the infant. Nevertheless, caution should be exercised when topical corticosteroids are prescribed for a nursing woman.

Pediatric Use: Data regarding use of DIPROLENE Ointment in pediatric patients are not available, so use of this product in patients under the age of 12 is not recommended. Pediatric patients may demonstrate greater susceptibility to topical corticosteroid-induced HPA axis suppression and Cushing's syndrome than mature patients because of a larger skin surface area to body weight ratio.

Hypothalamic-pituitary-adrenal (HPA) axis suppression, Cushing's syndrome, and intracranial hypertension have been reported in children receiving topical corticosteroids. Manifestations of adrenal suppression in children include linear growth retardation, delayed weight gain, low plasma cortisol levels, and absence of response to ACTH stimulation. Manifestations of intracranial hypertension include bulging fontanelles, headaches, and bilateral papilledema. Administration of topical corticosteroids to children should be limited to the least amount compatible with an effective therapeutic regimen. Chronic corticosteroid therapy may interfere with the growth and development of children.

ADVERSE REACTIONS

The local adverse reactions were reported with DIPROLENE Ointment applied either once or twice a day during clinical studies are as follows: erythema, 3 per 767 patients; folliculitis, 2 per 767 patients; pruritus, 2 per 767 patients; vesiculation, 1 per 767 patients.

The following local adverse reactions are reported infrequently when topical corticosteroids are used as recommended. These reactions are listed in an approximate decreasing order of occurrence: burning, itching, irritation, dryness, folliculitis, hypertrichosis, acneiform eruptions, hypopigmentation, perioral dermatitis, allergic contact dermatitis, maceration of the skin, secondary infection, skin atrophy, striae, miliaria.

Systemic absorption of topical corticosteroids has produced reversible HPA axis suppression, manifestations of Cushing's syndrome, hyperglycemia, and glucosuria in some patients.

OVERDOSAGE

Topically applied corticosteroids can be absorbed in sufficient amounts to produce systemic effects. (See **PRECAUTIONS.**)

DOSAGE AND ADMINISTRATION

Apply a thin film of DIPROLENE Ointment to the affected skin areas once or twice daily. Treatment with DIPROLENE Ointment should be limited to 45 g per week.

DIPROLENE Ointment is not to be used with occlusive dressings.

HOW SUPPLIED

DIPROLENE Ointment 0.05% is supplied in 15-g (NDC 0085-0575-02) and 50-g (NDC 0085-0575-05) tubes; boxes of one.

Store between 2° and 25°C (36° and 77°F).

Schering Corporation
Kenilworth, NJ 07033 USA
Rev. 1/00 **18670526T**

Shown in Product Identification Guide, page 334

DIPROSONE® ℞

[*dĭp-rō-sōne*]

brand of betamethasone dipropionate

Cream, USP 0.05%
Lotion, USP 0.05% w/w
Ointment, USP 0.05%
(potency expressed as betamethasone)

For Dermatologic Use Only—Not for Ophthalmic Use

DESCRIPTION

DIPROSONE products contain betamethasone dipropionate, USP, a synthetic adrenocorticosteroid, for dermatologic use. Betamethasone, an analog of prednisolone, has high corticosteroid activity and slight mineralocorticoid activity. Betamethasone dipropionate is the 17, 21-dipropionate ester of betamethasone.

Chemically, betamethasone dipropionate is 9-Fluoro-11β,17,21-trihydroxy-16β-methylpregna-1,4-diene-3,20-dione 17,21-dipropionate, with the empirical formula $C_{28}H_{37}FO_7$, a molecular weight of 504.6, and the following structural formula:

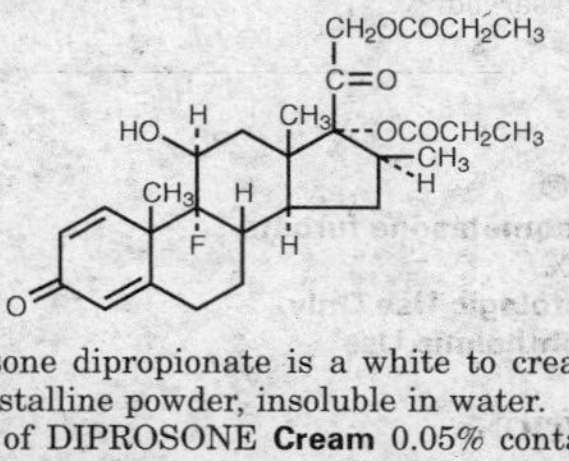

Betamethasone dipropionate is a white to creamy white, odorless crystalline powder, insoluble in water.

Each gram of DIPROSONE **Cream** 0.05% contains: 0.643 mg betamethasone dipropionate, USP (equivalent to 0.5 mg betamethasone) in a hydrophilic emollient cream consisting of purified water, USP; mineral oil, USP; white petrolatum, USP; ceteareth-30; cetearyl alcohol 70/30 (7.2%); sodium phosphate monobasic monohydrate R; and phosphoric acid, NF; chlorocresol, NF; and propylene glycol, USP as preservatives. May also contain sodium hydroxide R to adjust pH to approximately 5.0.

Each gram of DIPROSONE **Lotion** 0.05% w/w contains: 0.643 mg betamethasone dipropionate, USP (equivalent to 0.5 mg betamethasone) in a lotion base of isopropyl alcohol, USP (39.25%); and purified water, USP; slightly thickened with carbomer 974P; the pH is adjusted to approximately 4.7 with sodium hydroxide.

Each gram of DIPROSONE **Ointment** 0.05% contains: 0.643 mg betamethasone dipropionate, USP (equivalent to 0.5 mg betamethasone) in an ointment base of mineral oil, USP; and white petrolatum, USP.

CLINICAL PHARMACOLOGY

The corticosteroids are a class of compounds comprising steroid hormones, secreted by the adrenal cortex and their synthetic analogs. In pharmacologic doses corticosteroids are used primarily for their anti-inflammatory and/or immunosuppressive effects.

Topical corticosteroids, such as betamethasone dipropionate, are effective in the treatment of corticosteroid-responsive dermatoses primarily because of their anti-inflammatory, antipruritic, and vasoconstrictive actions. However, while the physiologic, pharmacologic, and clinical effects of the corticosteroids are well known, the exact mechanisms of their actions in each disease are uncertain. Betamethasone dipropionate, a corticosteroid, has been shown to have topical (dermatologic) and systemic pharmacologic and metabolic effects characteristic of this class of drugs.

Pharmacokinetics The extent of percutaneous absorption of topical corticosteroids is determined by many factors including the vehicle, the integrity of the epidermal barrier, and the use of occlusive dressings. (See **DOSAGE AND ADMINISTRATION.**)

Topical corticosteroids can be absorbed from normal intact skin. Inflammation and/or other disease processes in the skin increase percutaneous absorption. Occlusive dressings substantially increase the percutaneous absorption of topical corticosteroids. (See **DOSAGE AND ADMINISTRATION.**)

Once absorbed through the skin, topical corticosteroids are handled through pharmacokinetic pathways similar to systemically administered corticosteroids. Corticosteroids are bound to plasma proteins in varying degrees. Corticosteroids are metabolized primarily in the liver and are then excreted by the kidneys. Some of the topical corticosteroids and their metabolites are also excreted into the bile.

INDICATIONS AND USAGE

DIPROSONE products are indicated for relief of the inflammatory and pruritic manifestations of corticosteroid-responsive dermatoses.

CONTRAINDICATIONS

DIPROSONE products are contraindicated in patients who are hypersensitive to betamethasone dipropionate, to other corticosteroids, or to any ingredient in these preparations.

PRECAUTIONS

General Systemic absorption of topical corticosteroids has produced reversible hypothalamic-pituitary-adrenal (HPA) axis suppression, manifestations of Cushing's syndrome, hyperglycemia, and glucosuria in some patients.

Conditions which augment systemic absorption include the application of the more potent steroids, use over large surface areas, prolonged use, and the addition of occlusive dressings. (See **DOSAGE AND ADMINISTRATION.**)

Therefore, patients receiving a large dose of a potent topical steroid applied to a large surface area should be evaluated periodically for evidence of HPA axis suppression by using the urinary-free cortisol and ACTH stimulation tests. If HPA axis suppression is noted, an attempt should be made to withdraw the drug, to reduce the frequency of application, or to substitute a less potent steroid.

Recovery of HPA axis function is generally prompt and complete upon discontinuation of the drug. Infrequently, signs and symptoms of steroid withdrawal may occur, requiring supplemental systemic corticosteroids.

Pediatric patients may absorb proportionally larger amounts of topical corticosteroids and thus be more susceptible to systemic toxicity. (See **PRECAUTIONS—Pediatric Use.**)

If irritation develops, topical corticosteroids should be discontinued and appropriate therapy instituted.

In the presence of dermatological infections, the use of an appropriate antifungal or antibacterial agent should be instituted. If a favorable response does not occur promptly, the corticosteroid should be discontinued until the infection has been adequately controlled.

Information for Patients This information is intended to aid in the safe and effective use of this medication. It is not a disclosure of all possible adverse or intended effects.

Patients using topical corticosteroids should receive the following information and instructions:

1. This medication is to be used as directed by the physician. It is for external use only. Avoid contact with the eyes.
2. Patients should be advised not to use this medication for any disorder other than that for which it was prescribed.
3. The treated skin area should not be bandaged or otherwise covered or wrapped as to be occlusive. (See **DOSAGE AND ADMINISTRATION.**)
4. Patients should report any signs of local adverse reactions.
5. Parents of pediatric patients should be advised not to use tight-fitting diapers or plastic pants on a patient being treated in the diaper area, as these garments may constitute occlusive dressing. (See **DOSAGE AND ADMINISTRATION.**)

Laboratory Tests The following tests may be helpful in evaluating HPA axis suppression:

Urinary-free cortisol test
ACTH stimulation test

Carcinogenesis, Mutagenesis, and Impairment of Fertility Long-term animal studies have not been performed to evaluate the carcinogenic potential or the effect on fertility of topical corticosteroids.

Studies to determine mutagenicity with prednisolone have revealed negative results.

Pregnancy Category C Corticosteroids are generally teratogenic in laboratory animals when administered systemically at relatively low dosage levels. The more potent corticosteroids have been shown to be teratogenic after dermal application in laboratory animals. There are no adequate and well-controlled studies in pregnant women on teratogenic effects from topically applied corticosteroids. Therefore, topical corticosteroids should be used during pregnancy only if the potential benefit justifies the potential risk to the fetus. Drugs of this class should not be used extensively on pregnant patients, in large amounts, or for prolonged periods of time.

Nursing Mothers It is not known whether topical administration of corticosteroids could result in sufficient systemic absorption to produce detectable quantities in breast milk. Systemically administered corticosteroids are secreted into breast milk in quantities not likely to have a deleterious effect on the infant. Nevertheless, caution should be exercised when topical corticosteroids are prescribed for a nursing woman.

Pediatric Use Pediatric patients may demonstrate greater susceptibility to topical corticosteroid-induced HPA axis suppression and Cushing's syndrome than mature patients because of a larger skin surface area to body weight ratio.

Hypothalamic-pituitary-adrenal (HPA) axis suppression, Cushing's syndrome, and intracranial hypertension have been reported in pediatric patients receiving topical corticosteroids. Manifestations of adrenal suppression in pediatric patients include linear growth retardation, delayed weight gain, low plasma cortisol levels, and absence of response to ACTH stimulation. Manifestations of intracranial hypertension include bulging fontanelles, headaches, and bilateral papilledema.

Administration of topical corticosteroids to pediatric patients should be limited to the least amount compatible with an effective therapeutic regimen. Chronic corticosteroid therapy may interfere with the growth and development of pediatric patients.

ADVERSE REACTIONS

The following local adverse reactions are reported infrequently when DIPROSONE products are used as recommended in the **DOSAGE AND ADMINISTRATION** section. These reactions are listed in an approximate decreasing order of occurrence: burning, itching, irritation, dryness, folliculitis, hypertrichosis, acneiform eruptions, hypopigmentation, perioral dermatitis, allergic contact dermatitis, maceration of the skin, secondary infection, skin atrophy, striae, miliaria.

Systemic absorption of topical corticosteroids has produced reversible hypothalamic-pituitary-adrenal (HPA) axis suppression, manifestations of Cushing's syndrome, hyperglycemia, and glucosuria in some patients.

OVERDOSAGE

Topically applied corticosteroids can be absorbed in sufficient amounts to produce systemic effects. (See **PRECAUTIONS.**)

DOSAGE AND ADMINISTRATION

DIPROSONE **Cream:** Apply a thin film of DIPROSONE **Cream** 0.05% to the affected skin areas once daily. In some cases, a twice-daily dosage may be necessary.

DIPROSONE **Lotion:** Apply a few drops of DIPROSONE **Lotion** to the affected area and massage lightly until it disappears. Apply twice daily, in the morning and at night. For the most effective and economical use, apply nozzle very close to affected area and gently squeeze bottle.

DIPROSONE **Ointment:** Apply a thin film of DIPROSONE **Ointment** to the affected skin areas once daily. In some cases, a twice-daily dosage may be necessary.

DIPROSONE products are not to be used with occlusive dressings.

HOW SUPPLIED

DIPROSONE **Cream** 0.05% is supplied in 15-g (NDC 0085-0853-02) and 45-g (NDC 0085-0853-03) tubes; boxes of one.

DIPROSONE **Lotion** 0.05% w/w is available in 20-mL (18.7-g) (NDC 0085-0028-04) and 60-mL (56.2-g) (NDC 0085-0028-06) plastic squeeze bottles; boxes of one. **Protect from light. Store in carton until contents are used.**

DIPROSONE **Ointment** 0.05% is supplied in 15-g (NDC 0085-0510-04) and 45-g (NDC 0085-0510-06) tubes; boxes of one.

Continued on next page

Information on Schering products appearing on these pages is effective as of January 2000.

Diprosone—Cont.

Store all DIPROSONE preparations between 2° and 30°C (36° and 86°F).
Schering Corporation
Kenilworth, NJ 07033 USA
Rev. 2/99

20860510T

ELOCON® ℞

brand of mometasone furoate cream
Cream 0.1%
For Dermatologic Use Only
Not for Ophthalmic Use

DESCRIPTION

ELOCON® (mometasone furoate cream) Cream contains mometasone furoate for dermatologic use. Mometasone furoate is a synthetic corticosteroid with anti-inflammatory activity.

Chemically, mometasone furoate is 9α,21-Dichloro-11β,17-dihydroxy-16α-methylpregna-1,4-diene-3,20-dione 17-(2-furoate), with the empirical formula $C_{27}H_{30}Cl_2O_6$, a molecular weight of 521.4 and the following structural formula:

Mometasone furoate is a white to off-white powder practically insoluble in water, slightly soluble in octanol, and moderately soluble in ethyl alcohol.

Each gram of ELOCON Cream 0.1% contains: 1 mg mometasone furoate in a cream base of hexylene glycol, phosphoric acid, propylene glycol stearate, stearyl alcohol and ceteareth-20, titanium dioxide, aluminum starch octenylsuccinate, white wax, white petrolatum, and purified water.

CLINICAL PHARMACOLOGY

Like other topical corticosteroids, mometasone furoate has anti-inflammatory, antipruritic, and vasoconstrictive properties. The mechanism of the anti-inflammatory activity of the topical steroids, in general, is unclear. However, corticosteroids are thought to act by the induction of phospholipase A_2 inhibitory proteins, collectively called lipocortins. It is postulated that these proteins control the biosynthesis of potent mediators of inflammation such as prostaglandins and leukotrienes by inhibiting the release of their common precursor arachidonic acid. Arachidonic acid is released from membrane phospholipids by phospholipase A_2.

Pharmacokinetics The extent of percutaneous absorption of topical corticosteroids is determined by many factors including the vehicle and the integrity of the epidermal barrier. Occlusive dressings with hydrocortisone for up to 24 hours have not been demonstrated to increase penetration; however, occlusion of hydrocortisone for 96 hours markedly enhances penetration. Studies in humans indicate that approximately 0.4% of the applied dose of ELOCON Cream 0.1% enters the circulation after 8 hours of contact on normal skin without occlusion. Inflammation and/or other disease processes in the skin may increase percutaneous absorption.

Studies performed with ELOCON Cream indicate that it is in the medium range of potency as compared with other topical corticosteroids.

In a pediatric trial, 24 atopic dermatitis patients, of which 19 patients were age 2 to 12 years, were treated with ELOCON Cream 0.1% once daily. The majority of patients cleared within 3 weeks.

INDICATIONS AND USAGE

ELOCON Cream 0.1% is a medium potency corticosteroid indicated for the relief of the inflammatory and pruritic manifestations of corticosteroid-responsive dermatoses.

ELOCON (mometasone furoate cream) Cream may be used in pediatric patients 2 years of age or older, although the safety and efficacy of drug use for longer than 3 weeks have not been established (see **PRECAUTIONS – Pediatric Use**). Since safety and efficacy of ELOCON Cream have not been established in pediatric patients below 2 years of age, its use in this age group is not recommended.

CONTRAINDICATIONS

ELOCON Cream is contraindicated in those patients with a history of hypersensitivity to any of the components in the preparation.

PRECAUTIONS

General Systemic absorption of topical corticosteroids can produce reversible hypothalamic-pituitary-adrenal (HPA) axis suppression with the potential for glucocorticosteroid insufficiency after withdrawal of treatment. Manifestations of Cushing's syndrome, hyperglycemia, and glucosuria can also be produced in some patients by systemic absorption of topical corticosteroids while on treatment.

Patients applying a topical steroid to a large surface area or to areas under occlusion should be evaluated periodically for evidence of HPA axis suppression. This may be done by using the ACTH stimulation, A.M. plasma cortisol, and urinary free cortisol tests.

In a study evaluating the effects of mometasone furoate cream on the hypothalamic-pituitary-adrenal (HPA) axis, 15 grams were applied twice daily for 7 days to six adult patients with psoriasis or atopic dermatitis. The cream was applied without occlusion to at least 30% of the body surface. The results show that the drug caused a slight lowering of adrenal corticosteroid secretion.

If HPA axis suppression is noted, an attempt should be made to withdraw the drug, to reduce the frequency of application, or to substitute a less potent corticosteroid. Recovery of HPA axis function is generally prompt upon discontinuation of topical corticosteroids. Infrequently, signs and symptoms of glucocorticosteroid insufficiency may occur requiring supplemental systemic corticosteroids. For information on systemic supplementation, see Prescribing Information for those products.

Pediatric patients may be more susceptible to systemic toxicity from equivalent doses due to their larger skin surface to body mass ratios (see **PRECAUTIONS – Pediatric Use**).

If irritation develops, ELOCON Cream should be discontinued and appropriate therapy instituted. Allergic contact dermatitis with corticosteroids is usually diagnosed by observing a failure to heal rather than noting a clinical exacerbation as with most topical products not containing corticosteroids. Such an observation should be corroborated with appropriate diagnostic patch testing.

If concomitant skin infections are present or develop, an appropriate antifungal or antibacterial agent should be used. If a favorable response does not occur promptly, use of ELOCON Cream should be discontinued until the infection has been adequately controlled.

Information for Patients Patients using topical corticosteroids should receive the following information and instructions:

1. This medication is to be used as directed by the physician. It is for external use only. Avoid contact with the eyes.
2. This medication should not be used for any disorder other than that for which it was prescribed.
3. The treated skin area should not be bandaged or otherwise covered or wrapped so as to be occlusive unless directed by the physician.
4. Patients should report to their physician any signs of local adverse reactions.
5. Parents of pediatric patients should be advised not to use ELOCON Cream in the treatment of diaper dermatitis. ELOCON Cream should not be applied in the diaper area as diapers or plastic pants may constitute occlusive dressing (see **DOSAGE AND ADMINISTRATION**).
6. This medication should not be used on the face, underarms, or groin areas unless directed by the physician.
7. As with other corticosteroids, therapy should be discontinued when control is achieved. If no improvement is seen within 2 weeks, contact the physician.

Laboratory Tests The following tests may be helpful in evaluating patients for HPA axis suppression:

ACTH stimulation test
A.M. plasma cortisol test
Urinary free cortisol test

Carcinogenesis, Mutagenesis, and Impairment of Fertility In studies of the effect of mometasone furoate on fertility, pregnancy, and postnatal development in rats and rabbits, 25 rats were treated with doses up to 1.2 mg/kg of drug topically, and 15 rabbits with doses up to 0.3 mg/kg of drug topically. The drugs were left on the skin for 6 hours daily during gestation. At the highest dosage, the rat dams lost weight. One of the rabbit dams at the highest dosage had wrinkled skin, muscle wasting and aborted 5 fetuses.

Genetic toxicity studies with mometasone furoate, which included the Ames test, mouse lymphoma assay, and a micronucleus test did not reveal any mutagenic potential.

Long term animal studies have not been performed to evaluate the carcinogenic potential of ELOCON (mometasone furoate cream) Cream.

Pregnancy Teratogenic effects: Pregnancy Category C Corticosteroids have been shown to be teratogenic in laboratory animals when administered systemically at relatively low dosage levels. Some corticosteroids have been shown to be teratogenic after dermal application in laboratory animals.

Rat offspring of dams treated with 1.2 mg/kg of mometasone furoate topically (4 times the maximum dose in a 50 kg individual) displayed umbilical hernias, unossified sternebrae and vertebrae, and wavy ribs, as well as markedly depressed fetal growth. Rabbit offspring of dams treated with up to 0.3 mg/kg of mometasone furoate topically (the same dose as the maximum dose in a 50 kg individual) displayed flexed paws, umbilical hernias, and cleft palate. A 50 kg female using 1 gram of ELOCON Cream would apply approximately 0.023 mg/kg.

There are no adequate and well-controlled studies of the teratogenic potential of mometasone furoate in pregnant women. ELOCON Cream should be used during pregnancy only if the potential benefit justifies the potential risk to the fetus.

Nursing Mothers Systemically administered corticosteroids appear in human milk and could suppress growth, interfere with endogenous corticosteroid production, or cause other untoward effects. It is not known whether topical administration of corticosteroids could result in sufficient systemic absorption to produce detectable quantities in human milk. Because many drugs are excreted in human milk, caution should be exercised when ELOCON Cream is administered to a nursing woman.

Pediatric Use ELOCON Cream may be used with caution in pediatric patients 2 years of age or older, although the safety and efficacy of drug use for longer than 3 weeks have not been established. Use of ELOCON Cream is supported by results from adequate and well-controlled studies in pediatric patients with corticosteroid-responsive dermatoses. Since safety and efficacy of ELOCON Cream have not been established in pediatric patients below 2 years of age, its use in this age group is not recommended. Because of a higher ratio of skin surface area to body mass, pediatric patients are at a greater risk than adults of HPA axis suppression and Cushing's syndrome when they are treated with topical corticosteroids. They are, therefore, also at greater risk of adrenal insufficiency during and/or after withdrawal of treatment. Pediatric patients may be more susceptible than adults to skin atrophy, including striae, when they are treated with topical corticosteroids. Pediatric patients applying topical corticosteroids to greater than 20% of body surface are at higher risk of HPA axis suppression.

HPA axis suppression, Cushing's syndrome, linear growth retardation, delayed weight gain, and intracranial hypertension have been reported in pediatric patients receiving topical corticosteroids. Manifestations of adrenal suppression in children include low plasma cortisol levels, and an absence of response to ACTH stimulation. Manifestations of intracranial hypertension include bulging fontanelles, headaches, and bilateral papilledema.

ELOCON (mometasone furoate cream) Cream should not be used in the treatment of diaper dermatitis.

ADVERSE REACTIONS

In controlled clinical studies involving 319 patients, the incidence of adverse reactions associated with the use of ELOCON Cream was 1.6%. Reported reactions included burning, pruritus, and skin atrophy. Reports of rosacea associated with the use of ELOCON Cream have also been received. In controlled clinical studies (n=74) involving pediatric patients 2 to 12 years of age, the incidence of adverse experiences associated with the use of ELOCON Cream was approximately 7%. Reported reactions included stinging, pruritus, and furunculosis.

The following additional local adverse reactions have been reported infrequently with topical corticosteroids, but may occur more frequently with the use of occlusive dressings. These reactions are listed in an approximate decreasing order of occurrence: irritation, dryness, folliculitis, hypertrichosis, acneiform eruptions, hypopigmentation, perioral dermatitis, allergic contact dermatitis, secondary infection, striae, and miliaria.

OVERDOSAGE

Topically applied ELOCON Cream can be absorbed in sufficient amounts to produce systemic effects (see **PRECAUTIONS**).

DOSAGE AND ADMINISTRATION

Apply a thin film of ELOCON Cream to the affected skin areas once daily. ELOCON Cream may be used in pediatric patients 2 years of age or older. Safety and efficacy of ELOCON Cream in pediatric patients for more than 3 weeks of use have not been established. Use in pediatric patients under 2 years of age is not recommended.

As with other corticosteroids, therapy should be discontinued when control is achieved. If no improvement is seen within 2 weeks, reassessment of diagnosis may be necessary.

ELOCON Cream should not be used with occlusive dressings unless directed by a physician. ELOCON Cream should not be applied in the diaper area if the child still requires diapers or plastic pants as these garments may constitute occlusive dressing.

HOW SUPPLIED

ELOCON Cream 0.1% is supplied in 15 g (NDC 0085-0567-01) and 45 g (NDC 0085-0567-02) tubes; boxes of one.

Store ELOCON Cream between 2° and 25°C (36° and 77°F).
Schering Corporation
Kenilworth, NJ 07033 USA
Revised 8/95 14112839

18724308T

ELOCON® ℞

brand of mometasone furoate
Lotion 0.1%
For Dermatologic Use Only
Not for Ophthalmic Use

DESCRIPTION

ELOCON Lotion 0.1% contains mometasone furoate, USP, for dermatologic use. Mometasone furoate is a synthetic corticosteroid with anti-inflammatory activity.

Chemically, mometasone furoate is 9α, 21-Dichloro-11β, 17-dihydroxy-16α-methylpregna-1, 4-diene-3, 20 dione 17-(2-furoate), with the empirical formula $C_{27}H_{30}Cl_2O_6$, a molecular weight of 521.4 and the following structural formula:

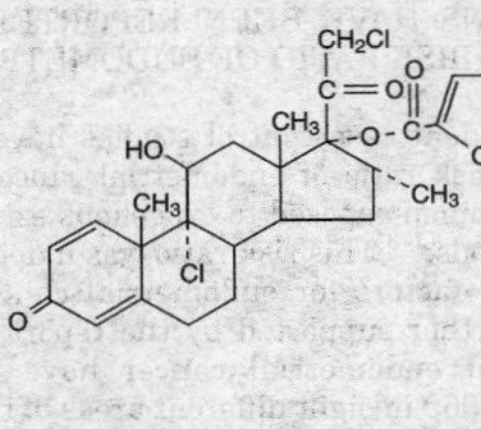

Mometasone furoate is a white to off-white powder practically insoluble in water, slightly soluble in octanol, and moderately soluble in ethyl alcohol.
Each gram of ELOCON Lotion 0.1% contains: 1 mg of mometasone furoate, USP, in a lotion base of isopropyl alcohol, USP (40%); propylene glycol, USP; hydyroxypropyl cellulose, NF; sodium phosphate monobasic monohydrate, R; and purified water, USP. May also contain phosphoric acid NF to adjust the pH to approximately 4.5.

CLINICAL PHARMACOLOGY

The corticosteroids are a class of compounds comprising steroid hormones secreted by the adrenal cortex and their synthetic analogs. In pharmacologic doses corticosteroids are used primarily for their anti-inflammatory and/or immunosuppressive effects.
Topical corticosteroids, such as mometasone furoate, are effective in the treatment of corticosteroid-responsive dermatoses primarily because of their anti-inflammatory, antipruritic, and vasoconstrictive actions. However, while the physiologic, pharmacologic, and clinical effects of the corticosteroids are well known, the exact mechanisms of their actions in each disease are uncertain. Mometasone furoate has been shown to have topical (dermatologic) and systemic pharmacologic and metabolic effects characteristic of this class of drugs.

Pharmacokinetics The extent of percutaneous absorption of topical corticosteroids is determined by many factors including the vehicle, the integrity of the epidermal barrier, and the use of occlusive dressings. (See **DOSAGE AND ADMINISTRATION**.) Topical corticosteroids can be absorbed from normal intact skin.
A study using a radio-labelled ^3H mometasone furoate ointment (0.1%) formulation was performed in man to measure systemic absorption and excretion. Results showed that approximately 0.7% of the steroid was absorbed during 8 hours of contact, without occlusion, with intact skin of normal volunteers. A similar minimal degree of absorption of the corticosteroid from the lotion formulation would be anticipated.
Inflammation and/or disease processes in the skin increase percutaneous absorption. Occlusive dressings substantially increase the percutaneous absorption of topical corticosteroids. (See **DOSAGE AND ADMINISTRATION**.)
Mometasone furoate lotion was applied at 15 mL twice daily (30 mL per day) to diseased skin (patients with scalp and body psoriasis) of four patients for seven days, to study its effects on the hypothalamic-pituitary-adrenal (HPA) axis. Plasma cortisol levels for each of the four patients remained well within the normal range and changed little from baseline.
Once absorbed through the skin, topical corticosteroids are handled through pharmacokinetic pathways similar to systemically administered corticosteroids. Corticosteroids are bound to plasma proteins in varying degrees. Corticosteroids are metabolized primarily in the liver and are then excreted by the kidneys. Some of the topical corticosteroids and their metabolites are also excreted into the bile.

INDICATIONS AND USAGE

ELOCON Lotion is indicated for the relief of the inflammatory and pruritic manifestations of corticosteroid-responsive dermatoses.

CONTRAINDICATIONS

ELOCON Lotion is contraindicated in patients who are hypersensitive to mometasone furoate, to other corticosteroids, or to any ingredient in this preparation.

PRECAUTIONS

General Systemic absorption of potent topical corticosteroids has produced reversible hypothalamic-pituitary-adrenal (HPA) axis suppression, manifestations of Cushing's syndrome, hyperglycemia, and glucosuria in some patients. Conditions which augment systemic absorption include application of more potent steroids, use over large surface areas, prolonged use, use in areas where the epidermal barrier is disrupted, and the use of occlusive dressings. (See **DOSAGE AND ADMINISTRATION**.)
Patients receiving a large dose of a potent topical steroid applied to a large surface area or under an occlusive dressing should be evaluated periodically for evidence of HPA axis suppression by using the urinary free cortisol and ACTH stimulation tests. If HPA axis suppression is noted, an attempt should be made to withdraw the drug, to reduce the frequency of application, or to substitute a less potent steroid.
Recovery of HPA axis function is generally prompt and complete upon discontinuation of the drug. Infrequently, signs and symptoms of steroid withdrawal may occur, requiring supplemental systemic corticosteroids.
Children may absorb proportionally larger amounts of topical corticosteroids and thus be more susceptible to systemic toxicity. (See **PRECAUTIONS—Pediatric Use**.)
If irritation develops, topical corticosteroids should be discontinued and appropriate therapy instituted.
In the presence of dermatological infections, use of an appropriate antifungal or antibacterial agent should be instituted. If a favorable response does not occur promptly, the corticosteroid should be discontinued until the infection has been adequately controlled.

Information for Patients Patients using topical corticosteroids should receive the following information and instructions. This information is intended to aid in the safe and effective use of this medication. It is not a disclosure of all possible adverse or intended effects.

1. This medication is to be used as directed by the physician. It is for external use only. Avoid contact with the eyes.
2. Patients should be advised not to use this medication for any disorder other than that for which it was prescribed.
3. The treated skin area should not be bandaged or otherwise covered or wrapped as to be occlusive unless directed by the physician. (See **DOSAGE AND ADMINISTRATION**.)
4. Patients should report any signs of local adverse reactions.
5. Parents of pediatric patients should be advised not to use tight-fitting diapers or plastic pants on a child being treated in the diaper area, as these garments may constitute occlusive dressing. (See **DOSAGE AND ADMINISTRATION**.)

Laboratory Tests The following tests may be helpful in evaluating HPA axis suppression:
Urinary free cortisol test
ACTH stimulation test

Carcinogenesis, Mutagenesis, and Impairment of Fertility Long-term animal studies have not been performed to evaluate the carcinogenic potential or the effect on fertility of topical corticosteroids.
Genetic toxicity studies with mometasone furoate, which included the Ames test, mouse lymphoma assay, and a micronucleus test, did not reveal any mutagenic potential.

Pregnancy Category C Corticosteroids are generally teratogenic in laboratory animals when administered systemically at relatively low dosage levels. Corticosteroids have been shown to be teratogenic after dermal application in laboratory animals. There are no adequate and well-controlled studies of teratogenic effects from topically applied corticosteroids in pregnant women. Therefore, topical corticosteroids should be used during pregnancy only if the potential benefit justifies the potential risk to the fetus. Drugs of this class should not be used extensively on pregnant patients, in large amounts, or for prolonged periods.

Nursing Mothers It is not known whether topical administration of corticosteroids could result in sufficient systemic absorption to produce detectable quantities in breast milk. Systemically administered corticosteroids are secreted into breast milk in quantities not likely to have a deleterious effect on the infant. Nevertheless, a decision should be made whether to discontinue nursing or to discontinue the drug, taking into account the importance of the drug to the mother.

Pediatric Use Pediatric patients may demonstrate greater susceptibility to topical corticosteroid-induced HPA axis suppression and Cushing's syndrome than mature patients because of a larger skin surface area to body weight ratio.
Hypothalamic-pituitary-adrenal (HPA) axis suppression, Cushing's syndrome, and intracranial hypertension have been reported in children receiving topical corticosteroids. Manifestations of adrenal suppression in children include linear growth retardation, delayed weight gain, low plasma cortisol levels, and absence of response to ACTH stimulation. Manifestations of intracranial hypertension include bulging fontanelles, headaches, and bilateral papilledema. Administration of topical corticosteroids to children should be limited to the least amount compatible with an effective therapeutic regimen. Chronic corticosteroid therapy may interfere with the growth and development of children.

ADVERSE REACTIONS

The following local adverse reactions were reported with ELOCON Lotion during clinical studies with 209 patients: acneiform reaction, 2; burning, 4; and itching, 1. In an irritation/sensitization study with 156 normal subjects, folliculitis was reported in 4.
The following local adverse reactions have been reported infrequently when other topical dermatologic corticosteroids have been used as recommended. These reactions are listed in an approximate decreasing order of occurrence: burning, itching, irritation, dryness, folliculitis, hypertrichosis, acneiform eruptions, hypopigmentation, perioral dermatitis, allergic contact dermatitis, maceration of the skin, secondary infection, skin atrophy, striae, miliaria.

OVERDOSAGE

Topically applied corticosteroids can be absorbed in sufficient amounts to produce systemic effects. (See **PRECAUTIONS**.)

DOSAGE AND ADMINISTRATION

Apply a few drops of ELOCON Lotion to the affected areas once daily and massage lightly until it disappears. For the most effective and economical use, hold the nozzle of the bottle very close to the affected areas and gently squeeze.

HOW SUPPLIED

ELOCON Lotion 0.1% is supplied in 30 mL (27.5 g) (NDC 0085-0854-01) and 60 mL (55 g) (NDC 0085-0854-02) bottles; boxes of one.
Store ELOCON Lotion between 2° and 30°C (36° and 86°F).
Schering Corporation
Kenilworth, NJ 07033 USA
Rev. 1/99 17980912

ELOCON® ℞
brand of mometasone furoate
ointment
Ointment 0.1%
For Dermatologic Use Only
Not for Ophthalmic Use

DESCRIPTION

ELOCON® (mometasone furoate ointment) Ointment contains mometasone furoate for dermatologic use. Mometasone furoate is a synthetic corticosteroid with anti-inflammatory activity.
Chemically, mometasone furoate is 9α,21-Dichloro-11β,17-dihydroxy-16α-methylpregna-1,4-diene-3,20-dione 17-(2-furoate), with the empirical formula $C_{27}H_{30}Cl_2O_6$, a molecular weight of 521.4 and the following structural formula:

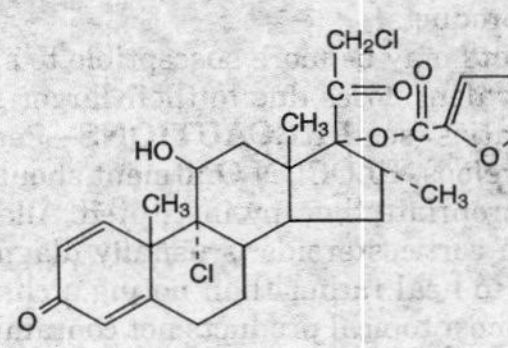

Mometasone furoate is a white to off-white powder practically insoluble in water, slightly soluble in octanol, and moderately soluble in ethyl alcohol.
Each gram of ELOCON Ointment 0.1% contains: 1 mg mometasone furoate in an ointment base of hexylene glycol, phosphoric acid, propylene glycol stearate, white wax, white petrolatum, and purified water.

CLINICAL PHARMACOLOGY

Like other topical corticosteroids, mometasone furoate has anti-inflammatory, anti-pruritic, and vasoconstrictive properties. The mechanism of the anti-inflammatory activity of the topical steroids, in general, is unclear. However, corticosteroids are thought to act by the induction of phospholipase A_2 inhibitory proteins, collectively called lipocortins. It is postulated that these proteins control the biosynthesis of potent mediators of inflammation such as prostaglandins and leukotrienes by inhibiting the release of their common precursor arachidonic acid. Arachidonic acid is released from membrane phospholipids by phospholipase A_2.

Pharmacokinetics The extent of percutaneous absorption of topical corticosteroids is determined by many factors including the vehicle and the integrity of the epidermal barrier. Occlusive dressings with hydrocortisone for up to 24 hours have not been demonstrated to increase penetration; however, occlusion of hydrocortisone for 96 hours markedly enhances penetration. Studies in humans indicate that approximately 0.7% of the applied dose of ELOCON Ointment 0.1% enters the circulation after 8 hours of contact on normal skin without occlusion. Inflammation and/or other disease processes in the skin may increase percutaneous absorption.
Studies performed with ELOCON Ointment indicate that it is in the medium range of potency as compared with other topical corticosteroids.
In a pediatric trial, 24 atopic dermatitis patients, of which 19 patients were age 2 to 12 years, were treated with ELOCON Cream 0.1% once daily. The majority of patients cleared within 3 weeks.

INDICATIONS AND USAGE

ELOCON Ointment 0.1% is a medium potency corticosteroid indicated for the relief of the inflammatory and pruritic manifestations of corticosteroid-responsive dermatoses.
ELOCON (mometasone furoate ointment) Ointment may be used in pediatric patients 2 years of age or older, although the safety and efficacy of drug use for longer than 3 weeks have not been established (see **PRECAUTIONS—Pediatric Use**). Since safety and efficacy of ELOCON Ointment have not been established in pediatric patients below 2 years of age, its use in this age group is not recommended.

Continued on next page

Information on Schering products appearing on these pages is effective as of January 2000.

Elocon Ointment—Cont.

CONTRAINDICATIONS

ELOCON Ointment is contraindicated in those patients with a history of hypersensitivity to any of the components in the preparation.

PRECAUTIONS

General Systemic absorption of topical corticosteroids can produce reversible hypothalamic-pituitary-adrenal (HPA) axis suppression with the potential for glucocorticosteroid insufficiency after withdrawal of treatment. Manifestations of Cushing's syndrome, hyperglycemia, and glucosuria can also be produced in some patients by systemic absorption of topical corticosteroids while on treatment.

Patients applying a topical steroid to a large surface area or areas under occlusion should be evaluated periodically for evidence of HPA axis suppression. This may be done by using the ACTH stimulation, A.M. plasma cortisol, and urinary free cortisol tests.

In a study evaluating the effects of mometasone furoate ointment on the hypothalamic-pituitary-adrenal (HPA) axis, 15 grams were applied twice daily for 7 days to six adult patients with psoriasis or atopic dermatitis. The ointment was applied without occlusion to at least 30% of the body surface. The results show that the drug caused a slight lowering of adrenal corticosteroid secretion.

If HPA axis suppression is noted, an attempt should be made to withdraw the drug, to reduce the frequency of application, or to substitute a less potent corticosteroid. Recovery of HPA axis function is generally prompt upon discontinuation of topical corticosteroids. Infrequently, signs and symptoms of glucocorticosteroid insufficiency may occur requiring supplemental systemic corticosteroids. For information on systemic supplementation, see Prescribing Information for those products.

Pediatric patients may be more susceptible to systemic toxicity from equivalent doses due to their larger skin surface to body mass ratios (see **PRECAUTIONS—Pediatric Use**).

If irritation develops, ELOCON Ointment should be discontinued and appropriate therapy instituted. Allergic contact dermatitis with corticosteroids is usually diagnosed by observing failure to heal rather than noting a clinical exacerbation as with most topical products not containing corticosteroids. Such an observation should be corroborated with appropriate diagnostic patch testing.

If concomitant skin infections are present or develop, an appropriate antifungal or antibacterial agent should be used. If a favorable response does not occur promptly, use of ELOCON Ointment should be discontinued until the infection has been adequately controlled.

Information for Patients Patients using topical corticosteroids should receive the following information and instructions:

1. This medication is to be used as directed by the physician. It is for external use only. Avoid contact with the eyes.
2. This medication should not be used for any disorder other than that for which it was prescribed.
3. The treated skin area should not be bandaged or otherwise covered or wrapped so as to be occlusive unless directed by the physician.
4. Patients should report to their physician any signs of local adverse reactions.
5. Parents of pediatric patients should be advised not to use ELOCON Ointment in the treatment of diaper dermatitis. ELOCON Ointment should not be applied in the diaper area as diapers or plastic pants may constitute occlusive dressing (see **DOSAGE AND ADMINISTRATION**).
6. This medication should not be used on the face, underarms, or groin areas unless directed by the physician.
7. As with other corticosteroids, therapy should be discontinued when control is achieved. If no improvement is seen within 2 weeks, contact the physician.

Laboratory Tests The following tests may be helpful in evaluating patients for HPA axis suppression:

ACTH stimulation test
A.M. plasma cortisol test
Urinary free cortisol test

Carcinogenesis, Mutagenesis, and Impairment of Fertility

In studies of the effect of mometasone furoate on fertility, pregnancy, and postnatal development in rats and rabbits, 25 rats were treated with doses up to 1.2 mg/kg of drug topically, and 15 rabbits with doses up to 0.3 mg/kg of drug topically. The drugs were left on the skin for 6 hours daily during gestation. At the highest dosage, the rat dams lost weight. One of the rabbit dams at the highest dosage had wrinkled skin, muscle wasting and aborted 5 fetuses.

Genetic toxicity studies with mometasone furoate, which included the Ames test, mouse lymphoma assay, and a micronucleus test did not reveal any mutagenic potential.

Long term animal studies have not been performed to evaluate the carcinogenic potential of ELOCON (mometasone furoate ointment) Ointment.

Pregnancy Teratogenic effects: Pregnancy Category C Corticosteroids have been shown to be teratogenic in laboratory animals when administered systemically at relatively low dosage levels. Some corticosteroids have been shown to be teratogenic after dermal application in laboratory animals.

Rat offspring of dams treated with 1.2 mg/kg of mometasone furoate topically (4 times the maximum dose in a 50 kg individual) displayed umbilical hernias, unossified sternebrae and vertebrae, and wavy ribs, as well as markedly depressed fetal growth. Rabbit offspring of dams treated with up to 0.3 mg/kg of mometasone furoate topically (the same dose as the maximum dose in a 50 kg individual) displayed flexed paws, umbilical hernias, and cleft palate. A 50 kg female using 1 gram of ELOCON Ointment would apply approximately 0.023 mg/kg.

There are no adequate and well-controlled studies of the teratogenic potential of mometasone furoate in pregnant women. Therefore, ELOCON Ointment should be used during pregnancy only if the potential benefit justifies the potential risk to the fetus.

Nursing Mothers Systemically administered corticosteroids appear in human milk and could suppress growth, interfere with endogenous corticosteroid production, or cause other untoward effects. It is not known whether topical administration of corticosteroids could result in sufficient systemic absorption to produce detectable quantities in human milk. Because many drugs are excreted in human milk, caution should be exercised when ELOCON Ointment is administered to a nursing woman.

Pediatric Use ELOCON Ointment may be used with caution in pediatric patients 2 years of age or older, although the safety and efficacy of drug use for longer than 3 weeks have not been established. Use of ELOCON Ointment is supported by results from adequate and well-controlled studies in pediatric patients with corticosteroid-responsive dermatoses. Since safety and efficacy of ELOCON Ointment have not been established in pediatric patients below 2 years of age, its use in this age group is not recommended. Because of a higher ratio of skin surface area to body mass, pediatric patients are at a greater risk than adults of HPA axis suppression and Cushing's syndrome when they are treated with topical corticosteroids. They are, therefore, also at greater risk of glucocorticosteroid insufficiency during and/or after withdrawal of treatment. Pediatric patients may be more susceptible than adults to skin atrophy, including striae, when they are treated with topical corticosteroids. Pediatric patients applying topical corticosteroids to greater than 20% of body surface are at higher risk of HPA axis suppression.

HPA axis suppression, Cushing's syndrome, linear growth retardation, delayed weight gain, and intracranial hypertension have been reported in children receiving topical corticosteroids. Manifestations of adrenal suppression in children include low plasma cortisol levels, and absence of response to ACTH stimulation. Manifestations of intracranial hypertension include bulging fontanelles, headaches, and bilateral papilledema.

ELOCON (mometasone furoate ointment) Ointment should not be used in the treatment of diaper dermatitis.

ADVERSE REACTIONS

In controlled clinical studies involving 812 patients, the incidence of adverse reactions associated with the use of ELOCON Ointment was 4.8%. Reported reactions included burning, pruritus, skin atrophy, tingling/stinging, and furunculosis. Reports of rosacea associated with the use of ELOCON Ointment have been received. In controlled clinical studies (n=74) involving pediatric patients 2 to 12 years of age, the incidence of adverse experiences associated with the use of ELOCON Cream is approximately 7%. Reported reactions included stinging, pruritus, and furunculosis.

The following additional local adverse reactions have been reported infrequently with topical corticosteroids, but may occur more frequently with the use of occlusive dressings. These reactions are listed in an approximate decreasing order of occurrence: irritation, dryness, folliculitis, hypertrichosis, acneiform eruptions, hypopigmentation, perioral dermatitis, allergic contact dermatitis, secondary infection, striae, and miliaria.

OVERDOSAGE

Topically applied ELOCON Ointment can be absorbed in sufficient amounts to produce systemic effects (see **PRECAUTIONS**).

DOSAGE AND ADMINISTRATION

Apply a thin film of ELOCON Ointment to the affected skin areas once daily. ELOCON Ointment may be used in pediatric patients 2 years of age or older. Safety and efficacy of ELOCON Ointment in pediatric patients for more than 3 weeks have not been established. Use in pediatric patients under 2 years of age is not recommended.

As with other corticosteroids, therapy should be discontinued when control is achieved. If no improvement is seen within 2 weeks, reassessment of diagnosis may be necessary.

ELOCON Ointment should not be used with occlusive dressings unless directed by a physician. ELOCON Ointment should not be applied in the diaper area if the child still requires diapers or plastic pants as these garments may constitute occlusive dressing.

HOW SUPPLIED

ELOCON Ointment 0.1% is supplied in 15 g (NDC 0085-0370-01) and 45 g (NDC 0085-0370-02) tubes; boxes of one.

Store ELOCON Ointment between 2° and 30°C (36° and 86°F).

Schering Corporation
Kenilworth, NJ 07033 USA
Revised 8/95 14112626
18724200T

ESTINYL® ℞
brand of ethinyl estradiol
Tablets, USP

WARNINGS

1. ESTROGENS HAVE BEEN REPORTED TO INCREASE THE RISK RATIO OF ENDOMETRIAL CARCINOMA.

Three independent case control studies have reported an increased risk ratio of endometrial cancer in postmenopausal women exposed to exogenous estrogens for prolonged periods.[1–3] This risk ratio was independent of the other risk factors for endometrial cancer. These studies are further supported by the report that incidence rates of endometrial cancer have increased sharply since 1969 in eight different areas of the United States with population-based cancer reporting systems, an increase which may be related to the rapidly expanding use of estrogens during the last decade.[4]

The three case control studies reported that the risk ratio of endometrial cancer in estrogen users was about 4.5 to 13.9 times greater than in nonusers. The risk ratio appears to depend on both duration of treatment[1] and on estrogen dose.[3] In view of these reports, when estrogens are used for the treatment of menopausal symptoms, the lowest dose that will control symptoms should be utilized and medication should be discontinued as soon as possible. When prolonged treatment is medically indicated, the patient should be reassessed on at least a semi-annual basis to determine the need for continued therapy. Although the evidence must be considered preliminary, one study suggests that cyclic administration of low doses of estrogen may carry less risk than continuous administration[3]; it therefore appears prudent to utilize such a regimen.

Close clinical surveillance of all women taking estrogens is important. In all cases of undiagnosed persistent or recurring abnormal vaginal bleeding, adequate diagnostic measures should be undertaken to rule out malignancy.

There is no evidence at present that "natural" estrogens are more or less hazardous than "synthetic" estrogens at equiestrogenic doses.

2. ESTROGENS SHOULD NOT BE USED DURING PREGNANCY.

The use of estrogens during early pregnancy may seriously damage the offspring. It has been reported that females exposed in utero to diethylstilbestrol, a nonsteroidal estrogen, may have an increased risk of developing in later life a form of vaginal or cervical cancer that is ordinarily extremely rare.[5,6] This risk has been estimated statistically as not greater than 4 per 1000 exposures.[7] In certain studies, a high percentage of such exposed women (from 30% to 90%) have been found to have vaginal adenosis,[8–11] epithelial changes of the vagina and cervix. Although these changes are histologically benign, it is not known whether they are precursors of malignancy. Although similar data are not available with the use of other estrogens, it cannot be presumed they would not induce similar changes. Exposure to diethylstilbestrol has also been associated with adverse effects on reproductive performance, including increased rates of spontaneous abortion, ectopic pregnancy, premature deliveries, and perinatal deaths.

Several reports suggest an association between intrauterine fetal exposure to female sex hormones and congenital anomalies, including congenital heart defects and limb reduction defects.[12–15] One case control study[15] estimated a 4.7-fold increased risk of limb reduction defects in infants exposed in utero to sex hormones (oral contraceptives, hormone withdrawal tests for pregnancy, or attempted treatment for threatened abortion). Some of these exposures were very short and involved only a few days of treatment. The data suggests that the risk of limb reduction defects in exposed fetuses is somewhat less than 1 per 1000.

In the past, estrogens have been used during pregnancy in an attempt to treat threatened or habitual abortion. There is considerable evidence that estrogens are ineffective for these indications.

If ESTINYL Tablets are used during pregnancy, or if the patient becomes pregnant while taking this drug, she should be apprised of the potential risks to the fetus, and the advisability of pregnancy continuation.

DESCRIPTION

ESTINYL Tablets contain ethinyl estradiol, USP, a potent synthetic estrogen, having the chemical name 19-Nor-17α-pregna-1,3,5(10)-trien-20-yne-3,17-diol; the chemical formula $C_{20}H_{24}O_2$; molecular weight of 296.41; and the following structural formula:

OH CH3 ---C≡CH H H H HO

Ethinyl estradiol is a white to creamy white, odorless, crystalline powder. It is insoluble in water, soluble in alcohol, chloroform, ether, and vegetable oils.

Biologically, estrogens may be defined as compounds capable of stimulating female secondary sex characteristics. Chemically, there are different groups of estrogens, depending on whether they are natural or synthetic, steroidal or nonsteroidal. Natural human estrogens are ultimately formed from either androstenedione or testosterone as immediate precursors. Ethinyl estradiol is a synthetic, steroidal estrogen.

ESTINYL, for oral administration, is available in tablets containing 0.02 or 0.05 mg ethinyl estradiol, USP.

The inactive ingredients for ESTINYL Tablets 0.02 mg include: acacia, butylparaben, calcium phosphate, calcium sulfate, carnauba wax, corn starch, FD&C Blue No. 2 Al Lake, FD&C Yellow No. 5, FD&C Yellow No. 5 Al Lake, FD&C Yellow No. 6 Al Lake, gelatin, lactose, magnesium stearate, potato starch, sodium phosphate, sugar, and white wax. May also contain talc.

The inactive ingredients for ESTINYL Tablets 0.05 mg include: acacia, butylparaben, calcium phosphate, calcium sulfate, carnauba wax, corn starch, FD&C Blue No. 1, FD&C Red No. 3, gelatin, lactose, magnesium stearate, potato starch, sodium phosphate, and white wax. May also contain talc.

CLINICAL PHARMACOLOGY

Ethinyl estradiol is a synthetic derivative of the natural estrogen, estradiol.

Ethinyl estradiol, like estradiol, promotes growth of the endometrium and thickening, stratification, and cornification of the vagina. It causes growth of the ducts of the mammary glands, but inhibits lactation. It also inhibits the anterior pituitary and causes capillary dilatation, fluid retention, and protein anabolism.

Estradiol is the major estrogen in premenopausal women, with up to 100 to 600 mcg being secreted daily by the ovary. Natural estrogens are poorly effective when given by mouth. Apparently this is due to rapid clearance of the endogenous hormone from blood, along with a "first-pass-effect" after oral administration. The addition of a 17-alpha-ethinyl group to estradiol increases potency and enhances oral activity by impeding hepatic degradation. The oral efficacy of ethinyl estradiol is related to slower elimination than estradiol from the circulation. A part of ingested ethinyl estradiol is excreted in glucuronide form via urine in animals and in man, but also extensive metabolism of the steroid nucleus occurs. The major metabolism takes place mainly in the liver. Large amounts of ethinyl estradiol metabolites are excreted via human bile, much similar to what has been reported for estradiol. However, unlike estradiol, ethinyl estradiol metabolites do not exclusively leave via urine. Urinary recovery is much less than that of estradiol and substantial amounts of ethinyl estradiol metabolites appear in human feces. Quantitatively, the major metabolic pathway for ethinyl estradiol, both in rats and in humans, is aromatic hydroxylation, as it is for the natural estrogens.

Rapid and complete absorption follows oral intake of ethinyl estradiol. Elimination of ethinyl estradiol from plasma proceeds slower than that of estradiol. After oral administration, an initial peak occurs in plasma at 2 to 3 hours, with a secondary peak at about 12 hours after dosing; the second peak is interpreted as evidence for extensive enterohepatic circulation of ethinyl estradiol.

INDICATIONS AND USAGE

ESTINYL Tablets are indicated in the treatment of: 1) Moderate to severe *vasomotor* symptoms associated with the menopause. (There is no evidence that estrogens are effective for nervous symptoms or depression which might occur during menopause, and they should not be used to treat these conditions.) 2) Female hypogonadism. 3) Prostatic carcinoma-palliative therapy of advanced disease. 4) Breast cancer (for palliation only) in appropriately selected women, such as those who are more than 5 years postmenopausal with progressing inoperable or radiation-resistant disease.

ETHINYL ESTRADIOL HAS NOT BEEN SHOWN TO BE EFFECTIVE FOR ANY PURPOSE DURING PREGNANCY AND ITS USE MAY CAUSE SEVERE HARM TO THE FETUS (SEE BOXED **WARNINGS**).

The lowest effective dose appropriate for the specific indication should be used. Studies of the addition of a progestin for 7 or more days of a cycle of estrogen administration have reported a lowered incidence of endometrial hyperplasia. Morphological and biochemical studies of endometrium suggest that 10 to 13 days of progestin are needed to provide maximal maturation of the endometrium and to eliminate any hyperplastic changes. Whether this will provide protection from endometrial carcinoma has not been clearly established. There are possible additional risks which may be associated with the inclusion of progestin in estrogen replacement regimens. The potential risks include adverse effects on carbohydrate and lipid metabolism. The choice of progestin and dosage may be important in minimizing these adverse effects.

CONTRAINDICATIONS

Estrogens should not be used in women (or men) with any of the following conditions:

1. Known or suspected cancer of the breast except in appropriately selected patients being treated for metastatic disease.
2. Known or suspected estrogen-dependent neoplasia.
3. Known or suspected pregnancy (see boxed **WARNINGS**).
4. Undiagnosed abnormal genital bleeding.
5. Active thrombophlebitis or thromboembolic disorders.
6. A past history of thrombophlebitis, thrombosis, or thromboembolic disorders associated with previous estrogen use (except when used in treatment of breast or prostatic malignancy).

WARNINGS

1. *Induction of malignant neoplasms.* Long-term continuous administration of natural and synthetic estrogens in certain animal species increases the frequency of carcinomas of the breast, cervix, vagina, and liver. There is now evidence that estrogens increase the risk of carcinoma of the endometrium in humans. (See boxed **WARNINGS**.)

At the present time there is no satisfactory evidence that estrogens given to postmenopausal women increase the risk of cancer of the breast,[16] although a recent long-term follow-up of a single physician's practice has raised this possibility.[17] Because of the animal data, there is a need for caution in prescribing estrogens for women with a strong family history of breast cancer or who have breast nodules, fibrocystic disease, or abnormal mammograms.

Estrogens have been reported to be associated with carcinoma of the male breast and suspicious lesions in males receiving estrogen therapy should be investigated accordingly.

2. *Gallbladder disease.* A recent study has reported a 2- to 3-fold increase in the risk of surgically confirmed gallbladder disease in women receiving postmenopausal estrogens,[16] similar to the 2-fold increase previously noted in users of oral contraceptives.[18,22] In the case of oral contraceptives, the increased risk appeared after 2 years of use.[22]

3. *Effects similar to those caused by estrogen-progestagen oral contraceptives.* There are several serious adverse effects of oral contraceptives, most of which have not, up to now, been documented as consequences of postmenopausal estrogen therapy. This may reflect the comparatively low doses of estrogen used in postmenopausal women. It would be expected that the larger doses of estrogen used to treat prostatic or breast cancer are more likely to result in these adverse effects, and, in fact, it has been shown that there is an increased risk of thrombosis in men receiving estrogens for prostatic cancer.[19–22]

a. *Thromboembolic disease.* It is now well established that users of oral contraceptives have an increased risk of various thromboembolic and thrombotic vascular diseases, such as thrombophlebitis, pulmonary embolism, stroke, and myocardial infarction.[22–29] Cases of retinal thrombosis, mesenteric thrombosis, and optic neuritis have been reported in oral contraceptive users. There is evidence that the risk of several of these adverse reactions is related to the dose of the drug.[30,31] An increased risk of postsurgery thromboembolic complications has also been reported in users of oral contraceptives.[32,33] If feasible, estrogen should be discontinued at least 4 weeks before surgery of the type associated with an increased risk of thromboembolism, or during periods of immobilization.

While an increased rate of thromboembolic and thrombotic disease in postmenopausal users of estrogen has not been found,[16,34] this does not rule out the possibility that such an increase may be present or that subgroups of women who have underlying risk factors or who are receiving relatively large doses of estrogens may have increased risk. Therefore, estrogens should not be used in persons with active thrombophlebitis or thromboembolic disorders, and they should not be used (except in treatment of malignancy) in persons with a history of such disorders in association with estrogen use. They should be used with caution in patients with cerebral vascular or coronary artery disease and only for those in whom estrogens are clearly needed.

Large doses of estrogen (5 mg conjugated estrogens per day), comparable to those used to treat cancer of the prostate and breast, have been shown in a large prospective clinical trial in men[35] to increase the risk of nonfatal myocardial infarction, pulmonary embolism and thrombophlebitis. When estrogen doses of this size are used, any of the thromboembolic and thrombotic adverse effects associated with oral contraceptive use should be considered a clear risk.

b. *Hepatic adenoma.* Benign hepatic adenomas appear to be associated with the use of oral contraceptives.[36,38] Although benign, and rare, these may rupture and may cause death through intra-abdominal hemorrhage. Such lesions have not yet been reported in association with other estrogen or progestagen preparations, but should be considered in estrogen users having abdominal pain and tenderness, abdominal mass, or hypovolemic shock. Hepatocellular carcinoma has also been reported in women taking estrogen-containing oral contraceptives.[37] The relationship of this malignancy to these drugs is not known at this time.

c. *Elevated blood pressure.* Increased blood pressure is not uncommon in women using oral contraceptives. There is now a report that this may occur with use of estrogens in the menopause[39] and blood pressure should be monitored with estrogen use, especially if high doses are used.

d. *Glucose tolerance.* A worsening of glucose tolerance has been observed in a significant percentage of patients on estrogen-containing oral contraceptives. For this reason, diabetic patients should be carefully observed while receiving estrogen.

4. *Hypercalcemia.* Administration of estrogens may lead to severe hypercalcemia in patients with breast cancer and bone metastases. If this occurs, the drug should be stopped and appropriate measures taken to reduce the serum calcium level.

PRECAUTIONS

General:

1. A complete medical and family history should be taken prior to the initiation of any estrogen therapy. The pretreatment and periodic physical examinations should include special reference to blood pressure, breasts, abdomen, and pelvic organs, and should include a Papanicolaou smear. As a general rule, estrogen should not be prescribed for longer than 1 year without another physical examination being performed.
2. Fluid retention—Because estrogens may cause some degree of fluid retention, conditions which might be influenced by this factor, such as epilepsy, migraine, and cardiac or renal dysfunction, require careful observation.
3. Certain patients may develop undesirable manifestations of excessive estrogenic stimulation, such as abnormal or excessive uterine bleeding, mastodynia, etc.
4. Oral contraceptives appear to be associated with an increased incidence of mental depression.[22] Although it is not clear whether this is due to the estrogenic or progestagenic component of the contraceptive, patients with a history of depression should be carefully observed.
5. Preexisting uterine leiomyomata may increase in size during estrogen use.
6. The pathologist should be advised of estrogen therapy when relevant specimens are submitted.
7. Patients with a past history of jaundice during pregnancy have an increased risk of recurrence of jaundice while receiving estrogen-containing oral contraceptive therapy. If jaundice develops in any patient receiving estrogen, the medication should be discontinued while the cause is investigated.
8. Estrogens may be poorly metabolized in patients with impaired liver function and they should be administered with caution in such patients.
9. Because estrogens influence the metabolism of calcium and phosphorus, they should be used with caution in patients with metabolic bone diseases that are associated with hypercalcemia or in patients with renal insufficiency.
10. Because of the effects of estrogens on epiphyseal closure, they should be used judiciously in young patients in whom bone growth is not complete.
11. ESTINYL Tablets, 0.02 mg, contain FD&C Yellow No. 5 (tartrazine) which may cause allergic-type reactions (including bronchial asthma) in certain susceptible individuals. Although the overall incidence of FD&C Yellow No. 5 (tartrazine) sensitivity in the general population is low, it is frequently seen in patients who also have aspirin hypersensitivity.

Information for the Patient: See text of Patient Package Insert.

Drug/Laboratory Test Interactions: Certain endocrine and liver function tests may be affected by estrogen-containing oral contraceptives. The following similar changes may be expected with larger doses of estrogen:

Increased sulfobromophthalein retention; increased prothrombin and factors VII, VIII, IX, and X; decreased antithrombin 3; increased norepinephrine-induced platelet aggregation; increased thyroid binding globulin (TBG) leading to increased circulating total thyroid hormone, as measured by PBI, T_4 by column, or T_4 by radioimmunoassay. Free T_3 resin uptake is decreased, reflecting the elevated TBG; free T_4 concentration is unaltered; impaired glucose tolerance; decreased pregnanediol excretion; reduced response to metyrapone test; reduced serum folate concentration; increased serum triglyceride and phospholipid concentration.

Carcinogenesis, Mutagenesis, Impairment of Fertility: See boxed **WARNINGS**.

Pregnancy Category X: See **CONTRAINDICATIONS** and boxed **WARNINGS**.

Nursing Mothers: Because of the potential for tumorigenicity shown for ethinyl estradiol in animal and human studies, a decision should be made whether to discontinue nursing or to discontinue the drug, taking into account the importance of the drug to the mother.

Pediatric Use: Safety and effectiveness in children have not been established.

ADVERSE REACTIONS

(See **WARNINGS** regarding induction of neoplasia, adverse effects on the fetus, increased incidence of gallbladder disease, the adverse effects similar to those of oral contraceptives, including thromboembolism.) The following additional adverse reactions have been reported with estrogenic therapy, including oral contraceptives:

Genitourinary system: Breakthrough bleeding, spotting, change in menstrual flow; dysmenorrhea; premenstrual-like syndrome; amenorrhea during and after treatment; increase in size of uterine fibromyomata; vaginal candidiasis; change in cervical eversion and in degree of cervical secretion; cystitis-like syndrome.

Breasts: Tenderness, enlargement, secretion.

Gastrointestinal: Nausea, vomiting; abdominal cramps, bloating; cholestatic jaundice.

Skin: Chloasma or melasma which may persist when drug is discontinued; erythema multiforme; erythema nodosum; hemorrhagic eruption; loss of scalp hair; hirsutism.

Eyes: Steepening of corneal curvature; intolerance to contact lenses.

CNS: Headache, migraine, dizziness; mental depression; chorea.

Continued on next page

Information on Schering products appearing on these pages is effective as of January 2000.

Estinyl—Cont.

Miscellaneous: Increase or decrease in weight; reduced carbohydrate tolerance; aggravation of porphyria; edema; changes in libido.

ACUTE OVERDOSAGE

Numerous reports of ingestion of large doses of estrogen-containing oral contraceptives by young children indicate that serious ill effects do not occur. Overdosage of estrogen may cause nausea, and withdrawal bleeding may occur in females.

DOSAGE AND ADMINISTRATION

1. *Given cyclically for short-term use only.*
For treatment of moderate to severe *vasomotor* symptoms associated with the menopause. The lowest dose that will control symptoms should be chosen and medication should be discontinued as promptly as possible. Administration should be cyclic (eg, 3 weeks on and 1 week off). Attempts to discontinue or taper medication should be made at 3- to 6-month intervals. The usual dosage range is 0.02 mg to 0.05 mg daily. In some instances, the effective dose may be as low as 0.02 mg every other day. A useful dosage schedule for early menopause, while spontaneous menstruation continues, is 0.05 mg once a day for 21 days and then a rest period for 7 days. For the initial treatment of the late menopause, the same regimen is indicated with a dose of 0.02 mg for the first few cycles, after which 0.05 mg dosage may be substituted. In more severe cases, such as those due to surgical and roentgenologic castration, a dose of 0.05 mg may be administered three times daily at the start of treatment. With adequate clinical improvement, usually obtainable in a few weeks, the dosage may be reduced to 0.05 mg daily and the patient continued thereafter on a maintenance dosage as in the average case.

2. *Given cyclically.*
Female hypogonadism: A dose of 0.05 mg is given one to three times daily during the first 2 weeks of a theoretical menstrual cycle. This is followed by progesterone during the last half of the arbitrary cycle. This regimen is continued for 3 to 6 months. The patient is then allowed to go untreated for 2 months to determine whether or not she can maintain the cycle without hormonal therapy. If not, additional courses of therapy may be prescribed.

3. *Given chronically.*
Inoperable progressing prostatic cancer: A dose ranging from 0.15 mg to 2.0 mg may be administered daily for palliation.
Inoperable progressing breast cancer in appropriately selected postmenopausal women (See **INDICATIONS AND USAGE**): A 1.0 mg dose three times daily for palliation.
Treated patients with an intact uterus should be monitored closely for signs of endometrial cancer and appropriate diagnostic measures should be taken to rule out malignancy in the event of persistent or recurring abnormal vaginal bleeding.

HOW SUPPLIED

ESTINYL Tablets 0.02 mg, beige, sugar-coated tablets branded in black with the Schering trademark and either product identification number 298, or letters ER; bottles of 100 (NDC 0085-0298-03) and 250 (NDC 0085-0298-06).
ESTINYL Tablets 0.05 mg, pink, sugar-coated tablets branded in black with the Schering trademark and either product identification number 070, or letters EM; bottles of 100 (NDC 0085-0070-03) and 250 (NDC 0085-0070-06).
Store between 2° and 30°C (36° and 86°F).

PHYSICIAN REFERENCES

1. Ziel, H. K. and W. D. Finkle, "Increased Risk of Endometrial Carcinoma Among Users of Conjugated Estrogens," *N Engl J Med.* 293:1167–1170, 1975.
2. Smith, D. C., R. Prentic, D. J. Thompson, and W. L. Hermann, "Association of Exogenous Estrogen and Endometrial Carcinoma," *N Engl J Med.* 293:1164–1167, 1975.
3. Mack, T. M., M. C. Pike, B. E. Henderson, et al. "Estrogens and Endometrial Cancer in a Retirement Community," *N Engl J Med.* 294:1262–1267, 1976.
4. Weiss, N. S., D. R. Szekely, and D. F. Austin, "Increasing Incidence of Endometrial Cancer in the United States," *N Engl J Med.* 294:1259–1262, 1976.
5. Herbst, A. L., H. Ulfelder, and D. C. Poskanzer, "Adenocarcinoma of Vagina," *N Engl J Med.* 284:878–881, 1971.
6. Greenwald, P., J. Barlow, P. Nasca, and W. Burnett, "Vaginal Cancer after Maternal Treatment with Synthetic Estrogens," *N Engl J Med.* 285:390–392, 1971.
7. Lanier, A., K. Noller, D. Decker, L. Elveback, and L. Kurland, "Cancer and Stilbestrol. A Follow-up of 1,719 Persons Exposed to Estrogens In Utero and Born 1943–1959," *Mayo Clin Proc.* 48:793–799, 1973.
8. Herbst, A., R. Kurman, and R. Scully, "Vaginal and Cervical Abnormalities After Exposure to Stilbestrol In Utero," *Obstet Gynecol.* 40:287–298, 1972.
9. Herbst, A., D. Poskanzer, S. Robboy, L. Friedlander, and R. Scully, "Prenatal Exposure to Stilbestrol, A Prospective Comparison of Exposed Female Offspring with Unexposed Controls," *N Engl J Med.* 292:334–339, 1975.
10. Stafl, A., R. Mattingly, D. Foley, and W. Fetherston, "Clinical Diagnosis of Vaginal Adenosis," *Obstet Gynecol.* 43:118–128, 1974.
11. Sherman, A. I., M. Goldrath, A. Berlin, et al. "Cervical-Vaginal Adenosis After *In Utero* Exposure to Synthetic Estrogens," *Obstet Gynecol.* 44:531–545, 1974.
12. Gal, I., B. Kirman, and J. Stern, "Hormone Pregnancy Tests and Congenital Malformation," *Nature.* 216:83, 1967.
13. Levy, E. P., A. Cohen, and F. C. Fraser, "Hormone Treatment During Pregnancy and Congenital Heart Defects," *Lancet.* 1:611, 1973.
14. Nora, J. and A. Nora, "Birth Defects and Oral Contraceptives," *Lancet.* 1:941–942, 1973.
15. Janerich, D. T., J. M. Piper, and D. M. Glebatis, "Oral Contraceptives and Congenital Limb-Reduction Defects," *N Engl J Med.* 291:697–700, 1974.
16. Boston Collaborative Drug Surveillance Program, "Surgically Confirmed Gallbladder Disease, Venous Thromboembolism and Breast Tumors in Relation to Post-Menopausal Estrogen Therapy," *N Engl J Med.* 290:15–19, 1974.
17. Hoover, R., L. A. Gray, Sr., P. Cole, and B. MacMahon, "Menopausal Estrogens and Breast Cancer," *N Engl J Med.* 295:401–405, 1976.
18. Boston Collaborative Drug Surveillance Program, "Oral Contraceptives and Venous Thromboembolic Disease, Surgically Confirmed Gallbladder Disease, and Breast Tumors," *Lancet.* 1:1399–1404, 1973.
19. The Veterans Administration Cooperative Urological Research Group, "Carcinoma of the Prostate: Treatment Comparisons," *J Urol.* 98:516–522, 1967.
20. Bailar, J. C., "Thromboembolism and Oestrogen Therapy," *Lancet.* 2:560, 1967.
21. Blackard, C., R. Doe, G. Mellinger, and D. Byar, "Incidence of Cardiovascular Disease and Death in Patients Receiving Diethylstilbestrol for Carcinoma of the Prostate," *Cancer.* 26:249–256, 1970.
22. Royal College of General Practitioners, "Oral Contraception and Thromboembolic Disease," *J R Coll Gen Pract.* 13:267–279, 1967.
23. Inman, W. H. W. and M. P. Vessey, "Investigation of Deaths from Pulmonary, Coronary, and Cerebral Thrombosis and Embolism in Women of Child-Bearing Age," *Br Med J.* 2:193–199, 1968.
24. Vessey, M. P. and R. Doll, "Investigation of Relation Between Use of Oral Contraceptives and Thromboembolic Disease. A Further Report," *Br Med J.* 2:651–657, 1969.
25. Sartwell, P. E., A. T. Masi, F. G. Arthes, G. R. Greene, and H. E. Smith, "Thromboembolism and Oral Contraceptives: An Epidemiological Case Control Study," *Am J Epidemiol.* 90:365–380, 1969.
26. Collaborative Group for the Study of Stroke in Young Women, "Oral Contraception and Increased Risk of Cerebral Ischemia or Thrombosis," *N Engl J Med.* 288:871–878, 1973.
27. Collaborative Group for the Study of Stroke in Young Women, "Oral Contraceptives and Stroke in Young Women: Associated Risk Factors," *JAMA.* 231:718–722, 1975.
28. Mann, J. I. and W. H. W. Inman, "Oral Contraceptives and Death from Myocardial Infarction," *Br Med J.* 2:245–248, 1975.
29. Mann, J. I., M. P. Vessey, M. Thorogood, and R. Doll, "Myocardial Infarction in Young Women with Special Reference to Oral Contraceptive Practice," *Br Med J.* 2:241–245, 1975.
30. Inman, W. H. W., M. P. Vessey, B. Westerholm, and A. Engelund, "Thromboembolic Disease and the Steroidal Content of Oral Contraceptives," *Br Med J.* 2:203–209, 1970.
31. Stolley, P. D., J. A. Tonascia, M. S. Tockman, P. E. Sartwell, A. H. Rutledge, and M. P. Jacobs, "Thrombosis With Low-Estrogen Oral Contraceptives," *Am J Epidemiol.* 102:197–208, 1975.
32. Vessey, M. P., R. Doll, A. S. Fairbairn, and G. Glober, "Post-Operative Thromboembolism and the Use of the Oral Contraceptives," *Br Med J.* 3:123–126, 1970.
33. Greene, G. R. and P. E. Sartwell, "Oral Contraceptive Use in Patients With Thromboembolism Following Surgery, Trauma or Infection," *Am J Public Health.* 62:680–685, 1972.
34. Rosenberg, L., M. B. Armstrong, and H. Jick, "Myocardial Infarction and Estrogen Therapy in Postmenopausal Women," *N Engl J Med.* 294:1256–1259, 1976.
35. Coronary Drug Project Research Group, "The Coronary Drug Project: Initial Findings Leading to Modifications of its Research Protocol," *JAMA.* 214:1303–1313, 1970.
36. Baum, J., F. Holtz, J. J. Bookstein, and E. W. Klein, "Possible Association Between Benign Hepatomas and Oral Contraceptives," *Lancet.* 2:926–928, 1973.
37. Mays, E. T., W. M. Christopherson, M. M. Mahr, and H. C. Williams, "Hepatic Changes in Young Women Ingesting Contraceptive Steroids: Hepatic Hemorrhage and Primary Hepatic Tumors," *JAMA.* 235:730–782, 1976.
38. Edmondson, H. A., B. Henderson, and B. Benton, "Liver Cell Adenomas Associated With the Use of Oral Contraceptives," *N Engl J Med.* 294:470–472, 1976.
39. Pfeffer, R. I. and S. Van Den Noort, "Estrogen Use and Stroke Risk in Postmenopausal Women," *Am J Epidemiol.* 103:445–456, 1976.

PATIENT LABELING

WHAT YOU SHOULD KNOW ABOUT ESTROGENS

Estrogens are female hormones produced by the ovaries. The ovaries make several different kinds of estrogens. In addition, scientists have been able to make a variety of synthetic estrogens. As far as we know, all these estrogens have similar properties and therefore much the same usefulness, side effects, and risks. This leaflet is intended to help you understand what estrogens are used for, the risks involved in their use, and how to use them as safely as possible.

This leaflet includes the most important information about estrogens, but not all the information. If you want to know more, you can ask your doctor or pharmacist to let you read the package insert prepared for the doctor.

USES OF ESTROGEN

Estrogens are prescribed by doctors for a number of purposes, including:
1. To provide estrogen during a period of adjustment when a woman's ovaries no longer produce it, in order to prevent certain uncomfortable symptoms of estrogen deficiency. (All women normally stop producing estrogens, generally between the ages of 45 and 55; this is called the menopause.)
2. To prevent symptoms of estrogen deficiency when a woman's ovaries have been removed surgically before the natural menopause.
3. To prevent pregnancy (estrogens are given along with a progestagen, another female hormone; these combinations are called oral contraceptives and they will not be discussed in this leaflet).
4. To treat certain cancers in women and men.

THERE IS NO PROPER USE OF ESTROGENS IN A PREGNANT WOMAN.

ESTROGENS IN THE MENOPAUSE

In the natural course of their lives, all women eventually experience a decrease in estrogen production. This usually occurs between ages 45 and 55 but may occur earlier or later. Sometimes the ovaries may need to be removed before natural menopause by an operation, producing a "surgical menopause."
When the amount of estrogen in the blood begins to decrease, many women may develop typical symptoms: feelings of warmth in the face, neck, and chest or sudden intense episodes of heat and sweating throughout the body (called "hot flashes" or "hot flushes"). These symptoms are sometimes very uncomfortable. A few women eventually develop changes in the vagina (called "atrophic vaginitis") which cause discomfort, especially during and after intercourse.
Estrogens can be prescribed to treat these symptoms of the menopause. It is estimated that considerably more than half of all women undergoing the menopause have only mild symptoms or no symptoms at all and therefore do not need estrogens. Other women may need estrogens for a few months, while their bodies adjust to lower estrogen levels. Sometimes the need will be for periods longer than 6 months. In an attempt to avoid overstimulation of the uterus (womb), estrogens are usually given cyclically during each month of use, that is, 3 weeks of pills followed by 1 week without pills.
Sometimes women experience nervous symptoms or depression during menopause. There is no evidence that estrogens are effective for such symptoms and they should not be used to treat them, although other treatment may be needed.
You may have heard that taking estrogens for long periods (years) after menopause will keep your skin soft and supple and keep you feeling young. There is no evidence that this is so, however, and such long-term treatment carries important risks.

THE DANGERS OF ESTROGENS

1. *Cancer of the uterus.* If estrogens are used in the postmenopausal period for more than a year, there is an increased risk of *endometrial cancer* (cancer of the uterus). Women taking estrogens have roughly 5 to 10 times as great a chance of getting this cancer as women who take no estrogens. To put this another way, while a postmenopausal woman not taking estrogens has one chance in 1,000 each year of getting cancer of the uterus, a woman taking estrogens has 5 to 10 chances in 1,000 each year. For this reason *it is important to take estrogens only when you really need them.*
The risk of this cancer is greater the longer estrogens are used and also seems to be greater when larger doses are taken. For this reason *it is important to take the lowest dose of estrogen that will control symptoms and to take it only as long as it is needed.* If estrogens are needed for longer periods of time, your doctor will want to reevaluate your need for estrogens at least every 6 months.
Women using estrogens should report any irregular vaginal bleeding to their doctors; such bleeding may be of no importance, but it can be an early warning of cancer of the uterus. If you have undiagnosed vaginal bleeding, you should not use estrogens until a diagnosis is made and you are certain there is no cancer of the uterus.
If you have had your uterus completely removed (total hysterectomy), there is no danger of developing cancer of the uterus.
2. *Other possible cancers.* Estrogens can cause development of other tumors in animals, such as tumors of the breast, cervix, vagina, or liver, when given for a long time. At present there is no good evidence that women using estrogens in the menopause have an increased risk of such tumors, but there is no way yet to be sure they do not; and one study raises the possibility that use of estrogens in the menopause may increase the risk of breast cancer many years later. This is a further reason to use estrogens only when clearly needed. While you are taking estrogens, it is important that you go to your doctor at least once a year for a physical examination.
Also, if members of your family have had breast cancer or if you have breast nodules or abnormal mammograms (breast x-rays), your doctor may wish to carry out more frequent examinations of your breasts.
3. *Gallbladder disease.* Women who use estrogens after menopause are more likely to develop gallbladder disease needing surgery than women who do not use estrogens. Birth control pills have a similar effect.

4. *Abnormal blood clotting.* Oral contraceptives increase the risk of blood clotting in various parts of the body. This can result in a stroke (if the clot is in the brain), a heart attack (clot in a blood vessel of the heart), or a pulmonary embolus (a clot which forms in the legs or pelvis, then breaks off and travels to the lungs). Any of these can be fatal.

At this time, use of estrogens in the menopause is not known to cause such blood clotting, but this has not been fully studied and there could still prove to be such a risk. It is recommended that if you have had clotting in the legs or lungs or a heart attack or stroke while you were using estrogens or birth control pills, you should not use estrogens (unless they are being used to treat cancer of the breast or prostate). If you have had a stroke or heart attack or if you have angina pectoris, estrogens should be used with great caution and only if clearly needed (for example, if you have severe symptoms of the menopause).

The larger doses of estrogen used to prevent swelling of the breasts after pregnancy have been reported to cause clotting in the legs and lungs.

SPECIAL WARNING ABOUT PREGNANCY

You should not receive estrogens if you are pregnant. If this should occur, there is a greater than usual chance that the developing child will be born with a birth defect, although the possibility remains fairly small. A female child may have an increased risk of developing cancer of the vagina or cervix later in life (in the teens or twenties). Every possible effort should be made to avoid exposure to estrogens during pregnancy. If exposure occurs, see your doctor.

OTHER EFFECTS OF ESTROGENS

In addition to the serious known risks of estrogens described above, estrogens have the following side effects and potential risks:

1. *Nausea and vomiting.* The most common side effect of estrogen therapy is nausea. Vomiting is less common.
2. *Effects on breasts.* Estrogens may cause breast tenderness or enlargement and may cause the breasts to secrete a liquid. These effects are not dangerous.
3. *Effects on the uterus.* Estrogens may cause benign fibroid tumors of the uterus to get larger. Some women will have menstrual bleeding when estrogens are stopped. But if the bleeding occurs on days you are still taking estrogens, you should report this to your doctor.
4. *Effects on liver.* Women taking oral contraceptives develop on rare occasions a tumor of the liver which can rupture and bleed into the abdomen. So far, these tumors have not been reported in women using estrogens in the menopause, but you should report any swelling or unusual pain or tenderness in the abdomen to your doctor immediately. Women with a past history of jaundice (yellowing of the skin and white parts of the eyes) may get jaundice again during estrogen use. If this occurs, stop taking estrogens and see your doctor.
5. *Other effects.* Estrogens may cause excess fluid to be retained in the body. This may make some conditions worse, such as epilepsy, migraine, heart disease, or kidney disease.

DOSAGE AND ADMINISTRATION

Use this medication as directed by your doctor. Generally, it may be prescribed one of three ways:

1. Cyclically for short-term use only.
   Administration is cyclic, that is, 3 weeks on and 1 week off. The usual dosage range is 0.02 mg or 0.05 mg daily.
2. Cyclically.
   0.05 mg taken one to three times daily for 2 weeks followed by progesterone (another kind of hormone) for 2 weeks. This schedule is maintained for several months.
3. Chronically.
   A dose ranging from 0.15 mg to 2.0 mg may be administered daily.
   The above dosages are intended as guidelines only. Your doctor will tell you how to take this medication to suit your particular needs.

SUMMARY

Estrogens have important uses, but they have serious risks as well. You must decide, with your doctor, whether the risks are acceptable to you in view of the benefits of treatment. Except where your doctor has prescribed estrogens for use in special cases of cancer of the breast or prostate, you should not use estrogens if you have cancer of the breast or uterus, are pregnant, have undiagnosed abnormal vaginal bleeding, clotting in the legs or lungs, or have had a stroke, heart attack or angina, or clotting in the legs or lungs in the past while you were taking estrogens.

You can use estrogens as safely as possible by understanding that your doctor will require regular physical examinations while you are taking them and will try to discontinue the drug as soon as possible and use the smallest dose possible. Be alert for signs of trouble including:

1. Abnormal bleeding from the vagina.
2. Pains in the calves or chest or sudden shortness of breath, or coughing blood (indicating possible clots in the legs, heart, or lungs).
3. Severe headache, dizziness, faintness, or changes in vision (indicating possible developing clots in the brain or eye).
4. Breast lumps (you should ask your doctor how to examine your own breasts).
5. Jaundice (yellowing of the skin).
6. Mental depression.

Based on his or her assessment of your medical needs, your doctor has prescribed this drug for you. Do not give the drug to anyone else.

HOW SUPPLIED

ESTINYL Tablets are available in two different strengths: ESTINYL 0.02 mg Tablets are beige in color and branded with either the number 298, or the letters ER.

These tablets contain FD&C Yellow No. 5 (tartrazine) which may cause allergic-type reactions (including bronchial asthma) in certain susceptible individuals. Although the overall incidence of FD&C Yellow No. 5 (tartrazine) sensitivity in the general population is low, it is frequently seen in patients who also have aspirin hypersensitivity.

ESTINYL 0.05 mg Tablets are pink in color and branded with either the number 070, or the letters EM.

ESTINYL Tablets should be stored between 2° and 30°C (36° and 86°F).

Schering Corporation
Kenilworth, NJ 07033 USA
Rev. 1/99 17406949

ETRAFON® ℞

brand of perphenazine and amitriptyline hydrochloride
ETRAFON 2-10 TABLETS (2-10), USP
ETRAFON TABLETS (2-25), USP
ETRAFON-FORTE TABLETS (4-25), USP

DESCRIPTION

ETRAFON Tablets contain perphenazine, USP and amitriptyline hydrochloride, USP. Perphenazine is a piperazinyl phenothiazine having the chemical formula, $C_{21}H_{26}ClN_3OS$. Amitriptyline hydrochloride is a dibenzocycloheptadiene derivative having the chemical formula, $C_{20}H_{23}N.HCl$.

ETRAFON Tablets are available in multiple strengths to afford dosage flexibility for optimum management. They are available as ETRAFON 2-10 Tablets, 2 mg perphenazine and 10 mg amitriptyline hydrochloride; ETRAFON Tablets, 2 mg perphenazine and 25 mg amitriptyline hydrochloride; ETRAFON-Forte Tablets, 4 mg perphenazine and 25 mg amitriptyline hydrochloride.

The inactive ingredients for ETRAFON 2–10 Tablets (2-10) include: acacia, butylparaben, calcium phosphate, calcium sulfate, carnauba wax, corn starch, D&C Yellow No. 10 Al Lake, FD&C Yellow No. 6 Al Lake, gelatin, lactose, magnesium stearate, potato starch, sugar, and white wax. May also contain talc.

The inactive ingredients for ETRAFON-Forte Tablets (4-25) include: acacia, butylparaben, calcium phosphate, calcium sulfate, carnauba wax, corn starch, FD&C Red No. 40 Al Lake, FD&C Yellow No. 6 Al Lake, gelatin, lactose, magnesium stearate, potato starch, sugar, and white wax. May also contain talc.

ACTIONS

ETRAFON Tablets combine the tranquilizing action of perphenazine with the antidepressant properties of amitriptyline hydrochloride. Perphenazine acts on the central nervous system, and has a greater behavioral potency than other phenothiazine derivatives whose side chains do not contain a piperazine moiety. Amitriptyline hydrochloride is a tricyclic antidepressant. While its mechanism of action in man is not known, it does not act primarily by stimulation of the central nervous system, and is not a monoamine oxidase (MAO) inhibitor.

INDICATIONS

ETRAFON Tablets are indicated for the treatment of patients with moderate to severe anxiety and/or agitation and depressed mood; patients with depression in whom anxiety and/or agitation are moderate or severe; patients with anxiety and depression associated with chronic physical disease; patients in whom depression and anxiety cannot be clearly differentiated.

Schizophrenic patients who have associated symptoms of depression should be considered for therapy with ETRAFON.

CONTRAINDICATIONS

ETRAFON Tablets are contraindicated in comatose or greatly obtunded patients and in patients receiving large doses of central nervous system depressants (barbiturates, alcohol, narcotics, analgesics, or antihistamines); in the presence of existing blood dyscrasias, bone marrow depression, or liver damage; and in patients who have shown hypersensitivity to ETRAFON Tablets, its components, or related compounds.

ETRAFON Tablets are also contraindicated in patients with suspected or established subcortical brain damage, with or without hypothalamic damage, since a hyperthermic reaction with temperatures in excess of 104°F may occur in such patients, sometimes not until 14 to 16 hours after drug administration. Total body ice-packing is recommended for such a reaction; antipyretics may also be useful.

ETRAFON Tablets should not be given concomitantly with a monoamine oxidase inhibiting compound. Hyperpyretic crises, severe convulsions, and deaths have occurred in patients receiving tricyclic antidepressant and monoamine oxidase inhibiting drugs simultaneously. In patients who have been receiving a monoamine oxidase inhibitor, it is recommended that 2 weeks or longer elapse before the start of treatment with ETRAFON Tablets to permit recovery from the effects of the MAO inhibitor and to avoid possible potentiation. Treatment with ETRAFON Tablets should be initiated cautiously in such patients, with gradual increase in dosage until a satisfactory response is obtained.

Amitriptyline hydrochloride is not recommended for use during the acute recovery phase following myocardial infarction.

WARNINGS

Tardive dyskinesia, a syndrome consisting of potentially irreversible, involuntary, dyskinetic movements, may develop in patients treated with neuroleptic (antipsychotic) drugs. Although the prevalence of the syndrome appears to be highest among the elderly, especially elderly women, it is impossible to rely upon prevalence estimates to predict, at the inception of neuroleptic treatment, which patients are likely to develop the syndrome. Whether neuroleptic drug products differ in their potential to cause tardive dyskinesia is unknown.

Both the risk of developing the syndrome and the likelihood that it will become irreversible are believed to increase as the duration of treatment and the total cumulative dose of neuroleptic drugs administered to the patient increase. However, the syndrome can develop, although much less commonly, after relatively brief treatment periods at low doses.

There is no known treatment for established cases of tardive dyskinesia, although the syndrome may remit, partially or completely, if neuroleptic treatment is withdrawn. Neuroleptic treatment itself, however, may suppress (or partially suppress) the signs and symptoms of the syndrome, and thereby may possibly mask the underlying disease process. The effect that symptomatic suppression has upon the long-term course of the syndrome is unknown.

Given these considerations, neuroleptics should be prescribed in a manner that is most likely to minimize the occurrence of tardive dyskinesia. Chronic neuroleptic treatment should generally be reserved for patients who suffer from a chronic illness that, 1) is known to respond to neuroleptic drugs, and, 2) for whom alternative, equally effective, but potentially less harmful treatments are not available or appropriate. In patients who do require chronic treatment, the smallest dose and the shortest duration of treatment producing a satisfactory clinical response should be sought. The need for continued treatment should be reassessed periodically.

If signs and symptoms of tardive dyskinesia appear in a patient on neuroleptics, drug discontinuation should be considered. However, some patients may require treatment despite the presence of the syndrome.

(For further information about the description of tardive dyskinesia and its clinical detection, please refer to **Information for Patients** and **ADVERSE REACTIONS**.)

NEUROLEPTIC MALIGNANT SYNDROME (NMS) A potentially fatal symptom complex, sometimes referred to as Neuroleptic Malignant Syndrome (NMS), has been reported in association with antipsychotic drugs. Clinical manifestations of NMS are hyperpyrexia, muscle rigidity, altered mental status, and evidence of autonomic instability (irregular pulse or blood pressure, tachycardia, diaphoresis, and cardiac dysrhythmias).

The diagnostic evaluation of patients with this syndrome is complicated. In arriving at a diagnosis, it is important to identify cases where the clinical presentation includes both serious medical illness (eg, pneumonia, systemic infection, etc.) and untreated or inadequately treated extrapyramidal signs and symptoms (EPS). Other important considerations in the differential diagnosis include central anticholinergic toxicity, heat stroke, drug fever, and primary central nervous system (CNS) pathology.

The management of NMS should include; 1) immediate discontinuation of antipsychotic drugs and other drugs not essential to concurrent therapy, 2) intensive symptomatic treatment and medical monitoring, and 3) treatment of any concomitant serious medical problems for which specific treatments are available. There is no general agreement about specific pharmacological treatment regimens for uncomplicated NMS.

If a patient requires antipsychotic drug treatment after recovery from NMS, the reintroduction of drug therapy should be carefully considered. The patient should be carefully monitored since recurrences of NMS have been reported.

Patients with cardiovascular disorders should be watched closely. Tricyclic antidepressant drugs, including amitriptyline hydrochloride, particularly when given in high doses, have been reported to produce arrhythmias, sinus tachycardia, and prolongation of the conduction time. Myocardial infarction and stroke have been reported with drugs of this class.

ETRAFON Tablets should not be given concomitantly with guanethidine or similarly acting compounds, since amitriptyline, like other tricyclic antidepressants, may block the antihypertensive effect of these compounds. If hypotension develops, epinephrine should not be administered since its action is blocked and partially reversed by perphenazine. If a vasopressor is needed, norepinephrine may be used. Severe, acute hypotension has occurred with the use of pheno-

Continued on next page

Information on Schering products appearing on these pages is effective as of January 2000.

Etrafon—Cont.

thiazines and is particularly likely to occur in patients with mitral insufficiency or pheochromocytoma. Rebound hypertension may occur in pheochromocytoma patients.

Perphenazine can lower the convulsive threshold in susceptible individuals; it should be used with caution in alcohol withdrawal and in patients with convulsive disorders. If the patient is being treated with an anticonvulsant agent, increased dosage of that agent may be required when ETRAFON Tablets are used concomitantly.

Because of the anticholinergic activity of amitriptyline hydrochloride, ETRAFON Tablets should be used with caution in patients with glaucoma, increased intraocular pressure, and those in whom urinary retention is present or anticipated. In patients with angle-closure glaucoma, even average doses may precipitate an attack.

Close supervision is required when amitriptyline hydrochloride is given to hyperthyroid patients or those receiving thyroid medication.

ETRAFON Tablets may impair the mental and/or physical abilities required for the performance of potentially hazardous tasks, such as driving a car or operating machinery; the patient should be warned accordingly.

Use in Pregnancy: Safe use of ETRAFON Tablets during pregnancy and lactation has not been established; therefore, in administering the drug to pregnant patients, nursing mothers, or women who may become pregnant, the possible benefits must be weighed against the possible hazards to mother and child.

PRECAUTIONS

The possibility of suicide in depressed patients remains during treatment and until significant remission occurs. This type of patient should not have access to large quantities of this drug.

Pediatric Use: Safety and effectiveness in pediatric patients have not been established.

Perphenazine

As with all phenothiazine compounds, perphenazine should not be used indiscriminately. Caution should be observed in giving it to patients who have previously exhibited severe adverse reactions to other phenothiazines. Some of the untoward actions of perphenazine tend to appear more frequently when high doses are used. However, as with other phenothiazine compounds, patients receiving perphenazine in any dosage should be kept under close supervision.

Neuroleptic drugs elevate prolactin levels; the elevation persists during chronic administration. Tissue culture experiments indicate that approximately one third of human breast cancers are prolactin dependent *in vitro*, a factor of potential importance if the prescription of these drugs is contemplated in a patient with a previously detected breast cancer. Although disturbances such as galactorrhea, amenorrhea, gynecomastia, and impotence have been reported, the clinical significance of elevated serum prolactin levels is unknown for most patients. An increase in mammary neoplasms has been found in rodents after chronic administration of neuroleptic drugs. Neither clinical studies nor epidemiologic studies conducted to date, however, have shown an association between chronic administration of these drugs and mammary tumorigenesis; the available evidence is considered too limited to be conclusive at this time.

The antiemetic effect of perphenazine may obscure signs of toxicity due to overdosage of other drugs, or render more difficult the diagnosis of disorders such as brain tumors or intestinal obstruction.

A significant, not otherwise explained, rise in body temperature may suggest individual intolerance to perphenazine, in which case ETRAFON Tablets should be discontinued.

Blood counts and hepatic and renal functions should be checked periodically. The appearance of signs of blood dyscrasias requires the discontinuance of the drug and institution of appropriate therapy. If abnormalities in hepatic tests occur, phenothiazine treatment should be discontinued. Renal function in patients on long-term therapy should be monitored; if blood urea nitrogen (BUN) becomes abnormal, treatment with the drug should be discontinued.

The use of phenothiazine derivatives in patients with diminished renal function should be undertaken with caution.

Use with caution in patients suffering from respiratory impairment due to acute pulmonary infections, or in chronic respiratory disorders such as severe asthma or emphysema.

In general, phenothiazines do not produce psychic dependence. Gastritis, nausea and vomiting, dizziness, and tremulousness have been reported following abrupt cessation of high-dose therapy. Reports suggest that these symptoms can be reduced by continuing concomitant antiparkinson agents for several weeks after the phenothiazine is withdrawn.

The possibility of liver damage, corneal and lenticular deposits, and irreversible dyskinesias should be kept in mind when patients are on long-term therapy.

Because photosensitivity has been reported, undue exposure to the sun should be avoided during phenothiazine treatment.

Information for Patients: This information is intended to aid in the safe and effective use of this medication. It is not a disclosure of all possible adverse or intended effects.

Given the likelihood that a substantial proportion of patients exposed chronically to neuroleptics will develop tardive dyskinesia, it is advised that all patients in whom chronic use is contemplated be given, if possible, full information about this risk. The decision to inform patients and/or their guardians must obviously take into account the clinical circumstances and the competency of the patient to understand the information provided.

Amitriptyline Hydrochloride

In manic-depressive psychosis, depressed patients may experience a shift toward the manic phase if they are treated with an antidepressant drug. Patients with paranoid symptomatology may have an exaggeration of such symptoms. The tranquilizing effect of ETRAFON Tablets has seemed to reduce the likelihood of this effect.

Both elevation and lowering of blood sugar levels have been reported.

The usefulness of amitriptyline in the treatment of depression has been amply demonstrated; however, it should be realized that abuse of amitriptyline among a narcotic-dependent population is not uncommon.

Drug Interactions: Drugs Metabolized by P450 2D6— The biochemical activity of the drug metabolizing isozyme cytochrome P450 2D6 (debrisoquin hydroxylase) is reduced in a subset of the Caucasian population (about 7%–10% of Caucasians are so-called "poor metabolizers"); reliable estimates of the prevalence of reduced P450 2D6 isozyme activity among Asian, African, and other populations are not yet available. Poor metabolizers have higher than expected plasma concentrations of tricyclic antidepressants (TCAs) when given usual doses. Depending on the fraction of drug metabolized by P450 2D6, the increase in plasma concentration may be small, or quite large (eight-fold increase in plasma AUC of the TCA).

In addition, certain drugs inhibit the activity of this isozyme and make normal metabolizers resemble poor metabolizers. An individual who is stable on a given dose of TCA may become abruptly toxic when given one of these inhibiting drugs as concomitant therapy. The drugs that inhibit cytochrome P450 2D6 include some that are not metabolized by the enzyme (quinidine; cimetidine) and many that are substrates for P450 2D6 (many other antidepressants, phenothiazines, and the Type 1C antiarrhythmics propafenone and flecainide). While all the selective serotonin reuptake inhibitors (SSRIs), eg, fluoxetine, sertraline, and paroxetine, inhibit P450 2D6, they may vary in the extent of inhibition. The extent to which SSRI TCA interactions may pose clinical problems will depend on the degree of inhibition and the pharmacokinetics of the SSRI involved. Nevertheless, caution is indicated in the coadministration of TCAs with any of the SSRIs and also in switching from one class to the other. Of particular importance, sufficient time must elapse before initiating TCA treatment in a patient being withdrawn from fluoxetine, given the long half-life of the parent and active metabolite (at least 5 weeks may be necessary).

Concomitant use of tricyclic antidepressants with drugs that can inhibit cytochrome P450 2D6 may require lower doses than usually prescribed for either the tricyclic antidepressant or the other drug. Furthermore, whenever one of these other drugs is withdrawn from co-therapy, an increased dose of tricyclic antidepressant may be required. It is desirable to monitor TCA plasma levels whenever a TCA is going to be coadministered with another drug known to be an inhibitor of P450 2D6.

Perphenazine

Patients on large doses of a phenothiazine drug who are undergoing surgery should be watched carefully for possible hypotensive phenomena. Moreover, reduced amounts of anesthetics or central nervous system depressants may be necessary.

Since phenothiazines and central nervous system depressants (opiates, analgesics, antihistamines, barbiturates) can potentiate each other, less than the usual dosage of the added drug is recommended and caution is advised when they are administered concomitantly.

Use with caution in patients who are receiving atropine or related drugs because of additive anticholinergic effects and also in patients who will be exposed to extreme heat or organic phosphate insecticides.

The use of alcohol should be avoided, since additive effects and hypotension may occur. Patients should be cautioned that their response to alcohol may be increased while they are being treated with ETRAFON Tablets. The risk of suicide and the danger of overdose may be increased in patients who use alcohol excessively due to its potentiation of the drug's effect.

Amitriptyline Hydrochloride

When amitriptyline hydrochloride is given with anticholinergic agents or sympathomimetic drugs, including epinephrine combined with local anesthetics, close supervision and careful adjustment of dosages are required.

Paralytic ileus may occur in patients taking tricyclic antidepressants in combination with anticholinergic-type drugs.

Concurrent use of large doses of ethchlorvynol should be used with caution, since transient delirium has been reported in patients receiving this drug in combination with amitriptyline hydrochloride.

This drug may enhance the response to alcohol and the effects of barbiturates and other CNS depressants.

Concurrent administration of amitriptyline hydrochloride and electroshock therapy may increase the hazards of therapy. Such treatment should be limited to patients for whom it is essential.

Discontinue the drug several days before elective surgery, if possible.

Concurrent administration of cimetidine and tricyclic antidepressants can produce clinically significant increases in the plasma concentrations of the tricyclic antidepressant. Serious anticholinergic symptoms (severe dry mouth, urinary retention, blurred vision) have been associated with elevations in the serum levels of the tricyclic antidepressant when cimetidine is added to the drug regimen. Additionally, higher than expected steady-state serum concentrations of the tricyclic antidepressant have been observed when therapy is initiated in patients taking cimetidine.

Alternatively, decreases in the steady-state serum concentration of the tricyclic antidepressant have been reported in well-controlled patients on concurrent therapy upon discontinuance of cimetidine. The therapeutic efficacy of the tricyclic antidepressant may be compromised in these patients as the cimetidine is discontinued.

ADVERSE REACTIONS

Adverse reactions to ETRAFON Tablets are the same as those to its components, perphenazine and amitriptyline hydrochloride. There have been no reports of effects peculiar to the combination of these components in ETRAFON Tablets.

Perphenazine

Not all of the following adverse reactions have been reported with perphenazine; however, pharmacological similarities among various phenothiazine derivatives require that each be considered. With the piperazine group (of which perphenazine is an example), the extrapyramidal symptoms are more common, and others (eg, sedative effects, jaundice, and blood dyscrasias) are less frequently seen.

CNS Effects: *Extrapyramidal reactions:* opisthotonus; trismus; torticollis; retrocollis; aching and numbness of the limbs; motor restlessness; oculogyric crisis; hyperreflexia; dystonia, including protrusion, discoloration, aching and rounding of the tongue; tonic spasm of the masticatory muscles; tight feeling in the throat; slurred speech; dysphagia; akathisia; dyskinesia; parkinsonism; and ataxia. Their incidence and severity usually increase with an increase in dosage, but there is considerable individual variation in the tendency to develop such symptoms. Extrapyramidal symptoms can usually be controlled by the concomitant use of effective antiparkinsonian drugs, such as benztropine mesylate, and/or by reduction in dosage. In some instances, however, these extrapyramidal reactions may persist after discontinuation of treatment with perphenazine.

Persistent tardive dyskinesia: As with all antipsychotic agents, tardive dyskinesia may appear in some patients on long-term therapy or may appear after drug therapy has been discontinued. Although the risk appears to be greater in elderly patients on high-dose therapy, especially females, it may occur in either sex and in pediatric patients. The symptoms are persistent and, in some patients, appear to be irreversible. The syndrome is characterized by rhythmical, involuntary movements of the tongue, face, mouth, or jaw (eg, protrusion of tongue, puffing of cheeks, puckering of mouth, chewing movements). Sometimes these may be accompanied by involuntary movements of the extremities. There is no known effective treatment for tardive dyskinesia; antiparkinsonism agents usually do not alleviate the symptoms of this syndrome. It is suggested that all antipsychotic agents be discontinued if these symptoms appear. Should it be necessary to reinstitute treatment, increase the dosage of the agent, or switch to a different antipsychotic agent, the syndrome may be masked. It has been reported that fine vermicular movements of the tongue may be an early sign of the syndrome, and if the medication is stopped at that time the syndrome may not develop.

Other CNS effects include cerebral edema; abnormality of cerebrospinal fluid proteins; convulsive seizures, particularly in patients with EEG abnormalities or a history of such disorders; and headaches.

Neuroleptic malignant syndrome has been reported in patients treated with neuroleptic drugs (see **WARNINGS** section for further information).

Drowsiness may occur, particularly during the first or second week, after which it generally disappears. If troublesome, lower the dosage. Hypnotic effects appear to be minimal, especially in patients who are permitted to remain active.

Adverse behavioral effects include paradoxical exacerbation of psychotic symptoms, catatonic-like states, paranoid reactions, lethargy, paradoxical excitement, restlessness, hyperactivity, nocturnal confusion, bizarre dreams, and insomnia.

Hyperreflexia has been reported in the newborn when a phenothiazine was used during pregnancy.

Autonomic Effects: dry mouth or salivation, nausea, vomiting, diarrhea, anorexia, constipation, obstipation, fecal impaction, urinary retention, frequency or incontinence, polyuria, bladder paralysis, nasal congestion, pallor, myosis, mydriasis, blurred vision, glaucoma, perspiration, hypertension, hypotension, and a change in pulse rate occasionally may occur. Significant autonomic effects have been infrequent in patients receiving less than 24 mg perphenazine daily.

Adynamic ileus occasionally occurs with phenothiazine therapy and, if severe, can result in complications and death. It is of particular concern in psychiatric patients, who may fail to seek treatment of the condition.

Allergic Effects: urticaria, erythema, eczema, exfoliative dermatitis, pruritus, photosensitivity, asthma, fever, anaphylactoid reactions, laryngeal edema, and angioneurotic edema; contact dermatitis in nursing personnel administering the drug; and, in extremely rare instances, individual idiosyncrasy or hypersensitivity to phenothiazines has resulted in cerebral edema, circulatory collapse, and death.

Endocrine Effects: lactation, galactorrhea, moderate breast enlargement in females and gynecomastia in males on large doses, disturbances in the menstrual cycle, amenorrhea, changes in libido, inhibition of ejaculation, false-positive pregnancy tests, hyperglycemia, hypoglycemia, glycosuria, syndrome of inappropriate ADH (antidiuretic hormone) secretion.
Cardiovascular Effects: postural hypotension, tachycardia (especially with sudden marked increase in dosage), bradycardia, cardiac arrest, faintness, and dizziness. Occasionally the hypotensive effect may produce a shock-like condition. ECG changes, nonspecific (quinidine-like effect), usually reversible, have been observed in some patients receiving phenothiazine tranquilizers.
Sudden death has occasionally been reported in patients who have received phenothiazines. In some cases, the death was apparently due to cardiac arrest; in others, the cause appeared to be asphyxia due to failure of the cough reflex. In some patients, the cause could not be determined nor could it be established that the death was due to the phenothiazine.
Hematological Effects: agranulocytosis, eosinophilia, leukopenia, hemolytic anemia, thrombocytopenic purpura, and pancytopenia. Most cases of agranulocytosis have occurred between the fourth and tenth weeks of therapy. Patients should be watched closely, especially during that period, for the sudden appearance of sore throat or signs of infection. If white blood cell and differential cell counts show significant cellular depression, discontinue the drug and start appropriate therapy. However, a slightly lowered white count is not in itself an indication to discontinue the drug.
Other Effects: Special considerations in long-term therapy include pigmentation of the skin, occurring chiefly in the exposed areas; ocular changes consisting of deposition of fine particulate matter in the cornea and lens, progressing in more severe cases to star-shaped lenticular opacities; epithelial keratopathies; and pigmentary retinopathy. Also noted: peripheral edema, reversed epinephrine effect, increase in PBI not attributable to an increase in thyroxine, parotid swelling (rare), hyperpyrexia, systemic lupus erythematosus-like syndrome, increases in appetite and weight, polyphagia, photophobia, and muscle weakness.
Liver damage (biliary stasis) may occur. Jaundice may occur, usually between the second and fourth weeks of treatment, and is regarded as a hypersensitivity reaction. Incidence is low. The clinical picture resembles infectious hepatitis but with laboratory features of obstructive jaundice. It is usually reversible; however, chronic jaundice has been reported.

Amitriptyline Hydrochloride

Although activation of latent schizophrenia has been reported with antidepressant drugs, including amitriptyline hydrochloride, it may be prevented with ETRAFON Tablets in some cases because of the antipsychotic effect of perphenazine. A few instances of epileptiform seizures have been reported in chronic schizophrenic patients during treatment with amitriptyline hydrochloride.
Note: Included in the listing which follows are a few adverse reactions which have not been reported with this specific drug. However, pharmacological similarities among the tricyclic antidepressant drugs require that each of the reactions be considered when amitriptyline hydrochloride is administered.
Allergic Effects: rash, pruritus, urticaria, photosensitization, edema of face and tongue.
Anticholinergic Effects: dry mouth, blurred vision, disturbance of accommodation, constipation, paralytic ileus, urinary retention, dilatation of urinary tract.
Cardiovascular Effects: hypotension, hypertension, tachycardia, palpitations, myocardial infarction, arrhythmias, heart block, stroke.
CNS and Neuromuscular Effects: confusional states; disturbed concentration; disorientation; delusions; hallucinations; excitement; jitteriness; anxiety; restlessness; insomnia; nightmares; numbness, tingling, and paresthesias of the extremities; peripheral neuropathy; incoordination; ataxia; tremors; seizures; alteration in EEG patterns; extrapyramidal symptoms; tinnitus.
Endocrine Effects: testicular swelling and gynecomastia in the male, breast enlargement and galactorrhea in the female, increased or decreased libido, elevation and lowering of blood sugar levels, syndrome of inappropriate ADH (antidiuretic hormone) secretion.
Gastrointestinal Effects: nausea, epigastric distress, heartburn, vomiting, anorexia, stomatitis, peculiar taste, diarrhea, jaundice, parotid swelling, black tongue. Rarely hepatitis has occurred (including altered liver function and jaundice).
Hematological Effects: bone marrow depression, including agranulocytosis, leukopenia, eosinophilia, purpura, thrombocytopenia.
Other Effects: dizziness, weakness, fatigue, headache, weight gain or loss, increased perspiration, urinary frequency, mydriasis, drowsiness, alopecia.
Withdrawal Symptoms: abrupt cessation of treatment after prolonged administration may produce nausea, headache, and malaise. These are not indicative of addiction.

DOSAGE AND ADMINISTRATION

Initial Dosage

In psychoneurotic patients whose anxiety and depression warrant combined therapy, one ETRAFON Tablet (2-25) or one ETRAFON-Forte Tablet (4-25) three or four times a day is recommended.
In elderly patients and adolescents, a lower initial dosage may be needed. The dosage may then be adjusted cautiously to produce an adequate response.
In more severely ill patients with schizophrenia, two ETRAFON-Forte Tablets (4-25) three times a day are recommended as the initial dosage. If necessary, a fourth dose may be given at bedtime. The total daily dosage should not exceed eight tablets of any strength.

Maintenance Dosage

Depending on the condition being treated, the onset of therapeutic response may vary from a few days to a few weeks or even longer. After a satisfactory response is noted, dosage should be reduced to the smallest dose which is effective for relief of the symptoms for which ETRAFON Tablets are being administered. A useful maintenance dosage is one ETRAFON Tablet (2-25) or one ETRAFON-Forte Tablet (4-25) two to four times a day. In some patients, maintenance dosage is required for many months.
ETRAFON 2-10 Tablets (2-10) can be used to increase flexibility in adjusting maintenance dosage to the lowest amount consistent with relief of symptoms.

OVERDOSAGE*

Deaths may occur from overdosage with this class of drugs. Multiple drug ingestion (including alcohol) is common in deliberate overdose. As the management is complex and changing, it is recommended that the physician contact a poison control center for current information on treatment. Signs and symptoms of toxicity develop rapidly after overdose; therefore, hospital monitoring is required as soon as possible.
Manifestations: Overdosage of ETRAFON Tablets may cause any of the adverse reactions listed for perphenazine or amitriptyline hydrochloride.
Overdosage of perphenazine usually produces extrapyramidal symptoms such as dyskinesia and dystonia as described under **ADVERSE REACTIONS**, but this may be masked by the anticholinergic effects of amitriptyline. Other symptoms may include stupor or coma; children may have convulsive seizures.
Critical manifestations of tricyclic antidepressant overdose includes: cardiac dysrhythmias, severe hypotension, convulsions, and CNS depression, including coma. Changes in the electrocardiogram, particularly in QRS axis or width, are clinically significant indicators of tricyclic antidepressant toxicity. Other signs of overdose may include: confusion, disturbed concentration, transient visual hallucinations, dilated pupils, agitation, hyperactive reflexes, stupor, drowsiness, muscle rigidity, vomiting, hypothermia, hyperpyrexia, or any of the symptoms listed under **ADVERSE REACTIONS**.
Management: *General:* Obtain an ECG and immediately initiate cardiac monitoring. Protect the patient's airway, establish an intravenous line, and initiate gastric decontamination. A minimum of 6 hours of observation with cardiac monitoring and observation for signs of CNS or respiratory depression, hypotension, cardiac dysrhythmias and/or conduction blocks, and seizures is necessary. If signs of toxicity occur at any time during this period, extended monitoring is required. There are case reports of patients succumbing to fatal dysrhythmias late after overdose; these patients had clinical evidence of significant poisoning prior to death and most received inadequate gastrointestinal decontamination. Monitoring of plasma drug levels should not guide management of the patient.
Gastrointestinal Decontamination: All patients suspected of tricyclic antidepressant overdose should receive gastrointestinal decontamination. This should include large volume gastric lavage followed by activated charcoal. If consciousness is impaired, the airway should be secured prior to lavage. Emesis is contraindicated.
Cardiovascular: A maximal limb-lead QRS duration of ≥ 0.10 seconds may be the best indication of the severity of the overdose. Intravenous sodium bicarbonate should be used to maintain the serum pH in the range of 7.45 to 7.55. If the pH response is inadequate, hyperventilation may also be used. Concomitant use of hyperventilation and sodium bicarbonate should be done with extreme caution, with frequent pH monitoring. A pH > 7.60 or a $pCO_2 < 20$ mm Hg is undesirable. Dysrhythmias unresponsive to sodium bicarbonate therapy/hyperventilation may respond to lidocaine, bretylium, or phenytoin. Type 1A and 1C anti-arrhythmics are generally contraindicated (eg, quinidine, disopyramide, and procainamide).
In rare instances, hemoperfusion may be beneficial in acute refractory cardiovascular instability in patients with acute toxicity. However, hemodialysis, peritoneal dialysis, exchange transfusions, and forced diuresis generally have been reported as ineffective in tricyclic antidepressant poisoning.
CNS: In patients with CNS depression, early intubation is advised because of the potential for abrupt deterioration. Seizures should be controlled with benzodiazepines, or if these are ineffective, other anticonvulsants (eg, phenobarbital, phenytoin). Physostigmine is not recommended except to treat life-threatening symptoms that have been unresponsive to other therapies, and then only in consultation with a poison control center.
Psychiatric Follow-up: Since overdosage is often deliberate, patients may attempt suicide by other means during the recovery phase. Psychiatric referral may be appropriate.
Pediatric Management: The principles of management of child and adult overdosages are similar. It is strongly recommended that the physician contact the local poison control center for specific pediatric treatment.

HOW SUPPLIED

ETRAFON 2-10 Tablets (perphenazine 2 mg and amitriptyline hydrochloride 10 mg): deep yellow, sugar-coated tablets branded in blue-black with the Schering trademark and either product identification letters ANA, or number 287; bottles of 100 (NDC 0085-0287-04) and box of 100 for unit-dose dispensing (10 strips of 10 tablets each) (NDC 0085-0287-08).
ETRAFON Tablets (perphenazine 2 mg and amitriptyline hydrochloride 25 mg): pink, sugar-coated tablets branded in red with the Schering trademark and either product identification letters ANC, or number 598; bottles of 100 (NDC 0085-0598-04) and box of 100 for unit-dose dispensing (10 strips of 10 tablets each) (NDC 0085-0598-08).
ETRAFON-Forte Tablets (perphenazine 4 mg and amitriptyline hydrochloride 25 mg): red, sugar-coated tablets branded in blue with the Schering trademark and either product identification letters ANE, or number 720; bottles of 100 (NDC 0085-0720-04) and box of 100 for unit-dose dispensing (10 strips of 10 tablets each) (NDC 0085-0720-08).
Store ETRAFON 2-10, 2-25, 4-25 Tablets between 2° and 25°C (36° and 77°F). In addition, protect unit-dose packages from excessive moisture.
* *Poisindex® Toxicologic Management.* Topic: Antidepressants, Tricyclic. Micromedex Inc. Vol 85.

ETRAFON®
brand of perphenazine and
amitriptyline hydrochloride
ETRAFON 2-10 TABLETS (2-10), USP
ETRAFON TABLETS (2-25), USP
ETRAFON-FORTE TABLETS (4-25), USP
Schering Corporation
Kenilworth, NJ 07033 USA
Rev. 1/00 23765004
23765101T

Shown in Product Identification Guide, page 334

EULEXIN® ℞
brand of flutamide
Capsules

WARNINGS

Hepatic Injury

There have been postmarketing reports of hospitalization and rarely death due to liver failure in patients taking flutamide. Evidence of hepatic injury included elevated serum transaminase levels, jaundice, hepatic encephalopathy, and death related to acute hepatic failure. The hepatic injury was reversible after discontinuation of therapy in some patients. Approximately half of the reported cases occurred within the initial 3 months of treatment with flutamide.
Serum transaminase levels should be measured prior to starting treatment with flutamide. Flutamide is not recommended in patients whose ALT values exceed twice the upper limit of normal. Serum transaminase levels should then be measured monthly for the first 4 months of therapy, and periodically thereafter. Liver function tests also should be obtained at the first signs and symptoms suggestive of liver dysfunction, eg, nausea, vomiting, abdominal pain, fatigue, anorexia, "flu-like" symptoms, hyperbilirubinuria, jaundice, or right upper quadrant tenderness. If at any time a patient has jaundice, or their ALT rises above 2 times the upper limit of normal, flutamide should be immediately discontinued with close follow-up of liver function tests until resolution.

DESCRIPTION

EULEXIN Capsules contain flutamide, an acetanilid, nonsteroidal, orally active antiandrogen having the chemical name, 2-methyl-*N*-[4-nitro-3-(trifluoromethyl)phenyl] propanamide.
Each capsule contains 125 mg flutamide. The compound is a buff to yellow powder with a molecular weight of 276.2 and the following structural formula:

CF_3
$CH_3CHCONH$—(ring)—NO_2
CH_3

The inactive ingredients for EULEXIN Capsules include: corn starch, lactose, magnesium stearate, povidone, and sodium lauryl sulfate. Gelatin capsule shells may contain methylparaben, propylparaben, butylparaben, and the fol-

Continued on next page

Information on Schering products appearing on these pages is effective as of January 2000.

Eulexin—Cont.

lowing dye systems: FD&C Blue 1, FD&C Yellow 6, and either FD&C Red 3 or FD&C Red 40 plus D&C Yellow 10, with titanium dioxide and other in active ingredients.

CLINICAL PHARMACOLOGY

General: In animal studies, flutamide demonstrates potent antiandrogenic effects. It exerts its antiandrogenic action by inhibiting androgen uptake and/or by inhibiting nuclear binding of androgen in target tissues or both. Prostatic carcinoma is known to be androgen-sensitive and responds to treatment that counteracts the effect of androgen and/or removes the source of androgen, eg, castration. Elevations of plasma testosterone and estradiol levels have been noted following flutamide administration.

Pharmacokinetics:

Absorption Analysis of plasma, urine, and feces following a single oral 200 mg dose of tritium-labeled flutamide to human volunteers showed that the drug is rapidly and completely absorbed. Following a single 250 mg oral dose to normal adult volunteers, the biologically active alpha-hydroxylated metabolite reaches maximum plasma concentrations in about 2 hours, indicating that it is rapidly formed from flutamide.

Distribution In male rats administered an oral 5 mg/kg dose of ^{14}C-flutamide neither flutamide nor any of its metabolites is preferentially accumulated in any tissue except the prostate. Total drug levels were highest 6 hours after drug administration in all tissues. Levels declined at roughly similar rates to low levels at 18 hours. The major metabolite was present at higher concentrations than flutamide in all tissues studied. Following a single 250 mg oral dose to normal adult volunteers, low plasma concentrations of flutamide were detected. The plasma half-life for the alpha-hydroxylated metabolite of flutamide is approximately 6 hours. Flutamide, *in vivo*, at steady-state plasma concentrations of 24 to 78 ng/mL is 94% to 96% bound to plasma proteins.The active metabolite of flutamide, *in vivo*, at steady-state plasma concentrations of 1556 to 2284 ng/mL, is 92% to 94% bound to plasma proteins.

Metabolism The composition of plasma radioactivity, following a single 200 mg oral dose of tritium-labeled flutamide to normal adult volunteers, showed that flutamide is rapidly and extensively metabolized, with flutamide comprising only 2.5% of plasma radioactivity 1 hour after administration. At least six metabolites have been identified in plasma. The major plasma metabolite is a biologically active alpha-hydroxylated derivative which accounts for 23% of the plasma tritium 1 hour after drug administration. The major urinary metabolite is 2-amino-5-nitro-4-(trifluoromethyl)phenol.

Excretion Flutamide and its metabolites are excreted mainly in the urine with only 4.2% of a single dose excreted in the feces over 72 hours.

[See first table above]

Special Populations:

Geriatric Following multiple oral dosing of 250 mg t.i.d. in normal geriatric volunteers, flutamide and its active metabolite approached steady-state plasma levels (based on pharmacokinetic simulations) after the fourth flutamide dose. The half-life of the active metabolite in geriatric volunteers after a single flutamide dose is about 8 hours and at steady state in 9.6 hours.

Race There are no known alterations in flutamide absorption, distribution, metabolism, or excretion due to race.

Renal Impairment Following a single 250 mg dose of flutamide administered to subjects with chronic renal insufficiency, there appeared to be no correlation between creatinine clearance and either C_{max} or AUC of flutamide. Renal impairment did not have an effect on the C_{max} or AUC of the biologically active alpha-hydroxylated metabolite of flutamide. In subjects with creatinine clearance of <29 mL/min, the half-life of the active metabolite was slightly prolonged. Flutamide and its active metabolite were not well dialyzed. Dose adjustment in patients with chronic renal insufficiency is not warranted.

Hepatic Impairment No information on the pharmacokinetics of flutamide in hepatic impairment is available (see **BOXED WARNING, Hepatic Injury**).

Women, Pediatrics Flutamide has not been studied in women or pediatric subjects.

Drug-Drug Interactions Interactions between EULEXIN Capsules and LHRH-agonists have not occurred. Increases in prothrombin time have been noted in patients receiving warfarin therapy (see **PRECAUTIONS**).

Clinical Studies Flutamide has been demonstrated to interfere with testosterone at the cellular level. This can complement medical castration achieved with LHRH-agonists which suppresses testicular androgen production by inhibiting luteinizing hormone secretion.

The effects of combination therapy have been evaluated in two studies. One study evaluated the effects of flutamide and an LHRH- agonist as neoadjuvant therapy to radiation in stage B_2-C prostatic carcinoma and the other study evaluated flutamide and an LHRH- agonist as the sole therapy in stage D_2 prostatic carcinoma.

Stage B_2-C Prostatic Carcinoma The effects of hormonal treatment combined with radiation was studied in 466 patients (231 EULEXIN + goserelin acetate implant + radiation, 235 radiation alone) with bulky primary tumors confined to the pros tate (stage B_2) or extending beyond the capsule (stage C), with or without pelvic node involvement.

Plasma Pharmacokinetics of Flutamide and Hydroxyflutamide in Geriatric Volunteers (mean ± SD)

	Single Dose		Steady State	
	Flutamide	Hydroxyflutamide	Flutamide	Hydroxyflutamide
C_{max} (ng/mL)	25.2 ± 34.2	894 ± 406	113 ± 213	1629 ± 586
Elimination half-life (hr)	—	8.1 ± 1.3	7.8	9.6 ± 2.5
T_{max} (hr)	1.9 ± 0.7	2.7 ± 1.0	1.3 ± 0.7	1.9 ± 0.6
C_{min} (ng/mL)	—	—	—	673 ± 316

Adverse Events During Acute Radiation Therapy (within first 90 days of radiation therapy)			Adverse Events During Late Radiation Phase (after 90 days of radiation therapy)		
	(n=231) Goserelin acetate implant + EULEXIN + Radiation % All	(n=235) Radiation Only % All		(n=231) Goserelin acetate implant + EULEXIN + Radiation % All	(n=235) Radiation Only % All
Rectum/Large Bowel	80	76	Diarrhea	36	40
Bladder	58	60	Cystitis	16	16
Skin	37	37	Rectal Bleeding	14	20
			Proctitis	8	8
			Hematuria	7	12

	(n=294) Flutamide + LHRH agonist % All	(n=285) Placebo + LHRH agonist % All
Hot Flashes	61	57
Loss of Libido	36	31
Impotence	33	29
Diarrhea	12	4
Nausea/Vomiting	11	10
Gynecomastia	9	11
Other	7	9
Other GI	6	4

In this multicentered, controlled trial, administration of EULEXIN Capsules (250 mg t.i.d.) and goserelin acetate (3.6 mg depot) prior to and during radiation was associated with a significantly lower rate of local failure compared to radiation alone (16% vs 33% at 4 years, P<0.001). The combination therapy also resulted in a trend toward reduction in the incidence of distant metastases (27% vs 36% at 4 years, P = 0.058). Median disease-free survival was significantly increased in patients who received complete hormonal therapy combined with radiation as compared to those patients who received radiation alone (4.4 vs 2.6 years, P<0.001). Inclusion of normal PSA level as a criterion for disease-free survival also resulted in significantly increased median disease-free survival in patients receiving the combination therapy (2.7 vs 1.5 years, P<0.001).

Stage D_2 Prostatic Carcinoma To study the effects of combination therapy in metastatic disease, 617 patients (311 leuprolide + flutamide, 306 leuprolide + placebo) with previously untreated advanced prostatic carcinoma were enrolled in a large multicentered, controlled clinical trial. Three and one-half years after the study was initiated, median survival had been reached. The median actuarial survival time was 34.9 months for patients treated with leuprolide and flutamide versus 27.9 months for patients treated with leuprolide alone. This 7-month increment represents a 25% improvement in overall survival time with the flutamide therapy. Analysis of progression-free survival showed a 2.6-month improvement in patients who received leuprolide plus flutamide, a 19% increment over leuprolide and placebo.

INDICATIONS AND USAGE

EULEXIN Capsules are indicated for use in combination with LHRH agonists for the management of locally confined Stage B_2-C and Stage D_2 metastatic carcinoma of the prostate.

Stage B_2-C Prostatic Carcinoma: Treatment with EULEXIN Capsules and the goserelin acetate implant should start 8 weeks prior to initiating radiation therapy and continue during radiation therapy.

Stage D_2 Metastatic Carcinoma: To achieve benefit from treatment, EULEXIN Capsules should be initiated with the LHRH-agonist and continued until progression.

CONTRAINDICATIONS

EULEXIN Capsules are contraindicated in patients who are hypersensitive to flutamide or any component of this preparation.

EULEXIN Capsules are contraindicated in patients with severe hepatic impairment (baseline hepatic enzymes should be evaluated prior to treatment).

WARNINGS

Hepatic Injury: SEE BOXED WARNING.

Use in Women: This product has no indication for women, and should not be used in this population, particularly for nonserious or nonlife-threatening conditions.

Fetal Toxicity: Flutamide may cause fetal harm when administered to a pregnant woman (see **Pregnancy**).

Aniline Toxicity: One metabolite of flutamide is 4-nitro-3-fluoro-methylaniline. Several toxicities consistent with aniline exposure, including methemoglobinemia, hemolytic anemia, and cholestatic jaundice have been observed in both animals and humans after flutamide administration. In patients susceptible to aniline toxicity (eg, persons with glucose-6-phosphate dehydrogenase deficiency, hemoglobin M disease, and smokers), monitoring of methemoglobin levels should be considered.

PRECAUTIONS

General: In clinical trials, gynecomastia occurred in 9% of patients receiving flutamide together with medical castration.

Information for Patients: Patients should be informed that EULEXIN Capsules and the drug used for medical castration should be administered concomitantly, and that they should not interrupt their dosing or stop taking these medications without consulting their physician.

Laboratory Tests: Regular assessment of serum Prostate Specific Antigen (PSA) may be helpful in monitoring the patient's response. If PSA levels rise significantly and consistently during EULEXIN therapy the patients should be evaluated for clinical progression. For patients who have objective progression of disease together with an elevated PSA, a treatment period free of antiandrogen while continuing the LHRH analogue may be considered.

Drug Interactions: Increases in prothrombin time have been noted in patients receiving long-term warfarin therapy after flutamide was initiated. Therefore, close monitoring of prothrombin time is recommended and adjustment of the anticoagulant dose may be necessary when EULEXIN Cap sules are administered concomitantly with warfarin.

Carcinogenesis, Mutagenesis, Impairment of Fertility: In a 1-year dietary study in male rats, interstitial cell adenomas of the testes were present in 49% to 75% of all treated rats (daily doses of 10, 30, and 50 mg/kg/day were administered). These produced plasma C_{max} values that are 1-, 2- to 3-, and 4-fold, respectively, those associated with therapeutic doses in humans. In male rats similarly dosed for 1 year, tumors were still present after 1 year of a drug-free period, but the incidences were 43% to 47%. In a 2-year carcinogenicity study in male rats, daily administration of flutamide at these same doses produced testicular interstitial cell adenomas in 91% to 95% of all treated rats as opposed to 11% of untreated control rats. Mammary adenomas, adenocarcinomas, and fibroadenomas were increased in treated male rats at exposure levels that were 1- to 4-fold those observed during therapeutic dosing in humans. There are likewise reports of malignant breast neoplasms in men treated with EULEXIN Capsules (see **ADVERSE REACTIONS** section).

Flutamide did not demonstrate DNA modifying activity in the Ames *Salmonella*/microsome Mutagenesis Assay. Dominant lethal tests in rats were negative.

Reduced sperm counts were observed during a 6-week study of flutamide monotherapy in normal human volunteers.

Flutamide did not affect estrous cycles or interfere with the mating behavior of male and female rats when the drug was administered at 25 and 75 mg/kg/day prior to mating. Males treated with 150 mg/kg/day (30 times the minimum effective antiandrogenic dose) failed to mate; mating behavior returned to normal after dosing was stopped. Conception rates were decreased in all dosing groups. Suppression of spermato genesis was observed in rats dosed for 52 weeks at approximately 3, 8, or 17 times the human dose and in dogs dosed for 78 weeks at 1.4, 2.3, and 3.7 times the human dose.

Animal Toxicology: Serious cardiac lesions were observed in 2/10 beagle dogs receiving 25 mg/kg/day for 78 weeks and

3/16 receiving 40 mg/kg/day for 2–4 years. These lesions, indicative of chronic injury and repair processes, included chronic myxomatous degeneration, intra-atrial fibrosis, myocardial acidophilic degeneration, vasculitis, and perivasculitis. The doses at which these lesions occurred were associated with 2-hydroxyflutamide levels that were 1- to 12-fold greater than those observed in humans at therapeutic levels.

Pregnancy: *Pregnancy Category D.* There was decreased 24-hour survival in the offspring of pregnant rats treated with flutamide at doses of 30, 100, or 200 mg/kg/day (approximately 3, 9, and 19 times the human dose). A slight increase in minor variations in the development of the sternebrae and vertebrae was seen in fetuses of rats treated with two higher doses. Feminization of the male rats also occurred at the two higher dose levels. There was a decreased survival rate in the offspring of rabbits receiving the highest dose (15 mg/kg/day, equal to 1.4 times the human dose).

ADVERSE REACTIONS

Stage B_2-C Prostatic Carcinoma: Treatment with EULEXIN Capsules and the goserelin acetate implant did not add substantially to the toxicity of radiation treatment alone. The following adverse experiences were reported during a multicenter clinical trial comparing flutamide + goserelin acetate implant + radiation versus radiation alone. The most frequently reported (greater than 5%) adverse experiences are listed below.

[See second table at top of previous page]

Additional adverse event data were collected for the combination therapy with radiation group over both the hormonal treatment and hormonal treatment plus radiation phases of the study. Adverse experiences occurring in more than 5% of patients in this group, over both parts of the study, were hot flashes (46%), diarrhea (40%), nausea (9%), and skin rash (8%).

Stage D_2 Metastatic Carcinoma: The following adverse experiences were reported during a multicenter clinical trial comparing flutamide + LHRH agonist versus placebo + LHRH agonist.

The most frequently reported (greater than 5%) adverse experiences during treatment with EULEXIN Capsules in combination with an LHRH agonist are listed in the table below. For comparison, adverse experiences seen with an LHRH agonist and placebo are also listed in the following table.

[See third table at top of previous page]

As shown in the table, for both treatment groups, the most frequently occurring adverse experiences (hot flashes, impotence, loss of libido) were those known to be associated with low serum androgen levels and known to occur with LHRH agonists alone.

The only notable difference was the higher incidence of diarrhea in the flutamide + LHRH agonist group (12%), which was severe in 5% as opposed to the placebo + LHRH agonist (4%), which was severe in less than 1%.

In addition, the following adverse reactions were reported during treatment with flutamide + LHRH agonist.

Cardiovascular System: hypertension in 1% of patients.

Central Nervous System: CNS (drowsiness/confusion/depression/anxiety/nervousness) reactions occurred in 1% of patients.

Gastrointestinal System: anorexia 4%, and other GI disorders occurred in 6% of patients.

Hematopoietic System: anemia occurred in 6%, leukopenia in 3%, and thrombocytopenia in 1% of patients.

Liver and Biliary System: hepatitis and jaundice in less than 1% of patients.

Skin: irritation at the injection site and rash occurred in 3% of patients.

Other: edema occurred in 4%, genitourinary and neuromuscular symptoms in 2%, and pulmonary symptoms in less than 1% of patients.

In addition, the following spontaneous adverse experiences have been reported during the marketing of flutamide: hemolytic anemia, macrocytic anemia, methemoglobinemia, sulfhemoglobinemia, photosensitivity reactions (including erythema, ulceration, bullous eruptions, and epidermal necrolysis), and urine discoloration. The urine was noted to change to an amber or yellow-green appearance which can be attributed to the flutamide and/or its metabolites. Also reported were cholestatic jaundice, hepatic encephalopathy, and hepatic necrosis. The hepatic conditions were often reversible after discontinuing therapy; however, there have been reports of death following severe hepatic injury associated with use of flutamide.

Malignant breast neoplasms have occurred rarely in male patients being treated with EULEXIN Capsules.

Abnormal Laboratory Test Values: Laboratory abnormalities including elevated SGOT, SGPT, bilirubin values, SGGT, BUN, and serum creatinine have been reported.

OVERDOSAGE

In animal studies with flutamide alone, signs of overdose included hypoactivity, piloerection, slow respiration, ataxia, and/or lacrimation, anorexia, tranquilization, emesis, and methemoglobinemia.

Clinical trials have been conducted with flutamide in doses up to 1500 mg per day for periods up to 36 weeks with no serious adverse effects reported. Those adverse reactions reported included gynecomastia, breast tenderness, and some increases in SGOT. The single dose of flutamide ordinarily associated with symptoms of overdose or considered to be life threatening has not been established.

Flutamide is highly protein bound and is not cleared by hemodialysis. As in the management of overdosage with any drug, it should be borne in mind that multiple agents may have been taken. If vomiting does not occur spontaneously, it should be induced if the patient is alert. General supportive care, including frequent monitoring of the vital signs and close observation of the patient, is indicated.

DOSAGE AND ADMINISTRATION

The recommended dosage is 2 capsules 3 times a day at 8-hour intervals for a total daily dose of 750 mg.

HOW SUPPLIED

EULEXIN Capsules, 125 mg, are available as opaque, two-toned brown capsules, imprinted with "Schering 525". They are supplied as follows:

NDC 0085-0525-05—Bottles of 500
NDC 0085-0525-03—Unit Dose packages of 100 (10 × 10's)
NDC 0085-0525-06—Bottles of 180

Store between 2° and 30°C (36° and 86°F).

Protect the Unit Dose packages from excessive moisture.

Schering Corporation
Kenilworth, NJ 07033 USA

Rev. 9/99 18822431

Shown in Product Identification Guide, page 334

INTRON® A ℞

Interferon alfa-2b, recombinant
For Injection

DESCRIPTION

INTRON A Interferon alfa-2b, recombinant for intramuscular, subcutaneous, intralesional, or intravenous Injection is a purified sterile recombinant interferon product.

Interferon alfa-2b, recombinant for Injection has been classified as an alfa interferon and is a water-soluble protein with a molecular weight of 19,271 daltons produced by recombinant DNA techniques. It is obtained from the bacterial fermentation of a strain of *Escherichia coli* bearing a genetically engineered plasmid containing an interferon alfa-2b gene from human leukocytes. The fermentation is carried out in a defined nutrient medium containing the antibiotic tetracycline hydrochloride at a concentration of 5 to 10 mg/L; the presence of this antibiotic is not detectable in the final product. The specific activity of Interferon alfa-2b, recombinant is approximately 2.6×10^8 IU/mg protein as measured by the HPLC assay.

[See first table at top of next page]

Prior to administration, the INTRON A Powder for Injection is to be reconstituted with the provided Diluent for INTRON A Interferon alfa-2b, recombinant for Injection (bacteriostatic water for injection) containing 0.9% benzyl alcohol as a preservative. (See **DOSAGE AND ADMINISTRATION.**) INTRON A Powder for Injection is a white to cream-colored powder.

[See second table at top of next page]
[See third table at top of next page]

CLINICAL PHARMACOLOGY

General The interferons are a family of naturally occurring small proteins and glycoproteins with molecular weights of approximately 15,000 to 2[7],600 daltons produced and secreted by cells in response to viral infections and to synthetic or biological inducers.

Preclinical Pharmacology Interferons exert their cellular activities by binding to specific membrane receptors on the cell surface. Once bound to the cell membrane, interferons initiate a complex sequence of intracellular events. *In vitro* studies demonstrated that these include the induction of certain enzymes, suppression of cell proliferation, immunomodulating activities such as enhancement of the phagocytic activity of macrophages and augmentation of the specific cytotoxicity of lymphocytes for target cells, and inhibition of virus replication in virus-infected cells.

In a study using human hepatoblastoma cell line, HB 611, the *in vitro* antiviral activity of alfa interferon was demonstrated by its inhibition of hepatitis B virus (HBV) replication.

The correlation between these *in vitro* data and the clinical results is unknown. Any of these activities might contribute to interferon's therapeutic effects.

Pharmacokinetics The pharmacokinetics of INTRON A Interferon alfa-2b, recombinant for Injection were studied in 12 healthy male volunteers following single doses of 5 million IU/m^2 administered intramuscularly, subcutaneously, and as a 30-minute intravenous infusion in a crossover design.

The mean serum INTRON A concentrations following intramuscular and subcutaneous injections were comparable. The maximum serum concentrations obtained via these routes were approximately 18 to 116 IU/mL and occurred 3 to 12 hours after administration. The elimination half-life of INTRON A Interferon alfa-2b, recombinant for Injection following both intramuscular and subcutaneous injections was approximately 2 to 3 hours. Serum concentrations were undetectable by 16 hours after the injections.

After intravenous administration, serum INTRON A concentrations peaked (135 to 273 IU/mL) by the end of the 30-minute infusion, then declined at a slightly more rapid rate than after intramuscular or subcutaneous drug administration, becoming undetectable 4 hours after the infusion. The elimination half-life was approximately 2 hours.

Urine INTRON A concentrations following a single dose (5 million IU/m^2) were not detectable after any of the parenteral routes of administration. This result was expected since preliminary studies with isolated and perfused rabbit kidneys have shown that the kidney may be the main site of interferon catabolism.

There are no pharmacokinetic data available for the intralesional route of administration.

Serum Neutralizing Antibodies In INTRON A treated patients tested for antibody activity in clinical trials, serum anti-interferon neutralizing antibodies were detected in 0% (0/90) of patients with hairy cell leukemia, 0.8% (2/260) of patients treated intralesionally for condylomata acuminata, and 4% (1/24) of patients with AIDS-Related Kaposi's Sarcoma. Serum neutralizing antibodies have been detected in <3% of patients treated with higher INTRON A doses in malignancies other than hairy cell leukemia or AIDS-Related Kaposi's Sarcoma. The clinical significance of the appearance of serum anti-interferon neutralizing activity in these indications is not known.

Serum anti-interferon neutralizing antibodies were detected in 7% (12/168) of patients either during treatment or after completing 12 to 48 weeks of treatment with 3 million IU TIW of INTRON A therapy for chronic hepatitis C and in 13% (6/48) of patients who received INTRON A therapy for chronic hepatitis B at 5 million IU QD for 4 months, and in 3% (1/33) of patients treated at 10 million IU TIW. Serum anti-interferon neutralizing antibodies were detected in 9% (5/53) of pediatric patients who received INTRON A therapy for chronic hepatitis B at 6 million IU/m^2 TIW. Among all chronic hepatitis B or C patients, pediatric and adults with detectable serum neutralizing antibodies, the titers detected were low (22/24 with titers ≤1:40 and 2/24 with titers ≤1:160). The appearance of serum anti-interferon neutralizing activity did not appear to affect safety or efficacy.

Hairy Cell Leukemia In clinical trials in patients with hairy cell leukemia, there was depression of hematopoiesis during the first 1 to 2 months of INTRON A treatment, resulting in reduced numbers of circulating red and white blood cells, and platelets. Subsequently, both splenectomized and nonsplenectomized patients achieved substantial and sustained improvements in granulocytes, platelets, and hemoglobin levels in 75% of treated patients and at least some improvement (minor responses) occurred in 90%. INTRON A treatment resulted in a decrease in bone marrow hypercellularity and hairy cell infiltrates. The hairy cell index (HCl), which represents the percent of bone marrow cellularity times the percent of hairy cell infiltrate, was ≥50% at the beginning of the study in 87% of patients. The percentage of patients with such an HCl decreased to 25% after 6 months and to 14% after 1 year. These results indicate that even though hematologic improvement had occurred earlier, prolonged INTRON A treatment may be required to obtain maximal reduction in tumor cell infiltrates in the bone marrow.

The percentage of patients with hairy cell leukemia who required red blood cell or platelet transfusions decreased significantly during treatment and the percentage of patients with confirmed and serious infections declined as granulocyte counts improved. Reversal of splenomegaly and of clinically significant hypersplenism was demonstrated in some patients.

A study was conducted to assess the effects of extended INTRON A treatment on duration of response for patients who responded to initial therapy. In this study, 126 responding patients were randomized to receive additional INTRON A treatment for 6 months or observation for a comparable period, after 12 months of initial INTRON A therapy. During this 6-month period, 3% (2/66) of INTRON A treated patients relapsed compared with 18% (11/60) who were not treated. This represents a significant difference in time to relapse in favor of continued INTRON A treatment (p=0.006/0.01, Log Rank/ Wilcoxon). Since a small proportion of the total population had relapsed, median time to relapse could not be estimated in either group. A similar pattern in relapses was seen when all randomized treatment, including that beyond 6 months, and available follow-up data were assessed. The 15% (10/66) relapses among INTRON A patients occurred over a significantly longer period of time than the 40% (24/60) with observation (p=0.0002/0.0001, Log Rank/Wilcoxon). Median time to relapse was estimated, using the Kaplan-Meier method, to be 6.8 months in the observation group but could not be estimated in the INTRON A group.

Subsequent follow-up with a median time of approximately 40 months demonstrated an overall survival of 87.8%. In a comparable historical control group followed for 24 months, overall median survival was approximately 40%.

Malignant Melanoma The safety and efficacy of INTRON A Interferon alfa-2b, recombinant for Injection was evaluated as adjuvant to surgical treatment in patients with melanoma who were free of disease (postsurgery) but at high risk for systemic recurrence. These included patients with lesions of Breslow thickness ≥4 mm, or patients with le-

Continued on next page

Information on Schering products appearing on these pages is effective as of January 2000.

Intron A—Cont.

sions of any Breslow thickness with primary or recurrent nodal involvement. In a randomized, controlled trial in 280 patients, 143 patients received INTRON A therapy at 20 million IU/m^2 intravenously five times per week for 4 weeks (induction phase) followed by 10 million IU/m^2 subcutaneously three times per week for 48 weeks (maintenance phase). INTRON A therapy was begun ≤56 days after surgical resection. The remaining 137 patients were observed. INTRON A therapy produced a significant increase in relapse-free and overall survival. Median time to relapse for the INTRON A treated patients vs observation patients was 1.72 years vs 0.98 years (p<0.01, stratified Log Rank). The estimated 5-year relapse-free survival rate, using the Kaplan-Meier method, was 37% for INTRON A treated patients vs 26% for observation patients. Median overall survival time for INTRON A treated patients vs observation patients was 3.82 years vs 2.78 years (p=0.047, stratified Log Rank). The estimated 5-year overall survival rate, using the Kaplan-Meier method, was 46% for INTRON A treated patients vs 37% for observation patients.

Follicular Lymphoma The safety and efficacy of INTRON A in conjunction with CHVP, a combination chemotherapy regimen, was evaluated as initial treatment in patients with clinically aggressive, large tumor burden, Stage III/IV follicular Non-Hodgkin's Lymphoma. Large tumor burden was defined by the presence of any one of the following: a nodal or extranodal tumor mass with a diameter of >7 cm; involvement of at least three nodal sites (each with a diameter of >3 cm); systemic symptoms; splenomegaly; serious effusion, orbital or epidural involvement; ureteral compression; or leukemia.

In a randomized, controlled trial, 130 patients received CHVP therapy and 135 patients received CHVP therapy plus INTRON A therapy at 5 million IU subcutaneously three times weekly for the duration of 18 months. CHVP chemotherapy consisted of cyclophosphamide 600 mg/m^2, doxorubicin 25 mg/m^2, and teniposide (VM-26) 60 mg/m^2, administered intravenously on Day 1 and prednisone at a daily dose of 40 mg/m^2 given orally on Days 1 to 5. Treatment consisted of six CHVP cycles administered monthly, followed by an additional six cycles administered every 2 months for 1 year. Patients in both treatment groups received a total of 12 CHVP cycles over 18 months.

The group receiving the combination of INTRON A therapy plus CHVP had a significantly longer progression-free survival (2.9 years vs 1.5 years, p=0.0001, Log Rank test). After a median follow-up of 6.1 years, the median survival for patients treated with CHVP alone was 5.5 years while median survival for patients treated with CHVP plus INTRON A therapy had not been reached (p=0.004, Log Rank test). In three additional published, randomized, controlled studies of the addition of interferon alfa to anthracycline-containing combination chemotherapy regimens,[1–3] the addition of interferon alfa was associated with significantly prolonged progression-free survival. Differences in overall survival were not consistently observed.

Condylomata Acuminata Condylomata acuminata (venereal or genital warts) are associated with infections of the human papilloma virus (HPV). The safety and efficacy of INTRON A Interferon alfa-2b, recombinant for Injection in the treatment of condylomata acuminata were evaluated in three controlled double-blind clinical trials. In these studies, INTRON A doses of 1 million IU per lesion were administered intralesionally three times a week (TIW), in ≤5 lesions per patient for 3 weeks. The patients were observed for up to 16 weeks after completion of the full treatment course.

INTRON A treatment of condylomata was significantly more effective than placebo, as measured by disappearance of lesions, decreases in lesion size, and by an overall change in disease status. Of 192 INTRON A treated patients and 206 placebo treated patients who were evaluable for efficacy at the time of best response during the course of the study, 42% of INTRON A patients vs 17% of placebo patients experienced clearing of all treated lesions. Likewise, 24% of INTRON A patients vs 8% of placebo patients experienced marked (≥75% to <100%) reduction in lesion size. 18% vs 9% experienced moderate (≥50% to ≤75%) reduction in lesion size, 10% vs 42% had a slight (<50%) reduction in lesion size, 5% vs 24% had no change in lesion size, and 0% vs 1% experienced exacerbation (p<0.001).

In one of these studies, 43% (54/125) of patients in whom multiple (≤3) lesions were treated, experienced complete clearing of all treated lesions during the course of the study. Of these patients, 81% remained cleared 16 weeks after treatment was initiated.

Patients who did not achieve total clearing of all their treated lesions had these same lesions treated with a second course of therapy. During this second course of treatment, 38% to 67% of patients had clearing of all treated lesions. The overall percentage of patients who had cleared all their treated lesions after two courses of treatment ranged from 57% to 85%.

INTRON A treated lesions showed improvement within 2 to 4 weeks after the start of treatment in the above study; maximal response to INTRON A therapy was noted 4 to 8 weeks after initiation of treatment.

The response to INTRON A therapy was better in patients who had condylomata for shorter durations than in patients with lesions for a longer duration.

Powder for Injection

Vial Strength	mL Diluent	Final Concentration after Reconstitution million IU/mL*	mg INTRON A† Interferon alfa-2b, recombinant	Route of Administration
3 MIU	1	3	0.012	IM, SC, IV
5 MIU	1	5	0.019	IM, SC, IV
10 MIU	2	5	0.038	IM, SC, IV, IL++
18 MIU	1	18	0.069	IM, SC, IV
25 MIU	5	5	0.096	IM, SC, IV
50 MIU	1	50	0.192	IM, SC, IV

*Each mL also contains 20 mg glycine, 2.3 mg sodium phosphate dibasic, 0.55 mg sodium phosphate monobasic, and 1.0 mg human albumin.
†Based on the specific activity of approximately 2.6 × 10^8 IU/mg protein, as measured by HPLC assay.
++The 10 MIU vial for intralesional use should be reconstituted with 1 mL of the provided diluent.

Solution Vials for Injection

Vial Strength	Final Concentration*	mg INTRON A† Interferon alfa-2b, recombinant	Route of Administration
3 MIU	3 million IU/0.5 mL	0.012	IM, SC
5 MIU	5 million IU/0.5 mL	0.019	IM, SC, IL
10 MIU	10 million IU/1.0 mL	0.038	IM, SC, IL
18‡ MIU multidose	3 million IU/0.5 mL	0.088	IM, SC
25¶ MIU multidose	5 million IU/0.5 mL	0.123	IM, SC, IL

*Each mL contains 7.5 mg sodium chloride, 1.8 mg sodium phosphate dibasic, 1.3 mg sodium phosphate monobasic, 0.1 mg edetate disodium, 0.1 mg polysorbate 80, and 1.5 mg m-cresol as a preservative.
† Based on the specific activity of approximately 2.6 × 10^8 IU/mg protein as measured by HPLC assay.
‡ This is a multidose vial which contains a total of 22.8 million IU of interferon alfa-2b, recombinant per 3.8 mL in order to provide the delivery of six 0.5-mL doses, each containing 3 million IU of INTRON A Interferon alfa-2b, recombinant for Injection (for a label strength of 18 million IU).
¶ This is a multidose vial which contains a total of 32.0 million IU of interferon alfa-2b, recombinant per 3.2 mL in order to provide the delivery of five 0.5-mL doses, each containing 5 million IU of INTRON A Interferon alfa-2b, recombinant for Injection (for a label strength of 25 million IU).

Solution in Multidose Pens for Injection

Pen Strength	Final Concentration*	INTRON A Dose Delivered (6 doses, 0.2 mL each)	mg INTRON A†	Route of Administration
18 MIU	22.5 MIU/1.5 mL	3 MIU/dose	0.087	SC
30 MIU	37.5 MIU/1.5 mL	5 MIU/dose	0.144	SC
60 MIU	75 MIU/1.5 mL	10 MIU/dose	0.288	SC

*Each mL also contains 7.5 mg sodium chloride, 1.8 mg sodium phosphate dibasic, 1.3 mg sodium phosphate monobasic, 0.1 mg edetate disodium, 0.1 mg polysorbate 80, and 1.5 mg m-cresol as a preservative.
† Based on the specific activity of approximately 2.6 × 10^8 IU/mg protein as measured by HPLC assay.
These packages do not require reconstitution prior to administration. (See **DOSAGE AND ADMINISTRATION**.)
INTRON A Solution for Injection is a clear, colorless solution.

Another study involved 97 patients in whom three lesions were treated with either an intralesional injection of 1.5 million IU of INTRON A Interferon alfa-2b, recombinant for Injection per lesion followed by a topical application of 25% podophyllin, or a topical application of 25% podophyllin alone. Treatment was given once a week for 3 weeks. The combined treatment of INTRON A Interferon alfa-2b, recombinant for Injection and podophyllin was shown to be significantly more effective than podophyllin alone, as determined by the number of patients whose lesions cleared. This significant difference in response was evident after the second treatment (Week 3) and continued through 8 weeks posttreatment. At the time of the patient's best response, 67% (33/49) of the INTRON A Interferon alfa-2b, recombinant for Injection and podophyllin treated patients had all three treated lesions clear while 42% (20/48) of the podophyllin treated patients had all three clear (p=0.003).

AIDS-Related Kaposi's Sarcoma The safety and efficacy of INTRON A Interferon alfa-2b, recombinant for Injection in the treatment of Kaposi's Sarcoma (KS), a common manifestation of the Acquired Immune Deficiency Syndrome (AIDS), were evaluated in clinical trials in 144 patients.

In one study, INTRON A doses of 30 million IU/m^2 were administered subcutaneously three times per week (TIW), to patients with AIDS-Related KS. Doses were adjusted for patient tolerance. The average weekly dose delivered in the first 4 weeks was 150 million IU; at the end of 12 weeks this averaged 110 million IU/week; and by 24 weeks averaged 75 million IU/week.

Forty-four percent of asymptomatic patients responded vs 7% of symptomatic patients. The median time to response was approximately 2 months and 1 month, respectively, for asymptomatic and symptomatic patients. The median duration of response was approximately 3 months and 1 month, respectively, for the asymptomatic and symptomatic patients. Baseline T4/T8 ratios were 0.46 for responders vs 0.33 for non-responders.

In another study, INTRON A doses of 35 million IU were administered subcutaneously, daily (QD), for 12 weeks. Maintenance treatment, with every other day dosing (QOD), was continued for up to 1 year in patients achieving antitumor and antiviral responses. The median time to response was 2 months and the median duration of response was 5 months in the asymptomatic patients.

In all studies, the likelihood of response was greatest in patients with relatively intact immune systems as assessed by baseline CD4 counts (interchangeable with T4 counts). Results at doses of 30 million IU/m^2 TIW and 35 million IU/QD were subcutaneously similar and are provided together in TABLE 1. This table demonstrates the relationship of response to baseline CD4 count in both asymptomatic and symptomatic patients in the 30 million IU/m^2 TIW and the 35 million IU/QD treatment groups.

In the 30 million IU study group, 7% (5/72) of patients were complete responders and 22% (16/72) of the patients were partial responders. The 35 million IU study had 13% (3/23 patients) complete responders and 17% (4/23) partial responders.

For patients who received 30 million IU TIW, the median survival time was longer in patients with CD4 >200 (30.7 months) than in patients with CD4 ≤200 (8.9 months). Among responders, the median survival time was 22.6 months vs 9.7 months in nonresponders.

Chronic Hepatitis C The safety and efficacy of INTRON A Interferon alfa-2b, recombinant for Injection in the treatment of chronic hepatitis C was evaluated in 5 randomized clinical studies in which an INTRON A dose of 3 million IU three times a week (TIW) was assessed. The initial three studies were placebo-controlled trials that evaluated a 6-month (24 week) course of therapy. In each of the three studies, INTRON A therapy resulted in a reduction in serum alanine aminotransferase (ALT) in a greater proportion of patients vs control patients at the end of 6 months of dosing. During the 6 months of follow-up, approximately 50% of the patients who responded maintained their ALT response. A combined analysis comparing pretreatment and posttreatment liver biopsies revealed histological improvement in a statistically significantly greater proportion of INTRON A treated patients compared to controls.

Two additional studies have investigated longer treatment durations (up to 24 months).[5,6] Patients in the two studies to evaluate longer duration of treatment had hepatitis with or without cirrhosis in the absence of decompensated liver disease. Complete response to treatment was defined as normalization of the final two serum ALT levels during the treatment period. A sustained response was defined as a complete response at the end of the treatment period with sustained normal ALT values lasting at least 6 months following discontinuation of therapy.

In Study 1, all patients were initially treated with INTRON-A 3 million IU TIW subcutaneously for 24 weeks (run-in-period). Patients who completed the initial 24-week treatment period were then randomly assigned to receive no further treatment, or to receive 3 million IU TIW for an additional 48 weeks. In Study 2, patients who met the entry criteria were randomly assigned to receive INTRON A 3 million IU TIW subcutaneously for 24 weeks or to receive INTRON A 3 million IU TIW subcutaneously for 96 weeks. In both studies, patient follow-up was variable and some data collection was retrospective.

Results show that longer durations of INTRON A therapy improved the sustained response rate (see TABLE 2). In patients with complete responses (CR) to INTRON A therapy after 6 months of treatment (149/352 [42%]), responses were less often sustained if drug was discontinued (21/70 [30%]) than if it was continued for 18 to 24 months (44/79 [56%]). Of all patients randomized, the sustained response rate in the patients receiving 18 or 24 months of therapy was 22% and 26%, respectively, in the two trials. In patients who did not have a CR by 6 months, additional therapy did not result in significantly more responses, since almost all patients who responded to therapy did so within the first 16 weeks of treatment.

A subset (<50%) of patients from the combined extended dosing studies had liver biopsies performed both before and after INTRON A treatment. Improvement in necroinflammatory activity as assessed retrospectively by the Knodell (Study 1) and Scheuer (Study 2) Histology Activity Indices was observed in both studies. A higher number of patients (58%, 45/78) improved with extended therapy than with shorter (6 months) therapy (38%, 34/89) in this subset.

REBETRON™ Combination Therapy containing INTRON A and REBETOL® (ribavirin, USP) Capsules has been shown to provide a significant reduction in virologic load and improved histologic response in patients with compensated liver disease who have relapsed following therapy with alfa interferon alone and in patients previously untreated with alfa interferon. See REBETRON Combination Therapy package insert for additional information.

Chronic Hepatitis B ***Adults*** The safety and efficacy of INTRON A Interferon alfa-2b, recombinant for Injection in the treatment of chronic hepatitis B were evaluated in three clinical trials in which INTRON A doses of 30 to 35 million IU per week were administered subcutaneously (SC), as either 5 million IU daily (QD), or 10 million IU three times a week (TIW) for 16 weeks vs no treatment. All patients were 18 years of age or older with compensated liver disease, and had chronic hepatitis B virus (HBV) infection (serum HBsAg positive for at least 6 months) and HBV replication (serum HBeAg positive). Patients were also serum HBV-DNA positive, an additional indicator of HBV replication, as measured by a research assay.[7,8] All patients had elevated serum alanine aminotransferase (ALT) and liver biopsy findings compatible with the diagnosis of chronic hepatitis. Patients with the presence of antibody to human immunodeficiency virus (anti-HIV) or antibody to hepatitis delta virus (anti-HDV) in the serum were excluded from the studies.

Virologic response to treatment was defined in these studies as a loss of serum markers of HBV replication (HBeAg and HBV DNA). Secondary parameters of response included loss of serum HBsAg, decreases in serum ALT, and improvement in liver histology.

In each of two randomized controlled studies, a significantly greater proportion of INTRON A treated patients exhibited a virologic response compared with untreated control patients (see TABLE 3). In a third study without a concurrent control group, a similar response rate to INTRON A therapy was observed. Pretreatment with prednisone, evaluated in two of the studies, did not improve the response rate and provided no additional benefit.

The response to INTRON A therapy was durable. No patient responding to INTRON A therapy at a dose of 5 million IU QD or 10 million IU, TIW, relapsed during the follow-up period which ranged from 2 to 6 months after treatment ended. The loss of serum HBeAg and HBV DNA was maintained in 100% of 19 responding patients followed for 3.5 to 36 months after the end of therapy.

In a proportion of responding patients, loss of HBeAg was followed by the loss of HBsAg. HBsAg was lost in 27% (4/15) of patients who responded to INTRON A therapy at a dose of 5 million IU QD, and 35% (8/23) of patients who responded to 10 million IU TIW. No untreated control patient lost HBsAg in these studies.

In an ongoing study to assess the long-term durability of virologic response, 64 patients responding to INTRON A therapy have been followed for 1.1 to 6.6 years after treatment; 95% (61/64) remain serum HBeAg negative and 49% (30/61) have lost serum HBsAg.

INTRON A therapy resulted in normalization of serum ALT in a significantly greater proportion of treated patients compared to untreated patients in each of two controlled studies

TABLE 2

SUSTAINED ALT RESPONSE RATE VS DURATION OF THERAPY

IN ***CHRONIC HEPATITIS C*** *PATIENTS*

INTRON A 3 Million IU TIW

Treatment Group—Number of Patients (%)*

Study Number	*INTRON A 3 million IU 24 weeks of treatment*		*INTRON A 3 million IU 72 or 96 weeks of treatment†*		*Difference (Extended - 24 weeks) (95% CI)‡*	
	ALT response at the end of follow-up					
1	12/101	(12%)	23/104	(22%)	10%	(-3, 24)
2	9/67	(13%)	21/80	(26%)	13%	(-4, 30)
Combined Studies	**21/168**	**(12.5%)**	**44/184**	**(24%)**	**11.4%**	**(2, 21)**
	ALT response at the end of treatment					
1	40/101	(40%)	51/104	(49%)	—	
2	32/67	(48%)	35/80	(44%)	—	

* Intent to treat groups.
† Study 1: 72 weeks of treatment; Study 2: 96 weeks of treatment.
‡ Confidence intervals adjusted for multiple comparisons due to 3 treatment arms in the study.

TABLE 3

*VIROLOGIC RESPONSE**

IN ***CHRONIC HEPATITIS B*** *PATIENTS*

Treatment Group†—Number of Patients (%)

Study Number	*INTRON A 5 million IU QD*		*INTRON A 10 million IU TIW*		*Untreated Controls*		*p‡ Value*
1[7]	15/38	(39%)	—	—	3/42	(7%)	0.0009
2	—	—	10/24	(42%)	1/22	(5%)	0.005
3[8]	—	—	13/24§	(54%)	2/27	(7%)§	NA§
All Studies	**15/38**	**(39%)**	**23/48**	**(48%)**	**6/91**	**(7%)**	**—**

* Loss of HBeAg and HBV DNA by 6 months posttherapy.
† Patients pretreated with prednisone not shown.
‡ INTRON A treatment group vs untreated control.
§ Untreated control patients evaluated after 24-week observation period. A subgroup subsequently received INTRON A therapy. A direct comparison is not applicable (NA).

(see TABLE 4). In a third study without a concurrent control group, normalization of serum ALT was observed in 50% (12/24) of patients receiving INTRON A therapy.

Virologic response was associated with a reduction in serum ALT to normal or near normal ($\leq 1.5 \times$ the upper limit of normal) in 87% (13/15) of patients responding to INTRON A therapy at 5 million IU QD, and 100% (23/23) of patients responding to 10 million IU TIW.

Improvement in liver histology was evaluated in Studies 1 and 3 by comparison of pretreatment and 6-month posttreatment liver biopsies using the semiquantitative Knodell Histology Activity Index.[9] No statistically significant difference in liver histology was observed in treated patients compared to control patients in Study 1. Although statistically significant histological improvement from baseline was observed in treated patients in Study 3 ($p \leq 0.01$), there was no control group for comparison. Of those patients exhibiting a virologic response following treatment with 5 million IU QD or 10 million IU TIW, histological improvement was observed in 85% (17/20) compared to 36% (9/25) of patients who were not virologic responders. The histological improvement was due primarily to decreases in severity of necrosis, degeneration, and inflammation in the periportal, lobular, and portal regions of the liver (Knodell Categories I + II + III). Continued histological improvement was observed in four responding patients who lost serum HBsAg and were followed 2 to 4 years after the end of INTRON A therapy.[10]

Pediatrics The safety and efficacy of INTRON A Interferon alfa-2b, recombinant for Injection in the treatment of chronic hepatitis B was evaluated in one randomized controlled trial of 149 patients ranging from 1 year to 17 years of age. Seventy-two patients were treated with 3 million IU/m^2 of INTRON A therapy administered subcutaneously three times a week (TIW) for 1 week; the dose was then escalated to 6 million IU/m^2 TIW for a minimum of 16 weeks up to 24 weeks. The maximum weekly dosage was 10 million IU TIW. Seventy-seven patients were untreated controls. Study entry and response criteria were identical to those described in the adult patient population.

Patients treated with INTRON A therapy had a better response (loss of HBV DNA and HBeAg at 24 weeks of follow up) compared to the untreated controls (24% [17/72] vs 10% [8/77] p=0.05). Sixteen of the 17 responders treated with INTRON A therapy remained HBV DNA and HBeAg negative and had a normal serum ALT 12 to 24 months after completion of treatment. Serum HBsAg became negative in 7 out of 17 patients who responded to INTRON A therapy. None of the control patients who had an HBV DNA and HBeAg response became HBsAg negative. At 24 weeks of follow up, normalization of serum ALT was similar in patients treated with INTRON A therapy (17%, 12/72) and in untreated control patients (16%, 12/77). Patients with a baseline HBV DNA <100 pg/mL were more likely to respond to INTRON A therapy than were patients with a baseline HBV DNA >100 pg/mL (35% vs 9%, respectively). Patients who contracted hepatitis B through maternal vertical transmission had lower response rates than those who contracted the disease by other means (5% vs 31%, respectively). There was no evidence that the effects of HBV DNA and HBeAg were limited to specific subpopulations based on age, gender, or race.

TABLE 1

*RESPONSE BY BASELINE CD4 COUNT**

IN ***AIDS-RELATED KS*** *PATIENTS*

30 million IU/m²

TIW, SC and 35 million IU QD, SC

	Asymptomatic			Symptomatic	
CD4<200	4/14	(29%)		0/19	(0%)
200≤CD4≤400	6/12	(50%)	} 58%	0/5	(0%)
CD4>400	5/7	(71%)		0/0	(0%)

* Data for CD4, and asymptomatic and symptomatic classification were not available for all patients.

[See table 2 above]
[See table 3 above]
[See table 4 at top of next page]

INDICATIONS AND USAGE

Hair Cell Leukemia

INTRON A Interferon alfa-2b, recombinant for Injection is indicated for the treatment of patients 18 years of age or older with hairy cell leukemia.

Malignant Melanoma

INTRON A Interferon alfa-2b, recombinant for Injection is indicated as adjuvant to surgical treatment in patients 18 years of age or older with malignant melanoma who are free of disease but at high risk for systemic recurrence, within 56 days of surgery.

Follicular Lymphoma

INTRON A Interferon alfa-2b, recombinant for Injection is indicated for the initial treatment of clinically aggressive (see **Clinical Experience**) follicular Non-Hodgkin's Lymphoma in conjunction with anthracycline-containing combination chemotherapy in patients 18 years of age or older. Efficacy of INTRON A in patients with low-grade, low-tumor burden follicular Non-Hodgkin's Lymphoma has not been demonstrated.

Condylomata Acuminata

INTRON A Interferon alfa-2b, recombinant for Injection is indicated for intralesional treatment of selected patients 18 years of age or older with condylomata acuminata involving external surfaces of the genital and perianal areas (see **DOSAGE AND ADMINISTRATION**).

The use of this product in adolescents has not been studied.

AIDS-Related Kaposi's Sarcoma INTRON A Interferon alfa-2b, recombinant for Injection is indicated for the treatment of selected patients 18 years of age or older with AIDS-

Continued on next page

Information on Schering products appearing on these pages is effective as of January 2000.

Intron A—Cont.

Related Kaposi's Sarcoma. The likelihood of response to INTRON A therapy is greater in patients who are without systemic symptoms, who have limited lymphadenopathy and who have a relatively intact immune system as indicated by total CD4 count.

Chronic Hepatitis C INTRON A Interferon alfa-2b, recombinant for Injection is indicated for the treatment of chronic hepatitis C in patients 18 years of age or older with compensated liver disease who have a history of blood or blood-product exposure and/or are HCV antibody positive. Studies in these patients demonstrated that INTRON A therapy can produce meaningful effects on this disease, manifested by normalization of serum alanine aminotransferase (ALT) and reduction in liver necrosis and degeneration.

A liver biopsy should be performed to establish the diagnosis of chronic hepatitis. Patients should be tested for the presence of antibody to HCV. Patients with other causes of chronic hepatitis, including autoimmune hepatitis, should be excluded. Prior to initiation of INTRON A therapy, the physician should establish that the patient has compensated liver disease. The following patient entrance criteria for compensated liver disease were used in the clinical studies and should be considered before INTRON A treatment of patients with chronic hepatitis C:

- No history of hepatic encephalopathy, variceal bleeding, ascites, or other clinical signs of decompensation
- Bilirubin ≤2 mg/dL
- Albumin Stable and within normal limits
- Prothrombin Time <3 seconds prolonged
- WBC ≥3000/mm³
- Platelets ≥70,000/mm³

Serum creatinine should be normal or near normal.

Prior to initiation of INTRON A therapy, CBC and platelet counts should be evaluated in order to establish baselines for monitoring potential toxicity. These tests should be repeated at weeks 1 and 2 following initiation of INTRON A therapy, and monthly thereafter. Serum ALT should be evaluated at approximately 3-month intervals to assess response to treatment (see **DOSAGE AND ADMINISTRATION**).

Patients with preexisting thyroid abnormalities may be treated if thyroid-stimulating hormone (TSH) levels can be maintained in the normal range by medication. TSH levels must be within normal limits upon initiation of INTRON A treatment and TSH testing should be repeated at 3 and 6 months (see **PRECAUTIONS – Laboratory Tests**).

INTRON A in combination with REBETOL (ribavirin, USP) Capsules is indicated for the treatment of chronic hepatitis C in patients with compensated liver disease previously untreated with alfa interferon therapy or who have relapsed following alfa interferon therapy. See REBETRON Combination Therapy package insert for additional information.

Chronic Hepatitis B INTRON A Interferon alfa-2b, recombinant for Injection is indicated for the treatment of chronic hepatitis B in patients 1 year of age or older with compensated liver disease. Patients who have been serum HBsAg positive for at least 6 months and have evidence of HBV replication (serum HBeAg positive) with elevated serum ALT are candidates for treatment. Studies in these patients demonstrated that INTRON A therapy can produce virologic remission of this disease (loss of serum HBeAg), and normalization of serum aminotransferases. INTRON A therapy resulted in the loss of serum HBsAg in some responding patients.

Prior to initiation of INTRON A therapy, it is recommended that a liver biopsy be performed to establish the presence of chronic hepatitis and the extent of liver damage. The physician should establish that the patient has compensated liver disease. The following patient entrance criteria for compensated liver disease were used in the clinical studies and should be considered before INTRON A treatment of patients with chronic hepatitis B:

- No history of hepatic encephalopathy, variceal bleeding, ascites, or other signs of clinical decompensation

• Bilirubin	Normal	
• Albumin	Stable and within normal limits	
• Prothrombin Time	*Adults* <3 seconds prolonged	*Pediatrics* ≤2 seconds prolonged
• WBC	≥4000/mm³	
• Platelets	*Adults* ≥100,000/mm³	*Pediatrics* ≥150,000/mm³

Patients with causes of chronic hepatitis other than chronic hepatitis B or chronic hepatitis C should be treated with INTRON A Interferon alfa-2b, recombinant for Injection. CBC and platelet counts should be evaluated prior to initiation of INTRON A therapy in order to establish baselines for monitoring potential toxicity. These tests should be repeated at treatment weeks 1, 2, 4, 8, 12, and 16. Liver function tests, including serum ALT, albumin, and bilirubin, should be evaluated at treatment weeks 1, 2, 4, 8, 12, and 16. HBeAg, HBsAg, and ALT should be evaluated at the end of therapy, as well as 3- and 6-months posttherapy, since patients may become virologic responders during the 6-month period following the end of treatment. In clinical studies in adults, 39% (15/38) of responding patients lost HBeAg 1 to 6 months following the end of INTRON A therapy. Of responding patients who lost HBsAg, 58% (7/12) did so 1- to 6-months posttreatment.

A transient increase in ALT ≥2 × baseline value (flare) can occur during INTRON A therapy for chronic hepatitis B. In

TABLE 4
*ALT RESPONSES**
IN ***CHRONIC HEPATITIS B*** *PATIENTS*

Study Number	*Treatment Group—Number of Patients (%)* INTRON A 5 million IU QD		INTRON A 10 million IU TIW		Untreated Controls		*P*† *Value*
1	16/38	(42%)	—	—	8/42	(19%)	0.03
2	—	—	10/24	(42%)	1/22	(5%)	0.0034
3	—	—	12/24‡	(50%)	2/27	(7%)‡	NA‡
All Studies	**16/38**	**(42%)**	**22/48**	**(46%)**	**11/91**	**(12%)**	—

* Reduction in serum ALT to normal by 6 months posttherapy.
† INTRON A treatment group vs untreated control.
‡ Untreated control patients evaluated after 24-week observation period. A subgroup subsequently received INTRON A therapy. A direct comparison is not applicable (NA).

clinical trials in adults and pediatrics, this flare generally occurred 8 to 12 weeks after initiation of therapy and was more frequent in INTRON A responders (*adults* 63%, 24/38; *pediatrics* 59%, 10/17) than in nonresponders (*adults* 27%, 13/48; *pediatrics* 35%, 19/55). However, in adults and pediatrics, elevations in bilirubin ≥3 mg/dL (≥2 times ULN) occurred infrequently (*adults* 2%, 2/86; *pediatrics* 3%, 2/72) during therapy. When ALT flare occurs, in general, INTRON A therapy should be continued unless signs and symptoms of liver failure are observed. During ALT flare, clinical symptomatology and liver function tests including ALT, prothrombin time, alkaline phosphatase, albumin, and bilirubin, should be monitored at approximately 2-week intervals (see **WARNINGS**).

DOSAGE AND ADMINISTRATION

IMPORTANT: INTRON A Interferon alfa-2b, recombinant for Injection dosing regimens are different for each of the following indications described in this section of the product information sheet. INTRON A Solution for Injection multidose pen contains a prefilled, multidose cartridge for subcutaneous administration. It is designed to deliver doses as required using a simple dial mechanism. The needles provided in the packaging should be used for the INTRON A Solution for Injection multidose pen only. A new needle is to be used each time as dose is delivered using the pen. Each INTRON A Solution for Injection multidose pen is for individual patient use only.

Hairy Cell Leukemia The recommended dosage of INTRON A Interferon alfa-2b, recombinant for Injection for the treatment of hairy cell leukemia is 2 million IU/m² administered intramuscularly (see **WARNINGS**) or subcutaneously 3 times a week for up to 6 months. The 50 million IU strength of the INTRON A Powder for Injection is not to be used for the treatment of hairy cell leukemia. Higher doses are not recommended. Responding patients may benefit from continued treatment.

If severe adverse reactions develop, the dosage should be modified (50% reduction) or therapy should be temporarily discontinued until the adverse reactions abate. If persistent or recurrent intolerance develops following adequate dosage adjustment, or disease progresses, INTRON A treatment should be discontinued. The minimum effective INTRON A dose has not been established.

Malignant Melanoma The recommended INTRON A treatment regimen includes induction treatment 5 consecutive days per week for 4 weeks as an intravenous (IV) infusion at a dose of 20 million IU/m², followed by maintenance treatment three times per week for 48 weeks as a subcutaneous (SC) injection, at a dose of 10 million IU/m².

In the clinical trial, the median daily INTRON A doses administered to patients were 19.1 million IU/m² during the induction phase and 9.1 million IU/m² during the maintenance phase.

Regular laboratory testing should be performed to monitor laboratory abnormalities for the purposes of dose modification (see **PRECAUTIONS – Laboratory Tests**). If adverse reactions develop during INTRON A treatment, particularly if granulocytes decrease to <500/mm³ or SGPT/SGOT rises to >5 × upper limit of normal, treatment should be temporarily discontinued until the adverse reactions abate. INTRON A treatment should be restarted at 50% of the previous dose. If intolerance persists after dose adjustments or if granulocytes decrease to <250/mm³ or SGPT/SGOT rises to > 10 × upper limit of normal, INTRON A therapy should be discontinued.

Follicular Lymphoma The recommended dosage of INTRON A Interferon alfa-2b, recombinant for Injection is 5 million IU subcutaneously three times per week for up to 18 months in conjunction with an anthracycline-containing chemotherapy regimen.

In published reports, the doses of myelosuppressive drugs were reduced by 25% from those utilized in a full-dose CHOP regimen, and cycle length increased by 33% (eg, from 21 to 28 days) when an alfa interferon was added to the regimen.[1,4] The dosing regimen should be modified for evidence of serious toxicity. The following dose modification guidelines for hematologic toxicity were used in the clinical trial: the chemotherapy regimen was delayed if either the neutrophil count was <1500/mm³ or the platelet count was <75,000/mm³. Administration of INTRON A was temporarily interrupted for a neutrophil count <1000/mm³, or a platelet count <50,000/mm³, or reduced by 50% to 2.5 MIU TIW for a neutrophil count >1000/mm³ but <1500/mm³. Reinstitution of the initial INTRON A dose (5 million IU TIW) was tolerated after resolution of hematologic toxicity (≥1500/mm³).

INTRON A therapy should be discontinued if SGOT exceeds >5 × the upper limit of normal or serum creatinine >2.0 mg/dL. (See **WARNINGS**.)

Condylomata Acuminata The 10 million IU vial of INTRON A Powder for Injection must be reconstituted with 1 mL of Diluent for INTRON A Interferon alfa-2b, recombinant for Injection (bacteriostatic water for injection). Do not reconstitute the 10 million IU vial of INTRON A Powder for Injection with more than 1 mL of diluent since the injection would be subpotent. Do not use the 3 million, 5 million, 18 million, 25 million, or 50 million IU vials of INTRON A Powder for Injection for the treatment of condylomata acuminata since the resulting reconstituted solution would be either hypertonic or an inappropriate concentration. Do not use the 3 million IU vial or the 18 million IU multidose vial of INTRON A Solution for Injection for the intralesional treatment of condylomata acuminata since the concentrations are inappropriate for such use.

Inject 1.0 million IU of INTRON A Interferon alfa-2b, recombinant for Injection (either 0.1 mL of reconstituted 10 million IU INTRON A Powder for Injection or 0.1 mL of the 5 million IU, 10 million IU, or 25 million IU strengths of INTRON A Solution for Injection, each having a final concentration of 10 million IU/mL) into each lesion three times per week on alternate days, for 3 weeks. The injection should be administered intralesionally using a Tuberculin or similar syringe and a 25- to 30-gauge needle. The needle should be directed at the center of the base of the wart and at an angle almost parallel to the plane of the skin (approximating that in the commonly used PPD test). This will deliver the interferon to the dermal core of the lesion, infiltrating the lesion and causing a small wheal. Care should be taken not to go beneath the lesion too deeply; subcutaneous injection should be avoided, since this area is below the base of the lesion. Do not inject too superficially since this will result in possible leakage, infiltrating only the keratinized layer, and not the dermal core. As many as five lesions can be treated at one time. To reduce side effects, INTRON A injections may be administered in the evening, when possible. Additionally, acetaminophen may be administered at the time of injection to alleviate some of the potential side effects.

The maximum response usually occurs 4 to 8 weeks after initiation of the first treatment course. If results at 12 to 16 weeks after the initial treatment course has concluded are not satisfactory, a second course of treatment using the above dosage schedule may be instituted providing that clinical symptoms and signs, or changes in laboratory parameters (liver function tests, WBC, and platelets) do not preclude such a course of action.

Patients with 6 to 10 condylomata may receive a second (sequential) course of treatment at the above dosage schedule, to treat up to five additional condylomata per course of treatment. Patients with greater than 10 condylomata may receive additional sequences depending on how large a number of condylomata are present.

AIDS-Related Kaposi's Sarcoma The recommended INTRON A dosage is 30 million IU/m² three times a week administered subcutaneously or intramuscularly. The 18 million and 25 million IU multidose strengths of the INTRON A Solution for Injection should not be used for the treatment of AIDS-Related Kaposi's Sarcoma since the concentrations are inappropriate.

The selected dosage regimen should be maintained unless the disease progresses rapidly or severe intolerance is manifested. If severe adverse reactions develop, the dosage should be modified (50% reduction) or therapy should be temporarily discontinued until the adverse reactions abate. When patients initiate therapy at 30 million IU/m² TW, the average dose tolerated at the end of 12 weeks of therapy is 110 million IU/week and 75 million IU/week at the end of 24 weeks of therapy.

When disease stabilization or a response to treatment occurs, treatment should continue until there is no further evidence of tumor or until discontinuation is required by evidence of a severe opportunistic infection or adverse effect.

Chronic Hepatitis C The recommended dosage of INTRON A Interferon alfa-2b, recombinant for Injection for the treatment of chronic hepatitis C is 3 million IU three times a week (TIW) administered subcutaneously or intramuscularly. In patients tolerating therapy with normalization of

ALT at 16 weeks of treatment, INTRON A therapy should be extended to 18 to 24 months (72 to 96 weeks) at 3 million IU TIW to improve the sustained response rate (see **CLINICAL PHARMACOLOGY – Chronic Hepatitis C**). Patients who do not normalize their ALTs after 16 weeks of therapy rarely achieve a sustained response with extension of treatment. Consideration should be given to discontinuing these patients from therapy.

If severe adverse reactions develop during INTRON A treatment, the dose should be modified (50% reduction) or therapy should be temporarily discontinued until the adverse reactions abate. If intolerance persists after dose adjustment, INTRON A therapy should be discontinued.

See REBETRON Combination Therapy package insert for dosing when used in combination with REBETOL (ribavirin, USP) Capsules.

Chronic Hepatitis B ***Adults*** The recommended dosage of INTRON A Interferon alfa-2b, recombinant for Injection for the treatment of chronic hepatitis B is 30 to 35 million IU per week, administered subcutaneously or intramuscularly, either as 5 million IU daily (QD) or as 10 million IU three times a week (TIW) for 16 weeks.

Pediatrics The recommended dosage of INTRON A Interferon alfa-2b, recombinant for Injection for the treatment of chronic hepatitis B is 3 million IU/m^2 three times a week (TIW) for the first week of therapy followed by dose escalation to 6 million IU/m^2 TIW (maximum of 10 million IU TIW) administered subcutaneously for a total therapy duration of 16 to 24 weeks.

If severe adverse reactions or laboratory abnormalities develop during INTRON A therapy, the dose should be modified (50% reduction), or discontinued if appropriate, until the adverse reactions abate. If intolerance persists after dose adjustment, INTRON A therapy should be discontinued.

For patients with decreases in white blood cell, granulocyte, or platelet counts, the following guidelines for dose modification should be followed:

INTRON A Dose	*White Blood Cell Count*	*Granulocyte Count*	*Platelet Count*
Reduce 50%	$<1.5 \times 10^9$/L	$<0.75 \times 10^9$/L	$<50 \times 10^9$/L
Permanently Discontinue	$<1.0 \times 10^9$/L	$<0.5 \times 10^9$/L	$<25 \times 10^9$/L

INTRON A therapy was resumed at up to 100% of the initial dose when white blood cell, granulocyte, and/or platelet counts returned to normal or baseline values.

At the discretion of the physician, the patient may self-administer the medication. (See illustrated **PATIENT INFORMATION SHEET** for instructions.)

Preparation and Administration of INTRON A Interferon alfa-2b, recombinant Powder for Injection for Intramuscular, Subcutaneous, or Intralesional Administration

Reconstitution of INTRON A Powder for Injection Inject the amount of Diluent for INTRON A Interferon alfa-2b, recombinant for Injection (bacteriostatic water for injection) stated in the chart below (diluent is supplied in either a vial or syringe, see **HOW SUPPLIED** below), into the INTRON A vial. Swirl gently to hasten complete dissolution of the powder. The appropriate INTRON A dose should then be withdrawn and injected intramuscularly, subcutaneously, or intralesionally. (See **PATIENT INFORMATION SHEET** for detailed instructions.) After preparation and administration of the INTRON A injection, it is essential to follow the procedure for proper disposal of syringes and needles. (See **PATIENT INFORMATION SHEET** for detailed instructions.)

INTRON A Powder for Injection is not indicated for use in infants and should not be used in pediatric patients in this age group because when reconstituted with the provided diluent it contains benzyl alcohol. (See **WARNINGS Chronic Hepatitis B.**)

Preparation and Administration of INTRON A Interferon alfa-2b, recombinant Powder for Injection for Intravenous Injection

The infusion solution should be prepared immediately prior to use. Based on the desired dose, the appropriate vial strength(s) of INTRON A Interferon alfa-2b, recombinant Powder for Injection should be reconstituted with the diluent provided. The appropriate INTRON A dose should then be withdrawn and injected into a 100-mL bag of 0.9% Sodium Chloride Injection, USP. The final concentration of INTRON A Interferon alfa-2b, recombinant for Injection should be not less than 10 million IU/100 mL. The prepared solution should be infused over a 20-minute period.

[See first table above]

Stability INTRON A Interferon alfa-2b, recombinant Powder for Injection provided in vials ranging from 3 to 50 million IU per vial, is stable at 45°C (113°F) for up to 7 days. After reconstitution with Diluent for INTRON A Interferon alfa-2b, recombinant for Injection (bacteriostatic water for injection) the solution is stable for 1 month at 2° to 8°C (36° to 46°F). The reconstituted solution is clear and colorless to light yellow.

Preparation and Administration of INTRON A Interferon alfa-2b, recombinant Solution for Injection

The 3 million IU, 5 million IU, and 10 million IU vials, and the 18 million and 25 million IU multidose vials of INTRON A Solution for Injection do not require reconstitution prior to administration. The solution is clear and colorless. The appropriate INTRON A dose should be withdrawn from the vial and injected intramuscularly, subcutaneously, or intralesionally (5 million IU and 10 million IU vials, and 25 million IU multidose vials only). After administration of INTRON A Solution for Injection, it is essential to follow the procedure for proper disposal of syringes and needles. (See **PATIENT INFORMATION SHEET** for detailed instructions.)

[See second table above]

INTRON A Interferon alfa-2b, recombinant Powder for Injection

	3 million IU	5 million IU	10 million IU	18 million IU	25 million IU	50 million IU‡
Chronic Hepatitis B		1 mL	1 mL			
Chronic Hepatitis C	1 mL					
Hairy Cell Leukemia	1 mL	1 mL	2 mL		5 mL	
AIDS-Related Kaposi's Sarcoma						1 mL
Condylomata Acuminata			1 mL**			
Malignant Melanoma induction phase†	1 mL*	1 mL	1 mL	1 mL	5 mL	1 mL
maintenance phase	1 mL*	1 mL	1 mL	1 mL		1 mL
Follicular Lymphoma	1 mL	1 mL	1 mL		5 mL	

*Use only for dose reduction.

**IMPORTANT: For patients with condylomata acuminata, reconstitute the 10 million IU vial with only 1 mL of the diluent provided to reach a final concentration of 10 million IU/mL to be administered intralesionally.

† Based on the desired dose, the appropriate vial strengths should be reconstituted and administered intravenously.

‡ This vial strength should be used only for the treatment of patients with AIDS-Related Kaposi's Sarcoma or malignant melanoma since the concentration is inappropriate for all other indications.

INTRON A Interferon alfa-2b, recombinant Solution for Injection

	3 million IU	5 million IU	10 million IU	18 million IU multidose*	25 million IU multidose†
Chronic Hepatitis B		✓	✓		✓§
Chronic Hepatitis C	✓			✓	
Hairy Cell Leukemia	✓	✓	✓	✓	✓
Condylomata Acuminata		✓	✓		✓
Malignant Melanoma	✓‡	✓	✓	✓‡	✓¶
Follicular Lymphoma		✓			✓

*This is a multidose vial which contains a total of 22.8 million IU of interferon alfa-2b, recombinant per 3.8 mL in order to provide the delivery of six 0.5-mL doses, each containing 3 million IU of INTRON A Interferon alfa-2b, recombinant for Injection (for a label strength of 18 million IU).

† This is a multidose vial which contains a total of 32 million IU of interferon alfa-2b, recombinant per 3.2 mL in order to provide the delivery of five 0.5-mL doses, each containing 5 million IU of INTRON A Interferon alfa-2b, recombinant for Injection (for a label strength of 25 million IU).

‡ Use only for dose reduction.

§ Use only for the 5 MIU daily regimen.

¶ Use only for maintenance treatment.

INTRON A Interferon alfa-2b, recombinant Solution in Multidose Pens

	3 million IU/0.2 mL*	5 million IU/0.2 mL**	10 million IU/0.2 mL***
Chronic Hepatitis B		✓	✓
Chronic Hepatitis C	✓		
Hairy Cell Leukemia	✓	✓	
Malignant Melanoma			✓
Follicular Lymphoma		✓	

* The 3 million IU multidose pen contains a total of 22.5 million IU of interferon alfa-2b, recombinant per 1.5 mL in order to provide delivery of six 0.2-mL doses each containing 3 million IU of interferon alfa-2b, recombinant Solution for Injection (for a label strength of 18 million IU).

** The 5 million IU multidose pen contains a total of 37.5 million IU of interferon alfa-2b, recombinant per 1.5 mL in order to provide delivery of six 0.2-mL doses each containing 5 million IU of interferon alfa-2b, recombinant Solution for Injection (for a label strength of 30 million IU).

*** The 10 million IU multidose pen contains a total of 75 million IU of interferon alfa-2b, recombinant per 1.5 mL in order to provide delivery of six 0.2-mL doses each containing 10 million IU of interferon alfa-2b, recombinant Solution for Injection (for a label strength of 60 million IU).

IMPORTANT: The 3 million IU vial and the 18 million IU multidose vial of INTRON A Solution for Injection are not to be used for chronic hepatitis B or condylomata acuminata. **The multidose pen should not be used for condylomata acuminata.** The 10 million IU vial of INTRON A Solution for Injection should not be used for chronic hepatitis C. INTRON A Solution for Injection should not be used for AIDS-Related Kaposi's Sarcoma since the concentrations are inappropriate. INTRON A Solution for Injection is not recommended for intravenous administration and should not be used for the induction phase of malignant melanoma. (See **DOSAGE AND ADMINISTRATION – Condylomata Acuminata; DOSAGE AND ADMINISTRATION – AIDS-Related Kaposi's Sarcoma.**)

Parenteral drug products should be inspected visually for particulate matter and discoloration prior to administration, whenever solution and container permit. INTRON A Interferon alfa-2b, recombinant for Injection may be administered using either sterilized glass or plastic disposable syringes.

Stability INTRON A Interferon alfa-2b, recombinant Solution for Injection multidose pens provided in strengths ranging from 18 to 60 million IU per pen is stable at 30°C (86°F) for up to 2 days. INTRON A Interferon alfa-2b, recombinant Solution for Injection provided in vials ranging from 3 to 25 million IU per vial, is stable at 35°C (95°F) for up to 7 days and at 30°C (86°F) for up to 14 days. The solution is clear and colorless.

Continued on next page

Information on Schering products appearing on these pages is effective as of January 2000.

Intron A—Cont.

INTRON A SOLUTION FOR INJECTION IS NOT RECOMMENDED FOR INTRAVENOUS ADMINISTRATION.

CONTRAINDICATIONS

INTRON A Interferon alfa-2b, recombinant for Injection is contraindicated in patients with a history of hypersensitivity to interferon alfa or any component of the injection. REBETRON Combination Therapy containing INTRON A and REBETOL (ribavirin, USP) Capsules must not be used by women who are pregnant or by men whose female partners are pregnant. Extreme care must be taken to avoid pregnancy in female patients and in female partners of patients taking combination INTRON A/REBETOL therapy. Patients with autoimmune hepatitis must not be treated with combination INTRON A/REBETOL therapy. See REBETRON Combination Therapy package insert for additional information.

WARNINGS

General Moderate to severe adverse experiences may require modification of the patient's dosage regimen, or in some cases termination of INTRON A therapy. Because of the fever and other "flu-like" symptoms associated with INTRON A administration, it should be used cautiously in patients with debilitating medical conditions, such as those with a history of pulmonary disease (eg, chronic obstructive pulmonary disease), or diabetes mellitus prone to ketoacidosis. Caution should also be observed in patients with coagulation disorders (eg, thrombophlebitis, pulmonary embolism) or severe myelosuppression.

Patients with platelet counts of less than 50,000/mm^3 should not be administered INTRON A Interferon alfa-2b, recombinant for Injection intramuscularly, but instead by subcutaneous administration.

INTRON A therapy should be used cautiously in patients with a history of cardiovascular disease. Those patients with a history of myocardial infarction and/or previous or current arrhythmic disorder who require INTRON A therapy should be closely monitored (see **Laboratory Tests**). Cardiovascular adverse experiences, which include hypotension, arrhythmia, or tachycardia of 150 beats per minute or greater, and rarely, cardiomyopathy and myocardial infarction have been observed in some INTRON A treated patients. Some patients with these adverse events had no history of cardiovascular disease. Transient cardiomyopathy was reported in approximately 2% of the AIDS-Related Kaposi's Sarcoma patients treated with INTRON A Interferon alfa-2b, recombinant for Injection. Hypotension may occur during INTRON A administration, or up to 2 days post-therapy, and may require supportive therapy including fluid replacement to maintain intravascular volume.

Supraventricular arrhythmias occurred rarely and appeared to be correlated with preexisting conditions and prior therapy with cardiotoxic agents. These adverse experiences were controlled by modifying the dose or discontinuing treatment, but may require specific additional therapy.

DEPRESSION AND SUICIDAL BEHAVIOR INCLUDING SUICIDAL IDEATION, SUICIDAL ATTEMPTS, AND COMPLETED SUICIDES HAVE BEEN REPORTED IN ASSOCIATION WITH TREATMENT WITH ALFA INTERFERONS, INCLUDING INTRON A THERAPY. Patients with a preexisting psychiatric condition, especially depression, or a history of severe psychiatric disorder should not be treated with INTRON A Interferon alfa-2b, recombinant for Injection.[11] INTRON A therapy should be discontinued for any patient developing severe depression or other psychiatric disorder during treatment. Obtundation and coma have also been observed in some patients, usually elderly, treated at higher doses. While these effects are usually rapidly reversible upon discontinuation of therapy, full resolution of symptoms has taken up to 3 weeks in a few severe episodes. Narcotics, hypnotics, or sedatives may be used concurrently with caution and patients should be closely monitored until the adverse effects have resolved.

Infrequently, patients receiving INTRON A therapy developed thyroid abnormalities, either hypothyroid or hyperthyroid. The mechanism by which INTRON A Interferon alfa-2b, recombinant for Injection may alter thyroid status is unknown. Patients with preexisting thyroid abnormalities whose thyroid function cannot be maintained in the normal range by medication should not be treated with INTRON A Interferon alfa-2b, recombinant for Injection. Prior to initiation of INTRON A therapy, serum TSH should be evaluated. Patients developing symptoms consistent with possible thyroid dysfunction during the course of INTRON A therapy should have their thyroid function evaluated and appropriate treatment instituted. Therapy should be discontinued for patients developing thyroid abnormalities during treatment whose thyroid function cannot be normalized by medication. Discontinuation of INTRON A therapy has not always reversed thyroid dysfunction occurring during treatment.

Hepatotoxicity, including fatality, has been observed in interferon alfa treated patients, including those treated with INTRON A Interferon alfa-2b, recombinant for Injection. Any patient developing liver function abnormalities during treatment should be monitored closely and if appropriate, treatment should be discontinued.

Pulmonary infiltrates, pneumonitis and pneumonia, including fatality, have been observed in interferon alfa treated patients, including those treated with INTRON A Interferon alfa-2b, recombinant for Injection. The etiologic explanation for these pulmonary findings has yet to be established. Any patient developing fever, cough, dyspnea, or other respiratory symptoms should have a chest x-ray taken. If the chest x-ray shows pulmonary infiltrates or there is evidence of pulmonary function impairment, the patient should be closely monitored, and, if appropriate, interferon alfa treatment should be discontinued. While this has been reported more often in patients with chronic hepatitis C treated with interferon alfa, it has also been reported in patients with oncologic diseases treated with interferon alfa.

Retinal hemorrhages, cotton-wool spots, and retinal artery or vein obstruction have been observed rarely in patients treated with interferon alfa, including those treated with INTRON A Interferon alfa-2b, recombinant for Injection. The etiologic explanation for these findings has not yet been established. These events appear to occur after use of the drug for several months, but also have been reported after shorter treatment periods. Diabetes mellitus or hypertension have been present in some patients. Any patient complaining of changes in visual acuity or visual fields, or reporting other ophthalmologic symptoms during treatment with INTRON A Interferon alfa-2b, recombinant for Injection, should have an eye examination. Because the retinal events may have to be differentiated from those seen with diabetic or hypertensive retinopathy, a baseline ocular examination is recommended prior to treatment with interferon in patients with diabetes mellitus or hypertension.

Rare cases of autoimmune diseases including thrombocytopenia, vasculitis, Raynaud's phenomenon, rheumatoid arthritis, lupus erythematosus, and rhabdomyolysis have been observed in patients treated with alfa interferons, including patients treated with INTRON A Interferon alfa-2b, recombinant for Injection. In very rare cases the event resulted in fatality. The mechanisms by which these events develop and their relationship to interferon alfa therapy is not clear. Any patient developing an autoimmune disorder during treatment should be closely monitored and, if appropriate, treatment should be discontinued.

Diabetes mellitus and hyperglycemia have been observed rarely in patients treated with INTRON A Interferon alfa-2b, recombinant for Injection. Symptomatic patients should have their blood glucose measured and followed up accordingly. Patients with diabetes mellitus may require adjustment of their antidiabetic regimen.

The 50 million IU strength of the INTRON A Powder for Injection is not to be used for the treatment of hairy cell leukemia, condylomata acuminata, follicular lymphoma, chronic hepatitis C, or chronic hepatitis B. The 3 million, 5 million, 18 million, and 25 million IU strengths of the INTRON A Powder for Injection are not to be used for the intralesional treatment of condylomata acuminata since the dilution required for the intralesional use would result in a hypertonic solution.

The INTRON A multidose pens, the 3 million IU vial, and the 18 million IU multidose vial of INTRON A Solution for Injection are not to be used for the treatment of condylomata acuminata. The INTRON A multidose pens and the 18 million and 25 million IU multidose vials of INTRON A Solution for Injection are not to be used for the treatment of AIDS-Related Kaposi's Sarcoma. INTRON A Solution for Injection is not recommended for the intravenous treatment of malignant melanoma.

The powder formulations of this product contain albumin, a derivative of human blood. Based on effective donor screening and product manufacturing processes, it carries an extremely remote risk for transmission of viral diseases. A theoretical risk for transmission of Creutzfeldt-Jakob disease (CJD) also is considered extremely remote. No cases of transmission of viral diseases or CJD have ever been identified for albumin.

AIDS-Related Kaposi's Sarcoma INTRON A therapy should not be used for patients with rapidly progressive visceral disease (see **CLINICAL PHARMACOLOGY**). Also of note, there may be synergistic adverse effects between INTRON A Interferon alfa-2b, recombinant for Injection and zidovudine. Patients receiving concomitant zidovudine have had a higher incidence of neutropenia than that expected with zidovudine alone. Careful monitoring of the WBC count is indicated in all patients who are myelosuppressed and in all patients receiving other myelosuppressive medications. The effects of INTRON A Interferon alfa-2b, recombinant for Injection when combined with other drugs used in the treatment of AIDS-Related disease are unknown.

Chronic Hepatitis C and Chronic Hepatitis B Patients with decompensated liver disease, autoimmune hepatitis or a history of autoimmune disease, and patients who are immunosuppressed transplant recipients should not be treated with INTRO A Interferon alfa-2b, recombinant for Injection. There are reports of worsening liver disease, including jaundice, hepatic encephalopathy, hepatic failure, and death following INTRON A therapy in such patients. Therapy should be discontinued for any patient developing signs and symptoms of liver failure.

Chronic hepatitis B patients with evidence of decreasing hepatic synthetic functions, such as decreasing albumin levels or prolongation of prothrombin time, who nevertheless meet the entry criteria to start therapy, may be at increased risk of clinical decompensation if a flare of aminotransferases occurs during INTRON A treatment. In such patients, if increases in ALT occur during INTRON A therapy for chronic hepatitis B, they should be followed carefully including close monitoring of clinical symptomatology and liver function tests, including ALT, prothrombin time, alkaline phosphatase, albumin, and bilirubin. In considering these patients for INTRON A therapy, the potential risks must be evaluated against the potential benefits of treatment.

INTRON A Interferon alfa-2b, recombinant Powder for Injection when reconstituted with the provided Diluent for INTRON A Interferon alfa-2b, recombinant for Injection (bacteriostatic water for injection) contains benzyl alcohol. There have been rare reports of death in infants associated with excessive exposure to benzyl alcohol. The amount of benzyl alcohol at which toxicity or adverse effects may occur in infants is not known. INTRON A **Powder for Injection** is not indicated for use in infants and should not be used in pediatric patients in this age group.

REBETRON Combination Therapy containing INTRON A and REBETOL (ribavirin, USP) Capsules was associated with hemolytic anemia. Hemoglobin <10 g/dL was observed in approximately 10% of patients in clinical trials. Anemia occurred within 1 to 2 weeks of initiation of ribavirin therapy. REBETRON Combination Therapy containing INTRON A and REBETOL is not recommended in patients with severe renal impairment and should be used with caution in patients with moderate renal impairment. See REBETRON Combination Therapy package insert for additional information.

PRECAUTIONS

General Acute serious hypersensitivity reactions (eg, urticaria, angioedema, bronchoconstriction, anaphylaxis) have been demonstrated rarely in INTRON A treated patients; if such an acute reaction develops, the drug should be discontinued immediately and appropriate medical therapy instituted. Transient rashes have occurred in some patients following injection, but have not necessitated treatment interruption.

While fever may be related to the flu-like syndrome reported commonly in patients treated with interferon, other causes of persistent fever should be ruled out.

There have been reports of interferon, including INTRON A Interferon alfa-2b, recombinant for Injection, exacerbating preexisting psoriasis; therefore, INTRON A therapy should be used in these patients only if the potential benefit justifies the potential risk.

Variations in dosage, routes of administration, and adverse reactions exist among different brands of interferon. Therefore, do not use different brands of interferon in any single treatment regimen.

Drug Interactions Interactions between INTRON A Interferon alfa-2b, recombinant for Injection and other drugs have not been fully evaluated. Caution should be exercised when administering INTRON A therapy in combination with other potentially myelosuppressive agents such as zidovudine. Concomitant use of alfa interferon and theophylline decreases theophylline clearance, resulting in a 100% increase in serum theophylline levels.

Information for Patients Patients receiving INTRON A treatment should be directed in its appropriate use, informed of benefits and risks associated with treatment, and referred to the **PATIENT INFORMATION SHEET**. This information is intended to aid in the safe and effective use of this medication. It is not a disclosure of all possible adverse or intended effects.

If home use is prescribed, a puncture-resistant container for the disposal of used syringes and needles should be supplied to the patient. Patients should be thoroughly instructed on the importance of proper disposal and cautioned against any reuse of needles and syringes. The full container should be disposed of according to the directions provided by the physician (see **PATIENT INFORMATION SHEET**).

Patients should be cautioned not to change brands of interferon without medical consultation as a change in dosage may result.

Patients receiving high INTRON A doses should be cautioned against performing tasks that would require complete mental alertness, such as operating machinery or driving a motor vehicle.

The most common adverse experiences occurring with INTRON A therapy are "flu-like" symptoms, such as fever, headache, fatigue, anorexia, nausea, or vomiting (see **ADVERSE REACTIONS**) and appear to decrease in severity as treatment continues. Some of these "flu-like" symptoms may be minimized by bedtime administration. Antipyretics may be used to prevent or partially alleviate the fever and headache. Another common adverse experience is thinning of the hair.

It is advised that patients be well hydrated, especially during the initial stages of treatment.

INTRON A in combination with REBETOL (ribavirin, USP) Capsules therapy must not be used by women who are pregnant or by men whose female partners are pregnant. Extreme care must be taken to avoid pregnancy in female patients and in female partners of patients taking INTRON A/REBETOL therapy. Combination INTRON A/REBETOL therapy should not be initiated until a report of a negative pregnancy test has been obtained immediately prior to initiation of therapy. See REBETRON Combination Therapy package insert for additional information.

Laboratory Tests In addition to those tests normally required for monitoring patients, the following laboratory tests are recommended for all patients on INTRON A therapy, prior to beginning treatment and then periodically thereafter.

- Standard hematologic tests – including hemoglobin, complete and differential white blood cell counts, and platelet count.
- Blood chemistries – electrolytes, liver function tests, and TSH.

TREATMENT-RELATED ADVERSE EXPERIENCES BY INDICATION
Dosing Regimens
*Percentage (%) of Patients**

	Malignant Melanoma	Follicular Lymphoma	Hairy Cell Leukemia	Condylomata Acuminata	AIDS-Related Kaposi's Sarcoma		Chronic Hepatitis C‖	Chronic Hepatitis B		
								Adults		Pediatrics
	20 MIU/m² Induction (IV) 10 MIU/m² Maintenance (SC)	5 MIU TIW/SC	2 MIU/m² TIW/SC	1 MIU lesion	30 MIU/m² TIW/SC	35 MIU QD/SC	3 MIU TIW	5 MIU QD	10 MIU TIW	6 MIU/m² TIW
ADVERSE EXPERIENCE	N=143	N=135	N=145	N=352	N=74	N=29	N=183	N=101	N=78	N=116
Application-Site Disorders			20							
injection site inflammation	—	1	—	—	—	—	5	3	—	—
other (≤5%)	burning, injection site bleeding, injection site pain, injection site reaction (5% in chronic hepatitis B pediatrics), itching									
Blood Disorders (<5%)	anemia, anemia hypochromic, granulocytopenia, hemolytic anemia, leukopenia, lymphocytosis, neutropenia (9% in chronic hepatitis C, 14% in chronic hepatitis B pediatrics), thrombocytopenia (10% in chronic hepatitis C) (bleeding 8% in malignant melanoma), thrombocytopenic purpura									
Body as a Whole										
facial edema	—	1	—	<1	—	10	<1	3	1	<1
weight decrease	3	13	<1	<1	5	3	10	2	5	3
other (≤5%)	allergic reaction, cachexia, dehydration, earache, hernia, edema, hypercalcemia, hyperglycemia, hypothermia, inflammation nonspecific, lymphadenitis, lymphadenopathy, mastitis, periorbital edema, poor peripheral circulation, peripheral edema (6% in follicular lymphoma), phlebitis superficial, scrotal/penile edema, thirst, weakness, weight increase									
Cardiovascular System Disorders (<5%)	angina, arrhythmia, atrial fibrillation, bradycardia, cardiac failure, cardiomegaly, cardiomyopathy, coronary artery disorder, extrasystoles, heart valve disorder, hematoma, hypertension (9% in chronic hepatitis C), hypotension, palpitations, phlebitis, postural hypotension, pulmonary embolism, Raynaud's disease, tachycardia, thrombosis, varicose vein									
Endocrine System Disorders (<5%)	aggravation of diabetes mellitus, goiter, gynecomastia, hyperglycemia, hyperthyroidism, hypertriglyceridemia, hypothyroidism, virilism									
Flu-like Symptoms										
fever	81	56	68	56	47	55	34	66	86	94
headache	62	21	39	47	36	21	43	61	44	57
chills	54	—	46	45	—	—	—	—	—	—
myalgia	75	16	39	44	34	28	43	59	40	27
fatigue	96	8	61	18	84	48	23	75	69	71
increased sweating	6	13	8	2	4	21	4	1	1	3
asthenia	—	63	7	—	11	—	40	5	15	5
rigors	2	7	—	—	30	14	16	38	42	30
arthralgia	6	8	8	9	—	3	16	19	8	15
dizziness	23	—	12	9	7	24	9	13	10	8
influenza-like symptoms	10	18	37	—	45	79	26	5	—	<1
back pain	—	15	19	6	1	3	—	—	—	—
dry mouth	1	2	19	—	22	28	5	6	5	—
chest pain	2	8	<1	<1	1	28	4	4	—	—
malaise	6	—	—	14	5	—	13	9	6	3
pain (unspecified)	15	9	18	3	3	3	—	—	—	—
other (<5%)	chest pain substernal, hyperthermia, rhinitis, rhinorrhea									
Gastrointestinal System Disorders										
diarrhea	35	19	18	2	18	45	13	19	8	12
anorexia	69	21	19	1	38	41	14	43	53	43
nausea	66	24	21	17	28	21	19	50	33	18
taste alteration	24	2	13	<1	5	7	2	10	—	—
abdominal pain	2	20	<5	1	5	21	16	5	4	23
loose stools	—	1	—	<1	—	10	2	2	—	2
vomiting	†	32	6	2	11	14	8	7	10	27
constipation	1	14	<1	—	1	10	4	5	—	2
gingivitis	2‡	7‡	—	—	—	14	—	1	—	—
dyspepsia	—	2	—	2	4	—	7	3	8	3
other (<5%)	abdominal ascites, abdominal distension, colitis, dysphagia, eructation, esophagitis, flatulence, gallstones, gastric ulcer, gastritis, gastroenteritis, gastrointestinal disorder (7% in follicular lymphoma), gastrointestinal hemorrhage, gastrointestinal mucosal discoloration, gingival bleeding, gum hyperplasia, halitosis, hemorrhoids, increased appetite, increased saliva, intestinal disorder, melena, mouth ulceration, mucositis, oral hemorrhage, oral leukoplakia, rectal bleeding after stool, rectal hemorrhage, stomatitis, stomatitis ulcerative, taste loss, tongue disorder, tooth disorder									
Liver and Biliary System Disorders (<5%)	abnormal hepatic function tests, biliary pain, bilirubinemia, hepatitis, increased lactate dehydrogenase, increased transaminases (SGOT/SGPT) (elevated SGOT 63% in malignant melanoma and 24% in follicular lymphoma), jaundice, right upper quadrant pain (15% in chronic hepatitis C), and very rarely, hepatic encephalopathy, hepatic failure, and death									

Those patients who have preexisting cardiac abnormalities and/or are in advanced stages of cancer should have electrocardiograms taken prior to and during the course of treatment.

Mild-to-moderate leukopenia and elevated serum liver enzyme (SGOT) levels have been reported with intralesional administration of INTRON A Interferon alfa-2b, recombinant for Injection (see **ADVERSE REACTIONS**); therefore, the monitoring of these laboratory parameters should be considered.

Baseline chest x-rays are suggested and should be repeated if clinically indicated.

For malignant melanoma patients, differential WBC count and liver function tests should be monitored weekly during the induction phase of therapy and monthly during the maintenance phase of therapy.

For specific recommendations in chronic hepatitis C and chronic hepatitis B, see **INDICATIONS AND USAGE**.

Carcinogenesis, Mutagenesis, Impairment of Fertility: Studies with INTRON A Interferon alfa-2b, recombinant for Injection have not been performed to determine carcinogenicity.

Interferon may impair fertility. In studies of interferon administration in nonhuman primates, menstrual cycle abnormalities have been observed. Decreases in serum estradiol and progesterone concentrations have been reported in women treated with human leukocyte interferon.[12] Therefore, fertile women should not receive INTRON A therapy unless they are using effective contraception during the therapy period. INTRON A therapy should be used with caution in fertile men.

Mutagenicity studies have demonstrated that INTRON A Interferon alfa-2b, recombinant for Injection is not mutagenic.

Studies in mice (0.1, 1.0 million IU/day), rats (4, 20, 100 million IU/kg/day), and cynomolgus monkeys (1.1 million IU/kg/day; 0.25, 0.75, 2.5 million IU/kg/day) injected with INTRON A Interferon alfa-2b, recombinant for Injection for up to 9 days, 3 months, and 1 month, respectively, have revealed no evidence of toxicity. However, if cynomolgus monkeys (4, 20, 100 million IU/kg/day) injected daily for 3 months with INTRON A Interferon alfa-2b, recombinant for Injection toxicity was observed at the mid and high doses and mortality was observed at the high dose.

However, due to the known species-specificity of interferon, the effects in animals are unlikely to be predictive of those in man.

INTRON A in combination with REBETOL (ribavirin, USP) Capsules should be used with caution in fertile men. See the REBETRON Combination Therapy package insert for additional information.

Pregnancy Category C INTRON A Interferon alfa-2b, recombinant for Injection has been shown to have abortifacient effects in *Macaca mulatta* (rhesus monkeys) at 7.5, 15, and 30 million IU/kg (90, 180, and 360 times the intramuscular or subcutaneous dose of 2 million IU/m²). Although abortion was observed in all dose groups, it was only statistically significant at the mid- and high-dose groups. There are no adequate and well-controlled studies in pregnant women. INTRON A therapy should be used during pregnancy only if the potential benefit justifies the potential risk to the fetus.

REBETRON Combination Therapy containing INTRON A and REBETOL (ribavirin, USP) Capsules

Pregnancy Category X applies to the REBETRON Combination Therapy containing Intron A and Rebetol (ribavirin, USP) (see **CONTRAINDICATIONS**). See Rebetron Combination Therapy package insert for additional information.

Nursing Mothers It is not known whether this drug is excreted in human milk. However, studies in mice have shown that mouse interferons are excreted into the milk. Because of the potential for serious adverse reactions from the drug to nursing infants, a decision should be made whether to discontinue nursing or to discontinue INTRON A therapy, taking into account the importance of the drug to the mother.

Continued on next page

Information on Schering products appearing on these pages is effective as of January 2000.

Intron A—Cont.

Pediatric Use *General* Safety and effectiveness in pediatric patients below the age of 18 years have not been established for indications other than chronic hepatitis B.

Chronic hepatitis B Safety and effectiveness in pediatric patients ranging in age from 1 to 17 years have been established based upon one controlled clinical trial (see **CLINICAL PHARMACOLOGY, INDICATIONS AND USAGE, DOSAGE AND ADMINISTRATION; Chronic Hepatitis B**). Safety and effectiveness in pediatric patients below the age of 1 year have not been established.

INTRON A Interferon alfa-2b, recombinant **Powder for Injection** when reconstituted with the provided Diluent for INTRON A Interferon alfa-2b, recombinant for Injection (bacteriostatic water for injection) contains benzyl alcohol and is not indicated for use in infants. There have been rare reports of death in infants associated with excessive exposure to benzyl alcohol. The amount of benzyl alcohol at which toxicity or adverse effects may occur in infants is not known. (See **WARNINGS Chronic Hepatitis B**.)

ADVERSE REACTIONS

General The adverse experiences listed below were reported to be possibly or probably related to INTRON A therapy during clinical trials. Most of these adverse reactions were mild to moderate in severity and were manageable. Some were transient and most diminished with continued therapy.

The most frequently reported adverse reactions were "flu-like" symptoms, particularly fever, headache, chills, myalgia, and fatigue. More severe toxicities are observed generally at higher doses and may be difficult for patients to tolerate.

In addition, the following spontaneous adverse experiences have been reported during the marketing surveillance of INTRON A Interferon alfa-2b, recombinant for Injection: nephrotic syndrome, pancreatitis, psychosis, including hallucinations, renal failure, and renal insufficiency.

[See table at top of previous page and below]

Hairy Cell Leukemia The adverse reactions most frequently reported during clinical trials in 145 patients with hairy cell leukemia were the "flu-like" symptoms of fever (68%), fatigue (61%), and chills (46%).

Malignant Melanoma The INTRON A dose was modified because of adverse events in 65% (n=93) of the patients. INTRON A therapy was discontinued because of adverse events in 8% of the patients during induction and 18% of the patients during maintenance. The most frequently reported adverse reaction was fatigue which was observed in 96% of patients. Other adverse reactions that were recorded in >20% of INTRON A treated patients included neutropenia (92%), fever (81%), myalgia (75%), anorexia (69%), vomiting/nausea (66%), increased SGOT (63%), headache (62%), chills (54%), depression (40%), diarrhea (35%), alopecia (29%), altered taste sensation (24%), dizziness/vertigo (23%), and anemia (22%).

Adverse reactions classified as severe or life threatening (ECOG Toxicity Criteria grade 3 or 4) were recorded in 66% and 14% of INTRON A treated patients, respectively. Severe adverse reactions recorded in >10% of INTRON A treated patients included neutropenia/leukopenia (26%), fatigue (23%), fever (18%), myalgia (17%), headache (17%), chills (16%), and increased SGOT (14%). Grade 4 fatigue was recorded in 4% and grade 4 depression was recorded in 2% of INTRON A treated patients. No other grade 4 AE was re-

TREATMENT-RELATED ADVERSE EXPERIENCES BY INDICATION
Dosing Regimens
*Percentage (%) of Patients**

	MALIGNANT MELANOMA	FOLLICULAR LYMPHOMA	HAIRY CELL LEUKEMIA	CONDYLOMATA ACUMINATA	AIDS-RELATED KAPOSI'S SARCOMA		CHRONIC HEPATITIS C‖	CHRONIC HEPATITIS B		
								Adults		Pediatrics
	20 MIU/m² Induction (IV) 10 MIU/m² Maintenance (SC)	*5 MIU TIW/SC*	*2 MIU/m² TIW/SC*	*1 MIU lesion*	*30 MIU/m² TIW/SC*	*35 MIU QD/SC*	*3 MIU TIW*	*5 MIU QD*	*10 MIU TIW*	*6 MIU/m² TIW*
ADVERSE EXPERIENCE	N=143	N=135	N=145	N=352	N=74	N=29	N=183	N=101	N=78	N=116
Musculoskeletal System Disorders										
musculoskeletal pain	—	18	—	—	—	—	21	9	1	10
other (<5%)	arteritis, arthritis, arthritis aggravated, arthrosis, bone disorder, bone pain, carpal tunnel syndrome, hyporeflexia, leg cramps, muscle atrophy, muscle weakness, polyarteritis nodosa, tendinitis, rheumatoid arthritis, spondylitis									
Nervous System and Psychiatric Disorders										
depression	40	9	6	3	9	28	19	17	6	4
paresthesia	13	13	6	1	3	21	5	6	3	<1
impaired concentration	—	1	—	<1	3	14	3	8	5	3
amnesia	§	1	<5	—	—	14	—	—	—	—
confusion	8	2	<5	4	12	10	1	—	—	2
hypoesthesia	—	1	<5	1	—	10	—	—	—	—
irritability	1	1	—	—	—	—	13	16	12	22
somnolence	1	2	<5	3	3	—	33¶	14	9	5
anxiety	1	9	5	<1	1	3	5	2	—	3
insomnia	5	4	—	<1	3	3	12	11	6	8
nervousness	1	1	—	1	—	3	2	3	—	3
decreased libido	1	1	<5	—	—	—	1	5	1	—
other (<5%)	abnormal coordination, abnormal dreaming, abnormal gait, abnormal thinking, aggravated depression, aggressive reaction, agitation (7% in chronic hepatitis B pediatrics) alcohol intolerance, apathy, aphasia, ataxia, Bell's palsy, CNS dysfunction, coma, convulsions, delirium, dysphonia, emotional lability, extrapyramidal disorder, feeling of ebriety, flushing, hearing disorder, hearing impairment, hot flashes, hyperesthesia, hyperkinesia, hypertonia, hypokinesia, impaired consciousness, labyrinthine disorder, loss of consciousness, manic depression, manic reaction, migraine, neuralgia, neuritis, neuropathy, neurosis, paresis, paroniria, parosmia, personality disorder, polyneuropathy, psychosis, speech disorder, stroke, suicidal ideation, suicide attempt, syncope, tinnitus, tremor, twitching, vertigo (8% in follicular lymphoma)									
Reproduction System Disorders (<5%)	amenorrhea (12% in follicular lymphoma), dysmenorrhea, impotence, leukorrhea, menorrhagia, menstrual irregularity, pelvic pain, penis disorder, sexual dysfunction, uterine bleeding, vaginal dryness									
Resistance Mechanism Disorders										
moniliasis	—	1	—	<1	—	17	—	—	—	—
herpes simplex	1	2	—	1	—	3	1	5	—	—
other (<5%)	abscess, conjunctivitis, fungal infection, hemophilus, herpes zoster, infection, infection bacterial, infection nonspecific (7% in follicular lymphoma), infection parasitic, otitis media, sepsis, stye, trichomonas, upper respiratory tract infection, viral infection (7% in chronic hepatitis C)									
Respiratory System Disorders										
dyspnea	15	14	<1	—	1	34	3	5	—	—
coughing	6	13	<1	—	—	31	1	4	—	5
pharyngitis	2	8	<5	1	1	31	3	7	1	7
sinusitis	1	4	—	—	—	21	2	—	—	—
nonproductive coughing	2	7	—	—	—	14	0	1	—	—
nasal congestion	1	7	—	1	—	10	<1	4	—	—
other (≤5%)	asthma, bronchitis (10% in follicular lymphoma), bronchospasm, cyanosis, epistaxis (7% in chronic hepatitis B pediatrics), hemoptysis, hypoventilation, laryngitis, lung fibrosis, pleural effusion, orthopnea, pleural pain, pneumonia, pneumonitis, pneumothorax, rales, respiratory disorder, respiratory insufficiency, sneezing, tonsillitis, tracheitis, wheezing									
Skin and Appendages Disorders										
dermatitis	1	—	8	—	—	—	2	1	—	—
alopecia	29	23	8	—	12	31	28	26	38	17
pruritus	—	10	11	1	7	—	9	6	4	3
rash	19	13	25	—	9	10	5	8	1	5
dry skin	1	3	9	—	9	10	4	3	—	<1
other (<5%)	abnormal hair texture, acne, cellulitis, cyanosis of the hand, cold and clammy skin, dermatitis lichenoides, eczema, epidermal necrolysis, erythema, erythema nodosum, folliculitis, furunculosis, increased hair growth, lacrimal gland disorder, lacrimation, lipoma, maculopapular rash, melanosis, nail disorders, nonherpetic cold sores, pallor, peripheral ischemia, photosensitivity, pruritus genital, psoriasis, psoriasis aggravated, purpura (5% in chronic hepatitis C), rash erythematous, sebaceous cyst, skin depigmentation, skin discoloration, skin nodule, urticaria, vitiligo									
Urinary System Disorders (<5%)	albumin/protein in urine, cystitis, dysuria, hematuria, incontinence, increased BUN, micturition disorder, micturition frequency, nocturia, polyuria (10% in follicular lymphoma), renal insufficiency, urinary tract infection (5% in chronic hepatitis C)									
Vision Disorders (<5%)	abnormal vision, blurred vision, diplopia, dry eyes, eye pain, nystagmus, photophobia									

* Dash (—) indicates not reported
† Vomiting was reported with nausea as a single term
‡ Includes stomatitis/mucositis
§ Amnesia was reported with confusion as a single term
‖ Percentages based upon a summary of all adverse events during 18 to 24 months of treatment
¶ Predominantly lethargy

ABNORMAL LABORATORY TEST VALUES BY INDICATION
Dosing Regimens
Percentage (%) of Patients

	Malignant Melanoma	Follicular Lymphoma	Hairy Cell Leukemia	Condylomata Acuminata	AIDS-Related Kaposi's Sarcoma		Chronic Hepatitis C	Chronic Hepatitis B Adults		Chronic Hepatitis B Pediatrics
	20 MIU/m² Induction (IV) 10 MIU/m² Maintenance (SC)	*5 MIU TIW/SC*	*2 MIU/m² TIW/SC*	*1 MIU/lesion*	*30 MIU/m² TIW/SC*	*35 MIU QD/SC*	*3 MIU TIW*	*5 MIU QD*	*10 MIU TIW*	*6 MIU/m² TIW*
Laboratory Tests	N=143	N=135	N=145	N=352	N=69–73	N=26–28	N=140–171	N=96–101	N=75–103	N=113–115
Hemoglobin	22	8	NA	—	1	15	26¶	32*	23*	17**
White Blood Cell Count	$\|$	—	NA	17	10	22	26†	68†	34†	9†
Platelet Count	15	13	NA	—	0	8	15‡	12‡	5‡	1‡
Serum Creatinine	3	2	0	—	—	—	6	3	0	3
Alkaline Phosphatase	13	—	4	—	—	—	—	8	4	0
Lactate Dehydrogenase	1	—	0	—	—	—	—		—	—
Serum Urea Nitrogen	12	4	0	—	—	—	—	2	0	2
SGOT	63	24	4	12	11	41	—	—		—
SGPT	2	—	13	—	10	15	—	—		
Granulocyte Count										
• Total	92	36	NA	—	31	39	45§	75§	61§	70§
• 1000 -<1500/mm³	66	—	—	—	—	—	32	30	32	43
• 750 -<1000/mm³	—	21	—	—	—	—	10	24	18	18
• 500 -<750/mm³	25	—	—	—	—	—	1	17	9	7
• <500/mm³	1	13	—	—	—	—	2	4	2	2

NA–Not Applicable - Patients' initial hematologic laboratory test values were abnormal due to their condition.
* Decrease of ≥2 g/dL
** Decrease of ≥2 g/dL; 14% 2-<3 g/dL; 3% ≥3g/dL
† Decrease to <3000/mm³
‡ Decrease to <70,000/mm³
§ Neutrophils plus bands
‖ White Blood Cell Count was reported as neutropenia
¶ Decrease of ≥2 g/dL; 20% 2-<3 g/dL; 6% ≥3 g/dL

ported in more than 2 INTRON A treated patients. Lethal hepatotoxicity occurred in 2 INTRON A treated patients early in the clinical trial. No subsequent lethal hepatotoxicities were observed with adequate monitoring of liver function tests (see **PRECAUTIONS – Laboratory Tests**).

Follicular Lymphoma Ninety-six percent of patients treated with CHVP plus INTRON A therapy and 91% of patients treated with CHVP alone reported an adverse event of any severity. Asthenia, fever, neutropenia, increased hepatic enzymes, alopecia, headache, anorexia, "flu-like" symptoms, myalgia, dyspnea, thrombocytopenia, paresthesia, and polyuria occurred more frequently in the CHVP plus INTRON A treated patients than in patients treated with CHVP alone. Adverse reactions classified as severe or life threatening (World Health Organization grade 3 or 4) recorded in >5% of CHVP plus INTRON A treated patients included neutropenia (34%), asthenia (10%), and vomiting (10%). The incidence of neutropenic infection was 6% in CHVP plus INTRON A vs 2% in CHVP alone. One patient in each treatment group required hospitalization.

Twenty-eight percent of CHVP plus INTRON A treated patients had a temporary modification/interruption of their INTRON A therapy, but only 13 patients (10%) permanently stopped INTRON A therapy because of toxicity. There were four deaths on study; two patients committed suicide in the CHVP plus INTRON A arm and two patients in the CHVP arm had unwitnessed sudden death. Three patients with hepatitis B (one of whom also had alcoholic cirrhosis) developed hepatoxicity leading to discontinuation of INTRON A. Other reasons for discontinuation included intolerable asthenia (5/135), severe flu symptoms (2/135), and one patient each with exacerbation of ankylosing spondylitis, psychosis, and decreased ejection fraction.

Condylomata Acuminata Eighty-eight percent (311/352) of patients treated with INTRON A Interferon alfa-2b, recombinant for Injection for condylomata acuminata who were evaluable for safety, reported an adverse reaction during treatment. The incidence of the adverse reactions reported increased when the number of treated lesions increased from one to five. All 40 patients who had five warts treated, reported some type of adverse reaction during treatment.

Adverse reactions and abnormal laboratory test values reported by patients who were untreated were qualitatively and quantitatively similar to those reported during the initial INTRON A treatment period.

AIDS-Related Kaposi's Sarcoma In patients with AIDS-Related Kaposi's Sarcoma, some type of adverse reaction occurred in 100% of the 74 patients treated with 30 million IU/m² three times a week and in 97% of the 29 patients treated with 35 million IU per day.

Of these adverse reactions, those classified as severe (World Health Organization grade 3 or 4) were reported in 27% to 55% of patients. Severe adverse reactions in the 30 million IU/m² TIW study included: fatigue (20%), influenza-like symptoms (15%), anorexia (12%), dry mouth (4%), headache (4%), confusion (3%), fever (3%), myalgia (3%), and nausea and vomiting (1% each). Severe adverse reactions for patients who received the 35 million IU QD included: fever (24%), fatigue (17%), influenza-like symptoms (14%), dyspnea (14%), headache (10%), pharyngitis (7%), and ataxia, confusion, dysphagia, GI hemorrhage, abnormal hepatic function, increased SGOT, myalgia, cardiomyopathy, face edema, depression, emotional lability, suicide attempt, chest pain, and coughing (1 patient each). Overall the incidence of severe toxicity was higher among patients who received the 35 million IU per day dose.

Chronic Hepatitis C Two studies of extended treatment (18 to 24 months) with INTRON A Interferon alfa-2b, recombinant for Injection show that approximately 95% of all patients treated experience some type of adverse event and that patients treated for extended duration continue to experience adverse events throughout treatment. Most adverse events reported are mild to moderate in severity. However, 29/152 (19%) of patients treated for 18 to 24 months experienced a serious adverse event compared to 11/163 (7%) of those treated for 6 months. Adverse events which occur or persist during extended treatment are similar in type and severity to those occurring during short-course therapy.

Of the patients achieving a complete response after 6 months of therapy, 12/79 (15%) subsequently discontinued INTRON A treatment during extended therapy because of adverse events, and 23/79 (29%) experienced severe adverse events (WHO grade 3 or 4) during extended therapy.

In patients using REBETRON Combination Therapy containing INTRON A and REBETOL (ribavirin, USP) Capsules, the primary toxicity observed was hemolytic anemia. Reductions in hemoglobin levels occurred within the first 1 to 2 weeks of therapy. Cardiac and pulmonary events associated with anemia occurred in approximately 10% of patients treated with INTRON A/REBETOL therapy. See REBETRON Combination Therapy package insert for additional information.

Chronic Hepatitis B *Adults* In patients with chronic hepatitis B, some type of adverse reaction occurred in 98% of the 101 patients treated at 5 million IU QD and 90% of the 78 patients treated at 10 million IU TIW. Most of these adverse reactions were mild to moderate in severity, were manageable, and were reversible following the end of therapy.

Adverse reactions classified as severe (causing a significant interference with normal daily activities or clinical state) were reported in 21% to 44% of patients. The severe adverse reactions reported most frequently were the "flu-like" symptoms of fever (28%), fatigue (15%), headache (5%), myalgia (4%), rigors (4%), and other severe "flu-like" symptoms which occurred in 1% to 3% of patients. Other severe adverse reactions occurring in more than one patient were alopecia (8%), anorexia (6%), depression (3%), nausea (3%), and vomiting (2%).

To manage side effects, the dose was reduced, or INTRON A therapy was interrupted in 25% to 38% of patients. Five percent of patients discontinued treatment due to adverse experiences.

Pediatrics In pediatric patients, the most frequently reported adverse events were those commonly associated with interferon treatment; flu-like symptoms (100%), gastrointestinal system disorders (46%), and nausea and vomiting (40%). Neutropenia (13%) and thrombocytopenia (3%) were also reported. None of the adverse events were life threatening. The majority were moderate to severe and resolved upon dose reduction or drug discontinuation.

[See table above]

HOW SUPPLIED

INTRON A Interferon alfa-2b, recombinant Powder for Injection INTRON A Interferon alfa-2b, recombinant Powder for Injection INTRON A, Pak-3, containing 6 INTRON A vials, 3 million IU per vial; 6 syringes of Diluent for INTRON A Interferon alfa-2b, recombinant for Injection (bacteriostatic water for injection) 1 mL per syringe for chronic hepatitis C; and 6 alcohol swabs (NDC 0085-0647-05).

INTRON A Interferon alfa-2b, recombinant Powder for Injection, 5 million IU per vial and Diluent for INTRON A Interferon alfa-2b, recombinant for Injection (bacteriostatic water for injection) 1 mL per vial; boxes containing INTRON A vial and 1 vial of INTRON A Diluent (NDC 0085-0120-02).

INTRON A Interferon alfa-2b, recombinant Powder for Injection, 10 million IU per vial and Diluent for INTRON A Interferon alfa-2b, recombinant for Injection (bacteriostatic water for injection) 2 mL per vial; boxes containing 1 INTRON A vial and 1 vial of INTRON A Diluent (NDC 0085-0571-02).

INTRON A Interferon alfa-2b, recombinant Powder for Injection, 18 million IU per vial and Diluent for INTRON A Interferon alfa-2b, recombinant for Injection (bacteriostatic water for injection) 1 mL per vial; boxes containing 1 vial of INTRON A and 1 vial of INTRON A Diluent (NDC 0085-1110-01).

INTRON A Interferon alfa-2b, recombinant Powder for Injection, 25 million IU per vial and Diluent for INTRON A Interferon alfa-2b, recombinant for Injection (bacteriostatic water for injection) 5 mL per vial; boxes containing 1 INTRON A vial and 1 vial of INTRON A Diluent (NDC 0085-0285-02).

INTRON A Interferon alfa-2b, recombinant Powder for Injection, 50 million IU per vial and Diluent for INTRON A Interferon alfa-2b, recombinant for Injection (bacteriostatic water for injection) 1 mL per vial; boxes containing 1 INTRON A vial and 1 vial of INTRON A Diluent (NDC 0085-0539-01).

Store INTRON A Interferon alfa-2b, recombinant Powder for Injection both before and after reconstitution between 2° and 8°C (36° and 46°F).

INTRON A Interferon alfa-2b, recombinant Solution for Injection INTRON A Interferon alfa-2b, recombinant Solution for Injection, 6 doses of 3 million IU (18 million IU) multidose pen (22.5 million IU per 1.5 mL per pen); boxes containing 1 INTRON A multidose pen, six disposable needles and alcohol swabs (NDC 0085-1242-01).

INTRON A Interferon alfa-2b, recombinant Solution for Injection, 6 doses of 5 million IU (30 million IU) multidose pen (37.5 million IU per 1.5 mL per pen); boxes containing 1 INTRON A multidose pen, six disposable needles and alcohol swabs (NDC 0085-1235-01).

INTRON A Interferon alfa-2b, recombinant Solution for Injection, 6 doses of 10 million IU (60 million IU) multidose pen (75 million IU per 1.5 mL per pen); boxes containing 1 INTRON A multidose pen, six disposable needles and alcohol swabs (NDC 0085-1254-01).

INTRON A Interferon alfa-2b, recombinant Solution for Injection INTRON A, Pak-3, containing 6 INTRON A vials, 3 million IU per vial; 6 syringes; and 6 alcohol swabs (NDC 0085-1184-02).

INTRON A Interferon alfa-2b, recombinant Solution for Injection INTRON A, Pak-5, containing 6 INTRON A vials, 5 million IU per vial; 6 syringes; and 6 alcohol swabs (NDC 0085-1191-02).

INTRON A Interferon alfa-2b, recombinant Solution for Injection INTRON A, Pak-10, containing 6 INTRON A vials, 10 million IU per vial; 6 syringes; and 6 alcohol swabs (NDC 0085-1179-02).

Continued on next page

Intron A—Cont.

INTRON A Interferon alfa-2b, recombinant Solution for Injection, 18 million IU multidose vial (22.8 million IU per 3.8 mL per vial); boxes containing 1 vial of INTRON A Solution for Injection (NDC 0085-1168-01).
INTRON A Interferon alfa-2b, recombinant Solution for Injection, 25 million IU multidose vial (32 million IU per 3.2 mL per vial); boxes containing 1 vial of INTRON A Solution for Injection (NDC 0085-1133-01).
Store INTRON A Interferon alfa-2b, recombinant Solution for Injection between 2° and 8°C (36° and 46°F).
Schering Corporation 18766183
Kenilworth, NJ 07033 USA
Rev. 8/99
U.S. Patents 4,530,901 & 4,496,537

REFERENCES

1. Smalley R, et al. *N Engl J Med.* 1992;327:1336–1341.
2. Aviles A, et al. *Leukemia and Lymphoma.* 1996;20:495–499.
3. Unterhalt M, et al. *Blood.* 1996;88 (10Suppl 1):1744A.
4. Schiller J, et al. *J Biol Response Mod.* 1989;8:252–261.
5. Poynard T, et al. *N Engl J Med.* 1995;332:(22)1457–1462.
6. Lin R, et al. *J Hepatol.* 1995;23:487–496.
7. Perrillo R, et al. *N Engl J Med.* 1990;323;295–301.
8. Perez V, et al. *J Hepatol.* 1990;11S113–S117.
9. Knodell R, et al. *Hepatology.* 1981;1:431–435.
10. Perrillo R, et al. *Ann Intern Med.* 1991;115:113–115.
11. Renault P, et al. *Arch Intern Med.* 1987;147:1577–1580.
12. Kauppila A, et al. *Int J Cancer.* 1982;29:291–294.

LOTRIMIN® ℞

brand of clotrimazole
Cream, USP 1%*
Lotion, USP 1%*
Topical Solution, USP 1%*
For Dermatologic Use Only—
Not For Ophthalmic Use
*These preparations are also available without a prescription as LOTRIMIN AF.

DESCRIPTION

LOTRIMIN products contain clotrimazole, USP, a synthetic antifungal agent having the chemical name 1-(*o*-Chloro-α,α-diphenylbenzyl)imidazole; the empirical formula, $C_{22}H_{17}ClN_2$; a molecular weight of 344.84; and the chemical structure:

Clotrimazole is an odorless, white crystalline substance. It is practically insoluble in water, sparingly soluble in ether, and very soluble in polyethylene glycol 400, ethanol, and chloroform.
Each gram of LOTRIMIN **Cream** contains 10 mg clotrimazole, USP in a vanishing cream base of benzyl alcohol NF (1%), cetearyl alcohol 70/30 (10%), cetyl esters wax NF, octyldodecanol NF, polysorbate 60 NF, sorbitan monostearate NF, and purified water USP.
Each gram of LOTRIMIN **Lotion** contains 10 mg clotrimazole, USP dispersed in an emulsion vehicle composed of benzyl alcohol NF (1%), cetearyl alcohol 70/30 (3.7%), cetyl esters wax NF, octyldodecanol NF, polysorbate 60 NF, sodium phosphate dibasic anhydrous R, sodium phosphate monobasic monohydrate USP, sorbitan monostearate NF, and purified water USP.
Each mL of LOTRIMIN **Topical Solution** contains 10 mg clotrimazole, USP in a nonaqueous vehicle of PEG 400 NF.

CLINICAL PHARMACOLOGY

Clotrimazole is a broad-spectrum antifungal agent that is used for the treatment of dermal infections caused by various pathogenic dermatophytes, yeasts, and *Malassezia furfur*. The primary action of clotrimazole is against dividing and growing organisms.
In vitro, clotrimazole exhibits fungistatic and fungicidal activity against isolates of *Trichophyton rubrum, Trichophyton mentagrophytes, Epidermophyton floccosum, Microsporum canis*, and *Candida* species, including *Candida albicans*. In general, the *in vitro* activity of clotrimazole corresponds to that of tolnaftate and griseofulvin against the mycelia of dermatophytes (*Trichophyton, Microsporum*, and *Epidermophyton*), and to that of the polyenes (amphotericin B and nystatin) against budding fungi (*Candida*). Using an *in vivo* (mouse) and an *in vitro* (mouse kidney homogenate) testing system, clotrimazole and miconazole were equally effective in preventing the growth of the pseudomycelia and mycelia of *Candida albicans.*
Strains of fungi having a natural resistance to clotrimazole are rare. Only a single isolate of *Candida guilliermondii* has been reported to have primary resistance to clotrimazole.
No single-step or multiple-step resistance to clotrimazole has developed during successive passages of *Candida albicans* and *Trichophyton mentagrophytes.* No appreciable change in sensitivity was detected after successive passages of isolates of *C. albicans, C. krusei*, or *C. pseudo-tropicalis* in liquid or solid media containing clotrimazole. Also, resistance could not be developed in chemically induced mutant strains of polyene-resistant isolates of *C. albicans.* Slight, reversible resistance was noted in three isolates of *C. albicans* tested by one investigator. There is a single report that records the clinical emergence of a *C. albicans* strain with considerable resistance to flucytosine and miconazole, and with cross-resistance to clotrimazole; the strain remained sensitive to nystatin and amphotericin B.
In studies of the mechanism of action, the minimum fungicidal concentration of clotrimazole caused leakage of intracellular phosphorus compounds into the ambient medium with concomitant breakdown of cellular nucleic acids and accelerated potassium efflux. Both these events began rapidly and extensively after addition of the drug.
Clotrimazole appears to be well absorbed in humans following oral administration and is eliminated mainly as inactive metabolites. Following topical and vaginal administration, however, clotrimazole appears to be minimally absorbed.
Six hours after the application of radioactive clotrimazole 1% cream and 1% solution onto intact and acutely inflamed skin, the concentration of clotrimazole varied from 100 mcg/cm^3 in the stratum corneum to 0.5 to 1 mcg/cm^3 in the stratum reticulare and 0.1 mcg/cm^3 in the subcutis. No measurable amount of radioactivity (≤0.001 mcg/mL) was found in the serum within 48 hours after application under occlusive dressing of 0.5 mL of the solution or 0.8 g of the cream. Only 0.5% or less of the applied radioactivity was excreted in the urine.
Following intravaginal administration of 100 mg ^{14}C-clotrimazole vaginal tablets to nine adult females, an average peak serum level, corresponding to only 0.03 μg equivalents/mL of clotrimazole, was reached 1 to 2 days after application. After intravaginal administration of 5 g of 1% ^{14}C-clotrimazole vaginal cream containing 50 mg active drug to five subjects (one with candidal colpitis), serum levels corresponding to approximately 0.01 μg equivalents/mL were reached between 8 and 24 hours after application.

INDICATIONS AND USAGE

Prescription LOTRIMIN (clotrimazole cream, lotion, and solution 1%) products are indicated for the topical treatment of candidiasis due to *Candida albicans* and tinea versicolor due to *Malassezia furfur.*
These formulations are also available as the LOTRIMIN AF (clotrimazole cream, lotion, and solution 1%) line of nonprescription products which are indicated for the topical treatment of the following dermal infections: tinea pedis, tinea cruris, and tinea corporis due to *Trichophyton rubrum, Trichophyton mentagrophytes, Epidermophyton floccosum*, and *Microsporum canis.*

CONTRAINDICATIONS

LOTRIMIN products are contraindicated in individuals who have shown hypersensitivity to any of their components.

WARNINGS

LOTRIMIN products are not for ophthalmic use.

PRECAUTIONS

General: If irritation or sensitivity develops with the use of clotrimazole, treatment should be discontinued and appropriate therapy instituted.
Information For Patients: This information is intended to aid in the safe and effective use of this medication. It is not a disclosure of all possible adverse or intended effects.
The patient should be advised to:
1. Use the medication for the full treatment time even though the symptoms may have improved. Notify the physician if there is no improvement after 4 weeks of treatment.
2. Inform the physician if the area of application shows signs of increased irritation (redness, itching, burning, blistering, swelling, oozing) indicative of possible sensitization.
3. Avoid sources of infection or reinfection.

Laboratory Tests: If there is lack of response to clotrimazole, appropriate microbiological studies should be repeated to confirm the diagnosis and rule out other pathogens before instituting another course of antimycotic therapy.
Drug Interactions: Synergism or antagonism between clotrimazole and nystatin, or amphotericin B, or flucytosine against strains of *C. albicans* has not been reported.
Carcinogenesis, Mutagenesis, Impairment of Fertility: An 18-month oral dosing study with clotrimazole in rats has not revealed any carcinogenic effect.
In tests for mutagenesis, chromosomes of the spermatophores of Chinese hamsters which had been exposed to clotrimazole were examined for structural changes during the metaphase. Prior to testing, the hamsters had received five oral clotrimazole doses of 100 mg/kg body weight. The results of this study showed that clotrimazole had no mutagenic effect.
Usage in Pregnancy: Pregnancy Category B: The disposition of ^{14}C-clotrimazole has been studied in humans and animals. Clotrimazole is very poorly absorbed following dermal application or intravaginal administration to humans. (See **CLINICAL PHARMACOLOGY.**)
In clinical trials, use of vaginally applied clotrimazole in pregnant women in their second and third trimesters has not been associated with ill effects. There are, however, no adequate and well-controlled studies in pregnant women during the first trimester of pregnancy.
Studies in pregnant rats with intravaginal doses up to 100 mg/kg have revealed no evidence of harm to the fetus due to clotrimazole.
High oral doses of clotrimazole in rats and mice ranging from 50 to 120 mg/kg resulted in embryotoxicity (possibly secondary to maternal toxicity), impairment of mating, decreased litter size and number of viable young and decreased pup survival to weaning. However, clotrimazole was not teratogenic in mice, rabbits, and rats at oral doses up to 200, 180, and 100 mg/kg, respectively. Oral absorption in the rat amounts to approximately 90% of the administered dose.
Because animal reproduction studies are not always predictive of human response, this drug should be used only if clearly indicated during the first trimester of pregnancy.
Nursing Mothers: It is not known whether this drug is excreted in human milk. Because many drugs are excreted in human milk, caution should be exercised when clotrimazole is used by a nursing woman.
Pediatric Use: Safety and effectiveness in children have been established for clotrimazole when used as indicated and in the recommended dosage.

ADVERSE REACTIONS

The following adverse reactions have been reported in connection with the use of clotrimazole: erythema, stinging, blistering, peeling, edema, pruritus, urticaria, burning, and general irritation of the skin.

OVERDOSAGE

Acute overdosage with topical application of clotrimazole is unlikely and would not be expected to lead to a life-threatening situation.

DOSAGE AND ADMINISTRATION

Gently massage sufficient LOTRIMIN into the affected and surrounding skin areas twice a day, in the morning and evening.
Clinical improvement, with relief of pruritus, usually occurs within the first week of treatment with LOTRIMIN. If the patient shows no clinical improvement after 4 weeks of treatment with LOTRIMIN, the diagnosis should be reviewed.

HOW SUPPLIED

LOTRIMIN Cream 1% is supplied in 15, 30, and 45-g tubes (NDC 0085-0613-02, 05, 04, respectively); boxes of one.
Store between 2° and 30°C (36° and 86°F).
LOTRIMIN Lotion 1% is supplied in 30-mL bottles (NDC 0085-0707-02); boxes of one.
Store between 2° and 25°C (36° and 77°F).
Shake well before using.
LOTRIMIN Topical Solution 1% is supplied in 10-mL and 30-mL plastic bottles (NDC 0085-0182-02, 04, respectively); boxes of one.
Store between 2° and 30°C (36° and 86°F).
Schering Corporation
Kenilworth, NJ 07033 USA
Rev. 1/99 17981013
22592203T

LOTRISONE® ℞

brand of clotrimazole and betamethasone dipropionate
Cream, USP
For Dermatologic Use Only –
Not for Ophthalmic Use

DESCRIPTION

LOTRISONE Cream contains a combination of clotrimazole, USP, a synthetic antifungal agent, and beta-methasone dipropionate, USP, a synthetic corticosteroid, for dermatologic use.
Chemically, clotrimazole is 1-(*o*-Chloro-α,α-diphenylbenzyl) imidazole, with the empirical formula $C_{22}H_{17}ClN_2$, a molecular weight of 344.8, and the following structural formula:

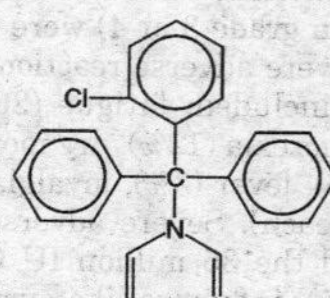

Clotrimazole is an odorless, white crystalline powder, insoluble in water and soluble in ethanol.
Betamethasone dipropionate has the chemical name 9-Fluoro-11β,17,21-trihydroxy-16β-methylpregna-1,4-di-

ene-3,20-dione 17,21-dipropionate, with the empirical formula $C_{28}H_{37}FO_7$, a molecular weight of 504.6, and the following structural formula:

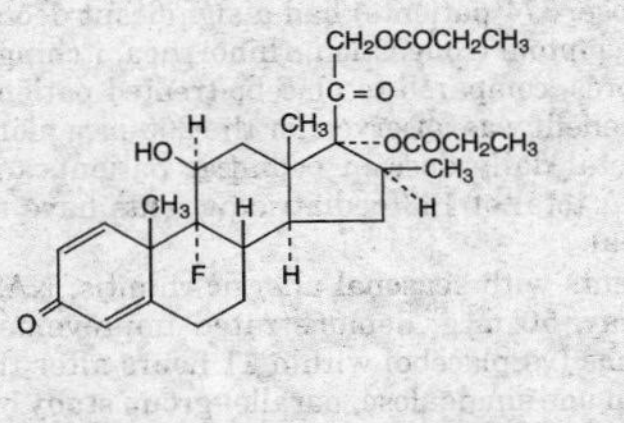

Betamethasone dipropionate is a white to creamy white, odorless crystalline powder, insoluble in water.
Each gram of LOTRISONE Cream contains 10.0 mg clotrim azole, USP and 0.64 mg betamethasone dipropionate, USP (equivalent to 0.5 mg betamethasone), in a hydrophilic emollient cream consisting of purified water, mineral oil, white petrolatum, cetearyl alcohol, ceteareth-30, propylene glycol, sodium phosphate monobasic, and phosphoric acid; benzyl alcohol as preservative.
LOTRISONE is a smooth, uniform, white to off-white cream.

CLINICAL PHARMACOLOGY

Clotrimazole

Clotrimazole is a broad-spectrum, antifungal agent that is used for the treatment of dermal infections caused by various species of pathogenic dermatophytes, yeasts, and *Malassezia furfur*. The primary action of clotrimazole is against dividing and growing organisms.
In vitro, clotrimazole exhibits fungistatic and fungicidal activity against isolates of *Trichophyton rubrum, Trichophyton mentagrophytes, Epidermophyton floccosum*, and *Microsporum canis*. In general, the *in vitro* activity of clotrimazole corresponds to that of tolnaftate and griseofulvin against the mycelia of dermatophytes (*Trichophyton, Microsporum*, and *Epidermophyton*).
In vivo studies in guinea pigs infected with *Trichophyton mentagrophytes* have shown no measurable loss of clotrimazole activity due to combination with betamethasone dipropionate.
Strains of fungi having a natural resistance to clotrimazole have not been reported.
No single-step or multiple-step resistance to clotrimazole has developed during successive passages of *Trichophyton mentagrophytes*.
In studies of the mechanism of action in fungal cultures, the minimum fungicidal concentration of clotrimazole caused leakage of intracellular phosphorous compounds into the ambient medium with concomitant breakdown of cellular nucleic acids, and accelerated potassium efflux. Both of these events began rapidly and extensively after addition of the drug to the cultures.
Clotrimazole appears to be minimally absorbed following topical application to the skin. Six hours after the application of radioactive clotrimazole 1% cream and 1% solution onto intact and acutely inflamed skin, the concentration of clotrimazole varied from 100 mcg/cm^3 in the stratum corneum, to 0.5 to 1 mcg/cm^3 in the stratum reticulare, and 0.1 mcg/cm^3 in the subcutis. No measurable amount of radioactivity (<0.001 mcg/mL) was found in the serum within 48 hours after application under occlusive dressing of 0.5 mL of the solution or 0.8 g of the cream.

Betamethasone dipropionate

Betamethasone dipropionate, a corticosteroid, is effective in the treatment of corticosteroid-responsive dermatoses primarily because of its anti-inflammatory, anti-pruritic, and vasoconstrictive actions. However, while the physiologic, pharmacologic, and clinical effects of corticosteroids are well known, the exact mechanisms of their actions in each disease are uncertain. Betamethasone dipropionate, a corticosteroid, has been shown to have topical (dermatologic) and systemic pharmacologic and metabolic effects characteristic of this class of drugs.
Pharmacokinetics: The extent of percutaneous absorption of topical corticosteroids is determined by many factors including the vehicle, the integrity of the epidermal barrier, and the use of occlusive dressings. (See **DOSAGE AND ADMINISTRATION** section.)
Topical corticosteroids can be absorbed from normal intact skin. Inflammation and/or other disease processes in the skin increase percutaneous absorption. Occlusive dressings substantially increase the percutaneous absorption of topical corticosteroids. (See **DOSAGE AND ADMINISTRATION** section.)
Once absorbed through the skin, topical corticosteroids are handled through pharmacokinetic pathways similar to systemically administered corticosteroids. Corticosteroids are bound to plasma proteins in varying degrees. Corticosteroids are metabolized primarily in the liver and are then excreted by the kidneys. Some of the topical corticosteroids and their metabolites are also excreted into the bile.

Clotrimazole and betamethasone dipropionate

In clinical studies of tinea corporis, tinea cruris, and tinea pedis, patients treated with LOTRISONE Cream showed a better clinical response at the first return visit than patients treated with clotrimazole cream. In tinea corporis and tinea cruris, the patient returned 3 days after starting treatment, and in tinea pedis, after 1 week. Mycological cure rates observed in patients treated with LOTRISONE Cream were as good as or better than in those patients treated with clotrimazole cream.
In these same clinical studies, patients treated with LOTRISONE Cream showed statistically significantly better clinical responses and mycological cure rates when compared with patients treated with betamethasone dipropionate cream.

INDICATIONS AND USAGE

LOTRISONE Cream is indicated for the topical treatment of the following dermal infections: tinea pedis, tinea cruris, and tinea corporis due to *Trichophyton rubrum, Trichophyton mentagrophytes, Epidermophyton floccosum*, and *Microsporum canis*.
NOT TO BE USED UNDER THE AGE OF 12 AND NOT TO BE USED IN DIAPER DERMATITIS.

CONTRAINDICATIONS

LOTRISONE Cream is contraindicated in patients who are sensitive to clotrimazole, betamethasone dipropionate, other corticosteroids or imidazoles, or to any ingredient in this preparation.

PRECAUTIONS

General:

Systemic absorption of topical corticosteroids has produced reversible hypothalamic-pituitary-adrenal (HPA) axis suppression, manifestations of Cushing's syndrome, hyperglycemia, and glucosuria in some patients.
Conditions which augment systemic absorption include the application of the more potent steroids, use over large surface areas, prolonged use, and the addition of occlusive dressings. (See **DOSAGE AND ADMINISTRATION** section.)
Therefore, patients receiving a large dose of a potent topical steroid applied to a large surface area should be evaluated periodically for evidence of HPA axis suppression by using the urinary free cortisol and ACTH stimulation tests. If HPA axis suppression is noted, an attempt should be made to withdraw the drug, to reduce the frequency of application, or to substitute a less potent steroid.
Recovery of HPA axis function is generally prompt and complete upon discontinuation of the drug. Infrequently, signs and symptoms of steroid withdrawal may occur, requiring supplemental systemic corticosteroids.
Children may absorb proportionally larger amounts of topical corticosteroids and thus be more susceptible to systemic toxicity. (See **PRECAUTIONS – Pediatric Use**.)
If irritation or hypersensitivity develops with the use of LOTRISONE Cream, treatment should be discontinued and appropriate therapy instituted.
Information for Patients: Patients using LOTRISONE Cream should receive the following information and instructions:

1. This medication is to be used as directed by the physician. It is for external use only. Avoid contact with the eyes.
2. The medication is to be used for the full prescribed treatment time, even though the symptoms may have improved. Notify the physician if there is no improvement after 1 week of treatment for tinea cruris or tinea corporis, or after 2 weeks for tinea pedis.
3. Patients should be advised not to use this medication for any disorder other than for which it was prescribed.
4. The treated skin areas should not be bandaged or otherwise covered or wrapped as to be occluded. (See **DOSAGE AND ADMINISTRATION** section.)
5. When using this medication in the groin area, patients should be advised to use the medication for 2 weeks only, and to apply the cream sparingly. The physician should be notified if the condition persists after 2 weeks. Patients should also be advised to wear loose fitting clothing. (See **DOSAGE AND ADMINISTRATION** section.)
6. Patients should report any signs of local adverse reactions.
7. Patients should avoid sources of infection or reinfection.

Laboratory Tests: If there is a lack of response to LOTRISONE Cream, appropriate microbiological studies should be repeated to confirm the diagnosis and rule out other pathogens before instituting another course of antimycotic therapy.
The following tests may be helpful in evaluating HPA axis suppression due to the corticosteroid component:

Urinary free cortisol test
ACTH stimulation test

Carcinogenesis, Mutagenesis, Impairment of Fertility: There are no animal or laboratory studies with the combination clotrimazole and betamethasone dipropionate to evaluate carcinogenesis, mutagenesis, or impairment of fertility.
An 18-month oral dosing study with clotrimazole in rats has not revealed any carcinogenic effect.
In tests for mutagenesis, chromosomes of the spermatophores of Chinese hamsters which had been exposed to clotrimazole were examined for structural changes during the metaphase. Prior to testing, the hamsters had received five oral clotrimazole doses of 100 mg/kg body weight. The results of this study showed that clotrimazole had no mutagenic effect.
Pregnancy Category C: There have been no teratogenic studies performed with the combination clotrimazole and betamethasone dipropionate.
Studies in pregnant rats with intravaginal doses up to 100 mg/kg have revealed no evidence of harm to the fetus due to clotrimazole.
High oral doses of clotrimazole in rats and mice ranging from 50 to 120 mg/kg resulted in embryotoxicity (possibly secondary to maternal toxicity), impairment of mating, decreased litter size and number of viable young and decreased pup survival to weaning. However, clotrimazole was not teratogenic in mice, rabbits, and rats at oral doses up to 200, 180, and 100 mg/kg, respectively. Oral absorption in the rat amounts to approximately 90% of the administered dose.
Corticosteroids are generally teratogenic in laboratory animals when administered systemically at relatively low dosage levels. The more potent corticosteroids have been shown to be teratogenic after dermal application in laboratory animals.
There are no adequate and well-controlled studies in pregnant women on teratogenic effects from a topically applied combination of clotrimazole and betamethasone dipropionate. Therefore, LOTRISONE Cream should be used during pregnancy only if the potential benefit justifies the potential risk to the fetus.
Drugs containing corticosteroids should not be used extensively on pregnant patients, in large amounts, or for prolonged periods of time.
Nursing Mothers: It is not known whether this drug is excreted in human milk. Because many drugs are excreted in human milk, caution should be exercised when LOTRISONE Cream is used by a nursing woman.
Pediatric Use: Safety and effectiveness in pediatric patients below the age of 12 have not been established with LOTRISONE Cream.
Pediatric patients may demonstrate greater susceptibility to topical corticosteroid-induced HPA axis suppression and Cushing's syndrome than mature patients because of a larger skin surface area to body weight ratio.
Hypothalamic-pituitary-adrenal (HPA) axis suppression, Cushing's syndrome, and intracranial hypertension have been reported in children receiving topical corticosteroids. Manifestations of adrenal suppression in children include linear growth retardation, delayed weight gain, low plasma cortisol levels, and absence of response to ACTH stimulation. Manifestations of intracranial hypertension include bulging fontanelles, headaches, and bilateral papilledema.
Administration of topical dermatologics containing a corticosteroid to pediatric patients should be limited to the least amount compatible with an effective therapeutic regimen. Chronic corticosteroid therapy may interfere with the growth and development of children.
NOT TO BE USED UNDER THE AGE OF 12 AND NOT TO BE USED IN DIAPER DERMATITIS.

ADVERSE REACTIONS

The following adverse reactions have been reported in connection with the use of LOTRISONE Cream: paresthesia in 5 of 270 patients, maculopapular rash, edema, and secondary infection, each in 1 of 270 patients.
Adverse reactions reported with the use of clotrimazole are as follows: erythema, stinging, blistering, peeling, edema, pruritus, urticaria, and general irritation of the skin.
The following local adverse reactions are reported infrequently when topical corticosteroids are used as recommended. These reactions are listed in an approximate decreasing order of occurrence: burning, itching, irritation, dryness, folliculitis, hypertrichosis, acneiform eruptions, hypo-pigmentation, perioral dermatitis, allergic contact dermatitis, maceration of the skin, secondary infection, skin atrophy, striae, and miliaria.

OVERDOSAGE

Acute overdosage with topical application of LOTRISONE Cream is unlikely and would not be expected to lead to a life-threatening situation.
Topically applied corticosteroids can be absorbed in sufficient amounts to produce systemic effects. (See **PRECAUTIONS**.)

DOSAGE AND ADMINISTRATION

Gently massage sufficient LOTRISONE Cream into the affected and surrounding skin areas twice a day, in the morning and evening, for 2 weeks in tinea cruris and tinea corporis and for 4 weeks in tinea pedis. The use of LOTRISONE Cream for longer than 4 weeks is not recommended.
Clinical improvement, with relief of erythema and pruritus, usually occurs within 3 to 5 days of treatment. If a patient with tinea cruris or tinea corporis shows no clinical improvement after 1 week of treatment with LOTRISONE Cream, the diagnosis should be reviewed. In tinea pedis, the treatment should be applied for 2 weeks prior to making that decision.
Treatment with LOTRISONE Cream should be discontinued if the condition persists after 2 weeks in tinea cruris and tinea corporis, and after 4 weeks in tinea pedis. Alternate therapy may then be instituted with LOTRIMIN Cream, a product containing an antifungal only.

Continued on next page

Information on Schering products appearing on these pages is effective as of January 2000.

Lotrisone—Cont.

LOTRISONE Cream should not be used with occlusive dressings.

HOW SUPPLIED

LOTRISONE Cream is supplied in 15-gram (NDC 0085-0924-01) and 45-gram tubes (NDC 0085-0924-02); boxes of one.

Store between 2° and 30°C (36° and 86°F).

Schering Corporation/Key Pharmaceuticals, Inc.
Kenilworth, NJ 07033 USA
Rev. 1/00 13182370
23847507T

NASONEX® ℞

(mometasone furoate monohydrate)
Nasal Spray, 50 mcg*
FOR INTRANASAL USE ONLY
*calculated on the anhydrous basis

DESCRIPTION

Mometasone furoate monohydrate, the active component of NASONEX Nasal Spray, 50 mcg, is an anti-inflammatory corticosteroid having the chemical name, 9,21-Dichloro-11β, 17-dihydroxy-16α-methylpregna-1,4-diene-3,20-dione 17-(2 furoate) monohydrate, and the following chemical structure:

Mometasone furoate monohydrate is a white powder, with an empirical formula of $C_{27}H_{30}Cl_2O_6 \bullet H_2O$, and a molecular weight of 539.45. It is practically insoluble in water; slightly soluble in methanol, ethanol, and isopropanol; soluble in acetone and chloroform; and freely soluble in tetrahydrofuran. Its partition coefficient between octanol and water is greater than 5000.

NASONEX Nasal Spray, 50 mcg is a metered-dose, manual pump spray unit containing an aqueous suspension of mometasone furoate monohydrate equivalent to 0.05% w/w mometasone furoate calculated on the anhydrous basis; in an aqueous medium containing glycerin, microcrystalline cellulose and carboxymethylcellulose sodium, sodium citrate, 0.25% w/w phenylethyl alcohol, citric acid, benzalkonium chloride, and polysorbate 80. The pH is between 4.3 and 4.9.

After initial priming (10 actuations), each actuation of the pump delivers a metered spray containing 100 mg of suspension containing mometasone furoate monohydrate equivalent to 50 mcg of mometasone furoate calculated on the anhydrous basis. Each bottle of NASONEX Nasal Spray, 50 mcg provides 120 sprays.

CLINICAL PHARMACOLOGY

NASONEX Nasal Spray, 50 mcg is a corticosteroid demonstrating anti-inflammatory properties. The precise mechanism of corticosteroid action on allergic rhinitis is not known. Corticosteroids have been shown to have a wide range of effects on multiple cell types (eg, mast cells, eosinophils, neutrophils, macrophages, and lymphocytes) and mediators (eg, histamine, eicosanoids, leukotrienes, and cytokines) involved in inflammation.

In two clinical studies utilizing nasal antigen challenge, NASONEX Nasal Spray, 50 mcg decreased some markers of the early- and late-phase allergic response. These observations included decreases (vs placebo) in histamine and eosinophil cationic protein levels, and reductions (vs baseline) in eosinophils, neutrophils, and epithelial cell adhesion proteins. The clinical significance of these findings is not known.

The effect of NASONEX Nasal Spray, 50 mcg on nasal mucosa following 12 months of treatment was examined in 46 patients with allergic rhinitis. There was no evidence of atrophy and there was a marked reduction in intraepithelial eosinophilia and inflammatory cell infiltration (eg, eosinophils, lymphocytes, monocytes, neutrophils, and plasma cells).

Pharmacokinetics: *Absorption:* Mometasone furoate monohydrate administered as a nasal spray is virtually undetectable in plasma from adult and pediatric subjects despite the use of a sensitive assay with a lower quantitation limit (LOQ) of 50 pcg/mL.

Distribution: The *in vitro* protein binding for mometasone furoate was reported to be 98% to 99% in concentration range of 5 to 500 ng/mL.

Metabolism: Studies have shown that any portion of a mometasone furoate dose which is swallowed and absorbed undergoes extensive metabolism to multiple metabolites. There are no major metabolites detectable in plasma. Upon *in vitro* incubation, one of the minor metabolites formed is 6β-hydroxy-mometasone furoate. In human liver microsomes, the formation of the metabolite is regulated by cytochrome P-450 3A4 (CYP3A4).

Elimination: Following intravenous administration, the effective plasma elimination half-life of mometasone furoate is 5.8 hours. Any absorbed drug is excreted as metabolites mostly via the bile, and to a limited extent, into the urine.

Special Populations: The effects of renal impairment, hepatic impairment, age, or gender on mometasone furoate pharmacokinetics have not been adequately investigated.

Pharmacodynamics: Three clinical pharmacology studies have been conducted in humans to assess the effect of NASONEX Nasal Spray, 50 mcg at various doses on adrenal function. In one study, daily doses of 200 and 400 mcg of NASONEX Nasal Spray, 50 mcg and 10 mg of prednisone were compared to placebo in 64 patients with allergic rhinitis. Adrenal function before and after 36 consecutive days of treatment was assessed by measuring plasma cortisol levels following a 6-hour Cortrosyn (ACTH) infusion and by measuring 24-hour urinary-free cortisol levels. NASONEX Nasal Spray, 50 mcg, at both the 200- and 400-mcg dose, was not associated with a statistically significant decrease in mean plasma cortisol levels post-Cortrosyn infusion or a statistically significant decrease in the 24-hour urinary-free cortisol levels compared to placebo. A statistically significant decrease in the mean plasma cortisol levels post-Cortrosyn infusion and 24-hour urinary-free cortisol levels was detected in the prednisone treatment group compared to placebo.

A second study assessed adrenal response to NASONEX Nasal Spray, 50 mcg (400 and 1600 mcg/day), predisone (10 mg/day), and placebo, administered for 29 days in 48 male volunteers. The 24-hour plasma cortisol area under the curve (AUC_{0-24}), during and after an 8-hour Cortrosyn infusion and 24-hour urinary-free cortisol levels were determined at baseline and after 29 days of treatment. No statistically significant differences of adrenal function were observed with NASONEX Nasal Spray, 50 mcg compared to placebo.

A third study evaluated single, rising doses of NASONEX Nasal Spray, 50 mcg (1000, 2000, and 4000 mcg/day), orally administered mometasone furoate (2000, 4000, and 8000 mcg/day), orally administered dexamethasone (200, 400, and 800 mcg/day), and placebo (administered at the end of each series of doses) in 24 male volunteers. Dose administrations were separated by at least 72 hours. Determination of serial plasma cortisol levels at 8 AM and for the 24-hour period following each treatment were used to calculate the plasma cortisol area under the curve (AUC_{0-24}). In addition, 24-hour urinary-free cortisol levels were collected prior to initial treatment administration and during the period immediately following each dose. No statistically significant decreases in the plasma cortisol AUC, 8 AM cortisol levels, or 24-hour urinary-free cortisol levels were observed in volunteers treated with either NASONEX Nasal Spray, 50 mcg or oral mometasone, as compared with placebo treatment. Conversely, nearly all volunteers treated with the three doses of dexamethasone demonstrated abnormal 8 AM cortisol levels (defined as a cortisol level <10 mcg/dL), reduced 24-hour plasma AUC values, and decreased 24-hour urinary-free cortisol levels, as compared to placebo treatment.

Two clinical pharmacology studies have been conducted in pediatric patients to assess the effect of mometasone furoate nasal spray, on the adrenal function at daily doses of 50, 100, and 200 mcg vs placebo. In one study, adrenal function before and after 7 consecutive days of treatment was assessed in 48 pediatric patients with allergic rhinitis (ages 6 to 11 years) by measuring morning plasma cortisol and 24-hour urinary-free cortisol levels. Mometasone furoate nasal spray, at all three doses, was not associated with a statistically significant decrease in mean plasma cortisol levels or a statistically significant decrease in the 24-hour urinary-free cortisol levels compared to placebo. In the second study, adrenal function before and after 14 consecutive days of treatment was assessed in 48 pediatric patients (ages 3 to 5 years) with allergic rhinitis by measuring plasma cortisol levels following a 30-minute Cortrosyn infusion. Mometasone furoate nasal spray, 50 mcg, at all three doses (50, 100, and 200 mcg/day), was not associated with a statistically significant decrease in mean plasma cortisol levels post-Cortrosyn infusion compared to placebo. All patients had a normal response to Cortrosyn.

Clinical Studies: The efficacy and safety of NASONEX Nasal Spray, 50 mcg in the prophylaxis and treatment of seasonal allergic rhinitis and the treatment of perennial allergic rhinitis have been evaluated in 18 controlled trials, and one uncontrolled clinical trial, in approximately 3000 adults (ages 17 to 85 years) and adolescents (ages 12 to 16 years). This included 1757 males and 1453 females, including a total of 283 adolescents (182 boys and 101 girls) with seasonal allergic or perennial allergic rhinitis, treated with NASONEX Nasal Spray, 50 mcg at doses ranging from 50 to 800 mcg/day. The majority of patients were treated with 200 mcg/day. These trials evaluated the total nasal symptom scores that included stuffiness, rhinorrhea, itching, and sneezing. Patients treated with NASONEX Nasal Spray, 50 mcg, 200 mcg/day had a significant decrease in total nasal symptom scores compared to placebo-treated patients. No additional benefit was observed for mometasone furoate doses greater than 200 mcg/day. A total of 350 patients have been treated with NASONEX Nasal Spray, 50 mcg for 1 year or longer.

The efficacy and safety of NASONEX Nasal Spray, 50 mcg in the treatment of seasonal allergic and perennial allergic rhinitis in pediatric patients (ages 3 to 11 years) have been evaluated in four controlled trials. This included approximately 990 pediatric patients ages 3 to 11 years (606 males and 384 females) with seasonal allergic or perennial allergic rhinitis treated with mometasone furoate nasal spray at doses ranging from 25 to 200 mcg/day. Pediatric patients treated with NASONEX Nasal Spray, 50 mcg (100 mcg total daily dose, 374 patients) had a significant decrease in total nasal symptom (congestion, rhinorrhea, itching, and sneezing) scores, compared to placebo-treated patients. No additional benefit was observed for the 200-mcg mometasone furoate total daily dose in pediatric patients (ages 3 to 11 years). A total of 163 pediatric patients have been treated for 1 year.

In patients with seasonal allergic rhinitis, NASONEX Nasal Spray, 50 mcg, demonstrated improvement in nasal symptoms (vs placebo) within 11 hours after the first dose based on one single-dose, parallel-group study of patients in an outdoor "park" setting (park study) and one environmental exposure unit (EEU) study, and within 2 days in two randomized, double-blind, placebo-controlled, parallel-group seasonal allergic rhinitis studies. Maximum benefit is usually achieved within 1 to 2 weeks after initiation of dosing.

Prophylaxis of seasonal allergic rhinitis for patients 12 years of age and older with NASONEX Nasal Spray, 50 mcg, given at a dose of 200 mcg/day, was evaluated in two clinical studies in 284 patients. These studies were designed such that patients received 4 weeks of prophylaxis with NASONEX Nasal Spray, 50 mcg prior to the anticipated onset of the pollen season; however, some patients received only 2 to 3 weeks of prophylaxis. Patients receiving 2 to 4 weeks of prophylaxis with NASONEX Nasal Spray, 50 mcg demonstrated a statistically significantly smaller mean increase in total nasal symptom scores with onset of the pollen season as compared to placebo patients.

INDICATIONS AND USAGE

NASONEX Nasal Spray, 50 mcg is indicated for the treatment of the nasal symptoms of seasonal allergic and perennial allergic rhinitis, in adults and pediatric patients 3 years of age and older. NASONEX Nasal Spray, 50 mcg is indicated for the prophylaxis of the nasal symptoms of seasonal allergic rhinitis in adult and adolescent patients 12 years and older. In patients with a known seasonal allergen that precipitates nasal symptoms of seasonal allergic rhinitis, initiation of prophylaxis with NASONEX Nasal Spray, 50 mcg is recommended 2 to 4 weeks prior to the anticipated start of the pollen season. Safety and effectiveness of NASONEX Nasal Spray, 50 mcg in pediatric patients less than 3 years of age have not been established.

CONTRAINDICATIONS

Hypersensitivity to any of the ingredients of this preparation contraindicates its use.

WARNINGS

The replacement of a systemic corticosteroid with a topical corticosteroid can be accompanied by signs of adrenal insufficiency and, in addition, some patients may experience symptoms of withdrawal; ie, joint and/or muscular pain, lassitude, and depression. Careful attention must be given when patients previously treated for prolonged periods with systemic corticosteroids are transferred to topical corticosteroids, with careful monitoring for acute adrenal insufficiency in response to stress. This is particularly important in those patients who have associated asthma or other clinical conditions where too rapid a decrease in systemic corticosteroid dosing may cause a severe exacerbation of their symptoms.

If recommended doses of intranasal corticosteroids are exceeded or if individuals are particularly sensitive or predisposed by virtue of recent systemic steroid therapy, symptoms of hypercorticism may occur, including very rare cases of menstrual irregularities, acneiform lesions, and cushingoid features. If such changes occur, topical corticosteroids should be discontinued slowly, consistent with accepted procedures for discontinuing oral steroid therapy.

Persons who are on drugs which suppress the immune system are more susceptible to infections than healthy individuals. Chickenpox and measles, for example, can have a more serious or even fatal course in nonimmune children or adults on corticosteroids. In such children or adults who have not had these diseases, particular care should be taken to avoid exposure. How the dose, route, and duration of corticosteroid administration affects the risk of developing a disseminated infection is not known. The contribution of the underlying disease and/or prior corticosteroid treatment to the risk is also not known. If exposed to chickenpox, prophylaxis with varicella zoster immune globin (VZIG) may be indicated. If exposed to measles, prophylaxis with pooled intramuscular immunoglobulin (IG) may be indicated. (See the respective package inserts for complete VZIG and IG prescribing information.) If chickenpox develops, treatment with antiviral agents may be considered.

PRECAUTIONS

General: Intranasal corticosteroids may cause a reduction in growth velocity when administered to pediatric patients (see **PRECAUTIONS, Pediatric Use** section). In clinical studies with NASONEX Nasal Spray, 50 mcg, the development of localized infections of the nose and pharynx with *Candida albicans* has occurred only rarely. When such an infection develops, use of NASONEX Nasal Spray, 50 mcg should be discontinued and appropriate local or systemic therapy instituted, if needed.

Nasal corticosteroids should be used with caution, if at all, in patients with active or quiescent tuberculous infection of the respiratory tract, or in untreated fungal, bacterial, systemic viral infections, or ocular herpes simplex.

Rarely, immediate hypersensitivity reactions may occur after the intranasal administration of mometasone furoate monohydrate. Extreme rare instances of wheezing have been reported.

Rare instances of nasal septum perforation and increased intraocular pressure have also been reported following the intranasal application of aerosolized corticosteroids. As with any long-term topical treatment of the nasal cavity, patients using NASONEX Nasal Spray, 50 mcg over several months or longer should be examined periodically for possible changes in the nasal mucosa.

Because of the inhibitory effect of corticosteroids on wound healing, patients who have experienced recent nasal septum ulcers, nasal surgery, or nasal trauma should not use a nasal corticosteroid until healing has occurred.

Glaucoma and cataract formation was evaluated in one controlled study of 12 weeks' duration and one uncontrolled study of 12 months' duration in patients treated with NASONEX Nasal Spray, 50 mcg at 200 mcg/day, using intraocular pressure measurements and slit lamp examination. No significant change from baseline was noted in the mean intraocular pressure measurements for the 141 NASONEX-treated patients in the 12-week study, as compared with 141 placebo-treated patients. No individual NASONEX-treated patient was noted to have developed a significant elevation in intraocular pressure or cataracts in this 12-week study. Likewise, no significant change from baseline was noted in the mean intraocular pressure measurements for the 139 NASONEX-treated patients in the 12-month study and again, no cataracts were detected in these patients. Nonetheless, nasal and inhaled corticosteroids have been associated with the development of glaucoma and/or cataracts. Therefore, close follow-up is warranted in patients with a change in vision and with a history of glaucoma and/or cataracts.

When nasal corticosteroids are used at excessive doses, systemic corticosteroid effects such as hypercorticism and adrenal suppression may appear. If such changes occur, NASONEX Nasal Spray, 50 mcg should be discontinued slowly, consistent with accepted procedures for discontinuing oral steroid therapy.

Information for Patients: Patients being treated with NASONEX Nasal Spray, 50 mcg should be given the following information and instructions. This information is intended to aid in the safe and effective use of this medication. It is not a disclosure of all intended or possible adverse effects. Patients should use NASONEX Nasal Spray, 50 mcg at regular intervals (once daily) since its effectiveness depends on regular use. Improvement in nasal symptoms of allergic rhinitis has been shown to occur within 11 hours after the first dose based on one single-dose, parallel-group study of patients in an outdoor "park" setting (park study) and one environmental exposure unit (EEU) study and within 2 days after the first dose in two randomized, double-blind, placebo-controlled, parallel-group seasonal allergic rhinitis studies. Maximum benefit is usually achieved within 1 to 2 weeks after initiation of dosing. Patients should take the medication as directed and should not increase the prescribed dosage by using it more than once a day in an attempt to increase its effectiveness. Patients should contact their physician if symptoms do not improve, or if the condition worsens. To assure proper use of this nasal spray, and to attain maximum benefit, patients should read and follow the accompanying Patient's Instructions for Use carefully.

Patients should be cautioned not to spray NASONEX Nasal Spray, 50 mcg into the eyes or directly onto the nasal septum.

Persons who are on immunosuppressant doses of corticosteroids should be warned to avoid exposure to chickenpox or measles, and patients should also be advised that if they are exposed, medical advice should be sought without delay.

Carcinogenesis, Mutagenesis, Impairment of Fertility: In a 2-year carcinogenicity study of Sprague Dawley rats, mometasone furoate demonstrated no statistically significant increase of tumors at inhalation doses up to 67 mcg/kg (approximately 3 and 2 times the maximum recommended daily intranasal dose in adults and children, respectively, on a mcg/m^2 basis). In a 19-month carcinogenicity study of Swiss CD-1 mice, mometasone furoate demonstrated no statistically significant increase in the incidence of tumors at inhalation doses up to 160 mcg/kg (approximately 4 and 3 times the maximum recommended daily intranasal dose in adults and children, respectively, on a mcg/m^2 basis).

At cytotoxic doses, mometasone furoate produced an increase in chromosome aberrations *in vitro* in Chinese hamster ovary-cell cultures in the nonactivation phase, but not in the presence of rat liver S9 fraction. Mometasone furoate was not mutagenic in the mouse-lymphoma assay and the *Salmonella/E. coli*/mammalian microsome mutation assay, a Chinese hamster lung cell (CHL) chromosomal-aberrations assay, an *in vivo* mouse bone-marrow erythrocyte-micronucleus assay, a rat bone-marrow clastogenicity assay, and the mouse male germ-cell clastogenicity assay. Mometasone furoate also did not induce unscheduled DNA synthesis *in vivo* in rat hepatocytes.

In reproductive studies in rats, impairment of fertility was not produced by subcutaneous doses up to 15 mcg/kg (less than the maximum recommended daily intranasal dose in adults on a mcg/m^2 basis). However, mometasone furoate caused prolonged gestation, prolonged and difficult labor, reduced offspring survival, and reduced maternal body weight gain at a dose of 15 mcg/kg.

Pregnancy: *Teratogenic Effects: Pregnancy Category C*: Mometasone furoate caused cleft palate in mice at subcutaneous doses of 60 mcg/kg and above (approximately 2 times the maximum recommended daily intranasal dose in adults on a mcg/m^2 basis). Offspring survival was reduced in the 180-mcg/kg group (approximately 4 times the maximum recommended daily intranasal dose in adults on a mcg/m^2 basis). No such effects were observed at 20 mcg/kg (less than the maximum recommended daily intranasal dose in adults on a mcg/m^2 basis).

In rabbits, mometasone furoate caused flexed front paws at a topical dermal dose of 150 mcg/kg (approximately 14 times the maximum recommended daily intranasal dose in adults on a mcg/m^2 basis).

In rats, mometasone furoate produced umbilical hernia, cleft palate, and delayed ossification at a topical dermal dose of 600 mcg/kg (approximately 30 times the maximum recommended daily intranasal dose in adults on a mcg/m^2 basis). At 1200 mcg/kg (approximately 60 times the maximum recommended daily intranasal dose in adults on a mcg/m^2 basis), microphthalmia, umbilical hernias, and delayed ossification were observed in rat pups.

In these developmental studies, there were also reductions in maternal body weight gain and effects on fetal growth (lower fetal body weights and/or delayed ossification) in mice (60 and 180 mcg/kg), rabbits (150 mcg/kg), and rats (600 mcg/kg).

In an oral developmental study in rabbits, at 700 mcg/kg, (approximately 70 times the maximum recommended daily intranasal dose in adults on a mcg/m^2 basis), increased incidences of resorptions and malformations, including cleft palate and/or head malformations (hydrocephaly or domed head) were observed. Pregnancy failure was observed in most rabbits at 2800 mcg/kg (approximately 270 times the maximum recommended daily intranasal dose in adults on a mcg/m^2 basis).

There are no adequate and well-controlled studies in pregnant women. NASONEX Nasal Spray, 50 mcg, like other corticosteroids, should be used during pregnancy only if the potential benefits justify the potential risk to the fetus. Experience with oral corticosteroids since their introduction in pharmacologic, as opposed to physiologic, doses suggests that rodents are more prone to teratogenic effects from corticosteroids than humans. In addition, because there is a natural increase in corticosteroid production during pregnancy, most women will require a lower exogenous corticosteroid dose and many will not need corticosteroid treatment during pregnancy.

Nonteratogenic Effects: Hypoadrenalism may occur in infants born to women receiving corticosteroids during pregnancy. Such infants should be carefully monitored.

Nursing Mothers: It is not known if mometasone furoate is excreted in human milk. Because other corticosteroids are excreted in human milk, caution should be used when NASONEX Nasal Spray, 50 mcg is administered to nursing women.

Pediatric Use: Controlled clinical studies have shown intranasal corticosteroids may cause a reduction in growth velocity in pediatric patients. This effect has been observed in the absence of laboratory evidence of hypothalamic-pituitary-adrenal (HPA) axis suppression, suggesting that growth velocity is a more sensitive indicator of systemic corticosteroid exposure in pediatric patients than some commonly used tests of HPA axis function. The long-term effects of this reduction in growth velocity associated with intranasal corticosteroids, including the impact on final adult height, are unknown. The potential for "catch up" growth following discontinuation of treatment with intranasal corticosteroids has not been adequately studied. The growth of pediatric patients receiving intranasal corticosteroids, including NASONEX Nasal Spray, 50 mcg should be monitored routinely (eg, via stadiometry). The potential growth effects of prolonged treatment should be weighed against clinical benefits obtained and the availability of safe and effective noncorticosteroid treatment alternatives. To minimize the systemic effects of intranasal corticosteroids, including NASONEX Nasal Spray, 50 mcg, each patient should be titrated to his/her lowest effective dose.

Seven hundred and twenty (720) patients 3 to 11 years of age were treated with mometasone furoate nasal spray, 50 mcg (100 mcg total daily dose) in controlled clinical trials. Safety and effectiveness in children less than 3 years of age have not been established.

A clinical study has been conducted for one year in pediatric patients (ages 3 to 9 years) to assess the effect of NASONEX Nasal Spray, 50 mcg (100 mcg total daily dose) on growth velocity. No statistically significant effect on growth velocity was observed for NASONEX Nasal Spray, 50 mcg compared to placebo. No evidence of clinically relevant HPA axis suppression was observed following a 30-minute Cosyntropin infusion.

The potential of NASONEX Nasal Spray to cause growth suppression in susceptible patients or when given at higher doses cannot be ruled out.

Geriatric Use: A total of 203 patients above 64 years of age (age range 64 to 85 years) have been treated with NASONEX Nasal Spray, 50 mcg for up to 3 months. The adverse reactions reported in this population were similar in type and incidence to those reported by younger patients.

ADVERSE REACTIONS

In controlled US and International clinical studies, a total of 3210 adult and adolescent patients aged 12 years and older received treatment with NASONEX Nasal Spray, 50 mcg at doses of 50 to 800 mcg/day. The majority of patients (n = 2103) were treated with 200 mcg/day. In controlled US and International studies, a total of 990 pediatric patients (ages 3 to 11 years) received treatment with NASONEX, 50 mcg, at doses of 25 to 200 mcg/day. The majority of pediatric patients (720) were treated with 100 mcg/day. A total of 513 adult, adolescent, and pediatric patients have been treated for 1 year or longer. The overall incidence of adverse events for patients treated with NASONEX Nasal Spray, 50 mcg was comparable to patients treated with the vehicle placebo. Also, adverse events did not differ significantly based on age, sex, or race. Three percent or less of patients in clinical trials discontinued treatment because of adverse events; this rate was similar for the vehicle and active comparators.

All adverse events (regardless of relationship to treatment) reported by 5% or more of adult and adolescent patients aged 12 years and older who received NASONEX Nasal Spray, 50 mcg, 200 mcg/day and by pediatric patients ages 3 to 11 years who received NASONEX Nasal Spray, 50 mcg, 100 mcg/day in clinical trials vs placebo and that were more common with NASONEX Nasal Spray, 50 mcg than placebo, are displayed in the table below.

[See table above]

ADVERSE EVENTS FROM CONTROLLED CLINICAL TRIALS IN SEASONAL ALLERGIC AND PERENNIAL ALLERGIC RHINITIS (PERCENT OF PATIENTS REPORTING)

	Adult and Adolescent Patients 12 years and older		Pediatric Patients Ages 3 to 11 years	
	NASONEX 200 mcg (N = 2103)	VEHICLE PLACEBO (N = 1671)	NASONEX 100 mcg (N = 374)	VEHICLE PLACEBO (N = 376)
Headache	26	22	17	18
Viral Infection	14	11	8	9
Pharyngitis	12	10	10	10
Epistaxis/Blood-Tinged Mucus	11	6	8	9
Coughing	7	6	13	15
Upper Respiratory Tract Infection	6	2	5	4
Dysmenorrhea	5	3	1	0
Musculoskeletal Pain	5	3	1	1
Sinusitis	5	3	4	4
Vomiting	1	1	5	4

Other adverse events which occurred in less than 5% but greater than or equal to 2% of mometasone furoate adult and adolescent patients (aged 12 years and older) treated with 200-mcg doses (regardless of relationship to treatment), and more frequently than in the placebo group included: arthralgia, asthma, bronchitis, chest pain, conjunctivitis, diarrhea, dyspepsia, earache, flu-like symptoms, myalgia, nausea, and rhinitis.

Other adverse events which occurred in less than 5% but greater or equal to 2% of mometasone furoate pediatric patients aged 3 to 11 years treated with 100-mcg doses vs placebo (regardless of relationship to treatment) and more frequently than in the placebo group included: diarrhea, nasal irritation, otitis media, and wheezing.

Rare cases of nasal ulcers and nasal and oral candidiasis were also reported in patients treated with NASONEX

Continued on next page

Information on Schering products appearing on these pages is effective as of January 2000.

Nasonex—Cont.

Nasal Spray, 50 mcg, primarily in patients treated for longer than 4 weeks.
In postmarketing surveillance of this product, cases of nasal burning and irritation and rare cases of nasal septal perforation have been reported.

OVERDOSAGE

There are no data available on the effects of acute or chronic overdosage with NASONEX Nasal Spray, 50 mcg. Because of low systemic bioavailability, and an absence of acute drug-related systemic findings in clinical studies, overdose is unlikely to require any therapy other than observation. Intranasal administration of 1600 mcg (8 times the recommended dose of NASONEX Nasal Spray, 50 mcg) daily for 29 days, to healthy human volunteers, was well tolerated with no increased incidence of adverse events. Single intranasal doses up to 4000 mcg have been studied in human volunteers with no adverse effects reported. Single oral doses up to 8000 mcg have been studied in human volunteers with no adverse effects reported. Chronic overdosage with any corticosteroid may result in signs or symptoms of hypercorticism (see **PRECAUTIONS**). Acute overdosage with this dosage form is unlikely since one bottle of NASONEX Nasal Spray, 50 mcg contains approximately 8500 mcg of mometasone furoate.

DOSAGE AND ADMINISTRATION

Adults and Children 12 Years of Age and Older: The usual recommended dose for prophylaxis and treatment of the nasal symptoms of seasonal allergic rhinitis and treatment of the nasal symptoms of perennial allergic rhinitis is two sprays (50 mcg of mometasone furoate in each spray) in each nostril once daily (total daily dose of 200 mcg).
In patients with a known seasonal allergen that precipitates nasal symptoms of seasonal allergic rhinitis, prophylaxis with NASONEX Nasal Spray, 50 mcg (200 mcg/day) is recommended 2 to 4 weeks prior to the anticipated start of the pollen season.
Children 3 to 11 Years of Age: The usual recommended dose for treatment of the nasal symptoms of seasonal allergic and perennial allergic rhinitis is one spray (50 mcg of mometasone furoate in each spray) in each nostril once daily (total daily dose of 100 mcg).
Improvement in nasal symptoms of allergic rhinitis has been shown to occur within 11 hours after the first dose based on one single-dose, parallel-group study of patients in an outdoor "park" setting (park study) and one environmental exposure unit (EEU) study and within 2 days after the first dose in two randomized, double-blind, placebo-controlled, parallel-group seasonal allergic rhinitis studies. Maximum benefit is usually achieved within 1 to 2 weeks. Patients should use NASONEX Nasal Spray, 50 mcg only once daily at a regular interval.
Prior to initial use of NASONEX Nasal Spray, 50 mcg, the pump must be primed by actuating ten times or until a fine spray appears. The pump may be stored unused for up to 1 week without repriming. If unused for more than 1 week, reprime by actuating two times, or until a fine spray appears.
Directions for Use: Illustrated Patient's Instructions for Use accompany each package of NASONEX Nasal Spray, 50 mcg.

HOW SUPPLIED

NASONEX (mometasone furoate monohydrate) Nasal Spray, 50 mcg is supplied in a white, high-density, polyethylene bottle fitted with a white metered-dose, manual spray pump, and teal-green cap. It contains 17 g of product formulation, 120 sprays, each delivering 50 mcg of mometasone furoate per actuation. Supplied with Patient's Instructions for Use (NDC 0085-1197-01).
Store between 2° and 25°C (36° and 77°F). Protect from light.
When NASONEX Nasal Spray, 50 mcg is removed from its cardboard container, prolonged exposure of the product to direct light should be avoided. Brief exposure to light, as with normal use, is acceptable.
SHAKE WELL BEFORE EACH USE.
Schering Corporation
Kenilworth, NJ 07033 USA
 Rev. 12/99
20109858T
Shown in Product Identification Guide, page 334

NITRO-DUR® ℞

[*nītrō-dur*]
(nitroglycerin)
Transdermal Infusion System

DESCRIPTION

Nitroglycerin is 1,2,3-propanetriol trinitrate, an organic nitrate whose structural formula is:

and whose molecular weight is 227.09. The organic nitrates are vasodilators, active on both arteries and veins.
The NITRO-DUR (nitroglycerin) Transdermal Infusion System is a flat unit designed to provide continuous controlled release of nitroglycerin through intact skin. The rate of release of nitroglycerin is linearly dependent upon the area of the applied system; each cm^2 of applied system delivers approximately 0.02 mg of nitroglycerin per hour. Thus, the 5-, 10-, 15-, 20-, 30-, and 40-cm^2 systems deliver approximately 0.1, 0.2, 0.3, 0.4, 0.6, and 0.8 mg of nitroglycerin per hour, respectively.
The remainder of the nitroglycerin in each system serves as a reservoir and is not delivered in normal use. After 12 hours, for example, each system has delivered approximately 6% of its original content of nitroglycerin.
The NITRO-DUR transdermal system contains nitroglycerin in acrylic-based polymer adhesives with a resinous cross-linking agent to provide a continuous source of active ingredient. Each unit is sealed in a paper polyethylene-foil pouch.

Cross section of the system.

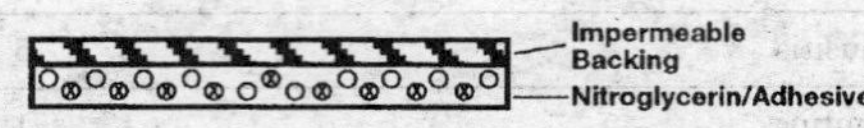

CLINICAL PHARMACOLOGY

The principal pharmacological action of nitroglycerin is relaxation of vascular smooth muscle and consequent dilatation of peripheral arteries and veins, especially the latter. Dilatation of the veins promotes peripheral pooling of blood and decreases venous return to the heart, thereby reducing left ventricular end-diastolic pressure and pulmonary capillary wedge pressure (preload). Arteriolar relaxation reduces systemic vascular resistance, systolic arterial pressure, and mean arterial pressure (afterload). Dilatation of the coronary arteries also occurs. The relative importance of preload reduction, afterload reduction, and coronary dilatation remains undefined.
Dosing regimens for most chronically used drugs are designed to provide plasma concentrations that are continuously greater than a minimally effective concentration. This strategy is inappropriate for organic nitrates. Several well-controlled clinical trials have used exercise testing to assess the antianginal efficacy of continuously delivered nitrates. In the large majority of these trials, active agents were indistinguishable from placebo after 24 hours (or less) of continuous therapy. Attempts to overcome nitrate tolerance by dose escalation, even to doses far in excess of those used acutely, have consistently failed. Only after nitrates have been absent from the body for several hours has their antianginal efficacy been restored.
Pharmacokinetics:
The volume of distribution of nitroglycerin is about 3 L/kg, and nitroglycerin is cleared from this volume at extremely rapid rates, with a resulting serum half-life of about 3 minutes. The observed clearance rates (close to 1 L/kg/min) greatly exceed hepatic blood flow; known sites of extrahepatic metabolism include red blood cells and vascular walls. The first products in the metabolism of nitroglycerin are inorganic nitrate and the 1,2- and 1,3-dinitro-glycerols. The dinitrates are less effective vasodilators than nitroglycerin, but they are longer-lived in the serum, and their net contribution to the overall effect of chronic nitroglycerin regimens is not known. The dinitrates are further metabolized to (nonvasoactive) mononitrates and, ultimately, to glycerol and carbon dioxide.
To avoid development of tolerance to nitroglycerine, drug-free intervals of 10 to 12 hours are known to be sufficient; shorter intervals have not been well studied. In one well-controlled clinical trial, subjects receiving nitroglycerin appeared to exhibit a rebound or withdrawal effect, so that their exercise tolerance at the end of the daily drug-free interval was *less* than that exhibited by the parallel group receiving placebo.
In healthy volunteers, steady-state plasma concentrations of nitroglycerin are reached by about 2 hours after application of a patch and are maintained for the duration of wearing the system (observations have been limited to 24 hours). Upon removal of the patch, the plasma concentration declines with a half-life of about an hour.
Clinical Trials:
Regimens in which nitroglycerin patches were worn for 12 hours daily have been studied in well-controlled trials up to 4 weeks in duration. Starting about 2 hours after application and continuing until 10 to 12 hours after application, patches that deliver at least 0.4 mg of nitroglycerin per hour have consistently demonstrated greater antianginal activity than placebo. Lower-dose patches have not been as well studied, but in one large, well-controlled trial in which higher-dose patches were also studied, patches delivering 0.2 mg/hr had significantly *less* antianginal activity than placebo.
It is reasonable to believe that the rate of nitroglycerin absorption from patches may vary with the site of application, but this relationship has not been adequately studied.

INDICATIONS AND USAGE

Transdermal nitroglycerin is indicated for the prevention of angina pectoris due to coronary artery disease. The onset of action of transdermal nitroglycerin is not sufficiently rapid for this product to be useful in aborting an acute attack.

CONTRAINDICATIONS

Allergic reactions to organic nitrates are extremely rare, but they do occur. Nitroglycerin is contraindicated in patients who are allergic to it. Allergy to the adhesives used in nitroglycerin patches has also been reported, and it similarly constitutes a contraindication to the use of this product.

WARNINGS

Amplification of the vasodilatory effects of the NITRO-DUR patch by sildenafil can result in severe hypotension. The time course and dose dependence of this interaction have not been studied. Appropriate supportive care has not been studied, but it seems reasonable to treat this as a nitrate overdose, with elevation of the extremities and with central volume expansion.
The benefits of transdermal nitroglycerin in patients with acute myocardial infarction or congestive heart failure have not been established. If one elects to use nitroglycerin in these conditions, careful clinical or hemodynamic monitoring must be used to avoid the hazards of hypotension and tachycardia.
A cardioverter/defibrillator should not be discharged through a paddle electrode that overlies a NITRO-DUR patch. The arcing that may be seen in this situation is harmless in itself, but it may be associated with local current concentration that can cause damage to the paddles and burns to the patient.

PRECAUTIONS

General:
Severe hypotension, particularly with upright posture, may occur with even small doses of nitroglycerin. This drug should therefore be used with caution in patients who may be volume depleted or who, for whatever reason, are already hypotensive. Hypotension induced by nitroglycerin may be accompanied by paradoxical bradycardia and increased angina pectoris.
Nitrate therapy may aggravate the angina caused by hypertrophic cardiomyopathy.
As tolerance to other forms of nitroglycerin develops, the effects of sublingual nitroglycerin on exercise tolerance, although still observable, is somewhat blunted.
In industrial workers who have had long-term exposure to unknown (presumably high) doses of organic nitrates, tolerance clearly occurs. Chest pain, acute myocardial infarction, and even sudden death have occurred during temporary withdrawal of nitrates from these workers, demonstrating the existence of true physical dependence.
Several clinical trials in patients with angina pectoris have evaluated nitroglycerin regimens which incorporated a 10- to 12-hour, nitrate-free interval. In some of these trials, an increase in the frequency of anginal attacks during the nitrate-free interval was observed in a small number of patients. In one trial, patients had decreased exercise tolerance at the end of the nitrate-free interval. Hemodynamic rebound has been observed only rarely; on the other hand, few studies were so designed that rebound, if it had occurred, would have been detected. The importance of these observations to the routine, clinical use of transdermal nitroglycerin is unknown.
Information for Patients:
Daily headaches sometimes accompany treatment with nitroglycerin. In patients who get these headaches, the headaches may be a marker of the activity of the drug. Patients should resist the temptation to avoid headaches by altering the schedule of their treatment with nitroglycerin, since loss of headache may be associated with simultaneous loss of antianginal efficacy.
Treatment with nitroglycerin may be associated with lightheadedness on standing, especially just after rising from a recumbent or seated position. This effect may be more frequent in patients who have also consumed alcohol.
After normal use, there is enough residual nitroglycerin in discarded patches that they are a potential hazard to children and pets.
A patient leaflet is supplied with the systems.
Drug Interactions:
The vasodilating effects of nitroglycerin may be additive with those of other vasodilators. Alcohol, in particular has been found to exhibit additive effects of this variety.
Carcinogenesis, Mutagenesis, Impairment of Fertility:
Animal carcinogenesis studies with topically applied nitroglycerin have not been performed.
Rats receiving up to 434 mg/kg/day of dietary nitroglycerin for 2 years developed dose-related fibrotic and neoplastic changes in liver, including carcinomas, and interstitial cell tumors in testes. At high dose, the incidences of hepatocellular carcinomas in both sexes were 52% vs 0% in controls, and incidences of testicular tumors were 52% vs 8% in controls. Lifetime dietary administration of up to 1058 mg/kg/day of nitroglycerin was not tumorigenic in mice.
Nitroglycerin was weakly mutagenic in Ames tests performed in two different laboratories. Nevertheless, there was no evidence of mutagenicity in an *in vivo* dominant lethal assay with male rats treated with doses up to about 363 mg/kg/day, po, or in *in vitro* cytogenetic tests in rat and dog tissues.
In a three-generation reproduction study, rats received dietary nitroglycerin at doses up to about 434 mg/kg/day for 6 months prior to mating of the F_0 generation with treatment continuing through successive F_1 and F_2 generations. The high dose was associated with decreased feed intake and body weight gain in both sexes at all matings. No specific effect on the fertility of the F_0 generation was seen. Infertility noted in subsequent generations, however, was attrib-

uted to increased interstitial cell tissue and aspermatogenesis in the high-dose males. In this three-genration study there was no clear evidence of teratogenicity.

Pregnancy: Pregnancy Category C:
Animal teratology studies have not been conducted with nitroglycerin transdermal systems. Teratology studies in rats and rabbits, however, were conducted with topically applied nitroglycerin ointment at doses up to 80 mg/kg/day and 240 mg/kg/day, respectively. No toxic effects on dams or fetuses were seen at any dose tested. There are no adequate and well-controlled studies in pregnant women. Nitroglycerin should be given to a pregnant woman only if clearly needed.

Nursing Mothers:
It is not known whether nitroglycerin is excreted in human milk. Because many drugs are excreted in human milk, caution should be exercised when nitroglycerin is administered to a nursing woman.

Pediatric Use:
Safety and effectiveness in pediatric patients have not been established.

ADVERSE REACTIONS

Adverse reactions to nitroglycerin are generally dose related, and almost all of these reactions are the result of nitroglycerin's activity as a vasodilator. Headache, which may be severe, is the most commonly reported side effect. Headache may be recurrent with each daily dose, especially at higher doses. Transient episodes of lightheadedness, occasionally related to blood pressure changes, may also occur. Hypotension occurs infrequently, but in some patients it may be severe enough to warrant discontinuation of therapy. Syncope, crescendo angina, and rebound hypertension have been reported but are uncommon.

Allergic reactions to nitroglycerin are also uncommon, and the great majority of those reported have been cases of contact dermatitis or fixed drug eruptions in patients receiving nitroglycerin in ointments or patches. There have been a few reports of genuine anaphylactoid reactions, and these reactions can probably occur in patients receiving nitroglycerin by any route.

Extremely rarely, ordinary doses of organic nitrates have caused methemoglobinemia in normal-seeming patients. Methemoglobinemia is so infrequent at these doses that further discussion of its diagnosis and treatment is deferred (see **OVERDOSAGE**).

Application-site irritation may occur but is rarely severe.

In two placebo-controlled trials of intermittent therapy with nitroglycerin patches at 0.2 to 0.8 mg/hr, the most frequent adverse reactions among 307 subjects were as follows:

	Placebo	Patch
Headache	18%	63%
Lightheadedness	4%	6%
Hypotension, and/or Syncope	0%	4%
Increased Angina	2%	2%

OVERDOSAGE

Hemodynamic Effects:
The ill effects of nitroglycerin overdose are generally the results of nitroglycerin's capacity to induce vasodilatation, venous pooling, reduced cardiac output, and hypotension. These hemodynamic changes may have protean manifestations, including increased intracranial pressure, with any or all of persistent throbbing headache, confusion, and moderate fever; vertigo; palpitations; visual disturbances; nausea and vomiting (possibly with colic and even bloody diarrhea); syncope (especially in the upright posture); air hunger and dyspnea, later followed by reduced ventilatory effort; diaphoresis, with the skin either flushed or cold and clammy; heart block and bradycardia; paralysis; coma; seizures; and death.

Laboratory determinations of serum levels of nitroglycerin and its metabolites are not widely available, and such determinations have, in any event, no established role in the management of nitroglycerin overdose.

No data are available to suggest physiological maneuvers (eg, maneuvers to change the pH of the urine) that might accelerate elimination of nitroglycerin and its active metabolites. Similarly, it is not known which – if any – of these substances can usefully be removed from the body by hemodialysis.

No specific antagonist to the vasodilator effects of nitroglycerin is known, and no intervention has been subject to controlled study as a therapy of nitroglycerin overdose. Because the hypotension associated with nitroglycerin overdose is the result of venodilatation and arterial hypovolemia, prudent therapy in this situation should be directed toward increase in central fluid volume. Passive elevation of the patient's legs may be sufficient, but intravenous infusion of normal saline or similar fluid may also be necessary.

The use of epinephrine or other arterial vasoconstrictors in this setting is likely to do more harm than good.

In patients with renal disease or congestive heart failure, therapy resulting in central volume expansion is not without hazard. Treatment of nitroglycerin overdose in these patients may be subtle and difficult, and invasive monitoring may be required.

Methemoglobinemia:
Nitrate ions liberated during metabolism of nitroglycerin can oxidize hemoglobin into methemoglobin. Even in patients totally without cytochrome b_5 reductase activity, however, and even assuming that the nitrate moieties of nitroglycerin are quantitatively applied to oxidation of hemoglobin, about 1 mg/kg of nitroglycerin should be required before any of these patients manifests clinically significant (≥10%) methemoglobinemia. In patients with normal reductase function, significant production of methemoglobin should require even larger doses of nitroglycerin. In one study in which 36 patients received 2 to 4 weeks of continuous nitroglycerin therapy at 3.1 to 4.4 mg/hr, the average methemoglobin level measured was 0.2%; this was comparable to that observed in parallel patients who received placebo.

Notwithstanding these observations, there are case reports of significant methemoglobinemia in association with moderate overdoses of organic nitrates. None of the affected patients had been thought to be unusually susceptible.

Methemoglobin levels are available from most clinical laboratories. The diagnosis should be suspected in patients who exhibit signs of impaired oxygen delivery despite adequate cardiac output and adequate arterial PO_2. Classically, methemoglobinemic blood is described as chocolate brown, without color change on exposure to air.

When methemoglobinemia is diagnosed, the treatment of choice is methylene blue, 1–2 mg/kg intravenously.

DOSAGE AND ADMINISTRATION

The suggested starting dose is between 0.2 mg/hr* and 0.4 mg/hr*. Doses between 0.4 mg/hr* and 0.8 mg/hr* have shown continued effectiveness for 10 to 12 hours daily for at least 1 month (the longest period studied) of intermittent administration. Although the minimum nitrate-free interval has not been defined, data show that a nitrate-free interval of 10 to 12 hours is sufficient (see **CLINICAL PHARMACOLOGY**). Thus, an appropriate dosing schedule for nitroglycerin patches would include a daily patch-on period of 12 to 14 hours and a daily patch-off period of 10 to 12 hours.

*Release rates were formerly described in terms of drug delivered per 24 hours. In these terms, the supplied NITRO-DUR systems would be rated at 2.5 mg/24 hours (0.1 mg/hour), 5 mg/24 hours (0.2 mg/hour), 7.5 mg/24 hours (0.3 mg/hour), 10 mg/24 hours (0.4 mg/hour), and 15 mg/24 hours (0.6 mg/hour).

Although some well-controlled clinical trials using exercise tolerance testing have shown maintenance of effectiveness when patches are worn continuously, the large majority of such controlled trials have shown the development of tolerance (ie, complete loss of effect) within the first 24 hours after therapy was initiated. Dose adjustment, even to levels much higher than generally used, did not restore efficacy.

HOW SUPPLIED

NITRO-DUR System Rated Release *In Vivo**	Total Nitroglycerin Content	System Size	Package Size
0.1 mg/hr	20 mg	5 cm²	Unit Dose 30 (NDC 0085-3305-30) Hospital Unit Dose 100 (NDC 0085-3305-01) Institutional Package 30 (NDC 0085-3305-35)
0.2 mg/hr	40 mg	10 cm²	Unit Dose 30 (NDC 0085-3310-30) Hospital Unit Dose 100 (NDC 0085-3310-01) Institutional Package 30 (NDC 0085-3310-35)
0.3 mg/hr	60 mg	15 cm²	Unit Dose 30 (NDC 0085-3315-30) Hospital Unit Dose 100 (NDC 0085-3315-01) Institutional Package 30 (NDC 0085-3315-35)
0.4 mg/hr	80 mg	20 cm²	Unit Dose 30 (NDC 0085-3320-30) Hospital Unit Dose 100 (NDC 0085-3320-01) Institutional Package 30 (NDC 0085-3320-35)
0.6 mg/hr	120 mg	30 cm²	Unit Dose 30 (NDC 0085-3330-30) Hospital Unit Dose 100 (NDC 0085-3330-01) Institutional Package 30 (NDC 0085-3330-35)
0.8 mg/hr	160 mg	40 cm²	Unit Dose 30 (NDC 0085-0819-30) Hospital Unit Dose 100 (NDC 0085-0819-01) Institutional Package 30 (NDC 0085-0819-35)

*Release rates were formerly described in terms of drug delivered per 24 hours. In these terms, the supplied NITRO-DUR systems would be rated at 2.5 mg/24 hours (0.1 mg/hour), 5 mg/24 hours (0.2 mg/hour), 7.5 mg/24 hours (0.3 mg/hour), 10 mg/24 hours (0.4 mg/hour), and 15 mg/24 hours (0.6 mg/hour).

Store between 15° and 30°C (59° and 86°F). Do not refrigerate.

CAUTION: Federal law prohibits dispensing without prescription.

Key Pharmaceuticals, Inc.
Kenilworth, NJ 07033 USA
Rev. 10/99 18143631
U.S. Patent No. 5,186,938

NORMODYNE® ℞

brand of labetalol hydrochloride, USP Injection

DESCRIPTION

NORMODYNE (labetalol HCl) is an adrenergic receptor blocking agent that has both selective $alpha_1$- and nonselective beta-adrenergic receptor blocking actions in a single substance.

Labetalol HCl is a racemate, chemically designated as 5-[1-hydroxy-2-[(1-methyl-3-phenylpropyl) amino] ethyl]salicylamide monohydrochloride, and has the following structure:

[Structure: phenyl–CH2CH2CHNHCH2CH(OH)– attached to a benzene ring bearing CONH2 and OH; CH3 on the CH; • HCl]

Labetalol HCl has the empirical formula $C_{19}H_{24}N_2O_3$ • HCl and a molecular weight of 364.9. It has two asymmetric centers and therefore exists as a molecular complex of two diastereoisomeric pairs. Dilevalol, the R,R′ stereoisomer, makes up 25% of racemic labetalol.

Labetalol HCl is a white or off-white crystalline powder, soluble in water.

NORMODYNE (labetalol HCl) Injection is a clear, colorless to light yellow aqueous sterile isotonic solution for intravenous injection. It has a pH range of 3.0 to 4.0. Each mL contains 5 mg labetalol HCl, USP; 45 mg anhydrous dextrose; 0.10 mg edetate disodium; 0.80 mg methylparaben and 0.10 mg propylparaben as preservatives; citric acid monohydrate and sodium hydroxide, as necessary, to bring the solution into the pH range.

CLINICAL PHARMACOLOGY

NORMODYNE (labetalol HCl) combines both selective, competitive $alpha_1$-adrenergic blocking and nonselective, competitive beta-adrenergic blocking activity in a single substance. In man, the ratios of alpha- to beta-blockade have been estimated to be approximately 1:3 and 1:7 following oral and intravenous administration, respectively. $Beta_2$-agonist activity has been demonstrated in animals with minimal $beta_1$-agonist (ISA) activity detected. In animals, at doses greater than those required for alpha- or beta-adrenergic blockade, a membrane-stabilizing effect has been demonstrated.

Pharmacodynamics The capacity of labetalol HCl to block alpha-receptors in man has been demonstrated by attenuation of the pressor effect of phenylephrine and by a significant reduction of the pressor response caused by immersing the hand in ice-cold water ("cold-pressor test"). Labetalol HCl's beta1-receptor blockade in man was demonstrated by a small decrease in the resting heart rate, attenuation of tachycardia produced by isoproterenol or exercise, and by attenuation of the reflex tachycardia to the hypotension produced by amyl nitrite. $Beta_2$-receptor blockade was demonstrated by inhibition of the isoproterenol-induced fall in diastolic blood pressure. Both the alpha- and beta-blocking actions of orally administered labetalol HCl contribute to a decrease in blood pressure in hypertensive patients. Labetalol HCl consistently, in dose-related fashion, blunted in-

Continued on next page

Information on Schering products appearing on these pages is effective as of January 2000.

Normodyne—Cont.

creases in exercise-induced blood pressure and heart rate, and in their double product. The pulmonary circulation during exercise was not affected by labetalol HCl dosing.

Single oral doses of labetalol HCl administered in patients with coronary artery disease had no significant effect on sinus rate, intraventricular conduction, or QRS duration. The AV conduction time was modestly prolonged in two of seven patients. In another study, intravenous labetalol HCl slightly prolonged AV nodal conduction time and atrial effective refractory period with only small changes in heart rate. The effects on AV nodal refractoriness were inconsistent.

Labetalol HCl produces dose-related falls in blood pressure without reflex tachycardia and without significant reduction in heart rate, presumably through a mixture of its alpha-blocking and beta-blocking effects. Hemodynamic effects are variable with small nonsignificant changes in cardiac output seen in some studies but not others, and small decreases in total peripheral resistance. Elevated plasma renins are reduced.

Doses of labetalol HCl that controlled hypertension did not affect renal function in mild to severe hypertensive patients with normal renal function.

Due to the alpha$_1$-receptor blocking activity of labetalol HCl, blood pressure is lowered more in the standing than in the supine position, and symptoms of postural hypotension can occur. During dosing with intravenous labetalol HCl, the contribution of the postural component should be considered when positioning patients for treatment, and patients should not be allowed to move to an erect position unmonitored until their ability to do so is established.

In a clinical pharmacologic study in severe hypertensives, an initial 0.25 mg/kg injection of labetalol HCl, administered to patients in the supine position, decreased blood pressure by an average of 11/7 mmHg. Additional injections of 0.5 mg/kg at 15-minute intervals up to a total cumulative dose of 1.75 mg/kg of labetalol HCl caused further dose-related decreases in blood pressure. Some patients required cumulative doses of up to 3.25 mg/kg. The maximal effect of each dose level occurred within 5 minutes. Following discontinuation of intravenous treatment with labetalol HCl, the blood pressure rose gradually and progressively, approaching pretreatment baseline values within an average of 16 to 18 hours in the majority of patients.

Similar results were obtained in the treatment of patients with severe hypertension requiring urgent blood pressure reduction with an initial dose of 20 mg (which corresponds to 0.25 mg/kg for an 80-kg patient) followed by additional doses of either 40 or 80 mg at 10-minute intervals to achieve the desired effect or up to a cumulative dose of 300 mg.

Labetalol HCl administered as a continuous intravenous infusion, with a mean dose of 136 mg (27 to 300 mg) over a period of 2 to 3 hours (mean of 2 hours and 39 minutes) lowered the blood pressure by an average of 60/35 mmHg.

Exacerbation of angina and, in some cases, myocardial infarction and ventricular dysrhythmias have been reported after abrupt discontinuation of therapy with beta-adrenergic blocking agents in patients with coronary artery disease. Abrupt withdrawal of these agents in patients without coronary artery disease has resulted in transient symptoms, including tremulousness, sweating, palpitation, headache, and malaise. Several mechanisms have been proposed to explain these phenomena, among them increased sensitivity to catecholamines because of increased numbers of beta-receptors.

Although beta-adrenergic receptor blockade is useful in the treatment of angina and hypertension, there are also situations in which sympathetic stimulation is vital. For example, in patients with severely damaged hearts, adequate ventricular function may depend on sympathetic drive. Beta-adrenergic blockade may worsen AV block by preventing the necessary facilitating effects of sympathetic activity on conduction. Beta$_2$-adrenergic blockade results in passive bronchial constriction by interfering with endogenous adrenergic bronchodilator activity in patients subject to bronchospasm and may also interfere with exogenous bronchodilators in such patients.

Pharmacokinetics and Metabolism Following intravenous infusion, the elimination half-life is about 5.5 hours and the total body clearance is approximately 33 mL/min/kg. The plasma half-life of labetalol following oral administration is about 6 to 8 hours. In patients with decreased hepatic or renal function, the elimination half-life of labetalol is not altered; however, the relative bioavailability in hepatically impaired patients is increased due to decreased "first-pass" metabolism.

The metabolism of labetalol is mainly through conjugation to glucuronide metabolites. These metabolites are present in plasma and are excreted in the urine and, via the bile, into the feces. Approximately 55% to 60% of a dose appears in the urine as conjugates or unchanged labetalol within the first 24 hours of dosing.

Labetalol has been shown to cross the placental barrier in humans. Only negligible amounts of the drug crossed the blood-brain barrier in animal studies. Labetalol is approximately 50% protein bound. Neither hemodialysis nor peritoneal dialysis removes a significant amount of labetalol HCl from the general circulation (<1%).

INDICATIONS AND USAGE

NORMODYNE (labetalol HCl) Injection is indicated for control of blood pressure in severe hypertension.

CONTRAINDICATIONS

NORMODYNE (labetalol HCl) Injection is contraindicated in bronchial asthma, overt cardiac failure, greater than first degree heart block, cardiogenic shock, severe bradycardia, other conditions associated with severe and prolonged hypotension, and in patients with a history of hypersensitivity to any component of the product (see **WARNINGS**). Beta-blockers, even those with apparent cardioselectivity, should not be used in patients with a history of obstructive airway disease, including asthma.

WARNINGS

Hepatic Injury Severe hepatocellular injury, confirmed by rechallenge in at least one case, occurs rarely with labetalol therapy. The hepatic injury is usually reversible, but hepatic necrosis and death have been reported. Injury has occurred after both short- and long-term treatment and may be slowly progressive despite minimal symptomatology. Similar hepatic events have been reported with a related compound, dilevalol HCl, including two deaths. Dilevalol HCl is one of the four isomers of labetalol HCl. Thus, for patients taking labetalol, periodic determination of suitable hepatic laboratory tests would be appropriate. Laboratory testing should also be done at the very first symptom or sign of liver dysfunction (eg, pruritus, dark urine, persistent anorexia, jaundice, right upper quadrant tenderness, or unexplained "flu-like" symptoms). If the patient has jaundice or laboratory evidence of liver injury, labetalol HCl should be stopped and not restarted.

Cardiac Failure Sympathetic stimulation is a vital component supporting circulatory function in congestive heart failure. Beta-blockade carries a potential hazard of further depressing myocardial contractility and precipitating more severe failure. Although beta-blockers should be avoided in overt congestive heart failure, if necessary, labetalol HCl can be used with caution in patients with a history of heart failure who are well compensated. Congestive heart failure has been observed in patients receiving labetalol HCl. Labetalol HCl does not abolish the inotropic action of digitalis on heart muscle.

In Patients Without a History of Cardiac Failure In patients with latent cardiac insufficiency, continued depression of the myocardium with beta-blocking agents over a period of time can lead, in some cases, to cardiac failure. At the first sign or symptom of impending cardiac failure, patients should be fully digitalized and/or be given a diuretic, and the response observed closely. If cardiac failure continues, despite adequate digitalization and diuretic, NORMODYNE (labetalol HCl) therapy should be withdrawn (gradually if possible).

Ischemic Heart Disease Angina pectoris has not been reported upon labetalol HCl discontinuation. However, following abrupt cessation of therapy with some beta-blocking agents in patients with coronary artery disease, exacerbations of angina pectoris and, in some cases, myocardial infarction have been reported. Therefore, such patients should be cautioned against interruption of therapy without the physician's advice. Even in the absence of overt angina pectoris, when discontinuation of NORMODYNE (labetalol HCl) is planned, the patient should be carefully observed and should be advised to limit physical activity. If angina markedly worsens or acute coronary insufficiency develops, NORMODYNE (labetalol HCl) administration should be reinstituted promptly, at least temporarily, and other measures appropriate for the management of unstable angina should be taken.

Nonallergic Bronchospasm (eg, chronic bronchitis and emphysema) Since NORMODYNE (labetalol HCl) Injection at the usual intravenous therapeutic doses has not been studied in patients with nonallergic bronchospastic disease, it should not be used in such patients.

Pheochromocytoma Intravenous labetalol HCl has been shown to be effective in lowering the blood pressure and relieving symptoms in patients with pheochromocytoma; higher than usual doses may be required. However, paradoxical hypertensive responses have been reported in a few patients with this tumor; therefore, use caution when administering labetalol HCl to patients with pheochromocytoma.

Diabetes Mellitus and Hypoglycemia Beta-adrenergic blockade may prevent the appearance of premonitory signs and symptoms (eg, tachycardia) of acute hypoglycemia. This is especially important with labile diabetics. Beta-blockade also reduces the release of insulin in response to hyperglycemia; it may therefore be necessary to adjust the dose of antidiabetic drugs.

Major Surgery The necessity or desirability of withdrawing beta-blocking therapy prior to major surgery is controversial. Protracted severe hypotension and difficulty in restarting or maintaining a heartbeat have been reported with beta-blockers. The effect of labetalol HCl's alpha-adrenergic activity has not been evaluated in this setting.

Several deaths have occurred when NORMODYNE (labetalol HCl) Injection was used during surgery (including when used in cases to control bleeding).

A synergism between labetalol HCl and halothane anesthesia has been shown (see **PRECAUTIONS—Drug Interactions**).

Rapid Decreases of Blood Pressure Caution must be observed when reducing severely elevated blood pressure. Although such findings have not been reported with intravenous labetalol HCl, a number of adverse reactions, including cerebral infarction, optic nerve infarction, angina, and ischemic changes in the electrocardiogram, have been reported with other agents when severely elevated blood pressure was reduced over time courses of several hours to as long as 1 or 2 days. The desired blood pressure lowering should therefore be achieved over as long a period of time as is compatible with the patient's status.

PRECAUTIONS

General: *Impaired Hepatic Function* may diminish metabolism of NORMODYNE (labetalol HCl) Injection.

Following Coronary Artery Bypass Surgery In one uncontrolled study, patients with low cardiac indices and elevated systemic vascular resistance following intravenous labetalol HCl experienced significant declines in cardiac output with little change in systemic vascular resistance. One of these patients developed hypotension following labetalol HCl treatment. Therefore, use of labetalol HCl should be avoided in such patients.

High-Dose Labetalol HCl Administration of up to 3 g/d as an infusion for up to 2 to 3 days has been anecdotally reported; several patients experienced hypotension or bradycardia (see **DOSAGE AND ADMINISTRATION**).

Hypotension Symptomatic postural hypotension (incidence 58%) is likely to occur if patients are tilted or allowed to assume the upright position within 3 hours of receiving NORMODYNE (labetalol HCl) Injection. Therefore, the patient's ability to tolerate an upright position should be established before permitting any ambulation.

Jaundice or Hepatic Dysfunction (see **WARNINGS**)

Information for Patients: The following information is intended to aid in the safe and effective use of this medication. It is not a disclosure of all possible adverse or intended effects. During and immediately following (for up to 3 hours) NORMODYNE (labetalol HCl) Injection, the patient should remain supine. Subsequently, the patient should be advised on how to proceed gradually to become ambulatory, and should be observed at the time of first ambulation.

When the patient is started on NORMODYNE (labetalol HCl) Tablets, following adequate control of blood pressure with NORMODYNE (labetalol HCl) Injection, appropriate directions for titration of dosage should be provided (see **DOSAGE AND ADMINISTRATION**).

As with all drugs with beta-blocking activity, certain advice to patients being treated with labetalol HCl is warranted: While no incident of the abrupt withdrawal phenomenon (exacerbation of angina pectoris) has been reported with labetalol HCl, dosing with NORMODYNE (labetalol HCl) Tablets should not be interrupted or discontinued without a physician's advice. Patients being treated with NORMODYNE (labetalol HCl) Tablets should consult a physician at any signs or symptoms of impending cardiac failure or hepatic dysfunction (see **WARNINGS**). Also, transient scalp tingling may occur, usually when treatment with NORMODYNE (labetalol HCl) Tablets is initiated (see **ADVERSE REACTIONS**).

Laboratory Tests: Routine laboratory tests are ordinarily not required before or after intravenous labetalol HCl. In patients with concomitant illnesses, such as impaired renal function, appropriate tests should be done to monitor these conditions.

Drug Interactions: Since NORMODYNE (labetalol HCl) Injection may be administered to patients already being treated with other medications, including other antihypertensive agents, careful monitoring of these patients is necessary to detect and treat promptly any undesired effect from concomitant administration.

In one survey, 2.3% of patients taking labetalol HCl orally in combination with tricyclic antidepressants experienced tremor as compared to 0.7% reported to occur with labetalol HCl alone. The contribution of each of the treatments to this adverse reaction is unknown but the possibility of a drug interaction cannot be excluded.

Drugs possessing beta-blocking properties can blunt the bronchodilator effect of beta-receptor agonist drugs in patients with bronchospasm; therefore, doses greater than the normal antiasthmatic dose of beta-agonist bronchodilator drugs may be required.

Cimetidine has been shown to increase the bioavailability of labetalol HCl administered orally. Since this could be explained either by enhanced absorption or by an alteration of hepatic metabolism of labetalol HCl, special care should be used in establishing the dose required for blood pressure control in such patients.

Synergism has been shown between halothane anesthesia and intravenously administered labetalol HCl. During controlled hypotensive anesthesia using labetalol HCl in association with halothane, high concentrations (3% or above) of halothane should not be used because the degree of hypotension will be increased and because of the possibility of a large reduction in cardiac output and an increase in central venous pressure. The anesthesiologist should be informed when a patient is receiving labetalol HCl.

Labetalol HCl blunts the reflex tachycardia produced by nitroglycerin without preventing its hypotensive effect. If labetalol HCl is used with nitroglycerin in patients with angina pectoris, additional antihypertensive effects may occur.

Care should be taken if labetalol HCl is used concomitantly with calcium antagonists of the verapamil type.

When drug products that are alkaline, such as furosemide, have been administered in combination with labetalol, a white precipitate has been noted. Therefore, these drugs should not be administered in the same infusion line.

Risk of Anaphylactic Reaction While taking beta-blockers, patients with a history of severe anaphylactic reactions to a variety of allergens may be more reactive to repeated challenge, either accidental, diagnostic, or therapeutic. Such patients may be unresponsive to the usual doses of epinephrine used to treat allergic reaction.

Drug/Laboratory Test Interactions: The presence of labetalol metabolites in the urine may result in falsely elevated levels of urinary catecholamines, metanephrine, normetanephrine, and vanillylmandelic acid (VMA) when measured by fluorimetric or photometric methods. In screening patients suspected of having a pheochromocytoma and being treated with labetalol HCl, a specific method, such as a high-performance liquid chromatographic assay with solid phase extraction (eg, *J Chromatogr.* 1987;385:241) should be employed in determining levels of catecholamines.

Labetalol HCl has also been reported to produce a false-positive test for amphetamine when screening urine for the presence of drugs using the commercially available assay methods Toxi-Lab A® (thin-layer chromatographic assay) and Emit-d.a.u.® (radioenzymatic assay). When patients being treated with labetalol HCl have a positive urine test for amphetamine using these techniques, confirmation should be made by using more specific methods, such as a gas chromatographic-mass spectrometer technique.

Carcinogenesis, Mutagenesis, Impairment of Fertility: Long-term oral dosing studies with labetalol HCl for 18 months in mice and for 2 years in rats showed no evidence of carcinogenesis. Studies with labetalol HCl, using dominant lethal assays in rats and mice, and exposing microorganisms according to modified Ames tests, showed no evidence of mutagenesis.

Pregnancy Category C: Teratogenic studies have been performed with labetalol HCl in rats and rabbits at oral doses up to approximately 6 and 4 times the maximum recommended human dose (MRHD), respectively. No reproducible evidence of fetal malformations was observed. Increased fetal resorptions were seen in both species at doses approximating the MRHD. A teratology study performed with labetalol HCl in rabbits at intravenous doses up to 1.7 times the MRHD revealed no evidence of drug-related harm to the fetus. There are no adequate and well-controlled studies in pregnant women. Labetalol HCl should be used during pregnancy only if the potential benefit justifies the potential risk to the fetus.

Nonteratogenic Effects: Hypotension, bradycardia, hypoglycemia, and respiratory depression have been reported in infants of mothers who were treated with labetalol HCl for hypertension during pregnancy. Oral administration of labetalol to rats during late gestation through weaning at doses of 2 to 4 times the MRHD caused a decrease in neonatal survival.

Labor and Delivery: Labetalol HCl given to pregnant women with hypertension did not appear to affect the usual course of labor and delivery.

Nursing Mothers: Small amounts of labetalol (approximately 0.004% of the maternal dose) are excreted in human milk. Caution should be exercised when NORMODYNE (labetalol HCl) Injection is administered to a nursing woman.

Pediatric Use: Safety and effectiveness in children have not been established.

ADVERSE REACTIONS

NORMODYNE (labetalol HCl) Injection is usually well tolerated. Most adverse effects have been mild and transient and in controlled trials involving 92 patients did not require labetalol HCl withdrawal. Symptomatic postural hypotension (incidence 58%) is likely to occur if patients are tilted or allowed to assume the upright position within 3 hours of receiving NORMODYNE (labetalol HCl) Injection. Moderate hypotension occurred in 1 of 100 patients while supine. Increased sweating was noted in 4 of 100 patients, and flushing occurred in 1 of 100 patients.

The following also were reported with NORMODYNE (labetalol HCl) Injection with the incidence per 100 patients as noted:

Cardiovascular System Ventricular arrhythmia in 1.

Central and Peripheral Nervous Systems Dizziness in 9; tingling of the scalp/skin 7; hypoesthesia (numbness) and vertigo, 1 each.

Gastrointestinal System Nausea in 13; vomiting 4; dyspepsia and taste distortion, 1 each.

Metabolic Disorders Transient increases in blood urea nitrogen and serum creatinine levels occurred in 8 of 100 patients; these were associated with drops in blood pressure, generally in patients with prior renal insufficiency.

Psychiatric Disorders Somnolence/yawning in 3.

Respiratory System Wheezing in 1.

Skin Pruritus in 1.

The incidence of adverse reactions depends upon the dose of labetalol HCl. The largest experience is with oral labetalol HCl (see NORMODYNE (labetalol HCl) Tablet Product Information for details). Certain of the side effects increased with increasing oral dose as shown in the table below which depicts the entire US therapeutic trials data base for adverse reactions that are clearly or possibly dose related.

[See table above]

In addition, a number of other less common adverse events have been reported:

Cardiovascular Hypotension, and rarely, syncope, bradycardia, heart block.

Liver and Biliary System Hepatic necrosis, hepatitis, cholestatic jaundice, elevated liver function tests.

Hypersensitivity Rare reports of hypersensitivity (eg, rash, urticaria, pruritus, angioedema, dyspnea) and anaphylactoid reactions.

Labetalol HCl Daily Dose (mg)	**200**	**300**	**400**	**600**	**800**	**900**	**1200**	**1600**	**2400**
Number of Patients	522	181	606	608	503	117	411	242	175
Dizziness (%)	2	3	3	3	5	1	9	13	16
Fatigue	2	1	4	4	5	3	7	6	10
Nausea	<1	0	1	2	4	0	7	11	19
Vomiting	0	0	<1	<1	<1	0	1	2	3
Dyspepsia	1	0	2	1	1	0	2	2	4
Paresthesias	2	0	2	2	1	1	2	5	5
Nasal Stuffiness	1	1	2	2	2	2	4	5	6
Ejaculation Failure	0	2	1	2	3	0	4	3	5
Impotence	1	1	1	1	2	4	3	4	3
Edema	1	0	1	1	1	0	1	2	2

The oculomucocutaneous syndrome associated with the beta-blocker practolol has not been reported with labetalol HCl during investigational use and extensive foreign marketing experience.

Clinical Laboratory Tests: Among patients dosed with NORMODYNE (labetalol HCl) Tablets, there have been reversible increases of serum transaminases in 4% of patients tested, and more rarely, reversible increases in blood urea.

OVERDOSAGE

Overdosage with NORMODYNE (labetalol HCl) Injection causes excessive hypotension that is posture sensitive, and sometimes, excessive bradycardia. Patients should be placed supine and their legs raised if necessary to improve the blood supply to the brain. If overdosage with labetalol HCl follows oral ingestion, gastric lavage or pharmaco logically induced emesis (using syrup of ipecac) may be useful for removal of the drug shortly after ingestion. The following additional measures should be employed if necessary: *Excessive bradycardia*—administer atropine or epinephrine. *Cardiac failure*—administer a digitalis glycoside and a diuretic. Dopamine or dobutamine may also be useful. *Hypotension*—administer vasopressors, eg, norepinephrine. There is pharmacological evidence that norepinephrine may be the drug of choice. *Bronchospasm*—administer epinephrine and/or an aerosolized beta$_2$-agonist. *Seizures*—administer diazepam.

In severe beta-blocker overdose resulting in hypotension and/or brady cardia, glucagon has been shown to be effective when administered in large doses (5–10 mg rapidly over 30 seconds, followed by continuous infusion of 5 mg/hr that can be reduced as the patient improves).

Neither hemodialysis nor peritoneal dialysis removes a significant amount of labetalol HCl from the general circulation (<1%).

The oral LD_{50} value of labetalol HCl in the mouse is approximately 600 mg/kg and in the rat is greater than 2 g/kg. The intravenous LD_{50} in these species is 50 to 60 mg/kg.

DOSAGE AND ADMINISTRATION

NORMODYNE (labetalol HCl) Injection is intended for intravenous use in hospitalized patients. DOSAGE MUST BE INDIVIDUALIZED depending upon the severity of hypertension and the response of the patient during dosing.

Patients should always be kept in a supine position during the period of intravenous drug administration. A substantial fall in blood pressure on standing should be expected in these patients. The patient's ability to tolerate an upright position should be established before permitting any ambulation, such as using toilet facilities.

Either of two methods of administration of NORMODYNE (labetalol HCl) Injection may be used: a) repeated intravenous injections, b) slow continuous infusion.

Repeated Intravenous Injection: Initially, NORMODYNE (labetalol HCl) Injection should be given in a dose of 20 mg labetalol HCl (which corresponds to 0.25 mg/kg for an 80 kg patient) by slow intravenous injection over a 2-minute period.

Immediately before the injection and at 5 and 10 minutes after injection, supine blood pressure should be measured to evaluate response. Additional injections of 40 mg or 80 mg can be given at 10-minute intervals until a desired supine blood pressure is achieved or a total of 300 mg labetalol HCl has been injected. The maximum effect usually occurs within 5 minutes of each injection.

Slow Continuous Infusion: NORMODYNE (labetalol HCl) Injection is prepared for intravenous continuous infusion by diluting the contents with commonly used intravenous fluids (see below). Examples of methods of preparing the infusion solution are:

The contents of either two 20-mL vials (40 mL), or one 40-mL vial, are added to 160 mL of a commonly used intravenous fluid such that the resultant 200 mL of solution contains 200 mg of labetalol HCl, 1 mg/mL. The diluted solution should be administered at a rate of 2 mL/min to deliver 2 mg/min.

Alternatively, the contents of either two 20-mL vials (40 mL), or one 40-mL vial, of NORMODYNE (labetalol HCl) Injection are added to 250 mL of a commonly used intravenous fluid. The resultant solution will contain 200 mg of labetalol HCl, approximately 2 mg/3 mL. The diluted solution should be administered at a rate of 3 mL/min to deliver approximately 2 mg/min.

The rate of infusion of the diluted solution may be adjusted according to the blood pressure response, at the discretion of the physician. To facilitate a desired rate of infusion, the diluted solution can be infused using a controlled administration mechanism, eg, graduated burette or mechanically driven infusion pump.

Since the half-life of labetalol is 5 to 8 hours, steady-state blood levels (in the face of a constant rate of infusion) would not be reached during the usual infusion time period. The infusion should be continued until a satisfactory response is obtained and should then be stopped and oral labetalol HCl started (see below). The effective intravenous dose is usually in the range of 50 to 200 mg. A total dose of up to 300 mg may be required in some patients.

Blood Pressure Monitoring: The blood pressure should be monitored during and after completion of the infusion or intravenous injections. Rapid or excessive falls in either systolic or diastolic blood pressure during intravenous treatment should be avoided. In patients with excessive systolic hypertension, the decrease in systolic pressure should be used as indicator of effectiveness in addition to the response of the diastolic pressure.

Initiation of Dosing with NORMODYNE (labetalol HCl) Tablets: Subsequent oral dosing with NORMODYNE (labetalol HCl) Tablets should begin when it has been established that the supine diastolic blood pressure has begun to rise. The recommended initial dose is 200 mg, followed in 6 to 12 hours by an additional dose of 200 or 400 mg, depending on the blood pressure response. Thereafter, *inpatient titration with NORMODYNE (labetalol HCl) Tablets* may proceed as follows:

Inpatient Titration Instructions

Regimen	Daily Dose*
200 mg bid	400 mg
400 mg bid	800 mg
800 mg bid	1600 mg
1200 mg bid	2400 mg

*If needed, the total daily dose may be given in three divided doses.

While in the hospital, the dosage of NORMODYNE (labetalol HCl) Tablets may be increased at 1-day intervals to achieve the desired blood pressure reduction.

For subsequent outpatient titration or maintenance dosing see NORMODYNE (labetalol HCl) Tablets Product Information **DOSAGE AND ADMINISTRATION** for additional recommendations.

Compatibility with commonly used intravenous fluids: Parenteral drug products should be inspected visually for particulate matter and discoloration prior to administration, whenever solution and container permit.

NORMODYNE (labetalol HCl) Injection was tested for compatibility with commonly used intravenous fluids at final concentrations of 1.25 mg to 3.75 mg labetalol HCl per mL of the mixture. NORMODYNE (labetalol HCl) Injection was found to be compatible with and stable (for 24 hours refrigerated or at room temperature) in mixtures with the following solutions:

Ringers Injection, USP
Lactated Ringers Injection, USP
5% Dextrose and Ringers Injection
5% Lactated Ringers and 5% Dextrose Injection
5% Dextrose Injection, USP
0.9% Sodium Chloride Injection, USP
5% Dextrose and 0.2% Sodium Chloride Injection, USP
2.5% Dextrose and 0.45% Sodium Chloride Injection, USP
5% Dextrose and 0.9% Sodium Chloride Injection, USP
5% Dextrose and 0.33% Sodium Chloride Injection, USP

NORMODYNE (labetalol HCl) Injection was NOT compatible with 5% Sodium Bicarbonate Injection, USP.

HOW SUPPLIED

NORMODYNE (labetalol HCl) Injection, 5 mg/mL, is supplied in:

20 mL (100 mg) (NDC 0085-0362-07) multi-dose vial, box of 1 and

40 mL (200 mg) (NDC 0085-0362-06) multi-dose vial, box of 1

4 mL (20 mg) (NDC 0085-0362-08) single-dose, prefilled, disposable syringe, box of 1 and

8 mL (40 mg) (NDC 0085-0362-09) single-dose, prefilled, disposable syringe, box of 1.

Store between 2° and 30°C (36° and 86°F). Protect from freezing. Protect syringe from light.

Note: To ensure patient safety, the needle and the prefilled syringes should be handled with care and should be destroyed and discarded if damaged in any manner. If the cannula is bent, no attempt should be made to straighten it. To prevent needle-stick injuries, needles should not be recapped, purposely bent, or broken by hand.

Continued on next page

Information on Schering products appearing on these pages is effective as of January 2000.

Normodyne—Cont.

Only the prefilled syringes are manufactured for Schering Corporation by:
Meridian Medical
Technologies, Inc.,
Columbia, MD 21046
Key Pharmaceuticals, Inc.
Kenilworth, NJ 07033 USA
Rev. 9/99 19881512

Shown in Product Identification Guide, page 334

NORMODYNE® ℞

brand of
labetalol hydrochloride
Tablets, USP

DESCRIPTION

NORMODYNE (labetalol HCl) is an adrenergic receptor blocking agent that has both selective alpha$_1$- and nonselective beta-adrenergic receptor blocking actions in a single substance.

Labetalol HCl is a racemate, chemically designated as 5-[1-hydroxy-2-[(1-methyl-3-phenylpropyl) amino] ethyl]salicylamide monohydrochloride, and has the following structure:

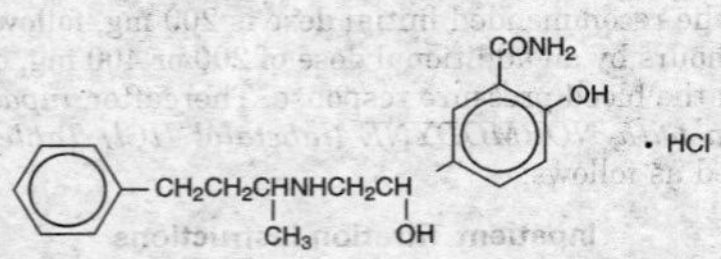

CONH$_2$
OH
CH$_2$CH$_2$CHNHCH$_2$CH • HCl
CH$_3$ OH

Labetalol HCl has the empirical formula $C_{19}H_{24}N_2O_3$•HCl and a molecular weight of 364.9. It has two asymmetric centers and therefore exists as a molecular complex of two diastereoisomeric pairs. Dilevalol, the R,R′ stereoisomer, makes up 25% of racemic labetalol.

Labetalol HCl is a white or off-white crystalline powder, soluble in water.

NORMODYNE Tablets contain 100 mg, 200 mg, or 300 mg labetalol HCl, USP and are taken orally.

The inactive ingredients for NORMODYNE Tablets, 100 mg, include: corn starch, FD&C Blue No. 2 Al Lake, FD&C Yellow No. 6 Al Lake, hydroxypropyl methylcellulose, lactose, magnesium stearate, methylparaben, PEG, and propylparaben. May also contain: potato starch and wheat starch.

The inactive ingredients for NORMODYNE Tablets, 200 mg, include: corn starch, hydroxypropyl methylcellulose, lactose, magnesium stearate, methylparaben, PEG, propylparaben, and titanium dioxide. May also contain: potato starch and wheat starch.

The inactive ingredients for NORMODYNE Tablets, 300 mg, include: corn starch, FD&C Blue No. 2 Al Lake, hydroxypropyl methylcellulose, lactose, magnesium stearate, methylparaben, PEG, and propylparaben. May also contain: potato starch and wheat starch.

CLINICAL PHARMACOLOGY

NORMODYNE (labetalol HCl) combines both selective, competitive alpha$_1$-adrenergic blocking and nonselective, competitive beta-adrenergic blocking activity in a single substance. In man, the ratios of alpha- to beta-blockade have been estimated to be approximately 1:3 and 1:7 following oral and intravenous administration, respectively. Beta$_2$-agonist activity has been demonstrated in animals with minimal beta$_1$-agonist (ISA) activity detected. In animals, at doses greater than those required for alpha- or beta-adrenergic blockade, a membrane-stabilizing effect has been demonstrated.

Pharmacodynamics The capacity of labetalol HCl to block alpha receptors in man has been demonstrated by attenuation of the pressor effect of phenylephrine and by a significant reduction of the pressor response caused by immersing the hand in ice-cold water ("cold-pressor test"). Labetalol HCl's beta$_1$-receptor blockade in man was demonstrated by a small decrease in the resting heart rate, attenuation of tachycardia produced by isoproterenol or exercise, and by attenuation of the reflex tachycardia to the hypotension produced by amyl nitrite. Beta$_2$-receptor blockade was demonstrated by inhibition of the isoproterenol-induced fall in diastolic blood pressure. Both the alpha- and beta-blocking actions of orally administered labetalol HCl contribute to a decrease in blood pressure in hypertensive patients. Labetalol HCl consistently, in dose-related fashion, blunted increases in exercise-induced blood pressure and heart rate, and in their double product. The pulmonary circulation during exercise was not affected by labetalol HCl dosing.

Single oral doses of labetalol HCl administered in patients with coronary artery disease has no significant effect on sinus rate, intraventricular conduction, or QRS duration. The AV conduction time was modestly prolonged in 2 of 7 patients. In another study, intravenous labetalol HCl slightly prolonged AV nodal conduction time and atrial effective refractory period with only small changes in heart rate. The effects on AV nodal refractoriness were inconsistent.

Labetalol HCl produces dose-related falls in blood pressure without reflex tachycardia and without significant reduction in heart rate, presumably through a mixture of its alpha-blocking and beta-blocking effects. Hemodynamic effects are variable with small nonsignificant changes in cardiac output seen in some studies but not others, and small decreases in total peripheral resistance. Elevated plasma renins are reduced.

Doses of labetalol HCl that controlled hypertension did not affect renal function in mild to severe hypertensive patients with normal renal function.

Due to the alpha$_1$-receptor blocking activity of labetalol HCl, blood pressure is lowered more in the standing than in the supine position, and symptoms of postural hypotension (2%), including rare instances of syncope, can occur. Following oral administration, when postural hypotension has occurred, it has been transient and is uncommon when the recommended starting dose and titration increments are closely followed (see **DOSAGE AND ADMINISTRATION**). Symptomatic postural hypotension is most likely to occur 2 to 4 hours after a dose, especially following the use of large initial doses or upon large changes in dose.

The peak effects of single oral doses of labetalol HCl occur within 2 to 4 hours. The duration of effect depends upon dose, lasting at least 8 hours following single oral doses of 100 mg and more than 12 hours following single oral doses of 300 mg. The maximum, steady-state blood pressure response upon oral, twice-a-day dosing occurs within 24 to 72 hours.

The antihypertensive effect of labetalol has a linear correlation with the logarithm of labetalol plasma concentration, and there is also a linear correlation between the reduction in exercise-induced tachycardia occurring at 2 hours after oral administration of labetalol HCl and the logarithm of the plasma concentration.

About 70% of the maximum beta-blocking effect is present for 5 hours after the administration of a single oral dose of 400 mg, with suggestion that about 40% remains at 8 hours.

The anti-anginal efficacy of labetalol HCl has not been studied. In 37 patients with hypertension and coronary artery disease, labetalol HCl did not increase the incidence or severity of angina attacks.

Exacerbation of angina and, in some cases, myocardial infarction and ventricular dysrhythmias have been reported after abrupt discontinuation of therapy with beta-adrenergic blocking agents in patients with coronary artery disease. Abrupt withdrawal of these agents in patients without coronary artery disease has resulted in transient symptoms, including tremulousness, sweating, palpitation, headache, and malaise. Several mechanisms have been proposed to explain these phenomena, among them increased sensitivity to catecholamines because of increased numbers of beta receptors.

Although beta-adrenergic receptor blockade is useful in the treatment of angina and hypertension, there are also situations in which sympathetic stimulation is vital. For example, in patients with severely damaged hearts, adequate ventricular function may depend on sympathetic drive. Beta-adrenergic blockade may worsen AV block by preventing the necessary facilitating effects of sympathetic activity on conduction. Beta$_2$-adrenergic blockade results in passive bronchial constriction by interfering with endogenous adrenergic bronchodilator activity in patients subject to bronchospasm and may also interfere with exogenous bronchodilators in such patients.

Pharmacokinetics and Metabolism Labetalol HCl is completely absorbed from the gastrointestinal tract with peak plasma levels occurring 1 to 2 hours after oral administration. The relative bioavailability of labetalol HCl tablets compared to an oral solution is 100%. The absolute bioavailability (fraction of drug reaching systemic circulation) of labetalol when compared to an intravenous infusion is 25%; this is due to extensive "first-pass" metabolism. Despite "first-pass" metabolism there is a linear relationship between oral doses of 100 to 3000 mg and peak plasma levels. The absolute bioavailability of labetalol is increased when administered with food.

The plasma half-life of labetalol following oral administration is about 6 to 8 hours. Steady-state plasma levels of labetalol during repetitive dosing are reached by about the third day of dosing. In patients with decreased hepatic or renal function, the elimination half-life of labetalol is not altered; however, the relative bioavailability in hepatically impaired patients is increased due to decreased "first-pass" metabolism.

The metabolism of labetalol is mainly through conjugation to glucuronide metabolites. These metabolites are present in plasma and are excreted in the urine and, via the bile, into the feces. Approximately 55% to 60% of a dose appears in the urine as conjugates or unchanged labetalol within the first 24 hours of dosing.

Labetalol has been shown to cross the placental barrier in humans. Only negligible amounts of the drug crossed the blood-brain barrier in animal studies. Labetalol is approximately 50% protein bound. Neither hemodialysis nor peritoneal dialysis removes a significant amount of labetalol HCl from the general circulation (<1%).

INDICATIONS AND USAGE

NORMODYNE (labetalol HCl) Tablets are indicated in the management of hypertension. NORMODYNE Tablets may be used alone or in combination with other antihypertensive agents, especially thiazide and loop diuretics.

CONTRAINDICATIONS

NORMODYNE (labetalol HCl) Tablets are contraindicated in bronchial asthma, overt cardiac failure, greater than first degree heart block, cardiogenic shock, severe bradycardia, other conditions associated with severe and prolonged hypotension, and in patients with a history of hypersensitivity to any component of the product (see **WARNINGS**). Beta-blockers, even those with apparent cardioselectivity, should not be used in patients with a history of obstructive airway disease, including asthma.

WARNINGS

Hepatic Injury Severe hepatocellular injury, confirmed by rechallenge in at least one case, occurs rarely with labetalol therapy. The hepatic injury is usually reversible, but hepatic necrosis and death have been reported. Injury has occurred after both short- and long-term treatment and may be slowly progressive despite minimal symptomatology. Similar hepatic events have been reported with a related compound, dilevalol HCl, including two deaths. Dilevalol HCl is one of the four isomers of labetalol HCl. Thus, for patients taking labetalol, periodic determination of suitable hepatic laboratory tests would be appropriate. Laboratory testing should also be done at the very first symptom or sign of liver dysfunction (eg, pruritus, dark urine, persistent anorexia, jaundice, right upper quadrant tenderness, or unexplained "flu-like" symptoms). If the patient has jaundice or laboratory evidence of liver injury, labetalol HCl should be stopped and not restarted.

Cardiac Failure Sympathetic stimulation is a vital component supporting circulatory function in congestive heart failure. Beta blockade carries a potential hazard of further depressing myocardial contractility and precipitating more severe failure. Although beta-blockers should be avoided in overt congestive heart failure, if necessary, labetalol HCl can be used with caution in patients with a history of heart failure who are well-compensated. Congestive heart failure has been observed in patients receiving labetalol HCl. Labetalol HCl does not abolish the inotropic action of digitalis on heart muscle.

In Patients Without a History of Cardiac Failure In patients with latent cardiac insufficiency, continued depression of the myocardium with beta-blocking agents over a period of time can, in some cases, lead to cardiac failure. At the first sign or symptom of impending cardiac failure, patients should be fully digitalized and/or be given a diuretic, and the response observed closely. If cardiac failure continues, despite adequate digitalization and diuretic, NORMODYNE (labetalol HCl) therapy should be withdrawn (gradually if possible).

Exacerbation of Ischemic Heart Disease Following Abrupt Withdrawal Angina pectoris has not been reported upon labetalol HCl discontinuation. However, hypersensitivity to catecholamines has been observed in patients withdrawn from beta-blocker therapy; exacerbation of angina and, in some cases, myocardial infarction have occurred after *abrupt* discontinuation of such therapy. When discontinuing chronically administered NORMODYNE (labetalol HCl), particularly in patients with ischemic heart disease, the dosage should be gradually reduced over a period of 1 to 2 weeks and the patient should be carefully monitored. If angina markedly worsens or acute coronary insufficiency develops, NORMODYNE (labetalol HCl) administration should be reinstituted promptly, at least temporarily, and other measures appropriate for the management of unstable angina should be taken. Patients should be warned against interruption or discontinuation of therapy without the physician's advice. Because coronary artery disease is common and may be unrecognized, it may be prudent not to discontinue NORMODYNE (labetalol HCl) therapy abruptly even in patients treated only for hypertension.

Nonallergic bronchospasm (eg, chronic bronchitis and emphysema) patients with bronchospastic disease should, in general, not receive beta-blockers. NORMODYNE (labetalol HCl) may be used with caution, however, in patients who do not respond to, or cannot tolerate, other antihypertensive agents. It is prudent, if NORMODYNE (labetalol HCl) is used, to use the smallest effective dose, so that inhibition of endogenous or exogenous beta-agonists is minimized.

Pheochromocytoma Labetalol HCl has been shown to be effective in lowering the blood pressure and relieving symptoms in patients with pheochromocytoma. However, paradoxical hypertensive responses have been reported in a few patients with this tumor; therefore, use caution when administering labetalol HCl to patients with pheochromocytoma.

Diabetes Mellitus and Hypoglycemia Beta-adrenergic blockade may prevent the appearance of premonitory signs and symptoms (eg, tachycardia) of acute hypoglycemia. This is especially important with labile diabetics. Beta-blockade also reduces the release of insulin in response to hyperglycemia; it may therefore be necessary to adjust the dose of antidiabetic drugs.

Major Surgery The necessity or desirability of withdrawing beta-blocking therapy prior to major surgery is controversial. Protracted severe hypotension and difficulty in restarting or maintaining a heartbeat have been reported with beta-blockers. The effect of labetalol HCl's alpha-adrenergic activity has not been evaluated in this setting.

A synergism between labetalol HCl and halothane anesthesia has been shown (see **PRECAUTIONS—Drug Interactions**).

PRECAUTIONS

General

Impaired Hepatic Function NORMODYNE (labetalol HCl) Tablets should be used with caution in patients with impaired hepatic function since metabolism of the drug may be diminished.

Jaundice or Hepatic Dysfunction (see **WARNINGS**).

Information for Patients

As with all drugs with beta-blocking activity, certain advice to patients being treated with labetalol HCl is warranted. This information is intended to aid in the safe and effective use of this medication. It is not a disclosure of all possible adverse or intended effects. While no incident of the abrupt withdrawal phenomenon (exacerbation of angina pectoris) has been reported with labetalol HCl, dosing with NORMODYNE (labetalol HCl) Tablets should not be interrupted or discontinued without a physician's advice. Patients being treated with NORMODYNE (labetalol HCl) Tablets should consult a physician at any signs or symptoms of impending cardiac failure or hepatic dysfunction (see **WARNINGS**). Also, transient scalp tingling may occur, usually when treatment with NORMODYNE (labetalol HCl) Tablets is initiated (see **ADVERSE REACTIONS**).

Laboratory Tests

As with any new drug given over prolonged periods, laboratory parameters should be observed over regular intervals. In patients with concomitant illnesses, such as impaired renal function, appropriate tests should be done to monitor these conditions.

Drug Interactions

In one survey, 2.3% of patients taking labetalol HCl in combination with tricyclic antidepressants experienced tremor as compared to 0.7% reported to occur with labetalol HCl alone. The contribution of each of the treatments to this adverse reactions is unknown but the possibility of a drug interaction cannot be excluded.

Drugs possessing beta-blocking properties can blunt the bronchodilator effect of beta-receptor agonist drugs in patients with bronchospasm; therefore, doses greater than the normal anti-asthmatic dose of beta-agonist bronchodilator drugs may be required.

Cimetidine has been shown to increase the bioavailability of labetalol HCl. Since this could be explained either by enhanced absorption or by an alteration of hepatic metabolism of labetalol HCl, special care should be used in establishing the dose required for blood pressure control in such patients.

Synergism has been shown between halothane anesthesia and intravenously administered labetalol HCl. During controlled hypotensive anesthesia using labetalol HCl in association with halothane, high concentrations (3% or above) of halothane should not be used because the degree of hypotension will be increased and because of the possibility of a large reduction in cardiac output and an increase in central venous pressure. The anesthesiologist should be informed when a patient is receiving labetalol HCl.

Labetalol HCl blunts the reflex tachycardia produced by nitroglycerin without preventing its hypotensive effect. If labetalol HCl is used with nitroglycerin in patients with angina pectoris, additional antihypertensive effects may occur. Care should be taken if labetalol HCl is used concomitantly with calcium antagonists of the verapamil type.

Risk of Anaphylactic Reaction While taking beta-blockers, patients with a history of severe anaphylactic reaction to a variety of allergens may be more reactive to repeated challenge, either accidental, diagnostic, or therapeutic. Such patients may be unresponsive to the usual doses of epinephrine used to treat allergic reaction.

Drug/Laboratory Test Interactions

The presence of labetalol metabolites in the urine may result in falsely elevated levels of urinary catecholamines, metanephrine, normetanephrine, and vanillylmandelic acid (VMA) when measured by fluorimetric or photometric methods. In screening patients suspected of having a pheochromocytoma and being treated with labetalol HCl, a specific method, such as a high performance liquid chromatographic assay with solid phase extraction (eg, *J Chromatogr* 385: 241, 1987) should be employed in determining levels of catecholamines.

Labetalol HCl has also been reported to produce a false-positive test for amphetamine when screening urine for the presence of drugs using the commercially available assay methods Toxi-Lab A® (thin-layer chromatographic assay) and Emit-d.a.u.® (radioenzymatic assay). When patients being treated with labetalol HCl have a positive urine test for amphetamine using these techniques, confirmation should be made by using more specific methods, such as a gas chromatographic-mass spectrometer technique.

Carcinogenesis, Mutagenesis, Impairment of Fertility

Long-term oral dosing studies with labetalol HCl for 18 months in mice and for 2 years in rats showed no evidence of carcinogenesis. Studies with labetalol HCl, using dominant lethal assays in rats and mice, and exposing microorganisms according to modified Ames tests, showed no evidence of mutagenesis.

Pregnant Category C

Teratogenic studies have been performed with labetalol HCl in rats and rabbits at oral doses up to approximately 6 and 4 times the maximum recommended human dose (MRHD), respectively. No reproducible evidence of fetal malformations was observed. Increased fetal resorptions were seen in both species at doses approximating the MRHD. A teratology study performed with labetalol HCl in rabbits at intravenous doses up to 1.7 times the MRHD revealed no evidence of drug-related harm to the fetus. There are no adequate and well-controlled studies in pregnant women. Labetalol HCl should be used during pregnancy only if the potential benefit justifies the potential risk to the fetus.

	Labetalol HCl (N=227) %	Placebo (N=98) %	Propranolol (N=84) %	Metoprolol (N=49) %
Body as a whole				
fatigue	5	0	12	12
asthenia	1	1	1	0
headache	2	1	1	2
Gastrointestinal				
nausea	6	1	1	2
vomiting	<1	0	0	0
dyspepsia	3	1	1	0
abdominal pain	0	0	1	2
diarrhea	<1	0	2	0
taste distortion	1	0	0	0
Central and Peripheral Nervous Systems				
dizziness	11	3	4	4
paresthesias	<1	0	0	0
drowsiness	<1	2	2	2
Autonomic Nervous System				
nasal stuffiness	3	0	0	0
ejaculation failure	2	0	0	0
impotence	1	0	1	3
increased sweating	<1	0	0	0
Cardiovascular				
edema	1	0	0	0
postural hypotension	1	0	0	0
bradycardia	0	0	5	12
Respiratory				
dyspnea	2	0	1	2
Skin				
rash	1	0	0	0
Special Senses				
vision abnormality	1	0	0	0
vertigo	2	1	0	0

Labetalol HCl Daily Dose (mg)	**200**	**300**	**400**	**600**	**800**	**900**	**1200**	**1600**	**2400**
Number of patients	522	181	606	608	503	117	411	242	175
Dizziness (%)	2	3	3	3	5	1	9	13	16
Fatigue	2	1	4	4	5	3	7	6	10
Nausea	<1	0	1	2	4	0	7	11	19
Vomiting	0	0	<1	<1	<1	0	1	2	3
Dyspepsia	1	0	2	1	1	0	2	2	4
Paresthesias	2	0	2	2	1	1	2	5	5
Nasal Stuffiness	1	1	2	2	2	2	4	5	6
Ejaculation Failure	0	2	1	2	3	0	4	3	5
Impotence	1	1	1	1	2	4	3	4	3
Edema	1	0	1	1	1	0	1	2	2

Nonteratogenic Effects

Hypotension, bradycardia, hypoglycemia, and respiratory depression have been reported in infants of mothers who were treated with labetalol HCl for hypertension during pregnancy. Oral administration of labetalol to rats during late gestation through weaning at doses of 2 to 4 times the MRHD caused a decrease in neonatal survival.

Labor and Delivery

Labetalol HCl given to pregnant women with hypertension did not appear to affect the usual course of labor and delivery.

Nursing Mothers

Small amounts of labetalol (approximately 0.004% of the maternal dose) are excreted in human milk. Caution should be exercised when NORMODYNE (labetalol HCl) Tablets are administered to a nursing woman.

Pediatric Use

Safety and effectiveness in children have not been established.

ADVERSE REACTIONS

Most adverse effects are mild, transient and occur early in the course of treatment. In controlled clinical trials of 3 to 4 months duration, discontinuation of NORMODYNE (labetalol HCl) Tablets due to one or more adverse effects was required in 7% of all patients. In these same trials, beta-blocker control agents led to discontinuation in 8% to 10% of patients, and a centrally acting alpha-agonist in 30% of patients.

The incidence rates of adverse reactions listed in the following table were derived from multicenter controlled clinical trials, comparing labetalol HCl, placebo, metoprolol, and propranolol, over treatment periods of 3 and 4 months. Where the frequency of adverse effects for labetalol HCl and placebo is similar, causal relationship is uncertain. The rates are based on adverse reactions considered probably drug related by the investigator. If all reports are considered, the rates are somewhat higher (eg, dizziness 20%, nausea 14%, fatigue 11%), but the overall conclusions are unchanged.

[See first table above]

The adverse effects were reported spontaneously and are representative of the incidence of adverse effects that may be observed in a properly selected hypertensive patient population, ie, a group excluding patients with bronchospastic disease, overt congestive heart failure, or other contraindications to beta-blocker therapy.

Clinical trials also included studies utilizing daily doses up to 2400 mg in more severely hypertensive patients. Certain of the side effects increased with increasing dose as shown in the table below which depicts the entire U.S. therapeutic trials data base for adverse reactions that are clearly or possibly drug related.

[See second table above]

In addition, a number of other less common adverse events have been reported:

Body as a Whole Fever.

Cardiovascular Hypotension, and rarely, syncope, bradycardia, heart block.

Central and Peripheral Nervous Systems Paresthesias, most frequently described as scalp tingling. In most cases, it was mild, transient and usually occurred at the beginning of treatment.

Collagen Disorders Systemic lupus erythematosus; positive antinuclear factor (ANF).

Eyes Dry eyes.

Immunological System Antimitochondrial antibodies.

Liver and Biliary System Hepatic necrosis; hepatitis; cholestatic jaundice; elevated liver function tests.

Musculoskeletal System Muscle cramps; toxic myopathy.

Respiratory System Bronchospasm.

Skin and Appendages Rashes of various types, such as generalized maculopapular; lichenoid; urticarial; bullous lichen planus; psoriaform; facial erythema; Peyronie's disease; reversible alopecia.

Urinary System Difficulty in micturition, including acute urinary bladder retention.

Hypersensitivity Rare reports of hypersensitivity (eg, rash, uritcaria, pruritus, angioedema, dyspnea) and anaphylactoid reactions.

Following approval for marketing in the United Kingdom, a monitored release survey involving approximately 6,800 patients was conducted for further safety and efficacy evaluation of this product. Results of this survey indicate that the type, severity, and incidence of adverse effects were comparable to those cited above.

Potential Adverse Effects

In addition, other adverse effects not listed above have been reported with other beta-adrenergic blocking agents.

Central Nervous System Reversible mental depression progressing to catatonia; an acute reversible syndrome characterized by disorientation for time and place, short-term memory loss, emotional lability, slightly clouded sensorium, and decreased performance on neuropsychometrics.

Cardiovascular Intensification of AV block (see **CONTRAINDICATIONS**).

Continued on next page

Information on Schering products appearing on these pages is effective as of January 2000.

Normodyne—Cont.

Allergic Fever combined with aching and sore throat; laryngospasm; respiratory distress.
Hematologic Agranulocytosis; thrombocytopenic or nonthrombocytopenic purpura.
Gastrointestinal Mesenteric artery thrombosis; ischemic colitis.
The oculomucocutaneous syndrome associated with the beta-blocker practolol has not been reported with labetalol HCl.

Clinical Laboratory Tests
There have been reversible increases of serum transaminases in 4% of patients treated with labetalol HCl and tested, and more rarely, reversible increases in blood urea.

OVERDOSAGE

Overdosage with NORMODYNE (labetalol HCl) Tablets causes excessive hypotension that is posture sensitive, and sometimes, excessive bradycardia. Patients should be placed supine and their legs raised if necessary to improve the blood supply to the brain. If overdosage with labetalol HCl follows oral ingestion, gastric lavage or pharmacologically induced emesis (using syrup of ipecac) may be useful for removal of the drug shortly after ingestion. The following additional measures should be employed if necessary: *Excessive bradycardia*—administer atropine or epinephrine. *Cardiac failure*—administer a digitalis glycoside and a diuretic. Dopamine or dobutamine may also be useful. *Hypotension*—administer vasopressors, eg, norepinephrine. There is pharmacological evidence that norepinephrine may be the drug of choice. *Bronchospasm*—administer epinephrine and/or an aerosolized beta$_2$-agonist. *Seizures*—administer diazepam.
In severe beta-blocker overdose resulting in hypotension and/or bradycardia, glucagon has been shown to be effective when administered in large doses (5 to 10 mg rapidly over 30 seconds, followed by continuous infusion of 5 mg/hr that can be reduced as the patient improves).
Neither hemodialysis nor peritoneal dialysis removes a significant amount of labetalol HCl from the general circulation (<1%).
The oral LD$_{50}$ value of labetalol HCl in the mouse is approximately 600 mg/kg and in the rat is greater than 2 g/kg. The intravenous LD$_{50}$ in these species is 50 to 60 mg/kg.

DOSAGE AND ADMINISTRATION

DOSAGE MUST BE INDIVIDUALIZED. The recommended initial dose is 100 mg twice daily whether used alone or added to a diuretic regimen. After 2 or 3 days, using standing blood pressure as an indicator, dosage may be titrated in increments of 100 mg b.i.d. every 2 or 3 days. The usual maintenance dosage of labetalol HCl is between 200 and 400 mg twice daily.
Since the full antihypertensive effect of labetalol HCl is usually seen within the first 1 to 3 hours of the initial dose or dose increment, the assurance of a lack of an exaggerated hypotensive response can be clinically established in the office setting. The antihypertensive effects of continued dosing can be measured at subsequent visits, approximately 12 hours after a dose, to determine whether further titration is necessary.
Patients with severe hypertension may require from 1200 mg to 2400 mg per day, with or without thiazide diuretics. Should side effects (principally nausea or dizziness) occur with these doses administered b.i.d., the same total daily dose administered t.i.d. may improve tolerability and facilitate further titration. Titration increments should not exceed 200 mg b.i.d.
When a diuretic is added, an additive antihypertensive effect can be expected. In some cases this may necessitate a labetalol HCl dosage adjustment. As with most antihypertensive drugs, optimal dosages of NORMODYNE (labetalol HCl) Tablets are usually lower in patients also receiving a diuretic.
When transferring patients from other antihypertensive drugs, NORMODYNE (labetalol HCl) Tablets should be introduced as recommended and the dosage of the existing therapy progressively decreased.

HOW SUPPLIED

NORMODYNE (labetalol HCl) Tablets, 100 mg, light-brown, round, scored, film-coated tablets engraved on one side with Schering and product identification number 244, and on the other side the number 100 for the strength and "NORMODYNE"; bottles of 100 (NDC-0085-0244-04), bottles of 500 (NDC-0085-0244-05), bottles of 1000 (NDC-0085-0244-07), and box of 100 for unit-dose dispensing (NDC-0085-0244-08).
NORMODYNE (labetalol HCl) Tablets, 200 mg, white, round, scored, film-coated tablets engraved on one side with Schering and product identification numbers 752, and on the other side the number 200 for the strength and "NORMODYNE"; bottles of 100 (NDC-0085-0752-04), bottles of 500 (NDC-0085-0752-05), bottles of 1000 (NDC-0085-0752-07), box of 100 for unit-dose dispensing (NDC-0085-0752-08).
NORMODYNE (labetalol HCl) Tablets, 300 mg, blue, round, film-coated tablets engraved on one side with Schering and product identification numbers 438, and on the other side the number 300 for the strength and "NORMODYNE"; bottles of 100 (NDC-0085-0438-03), bottles of 500 (NDC-0085-0438-05), box of 100 for unit-dose dispensing (NDC-0085-0438-06).
NORMODYNE (labetalol HCl) Tablets should be stored between 2° and 30°C (36° and 86°F).
NORMODYNE (labetalol HCl) Tablets in the unit-dose boxes should be protected from excessive moisture.
Key Pharmaceuticals, Inc.
Kenilworth, NJ 07033 USA
Rev. 6/99

16833533
23116707T

Shown in Product Identification Guide, page 334

PROVENTIL® ℞

brand of albuterol, USP
Inhalation Aerosol
Bronchodilator Aerosol
FOR ORAL INHALATION ONLY

DESCRIPTION

The active component of PROVENTIL Inhalation Aerosol is albuterol, USP racemic α^1-[(*tert*-butylamino)methyl]-4-hydroxy-*m*-xylene-α,α'-diol), a relatively selective beta$_2$-adrenergic bronchodilator, having the chemical structure:

HOCH$_2$
HO—[ring]—CHCH$_2$NHC(CH$_3$)$_3$
OH

The molecular weight of albuterol is 239.3, and the empirical formula is $C_{13}H_{21}NO_3$. Albuterol is a white to off-white crystalline solid. It is soluble in ethanol, sparingly soluble in water, and very soluble in chloroform. The World Health Organization recommended name for albuterol base is salbutamol.
PROVENTIL Inhalation Aerosol is a pressurized metered-dose aerosol unit for oral inhalation. It contains a microcrystalline suspension of albuterol in propellants (trichloromonofluoromethane and dichlorodifluoromethane) with oleic acid. Each actuation delivers 100 mcg albuterol, USP from the valve and 90 mcg of albuterol, USP from the mouthpiece. Each 17.0 g canister provides 200 oral inhalations.

CLINICAL PHARMACOLOGY

The primary action of beta-adrenergic drugs, including albuterol, is to stimulate adenyl cyclase, the enzyme which catalyzes the formation of cyclic-3',5'-adenosine monophosphate (cyclic AMP) from adenosine triphosphate (ATP) is beta-adrenergic cells. The cyclic AMP thus formed mediates the cellular responses. Increased cyclic AMP levels are associated with relaxation of bronchial smooth muscle and inhibition of release of mediators of immediate hypersensitivity from cells, especially from mast cells.
In vitro studies and *in vivo* pharmacologic studies have demonstrated that albuterol has a preferential effect on beta$_2$-adrenergic receptors compared with isoproterenol. While it is recognized that beta$_2$-adrenergic receptors are the predominant receptors in bronchial smooth muscle, data indicate that there is a population of beta$_2$-receptors in the human heart existing in a concentration between 10% and 50%. The precise function of these receptors has not been established.
In controlled clinical trials, albuterol has been shown to have more effect on the respiratory tract, in the form of bronchial smooth muscle relaxation than isoproterenol at comparable doses while producing fewer cardiovascular effects. Controlled clinical studies and other clinical experience have shown that inhaled albuterol, like other beta-adrenergic agonist drugs, can produce a significant cardiovascular effect in some patients, as measured by pulse rate, blood pressure, symptoms, and/or ECG changes.
Albuterol is longer acting than isoproterenol in most patients by any route of administration because it is not a substrate for the cellular uptake processes for catecholamines nor for catechol-*O*-methyl transferase.
The effects of rising doses of albuterol and isoproterenol aerosols were studied in volunteers and asthmatic patients. Results in normal volunteers indicated that the propensity for increase in heart rate for albuterol is ½ to ¼ that of isoproterenol. In asthmatic patients similar cardiovascular differentiation between the two drugs was also seen.
Preclinical: Intravenous studies in rats with albuterol sulfate have demonstrated that albuterol crosses the blood-brain barrier and reaches brain concentrations that are amounting to approximately 5.0% of the plasma concentrations. In structures outside the blood-brain barrier (pineal and pituitary glands), albuterol concentrations were found to be 100 times those in the whole brain.
Studies in laboratory animals (minipigs, rodents, and dogs) have demonstrated the occurrence of cardiac arrhythmias and sudden death (with histologic evidence of myocardial necrosis) when beta-agonists and methylxanthines are administered concurrently. The clinical significance of these findings is unknown.
Pharmacokinetics: Because of its gradual absorption from the bronchi, systemic levels of albuterol are low after inhalation at recommended doses.
Administration of tritiated albuterol by inhalation to four subjects resulted in maximum plasma concentrations within 2 to 4 hours. Due to the insensitivity of the assay method, the metabolic rate and half-life of elimination of albuterol in plasma could not be determined. However, data from urinary excretion studies indicated that albuterol has an elimination half-life of 3.8 hours. Approximately 72% of the inhaled dose is excreted in the urine within 24 hours, 28% as unchanged drug and 44% as metabolite.
Clinical Trials: In controlled clinical trials the onset of improvement in pulmonary function was within 15 minutes, as determined by both maximal midexpiratory flow rate (MMEF) and FEV$_1$. MMEF measurements also showed that near maximum improvement in pulmonary function generally occurs within 60 to 90 minutes, following 2 inhalations of albuterol and that clinically significant improvement generally continues for 3 to 4 hours in most patients. In clinical trials, some patients with asthma showed a therapeutic response (defined by maintaining FEV$_1$ values 15% or more above baseline) which was still apparent at 6 hours. Continued effectiveness of albuterol was demonstrated over a 13-week period in these same trials.
In clinical trials, 2 inhalations of albuterol taken approximately 15 minutes prior to exercise prevented exercise-induced bronchospasm, as demonstrated by the maintenance of FEV$_1$ within 80% of baseline values in the majority of patients. One of these studies also evaluated the duration of the prophylactic effect to repeated exercise challenges, which was evident at 4 hours in the majority of patients, and at 6 hours in approximately one third of the patients.

INDICATIONS AND USAGE

PROVENTIL Inhalation Aerosol is indicated in patients 12 years of age and older, for the prevention and relief of bronchospasm in patients with reversible obstructive airway disease, and for the prevention of exercise-induced bronchospasm.

CONTRAINDICATIONS

PROVENTIL Inhalation Aerosol is contraindicated in patients with a history of hypersensitivity to albuterol or any of its components.

WARNINGS

Deterioration of Asthma: Asthma may deteriorate acutely over a period of hours, or chronically over several days or longer. If the patient needs more doses of PROVENTIL Inhalation Aerosol than usual, this may be a marker of destabilization of asthma and requires re-evaluation of the patient and the treatment regimen, giving special consideration to the possible need for anti-inflammatory treatment, eg, corticosteroids.
Use of Anti-inflammatory Agents: The use of beta-adrenergic agonist bronchodilators alone may not be adequate to control asthma in many patients. Early consideration should be given to adding anti-inflammatory agents, eg, corticosteroids.
Paradoxical Bronchospasm: PROVENTIL Inhalation Aerosol can produce paradoxical bronchospasm, which may be life threatening. If paradoxical bronchospasm occurs, PROVENTIL Inhalation Aerosol should be discontinued immediately and alternative therapy instituted. It should be recognized that paradoxical bronchospasm, when associated with inhaled formulations, frequently occurs with the first use of a new canister or vial.
Cardiovascular Effects: PROVENTIL Inhalation Aerosol, like all other beta-adrenergic agonists, can produce a clinically significant cardiovascular effect in some patients as measured by pulse rate, blood pressure, and/or symptoms. Although such effects are uncommon after administration of PROVENTIL Inhalation Aerosol at recommended doses, if they occur, the drug may need to be discontinued. In addition, beta-agonists have been reported to produce electrocardiogram (ECG) changes, such as flattening of the T wave, prolongation of the QT$_c$ interval, and ST segment depression. The clinical significance of these findings is unknown. Therefore, PROVENTIL Inhalation Aerosol, like all sympathomimetic amines, should be used with caution in patients with cardiovascular disorders, especially coronary insufficiency, cardiac arrhythmias, and hypertension.
Immediate Hypersensitivity Reactions: Immediate hypersensitivity reactions may occur after administration of albuterol, as demonstrated by rare cases of urticaria, angioedema, rash, bronchospasm, anaphylaxis, and oropharyngeal edema.

PRECAUTIONS

General: Albuterol, as with all sympathomimetic amines, should be used with caution in patients with cardiovascular disorders, especially coronary insufficiency, cardiac arrhythmias, and hypertension; in patients with convulsive disorders, hyperthyroidism, or diabetes mellitus; and in patients who are unusually responsive to sympathomimetic amines. Clinically significant changes in systolic and diastolic blood pressure have been seen and could be expected to occur in some patients after use of any beta-adrenergic bronchodilator.

Large doses of intravenous albuterol have been reported to aggravate pre-existing diabetes mellitus and ketoacidosis. As with other beta-agonists, albuterol may produce significant hypokalemia in some patients, possibly through intracellular shunting, which has the potential to produce adverse cardiovascular effects. The decrease is usually transient, not requiring supplementation.

Information For Patients: The action of PROVENTIL Inhalation Aerosol may last up to 6 hours or longer. PROVENTIL Inhalation Aerosol should not be used more frequently than recommended. Do not increase the dose or frequency of doses of PROVENTIL Inhalation Aerosol without consulting your physician. If you find that treatment with PROVENTIL Inhalation becomes less effective for symptomatic relief, your symptoms become worse, and/or you need to use the product more frequently than usual, you should seek medical attention immediately. While you are using PROVENTIL Inhalation Aerosol, other inhaled drugs and asthma medications should be taken only as directed by your physician. Common adverse effects include palpitations, chest pain, rapid heart rate, tremor, or nervousness. If you are pregnant or nursing, contact your physician about the use of PROVENTIL Inhalation Aerosol. Effective and safe use of PROVENTIL Inhalation Aerosol includes an understanding of the way that it should be administered. See illustrated **Patient's Instructions For Use.**

The contents of PROVENTIL Inhalation Aerosol are under pressure. Do not puncture. Do not use or store near heat or open flame. Exposure to temperatures above 120°F may cause bursting. Never throw container into fire or incinerator. Keep out of reach of children. Avoid spraying in eyes.

Drug Interactions: Other short-acting sympathomimetic aerosol bronchodilators should not be used concomitantly with albuterol. If additional adrenergic drugs are to be administered by any route, they should be used with caution to avoid deleterious cardiovascular effects.

Beta Blockers: Beta-adrenergic receptor blocking agents not only block the pulmonary effect of beta-agonists, such as PROVENTIL Inhalation Aerosol but may produce severe bronchospasm in asthmatic patients. Therefore, patients with asthma should not normally be treated with beta-blockers. However, under certain circumstances, eg, as prophylaxis after myocardial infarction, there may be no acceptable alternatives to the use of beta-adrenergic blocking agents in patients with asthma. In this setting, cardioselective beta-blockers could be considered, although they should be administered with caution.

Diuretics: The ECG changes and/or hypokalemia that may result from the administration of nonpotassium-sparing diuretics (such as loop or thiazide diuretics) can be acutely worsened by beta-agonist, especially when the recommended dose of the beta-agonist is exceeded. Although the clinical significance of these effects is not known, caution is advised in the coadministration of beta-agonists with nonpotassium-sparing diuretics.

Digoxin: Mean decreases of 16% to 22% in serum digoxin levels were demonstrated after single dose intravenous and oral administration of albuterol, respectively, to normal volunteers who had received digoxin for 10 days. The clinical significance of this finding for patients with obstructive airway disease who are receiving albuterol and digoxin on a chronic basis is unclear. Nevertheless, it would be prudent to carefully evaluate the serum digoxin levels in patients who are currently receiving digoxin and albuterol.

Monoamine Oxidase Inhibitors or Tricyclic Antidepressants: Albuterol should be administered with extreme caution to patients being treated with monoamine oxidase inhibitors or tricyclic antidepressants, or within 2 weeks of discontinuation of such agents, because the action of albuterol on the vascular system may be potentiated.

Carcinogenesis, Mutagenesis, and Impairment of Fertility: In a 2-year study in Sprague-Dawley rats, albuterol sulfate caused a significant dose-related increase in the incidence of benign leiomyomas of the mesovarium at and above dietary doses of 2.0 mg/kg (approximately 15 times the maximum recommended daily inhalation dose for adults on a mg/m^2 basis). In another study this effect was blocked by the coadministration of propranolol, a non-selective beta-adrenergic antagonist.

In an 18-month study in CD-1 mice, albuterol sulfate showed no evidence of tumorigenicity at dietary doses up to 500 mg/kg (approximately 1700 times the maximum recommended daily inhalation dose for adults on an mg/m^2 basis). In a 22-month study in the Golden Hamster, albuterol sulfate showed no evidence of tumorigenicity at dietary doses up to 50 mg/kg (approximately 230 times the maximum recommended daily inhalation dose for adults on an mg/m^2 basis).

Albuterol sulfate was not mutagenic in the Ames test with or without metabolic activation using tester strains *S. typhimurium* TA1537, TA1538, and TA98 or *E. coli* WP2, WP2uvrA, and WP67. No forward mutation was seen in yeast strain *S. cerevisiae* S9 nor any mitotic gene conversion in yeast strain *S. cerevisiae* JD1 with or without metabolic activation. Fluctuation assays in *S. typhimurium* TA98 and *E. coli* WP2, both with metabolic activation, were negative. Albuterol sulfate was not clastogenic in a human peripheral lymphocyte assay or in an AH1 strain mouse micronucleus assay.

Reproduction studies in rats demonstrated no evidence of impaired fertility at oral doses of albuterol sulfate up to 50 mg/kg (approximately 340 times the maximum recommended daily inhalation dose for adults on an mg/m^2 basis).

Teratogenic Effects—Pregnancy Category C: Albuterol sulfate has been shown to be teratogenic in mice. A study in CD-1 mice at subcutaneous (sc) doses at and above 0.25 mg/kg (approximately equal to the maximum recommended daily inhalation dose for adults on an mg/m^2 basis), induced cleft palate formation in 5 of 111 (4.5%) fetuses. At an sc dose of 2.5 mg/kg (approximately 8 times the maximum recommended daily inhalation dose for adults on an mg/m^2 basis) albuterol sulfate induced cleft palate formation in 10 of 108 (9.3%) fetuses. The drug did not induce cleft palate formation when administered at an sc dose of 0.025 mg/kg (significantly less than the maximum recommended daily inhalation dose for adults on an mg/m^2 basis). Cleft palate also occurred in 22 of 72 (30.5%) fetuses from females treated with 2.5 mg/kg isoproterenol (positive control) administered subcutaneously.

A reproduction study in Stride Dutch rabbits revealed cranioschisis in 7 of 19 (37%) fetuses when albuterol sulfate was administered orally at a dose of 50 mg/kg (approximately 680 times the maximum recommended daily inhalation dose for adults on an mg/m^2 basis).

Studies in pregnant rats with tritiated albuterol demonstrated that approximately 10% of the circulating maternal drug is transferred to the fetus. Disposition in the fetal lungs is comparable to maternal lungs, but fetal liver disposition is 1% of the maternal liver levels.

There are no adequate and well-controlled studies in pregnant women. Because animal reproduction studies are not always predictive of human response, albuterol should be used during pregnancy only if the potential benefit justifies the potential risk to the fetus.

During worldwide marketing experience, various congenital anomalies, including cleft palate and limb defects, have been reported in the offspring of patients being treated with albuterol. Some of the mothers were taking multiple medications during their pregnancies. Because no consistent pattern of defects can be discerned, a relationship between albuterol use and congenital anomalies has not been established.

Use in Labor and Delivery—Use in Labor: Because of the potential for beta-agonist interference with uterine contractility, use of PROVENTIL Inhalation Aerosol for relief of bronchospasm during labor should be restricted to those patients in whom the benefits clearly outweigh the risk.

Tocolysis: Albuterol has not been approved for the management of preterm labor. The benefit:risk ratio when albuterol is administered for tocolysis has not been established. Serious adverse reactions, including maternal pulmonary edema, have been reported during or following treatment of premature labor with beta$_2$-agonists, including albuterol.

Nursing Mothers: It is not known whether this drug is excreted in human milk. Because of the potential for tumorigenicity shown for albuterol in some animal studies, a decision should be made whether to discontinue nursing or to discontinue the drug, taking into account the importance of the drug to the mother.

Pediatric Use: Safety and effectiveness in children below the age of 12 years have not been established.

ADVERSE REACTIONS

The adverse reactions of albuterol are similar in nature to those of other sympathomimetic agents, although the incidence of certain cardiovascular effects is less with albuterol.

Percent Incidence of Adverse Reactions in Patients ≥ 12 Years of Age in a 13-Week Clinical Trial* (n=147)

Adverse Event	PROVENTIL Inhalation Aerosol	Isoproterenol Inhaler
Tremor	<15	<15
Nausea	<15	<15
Tachycardia	10	10
Palpitations	<10	<15
Nervousness	<10	<15
Increased Blood Pressure	<5	<5
Dizziness	<5	<5
Heartburn	<5	<5

*A 13-week, double-blind study compared albuterol and isoproterenol aerosols in 147 asthmatic patients.

Cases of urticaria, angioedema, rash, bronchospasm, hoarseness, oropharyngeal edema, and arrhythmias (including atrial fibrillation, supraventricular tachycardia, and extrasystoles) have also been reported after the use of inhaled albuterol. In addition, albuterol, like other sympathomimetic agents, can cause adverse reactions such as hypertension, angina, vomiting, vertigo, central nervous system stimulation, insomnia, headache, unusual taste, and drying or irritation of the oropharynx.

OVERDOSAGE

The expected symptoms with overdosage are those of excessive beta-adrenergic stimulation and/or occurrence or exaggeration of any of the symptoms listed under **ADVERSE REATIONS**, eg, angina, hypertension, tachycardia with rates up to 200 beats per minute, nervousness, headache, tremor, dry mouth, palpitation, nausea, dizziness, and insomnia. In addition, seizures, hypotension, arrhythmias, fatigue, malaise, and hypokalemia may also occur. As with all sympathomimetic aerosol medications, cardiac arrest and even death may be associated with abuse of PROVENTIL Inhalation Aerosol. Treatment consists of discontinuation of PROVENTIL Inhalation Aerosol together with appropriate symptomatic therapy. The judicious use of a cardioselective beta-receptor blocker may be considered, bearing in mind that such medication can produce bronchospasm. There is insufficient evidence to determine if dialysis is beneficial for overdosage of PROVENTIL Inhalation Aerosol.

The oral median lethal dose of albuterol sulfate in mice is greater than 2000 mg/kg (approximately 6800 times the maximum recommended daily inhalation dose for adults on an mg/m^2 basis). In mature rats, the subcutaneous median lethal dose of albuterol sulfate is approximately 450 mg/kg (approximately 3000 times the maximum recommended daily inhalation dose for adults on an mg/m^2 basis). In small young rats, the subcutaneous median lethal dose is approximately 2000 mg/kg (approximately 14,000 times the maximum recommended daily inhalation dose for adults and children on an mg/m^2 basis). The inhalation median lethal dose has not been determined in animals.

DOSAGE AND ADMINISTRATION

Treatment of acute episodes of bronchospasm or prevention of asthmatic symptoms: The usual dosage for adults and children 12 years of age and older is 2 inhalations repeated every 4 to 6 hours; in some patients, 1 inhalation every 4 hours may be sufficient. More frequent administration or a larger number of inhalations is not recommended. For maintenance therapy or prevention of exacerbation of bronchospasm, 2 inhalations, 4 times a day should be sufficient.

The use of PROVENTIL Inhalation Aerosol can be continued as medically indicated to control recurring bouts of bronchospasm. During this time most patients gain optimal benefit from regular use of the inhaler. Safe usage for periods extending over several years has been documented.

If a previously effective dosage regimen fails to provide the usual response, this may be a marker of destabilization of asthma and requires re-evaluation of the patient and treatment regimen, giving special consideration to the possible need for anti-inflammatory treatment, eg, corticosteroids.

Exercise-Induced Bronchospasm Prevention: The usual dosage for adults and children 12 years and older is 2 inhalations, 15 minutes prior to exercise. For treatment, see above.

It is recommended to "test spray" PROVENTIL Inhalation Aerosol into the air before using for the first time and in cases where the aerosol has not been used for a prolonged period of time.

HOW SUPPLIED

PROVENTIL Inhalation Aerosol, 17.0 g canister contains 200 metered inhalations, box of one (NDC 0085-0614-02). Each actuation delivers 100 mcg of albuterol from the valve and 90 mcg of albuterol from the mouthpiece. Each canister is supplied with a yellow plastic actuator with orange dust cap, and Patient's Instructions.

PROVENTIL Inhalation Aerosol REFILL canister, 17.0 g, contains 200 metered inhalations, with Patient's Instructions; box of one (NDC 0085-0614-03).

The correct amount of medication in each inhalation cannot be assured after 200 actuations from the 17.0 g canister even though the canister is not completely empty. The canister should be discarded when the labeled number of actuations have been used.

Store between 15° and 30°C (59° and 86°F). Failure to use the product within this temperature range may result in improper dosing. For optimal results, the canister should be at room temperature before use. Shake well before using.

PROVENTIL Inhalation Aerosol canister should be used only with the actuator provided. The yellow actuator should not be used with other aerosol medication canisters.

NOTE: The indented statement below is required by the Federal government's Clean Air Act for all products containing or manufactured with chlorofluorocarbons (CFCs).

> **WARNING:** Contains dichlorodifluoromethane (CFC-12) and trichloromonofluoromethane (CFC-11), substances which harm public health and the environment by destroying ozone in the upper atmosphere.

A notice similar to the above WARNING has been placed in the "Patient's Instructions for Use" portion of this package insert under the Environmental Protection Agency's (EPA's) regulations. The patient's warning states that the patient should consult his or her physician if there are questions about alternatives.

Schering Corporation
Kenilworth, NJ 07033 USA
Rev. 8/99 19529320

Continued on next page

Information on Schering products appearing on these pages is effective as of January 2000.

Proventil Aerosol—Cont.

PROVENTIL®
brand of albuterol, USP
Inhalation Aerosol
FOR ORAL INHALATION ONLY
Patient's Instructions
For Use

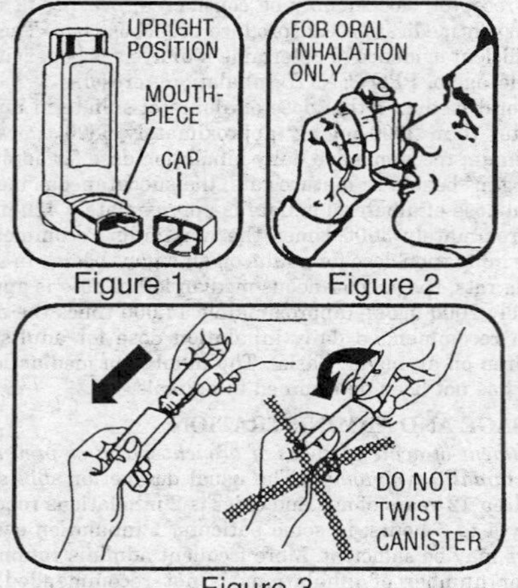

Figure 1 Figure 2

Figure 3

Before using your PROVENTIL Inhalation Aerosol, read complete instructions carefully.

1. SHAKE THE INHALER WELL immediately before each use. **Then remove the cap from the mouthpiece. Check mouthpiece for foreign objects prior to use.** Make sure the canister is fully and firmly inserted into the actuator. The PROVENTIL Inhalation Aerosol canister should only be used with the yellow PROVENTIL Inhalation Aerosol mouthpiece. This yellow mouthpiece should not be used with any other inhalation drug product. Similarly, the canister should not be used with any other mouthpieces.

2. As with all aerosol medications, it is recommended to "test spray" into the air before using for the first time and in cases where the aerosol has not been used for a prolonged period of time.

3. BREATHE OUT FULLY THROUGH THE MOUTH, expelling as much air from your lungs as possible. Place the mouthpiece fully into the mouth, holding the inhaler in its upright position (See Figure 1) and closing the lips around it.

4. WHILE BREATHING IN DEEPLY AND SLOWLY THROUGH THE MOUTH, FULLY DEPRESS THE TOP OF THE METAL CANISTER with your index finger. (See Figure 2.)

5. HOLD YOUR BREATH AS LONG AS POSSIBLE. Before breathing out, remove the inhaler from your mouth and release your finger from the canister.

6. Wait one minute and SHAKE the inhaler again. Repeat steps 2 through 4 for each inhalation prescribed by your physician.

7. CLEANSE THE INHALER THOROUGHLY AND FREQUENTLY. Remove the metal canister and cleanse the plastic case and cap by rinsing thoroughly in warm running water, at least once a day. After thoroughly drying the plastic case and cap, gently replace the canister downward into the case **without using a twisting motion.** (See Figure 3.) Replace the cap.

DOSAGE: Use only as directed by your physician.
The correct amount of medication in each inhalation cannot be assured after 200 actuations from the 17.0 g canister even though the canister is not completely empty. The canister should be discarded when the labeled number of actuations have been used. Before you reach the specified number of actuations, you should consult your physician to determine whether a refill is needed. Just as you should not take extra doses without consulting your physician, you also should not stop using PROVENTIL Inhalation Aerosol without consulting your physician.

WARNINGS: The action of PROVENTIL Inhalation Aerosol may last up to 6 hours or longer. PROVENTIL Inhalation Aerosol should not be used more frequently than recommended. Do not increase the dose or frequency of PROVENTIL Inhalation Aerosol without consulting your physician. If you find that treatment with PROVENTIL Inhalation Aerosol becomes less effective for symptomatic relief, your symptoms become worse, and/or you need to use the product more frequently than usual, you should seek immediate medical attention. While taking PROVENTIL Inhalation Aerosol, other asthma drugs and inhaled medicines should be used only as prescribed by your physician.

Contents Under Pressure. Do not puncture. Do not store near heat or open flame. Exposure to temperatures above 120°F may cause bursting. Never throw container into fire or incinerator. Keep out of reach of children. Avoid spraying in eyes.

Store between 15° and 30°C (59° and 86°F). Failure to use the product within this temperature range may result in improper dosing. Shake well before using. For optimal results, the canister should be at room temperature before use.

NOTE: The indented statement below is required by the Federal government's Clean Air Act for all products containing or manufactured with chlorofluorocarbons (CFCs).

> This product contains dichlorodifluoromethane (CFC-12) and trichloromonofluoromethane (CFC-11), substances which harm the environment by destroying ozone in the upper atmosphere.

Your physician has determined that this product is likely to help your personal health. USE THIS PRODUCT AS DIRECTED, UNLESS INSTRUCTED TO DO OTHERWISE BY YOUR PHYSICIAN. If you have any questions about alternatives, consult with your physician.
Schering Corporation
Kenilworth, NJ 07033 USA

19529320 Rev. 8/99

PROVENTIL® ℞
brand of albuterol sulfate, USP
Solution for Inhalation 0.5%*
(*Potency expressed as albuterol)

DESCRIPTION

PROVENTIL Solution for Inhalation contains albuterol sulfate, USP, the racemic form of albuterol and a relatively selective beta$_2$-adrenergic bronchodilator. Albuterol sulfate has the chemical name α^1-[(*tert*-Butylamino) methyl]-4-hydroxy-*m*-xylene-α,α'-diol sulfate (2:1) (salt), and the following chemical structure:

[HOCH$_2$ / HO– benzene ring –CHCH$_2$NHC(CH$_3$)$_3$ / OH]$_2$ •H$_2$SO$_4$

The molecular weight of albuterol sulfate is 576.7, and the empirical formula is $(C_{13}H_{21}NO_3)_2 \cdot H_2SO_4$. Albuterol sulfate is a white crystalline powder, soluble in water and slightly soluble in ethanol. The World Health Organization's recommended name for albuterol base in salbutamol.
PROVENTIL Solution for Inhalation 0.5% is in concentrated form. Dilute 0.5 mL of the solution to 3 mL with sterile normal saline solution prior to administration.
Each mL of PROVENTIL Solution for Inhalation 0.5% contains 5 mg of albuterol (as 6.0 mg of albuterol sulfate, USP) in an aqueous solution containing benzalkonium chloride NF; sulfuric acid R is used to adjust the pH between 3 and 5. PROVENTIL Solution for Inhalation 0.5% contains no sulfiting agents. It is supplied in 20 mL amber glass bottles. PROVENTIL Solution for Inhalation is a clear, colorless to light yellow solution.

CLINICAL PHARMACOLOGY

The primary action of beta-adrenergic drugs, including albuterol, is to stimulate adenyl cyclase, the enzyme which catalyzes the formation of cyclic-3′,5′-adenosine monophosphate (cyclic AMP) from adenosine triphosphate (ATP) in beta-adrenergic cells. The cyclic AMP thus formed mediates the cellular responses. Increased cyclic AMP levels are associated with relaxation of bronchial smooth muscle and inhibition of release of mediators of immediate hypersensitivity from cells, especially from mast cells.
In vitro studies and *in vivo* pharmacologic studies have demonstrated that albuterol has a preferential effect on beta$_2$-adrenergic receptors compared with isoproterenol. While it is recognized that beta$_2$-adrenergic receptors are the predominant receptors in bronchial smooth muscle, data indicate that there is a population of beta$_2$-receptors in the human heart existing in a concentration between 10% and 50%. The precise function of these receptors has not been established.
In controlled clinical trials, albuterol has been shown to have more effect on the respiratory tract in the form of bronchial smooth muscle relaxation, than isoproterenol at comparable doses while producing fewer cardiovascular effects. Controlled clinical studies and other clinical experience have shown that inhaled albuterol, like other beta-adrenergic agonist drugs, can produce a significant cardiovascular effect in some patients, as measured by pulse rate, blood pressure, symptoms, and/or ECG changes.
Albuterol is longer acting than isoproterenol in most patients by any route of administration because it is not a substrate for the cellular uptake processes for catecholamines nor for catechol-*O*-methyl transferase.
The effects of rising doses of albuterol and isoproterenol aerosols were studied in volunteers and asthmatic patients. Results in normal volunteers indicated that the propensity for increase in heart rate for albuterol is $^1/_2$ to $^1/_4$ that of isoproterenol. In asthmatic patients similar cardiovascular differentiation between the two drugs was also seen.

Preclinical: Intravenous studies in rats with albuterol sulfate have demonstrated that albuterol crosses the blood-brain barrier and reaches brain concentrations that are amounting to approximately 5.0% of the plasma concentrations. In structures outside the blood-brain barrier (pineal and pituitary glands), albuterol concentrations were found to be 100 times those in the whole brain.
Studies in laboratory animals (minipigs, rodents, and dogs) have demonstrated the occurrence of cardiac arrhythmias and sudden death (with histologic evidence of myocardial necrosis) when beta-agonists and methylxanthines are administered concurrently. The clinical significance of these findings is unknown.

Pharmacokinetics: After either IPPB or nebulizer administration in asthmatic patients, less than 20% of a single albuterol dose was absorbed; the remaining amount was recovered from the nebulizer and apparatus and expired air. Most of the absorbed dose was recovered in the urine 24 hours after drug administration. Following a 3.0 mg dose of nebulized albuterol, the maximum albuterol plasma level at 0.5 hour was 2.1 ng/mL (range 1.4 to 3.2 ng/mL). It has been demonstrated that following oral administration of 4 mg of albuterol, the elimination half-life was 5 to 6 hours.

Clinical Trials: In controlled clinical trials, most patients exhibited an onset of improvement in pulmonary function within 5 minutes as determined by FEV$_1$. FEV$_1$ measurements also showed that the maximum average improvement in pulmonary function usually occurred at approximately 1 hour following inhalation of 2.5 mg of albuterol by compressor-nebulizer, and remained close to peak for 2 hours. Clinically significant improvement in pulmonary function (defined as maintenance of a 15% or more increase in FEV$_1$ over baseline values) continued for 3 to 4 hours in most patients and in some patients continued up to 6 hours.

INDICATIONS AND USAGE

PROVENTIL Solution for Inhalation is indicated for the relief of bronchospasm in patients 12 years of age and older with reversible obstructive airway disease and acute attacks of bronchospasm.

CONTRAINDICATIONS

PROVENTIL Solution for Inhalation is contraindicated in patients with a history of hypersensitivity to albuterol or any of its components.

WARNINGS

Deterioration of Asthma: Asthma may deteriorate acutely over a period of hours, or chronically over several days or longer. If the patient needs more doses of PROVENTIL Solution for Inhalation than usual, this may be a marker of destabilization of asthma and requires re-evaluation of the patient and the treatment regimen, giving special consideration to the possible need for anti-inflammatory treatment, eg, corticosteroids.

Use of Anti-inflammatory Agents: The use of beta-adrenergic agonist bronchodilators alone may not be adequate to control asthma in many patients. Early consideration should be given to adding anti-inflammatory agents, eg, corticosteroids.

Paradoxical Bronchospasm: PROVENTIL Solution for Inhalation can produce paradoxical bronchospasm, which may be life-threatening. If paradoxical bronchospasm occurs, PROVENTIL Solution for Inhalation should be discontinued immediately and alternative therapy instituted. It should be recognized that paradoxical bronchospasm, when associated with inhaled formulations, frequently occurs with the first use of a new vial.

Cardiovascular Effects: PROVENTIL Solution for Inhalation, like all other beta-adrenergic agonists, can produce a clinically significant cardiovascular effect in some patients as measured by pulse rate, blood pressure, and/or symptoms. Although such effects are uncommon after administration of PROVENTIL Solution for Inhalation at recommended doses, if they occur, the drug may need to be discontinued. In addition, beta-agonists have been reported to produce electrocardiogram (ECG) changes, such as flattening of the T wave, prolongation of the QT$_c$ interval, and ST segment depression. The clinical significance of these findings is unknown. Therefore, PROVENTIL Solution for Inhalation, like all sympathomimetic amines, should be used with caution in patients with cardiovascular disorders, especially coronary insufficiency, cardiac arrhythmias, and hypertension.

Immediate Hypersensitivity Reactions: Immediate hypersensitivity reactions may occur after administration of albuterol, as demonstrated by rare cases of urticaria, angioedema, rash, bronchospasm, anaphylaxis, and oropharyngeal edema.

Microbial Contamination: To avoid microbial contamination, proper aseptic technique should be used each time the bottle is opened. Precautions should be taken to prevent contact of the dropper tip of the bottle with any surface, including the nebulizer reservoir and associated ventilatory equipment. In addition, if the solution changes color or becomes cloudy, it should not be used.

PRECAUTIONS

General: Albuterol, as with all sympathomimetic amines, should be used with caution in patients with cardiovascular disorders, especially coronary insufficiency, cardiac arrhythmias, and hypertension; in patients with convulsive disorders, hyperthyroidism or diabetes mellitus; and in patients who are unusually responsive to sympathomimetic amines. Clinically significant changes in systolic and diastolic blood pressure have been seen in individual patients and could be expected to occur in some patients after use of any beta-adrenergic bronchodilator.

Large doses of intravenous albuterol have been reported to aggravate pre-existing diabetes mellitus and ketoacidosis. As with other beta-agonist medications, albuterol may produce significant hypokalemia in some patients, possibly through intracellular shunting, which has the potential to produce adverse cardiovascular effects. The decrease is usually transient, not requiring potassium supplementation.

To avoid contaminating the multi-dose bottle of PROVENTIL Solution for Inhalation, proper aseptic technique should be used when withdrawing and delivering the dose into the nebulizer.

Information for Patients: The action of PROVENTIL Solution for Inhalation may last up to 6 hours or longer. PROVENTIL Solution for Inhalation should not be used more frequently than recommended. Do not increase the dose or frequency of doses of PROVENTIL Solution for Inhalation without consulting your physician. If you find that treatment with PROVENTIL Solution for Inhalation becomes less effective for symptomatic relief, your symptoms become worse, and/or you need to use the product more frequently than usual, you should seek medical attention immediately. While you are using PROVENTIL Solution for Inhalation, other inhaled drugs and asthma medications should be taken only as directed by your physician. Common adverse effects include palpitations, chest pain, rapid heart rate, tremor, or nervousness. If you are pregnant or nursing, contact your physician about the use of PROVENTIL Solution for Inhalation. Effective use of PROVENTIL Solution for Inhalation includes an understanding of the way that it should be administered. See illustrated **Patient's Instructions for Use**.

Microbial Contamination: To avoid microbial contamination, proper aseptic technique should be used each time the bottle is opened. Precautions should be taken to prevent contact of the dropper tip of the bottle with any surface, including the nebulizer reservoir and associated ventilatory equipment. In addition, if the solution changes color or becomes cloudy it should not be used.

Mixing Different Inhalation Solutions: Drug compatibility (physical and chemical), efficacy, and safety of PROVENTIL Solution for Inhalation when mixed with other drugs in a nebulizer have not been established.

Drug Interactions: Other short-acting sympathomimetic aerosol bronchodilators or epinephrine should not be used concomitantly with albuterol.

Beta Blockers: Beta-adrenergic receptor blocking agents not only block the pulmonary effect of beta-agonists, such as PROVENTIL Solution for Inhalation, but may produce severe bronchospasm in asthmatic patients. Therefore, patients with asthma should not normally be treated with beta blockers. However, under certain circumstances, eg, as prophylaxis after myocardial infarction, there may be no acceptable alternatives to the use of beta-adrenergic blocking agents in patients with asthma. In this setting, cardioselective beta blockers could be considered, although they should be administered with caution.

Diuretics: The ECG changes and/or hypokalemia that may result from the administration of nonpotassium-sparing diuretics (such as loop or thiazide diuretics) can be acutely worsened by beta-agonists, especially when the recommended dose of the beta-agonist is exceeded. Although the clinical significance of these effects is not known, caution is advised in the coadministration of beta-agonists with nonpotassium-sparing diuretics.

Digoxin: Mean decreases of 16% to 22% in serum digoxin levels were demonstrated after single dose intravenous and oral administration of albuterol, respectively, to normal volunteers who had received digoxin for 10 days. The clinical significance of this finding for patients with obstructive airway disease who are receiving albuterol and digoxin on a chronic basis is unclear. Nevertheless, it would be prudent to carefully evaluate the serum digoxin levels in patients who are currently receiving digoxin and albuterol.

Monoamine Oxidase Inhibitors or Tricyclic Antidepressants: Albuterol should be administered with extreme caution to patients being treated with monoamine oxidase inhibitors or tricyclic antidepressants, or within 2 weeks of discontinuation of such agents, because the action of albuterol on the vascular system may be potentiated.

Carcinogenesis, Mutagenesis, and Impairment of Fertility: In a 2-year study in Sprague-Dawley rats, albuterol sulfate caused a significant dose-related increase in the incidence of benign leiomyomas of the mesovarium at and above dietary doses of 2 mg/kg (approximately 2 times the maximum recommended daily inhalation dose for adults on an mg/m^2 basis). In another study, this effect was blocked by the coadministration of propranolol, a nonselective beta-adrenergic antagonist.

In an 18-month study in CD-1 mice, albuterol sulfate showed no evidence of tumorigenicity at dietary doses up to 500 mg/kg (approximately 200 times the maximum recommended daily inhalation dose for adults on an mg/m^2 basis). In a 22-month study in the Golden Hamster, albuterol sulfate showed no evidence of tumorigenicity at dietary doses of up to 50 mg/kg (approximately 25 times the maximum recommended daily inhalation dose for adults on an mg/m^2 basis).

Albuterol sulfate was not mutagenic in the Ames test with or without metabolic activation using tester strains *S. typhimurium* TA1537, TA1538, and TA98 or *E. coli* WP2, WP2uvrA, and WP67. No forward mutation was seen in yeast strain *S. cerevisiae* S9 nor any mitotic gene conversion in yeast strain *S. cerevisiae* JD1 with or without metabolic activation. Fluctuation assays in *S. typhimurium* TA98 and *E. coli* WP2, both with metabolic activation, were negative. Albuterol sulfate was not clastogenic in a human peripheral lymphocyte assay or in an AH1 strain mouse micronucleus assay.

Reproduction studies in rats demonstrated no evidence of impaired fertility at oral doses of albuterol sulfate up to 50 mg/kg (approximately 40 times the maximum recommended daily inhalation dose for adults on an mg/m^2 basis).

Teratogenic Effects—Pregnancy Category C: Albuterol sulfate has been shown to be teratogenic in mice. A study in CD-1 mice at subcutaneous (sc) doses at and above 0.25 mg/kg (corresponding to less than the maximum recommended daily inhalation dose for adults on an mg/m^2 basis), induced cleft palate formation in 5 of 111 (4.5%) fetuses. At an sc dose of 2.5 mg/kg (approximately equal to the maximum recommended daily inhalation dose for adults on an mg/m^2 basis), albuterol sulfate induced cleft palate formation in 10 of 108 (9.3%) fetuses. The drug did not induce cleft palate formation when administered at an sc dose of 0.025 mg/kg (corresponding to less than the maximum recommended daily inhalation dose for adults on an mg/m^2 basis). Cleft palate also occurred in 22 of 72 (30.5%) fetuses from females treated with 2.5 mg/kg isoproterenol (positive control) administered subcutaneously.

A reproduction study in Stride Dutch rabbits revealed cranioschisis in 7 of 19 (37%) fetuses when albuterol was administered orally at a dose of 50 mg/kg (approximately 80 times the maximum recommended daily inhalation dose for adults on a mg/m^2 basis).

Studies in pregnant rats with tritiated albuterol demonstrated that approximately 10% of the circulating maternal drug is transferred to the fetus. Disposition in the fetal lungs is comparable to maternal lungs, but fetal liver disposition is 1% of the maternal liver levels.

There are no adequate and well-controlled studies in pregnant women. Because animal reproduction studies are not always predictive of human response, albuterol should be used during pregnancy only if the potential benefit justifies the potential risk to the fetus.

During worldwide marketing experience, various congenital anomalies, including cleft palate and limb defects, have been reported in the offspring of patients being treated with albuterol. Some of the mothers were taking multiple medications during their pregnancies. Because no consistent pattern of defects can be discerned, a relationship between albuterol use and congenital anomalies has not been established.

Use in Labor and Delivery—Use in Labor: Because of the potential for beta-agonist interference with uterine contractility, use of PROVENTIL Solution for Inhalation for relief of bronchospasm during labor should be restricted to those patients in whom the benefits clearly outweigh the risk.

Tocolysis: Albuterol has not been approved for the management of preterm labor. The benefit:risk ratio when albuterol is administered for tocolysis has not been established. Serious adverse reactions, including maternal pulmonary edema, have been reported during or following treatment of premature labor with beta-agonists, including albuterol.

Nursing Mothers: It is not known whether this drug is excreted in human milk. Because of the potential for tumorigenicity shown for albuterol in some animal studies, a decision should be made whether to discontinue nursing or to discontinue the drug, taking into account the importance of the drug to the mother.

Pediatric Use: Safety and effectiveness of albuterol inhalation solution and solution for inhalation in children below the age of 12 years have not been established.

ADVERSE REACTIONS

The results of clinical trials with PROVENTIL Solution for Inhalation in 135 patients showed the following side effects which were considered probably or possibly drug related:

Percent Incidence of Adverse Reactions

Reaction	Percent Incidence
Central Nervous System	
Tremors	20
Dizziness	7
Nervousness	4
Headache	3
Insomnia	1
Gastrointestinal	
Nausea	4
Dyspepsia	1
Ear, Nose, and Throat	
Nasal congestion	1
Pharyngitis	<1
Cardiovascular	
Tachycardia	1
Hypertension	1
Respiratory	
Bronchospasm	8
Cough	4
Bronchitis	4
Wheezing	1

No clinically relevant laboratory abnormalities related to PROVENTIL Solution for Inhalation were determined in these studies.

Cases of urticaria, angioedema, rash, bronchospasm, hoarseness, oropharyngeal edema, and arrhythmias (including atrial fibrillation, supraventricular tachycardia, and extrasystoles) have also been reported after the use of inhaled albuterol.

OVERDOSAGE

The expected symptoms with overdosage are those of excessive beta-adrenergic stimulation and/or occurrence of exaggeration of any of the symptoms listed under **ADVERSE REACTIONS**, eg, angina, hypertension, tachycardia with rates up to 200 beats per minute, arrhythmias, nervousness, headache, tremor, dry mouth, palpitation, nausea, dizziness, malaise, and insomnia. In addition, seizures, hypotension, fatigue, and hypokalemia may also occur. As with all sympathomimetic aerosol medications, cardiac arrest and even death may be associated with abuse of PROVENTIL Solution for Inhalation. Treatment consists of discontinuation of PROVENTIL Solution for Inhalation together with appropriate symptomatic therapy. The judicious use of a cardioselective beta-receptor blocker may be considered, bearing in mind that such medication can produce bronchospasm. There is insufficient evidence to determine if dialysis is beneficial for overdosage of PROVENTIL Solution for Inhalation.

The oral median lethal dose of albuterol sulfate in mice is greater than 2000 mg/kg (approximately 810 times the maximum recommended daily inhalation dose for adults on an mg/m^2 basis). In mature rats, the subcutaneous (sc) median lethal dose of albuterol sulfate is approximately 450 mg/kg (approximately 360 times the maximum recommended daily inhalation dose for adults on an mg/m^2 basis). In small young rats, the sc median lethal dose is approximately 2000 mg/kg (approximately 1600 times the maximum recommended daily inhalation dose for adults on an mg/m^2 basis). The inhalation median lethal dose has not been determined in animals.

DOSAGE AND ADMINISTRATION

The usual dosage for adults and pediatric patients 12 years of age and older is 2.5 mg of albuterol administered 3 to 4 times daily by nebulization. More frequent administration or higher doses are not recommended. To administer 2.5 mg of albuterol, dilute 0.5 mL of the 0.5% solution for inhalation to a total volume of 3 mL with sterile normal saline solution and administer by nebulization. The flow rate is regulated to suit the particular nebulizer so that the PROVENTIL Solution for Inhalation will be delivered over approximately 5 to 15 minutes.

Drug compatibility (physical and chemical), efficacy, and safety of PROVENTIL Solution for Inhalation when mixed with other drugs in a nebulizer have not been established.

The use of PROVENTIL Solution for Inhalation can be continued as medically indicated to control recurring bouts of bronchospasm. During treatment, most patients gain optimum benefit from regular use of the nebulizer solution.

If a previously effective dosage regimen fails to provide the usual relief, medical advice should be sought immediately, as this is often a sign of seriously worsening asthma which would require reassessment of therapy.

Microbial Contamination: To avoid microbial contamination, proper aseptic technique should be used each time the bottle is opened. Precautions should be taken to prevent contact of the dropper tip of the bottle with any surface, including the nebulizer reservoir and associated ventilatory equipment. In addition, if the solution changes color or becomes cloudy, it should not be used.

The nebulizer should be cleaned in accordance with the manufacturer's instructions. Failure to do so could lead to bacterial contamination of the nebulizer and possible infection.

HOW SUPPLIED

PROVENTIL Solution for Inhalation 0.5% is a clear, colorless to light yellow solution and is supplied in amber glass bottles of 20 mL fill (NDC 0085-0208-02) with accompanying calibrated dropper; boxes of one. **Store between 2° and 25°C (36° and 77°F).**

Schering Corporation,
Kenilworth, NJ 07033 USA.

Rev. 5/99 17979930

Patient's Instructions For Use

PROVENTIL®
brand of albuterol sulfate, USP
Solution for Inhalation 0.5%*

*Potency expressed as albuterol

Note: The PROVENTIL Solution contained in the 20 mL multiple-dose bottle is concentrated and must be diluted. Read complete instructions carefully before using.

Continued on next page

Information on Schering products appearing on these pages is effective as of January 2000.

Proventil Solution—Cont.

1. Draw 0.5 mL of PROVENTIL Solution into the specially marked dropper that comes with each multi-dose bottle (Figure 1).

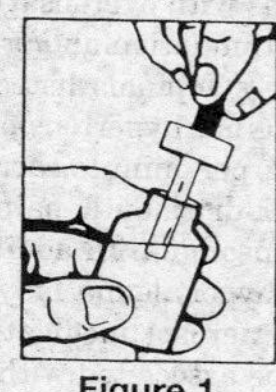

Figure 1

2. Squeeze the solution into the nebulizer reservoir through the appropriate opening (Figure 2).

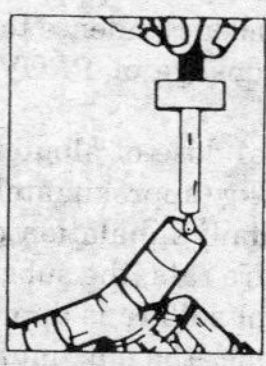

Figure 2

3. Add 2.5 mL of diluting fluid—sterile normal saline solution (as your physician has directed).
4. Gently swirl the nebulizer to mix the contents and connect it with the mouthpiece or face mask (Figure 3).

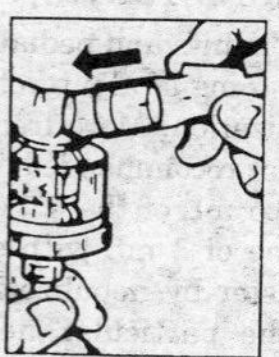

Figure 3

5. Connect the nebulizer to the compressor.
6. Sit in a comfortable, upright position; place the mouthpiece in your mouth (Figure 4) (or put the face mask on); and turn the compressor on.

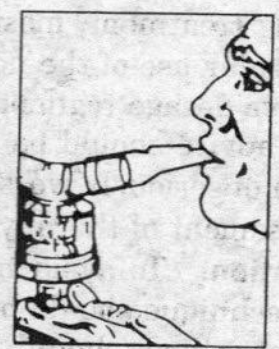

Figure 4

7. Breathe as calmly, deeply, and evenly as possible until no more mist is formed in the nebulizer chamber (about 5–15 minutes). At this point, the treatment is finished.
8. Clean the nebulizer (see manufacturer's instructions). Failure to clean the nebulizer in accordance with the manufacturer's instructions could lead to bacterial contamination of the nebulizer, and possible infection.

Note: Use only as directed by your physician. More frequent administration or higher doses are not recommended. To avoid microbial contamination of PROVENTIL Solution for Inhalation, you should be careful not to touch the dropper tip on any surface, including the nebulizer reservoir or other nebulizer parts. If the liquid changes color or becomes cloudy, this may be a sign of contamination, and it should not be used.

Mixing Compatibility: The safety and effectiveness of PROVENTIL Solution for Inhalation have not been determined when one or more drugs are mixed with it in a nebulizer. Check with your physician before mixing any medications in your nebulizer. **Store PROVENTIL® Solution for Inhalation 0.5% between 2° and 25°C (36° and 77°F).**

ADDITIONAL INSTRUCTIONS:

Rev. 5/99 17979930

PROVENTIL® ℞
brand of albuterol sulfate, USP
Inhalation Solution 0.083%*
(*Potency expressed as albuterol)

DESCRIPTION

PROVENTIL Inhalation Solution contains albuterol sulfate, USP, the racemic form of albuterol, a relatively selective beta$_2$-adrenergic bronchodilator. Albuterol sulfate has the chemical name α′-[(*tert*-Butylamino)methyl]-4-hydroxy-*m*-xylene-α, α′-diol sulfate (2:1) (salt), and the following chemical structure:

$$\left[HO-C_6H_3(CH_2OH)-CHCH_2NHC(CH_3)_3 \text{ (OH on CH)} \right]_2 \cdot H_2SO_4$$

The molecular weight of albuterol sulfate is 576.7, and the empirical formula is $(C_{13}H_{21}NO_3)_2 \bullet H_2SO_4$. Albuterol sulfate is a white crystalline powder, soluble in water and slightly soluble in ethanol. The World Health Organization recommended name for albuterol base is salbutamol.

Each mL of PROVENTIL Inhalation Solution 0.083% contains 0.83 mg of albuterol (as 1.0 mg of albuterol sulfate, USP) in an isotonic aqueous solution containing sodium chloride, USP and benzalkonium chloride, NF; sulfuric acid R is used to adjust the pH between 3 and 5. The 0.083% solution requires no dilution prior to administration by nebulization. PROVENTIL Inhalation Solution 0.083% contains no sulfiting agents. It is supplied in 3 mL HDPE bottles for unit-dose dispensing.

PROVENTIL Inhalation Solution is a clear, colorless to light yellow solution.

CLINICAL PHARMACOLOGY

The primary action of beta-adrenergic drugs, including albuterol, is to stimulate adenyl cyclase, the enzyme which catalyzes the formation of cyclic-3′-5′-adenosine monophosphate (cyclic AMP) from adenosine triphosphate (ATP) in beta-adrenergic cells. The cyclic AMP thus formed mediates the cellular responses. Increased cyclic AMP levels are associated with relaxation of bronchial smooth muscle and inhibition of release of mediators of immediate hypersensitivity from cells, especially from mast cells.

In vitro studies and *in vivo* pharmacologic studies have demonstrated that albuterol has a preferential effect on beta$_2$-adrenergic receptors compared with isoproterenol. While it is recognized that beta-$_2$-adrenergic receptors are the predominant receptors in bronchial smooth muscle, data indicate that there is a population of beta-$_2$ receptors in the human heart existing in a concentration between 10% and 50%. The precise function of these receptors has not been established.

In controlled clinical trials, albuterol has been shown to have more effect on the respiratory tract, in the form of bronchial smooth muscle relaxation, than isoproterenol at comparable doses while producing fewer cardiovascular effects. Controlled clinical studies and other clinical experience have shown that inhaled albuterol, like other beta-adrenergic agonist drugs, can produce a significant cardiovascular effect in some patients, as measured by pulse rate, blood pressure, symptoms, and/or ECG changes.

Albuterol is longer acting than isoproterenol in most patients by any route of administration because it is not a substrate for the cellular uptake processes for catecholamines nor for catechol-*O*-methyl transferase.

The effects of rising doses of albuterol and isoproterenol aerosols were studied in volunteers and asthmatic patients. Results in normal volunteers indicated that the propensity for increase in heart rate for albuterol is $^1/_2$ to $^1/_4$ that of isoproterenol. In asthmatic patients similar cardiovascular differentiation between the two drugs was also seen.

Preclinical: Intravenous studies in rats with albuterol sulfate have demonstrated that albuterol crosses the blood-brain barrier and reaches brain concentrations that are amounting to approximately 5.0% of the plasma concentrations. In structures outside the blood-brain barrier (pineal and pituitary glands), albuterol concentrations were found to be 100 times those in the whole brain.

Studies in laboratory animals (minipigs, rodents, and dogs) have demonstrated the occurrence of cardiac arrhythmias and sudden death (with histologic evidence of myocardial necrosis) when beta-agonists and methylxanthines are administered concurrently. The clinical significance of these findings is unknown.

Pharmacokinetics: After either IPPB or nebulizer administration in asthmatic patients, less than 20% of a single albuterol dose was absorbed; the remaining amount was recovered from the nebulizer and apparatus and expired air. Most of the absorbed dose was recovered in the urine 24 hours after drug administration. Following a 3.0-mg dose of nebulized albuterol, the maximum albuterol plasma level at 0.5 hour was 2.1 ng/mL (range 1.4-3.2 ng/mL). It has been demonstrated that following oral administration of 4 mg of albuterol, the elimination half-life was 5 to 6 hours.

Clinical Trials: In controlled clinical trials, most patients exhibited an onset of improvement in pulmonary function within 5 minutes as determined by FEV$_1$. FEV$_1$ measurements also showed that the maximum average improvement in pulmonary function usually occurred at approximately 1 hour following inhalation of 2.5 mg of albuterol by compressor-nebulizer, and remained close to peak for 2 hours. Clinically significant improvement in pulmonary function (defined as maintenance of a 15% or more increase in FEV$_1$ over baseline values) continued for 3 to 4 hours in most patients and in some patients continued up to 6 hours.

INDICATIONS AND USAGE

PROVENTIL Inhalation Solution is indicated for the relief of bronchospasm in patients 12 years of age and older with reversible obstructive airway disease and acute attacks of bronchospasm.

CONTRAINDICATIONS

PROVENTIL Inhalation Solution is contraindicated in patients with a history of hypersensitivity to albuterol or any of its components.

WARNINGS

Deterioration of Asthma: Asthma may deteriorate acutely over a period of hours, or chronically over several days or longer. If the patient needs more doses of PROVENTIL Inhalation Solution than usual, this may be a marker of destabilization of asthma and requires re-evaluation of the patient and the treatment regimen, giving special consideration to the possible need for anti-inflammatory treatment, eg, corticosteroids.

Use of Anti-inflammatory Agents: The use of beta-adrenergic agonist bronchodilators alone may not be adequate to control asthma in many patients. Early consideration should be given to adding anti-inflammatory agents, eg, corticosteroids.

Paradoxical Bronchospasm: PROVENTIL Inhalation Solution can produce paradoxical bronchospasm, which may be life-threatening. If paradoxical bronchospasm occurs, PROVENTIL Inhalation Solution should be discontinued immediately and alternative therapy instituted. It should be recognized that paradoxical bronchospasm, when associated with inhaled formulations, frequently occurs with the first use of a new vial.

Cardiovascular Effects: PROVENTIL Inhalation Solution, like all other beta-adrenergic agonists, can produce a significant cardiovascular effect in some patients as measured by pulse rate, blood pressure, and/or symptoms. Although such effects are uncommon after administration of PROVENTIL Inhalation Solution at recommended doses, if they occur, the drug may need to be discontinued. In addition, beta-agonists have been reported to produce electrocardiogram (ECG) changes, such as flattening of the T wave, prolongation of the QTc interval, and ST segment depression. The clinical significance of these findings is unknown. Therefore, PROVENTIL Inhalation Solution, like all sympathomimetic amines, should be used with caution in patients with cardiovascular disorders, especially coronary insufficiency, cardiac arrhythmias, and hypertension.

Immediate Hypersensitivity Reactions: Immediate hypersensitivity reactions may occur after administration of albuterol, as demonstrated by rare cases of urticaria, angioedema, rash, bronchospasm, anaphylaxis, and oropharyngeal edema.

Microbial Contamination: To avoid microbial contamination, the entire contents of the unit-dose vial should be administered immediately after the vial has been opened for the first time.

PRECAUTIONS

General: Albuterol, as with all sympathomimetic amines, should be used with caution in patients with cardiovascular disorders, especially coronary insufficiency, cardiac arrhythmias, and hypertension; in patients with convulsive disorders, hyperthyroidism, or diabetes mellitus; and in patients who are unusually responsive to sympathomimetic amines. Clinically significant changes in systolic and diastolic blood pressure have been seen and could be expected to occur in some patients after use of any beta-adrenergic bronchodilator.

Large doses of intravenous albuterol have been reported to aggravate pre-existing diabetes and ketoacidosis. As with other beta-agonist medications, albuterol may produce significant hypokalemia in some patients, possibly through intracellular shunting, which has the potential to produce adverse cardiovascular effects. The decrease is usually transient, not requiring potassium supplementation.

Information for Patients: See illustrated **Patient's Instructions for Use.**

General: The action of PROVENTIL Inhalation Solution may last up to 6 hours or longer. PROVENTIL Inhalation Solution should not be used more frequently than recommended. Do not increase the dose or frequency of doses of PROVENTIL Inhalation Solution without consulting your physician. If you find that treatment with PROVENTIL Inhalation Solution becomes less effective for symptomatic relief, your symptoms become worse, and/or you need to use the product more frequently than usual, you should seek medical attention immediately. While you are using PROVENTIL Inhalation Solution, other inhaled drugs and asthma medications should be taken only as directed by your physician. Common adverse effects include palpitations, chest pain, rapid heart rate, tremor, or nervousness. If you are pregnant or nursing, contact your physician about the use of PROVENTIL Inhalation Solution. Effective use of PROVENTIL Inhalation Solution includes an understanding of the way that it should be administered. See illustrated **Patient's Instructions for Use.**

Microbial Contamination: To avoid microbial contamination, the entire contents of the unit-dose vial should be administered immediately after the vial has been opened for the first time.

Mixing Different Inhalation Solutions: Drug compatibility (physical and chemical), efficacy, and safety of PROVENTIL Inhalation Solution when mixed with other drugs in a nebulizer have not been established.

Drug Interactions: Other short-acting sympathomimetic aerosol bronchodilators or epinephrine should not be used concomitantly with albuterol.

Beta Blockers: Beta-adrenergic receptor blocking agents not only block the pulmonary effect of beta-agonists, such as PROVENTIL Inhalation Solution, but may produce severe bronchospasm in asthmatic patients. Therefore, patients with asthma should not normally be treated with beta blockers. However, under certain circumstances, eg, as prophylaxis after myocardial infarction, there may be no acceptable alternatives to the use of beta-adrenergic blocking agents in patients with asthma. In this setting, cardioselective beta blockers could be considered, although they should be administered with caution.

Diuretics: The ECG changes and/or hypokalemia that may result from the administration of nonpotassium-sparing diuretics (such as loop or thiazide diuretics) can be acutely worsened by beta-agonists, especially when the recommended dose of beta-agonist is exceeded. Although the clinical significance of these effects is not known, caution is advised in the coadministration of beta-agonists with nonpotassium-sparing diuretics.

Digoxin: Mean decreases of 16% to 22% in serum digoxin levels were demonstrated after single dose intravenous and oral administration of albuterol, respectively, to normal volunteers who had received digoxin for 10 days. The clinical significance of this finding for patients with obstructive airway disease who are receiving albuterol and digoxin on a chronic basis is unclear. Nevertheless, it would be prudent to carefully evaluate the serum digoxin levels in patients who are currently receiving digoxin and albuterol.

Monoamine Oxidase Inhibitors or Tricyclic Antidepressants: Albuterol should be administered with extreme caution to patients being treated with monoamine oxidase inhibitors or tricyclic antidepressants, or within 2 weeks of discontinuation of such agents, because the action of albuterol on the vascular system may be potentiated.

Carcinogenesis, Mutagenesis, and Impairment of Fertility: In a 2-year study in Sprague-Dawley rats, albuterol sulfate caused a significant dose-related increase in the incidence of benign leiomyomas of the mesovarium at the above dietary doses of 2 mg/kg (approximately two times the maximum recommended daily inhalation dose for adults on an mg/m^2 basis). In another study, this effect was blocked by the coadministration of a propranolol, a nonselective beta-adrenergic antagonist.

In an 18-month study in CD-1 mice, albuterol sulfate showed no evidence of tumorigenicity at dietary doses up to 500 mg/kg (approximately 200 times the maximum recommended daily inhalation dose for adults on an mg/m^2 basis). In a 22-month study in the Golden Hamster, albuterol sulfate showed no evidence of tumorigenicity at dietary doses up to 50 mg/kg (approximately 25 times the maximum recommended daily inhalation dose for adults on an mg/m^2 basis).

Albuterol sulfate was not mutagenic in the Ames test with or without metabolic activation using tester strains *S. typhimurium* TA1537, TA1538, and TA98 or *E. coli* WP2, WP2uvrA, and WP67. No forward mutation was seen in yeast strain *S. cerevisiae* S9 nor any mitotic gene conversion in yeast strain *S. cerevisiae* JD1 with or without metabolic activation. Fluctuation assays in *S. typhimurium* TA98 and *E. coli* WP2, both with metabolic activation, were negative. Albuterol sulfate was not clastogenic in a human peripheral lymphocyte assay or in an AH1 strain mouse micronucleus assay.

Reproduction studies in rats demonstrated no evidence of impaired fertility at oral doses of albuterol sulfate up to 50 mg/kg (approximately 40 times the maximum recommended daily inhalation dose for adults on an mg/m^2 basis).

Teratogenic Effects—Pregnancy Category C: Albuterol sulfate has been shown to be teratogenic in mice. A study in CD-1 mice at subcutaneous (sc) doses at and above 0.25 mg/kg (corresponding to less than the maximum recommended daily inhalation dose for adults on an mg/m^2 basis), induced cleft palate formation in 5 of 111 (4.5%) fetuses. At an sc dose of 2.5 mg/kg (approximately equal to the maximum recommended daily inhalation dose for adults on an mg/m^2 basis) albuterol sulfate induced cleft palate formation in 10 of 108 (9.3%) fetuses. The drug did not induce cleft palate formation when administered at an sc dose of 0.025 mg/kg (corresponding to less than the maximum recommended daily inhalation dose for adults on an mg/m^2 basis). Cleft palate also occurred in 22 of 72 (30.5%) fetuses from females treated with 2.5 mg/kg isoproterenol (positive control) administered subcutaneously.

A reproduction study in Stride Dutch rabbits revealed cranioschisis in 7 of 19 (37%) fetuses when albuterol was administered orally at a dose of 50 mg/kg (approximately 80 times the maximum recommended daily inhalation dose for adults on an mg/m^2 basis).

Studies in pregnant rats with tritiated albuterol demonstrated that approximately 10% of the circulating maternal drug is transferred to the fetus. Disposition in the fetal lungs is comparable to maternal lungs, but fetal liver disposition is 1% of the maternal liver levels.

There are no adequate and well-controlled studies in pregnant women. Because animal reproduction studies are not always predictive of human response, albuterol should be used during pregnancy only if the potential benefit justifies the potential risk to the fetus.

During worldwide marketing experience, various congenital anomalies, including cleft palate and limb defects, have been reported in the offspring of patients being treated with albuterol. Some of the mothers were taking multiple medications during their pregnancies. Because no consistent pattern of defects can be discerned, a relationship between albuterol use and congenital anomalies has not been established.

Use in Labor and Delivery—Use in Labor: Because of the potential for beta-agonist interference with uterine contractility, use of PROVENTIL Inhalation Solution for relief of bronchospasm during labor should be restricted to those patients in whom the benefits clearly outweigh the risk.

Tocolysis: Albuterol has not been approved for the management of preterm labor. The benefit:risk ratio when albuterol is administered for tocolysis has not been established. Serious adverse reactions, including maternal pulmonary edema, have been reported during or following treatment of premature labor with beta-agonists, including albuterol.

Nursing Mothers: It is not known whether this drug is excreted in human milk. Because of the potential for tumorigenicity shown for albuterol in some animal studies, a decision should be made whether to discontinue nursing or to discontinue the drug, taking into account the importance of the drug to the mother.

Pediatric Use: Safety and effectiveness of albuterol inhalation solution and solution for inhalation in children below the age of 12 years have not been established.

ADVERSE REACTIONS

The results of clinical trials with PROVENTIL Inhalation Solution in 135 patients showed the following side effects which were considered probably or possibly drug related:

Percent Incidence of Adverse Reactions

Reaction	Percent Incidence
Central Nervous System	
Tremors	20
Dizziness	7
Nervousness	4
Headache	3
Insomnia	1
Gastrointestinal	
Nausea	4
Dyspepsia	1
Ear, Nose, and Throat	
Nasal congestion	1
Pharyngitis	<1
Cardiovascular	
Tachycardia	1
Hypertension	1
Respiratory	
Bronchospasm	8
Cough	4
Bronchitis	4
Wheezing	1

No clinically relevant laboratory abnormalities related to PROVENTIL Inhalation Solution were determined in these studies.

Cases of urticaria, angioedema, rash, bronchospasm, hoarseness, oropharyngeal edema, and arrhythmias (including atrial fibrillation, supraventricular tachycardia, and extrasystoles) have also been reported after the use of inhaled albuterol.

OVERDOSAGE

The expected symptoms with overdosage are those of excessive beta-adrenergic stimulation and/or occurrence or exaggeration of any of the symptoms listed under **ADVERSE REACTIONS** eg, angina, hypertension, tachycardia with rates up to 200 beats per minute, arrhythmias, nervousness, headache, tremor, dry mouth, palpitation, nausea, dizziness, malaise, and insomnia. In addition, seizures, hypotension, fatigue, and hypokalemia may also occur. As with all sympathomimetic aerosol medications, cardiac arrest and even death may be associated with abuse of PROVENTIL Inhalation Solution. Treatment consists of discontinuation of PROVENTIL Inhalation Solution together with appropriate symptomatic therapy. The judicious use of a cardioselective beta-receptor blocker may be considered, bearing in mind that such medication can produce bronchospasm. There is insufficient evidence to determine if dialysis is beneficial for overdosage of PROVENTIL Inhalation Solution.

The oral median lethal dose of albuterol sulfate in mice is greater than 2000 mg/kg (approximately 810 times the maximum recommended daily inhalation dose for adults on an mg/m^2 basis). In mature rats, the subcutaneous (sc) median lethal dose of albuterol sulfate is approximately 450 mg/kg (approximately 360 times the maximum recommended daily inhalation dose for adults on an mg/m^2 basis). In small young rats, the sc median lethal dose is approximately 2000 mg/kg (approximately 1600 times the maximum recommended daily inhalation dose for adults on an mg/m^2 basis). The inhalational median lethal dose has not been determined in animals.

DOSAGE AND ADMINISTRATION

The usual dosage for adults and pediatric patients 12 years of age and older is 2.5 mg of albuterol administered three to four times daily by nebulization. More frequent administration or higher doses are not recommended. To administer 2.5 mg of albuterol, administer the entire contents of one unit-dose bottle (3 mL of 0.083% nebulizer solution) by nebulization. The flow rate is regulated to suite the particular nebulizer so that the PROVENTIL Inhalation Solution will be delivered over approximately 5 to 15 minutes.

Drug compatibility (physical and chemical), efficacy, and safety of PROVENTIL Inhalation Solution when mixed with other drugs in a nebulizer have not been established.

The use of PROVENTIL Inhalation Solution can be continued as medically indicated to control recurring bouts of bronchospasm. During treatment, most patients gain optimum benefit from regular use of the nebulizer solution.

If a previously effective dosage regimen fails to provide the usual relief, medical advice should be sought immediately, as this is often a sign of seriously worsening asthma which would require reassessment of therapy.

Microbial Contamination: To avoid microbial contamination, the entire contents of the unit-dose vial should be administered immediately after the vial has been opened for the first time.

The nebulizer should be cleaned in accordance with the manufacturer's instructions. Failure to do so could lead to bacterial contamination of the nebulizer and possible infection.

HOW SUPPLIED

PROVENTIL Inhalation Solution 0.083% is a clear, colorless to light yellow solution, and is supplied in unit-dose HDPE (high-density polyethylene) bottles of 3 mL fill each, boxes of 25 (NDC 0085-0209-01). **Store between 2° and 25°C (36° and 77°F).**

Schering Corporation
Kenilworth, NJ 07033 USA.
Rev. 8/99 23348101

Patient's Instructions for Use

PROVENTIL® Inhalation Solution 0.083%*
brand of albuterol sulfate, USP
*Potency expressed as albuterol
Note: This is a unit-dose bottle.
No dilution is required.
Read complete instructions carefully before using.

UNIT DOSE

1. Twist open the top of one bottle and pour the entire contents into the nebulizer reservoir (Figure 1).

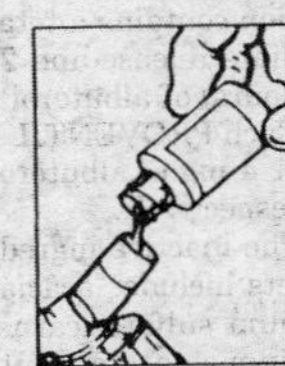

Figure 1

2. Connect the nebulizer reservoir to the mouthpiece or face mask (Figure 2).
3. Connect the nebulizer to the compressor.

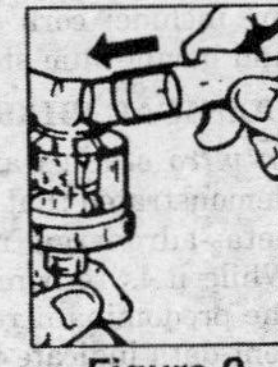

Figure 2

4. Sit in a comfortable, upright position; place the mouthpiece in your mouth (Figure 3) (or put the face mask on); and turn the compressor on.
5. Breathe as calmly, deeply, and evenly as possible until no more mist is formed in the nebulizer chamber (about 5-15 minutes). At this point, the treatment is finished.
6. Clean the nebulizer (see manufacturer's instructions). Failure to clean the nebulizer in accordance with the manufacturer's instructions could lead to bacterial contamination of the nebulizer and possible infection.

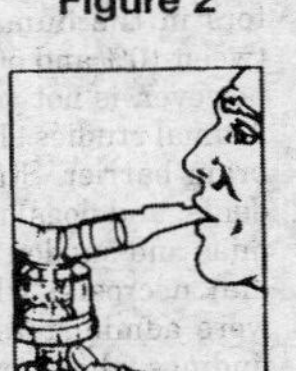

Figure 3

Note: Use only as directed by your physician. More frequent administration or higher doses are not recommended.

Mixing Compatibility: The safety and effectiveness of PROVENTIL Inhalation Solution have not been determined when one or more drugs are mixed with it in a nebulizer. Check with your physician before mixing any medications in your nebulizer.

Microbial Contamination: To avoid microbial contamination, the entire contents of the unit-dose vial should be administered immediately after the vial has been opened for

Continued on next page

Information on Schering products appearing on these pages is effective as of January 2000.

Proventil Solution—Cont.

the first time. **Store PROVENTIL® Inhalation Solution 0.083% between 2° and 25°C (36° and 77°F).**
ADDITIONAL INSTRUCTIONS:

PROVENTIL® ℞
brand of albuterol sulfate, USP
REPETABS® brand of
extended-release Tablets

PROVENTIL®
brand of albuterol sulfate, USP
Tablets

DESCRIPTION

PROVENTIL REPETABS Tablets and PROVENTIL Tablets contain albuterol sulfate, USP, the racemic form of albuterol and a relatively selective beta$_2$-adrenergic bronchodilator. Albuterol sulfate has the chemical name α^1-[(*tert*-Butylamino)methyl]-4-hydroxy-*m*-xylene-α, α′-diol sulfate (2:1) (salt), and the following chemical structure:

[HOCH$_2$; HO; CHCH$_2$NHC(CH$_3$)$_3$; OH]$_2$ • H_2SO_4

The molecular weight of albuterol sulfate is 576.7, and the empirical formula $(C_{13}H_{21}NO_3)_2 \bullet H_2SO_4$. Albuterol sulfate is a white crystalline powder, soluble in water and slightly soluble in ethanol. The World Health Organization recommended name for albuterol base is salbutamol.
Each PROVENTIL REPETABS Tablet for oral administration contains a total of 4 mg (2 mg in the coating for immediate release and 2 mg in the core for release after several hours) of albuterol as 4.8 mg of albuterol sulfate.
Each PROVENTIL Tablet for oral administration contains 2 or 4 mg of albuterol as 2.4 and 4.8 mg of albuterol sulfate, respectively.
The inactive ingredients for PROVENTIL REPETABS Tablets include: acacia, butylparaben, calcium phosphate, calcium sulfate, carnauba wax, corn starch, lactose, magnesium stearate, neutral soap, oleic acid, rosin, sugar, talc, titanium dioxide, white wax, and zein.
The inactive ingredients for PROVENTIL Tablets, 2 and 4 mg include: corn starch food grade, lactose monohydrate, and magnesium stearate, NF.

CLINICAL PHARMACOLOGY

In vitro studies and *in vivo* pharmacologic studies have demonstrated that PROVENTIL has a preferential effect on beta$_2$-adrenergic receptors compared with isoproterenol. While it is recognized that beta$_2$-adrenergic receptors are the predominant receptors in bronchial smooth muscle, recent data indicate that there is a population of beta$_2$-receptors in the human heart, existing in a concentration between 10% and 50%. The precise function of these receptors, however, is not yet established.
Animal studies show that albuterol does not pass the blood-brain barrier. Studies in laboratory animals (minipigs, rodents, and dogs) recorded the occurrence of cardiac arrhythmias and sudden death (with histologic evidence of myocardial necrosis) when beta-agonists and methylxanthines were administered concurrently. The significance of these findings when applied to humans is currently unknown.
Albuterol is longer acting than isoproterenol in most patients by any route of administration because it is not a substrate for the cellular uptake processes for catecholamines nor for catechol-*O*-methyl transferase.
Pharmacokinetics and Disposition: Albuterol is rapidly and well absorbed following oral administration. In studies involving normal volunteers, the mean steady-state peak and trough plasma levels of albuterol were 6.7 and 3.8 ng/mL, respectively, following dosing with a 2 mg PROVENTIL Tablet every 6 hours and 14.8 and 8.6 ng/mL, respectively, following dosing with a 4 mg PROVENTIL Tablet every 6 hours. Maximum albuterol plasma levels are usually obtained between 2 and 3 hours after dosing and the elimination half-life is 5 to 6 hours. These data indicate that albuterol, administered orally, is dose proportional and exhibits dose independent pharmacokinetics.
PROVENTIL REPETABS Tablets have been formulated to provide a duration of action of up to 12 hours. In studies conducted in normal adult volunteers, the mean steady-state peak and trough plasma levels of albuterol were 6.5 and 3.0 ng/mL, respectively, following dosing with a 4 mg PROVENTIL REPETABS Tablet every 12 hours. In addition, it has been shown that administration of a 4 mg PROVENTIL REPETABS Tablet every 12 hours, and a 2 mg PROVENTIL Tablet every 6 hours for 5 days gave comparable peak albuterol levels and similar extent of absorption at steady state.
In other studies, the analysis of urine samples of subjects given tritiated albuterol (4 to 10 mg) orally showed that 65% to 90% of the dose was excreted over 3 days, with the majority of the dose being excreted within the first 24 hours. Sixty percent of this radioactivity was shown to be the metabolite of albuterol. Feces collected over this period contained 4% of the administered dose.
Clinical Studies: In controlled clinical trials in patients with asthma, the onset of improvement in pulmonary function, as measured by maximal mid-expiratory flow rate, MMEF, was noted within 30 minutes after a dose of PROVENTIL Tablets with peak improvement occurring between 2 and 3 hours. In controlled clinical trials, in which measurements were conducted for 6 hours, significant clinical improvement in pulmonary function (defined as maintaining a 15% or more increase in FEV_1 and a 20% or more increase in MMEF over baseline values) was observed in 60% of patients at 4 hours and in 40% at 6 hours. In other single-dose, controlled clinical trials, clinically significant improvement was observed in at least 40% of the patients at 8 hours with the 4 mg PROVENTIL Tablet. No decrease in the effectiveness of PROVENTIL Tablets has been reported in patients who received long-term treatment with the drug in uncontrolled studies for periods up to 6 months.
In another controlled clinical study in adult asthmatic patients, it has been demonstrated that the initiation of therapy with either the 4 mg PROVENTIL REPETABS Tablet dosed every 12 hours, or the 2 mg PROVENTIL Tablet dosed every 6 hours, achieve therapeutically equivalent effects.

INDICATIONS AND USAGE

PROVENTIL REPETABS Tablets and PROVENTIL Tablets are indicated for the relief of bronchospasm in patients 6 years of age or older with reversible obstructive airway disease.

CONTRAINDICATIONS

PROVENTIL REPETABS Tablets and PROVENTIL Tablets are contraindicated in patients with a history of hypersensitivity to any of their components.

PRECAUTIONS

General: Since albuterol is a sympathomimetic amine, it should be used with caution in patients with cardiovascular disorders, including ischemic heart disease, hypertension, or cardiac arrhythmias, in patients with hyperthyroidism or diabetes mellitus, and in patients who are unusually responsive to sympathomimetic amines or who have convulsive disorders. Significant changes in systolic and diastolic blood pressure could be expected to occur in some patients after use of any beta adrenergic bronchodilator.
Large doses of intravenous albuterol have been reported to aggravate preexisting diabetes mellitus and ketoacidosis. Additionally, albuterol and other beta agonists, when given intravenously, may cause a decrease in serum potassium, possibly through intracellular shunting. The decrease is usually transient not requiring supplementation. The relevance of these observations to the use of PROVENTIL REPETABS Tablets and PROVENTIL Tablets is unknown.
Information for Patients: Patients being treated with PROVENTIL REPETABS Tablets or PROVENTIL Tablets should receive the following information and instructions. This information is intended to aid in the safe and effective use of this medication. It is not a disclosure of all possible adverse or intended effects.
PROVENTIL REPETABS Tablets should not be chewed, crushed, or mixed in food.
PROVENTIL REPETABS Tablets and PROVENTIL Tablets should not be taken more frequently than recommended. Do not increase the dose or frequency of either medication, or add other medications to your therapy without medical consultation. If symptoms get worse, medical consultation should be sought promptly. If pregnant or nursing, consult with your physician.
Drug Interactions: The concomitant use of PROVENTIL REPETABS Tablets or PROVENTIL Tablets and other oral sympathomimetic agents is not recommended since such combined use may lead to deleterious cardiovascular effects. This recommendation does not preclude the judicious use of an aerosol bronchodilator of the adrenergic stimulant type in patients receiving PROVENTIL REPETABS Tablets or PROVENTIL Tablets. Such concomitant use, however, should be individualized and not given on a routine basis. If regular coadministration is required, then alternative therapy should be considered.
Albuterol should be administered with extreme caution to patients being treated with monoamine oxidase inhibitors or tricyclic antidepressants, since the action of albuterol on the vascular system may be potentiated.
Beta-receptor blocking agents and albuterol inhibit the effect of each other.
Since albuterol may lower serum potassium, care should be taken in patients also using other drugs which lower serum potassium as the effects may be additive.
After single-dose administration of albuterol to normal volunteers who had received digoxin for 10 days, a 16% to 22% decrease in serum digoxin levels was demonstrated. The clinical significance of these findings for patients with obstructive airway disease who are receiving albuterol and digoxin on a chronic basis is unclear. Nevertheless, it would be prudent to carefully evaluate the serum digoxin levels in patients who are concurrently receiving digoxin and albuterol.
Carcinogenesis, Mutagenesis, and Impairment of Fertility: Albuterol sulfate, like other agents in its class, caused a significant dose-related increase in the incidence of benign leiomyomas of the mesovarium in a 2-year study in the rat, at doses corresponding to 3, 16 and 78 times the maximum human oral dose. In another study this effect was blocked by the coadministration of propranolol. The relevance of these findings to humans is not known. An 18-month study in mice and a lifetime study in hamsters revealed no evidence of tumorigenicity.
Studies with albuterol revealed no evidence of mutagenesis. Reproduction studies in rats revealed no evidence of impaired fertility.
Teratogenic Effects—Pregnancy Category C: Albuterol has been shown to be teratogenic in mice when given subcutaneously in doses corresponding to 0.4 times the maximum human oral dose. There are no adequate and well-controlled studies in pregnant women. Albuterol should be used during pregnancy only if the potential benefit justifies the potential risk to the fetus. A reproduction study in CD-1 mice with albuterol showed cleft palate formation in 5 of 111 (4.5%) fetuses at 0.25 mg/kg and in 10 of 108 (9.3%) fetuses at 2.5 mg/kg; none were observed at 0.025 mg/kg. Cleft palate also occurred in 22 of 72 (30.5%) fetuses treated with 2.5 mg/kg isoproterenol (positive control). A reproduction study in Stride Dutch rabbits revealed cranioschisis in 7 of 19 (37%) fetuses of 50 mg/kg, corresponding to 78 times the maximum human oral dose of albuterol.
During marketing, various congenital anomalies, including cleft palate and limb defects, have been reported in the offspring of patients being treated with albuterol. Some of the mothers were taking multiple medications during their pregnancies. Because no consistent pattern of defects can be discerned a relationship between albuterol use and congenital anomalies cannot be established.
Labor and Delivery: Oral albuterol has been shown to delay preterm labor in some reports. There are presently no well-controlled studies which demonstrate what it will stop preterm labor or prevent labor at term. Therefore, cautious use of PROVENTIL REPETABS Tablets or PROVENTIL Tablets is required in pregnant patients when given for relief of bronchospasm so as to avoid interference with uterine contractibility.
Nursing Mothers: It is not known whether this drug is excreted in human milk. Because of the potential for tumorigenicity shown for albuterol in some animal studies, a decision should be made whether to discontinue nursing or to discontinue the drug, taking into account the importance of the drug to the mother.
Pediatric Use: The safety and effectiveness of PROVENTIL Tablets and PROVENTIL REPETABS Tablets have been established in pediatric patients 6 years of age and older. Use of PROVENTIL REPETABS Tablets in these age groups is supported by evidence from adequate and well-controlled studies of PROVENTIL REPETABS Tablets in adults; the likelihood that the disease course, pathophysiology, and the drug's effect in pediatric and adult patients are substantially similar; the established safety and effectiveness of PROVENTIL Tablets in pediatric patients 6 years of age and older; and one clinical trial that provides evidence of the safety of PROVENTIL REPETABS Tablets in pediatric patients aged 6 to 12 years. The recommended dose of PROVENTIL REPETABS Tablets for the pediatric population is based upon the recommended pediatric dosing of PROVENTIL Tablets and pharmacokinetic studies in adults showing PROVENTIL REPETABS Tablets to have similar peak albuterol levels (ie, C_{max}) and exposures (ie, AUC) as PROVENTIL Tablets administered every 6 hours at one-half of the PROVENTIL REPETABS Tablets dose.
Safety and effectiveness in pediatric patients below the age of 6 years have not been established for PROVENTIL Tablets and PROVENTIL REPETABS Tablets.

ADVERSE REACTIONS

The adverse reactions to albuterol are similar in nature to those of other sympathomimetic agents. The most frequent adverse reactions to PROVENTIL Tablets were nervousness and tremor, with each occurring in approximately 20 of 100 patients (20%). Other reported reactions were headache, 7 of 100 patients (7%); tachycardia and palpitations, 5 of 100 patients (5%); muscle cramps, 3 of 100 patients (3%); insomnia, nausea, weakness, and dizziness, each occurred in 2 of 100 patients (2%). Drowsiness, flushing, restlessness, irritability, chest discomfort, and difficulty in micturition each occurred in less than 1 of 100 patients (less than 1%).
In a clinical study of 1 week duration in adults, comparing a 4 mg PROVENTIL REPETABS Tablet administered every 12 hours to a 2 mg PROVENTIL Tablet administered every 6 hours, the following adverse reactions considered to be possibly or probably treatment related were reported: nervousness in 1 of 50 (2%) and 3 of 50 patients (6%) for PROVENTIL REPETABS Tablets and PROVENTIL Tablets, respectively; nausea in 2 of 50 (4%) for both; vomiting in 1 of 50 (2%) and 2 of 50 (4%) for PROVENTIL REPETABS Tablets and PROVENTIL Tablets, respectively; somnolence in 1 of 50 (2%) for both. The following adverse reactions were reported for PROVENTIL Tablets only: tremor in 3 of 50 patients (6%); tinnitus, dyspepsia, and rash each occurred in 1 of 50 patients (2%).

Although not reported for PROVENTIL REPETABS Tablets in the above study in adults, there have been reports of tremor in other trials. When all clinical experience is considered, the incidence of tremor is approximately the same as that seen with PROVENTIL Tablets.

A placebo-controlled trial of 4 weeks duration in 157 mild-to-moderate asthmatic children aged 6 to 12 years, demonstrated the safety of escalating doses of PROVENTIL REPETABS Tablets. In this study, the starting dose of PROVENTIL REPETABS Tablets was 4 mg twice daily. Patients were advanced to a maximum of 12 mg PROVENTIL REPETABS Tablets twice daily by the investigator, based on patient tolerance and response. Only one of the 79 children treated with PROVENTIL REPETABS Tablets was advanced to the maximum daily dose of 12 mg twice daily. The following treatment-related adverse events occurred in more than 5% of treated patients and were greater in PROVENTIL REPETABS Tablets patients when compared to placebo: headache (22% PROVENTIL REPETABS Tablets, 9% placebo); tremor (10% PROVENTIL REPETABS Tablets, 1% placebo); tachycardia and palpitations (8% PROVENTIL REPETABS Tablets, 1% placebo); insomnia (11% PROVENTIL REPETABS Tablets, 5% placebo); and nervousness (13% PROVENTIL REPETABS Tablets, 6% placebo). Other adverse events were noted in 5% or fewer patients, or had equal or greater rates of occurrence in placebo patients than in PROVENTIL REPETABS Tablets patients.

In addition to those adverse reactions reported above, albuterol, like other sympathomimetic agents, can cause adverse reactions such as hypertension, angina, vomiting, vertigo, central nervous system stimulation, unusual taste, and drying or irritation of the oropharynx.

The reactions are generally transient in nature, and it is usually not necessary to discontinue treatment with PROVENTIL REPETABS Tablets or PROVENTIL Tablets. In selected cases, however, dosage may be reduced temporarily; after the reaction has subsided, dosage should be increased in small increments to the optimal dosage.

OVERDOSAGE

Manifestations of overdosage include anginal pain, hypertension, hypokalemia, and exaggeration of the pharmacological effects listed in **ADVERSE REACTIONS.**

The oral LD_{50} in rats and mice was greater than 2,000 mg/kg.

There is insufficient evidence to determine if dialysis is beneficial for overdosage of PROVENTIL REPETABS Tablets or PROVENTIL Tablets.

DOSAGE AND ADMINISTRATION

The following dosages of PROVENTIL REPETABS Tablets and PROVENTIL Tablets are expressed in terms of albuterol base.

PROVENTIL REPETABS Tablets

Usual Dose: **Pediatric Patients 6 to 11 years of age:** The usual starting dosage of PROVENTIL REPETABS Tablets is 4 mg (one tablet) every 12 hours.

Adults and Pediatric Patients 12 years and over: The usual starting dosage of PROVENTIL REPETABS Tablets is 4 or 8 mg (one or two tablets) every 12 hours.

Dosage Adjustment in Pediatric Patients aged 6 to 11 years: Doses of PROVENTIL REPETABS Tablets above 4 mg twice a day should be used only when the patient fails to respond to this dose while on otherwise optimized asthma therapy. In such instances, the PROVENTIL REPETABS Tablets dose may be increased cautiously stepwise as tolerated if a favorable response does not occur with the 4 mg twice daily initial dose. The maximum recommended dose of PROVENTIL REPETABS Tablets in pediatric patients aged 6 to 11 years is 12 mg twice a day.

Dosage Adjustment in Adults and Pediatric Patients 12 years of age and over: Doses of PROVENTIL REPETABS Tablets above 8 mg twice a day should be used only when the patient fails to respond to this dose while on otherwise optimized asthma therapy. The PROVENTIL REPETABS Tablets dose may be increased cautiously stepwise as tolerated if a favorable response does not occur with the 8 mg twice daily dose. The maximum recommended dose of PROVENTIL REPETABS Tablets in adults and pediatric patients over 12 years of age is 16 mg twice a day.

Switching to PROVENTIL REPETABS Tablets: Patients currently maintained on PROVENTIL Tablets can be switched to PROVENTIL REPETABS Tablets. For example, the administration of a 4 mg PROVENTIL REPETABS Tablet every 12 hours is clinically comparable to one 2 mg PROVENTIL Tablet every 6 hours. Multiples of this regimen up to the maximum recommended daily dose also apply.

PROVENTIL Tablets

Usual Dose: **Pediatric Patients 6 to 12 years of age:** The usual starting dosage for pediatric patients 6 to 12 years of age is 2 mg three or four times a day.

Adults and Pediatric Patients 12 years and over: The usual starting dosage for adults and pediatric patients 12 years and over is 2 mg or 4 mg three or four times a day.

Dosage Adjustment: For pediatric patients from 6 to 12 years of age who fail to respond to the initial starting dosage of 2 mg four times a day, the dosage may be cautiously increased stepwise, but not to exceed 24 mg per day (given in divided doses).

For adults and pediatric patients 12 years and over, a dosage above 4 mg four times a day should be used only when the patient fails to respond to lower doses. The dose should be increased cautiously stepwise up to a maximum of 8 mg four times a day as tolerated if a favorable response does not occur with the 4 mg initial dose.

Elderly Patients and Those Sensitive to Beta-Adrenergic Stimulators: An initial dosage of 2 mg three or four times a day is recommended for elderly patients and for those with a history of unusual sensitivity to beta-adrenergic stimulators. If adequate bronchodilation is not obtained, dosage may be increased gradually to as much as 8 mg three or four times a day.

The total daily dose should not exceed 24 mg per day in pediatric patients from 6 to 12 years of age, and 32 mg per day in adults and pediatric patients 12 years and over.

HOW SUPPLIED

PROVENTIL REPETABS Tablets, 4 mg albuterol as the sulfate (2 mg in the coating for immediate release and 2 mg in the core for release after several hours), white, round, coated tablets, branded in red on one side with the Schering trademark and product identification numbers, 431, bottles of 100 (NDC 0085-0431-02) and 500 (NDC 0085-0431-03) and boxes of 100 for unit dose dispensing (NDC 0085-0431-04).

PROVENTIL Tablets, 2 mg albuterol as the sulfate, white, round, compressed tablets, impressed with the product name (PROVENTIL) and the number 2 on one side, and product identification numbers, 252, and scored on the other, bottles of 100 (NDC 0085-0252-02) and 500 (NDC 0085-0252-03).

PROVENTIL Tablets, 4 mg albuterol as the sulfate, white, round, compressed tablets, impressed with the product name (PROVENTIL) and the number 4 on one side, and product identification numbers, 573, and scored on the other, bottles of 100 (NDC 0085-0573-02) and 500 (NDC 0085-0573-03).

Store PROVENTIL REPETABS Tablets between 2° and 25°C (36° and 77°F), and PROVENTIL Tablets between 2° and 30°C (36° and 86°F). Protect PROVENTIL REPETABS Tablets in the unit dose box from excessive moisture.

Schering Corporation
Kenilworth, NJ 07033 USA

Rev. 10/97 17543342

Shown in Product Identification Guide, page 334

PROVENTIL® HFA ℞

(albuterol sulfate)
Inhalation Aerosol
FOR ORAL INHALATION ONLY
Prescribing Information

DESCRIPTION

The active component of PROVENTIL HFA (albuterol sulfate) Inhalation Aerosol is albuterol sulfate, USP racemic α[1][(*tert*-Butylamino)methyl]-4-hydroxy-*m*-xylene-α,α′-diol sulfate (2:1)(salt), a relatively selective $beta_2$-adrenergic bronchodilator having the following chemical structure:

Albuterol sulfate is the official generic name in the United States. The World Health Organization recommended name for the drug is salbutamol sulfate. The molecular weight of albuterol sulfate is 576.7, and the empirical formula is $(C_{13}H_{21}NO_3)_2 \bullet H_2SO_4$. Albuterol sulfate is a white to off-white crystalline solid. It is soluble in water and slightly soluble in ethanol. PROVENTIL HFA Inhalation Aerosol is a pressurized metered-dose aerosol unit for oral inhalation. It contains a microcrystalline suspension of albuterol sulfate in propellant HFA-134a (1,1,1,2-tetrafluoroethane), ethanol, and oleic acid.

Each actuation delivers 120 mcg albuterol sulfate, USP from the valve and 108 mcg albuterol sulfate, USP from the mouthpiece (equivalent to 90 mcg of albuterol base from the mouthpiece). Each canister provides 200 inhalations. It is recommended to prime the inhaler before using for the first time and in cases where the inhaler has not been used for more than 2 weeks by releasing four "test sprays" into the air, away from the face.

This product does not contain chlorofluorocarbons (CFCs) as the propellant.

CLINICAL PHARMACOLOGY

Mechanism of Action *In vitro* studies and *in vivo* pharmacologic studies have demonstrated that albuterol has a preferential effect on $beta_2$-adrenergic receptors compared with isoproterenol. While it is recognized that $beta_2$-adrenergic receptors are the predominant receptors on bronchial smooth muscle, data indicate that there is a population of $beta_2$ receptors in the human heart existing in a concentration between 10% and 50% of cardiac beta-adrenergic receptors. The precise function of these receptors has not been established. (See **WARNINGS** for **Cardiovascular Effects.**)

Activation of $beta_2$-adrenergic receptors on airway smooth muscle leads to the activation of adenylcyclase and to an increase in the intracellular concentration of cyclic-3′,5′-adenosine monophosphate (cyclic AMP). This increase of cyclic AMP leads to the activation of protein kinase A, which inhibits the phosphorylation of myosin and lowers intracellular ionic calcium concentrations, resulting in relaxation. Albuterol relaxes the smooth muscles of all airways, from the trachea to the terminal bronchioles. Albuterol acts as a functional antagonist to relax the airway irrespective of the spasmogen involved, thus protecting against all bronchoconstrictor challenges. Increased cyclic AMP concentrations are also associated with the inhibition of release of mediators from mast cells in the airway.

Albuterol has been shown in most clinical trials to have more effect on the respiratory tract, in the form of bronchial smooth muscle relaxation, than isoproterenol at comparable doses while producing fewer cardiovascular effects. Controlled clinical studies and other clinical experience have shown that inhaled albuterol, like other beta-adrenergic agonist drugs, can produce a significant cardiovascular effect in some patients, as measured by pulse rate, blood pressure, symptoms, and/or electrocardiographic changes.

Preclinical Intravenous studies in rats with albuterol sulfate have demonstrated that albuterol crosses the blood-brain barrier and reaches brain concentrations amounting to approximately 5% of the plasma concentrations. In structures outside the blood-brain barrier (pineal and pituitary glands), albuterol concentrations were found to be 100 times those in the whole brain.

Studies in laboratory animals (minipigs, rodents, and dogs) have demonstrated the occurrence of cardiac arrhythmias and sudden death (with histologic evidence of myocardial necrosis) when β-agonists and methylxanthines were administered concurrently. The clinical significance of these findings is unknown.

Propellant HFA-134a is devoid of pharmacological activity except at very high doses in animals (380–1300 times the maximum human exposure based on comparisons of AUC values), primarily producing ataxia, tremors, dyspnea, or salivation. These are similar to effects produced by the structurally related chlorofluorocarbons (CFCs), which have been used extensively in metered dose inhalers.

In animals and humans, propellant HFA-134a was found to be rapidly absorbed and rapidly eliminated, with an elimination half-life of 3 to 27 minutes in animals and 5 to 7 minutes in humans. Time to maximum plasma concentration (Tmax) and mean residence time are both extremely short leading to a transient appearance of HFA-134a in the blood with no evidence of accumulation.

Pharmacokinetics In a single-dose bioavailability study which enrolled six healthy, male volunteers, transient low albuterol levels (close to the lower limit of quantitation) were observed after administration of two puffs from both PROVENTIL HFA Inhalation Aerosol and a CFC 11/12 propelled albuterol inhaler. No formal pharmacokinetic analyses were possible for either treatment, but systemic albuterol levels appeared similar.

Clinical Trials In a 12-week, randomized, double-blind, double-dummy, active- and placebo-controlled trial, 565 patients with asthma were evaluated for the bronchodilator efficacy of PROVENTIL HFA Inhalation Aerosol (193 patients) in comparison to a CFC 11/12 propelled albuterol inhaler (186 patients) and an HFA-134a placebo inhaler (186 patients).

Serial FEV_1 measurements (shown below as percent change from test-day baseline) demonstrated that two inhalations of PROVENTIL HFA Inhalation Aerosol produced significantly greater improvement in pulmonary function than placebo and produced outcomes which were clinically comparable to a CFC 11/12 propelled albuterol inhaler.

The mean time to onset of a 15% increase in FEV_1 was 6 minutes and the mean time to peak effect was 50 to 55 minutes. The mean duration of effect as measured by a 15% increase in FEV_1 was 3 hours. In some patients, duration of effect was as long as 6 hours.

In another clinical study in adults, two inhalations of PROVENTIL HFA Inhalation Aerosol taken 30 minutes before exercise prevented exercise-induced bronchospasm as demonstrated by the maintenance of FEV_1 within 80% of baseline values in the majority of patients.

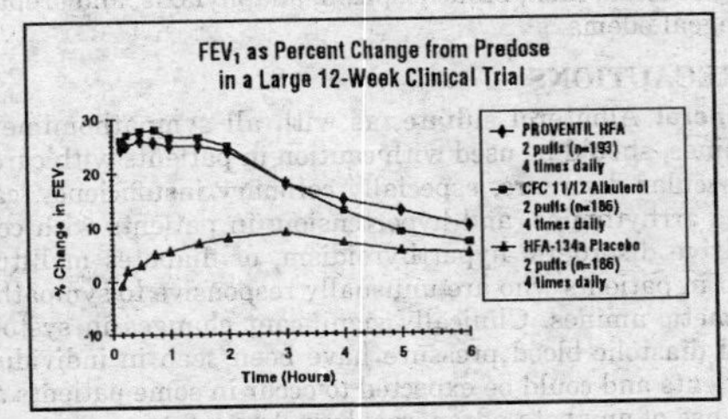

Continued on next page

Information on Schering products appearing on these pages is effective as of January 2000.

Proventil HFA—Cont.

In a 4-week, randomized, open-label trial, 63 children, 4 to 11 years of age, with asthma were evaluated for the bronchodilator efficacy of PROVENTIL HFA Inhalation Aerosol (33 pediatric patients) in comparison to a CFC 11/12 propelled albuterol inhaler (30 pediatric patients).

Serial FEV_1 measurements as percent change from test-day baseline demonstrated that two inhalations of PROVENTIL HFA Inhalation Aerosol produced outcomes which were clinically comparable to a CFC 11/12 propelled albuterol inhaler.

The mean time to onset of a 12% increase in FEV_1 for PROVENTIL HFA Inhalation Aerosol was 7 minutes and the mean time to peak effect was approximately 50 minutes. The mean duration of effect as measured by a 12% increase in FEV_1 was 2.3 hours. In some pediatric patients, duration of effect was as long as 6 hours.

In another clinical study in pediatric patients, two inhalations of PROVENTIL HFA Inhalation Aerosol taken 30 minutes before exercise provided comparable protection against exercise-induced bronchospasm as a CFC 11/12 propelled albuterol inhaler.

INDICATIONS AND USAGE

PROVENTIL HFA Inhalation Aerosol is indicated in adults and children 4 years of age and older for the treatment or prevention of bronchospasm with reversible obstructive airway disease and for the prevention of exercise-induced bronchospasm.

CONTRAINDICATIONS

PROVENTIL HFA Inhalation Aerosol is contraindicated in patients with a history of hypersensitivity to albuterol or any other PROVENTIL HFA components.

WARNINGS

1. Paradoxical Bronchospasm: Inhaled albuterol sulfate can produce paradoxical bronchospasm that may be life threatening. If paradoxical bronchospasm occurs, PROVENTIL HFA Inhalation Aerosol should be discontinued immediately and alternative therapy instituted. It should be recognized that paradoxical bronchospasm, when associated with inhaled formulations, frequently occurs with the first use of a new canister.

2. Deterioration of Asthma: Asthma may deteriorate acutely over a period of hours or chronically over several days or longer. If the patient needs more doses of PROVENTIL HFA Inhalation Aerosol than usual, this may be a marker of destabilization of asthma and requires reevaluation of the patient and treatment regimen, giving special consideration to the possible need for anti-inflammatory treatment, eg, corticosteroids.

3. Use of Anti-inflammatory Agents: The use of beta-adrenergic-agonist bronchodilators alone may not be adequate to control asthma in many patients. Early consideration should be given to adding anti-inflammatory agents, eg, corticosteroids, to the therapeutic regimen.

4. Cardiovascular Effects: PROVENTIL HFA Inhalation Aerosol, like other beta-adrenergic agonists, can produce clinically significant cardiovascular effects in some patients as measured by pulse rate, blood pressure, and/or symptoms. Although such effects are uncommon after administration of PROVENTIL HFA Inhalation Aerosol at recommended doses, if they occur, the drug may need to be discontinued. In addition, beta agonists have been reported to produce ECG changes, such as flattening of the T wave, prolongation of the QT_c interval, and ST segment depression. The clinical significance of these findings is unknown. Therefore, PROVENTIL HFA Inhalation Aerosol, like all sympathomimetic amines, should be used with caution in patients with cardiovascular disorders, especially coronary insufficiency, cardiac arrhythmias, and hypertension.

5. Do Not Exceed Recommended Dose: Fatalities have been reported in association with excessive use of inhaled sympathomimetic drugs in patients with asthma. The exact cause of death is unknown, but cardiac arrest following an unexpected development of a severe acute asthmatic crisis and subsequent hypoxia is suspected.

6. Immediate Hypersensitivity Reactions: Immediate hypersensitivity reactions may occur after administration of albuterol sulfate, as demonstrated by rare cases of urticaria, angioedema, rash, bronchospasm, anaphylaxis, and oropharyngeal edema.

PRECAUTIONS

General Albuterol sulfate, as with all sympathomimetic amines, should be used with caution in patients with cardiovascular disorders, especially coronary insufficiency, cardiac arrhythmias, and hypertension; in patients with convulsive disorders, hyperthyroidism, or diabetes mellitus; and in patients who are unusually responsive to sympathomimetic amines. Clinically significant changes in systolic and diastolic blood pressure have been seen in individual patients and could be expected to occur in some patients after use of any beta-adrenergic bronchodilator.

Large doses of intravenous albuterol have been reported to aggravate preexisting diabetes mellitus and ketoacidosis. As with other beta-agonists, albuterol may produce significant hypokalemia in some patients, possibly through intracellular shunting, which has the potential to produce adverse cardiovascular effects. The decrease is usually transient, not requiring supplementation.

Information for Patients See illustrated **Patient's Instructions for Use**. SHAKE WELL BEFORE USING. Patients should be given the following information:

It is recommended to prime the inhaler before using for the first time and in cases where the inhaler has not been used for more than 2 weeks by releasing four "test sprays" into the air, away from the face.

KEEPING THE PLASTIC MOUTHPIECE CLEAN IS VERY IMPORTANT TO PREVENT MEDICATION BUILD-UP AND BLOCKAGE. THE MOUTHPIECE SHOULD BE WASHED, SHAKEN TO REMOVE EXCESS WATER, AND AIR DRIED THOROUGHLY AT LEAST ONCE A WEEK. INHALER MAY CEASE TO DELIVER MEDICATION IF NOT PROPERLY CLEANED.

The mouthpiece should be cleaned (with the canister removed) by running warm water through the top and bottom for 30 seconds at least once a week. The mouthpiece must be shaken to remove excess water, then air dried thoroughly (such as overnight). Blockage from medication build-up or improper medication delivery may result from failure to thoroughly air dry the mouthpiece.

If the mouthpiece should become blocked (little or no medication coming out of the mouthpiece), the blockage may be removed by washing as described above.

If it is necessary to use the inhaler before it is completely dry, shake off excess water, replace canister, test spray twice away from face, and take the prescribed dose. After such use, the mouthpiece should be rewashed and allowed to air dry thoroughly.

The action of PROVENTIL HFA Inhalation Aerosol should last up to 4 to 6 hours. PROVENTIL HFA Inhalation Aerosol should not be used more frequently than recommended. Do not increase the dose or frequency of doses of PROVENTIL HFA Inhalation Aerosol without consulting your physician. If you find that treatment with PROVENTIL HFA Inhalation Aerosol becomes less effective for symptomatic relief, your symptoms become worse, and/or you need to use the product more frequently than usual, medical attention should be sought immediately. While you are taking PROVENTIL HFA Inhalation Aerosol, other inhaled drugs and asthma medications should be taken only as directed by your physician.

Common adverse effects of treatment with inhaled albuterol include palpitations, chest pain, rapid heart rate, tremor, or nervousness. If you are pregnant or nursing, contact your physician about use of PROVENTIL HFA Inhalation Aerosol. Effective and safe use of PROVENTIL HFA Inhalation Aerosol includes an understanding of the way that it should be administered. Use PROVENTIL HFA Inhalation Aerosol only with the actuator supplied with the product. Discard the canister after 200 sprays have been used.

In general, the technique for administering PROVENTIL HFA Inhalation Aerosol to children is similar to that for adults. Children should use PROVENTIL HFA Inhalation Aerosol under adult supervision, as instructed by the patient's physician. (See **Patient's Instructions for Use**).

Drug Interactions

1. Beta Blockers: Beta-adrenergic-receptor blocking agents not only block the pulmonary effect of beta agonists, such as PROVENTIL HFA Inhalation Aerosol, but may produce severe bronchospasm in asthmatic patients. Therefore, patients with asthma should not normally be treated with beta blockers. However, under certain circumstances, eg, as prophylaxis after myocardial infarction, there may be no acceptable alternatives to the use of beta-adrenergic-blocking agents in patients with asthma. In this setting, cardioselective beta blockers should be considered, although they should be administered with caution.

2. Diuretics: The ECG changes and/or hypokalemia which may result from the administration of nonpotassium sparing diuretics (such as loop or thiazide diuretics) can be acutely worsened by beta agonists, especially when the recommended dose of the beta agonist is exceeded. Although the clinical significance of these effects is not known, caution is advised in the coadministration of beta agonists with nonpotassium sparing diuretics.

3. Albuterol-Digoxin: Mean decreases of 16% and 22% in serum digoxin levels were demonstrated after single-dose intravenous and oral administration of albuterol, respectively, to normal volunteers who had received digoxin for 10 days. The clinical significance of these findings for patients with obstructive airway disease who are receiving albuterol and digoxin on a chronic basis is unclear; nevertheless, it would be prudent to carefully evaluate the serum digoxin levels in patients who are currently receiving digoxin and albuterol.

4. Monoamine Oxidase Inhibitors or Tricyclic Antidepressants: PROVENTIL HFA Inhalation Aerosol should be administered with extreme caution to patients being treated with monoamine oxidase inhibitors or tricyclic antidepressants, or within 2 weeks of discontinuation of such agents, because the action of albuterol on the cardiovascular system may be potentiated.

Carcinogenesis, Mutagenesis, and Impairment of Fertility

In a 2-year study in Sprague-Dawley rats, albuterol sulfate caused a dose-related increase in the incidence of benign leiomyomas of the mesovarium at and above dietary doses of 2 mg/kg (approximately 10 times the maximum recommended daily inhalation dose for adults on a mg/m^2 basis and approximately 5 times the maximum recommended daily inhalation dose for children on a mg/m^2 basis). In another study this effect was blocked by the coadministration of propranolol, a nonselective beta-adrenergic antagonist. In an 18-month study in CD-1 mice, albuterol sulfate showed no evidence of tumorigenicity at dietary doses of up to 500 mg/kg (approximately 1400 times the maximum recommended daily inhalation dose for adults on a mg/m^2 basis and approximately 670 times the maximum recommended daily inhalation dose for children on a mg/m^2 basis). In a 22-month study in Golden Hamsters, albuterol sulfate showed no evidence of tumorigenicity at dietary doses of up to 50 mg/kg (approximately 190 times the maximum recommended daily inhalation dose for adults on a mg/m^2 basis and approximately 90 times the maximum recommended daily inhalation dose for children on a mg/m^2 basis).

Albuterol sulfate was not mutagenic in the Ames test or a mutation test in yeast. Albuterol sulfate was not clastogenic in a human peripheral lymphocyte assay or in an AH1 strain mouse micronucleus assay.

Reproduction studies in rats demonstrated no evidence of impaired fertility at oral doses up to 50 mg/kg (approximately 280 times the maximum recommended daily inhalation dose for adults on a mg/m^2 basis).

Teratogenic Effects — Pregnancy Category C

Albuterol sulfate has been shown to be teratogenic in mice. A study in CD-1 mice given albuterol sulfate subcutaneously showed cleft palate formation in 5 of 111 (4.5%) fetuses at 0.25 mg/kg (less than the maximum recommended daily inhalation dose for adults on a mg/m^2 basis) and in 10 of 108 (9.3%) fetuses at 2.5 mg/kg (approximately 7 times the maximum recommended daily inhalation dose for adults on a mg/m^2 basis). The drug did not induce cleft palate formation at a dose of 0.025 mg/kg (less than the maximum recommended daily inhalation dose for adults on a mg/m^2 basis). Cleft palate also occurred in 22 of 72 (30.5%) fetuses from females treated subcutaneously with 2.5 mg/kg isoproterenol (positive control).

A reproduction study in Stride Dutch rabbits revealed cranioschisis in 7 of 19 (37%) fetuses when albuterol sulfate was administered orally at 50 mg/kg dose (approximately 560 times the maximum recommended daily inhalation dose for adults on a mg/m^2 basis).

In an inhalation reproduction study in Sprague-Dawley rats, the albuterol sulfate/HFA-134a formulation did not exhibit any teratogenic effects at 10.5 mg/kg (approximately 60 times the maximum recommended daily inhalation dose for adults on a mg/m^2 basis).

A study in which pregnant rats were dosed with radiolabeled albuterol sulfate demonstrated that drug-related material is transferred from the maternal circulation to the fetus.

There are no adequate and well-controlled studies of PROVENTIL HFA Inhalation Aerosol or albuterol sulfate in pregnant women. PROVENTIL HFA Inhalation Aerosol should be used during pregnancy only if the potential benefit justifies the potential risk to the fetus.

During worldwide marketing experience, various congenital anomalies, including cleft palate and limb defects, have been reported in the offspring of patients being treated with albuterol. Some of the mothers were taking multiple medications during their pregnancies. Because no consistent pattern of defects can be discerned, a relationship between albuterol use and congenital anomalies has not been established.

Use in Labor and Delivery

Because of the potential for beta-agonist interference with uterine contractility, use of PROVENTIL HFA Inhalation Aerosol for relief of bronchospasm during labor should be restricted to those patients in whom the benefits clearly outweigh the risk.

Tocolysis: Albuterol has not been approved for the management of preterm labor. The benefit:risk ratio when albuterol is administered for tocolysis has not been established. Serious adverse reactions, including pulmonary edema, have been reported during or following treatment of premature labor with $beta_2$-agonists, including albuterol.

Nursing Mothers

Plasma levels of albuterol sulfate and HFA-134a after inhaled therapeutic doses are very low in humans, but it is not known whether the components of PROVENTIL HFA Inhalation Aerosol are excreted in human milk.

Because of the potential for tumorigenicity shown for albuterol in animal studies and lack of experience with the use of PROVENTIL HFA Inhalation Aerosol by nursing mothers, a decision should be made whether to discontinue nursing or to discontinue the drug, taking into account the importance of the drug to the mother. Caution should be exercised when albuterol sulfate is administered to a nursing woman.

Pediatrics

The safety and effectiveness of PROVENTIL HFA Inhalation Aerosol in pediatric patients below the age of 4 years have not been established.

Geriatrics

PROVENTIL HFA Inhalation Aerosol has not been studied in a geriatric population. As with other $beta_2$-agonists, special caution should be observed when using PROVENTIL HFA Inhalation Aerosol in elderly patients who have concomitant cardiovascular disease that could be adversely affected by this class of drug.

ADVERSE REACTIONS

Adverse reaction information concerning PROVENTIL HFA Inhalation Aerosol is derived from a 12-week, double-blind, double-dummy study which compared PROVENTIL HFA Inhalation Aerosol, a CFC 11/12 propelled albuterol inhaler, and an HFA-134a placebo inhaler in 565 asthmatic patients. The following table lists the incidence of all adverse events (whether considered by the investigator drug related or unrelated to drug) from this study which occurred at a rate of 3% or greater in the PROVENTIL HFA Inhalation Aerosol treatment group and more frequently in the PROVENTIL HFA Inhalation Aerosol treatment group than in the placebo group. Overall, the incidence and nature of the adverse reactions reported for PROVENTIL HFA Inhalation Aerosol and a CFC 11/12 propelled albuterol inhaler were comparable.

[See table at right]

Adverse events reported by less than 3% of the patients receiving PROVENTIL HFA Inhalation Aerosol, and by a greater proportion of PROVENTIL HFA Inhalation Aerosol patients than placebo patients, which have the potential to be related to PROVENTIL HFA Inhalation Aerosol include: dysphonia, increased sweating, dry mouth, chest pain, edema, rigors, ataxia, leg cramps, hyperkinesia, eructation, flatulence, tinnitus, diabetes mellitus, anxiety, depression, somnolence, rash. Palpitation and dizziness have also been observed with PROVENTIL HFA Inhalation Aerosol.

Adverse events reported in a 4-week pediatric clinical trial comparing PROVENTIL HFA Inhalation Aerosol and a CFC 11/12 propelled albuterol inhaler occurred at a low incidence rate and were similar to those seen in the adult trials.

In small, cumulative dose studies, tremor, nervousness, and headache appeared to be dose related.

Rare cases of urticaria, angioedema, rash, bronchospasm, and oropharyngeal edema have been reported after the use of inhaled albuterol. In addition, albuterol, like other sympathomimetic agents, can cause adverse reactions such as hypertension, angina, vertigo, central nervous system stimulation, insomnia, headache, and drying or irritation of the oropharynx.

Adverse Experience Incidences (% of patients) in a Large 12-week Clinical Trial*

Body System/ Adverse Event (Preferred Term)		PROVENTIL HFA Inhalation Aerosol (N = 193)	CFC 11/12 Propelled Albuterol Inhaler (N = 186)	HFA-134a Placebo Inhaler (N = 186)
Application Site Disorders	Inhalation Site Sensation	6	9	2
	Inhalation Taste Sensation	4	3	3
Body as a Whole	Allergic Reaction/Symptoms	6	4	< 1
	Back Pain	4	2	3
	Fever	6	2	5
Central and Peripheral Nervous System	Tremor	7	8	2
Gastrointestinal System	Nausea	10	9	5
	Vomiting	7	2	3
Heart Rate and Rhythm Disorder	Tachycardia	7	2	< 1
Psychiatric Disorders	Nervousness	7	9	3
Respiratory System Disorders	Respiratory Disorder (unspecified)	6	4	5
	Rhinitis	16	22	14
	Upper Resp Tract Infection	21	20	18
Urinary System Disorder	Urinary Tract Infection	3	4	2

*This table includes all adverse events (whether considered by the investigator drug related or unrelated to drug) which occurred at an incidence rate of at least 3.0% in the PROVENTIL HFA Inhalation Aerosol group and more frequently in the PROVENTIL HFA Inhalation Aerosol group than in the HFA-134a placebo inhaler group.

OVERDOSAGE

The expected symptoms with overdosage are those of excessive beta-adrenergic stimulation and/or occurrence or exaggeration of any of the symptoms listed under **ADVERSE REACTIONS**, eg, seizures, angina, hypertension or hypotension, tachycardia with rates up to 200 beats per minute, arrhythmias, nervousness, headache, tremor, dry mouth, palpitation, nausea, dizziness, fatigue, malaise, and insomnia.

Hypokalemia may also occur. As with all sympathomimetic medications, cardiac arrest and even death may be associated with abuse of PROVENTIL HFA Inhalation Aerosol. Treatment consists of discontinuation of PROVENTIL HFA Inhalation Aerosol together with appropriate symptomatic therapy. The judicious use of a cardioselective beta-receptor blocker may be considered, bearing in mind that such medication can produce bronchospasm. There is insufficient evidence to determine if dialysis is beneficial for overdosage of PROVENTIL HFA Inhalation Aerosol.

The oral median lethal dose of albuterol sulfate in mice is greater than 2000 mg/kg (approximately 5600 times the maximum recommended daily inhalation dose for adults on a mg/m^2 basis and approximately 2700 times the maximum recommended daily inhalation dose for children on a mg/m^2 basis). In mature rats, the subcutaneous median lethal dose of albuterol sulfate is approximately 450 mg/kg (approximately 2500 times the maximum recommended daily inhalation dose for adults on a mg/m^2 basis and approximately 1200 times the maximum recommended daily inhalation dose for children on a mg/m^2 basis). In young rats, the subcutaneous median lethal dose is approximately 2000 mg/kg (approximately 11,000 times the maximum recommended daily inhalation dose for adults on a mg/m^2 basis and approximately 5300 times the maximum recommended daily inhalation dose for children on a mg/m^2 basis). The inhalation median lethal dose has not been determined in animals.

DOSAGE AND ADMINISTRATION

For treatment of acute episodes of bronchospasm or prevention of asthmatic symptoms, the usual dosage for adults and children 4 years of age and older is two inhalations repeated every 4 to 6 hours. More frequent administration or a larger number of inhalations is not recommended. In some patients, one inhalation every 4 hours may be sufficient. Each actuation of PROVENTIL HFA Inhalation Aerosol delivers 108 mcg of albuterol sulfate (equivalent to 90 mcg of albuterol base) from the mouthpiece. It is recommended to prime the inhaler before using for the first time and in cases where the inhaler has not been used for more than 2 weeks by releasing four "test sprays" into the air, away from the face.

Exercise Induced Bronchospasm Prevention: The usual dosage for adults and children 4 years of age and older is two inhalations 15 to 30 minutes before exercise.

To maintain proper use of this product, it is important that the mouthpiece be washed and dried thoroughly at least once a week. The inhaler may cease to deliver medication if not properly cleaned and dried thoroughly. See **Information for Patients**. Keeping the plastic mouthpiece clean is very important to prevent medication build-up and blockage. The inhaler may cease to deliver medication if not properly cleaned and air dried thoroughly. If the mouthpiece becomes blocked, washing the mouthpiece will remove the blockage.

If a previously effective dose regimen fails to provide the usual response, this may be a marker of destabilization of asthma and requires reevaluation of the patient and the treatment regimen, giving special consideration to the possible need for anti-inflammatory treatment, eg, corticosteroids.

HOW SUPPLIED

PROVENTIL HFA (albuterol sulfate) Inhalation Aerosol is supplied as a pressurized aluminum canister with a yellow plastic actuator and orange dust cap each in boxes of one. Each actuation delivers 120 mcg of albuterol sulfate from the valve and 108 mcg of albuterol sulfate from the mouthpiece (equivalent to 90 mcg of albuterol base). Canisters with a labeled net weight of 6.7 g contain 200 inhalations (NDC 0085-1132-01).

Rx only. Store between 15° and 25°C (59° and 77°F). For best results, canister should be at room temperature before use.

SHAKE WELL BEFORE USING.

The yellow actuator supplied with PROVENTIL HFA Inhalation Aerosol should not be used with any other product canisters, and actuator from other products should not be used with a PROVENTIL HFA Inhalation Aerosol canister. The correct amount of medication in each canister cannot be assured after 200 actuations, even though the canister is not completely empty. The canister should be discarded when the labeled number of actuations have been used.

WARNING: Avoid spraying in eyes. Contents under pressure. Do not puncture or incinerate. Exposure to temperatures above 120°F may cause bursting. Keep out of reach of children.

PROVENTIL HFA Inhalation Aerosol does not contain chlorofluorocarbons (CFCs) as the propellant.

Developed and Manufactured by
3M Health Care Limited
Loughborough UK
or
3M Pharmaceuticals,
Northridge, CA 91324
for
Key Pharmaceuticals, Inc.
Kenilworth, NJ 07033 USA

B03085

 23800101T
Rev. 1/00 23549611

PROVENTIL® HFA
(albuterol sulfate)
Inhalation Aerosol
FOR ORAL INHALATION ONLY
Patient's Instructions for Use

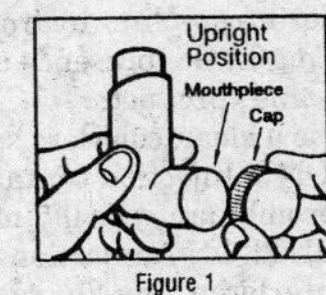

Figure 1

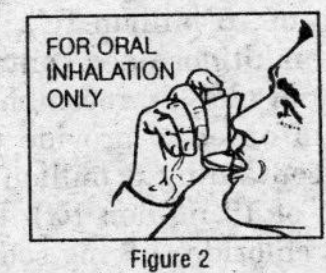

Figure 2

Before using your PROVENTIL HFA (albuterol sulfate) Inhalation Aerosol, read complete instructions carefully. Children should use PROVENTIL HFA Inhalation Aerosol under adult supervision, as instructed by the patient's doctor. Please note that (CFC) indicates that this inhalation aerosol does not contain chlorofluorocarbons (CFCs) as the propellant.

1. SHAKE THE INHALER WELL immediately before each use. **Then remove the cap from the mouthpiece** (see Figure 1). **Check mouthpiece for foreign objects prior to use.** Make sure the canister is fully inserted into the actuator.
2. As with all aerosol medications, it is recommended to prime the inhaler before using for the first time and in cases where the inhaler has not been used for more than 2 weeks. Prime by releasing four "test sprays" into the air, away from your face.
3. BREATHE OUT FULLY THROUGH THE MOUTH, expelling as much air from your lungs as possible. Place the mouthpiece fully into the mouth holding the inhaler in its upright position (see Figure 2) and closing the lips around it.
4. WHILE BREATHING IN DEEPLY AND SLOWLY THROUGH THE MOUTH, FULLY DEPRESS THE TOP OF THE METAL CANISTER with your index finger (see Figure 2).
5. HOLD YOUR BREATH AS LONG AS POSSIBLE, up to 10 seconds. Before breathing out, remove the inhaler from your mouth and release your finger from the canister.
6. If your physician has prescribed additional puffs, wait 1 minute, shake the inhaler again, and repeat steps 2 through 4. Replace the cap after use.
7. KEEPING THE PLASTIC MOUTHPIECE CLEAN IS EXTREMELY IMPORTANT TO PREVENT MEDICATION BUILD-UP AND BLOCKAGE. THE MOUTHPIECE SHOULD BE WASHED, SHAKEN TO REMOVE EXCESS WATER, AND AIR DRIED THOROUGHLY AT LEAST ONCE A WEEK. INHALER MAY STOP SPRAYING IF NOT PROPERLY CLEANED.

Routine cleaning instructions:

Step 1. To clean, remove the canister and mouthpiece cap. Wash the mouthpiece through the top and bottom with warm running water for 30 seconds at least once a week (see Figure A). **Never immerse the metal canister in water.**

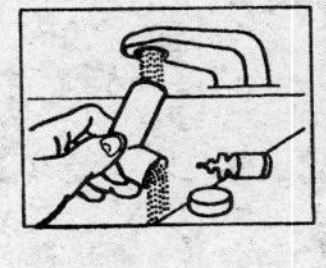
Figure A Wash mouthpiece under warm running water.

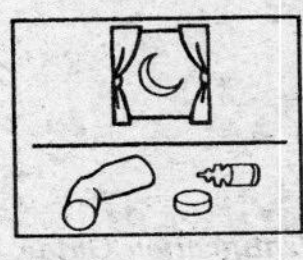
Figure B Allow mouthpiece to air dry, such as overnight.

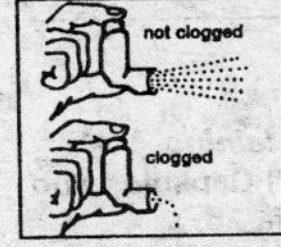

Figure C When blocked, little or no medicine comes out.

Step 2. To dry, shake off excess water and let the mouthpiece air dry thoroughly, such as overnight (see

Continued on next page

Information on Schering products appearing on these pages is effective as of January 2000.

Proventil HFA—Cont.

Figure B). When the mouthpiece is dry, replace the canister and the mouthpiece cap. Blockage from medication build-up is more likely to occur if the mouthpiece is not allowed to air dry thoroughly.

IF YOUR INHALER HAS BECOME BLOCKED (little or no medication coming out of the mouthpiece, see Figure C), wash the mouthpiece as described in Step 1 and air dry thoroughly as described in Step 2. **IF YOU NEED TO USE YOUR INHALER BEFORE IT IS COMPLETELY DRY, SHAKE OFF EXCESS WATER,** replace the canister, and test spray twice into the air, away from your face, to remove most of the water remaining in the mouthpiece. Then take your dose as prescribed. **After such use, rewash and air dry thoroughly as described in Steps 1 and 2.**

8. The correct amount of medication in each inhalation cannot be assured after 200 actuations, even though the canister is not completely empty. The canister should be discarded when the labeled number of actuations have been used. Before you reach the specific number of actuations, you should consult your physician to determine whether a refill is needed. Just as you should not take extra doses without consulting your physician, you also should not stop using PROVENTIL HFA Inhalation Aerosol without consulting your physician.

You may notice a slightly different taste or spray force than you are used to with PROVENTIL HFA Inhalation Aerosol, compared to other albuterol inhalation aerosol products.

DOSAGE

Use only as directed by your physician.

WARNINGS

The action of PROVENTIL HFA Inhalation Aerosol should last up to 4 to 6 hours. PROVENTIL HFA Inhalation Aerosol should not be used more frequently than recommended. Do not increase the number of puffs or frequency of doses of PROVENTIL HFA Inhalation Aerosol without consulting your physician. If you find that treatment with PROVENTIL HFA Inhalation Aerosol becomes less effective for symptomatic relief, your symptoms become worse, and/or you need to use the product more frequently than usual, medical attention should be sought immediately. While you are taking PROVENTIL HFA Inhalation Aerosol, other inhaled drugs should be taken only as directed by your physician. If you are pregnant or nursing, contact your physician about the use of PROVENTIL HFA Inhalation Aerosol.

Common adverse effects of treatment with PROVENTIL HFA Inhalation Aerosol include palpitations, chest pain, rapid heart rate, tremor, or nervousness. Effective and safe use of PROVENTIL HFA Inhalation Aerosol includes an understanding of the way that it should be administered. Use PROVENTIL HFA Inhalation Aerosol only with the yellow actuator supplied with the product. The PROVENTIL HFA Inhalation Aerosol actuator should not be used with other aerosol medications.

For best results, use at room temperature. Avoid exposing product to extreme heat and cold.

Shake well before use.

Contents Under Pressure.

Do not puncture. Do not store near heat or open flame. Exposure to temperatures above 120°F may cause bursting. Never throw container into fire or incinerator. Store between 15° and 25°C (59° and 77°F). Avoid spraying in eyes. Keep out of reach of children.

Further Information: Your PROVENTIL HFA (albuterol sulfate) Inhalation Aerosol does not contain chlorofluorocarbons (CFCs) as the propellant. Instead, the inhaler contains a hydrofluoroalkane (HFA-134a) as the propellant.

Developed and Manufactured by
3M Health Care Limited
Loughborough UK
or
3M Pharmaceuticals
Northridge, CA 91324
for
Key Pharmaceuticals, Inc.
Kenilworth, NJ 07033 USA
Rev. 1/00 23549611
U.S. Patent No. 5,225,183

Shown in Product Identification Guide, page 334

REBETRON™ ℞

Combination Therapy *containing* REBETOL® (ribavirin, USP) Capsules *and* INTRON® A (interferon alfa-2b, recombinant) Injection

CONTRAINDICATIONS AND WARNINGS

Combination REBETOL/INTRON A therapy is contraindicated in women who are pregnant and in the male partners of women who are pregnant. Extreme care must be taken to avoid pregnancy during therapy and for 6 months after completion of treatment in female patients, and in female partners of male patients who are taking combination REBETOL/INTRON A therapy. Women of childbearing potential and men must use two reliable forms of effective contraception during treatment and during the 6-month posttreatment follow-up period. Significant teratogenic and/or embryocidal effects have been demonstrated for ribavirin in all animal species studied. See CONTRAINDICATIONS and WARNINGS. REBETOL monotherapy is not effective for the treatment of chronic hepatitis C and should not be used for this indication. See WARNINGS.

TABLE 1. Mean (% CV) Pharmacokinetic Parameters for INTRON A and REBETOL When Administered Individually to Adults with Chronic Hepatitis C

Parameter	INTRON A (N=12)		REBETOL (N=12)	
	Single Dose 3 MIU	Multiple Dose 3 MIU TIW	Single Dose 600 mg	Multiple Dose 600 mg BID
T_{max} (hr)	7 (44)	5 (37)	1.7 (46)***	3 (60)
C_{max} *	13.9 (32)	29.7 (33)	782 (37)	3680 (85)
AUC_{tf} **	142 (43)	333 (39)	13400 (48)	228000 (25)
$T_{1/2}$ (hr)	6.8 (24)	6.5 (29)	43.6 (47)	298 (30)
Apparent Volume of Distribution (L)			2825 (9)†	
Apparent Clearance (L/hr)	14.3 (17)		38.2 (40)	
Absolute Bioavailability			64% (44)††	

* IU/mL for INTRON A and ng/mL for REBETOL
** IU.hr/mL for INTRON A and ng.hr/mL for REBETOL
† Data obtained from a single-dose pharmacokinetic study using ^{14}C labeled ribavirin; N=5
†† N=6
*** N=11

DESCRIPTION

REBETOL®

REBETOL is Schering Corporation's brand name for ribavirin, a nucleoside analog with antiviral activity. The chemical name of ribavirin is 1-β-D-ribofuranosyl-1*H*-1,2,4-triazole-3-carboxamide and has the following structural formula:

Ribavirin is a white, crystalline powder. It is freely soluble in water and slightly soluble in anhydrous alcohol. The empirical formula is $C_8H_{12}N_4O_5$ and the molecular weight is 244.21.

REBETOL Capsules consist of a white powder in a white, opaque, gelatin capsule. Each capsule contains 200 mg ribavirin and the inactive ingredients microcrystalline cellulose, lactose monohydrate, croscarmellose sodium, and magnesium stearate. The capsule shell consists of gelatin, sodium lauryl sulfate, silicon dioxide, and titanium dioxide. The capsule is printed with edible blue pharmaceutical ink which is made of shellac, anhydrous ethyl alcohol, isopropyl alcohol, n-butyl alcohol, propylene glycol, ammonium hydroxide, and FD&C Blue #2 aluminum lake.

INTRON® A

INTRON A is Schering Corporation's brand name for interferon alfa-2b, recombinant, a purified, sterile, recombinant interferon product.

Interferon alfa-2b, recombinant has been classified as an alpha interferon and is a water-soluble protein composed of 165 amino acids with a molecular weight of 19,271 daltons produced by recombinant DNA techniques. It is obtained from the bacterial fermentation of a strain of *Escherichia coli* bearing a genetically engineered plasmid containing an interferon alfa-2b gene from human leukocytes. The fermentation is carried out in a defined nutrient medium containing the antibiotic tetracycline hydrochloride at a concentration of 5 to 10 mg/L; the presence of this antibiotic is not detectable in the final product.

INTRON A Injection is a clear, colorless solution. The 3 million IU vial of INTRON A Injection contains 3 million IU of interferon alfa-2b, recombinant per 0.5 mL. The 18 million IU multidose vial of INTRON A Injection contains a total of 22.8 million IU of interferon alfa-2b, recombinant per 3.8 mL (3 million IU/0.5 mL) in order to provide the delivery of six 0.5-mL doses, each containing 3 million IU of INTRON A (for a label strength of 18 million IU). The 18 million IU INTRON A Injection multidose pen contains a total of 22.5 million IU of interferon alfa-2b, recombinant per 1.5 mL (3 million IU/0.2 mL) in order to provide the delivery of six 0.2-mL doses, each containing 3 million IU of INTRON A (for a label strength of 18 million IU). Each mL also contains 7.5 mg sodium chloride, 1.8 mg sodium phosphate dibasic, 1.3 mg sodium phosphate monobasic, 0.1 mg edetate disodium, 0.1 mg polysorbate 80, and 1.5 mg m-cresol as a preservative.

Based on the specific activity of approximately 2.6×10^8 IU/mg protein as measured by HPLC assay, the corresponding quantities of interferon alfa-2b, recombinant in the vials and pen described above are approximately 0.012 mg, 0.088 mg, and 0.087 mg protein, respectively.

Mechanism of Action

Ribavirin/Interferon alfa-2b, recombinant The mechanism of inhibition of hepatitis C virus (HCV) RNA by combination therapy with REBETOL and INTRON A has not been established.

CLINICAL PHARMACOLOGY

Pharmacokinetics

Interferon alfa-2b, recombinant Single- and multiple-dose pharmacokinetic properties of INTRON A (interferon alfa-2b, recombinant) are summarized in **TABLE 1.** Following a single 3 million IU (MIU) subcutaneous dose in 12 patients with chronic hepatitis C, mean (% CV*) serum concentrations peaked at 7 (44%) hours. Following 4 weeks of subcutaneous dosing with 3 MIU three times a week (TIW), interferon serum concentrations were undetectable predose. However, a twofold increase in bioavailability was noted upon multiple dosing of interferon; the reason for this is unknown. Mean half-life values following single- and multiple-dose administrations were 6.8 (24%) hours and 6.5 (29%) hours, respectively.

Ribavirin Single- and multiple-dose pharmacokinetic properties in adults with chronic hepatitis C are summarized in **TABLE 1.** Ribavirin was rapidly and extensively absorbed following oral administration. However, due to first-pass metabolism, the absolute bioavailability averaged 64% (44%). There was a linear relationship between dose and AUC_{tf} (AUC from time zero to last measurable concentration) following single doses of 200–1200 mg ribavirin. The relationship between dose and C_{max} was curvilinear, tending to asymptote above single doses of 400–600 mg.

Upon multiple oral dosing, based on $AUC12_{hr}$, a sixfold accumulation of ribavirin was observed in plasma. Following oral dosing with 600 mg BID, steady-state was reached by approximately 4 weeks, with mean steady-state plasma concentrations of 2200 (37%) ng/mL. Upon discontinuation of dosing, the mean half-life was 298 (30%) hours, which probably reflects slow elimination from nonplasma compartments.

Effect of Food on Absorption of Ribavirin Both AUC_{tf} and C_{max} increased by 70% when REBETOL Capsules were administered with a high-fat meal (841 kcal, 53.8 g fat, 31.6 g protein, and 57.4 g carbohydrate) in a single-dose pharmacokinetic study. There are insufficient data to address the clinical relevance of these results. Clinical efficacy studies were conducted without instructions with respect to food consumption. (See **DOSAGE AND ADMINISTRATION.**)

Effect of Antacid on Absorption of Ribavirin Coadministration with an antacid containing magnesium, aluminum, and simethicone (Mylanta®) resulted in a 14% decrease in mean ribavirin AUC_{tf}. The clinical relevance of results from this single-dose study is unknown.

[See table above]

Ribavirin transport into nonplasma compartments has been most extensively studied in red blood cells, and has been identified to be primarily via an e_s-type equilibrative nucleoside transporter. This type of transporter is present on virtually all cell types and may account for the extensive volume of distribution. Ribavirin does not bind to plasma proteins.

Ribavirin has two pathways of metabolism: (i) a reversible phosphorylation pathway in nucleated cells; and (ii) a degradative pathway involving deribosylation and amide hydrolysis to yield a triazole carboxylic acid metabolite. Ribavirin and its triazole carboxamide and triazole carboxylic acid metabolites are excreted renally. After oral administration of 600 mg of ^{14}C-ribavirin, approximately 61% and 12% of the radioactivity was eliminated in the urine and feces, respectively, in 336 hours. Unchanged ribavirin accounted for 17% of the administered dose.

Results of *in vitro* studies using both human and rat liver microsome preparations indicated little or no cytochrome P450 enzyme-mediated metabolism of ribavirin, with minimal potential for P450 enzyme-based drug interactions.

No pharmacokinetic interactions were noted between INTRON A Injection and REBETOL Capsules in a multiple-dose pharmacokinetic study.

Special Populations

Renal Dysfunction The pharmacokinetics of ribavirin were assessed after administration of a single oral dose (400 mg) of ribavirin to subjects with varying degrees of renal dysfunction. The mean AUC_{tf} value was threefold greater in subjects with creatinine clearance values between 10 to 30 mL/min when compared to control subjects (creatinine clearance >90 mL/min). This appears to be due to reduction of apparent clearance in these patients. Ribavirin was not removed by hemodialysis. REBETOL is not recommended for patients with severe renal impairment (see **WARNINGS**).

Hepatic Dysfunction The effect of hepatic dysfunction was assessed after a single oral dose of ribavirin (600 mg). The mean AUC_{tf} values were not significantly different in subjects with mild, moderate, or severe hepatic dysfunction (Child-Pugh Classification A, B, or C) when compared to control subjects. However, the mean C_{max} values increased with severity of hepatic dysfunction and was twofold greater in subjects with severe hepatic dysfunction when compared to control subjects.

Pediatric Patients Pharmacokinetic evaluations for pediatric subjects have not been performed.

Elderly Patients Pharmacokinetic evaluations for elderly subjects have not been performed.

Gender There were no clinically significant pharmacokinetic differences noted in a single-dose study of eighteen male and eighteen female subjects.

In this section of the label, numbers in parenthesis indicate % coefficient of variation.

INDICATIONS AND USAGE

REBETOL (ribavirin, USP) Capsules is indicated in combination with INTRON A (interferon alfa-2b, recombinant) Injection for the treatment of chronic hepatitis C in patients with compensated liver disease previously untreated with alpha interferon or who have relapsed following alpha interferon therapy.

Description of Clinical Studies

Previously Untreated Patients Adults with compensated chronic hepatitis C and detectable HCV RNA (assessed by a central laboratory using a research-based RT-PCR assay) who were previously untreated with alpha interferon therapy were enrolled into two multicenter, double-blind trials (US and International) and randomized to receive REBETOL Capsules 1200 mg/day (1000 mg/day for patients weighing ≤75 kg) plus INTRON A Injection 3 MIU TIW or INTRON A Injection plus placebo for 24 or 48 weeks followed by 24 weeks of off-therapy follow-up. The International study did not contain a 24-week INTRON A plus placebo treatment arm. The US study enrolled 912 patients who, at baseline, were 67% male, 89% caucasian with a mean Knodell HAI score (I+II+III) of 7.5, and 72% genotype 1. The International study, conducted in Europe, Israel, Canada, and Australia, enrolled 799 patients (65% male, 95% caucasian, mean Knodell score 6.8, and 58% genotype 1). Study results are summarized in **TABLE 2.**

[See table 2 above]

TABLE 2. Virologic and Histologic Responses: Previously Untreated Patients*

	US Study				International Study		
	24 weeks of treatment		48 weeks of treatment		24 weeks of treatment	48 weeks of treatment	
	INTRON A plus REBETOL (N=228)	**INTRON A plus Placebo (N=231)**	**INTRON A plus REBETOL (N=228)**	**INTRON A plus Placebo (N=225)**	**INTRON A plus REBETOL (N=265)**	**INTRON A plus REBETOL (N=268)**	**INTRON A plus Placebo (N=266)**
Virologic Response							
–Responder[1]	65 (29)	13 (6)	85 (37)	27 (12)	86 (32)	113 (42)	46 (17)
–Nonresponder	147 (64)	194 (84)	110 (48)	168 (75)	158 (60)	120 (45)	196 (74)
–Missing data	16 (7)	24 (10)	33 (14)	30 (13)	21 (8)	35 (13)	24 (9)
Histologic Response							
–Improvement[2]	102 (45)	77 (33)	96 (42)	65 (29)	103 (39)	102 (38)	69 (26)
–No improvement	77 (34)	99 (43)	61 (27)	93 (41)	85 (32)	58 (22)	111 (41)
–Missing data	49 (21)	55 (24)	71 (31)	67 (30)	77 (29)	108 (40)	86 (32)

* Number (%) of patients

[1] Defined as HCV RNA below limit of detection using a research-based RT-PCR assay at end of treatment and during follow-up period.

[2] Defined as posttreatment (end of follow-up) minus pretreatment liver biopsy Knodell HAI score (I+II+III) improvement of ≥2 points.

Of patients who had not achieved HCV RNA below the limit of detection of the research-based assay by week 24 of REBETOL/INTRON A treatment, less than 5% responded to an additional 24 weeks of combination treatment.

Among patients with HCV genotype 1 treated with REBETOL/INTRON A therapy who achieved HCV RNA below the detection limit of the research-based assay by 24 weeks, those randomized to 48 weeks of treatment had higher virologic responses compared to those in the 24-week treatment group. There was no observed increase in response rates for patients with HCV nongenotype 1 randomized to REBETOL/INTRON A therapy for 48 weeks compared to 24 weeks.

Relapse Patients Patients with compensated chronic hepatitis C and detectable HCV RNA (assessed by a central laboratory using a research-based RT-PCR assay) who had relapsed following one or two courses of interferon therapy (defined as abnormal serum ALT levels) were enrolled into two multicenter, double-blind trials (US and International) and randomized to receive REBETOL 1200 mg/day (1000 mg/day for patients weighing ≤75 kg) plus INTRON A 3 MIU TIW or INTRON A plus placebo for 24 weeks followed by 24 weeks of off-therapy follow-up. The US study enrolled 153 patients who, at baseline, were 67% male, 92% caucasian with a mean Knodell HAI score (I+II+III) of 6.8, and 58% genotype 1. The International study, conducted in Europe, Israel, Canada, and Australia, enrolled 192 patients (64% male, 95% caucasian, mean Knodell score 6.6, and 56% genotype 1).

Study results are summarized in **TABLE 3.**

[See table 3 above]

TABLE 3. Virologic and Histologic Responses: Relapse Patients*

	US Study		International Study	
	INTRON A plus REBETOL (N=77)	**INTRON A plus Placebo (N=76)**	**INTRON A plus REBETOL (N=96)**	**INTRON A plus Placebo (N=96)**
Virologic Response				
–Responder[1]	33 (43)	3 (4)	46 (48)	5 (5)
–Nonresponder	36 (47)	66 (87)	45 (47)	91 (95)
–Missing data	8 (10)	7 (9)	5 (5)	0 (0)
Histologic Response	38 (49)	27 (36)	49 (51)	30 (31)
–Improvement[2]	23 (30)	37 (49)	29 (30)	44 (46)
–No improvement	16 (21)	12 (16)	18 (19)	22 (23)
–Missing data				

* Number (%) of patients

[1] Defined as HCV RNA below limit of detection using a research-based RT-PCR assay at end of treatment and during follow-up period.

[2] Defined as posttreatment (end of follow-up) minus pretreatment liver biopsy Knodell HAI score (I+II+III) improvement of ≥2 points.

Virologic and histologic responses were similar among male and female patients in both the previously untreated and relapse studies.

CONTRAINDICATIONS

Combination REBETOL/INTRON A therapy must not be used by women who are pregnant or by men whose female partners are pregnant. Extreme care must be taken to avoid pregnancy in female patients and in female partners of male patients taking combination REBETOL/INTRON A therapy. Combination REBETOL/INTRON A therapy should not be initiated until a report of a negative pregnancy test has been obtained immediately prior to initiation of therapy. Women of childbearing potential and men must use two forms of effective contraception during treatment and during the 6 months after treatment has been concluded. Significant teratogenic and/or embryocidal effects have been demonstrated for ribavirin in all animal species in which adequate studies have been conducted. These effects occurred at doses as low as one twentieth of the recommended human dose of REBETOL Capsules. If pregnancy occurs in a patient or partner of a patient during treatment or during the 6 months after treatment stops, physicians are encouraged to report such cases by calling (800) 727-7064. **See boxed CONTRAINDICATIONS AND WARNINGS. See WARNINGS.**

REBETOL Capsules in combination with INTRON A Injection is contraindicated in patients with a history of hypersensitivity to ribavirin and/or alpha interferon or any component of the capsule and/or injection.

Patients with autoimmune hepatitis must not be treated with combination REBETOL/INTRON A therapy.

WARNINGS

Pregnancy

Category X, may cause birth defects. See boxed CONTRAINDICATIONS AND WARNINGS. See CONTRAINDICATIONS.

Anemia

HEMOLYTIC ANEMIA (HEMOGLOBIN <10 G/DL) WAS OBSERVED IN APPROXIMATELY 10% OF REBETOL/INTRON A-TREATED PATIENTS IN CLINICAL TRIALS (SEE ADVERSE REACTIONS LABORATORY VALUES – *HEMOGLOBIN*). ANEMIA OCCURRED WITHIN 1–2 WEEKS OF INITIATION OF RIBAVIRIN THERAPY. BECAUSE OF THIS INITIAL ACUTE DROP IN HEMOGLOBIN, IT IS ADVISED THAT COMPLETE BLOOD COUNTS (CBC) SHOULD BE OBTAINED PRETREATMENT AND AT WEEK 2 AND WEEK 4 OF THERAPY OR MORE FREQUENTLY IF CLINICALLY INDICATED. PATIENTS SHOULD THEN BE FOLLOWED AS CLINICALLY APPROPRIATE.

The anemia associated with REBETOL/INTRON A therapy may result in deterioration of cardiac function and/or exacerbation of the symptoms of coronary disease. Patients should be assessed before initiation of therapy and should be appropriately monitored during therapy. If there is any deterioration of cardiovascular status, therapy should be suspended or discontinued. (See **DOSAGE AND ADMINISTRATION.**) Because cardiac disease may be worsened by drug induced anemia, patients with a history of significant or unstable cardiac disease should not use combination REBETOL/INTRON A therapy. (See **ADVERSE REACTIONS.**)

Similarly, patients with hemoglobinopathies (eg, thalassemia, sickle-cell anemia) should not be treated with combination REBETOL/INTRON A therapy.

Psychiatric

Severe psychiatric adverse events, including depression, psychoses, aggressive behavior, hallucinations, violent behavior (suicidal ideation, suicidal attempts, suicides), and rare instances of homicidal ideation have occurred during combination REBETOL/INTRON A therapy, both in patients with and without a previous psychiatric disorder. REBETOL/INTRON A therapy should be used with extreme caution in patients with a history of pre-existing psychiatric disorders, and all patients should be carefully monitored for evidence of depression and other psychiatric symptoms. Suspension of REBETOL/INTRON A therapy should be considered if psychiatric intervention and/or dose reduction is unsuccessful in controlling psychiatric symptoms. In severe cases, therapy should be stopped immediately and psychiatric intervention sought. (See ADVERSE REACTIONS.)

Pulmonary

Pulmonary symptoms, including dyspnea, pulmonary infiltrates, pneumonitis and pneumonia, including fatality, have been reported during therapy with REBETOL/INTRON A. If there is evidence of pulmonary infiltrates or pulmonary function impairment, the patient should be closely monitored, and, if appropriate, combination REBETOL/INTRON A treatment should be discontinued.

Other

- REBETOL Capsule monotherapy is not effective for the treatment of chronic hepatitis C and should not be used for this indication.
- Fatal and nonfatal pancreatitis has been observed in patients treated with REBETOL/INTRON A therapy. REBETOL/INTRON A therapy should be suspended in patients with signs and symptoms of pancreatitis and discontinued in patients with confirmed pancreatitis.
- Combination REBETOL/INTRON A therapy should be used with caution in patients with creatinine clearance <50 mL/min.
- Diabetes mellitus and hyperglycemia have been observed in patients treated with INTRON A.
- Ophthalmologic disorders have been reported with treatment with alpha interferons (including INTRON A therapy). Investigators using alpha interferons have reported the occurrence of retinal hemorrhages, cotton wool spots, and retinal artery or vein obstruction in rare instances. Any patient complaining of loss of visual acuity or visual field should have an eye examination. Because these ocular events may occur in conjunction with other disease states, a visual exam prior to initiation of combination REBETOL/INTRON A therapy is recommended in patients with diabetes mellitus or hypertension.

Continued on next page

Information on Schering products appearing on these pages is effective as of January 2000.

Rebetron—Cont.

- Acute serious hypersensitivity reactions (eg, urticaria, angioedema, bronchoconstriction, anaphylaxis) have been observed in INTRON A-treated patients; if such an acute reaction develops, combination REBETOL/INTRON A therapy should be discontinued immediately and appropriate medical therapy instituted.
- Combination REBETOL/INTRON A therapy should be discontinued for patients developing thyroid abnormalities during treatment whose thyroid function cannot be controlled by medication.

PRECAUTIONS

Exacerbation of autoimmune disease has been reported in patients receiving alpha interferon therapy (including INTRON A therapy). REBETOL/INTRON A therapy should be used with caution in patients with other autoimmune disorders.

There have been reports of interferon, including INTRON A (interferon alfa-2b, recombinant) exacerbating pre-existing psoriasis; therefore, combination REBETOL/INTRON A therapy should be used in these patients only if the potential benefit justifies the potential risk.

The safety and efficacy of REBETOL/INTRON A therapy has not been established in liver or other organ transplant patients, decompensated hepatitis C patients, patients who are nonresponders to interferon therapy, or patients coinfected with HBV or HIV.

The safety and efficacy of REBETOL Capsule monotherapy for the treatment of HIV infection, adenovirus, early RSV infection, parainfluenza, or influenza have not been established and REBETOL Capsules should not be used for these indications.

There is no information regarding the use of REBETOL Capsules with other interferons.

Information for Patients Combination REBETOL/INTRON A therapy must not be used by women who are pregnant or by men whose female partners are pregnant. Extreme care must be taken to avoid pregnancy in female patients and in female partners of male patients taking combination REBETOL/INTRON A therapy. Combination REBETOL/INTRON A therapy should not be initiated until a report of a negative pregnancy test has been obtained immediately prior to initiation of therapy. Patients must perform a pregnancy test monthly during therapy and for 6 months posttherapy. Women of childbearing potential must be counseled about use of effective contraception (two reliable forms) prior to initiating therapy. Patients (male and female) must be advised of the teratogenic/embryocidal risks and must be instructed to practice effective contraception during combination REBETOL/INTRON A therapy and for 6 months posttherapy. Patients (male and female) should be advised to notify the physician immediately in the event of a pregnancy. (See **CONTRAINDICATIONS**.)

If pregnancy does occur during treatment or during 6 months posttherapy, the patient must be advised of the significant teratogenic risk of REBETOL therapy to the fetus. Patients, or partners of patients, should immediately report any pregnancy that occurs during treatment or within 6 months after treatment cessation to their physician. Physicians are encouraged to report such cases by calling (800) 727-7064.

Patients receiving combination REBETOL/INTRON A treatment should be directed in its appropriate use, informed of the benefits and risks associated with treatment, and referred to the patient **MEDICATION GUIDE**. There are no data evaluating whether REBETOL/ INTRON A therapy will prevent transmission of infection to others. Also, it is not known if treatment with REBETOL/INTRON A therapy will cure hepatitis C or prevent cirrhosis, liver failure, or liver cancer that may be the result of infection with the hepatitis C virus.

If home use is prescribed, a puncture-resistant container for the disposal of used syringes and needles should be supplied to the patient. Patients should be thoroughly instructed in the importance of proper disposal and cautioned against any reuse of needles and syringes. The full container should be disposed of according to the directions provided by the physician (see **MEDICATION GUIDE**).

The most common adverse experiences occurring with combination REBETOL/INTRON A therapy are "flu-like" symptoms, such as headache, fatigue, myalgia, and fever (see **ADVERSE REACTIONS**) and appear to decrease in severity as treatment continues. Some of these "flu-like" symptoms may be minimized by bedtime administration of INTRON A therapy. Antipyretics should be considered to prevent or partially alleviate the fever and headache. Another common adverse experience associated with INTRON A therapy is thinning of the hair.

Patients should be advised that laboratory evaluations are required prior to starting therapy and periodically thereafter (see **Laboratory Tests**). It is advised that patients be well hydrated, especially during the initial stages of treatment.

Laboratory Tests The following laboratory tests are recommended for all patients on combination REBETOL/INTRON A therapy, prior to beginning treatment and then periodically thereafter.

- Standard hematologic tests—including hemoglobin (pretreatment, week 2 and week 4 of therapy, and as clinically appropriate [see **WARNINGS**]), complete and differential white blood cell counts, and platelet count.
- Blood chemistries—liver function tests and TSH.

TABLE 4. Selected Treatment-Emergent Adverse Events: Previously Untreated and Relapse Patients

	Percentage of Patients					
	US Previously Untreated Study				US Relapse Study	
	24 weeks of treatment		48 weeks of treatment		24 weeks of treatment	
Patients Reporting Adverse Events*	**INTRON A plus REBETOL (N=228)**	**INTRON A plus Placebo (N=231)**	**INTRON A plus REBETOL (N=228)**	**INTRON A plus Placebo (N=225)**	**INTRON A plus REBETOL (N=77)**	**INTRON A plus Placebo (N=76)**
Application Site Disorders						
injection site inflammation	13	10	12	14	6	8
injection site reaction	7	9	8	9	5	3
Body as a Whole – General Disorders						
headache	63	63	66	67	66	68
fatigue	68	62	70	72	60	53
rigors	40	32	42	39	43	37
fever	37	35	41	40	32	36
influenza-like symptoms	14	18	18	20	13	13
asthenia	9	4	9	9	10	4
chest pain	5	4	9	8	6	7
Central & Peripheral Nervous System Disorders						
dizziness	17	15	23	19	26	21
Gastrointestinal System Disorders						
nausea	38	35	46	33	47	33
anorexia	27	16	25	19	21	14
dyspepsia	14	6	16	9	16	9
vomiting	11	10	9	13	12	8
Musculoskeletal System Disorders						
myalgia	61	57	64	63	61	58
arthralgia	30	27	33	36	29	29
musculoskeletal pain	20	26	28	32	22	28
Psychiatric Disorders						
insomnia	39	27	39	30	26	25
irritability	23	19	32	27	25	20
depression	32	25	36	37	23	14
emotional lability	7	6	11	8	12	8
concentration impaired	11	14	14	14	10	12
nervousness	4	2	4	4	5	4
Respiratory System Disorders						
dyspnea	19	9	18	10	17	12
sinusitis	9	7	10	14	12	7
Skin and Appendages Disorders						
alopecia	28	27	32	28	27	26
rash	20	9	28	8	21	5
pruritus	21	9	19	8	13	4
Special Senses, Other Disorders						
taste perversion	7	4	8	4	6	5

* Patients reporting one or more adverse events. A patient may have reported more than one adverse event within a body system/organ class category.

- Pregnancy—including monthly monitoring for women of childbearing potential.

Carcinogenesis and Mutagenesis Carcinogenicity studies with interferon alfa-2b, recombinant have not been performed because neutralizing activity appears in the serum after multiple dosing in all of the animal species tested.

Adequate studies to assess the carcinogenic potential of ribavirin in animals have not been conducted. However, ribavirin is a nucleoside analog that has produced positive findings in multiple *in vitro* and animal *in vivo* genotoxicity assays, and should be considered a potential carcinogen. Further studies to assess the carcinogenic potential of ribavirin in animals are ongoing.

Mutagenicity studies have demonstrated that interferon alfa-2b, recombinant is not mutagenic. Ribavirin demonstrated increased incidences of mutation and cell transformation in multiple genotoxicity assays. Ribavirin was active in the Balb/3T3 *In Vitro* Cell Transformation Assay. Mutagenic activity was observed in the mouse lymphoma assay, and at doses of 20–200 mg/kg (estimated human equivalent of 1.67 – 16.7 mg/kg, based on body surface area adjustment for a 60 kg adult; 0.1 – 1 X the maximum recommended human 24-hour dose of ribavirin) in a mouse micronucleus assay. A dominant lethal assay in rats was negative, indicating that if mutations occurred in rats they were not transmitted through male gametes.

Impairment of Fertility No reproductive toxicology studies have been performed using interferon alfa-2b, recombinant in combination with ribavirin. However, evidence provided below for interferon alfa-2b, recombinant and ribavirin when administered alone indicate that both agents have adverse effects on reproduction. It should be assumed that the effects produced by either agent alone will also be caused by the combination of the two agents. Interferons may impair human fertility. In studies of interferon alfa-2b, recombinant administration in nonhuman primates, menstrual cycle abnormalities have been observed. Decreases in serum estradiol and progesterone concentrations have been reported in women treated with human leukocyte interferon. In addition, ribavirin demonstrated significant embryocidal and/or teratogenic effects at doses well below the recommended human dose in all animal species in which adequate studies have been conducted.

Fertile women and partners of fertile women should not receive combination REBETOL/INTRON A therapy unless the patient and his/her partner are using effective contraception (two reliable forms). Based on a multiple dose half-life ($t_{1/2}$) of ribavirin of 12 days, effective contraception must be utilized for 6 months posttherapy (eg, 15 half-lives of clearance for ribavirin).

Combination REBETOL/INTRON A therapy should be used with caution in fertile men. In studies in mice to evaluate the time course and reversibility of ribavirin-induced testicular degeneration at doses of 15 to 150 mg/kg/day (estimated human equivalent of 1.25–12.5 mg/kg/day, based on body surface area adjustment for a 60 kg adult; 0.1–0.8 × the maximum human 24-hour dose of ribavirin) administered for 3 or 6 months, abnormalities in sperm occurred. Upon cessation of treatment, essentially total recovery from ribavirin-induced testicular toxicity was apparent within 1 or 2 spermatogenesis cycles.

Animal Toxicology Long-term studies in the mouse and rat (18–24 months; doses of 20–75 and 10–40 mg/kg/day, respectively [estimated human equivalent doses of 1.67–6.25 and 1.43–5.71 mg/kg/day, respectively, based on body surface area adjustment for a 60 kg adult; approximately 0.1–0.4 × the maximum human 24-hour dose of ribavirin]) have demonstrated a relationship between chronic ribavirin exposure and increased incidences of vascular lesions (microscopic hemorrhages) in mice. In rats, retinal degeneration

TABLE 5. Selected Hematologic Values During Treatment with REBETOL plus INTRON A: Previously Untreated and Relapse Patients

	Percentage of Patients					
	US Previously Untreated Study				US Relapse Study	
	24 weeks of treatment		48 weeks of treatment		24 weeks of treatment	
	INTRON A plus REBETOL (N=228)	**INTRON A plus Placebo (N=231)**	**INTRON A plus REBETOL (N=228)**	**INTRON A plus Placebo (N=225)**	**INTRON A plus REBETOL (N=77)**	**INTRON A plus Placebo (N=76)**
Hemoglobin (g/dL)						
9.5–10.9	24	1	32	1	21	3
8.0–9.4	5	0	4	0	4	0
6.5–7.9	0	0	0	0.4	0	0
<6.5	0	0	0	0	0	0
Leukocytes ($\times 10^9$/L)						
2.0–2.9	40	20	38	23	45	26
1.5–1.9	4	1	9	2	5	3
1.0–1.4	0.9	0	2	0	0	0
<1	0	0	0	0	0	0
Neutrophils ($\times 10^9$/L)						
1.0–1.49	30	32	31	44	42	34
0.75–0.99	14	15	14	11	16	18
0.5–0.74	9	9	14	7	8	4
<5	11	8	11	5	5	8
Platelets ($\times 10^9$/L)						
70–99	9	11	11	14	6	12
50–69	2	3	2	3	0	5
30–49	0	0.4	0	0.4	0	0
<30	0.9	0	1	0.9	0	0
Total Bilirubin (mg/dL)						
1.5–3.0	27	13	32	13	21	7
3.1–6.0	0.9	0.4	2	0	3	0
6.1–12.0	0	0	0.4	0	0	0
>12.0	0	0	0	0	0	0

TABLE 6. Recommended Dosing

Body weight	REBETOL Capsules	INTRON A Injection
≤75 kg	2 × 200-mg capsules AM, 3 × 200-mg capsules PM daily p.o.	3 million IU 3 times weekly s.c.
>75 kg	3 × 200-mg capsules AM, 3 × 200-mg capsules PM daily p.o.	3 million IU 3 times weekly s.c.

TABLE 7. Guidelines for Dose Modifications

	Dose Reduction* REBETOL – 600 mg daily INTRON A – 1.5 million IU TIW	Permanent Discontinuation of Treatment REBETOL and INTRON A
Hemoglobin	<10 g/dL (REBETOL) **Cardiac History Patients Only. ≥2 g/dL decrease during any 4-week period during treatment (REBETOL/INTRON A)**	<8.5 g/dL **Cardiac History Patients Only. <12 g/dL after 4 weeks of dose reduction**
White blood count	$<1.5 \times 10^9$/L (INTRON A)	$<1.0 \times 10^9$/L
Neutrophil count	$<0.75\times 10^9$/L (INTRON A)	$<0.5 \times 10^9$/L
Platelet count	$<50 \times 10^9$/L (INTRON A)	$<25 \times 10^9$/L

*Study medication to be dose reduced is shown in parenthesis.

Vial/Pen Label Strength	Fill Volume	Concentration
3 million IU vial	0.5 mL	3 million IU/0.5 mL
18 million IU multidose vial†	3.8 mL	3 million IU/0.5 mL
18 million IU multidose pen††	1.5 mL	3 million IU/0.2 mL

† This is a multidose vial which contains a total of 22.8 million IU of interferon alfa-2b, recombinant per 3.8 mL in order to provide the delivery of six 0.5-mL doses, each containing 3 million IU of interferon alfa-2b, recombinant (for a label strength of 18 million IU).

†† This is a multidose pen which contains a total of 22.5 million IU of interferon alfa-2b, recombinant per 1.5 mL in order to provide the delivery of six 0.2-mL doses, each containing 3 million IU of interferon alfa-2b, recombinant (for a label strength of 18 million IU).

occurred in controls, but the incidence was increased in ribavirin-treated rats.

Pregnancy Category X (see **CONTRAINDICATIONS**) Interferon alfa-2b, recombinant has been shown to have abortifacient effects in *Macaca mulatta* (rhesus monkeys) at 15 and 30 million IU/kg (estimated human equivalent of 5 and 10 million IU/kg, based on body surface area adjustment for a 60 kg adult). There are no adequate and well-controlled studies in pregnant women.

Ribavirin produced significant embryocidal and/or teratogenic effects in all animal species in which adequate studies have been conducted. Malformations of the skull, palate, eye, jaw, limbs, skeleton, and gastrointestinal tract were noted. The incidence and severity of teratogenic effects increased with escalation of the drug dose. Survival of fetuses and offspring was reduced. In conventional embryotoxicity/teratogenicity studies in rats and rabbits, observed no effect dose levels were well below those for proposed clinical use (0.3 mg/kg/day for both the rat and rabbit; approximately 0.06 × the recommended human 24-hour dose of ribavirin). No maternal toxicity or effects on offspring were observed in a peri/postnatal toxicity study in rats dosed orally at up to 1 mg/kg/day (estimated human equivalent dose of 0.17 mg/kg based on body surface area adjustment for a 60 kg adult; approximately 0.01 × the maximum recommended human 24-hour dose of ribavirin).

Treatment and Posttreatment: Potential Risk to the Fetus Ribavirin is known to accumulate in intracellular components from where it is cleared very slowly. It is not known whether ribavirin contained in sperm will exert a potential teratogenic effect upon fertilization of the ova. In a study in rats, it was concluded that dominant lethality was not induced by ribavirin at doses up to 200 mg/kg for 5 days (estimated human equivalent doses of 7.14–28.6 mg/kg, based on body surface area adjustment for a 60 kg adult; up to 1.7 × the maximum recommended human dose of ribavirin). However, because of the potential human teratogenic effects of ribavirin, male patients should be advised to take every precaution to avoid risk of pregnancy for their female partners.

Women of childbearing potential should not receive combination REBETOL/INTRON A therapy unless they are using effective contraception (two reliable forms) during the therapy period. In addition, effective contraception should be utilized for 6 months posttherapy based on a multiple dose half-life ($t_{1/2}$) of ribavirin of 12 days.

Male patients and their female partners must practice effective contraception (two reliable forms) during treatment with combination REBETOL/INTRON A therapy and for the 6-month posttherapy period (eg, 15 half-lives for ribavirin clearance from the body).

If pregnancy occurs in a patient or partner of a patient during treatment or during the 6 months after treatment cessation, physicians are encouraged to report such cases by calling (800) 727-7064.

Nursing Mothers It is not known whether REBETOL and INTRON A are excreted in human milk. However, studies in mice have shown that mouse interferons are excreted into the milk. Because of the potential for serious adverse reactions from the drugs in nursing infants, a decision should be made whether to discontinue nursing or to discontinue combination REBETOL/INTRON A therapy, taking into account the importance of the therapy to the mother.

Pediatric Use Safety and effectiveness in pediatric patients below the age of 18 years have not been established.

ADVERSE REACTIONS

The safety of combination REBETOL/INTRON A therapy was evaluated in controlled trials of 1010 HCV-infected adults who were previously untreated with interferon therapy and were subsequently treated for 24 or 48 weeks with combination REBETOL/INTRON A therapy and in 173 HCV-infected patients who had relapsed after interferon therapy and were subsequently treated for 24 weeks with combination REBETOL/INTRON A therapy. (See **Description of Clinical Studies.**) Overall, 19% and 6% of previously untreated and relapse patients, respectively, discontinued therapy due to adverse events in the combination arms compared to 13% and 3% in the interferon arms.

The primary toxicity of ribavirin is hemolytic anemia. Reductions in hemoglobin levels occurred within the first 1–2 weeks of therapy (see WARNINGS). Cardiac and pulmonary events associated with anemia occurred in approximately 10% of patients treated with REBETOL/INTRON A therapy. (See WARNINGS.)

The most common psychiatric events occurring in US studies of previously untreated and relapse patients treated with REBETOL/INTRON A therapy, respectively, were insomnia (39%, 26%), depression (34%, 23%), and irritability (27%, 25%). Suicidal behavior (ideation, attempts, and suicides) occurred in 1% of patients. (See **WARNINGS**.) In addition, the following spontaneous adverse events have been reported during the marketing surveillance of REBETOL/INTRON A therapy: hearing disorder and vertigo. Very rarely, combination REBETOL/INTRON A therapy may be associated with aplastic anemia.

Selected treatment-emergent adverse events that occurred in the US studies with ≥5% incidence are provided in **TABLE 4** by treatment group. In general, the selected treatment-emergent adverse events reported with lower incidence in the international studies as compared to the US studies with the exception of asthenia, influenza-like symptoms, nervousness, and pruritus.

[See table 4 at top of previous page]

Laboratory Values

Changes in selected hematologic values (hemoglobin, white blood cells, neutrophils, and platelets) during combination REBETOL/INTRON A treatment are described in **TABLE 5**.

Hemoglobin Hemoglobin decreases among patients on combination therapy began at Week 1, with stabilization by Week 4. In previously untreated patients treated for 48 weeks, the mean maximum decrease from baseline was 3.1 g/dL in the US study and 2.9 g/dL in the International study. In relapse patients, the mean maximum decrease from baseline was 2.8 g/dL in the US study and 2.6 g/dL in the International study. Hemoglobin values returned to pretreatment levels within 4 to 8 weeks of cessation of therapy in most patients.

Neutrophils There were decreases in neutrophil counts in both the combination REBETOL/INTRON A and INTRON A plus placebo dose groups. In previously untreated patients treated for 48 weeks, the mean maximum decrease in neutrophil count in the US study was 1.3×10^9/L and in the International study was 1.5×10^9/L. In relapse patients the mean maximum decrease in neutrophil count in the US study was 1.3×10^9/L and in the International study was 1.6×10^9/L. Neutrophil counts returned to pretreatment levels within 4 weeks of cessation of therapy in most patients.

Platelets In both previously untreated and relapse patients mean platelet counts generally remained in the normal range in all treatment groups; however, mean platelet counts were 10% to 15% lower in the INTRON A plus placebo group than the REBETOL/INTRON A group. Mean platelet counts returned to baseline levels within 4 weeks after treatment discontinuation.

Continued on next page

Information on Schering products appearing on these pages is effective as of January 2000.

Rebetron—Cont.

Thyroid Function Of patients who entered the previously untreated (24 and 48 week treatments) and relapse (24 week treatment) studies without thyroid abnormalities, approximately 3% to 6% and 1% to 2%, respectively, developed thyroid abnormalities requiring clinical intervention.

Bilirubin and Uric Acid Increases in both bilirubin and uric acid, associated with hemolysis, were noted in clinical trials. Most were moderate biochemical changes and were reversed within 4 weeks after treatment discontinuation. This observation occurs most frequently in patients with a previous diagnosis of Gilbert's syndrome. This has not been associated with hepatic dysfunction or clinical morbidity.

[See table 5 at top of previous page]

OVERDOSAGE

In combination REBETOL/INTRON A clinical trials, the maximum overdose reported was a dose of 39 million units of INTRON A (13 subcutaneous injections of 3 million IU each) taken with 10 g of REBETOL (fifty 200-mg capsules) in an investigator-initiated trial. The patient was observed for 2 days in the emergency room during which time no adverse event from the overdose was noted.

DOSAGE AND ADMINISTRATION

INTRON A Injection should be administered subcutaneously and REBETOL Capsules should be administered orally (see **TABLE 6**).

The recommended dose of REBETOL Capsules depends on the patient's body weight. The recommended doses of REBETOL and INTRON A are given in **TABLE 6**.

The recommended duration of treatment for patients previously untreated with interferon is 24 to 48 weeks. The duration of treatment should be individualized to the patient depending on baseline disease characteristics, response to therapy, and tolerability of the regimen (see **Description of Clinical Studies** and **ADVERSE REACTIONS**). After 24 weeks of treatment virologic response should be assessed. Treatment discontinuation should be considered in any patient who has not achieved an HCV RNA below the limit of detection of the assay by 24 weeks. There are no safety and efficacy data on treatment for longer than 48 weeks in the previously untreated patient population.

In patients who relapse following interferon therapy, the recommended duration of treatment is 24 weeks. There are no safety and efficacy data on treatment for longer than 24 weeks in the relapse patient populations.

[See table 6 at top of previous page]

REBETOL may be administered without regard to food, but should be administered in a consistent manner. (See **CLINICAL PHARMACOLOGY**.)

Dose Modifications **(TABLE 7)**

In clinical trials, approximately 26% of patients required modification of their dose of REBETOL Capsules, INTRON A Injection, or both agents. If severe adverse reactions or laboratory abnormalities develop during combination REBETOL/INTRONA therapy, the dose should be modified, or discontinued if appropriate, until the adverse reactions abate. If intolerance persists after dose adjustment, REBETOL/INTRON A therapy should be discontinued.

REBETOL/INTRON A therapy should be administered with caution to patients with pre-existing cardiac disease. Patients should be assessed before commencement of therapy and should be appropriately monitored during therapy. If there is any deterioration of cardiovascular status, therapy should be stopped. (See **WARNINGS**.)

For patients with a history of stable cardiovascular disease, a permanent dose reduction is required if the hemoglobin decreases by ≥2 g/dL during any 4-week period. In addition, for these cardiac history patients, if the hemoglobin remains <12 g/dL after 4 weeks on a reduced dose, the patient should discontinue combination REBETOL/INTRON A therapy.

It is recommended that a patient whose hemoglobin level falls below 10 g/dL have his/her REBETOL dose reduced to 600 mg daily (1 × 200-mg capsule AM, 2 × 200-mg capsules PM). A patient whose hemoglobin level falls below 8.5 g/dL should be permanently discontinued from REBETOL/INTRON A therapy (See **WARNINGS**.)

It is recommended that a patient who experiences moderate depression (persistent low mood, loss of interest, poor self image, and/or hopelessness) have his/her INTRON A dose temporarily reduced and/or be considered for medical therapy. A patient experiencing severe depression or suicidal ideation/attempt should be discontinued from REBETOL/INTRON A therapy and followed closely with appropriate medical management. (See **WARNINGS**.)

[See table 7 at top of previous page]

Administration of INTRON A Injection

At the discretion of the physician, the patient may self-administer the INTRON A. (See illustrated **MEDICATION GUIDE** for instructions.)

The INTRON A Injection is supplied as a clear and colorless solution. The appropriate INTRON A dose should be withdrawn from the vial or set on the multidose pen and injected subcutaneously. After administration of INTRON A Injection, it is essential to follow the procedure for proper disposal of syringes and needles. (See **MEDICATION GUIDE** for detailed instructions.)

[See last table on previous page]

Parenteral drug products should be inspected visually for particulate matter and discoloration prior to administration, whenever solution and container permit. INTRON A Injection may be administered using either sterilized glass or plastic disposable syringes.

Stability INTRON A Injection provided in vials is stable at 35°C (95°F) for up to 7 days and at 30°C (86°F) for up to 14 days. INTRON A Injection provided in a multidose pen is stable at 30°C (86°F) for up to 2 days. The solution is clear and colorless.

HOW SUPPLIED

REBETOL 200-mg Capsules are white, opaque capsules with REBETOL, 200 mg, and the Schering Corporation logo imprinted on the capsule shell; the capsules are packaged in a bottle.

INTRON A Injection is a clear, colorless solution packaged in single-dose and multidose vials, and a multidose pen.

INTRON A Injection and REBETOL Capsules are available in the following combination package presentations:

[See table below]

STORAGE CONDITIONS

Store the REBETOL Capsules plus INTRON A Injection combination package refrigerated between 2° and 8°C (36° and 46°F).

When separated, the individual bottle of REBETOL Capsules should be stored refrigerated between 2° and 8°C (36° and 46°F) or at 25° (77°F); excursions are permitted between 15° and 30°C (59° and 86°F).

When separated, the individuals vials of INTRON A Injection and the INTRON A multidose pen should be stored refrigerated between 2° and 8°C (36° and 46°F).

Schering Corporation
Kenilworth, NJ 07033 USA
U.S. Patents 4,530,901 & 4,211,771

21617679 Rev. 5/00

	Each REBETRON Combination Package Consists of:	
For Patients ≤75 kg	A box containing 6 vials of INTRON A Injection (3 million IU in 0.5 mL per vial), 6 syringes, alcohol swabs, and one bottle containg 70 REBETOL Capsules.	(NDC 0085-1241-02)
	One 18 million IU multidose vial of INTRON A Injection (22.8 million IU per 3.8 mL; 3 million IU/0.5 mL), 6 syringes, alcohol swabs, and one bottle containing 70 REBETOL Capsules.	(NDC 0085-1236-02)
	One 18 million IU INTRON A Injection multidose pen (22.5 million IU per 1.5 mL; 3 million IU/0.2 mL), 6 disposable needles, alcohol swabs, and one bottle containing 70 REBETOL Capsules.	(NDC 0085-1258-02)
For Patients >75 kg	A box containing 6 vials of INTRON A Injection (3 million IU in 0.5 mL per vial), 6 syringes, alcohol swabs, and one bottle containing 84 REBETOL Capsules.	(NDC 0085-1241-01)
	One 18 million IU multidose vial of INTRON A Injection (22.8 million IU per 3.8 mL; 3 million IU/0.5 mL), 6 syringes, alcohol swabs, and one bottle containing 84 REBETOL Capsules.	(NDC 0085-1236-01)
	One 18 million IU INTRON A Injection multidose pen (22.5 million IU per 1.5 mL; 3 million IU/0.2 mL), 6 disposable needles, alcohol swabs, and one bottle containing 84 REBETOL Capsules.	(NDC 0085-1258-01)
For REBETOL Dose Reduction	A box containing 6 vials of INTRON A Injection (3 million IU in 0.5 mL per vial), 6 syringes, alcohol swabs, and one bottle containing 42 REBETOL Capsules.	(NDC 0085-1241-03)
	One 18 million IU multidose of INTRON A Injection (22.8 million IU per 3.8 mL; 3 million IU/0.5 mL), 6 syringes, alcohol swabs, and one bottle containing 42 REBETOL Capsules.	(NDC 0085-1236-03)
	One 18 million IU INTRON A Injection multidose pen (22.5 million IU per 1.5 mL; 3 million IU/0.2 mL), 6 disposable needles, alcohol swabs, and one bottle containing 42 REBETOL Capsules.	(NDC 0085-1258-03)

TEMODAR™ ℞

[těm-ō-dăr]
(temozolomide)
CAPSULES

DESCRIPTION

TEMODAR Capsules for oral administration contain temozolomide, an imidazotetrazine derivative. The chemical name of temozolomide is 3,4-dihydro-3-methyl-4-oxoimidazo[5,1-d]-*as*-tetrazine-8-carboxamide. The structural formula is:

The material is a white to light tan/light pink powder with a molecular formula of $C_6H_6N_6O_2$ and a molecular weight of 194.15. The molecule is stable at acidic pH (<5), and labile at pH >7, hence can be administered orally. The prodrug, temozolomide, is rapidly hydrolysed to the active 5-(3-methyltriazen-1-yl)imidazole-4-carboxamide (MTIC) at neutral and alkaline pH values, with hydrolysis taking place even faster at alkaline pH.

Each capsule contains either 5 mg, 20 mg, 100 mg, or 250 mg of temozolomide. The inactive ingredients for TEMODAR Capsules are lactose anhydrous, colloidal silicon dioxide, sodium starch glycolate, tartaric acid, and stearic acid. Gelatin capsule shells contain titanium dioxide. The capsules are imprinted with pharmaceutical ink.

TEMODAR 5 mg: green imprint contains pharmaceutical grade shellac, anhydrous ethyl alcohol, isopropyl alcohol, n-butyl alcohol, propylene glycol, ammonium hydroxide, titanium dioxide, yellow iron oxide, and FD&C Blue #2 aluminum lake.

TEMODAR 20 mg: brown imprint also contains pharmaceutical grade shellac, anhydrous ethyl alcohol, isopropyl alcohol, n-butyl alcohol, propylene glycol, purified water, ammonium hydroxide, potassium hydroxide, titanium dioxide, black iron oxide, yellow iron oxide, brown iron oxide, and red iron oxide.

TEMODAR 100 mg: blue imprint contains pharmaceutical glaze (modified) in an ethanol/shellac mixture, isopropyl alcohol, n-butyl alcohol, propylene glycol, titanium dioxide, and FD&C Blue #2 aluminum lake.

TEMODAR 250 mg: black, imprint contains pharmaceutical grade shellac, anhydrous ethyl alcohol, isopropyl alcohol, n-butyl alcohol, propylene glycol, purified water, ammonium hydroxide, potassium hydroxide, and black iron oxide.

CLINICAL PHARMACOLOGY

Mechanism of Action: Temozolomide is not directly active but undergoes rapid nonenzymatic conversion at physiologic pH to the reactive compound MTIC. The cytotoxicity of MTIC is thought to be primarily due to alkylation of DNA. Alkylation (methylation) occurs mainly at the O^6 and N^7 positions at guanine.

Pharmacokinetics: Temozolomide is rapidly and completely absorbed after oral administration; peak plasma concentrations occur in 1 hour. Food reduces the rate and extent of temozolomide absorption. Mean peak plasma concentration and AUC decreased by 32% and 9%, respectively, and T_{max} increased 2-fold (from 1.1 to 2.25 hours) when temozolomide was administered after a modified high-fat breakfast. Temozolomide is rapidly eliminated with a mean elimination half-life of 1.8 hours and exhibits linear kinetics over the therapeutic dosing range. Temozolomide has a mean apparent volume of distribution of 0.4 L/kg (%CV=13%). It is weakly bound to human plasma proteins; the mean percent bound of drug-related total radioactivity is 15%.

Metabolism and Elimination: Temozolomide is spontaneously hydrolyzed at physiologic pH to the active species, 3-methyl-(triazen-1-yl)imidazole-4-carboxamide (MTIC) and to temozolomide acid metabolite. MTIC is further hydrolyzed to 5-amino-imidazole-4-carboxamide (AIC) which is known to be an intermediate in purine and nucleic acid biosynthesis and to methylhydrazine, which is believed to be the active alkylating species. Cytochrome P450 enzymes play only a minor role in the metabolism of temozolomide and MTIC. Relative to the AUC of temozolomide, the exposure to MTIC and AIC is 2.4% and 23%, respectively. About 38% of the administered temozolomide total radioactive dose is recovered over 7 days; 37.7% in urine and 0.8% in feces. The majority of the recovery of radioactivity in urine is as unchanged temozolomide (5.6%), AIC (12%), temozolomide acid metabolite (2.3%), and unidentified polar metabolite(s) (17%). Overall clearance of temozolomide is about 5.5 L/hr/m^2.

Special Populations: *Age* Population pharmacokinetic analysis indicates that age (range 19 to 78 years) has no influence on the pharmacokinetics of temozolomide. In the anaplastic astrocytoma study population, patients 70 years of age or older had a higher incidence of Grade 4 neutropenia and Grade 4 thrombocytopenia in the first cycle of therapy than patients under 70 years of age (see **PRECAUTIONS**). In the entire safety database, however, there did not appear to be a higher incidence in patients 70 years of age or older (see **ADVERSE REACTIONS**).

Gender Population pharmacokinetic analysis indicates that women have an approximately 5% lower clearance (adjusted for body surface area) for temozolomide than men. Women have higher incidences of Grade 4 neutropenia and thrombocytopenia in the first cycle of therapy than men (see **ADVERSE REACTIONS**).

Race The effect of race on the pharmacokinetics of temozolomide has not been studied.

Tobacco Use Population pharmacokinetic analysis indicates that the oral clearance of temozolomide is similar in smokers and nonsmokers.

Creatinine Clearance Population pharmacokinetic analysis indicates that creatinine clearance over the range of 36-130 mL/min/m^2 has no effect on the clearance of temozolomide after oral administration. The pharmacokinetics of temozolomide have not been studied in patients with severely impaired renal function (CLcr < 36 mL/min/m^2). Caution should be exercised when TEMODAR is administered to patients with severe renal impairment. TEMODAR has not been studied in patients on dialysis.

Hepatically Impaired Patients In a pharmacokinetic study, the pharmacokinetics of temozolomide in patients with mild-to-moderate hepatic impairment (Child's-Pugh Class I - II) were similar to those observed in patients with normal hepatic function. Caution should be exercised when temozolomide is administered to patients with severe hepatic impairment.

Pediatrics Pediatric patients (3 to 17 years of age) and adult patients have similar clearance and half-life values for temozolomide. There is no clinical experience with the use of TEMODAR in children under the age of 3 years.

Drug-Drug Interactions In a multiple-dose study, administration of TEMODAR with ranitidine did not change the C_{max} or AUC values for temozolomide or MTIC.

Population analysis indicates that administration of valproic acid decreases the clearance of temozolomide by about 5% (see **PRECAUTIONS**).

Population analysis failed to demonstrate any influence of coadministered dexamethasone, prochlorperazine, phenytoin, carbamazepine, ondansetron, H_2-receptor antagonists, or phenobarbital on the clearance of orally administered temozolomide.

Clinical Studies: A single-arm, multicenter study was conducted in 162 patients who had anaplastic astrocytoma at first release and who had a baseline Karnofsky performance status of 70 or greater. Patients had previously received radiation therapy and may also have previously received a nitrosourea with or without other chemotherapy. Fifty-four patients had disease progression on prior therapy with both a nitrosourea and procarbazine and their malignancy was considered refractory to chemotherapy (refractory anaplastic astrocytoma population). Median age of this subgroup of 54 patients was 42 years (19 to 76). Sixty-five percent were male. Seventy-two percent of patients had a KPS of ≥80. Sixty-three percent of patients had surgery other than a biopsy at the time of initial diagnosis. Of those patients undergoing resection, 73% underwent a subtotal resection and 27% underwent a gross total resection. Eighteen percent of patients had surgery at the time of first relapse. The median time from initial diagnosis to first relapse was 13.8 months (4.2 to 75.4).

TEMODAR was given for the first 5 consecutive days of a 28-day cycle at a starting dose of 150 mg/m^2/day. If the nadir and day of dosing (Day 29, Day 1 of next cycle) absolute neutrophil count was ≥1.5 × 10^9/L (1,500/µL) and the nadir and Day 29, Day 1 of next cycle, platelet count was ≥100 × 10^9/L (100,000/µL), the TEMODAR dose was increased to 200 mg/m^2/day for the first 5 consecutive days of a 28-day cycle.

In the refractory anaplastic astrocytoma population the overall tumor response rate (CR + PR) was 22% (12/54 patients) and the complete response rate was 9% (5/54 patients). The median duration of all responses was 50 weeks (range of 16 to 114 weeks) and the median duration of complete responses was 64 weeks (range of 52 to 114 weeks). In this population, progression-free survival at 6 months was 45% (95% confidence interval 31% to 58%) and progression-free survival at 12 months was 29% (95% confidence interval 16% to 42%). Median progression-free survival was 4.4 months. Overall survival at 6 months was 74% (95% confidence interval 62% to 86%) and 12-month overall survival was 65% (95% confidence interval 52% to 78%). Median overall survival was 15.9 months.

INDICATIONS AND USAGE

TEMODAR (temozolomide) Capsules are indicated for the treatment of adult patients with refractory anaplastic astrocytoma, ie, patients at first relapse who have experienced disease progression on a drug regimen containing a nitrosourea and procarbazine.

This indication is based on the response rate in the indicated population. No results are available from randomized controlled trials in recurrent anaplastic astrocytoma that demonstrate a clinical benefit resulting from treatment, such as improvement in disease-related symptoms, delayed disease progression, or improved survival.

CONTRAINDICATIONS

TEMODAR (temozolomide) Capsules are contraindicated in patients who have a history of hypersensitivity reaction to any of its components. TEMODAR is also contraindicated in patients who have a history of hypersensitivity to DTIC, since both drugs are metabolized to MTIC.

WARNINGS

Patients treated with TEMODAR may experience myelosuppression. Prior to dosing, patients must have an absolute neutrophil count (ANC) ≥1.5 × 10^9/L and a platelet count ≥100 × 10^9/L. A complete blood count should be obtained on Day 22 (21 days after the first dose) or within 48 hours of that day, and weekly until the ANC is above 1.5 × 10^9/L and platelet count exceeds 100 × 10^9/L. In the clinical trials, if the ANC fell to <1.0 ×10^9/L or the platelet count was <50 × 10^9/L during any cycle, the next cycle was reduced by 50 mg/m^2, but not below 100 mg/m^2. Patients who do not tolerate 100 mg/m^2 should not receive TEMODAR. Geriatric patients and women have been shown in clinical trials to have a higher risk of developing myelosuppression. Myelosuppression generally occurred late in the treatment cycle. The median nadirs occurred at 26 days for platelets (range 21 to 40 days) and 28 days for neutrophils (range 1 to 44 days). Only 14% (22/158) of patients had a neutrophil nadir and 20% (32/158) of patients had a platelet nadir which may have delayed the start of the next cycle. Neutrophil and platelet counts returned to normal, on average, within 14 days of nadir counts (see **PRECAUTIONS**).

Pregnancy: Temozolomide may cause fetal harm when administered to a pregnant woman. Five consecutive days of oral administration of 75 mg/m^2/day in rats and 150 mg/m^2/day in rabbits during the period of organogenesis (3/8 and 3/4 the maximum recommended human dose, respectively) caused numerous malformations of the external organs, soft tissues, and skeleton in both species. Doses of 150 mg/m^2/day in rats and rabbits also caused embryolethality as indicated by increased resorptions. There are no adequate and well-controlled studies in pregnant women. If this drug is used during pregnancy, or if the patient becomes pregnant while taking this drug, the patient should be apprised of the potential hazard to the fetus. Women of childbearing potential should be advised to avoid becoming pregnant during therapy with TEMODAR.

PRECAUTIONS

Information for Patients: In clinical trials, the most frequently occurring adverse effects were nausea and vomiting. These were usually either self-limiting or readily controlled with standard antiemetic therapy. Capsules should not be opened. If capsules are accidentally opened or damaged, rigorous precautions should be taken with the capsule contents to avoid inhalation or contact with the skin or mucous membranes. The medication should be kept away from children and pets.

Drug Interaction: Administration of valproic acid decreases oral clearance of temozolomide by about 5%. The clinical implication of this effect is not known.

Patients with Severe Hepatic or Renal Impairment: Caution should be exercised when TEMODAR is administered to patients with severe hepatic or renal impairment (see **Special Populations**).

Geriatrics: Clinical studies of temozolomide did not include sufficient numbers of subjects aged 65 and over to determine whether they responded differently from younger subjects. Other reported clinical experience has not identified differences in responses between the elderly and younger patients. Caution should be exercised when treating elderly patients.

In the anaplastic astrocytoma study population, patients 70 years of age or older had a higher incidence of Grade 4 neutropenia and Grade 4 thrombocytopenia (2/8; 25%, p=.31 and 2/10; 20%, p=.09, respectively) in the first cycle of therapy than patients under 70 years of age (see **ADVERSE REACTIONS**).

Laboratory Tests: A complete blood count should be obtained on Day 22 (21 days after the first dose). Blood counts should be performed weekly until recovery if the ANC falls below 1.5 × 10^9/L and the platelet count falls below 100 × 10^9/L.

Carcinogenesis, Mutagenesis, and Impairment of Fertility: Standard carcinogenicity studies were not conducted with temozolomide. In rats treated with 200 mg/m^2 temozolomide (equivalent to the maximum recommended daily human dose) on 5 consecutive days every 28 days for 3 cycles, mammary carcinomas were found in both males and females. With 6 cycles of treatment at 25, 50, and 125 mg/m^2 (about 1/8 to 1/2 the maximum recommended daily human dose), mammary carcinomas were observed at all doses and fibrosarcomas of the heart, eye, seminal vesicles, salivary glands, abdominal cavity, uterus, and prostate; carcinoma of the seminal vesicles, schwannoma of the heart, optic nerve, and harderian gland; and adenomas of the skin, lung, pituitary, and thyroid were observed at the high dose.

Temozolomide was mutagenic *in vitro* in bacteria (Ames assay) and clastogenic in mammalian cells (human peripheral blood lymphocyte assays).

Reproductive function studies have not been conducted with temozolomide. However, multicycle toxicology studies in rats and dogs have demonstrated testicular toxicity (syncytial cells/immature sperm, testicular atrophy) at doses of 50 mg/m^2 in rats and 125 mg/m^2 in dogs (1/4 and 5/8, respectively, of the maximum recommended human dose on a body surface area basis).

Pregnancy Category D: See **WARNINGS** section.

Nursing Mothers: It is not known whether this drug is excreted in human milk. Because many drugs are excreted in human milk and because of the potential for serious adverse reactions in nursing infants from TEMODAR, patients receiving TEMODAR should discontinue nursing.

Pediatric Use: Safety and effectiveness in pediatric patients have not been established.

ADVERSE REACTIONS

Tables 1 and **2** show the incidence of adverse events in the 158 patients in the anaplastic astrocytoma study for whom data are available. In the absence of a control group, it is not clear in many cases whether these events should be attributed to temozolomide or the patients' underlying conditions, but nausea, vomiting, fatigue, and hematologic effects appear to be clearly drug related. The most frequently occurring side effects were nausea, vomiting, headache, and fatigue. The adverse events were usually NCI Common Toxicity Criteria (CTC) Grade 1 or 2 (mild to moderate in severity) and were self-limiting, with nausea and vomiting readily controlled with antiemetics. The incidence of severe nausea and vomiting (CTC Grade 3 or 4) was 10% and 6%, respectively. Myelosuppression (thrombocytopenia and neutropenia) was the dose-limiting adverse event. It usually occurred within the first few cycles of therapy and was not cumulative.

Myelosuppression occurred late in the treatment cycle and returned to normal, on average, within 14 days of nadir counts. The median nadirs occurred at 26 days for platelets (range 21 to 40 days) and 28 days for neutrophils (range 1 to 44 days). Only 14% (22/158) of patients had a neutrophil nadir and 20% (32/158) of patients had platelet nadir which may have delayed the start of the next cycle (see **WARNINGS**). Less than 10% of patients required hospitalization, blood transfusion, or discontinuation of therapy due to myelosuppression.

In clinical trial experience with 110 to 111 women and 169 to 174 men (depending on measurements), there were higher rates of Grade 4 neutropenia (ANC < 500 cells/µL) and thrombocytopenia (< 20,000 cells/µL) in women than men in the first cycle of therapy: (12% versus 5% and 9% versus 3%, respectively).

In the entire safety database for which hematologic data exist (N=932), 7% (4/61) and 9.5% (6/63) of patients over age 70 experienced Grade 4 neutropenia or thrombocytopenia in the first cycle, respectively. For patients less than or equal to age 70, 7% (62/871) and 5.5% (48/879) experienced Grade 4 neutropenia or thrombocytopenia in the first cycle, respectively.

Table 1
Adverse Events in the Anaplastic Astrocytoma Trial (≥5%)

	No. (%) of TEMODAR Patients (N=158)	
	All Events	**Grade 3/4**
Any Adverse Event	**153 (97)**	**79 (50)**
Body as a Whole		
Headache	65 (41)	10 (6)
Fatigue	54 (34)	7 (4)
Asthenia	20 (13)	9 (6)
Fever	21 (13)	3 (2)
Back pain	12 (8)	4 (3)
Cardiovascular		
Edema peripheral	17 (11)	1 (1)
Central and Peripheral Nervous System		
Convulsions	36 (23)	8 (5)
Hemiparesis	29 (18)	10 (6)
Dizziness	19 (12)	1 (1)
Coordination abnormal	17 (11)	2 (1)
Amnesia	16 (10)	6 (4)
Insomnia	16 (10)	0

Continued on next page

Information on Schering products appearing on these pages is effective as of January 2000.

Temodar—Cont.

Paresthesia	15 (9)	1 (1)
Somnolence	15 (9)	5 (3)
Paresis	13 (8)	4 (3)
Urinary incontinence	13 (8)	3 (2)
Ataxia	12 (8)	3 (2)
Dysphasia	11 (7)	1 (1)
Convulsions local	9 (6)	0
Gait abnormal	9 (6)	1 (1)
Confusion	8 (5)	0
Endocrine		
Adrenal hypercorticism	13 (8)	0
Gastrointestinal System		
Nausea	84 (53)	16 (10)
Vomiting	66 (42)	10 (6)
Constipation	52 (33)	1 (1)
Diarrhea	25 (16)	3 (2)
Abdominal pain	14 (9)	2 (1)
Anorexia	14 (9)	1 (1)
Metabolic		
Weight increase	8 (5)	0
Musculoskeletal System		
Myalgia	8 (5)	
Psychiatric Disorders		
Anxiety	11 (7)	1 (1)
Depression	10 (6)	0
Reproductive Disorders		
Breast pain, female	4 (6)	
Resistance Mechanism Disorders		
Infection viral	17 (11)	0
Respiratory System		
Upper respiratory tract infection	13 (8)	0
Pharyngitis	12 (8)	0
Sinusitis	10 (6)	0
Coughing	8 (5)	0
Skin and Appendages		
Rash	13 (8)	0
Pruritus	12 (8)	2 (1)
Urinary System		
Urinary tract infection	12 (8)	0
Micturition increased frequency	9 (6)	0
Vision		
Diplopia	8 (5)	0
Vision Abnormal*	8 (5)	

*Blurred vision, visual deficit, vision changes, vision troubles.

Table 2
Adverse Hematologic Effects (Grade 3 to 4) in the Anaplastic Astrocytoma Trial

	TEMODAR[a]
Hemoglobin	7/158 (4%)
Neutrophils	20/142 (14%)
Platelets	29/156 (19%)
WBC	18/158 (11%)

[a]Change from Grade 0 to 2 at baseline to Grade 3 or 4 during treatment.

OVERDOSAGE

Doses of 500, 750, 1,000, 1,250 mg/m² (total dose per cycle over 5 days) have been evaluated clinically in patients. Dose-limiting toxicity was hematologic and was reported at 1,000 mg/m² and at 1,250 mg/m². Up to 1,000 mg/m² has been taken as a single dose, with only the expected effects of neutropenia and thrombocytopenia resulting. In the event of an overdose, hematologic evaluation is needed. Supportive measures should be provided as necessary.

DOSAGE AND ADMINISTRATION

Dosage of TEMODAR must be adjusted according to nadir neutrophil and platelet counts in the previous cycle and neutrophil and platelet counts at the time of initiating the next cycle. The initial dose is 150 mg/m² orally once daily for 5 consecutive days per 28-day treatment cycle. If both the nadir and day of dosing (Day 29, Day 1 of next cycle) absolute neutrophil counts (ANC) are $\geq 1.5 \times 10^9$/L (1,500/µL) and both the nadir and Day 29, Day 1 of next cycle platelet counts are $\geq 100 \times 10^9$/L (100,000/µL), the TEMODAR dose may be increased to 200 mg/m²/day for 5 consecutive days per 28-day treatment cycle. During treatment, a complete blood count should be obtained on Day 22 (21 days after the first dose) or within 48 hours of that day, and weekly until the ANC is above 1.5×10^9/L (1,500/µL) and the platelet count exceeds 100×10^9/L (100,000/µL). The next cycle of TEMODAR should not be started until the ANC and platelet count exceed these levels. If the ANC falls to $<1.0 \times 10^9$/L (1,000/µL) or the platelet count is $<50 \times 10^9$/L (50,000/µL) during any cycle, the next cycle should be reduced by 50 mg/m², but not below 100 mg/m², the lowest recommended dose (see **Table 3**) (see **WARNINGS**). TEMODAR therapy can be continued until disease progression. In the clinical trial, treatment could be continued for a maximum of 2 years; but the optimum duration of therapy is not known. For TEMODAR dosage calculations based on body surface area (BSA), see **Table 4**. For suggested capsule combinations based on daily dose, see **Table 5**.

Table 3 Dosing Modification Table

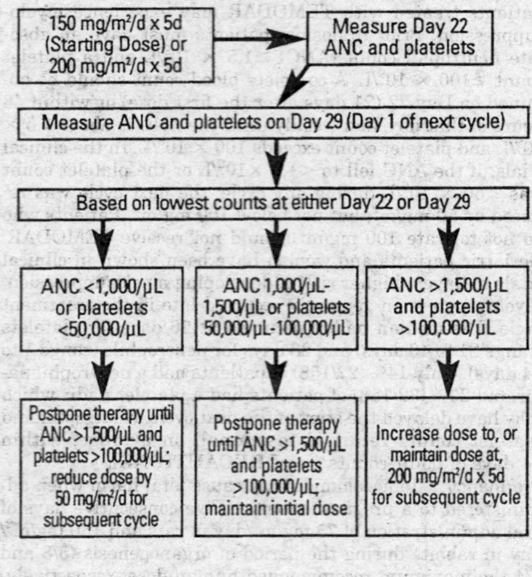

Table 4
Daily Dose Calculations by Body Surface Area (BSA) for 5 consecutive days per 28-day treatment cycle for the initial chemotherapy cycle (150 mg/m²) and for subsequent chemotherapy cycles (200 mg/m²) for patients whose nadir and day of dosing (Day 29, Day 1 of next cycle) absolute neutrophil count (ANC) is >1.5 × 10⁹/L (1,500/µL) and whose nadir and Day 29, Day 1 of next cycle platelet count is >100× 10⁹/L (100,000/µL).

Total BSA (m²)	150 mg/m² (mg daily)	200 mg/m² (mg daily)
0.5	75	100
0.6	90	120
0.7	105	140
0.8	120	160
0.9	135	180
1.0	150	200
1.1	165	220
1.2	180	240
1.3	195	260
1.4	210	280
1.5	225	300
1.6	240	320
1.7	255	340
1.8	270	360
1.9	285	380
2.0	300	400
2.1	315	420
2.2	330	440
2.3	345	460
2.4	360	480
2.5	375	500

Table 5
Suggested Capsule Combinations Based on Daily Dose

	Number of Daily Capsules by Strength (mg)			
Total Daily Dose (mg)	250	100	20	5
200	0	2	0	0
205	0	2	0	1
210	0	2	0	2
215	0	2	0	3
220	0	2	1	0
225	0	2	1	1
230	0	2	1	2
235	0	2	1	3
240	0	2	2	0
245	0	2	2	1
250	1	0	0	0
255	1	0	0	1
260	1	0	0	2
265	1	0	0	3
270	1	0	1	0
275	1	0	1	1
280	1	0	1	2
285	1	0	1	3
290	1	0	2	0
295	1	0	2	1
300	0	3	0	0
305	0	3	0	1
310	0	3	0	2
315	0	3	0	3
320	0	3	1	0
325	0	3	1	1
330	1	0	4	0
335	1	0	4	1
340	0	3	2	0
345	0	3	2	1
350	1	1	0	0
355	1	1	0	1
360	1	1	0	2
365	1	1	0	3
370	1	1	1	0
375	1	1	1	1
380	1	1	1	2
385	1	1	1	3
390	1	1	2	0
395	1	1	2	1
400	0	4	0	0
405	0	4	0	1
410	0	4	0	2
415	0	4	0	3
420	0	4	1	0
425	0	4	1	1
430	1	1	4	0
435	0	4	1	3
440	0	4	2	0
445	0	4	2	1
450	1	2	0	0
455	1	2	0	1
460	1	2	0	2
465	1	2	0	3
470	1	2	1	0
475	1	2	1	1
480	1	2	1	2
485	1	2	1	3
490	1	2	2	0
495	1	2	2	1
500	2	0	0	0

In the clinical trial, TEMODAR was administered under both fasting and nonfasting conditions; however, absorption is affected by food (see **CLINICAL PHARMACOLOGY**) and consistency of administration with respect to food is recommended. There are no dietary restrictions with temozolomide. To reduce nausea and vomiting, temozolomide should be taken on an empty stomach. Bedtime administration may be advised. Antiemetic therapy may be administered to and/or following administration of TEMODAR.
TEMODAR (temozolomide) Capsules should not be opened or chewed. They should be swallowed whole with a glass of water.

Handling and Disposal: Temozolomide causes the rapid appearance of malignant tumors in rats. Capsules should not be opened. If capsules are accidentally opened or damaged, rigorous precautions should be taken with the capsule contents to avoid inhalation or contact with the skin or mucous membranes. Procedures for proper handling and disposal of anticancer drugs should be considered.[1–7] Several guidelines on this subject have been published. There is no general agreement that all of the procedures recommended in the guidelines are necessary or appropriate.

HOW SUPPLIED

TEMODAR (temozolomide) Capsules are supplied in amber glass bottles with child-resistant polypropylene caps containing the following capsule strengths:
TEMODAR (temozolomide) Capsules 5 mg: 5 and 20 capsule bottles.
5 count — NDC 0085-1248-01
20 count — NDC 0085-1248-02
TEMODAR (temozolomide) Capsules 20 mg: 5 and 20 capsule bottles.
5 count — NDC 0085-1244-01
20 count — NDC 0085-1244-02
TEMODAR (temozolomide) Capsules 100 mg: 5 and 20 capsule bottles.
5 count — NDC 0085-1259-01
20 count — NDC 0085-1259-02
TEMODAR (temozolomide) Capsules 250 mg: 5 and 20 capsule bottles.
5 count — NDC 0085-1252-01
20 count — NDC 0085-1252-02

Store at 25°C (77°F); excursions permitted to 15°-30°C (59°-86°F).
[See USP Controlled Room Temperature]

REFERENCES
1. Recommendations for the Safe Handling of Parenteral Antineoplastic Drugs, NIH Publication No. 83-2621. For sale by the Superintendent of Documents, U.S. Government Printing Office, Washington, DC 20402.
2. AMA Council Report, Guidelines for Handling Parenteral Antineoplastics. *JAMA*. 1985;2:53(11):1590-1592.
3. National Study Commission on Cytotoxic Exposure—Recommendations for Handling Cytotoxic Agents. Available from Louis P. Jeffrey, ScD., Chairman, National Study Commission on Cytotoxic Exposure, Massachusetts College of Pharmacy and Allied Health Sciences, 179 Longwood Avenue, Boston, Massachusetts 02115.
4. Clinical Oncological Society of Australia, Guidelines and Recommendations for Safe Handling of Antineoplastic Agents. *Med J Australia*. 1983;1:426-428.
5. Jones RB, et al. Safe Handling Of Chemotherapeutic Agents: A Report from the Mount Sinai Medical Center. CA — *A Cancer Journal for Clinicians*. 1983;(Sept/Oct):258-263.
6. American Society of Hospital Pharmacists Technical Assistance Bulletin on Handling Cytotoxic and Hazardous Drugs. *Am J Hosp Pharm*. 1990;47:1033-1049.
7. Controlling Occupational Exposure to Hazardous Drugs. (OSHA Work-Practice Guidelines), *Am J Health-Syst Pharm*. 1996;53:1669-1685.

Schering Corporation
Kenilworth, NJ 07033 USA
8/99 22487809

TRILAFON® ℞
brand of perphenazine, USP
Tablets,
Injection

DESCRIPTION
TRILAFON products contain perphenazine, USP (4-[3-(2-chlorophenothiazin-10-yl)propyl]-1-piper-azineethanol), a piperazinyl phenothiazine having the chemical formula, $C_{21}H_{26}ClN_3OS$. They are available as **Tablets**, 2, 4, 8, and 16 mg; and **Injection**, perphenazine 5 mg per 1 mL.
The inactive ingredients for TRILAFON **Tablets**, 2, 4, 8, and 16 mg, include: acacia, black iron oxide, butylparaben, calcium phosphate, calcium sulfate, carnauba wax, corn starch, gelatin, lactose, magnesium stearate, potato starch, sugar, titanium dioxide, white wax, and other ingredients. May also contain talc.
The inactive ingredients for TRILAFON **Injection** include: citric acid, sodium bisulfite, sodium hydroxide, and water.

ACTIONS
Perphenazine has actions at all levels of the central nervous system, particularly the hypothalamus. However, the site and mechanism of action of therapeutic effect are not known.

INDICATIONS
Perphenazine is indicated for use in the management of the manifestations of psychotic disorders; and for the control of severe nausea and vomiting in adults.
TRILAFON has not been shown effective for the management of behavioral complications in patients with mental retardation.

CONTRAINDICATIONS
TRILAFON products are contraindicated in comatose or greatly obtunded patients and in patients receiving large doses of central nervous system depressants (barbiturates, alcohol, narcotics, analgesics, or antihistamines); in the presence of existing blood dyscrasias, bone marrow depression, or liver damage; and in patients who have shown hypersensitivity to TRILAFON products, their components, or related compounds.
TRILAFON products are also contraindicated in patients with suspected or established subcortical brain damage, with or without hypothalamic damage, since a hyperthermic reaction with temperatures in excess of 104°F may occur in such patients, sometimes not until 14 to 16 hours after drug administration. Total body ice-packing is recommended for such a reaction; antipyretics may also be useful.

WARNINGS
Tardive dyskinesia, a syndrome consisting of potentially irreversible, involuntary, dyskinetic movements, may develop in patients treated with neuroleptic (antipsychotic) drugs. Although the prevalence of the syndrome appears to be highest among the elderly, especially elderly women, it is impossible to rely upon prevalence estimates to predict, at the inception of neuroleptic treatment, which patients are likely to develop the syndrome. Whether neuroleptic drug products differ in their potential to cause tardive dyskinesia is unknown.
Both the risk of developing the syndrome and the likelihood that it will become irreversible are believed to increase as the duration of treatment and the total cumulative dose of neuroleptic drugs administered to the patient increase. However, the syndrome can develop, although much less commonly, after relatively brief treatment periods at low doses.
There is no known treatment for established cases of tardive dyskinesia, although the syndrome may remit, partially or completely, if neuroleptic treatment is withdrawn. Neuroleptic treatment itself, however, may suppress (or partially suppress) the signs and symptoms of the syndrome, and thereby may possibly mask the underlying disease process. The effect that symptomatic suppression has upon the long-term course of the syndrome is unknown.
Given these considerations, neuroleptics should be prescribed in a manner that is most likely to minimize the occurrence of tardive dyskinesia. Chronic neuroleptic treatment should generally be reserved for patients who suffer from a chronic illness that 1) is known to respond to neuroleptic drugs, and 2) for whom alternative, equally effective, but potentially less harmful treatments are not available or appropriate. In patients who do require chronic treatment, the smallest dose and the shortest duration of treatment producing a satisfactory clinical response should be sought. The need for continued treatment should be reassessed periodically.
If signs and symptoms of tardive dyskinesia appear in a patient on neuroleptics, drug discontinuation should be considered. However, some patients may require treatment despite the presence of the syndrome.
(For further information about the description of tardive dyskinesia and its clinical detection, please refer to **Information for Patients** and **ADVERSE REACTIONS.**)
TRILAFON **Injection** contains sodium bisulfite, a sulfite that may cause allergic-type reactions including anaphylactic symptoms and life-threatening or less severe asthmatic episodes in certain susceptible people. The overall prevalence of sulfite sensitivity is seen more frequently in asthmatic than in nonasthmatic people.

NEUROLEPTIC MALIGNANT SYNDROME (NMS)
A potentially fatal symptom complex, sometimes referred to as Neuroleptic Malignant Syndrome (NMS), has been reported in association with antipsychotic drugs. Clinical manifestations of NMS are hyperpyrexia, muscle rigidity, altered mental status and evidence of autonomic instability (irregular pulse or blood pressure, tachycardia, diaphoresis, and cardiac dysrhythmias).
The diagnostic evaluation of patients with this syndrome is complicated. In arriving at a diagnosis, it is important to identify cases where the clinical presentation includes both serious medical illness (eg, pneumonia, systemic infection, etc) and untreated or inadequately treated extrapyramidal signs and symptoms (EPS). Other important considerations in the differential diagnosis include central anticholinergic toxicity, heat stroke, drug fever, and primary central nervous system (CNS) pathology.
The management of NMS should include 1) immediate discontinuation of antipsychotic drugs and other drugs not essential to concurrent therapy, 2) intensive symptomatic treatment and medical monitoring, and 3) treatment of any concomitant serious medical problems for which specific treatments are available. There is no general agreement about specific pharmacological treatment regimens for uncomplicated NMS.
If a patient requires antipsychotic drug treatment after recovery from NMS, the reintroduction of drug therapy should be carefully considered. The patient should be carefully monitored, since recurrences of NMS have been reported.
If hypotension develops, epinephrine should not be administered since its action is blocked and partially reversed by perphenazine. If a vasopressor is needed, norepinephrine may be used. Severe, acute hypotension has occurred with the use of phenothiazines and is particularly likely to occur in patients with mitral insufficiency or pheochromocytoma. Rebound hypertension may occur in pheochromocytoma patients.
TRILAFON products can lower the convulsive threshold in susceptible individuals; they should be used with caution in alcohol withdrawal and in patients with convulsive disorders. If the patient is being treated with an anti-convulsant agent, increased dosage of that agent may be required when TRILAFON products are used concomitantly.
TRILAFON products should be used with caution in patients with psychic depression.
Perphenazine may impair the mental and/or physical abilities required for the performance of hazardous tasks such as driving a car or operating machinery; therefore, the patient should be warned accordingly.
TRILAFON products are not recommended for children under 12 years of age.
Usage in Pregnancy: Safe use of TRILAFON during pregnancy and lactation has not been established; therefore, in administering the drug to pregnant patients, nursing mothers, or women who may become pregnant, the possible benefits must be weighed against the possible hazards to mother and child.

PRECAUTIONS
The possibility of suicide in depressed patients remains during treatment and until significant remission occurs. This type of patient should not have access to large quantities of this drug.
As with all phenothiazine compounds, perphenazine should not be used indiscriminately. Caution should be observed in giving it to patients who have previously exhibited severe adverse reactions to other phenothiazines. Some of the untoward actions of perphenazine tend to appear more frequently when high doses are used. However, as with other phenothiazine compounds, patients receiving TRILAFON products in any dosage should be kept under close supervision.
Neuroleptic drugs elevate prolactin levels; the elevation persists during chronic administration. Tissue culture experiments indicate that approximately one-third of human breast cancers are prolactin dependent *in vitro*, a factor of potential importance if the prescription of these drugs is contemplated in a patient with a previously detected breast cancer. Although disturbances such as galactorrhea, amenorrhea, gynecomastia, and impotence have been reported, the clinical significance of elevated serum prolactin levels is unknown for most patients. An increase in mammary neoplasms has been found in rodents after chronic administration of neuroleptic drugs. Neither clinical studies nor epidemiologic studies conducted to date, however, have shown an association between chronic administration of these drugs and mammary tumorigenesis; the available evidence is considered too limited to be conclusive at this time.
The antiemetic effect of perphenazine may obscure signs of toxicity due to overdosage of other drugs, or render more difficult the diagnosis of disorders such as brain tumors or intestinal obstruction.
A significant, not otherwise explained, rise in body temperature may suggest individual intolerance to perphenazine, in which case it should be discontinued.
Patients on large doses of a phenothiazine drug who are undergoing surgery should be watched carefully for possible hypotensive phenomena. Moreover, reduced amounts of anesthetics or central nervous system depressants may be necessary.
Since phenothiazines and central nervous system depressants (opiates, analgesics, antihistamines, barbiturates) can potentiate each other, less than the usual dosage of the added drug is recommended and caution is advised when they are administered concomitantly.
Use with caution in patients who are receiving atropine or related drugs because of additive anticholinergic effects and also in patients who will be exposed to extreme heat or phosphorus insecticides.
The use of alcohol should be avoided, since additive effects and hypotension may occur. Patients should be cautioned that their response to alcohol may be increased while they are being treated with TRILAFON products. The risk of suicide and the danger of overdose may be increased in patients who use alcohol excessively due to its potentiation of the drug's effect.
Blood counts and hepatic and renal functions should be checked periodically. The appearance of signs of blood dyscrasias requires the discontinuance of the drug and institution of appropriate therapy. If abnormalities in hepatic tests occur, phenothiazine treatment should be discontinued. Renal function in patients on long-term therapy should be monitored; if blood urea nitrogen (BUN) becomes abnormal, treatment with the drug should be discontinued.
The use of phenothiazine derivatives in patients with diminished renal function should be undertaken with caution.
Use with caution in patients suffering from respiratory impairment due to acute pulmonary infections, or in chronic respiratory disorders such as severe asthma or emphysema.
In general, phenothiazines, including perphenazine, do not produce psychic dependence. Gastritis, nausea and vomiting, dizziness, and tremulousness have been reported following abrupt cessation of high-dose therapy. Reports suggest that these symptoms can be reduced by continuing concomitant antiparkinson agents for several weeks after the phenothiazine is withdrawn.
The possibility of liver damage, corneal and lenticular deposits, and irreversible dyskinesias should be kept in mind when patients are on long-term therapy.
Because photosensitivity has been reported, undue exposure to the sun should be avoided during phenothiazine treatment.
Information for Patients: This information is intended to aid in the safe and effective use of this medication. It is not a disclosure of all possible adverse or intended effects.
Given the likelihood that a substantial proportion of patients exposed chronically to neuroleptics will develop tardive dyskinesia, it is advised that all patients in whom chronic use is contemplated be given, if possible, full information about this risk. The decision to inform patients and/or their guardians must obviously take into account the clinical circumstances and the competency of the patient to understand the information provided.

ADVERSE REACTIONS
Not all of the following adverse reactions have been reported with this specific drug; however, pharmacological similarities among various phenothiazine derivatives require that each be considered. With the piperazine group (of which perphenazine is an example), the extrapyramidal symptoms are more common, and others (eg, sedative effects, jaundice, and blood dyscrasias) are less frequently seen.
CNS Effects: *Extrapyramidal reactions:* opisthotonus, trismus, torticollis, retrocollis, aching and numbness of the limbs, motor restlessness, oculogyric crisis, hyperreflexia,

Continued on next page

Information on Schering products appearing on these pages is effective as of January 2000.

Trilafon—Cont.

dystonia, including protrusion, discoloration, aching and rounding of the tongue, tonic spasm of the masticatory muscles, tight feeling in the throat, slurred speech, dysphagia, akathisia, dyskinesia, parkinsonism, and ataxia. Their incidence and severity usually increase with an increase in dosage, but there is considerable individual variation in the tendency to develop such symptoms. Extrapyramidal symptoms can usually be controlled by the concomitant use of effective antiparkinsonian drugs, such as benztropine mesylate, and/or by reduction in dosage. In some instances, however, these extrapyramidal reactions may persist after discontinuation of treatment with perphenazine.

Persistent tardive dyskinesia: As with all antipsychotic agents, tardive dyskinesia may appear in some patients on long-term therapy or may appear after drug therapy has been discontinued. Although the risk appears to be greater in elderly patients on high-dose therapy, especially females, it may occur in either sex and in children. The symptoms are persistent and in some patients appear to be irreversible. The syndrome is characterized by rhythmical, involuntary movements of the tongue, face, mouth, or jaw (eg, protrusion of tongue, puffing of cheeks, puckering of mouth, chewing movements). Sometimes these may be accompanied by involuntary movements of the extremities. There is no known effective treatment for tardive dyskinesia; antiparkinsonism agents usually do not alleviate the symptoms of this syndrome. It is suggested that all antipsychotic agents be discontinued if these symptoms appear. Should it be necessary to reinstitute treatment, or increase the dosage of the agent, or switch to a different antipsychotic agent, the syndrome may be masked. It has been reported that fine, vermicular movements of the tongue may be an early sign of the syndrome, and if the medication is stopped at that time the syndrome may not develop.

Other CNS effects include cerebral edema; abnormality of cerebrospinal fluid proteins; convulsive seizures, particularly in patients with EEG abnormalities or a history of such disorders; and headaches.

Neuroleptic malignant syndrome has been reported in patients treated with neuroleptic drugs (see **WARNINGS** section for further information).

Drowsiness may occur, particularly during the first or second week, after which it generally disappears. If troublesome, lower the dosage. Hypnotic effects appear to be minimal, especially in patients who are permitted to remain active.

Adverse behavioral effects include paradoxical exacerbation of psychotic symptoms, catatonic-like states, paranoid reactions, lethargy, paradoxical excitement, restlessness, hyperactivity, nocturnal confusion, bizarre dreams, and insomnia.

Hyperreflexia has been reported in the newborn when a phenothiazine was used during pregnancy.

Autonomic Effects: dry mouth or salivation, nausea, vomiting, diarrhea, anorexia, constipation, obstipation, fecal impaction, urinary retention, frequency or incontinence, bladder paralysis, polyuria, nasal congestion, pallor, myosis, mydriasis, blurred vision, glaucoma, perspiration, hypertension, hypotension, and change in pulse rate occasionally may occur. Significant autonomic effects have been infrequent in patients receiving less than 24 mg perphenazine daily.

Adynamic ileus occasionally occurs with phenothiazine therapy and if severe can result in complications and death. It is of particular concern in psychiatric patients, who may fail to seek treatment of the condition.

Allergic Effects: urticaria, erythema, eczema, exfoliative dermatitis, pruritus, photosensitivity, asthma, fever, anaphylactoid reactions, laryngeal edema, and angioneurotic edema; contact dermatitis in nursing personnel administering the drug; and in extremely rare instances, individual idiosyncrasy or hypersensitivity to phenothiazines has resulted in cerebral edema, circulatory collapse, and death.

Endocrine Effects: lactation, galactorrhea, moderate breast enlargement in females and gynecomastia in males on large doses, disturbances in the menstrual cycle, amenorrhea, changes in libido, inhibition of ejaculation, syndrome of inappropriate ADH (antidiuretic hormone) secretion, false positive pregnancy tests, hyperglycemia, hypoglycemia, glycosuria.

Cardiovascular Effects: postural hypotension, tachycardia (especially with sudden marked increase in dosage), bradycardia, cardiac arrest, faintness, and dizziness. Occasionally the hypotensive effect may produce a shock-like condition. ECG changes, nonspecific (quinidinelike effect) usually reversible, have been observed in some patients receiving phenothiazine tranquilizers.

Sudden death has occasionally been reported in patients who have received phenothiazines. In some cases the death was apparently due to cardiac arrest; in others, the cause appeared to be asphyxia due to failure of the cough reflex. In some patients, the cause could not be determined nor could it be established that the death was due to the phenothiazine.

Hematological Effects: agranulocytosis, eosinophilia, leukopenia, hemolytic anemia, thrombocytopenic purpura, and pancytopenia. Most cases of agranulocytosis have occurred between the fourth and tenth weeks of therapy. Patients should be watched closely, especially during that period, for the sudden appearance of sore throat or signs of infection. If white blood cell and differential cell counts show significant cellular depression, discontinue the drug and start appropriate therapy. However, a slightly lowered white count is not in itself an indication to discontinue the drug.

Other Effects: Special considerations in long-term therapy include pigmentation of the skin, occurring chiefly in the exposed areas; ocular changes consisting of deposition of fine particulate matter in the cornea and lens, progressing in more severe cases to star-shaped lenticular opacities; epithelial keratopathies; and pigmentary retinopathy. Also noted: peripheral edema, reversed epinephrine effect, increase in PBI not attributable to an increase in thyroxine, parotid swelling (rare), hyperpyrexia, systemic lupus erythematosuslike syndrome, increases in appetite and weight, polyphagia, photophobia, and muscle weakness.

Liver damage (biliary stasis) may occur. Jaundice may occur, usually between the second and fourth weeks of treatment, and is regarded as a hypersensitivity reaction. Incidence is low. The clinical picture resembles infectious hepatitis but with laboratory features of obstructive jaundice. It is usually reversible; however, chronic jaundice has been reported.

Side effects with intramuscular TRILAFON Injection have been infrequent and transient. Dizziness or significant hypotension after treatment with TRILAFON Injection is a rare occurrence.

DOSAGE AND ADMINISTRATION

Dosage must be individualized and adjusted according to the severity of the condition and the response obtained. As with all potent drugs, the best dose is the lowest dose that will produce the desired clinical effect. Since extrapyramidal symptoms increase in frequency and severity with increased dosage, it is important to employ the lowest effective dose. These symptoms have disappeared upon reduction of dosage, withdrawal of the drug, or administration of an antiparkinsonian agent.

Prolonged administration of doses exceeding 24 mg daily should be reserved for hospitalized patients or patients under continued observation for early detection and management of adverse reactions. An antiparkinsonian agent, such as trihexyphenidyl hydrochloride or benztropine mesylate, is valuable in controlling drug-induced extrapyramidal symptoms.

TRILAFON **Tablets**

Suggested dosages for **Tablets** for various conditions follow:

Moderately disturbed nonhospitalized psychotic patients: **Tablets** 4 to 8 mg t.i.d. initially; reduce as soon as possible to minimum effective dosage.

Hospitalized psychotic patients: **Tablets** 8 to 16 mg b.i.d. to q.i.d.; avoid dosages in excess of 64 mg daily.

Severe nausea and vomiting in adults: **Tablets** 8 to 16 mg daily in divided doses; 24 mg occasionally may be necessary; early dosage reduction is desirable.

TRILAFON **Injection**

Intramuscular Administration

The injection is used when rapid effect and prompt control of acute or intractable conditions is required or when oral administration is not feasible. TRILAFON Injection, administered by deep intramuscular injection, is well tolerated. The injection should be given with the patient seated or recumbent, and the patient should be observed for a short period after administration.

Therapeutic effect is usually evidenced in 10 minutes and is maximal in 1 to 2 hours. The average duration of effective action is 6 hours, occasionally 12 to 24 hours.

Pediatric dosage has not yet been established. Children over 12 years may receive the lowest limit of adult dosage.

The usual initial dose is 5 mg (1 mL). This may be repeated every 6 hours. Ordinarily, the total daily dosage should not exceed 15 mg in ambulatory patients or 30 mg in hospitalized patients. When required for satisfactory control of symptoms in severe conditions, an initial 10-mg intramuscular dose may be given. Patients should be placed on oral therapy as soon as practicable. Generally, this may be achieved within 24 hours. In some instances, however, patients have been maintained on injectable therapy for several months. It has been established that TRILAFON Injection is more potent than TRILAFON Tablets. Therefore, equal or higher dosage should be used when the patient is transferred to oral therapy after receiving the injection.

Psychotic conditions: While 5 mg of the injection has a definite tranquilizing effect, it may be necessary to use 10-mg doses to initiate therapy in severely agitated states. Most patients will be controlled and amenable to oral therapy within a maximum of 24 to 48 hours. Acute conditions (hysteria, panic reaction) often respond well to a single dose, whereas in chronic conditions, several injections may be required. When transferring patients to oral therapy, it is suggested that increased dosage be employed to maintain adequate clinical control. This should be followed by gradual reduction to the minimal maintenance dose which is effective.

Severe nausea and vomiting in adults: To obtain rapid control of vomiting, administer 5 mg (1 mL); in rare instances it may be necessary to increase the dose to 10 mg; in general, higher doses should be given only to hospitalized patients.

Intravenous Administration

The intravenous administration of TRILAFON Injection is seldom required. This route of administration should be used with particular caution and care, and only when absolutely necessary to control severe vomiting, intractable hiccoughs, or acute conditions, such as violent retching during surgery. Its use should be limited to recumbent hospitalized adults in doses not exceeding 5 mg. When employed in this manner, intravenous injection ordinarily should be given as a diluted solution by either fractional injection or a slow drip infusion. In the surgical patient, slow infusion of not more than 5 mg is preferred. When administered in divided doses, TRILAFON Injection should be diluted to 0.5 mg/mL (1 mL mixed with 9 mL of physiologic saline solution), and not more than 1 mg per injection given at not less than one- to two-minute intervals. Intravenous injection should be discontinued as soon as symptoms are controlled and should not exceed 5 mg. The possibility of hypotensive and extrapyramidal side effects should be considered and appropriate means for management kept available. Blood pressure and pulse should be monitored continuously during intravenous administration. Pharmacologic and clinical studies indicate that intravenous administration of norepinephrine should be useful in alleviating the hypotensive effect.

OVERDOSAGE

In the event of overdosage, emergency treatment should be started immediately. All patients suspected of having taken an overdose should be hospitalized as soon as possible.

Manifestations Overdosage of perphenazine primarily involves the extrapyramidal mechanism and produces the same side effects described under **ADVERSE REACTIONS**, but to a more marked degree. It is usually evidenced by stupor or coma; children may have convulsive seizures.

Treatment Treatment is symptomatic and supportive. There is no specific antidote. The patient should be induced to vomit even if emesis has occurred spontaneously. Pharmacologic vomiting by the administration of ipecac syrup is a preferred method. It should be noted that ipecac has a central mode of action in addition to its local gastric irritant properties, and the central mode of action may be blocked by the antiemetic effect of TRILAFON products. Vomiting should not be induced in patients with impaired consciousness. The action of ipecac is facilitated by physical activity and by the administration of 8 to 12 fluid ounces of water. If emesis does not occur within 15 minutes, the dose of ipecac should be repeated. Precautions against aspiration must be taken, especially in infants and children. Following emesis, any drug remaining in the stomach may be adsorbed by activated charcoal administered as a slurry with water. If vomiting is unsuccessful or contraindicated, gastric lavage should be performed. Isotonic and one-half isotonic saline are the lavage solutions of choice. Saline cathartics, such as milk of magnesia, draw water into the bowel by osmosis and therefore, may be valuable for their action in rapid dilution of bowel content.

Standard measures (oxygen, intravenous fluids, corticosteroids) should be used to manage circulatory shock or metabolic acidosis. An open airway and adequate fluid intake should be maintained. Body temperature should be regulated. Hypothermia is expected, but severe hyperthermia may occur and must be treated vigorously. (See **CONTRAINDICATIONS.**)

An electrocardiogram should be taken and close monitoring of cardiac function instituted if there is any sign of abnormality. Cardiac arrhythmias may be treated with neostigmine, pyridostigmine, or propranolol. Digitalis should be considered for cardiac failure. Close monitoring of cardiac function is advisable for not less than five days. Vasopressors such as norepinephrine may be used to treat hypotension, but epinephrine should NOT be used.

Anticonvulsants (an inhalation anesthetic, diazepam, or paraldehyde) are recommended for control of convulsions, since perphenazine increases the central nervous system depressant action, but not the anticonvulsant action of barbiturates.

If acute parkinson like symptoms result from perphenazine intoxication, benztropine mesylate or diphenhydramine may be administered.

Central nervous system depression may be treated with nonconvulsant doses of CNS stimulants. Avoid stimulants that may cause convulsions (eg, picrotoxin and pentylenetetrazol).

Signs of arousal may not occur for 48 hours.

Dialysis is of no value because of low plasma concentrations of the drug.

Since overdosage is often deliberate, patients may attempt suicide by other means during the recovery phase. Deaths by deliberate or accidental overdosage have occurred with this class of drugs.

HOW SUPPLIED

TRILAFON **Tablets** (2 mg): gray, sugar-coated tablets branded in black with the Schering trademark and either product identification letters, ADH, or numbers, 705; bottles of 100 (NDC 0085-0705-04). **Store between 2° and 25°C (36° and 77°F).**

TRILAFON **Tablets** (4 mg): gray, sugar-coated tablets branded in green with the Schering trademark and either product identification letters, ADK, or numbers, 940; bottles of 100 (NDC 0085-0940-05). **Store between 2° and 25°C (36° and 77°F).**

TRILAFON **Tablets** (8 mg): gray, sugar-coated tablets branded in blue with the Schering trademark and either product identification letters, ADJ, or numbers, 313; bottles of 100 (NDC 0085-0313-05). **Store between 2° and 25°C (36° and 77°F).**

TRILAFON **Tablets** (16 mg): gray, sugar-coated tablets branded in red with the Schering trademark and either product identification letters, ADM, or numbers, 077; bottles of 100 (NDC 0085-0077-05). **Store between 2° and 25°C (36° and 77°F).**

TRILAFON **Injection**, 5 mg per mL, 1-mL ampule for intramuscular or intravenous use, box of 100 (NDC 0085-0012-04). **Store between 2° and 30°C (36° and 86°F).** Keep package closed to protect from light. Exposure may cause discoloration. Slight yellowish discoloration will not alter potency or therapeutic efficacy; if markedly discolored, ampule should be discarded. **Protect from light. Store in carton until completely used.**

Schering Corporation
Kenilworth, NJ 07033 USA
Rev. 3/00 22728016
22728210T

Shown in Product Identification Guide, page 334

VANCENASE® POKETHALER® ℞

(beclomethasone dipropionate nasal aerosol)
For Nasal Inhalation Only

DESCRIPTION

Beclomethasone dipropionate, USP, the active component of VANCENASE POCKETHALER (beclomethasone dipropionate nasal aerosol) is an anti-inflammatory steroid having the chemical name, 9-Chloro-11β,17,21-trihydroxy-16β-methylpregna-1,4-diene-3,20-dione 17,21-dipropionate, and the following formula:

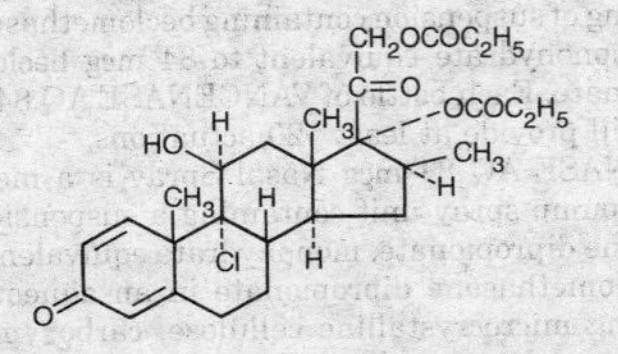

Beclomethasone dipropionate is a white to creamy-white, odorless powder with a molecular weight of 521.25. It is very slightly soluble in water, very soluble in chloroform, and freely soluble in acetone and in alcohol.

VANCENASE POCKETHALER (beclomethasone dipropionate nasal aerosol) is a metered-dose aerosol unit containing a microcrystalline suspension of beclomethasonedipropionate-trichloromonofluoromethane clathrate in a mixture of propellants (trichloromonofluoromethane and dichlorodifluoromethane) with oleic acid. Each canister contains beclomethasone dipropionate-trichloromonofluoromethane clathrate having a molecular proportion of beclomethasone dipropionate to trichloromonofluoro methane between 3:1 and 3:2. Each actuation delivers from the nasal adapter a quantity of clathrate equivalent to 42 mcg of beclomethasone dipropionate, USP. The contents of one canister provide at least 200 metered doses.

CLINICAL PHARMACOLOGY

Beclomethasone 17,21-dipropionate is a diester of beclomethasone, a synthetic halogenated corticosteroid. Animal studies showed that beclomethasone dipropionate has potent glucocorticoid and weak mineralocorticoid activity. The mechanisms for the anti-inflammatory action of beclomethasone dipropionate are unknown. The precise mechanism of the aerosolized drug's action in the nose is also unknown. Biopsies of nasal mucosa obtained during clinical studies showed no histopathologic changes when beclomethasone dipropionate was administered intranasally.

The effects of beclomethasone dipropionate on hypothalamic-pituitary-adrenal (HPA) function have been evaluated in adult volunteers by other routes of administration. Studies are currently being undertaken with beclomethasone dipropionate by the intranasal route, which may demonstrate that there is more or that there is less absorption by this route of administration. There was no suppression of early morning plasma cortisol concentrations when beclomethasone dipropionate was administered in a dose of 1000 mcg/day for 1 month as an oral aerosol or for 3 days by intramuscular injection. However, partial suppression of plasma cortisol concentration was observed when beclomethasone dipropionate was administered in doses of 2000 mcg/day either by oral aerosol or intramuscularly. Immediate suppression of plasma cortisol concentrations was observed after single doses of 4000 mcg of beclomethasone dipropionate. Suppression of HPA function (reduction of early morning plasma cortisol levels) has been reported in adult patients who received 1600 mcg daily doses of oral beclomethasone dipropionate for 1 month. In clinical studies using beclomethasone dipropionate intranasally, there was no evidence of adrenal insufficiency.

Beclomethasone dipropionate is sparingly soluble. When given by nasal inhalation in the form of an aqueous or aerosolized suspension, the drug is deposited primarily in the nasal passages. A portion of the drug is swallowed. Absorption occurs rapidly from all respiratory and gastrointestinal tissues. There is no evidence of tissue storage of beclomethasone dipropionate or its metabolites. *In vitro* studies have shown that tissue other than the liver (lung slices) can rapidly metabolize beclomethasone dipropionate to beclomethasone 17-monopropionate and more slowly to free beclomethasone (which has very weak anti-inflammatory activity). However, irrespective of the route of entry, the principal route of excretion of the drug and its metabolites is the feces. In humans, 12% to 15% of an orally administered dose of beclomethasone dipropionate is excreted in the urine as both conjugated and free metabolites of the drug.

Studies have shown that the degree of binding to plasma proteins is 87%.

INDICATIONS AND USAGE

VANCENASE POCKETHALER (beclomethasone dipropionate nasal aerosol) is indicated for the relief of the symptoms of seasonal or perennial rhinitis in those cases poorly responsive to conventional treatment.

VANCENASE POCKETHALER (beclomethasone dipropionate nasal aerosol) is also indicated for the prevention of recurrence of nasal polyps following surgical removal.

Clinical studies in seasonal and perennial rhinitis have shown that improvement is usually apparent within a few days. However, symptomatic relief may not occur in some patients for as long as 2 weeks. Although systemic effects are minimal at recommended doses, VANCENASE treatment should not be continued beyond 3 weeks in the absence of significant symptomatic improvement. VANCENASE treatment should not be used in the presence of untreated, localized infection involving the nasal mucosa.

Clinical studies have shown that treatment of the symptoms associated with nasal polyps may have to be continued for several weeks or more before a therapeutic result can be fully assessed. Recurrence of symptoms due to polyps can occur after stopping treatment, depending on the severity of the disease.

CONTRAINDICATIONS

Hypersensitivity to any of the ingredients of this preparation contraindicates its use.

WARNINGS

The replacement of a systemic corticosteroid with VANCENASE POCKETHALER (beclomethasone dipropionate nasal aerosol) can be accompanied by signs of adrenal insufficiency.

Careful attention must be given when patients, previously treated for prolonged periods with systemic corticosteroids, are transferred to VANCENASE POCKETHALER (beclomethasone dipropionate nasal aerosol). This is particularly important in those patients who have associated asthma or other clinical conditions, where too rapid a decrease in systemic corticosteroids may cause a severe exacerbation of their symptoms.

Studies have shown that the combined administration of alternate day prednisone systemic treatment and orally inhaled beclomethasone increased the likelihood of HPA suppression compared to a therapeutic dose of either one alone. Therefore, VANCENASE treatment should be used with caution in patients already on alternate day prednisone regimens for any disease.

If recommended doses of intranasal beclomethasone are exceeded or if individuals are particularly sensitive or predisposed by virtue of recent systemic steroid therapy, symptoms of hypercorticism may occur, including very rare cases of menstrual irregularities, acneiform lesions, and cushingoid features. If such changes occur, VANCENASE POCKETHALER (beclomethasone dipropionate nasal aerosol) should be discontinued slowly, consistent with accepted procedures for dis continuing oral steroid therapy.

Persons who are on drugs which suppress the immune system are more susceptible to infections than healthy individuals. Chickenpox and measles, for example, can have a more serious or even fatal course in nonimmune pediatric patients or adults on corticosteroids. In such pediatric patients or adults who have not had these diseases, particular care should be taken to avoid exposure. How the dose, route, and duration of cortico steroid administration affects the risk of developing a disseminated infection is not known. The contribution of the underlying disease and/or prior corticosteroid treatment to the risk is also not known. If exposed to chickenpox, prophylaxis with varicella-zoster immune globulin (VZIG) may be indicated. If exposed to measles, prophylaxis with pooled intramuscular immunoglobulin (IG) may be indicated. (See the respective package inserts for complete VZIG and IG prescribing information.) If chickenpox develops, treatment with antiviral agents may be considered.

PRECAUTIONS

General: During withdrawal from oral steroids, some patients may experience symptoms of withdrawal, eg, joint and/or muscular pain, lassitude, and depression.

Extremely rare instances of nasal septum perforation and increased intraocular pressure have been reported following the intranasal application of aerosolized corticosteroids.

In clinical studies with beclomethasone dipropionate administered intranasally, the development of localized infections of the nose and pharynx with *Candida albicans* has occurred only rarely. When such an infection develops, it may require treatment with appropriate local therapy or discontinuance of treatment with VANCENASE POCKETHALER (beclomethasone dipropionate nasal aerosol).

Beclomethasone dipropionate is absorbed into the circulation. Use of excessive doses of VANCENASE POCKETHALER (beclomethasone dipropionate nasal aerosol) may suppress HPA function.

VANCENASE treatment should be used with caution, if at all, in patients with active or quiescent tuberculous infections of the respiratory tract, or in untreated fungal, bacterial, systemic viral infections, or ocular herpes simplex.

For VANCENASE POCKETHALER (beclomethasone dipropionate nasal aerosol) to be effective in the treatment of nasal polyps, the aerosol must be able to enter the nose. Therefore, treatment of nasal polyps with VANCENASE POCKETHALER (beclomethasone dipropionate nasal aerosol) should be considered adjunctive therapy to surgical removal and/or the use of other medications which will permit effective penetration of the VANCENASE product into the nose. Nasal polyps may recur after any form of treatment.

As with any long-term treatment, patients using VANCENASE treatment over several months or longer should be examined periodically for possible changes in the nasal mucosa.

Because of the inhibitory effect of corticosteroids on wound healing, patients who have experienced recent nasal septum ulcers, nasal surgery, or trauma should not use a nasal corticosteroid until healing has occurred.

Nasal and inhaled corticosteroids have been associated with the development of glaucoma and/or cataracts. Therefore, close follow-up is warranted in patients with a change in vision and with a history of glaucoma and/or cataracts.

Although systemic effects have been minimal with recommended doses, this potential increases with excessive doses. Therefore, larger than recommended doses should be avoided.

Information for Patients: Patients should use VANCENASE POCKETHALER (beclomethasone dipropionate nasal aerosol) at regular intervals since its effectiveness depends on its regular use. The patient should take the medication as directed. It is not acutely effective and the prescribed dosage should not be increased. Instead, nasal vasoconstrictors or oral antihistamines may be needed until the effects of VANCENASE POCKETHALER (beclomethasone dipropionate nasal aerosol) are fully manifested. One to 2 weeks may pass before full relief is obtained. The patient should contact the doctor if symptoms do not improve, if the condition worsens, or if sneezing or nasal irritation occurs. For the proper use of this unit and to attain maximum improvement, the patient should read and follow the accompanying PATIENT'S INSTRUCTIONS carefully.

Persons who are on immunosuppressant doses of corticosteroids should be warned to avoid exposure to chickenpox or measles. Patients should also be advised that if they are exposed, medical advice should be sought without delay.

Carcinogenesis, Mutagenesis, Impairment of Fertility: Treatment of rats for a total of 95 weeks, 13 weeks by inhalation and 82 weeks by the oral route, resulted in no evidence of carcinogenic activity. Mutagenic studies have not been performed.

Impairment of fertility, as evidenced by inhibition of the estrous cycle in dogs, was observed following treatment by the oral route. No inhibition of the estrous cycle in dogs was seen following treatment with beclomethasone dipropionate by the inhalation route.

Pregnancy Category C: Like other corticoids, parenteral (subcutaneous) beclomethasone dipropionate has been shown to be teratogenic and embryocidal in the mouse and rabbit when given in doses approximately ten times the human dose. In these studies, beclomethasone was found to produce fetal resorption, cleft palate, agnathia, microstomia, absence of tongue, delayed ossification, and agenesis of the thymus. No teratogenic or embryocidal effects have been seen in the rat when beclomethasone dipropionate was administered by inhalation at ten times the human dose or orally at 1000 times the human dose. There are no adequate and well-controlled studies in pregnant women. Beclomethasone dipropionate should be used during pregnancy only if the potential benefit justifies the potential risk to the fetus.

Nonteratogenic Effects: Hypoadrenalism may occur in infants born of mothers receiving corticosteroids during pregnancy. Such infants should be carefully observed.

Nursing Mothers: It is not known whether beclomethasone dipropionate is excreted in human milk. Because other corticosteroids are excreted in human milk, caution should be exercised when VANCENASE POCKETHALER (beclomethasone dipropionate nasal aerosol) is administered to nursing women.

Pediatric Use: Safety and effectiveness in pediatric patients below the age of 6 years have not been established.

ADVERSE REACTIONS

In general, side effects in clinical studies have been primarily associated with the nasal mucous membranes. Adverse reactions reported in controlled clinical trials and in long-term open studies in patients treated with VANCENASE Nasal Inhaler are described below.

Sensations of irritation and burning in the nose (11 per 100 patients) following the use of VANCENASE Nasal Inhaler have been reported. Also, occasional sneezing attacks (10 per 100 patients) have occurred immediately following the use of the intranasal inhaler. This symptom may be more common in children.

Rhinorrhea may occur occasionally (1 per 100 patients). Localized infections of the nose and pharynx with Candida albicans have occurred rarely. (See **PRECAUTIONS**.)

Transient episodes of epistaxis or bloody discharge from the nose have been reported in 2 per 100 patients.

Continued on next page

Information on Schering products appearing on these pages is effective as of January 2000.

Vancenase Pockethaler—Cont.

Ulceration of the nasal mucosa has been reported rarely. Extremely rare instances of nasal septum perforation have been reported following the intranasal application of aerosolized corticosteroids. Rare cases of immediate and delayed hypersensitivity reactions, including urticaria, angioedema, rash, and bronchospasm have been reported following the oral and intranasal inhalation of beclomethasone.
Increased intraocular pressure has been reported rarely. (See **PRECAUTIONS**.)
Systemic corticosteroid side effects were not reported during controlled clinical trials. If recommended doses are exceeded, however, or if individuals are particularly sensitive, symptoms of hypercorticism, ie, Cushing's syndrome could occur.

DOSAGE AND ADMINISTRATION

Adults and Pediatric Patients 12 Years of Age and Over: The usual dosage is one inhalation (42 mcg) in each nostril two to four times a day (total dose 168-336 mcg/day). Patients can often be maintained on a maximum dose of one inhalation in each nostril three times a day (252 mcg/day).
Pediatric Patients 6 to 12 Years of Age: The usual dosage is one inhalation in each nostril three times a day (252 mcg/day). VANCENASE POCKETHALER (beclomethasone dipropionate nasal aerosol) is not recommended for pediatric patients below 6 years of age since safety and efficacy studies have not been conducted in this age group.
In patients who respond to VANCENASE POCKETHALER (beclomethasone dipropionate nasal aerosol), an improvement of the symptoms of seasonal or perennial rhinitis usually becomes apparent within a few days after the start of VANCENASE POCKETHALER (beclomethasone dipropionate nasal aerosol) therapy. However, symptomatic relief may not occur in some patients for as long as 2 weeks. VANCENASE POCKETHALER (beclomethasone dipropionate nasal aerosol) should not be continued beyond 3 weeks in the absence of significant symptomatic improvement.
The therapeutic effects of corticosteroids, unlike those of decongestants, on seasonal or perennial rhinitis or on nasal polyps are not immediate. This should be explained to the patient in advance in order to ensure cooperation and continuation of treatment with the prescribed dosage regimen.
VANCENASE POCKETHALER (beclomethasone dipropionate nasal aerosol) is not recommended for pediatric patients below 6 years of age.
In the presence of excessive nasal mucus secretion or edema of the nasal mucosa, the drug may fail to reach the site of intended action. In such cases it is advisable to use a nasal vasoconstrictor during the first 2 to 3 days of VANCENASE POCKETHALER (beclomethasone dipropionate nasal aerosol) therapy.
Directions for Use: Illustrated PATIENT'S INSTRUCTIONS for proper use accompany each package of VANCENASE POCKETHALER (beclomethasone dipropionate nasal aerosol).
CONTENTS UNDER PRESSURE. Do not puncture. Do not use or store near heat or open flame. Exposure to temperatures above 120°F may cause bursting. Never throw container into fire or incinerator. Keep out of reach of children.

OVERDOSAGE

When used at excessive doses, systemic corticosteroid effects such as hypercorticism and adrenal suppression may appear. If such changes occur, VANCENASE POCKETHALER (beclomethasone dipropionate nasal aerosol) should be discontinued slowly consistent with accepted procedures for discontinuing oral steroid therapy.
The oral LD_{50} of beclomethasone dipropionate is greater than 1 g/kg in rodents. One canister of VANCENASE POCKETHALER (beclomethasone dipropionate nasal aerosol) contains 8.4 mg of beclomethasone dipropionate; therefore acute overdosage is unlikely.

HOW SUPPLIED

VANCENASE POCKETHALER (beclomethasone dipropionate nasal aerosol), 7 g canister; box of one. Supplied with nasal adapter and PATIENT'S INSTRUCTIONS (NDC 0085-0649-02).
Store between 15° and 30°C (59° and 86°F). Protect from moisture and unusual temperature fluctuations. Shake well before using. Failure to use the product within this temperature range may result in improper dosing.
Note: The indented statement below is required by the Federal government's Clean Air Act for all products containing or manufactured with chlorofluorocarbons (CFCs).
WARNING: Contains dichlorodifluoromethane (CFC-12) and trichloromonofluoromethane (CFC-11), substances which harm public health and the environment by destroying ozone in the upper atmosphere.
A notice similar to the above WARNING has been placed in the Patient's Instructions for Use portion of this package insert pursuant to EPA regulations.
Schering Corporation
Kenilworth, NJ 07033 USA
Rev. 10/99 19529649

VANCENASE® POCKETHALER®

(beclomethasone dipropionate nasal aerosol)
PATIENT'S INSTRUCTIONS FOR USE

SHAKE WELL BEFORE USE
Read complete instructions carefully and use only as directed by your physician.
Before using your VANCENASE® POCKETHALER® (beclomethasone dipropionate nasal aerosol), read complete instructions carefully.
1. Gently blow your nose to clear the nostrils.
2. SHAKE THE INHALER WELL immediately before each use (Figure 1).

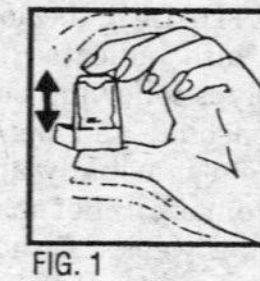
FIG. 1

3. Remove the cap to uncover the plastic nasal piece. Hold the inhaler as shown in Figure 2.

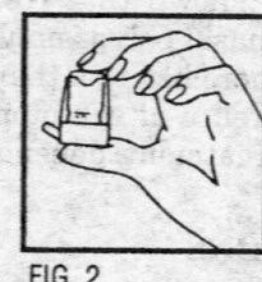
FIG. 2

4. Tilt the head back. Carefully insert the opening of the plastic nasal piece into one nostril and close the other nostril with one finger (Figure 3).

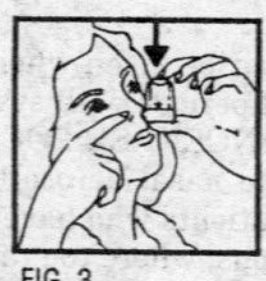
FIG. 3

5. While gently breathing in through the nostril, press the canister down firmly between finger and thumb to release the medication (Figure 3).
6. Now breathe out through the mouth (Figure 4).

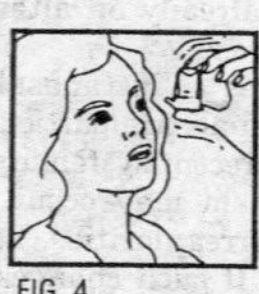
FIG. 4

7. SHAKE THE INHALER AGAIN and then repeat steps 4 through 7 in the other nostril.
8. Replace the cap.
Cleaning: Remove the metal canister from the plastic nasal inhaler unit. Remove the maroon protective cap. Rinse the plastic nasal inhaler and cap in warm running water once a day. Dry thoroughly. Replace the metal canister into the nasal inhaler unit. Replace the maroon protective cap.
CAUTION: VANCENASE POCKETHALER (beclomethasone dipropionate nasal aerosol) is not intended to give immediate relief of your nasal symptoms. Improvement with VANCENASE POCKETHALER (beclomethasone dipropionate nasal aerosol) may take a few days to develop, and it is important that you use it regularly at the times recommended by your physician.
Contents under pressure. Do not puncture. Do not use or store near heat or open flame. Exposure to temperatures above 120°F may cause bursting. Never throw container into fire or incinerator. Keep out of reach of children.
Store between 15° and 30°C (59° and 86°F). Protect from moisture and unusual temperature fluctuations. Shake well before using. Failure to use the product within this temperature range may result in improper dosing.
Note: The indented statement below is required by the Federal government's Clean Air Act for all products containing or manufactured with chlorofluorocarbons (CFCs).
This product contains dichlorodifluoromethane (CFC-12) and trichloromonofluoromethane (CFC-11), substances which harm the environment by destroying ozone in the upper atmosphere.
Your physician has determined that this product is likely to help your personal health. USE THIS PRODUCT AS DIRECTED, UNLESS INSTRUCTED TO DO OTHERWISE BY YOUR PHYSICIAN. If you have any questions about alternatives, consult with your physician.
Schering Corporation
Kenilworth, NJ 07033 USA

19529649 Rev. 10/99
Shown in Product Identification Guide, page 334

VANCENASE® AQ 84 mcg ℞

(beclomethasone dipropionate, monohydrate)
Nasal Spray
FOR INTRANASAL USE ONLY

DESCRIPTION

Beclomethasone dipropionate, monohydrate, the active component of VANCENASE AQ 84 mcg Nasal Spray, is an anti-inflammatory steroid having the chemical name, 9-Chloro-11β, 17,21-trihydroxy-16β-methylpregna-1, 4-diene-3, 20-dione 17,21-dipropionate, monohydrate and the following chemical structure:

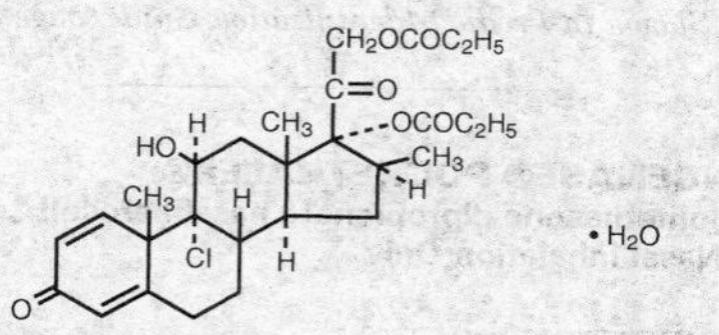

Beclomethasone dipropionate, monohydrate, is a white to creamy-white, odorless powder with a molecular formula of $C_{28}H_{37}ClO_7 \bullet H_2O$ and a molecular weight of 539.06. It is very slightly soluble in water; very soluble in chloroform; and freely soluble in acetone and in alcohol.
After initial priming (at least 6 actuations) of VANCENASE AQ 84 mcg Nasal Spray, each actuation of the pump delivers 100 mg of suspension containing beclomethasone dipropionate, monohydrate equivalent to 84 mcg beclomethasone dipropionate. Each bottle of VANCENASE AQ 84 mcg Nasal Spray will provide at least 120 actuations.
VANCENASE AQ 84 mcg Nasal Spray is a metered-dose, manual pump spray unit containing a suspension of beclomethasone dipropionate, monohydrate equivalent to 0.084% w/w beclomethasone dipropionate in an aqueous medium containing microcrystalline cellulose, carboxymethylcellulose sodium, dextrose, benzalkonium chloride, polysorbate 80, and phenylethyl alcohol. The suspension is formulated at a target pH of 6.4, with a range of 5.5 to 6.8 over its shelf life.

CLINICAL PHARMACOLOGY

Beclomethasone 17,21-dipropionate is a diester of beclomethasone, a synthetic halogenated corticosteroid. Animal studies show that beclomethasone dipropionate has potent glucocorticosteroid and weak mineralcorticosteroid activity. The mechanisms for the anti-inflammatory action of beclomethasone dipropionate are unknown. The precise mechanism of the aerosolized drug's action in the nose is also unknown. Biopsies of nasal mucosa obtained during clinical studies (duration of treatment from 1 to 6 years at doses up to 336 mcg/day) showed no histopathologic changes when beclomethasone dipropionate was administered intranasally.
In a study evaluating the hypothalamic-pituitary-adrenal (HPA) effects of 336 mcg/day beclomethasone dipropionate administered intranasally for 36 consecutive days via aqueous suspension, there was no statistically significant difference in cortisol suppression between beclomethasone dipropionate 336 mcg once daily, beclomethasone dipropionate 168 mcg twice daily, and placebo. Plasma cortisol response to 6-hour cosyntropin stimulation was attenuated in control patients who received oral prednisone 10 mg daily.
The effects of beclomethasone dipropionate on HPA function have also been evaluated in adult volunteers by other routes of administration. There was no suppression of early morning plasma cortisol concentrations when beclomethasone dipropionate was administered in a dose of 1000 mcg/day for 1 month as an oral aerosol or for 3 days by intramuscular injection. However, partial suppression of plasma cortisol concentration was observed when beclomethasone dipropionate was administered in doses of 2000 mcg/day either by oral aerosol or intramuscular injection. Immediate suppression of plasma cortisol concentrations was observed after single doses of 4000 mcg of beclomethasone dipropionate. Suppression of HPA function (reduction of early morning plasma cortisol levels) has been reported in adult patients who received 1600 mcg daily doses of oral beclomethasone dipropionate for 1 month.
In one study of pediatric patients with asthma, the administration of inhaled beclomethasone dipropionate at recommended daily doses for at least 1 year was associated with a reduction in nocturnal cortisol secretion. The clinical significance of this finding is not clear. It reinforces other evidence, however, that topical beclomethasone dipropionate may be absorbed in amounts that can have systemic effects and that physicians should be alert for evidence of systemic effects, especially in chronically treated patients (see **PRECAUTIONS**).
Beclomethasone dipropionate is sparingly soluble. When given by nasal inhalation in the form of an aqueous or aerosolized suspension, the drug is deposited primarily in the nasal passages. A portion of the drug is swallowed. Absorption occurs rapidly from all respiratory and gastrointestinal tissues. There is no evidence of tissue storage of beclomethasone dipropionate or its metabolites. *In vitro* studies have shown that tissue other than the liver (lung slices) can rapidly metabolize beclomethasone dipropionate to beclomethasone 17-monopropionate and more slowly to free beclomethasone (which has very weak anti-inflammatory activity). However, irrespective of the route of entry, the principal

route of excretion is the feces. In humans, 12% to 15% of an orally administered dose of beclomethasone dipropionate is excreted in the urine. The drug is excreted in both urine and feces as free and conjugated polar metabolites.
Studies have shown that the degree of binding to plasma proteins is 87%.
In clinical trials with VANCENASE AQ 84 mcg Nasal Spray in patients with seasonal allergic rhinitis, 336 mcg of beclomethasone dipropionate once daily was superior to placebo with respect to effects on nasal symptoms. In a study comparing VANCENASE AQ 84 mcg Nasal Spray once daily with beclomethasone dipropionate 42 mcg nasal spray twice daily, each delivering a total daily dose of 336 mcg beclomethasone dipropionate, both regimens were comparable with respect to effects on physician-rated nasal symptoms. In this study, a significant advantage over placebo was observed for both regimens within 3 days of the start of treatment.

INDICATIONS AND USAGE

VANCENASE AQ 84 mcg Nasal Spray is indicated for the relief of symptoms of allergic and nonallergic (vasomotor) rhinitis. Results from clinical trials of intranasal beclomethasone dipropionate in patients with seasonal allergic rhinitis have shown that significant symptom relief was obtained in most patients within 3 days. However, symptom relief may not occur in some patients for as long as 2 weeks. VANCENASE AQ 84 mcg Nasal Spray should not be continued beyond 3 weeks in the absence of significant symptom improvement. VANCENASE AQ 84 mcg Nasal Spray should not be used in the presence of untreated localized infection involving the nasal mucosa.
VANCENASE AQ 84 mcg Nasal Spray is also indicated for the prevention of recurrence of nasal polyps following surgical removal.
Clinical studies with beclomethasone dipropionate 42 mcg nasal spray have shown that treatment of the symptoms associated with nasal polyps may have to be continued for several weeks or more before a therapeutic result can be fully assessed. Recurrence of symptoms due to polyps can occur after stopping treatment, depending on the severity of the disease.

CONTRAINDICATIONS

Hypersensitivity to any of the ingredients of this preparation contraindicates its use.

WARNINGS

The replacement of a systemic corticosteroid with VANCENASE AQ 84 mcg Nasal Spray can be accompanied by signs of adrenal insufficiency.
When transferred to VANCENASE AQ 84 mcg Nasal Spray, careful attention must be given to patients previously treated for prolonged periods with systemic corticosteroids. This is particularly important in those patients who have associated asthma or other clinical conditions, where too rapid a decrease in systemic corticosteroids may cause a severe exacerbation of their symptoms.
If recommended doses of intranasal beclomethasone dipropionate are exceeded or if individuals are particularly sensitive or predisposed by virtue of recent systemic steroid therapy, symptoms of hypercorticism may occur, including very rare cases of menstrual irregularities, acneiform lesions, and cushingoid features. If such changes occur, VANCENASE AQ 84 mcg Nasal Spray should be discontinued slowly, consistent with accepted procedures for discontinuing oral steroid therapy.
Persons who are on drugs which suppress the immune system are more susceptible to infections than healthy individuals. Chickenpox and measles, for example, can have a more serious or even fatal course in nonimmune pediatric or adult patients on corticosteroids. In such pediatric or adult patients who have not had these diseases, particular care should be taken to avoid exposure. How the dose, route, and duration of corticosteroid administration affects the risk of developing a disseminated infection is not known. The contribution of the underlying disease and/or prior corticosteroid treatment to the risk is also not known. If exposed to chickenpox, prophylaxis with varicella-zoster immune globulin (VZIG) may be indicated. If exposed to measles, prophylaxis with pooled intramuscular immunoglobulin (IG) may be indicated. (See the respective package inserts for complete VZIG and IG prescribing information.) If chickenpox develops, treatment with antiviral agents may be considered.

PRECAUTIONS

General: During withdrawal from oral steroids, some patients may experience symptoms of withdrawal, eg, joint and/or muscular pain, lassitude, and depression.
Rarely, immediate hypersensitivity reactions may occur after the intranasal administration of beclomethasone. Rare instances of nasal septum perforation have been reported. Rare instances of wheezing and increased intraocular pressure have been reported following the intranasal application of aerosolized corticosteroids. Although these have not been observed in clinical trials with VANCENASE AQ 84 mcg Nasal Spray, vigilance should be maintained.
In clinical studies with beclomethasone dipropionate administered intranasally, the development of localized infections of the nose and pharynx with *Candida albicans* has occurred only rarely. When such an infection develops, use of VANCENASE AQ 84 mcg Nasal Spray should be discontinued and appropriate local or systemic therapy instituted, if needed.
If persistent nasopharyngeal irritation occurs, VANCENASE AQ 84 mcg Nasal Spray should be discontinued.
Beclomethasone dipropionate is absorbed into the circulation. Use of excessive doses of VANCENASE AQ 84 mcg Nasal Spray may suppress HPA function.
VANCENASE AQ 84 mcg Nasal Spray should be used with caution, if at all, in patients with active or quiescent tuberculous infections of the respiratory tract, or in untreated fungal, bacterial, systemic viral infections, or ocular herpes simplex.
For VANCENASE AQ 84 mcg Nasal Spray to be effective in the treatment of nasal polyps, the spray must be able to enter the nose. Therefore, treatment of nasal polyps with VANCENASE AQ 84 mcg Nasal Spray should be considered adjunctive therapy to surgical removal and/or the use of other medications which will permit effective penetration of VANCENASE AQ 84 mcg Nasal Spray into the nose. Nasal polyps may recur after any form of treatment.
As with any long-term treatment, patients using VANCENASE AQ 84 mcg Nasal Spray over several months or longer should be examined periodically for possible changes in the nasal mucosa.
Because of the inhibitory effect of corticosteroids on wound healing, patients who have experienced recent nasal septum ulcers, nasal surgery, or trauma should not use a corticosteroid intranasally until healing has occurred.
Although systemic effects have been minimal with recommended doses, this potential increases with excessive doses. Therefore, larger than recommended doses should be avoided.
Information for Patients: Patients being treated with VANCENASE AQ 84 mcg Nasal Spray should receive the following information and instructions. This information is intended to aid in the safe and effective use of this medication. It is not a disclosure of all possible adverse or intended effects. Patients should use VANCENASE AQ 84 mcg Nasal Spray ONLY once daily at a regular interval. Improvement usually becomes apparent within 3 days after the start of therapy. However, 1 to 2 weeks may pass before full relief is obtained. Since VANCENASE AQ 84 mcg Nasal Spray is not immediately effective, the prescribed dosage of VANCENASE AQ 84 mcg Nasal Spray should not be increased by using it more often than once a day in an attempt to increase its efficacy. Instead, nasal vasoconstrictors or oral antihistamines may be needed until the effects of VANCENASE AQ 84 mcg Nasal Spray are fully manifested. The patient should contact the physician if symptoms do not improve, or if the condition worsens, or if sneezing or nasal irritation occurs. For the proper use of this unit and to attain maximum benefit, the patient should read and follow the accompanying Patient's Instructions carefully.
Patients should be warned not to spray VANCENASE AQ 84 mcg Nasal Spray into the eyes.
Persons who are on immunosuppressant doses of corticosteroids should be warned to avoid exposure to chickenpox or measles, and patients should also be advised that if they are exposed, medical advice should be sought without delay.
Carcinogenesis, Mutagenesis, Impairment of Fertility: The carcinogenicity of beclomethasone dipropionate was evaluated in rats which were treated for a total of 95 weeks, 13 weeks at inhalation doses up to 0.4 mg/kg/day and the remaining 82 weeks at combined oral and inhalation doses up to 2.4 mg/kg/day (approximately 40 times the maximum recommended human daily intranasal dose on a mg/m^2 basis). There was no evidence of carcinogenicity in this study. Studies to assess the mutagenic potential of beclomethasone dipropionate have not been conducted. Impairment of fertility, as evidenced by inhibition of the estrous cycle in dogs, was observed following treatment by the oral route at a dose of 0.5 mg/kg/day (approximately 40 times the maximum recommended human daily intranasal dose on a mg/m^2 basis). No inhibition of the estrous cycle in dogs was seen following 12 months of exposure to beclomethasone dipropionate by the inhalation route at an estimated weekly dose of 2.3 mg/kg (approximately 26 times the maximum recommended human weekly intranasal dose on a mg/m^2 basis).
Pregnancy Category C: Like other corticosteroids, parenteral (subcutaneous) beclomethasone dipropionate has been shown to be teratogenic and embryocidal in the mouse and rabbit when given at a dose of 0.1 mg/kg/day in mice and at a dose of 0.025 mg/kg/day in rabbits (approximately 1.2 times the maximum recommended human daily intranasal dose on a mg/m^2 basis). No teratogenic or embryocidal effects have been seen in rats treated with beclomethasone by combined inhalation and oral administration at doses of 0.1 mg/kg/day and 10 mg/kg/day, respectively (approximately 250 times the maximum recommended human daily intranasal dose on a mg/m^2 basis). There are no adequate and well-controlled studies in pregnant women. Beclomethasone dipropionate should be used during pregnancy only if the potential benefit justifies the potential risk to the fetus.
Nonteratogenic Effects: Hypoadrenalism may occur in infants born of mothers receiving corticosteroids during pregnancy. Such infants should be carefully observed.
Nursing Mothers: It is not known whether beclomethasone dipropionate is excreted in human milk. Because other corticosteroids are excreted in human milk, caution should be exercised when VANCENASE AQ 84 mcg Nasal Spray is administered to nursing women.
Pediatric Use: Safety and effectiveness of VANCENASE AQ 84 mcg Nasal Spray in pediatric patients below the age of 6 years have not been established.

ADVERSE REACTIONS

In clinical studies with intranasally administered beclomethasone dipropionate, adverse effects have primarily been related to irritation of the nasal mucous membranes. Rarely, immediate hypersensitivity reactions may occur after intranasal administration of beclomethasone dipropionate.
Clinical trials of VANCENASE AQ 84 mcg Nasal Spray included 187 patients who received VANCENASE AQ 84 mcg Nasal Spray, 127 patients who received beclomethasone dipropionate 42 mcg nasal spray, and 192 patients who received vehicle placebo. The incidence and nature of adverse events with VANCENASE AQ 84 mcg Nasal Spray (336 mcg beclomethasone dipropionate once daily) was comparable to that seen with beclomethasone dipropionate 42 mcg nasal spray (168 mcg beclomethasone dipropionate twice daily) and with vehicle placebo. Adverse events reported by 2% or more of patients (regardless of relationship to treatment) who received VANCENASE AQ 84 mcg Nasal Spray in clinical trials and that were more common with VANCENASE AQ 84 mcg Nasal Spray than with placebo are displayed in the table below.

ADVERSE EVENTS FROM CONTROLLED CLINICAL TRIALS IN SEASONAL ALLERGIC RHINITIS

	VANCENASE AQ 84 mcg Once daily (N=187)	BECLOMETHASONE DIPROPIONATE 42 mcg Twice daily (N=127)	VEHICLE PLACEBO (N=192)
Headache	34%	33%	32%
Pharyngitis	12%	11%	6%
Coughing	6%	6%	5%
Epistaxis	5%	2%	4%
Nasal burning	5%	4%	3%
Pain	4%	2%	1%
Conjunctivitis	2%	2%	1%
Myalgia	2%	1%	1%
Tinnitus	2%	3%	0%

Rare cases of ulceration of the nasal mucosa and instances of nasal septum perforation have been reported following the intranasal administration of beclomethasone dipropionate (see **PRECAUTIONS**).
Rare instances of wheezing and increased intraocular pressure have been reported following the intranasal administration of aerosolized corticosteroids (see **PRECAUTIONS**).
Single cases each of aseptic necrosis of the femoral head and of nasal fungal infection with erosion through the cribriform plate have been reported after long-term administration of beclomethasone dipropionate nasal spray.

OVERDOSAGE

When used at excessive doses, systemic corticosteroid effects such as hypercorticism and adrenal suppression may appear. If such changes occur, VANCENASE AQ 84 mcg Nasal Spray should be discontinued slowly consistent with accepted procedures for discontinuing oral steroid therapy.
The oral median lethal dose of beclomethasone dipropionate is greater than 1 g/kg in mice and rats (approximately 7000 times and 14,000 times, respectively, the maximum recommended human daily intranasal dose on a mg/m^2 basis).
One bottle of VANCENASE AQ 84 mcg Nasal Spray contains beclomethasone dipropionate, monohydrate equivalent to 16.0 mg of beclomethasone dipropionate; therefore, acute overdosage is unlikely.

DOSAGE AND ADMINISTRATION

Adults and Pediatric Patients 6 Years of Age and Over: The usual dosage of VANCENASE AQ 84 mcg Nasal Spray is 1 or 2 inhalations in each nostril once daily (total dose 168–336 mcg/day).
In patients who respond to VANCENASE AQ 84 mcg Nasal Spray, an improvement of the symptoms of allergic rhinitis usually becomes apparent within a few days after the start of therapy. Patients should use VANCENASE AQ 84 mcg Nasal Spray ONLY once daily at a regular interval. VANCENASE AQ 84 mcg Nasal Spray is not acutely effective, therefore, the prescribed dosage of VANCENASE AQ 84 mcg Nasal Spray should not be increased by using it more often than once daily. Symptom relief may not occur in some patients for as long as 2 weeks. VANCENASE AQ 84 mcg Nasal Spray should not be continued beyond 3 weeks in the absence of significant symptom improvement.
Since the therapeutic effects of corticosteroids, unlike those of a decongestant on allergic rhinitis or on nasal polyps, are not immediate, this should be explained to the patient in advance in order to ensure cooperation and continuation of treatment with the prescribed dosage regimen.
VANCENASE AQ 84 mcg Nasal Spray is not recommended for pediatric patients below 6 years of age.
In the presence of excessive nasal mucus secretion or edema of the nasal mucosa, the drug may fail to reach the sites of intended action. In such cases it is advisable to use a topical or oral nasal vasoconstrictor/decongestant during the first 2 to 3 days of VANCENASE AQ 84 mcg Nasal Spray therapy.

Continued on next page

Information on Schering products appearing on these pages is effective as of January 2000.

Vancenase AQ—Cont.

Prior to initial use of VANCENASE AQ 84 mcg Nasal Spray, the pump must be primed by actuating six times or until a fine spray appears. If the pump is unused for more than 4 days, repriming may be necessary. To reprime the unit, spray once or until a fine spray appears.

Directions for Use: Illustrated Patient's Instructions for proper use accompany each package of VANCENASE AQ 84 mcg Nasal Spray.

HOW SUPPLIED

VANCENASE AQ 84 mcg (beclomethasone dipropionate, monohydrate) Nasal Spray, 19 g net weight, 120 actuations, white high-density polyethylene bottle fitted with a white metered-dose nasal spray pump, maroon safety clip, and white dust cap; box of one. Supplied with Patient's Instructions for Use (NDC 0085-1049-01).

Store between 2° and 25°C (36° and 77°F).
SHAKE WELL BEFORE EACH USE.

Schering Corporation
Kenilworth, NJ 07033 USA

 Rev. 4/97
18802333
18780941T

Shown in Product Identification Guide, page 334

VANCERIL® 42 mcg ℞
(beclomethasone dipropionate, 42 mcg)
Inhalation Aerosol

For Oral Inhalation Only

DESCRIPTION

Beclomethasone dipropionate, USP, the active component of VANCERIL 42 mcg Inhalation Aerosol, is an anti-inflammatory steroid having the chemical name 9-Chloro-11β,17,21-trihydroxy-16β-methylpregna-1,4-diene-3,20-dione 17,21-dipropionate.

VANCERIL 42 mcg Inhalation Aerosol is a metered-dose aerosol unit containing a microcrystalline suspension of beclomethasone dipropionate-trichloromonofluoromethane clathrate in a mixture of propellants (trichloromonofluoromethane and dichlorodifluoromethane) with oleic acid. Each canister contains beclomethasone dipropionate-trichloromonofluoromethane clathrate having a molecular proportion of beclomethasone dipropionate, USP, to trichloromonofluoromethane between 3:1 and 3:2. Each actuation delivers from the mouthpiece a quantity of clathrate equivalent to 42 mcg of beclomethasone dipropionate, USP. The contents of one canister provide at least 200 oral inhalations.

CLINICAL PHARMACOLOGY

Beclomethasone 17, 21-dipropionate is a diester of beclomethasone, a synthetic corticosteroid which is chemically related to dexamethasone. Beclomethasone differs from dexamethasone only in having a chlorine at the 9-alpha in place of a fluorine and in having a 16β-methyl group instead of a 16 alpha-methyl group. Animal studies show that beclomethasone dipropionate has potent anti-inflammatory activity. When administered systemically to mice, the anti-inflammatory activity was accompanied by other typical features of glucocorticoid action including thymic involution, liver glycogen deposition, and pituitary-adrenal suppression. However, after systemic administration to rats, the anti-inflammatory action was associated with little or no effect on other tests of glucocorticoid activity.

Beclomethasone dipropionate is sparingly soluble and is poorly mobilized from subcutaneous or intramuscular injection sites. However, systemic absorption occurs after all routes of administration. When given to animals in the form of an aerosolized suspension of the trichloromonofluoromethane clathrate, the drug is deposited in the mouth and nasal passages, the trachea and principal bronchi, and in the lung; a considerable portion of the drug is also swallowed. Absorption occurs rapidly from all respiratory and gastrointestinal tissues, as indicated by the rapid clearance of radioactivity labeled drug from local tissues and appearance of tracer in the circulation. There is no evidence of tissue storage of beclomethasone dipropionate or its metabolites. Lung slices can metabolize beclomethasone dipropionate rapidly to beclomethasone 17-monopropionate and more slowly to free beclomethasone (which has very weak anti-inflammatory activity). However, irrespective of the route of administration (injection, oral, or aerosol), the principal route of excretion of the drug and its metabolites is the feces. Less than 10% of the drug and its metabolites is excreted in the urine. In humans, 12% to 15% of an orally administered dose of beclomethasone dipropionate is excreted in the urine as both conjugated and free metabolites of the drug.

The mechanisms responsible for the anti-inflammatory action of beclomethasone dipropionate are unknown. The precise mechanism of the aerosolized drug's action in the lung is also unknown.

INDICATIONS

VANCERIL 42 mcg Inhalation Aerosol is indicated only for patients who required chronic treatment with corticosteroids for control of the symptoms of bronchial asthma. Such patients would include those already receiving systemic corticosteroids, and selected patients who are inadequately controlled on a nonsteroid regimen and in whom steroid therapy has been withheld because of concern over potential adverse effects.

VANCERIL 42 mcg Inhalation Aerosol is NOT indicated:

1. For relief of asthma which can be controlled by bronchodilators and other nonsteroid medications.
2. In patients who require systemic corticosteroid treatment infrequently.
3. In the treatment of nonasthmatic bronchitis.

CONTRAINDICATIONS

VANCERIL 42 mcg Inhalation Aerosol is contraindicated in the primary treatment of status asthmaticus or other acute episodes of asthma where intensive measures are required.

Hypersensitivity to any of the ingredients of this preparation contraindicates its use.

WARNINGS

Particular care is needed in patients who are transferred from systemically active corticosteroids to VANCERIL 42 mcg Inhalation Aerosol because deaths due to adrenal insufficiency have occurred in asthmatic patients during and after transfer from systemic corticosteroids to aerosol beclomethasone dipropionate. After withdrawal from systemic corticosteroids, a number of months are required for recovery of hypothalamic-pituitary-adrenal (HPA) function. During this period of HPA suppression, patients may exhibit signs and symptoms of adrenal insufficiency when exposed to trauma, surgery, or infections, particularly gastroenteritis. Although VANCERIL 42 mcg Inhalation Aerosol may provide control of asthmatic symptoms during these episodes, it does NOT provide the systemic steroid which is necessary for coping with these emergencies.

During periods of stress or a severe asthmatic attack, patients who have been withdrawn from systemic corticosteroids should be instructed to resume systemic steroids (in large doses) immediately and to contact their physician for further instruction. These patients should also be instructed to carry a warning card indicating that they may need supplementary systemic steroids during periods of stress or a severe asthma attack. To assess the risk of adrenal insufficiency in emergency situations, routine tests of adrenal cortical function, including measurement of early morning resting cortisol levels, should be performed periodically in all patients. An early morning resting cortisol level may be accepted as normal only if it falls at or near the normal mean level.

Localized infections with *Candida albicans* or *Aspergillus niger* have occurred frequently in the mouth and pharynx and occasionally in the larynx. Positive cultures for oral *Candida* may be present in up to 75% of patients. Although the frequency of clinically apparent infection is considerably lower, these infections may require treatment with appropriate antifungal therapy or discontinuance of treatment with VANCERIL 42 mcg Inhalation Aerosol.

VANCERIL 42 mcg Inhalation Aerosol is not to be regarded as a bronchodilator and is not indicated for rapid relief of bronchospasm.

Patients should be instructed to contact their physician immediately when episodes of asthma which are not responsive to bronchodilators occur during the course of treatment with VANCERIL 42 mcg Inhalation Aerosol. During such episodes, patients may require therapy with systemic corticosteroids.

There is no evidence that control of asthma can be achieved by the administration of VANCERIL 42 mcg Inhalation Aerosol in amounts greater than the recommended doses.

Transfer of patients from systemic steroid therapy to VANCERIL 42 mcg Inhalation Aerosol may unmask allergic conditions previously suppressed by the systemic steroid therapy, eg, rhinitis, conjunctivitis, and eczema.

Persons who are on drugs which suppress the immune system are more susceptible to infections than healthy individuals. Chickenpox and measles, for example, can have a more serious or even fatal course in nonimmune children or adults on corticosteroids. In such children or adults who have not had these diseases, particular care should be taken to avoid exposure. How the dose, route, and duration of corticosteroid administration affects the risk of developing a disseminated infection is not known. The contribution of the underlying disease and/or prior corticosteroid treatment to the risk is also not known. If exposed to chickenpox, prophylaxis with varicella-zoster immune globulin (VZIG) may be indicated. If exposed to measles, prophylaxis with pooled intramuscular immunoglobulin (IG) may be indicated. (See the respective package inserts for complete VZIG and IG prescribing information.) If chickenpox develops, treatment with antiviral agents may be considered.

PRECAUTIONS

During withdrawal from oral steroids, some patients may experience symptoms of systemically active steroid withdrawal, eg, joint and/or muscular pain, lassitude and depression, despite maintenance or even improvement of respiratory function. (See **DOSAGE AND ADMINISTRATION** for details.)

In responsive patients, beclomethasone dipropionate may permit control of asthmatic symptoms without suppression of HPA function, as discussed below. (See **CLINICAL STUDIES.**) Since beclomethasone dipropionate is absorbed into the circulation and can be systemically active, the beneficial effects of VANCERIL 42 mcg Inhalation Aerosol in minimizing or preventing HPA dysfunction may be expected only when recommended dosages are not exceeded.

The long-term effects of beclomethasone dipropionate in human subjects are still unknown. In particular, the local effects of the agent on developmental or immunologic processes in the mouth, pharynx, trachea, and lung are unknown. There is also no information about the possible long-term systemic effects of the agent.

The potential effects of VANCERIL 42 mcg Inhalation Aerosol on acute, recurrent, or chronic pulmonary infections, including active or quiescent tuberculosis, are not known. Similarly, the potential effects of long-term administration of the drug on lung or other tissues are unknown.

Pulmonary infiltrates with eosinophilia may occur in patients on VANCERIL 42 mcg Inhalation Aerosol therapy. Although it is possible that in some patients this state may become manifest because of systemic steroid withdrawal when inhalational steroids are administered, a causative role for beclomethasone dipropionate and/or its vehicle cannot be ruled out.

Use in Pregnancy: Glucocorticoids are known teratogens in rodent species and beclomethasone dipropionate is no exception.

Teratology studies were done in rats, mice, and rabbits treated with subcutaneous beclomethasone dipropionate. Beclomethasone dipropionate was found to produce fetal resorptions, cleft palate, agnathia, microstomia, absence of tongue, delayed ossification, and partial agenesis of the thymus. Well-controlled trials relating to fetal risk in humans are not available. Glucocorticoids are secreted in human milk. It is not known whether belcomethasone dipropionate would be secreted in human milk but it is safe to assume that it is likely. The use of beclomethasone dipropionate in pregnancy, nursing mothers, or women of childbearing potential requires that the possible benefits of the drug be weighed against the potential hazards to the mother, embryo, or fetus. Infants born of mothers who have received substantial doses of corticosteroids during pregnancy should be carefully observed for hypoadrenalism.

Information for Patients: Persons who are on immunosuppressant doses of corticosteroids should be warned to avoid exposure to chickenpox or measles. Patients should also be advised that if they are exposed, medical advice should be sought without delay.

ADVERSE REACTIONS

Deaths due to adrenal insufficiency have occurred in asthmatic patients during and after transfer from systemic corticosteroids to aerosol beclomethasone dipropionate. (See **WARNINGS.**)

Suppression of HPA function (reduction of early morning plasma cortisol levels) has been reported in adult patients who received 1600 mcg daily doses of VANCERIL 42 mcg Inhalation Aerosol for 1 month. A few patients on VANCERIL 42 mcg Inhalation Aerosol have complained of hoarseness or dry mouth.

Rare cases of immediate and delayed hypersensitivity reactions, including urticaria, angioedema, rash, and bronchospasm have been reported following the oral and intranasal inhalation of beclomethasone.

DOSAGE AND ADMINISTRATION

Adults: The usual recommended dosage is two inhalations (84 mcg) given three or four times a day. Alternatively, four inhalations (168 mcg) given twice daily has been shown to be effective in some patients. In patients with severe asthma, it is advisable to start with 12 to 16 inhalations a day and adjust the dosage downward according to the response of the patient. The maximal daily intake should not exceed 20 inhalations, 840 mcg (0.84 mg), in adults.

Children 6 to 12 Years of Age: The usual recommended dosage is one or two inhalations (42 to 84 mcg) given three or four times a day according to the response of the patient. Alternatively, four inhalations (168 mcg) given twice daily has been shown to be effective in some patients. The maximal daily intake should not exceed ten inhalations, 420 mcg (0.42 mcg), in children 6 to 12 years of age. Insufficient clinical data exist with respect to the administration of VANCERIL 42 mcg Inhalation Aerosol in children below the age of 6.

Rinsing the mouth after inhalation is advised.

Patients receiving bronchodilators by inhalation should be advised to use the bronchodilator before VANCERIL 42 mcg Inhalation Aerosol in order to enhance penetration of beclomethasone dipropionate into the bronchial tree. After use of an aerosol bronchodilator, several minutes should elapse before use of the VANCERIL 42 mcg Inhalation Aerosol to reduce the potential toxicity from the inhaled fluorocarbon propellants in the two aerosols.

Different considerations must be given to the following groups of patients in order to obtain the full therapeutic benefit of VANCERIL 42 mcg Inhalation Aerosol.

Patients Not Receiving Systemic Steroids: The use of VANCERIL 42 mcg Inhalation Aerosol is straightforward in patients who are inadequately controlled with nonsteroid medications but in whom systemic steroid therapy has been withheld because of concern over potential adverse reactions. In patients who respond to VANCERIL, an improvement in pulmonary function is usually apparent within 1 to 4 weeks after the start of VANCERIL 42 mcg Inhalation Aerosol.

Patients Receiving Systemic Steroids: In those patients dependent on systemic steroids, transfer to VANCERIL 42 mcg Inhalation Aerosol and subsequent management may be more difficult because of recovery from impaired adrenal function is usually slow. Such suppression has been known to last for up to 12 months. Clinical studies, however, have demonstrated that VANCERIL may be effective in the management of these asthmatic patients and may permit replacement or significant reduction in the dosage of systemic corticosteroids.

The patient's asthma should be reasonably stable before treatment with VANCERIL 42 mcg Inhalation Aerosol is started. Initially, the aerosol should be used concurrently with the patient's usual maintenance dose of systemic steroid. After approximately 1 week, gradual withdrawal of the systemic steroid is started by reducing the daily or alternate daily dose. The next reduction is made after an interval of 1 or 2 weeks, depending on the response of the patient. Generally, these decrements should not exceed 2.5 mg of prednisone or its equivalent. A slow rate of withdrawal cannot be overemphasized. During withdrawal, some patients may experience symptoms of systemically active steroid withdrawal, eg, joint and/or muscular pain, lassitude and depression, despite maintenance or even improvement of respiratory function. Such patients should be encouraged to continue with the inhaler but should be watched carefully for objective signs of adrenal insufficiency, such as hypotension and weight loss. If evidence of adrenal insufficiency occurs, the systemic steroid dose should be boosted temporarily and thereafter further withdrawal should continue more slowly.

During periods of stress or a severe asthma attack, transfer patients will require supplementary treatment with systemic steroids. Exacerbations of asthma which occur during the course of treatment with VANCERIL 42 mcg Inhalation Aerosol should be treated with a short course of systemic steroid which is gradually tapered as these symptoms subside. There is no evidence that control of asthma can be achieved by administration of VANCERIL in amounts greater than the recommended doses.

Directions for Use: Illustrated Patient's Instructions for proper use accompany each package of VANCERIL 42 mcg Inhalation Aerosol.

CONTENTS UNDER PRESSURE. Do not puncture. Do not use or store near heat or open flame. Exposure to temperatures above 120°F may cause bursting. Never throw container into fire or incinerator. Keep out of reach of children.

HOW SUPPLIED

VANCERIL 42 mcg Inhalation Aerosol 16.8 g canister supplied with an oral adapter and Patient's Instructions; box of one (NDC 0085-0736-04). Institutional Pack for Inpatient Use Only: VANCERIL 42 mcg Inhalation Aerosol 6.7 g canister supplied with an oral adapter and Patient's Instructions; box of one (NDC 0085-0738-01).

Store between 15° and 30°C (59° and 86°F). Protect from moisture and unusual temperature fluctuations. Shake well before using. Failure to use the product within this temperature range may result in improper dosing.

Note: The indented statement below is required by the Federal government's Clean Air Act for all products containing or manufactured with chlorofluorocarbons (CFCs).

> **WARNING:** Contains dichlorodifluoromethane (CFC-11) and trichloromonofluoromethane (CFC-12), substances which harm public health and the environment by destroying ozone in the upper atmosphere.

A notice similar to the above WARNING has been placed in the "Patient's Instructions" portion of this package insert pursuant to EPA regulations.

ANIMAL PHARMACOLOGY AND TOXICOLOGY

Studies in a number of animal species including rats, rabbits, and dogs have shown no unusual toxicity during acute experiments. However, the effects of beclomethasone dipropionate in producing signs of glucocorticoid excess during chronic administration by various routes were dose related.

CLINICAL STUDIES

The effects of beclomethasone dipropionate on hypothalamic-pituitary-adrenal (HPA) function have been evaluated in adult volunteers. There was no suppression of early morning plasma cortisol concentrations when beclomethasone dipropionate was administered at a dose of 1000 mcg/day for 1 month as an aerosol or for 3 days by intramuscular injection. However, partial suppression of plasma cortisol concentration was observed when beclomethasone dipropionate was administered at doses of 2000 mcg/day either intramuscularly or by aerosol. Immediate suppression of plasma cortisol concentrations was observed after single doses of 4000 mcg of beclomethasone dipropionate.

In one study, the effects of beclomethasone dipropionate on HPA function were examined in patients with asthma. There was no change in basal early morning plasma cortisol concentrations or in the cortisol responses to tetracosactrin (ACTH 1:24) stimulation after daily administration of 400, 800, or 1200 mcg of beclomethasone dipropionate for 28 days. After daily administration of 1600 mcg each day for 28 days, there was a slight reduction in basal cortisol concentrations and a statistically significant ($p < .01$) reduction in plasma cortisol responses to tetracosactrin stimulation. The effects of a more prolonged period of beclomethasone dipropionate administration on HPA function have not been evaluated. However, a number of investigators have noted that when systemic corticosteroid therapy in asthmatic subjects can be replaced with recommended doses of beclomethasone dipropionate, there is gradual recovery of endogenous cortisol concentrations to the normal range. There is still no documented evidence of recovery from other adverse systemic corticosteroid-induced reactions during prolonged therapy of patients with beclomethasone dipropionate.

Clinical experience has shown that some patients with bronchial asthma who require corticosteroid therapy for control of symptoms can be partially or completely withdrawn from systemic corticosteroid if therapy with beclomethasone dipropionate aerosol is substituted. Beclomethasone dipropionate aerosol is not effective for all patients with bronchial asthma or at all stages of the disease in a given patient.

The early clinical experience has revealed several new problems which may be associated with the use of beclomethasone dipropionate by inhalation for treatment of patients with bronchial asthma:

1. There is a risk of adrenal insufficiency when patients are transferred from systemic corticosteroids to aerosol beclomethasone dipropionate. Although the aerosol may provide adequate control of asthma during the transfer period, it does not provide the systemic steroid which is needed during acute stress situations. Deaths due to adrenal insufficiency have occurred in asthmatic patients during and after transfer from systemic corticosteroids to aerosol beclomethasone dipropionate. (See **WARNINGS.**)
2. Transfer of patients from systemic steroid therapy to beclomethasone dipropionate aerosol may unmask allergic conditions which were previously controlled by the systemic steroid therapy, eg, rhinitis, conjunctivitis, and eczema.
3. Localized infections with *Candida albicans* or *Aspergillus niger* have occurred frequently in the mouth and pharynx and occasionally in the larynx. It has been reported that up to 75% of the patients who receive prolonged treatment with beclomethasone dipropionate have positive oral cultures for *Candida albicans*. The incidence of clinically apparent infection is considerably lower but may require therapy with appropriate antifungal agents or discontinuation of treatment with beclomethasone dipropionate aerosol.

The long-term effects of beclomethasone dipropionate in human subjects are still unknown. In particular, the local effects of the agent on developmental or immunologic processes in the mouth, pharynx, trachea, and lung are unknown. There is also no information about the possible long-term systemic effects of the agent. The possible relevance of the data in animal studies to results in human subjects cannot be evaluated.

Schering Corporation
Kenilworth, NJ 07033 USA

Rev. 4/97 20108908

VANCERIL® 42 mcg
(beclomethasone dipropionate, 42 mcg) Inhalation Aerosol

For Oral Inhalation Only

PATIENT'S INSTRUCTIONS

It is important that you read these instructions before using your VANCERIL 42 mcg Inhalation Aerosol. Correct and regular use of the inhaler will prevent or lessen the severity of asthma attacks.

1. SHAKE THE INHALER WELL and remove the plastic cap (see Figure 1).

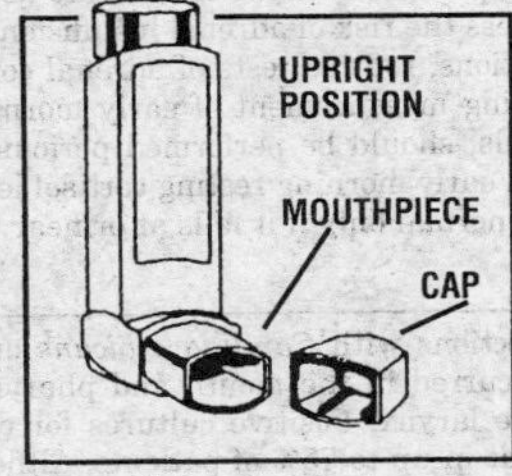

Figure 1

2. As with all aerosol medications, it is recommended to "test spray" into the air before using for the first time and in cases where the aerosol has not been used for a prolonged period of time.
3. BREATHE OUT AS FULLY AS YOU COMFORTABLY CAN. Hold the inhaler in the upright position and put the mouthpiece into your mouth (see Figure 2). Close your lips around the mouthpiece, *keeping your tongue below it.*

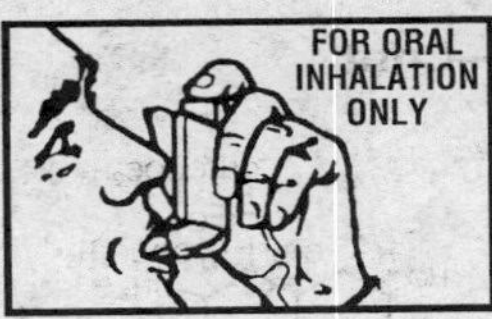

Figure 2

4. WHILE BREATHING IN DEEPLY, PRESS DOWN ON THE CAN WITH YOUR FIRST FINGER. When you have finished breathing in, hold your breath as long as you comfortably can.
5. TAKE YOUR FINGER OFF THE CAN and remove the inhaler from your mouth. Breathe out gently.
6. If your physician has told you to take more than one inhalation per treatment, wait 1 minute between puffs. Shake the inhaler well and repeat steps 3 through 5.
7. It is recommended that you rinse your mouth thoroughly with water, gargle, or drink water after inhalation(s), whenever possible.
8. CLEAN YOUR INHALER AT LEAST ONCE A DAY. Remove the can and rinse the plastic case and cap in warm running water. Dry the case and cap and gently replace the metal canister into the case with a twisting motion. Put the cap on the mouthpiece.
9. DISCARD THE CANISTER AFTER the date calculated by your physician or pharmacist. The correct amount of medication in each inhalation cannot be assured after a specified number of inhalations even though the canister is not completely empty. Before the discard date you should consult your physician to determine whether a refill is needed. Just as you should not take extra doses without consulting your physician, you also should not stop VANCERIL without consulting your physician.

IMPORTANT: VANCERIL 42 mcg Inhalation Aerosol is preventive therapy for asthma and must be used regularly and at the times your physician has prescribed. DO NOT CONFUSE VANCERIL 42 mcg Inhalation Aerosol WITH OTHER ASTHMA MEDICATION. VANCERIL 42 mcg Inhalation Aerosol WILL NOT PROVIDE IMMEDIATE RELIEF IF YOU ARE HAVING AN ATTACK. Your physician will decide whether other medication is needed should you require immediate relief. If you also use another medicine by inhalation, you should consult your physician for instructions on when to use it in relation to using VANCERIL. If this is the first time you will be using VANCERIL 42 mcg Inhalation Aerosol, it may take from 1 to 4 weeks before you feel the full benefits.

Dosage: Use only as directed by your physician.

Contents under pressure. Do not puncture. Do not use or store near heat or open flame. Exposure to temperatures above 120°F may cause bursting. Never throw container into fire or incinerator. Keep out of reach of children.

Store between 15° and 30°C (59° and 86°F). Protect from moisture and unusual temperature fluctuations. Shake well before using. Failure to use the product within this temperature range may result in improper dosing.

Note: The indented statement below is required by the Federal government's Clean Air Act for all products containing or manufactured with chlorofluorocarbons (CFCs).

> This product contains dichlorodifluromethane (CFC-11) and trichloromonofluoromethane (CFC-12), substances which harm the environment by destroying ozone in the upper atmosphere.

Your physician has determined that this product is likely to help your personal health. USE THIS PRODUCT AS DIRECTED, UNLESS INSTRUCTED TO DO OTHERWISE BY YOUR PHYSICIAN. If you have any questions about alternatives, consult with your physician.

Schering Corporation
Kenilworth, NJ 07033 USA
 Rev. 4/97

VANCERIL® 84 mcg DOUBLE STRENGTH ℞
(beclomethasone dipropionate, 84 mcg)
Inhalation Aerosol

DESCRIPTION

Beclomethasone dipropionate, USP, the active component of VANCERIL 84 mcg DOUBLE STRENGTH Inhalation Aerosol, is an anti-inflammatory corticosteroid having the chemical name 9-Chloro-11β,17,21-trihydroxy-16β-methylpregna-1,4-diene-3,20-dione 17,21-dipropionate. Beclomethasone 17,21-dipropionate is a diester of beclomethasone, a synthetic corticosteroid which is chemically related to dexamethasone. Beclomethasone differs from dexamethasone only in having a chlorine at the 9α carbon in place of fluorine and in having a 16β-methyl group instead of a 16α-methyl group.

[See chemical structure at top of next column]

Continued on next page

Information on Schering products appearing on these pages is effective as of January 2000.

Vanceril—Cont.

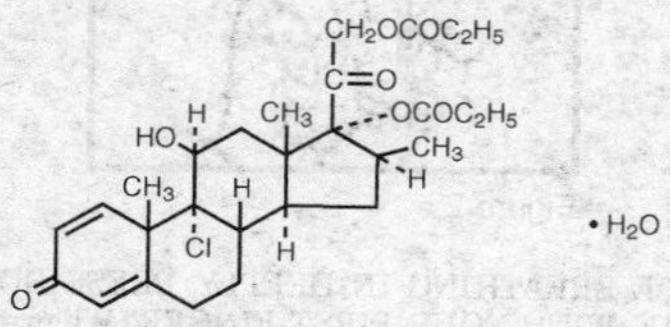

Beclomethasone dipropionate is a white to creamy white, odorless powder with a molecular formula of $C_{28}H_{37}ClO_7$, and a molecular weight of 521.05. It is very slightly soluble in water, very soluble in chloroform, and freely soluble in acetone and in alcohol.

VANCERIL 84 mcg DOUBLE STRENGTH Inhalation Aerosol is a pressurized metered-dose aerosol unit containing a microcrystalline suspension of beclomethasone dipropionate-trichloromonofluoromethane clathrate in a mixture of propellants (trichloromonofluoromethane and dichlorodifluoromethane) with oleic acid. Each canister contains beclomethasone dipropionate-trichloromonofluoromethane clathrate having a molecular proportion of beclomethasone dipropionate, USP, to trichloromonofluoromethane between 3:1 and 3:2. Each actuation delivers a quantity of clathrate equivalent to 84 mcg of beclomethasone dipropionate, USP from the mouthpiece and 100 mcg of beclomethasone dipropionate from the valve. The contents of the 5.4 g and 12.2 g canisters provide 40 and 120 oral inhalations, respectively (see **HOW SUPPLIED**).

CLINICAL PHARMACOLOGY

Animal studies showed that beclomethasone dipropionate has potent anti-inflammatory activity. When administered systemically to mice, the anti-inflammatory activity was accompanied by other typical features of glucocorticoid action including thymic involution, liver glycogen deposition, and pituitary-adrenal suppression. However, after systemic administration to rats, the anti-inflammatory action was associated with little or no effect on other tests of glucocorticoid activity.

Beclomethasone dipropionate is sparingly soluble and is poorly mobilized from subcutaneous or intramuscular injection sites. However, systemic absorption occurs after all routes of administration. When given to animals in the form of an aerosolized suspension of the trichloromonofluoromethane clathrate, the drug is deposited in the mouth and nasal passages, the trachea and principal bronchi, and in the lung; a considerable portion of the drug is also swallowed. Absorption occurs rapidly from all respiratory and gastrointestinal tissues, as indicated by the rapid clearance of radioactively labeled drug from local tissues and appearance of tracer in the circulation. There is no evidence of tissue storage of beclomethasone dipropionate or its metabolites. Lung slices can metabolize beclomethasone dipropionate rapidly to beclomethasone 17-monopropionate and more slowly to free beclomethasone (which has very weak anti-inflammatory activity). However, irrespective of the route of administration (injection, oral, or aerosol), the principal route of excretion of the drug and its metabolites is the feces. Less than 10% of the drug and its metabolites is excreted in the urine. In humans, 12% to 15% of an orally administered dose of beclomethasone dipropionate was excreted in the urine as both conjugated and free metabolites of the drug.

The mechanisms responsible for the anti-inflammatory action of beclomethasone dipropionate are unknown. The precise mechanism of the aerosolized drug's action in the lung is also unknown.

Clinical Trials: The efficacy of VANCERIL 84 mcg DOUBLE STRENGTH Inhalation Aerosol was compared with VANCERIL Inhaler (42 mcg/actuation) in a 28-day, randomized, parallel-group, double-blind, placebo-controlled study in patients with moderate to severe asthma. A total of 336 mcg/day of each VANCERIL formulation or placebo was administered based on BID dosing. FEV_1 at endpoint (last valid visit for each patient) was regarded as the primary measure of efficacy. VANCERIL 84 mcg DOUBLE STRENGTH Inhalation Aerosol and VANCERIL Inhaler were both significantly more effective ($p \leq 0.01$) than placebo in improving FEV_1 at all time points, but were not significantly different from each other at any time point ($p > 0.05$). Thus VANCERIL 84 mcg DOUBLE STRENGTH Inhalation Aerosol administered twice daily to give a total daily dose of 336 mcg was comparable in efficacy to VANCERIL Inhaler when administered at the same total daily dose.

The effects of beclomethasone dipropionate on hypothalamic pituitary-adrenal (HPA) function have been evaluated in adult volunteers. There was no suppression of early morning plasma cortisol concentrations when beclomethasone dipropionate was administered at a dose of 840 mcg/day for 1 month as an aerosol or 1000 mcg/day for 3 days by intramuscular injection. However, partial suppression of plasma cortisol concentration was observed when beclomethasone dipropionate was administered at doses of 2000 mcg/day intramuscularly or 1680 mcg/day by aerosol. Immediate suppression of plasma cortisol concentrations was observed after single doses of 4000 mcg of beclomethasone dipropionate intramuscularly.

The potential for VANCERIL 84 mcg DOUBLE STRENGTH Inhalation Aerosol (84 mcg/actuation) to cause HPA axis suppression was compared with VANCERIL Inhaler (42 mcg/actuation) in a randomized, parallel, placebo- and positive-controlled study. Sixty-four adult patients with moderate asthma received doses of either: 1) 420 mcg twice daily of VANCERIL 84 mcg DOUBLE STRENGTH; 2) 420 mcg twice daily of VANCERIL Inhaler; 3) 10 mg of prednisone orally; or 4) placebo, for 35.5 days. The potential for HPA axis suppression was evaluated via a cosyntropin stimulation test administered on the 36th day. In response to a 6-hour cosyntropin 250 mcg infusion, there was no evidence of HPA axis suppression associated with either VANCERIL 84 mcg DOUBLE STRENGTH Inhalation Aerosol or VANCERIL Inhaler preparations as compared with placebo. However, there were significant ($p \leq 0.01$) attenuations of the plasma cortisol concentration responses to cosyntropin stimulation in the prednisone-treated group compared with the placebo-treated group.

In another study with VANCERIL Inhaler, the effects of beclomethasone dipropionate on HPA function were examined in patients with asthma. There was no change in basal early morning plasma cortisol concentrations or in the cortisol responses to tetracosactrin (ACTH 1:24) stimulation after daily aerosol administration of 336, 672, or 1008 mcg of beclomethasone dipropionate for 28 days. After daily aerosol administration of 1344 mcg for 28 days, there was a slight reduction in basal cortisol concentrations and a statistically significant ($p < 0.01$) reduction in plasma cortisol responses to tetracosactrin stimulation. The effects of a more prolonged period of beclomethasone dipropionate administration on HPA function have not been evaluated.

Clinical experience has shown that some patients with asthma who require corticosteroid therapy for control of symptoms can be partially or completely withdrawn from systemic corticosteroid if therapy with beclomethasone dipropionate aerosol is substituted. Beclomethasone dipropionate aerosol is not effective for all patients with asthma or at all stages of the disease in a given patient.

INDICATIONS

VANCERIL 84 mcg DOUBLE STRENGTH Inhalation Aerosol is indicated in the maintenance treatment of asthma as prophylactic therapy. VANCERIL 84 mcg DOUBLE STRENGTH Inhalation Aerosol is also indicated for asthma patients who require systemic corticosteroid administration, where adding VANCERIL 84 mcg DOUBLE STRENGTH Inhalation Aerosol may reduce or eliminate the need for systemic corticosteroids.

VANCERIL 84 mcg DOUBLE STRENGTH Inhalation Aerosol is NOT indicated for the relief of acute bronchospasm.

CONTRAINDICATIONS

VANCERIL 84 mcg DOUBLE STRENGTH Inhalation Aerosol is contraindicated in the primary treatment of status asthmaticus or other acute episodes of asthma where intensive measures are required.

Hypersensitivity to any of the ingredients of this preparation contraindicates its use.

WARNINGS

Particular care is needed in patients who are transferred from systemically active corticosteroids to VANCERIL 84 mcg DOUBLE STRENGTH Inhalation Aerosol because deaths due to adrenal insufficiency have occurred in asthmatic patients during and after transfer from systemic corticosteroids to aerosol beclomethasone dipropionate. After withdrawal from systemic corticosteroids, a number of months are required for recovery of hypothalamic-pituitary-adrenal (HPA) function. During this period of HPA suppression, patients may exhibit signs and symptoms of adrenal insufficiency when exposed to trauma, surgery, or infections, particularly gastroenteritis. Although VANCERIL 84 mcg DOUBLE STRENGTH Inhalation Aerosol may provide control of asthmatic symptoms during these episodes, it does NOT provide the systemic steroid which is necessary for coping with these emergencies.

During periods of stress or a severe asthmatic attack, patients who have been withdrawn from systemic corticosteroids should be instructed to resume systemic corticosteroids (in large doses) immediately and to contact their physician for further instruction. These patients should also be instructed to carry a warning card indicating that they may need supplementary systemic steroids during periods of stress or a severe asthmatic attack. To assess the risk of adrenal insufficiency in emergency situations, routine tests of adrenal cortical function, including measurement of early morning resting cortisol levels, should be performed periodically in all patients. An early morning resting cortisol level may be accepted as normal only if it falls at or near the normal mean level.

Localized infections with *Candida albicans* or *Aspergillus niger* have occurred in the mouth and pharynx and occasionally in the larynx. Positive cultures for oral *Candida* may be present in up to 75% of patients. Although the frequency of clinically apparent infection is considerably lower, these infections can develop with any inhaled corticosteroid and may require treatment with appropriate antifungal therapy or discontinuance of treatment with VANCERIL 84 mcg DOUBLE STRENGTH Inhalation Aerosol.

VANCERIL 84 mcg DOUBLE STRENGTH Inhalation Aerosol is not a bronchodilator and is, therefore, not indicated for rapid relief of bronchospasm.

Patients should be instructed to contact their physician immediately when episodes of asthma which are not responsive to bronchodilators occur during the course of treatment with VANCERIL 84 mcg DOUBLE STRENGTH Inhalation Aerosol. During such episodes, patients may require therapy with systemic corticosteroids.

Transfer of patients from systemic corticosteroid therapy to VANCERIL 84 mcg DOUBLE STRENGTH Inhalation Aerosol may unmask allergic conditions previously suppressed by the systemic corticosteroid therapy, eg, rhinitis, conjunctivitis, and eczema.

Patients who are on drugs which suppress the immune system are more susceptible to infections than healthy individuals. Chicken-pox and measles, for example, can have a more serious or even fatal course in non-immune children or adults on corticosteroids. In children or adults who have not had these diseases, particular care should be taken to avoid exposure to these infectious agents. How the dose, route, and duration of corticosteroid administration affects the risk of developing disseminated infection is not known. The contribution of underlying disease and/or prior corticosteroid treatment to the risk of developing more severe infection is also not known. If exposed to chickenpox, prophylaxis with varicella-zoster immune globulin (VZIG) may be indicated. If exposed to measles, prophylaxis with pooled intramuscular immunoglobulin (IG) may be indicated. (See the respective package inserts for complete VZIG and IG prescribing information.) If chickenpox develops, treatment with antiviral agents may be considered.

Avoid spraying in eyes.

PRECAUTIONS

During withdrawal from oral corticosteroids, some patients may experience symptoms of systemically active corticosteroid withdrawal, eg, joint and/or muscular pain, lassitude and depression, despite maintenance or even improvement of respiratory function. (See **DOSAGE AND ADMINISTRATION** for details.)

In responsive patients, beclomethasone dipropionate may permit control of asthmatic symptoms without suppression of HPA function, as discussed above. (See **CLINICAL PHARMACOLOGY**.) Since inhaled beclomethasone dipropionate is absorbed into the circulation and can be systemically active, lack of HPA suppression by VANCERIL 84 mcg DOUBLE STRENGTH Inhalation Aerosol may be expected only when recommended dosages are not exceeded.

The long-term local and systemic effects of VANCERIL 84 mcg DOUBLE STRENGTH Inhalation Aerosol in human subjects are still not fully known. In particular, the effects resulting from chronic use of the agent on developmental or immunologic processes in the mouth, pharynx, trachea, and lung are unknown.

Inhaled corticosteroids should be used with caution, if at all, in patients with active or quiescent tuberculous infection of the respiratory tract; untreated systemic fungal, bacterial, parasitic, or viral infections; or ocular herpes simplex.

Pulmonary infiltrates with eosinophilia may occur in patients receiving orally inhaled beclomethasone dipropionate. Although it is possible that in some patients this state may become manifest because of systemic corticosteroid withdrawal when inhalational corticosteroids are administered, a causative role for beclomethasone dipropionate and/or its vehicle cannot be ruled out.

Carcinogenesis, Mutagenesis, Impairment of Fertility: The carcinogenicity of beclomethasone dipropionate was evaluated in rats which were exposed for a total of 95 weeks, 13 weeks at inhalation doses up to 0.4 mg/kg/day and the remaining 82 weeks at combined oral and inhalation doses up to 2.4 mg/kg/day. There was no evidence of carcinogenicity in this study at the highest dose which is approximately 23 times the maximum recommended human daily inhalation dose on an mg/m^2 basis. Impairment of fertility, as evidenced by inhibition of the estrous cycle in dogs, was observed following treatment by the oral route at a dose of 0.5 mg/kg/day which is approximately 16 times the maximum recommended human daily inhalation dose on an mg/m^2 basis. No inhibition of the estrous cycle in dogs was seen following 12 months of exposure to beclomethasone dipropionate by the inhalation route at an estimated daily dose of 0.33 mg/kg (approximately 11 times the maximum recommended human daily inhalation dose on an mg/m^2 basis).

Pregnancy Category C: Like other corticosteroids, parenteral (subcutaneous) beclomethasone dipropionate was teratogenic and embryocidal in the mouse and rabbit when given at a dose of 0.1 mg/kg/day in mice or at a dose of 0.025 mg/kg/day in rabbits.

These doses in mice and rabbits were approximately one-half the maximum recommended human daily inhalation dose on an mg/m^2 basis. No teratogenicity or embryocidal effects were seen in rats when exposed to an inhalation dose of 0.1 mg/kg plus oral doses of up to 10 mg/kg/day for a combined daily dose of 10.1 mg/kg (approximately 97 times the maximum recommended human daily inhalation dose on an mg/m^2 basis). There are no adequate and well-controlled studies in pregnant women. Beclomethasone dipropionate should be used during pregnancy only if the potential benefit justifies the potential risk to the fetus.

Nursing Mothers: Corticosteroids are secreted in human milk. Because of the potential for serious adverse reactions in nursing infants from VANCERIL 84 mcg DOUBLE STRENGTH Inhalation Aerosol, a decision should be made whether to discontinue nursing or to discontinue the drug, taking into account the importance of the drug to the mother.

Pediatric Use: Safety and effectiveness in pediatric patients below the age of 6 years have not been established.

Information for Patients: Patients being treated with VANCERIL 84 mcg DOUBLE STRENGTH Inhalation Aerosol should receive the following information and instructions. This information is intended to aid them in the safe and effective use of this medication. It is not a disclosure of all possible adverse or intended effects.

Patients should use VANCERIL 84 mcg DOUBLE STRENGTH Inhalation Aerosol at regular intervals as directed. Results of clinical trials indicated significant improvement may occur within the first day or two of treatment; however, the full benefit may not be achieved until treatment has been administered for 1 to 2 weeks or longer. The patient should not increase the prescribed dosage but should contact the physician if symptoms do not improve or if the condition worsens.

Patients should be warned to avoid exposure to chickenpox or measles. Patients should be advised that if they are exposed, medical advice should be sought without delay.

Patients should also be advised that VANCERIL 84 mcg DOUBLE STRENGTH Inhalation Aerosol is not intended for use in the treatment of acute asthma. Patients should be instructed to contact their physician immediately if there is any deterioration of their asthma.

Patients should be advised to rinse his/her mouth each time after using VANCERIL 84 mcg DOUBLE STRENGTH Inhalation Aerosol.

VANCERIL 84 mcg DOUBLE STRENGTH Inhalation Aerosol should not be stopped abruptly. If discontinuing use of VANCERIL 84 mcg DOUBLE STRENGTH Inhalation Aerosol is necessary, the patient's physician should be contacted immediately.

ADVERSE REACTIONS

In a 4-week, randomized, double-blind, placebo-controlled clinical trial, the incidence of adverse events reported for VANCERIL 84 mcg DOUBLE STRENGTH Inhalation Aerosol was similar to that reported for placebo. Adverse event rates did not appear to differ significantly based on age, sex, or race. Adverse events that were reported by 2% or more of patients receiving VANCERIL 84 mcg DOUBLE STRENGTH Inhalation Aerosol (regardless of relationship to treatment) and that occurred more frequently than placebo are displayed in the following table.

ADVERSE EVENTS FROM A 4-WEEK PLACEBO-CONTROLLED CLINICAL TRIAL IN PATIENTS WITH ASTHMA

	PERCENT OF PATIENTS REPORTING		
	VANCERIL 84 mcg DOUBLE STRENGTH Inhalation Aerosol (336 mcg/day) n = 103	**VANCERIL Inhaler (336 mcg/day) n = 104**	**Vehicle Placebo n = 109**
Headache	22	27	18
Pharyngitis	14	11	8
Coughing	9	7	4
Infection (Viral)	8	5	6
Nasal Congestion	6	5	2
Dysmenorrhea	4	0	3
Sinusitis	4	3	3
Dyspepsia	3	6	2
Fatigue	3	2	2
Influenza-like Symptoms	3	<1	0
Sneezing	3	2	0
Eczema	2	0	0
Pruritus	2	0	<1
Respiratory Disorder	2	0	0

In a 4-week, randomized, double-blind clinical study, there were no reports of oral candidiasis in patients receiving VANCERIL 84 mcg DOUBLE STRENGTH Inhalation Aerosol (0/103) (see **WARNINGS**).

[See table above]

In addition to those adverse events reported in the table above, the following adverse events have been reported in fewer than 2% of patients (regardless of relationship to treatment).

Autonomic Nervous System: Lacrimation.
Body as a Whole: Increased allergy symptoms, chest pain, fever, rigors.
Gastrointestinal System: Diarrhea, nausea, rectal hemorrhage.
Hearing and Vestibular: Earache.
Heart Rate and Rhythm: Tachycardia.
Musculoskeletal: Arthralgia, pain.
Psychiatric: Depression, insomnia.
Respiratory System: Bronchitis, bronchospasm, chest congestion, dysphonia, upper respiratory infection.
Skin and Appendages: Rash, skin discoloration, urticaria.
Special Senses: Taste perversion.
Urinary System: Urinary tract infection.
Vascular (Extracardiac): Migraine.
White Cell and Reticuloendothelial System: Lymphadenopathy.

Deaths due to adrenal insufficiency have occurred in asthmatic patients during and after transfer from systemic corticosteroids to aerosol beclomethasone dipropionate. (See **WARNINGS**.)

Suppression of HPA function (reduction of early morning plasma cortisol levels) has been reported in adult patients who received 1344 mcg daily doses (approximately twice the maximum recommended daily dose) of beclomethasone dipropionate by oral inhalation for 1 month. Some patients receiving orally inhaled beclomethasone dipropionate have complained of hoarseness or dry mouth.

Rare cases of immediate and delayed hypersensitivity reactions, including urticaria, angioedema, rash, and bronchospasm have been reported following the oral and intranasal inhalation of beclomethasone.

Rare cases of hypercorticism, adrenal insufficiency, growth inhibitory effects, cataracts, glaucoma, and hyperglycemia have been reported with inhaled corticosteroids.

OVERDOSAGE

There were no deaths over 15 days following the oral administration of a single dose of 3000 mg/kg in mice, 2000 mg/kg in rats, and 1000 mg/kg in rabbits. The doses in mice, rats, and rabbits were 14,500, 19,300 times, respectively, the maximum recommended human daily inhalation dose on an mg/m^2 basis.

DOSAGE AND ADMINISTRATION

VANCERIL 84 mcg DOUBLE STRENGTH Inhalation Aerosol should be test sprayed 2 times into the air before using for the first time and in cases where the product has not been used for more than 7 days.

Adults: The usual recommended dosage is two inhalations (168 mcg) given twice daily. In patients with severe asthma, it is advisable to start with 6 to 8 inhalations a day and adjust the dosage downward according to the response of the patient. The maximal daily intake should not exceed 10 inhalations, 840 mcg (0.84 mg), in adults.

Children 6 to 12 Years of Age: The usual recommended dosage is two inhalations (168 mcg) given twice daily. The maximal daily intake should not exceed 5 inhalations, 420 mcg (0.42 mg), in children 6 to 12 years of age. Insufficient clinical data exist with respect to the administration of VANCERIL 84 mcg DOUBLE STRENGTH Inhalation Aerosol in children below the age of 6.

Rinsing the mouth after inhalation is advised.

Different considerations must be given to the following groups of patients in order to obtain the full therapeutic benefit of VANCERIL 84 mcg DOUBLE STRENGTH Inhalation Aerosol.

Patients Not Receiving Systemic Corticosteroids Patients who require maintenance therapy of their asthma may benefit from treatment with VANCERIL 84 mcg DOUBLE STRENGTH Inhalation Aerosol at the doses recommended above. In patients who respond to VANCERIL 84 mcg DOUBLE STRENGTH Inhalation Aerosol, improvement in pulmonary function is usually apparent within 1 to 4 weeks after the start of therapy. Once the desired effect is achieved, consideration should be given to tapering to the lowest effective dose.

Patients Maintained on Systemic Corticosteroids Clinical studies have shown that beclomethasone dipropionate may be effective in the management of asthmatics dependent or maintained on systemic corticosteroids and may permit replacement or significant reduction in the dosage of systemic corticosteroids.

The patient's asthma should be reasonably stable before treatment with VANCERIL 84 mcg DOUBLE STRENGTH Inhalation Aerosol is started. Initially, VANCERIL 84 mcg DOUBLE STRENGTH Inhalation Aerosol should be used concurrently with the patient's usual maintenance dose of systemic corticosteroid. After approximately 1 week, gradual withdrawal of the systemic corticosteroid is started by reducing the daily or alternate daily dose. Reductions may be made after an interval of 1 or 2 weeks, depending on the response of the patient. A slow rate of withdrawal is strongly recommended. Generally, these decrements should not exceed 2.5 mg of prednisone or its equivalent. During withdrawal, some patients may experience symptoms of systemic corticosteroid withdrawal, eg, joint and/or muscular pain, lassitude and depression, despite maintenance or even improvement in pulmonary function. Such patients should be encouraged to continue with the inhaler but should be monitored for objective signs of adrenal insufficiency. If evidence of adrenal insufficiency occurs, the systemic corticosteroid doses should be increased temporarily and thereafter withdrawal should continue more slowly.

During periods of stress or a severe asthma attack, transfer patients may require supplementary treatment with systemic corticosteroids.

Directions for Use: Illustrated Patient's Instructions for Use accompany each package of VANCERIL 84 mcg DOUBLE STRENGTH Inhalation Aerosol.

CONTENTS UNDER PRESSURE. Do not puncture. Do not use or store near heat or open flame. Exposure to temperatures above 120°F may cause bursting. Never throw container into fire or incinerator. Keep out of reach of children.

HOW SUPPLIED

VANCERIL 84 mcg DOUBLE STRENGTH Inhalation Aerosol 12.2 g canisters containing 120 metered inhalations, in boxes of one (NDC 0085-1112-01); 5.4 g canisters containing 40 metered inhalations for Institutional Use only, in boxes of one (NDC 0085-1112-02); and 5.4 g canisters containing 40 metered inhalations, in boxes of three (NDC 0085-1112-03). Each canister is supplied with a dark-pink plastic actuator with a maroon cap and each package contains a Patient's Instructions for Use. Each actuation delivers an amount of beclomethasone dipropionate-trichloromonofluoromethane clathrate equivalent to 84 mcg of beclomethasone dipropionate from the mouthpiece and 100 mcg of beclomethasone dipropionate from the valve.

The VANCERIL 84 mcg DOUBLE STRENGTH Inhalation Aerosol canister should only be used with the VANCERIL 84 mcg DOUBLE STRENGTH Inhalation Aerosol mouthpiece and this mouthpiece should not be used with any other inhalation drug product.

The correct amount of medication in each inhalation cannot be assured after 120 actuations from the 12.2 g canister or 40 actuations from the 5.4 g canister even though the canister is not completely empty. The canister should be discarded when the labeled number of actuations have been used.

Store at 15°–30°C (59°–86°F). Protect from moisture and unusual temperature fluctuations. Failure to use the product within this temperature range may result in improper dosing. For optimal results, the canister should be at room temperature before use. Shake well before using. If the canister is enclosed in a moisture protective package, the canister must be used within 6 months after removal.

Note: The indented statement below is required by the Federal government's Clean Air Act for all products containing or manufactured with chlorofluorocarbons (CFCs).

WARNING: Contains dichlorodifluoromethane (CFC-12) and trichloromonofluoromethane (CFC-11) and is manufactured with dichlorodifluoromethane (CFC-12), substances which harm public health and the environment by destroying ozone in the upper atmosphere.

A notice similar to the above **WARNING** has been placed in the "Patient's Instructions for Use" portion of this package insert pursuant to Environmental Protection Agency (EPA) regulations. The patient's warning states that the patient should consult his or her physician if there are questions about alternatives.

Schering/Key
Kenilworth, NJ 07033 USA

Rev. 8/99 18682141
18691450T

VANCERIL® 84 mcg
DOUBLE STRENGTH
(beclomethasone dipropionate, 84 mcg)
Inhalation Aerosol

For Oral Inhalation Only

PATIENT'S INSTRUCTIONS FOR USE

It is important that you read these instructions before using your VANCERIL 84 mcg DOUBLE STRENGTH Inhalation Aerosol. Correct and regular use of the inhaler may prevent or lessen the severity of asthma attacks.

1. Make sure the canister is fully and firmly inserted into the mouthpiece. SHAKE THE INHALER WELL before each use and remove the plastic cap (see Figure 1). If cap is not present, the inhaler mouthpiece should be inspected for the presence of foreign objects.

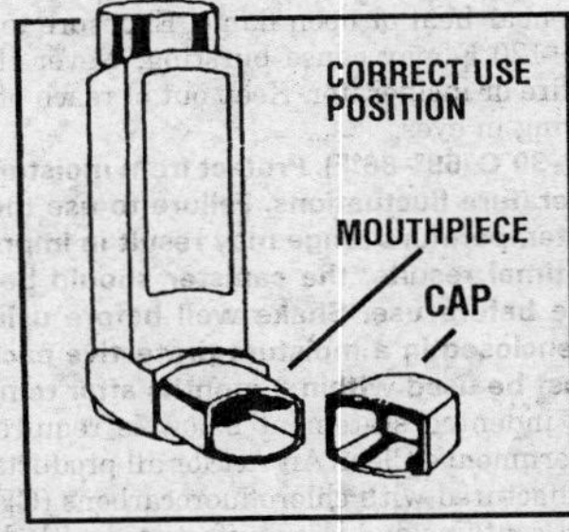

Figure 1

The VANCERIL 84 mcg DOUBLE STRENGTH Inhalation Aerosol canister should only be used with the VANCERIL

Continued on next page

Information on Schering products appearing on these pages is effective as of January 2000.

Vanceril—Cont.

84 mcg DOUBLE STRENGTH Inhalation Aerosol mouthpiece. This mouthpiece should not be used with any other inhalation drug product. Similarly, the canister should not be used with other mouthpieces.
2. It is recommended to "test spray" two times into the air before using for the first time and in cases where the product has not been used for more than 7 days.
3. Avoid spraying in eyes.
4. BREATHE OUT THROUGH THE MOUTH AS FULLY AS YOU COMFORTABLY CAN. Hold the inhaler in the valve down position (see Figure 1) and put the mouthpiece into your mouth (see Figure 2). Close your lips around the mouthpiece, *keeping your tongue below it.*

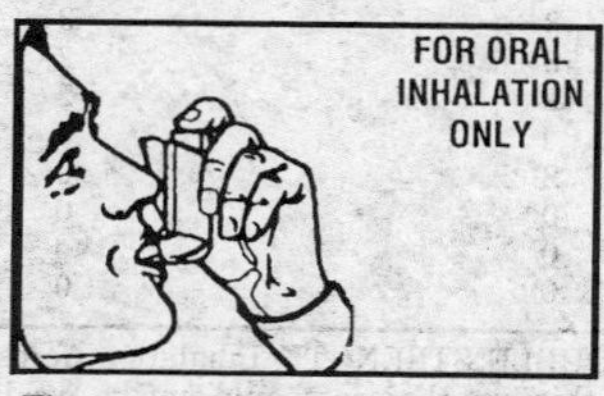

Figure 2

5. WHILE BREATHING IN DEEPLY AND SLOWLY THROUGH THE MOUTH, PRESS DOWN FIRMLY AND FULLY ON THE CANISTER WITH YOUR INDEX FINGER. When you have finished breathing in, hold your breath as long as you comfortably can.
6. TAKE YOUR FINGER OFF THE CANISTER and remove the inhaler from your mouth. Breathe out gently.
7. If your physician has told you to take more than one inhalation per treatment, wait 1 minute between puffs. Shake the inhaler well and repeat steps 4 through 6.
8. It is recommended that you rinse your mouth thoroughly with water, gargle, or drink water after inhalation(s), whenever possible.
9. CLEAN YOUR INHALER AT LEAST ONCE A DAY. Remove the canister and rinse the plastic actuator and cap in warm running water. Dry the actuator and cap thoroughly and gently replace the metal canister into the actuator with a twisting motion. Put the cap on the mouthpiece.
10. If the canister is enclosed in a moisture protective package, the canister must be used within 6 months after removal. The correct amount of medication in each inhalation cannot be assured after 120 actuations from the 12.2 g canister or 40 actuations from the 5.4 g canister even though the canister is not completely empty. You should keep track of the number of actuations used from each canister of VANCERIL 84 mcg DOUBLE STRENGTH Inhalation Aerosol, and discard the canister after 120 actuations from the 12.2 g canister or 40 actuations from the 5.4 g canister. Before you reach the specified number of actuations, you should consult your physician to determine whether a refill is needed. Just as you should not take extra doses without consulting your physician, you should not stop using VANCERIL 84 mcg DOUBLE STRENGTH Inhalation Aerosol without consulting your physician.
IMPORTANT: VANCERIL 84 mcg DOUBLE STRENGTH Inhalation Aerosol is preventive therapy for asthma and must be used regularly and at the times your physician has prescribed. DO NOT CONFUSE VANCERIL 84 mcg DOUBLE STRENGTH Inhalation Aerosol WITH OTHER ASTHMA MEDICATION. VANCERIL 84 mcg DOUBLE STRENGTH Inhalation Aerosol WILL NOT PROVIDE IMMEDIATE RELIEF IF YOU ARE HAVING AN ASTHMA ATTACK. Your physician will decide whether other medication is needed should you require immediate relief. If you also use another medicine by inhalation, you should consult your physician for instructions on when to use it in relation to using VANCERIL 84 mcg DOUBLE STRENGTH Inhalation Aerosol. If this is the first time you will be using VANCERIL 84 mcg DOUBLE STRENGTH Inhalation Aerosol, it may take from 1 to 4 weeks before you feel the full benefits.
Dosage: Use only as directed by your physician.
CONTENTS UNDER PRESSURE. Do not puncture. Do not use or store near heat or open flame. Exposure to temperatures above 120°F may cause bursting. Never throw container into fire or incinerator. Keep out of reach of children. Avoid spraying in eyes.
Store at 15°–30°C (59°–86°F). Protect from moisture and unusual temperature fluctuations. Failure to use the product within this temperature range may result in improper dosing. For optimal results, the canister should be at room temperature before use. Shake well before using. If the canister is enclosed in a moisture protective package, the canister must be used within 6 months after removal.
Note: The indented statement below is required by the Federal government's Clean Air Act for all products containing or manufactured with chlorofluorocarbons (CFCs).
This product contains and is manufactured with dichlorodifluoromethane (CFC-12) and contains trichloromonofluoromethane (CFC-11), substances which harm the environment by destroying ozone in the upper atmosphere.
Your physician has determined that this product is likely to help your personal health. USE THIS PRODUCT AS DIRECTED, UNLESS INSTRUCTED TO DO OTHERWISE BY YOUR PHYSICIAN. If you have any questions about alternatives, consult with your physician.
Schering/Key
Kenilworth, NJ 07033 USA

Rev. 8/99 18682141
Shown in Product Identification Guide, page 334

Schwarz Pharma, Inc.
6140 W. Executive Drive
MEQUON, WI 53092

For Medical Information Contact:
Schwarz Pharma, Inc.
Professional Services
(262) 238-9994
(800) 558-5114

CALCIFEROL™ Products
[kal-si 'fur-ol]
CALCIFEROL™ Drops OTC
(ergocalciferol oral solution USP)
8,000 USP Units/mL
CALCIFEROL™ in Oil Injection ℞
(ergocalciferol)
500,000 Units/mL

COLYTE® ℞
(PEG-3350 & ELECTROLYTES for Oral Solution)
For Gastrointestinal Lavage
Rx Only

DESCRIPTION
COLYTE® is a colon lavage preparation provided as water-soluble components for solution. In solution each COLYTE preparation delivers the following, in grams per liter.

Polyethylene Glycol 3350	60.00
Sodium Chloride	1.46
Potassium Chloride	0.745
Sodium Bicarbonate	1.68
Sodium Sulfate	5.68

When dissolved in sufficient water to make 4 liters, the final solution contains 125 mEq/L sodium, 10 mEq/L potassium, 20 mEq/L bicarbonate, 80 mEq/L sulfate, 35 mEq/L chloride and 18 mEq/L polyethylene glycol 3350. The reconstituted solution is isosmotic and has a mildly salty taste. COLYTE is administered orally or via nasogastric tube.

HOW SUPPLIED
COLYTE® is supplied in 4 liter and 18 oz. bottles. Each **4 liter** bottle contains polyethylene glycol 3350 240 g, sodium chloride 5.84 g, potassium chloride 2.98 g, sodium bicarbonate 6.72 g, sodium sulfate (anhydrous) 22.72 g. Each **18 oz.** bottle contains polyethylene glycol 3350 227.10 g, sodium chloride 5.53 g, potassium chloride 2.82 g, sodium bicarbonate 6.36 g, sodium sulfate (anhydrous) 21.50 g. Each preparation is supplied in powdered form, for oral administration as a solution.

COLYTE®	4 liter	NDC 0091-4401-23
	18 oz.	NDC 0091-4401-49

Store powder at controlled room temperature 15°–30°C (59°–86°F).
KEEP RECONSTITUTED SOLUTION REFRIGERATED. USE WITHIN 48 HOURS. DISCARD UNUSED PORTION.
Also available as:

COLYTE®-FLAVORED	4 liter	NDC 0091-4403-05
	18 oz.	NDC 0091-4403-13
Colyte® with Flavor Packs	4 liter	NDC 0091-7036-23

PCL2109B
Rev. 11/98

COLYTE®-FLAVORED ℞
(PEG-3350 & ELECTROLYTES for Oral Solution)
For Gastrointestinal Lavage
Rx Only

DESCRIPTION
COLYTE®-FLAVORED is a colon lavage preparation provided as water-soluble components for solution. In solution each COLYTE-FLAVORED preparation delivers the following, in grams per liter.

Polyethylene Glycol 3350	60.00
Sodium Chloride	1.46
Potassium Chloride	0.745
Sodium Bicarbonate	1.68
Sodium Sulfate	5.68
Flavor ingredients	0.463

When dissolved in sufficient water to make 4 liters, the final solution contains 125 mEq/L sodium, 10 mEq/L potassium, 20 mEq/L bicarbonate, 80 mEq/L sulfate, 35 mEq/L chloride and 18 mEq/L polyethylene glycol 3350. The reconstituted solution is isosmotic and has a mildly salty taste. COLYTE-FLAVORED is administered orally or via nasogastric tube.

HOW SUPPLIED
COLYTE®-FLAVORED is supplied in 4 liter and 18 oz. bottles. Each **4 liter** bottle contains polyethylene glycol 3350 240 g, sodium chloride 5.84 g, potassium chloride 2.98 g, sodium bicarbonate 6.72 g, sodium sulfate (anhydrous) 22.72 g, flavor ingredients 1.85 g. Each **18 oz.** bottle contains polyethylene glycol 3350 227.10 g, sodium chloride 5.53 g, potassium chloride 2.82 g, sodium bicarbonate 6.36 g, sodium sulfate (anhydrous) 21.50 g, flavor ingredients 1.75 g. Each preparation is supplied in powdered form, for oral administration as a solution.

COLYTE®-FLAVORED	4 liter	NDC 0091-4403-05
	18 oz.	NDC 0091-4403-13

Store powder at controlled room temperature 15°–30°C (59°–86°F).
KEEP RECONSTITUTED SOLUTION REFRIGERATED. USE WITHIN 48 HOURS. DISCARD UNUSED PORTION.
Also available as:

COLYTE®	4 liter	NDC 0091-4401-23
	18 oz.	NDC 0091-4401-49
Colyte® with Flavor Packs	4 liter	NDC 0091-7036-23

PCL2107A
Rev. 11/98

COLYTE® WITH FLAVOR PACKS ℞
(PEG-3350 & ELECTROLYTES for Oral Solution
For Gastrointestinal Lavage
Rx Only

DESCRIPTION
Colyte® with Flavor Packs is a colon lavage preparation provided as water-soluble components for solution. In solution this preparation with one Flavor Pack added delivers the following, in grams per liter.

Polyethylene Glycol 3350	60.00
Sodium Chloride	1.46
Potassium Chloride	0.745
Sodium Bicarbonate	1.68
Sodium Sulfate	5.68
Flavor Ingredients	0.805

When dissolved in sufficient water to make 4 liters, the final solution contains 125 mEq/L sodium, 10 mEq/L potassium, 20 mEq/L bicarbonate, 80 mEq/L sulfate, 35 mEq/L chloride and 18 mEq/L polyethylene glycol 3350. The reconstituted solution is isosmotic and has a mild salty taste. *Colyte*® Flavor Packs are available in citrus berry, lemon lime, cherry, and pineapple. This preparation can be used without the *Colyte*® Flavor Packs and is administered orally or via nasogastric tube.
Each Citrus Berry *Colyte*® Flavor Pack (3.22g) contains hydroxypropyl methylcellulose 2910, citrus berry powder, saccharin sodium, colloidal silicon dioxide. Each Lemon Lime *Colyte*® Flavor Pack (3.22g) contains lemon lime NTA powder, hydroxypropyl methylcellulose 2910, Prosweet® Powder Natural, saccharin sodium, colloidal silicon dioxide. Each Cherry *Colyte*® Flavor Pack (3.22g) contains hydroxypropyl methylcellulose 2910, artificial cherry powder, saccharin sodium, colloidal silicon dioxide. Each Pineapple *Colyte*® Flavor Pack (3.22g) contains hydroxypropyl methylcellulose 2910, pineapple flavor powder, Magna Sweet™, saccharin sodium, colloidal silicon dioxide.

CLINICAL PHARMACOLOGY
Colyte® with Flavor Packs cleanses the bowel by induction of diarrhea. The osmotic activity of Polyethylene Glycol 3350, in combination with the electrolyte concentration, results in virtually no net absorption or excretion of ions or water. Accordingly, large volumes may be administered without significant changes in fluid and electrolyte balance.

INDICATIONS AND USAGE
Colyte® with Flavor Packs is indicated for bowel cleansing prior to colonoscopy or barium enema X-ray examination.

CONTRAINDICATIONS
Colyte® with Flavor Packs is contraindicated in patients with ileus, gastric retention, gastrointestinal obstruction, bowel perforation, toxic colitis and toxic megacolon.

WARNINGS
Colyte® Flavor Packs are for use only in combination with the contents of the accompanying 4 liter container. No other additional ingredients (e.g., flavorings) should be added to the solution. Colyte® with Flavor Packs should be used with caution in patients with severe ulcerative colitis.

PRECAUTIONS
General: Patients with impaired gag reflex, unconscious or semiconscious patients and patients prone to regurgitation or aspiration should be observed during the administration of Colyte® with Flavor Packs, especially if it is administered via nasogastric tube.
If gastrointestinal obstruction or perforation is suspected appropriate studies should be performed to rule out these conditions before administration of Colyte® with Flavor Packs.
INFORMATION FOR PATIENTS
Colyte® with Flavor Packs produces a watery stool which cleanses the bowel prior to examination.
For best results, no solid food should be ingested during the 3 to 4 hour period prior to the initiation of Colyte® with Flavor Packs administration. In no case should solid foods be eaten within 2 hours of drinking Colyte® with Flavor Packs.
The rate of administration is 240 mL (8 fl. oz.) every 10 minutes. Rapid drinking of each portion is preferred rather than drinking small amounts continuously.
The first bowel movement should occur approximately one hour after the start of Colyte® with Flavor Packs administration.

Administration of Colyte® with Flavor Packs should be continued until the watery stool is clear and free of solid matter. This normally requires the consumption of approximately 3–4 liters (3–4 quarts), although more or less may be required in some patients. The unused portion should be discarded.

DRUG INTERACTIONS

Oral medication administered within one hour of the start of administration of Colyte® with Flavor Packs may be flushed from the gastrointestinal tract and not absorbed.

CARCINOGENESIS, MUTAGENESIS, IMPAIRMENT OF FERTILITY

Studies to evaluate carcinogenic or mutagenic potential or potential to adversely affect male or female fertility have not been performed.

PREGNANCY

Category C. Animal reproduction studies have not been conducted with Colyte® with Flavor Packs, and it is not known whether Colyte® with Flavor Packs can affect reproductive capacity or harm the fetus when administered to a pregnant patient. Colyte® with Flavor Packs should be given to a pregnant patient only if clearly needed.

PEDIATRIC USE

Safety and effectiveness in pediatric patients have not been established.

ADVERSE REACTIONS

Nausea, abdominal fullness and bloating are the most frequent adverse reactions, occurring in up to 50% of patients. Abdominal cramps, vomiting and anal irritation occur less frequently. These adverse reactions are transient. Isolated cases of urticaria, rhinorrhea and dermatitis have been reported which may represent allergic reactions.

DOSAGE AND ADMINISTRATION

Colyte® with Flavor Packs can be administered orally or by nasogastric tube. Patients should fast at least 3 hours prior to administration. A one hour waiting period after the appearance of clear liquid stool should be allowed prior to examination to complete bowel evacuation. No foods except clear liquids should be permitted prior to examination after Colyte® with Flavor Packs administration.

ORAL: The recommended adult oral dose is 240 mL (8 fl. oz.) every 10 minutes (see INFORMATION FOR PATIENTS). Lavage is complete when fecal discharge is clear. Lavage is usually complete after the ingestion of 3–4 liters.

NASOGASTRIC TUBE: Colyte® with Flavor Packs is administered at a rate of 20–30 mL per minute (1.2–1.8 L/hour).

PREPARATION OF COLYTE® WITH FLAVOR PACKS SOLUTION:

This preparation can be used without the *Colyte*® Flavor Packs.

1. To add flavor, tear open one *Colyte*® Flavor Pack at the indicated marking and pour contents into the bottle BEFORE reconstitution. Discard unused flavor packs.
2. SHAKE WELL to incorporate flavoring into the powder.
3. Add tap water to FILL line. Replace cap tightly and mix or shake well until all ingredients have dissolved. (No other additional ingredients, e.g. flavorings, should be added to the solution.)

Note: If not using *Colyte*® Flavor Packs, omit steps one and two, above.

HOW SUPPLIED

Colyte® with Flavor Packs is supplied in 4 liter bottles with an attached package containing 4 *Colyte*® Flavor Packs; one each of Citrus Berry, Lemon Lime, Cherry and Pineapple. Each 4 liter bottle contains polyethylene glycol 3350 240 g, sodium chloride 5.84 g, potassium chloride 2.98 g, sodium bicarbonate 6.72 g, sodium sulfate (anhydrous) 22.72 g. This preparation is supplied in powdered form, for oral administration as a solution.

Colyte® with Flavor Packs 4 liter NDC 0091-7036-23

Store powder at controlled room temperature 15°–30°C (59°–86°F).

KEEP RECONSTITUTED SOLUTION REFRIGERATED. USE WITHIN 48 HOURS. DISCARD UNUSED PORTION.

Also available as:

COLYTE®	4 liter	NDC 0091-4401-23
	18 oz.	NDC 0091-4401-49
COLYTE® -FLAVORED	4 liter	NDC 0091-4403-05
	18 oz.	NDC 0091-4403-13

PCL3827 Rev. 11/98

Shown in Product Identification Guide, page 334

CORTIFOAM® ℞

(hydrocortisone acetate) 10%
Rectal Foam
Rx Only

DESCRIPTION

CORTIFOAM® (hydrocortisone acetate) 10% Rectal Foam contains hydrocortisone acetate 10% in a base containing propylene glycol, emulsifying wax, polyoxyethylene-10-stearyl ether, cetyl alcohol, methylparaben, propylparaben, trolamine, purified water and inert propellants: isobutane and propane.

Each application delivers approximately 900 mg of foam containing 80 mg of hydrocortisone (90 mg of hydrocortisone acetate).

Molecular weight: Hydrocortisone acetate 404.51

Solubility of hydrocortisone acetate in water: 1 mg/100 mL

Chemical name: Pregn-4-ene-3,20-dione, 21-(acetyloxy)-11, 17-dihydroxy-, (11β)-.

CLINICAL PHARMACOLOGY

CORTIFOAM provides effective topical administration of an anti-inflammatory corticosteroid as adjunctive therapy of ulcerative proctitis.

INDICATIONS AND USAGE

CORTIFOAM is indicated as adjunctive therapy in the topical treatment of ulcerative proctitis of the distal portion of the rectum in patients who cannot retain hydrocortisone or other corticosteroid enemas. Direct observations of methylene blue-containing foam have shown staining about 10 centimeters into the rectum.

CONTRAINDICATIONS

Local contraindications to the use of intrarectal steroids include obstruction, abscess, perforation, peritonitis, fresh intestinal anastomoses, extensive fistulas and sinus tracts. Tuberculosis (active, latent or questionably healed), ocular herpes simplex and acute psychosis are usually considered absolute contraindications to the use of corticosteroids. Relative contraindications include active peptic ulcer, acute glomerulonephritis, myasthenia gravis, osteoporosis, diverticulitis, thrombophlebitis, psychic disturbances, pregnancy, diabetes, hyperthyroidism, acute coronary disease, hypertension, limited cardiac reserve, and local or systemic infections, including fungal or exanthematous diseases. Where these conditions exist, the expected benefits from steroid therapy must be weighed against the risks involved in its use. Pregnancy is a relative contraindication to corticosteroids, particularly during third trimester. If corticosteroids must be administered in pregnancy, watch newborn infant closely for signs of hypoadrenalism, and administer appropriate therapy if needed.

WARNINGS

Do not insert any part of the aerosol container directly into the anus. Contents of the container are under pressure. Do not burn or puncture the aerosol container. Do not store at temperature above 120°F. Because CORTIFOAM is not expelled, systemic hydrocortisone absorption may be greater from CORTIFOAM than from corticosteroid enema formulations. If there is not evidence of clinical or proctologic improvement within two or three weeks after starting CORTIFOAM therapy, or if the patient's condition worsens, discontinue the drug.

Persons who are on drugs which suppress the immune system are more susceptible to infections than healthy individuals. Chickenpox and measles, for example, can have a more serious or even fatal course in non-immune pediatric patients or adults on corticosteroids. In such pediatric patients or adults who have not had these diseases, particular care should be taken to avoid exposure. How the dose, route and duration of corticosteroid administration affects the risk of developing a disseminated infection is not known. The contribution of the underlying disease and/or prior corticosteroid treatment to the risk is also not known. If exposed to chickenpox, prophylaxis with varicella zoster immune globulin (VZIG) may be indicated. If exposed to measles, prophylaxis with pooled intramuscular immunoglobulin (IG) may be indicated. (See the respective package inserts for complete VZIG and IG prescribing information.) If chickenpox develops, treatment with antiviral agents may be considered.

PRECAUTIONS

General

Steroid therapy should be administered with caution in patients with severe ulcerative disease because these patients are predisposed to perforation of the bowel wall. Where surgery is imminent, it is hazardous to wait more than a few days for a satisfactory response to medical treatment. General precautions common to all corticosteroid therapy should be observed during treatment with CORTIFOAM. These include gradual withdrawal of therapy to allow for possible adrenal insufficiency and awareness to possible growth suppression in pediatric patients. Patients should be kept under close observation for, as with all drugs, rare individuals may react unfavorably under certain conditions. If severe reactions or idiosyncrasies occur, steroids should be discontinued immediately and appropriate measures instituted. Do not employ in immediate or early postoperative period following ileorectostomy.

Information for Patients

Persons who are on immunosuppressant doses of corticosteroids should be warned to avoid exposure to chickenpox or measles. Patients should also be advised that if they are exposed, medical advice should be sought without delay.

Pediatric Use

Safety and effectiveness in pediatric patients have not been established. (Please see **WARNINGS** and **ADVERSE REACTIONS** for additional information.)

ADVERSE REACTIONS

Corticosteroid therapy may produce side effects which include moon face, fluid retention, excessive appetite and weight gain, abnormal fat deposits, mental symptoms, hypertrichosis, acne, ecchymosis, increased sweating, pigmentation, dry scaly skin, thinning scalp hair, thrombophlebitis, decreased resistance to infection, negative nitrogen balance with delayed bone and wound healing, menstrual disorders, neuropathy, peptic ulcer, decreased glucose tolerance, hypopotassemia, adrenal insufficiency, necrotizing angiitis, hypertension, pancreatitis and increased intraocular pressure. In pediatric patients, suppression of growth may occur. Increased intracranial pressure may occur and possibly account for headache, insomnia and fatigue. Subcapsular cataracts may result from prolonged usage. Long-term use of all corticosteroids results in catabolic effects characterized by negative protein and calcium balance. Osteoporosis, spontaneous fractures and aseptic necrosis of the hip and humerus may occur as part of this catabolic phenomenon. Where hypopotassemia and other symptoms associated with fluid and electrolyte imbalance call for potassium supplementation and salt poor or salt-free diets, these may be instituted and are compatible with diet requirements for ulcerative proctitis.

DOSAGE AND ADMINISTRATION

Usual dose is one applicatorful once or twice daily for two or three weeks, and every second day thereafter, administered rectally. Directions for use, below and on the carton, describe how to use the aerosol container and applicator. Satisfactory response usually occurs within five to seven days marked by a decrease in symptoms. Symptomatic improvement in ulcerative proctitis should not be used as the sole criterion for evaluating efficacy. Sigmoidoscopy is also recommended to judge dosage adjustment, duration of therapy and rate of improvement.

Directions For Use

1) Shake foam container vigorously for 5–10 seconds before each use. **Do not remove container cap during use of the product. 2)** Hold container upright on a level surface and gently place the tip of the applicator onto the nose of the container cap. CONTAINER MUST BE HELD UPRIGHT TO OBTAIN PROPER FLOW OF MEDICATION. **3)** Gently withdraw applicator plunger past the fill line on the applicator barrel. **4)** To fill applicator barrel, press down slowly on cap flanges and release, pause, and allow foam to enter and expand in applicator barrel. Repeat until foam in the applicator reaches fill line. Remove applicator from container cap. Allow some foam to remain on the applicator tip. **5)** Hold applicator firmly by barrel, making sure thumb and middle finger are positioned securely underneath and resting against barrel wings. Place index finger over the plunger. Gently insert tip into anus. Once in place, push plunger to expel foam, then withdraw applicator. **CAUTION:** Do not insert any part of the aerosol container directly into the anus. Apply to anus only with enclosed applicator. **6)** After each use, applicator parts should be pulled apart for thorough cleaning with warm water. The container cap and underlying tip should also be pulled apart and rinsed to help prevent build-up of foam and possible blockage.

HOW SUPPLIED

CORTIFOAM is supplied in an aerosol container with a special rectal applicator. Each applicator delivers approximately 900 mg of foam containing approximately 80 mg of hydrocortisone as 90 mg of hydrocortisone acetate. When used correctly, the aerosol container will deliver a minimum of 14 applications.

NDC 0091-0695-20 15 g

Store upright at controlled room temperature 15°–30°C (59°–86°F).

DO NOT REFRIGERATE.

PC2080B Rev. 8/99

Shown in Product Identification Guide, page 335

DILATRATE®-SR ℞

[*dī 'lă-trāt*]
(isosorbide dinitrate)
Sustained Release Capsules
40 mg
Rx Only

DESCRIPTION

Isosorbide dinitrate (ISDN) is 1,4:3,6-dianhydro-D-glucitol 2,5 dinitrate, an organic nitrate whose structural formula is

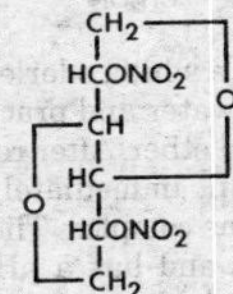

and whose molecular weight is 236.14. The organic nitrates are vasodilators, active on both arteries and veins. Each Di-

Continued on next page

Dilatrate-SR—Cont.

latrate-SR sustained release capsule contains 40 mg of isosorbide dinitrate, in a microdialysis delivery system that causes the active drug to be released over an extended period. Each capsule also contains ethylcellulose, lactose, pharmaceutical glaze, starch, sucrose and talc. The capsule shells contain D&C Red 33, D&C Yellow 10, gelatin and titanium dioxide.

HOW SUPPLIED

Dilatrate®-SR (isosorbide dinitrate) 40 mg Sustained Release Capsules are opaque pink and colorless capsules with white beadlets and are imprinted "Schwarz" and "0920". They are supplied as follows:

Bottles of 100 NDC 0091-0920-01

Store at controlled room temperature 15°–30°C (59°–86°F) in a dry place.

PC2088C Rev. 9/98

EDEX® ℞

[*ē-'deks*]

(alprostadil for injection)
For Intracavernous Use Only
Sterile Powder in Vials
Sterile Powder and Diluent in Cartridges
Rx Only

DESCRIPTION

EDEX (alprostadil for injection) is a sterile, pyrogen-free powder for intracavernous administration after reconstitution with sterile 0.9% sodium chloride. EDEX is lyophilized in single-dose vials containing either 12.45, 24.90 or 49.80 mcg (micrograms) of alprostadil, also known as prostaglandin E_1 (PGE_1), an endogenous substance, in an alfadex (α-cyclodextrin) inclusion complex. Lactose comprises the remainder of the dry powder in each vial. The EDEX vials are supplied in three strengths: 10 mcg vial (12.45 mcg alprostadil, 402.55 mcg α-cyclodextrin, 56.3 mg lactose anhydrous); 20 mcg vial (24.90 mcg alprostadil, 805.10 mcg α-cyclodextrin, 56.3 mg lactose anhydrous); 40 mcg vial (49.80 mcg alprostadil, 1610.2 mcg α-cyclodextrin, 56.3 mg lactose anhydrous).

EDEX is also lyophilized in single-dose, dual-chamber cartridges intended for use with the reusable EDEX injection device. One chamber of the cartridge contains alprostadil, alfadex and lactose as a sterile, pyrogen-free powder. The other chamber contains 1.075 mL of sterile 0.9% sodium chloride. The EDEX cartridges are supplied in three strengths: 10 mcg cartridge (10.75 mcg alprostadil, 347.55 mcg α-cyclodextrin, 51.06 mg lactose); 20 mcg cartridge (21.5 mcg alprostadil, 695.2 mcg α-cyclodextrin, 51.06 mg lactose); 40 mcg cartridge (43.0 mcg alprostadil, 1,390.3 mcg α-cyclodextrin, 51.06 mg lactose). The EDEX injection device is used to reconstitute the sterile powder in one chamber with the sterile 0.9% sodium chloride in the other chamber. After reconstitution, the EDEX injection device is used to administer the intracavernous injection of alprostadil.

The chemical name for alprostadil is (1R,2R,3R)-3-Hydroxy-2-[(E)-(3S)-3-hydroxy-1-octenyl]-5-oxocyclopentane heptanoic acid. The empirical formula is $C_{20}H_{34}O_5$ and the molecular weight is 354.49. The chemical structure is:

The α-cyclodextrin inclusion complex improves the water solubility of alprostadil. The empirical formula of α-cyclodextrin is $C_{36}H_{60}O_{30}$ and the molecular weight is 972.85. The chemical structure is:

Alprostadil alfadex is a white, odorless, hygroscopic powder. It is freely soluble in water and practically insoluble in ethanol, ethyl acetate and ether. After reconstitution, the active ingredient, alprostadil, immediately dissociates from the α-cyclodextrin inclusion complex. The reconstituted solution is clear and colorless and has a pH between 4.0 and 8.0. When the single-dose vials containing either 12.45, 24.90, or 49.80 mcg of alprostadil are reconstituted with 1.2 mL of sterile 0.9% sodium chloride, the deliverable amount of alprostadil in each milliliter is 10, 20, or 40 micrograms, respectively. When the single-dose, dual-chamber cartridge containing either 10.75, 21.5 or 43.0 mcg of alprostadil is placed into the EDEX injection device and reconstituted, the deliverable amount of alprostadil in each milliliter is 10, 20, or 40 micrograms, respectively.

HOW SUPPLIED

EDEX (alprostadil for injection) is supplied as a white, sterile, lyophilized powder in single-dose vials containing either 12.45, 24.90 or 49.80 mcg of alprostadil. When reconstituted with 1.2 mL of sterile 0.9% sodium chloride, the deliverable amount of alprostadil in each milliliter is 10, 20 or 40 micrograms, respectively. The single-dose vials are supplied individually in a package of six or in a kit which also contains a syringe pre-filled with 1.2 mL of sterile 0.9% sodium chloride, one plunger rod, a 1/2 inch 27 gauge needle, a 1/2 inch 30 gauge needle, one alcohol swab for the top of the vial, one alcohol swab for the injection site and tape to secure the kit after use.

EDEX is supplied in the following packages:

Individual Vials

10 mcg	6 Individual Vials	NDC 0091-1010-06
20 mcg	6 Individual Vials	NDC 0091-1020-06
40 mcg	6 Individual Vials	NDC 0091-1040-06

Kits (include one EDEX vial, one pre-filled diluent syringe, two needles and two alcohol swabs)

10 mcg	4 Kits	NDC 0091-1010-44
20 mcg	4 Kits	NDC 0091-1020-44
40 mcg	4 Kits	NDC 0091-1040-44

EDEX is also available in single-dose, dual-chamber cartridges intended for use with the reusable EDEX injection device. One chamber of the cartridge contains 10.75, 21.5 or 43.0 mcg of alprostadil as a white, sterile, lyophilized powder. The other chamber contains 1.075 mL of sterile 0.9% sodium chloride. When the cartridge is placed into the EDEX injection device and reconstituted, the deliverable amount of alprostadil in each milliliter is 10, 20, or 40 micrograms, respectively. EDEX Cartridge Starter Pack contains one reusable EDEX injection device, two single-dose, dual-chamber cartridges, two ½ inch, 29 gauge (0.33 mm x 12.7 mm) needles, and four alcohol swabs. EDEX Cartridge Refill Pack contains two single-dose, dual-chamber cartridges, two ½ inch, 29 gauge (0.33 mm x 12.7 mm) needles, and four alcohol swabs.

The EDEX cartridges are supplied in the following packages:

EDEX Cartridge Starter Pack (includes one injection device, two cartridges, two needles and four alcohol swabs)

10 mcg	1 Starter Pack	NDC 0091-1110-11
20 mcg	1 Starter Pack	NDC 0091-1120-11
40 mcg	1 Starter Pack	NDC 0091-1140-11

EDEX Cartridge Refill Pack (includes two cartridges, two needles and four alcohol swabs)

10 mcg	1 Refill Pack	NDC 0091-1027-22
20 mcg	1 Refill Pack	NDC 0091-1029-22
40 mcg	1 Refill Pack	NDC 0091-1032-22

Store at 25°C (77°F); excursions permitted between 15°–30°C (59°–86°F).

Shown in Product Identification Guide, page 335

EPIFOAM® ℞

topical aerosol
(hydrocortisone acetate 1% and pramoxine hydrochloride 1%)
Rx Only

DESCRIPTION

A topical corticosteroid in an aerosol foam containing hydrocortisone acetate 1% and pramoxine hydrochloride 1% in a base containing: propylene glycol, cetyl alcohol, glyceryl monostearate and PEG 100 stearate blend, laureth-23, polyoxyl-40 stearate, methylparaben, propylparaben, trolamine, hydrochloric acid to adjust pH, purified water, propellants (inert): isobutane and propane.

EPIFOAM® contains a synthetic steroid used as an anti-inflammatory and antipruritic agent, and a local anesthetic.

Hydrocortisone acetate

Molecular weight: 404.51. Solubility of hydrocortisone acetate in water: 1 mg/100 ml. Chemical name: Pregn-4-ene-3,20-dione, 21-(acetyloxy)-11, 17-dihydroxy- (11β).

Pramoxine hydrochloride

Molecular weight: 329.87. Pramoxine hydrochloride is freely soluble in water. Chemical name: Morpholine, 4-[3-(4-butoxyphenoxy) propyl]-, hydrochloride, 4-[3-(*p*-butoxyphenoxy) propyl] morpholine hydrochloride.

HOW SUPPLIED

EPIFOAM® is supplied in 10 g pressurized cans.

10 g (NDC 0091-0740-10)

Store upright at controlled room temperature 15°–30°C (59°–86°F). Do not refrigerate.

PC2202B Rev. 8/98

Shown in Product Identification Guide, page 335

KUTRASE® Capsules ℞

[*qū 'trās*]

Rx Only

DESCRIPTION

KUTRASE® Capsules contain three standardized digestive enzymes: lipase, amylase and protease. The source of the enzymes is pancreatin and they are designed for oral digestive enzyme supplement therapy. Each capsule provides the following enzymatic activity:

lipase	2,400 USP Units
amylase	30,000 USP Units
protease	30,000 USP Units

Each capsule also contains as inactive ingredients: colloidal silicon dioxide, D&C yellow #10, FD&C green #3, FD&C yellow #6, gelatin, sodium lauryl sulfate and titanium dioxide.

HOW SUPPLIED

KUTRASE Capsules are green and white capsules and are imprinted "SCHWARZ" and "4175".

Bottles of 100 capsules NDC 0091-4175-01

Store at controlled room temperature 15°–30°C (59°–86°F). Protect from high humidity.

PC4164 Rev. 10/99

KU-ZYME® Capsules ℞

[*qū ' zīm*]

Rx Only

DESCRIPTION

KU-ZYME® Capsules contain three standardized digestive enzymes: lipase, amylase and protease. The source of the enzymes is pancreatin and they are designed for oral digestive enzyme supplement therapy. Each capsule provides the following enzymatic activity:

lipase	1,200 USP Units
amylase	15,000 USP Units
protease	15,000 USP Units

Each capsule also contains as inactive ingredients: colloidal silicon dioxide, D&C yellow #10, FD&C yellow #6, gelatin, sodium lauryl sulfate and titanium dioxide.

HOW SUPPLIED

KU-ZYME Capsules are yellow and white capsules and are imprinted "SCHWARZ" and "4122".

Bottles of 100 capsules NDC 0091-4122-01

Store at controlled room temperature 15°–30°C (59°–86°F). Protect from high humidity.

PC4166 Rev. 10/99

KU-ZYME® HP Capsules ℞

[*qū ' zīm*]

(pancrelipase capsules USP)
Rx Only

DESCRIPTION

KU-ZYME® HP Capsules (pancrelipase capsules USP) contain standardized lipase, amylase and protease obtained from hog pancreas and are designed for oral digestive enzyme replacement therapy. Each capsule contains:

lipase	8,000 USP Units
protease	30,000 USP Units
amylase	30,000 USP Units

Each capsule also contains as inactive ingredients: gelatin, lactose, magnesium stearate, titanium dioxide and other ingredients.

HOW SUPPLIED

KU-ZYME® HP Capsules (pancrelipase capsules USP) are white opaque capsules and are imprinted "SCHWARZ" and "525."

Bottles of 100 capsules NDC 0091-3525-01

Store at a temperature not exceeding 25°C (77°F). Protect from high humidity.

PC3752 Rev. 9/98

LEVATOL® ℞

[*lev 'a-tol*]

(penbutolol sulfate) 20 mg
TABLETS

DESCRIPTION

Levatol® (penbutolol sulfate) is a synthetic β-receptor antagonist for oral administration. The chemical name of penbutolol sulfate is (S)-1-tert-butylamino-3-(o-cyclopentylphenoxy)-2-propanol sulfate. It is provided as the levorotatory isomer. The empirical formula for penbutolol sulfate is $C_{36}H_{60}N_2O_8S$. Its molecular weight is 680.94. A dose of 20 mg is equivalent to 29.4 μmol. The structural formula is as follows:

$$\left[\text{OCH}_2-\text{CH}(\text{OH})-\text{CH}_2-\overset{+}{\text{N}}\text{H}_2\text{C}(\text{CH}_3)_3 \right]_2 \ SO_4^{--}$$

Penbutolol is a white, odorless, crystalline powder. Levatol is available as tablets for oral administration. Each tablet contains 20 mg of penbutolol sulfate. It also contains corn starch, D&C Yellow No. 10, lactose, magnesium stearate, povidone, silicon dioxide, talc, titanium dioxide, and other inactive ingredients.

HOW SUPPLIED

Levatol® (penbutolol sulfate) 20 mg tablets are yellow, scored, capsule-shaped and engraved "RC22". They are supplied as follows:

Bottles of 100 NDC 0091-4500-15

Store at controlled room temperature 15°–30°C (59°–86°F). Keep tightly closed and protect from light.

CAUTION: Federal law prohibits dispensing without prescription.

PC2077 Rev. 7/95

LEVSIN® PRODUCTS ℞

[lev´sin]

(hyoscyamine sulfate USP)

LEVBID® Extended-Release Tablets

LEVSIN®/SL Tablets

LEVSIN® Tablets

LEVSIN® Elixir

LEVSIN® Drops (Oral Solution)

LEVSIN® Injection

LEVSINEX® TIMECAPS™

Rx Only

DESCRIPTION

LEVSIN® (hyoscyamine sulfate USP) is one of the principal anticholinergic/antispasmodic components of belladonna alkaloids. The empirical formula is $(C_{17}H_{23}NO_3)_2 \cdot H_2SO_4 \cdot 2H_2O$ and the molecular weight is 712.85. Chemically, it is benzeneacetic acid, α-(hydroxymethyl)-,8-methyl-8-azabicyclo [3.2.1.] oct-3-yl ester, [3(S)-endo]-, sulfate (2:1), dihydrate.

LEVBID Extended-Release Tablets contain 0.375 mg of hyoscyamine sulfate in a formulation designed for oral b.i.d. dosage. Each LEVBID Extended-Release Tablet also contains as inactive ingredients: lactose, magnesium stearate, FD&C yellow #6 and other ingredients.

LEVSIN/SL Tablets contain 0.125 mg hyoscyamine sulfate formulated for sublingual administration. However, the tablets may be chewed or taken orally. Each tablet also contains as inactive ingredients: colloidal silicon dioxide, dextrates, flavor, mannitol, and stearic acid.

LEVSIN Tablets contain 0.125 mg hyoscyamine sulfate formulated for oral administration. Each tablet also contains as inactive ingredients: acacia, confectioner's sugar, corn starch, lactose, powdered cellulose and stearic acid.

LEVSIN Elixir contains 0.125 mg hyoscyamine sulfate per 5 mL with 20% alcohol for oral administration. LEVSIN Elixir also contains as inactive ingredients: FD&C Red #40, FD&C Yellow #6, flavor, glycerin, purified water, sorbitol solution and sucrose.

LEVSIN Drops contain 0.125 mg hyoscyamine sulfate per mL with 5% alcohol for oral administration. LEVSIN Drops also contain as inactive ingredients: FD&C Red #40, FD&C Yellow #6, flavor, glycerin, purified water, sodium citrate, sorbitol solution, and sucrose.

LEVSIN Injection is a sterile solution containing 0.5 mg hyoscyamine sulfate per mL. The 1 mL ampuls contain as inactive ingredients: water for injection, pH is adjusted with hydrochloric acid when necessary.

LEVSINEX TIMECAPS contain 0.375 mg hyoscyamine sulfate in an extended-release formulation designed for oral b.i.d. dosage. Each capsule also contains as inactive ingredients: FD&C blue #1, D&C red #28, FD&C red #40, FD&C yellow #6, gelatin, lactose monohydrate, sodium lauryl sulfate, magnesium stearate, silicon dioxide, titanium dioxide and other ingredients.

CLINICAL PHARMACOLOGY

LEVSIN inhibits specifically the actions of acetylcholine on structures innervated by postganglionic cholinergic nerves and on smooth muscles that respond to acetylcholine but lack cholinergic innervation. These peripheral cholinergic receptors are present in the autonomic effector cells of the smooth muscle, the cardiac muscle, the sinoatrial node, the atrioventricular node, and the exocrine glands. At therapeutic doses, it is completely devoid of any action on autonomic ganglia. LEVSIN inhibits gastrointestinal propulsive motility and decreases gastric acid secretion. LEVSIN also controls excessive pharyngeal, tracheal and bronchial secretions.

LEVSIN is absorbed totally and completely by sublingual administration as well as oral administration. Once absorbed, LEVSIN disappears rapidly from the blood and is distributed throughout the entire body. The half-life of LEVSIN is 2 to $3^1/_2$ hours. LEVSIN is partly hydrolyzed to tropic acid and tropine but the majority of the drug is excreted in the urine unchanged within the first 12 hours. Only traces of this drug are found in breast milk. LEVSIN passes the blood brain barrier and the placental barrier.

LEVBID releases 0.375 mg hyoscyamine sulfate at a controlled and predictable rate for 12 hours. The mean peak plasma concentration occurred at 4.20 hours. The mean (±SEM) apparent plasma elimination half-life is 7.47 hours (±0.60). Tablets may not completely disintegrate and may be excreted by some patients.

LEVSINEX TIMECAPS release 0.375 mg hyoscyamine sulfate at a controlled and predictable rate for 12 hours. The mean peak plasma concentration occurred at 4.66 hours. The mean (±SEM) apparent plasma elimination half-life is 6.21 hours (±0.43). Capsule contents may not completely disintegrate and may be excreted by some patients.

INDICATIONS AND USAGE

LEVSIN is effective as adjunctive therapy in the treatment of peptic ulcer. It can also be used to control gastric secretion, visceral spasm, and hypermotility in spastic colitis, spastic bladder, cystitis, pylorospasm, and associated abdominal cramps. May be used in functional intestinal disorders to reduce symptoms such as those seen in mild dysenteries, diverticulitis, and acute enterocolitis. For use as adjunctive therapy in the treatment of irritable bowel syndrome (irritable colon, spastic colon, mucous colitis) and functional gastrointestinal disorders. Also used as adjunctive therapy in the treatment of neurogenic bladder and neurogenic bowel disturbances (including the splenic flexure syndrome and neurogenic colon). Also used in the treatment of infant colic (elixir and drops). LEVSIN is indicated along with morphine or other narcotics in symptomatic relief of biliary and renal colic; as a "drying agent" in the relief of symptoms of acute rhinitis; in the therapy of parkinsonism to reduce rigidity and tremors and to control associated sialorrhea and hyperhidrosis. May be used in the therapy of poisoning by anticholinesterase agents.

Parenterally administered LEVSIN is also effective in reducing gastrointestinal motility to facilitate diagnostic procedures such as endoscopy or hypotonic duodenography. LEVSIN may be used to reduce pain and hypersecretion in pancreatitis. LEVSIN may also be used in certain cases of partial heart block associated with vagal activity.

IN ANESTHESIA:

LEVSIN Injection is indicated as a pre-operative antimuscarinic to reduce salivary, tracheobronchial, and pharyngeal secretions; to reduce the volume and acidity of gastric secretions, and to block cardiac vagal inhibitory reflexes during induction of anesthesia and intubation. LEVSIN protects against the peripheral muscarinic effects such as bradycardia and excessive secretions produced by halogenated hydrocarbons and cholinergic agents such as physostigmine, neostigmine, and pyridostigmine given to reverse the actions of curariform agents.

IN UROLOGY:

LEVSIN Injection may also be used intravenously to improve radiologic visibility of the kidneys. It is also indicated along with morphine or other narcotics in symptomatic relief of biliary and renal colic.

CONTRAINDICATIONS

Glaucoma; obstructive uropathy (for example, bladder neck obstruction due to prostatic hypertrophy); obstructive disease of the gastrointestinal tract (as in achalasia, pyloroduodenal stenosis); paralytic ileus, intestinal atony of elderly or debilitated patients; unstable cardiovascular status in acute hemorrhage; severe ulcerative colitis; toxic megacolon complicating ulcerative colitis; myasthenia gravis.

WARNINGS

In the presence of high environmental temperature, heat prostration can occur with drug use (fever and heat stroke due to decreased sweating). Diarrhea may be an early symptom of incomplete intestinal obstruction, especially in patients with ileostomy or colostomy. In this instance, treatment with this drug would be inappropriate and possibly harmful. Like other anticholinergic agents, LEVSIN may produce drowsiness, dizziness or blurred vision. In this event, the patient should be warned not to engage in activities requiring mental alertness such as operating a motor vehicle or other machinery or to perform hazardous work while taking this drug.

Psychosis has been reported in sensitive individuals given anticholinergic drugs. CNS signs and symptoms inlude confusion, disorientation, short term memory loss, hallucinations, dysarthria, ataxia, coma, euphoria, decreased anxiety, fatigue, insomnia, agitation and mannerisms, and inappropriate affect. These CNS signs and symptoms usually resolve within 12 to 48 hours after discontinuation of the drug.

PRECAUTIONS

General:

Use with caution in patients with: autonomic neuropathy, hyperthyroidism, coronary heart disease, congestive heart failure, cardiac arrhythmias, hypertension and renal disease. Investigate any tachycardia before giving any anticholinergic drug since they may increase the heart rate. Use with caution in patients with hiatal hernia associated with reflux esophagitis.

Information for Patients:

Like other anticholinergic agents, LEVSIN may produce drowsiness, dizziness or blurred vision. In this event, the patient should be warned not to engage in activities requiring mental alertness such as operating a motor vehicle or other machinery or to perform hazardous work while taking this drug.

Use of LEVSIN may decrease sweating resulting in heat prostration, fever or heat stroke; febrile patients or those who may be exposed to elevated environmental temperatures should use caution.

LEVBID Tablets may not completely disintegrate and may be excreted by some patients.

LEVSINEX capsule contents may not completely disintegrate and may be excreted by some patients.

Drug Interactions:

Additive adverse effects resulting from cholinergic blockade may occur when LEVSIN is administered concomitantly with other antimuscarinics, amantadine, haloperidol, phenothiazines, monoamine oxidase (MAO) inhibitors, tricyclic antidepressants or some antihistamines.

Antacids may interfere with the absorption of LEVSIN. Administer LEVSIN before meals; antacids after meals.

Carcinogenesis, Mutagenesis, Impairment of Fertility:

No long-term studies in animals have been performed to determine the carcinogenic, mutagenic or impairment of fertility potential of LEVSIN; however, 40 years of marketing experience with hyoscyamine sulfate shows no demonstrable evidence of a problem.

Pregnancy—Pregnancy Category C:

Animal reproduction studies have not been conducted with LEVSIN. It is also not known whether LEVSIN can cause fetal harm when administered to a pregnant woman or can affect reproduction capacity. LEVSIN should be given to a pregnant woman only if clearly needed.

Nursing Mothers:

LEVSIN is excreted in human milk. Caution should be exercised when LEVSIN is administered to a nursing woman.

ADVERSE REACTIONS

Not all of the following adverse reactions have been reported with hyoscyamine sulfate. The following adverse reactions have been reported for pharmacologically similar drugs with anticholinergic/antispasmodic action. Adverse reactions may include dryness of the mouth; urinary hesitancy and retention; blurred vision; tachycardia; palpitations; mydriasis; cycloplegia; increased ocular tension; loss of taste; headache; nervousness; drowsiness; weakness; dizziness; insomnia; nausea; vomiting; impotence; suppression of lactation; constipation; bloated feeling; allergic reactions or drug idiosyncrasies; urticaria and other dermal manifestations; ataxia; speech disturbance; some degree of mental confusion and/or excitement (especially in elderly persons); and decreased sweating.

OVERDOSAGE

The signs and symptoms of overdose are headache, nausea, vomiting, blurred vision, dilated pupils, hot dry skin, dizziness, dryness of the mouth, difficulty in swallowing and CNS stimulation.

Measures to be taken are immediate lavage of the stomach and injection of physostigmine 0.5 to 2 mg intravenously and repeated as necessary up to a total of 5 mg. Fever may be treated symptomatically (tepid water sponge baths, hypothermic blanket). Excitement to a degree which demands attention may be managed with sodium thiopental 2% solution given slowly intravenously or chloral hydrate (100–200 mL of a 2% solution) by rectal infusion. In the event of progression of the curare-like effect to paralysis of the respiratory muscles, artificial respiration should be instituted and maintained until effective respiratory action returns.

In rats, the LD_{50} for LEVSIN is 375 mg/kg. LEVSIN is dialyzable.

DOSAGE AND ADMINISTRATION

Dosage may be adjusted according to the conditions and severity of symptoms.

LEVBID Extended-Release Tablets: *Adults and pediatric patients 12 years of age and older:* 1 to 2 tablets every 12 hours. Tablets are scored and may be broken to allow for dose titration if needed. Do not crush or chew tablets. Do not exceed 4 tablets in 24 hours.

LEVSIN/SL Tablets: The tablets may be taken sublingually, orally or chewed. *Adults and pediatric patients 12 years of age and older:* 1 to 2 tablets every four hours or as needed. Do not exceed 12 tablets in 24 hours. *Pediatric patients 2 to under 12 years of age:* $^1/_2$ to 1 tablet every four hours or as needed. Do not exceed 6 tablets in 24 hours.

LEVSIN Tablets: *Adults and pediatric patients 12 years of age and older:* 1 to 2 tablets every four hours or as needed. Do not exceed 12 tablets in 24 hours.

Pediatric patients 2 to under 12 years of age: $^1/_2$ to 1 tablet every four hours or as needed. Do not exceed 6 tablets in 24 hours.

LEVSIN Elixir: *Adults and pediatric patients 12 years of age and older:* 1 to 2 teaspoonfuls every four hours or as needed. Do not exceed 12 teaspoonfuls in 24 hours.

Continued on next page

Levsin/Levbid/Levsinex—Cont.

Pediatric patients 2 to under 12 years of age: Please see the following dosage guide based on body weight. The doses may be repeated every four hours or as needed. Do not exceed 6 teaspoonfuls in 24 hours.

Body Weight	Usual Dose
10 kg (22 lb)	1/4 tsp (1.25 mL)
20 kg (44 lb)	1/2 tsp (2.5 mL)
40 kg (88 lb)	3/4 tsp (3.75 mL)
50 kg (110 lb)	1 tsp (5 mL)

LEVSIN Drops: *Adults and pediatric patients 12 years of age and older:* 1 to 2 mL every four hours or as needed. Do not exceed 12 mL in 24 hours.

Pediatric patients 2 to under 12 years of age: 1/4 to 1 mL every four hours or as needed. Do not exceed 6 mL in 24 hours.

Pediatric patients under 2 years of age: The following dosage guide is based upon body weight. The doses may be repeated every four hours or as needed.

Body Weight	Usual Dose	Do Not Exceed in 24 Hours
3.4 kg (7.5 lb)	4 drops	24 drops
5 kg (11 lb)	5 drops	30 drops
7 kg (15 lb)	6 drops	36 drops
10 kg (22 lb)	8 drops	48 drops

LEVSIN Injection: The dose may be administered subcutaneously, intramuscularly, or intravenously without dilution. As with all parenteral drug products, LEVSIN Injection should be inspected visually for particulate matter and discoloration prior to administration whenever solution and container permit.

Gastrointestinal Disorders: The usual adult recommended dose is 0.5 to 1 mL (0.25 to 0.5 mg). Some patients may need only a single dose; others may require administration two, three, or four times a day at four hour intervals.

Diagnostic Procedures: The usual adult recommended dose is 0.5 to 1 mL (0.25 to 0.5 mg) administered intravenously 5 to 10 minutes prior to the diagnostic procedure.

Anesthesia: Adults and pediatric patients over 2 years of age: As a pre-anesthetic medication, the recommended dose is 5 µg (0.005 mg) per kg of body weight. This dose is usually given 30 to 60 minutes prior to the anticipated time of induction of anesthesia or at the time the pre-anesthetic narcotic or sedatives are administered.

LEVSIN Injection may be used during surgery to reduce drug-induced bradycardia. It should be administered intravenously in increments of 0.25 mL and repeated as needed. To achieve reversal of neuromuscular blockade, the recommended dose is 0.2 mg (0.4 mL) LEVSIN Injection for every 1 mg neostigmine or the equivalent dose of physostigmine or pyridostigmine.

LEVSINEX TIMECAPS: *Adults and pediatric patients 12 years of age and older:* 1 to 2 capsules every 12 hours. Dosage may be adjusted to 1 capsule every 8 hours if needed. Do not crush or chew capsules. Do not exceed 4 capsules in 24 hours.

HOW SUPPLIED

LEVBID Extended-Release Tablets (hyoscyamine sulfate, 0.375 mg) are light orange, capsule-shaped, scored tablets. They are coded SP538.

Bottles of 100 tablets	NDC 0091-3538-01
Bottles of 500 tablets	NDC 0091-3538-05

LEVSIN/SL Tablets (hyoscyamine sulfate tablets USP, 0.125 mg) are white, peppermint-flavored, octagonal shaped, scored, and imprinted with "SCHWARZ" on one side and "532" on the other.

Bottles of 100 tablets	NDC 0091-3532-01
Bottles of 500 tablets	NDC 0091-3532-05

LEVSIN Tablets (hyoscyamine sulfate tablets USP, 0.125 mg) are white, scored and imprinted with "SCHWARZ" on one side and "531" on the other.

Bottles of 100 tablets	NDC 0091-3531-01
Bottles of 500 tablets	NDC 0091-3531-05

LEVSIN Elixir (hyoscyamine sulfate elixir USP, 0.125 mg/ 5 mL) is orange colored and flavored and contains 20% alcohol.

Pint (473 mL) bottles	NDC 0091-4532-16

LEVSIN Drops (hyoscyamine sulfate oral solution USP, 0.125 mg/mL) are orange colored and flavored.

15 mL Dropper bottles	NDC 0091-4538-15

LEVSIN Injection (hyoscyamine sulfate injection USP, 0.5 mg/mL) is a clear, colorless and sterile solution.

1 mL ampuls-Box of 5	NDC 0091-1536-05

LEVSINEX TIMECAPS (hyoscyamine sulfate, 0.375 mg) Extended-Release Capsules are brown and white capsules imprinted "SCHWARZ" and "537."

Bottles of 100 capsules	NDC 0091-3537-01
Bottles of 500 capsules	NDC 0091-3537-05

Store at controlled room temperature 15°–30°C (59°–86°F).

Shown in Product Identification Guide, page 335

MONOKET® TABLETS ℞

[*män'-o-ket*]

(isosorbide mononitrate)

Rx Only

DESCRIPTION

MONOKET, an organic nitrate, is a vasodilator with effects on both arteries and veins. The empirical formula is $C_6H_9NO_6$ and the molecular weight is 191.14. The chemical name for MONOKET is 1,4:3,6-Dianhydro-D-glucitol 5-nitrate and the compound has the following structural formula:

MONOKET is available in 10 mg and 20 mg tablets. Each tablet also contains as inactive ingredients: lactose, talc, colloidal silicon dioxide, starch, microcrystalline cellulose and aluminum stearate.

HOW SUPPLIED

MONOKET® (isosorbide mononitrate) 10mg Tablets are white, round, scored and engraved "10" on one side and engraved "SCHWARZ 610" on the other. They are supplied as follows:

Bottles of 100	NDC 0091-3610-01

MONOKET® (isosorbide mononitrate) 20 mg Tablets are white, round, scored and engraved "20" on one side and engraved "SCHWARZ 620" on the other. They are supplied as follows:

Bottles of 100	NDC 0091-3620-01
Bottles of 180	NDC 0091-3620-18
Unit Dose Packages of 100	NDC 0091-3620-11

Store at controlled room temperature 15°–30°C (59°–86°F).
Keep tightly closed.

PC3734 Rev. 9/98

Shown in Product Identification Guide, page 335

NASCOBAL® ℞

[*nās'cobal*]

(Cyanocobalamin, USP)

Gel for Intranasal Administration

Rx Only

DESCRIPTION

Cyanocobalamin is a synthetic form of vitamin B_{12} with equivalent vitamin B_{12} activity. The chemical name is 5,6-dimethyl-benzimidazolyl cyanocobamide. The cobalt content is 4.35%. The molecular formula is $C_{63}H_{88}CoN_{14}O_{14}P$, which corresponds to a molecular weight of 1355.38 and the following structural formula:

Cyanocobalamin occurs as dark red crystals or orthorhombic needles or crystalline red powder. It is very hygroscopic in the anhydrous form, and sparingly to moderately soluble in water (1:80). Its pharmacologic activity is destroyed by heavy metals (iron) and strong oxidizing or reducing agents (vitamin C), but not by autoclaving for short periods of time (15–20 minutes) at 121°C. The vitamin B_{12} coenzymes are very unstable in light.

NASCOBAL® (Cyanocobalamin, USP) Gel for Intranasal Administration is a solution of Cyanocobalamin, USP (vitamin B_{12}) for administration as a metered gel to the nasal mucosa. Each bottle of NASCOBAL® contains 2.3 mL of a 500 mcg/0.1 mL gel solution of cyanocobalamin with methylcellulose, sodium citrate, citric acid, glycerin and benzalkonium chloride in purified water. The gel solution has a pH between 4.5 and 5.5. The gel pump unit must be fully primed (see Patient Instructions) prior to initial use. After initial priming, each metered gel delivers an average of 500 mcg of cyanocobalamin and the 2.3 mL of gel contained in the bottle will deliver 8 doses of NASCOBAL®. If the unit is kept upright, repriming between doses should not be necessary (see Patient Instructions).

CLINICAL PHARMACOLOGY

GENERAL PHARMACOLOGY AND MECHANISM OF ACTION

Vitamin B_{12} is essential to growth, cell reproduction, hematopoiesis, and nucleoprotein and myelin synthesis. Cells characterized by rapid division (e.g., epithelial cells, bone marrow, myeloid cells) appear to have the greatest requirement for vitamin B_{12}. Vitamin B_{12} can be converted to coenzyme B_{12} in tissues, and as such is essential for conversion of methylmalonate to succinate and synthesis of methionine from homocysteine, a reaction which also requires folate. In the absence of coenzyme B_{12}, tetrahydrofolate cannot be regenerated from its inactive storage form, 5-methyl tetrahydrofolate, and a functional folate deficiency occurs. Vitamin B_{12} also may be involved in maintaining sulfhydryl (SH) groups in the reduced form required by many SH-activated enzyme systems. Through these reactions, vitamin B_{12} is associated with fat and carbohydrate metabolism and protein synthesis. Vitamin B_{12} deficiency results in megaloblastic anemia, GI lesions, and neurologic damage that begins with an inability to produce myelin and is followed by gradual degeneration of the axon and nerve head.

Cyanocobalamin is the most stable and widely used form of vitamin B_{12}, and has hematopoietic activity apparently identical to that of the antianemia factor in purified liver extract. The information below, describing the clinical pharmacology of cyanocobalamin, has been derived from studies with injectable vitamin B_{12}.

Vitamin B_{12} is quantitatively and rapidly absorbed from intramuscular and subcutaneous sites of injection. It is bound to plasma proteins and stored in the liver. Vitamin B_{12} is excreted in the bile and undergoes some enterohepatic recycling. Absorbed vitamin B_{12} is transported via specific B_{12} binding proteins, transcobalamin I and II, to the various tissues. The liver is the main organ for vitamin B_{12} storage.

Parenteral (intramuscular) administration of vitamin B_{12} completely reverses the megaloblastic anemia and GI symptoms of vitamin B_{12} deficiency; the degree of improvement in neurologic symptoms depends on the duration and severity of the lesions, although progression of the lesions is immediately arrested.

Gastrointestinal absorption of vitamin B_{12} depends on the presence of sufficient intrinsic factor and calcium ions. Intrinsic factor deficiency causes pernicious anemia, which may be associated with subacute combined degeneration of the spinal cord. Prompt parenteral administration of vitamin B_{12} prevents progression of neurologic damage.

The average diet supplies about 4 to 15 mcg/day of vitamin B_{12} in a protein-bound form that is available for absorption after normal digestion. Vitamin B_{12} is not present in foods of plant origin, but is abundant in foods of animal origin. In people with normal absorption, deficiencies have been reported only in strict vegetarians who consume no products of animal origin (including no milk products or eggs).

Vitamin B_{12} is bound to intrinsic factor during transit through the stomach; separation occurs in the terminal ileum in the presence of calcium, and vitamin B_{12} enters the mucosal cell for absorption. It is then transported by the transcobalamin binding proteins. A small amount (approximately 1% of the total amount ingested) is absorbed by simple diffusion, but this mechanism is adequate only with very large doses. Oral absorption is considered too undependable to rely on in patients with pernicious anemia or other conditions resulting in malabsorption of vitamin B_{12}.

Colchicine, para-aminosalicylic acid, and heavy alcohol intake for longer than 2 weeks may produce malabsorption of vitamin B_{12}.

PHARMACOKINETICS

Absorption

In a bioavailability study in 24 pernicious anemia patients comparing B_{12} nasal gel to intramuscular B_{12}, peak concentrations of B_{12} after intranasal administration were reached in 1–2 hours. The average peak concentration of B_{12} after intranasal administration was 1,414 ± 1,003 pg/mL. The bioavailability of the nasal gel relative to an intramuscular injection was found to be 8.9% (90% confidence intervals 7.1–11.2%).

In pernicious anemia patients, once weekly intranasal dosing with 500 mcg B_{12} resulted in a consistent increase in pre-dose serum B_{12} levels during one month of treatment ($p < 0.003$) above that seen one month after 100 mcg intramuscular dose (Figure).

Distribution

In the blood, B_{12} is bound to transcobalamin II, a specific B-globulin carrier protein, and is distributed and stored primarily in the liver and bone marrow.

Elimination

About 3–8 mcg of B_{12} is secreted into the GI tract daily via the bile; in normal subjects with sufficient intrinsic factor, all but about 1 mcg is re-absorbed. When B_{12} is administered in doses which saturate the binding capacity of plasma proteins and the liver, the unbound B_{12} is rapidly eliminated in the urine. Retention of B_{12} in the body is dose-dependent. About 80–90% of an intramuscular dose up to 50 mcg is retained in the body; this percentage drops to 55% for a 100 mcg dose, and decreases to 15% when a 1000 mcg dose is given.

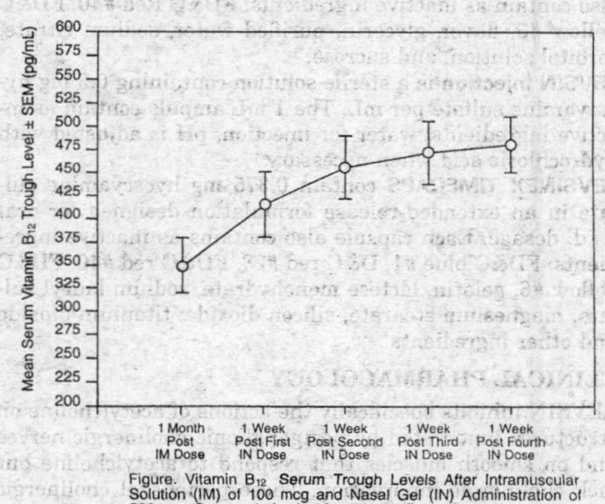

Figure. Vitamin B_{12} Serum Trough Levels After Intramuscular Solution (IM) of 100 mcg and Nasal Gel (IN) Administration of 500 mcg Cyanocobalamin After Weekly Doses.

INDICATIONS AND USAGE

NASCOBAL® (Cyanocobalamin, USP) Gel for Intranasal Administration is indicated for the maintenance of the hematologic status of patients who are in remission following intramuscular vitamin B_{12} therapy for the following conditions:

I. Pernicious anemia. Indicated only in patients who are in hematologic remission with no nervous system involvement.
II. Dietary deficiency of vitamin B_{12} occurring in strict vegetarians. (Isolated vitamin B_{12} deficiency is very rare).
III. Malabsorption of vitamin B_{12} resulting from structural or functional damage to the stomach, where intrinsic factor is secreted or to the ileum, where intrinsic factor facilitates vitamin B_{12} absorption. These conditions include tropical sprue, and nontropical sprue (Idiopathic steatorrhea, gluten-induced enteropathy). Folate deficiency in these patients is usually more severe than vitamin B_{12} deficiency.
IV. Inadequate secretion of intrinsic factor, resulting from lesions that destroy the gastric mucosa (ingestion of corrosives, extensive neoplasia), and a number of conditions associated with a variable degree of gastric atrophy (such as multiple sclerosis, certain endocrine disorders, iron deficiency, and subtotal gastrectomy). Total gastrectomy always produces vitamin B_{12} deficiency. Structural lesions leading to vitamin B_{12} deficiency include regional ileitis, ileal resections, malignancies, etc.
V. Competition for vitamin B_{12} by intestinal parasites or bacteria.
The fish tapeworm (Diphyllobothrium latum) absorbs huge quantities of vitamin B_{12} and infested patients often have associated gastric atrophy. The blind-loop syndrome may produce deficiency of vitamin B_{12} or folate.
VI. Inadequate utilization of vitamin B_{12}. This may occur if antimetabolites for the vitamin are employed in the treatment of neoplasia.

It may be possible to treat the underlying disease by surgical correction of anatomic lesions leading to small bowel bacterial overgrowth, expulsion of fish tapeworm, discontinuation of drugs leading to vitamin malabsorption (see "Drug/Laboratory Test Interactions"), use of a gluten-free diet in nontropical sprue, or administration of antibiotics in tropical sprue. Such measures remove the need for long-term administration of vitamin B_{12}.

Requirements of vitamin B_{12} in excess of normal (due to pregnancy, thyrotoxicosis, hemolytic anemia, hemorrhage, malignancy, hepatic and renal disease) can usually be met with intranasal or oral supplementation.

NASCOBAL® (Cyanocobalamin, USP) Gel for Intranasal Administration has only been tested in patients with vitamin B_{12} malabsorption who have received prior intramuscular cyanocobalamin treatment and are in hematologic remission.

NASCOBAL® (Cyanocobalamin, USP) Gel for Intranasal Administration is not suitable for the vitamin B_{12} absorption test (Schilling Test).

CONTRAINDICATION

Sensitivity to cobalt and/or vitamin B_{12} or any component of the medication is a contraindication.

WARNINGS

Patients with early Leber's disease (hereditary optic nerve atrophy) who were treated with vitamin B_{12} suffered severe and swift optic atrophy.

Hypokalemia and sudden death may occur in severe megaloblastic anemia which is treated intensely with vitamin B_{12}. Folic acid is not a substitute for vitamin B_{12} although it may improve vitamin B_{12}-deficient megaloblastic anemia. Exclusive use of folic acid in treating vitamin B_{12}-deficient megaloblastic anemia could result in progressive and irreversible neurologic damage.

Anaphylactic shock and death have been reported after parenteral vitamin B_{12} administration. No such reactions have been reported in clinical trials with NASCOBAL® (Cyanocobalamin, USP) Gel for Intranasal Administration.

Blunted or impeded therapeutic response to vitamin B_{12} may be due to such conditions as infection, uremia, drugs having bone marrow suppressant properties such as chloramphenicol, and concurrent iron or folic acid deficiency.

PRECAUTIONS

1. GENERAL

An intradermal test dose of parenteral vitamin B_{12} is recommended before NASCOBAL® (Cyanocobalamin, USP) Gel for Intranasal Administration is administered to patients suspected of cyanocobalamin sensitivity. Vitamin B_{12} deficiency that is allowed to progress for longer than three months may produce permanent degenerative lesions of the spinal cord. Doses of folic acid greater than 0.1 mg per day may result in hematologic remission in patients with vitamin B_{12} deficiency. Neurologic manifestations will not be prevented with folic acid, and if not treated with vitamin B_{12}, irreversible damage will result.

Doses of vitamin B_{12} exceeding 10 mcg daily may produce hematologic response in patients with folate deficiency. Indiscriminate administration may mask the true diagnosis. The validity of diagnostic vitamin B_{12} or folic acid blood assays could be compromised by medications, and this should be considered before relying on such tests for therapy.

Vitamin B_{12} is not a substitute for folic acid and since it might improve folic acid deficient megaloblastic anemia, indiscriminate use of vitamin B_{12} could mask the true diagnosis.

Hypokalemia and thrombocytosis could occur upon conversion of severe megaloblastic to normal erythropoiesis with vitamin B_{12} therapy. Therefore, serum potassium levels and the platelet count should be monitored carefully during therapy.

Vitamin B_{12} deficiency may suppress the signs of polycythemia vera. Treatment with vitamin B_{12} may unmask this condition.

If a patient is not properly maintained with NASCOBAL® (Cyanocobalamin, USP) Gel for Intranasal Administration, intramuscular vitamin B_{12} is necessary for adequate treatment of the patient. No single regimen fits all cases, and the status of the patient observed in follow-up is the final criterion for adequacy of therapy.

The effectiveness of NASCOBAL® (Cyanocobalamin, USP) Gel for Intranasal Administration in patients with nasal congestion, allergic rhinitis and upper respiratory infections has not been determined. Therefore, treatment with NASCOBAL® should be deferred until symptoms have subsided.

2. INFORMATION FOR PATIENTS

Patients with pernicious anemia should be instructed that they will require weekly intranasal administration of NASCOBAL® (Cyanocobalamin, USP) Gel for Intranasal Administration for the remainder of their lives. Failure to do so will result in return of the anemia and in development of incapacitating and irreversible damage to the nerves of the spinal cord. Also, patients should be warned about the danger of taking folic acid in place of vitamin B_{12}, because the former may prevent anemia but allow progression of subacute combined degeneration of the spinal cord.

(Hot foods may cause nasal secretions and a resulting loss of medication; therefore, patients should be told to administer NASCOBAL® at least one hour before or one hour after ingestion of hot foods or liquids.)

A vegetarian diet which contains no animal products (including milk products or eggs) does not supply any vitamin B_{12}. Therefore, patients following such a diet should be advised to take NASCOBAL® (Cyanocobalamin, USP) Gel for Intranasal Administration weekly. The need for vitamin B_{12} is increased by pregnancy and lactation. Deficiency has been recognized in infants of vegetarian mothers who were breast fed, even though the mothers had no symptoms of deficiency at the time.

The patient should also understand the importance of returning for follow-up blood tests every 3 to 6 months to confirm adequacy of the therapy. Careful instructions on the actuator assembly, priming of the actuator and nasal administration of NASCOBAL® (Cyanocobalamin, USP) Gel for Intranasal Administration should be given to the patient. Although instructions for patients are supplied with individual bottles, procedures for use should be demonstrated to each patient.

3. LABORATORY TESTS

Hematocrit, reticulocyte count, vitamin B_{12}, folate and iron levels should be obtained prior to treatment. If folate levels are low, folic acid should also be administered. All hematologic parameters should be normal when beginning treatment with NASCOBAL® (Cyanocobalamin, USP) Gel for Intranasal Administration.

Vitamin B_{12} blood levels and peripheral blood counts must be monitored initially at one month after the start of treatment with NASCOBAL®, and then at intervals of 3 to 6 months.

A decline in the serum levels of B_{12} after one month of treatment with B_{12} nasal gel may indicate that the dose may need to be adjusted upward. Patients should be seen one month after each dose adjustment; continued low levels of serum B_{12} may indicate that the patient is not a candidate for this mode of administration.

Patients with pernicious anemia have about 3 times the incidence of carcinoma of the stomach as in the general population, so appropriate tests for this condition should be carried out when indicated.

4. DRUG/LABORATORY TEST INTERACTIONS

Persons taking most antibiotics, methotrexate or pyrimethamine invalidate folic acid and vitamin B_{12} diagnostic blood assays.

Colchicine, para-aminosalicylic acid and heavy alcohol intake for longer than 2 weeks may produce malabsorption of vitamin B_{12}.

5. CARCINOGENESIS, MUTAGENESIS, IMPAIRMENT OF FERTILITY

Long-term studies in animals to evaluate carcinogenic potential have not been done. There is no evidence from long-term use in patients with pernicious anemia that vitamin B_{12} is carcinogenic. Pernicious anemia is associated with an increased incidence of carcinoma of the stomach, but this is believed to be related to the underlying pathology and not to treatment with vitamin B_{12}.

6. PREGNANCY

Pregnancy Category C: Animal reproduction studies have not been conducted with vitamin B_{12}. It is also not known whether vitamin B_{12} can cause fetal harm when administered to a pregnant woman or can affect reproduction capac-

Table. **Adverse Experiences by Body System, Number of Patients and Number of Occurrences by Treatment Following Intramuscular and Intranasal Administration of Cyanocobalamin.**

Body System	Adverse Experience	Number of Patients (Occurrences)	
		Vitamin B_{12} Nasal Gel, 500 mcg N=24	Intramuscular Vitamin B_{12}, 100 mcg N=25
Body as a Whole	Asthenia	1 (1)	4 (4)
	Back Pain	0 (0)	1 (1)
	Generalized Pain	0 (0)	2 (3)
	Headache	1 (2)*	5 (11)
	Infection[a]	3 (4)	3 (3)
Cardiovascular System	Peripheral Vascular Disorder	0 (0)	1 (1)
Digestive System	Dyspepsia	0 (0)	1 (2)
	Glossitis	1 (1)	0 (0)
	Nausea	1 (1)*	1 (1)
	Nausea & Vomiting	0 (0)	1 (1)
	Vomiting	0 (0)	1 (1)
Musculoskeletal System	Arthritis	0 (0)	2 (2)
	Myalgia	0 (0)	1 (1)
Nervous System	Abnormal Gait	0 (0)	1 (1)
	Anxiety	0 (0)	1 (1)*
	Dizziness	0 (0)	3 (3)
	Hypoesthesia	0 (0)	1 (1)
	Incoordination	0 (0)	1 (2)*
	Nervousness	0 (0)	1 (3)*
	Paresthesia	1 (1)	1 (1)
Respiratory System	Dyspnea	0 (0)	1 (1)
	Rhinitis	1 (1)*	2 (2)

[a] Sore throat, common cold
* There may be a possible relationship between these adverse experiences and the study drugs. These adverse experiences could have also been produced by the patient's clinical state or other concomitant therapy.

Continued on next page

Nascobal—Cont.

ity. Adequate and well-controlled studies have not been done in pregnant women. However, vitamin B_{12} is an essential vitamin and requirements are increased during pregnancy. Amounts of vitamin B_{12} that are recommended by the Food and Nutrition Board, National Academy of Science-National Research Council for pregnant women should be consumed during pregnancy.

7. NURSING MOTHERS

Vitamin B_{12} appears in the milk of nursing mothers in concentrations which approximate the mother's vitamin B_{12} blood level. Amounts of vitamin B_{12} that are recommended by the Food and Nutrition Board, National Academy of Science-National Research Council for lactating women should be consumed during lactation.

8. PEDIATRIC USE

Intake in pediatric patients should be in the amount recommended by the Food and Nutrition Board, National Academy of Science-National Research Council.

ADVERSE REACTIONS

The incidence of adverse experiences described in the Table below are based on data from a short-term clinical trial in vitamin B_{12} deficient patients in hematologic remission receiving NASCOBAL® (Cyanocobalamin, USP) Gel for Intranasal Administration (N=24) and intramuscular vitamin B_{12} (N=25).

[See table at top of previous page]

The intensity of the reported adverse experiences following the administration of NASCOBAL® (Cyanocobalamin, USP) Gel for Intranasal Administration and intramuscular vitamin B_{12} were generally mild. One patient reported severe headache following intramuscular dosing. Similarly, a few adverse experiences of moderate intensity were reported following intramuscular dosing (two headaches and rhinitis; one dyspepsia, arthritis, and dizziness), and dosing with NASCOBAL® (Cyanocobalamin, USP) Gel for Intranasal Administration (one headache, infection, and paresthesia).

The majority of the reported adverse experiences following dosing with NASCOBAL® (Cyanocobalamin, USP) Gel for Intranasal Administration and intramuscular vitamin B_{12} were judged to be intercurrent events. For the other reported adverse experiences, the relationship to study drug was judged as "possible" or "remote". Of the adverse experiences judged to be of "possible" relationship to the study drug, anxiety, incoordination, and nervousness were reported following intramuscular vitamin B_{12} and headache, nausea, and rhinitis were reported following dosing with NASCOBAL® (Cyanocobalamin, USP) Gel for Intranasal Administration.

The following adverse reactions have been reported with parenteral vitamin B_{12}:

Generalized:	Anaphylactic shock and death (See Warnings and Precautions).
Cardiovascular:	Pulmonary edema and congestive heart failure early in treatment; peripheral vascular thrombosis.
Hematological:	Polycythemia vera.
Gastrointestinal:	Mild transient diarrhea.
Dermatological:	Itching; transitory exanthema.
Miscellaneous:	Feeling of swelling of the entire body.

OVERDOSAGE

No overdosage has been reported with NASCOBAL® (Cyanocobalamin, USP) Gel for Intranasal Administration or parenteral vitamin B_{12}.

DOSAGE AND ADMINISTRATION

The recommended initial dose of NASCOBAL® (Cyanocobalamin, USP) Gel for Intranasal Administration in patients with vitamin B_{12} malabsorption who are in remission following injectable vitamin B_{12} therapy is 500 mcg administered intranasally once weekly. Patients should be in hematologic remission before treatment with NASCOBAL® (Cyanocobalamin, USP) Gel for Intranasal Administration. See LABORATORY TESTS for monitoring B_{12} levels and adjustment of dosage.

HOW SUPPLIED

NASCOBAL® (Cyanocobalamin, USP) Gel for Intranasal Administration is available as a metered dose gel in 5 mL glass bottles containing 2.3 mL of gel. It is available in a dosage strength of 500 mcg per actuation (0.1 mL/actuation). A screw-on actuator is provided. This actuator, following priming, will deliver 0.1 mL of the gel. NASCOBAL® (Cyanocobalamin, USP) Gel for Intranasal Administration is provided in a sealed prescription vial containing a metered dose nasal gel actuator with dust cover, a bottle of nasal gel solution, and a patient instruction leaflet. One bottle will deliver 8 doses (NDC 0091-7033-13).

PHARMACIST ASSEMBLY INSTRUCTIONS FOR NASCOBAL® (CYANOCOBALAMIN, USP) GEL FOR INTRANASAL ADMINISTRATION

The pharmacist should assemble NASCOBAL® (Cyanocobalamin, USP) Gel for Intranasal Administration prior to dispensing to the patient, according to the following instructions:

1. Break the protective seal, open the prescription vial, and remove the gel actuator and gel solution bottle.
2. Assemble NASCOBAL® by first unscrewing the white cap from the gel solution bottle and screwing the actuator unit tightly onto the bottle. Make sure the clear dust cover is on the pump unit.
3. Return the NASCOBAL® bottle to the prescription vial for dispensing to the patient.

STORAGE CONDITIONS

Protect from light. Keep covered in prescription vial until ready to use. Store upright at controlled room temperature 15°C to 30°C (59°F to 86°F). Protect from freezing.

PC3137B Rev. 2/99

Shown in Product Identification Guide, page 335

NIFEREX® TABLETS/ELIXIR OTC

[ni 'fer "ex]

(polysaccharide-iron complex, as cell-contracted akaganéite)

DESCRIPTION

NIFEREX Film Coated Tablets contain 50 mg elemental iron. Each 5 mL (teaspoonful) NIFEREX Elixir contains 100 mg elemental iron.

Each tablet also contains as inactive ingredients: Castor Oil, Hydroxypropyl Cellulose, FD&C Blue #1 Aluminum Lake, FD&C Red #40 Aluminum Lake, FD&C Yellow #6 Aluminum Lake, Hydroxypropyl Methylcellulose, Lactose, Magnesium Stearate, Microcrystalline Cellulose, Pharmaceutical Glaze, Polyethylene Glycol, Povidone, Propylene Glycol, Sodium Starch Glycolate, Titanium Dioxide.

The elixir also contains as inactive ingredients: Alcohol 10%, Flavor, Hydrochloric Acid, Purified Water, Sorbitol. May also contain: Sodium Hydroxide.

INDICATIONS AND USAGE

For treatment of uncomplicated iron deficiency anemias.

WARNINGS

WARNING: Accidental overdose of iron-containing products is a leading cause of fatal poisoning in children under 6. Keep this product out of reach of children. In case of accidental overdose, call a doctor or poison control center immediately.

DOSAGE AND ADMINISTRATION

Adults: 1 or 2 tablets twice daily, *or* 1 or 2 teaspoonfuls elixir daily. *Pediatric patients age 6 and older:* 1 or 2 tablets daily, or 1 teaspoonful elixir daily; *under 6 years of age,* as directed by a physician.

HOW SUPPLIED

NIFEREX Tablets Unit Dose 100 NDC 0131-2200-86
NIFEREX Elixir Bottles of 8 ounces NDC 0131-5066-68
Store at controlled room temperature 15°–30°C (59°–86°F).

NIFEREX®-150 CAPSULES OTC

[ni ' fer " ex]

(polysaccharide-iron complex, as cell-contracted akaganéite)

DESCRIPTION

Each bead–filled NIFEREX-150 Capsule contains 150 mg elemental iron as polysaccharide-iron complex, as cell–contracted akaganéite.

Each capsule also contains as inactive ingredients: D&C Red #7, D&C Red #28, D&C Yellow #10, FD&C Blue #1, FD&C Red #40, FD&C Yellow #6, Gelatin, Hydrogenated Castor Oil, Pharmaceutical Glaze, Povidone, Sodium Lauryl Sulfate, Starch, Sucrose, Titanium Dioxide. May contain: Silicon Dioxide.

INDICATIONS AND USAGE

For treatment of uncomplicated iron deficiency anemias.

WARNINGS

WARNING: Accidental overdose of iron-containing products is a leading cause of fatal poisoning in children under 6. Keep this product out of reach of children. In case of accidental overdose, call a doctor or poison control center immediately.

DOSAGE AND ADMINISTRATION

Adults: 1 or 2 capsules daily.

HOW SUPPLIED

NIFEREX-150 Capsules are orange and clear capsules containing brown beads. The capsules are imprinted "SP" and "4220". They are supplied as follows:

Unit Dose 100 NDC 0131-4220-09
Store at controlled room temperature 15°–30°C (59°–86°F).
CR2912B 3/99

Shown in Product Identification Guide, page 335

NIFEREX®-150 FORTE CAPSULES ℞

[ni 'fer "ex for 'ta]

Rx Only

DESCRIPTION

Each bead-filled capsule for oral administration contains:

Iron (elemental) .... 150 mg
(polysaccharide-iron complex, as cell-contracted akaganéite)
Folic Acid .... 1 mg
Vitamin B_{12} (cyanocobalamin) .... 25 mcg

Each capsule also contains the following inactive ingredients: corn starch, D&C Red #7, D&C Red #28, FD&C Blue #1, FD&C Red #40, FD&C Yellow #6, gelatin, hydrogenated castor oil, pharmaceutical glaze, povidone, sodium lauryl sulfate, sucrose, and titanium dioxide. It may contain: silicon dioxide.

NIFEREX® (polysaccharide-iron complex, as cell-contracted akaganéite) is the product of ferric iron complexed to a low molecular weight polysaccharide. This polysaccharide is produced by the extensive hydrolysis of starch. NIFEREX® is a dark brown powder which dissolves in water to form a very dark brown solution. It is virtually tasteless and odorless. Because it is an organic complex, it contains no free ions.

CLINICAL PHARMACOLOGY

Iron is an essential component in the formation of hemoglobin. Adequate amounts of iron are necessary for effective erythropoiesis. Iron also serves as a cofactor of several essential enzymes, including cytochromes that are involved in electron transport. A radioisotope tracer study in man demonstrated that absorption of NIFEREX® Elixir is comparable to ferrous sulfate elixir. Clinical studies demonstrate that NIFEREX® produces good hematopoietic response as shown by increases in hemoglobin and hematocrit in pediatric and elderly patients. NIFEREX® is effective in maintaining the hematopoietic status in end-stage renal disease patients receiving epoetin alfa therapy.

Folic acid is required for nucleoprotein synthesis and the maintenance of normal erythropoiesis. Folic acid is converted in the liver and plasma to its metabolically active form, tetrahydrofolic acid, by dihydrofolate reductase.

Vitamin B_{12} is required for the maintenance of normal erythropoiesis, nucleoprotein and myelin synthesis, cell reproduction and normal growth. Intrinsic factor, a glycoprotein secreted by the gastric mucosa, is required for active absorption of Vitamin B_{12} from the gastrointestinal tract.

INDICATIONS AND USAGE

NIFEREX®-150 FORTE is indicated for the prevention and treatment of iron deficiency anemia and/or nutritional megaloblastic anemias.

CONTRAINDICATIONS

NIFEREX®-150 FORTE is contraindicated in patients with a known hypersensitivity to any of the components of this product. Hemochromatosis and hemosiderosis are contraindications to iron therapy.

WARNINGS

WARNING: Accidental overdose of iron-containing products is a leading cause of fatal poisoning in children under 6. Keep this product out of reach of children. In case of accidental overdose, call a doctor or poison control center immediately.

Folic acid alone is improper therapy in the treatment of pernicious anemia and other megaloblastic anemias where Vitamin B_{12} is deficient.

PRECAUTIONS

General:

The type of anemia and the underlying cause or causes should be determined before starting therapy with NIFEREX®-150 FORTE. Since the anemia may be a result of a systemic disturbance, such as recurrent blood loss, the underlying cause or causes should be corrected, if possible. Folic acid in doses above 0.1 mg daily may obscure pernicious anemia in that hematologic remission can occur while neurological manifestations remain progressive.

Information for Patients:

As with all oral iron preparations, NIFEREX®-150 FORTE should be stored out of the reach of children to guard against accidental iron poisoning. Patients should not exceed the recommended dosage unless directed by the physician. Patients should be informed that iron therapy can cause black or dark stools.

ADVERSE REACTIONS

Adverse reactions with iron therapy may include constipation, diarrhea, nausea, vomiting, dark stools and abdominal pain. Adverse reactions with iron therapy are usually transient. Allergic sensitization has been reported following both oral and parenteral administration of folic acid.

OVERDOSAGE

ACCIDENTAL OVERDOSE OF IRON-CONTAINING PRODUCTS IS A LEADING CAUSE OF FATAL POISONING IN CHILDREN UNDER 6. KEEP THIS PRODUCT OUT OF REACH OF CHILDREN. IN CASE OF ACCIDENTAL OVERDOSE, CALL A DOCTOR OR POISON CONTROL CENTER IMMEDIATELY.

The clinical course of acute iron overdosage can be variable. Initial symptoms may include abdominal pain, nausea, vomiting, diarrhea, tarry stools, melena, hematemesis, hypotension, tachycardia, metabolic acidosis, hyperglycemia, dehydration, drowsiness, pallor, cyanosis, lassitude, seizures, shock and coma.

The oral LD_{50} of polysaccharide-iron complex was estimated to be greater than 5000 mg iron/kg in the rat. Chronic toxicity studies in rats and dogs administered polysaccharide-iron complex showed that a daily dosage of 250 mg iron/kg for three months had no adverse effects.

DOSAGE AND ADMINISTRATION

Adults: 1 capsule daily or as directed by a physician.

HOW SUPPLIED

NIFEREX®-150 FORTE Capsules are red and clear capsules containing brown beads. The capsules are imprinted "SP" and "4330". They are supplied as follows:

Unit Dose 100 NDC 0131-4330-86

Store at controlled room temperature 15°–30°C (59°–86°F).

PC2621C Rev. 7/99

Shown in Product Identification Guide, page 335

NIFEREX®-PN TABLETS ℞

[ni 'fer "ex]

Rx Only

DESCRIPTION

NIFEREX®-PN Tablets contain ingredients of the following classes: vitamins and minerals. Each blue, film-coated tablet for oral administration contains:

Iron (elemental)	60 mg
(polysaccharide-iron complex, as cell-contracted akaganéite)	
Folic Acid	1 mg
Vitamin C (as sodium ascorbate)	50 mg
Vitamin B_{12} (cyanocobalamin)	3 mcg
Vitamin A	4000 IU
Vitamin D	400 IU
Vitamin B_1 (as thiamine mononitrate)	2.43 mg
Vitamin B_2 (riboflavin)	3 mg
Vitamin B_6 (as pyridoxine hydrochloride)	1.64 mg
Niacinamide	10 mg
Calcium (as calcium carbonate)	125 mg
Zinc (as zinc sulfate)	18 mg

Each tablet also contains the following inactive ingredients: castor oil, corn starch, FD&C Blue #1 (Lake), gelatin, hydrogenated vegetable oil, hydroxypropyl cellulose, hydroxypropyl methylcellulose, magnesium stearate, microcrystalline cellulose, pharmaceutical glaze, polyethylene glycol, povidone, propylene glycol and titanium dioxide.

NIFEREX® (polysaccharide-iron complex, as cell-contracted akaganéite) is the product of ferric iron complexed to a low molecular weight polysaccharide. This polysaccharide is produced by the extensive hydrolysis of starch. NIFEREX® is a dark brown powder which dissolves in water to form a very dark brown solution. It is virtually tasteless and odorless. Because it is an organic complex, it contains no free ions.

CLINICAL PHARMACOLOGY

This product is formulated to meet the vitamin and mineral needs of the pregnant or lactating patient with special consideration given to adequate amounts of the hematopoietic factors: iron, folic acid and cyanocobalamin. Calcium is included in the formula to help supply the increased requirements of this mineral. Sixty (60) mg of elemental iron is available in the form of NIFEREX® (polysaccharide-iron complex, as cell–contracted akaganéite). A radioisotope tracer study in man demonstrated that absorption of NIFEREX® Elixir is comparable to that of ferrous sulfate elixir. In addition, folic acid and cyanocobalamin are included to prevent or treat pregnancy-related megaloblastic anemia.

INDICATIONS AND USAGE

NIFEREX®-PN is indicated for the prevention and/or treatment of dietary vitamin and mineral deficiencies associated with pregnancy and lactation.

CONTRAINDICATIONS

NIFEREX®-PN is contraindicated in patients with a known hypersensitivity to any of the components of this product. Hemochromatosis and hemosiderosis are contraindications to iron therapy.

WARNINGS

WARNING: Accidental overdose of iron-containing products is a leading cause of fatal poisoning in children under 6. Keep this product out of reach of children. In case of accidental overdose, call a doctor or poison control center immediately.

Folic acid alone is improper therapy in the treatment of pernicious anemia and other megaloblastic anemias where Vitamin B_{12} is deficient.

PRECAUTIONS

General:

Folic acid in doses above 0.1 mg daily may obscure pernicious anemia, in that hematologic remission can occur while neurological manifestations remain progressive. Vitamin A, in high doses, may be associated with birth defects.

Information for Patients:

As with all oral iron preparations, NIFEREX®-PN should be stored out of the reach of children to guard against accidental iron poisoning. Patients should not exceed the recommended dosage unless directed by the physician. Patients should be informed that iron therapy can cause black or dark stools.

ADVERSE REACTIONS

Adverse reactions with iron therapy may include constipation, diarrhea, nausea, vomiting, dark stools and abdominal pain. Adverse reactions with iron therapy are usually transient. Allergic sensitization has been reported following both oral and parenteral administration of folic acid.

OVERDOSAGE

ACCIDENTAL OVERDOSE OF IRON-CONTAINING PRODUCTS IS A LEADING CAUSE OF FATAL POISONING IN CHILDREN UNDER 6. KEEP THIS PRODUCT OUT OF REACH OF CHILDREN. IN CASE OF ACCIDENTAL OVERDOSE, CALL A DOCTOR OR POISON CONTROL CENTER IMMEDIATELY.

The clinical course of acute iron overdosage can be variable. Initial symptoms may include abdominal pain, nausea, vomiting, diarrhea, tarry stools, melena, hematemesis, hypotension, tachycardia, metabolic acidosis, hyperglycemia, dehydration, drowsiness, pallor, cyanosis, lassitude, seizures, shock and coma.

The oral LD_{50} of polysaccharide-iron complex was estimated to be greater than 5000 mg iron/kg in the rat. Chronic toxicity studies in rats and dogs administered polysaccharide-iron complex showed that a daily dosage of 250 mg iron/kg for three months had no adverse effects.

DOSAGE AND ADMINISTRATION

Adults: 1 tablet daily or as directed by a physician.

HOW SUPPLIED

NIFEREX®-PN Tablets are blue, oval, film-coated tablets debossed with "131/05" on one side and "SP2209" on the other. They are supplied as follows:

Unit Dose 100 NDC 0131-2209-09

Store at controlled room temperature 15°–30°C (59°–86°F).

PC2622C Rev. 5/98

Shown in Product Identification Guide, page 335

NIFEREX®-PN FORTE TABLETS ℞

[ni 'fer "ex]

Rx Only

DESCRIPTION

NIFEREX®-PN FORTE Tablets contain ingredients of the following classes: vitamins and minerals. Each white, film-coated tablet for oral administration contains:

Iron (elemental)	60 mg
(polysaccharide-iron complex, as cell-contracted akaganéite)	
Vitamin A	5000 IU
Vitamin D	400 IU
Vitamin E (as dl-alpha-tocopheryl acetate)	30 IU
Vitamin C (ascorbic acid)	80 mg
Folic acid	1 mg
Vitamin B_1 (as thiamine mononitrate)	3 mg
Vitamin B_2 (riboflavin)	3.4 mg
Vitamin B_6 (as pyridoxine hydrochloride)	4 mg
Niacinamide	20 mg
Vitamin B_{12} (cyanocobalamin)	12 mcg
Calcium (as calcium carbonate)	250 mg
Iodine (as potassium iodide)	200 mcg
Magnesium (as magnesium oxide)	10 mg
Copper (as cupric oxide)	2 mg
Zinc (as zinc sulfate)	25 mg

Each tablet also contains the following inactive ingredients: castor oil, corn starch, ethyl cellulose, flavor, gelatin, hydrogenated vegetable oil, hydroxypropyl cellulose, hydroxypropyl methylcellulose, magnesium stearate, microcrystalline cellulose, pharmaceutical glaze, polyethylene glycol, povidone, propylene glycol, silicon dioxide, sodium benzoate, sorbic acid and titanium dioxide.

NIFEREX® (polysaccharide-iron complex, as cell-contracted akaganéite) is the product of ferric iron complexed to a low molecular weight polysaccharide. This polysaccharide is produced by the extensive hydrolysis of starch. NIFEREX® is a dark brown powder which dissolves in water to form a very dark brown solution. It is virtually tasteless and odorless. Because it is an organic complex, it contains no free ions.

CLINICAL PHARMACOLOGY

This product is formulated to meet the vitamin and mineral needs of the pregnant or lactating patient with special consideration given to adequate amounts of the hematopoietic factors: iron, folic acid and cyanocobalamin. Calcium is included in the formula to help supply the increased requirements of this mineral. Sixty (60) mg of elemental iron is available in the form of NIFEREX® (polysaccharide-iron complex, as cell–contracted akaganéite). A radioisotope tracer study in man demonstrated that absorption of NIFEREX® Elixir is comparable to ferrous sulfate elixir. In addition, folic acid and cyanocobalamin are included to prevent or treat pregnancy-related megaloblastic anemia.

INDICATIONS AND USAGE

NIFEREX®-PN FORTE is indicated for the prevention and/or treatment of dietary vitamin and mineral deficiencies associated with pregnancy and lactation.

CONTRAINDICATIONS

NIFEREX®-PN FORTE is contraindicated in patients with a known hypersensitivity to any of the components of this product. Hemochromatosis and hemosiderosis are contraindications to iron therapy.

WARNINGS

WARNING: Accidental overdose of iron-containing products is a leading cause of fatal poisoning in children under 6. Keep this product out of reach of children. In case of accidental overdose, call a doctor or poison control center immediately.

Folic acid alone is improper therapy in the treatment of pernicious anemia and other megaloblastic anemias where Vitamin B_{12} is deficient.

PRECAUTIONS

General:

Folic acid in doses above 0.1 mg daily may obscure pernicious anemia in that hematologic remission can occur while neurological manifestations remain progressive. Vitamin A, in high doses, may be associated with birth defects.

Information for Patients:

As with all oral iron preparations, NIFEREX®-PN FORTE should be stored out of the reach of children to guard against accidental poisoning. Patients should not exceed the recommended dosage unless directed by the physician. Patients should be informed that iron therapy can cause black or dark stools.

ADVERSE REACTIONS

Adverse reactions with iron therapy may include constipation, diarrhea, nausea, vomiting, dark stools and abdominal pain. Adverse reactions with iron therapy are usually transient. Allergic sensitization has been reported following both oral and parenteral administration of folic acid.

OVERDOSAGE

ACCIDENTAL OVERDOSE OF IRON-CONTAINING PRODUCTS IS A LEADING CAUSE OF FATAL POISONING IN CHILDREN UNDER 6. KEEP THIS PRODUCT OUT OF REACH OF CHILDREN. IN CASE OF ACCIDENTAL OVERDOSE, CALL A DOCTOR OR POISON CONTROL CENTER IMMEDIATELY.

The clinical course of acute iron overdosage can be variable. Initial symptoms may include abdominal pain, nausea, vomiting, diarrhea, tarry stools, melena, hematemesis, hypotension, tachycardia, metabolic acidosis, hyperglycemia, dehydration, drowsiness, pallor, cyanosis, lassitude, seizures, shock and coma.

The oral LD_{50} of polysaccharide-iron complex was estimated to be greater than 5000 mg iron/kg in the rat. Chronic toxicity studies in rats and dogs administered polysaccharide-iron complex showed that a daily dosage of 250 mg iron/kg for three months had no adverse effects.

DOSAGE AND ADMINISTRATION

Adults: 1 tablet daily or as directed by a physician.

HOW SUPPLIED

NIFEREX®-PN FORTE Tablets are white, capsule shaped, scored, film-coated tablets debossed with "SP2309" on the unscored side and 1/0 on the scored side. They are supplied as follows:

Unit Dose 100 NDC 0131-2309-09

Store at controlled room temperature 15°–30°C (59°–86°F).

PC2623C Rev. 5/98

Shown in Product Identification Guide, page 335

PROCTOCREAM®•HC 2.5% ℞

(hydrocortisone cream USP, 2.5%)

[topical]

Rx Only

DESCRIPTION

proctoCream®•HC 2.5% contains Hydrocortisone [Pregn-4-ene-3, 20-dione, 11, 17,21-trihydroxy-, (11β)-] with the molecular formula $C_{21}H_{30}O_5$ and a molecular weight of 362.47, CAS 50-23-7. Each gram for topical administration contains: 25 mg of hydrocortisone in a base of glyceryl monostearate, polyoxyl 40 stearate, glycerin, paraffin, stearyl alcohol, isopropyl palmitate, sorbitan monostearate, benzyl alcohol, potassium sorbate, lactic acid, and purified water.

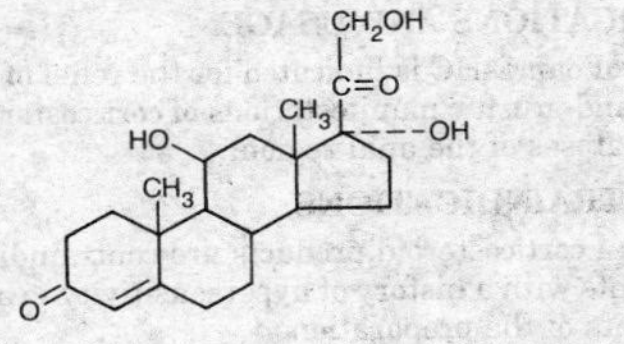

HOW SUPPLIED

proctoCream®•HC 2.5% (hydrocortisone cream USP, 2.5%) is supplied in 30 gram tubes.

30 g NDC 0091-4640-24

Store at controlled room temperature 15°-30°C (59°-86°F).

PC2178A Rev. 3/99

Shown in Product Identification Guide, page 335

PROCTOFOAM®–HC ℞

(hydrocortisone acetate 1%
and pramoxine hydrochloride 1%)
TOPICAL AEROSOL
Rx Only

DESCRIPTION

ProctoFoam®-HC (hydrocortisone acetate 1% and pramoxine hydrochloride 1%) is a topical aerosol foam for anal use

Continued on next page

Proctofoam-HC—Cont.

containing hydrocortisone acetate 1% and pramoxine hydrochloride 1% in a hydrophilic base containing cetyl alcohol, emulsifying wax, methylparaben, polyoxyethylene-10 stearyl ether, propylene glycol, propylparaben, purified water, trolamine, and inert propellants: isobutane and propane.
ProctoFoam®-HC contains a synthetic corticosteroid used as an anti-inflammatory/antipruritic agent and a local anesthetic.
Hydrocortisone acetate
Molecular weight: 404.51. Solubility of hydrocortisone acetate in water: 1mg/100mL.
Chemical name: Pregn-4-ene-3,20-dione, 21-(acetyloxy)-11, 17-dihydroxy-,(11β)-.

Pramoxine hydrochloride
Molecular weight: 329.87. Pramoxine hydrochloride is freely soluble in water.
Chemical name: Morpholine, 4-[3-(4-butoxyphenoxy) propyl]-, hydrochloride.

$CH_3CH_2CH_2CH_2O$—⟨phenyl⟩—$OCH_2CH_2CH_2N$⟨morpholine⟩ • HCl

CLINICAL PHARMACOLOGY

Topical corticosteroids share anti-inflammatory, antipruritic and vasoconstrictive actions.
The mechanism of anti-inflammatory activity of the topical corticosteroids is unclear. Various laboratory methods, including vasoconstrictor assays, are used to compare and predict potencies and/or clinical efficacies of the topical corticosteroids. There is some evidence to suggest that a recognizable correlation exists between vasoconstrictor potency and therapeutic efficacy in man.
Pramoxine hydrochloride is a surface or local anesthetic which is not chemically related to the "caine" types of local anesthetics. Its unique chemical structure is likely to minimize the danger of cross-sensitivity reactions in patients allergic to other local anesthetics.
Pharmacokinetics: The extent of percutaneous absorption of topical corticosteroids is determined by many factors including the vehicle, the integrity of the epidermal barrier, and the use of occlusive dressings.
Topical corticosteroids can be absorbed through normal intact skin. Inflammation and/or other disease processes in the skin increase the percutaneous absorption of topical corticosteroids. Occlusive dressings substantially increase the percutaneous absorption of topical corticosteroids. Thus, occlusive dressings may be a valuable therapeutic adjunct for treatment of resistant dermatoses. (See DOSAGE AND ADMINISTRATION.)
Once absorbed through the skin, topical corticosteroids are handled through pharmacokinetic pathways similar to systemically administered corticosteroids. Corticosteroids are bound to plasma proteins in varying degrees. Corticosteroids are metabolized primarily in the liver and are then excreted by the kidneys. Some of the topical corticosteroids and their metabolites are also excreted into the bile.

INDICATIONS AND USAGE

ProctoFoam®-HC is indicated for the relief of the inflammatory and pruritic manifestations of corticosteroid-responsive dermatoses of the anal region.

CONTRAINDICATIONS

Topical corticosteroid products are contraindicated in those patients with a history of hypersensitivity to any of the components of the preparation.

WARNINGS

Do not insert any part of the aerosol container directly into the anus. Avoid contact with the eyes. Contents of the container are under pressure. Do not incinerate or puncture the aerosol container. Do not store at temperature above 120°F. If there is no evidence of clinical improvement within two or three weeks after starting ProctoFoam®-HC therapy, or if the patient's condition worsens, discontinue the drug. Keep this and all medicines out of the reach of children.

PRECAUTIONS

General: Systemic absorption of topical corticosteroids has produced reversible hypothalamic-pituitary-adrenal (HPA) axis suppression, manifestations of Cushing's syndrome, hyperglycemia, and glucosuria in some patients.
Conditions which augment systemic absorption include the application of the more potent steroids, use over large surface areas, prolonged use, and the addition of occlusive dressings. Therefore, patients receiving a large dose of a potent topical steroid applied to a large surface area or under an occlusive dressing should be evaluated periodically for evidence of HPA axis suppression by using the urinary free cortisol and ACTH stimulation tests. If HPA axis suppression is noted, an attempt should be made to withdraw the drug, to reduce the frequency of application, or to substitute a less potent steroid.
Recovery of HPA axis function is generally prompt and complete upon discontinuation of the drug. Infrequently, signs and symptoms of steroid withdrawal may occur, requiring supplemental systemic corticosteroids.
Pediatric patients may absorb proportionally larger amounts of topical corticosteroids and thus be more susceptible to systemic toxicity. (see PRECAUTIONS – *Pediatric Use.*)
If irritation develops, topical corticosteroids should be discontinued and appropriate therapy instituted.
In the presence of dermatological infections, the use of an appropriate antifungal or antibacterial agent should be instituted. If a favorable response does not occur promptly, the corticosteroid should be discontinued until the infection has been adequately controlled.
Information for the Patient: Patients using topical corticosteroids should receive the following information and instructions:

1. This medication is to be used as directed by the physician. It is for anal or perianal use only. Avoid contact with the eyes.
2. Be advised not to use this medication for any disorder other than for which it has been prescribed.
3. Report any signs of adverse reactions.

Laboratory Tests: The following tests may be helpful in evaluating the HPA axis suppression:
Urinary free cortisol test
ACTH stimulation test
Carcinogenesis, Mutagenesis, Impairment of Fertility: Long-term animal studies have not been performed to evaluate the carcinogenic potential or the effect on fertility of topical corticosteroids.
Studies to determine mutagenicity with prednisolone and hydrocortisone have revealed negative results.
Pregnancy: Teratogenic Effects. Pregnancy Category C. Corticosteroids are generally teratogenic in laboratory animals when administered systemically at relatively low dosage levels. The more potent corticosteroids have been shown to be teratogenic after dermal application in laboratory animals. There are no adequate, well-controlled studies of teratogenic effects from topically applied corticosteroids in pregnant women. Therefore, topical corticosteroids should be used during pregnancy only if the potential benefit justifies the potential risk to the fetus. Drugs of this class should not be used extensively on pregnant patients, in large amounts, or for prolonged periods of time.
Nursing Mothers: It is not known whether topical administration of corticosteroids could result in sufficient systemic absorption to produce detectable quantities in breast milk. Systemically administered corticosteroids are secreted into breast milk in quantities *not* likely to have a deleterious effect on the infant. Nevertheless, caution should be exercised when topical corticosteroids are administered to a nursing woman.
Pediatric Use: Pediatric patients may demonstrate greater susceptibility to topical corticosteroid-induced HPA axis suppression and Cushing's syndrome than mature patients because of a larger skin surface area to body weight ratio.
Hypothalamic-pituitary-adrenal (HPA) axis suppression, Cushing's syndrome, and intracranial hypertension have been reported in pediatric patients receiving topical corticosteroids. Manifestations of adrenal suppression in pediatric patients include linear growth retardation, delayed weight gain, low plasma cortisol levels, and absence of response to ACTH stimulation. Manifestations of intracranial hypertension include bulging fontanelles, headaches, and bilateral papilledema.
Administration of topical corticosteroids to pediatric patients should be limited to the least amount compatible with an effective therapeutic regimen. Chronic corticosteroid therapy may interfere with the growth and development of pediatric patients.

ADVERSE REACTIONS

The following local adverse reactions are reported infrequently with topical corticosteroids, but may occur more frequently with the use of occlusive dressings. These reactions are listed in an approximate decreasing order of occurrence: burning, itching, irritation, dryness, folliculitis, hypertrichosis, acneiform eruptions, hypopigmentation, perioral dermatitis, allergic contact dermatitis, maceration of the skin, secondary infection, skin atrophy, striae and miliaria.

OVERDOSAGE

Topically applied corticosteroids can be absorbed in sufficient amounts to produce systemic effects. (See PRECAUTIONS.)

DOSAGE AND ADMINISTRATION

Apply to affected area 3 to 4 times daily. Use the applicator supplied for anal administration. For perianal use, transfer a small quantity to a tissue and rub in gently.
Directions for Use.

1. Place cap on top of container. Shake foam container vigorously for 5–10 seconds before each use. **Do not remove container cap during use of the product.**
2. Hold container upright on a level surface and gently place the tip of the applicator onto the nose of the container cap. **CONTAINER MUST BE HELD UPRIGHT TO OBTAIN PROPER FLOW OF MEDICATION.**
3. Pull plunger past the fill line on the applicator barrel.
4. Hold the container and applicator at eye level. Place the index and middle fingers on the container cap flanges and the thumb beneath the container. Support the container and applicator with your other hand. Prime the container by pressing down firmly on flanges and then release. With initial priming, a burst of air may come out of the container. It usually requires 1–2 pumps for foam to appear.
5. To fill applicator barrel, **press down firmly** on cap flanges, hold for 1–2 seconds, and release. **Wait 5–10 seconds to allow foam to expand in applicator barrel. Repeat until foam reaches fill line.** It usually requires **3–4 pumps** for foam to reach fill line. Remove applicator from container cap. **Note:** If foam goes beyond fill line, it will continue to expand and flow backwards resulting in foam build-up under cap.
6. Hold applicator firmly by barrel, making sure thumb and middle finger are positioned securely underneath and resting against barrel wings. Place index finger over the plunger. Gently insert tip into anus. Once in place, push plunger to expel foam, then withdraw applicator. **CAUTION:** Do not insert any part of the aerosol container directly into the anus. Apply to anus only with enclosed applicator. Do not insert any part of applicator past the anus into rectum.
7. After each use, applicator parts should be pulled apart for thorough cleaning with warm water. Since some foam will appear under the cap, the cap and underlying tip should be pulled apart and rinsed to help prevent build-up of foam and possible blockage.

HOW SUPPLIED

ProctoFoam®-HC is supplied in an aerosol container with a special anal applicator. When used correctly, the aerosol container will deliver a minimum of 14 applications. **Store upright at controlled room temperature 15°–30°C (59°–86°F). Do not refrigerate.**
NDC 0091-0690-10 10g
PC2585D Rev. 6/99
Shown in Product Identification Guide, page 335

UNIRETIC™ ℞

[yü-nə-retic]
(moexipril hydrochloride/hydrochlorothiazide)
Tablets
7.5 mg/12.5 mg
15 mg/25 mg
Rx only

> **USE IN PREGNANCY**
> **When used in pregnancy during the second and third trimesters, ACE inhibitors can cause injury and even death to the developing fetus.** When pregnancy is detected, UNIRETIC should be discontinued as soon as possible. **See WARNINGS, Fetal/Neonatal Morbidity and Mortality.**

DESCRIPTION

UNIRETIC (moexipril hydrochloride/hydrochlorothiazide) is a combination of an angiotensin-converting enzyme (ACE) inhibitor, moexipril hydrochloride, and a diuretic, hydrochlorothiazide. Moexipril hydrochloride is a fine white to off-white powder. It is soluble (about 10% weight-to-volume) in distilled water at room temperature. It has the empirical formula $C_{27}H_{34}N_2O_7$·HCl and a molecular weight of 535.04. It is chemically described as [3S-[2[R*(R*)],3R*]]-2- [2-[[1-(Ethoxycarbonyl)-3-phenylpropyl]amino]-1-oxopropyl]-1,2,3,4-tetrahydro-6,7-dimethoxy-3-isoquinolinecarboxylic acid, monohydrochloride. Moexipril hydrochloride is a non-sulfhydryl containing precursor of the active ACE inhibitor moexiprilat and its structural formula is:

Hydrochlorothiazide is a white, or practically white, crystalline powder. It is slightly soluble in water, freely soluble in sodium hydroxide solution, in n-butylamine and in dimethylformamide. Hydrochlorothiazide has the empirical formula $C_7H_8ClN_3O_4S_2$ and a molecular weight of 297.75. It is chemically described as 2*H*-1,2,4-Benzothiadiazine-7-sulfonamide, 6-chloro-3,4-dihydro-, 1,1-dioxide. Hydrochlorothiazide is a thiazide diuretic and its structural formula is:

UNIRETIC is available for oral administration in two tablet strengths. The inactive ingredients in both strengths are lactose, magnesium oxide, crospovidone, magnesium stearate and gelatin. The film coating in both strengths contains hydroxypropyl methylcellulose, hydroxypropyl cellulose, polyethylene glycol 6000, magnesium stearate, titanium dioxide and ferric oxide.

CLINICAL PHARMACOLOGY

Mechanism of Action

Moexipril Hydrochloride

Moexipril hydrochloride is a prodrug for moexiprilat, which inhibits ACE in humans and animals. The mechanism through which moexiprilat lowers blood pressure is believed to be primarily inhibition of ACE activity. ACE is a peptidyl dipeptidase that catalyzes the conversion of the inactive decapeptide angiotensin I to the vasoconstrictor substance angiotensin II. Angiotensin II is a potent peripheral vasoconstrictor that also stimulates aldosterone secretion by the adrenal cortex and provides negative feedback on renin secretion. ACE is identical to kininase II, an enzyme that degrades bradykinin, an endothelium-dependent vasodilator. Moexiprilat is about 1000 times as potent as moexipril in inhibiting ACE and kininase II. Inhibition of ACE results in decreased angiotensin II formation, leading to decreased vasoconstriction, increased plasma renin activity, and decreased aldosterone secretion. The latter results in diuresis and natriuresis and a small increase in serum potassium concentration (mean increases of about 0.25 mEq/L were seen when moexipril was used alone).

Whether increased levels of bradykinin, a potent vasodepressor peptide, play a role in the therapeutic effects of moexipril remains to be elucidated. Although the principal mechanism of moexipril in blood pressure reduction is believed to be through the renin-angiotensin-aldosterone system, ACE inhibitors have some effect on blood pressure even in apparent low-renin hypertension. As is the case with other ACE inhibitors, however, the antihypertensive effect of moexipril is smaller in black patients, a predominantly low-renin population, than in nonblack hypertensive patients. Although moexipril monotherapy is less effective in blacks than in nonblacks, the efficacy of combination therapy appears to be independent of race.

Hydrochlorothiazide

Hydrochlorothiazide is a thiazide diuretic and antihypertensive. Thiazides affect the distal renal tubular mechanisms of electrolyte reabsorption, directly increasing excretion of sodium and chloride in approximately equivalent amounts. Indirectly, the diuretic action of hydrochlorothiazide reduces plasma volume, with consequent increases in plasma renin activity, increases in aldosterone secretion, increases in urinary potassium loss, and decreases in serum potassium. The renin-aldosterone link is mediated by angiotensin, so coadministration of an ACE inhibitor tends to reverse the potassium loss associated with these diuretics. The mechanism of the antihypertensive effect of thiazides is unknown.

Pharmacokinetics

Moexipril-Hydrochlorothiazide

Following oral administration of UNIRETIC, the moexipril peak plasma concentration was reached within 0.8 hour and the peak plasma concentration of moexiprilat occurred 1.6 hours after administration. After reaching the peak plasma level (C_{max}), moexiprilat plasma concentrations decreased biphasically. After administration of UNIRETIC, renal excretion of unchanged hydrochlorothiazide is about 60% in 24 hours. The pharmacokinetics of moexipril and hydrochlorothiazide after administration of UNIRETIC are not different, respectively, from the pharmacokinetics of moexipril and hydrochlorothiazide from immediate-release monotherapy formulations.

Moexipril Hydrochloride

Moexipril's antihypertensive activity is almost entirely due to its deesterified metabolite, moexiprilat. Bioavailability of oral moexipril is about 13% compared to intravenous (I.V.) moexipril (both measuring the metabolite moexiprilat), and is markedly affected by food, which reduces C_{max} and AUC (see Absorption). Moexipril should therefore be taken in a fasting state. The time of peak plasma concentration (T_{max}) of moexiprilat is about $1^1/_2$ hours and elimination half-life ($t_{1/2}$) is estimated at 2 to 9 hours in various studies, the variability reflecting a complex elimination pattern that is not simply exponential. Like all ACE inhibitors, moexiprilat has a prolonged terminal elimination phase, presumably reflecting slow release of drug bound to the ACE. Accumulation of moexiprilat with repeated dosing is minimal, about 30%, compatible with a functional elimination $t_{1/2}$ of about 12 hours. Over the dose range of 7.5 to 30 mg, pharmacokinetics are approximately dose proportional.

Absorption: Moexipril is incompletely absorbed, with bioavailability as moexiprilat of about 13%. Bioavailability varies with formulation and food intake which reduces C_{max} and AUC of moexiprilat by about 70% and 40% respectively after the ingestion of a low-fat breakfast or by 80% and 50% respectively after the ingestion of a high-fat breakfast.

Distribution: The clearance (CL) for moexipril is 441 mL/min and for moexiprilat 232 mL/min with a $t_{1/2}$ of 1.3 and 9.8 hours, respectively. Moexiprilat is about 50% protein bound. The volume of distribution of moexiprilat is about 2.8 L/kg.

Metabolism and Excretion: Moexipril is relatively rapidly converted to its active metabolite moexiprilat, but persists longer than some other ACE inhibitor prodrugs, such that its $t_{1/2}$ is over one hour and it has a significant AUC. Both moexipril and moexiprilat are converted to diketopiperazine derivatives and unidentified metabolites. After I.V. administration of moexipril, about 40% of the dose appears in urine as moexiprilat, about 26% as moexipril, with small amounts of the metabolites; about 20% of the I.V. dose appears in feces, principally as moexiprilat. After oral administration, only about 7% of the dose appears in urine as moexiprilat, about 1% as moexipril, with about 5% as other metabolites. Fifty-two percent of the dose is recovered in feces as moexiprilat and 1% as moexipril.

Special Populations:

Decreased Renal Function: The effective elimination $t_{1/2}$ and AUC of both moexipril and moexiprilat are increased with decreasing renal function. There is insufficient information available to characterize this relationship fully, but at creatinine clearances in the range of 10 to 40 mL/min, the $t_{1/2}$ of moexiprilat is increased by a factor of 3 to 4.

Decreased Hepatic Function: In patients with mild to moderate cirrhosis given single 15-mg doses of moexipril, the C_{max} of moexipril was increased by about 50% and the AUC increased by about 120%, while the C_{max} for moexiprilat was decreased by about 50% and the AUC increased by almost 300%.

Elderly Patients: In elderly male subjects (65–80 years old) with clinically normal renal and hepatic function, the AUC and C_{max} of moexiprilat are about 30% greater than in younger subjects (19–42 years old).

Pharmacokinetic Interactions With Other Drugs: No clinically important pharmacokinetic interactions occurred when moexipril was administered concomitantly with hydrochlorothiazide, digoxin, or cimetidine.

Hydrochlorothiazide

Absorption: After oral administration, 60–80% of a single dose of hydrochlorothiazide is absorbed. The reported studies of food effects on hydrochlorothiazide absorption have been inconclusive. The absorption of hydrochlorothiazide is reported to be reduced by 50% in patients with congestive heart failure. Hydrochlorothiazide exhibits dose proportionality over the dose range of 12.5 to 75 mg.

Distribution: The apparent volume of distribution has been observed to vary between 1.5–4.2 L/kg. Hydrochlorothiazide accumulates in red blood cells, so that whole blood levels are higher than those measured in plasma. Equilibrium between whole blood levels and plasma levels is reached 4 hours after oral administration. Hydrochlorothiazide crosses the placental barrier. Hydrochlorothiazide has a protein binding of 21–24%.

Metabolism and Excretion: Hydrochlorothiazide is not metabolized. Hydrochlorothiazide is eliminated rapidly by the kidney. More than 60 percent of the oral dose is eliminated unchanged within 24 hours. When plasma levels have been followed for at least 24 hours, the plasma half-life has been observed to vary between 5.6 and 14.8 hours. The renal clearance has been observed to vary between 3.1–5.5 mL/min/kg.

Special Populations:

Decreased Renal Function: In a study of patients with impaired renal function (mean creatinine clearance of 19 mL/min), the elimination half-life of hydrochlorothiazide was increased to 21 hours.

Pharmacokinetic Interactions With Other Drugs: Coadministration of propantheline or guanabenz increased the absorption of hydrochlorothiazide and coadministration of cholestyramine or colestipol decreased the absorption of hydrochlorothiazide.

Pharmacodynamics and Clinical Effect

Moexipril—Hydrochlorothiazide

In UNIRETIC clinical trials using moexipril doses of 3.75–30 mg and hydrochlorothiazide doses of 3.125–50 mg, the antihypertensive effects were sustained for at least 24 hours and they increased with increasing dose of either component. The extent of blood pressure reduction seen with UNIRETIC was approximately additive as compared to monotherapy of each component. The antihypertensive effects of UNIRETIC continue during therapy for up to 24 months. The effectiveness of UNIRETIC was not significantly influenced by patient age or gender. Although moexipril monotherapy is less effective in blacks than in nonblacks, the efficacy of UNIRETIC appears to be independent of race.

By blocking the renin-angiotensin-aldosterone axis, administration of moexipril tends to reduce the potassium loss associated with hydrochlorothiazide. In UNIRETIC controlled clinical trials, the average change in serum potassium was near zero in subjects who received 3.75/6.25 mg or 7.5/12.5 mg, but subjects who received 15/25 mg experienced a mild decrease in serum potassium, similar to that experienced by subjects who received hydrochlorothiazide 25 mg monotherapy.

Moexipril Hydrochloride

Single and multiple doses of 15 mg or more of moexipril give sustained inhibition of plasma ACE activity of 80–90%, beginning within 2 hours and lasting 24 hours (80%).

In controlled trials, the peak effects of orally administered moexipril increased with the dose administered over a dose range of 7.5 to 60 mg, given once a day. Antihypertensive effects were first detectable about 1 hour after dosing, with a peak effect between 3 and 6 hours after dosing. Just before dosing (i.e., at trough), the antihypertensive effects were less prominently related to dose and the antihypertensive effect tended to diminish during the 24-hour dosing interval when the drug was administered once a day.

In multiple-dose studies in the dose range of 7.5 to 30 mg once daily, moexipril lowered sitting blood pressure at trough by 4-11/3-6 mmHg more than placebo, a tendency toward increased response with higher doses. These effects are typical of ACE inhibitors; there are no trials of adequate size comparing moexipril with other antihypertensive agents.

Higher doses of moexipril generally leave a greater fraction of the peak blood pressure effect still present at trough. During dose titration, any decision as to the adequacy of a dosing regimen should be based on trough blood pressure measurements. If diastolic blood pressure control is not adequate at the end of the dosing interval, the dose can be increased or given as a divided (BID) regimen.

During chronic therapy, the antihypertensive effect of any dose of moexipril is generally evident within 2 weeks of treatment, with maximal reduction after 4 weeks. The antihypertensive effects of moexipril have been proven to continue during therapy for up to 24 months.

Moexipril, like other ACE inhibitors, is less effective in decreasing trough blood pressures in blacks than in nonblacks. Placebo-corrected trough group diastolic blood pressure effects in blacks in the proposed dose range were +1 to −3 mmHg compared with responses in nonblacks of −4 to −6 mmHg.

The effectiveness of moexipril was not significantly influenced by patient age, gender, or weight. Moexipril has been shown to have antihypertensive activity in both pre- and postmenopausal women who have participated in placebo-controlled clinical trials.

INDICATIONS AND USAGE

UNIRETIC is indicated for treatment of patients with hypertension. **This fixed combination is not indicated for the initial therapy of hypertension (see DOSAGE AND ADMINISTRATION).**

In using UNIRETIC, consideration should be given to the fact that another ACE inhibitor, captopril, has caused agranulocytosis, particularly in patients with renal impairment or collagen-vascular disease. Available data are insufficient to show that UNIRETIC does not have a similar risk (see WARNINGS, Neutropenia/Agranulocytosis). In addition, ACE inhibitors, for which adequate data are available, cause a higher rate of angioedema in black than in nonblack patients (see WARNINGS, Angioedema).

CONTRAINDICATIONS

UNIRETIC is contraindicated in patients who are hypersensitive to any component of this product and in patients with a history of angioedema related to previous treatment with an ACE inhibitor. Because of the hydrochlorothiazide component, this product is contraindicated in patients with anuria or hypersensitivity to other sulfonamide-derived drugs. Hypersensitivity reactions are more likely to occur in patients with a history of allergy or bronchial asthma.

WARNINGS

Anaphylactoid and Possibly Related Reactions

Presumably because angiotensin-converting enzyme inhibitors affect the metabolism of eicosanoids and polypeptides, including endogenous bradykinin, patients receiving ACE inhibitors, including UNIRETIC, may be subject to a variety of adverse reactions, some of them serious.

Angioedema: Angioedema involving the face, extremities, lips, tongue, glottis, and/or larynx has been reported in patients treated with ACE inhibitors, including moexipril. Symptoms suggestive of angioedema or facial edema occurred in <0.5% of moexipril-treated patients in placebo-controlled trials. None of the cases were considered life-threatening and all resolved either without treatment or with medication (antihistamines or glucocorticoids). One patient treated with hydrochlorothiazide alone experienced laryngeal edema. No instances of angioedema were reported in placebo-treated patients.

In cases of angioedema, treatment with UNIRETIC should be promptly discontinued and the patient carefully observed until the swelling disappears. In instances where swelling has been confined to the face and lips, the condition has generally resolved without treatment, although antihistamines have been useful in relieving symptoms.

Angioedema associated with involvement of the tongue, glottis, or larynx may be fatal due to airway obstruction. Appropriate therapy, e.g., subcutaneous epinephrine solution 1:1000 (0.3 to 0.5 mL) and/or measures to ensure a patent airway, should be promptly provided (see ADVERSE REACTIONS).

Anaphylactoid Reactions During Desensitization: Two patients undergoing desensitizing treatment with hymenoptera venom while receiving ACE inhibitors sustained life-threatening anaphylactoid reactions. In the same patients, these reactions did not occur when ACE inhibitors were temporarily withheld, but they reappeared when the ACE inhibitors were inadvertently readministered.

Anaphylactoid Reactions During Membrane Exposure: Anaphylactoid reactions have been reported in patients dialyzed with high-flux membranes and treated concomitantly with an ACE inhibitor. Anaphylactoid reactions have also been reported in patients undergoing low-density lipoprotein apheresis with dextran sulfate absorption.

Hypotension

UNIRETIC can cause symptomatic hypotension, although, as with other ACE inhibitors, this is unusual in uncomplicated hypertensive patients treated with UNIRETIC alone. Symptomatic hypotension is most likely to occur in patients who have been salt- and/or volume-depleted as a result of prolonged diuretic therapy, dietary salt restriction, dialysis, diarrhea, or vomiting. Volume- and/or salt-depletion should be corrected before initiating therapy with UNIRETIC (see ADVERSE REACTIONS).

The thiazide component of UNIRETIC may potentiate the action of other antihypertensive drugs, especially ganglionic

Continued on next page

Uniretic—Cont.

or peripheral adrenergic-blocking drugs. The antihypertensive effects of the thiazide component may also be enhanced in the postsympathectomy patient.
In patients with congestive heart failure, with or without associated renal insufficiency, ACE inhibitor therapy may cause excessive hypotension, which may be associated with oliguria or progressive azotemia, and rarely, with acute renal failure and death. In these patients, UNIRETIC therapy should be started under close medical supervision, and patients should be followed closely for the first two weeks of treatment and whenever the dose of UNIRETIC is increased. Care in avoiding hypotension should also be taken in patients with ischemic heart disease, aortic stenosis, or cerebrovascular disease, in whom an excessive decrease in blood pressure could result in a myocardial infarction or a cerebrovascular accident.
If hypotension occurs, the patient should be placed in a supine position and, if necessary, treated with an intravenous infusion of normal saline. UNIRETIC treatment usually can be continued following restoration of blood pressure and volume.

Impaired Renal Function
UNIRETIC should be used with caution in patients with severe renal disease. Thiazide diuretics may precipitate azotemia in such patients and the effects of repeated dosing may be cumulative.
As a consequence of inhibition of the renin-angiotensin-aldosterone system, changes in renal function may be anticipated in susceptible individuals. There is no clinical experience of UNIRETIC in the treatment of hypertension in patients with renal failure.
Some hypertensive patients with no apparent preexisting renal vascular disease have developed increases in blood urea nitrogen and serum creatinine, usually minor and transient, especially when moexipril has been given concomitantly with a thiazide diuretic. This is more likely to occur in patients with preexisting renal impairment. There may be a need for dose adjustment of UNIRETIC. **Evaluation of hypertensive patients should always include assessment of renal function** (see DOSAGE AND ADMINISTRATION).
In hypertensive patients with severe congestive heart failure, whose renal function may depend on the activity of the renin-angiotensin-aldosterone system, treatment with ACE inhibitors, including moexipril, may be associated with oliguria and/or progressive azotemia and, rarely, acute renal failure and/or death.
In hypertensive patients with unilateral or bilateral renal artery stenosis, increases in blood urea nitrogen and serum creatinine have been observed in some patients following ACE inhibitor therapy. These increases were almost always reversible upon discontinuation of the ACE inhibitor and/or diuretic therapy. In such patients, renal function should be monitored during the first few weeks of therapy.

Neutropenia/Agranulocytosis
Another ACE inhibitor, captopril, has been shown to cause agranulocytosis and bone marrow depression, rarely in patients with uncomplicated hypertension, but more frequently in hypertensive patients with renal impairment, especially if they also have a collagen-vascular disease such as systemic lupus erythematosus or scleroderma. Although there were no instances of severe neutropenia (absolute neutrophil count <500/mm^3) among patients given moexipril, as with other ACE inhibitors, monitoring of white blood cell counts should be considered for patients who have collagen-vascular disease, especially if the disease is associated with impaired renal function. Available data from clinical trials of moexipril are insufficient to show that moexipril does not cause agranulocytosis at rates similar to captopril.

Fetal/Neonatal Morbidity and Mortality
ACE inhibitors can cause fetal and neonatal morbidity and death when administered to pregnant women. Several dozen cases have been reported in the world literature. When pregnancy is detected, ACE inhibitors should be discontinued as soon as possible.
The use of ACE inhibitors during the second and third trimesters of pregnancy has been associated with fetal and neonatal injury, including hypotension, neonatal skull hypoplasia, anuria, reversible or irreversible renal failure, and death. Oligohydramnios has also been reported, presumably resulting from decreased fetal renal function; oligohydramnios in this setting has been associated with fetal limb contractures, craniofacial deformation, and hypoplastic lung development. Prematurity, intrauterine growth retardation, and patent ductus arteriosus have also been reported, although it is not clear whether these were caused by the ACE inhibitor exposure.
Fetal and neonatal morbidity do not appear to have resulted from intrauterine ACE inhibitor exposure limited to the first trimester. Mothers who have used ACE inhibitors only during the first trimester should be informed of this. Nonetheless, when patients become pregnant, physicians should make every effort to discontinue the use of UNIRETIC as soon as possible.
Rarely (probably less often than once in every thousand pregnancies), no alternative to ACE inhibitors will be found. In these rare cases, the mothers should be apprised of the potential hazards to their fetuses, and serial ultrasound examinations should be performed to assess the intraamniotic environment.
If oligohydramnios is observed, UNIRETIC should be discontinued unless it is considered life-saving for the mother. Contraction stress testing (CST), a non-stress test (NST), or biophysical profiling (BPP) may be appropriate, depending upon the week of pregnancy. Patients and physicians should be aware, however, that oligohydramnios may not be detected until after the fetus has sustained irreversible injury.
Infants with histories of *in utero* exposure to ACE inhibitors should be closely observed for hypotension, oliguria, and hyperkalemia. If oliguria occurs, attention should be directed toward support of blood pressure and renal perfusion. Exchange transfusion or peritoneal dialysis may be required as means of reversing hypotension and/or substituting for disordered renal function. Theoretically, the ACE inhibitor could be removed from the neonatal circulation by exchange transfusion, but no experience with this procedure has been reported.
Intrauterine exposure to thiazide diuretics is associated with fetal or neonatal jaundice, thrombocytopenia, and possibly other adverse reactions that have occurred in adults.
Reproduction studies with the combination of moexipril hydrochloride and hydrochlorothiazide (ratio 7.5:12.5) indicated that the combination possessed no teratogenic properties up to the lethal dose of 800 mg/kg/day in rats and up to the maternotoxic dose of 160 mg/kg/day in rabbits.

Hepatic Failure
Rarely, ACE inhibitors have been associated with a syndrome that starts with cholestatic jaundice and progresses to fulminant hepatic necrosis and sometimes death. The mechanism of this syndrome is not understood. Patients receiving ACE inhibitors who develop jaundice or marked elevations of hepatic enzymes should discontinue the ACE inhibitor and receive appropriate medical follow-up.

Impaired Hepatic Function
UNIRETIC should be used with caution in patients with impaired hepatic function or progressive liver disease, since minor alterations of fluid and electrolyte balance may precipitate hepatic coma. In patients with mild to moderate cirrhosis given single 15 mg doses of moexipril, the C_{max} of moexipril was increased by about 50% and the AUC increased by about 120%, while the C_{max} for moexiprilat was decreased by about 50% and the AUC increased by almost 300%. No formal pharmacokinetic studies have been carried out with UNIRETIC in hypertensive patients with impaired liver function.

Systemic Lupus Erythematosus
Thiazide diuretics have been reported to cause exacerbation or activation of systemic lupus erythematosus.

PRECAUTIONS

General
Serum Electrolyte Imbalances: In clinical trials with moexipril monotherapy, persistent hyperkalemia (serum potassium above 5.4 mEq/L) occurred in approximately 1.3% of hypertensive patients receiving moexipril. Risk factors for the development of hyperkalemia with ACE inhibitors include renal insufficiency, diabetes mellitus, and the concomitant use of potassium-sparing diuretics, potassium supplements, and/or potassium-containing salt substitutes.
Treatment with thiazide diuretics has been associated with hypokalemia, hyponatremia, and hypochloremic alkalosis. These disturbances sometimes manifest as one or more of the following: dryness of mouth, thirst, weakness, lethargy, drowsiness, restlessness, muscle pains or cramps, muscular fatigue, hypotension, oliguria, tachycardia, nausea, and vomiting. Hypokalemia has also been reported to sensitize or exaggerate the response of the heart to the toxic effects of digitalis. The risk of hypokalemia is greatest in patients with cirrhosis of the liver, in patients experiencing a brisk diuresis, in patients who are receiving inadequate oral intake of electrolytes, and in patients receiving concomitant therapy with corticosteroids or ACTH.
The opposite effects of moexipril and hydrochlorothiazide on serum potassium will approximately counterbalance each other in many patients, so that little net effect upon serum potassium will be seen. Initial and periodic determinations of serum electrolytes to detect possible electrolyte imbalance should be performed at appropriate intervals.
Chloride deficits generally are mild and require specific treatment only under extraordinary circumstances (e.g., in liver disease or renal disease). Dilutional hyponatremia may occur in edematous patients; appropriate therapy is water restriction rather than administration of salt, except in rare instances when the hyponatremia is life-threatening. In actual salt depletion, appropriate replacement is the therapy of choice.
Calcium excretion is reduced by thiazides. In a few patients on prolonged thiazide therapy, pathological changes in the parathyroid gland have been seen, with hypercalcemia and hypophosphatemia. More serious complications of hyperparathyroidism (renal lithiasis, bone resorption, and peptic ulceration) have not been seen.
Thiazides enhance urinary excretion of magnesium and hypomagnesemia may result.
Other Metabolic Disturbances: Thiazide diuretics may reduce glucose tolerance and may raise serum levels of cholesterol, triglycerides, and uric acid. These effects are usually minor, but frank gout or overt diabetes may be precipitated in susceptible patients.
Surgery/Anesthesia: In patients undergoing major surgery or during anesthesia with agents that produce hypotension, moexipril may block the effects of compensatory renin release. If hypotension occurs in this setting and is considered to be due to this mechanism, it can be corrected by volume expansion.
Cough: Presumably due to the inhibition of the degradation of endogenous bradykinin, persistent nonproductive cough has been reported with all ACE inhibitors, always resolving after discontinuation of therapy. ACE inhibitor-induced cough should be considered in the differential diagnosis of cough. In placebo-controlled trials with UNIRETIC, cough was present in 3% of UNIRETIC patients and 1% of patients given placebo.

Information for Patients
Food: Patients should be advised to take UNIRETIC one hour before a meal (see CLINICAL PHARMACOLOGY and DOSAGE AND ADMINISTRATION).
Angioedema: Angioedema, including laryngeal edema, may occur with treatment with ACE inhibitors, usually occurring early in therapy (within the first month). Patients should be so advised and told to report immediately any signs or symptoms suggesting angioedema (swelling of the face, extremities, eyes, lips, tongue, difficulty in breathing) and to take no more drug until they have consulted with the prescribing physician.
Symptomatic Hypotension: Patients should be cautioned that lightheadedness can occur with UNIRETIC, especially during the first few days of therapy. If fainting occurs, the patient should stop taking UNIRETIC and consult the prescribing physician.
All patients should be cautioned that excessive perspiration and dehydration may lead to an excessive fall in blood pressure because of reduction in fluid volume. Other causes of volume depletion such as vomiting or diarrhea may also lead to a fall in blood pressure; patients should be advised to consult their physician if they develop these conditions.
Hyperkalemia: Patients should be told not to use potassium supplements or salt substitutes containing potassium without consulting their physician.
Neutropenia: Patients should be told to report promptly any indication of infection (e.g., sore throat, fever) that could be a sign of neutropenia.
Pregnancy: Female patients of childbearing age should be told about the consequences of second- and third-trimester exposure to ACE inhibitors and should also be told that these consequences do not appear to have resulted from intrauterine ACE inhibitor exposure that has been limited to the first trimester. Patients should be asked to report pregnancies to their physicians as soon as possible.

Drug Interactions
Potassium Supplements and Potassium-Sparing Diuretics: As noted above (*Serum Electrolyte Imbalances*), the net effect of UNIRETIC may be to elevate a patient's serum potassium (at low doses of hydrochlorothiazide), to reduce it (at high doses of hydrochlorothiazide), or to leave it unchanged. Potassium-sparing diuretics (spironolactone, amiloride, triamterene) or potassium supplements can increase the risk of hyperkalemia. If concomitant use of such agents is indicated, they should be given with caution, and the patient's serum potassium should be monitored.
Oral Anticoagulants: Interaction studies with warfarin failed to identify any clinically important effect of moexipril monotherapy on the serum concentrations of the anticoagulant or on its anticoagulant effect.
Lithium: Increased serum lithium levels and symptoms of lithium toxicity have been reported in patients receiving ACE inhibitors during therapy with lithium. Because renal clearance of lithium is reduced by thiazides, the risk of lithium toxicity is presumably raised further when, as in therapy with UNIRETIC, a thiazide diuretic is coadministered with the ACE inhibitor. These drugs should be coadministered with caution, and frequent monitoring of serum lithium levels is recommended.
Alcohol, Barbiturates, or Narcotics: Potentiation of orthostatic hypotension may occur in patients on thiazide diuretic therapy with concomitant use of alcohol, barbiturates, or narcotics.
Antidiabetic Agents: Use of thiazide diuretics concomitantly with antidiabetic agents (oral agents and insulin) may require dosage adjustment of the antidiabetic agent. Moexipril has been used in clinical trials concomitantly with oral hypoglycemic agents and there was no evidence of any clinically important adverse interactions.
Cholestyramine and Colestipol Resins: Absorption of hydrochlorothiazide is impaired in the presence of anionic exchange resins. Single doses of either cholestyramine or colestipol resins bind the hydrochlorothiazide and reduce its absorption from the gastrointestinal tract by up to 85% and 43%, respectively.
Corticosteroids, ACTH: Use of thiazide diuretics concomitantly with corticosteroids or ACTH may intensify electrolyte depletion, particularly hypokalemia.
Pressor Amines: Thiazide diuretics may decrease arterial responsiveness to pressor amines (eg. norepinephrine), but not enough to preclude effectiveness of the pressor agent for therapeutic use.
Skeletal Muscle Relaxants, Nondepolarizing: Thiazide diuretics may increase the responsiveness to tubocurarine.
Non-steroidal Anti-inflammatory Drugs: In some patients, the administration of a non-steroidal anti-inflammatory agent can reduce the diuretic, natriuretic, and antihypertensive effects of loop, potassium-sparing and thiazide diuretics. Thus, when UNIRETIC and non-steroidal anti-inflammatory agents are used concomitantly, the patient should be observed closely to determine if the desired effect of the diuretic is obtained.

Other Agents: No clinically important pharmacokinetic interactions occurred when moexipril was administered concomitantly with digoxin or cimetidine.

Moexipril has been used in clinical trials concomitantly with calcium-channel-blocking agents, diuretics, H_2 blockers, digoxin, and cholesterol-lowering agents. There was no evidence of clinically important adverse interactions. In general, ACE inhibitors have less than additive effects with beta-adrenergic blockers, presumably because both work by inhibiting the renin-angiotensin system.

Coadministration of propantheline or guanabenz increased the absorption of hydrochlorothiazide.

Carcinogenesis, Mutagenesis, Impairment of Fertility

Moexipril Hydrochloride

No evidence of carcinogenicity was detected in long-term studies when moexipril was administered to mice and rats at doses up to 14 or 27.3 times the Maximum Recommended Human Dose (MRHD) on a mg/m^2 basis. No mutagenicity was detected in the Ames test and microbial reverse mutation assay, with and without metabolic activation, or in an *in vivo* nucleus anomaly test. However, increased chromosomal aberration frequency in Chinese hamster ovary (CHO) cells was detected under metabolic activation conditions at a 20-hour harvest time. Reproduction studies have been performed in rabbits at oral doses up to 0.7 times the MRHD on a mg/m^2 basis, and in rats up to 90.9 times the MRHD on a mg/m^2 basis. No indication of impaired fertility, reproductive toxicity, or teratogenicity was observed.

Hydrochlorothiazide

Under the auspices of the National Toxicology Program, rats and mice received hydrochlorothiazide in their feed for two years, at doses up to 600 mg/kg/day in mice and up to 100 mg/kg/day in rats. These studies uncovered no evidence of a carcinogenic potential of hydrochlorothiazide in rats or female mice, but there was equivocal evidence of hepatocarcinogenicity in male mice. Hydrochlorothiazide was not genotoxic in *in vitro* assays using strains TA 98, TA 100, TA 1535, TA 1537, and TA 1538 of *Salmonella typhimurium* (the Ames test); in the CHO test for chromosomal aberrations; or in *in vivo* assays using mouse germinal cell chromosomes, Chinese hamster bone marrow chromosomes; and the *Drosophila* sex-linked recessive lethal trait gene. Positive test results were obtained in the *in vitro* CHO Sister Chromatid Exchange (clastogenicity) test and in the Mouse Lymphoma Cell (mutagenicity) assays, using concentrations of hydrochlorothiazide of 43-1300 mcg/mL. Positive test results were also obtained in the *Aspergillus nidulans* nondisjunction assay, using an unspecified concentration of hydrochlorothiazide.

Hydrochlorothiazide had no adverse effects on the fertility of mice and rats of either sex in studies wherein these species were exposed, via their diets, to doses up to 100 and 4 mg/kg/day, respectively, prior to mating and throughout gestation.

Pregnancy

Pregnancy Categories C (first trimester) and D (second and third trimesters).

See WARNINGS, Fetal/Neonatal Morbidity and Mortality.

Nursing Mothers

It is not known whether moexipril or moexiprilat is excreted in human milk. Thiazides are excreted in human milk. Because of the potential for serious adverse reactions in nursing infants from hydrochlorothiazide and the unknown effects of moexipril or moexiprilat in infants, a decision should be made whether to discontinue nursing or to discontinue UNIRETIC, taking into account the importance of the drug to the mother.

Geriatric Use

Of the patients who received UNIRETIC in controlled clinical studies, 24% were 65 years of age or older. No overall differences in effectiveness or safety were observed between these patients and younger patients. In elderly patients receiving moexipril, plasma levels of drug are slightly higher and renal clearance is reduced when compared to younger patients, but these effects did not have detectable consequences.

Pediatric Use

Safety and effectiveness of UNIRETIC in pediatric patients have not been established.

ADVERSE REACTIONS

UNIRETIC has been evaluated for safety in more than 1140 patients with hypertension with more than 120 treated for more than one year. UNIRETIC has not demonstrated a potential for causing adverse experiences different from those previously associated with other ACE inhibitor/diuretic combinations. The overall incidence of reported adverse events was slightly less in patients treated with UNIRETIC than patients treated with placebo.

Adverse experiences were usually mild and transient, and there was no relationship between adverse experiences and gender, race, age, or total daily dosage (except for serum potassium decreases at 50 mg hydrochlorothiazide) within the moexipril/hydrochlorothiazide dosage range of 3.75 mg/3.125 mg to 30 mg/50 mg. Discontinuation of therapy due to adverse experiences was required in 5.3% of patients treated with UNIRETIC and in 8.4% of patients treated with placebo. The most common reasons for discontinuation of therapy with UNIRETIC were cough (0.5%) and dizziness (0.5%).

All adverse experiences considered at least possibly related to treatment that occurred at any dose in placebo-controlled trials of once-daily dosing in more than 1% of patients treated with UNIRETIC and that were at least as frequent in the UNIRETIC group as in the placebo group are shown in the following table.

Adverse Events in Placebo-Controlled Trials

ADVERSE EVENT	UNIRETIC (N = 506) N (%)	PLACEBO (N = 202) N (%)
Cough	15 (3)	2 (1)
Dizziness	7 (1.4)	2 (1)
Fatigue	5 (1)	1 (0.5)

Other adverse experiences occurring in more than 1% of patients treated with UNIRETIC in controlled or uncontrolled trials, some of which were of uncertain drug relationship, listed in decreasing frequency include: upper respiratory infection, headache, pain, flu syndrome, pharyngitis, hyperuricemia, diarrhea, back pain, rhinitis, sinusitis, abnormal ECG, infection, abdominal pain, chest pain, dyspepsia, hyperglycemia, hypokalemia, rash, vertigo, nausea, hypertonia, increased SGPT, urinary tract infection, impotence, peripheral edema, pyuria, bronchitis, and fever. See WARNINGS and PRECAUTIONS for discussion of anaphylactoid reactions, angioedema, hypotension, neutropenia/agranulocytosis, fetal/neonatal morbidity and mortality, serum electrolyte imbalances, and cough.

The following adverse experiences, some of which are of uncertain drug relationship, were reported in UNIRETIC controlled or uncontrolled clinical trials in less than 1% of patients or have been attributed to other ACE inhibitors. Within each organ system, adverse experiences are listed in decreasing frequency.

Cardiovascular: palpitation, flushing, syncope, tachycardia, myocardial infarct, hypotension, postural hypotension, arrhythmia, first degree AV block, ventricular extrasystoles, atrial fibrillation, migraine, hemorrhage, sinus bradycardia, bigeminy, bradycardia, bundle branch block, heart arrest, myocardial ischemia, peripheral vascular disorder, prolonged QT interval, inverted T wave, ventricular fibrillation

Dermatologic: eczema, pruritus, sweating, acne, dry skin, herpes simplex, contact dermatitis, herpes zoster, psoriasis, alopecia, angioedema, erythema nodosum, fungal dermatitis, furunculosis, maculopapular rash, purpuric rash, skin carcinoma, subcutaneous nodule, urticaria, pemphigus

Gastrointestinal: vomiting, constipation, gastroenteritis, periodontal abscess, cholelithiasis, gastritis, gingivitis, esophagitis, flatulence, anorexia, colitis, dysphagia, tooth caries, cheilitis, enteritis, eructation, gastrointestinal carcinoma, gastrointestinal hemorrhage, glossitis, increased appetite, jaundice, melena, rectal hemorrhage, stomatitis, tongue discoloration, tongue edema

Hematologic: anemia, hypochromic anemia, leukopenia, abnormal erythrocytes, ecchymosis, lymphocytosis, hemolysis, lymphadenopathy, eosinophilia, petechia, abnormal WBC, hemolytic anemia

Metabolic: hyperlipemia, increased SGOT, gout, bilirubinemia, increased creatinine, hypercholesterolemia, increased BUN, increased CPK, diabetes mellitus, hyponatremia, thirst, edema, increased alkaline phosphatase, increased amylase, dehydration, decreased glucose tolerance, goiter, hypercalcemia, hyperkalemia, hypocalcemia, hypochloremia, hypoproteinemia, weight gain

Neurologic/Psychiatric: insomnia, postural dizziness, somnolence, dry mouth, anxiety, nervousness, paresthesia, depression, neuritis, hypesthesia, decreased libido, neuralgia, amnesia, ataxia, cerebral infarct, emotional lability, facial paralysis, hypokinesia, neurosis, vocal cord paralysis

Renal: albuminuria, urinary frequency, hematuria, glycosuria, cystitis, dysuria, nocturia, polyuria, kidney calculus, pyelonephritis, urate crystalluria, urinary casts, urinary retention

Respiratory: epistaxis, pneumonia, dyspnea, asthma, lung carcinoma, hemoptysis, laryngitis, voice alteration, eosinophilic pneumonitis

Urogenital: vaginal hemorrhage, breast carcinoma, scrotal edema, vaginitis, breast enlargement, breast pain, dysmenorrhea, leukorrhea

Other: asthenia, conjunctivitis, myalgia, arthralgia, arthrosis, hernia, neck pain, cyst, tenosynovitis, abnormal vision, allergic reaction, arthritis, cataract, cellulitis, moniliasis, otitis media, eye hemorrhage, chills, abscess, bursitis, deafness, ear pain, glaucoma, iritis, neck rigidity, photosensitivity, retinal degeneration, tinnitus

Monotherapy with moexipril has been evaluated for safety in over 3000 patients. In clinical trials, the observed adverse experiences with moexipril were similar to those seen in the UNIRETIC trials.

Hydrochlorothiazide: The following adverse reactions have been reported with hydrochlorothiazide and, within each organ system, are listed by decreasing severity.

Cardiovascular: orthostatic hypotension (may be potentiated by alcohol, barbiturates, or narcotics)

Gastrointestinal: pancreatitis, jaundice (intrahepatic cholestatic, see WARNINGS), sialadenitis, vomiting, diarrhea, cramping, nausea, gastric irritation, constipation, anorexia

Neurologic/Psychiatric: vertigo, dizziness, transient blurred vision, headache, paresthesia, xanthopsia, weakness, restlessness

Musculoskeletal: muscle spasm

Hematologic: aplastic anemia, agranulocytosis, leukopenia, thrombocytopenia

Metabolic: hyperglycemia, glycosuria, hyperuricemia

Hypersensitivity: necrotizing angiitis, Stevens-Johnson syndrome, respiratory distress including pneumonitis and pulmonary edema, purpura, urticaria, rash, photosensitivity

Clinical Laboratory Test Findings

Serum Electrolytes: See PRECAUTIONS, General.

Creatinine and Blood Urea Nitrogen: As with other ACE inhibitors, minor increases in blood urea nitrogen or serum creatinine, reversible upon discontinuation of therapy, were observed in less than 1% of patients with essential hypertension who were treated with UNIRETIC. Increases are more likely to occur in patients with compromised renal function (see PRECAUTIONS, General).

Other (causal relationship unknown): Clinically important changes in standard laboratory tests were rarely associated with UNIRETIC administration.

OVERDOSAGE

No specific information is available on the treatment of overdosage with UNIRETIC. Treatment should be symptomatic and supportive. Therapy with UNIRETIC should be discontinued and the patient observed closely. Suggested measures include induction of emesis and/or gastric lavage and correction of dehydration, electrolyte imbalance and hypotension by established procedures.

Single oral doses of 2 g/kg moexipril were associated with significant lethality in mice. Rats, however, tolerated single oral doses of up to 3 g/kg. The oral LD_{50} of hydrochlorothiazide is greater than 10 g/kg in mice and rats. For the combination of moexipril hydrochloride and hydrochlorothiazide (ratio 7.5:12.5), the approximate LD_{50} was around 10 g/kg for mice and above 10 g/kg for rats. Addition of hydrochlorothiazide to moexipril hydrochloride did not increase the acute toxicity due to moexipril hydrochloride.

Human overdoses of moexipril have not been reported. In case reports of overdoses with other ACE inhibitors, hypotension has been the principal adverse effect noted. The most common signs and symptoms observed with an overdose of hydrochlororthiazide have been those of dehydration and electrolyte depletion (hypokalemia, hypochloremia, hyponatremia). If digitalis has also been administered, hypokalemia may accentuate cardiac arrhythmias.

No data are available to suggest that physiological maneuvers (e.g., maneuvers to change the pH of the urine) would accelerate elimination of moexipril and its metabolites. The dialyzability of moexipril is not known.

Angiotensin II could presumably serve as a specific antagonist-antidote in the setting of moexipril overdose, but angiotensin II is essentially unavailable outside of research facilities. Because the hypotensive effect of moexipril is achieved through vasodilation and effective hypovolemia, it is reasonable to treat moexipril overdose by infusion of normal saline solution. In addition, renal function and serum potassium should be monitored.

DOSAGE AND ADMINISTRATION

Moexipril and hydrochlorothiazide are effective treatments for hypertension. The recommended dosage range of moexipril is 7.5 to 30 mg daily, administered in a single or two divided doses one hour before meals, while hydrochlorothiazide is effective in a dosage of 12.5 to 50 mg daily.

The side effects (see WARNINGS) of moexipril are generally rare and apparently independent of dose; those of hydrochlorothiazide are a mixture of dose-dependent phenomena (primarily hypokalemia) and dose-independent phenomena (e.g., pancreatitis), the former much more common than the latter. Therapy with any combination of moexipril and hydrochlorothiazide will be associated with both sets of dose-independent side effects, but regimens in which moexipril is combined with low doses of hydrochlorothiazide produce minimal effects on serum potassium. In UNIRETIC controlled clinical trials, the average change in serum potassium was near zero in subjects who received 3.75/6.25 mg or 7.5/12.5 mg, but subjects who received 15/25 mg experienced a mild decrease in serum potassium, similar to that experienced by subjects who received hydrochlorothiazide 25 mg monotherapy. To minimize dose-independent side effects, it is usually appropriate to begin combination therapy only after a patient has failed to achieve the desired effect with monotherapy.

Dose Titration Guided by Clinical Effect: A patient whose blood pressure is not adequately controlled with either moexipril or hydrochlorothiazide monotherapy may be given UNIRETIC 7.5/12.5 or UNIRETIC 15/25 one hour before a meal. Further increases of moexipril, hydrochlorothiazide or both depend on clinical response. The hydrochlorothiazide dose should generally not be increased until 2–3 weeks have elapsed.

Total daily doses above 30 mg/50 mg a day have not been studied in hypertensive patients. Patients whose blood pressures are adequately controlled with 25 mg of hydrochlorothiazide daily, but who experience significant potassium loss with this regimen, may achieve blood-pressure control without electrolyte disturbance if they are switched to moexipril 3.75 mg/hydrochlorothiazide 6.25 mg (one-half of the UNIRETIC 7.5/12.5 tablet). For patients who experience an excessive reduction in blood pressure with UNIRETIC 7.5/12.5, the physician may consider prescribing moexipril 3.75 mg/hydrochlorothiazide 6.25 mg.

Continued on next page

Uniretic—Cont.

Replacement Therapy: The combination may be substituted for the titrated individual active ingredients.

Use in Renal Impairment: The usual dosage regimen of UNIRETIC does not need to be adjusted as long as the patient's creatinine clearance is > 40 mL/min/1.73 m^2 (serum creatinine approximately ≤ 3 mg/dL or 265 μmol/L). In patients with more severe renal impairment, loop diuretics are preferred to thiazides, so UNIRETIC is not recommended (see PRECAUTIONS, General).

HOW SUPPLIED

UNIRETIC (moexipril hydrochloride/hydrochlorothiazide) 7.5/12.5 tablets are yellow, oval, film-coated and scored with engraved code 712 on the unscored side and S and P on either side of the score. They are supplied as follows:

Bottles of 100 NDC 0091-3712-01

UNIRETIC (moexipril hydrochloride/hydrochlorothiazide) 15/25 tablets are yellow, oval, film-coated and scored with engraved code 725 on the unscored side and S and P on either side of the score. They are supplied as follows:

Bottles of 100 NDC 0091-3725-01

Store, tightly closed, at controlled room temperature 20°–25°C (68°–77°F). Protect from excessive moisture.

If product package is subdivided, dispense in tight containers as described in USP-NF.

PC2459B Rev. 5/98

Shown in Product Identification Guide, page 335

UNIVASC® ℞

[yū-nə-vask]

(moexipril hydrochloride)

Tablets

℞ Only

USE IN PREGNANCY

When used in pregnancy during the second and third trimesters, ACE inhibitors can cause injury and even death to the developing fetus. When pregnancy is detected, UNIVASC should be discontinued as soon as possible. **See WARNINGS, Fetal/Neonatal Morbidity and Mortality.**

DESCRIPTION

UNIVASC (moexipril hydrochloride), the hydrochloride salt of moexipril, has the empirical formula $C_{27}H_{34}N_2O_7$·HCl and a molecular weight of 535.04. It is chemically described as [3S-[2[R*(R*)],3R*]]-2-[2-[[1-(ethoxycarbonyl)-3-phenylpropyl]amino]-1-oxopropyl]-1,2,3,4-tetrahydro-6,7-dimethoxy-3-isoquinolinecarboxylic acid, monohydrochloride. It is a non-sulfhydryl containing precursor of the active angiotensin-converting enzyme (ACE) inhibitor moexiprilat and its structural formula is:

Moexipril hydrochloride is a fine white to off-white powder. It is soluble (about 10% weight-to-volume) in distilled water at room temperature.

UNIVASC is supplied as scored, coated tablets containing 7.5 mg and 15 mg of moexipril hydrochloride for oral administration. In addition to the active ingredient, moexipril hydrochloride, the tablet core contains the following inactive ingredients: lactose, magnesium oxide, crospovidone, magnesium stearate and gelatin. The film coating contains hydroxypropyl methylcellulose, hydroxypropyl cellulose, polyethylene glycol 6000, magnesium stearate, titanium dioxide, and ferric oxide.

CLINICAL PHARMACOLOGY

Mechanism of Action

Moexipril hydrochloride is a prodrug for moexiprilat, which inhibits ACE in humans and animals. The mechanism through which moexiprilant lowers blood pressure is believed to be primarily inhibition of ACE activity. ACE is a peptidyl dipeptidase that catalyzes the conversion of the inactive decapeptide angiotensin I to the vasoconstrictor substance angiotensin II. Angiotensin II is a potent peripheral vasoconstrictor that also stimulates aldosterone secretion by the adrenal cortex and provides negative feedback on renin secretion. ACE is identical to kininase II, an enzyme that degrades bradykinin, an endothelium-dependent vasodilator. Moexiprilat is about 1000 times as potent as moexipril in inhibiting ACE and kininase II. Inhibition of ACE results in decreased angiotensin II formation, leading to decreased vasoconstriction, increased plasma renin activity, and decreased aldosterone secretion. The latter results in diuresis and natriuresis and a small increase in serum potassium concentration (mean increases of about 0.25 mEq/L were seen when moexipril was used alone, see PRECAUTIONS).

Whether increased levels of bradykinin, a potent vasodepressor peptide, play a role in the therapeutic effects of moexipril remains to be elucidated. Although the principal mechanism of moexipril in blood pressure reduction is believed to be through the renin-angiotensin-aldosterone system, ACE inhibitors have some effect on blood pressure even in apparent low-renin hypertension. As is the case with other ACE inhibitors, however, the antihypertensive effect of moexipril is considerably smaller in black patients, a predominantly low-renin population, than in non-black hypertensive patients.

Pharmacokinetics and Metabolism

Pharmacokinetics: Moexipril's antihypertensive activity is almost entirely due to its deesterified metabolite, moexiprilat. Bioavailability of oral moexipril is about 13% compared to intravenous (I.V.) moexipril (both measuring the metabolite moexiprilat), and is markedly affected by food, which reduces the peak plasma level (C_{max}) and AUC (see Absorption). Moexipril should therefore be taken in a fasting state. The time of peak plasma concentration (T_{max}) of moexiprilat is about 1½ hours and elimination half-life (t½) is estimated at 2 to 9 hours in various studies, the variability reflecting a complex elimination pattern that is not simply exponential. Like all ACE inhibitors, moexiprilat has a prolonged terminal elimination phase, presumably reflecting slow release of drug bound to the ACE. Accumulation of moexiprilat with repeated dosing is minimal, about 30%, compatible with a functional elimination t½ of about 12 hours. Over the dose range of 7.5 to 30 mg, pharmacokinetics are approximately dose proportional.

Absorption: Moexipril is incompletely absorbed, with bioavailability as moexiprilat of about 13%. Bioavailability varies with formulation and food intake which reduces C_{max} and AUC by about 70% and 40% respectively after the ingestion of a low-fat breakfast or by 80% and 50% respectively after the ingestion of a high-fat breakfast.

Distribution: The clearance (CL) for moexipril is 441 mL/min and for moexiprilat 232 mL/min with a t½ of 1.3 and 9.8 hours, respectively. Moexiprilat is about 50% protein bound. The volume of distribution of moexiprilat is about 183 liters.

Metabolism and Excretion: Moexipril is relatively rapidly converted to its active metabolite moexiprilat, but persists longer than some other ACE inhibitor prodrugs, such that its t½ is over one hour and it has a significant AUC. Both moexipril and moexiprilat are converted to diketopiperazine derivatives and unidentified metabolites. After I.V. administration of moexipril, about 40% of the dose appears in urine as moexiprilat, about 26% as moexipril, with small amounts of the metabolites; about 20% of the I.V. dose appears in feces, principally as moexiprilat. After oral administration, only about 7% of the dose appears in urine as moexiprilat, about 1% as moexipril, with about 5% as other metabolites. Fifty-two percent of the dose is recovered in feces as moexiprilat and 1% as moexipril.

Special Populations:

Decreased Renal Function: The effective elimination t½ and AUC of both moexipril and moexiprilat are increased with decreasing renal function. There is insufficient information available to characterize this relationship fully, but at creatinine clearances in the range of 10 to 40 mL/min, the t½ of moexiprilat increased by a factor of 3 to 4.

Decreased Hepatic Function: In patients with mild to moderate cirrhosis given single 15 mg doses of moexipril, the C_{max} of moexipril was increased by about 50% and the AUC increased by about 120%, while the C_{max} for moexiprilat was decreased by about 50% and the AUC increased by almost 300%.

Elderly Patients: In elderly male subjects (65–80 years old) with clinically normal renal and hepatic function, the AUC and C_{max} of moexiprilat is about 30% greater than those of younger subjects (19–42 years old).

Pharmacokinetic Interactions With Other Drugs:

No clinically important pharmacokinetic interactions occurred when UNIVASC was administered concomitantly with hydrochlorothiazide, digoxin, or cimetidine.

Pharmacodynamics and Clinical Effect

Single and multiple doses of 15 mg or more of UNIVASC gives sustained inhibition of plasma ACE activity of 80–90%, beginning within 2 hours and lasting 24 hours (80%).

In controlled trials, the peak effects of orally administered moexipril increased with the dose administered over a dose range of 7.5 to 60 mg, given once a day. Antihypertensive effects were first detectable about 1 hour after dosing, with a peak effect between 3 and 6 hours after dosing. Just before dosing (i.e., at trough), the antihypertensive effects were less prominently related to dose and the antihypertensive effect tended to diminish during the 24-hour dosing interval when the drug was administered once a day.

In multiple dose studies in the dose range of 7.5 to 30 mg once daily, UNIVASC lowered sitting diastolic and systolic blood pressure effects at trough by 3 to 6 mmHg and 4 to 11 mmHg more than placebo, respectively. There was a tendency toward increased response with higher doses over this range. These effects are typical of ACE inhibitors but, to date, there are no trials of adequate size comparing moexipril with other antihypertensive agents.

The trough diastolic blood pressure effects of moexipril were approximately 3 to 6 mmHg in various studies. Generally, higher doses of moexipril leave a greater fraction of the peak blood pressure effect still present at trough. During dose titration, any decision as to the adequacy of a dosing regimen should be based on trough blood pressure measurements. If diastolic blood pressure control is not adequate at the end of the dosing interval, the dose can be increased or given as a divided (BID) regimen.

During chronic therapy, the antihypertensive effect of any dose of UNIVASC is generally evident within 2 weeks of treatment, with maximal reduction after 4 weeks. The antihypertensive effects of UNIVASC have been proven to continue during therapy for up to 24 months.

UNIVASC, like other ACE inhibitors, is less effective in decreasing trough blood pressures in blacks than in non-blacks. Placebo-corrected trough group mean diastolic blood pressure effects in blacks in the proposed dose range varied between +1 to −3 mmHg compared with responses in non-blacks of −4 to −6 mmHg.

The effectiveness of UNIVASC was not significantly influenced by patient age, gender, or weight. UNIVASC has been shown to have antihypertensive activity in both pre- and postmenopausal women who have participated in placebo-controlled clinical trials.

Formal interaction studies with moexipril have not been carried out with anithypertensive agents other than thiazide diuretics. In these studies, the added effect of moexipril was similar to its effect as monotherapy. In general, ACE inhibitors have less than additive effects with beta-adrenergic blockers, presumably because both work by inhibiting the renin-angiotensin system.

INDICATIONS AND USAGE

UNIVASC is indicated for treatment of patients with hypertension. It may be used alone or in combination with thiazide diuretics.

In using UNIVASC, consideration should be given to the fact that another ACE inhibitor, captopril, has caused agranulocytosis, particularly in patients with renal impairment or collagen-vascular disease. Available data are insufficient to show that UNIVASC does not have a similar risk (see WARNINGS).

In considering use of UNIVASC, it should be noted that in controlled trials ACE inhibitors have an effect on blood pressure that is less in black patients than in non-blacks. In addition, ACE inhibitors (for which adequate data are available) cause a higher rate of angioedema in black than in non-black patients (see WARNINGS, Angioedema).

CONTRAINDICATIONS

UNIVASC is contraindicated in patients who are hypersensitive to this product and in patients with a history of angioedema related to previous treatment with an ACE inhibitor.

WARNINGS

Anaphylactoid and Possibly Related Reactions

Presumably because angiotensin-converting enzyme inhibitors affect the metabolism of eicosanoids and polypeptides, including endogenous bradykinin, patients receiving ACE inhibitors, including UNIVASC, may be subject to a variety of adverse reactions, some of them serious.

Angioedema: Angioedema involving the face, extremities, lips, tongue, glottis, and/or larynx has been reported in patients treated with ACE inhibitors, including UNIVASC. Symptoms suggestive of angioedema or facial edema occurred in <0.5% of moexipril-treated patients in placebo-controlled trials. None of the cases were considered life-threatening and all resolved either without treatment or with medication (antihistamines or glucocorticoids). One patient treated with hydrochlorothiazide alone experienced laryngeal edema. No instances of angioedema were reported in placebo-treated patients.

In cases of angioedema, treatment should be promptly discontinued and the patient carefully observed until the swelling disappears. In instances where swelling has been confined to the face and lips, the condition has generally resolved without treatment, although antihistamines have been useful in relieving symptoms.

Angioedema associated with involvement of the tongue, glottis, or larynx, may be fatal due to airway obstruction. Appropriate therapy, e.g., subcutaneous epinephrine solution 1:1000 (0.3 to 0.5 mL) and/or measures to ensure a patent airway, should be promptly provided (see ADVERSE REACTIONS).

Anaphylactoid Reactions During Desensitization: Two patients undergoing desensitizing treatment with hymenoptera venom while receiving ACE inhibitors sustained life-threatening anaphylactoid reactions. In the same patients, these reactions did not occur when ACE inhibitors were temporarily withheld, but they reappeared when the ACE inhibitors were inadvertently readministered.

Anaphylactoid Reactions During Membrane Exposure: Anaphylactoid reactions have been reported in patients dialyzed with high-flux membranes and treated concomitantly with an ACE inhibitor. Anaphylactoid reactions have also been reported in patients undergoing low-density lipoprotein apheresis with dextran sulfate absorption.

Hypotension

UNIVASC can cause symptomatic hypotension, although, as with other ACE inhibitors, this is unusual in uncomplicated hypertensive patients treated with UNIVASC alone. Symptomatic hypotension was seen in 0.5% of patients given moexipril and led to discontinuation of therapy in about 0.25%. Symptomatic hypotension is most likely to occur in patients who have been salt- and volume-depleted as a result of prolonged diuretic therapy, dietary salt restriction, dialysis, diarrhea, or vomiting. Volume- and salt-depletion should be corrected and, in general, diuretics stopped, be-

fore initiating therapy with UNIVASC (see PRECAUTIONS, Drug Interactions, and ADVERSE REACTIONS).
In patients with congestive heart failure, with or without associated renal insufficiency, ACE inhibitor therapy may cause excessive hypotension, which may be associated with oliguria or progressive azotemia, and rarely, with acute renal failure and death. In these patients, UNIVASC therapy should be started under close medical supervision, and patients should be followed closely for the first two weeks of treatment and whenever the dose of moexipril or an accompanying diuretic is increased. Care in avoiding hypotension should also be taken in patients with ischemic heart disease, aortic stenosis, or cerebrovascular disease, in whom an excessive decrease in blood pressure could result in a myocardial infarction or a cerebrovascular accident.
If hypotension occurs, the patient should be placed in a supine position and, if necessary, treated with an intravenous infusion of normal saline. UNIVASC treatment usually can be continued following restoration of blood pressure and volume.

Neutropenia/Agranulocytosis

Another ACE inhibitor, captopril, has been shown to cause agranulocytosis and bone marrow depression, rarely in patients with uncomplicated hypertension, but more frequently in hypertensive patients with renal impairment, especially if they also have a collagen-vascular disease such as systemic lupus erythematosus or scleroderma. Although there were no instances of severe neutropenia (absolute neutrophil count $<500/mm^3$) among patients given UNIVASC, as with other ACE inhibitors, monitoring of white blood cell counts should be considered for patients who have collagen-vascular disease, especially if the disease is associated with impaired renal function. Available data from clinical trials of UNIVASC are insufficient to show that UNIVASC does not cause agranulocytosis at rates similar to captopril.

Fetal/Neonatal Morbidity and Mortality

ACE inhibitors can cause fetal and neonatal morbidity and death when administered to pregnant women. Several dozen cases have been reported in the world literature. When pregnancy is detected, ACE inhibitors should be discontinued as soon as possible.
The use of ACE inhibitors during the second and third trimesters of pregnancy has been associated with fetal and neonatal injury, including hypotension, neonatal skull hypoplasia, anuria, reversible or irreversible renal failure, and death.
Oligohydramnios has also been reported, presumably resulting from decreased fetal renal function; oligohydramnios in this setting has been associated with fetal limb contractures, craniofacial deformation, and hypoplastic lung development. Prematurity, intrauterine growth retardation, and patent ductus arteriosus have also been reported, although it is not clear whether these were caused by the ACE inhibitor exposure.
Fetal and neonatal morbidity do not appear to have resulted from intrauterine ACE inhibitor exposure limited to the first trimester. Mothers who have used ACE inhibitors only during the first trimester should be informed of this. Nonetheless, when patients become pregnant, physicians should make every effort to discontinue the use of moexipril as soon as possible. Rarely (probably less often than once in every thousand pregnancies), no alternative to ACE inhibitors will be found. In these rare cases, the mothers should be apprised of the potential hazards to their fetuses, and serial ultrasound examinations should be performed to assess the intraamniotic environment.
If oligohydramnios is observed, moexipril should be discontinued unless it is considered life-saving for the mother. Contractions stress testing (CST), a non-stress test (NST), or biophysical profiling (BPP) may be appropriate, depending upon the week of pregnancy. Patients and physicians should be aware, however, that oligohydramnios may not be detected until after the fetus has sustained irreversible injury.
Infants with histories of *in utero* exposure to ACE inhibitors should be closely observed for hypotension, oliguria, and hyperkalemia. If oliguria occurs, attention should be directed toward support of blood pressure and renal perfusion. Exchange transfusion or peritoneal dialysis may be required as means of reversing hypotension and/or substituting for disordered renal function.
Theoretically, the ACE inhibitor could be removed from the neonatal circulation by exchange transfusion, but no experience with this procedure has been reported.
No embryotoxic, fetotoxic, or teratogenic effects were seen in rats or in rabbits treated with up to 90.9 and 0.7 times, respectively, the Maximum Recommended Human Dose (MRHD) on a mg/m^2 basis.

Hepatic Failure

Rarely, ACE inhibitors have been associated with a syndrome that starts with cholestatic jaundice and progresses to fulminant hepatic necrosis and sometimes death. The mechanism of this syndrome is not understood. Patients receiving ACE inhibitors who develop jaundice or marked elevations of hepatic enzymes should discontinue the ACE inhibitor and receive appropriate medical follow-up.

PRECAUTIONS

General

Impaired Renal Function: As a consequence of inhibition of the renin-angiotensin-aldosterone system, changes in renal function may be anticipated in susceptible individuals. There is no clinical experience of UNIVASC in the treatment of hypertension in patients with renal failure.
Some hypertensive patients with no apparent preexisting renal vascular disease have developed increases in blood urea nitrogen and serum creatinine, usually minor and transient, especially when UNIVASC has been given concomitantly with a thiazide diuretic. This is more likely to occur in patients with preexisting renal impairment. There may be a need for dose adjustment of UNIVASC and/or the discontinuation of the thiazide diuretic.
Evaluation of hypertensive patients should always include assessment of renal function (see DOSAGE AND ADMINISTRATION).
Hypertensive Patients With Congestive Heart Failure: In hypertensive patients with severe congestive heart failure, whose renal function may depend on the activity of the renin-angiotensin-aldosterone system, treatment with ACE inhibitors, including UNIVASC, may be associated with oliguria and/or progressive azotemia and, rarely, acute renal failure and/or death.
Hypertensive Patients With Renal Artery Stenosis: In hypertensive patients with unilateral or bilateral renal artery stenosis, increase in blood urea nitrogen and serum creatinine have been observed in some patients following ACE inhibitor therapy. These increases were almost always reversible upon discontinuation of the ACE inhibitor and/or diuretic therapy. In such patients, renal function should be monitored during the first few weeks of therapy.
Hyperkalemia: In clinical trials, persistent hyperkalemia (serum potassium above 5.4 mEq/L) occurred in approximately 1.3% of hypertensive patients receiving UNIVASC. Risk factors for the development of hyperkalemia with ACE inhibitors include renal insufficiency, diabetes mellitus, and the concomitant use of potassium-sparing diuretics, potassium supplements, and/or potassium-containing salt substitutes, which should be used cautiously, if at all, with UNIVASC (see PRECAUTIONS, Drug Interactions).
Surgery/Anesthesia: In patients undergoing major surgery or during anesthesia with agents that produce hypotension, moexipril may block the effects of compensatory renin release. If hypotension occurs in this setting and is considered to be due to this mechanism, it can be corrected by volume expansion.
Cough: Presumably due to the inhibition of the degradation of endogenous bradykinin, persistent nonproductive cough has been reported with all ACE inhibitors, always resolving after discontinuation of therapy. ACE inhibitor-induced cough should be considered in the differential diagnosis of cough. In controlled trials with moexipril, cough was present in 6.1% of moexipril patients and 2.2% of patients given placebo.

Information for Patients

Food: Patients should be advised to take moexipril one hour before meals (see CLINICAL PHARMACOLOGY and DOSAGE AND ADMINISTRATION).
Angioedema: Angioedema, including laryngeal edema, may occur with treatment with ACE inhibitors, usually occurring early in therapy (within the first month). Patients should be so advised and told to report immediately any signs or symptoms suggesting angioedema (swelling of the face, extremities, eyes, lips, tongue, difficulty in breathing) and to take no more UNIVASC until they have consulted with the prescribing physician.
Symptomatic Hypotension: Patients should be cautioned that lightheadedness can occur with UNIVASC, especially during the first few days of therapy. If fainting occurs, the patient should stop taking UNIVASC and consult the prescribing physician.
All patients should be cautioned that excessive perspiration and dehydration may lead to an excessive fall in blood pressure because of reduction in fluid volume. Other causes of volume depletion such as vomiting or diarrhea may also lead to a fall in blood pressure; patients should be advised to consult their physician if they develop these conditions.
Hyperkalemia: Patients should be told not to use potassium supplements or salt substitutes containing potassium without consulting their physician.
Neutropenia: Patients should be told to report promptly any indication of infection (e.g., sore throat, fever) that could be a sign of neutropenia.
Pregnancy: Female patients of childbearing age should be told about the consequences of second- and third-trimester exposure to ACE inhibitors and should also be told that these consequences do not appear to have resulted from intrauterine ACE inhibitor exposure that has been limited to the first trimester. Patients should be asked to report pregnancies to their physicians as soon as possible.

Drug Interactions

Diuretics: Excessive reductions in blood pressure may occur in patients on diuretic therapy when ACE inhibitors are started. The possibility of hypotensive effects with UNIVASC can be minimized by discontinuing diuretic therapy for several days or cautiously increasing salt intake before initiation of treatment with UNIVASC. If this is not possible, the starting dose of moexipril should be reduced. (See WARNINGS and DOSAGE AND ADMINISTRATION).
Potassium Supplements and Potassium-Sparing Diuretics: UNIVASC can increase serum potassium because it decreases aldosterone secretion. Use of potassium-sparing diuretics (spironolactone, triamterene, amiloride) or potassium supplements concomitantly with ACE inhibitors can increase the risk of hyperkalemia. Therefore, if concomitant use of such agents is indicated, they should be given with caution and the patient's serum potassium should be monitored.
Oral Anticoagulants: Interaction studies with warfarin failed to identify any clinically important effect on the serum concentrations of the anticoagulant or on its anticoagulant effect.
Lithium: Increased serum lithium levels and symptoms of lithium toxicity have been reported in patients receiving ACE inhibitors during therapy with lithium. These drugs should be coadministered with caution, and frequent monitoring of serum lithium levels is recommended. If a diuretic is also used, the risk of lithium toxicity may be increased.
Other Agents: No clinically important pharmacokinetic interactions occurred when UNIVASC was administered concomitantly with hydrochlorothiazide, digoxin, or cimetidine. UNIVASC has been used in clinical trials concomitantly with calcium-channel-blocking agents, diuretics, H_2 blockers, digoxin, oral hypoglycemic agents, and cholesterol-lowering agents. There was no evidence of clinically important adverse interactions.

Carcinogenesis, Mutagenesis, Impairment of Fertility

No evidence of carcinogenicity was detected in long-term studies in mice and rats at doses up to 14 or 27.3 times the Maximum Recommended Human Dose (MRHD) on a mg/m^2 basis.
No mutagenicity was detected in the Ames test and microbial reverse mutation assay, with and without metabolic activation, or in an *in vivo* nucleus anomaly test. However, increased chromosomal aberration frequency in Chinese hamster ovary cells was detected under metabolic activation conditions at a 20-hour harvest time.
Reproduction studies have been performed in rabbits at oral doses up to 0.7 times the MRHD on a mg/m^2 basis, and in rats up to 90.9 times the MRHD on a mg/m^2 basis. No indication of impaired fertility, reproductive toxicity, or teratogenicity was observed.

Pregnancy

Pregnancy Categories C (first trimester) and D (second and third trimesters). See WARNINGS, Fetal/Neonatal Morbidity and Mortality.

Nursing Mothers

It is not known whether UNIVASC is excreted in human milk. Because many drugs are excreted in human milk, caution should be exercised when UNIVASC is given to a nursing mother.

Pediatric Use

Safety and effectiveness of UNIVASC in pediatric patients have not been established.

Geriatric Use

Clinical studies of UNIVASC did not include sufficient numbers of subjects aged 65 and over to determine whether they respond differently from younger subjects. Other reported clinical experience has not identified differences in responses between the elderly and younger patients. In general, dose selection for an elderly patient should be cautious, usually starting at the low end of the dosing range, reflecting the greater frequency of decreased hepatic, renal, or cardiac function, and of concomitant disease or other drug therapy.

ADVERSE REACTIONS

UNIVASC has been evaluated for safety in more than 2500 patients with hypertension; more than 250 of these patients were treated for approximately one year. The overall incidence of reported adverse events was only slightly greater in patients treated with UNIVASC than patients treated with placebo.
Reported adverse experiences were usually mild and transient, and there were no differences in adverse reaction rates related to gender, race, age, duration of therapy, or total daily dosage within the range of 3.75 mg to 60 mg. Discontinuation of therapy because of adverse experiences was required in 3.4% of patients treated with UNIVASC and in 1.8% of patients treated with placebo. The most common reasons for discontinuation in patients treated with UNIVASC were cough (0.7%) and dizziness (0.4%).
All adverse experiences considered at least possibly related to treatment that occurred at any dose in placebo-controlled trials of once-daily dosing in more than 1% of patients treated with UNIVASC alone and that were at least as frequent in the UNIVASC group as in the placebo group are shown in the following table:

ADVERSE EVENTS IN PLACEBO-CONTROLLED STUDIES

ADVERSE EVENT	UNIVASC (N=674)		PLACEBO (N=226)	
	N	(%)	N	(%)
Cough Increased	41	(6.1)	5	(2.2)
Dizziness	29	(4.3)	5	(2.2)
Diarrhea	21	(3.1)	5	(2.2)
Flu Syndrome	21	(3.1)	0	(0)
Fatigue	16	(2.4)	4	(1.8)
Pharyngitis	12	(1.8)	2	(0.9)
Flushing	11	(1.6)	0	(0)
Rash	11	(1.6)	2	(0.9)
Myalgia	9	(1.3)	0	(0)

Other adverse events occurring in more than 1% of patients on moexipril that were at least as frequent on placebo in-

Continued on next page

Univasc—Cont.

clude: headache, upper respiratory infection, pain, rhinitis, dyspepsia, nausea, peripheral edema, sinusitis, chest pain, and urinary frequency. See WARNINGS and PRECAUTIONS for discussion of anaphylactoid reactions, angioedema, hypotension, neutropenia/agranulocytosis, second and third trimester fetal/neonatal morbidity and mortality, hyperkalemia, and cough.

Other potentially important adverse experiences reported in controlled or uncontrolled clinical trials in less than 1% of moexipril patients or that have been attributed to other ACE inhibitors include the following:

Cardiovascular: Symptomatic hypotension, postural hypotension, or syncope were seen in 9/1750 (0.51%) patients; these reactions led to discontinuation of therapy in controlled trials in 3/1254 (0.24%) patients who had received UNIVASC monotherapy and in 1/344 (0.3%) patients who had received UNIVASC with hydrochlorothiazide (see PRECAUTIONS and WARNINGS). Other adverse events included angina/myocardial infarction, palpitations, rhythm disturbances, and cerebrovascular accident.

Renal: Of hypertensive patients with no apparent preexisting renal disease, 1% of patients receiving UNIVASC alone and 2% of patients receiving UNIVASC with hydrochlorothiazide experienced increases in serum creatinine to at least 140% of their baseline values (see PRECAUTIONS and DOSAGE AND ADMINISTRATION).

Gastrointestinal: Abdominal pain, constipation, vomiting, appetite/weight change, dry mouth, pancreatitis, hepatitis.

Respiratory: Bronchospasm, dyspnea, eosinophilic pneumonitis.

Urogenital: Renal insufficiency, oliguria.

Dermatologic: Apparent hypersensitivity reactions manifested by urticaria, rash, pemphigus, pruritus, photosensitivity.

Neurological and Psychiatric: Drowsiness, sleep disturbances, nervousness, mood changes, anxiety.

Other: Angioedema (see WARNINGS), taste disturbances, tinnitus, sweating, malaise, arthralgia, hemolytic anemia.

Clinical Laboratory Test Findings

Creatinine and Blood Urea Nitrogen: As with other ACE inhibitors, minor increases in blood urea nitrogen or serum creatinine, reversible upon discontinuation of therapy, were observed in approximately 1% of patients with essential hypertension who were treated with UNIVASC. Increases are more likely to occur in patients receiving concomitant diuretics and in patients with compromised renal function (see PRECAUTIONS, General).

Other (causal relationship unknown): Clinically important changes in standard laboratory tests were rarely associated with UNIVASC administration.

Elevations of liver enzymes and uric acid have been reported. In trials, less than 1% of moexipril-treated patients discontinued UNIVASC treatment because of laboratory abnormalities. The incidence of abnormal laboratory values with moexipril was similar to that in the placebo-treated group.

OVERDOSAGE

Human overdoses of moexipril have not been reported. In case reports of overdoses with other ACE inhibitors, hypotension has been the principal adverse effect noted. Single oral doses of 2 g/kg moexipril were associated with significant lethality in mice. Rats, however, tolerated single oral doses of up to 3 g/kg.

No data are available to suggest that physiological maneuvers (e.g., maneuvers to change the pH of the urine) would accelerate elimination of moexipril and its metabolites. The dialyzability of moexipril is not known.

Angiotensin II could presumably serve as a specific antagonist-antidote in the setting of moexipril overdose, but angiotensin II is essentially unavailable outside of research facilities. Because the hypotensive effect of moexipril is achieved through vasodilation and effective hypovolemia, it is reasonable to treat moexipril overdose by infusion of normal saline solution. In addition, renal function and serum potassium should be monitored.

DOSAGE AND ADMINISTRATION

Hypertension

The recommended initial dose of UNIVASC in patients not receiving diuretics is 7.5 mg, one hour prior to meals, once daily. Dosage should be adjusted according to blood pressure response. The antihypertensive effect of UNIVASC may diminish towards the end of the dosing interval. Blood pressure should, therefore, be measured just prior to dosing to determine whether satisfactory blood pressure control is obtained. If control is not adequate, increased dose or divided dosing can be tried. The recommended dose range is 7.5 to 30 mg daily, administered in one or two divided doses one hour before meals. Total daily doses above 60 mg a day have not been studied in hypertensive patients.

In patients who are currently being treated with a diuretic, symptomatic hypotension may occasionally occur following the initial dose of UNIVASC. The diuretic should, if possible, be discontinued for 2 to 3 days before therapy with UNIVASC is begun, to reduce the likelihood of hypotension (see WARNINGS). If the patient's blood pressure is not controlled with UNIVASC alone, diuretic therapy may then be reinstituted. If diuretic therapy cannot be discontinued, an initial dose of 3.75 mg of UNIVASC should be used with medical supervision until blood pressure has stabilized (see WARNINGS and PRECAUTIONS, Drug Interactions).

Dosage Adjustment in Renal Impairment

For patients with a creatinine clearance ≤40 mL/min/1.73 m^2, an initial dose of 3.75 mg once daily should be given cautiously. Doses may be titrated upward to a maximum daily dose of 15 mg.

HOW SUPPLIED

UNIVASC (moexipril hydrochloride) 7.5 mg tablets are pink colored, biconvex, film-coated and scored with engraved code **707** on the unscored side and **SP** above and **7.5** below the score. They are supplied as follows:

Bottles of 90 (Unit-of-Use)	NDC 0091-3707-09
Bottles of 100	NDC 0091-3707-01

UNIVASC (moexipril hydrochloride) 15 mg tablets are salmon colored, biconvex, film-coated, and scored with engraved code **715** on the unscored side and **SP** above and **15** below the score. They are supplied as follows:

Bottles of 90 (Unit-of-Use)	NDC 0091-3715-09
Bottles of 100	NDC 0091-3715-01

Store, tightly closed, at controlled room temperature. Protect from excessive moisture.

If product package is subdivided, dispense in tight containers as described in USP-NF.

SCHWARZ PHARMA
Milwaukee, Wisconsin 53201

PC 1879G
Rev. 2/00

Shown in Product Identification Guide, page 335

VERELAN® ℞

[*vĕr′ă-lăn*]
(Verapamil HCl)
Sustained-Release Pellet Filled Capsules
Rx Only

DESCRIPTION

VERELAN (verapamil hydrochloride capsules) is a calcium ion influx inhibitor (slow channel blocker or calcium ion antagonist). VERELAN is available for oral administration as a 360 mg hard gelatin capsule (lavender cap/yellow body), a 240 mg hard gelatin capsule (dark blue cap/yellow body), a 180 mg hard gelatin capsule (light grey cap/yellow body), and a 120 mg hard gelatin capsule (yellow cap/yellow body). These pellet filled capsules provide a sustained-release of the drug in the gastrointestinal tract.

The structural formula of verapamil HCl is given below:

$C_{27}H_{38}N_2O_4$•HCl M.W. 491.07

Chemical name: Benzeneacetonitrile, α-[3-[[2-(3,4-dimethoxyphenyl)-ethyl]methylamino]propyl]-3,4-dimethoxy-α-(1-methylethyl) monohydrochloride.

Verapamil HCl is an almost white, crystalline powder, practically free of odor, with a bitter taste. It is soluble in water, chloroform, and methanol. Verapamil HCl is not structurally related to other cardioactive drugs.

In addition to verapamil HCl the VERELAN capsule contains the following inactive ingredients: fumaric acid, talc, sugar spheres, povidone, shellac, gelatin, FD&C red #40, yellow iron oxide, titanium dioxide, methylparaben, propylparaben, silicon dioxide, and sodium lauryl sulfate. In addition, the VERELAN 240 mg and 360 mg capsules contain FD&C blue #1 and D&C red #28; and the VERELAN 180 mg capsule contains black iron oxide.

CLINICAL PHARMACOLOGY

VERELAN is a calcium ion influx inhibitor (slow channel blocker or calcium ion antagonist) which exerts its pharmacologic effects by modulating the influx of ionic calcium across the cell membrane of the arterial smooth muscle as well as in conductile and contractile myocardial cells.

Normal sinus rhythm is usually not affected by verapamil HCl. However in patients with sick sinus syndrome, verapamil HCl may interfere with sinus node impulse generation and may induce sinus arrest or sinoatrial block. Atrioventricular block can occur in patients without preexisting conduction defects. (See **WARNINGS.**) Verapamil HCl does not alter the normal atrial action potential or intraventricular conduction time, but depresses amplitude, velocity of depolarization and conduction in depressed atrial fibers. Verapamil HCl may shorten the antegrade effective refractory period of accessory bypass tracts. Acceleration of ventricular rate and/or ventricular fibrillation has been reported in patients with atrial flutter or atrial fibrillation and a coexisting accessory AV pathway following administration of verapamil. (See **WARNINGS.**)

Verapamil HCl has a local anesthetic action that is 1.6 times that of procaine on an equimolar basis. It is not known whether this action is important at the doses used in man.

Mechanism of Action

Essential Hypertension

Verapamil HCl exerts antihypertensive effects by decreasing systemic vascular resistance, usually without orthostatic decreases in blood pressure or reflex tachycardia; bradycardia (rate less than 50 beats/minute is uncommon). Verapamil HCl regularly reduces arterial pressure at rest and at a given level of exercise by dilating peripheral arterioles and reducing the total peripheral resistance (afterload) against which the heart works.

Pharmacokinetics and Metabolism

With the immediate release formulations, more than 90% of the orally administered dose is absorbed, and peak plasma concentrations of verapamil are observed 1 to 2 hours after dosing. Because of rapid biotransformation of verapamil during its first pass through the portal circulation, the absolute bioavailability ranges from 20% to 35%. Chronic oral administration of the highest recommended dose (120 mg every 6 hours) resulted in plasma verapamil levels ranging from 125 to 400 ng/mL with higher values reported occasionally. A nonlinear correlation between the verapamil HCl dose administered and verapamil plasma levels does exist. During initial dose titration with verapamil a relationship exists between verapamil plasma concentrations and the prolongation of the PR interval. However, during chronic administration this relationship may disappear. The quantitative relationship between plasma verapamil concentrations and blood pressure reduction has not been fully characterized.

In a multiple dose pharmacokinetic study, peak concentrations for a single daily dose of VERELAN 240 mg were approximately 65% of those obtained with an 80 mg t.i.d. dose of the conventional immediate-release tablets, and the 24-hour post-dose concentrations were approximately 30% higher. At a total daily dose of 240 mg, VERELAN was shown to have a similar extent of verapamil bioavailability based on the AUC-24 as that obtained with the conventional immediate-release tablets. In this same study VERELAN doses of 120 mg, 240 mg and 360 mg once daily were compared after multiple doses. The ratios of the verapamil and norverapamil AUCs for the VERELAN 120 mg, 240 mg, and 360 mg once daily doses are 1 (565 ng·hr/mL):3 (1660 ng·hr/mL):5 (2729 ng·hr/mL) and 1 (621 ng·hr/mL):3 (1614 ng·hr/mL):4 (2535 ng·hr/mL) respectively, indicating that the AUC increased non-proportionately with increasing doses. Food does not affect the extent or rate of the absorption of verapamil from the controlled release VERELAN capsule. The VERELAN 240 mg capsule when administered with food had a C_{max} of 77 ng/mL which occurred 9.0 hours after dosing, and an AUC(0-inf) of 1387 ng·hr/mL. VERELAN 240 mg under fasting conditions had a C_{max} of 77 ng/mL which occurred 9.8 hours after dosing, and an AUC(0-inf) of 1541 ng·hr/mL.

The bioequivalence of VERELAN 240 mg, administered as the pellets sprinkled on applesauce and as the intact capsule, was demonstrated in a single-dose, cross-over study in 32 healthy adults. Comparative ratios (sprinkled/intact) of verapamil were 0.95, 1.02, and 1.01 for C_{max}, T_{max}, and AUC (O-inf) respectively. Similar results were observed with norverapamil.

The time to reach maximum verapamil concentrations (T_{max}) with VERELAN has been found to be approximately 7–9 hours in each of the single dose (fasting), single dose (fed), the multiple dose (steady state) studies and dose proportionality pharmacokinetic studies. Similarly the apparent half-life ($t_{1/2}$) has been found to be approximately 12 hours independent of dose. Aging may affect the pharmacokinetics of verapamil. Elimination half-life may be prolonged in the elderly.

In healthy man, orally administered verapamil HCl undergoes extensive metabolism in the liver. Twelve metabolites have been identified in plasma; all except norverapamil are present in trace amounts only. Norverapamil can reach steady-state plasma concentrations approximately equal to those of verapamil itself. The biologic activity of norverapamil appears to be approximately 20% that of verapamil. Approximately 70% of an administered dose of verapamil HCl is excreted as metabolites in the urine and 16% or more in the feces within 5 days. About 3% to 4% is excreted in the urine as unchanged drug. Approximately 90% is bound to plasma proteins. In patients with hepatic insufficiency, metabolism is delayed and elimination half-life prolonged up to 14 to 16 hours (see **PRECAUTIONS**), the volume of distribution is increased and plasma clearance reduced to about 30% of normal. Verapamil clearance values suggest that patients with liver dysfunction may attain therapeutic verapamil plasma concentrations with one-third of the oral daily dose required for patients with normal liver function.

After four weeks of oral dosing (120 mg q.i.d.), verapamil and norverapamil levels were noted in the cerebrospinal fluid with estimated partition coefficient of 0.06 for verapamil and 0.04 for norverapamil.

In 10 healthy males, administration of oral verapamil (80 mg every 8 hours for 6 days) and a single oral dose of ethanol (0.8 g/kg), resulted in a 17% increase in mean peak ethanol concentrations (106.45±21.40 to 124.23±24.74 mg/dL) compared with placebo. (See **PRECAUTIONS—Drug Interactions.)**

The area under the blood ethanol concentration versus time curve (AUC over 12 hours) increased by 30% (365.67±93.52 to 475.07±97.24 mg·hr/dL). Verapamil AUCs were positively correlated (r=0.71) to increased ethanol blood AUC values.

Hemodynamics and Myocardial Metabolism

Verapamil HCl reduces afterload and myocardial contractility. Improved left ventricular diastolic function in patients with IHSS and those with coronary heart disease has also been observed with verapamil HCl therapy. In most patients, including those with organic cardiac disease, the negative inotropic action of verapamil HCl is countered by reduction of afterload and cardiac index is usually not reduced. In patients with severe left ventricular dysfunction however, (e.g., pulmonary wedge pressure above 20 mmHg or ejection fraction lower than 30%), or in patients on beta-adrenergic blocking agents or other cardiodepressant drugs, deterioration of ventricular function may occur. (See **DRUG INTERACTIONS.**)

Pulmonary Function

Verapamil HCl does not induce broncho-constriction and hence, does not impair ventilatory function.

INDICATIONS AND USAGE

VERELAN (verapamil HCl) is indicated for the management of essential hypertension.

CONTRAINDICATIONS

Verapamil HCl is contraindicated in:

1. Severe left ventricular dysfunction. (See **WARNINGS.**)
2. Hypotension (less than 90 mm Hg systolic pressure) or cardiogenic shock.
3. Sick sinus syndrome (except in patients with a functioning artificial ventricular pacemaker).
4. Second- or third-degree AV block (except in patients with a functioning artificial ventricular pacemaker).
5. Patients with atrial flutter or atrial fibrillation and an accessory bypass tract (e.g., Wolff-Parkinson-White, Lown-Ganong-Levine syndromes). (See **WARNINGS.**)
6. Patients with known hypersensitivity to verapamil hydrochloride.

WARNINGS

Heart Failure

Verapamil has a negative inotropic effect which, in most patients, is compensated by its afterload reduction (decreased systemic vascular resistance) properties without a net impairment of ventricular performance. In clinical experience with 4,954 patients, 87 (1.8%) developed congestive heart failure or pulmonary edema. Verapamil should be avoided in patients with severe left ventricular dysfunction (e.g., ejection fraction less than 30% or moderate to severe symptoms of cardiac failure) and in patients with any degree of ventricular dysfunction if they are receiving a beta-adrenergic blocker. (See **Drug Interactions.**) Patients with milder ventricular dysfunction should, if possible, be controlled with optimum doses of digitalis and/or diuretics before verapamil treatment (note interactions with digoxin under: **PRECAUTIONS**).

Hypotension

Occasionally, the pharmacologic action of verapamil may produce a decrease in blood pressure below normal levels which may result in dizziness or symptomatic hypotension. The incidence of hypotension observed in 4,954 patients enrolled in clinical trials was 2.5%. In hypertensive patients, decreases in blood pressure below normal are unusual. Tilt table testing (60 degrees) was not able to induce orthostatic hypotension.

Elevated Liver Enzymes

Elevations of transaminases with and without concomitant elevations in alkaline phosphatase and bilirubin have been reported. Such elevations have sometimes been transient and may disappear even in the face of continued verapamil treatment. Several cases of hepatocellular injury related to verapamil have been proven by rechallenge; half of these had clinical symptoms (malaise, fever, and/or right upper quadrant pain) in addition to elevations of SGOT, SGPT, and alkaline phosphatase. Periodic monitoring of liver function in patients receiving verapamil is therefore prudent.

Accessory Bypass Tract (Wolff-Parkinson-White or Lown-Ganong-Levine)

Some patients with paroxysmal and/or chronic atrial flutter or atrial fibrillation and a coexisting accessory AV pathway have developed increased antegrade conduction across the accessory pathway bypassing the AV node, producing a very rapid ventricular response or ventricular fibrillation after receiving intravenous verapamil (or digitalis). Although a risk of this occurring with oral verapamil has not been established, such patients receiving oral verapamil may be at risk and its use in these patients is contraindicated. (See **CONTRAINDICATIONS.**)

Treatment is usually DC-cardioversion. Cardioversion has been used safely and effectively after oral verapamil.

Atrioventricular Block

The effect of verapamil on AV conduction and the SA node may lead to asymptomatic first-degree AV block and transient bradycardia, sometimes accompanied by nodal escape rhythms. PR interval prolongation is correlated with verapamil plasma concentrations, especially during the early titration phase of therapy. Higher degrees of AV block, however, were infrequently (0.8%) observed.

Marked first-degree block or progressive development to second- or third-degree AV block requires a reduction in dosage or, in rare instances, discontinuation of verapamil HCl and institution of appropriate therapy depending upon the clinical situation.

Patients with Hypertrophic Cardiomyopathy (IHSS)

In 120 patients with hypertrophic cardiomyopathy (most of them refractory or intolerant to propranolol) who received therapy with verapamil at doses up to 720 mg/day, a variety of serious adverse effects were seen. Three patients died in pulmonary edema; all had severe left ventricular outflow obstruction and a past history of left ventricular dysfunction. Eight other patients had pulmonary edema and/or severe hypotension; abnormally high (over 20 mm Hg) capillary wedge pressure and a marked left ventricular outflow obstruction were present in most of these patients. Concomitant administration of quinidine (see **Drug Interactions**) preceded the severe hypotension in 3 of the 8 patients (2 of whom developed pulmonary edema). Sinus bradycardia occurred in 11% of the patients, second-degree AV block in 4% and sinus arrest in 2%. It must be appreciated that this group of patients had a serious disease with a high mortality rate. Most adverse effects responded well to dose reduction and only rarely did verapamil have to be discontinued.

PRECAUTIONS

THE CONTENTS OF THE VERELAN CAPSULE SHOULD NOT BE CRUSHED OR CHEWED.

General

Use in Patients with Impaired Hepatic Function

Since verapamil is highly metabolized by the liver, it should be administered cautiously to patients with impaired hepatic function. Severe liver dysfunction prolongs the elimination half-life of immediate-release verapamil to about 14 to 16 hours; hence, approximately 30% of the dose given to patients with normal liver function should be administered to these patients. Careful monitoring for abnormal prolongation of the PR interval or other signs of excessive pharmacologic effects (see **OVERDOSAGE**) should be carried out.

Use in Patients with Attenuated (Decreased) Neuromuscular Transmission

It has been reported that verapamil decreases neuromuscular transmission in patients with Duchenne's muscular dystrophy, and that verapamil prolongs recovery from the neuromuscular blocking agent, vecuronium. It may be necessary to decrease the dosage of verapamil when it is administered to patients with attenuated neuromuscular transmission.

Use in Patients with Impaired Renal Function

About 70% of an administered dose of verapamil is excreted as metabolites in the urine. Until further data are available, verapamil should be administered cautiously to patients with impaired renal function. These patients should be carefully monitored for abnormal prolongation of the PR interval or other signs of overdosage (See **OVERDOSAGE.**)

Information for Patients

When the sprinkle method of administration is prescribed, details of the proper technique should be explained to the patient. (See **DOSAGE AND ADMINISTRATION.**)

Drug Interactions

Beta Blockers

Concomitant therapy with beta-adrenergic blockers and verapamil may result in additive negative effects on heart rate, atrioventricular conduction, and/or cardiac contractility. The combination of sustained-release verapamil and beta-adrenergic blocking agents has not been studied. However, there have been reports of excess bradycardia and AV block, including complete heart block, when the combination has been used for the treatment of hypertension.

For hypertensive patients, the risk of combined therapy may outweigh the potential benefits. The combination should be used only with caution and close monitoring.

Asymptomatic bradycardia (36 beats/min) with a wandering atrial pacemaker has been observed in a patient receiving concomitant timolol (a beta-adrenergic blocker) eyedrops and oral verapamil.

A decrease in metoprolol clearance has been reported when verapamil and metoprolol were administered together. A similar effect has not been observed when verapamil and atenolol are given together.

Digitalis

Clinical use of verapamil in digitalized patients has shown the combination to be well tolerated if digoxin doses are properly adjusted. Chronic verapamil treatment can increase serum digoxin levels by 50% to 75% during the first week of therapy, and this can result in digitalis toxicity. In patients with hepatic cirrhosis the influence of verapamil on digoxin kinetics is magnified. Maintenance digitalis doses should be reduced when verapamil is administered, and the patient should be carefully monitored to avoid over- or underdigitalization. Whenever overdigitalization is suspected, the daily dose of digoxin should be reduced or temporarily discontinued. Upon discontinuation of verapamil HCl, the patient should be reassessed to avoid underdigitalization.

Antihypertensive Agents

Verapamil administered concomitantly with oral antihypertensive agents (e.g., vasodilators, angiotensin-converting enzyme inhibitors, diuretics, beta blockers) will usually have an additive effect on lowering blood pressure. Patients receiving these combinations should be appropriately monitored. Concomitant use of agents that attenuate alpha-adrenergic function with verapamil may result in reduction in blood pressure that is excessive in some patients. Such an effect was observed in one study following the concomitant administration of verapamil and prazosin.

Antiarrhythmic Agents

Disopyramide: Until data on possible interactions between verapamil and disopyramide phosphate are obtained, disopyramide should not be administered within 48 hours before or 24 hours after verapamil administration.

Flecainide: A study in healthy volunteers showed that the concomitant administration of flecainide and verapamil may have additive effects on myocardial contractility, AV conduction, and repolarization. Concomitant therapy with flecainide and verapamil may result in additive negative inotropic effect and prolongation of atrioventricular conduction.

Quinidine: In a small number of patients with hypertrophic cardiomyopathy (IHSS), concomitant use of verapamil and quinidine resulted in significant hypotension. Until further data are obtained, combined therapy of verapamil and quinidine in patients with hypertrophic cardiomyopathy should probably be avoided.

The electrophysiological effects of quinidine and verapamil on AV conduction were studied in 8 patients. Verapamil significantly counteracted the effects of quinidine on AV conduction. There has been a report of increased quinidine levels during verapamil therapy.

Nitrates: Verapamil has been given concomitantly with short- and long-acting nitrates without any undesirable drug interactions. The pharmacologic profile of both drugs and the clinical experience suggest beneficial interactions.

Alcohol: Verapamil has been found to significantly inhibit ethanol elimination resulting in elevated blood ethanol concentrations that may prolong the intoxicating effects of alcohol. (See **CLINICAL PHARMACOLOGY—Pharmacokinetics and Metabolism.**)

Other

Aspirin: In a few reported cases, coadministration of verapamil with aspirin has led to increased bleeding times greater than observed with aspirin alone.

Cimetidine: The interaction between cimetidine and chronically administered verapamil has not been studied. Variable results on clearance have been obtained in acute studies of healthy volunteers; clearance of verapamil was either reduced or unchanged.

Lithium: Pharmacokinetic and pharmacodynamic interactions between oral verapamil and lithium have been reported. The former may result in a lowering of serum lithium levels in patients receiving chronic stable oral lithium therapy. The latter may result in an increased sensitivity to the effects of lithium. Patients receiving both drugs must be monitored carefully.

Carbamazepine: Verapamil therapy may increase carbamazepine concentrations during combined therapy. This may produce carbamazepine side effects such as diplopia, headache, ataxia, or dizziness.

Rifampin: Therapy with rifampin may markedly reduce oral verapamil bioavailability.

Phenobarbital: Phenobarbital therapy may increase verapamil clearance.

Cyclosporine: Verapamil therapy may increase serum levels of cyclosporine.

Inhalation Anesthetics: Animal experiments have shown that inhalation anesthetics depress cardiovascular activity by decreasing the inward movement of calcium ions. When used concomitantly, inhalation anesthetics and calcium antagonists, such as verapamil, should be titrated carefully to avoid excessive cardiovascular depression.

Neuromuscular Blocking Agents: Clinical data and animal studies suggest that verapamil may potentiate the activity of neuromuscular blocking agents (curare-like and depolarizing). It may be necessary to decrease the dose of verapamil and/or the dose of the neuromuscular blocking agent when the drugs are used concomitantly.

Carcinogenesis, Mutagenesis, Impairment of Fertility

An 18-month toxicity study in rats, at a low multiple (6-fold) of the maximum recommended human dose, and not the maximum tolerated dose, did not suggest a tumorigenic potential. There was no evidence of a carcinogenic potential of verapamil administered in the diet of rats for two years at doses of 10, 35 and 120 mg/kg per day or approximately 1x, 3.5x, and 12x, respectively, the maximum recommended human daily dose (480 mg per day or 9.6 mg/kg/day).

Verapamil was not mutagenic in the Ames test in 5 test strains at 3 mg per plate, with or without metabolic activation.

Studies in female rats at daily dietary doses up to 5.5 times (55 mg/kg/day) the maximum recommended human dose did not show impaired fertility. Effects on male fertility have not been determined.

Pregnancy

Pregnancy Category C. Reproduction studies have been performed in rabbits and rats at oral doses up to 1.5 (15 mg/kg/day) and 6 (60 mg/kg/day) times the maximum recommended human daily dose, respectively, and have revealed no evidence of teratogenicity. In the rat, however, this multiple of the human dose was embryocidal and retarded fetal growth and development, probably because of adverse maternal effects reflected in reduced weight gains of the dams. This oral dose has also been shown to cause hypotension in rats. There are no adequate and well-controlled studies in pregnant women. Because animal reproduction studies are not always predictive of human response, this drug should be used during pregnancy only if clearly needed. Verapamil crosses the placental barrier and can be detected in umbilical vein blood at delivery.

Labor and Delivery

It is not known whether the use of verapamil during labor or delivery has immediate or delayed adverse effects on the fetus, or whether it prolongs the duration of labor or increases the need for forceps delivery or other obstetric intervention. Such adverse experiences have not been reported in the literature, despite a long history of use of verapamil HCl in Europe in the treatment of cardiac side effects of beta-adrenergic agonist agents used to treat premature labor.

Continued on next page

Verelan—Cont.

Nursing Mothers
Verapamil is excreted in human milk. Because of the potential for adverse reactions in nursing infants from verapamil, nursing should be discontinued while verapamil is administered.
Pediatric Use
Safety and efficacy of verapamil in children below the age of 18 years have not been established.
Geriatric Use
Clinical studies of verapamil did not include sufficient numbers of subjects aged 65 and over to determine whether they respond differently from younger subjects. Other reported clinical experience has not identified differences in responses between the elderly and younger patients. In general, dose selection for an elderly patient should be cautious, usually starting at the low end of the dosing range, reflecting the greater frequency of decreased hepatic, renal, or cardiac function, and of concomitant disease or other drug therapy.
Animal Pharmacology and/or Animal Toxicology
In chronic animal toxicology studies verapamil causes lenticular and/or suture line changes at 30 mg/kg/day or greater and frank cataracts at 62.5 mg/kg/day or greater in the beagle dog but not the rat. Development of cataracts due to verapamil has not been reported in man.

ADVERSE REACTIONS

Serious adverse reactions are uncommon when verapamil HCl therapy is initiated with upward dose titration within the recommended single and total daily dose. See **WARNINGS** for discussion of heart failure, hypotension, elevated liver enzymes, AV block, and rapid ventricular response.
Reversible (upon discontinuation of verapamil) non-obstructive, paralytic ileus has been infrequently reported in association with the use of verapamil.
In clinical trials involving 285 hypertensive patients on VERELAN for greater than 1 week the following adverse reactions were reported in greater than 1.0% of the patients:

Constipation	7.4%
Headache	5.3%
Dizziness	4.2%
Lethargy	3.2%
Dyspepsia	2.5%
Rash	1.4%
Ankle Edema	1.4%
Sleep Disturbance	1.4%
Myalgia	1.1%

In clinical trials of other formulations of verapamil HCl (N=4,954) the following reactions have occurred at rates greater than 1.0%:

Constipation	7.3%
Dizziness	3.3%
Nausea	2.7%
Hypotension	2.5%
Edema	1.9%
Headache	2.2%
Rash	1.2%
CHF/Pulmonary Edema	1.8%
Fatigue	1.7%
Bradycardia (HR<50/min)	1.4%
AV block-total	
1°, 2°, 3°	1.2%
2° and 3°	0.8%
Flushing	0.6%
Elevated Liver Enzymes (see WARNINGS)	

In clinical trials related to the control of ventricular response in digitalized patients who had atrial fibrillation or atrial flutter, ventricular rate below 50/min at rest occurred in 15% of patients and asymptomatic hypotension occurred in 5% of patients.
The following reactions, reported in 1.0% or less of patients, occurred under conditions (open trials, marketing experience) where a causal relationship is uncertain; they are listed to alert the physician to a possible relationship:
Cardiovascular: angina pectoris, atrioventricular dissociation, chest pain, claudication, myocardial infarction, palpitations, purpura (vasculitis), syncope.
Digestive System: diarrhea, dry mouth, gastrointestinal distress, gingival hyperplasia.
Hemic and Lymphatic: ecchymosis or bruising.
Nervous System: cerebrovascular accident, confusion, equilibrium disorders, insomnia, muscle cramps, paresthesia, psychotic symptoms, shakiness, somnolence.
Respiratory: dyspnea.
Skin: arthralgia and rash, exanthema, hair loss, hyperkeratosis, maculae, sweating, urticaria, Stevens-Johnson syndrome, erythema multiforme.
Special Senses: blurred vision, tinnitus.
Urogenital: gynecomastia, impotence, increased urination, spotty menstruation.
Treatment of Acute Cardiovascular Adverse Reactions
The frequency of cardiovascular adverse reactions which require therapy is rare; hence, experience with their treatment is limited. Whenever severe hypotension or complete AV block occurs following oral administration of verapamil, the appropriate emergency measures should be applied immediately, e.g., intravenously administered isoproterenol HCl, levarterenol bitartrate, atropine (all in the usual doses), or calcium gluconate (10% solution). In patients with hypertrophic cardiomyopathy (IHSS), alpha-adrenergic agents (phenylephrine, metaraminol bitartrate or methoxamine) should be used to maintain blood pressure, and isoproterenol and levarterenol should be avoided. If further support is necessary, inotropic agents (dopamine or dobutamine) may be administered. Actual treatment and dosage should depend on the severity and the clinical situation and the judgment and experience of the treating physician.

OVERDOSAGE

There is no specific antidote for verapamil overdosage; treatment should be supportive. Delayed pharmacodynamic consequences may occur with sustained-release formulations, and patients should be observed for at least 48 hours, preferably under continuous hospital care. Reported effects include hypotension, bradycardia, cardiac conduction defects, arrhythmias, hyperglycemia, and decreased mental status. In addition, there have been literature reports of noncardiogenic pulmonary edema in patients taking large overdoses of verapamil (up to approximately 9g).
In acute overdosage, gastrointestinal decontamination with cathartics and whole bowel irrigation should be considered. Calcium, inotropes (i.e., isoproterenol, dopamine, and glucagon), atropine, vasopressors (i.e., norepinephrine, and epinephrine), and cardiac pacing have been used with variable results to reverse hypotension and myocardial depression. In a few reported cases, overdose with calcium channel blockers that was initially refractory to atropine became more responsive to this treatment when the patients received large doses (close to 1g/hour for more than 24 hours) of calcium chloride. Calcium chloride is preferred to calcium gluconate since it provides 3 times more calcium per volume. Asystole should be handled by the usual measures including cardiopulmonary resuscitation. Verapamil cannot be removed by hemodialysis.

DOSAGE AND ADMINISTRATION

Essential Hypertension
The dose of VERELAN should be individualized by titration. The usual daily dose of sustained-release verapamil, VERELAN, in clinical trials has been 240 mg given by mouth once daily in the morning. However, initial doses of 120 mg a day may be warranted in patients who may have an increased response to verapamil (e.g., elderly, small people, etc.). Upward titration should be based on therapeutic efficacy and safety evaluated approximately 24 hours after dosing. The antihypertensive effects of VERELAN are evident within the first week of therapy.
If adequate response is not obtained with 120 mg of VERELAN, the dose may be titrated upward in the following manner:
(a) 180 mg in the morning.
(b) 240 mg in the morning.
(c) 360 mg in the morning.
(d) 480 mg in the morning.
VERELAN sustained-release capsules are for once-a-day administration. When switching from immediate-release verapamil to VERELAN capsules, the same total daily dose of VERELAN capsules can be used.
As with immediate-release verapamil, dosages of VERELAN capsules should be individualized and titration may be needed in some patients.
Sprinkling the Capsule Contents on Food
VERELAN Pellet Filled Capsules may also be administered by carefully opening the capsule and sprinkling the pellets on a spoonful of applesauce. The applesauce should be swallowed immediately without chewing and followed with a glass of cool water to ensure complete swallowing of the pellets. The applesauce used should not be hot, and it should be soft enough to be swallowed without chewing. Any pellet/applesauce mixture should be used immediately and not stored for future use. Subdividing the contents of a VERELAN capsule is not recommended.

HOW SUPPLIED

VERELAN® verapamil HCl sustained-release pellet filled capsules are supplied in four dosage strengths:
120 mg—Two-piece, size 2 hard gelatin capsule (yellow cap/yellow body), printed with SCHWARZ above 2490 on left and VERELAN above 120 mg on right side of the capsule in black ink, supplied as follows:
NDC 0091-2490-23—Bottle of 100s
180 mg—Two-piece, size 1 elongated hard gelatin capsule (light grey cap/yellow body), printed with SCHWARZ above 2489 on left and VERELAN above 180 mg on right side of the capsule in black ink, supplied as follows:
NDC 0091-2489-23–Bottle of 100s
240 mg—Two-piece, size 0 hard gelatin capsule (dark blue cap/yellow body), printed with SCHWARZ above 2491 on left and VERELAN above 240 mg on right side of the capsule in black ink, supplied as follows:
NDC 0091-2491-23—Bottle of 100s
360 mg—Two-piece, size 00 hard gelatin capsule (lavender cap/yellow body), printed with SCHWARZ above 2495 on left and VERELAN above 360 mg on right side of the capsule in black ink, supplied as follows:
NDC 0091-2495-23—Bottle of 100s.
Store at controlled room temperature 20°–25°C (68°–77°F) [See USP]. Avoid excessive heat. Brief digressions above 25°C, while not detrimental, should be avoided. Protect from moisture.
Dispense in tight, light-resistant container as defined in USP.
Manufactured for:
SCHWARZ
PHARMA
Milwaukee, WI 53201
by
ELAN HOLDINGS, INC.
Gainesville, GA 30504
PC3799A Rev. 6/99
Shown in Product Identification Guide, page 335

VERELAN® PM ℞

[vĕr'ă-lăn]
(verapamil HCl)
Extended-Release Capsules
Controlled-Onset
Rx Only

DESCRIPTION

VERELAN® PM (verapamil hydrochloride) is a calcium ion influx inhibitor (slow channel blocker or calcium ion antagonist). VERELAN® PM is available for oral administration as a 100 mg hard gelatin capsule (white opaque cap/amethyst body), a 200 mg hard gelatin capsule (amethyst opaque cap/amethyst body), and as a 300 mg hard gelatin capsule (lavender opaque cap/amethyst body). Verapamil is administered as a racemic mixture of the R and S enantiomers.
This structural formulae of the verapamil HCl enantiomers are:

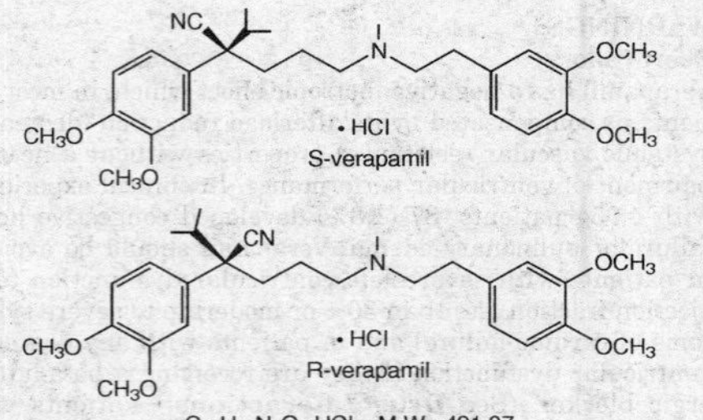

S-verapamil

R-verapamil

$C_{27}H_{38}N_2O_4$•HCl M.W.=491.07

Chemical name: Benzeneacetonitrile, α-[3-[[2-(3,4-dimethoxyphenyl)ethyl]methylamino]propyl]-3,4-dimethoxy-α-(1-methylethyl)-, monohydrochloride, (±)-.
Verapamil HCl is an almost white, crystalline powder, practically free of odor, with a bitter taste. It is soluble in water, chloroform and methanol. Verapamil HCl is not structurally related to other cardioactive drugs.
In addition to verapamil HCl the VERELAN® PM capsule contains the following inactive ingredients: D&C Red #28, FD & C Blue #1, FD&C red #40, fumaric acid, gelatin, povidone, shellac, silicon dioxide, sodium lauryl sulfate, starch, sugar spheres, talc, and titanium dioxide.

CLINICAL PHARMACOLOGY

Verapamil is a calcium ion influx inhibitor (L-type calcium channel blocker or calcium channel antagonist). Verapamil exerts its pharmacologic effects by selectively inhibiting the transmembrane influx of ionic calcium into arterial smooth muscle as well as in conductile and contractile myocardial cells without altering serum calcium concentrations.
System Components and Performance: VERELAN® PM uses the proprietary CODAS™ (Chronotherapeutic Oral Drug Absorption System) technology, which is designed for bedtime dosing, incorporating a 4 to 5-hour delay in drug delivery. The controlled-onset delivery system results in a maximum plasma concentration (C_{max}) of verapamil in the morning hours. These pellet filled capsules provide for extended-release of the drug in the gastrointestinal tract. The VERELAN® PM formulation has been designed to initiate the release of verapamil 4–5 hours after ingestion. This delay is introduced by the level of non-enteric release-controlling polymer applied to drug loaded beads. The release-controlling polymer is a combination of water soluble and water insoluble polymers. As water from the gastrointestinal tract comes into contact with the polymer coated beads, the water soluble polymer slowly dissolves and the drug diffuses through the resulting pores in the coating. The water insoluble polymer continues to act as a barrier, maintaining the controlled release of the drug. The rate of release is essentially independent of pH, posture and food. Multiparticulate systems such as VERELAN® PM have been shown to be independent of gastrointestinal motility.
Mechanism of Action
In vitro: Verapamil binding is voltage-dependent with affinity increasing as the vascular smooth muscle membrane potential is reduced. In addition, verapamil binding is frequency dependent and apparent affinity increases with increased frequency of depolarizing stimulus.
The L-type calcium channel is an oligomeric structure consisting of five putative subunits designated alpha-1, alpha-2, beta, tau, and epsilon. Biochemical evidence points to separate binding sites for 1,4-dihydropyridines, phenylalkylamines, and the benzothiazepines (all located on the alpha-1 subunit). Although they share a similar mechanism of action, calcium channel blockers represent three heterogeneous categories of drugs with differing vascular-cardiac selectivity ratios.
Essential hypertension: Verapamil produces its antihypertensive effect by a combination of vascular and cardiac effects. It acts as a vasodilator with selectivity for the arterial portion of the peripheral vasculature. As a result the sys-

temic vascular resistance is reduced and usually without orthostatic hypotension or reflex tachycardia. Bradycardia (rate less than 50 beats/min) is uncommon. During isometric or dynamic exercise verapamil does not alter systolic cardiac function in patients with normal ventricular function. Verapamil does not alter total serum calcium levels. However, one report has suggested that calcium levels above the normal range may alter the therapeutic effect of verapamil. Verapamil regularly reduces the total systemic resistance (afterload) against which the heart works both at rest and at a given level of exercise by dilating peripheral arterioles.

Effects in hypertension: VERELAN® PM was evaluated in two placebo-controlled, parallel design, double-blind studies of patients with mild to moderate hypertension. In the clinical trials, 413 evaluable patients were randomized to either placebo, 100 mg, 200 mg, 300 mg, or 400 mg and treated for up to 8 weeks. VERELAN® PM or placebo was given once daily between 9 pm and 11 pm (nighttime) and blood pressure changes were measured with 36-hour ambulatory blood pressure monitoring (ABPM). The results of these studies demonstrate that VERELAN® PM, at 200, 300 and 400 mg, is a consistently and significantly more effective antihypertensive agent than placebo in reducing ambulatory blood pressures. Over this dose range, the placebo-subtracted net decreases in diastolic BP at trough (averaged over 6–10 pm) were dose-related, and ranged from 3.8 to 10.0 mm Hg after 8 weeks of therapy. Although VERELAN® PM 100 mg was not effective in reducing diastolic BP at trough when measured by ABPM, efficacy was demonstrated in reducing diastolic BP when measured manually at trough and peak and, from 6 am to 12 noon and over 24 hours when measured by ABPM (See *Dosage and Administration for titration schedule*).

There were no apparent differences between patient subgroups of different age (older or younger than 65 years), sex and race. For severity of hypertension, "moderate" hypertensives (mean daytime diastolic BP ≥ 105 mm Hg and ≤ 114 mm Hg) appeared to respond better than "mild" hypertensives (mean daytime diastolic BP ≥ 90 mm Hg and ≤ 104 mm Hg). However, sample size for the sub-group comparisons were limited.

Electrophysiologic effects: Electrical activity through the AV node depends, to a significant degree, upon the transmembrane influx of extracellular calcium through the L-type (slow) channel. By decreasing the influx of calcium, verapamil prolongs the effective refractory period within the AV node and slows AV conduction in a rate-related manner.

Normal sinus rhythm is usually not affected, but in patients with sick sinus syndrome, verapamil may interfere with sinus-node impulse generation and may induce sinus arrest or sinoatrial block. Atrioventricular block can occur in patients without pre-existing conduction defects (See *WARNINGS*).

Verapamil does not alter the normal atrial action potential or intraventricular conduction time, but depresses amplitude, velocity of depolarization, and conduction in depressed atrial fibers. Verapamil may shorten the antegrade effective refractory period of the accessory bypass tract. Acceleration of ventricular rate and/or ventricular fibrillation has been reported in patients with atrial flutter or atrial fibrillation and a coexisting accessory AV pathway following administration of verapamil (See *WARNINGS*).

Verapamil has a local anesthetic action that is 1.6 times that of procaine on an equimolar basis. It is not known whether this action is important at the doses used in man.

Pharmacokinetics and metabolism: Verapamil is administered as a racemic mixture of the R and S enantiomers. The systemic concentrations of R and S enantiomers, as well as overall bioavailability, are dependent upon the route of administration and the rate and extent of release from the dosage forms. Upon oral administration, there is rapid stereoselective biotransformation during the first pass of verapamil through the portal circulation. In a study in 5 subjects with oral immediate-release verapamil, the systemic bioavailability was from 33% to 65% for the R enantiomer and from 13% to 34% for the S enantiomer. Following oral administration of an immediately releasing formulation every 8 hours in 24 subjects, the relative systemic availability of the S enantiomer compared to the R enantiomer was approximately 13% following a single day's administration and approximately 18% following administration to steady-state. The degree of stereoselectivity of metabolism for VERELAN® PM was similar to that for the immediately releasing formulation. The R and S enantiomers have differing levels of pharmacologic activity. In studies in animals and humans, the S enantiomer has 8 to 20 times the activity of the R enantiomer in slowing AV conduction. In animal studies, the S enantiomer has 15 to 50 times the activity of the R enantiomer in reducing myocardial contractility in isolated blood-perfused dog papillary muscle, respectively, and twice the effect in reducing peripheral resistance. In isolated septal strip preparations from 5 patients, the S enantiomer was 8 times more potent than the R in reducing myocardial contractility. Dose escalation study data indicate that verapamil concentrations increase disproportionally to dose as measured by relative peak plasma concentrations (C_{max}) or areas under the plasma concentration vs time curves (AUC).

Although some evidence of lack of dose linearity was observed for VERELAN® PM, this non-linearity was enantiomer specific, with the R enantiomer showing the greatest degree of non-linearity.

Pharmacokinetic Characteristics of Verapamil Enantiomers After Administration of Escalating Doses of VERELAN® PM

	ISOMER	200	300	400
Dose Ratio		1	1.5	2
Relative C_{max}	R	1	1.89	2.34
	S	1	1.88	2.5
Relative AUC	R	1	1.67	2.34
	S	1	1.35	2.20

[See table above]

Racemic verapamil is released from VERELAN® PM by diffusion following the gradual solubilization of the water soluble polymer. The rate of solubilization of the water soluble polymer produces a lag period in drug release for approximately 4–5 hours. The drug release phase is prolonged with the peak plasma concentration (C_{max}) occurring approximately 11 hours after administration. Trough concentrations occur approximately 4 hours after bedtime dosing while the patient is sleeping. Steady-state pharmacokinetics were determined in healthy volunteers. Steady-state concentration is achieved by day 5 of dosing.

In healthy volunteers, following administration of VERELAN® PM (200 mg per day), steady-state pharmacokinetics of the R and S enantiomers of verapamil is as follows: Mean C_{max} of the R isomer was 77.8 ng/ml and 16.8 ng/ml for the S isomer; AUC (0–24h) of the R isomer was 1037 ng.h/ml and 195 ng.h/ml for the S isomer.

In general, bioavailability of verapamil is higher and half life longer in older (>65 yrs) subjects. Lean body weight also affects its pharmacokinetics inversely. It was not possible to observe a gender difference in the clinical trials of VERELAN® PM due to the small sample size. However, there are conflicting data in the literature suggesting that verapamil clearance decreased with age in women to a greater degree than in men.

Consumption of a high fat meal just prior to dosing in the morning had no effect on the extent of absorption and a modest effect on the rate of absorption from VERELAN® PM. The rate of absorption was not affected by whether the volunteers were supine two hours after night-time dosing or non-supine for four hours following morning dosing. Administering VERELAN® PM in the morning increased the extent of absorption of verapamil and/or decreased the metabolism to norverapamil.

Orally administered verapamil undergoes extensive metabolism in the liver. Verapamil is metabolized by O-demethylation (25%) and N-dealkylation (40%), and is subject to presystemic hepatic metabolism with elimination of up to 80% of the dose. The metabolism is mediated by hepatic cytochrome P_{450}, and animal studies have implied that the mono-oxygenase is the specific isoenzyme of the P_{450} family. Thirteen metabolites have been identified in urine. Norverapamil enantiomers can reach steady-state plasma concentrations approximately equal to those of the enantiomers of the parent drug. For VERELAN® PM, the norverapamil R enantiomer reached steady-state plasma concentrations similar to the verapamil R enantiomer, but the norverapamil S enantiomer concentrations were approximately twice that of the verapamil S enantiomer concentrations. The cardiovascular activity of norverapamil appears to be approximately 20% that of verapamil. Approximately 70% of an administered dose is excreted as metabolites in the urine and 16% or more in the feces within 5 days. About 3% to 4% is excreted in the urine as unchanged drug.

R verapamil is 94% bound to plasma albumin, while S verapamil is 88% bound. In addition, R verapamil is 92% and S verapamil 86% bound to alpha-1 acid glycoprotein. In patients with hepatic insufficiency, metabolism of immediate-release verapamil is delayed and elimination half-life prolonged up to 14 to 16 hours because of the extensive hepatic metabolism (See *PRECAUTIONS*). In addition, in these patients there is a reduced first pass effect, and verapamil is more bioavailable. Verapamil clearance values suggest that patients with liver dysfunction may attain therapeutic verapamil plasma concentrations with one third of the oral daily dose required for patients with normal liver function.

After four weeks of oral dosing of immediate-release verapamil (120 mg q.i.d.), verapamil and norverapamil levels were noted in the cerebrospinal fluid with estimated partition coefficient of 0.06 for verapamil and 0.04 for norverapamil.

Hemodynamics: Verapamil reduces afterload and myocardial contractility. In most patients, including those with organic cardiac disease, the negative inotropic action of verapamil is countered by reduction of afterload and cardiac index remains unchanged. During isometric or dynamic exercise, verapamil does not alter systolic cardiac function in patients with normal ventricular function. Improved left ventricular diastolic function in patients with IHSS and those with coronary heart disease has also been observed with verapamil. In patients with severe left ventricular dysfunction (e.g., pulmonary wedge pressure above 20 mm Hg or ejection fraction less than 30%), or in patients taking beta-adrenergic blocking agents or other cardiodepressant drugs, deterioration of ventricular function may occur (See *Drug Interactions*).

Pulmonary function: Verapamil does not induce bronchoconstriction and, hence, does not impair ventilatory function. Verapamil has been shown to have either a neutral or relaxant effect on bronchial smooth muscle.

INDICATIONS AND USAGE

VERELAN® PM is indicated for the management of essential hypertension.

CONTRAINDICATIONS

Verapamil is contraindicated in:

1. Severe left ventricular dysfunction (See *WARNINGS*).
2. Hypotension (less than 90 mm Hg systolic pressure) or cardiogenic shock.
3. Sick sinus syndrome (except in patients with a functioning artificial ventricular pacemaker).
4. Second- or third-degree AV block (except in patients with a functioning artificial ventricular pacemaker).
5. Patients with atrial flutter or atrial fibrillation and an accessory bypass tract (e.g., Wolff-Parkinson-White, Lown-Ganong-Levine syndromes) (See *WARNINGS*).
6. Patients with known hypersensitivity to verapamil hydrochloride.

WARNINGS

Heart failure: Verapamil has a negative inotropic effect which, in most patients, is compensated by its afterload reduction (decreased systemic vascular resistance) properties without a net impairment of ventricular performance. In previous clinical experience with 4,954 patients primarily with immediate-release verapamil, 87 (1.8%) developed congestive heart failure or pulmonary edema. Verapamil should be avoided in patients with severe left ventricular dysfunction (e.g., ejection fraction less than 30% or moderate to severe symptoms of cardiac failure) and in patients with any degree of ventricular dysfunction if they are receiving a beta-adrenergic blocker (See *Drug Interactions*). Patients with milder ventricular dysfunction should, if possible, be controlled with optimum doses of digitalis and/or diuretics before verapamil treatment is started (See *PRECAUTIONS, Drug Interactions, Digitalis*).

Hypotension: Occasionally, the pharmacologic action of verapamil may produce a decrease in blood pressure below normal levels which may result in dizziness or symptomatic hypotension. The incidence of hypotension observed in 4,954 patients enrolled in clinical trials was 2.5%. In hypertensive patients, decreases in blood pressure below normal are unusual. Tilt table testing (60 degrees) was not able to induce orthostatic hypotension. In clinical studies of VERELAN® PM, 1.7% of the patients developed significant hypotension.

Elevated liver enzymes: Elevations of transaminases with and without concomitant elevations in alkaline phosphatase and bilirubin have been reported. Such elevations have sometimes been transient and may disappear even in the face of continued verapamil treatment.

Several cases of hepatocellular injury related to verapamil have been proven by rechallenge; half of these had clinical symptoms (malaise, fever, and/or right upper quadrant pain) in addition to elevations of SGOT, SGPT and alkaline phosphatase. Periodic monitoring of liver function in patients receiving verapamil is therefore prudent.

Accessory bypass tract (Wolff-Parkinson-White or Lown-Ganong Levine): Some patients with paroxysmal and/or chronic atrial flutter or atrial fibrillation and a coexisting accessory AV pathway have developed increased antegrade conduction across the accessory pathway bypassing the AV node, producing a very rapid ventricular response or ventricular fibrillation after receiving intravenous verapamil (or digitalis). Although a risk of this occurring with oral verapamil has not been established, such patients receiving oral verapamil may be at risk and its use in these patients is contraindicated (See *CONTRAINDICATIONS*).

Treatment is usually DC-cardioversion. Cardioversion has been used safely and effectively after oral verapamil.

Atrioventricular block

The effect of verapamil on AV conduction and the SA node may lead to asymptomatic first-degree AV block and transient bradycardia, sometimes accompanied by nodal escape rhythms PR interval prolongation is correlated with verapamil plasma concentrations, especially during the early titration phase of therapy. Higher degrees of AV block, however, were infrequently (0.8%) observed in previous verapamil clinical trials.

Marked first-degree block or progressive development to second- or third-degree AV block requires a reduction in dosage or, in rare instances, discontinuation of verapamil and institution of appropriate therapy depending upon the clinical situation.

Patients with hypertrophic cardiomyopathy (IHSS)

In 120 patients with hypertrophic cardiomyopathy (most of them refractory or intolerant to propranolol) who received therapy with verapamil at doses up to 720 mg/day, a variety

Continued on next page

Verelan PM—Cont.

of serious adverse effects were seen. Three patients died in pulmonary edema; all had severe left ventricular outflow obstruction and a past history of left ventricular dysfunction. Eight other patients had pulmonary edema and/or severe hypotension; abnormally high (over 20 mm Hg) pulmonary capillary wedge pressure and a marked left ventricular outflow obstruction were present in most of these patients. Concomitant administration of quinidine (See *Drug Interactions*) preceded the severe hypotension in 3 of the 8 patients (2 of whom developed pulmonary edema). Sinus bradycardia occurred in 11% of the patients, second-degree AV block in 4% and sinus arrest in 2%. It must be appreciated that this group of patients had a serious disease with a high mortality rate. Most adverse effects responded well to dose reduction and only rarely did verapamil have to be discontinued.

PRECAUTIONS

THE CONTENTS OF THE VERELAN® PM CAPSULE SHOULD NOT BE CRUSHED OR CHEWED.

General

Use in patients with impaired hepatic function: Since verapamil is highly metabolized by the liver, it should be administered cautiously to patients with impaired hepatic function. Severe liver dysfunction prolongs the elimination half-life of immediate-release verapamil to about 14 to 16 hours; hence, approximately 30% of the dose given to patients with normal liver function should be administered to these patients. Careful monitoring for abnormal prolongation of the PR interval or other signs of excessive pharmacologic effects (See *OVERDOSAGE*) should be carried out.

Use in patients with attenuated (decreased) neuromuscular transmission: It has been reported that verapamil decreases neuromuscular transmission in patients with Duchenne's muscular dystrophy, and that verapamil prolongs recovery from the neuromuscular blocking agent vecuronium. It may be necessary to decrease the dosage of verapamil when it is administered to patients with attenuated neuromuscular transmission.

Use in patients with impaired renal function: About 70% of an administered dose of verapamil is excreted as metabolites in the urine. Until further data are available, verapamil should be administered cautiously to patients with impaired renal function. These patients should be carefully monitored for abnormal prolongation of the PR interval or other signs of overdosage (See *OVERDOSAGE*).

Drug Interactions

Verapamil undergoes biotransformation by predominantly CYP3A4, however CYP1A2 and members of the CYP2C subfamily are involved in its metabolism. Coadministration of verapamil with other drugs metabolized by the above-mentioned enzymes may alter the bioavailability of either verapamil and/or the other drugs. Therefore, coadministration of narrow therapeutic index drugs with similar metabolic pathways as verapamil should be carefully monitored. Similarly, verapamil plasma levels in patients with hepatic dysfunction should be carefully monitored, due to decreased clearance of verapamil in these patients.

Alcohol: Verapamil has been found to significantly inhibit ethanol elimination resulting in elevated blood ethanol concentrations that may prolong the intoxicating effects of alcohol.

Antineoplastic agents: Verapamil can increase the efficacy of doxorubicin both in tissue culture systems and in patients. It raises the serum doxorubicin levels. The absorption of verapamil can be reduced by the cyclophosphamide, oncovin, procarbazine, prednisone (COPP) and the vindesine, adriamycin, cisplatin (VAC) cytotoxic drug regimens. Concomitant administration of R verapamil can decrease the clearance of paclitaxel.

Aspirin: In a few reported cases, coadministration of verapamil with aspirin has led to increased bleeding times greater than observed with aspirin alone.

Beta blockers: Concomitant therapy with beta-adrenergic blockers and verapamil may result in additive negative effects on heart rate, atrioventricular conduction, and/or cardiac contractility. The combination of extended-release verapamil and beta-adrenergic blocking agents has not been studied. However, there have been reports of excess bradycardia and AV block, including complete heart block, when the combination has been used for the treatment of hypertension. For hypertensive patients, the risk of combined therapy may outweigh the potential benefits. The combination should be used only with caution and close monitoring. Asymptomatic bradycardia (36 beats/min) with a wandering atrial pacemaker has been observed in a patient receiving concomitant timolol (a beta-adrenergic blocker) eyedrops and oral verapamil.

A decrease in metoprolol and propranolol clearance has been observed when either drug is administered concomitantly with verapamil. A variable effect has been seen when verapamil and atenolol were given together.

Digitalis: Clinical use of verapamil in digitalized patients has shown the combination to be well tolerated if digoxin doses are properly adjusted. However, chronic verapamil treatment can increase serum digoxin levels by 50% to 75% during the first week of therapy, and this can result in digitalis toxicity. In patients with hepatic cirrhosis the influence of verapamil on digoxin kinetics is magnified. Verapamil may reduce total body clearance and extrarenal clearance of digitoxin by 27% and 29%, respectively.

	Placebo N = 116	All Doses Studied N = 297
	%	%
Headache	11.2	12.1
Infection	6.9	12.1*
Constipation	0.9	8.8*
Flu Syndrome	2.6	3.7
Peripheral edema	0.9	3.7
Dizziness	0.9	3.0
Pharyngitis	2.6	3.0
Sinusitis	2.6	3.0
Dyspepsia	1.7	2.7
Rhinitis	2.6	2.7
Diarrhea	1.7	2.4
Pain	1.7	2.4
Rash	2.6	2.4
Asthenia	3.4	2.0
ECG Abnormal	3.4	2.0
Hypertension	2.0	1.7
Edema	0.0	1.7
Nausea	0.0	1.7
Accidental Injury	0.0	1.5

*Infection, primarily upper respiratory infection (URI) and unrelated to study medication. Constipation was typically mild and easily manageable. At the usual once-daily dose of 200 mg, the observed incidence of constipation was 3.9%.

Constipation	7.3%
Dizziness	3.3%
Nausea	2.7%
Hypotension	2.5%
Headache	2.2%
Edema	1.9%
CHF/Pulmonary Edema	1.8%
Fatigue	1.7%
Bradycardia (HR<50/min)	1.4%
Rash	1.2%
AV block (total 1°, 2°, 3°)	1.2%
AV block (2° and 3°)	0.8%
Flushing	0.6%
Elevated Liver Enzymes (See *WARNINGS*)	

Maintenance and digitalization doses should be reduced when verapamil is administered, and the patient should be reassessed to avoid over- or underdigitalization. Whenever overdigitalization is suspected, the daily dose of digoxin should be reduced or temporarily discontinued. On discontinuation of verapamil use, the patient should be reassessed to avoid underdigitalization. In previous clinical trials with other verapamil formulations related to the control of ventricular response in digitalized patients who had atrial fibrillation or atrial flutter, ventricular rates below 50/min at rest occurred in 15% of patients, and asymptomatic hypotension occurred in 5% of patients.

Antihypertensive agents

Verapamil administered concomitantly with oral antihypertensive agents (e.g., vasodilators, angiotensin-converting enzyme inhibitors, diuretics, beta blockers) will usually have an additive effect on lowering blood pressure. Patients receiving these combinations should be appropriately monitored. Concomitant use of agents that attenuate alpha-adrenergic function with verapamil may result in reduction in blood pressure that is excessive in some patients. Such an effect was observed in one study following the concomitant administration of verapamil and prazosin.

Antiarrhythmic agents

Disopyramide: Until data on possible interactions between verapamil and disopyramide are obtained, disopyramide should not be administered within 48 hours before or 24 hours after verapamil administration.

Flecainide: A study of healthy volunteers showed that the concomitant administration of flecainide and verapamil may have additive effects on myocardial contractility, AV conduction, and repolarization. Concomitant therapy with flecainide and verapamil may result in additive negative inotropic effect and prolongation of atrioventricular conduction.

Quinidine: In a small number of patients with hypertrophic cardiomyopathy (IHSS), concomitant use of verapamil and quinidine resulted in significant hypotension. Until further data are obtained, combined therapy of verapamil and quinidine in patients with hypertrophic cardiomyopathy should probably be avoided.

The electrophysiological effects of quinidine and verapamil on AV conduction were studied in 8 patients. Verapamil significantly counteracted the effects of quinidine on AV conduction. There has been a report of increased quinidine levels during verapamil therapy.

Other

Nitrates: Verapamil has been given concomitantly with short- and long-acting nitrates without any undesirable drug interactions. The pharmacologic profile of both drugs and the clinical experience suggest beneficial interactions.

Cimetidine: The interaction between cimetidine and chronically administered verapamil has not been studied. Variable results on clearance have been obtained in acute studies of healthy volunteers; clearance of verapamil was either reduced or unchanged.

Lithium: Increased sensitivity to the effects of lithium (neurotoxicity) has been reported during concomitant verapamil-lithium therapy with either no change or an increase in serum lithium levels. However, the addition of verapamil has also resulted in the lowering of serum lithium levels in patients receiving chronic stable oral lithium. Patients receiving both drugs must be monitored carefully.

Carbamazepine: Verapamil therapy may increase carbamazepine concentrations during combined therapy. This may produce carbamazepine side effects such as diplopia, headache, ataxia, or dizziness.

Rifampin: Therapy with rifampin may markedly reduce oral verapamil bioavailability.

Phenobarbital: Phenobarbital therapy may increase verapamil clearance.

Cyclosporine: Verapamil therapy may increase serum levels of cyclosporine.

Theophylline: Verapamil may inhibit the clearance and increase the plasma levels of theophylline.

Inhalation anesthetics: Animal experiments have shown that inhalation anesthetics depress cardiovascular activity by decreasing the inward movement of calcium ions. When used concomitantly, inhalation anesthetics and calcium antagonists, such as verapamil, should each be titrated carefully to avoid excessive cardiovascular depression.

Neuromusucular blocking agents: Clinical data and animal studies suggest that verapamil may potentiate the activity of neuromuscular blocking agents (curare-like and depolarizing). It may be necessary to decrease the dose of verapamil and/or the dose of the neuromuscular blocking agent when the drugs are used concomitantly.

Carcinogenesis, Mutagenesis, Impairment of Fertility

An 18-month toxicity study in rats, at a low multiple (6-fold) of the maximum recommended human dose, and not the maximum tolerated dose, did not suggest a tumorigenic potential. There was no evidence of a carcinogenic potential of verapamil administered in the diet of rats for two years at doses of 10, 35 and 120 mg/kg/day or approximately 1.3, 4.4 and 15 times, respectively, the maximum recommended human daily dose (400 mg/day or 8 mg/kg/day).

Verapamil was not mutagenic in the Ames test in 5 test strains at 3 mg per plate, with or without metabolic activation.

Studies in female rats at daily dietary doses up to 6.9 times (55 mg/kg/day) the maximum recommended human dose did not show impaired fertility. Effects on male fertility have not been determined.

Pregnancy

Pregnancy Category C. Reproduction studies have been performed in rabbits and rats at oral doses up to 1.9 (15 mg/kg/day) and 7.5 (60 mg/kg/day) times the human oral daily dose, respectively, and have revealed no evidence of teratogenicity. In the rat, however, this multiple of the human dose was embryocidal and retarded fetal growth and development, probably because of adverse maternal effects reflected in reduced weight gains of the dams. This oral dose has also been shown to cause hypotension in rats. There are no adequate and well-controlled studies in pregnant women. Because animal reproduction studies are not always predictive of human response, this drug should be used during pregnancy only if clearly needed. Verapamil crosses the placental barrier and can be detected in umbilical vein blood at delivery.

Labor and Delivery

It is not known whether the use of verapamil during labor or delivery has immediate or delayed adverse effects on the fetus, or whether it prolongs the duration of labor or increases the need for forceps delivery or other obstetric intervention. Such adverse experiences have not been reported in the literature, despite a long history of use of verapamil in Europe in the treatment of cardiac side effects of beta-adrenergic agonist agents used to treat premature labor.

Nursing Mothers

Verapamil is excreted in human milk. Because of the potential for adverse reactions in nursing infants from verapamil, nursing should be discontinued while verapamil is administered.

Pediatric Use

Safety and effectiveness in pediatric patients have not been established.

Geriatric Use

Clinical studies of VERELAN® PM were not adequate to determine if subjects aged 65 or over respond differently from younger patients. Other reported clinical experience has not identified differences in response between the elderly and younger patients; however, greater sensitivity to VERELAN® PM by some older individuals cannot be ruled out.

Aging, may affect the pharmacokinetics of verapamil. Elimination half-life may be prolonged in the elderly (See *CLINICAL PHARMACOLOGY, Pharmacokinetics and metabolism*).

Verapamil is highly metabolized by the liver, and about 70% of the administered dose is excreted as metabolites in the urine. Clinical circumstances, some of which may be more common in the elderly, such as hepatic or renal impairment, should be considered (See *PRECAUTIONS, General*). In general, lower initial doses of VERELAN® PM may be warranted in the elderly (See *DOSAGE AND ADMINISTRATION, Essential Hypertension*).

Animal Pharmacology and/or Animal Toxicology

In chronic animal toxicology studies verapamil caused lenticular and/or suture line changes at 30 mg/kg/day or greater and frank cataracts at 62.5 mg/kg/day or greater in the beagle dog but not in the rat. Development of cataracts due to verapamil has not been reported in man.

ADVERSE REACTIONS

Serious adverse reactions are uncommon when verapamil therapy is initiated with upward dose titration within the recommended single and total daily dose.

The following reactions to orally administered VERELAN® PM occurred at rates of 2.0% or greater or occurred at lower rates but appeared to be drug-related in clinical trials in hypertension.

[See first table at top of previous page]

See *WARNINGS* for discussion of heart failure, hypotension, elevated liver enzymes, AV block, and rapid ventricular response. Reversible (upon discontinuation of verapamil) non-obstructive, paralytic ileus has been infrequently reported in association with the use of verapamil.

In previous experience with other formulations of verapamil (N=4,954) the following reactions have occurred at rates greater than 1.0% or occurred at lower rates but appeared clearly drug related in clinical trials in 4,954 patients.

[See second table at top of previous page]

In clinical trials related to the control of ventricular response in digitalized patients who had atrial fibrillation or atrial flutter, ventricular rate below 50/min at rest occurred in 15% of patients and asymptomatic hypotension occurred in 5% of patients.

The following reactions, reported with orally administered verapamil in 2.0% or less of patients, occurred under conditions (open trials, marketing experience) where a causal relationship is uncertain; they are listed to alert the physician to a possible relationship:

Cardiovascular: angina pectoris, atrioventricular dissociation, chest pain, claudication, myocardial infarction, palpitations, purpura (vasculitis), syncope.

Digestive System: diarrhea, dry mouth, gastrointestinal distress, gingival hyperplasia.

Hemic and Lymphatic: ecchymosis or bruising.

Nervous System: cerebrovascular accident, confusion, equilibrium disorders, insomnia, muscle cramps, paresthesia, psychotic symptoms, shakiness, somnolence.

Respiratory: dyspnea.

Skin: arthralgia and rash, exanthema, hair loss, hyperkeratosis, macules, sweating, urticaria, Stevens-Johnson syndrome, erythema multiforme.

Special Senses: blurred vision, tinnitus.

Urogenital: gynecomastia, galactorrhea/hyperprolactinemia, impotence, increased urination, spotty menstruation.

Other: allergy aggravated.

Treatment of Acute Cardiovascular Adverse Reactions

The frequency of cardiovascular adverse reactions that require therapy is rare; hence, experience with their treatment is limited. Whenever severe hypotension or complete AV block occurs following oral administration of verapamil, the appropriate emergency measures should be applied immediately; e.g., intravenously administered norepinephrine bitartrate, atropine sulfate, isoproterenol HCl (all in the usual doses), or calcium gluconate (10% solution). In patients with hypertrophic cardiomyopathy (IHSS), alpha-adrenergic agents (phenylephrine HCl, metaraminol bitartrate, or methoxamine HCl) should be used to maintain blood pressure, and isoproterenol and norepinephrine should be avoided. If further support is necessary, inotropic agents (dopamine HCl or dobutamine HCl) may be administered. Actual treatment and dosage should depend on the severity of the clinical situation and the judgment and experience of the treating physician.

OVERDOSAGE

There is no specific antidote for verapamil overdosage; treatment should be supportive. Delayed pharmacodynamic consequences may occur with sustained-release formulations, and patients should be observed for at least 48 hours, preferably under continuous hospital care. Reported effects include hypotension, bradycardia, cardiac conduction defects, arrhythmias, hyperglycemia, and decreased mental status. In addition, there have been literature reports of noncardiogenic pulmonary edema in patients taking large overdoses of verapamil (up to approximately 9g).

In acute overdosage, gastrointestinal decontamination with cathartics and whole bowel irrigation should be considered. Calcium, inotropes (i.e., isoproterenol HCl, dopamine HCl, and glucagon), atropine sulfate, vasopressors (i.e., norepinephrine, and epinephrine), and cardiac pacing have been used with variable results to reverse hypotension and myocardial depression. In a few reported cases, overdose with calcium channel blockers that was initially refractory to atropine became more responsive to this treatment when the patients received large doses (close to 1 gram/hour for more than 24 hours) of calcium chloride.

Calcium chloride is preferred to calcium gluconate since it provides 3 times more calcium per volume. Asystole should be handled by the usual measures including cardiopulmonary resuscitation. Verapamil cannot be removed by hemodialysis.

DOSAGE AND ADMINISTRATION

Essential Hypertension

VERELAN® PM should be administered once daily at bedtime. Clinical trials studied doses of 100 mg, 200 mg, 300 mg and 400 mg. The usual daily dose of extended-release VERELAN® PM in clinical trials has been 200 mg given by mouth once daily at bedtime. In rare instances, initial doses of 100 mg a day may be warranted in patients who have an increased response to verapamil [e.g. patients with impaired renal function (See *PRECAUTIONS*), impaired hepatic function, elderly, small people, etc.]. Upward titration should be based on therapeutic efficacy and safety evaluated approximately 24 hours after dosing. The antihypertensive effects of VERELAN® PM are evident within the first week of therapy.

If an adequate response is not obtained with 200 mg of VERELAN® PM, the dose may be titrated upward in the following manner:

a) 300 mg each evening

b) 400 mg each evening (2 × 200 mg)

When VERELAN® PM is administered at bedtime, office evaluation of blood pressure during morning and early afternoon hours is essentially a measure of peak effect. The usual evaluation of trough effect, which sometimes might be needed to evaluate the appropriateness of any given dose of VERELAN® PM would be just prior to bedtime.

As with immediate-release and sustained-release verapamil, dosages of VERELAN® PM capsules should be individualized and titration may be needed in some patients.

HOW SUPPLIED

VERELAN® PM (verapamil HCl) extended-release pellet filled capsules are supplied in three dosage strengths:

100 mg: Two piece size 2 hard gelatin capsule, white opaque cap imprinted SCHWARZ/4085 and amethyst body imprinted with 100 mg. Product identification printed in black ink, supplied as follows:
NDC 0091-4085-01 Bottle of 100s

200 mg: Two piece size 0 hard gelatin capsule, amethyst opaque cap imprinted SCHWARZ/4086 and amethyst body imprinted with 200 mg. Product identification printed in black ink, supplied as follows:
NDC 0091-4086-01 Bottle of 100s

300 mg: Two piece size 00 hard gelatin capsule, lavender opaque cap imprinted SCHWARZ/4087 and amethyst body imprinted with 300 mg. Product identification printed in black ink, supplied as follows:
NDC 0091-4087-01 Bottle of 100s

Store at 25°C (77°F); excursions permitted to 15–30°C (59–86°F). [See USP Controlled Room Temperature]. Protect from moisture.

Dispense in tight, light-resistant container as defined in USP.

Manufactured for:
SCHWARZ
PHARMA
Milwaukee, WI 53201
by
ELAN HOLDINGS, INC.
Gainesville, GA 30504
PC3810 11/98

Shown in Product Identification Guide, page 335

SCS Pharmaceuticals

BOX 5110
CHICAGO, IL 60680

Direct Inquiries to:
(800) 323-1603

For Medical Information Contact:
Generally:
G.D. Searle & Co.
Healthcare Information Services
5200 Old Orchard Road
Skokie, IL 60077
In Emergencies:
Outside IL:
(800) 323-4204 (business hours)
(847) 982-7000 (at other times)
Within IL:
(847) 982-7000

Sales and Ordering:
(800) 323-1603

Alphabetic Product Listing

Product, ID #, (NDC*), Form, Strength
Flagyl, I.V., 1804, Vial (partial fill, lyoph. pwd.), 500 mg
Piroxicam USP, 5752, Tablet, 10 mg
Piroxicam USP, 5762, Tablet, 20 mg

*When the product ID # is not the same as the NDC #, the NDC # appears in parentheses.

Product Information Available on Request
Piroxicam Tablets USP ℞

*When the product ID # is not the same as the NDC #, the NDC # appears in parentheses.

FLAGYL® I.V. ℞

[flaj 'yl]
(metronidazole hydrochloride)
STERILE
For Intravenous Infusion Only

WARNING

Metronidazole has been shown to be carcinogenic in mice and rats (see *Precautions*). Its use, therefore, should be reserved for the conditions described in the *Indications and Usage* section below.

DESCRIPTION

Flagyl I.V., sterile (metronidazole hydrochloride), is a parenteral dosage form of the synthetic antibacterial agent 1-(β-hydroxyethyl)-2-methyl-5-nitroimidazole hydrochloride.

Cl⁻ H CH₂CH₂OH
O₂N N⁺ CH₃
N

metronidazole hydrochloride

Each single-dose vial of lyophilized Flagyl I.V. contains sterile, nonpyrogenic metronidazole hydrochloride, equivalent to 500 mg metronidazole, and 415 mg mannitol.

CLINICAL PHARMACOLOGY

Metronidazole is a synthetic antibacterial compound. Disposition of metronidazole in the body is similar for both oral and intravenous dosage forms, with an average elimination half-life in healthy humans of 8 hours.

The major route of elimination of metronidazole and its metabolites is via the urine (60–80% of the dose), with fecal excretion accounting for 6–15% of the dose. The metabolites that appear in the urine result primarily from side-chain oxidation [1-(β-hydroxyethyl) -2- hydroxymethyl-5-nitroimidazole and 2-methyl-5-nitroimidazole-1-yl-acetic acid] and glucuronide conjugation, with unchanged metronidazole accounting for approximately 20% of the total. Renal clearance of metronidazole is approximately 10 mL/min/1.73 m^2.

Metronidazole is the major component appearing in the plasma, with lesser quantities of the 2-hydroxymethyl metabolite also being present. Less than 20% of the circulating metronidazole is bound to plasma proteins. Both the parent compound and the metabolite possess *in vitro* bactericidal activity against most strains of anaerobic bacteria.

Metronidazole appears in cerebrospinal fluid, saliva, and breast milk in concentrations similar to those found in plasma. Bactericidal concentrations of metronidazole have also been detected in pus from hepatic abscesses.

Plasma concentrations of metronidazole are proportional to the administered dose. An 8-hour intravenous infusion of 100–4,000 mg of metronidazole in normal subjects showed a linear relationship between dose and peak plasma concentration.

In patients treated with Flagyl I.V., using a dosage regimen of 15 mg/kg loading dose followed 6 hours later by 7.5 mg/kg every six hours, peak steady-state plasma concentrations of metronidazole averaged 25 mcg/mL with trough (minimum) concentrations averaging 18 mcg/mL.

Decreased renal function does not alter the single-dose pharmacokinetics of metronidazole. However, plasma clearance of metronidazole is decreased in patients with decreased liver function.

In one study newborn infants appeared to demonstrate diminished capacity to eliminate metronidazole. The elimination half-life, measured during the first 3 days of life, was inversely related to gestational age. In infants whose gestational ages were between 28 and 40 weeks, the corresponding elimination half-lives ranged from 109 to 22.5 hours.

Microbiology: Metronidazole is active *in vitro* against most obligate anaerobes, but does not appear to possess any clinically relevant activity against facultative anaerobes or obligate aerobes. Against susceptible organisms, metronidazole is generally bactericidal at concentrations equal to or slightly higher than the minimal inhibitory concentrations. Metronidazole has been shown to have *in vitro* and clinical activity against the following organisms:

- Anaerobic gram-negative bacilli, including:
  - *Bacteroides* species, including the *Bacteroides fragilis* group (*B. fragilis, B. distasonis, B. ovatus, B. thetaiotaomicron, B. vulgatus*)
  - *Fusobacterium* species
- Anaerobic gram-positive bacilli, including:
  - *Clostridium* species and susceptible strains of *Eubacterium*
- Anaerobic gram-positive cocci, including:
  - *Peptococcus* species
  - *Peptostreptococcus* species

Susceptibility Tests: Bacteriologic studies should be performed to determine the causative organisms and their susceptibility to metronidazole; however, the rapid, routine susceptibility testing of individual isolates of anaerobic bacteria is not always practical, and therapy may be started while awaiting these results.

Continued on next page

Flagyl I.V.—Cont.

Quantitative methods give the most accurate estimates of susceptibility to antibacterial drugs. A standardized agar dilution method and a broth microdilution method are recommended.[1]

Control strains are recommended for standardized susceptibility testing. Each time the test is performed, one or more of the following strains should be included: *Clostridium perfringens* ATCC 13124, *Bacteroides fragilis* ATCC 25285, and *Bacteroides thetaiotaomicron* ATCC 29741. The mode metronidazole MICs for those three strains are reported to be 0.25, 0.25, and 0.5 mcg/mL, respectively.

A clinical laboratory test is considered under acceptable control if the results of the control strains are within one doubling dilution of the mode MICs reported for metronidazole.

A bacterial isolate may be considered susceptible if the MIC value for metronidazole is not more than 16 mcg/mL. An organism is considered resistant if the MIC is greater than 16 mcg/mL. A report of "resistant" from the laboratory indicates that the infecting organism is not likely to respond to therapy.

INDICATIONS AND USAGE

Treatment of Anaerobic Infections

Flagyl I.V. (metronidazole hydrochloride) is indicated in the treatment of serious infections caused by susceptible anaerobic bacteria. Indicated surgical procedures should be performed in conjunction with Flagyl I.V. therapy. In a mixed aerobic and anaerobic infection, antibiotics appropriate for the treatment of the aerobic infection should be used in addition to Flagyl I.V.

Flagyl I.V. is effective in *Bacteroides fragilis* infections resistant to clindamycin, chloramphenicol, and penicillin.

INTRA-ABDOMINAL INFECTIONS, including peritonitis, intra-abdominal abscess, and liver abscess, caused by *Bacteroides* species including the *B. fragilis* group *(B. fragilis, B. distasonis, B. ovatus, B. thetaiotaomicron, B. vulgatus), Clostridium* species, *Eubacterium* species, *Peptococcus* species, and *Peptostreptococcus* species.

SKIN AND SKIN STRUCTURE INFECTIONS caused by *Bacteroides* species including the *B. fragilis* group, *Clostridium* species, *Peptococcus* species, *Peptostreptococcus* species, and *Fusobacterium* species.

GYNECOLOGIC INFECTIONS, including endometritis, endomyometritis, tubo-ovarian abscess, and postsurgical vaginal cuff infection, caused by *Bacteroides* species including the *B. fragilis* group, *Clostridium* species, *Peptococcus* species, and *Peptostreptococcus* species.

BACTERIAL SEPTICEMIA caused by *Bacteroides* species including the *B. fragilis* group, and *Clostridium* species.

BONE AND JOINT INFECTIONS, as adjunctive therapy, caused by *Bacteroides* species including the *B. fragilis* group.

CENTRAL NERVOUS SYSTEM (CNS) INFECTIONS, including meningitis and brain abscess, caused by *Bacteroides* species including the *B. fragilis* group.

LOWER RESPIRATORY TRACT INFECTIONS, including pneumonia, empyema, and lung abscess, caused by *Bacteroides* species including the *B. fragilis* group.

ENDOCARDITIS caused by *Bacteroides* species including the *B. fragilis* group.

Prophylaxis

The prophylactic administration of Flagyl I.V. preoperatively, intraoperatively, and postoperatively may reduce the incidence of postoperative infection in patients undergoing elective colorectal surgery which is classified as contaminated or potentially contaminated.

Prophylactic use of Flagyl I.V. should be discontinued within 12 hours after surgery. If there are signs of infection, specimens for cultures should be obtained for the identification of the causative organism(s) so that appropriate therapy may be given (see *Dosage and Administration*).

CONTRAINDICATIONS

Flagyl I.V. is contraindicated in patients with a prior history of hypersensitivity to metronidazole or other nitroimidazole derivatives.

WARNINGS

Convulsive Seizures and Peripheral Neuropathy: Convulsive seizures and peripheral neuropathy, the latter characterized mainly by numbness or paresthesia of an extremity, have been reported in patients treated with metronidazole. The appearance of abnormal neurologic signs demands the prompt evaluation of the benefit/risk ratio of the continuation of therapy.

PRECAUTIONS

General: Patients with severe hepatic disease metabolize metronidazole slowly, with resultant accumulation of metronidazole and its metabolites in the plasma. Accordingly, for such patients, doses below those usually recommended should be administered cautiously.

Administration of solutions containing sodium ions may result in sodium retention.

Known or previously unrecognized candidiasis may present more prominent symptoms during therapy with Flagyl I.V. and requires treatment with a candidacidal agent.

Laboratory Tests: Metronidazole is a nitroimidazole, and Flagyl I.V. should be used with care in patients with evidence of or history of blood dyscrasia. A mild leukopenia has been observed during its administration; however, no persistent hematologic abnormalities attributable to metronidazole have been observed in clinical studies. Total and differential leukocyte counts are recommended before and after therapy.

Drug Interactions: Metronidazole has been reported to potentiate the anticoagulant effect of warfarin and other oral coumarin anticoagulants, resulting in a prolongation of prothrombin time. This possible drug interaction should be considered when Flagyl I.V. is prescribed for patients on this type of anticoagulant therapy.

The simultaneous administration of drugs that induce microsomal liver enzymes, such as phenytoin or phenobarbital, may accelerate the elimination of metronidazole, resulting in reduced plasma levels; impaired clearance of phenytoin has also been reported.

The simultaneous administration of drugs that decrease microsomal liver enzyme activity, such as cimetidine, may prolong the half-life and decrease plasma clearance of metronidazole.

Alcoholic beverages should not be consumed during metronidazole therapy because abdominal cramps, nausea, vomiting, headaches, and flushing may occur.

Psychotic reactions have been reported in alcoholic patients who are using metronidazole and disulfiram concurrently. Metronidazole should not be given to patients who have taken disulfiram within the last two weeks.

Drug/Laboratory Test Interactions: Metronidazole may interfere with certain types of determinations of serum chemistry values, such as aspartate aminotransferase (AST, SGOT), alanine aminotransferase (ALT, SGPT), lactate dehydrogenase (LDH), triglycerides, and hexokinase glucose. Values of zero may be observed. All of the assays in which interference has been reported involve enzymatic coupling of the assay to oxidation-reduction of nicotine adenine dinucleotide ($NAD^+ \rightleftarrows NADH$). Interference is due to the similarity in absorbance peaks of NADH (340 nm) and metronidazole (322 nm) at pH 7.

Carcinogenesis, Mutagenesis, Impairment of Fertility: Tumorigenicity in Rodents—Metronidazole has shown evidence of carcinogenic activity in studies involving chronic, oral administration in mice and rats, but similar studies in the hamster gave negative results. Also, metronidazole has shown mutagenic activity in a number of *in vitro* assay systems, but studies in mammals (*in vivo*) failed to demonstrate a potential for genetic damage.

Pregnancy: Teratogenic Effects—Pregnancy Category B. Metronidazole crosses the placental barrier and enters the fetal circulation rapidly. Reproduction studies have been performed in rats at doses up to five times the human dose and have revealed no evidence of impaired fertility or harm to the fetus due to metronidazole. Metronidazole administered intraperitoneally to pregnant mice at approximately the human dose caused fetotoxicity; administered orally to pregnant mice, no fetotoxicity was observed. There are, however, no adequate and well-controlled studies in pregnant women. Because animal reproduction studies are not always predictive of human response, and because metronidazole is a carcinogen in rodents, these drugs should be used during pregnancy only if clearly needed.

Nursing Mothers: Because of the potential for tumorigenicity shown for metronidazole in mouse and rat studies, a decision should be made whether to discontinue nursing or to discontinue the drug, taking into account the importance of the drug to the mother. Metronidazole is secreted in breast milk in concentrations similar to those found in plasma.

Pediatric Use: Safety and effectiveness in pediatric patients have not been established.

ADVERSE REACTIONS

Two serious adverse reactions reported in patients treated with Flagyl I.V. have been convulsive seizures and peripheral neuropathy, the latter characterized mainly by numbness or paresthesia of an extremity. Since persistent peripheral neuropathy has been reported in some patients receiving prolonged oral administration of Flagyl® (metronidazole), patients should be observed carefully if neurologic symptoms occur and a prompt evaluation made of the benefit/risk ratio of the continuation of therapy.

The following reactions have also been reported during treatment with Flagyl I.V. (metronidazole hydrochloride):

Gastrointestinal: Nausea, vomiting, abdominal discomfort, diarrhea, and an unpleasant metallic taste.

Hematopoietic: Reversible neutropenia (leukopenia).

Dermatologic: Erythematous rash and pruritus.

Central Nervous System: Headache, dizziness, syncope, ataxia, and confusion.

Local Reactions: Thrombophlebitis after intravenous infusion. This reaction can be minimized or avoided by avoiding prolonged use of indwelling intravenous catheters.

Other: Fever. Instances of a darkened urine have also been reported, and this manifestation has been the subject of a special investigation. Although the pigment which is probably responsible for this phenomenon has not been positively identified, it is almost certainly a metabolite of metronidazole and seems to have no clinical significance.

The following adverse reactions have been reported during treatment with oral Flagyl (metronidazole):

Gastrointestinal: Nausea, sometimes accompanied by headache, anorexia, and occasionally vomiting; diarrhea, epigastric distress, abdominal cramping, and constipation.

Mouth: A sharp, unpleasant metallic taste is not unusual. Furry tongue, glossitis, and stomatitis have occurred; these may be associated with a sudden overgrowth of *Candida* which may occur during effective therapy.

Hematopoietic: Reversible neutropenia (leukopenia); rarely, reversible thrombocytopenia.

Cardiovascular: Flattening of the T-wave may be seen in electrocardiographic tracings.

Central Nervous System: Convulsive seizures, peripheral neuropathy, dizziness, vertigo, incoordination, ataxia, confusion, irritability, depression, weakness, and insomnia.

Hypersensitivity: Urticaria, erythematous rash, flushing, nasal congestion, dryness of the mouth (or vagina or vulva), and fever.

Renal: Dysuria, cystitis, polyuria, incontinence, a sense of pelvic pressure, and darkened urine.

Other: Proliferation of *Candida* in the vagina, dyspareunia, decrease of libido, proctitis, and fleeting joint pains sometimes resembling "serum sickness." If patients receiving metronidazole drink alcoholic beverages, they may experience abdominal distress, nausea, vomiting, flushing, or headache. A modification of the taste of alcoholic beverages has also been reported. Rare cases of pancreatitis, which abated on withdrawal of the drug, have been reported.

Crohn's disease patients are known to have an increased incidence of gastrointestinal and certain extraintestinal cancers. There have been some reports in the medical literature of breast and colon cancer in Crohn's disease patients who have been treated with metronidazole at high doses for extended periods of time. A cause and effect relationship has not been established. Crohn's disease is not an approved indication for Flagyl I.V.

OVERDOSAGE

Use of dosages of Flagyl I.V. (metronidazole hydrochloride) higher than those recommended has been reported. These include the use of 27 mg/kg three times a day for 20 days, and the use of 75 mg/kg as a single loading dose followed by 7.5 mg/kg maintenance doses. No adverse reactions were reported in either of the two cases.

Single oral doses of metronidazole, up to 15 g, have been reported in suicide attempts and accidental overdoses. Symptoms reported include nausea, vomiting, and ataxia.

Oral metronidazole has been studied as a radiation sensitizer in the treatment of malignant tumors. Neurotoxic effects, including seizures and peripheral neuropathy, have been reported after 5 to 7 days of doses of 6 to 10.4 g every other day.

Treatment: There is no specific antidote for overdose; therefore, management of the patient should consist of symptomatic and supportive therapy.

DOSAGE AND ADMINISTRATION

In elderly patients the pharmacokinetics of metronidazole may be altered and therefore monitoring of serum levels may be necessary to adjust the metronidazole dosage accordingly.

Treatment of Anaerobic Infections

The recommended dosage schedule for *adults* is:

Loading Dose

15 mg/kg infused over 1 hour (approximately 1 g for a 70-kg adult).

Maintenance Dose

7.5 mg/kg infused over one hour every 6 hours (approximately 500 mg for a 70-kg adult). The first maintenance dose should be instituted 6 hours following the initiation of the loading dose.

Parenteral therapy may be changed to oral Flagyl (metronidazole) when conditions warrant, based upon the severity of the disease and the response of the patient to Flagyl I.V. treatment. The usual adult oral dosage is 7.5 mg/kg every 6 hours.

A maximum of 4 g should not be exceeded during a 24-hour period.

Patients with severe hepatic disease metabolize metronidazole slowly, with resultant accumulation of metronidazole and its metabolites in the plasma. Accordingly, for such patients, doses below those usually recommended should be administered cautiously. Close monitoring of plasma metronidazole levels[2] and toxicity is recommended.

In patients receiving Flagyl I.V. in whom gastric secretions are continuously removed by nasogastric aspiration, sufficient metronidazole may be removed in the aspirate to cause a reduction in serum levels.

The dose of Flagyl I.V. should not be specifically reduced in anuric patients since accumulated metabolites may be rapidly removed by dialysis.

The usual duration of therapy is 7 to 10 days; however, infections of the bone and joint, lower respiratory tract, and endocardium may require longer treatment.

Prophylaxis

For surgical prophylactic use, to prevent postoperative infection in contaminated or potentially contaminated colorectal surgery, the recommended dosage schedule for adults is:

a. 15 mg/kg infused over 30 to 60 minutes and completed approximately 1 hour before surgery; followed by

b. 7.5 mg/kg infused over 30 to 60 minutes at 6 and 12 hours after the initial dose.

It is important that (1) administration of the initial preoperative dose be completed approximately one hour before surgery so that adequate drug levels are present in the serum and tissues at the time of initial incision, and (2) Flagyl I.V. be administered, if necessary, at 6-hour intervals to maintain effective drug levels. Prophylactic use of Flagyl I.V. should be limited to the day of surgery only, following the above guidelines.

CAUTION: Flagyl I.V. (metronidazole hydrochloride) is to be administered by slow intravenous drip infusion only, either as a continuous or intermittent infusion. I.V. admixtures containing metronidazole and other drugs should be avoided. If used with a primary intravenous fluid system, the primary solution should be discontinued during metronidazole infusion. DO NOT USE EQUIPMENT CONTAINING ALUMINUM (EG, NEEDLES, CANNULAE) THAT WOULD COME IN CONTACT WITH THE DRUG SOLUTION.

FLAGYL I.V.

Flagyl I.V. cannot be given by direct intravenous injection (I.V. bolus) because of the low pH (0.5 to 2.0) of the reconstituted product. FLAGYL I.V. MUST BE FURTHER DILUTED AND NEUTRALIZED FOR I.V. INFUSION.

Flagyl I.V. is prepared for use in two steps:
NOTE: ORDER OF MIXING IS IMPORTANT

A. Reconstitution
B. Dilution in intravenous solution followed by pH neutralization with sodium bicarbonate injection into the dilution.

Reconstitution: To prepare the solution, add 4.4 mL of one of the following diluents and mix thoroughly: Sterile Water for Injection, USP; Bacteriostatic Water for Injection, USP; 0.9% Sodium Chloride Injection, USP; or Bacteriostatic 0.9% Sodium Chloride Injection, USP. The resultant approximate withdrawal volume is 5.0 mL with an approximate concentration of 100 mg/mL.

The pH of the reconstituted product will be in the range of 0.5 to 2.0. Reconstituted Flagyl I.V. is clear, and pale yellow to yellow-green in color.

Dilution in Intravenous Solutions: Properly reconstituted Flagyl I.V. (metronidazole hydrochloride) may be added to a glass or plastic I.V. container not to exceed a concentration of 8 mg/mL. Any of the following intravenous solutions may be used: 0.9% Sodium Chloride Injection, USP; 5% Dextrose Injection, USP; or Lactated Ringer's Injection, USP.

NEUTRALIZATION IS REQUIRED PRIOR TO ADMINISTRATION. The final product should be mixed thoroughly and used within 24 hours.

Neutralization For Intravenous Infusion: Neutralize the intravenous solution containing Flagyl I.V. with approximately 5 mEq of sodium bicarbonate injection for each 500 mg of Flagyl I.V. used. Mix thoroughly. The pH of the neutralized intravenous solution will be approximately 6.0 to 7.0. Carbon dioxide gas will be generated with neutralization. It may be necessary to relieve gas pressure within the container.

Note: When the contents of one vial (500 mg) are diluted and neutralized to 100 mL, the resultant concentration is 5 mg/mL. Do not exceed an 8 mg/mL concentration of Flagyl I.V. in the neutralized intravenous solution, since neutralization will decrease the aqueous solubility and precipitation may occur. DO NOT REFRIGERATE NEUTRALIZED SOLUTIONS; otherwise, precipitation may occur.

Storage and Stability: Reconstituted vials of Flagyl I.V. are chemically stable for 96 hours when stored below 86°F (30°C) in room light.

Use diluted and neutralized intravenous solutions containing Flagyl I.V. within 24 hours of mixing.

Parenteral drug products should be inspected visually for particulate matter and discoloration prior to administration, whenever solution and container permit. Do not use if cloudy or precipitated or if the seal is not intact.

Use sterile equipment. It is recommended that the intravenous administration apparatus be replaced at least once every 24 hours.

HOW SUPPLIED

FLAGYL I.V.

Flagyl I.V., sterile (metronidazole hydrochloride), is supplied in single-dose lyophilized vials each containing 500 mg metronidazole equivalent, individually packaged in cartons of 10 vials.

Flagyl I.V., prior to reconstitution, should be stored below 77°F (25°C) and protected from light.

1. Proposed standard: PSM-11—Proposed Reference Dilution Procedure for Antimicrobic Susceptibility Testing of Anaerobic Bacteria, National Committee for Clinical Laboratory Standards; and Sutter, et al.: Collaborative Evaluation of a Proposed Reference Dilution Method of Susceptibility Testing of Anaerobic Bacteria, Antimicrob. Agents Chemother. *16:* 495–502 (Oct.) 1979; and Tally, et al.: *In Vitro* Activity of Thienamycin, Antimicrob. Agents Chemother. *14:* 436–438 (Sept.) 1978.

2. Ralph, E.D., and Kirby, W.M.M.: Bioassay of Metronidazole With Either Anaerobic or Aerobic Incubation, J. Infect. Dis. *132:* 587–591 (Nov.) 1975; or Gulaid, et al.: Determination of Metronidazole and Its Major Metabolites in Biological Fluids by High Pressure Liquid Chromatography, Br. J. Clin. Pharmacol. *6:* 430–432, 1978.

Rx only 7/23/99•A05040

G.D. Searle & Co.

BOX 5110
CHICAGO, IL 60680-5110

Direct Inquiries to:
(800) 323-1603

For Medical Information Contact:
Generally:
G.D. Searle & Co.
Healthcare Information Services
5200 Old Orchard Road
Skokie, IL 60077
In Emergencies:
Outside IL:
(800) 323-4204 (business hours)
(847) 982-7000 (at other times)
Within IL:
(847) 982-7000

Sales and Ordering:
(800) 323-1603

Alphabetic Product Listing
Product, ID# (NDC*), Form, Strength

Aldactazide, 1011, Tablet, 25 mg/25 mg
Aldactazide, 1021, Tablet, 50 mg/50 mg
Aldactone, 1001, Tablet, 25 mg
Aldactone, 1041, Tablet, 50 mg
Aldactone, 1031, Tablet, 100 mg
Ambien Ⓒ, 5401, Tablet, 5 mg
Ambien Ⓒ, 5421, Tablet, 10 mg
Arthrotec, 1141, Tablet, 50 mg/200 mcg
Arthrotec, 1421, Tablet, 75 mg/200 mcg
Calan, 40 (1771), Tablet, 40 mg
Calan, 80 (1851), Tablet, 80 mg
Calan, 120 (1861), Tablet, 120 mg
Calan SR, 120 (1901), Caplet, 120 mg
Calan SR, 180 (1911), Caplet, 180 mg
Calan SR, 240 (1891), Caplet, 240 mg
Celebrex, 7767, (1520), Capsule, 100 mg
Celebrex, 7767, (1525), Capsule, 200 mg
Covera-HS 180, (2011), Tablets, 180 mg
Covera-HS 240, (2021), Tablets, 240 mg
Cytotec, 1451, Tablet, 100 mcg
Cytotec, 1461, Tablet, 200 mcg
Daypro, 1381, Caplet, 600 mg
Demulen 1/35-21, Compack, 151, Tablet, 1 mg/35 mcg
Demulen 1/35-28, Compack, 151 (0161), Tablet, 1 mg/35 mcg
Demulen 1/50-21, Compack, 71, Tablet, 1 mg/50 mcg
Demulen 1/50-28, Compack, 71 (0081), Tablet, 1 mg/50 mcg
Flagyl, 1831, Tablet, 250 mg
Flagyl 500 (1821), Tablet, 500 mg
Flagyl 375, (1942), Capsule, 375 mg
Flagyl ER, 1961, Tablet, 750 mg
Kerlone, 10 (5101), Tablet, 10 mg
Kerlone, 20 (5201), Tablet, 20 mg
Lomotil Ⓒ, 61, Tablet, 2.5 mg/0.025 mg
Lomotil Ⓒ, Liquid, 66, 2.5 mg/0.025 mg per 5 ml
Norpace, 2752, Capsule, 100 mg
Norpace, 2762, Capsule, 150 mg
Norpace CR, 2732, Capsule, 100 mg
Norpace CR, 2742, Capsule, 150 mg
Synarel, Liquid, (0166), Bottle, 2 mg/ml

*When the product ID # is not the same as the NDC #, the NDC # appears in parentheses.

Product Information Available on Request
Flagyl Tablets

Various educational materials are available for physicians, pharmacists, nurses, physicians' assistants, and patients (through the physician). Please ask your Searle representative for information about these materials.

ALDACTAZIDE® ℞

[*al-dac 'tuh "zīde*]
(spironolactone with hydrochlorothiazide)

> *WARNING*
> Spironolactone, an ingredient of Aldactazide, has been shown to be a tumorigen in chronic toxicity studies in rats (see *Precautions*). Aldactazide should be used only in those conditions described under *Indications and Usage.* Unnecessary use of this drug should be avoided.
> Fixed-dose combination drugs are not indicated for initial therapy of edema or hypertension. Edema or hypertension requires therapy titrated to the individual patient. If the fixed combination represents the dosage so determined, its use may be more convenient in patient management. The treatment of hypertension and edema is not static but must be reevaluated as conditions in each patient warrant.

DESCRIPTION

Aldactazide oral tablets contain:

spironolactone	25 mg
hydrochlorothiazide	25 mg
or	
spironolactone	50 mg
hydrochlorothiazide	50 mg

Spironolactone (Aldactone®), an aldosterone antagonist, is 17- hydroxy-7α-mercapto-3-oxo-17α-pregn-4-ene- 21- carboxylic acid γ-lactone acetate and has the following structural formula:

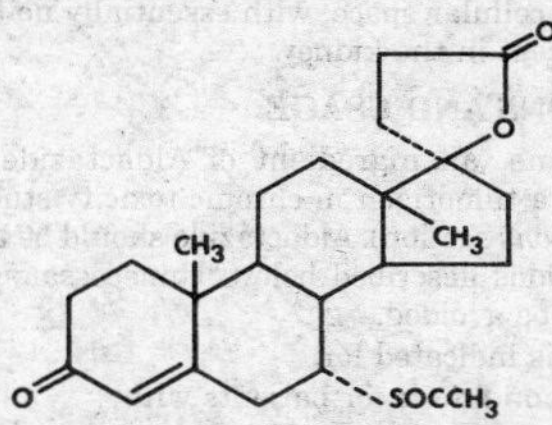

Spironolactone is practically insoluble in water, soluble in alcohol, and freely soluble in benzene and in chloroform.

Hydrochlorothiazide, a diuretic and antihypertensive, is 6-chloro-3, 4-dihydro-2H-1,2,4-benzothiadiazine-7-sulfonamide 1,1-dioxide and has the following structural formula:

Hydrochlorothiazide is slightly soluble in water and freely soluble in sodium hydroxide solution.

Inactive ingredients include calcium sulfate, corn starch, flavor, hydroxypropyl cellulose, hydroxypropyl methylcellulose, iron oxide, magnesium stearate, polyethylene glycol, povidone, and titanium dioxide.

ACTIONS/CLINICAL PHARMACOLOGY

Mechanism of action: Aldactazide is a combination of two diuretic agents with different but complementary mechanisms and sites of action, thereby providing additive diuretic and antihypertensive effects. Additionally, the spironolactone component helps to minimize the potassium loss characteristically induced by the thiazide component.

The diuretic effect of spironolactone is mediated through its action as a specific pharmacologic antagonist of aldosterone, primarily by competitive binding of receptors at the aldosterone-dependent sodium-potassium exchange site in the distal convoluted renal tubule. Hydrochlorothiazide promotes the excretion of sodium and water primarily by inhibiting their reabsorption in the cortical diluting segment of the distal renal tubule.

Aldactazide is effective in significantly lowering the systolic and diastolic blood pressure in many patients with essential hypertension, even when aldosterone secretion is within normal limits.

Both spironolactone and hydrochlorothiazide reduce exchangeable sodium, plasma volume, body weight, and blood pressure. The diuretic and antihypertensive effects of the individual components are potentiated when spironolactone and hydrochlorothiazide are given concurrently.

Pharmacokinetics: Spironolactone is rapidly and extensively metabolized. Sulfur-containing products are the predominant metabolites and are thought to be primarily responsible, together with spironolactone, for the therapeutic effects of the drug. The following pharmacokinetic data were obtained from 12 healthy volunteers following the administration of 100 mg of spironolactone (Aldactone film-coated tablets) daily for 15 days. On the 15th day, spironolactone was given immediately after a low-fat breakfast and blood was drawn thereafter.

[See table at top of next page]

The pharmacological activity of spironolactone metabolites in man is not known. However, in the adrenalectomized rat the antimineralocorticoid activities of the metabolites C, TMS, and HTMS, relative to spironolactone, were 1.10, 1.28, and 0.32, respectively. Relative to spironolactone, their binding affinities to the aldosterone receptors in rat kidney slices were 0.19, 0.86, and 0.06, respectively.

In humans the potencies of TMS and 7-α-thiospirolactone in reversing the effects of the synthetic mineralocorticoid, fludrocortisone, on urinary electrolyte composition were 0.33 and 0.26, respectively, relative to spironolactone. However, since the serum concentrations of these steroids were not determined, their incomplete absorption and/or first-pass metabolism could not be ruled out as a reason for their reduced *in vivo* activities.

Spironolactone and its metabolites are more than 90% bound to plasma proteins. The metabolites are excreted primarily in the urine and secondarily in bile.

The effect of food on spironolactone absorption (two 100-mg Aldactone tablets) was assessed in a single dose study of 9 healthy, drug-free volunteers. Food increased the bioavailability of unmetabolized spironolactone by almost 100%. The clinical importance of this finding is not known.

Hydrochlorothiazide is rapidly absorbed following oral administration. Onset of action of hydrochlorothiazide is ob-

Continued on next page

Aldactazide—Cont.

served within one hour and persists for 6 to 12 hours. Hydrochlorothiazide plasma concentrations attain peak levels at one to two hours and decline with a half-life of four to five hours. Hydrochlorothiazide undergoes only slight metabolic alteration and is excreted in urine. It is distributed throughout the extracellular space, with essentially no tissue accumulation except in the kidney.

	Accumulation Factor: AUC (0–24 hr, day 15)/AUC (0–24 hr, day 1)	Mean Peak Serum Concentration	Mean (SD) Post-Steady State Half-life
7-α-(thiomethyl) spirolactone (TMS)	1.25	391 ng/mL at 3.2 hr	13.8 hr (6.4) (terminal)
6-β-hydroxy-7-α-(thiomethyl) spirolactone (HTMS)	1.50	125 ng/mL at 5.1 hr	15.0 hr (4.0) (terminal)
Canrenone (C)	1.41	181 ng/mL at 4.3 hr	16.5 hr (6.3) (terminal)
Spironolactone	1.30	80 ng/mL at 2.6 hr	Approximately 1.4 hr (0.5) (β half-life)

INDICATIONS AND USAGE

Spironolactone, an ingredient of Aldactazide, has been shown to be a tumorigen in chronic toxicity studies in rats (see *Precautions* section). Aldactazide should be used only in those conditions described below. Unnecessary use of this drug should be avoided.

Aldactazide is indicated for:

Edematous conditions for patients with:

Congestive heart failure: For the management of edema and sodium retention when the patient is only partially responsive to, or is intolerant of, other therapeutic measures. The treatment of diuretic-induced hypokalemia in patients with congestive heart failure when other measures are considered inappropriate. The treatment of patients with congestive heart failure taking digitalis when other therapies are considered inadequate or inappropriate.

Cirrhosis of the liver accompanied by edema and/or ascites: Aldosterone levels may be exceptionally high in this condition. Aldactazide is indicated for maintenance therapy together with bed rest and the restriction of fluid and sodium.

The nephrotic syndrome: For nephrotic patients when treatment of the underlying disease, restriction of fluid and sodium intake, and the use of other diuretics do not provide an adequate response.

Essential hypertension

For patients with essential hypertension in whom other measures are considered inadequate or inappropriate. In hypertensive patients for the treatment of a diuretic-induced hypokalemia when other measures are considered inappropriate.

Usage in Pregnancy. The routine use of diuretics in an otherwise healthy woman is inappropriate and exposes mother and fetus to unnecessary hazard. Diuretics do not prevent development of toxemia of pregnancy, and there is no satisfactory evidence that they are useful in the treatment of developing toxemia.

Edema during pregnancy may arise from pathologic causes or from the physiologic and mechanical consequences of pregnancy. Aldactazide is indicated in pregnancy when edema is due to pathologic causes just as it is in the absence of pregnancy (however, see *: Pregnancy*). Dependent edema in pregnancy, resulting from restriction of venous return by the expanded uterus, is properly treated through elevation of the lower extremities and use of support hose; use of diuretics to lower intravascular volume in this case is unsupported and unnecessary. There is hypervolemia during normal pregnancy which is not harmful to either the fetus or the mother (in the absence of cardiovascular disease), but which is associated with edema, including generalized edema, in the majority of pregnant women. If this edema produces discomfort, increased recumbency will often provide relief. In rare instances, this edema may cause extreme discomfort which is not relieved by rest. In these cases, a short course of diuretics may provide relief and may be appropriate.

CONTRAINDICATIONS

Aldactazide is contraindicated in patients with anuria, acute renal insufficiency, significant impairment of renal excretory function, or hyperkalemia, and in patients who are allergic to thiazide diuretics or to other sulfonamide-derived drugs. Aldactazide may also be contraindicated in acute or severe hepatic failure.

WARNINGS

Potassium supplementation, either in the form of medication or as a diet rich in potassium, should not ordinarily be given in association with Aldactazide therapy. Excessive potassium intake may cause hyperkalemia in patients receiving Aldactazide (see *Precautions: General*). Aldactazide should not be administered concurrently with other potassium-sparing diuretics. Spironolactone, when used with ACE inhibitors or indomethacin, even in the presence of a diuretic, has been associated with severe hypokalemia. Extreme caution should be exercised when Aldactazide is given concomitantly with these drugs (see *Precautions: Drug interactions*).

Aldactazide should be used with caution in patients with impaired hepatic function because minor alterations of fluid and electrolyte balance may precipitate hepatic coma.

Lithium generally should not be given with diuretics (see *Precautions: Drug interactions.)*

Thiazides should be used with caution in severe renal disease. In patients with renal disease, thiazides may precipitate azotemia. Cumulative effects of the drug may develop in patients with impaired renal function.

Thiazides may add to or potentiate the action of other antihypertensive drugs.

Sensitivity reactions to thiazides may occur in patients with or without a history of allergy or bronchial asthma.

Sulfonamide derivatives, including thiazides, have been reported to exacerbate or activate systemic lupus erythematosus.

PRECAUTIONS

General: All patients receiving diuretic therapy should be observed for evidence of fluid or electrolyte imbalance, eg, hypomagnesemia, hyponatremia, hypochloremic alkalosis, and hypokalemia or hyperkalemia.

Serum and urine electrolyte determinations are particularly important when the patient is vomiting excessively or receiving parenteral fluids. Warning signs or symptoms of fluid and electrolyte imbalance, irrespective of cause, include dryness of the mouth, thirst, weakness, lethargy, drowsiness, restlessness, muscle pains or cramps, muscular fatigue, hypotension, oliguria, tachycardia, and gastrointestinal disturbances such as nausea and vomiting. Hyperkalemia may occur in patients with impaired renal function or excessive potassium intake and can cause cardiac irregularities, which may be fatal. Consequently, no potassium supplement should ordinarily be given with Aldactazide.

Concomitant administration of potassium-sparing diuretics and ACE inhibitors or nonsteroidal anti-inflammatory drugs (NSAIDs), eg, indomethacin, has been associated with severe hyperkalemia.

If hyperkalemia is suspected (warning signs include paresthesia, muscle weakness, fatigue, flaccid paralysis of the extremities, bradycardia and shock) an electrocardiogram (ECG) should be obtained. However, it is important to monitor serum potassium levels because mild hyperkalemia may not be associated with ECG changes.

If hyperkalemia is present, Aldactazide should be discontinued immediately. With severe hyperkalemia, the clinical situation dictates the procedures to be employed. These include the intravenous administration of calcium chloride solution, sodium bicarbonate solution and/or the oral or parenteral administration of glucose with a rapid-acting insulin preparation. These are temporary measures to be repeated as required. Cationic exchange resins such as sodium polystyrene sulfonate may be orally or rectally administered. Persistent hyperkalemia may require dialysis.

Hypokalemia may develop as a result of profound diuresis, particularly when Aldactazide is used concomitantly with loop diuretics, glucocorticoids, or ACTH, when severe cirrhosis is present or after prolonged therapy. Interference with adequate oral electrolyte intake will also contribute to hypokalemia. Hypokalemia may cause cardiac arrhythmias and may exaggerate the effects of digitalis therapy. Potassium depletion may induce signs of digitalis intoxication at previously tolerated dosage levels. Although any chloride deficit is generally mild and usually does not require specific treatment except under extraordinary circumstances (as in liver disease or renal disease), chloride replacement may be required in the treatment of metabolic alkalosis.

Aldactazide therapy may cause a transient elevation of BUN. This appears to represent a concentration phenomenon rather than renal toxicity, since the BUN level returns to normal after use of Aldactazide is discontinued. Progressive elevation of BUN is suggestive of the presence of preexisting renal impairment.

Reversible hyperchloremic metabolic acidosis, usually in association with hyperkalemia, has been reported to occur in some patients with decompensated hepatic cirrhosis, even in the presence of normal renal function.

Dilutional hyponatremia, manifested by dryness of the mouth, thirst, lethargy, and drowsiness, and confirmed by a low serum sodium level, may be induced, especially when Aldactazide is administered in combination with other diuretics, and dilutional hyponatremia may occur in edematous patients in hot weather; appropriate therapy is water restriction rather than administration of sodium, except in rare instances when the hyponatremia is life-threatening. A true low-salt syndrome may rarely develop with Aldactazide therapy and may be manifested by increasing mental confusion similar to that observed with hepatic coma. This syndrome is differentiated from dilutional hyponatremia in that it does not occur with obvious fluid retention. Its treatment requires that diuretic therapy be discontinued and sodium administered.

Hyperuricemia may occur or acute gout may be precipitated in certain patients receiving thiazides. Thiazides have been shown to increase the urinary excretion of magnesium; this may result in hypomagnesemia. Increases in cholesterol and triglyceride levels may be associated with thiazide diuretic therapy.

In diabetic patients, dosage adjustments of insulin or oral hypoglycemic agents may be required. Hyperglycemia may occur with thiazide diuretics. Thus, latent diabetes mellitus may become manifest during thiazide therapy.

The antihypertensive effects of Aldactazide may be enhanced in the post-sympathetectomy patient. If progressive renal impairment become evident, consider withholding or discontinuing diuretic therapy.

Thiazides may decrease urinary calcium excretion. Thiazides may cause intermittent and slight elevation of serum calcium in the absence of known disorders of calcium metabolism. Marked hypercalcemia may be evidence of hidden hyperparathyroidism. Thiazides should be discontinued before carrying out tests for parathyroid function. Pathologic changes in the parathyroid gland with hypercalcemia and hypophosphatemia have been observed in patients on prolonged thiazide therapy.

Gynecomastia may develop in association with the use of spironolactone; physicians should be alert to its possible onset. The development of gynecomastia appears to be related to both dosage level and duration of therapy and is normally reversible when Aldactazide is discontinued. In rare instances some breast enlargement may persist when Aldactazide is discontinued.

Information for patients: Patients who receive Aldactazide should be advised to avoid potassium supplements and foods containing high levels of potassium including salt substitutes.

Laboratory tests: Periodic determination of serum electrolytes to detect possible electrolyte imbalance should be done at appropriate intervals, particularly in the elderly and those with significant renal or hepatic impairments.

Drug interactions:

ACE inhibitors: Concomitant administration of ACE inhibitors with potassium-sparing diuretics has been associated with severe hyperkalemia.

Alcohol, barbiturates, or narcotics: Potentiation of orthostatic hypotension may occur.

Antidiabetic drugs (eg, oral agents, insulin): Dosage adjustment of the antidiabetic drug may be required.

Corticosteroids, ACTH: Intensified electrolyte depletion, particularly hypokalemia, may occur.

Pressor amines (eg, norepinephrine): Both spironolactone and hydrochlorothiazide reduce the vascular responsiveness to norepinephrine. Therefore, caution should be exercised in the management of patients subjected to regional or general anesthesia while they are being treated with Aldactazide.

Skeletal muscle relaxants, nondepolarizing (eg, tubocurarine): Possible increased reponsiveness to the muscle relaxant may result.

Lithium: Lithium generally should not be given with diuretics. Diuretic agents reduce the renal clearance of lithium and add a high risk of lithium toxicity.

Nonsteroidal anti-inflammatory drugs (NSAIDs): In some patients, the administration of an NSAID can reduce the diuretic, natriuretic, and antihypertensive effect of loop, potassium-sparing and thiazide diuretics. Combination of NSAIDs, eg, indomethacin, with potassium-sparing diuretics has been associated with severe hyperkalemia. Therefore, when Aldactazide and NSAIDs are used concomitantly, the patient should be observed closely to determine if the desired effect of the diuretic is obtained.

Digoxin: Spironolactone has been shown to increase the half-life of digoxin. This may result in increased serum digoxin levels and subsequent digitalis toxicity. It may be necessary to reduce the maintenance and digitalization doses when spironolactone is administered, and the patient should be carefully monitored to avoid over- or underdigitalization.

Drug/Laboratory test interactions: Thiazides should be discontinued before carrying out tests for parathyroid function (see *Precautions: General*). Thiazides may also decrease serum PBI levels without evidence of alteration of thyroid function.

Several reports of possible interference with digoxin radioimmunoassays by spironolactone or its metabolites have appeared in the literature. Neither the extent nor the potential clinical significance of its interference (which may be assay specific) has been fully established.

Carcinogenesis, mutagenesis, impairment of fertility:
Spironolactone: Orally administered spironolactone has been shown to be a tumorigen in dietary administration studies performed in rats, with its proliferative effects manifested on endocrine organs and the liver. In an 18-

month study using doses of about 50, 150 and 500 mg/kg/day, there were statistically significant increases in benign adenomas of the thyroid and testes and, in male rats, a dose-related increase in proliferative changes in the liver (including hepatocytomegaly and hyperplastic nodules). In a 24-month study in which the same strain of rat was administered doses of about 10, 30, 100 and 150 mg spironolactone/kg/day, the range of proliferative effects included significant increases in hepatocellular adenomas and testicular interstitial cell tumors in males, and significant increases in thyroid follicular cell adenomas and carcinomas in both sexes. There was also a statistically significant, but not dose-related, increase in benign uterine endometrial stromal polyps in females.

A dose-related (above 20 mg/kg/day) incidence of myelocytic leukemia was observed in rats fed daily doses of potassium canrenoate (a compound chemically similar to spironolactone and whose primary metabolite, canrenone, is also a major product of spironolactone in man) for a period of one year. In two year studies in the rat, oral administration of potassium canrenoate was associated with myelocytic leukemia and hepatic, thyroid, testicular and mammary tumors.

Neither spironolactone nor potassium canrenoate produced mutagenic effects in tests using bacteria or yeast. In the absence of metabolic activation, neither spironolactone nor potassium canrenoate has been shown to be mutagenic in mammalian tests *in vitro*. In the presence of metabolic activation, spironolactone has been reported to be negative in some mammalian mutagenicity tests *in vitro* and inconclusive (but slightly positive) for mutagenicity in other mammalian tests *in vitro*. In the presence of metabolic activation, potassium canrenoate has been reported to test positive for mutagenicity in some mammalian tests *in vitro*, inconclusive in others, and negative in still others.

In a three-litter reproduction study in which female rats received dietary doses of 15 and 50 mg spironolactone/kg/day, there were no effects on mating and fertility, but there was a small increase in incidence of stillborn pups at 50 mg/kg/day. When injected into female rats (100 mg/kg/day for 7 days, i.p.), spironolactone was found to increase the length of the estrous cycle by prolonging diestrus during treatment and inducing constant diestrus during a two week post-treatment observation period. These effects were associated with retarded ovarian follicle development and a reduction in circulating estrogen levels, which would be expected to impair mating, fertility and fecundity. Spironolactone (100 mg/kg/day), administered i.p. to female mice during a two week cohabitation period with untreated males, decreased the number of mated mice that conceived (effect shown to be caused by an inhibition of ovulation) and decreased the number of implanted embryos in those that became pregnant (effect shown to be caused by an inhibition of implantation), and at 200 mg/kg, also increased the latency period to mating.

Hydrochlorothiazide: Two-year feeding studies in mice and rats conducted under the auspices of the National Toxicology Program (NTP) uncovered no evidence of a carcinogenic potential of hydrochlorothiazide in female mice (at doses of up to approximately 600 mg/kg/day) or in male and female rats (at doses of up to approximately 100 mg/kg/day). The NTP, however, found equivocal evidence for hepatocarcinogenicity in male mice.

Hydrochlorothiazide was not genotoxic in *in vitro* assays using strains TA 98, TA 100, TA 1535, TA 1537 and TA 1538 of *Salmonella typhimurium* (Ames assay) and in the Chinese Hamster Ovary (CHO) test for chromosomal aberrations, or in *in vivo* assays using mouse germinal cell chromosomes, Chinese hamster bone marrow chromosomes, and the *Drosophila* sex-linked recessive lethal trait gene. Positive test results were obtained only in the *in vitro* CHO Sister Chromatid Exchange (clastogenicity) and in the Mouse Lymphoma Cell (mutagenicity) assays, using concentrations of hydrochlorothiazide from 43 to 133 µg/ml, and in the *Aspergillus nidulans* non-disjunction assay at an unspecified concentration.

Hydrochlorothiazide had no adverse effects on the fertility of mice and rats of either sex in studies wherein these species were exposed, via their diet, to doses of up to 100 and 4 mg/kg, respectively, prior to mating and throughout gestation.

Pregnancy: Teratogenic effects. Pregnancy Category C. *Hydrochlorothiazide:* Studies in which hydrochlorothiazide was orally administered to pregnant mice and rats during their respective periods of major organogenesis at doses up to 3000 and 1000 mg hydrochlorothiazide/kg, respectively, provided no evidence of harm to the fetus. There are, however, no adequate and well controlled studies in pregnant women.

Spironolactone: Teratology studies with spironolactone have been carried out in mice and rabbits at doses of up to 20 mg/kg/day. On a body surface area basis, this dose in the mouse is substantially below the maximum recommended human dose and, in the rabbit, approximates the maximum recommended human dose. No teratogenic or other embryotoxic effects were observed in mice, but the 20 mg/kg dose caused an increased rate of resorption and a lower number of live fetuses in rabbits. Because of its anti-androgenic activity and the requirement of testosterone for male morphogenesis, spironolactone may have the potential for adversely affecting sex differentiation of the male during embryogenesis. When administered to rats at 200 mg/kg/day between gestation days 13 and 21 (late embryogenesis and fetal development), feminization of male fetuses was observed. Offspring exposed during late pregnancy to 50 and 100 mg/kg/day doses of spironolactone exhibited changes in the reproductive tract including dose-dependent decreases in weights of the ventral prostate and seminal vesicle in males, ovaries and uteri that were enlarged in females, and other indications of endocrine dysfunction, that persisted into adulthood. There are no adequate and well-controlled studies with Aldactazide in pregnant women. Spironolactone has known endocrine effects in animals including progestational and antiandrogenic effects. The antiandrogenic effects can result in apparent estrogenic side effects in humans, such as gynecomastia. Therefore, the use of Aldactazide in pregnant women requires that the anticipated benefit be weighed against the possible hazards to the fetus.

Non-teratogenic effects: Spironolactone or its metabolites may, and hydrochlorothiazide does, cross the placental barrier and appear in cord blood. Therefore, the use of Aldactazide in pregnant women requires that the anticipated benefit be weighed against possible hazards to the fetus. The hazards include fetal or neonatal jaundice, thrombocytopenia, and possibly other adverse reactions that have occurred in adults.

Nursing mothers: Canrenone, a major (and active) metabolite of spironolactone, appears in human breast milk. Because spironolactone has been found to be tumorigenic in rats, a decision should be made whether to discontinue the drug, taking into account the importance of the drug to the mother. If use of the drug is deemed essential, an alternative method of infant feeding should be instituted.

Pediatric use: Safety and effectiveness in pediatric patients have not been established.

ADVERSE REACTIONS

The following adverse reactions have been reported and, within each category (body system), are listed in order of decreasing severity.

Hydrochlorothiazide:

Body as a whole: Weakness.

Cardiovascular: Hypotension including orthostatic hypotension (may be aggravated by alchohol, barbiturates, narcotics or antihypertensive drugs).

Digestive: Pancreatitis, jaundice (intrahepatic cholestatic jaundice), diarrhea, vomiting, sialoadenitis, cramping, constipation, gastric irritation, nausea, anorexia.

Hematologic: Aplastic anemia, agranulocytosis, leukopenia, hemolytic anemia, thrombocytopenia.

Hypersensitivity: Anaphylactic reactions, necrotizing angitis (vasculitis and cutaneous vasculitis), respiratory distress including pneumonitis and pulmonary edema, photosensitivity, fever, urticaria, rash, purpura.

Metabolic: Electrolyte imbalance (see *Precautions*), hyperglycemia, glycosuria, hyperuricemia.

Musculoskeletal: Muscle spasm.

Nervous system/psychiatric: Vertigo, paresthesias, dizziness, headache, restlessness.

Renal: Renal failure, renal dysfunction, interstitial nephritis (see *Warnings*).

Skin: Erythema multiforme, pruritus.

Special senses: Transient blurred vision, xanthopsia.

Spironolactone:

Digestive: Gastric bleeding, ulceration, gastritis, diarrhea and cramping, nausea, vomiting.

Endocrine: Gynecomastia (see *Precautions*), inability to achieve or maintain erection, irregular menses or amenorrhea, postmenopausal bleeding. Carcinoma of the breast has been reported in patients taking spironolactone but a cause and effect relationship has not been established.

Hematologic: Agranulocytosis.

Hypersensitivity: Fever, urticaria, maculopapular or erythematous cutaneous eruptions, anaphylactic reactions, vasculitis.

Nervous system/psychiatric: Mental confusion, ataxia, headache, drowsiness, lethargy.

Liver/biliary: A very few cases of mixed cholestatic/hepatocellular toxicity, with one reported fatality, have been reported with spironolactone administration.

Renal: Renal dysfunction (including renal failure).

OVERDOSAGE

The oral LD_{50} of spironolactone is greater than 1,000 mg/kg in mice, rats, and rabbits. The oral LD_{50} of hydrochlorothiazide is greater than 10 g/kg in both mice and rats.

Acute overdosage of spironolactone may be manifested by drowsiness, mental confusion, maculopapular or erythematous rash, nausea, vomiting, dizziness, or diarrhea. Rarely, instances of hyponatremia, hyperkalemia (less commonly seen with Aldactazide because the hydrochlorothiazide component tends to produce hypokalemia), or hepatic coma may occur in patients with severe liver disease, but these are unlikely due to acute overdosage.

However, because Aldactazide contains both spironolactone and hydrochlorothiazide, the toxic effects may be intensified, and signs of thiazide overdosage may be present. These include electrolyte imbalance such as hypokalemia and/or hyponatremia. The potassium-sparing action of spironolactone may predominate and hyperkalemia may occur, especially in patients with impaired renal function. BUN determinations have been reported to rise transiently with hydrochlorothiazide. There may be CNS depression with lethargy or even coma.

Treatment: Induce vomiting or evacuate the stomach by lavage. There is no specific antidote. Treatment is supportive to maintain hydration, electrolyte balance, and vital functions.

Patients who have renal impairment may develop spironolactone-induced hyperkalemia. In such cases, Aldactazide should be discontinued immediately. With severe hyperkalemia, the clinical situation dictates the procedures to be employed. These include the intravenous administration of calcium chloride solution, sodium bicarbonate solution and/or the oral or parenteral administration of glucose with a rapid-acting insulin preparation. These are temporary measures to be repeated as required. Cationic exchange resins such as sodium polystyrene sulfonate may be orally or rectally administered. Persistent hyperkalemia may require dialysis.

DOSAGE AND ADMINISTRATION

Optimal dosage should be established by individual titration of the components (see boxed ***Warning***).

Edema in adults *(congestive heart failure, hepatic cirrhosis, or nephrotic syndrome).* The usual maintenance dose of Aldactazide is 100 mg each of spironolactone and hydrochlorothiazide daily, administered in a single dose or in divided doses, but may range from 25 mg to 200 mg of each component daily depending on the response to the initial titration. In some instances it may be desirable to administer separate tablets of either Aldactone (spironolactone) or hydrochlorothiazide in addition to Aldactazide in order to provide optimal individual therapy.

The onset of diuresis with Aldactazide occurs promptly and, due to prolonged effect of the spironolactone component, persists for two to three days after Aldactazide is discontinued.

Essential hypertension. Although the dosage will vary depending on the results of titration of the individual ingredients, many patients will be found to have an optimal response to 50 mg to 100 mg each of spironolactone and hydrochlorothiazide daily, given in a single dose or in divided doses.

Concurrent potassium supplementation is not recommended when Aldactazide is used in the long-term management of hypertension or in the treatment of most edematous conditions, since the spironolactone content of Aldactazide is usually sufficient to minimize loss induced by the hydrochlorothiazide component.

HOW SUPPLIED

Aldactazide tablets containing 25 mg of spironolactone (Aldactone) and 25 mg of hydrochlorothiazide are round, tan, film coated, with SEARLE and 1011 debossed on one side and ALDACTAZIDE and 25 on the other side, supplied as:

NDC Number	Size
0025-1011-31	bottle of 100
0025-1011-55	bottle of 2500

Aldactazide tablets containing 50 mg of spironolactone (Aldactone) and 50 mg of hydrochlorothiazide are oblong, tan, scored, film coated, with SEARLE and 1021 debossed on the scored side and ALDACTAZIDE and 50 on the other side, supplied as:

NDC Number	Size
0025-1021-31	bottle of 100

Store below 77°F (25°C).

Rx only

Oct. 15, 1998

 A05456

Shown in Product Identification Guide, page 335

ALDACTONE® ℞

[al-dac 'tone]

(spironolactone)

> **WARNING**
> Spironolactone has been shown to be a tumorigen in chronic toxicity studies in rats (see *Precautions*). Aldactone should be used only in those conditions described under *Indications and Usage*. Unnecessary use of this drug should be avoided.

DESCRIPTION

Aldactone oral tablets contain 25 mg, 50 mg, or 100 mg of the aldosterone antagonist spironolactone, 17- hydroxy-7α -mercapto-3-oxo-17α -pregn-4-ene-21-carboxylic acid γ-lactone acetate, which has the following structural formula:

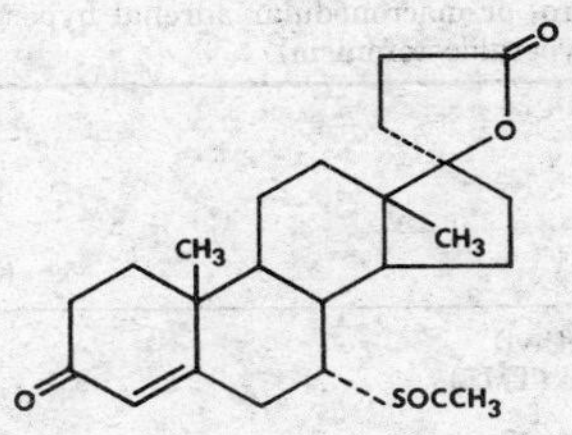

Spironolactone is practically insoluble in water, soluble in alcohol, and freely soluble in benzene and in chloroform.

Inactive ingredients include calcium sulfate, corn starch, flavor, hydroxypropyl methylcellulose, iron oxide, magnesium stearate, polyethylene glycol, povidone, and titanium dioxide.

Continued on next page

Aldactone—Cont.

ACTIONS/CLINICAL PHARMACOLOGY

Mechanism of action: Aldactone (spironolactone) is a specific pharmacologic antagonist of aldosterone, acting primarily through competitive binding of receptors at the aldosterone-dependent sodium-potassium exchange site in the distal convoluted renal tubule. Aldactone causes increased amounts of sodium and water to be excreted, while potassium is retained. Aldactone acts both as a diuretic and as an antihypertensive drug by this mechanism. It may be given alone or with other diuretic agents which act more proximally in the renal tubule.

Aldosterone antagonist activity: Increased levels of the mineralocorticoid, aldosterone, are present in primary and secondary hyperaldosteronism. Edematous states in which secondary aldosteronism is usually involved include congestive heart failure, hepatic cirrhosis, and the nephrotic syndrome. By competing with aldosterone for receptor sites, Aldactone provides effective therapy for the edema and ascites in those conditions. Aldactone counteracts secondary aldosteronism induced by the volume depletion and associated sodium loss caused by active diuretic therapy.

Aldactone is effective in lowering the systolic and diastolic blood pressure in patients with primary hyperaldosteronism. It is also effective in most cases of essential hypertension, despite the fact that aldosterone secretion may be within normal limits in benign essential hypertension.

Through its action in antagonizing the effect of aldosterone, Aldactone inhibits the exchange of sodium for potassium in the distal renal tubule and helps to prevent potassium loss.

Aldactone has not been demonstrated to elevate serum uric acid, to precipitate gout, or to alter carbohydrate metabolism.

Pharmacokinetics: Spironolactone is rapidly and extensively metabolized. Sulfur-containing products are the predominant metabolites and are thought to be primarily responsible, together with spironolactone, for the therapeutic effects of the drug. The following pharmacokinetic data were obtained from 12 healthy volunteers following the administration of 100 mg of spironolactone (Aldactone film-coated tablets) daily for 15 days. On the 15th day, spironolactone was given immediately after a low-fat breakfast and blood was drawn thereafter.

[See table below]

The pharmacological activity of spironolactone metabolites in man is not known. However, in the adrenalectomized rat the antimineralocorticoid activities of the metabolites C, TMS, and HTMS, relative to spironolactone, were 1.10, 1.28, and 0.32, respectively. Relative to spironolactone, their binding affinities to the aldosterone receptors in rat kidney slices were 0.19, 0.86, and 0.06, respectively.

In humans the potencies of TMS and 7-α-thiospirolactone in reversing the effects of the synthetic mineralocorticoid, fludrocortisone, on urinary electrolyte composition were 0.33 and 0.26, respectively, relative to spironolactone. However, since the serum concentrations of these steroids were not determined, their incomplete absorption and/or first-pass metabolism could not be ruled out as a reason for their reduced *in vivo* activities.

Spironolactone and its metabolites are more than 90% bound to plasma proteins. The metabolites are excreted primarily in the urine and secondarily in bile.

The effect of food on spironolactone absorption (two 100-mg Aldactone tablets) was assessed in a single dose study of 9 healthy, drug-free volunteers. Food increased the bioavailability of unmetabolized spironolactone by almost 100%. The clinical importance of this finding is not known.

INDICATIONS AND USAGE

Aldactone (spironolactone) is indicated in the management of:

Primary hyperaldosteronism for:

Establishing the diagnosis of primary hyperaldosteronism by therapeutic trial.

Short-term preoperative treatment of patients with primary hyperaldosteronism.

Long-term maintenance therapy for patients with discrete aldosterone-producing adrenal adenomas who are judged to be poor operative risks or who decline surgery.

Long-term maintenance therapy for patients with bilateral micro- or macronodular adrenal hyperplasia (idiopathic hyperaldosteronism).

Edematous conditions for patients with:

Congestive heart failure: For the management of edema and sodium retention when the patient is only partially responsive to, or is intolerant of, other therapeutic measures. Aldactone is also indicated for patients with congestive heart failure taking digitalis when other therapies are considered inappropriate.

Cirrhosis of the liver accompanied by edema and/or ascites: Aldosterone levels may be exceptionally high in this condition. Aldactone is indicated for maintenance therapy together with bed rest and the restriction of fluid and sodium.

The nephrotic syndrome: For nephrotic patients when treatment of the underlying disease, restriction of fluid and sodium intake, and the use of other diuretics do not provide an adequate response.

Essential hypertension

Usually in combination with other drugs, Aldactone is indicated for patients who cannot be treated adequately with other agents or for whom other agents are considered inappropriate.

Hypokalemia

For the treatment of patients with hypokalemia when other measures are considered inappropriate or inadequate. Aldactone is also indicated for the prophylaxis of hypokalemia in patients taking digitalis when other measures are considered inadequate or inappropriate.

Usage in Pregnancy. The routine use of diuretics in an otherwise healthy woman is inappropriate and exposes mother and fetus to unnecessary hazard. Diuretics do not prevent development of toxemia of pregnancy, and there is no satisfactory evidence that they are useful in the treatment of developing toxemia.

Edema during pregnancy may arise from pathologic causes or from the physiologic and mechanical consequences of pregnancy.

Aldactone is indicated in pregnancy when edema is due to pathologic causes just as it is in the absence of pregnancy (however, see *Precautions: Pregnancy*). Dependent edema in pregnancy, resulting from restriction of venous return by the expanded uterus, is properly treated through elevation of the lower extremities and use of support hose; use of diuretics to lower intravascular volume in this case is unsupported and unnecessary. There is hypervolemia during normal pregnancy which is not harmful to either the fetus or the mother (in the absence of cardiovascular disease), but which is associated with edema, including generalized edema, in the majority of pregnant women. If this edema produces discomfort, increased recumbency will often provide relief. In rare instances, this edema may cause extreme discomfort which is not relieved by rest. In these cases, a short course of diuretics may provide relief and may be appropriate.

CONTRAINDICATIONS

Aldactone is contraindicated for patients with anuria, acute renal insufficiency, significant impairment of renal excretory function, or hyperkalemia.

WARNINGS

Potassium supplementation, either in the form of medication or as a diet rich in potassium, should not ordinarily be given in association with Aldactone therapy. Excessive potassium intake may cause hyperkalemia in patients receiving Aldactone (see *Precautions: General*). Aldactone should not be administered concurrently with other potassium-sparing diuretics. Aldactone, when used with ACE inhibitors or indomethacin, even in the presence of a diuretic, has been associated with severe hyperkalemia. Extreme caution should be exercised when Aldactone is given concomitantly with these drugs.

Aldactone should be used with caution in patients with impaired hepatic function because minor alterations of fluid and electrolyte balance may precipitate hepatic coma.

Lithium generally should not be given with diuretics (see *Precautions: Drug interactions*).

PRECAUTIONS

General: All patients receiving diuretic therapy should be observed for evidence of fluid or electrolyte imbalance, eg, hypomagnesemia, hyponatremia, hypochloremic alkalosis, and hyperkalemia.

Serum and urine electrolyte determinations are particularly important when the patient is vomiting excessively or receiving parenteral fluids. Warning signs or symptoms of fluid and electrolyte imbalance, irrespective of cause, include dryness of the mouth, thirst, weakness, lethargy, drowsiness, restlessness, muscle pains or cramps, muscular fatigue, hypotension, oliguria, tachycardia, and gastrointestinal disturbances such as nausea and vomiting. Hyperkalemia may occur in patients with impaired renal function or excessive potassium intake and can cause cardiac irregularities, which may be fatal. Consequently, no potassium supplement should ordinarily be given with Aldactone.

Concomitant administration of potassium-sparing diuretics and ACE inhibitors or nonsteroidal anti-inflammatory drugs (NSAIDs), eg, indomethacin, has been associated with severe hyperkalemia.

If hyperkalemia is suspected (warning signs include paresthesia, muscle weakness, fatigue, flaccid paralysis of the extremities, bradycardia and shock) an electrocardiogram (ECG) should be obtained. However, it is important to monitor serum potassium levels because mild hyperkalemia may not be associated with ECG changes.

If hyperkalemia is present, Aldactone should be discontinued immediately. With severe hyperkalemia, the clinical situation dictates the procedures to be employed. These include the intravenous administration of calcium chloride solution, sodium bicarbonate solution and/or the oral or parenteral administration of glucose with a rapid-acting insulin preparation. These are temporary measures to be repeated as required. Cationic exchange resins such as sodium polystyrene sulfonate may be orally or rectally administered. Persistent hyperkalemia may require dialysis.

Reversible hyperchloremic metabolic acidosis, usually in association with hyperkalemia, has been reported to occur in some patients with decompensated hepatic cirrhosis, even in the presence of normal renal function.

Dilutional hyponatremia, manifested by dryness of the mouth, thirst, lethargy, and drowsiness, and confirmed by a low serum sodium level, may be caused or aggravated, especially when Aldactone is administered in combination with other diuretics, and dilutional hyponatremia may occur in edematous patients in hot weather; appropriate therapy is water restriction rather than administration of sodium, except in rare instances when the hyponatremia is life-threatening.

Aldactone therapy may cause a transient elevation of BUN, especially in patients with preexisting renal impairment. Aldactone may cause mild acidosis.

Gynecomastia may develop in association with the use of spironolactone; physicians should be alert to its possible onset. The development of gynecomastia appears to be related to both dosage level and duration of therapy and is normally reversible when Aldactone is discontinued. In rare instances some breast enlargement may persist when Aldactone is discontinued.

Information for patients: Patients who receive Aldactone should be advised to avoid potassium supplements and foods containing high levels of potassium including salt substitutes.

Laboratory tests: Periodic determination of serum electrolytes to detect possible electrolyte imbalance should be done at appropriate intervals, particularly in the elderly and those with significant renal or hepatic impairments.

Drug interactions:

ACE inhibitors: Concomitant administration of ACE inhibitors with potassium-sparing diuretics has been associated with severe hyperkalemia.

Alcohol, barbiturates, or narcotics: Potentiation of orthostatic hypotension may occur.

Corticosteroids, ACTH: Intensified electrolyte depletion, particularly hypokalemia, may occur.

Pressor amines (eg, norepinephrine): Spironolactone reduces the vascular responsiveness to norepinephrine. Therefore, caution should be exercised in the management of patients subjected to regional or general anesthesia while they are being treated with Aldactone.

Skeletal muscle relaxants, nondepolarizing (eg, tubocurarine): Possible increased responsiveness to the muscle relaxant may result.

Lithium: Lithium generally should not be given with diuretics. Diuretic agents reduce the renal clearance of lithium and add a high risk of lithium toxicity.

Nonsteroidal anti-inflammatory drugs (NSAIDs): In some patients, the administration of an NSAID can reduce the diuretic, natriuretic, and antihypertensive effect of loop, potassium-sparing and thiazide diuretics. Combination of NSAIDs, eg, indomethacin, with potassium-sparing diuretics has been associated with severe hyperkalemia. Therefore, when Aldactone and NSAIDs are used concomitantly, the patient should be observed closely to determine if the desired effect of the diuretic is obtained.

Digoxin: Spironolactone has been shown to increase the half-life of digoxin. This may result in increased serum digoxin levels and subsequent digitalis toxicity. It may be necessary to reduce the maintenance and digitalization doses when spironolactone is administered, and the patient should be carefully monitored to avoid over- or underdigitalization.

Drug/Laboratory test interactions: Several reports of possible interference with digoxin radioimmunoassays by spironolactone, or its metabolites, have appeared in the literature. Neither the extent nor the potential clinical significance of its interference (which may be assay-specific) has been fully established.

Carcinogenesis, mutagenesis, impairment of fertility: Orally administered spironolactone has been shown to be a tumorigen in dietary administration studies performed in rats, with its proliferative effects manifested on endocrine organs and the liver. In an 18-month study using doses of

	Accumulation Factor: AUC (0–24 hr, day 15)/AUC (0–24 hr, day 1)	Mean Peak Serum Concentration	Mean (SD) Post-Steady State Half-life
7-α-(thiomethyl) spirolactone (TMS)	1.25	391 ng/mL at 3.2 hr	13.8 hr (6.4) (terminal)
6-β-hydroxy-7-α-(thiomethyl) spirolactone (HTMS)	1.50	125 ng/mL at 5.1 hr	15.0 hr (4.0) (terminal)
Canrenone (C)	1.41	181 ng/mL at 4.3 hr	16.5 hr (6.3) (terminal)
Spironolactone	1.30	80 ng/mL at 2.6 hr	Approximately 1.4 hr (0.5) (β half-life)

about 50, 150 and 500 mg/kg/day, there were statistically significant increases in benign adenomas of the thyroid and testes and, in male rats, a dose-related increase in proliferative changes in the liver (including hepatocytomegaly and hyperplastic nodules). In a 24-month study in which the same strain of rat was administered doses of about 10, 30, 100 and 150 mg spironolactone/kg/day, the range of proliferative effects included significant increases in hepatocellular adenomas and testicular interstitial cell tumors in males, and significant increases in thyroid follicular cell adenomas and carcinomas in both sexes. There was also a statistically significant, but not dose-related, increase in benign uterine endometrial stromal polyps in females.

A dose-related (above 20 mg/kg/day) incidence of myelocytic leukemia was observed in rats fed daily doses of potassium canrenoate (a compound chemically similar to spironolactone and whose primary metabolite, canrenone, is also a major product of spironolactone in man) for a period of one year. In two year studies in the rat, oral administration of potassium canrenoate was associated with myelocytic leukemia and hepatic, thyroid, testicular and mammary tumors.

Neither spironolactone nor potassium canrenoate produced mutagenic effects in tests using bacteria or yeast. In the absence of metabolic activation, neither spironolactone nor potassium canrenoate has been shown to be mutagenic in mammalian tests *in vitro*. In the presence of metabolic activation, spironolactone has been reported to be negative in some mammalian mutagenicity tests *in vitro* and inconclusive (but slightly positive) for mutagenicity in other mammalian tests *in vitro*. In the presence of metabolic activation, potassium canrenoate has been reported to test positive for mutagenicity in some mammalian tests *in vitro*, inconclusive in others, and negative in still others.

In a three-litter reproduction study in which female rats received dietary doses of 15 and 50 mg spironolactone/kg/day, there were no effects on mating and fertility, but there was a small increase in incidence of stillborn pups at 50 mg/kg/day. When injected into female rats (100 mg/kg/day for 7 days, i.p.), spironolactone was found to increase the length of the estrous cycle by prolonging diestrus during treatment and inducing constant diestrus during a two week post-treatment observation period. These effects were associated with retarded ovarian follicle development and a reduction in circulating estrogen levels, which would be expected to impair mating, fertility and fecundity. Spironolactone (100 mg/kg/day), administered i.p. to female mice during a two week cohabitation period with untreated males, decreased the number of mated mice that conceived (effect shown to be caused by an inhibition of ovulation) and decreased the number of implanted embryos in those that became pregnant (effect shown to be caused by an inhibition of implantation), and at 200 mg/kg, also increased the latency period to mating.

Pregnancy: Teratogenic effects. Pregnancy Category C. Teratology studies with spironolactone have been carried out in mice and rabbits at doses of up to 20 mg/kg/day. On a body surface area basis, this dose in the mouse is substantially below the maximum recommended human dose and, in the rabbit, approximates the maximum recommended human dose. No teratogenic or other embryotoxic effects were observed in mice, but the 20 mg/kg dose caused an increased rate of resorption and a lower number of live fetuses in rabbits. Because of its anti-androgenic activity and the requirement of testosterone for male morphogenesis, Aldactone may have the potential for adversely affecting sex differentiation of the male during embryogenesis. When administered to rats at 200 mg/kg/day between gestation days 13 and 21 (late embryogenesis and fetal development), feminization of male fetuses was observed. Offspring exposed during late pregnancy to 50 and 100 mg/kg/day doses of spironolactone exhibited changes in the reproductive tract including dose-dependent decreases in weights of the ventral prostate and seminal vesicle in males, ovaries and uteri that were enlarged in females, and other indications of endocrine dysfunction, that persisted into adulthood. There are no adequate and well-controlled studies with Aldactone in pregnant women. Spironolactone has known endocrine effects in animals including progestational and antiandrogenic effects. The anti-androgenic effects can result in apparent estrogenic side effects in humans, such as gynecomastia. Therefore, the use of Aldactone in pregnant women requires that the anticipated benefit be weighed against the possible hazards to the fetus.

Nursing mothers: Canrenone, a major (and active) metabolite of spironolactone, appears in human breast milk. Because spironolactone has been found to be tumorigenic in rats, a decision should be made whether to discontinue the drug, taking into account the importance of the drug to the mother. If use of the drug is deemed essential, an alternative method of infant feeding should be instituted.

Pediatric use: Safety and effectiveness in pediatric patients have not been established.

ADVERSE REACTIONS

The following adverse reactions have been reported and, within each category (body system), are listed in order of decreasing severity.

Digestive: Gastric bleeding, ulceration, gastritis, diarrhea and cramping, nausea, vomiting.

Endocrine: Gynecomastia (see *Precautions*), inability to achieve or maintain erection, irregular menses or amenorrhea, postmenopausal bleeding. Carcinoma of the breast has been reported in patients taking spironolactone but a cause and effect relationship has not been established.

Hematologic: Agranulocytosis.

Hypersensitivity: Fever, urticaria, maculopapular or erythematous cutaneous eruptions, anaphylactic reactions, vasculitis.

Nervous system/psychiatric: Mental confusion, ataxia, headache, drowsiness, lethargy.

Liver/biliary: A very few cases of mixed cholestatic/hepatocellular toxicity, with one reported fatality, have been reported with spironolactone administration.

Renal: Renal dysfunction (including renal failure).

OVERDOSAGE

The oral LD_{50} of spironolactone is greater than 1,000 mg/kg in mice, rats, and rabbits.

Acute overdosage of spironolactone may be manifested by drowsiness, mental confusion, maculopapular or erythematous rash, nausea, vomiting, dizziness, or diarrhea. Rarely, instances of hyponatremia, hyperkalemia, or hepatic coma may occur in patients with severe liver disease, but these are unlikely due to acute overdosage. Hyperkalemia may occur, especially in patients with impaired renal function.

Treatment: Induce vomiting or evacuate the stomach by lavage. There is no specific antidote. Treatment is supportive to maintain hydration, electrolyte balance, and vital functions.

Patients who have renal impairment may develop spironolactone-induced hyperkalemia. In such cases, Aldactone should be discontinued immediately. With severe hyperkalemia, the clinical situation dictates the procedures to be employed. These include the intravenous administration of calcium chloride solution, sodium bicarbonate solution and/or the oral or parenteral administration of glucose with a rapid-acting insulin preparation. These are temporary measures to be repeated as required. Cationic exchange resins such as sodium polystyrene sulfonate may be orally or rectally administered. Persistent hyperkalemia may require dialysis.

DOSAGE AND ADMINISTRATION

Primary hyperaldosteronism. Aldactone may be employed as an initial diagnostic measure to provide presumptive evidence of primary hyperaldosteronism while patients are on normal diets.

Long test: Aldactone is administered at a daily dosage of 400 mg for three to four weeks. Correction of hypokalemia and of hypertension provides presumptive evidence for the diagnosis of primary hyperaldosteronism.

Short test: Aldactone is administered at a daily dosage of 400 mg for four days. If serum potassium increases during Aldactone administration but drops when Aldactone is discontinued, a presumptive diagnosis of primary hyperaldosteronism should be considered.

After the diagnosis of hyperaldosteronism has been established by more definitive testing procedures, Aldactone may be administered in doses of 100 to 400 mg daily in preparation for surgery. For patients who are considered unsuitable for surgery, Aldactone may be employed for long-term maintenance therapy at the lowest effective dosage determined for the individual patient.

Edema in adults *(congestive heart failure, hepatic cirrhosis, or nephrotic syndrome)*. An initial daily dosage of 100 mg of Aldactone administered in either single or divided doses is recommended, but may range from 25 to 200 mg daily. When given as the sole agent for diuresis, Aldactone should be continued for at least five days at the initial dosage level, after which it may be adjusted to the optimal therapeutic or maintenance level administered in either single or divided daily doses. If, after five days, an adequate diuretic response to Aldactone has not occurred, a second diuretic which acts more proximally in the renal tubule may be added to the regimen. Because of the additive effect of Aldactone when administered concurrently with such diuretics, an enhanced diuresis usually begins on the first day of combined treatment; combined therapy is indicated when more rapid diuresis is desired. The dosage of Aldactone should remain unchanged when other diuretic therapy is added.

Essential hypertension. For adults, an initial daily dosage of 50 to 100 mg of Aldactone administered in either single or divided doses is recommended. Aldactone may also be given with diuretics which act more proximally in the renal tubule or with other antihypertensive agents. Treatment with Aldactone should be continued for at least two weeks, since the maximum response may not occur before this time. Subsequently, dosage should be adjusted according to the response of the patient.

Hypokalemia. Aldactone in a dosage ranging from 25 mg to 100 mg daily is useful in treating a diuretic-induced hypokalemia, when oral potassium supplements or other potassium-sparing regimens are considered inappropriate.

HOW SUPPLIED

Aldactone 25-mg tablets are round, light yellow, film coated, with SEARLE and 1001 debossed on one side and ALDACTONE and 25 on the other side, supplied as:

NDC Number	Size
0025-1001-31	bottle of 100
0025-1001-51	bottle of 500
0025-1001-55	bottle of 2500

Aldactone 50-mg tablets are oval, light orange, scored, film coated, with SEARLE and 1041 debossed on the scored side and ALDACTONE and 50 on the other side, supplied as:

NDC Number	Size
0025-1041-31	bottle of 100
0025-1041-34	carton of 100 unit dose

Aldactone 100-mg tablets are round, peach colored, scored, film coated, with SEARLE and 1031 debossed on the scored side and ALDACTONE and 100 on the other side, supplied as:

NDC Number	Size
0025-1031-31	bottle of 100
0025-1031-34	carton of 100 unit dose

Store below 77°F (25°C).

Rx only 10/15/98

A05455

Shown in Product Identification Guide, page 335

AMBIEN® Ⓒ℞

[am 'bē-ən]

(zolpidem tartrate)

DESCRIPTION

Ambien (zolpidem tartrate), is a non-benzodiazepine hypnotic of the imidazopyridine class and is available in 5-mg and 10-mg strength tablets for oral administration.

Chemically, zolpidem is N,N,6-trimethyl-2-p-tolyl-imidazo[1,2-a]pyridine-3-acetamide L-(+)-tartrate (2:1). It has the following structure:

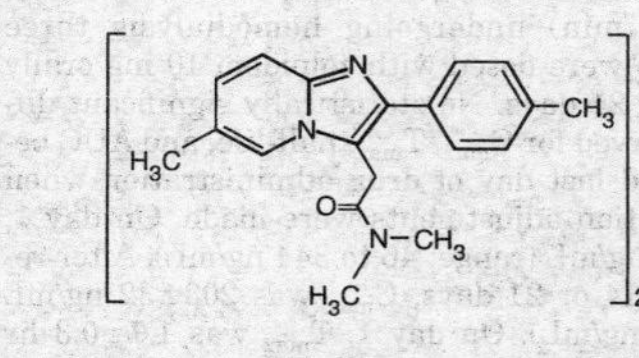

Zolpidem tartrate is a white to off-white crystalline powder that is sparingly soluble in water, alcohol, and propylene glycol. It has a molecular weight of 764.88.

Each Ambien tablet includes the following inactive ingredients: hydroxypropyl methylcellulose, lactose, magnesium stearate, microcrystalline cellulose, polyethylene glycol, sodium starch glycolate, and titanium dioxide; the 5-mg tablet also contains FD&C Red No. 40, iron oxide colorant, and polysorbate 80.

CLINICAL PHARMACOLOGY

Pharmacodynamics: Subunit modulation of the $GABA_A$ receptor chloride channel macromolecular complex is hypothesized to be responsible for sedative, anticonvulsant, anxiolytic, and myorelaxant drug properties. The major modulatory site of the $GABA_A$ receptor complex is located on its alpha (α) subunit and is referred to as the benzodiazepine (BZ) or omega (ω) receptor. At least three subtypes of the (ω) receptor have been identified.

While zolpidem is a hypnotic agent with a chemical structure unrelated to benzodiazepines, barbiturates, or other drugs with known hypnotic properties, it interacts with a GABA-BZ receptor complex and shares some of the pharmacological properties of the benzodiazepines. In contrast to the benzodiazepines, which nonselectively bind to and activate all omega receptor subtypes, zolpidem in vitro binds the (ω_1) receptor preferentially with a high affinity ratio of the $alpha_1/alpha_5$ subunits. The (ω_1) receptor is found primarily on the Lamina IV of the sensorimotor cortical regions, substantia nigra (pars reticulata), cerebellum molecular layer, olfactory bulb, ventral thalamic complex, pons, inferior colliculus, and globus pallidus. This selective binding of zolpidem on the (ω_1) receptor is not absolute, but it may explain the relative absence of myorelaxant and anticonvulsant effects in animal studies as well as the preservation of deep sleep (stages 3 and 4) in human studies of zolpidem at hypnotic doses.

Pharmacokinetics: The pharmacokinetic profile of Ambien is characterized by rapid absorption from the GI tract and a short elimination half-life ($T_{1/2}$) in healthy subjects. In a single-dose crossover study in 45 healthy subjects administered 5- and 10-mg zolpidem tartrate tablets, the mean peak concentrations (C_{max}) were 59 (range: 29 to 113) and 121 (range: 58 to 272) ng/mL, respectively, occurring at a mean time (T_{max}) of 1.6 hours for both. The mean Ambien elimination half-life was 2.6 (range: 1.4 to 4.5) and 2.5 (range: 1.4 to 3.8) hours, for the 5- and 10-mg tablets, respectively. Ambien is converted to inactive metabolites that are eliminated primarily by renal excretion. Ambien demonstrated linear kinetics in the dose range of 5 to 20 mg. Total protein binding was found to be 92.5±0.1% and remained constant, independent of concentration between 40 and 790 ng/mL. Zolpidem did not accumulate in young adults following nightly dosing with 20-mg zolpidem tartrate tablets for 2 weeks.

A food-effect study in 30 healthy male volunteers compared the pharmacokinetics of Ambien 10 mg when administered while fasting or 20 minutes after a meal. Results demonstrated that with food, mean AUC and C_{max} were decreased by 15% and 25%, respectively, while mean T_{max} was prolonged by 60% (from 1.4 to 2.2 hr). The half-life remained unchanged. These results suggest that, for faster sleep onset, Ambien should not be administered with or immediately after a meal.

Continued on next page

Ambien—Cont.

In the elderly, the dose for Ambien should be 5 mg (see *Precautions* and *Dosage and Administration*). This recommendation is based on several studies in which the mean C_{max}, $T_{1/2}$, and AUC were significantly increased when compared to results in young adults. In one study of eight elderly subjects (>70 years), the means for C_{max}, $T_{1/2}$, and AUC significantly increased by 50% (255 vs 384 ng/mL), 32% (2.2 vs 2.9 hr), and 64% (955 vs 1,562 ng·hr/mL), respectively, as compared to younger adults (20 to 40 years) following a single 20-mg oral zolpidem dose. Ambien did not accumulate in elderly subjects following nightly oral dosing of 10 mg for 1 week.

The pharmacokinetics of Ambien in eight patients with chronic hepatic insufficiency were compared to results in healthy subjects. Following a single 20-mg oral zolpidem dose, mean C_{max} and AUC were found to be two times (250 vs 499 ng/mL) and five times (788 vs 4,203 ng·hr/mL) higher, respectively, in hepatically compromised patients. T_{max} did not change. The mean half-life in cirrhotic patients of 9.9 hr (range: 4.1 to 25.8 hr) was greater than that observed in normals of 2.2 hr (range: 1.6 to 2.4 hr). Dosing should be modified accordingly in patients with hepatic insufficiency (see *Precautions* and *Dosage and Administration*).

The pharmacokinetics of zolpidem tartrate were studied in 11 patients with end-stage renal failure (mean Cl_{Cr}=6.5±1.5 mL/min) undergoing hemodialysis three times a week, who were dosed with zolpidem 10 mg orally each day for 14 or 21 days. No statistically significant differences were observed for C_{max}, T_{max}, half-life, and AUC between the first and last day of drug administration when baseline concentration adjustments were made. On day 1, C_{max} was 172±29 ng/mL (range: 46 to 344 ng/mL). After repeated dosing for 14 or 21 days, C_{max} was 203±32 ng/mL (range: 28 to 316 ng/mL). On day 1, T_{max} was 1.7±0.3 hr (range: 0.5 to 3.0 hr); after repeated dosing T_{max} was 0.8±0.2 hr (range: 0.5 to 2.0 hr). This variation is accounted for by noting that last-day serum sampling began 10 hours after the previous dose, rather than after 24 hours. This resulted in residual drug concentration and a shorter period to reach maximal serum concentration. On day 1, $T_{1/2}$ was 2.4±0.4 hr (range: 0.4 to 5.1 hr). After repeated dosing, $T_{1/2}$ was 2.5±0.4 hr (range: 0.7 to 4.2 hr). AUC was 796±159 ng·hr/mL after the first dose and 818±170 ng·hr/mL after repeated dosing. Zolpidem was not hemodialyzable. No accumulation of unchanged drug appeared after 14 or 21 days. Ambien (zolpidem tartrate) pharmacokinetics were not significantly different in renally impaired patients. No dosage adjustment is necessary in patients with compromised renal function. As a general precaution, these patients should be closely monitored.

Postulated relationship between elimination rate of hypnotics and their profile of common untoward effects: The type and duration of hypnotic effects and the profile of unwanted effects during administration of hypnotic drugs may be influenced by the biologic half-life of administered drug and any active metabolites formed. When half-lives are long, drug or metabolites may accumulate during periods of nightly administration and be associated with impairment of cognitive and/or motor performance during waking hours; the possibility of interaction with other psychoactive drugs or alcohol will be enhanced. In contrast, if half-lives, including half-lives of active metabolites, are short, drug and metabolites will be cleared before the next dose is ingested, and carryover effects related to excessive sedation or CNS depression should be minimal or absent. Ambien has a short half-life and no active metabolites. During nightly use for an extended period, pharmacodynamic tolerance or adaptation to some effects of hypnotics may develop. If the drug has a short elimination half-life, it is possible that a relative deficiency of the drug or its active metabolites (ie, in relationship to the receptor site) may occur at some point in the interval between each night's use. This sequence of events may account for two clinical findings reported to occur after several weeks of nightly use of other rapidly eliminated hypnotics, namely, increased wakefulness during the last third of the night, and the appearance of increased signs of daytime anxiety. Increased wakefulness during the last third of the night as measured by polysomnography has not been observed in clinical trials with Ambien.

Controlled trials supporting safety and efficacy

Transient insomnia: Normal adults experiencing transient insomnia (n=462) during the first night in a sleep laboratory were evaluated in a double-blind, parallel group, single-night trial comparing two doses of zolpidem (7.5 and 10 mg) and placebo. Both zolpidem doses were superior to placebo on objective (polysomnographic) measures of sleep latency, sleep duration, and number of awakenings.

Normal elderly adults (mean age 68) experiencing transient insomnia (n=35) during the first two nights in a sleep laboratory were evaluated in a double-blind, crossover, 2-night trial comparing four doses of zolpidem (5, 10, 15 and 20 mg) and placebo. All zolpidem doses were superior to placebo on the two primary PSG parameters (sleep latency and efficiency) and all four subjective outcome measures (sleep duration, sleep latency, number of awakenings, and sleep quality).

Chronic insomnia: Zolpidem was evaluated in two controlled studies for the treatment of patients with chronic insomnia (most closely resembling primary insomnia, as defined in the APA Diagnostic and Statistical Manual of Mental Disorders, DSM-IV™). Adult outpatients with chronic insomnia (n=75) were evaluated in a double-blind, parallel group, 5-week trial comparing two doses of zolpidem tartrate (10 and 15 mg) and placebo. On objective (polysomnographic) measures of sleep latency and sleep efficiency, zolpidem 15 mg was superior to placebo for all 5 weeks; zolpidem 10 mg was superior to placebo on sleep latency for the first 4 weeks and on sleep efficiency for weeks 2 and 4. Zolpidem was comparable to placebo on number of awakenings at both doses studied.

Adult outpatients (n=141) with chronic insomnia were also evaluated in a double-blind, parallel group, 4-week trial comparing two doses of zolpidem (10 and 15 mg) and placebo. Zolpidem 10 mg was superior to placebo on a subjective measure of sleep latency for all 4 weeks, and on subjective measures of total sleep time, number of awakenings, and sleep quality for the first treatment week. Zolpidem 15 mg was superior to placebo on a subjective measure of sleep latency for the first 3 weeks, on a subjective measure of total sleep time for the first week, and on number of awakenings and sleep quality for the first 2 weeks.

Next-day residual effects: Next-day residual effects of Ambien were evaluated in seven studies involving normal volunteers. In three studies in adults (including one study in a phase advance model of transient insomnia) and in one study in elderly subjects, a small but statistically significant decrease in performance was observed in the Digit Symbol Substitution Test (DSST) when compared to placebo. Studies of Ambien in non-elderly patients with insomnia did not detect evidence of next-day residual effects using the DSST, the Multiple Sleep Latency Test (MSLT), and patient ratings of alertness.

Rebound effects: There was no objective (polysomnographic) evidence of rebound insomnia at recommended doses seen in studies evaluating sleep on the nights following discontinuation of Ambien (zolpidem tartrate). There was subjective evidence of impaired sleep in the elderly on the first posttreatment night at doses above the recommended elderly dose of 5 mg.

Memory impairment: Controlled studies in adults utilizing objective measures of memory yielded no consistent evidence of next-day memory impairment following the administration of Ambien. However, in one study involving zolpidem doses of 10 and 20 mg, there was a significant decrease in next-morning recall of information presented to subjects during peak drug effect (90 minutes post-dose), ie, these subjects experienced anterograde amnesia. There was also subjective evidence from adverse event data for anterograde amnesia occurring in association with the administration of Ambien, predominantly at doses above 10 mg.

Effects on sleep stages: In studies that measured the percentage of sleep time spent in each sleep stage, Ambien has generally been shown to preserve sleep stages. Sleep time spent in stages 3 and 4 (deep sleep) was found comparable to placebo with only inconsistent, minor changes in REM (paradoxical) sleep at the recommended dose.

INDICATIONS AND USAGE

Ambien (zolpidem tartrate) is indicated for the short-term treatment of insomnia. Ambien has been shown to decrease sleep latency and increase the duration of sleep for up to 35 days in controlled clinical studies (see *Clinical Pharmacology*: *Controlled trials supporting safety and efficacy*).

Hypnotics should generally be limited to 7 to 10 days of use, and reevaluation of the patient is recommended if they are to be taken for more than 2 to 3 weeks. Ambien should not be prescribed in quantities exceeding a 1-month supply (see *Warnings*).

CONTRAINDICATIONS

None known.

WARNINGS

Since sleep disturbances may be the presenting manifestation of a physical and/or psychiatric disorder, symptomatic treatment of insomnia should be initiated only after a careful evaluation of the patient. The failure of insomnia to remit after 7 to 10 days of treatment may indicate the presence of a primary psychiatric and/or medical illness which should be evaluated. Worsening of insomnia or the emergence of new thinking or behavior abnormalities may be the consequence of an unrecognized psychiatric or physical disorder. Such findings have emerged during the course of treatment with sedative/hypnotic drugs, including Ambien. Because some of the important adverse effects of Ambien appear to be dose related (see *Precautions* and *Dosage and Administration*), it is important to use the smallest possible effective dose, especially in the elderly.

A variety of abnormal thinking and behavior changes have been reported to occur in association with the use of sedative/hypnotics. Some of these changes may be characterized by decreased inhibition (eg, aggressiveness and extroversion that seemed out of character), similar to effects produced by alcohol and other CNS depressants. Other reported behavioral changes have included bizarre behavior, agitation, hallucinations, and depersonalization. Amnesia and other neuropsychiatric symptoms may occur unpredictably. In primarily depressed patients, worsening of depression, including suicidal thinking, has been reported in association with the use of sedative/hypnotics.

It can rarely be determined with certainty whether a particular instance of the abnormal behaviors listed above is drug induced, spontaneous in origin, or a result of an underlying psychiatric or physical disorder. Nonetheless, the emergence of any new behavioral sign or symptom of concern requires careful and immediate evaluation.

Following the rapid dose decrease or abrupt discontinuation of sedative/hypnotics, there have been reports of signs and symptoms similar to those associated with withdrawal from other CNS-depressant drugs (see *Drug Abuse and Dependence*).

Ambien, like other sedative/hypnotic drugs, has CNS-depressant effects. Due to the rapid onset of action, Ambien should only be ingested immediately prior to going to bed. Patients should be cautioned against engaging in hazardous occupations requiring complete mental alertness or motor coordination such as operating machinery or driving a motor vehicle after ingesting the drug, including potential impairment of the performance of such activities that may occur the day following ingestion of Ambien. Ambien showed additive effects when combined with alcohol and should not be taken with alcohol. Patients should also be cautioned about possible combined effects with other CNS-depressant drugs. Dosage adjustments may be necessary when Ambien is administered with such agents because of the potentially additive effects.

PRECAUTIONS

General

Use in the elderly and/or debilitated patients: Impaired motor and/or cognitive performance after repeated exposure or unusual sensitivity to sedative/hypnotic drugs is a concern in the treatment of elderly and/or debilitated patients. Therefore, the recommended Ambien dosage is 5 mg in such patients (see *Dosage and Administration*) to decrease the possibility of side effects. These patients should be closely monitored.

Use in patients with concomitant illness: Clinical experience with Ambien (zolpidem tartrate) in patients with concomitant systemic illness is limited. Caution is advisable in using Ambien in patients with diseases or conditions that could affect metabolism or hemodynamic responses. Although studies did not reveal respiratory depressant effects at hypnotic doses of Ambien in normals or in patients with mild to moderate chronic obstructive pulmonary disease (COPD), a reduction in the Total Arousal Index together with a reduction in lowest oxygen saturation and increase in the times of oxygen desaturation below 80% and 90% was observed in patients with mild-to-moderate sleep apnea when treated with Ambien (10 mg) when compared to placebo. However, precautions should be observed if Ambien is prescribed to patients with compromised respiratory function, since sedative/hypnotics have the capacity to depress respiratory drive. Post-marketing reports of respiratory insufficiency, most of which involved patients with pre-existing respiratory impairment, have been received. Data in end-stage renal failure patients repeatedly treated with Ambien did not demonstrate drug accumulation or alterations in pharmacokinetic parameters. No dosage adjustment in renally impaired patients is required; however, these patients should be closely monitored (see *Pharmacokinetics*). A study in subjects with hepatic impairment did reveal prolonged elimination in this group; therefore, treatment should be initiated with 5 mg in patients with hepatic compromise, and they should be closely monitored.

Use in depression: As with other sedative/hypnotic drugs, Ambien should be administered with caution to patients exhibiting signs or symptoms of depression. Suicidal tendencies may be present in such patients and protective measures may be required. Intentional overdosage is more common in this group of patients; therefore, the least amount of drug that is feasible should be prescribed for the patient at any one time.

Information for patients: Patient information is printed at the end of this insert. To assure safe and effective use of Ambien, this information and instructions provided in the patient information section should be discussed with patients.

Laboratory tests: There are no specific laboratory tests recommended.

Drug Interactions

CNS-active drugs: Ambien was evaluated in healthy volunteers in single-dose interaction studies for several CNS drugs. A study involving haloperidol and zolpidem revealed no effect of haloperidol on the pharmacokinetics or pharmacodynamics of zolpidem. Imipramine in combination with zolpidem produced no pharmacokinetic interaction other than a 20% decrease in peak levels of imipramine, but there was an additive effect of decreased alertness. Similarly, chlorpromazine in combination with zolpidem produced no pharmacokinetic interaction, but there was an additive effect of decreased alertness and psychomotor performance. The lack of a drug interaction following single-dose administration does not predict a lack following chronic administration.

An additive effect on psychomotor performance between alcohol and zolpidem was demonstrated.

A single-dose interaction study with zolpidem 10 mg and fluoxetine 20 mg at steady-state levels in male volunteers did not demonstrate any clinically significant pharmacokinetic or pharmacodynamic interactions. When multiple doses of zolpidem and fluoxetine at steady-state concentrations were evaluated in healthy females, the only significant change was a 17% increase in the zolpidem half-life. There was no evidence of an additive effect in psychomotor performance.

Following five consecutive nightly doses of zolpidem 10 mg in the presence of sertraline 50 mg (17 consecutive daily doses, at 7:00 am, in healthy female volunteers), zolpidem C_{max} was significantly higher (43%) and T_{max} was significantly decreased (53%). Pharmacokinetics of sertraline and N-desmethylsertraline were unaffected by zolpidem.

Since the systematic evaluations of Ambien (zolpidem tartrate) in combination with other CNS-active drugs have been limited, careful consideration should be given to the pharmacology of any CNS-active drug to be used with zolpidem. Any drug with CNS-depressant effects could potentially enhance the CNS-depressant effects of zolpidem.

Drugs that affect drug metabolism via cytochrome P450: A randomized, double-blind, crossover interaction study in ten healthy volunteers between itraconazole (200 mg once daily for 4 days) and a single dose of zolpidem (10 mg) given 5 hours after the last dose of itraconazole resulted in a 34% increase in $AUC_{0\to\infty}$ of zolpidem. There were no significant pharmacodynamic effects of zolpidem on subjective drowsiness, postural sway, or psychomotor performance.

A randomized, placebo-controlled, crossover interaction study in eight healthy female volunteers between 5 consecutive daily doses of rifampin (600 mg) and a single dose of zolpidem (20 mg) given 17 hours after the last dose of rifampin showed significant reductions of the AUC (−73%), C_{max} (−58%), and $T_{1/2}$ (−36%) of zolpidem together with significant reductions in the pharmacodynamic effects of zolpidem.

Other drugs: A study involving cimetidine/zolpidem and ranitidine/zolpidem combinations revealed no effect of either drug on the pharmacokinetics or pharmacodynamics of zolpidem. Zolpidem had no effect on digoxin kinetics and did not affect prothrombin time when given with warfarin in normal subjects. Zolpidem's sedative/hypnotic effect was reversed by flumazenil; however, no significant alterations in zolpidem pharmacokinetics were found.

Drug/Laboratory test interactions: Zolpidem is not known to interfere with commonly employed clinical laboratory tests. In addition, clinical data indicate that zolpidem does not cross-react with benzodiazepines, opiates, barbiturates, cocaine, cannabinoids, or amphetamines in two standard urine drug screens.

Carcinogenesis, mutagenesis, impairment of fertility

Carcinogenesis: Zolpidem was administered to rats and mice for 2 years at dietary dosages of 4, 18, and 80 mg/kg/day. In mice, these doses are 26 to 520 times or 2 to 35 times the maximum 10-mg human dose on a mg/kg or mg/m^2 basis, respectively. In rats these doses are 43 to 876 times or 6 to 115 times the maximum 10-mg human dose on a mg/kg or mg/m^2 basis, respectively. No evidence of carcinogenic potential was observed in mice. Renal liposarcomas were seen in 4/100 rats (3 males, 1 female) receiving 80 mg/kg/day and a renal lipoma was observed in one male rat at the 18 mg/kg/day dose. Incidence rates of lipoma and liposarcoma for zolpidem were comparable to those seen in historical controls and the tumor findings are thought to be a spontaneous occurrence.

Mutagenesis: Zolpidem did not have mutagenic activity in several tests including the Ames test, genotoxicity in mouse lymphoma cells in vitro, chromosomal aberrations in cultured human lymphocytes, unscheduled DNA synthesis in rat hepatocytes in vitro, and the micronucleus test in mice.

Impairment of fertility: In a rat reproduction study, the high dose (100 mg base/kg) of zolpidem resulted in irregular estrus cycles and prolonged precoital intervals, but there was no effect on male or female fertility after daily oral doses of 4 to 100 mg base/kg or 5 to 130 times the recommended human dose in mg/m^2. No effects on any other fertility parameters were noted.

Pregnancy

Teratogenic effects: Pregnancy Category B. Studies to assess the effects of zolpidem on human reproduction and development have not been conducted.

Teratology studies were conducted in rats and rabbits.

In rats, adverse maternal and fetal effects occurred at 20 and 100 mg base/kg and included dose-related maternal lethargy and ataxia and a dose-related trend to incomplete ossification of fetal skull bones. Underossification of various fetal bones indicates a delay in maturation and is often seen in rats treated with sedative/hypnotic drugs. There were no teratogenic effects after zolpidem administration. The no-effect dose for maternal or fetal toxicity was 4 mg base/kg or 5 times the maximum human dose on a mg/m^2 basis.

In rabbits, dose-related maternal sedation and decreased weight gain occurred at all doses tested. At the high dose, 16 mg base/kg, there was an increase in postimplantation fetal loss and underossification of sternebrae in viable fetuses. These fetal findings in rabbits are often secondary to reductions in maternal weight gain. There were no frank teratogenic effects. The no-effect dose for fetal toxicity was 4 mg base/kg or 7 times the maximum human dose on a mg/m^2 basis.

Because animal reproduction studies are not always predictive of human response, this drug should be used during pregnancy only if clearly needed.

Nonteratogenic effects: Studies to assess the effects on children whose mothers took zolpidem during pregnancy have not been conducted. However, children born of mothers taking sedative/hypnotic drugs may be at some risk for withdrawal symptoms from the drug during the postnatal period. In addition, neonatal flaccidity has been reported in infants born of mothers who received sedative/hypnotic drugs during pregnancy.

Incidence of Treatment-Emergent Adverse Experiences in Short-term Placebo-Controlled Clinical Trials
(Percentage of patients reporting)

Body System/ Adverse Event*	Zolpidem (≤10 mg) (N=685)	Placebo (N=473)
Central and Peripheral Nervous System		
Headache	7	6
Drowsiness	2	–
Dizziness	1	–
Gastrointestinal System		
Nausea	2	3
Diarrhea	1	–
Musculoskeletal System		
Myalgia	1	2

*Events reported by at least 1% of Ambien patients are included.

Labor and delivery: Ambien (zolpidem tartrate) has no established use in labor and delivery.

Nursing mothers: Studies in lactating mothers indicate that the half-life of zolpidem is similar to that in young normal volunteers (2.6±0.3 hr). Between 0.004 and 0.019% of the total administered dose is excreted into milk, but the effect of zolpidem on the infant is unknown.

In addition, in a rat study, zolpidem inhibited the secretion of milk. The no-effect dose was 4 mg base/kg or 6 times the recommended human dose in mg/m^2.

The use of Ambien in nursing mothers is not recommended.

Pediatric use: Safety and effectiveness in pediatric patients below the age of 18 have not been established.

Geriatric use: A total of 154 patients in U.S. controlled clinical trials and 897 patients in non-U.S. clinical trials who received zolpidem were ≥60 years of age. For a pool of U.S. patients receiving zolpidem at doses of ≤10 mg or placebo, there were three adverse events occurring at an incidence of at least 3% for zolpidem and for which the zolpidem incidence was at least twice the placebo incidence (ie, they could be considered drug related).

Adverse Event	Zolpidem	Placebo
Dizziness	3%	0%
Drowsiness	5%	2%
Diarrhea	3%	1%

A total of 30/1,959 (1.5%) non-U.S. patients receiving zolpidem reported falls, including 28/30 (93%) who were ≥70 years of age. Of these 28 patients, 23 (82%) were receiving zolpidem doses >10 mg. A total of 24/1,959 (1.2%) non-U.S. patients receiving zolpidem reported confusion, including 18/24 (75%) who were ≥70 years of age. Of these 18 patients, 14 (78%) were receiving zolpidem doses >10 mg.

ADVERSE REACTIONS

Associated with discontinuation of treatment: Approximately 4% of 1,701 patients who received zolpidem at all doses (1.25 to 90 mg) in U.S. premarketing clinical trials discontinued treatment because of an adverse clinical event. Events most commonly associated with discontinuation from U.S. trials were daytime drowsiness (0.5%), dizziness (0.4%), headache (0.5%), nausea (0.6%), and vomiting (0.5%).

Approximately 4% of 1,959 patients who received zolpidem at all doses (1 to 50 mg) in similar foreign trials discontinued treatment because of an adverse event. Events most commonly associated with discontinuation from these trials were daytime drowsiness (1.1%), dizziness/vertigo (0.8%), amnesia (0.5%), nausea (0.5%), headache (0.4%), and falls (0.4%).

Data from a clinical study in which selective serotonin reuptake inhibitor- (SSRI) treated patients were given zolpidem revealed that four of the seven discontinuations during double-blind treatment with zolpidem (n=95) were associated with impaired concentration, continuing or aggravated depression, and manic reaction; one patient treated with placebo (n=97) was discontinued after an attempted suicide.

Incidence in controlled clinical trials

Most commonly observed adverse events in controlled trials: During short-term treatment (up to 10 nights) with Ambien at doses up to 10 mg, the most commonly observed adverse events associated with the use of zolpidem and seen at statistically significant differences from placebo-treated patients were drowsiness (reported by 2% of zolpidem patients), dizziness (1%), and diarrhea (1%). During longer-term treatment (28 to 35 nights) with zolpidem at doses up to 10 mg, the most commonly observed adverse events associated with the use of zolpidem and seen at statistically significant differences from placebo-treated patients were dizziness (5%) and drugged feelings (3%).

Adverse events observed at an incidence of ≥1% in controlled trials: The following tables enumerate treatment-emergent adverse event frequencies that were observed at an incidence equal to 1% or greater among patients with insomnia who received Ambien in U.S. placebo-controlled trials. Events reported by investigators were classified utilizing a modified World Health Organization (WHO) dictionary of preferred terms for the purpose of establishing event frequencies. The prescriber should be aware that these figures cannot be used to predict the incidence of side effects in the course of usual medical practice, in which patient characteristics and other factors differ from those that prevailed in these clinical trials. Similarly, the cited frequencies cannot be compared with figures obtained from other clinical investigators involving related drug products and uses, since each group of drug trials is conducted under a different set of conditions. However, the cited figures provide the physician with a basis for estimating the relative contribution of drug and nondrug factors to the incidence of side effects in the population studied.

The following table was derived from a pool of 11 placebo-controlled short-term U.S. efficacy trials involving zolpidem in doses ranging from 1.25 to 20 mg. The table is limited to data from doses up to and including 10 mg, the highest dose recommended for use.

[See table above]

The following table was derived from a pool of three placebo-controlled long-term efficacy trials involving Ambien (zolpidem tartrate). These trials involved patients with chronic insomnia who were treated for 28 to 35 nights with zolpidem at doses of 5, 10, or 15 mg. The table is limited to data from doses up to and including 10 mg, the highest dose recommended for use. The table includes only adverse events occurring at an incidence of at least 1% for zolpidem patients.

Incidence of Treatment-Emergent Adverse Experiences in Long-term Placebo-Controlled Clinical Trials
(Percentage of patients reporting)

Body System/ Adverse Event*	Zolpidem (≤10 mg) (N=152)	Placebo (N=161)
Autonomic Nervous System		
Dry mouth	3	1
Body as a Whole		
Allergy	4	1
Back pain	3	2
Influenza-like symptoms	2	–
Chest pain	1	–
Fatigue	1	2
Cardiovascular System		
Palpitation	2	–
Central and Peripheral Nervous System		
Headache	19	22
Drowsiness	8	5
Dizziness	5	1
Lethargy	3	1
Drugged feeling	3	–
Lightheadedness	2	1
Depression	2	1
Abnormal dreams	1	–
Amnesia	1	–
Anxiety	1	1
Nervousness	1	3
Sleep disorder	1	–
Gastrointestinal System		
Nausea	6	6
Dyspepsia	5	6
Diarrhea	3	2
Abdominal pain	2	2
Constipation	2	1
Anorexia	1	1
Vomiting	1	1
Immunologic System		
Infection	1	1
Musculoskeletal System		
Myalgia	7	7
Arthralgia	4	4
Respiratory System		
Upper respiratory infection	5	6
Sinusitis	4	2
Pharyngitis	3	1
Rhinitis	1	3
Skin and Appendages		
Rash	2	1
Urogenital System		
Urinary tract infection	2	2

*Events reported by at least 1% of patients treated with Ambien.

Dose relationship for adverse events: There is evidence from dose comparison trials suggesting a dose relationship for many of the adverse events associated with zolpidem

Continued on next page

Ambien—Cont.

use, particularly for certain CNS and gastrointestinal adverse events.

Adverse event incidence across the entire preapproval database: Ambien (zolpidem tartrate) was administered to 3,660 subjects in clinical trials throughout the U.S., Canada, and Europe. Treatment-emergent adverse events associated with clinical trial participation were recorded by clinical investigators using terminology of their own choosing. To provide a meaningful estimate of the proportion of individuals experiencing treatment-emergent adverse events, similar types of untoward events were grouped into a smaller number of standardized event categories and classified utilizing a modified World Health Organization (WHO) dictionary of preferred terms. The frequencies presented, therefore, represent the proportions of the 3,660 individuals exposed to zolpidem, at all doses, who experienced an event of the type cited on at least one occasion while receiving zolpidem. All reported treatment-emergent adverse events are included, except those already listed in the table above of adverse events in placebo-controlled studies, those coding terms that are so general as to be uninformative, and those events where a drug cause was remote. It is important to emphasize that, although the events reported did occur during treatment with Ambien, they were not necessarily caused by it.

Adverse events are further classified within body system categories and enumerated in order of decreasing frequency using the following definitions: frequent adverse events are defined as those occurring in greater than 1/100 subjects; infrequent adverse events are those occurring in 1/100 to 1/1,000 patients; rare events are those occurring in less than 1/1,000 patients.

Autonomic nervous system: Infrequent: increasing sweating, pallor, postural hypotension, syncope. Rare: abnormal accommodation, altered saliva, flushing, glaucoma, hypotension, impotence, increased saliva, tenesmus.

Body as a whole: Frequent: asthenia. Infrequent: edema, falling, fever, malaise, trauma. Rare: allergic reaction, allergy aggravated, abdominal body sensation, anaphylactic shock, face edema, hot flashes, increased ESR, pain, restless legs, rigors, tolerance increased, weight decrease.

Cardiovascular system: Infrequent: cerebrovascular disorder, hypertension, tachycardia. Rare: angina pectoris, arrhythmia, arteritis, circulatory failure, extrasystoles, hypertension aggravated, myocardial infarction, phlebitis, pulmonary embolism, pulmonary edema, varicose veins, ventricular tachycardia

Central and peripheral nervous system: Frequent: ataxia, confusion, euphoria, insomnia, vertigo. Infrequent: agitation, decreased cognition, detached, difficulty concentrating, dysarthria, emotional lability, hallucination, hypoesthesia, illusion, leg cramps, migraine, paresthesia, sleeping (after daytime dosing), speech disorder, stupor, tremor. Rare: abnormal gait, abnormal thinking, aggressive reaction, apathy, appetite increased, decreased libido, delusion, dementia, depersonalization, dysphasia, feeling strange, hypokinesia, hypotonia, hysteria, intoxicated feeling, manic reaction, neuralgia, neuritis, neuropathy, neurosis, panic attacks, paresis, personality disorder, somnambulism, suicide attempts, tetany, yawning.

Gastrointestinal system: Frequent: hiccup. Infrequent: constipation, dysphagia, flatulence, gastroenteritis. Rare: enteritis, eructation, esophagospasm, gastritis, hemorrhoids, intestinal obstruction, rectal hemorrhage, tooth caries.

Hematologic and lymphatic system: Rare: anemia, hyperhemoglobinemia, leukopenia, lymphadenopathy, macrocytic anemia, purpura, thrombosis.

Immunologic system: Rare: abscess, herpes simplex, herpes zoster, otitis externa, otitis media.

Liver and biliary system: Infrequent: abnormal hepatic function, increased SGPT. Rare: bilirubinemia, increased SGOT.

Metabolic and nutritional: Infrequent: hyperglycemia, thirst. Rare: gout, hypercholesteremia, hyperlipidemia, increased alkaline phosphatase, increased BUN, periorbital edema.

Musculoskeletal system: Infrequent: arthritis. Rare: arthrosis, muscle weakness, sciatica, tendinitis.

Reproductive system: Infrequent: menstrual disorder, vaginitis. Rare: breast fibroadenosis, breast neoplasm, breast pain.

Respiratory system: Infrequent: bronchitis, coughing, dyspnea. Rare: bronchospasm, epistaxis, hypoxia, laryngitis, pneumonia.

Skin and appendages: Infrequent: pruritus. Rare: acne, bullous eruption, dermatitis, furunculosis, injection-site inflammation, photosensitivity reaction, urticaria.

Special senses: Frequent: diplopia, vision abnormal. Infrequent: eye irritation, eye pain, scleritis, taste perversion, tinnitus. Rare: conjunctivitis, corneal ulceration, lacrimation abnormal, parosmia, photopsia.

Urogenital system: Infrequent: cystitis, urinary incontinence. Rare: acute renal failure, dysuria, micturition frequency, nocturia, polyuria, pyelonephritis, renal pain, urinary retention.

DRUG ABUSE AND DEPENDENCE

Controlled substance: Zolpidem tartrate is classified as a Schedule IV controlled substance by federal regulation.

Abuse and dependence: Studies of abuse potential in former drug abusers found that the effects of single doses of Ambien (zolpidem tartrate) 40 mg were similar, but not identical, to diazepam 20 mg, while zolpidem tartrate 10 mg was difficult to distinguish from placebo.

Sedative/hypnotics have produced withdrawal signs and symptoms following abrupt discontinuation. These reported symptoms range from mild dysphoria and insomnia to a withdrawal syndrome that may include abdominal and muscle cramps, vomiting, sweating, tremors, and convulsions. The U.S. clinical trial experience from zolpidem does not reveal any clear evidence for withdrawal syndrome. Nevertheless, the following adverse events included in DSM-III-R criteria for uncomplicated sedative/hypnotic withdrawal were reported during U.S. clinical trials following placebo substitution occurring within 48 hours following last zolpidem treatment: fatigue, nausea, flushing, lightheadedness, uncontrolled crying, emesis, stomach cramps, panic attack, nervousness, and abdominal discomfort. These reported adverse events occurred at an incidence of 1% or less. However, available data cannot provide a reliable estimate of the incidence, if any, of dependence during treatment at recommended doses. Rare post-marketing reports of abuse, dependence and withdrawal have been received.

Because persons with a history of addiction to, or abuse of, drugs or alcohol are at increased risk of habituation and dependence, they should be under careful surveillance when receiving zolpidem or any other hypnotic.

OVERDOSAGE

Signs and symptoms: In European postmarketing reports of overdose with zolpidem alone, impairment of consciousness has ranged from somnolence to light coma. There was one case each of cardiovascular and respiratory compromise. Individuals have fully recovered from zolpidem tartrate overdoses up to 400 mg (40 times the maximum recommended dose). Overdose cases involving multiple CNS-depressant agents, including zolpidem, have resulted in more severe symptomatology, including fatal outcomes.

Recommended treatment: General symptomatic and supportive measures should be used along with immediate gastric lavage where appropriate. Intravenous fluids should be administered as needed. Flumazenil may be useful. As in all cases of drug overdose, respiration, pulse, blood pressure, and other appropriate signs should be monitored and general supportive measures employed. Hypotension and CNS depression should be monitored and treated by appropriate medical intervention. Sedating drugs should be withheld following zolpidem overdosage, even if excitation occurs. The value of dialysis in the treatment of overdosage has not been determined, although hemodialysis studies in patients with renal failure receiving therapeutic doses have demonstrated that zolpidem is not dialyzable.

Poison control center: As with the management of all overdosage, the possibility of multiple drug ingestion should be considered. The physician may wish to consider contacting a poison control center for up-to-date information on the management of hypnotic drug product overdosage.

DOSAGE AND ADMINISTRATION

The dose of Ambien should be individualized.

The recommended dose for adults is 10 mg immediately before bedtime.

Downward dosage adjustment may be necessary when Ambien is administered with agents having known CNS-depressant effects because of the potentially additive effects.

Elderly or debilitated patients may be especially sensitive to the effects of Ambien (zolpidem tartrate). Patients with hepatic insufficiency do not clear the drug as rapidly as normals. An initial 5-mg dose is recommended in these patients (see *Precautions*).

The total Ambien dose should not exceed 10 mg.

HOW SUPPLIED

Ambien 5-mg tablets are capsule-shaped, pink, film coated, with AMB 5 debossed on one side and 5401 on the other and supplied as:

NDC Number	Size
0025-5401-31	bottle of 100
0025-5401-34	carton of 100 unit dose

Ambien 10-mg tablets are capsule-shaped, white, film coated, with AMB 10 debossed on one side and 5421 on the other and supplied as:

NDC Number	Size
0025-5421-31	bottle of 100
0025-5421-34	carton of 100 unit dose

Store at controlled room temperature 20°–25°C (68°–77°F).

Rx only

INFORMATION FOR PATIENTS TAKING AMBIEN

Your doctor has prescribed Ambien to help you sleep. The following information is intended to guide you in the safe use of this medicine. It is not meant to take the place of your doctor's instructions. If you have any questions about Ambien tablets be sure to ask your doctor or pharmacist.

Ambien is used to treat different types of sleep problems, such as:

- trouble falling asleep
- waking up too early in the morning
- waking up often during the night

Some people may have more than one of these problems.

Ambien belongs to a group of medicines known as the "sedative/hpnotics," or simply, sleep medicines. There are many different sleep medicines available to help people sleep better. Sleep problems are usually temporary, requiring treatment for only a short time, usually 1 or 2 days up to 1 or 2 weeks. Some people have chronic sleep problems that may require more prolonged use of sleep medicine. However, you should not use these medicines for long periods without talking with your doctor about the risks and benefits of prolonged use.

SIDE EFFECTS

Most common side effects: All medicines have side effects. Most common side effects of sleep medicines include:

- drowsiness
- dizziness
- lightheadedness
- difficulty with coordination

You may find that these medicines make you sleepy during the day. How drowsy you feel depends upon how your body reacts to the medicine, which sleep medicine you are taking, and how large a dose your doctor has prescribed. Daytime drowsiness is best avoided by taking the lowest dose possible that will still help you sleep at night. Your doctor will work with you to find the dose of Ambien that is best for you.

To manage these side effects while you are taking this medicine:

- When you first start taking Ambien or any other sleep medicine until you know whether the medicine will still have some carryover effect in you the next day, use extreme care while doing anything that requires complete alertness, such as driving a car, operating machinery, or piloting an aircraft.
- NEVER drink alcohol while you are being treated with Ambien or any sleep medicine. Alcohol can increase the side effects of Ambien or any other sleep medicine.
- Do not take any other medicines without asking your doctor first. This includes medicines you can buy without a prescription. Some medicines can cause drowsiness and are best avoided while taking Ambien.
- Always take the exact dose of Ambien prescribed by your doctor. Never change your dose without talking to your doctor first.

SPECIAL CONCERNS

There are some special problems that may occur while taking sleep medicines.

Memory problems: Sleep medicines may cause a special type of memory loss or "amnesia." When this occurs, a person may not remember what has happened for several hours after taking the medicine. This is usually not a problem since most people fall asleep after taking the medicine.

Memory loss can be a problem, however, when sleep medicines are taken while traveling, such as during an airplane flight and the person wakes up before the effect of the medicine is gone. This has been called "traveler's amnesia."

Memory problems are not common while taking Ambien. In most instances memory problems can be avoided if you take Ambien only when you are able to get a full night's sleep (7 to 8 hours) before you need to be active again. Be sure to talk to your doctor if you think you are having memory problems.

Tolerance: When sleep medicines are used every night for more than a few weeks, they may lose their effectiveness to help you sleep. This is known as "tolerance." Sleep medicines should, in most cases, be used only for short periods of time, such as 1 or 2 days and generally no longer than 1 or 2 weeks. If your sleep problems continue, consult your doctor, who will determine whether other measures are needed to overcome your sleep problems.

Dependence: Sleep medicines can cause dependence, especially when these medicines are used regularly for longer than a few weeks or at high doses. Some people develop a need to continue taking their medicines. This is known as dependence or "addiction."

When people develop dependence, they may have difficulty stopping the sleep medicine. If the medicine is suddenly stopped, the body is not able to function normally and unpleasant symptoms (see *Withdrawal*) may occur. They may find they have to keep taking the medicine either at the prescribed dose or at increasing doses just to avoid withdrawal symptoms.

All people taking sleep medicines have some risk of becoming dependent on the medicine. However, people who have been dependent on alcohol or other drugs in the past may have a higher chance of becoming addicted to sleep medicines. This possibility must be considered before using these medicines for more than a few weeks.

If you have been addicted to alcohol or drugs in the past, it is important to tell your doctor before starting Ambien or any sleep medicine.

Withdrawal: Withdrawal symptoms may occur when sleep medicines are stopped suddenly after being used daily for a long time. In some cases, these symptoms can occur even if the medicine has been used for only a week or two.

In mild cases, withdrawal symptoms may include unpleasant feelings. In more severe cases, abdominal and muscle cramps, vomiting, sweating, shakiness, and rarely, seizures may occur. These more severe withdrawal symptoms are very uncommon.

Another problem that may occur when sleep medicines are stopped is known as "rebound insomnia." This means that a person may have more trouble sleeping the first few nights after the medicine is stopped than before starting the medicine. If you should experience rebound insomnia, do not get discouraged. This problem usually goes away on its own after 1 or 2 nights.

If you have been taking Ambien or any other sleep medicine for more than 1 or 2 weeks, do not stop taking it on your own. Always follow your doctor's directions.

Changes in behavior and thinking: Some people using sleep medicines have experienced unusual changes in their thinking and/or behavior. These effects are not common. However, they have included:

- more outgoing or aggressive behavior than normal
- loss of personal identity
- confusion
- strange behavior
- agitation
- hallucinations
- worsening of depression
- suicidal thoughts

How often these effects occur depends on several factors, such as a person's general health, the use of other medicines, and which sleep medicine is being used. Clinical experience with Ambien suggests that it is uncommonly associated with these behavior changes.

It is also important to realize that it is rarely clear whether these behavior changes are caused by the medicine, an illness, or occur on their own. In fact, sleep problems that do not improve may be due to illnesses that were present before the medicine was used. If you or your family notice any changes in your behavior, or if you have any unusual or disturbing thoughts, call your doctor immediately.

Pregnancy: Sleep medicines may cause sedation of the unborn baby when used during the last weeks of pregnancy. Be sure to tell your doctor if you are pregnant, if you are planning to become pregnant, or if you become pregnant while taking Ambien.

SAFE USE OF SLEEPING MEDICINES

To ensure the safe and effective use of Ambien or any other sleep medicine, you should observe the following cautions:

1. Ambien is a prescription medicine and should be used ONLY as directed by your doctor. Follow your doctor's instructions about how to take, when to take, and how long to take Ambien.
2. Never use Ambien or any other sleep medicine for longer than directed by your doctor.
3. If you notice any unusual and/or disturbing thoughts or behavior during treatment with Ambien or any other sleep medicine, contact your doctor.
4. Tell your doctor about any medicines you may be taking, including medicines you may buy without a prescription. You should also tell your doctor if you drink alcohol. DO NOT use alcohol while taking Ambien or any other sleep medicine.
5. Do not take Ambien unless you are able to get a full night's sleep before you must be active again. For example, Ambien should not be taken on an overnight airplane flight of less than 7 to 8 hours since "traveler's amnesia" may occur.
6. Do not increase the prescribed dose of Ambien or any other sleep medicine unless instructed by your doctor.
7. When you first start taking Ambien or any other sleep medicine until you know whether the medicine will still have some carryover effect in you the next day, use extreme care while doing anything that requires complete alertness, such as driving a car, operating machinery, or piloting an aircraft.
8. Be aware that you may have more sleeping problems the first night or two after stopping Ambien or any other sleep medicine.
9. Be sure to tell your doctor if you are pregnant, if you are planning to become pregnant, or if you become pregnant while taking Ambien.
10. As with all prescription medicines, never share Ambien or any other sleep medicine with anyone else. Always store Ambien or any other sleep medicine in the original container out of reach of children.
11. Ambien works very quickly. You should only take Ambien right before going to bed and are ready to go to sleep.

Revised: Dec. 13, 1999

Manufactured and distributed by
G.D. Searle & Co.
Chicago IL 60680 USA
by agreement with
Lorex Pharmaceuticals
Skokie IL USA
Address medical inquiries to:
G.D. Searle & Co.
Healthcare Information Services
5200 Old Orchard Road
Skokie IL 60077 USA

Ambien is a registered trademark of Sanofi~Synthelabo, Inc.

Shown in Product Identification Guide, page 335

ARTHROTEC® ℞
[*ă 'thrŏ tek*]
(diclofenac sodium and misoprostol)
Tablets

CONTRAINDICATIONS AND WARNINGS

ARTHROTEC, because of the abortifacient property of the misoprostol component, is contraindicated in women who are pregnant. (See *PRECAUTIONS*). Reports, primarily from Brazil, of congenital anomalies and reports of fetal death subsequent to misuse of misoprostol alone, as an abortifacient, have been received. Patients must be advised of the abortifacient property and warned not to give the drug to others. ARTHROTEC should not be used in women of childbearing potential unless the patient requires nonsteroidal anti-inflammatory drug (NSAID) therapy and is at high risk of developing gastric or duodenal ulceration or for developing complications from gastric or duodenal ulcers associated with the use of the NSAID. (See *WARNINGS*). In such patients, ARTHROTEC may be prescribed if the patient:

- has had a negative serum pregnancy test within 2 weeks prior to beginning therapy.
- is capable of complying with effective contraceptive measures.
- has received both oral and written warnings of the hazards of misoprostol, the risk of possible contraception failure, and the danger to other women of childbearing potential should the drug be taken by mistake.
- will begin ARTHROTEC only on the second or third day of the next normal menstrual period.

DESCRIPTION

ARTHROTEC is a combination product containing diclofenac sodium, a nonsteroidal anti-inflammatory drug (NSAID) with analgesic properties, and misoprostol, a gastrointestinal (GI) mucosal protective prostaglandin E_1 analog. ARTHROTEC oral tablets are white to off-white, round, biconvex and approximately 11 mm in diameter. Each tablet consists of an enteric-coated core containing 50 mg (ARTHROTEC 50) or 75 mg (ARTHROTEC 75) diclofenac sodium surrounded by an outer mantle containing 200 mcg misoprostol.

Diclofenac sodium is a phenylacetic acid derivative that is a white to off-white, virtually odorless, crystalline powder. Diclofenac sodium is freely soluble in methanol, soluble in ethanol and practically insoluble in chloroform and in dilute acid. Diclofenac sodium is sparingly soluble in water. Its chemical formula and name are:

$C_{14}H_{10}Cl_2NO_2Na$ [M.W. = 318.14] 2-[(2,6-dichlorophenyl) amino]benezeneacetic acid, monosodium salt.

Misoprostol is a water-soluble, viscous liquid that contains approximately equal amounts of two diastereomers. Its chemical formula and name are:

$C_{22}H_{38}O_5$ [M.W. = 382.54] (±) methyl 11α, 16-dihydroxy-16-methyl-9-oxoprost-13E-en-1-oate.

Inactive ingredients in ARTHROTEC include: colloidal silicon dioxide; crospovidone; hydrogenated castor oil; hydroxypropyl methylcellulose; lactose; magnesium stearate; methacrylic acid copolymer; microcrystalline cellulose; povidone (polyvidone) K-30; sodium hydroxide; starch (corn); talc; triethyl citrate.

CLINICAL PHARMACOLOGY

Pharmacodynamics and pharmacokinetics of diclofenac sodium

Diclofenac sodium is a nonsteroidal anti-inflammatory drug (NSAID). In pharmacologic studies, diclofenac sodium has shown anti-inflammatory, analgesic and antipyretic properties. The mechanism of action of diclofenac sodium, like other NSAIDs, is not completely understood but may be related to prostaglandin synthetase inhibition.

Diclofenac sodium is completely absorbed from the GI tract after fasting, oral administration. The diclofenac sodium in ARTHROTEC is in a pharmaceutical formulation that resists dissolution in the low pH of gastric fluid but allows a rapid release of drug in the higher pH environment of the duodenum. Only 50% of the absorbed dose is systemically available due to first pass metabolism. Peak plasma levels are achieved in 2 hours (range 1–4 hours), and the area under the plasma concentration curve (AUC) is dose proportional within the range of 25 mg to 150 mg. Peak plasma levels are less than dose proportional and are approximately 1.5 and 2.0 mcg/mL for 50 mg and 75 mg doses, respectively.

Plasma concentrations of diclofenac sodium decline from peak levels in a biexponential fashion, with the terminal phase having a half-life of approximately 2 hours. Clearance and volume of distribution are about 350 mL/min and 550 mL/kg, respectively. More than 99% of diclofenac sodium is reversibly bound to human plasma albumin.

Diclofenac sodium is eliminated through metabolism and subsequent urinary and biliary excretion of the glucuronide and the sulfate conjugates of the metabolites. Approximately 65% of the dose is excreted in the urine and 35% in the bile.

Conjugates of unchanged diclofenac account for 5–10% of the dose excreted in the urine and for less than 5% excreted in the bile. Little or no unchanged unconjugated drug is excreted. Conjugates of the principal metabolite account for 20–30% of the dose excreted in the urine and for 10–20% of the dose excreted in the bile.

Conjugates of three other metabolites together account for 10–20% of the dose excreted in the urine and for small amounts excreted in the bile. The elimination half-life values for these metabolites are shorter than those for the parent drug. Urinary excretion of an additional metabolite (half-life = 80 hours) accounts for only 1.4% of the oral dose. The degree of accumulation of diclofenac metabolites is unknown. Some of the metabolites may have activity.

Pharmacodynamics and pharmacokinetics of misoprostol

Misoprostol is a synthetic prostaglandin E_1 analog with gastric antisecretory and (in animals) muscosal protective properties. NSAIDs inhibit prostaglandin synthesis. A deficiency of prostaglandins within the gastric and duodenal mucosa may lead to diminishing bicarbonate and mucus secretion and may contribute to the mucosal damage caused by NSAIDs.

Misoprostol can increase bicarbonate and mucus production, but in humans this has been shown at doses 200 mcg and above that are also antisecretory. It is therefore not possible to tell whether the ability of misoprostol to prevent gastric and duodenal ulcers is the result of its antisecretory effect, its mucosal protective effect, or both.

In vitro studies on canine parietal cells using tritiated misoprostol acid as the ligand have led to the identification and characterization of specific prostaglandin receptors. Receptor binding is saturable, reversible, and stereospecific. The sites have a high affinity for misoprostol, for its acid metabolite, and for other E type prostaglandins, but not for F or I prostaglandins and other unrelated compounds, such as histamine or cimetidine. Receptor-site affinity for misoprostol correlates well with an indirect index of antisecretory activity. It is likely that these specific receptors allow misoprostol taken with food to be effective topically, despite the lower serum concentrations attained.

Misoprostol produces a moderate decrease in pepsin concentration during basal conditions, but not during histamine stimulation. It has no significant effect on fasting or postprandial gastrin nor intrinsic factor output.

Effects on gastric acid secretion: Misoprostol, over the range of 50–200 mcg, inhibits basal and nocturnal gastric acid secretion, and acid secretion in response to a variety of stimuli, including meals, histamine, pentagastrin, and coffee. Activity is apparent 30 minutes after oral administration and persists for at least 3 hours. In general, the effects of 50 mcg were modest and shorter lived, and only the 200-mcg dose had substantial effects on nocturnal secretion or on histamine- and meal-stimulated secretion.

Orally administered misoprostol is rapidly and extensively absorbed, and it undergoes rapid metabolism to its biologically active metabolite, misoprostol acid. Misoprostol acid in ARTHROTEC reaches a maximum plasma concentration in about 20 minutes and is, thereafter, quickly eliminated with an elimination $t_{1/2}$ of about 30 minutes. There is high variability in plasma levels of misoprostol acid between and within studies, but mean values after single doses show a linear relationship with dose of misoprostol over the range of 200 to 400 mcg. No accumulation of misoprostol acid was found in multiple dose studies, and plasma steady state was achieved within 2 days. The serum protein binding of misoprostol acid is less than 90% and is concentration-independent in the therapeutic range.

After oral administration of radiolabeled misoprostol, about 70% of detected radioactivity appears in the urine. Maximum plasma concentrations of misoprostol acid are diminished when the dose is taken with food, and total availability of misoprostol acid is reduced by use of concomitant antacid. Clinical trials were conducted with concomitant antacid; this effect does not appear to be clinically important.

Pharmacokinetic studies also showed a lack of drug interaction with antipyrine or propranolol given with misoprostol. Misoprostol given for 1 week had no effect on the steady state pharmacokinetics of diazepam when the two drugs were administered 2 hours apart.

Pharmacokinetics of ARTHROTEC

The pharmacokinetics following oral administration of a single dose (see Table 1) or multiple doses of ARTHROTEC (diclofenac sodium/misoprostol) to healthy subjects under fasted conditions are similar to the pharmacokinetics of the two individual components.

[See table 1 at top of next page]

The rate and extent of absorption of both diclofenac sodium and misoprostol acid from ARTHROTEC 50 and ARTHROTEC 75 are similar to those from diclofenac sodium and misoprostol formulations each administered alone.

Neither diclofenac sodium nor misoprostol acid accumulated in plasma following repeated doses of ARTHROTEC given every 12 hours under fasted conditions. Food decreases the multiple-dose bioavailability profile of ARTHROTEC 50 and ARTHROTEC 75.

Special populations

A 4-week study, comparing plasma level profiles of diclofenac (50 mg bid) in younger (26–46 years) versus older (66–81 years) adults, did not show differences between age groups (10 patients per age group). In a multiple-dose (bid) crossover study of 24 people aged 65 years or older, the misoprostol contained in ARTHROTEC did not affect the pharmacokinetics of diclofenac sodium.

Differences in the pharmacokinetics of diclofenac have not been detected in studies of patients with renal (50 mg intravenously) or hepatic impairment (100 mg oral solution). In patients with renal impairment (N = 5, creatinine clearance 3 to 42 mL/min), AUC values and elimination rates were comparable to those in healthy people. In patients with biopsy-confirmed cirrhosis or chronic active hepatitis (variably elevated transaminases and mildly elevated bilirubins, N = 10), diclofenac concentrations and urinary elimination values were comparable to those in healthy people.

Continued on next page

Arthrotec—Cont.

Pharmacokinetic studies with misoprostol in patients with varying degrees of renal impairment showed an approximate doubling of $t_{1/2}$, C_{max} and AUC compared to healthy people. In people over 64 years of age, the AUC for misoprostol acid is increased.
Misoprostol does not affect the hepatic mixed function oxidase (cytochrome P-450) enzyme system in animals. In a study of people with mild to moderate hepatic impairment, mean misoprostol acid AUC and C_{max} showed approximately double the mean values obtained in healthy people. Three people who had the lowest antipyrine and lowest indocyanine green clearance values had the highest misoprostol acid AUC and C_{max} values.

CLINICAL STUDIES

Osteoarthritis
Diclofenac sodium, as a single ingredient or in combination with misoprostol, has been shown to be effective in the management of the signs and symptoms of osteoarthritis.

Rheumatoid arthritis
Diclofenac sodium, as a single ingredient or in combination with misoprostol, has been shown to be effective in the management of the signs and symptoms of rheumatoid arthritis.

Upper gastrointestinal safety
Diclofenac, and other NSAIDs, have caused serious gastrointestinal toxicity, such as bleeding, ulceration and perforation of the stomach, small intestine or large intestine. Misoprostol has been shown to reduce the incidence of endoscopically diagnosed NSAID-induced gastric and duodenal ulcers. In a 12-week, randomized, double-blind, dose response study, misoprostol 200 mcg administered qid, tid or bid, was significantly more effective than placebo in reducing the incidence of gastric ulcer in OA and RA patients using a variety of NSAIDs. The tid regimen was therapeutically equivalent to misoprostol 200 mcg qid with respect to the prevention of gastric ulcers. Misoprostol 200 mcg given bid was less effective than 200 mcg given tid or qid. The incidence of NSAID-induced duodenal ulcer was also significantly reduced with all three regimens of misoprostol compared to placebo (see Table 2).

Table 2.
Misoprostol 200 mcg Dosage Regimen

	Placebo	bid	tid	qid
Gastric ulcer	11%	6%*	3%*	3%*
Duodenal ulcer	6%	2%*	3%*	1%*

N = 1623; 12 weeks.
* Misoprostol significantly different from placebo ($p<0.05$)

Results of a study in 572 patients with osteoarthritis demonstrate that patients receiving ARTHROTEC have a lower incidence of endoscopically defined gastric ulcers compared to patients receiving diclofenac sodium (see Table 3).
[See table 3 above]

Table 1.
MISOPROSTOL ACID Mean (SD)

Treatment (n=36)	C_{max} (pg/mL)	t_{max} (hr)	AUC (0–4h) (pg·hr/mL)
ARTHROTEC 50	441 (137)	0.30 (0.13)	266 (95)
Cytotec®	478 (201)	0.30 (0.10)	295 (143)
ARTHROTEC 75	304 (110)	0.26 (0.09)	177 (49)
Cytotec	290 (130)	0.35 (0.12)	176 (58)

DICLOFENAC Mean (SD)

Treatment (n=36)	C_{max} (ng/mL)	t_{max} (hr)	AUC (0–12h) (ng·hr/mL)
ARTHROTEC 50	1207 (364)	2.4 (1.0)	1380 (272)
Voltaren®	1298 (441)	2.4 (1.0)	1357 (290)
ARTHROTEC 75	2025 (2005)	2.0 (1.4)	2773 (1347)
Voltaren	2367 (1318)	1.9 (0.7)	2609 (1185)

SD: Standard deviation of the mean
AUC: Area under the curve
C_{max}: Peak concentration
t_{max}: Time to peak concentration

Table 3.

Osteoarthritis patients with a history of ulcer or erosive disease (N=572), 6 weeks	Incidence of ulcers	
	Gastric	Duodenal
ARTHROTEC 50 tid	3%*	6%
ARTHROTEC 75 bid	4%*	3%
diclofenac sodium 75 mg bid	11%	7%
placebo	3%	1%

* Statistically significantly different from diclofenac ($p<0.05$)

INDICATIONS AND USAGE

ARTHROTEC is indicated for treatment of the signs and symptoms of osteoarthritis or rheumatoid arthritis in patients at high risk of developing NSAID-induced gastric and duodenal ulcers and their complications. See *WARNINGS—Gastrointestinal effects* for a list of factors that may increase the risk of NSAID-induced gastric and duodenal ulcers and their complications.

CONTRAINDICATIONS

See boxed ***CONTRAINDICATIONS AND WARNINGS*** related to misoprostol.
ARTHROTEC is contraindicated in patients with hypersensitivity to diclofenac or to misoprostol or other prostaglandins. ARTHROTEC should not be given to patients who have experienced asthma, urticaria, or other allergic-type reactions after taking aspirin or other NSAIDs. Severe, rarely fatal, anaphylactic-like reactions to diclofenac sodium have been reported.

WARNINGS

Regarding misoprostol:
See boxed ***CONTRAINDICATIONS AND WARNINGS***.
Regarding diclofenac:

Gastrointestinal (GI) effects—risk of GI ulceration, bleeding and perforation
Serious GI toxicity, such as inflammation, bleeding, ulceration and perforation of the stomach, small intestine or large intestine, can occur at any time, with or without warning symptoms, in patients treated with NSAIDs. Minor upper GI problems, such as dyspepsia, are common and may also occur at any time during NSAID therapy. Therefore, physicians and patients should remain alert for ulceration and bleeding, even in the absence of previous GI tract symptoms. Patients should be informed about the signs and/or symptoms and the steps to take if they occur. The utility of periodic laboratory monitoring has not been demonstrated, nor has it been adequately assessed. Only 1 in 5 patients who develop a serious upper GI adverse event on NSAID therapy is symptomatic. It has been demonstrated that upper GI ulcers, gross bleeding, or perforation, caused by NSAIDs, appear to occur in approximately 1% of patients treated for 3–6 months, and in 2–4% of patients treated for 1 year. These trends continue thus, increasing the likelihood of developing a serious GI event at some time during the course of therapy. However, even short-term therapy has risk.
NSAIDs should be prescribed with extreme caution in those with a prior history of ulcer disease or GI bleeding. Most spontaneous reports of fatal GI events are in elderly or debilitated patients and therefore special care should be taken in treating this population. **To minimize the potential risk for an adverse event, the lowest effective dose should be used for the shortest possible duration.** For very high-risk patients, alternate therapies that do not involve NSAIDs should be considered.
Studies have shown that patients with a history of peptic ulcer disease and/or GI bleeding, and who use NSAIDs, have a greater than 10-fold risk for developing a GI bleed than patients with neither of these risk factors. In addition to a past history of ulcer disease, pharmacoepidemiological studies have identified several other conditions or co-therapies that may increase the risk for GI bleeding, such as: treatment with oral corticosteroids, treatment with anticoagulants, longer duration of NSAID therapy, older age, smoking, alcoholism, poor general health and *Helicobacter pylori* positive status.

Hepatic effects
Elevations of one or more liver tests may occur during ARTHROTEC therapy. These laboratory abnormalities may progress, may remain unchanged, or may be transient with continued therapy. Borderline elevations (ie, less than 3 times the ULN [ULN = the upper limit of the normal range]), or greater elevations of transaminases occurred in about 15% of diclofenac-treated patients. Of the hepatic enzymes, ALT (SGPT) is the one recommended for the monitoring of liver injury.
In clinical trials, meaningful elevations (ie, more than 3 times the ULN) of AST (SGOT) (ALT was not measured in all studies) occurred in about 2% of approximately 5,700 patients at some time during diclofenac treatment. In a large, open, controlled trial, meaningful elevations of ALT and/or AST occurred in about 4% of 3,700 patients treated for 2–6 months, including marked elevations (ie, more than 8 times the ULN) in about 1% of the 3,700 patients. In that open-label study, a higher incidence of borderline (less than 3 times the ULN), moderate (3–8 times the ULN), and marked (>8 times the ULN) elevations of ALT or AST was observed in patients receiving diclofenac when compared to other NSAIDs. Transaminase elevations were seen more frequently in patients with osteoarthritis than in those with rheumatoid arthritis.
In addition to enzyme elevations seen in clinical trials, postmarketing surveillance has found rare cases of severe hepatic reactions, including liver necrosis, jaundice, and fulminant fatal hepatitis with and without jaundice. Some of these rare reported cases underwent liver transplantation.
Physicians should measure transaminases periodically in patients receiving long-term therapy with diclofenac, because severe hepatotoxicity may develop without a prodrome of distinguishing symptoms. The optimum times for making the first and subsequent transaminase measurements are not known. In the largest U.S. trial (open-label) that involved 3,700 patients monitored first at 8 weeks and 1,200 patients monitored again at 24 weeks, almost all meaningful elevations in transaminases were detected before patients became symptomatic. In 42 of the 51 patients in all trials who developed marked transaminase elevations, abnormal tests occurred during the first 2 months of therapy with diclofenac. Postmarketing experience has shown severe hepatic reactions can occur at any time during treatment with diclofenac. Cases of drug-induced hepatotoxicity have been reported in the first month, and in some cases, the first 2 months of therapy. Based on these experiences, transaminases should be monitored within 4 to 8 weeks after initiating treatment with diclofenac (see *PRECAUTIONS—Laboratory tests*).
In clinical trials with ARTHROTEC, meaningful elevation of ALT (SGPT, more than 3 times the ULN) occurred in 1.6% of 2,184 patients treated with ARTHROTEC, and in 1.4% of 1,691 patients treated with diclofenac sodium. These increases were generally transient, and enzyme levels returned to within the normal range upon discontinuation of ARTHROTEC therapy. The misoprostol component of ARTHROTEC does not appear to exacerbate the hepatic effects caused by the diclofenac sodium component. As with other NSAID containing products, if abnormal liver tests persist or worsen, if clinical signs and/or symptoms consistent with liver disease develop, or if systemic manifestations occur (eg, eosinophilia, rash, etc), ARTHROTEC should be discontinued immediately.
To minimize the possibility that hepatic injury will become severe between transaminase measurements, physicians should inform patients of the warning signs and symptoms of hepatotoxicity (eg, nausea, fatigue, lethargy, pruritus, jaundice, right upper quadrant tenderness, and "flu-like" symptoms), and the appropriate action patients should take if these signs and symptoms appear.

Anaphylactoid reactions
As with other NSAID containing products, anaphylactoid reactions may occur in patients without known prior exposure to ARTHROTEC or its components. ARTHROTEC should not be given to patients with the aspirin triad. The triad typically occurs in asthmatic patients who experience rhinitis with or without nasal polyps, or who exhibit severe, potentially fatal bronchospasm after taking aspirin or other NSAIDs (see *CONTRAINDICATIONS* and *PRECAUTIONS—Preexisting asthma*). Emergency help should be sought in cases where an anaphylactoid reaction occurs. Allergic reactions have been reported by less than 0.1% of patients who received ARTHROTEC in clinical trials, and there have been rare reports of anaphylaxis in the marketed use of ARTHROTEC outside of the United States.

Advanced renal disease
In patients with advanced kidney disease, treatment with ARTHROTEC is not recommended. If NSAID therapy must be initiated however, close monitoring of the patient's kidney function is advisable (see *PRECAUTIONS—Renal effects*).

PRECAUTIONS

Information for patients
See *PATIENT INFORMATION* at the end of this labeling for important information to discuss with the patient.
ARTHROTEC is available only as a unit-of-use package that includes a leaflet containing patient information. The patient should read the leaflet before taking ARTHROTEC and each time the prescription is renewed because the leaflet may have been revised. Keep ARTHROTEC out of the reach of children.

General
ARTHROTEC cannot be used to substitute for corticosteroids or to treat for corticosteroid insufficiency. Abrupt dis-

continuation of corticosteroids may lead to disease exacerbation. Patients on prolonged corticosteroid therapy should have their therapy tapered slowly if a decision is made to discontinue corticosteroids.
The pharmacological activity of ARTHROTEC in reducing inflammation may diminish the utility of this diagnostic sign in detecting complications of presumed noninfectious, painful conditions.

Renal effects

Caution should be used when initiating treatment with ARTHROTEC in patients with considerable dehydration. It is advisable to rehydrate patients first and then start therapy with ARTHROTEC. Caution is also recommended in patients with preexisting kidney disease (see *WARNINGS—Advanced renal disease*).
As with other NSAIDs, long-term administration of diclofenac has resulted in renal papillary necrosis and other renal medullary changes. Renal toxicity has also been seen in patients in which renal prostaglandins have a compensatory role in the maintenance of renal perfusion. In these patients, administration of an NSAID may cause a dose-dependent reduction in prostaglandin formation and, secondarily, in renal blood flow, which may precipitate overt renal decompensation. Patients at greatest risk of this reaction are those with impaired renal function, heart failure, or liver dysfunction, those taking diuretics and ACE inhibitors, and the elderly. Discontinuation of NSAID therapy is usually followed by recovery to the pretreatment state.
Diclofenac metabolites are eliminated primarily by the kidneys. The extent to which the metabolites may accumulate in patients with renal failure has not been studied. As with other NSAIDs, metabolites of which are excreted by the kidney, patients with significantly impaired renal function should be more closely monitored.

Hematologic effects

Anemia is sometimes seen in patients receiving diclofenac or other NSAIDs. This may be due to fluid retention, GI blood loss, or an incompletely described effect upon erythropoiesis. Patients on long-term treatment with NSAIDs, including ARTHROTEC, should have their hemoglobin or hematocrit checked if they exhibit any signs or symptoms of anemia.
All drugs that inhibit the biosynthesis of prostaglandins may interfere to some extent with platelet function and vascular responses to bleeding.
NSAIDs inhibit platelet aggregation and, unlike aspirin, their effect on platelet function is reversible, quantitatively less, and of shorter duration. ARTHROTEC does not generally affect platelet counts, prothrombin time (PT), or partial thromboplastin time (PTT). Patients receiving ARTHROTEC who may be adversely affected by alterations in platelet function, such as those with coagulation disorders or patients receiving anticoagulants, should be carefully monitored.

Aseptic meningitis

As with other NSAIDs, aseptic meningitis with fever and coma has been observed on rare occasions in patients on diclofenac therapy. Although it is probably more likely to occur in patients with systemic lupus and related connective tissue diseases, it has been reported in patients who do not have an underlying chronic disease. If signs or symptoms of meningitis develop in a patient on diclofenac, the possibility of its being related to diclofenac should be considered.

Fluid retention and edema

Fluid retention and edema have been observed in some patients taking NSAID containing products, including ARTHROTEC. Therefore, as with other NSAID containing products, ARTHROTEC should be used with caution in patients with a history of cardiac decompensation, hypertension, or other conditions predisposing to fluid retention.

Preexisting asthma

Patients with asthma may have aspirin-sensitive asthma. The use of aspirin in patients with aspirin-sensitive asthma has been associated with severe bronchospasm, which can be fatal. Since cross-reactivity, including bronchospasm, between aspirin and other NSAIDs has been reported in such aspirin-sensitive patients. ARTHROTEC should not be administered to patients with this form of aspirin sensitivity and should be used with caution in patients with preexisting asthma.

Porphyria

The use of ARTHROTEC in patients with hepatic porphyria should be avoided. To date, one patient has been described in whom diclofenac sodium probably triggered a clinical attack of porphyria. The postulated mechanism, demonstrated in rats, for causing such attacks by diclofenac sodium, as well as some other NSAIDs, is through stimulation of the porphyrin precursor delta-aminolevulinic acid (ALA).

Laboratory tests

Patients on long-term treatment with NSAIDs should have their CBC and a chemistry profile checked periodically. If clinical signs and symptoms consistent with liver or renal disease develop, systemic manifestations occur (eg, eosinophilia, rash, etc) or if abnormal liver tests persist or worsen, ARTHROTEC should be discontinued.
Effect on blood coagulation: Diclofenac sodium impairs platelet aggregation but does not affect bleeding time, plasma thrombin clotting time, plasma fibrinogen, or factors V and VII to XII. Statistically significant changes in prothrombin and partial thromboplastin times have been reported in normal volunteers. The mean changes were observed to be less than 1 second in both instances, however, and are unlikely to be clinically important. Diclofenac sodium is a prostaglandin synthetase inhibitor, however, and all drugs that inhibit prostaglandin synthesis interfere with platelet function to some degree; therefore, patients who may be adversely affected by such an action should be carefully observed. Misoprostol has not been shown to exacerbate the effects of diclofenac on platelet activity.

Drug interactions

Aspirin: Concomitant administration of ARTHROTEC and aspirin is not recommended because diclofenac sodium is displaced from its binding sites by aspirin, resulting in lower plasma concentrations, peak plasma levels and AUC values.
Digoxin: Elevated digoxin levels have been reported in patients receiving digoxin and diclofenac sodium. Patients receiving digoxin and ARTHROTEC should be monitored for possible digoxin toxicity.
Antihypertensive agents: NSAIDs can inhibit the activity of antihypertensives, including ACE inhibitors. Thus, caution should be taken when administering ARTHROTEC with such agents.
Warfarin: The effects of warfarin and NSAIDs on GI bleeding are synergistic, such that users of both drugs together have a risk of serious bleeding greater than users of either drug alone.
Oral hypoglycemics: Diclofenac sodium does not alter glucose metabolism in healthy people nor does it alter the effects of oral hypoglycemic agents. There are rare reports, however, from marketing experience, of changes in effects of insulin or oral hypoglycemic agents in the presence of diclofenac sodium that necessitated change in the doses of such agents. Both hypo- and hyperglycemic effects have been reported. A direct causal relationship has not been established, but physicians should consider the possibility that diclofenac sodium may alter a diabetic patient's response to insulin or oral hypoglycemic agents.
Methotrexate and cyclosporine: ARTHROTEC, like other NSAID containing products, may affect renal prostaglandins and increase the toxicity of certain drugs. Ingestion of ARTHROTEC may increase serum concentrations of methotrexate and increase cyclosporine nephrotoxicity. Patients who begin taking ARTHROTEC or who increase their dose of ARTHROTEC or any other NSAID containing product while taking methotrexate or cyclosporine may develop toxicity characteristic for these drugs. They should be observed closely, particularly if renal function is impaired.
Lithium: NSAIDs have produced an elevation of plasma lithium levels and a reduction in renal lithium clearance. The mean minimum lithium concentration increased 15% and the renal clearance was decreased by approximately 20%. These effects have been attributed to inhibition of renal prostaglandin synthesis by the NSAID. Thus, when NSAIDs and lithium are administered concurrently, subjects should be observed carefully for signs of lithium toxicity.
Antacids: Antacids reduce the bioavailability of misoprostol acid. Antacids may also delay absorption of diclofenac sodium. Magnesium-containing antacids exacerbate misoprostol-associated diarrhea. Thus, it is not recommended that ARTHROTEC be coadministered with magnesium-containing antacids.
Diuretics: The diclofenac sodium component of ARTHROTEC, like other NSAIDs, can inhibit the activity of diuretics. Concomitant therapy with potassium-sparing diuretics may be associated with increased serum potassium levels.
Other drugs: In small groups of patients (7–10 patients/interaction study), the concomitant administration of azathioprine, gold, chloroquine, D-penicillamine, prednisolone, doxycycline or digitoxin did not significantly affect the peak levels and AUC levels of diclofenac sodium. Phenobarbital toxicity has been reported to have occurred in a patient on chronic phenobarbital treatment following the initiation of diclofenac therapy. *In vitro*, diclofenac interferes minimally with the protein binding of prednisolone (10% decrease in binding). Benzylpenicillin, ampicillin, oxacillin, chlortetracycline, doxycycline, cephalothin, erythromycin, and sulfamethoxazole have no influence, *in vitro*, on the protein binding of diclofenac in human serum.

Animal toxicology

A reversible increase in the number of normal surface gastric epithelial cells occurred in the dog, rat, and mouse during long-term toxicology studies with misoprostol. No such increase has been observed in humans administered misoprostol for up to 1 year. An apparent response of the female mouse to misoprostol in long-term studies at 100 to 1000 times the human dose was hyperostosis, mainly of the medulla of sternebrae. Hyperostosis did not occur in long-term studies in the dog and rat and has not been seen in humans treated with misoprostol.

Carcinogenesis, mutagenesis, impairment of fertility

Long-term animal studies to evaluate the potential for carcinogenesis and animal studies to evaluate the effects on fertility have been performed with each component of ARTHROTEC given alone. ARTHROTEC itself (diclofenac sodium and misoprostol combinations in 250:1 ratio) was not genotoxic in the Ames test, the Chinese hamster ovary cell (CHO/HGPRT) forward mutation test, the rat lymphocyte chromosome aberration test or the mouse micronucleus test.

In a 24-month rat carcinogenicity study, oral misoprostol at doses up to 2.4 mg/kg/day (14.4 mg/m^2/day, 24 times the recommended maximum human dose of 0.6 mg/m^2/day) was not tumorigenic. In a 21-month mouse carcinogenicity study, oral misoprostol at doses up to 16 mg/kg/day (48 mg/m^2/day), 80 times the recommended maximum human dose based on body surface area, was not tumorigenic. Misoprostol, when administered to male and female breeding rats in an oral dose-range of 0.1 to 10 mg/kg/day (0.6 to 60 mg/m^2/day, 1 to 100 times the recommended maximum human dose based on body surface area) produced dose-related pre- and post-implantation losses and a significant decrease in the number of live pups born at the highest dose. These findings suggest the possibility of a general adverse effect on fertility in males and females.
In a 24-month rat carcinogenicity study, oral diclofenac sodium up to 2 mg/kg/day (12 mg/m^2/day) was not tumorigenic. For a 50-kg person of average height (1.46m^2 body surface area), this dose represents 0.08 times the recommended maximum human dose (148 mg/m^2) on a body surface area basis. In a 24-month mouse carcinogenicity study, oral diclofenac sodium at doses up to 0.3 mg/kg/day (0.9 mg/m^2/day, 0.006 times the recommended maximum human dose based on body surface area) in males and 1 mg/kg/day (3 mg/m^2/day, 0.02 times the recommended maximum human dose based on body surface area) in females was not tumorigenic. Diclofenac sodium at oral doses up to 4 mg/kg/day (24 mg/m^2/day, 0.16 times the recommended maximum human dose based on body surface area) was found to have no effect on fertility and reproductive performance of male and female rats.

Pregnancy

Pregnancy category X: See boxed ***CONTRAINDICATIONS AND WARNINGS*** regarding misoprostol. ARTHROTEC is contraindicated in pregnancy.

Non-teratogenic effects

Misoprostol may endanger pregnancy (may cause miscarriage) and thereby cause harm to the fetus when administered to a pregnant woman. Misoprostol produces uterine contractions, uterine bleeding, and expulsion of the products of conception. Miscarriages caused by misoprostol may be incomplete. In studies in women undergoing elective termination of pregnancy during the first trimester, misoprostol caused partial or complete expulsion of the products of conception in 11% of the subjects and increased uterine bleeding in 41%.
Reports, primarily from Brazil, of congenital anomalies and reports of fetal death subsequent to misuse of misoprostol alone, as an abortifacient, have been received (see boxed ***CONTRAINDICATIONS AND WARNINGS***). If a woman is or becomes pregnant while taking this drug, the drug should be discontinued and the patient apprised of the potential hazard to the fetus.
The diclofenac sodium component of ARTHROTEC, like other NSAIDs which are prostaglandin-inhibiting drugs, may affect the fetal cardiovascular system causing premature closure of the ductus arteriosus. NSAIDs may also inhibit uterine contractions.

Teratogenic effects

An oral teratology study has been performed in pregnant rabbits at dose combinations (250:1 ratio) up to 10 mg/kg/day diclofenac sodium (120 mg/m^2/day, 0.8 times the recommended maximum human dose based on body surface area) and 0.04 mg/kg/day misoprostol (0.48 mg/m^2/day, 0.8 times the recommended maximum human dose based on body surface area) and has revealed no evidence of teratogenic potential for ARTHROTEC.
Oral teratology studies have been performed in pregnant rats at doses up to 1.6 mg/kg/day (9.6 mg/m^2/day, 16 times the recommended maximum human dose based on body surface area) and pregnant rabbits at doses up to 1.0 mg/kg/day (12 mg/m^2/day, 20 times the recommended maximum human dose based on body surface area) and have revealed no evidence of teratogenic potential for misoprostol.
Oral teratology studies have been performed in pregnant mice at doses up to 20 mg/kg/day (60 mg/m^2/day, 0.4 times the recommended maximum human dose based on body surface area), pregnant rats at doses up to 10 mg/kg/day (60 mg/m^2/day. 0.4 times the recommended maximum human dose based on body surface area) and pregnant rabbits at doses up to 10 mg/kg/day (120 mg/m^2/day, 0.8 times the recommended maximum human dose based on body surface area) and have revealed no evidence of teratogenic potential for diclofenac sodium.

Nursing mothers

Diclofenac sodium has been found in the milk of nursing mothers. It is unlikely that misoprostol is excreted into milk since the drug is rapidly metabolized throughout the body. Excretion of the active metabolite (misoprostol acid) into milk is possible, but has not been studied. Because of the potential for serious adverse reactions in nursing infants, ARTHROTEC is not recommended for use by nursing mothers.

Pediatric use

Safety and effectiveness of ARTHROTEC in pediatric patients have not been established.

Geriatric use

Of the more than 2100 subjects in clinical studies with ARTHROTEC, 25% were 65 and over, while 6% wre 75 and over. In studies with diclofenac, 31% of subjects were 65 and over. No overall differences in safety or effectiveness were observed between these subjects and younger subjects, and other reported clinical experience has not identified differences in repsonses between the elderly and younger patients, but greater sensitivity of some older individuals cannot be ruled out. As with any NSAID, the elderly are likely to tolerate adverse events less well than younger patients
Diclofenac is known to be substantially excreted by the kidney, and the risk of toxic reactions to ARTHROTEC may be greater in patients with impaired renal function. Because elderly patients are more likely to have decreased renal function, care should be taken in dose selection, and it may

Continued on next page

Arthrotec—Cont.

be useful to monitor renal function (See *PRECAUTIONS—Renal Effects*).
Based on studies in the elderly, no adjustment of the dose of ARTHROTEC is necessary in the elderly for pharmacokinetic reasons. (See *Pharmacokinetics of ARTHROTEC—Special populations*), although many elderly may need to receive a reduced dose because of low body weight or disorders associated with aging.

ADVERSE REACTIONS

Adverse reactions associated with ARTHROTEC

Adverse reaction information for ARTHROTEC is derived from Phase III multinational controlled clinical trials in over 2,000 patients receiving ARTHROTEC 50 or ARTHROTEC 75, as well as from blinded, controlled trials of Voltaren® Delayed-Release Tablets (diclofenac) and Cytotec® Tablets (misoprostol).

Gastrointestinal

GI disorders had the highest reported incidence of adverse events for patients receiving ARTHROTEC. These events were generally minor, but let to discontinuation of therapy in 9% of patients on ARTHROTEC and 5% of patients on diclofenac. For GI ulcer rates, see *CLINICAL STUDIES—Upper gastrointestinal safety.*

GI disorder	ARTHROTEC	Diclofenac
Abdominal pain	21%	15%
Diarrhea	19%	11%
Dyspepsia	14%	11%
Nausea	11%	6%
Flatulence	9%	4%

ARTHROTEC can cause more abdominal pain, diarrhea and other GI symptoms than diclofenac alone.
Diarrhea and abdominal pain developed early in the course of therapy, and were usually self-limited (resolved after 2 to 7 days). Rare instances of profound diarrhea leading to severe dehydration have been reported in patients receiving misoprostol. Patients with an underlying condition such as inflammatory bowel disease, or those in whom dehydration, were it to occur, would be dangerous, should be monitored carefully if ARTHROTEC is prescribed. The incidence of diarrhea can be minimized by administering ARTHROTEC with food and by avoiding coadministration with magnesium-containing antacids.

Gynecological

Gynecological disorders previously reported with misoprostol use have also been reported for women receiving ARTHROTEC (see below). Postmenopausal vaginal bleeding may be related to ARTHROTEC administration. If it occurs, diagnostic workup should be undertaken to rule out gynecological pathology.

Elderly

Overall, there were no significant differences in the safety profile of ARTHROTEC in over 500 patients 65 years of age or older compared with younger patients.
Other adverse experiences reported occasionally or rarely with ARTHROTEC, diclofenac or other NSAIDs, or misoprostol are:
Body as a Whole: Asthenia, death, fatigue, fever, infection, malaise, sepsis.
Cardiovascular system: Arrhythmia, atrial fibrillation, congestive heart failure, hypertension, hypotension, increased CPK, increased LDH, myocardial infarction, palpitations, phlebitis, premature ventricular contractions, syncope, tachycardia, vasculitis.
Central and peripheral nervous system: Coma, convulsions, dizziness, drowsiness, headache, hyperesthesia, hypertonia, hypoesthesia, insomnia, meningitis, migraine, neuralgia, paresthesia, somnolence, tremor, vertigo.
Digestive: Anorexia, appetite changes, constipation, dry mouth, dysphagia, enteritis, esophageal ulceration, esophagitis, eructation, gastritis, gastroesophageal reflux, GI bleeding, GI neoplasm benign, glossitis, heartburn, hematemesis, hemorrhoids, intestinal perforation, peptic ulcer, stomatitis and ulcerative stomatitis, tenesmus, vomiting.
Female reproductive disorders: Breast pain, dysmenorrhea, intermenstrual bleeding, leukorrhea, menstrual disorder, menorrhagia, vaginal hemorrhage.
Hemic and lymphatic system: Agranulocytosis, anemia, aplastic anemia, coagulation time increased, ecchymosis, eosinophilia, epistaxis, hemolytic anemia, leukocytosis, leukopenia, lymphadenopathy, melena, pancytopenia, pulmonary embolism, purpura, rectal bleeding, thrombocythemia, thrombocytopenia.
Hypersensitivity: Angioedema, laryngeal/pharyngeal edema, urticaria.
Liver and biliary system: Abnormal hepatic function, bilirubinemia, hepatitis, jaundice, liver failure, pancreatitis.
Male reproductive disorders: Impotence, perineal pain.
Metabolic and nutritional: Alkaline phosphatase increased, BUN increased, dehydration, glycosuria, gout, hypercholesterolemia, hyperglycemia, hyperuricemia, hypoglycemia, hyponatremia, periorbital edema, porphyria, weight changes.
Musculoskeletal system: Arthralgia, myalgia.
Psychiatric: Anxiety, concentration impaired, confusion, depression, disorientation, dream abnormalities, hallucinations, irritability, nervousness, paranoia, psychotic reaction.
Respiratory system: Asthma, coughing, dyspnea, hyperventilation, pneumonia, respiratory depression.
Skin and appendages: Acne, alopecia, bruising, eczema, erythema multiforme, exfoliative dermatitis, pemphigoid reaction, photosensitivity, pruritus, pruritus ani, rash, skin ulceration, Stevens-Johnson syndrome, sweating increased, toxic epidermal necrolysis.
Special senses: Hearing impairment, taste loss, taste perversion, tinnitus.
Urinary system: Cystitis, dysuria, hematuria, interstitial nephritis, micturition frequency, nocturia, nephrotic syndrome, oliguria/polyuria, papillary necrosis, proteinuria, renal failure, urinary tract infection.
Vision: Amblyopia, blurred vision, conjunctivitis, diplopia, glaucoma, iritis, lacrimation abnormal, night blindness, vision abnormal.

OVERDOSAGE

The toxic dose of ARTHROTEC has not been determined. However, signs of overdosage from the components of the product have been described.

Diclofenac sodium

Clinical signs that may suggest diclofenac sodium overdose include GI complaints, confusion, drowsiness or general hypotonia. Reports of overdosage with diclofenac cover 66 cases. In approximately one-half of these reports of overdosage, concomitant medications were also taken. The highest dose of diclofenac was 5.0 g in a 17-year-old man who suffered loss of consciousness, increased intracranial pressure, and aspiration pneumonitis, and died 2 days after overdose. A 24-year-old woman who took 4.0 g and the 28- and 42-year-old women, each of whom took 3.75 g, did not develop any clinically significant signs or symptoms. However, there was a report of a 17-year-old female who experienced vomiting and drowsiness after an overdose of 2.37 g of diclofenac.
Animal studies show a wide range of susceptibilities to acute overdosage, with primates being more resistant to acute toxicity than rodents (LD_{50} in mg/kg: rats, 55; dogs, 500; monkeys, 3200).

Misoprostol

The toxic dose of misoprostol in humans has not been determined. Cumulative total daily doses of 1600 mcg have been tolerated, with only symptoms of GI discomfort being reported. In animals, the acute toxic effects are diarrhea, GI lesions, focal cardiac necrosis, hepatic necrosis, renal tubular necrosis, testicular atrophy, respiratory difficulties, and depression of the central nervous system. Clinical signs that may indicate an overdose are sedation, tremor, convulsions, dyspnea, abdominal pain, diarrhea, fever, palpitations, hypotension, or bradycardia.

ARTHROTEC

Symptoms of ARTHROTEC overdosage should be treated with supportive therapy. In case of acute overdosage, gastric lavage is recommended. Induced diuresis may be beneficial because diclofenac sodium and misoprostol metabolites are excreted in the urine. The effect of dialysis or hemoperfusion on the elimination of diclofenac sodium (99% protein bound) and misoprostol acid remains unproven. The use of oral activated charcoal may help to reduce the absorption of diclofenac sodium and misoprostol.

DOSAGE AND ADMINISTRATION

ARTHROTEC is administered as ARTHROTEC 50 (50 mg diclofenac sodium/200 mcg misoprostol) or as ARTHROTEC 75 (75 mg diclofenac sodium/200 mcg misoprostol).
Note: See *SPECIAL DOSING CONSIDERATIONS* section, below.
Osteoarthritis: The recommended dosage for maximal GI mucosal protection is ARTHROTEC 50 tid. For patients who experience intolerance, ARTHROTEC 75 bid or ARTHROTEC 50 bid can be used, but are less effective in preventing ulcers. This fixed combination product, ARTHROTEC, is not appropriate for patients who would not receive the appropriate dose of both ingredients. Doses of the components delivered with these regimens are as follows:

	OA regimen	Diclofenac sodium (mg/day)	Misoprostol (mcg/day)
ARTHROTEC 50	tid	150	600
	bid	100	400
ARTHROTEC 75	bid	150	400

Rheumatoid Arthritis: The recommended dosage is ARTHROTEC 50 tid or qid. For patients who experience intolerance, ARTHROTEC 75 bid or ARTHROTEC 50 bid can be used, but are less effective in preventing ulcers. This fixed combination product, ARTHROTEC, is not appropriate for patients who would not receive the appropriate dose of both ingredients. Doses of the components delivered with these regimens are as follows:

	RA regimen	Diclofenac sodium (mg/day)	Misoprostol (mcg/day)
ARTHROTEC 50	qid	200	800
	tid	150	600
	bid	100	400
ARTHROTEC 75	bid	150	400

SPECIAL DOSING CONSIDERATIONS: ARTHROTEC contains misoprostol, which provides protection against gastric and duodenal ulcers (see *CLINICAL STUDIES*). For gastric ulcer prevention, the 200 mcg qid and tid regimens are therapeutically equivalent, but more protective than the bid regimen. For duodenal ulcer prevention, the qid regimen is more protective than the tid or bid regimens. However, the qid regimen is less well tolerated than the tid regimen because of usually self-limited diarrhea related to the misoprostol dose (see *ADVERSE REACTIONS—Gastrointestinal*), and the bid regimen may be better tolerated than tid in some patients.

Dosages may be individualized using the separate products (misoprostol and diclofenac), after which the patient may be changed to the appropriate ARTHROTEC dose. If clinically indicated, misoprostol co-therapy with ARTHROTEC, or use of the individual components to optimize the misoprostol dose and/or frequency of administration, may be appropriate. The total dose of misoprostol should not exceed 800 mcg/day, and no more than 200 mcg of misoprostol should be administered at any one time. Doses of diclofenac higher than 150 mcg/day in osteoarthritis or higher than 225 mg/day in rheumatoid arthritis are not recommended.
For additional information, it may be helpful to refer to the package inserts for Cytotec® tablets and Voltaren® tablets.

HOW SUPPLIED

ARTHROTEC (diclofenac sodium/misoprostol) is supplied as a film-coated tablet in dosage strengths of either 50 mg diclofenac sodium/200 mcg misoprostol or 75 mg diclofenac sodium/200 mcg misoprostol. The 50 mg/200 mcg dosage strength is a round, biconvex, white to off-white tablet imprinted with four "A's" encircling a "50" in the middle on one side and "SEARLE" and "1411" on the other. The 75 mg/200 mcg dosage strength is a round, biconvex, white to off-white tablet imprinted with four "A's" encircling a "75" in the middle on one side and "SEARLE" and "1421" on the other.
The dosage strengths are supplied in:

Strength	NDC Number	Size
50/200	0025-1411-60	bottle of 60
	0025-1411-90	bottle of 90
	0025-1411-34	carton of 100 unit dose
75/200	0025-1421-60	bottle of 60
	0025-1421-34	carton of 100 unit dose

Store at or below 25°C (77°F), in a dry area.

PATIENT INFORMATION

Read this leaflet before taking ARTHROTEC (diclofenac sodium 50 or 75 mg/misoprostol 200 mcg) and each time your prescription is renewed, because the leaflet may be changed.

ARTHROTEC is being prescribed by your doctor for treatment of your arthritis symptoms while at the same time providing protection from the development of stomach and intestinal ulcers due to the arthritis medication. ARTHROTEC contains diclofenac, an arthritis medication. ARTHROTEC also contains misoprostol to decrease the chance of getting stomach and intestinal ulcers that sometimes develop with NSAID medications. Serious side effects are still possible, however, and you should report to your physician any signs or symptoms of gastrointestinal ulceration or bleeding, skin rash, weight gain or swelling. If signs of liver toxicity occur (nausea, fatigue, lethargy, itching, jaundice, right upper quadrant tenderness, and "flu-like" symptoms) you should stop therapy and seek immediate medical attention.
Do not take ARTHROTEC if you are pregnant and do not become pregnant while taking this medication. ARTHROTEC can cause miscarriage, often associated with potentially dangerous bleeding. Such miscarriages may result in hospitalization, surgery, infertility or death.
If you become pregnant during ARTHROTEC therapy, stop taking ARTHROTEC and contact your doctor immediately. Remember that even if you are using a means of birth control, it is still possible to become pregnant. Should this occur, stop taking ARTHROTEC and consult your physician immediately.
ARTHROTEC may cause diarrhea, abdominal pain, upset stomach and/or nausea in some people. In most cases these problems develop during the first few weeks of therapy and stop after about a week with continued treatment. You can minimize possible diarrhea by making sure you take ARTHROTEC with meals and by avoiding the use of antacids containing magnesium (if needed, use one containing aluminum or calcium instead). ARTHROTEC tablets should be swallowed whole, and not chewed, crushed or dissolved.

Because these side effects are usually mild to moderate and usually go away in a matter of days, most patients can continue to take ARTHROTEC. If you have prolonged difficulty (more than 7 days), or if you have severe diarrhea, cramping and/or nausea, call your doctor.
Take ARTHROTEC only according to the directions given by your doctor. Changes in dose should be made only with your doctor's approval.
Do not give ARTHROTEC to anyone else. It has been prescribed for your specific condition, may not be the correct treatment for another person, and could be dangerous for another person, especially a woman who may be, or could become, pregnant.
This information sheet does not cover all possible side effects of ARTHROTEC. See your doctor if you have questions.
Keep out of reach of children.
Rx only **Revised: Jan. 17, 2000**

Packaged by G.D. Searle & Co., San Juan PR 00936
Manufactured by Searle, Morpeth, England
For G.D. Searle & Co.
Chicago IL 60680 USA

Address medical inquiries to:
G.D. Searle & Co.
Healthcare Information Services
5200 Old Orchard Road
Skokie IL 60077

SEARLE

A05440-4

Shown in Product Identification Guide, page 335

CALAN® Tablets ℞
[*cal 'an*]
(verapamil hydrochloride)

PRODUCT OVERVIEW

KEY FACTS

Calan, a calcium ion antagonist, exerts its pharmacologic effects by modulating the influx of ionic calcium across the cell membrane of the arterial smooth muscle as well as in conductile and contractile myocardial cells. Calan increases myocardial oxygen supply, reduces myocardial oxygen consumption, and is a potent inhibitor of coronary artery spasm, making it an effective antianginal agent. By decreasing the influx of calcium, Calan prolongs the effective refractory period within the AV node and slows AV conduction in a rate-related manner, thereby slowing the ventricular rate in patients with chronic atrial flutter or fibrillation. Calan exerts antihypertensive effects by decreasing systemic vascular resistance, usually without orthostatic decreases in blood pressure or reflex tachycardia.

MAJOR USES

Calan Tablets are indicated for: angina at rest, including vasospastic and unstable angina; chronic stable angina; control (in association with digitalis) of ventricular rate at rest and during stress in patients with chronic atrial flutter and/or atrial fibrillation; prophylaxis of repetitive paroxysmal supraventricular tachycardia; management of essential hypertension.

SAFETY INFORMATION

See complete safety information set forth below.

PRESCRIBING INFORMATION

CALAN® Tablets ℞
[*cal 'an*]
(verapamil hydrochloride)

DESCRIPTION

Calan (verapamil HCl) is a calcium ion influx inhibitor (slow-channel blocker or calcium ion antagonist) available for oral administration in film-coated tablets containing 40 mg, 80 mg, or 120 mg of verapamil hydrochloride.
The structural formula of verapamil HCl is

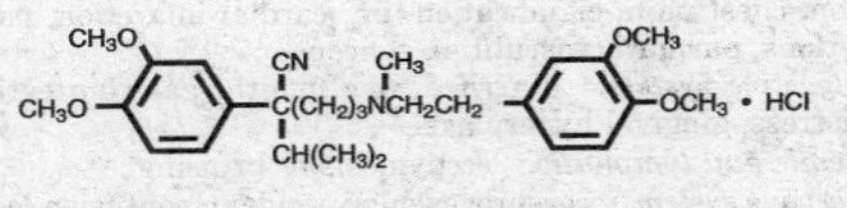

$C_{27}H_{38}N_2O_4 \cdot HCl$ M. W. = 491.08

Benzeneacetonitrile, α-[3-[[2-(3,4-dimethoxyphenyl) ethyl] methylamino]propyl]-3,4-dimethoxy-α-(1-methylethyl) hydrochloride

Verapamil HCl is an almost white, crystalline powder, practically free of odor, with a bitter taste. It is soluble in water, chloroform, and methanol. Verapamil HCl is not chemically related to other cardioactive drugs.
Inactive ingredients include microcrystalline cellulose, corn starch, gelatin, hydroxypropyl cellulose, hydroxypropyl methylcellulose, iron oxide colorant, lactose, magnesium stearate, polyethylene glycol, talc, and titanium dioxide.

CLINICAL PHARMACOLOGY

Calan is a calcium ion influx inhibitor (slow-channel blocker or calcium ion antagonist) that exerts its pharmacologic effects by modulating the influx of ionic calcium across the cell membrane of the arterial smooth muscle as well as in conductile and contractile myocardial cells.

Mechanism of action

Angina: The precise mechanism of action of Calan as an antianginal agent remains to be fully determined, but includes the following two mechanisms:

1. *Relaxation and prevention of coronary artery spasm:* Calan dilates the main coronary arteries and coronary arterioles, both in normal and ischemic regions, and is a potent inhibitor of coronary artery spasm, whether spontaneous or ergonovine-induced. This property increases myocardial oxygen delivery in patients with coronary artery spasm and is responsible for the effectiveness of Calan in vasospastic (Prinzmetal's or variant) as well as unstable angina at rest. Whether this effect plays any role in classical effort angina is not clear, but studies of exercise tolerance have not shown an increase in the maximum exercise rate–pressure product, a widely accepted measure of oxygen utilization. This suggests that, in general, relief of spasm or dilation of coronary arteries is not an important factor in classical angina.
2. *Reduction of oxygen utilization:* Calan regularly reduces the total peripheral resistance (afterload) against which the heart works both at rest and at a given level of exercise by dilating peripheral arterioles. This unloading of the heart reduces myocardial energy consumption and oxygen requirements and probably accounts for the effectiveness of Calan in chronic stable effort angina.

Arrhythmia: Electrical activity through the AV node depends, to a significant degree, upon calcium influx through the slow channel. By decreasing the influx of calcium, Calan prolongs the effective refractory period within the AV node and slows AV conduction in a rate-related manner. This property accounts for the ability of Calan to slow the ventricular rate in patients with chronic atrial flutter or atrial fibrillation.
Normal sinus rhythm is usually not affected, but in patients with sick sinus syndrome, Calan may interfere with sinus-node impulse generation and may induce sinus arrest or sinoatrial block. Atrioventricular block can occur in patients without preexisting conduction defects (see *Warnings*). Calan decreases the frequency of episodes of paroxysmal supraventricular tachycardia.
Calan does not alter the normal atrial action potential or intraventricular conduction time, but in depressed atrial fibers it decreases amplitude, velocity of depolarization, and conduction velocity. Calan may shorten the antegrade effective refractory period of the accessory bypass tract. Acceleration of ventricular rate and/or ventricular fibrillation has been reported in patients with atrial flutter or atrial fibrillation and a coexisting accessory AV pathway following administration of verapamil (see *Warnings*).
Calan has a local anesthetic action that is 1.6 times that of procaine on an equimolar basis. It is not known whether this action is important at the doses used in man.

Essential hypertension: Calan exerts antihypertensive effects by decreasing systemic vascular resistance, usually without orthostatic decreases in blood pressure or reflex tachycardia; bradycardia (rate less than 50 beats/min) is uncommon (1.4%). During isometric or dynamic exercise Calan does not alter systolic cardiac function in patients with normal ventricular function.
Calan does not alter total serum calcium levels. However, one report suggested that calcium levels above the normal range may alter the therapeutic effect of Calan.

Pharmacokinetics and metabolism: More than 90% of the orally administered dose of Calan is absorbed. Because of rapid biotransformation of verapamil during its first pass through the portal circulation, bioavailability ranges from 20% to 35%. Peak plasma concentrations are reached between 1 and 2 hours after oral administration. Chronic oral administration of 120 mg of verapamil HCl every 6 hours resulted in plasma levels of verapamil ranging from 125 to 400 ng/ml, with higher values reported occasionally. A nonlinear correlation between the verapamil dose administered and verapamil plasma levels does exist. No relationship has been established between the plasma concentration of verapamil and a reduction in blood pressure. In early dose titration with verapamil a relationship exists between verapamil plasma concentration and prolongation of the PR interval. However, during chronic administration this relationship may disappear. The mean elimination half-life in single-dose studies ranged from 2.8 to 7.4 hours. In these same studies, after repetitive dosing, the half-life increased to a range from 4.5 to 12.0 hours (after less than 10 consecutive doses given 6 hours apart). Half-life of verapamil may increase during titration. Aging may affect the pharmacokinetics of verapamil. Elimination half-life may be prolonged in the elderly. In healthy men, orally administered Calan undergoes extensive metabolism in the liver. Twelve metabolites have been identified in plasma; all except norverapamil are present in trace amounts only. Norverapamil can reach steady-state plasma concentrations approximately equal to those of verapamil itself. The cardiovascular activity of norverapamil appears to be approximately 20% that of verapamil. Approximately 70% of an administered dose is excreted as metabolites in the urine and 16% or more in the feces within 5 days. About 3% to 4% is excreted in the urine as unchanged drug. Approximately 90% is bound to plasma proteins. In patients with hepatic insufficiency, metabolism is delayed and elimination half-life prolonged up to 14 to 16 hours (see *Precautions*); the volume of distribution is increased and plasma clearance reduced to about 30% of normal. Verapamil clearance values suggest that patients with liver dysfunction may attain therapeutic verapamil plasma concentrations with one third of the oral daily dose required for patients with normal liver function.
After four weeks of oral dosing (120 mg q.i.d.), verapamil and norverapamil levels were noted in the cerebrospinal fluid with estimated partition coefficient of 0.06 for verapamil and 0.04 for norverapamil.

Hemodynamics and myocardial metabolism: Calan reduces afterload and myocardial contractility. Improved left ventricular diastolic function in patients with IHSS and those with coronary heart disease has also been observed with Calan therapy. In most patients, including those with organic cardiac disease, the negative inotropic action of Calan is countered by reduction of afterload, and cardiac index is usually not reduced. However, in patients with severe left ventricular dysfunction (eg, pulmonary wedge pressure above 20 mm Hg or ejection fraction less than 30%), or in patients taking beta-adrenergic blocking agents or other cardiodepressant drugs, deterioration of ventricular function may occur (see *Drug interactions*).

Pulmonary function: Calan does not induce bronchoconstriction and, hence, does not impair ventilatory function.

INDICATIONS AND USAGE

Calan tablets are indicated for the treatment of the following:

Angina

1. Angina at rest, including:
   — Vasospastic (Prinzmetal's variant) angina
   — Unstable (crescendo, pre-infarction) angina
2. Chronic stable angina (classic effort-associated angina)

Arrhythmias

1. In association with digitalis for the control of ventricular rate at rest and during stress in patients with chronic atrial flutter and/or atrial fibrillation (see *Warnings: Accessory bypass tract*)
2. Prophylaxis of repetitive paroxysmal supraventricular tachycardia

Essential hypertension

CONTRAINDICATIONS

Verapamil HCl tablets are contraindicated in:

1. Severe left ventricular dysfunction (see *Warnings*)
2. Hypotension (systolic pressure less than 90 mm Hg) or cardiogenic shock
3. Sick sinus syndrome (except in patients with a functioning artificial ventricular pacemaker)
4. Second- or third-degree AV block (except in patients with a functioning artificial ventricular pacemaker)
5. Patients with atrial flutter or atrial fibrillation and an accessory bypass tract (eg, Wolff-Parkinson-White, Lown-Ganong-Levine syndromes). (See *Warnings.*)
6. Patients with known hypersensitivity to verapamil hydrochloride.

WARNINGS

Heart failure: Verapamil has a negative inotropic effect, which in most patients is compensated by its afterload reduction (decreased systemic vascular resistance) properties without a net impairment of ventricular performance. In clinical experience with 4,954 patients, 87 (1.8%) developed congestive heart failure or pulmonary edema. Verapamil should be avoided in patients with severe left ventricular dysfunction (eg, ejection fraction less than 30%) or moderate to severe symptoms of cardiac failure and in patients with any degree of ventricular dysfunction if they are receiving a beta-adrenergic blocker (see *Drug interactions*). Patients with milder ventricular dysfunction should, if possible, be controlled with optimum doses of digitalis and/or diuretics before verapamil treatment. **(Note interactions with digoxin under *Precautions.*)**

Hypotension: Occasionally, the pharmacologic action of verapamil may produce a decrease in blood pressure below normal levels, which may result in dizziness or symptomatic hypotension. The incidence of hypotension observed in 4,954 patients enrolled in clinical trials was 2.5%. In hypertensive patients, decreases in blood pressure below normal are unusual. Tilt-table testing (60 degrees) was not able to induce orthostatic hypotension.

Elevated liver enzymes: Elevations of transaminases with and without concomitant elevations in alkaline phosphatase and bilirubin have been reported. Such elevations have sometimes been transient and may disappear even with continued verapamil treatment. Several cases of hepatocellular injury related to verapamil have been proven by rechallenge; half of these had clinical symptoms (malaise, fever, and/or right upper quadrant pain), in addition to elevation of SGOT, SGPT, and alkaline phosphatase. Periodic monitoring of liver function in patients receiving verapamil is therefore prudent.

Accessory bypass tract (Wolff-Parkinson-White or Lown-Ganong-Levine): Some patients with paroxysmal and/or chronic atrial fibrillation or atrial flutter and a coexisting accessory AV pathway have developed increased antegrade conduction across the accessory pathway bypassing the AV node, producing a very rapid ventricular response or ventricular fibrillation after receiving intravenous verapamil (or digitalis). Although a risk of this occurring with oral verapamil has not been established, such patients receiving oral verapamil may be at risk and its use in these patients is contraindicated (see *Contraindications*). Treatment is usually DC-cardioversion. Cardioversion has been used safely and effectively after oral Calan.

Atrioventricular block: The effect of verapamil on AV conduction and the SA node may cause asymptomatic first-degree AV block and transient bradycardia, sometimes accompanied by nodal escape rhythms. PR-interval prolongation is correlated with verapamil plasma concentrations especially during the early titration phase of therapy. Higher degrees of AV block, however, were infrequently (0.8%) observed. Marked first-degree block or progressive development to second- or third-degree AV block requires a reduction in dosage or, in rare instances, discontinuation of verapamil HCl and institution of appropriate therapy, depending on the clinical situation.

Patients with hypertrophic cardiomyopathy (IHSS): In 120 patients with hypertrophic cardiomyopathy (most of them refractory or intolerant to propranolol) who received therapy with verapamil at doses up to 720 mg/day, a variety of serious adverse effects were seen. Three patients died in

Continued on next page

Calan—Cont.

pulmonary edema; all had severe left ventricular outflow obstruction and a past history of left ventricular dysfunction. Eight other patients had pulmonary edema and/or severe hypotension; abnormally high (greater than 20 mm Hg) pulmonary wedge pressure and a marked left ventricular outflow obstruction were present in most of these patients. Concomitant administration of quinidine (see *Drug interactions*) preceded the severe hypotension in 3 of the 8 patients (2 of whom developed pulmonary edema). Sinus bradycardia occurred in 11% of the patients, second-degree AV block in 4%, and sinus arrest in 2%. It must be appreciated that this group of patients had a serious disease with a high mortality rate. Most adverse effects responded well to dose reduction, and only rarely did verapamil use have to be discontinued.

PRECAUTIONS

General

Use in patients with impaired hepatic function: Since verapamil is highly metabolized by the liver, it should be administered cautiously to patients with impaired hepatic function. Severe liver dysfunction prolongs the elimination half-life of verapamil to about 14 to 16 hours; hence, approximately 30% of the dose given to patients with normal liver function should be administered to these patients. Careful monitoring for abnormal prolongation of the PR interval or other signs of excessive pharmacologic effects (see *Overdosage*) should be carried out.

Use in patients with attenuated (decreased) neuromuscular transmission: It has been reported that verapamil decreases neuromuscular transmission in patients with Duchenne's muscular dystrophy, and that verapamil prolongs recovery from the neuromuscular blocking agent vecuronium. It may be necessary to decrease the dosage of verapamil when it is administered to patients with attenuated neuromuscular transmission.

Use in patients with impaired renal function: About 70% of an administered dose of verapamil is excreted as metabolites in the urine. Verapamil is not removed by hemodialysis. Until further data are available, verapamil should be administered cautiously to patients with impaired renal function. These patients should be carefully monitored for abnormal prolongation of the PR interval or other signs of overdosage (see *Overdosage*).

Drug interactions

Alcohol: Verapamil may increase blood alcohol concentrations and prolong its effects.

Beta-blockers: Controlled studies in small numbers of patients suggest that the concomitant use of Calan and oral beta-adrenergic blocking agents may be beneficial in certain patients with chronic stable angina or hypertension, but available information is not sufficient to predict with confidence the effects of concurrent treatment in patients with left ventricular dysfunction or cardiac conduction abnormalities. Concomitant therapy with beta-adrenergic blockers and verapamil may result in additive negative effects on heart rate, atrioventricular conduction and/or cardiac contractility.

In one study involving 15 patients treated with high doses of propranolol (median dose, 480 mg/day; range, 160 to 1,280 mg/day) for severe angina, with preserved left ventricular function (ejection fraction greater than 35%), the hemodynamic effects of additional therapy with verapamil HCl were assessed using invasive methods. The addition of verapamil to high-dose beta-blockers induced modest negative inotropic and chronotropic effects that were not severe enough to limit short-term (48 hours) combination therapy in this study. These modest cardiodepressant effects persisted for greater than 6 but less than 30 hours after abrupt withdrawal of beta-blockers and were closely related to plasma levels of propranolol. The primary verapamil/beta-blocker interaction in this study appeared to be hemodynamic rather than electrophysiologic.

In other studies verapamil did not generally induce significant negative inotropic, chronotropic, or dromotropic effects in patients with preserved left ventricular function receiving low or moderate doses of propranolol (less than or equal to 320 mg/day); in some patients, however, combined therapy did produce such effects. Therefore, if combined therapy is used, close surveillance of clinical status should be carried out. Combined therapy should usually be avoided in patients with atrioventricular conduction abnormalities and those with depressed left ventricular function.

Asymptomatic bradycardia (36 beats/min) with a wandering atrial pacemaker has been observed in a patient receiving concomitant timolol (a beta-adrenergic blocker) eyedrops and oral verapamil.

A decrease in metoprolol and propranolol clearance has been observed when either drug is administered concomitantly with verapamil. A variable effect has been seen when verapamil and atenolol were given together.

Digitalis: Clinical use of verapamil in digitalized patients has shown the combination to be well tolerated if digoxin doses are properly adjusted. However, chronic verapamil treatment can increase serum digoxin levels by 50% to 75% during the first week of therapy, and this can result in digitalis toxicity. In patients with hepatic cirrhosis the influence of verapamil on digoxin kinetics is magnified. Verapamil may reduce total body clearance and extrarenal clearance of digitoxin by 27% and 29%, respectively. Maintenance and digitalization doses should be reduced when verapamil is administered, and the patient should be reassessed to avoid over- or underdigitalization. Whenever overdigitalization is suspected, the daily dose of digitalis should be reduced or temporarily discontinued. On discontinuation of Calan use, the patient should be reassessed to avoid underdigitalization.

Antihypertensive agents: Verapamil administered concomitantly with oral antihypertensive agents (eg, vasodilators, angiotensin-converting enzyme inhibitors, diuretics, beta-blockers) will usually have an additive effect on lowering blood pressure. Patients receiving these combinations should be appropriately monitored. Concomitant use of agents that attenuate alpha-adrenergic function with verapamil may result in a reduction in blood pressure that is excessive in some patients. Such an effect was observed in one study following the concomitant administration of verapamil and prazosin.

Antiarrhythmic agents:

Disopyramide: Until data on possible interactions between verapamil and disopyramide are obtained, disopyramide should not be administered within 48 hours before or 24 hours after verapamil administration.

Flecainide: A study in healthy volunteers showed that the concomitant administration of flecainide and verapamil may have additive effects on myocardial contractility, AV conduction, and repolarization. Concomitant therapy with flecainide and verapamil may result in additive negative inotropic effect and prolongation of atrioventricular conduction.

Quinidine: In a small number of patients with hypertrophic cardiomyopathy (IHSS), concomitant use of verapamil and quinidine resulted in significant hypotension. Until further data are obtained, combined therapy of verapamil and quinidine in patients with hypertrophic cardiomyopathy should probably be avoided.

The electrophysiologic effects of quinidine and verapamil on AV conduction were studied in 8 patients. Verapamil significantly counteracted the effects of quinidine on AV conduction. There has been a report of increased quinidine levels during verapamil therapy.

Other:

Nitrates: Verapamil has been given concomitantly with short- and long-acting nitrates without any undesirable drug interactions. The pharmacologic profile of both drugs and the clinical experience suggest beneficial interactions.

Cimetidine: The interaction between cimetidine and chronically administered verapamil has not been studied. Variable results on clearance have been obtained in acute studies of healthy volunteers; clearance of verapamil was either reduced or unchanged.

Lithium: Increased sensitivity to the effects of lithium (neurotoxicity) has been reported during concomitant verapamil-lithium therapy; lithium levels have been observed sometimes to increase, sometimes to decrease, and sometimes to be unchanged. Patients receiving both drugs must be monitored carefully.

Carbamazepine: Verapamil therapy may increase carbamazepine concentrations during combined therapy. This may produce carbamazepine side effects such as diplopia, headache, ataxia, or dizziness.

Rifampin: Therapy with rifampin may markedly reduce oral verapamil bioavailability.

Phenobarbital: Phenobarbital therapy may increase verapamil clearance.

Cyclosporin: Verapamil therapy may increase serum levels of cyclosporin.

Theophylline: Verapamil may inhibit the clearance and increase the plasma levels of theophylline.

Inhalation anesthetics: Animal experiments have shown that inhalation anesthetics depress cardiovascular activity by decreasing the inward movement of calcium ions. When used concomitantly, inhalation anesthetics and calcium antagonists, such as verapamil, should each be titrated carefully to avoid excessive cardiovascular depression.

Neuromuscular blocking agents: Clinical data and animal studies suggest that verapamil may potentiate the activity of neuromuscular blocking agents (curare-like and depolarizing). It may be necessary to decrease the dose of verapamil and/or the dose of the neuromuscular blocking agent when the drugs are used concomitantly.

Carcinogenesis, mutagenesis, impairment of fertility: An 18-month toxicity study in rats, at a low multiple (6-fold) of the maximum recommended human dose, and not the maximum tolerated dose, did not suggest a tumorigenic potential. There was no evidence of a carcinogenic potential of verapamil administered in the diet of rats for two years at doses of 10, 35, and 120 mg/kg/day or approximately 1, 3.5, and 12 times, respectively, the maximum recommended human daily dose (480 mg/day or 9.6 mg/kg/day).

Verapamil was not mutagenic in the Ames test in 5 test strains at 3 mg per plate with or without metabolic activation.

Studies in female rats at daily dietary doses up to 5.5 times (55 mg/kg/day) the maximum recommended human dose did not show impaired fertility. Effects on male fertility have not been determined.

Pregnancy: Pregnancy Category C. Reproduction studies have been performed in rabbits and rats at oral doses up to 1.5 (15 mg/kg/day) and 6 (60 mg/kg/day) times the human oral daily dose, respectively, and have revealed no evidence of teratogenicity. In the rat, however, this multiple of the human dose was embryocidal and retarded fetal growth and development, probably because of adverse maternal effects reflected in reduced weight gains of the dams. This oral dose has also been shown to cause hypotension in rats. There are no adequate and well-controlled studies in pregnant women. Because animal reproduction studies are not always predictive of human response, this drug should be used during pregnancy only if clearly needed. Verapamil crosses the placental barrier and can be detected in umbilical vein blood at delivery.

Labor and delivery: It is not known whether the use of verapamil during labor or delivery has immediate or delayed adverse effects on the fetus, or whether it prolongs the duration of labor or increases the need for forceps delivery or other obstetric intervention. Such adverse experiences have not been reported in the literature, despite a long history of use of verapamil in Europe in the treatment of cardiac side effects of beta-adrenergic agonist agents used to treat premature labor.

Nursing mothers: Verapamil is excreted in human milk. Because of the potential for adverse reactions in nursing infants from verapamil, nursing should be discontinued while verapamil is administered.

Pediatric use: Safety and effectiveness in pediatric patients have not been established.

Animal pharmacology and/or animal toxicology: In chronic animal toxicology studies verapamil caused lenticular and/or suture line changes at 30 mg/kg/day or greater, and frank cataracts at 62.5 mg/kg/day or greater in the beagle dog but not in the rat. Development of cataracts due to verapamil has not been reported in man.

ADVERSE REACTIONS

Serious adverse reactions are uncommon when Calan therapy is initiated with upward dose titration within the recommended single and total daily dose. See *Warnings* for discussion of heart failure, hypotension, elevated liver enzymes, AV block, and rapid ventricular response. Reversible (upon discontinuation of verapamil) non-obstructive, paralytic ileus has been infrequently reported in association with the use of verapamil. The following reactions to orally administered verapamil occurred at rates greater than 1.0% or occurred at lower rates but appeared clearly drug-related in clinical trials in 4,954 patients:

Constipation	7.3%	Dyspnea	1.4%
Dizziness	3.3%	Bradycardia	
Nausea	2.7%	(HR<50/min)	1.4%
Hypotension	2.5%	AV block	
Headache	2.2%	total (1°, 2°, 3°)	1.2%
Edema	1.9%	2° and 3°	0.8%
CHF/Pulmonary		Rash	1.2%
edema	1.8%	Flushing	0.6%
Fatigue	1.7%		

Elevated liver enzymes (see *Warnings*)

In clinical trials related to the control of ventricular response in digitalized patients who had atrial fibrillation or flutter, ventricular rates below 50 at rest occurred in 15% of patients and asymptomatic hypotension occurred in 5% of patients.

The following reactions, reported in 1.0% or less of patients, occurred under conditions (open trials, marketing experience) where a causal relationship is uncertain; they are listed to alert the physician to a possible relationship:

Cardiovascular: angina pectoris, atrioventricular dissociation, chest pain, claudication, myocardial infarction, palpitations, purpura (vasculitis), syncope.

Digestive system: diarrhea, dry mouth, gastrointestinal distress, gingival hyperplasia.

Hemic and lymphatic: ecchymosis or bruising.

Nervous system: cerebrovascular accident, confusion, equilibrium disorders, insomnia, muscle cramps, paresthesia, psychotic symptoms, shakiness, somnolence.

Skin: arthralgia and rash, exanthema, hair loss, hyperkeratosis, macules, sweating, urticaria, Stevens-Johnson syndrome, erythema multiforme.

Special senses: blurred vision, tinnitus.

Urogenital: gynecomastia, galactorrhea/hyperprolactinemia, increased urination, spotty menstruation, impotence.

Treatment of acute cardiovascular adverse reactions: The frequency of cardiovascular adverse reactions that require therapy is rare; hence, experience with their treatment is limited. Whenever severe hypotension or complete AV block occurs following oral administration of verapamil, the appropriate emergency measures should be applied immediately; eg, intravenously administered norepinephrine bitartrate, atropine sulfate, isoproterenol HCl (all in the usual doses), or calcium gluconate (10% solution). In patients with hypertrophic cardiomyopathy (IHSS), alpha-adrenergic agents (phenylephrine HCl, metaraminol bitartrate, or methoxamine HCl) should be used to maintain blood pressure, and isoproterenol and norepinephrine should be avoided. If further support is necessary, dopamine HCl or dobutamine HCl may be administered. Actual treatment and dosage should depend on the severity of the clinical situation and the judgment and experience of the treating physician.

OVERDOSAGE

Treat all verapamil overdoses as serious and maintain observation for at least 48 hours (especially Calan SR), preferably under continuous hospital care. Delayed pharmacodynamic consequences may occur with the sustained-release formulation. Verapamil is known to decrease gastrointestinal transit time.

Treatment of overdosage should be supportive. Beta adrenergic stimulation or parenteral administration of calcium solutions may increase calcium ion flux across the slow channel, and have been used effectively in treatment of deliberate overdosage with verapamil. In a few reported cases, overdose with calcium channel blockers has been associated with hypotension and bradycardia, initially refractory to atropine but becoming more responsive to this treatment when the patients received large doses (close to 1 gram/hour for more than 24 hours) of calcium chloride. Verapamil cannot be removed by hemodialysis. Clinically significant hypotensive reactions or high degree AV block should be treated with vasopressor agents or cardiac pacing, respectively. Asystole should be handled by the usual measures including cardiopulmonary resuscitation.

DOSAGE AND ADMINISTRATION

The dose of verapamil must be individualized by titration. The usefulness and safety of dosages exceeding 480 mg/day have not been established; therefore, this daily dosage should not be exceeded. Since the half-life of verapamil increases during chronic dosing, maximum response may be delayed.

Angina: Clinical trials show that the usual dose is 80 mg to 120 mg three times a day. However, 40 mg three times a day may be warranted in patients who may have an increased response to verapamil (eg, decreased hepatic function, elderly, etc). Upward titration should be based on therapeutic efficacy and safety evaluated approximately eight hours after dosing. Dosage may be increased at daily (eg, patients with unstable angina) or weekly intervals until optimum clinical response is obtained.

Arrhythmias: The dosage in digitalized patients with chronic atrial fibrillation (see *Precautions*) ranges from 240 to 320 mg/day in divided (t.i.d. or q.i.d.) doses. The dosage for prophylaxis of PSVT (non-digitalized patients) ranges from 240 to 480 mg/day in divided (t.i.d or q.i.d.) doses. In general, maximum effects for any given dosage will be apparent during the first 48 hours of therapy.

Essential hypertension: Dose should be individualized by titration. The usual initial monotherapy dose in clinical trials was 80 mg three times a day (240 mg/day). Daily dosages of 360 and 480 mg have been used but there is no evidence that dosages beyond 360 mg provided added effect. Consideration should be given to beginning titration at 40 mg three times per day in patients who might respond to lower doses, such as the elderly or people of small stature. The antihypertensive effects of Calan are evident within the first week of therapy. Upward titration should be based on therapeutic efficacy, assessed at the end of the dosing interval.

HOW SUPPLIED

Calan 40-mg tablets are round, pink, film coated, with CALAN debossed on one side and 40 on the other, supplied as:

NDC Number	Size
0025-1771-31	bottle of 100

Calan 80-mg tablets are oval, peach colored, scored, film coated, with CALAN debossed on one side and 80 on the other, supplied as:

NDC Number	Size
0025-1851-31	bottle of 100
0025-1851-51	bottle of 500
0025-1851-52	bottle of 1,000

Calan 120-mg tablets are oval, brown, scored, film coated, with CALAN 120 debossed on one side, supplied as:

NDC Number	Size
0025-1861-31	bottle of 100
0025-1861-52	bottle of 1,000

Store at 59° to 77°F (15° to 25°C) and protect from light. Dispense in tight, light-resistant containers.

Rx only

5/18/99 • A05315-3

Shown in Product Identification Guide, page 335

CALAN® SR ℞

[cal 'an ess ar]

(verapamil hydrochloride)

Sustained-Release Oral Caplets

PRODUCT OVERVIEW

KEY FACTS

Calan SR, a calcium ion antagonist designed for sustained release in the gastrointestinal tract, exerts an antihypertensive effect by decreasing systemic vascular resistance, usually without orthostatic decreases in blood pressure or reflex tachycardia.

MAJOR USE

Calan SR is indicated for the management of essential hypertension.

SAFETY INFORMATION

See complete safety information set forth below.

PRESCRIBING INFORMATION

CALAN® SR ℞

[cal 'an ess ar]

(verapamil hydrochloride)

Sustained-Release Oral Caplets

DESCRIPTION

Calan SR (verapamil hydrochloride) is a calcium ion influx inhibitor (slow-channel blocker or calcium ion antagonist). Calan SR is available for oral administration as light green, capsule-shaped, scored, film-coated tablets (caplets) containing 240 mg of verapamil hydrochloride; as light pink, oval, scored, film-coated tablets (caplets) containing 180 mg of verapamil hydrochloride; and as light violet, oval, film-coated tablets (caplets) containing 120 mg of verapamil hydrochloride. The caplets are designed for sustained release of the drug in the gastrointestinal tract; sustained-release characteristics are not altered when the caplet is divided in half.

The structural formula of verapamil HCl is

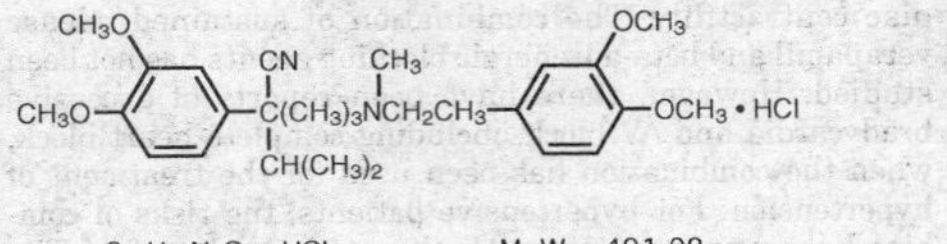

$C_{27}H_{38}N_2O_4 \cdot HCl$ M. W. - 491.08

Benzeneacetonitrile, α-[3-[[2-(3, 4-dimethoxyphenyl) ethyl] methylamino]propyl]-3,4-dimethoxy-α- (1-methylethyl) hydrochloride

Verapamil HCl is an almost white, crystalline powder, practically free of odor, with a bitter taste. It is soluble in water, chloroform, and methanol. Verapamil HCl is not chemically related to other cardioactive drugs.

Inactive ingredients include alginate, carnauba wax, hydroxypropyl methylcellulose, magnesium stearate, microcrystalline cellulose, polyethylene glycol, polyvinyl pyrrolidone, talc, titanium dioxide, and coloring agents: 240-mg—D&C Yellow No. 10 Lake and FD&C Blue No. 2 Lake; 120- and 180-mg—iron oxide.

CLINICAL PHARMACOLOGY

Calan (verapamil HCl) is a calcium ion influx inhibitor (slow-channel blocker or calcium ion antagonist) that exerts its pharmacologic effects by modulating the influx of ionic calcium across the cell membrane of the arterial smooth muscle as well as in conductile and contractile myocardial cells.

Mechanism of action

Essential hypertension: Verapamil exerts antihypertensive effects by decreasing systemic vascular resistance, usually without orthostatic decreases in blood pressure or reflex tachycardia; bradycardia (rate less than 50 beats/min) is uncommon (1.4%). During isometric or dynamic exercise Calan does not alter systolic cardiac function in patients with normal ventricular function.

Calan does not alter total serum calcium levels. However, one report suggested that calcium levels above the normal range may alter the therapeutic effect of Calan.

Other pharmacologic actions of Calan include the following: Calan dilates the main coronary arteries and coronary arterioles, both in normal and ischemic regions, and is a potent inhibitor of coronary artery spasm, whether spontaneous or ergonovine-induced. This property increases myocardial oxygen delivery in patients with coronary artery spasm and is responsible for the effectiveness of Calan in vasospastic (Prinzmetal's or variant) as well as unstable angina at rest. Whether this effect plays any role in classical effort angina is not clear, but studies of exercise tolerance have not shown an increase in the maximum exercise rate–pressure product, a widely accepted measure of oxygen utilization. This suggests that, in general, relief of spasm or dilation of coronary arteries is not an important factor in classical angina.

Calan regularly reduces the total systemic resistance (afterload) against which the heart works both at rest and at a given level of exercise by dilating peripheral arterioles.

Electrical activity through the AV node depends, to a significant degree, upon calcium influx through the slow channel. By decreasing the influx of calcium, Calan prolongs the effective refractory period within the AV node and slows AV conduction in a rate-related manner.

Normal sinus rhythm is usually not affected, but in patients with sick sinus syndrome, Calan may interfere with sinus-node impulse generation and may induce sinus arrest or sinoatrial block. Atrioventricular block can occur in patients without preexisting conduction defects (see *Warnings*).

Calan does not alter the normal atrial action potential or intraventricular conduction time, but depresses amplitude, velocity of depolarization, and conduction in depressed atrial fibers. Calan may shorten the antegrade effective refractory period of the accessory bypass tract. Acceleration of ventricular rate and/or ventricular fibrillation has been reported in patients with atrial flutter or atrial fibrillation and a coexisting accessory AV pathway following administration of verapamil (see *Warnings*).

Calan has a local anesthetic action that is 1.6 times that of procaine on an equimolar basis. It is not known whether this action is important at the doses used in man.

Pharmacokinetics and metabolism: With the immediate-release formulation, more than 90% of the orally administered dose of Calan is absorbed. Because of rapid biotransformation of verapamil during its first pass through the portal circulation, bioavailability ranges from 20% to 35%. Peak plasma concentrations are reached between 1 and 2 hours after oral administration. Chronic oral administration of 120 mg of verapamil HCl every 6 hours resulted in plasma levels of verapamil ranging from 125 to 400 ng/ml, with higher values reported occasionally. A nonlinear correlation between the verapamil dose administered and verapamil plasma level does exist. In early dose titration with verapamil a relationship exists between verapamil plasma concentration and prolongation of the PR interval. However, during chronic administration this relationship may disappear. The mean elimination half-life in single-dose studies ranged from 2.8 to 7.4 hours. In these same studies, after repetitive dosing, the half-life increased to a range from 4.5 to 12.0 hours (after less than 10 consecutive doses given 6 hours apart). Half-life of verapamil may increase during titration. No relationship has been established between the plasma concentraton of verapamil and a reduction in blood pressure.

Aging may affect the pharmacokinetics of verapamil. Elimination half-life may be prolonged in the elderly. In multiple-dose studies under fasting conditions, the bioavailability, measured by AUC, of Calan SR was similar to Calan (immediate release); rates of absorption were of course different.

In a randomized, single-dose, crossover study using healthy volunteers, administration of 240 mg Calan SR with food produced peak plasma verapamil concentrations of 79 ng/ml; time to peak plasma verapamil concentration of 7.71 hours; and AUC (0–24 hr) of 841 ng·hr/ml). When Calan SR was administered to fasting subjects, peak plasma verapamil concentration was 164 ng/ml; time to peak plasma verapamil concentration was 5.21 hours; and AUC (0–24 hr) was 1,478 ng·hr/ml. Similar results were demonstrated for plasma norverapamil. Food thus produces decreased bioavailability (AUC) but a narrower peak-to-trough ratio. Good correlation of dose and response is not available, but controlled studies of Calan SR have shown effectiveness of doses similar to the effective doses of Calan (immediate release).

In healthy men, orally administered Calan undergoes extensive metabolism in the liver. Twelve metabolites have been identified in plasma; all except norverapamil are present in trace amounts only. Norverapamil can reach steady-state plasma concentrations approximately equal to those of verapamil itself. The cardiovascular activity of norverapamil appears to be approximately 20% that of verapamil. Approximately 70% of an administered dose is excreted as metabolites in the urine and 16% or more in the feces within 5 days. About 3% to 4% is excreted in the urine as unchanged drug. Approximately 90% is bound to plasma proteins. In patients with hepatic insufficiency, metabolism of immediate-release verapamil is delayed and elimination half-life prolonged up to 14 to 16 hours (see *Precautions*); the volume of distribution is increased and plasma clearance reduced to about 30% of normal. Verapamil clearance values suggest that patients with liver dysfunction may attain therapeutic verapamil plasma concentrations with one third of the oral daily dose required for patients with normal liver function.

After four weeks of oral dosing (120 mg q.i.d.), verapamil and norverapamil levels were noted in the cerebrospinal fluid with estimated partition coefficient of 0.06 for verapamil and 0.04 for norverapamil.

In ten healthy males, administration of oral verapamil (80 mg every 8 hours for 6 days) and a single oral dose of ethanol (0.8 g/kg) resulted in a 17% increase in mean peak ethanol concentrations (106.45 ± 21.40 to 124.23 ± 24.74 mg•hr/dL) compared to placebo. The area under the blood ethanol concentration versus time curve (AUC over 12 hours) increased by 30% (365.67 ± 93.52 to 475.07 ± 97.24 mg•hr/dL). Verapamil AUCs were positively correlated (r=0.71) to increased ethanol blood AUC values (see *Precautions: Drug interactions*).

Hemodynamics and myocardial metabolism: Calan reduces afterload and myocardial contractility. Improved left ventricular diastolic function in patients with IHSS and those with coronary heart disease has also been observed with Calan. In most patients, including those with organic cardiac disease, the negative inotropic action of Calan is countered by reduction of afterload, and cardiac index is usually not reduced. However, in patients with severe left ventricular dysfunction (eg, pulmonary wedge pressure above 20 mm Hg or ejection fraction less than 30%), or in patients taking beta-adrenergic blocking agents or other cardiodepressant drugs, deterioration of ventricular function may occur (see *Drug interactions*).

Pulmonary function: Calan does not induce bronchoconstriction and, hence, does not impair ventilatory function.

INDICATIONS AND USAGE

Calan SR is indicated for the management of essential hypertension.

CONTRAINDICATIONS

Verapamil HCl caplets are contraindicated in:

1. Severe left ventricular dysfunction (see *Warnings*)
2. Hypotension (systolic pressure less than 90 mm Hg) or cardiogenic shock
3. Sick sinus syndrome (except in patients with a functioning artificial ventricular pacemaker)
4. Second- or third-degree AV block (except in patients with a functioning artificial ventricular pacemaker)
5. Patients with atrial flutter or atrial fibrillation and an accessory bypass tract (eg, Wolff-Parkinson-White, Lown-Ganong-Levine syndromes). (See *Warnings.*)

Continued on next page

Calan SR—Cont.

6. Patients with known hypersensitivity to verapamil hydrochloride.

WARNINGS

Heart failure: Verapamil has a negative inotropic effect, which in most patients is compensated by its afterload reduction (decreased systemic vascular resistance) properties without a net impairment of ventricular performance. In clinical experience with 4,954 patients, 87 (1.8%) developed congestive heart failure or pulmonary edema. Verapamil should be avoided in patients with severe left ventricular dysfunction (eg, ejection fraction less than 30%) or moderate to severe symptoms of cardiac failure and in patients with any degree of ventricular dysfunction if they are receiving a beta-adrenergic blocker (see *Drug interactions*). Patients with milder ventricular dysfunction should, if possible, be controlled with optimum doses of digitalis and/or diuretics before verapamil treatment. **(Note interactions with digoxin under *Precautions*.)**

Hypotension: Occasionally, the pharmacologic action of verapamil may produce a decrease in blood pressure below normal levels, which may result in dizziness or symptomatic hypotension. The incidence of hypotension observed in 4,954 patients enrolled in clinical trials was 2.5%. In hypertensive patients, decreases in blood pressure below normal are unusual. Tilt-table testing (60 degrees) was not able to induce orthostatic hypotension.

Elevated liver enzymes: Elevations of transaminases with and without concomitant elevations in alkaline phosphatase and bilirubin have been reported. Such elevations have sometimes been transient and may disappear even in the face of continued verapamil treatment. Several cases of hepatocellular injury related to verapamil have been proven by rechallenge; half of these had clinical symptoms (malaise, fever, and/or right upper quadrant pain) in addition to elevation of SGOT, SGPT, and alkaline phosphatase. Periodic monitoring of liver function in patients receiving verapamil is therefore prudent.

Accessory bypass tract (Wolff-Parkinson-White or Lown-Ganong-Levine): Some patients with paroxysmal and/or chronic atrial fibrillation or atrial flutter and a coexisting accessory AV pathway have developed increased antegrade conduction across the accessory pathway bypassing the AV node, producing a very rapid ventricular response or ventricular fibrillation after receiving intravenous verapamil (or digitalis). Although a risk of this occurring with oral verapamil has not been established, such patients receiving oral verapamil may be at risk and its use in these patients is contraindicated (see *Contraindications*). Treatment is usually DC-cardioversion. Cardioversion has been used safely and effectively after oral Calan.

Atrioventricular block: The effect of verapamil on AV conduction and the SA node may cause asymptomatic first-degree AV block and transient bradycardia, sometimes accompanied by nodal escape rhythms. PR-interval prolongation is correlated with verapamil plasma concentrations, especially during the early titration phase of therapy. Higher degrees of AV block, however, were infrequently (0.8%) observed. Marked first-degree block or progressive development to second- or third-degree AV block requires a reduction in dosage or, in rare instances, discontinuation of verapamil HCl and institution of appropriate therapy, depending upon the clinical situation.

Patients with hypertrophic cardiomyopathy (IHSS): In 120 patients with hypertrophic cardiomyopathy (most of them refractory or intolerant to propranolol) who received therapy with verapamil at doses up to 720 mg/day, a variety of serious adverse effects were seen. Three patients died in pulmonary edema; all had severe left ventricular outflow obstruction and a past history of left ventricular dysfunction. Eight other patients had pulmonary edema and/or severe hypotension; abnormally high (greater than 20 mm Hg) pulmonary wedge pressure and a marked left ventricular outflow obstruction were present in most of these patients. Concomitant administration of quinidine (see *Drug interactions*) preceded the severe hypotension in 3 of the 8 patients (2 of whom developed pulmonary edema). Sinus bradycardia occurred in 11% of the patients, second-degree AV block in 4%, and sinus arrest in 2%. It must be appreciated that this group of patients had a serious disease with a high mortality rate. Most adverse effects responded well to dose reduction, and only rarely did verapamil use have to be discontinued.

PRECAUTIONS

General

Use in patients with impaired hepatic function: Since verapamil is highly metabolized by the liver, it should be administered cautiously to patients with impaired hepatic function. Severe liver dysfunction prolongs the elimination half-life of immediate-release verapamil to about 14 to 16 hours; hence, approximately 30% of the dose given to patients with normal liver function should be administered to these patients. Careful monitoring for abnormal prolongation of the PR interval or other signs of excessive pharmacologic effects (see *Overdosage*) should be carried out.

Use in patients with attenuated (decreased) neuromuscular transmission: It has been reported that verapamil decreases neuromuscular transmission in patients with Duchenne's muscular dystrophy, and that verapamil prolongs recovery from the neuromuscular blocking agent vecuronium. It may be necessary to decrease the dosage of verapamil when it is administered to patients with attenuated neuromuscular transmission.

Use in patients with impaired renal function: About 70% of an administered dose of verapamil is excreted as metabolites in the urine. Verapamil is not removed by hemodialysis. Until further data are available, verapamil should be administered cautiously to patients with impaired renal function. These patients should be carefully monitored for abnormal prolongation of the PR interval or other signs of overdosage (see *Overdosage*).

Drug interactions

Beta-blockers: Concomitant therapy with beta-adrenergic blockers and verapamil may result in additive negative effects on heart rate, atrioventricular conduction and/or cardiac contractility. The combination of sustained-release verapamil and beta-adrenergic blocking agents has not been studied. However, there have been reports of excessive bradycardia and AV block, including complete heart block, when the combination has been used for the treatment of hypertension. For hypertensive patients, the risks of combined therapy may outweigh the potential benefits. The combination should be used only with caution and close monitoring.

Asymptomatic bradycardia (36 beats/min) with a wandering atrial pacemaker has been observed in a patient receiving concomitant timolol (a beta-adrenergic blocker) eyedrops and oral verapamil.

A decrease in metroprolol and propranolol clearance has been observed when either drug is administered concomitantly with verapamil. A variable effect has been seen when verapamil and atenolol were given together.

Digitalis: Clinical use of verapamil in digitalized patients has shown the combination to be well tolerated if digoxin doses are properly adjusted. However, chronic verapamil treatment can increase serum digoxin levels by 50% to 75% during the first week of therapy, and this can result in digitalis toxicity. In patients with hepatic cirrhosis the influence of verapamil on digoxin kinetics is magnified. Verapamil may reduce total body clearance and extrarenal clearance of digitoxin by 27% and 29%, respectively. Maintenance and digitalization doses should be reduced when verapamil is administered, and the patient should be carefully monitored to avoid over- or underdigitalization. Whenever overdigitalization is suspected, the daily dose of digitalis should be reduced or temporarily discontinued. On discontinuation of Calan use, the patient should be reassessed to avoid underdigitalization.

Antihypertensive agents: Verapamil administered concomitantly with oral antihypertensive agents (eg, vasodilators, angiotensin-converting enzyme inhibitors, diuretics, beta-blockers) will usually have an additive effect on lowering blood pressure. Patients receiving these combinations should be appropriately monitored. Concomitant use of agents that attenuate alpha-adrenergic function with verapamil may result in a reduction in blood pressure that is excessive in some patients. Such an effect was observed in one study following the concomitant administration of verapamil and prazosin.

Antiarrhythmic agents:

Disopyramide: Until data on possible interactions between verapamil and disopyramide phosphate are obtained, disopyramide should not be administered within 48 hours before or 24 hours after verapamil administration.

Flecainide: A study in healthy volunteers showed that the concomitant administration of flecainide and verapamil may have additive effects on myocardial contractility, AV conduction, and repolarization. Concomitant therapy with flecainide and verapamil may result in additive negative inotropic effect and prolongation of atrioventricular conduction.

Quinidine: In a small number of patients with hypertrophic cardiomyopathy (IHSS), concomitant use of verapamil and quinidine resulted in significant hypotension. Until further data are obtained, combined therapy of verapamil and quinidine in patients with hypertrophic cardiomyopathy should probably be avoided.

The electrophysiologic effects of quinidine and verapamil on AV conduction were studied in 8 patients. Verapamil significantly counteracted the effects of quinidine on AV conduction. There has been a report of increased quinidine levels during verapamil therapy.

Other:

Alcohol: Verapamil has been found to inhibit ethanol elimination significantly, resulting in elevated blood ethanol concentrations that may prolong the intoxicating effects of alcohol (see *Clinical Pharmacology: Pharmacokinetics and metabolism*).

Nitrates: Verapamil has been given concomitantly with short- and long-acting nitrates without any undesirable drug interactions. The pharmacologic profile of both drugs and the clinical experience suggest beneficial interactions.

Cimetidine: The interaction between cimetidine and chronically administered verapamil has not been studied. Variable results on clearance have been obtained in acute studies of healthy volunteers; clearance of verapamil was either reduced or unchanged.

Lithium: Increased sensitivity to the effects of lithium (neurotoxicity) has been reported during concomitant verapamil-lithium therapy; lithium levels have been observed sometimes to increase, sometimes to decrease, and sometimes to be unchanged. Patients receiving both drugs must be monitored carefully.

Carbamazepine: Verapamil therapy may increase carbamazepine concentrations during combined therapy. This may produce carbamazepine side effects such as diplopia, headache, ataxia, or dizziness.

Rifampin: Therapy with rifampin may markedly reduce oral verapamil bioavailability.

Phenobarbital: Phenobarbital therapy may increase verapamil clearance.

Cyclosporin: Verapamil therapy may increase serum levels of cyclosporin.

Theophylline: Verapamil may inhibit the clearance and increase the plasma levels of theophylline.

Inhalation anesthetics: Animal experiments have shown that inhalation anesthetics depress cardiovascular activity by decreasing the inward movement of calcium ions. When used concomitantly, inhalation anesthetics and calcium antagonists, such as verapamil, should each be titrated carefully to avoid excessive cardiovascular depression.

Neuromuscular blocking agents: Clinical data and animal studies suggest that verapamil may potentiate the activity of neuromuscular blocking agents (curare-like and depolarizing). It may be necessary to decrease the dose of verapamil and/or the dose of the neuromuscular blocking agent when the drugs are used concomitantly.

Carcinogenesis, mutagenesis, impairment of fertility: An 18-month toxicity study in rats, at a low multiple (6-fold) of the maximum recommended human dose, and not the maximum tolerated dose, did not suggest a tumorigenic potential. There was no evidence of a carcinogenic potential of verapamil administered in the diet of rats for two years at doses of 10, 35, and 120 mg/kg/day or approximately 1, 3.5, and 12 times, respectively, the maximum recommended human daily dose (480 mg/day or 9.6 mg/kg/day).

Verapamil was not mutagenic in the Ames test in 5 test strains at 3 mg per plate with or without metabolic activation.

Studies in female rats at daily dietary doses up to 5.5 times (55 mg/kg/day) the maximum recommended human dose did not show impaired fertility. Effects on male fertility have not been determined.

Pregnancy: Pregnancy Category C. Reproduction studies have been performed in rabbits and rats at oral doses up to 1.5 (15 mg/kg/day) and 6 (60 mg/kg/day) times the human oral daily dose, respectively, and have revealed no evidence of teratogenicity. In the rat, however, this multiple of the human dose was embryocidal and retarded fetal growth and development, probably because of adverse maternal effects reflected in reduced weight gains of the dams. This oral dose has also been shown to cause hypotension in rats. There are no adequate and well-controlled studies in pregnant women. Because animal reproduction studies are not always predictive of human response, this drug should be used during pregnancy only if clearly needed. Verapamil crosses the placental barrier and can be detected in umbilical vein blood at delivery.

Labor and delivery: It is not known whether the use of verapamil during labor or delivery has immediate or delayed adverse effects on the fetus, or whether it prolongs the duration of labor or increases the need for forceps delivery or other obstetric intervention. Such adverse experiences have not been reported in the literature, despite a long history of use of verapamil in Europe in the treatment of cardiac side effects of beta-adrenergic agonist agents used to treat premature labor.

Nursing mothers: Verapamil is excreted in human milk. Because of the potential for adverse reactions in nursing infants from verapamil, nursing should be discontinued while verapamil is administered.

Pediatric use: Safety and efficacy of Calan SR in pediatric patients below the age of 18 years have not been established.

Animal pharmacology and/or animal toxicology: In chronic animal toxicology studies verapamil caused lenticular and/or suture line changes at 30 mg/kg/day or greater, and frank cataracts at 62.5 mg/kg/day or greater in the beagle dog but not in the rat. Development of cataracts due to verapamil has not been reported in man.

ADVERSE REACTIONS

Serious adverse reactions are uncommon when verapamil therapy is initiated with upward dose titration within the recommended single and total daily dose. See *Warnings* for discussion of heart failure, hypotension, elevated liver enzymes, AV block, and rapid ventricular response. Reversible (upon discontinuation of verapamil) non-obstructive, paralytic ileus has been infrequently reported in association with the use of verapamil. The following reactions to orally administered verapamil occurred at rates greater than 1.0% or occurred at lower rates but appeared clearly drug-related in clinical trials in 4,954 patients:

Constipation	7.3%	Dyspnea	1.4%
Dizziness	3.3%	Bradycardia	
Nausea	2.7%	(HR<50/min)	1.4%
Hypotension	2.5%	AV block	
Headache	2.2%	total (1°, 2°, 3°)	1.2%
Edema	1.9%	2° and 3°	0.8%
CHF, Pulmonary		Rash	1.2%
edema	1.8%	Flushing	0.6%
Fatigue	1.7%		

Elevated liver enzymes (see *Warnings*)

In clinical trials related to the control of ventricular response in digitalized patients who had atrial fibrillation or

flutter, ventricular rates below 50/min at rest occurred in 15% of patients and asymptomatic hypotension occurred in 5% of patients.
The following reactions, reported in 1% or less of patients, occurred under conditions (open trials, marketing experience) where a causal relationship is uncertain; they are listed to alert the physician to a possible relationship:
Cardiovascular: angina pectoris, atrioventricular dissociation, chest pain, claudication, myocardial infarction, palpitations, purpura (vasculitis), syncope.
Digestive system: diarrhea, dry mouth, gastrointestinal distress, gingival hyperplasia.
Hemic and lymphatic: ecchymosis or bruising.
Nervous system: cerebrovascular accident, confusion, equilibrium disorders, insomnia, muscle cramps, paresthesia, psychotic symptoms, shakiness, somnolence.
Skin: arthralgia and rash, exanthema, hair loss, hyperkeratosis, macules, sweating, urticaria, Stevens-Johnson syndrome, erythema multiforme.
Special senses: blurred vision, tinnitus.
Urogenital: gynecomastia, galactorrhea/hyperprolactinemia, increased urination, spotty menstruation, impotence.
Treatment of acute cardiovascular adverse reactions: The frequency of cardiovascular adverse reactions that require therapy is rare; hence, experience with their treatment is limited. Whenever severe hypotension or complete AV block occurs following oral administration of verapamil, the appropriate emergency measures should be applied immediately; eg, intravenously administered norepinephrine bitartrate, atropine sulfate, isoproterenol HCl (all in the usual doses), or calcium gluconate (10% solution). In patients with hypertrophic cardiomyopathy (IHSS), alpha-adrenergic agents (phenylephrine HCl, metaraminol bitartrate, or methoxamine HCl) should be used to maintain blood pressure, and isoproterenol and norepinephrine should be avoided. If further support is necessary, dopamine HCl or dobutamine HCl may be administered. Actual treatment and dosage should depend on the severity of the clinical situation and the judgment and experience of the treating physician.

OVERDOSAGE

Overdosage with verapamil may lead to pronounced hypotension, bradycardia, and conduction system abnormalities (eg, junctional rhythm with AV dissociation and high degree AV block, including asystole). Other symptoms secondary to hypoperfusion (eg, metabolic acidosis, hyperglycemia, hyperkalemia, renal dysfunction, and convulsions) may be evident.
Treat all verapamil overdoses as serious and maintain observation for at least 48 hours (especially Calan SR), preferably under continuous hospital care. Delayed pharmacodynamic consequences may occur with the sustained-release formulation. Verapamil is known to decrease gastrointestinal transit time.
In overdose, caplets of Calan SR have occasionally been reported to form concretions within the stomach or intestines. These concretions have not been visible on plain radiographs of the abdomen, and no medical means of gastrointestinal emptying is of proven efficacy in removing them. Endoscopy might reasonably be considered in cases of massive overdose when symptoms are unusually prolonged.
Treatment of overdosage should be supportive. Beta adrenergic stimulation or parenteral administration of calcium solutions may increase calcium ion flux across the slow channel, and have been used effectively in treatment of deliberate overdosage with verapamil. Continued treatment with large doses of calcium may produce a response. In a few reported cases, overdose with calcium channel blockers that was initially refractory to atropine became more responsive to this treatment when the patients received large doses (close to 1 g/hr for more than 24 hr) of calcium chloride. Verapamil cannot be removed by hemodialysis. Clinically significant hypotensive reactions or high degree AV block should be treated with vasopressor agents or cardiac pacing, respectively. Asystole should be handled by the usual measures including cardiopulmonary resuscitation.

DOSAGE AND ADMINISTRATION

Essential hypertension: The dose of Calan SR should be individualized by titration and the drug should be administered with food. Initiate therapy with 180 mg of sustained-release verapamil HCl, Calan SR, given in the morning. Lower initial doses of 120 mg a day may be warranted in patients who may have an increased response to verapamil (eg, the elderly or small people). Upward titration should be based on therapeutic efficacy and safety evaluated weekly and approximately 24 hours after the previous dose. The antihypertensive effects of Calan SR are evident within the first week of therapy.
If adequate response is not obtained with 180 mg of Calan SR, the dose may be titrated upward in the following manner:
a) 240 mg each morning,
b) 180 mg each morning plus
 180 mg each evening; or
 240 mg each morning plus
 120 mg each evening,
c) 240 mg every 12 hours.
When switching from immediate-release Calan to Calan SR the total daily dose in milligrams may remain the same.

HOW SUPPLIED

Calan SR 240-mg caplets are light green, capsule shaped, scored, film coated, with CALAN debossed on one side and SR 240 on the other, supplied as:

NDC Number	Size
0025-1891-31	bottle of 100
0025-1891-51	bottle of 500
0025-1891-34	carton of 100 unit dose

Calan SR 180-mg caplets are light pink, oval, scored, film coated, with CALAN debossed on one side and SR 180 on the other, supplied as:

NDC Number	Size
0025-1911-31	bottle of 100
0025-1911-34	carton of 100 unit dose

Calan SR 120-mg caplets are light violet, oval, film-coated, with CALAN debossed on one side and SR 120 on the other, supplied as:

NDC Number	Size
0025-1901-31	bottle of 100
0025-1901-34	carton of 100 unit dose

Store at 59° to 77°F (15° to 25°C) and protect from light and moisture. Dispense in tight, light-resistant containers.
Rx only

4/2/98 • A05298-4

Shown in Product Identification Guide, page 335

CELEBREX™ ℞
(celecoxib capsules)

DESCRIPTION

CELEBREX (celecoxib) is chemically designated as 4-[5-(4-methylphenyl)-3-(trifluoromethyl)-1H-pyrazol-1-yl] benzenesulfonamide and is a diaryl substituted pyrazole. It has the following chemical structure:

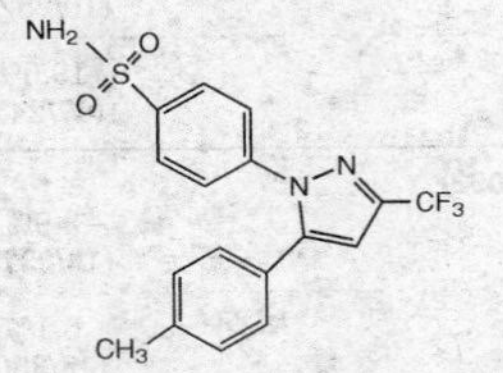

The empirical formula for celecoxib is $C_{17}H_{14}F_3N_3O_2S$, and the molecular weight is 381.38.
CELEBREX oral capsules contain 100 mg and 200 mg of celecoxib.
The inactive ingredients in CELEBREX capsules include: croscarmellose sodium, edible inks, gelatin, lactose monohydrate, magnesium stearate, povidone, sodium lauryl sulfate and titanium dioxide.

CLINICAL PHARMACOLOGY

Mechanism of Action: CELEBREX is a nonsteroidal anti-inflammatory drug that exhibits anti-inflammatory, analgesic, and antipyretic activities in animal models. The mechanism of action of CELEBREX is believed to be due to inhibition of prostaglandin synthesis, primarily via inhibition of cyclooxygenase-2 (COX-2), and at therapeutic concentrations in humans, CELEBREX does not inhibit the cyclooxygenase-1 (COX-1) isoenzyme. In animal colon tumor models, celecoxib reduced the incidence and multiplicity of tumors.
Pharmacokinetics:
Absorption
Peak plasma levels of celecoxib occur approximately 3 hrs after an oral dose. Under fasting conditions, both peak plasma levels (C_{max}) and area under the curve (AUC) are roughly dose proportional up to 200 mg BID; at higher doses there are less than proportional changes in C_{max} and AUC (see Food Effects). Absolute bioavailability studies have not been conducted. With multiple dosing, steady state conditions are reached on or before Day 5.
The pharmacokinetic parameters of celecoxib in a group of healthy subjects are shown in Table 1.
[See table 1 at top of next page]
Food Effects
When CELEBREX capsules were taken with a high fat meal, peak plasma levels were delayed for about 1 to 2 hours with an increase in total absorption (AUC) of 10% to 20%. Under fasting conditions, at doses above 200 mg, there is less than a proportional increase in C_{max} and AUC, which is thought to be due to the low solubility of the drug in aqueous media. Coadministration of CELEBREX with an aluminum- and magnesium-containing antacid resulted in a reduction in plasma celecoxib concentrations with a decrease of 37% in C_{max} and 10% in AUC. CELEBREX, at doses up to 200 mg BID can be administered without regard to the timing of meals. Higher doses (400 mg BID) should be administered with food.
Distribution
In healthy subjects, celecoxib is highly protein bound (~97%) within the clinical dose range. *In vitro* studies indicate that celecoxib binds primarily to albumin and, to a lesser extent, α_1-acid glycoprotein. The apparent volume of distribution at steady state (V_{ss}/F) is approximately 400 L, suggesting extensive distribution into the tissues. Celecoxib is not preferentially bound to red blood cells.
Metabolism
Celecoxib metabolism is primarily mediated via cytochrome P450 2C9. Three metabolites, a primary alcohol, the corresponding carboxylic acid and its glucuronide conjugate, have been identified in human plasma. These metabolites are inactive as COX-1 or COX-2 inhibitors. Patients who are known or suspected to be P450 2C9 poor metabolizers based on a previous history should be administered celecoxib with caution as they may have abnormally high plasma levels due to reduced metabolic clearance.
Excretion
Celecoxib is eliminated predominantly by hepatic metabolism with little (<3%) unchanged drug recovered in the urine and feces. Following a single oral dose of radiolabeled drug, approximately 57% of the dose was excreted in the feces and 27% was excreted into the urine. The primary metabolite in both urine and feces was the carboxylic acid metabolite (73% of dose) with low amounts of the glucuronide also appearing in the urine. It appears that the low solubility of the drug prolongs the absorption process making terminal half-life ($t_{1/2}$) determinations more variable. The effective half-life is approximately 11 hours under fasted conditions. The apparent plasma clearance (CL/F) is about 500 mL/min.
Special Populations
Geriatric: At steady state, elderly subjects (over 65 years old) had a 40% higher C_{max} and a 50% higher AUC compared to the young subjects. In elderly females, celecoxib C_{max} and AUC are higher than those for elderly males, but these increases are predominantly due to lower body weight in elderly females. Dose adjustment in the elderly is not generally necessary. However, for patients of less than 50 kg in body weight, initiate therapy at the lowest recommended dose.
Pediatric: CELEBREX capsules have not been investigated in pediatric patients below 18 years of age.
Races: Meta-analysis of pharmacokinetic studies has suggested an approximately 40% higher AUC of celecoxib in Blacks compared to Caucasians. The cause and clinical significance of this finding is unknown.
Hepatic Insufficiency: A pharmacokinetic study in subjects with mild (Child-Pugh Class I) and moderate (Child-Pugh Class II) hepatic impairment has shown that steady-state celecoxib AUC is increased about 40% and 180%, respectively, above that seen in healthy control subjects. Therefore, the recommended daily dose of CELEBREX capsules should be reduced by approximately 50% in patients with moderate (Child-Pugh Class II) hepatic impairment. Patients with severe hepatic impairment have not been studied. The use of CELEBREX in patients with severe hepatic impairment is not recommended.
Renal Insufficiency: In a cross-study comparison, celecoxib AUC was approximately 40% lower in patients with chronic renal insufficiency (GFR 35–60 mL/min) than that seen in subjects with normal renal function. No significant relationship was found between GFR and celecoxib clearance. Patients with severe renal insufficiency have not been studied.
Drug Interactions
Also see PRECAUTIONS —Drug Interactions.
General: Significant interactions may occur when celecoxib is administered together with drugs that inhibit P450 2C9. *In vitro* studies indicate that celecoxib is not an inhibitor of cytochrome P450 2C9, 2C19 or 3A4.
Clinical studies with celecoxib have identified potentially significant interactions with fluconazole and lithium. Experience with nonsteroidal anti-inflammatory drugs (NSAIDs) suggests the potential for interactions with furosemide and ACE inhibitors. The effects of celecoxib on the pharmacokinetics and/or pharmacodynamics of glyburide, ketoconazole, methotrexate, phenytoin, and tolbutamide have been studied *in vivo* and clinically important interactions have not been found.

CLINICAL STUDIES

Osteoarthritis (OA): CELEBREX has demonstrated significant reduction in joint pain compared to placebo. CELEBREX was evaluated for treatment of the signs and the symptoms of OA of the knee and hip in approximately 4,200 patients in placebo- and active-controlled clinical trials of up to 12 weeks duration. In patients with OA, treatment with CELEBREX 100 mg BID or 200 mg QD resulted in improvement in WOMAC (Western Ontario and McMaster Universities) osteoarthritis index, a composite of pain, stiffness, and functional measures in OA. In three 12-week studies of pain accompanying OA flare, CELEBREX doses of 100 mg BID and 200 mg BID provided significant reduction of pain within 24–48 hours of initiation of dosing. At doses of 100 mg BID or 200 mg BID the effectiveness of CELEBREX was shown to be similar to that of naproxen 500 mg BID. Doses of 200 mg BID provided no additional benefit above that seen with 100 mg BID. A total daily dose of 200 mg has been shown to be equally effective whether administered as 100 mg BID or 200 mg QD.
Rheumatoid Arthritis (RA): CELEBREX has demonstrated significant reduction in joint tenderness/pain and joint swelling compared to placebo. CELEBREX was evaluated for treatment of the signs and symptoms of RA in approximately 2,100 patients in placebo- and active-controlled clinical trials of up to 24 weeks in duration. CELEBREX was shown to be superior to placebo in these studies, using the ACR20 Responder Index, a composite of clinical, laboratory, and functional measures in RA. CELEBREX doses of 100 mg BID and 200 mg BID were similar in effectiveness and both were comparable to naproxen 500 mg BID.
Although CELEBREX 100 mg BID and 200 mg BID provided similar overall effectiveness, some patients derived

Continued on next page

Celebrex—Cont.

additional benefit from the 200 mg BID dose. Doses of 400 mg BID provided no additional benefit above that seen with 100–200 mg BID.

Familial Adenomatous Polyposis (FAP): CELEBREX was evaluated to reduce the number of adenomatous colorectal polyps. A randomized double-blind placebo-controlled study was conducted in 83 patients with FAP. The study population included 58 patients with a prior subtotal or total colectomy and 25 patients with an intact colon. Thirteen patients had the attenuated FAP phenotype.

One area in the rectum and up to four areas in the colon were identified at baseline for specific follow-up, and polyps were counted at baseline and following six months of treatment. The mean reduction in the number of colorectal polyps was 28% for CELEBREX 400 mg BID, 12% for CELEBREX 100 mg BID, and 5% for placebo. The reduction in polyps observed with CELEBREX 400 mg BID was statistically superior to placebo at the six-month timepoint (p=0.003). (See Figure 1.)

Figure 1
Percent Change from Baseline in Number of Colorectal Polyps (FAP Patients)

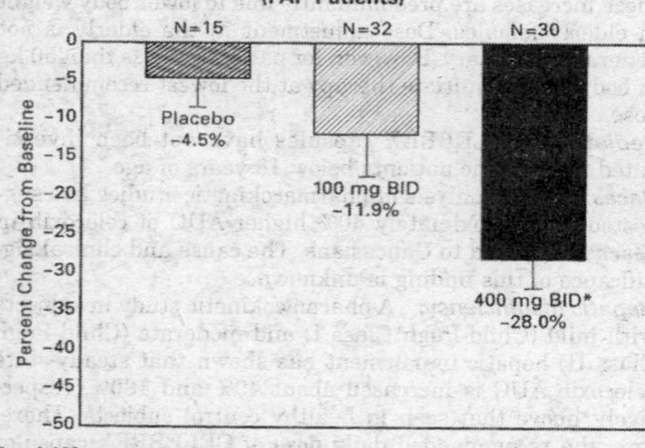

*p=0.003 versus placebo.

Special Studies

Gastrointestinal: Scheduled upper GI endoscopic evaluations were performed in over 4,500 arthritis patients who were enrolled in five controlled randomized 12–24 week trials using active comparators, two of which also included placebo controls. Twelve-week endoscopic ulcer data are available on approximately 1,400 patients and 24 week endoscopic ulcer data are available on 184 patients on CELEBREX at doses ranging from 50–400 mg BID. In all three studies that included naproxen 500 mg BID, and in the study that included ibuprofen 800 mg TID, CELEBREX was associated with a statistically significantly lower incidence of endoscopic ulcers over the study period. Two studies compared CELEBREX with diclofenac 75 mg BID; one study revealed a statistically significantly higher prevalence of endoscopic ulcers in the diclofenac group at the study endpoint (6 months on treatment), and one study revealed no statistically significant difference between cumulative endoscopic ulcer incidence rates in the diclofenac and CELEBREX groups after 1, 2, and 3 months of treatment. There was no consistent relationship between the incidence of gastroduodenal ulcers and the dose of CELEBREX over the range studied.

Figure 2 and Table 2 summarize the incidence of endoscopic ulcers in two 12-week studies that enrolled patients in whom baseline endoscopies revealed no ulcers.

Figure 2
Incidence of Endoscopically Observed Gastroduodenal Ulcers after Twelve Weeks of Treatment

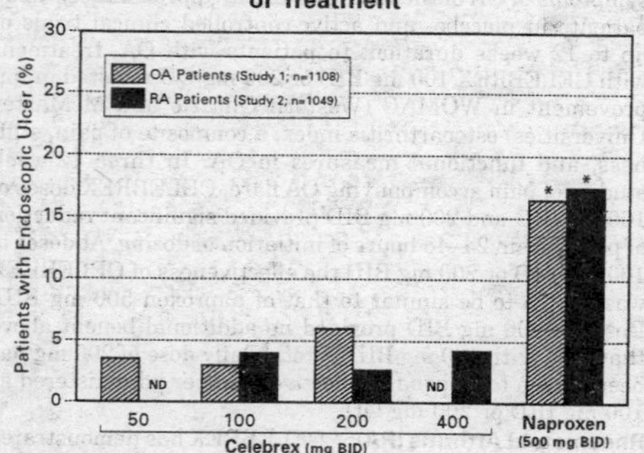

ND=Not Done
*Significantly different from all other treatments; p<0.05.
Celebrex 100 mg BID and 200 mg QD, BID are the recommended doses.
These studies were not powered to compare the endoscopic ulcer rates of Celebrex vs. placebo.
Study 1: placebo ulcer rate = 2.3%
Study 2: placebo ulcer rate = 2.0%

[See table 2 above]

Figure 3 and Table 3 summarize data from two 12-week studies that enrolled patients in whom baseline endoscopies revealed no ulcers. Patients underwent interval endoscopies every 4 weeks to give information on ulcer risk over time.

[See figure 3 at top of next column]

Table 1
Summary of Single Dose (200 mg) Disposition Kinetics of Celecoxib in Healthy Subjects[1]
Mean (%CV) PK Parameter Values

C_{max}, ng/mL	T_{max}, hr	Effective $t_{1/2}$, hr	Vss/F, L	CL/F, L/hr
705 (38)	2.8 (37)	11.2 (31)	429 (34)	27.7 (28)

[1]Subjects under fasting conditions (n=36, 19–52 yrs.)

Table 2
Incidence of Gastroduodenal Ulcers from Endoscopic Studies in OA and RA Patients

	3 Month Studies	
	Study 1 (n=1108)	**Study 2 (n=1049)**
Placebo	2.3% (5/217)	2.0% (4/200)
Celebrex 50 mg BID	3.4% (8/233)	
Celebrex 100 mg BID	3.1% (7/227)	4.0% (9/223)
Celebrex 200 mg BID	5.9% (13/221)	2.7% (6/219)
Celebrex 400 mg BID		4.1% (8/197)
Naproxen 500 mg BID	16.2% (34/210)*	17.6% (37/210)*

*p≤0.05 vs all other treatments

Table 3
Incidence of Gastroduodenal Ulcers from 3-Month Serial Endoscopy Studies in OA and RA Patients

	Week 4	Week 8	Week 12	Final
Study 3 (n=523)				
Celebrex 200 mg BID	4.0% (10/252)*	2.2% (5/227)*	1.5% (3/196)*	7.5% (20/266)*
Naproxen 500 mg BID	19.0% (47/247)	14.2% (26/182)	9.9% (14/141)	34.6% (89/257)
Study 4 (n=1062)				
Celebrex 200 mg BID	3.9% (13/337)†	2.4% (7/296)†	1.8% (5/274)†	7.0% (25/356)†
Diclofenac 75 mg BID	5.1% (18/350)	3.3% (10/306)	2.9% (8/278)	9.7% (36/372)
Ibuprofen 800 mg TID	13.0% (42/323)	6.2% (15/241)	9.6% (21/219)	23.3% (78/334)

*p≤0.05 Celebrex vs. naproxen based on interval and cumulative analyses
†p≤0.05 Celebrex vs. ibuprofen based on interval and cumulative analyses

Figure 3
Cumulative Incidence of Gastroduodenal Ulcers Based on 4 Serial Endoscopies over 12 Weeks

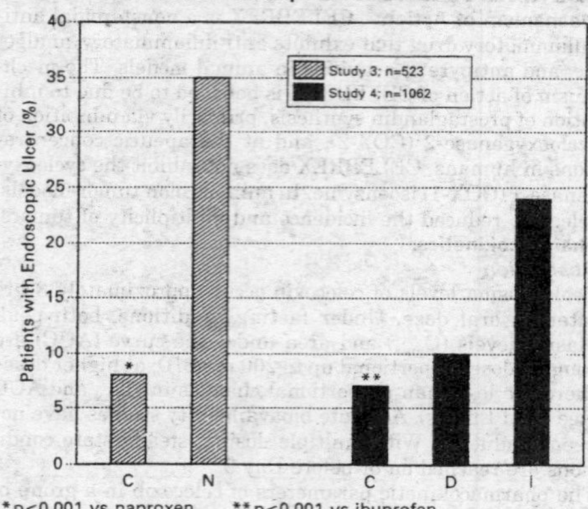

*p<0.001 vs naproxen **p<0.001 vs ibuprofen
C = Celecoxib 200 mg BID D = Diclofenac 75 mg BID
N = Naproxen 500 mg BID I = Ibuprofen 800 mg TID

[See table 3 above]

One randomized and double-blinded 6-month study in 430 RA patients was conducted in which an endoscopic examination was performed at 6 months. The results are shown in Figure 4.

[See figure 4 at top of next column]

The correlation between findings of endoscopic studies, and the relative incidence of clinically serious upper GI events that may be observed with different products, has not been fully established. Serious clinically significant upper GI bleeding has been observed in patients receiving CELEBREX in controlled and open-labeled trials, albeit infrequently (see WARNINGS—Gastrointestinal [GI] effects). Prospective, long-term studies required to compare the incidence of serious, clinically significant upper GI adverse events in patients taking CELEBREX vs. comparator NSAID products have not been performed.

Use with Aspirin: Approximately 11% of patients (440/4,000) enrolled in 4 of the 5 endoscopic studies were taking aspirin (≤325 mg/day). In the CELEBREX groups, the endoscopic ulcer rate appeared to be higher in aspirin users than in non-users. However, the increased rate of ulcers in these aspirin users was less than the endoscopic ulcer rates observed in the active comparator groups, with or without aspirin.

Figure 4
Prevalence of Endoscopically Observed Gastroduodenal Ulcers after Six Months of Treatment in Patients with Rheumatoid Arthritis

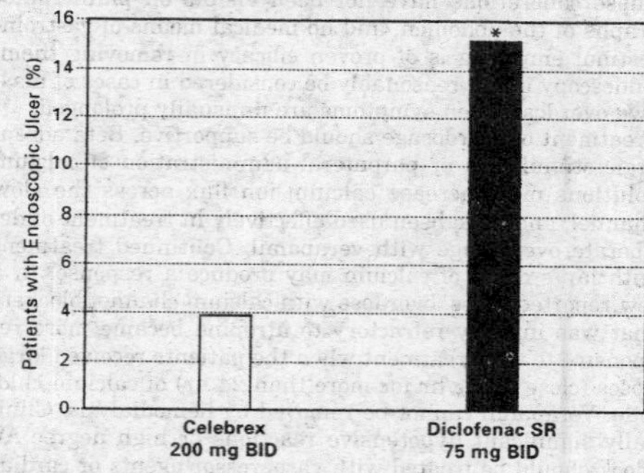

*Significantly different from Celebrex; p<0.001

Platelets: In clinical trials, CELEBREX at single doses up to 800 mg and multiple doses of 600 mg BID for up to 7 days duration (higher than recommended therapeutic doses) had no effect on platelet aggregation and bleeding time. Comparators (naproxen 500 mg BID, ibuprofen 800 mg TID, diclofenac 75 mg BID) significantly reduced platelet aggregation and prolonged bleeding time.

INDICATIONS AND USAGE

CELEBREX is indicated:

1) For relief of the signs and symptoms of osteoarthritis.
2) For relief of the signs and symptoms of rheumatoid arthritis in adults.
3) To reduce the number of adenomatous colorectal polyps in familial adenomatous polyposis (FAP), as an adjunct to usual care (e.g., endoscopic surveillance, surgery). It is not known whether there is a clinical benefit from a reduction in the number of colorectal polyps in FAP patients. It is also not known whether the effects of CELEBREX treatment will persist after CELEBREX is discontinued. The efficacy and safety of CELEBREX treatment in patients with FAP beyond six months have not been studied (see CLINICAL STUDIES, WARNINGS, and PRECAUTIONS sections).

CONTRAINDICATIONS

CELEBREX is contraindicated in patients with known hypersensitivity to celecoxib.

CELEBREX should not be given to patients who have demonstrated allergic-type reactions to sulfonamides.
CELEBREX should not be given to patients who have experienced asthma, urticaria, or allergic-type reactions after taking aspirin or other NSAIDs. Severe, rarely fatal, anaphylactic-like reactions to NSAIDs have been reported in such patients (see WARNINGS—Anaphylactoid Reactions, and PRECAUTIONS—Preexisting Asthma).

WARNINGS

Gastrointestinal (GI) Effects—Risk of GI Ulceration, Bleeding, and Perforation

Serious gastrointestinal toxicity such as bleeding, ulceration, and perforation of the stomach, small intestine or large intestine, can occur at any time, with or without warning symptoms, in patients treated with nonsteroidal anti-inflammatory drugs (NSAIDs). Minor upper gastrointestinal problems, such as dyspepsia, are common and may also occur at any time during NSAID therapy. Therefore, physicians and patients should remain alert for ulceration and bleeding, even in the absence of previous GI tract symptoms. Patients should be informed about the signs and/or symptoms of serious GI toxicity and the steps to take if they occur. The utility of periodic laboratory monitoring has not been demonstrated, nor has it been adequately assessed. Only one in five patients who develop a serious upper GI adverse event on NSAID therapy is symptomatic. It has been demonstrated that upper GI ulcers, gross bleeding or perforation, caused by NSAIDs, appear to occur in approximately 1% of patients treated for 3–6 months, and in about 2–4% of patients treated for one year. These trends continue thus, increasing the likelihood of developing a serious GI event at some time during the course of therapy. However, even short-term therapy is not without risk.
It is unclear, at the present time, how the above rates apply to CELEBREX (See CLINICAL STUDIES—Special Studies). Among 5,285 patients who received CELEBREX in controlled clinical trials of 1 to 6 months duration (most were 3 month studies) at a daily dose of 200 mg or more, 2 (0.04%) experienced significant upper GI bleeding, at 14 and 22 days after initiation of dosing. Approximately 40% of these 5,285 patients were in studies that required them to be free of ulcers by endoscopy at study entry. Thus it is unclear if this study population is representative of the general population. Prospective, long-term studies required to compare the incidence of serious, clinically significant upper GI adverse events in patients taking CELEBREX vs. comparator NSAID products have not been performed.
NSAIDs should be prescribed with extreme caution in patients with a prior history of ulcer disease or gastrointestinal bleeding. Most spontaneous reports of fatal GI events are in elderly or debilitated patients and therefore special care should be taken in treating this population. **To minimize the potential risk for an adverse GI event, the lowest effective dose should be used for the shortest possible duration.** For high risk patients, alternate therapies that do not involve NSAIDs should be considered.
Studies have shown that patients with a *prior history of peptic ulcer disease and/or gastrointestinal bleeding* and who use NSAIDs, have a greater than 10-fold higher risk for developing a GI bleed than patients with neither of these risk factors. In addition to a past history of ulcer disease, pharmacoepidemiological studies have identified several other co-therapies or co-morbid conditions that may increase the risk for GI bleeding such as: treatment with oral corticosteroids, treatment with anticoagulants, longer duration of NSAID therapy, smoking, alcoholism, older age, and poor general health status.

Anaphylactoid Reactions

As with NSAIDs in general, anaphylactoid reactions have occurred in patients without known prior exposure to CELEBREX. In post-marketing experience, rare cases of anaphylactic reactions and angioedema have been reported in patients receiving CELEBREX. CELEBREX should not be given to patients with the aspirin triad. This symptom complex typically occurs in asthmatic patients who experience rhinitis with or without nasal polyps, or who exhibit severe, potentially fatal bronchospasm after taking aspirin or other NSAIDs (see CONTRAINDICATIONS and PRECAUTIONS—Preexisting Asthma). Emergency help should be sought in cases where an anaphylactoid reaction occurs.

Advanced Renal Disease

No information is available regarding the use of CELEBREX in patients with advanced kidney disease. Therefore, treatment with CELEBREX is not recommended in these patients. If CELEBREX therapy must be initiated, close monitoring of the patient's kidney function is advisable (see PRECAUTIONS—Renal Effects).

Pregnancy

In late pregnancy CELEBREX should be avoided because it may cause premature closure of the ductus arteriosus.

Familial Adenomatous Polyposis (FAP): Treatment with CELEBREX in FAP has not been shown to reduce the risk of gastrointestinal cancer or the need for prophylactic colectomy or other FAP-related surgeries. Therefore, the usual care of FAP patients should not be altered because of the concurrent administration of CELEBREX. In particular, the frequency of routine endoscopic surveillance should not be decreased and prophylactic colectomy or other FAP-related surgeries should not be delayed.

PRECAUTIONS

General: CELEBREX cannot be expected to substitute for corticosteroids or to treat corticosteroid insufficiency. Abrupt discontinuation of corticosteroids may lead to exacerbation of corticosteroid-responsive illness. Patients on prolonged corticosteroid therapy should have their therapy tapered slowly if a decision is made to discontinue corticosteroids.
The pharmacological activity of CELEBREX in reducing inflammation, and possibly fever, may diminish the utility of these diagnostic signs in detecting infectious complications of presumed noninfectious, painful conditions.

Hepatic Effects: Borderline elevations of one or more liver tests may occur in up to 15% of patients taking NSAIDs, and notable elevations of ALT or AST (approximately three or more times the upper limit of normal) have been reported in approximately 1% of patients in clinical trials with NSAIDs. These laboratory abnormalities may progress, may remain unchanged, or may be transient with continuing therapy. Rare cases of severe hepatic reactions, including jaundice and fatal fulminant hepatitis, liver necrosis and hepatic failure (some with fatal outcome) have been reported with NSAIDs, including CELEBREX (See ADVERSE REACTIONS—post-marketing experience.) In controlled clinical trials of CELEBREX, the incidence of borderline elevations of liver tests was 6% for CELEBREX and 5% for placebo, and approximately 0.2% of patients taking CELEBREX and 0.3% of patients taking placebo had notable elevations of ALT and AST.
A patient with symptoms and/or signs suggesting liver dysfunction, or in whom an abnormal liver test has occurred, should be monitored carefully for evidence of the development of a more severe hepatic reaction while on therapy with CELEBREX. If clinical signs and symptoms consistent with liver disease develop, or if systemic manifestations occur (e.g., eosinophilia, rash, etc.), CELEBREX should be discontinued.

Renal Effects: Long-term administration of NSAIDs has resulted in renal papillary necrosis and other renal injury. Renal toxicity has also been seen in patients in whom renal prostaglandins have a compensatory role in the maintenance of renal perfusion. In these patients, administration of a nonsteroidal anti-inflammatory drug may cause a dose-dependent reduction in prostaglandin formation and, secondarily, in renal blood flow, which may precipitate overt renal decompensation. Patients at greatest risk of this reaction are those with impaired renal function, heart failure, liver dysfunction, those taking diuretics and ACE inhibitors, and the elderly. Discontinuation of NSAID therapy is usually followed by recovery to the pretreatment state. Clinical trials with CELEBREX have shown renal effects similar to those observed with comparator NSAIDs.
Caution should be used when initiating treatment with CELEBREX in patients with considerable dehydration. It is advisable to rehydrate patients first and then start therapy with CELEBREX. Caution is also recommended in patients with pre-existing kidney disease (see WARNINGS–Advanced Renal Disease).

Hematological Effects: Anemia is sometimes seen in patients receiving CELEBREX. In controlled clinical trials the incidence of anemia was 0.6% with CELEBREX and 0.4% with placebo. Patients on long-term treatment with CELEBREX should have their hemoglobin or hematocrit checked if they exhibit any signs or symptoms of anemia or blood loss. CELEBREX does not generally affect platelet counts, prothrombin time (PT), or partial thromboplastin time (PTT), and does not appear to inhibit platelet aggregation at indicated dosages (See CLINICAL STUDIES—Special Studies—Platelets).

Fluid Retention and Edema: Fluid retention and edema have been observed in some patients taking CELEBREX (see ADVERSE REACTIONS). Therefore, CELEBREX should be used with caution in patients with fluid retention, hypertension, or heart failure.

Preexisting Asthma: Patients with asthma may have aspirin-sensitive asthma. The use of aspirin in patients with aspirin-sensitive asthma has been associated with severe bronchospasm which can be fatal. Since cross reactivity, including bronchospasm, between aspirin and other nonsteroidal anti-inflammatory drugs has been reported in such aspirin-sensitive patients, CELEBREX should not be administered to patients with this form of aspirin sensitivity and should be used with caution in patients with preexisting asthma.

Information for Patients: CELEBREX can cause discomfort and, rarely, more serious side effects, such as gastrointestinal bleeding, which may result in hospitalization and even fatal outcomes. Although serious GI tract ulcerations and bleeding can occur without warning symptoms, patients should be alert for the signs and symptoms of ulcerations and bleeding, and should ask for medical advice when observing any indicative signs or symptoms. Patients should be apprised of the importance of this follow-up (see WARNINGS—Risk of Gastrointestinal Ulceration, Bleeding and Perforation).
Patients should promptly report signs or symptoms of gastrointestinal ulceration or bleeding, skin rash, unexplained weight gain, or edema to their physicians.
Patients should be informed of the warning signs and symptoms of hepatotoxicity (e.g., nausea, fatigue, lethargy, pruritus, jaundice, right upper quadrant tenderness, and "flu-like" symptoms). If these occur, patients should be instructed to stop therapy and seek immediate medical therapy.
Patients should also be instructed to seek immediate emergency help in the case of an anaphylactoid reaction (see WARNINGS).
In late pregnancy CELEBREX should be avoided because it may cause premature closure of the ductus arteriosus.
Patients with familial adenomatous polyposis (FAP) should be informed that CELEBREX has not been shown to reduce colorectal, duodenal or other FAP-related cancers, or the need for endoscopic surveillance, prophylactic or other FAP-related surgery. Therefore, all patients with FAP should be instructed to continue their usual care while receiving CELEBREX.

Laboratory Tests: Because serious GI tract ulcerations and bleeding can occur without warning symptoms, physicians should monitor for signs or symptoms of GI bleeding.
During the controlled clinical trials, there was an increased incidence of hyperchloremia in patients receiving celecoxib compared with patients on placebo. Other laboratory abnormalities that occurred more frequently in the patients receiving celecoxib included hypophosphatemia, and elevated BUN. These laboratory abnormalities were also seen in patients who received comparator NSAIDs in these studies. The clinical significance of these abnormalities has not been established.

Drug Interactions

General: Celecoxib metabolism is predominantly mediated via cytochrome P450 2C9 in the liver. Co-administration of celecoxib with drugs that are known to inhibit 2C9 should be done with caution.
In vitro studies indicate that celecoxib, although not a substrate, is an inhibitor of cytochrome P450 2D6. Therefore, there is a potential for an *in vivo* drug interaction with drugs that are metabolized by P450 2D6.

ACE-inhibitors: Reports suggest that NSAIDs may diminish the antihypertensive effect of Angiotensin Converting Enzyme (ACE) inhibitors. This interaction should be given consideration in patients taking CELEBREX concomitantly with ACE-inhibitors.

Furosemide: Clinical studies, as well as post marketing observations, have shown that NSAIDs can reduce the natriuretic effect of furosemide and thiazides in some patients. This response has been attributed to inhibition of renal prostaglandin synthesis.

Aspirin: CELEBREX can be used with low dose aspirin. However, concomitant administration of aspirin with CELEBREX may result in an increased rate of GI ulceration or other complications, compared to use of CELEBREX alone (see CLINICAL STUDIES—Special Studies—Gastrointestinal). Because of its lack of platelet effects, CELEBREX is not a substitute for aspirin for cardiovascular prophylaxis.

Fluconazole: Concomitant administration of fluconazole at 200 mg QD resulted in a two-fold increase in celecoxib plasma concentration. This increase is due to the inhibition of celecoxib metabolism via P450 2C9 by fluconazole (see Pharmacokinetics—Metabolism). CELEBREX should be introduced at the lowest recommended dose in patients receiving fluconazole.

Lithium: In a study conducted in healthy subjects, mean steady-state lithium plasma levels increased approximately 17% in subjects receiving lithium 450 mg BID with CELEBREX 200 mg BID as compared to subjects receiving lithium alone. Patients on lithium treatment should be closely monitored when CELEBREX is introduced or withdrawn.

Methotrexate: In an interaction study of rheumatoid arthritis patients taking methotrexate, CELEBREX did not have a significant effect on the pharmacokinetics of methotrexate.

Warfarin: Anticoagulant activity should be monitored, particularly in the first few days, after initiating or changing CELEBREX therapy in patients receiving warfarin or similar agents, since these patients are at an increased risk of bleeding complications. The effect of celecoxib on the anticoagulant effect of warfarin was studied in a group of healthy subjects receiving daily doses of 2 to 5 mg of warfarin. In these subjects, celecoxib did not alter the anticoagulant effect of warfarin as determined by prothrombin time. However, in post-marketing experience, bleeding events have been reported, predominantly in the elderly, in association with increases in prothrombin time in patients receiving CELEBREX concurrently with warfarin.

Carcinogenesis, mutagenesis, impairment of fertility: Celecoxib was not carcinogenic in rats given oral doses up to 200 mg/kg for males and 10 mg/kg for females (approximately 2- to 4-fold the human exposure as measured by the AUC_{0-24} at 200 mg BID) or in mice given oral doses up to 25 mg/kg for males and 50 mg/kg for females (approximately equal to human exposure as measured by the AUC_{0-24} at 200 mg BID) for two years.
Celecoxib was not mutagenic in an Ames test and a mutation assay in Chinese hamster ovary (CHO) cells, nor clastogenic in a chromosome aberration assay in CHO cells and an *in vivo* micronucleus test in rat bone marrow.
Celecoxib did not impair male and female fertility in rats at oral doses up to 600 mg/kg/day (approximately 11-fold human exposure at 200 mg BID based on the AUC_{0-24}).

Pregnancy

Teratogenic effects: Pregnancy Category C. Celecoxib was not teratogenic in rabbits up to an oral dose of 60 mg/kg/day (equal to human exposure at 200 mg BID as measured by AUC_{0-24}); however, at oral doses ≥150 mg/kg/day (approximately 2-fold human exposure at 200 mg BID as measured by AUC_{0-24}), an increased incidence of fetal alterations, such as ribs fused, sternebrae fused and sternebrae misshapen, was observed. A dose-dependent increase in diaphragmatic hernias was observed in one of two rat studies

Continued on next page

Celebrex—Cont.

at oral doses ≥30 mg/kg/day (approximately 6-fold human exposure based on the AUC_{0-24} at 200 mg BID). There are no studies in pregnant women. CELEBREX should be used during pregnancy only if the potential benefit justifies the potential risk to the fetus.

Nonteratogenic effects: Celecoxib produced pre-implantation and post-implantation losses and reduced embryo/fetal survival in rats at oral dosages ≥50 mg/kg/day (approximately 6-fold human exposure based on the AUC_{0-24} at 200 mg BID). These changes are expected with inhibition of prostaglandin synthesis and are not the result of permanent alteration of female reproductive function, nor are they expected at clinical exposures. No studies have been conducted to evaluate the effect of celecoxib on the closure of the ductus arteriosus in humans. Therefore, use of CELEBREX during the third trimester of pregnancy should be avoided.

Labor and delivery: Celecoxib produced no evidence of delayed labor or parturition at oral doses up to 100 mg/kg in rats (approximately 7-fold human exposure as measured by the AUC_{0-24} at 200 mg BID). The effects of CELEBREX on labor and delivery in pregnant women are unknown.

Nursing mothers: Celecoxib is excreted in the milk of lactating rats at concentrations similar to those in plasma. It is not known whether this drug is excreted in human milk. Because many drugs are excreted in human milk and because of the potential for serious adverse reactions in nursing infants from CELEBREX, a decision should be made whether to discontinue nursing or to discontinue the drug, taking into account the importance of the drug to the mother.

Pediatric Use

Safety and effectiveness in pediatric patients below the age of 18 years have not been evaluated.

Geriatric Use

Of the total number of patients who received CELEBREX in clinical trials, more than 2,100 were 65–74 years of age, while approximately 800 additional patients were 75 years and over. While the incidence of adverse experiences tended to be higher in elderly patients, no substantial differences in safety and effectiveness were observed between these subjects and younger subjects. Other reported clinical experience has not identified differences in response between the elderly and younger patients, but greater sensitivity of some older individuals cannot be ruled out.

In clinical studies comparing renal function as measured by the GFR, BUN and creatinine, and platelet function as measured by bleeding time and platelet aggregation, the results were not different between elderly and young volunteers.

ADVERSE REACTIONS

Of the CELEBREX treated patients in controlled trials, approximately 4,250 were patients with OA, approximately 2,100 were patients with RA, and approximately 1,050 were patients with post-surgical pain. More than 8,500 patients have received a total daily dose of CELEBREX of 200 mg (100 mg BID or 200 mg QD) or more, including more than 400 treated at 800 mg (400 mg BID). Approximately 3,900 patients have received CELEBREX at these doses for 6 months or more; approximately 2,300 of these have received it for 1 year or more and 124 of these have received it for 2 years or more.

Adverse events from controlled trials: Table 4 lists all adverse events, regardless of causality, occurring in ≥2% of patients receiving CELEBREX from 12 controlled studies conducted in patients with OA or RA that included a placebo and/or a positive control group.

[See table below]

In placebo- or active-controlled clinical trials, the discontinuation rate due to adverse events was 7.1% for patients receiving CELEBREX and 6.1% for patients receiving placebo. Among the most common reasons for discontinuation due to adverse events in the CELEBREX treatment groups were dyspepsia and abdominal pain (cited as reasons for discontinuation in 0.8% and 0.7% of CELEBREX patients, respectively). Among patients receiving placebo, 0.6% discontinued due to dyspepsia and 0.6% withdrew due to abdominal pain.

The following adverse events occurred in 0.1–1.9% of patients regardless of causality.

Celebrex
(100–200 mg BID or 200 mg QD)

Gastrointestinal: Constipation, diverticulitis, dysphagia, eructation, esophagitis, gastritis, gastroenteritis, gastroesophageal reflux, hemorrhoids, hiatal hernia, melena, dry mouth, stomatitis, tenesmus, tooth disorder, vomiting

Cardiovascular: Aggravated hypertension, angina pectoris, coronary artery disorder, myocardial infarction

General: Allergy aggravated, allergic reaction, asthenia, chest pain, cyst NOS, edema generalized, face edema, fatigue, fever, hot flushes, influenza-like symptoms, pain, peripheral pain

Resistance mechanism disorders: Herpes simplex, herpes zoster, infection bacterial, infection fungal, infection soft tissue, infection viral, moniliasis, moniliasis genital, otitis media

Central, peripheral nervous system: Leg cramps, hypertonia, hypoesthesia, migraine, neuralgia, neuropathy, paresthesia, vertigo

Female reproductive: Breast fibroadenosis, breast neoplasm, breast pain, dysmenorrhea, menstrual disorder, vaginal hemorrhage, vaginitis

Male reproductive: Prostatic disorder

Hearing and vestibular: Deafness, ear abnormality, earache, tinnitus

Heart rate and rhythm: Palpitation, tachycardia

Liver and biliary system: Hepatic function abnormal, SGOT increased, SGPT increased

Metabolic and nutritional: BUN increased, CPK increased, diabetes mellitus, hypercholesterolemia, hyperglycemia, hypokalemia, NPN increase, creatinine increased, alkaline phosphatase increased, weight increase

Musculoskeletal: Arthralgia, arthrosis, bone disorder, fracture accidental, myalgia, neck stiffness, synovitis, tendinitis

Platelets (bleeding or clotting): Ecchymosis, epistaxis, thrombocythemia

Psychiatric: Anorexia, anxiety, appetite increased, depression, nervousness, somnolence

Hemic: Anemia

Respiratory: Bronchitis, bronchospasm, bronchospasm aggravated, coughing, dyspnea, laryngitis, pneumonia

Skin and appendages: Alopecia, dermatitis, nail disorder, photosensitivity reaction, pruritus, rash erythematous, rash maculopapular, skin disorder, skin dry, sweating increased, urticaria

Application site disorders: Cellulitis, dermatitis contact, injection site reaction, skin nodule

Special senses: Taste perversion

Urinary system: Albuminuria, cystitis, dysuria, hematuria, micturition frequency, renal calculus, urinary incontinence, urinary tract infection

Vision: Blurred vision, cataract, conjunctivitis, eye pain, glaucoma

Other serious adverse reactions which occur rarely (<0.1%), regardless of causality: The following serious adverse events have occurred rarely in patients, taking CELEBREX. Cases reported only in the post-marketing experience are indicated in italics.

Cardiovascular: Syncope, congestive heart failure, ventricular fibrillation, pulmonary embolism, cerebrovascular accident, peripheral gangrene, thrombophlebitis, *vasculitis*

Gastrointestinal: Intestinal obstruction, intestinal perforation, gastrointestinal bleeding, colitis with bleeding, esophageal perforation, pancreatitis, cholelithiasis, ileus

Liver and biliary system: Cholelithiasis, *hepatitis, jaundice, liver failure*

Hemic and lymphatic: Thrombocytopenia, *agranulocytosis, aplastic anemia, pancytopenia, leukopenia*

Metabolic: *Hypoglycemia*

Nervous system: Ataxia, suicide

Renal: Acute renal failure, *interstitial nephritis*

Skin: *Erythema multiforme, exfoliative dermatitis, Stevens-Johnson syndrome, toxic epidermal necrolysis*

General: Sepsis, sudden death, *anaphylactoid reaction, angioedema*

Adverse events from the controlled trial in familial adenomatous polyposis: The adverse event profile reported for the 83 patients with familial adenomatous polyposis enrolled in the randomized, controlled clinical trial was similar to that reported for patients in the arthritis controlled trials. Intestinal anastomotic ulceration was the only new adverse event reported in the FAP trial, regardless of causality, and was observed in 3 of 58 patients (one at 100 mg BID, and two at 400 mg BID) who had prior intestinal surgery.

OVERDOSAGE

Symptoms following acute NSAID overdoses are usually limited to lethargy, drowsiness, nausea, vomiting, and epigastric pain, which are generally reversible with supportive care. Gastrointestinal bleeding can occur. Hypertension, acute renal failure, respiratory depression and coma may occur, but are rare. Anaphylactoid reactions have been reported with therapeutic ingestion of NSAIDs, and may occur following an overdose.

Patients should be managed by symptomatic and supportive care following an NSAID overdose. There are no specific antidotes. No information is available regarding the removal of celecoxib by hemodialysis, but based on its high degree of plasma protein binding (>97%) dialysis is unlikely to be useful in overdose. Emesis and/or activated charcoal (60 to 100 g in adults, 1 to 2 g/kg in children) and/or osmotic cathartic may be indicated in patients seen within 4 hours of ingestion with symptoms or following a large overdose. Forced diuresis, alkalinization of urine, hemodialysis, or hemoperfusion may not be useful due to high protein binding.

DOSAGE AND ADMINISTRATION

For osteoarthritis and rheumatoid arthritis, the lowest dose of CELEBREX should be sought for each patient. These doses can be given without regard to timing of meals.

Osteoarthritis: For relief of the signs and symptoms of osteoarthritis the recommended oral dose is 200 mg per day administered as a single dose or as 100 mg twice per day.

Rheumatoid arthritis: For relief of the signs and symptoms of rheumatoid arthritis the recommended oral dose is 100 to 200 mg twice per day.

Familial adenomatous polyposis (FAP): Usual medical care for FAP patients should be continued while on CELEBREX. To reduce the number of adenomatous colorectal polyps in patients with FAP, the recommended oral dose is 400 mg (2 × 200 mg capsules) twice per day to be taken with food.

Hepatic Insufficiency: The daily recommended dose of CELEBREX capsules in patients with moderate hepatic impairment (Child-Pugh Class II) should be reduced by approximately 50% (see CLINICAL PHARMACOLOGY—Special popoulations).

HOW SUPPLIED

CELEBREX 100-mg capsules are white, reverse printed white on blue band of body and cap with markings of 7767 on the cap and 100 on the body, supplied as:

NDC Number	Size
0025-1520-31	bottle of 100
0025-1520-51	bottle of 500
0025-1520-34	carton of 100 unit dose

CELEBREX 200-mg capsules are white, with reverse printed white on gold band with markings of 7767 on the cap and 200 on the body, supplied as:

NDC Number	Size
0025-1525-31	bottle of 100
0025-1525-51	bottle of 500
0025-1525-34	carton of 100 unit dose

Store at 25°C (77°F); excursions permitted to 15–30°C (59–86°F). [See USP Controlled Room Temperature]

Rx only **A05264-5 • 12/23/99**

Mfd. for Searle Ltd.
Caguas PR 00725
By Searle & Co.
San Juan PR 00936

Marketed by:
G.D. Searle & Co.
Chicago IL 60680 USA
Pfizer Inc.
New York NY 10017 USA

Address medical inquiries to:
G.D. Searle & Co.
Healthcare Information Services
5200 Old Orchard Rd.
Skokie IL 60077

Shown in Product Identification Guide, page 335

Table 4
Adverse Events Occurring in ≥2% of Celebrex Patients From Controlled Arthritis Trials

	Celebrex (100–200 mg BID or 200 mg QD) (N=4146)	Placebo (N=1864)	Naproxen 500 mg BID (N=1366)	Ibuprofen 800 mg TID (N=387)	Diclofenac 75 mg BID (N=345)
Gastrointestinal					
Abdominal pain	4.1%	2.8%	7.7%	9.0%	9.0%
Diarrhea	5.6%	3.8%	5.3%	9.3%	5.8%
Dyspepsia	8.8%	6.2%	12.2%	10.9%	12.8%
Flatulence	2.2%	1.0%	3.6%	4.1%	3.5%
Nausea	3.5%	4.2%	6.0%	3.4%	6.7%
Body as a whole					
Back pain	2.8%	3.6%	2.2%	2.6%	0.9%
Peripheral edema	2.1%	1.1%	2.1%	1.0%	3.5%
Injury-accidental	2.9%	2.3%	3.0%	2.6%	3.2%
Central and peripheral nervous system					
Dizziness	2.0%	1.7%	2.6%	1.3%	2.3%
Headache	15.8%	20.2%	14.5%	15.5%	15.4%
Psychiatric					
Insomnia	2.3%	2.3%	2.9%	1.3%	1.4%
Respiratory					
Pharyngitis	2.3%	1.1%	1.7%	1.6%	2.6%
Rhinitis	2.0%	1.3%	2.4%	2.3%	0.6%
Sinusitis	5.0%	4.3%	4.0%	5.4%	5.8%
Upper respiratory tract infection	8.1%	6.7%	9.9%	9.8%	9.9%
Skin					
Rash	2.2%	2.1%	2.1%	1.3%	1.2%

COVERA-HS™ ℞

[*Cō-ver ´-ə*]
(verapamil hydrochloride)
Extended-Release Tablets
Controlled-Onset

DESCRIPTION

Covera-HS (verapamil hydrochloride) is a calcium ion influx inhibitor (slow-channel blocker or calcium ion antagonist). Covera-HS is available for oral administration as pale yellow, round, film-coated tablets containing 240 mg of verapamil hydrochloride and as lavender, round, film-coated tablets containing 180 mg of verapamil hydrochloride. Verapamil is administered as a racemic mixture of the R and S enantiomers. The structural formulae of the verapamil HCl enantiomers are:

S-verapamil

R-verapamil

$C_{27}H_{38}N_2O_4 \cdot HCl$ M.W.=491.07

Benzeneacetonitrile, (±)-α[3[[2-(3,4-dimethoxyphenyl) ethyl]methylamino]propyl]-3,4-dimethoxy-α-(1-methylethyl) hydrochloride

Verapamil HCl is an almost white, crystalline powder, practically free of odor, with a bitter taste. It is soluble in water, chloroform, and methanol. Verapamil HCl is not chemically related to other cardioactive drugs.

Inactive ingredients are black ferric oxide, BHT, cellulose acetate, hydroxyethyl cellulose, hydroxypropyl cellulose, hydroxypropyl methylcellulose, magnesium stearate, polyethylene glycol, polyethylene oxide, polysorbate 80, povidone, sodium chloride, titanium dioxide, and coloring agents: 240-mg—FD&C Blue No. 2 Lake and D&C Yellow No. 10 Lake; 180-mg—FD&C Blue No. 2 Lake and D&C Red No. 30 Lake.

System components and performance: The Covera-HS formulation has been designed to initiate the release of verapamil 4–5 hours after ingestion. This delay is introduced by a layer between the active drug core and outer semipermeable membrane. As water from the gastrointestinal tract enters the tablet, this delay coating is solubilized and released. As tablet hydration continues, the osmotic layer expands and pushes against the drug layer, releasing drug through precision laser-drilled orifices in the outer membrane at a constant rate. This controlled rate of drug delivery in the gastrointestinal lumen is independent of posture, pH, gastrointestinal motility, and fed or fasting conditions.

The biologically inert components of the delivery system remain intact during GI transit and are eliminated in the feces as an insoluble shell.

CLINICAL PHARMACOLOGY

Covera-HS has a unique delivery system, designed for bedtime dosing, incorporating a 4 to 5-hour delay in drug delivery. The unique controlled-onset, extended-release (COER) delivery system, which is designed for bedtime dosing, results in a maximum plasma concentration (C_{max}) of verapamil in the morning hours.

Verapamil is a calcium ion influx inhibitor (L-type calcium channel blocker or calcium channel antagonist). Verapamil exerts its pharmacologic effects by selectively inhibiting the transmembrane influx of ionic calcium into arterial smooth muscle as well as in conductile and contractile myocardial cells without altering serum calcium concentrations.

Mechanism of Action

In vitro: Verapamil binding is voltage-dependent with affinity increasing as the vascular smooth muscle membrane potential is reduced. In addition, verapamil binding is frequency dependent and apparent affinity increases with increased frequency of depolarizing stimulus.

The L-type calcium channel is an oligomeric structure consisting of five putative subunits designated alpha-1, alpha-2, beta, tau, and epsilon. Biochemical evidence points to separate binding sites for 1,4-dihydropyridines, phenylalkylamines, and the benzothiazepines (all located on the alpha-1 subunit). Although they share a similar mechanism of action, calcium channel blockers represent three heterogeneous categories of drugs with differing vascular-cardiac selectivity ratios.

Essential hypertension: Verapamil produces its antihypertensive effect by a combination of vascular and cardiac effects. It acts as a vasodilator with selectivity for the arterial portion of the peripheral vasculature. As a result the systemic vascular resistence is reduced and usually without orthostatic hypotension or reflex tachycardia. Bradycardia (rate less than 50 beats/min) is uncommon (<1% with Covera-HS as assessed by ECG). During isometric or dynamic exercise Covera-HS does not alter systolic cardiac function in patients with normal ventricular function.

Covera-HS does not alter total serum calcium levels. However, one report has suggested that calcium levels above the normal range may alter the therapeutic effect of verapamil.

Covera-HS regularly reduces the total systemic resistance (afterload) against which the heart works both at rest and at a given level of exercise by dilating peripheral arterioles.

Effects in hypertension: Covera-HS was evaluated in two placebo-controlled, parallel design, double-blind studies of 382 patients with mild to moderate hypertension.

In clinical trials 287 patients were randomized to placebo, 120 mg, 180 mg, 360 mg, or 540 mg and treated for 8 weeks (the two higher doses were titrated from low doses and maintained for 6 and 4 weeks, respectively). Covera-HS or placebo was given once daily at 10 pm and blood pressure changes were measured with 36-hour ambulatory blood pressure monitoring (ABPM). The results of these studies demonstrate that Covera-HS, at 180–540 mg, is a consistently and significantly more effective antihypertensive agent than placebo in reducing ambulatory blood pressures. Over this dose range, the placebo-subtracted net decreases in diastolic BP at trough (averaged over 6–10 pm) were dose-related, ranged from 4.5 to 11.2 mm Hg after 4–8 weeks of therapy, and correlated well with sitting cuff blood pressures.

These studies demonstrate that clinically and statistically significant blood pressure reductions are achieved with Covera-HS throughout the 24-hour dosing period.

There were no significant treatment differences between patient subgroups of different age (older or younger than 65 years), sex, race (Caucasian and non-Caucasian) and severity of hypertension at baseline (cuff BP below and above 105 mm Hg).

Angina: Verapamil dilates the main coronary arteries and coronary arterioles, both in normal and ischemic regions, and is a potent inhibitor of coronary artery spasm, whether spontaneous or ergonovine-induced. This property increases myocardial oxygen delivery in patients with coronary artery spasm and is responsible for the effectiveness of verapamil in vasospastic (Prinzmetal's or variant) as well as unstable angina at rest. Whether this effect plays any role in classical effort angina is not clear, but studies of exercise tolerance have not shown an increase in the maximum exercise rate-pressure product, a widely accepted measure of oxygen utilization. This suggests that, in general, relief of spasm or dilation of coronary arteries is not an important factor in classical angina.

Verapamil regularly reduces the total systemic resistance (afterload) against which the heart works both at rest and at a given level of exercise by dilating peripheral arterioles.

Effect in chronic stable angina: Covera-HS was evaluated in two placebo-controlled, parallel design, double-blind studies of 453 patients with chronic stable angina.

In the first clinical trial 277 patients were randomized to placebo, 180 mg, 360 mg, or 540 mg and treated for 4 weeks (the two higher doses were titrated from low doses and maintained for 3 and 2 weeks, respectively). A single dose of 240 mg was compared to placebo in a separate study of 176 patients. In these studies Covera-HS was significantly more effective than placebo in improvement of exercise tolerance. Placebo-adjusted net increases in median exercise times at the end of the dosing interval were 0.1 to 1.0 minute for symptom limited duration, 0.3 to 1.4 minutes for time to angina, and 0.1 to 1.1 minutes for time to ST change. Increases in exercise tolerance were in general greater at higher doses, but dose-response relationship was not well defined due to shorter treatment duration for high doses.

In addition, in the first study, 24 to 34% of patients treated with Covera-HS did not experience exercise-limiting angina on exercise treadmill testing (ETT) versus 12% of patients on placebo.

Electrophysiologic effects: Electrical activity through the AV node depends, to a significant degree, upon the transmembrane influx of extracellular calcium through the L-type (slow) channel. By decreasing the influx of calcium, verapamil prolongs the effective refractory period within the AV node and slows AV conduction in a rate-related manner.

Normal sinus rhythm is usually not affected, but in patients with sick sinus syndrome, verapamil may interfere with sinus-node impulse generation and may induce sinus arrest or sinoatrial block. Atrioventricular block can occur in patients without preexisting conduction defects (see *Warnings*).

Covera-HS does not alter the normal atrial action potential or intra-ventricular conduction time, but depresses amplitude, velocity of depolarization, and conduction in depressed atrial fibers. Verapamil may shorten the antegrade effective refractory period of the accessory bypass tract. Acceleration of ventricular rate and/or ventricular fibrillation has been reported in patients with atrial flutter or atrial fibrillation and a coexisting accessory AV pathway following administration of verapamil (see *Warnings*).

Verapamil has a local anesthetic action that is 1.6 times that of procaine on an equimolar basis. It is not known whether this action is important at the doses used in man.

Pharmacokinetics and metabolism: Verapamil is administered as a racemic mixture of the R and S enantiomers. The systemic concentrations of R and S enantiomers, as well as overall bioavailability, are dependent upon the route of administration and the rate and extent of release from the dosage forms. Upon oral administration, there is rapid stereoselective biotransformation during the first pass of verapamil through the portal circulation. In a study in 5 subjects with oral immediate-release verapamil, the systemic bioavailability was from 33% to 65% for the R enantiomer and from 13% to 34% for the S enantiomer. The R and S enantiomers have differing levels of pharmacologic activity. In studies in animals and humans, the S enantiomer has 8 to 20 times the activity of the R enantiomer in slowing AV conduction. In animal studies, the S enantiomer has 15 and 50 times the activity of the R enantiomer in reducing myocardial contractility in isolated blood-perfused dog papillary muscle and isolated rabbit papillary muscle, respectively, and twice the effect in reducing peripheral resistance. In isolated septal strip preparations from 5 patients, the S enantiomer was 8 times more potent than the R in reducing myocardial contractility. Dose escalation study data indicate that verapamil concentrations increase disproportionally to dose as measured by relative peak plasma concentrations (C_{max}) or areas under the plasma concentration vs time curves (AUC).

Pharmacokinetic Characteristics of Verapamil Enantiomers After Administration of Escalating Doses

		Total Dose of Racemic Verapamil (mg)			
	Isomer	**120**	**180**	**360**	**540**
Dose Ratio	—	1	1.5	3	4.5
Relative C_{max}	R	1	1.55	4.47	7.06
	S	1	1.62	5.17	9.21
Relative AUC	R	1	1.59	6.14	11.1
	S	1	1.89	8.17	15.9

Pharmacokinetic Characteristics of Verapamil Enantiomers After Administration of a Single 180 mg Dose and at Steady State

	Isomer	First Dose (Verapamil-naive subject)	Steady State (Current verapamil exposure)
C_{max} (ng/ml)	R	59.4	90.5
	S	11.7	21.2
AUC (0–24h) (ng·hr/ml)	R	644	1,223
	S	111	266

Racemic verapamil is released from Covera-HS at a constant rate following solubilization and release of the delay coat through the tablet orifices. This delay coat produces a lag period in drug release for approximately 4–5 hours. The drug release phase is prolonged with the peak plasma concentration (C_{max}) occurring approximately 11 hours after administration. Trough concentrations occur approximately 4 hours after bedtime dosing while the patient is sleeping. Steady-state pharmacokinetics were determined in healthy volunteers. Steady-state concentration is reached by the third or fourth day of dosing.

Steady-State Pharmacokinetics of Verapamil Enantiomers in Healthy Humans

		Verapamil Dose (mg)	
	Isomer	**180**	**240**
Mean C_{max} (ng/ml)	R	90.5	120
	S	21.2	28.7
AUC (0–24h) (ng·hr/ml)	R	1,223	1,470
	S	266	322

In general, bioavailability of Covera-HS is higher and half life longer in older (>65 yrs) subjects. Lean body weight also affects its pharmacokinetics inversely, but no gender difference was observed in the clinical trials of Covera-HS. However, there are conflicting data in literature suggesting that verapamil clearance decreased with age in women to a greater degree than in men.

Consumption of a high fat meal just prior to dosing at night had no effect on the pharmacokinetics of Covera-HS. The pharmacokinetics were also not affected by whether the volunteers were supine or ambulatory for the 8 hours following dosing. Administering Covera-HS in the morning led to a slower rate of absorption and/or elimination, but did not affect the extent of absorption or extent of metabolism to norverapamil.

Orally administered verapamil undergoes extensive metabolism in the liver. Thirteen metabolites have been identified in urine. Norverapamil enantiomers can reach steady-state plasma concentrations approximately equal to those of the enantiomers of the parent drug. The cardiovascular activity of norverapamil appears to be approximately 20% that of verapamil. Approximately 70% of an administered dose is excreted as metabolites in the urine and 16% or more in the feces within 5 days. About 3% to 4% is excreted in the urine as unchanged drug. R-verapamil is 94% bound to plasma albumin, while S-verapamil is 88% bound. In addition, R-verapamil is 92% and S-verapamil 86% bound to alpha-1

Continued on next page

Covera-HS—Cont.

acid glycoprotein. In patients with hepatic insufficiency, metabolism of immediate-release verapamil is delayed and elimination half-life prolonged up to 14 to 16 hours because of the extensive hepatic metabolism (see *Precautions*). In addition, in these patients there is a reduced first pass effect, and verapamil is more bioavailable. Verapamil clearance values suggest that patients with liver dysfunction may attain therapeutic verapamil plasma concentrations with one third of the oral daily dose required for patients with normal liver function.

After four weeks of oral dosing of immediate release verapamil (120 mg q.i.d.), verapamil and norverapamil levels were noted in the cerebrospinal fluid with estimated partition coefficient of 0.06 for verapamil and 0.04 for norverapamil.

Hemodynamics: Verapamil reduces afterload and myocardial contractility. In most patients, including those with organic cardiac disease, the negative inotropic action of verapamil is countered by reduction of afterload and cardiac index remains unchanged. During isometric or dynamic exercise, verapamil does not alter systolic cardiac function in patients with normal ventricular function. Improved left ventricular diastolic function in patients with IHSS and those with coronary heart disease has also been observed with verapamil. In patients with severe left ventricular dysfunction (eg, pulmonary wedge pressure above 20 mm Hg or ejection fraction less than 30%), or in patients taking beta-adrenergic blocking agents or other cardio-depressant drugs, deterioration of ventricular function may occur (see *Drug interactions*).

Pulmonary function: Verapamil does not induce bronchoconstriction and, hence, does not impair ventilatory function.

Verapamil has been shown to have either a neutral or relaxant effect on bronchial smooth muscle.

INDICATIONS AND USAGE

Covera-HS is indicated for the management of hypertension and angina.

CONTRAINDICATIONS

Covera-HS is contraindicated in:

1. Severe left ventricular dysfunction (see *Warnings*)
2. Hypotension (systolic pressure less than 90 mm Hg) or cardiogenic shock
3. Sick sinus syndrome (except in patients with a functioning artificial ventricular pacemaker)
4. Second- or third-degree AV block (except in patients with a functioning artificial ventricular pacemaker)
5. Patients with atrial flutter or atrial fibrillation and an accessory bypass tract (eg, Wolff-Parkinson-White, Lown-Ganong-Levine syndromes). (See *Warnings.*)
6. Patients with known hypersensitivity to verapamil hydrochloride.

WARNINGS

Heart failure: Verapamil has a negative inotropic effect, which in most patients is compensated by its afterload reduction (decreased systemic vascular resistance) properties without a net impairment of ventricular performance. In previous clinical experience with 4,954 patients primarily with immediate-release verapamil, 1.8% developed congestive heart failure or pulmonary edema. Verapamil should be avoided in patients with severe left ventricular dysfunction (eg, ejection fraction less than 30%) or moderate to severe symptoms of cardiac failure and in patients with any degree of ventricular dysfunction if they are receiving a beta-adrenergic blocker (see *Drug Interactions*). Patients with milder ventricular dysfunction should, if possible, be controlled with optimum doses of digitalis and/or diuretics before verapamil treatment is started. (**Note interactions with digoxin under *Precautions*.**)

Hypotension: Occasionally, the pharmacologic action of verapamil may produce a decrease in blood pressure below normal levels, which may result in dizziness or symptomatic hypotension. In previous verapamil clinical trials the incidence observed in 4,954 patients was 2.5%. In clinical studies of Covera-HS, 0.4% of hypertensive patients and 1.0% of angina patients developed significant hypotension. In hypertensive patients, decreases in blood pressure below normal are unusual. Tilt-table testing (60 degrees) was not able to induce orthostatic hypotension.

Elevated liver enzymes: Elevations of transaminases with and without concomitant elevations in alkaline phosphatase and bilirubin have been reported. Such elevations have sometimes been transient and may disappear even in the face of continued verapamil treatment. Several cases of hepatocellular injury related to verapamil have been proven by rechallenge; half of these had clinical symptoms (malaise, fever, and/or right upper quadrant pain) in addition to elevation of SGOT, SGPT, and alkaline phosphatase. Periodic monitoring of liver function in patients receiving verapamil is therefore prudent.

Accessory bypass tract (Wolff-Parkinson-White or Lown-Ganong-Levine): Some patients with paroxysmal and/or chronic atrial fibrillation or atrial flutter and a coexisting accessory AV pathway have developed increased antegrade conduction across the accessory pathway bypassing the AV node, producing a very rapid ventricular response or ventricular fibrillation after receiving intravenous verapamil (or digitalis). Although a risk of this occurring with oral verapamil has not been established, such patients receiving oral verapamil may be at risk and its use in these patients is contraindicated (see *Contraindications*). Treatment is usually DC-cardioversion. Cardioversion has been used safely and effectively after oral verapamil.

Atrioventricular block: The effect of verapamil on AV conduction and the SA node may cause asymptomatic first-degree AV block and transient bradycardia, sometimes accompanied by nodal escape rhythms. PR-interval prolongation is correlated with verapamil plasma concentrations, especially during the early titration phase of therapy. Higher degrees of AV block, however, were infrequently (0.8%) observed in previous verapamil clinical trials. Marked first-degree block or progressive development to second- or third-degree AV block requires a reduction in dosage or, in rare instances, discontinuation of verapamil HCl and institution of appropriate therapy, depending upon the clinical situation.

Patients with hypertrophic cardiomopathy (IHSS): In 120 patients with hypertrophic cardiomyopathy (most of them refractory or intolerant to propranolol) who received therapy with verapamil at doses up to 720 mg/day, a variety of serious adverse effects were seen. Three patients died in pulmonary edema; all had severe left ventricular outflow obstruction and a past history of left ventricular dysfunction. Eight other patients had pulmonary edema and/or severe hypotension; abnormally high (greater than 20 mm Hg) pulmonary wedge pressure and a marked left ventricular outflow obstruction were present in most of these patients. Concomitant administration of quinidine (see *Drug interactions*) preceded the severe hypotension in 3 of the 8 patients (2 of whom developed pulmonary edema). Sinus bradycardia occurred in 11% of the patients, second-degree AV block in 4%, and sinus arrest in 2%. It must be appreciated that this group of patients had a serious disease with a high mortality rate. Most adverse efffects responded well to dose reduction, and only rarely did verapamil use have to be discontinued.

PRECAUTIONS

General

Formulation specific: As with any other non-deformable dosage form caution should be used when administering Covera-HS in patients with preexisting severe gastrointestinal narrowing (pathologic or iatrogenic). In patients with extremely short GI transit time (<7 hrs), pharmacokinetic data are not available and dosage adjustment may be required.

Use in patients with impaired hepatic function: Since verapamil is highly metabolized by the liver, it should be administered cautiously to patients with impaired hepatic function. Severe liver dysfunction prolongs the elimination half-life of immediate-release verapamil to about 14 to 16 hours; hence, approximately 30% of the dose given to patients with normal liver function should be administered to these patients. Careful monitoring for abnormal prolongation of the PR interval or other signs of excessive pharmacologic effects (see *Overdosage*) should be carried out.

Use in patients with attenuated (decreased) neuromuscular transmission: It has been reported that verapamil decreases neuromuscular transmission in patients with Duchenne's muscular dystrophy, and that verapamil prolongs recovery from the neuromuscular blocking agent vecuronium. It may be necessary to decrease the dosage of verapamil when it is administered to patients with attenuated neuromuscular transmission.

Use in patients with impaired renal function: About 70% of an administered dose of verapamil is excreted as metabolites in the urine. Verapamil is not removed by hemodialysis. Until further data are available, verapamil should be admiministered cautiously to patients with impaired renal function. These patients should be carefully monitored for abnormal prolongation of the PR interval or other signs of overdosage (see *Overdosage*).

Information for patients: Covera-HS tablets should be swallowed whole; do not break, crush, or chew. The medication in the Covera-HS tablet is released slowly through an outer shell that does not dissolve. The patient should not be concerned if they occasionally observe this outer shell in their stool as it passes from the body.

Drug interactions

Alcohol: Verapamil may increase blood alcohol concentrations and prolong its effects.

Beta-blockers: Concomitant therapy with beta-adrenergic blockers and verapamil may result in additive negative effects on heart rate, atrioventricular conduction and/or cardiac contractility. The combination of sustained-release verapamil and beta-adrenergic blocking agents has not been studied. However, there have been reports of excessive bradycardia and AV block, including complete heart block, when the combination has been used for the treatment of hypertension. For hypertensive patients, the risks of combined therapy may outweigh the potential benefits. The combination should be used only with caution and close monitoring.

Asymptomatic bradycardia (36 beats/min) with a wandering atrial pacemaker has been observed in a patient receiving concomitant timolol (a beta-adrenergic blocker) eyedrops and oral verapamil.

A decrease in metoprolol and propranolol clearance has been observed when either drug is administered concomitantly with verapamil. A variable effect has been seen when verapamil and atenolol were given together.

Digitalis: Clinical use of verapamil in digitalized patients has shown the combination to be well tolerated if digoxin doses are properly adjusted. However, chronic verapamil treatment can increase serum digoxin levels by 50% to 75% during the first week of therapy, and this can result in digitalis toxicity. In patients with hepatic cirrhosis the influence of verapamil on digoxin kinetics is magnified. Verapamil may reduce total body clearance and extrarenal clearance of digitoxin by 27% and 29%, respectively. Maintenance and digitalization doses should be reduced when verapamil is administered, and the patient should be reassessed to avoid over- to underdigitalization. Whenever overdigitalization is suspected, the daily dose of digitalis should be reduced or temporarily discontinued. On discontinuation of verapamil use, the patient should be reassessed to avoid underdigitalization. In previous clinical trials with other verapamil formulations related to the control of ventricular response in digitalized patients who had atrial fibrillation or atrial flutter, ventricular rates below 50/min at rest occurred in 15% of patients, and asymptomatic hypotension occurred in 5% of patients.

Antihypertensive agents: Verapamil administered concomitantly with oral antihypertensive agents (eg, vasodilators, angiotensin-converting enzyme inhibitors, diuretics, beta-blockers) will usually have an additive effect on lowering blood pressure. Patients receiving these combinations should be appropriately monitored. Concomitant use of agents that attenuate alpha-adrenergic function with verapamil may result in a reduction in blood pressure that is excessive in some patients. Such an effect was observed in one study following the concomitant administration of verapamil and prazosin.

Antiarrhythmic agents:

Disopyramide: Until data on possible interactions between verapamil and disopyramide are obtained, disopyramide should not be administered within 48 hours before or 24 hours after verapamil administration.

Flecainide: A study in healthy volunteers showed that the concomitant administration of flecainide and verapamil may have additive effects on myocardial contractility, AV conduction, and repolarization. Concomitant therapy with flecainide and verapamil may result in additive negative inotropic effect and prolongation of atrioventricular conduction.

Quinidine: In a small number of patients with hypertrophic cardiomyopathy (IHSS), concomitant use of verapamil and quinidine resulted in significant hypotension. Until further data are obtained, combined therapy of verapamil and quinidine in patients with hypertrophic cardiomyopathy should probably be avoided.

The electrophysiologic effects of quinidine and verapamil on AV conduction were studied in 8 patients. Verapamil significantly counteracted the effects of quinidine on AV conduction. There has been a report of increased quinidine levels during verapamil therapy.

Other:

Nitrates: Verapamil has been given concomitantly with short- and long-acting nitrates without any undesirable drug interactions. The pharmacologic profile of both drugs and clinical experience suggest beneficial interactions.

Cimetidine: The interaction between cimetidine and chronically administered verapamil has not been studied. Variable results on clearance have been obtained in acute studies of healthy volunteers; clearance of verapamil was either reduced or unchanged.

Lithium: Increased sensitivity to the effects of lithium (neurotoxicity) has been reported during concomitant verapamil-lithium therapy; lithium levels have been observed sometimes to increase, sometimes to decrease, and sometimes to be unchanged. Patients receiving both drugs must be monitored carefully.

Carbamazepine: Verapamil therapy may increase carbamazepine concentrations during combined therapy. This may produce carbamazepine side effects such as diplopia, headache, ataxia, or dizziness.

Rifampin: Therapy with rifampin may markedly reduce oral verapamil bioavailability.

Phenobarbital: Phenobarbital therapy may increase verapamil clearance.

Cyclosporin: Verapamil therapy may increase serum levels of cyclosporin.

Theophylline: Verapamil may inhibit the clearance and increase the plasma levels of theophylline.

Inhalation anesthetics: Animal experiments have shown that inhalation anesthetics depress cardiovascular activity by decreasing the inward movement of calcium ions. When used concomitantly, inhalation anesthetics and calcium channel blocking agents, such as verapamil, should each be titrated carefully to avoid excessive cardiovascular depression.

Neuromuscular blocking agents: Clinical data and animal studies suggest that verapamil may potentiate the activity of neuromuscular blocking agents (curare-like and depolarizing). It may be necessary to decrease the dose of verapamil and/or the dose of the neuromuscular blocking agent when the drugs are used concomitantly.

Carcinogenesis, mutagenesis, impairment of fertility: An 18-month toxicity study in rats, at a low multiple (6-fold) of the maximum recommended human dose, not the maximum tolerated dose, did not suggest a tumorigenic potential. There was no evidence of a carcinogenic potential of verapamil administered in the diet of rats for two years at doses of 10, 35, and 120 mg/kg/day or approximately 1, 3.5 and 12 times, respectively, the maximum recommended human daily dose (480 mg/day or 9.6 mg/kg/day).

Verapamil was not mutagenic in the Ames test in 5 test strains at 3 mg per plate with or without metabolic activation.

Studies in female rats at daily dietary doses up to 5.5 times (55 mg/kg/day) the maximum recommended human dose did not show impaired fertility. Effects on male fertility have not been determined.

Pregnancy: Pregnancy Category C. Reproduction studies have been performed in rabbits and rats at oral doses up to 1.5 (15 mg/kg/day) and 6 (60 mg/kg/day) times the human oral daily dose, respectively, and have revealed no evidence of teratogenicity. In the rat, however, this multiple of the human dose was embryocidal and retarded fetal growth and development, probably because of adverse maternal effects reflected in reduced weight gains of the dams. This oral dose has also been shown to cause hypotension in rats. There are no adequate and well-controlled studies in pregnant women. Because animal reproduction studies are not always predictive of human response, this drug should be used during pregnancy only if clearly needed. Verapamil crosses the placental barrier and can be detected in umbilical vein blood at delivery.

Labor and delivery: It is not known whether the use of verapamil during labor or delivery has immediate or delayed adverse effects on the fetus, or whether it prolongs the duration of labor or increases the need for forceps delivery or other obstetric intervention. Such adverse experiences have not been reported in the literature, despite a long history of use of verapamil in Europe in the treatment of cardiac side effects of beta-adrenergic agonist agents used to treat premature labor.

Nursing mothers: Verapamil is excreted in human milk. Because of the potential for adverse reactions in nursing infants from verapamil, nursing should be discontinued while verapamil is administered.

Pediatric use: Safety and effectiveness in pediatric patients have not been established.

Elderly use: Dosage adjustment may be required in elderly patients with impaired renal function. Verapamil should be administered cautiously in patients with impaired renal function.

Animal pharmacology and/or animal toxicology: In chronic animal toxicology studies verapamil caused lenticular and/or suture line changes at 30 mg/kg/day or greater, and frank cataracts at 62.5 mg/kg/day or greater in the beagle dog but not in the rat. Development of cataracts due to verapamil has not been reported in man.

ADVERSE REACTIONS

Serious adverse reactions are uncommon when verapamil therapy is initiated with upward dose titration within the recommended single and total daily dose. See *Warnings* for discussion of heart failure, hypotension, elevated liver enzymes, AV block, and rapid ventricular response. Reversible (upon discontinuation of verapamil) non-obstructive, paralytic ileus has been infrequently reported in association with the use of verapamil. The following reactions to orally administered Covera-HS occurred at rates greater than 2.0% or occurred at lower rates but appeared drug-related in clinical trials in hypertension and angina:

	Placebo n=261 %	All doses studied n=572 %
Constipation	2.7	11.7*
Headache	7.3	6.6
Upper respiratory infection	4.6	5.4
Dizziness	2.7	4.7
Fatigue	3.8	4.5
Edema	3.1	3.0
Nausea	1.9	2.1
AV block (1°)	0.0	1.7
Elevated liver enzymes (see *Warnings*)	0.8	1.4
Bradycardia	0.4	1.4
Paresthesia	0.0	1.0
Flushing	0.3	0.8
Hypotension	0.0	0.7
Postural hypotension	0.3	0.4

* Constipation was typically mild, easily manageable, and the incidence usually diminished within about one week. At a typical once-daily dose of 240 mg, the observed incidence was 7.2%.

In previous experience with other formulations of verapamil, the following reactions occurred at rates greater than 1.0% or occurred at lower rates but appeared clearly drug related in clinical trials in 4,954 patients.

Constipation	7.3%
Dizziness	3.3%
Nausea	2.7%
Hypotension	2.5%
Headache	2.2%
Edema	1.9%
CHF/Pulmonary Edema	1.8%
Fatigue	1.7%
Dyspnea	1.4%
Bradycardia (HR<50/min)	1.4%
AV Block (total 1°,2°,3°)	1.2%
AV Block (2° and 3°)	0.8%
Rash	1.2%
Flushing	0.6%
Elevated liver enzymes (see *Warnings*)	

The following reactions, reported with orally administered verapamil in 2% or less of patients, occurred under conditions (open trials, marketing experience) where a causal relationship is uncertain; they are listed to alert the physician to a possible relationship:

Cardiovascular: angina pectoris, AV block (2° & 3°), atrioventricular dissociation, CHF, pulmonary edema, chest pain, claudication, myocardial infarction, palpitations, purpura (vasculitis), syncope.

Digestive system: diarrhea, dry mouth, gastrointestinal distress, gingival hyperplasia.

Hemic and lymphatic: ecchymosis or bruising.

Nervous system: cerebrovascular accident, confusion, equilibrium disorders, insomnia, muscle cramps, psychotic symptoms, shakiness, somnolence.

Skin: arthralgia and rash, exanthema, hair loss, hyperkeratosis, macules, sweating, urticaria, Stevens-Johnson syndrome, erythema multiforme.

Special senses: blurred vision, tinnitus.

Urogenital: gynecomastia, galactorrhea/hyperprolactinemia, increased urination, spotty menstruation, impotence.

Other: allergy aggravated, dyspnea.

Treatment of acute cardiovascular adverse reactions: The frequency of cardiovascular adverse reactions that require therapy is rare; hence, experience with their treatment is limited. Whenever severe hypotension or complete AV block occurs following oral administration of verapamil, the appropriate emergency measures should be applied immediately; eg, intravenously administered norepinephrine bitartrate, atropine sulfate, isoproterenol HCl (all in usual doses), or calcium gluconate (10% solution). In patients with hypertrophic cardiomyopathy (IHSS), alpha-adrenergic agents (phenylephrine HCl, metaraminol bitartrate, or methoxamine HCl) should be used to maintain blood pressure, and isoproterenol and norepinephrine should be avoided. If further support is necessary, dopamine HCl or dobutamine HCl may be administered. Actual treatment and dosage should depend on the severity of the clinical situation and the judgement and experience of the treating physician.

OVERDOSAGE

Treat all verapamil overdoses as serious and maintain observation for at least 48 hours (especially sustained-release verapamil products), preferably under continuous hospital care. Delayed pharmacodynamic consequences may occur with the sustained-release formulations. Verapamil is known to decrease gastrointestinal transit time.

Treatment of overdosage should be supportive. Beta-adrenergic stimulation or parenteral administration of calcium solutions may increase calcium ion flux across the slow channel and have been used effectively in treatment of deliberate overdosage with verapamil. In a few reported cases, overdose with calcium channel blockers has been associated with hypotension and bradycardia, initially refractory to atropine but becoming more responsive to this treatment when the patients received large doses (close to 1 gram/hour for more than 24 hours) of calcium chloride. Verapamil cannot be removed by hemodialysis. Clinically significant hypotensive reactions or high degree AV block should be treated with vasopressor agents or cardiac pacing, respectively. Asystole should be handled by the usual measures including cardiopulmonary resuscitation.

DOSAGE AND ADMINISTRATION

Covera-HS should be administered once daily at bedtime. Clinical trials explored dose ranges between 180 mg and 540 mg given at bedtime and found effects to persist throughout the dosing interval.

Covera-HS tablets should be swallowed whole and not chewed, broken, or crushed.

For both hypertension and angina the dose of Covera-HS should be individualized by titration. Initiate therapy with 180 mg of Covera-HS.

If an adequate response is not obtained with 180 mg of Covera-HS, the dose may be titrated upward in the following manner:

a) 240 mg each evening
b) 360 mg each evening (2 × 180 mg)
c) 480 mg each evening (2 × 240 mg)

When Covera-HS is administered at bedtime, office evaluation of blood pressure during morning and early afternoon hours is essentially a measure of peak effect. The usual evaluation of trough effect, which sometimes might be needed to evaluate the appropriateness of any given dose of Covera-HS, would be just prior to bedtime.

HOW SUPPLIED

Covera-HS 240-mg tablets are pale yellow, round, film coated with COVERA-HS 2021 printed on one side, supplied as:

NDC Number	Size
0025-2021-31	bottle of 100
0025-2021-34	carton of 100 unit dose

Covera-HS 180-mg tablets are lavender, round, film coated, with COVERA-HS 2011 printed on one side, supplied as:

NDC Number	Size
0025-2011-31	bottle of 100
0025-2011-34	carton of 100 unit dose

Store at controlled room temperature 20°–25°C (68°–77°F) [see USP]. Dispense in tight, light-resistant containers.

Caution: Federal law prohibits dispensing without prescription.

5/1/97 • A05351-1

Manufactured for
G.D. Searle & Co.
Chicago IL 60680 USA
By Alza Corporation
Palo Alto CA USA
Address medical inquiries to:
G.D. Searle & Co.
Healthcare Information Services
5200 Old Orchard Road
Skokie IL 60077

Shown in Product Identification Guide, page 335

CYTOTEC® ℞

[sī-tō-tĕc]
(misoprostol)

CONTRAINDICATIONS AND WARNINGS

Cytotec (misoprostol) is contraindicated, because of its abortifacient property, in women who are pregnant. (See *Precautions.*) Patients must be advised of the abortifacient property and warned not to give the drug to others. Anecdotal reports, primarily from Brazil, of congenital anomalies and reports of fetal death subsequent to misuse of misoprostol as an abortifacient have been received. Cytotec should not be used in women of childbearing potential unless the patient requires nonsteroidal anti-inflammatory drug (NSAID) therapy and is at high risk of complications from gastric ulcers associated with use of the NSAID, or is at high risk of developing gastric ulceration. In such patients, Cytotec may be prescribed if the patient

- has had a negative serum pregnancy test within 2 weeks prior to beginning therapy.
- is capable of complying with effective contraceptive measures.
- has received both oral and written warnings of the hazards of misoprostol, the risk of possible contraception failure, and the danger to other women of childbearing potential should the drug be taken by mistake.
- will begin Cytotec only on the second or third day of the next normal menstrual period.

DESCRIPTION

Cytotec oral tablets contain either 100 mcg or 200 mcg of misoprostol, a synthetic prostaglandin E_1 analog.

Misoprostol contains approximately equal amounts of the two diastereomers presented below with their enantiomers indicated by (±):

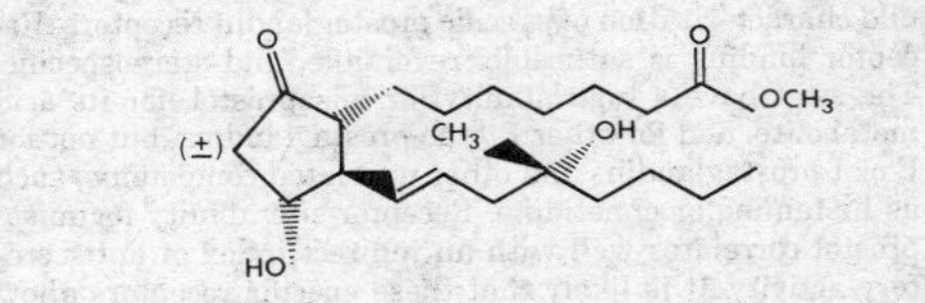

and

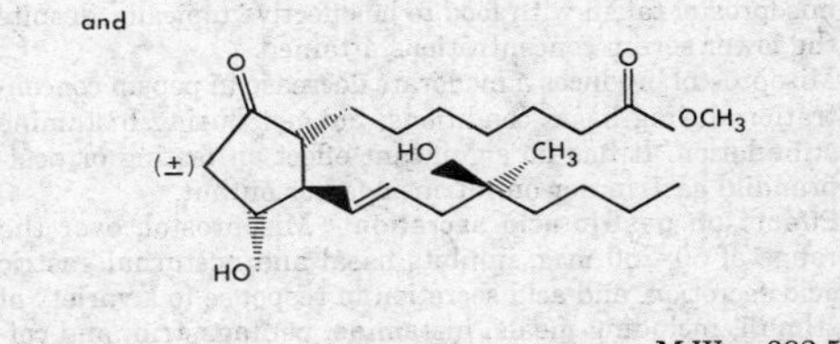

$C_{22}H_{38}O_5$ M.W. = 382.5

(±) methyl 11α, 16-dihydroxy-16-methyl-9-oxoprost-13E-en-1-oate

Misoprostol is a water-soluble, viscous liquid.

Inactive ingredients of tablets are hydrogenated castor oil, hydroxypropyl methylcellulose, microcrystalline cellulose, and sodium starch glycolate.

CLINICAL PHARMACOLOGY

Pharmacokinetics: Misoprostol is extensively absorbed, and undergoes rapid de-esterification to its free acid, which is responsible for its clinical activity and, unlike the parent compound, is detectable in plasma. The alpha side chain undergoes beta oxidation and the beta side chain undergoes omega oxidation followed by reduction of the ketone to give prostaglandin F analogs.

In normal volunteers, Cytotec (misoprostol) is rapidly absorbed after oral administration with a T_{max} of misoprostol acid of 12 ± 3 minutes and a terminal half-life of 20–40 minutes.

There is high variability of plasma levels of misoprostol acid between and within studies but mean values after single doses show a linear relationship with dose over the range of 200–400 mcg. No accumulation of misoprostol acid was noted in multiple dose studies; plasma steady state was achieved within two days.

Maximum plasma concentrations of misoprostol acid are diminished when the dose is taken with food and total avail-

Continued on next page

Cytotec—Cont.

ability of misoprostol acid is reduced by use of concomitant antacid. Clinical trials were conducted with concomitant antacid, however, so this effect does not appear to be clinically important.

Mean ± SD	C_{max}(pg/ml)	AUC (0-4) (pg·hr/ml)	T_{max}(min)
Fasting	811 ± 317	417 ± 135	14 ± 8
With Antacid	689 ± 315	349 ± 108*	20 ± 14
With High Fat Breakfast	303 ± 176*	373 ± 111	64 ± 79*

* Comparisons with fasting results statistically significant, $p<0.05$.

After oral administration of radiolabeled misoprostol, about 80% of detected radioactivity appears in urine. Pharmacokinetic studies in patients with varying degrees of renal impairment showed an approximate doubling of $T_{1/2}$, C_{max}, and AUC compared to normals, but no clear correlation between the degree of impairment and AUC. In subjects over 64 years of age, the AUC for misoprostol acid is increased. No routine dosage adjustment is recommended in older patients or patients with renal impairment, but dosage may need to be reduced if the usual dose is not tolerated.

Cytotec does not affect the hepatic mixed function oxidase (cytochrome P-450) enzyme systems in animals.

Drug interaction studies between misoprostol and several nonsteroidal anti-inflammatory drugs showed no effect on the kinetics of ibuprofen or diclofenac, and a 20% decrease in aspirin AUC, not thought to be clinically significant.

Pharmacokinetic studies also showed a lack of drug interaction with antipyrine and propranolol when these drugs were given with misoprostol. Misoprostol given for 1 week had no effect on the steady state pharmacokinetics of diazepam when the two drugs were administered 2 hours apart. The serum protein binding of misoprostol acid is less than 90% and is concentration-independent in the therapeutic range.

Pharmacodynamics: Misoprostol has both antisecretory (inhibiting gastric acid secretion) and (in animals) mucosal protective properties. NSAIDs inhibit prostaglandin synthesis, and a deficiency of prostaglandins within the gastric mucosa may lead to diminishing bicarbonate and mucus secretion and may contribute to the mucosal damage caused by these agents. Misoprostol can increase bicarbonate and mucus production, but in man this has been shown at doses 200 mcg and above that are also antisecretory. It is therefore not possible to tell whether the ability of misoprostol to prevent gastric ulcer is the result of its antisecretory effect, its mucosal protective effect, or both.

In vitro studies on canine parietal cells using tritiated misoprostol acid as the ligand have led to the identification and characterization of specific prostaglandin receptors. Receptor binding is saturable, reversible, and stereospecific. The sites have a high affinity for misoprostol, for its acid metabolite, and for other E type prostaglandins, but not for F or I prostaglandins and other unrelated compounds, such as histamine or cimetidine. Receptor-site affinity for misoprostol correlates well with an indirect index of antisecretory activity. It is likely that these specific receptors allow misoprostol taken with food to be effective topically, despite the lower serum concentrations attained.

Misoprostol produces a moderate decrease in pepsin concentration during basal conditions, but not during histamine stimulation. It has no significant effect on fasting or postprandial gastrin nor on intrinsic factor output.

Effects on gastric acid secretion: Misoprostol, over the range of 50–200 mcg, inhibits basal and nocturnal gastric acid secretion, and acid secretion in response to a variety of stimuli, including meals, histamine, pentagastrin, and coffee. Activity is apparent 30 minutes after oral administration and persists for at least 3 hours. In general, the effects of 50 mcg were modest and shorter lived, and only the 200-mcg dose had substantial effects on nocturnal secretion or on histamine and meal-stimulated secretion.

Uterine effects: Cytotec has been shown to produce uterine contractions that may endanger pregnancy. (See *Contraindications* and *Warnings*.) In studies in women undergoing elective termination of pregnancy during the first trimester, Cytotec caused partial or complete expulsion of the uterine contents in 11% of the subjects and increased uterine bleeding in 41%.

Other pharmacologic effects: Cytotec does not produce clinically significant effects on serum levels of prolactin, gonadotropins, thyroid-stimulating hormone, growth hormone, thyroxine, cortisol, gastrointestinal hormones (somatostatin, gastrin, vasoactive intestinal polypeptide, and motilin), creatinine, or uric acid. Gastric emptying, immunologic competence, platelet aggregation, pulmonary function, or the cardiovascular system are not modified by recommended doses of Cytotec.

Clinical studies: In a series of small short-term (about 1 week) placebo-controlled studies in healthy human volunteers, doses of misoprostol were evaluated for their ability to prevent NSAID-induced mucosal injury. Studies of 200 mcg q.i.d. of misoprostol with tolmetin and naproxen, and of 100 and 200 mcg q.i.d. with ibuprofen, all showed reduction of the rate of significant endoscopic injury from about 70–75% on placebo to 10–30% on misoprostol. Doses of 25–200 mcg q.i.d. reduced aspirin-induced mucosal injury and bleeding.

Prevention of Gastric Ulcers Induced by Ibuprofen, Piroxicam, or Naproxen
[No. of patients with ulcer(s) (%)]

Therapy	Therapy Duration 4 weeks	8 weeks	12 weeks	
Study No. 1				
Cytotec 200 mcg q.i.d. (n=74)	1 (1.4)	0	0	1 (1.4)*
Cytotec 100 mcg q.i.d. (n=77)	3 (3.9)	1 (1.3)	1 (1.3)	5 (6.5)*
Placebo (n=76)	11 (14.5)	4 (5.3)	4 (5.3)	19 (25.0)
Study No. 2				
Cytotec 200 mcg q.i.d. (n=65)	1 (1.5)	1 (1.5)	0	2 (3.1)*
Cytotec 100 mcg q.i.d. (n=66)	2 (3.0)	2 (3.0)	1 (1.5)	5 (7.6)
Placebo (n=62)	6 (9.7)	2 (3.2)	3 (4.8)	11 (17.7)
*Studies No. 1 & No. 2***				
Cytotec 200 mcg q.i.d. (n=139)	2 (1.4)	1 (0.7)	0	3 (2.2)*
Cytotec 100 mcg q.i.d. (n=143)	5 (3.5)	3 (2.1)	2 (1.4)	10 (7.0)*
Placebo (n=138)	17 (12.3)	6 (4.3)	7 (5.1)	30 (21.7)

* Statistically significantly different from placebo at the 5% level.
** Combined data from Study No. 1 and Study No. 2.

Preventing gastric ulcers caused by nonsteroidal anti-inflammatory drugs (NSAIDs): Two 12-week, randomized, double-blind trials in osteoarthritic patients who had gastrointestinal symptoms but no ulcer on endoscopy while taking an NSAID compared the ability of 200 mcg of Cytotec, 100 mcg of Cytotec, and placebo to prevent gastric ulcer (GU) formation. Patients were approximately equally divided between ibuprofen, piroxicam, and naproxen, and continued this treatment throughout the 12 weeks. The 200-mcg dose caused a marked, statistically significant reduction in gastric ulcers in both studies. The lower dose was somewhat less effective, with a significant result in only one of the studies.

[See table above]

In these trials there were no significant differences between Cytotec and placebo in relief of day or night abdominal pain. No effect of Cytotec in preventing duodenal ulcers was demonstrated, but relatively few duodenal lesions were seen.

In another clinical trial, 239 patients receiving aspirin 650–1300 mg q.i.d. for rheumatoid arthritis who had endoscopic evidence of duodenal and/or gastric inflammation were randomized to misoprostol 200 mcg q.i.d. or placebo for eight weeks while continuing to receive aspirin. The study evaluated the possible interference of Cytotec on the efficacy of aspirin in these patients with rheumatoid arthritis by analyzing joint tenderness, joint swelling, physician's clinical assessment, patient's assessment, change in ARA classification, change in handgrip strength, change in duration of morning stiffness, patient's assessment of pain at rest, movement, interference with daily activity, and ESR. Cytotec did not interfere with the efficacy of aspirin in these patients with rheumatoid arthritis.

INDICATIONS AND USAGE

Cytotec (misoprostol) is indicated for the prevention of NSAID (nonsteroidal anti-inflammatory drugs, including aspirin)-induced gastric ulcers in patients at high risk of complications from gastric ulcer, eg, the elderly and patients with concomitant debilitating disease, as well as patients at high risk of developing gastric ulceration, such as patients with a history of ulcer. Cytotec has not been shown to prevent duodenal ulcers in patients taking NSAIDs. Cytotec should be taken for the duration of NSAID therapy. Cytotec has been shown to prevent gastric ulcers in controlled studies of three months' duration. It had no effect, compared to placebo, on gastrointestinal pain or discomfort associated with NSAID use.

CONTRAINDICATIONS

See boxed *CONTRAINDICATIONS AND WARNINGS.*

Cytotec should not be taken by anyone with a history of allergy to prostaglandins.

WARNINGS

See boxed *CONTRAINDICATIONS AND WARNINGS.*

PRECAUTIONS

Information for patients: Cytotec is contraindicated in women who are pregnant, and should not be used in women of childbearing potential unless the patient requires nonsteroidal anti-inflammatory drug (NSAID) therapy and is at high risk of complications from gastric ulcers associated with the use of the NSAID, or is at high risk of developing gastric ulceration. Women of childbearing potential should be told that they must not be pregnant when Cytotec therapy is initiated, and that they must use an effective contraception method while taking Cytotec.

See boxed *CONTRAINDICATIONS AND WARNINGS.*

Patients should be advised of the following:

Cytotec is intended for administration along with nonsteroidal anti-inflammatory drugs (NSAIDs), including aspirin, to decrease the chance of developing an NSAID-induced gastric ulcer.

Cytotec should be taken only according to the directions given by a physician.

If the patient has questions about or problems with Cytotec, the physician should be contacted promptly.

THE PATIENT SHOULD NOT GIVE CYTOTEC TO ANYONE ELSE. Cytotec has been prescribed for the patient's specific condition, may not be the correct treatment for another person, and may be dangerous to the other person if she were to become pregnant.

The Cytotec package the patient receives from the pharmacist will include a leaflet containing patient information. The patient should read the leaflet before taking Cytotec and each time the prescription is renewed because the leaflet may have been revised.

Keep Cytotec out of the reach of children.

SPECIAL NOTE FOR WOMEN: Cytotec must not be used by pregnant women. Cytotec may cause miscarriage. Miscarriages caused by Cytotec may be incomplete, which could lead to potentially dangerous bleeding, hospitalization, surgery, infertility, or maternal or fetal death.

Cytotec is available only as a unit-of-use package that includes a leaflet containing patient information. See *Patient Information* at the end of this labeling.

Drug interactions: See *Clinical Pharmacology.* Cytotec has not been shown to interfere with the beneficial effects of aspirin on signs and symptoms of rheumatoid arthritis. Cytotec does not exert clinically significant effects on the absorption, blood levels, and antiplatelet effects of therapeutic doses of aspirin. Cytotec has no clinically significant effect on the kinetics of diclofenac or ibuprofen.

Animal toxicology: A reversible increase in the number of normal surface gastric epithelial cells occurred in the dog, rat, and mouse. No such increase has been observed in humans administered Cytotec for up to 1 year.

An apparent response of the female mouse to Cytotec in long-term studies at 100 to 1000 times the human dose was hyperostosis, mainly of the medulla of sternebrae. Hyperostosis did not occur in long-term studies in the dog and rat and has not been seen in humans treated with Cytotec.

Carcinogenesis, mutagenesis, impairment of fertility: There was no evidence of an effect of Cytotec on tumor occurrence or incidence in rats receiving daily doses up to 150 times the human dose for 24 months. Similarly, there was no effect of Cytotec on tumor occurrence or incidence in mice receiving daily doses up to 1000 times the human dose for 21 months. The mutagenic potential of Cytotec was tested in several *in vitro* assays, all of which were negative.

Misoprostol, when administered to breeding male and female rats at doses 6.25 times to 625 times the maximum recommended human therapeutic dose, produced dose-related pre- and post-implantation losses and a significant decrease in the number of live pups born at the highest dose. These findings suggest the possibility of a general adverse effect on fertility in males and females.

Pregnancy: Pregnancy Category X. See boxed *CONTRAINDICATIONS AND WARNINGS.*

Nonteratogenic effects: Cytotec may endanger pregnancy (may cause miscarriage) and thereby cause harm to the fetus when administered to a pregnant woman. Cytotec produces uterine contractions, uterine bleeding, and expulsion of the products of conception. Miscarriages caused by Cytotec may be incomplete. In studies in women undergoing elective termination of pregnancy during the first trimester, Cytotec caused partial or complete expulsion of the products of conception in 11% of the subjects and increased uterine bleeding in 41%. Anecdotal reports, primarily from Brazil, of congenital anomalies and reports of fetal death subsequent to misuse of misoprostol as an abortifacient have been received (see *Contraindications and Warnings*). If a woman is or becomes pregnant while taking this drug, the drug should be discontinued and the patient apprised of the potential hazard to the fetus.

Teratogenic effects: Cytotec is not fetotoxic or teratogenic in rats and rabbits at doses 625 and 63 times the human dose, respectively.

Nursing mothers: See *Contraindications.* It is unlikely that Cytotec is excreted in human milk since it is rapidly metabolized throughout the body. However, it is not known if the active metabolite (misoprostol acid) is excreted in human milk. Therefore, Cytotec should not be administered to nursing mothers because the potential excretion of misoprostol acid could cause significant diarrhea in nursing infants.

Pediatric use: Safety and effectiveness of Cytotec in pediatric patients have not been established.

ADVERSE REACTIONS

The following have been reported as adverse events in subjects receiving Cytotec:

Gastrointestinal: In subjects receiving Cytotec 400 or 800 mcg daily in clinical trials, the most frequent gastrointestinal adverse events were diarrhea and abdominal pain. The incidence of diarrhea at 800 mcg in controlled trials in patients on NSAIDs ranged from 14–40% and in all studies (over 5,000 patients) averaged 13%. Abdominal pain occurred in 13–20% of patients in NSAID trials and about 7% in all studies, but there was no consistent difference from placebo.

Diarrhea was dose related and usually developed early in the course of therapy (after 13 days), usually was self-limiting (often resolving after 8 days), but sometimes required discontinuation of Cytotec (2% of the patients). Rare instances of profound diarrhea leading to severe dehydration have been reported. Patients with an underlying condition such as inflammatory bowel disease, or those in whom dehydration, were it to occur, would be dangerous, should be monitored carefully if Cytotec is prescribed. The incidence of diarrhea can be minimized by administering after meals and at bedtime, and by avoiding coadministration of Cytotec with magnesium-containing antacids.

Gynecological: Women who received Cytotec during clinical trials reported the following gynecological disorders: spotting (0.7%), cramps (0.6%), hypermenorrhea (0.5%), menstrual disorder (0.3%) and dysmenorrhea (0.1%). Postmenopausal vaginal bleeding may be related to Cytotec administration. If it occurs, diagnostic workup should be undertaken to rule out gynecological pathology.

Elderly: There were no significant differences in the safety profile of Cytotec in approximately 500 ulcer patients who were 65 years of age or older compared with younger patients.

Additional adverse events which were reported are categorized as follows:

Incidence greater than 1%: In clinical trials, the following adverse reactions were reported by more than 1% of the subjects receiving Cytotec and may be causally related to the drug: nausea (3.2%), flatulence (2.9%), headache (2.4%), dyspepsia (2.0%), vomiting (1.3%), and constipation (1.1%). However, there were no significant differences between the incidences of these events for Cytotec and placebo.

Causal relationship unknown: The following adverse events were infrequently reported. Causal relationships between Cytotec and these events have not been established but cannot be excluded:

Body as a whole: aches/pains, asthenia, fatigue, fever, rigors, weight changes.

Skin: rash, dermatitis, alopecia, pallor, breast pain.

Special senses: abnormal taste, abnormal vision, conjunctivitis, deafness, tinnitus, earache.

Respiratory: upper respiratory tract infection, bronchitis, bronchospasm, dyspnea, pneumonia, epistaxis.

Cardiovascular: chest pain, edema, diaphoresis, hypotension, hypertension, arrhythmia, phlebitis, increased cardiac enzymes, syncope.

Gastrointestinal: GI bleeding, GI inflammation/infection, rectal disorder, abnormal hepatobiliary function, gingivitis, reflux, dysphagia, amylase increase.

Hypersensitivity: Anaphylaxis.

Metabolic: glycosuria, gout, increased nitrogen, increased alkaline phosphatase.

Genitourinary: polyuria, dysuria, hematuria, urinary tract infection.

Nervous system/Psychiatric: anxiety, change in appetite, depression, drowsiness, dizziness, thirst, impotence, loss of libido, sweating increase, neuropathy, neurosis, confusion.

Musculoskeletal: arthralgia, myalgia, muscle cramps, stiffness, back pain.

Blood/Coagulation: anemia, abnormal differential, thrombocytopenia, purpura, ESR increased.

OVERDOSAGE

The toxic dose of Cytotec in humans has not been determined. Cumulative total daily doses of 1600 mcg have been tolerated, with only symptoms of gastrointestinal discomfort being reported. In animals, the acute toxic effects are diarrhea, gastrointestinal lesions, focal cardiac necrosis, hepatic necrosis, renal tubular necrosis, testicular atrophy, respiratory difficulties, and depression of the central nervous system. Clinical signs that may indicate an overdose are sedation, tremor, convulsions, dyspnea, abdominal pain, diarrhea, fever, palpitations, hypotension, or bradycardia. Symptoms should be treated with supportive therapy.

It is not known if misoprostol acid is dialyzable. However, because misoprostol is metabolized like a fatty acid, it is unlikely that dialysis would be appropriate treatment for overdosage.

DOSAGE AND ADMINISTRATION

The recommended adult oral dose of Cytotec for the prevention of NSAID-induced gastric ulcers is 200 mcg four times daily with food. If this dose cannot be tolerated, a dose of 100 mcg can be used. (See *Clinical Pharmacology: Clinical studies.*) Cytotec should be taken for the duration of NSAID therapy as prescribed by the physician. Cytotec should be taken with a meal, and the last dose of the day should be at bedtime.

Renal impairment: Adjustment of the dosing schedule in renally impaired patients is not routinely needed, but dosage can be reduced if the 200-mcg dose is not tolerated. (See *Clinical Pharmacology.*)

HOW SUPPLIED

Cytotec 100-mcg tablets are white, round, with SEARLE debossed on one side and 1451 on the other side; supplied as:

NDC Number	Size
0025-1451-60	unit-of-use bottle of 60
0025-1451-20	unit-of-use bottle of 120
0025-1451-34	carton of 100 unit dose

Cytotec 200-mcg tablets are white, hexagonal, with SEARLE debossed above and 1461 debossed below the line on one side and a double stomach debossed on the other side; supplied as:

NDC Number	Size
0025-1461-60	unit-of-use bottle of 60
0025-1461-31	unit-of-use bottle of 100
0025-1461-34	carton of 100 unit dose

Store at or below 25°C (77°F) in a dry area.

Rx only

PATIENT INFORMATION

Read this leaflet before taking Cytotec® (misoprostol) and each time your prescription is renewed, because the leaflet may be changed.

Cytotec (misoprostol) is being prescribed by your doctor to decrease the chance of getting stomach ulcers related to the arthritis/pain medication that you take.

Cytotec can cause miscarriage, often associated with potentially dangerous bleeding. This may result in hospitalization, surgery, infertility, or death. **Do not take it if you are pregnant and do not become pregnant while taking this medicine.**

If you become pregnant during Cytotec therapy, stop taking Cytotec and contact your physician immediately. Remember that even if you are on a means of birth control it is still possible to become pregnant. Should this occur, stop taking Cytotec and contact your physician immediately.

Cytotec may cause diarrhea, abdominal cramping, and/or nausea in some people. In most cases these problems develop during the first few weeks of therapy and stop after about a week. You can minimize possible diarrhea by making sure you take Cytotec with food.

Because these side effects are usually mild to moderate and usually go away in a matter of days, most patients can continue to take Cytotec. If you have prolonged difficulty (more than 8 days), or if you have severe diarrhea, cramping and/or nausea, call your doctor.

Take Cytotec only according to the directions given by your physician.

Do not give Cytotec to anyone else. It has been prescribed for your specific condition, may not be the correct treatment for another person, and would be dangerous if the other person were pregnant.

This information sheet does not cover all possible side effects of Cytotec. This patient information leaflet does not address the side effects of your arthritis/pain medication. See your doctor if you have questions.

Keep out of reach of children.

11/4/98 • A05450-2

Shown in Product Identification Guide, page 335

DAYPRO® ℞

[dā-prō]

(oxaprozin)

DESCRIPTION

Daypro (oxaprozin) is a nonsteroidal anti-inflammatory drug (NSAID), chemically designated as 4,5-diphenyl-2-oxazole-propionic acid, and has the following chemical structure:

The empirical formula for oxaprozin is $C_{18}H_{15}NO_3$, and the molecular weight is 293. Oxaprozin is a white to off-white powder with a slight odor and a melting point of 162°C to 163°C. It is slightly soluble in alcohol and insoluble in water, with an octanol/water partition coefficient of 4.8 at physiologic pH (7.4). The pK_a in water is 4.3.

Daypro oral caplets contain 600 mg of oxaprozin.

Inactive ingredients in Daypro oral caplets are microcrystalline cellulose, hydroxypropyl methylcellulose, methylcellulose, magnesium stearate, polacrilin potassium, starch, polyethylene glycol, and titanium dioxide.

CLINICAL PHARMACOLOGY

Oxaprozin is a nonsteroidal anti-inflammatory drug (NSAID) that has been shown to have anti-inflammatory, analgesic, and antipyretic properties in animal models. As with other nonsteroidal anti-inflammatory agents, all of the modes of action of oxaprozin are not fully established. Oxaprozin is an inhibitor of several steps along the arachidonic acid pathway of prostaglandin synthesis, and one of its modes of action is presumed to be due to the inhibition of prostaglandin synthesis at the site of inflammation.

Pharmacodynamics: Acute analgesic effects are demonstrable in humans after a single 1200-mg dose of oxaprozin, but anti-inflammatory effects are not reliably achieved after a single dose. Because of the long half-life of oxaprozin, it takes several days of dosing to reach steady state (see *Pharmacokinetics*).

Pharmacokinetics: The pharmacokinetics of oxaprozin have been evaluated in approximately 400 individuals, which have included patients with rheumatoid arthritis, osteoarthritis, healthy elderly volunteers, and patients with cardiac, renal, and hepatic disease.

Oxaprozin demonstrates high oral bioavailability (95%), with peak plasma concentrations occurring between 3 and 5 hours after dosing. Food may reduce the rate of absorption of oxaprozin, but the extent of absorption is unchanged. Antacids have no effect on the rate or extent of oxaprozin absorption.

As is true for most NSAIDs, approximately 99.9% of the oxaprozin present in plasma is bound to albumin. The fraction of the drug present in the tissues across the therapeutic dosage range ranges between 40% and 60% of the total drug in the body and is proportional to dose, since the tissue sites are not saturated with the usual clinical doses.

Figure 1 shows the amount of oxaprozin in the plasma and in the tissue as a function of dose and the concentration of the free drug.

Figure 1.
Amount of oxaprozin in plasma and tissue as a function of dose and free (unbound) oxaprozin concentration.

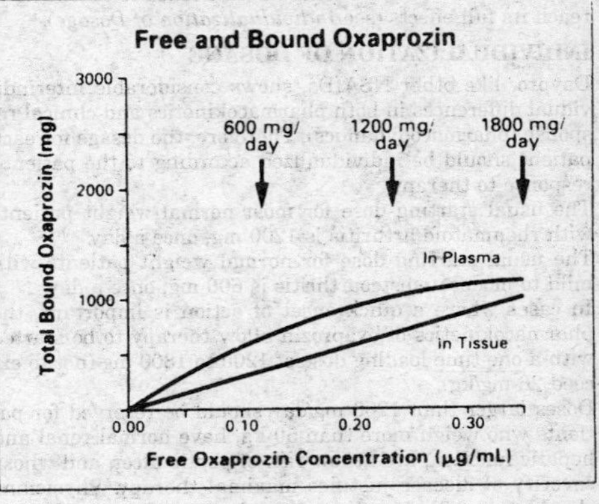

Unbound oxaprozin is the pharmacologically active component; it is able to distribute into tissues and to be cleared from the body. The average unbound concentration is a function of the tissue-bound and plasma-bound drug, and it increases proportionally with dose.

As the amount of oxaprozin in the tissues increases at higher dose, the plasma concentration of oxaprozin is limited by saturation of plasma protein binding. In addition, the increase in free (unbound) oxaprozin results in an increase in clearance. Both of these contribute to the total plasma concentration of oxaprozin increasing less than proportionately with dose.

Oxaprozin kinetics were modeled using a two-compartment model with first-order absorption and protein binding that becomes saturable in the clinical dosage range. As the dose is increased from 600 to 1200 mg daily, the steady state clearance of total oxaprozin increases from 0.25 to 0.34 L/hr, the steady state apparent volume of distribution increases from 10 to 12.5 L, and the accumulation half-life decreases from 25 to 21 hours. The terminal elimination half-life is approximately twice as long as the accumulation half-life because of the increased binding and decreased clearance at lower concentrations. Steady state concentrations in clinical usage are achieved in 4 to 7 days.

Plasma levels of total oxaprozin (free and bound drug) in studies of patients taking 600 to 1200 mg/day for several months ranged from 98 to 230 µg/mL, corresponding to estimated levels of free drug ranging from about 0.10 to 0.40 µg/mL.

Oxaprozin is primarily metabolized in the liver, by both microsomal oxidation (65%) and glucuronic acid conjugation (35%). A small amount (<5%) of active phenolic metabolites is produced, but the contribution to overall activity is minimal. All conjugated metabolites are inactive.

Biliary excretion of unchanged oxaprozin is a minor elimination pathway, and enterohepatic recycling of oxaprozin is insignificant. The glucuronide metabolites can be recovered from the urine (65%) and feces (35%), while unchanged oxaprozin is poorly excreted.

Renal dysfunction appears to alter oxaprozin binding and to reduce unbound clearance and unbound volume of distribution; dosage reductions should be made (see *Precautions: General*).

Age, gender, and well-compensated cardiac failure do not affect the plasma protein binding or the pharmacokinetics of oxaprozin.

Like other NSAIDs exhibiting a high degree of protein binding and a primarily metabolic route of elimination, oxaprozin has the potential for drug-drug interactions (see *Precautions: Drug interactions*).

Continued on next page

Daypro—Cont.

CLINICAL STUDIES

Rheumatoid arthritis: Daypro was evaluated for managing the signs and symptoms of rheumatoid arthritis in placebo and active controlled clinical trials in a total of 646 patients. Daypro was given in single or divided daily doses of 600 to 1800 mg/day and was found to be comparable to 2600 to 3900 mg/day of aspirin. At these doses there was a trend (over all trials) for oxaprozin to be more effective and cause fewer gastrointestinal side effects than aspirin.

Daypro was given as a once-a-day dose of 1200 mg in most of the clinical trials, but larger doses (up to 26 mg/kg or 1800 mg/day) were used in selected patients. In some patients, Daypro may be better tolerated in divided doses. Due to its long half-life, several days of Daypro therapy were needed for the drug to reach its full effect (see *Individualization of Dosage*).

Osteoarthritis: Daypro was evaluated for the management of the signs and symptoms of osteoarthritis in a total of 616 patients in active controlled clinical trials against aspirin (N=464), piroxicam (N=102), and other NSAIDs. Daypro was given both in variable (600 to 1200 mg/day) and in fixed (1200 mg/day) dosing schedules in either single or divided doses. In these trials, oxaprozin was found to be comparable to 2600 to 3200 mg/day doses of aspirin or 20 mg/day doses of piroxicam. Oxaprozin was effective both in once-daily and in divided dosing schedules. In controlled clinical trials several days of oxaprozin therapy were needed for the drug to reach its full effects (see *Individualization of Dosage*).

INDIVIDUALIZATION OF DOSAGE

Daypro, like other NSAIDs, shows considerable interindividual differences in both pharmacokinetics and clinical response (pharmacodynamics). Therefore, the dosage for each patient should be individualized according to the patient's response to therapy.

The usual starting dose for most normal weight patients with rheumatoid arthritis is 1200 mg, once a day.

The usual starting dose for normal weight patients with mild to moderate osteoarthritis is 600 mg, once a day.

In cases where a quick onset of action is important, the pharmacokinetics of oxaprozin allow therapy to be started with a one-time loading dose of 1200 to 1800 mg (not to exceed 26 mg/kg).

Doses larger than 1200 mg/day should be reserved for patients who weigh more than 50 kg, have normal renal and hepatic function, are at low risk of peptic ulcer, and whose severity of disease justifies maximal therapy. Physicians should ensure that patients are tolerating doses in the 600 to 1200 mg/day range without gastroenterologic, renal, hepatic, or dermatologic adverse effects before advancing to the larger doses.

The maximum recommended total daily dosage is 1800 mg in divided doses.

Most patients will tolerate once-a-day dosing with Daypro, although divided doses may be tried in patients unable to tolerate single doses. As with all drugs of this class, the frequency and severity of adverse events will depend on the dose of the drug, the age and physical condition of the patient, any concurrent medical diagnoses, individual vulnerability, and the duration of therapy. In clinical trials of oxaprozin, no clear dose-response relationship was seen for serious adverse effects, but physicians are cautioned that the reported safety data were developed in patients who had successfully taken lower doses of Daypro before being advanced above 1200 mg/day.

Experience with other NSAIDs has shown that starting therapy with maximal doses in patients at increased risk due to renal or hepatic disease, low body weight, advanced age, a known ulcer diathesis, or known sensitivity to NSAID effects is likely to increase the frequency of adverse events and is not recommended (see *Precautions*).

INDICATIONS AND USAGE

Daypro is indicated for acute and long-term use in the management of the signs and symptoms of osteoarthritis and rheumatoid arthritis.

CONTRAINDICATIONS

Daypro should not be used in patients with previously demonstrated hypersensitivity to oxaprozin or any of its components or in individuals with the complete or partial syndrome of nasal polyps, angioedema, and bronchospastic reactivity to aspirin or other nonsteroidal anti-inflammatory drugs (NSAIDs).

Severe and occasionally fatal asthmatic and anaphylactic reactions have been reported in patients receiving NSAIDs, and there have been rare reports of anaphylaxis in patients taking oxaprozin.

WARNINGS

RISK OF GASTROINTESTINAL (GI) ULCERATION, BLEEDING, AND PERFORATION WITH NONSTEROIDAL ANTI-INFLAMMATORY DRUG THERAPY: Serious gastrointestinal toxicity, such as bleeding, ulceration, and perforation, can occur at any time, with or without warning symptoms, in patients treated with NSAIDs. Although minor upper gastrointestinal problems, such as dyspepsia, are common, and usually develop early in therapy, physicians should remain alert for ulceration and bleeding in patients treated chronically with NSAIDs, even in the absence of previous GI tract symptoms. In patients observed in clinical trials for several months to 2 years, symptomatic upper GI ulcers, gross bleeding, or perforation appear to occur in approximately 1% of patients treated for 3 to 6 months, and in about 2% to 4% of patients treated for 1 year. Physicians should inform patients about the signs and/or symptoms of serious GI toxicity and what steps to take if they occur.

Patients at risk for developing peptic ulceration and bleeding are those with a prior history of serious GI events, alcoholism, smoking, or other factors known to be associated with peptic ulcer disease. Elderly or debilitated patients seem to tolerate ulceration or bleeding less well than other individuals, and most spontaneous reports of fatal GI events are in these populations. Studies to date are inconclusive concerning the relative risk of various nonsteroidal anti-inflammatory drugs (NSAIDs) in causing such reactions. High doses of any NSAID probably carry a greater risk of these reactions, and substantial benefit should be anticipated to patients prior to prescribing maximal doses of Daypro.

PRECAUTIONS

General

Hepatic effects: As with other nonsteroidal anti-inflammatory drugs, borderline elevations of one or more liver tests may occur in up to 15% of patients. These abnormalities may progress, remain essentially unchanged, or resolve with continued therapy. The SGPT (ALT) test is probably the most sensitive indicator of liver dysfunction. Meaningful (3 times the upper limit of normal) elevations of SGOT (AST) occurred in controlled clinical trials of Daypro in just under 1% of patients. A patient with symptoms and/or signs suggesting liver dysfunction or in whom an abnormal liver test has occurred should be evaluated for evidence of the development of more severe hepatic reaction while on therapy with this drug. Severe hepatic reactions including jaundice have been reported with Daypro, and there may be a risk of fatal hepatitis with oxaprozin, such as has been seen with other NSAIDs. Although such reactions are rare, if abnormal liver tests persist or worsen, clinical signs and symptoms consistent with liver disease develop, or systemic manifestations occur (eosinophilia, rash, fever), Daypro should be discontinued.

Well-compensated hepatic cirrhosis does not appear to alter the disposition of unbound oxaprozin, so dosage adjustment is not necessary. However, the primary route of elimination of oxaprozin is hepatic metabolism, so caution should be observed in patients with severe hepatic dysfunction.

Renal effects: Acute interstitial nephritis, hematuria, and proteinuria have been reported with Daypro as with other NSAIDs. Long-term administration of some nonsteroidal anti-inflammatory drugs to animals has resulted in renal papillary necrosis and other abnormal renal pathology. This was not observed with oxaprozin, but the clinical significance of this difference is unknown.

A second form of renal toxicity has been seen in patients with preexisting conditions leading to a reduction in renal blood flow, where the renal prostaglandins have a supportive role in the maintenance of renal perfusion. In these patients administration of a nonsteroidal anti-inflammatory drug may cause a dose-dependent reduction in prostaglandin formation and may precipitate overt renal decompensation. Patients at greatest risk of this reaction are those with previously impaired renal function, heart failure, or liver dysfunction, those taking diuretics, and the elderly. Discontinuation of nonsteroidal anti-inflammatory drug therapy is often followed by recovery to the pretreatment state. Those patients at high risk who chronically take oxaprozin should have renal function monitored if they have signs or symptoms that may be consistent with mild azotemia, such as malaise, fatigue, or loss of appetite. As with all NSAID therapy, patients may occasionally develop some elevation of serum creatinine and BUN levels without any signs or symptoms.

The pharmacokinetics of oxaprozin may be significantly altered in patients with renal insufficiency or in patients who are undergoing hemodialysis. Such patients should be started on doses of 600 mg/day, with cautious dosage increases if the desired effect is not obtained. Oxaprozin is not dialyzed because of its high degree of protein binding.

Like other NSAIDs, Daypro may worsen fluid retention by the kidneys in patients with uncompensated cardiac failure due to its effect on prostaglandins. It should be used with caution in patients with a history of hypertension, cardiac decompensation, in patients on chronic diuretic therapy, or in those with other conditions predisposing to fluid retention.

Photosensitivity: Oxaprozin has been associated with rash and/or mild photosensitivity in dermatologic testing. An increased incidence of rash on sun-exposed skin was seen in some patients in the clinical trials.

Recommended laboratory testing: Because serious GI tract ulceration and bleeding can occur without warning symptoms, physicians should follow chronically treated patients for the signs and symptoms of ulceration and bleeding and should inform them of the importance of this follow-up (see *Warnings*).

Anemia may occur in patients receiving oxaprozin or other NSAIDs. This may be due to fluid retention, gastrointestinal blood loss, or an incompletely described effect upon erythrogenesis. Patients on long-term treatment with Daypro should have their hemoglobin or hematocrit values determined at appropriate intervals as determined by the clinical situation.

Oxaprozin, like other NSAIDs, can affect platelet aggregation and prolong bleeding time. Daypro should be used with caution in patients with underlying hemostatic defects or in those who are undergoing surgical procedures where a high degree of hemostasis is needed.

Information for patients: Daypro, like other drugs of its class, nonsteroidal anti-inflammatory drugs (NSAIDs), is not free of side effects. The side effects of these drugs can cause discomfort and, rarely, serious side effects, such as gastrointestinal bleeding, which may result in hospitalization and even fatal outcomes.

NSAIDs are often essential agents in the management of arthritis, but they may also be commonly employed for conditions that are less serious.

Physicians may wish to discuss with their patients the potential risks (see *Warnings, Precautions,* and *Adverse Reactions*) and likely benefits of Daypro treatment, particularly in less-serious conditions where treatment without Daypro may represent an acceptable alternative to both the patient and the physician.

Patients receiving Daypro may benefit from physician instruction in the symptoms of the more common or serious gastrointestinal, renal, hepatic, hematologic, and dermatologic adverse effects.

Laboratory test interactions: False-positive urine immunoassay screening tests for benzodiazepines have been reported in patients taking Daypro. This is due to lack of specificity of the screening tests. False-positive test results may be expected for several days following discontinuation of Daypro therapy. Confirmatory tests, such as gas chromatography/mass spectrometry, will distinguish Daypro from benzodiazepines.

Drug interactions

Aspirin: Concomitant administration of Daypro and aspirin is not recommended because oxprozin displaces salicylates from plasma protein binding sites. Coadministration would be expected to increase the risk of salicylate toxicity.

Oral anticoagulants: The anticoagulant effects of warfarin were not affected by the coadministration of 1200 mg/day of Daypro. Nevertheless, caution should be exercised when adding any drug that affects platelet function to the regimen of patients receiving oral anticoagulants.

H_2-receptor antagonists: The total body clearance of oxaprozin was reduced by 20% in subjects who concurrently received therapeutic doses of cimetidine or ranitidine; no other pharmacokinetic parameter was affected. A change of clearance of this magnitude lies within the range of normal variation and is unlikely to produce a clinically detectable difference in the outcome of therapy.

Beta-blockers: Subjects receiving 1200 mg Daypro qd with 100 mg metoprolol bid exhibited statistically significant but transient increases in sitting and standing blood pressures after 14 days. Therefore, as with all NSAIDs, routine blood pressure monitoring should be considered in these patients when starting Daypro therapy.

Other drugs: The coadministration of oxaprozin and antacids, acetaminophen, or conjugated estrogens resulted in no statistically significant changes in pharmacokinetic parameters in single- and/or multiple-dose studies. The interaction of oxaprozin with lithium and cardiac glycosides has not been studied.

Carcinogenesis, mutagenesis, impairment of fertility: In oncogenicity studies, oxaprozin administration for 2 years was associated with the exacerbation of liver neoplasms (hepatic adenomas and carcinomas) in male CD mice, but not in female CD mice or rats. The significance of this species-specific finding to man is unknown.

Oxaprozin did not display mutagenic potential. Results from the Ames test, forward mutation in yeast and Chinese hamster ovary (CHO) cells, DNA repair testing in CHO cells, micronucleus testing in mouse bone marrow, chromosomal aberration testing in human lymphocytes, and cell transformation testing in mouse fibroblast all showed no evidence of genetic toxicity or cell-transforming ability.

Oxaprozin administration was not associated with impairment of fertility in male and female rats at oral doses up to 200 mg/kg/day (1180 mg/m^2); the usual human dose is 17 mg/kg/day (629 mg/m^2). However, testicular degeneration was observed in beagle dogs treated with 37.5 to 150 mg/kg/day (750 to 3000 mg/m^2) of oxaprozin for 6 months, or 37.5 mg/kg/day for 42 days, a finding not confirmed in other species. The clinical relevance of this finding is not known.

Pregnancy: Teratogenic Effects—Pregnancy Category C. There are no adequate or well-controlled studies in pregnant women. Teratology studies with oxaprozin were performed in mice, rats, and rabbits. In mice and rats, no drug-related developmental abnormalities were observed at 50 to 200 mg/kg/day of oxaprozin (225 to 900 mg/m^2). However, in rabbits, infrequent malformed fetuses were observed in dams treated with 7.5 to 30 mg/kg/day of oxaprozin (the usual human dosage range). Oxaprozin should be used during pregnancy only if the potential benefits justify the potential risks to the fetus.

Labor and delivery: The effect of oxaprozin in pregnant women is unknown. NSAIDs are known to delay parturition, to accelerate closure of the fetal ductus arteriosus, and to be associated with dystocia. Oxaprozin is known to have caused decreases in pup survival in rat studies. Accordingly, the use of oxaprozin during late pregnancy should be avoided.

Nursing mothers: Studies of oxaprozin excretion in human milk have not been conducted; however, oxaprozin was found in the milk of lactating rats. Since the effects of oxaprozin on infants are not known, caution should be exercised if oxaprozin is administered to nursing women.

Pediatric use: Safety and effectiveness of Daypro in pediatric patients have not been established.
Geriatric use: No adjustment of the dose of Daypro is necessary in the elderly for *pharmacokinetic* reasons, although many elderly may need to receive a reduced dose because of low body weight or disorders associated with aging. No significant differences in the pharmacokinetic profile for oxaprozin were seen in studies in the healthy elderly.
Although selected elderly patients in controlled clinical trials tolerated Daypro as well as younger patients, caution should be exercised in treating the elderly, and extra care should be taken when choosing a dose. As with any NSAID, the elderly are likely to tolerate adverse reactions less well than younger patients.

ADVERSE REACTIONS

Adverse reaction data were derived from patients who received Daypro in multidose, controlled, and open-label clinical trials, and from worldwide marketing experience. Rates for events occurring in more than 1% of patients, and for most of the less common events, are based on 2253 patients who took 1200 to 1800 mg Daypro per day in clinical trials. Of these, 1721 were treated for at least 1 month, 971 for at least 3 months, and 366 for more than 1 year. Rates for the rarer events and for events reported from worldwide marketing experience are difficult to estimate accurately and are only listed as less than 1%.
The adverse event rates below refer to the incidence in the first month of use. Most of the events were seen by this time for common adverse reactions. However, the cumulative incidence can be expected to rise with continued therapy, and some events, such as gastrointestinal bleeding (see *Warnings*), seem to occur at a constant or possibly increasing rate over time.
The most frequently reported adverse reactions were related to the gastrointestinal tract. They were nausea (8%) and dyspepsia (8%).
INCIDENCE GREATER THAN 1%: In clinical trials the following adverse reactions occurred at an incidence greater than 1% and are probably related to treatment. Reactions occurring in 3% to 9% of patients treated with Daypro are indicated by an asterisk(*); those reactions occurring in less than 3% of patients are unmarked.
Digestive system: abdominal pain/distress, anorexia, constipation*, diarrhea*, dyspepsia*, flatulence, nausea*, vomiting.
Nervous system: CNS inhibition (depression, sedation, somnolence, or confusion), disturbance of sleep.
Skin and appendages: rash*.
Special senses: tinnitus.
Urogenital system: dysuria or frequency.
INCIDENCE LESS THAN 1%:
Probable causal relationship: *The following adverse reactions were reported in clinical trials or from worldwide marketing experience at an incidence of less than 1%. Those reactions reported only from worldwide marketing experience are in italics.* The probability of a causal relationship exists between the drug and these adverse reactions.
Body as a whole: drug hypersensitivity reactions including anaphylaxis *and serum sickness.*
Cardiovascular system: edema, blood pressure changes.
Digestive system: peptic ulceration and/or GI bleeding (see *Warnings*), liver function abnormalities including *hepatitis* (see *Precautions*), stomatitis, hemorrhoidal or rectal bleeding, *pancreatitis.*
Hematologic system: anemia, thrombocytopenia, leukopenia, ecchymoses, *agranulocytosis, pancytopenia.*
Metabolic system: weight gain, weight loss.
Nervous system: weakness, malaise.
Respiratory system: symptoms of upper respiratory tract infection.
Skin: pruritus, urticaria, photosensitivity, *pseudoporphyria, exfoliative dermatitis, erythema multiforme, Stevens-Johnson syndrome, toxic epidermal necrolysis (Lyell's syndrome).*
Special senses: blurred vision, conjunctivitis.
Urogenital: *acute interstitial nephritis, nephrotic syndrome,* hematuria, renal insufficiency, *acute renal failure,* decreased menstrual flow.
Causal relationship unknown: The following adverse reactions occurred at an incidence of less than 1% in clinical trials, or were suggested from marketing experience, under circumstances where a causal relationship could not be definitely established. They are listed as alerting information for the physician.
Cardiovascular system: palpitations.
Digestive system: alteration in taste.
Respiratory system: sinusitis, pulmonary infections.
Skin and appendages: alopecia.
Special senses: hearing decrease.
Urogenital system: increase in menstrual flow.

DRUG ABUSE AND DEPENDENCE

Daypro is a non-narcotic drug. Usually reliable animal studies have indicated that Daypro has no known addiction potential in humans.

OVERDOSAGE

No patient experienced either an accidental or intentional overdosage of Daypro in the clinical trials of the drug. Symptoms following acute overdose with other NSAIDs are usually limited to lethargy, drowsiness, nausea, vomiting, and epigastric pain and are generally reversible with supportive care. Gastrointestinal bleeding and coma have occurred following NSAID overdose. Hypertension, acute renal failure, and respiratory depression are rare.
Patients should be managed by symptomatic and supportive care following an NSAID overdose. There are no specific antidotes. Gut decontamination may be indicated in patients seen within 4 hours of ingestion with symptoms or following a large overdose (5 to 10 times the usual dose). This should be accomplished via emesis and/or activated charcoal (60 to 100 g in adults, 1 to 2 g/kg in children) with an osmotic cathartic. Forced diuresis, alkalization of the urine, or hemoperfusion would probably not be useful due to the high degree of protein binding of oxaprozin.

DOSAGE AND ADMINISTRATION

Rheumatoid arthritis: The usual daily dose of Daypro in the management of the signs and symptoms of rheumatoid arthritis is 1200 mg (two 600-mg caplets) once a day. Both smaller and larger doses may be required in individual patients (see *Individualization of Dosage*).
Osteoarthritis: The usual daily dose of Daypro for the management of the signs and symptoms of moderate to severe osteoarthritis is 1200 mg (two 600-mg caplets) once a day. For patients of low body weight or with milder disease, an initial dosage of one 600-mg caplet once a day may be appropriate (see *Individualization of Dosage*).
Regardless of the indication, the dosage should be individualized to the lowest effective dose of Daypro to minimize adverse effects, and the maximum recommended total daily dose is 1800 mg (or 26 mg/kg, whichever is lower) in divided doses.

SAFETY AND HANDLING

Daypro is supplied as a solid dosage form in closed containers, is not known to produce contact dermatitis, and poses no known risk to healthcare workers. It may be disposed of in accordance with applicable local regulations governing the disposal of pharmaceuticals.

HOW SUPPLIED

Daypro 600-mg caplets are white, capsule-shaped, scored, film-coated, with DAYPRO debossed on one side and 1381 on the other side.

NDC Number	Size
0025-1381-31	bottle of 100
0025-1381-51	bottle of 500
0025-1381-34	carton of 100 unit dose

Keep bottles tightly closed and store below 77°F (25°C). Dispense in a tight, light-resistant container with a child-resistant closure. Protect the unit dose from light.
Caution: **Rx only**

4/29/98 • A05222-7

Shown in Product Identification Guide, page 335

DEMULEN® 1/35–21 ℞
DEMULEN® 1/35–28 ℞
DEMULEN® 1/50–21 ℞
DEMULEN® 1/50–28 ℞
[*dem 'ū-len*]
(ethynodiol diacetate with ethinyl estradiol)

PRODUCT OVERVIEW

KEY FACTS

The Searle line of oral contraceptives contains two fixed-dose combination oral contraceptives (DEMULEN 1/35-21 and DEMULEN 1/35-28) containing ethynodiol diacetate (1 mg) with ethinyl estradiol (35 mcg) and two fixed-dose combination oral contraceptives (DEMULEN 1/50-21 and DEMULEN 1/50-28) containing ethynodiol diacetate (1 mg) with ethinyl estradiol (50 mcg). DEMULEN 1/35-21 and DEMULEN 1/50-21 are 21-day dosage regimens. DEMULEN 1/35-28 and DEMULEN 1/50-28 are 28-day dosage regimens (including 7 days of inert tablets). These forms are packaged in Compack® tablet dispensers.

MAJOR USE

DEMULEN 1/35 and DEMULEN 1/50 are highly effective in preventing pregnancy.

SAFETY INFORMATION

See complete safety information set forth below.

PRESCRIBING INFORMATION

DEMULEN® 1/35–21 ℞
DEMULEN® 1/35–28 ℞
DEMULEN® 1/50–21 ℞
DEMULEN® 1/50–28 ℞
[*dem 'ū-len*]
(ethynodiol diacetate with ethinyl estradiol)

Patients should be counseled that this product does not protect against HIV infection (AIDS) and other sexually transmitted diseases.

DESCRIPTION

Demulen 1/35-21 and Demulen 1/35-28. Each white tablet contains 1 mg of ethynodiol diacetate and 35 mcg of ethinyl estradiol, and the inactive ingredients include calcium acetate, calcium phosphate, corn starch, hydrogenated castor oil, and povidone. Each blue tablet in the Demulen 1/35-28 package is a placebo containing no active ingredients, and the inactive ingredients include lactose monohydrate, microcrystalline cellulose, anhydrous lactose, FD&C Blue No. 1 Lake, and magnesium stearate.
Demulen 1/50-21 and Demulen 1/50-28. Each white tablet contains 1 mg of ethynodiol diacetate and 50 mcg of ethinyl estradiol, and the inactive ingredients include calcium acetate, calcium phosphate, corn starch, hydrogenated castor oil, and povidone. Each pink tablet in the Demulen 1/50-28 package is a placebo containing no active ingredients, and the inactive ingredients include lactose monohydrate, microcrystalline cellulose, anhydrous lactose, FD&C Yellow No. 6 Lake, and magnesium stearate.
The chemical name for ethynodiol diacetate is 19-nor-17α-pregn-4-en-20-yne-3β,17-diol diacetate, and for ethinyl estradiol it is 19-nor-17α-pregna-1,3,5(10)-trien-20-yne-3, 17-diol. The structural formulas are as follows:

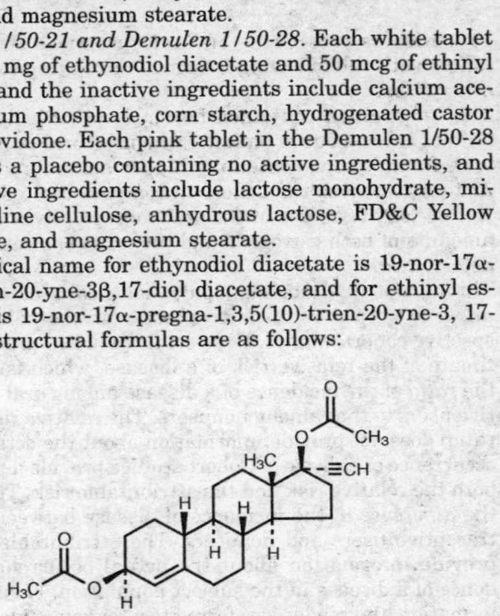

ethynodiol diacetate

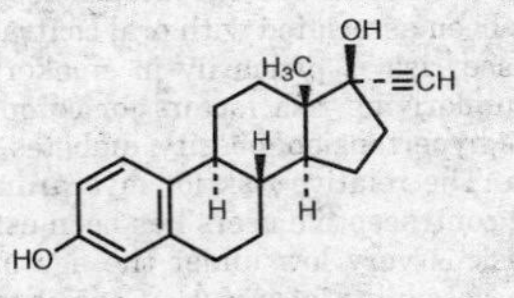

ethinyl estradiol

Therapeutic class: Oral contraceptive.

CLINICAL PHARMACOLOGY

Combination oral contraceptives act primarily by suppression of gonadotropins. Although the primary mechanism of this action is inhibition of ovulation, other alterations in the genital tract, including changes in the cervical mucus (which increase the difficulty of sperm entry into the uterus) and the endometrium (which may reduce the likelihood of implantation) may also contribute to contraceptive effectiveness.

INDICATIONS AND USAGE

Demulen 1/35 and Demulen 1/50 are indicated for the prevention of pregnancy in women who elect to use oral contraceptives as a method of contraception. Oral contraceptive products such as Demulen 1/50, which contain 50 mcg of estrogen, should not be used unless medically indicated.
Oral contraceptives are highly effective. Table 1 lists the typical accidental pregnancy rates for users of combination oral contraceptives and other methods of contraception. The efficacy of these contraceptive methods, except sterilization and progestogen implants and injections, depends upon the reliability with which they are used. Correct and consistent use of methods can result in lower failure rates.
[See table at top of next page]

CONTRAINDICATIONS

Oral contraceptives should not be used in women who have the following conditions:

- Thrombophlebitis or thromboembolic disorders
- A past history of deep vein thrombophlebitis or thromboembolic disorders
- Cerebral vascular disease, myocardial infarction, or coronary artery disease, or a past history of these conditions
- Known or suspected carcinoma of the breast, or a history of this condition
- Known or suspected carcinoma of the female reproductive organs or suspected estrogen-dependent neoplasia, or a history of these conditions
- Undiagnosed abnormal genital bleeding
- History of cholestatic jaundice of pregnancy or jaundice with prior oral contraceptive use
- Past or present, benign or malignant liver tumors
- Known or suspected pregnancy

WARNINGS

Cigarette smoking increases the risk of serious cardiovascular side effects from oral contraceptive use. This risk increases with age and with heavy smoking (15 or more cigarettes per day) and is quite marked in women over 35 years of age. Women who use oral contraceptives should be strongly advised not to smoke.

The use of oral contraceptives is associated with increased risk of several serious conditions including venous and arterial thromboembolism. thrombotic and hemorrhagic stroke, myocardial infarction, liver tumors or other liver lesions, and gallbladder disease. The risk of morbidity and mortality increases significantly in the presence of other risk factors such as hypertension, hyperlipidemia, obesity, and diabetes mellitus.

Continued on next page

Demulen—Cont.

Practitioners prescribing oral contraceptives should be familiar with the following information relating to these and other risks.

The information contained herein is principally based on studies carried out in patients who used oral contraceptives with formulations containing higher amounts of estrogens and progestogens than those in common use today. The effect on long-term use of the oral contraceptives with lesser amounts of both estrogens and progestogens remains to be determined.

Throughout this labeling, epidemiological studies reported are of two types: retrospective case-control studies and prospective cohort studies. Case-control studies provide an estimate of the relative risk of a disease, which is defined as the *ratio* of the incidence of a disease among oral contraceptive users to that among nonusers. The relative risk (or odds ratio) does not provide information about the actual clinical occurrence of a disease. Cohort studies provide a measure of both the relative risk and the attributable risk. The latter is the *difference* in the incidence of disease between oral contraceptive users and nonusers. The attributable risk does provide information about the actual occurrence or incidence of a disease in the subject population. For further information, the reader is referred to a text on epidemiological methods.

1. Thromboembolic disorders and other vascular problems.
a. Myocardial infarction. An increased risk of myocardial infarction has been associated with oral contraceptive use.[2–21] This increased risk is primarily in smokers or in women with other underlying risk factors for coronary artery disease such as hypertension, obesity, diabetes, and hypercholesterolemia. The relative risk for myocardial infarction in current oral contraceptive users has been estimated to be 2 to 6. The risk is very low under the age of 30. However, there is the possibility of a risk of cardiovascular disease even in very young women who take oral contraceptives.

Smoking in combination with oral contraceptive use has been reported to contribute substantially to the risk of myocardial infarction in women in their mid-thirties or older, with smoking accounting for the majority of excess cases.[22]

Mortality rates associated with circulatory disease have been shown to increase substantially in smokers, especially in those 35 years of age and older among women who use oral contraceptives (see Figure 1, Table 2).

Figure 1. Circulatory disease mortality rates per 100,000 woman-years by age, smoking status, and oral contraceptive use.[14]

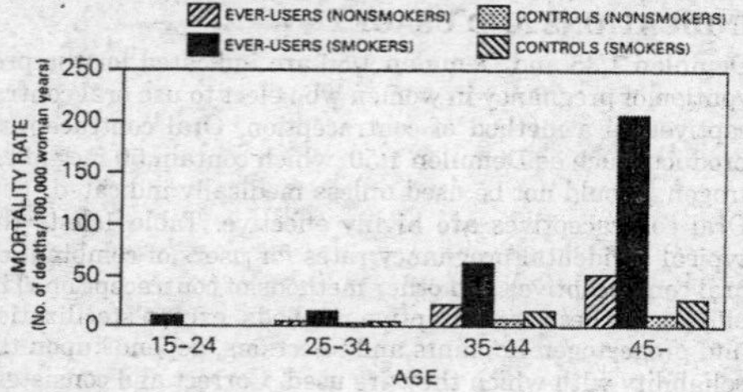

Adapted from Layde and Beral.[14]

Oral contraceptives may compound the effects of well-known cardiovascular risk factors such as hypertension, diabetes, hyperlipidemias, hypercholesterolemia, age, cigarette smoking, and obesity. In particular, some progestogens decrease HDL cholesterol[23–31] and cause glucose intolerance, while estrogens may create a state of hyperinsulinism.[32] Oral contraceptives have been shown to increase blood pressure among some users (see *Warning* No. 9). Similar effects on risk factors have been associated with an increased risk of heart disease.

b. Thromboembolism. An increased risk of thromboembolic and thrombotic disease associated with the use of oral contraceptives is well established.[17,33–51] Case-control studies have estimated the relative risk to be 3 for the first episode of superficial venous thrombosis, 4 to 11 for deep vein thrombosis or pulmonary embolism, and 1.5 to 6 for women with predisposing conditions for venous thromboemoblic disease.[34–37,45,46] Cohort studies have shown the relative risk to be somewhat lower, about 3 for new cases (subjects with no past history of venous thrombosis or varicose veins) and about 4.5 for new cases requiring hospitalization.[42,47,48] The risk of venous thromboembolic disease associated with oral contraceptives is not related to duration of use.

A two- to seven-fold increase in relative risk of postoperative thromboembolic complications has been reported with the use of oral contraceptives.[38,39] The relative risk of venous thrombosis in women who have predisposing conditions is about twice that of women without such medical conditions.[43] If feasible, oral contraceptives should be discontinued at least 4 weeks prior to and for 2 weeks after elective surgery of a type associated with an increased risk of thromboembolism, and also during and following prolonged immobilization. Since the immediate postpartum period is also associated with an increased risk of thromboembolism, oral contraceptives should be started no earlier than 4 to 6 weeks after delivery in women who elect not to breast feed.

c. Cerebrovascular diseases. Both the relative and attributable risks of cerebrovascular events (thrombotic and hemorrhagic strokes) have been reported to be increased with oral contraceptive use,[14,17,18,34,42,46,52–59] although, in general, the risk was greatest among older (over 35 years), hypertensive women who also smoked. Hypertension was reported to be a risk factor for both users and nonusers, for both types of strokes, while smoking increased the risk for hemorrhagic strokes.

In one large study,[52] the relative risk for thrombotic stroke was reported as 9.5 times greater in users than in nonusers. It ranged from 3 for normotensive users to 14 for users with severe hypertension.[54] The relative risk for hemorrhagic stroke was reported to be 1.2 for nonsmokers who used oral contraceptives, 1.9 to 2.6 for smokers who did not use oral contraceptives, 6.1 to 7.6 for smokers who used oral contraceptives, 1.8 for normotensive users, and 25.7 for users with severe hypertension. The risk is also greater in older women and among smokers.

d. Dose-related risk of vascular disease with oral contraceptives. A positive association has been reported between the amount of estrogen and progestogen in oral contraceptives and the risk of vascular disease.[41,43,53,59–64] A decline in serum high density lipoproteins (HDL) has been reported with many progestogens.[23–31] A decline in serum high density lipoproteins has been associated with an increased incidence of ischemic heart disease.[65] Because estrogens increase HDL-cholesterol, the net effect of an oral contraceptive depends on the balance achieved between doses of estrogen and progestogen and the nature and absolute amount of progestogens used in the contraceptives. The amount of both steroids should be considered in the choice of an oral contraceptive.

Minimizing exposure to estrogen and progestogen is in keeping with good principles of therapeutics. For any particular estrogen-progestogen combination, the dosage regimen prescribed should be one that contains the least amount of estrogen and progestogen that is compatible with a low failure rate and the needs of the individual patient. New acceptors of oral contraceptives should be started on preparations containing the lowest estrogen content that produces satisfactory results in the individual.

Products containing 50 mcg estrogen should be used only when medically indicated.

e. Persistence of risk of vascular disease. There are three studies that have shown persistence of risk of vascular disease for users of oral contraceptives. In a study in the United States, the risk of developing myocardial infarction after discontinuing oral contraceptives persisted for at least 9 years for women 40–49 years old who had used oral contraceptives for 5 or more years, but this increased risk was not demonstrated in other age groups.[16] Another American study reported former use of oral contraceptives was significantly associated with increased risk of subarachnoid hemorrhage.[57] In another study, in Great Britain, the risk of developing nonrheumatic heart disease plus hypertension, subarachnoid hemorrhage, cerebral thrombosis, and transient ischemic attacks persisted for at least 6 years after discontinuation of oral contraceptives, although the excess risk was small.[14, 18, 66] It should be noted that these studies were performed with oral contraceptive formulations containing 50 mcg or more of estrogens.

2. Estimates of mortality from contraceptive use. One study[67] gathered data from a variety of sources that have estimated the mortality rates associated with different methods of contraception at different ages (Table 2). These estimates include the combined risk of death associated with contraceptive methods plus the risk attributable to pregnancy in the event of method failure. Each method of contraception has its specific benefits and risks. The study concluded that, with the exception of oral contraceptive us-

Table 1. Percentage of women experiencing an unintended pregnancy during the first year of typical use and the first year of perfect use of contraception and the percentage continuing use at the end of the first year. United States.

Method (1)	% of women experiencing an unintended pregnancy within the first year of use: Typical use[A] (2)	Perfect use[B] (3)	% of women continuing use at one year[C] (4)
Chance[D]	85	85	
Spermicides[E]	26	6	40
Periodic abstinence	25		63
Calendar		9	
Ovulation method		3	
Sympto-thermal[F]		2	
Post-ovulation		1	
Withdrawal	19	4	
Cap[G]			
Parous women	40	26	42
Nulliparous women	20	9	56
Sponge			
Parous women	40	20	42
Nulliparous women	20	9	56
Diaphragm[G]	20	6	56
Condom[H]			
Female (Reality)	21	5	56
Male	14	3	61
Pill	5		71
Progestin only		0.5	
Combined		0.1	
IUD			
Progesterone T	2.0	1.5	81
Copper T 380A	0.8	0.6	78
LNg 20	0.1	0.1	81
Injection (Depo-Provera)	0.3	0.3	70
Implant (Norplant and Norplant-2)	0.05	0.05	88
Female sterilization	0.5	0.5	100
Male sterilization	0.15	0.10	100

Emergency Contraceptive Pills: Treatment initiated within 72 hours after unprotected intercourse reduces the risk of pregnancy by at least 75%.[I]

Lactational Amenorrhea Method: LAM is a highly effective, *temporary* method of contraception.[J]

Source: Trussell J, Contraceptive efficacy. In Hatcher RA, Trussell J, Stewart F, Cates W, Stewart GK, Kowal D, Guest F, *Contraceptive Technology: Seventeenth Revised Edition.* New York NY: Irvington Publishers, 1998, in press.[1]

[A] Among *typical* couples who initiate use of a method (not necessarily for the first time), the percentage who experience an accidental pregnancy during the first year if they do not stop use for any other reason.
[B] Among couples who initiate use of a method (not necessarily for the first time) and who use it *perfectly* (both consistently and correctly), the percentage who experience an accidental pregnancy during the first year if they do not stop use for any other reason.
[C] Among couples attempting to avoid pregnancy, the percentage who continue to use a method for one year.
[D] The percents becoming pregnant in columns (2) and (3) are based on data from populations where contraception is not used and from women who cease using contraception in order to become pregnant. Among such populations, about 89% become pregnant within one year. This estimate was lowered slightly (to 85%) to represent the percent who would become pregnant within one year among women now relying on reversible methods of contraception if they abandoned contraception altogether.
[E] Foams, creams, gels, vaginal suppositories, and vaginal film.
[F] Cervical mucus (ovulation) method supplemented by calendar in the pre-ovulatory and basal body temperature in the post-ovulatory phases.
[G] With spermicidal cream or jelly.
[H] Without spermicides.
[I] The treatment schedule is one dose within 72 hours after unprotected intercourse, and a second dose 12 hours after the first dose. The Food and Drug Administration has declared the following brands of oral contraceptives to be safe and effective for emergency contraception: Ovral (1 dose is 2 white pills), Alesse (1 dose is 5 pink pills), Nordette or Levlen (1 dose is 2 light-orange pills), Lo/Ovral (1 dose is 4 white pills), Triphasil or Tri-Levlen (1 dose is 4 yellow pills).
[J] However, to maintain effective protection against pregnancy, another method of contraception must be used as soon as menstruation resumes, the frequency or duration of breastfeeds is reduced, bottle feeds are introduced or the baby reaches six months of age.

ers 35 and older who smoke and 40 or older who do not smoke, mortality associated with all methods of birth control is low and below that associated with childbirth. The observation of a possible increase in risk of mortality with age for oral contraceptive users is based on data gathered in the 1970's, but not reported until 1983.[67] However, current clinical practice involves the use of lower estrogen dose formulations combined with careful restriction of oral contraceptive use to women who do not have the various risk factors listed in this labeling.

Because of these changes in practice and, also, because of some limited new data that suggest that the risk of cardiovascular disease with the use of oral contraceptives may now be less than previously observed,[48, 152] the Fertility and Maternal Health Drugs Advisory Committee was asked to review the topic in 1989. The Committee concluded that, although cardiovascular disease risks may be increased with oral contraceptive use after age 40 in healthy nonsmoking women (even with the newer low-dose formulations), there are greater potential health risks associated with pregnancy in older women and with the alternative surgical and medical procedures that may be necessary if such women do not have access to effective and acceptable means of contraception.

Therefore, the Committee recommended that the benefits of oral contraceptive use by healthy nonsmoking women over 40 may outweigh the possible risks. Of course, older women, as all women who take oral contraceptives, should take the lowest possible dose formulation that is effective.

[See table above]

Table 2. Annual number of birth-related or method-related deaths associated with control of fertility per 100,000 nonsterile women, by fertility control method according to age.[67]

	Age					
Method of control	**15–19**	**20–24**	**25–29**	**30–34**	**35–39**	**40–44**
No fertility control methods*	7.0	7.4	9.1	14.8	25.7	28.2
Oral contraceptives						
nonsmoker**	0.3	0.5	0.9	1.9	13.8	31.6
smoker**	2.2	3.4	6.6	13.5	51.1	117.2
IUD**	0.8	0.8	1.0	1.0	1.4	1.4
Condom*	1.1	1.6	0.7	0.2	0.3	0.4
Diaphragm/ spermicide*	1.9	1.2	1.2	1.3	2.2	2.8
Periodic abstinence*	2.5	1.6	1.6	1.7	2.9	3.6

* Deaths are birth-related
** Deaths are method-related
Adapted from Ory.[67]

3. Carcinoma of the breast and reproductive organs. Numerous epidemiological studies have been performed on the incidence of breast, endometrial, ovarian, and cervical cancer in women using oral contraceptives. While there are conflicting reports, many studies suggest that the use of oral contraceptives is not associated with an overall increase in the risk of developing breast cancer.[17,40,68–78] Other studies, however, have reported an increased risk overall,[153–155] or in certain subgroups. In these studies, increased risk has been associated with long duration of use, use beginning at a young age, use before the first term pregnancy, use by those who had an early menarche, those who had a positive family history of breast cancer, or in nulliparas.[79–102, 151, 156–162] These risks have been surveyed in two books[163–164] and in review articles.[85,99,153, 165–167]

Some studies suggested that oral contraceptive use was associated with an increase in the risk of cervical intraepithelial neoplasia, dysplasia, erosion, carcinoma, or microglandular dysplasia in some populations of women.[17,50, 103–115] However, there continues to be controversy about the extent to which such findings may be due to differences in sexual behavior and other factors.

In spite of many studies of the relationship between oral contraceptive use and breast and cervical cancers, a cause and effect relationship has not been established.

4. Hepatic neoplasia. Benign hepatic adenomas and other hepatic lesions have been associated with oral contraceptive use.[116–121] although the incidence of such benign tumors is rare in the United States. Indirect calculations have estimated the attributable risk to be in the range of 3.3 cases per 100,000 for users, a risk that increases after 4 or more years of use.[120] Rupture of benign, hepatic adenomas or other lesions may cause death through intra-abdominal hemorrhage. Therefore, such lesions should be considered in women presenting with abdominal pain and tenderness, abdominal mass, or shock. About one quarter of the cases presented because of abdominal masses; up to one half had signs and symptoms of acute intraperitoneal hemorrhage.[121] Diagnosis may prove difficult.

Studies from the U.S.,[122, 150] Great Britain,[123, 124] and Italy[125] have shown an increased risk of hepatocellular carcinoma in long-term (>8 years; relative risk of 7–20) oral contraceptive users. However, these cancers are rare in the United States, and the attributable risk (the excess incidence) of liver cancers in oral contraceptive users approaches less than 1 per 1,000,000 users.

5. Ocular lesions. There have been reports of retinal thrombosis and other ocular lesions associated with the use of oral contraceptives. Oral contraceptives should be discontinued if there is unexplained, gradual or sudden, partial or complete loss of vision; onset of proptosis or diplopia; papilledema; or any evidence of retinal vascular lesions. Appropriate diagnostic and therapeutic measures should be undertaken immediately.

6. Oral contraceptive use before or during pregnancy. Extensive epidemiological studies have revealed no increased risk of birth defects in women who have used oral contraceptives prior to pregnancy.[126, 129] The majority of recent studies also do not suggest a teratogenic effect, particularly insofar as cardiac anomalies and limb reduction defects are concerned,[126–129] when the pill is taken inadvertently during early pregnancy.

The administration of oral contraceptives to induce withdrawal bleeding should not be used as a test for pregnancy. Oral contraceptives should not be used during pregnancy to treat threatened or habitual abortion. It is recommended that for any patient who has missed two consecutive periods, pregnancy should be ruled out before continuing oral contraceptive use. If the patient has not adhered to the prescribed schedule, the possibility of pregnancy should be considered at the time of the first missed period and further use of oral contraceptives should be withheld until pregnancy has been ruled out. Oral contraceptive use should be discontinued if pregnancy is confirmed.

7. Gallbladder disease. Earlier studies reported an increased lifetime relative risk of gallbladder surgery in users of oral contraceptives and estrogens.[40,42,53,70] More recent studies, however, have shown that the relative risk of developing gallbladder disease among oral contraceptive users may be minimal.[130–132] The recent findings of minimal risk may be related to the use of oral contraceptive formulations containing lower doses of estrogens and progestogens.

8. Carbohydrate and lipid metabolic effects. Oral contraceptives have been shown to cause a decrease in glucose tolerance in a significant percentage of users.[32] This effect has been shown to be directly related to estrogen dose.[133] Progestogens increase insulin secretion and create insulin resistance, the effect varying with different progestational agents.[32, 134] However, in the nondiabetic woman, oral contraceptives appear to have no effect on fasting blood glucose. Because of these demonstrated effects, prediabetic and diabetic women should be carefully observed while taking oral contraceptives.

Some women may have persistent hypertriglyceridemia while on the pill. As discussed earlier (see *WARNINGS* 1a and 1d), changes in serum triglycerides and lipoprotein levels have been reported in oral contraceptive users.[23–31, 135, 136]

9. Elevated blood pressure. An increase in blood pressure has been reported in women taking oral contraceptives[50, 53, 137–139] and this increase is more likely in older oral contraceptive users[137] and with extended duration of use.[53] Data from the Royal College of General Practitioners[138] and subsequent randomized trials have shown that the incidence of hypertension increases with increasing concentrations of progestogens.

Women with a history of hypertension or hypertension-related diseases, or renal disease[139] should be encouraged to use another method of contraception. If such women elect to use oral contraceptives, they should be monitored closely and if significant elevation of blood pressure occurs, oral contraceptives should be discontinued. For most women, elevated blood pressure will return to normal after stopping oral contraceptives,[137] and there is no difference in the occurrence of hypertension among ever- and never-users.[140]

10. Headache. The onset or exacerbation of migraine or the development of headache of a new pattern that is recurrent, persistent, or severe requires discontinuation of oral contraceptives and evaluation of the cause.

11. Bleeding irregularities. Breakthrough bleeding and spotting are sometimes encountered in patients on oral contraceptives, especially during the first three months of use. Nonhormonal causes should be considered and adequate diagnostic measures taken to rule out malignancy or pregnancy in the event of breakthrough bleeding, as in the case of any abnormal vaginal bleeding. If a pathologic basis has been excluded, time alone or a change to another formulation may solve the problem. In the event of amenorrhea, pregnancy should be ruled out. Some women may encounter post-pill amenorrhea or oligomenorrhea, especially when such a condition was pre-existent.

PRECAUTIONS

1. Physical examination and follow-up. It is good medical practice for all women to have annual history and physical examinations, including women using oral contraceptives. The physical examination, however, may be deferred until after initiation of oral contraceptives if requested by the woman and judged appropriate by the clinician. The physical examination should include special reference to blood pressure, breasts, abdomen, and pelvic organs, including cervical cytology, and relevant laboratory tests. In case of undiagnosed, persistent, or recurrent abnormal vaginal bleeding, appropriate measures should be conducted to rule out malignancy. Women with a strong family history of breast cancer or who have breast nodules should be monitored with particular care.

2. Lipid disorders. Women who are being treated for hyperlipidemias should be followed closely if they elect to use oral contraceptives. Some progestogens may elevate LDL levels and may render the control of hyperlipidemias more difficult.

3. Liver function. If jaundice develops in any woman receiving oral contraceptives, they should be discontinued. Steroids may be poorly metabolized in patients with impaired liver function and should be administered with caution in such patients. Cholestatic jaundice has been reported after combined treatment with oral contraceptives and troleandomycin. Hepatotoxicity following a combination of oral contraceptives and cyclosporine has also been reported.

4. Fluid retention. Oral contraceptives may cause some degree of fluid retention. They should be prescribed with caution, and only with careful monitoring, in patients with conditions that might be aggravated by fluid retention, such as convulsive disorders, migraine syndrome, asthma, or cardiac, hepatic, or renal dysfunction.

5. Emotional disorders. Women with a history of depression should be carefully observed and the drug discontinued if depression recurs to a serious degree.

6. Contact lenses. Contact lens wearers who develop visual changes or changes in lens tolerance should be assessed by an ophthalmologist.

7. Drug Interactions. Reduced efficacy and increased incidence of breakthrough bleeding and menstrual irregularities have been associated with concomitant use of rifampin. A similar association, though less marked, has been suggested for barbiturates, phenylbutazone, phenytoin sodium, and possibly with griseofulvin, ampicillin, and tetracyclines. Administration of troglitazone concomitantly with a combination oral contraceptive (estrogen and progestin) reduced the plasma concentrations of both hormones by approximately 30% This could result in loss of contraceptive efficacy.

8. Laboratory test interactions. Certain endocrine and liver function tests and blood components may be affected by oral contraceptives:

a. Increased prothrombin and factors VII, VIII, IX, and X; decreased antithrombin III; increased platelet aggregability.
b. Increased thyroid binding globulin (TBG), leading to increased circulating total thyroid hormone as measured by protein-bound iodine (PBI), T_4 by column or by radio-immunoassay. Free T_3 resin uptake is decreased, reflecting the elevated TBG; free T_4 concentration is unaltered.
c. Other binding proteins may be elevated in the serum.
d. Sex-steroid binding globulins are increased and result in elevated levels of total circulating sex steroids and corticoids; however, free or biologically active levels remain unchanged.
e. Triglycerides and phospholipids may be increased.
f. Glucose tolerance may be decreased.
g. Serum folate levels may be depressed. This may be of clinical significance if a woman becomes pregnant shortly after discontinuing oral contraceptives.
h. Increased sulfobromophthalein and other abnormalities in liver function tests may occur.
i. Plasma levels of trace minerals may be altered.
j. Response to the metyrapone test may be reduced.

9. Carcinogenesis. See *WARNINGS*.

10. Pregnancy. Pregnancy Category X. See *CONTRAINDICATIONS* and *WARNINGS*.

11. Nursing mothers. Small amounts of oral contraceptive steroids have been identified in the milk of nursing mothers[141–143] and a few adverse effects on the child have been reported, including jaundice and breast enlargement. In addition, oral contraceptives given in the postpartum period may interfere with lactation by decreasing the quantity and quality of breast milk. If possible, the nursing mother should be advised not to use oral contraceptives, but to use other forms of contraception until she has completely weaned her child.

12. Pediatric use. Safety and efficacy of Demulen have been established in women of reproductive age. Safety and efficacy are expected to be the same for postpubertal adolescents under the age of 16 and for users 16 years and older. Use of this product before menarche is not indicated.

13. Venereal diseases. Oral contraceptives are of no value in the prevention or treatment of veneral disease. The prevalence of cervical *Chlamydia trachomatis* and *Neisseria gonorrhoeae* in oral contraceptive users is increased severalfold.[144, 145] It should not be assumed that oral contraceptives afford prtoection against pelvic inflammatory disease from chlamydia.[144] Patients should be counseled that this product does not protect against HIV infection (AIDS) and other sexually transmitted diseases.

Continued on next page

Demulen—Cont.

14. General.

a. The pathologist should be advised of oral contraceptive therapy when relevant specimens are submitted.

b. Treatment with oral contraceptives may mask the onset of the climacteric. (See *WARNINGS* regarding risks in this age group.)

INFORMATION FOR THE PATIENT

See patient labeling printed below.

ADVERSE REACTIONS

An increased risk of the following serious adverse reactions has been associated with the use of oral contraceptives (see *WARNINGS*):

- Thrombophlebitis and thrombosis
- Arterial thromboembolism
- Pulmonary embolism
- Myocardial infarction and coronary thrombosis
- Cerebral hemorrhage
- Cerebral thrombosis
- Hypertension
- Gallbladder disease
- Benign and malignant liver tumors, and other hepatic lesions

There is evidence of an association between the following conditions and the use of oral contraceptives, although additional confirmatory studies are needed:

- Mesenteric thrombosis
- Neuro-ocular lesions (eg, retinal thrombosis and optic neuritis)

The following adverse reactions have been reported in patients receiving oral contraceptives and are believed to be drug-related:

- Nausea
- Vomiting
- Gastrointestinal symptoms (such as abdominal cramps and bloating)
- Breakthrough bleeding
- Spotting
- Change in menstrual flow
- Amenorrhea during or after use
- Temporary infertility after discontinuation of use
- Edema
- Chloasma or melasma, which may persist
- Breast changes: tenderness, enlargement, secretion
- Change in weight (increase or decrease)
- Change in cervical erosion or secretion
- Diminution in lactation when given immediately postpartum
- Cholestatic jaundice
- Migraine
- Rash (allergic)
- Mental depression
- Reduced tolerance to carbohydrates
- Vaginal candidiasis
- Change in corneal curvature (steepening)
- Intolerance to contact lenses

The following adverse reactions or conditions have been reported in users of oral contraceptives and the association has been neither confirmed nor refuted:

- Premenstrual syndrome
- Cataracts
- Changes in appetite
- Cystitis-like syndrome
- Headache
- Nervousness
- Dizziness
- Hirsutism
- Loss of scalp hair
- Erythema multiforme
- Erythema nodosum
- Hemorrhagic eruption
- Vaginitis
- Porphyria
- Impaired renal function
- Hemolytic uremic syndrome
- Acne
- Changes in libido
- Colitis
- Budd-Chiari syndrome
- Endocervical hyperplasia or ectropion

OVERDOSAGE

Serious ill effects have not been reported following acute ingestion of large doses of oral contraceptives by young children.[180, 181] Overdosage may cause nausea, and withdrawal bleeding may occur in females.

NON-CONTRACEPTIVE HEALTH BENEFITS

The following non-contraceptive health benefits related to the use of oral contraceptives are supported by epidemiological studies that largely utilized oral contraceptive formulations containing estrogen doses exceeding 35 mcg of ethinyl estradiol or 50 mcg of mestranol.[148,149]

Effects on menses:

- Increased menstrual cycle regularity
- Decreased blood loss and decreased risk of iron-deficiency anemia
- Decreased frequency of dysmenorrhea

Effects related to inhibition of ovulation:

- Decreased risk of functional ovarian cysts
- Decreased risk of ectopic pregnancies

Effects from long-term use:

- Decreased risk of fibroadenomas and fibrocystic disease of the breast
- Decreased risk of acute pelvic inflammatory disease
- Decreased risk of endometrial cancer
- Decreased risk of ovarian cancer
- Decreased risk of uterine fibroids

DOSAGE AND ADMINISTRATION

To achieve maximum contraceptive effectiveness, oral contraceptives must be taken exactly as directed and at intervals of 24 hours.

IMPORTANT: If the Sunday start schedule is selected, the patient should be instructed to use an additional method of protection until after the first week of administration *in the initial cycle*. The possibility of ovulation and conception prior to initiation of use should be considered.

Demulen 1/35-21, Demulen 1/35-28, Demulen 1/50-21, and Demulen 1/50-28 Dosage Schedules

The Demulen 1/35-21 and Demulen 1/50-21 Compack® tablet dispensers contain 21 tablets arranged in three numbered rows of 7 tablets each.

The Demulen 1/35-28 and Demulen 1/50-28 tablet dispensers contain 21 white active tablets arranged in three numbered rows of 7 tablets each, followed by a fourth row of 7 pink (blue for Demulen 1/35-28) placebo tablets.

Days of the week are printed above the tablets, starting with Sunday on the left.

Two dosage schedules are described, one of which may be more convenient or suitable than the other for an individual patient.

21-Day Schedule: For a DAY 1 START, count the first day of menstrual flow as Day 1 and the first tablet is then taken on Day 1. For a SUNDAY START when menstrual flow begins on or before Sunday, the first tablet is taken on that day. With either a DAY 1 START or SUNDAY START, 1 tablet is taken each day at the same time for 21 days. No tablets are taken for 7 days, then, whether bleeding has stopped or not, a new course is started of 1 tablet a day for 21 days. This institutes a 3 weeks on, 1 week off dosage regimen.

28-Day Schedule: For a DAY 1 START, count the first day of menstrual flow as Day 1 and the first tablet (white) is then taken on Day 1. For a SUNDAY START when menstrual flow begins on or before Sunday, the first tablet (white) is taken on that day. With either a DAY 1 START or SUNDAY START, 1 tablet (white) is taken each day at the same time for 21 days. Then the pink or blue tablets are taken for 7 days, whether bleeding has stopped or not. After all 28 tablets have been taken, whether bleeding has stopped or not, the same dosage schedule is repeated beginning on the following day.

Special notes

Spotting, breakthrough bleeding, or nausea: If spotting (bleeding insufficient to require a pad), breakthrough bleeding (heavier bleeding similar to a menstrual flow), or nausea occurs the patient should continue taking her tablets as directed. The incidence of spotting, breakthrough bleeding, or nausea is minimal, most frequently occurring in the first cycle. Ordinarily spotting or breakthrough bleeding will stop within a week. Usually the patient will begin to cycle regularly within two or three courses of tablet-taking. In the event of spotting or breakthrough bleeding organic causes should be borne in mind. (See *Warning* No. 11.)

Missed menstrual periods. Withdrawal flow will normally occur 2 or 3 days after the last active tablet is taken. Failure of withdrawal bleeding ordinarily does not mean that the patient is pregnant, providing the dose schedule has been correctly followed (See *Warning* No. 6.)

If the patient has *not* adhered to the prescribed dosage regimen, the possibility of pregnancy should be considered after the first missed period, and oral contraceptives should be withheld until pregnancy has been ruled out.

If the patient has adhered to the prescribed regimen and misses two consecutive periods, pregnancy should be ruled out before continuing the contraceptive regimen.

The first intermenstrual interval after discontinuing the tablets is usually prolonged; consequently, a patient for whom a 28-day cycle is usual might not begin to menstruate for 35 days or longer. Ovulation in such prolonged cycles will occur correspondingly later in the cycle. Posttreatment cycles after the first one, however, are usually typical for the individual woman prior to taking tablets. (See *Warning* No. 11.)

Missed tablets: If a woman misses taking one active tablet the missed tablet should be taken as soon as it is remembered. In addition, the next tablet should be taken at the usual time. If two consecutive active tablets are missed in week 1 or week 2 of the pack, the dosage should be doubled for the next 2 days. The regular schedule should then be resumed, but an additional method of protection must be used as a backup for the next 7 days if she has sex during that time or she may become pregnant.

If two consecutive active tablets are missed in week 3 of the pack or three consecutive active tablets are missed during any of the first 3 weeks of the pack, direct the patient to do one of the following: Day 1 Starters should discard the rest of the pack and begin a new pack that same day: Sunday Starters should continue to take 1 tablet daily until Sunday, discard the rest of the pack, and begin a new pack that same day. The patient may not have a period this month; however, if she has missed two consecutive periods, pregnancy should be ruled out. An additional method of protection must be used as a backup for the next 7 days after the tablets are missed if she has sex during that time or she may become pregnant.

While there is little likelihood of ovulation if only one active tablet is missed, the possibility of spotting or breakthrough bleeding is increased and should be expected if two or more successive active tablets are missed. However, the possibility of ovulation increases with each successive day that scheduled active tablets are missed.

If one or more placebo tablets of Demulen 1/35-28 or Demulen 1/50-28 are missed, the Demulen 1/35-28 or Demulen 1/50-28 schedule should be resumed on the eighth day after the last white tablet was taken. Omission of placebo tablets in the 28-tablet courses does not increase the possibility of conception provided that this schedule is followed.

HOW SUPPLIED

Demulen 1/35:

Each white Demulen 1/35 tablet is round in shape, with a debossed SEARLE on one side and 151 and design on the other side, and contains 1 mg of ethynodiol diacetate and 35 mcg of ethinyl estradiol.

Demulen 1/35-21 is packaged in cartons of 6 and 24 Compack tablet dispensers of 21 tablets each.

Demulen 1/35-28 is packaged in cartons of 6 and 24 Compack tablet dispensers. Each Compack contains 21 white Demulen 1/35 tablets and 7 blue placebo tablets. (Placebo tablets have a debossed SEARLE on one side and a "P" on the other side.)

Demulen 1/50:

Each white Demulen 1/50 tablet is round in shape, with a debossed SEARLE on one side and 71 on the other side, and contains 1 mg of ethynodiol diacetate and 50 mcg of ethinyl estradiol.

Demulen 1/50-21 is packaged in cartons of 6 and 24 Compack tablet dispensers of 21 tablets each.

Demulen 1/50-28 is packaged in cartons of 6 and 24 Compack tablet dispensers. Each Compack contains 21 white Demulen 1/50 tablets and 7 pink placebo tablets. (Placebo tablets have a debossed SEARLE on one side and a "P" on the other side.)

Store below 77°F (25°C).

REFERENCES

1. Hatcher RA, et al. *Contraceptive Technology: Seventeenth Revised Edition.* New York, NY, 1998. **1a.** *Physicians' Desk Reference.* 47th ed. Oradell, NJ: Medical Economics Co Inc; 1993:2598-2601. **2.** Mann JI, et al. *Br Med J.* 1975;2(May 3):241. **3.** Mann JI, et al. *Br Med J.* 1975;3(Sept 13):631. **4.** Mann JI, et al. *Br Med J.* 1975;2(May 3):245. **5.** Mann JI, et al. *Br Med J.* 1976;2(Aug 21):445. **6.** Arthes FG, et al. *Chest.* 1976;70(Nov):574. **7.** Jain AK. *Am J Obstet Gynecol.* 1976;301(Oct 1):126; and *Stud Fam Plann.* 1977;8(March): 50. **8.** Ory HW. *JAMA.* 1977;237(June 13):2619. **9.** Jick H, et al. *JAMA.* 1978;239(April 3):1403, 1407. **10.** Jick H, et al. *JAMA.* 1978;240(Dec 1):2548. **11.** Shapiro S, et al. *Lancet.* 1979;1(April 7):743. **12.** Rosenberg L, et al. *Am J Epidemiol.* 1980;111(Jan):59.**13.** Krueger DE, et al. *Am J Epidemiol.* 1980;111(June):655.**14.** Layde P, et al. *Lancet.* 1981;1(March 7):541. **15.** Adam SA, et al. *Br J Obstet Gynaecol.* 1981;88(Aug):838. **16.** Slone D, et al. *N Engl J Med.* 1981;305(Aug 20):420. **17.** Ramcharan S, et al. *The Walnut Creek Contraceptive Drug Study.* Vol 3. US Govt Ptg Off; 1981; and *J Reprod Med.* 1980;25(Dec):346. **18.** Layde PM, et al. *J R Coll Gen Pract.* 1983;33(Feb):75. **19.** Rosenberg L, et al. *JAMA.* 1985;253(May 24/31):2965. **20.** Mant D, et al. *J Epidemiol Community Health.* 1987;41(Sept):215. **21.** Croft P, et al. *Br Med J.* 1989;298(Jan 21):165. **22.** Goldbaum GM, et al. *JAMA.* 1987;258(Sept 11):1339. **23.** Bradley DD, et al. *N Engl J Med.* 1978;299(July 6):17. **24.** Tikkanen MJ. *J Reprod Med.* 1986;31(Sept suppl):898. **25.** Lipson A, et al. *Contraception.* 1986;34(Aug):121. **26.** Burkman RT, et al. *Obstet Gynecol.* 1988;71(Jan):33. **27.** Knopp RH, *J Reprod Med.* 1986;31(Sept suppl):913. **28.** Krauss RM, et al. *Am J Obstet Gynecol.* 1983; 145(Feb 15):446. **29.** Wahl P, et al. *N Engl J Med.* 1983;308(April 14):862. **30.** Wynn V, et al. *Am J Obstet Gynecol.* 1982;142(March 15):766. **31.** LaRosa JC. *J Reprod Med.* 1986;31(Sept suppl):906. **32.** Wynn V, et al. *J Reprod Med.* 1986;31(Sept suppl):892. **33.** Royal College of General Practitioners. *J R Coll Gen Pract.* 1967;13(May):267. **34.** Inman WHW, et al. *Br Med J.* 1968;2(April 27):193. **35.** Vessey MP, et al. *Br Med J.* 1968;2(April 27):199. **36.** Vessey MP, et al. *Br Med J.* 1969;2(June 14):651. **37.** Sartwell PE, et al. *Am J Epidemiol.* 1969;90(Nov):365. **38.** Vessey MP, et al. *Br Med J.* 1970;3(July 18):123. **39.** Greene GR, et al. *Am J Public Health.* 1972;62(May):680. **40.** Boston Collaborative Drug Surveillance Programme. *Lancet.* 1973;1(June 23): 1399. **41.** Stolley PD, et al. *Am J Epidemiol.* 1975;102(Sept): 197. **42.** Vessey MP, et al. *J Biosoc Sci.* 1976;8(Oct):373. **43.** Kay CR, *J R Coll Gen Pract.* 1978;28(July):393. **44.** Petitti DB, et al. *Am J Epidemiol.* 1978;108(Dec):480. **45.** Maguire MG, et al. *Am J Epidemiol.* 1979;110(Aug):188. **46.** Petitti DB, et al. *JAMA.* 1979;242(Sept 14):1150. **47.** Porter JB, et al. *Obstet Gynecol.* 1982;59(March):299. **48.** Porter JB, et al. *Obstet Gynecol.* 1985;66(July):1. **49.** Vessey MP, et al. *Br Med J.* 1986;292(Feb 22):526. **50.** Hoover R, et al. *Am J Public Health.* 1978;68(April):335. **51.** Vessey MP. *Br J Fam Plann.* 1980;6(Oct suppl):1. **52.** Collaborative Group for the Study of Stroke in Young Women. *N Engl J Med.* 1973;288(April 26):871. **53.** Royal College of General Practitioners. *Oral Contraceptives and Health.* New York, NY: Pitman Publ Corp; May 1974. **54.** Collaborative Group for the Study of Stroke in Young Women. *JAMA.* 1975;231(Feb 17):

718. **55.** Beral V. *Lancet.* 1976;2(Nov 13):1047. **56.** Vessey MP, et al. *Lancet.* 1977;2(Oct 8):731; and 1981;1(March 7): 549. **57.** Petitti DB, et al. *Lancet.* 1978;2(July 29):234. **58.** Inman WHW. *Br Med J.* 1979;2(Dec 8):1468. **59.** Vessey MP, et al. *Br Med J.* 1984;289(Sept 1):530. **60.** Inman WHW, et al. *Br Med J.* 1970;2(April 25):203. **61.** Meade TW, et al. *Br Med J.* 1980;280(May 10):1157. **62.** Böttiger LE, et al. *Lancet.* 1980;1(May 24):1097. **63.** Kay CR, *Am J Obstet Gynecol.* 1982;142(March 15):762. **64.** Vessey MP, et al. *Br Med J.* 1986;292(Feb 22):526. **65.** Gordon T, et al. *Am J Med.* 1977;62(May): 707. **66.** Beral V, et al. *Lancet.* 1977;2(Oct 8): 727. **67.** Ory H. *Fam Plann Perspect.* 1983;15(March-April): 57. **68.** Arthes FG, et al. *Cancer.* 1971;28(Dec):1391. **69.** Vessey MP, et al. *Br Med J.* 1972;3(Sept 23):719. **70.** Boston Collaborative Drug Surveillance Program. *N Engl J Med.* 1974;290(Jan 3):15. **71.** Vessey MP, et al. *Lancet.* 1975; 1(April 26):941. **72.** Casagrande J, et al. *J Natl Cancer Inst.* 1976;56(April):839. **73.** Kelsey JL, et al. *Am J Epidemiol.* 1978;107(March):236. **74.** Kay CR, *Br Med J.* 1981;282(June 27):2089. **75.** Vessey MP, et al. *Br Med J.* 1981;282(June 27): 2093. **76.** The Cancer and Steroid Hormone Study of the Centers for Disease Control and the National Institute of Child Health and Human Development. Oral contraceptive use and the risk of breast cancer. *N Engl J Med.* 1986;315(Aug 14):405. **77.** Paul C, et al. *Br Med J.* 1986;293(Sept 20):723. **78.** Miller DR, et al. *Obstet Gynecol.* 1986;68(Dec):863. **79.** Pike MC, et al. *Lancet.* 1983;2(Oct 22):926. **80.** McPherson K, et al. *Br J Cancer.* 1987;56(Nov): 653. **81.** Hoover R, et al. *N Engl J Med.* 1976;295(Aug 19): 401. **82.** Lees AW, et al. *Int J Cancer.* 1978;22(Dec):700. **83.** Brinton LA, et al. *J Natl Cancer Inst.* 1979;62(Jan):37. **84.** Black MM. *Pathol Res Pract.* 1980;166:491; and *Cancer.* 1980;46(Dec):2747; and *Cancer.* 1983;51(June):2147. **85.** Thomas DB. *JNCI.* 1993;85(March 3):359. **86.** Brinton LA, et al. *Int J Epidemiol.* 1982;11(Dec):316. **87.** Harris NV, et al. *Am J Epidemiol.* 1982;116(Oct):643. **88.** Jick H, et al. *Am J Epidemiol.* 1980;112(Nov):577. **89.** McPherson K, et al. *Lancet.* 1983;2(Dec 17):1414. **90.** Hoover R, et al. *J Natl Cancer Inst.* 1981;67(Oct):815. **91.** Jick H, et al. *Am J Epidemiol.* 1980;112(Nov):586. **92.** Meirik O, et al. *Lancet.* 1986;2(Sept 20):650. **93.** Fasal E, et al. *J Natl Cancer Inst.* 1975;55(Oct):767. **94.** Paffenbarger RS, et al. *Cancer.* 1977;39(April suppl):1887. **95.** Stadel BV, et al. *Contraception.* 1988;38(Sept):287. **96.** Miller DR, et al. *Am J Epidemiol.* 1989;129(Feb):269. **97.** Kay CR, et al. *Br J Cancer.* 1988;58(Nov):675. **98.** Miller DR, et al. *Obstet Gynecol.* 1986;68(Dec):863. **99.** Hulka BS, et al. *Cancer.* 1994;74(August 1 suppl):1111. **100.** Chilver CED, et al. *Br J Cancer.* 1994;67(May):922. **101.** Huggins GR, et al. *Fertil Steril.* 1987;47(May):733. **102.** Pike MC, et al. *Br J Cancer.* 1981;43(Jan):72. **103.** Ory H, et al. *Am J Obstet Gynecol.* 1976;124(March 15):573. **104.** Stern E, et al. *Science.* 1977;196(June 24):1460. **105.** Peritz E, et al. *Am J Epidemiol.* 1977;106(Dec):462. **106.** Ory HW, et al. In: Garattini S, Berendes H, eds. *Pharmacology of Steroid Contraceptive Drugs.* New York, NY: Raven Press; 1977:211–224. **107.** Meisels A, et al. *Cancer.* 1977;40(Dec):3076. **108.** Goldacre MJ, et al. *Br Med J.* 1978;1(March 25):748. **109.** Swan SH, et al. *Am J Obstet Gynecol.* 1981;139(Jan 1):52. **110.** Vessey MP, et al. *Lancet.* 1983;2(Oct 22):930. **111.** Dallenbach-Hellweg G. *Pathol Res Pract.* 1984;179:38. **112.** Thomas DB, et al. *Br Med J.* 1985;290(March 30):961. **113.** Brinton LA, et al. *Int J Cancer.* 1986;38(Sept):339. **114.** Ebeling K, et al. *Int J Cancer.* 1987;39(April):427. **115.** Beral V. et al. *Lancet.* 1988;2(Dec 10):1331. **116.** Baum JK, et al. *Lancet.* 1973;2(Oct 27):926. **117.** Edmondson HA, et al. *N Engl J Med.* 1976;294(Feb 26):470. **118.** Bein NN, et al. *Br J Surg.* 1977;64(June):433. **119.** Klatskin G. *Gastroenterology.* 1977;73(Aug):386. **120.** Rooks JB, et al. *JAMA.* 1979;242(Aug 17):644. **121.** Sturtevant FM. In: Moghissi K, ed. *Controversies in Contraception,* Baltimore, MD; Williams & Wilkins; 1979:93–150. **122.** Henderson BE, et al. *Br J Cancer.* 1983;48(July):437. **123.** Neuberger J, et al. *Br Med J.* 1986;292(May 24):1355. **124.** Forman D, et al. *Br Med J.* 1986;292(May 24):1357. **125.** La Vecchia C, et al. *Br J Cancer.* 1989;59(March):460. **126.** Savolainen E, et al. *Am J Obstet Gynecol.* 1981;140(July 1):521. **127.** Ferencz C, et al. *Teratology.* 1980;21(April):225. **128.** Rothman KJ, et al. *Am J Epidemiol.* 1979;109(April):433. **129.** Harlap S, et al. *Obstet Gynecol.* 1980;55(April):447. **130.** Layde PM, et al. *J Epidemiol Community Health.* 1982;36(Dec):274. **131.** Rome Group for the Epidemiology and Prevention of Cholelithiasis (GREPCO). *Am J Epidemiol.* 1984;119(May):796. **132.** Strom BL, et al. *Clin Pharmacol Ther.* 1986;39(March):335. **133.** Wynn V. In: Bardin CE, et al. eds. *Progesterone and Progestins.* New York, NY: Raven Press; 1983:395–410. **134.** Perlman JA, et al. *J Chron Dis.* 1985;38(Oct):857. **135.** Powell MG, et al. *Obstet Gynecol.* 1984;63(June):764. **136.** Wynn V, et al. *Lancet.* 1966;2(Oct 1):720. **137.** Fisch IR, et al. *JAMA.* 1977;237(June 6):2499. **138.** Kay CR, *Lancet.* 1977;1(March 19):624. **139.** Laragh JH. *Am J Obstet Gynecol.* 1976;126(Sept 1):141. **140.** Ramcharan S. In: Garattini S. Berendes HW, eds. *Pharmacology of Steroid Contraceptive Drugs.* New York, NY: Raven Press; 1977:277–288. **141.** Laumas KR, et al. *Am J Obstet Gynecol.* 1967;98(June 1):411. **142.** Saxena BN, et al. *Contraception.* 1977;16(Dec): 605. **143.** Nilsson S, et al. *Contraception.* 1978;17(Feb):131. **144.** Washington AE, et al. *JAMA.* 1985;253(April 19):2246. **145.** Louv WC, et al. *Am J Obstet Gynecol.* 1989;160(Feb): 396. **146.** Francis WG, et al. *Can Med Assoc J.* 1965;92(Jan 23):191. **147.** Verhulst HL, et al. *J Clin Pharmacol.* 1967;7(Jan-Feb):9. **148.** Ory HW. *Fam Plann Perspect.* 1982;14(July-Aug):182. **149.** Ory HW, et al. *Making Choices: Evaluating the Health Risks and Benefits of Birth Control Methods.* New York, NY: The Alan Guttmacher Institute; 1983. **150.** Palmer JR, et al. *Am J Epidemiol.* 1989;130(Nov):878. **151.** Romieu I, et al. *J Natl Cancer Inst.* 1989;81(Sept):1313. **152.** Porter JB, et al. *Obstet Gynecol.* 1987;70(July):29. **153.** Olsson H, et al. *Cancer Detect Prev.* 1991;15:265. **154.** Delgado-Rodriguez M, et al. *Rev Epidém Santé Publ.* 1991;39:165 **155.** Clavel F, et al. *Int J Epidemiol.* 1991;20(March):32 **156.** Brinton LA, et al. *JNCI.* 1995;87(June 7):827. **157.** Thomas DB, et al. *Br J Cancer.* 1992;65(January):108. **158.** Thomas DB, et al. *Cancer Causes Cont.* 1991;2(Nov):389 **159.** Weinstein AL, et al. *Epidemiology.* 1991;2(Sept):353. **160.** Ranstam J, et al. *Anticancer Res.* 1991;11(Nov-Dec):2043. **161.** Ursin G. et al. *Epidemiology.* 1992;3(Sept):414. **162.** White E, et al. *JNCI.* 1994;86(April 6):505. **163.** Mann R, et al. *Oral contraceptives and Breast Cancer. Park Ridge, NJ: The Parthenon Publishing Group Inc.; 1980.* **164.** Institute of Medicine. Committee on the Relationship Between Oral Contraceptives and Breast Cancer. *Oral Contraceptives and Breast Cancer.* Washington, DC: National Academy Press; 1991. **165.** Harlap S. *J Reprod Med.* 1991;36(May):374. **166.** Rushton L, et al. *Br J Obstet Gynaecol.* 1992;99(March):239. **167.** Colditz G. *Cancer.* 1993;71(Feb 15 suppl):1480.

BRIEF SUMMARY OF PATIENT WARNINGS

This product (like all oral contraceptives) is intended to prevent pregnancy. It does not protect against HIV infection (AIDS) and other sexually transmitted diseases.

Cigarette smoking increases the risk of serious adverse effects on the heart and blood vessels from oral contraceptive use. This risk increases with age and with heavy smoking (15 or more cigarettes per day) and is quite marked in women over 35 years of age. Women who use oral contraceptives are strongly advised not to smoke.

In the detailed leaflet, "What You Should Know About Oral Contraceptives," which you have received, the risks and benefits of oral contraceptives are discussed in much more detail. That leaflet also provides information on other forms of contraception. ***Please take time to read it carefully for it may have been recently revised.***

If you have any questions or problems regarding this information, contact your doctor.

Oral contraceptives, also known as "birth control pills" or "the pill," are taken to prevent pregnancy and, when taken correctly, have a failure rate of about 1% per year when used without missing any pills. The typical failure rate of large numbers of pill users is less than 3% per year when women who miss pills are included. However, forgetting to take pills considerably increases the chances of pregnancy.

For most women, oral contraceptives are free of serious or unpleasant side effects. However, oral contraceptive use is associated with certain serious diseases or conditions that can cause severe disability or death, though rarely. There are some women who are at high risk of developing certain serious diseases that can be life-threatening or may cause temporary or permanent disability. The risks associated with taking oral contraceptives increase significantly if you:

- smoke, or
- have high blood pressure, diabetes, high cholesterol, or are overweight, or
- have or have had clotting disorders, heart attack, stroke, angina pectoris (chest pains on exertion), cancer of the breast or sex organs, jaundice (yellowing of the skin or whites of the eyes), or malignant (cancerous) or benign (noncancerous) liver tumors.

Women should not use oral contraceptives if they suspect they are pregnant or if they have unexplained vaginal bleeding.

Most side effects of the pill are not serious. The most common effects are nausea, vomiting, bleeding between menstrual periods, weight gain, breast tenderness, and difficulty wearing contact lenses. These side effects, especially nausea and vomiting, may subside within the first three months of use.

Proper use of oral contraceptives requires that they be taken under your doctor's continuing supervision, because they can be associated with serious side effects. The serious side effects of the pill occur very infrequently, especially if you are in good health and are young. However, you should know that the following medical conditions have been associated with or made worse by the pill, and that certain of the risks may persist after use of the pill has been discontinued:

1. Blood clots in the legs, arms, lungs, heart (heart attack), eyes, abdomen, or elsewhere in the body. As mentioned above, smoking increases the risk of heart attacks and strokes and subsequent serious medical consequences.
2. Stroke, due to a blood clot, or to bleeding in the brain (hemorrhage) as a result of bursting of a blood vessel. Stroke can lead to paralysis in all or part of the body, or to death.
3. Liver tumors, which may rupture and cause severe bleeding and death. A possible, but not definite, association has also been found with the pill and liver cancer. However, with or without use of the pill, liver cancers are extremely rare in the United States.
4. High blood pressure, although blood pressure ordinarily, but not always, returns to original levels when the pill is stopped.
5. Gallbladder disease, which might require surgery.

The symptoms associated with these serious side effects are discussed in the detailed leaflet given to you with your supply of pills. Notify your doctor or health care provider if you notice any unusual physical disturbances while taking the pill. In addition, you should be aware that drugs such as antiepileptics, antibiotics (especially rifampin), as well as certain other drugs, may decrease oral contraceptive effectiveness.

There is a conflict among studies regarding breast cancer and oral contraceptive use. Some studies have reported an increase in the risk of developing breast cancer, particularly at a younger age. This increased risk appears to be related to duration of use. The majority of studies have found no overall increase in the risk of developing breast cancer. Some studies have found an increase in the incidence of cancer of the cervix in women who use oral contraceptives. However, this finding may be related to factors other than the use of oral contraceptives. There is insufficient evidence to rule out the possibility that pills may cause such cancers.

Taking the pill may provide some important non-contraceptive benefits. These include less painful menstruation, less menstrual blood loss and anemia, less risk of fibroids, pelvic infections, and noncancerous breast diseases, and less risk of cancer of the ovary and of the lining of the uterus (womb).

Be sure to discuss any medical condition you may have with your health care provider. He or she will take a medical and family history before prescribing oral contraceptives and will also examine you. The physical examination may be delayed to another time if you request it and the health care provider believes that it is a good medical practice to postpone it. You should be reexamined at least once a year while taking oral contraceptives. The detailed patient information leaflet gives you further information that you should read and discuss with your health care provider.

DETAILED PATIENT LABELING

What you should know about oral contraceptives

This product (like all oral contraceptives) is intended to prevent pregnancy. It does not protect against HIV infection (AIDS) and other sexually transmitted diseases.

INTRODUCTION

You should not use Demulen 1/50, which contains higher doses of estrogen than other oral contraceptives, unless specifically recommended by your health care provider.

It is important that any woman who considers using an oral contraceptive understand the risks involved. Although the oral contraceptives have important advantages over other methods of contraception, they have certain risks that no other method has. Only you and your physician can decide whether the advantages are worth these risks. This leaflet will tell you about the most important risks. It will explain how you can help your doctor prescribe the pill as safely as possible by telling him/her about yourself and being alert for the earliest signs of trouble. And it will tell you how to use the pill properly so that it will be as effective as possible. THERE IS MORE DETAILED INFORMATION AVAILABLE IN THE LEAFLET PREPARED FOR DOCTORS. Your pharmacist can show you a copy or you can request one from the manufacturer by phoning toll-free 1-800-323-4204; you may need your doctor's help in understanding parts of it.

This leaflet is not a replacement for a careful discussion between you and your health care provider. You should discuss the information provided in this leaflet with him or her, both when you first start taking the pill and during your revisits. You should also follow your health care provider's advice with regard to regular check-ups while you are on the pill.

If you do not have any of the conditions listed below and are thinking about using oral contraceptives, to help you decide, you need information about the advantages and risks of oral contraceptives and of other contraceptive methods as well. This leaflet describes the advantages and risks of oral contraceptives. Except for sterilization, the intrauterine device (IUD), and abortion, which have their own specific risks, the only risks of other methods are those due to pregnancy should the method fail. Your doctor can answer questions you may have with respect to other methods of contraception, and further questions you may have on oral contraceptives after reading this leaflet.

WHAT ARE ORAL CONTRACEPTIVES?

The most common type of oral contraceptive, often simply called "the pill," is a combination of estrogen and progestogen, the two kinds of female hormones. The amount of estrogen and progestogen can vary, but the amount of estrogen is more important because both the effectiveness and some of the dangers of the pill have been related to the amount of estrogen. The pill works principally by preventing release of an egg from the ovary during the cycle in which the pills are taken.

EFFECTIVENESS OF ORAL CONTRACEPTIVES

The pill is one of the most effective methods of birth control. When they are taken correctly, without missing any pills, the chance of becoming pregnant is less than 1% (1 pregnancy per 100 women per year of use) when used perfectly, without missing any pills. Typical failure rates are actually about 3% per year. The chance of becoming pregnant increases with each missed pill during a menstrual cycle.

Continued on next page

Demulen—Cont.

In comparison, typical failure rates for other methods of birth control during the first year of use are as follows:
[See table below]

WHO SHOULD NOT TAKE ORAL CONTRACEPTIVES

Cigarette smoking increases the risk of serious adverse effects on the heart and blood vessels from oral contraceptive use. This risk increases with age and with heavy smoking (15 or more cigarettes per day) and is quite marked in women over 35 years of age. Women who use oral contraceptives are strongly advised not to smoke.

Some women should not use the pill. For example, you should not take the pill if you are pregnant or think you may be pregnant. You should also not use the pill if you have any of the following conditions:

- Heart attack or stroke (blood clot or hemorrhage in the brain), currently or in the past.
- Blood clots in the legs (thrombophlebitis), lungs (pulmonary embolism), eyes, or elsewhere in the body, currently or in the past.
- Chest pain (angina pectoris), currently or in the past.
- Known or suspected breast cancer or cancer of the lining of the uterus (womb), cervix, or vagina, currently or in the past.
- Unexplained vaginal bleeding (until a diagnosis is reached by your doctor).
- Yellowing of the whites of the eyes or of the skin (jaundice) during pregnancy or during previous use of the pill.
- Liver tumor (whether cancerous or not), currently or in the past.
- Known or suspected pregnancy (one or more menstrual periods missed).

Tell your health care provider if you have ever had any of these conditions. He or she can recommend a safer method of birth control.

OTHER CONSIDERATIONS BEFORE TAKING ORAL CONTRACEPTIVES

Tell your health care provider if you have or have had any of the following conditions, as he or she will want to watch them closely or they might cause him or her to suggest using another method of contraception:

- Breast nodules (lumps), fibrocystic disease (breast cysts), abnormal mammograms (x-ray pictures of the breast), or abnormal Pap smears
- Diabetes
- High blood pressure
- High blood cholesterol or triglycerides
- Migraine or other headaches or epilepsy
- Mental depression
- Gallbladder, heart, or kidney disease
- History of scanty or irregular menstrual periods
- Problems during a prior pregnancy
- Fibroid tumors of the womb
- History of jaundice (yellowing of the whites of the eyes or of the skin)
- Varicose veins
- Tuberculosis
- Plans for elective surgery

Women with any of these conditions should be checked often by their health care provider if they choose to use oral contraceptives.

Percentage of women experiencing an unintended pregnancy during the first year of typical use and the first year of perfect use of contraception and the percentage continuing use at the end of the first year. United States.

Method (1)	% of women experiencing an unintended pregnancy within the first year of use: Typical use[A] (2)	Perfect use[B] (3)	% of women continuing use at one year[C] (4)
Chance[D]	85	85	
Spermicides[E]	26	6	40
Periodic abstinence	25		63
Calendar		9	
Ovulation method		3	
Sympto-thermal[F]		2	
Post-ovulation		1	
Withdrawal	19	4	
Cap[G]			
Parous women	40	26	42
Nulliparous women	20	9	56
Sponge			
Parous women	40	20	42
Nulliparous women	20	9	56
Diaphragm[G]	20	6	56
Condom[H]			
Female (Reality)	21	5	56
Male	14	3	61
Pill	5		71
Progestin only		0.5	
Combined		0.1	
IUD			
Progesterone T	2.0	1.5	81
Copper T 380A	0.8	0.6	78
LNg 20	0.1	0.1	81
Injection (Depo-Provera)	0.3	0.3	70
Implant (Norplant and Norplant-2)	0.05	0.05	88
Female sterilization	0.5	0.5	100
Male sterilization	0.15	0.10	100

Emergency Contraceptive Pills: Treatment initiated within 72 hours after unprotected intercourse reduces the risk of pregnancy by at least 75%.[I]

Lactational Amenorrhea Method: LAM is a highly effective, *temporary* method of contraception.[J]

Source: Trussell J, Contraceptive efficacy. In Hatcher RA, Trussell J, Stewart F, Cates W, Stewart GK, Kowal D, Guest F, *Contraceptive Technology: Seventeenth Revised Edition.* New York NY: Irvington Publishers, 1998, in press.[1]

[A] Among *typical* couples who initiate use of a method (not necessarily for the first time), the percentage who experience an accidental pregnancy during the first year if they do not stop use for any other reason.

[B] Among couples who initiate use of a method (not necessarily for the first time) and who use it *perfectly* (both consistently and correctly), the percentage who experience an accidental pregnancy during the first year if they do not stop use for any other reason.

[C] Among couples attempting to avoid pregnancy, the percentage who continue to use a method for one year.

[D] The percents becoming pregnant in columns (2) and (3) are based on data from populations where contraception is not used and from women who cease using contraception in order to become pregnant. Among such populations, about 89% become pregnant within one year. This estimate was lowered slightly (to 85%) to represent the percent who would become pregnant within one year among women now relying on reversible methods of contraception if they abandoned contraception altogether.

[E] Foams, creams, gels, vaginal suppositories, and vaginal film.

[F] Cervical mucus (ovulation) method supplemented by calendar in the pre-ovulatory and basal body temperature in the post-ovulatory phases.

[G] With spermicidal cream or jelly.

[H] Without spermicides.

[I] The treatment schedule is one dose within 72 hours after unprotected intercourse, and a second dose 12 hours after the first dose. The Food and Drug Administration has declared the following brands of oral contraceptives to be safe and effective for emergency contraception: Ovral (1 dose is 2 white pills), Alesse (1 dose is 5 pink pills), Nordette or Levlen (1 dose is 2 light-orange pills), Lo/Ovral (1 dose is 4 white pills), Triphasil or Tri-Levlen (1 dose is 4 yellow pills).

[J] However, to maintain effective protection against pregnancy, another method of contraception must be used as soon as menstruation resumes, the frequency or duration of breastfeeds is reduced, bottle feeds are introduced or the baby reaches six months of age.

Also, be sure to tell your doctor if you smoke or are on any medications.

RISKS OF TAKING ORAL CONTRACEPTIVES

1. Risk of developing blood clots. Blood clots and blockage of blood vessels are the most serious side effects of taking oral contraceptives. In particular, a clot in the legs can cause thrombophlebitis and a clot that travels to the lungs can cause a sudden blocking of the vessel carrying blood to the lungs. Rarely, clots occur in the blood vessels of the eye and may cause blindness, double vision, or impaired vision.

If you take oral contraceptives and need elective surgery, need to stay in bed for a prolonged illness, or have recently delivered a baby, you may be at risk of developing blood clots. You should consult your doctor about stopping oral contraceptives 3 to 4 weeks before surgery and not taking oral contraceptives for 2 weeks after surgery or during bed rest. You should also not take oral contraceptives soon after delivery of a baby. It is advisable to wait for at least 4 weeks after delivery if you are not breast feeding. If you are breast feeding, you should wait until you have weaned your child before using the pill. (See also the section on Breast feeding in General Precautions.)

The risk of circulatory disease in oral contraceptive users may be higher in users of high-dose pills and may be greater with longer duration of oral contraceptive use. In addition, some of these increased risks may continue for a number of years after stopping oral contraceptives. The risk of abnormal blood clotting increases with age in both users and nonusers of oral contraceptives, but the increased risk from the oral contraceptive appears to be present at all ages. For women aged 20 to 44 it is estimated that about 1 in 2,000 using oral contraceptives will be hospitalized each year because of abnormal clotting. Among nonusers in the same age group, about 1 in 20,000 would be hospitalized each year. For oral contraceptive users in general, it has been estimated that in women between the ages of 15 and 34, the risk of death due to a circulatory disorder is about 1 in 12,000 per year, whereas for nonusers the rate is about 1 in 50,000 per year. In the age group 35 to 44, the risk is estimated to be about 1 in 2,500 per year for oral contraceptive users and about 1 in 10,000 per year for nonusers.

2. Heart attacks and strokes. Oral contraceptives may increase the tendency to develop strokes (stoppage by blood clots or rupture of blood vessels of the brain) and angina pectoris and heart attacks (blockage of blood vessels of the heart). Any of these conditions can cause death or permanent disability.

Smoking greatly increases the possibility of suffering heart attacks and strokes. Furthermore, smoking and the use of oral contraceptives greatly increases the chances of developing and dying of heart disease.

3. Gallbladder disease. Oral contraceptive users probably have a greater risk than nonusers of having gallbladder disease, although this risk may be related to pills containing high doses of estrogens.

4. Liver tumors. In rare cases, oral contraceptives can cause benign but dangerous liver tumors. These benign tumors can rupture and cause fatal internal bleeding. In addition, a possible but not definite association has been found with the pill and liver cancers in several studies, in which a few women who developed these very rare cancers were found to have used oral contraceptives for long periods. However, liver cancers are rare.

5. Cancer of the reproductive organs and breasts. There is conflict among studies regarding breast cancer and oral contraceptive use. Some studies have reported an increase in the risk of developing breast cancer, particularly at a younger age. This increased risk appears to be related to duration of use. The majority of studies have found no overall increase in the risk of developing breast cancer. Women who use oral contraceptives and have a strong family history of breast cancer or who have had breast nodules or abnormal mammograms should be closely followed by their doctors.

Some studies have found an increase in the incidence of cancer of the cervix in women who use oral contraceptives. However, this finding may be related to factors other than the use of oral contraceptives. There is insufficient evidence to rule out the possibility that pills may cause such cancers.

ESTIMATED RISK OF DEATH FROM A BIRTH CONTROL METHOD OR PREGNANCY

All methods of birth control and pregnancy are associated with a risk of developing certain diseases that may lead to disability or death. An estimate of the number of deaths associated with different methods of birth control and pregnancy has been calculated and is shown in the following table.

[See table at bottom of next page]

In the above table, the risk of death from any birth control method is less than the risk of childbirth, except for oral contraceptive users over the age of 35 who smoke and pill users over the age of 40 even if they do not smoke. It can be seen in the table that for women aged 15 to 39, the risk of death was highest with pregnancy (7–26 deaths per 100,000 women, depending on age). Among pill users who do not smoke, the risk of death was always lower than that associated with pregnancy for any age group, although over the age of 40, the risk increases to 32 deaths per 100,000 women, compared to 28 associated with pregnancy at that age. However, for pill users who smoke and are over the age of 35, the estimated number of deaths exceeds those for other methods of birth control. If a woman is over the age of 40 and smokes, her estimated risk of death is four times higher (117/100,000 women) than the estimated risk associated with pregnancy (28/100,000) in that age group.

The suggestion that women over 40 who don't smoke should not take oral contraceptives is based on information from older high-dose pills and on less selective use of pills than is practiced today. An Advisory Committee of the FDA discussed this issue in 1989 and recommended that the benefits of oral contraceptive use by healthy, nonsmoking women over 40 years of age may outweigh the possible risks. However, all women, especially older women, are cautioned to use the lowest dose pill that is effective.

WARNING SIGNALS

If any of these adverse effects occur while you are taking oral contraceptives, call your doctor immediately:

- Sharp chest pain, coughing up of blood, or sudden shortness of breath (indicating a possible blood clot in the lung)
- Pain in the calf (indicating a possible blood clot in the leg)
- Crushing chest pain or heaviness in the chest (indicating a possible heart attack)
- Sudden severe headache or vomiting, dizziness or fainting, disturbances of vision or speech, or numbness in an arm or leg (indicating a possible stroke)
- Sudden partial or complete loss of vision (indicating a possible blood clot in the blood vessels of the eye)
- Breast lumps (indicating possible breast cancer or fibrocystic disease of the breast). Ask your doctor or health care provider to show you how to examine your own breasts
- Severe pain or tenderness or a mass in the stomach area (indicating a possibly ruptured liver tumor)
- Difficulty in sleeping, weakness, lack of energy, fatigue, or change in mood (possibly indicating severe depression)
- Jaundice or a yellowing of the skin or eyeballs, accompanied frequently by fever, fatigue, loss of appetite, dark-colored urine, or light-colored bowel movements (indicating possible liver problems)
- Unusual swelling
- Other unusual conditions

SIDE EFFECTS OF ORAL CONTRACEPTIVES

1. Vaginal bleeding

Spotting. This is a slight staining between your menstrual periods that may not even require a pad. Some women spot even though they take their pills exactly as directed. Many women spot although they have never taken the pills. Spotting does not mean that your ovaries are releasing an egg. Spotting may be the result of irregular pill-taking. Getting back on schedule will usually stop it.

If you should spot while taking the pills, you should not be alarmed, because spotting usually stops by itself within a few days. It seldom occurs after the first pill cycle. Consult your doctor if spotting persists for more than a few days or if it occurs after the second cycle.

Unexpected (breakthrough) bleeding. Unexpected (breakthrough) bleeding does not mean that your ovaries have released an egg. It seldom occurs, but when it does happen it is most common in the first pill cycle. It is a flow much like a regular period, requiring the use of a pad or tampon.

If you experience breakthrough bleeding use a pad or tampon and continue with your schedule. Usually your periods will become regular within a few cycles. Breakthrough bleeding will seldom bother you again.

Consult your doctor or health care provider if breakthrough bleeding is heavy, does not stop within a week, or if it occurs after the second cycle.

2. Contact lenses. If you wear contact lenses and notice a change in vision or an inability to wear your lenses, contact your doctor or health care provider.

3. Fluid retention or raised blood pressure. Oral contraceptives may cause edema (fluid retention), with swelling of the fingers or ankles. If you experience fluid retention, contact your doctor or health care provider. Some women develop high blood pressure while on the pill, which ordinarily, but not always, returns to the original levels when the pill is stopped. High blood pressure predisposes one to strokes, heart attacks, kidney disease, and other diseases of the blood vessels.

4. Melasma. A spotty darkening of the skin is possible, particularly of the face. This may persist after the pill is discontinued.

5. Other side effects. Other side effects may include nausea and vomiting, change in appetite, headache, nervousness, depression, dizziness, loss of scalp hair, rash, and vaginal infections.

If any of these, or other, side effects occur, call your doctor or health care provider.

GENERAL PRECAUTIONS

1. Missed periods and use of oral contraceptives before or during early pregnancy. Occasionally women who are taking the pill miss periods. It has been reported to occur as frequently as several times each year in some women, depending on various factors such as age and prior history. (Your doctor is the best source of information about this.) The pill should not be used when you are pregnant or suspect you may be pregnant. Very rarely, women who are using the pill as directed become pregnant. The likelihood of becoming pregnant is higher if you occasionally miss one or two pills. Therefore, if you miss a period you should consult your physician before continuing to take the pill. If you miss a period, especially if you have not taken the pill regularly, you should use an alternative method of contraception until pregnancy has been ruled out; if you have missed more than one pill at any time, you should immediately start using an additional method of contraception and complete your pill cycle.

There is no conclusive evidence that oral contraceptive use is associated with an increase in birth defects when taken inadvertently during early pregnancy. Previously, a few studies had reported that oral contraceptives might be associated with birth defects, but these findings have not been seen in more recent studies. Nevertheless, oral contraceptives or any other drugs should not be used during pregnancy unless clearly necessary and prescribed by your doctor. You should check with your doctor about risks to your unborn child of any medication taken during pregnancy.

2. Breast feeding. If you are breast feeding, consult your doctor before starting oral contraceptives. Some of the drug will be passed on to the child in the milk. A few adverse effects on the child have been reported, including yellowing of the skin (jaundice) and breast enlargement. In addition, oral contraceptives may decrease the amount and quality of your milk. If possible, do not use oral contraceptives while breast feeding. You should use another method of contraception since breast feeding provides only partial protection from becoming pregnant and this partial protection decreases significantly as you breast feed for longer periods of time. You should consider starting oral contraceptives only after you have weaned your child completely.

3. Laboratory tests. If you are scheduled for any laboratory tests, tell your doctor you are taking birth control pills. Certain blood tests may be affected by birth control pills.

4. Drug interactions. Certain drugs may interact with birth control pills to make them less effective in preventing pregnancy or cause an increase in breakthrough bleeding. Such drugs include rifampin, drugs used for epilepsy such as barbiturates (for example, phenobarbital) and phenytoin (Dilantin is one brand of this drug), phenylbutazone (Butazolidin is one brand), Rezulin (troglitazone) a hypoglycemic, and possibly certain antibiotics. You may need to use additional contraception when you take drugs that can make oral contraceptives less effective.

Oral contraceptives may have an influence upon the way other drugs act. Check with your doctor if you are taking *any* other drugs while you are on the pill.

HOW TO TAKE THE PILL

IMPORTANT POINTS TO REMEMBER

BEFORE YOU START TAKING YOUR PILLS:

1. BE SURE TO READ THESE DIRECTIONS:
   - Before you start taking your pills.
   - Anytime you are not sure what to do.
2. THE RIGHT WAY TO TAKE THE PILL IS TO TAKE ONE PILL EVERY DAY AT THE SAME TIME.
   If you miss pills you could get pregnant. This includes starting the pack late.
   The more pills you miss, the more likely you are to get pregnant.
3. MANY WOMEN HAVE SPOTTING OR LIGHT BLEEDING, OR MAY FEEL SICK TO THEIR STOMACH DURING THE FIRST 1–3 PACKS OF PILLS.
   If you feel sick to your stomach, do not stop taking the pill. The problem will usually go away. If it doesn't go away, check with your doctor or clinic.
4. MISSING PILLS CAN ALSO CAUSE SPOTTING OR LIGHT BLEEDING, even when you make up these missed pills. On the days you take 2 pills to make up to for missed pills, you could also feel a little sick to your stomach.
5. IF YOU HAVE VOMITING OR DIARRHEA, for any reason, or IF YOU TAKE SOME MEDICINES, including some antibiotics, your pills may not work as well.
   Use a backup method (such as condoms, foam, or sponge) until you check with your doctor or clinic.
6. IF YOU HAVE TROUBLE REMEMBERING TO TAKE THE PILL, talk to your doctor or clinic about how to make pill-taking easier or about using another method of birth control.
7. IF YOU HAVE ANY QUESTIONS OR ARE UNSURE ABOUT THE INFORMATION IN THIS LEAFLET, call your doctor or clinic.

Annual number of birth-related or method-related deaths associated with control of fertility per 100,000 nonsterile women, by fertility control method according to age.

	Age					
Method of control	**15–19**	**20–24**	**25–29**	**30–34**	**35–39**	**40–44**
No fertility control methods*	7.0	7.4	9.1	14.8	25.7	28.2
Oral contraceptives						
nonsmoker**	0.3	0.5	0.9	1.9	13.8	31.6
smoker**	2.2	3.4	6.6	13.5	51.1	117.2
IUD**	0.8	0.8	1.0	1.0	1.4	1.4
Condom*	1.1	1.6	0.7	0.2	0.3	0.4
Diaphragm/ spermicide*	1.9	1.2	1.2	1.3	2.2	2.8
Periodic abstinence*	2.5	1.6	1.6	1.7	2.9	3.6

* Deaths are birth-related
** Deaths are method-related

BEFORE YOU START TAKING YOUR PILLS

1. DECIDE WHAT TIME OF DAY YOU WANT TO TAKE YOUR PILL.
   It is important to take it at about the same time every day.
2. LOOK AT YOUR PILL PACK TO SEE IF IT HAS 21 OR 28 PILLS:
   Your Compack tablet dispenser consists of a case and a pill pack containing 21 or 28 pills. They are arranged in three or four numbered rows with the days of the week printed above them. The 21-pill pack has 21 "active" white pills (with hormones) to take for 3 weeks, followed by 1 week without pills. The 28-pill pack has 21 "active" white pills (with hormones) to take for 3 weeks, followed by 1 week of reminder blue or pink pills (without hormones). To remove a pill press down on it with the flat of your finger. The pill will drop through a hole in the bottom of the Compack.
3. ALSO FIND:
   - Where on the pack to start taking pills.
   - In what order to take the pills (follow the arrows).

Begin the **21-pill pack** with the pill in Row 1 under the day that your doctor or clinic told you to start and continue (→) across Row 1 and then follow the arrow down to the far left of Row 2 and continue across and then down to the far left of Row 3, and finally back up to the far left of Row 1 if any pills remain.

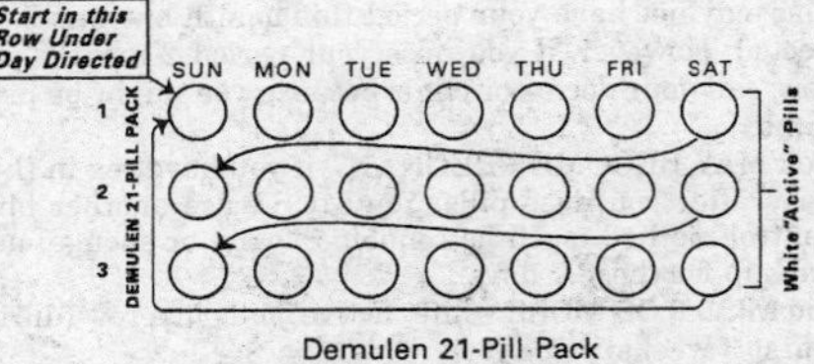

Demulen 21-Pill Pack

Begin the **28-pill pack** with the pill in Row 1 and continue (→) across Row 1 (Week 1). Follow the arrows and repeat for Row 2, Row 3, and finally Row 4. Take all white active pills before starting Row 4.

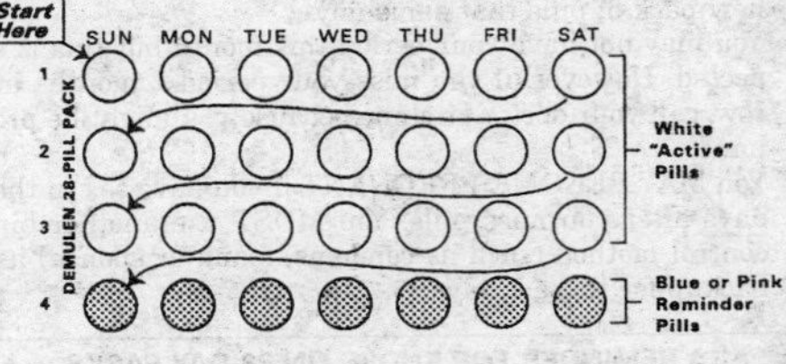

Demulen 28-Pill Pack

- BE SURE YOU HAVE READY AT ALL TIMES:
  - ANOTHER KIND OF BIRTH CONTROL (such as condoms, foam, or sponge) to use as backup in case you miss pills.
  - AN EXTRA, FULL PILL PACK.

WHEN TO START THE FIRST PACK OF PILLS

You have a choice of which day to start taking your first pack of pills. Decide with your doctor or clinic which is the best day for you. Pick a time of day which will be easy to remember.

DAY 1 START:

1. Take the first "active" white pill of the first pack during the first 24 hours of your period.
2. You will not need to use a backup method of birth control, since you are starting the pill at the beginning of your period.

SUNDAY START:

1. Take the first "active" white pill of the first pack on the Sunday after your period starts, even if you are still bleeding. If your period begins on Sunday, start the pack that same day.
2. Use another method of birth control as a backup method if you have sex anytime from the Sunday you start your

Continued on next page

Demulen—Cont.

first pack until the next Sunday (7 days). Condoms, foam, or the sponge are good backup methods of birth control.

WHAT TO DO DURING THE MONTH

1. **TAKE ONE PILL AT THE SAME TIME EVERY DAY UNTIL THE PACK IS EMPTY.**
   - Do not skip pills even if you are spotting or bleeding between monthly periods or feel sick to your stomach (nausea).
   - Do not skip pills even if you do not have sex very often.
2. **WHEN YOU FINISH A PACK OR SWITCH YOUR BRAND OF 21-DAY PILLS:** Wait 7 days to start the next pack. You will probably have your period during that week. Be sure that no more than 7 days pass between 21-day packs.
   WHEN YOU FINISH A PACK OR SWITCH YOUR BRAND OF 28-DAY PILLS: Start the next pack on the day after your last "reminder" pill. Do not wait any days between 28-day packs.

WHAT TO DO IF YOU MISS PILLS

If you **MISS 1** white "active" pill:
1. Take it as soon as you remember. Take the next pill at your regular time. This means you may take 2 pills in 1 day.
2. You do not need to use a backup birth control method if you have sex.

If you **MISS 2** white "active" pills in a row in **WEEK 1 OR WEEK 2** of your pack:
1. Take 2 pills on the day you remember and 2 pills the next day.
2. Then take 1 pill a day until you finish the pack.
3. You MAY BECOME PREGNANT if you have sex in the 7 days after you miss pills. You MUST use another birth control method (such as condoms, foam, or sponge) as a backup for those 7 days.

If you **MISS 2** white "active" pills in a row in **THE 3rd WEEK:**
1. ***If you are a Day 1 Starter:***
   THROW OUT the rest of the pill pack and start a new pack that same day.
   If you are a Sunday Starter:
   Keep taking 1 pill every day until Sunday.
   On Sunday, THROW OUT the rest of the pack and start a new pack of pills that same day.
2. You may not have your period this month but this is expected. However, if you miss your period 2 months in a row, call your doctor or clinic because you might be pregnant.
3. You MAY BECOME PREGNANT if you have sex in the 7 days after you miss pills. You MUST use another birth control method (such as condoms, foam, or sponge) as a backup for those 7 days.

If you **MISS 3 OR MORE** white "active" pills in a row (during the first 3 weeks):
1. ***If you are a Day 1 Starter:***
   THROW OUT the rest of the pill pack and start a new pack of pills that same day.
   If you are a Sunday Starter:
   Keep taking 1 pill every day until Sunday.
   On Sunday, THROW OUT the rest of the pack and start a new pack of pills that same day.
2. You may not have your period this month but this is expected. However, if you miss your period 2 months in a row, call your doctor or clinic because you might be pregnant.
3. You MAY BECOME PREGNANT if you have sex in the 7 days after you miss pills. You MUST use another birth control method (such as condoms, foam, or sponge) as a backup for those 7 days.

A REMINDER FOR THOSE ON 28-DAY PACKS

If you forget any of the 7 blue or pink "reminder" pills in Week 4:
- THROW AWAY the pills you missed.
- Keep taking 1 pill each day until the pack is empty.
- You do not need a backup method.

FINALLY, IF YOU ARE STILL NOT SURE WHAT TO DO ABOUT THE PILLS YOU HAVE MISSED

- Use a BACKUP METHOD of birth control anytime you have sex.
- KEEP TAKING ONE "ACTIVE" PILL EACH DAY until you can reach your doctor or clinic.

PREGNANCY DUE TO PILL FAILURE

The incidence of pill failure resulting in pregnancy is approximately 1% (ie, one pregnancy per 100 women per year) if taken every day as directed, but, because some women fail to follow the daily schedule, more typical failure rates are about 3%. If you become pregnant, you should discuss your pregnancy with your doctor.

PREGNANCY AFTER STOPPING THE PILL

There may be some delay in becoming pregnant after you stop using oral contraceptives, especially if you had irregular menstrual cycles before you used oral contraceptives. It may be advisable to postpone conception until you begin menstruating regularly once you have stopped taking the pill and desire pregnancy.

There does not appear to be any increase in birth defects in newborn babies when pregnancy occurs after stopping the pill.

OVERDOSAGE

Serious ill effects have not been reported following ingestion of large doses of oral contraceptives by young children. Overdosage may cause nausea and withdrawal bleeding in females. In case of overdosage, contact your health care provider, pharmacist, or Poison Control Center.

OTHER INFORMATION

Your health care provider will take a medical and family history before prescribing oral contraceptives and will also examine you. The physical examination may be delayed to another time if you request it and the health care provider believes that it is a good medical practice to postpone it. You should be reexamined at least once a year. Certain health problems or conditions in your medical or family history may require that your doctor see you more frequently while you are taking the pill. Be sure to keep all appointments with your health care provider because this is a time to determine if there are early signs of side effects of oral contraceptive use.

Do not use the drug for any condition other than the one for which it was prescribed. This drug has been prescribed specifically for you; do not give it to others who may want birth control pills.

This product (like all oral contraceptives) is intended to prevent pregnancy. It does not protect against transmission of HIV (AIDS) and other sexually transmitted diseases such as chlamydia, genital herpes, genital warts, gonorrhea, hepatitis B, and syphilis.

HEALTH BENEFITS FROM ORAL CONTRACEPTIVES

In addition to preventing pregnancy, use of oral contraceptives may provide certain benefits. They are:
- Menstrual cycles may become more regular
- Blood flow during menstruation may be lighter and less iron may be lost. Therefore, anemia due to iron deficiency is less likely to occur.
- Pain or other symptoms during menstruation may be encountered less frequently
- Ectopic (tubal) pregnancy may occur less frequently
- Noncancerous cysts or lumps in the breast may occur less frequently
- Acute pelvic inflammatory disease may occur less frequently
- Fibroids of the uterus (womb) may occur less frequently
- Oral contraceptive use may provide some protection against developing two forms of cancer: cancer of the ovaries and cancer of the lining of the uterus (womb)

If you want more information about birth control pills, ask your doctor or pharmacist. They have a more technical leaflet called the Professional Labeling, which you may wish to read. The Professional Labeling is also published in a book entitled *Physicians' Desk Reference,* available in many book stores and public libraries.

Be certain to read new revisions of this leaflet. You may check the date of the most recent revision by phoning the manufacturer toll-free at 1-800-323-4204 or by writing to the address below.

Keep this and all medications out of the reach of children.
Store below 77°F (25°C).

Rx only 4/29/98

G.D. Searle & Co.
Chicago IL 60680 USA
©1998, G.D. Searle & Co.

Shown in Product Identification Guide, page 335

FLAGYL® 375 ℞

[flaj 'yl]
(metronidazole capsules)

WARNING
Metronidazole has been shown to be carcinogenic in mice and rats. (See **PRECAUTIONS.**) Unnecessary use of the drug should be avoided. Its use should be reserved for the conditions described in the **INDICATIONS AND USAGE** section below.

DESCRIPTION

Metronidazole is an oral synthetic antiprotozoal and antibacterial agent, 2-Methyl-5-nitroimidazole-1-ethanol, which has the following structural formula:

CH_2CH_2OH / O_2N / N / CH_3 / N

Flagyl® 375 capsules contain 375 mg of metronidazole USP. Inactive ingredients include corn starch, magnesium stearate, gelatin, black iron oxide, titanium dioxide, FD&C Green No. 3, and D&C Yellow No. 10.

CLINICAL PHARMACOLOGY

Disposition of metronidazole in the body is similar for both oral and intravenous dosage forms, with an average elimination half-life in healthy humans of 8 hours.

The major route of elimination of metronidazole and its metabolites is via the urine (60% to 80% of the dose), with fecal excretion accounting for 6% to 15% of the dose. The metabolites that appear in the urine result primarily from side-chain oxidation (1-(β-hydroxyethyl)-2-hydroxymethyl-5-nitroimidazole and 2-methyl-5-nitroimidazole-1-yl-acetic acid] and glucuronide conjugation, with unchanged metronidazole accounting for approximately 20% of the total. Renal clearance of metronidazole is approximately 10 mL/min/1.73m^2.

Metronidazole is the major component appearing in the plasma, with lesser quantities of the 2-hydroxymethyl metabolite also being present. Less than 20% of the circulating metronidazole is bound to plasma proteins. Both the parent compound and the metabolite possess *in vitro* bactericidal activity against most strains of anaerobic bacteria and *in vitro* trichomonacidal activity.

Metronidazole appears in cerebrospinal fluid, saliva, and human milk in concentrations similar to those found in plasma. Bactericidal concentrations of metronidazole have also been detected in pus from hepatic abscesses.

Flagyl® 375 capsules have been shown to have a rate and extent of absorption similar to metronidazole tablets (Flagyl®) and were bioequivalent at an equal single dose of 750 mg. In a study conducted with 23 adult, healthy, female volunteers, oral administration of two 375-mg Flagyl® capsules under fasted conditions produced a mean (± 1 SD) peak plasma concentration (C_{max}) of 21.4 (±2.8) mcg/mL with a mean T_{max} of 1.6 (± 0.7) hours and a mean area under the plasma concentration-time curve (AUC) of 223 (± 44) mcg·hr/mL. In the same study, three 250-mg Flagyl® tablets produced a mean C_{max} of 20.4 (± 3.8) mcg/mL with a mean T_{max} of 1.4 (± 0.4) hours and a mean AUC of 218 (± 50) mcg·hr/mL.

Administration of Flagyl® 375 capsules with food does not affect the extent of absorption of metronidazole; however, the presence of food results in a lower C_{max} and a delayed T_{max} compared to fasted conditions. In a study of 14 healthy, adult, female volunteers, administration of Flagyl® 375 capsules under fasting conditions produced a mean C_{max} of 10.9 (± 1.5) mcg/mL, a mean T_{max} of 1.5 (± 1.4) hours, and a mean AUC of 110 (± 34) mcg·hr/mL compared to a mean C_{max} of 8.6 (± 1.6) mcg/mL, a mean T_{max} of 4.2 (± 1.7) hours, and a mean AUC of 99 (±14) mcg·hr/mL under fed conditions.

Decreased renal function does not alter the single-dose pharmacokinetics of metronidazole. However, plasma clearance of metronidazole is decreased in patients with decreased liver function.

Microbiology:

Metronidazole exerts antimicrobial effects in an anaerobic environment by the following possible mechanism: Once metronidazole enters the organism, the drug is reduced by intracellular electron transport proteins. Because of this alteration to the metronidazole molecule, a concentration gradient is maintained which promotes the drug's intracellular transport. Presumably, free radicals are formed which, in turn, react with cellular components resulting in death of the microorganism.

Metronidazole has been shown to be active against most strains of the following microorganisms both *in vitro* and in clinical infections as described in the **INDICATIONS AND USAGE** section.

Gram-positive anaerobes:
Clostridium species
Eubacterium species
Peptococcus niger
Peptostreptococcus species

Gram-negative anaerobes:
Bacteroides fragilis group (*B. fragilis, B. distasonis, B. ovatus, B. thetaiotaomicron, B. vulgatus*)
Fusobacterium species

Protozoal parasites:
Entamoeba histolytica
Trichomonas vaginalis

The following *in vitro* data are available, **but their clinical significance is unknown:**

Metronidazole exhibits *in vitro* minimal inhibitory concentrations (MIC's) of 8 µg/mL or less against most (≥90%) strains of the following microorganisms; however, the safety and effectiveness of metronidazole in treating clinical infections due to these microorganisms have not been established in adequate and well-controlled clinical trials.

Gram-negative anaerobes:
Bacteroides fragilis group (*B. caccae, B. uniformis*)
Prevotella species (*P. bivia, P. buccae, P. disiens*)

Metronidazole is active against most obligate anaerobes, but does not possess any clinically relevant activity against facultative anaerobes or obligate aerobes.

Susceptibility Tests:

Dilution techniques:

Quantitative methods that are used to determine minimum inhibitory concentrations provide reproducible estimates of the susceptibility of bacteria to antimicrobial compounds. For anaerobic bacteria, the susceptibility to metronidazole can be determined by the reference agar dilution method or by alternate standardized test methods[1]. The MIC values obtained should be interpreted according to the following criteria:

MIC (µg/mL)	Interpretation
≤8	Susceptible (S)
16	Intermediate (I)
≥32	Resistant (R)

For protozoal parasites: Standardized tests do not exist for use in clinical microbiology laboratories.

A report of "Susceptible" indicates that the pathogen is likely to be inhibited by usually achievable concentrations of the antimicrobial compound in the blood. A report of "Intermediate" indicates that the result should be considered equivocal, and, if the microorganism is not fully susceptible to alternative, clinically feasible drugs, the test should be repeated. This category implies possible clinical applicability in body sites where the drug is physiologically concentrated or in situations where high dosage of drug can be used. This category also provides a buffer zone which prevents small uncontrolled technical factors from causing major discrepancies in interpretation. A report of "Resistant" indicates that usually achievable concentrations of the antimicrobial compound in the blood are unlikely to be inhibitory and other therapy should be selected.
Standardized susceptibility test procedures require the use of laboratory control microorganisms that are used to control the technical aspects of the laboratory procedures. Standard metronidazole powder should provide the following MIC values:

Microorganism	MIC (μg/mL)
Bacteroides fragilis ATCC 25285	0.25-1.0
Bacteroides thetaiotaomicron ATCC 29741	0.5-2.0

INDICATIONS AND USAGE

Symptomatic Trichomoniasis. Flagyl® 375 capsules are indicated for the treatment of symptomatic trichomoniasis in females and males when the presence of the trichomonad has been confirmed by appropriate laboratory procedures (wet smears and/or cultures).
Asymptomatic Trichomoniasis. Flagyl® 375 capsules are indicated in the treatment of asymptomatic females when the organism is associated with endocervicitis, cervicitis, or cervical erosion. Since there is evidence that presence of the trichomonad can interfere with accurate assessment of abnormal cytological smears, additional smears should be performed after eradication of the parasite.
Treatment of Asymptomatic Consorts. T. vaginalis infection is a venereal disease. Therefore, asymptomatic sexual partners of treated patients should be treated simultaneously if the organism has been found to be present, in order to prevent reinfection of the partner. The decision as to whether to treat an asymptomatic male partner who has a negative culture or one for whom no culture has been attempted is an individual one. In making this decision, it should be noted that there is evidence that a woman may become reinfected if her consort is not treated. Also, since there can be considerable difficulty in isolating the organism from the asymptomatic male carrier, negative smears and cultures cannot be relied upon in this regard. In any event, the consort should be treated with metronidazole in cases of reinfection.
Amebiasis. Flagyl® 375 capsules are indicated in the treatment of acute intestinal amebiasis (amebic dysentery) and amebic liver abscess.
In amebic liver abscess, metronidazole therapy does not obviate the need for aspiration or drainage of pus.
Anaerobic Bacterial Infections. Flagyl® 375 capsules are indicated in the treatment of serious infections caused by susceptible anaerobic bacteria. Indicated surgical procedures should be performed in conjunction with metronidazole therapy. In a mixed aerobic and anaerobic infection, antimicrobials appropriate for the treatment of the aerobic infection should be used in addition to Flagyl® 375 capsules.
In the treatment of most serious anaerobic infections, intravenous metronidazole is usually administered initially. This may be followed by oral therapy with Flagyl® 375 capsules at the discretion of the physician.
INTRA-ABDOMINAL INFECTIONS, including peritonitis, intra-abdominal abscess, and liver abscess, caused by *Bacteroides* species including the *B, fragilis* group (*B. fragilis, B. distasonis, B. ovatus, B. thetaiotaomicron, B. vulgatus*), *Clostridium* species, *Eubacterium* species, *Peptococcus niger*, or *Peptostreptococcus* species.
SKIN AND SKIN STRUCTURE INFECTIONS caused by *Bacteroides* species including the *B. fragilis* group, *Clostridium* species, *Peptococcus niger, Peptostreptococcus* species, or *Fusobacterium* species.
GYNECOLOGIC INFECTIONS, including endometritis, endomyometritis, tubo-ovarian abscess, and postsurgical vaginal cuff infection, caused by *Bacteroides* species including the *B. fragilis* group, *Clostridium* species, *Peptococcus niger*, or *Peptostreptococcus* species.
BACTERIAL SEPTICEMIA caused by *Bacteroides* species including the *B. fragilis* group or *Clostridium* species.
BONE AND JOINT INFECTIONS (as adjunctive therapy) caused by *Bacteroides* species including the *B. fragilis* group.
CENTRAL NERVOUS SYSTEM (CNS) INFECTIONS, including meningitis and brain abscess, caused by *Bacteroides* species including the *B. fragilis* group.
LOWER RESPIRATORY TRACT INFECTIONS, including pneumonia, empyema, and lung abscess, caused by *Bacteroides* species including the *B. fragilis* group.
ENDOCARDITIS caused by *Bacteroides* species including the *B. fragilis* group.

CONTRAINDICATIONS

Flagyl® 375 capsules are contraindicated in patients with a prior history of hypersensitivity to metronidazole or other nitroimidazole derivatives.
In patients with trichomoniasis, Flagyl® 375 capsules are contraindicated during the first trimester of pregnancy. (See **PRECAUTIONS.**)

WARNINGS

Convulsive seizures and peripheral neuropathy: Convulsive seizures and peripheral neuropathy, the latter characterized mainly by numbness or paresthesia of an extremity, have been reported in patients treated with metronidazole. The appearance of abnormal neurologic signs demands the prompt discontinuation of metronidazole therapy. Metronidazole should be administered with caution to patients with central nervous system diseases.

PRECAUTIONS

General: Patients with severe hepatic disease metabolize metronidazole slowly, with resultant accumulation of metronidazole and its metabolites in the plasma. Accordingly, for such patients, doses below those usually recommended should be administered cautiously. Known or previously unrecognized candidiasis may present more prominent symptoms during therapy with metronidazole and requires treatment with a candidacidal agent.
Information for patients: Alcoholic beverages should be avoided while taking Flagyl® 375 capsules and for at least three days afterward. (See **Drug interactions.**)
Laboratory tests: Metronidazole is a nitroimidazole and should be used with caution in patients with evidence of or history of blood dyscrasia. A mild leukopenia has been observed during its administration; however, no persistent hematologic abnormalities attributable to metronidazole have been observed in clinical studies. Total and differential leukocyte counts are recommended before and after therapy for trichomoniasis and amebiasis, especially if a second course of therapy is necessary, and before and after therapy for anaerobic infections.
Drug interactions: Metronidazole has been reported to potentiate the anticoagulant effect of warfarin and other oral coumarin anticoagulants, resulting in a prolongation of prothrombin time. This possible drug interaction should be considered when metronidazole is prescibed for patients on this type of anticoagulant therapy.
The simultaneous administration of drugs that induce microsomal liver enzymes, such as phenytoin or phenobarbital, may accelerate the elimination of metronidazole, resulting in reduced plasma levels; impaired clearance of phenytoin has also been reported.
The simultaneous administration of drugs that decrease microsomal liver enzyme activity, such as cimetidine, may prolong the half-life and decrease plasma clearance of metronidazole. In patients stabilized on relatively high doses of lithium, short-term metronidazole therapy has been associated with elevation of serum lithium and, in a few cases, signs of lithium toxicity. Serum lithium and serum creatinine levels should be obtained several days after beginning metronidazole to detect any increase that may precede clinical symptoms of lithium intoxication.
Alcoholic beverages should not be consumed during metronidazole therapy and for at least three days afterward because abdominal cramps, nausea, vomiting, headaches, and flushing may occur.
Psychotic reactions have been reported in alcoholic patients who are using metronidazole and disulfiram concurrently. Metronidazole should not be given to patients who have taken disulfiram within the last 2 weeks.
Drug/Laboratory test interactions: Metronidazole may interfere with certain types of determinations of serum chemistry values, such as aspartate aminotransferase (AST, SGOT), alanine aminotransferase (ALT, SGPT), lactate dehydrogenase (LDH), triglycerides, and hexokinase glucose. Values of zero may be observed. All of the assays in which interference has been reported involve enzymatic coupling of the assay to oxidation-reduction of nicotinamide adenine dinucleotide ($NAD^+ \rightleftarrows NADH$). Interference is due to the similarity in absorbance peaks of NADH (340 nm) and metronidazole (322 nm) at pH 7.
Carcinogenesis, mutagenesis, impairment of fertility: Metronidazole has shown evidence of carcinogenic activity in a number of studies involving chronic, oral administration in mice and rats, but similar studies in the hamster gave negative results.
Prominent among the effects in the mouse was the promotion of pulmonary tumorigenesis. This has been observed in all six reported studies in that species, including one study in which the animals were dosed on an intermittent schedule (administration during every fourth week only). At very high dose levels (approximately 1500 mg/m^2 which is approximately 3 times the most frequently recommended human dose for a 50 kg adult based on mg/m^2) there was a statistically significant increase in the incidence of malignant liver tumors in males. Also, the published results of one of the mouse studies indicate an increase in the incidence of malignant lymphomas as well as pulmonary neoplasms associated with lifetime feeding of the drug. All these effect are statistically significant.
Several long-term, oral-dosing studies in the rat have been completed. There were statistically significant increases in the incidence of various neoplasms, particularly in mammary and hepatic tumors, among female rats administered metronidazole over those noted in the concurrent female control groups.
Two lifetime tumorigenicity studies in hamsters have been performed and reported to be negative.
Metronidazole has shown mutagenic activity in a number of *in vitro* assay systems. *In vivo* studies have failed to demonstrate a potential for genetic damage.
Fertility studies have been performed in mice at doses up to six times the maximum recommended human dose based on mg/m^2 and have revealed no evidence of impaired fertility.
Pregnancy:
Teratogenic effects: Pregnancy Category B. Metronidazole crosses the placental barrier and enters the fetal circulation rapidly. Reproduction studies have been performed in rats at doses up to five times the human dose and have revealed no evidence of impaired fertility or harm to the fetus due to metronidazole. No fetotoxicity was observed when metronidazole was administered orally to pregnant mice at 60 mg/m^2/day, which is approximately 10% of the human dose when expressed as mg/m^2. However, in a single small study where the drug was administered intraperitoneally, some intrauterine deaths were observed. The relationship of these findings to the drug is unknown. There are, however, no adequate and well-controlled studies in pregnant women. Because animal reproduction studies are not always predictive of human response, and because metronidazole is a carcinogen in rodents, this drug should be used during pregnancy only if clearly needed. (See **CONTRAINDICATIONS.**)
Metronidazole use in the second and third trimesters of pregnancy should be restricted to those patients in whom alternative treatment has been inadequate. Use of metronidazole in the first trimester should be carefully evaluated because metronidazole crosses the placental barrier and its effects on human fetal organogenesis are not known. (See above.)
Nursing mothers: Because of the potential for tumorigenicity shown for metronidazole in mouse and rat studies, a decision should be made whether to discontinue nursing or to discontinue the drug, taking into account the importance of the drug to the mother. Metronidazole is secreted in human milk in concentrations similar to those found in plasma.
Geriatric use: Decreased renal function does not alter the single-dose pharmacokinetics of metronidazole. However, plasma clearance of metronidazole is decreased in patients with decreased liver function. Therefore, in elderly patients, monitoring of serum levels may be necessary to adjust the metronidazole dosage accordingly.
Pediatric use: Safety and effectiveness in pediatric patients have not been established, except in the treatment of amebiasis.

ADVERSE REACTIONS

The following reactions have also been reported during treatment with metronidazole:
Central Nervous System: Two serious adverse reactions reported in patients treated with metronidazole have been convulsive seizures and peripheral neuropathy, the latter characterized mainly by numbness or paresthesia of an extremity. Since persistent peripheral neuropathy has been reported in some patients receiving prolonged administration of metronidazole, patients should be specifically warned about these reactions and should be told to stop the drug and report immediately to their physicians if any neurologic symptoms occur. In addition, patients have reported dizziness, vertigo, incoordination, ataxia, confusion, irritability, depression, weakness, and insomnia. (See **WARNINGS.**)
Gastrointestinal: The most common adverse reactions reported have been referable to the gastrointestinal tract, particularly nausea reported by about 12% of patients, sometimes accompanied by headache, anorexia, and occasionally vomiting; diarrhea; epigastric distress; and abdominal cramping. Constipation has also been reported.
A sharp, unpleasant metallic taste is not unusual. Furry tongue, glossitis, and stomatitis have occurred; these may be associated with a sudden overgrowth of *Candida* which may occur during therapy. Rare cases of pancreatitis, which generally abated on withdrawal of the drug, have been reported.
Hematopoietic: Reversible neutropenia (leukopenia); rarely, reversible thrombocytopenia.
Cardiovascular: Flattening of the T-wave may be seen in electrocardiographic tracings.
Hypersensitivity: Urticaria, erythematous rash, flushing, nasal congestion, dryness of the mouth (or vagina or vulva), and fever.
Renal: Dysuria, cystitis, polyuria, incontinence, and a sense of pelvic pressure. Instances of darkened urine have been reported by approximately one patient in 100,000. Although the pigment which is probably responsible for this phenomenon has not been positively identified, it is almost certainly a metabolite of metronidazole and seems to have no clinical significance.
Other: Proliferation of *Candida* in the vagina, dyspareunia, decrease of libido, proctitis, and fleeting joint pains sometimes resembling "serum sickness." If patients receiving metronidazole drink alcoholic beverages, they may experience abdominal distress, nausea, vomiting, flushing, or headache. A modification of the taste of alcoholic beverages has also been reported.
Patients with Crohn's disease are known to have an increased incidence of gastrointestinal and certain extraintestinal cancers. There have been some reports in the medical literature of breast and colon cancer in Crohn's disease pa-

Continued on next page

Flagyl 375—Cont.

tients who have been treated with metronidazole at high doses for extended periods of time. A cause and effect relationship has not been established. Crohn's disease is not an approved indication for Flagyl® 375 capsules.

OVERDOSAGE

Single oral doses of metronidazole, up to 15 g, have been reported in suicide attempts and accidental overdoses. Symptoms reported include nausea, vomiting, and ataxia.
Oral metronidazole has been studied as a radiation sensitizer in the treatment of malignant tumors. Neurotoxic effects, including seizures and peripheral neuropathy, have been reported after 5 to 7 days of doses of 6 to 10.4 g every other day.
Treatment: There is no specific antidote for metronidazole overdose; therefore, management of the patient should consist of symptomatic and supportive therapy.

DOSAGE AND ADMINISTRATION

In elderly patients, the pharmacokinetics of metronidazole may be altered, and, therefore, monitoring of serum levels may be necessary to adjust the metronidazole dosage accordingly.
Trichomoniasis:
In the Female:
Seven-day course of treatment—375 mg two times daily for seven consecutive days.
A seven-day course of treatment may minimize reinfection by protecting the patient long enough for the sexual contacts to obtain treatment. Pregnant patients should not be treated during the first trimester. (See **CONTRAINDICATIONS** and **PRECAUTIONS.**)
When repeat courses of the drug are required, it is recommended that an interval of four to six weeks elapse between courses and that the presence of the trichomonad be reconfirmed by appropriate laboratory measures. Total and differential leukocyte counts should be made before and after re-treatments.
In the Male: Treatment should be individualized as for the female.
Amebiasis:
Adults:
For acute intestinal amebiasis (acute amebic dysentery): 750 mg orally three times daily for 5 to 10 days.
For amebic liver abscess: 750 mg orally three times daily for 5 to 10 days.
Pediatric Patients: 35 to 50 mg/kg/24 hours, divided into three doses, orally for 10 days.
Anaerobic Bacterial Infections: In the treatment of most serious anaerobic infections, intravenous metronidazole is usually administered initially.
The usual adult oral dosage is 7.5 mg/kg every 6 hours. A maximum of 4 g should not be exceeded during a 24-hour period.
The usual duration of therapy is 7 to 10 days; however, infections of the bone and joint, lower respiratory tract, and endocardium may require longer treatment.
Patients with severe hepatic disease metabolize metronidazole slowly, with resultant accumulation of metronidazole and its metabolites in the plasma. Accordingly, for such patients, doses below those usually recommended should be administered cautiously. Close monitoring of plasma metronidazole levels[2] and toxicity is recommended.
The dose of metronidazole should not be specifically reduced in anuric patients because accumulated metabolites may be rapidly removed by dialysis.

HOW SUPPLIED

Flagyl® 375 capsules have an iron gray opaque body imprinted with 375 mg and a light green opaque cap imprinted with FLAGYL, supplied as:

NDC Number	Size
0025-1942-50	Bottle of 50
0025-1942-34	Carton of 100 unit dose

Storage and Stability: Store at controlled room temperature 15–25°C (59–77°F). Dispense in a well-closed container with a child-resistant closure.

REFERENCES

1. National Committee for Clinical Laboratory Standards, Methods for Antimicrobial Susceptibility Testing of Anaerobic Bacteria—Third Edition. Approved Standard NCCLS Document M11-A3, Vol. 13, No. 26, NCCLS, Villanova, PA, December, 1993.
2. Ralph ED, Kirby WMM. Bioassay of metronidazole with either anaerobic or aerobic incubation, *J. Infect. Dis.* 1975; 132(Nov): 587-591 or Gulaid et al. Determination of metronidazole and its major metabolites in biological fluids by high pressure liquid chromatography, *Br. J. Clin. Pharmacol.* 1978; 6:430-432.

Rx only

Manufactured by
G.D. Searle & Co.
Box 5110
Chicago IL 60680
Address medical inquiries to:
G.D. Searle & Co.
Healthcare Information Services
5200 Old Orchard Road
Skokie IL 60077

5/5/99 • A05712-4

Shown in Product Identification Guide, page 336

FLAGYL® ER ℞
[flaj 'yl ER]
(metronidazole extended release tablets)
750 mg

> **WARNING**
> Metronidazole has been shown to be carcinogenic in mice and rats. (See **PRECAUTIONS.**) Unnecessary use of the drug should be avoided. Its use should be reserved for conditions described in the **INDICATIONS AND USAGE** section below.

DESCRIPTION

Metronidazole is an oral synthetic antiprotozoal and antibacterial agent, 2-methyl-5-nitroimidazole-1-ethanol, which has the following structural formula:

Flagyl ER 750 mg tablets contain 750 mg of metronidazole USP. Inactive ingredients include hydroxypropyl methylcellulose, lactose, magnesium stearate, polyethylene glycol, poly (meth) acrylic acid ester copolymers, polysorbate 80, silicon dioxide, simethicone emulsion, talc, titanium dioxide, FD&C Blue No. 2 Aluminum Lake.

CLINICAL PHARMACOLOGY

Pharmacokinetics: Disposition of metronidazole in the body is similar for both oral and intravenous dosage forms, with an average elimination half-life in healthy humans of 8 hours.
The major route of elimination of metronidazole and its metabolites is via the urine (60% to 80% of the dose), with fecal excretion accounting for 6% to 15% of the dose. The metabolites that appear in the urine result primarily from side-chain oxidation [1-(β-hydroxyethyl)-2-hydroxymethyl-5-nitroimidazole and 2-methyl-5-nitroimidazole-1-yl-acetic acid] and glucuronide conjugation, with unchanged metronidazole accounting for approximately 20% of the total. Renal clearance of metronidazole is approximately 10 mL/min/1.73 m^2.[1]
Flagyl ER 750 mg tablets contain 750 mg of metronidazole in an extended release formulation which allows for once-daily dosing. The steady state pharmacokinetics were determined in 24 healthy adult female subjects with a mean ± SD age of 28.8 ± 8.8 years (range: 19 – 46).[2] The pharmacokinetic parameters of metronidazole after administration of Flagyl ER 750 mg under fed and fasting conditions are summarized in the following table.

Steady State Pharmacokinetic Parameters of Metronidazole after 750 mg of Flagyl ER Given Once a Day for 7 Days

	Flagyl ER 750 mg daily Mean ± SD (N=24)	
Parameter	fed	fasted
$AUC_{(0-24)}$ (μg·hr/mL)	211 ± 60.0	198 ± 75.3
C_{max} (μg/mL)	19.4 ± 4.7	12.5 ± 4.8
C_{min} (μg/mL)	3.4 ± 2.0	4.2 ± 2.2
T_{max} (hrs)	4.6 ± 2.4	6.8 ± 2.8
$T_{1/2}$ (hrs)	7.4 ± 1.6	8.7 ± 2.2

Relative to the fasting state, the rate of metronidazole absorption from the extended release tablet is increased in the fed state resulting in alteration of the extended release characteristics.
Decreased renal function does not alter the single-dose pharmacokinetics of metronidazole. However, plasma clearance of metronidazole is decreased in patients with decreased liver function.
Microbiology: Metronidazole exerts an antimicrobial effect in an anaerobic environment by the following possible mechanism: Once metronidazole enters the organism, the drug is reduced by intracellular electron transport proteins. Because of this alteration to the metronidazole molecule, a concentration gradient is maintained which promotes the drug's intracellular transport. Presumably, free radicals are formed which, in turn, react with cellular components resulting in death of the microorganism.
The following *in vitro* data are available, **but their clinical significance is unknown:**
Metronidazole exhibits *in vitro* minimal inhibitory concentrations (MIC's) of 8 μg/mL or less against most (≥90%) strains of the following microorganisms; however, the safety and effectiveness of metronidazole in treating clinical infections due to these microorganisms have not been established in adequate and well-controlled clinical trials.
Gram-positive anaerobes:
Clostridium species
Eubacterium species
Peptococcus niger
Peptostreptococcus species
Gram-negative anaerobes:
Bacteroides fragilis group (*B. fragilis, B. distasonis, B. ovatus, B. thetaiotaomicron, B. vulgatus*)
Fusobacterium species.
Prevotella species (*P. bivia, P. buccae, P. disiens*)
Porphyromonas species
Protozoal parasites:
Entamoeba histolytica
Trichomonas vaginalis
Metronidazole has shown minimal to no activity against clinically relevant facultative anaerobes or obligate aerobes. Metronidazole has minimal activity against *Lactobacillus* spp and other aerobic microorganisms commonly isolated from the vaginal tract.
Susceptibility Tests:
Dilution techniques:
Quantitative methods that are used to determine minimum inhibitory concentrations provide reproducible estimates of the susceptibility of bacteria to antimicrobial compounds. For anaerobic bacteria, the susceptibility to metronidazole can be determined by the reference agar dilution method or by alternate standardized test methods.[3] The MIC values obtained should be interpreted according to the following criteria:

MIC (μg/mL)	Interpretation
≤ 8	Susceptible (S)
16	Intermediate (I)
≥ 32	Resistant (R)

For protozoal parasites: Standardized tests do not exist for use in clinical microbiology laboratories.
A report of "Susceptible" indicates that the pathogen is likely to be inhibited by usually achievable concentrations of the antimicrobial compound in the blood. A report of "Intermediate" indicates that the result should be considered equivocal, and if the microorganism is not fully susceptible to alternative, clinically feasible drugs, the test should be repeated. This category implies possible clinical applicability in body sites where the drug is physiologically concentrated or in situations where high dosage of drug can be used. This category also provides a buffer zone which prevents small uncontrolled technical factors from causing major discrepancies in interpretation. A report of "Resistant" indicates that usually achievable concentrations of the antimicrobial compound in the blood are unlikely to be inhibitory and other therapy should be selected.
Standardized susceptibility test procedures require the use of laboratory control microorganisms that are used to control the technical aspects of the laboratory procedures. Standard metronidazole powder should provide the following MIC values:

Microorganism	MIC (μg/mL)
Bacteroides fragilis ATCC 25285	0.25–1.0
Bacteroides thetaiotaomicron ATCC 29741	0.5–2.0

INDICATIONS AND USAGE

Bacterial Vaginosis (BV). Flagyl ER 750 mg tablets are indicated in the treatment of women with BV.

CONTRAINDICATIONS

Flagyl ER 750 mg tablets are contraindicated in patients with a prior history of hypersensitivity to metronidazole or other nitroimidazole derivatives.
Flagyl ER, like other formulations of metronidazole-containing products, is contraindicated during the first trimester of pregnancy (See **PRECAUTIONS.**)

WARNINGS

Convulsive seizures and peripheral neuropathy: Convulsive seizures and peripheral neuropathy, the latter characterized mainly by numbness or paresthesia of an extremity, have been reported in patients treated with metronidazole. The appearance of abnormal neurologic signs demands the prompt discontinuation of metronidazole therapy. Metronidazole should be administered with caution to patients with central nervous system diseases.

PRECAUTIONS

General: Patients with severe hepatic disease metabolize metronidazole slowly, with resultant accumulation of metronidazole and its metabolites in the plasma. Accordingly, for such patients, doses below those usually recommended should be administered cautiously. Known or previously unrecognized candidiasis may present more prominent symptoms during therapy with metronidazole and requires treatment with a candidacidal agent.
Information for patients: Alcoholic beverages should be avoided while taking metronidazole and for at least three days afterward. (See **Drug Interactions.**)
Laboratory tests: Metronidazole is a nitroimidazole and should be used with caution in patients with evidence of or history of blood dyscrasia. A mild leukopenia has been observed during its administration; however, no persistent hematologic abnormalities attributable to metronidazole have been observed in clinical studies. Total and differential leukocyte counts should be made before and after re-treatments.
Drug interactions: Metronidazole has been reported to potentiate the anticoagulant effect of warfarin and other oral coumarin anticoagulants, resulting in a prolongation of prothrombin time. This possible drug interaction should be considered when metronidazole is prescribed for patients on this type of anticoagulant therapy.

The simultaneous administration of drugs that induce microsomal liver enzymes, such as phenytoin or phenobarbital, may accelerate the elimination of metronidazole, resulting in reduced plasma levels; impaired clearance of phenytoin has been reported.

The simultaneous administration of drugs that decrease microsomal liver enzyme activity, such as cimetidine, may prolong the half-life and decrease plasma clearance of metronidazole. In patients stabilized on relatively high doses of lithium, short-term metronidazole therapy has been associated with elevation of serum lithium and, in a few cases, signs of lithium toxicity. Serum lithium and serum creatinine levels should be obtained several days after beginning metronidazole to detect any increase that may precede clinical symptoms of lithium intoxication.

Alcoholic beverages should not be consumed during metronidazole therapy and for at least three days afterward because abdominal cramps, nausea, vomiting, headaches, and flushing may occur.

Psychotic reactions have been reported in alcoholic patients who are using metronidazole and disulfiram concurrently. Metronidazole should not be given to patients who have taken disulfiram within the last 2 weeks.

Drug/Laboratory test interactions: Metronidazole may interfere with certain types of determinations of serum chemistry values, such as aspartate aminotransferase (AST, SGOT), alanine aminotransferase (ALT, SGPT), lactate dehydrogenase (LDH), triglycerides, and hexokinase glucose. Values of zero may be observed. All of the assays in which interference has been reported involve enzymatic coupling of the assay to oxidation-reduction of nicotinamide adenine dinucleotide ($NAD^+ \rightleftarrows NADH$). Interference is due to the similarity in absorbance peaks of NADH (340 nm) and metronidazole (322 nm) at pH 7.

Carcinogenesis, mutagenesis, impairment of fertility: Pulmonary tumors have been observed in all six reported studies in the mouse, including one study in which the animals were dosed on an intermittent schedule (administration during every fourth week only).

Malignant liver tumors were increased in male mice treated at approximately 1500 mg/m^2. This dose is approximately 3 times the recommended dose.

Malignant lymphomas and pulmonary neoplasms are also increased with lifetime feeding of the drug to mice (published data).

Mammary and hepatic tumors were increased among female rats administered oral metronidazole compared to concurrent controls.

Two lifetime tumorigenicity studies in hamsters have been performed and reported to be negative.

Metronidazole has shown mutagenic activity in *in vitro* assay systems including the Ames test. Studies in mammals *in vivo* have failed to demonstrate a potential for genetic damage. Fertility studies have been performed in mice at doses up to six times the maximum recommended human dose based on mg/m^2 and have revealed no evidence of impaired fertility.

Pregnancy:

Teratogenic effects: Pregnancy Category B.

Flagyl ER has not been studied in pregnant women. Since metronidazole crosses the placental barrier and enters the fetal circulation rapidly, it should not be administered to pregnant patients during the first trimester. No fetotoxicity was observed when metronidazole was administered orally to pregnant mice at 60 mg/m^2/day, which is approximately 10% of the human dose when expressed as mg/m^2. However, in a single small study where the drug was administered intraperitoneally, some intrauterine deaths were observed. The relationship of these findings to the drug is unknown. There are, however, no adequate and well-controlled studies in pregnant women. (See **CONTRAINDICATIONS**.)

Because animal reproduction studies are not always predictive of human response, and because metronidazole is a carcinogen in rodents, this drug should be used during pregnancy only if clearly needed.

Nursing mothers: Since metronidazole is secreted in human milk in concentrations similar to those found in plasma, and since tumors were increased in rats and mice treated with metronidazole, a decision should be made whether to discontinue nursing or to discontinue the drug, taking into account the importance of the drug to the mother.

Geriatric use: Decreased renal function does not alter the single-dose pharmacokinetics of metronidazole. However, plasma clearance of metronidazole is decreased in patients with decreased liver function. Therefore, in elderly patients, monitoring of serum levels may be necessary to adjust the metronidazole dosage accordingly.

Pediatric use: Safety and effectiveness of this dosage form of metronidazole in pediatric patients have not been established.

ADVERSE REACTIONS

In two multicenter clinical trials, a total of 270 patients received 750 mg Flagyl ER tablets orally once daily for 7 days, and 287 were treated with a comparator agent administered intravaginally once daily for 7 days. (See **CLINICAL STUDIES**.)[4,5]

Most adverse events were described as being of mild or moderate severity. Among patients taking Flagyl ER who reported headaches, 10% considered them severe, and less than 2% of reported episodes of nausea were considered severe. Metallic taste was reported by 9% of patients taking Flagyl ER.

Adverse Events
(≥2% Incidence Rate)—Irrespective of Treatment Causality

	Flagyl ER 7 days (N=267)	Vaginal Preparation (N=285)
Headache	48 (18%)	44 (15%)
Vaginitis	39 (15%)	32 (12%)
Nausea	28 (10%)	8 (3%)
Taste Perversion (metallic taste)	23 (9%)	1 (0%)
Infection Bacterial	19 (7%)	17 (6%)
Influenza-like Symptoms	17 (6%)	20 (7%)
Pruritus Genital	14 (5%)	25 (9%)
Abdominal Pain	10 (4%)	13 (5%)
Dizziness	11 (4%)	3 (1%)
Diarrhea	11 (4%)	3 (1%)
Upper Respiratory Tract Infection	11 (4%)	10 (4%)
Rhinitis	12 (4%)	10 (4%)
Sinusitis	7 (3%)	6 (2%)
Urine Abnormal	7 (3%)	4 (1%)
Pharyngitis	8 (3%)	4 (1%)
Dysmenorrhea	9 (3%)	7 (2%)
Moniliasis	9 (3%)	8 (3%)
Mouth Dry	5 (2%)	2 (1%)
Urinary Tract Infection	6 (2%)	16 (6%)

Clinical Cure Rates at One Month

	Flagyl ER % (n/N)	2% clindamycin cream % (n/N)
Study 1	61% (77/126)	59% (80/135)
Study 2	62% (74/119)*	43% (50/117)

* $p<0.05$ versus clindamycin cream

Adverse events reported at ≥2% incidence for either treatment group, irrespective of treatment causality, are summarized in the table below.

[See first table above]

Vulvovaginal candidiasis is a recognized consequence of treatment with many anti-infective agents. In these multicenter clinical trials, there were no statistically significant differences in the incidence rates of yeast vaginitis for groups of patients treated with Flagyl ER or the vaginal comparator.

The following reactions have also been reported during treatment with metronidazole:

Central Nervous System: Two serious adverse reactions reported in patients treated with metronidazole have been convulsive seizures and peripheral neuropathy, the latter characterized mainly by numbness or paresthesia of an extremity. Since persistent peripheral neuropathy has been reported in some patients receiving prolonged administration of metronidazole, patients should be specifically warned about these reactions and should be told to stop the drug and report immediately to their physicians if any neurologic symptoms occur. In addition, patients have reported dizziness, vertigo, incoordination, ataxia, confusion, irritability, depression, weakness, and insomnia. (See **WARNINGS**.)

Gastrointestinal: The most common adverse reactions reported have been referable to the gastrointestinal tract, particularly nausea reported by about 12% of patients, sometimes accompanied by headache, anorexia, and occasionally vomiting, diarrhea, epigastric distress, and abdominal cramping. Constipation has also been reported.

Furry tongue, glossitis, and stomatitis have occurred; these may be associated with a sudden overgrowth of *Candida* which may occur during therapy. Rare cases of pancreatitis, which generally abated on withdrawal of the drug, have been reported.

Hematopoietic: Reversible neutropenia (leukopenia); rarely, reversible thrombocytopenia.

Cardiovascular: Flattening of the T-wave may be seen in electrocardiographic tracings.

Hypersensitivity: Urticaria, erythematous rash, flushing, nasal congestion, dryness of the mouth (or vagina or vulva), and fever.

Renal: Dysuria, cystitis, polyuria, incontinence, and a sense of pelvic pressure. Instances of darkened urine have been reported by approximately one patient in 100,000. Although the pigment which is probably responsible for this phenomenon has not been positively identified, it is almost certainly a metabolite of metronidazole and seems to have no clinical significance.

Other: Proliferation of *Candida* in the vagina, dyspareunia, decrease of libido, proctitis, and fleeting joint pains sometimes resembling "serum sickness." If patients receiving metronidazole drink alcoholic beverages, they may experience abdominal distress, nausea, vomiting, flushing, or headache. A modification of the taste of alcoholic beverages has also been reported.

Patients with Crohn's disease are known to have an increased incidence of gastrointestinal and certain extraintestinal cancers. There have been some reports in the medical literature of breast and colon cancer in Crohn's disease patients who have been treated with metronidazole at high doses for extended periods of time. A cause and effect relationship has not been established. Crohn's disease is not an approved indication for Flagyl ER 750 mg tablets.

OVERDOSAGE

Single oral doses of metronidazole, up to 15 g, have been reported in suicide attempts and accidental overdoses. Symptoms reported include nausea, vomiting, and ataxia.

Oral metronidazole has been studied as a radiation sensitizer in the treatment of malignant tumors. Neurotoxic effects, including seizures and peripheral neuropathy, have been reported after 5 to 7 days of doses of 6 g to 10.4 g every other day.

Treatment: There is no specific antidote for metronidazole overdose; therefore, management of the patient should consist of symptomatic and supportive therapy.

DOSAGE AND ADMINISTRATION

Bacterial Vaginosis:

Seven-day course of treatment—750 mg once daily by mouth for seven consecutive days.

Flagyl ER 750 mg tablets should be taken under fasting conditions, at least one hour before or two hours after meals. The optimum extended-release characteristics of Flagyl ER 750 mg are obtained when the drug is taken under fasting conditions. (See **CLINICAL PHARMACOLOGY—Pharmacokinetics.**)

Pregnant patients should not be treated during the first trimester. (See **CONTRAINDICATIONS** and **PRECAUTIONS**.)

Patients with severe hepatic disease metabolize metronidazole slowly, with resultant accumulation of metronidazole and its metabolites in the plasma. Accordingly, for such patients, doses below those usually recommended should be administered cautiously. Close monitoring of plasma metronidazole levels[6] and toxicity is recommended.

The dose of metronidazole should not be specifically reduced in anuric patients because accumulated metabolites may be rapidly removed by dialysis.

In elderly patients, the pharmacokinetics of metronidazole may be altered and therefore, monitoring of serum levels may be necessary to adjust the metronidazole dosage accordingly.

HOW SUPPLIED

Flagyl ER 750 mg tablets are oval, blue, film coated, with SEARLE and 1961 embossed on one side and FLAGYL and ER on the other side, supplied as:

NDC Number	Size
0025-1961-30	Bottle of 30

Storage and Stability: Store in a dry place at 25°C (77°F); excursions permitted to 15°–30°C (59°–86°F). [See USP Controlled Room Temperature.] Dispense in a well-closed container with a child-resistant closure.

CLINICAL STUDIES

BV is a clinical syndrome that results from a replacement of the normal, *Lactobacillus*-dominant flora with several other organisms including *Gardnerella vaginalis, Mobiluncus* spp, *Mycoplasma hominis* and anaerobes (*Peptostreptococcus* spp and *Bacteroides* spp).

Flagyl ER was studied in patients with BV in two randomized, multicenter, well-controlled, investigator blind clinical trials.[4,5] A total of 557 otherwise healthy nonpregnant patients with BV were randomized to treatment with Flagyl ER once a day for 7 days (n = 270) or 2% clindamycin vaginal cream one applicator full (5 grams) once a day for 7 days (n = 287).

Continued on next page

Flagyl ER—Cont.

The primary efficacy endpoint for each treatment regimen was defined as clinical cure assessed at 28–32 days post-therapy. Clinical cure was defined as a return to normal of the vaginal pH (≤4.5), absence of a "fishy" amine odor, and absence of clue cells.
The study results are presented in the table below:
[See second table at top of previous page]
At one month post-therapy the pH of the vagina returned to normal earlier and in a greater percentage of patients in the Flagyl ER treatment group when compared to the 2% clindamycin vaginal cream group; 72% vs 65%, respectively. Likewise, Flagyl ER restored the normal *Lactobacillus*-predominant vaginal flora in a larger percentage of patients at one month post-therapy when compared to the 2% clindamycin treated group; 74% vs 63%, respectively.

REFERENCES

1. Salas-Herrera IG, Pearson RM, Johnston A, and Turner P. Concentration of metronidazole in cervical mucus and serum after single and repeated oral doses. *J Antimicrobial Chemotherapy* 1991; 28:283–289. **2.** Metronidazole modified-release tablet multiple-dose bioequivalency study (fed/fasting). G.D. Searle & Co., Protocol No. S13-94-02-014; Report No. S13-95-06-014, 11 July 1995. **3.** National Committee for Clinical Laboratory Standards, Methods for Antimicrobial Susceptibility Testing of Anaerobic Bacteria—Third Edition. Approved Standard NCCLS Document M11-A3, Vol. 13, No. 26, NCCLS, Villanova, PA, December, 1993. **4.** Integrated clinical and statistical report for the treatment of bacterial vaginosis with metronidazole modified release tablet—a dose duration study. G.D. Searle & Co., Protocol No. N13-95-02-015; Report No. N13-96-06-015, 19 Nov 1996. **5.** Integrated clinical and statistical report for the treatment of bacterial vaginosis with metronidazole modified release tablet. G.D. Searle & Co., Protocol No. N13-95-02-017; Report No. N13-96-06-017, 11 Nov 1996. **6.** Ralph ED, Kirby WMM. Bioassay of metronidazole with either anaerobic or aerobic incubation. *J Infect Dis* 1975; 132: 587–591 or Gulaid et al. Determination of metronidazole and its major metabolites in biological fluids by high pressure liquid chromatography. *Br J Clin Pharmacol* 1978; 6:430–432.

Rx only Revised: Mar. 26, 1998

Manufactured by
MOVA Pharmaceuticals, Inc.
P.O. Box 8639
Caguas, Puerto Rico 00726
for G.D. Searle & Co.
Box 5110
Chicago IL 60680 USA

Address medical inquiries to:
G.D. Searle & Co.
Healthcare Information Services
5200 Old Orchard Road
Skokie IL 60077
SEARLE

633702MV

Shown in Product Identification Guide, page 336

KERLONE® ℞

[kur 'lōn]
(betaxolol hydrochloride)

DESCRIPTION

Kerlone (betaxolol hydrochloride) is a β_1-selective (cardioselective) adrenergic receptor blocking agent available as 10-mg and 20-mg tablets for oral administration. Kerlone is chemically described as 2-propanol, 1-[4-[2-(cyclopropylmethoxy)ethyl]phenoxy]-3-[(1-methylethyl)amino]-, hydrochloride, (±). It has the following chemical structure:

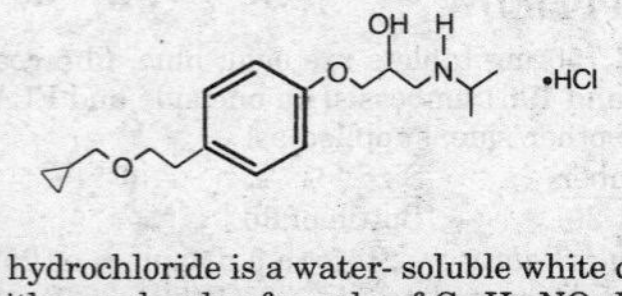

Betaxolol hydrochloride is a water- soluble white crystalline powder with a molecular formula of $C_{18}H_{29}NO_3 \cdot HCl$ and a molecular weight of 343.9. It is freely soluble in water, ethanol, chloroform, and methanol, and has a pKa of 9.4.
The inactive ingredients are hydroxypropyl methylcellulose, lactose, magnesium stearate, polyethylene glycol 400, microcrystalline cellulose, colloidal silicon dioxide, sodium starch glycolate, and titanium dioxide.

CLINICAL PHARMACOLOGY

Kerlone is a β_1-selective (cardioselective) adrenergic receptor blocking agent that has weak membrane-stabilizing activity and no intrinsic sympathomimetic (partial agonist) activity. The preferential effect on β_1 receptors is not absolute, however, and some inhibitory effects on β_2 receptors (found chiefly in the bronchial and vascular musculature) can be expected at higher doses.
Pharmacokinetics and metabolism: In man, absorption of an oral dose is complete. There is a small and consistent first-pass effect resulting in an absolute bioavailability of 89% ± 5% that is unaffected by the concomitant ingestion of food or alcohol. Mean peak blood concentrations of 21.6 ng/ml (range 16.3 to 27.9 ng/ml) are reached between 1.5 and 6 (mean about 3) hours after a single oral dose, in healthy volunteers, of 10 mg of Kerlone. Peak concentrations for 20-mg and 40-mg doses are 2 and 4 times that of a 10-mg dose and have been shown to be linear over the dose range of 5 to 40 mg. The peak to trough ratio of plasma concentrations over 24 hours is 2.7. The mean elimination half-life in various studies in normal volunteers ranged from about 14 to 22 hours after single oral doses and is similar in chronic dosing. Steady state plasma concentrations are attained after 5 to 7 days with once-daily dosing in persons with normal renal function.
Kerlone is approximately 50% bound to plasma proteins. It is eliminated primarily by liver metabolism and secondarily by renal excretion. Following oral administration, greater than 80% of a dose is recovered in the urine as betaxolol and its metabolites. Approximately 15% of the dose administered is excreted as unchanged drug, the remainder being metabolites whose contribution to the clinical effect is negligible.
Steady state studies in normal volunteers and hypertensive patients found no important differences in kinetics. In patients with hepatic disease, elimination half-life was prolonged by about 33%, but clearance was unchanged, leading to little change in AUC. Dosage reductions have not routinely been necessary in these patients. In patients with chronic renal failure undergoing dialysis, mean elimination half-life was approximately doubled, as was AUC, indicating the need for a lower initial dosage (5 mg) in these patients. The clearance of betaxolol by hemodialysis was 0.015 L/h/kg and by peritoneal dialysis, 0.010 L/h/kg. In one study (n=8), patients with stable renal failure, not on dialysis, with mean creatinine clearance of 27 ml/min showed slight increases in elimination half-life and AUC, but no change in C_{max}. In a second study of 30 hypertensive patients with mild to severe renal impairment, there was a reduction in clearance of betaxolol with increasing degrees of renal insufficiency. Inulin clearance (mL/min/1.73 m^2) ranged from 70 to 107 in 7 patients with mild impairment, 41 to 69 in 14 patients with moderate impairment, and 8 to 37 in 9 patients with severe impairment. Clearance following oral dosing was reduced significantly in patients with moderate and severe renal impairment (26% and 35%, respectively) when compared with those with mildly impaired renal function. In the severely impaired group, the mean C_{max} and the mean elimination half-life tended to increase (28% and 24%, respectively) when compared with the mildly impaired group. A starting dose of 5 mg is recommended in patients with severe renal impairment. (See *Dosage and Administration.*)
Studies in elderly patients (n=10) gave inconsistent results but suggest some impairment of elimination, with one small study (n=4) finding a mean half-life of 30 hours. A starting dose of 5 mg is suggested in older patients.
Pharmacodynamics: Clinical pharmacology studies have demonstrated the beta-adrenergic receptor blocking activity of Kerlone by (1) reduction in resting and exercise heart rate, cardiac output, and cardiac work load, (2) reduction of systolic and diastolic blood pressure at rest and during exercise, (3) inhibition of isoproterenol-induced tachycardia, and (4) reduction of reflex orthostatic tachycardia.
The β_1 selectivity of Kerlone in man was shown in three ways: (1) In normal subjects, 10- and 40-mg oral doses of Kerlone, which reduced resting heart rate at least as much as 40 mg of propranolol, produced less inhibition of isoproterenol-induced increases in forearm blood flow and finger tremor than propranolol. In this study, 10 mg of Kerlone was at least comparable to 50 mg of atenolol. Both doses of Kerlone, and the one dose of atenolol, however, had more effect on the isoproterenol-induced changes than placebo (indicating some β_2 effect at clinical doses) and the higher dose of Kerlone was more inhibitory than the lower. (2) In normal subjects, single intravenous doses of betaxolol and propranolol, which produced equal effects on exercise-induced tachycardia, had differing effects on insulin-induced hypoglycemia, with propranolol, but not betaxolol, prolonging the hypoglycemia compared with placebo. Neither drug affected the maximum extent of the hypoglycemic response. (3) In a single-blind crossover study in asthmatics (n=10), intravenous infusion over 30 minutes of low doses of betaxolol (1.5 mg) and propranolol (2 mg) had similar effects on resting heart rate but had differing effects on FEV_1 and forced vital capacity, with propranolol causing statistically significant (10% to 20%) reductions from baseline in mean values for both parameters while betaxolol had no effect on mean values. While blood levels were not measured, the dose of betaxolol used in this study would be expected to produce blood concentrations, at the time of the pulmonary function studies, considerably lower than those achieved during antihypertensive therapy with recommended doses of Kerlone. In a randomized double-blind, placebo-controlled crossover (4×4 Latin Square) study in 10 asthmatics, betaxolol (about 5 or 10 mg IV) had little effect on isoproterenol-induced increases in FEV_1; in contrast, propranolol (about 7 mg IV) inhibited the response.
Consistent with its negative chronotropic effect, due to beta-blockade of the SA node, and lack of intrinsic sympathomimetic activity, Kerlone increases sinus cycle length and sinus node recovery time. Conduction in the AV node is also prolonged.
Significant reductions in blood pressure and heart rate were observed 24 hours after dosing in double-blind, placebo-controlled trials with doses of 5 to 40 mg administered once daily. The antihypertensive response to betaxolol was similar at peak blood levels (3 to 4 hours) and at trough (24 hours). In a large randomized, parallel dose-response study of 5, 10, and 20 mg, the antihypertensive effects of the 5-mg dose were roughly half of the effects of the 20-mg dose (after adjustment for placebo effects) and the 10-mg dose gave more than 80% of the antihypertensive response to the 20-mg dose. The effect of increasing the dose from 10 mg to 20 mg was thus small. In this study, while the antihypertensive response to betaxolol showed a dose-response relationship, the heart rate response (reduction in HR) was not dose related. In other trials, there was little evidence of a greater antihypertensive response to 40 mg than to 20 mg. The maximum effect of each dose was achieved within 1 or 2 weeks. In comparative trials against propranolol, atenolol, and chlorthalidone, betaxolol appeared to be at least as effective as the comparative agent.
Kerlone has been studied in combination with thiazide-type diuretics and the blood pressure effects of the combination appear additive. Kerlone has also been used concurrently with methyldopa, hydralazine, and prazosin.
The mechanism of the antihypertensive effects of beta-adrenergic receptor blocking agents has not been established. Several possible mechanisms have been proposed, however, including: (1) competitive antagonism of catecholamines at peripheral (especially cardiac) adrenergic-neuronal sites, leading to decreased cardiac output, (2) a central effect leading to reduced sympathetic outflow to the periphery, and (3) suppression of renin activity.
The results from long-term studies have not shown any diminution of the antihypertensive effect of Kerlone with prolonged use.

INDICATIONS AND USAGE

Kerlone is indicated in the management of hypertension. It may be used alone or concomitantly with other antihypertensive agents, particularly thiazide-type diuretics.

CONTRAINDICATIONS

Kerlone is contraindicated in patients with known hypersensitivity to the drug.
Kerlone is contraindicated in patients with sinus bradycardia, heart block greater than first degree, cardiogenic shock, and overt cardiac failure (see *Warnings*).

WARNINGS

Cardiac failure: Sympathetic stimulation may be a vital component supporting circulatory function in congestive heart failure, and beta-adrenergic receptor blockade carries the potential hazard of further depressing myocardial contractility and precipitating more severe heart failure. In hypertensive patients who have congestive heart failure controlled by digitalis and diuretics, beta-blockers should be administered cautiously. Both digitalis and beta-adrenergic receptor blocking agents slow AV conduction.
In patients without a history of cardiac failure: Continued depression of the myocardium with beta-blocking agents over a period of time can, in some cases, lead to cardiac failure. Therefore, at the first sign or symptom of cardiac failure, discontinuation of Kerlone should be considered. In some cases beta-blocker therapy can be continued while cardiac failure is treated with cardiac glycosides, diuretics, and other agents, as appropriate.
Exacerbation of angina pectoris upon withdrawal: Abrupt cessation of therapy with certain beta-blocking agents in patients with coronary artery disease has been followed by exacerbations of angina pectoris and, in some cases, myocardial infarction has been reported. Therefore, such patients should be warned against interruption of therapy without the physician's advice. Even in the absence of overt angina pectoris, when discontinuation of Kerlone is planned, the patient should be carefully observed and therapy should be reinstituted, at least temporarily, if withdrawal symptoms occur.
Bronchospastic diseases: PATIENTS WITH BRONCHOSPASTIC DISEASE SHOULD NOT IN GENERAL RECEIVE BETA-BLOCKERS. Because of its relative β_1 selectivity (cardioselectivity), low doses of Kerlone may be used with caution in patients with bronchospastic disease who do not respond to or cannot tolerate alternative treatment. Since β_1 selectivity is not absolute and is inversely related to dose, the lowest possible dose of Kerlone should be used (5 to 10 mg once daily) and a bronchodilator should be made available. If dosage must be increased, divided dosage should be considered to avoid the higher peak blood levels associated with once-daily dosing.
Anesthesia and major surgery: The necessity, or desirability, of withdrawal of a beta-blocking therapy prior to major surgery is controversial. Beta-adrenergic receptor blockade impairs the ability of the heart to respond to beta-adrenergically mediated reflex stimuli. While this might be of benefit in preventing arrhythmic response, the risk of excessive myocardial depression during general anesthesia may be increased and difficulty in restarting and maintaining the heart beat has been reported with beta-blockers. If treatment is continued, particular care should be taken when using anesthetic agents which depress the myocardium, such as ether, cyclopropane, and trichloroethylene, and it is prudent to use the lowest possible dose of Kerlone. Kerlone, like other beta-blockers, is a competitive inhibitor of beta-receptor agonists and its effect on the heart can be reversed by cautious administration of such agents (eg, dobutamine or isoproterenol—see *Overdosage*). Manifestations of exces-

sive vagal tone (eg, profound bradycardia, hypotension) may be corrected with atropine 1 to 3 mg IV in divided doses.

Diabetes and hypoglycemia: Beta-blockers should be used with caution in diabetic patients. Beta-blockers may mask tachycardia occurring with hypoglycemia (patients should be warned of this), although other manifestations such as dizziness and sweating may not be significantly affected. Unlike nonselective beta-blockers, Kerlone does not prolong insulin-induced hypoglycemia.

Thyrotoxicosis: Beta-adrenergic blockade may mask certain clinical signs of hyperthyroidism (eg, tachycardia). Abrupt withdrawal of beta-blockade might precipitate a thyroid storm; therefore, patients known or suspected of being thyrotoxic from whom Kerlone is to be withdrawn should be monitored closely (see *Dosage and Administration: Cessation of therapy*).

PRECAUTIONS

General: Beta-adrenoceptor blockade can cause reduction of intraocular pressure. Since betaxolol hydrochloride is marketed as an ophthalmic solution for treatment of glaucoma, patients should be told that Kerlone may interfere with the glaucoma-screening test. Withdrawal may lead to a return of increased intraocular pressure. Patients receiving beta-adrenergic blocking agents orally and beta-blocking ophthalmic solutions should be observed for potential additive effects either on the intraocular pressure or on the known systemic effects of beta-blockade.

Impaired hepatic or renal function: Kerlone is primarily metabolized in the liver to metabolites that are inactive and then excreted by the kidneys; clearance is somewhat reduced in patients with renal failure but little changed in patients with hepatic disease. Dosage reductions have not routinely been necessary when hepatic insufficiency is present (see *Dosage and Administration*) but patients should be observed. Patients with severe renal impairment and those on dialysis require a reduced dose. (See *Dosage and Administration.*)

Information for patients: Patients, especially those with evidence of coronary artery insufficiency, should be warned against interruption or discontinuation of Kerlone therapy without the physician's advice.

Although cardiac failure rarely occurs in appropriately selected patients, patients being treated with beta-adrenergic blocking agents should be advised to consult a physician at the first sign or symptom of failure.

Patients should know how they react to this medicine before they operate automobiles and machinery or engage in other tasks requiring alertness. Patients should contact their physician if any difficulty in breathing occurs, and before surgery of any type. Patients should inform their physicians or dentists that they are taking Kerlone. Patients with diabetes should be warned that beta-blockers may mask tachycardia occurring with hypoglycemia.

Drug interactions: The following drugs have been coadministered with Kerlone and have not altered its pharmacokinetics: cimetidine, nifedipine, chlorthalidone, and hydrochlorothiazide. Concomitant administration of Kerlone with the oral anticoagulant warfarin has been shown not to potentiate the anticoagulant effect of warfarin.

Catecholamine-depleting drugs (eg, reserpine) may have an additive effect when given with beta-blocking agents. Patients treated with a beta-adrenergic receptor blocking agent plus a catecholamine depletor should therefore be closely observed for evidence of hypotension or marked bradycardia, which may produce vertigo, syncope, or postural hypotension.

Should it be decided to discontinue therapy in patients receiving beta-blockers and clonidine concurrently, the beta-blocker should be discontinued slowly over several days before the gradual withdrawal of clonidine.

Literature reports suggest that oral calcium antagonists may be used in combination with beta-adrenergic blocking agents when heart function is normal, but should be avoided in patients with impaired cardiac function. Hypotension, AV conduction disturbances, and left ventricular failure have been reported in some patients receiving beta-adrenergic blocking agents when an oral calcium antagonist was added to the treatment regimen. Hypotension was more likely to occur if the calcium antagonist were a dihydropyridine derivative, eg, nifedipine, while left ventricular failure and AV conduction disturbances, including complete heart block, were more likely to occur with either verapamil or diltiazem.

Risk of anaphylactic reaction: Although it is known that patients on beta-blockers may be refractory to epinephrine in the treatment of anaphylactic shock, beta-blockers can, in addition, interfere with the modulation of allergic reaction and lead to an increased severity and/or frequency of attacks. Severe allergic reactions including anaphylaxis have been reported in patients exposed to a variety of allergens either by repeated challenge, or accidental contact, and with diagnostic or therapeutic agents while receiving beta-blockers. Such patients may be unresponsive to the usual doses of epinephrine used to treat allergic reaction.

Carcinogenesis, mutagenesis, impairment of fertility: Lifetime studies with betaxolol HCl in mice at oral dosages of 6, 20, and 60 mg/kg/day (up to 90 × the maximum recommended human dose [MRHD] based on 60-kg body weight) and in rats at 3, 12, or 48 mg/kg/day (up to 72 × MRHD) showed no evidence of a carcinogenic effect. In a variety of *in vitro* and *in vivo* bacterial and mammalian cell assays, betaxolol HCl was nonmutagenic. Betaxolol did not adversely affect fertility or mating performance of male or female rats at doses up to 256 mg/kg/day (380 × MRHD).

Pregnancy: Pregnancy Category C. In a study in which pregnant rats received betaxolol at doses of 4, 40, or 400 mg/kg/day, the highest dose (600 × MRHD) was associated with increased postimplantation loss, reduced litter size and weight, and an increased incidence of skeletal and visceral abnormalities, which may have been a consequence of drug-related maternal toxicity. Other than a possible increased incidence of incomplete descent of testes and sternebral reductions, betaxolol at 4 mg/kg/day and 40 mg/kg/day (6 × MRHD and 60 × MRHD) caused no fetal abnormalities. In a second study with a different strain of rat, 200 mg betaxolol/kg/day (300 × MRHD) was associated with maternal toxicity and an increase in resorptions, but no teratogenicity. In a study in which pregnant rabbits received doses of 1, 4, 12, or 36 mg betaxolol/kg/day (54 × MRHD), a marked increase in postimplantation loss occurred at the highest dose, but no drug-related teratogenicity was observed. The rabbit is more sensitive to betaxolol than other species because of higher bioavailability resulting from saturation of the first-pass effect. In a peri- and postnatal study in rats at doses of 4, 32, and 256 mg betaxolol/kg/day (380 ×MRHD), the highest dose was associated with a marked increase in total litter loss within 4 days postpartum. In surviving offspring, growth and development were also affected.

There are no adequate and well-controlled studies in pregnant women. Kerlone should be used during pregnancy only if the potential benefit justifies the potential risk to the fetus.

Nursing mothers: Since Kerlone is excreted in human milk in sufficient amounts to have pharmacological effects in the infant, caution should be exercised when Kerlone is administered to a nursing mother.

Pediatric use: Safety and effectiveness in pediatric patients have not been established.

Elderly patients: Kerlone may produce bradycardia more frequently in elderly patients. In general, patients 65 years of age and older had a higher incidence rate of bradycardia (heart rate <50 BPM) than younger patients in U.S. clinical trials. In a double-blind study in Europe, 19 elderly patients (mean age = 82) received betaxolol 20 mg daily. Dosage reduction to 10 mg or discontinuation was required for 6 patients due to bradycardia (See *Dosage and Administration*).

ADVERSE REACTIONS

Most adverse reactions have been mild and transient and are typical of beta-adrenergic blocking agents, eg, bradycardia, fatigue, dyspnea, and lethargy. Withdrawal of therapy in U.S. and European controlled clinical trials has been necessary in about 3.5% of patients, principally because of bradycardia, fatigue, dizziness, headache, and impotence.

Frequency estimates of adverse events were derived from controlled studies in which adverse reactions were volunteered and elicited in U.S. studies and volunteered and/or elicited in European studies.

In the U.S., the placebo-controlled hypertension studies lasted for 4 weeks, while the active-controlled hypertension studies had a 22- to 24-week double-blind phase. The following doses were studied: betaxolol—5, 10, 20, and 40 mg once daily; atenolol—25, 50, and 100 mg once daily; and propranolol—40, 80, and 160 mg b.i.d.

Kerlone, like other beta-blockers, has been associated with the development of antinuclear antibodies (ANA). In controlled clinical studies, conversion of ANA from negative to positive occurred in 5.3% of the patients treated with betaxolol, 6.3% of the patients treated with atenolol, 4.9% of the patients treated with propranolol, and 3.2% of the patients treated with placebo.

Betaxolol adverse events reported with a 2% or greater frequency, and selected events with lower frequency, in U.S. controlled studies are:

[See table 1 above]

Table 1

Body System/Adverse Reaction	Betaxolol (N=509) 5–40 mg q.d.* (%)	Propranolol (N=73) 40–160 mg b.i.d. (%)	Atenolol (N=75) 25–100 mg q.d. (%)	Placebo (N=109) (%)
Dose Range	5–40 mg q.d.*	40–160 mg b.i.d.	25–100 mg q.d.	
Cardiovascular				
Bradycardia (heart rate <50 BPM)	8.1	4.1	12.0	0
Symptomatic bradycardia	0.8	1.4	0	0
Edema	1.8	0	0	1.8
Central Nervous System				
Headache	6.5	4.1	5.3	15.6
Dizziness	4.5	11.0	2.7	5.5
Fatigue	2.9	9.6	4.0	0
Lethargy	2.8	4.1	2.7	0.9
Psychiatric				
Insomnia	1.2	8.2	2.7	0
Nervousness	0.8	1.4	2.7	0
Bizarre dreams	1.0	2.7	1.3	0
Depression	0.8	2.7	4.0	0
Autonomic				
Impotence	1.2†	0	0	0
Respiratory				
Dyspnea	2.4	2.7	1.3	0.9
Pharyngitis	2.0	0	4.0	0.9
Rhinitis	1.4	0	4.0	0.9
Upper respiratory infection	2.6	0	0	5.5
Gastrointestinal				
Dyspepsia	4.7	6.8	2.7	0.9
Nausea	1.6	1.4	4.0	0
Diarrhea	2.0	6.8	8.0	0.9
Musculoskeletal				
Chest pain	2.4	1.4	2.7	0.9
Arthralgia	3.1	0	4.0	1.8
Skin				
Rash	1.2	0	0	0

* Five patients received 80 mg q.d.

† N = 336 males; impotence is a known possible adverse effect of this pharmacological class.

Table 2

Body System/Adverse Reaction	Betaxolol (N=155) 20–40 mg q.d. (%)	Atenolol (N=81) 100 mg q.d. (%)	Placebo (N=60) (%)
Dose Range	20–40 mg q.d.	100 mg q.d.	
Cardiovascular			
Bradycardia (heart rate <50 BPM)	5.8	5.0	0
Symptomatic bradycardia	1.9	2.5	0
Palpitation	1.9	3.7	1.7
Edema	1.3	1.2	0
Cold extremities	1.9	0	0
Central Nervous System			
Headache	14.8	9.9	23.3
Dizziness	14.8	17.3	15.0
Fatigue	9.7	18.5	0
Asthenia	7.1	0	16.7
Insomnia	5.0	3.7	3.3
Paresthesia	1.9	2.5	0
Gastrointestinal			
Nausea	5.8	1.2	0
Dyspepsia	3.9	7.4	3.3
Diarrhea	1.9	3.7	0
Musculoskeletal			
Chest pain	7.1	6.2	5.0
Joint pain	5.2	4.9	1.7
Myalgia	3.2	3.7	3.3

Continued on next page

Kerlone—Cont.

Of the above adverse reactions [listed in Table 1] associated with the use of betaxolol, only bradycardia was clearly dose related, but there was a suggestion of dose relatedness for fatigue, lethargy, and dyspepsia.

In Europe, the placebo-controlled study lasted for 4 weeks, while the comparative studies had a 4- to 52-week double-blind phase. The following doses were studied: betaxolol 20 and 40 mg once daily and atenolol 100 mg once daily.

From European controlled hypertension clinical trials, the following adverse events reported by 2% or more patients and selected events with lower frequency are presented:

[See table 2 at top of previous page]

The only adverse event whose frequency clearly rose with increasing dose was bradycardia. Elderly patients were especially susceptible to bradycardia, which in some cases responded to dose-reduction (see *Precautions*).

The following selected (potentially important) adverse events have been reported at an incidence of less than 2% in U.S. controlled and open, long-term clinical studies, European controlled clinical trials, or in marketing experience. It is not known whether a causal relationship exists between betaxolol and these events; they are listed to alert the physician to a possible relationship:

Autonomic: flushing, salivation, sweating.

Body as a whole: allergy, fever, malaise, pain, rigors.

Cardiovascular: angina pectoris, arrhythmia, atrioventricular block, heart failure, hypertension, hypotension, myocardial infarction, thrombosis, syncope.

Central and peripheral nervous system: ataxia, neuralgia, neuropathy, numbness, speech disorder, stupor, tremor, twitching.

Gastrointestinal: anorexia, constipation, dry mouth, increased appetite, mouth ulceration, rectal disorders, vomiting, dysphagia.

Hearing and vestibular: earache, labyrinth disorders, tinnitus, deafness.

Hematologic: anemia, leucocytosis, lymphadenopathy, purpura, thrombocytopenia.

Liver and biliary: increased AST, increased ALT.

Metabolic and nutritional: acidosis, diabetes, hypercholesterolemia, hyperglycemia, hyperkalemia, hyperlipemia, hyperuricemia, hypokalemia, weight gain, weight loss, thirst, increased LDH.

Musculoskeletal: arthropathy, neck pain, muscle cramps, tendonitis.

Psychiatric: abnormal thinking, amnesia, impaired concentration, confusion, emotional lability, hallucinations, decreased libido.

Reproductive disorders: Female: breast pain, breast fibroadenosis, menstrual disorder; Male: Peyronie's disease, prostatitis.

Respiratory: bronchitis, bronchospasm, cough, epistaxis, flu, pneumonia, sinusitis.

Skin: alopecia, eczema, erythematous rash, hypertrichosis, pruritus, skin disorders.

Special senses: abnormal taste, taste loss.

Urinary system: cystitis, dysuria, micturition disorder, oliguria, proteinuria, abnormal renal function, renal pain.

Vascular: cerebrovascular disorder, intermittent claudication, leg cramps, peripheral ischemia, thrombophlebitis.

Vision: abnormal lacrimation, abnormal vision, blepharitis, ocular hemorrhage, conjunctivitis, dry eyes, iritis, cataract, scotoma.

Potential adverse effects: Although not reported in clinical studies with betaxolol, a variety of adverse effects have been reported with other beta-adrenergic blocking agents and may be considered potential adverse effects of betaxolol:

Central nervous system: Reversible mental depression progressing to catatonia, an acute reversible syndrome characterized by disorientation for time and place, short-term memory loss, emotional lability with slightly clouded sensorium, and decreased performance on neuropsychometric tests.

Allergic: Fever combined with aching and sore throat, laryngospasm, respiratory distress.

Hematologic: Agranulocytosis, thrombocytopenic purpura, and nonthrombocytopenic purpura.

Gastrointestinal: Mesenteric arterial thrombosis, ischemic colitis.

Miscellaneous: Raynaud's phenomena. There have been reports of skin rashes and/or dry eyes associated with the use of beta-adrenergic blocking drugs. The reported incidence is small, and in most cases, the symptoms have cleared when treatment was withdrawn. Discontinuation of the drug should be considered if any such reaction is not otherwise explicable. Patients should be closely monitored following cessation of therapy.

The oculomucocutaneous syndrome associated with the beta-blocker practolol has not been reported with Kerlone during investigational use and extensive foreign experience. However, dry eyes have been reported.

OVERDOSAGE

No specific information on emergency treatment of overdosage with Kerlone is available. The most common effects expected are bradycardia, congestive heart failure, hypotension, bronchospasm, and hypoglycemia. In one acute overdosage of betaxolol, a 16-year-old female recovered fully after ingesting 460 mg.

Oral LD_{50}s are 350 to 400 mg betaxolol/kg in mice and 860 to 980 mg/kg in rats.

In the case of overdosage, treatment with Kerlone should be stopped and the patient carefully observed. Hemodialysis or peritoneal dialysis does not remove substantial amounts of the drug. In addition to gastric lavage, the following therapeutic measures are suggested if warranted:

Hypotension: Use sympathomimetic pressor drug therapy, such as dopamine, dobutamine, or norepinephrine. In refractory cases of overdosage of other beta-blockers, the use of glucagon hydrochloride has been reported to be useful.

Bradycardia: Atropine should be administered. If there is no response to vagal blockade, isoproterenol should be administered cautiously. In refractory cases the use of a transvenous cardiac pacemaker may be considered.

Acute cardiac failure: Conventional therapy including digitalis, diuretics, and oxygen should be instituted immediately.

Bronchospasm: Use a β_2-agonist. Additional therapy with aminophylline may be considered.

Heart block (2nd- or 3rd-degree): Use isoproterenol or a transvenous cardiac pacemaker.

DOSAGE AND ADMINISTRATION

The initial dose of Kerlone in hypertension is ordinarily 10 mg once daily either alone or added to diuretic therapy. The full antihypertensive effect is usually seen within 7 to 14 days. If the desired response is not achieved the dose can be doubled after 7 to 14 days. Increasing the dose beyond 20 mg has not been shown to produce a statistically significant additional antihypertensive effect; but the 40-mg dose has been studied and is well tolerated. An increased effect (reduction) on heart rate should be anticipated with increasing dosage. If monotherapy with Kerlone does not produce the desired response, the addition of a diuretic agent or other antihypertensive should be considered (see *Drug interactions*).

Dosage adjustments for specific patients

Patients with renal failure: In patients with renal impairment, clearance of betaxolol declines with decreasing renal function.

In patients with severe renal impairment and those undergoing dialysis the initial dose of Kerlone is 5 mg once daily. If the desired response is not achieved, dosage may be increased by 5 mg/day increments every 2 weeks to a maximum dose of 20 mg/day.

Patients with hepatic disease: Patients with hepatic disease do not have significantly altered clearance. Dosage adjustments are not routinely needed.

Elderly patients: Consideration should be given to reduction in the starting dose to 5 mg in elderly patients. These patients are especially prone to beta-blocker–induced bradycardia, which appears to be dose related and sometimes responds to reductions in dose.

Cessation of therapy: If withdrawal of Kerlone therapy is planned, it should be achieved gradually over a period of about 2 weeks. Patients should be carefully observed and advised to limit physical activity to a minimum.

HOW SUPPLIED

Kerlone 10-mg tablets are round, white, film coated, with KERLONE 10 debossed on one side and scored on the other, supplied as:

NDC Number	Size
0025-5101-31	bottle of 100

Kerlone 20-mg tablets are round, white, film coated, with KERLONE 20 debossed on one side and β on the other, supplied as:

NDC Number	Size
0025-5201-31	bottle of 100

Store at controlled room temperature 15°-25°C (59°-77°F).

Rx only

Manufactured and distributed by
G.D. Searle & Co.
Chicago, IL 60680
by agreement with
Lorex Pharmaceuticals
Skokie, IL

Kerlone is a registered trademark of Synthelabo.

5/19/99 • A05426-3

Shown in Product Identification Guide, page 336

LOMOTIL® Liquid Ⓒ
LOMOTIL® Tablets Ⓒ

[lō-mō 'til]

(diphenoxylate hydrochloride with atropine sulfate)

DESCRIPTION

Each Lomotil tablet and each 5 ml of Lomotil liquid for oral use contains:

diphenoxylate hydrochloride .... 2.5 mg
(Warning—May be habit forming.)
atropine sulfate .... 0.025 mg

Diphenoxylate hydrochloride, an antidiarrheal, is ethyl 1-(3-cyano-3,3-diphenylpropyl)-4-phenylisonipecotate monohydrochloride and has the following structural formula:

Atropine sulfate, an anticholinergic, is endo-(±)-α-(hydroxymethyl) benzeneacetic acid 8-methyl-8-azabicyclo[3.2.1] oct-3-yl ester sulfate (2:1) (salt) monohydrate and has the following structural formula:

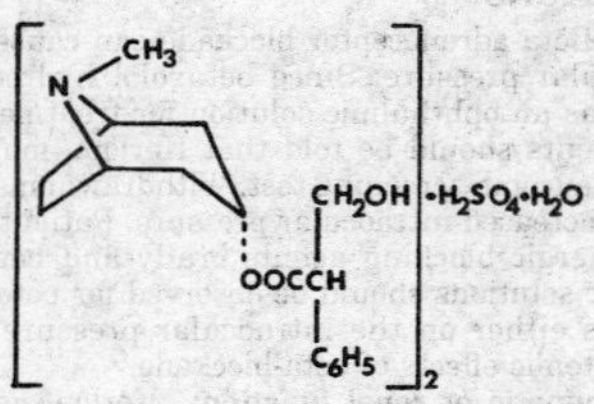

A subtherapeutic amount of atropine sulfate is present to discourage deliberate overdosage.

Inactive ingredients of Lomotil tablets include acacia, corn starch, magnesium stearate, sorbitol, sucrose, and talc. Inactive ingredients of Lomotil liquid include cherry flavor, citric acid, ethyl alcohol 15%, FD&C Yellow No. 6, glycerin, sodium phosphate, sorbitol, and water.

CLINICAL PHARMACOLOGY

Diphenoxylate is rapidly and extensively metabolized in man by ester hydrolysis to diphenoxylic acid (difenoxine), which is biologically active and the major metabolite in the blood. After a 5-mg oral dose of carbon-14 labeled diphenoxylate hydrochloride in ethanolic solution was given to three healthy volunteers, an average of 14% of the drug plus its metabolites was excreted in the urine and 49% in the feces over a four-day period. Urinary excretion of the unmetabolized drug constituted less than 1% of the dose, and diphenoxylic acid plus its glucuronide conjugate constituted about 6% of the dose. In a 16-subject crossover bioavailability study, a linear relationship in the dose range of 2.5 to 10 mg was found between the dose of diphenoxylate hydrochloride (given as Lomotil liquid) and the peak plasma concentration, the area under the plasma concentration-time curve, and the amount of diphenoxylic acid excreted in the urine. In the same study the bioavailability of the tablet compared with an equal dose of the liquid was approximately 90%. The average peak plasma concentration of diphenoxylic acid following ingestion of four 2.5-mg tablets was 163 ng/ml at about 2 hours, and the elimination half-life of diphenoxylic acid was approximately 12 to 14 hours.

In dogs, diphenoxylate hydrochloride has a direct effect on circular smooth muscle of the bowel that conceivably results in segmentation and prolongation of gastrointestinal transit time. The clinical antidiarrheal action of diphenoxylate hydrochloride may thus be a consequence of enhanced segmentation that allows increased contact of the intraluminal contents with the intestinal mucosa.

INDICATIONS AND USAGE

Lomotil is effective as adjunctive therapy in the management of diarrhea.

CONTRAINDICATIONS

Lomotil is contraindicated in patients with

1. Known hypersensitivity to diphenoxylate or atropine.
2. Obstructive jaundice.
3. Diarrhea associated with pseudomembranous enterocolitis or enterotoxin-producing bacteria.

WARNINGS

LOMOTIL IS *NOT* AN INNOCUOUS DRUG AND DOSAGE RECOMMENDATIONS SHOULD BE STRICTLY ADHERED TO, ESPECIALLY IN CHILDREN. LOMOTIL IS NOT RECOMMENDED FOR CHILDREN UNDER 2 YEARS OF AGE. OVERDOSAGE MAY RESULT IN SEVERE RESPIRATORY DEPRESSION AND COMA, POSSIBLY LEADING TO PERMANENT BRAIN DAMAGE OR DEATH (SEE *OVERDOSAGE*). THEREFORE, KEEP THIS MEDICATION OUT OF THE REACH OF CHILDREN.

THE USE OF LOMOTIL SHOULD BE ACCOMPANIED BY APPROPRIATE FLUID AND ELECTROLYTE THERAPY, WHEN INDICATED. IF SEVERE DEHYDRATION OR ELECTROLYTE IMBALANCE IS PRESENT, LOMOTIL SHOULD BE WITHHELD UNTIL APPROPRIATE CORRECTIVE THERAPY HAS BEEN INITIATED. DRUG-INDUCED INHIBITION OF PERISTALSIS MAY RESULT IN FLUID RETENTION IN THE INTESTINE, WHICH MAY FURTHER AGGRAVATE DEHYDRATION AND ELECTROLYTE IMBALANCE.

LOMOTIL SHOULD BE USED WITH SPECIAL CAUTION IN YOUNG CHILDREN BECAUSE THIS AGE GROUP MAY BE PREDISPOSED TO DELAYED DIPHENOXYLATE TOXICITY AND BECAUSE OF THE GREATER VARIABILITY OF RESPONSE IN THIS AGE GROUP.

Antiperistaltic agents may prolong and/or worsen diarrhea associated with organisms that penetrate the intestinal mucosa (toxigenic *E. coli, Salmonella, Shigella*), and pseudomembranous enterocolitis associated with broad-spectrum antibiotics. Antiperistaltic agents should not be used in these conditions.

In some patients with acute ulcerative colitis, agents that inhibit intestinal motility or prolong intestinal transit time have been reported to induce toxic megacolon. Consequently, patients with acute ulcerative colitis should be carefully observed and Lomotil therapy should be discontinued promptly if abdominal distention occurs or if other untoward symptoms develop.

Since the chemical structure of diphenoxylate hydrochloride is similar to that of meperidine hydrochloride, the concurrent use of Lomotil with monoamine oxidase (MAO) inhibitors may, in theory, precipitate hypertensive crisis.

Lomotil should be used with extreme caution in patients with advanced hepatorenal disease and in all patients with abnormal liver function since hepatic coma may be precipitated.

Diphenoxylate hydrochloride may potentiate the action of barbiturates, tranquilizers, and alcohol. Therefore, the patient should be closely observed when any of these are used concomitantly.

PRECAUTIONS

General: Since a subtherapeutic dose of atropine has been added to the diphenoxylate hydrochloride, consideration should be given to the precautions relating to the use of atropine. In children, Lomotil should be used with caution since signs of atropinism may occur even with recommended doses, particularly in patients with Down's syndrome.

Information for patients: INFORM THE PATIENT (PARENT OR GUARDIAN) NOT TO EXCEED THE RECOMMENDED DOSAGE AND TO KEEP LOMOTIL OUT OF THE REACH OF CHILDREN AND IN A CHILD-RESISTANT CONTAINER. INFORM THE PATIENT OF THE CONSEQUENCES OF OVERDOSAGE, INCLUDING SEVERE RESPIRATORY DEPRESSION AND COMA, POSSIBLY LEADING TO PERMANENT BRAIN DAMAGE OR DEATH. Lomotil may produce drowsiness or dizziness. The patient should be cautioned regarding activities requiring mental alertness, such as driving or operating dangerous machinery. Potentiation of the action of alcohol, barbiturates, and tranquilizers with concomitant use of Lomotil should be explained to the patient. The physician should also provide the patient with other information in this labeling, as appropriate.

Drug interactions: Known drug interactions include barbiturates, tranquilizers, and alcohol. Lomotil may interact with MAO inhibitors (see *Warnings*).

In studies with male rats, diphenoxylate hydrochloride was found to inhibit the hepatic microsomal enzyme system at a dose of 2 mg/kg/day. Therefore, diphenoxylate has the potential to prolong the biological half-lives of drugs for which the rate of elimination is dependent on the microsomal drug metabolizing enzyme system.

Carcinogenesis, mutagenesis, impairment of fertility: No long-term study in animals has been performed to evaluate carcinogenic potential. Diphenoxylate hydrochloride was administered to male and female rats in their diets to provide dose levels of 4 and 20 mg/kg/day throughout a three-litter reproduction study. At 50 times the human dose (20 mg/kg/day), female weight gain was reduced and there was a marked effect on fertility as only 4 of 27 females became pregnant in three test breedings. The relevance of this finding to usage of Lomotil in humans is unknown.

Pregnancy: Pregnancy Category C. Diphenoxylate hydrochloride has been shown to have an effect on fertility in rats when given in doses 50 times the human dose (see above discussion). Other findings in this study include a decrease in maternal weight gain of 30% at 20 mg/kg/day and of 10% at 4 mg/kg/day. At 10 times the human dose (4 mg/kg/day), average litter size was slightly reduced.

Teratology studies were conducted in rats, rabbits, and mice with diphenoxylate hydrochloride at oral doses of 0.4 to 20 mg/kg/day. Due to experimental design and small numbers of litters, embryotoxic, fetotoxic, or teratogenic effects cannot be adequately assessed. However, examination of the available fetuses did not reveal any indication of teratogenicity.

There are no adequate and well-controlled studies in pregnant women. Lomotil should be used during pregnancy only if the anticipated benefit justifies the potential risk to the fetus.

Nursing mothers: Caution should be exercised when Lomotil is administered to a nursing woman, since the physicochemical characteristics of the major metabolite, diphenoxylic acid, are such that it may be excreted in breast milk and since it is known that atropine is excreted in breast milk.

Pediatric use: Lomotil may be used as an adjunct to the treatment of diarrhea but should be accompanied by appropriate fluid and electrolyte therapy, if needed. LOMOTIL IS NOT RECOMMENDED FOR CHILDREN UNDER 2 YEARS OF AGE. Lomotil should be used with special caution in young children because of the greater variability of response in this age group. See *Warnings* and *Dosage and Administration.* In case of accidental ingestion by children, see *Overdosage* for recommended treatment.

ADVERSE REACTIONS

At *therapeutic* doses, the following have been reported; they are listed in decreasing order of severity, but not of frequency:

Nervous system: numbness of extremities, euphoria, depression, malaise/lethargy, confusion, sedation/drowsiness, dizziness, restlessness, headache.

Allergic: anaphylaxis, angioneurotic edema, urticaria, swelling of the gums, pruritus.

Gastrointestinal system: toxic megacolon, paralytic ileus, pancreatitis, vomiting, nausea, anorexia, abdominal discomfort.

The following atropine sulfate effects are listed in decreasing order of severity, but not of frequency: hyperthermia, tachycardia, urinary retention, flushing, dryness of the skin and mucous membranes. These effects may occur, especially in children.

THIS MEDICATION SHOULD BE KEPT IN A CHILD-RESISTANT CONTAINER AND OUT OF THE REACH OF CHILDREN SINCE AN OVERDOSAGE MAY RESULT IN SEVERE RESPIRATORY DEPRESSION AND COMA, POSSIBLY LEADING TO PERMANENT BRAIN DAMAGE OR DEATH.

DRUG ABUSE AND DEPENDENCE

Controlled substance: Lomotil is classified as a Schedule V controlled substance by federal regulation. Diphenoxylate hydrochloride is chemically related to the narcotic analgesic meperidine.

Drug abuse and dependence: In doses used for the treatment of diarrhea, whether acute or chronic, diphenoxylate has not produced addiction.

Diphenoxylate hydrochloride is devoid of morphine-like subjective effects at therapeutic doses. At high doses it exhibits codeine-like subjective effects. The dose which produces antidiarrheal action is widely separated from the dose which causes central nervous system effects. The insolubility of diphenoxylate hydrochloride in commonly available aqueous media precludes intravenous self-administration. A dose of 100 to 300 mg/day, which is equivalent to 40 to 120 tablets, administered to humans for 40 to 70 days, produced opiate withdrawal symptoms. Since addiction to diphenoxylate hydrochloride is possible at high doses, the recommended dosage should not be exceeded.

OVERDOSAGE

RECOMMENDED DOSAGE SCHEDULES SHOULD BE STRICTLY FOLLOWED. THIS MEDICATION SHOULD BE KEPT IN A CHILD-RESISTANT CONTAINER AND OUT OF THE REACH OF CHILDREN, SINCE AN OVERDOSAGE MAY RESULT IN SEVERE, EVEN FATAL, RESPIRATORY DEPRESSION.

Diagnosis: Initial signs of overdosage may include dryness of the skin and mucous membranes, mydriasis, restlessness, flushing, hyperthermia, and tachycardia followed by lethargy or coma, hypotonic reflexes, nystagmus, pinpoint pupils, and respiratory depression. Respiratory depression may be evidenced as late as 30 hours after ingestion and may recur despite an initial response to narcotic antagonists. TREAT ALL POSSIBLE LOMOTIL OVERDOSAGES AS SERIOUS AND MAINTAIN MEDICAL OBSERVATION FOR AT LEAST 48 HOURS, PREFERABLY UNDER CONTINUOUS HOSPITAL CARE.

Treatment: In the event of overdose, induction of vomiting, gastric lavage, establishment of a patent airway, and possibly mechanically assisted respiration are advised. *In vitro* and animal studies indicate that activated charcoal may significantly decrease the bioavailability of diphenoxylate. In noncomatose patients, a slurry of 100 g of activated charcoal can be administered immediately after the induction of vomiting or gastric lavage.

A pure narcotic antagonist (eg, naloxone) should be used in the treatment of respiratory depression caused by Lomotil. When a narcotic antagonist is administered intravenously, the onset of action is generally apparent within two minutes. It may also be administered subcutaneously or intramuscularly, providing a slightly less rapid onset of action but a more prolonged effect.

To counteract respiratory depression caused by Lomotil overdosage, the following dosage schedule for the narcotic antagonist naloxone hydrochloride should be followed:

Adult dosage: An initial dose of 0.4 mg to 2 mg of naloxone hydrochloride may be administered intravenously. If the desired degree of counteraction and improvement in respiratory function is not obtained, it may be repeated at 2- to 3-minute intervals. If no response is observed after 10 mg of naloxone hydrochloride has been administered, the diagnosis of narcotic-induced or partial narcotic-induced toxicity should be questioned. Intramuscular or subcutaneous administration may be necessary if the intravenous route is not available.

Children: The usual initial dose in children is 0.01 mg/kg body weight given I.V. If this dose does not result in the desired degree of clinical improvement, a subsequent dose of 0.1 mg/kg body weight may be administered. If an I.V. route of administration is not available, naloxone hydrochloride may be administered I.M. or S.C. in divided doses. If necessary, naloxone hydrochloride can be diluted with sterile water for injection.

Following initial improvement of respiratory function, repeated doses of naloxone hydrochloride may be required to counteract recurrent respiratory depression. Supplemental intramuscular doses of naloxone hydrochloride may be utilized to produce a longer-lasting effect.

Since the duration of action of diphenoxylate hydrochloride is longer than that of naloxone hydrochloride, improvement of respiration following administration may be followed by recurrent respiratory depression. Consequently, continuous observation is necessary until the effect of diphenoxylate hydrochloride on respiration has passed. This effect may persist for many hours. The period of observation should extend over at least 48 hours, preferably under continuous hospital care. Although signs of overdosage and respiratory depression may not be evident soon after ingestion of diphenoxylate hydrochloride, respiratory depression may occur from 12 to 30 hours later.

DOSAGE AND ADMINISTRATION

DO NOT EXCEED RECOMMENDED DOSAGE.

Adults: The recommended initial dosage is two Lomotil tablets four times daily or 10 ml (two regular teaspoonfuls) of Lomotil liquid four times daily (20 mg per day). Most patients will require this dosage until initial control has been achieved, after which the dosage may be reduced to meet individual requirements. Control may often be maintained with as little as 5 mg (two tablets or 10 ml of liquid) daily.

Clinical improvement of acute diarrhea is usually observed within 48 hours. If clinical improvement of chronic diarrhea after treatment with a maximum daily dose of 20 mg of diphenoxylate hydrochloride is not observed within 10 days, symptoms are unlikely to be controlled by further administration.

Children: Lomotil is not recommended in children under 2 years of age and should be used with special caution in young children (see *Warnings* and *Precautions*). *The nutritional status and degree of dehydration must be considered. In children under 13 years of age, use Lomotil liquid. Do not use Lomotil tablets for this age group.*

Only the plastic dropper should be used when measuring Lomotil liquid for administration to children.

Dosage schedule for children: The recommended initial total daily dosage of Lomotil liquid for children is 0.3 to 0.4 mg/kg, administered in four divided doses. The following table provides an *approximate* initial daily dosage recommendation for children.

Age (years)	Approximate weight (kg)	(lb)	Dosage in ml (four times daily)
2	11–14	24–31	1.5–3.0
3	12–16	26–35	2.0–3.0
4	14–20	31–44	2.0–4.0
5	16–23	35–51	2.5–4.5
6–8	17–32	38–71	2.5–5.0
9–12	23–55	51–121	3.5–5.0

The recommended dosage for children 13–16 years: 2 tablets or two 5ml liquid measures three times daily.

These pediatric schedules are the best approximation of an average dose recommendation which may be adjusted downward according to the overall nutritional status and degree of dehydration encountered in the sick child. Reduction of dosage may be made as soon as initial control of symptoms has been achieved. Maintenance dosage may be as low as one-fourth of the initial daily dosage. If no response occurs within 48 hours, Lomotil is unlikely to be effective.

KEEP THIS AND ALL MEDICATIONS OUT OF THE REACH OF CHILDREN.

HOW SUPPLIED

Tablets—round, white, with SEARLE debossed on one side and 61 on the other side and containing 2.5 mg of diphenoxylate hydrochloride and 0.025 mg of atropine sulfate, supplied as:

NDC Number	Size
0025-0061-31	bottle of 100
0025-0061-51	bottle of 500
0025-0061-52	bottle of 1,000
0025-0061-55	bottle of 2,500
0025-0061-34	carton of 100 unit dose

Liquid—containing 2.5 mg of diphenoxylate hydrochloride and 0.025 mg of atropine sulfate per 5 ml; bottles of 2 fl oz (NDC Number 0025-0066-02). Dispense only in original container.

A plastic dropper calibrated in increments of $^1/_2$ ml ($^1/_4$ mg) with a capacity of 2 ml (1 mg) accompanies each 2-oz bottle of Lomotil liquid. Only this plastic dropper should be used when measuring Lomotil liquid for administration to children.

Rx only 12/15/98 • A05758-5

Shown in Product Identification Guide, page 336

NORPACE® Capsules ℞
[*nor 'pāce*]
(disopyramide phosphate)

NORPACE® CR Capsules ℞
(disopyramide phosphate extended-release)

DESCRIPTION

Norpace (disopyramide phosphate) is an antiarrhythmic drug available for oral administration in immediate-release and controlled-release capsules containing 100 mg or 150

Continued on next page

Norpace/Norpace CR—Cont.

mg of disopyramide base, present as the phosphate. The base content of the phosphate salt is 77.6%. The structural formula of Norpace is:

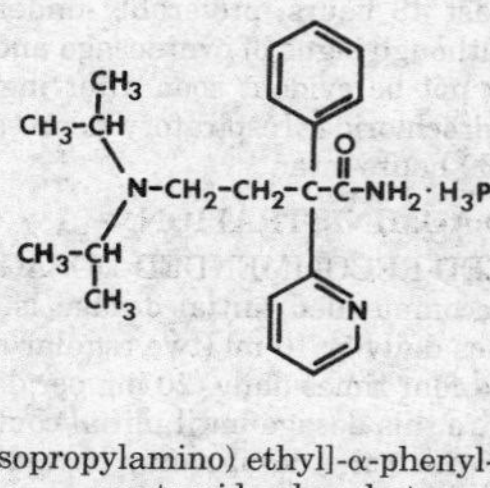

α-[2-(diisopropylamino) ethyl]-α-phenyl-2-pyridine-acetamide phosphate

Norpace is freely soluble in water, and the free base (pKa 10.4) has an aqueous solubility of 1 mg/ml. The chloroform: water partition coefficient of the base is 3.1 at pH 7.2.

Norpace is a racemic mixture of *d* - and *l*-isomers. This drug is not chemically related to other antiarrhythmic drugs.

Norpace CR (controlled-release) capsules are designed to afford a gradual and consistent release of disopyramide. Thus, for maintenance therapy, Norpace CR provides the benefit of less-frequent dosing (every 12 hours) as compared with the every-6-hour dosage schedule of immediate-release Norpace capsules.

Inactive ingredients of Norpace include corn starch, edible ink, FD&C Red No. 3, FD&C Yellow No. 6, gelatin, lactose, talc, and titanium dioxide; the 150-mg capsule also contains FD&C Blue No. 1.

Inactive ingredients of Norpace CR include corn starch, D&C Yellow No. 10, edible ink, ethylcellulose, FD&C Blue No. 1, gelatin, shellac, sucrose, talc, and titanium dioxide; the 150-mg capsule also contains FD&C Red No. 3 and FD&C Yellow No. 6.

CLINICAL PHARMACOLOGY

Mechanisms of Action

Norpace (disopyramide phosphate) is a Type 1 antiarrhythmic drug (ie, similar to procainamide and quinidine). *In animal studies* Norpace decreases the rate of diastolic depolarization (phase 4) in cells with augmented automaticity, decreases the upstroke velocity (phase 0) and increases the action potential duration of normal cardiac cells, decreases the disparity in refractoriness between infarcted and adjacent normally perfused myocardium, and has no effect on alpha- or beta-adrenergic receptors.

Electrophysiology

In man, Norpace at therapeutic plasma levels shortens the sinus node recovery time, lengthens the effective refractory period of the atrium, and has a minimal effect on the effective refractory period of the AV node. Little effect has been shown on AV-nodal and His-Purkinje conduction times or QRS duration. However, prolongation of conduction in accessory pathways occurs.

Hemodynamics

At recommended oral doses, Norpace rarely produces significant alterations of blood pressure in patients without congestive heart failure (see *Warnings*). With intravenous Norpace, either increases in systolic/diastolic or decreases in systolic blood pressure have been reported, depending on the infusion rate and the patient population. Intravenous Norpace may cause cardiac depression with an approximate mean 10% reduction of cardiac output, which is more pronounced in patients with cardiac dysfunction.

The *in vitro* anticholinergic activity of Norpace is approximately 0.06% that of atropine; however, the usual dose for Norpace is 150 mg every 6 hours and for Norpace CR 300 mg every 12 hours, compared to 0.4 to 0.6 mg for atropine (see *Warnings* and *Adverse Reactions* for anticholinergic side effects).

Pharmacokinetics

Following oral administration of immediate-release Norpace, disopyramide phosphate is rapidly and almost completely absorbed, and peak plasma levels are usually attained within 2 hours. The usual therapeutic plasma levels of disopyramide base are 2 to 4 mcg/ml, and at these concentrations protein binding varies from 50% to 65%. Because of concentration-dependent protein binding, it is difficult to predict the concentration of the free drug when total drug is measured.

The mean plasma half-life of disopyramide in healthy humans is 6.7 hours (range of 4 to 10 hours). In six patients with impaired renal function (creatinine clearance less than 40 ml/min), disopyramide half-life values were 8 to 18 hours.

After the oral administration of 200 mg of disopyramide to 10 cardiac patients with borderline to moderate heart failure, the time to peak serum concentration of 2.3 ± 1.5 hours (mean ± SD) was increased, and the mean peak serum concentration of 4.8 ± 1.6 mcg/ml was higher than in healthy volunteers. After intravenous administration in these same patients, the mean elimination half-life was 9.7 ± 4.2 hours (range in healthy volunteers of 4.4 to 7.8 hours). In a second study of the oral administration of disopyramide to 7 patients with heart disease, including left ventricular dysfunction, the mean plasma half-life was slightly prolonged to 7.8 ± 1.9 hours (range of 5 to 9.5 hours).

In healthy men, about 50% of a given dose of disopyramide is excreted in the urine as the unchanged drug, about 20% as the mono-N-dealkylated metabolite, and 10% as the other metabolites. The plasma concentration of the major metabolite is approximately one tenth that of disopyramide. Altering the urinary pH in man does not affect the plasma half-life of disopyramide.

In a crossover study in healthy subjects, the bioavailability of disopyramide from Norpace CR capsules was similar to that from the immediate-release capsules. With a single 300-mg oral dose, peak disopyramide plasma concentrations of 3.23 ± 0.75 mcg/ml (mean ± SD) at 2.5 ± 2.3 hours were obtained with two 150-mg immediate-release capsules and 2.22 ± 0.47 mcg/ml at 4.9 ± 1.4 hours with two 150-mg Norpace CR capsules. The elimination half-life of disopyramide was 8.31 ± 1.83 hours with the immediate-release capsules and 11.65 ± 4.72 hours with Norpace CR capsules. The amount of disopyramide and mono-N-dealkylated metabolite excreted in the urine in 48 hours was 128 and 48 mg, respectively, with the immediate-release capsules, and 112 and 33 mg, respectively, with Norpace CR capsules. The differences in the urinary excretion of either constituent were not statistically significant.

Following multiple doses, steady-state plasma levels of between 2 and 4 mcg/ml were attained following either 150 mg every-6-hour dosing with immediate-release capsules or 300 mg every-12-hour dosing with Norpace CR capsules.

Drug Interactions

Effects of other drugs on disopyramide pharmacokinetics: In vitro metabolic studies indicated that disopyramide is metabolized by cytochrome P450 3A4 and that inhibitors of this enzyme may result in elevation of plasma levels of disopyramide. Although specific drug interaction studies have not been done, cases of life-threatening interactions have been reported for disopyramide when given with clarithromycin and erythromycin.

INDICATIONS AND USAGE

Norpace and Norpace CR are indicated for the treatment of documented ventricular arrhythmias, such as sustained ventricular tachycardia, that, in the judgment of the physician, are life-threatening. Because of the proarrhythmic effects of Norpace and Norpace CR, their use with lesser arrhythmias is generally not recommended. Treatment of patients with asymptomatic ventricular premature contractions should be avoided.

Initiation of Norpace or Norpace CR treatment, as with other antiarrhythmic agents used to treat life-threatening arrhythmias, should be carried out in the hospital. Norpace CR should not be used initially if rapid establishment of disopyramide plasma levels is desired.

Antiarrhythmic drugs have not been shown to enhance survival in patients with ventricular arrhythmias.

CONTRAINDICATIONS

Norpace and Norpace CR are contraindicated in the presence of cardiogenic shock, preexisting second- or third-degree AV block (if no pacemaker is present), congenital Q-T prolongation, or known hypersensitivity to the drug.

WARNINGS

Mortality

In the National Heart, Lung and Blood Institute's Cardiac Arrhythmia Suppression Trial (CAST), a long-term, multi-center, randomized, double-blind study in patients with asymptomatic non-life-threatening ventricular arrhythmias who had had a myocardial infarction more than 6 days but less than 2 years previously, an excessive mortality or non-fatal cardiac arrest rate (7.7%) was seen in patients treated with encainide or flecainide compared with that seen in patients assigned to carefully matched placebo-treated groups (3.0%). The average duration of treatment with encainide or flecainide in this study was 10 months.

The applicability of the CAST results to other populations (eg, those without recent myocardial infarction) is uncertain. Considering the known proarrhythmic properties of Norpace or Norpace CR and the lack of evidence of improved survival for any antiarrhythmic drug in patients without life-threatening arrhythmias, the use of Norpace or Norpace CR as well as other antiarrhythmic agents should be reserved for patients with life-threatening ventricular arrhythmias.

Negative Inotropic Properties:
Heart Failure/Hypotension

Norpace or Norpace CR may cause or worsen congestive heart failure or produce severe hypotension as a consequence of its negative inotropic properties. Hypotension has been observed primarily in patients with primary cardiomyopathy or inadequately compensated congestive heart failure. Norpace or Norpace CR should not be used in patients with uncompensated or marginally compensated congestive heart failure or hypotension unless the congestive heart failure or hypotension is secondary to cardiac arrhythmia. Patients with a history of heart failure may be treated with Norpace or Norpace CR, but careful attention must be given to the maintenance of cardiac function, including optimal digitalization. If hypotension occurs or congestive heart failure worsens, Norpace or Norpace CR should be discontinued and, if necessary, restarted at a lower dosage only after adequate cardiac compensation has been established.

QRS Widening

Although it is unusual, significant widening (greater than 25%) of the QRS complex may occur during Norpace or Norpace CR administration; in such cases Norpace or Norpace CR should be discontinued.

Q-T Prolongation

As with other Type 1 antiarrhythmic drugs, prolongation of the Q-T interval (corrected) and worsening of the arrhythmia, including ventricular tachycardia and ventricular fibrillation, may occur. Patients who have evidenced prolongation of the Q-T interval in response to quinidine may be at particular risk. As with other Type 1A antiarrhythmics, disopyramide phosphate has been associated with torsade de pointes.

If a Q-T prolongation of greater than 25% is observed and if ectopy continues, the patient should be monitored closely, and consideration be given to discontinuing Norpace or Norpace CR.

Hypoglycemia

In rare instances significant lowering of blood glucose values has been reported during Norpace administration. The physician should be alert to this possibility, especially in patients with congestive heart failure, chronic malnutrition, hepatic, renal, or other diseases, or drugs (eg, beta adrenoceptor blockers, alcohol) which could compromise preservation of the normal glucoregulatory mechanisms in the absence of food. In these patients the blood glucose levels should be carefully followed.

Concomitant Antiarrhythmic Therapy

The concomitant use of Norpace or Norpace CR with other Type 1A antiarrhythmic agents (such as quinidine or procainamide), Type 1C antiarrhythmics (such as encainide, flecainide or propafenone), and/or propranolol should be reserved for patients with life-threatening arrhythmias who are demonstrably unresponsive to single-agent antiarrhythmic therapy. Such use may produce serious negative inotropic effects, or may excessively prolong conduction. This should be considered particularly in patients with any degree of cardiac decompensation or those with a prior history thereof. Patients receiving more than one antiarrhythmic drug must be carefully monitored.

Heart Block

If first-degree heart block develops in a patient receiving Norpace or Norpace CR, the dosage should be reduced. If the block persists despite reduction of dosage, continuation of the drug must depend upon weighing the benefit being obtained against the risk of higher degrees of heart block. Development of second- or third-degree AV block or unifascicular, bifascicular, or trifascicular block requires discontinuation of Norpace or Norpace CR therapy, unless the ventricular rate is adequately controlled by a temporary or implanted ventricular pacemaker.

Anticholinergic Activity

Because of its anticholinergic activity, disopyramide phosphate should not be used in patients with glaucoma, myasthenia gravis, or urinary retention unless adequate overriding measures are taken; these consist of the topical application of potent miotics (eg, pilocarpine) for patients with glaucoma, and catheter drainage or operative relief for patients with urinary retention. Urinary retention may occur in patients of either sex as a consequence of Norpace or Norpace CR administration, but males with benign prostatic hypertrophy are at particular risk. In patients with a family history of glaucoma, intraocular pressure should be measured before initiating Norpace or Norpace CR therapy. Disopyramide phosphate should be used with special care in patients with myasthenia gravis since its anticholinergic properties could precipitate a myasthenic crisis in such patients.

PRECAUTIONS

General

Atrial Tachyarrhythmias

Patients with atrial flutter or fibrillation should be digitalized prior to Norpace or Norpace CR administration to ensure that drug-induced enhancement of AV conduction does not result in an increase of ventricular rate beyond physiologically acceptable limits.

Conduction Abnormalities

Care should be taken when prescribing Norpace or Norpace CR for patients with sick sinus syndrome (bradycardia-tachycardia syndrome), Wolff-Parkinson-White syndrome (WPW), or bundle branch block. The effect of disopyramide phosphate in these conditions is uncertain at present.

Cardiomyopathy

Patients with myocarditis or other cardiomyopathy may develop significant hypotension in response to the usual dosage of disopyramide phosphate, probably due to cardiodepressant mechanisms. Therefore, a loading dose of Norpace should not be given to such patients, and initial dosage and subsequent dosage adjustments should be made under close supervision (see *Dosage and Administration*).

Renal Impairment

More than 50% of disopyramide is excreted in the urine unchanged. Therefore Norpace dosage should be reduced in patients with impaired renal function (see *Dosage and Administration*). The electrocardiogram should be carefully monitored for prolongation of PR interval, evidence of QRS widening, or other signs of overdosage (see *Overdosage*).

Norpace CR is not recommended for patients with severe renal insufficiency (creatinine clearance 40 ml/min or less).

Hepatic Impairment

Hepatic impairment also causes an increase in the plasma half-life of disopyramide. Dosage should be reduced for patients with such impairment. The electrocardiogram should be carefully monitored for signs of overdosage (see *Overdosage*).

Patients with cardiac dysfunction have a higher potential for hepatic impairment; this should be considered when administering Norpace or Norpace CR.

Potassium Imbalance

Antiarrhythmic drugs may be ineffective in patients with hypokalemia, and their toxic effects may be enhanced in patients with hyperkalemia. Therefore, potassium abnormalities should be corrected before starting Norpace or Norpace CR therapy.

Drug Interactions

If phenytoin or other hepatic enzyme inducers are taken concurrently with Norpace or Norpace CR, lower plasma levels of disopyramide may occur. Monitoring of disopyramide plasma levels is recommended in such concurrent use to avoid ineffective therapy. Other antiarrhythmic drugs (eg, quinidine, procainamide, lidocaine, propranolol) have occasionally been used concurrently with Norpace. Excessive widening of the QRS complex and/or prolongation of the Q-T interval may occur in these situations (see *Warnings*).

In healthy subjects, no significant drug-drug interaction was observed when Norpace was coadministered with either propranolol or diazepam. Concomitant administration of Norpace and quinidine resulted in slight increases in plasma disopyramide levels and slight decreases in plasma quinidine levels. Norpace does not increase serum digoxin levels.

Until data on possible interactions between verapamil and disopyramide phosphate are obtained, disopyramide should not be administered within 48 hours before or 24 hours after verapamil administration.

Although potent inhibitors of cytochrome P450 3A4 (eg, ketoconazole) have not been studied clinically, in vitro studies have shown that erythromycin and oleandomycin inhibit the metabolism of disopyramide. Cases of life-threatening interactions have been reported for disopyramide when given with clarithromycin and erythromycin indicating that coadministration of disopyramide with inhibitors of cytochrome P450 3A4 could result in potentially fatal interaction.

Carcinogenesis, Mutagenesis, Impairment of Fertility

Eighteen months of Norpace administration to rats, at oral doses up to 400 mg/kg/day (about 30 times the usual daily human dose of 600 mg/day, assuming a patient weight of at least 50 kg), revealed no evidence of carcinogenic potential. An evaluation of mutagenic potential by Ames test was negative. Norpace, at doses up to 250 mg/kg/day, did not adversely affect fertility of rats.

Pregnancy

Teratogenic Effects: Pregnancy Category C. Norpace was associated with decreased numbers of implantation sites and decreased growth and survival of pups when administered to pregnant rats at 250 mg/kg/day (20 or more times the usual daily human dose of 12 mg/kg, assuming a patient weight of at least 50 kg), a level at which weight gain and food consumption of dams were also reduced. Increased resorption rates were reported in rabbits at 60 mg/kg/day (5 or more times the usual daily human dose). Effects on implantation, pup growth, and survival were not evaluated in rabbits. There are no adequate and well-controlled studies in pregnant women. Norpace or Norpace CR should be used during pregnancy only if the potential benefit justifies the potential risk to the fetus.

Nonteratogenic Effects: **Norpace has been reported to stimulate contractions of the pregnant uterus.** Disopyramide has been found in human fetal blood.

Labor and Delivery

It is not known whether the use of Norpace or Norpace CR during labor or delivery has immediate or delayed adverse effects on the fetus, or whether it prolongs the duration of labor or increases the need for forceps delivery or other obstetric intervention.

Nursing Mothers

Studies in rats have shown that the concentration of disopyramide and its metabolites is between one and three times greater in milk than it is in plasma. Following oral administration, disopyramide has been detected in human milk at a concentration not exceeding that in plasma. Because of the potential for serious adverse reactions in nursing infants from Norpace or Norpace CR, a decision should be made whether to discontinue nursing or to discontinue the drug, taking into account the importance of the drug to the mother.

Pediatric Use

Safety and effectiveness in pediatric patients have not been established (see *Dosage and Administration*).

Geriatric Use

Clinical studies of Norpace/Norpace CR did not include sufficient numbers of subjects aged 65 and over to determine whether they respond differently from younger subjects. Other reported clinical experience has not identified differences in responses between the elderly and younger patients. In general, dose selection for an elderly patient should be cautious, usually starting at the low end of the dosing range, reflecting the greater frequency of decreased hepatic, renal, or cardiac function, and of concomitant disease or other drug therapy.

Because of its anticholinergic activity, disopyramide phosphate should not be used in patients with glaucoma, urinary retention, or benign prostatic hypertrophy (medical conditions commonly associated with the elderly) unless adequate overriding measures are taken (see *Warnings: Anticholinergic Activity*). In the event of increased anticholinergic side effects, plasma levels of disopyramide should be monitored and the dose of the drug adjusted accordingly. A reduction of the dose by one third, from the recommended 600 mg/day to 400 mg/day, would be reasonable, without changing the dosing interval. This drug is known to be substantially excreted by the kidney, and the risk of toxic reactions to this drug may be greater in patients with impaired renal function. Because elderly patients are more likely to have decreased renal function, care should be taken in dose selection, and it may be useful to monitor renal function (see *Precautions: Renal Impairment* and *Dosage and Administration*).

ADVERSE REACTIONS

The adverse reactions which were reported in Norpace clinical trials encompass observations in 1,500 patients, including 90 patients studied for at least 4 years. The most serious adverse reactions are hypotension and congestive heart failure. The most common adverse reactions, which are dose dependent, are associated with the anticholinergic properties of the drug. These may be transitory, but may be persistent or can be severe. Urinary retention is the most serious anticholinergic effect.

The following reactions were reported in 10% to 40% of patients:

Anticholinergic: dry mouth (32%), urinary hesitancy (14%), constipation (11%)

The following reactions were reported in 3% to 9% of patients:

Anticholinergic: blurred vision, dry nose/eyes/throat

Genitourinary: urinary retention, urinary frequency and urgency

Gastrointestinal: nausea, pain/bloating/gas

General: dizziness, general fatigue/muscle weakness, headache, malaise, aches/pains

The following reactions were reported in 1% to 3% of patients:

Genitourinary: impotence

Cardiovascular: hypotension with or without congestive heart failure, increased congestive heart failure (see *Warnings*), cardiac conduction disturbances (see *Warnings*), edema/weight gain, shortness of breath, syncope, chest pain

Gastrointestinal: anorexia, diarrhea, vomiting

Dermatologic: generalized rash/dermatoses, itching

Central nervous system: nervousness

Other: hypokalemia, elevated cholesterol/triglycerides

The following reactions were reported in less than 1%:

Depression, insomnia, dysuria, numbness/tingling, elevated liver enzymes, AV block, elevated BUN, elevated creatinine, decreased hemoglobin/hematocrit

Hypoglycemia has been reported in association with Norpace administration (see *Warnings*).

Infrequent occurrences of reversible cholestatic jaundice, fever, and respiratory difficulty have been reported in association with disopyramide therapy, as have rare instances of thrombocytopenia, reversible agranulocytosis, and gynecomastia. Some cases of LE (lupus erythematosus) symptoms have been reported; most cases occurred in patients who had been switched to disopyramide from procainamide following the development of LE symptoms. Rarely, acute psychosis has been reported following Norpace therapy, with prompt return to normal mental status when therapy was stopped. The physician should be aware of these possible reactions and should discontinue Norpace or Norpace CR therapy promptly if they occur.

OVERDOSAGE

Symptoms

Deliberate or accidental overdosage of oral disopyramide may be followed by apnea, loss of consciousness, cardiac arrhythmias, and loss of spontaneous respiration. Death has occurred following overdosage.

Toxic plasma levels of disopyramide produce excessive widening of the QRS complex and Q-T interval, worsening of congestive heart failure, hypotension, varying kinds and degrees of conduction disturbance, bradycardia, and finally asystole. Obvious anticholinergic effects are also observed.

The approximate oral LD_{50} of disopyramide phosphate is 580 and 700 mg/kg for rats and mice, respectively.

Treatment

Experience indicates that prompt and vigorous treatment of overdosage is necessary, even in the absence of symptoms. Such treatment may be lifesaving. No specific antidote for disopyramide phosphate has been identified. Treatment should be symptomatic and may include induction of emesis or gastric lavage, administration of a cathartic followed by activated charcoal by mouth or stomach tube, intravenous administration of isoproterenol and dopamine, insertion of an intra-aortic balloon for counterpulsation, and mechanically assisted ventilation. Hemodialysis or, preferably, hemoperfusion with charcoal may be employed to lower serum concentration of the drug.

The electrocardiogram should be monitored, and supportive therapy with cardiac glycosides and diuretics should be given as required.

If progressive AV block should develop, endocardial pacing should be implemented. In case of any impaired renal function, measures to increase the glomerular filtration rate may reduce the toxicity (disopyramide is excreted primarily by the kidney).

The anticholinergic effects can be reversed with neostigmine at the discretion of the physician.

Altering the urinary pH in humans does not affect the plasma half-life or the amount of disopyramide excreted in the urine.

DOSAGE AND ADMINISTRATION

The dosage of Norpace or Norpace CR must be individualized for each patient on the basis of response and tolerance. The usual adult dosage of Norpace or Norpace CR is 400 to 800 mg per day given in divided doses. The recommended dosage for most adults is 600 mg/day given in divided doses (either 150 mg every 6 hours for immediate-release Norpace or 300 mg every 12 hours for Norpace CR). For patients whose body weight is less than 110 pounds (50 kg), the recommended dosage is 400 mg/day given in divided doses (either 100 mg every 6 hours for immediate-release Norpace or 200 mg every 12 hours for Norpace CR). In the event of increased anticholinergic side effects, plasma levels of disopyramide should be monitored and the dose of the drug adjusted accordingly. A reduction of the dose by one third, from the recommended 600 mg/day to 400 mg/day, would be reasonable, without changing the dosing interval.

For patients with cardiomyopathy or possible cardiac decompensation, a loading dose, as discussed below, should not be given, and initial dosage should be limited to 100 mg of immediate-release Norpace every 6 to 8 hours. Subsequent dosage adjustments should be made gradually, with close monitoring for the possible development of hypotension and/or congestive heart failure (see *Warnings*).

For patients with moderate renal insufficiency (creatinine clearance greater than 40 ml/min) or hepatic insufficiency, the recommended dosage is 400 mg/day given in divided doses (either 100 mg every 6 hours for immediate-release Norpace or 200 mg every 12 hours for Norpace CR).

For patients with severe renal insufficiency (C_{cr} 40 ml/min or less), the recommended dosage regimen of immediate-release Norpace is 100 mg at intervals shown in the table below, with or without an initial loading dose of 150 mg.

IMMEDIATE-RELEASE NORPACE DOSAGE INTERVAL FOR PATIENTS WITH RENAL INSUFFICIENCY

Creatinine clearance (ml/min)	40–30	30–15	less than 15
Approximate maintenance dosing interval	q 8 hr	q 12 hr	q 24 hr

The above dosing schedules are for Norpace immediate-release capsules; Norpace CR is not recommended for patients with severe renal insufficiency.

For patients in whom rapid control of ventricular arrhythmia is essential, an initial loading dose of 300 mg of immediate-release Norpace (200 mg for patients whose body weight is less than 110 pounds) is recommended, followed by the appropriate maintenance dosage. Therapeutic effects are usually attained 30 minutes to 3 hours after administration of a 300-mg loading dose. If there is no response or evidence of toxicity within 6 hours of the loading dose, 200 mg of immediate-release Norpace every 6 hours may be prescribed instead of the usual 150 mg. If there is no response to this dosage within 48 hours, either Norpace should then be discontinued or the physician should consider hospitalizing the patient for careful monitoring while subsequent immediate-release Norpace doses of 250 mg or 300 mg every 6 hours are given. A limited number of patients with severe refractory ventricular tachycardia have tolerated daily doses of Norpace up to 1600 mg per day (400 mg every 6 hours), resulting in disopyramide plasma levels up to 9 mcg/ml. If such treatment is warranted, it is essential that patients be hospitalized for close evaluation and continuous monitoring.

Norpace CR should not be used initially if rapid establishment of disopyramide plasma levels is desired.

Transferring to Norpace or Norpace CR

The following dosage schedule based on theoretical considerations rather than experimental data is suggested for transferring patients with normal renal function from either quinidine sulfate or procainamide therapy (Type 1 antiarrhythmic agents) to Norpace or Norpace CR therapy:

Norpace or Norpace CR should be started using the regular maintenance schedule **without a loading dose** 6 to 12 hours after the last dose of quinidine sulfate or 3 to 6 hours after the last dose of procainamide.

In patients in whom withdrawal of quinidine sulfate or procainamide is likely to produce life-threatening arrhythmias, the physician should consider hospitalization of the patient.

When transferring a patient from immediate-release Norpace to Norpace CR, the maintenance schedule of Norpace CR may be started 6 hours after the last dose of immediate-release Norpace.

Continued on next page

Norpace/Norpace CR—Cont.

Pediatric Dosage

Controlled clinical studies have not been conducted in pediatric patients; however, the following suggested dosage table is based on published clinical experience.

Total daily dosage should be divided and equal doses administered orally every 6 hours or at intervals according to individual patient needs. Disopyramide plasma levels and therapeutic response must be monitored closely. Patients should be hospitalized during the initial treatment period, and dose titration should start at the lower end of the ranges provided below.

SUGGESTED TOTAL DAILY DOSAGE*

Age (years)	Disopyramide (mg/kg body weight/day)
Under 1	10 to 30
1 to 4	10 to 20
4 to 12	10 to 15
12 to 18	6 to 15

* Dosage is expressed in milligrams of disopyramide base. Since Norpace (disopyramide phosphate) 100-mg capsules contain 100 mg of disopyramide base, the pharmacist can readily prepare a 1-mg/ml to 10-mg/ml liquid suspension by adding the entire contents of Norpace capsules to cherry syrup. (Prepare cherry syrup as follows: cherry juice, 475 mL; sucrose 800g; alcohol 20mL; purified water, a sufficient quantity to make 1000 mL.) The resulting suspension, when refrigerated, is stable for one month and should be thoroughly shaken before the measurement of each dose. The suspension should be dispensed in an amber glass bottle with a child-resistant closure.

Norpace CR capsules should not be used to prepare the above suspension.

HOW SUPPLIED

Norpace (disopyramide phosphate) is supplied in hard gelatin capsules containing either 100 mg or 150 mg of disopyramide base, present as the phosphate.

Norpace 100-mg capsules are white and orange, with markings SEARLE, 2752, NORPACE, and 100 MG.

NDC Number	Size
0025-2752-31	bottle of 100
0025-2752-52	bottle of 1,000

Norpace 150-mg capsules are brown and orange, with markings SEARLE, 2762, NORPACE, and 150 MG.

NDC Number	Size
0025-2762-31	bottle of 100
0025-2762-52	bottle of 1,000

Norpace CR (disopyramide phosphate) Controlled-Release is supplied as specially prepared controlled-release beads in hard gelatin capsules containing either 100 mg or 150 mg of disopyramide base, present as the phosphate.

Norpace CR 100-mg capsules are white and light green, with markings SEARLE, 2732, NORPACE CR, and 100 mg.

NDC Number	Size
0025-2732-31	bottle of 100
0025-2732-51	bottle of 500
0025-2732-34	carton of 100 unit dose

Norpace CR 150-mg capsules are brown and light green, with markings SEARLE, 2742, NORPACE CR, and 150 mg.

NDC Number	Size
0025-2742-31	bottle of 100
0025-2742-51	bottle of 500
0025-2742-34	carton of 100 unit dose

Store at 25°C (77°F); excursions permitted to 15–30°C (59–86°F). [See USP Controlled Room Temperature.]

Rx only.

4/15/99 • A05855-5

Shown in Product Identification Guide, page 336

SYNAREL® ℞

[sin 'er-el]

(nafarelin acetate)
Nasal Solution 2 mg/mL
(as nafarelin base)

CENTRAL PRECOCIOUS PUBERTY (FOR ENDOMETRIOSIS, SEE ENDOMETRIOSIS SECTION)

DESCRIPTION

SYNAREL (nafarelin acetate) Nasal Solution is intended for administration as a spray to the nasal mucosa. Nafarelin acetate, the active component of SYNAREL Nasal Solution, is a decapeptide with the chemical name: 5-oxo-L-prolyl-L-histidyl-L-tryptophyl-L-seryl-L-tyrosyl -3- (2-naphthyl)-D-alanyl-L-leucyl-L-arginyl-L-prolyl-glycinamide acetate. Nafarelin acetate is a synthetic analog of the naturally occurring gonadotropin-releasing hormone (GnRH).

Nafarelin acetate has the following chemical structure:

$\cdot x\,CH_3COOH \cdot y\,H_2O \quad (1 < x < 2; 2 < y < 8)$

SYNAREL Nasal Solution contains nafarelin acetate (2 mg/mL, content expressed as nafarelin base) in a solution of benzalkonium chloride, glacial acetic acid, sodium hydroxide or hydrochloric acid (to adjust pH), sorbitol, and purified water.

After priming the pump unit for SYNAREL, each actuation of the unit delivers approximately 100 µL of the spray containing approximately 200 µg nafarelin base. The contents of one spray bottle are intended to deliver at least 60 sprays.

CLINICAL PHARMACOLOGY

Nafarelin acetate is a potent agonistic analog of gonadotropin-releasing hormone (GnRH). At the onset of administration, nafarelin stimulates the release of the pituitary gonadotropins, LH and FSH, resulting in a temporary increase of gonadal steroidogenesis. Repeated dosing abolishes the stimulatory effect on the pituitary gland. Twice daily administration leads to decreased secretion of gonadal steroids by about 4 weeks; consequently, tissues and functions that depend on gonadal steroids for their maintenance become quiescent.

In **children**, nafarelin acetate was rapidly absorbed into the systemic circulation after intranasal administration. Maximum serum concentrations (measured by RIA) were achieved between 10 and 45 minutes. Following a single dose of 400 µg base, the observed peak concentration was 2.2 ng/mL, whereas following a single dose of 600 µg base, the observed peak concentration was 6.6 ng/mL. The average serum half-life of nafarelin following intranasal administration of a 400 µg dose was approximately 2.5 hours. It is not known and cannot be predicted what the pharmacokinetics of nafarelin will be in children given a dose above 600 µg.

In **adult women**, nafarelin acetate was rapidly absorbed into the systemic circulation after intranasal administration. Maximum serum concentrations (measured by RIA) were achieved between 10 and 40 minutes. Following a single dose of 200 µg base, the observed average peak concentration was 0.6 ng/mL (range 0.2 to 1.4 ng/mL), whereas following a single dose of 400 µg base, the observed average peak concentration was 1.8 ng/mL (range 0.5 to 5.3 ng/mL). Bioavailability from a 400 µg dose averaged 2.8% (range 1.2 to 5.6%). The average serum half-life of nafarelin following intranasal administration was approximately 3 hours. About 80% of nafarelin acetate was bound to plasma proteins at 4°C. Twice daily intranasal administration of 200 or 400 µg of SYNAREL in 18 healthy women for 22 days did not lead to significant accumulation of the drug. Based on the mean C_{min} levels on Days 15 and 22, there appeared to be dose proportionality across the two dose levels.

After subcutaneous administration of ^{14}C-nafarelin acetate to men, 44-55% of the dose was recovered in urine and 18.5-44.2% was recovered in feces. Approximately 3% of the administered dose appeared as unchanged nafarelin in urine. The ^{14}C serum half-life of the metabolites was about 85.5 hours. Six metabolites of nafarelin have been identified of which the major metabolite is Tyr-D(2)-Nal-Leu-Arg-Pro-Gly-NH_2(5–10). The activity of the metabolites, the metabolism of nafarelin by nasal mucosa, and the pharmacokinetics of the drug in hepatically- and renally-impaired patients have not been determined.

There appeared to be no significant effect of rhinitis, i.e., nasal congestion, on the systemic bioavailability of SYNAREL; however, if the use of a nasal decongestant for rhinitis is necessary during treatment with SYNAREL, the decongestant should not be used until at least 2 hours following dosing with SYNAREL.

When used regularly in girls and boys with **central precocious puberty (CPP)** at the recommended dose, SYNAREL suppresses LH and sex steroid hormone levels to prepubertal levels, affects a corresponding arrest of secondary sexual development, and slows linear growth and skeletal maturation. In some cases, initial estrogen withdrawal bleeding may occur, generally within 6 weeks after initiation of therapy. Thereafter, menstruation should cease.

In clinical studies the peak response of LH to GnRH stimulation was reduced from a pubertal response to a prepubertal response (<15 mIU/mL) within one month of treatment.

Linear growth velocity, which is commonly pubertal in children with CPP, is reduced in most children within the first year of treatment to values of 5 to 6 cm/year or less. Children with CPP are frequently taller than their chronological age peers; height for chronological age approaches normal in most children during the second or third year of treatment with SYNAREL. Skeletal maturation rate (bone age velocity—change in bone age divided by change in chronological age) is usually abnormal (greater than 1) in children with CPP; in most children, bone age velocity approaches normal (1) during the first year of treatment. This results in a narrowing of the gap between bone age and chronological age, usually by the second or third year of treatment. The mean predicted adult height increases.

In clinical trials, breast development was arrested or regressed in 82% of girls, and genital development was arrested or regressed in 100% of boys. Because pubic hair growth is largely controlled by adrenal androgens, which are unaffected by nafarelin, pubic hair development was arrested or regressed only in 54% of girls and boys.

Reversal of the suppressive effects of SYNAREL has been demonstrated to occur in all children with CPP for whom one-year post- treatment follow-up is available (n=69). This demonstration consisted of the appearance or return of menses, the return of pubertal gonadotropin and gonadal sex steroid levels, and/or the advancement of secondary sexual development. Semen analysis was normal in the two ejaculated specimens obtained thus far from boys who have been taken off therapy to resume puberty. Fertility has not been documented by pregnancies and the effect of long-term use of the drug on fertility is not known.

INDICATIONS AND USAGE FOR CENTRAL PRECOCIOUS PUBERTY

(For Endometriosis, See Endometriosis section)

SYNAREL is indicated for treatment of **central precocious puberty (CPP)** (gonadotropin-dependent precocious puberty) in children of both sexes.

The diagnosis of **central precocious puberty (CPP)** is suspected when premature development of secondary sexual characteristics occurs at or before the age of 8 years in girls and 9 years in boys, and is accompanied by significant advancement of bone age and/or a poor adult height prediction. The diagnosis should be confirmed by pubertal gonadal sex steroid levels and a pubertal LH response to stimulation by native GnRH. Pelvic ultrasound assessment in girls usually reveals enlarged uterus and ovaries, the latter often with multiple cystic formations. Magnetic resonance imaging or CT-scanning of the brain is recommended to detect hypothalamic or pituitary tumors, or anatomical changes associated with increased intracranial pressure. Other causes of sexual precocity, such as congenital adrenal hyperplasia, testotoxicosis, testicular tumors and/or other autonomous feminizing or masculinizing disorders, must be excluded by proper clinical hormonal and diagnostic imaging examinations.

CONTRAINDICATIONS

1. Hypersensitivity to GnRH, GnRH agonist analogs or any of the excipients in SYNAREL;
2. Undiagnosed abnormal vaginal bleeding;
3. Use in pregnancy or in women who may become pregnant while receiving the drug. SYNAREL may cause fetal harm when administered to a pregnant woman. Major fetal abnormalities were observed in rats, but not in mice or rabbits after administration of SYNAREL during the period of organogenesis. There was a dose-related increase in fetal mortality and a decrease in fetal weight in rats (see ***Pregnancy*** Section). The effects on rat fetal mortality are expected consequences of the alterations in hormonal levels brought about by the drug. If this drug is used during pregnancy or if the patient becomes pregnant while taking this drug, she should be apprised of the potential hazard to the fetus;
4. Use in women who are breast-feeding (see ***Nursing Mothers*** Section).

WARNINGS

The diagnosis of central precocious puberty (CPP) must be established before treatment is initiated. Regular monitoring of CPP patients is needed to assess both patient response as well as compliance. This is particularly important during the first 6 to 8 weeks of treatment to assure that suppression of pituitary-gonadal function is rapid. Testing may include LH response to GnRH stimulation and circulating gonadal sex steroid levels. Assessment of growth velocity and bone age velocity should begin within 3 to 6 months of treatment initiation.

Some patients may not show suppression of the pituitary-gonadal axis by clinical and/or biochemical parameters. This may be due to lack of compliance with the recommended treatment regimen and may be rectified by recommending that the dosing be done by caregivers. If compliance problems are excluded, the possibility of gonadotropin independent sexual precocity should be reconsidered and appropriate examinations should be conducted. If compliance problems are excluded and if gonadotropin independent sexual precocity is not present, the dose of SYNAREL may be increased to 1800 µg/day administered as 600 µg TID.

PRECAUTIONS

General

As with other drugs that stimulate the release of gonadotropins or that induce ovulation, in adult women with endometriosis ovarian cysts have been reported to occur in the first two months of therapy with SYNAREL. Many, but not all, of these events occurred in women with polycystic ovarian disease. These cystic enlargements may resolve spontaneously, generally by about four to six weeks of therapy, but in some cases may require discontinuation of drug and/or surgical intervention. The relevance, if any, of such events in children is unknown.

Information for Patients, Patients' Parents or Guardians
An information pamphlet for patients is included with the product. Patients and their caregivers should be aware of the following information:

1. Reversibility of the suppressive effects of nafarelin has been demonstrated by the appearance or return of menses, by the return of pubertal gonadotropin and gonadal sex steroid levels, and/or by advancement of secondary sexual development. Semen analysis was normal in the two ejaculated specimens obtained thus far from boys who have been taken off therapy to resume puberty. Fertility has not been documented by pregnancies and the effect of long-term use of the drug on fertility is not known.
2. Patients and their caregivers should be adequately counseled to assure full compliance; irregular or incomplete daily doses may result in stimulation of the pituitary-gonadal axis.
3. During the first month of treatment with SYNAREL, some signs of puberty, e.g., vaginal bleeding or breast enlargement, may occur. This is the expected initial effect of the drug. Such changes should resolve soon after the first month. If such resolution does not occur within the first two months of treatment, this may be due to lack of compliance or the presence of gonadotropin independent sexual precocity. If both possibilities are definitively excluded, the dose of SYNAREL may be increased to 1800 µg/day administered as 600 µg TID.
4. Patients with intercurrent rhinitis should consult their physician for the use of a topical nasal decongestant. If the use of a topical nasal decongestant is required during treatment with SYNAREL, the decongestant should not be used until at least 2 hours following dosing with SYNAREL.
   Sneezing during or immediately after dosing with SYNAREL should be avoided, if possible, since this may impair drug absorption.

Drug Interactions
No pharmacokinetic-based drug-drug interaction studies have been conducted with SYNAREL. However, because nafarelin acetate is a peptide that is primarily degraded by peptidase and not by cytochrome P-450 enzymes, and the drug is only about 80% bound to plasma proteins at 4°C, drug interactions would not be expected to occur.

Carcinogenesis, Mutagenesis, Impairment of Fertility
Carcinogenicity studies of nafarelin were conducted in rats (24 months) at doses up to 100 µg/kg/day and mice (18 months) at doses up to 500 µg/kg/day using intramuscular doses (up to 110 times and 560 times the maximum recommended human intranasal dose, respectively). These multiples of the human dose are based on the relative bioavailability of the drug by the two routes of administration. As seen with other GnRH agonists, nafarelin acetate given to laboratory rodents at high doses for prolonged periods induced proliferative responses (hyperplasia and/or neoplasia) of endocrine organs. At 24 months, there was an increase in the incidence of pituitary tumors (adenoma/carcinoma) in high-dose female rats and a dose-related increase in male rats. There was an increase in pancreatic islet cell adenomas in both sexes, and in benign testicular and ovarian tumors in the treated groups. There was a dose-related increase in benign adrenal medullary tumors in treated female rats. In mice, there was a dose-related increase in Harderian gland tumors in males and an increase in pituitary adenomas in high-dose females. No metastases of these tumors were observed. It is known that tumorigenicity in rodents is particularly sensitive to hormonal stimulation.
Mutagenicity studies were performed with nafarelin acetate using bacterial, yeast, and mammalian systems. These studies provided no evidence of mutagenic potential.
Reproduction studies in male and female rats have shown full reversibility of fertility suppression when drug treatment was discontinued after continuous administration for up to 6 months. The effect of treatment of prepubertal rats on the subsequent reproductive performance of mature animals has not been investigated.

Pregnancy, Teratogenic Effects
Pregnancy Category X. See '***CONTRAINDICATIONS***.' Intramuscular SYNAREL was administered to rats during the period of organogenesis at 0.4, 1.6, and 6.4 µg/kg/day (about 0.5, 2, and 7 times the maximum recommended human intranasal dose based on the relative bioavailability by the two routes of administration). An increase in major fetal abnormalities was observed in 4/80 fetuses at the highest dose. A similar, repeat study at the same doses in rats and studies in mice and rabbits at doses up to 600 µg/kg/day and 0.18 µg/kg/day, respectively, failed to demonstrate an increase in fetal abnormalities after administration during the period of organogenesis. In rats and rabbits, there was a dose-related increase in fetal mortality and a decrease in fetal weight with the highest dose.

Nursing Mothers
It is not known whether SYNAREL is excreted in human milk. Because many drugs are excreted in human milk, and because the effects of SYNAREL on lactation and/or the breastfed child have not been determined, SYNAREL should not be used by nursing mothers.

ADVERSE REACTIONS

In clinical trials of 155 pediatric patients, 2.6% reported symptoms suggestive of drug sensitivity, such as shortness of breath, chest pain, urticaria, rash, and pruritus.
In these 155 patients treated for an average of 41 months and as long as 80 months (6.7 years), adverse events most frequently reported (>3% of patients) consisted largely of episodes occurring during the first 6 weeks of treatment as a result of the transient stimulatory action of nafarelin upon the pituitary-gonadal axis:

- acne (10%)
- transient breast enlargement (8%)
- vaginal bleeding (8%)
- emotional lability (6%)
- transient increase in pubic hair (5%)
- body odor (4%)
- seborrhea (3%)

Hot flashes, common in adult women treated for endometriosis, occurred in only 3% of treated children and were transient. Other adverse events thought to be drug-related, and occurring in >3% of patients were rhinitis (5%) and white or brownish vaginal discharge (3%). Approximately 3% of patients withdrew from clinical trials due to adverse events.

In one male patient with concomitant congenital adrenal hyperplasia, and who had discontinued treatment 8 months previously to resume puberty, adrenal rest tumors were found in the left testis. Relationship to SYNAREL is unlikely.
Regular examinations of the pituitary gland by magnetic resonance imaging (MRI) or computer assisted tomography of children during long-term nafarelin therapy as well as during the post-treatment period have occasionally revealed changes in the shape and size of the pituitary gland. These changes include asymmetry and enlargement of the pituitary gland, and a pituitary micro-adenoma has been suspected in a few children. The relationship of these findings to SYNAREL is not known.

OVERDOSAGE

In experimental animals, a single subcutaneous administration of up to 60 times the recommended human dose (on a µg/kg basis, not adjusted for bioavailability) had no adverse effects. At present, there is no clinical evidence of adverse effects following overdosage of GnRH analogs.
Based on studies in monkeys, SYNAREL is not absorbed after oral administration.

DOSAGE AND ADMINISTRATION

For the treatment of **central precocious puberty (CPP)**, the recommended daily dose of SYNAREL is 1600 µg. The dose can be increased to 1800 µg daily if adequate suppression cannot be achieved at 1600 µg/day.
The 1600 µg dose is achieved by two sprays (400 µg) into each nostril in the morning (4 sprays) and two sprays into each nostril in the evening (4 sprays), a total of 8 sprays per day. The 1800 µg dose is achieved by 3 sprays (600 µg) into alternating nostrils three times a day, a total of 9 sprays per day. The patient's head should be tilted back slightly, and 30 seconds should elapse between sprays.
If the prescribed therapy has been well tolerated by the patient, treatment of CPP with SYNAREL should continue until resumption of puberty is desired.
There appeared to be no significant effect of rhinitis, i.e., nasal congestion, on the systemic bioavailability of SYNAREL; however, if the use of a nasal decongestant for rhinitis is necessary during treatment with SYNAREL, the decongestant should not be used until at least 2 hours following dosing with SYNAREL.
Sneezing during or immediately after dosing with SYNAREL should be avoided, if possible, since this may impair drug absorption.
At 1600 µg/day, a bottle of SYNAREL provides about a 7-day supply (about 56 sprays). If the daily dose is increased, increase the supply to the patient to ensure uninterrupted treatment for the duration of therapy.

HOW SUPPLIED

Each 0.5 ounce bottle (NDC 0025-0166-08) contains 8mL SYNAREL (nafarelin acetate) Nasal Solution 2 mg/mL (as nafarelin base), and is supplied with a metered spray pump that delivers 200 µg of nafarelin per spray. A dust cover and a leaflet of patient instructions are also included.
Store upright at 25°C (77°F); excursions permitted to 15–30°C (59–86°F). [See USP Controlled Room Temperature]. Protect from light.
Rx only
U.S. Patent No. 4,234,571.

SEARLE

G.D. Searle & Co.
Chicago IL 60680 USA 10/1/99 • A05579

SYNAREL® ℞

[sin 'er-el]
(nafarelin acetate)
Nasal Solution 2 mg/mL
(as nafarelin base)

ENDOMETRIOSIS
(FOR CENTRAL PRECOCIOUS PUBERTY, SEE CENTRAL PRECOCIOUS PUBERTY SECTION)

DESCRIPTION

SYNAREL (nafarelin acetate) Nasal Solution is intended for administration as a spray to the nasal mucosa. Nafarelin acetate, the active component of SYNAREL Nasal Solution, is a decapeptide with the chemical name: 5-oxo-L-prolyl-L-histidyl-L-tryptophyl-L-seryl-L-tyrosyl- 3- (2-naphthyl) -D-alanyl-L-leucyl-L-arginyl-L-prolyl-glycinamide acetate. Nafarelin acetate is a synthetic analog of the naturally occurring gonadotropin-releasing hormone (GnRH).
Nafarelin acetate has the following chemical structure:

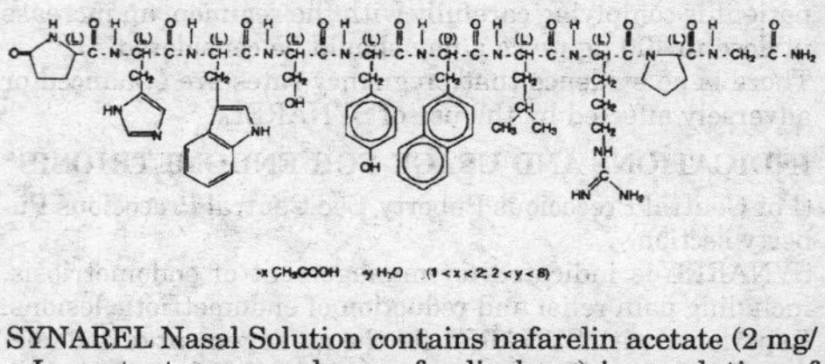

•x CH_3COOH •y H_2O (1<x<2; 2<y<8)

SYNAREL Nasal Solution contains nafarelin acetate (2 mg/mL, content expressed as nafarelin base) in a solution of benzalkonium chloride, glacial acetic acid, sodium hydroxide or hydrochloric acid (to adjust pH), sorbitol, and purified water.
After priming the pump unit for SYNAREL, each actuation of the unit delivers approximately 100 µL of the spray containing approximately 200 µg nafarelin base. The contents of one spray bottle are intended to deliver at least 60 sprays.

CLINICAL PHARMACOLOGY

Nafarelin acetate is a potent agonistic analog of gonadotropin-releasing hormone (GnRH). At the onset of administration, nafarelin stimulates the release of the pituitary gonadotropins, LH and FSH, resulting in a temporary increase of ovarian steroidogenesis. Repeated dosing abolishes the stimulatory effect on the pituitary gland. Twice daily administration leads to decreased secretion of gonadal steroids by about 4 weeks; consequently, tissues and functions that depend on gonadal steroids for their maintenance become quiescent.
Nafarelin acetate is rapidly absorbed into the systemic circulation after intranasal administration. Maximum serum concentrations (measured by RIA) were achieved between 10 and 40 minutes. Following a single dose of 200 µg base, the observed average peak concentration was 0.6 ng/mL (range 0.2 to 1.4 ng/mL), whereas following a single dose of 400 µg base, the observed average peak concentration was 1.8 ng/mL (range 0.5 to 5.3 ng/mL). Bioavailability from a 400 µg dose averaged 2.8% (range 1.2 to 5.6%). The average serum half-life of nafarelin following intranasal administration is approximately 3 hours. About 80% of nafarelin acetate is bound to plasma proteins at 4°C. Twice daily intranasal administration of 200 or 400 µg of SYNAREL in 18 healthy women for 22 days did not lead to significant accumulation of the drug. Based on the mean C_{min} levels on Days 15 and 22, there appeared to be dose proportionality across the two dose levels.
After subcutaneous administration of ^{14}C-nafarelin acetate to men, 44-55% of the dose was recovered in urine and 18.5-44.2% was recovered in feces. Approximately 3% of the administered dose appeared as unchanged nafarelin in urine. The ^{14}C serum half-life of the metabolites was about 85.5 hours. Six metabolites of nafarelin have been identified of which the major metabolite is Tyr-D(2)-Nal-Leu-Arg-Pro-Gly-NH_2(5-10). The activity of the metabolites, the metabolism of nafarelin by nasal mucosa, and the pharmacokinetics of the drug in hepatically- and renally-impaired patients have not been determined.
There appeared to be no significant effect of rhinitis, i.e., nasal congestion, on the systemic bioavailability of SYNAREL; however, if the use of a nasal decongestant for rhinitis is necessary during treatment with SYNAREL, the decongestant should not be used until at least 2 hours following dosing of SYNAREL.
In controlled clinical studies, SYNAREL at doses of 400 and 800 µg/day for 6 months was shown to be comparable to danazol, 800 mg/day, in relieving the clinical symptoms of endometriosis (pelvic pain, dysmenorrhea, and dyspareunia) and in reducing the size of endometrial implants as determined by laparoscopy. The clinical significance of a decrease in endometriotic lesions is not known at this time and, in addition, laparoscopic staging of endometriosis does not necessarily correlate with severity of symptoms.
In a single controlled clinical trial, intranasal Synarel (nafarelin acetate) at a dose of 400 mg per day was shown to be clinically comparable to intramuscular leuprolide depot, 3.75 mg monthly, for the treatment of the symptoms (dysmenorrhea, dyspareunia and pelvic pain), associated with endometriosis.
SYNAREL 400 µg daily induced amenorrhea in approximately 65%, 80%, and 90% of the patients after 60, 90, and 120 days, respectively. In the first, second, and third post-treatment months, normal menstrual cycles resumed in 4%, 82%, and 100%, respectively, of those patients who did not become pregnant.
At the end of treatment, 60% of patients who received SYNAREL, 400 µg/day, were symptom free, 32% had mild symptoms, 7% had moderate symptoms, and 1% had severe symptoms. Of the 60% of patients who had complete relief of symptoms at the end of treatment, 17% had moderate symptoms 6 months after treatment was discontinued, 33% had mild symptoms, 50% remained symptom free, and no patient had severe symptoms.
During the first two months use of SYNAREL, some women experience vaginal bleeding of variable duration and inten-

Continued on next page

Synarel—Cont.

sity. In all likelihood, this bleeding represents estrogen withdrawal bleeding and is expected to stop spontaneously. If vaginal bleeding continues, the possibility of lack of compliance with the dosing regimen should be considered. If the patient is complying carefully with the regimen, an increase in dose to 400 µg twice a day should be considered.

There is no evidence that pregnancy rates are enhanced or adversely affected by the use of SYNAREL.

INDICATIONS AND USAGE FOR ENDOMETRIOSIS

(For Central Precocious Puberty, See Central Precocious Puberty section)

SYNAREL is indicated for management of endometriosis, including pain relief and reduction of endometriotic lesions. Experience with SYNAREL for the management of endometriosis has been limited to women 18 years of age and older treated for 6 months.

CONTRAINDICATIONS

1. Hypersensitivity to GnRH, GnRH agonist analogs or any of the excipients in SYNAREL;
2. Undiagnosed abnormal vaginal bleeding;
3. Use in pregnancy or in women who may become pregnant while receiving the drug. SYNAREL may cause fetal harm when administered to a pregnant woman. Major fetal abnormalities were observed in rats, but not in mice or rabbits after administration of SYNAREL during the period of organogenesis. There was a dose-related increase in fetal mortality and a decrease in fetal weight in rats (see ***Pregnancy*** Section). The effects on rat fetal mortality are expected consequences of the alterations in hormonal levels brought about by the drug. If this drug is used during pregnancy or if the patient becomes pregnant while taking this drug, she should be apprised of the potential hazard to the fetus;
4. Use in women who are breast-feeding (see ***Nursing Mothers*** Section).

WARNINGS

Safe use of nafarelin acetate in pregnancy has not been established clinically. Before starting treatment with SYNAREL, pregnancy must be excluded.

When used regularly at the recommended dose, SYNAREL usually inhibits ovulation and stops menstruation. Contraception is not insured, however, by taking SYNAREL, particularly if patients miss successive doses. Therefore, patients should use nonhormonal methods of contraception. Patients should be advised to see their physician if they believe they may be pregnant. If a patient becomes pregnant during treatment, the drug must be discontinued and the patient must be apprised of the potential risk to the fetus.

PRECAUTIONS

General

As with other drugs that stimulate the release of gonadotropins or that induce ovulation, ovarian cysts have been reported to occur in the first two months of therapy with SYNAREL. Many, but not all, of these events occurred in patients with polycystic ovarian disease. These cystic enlargements may resolve spontaneously, generally by about four to six weeks of therapy, but in some cases may require discontinuation of drug and/or surgical intervention.

Information for Patients

An information pamphlet for patients is included with the product. Patients should be aware of the following information:

1. Since menstruation should stop with effective doses of SYNAREL, the patient should notify her physician if regular menstruation persists. The cause of vaginal spotting, bleeding or menstruation could be noncompliance with the treatment regimen, or it could be that a higher dose of the drug is required to achieve amenorrhea. The patient should be questioned regarding her compliance. If she is careful and compliant, and menstruation persists to the second month, consideration should be given to doubling the dose of SYNAREL. If the patient has missed several doses, she should be counseled on the importance of taking SYNAREL regularly as prescribed.
2. Patients should not use SYNAREL if they are pregnant, breast-feeding, have undiagnosed abnormal vaginal bleeding, or are allergic to any of the ingredients in SYNAREL.
3. Safe use of the drug in pregnancy has not been established clinically. Therefore, a nonhormonal method of contraception should be used during treatment. Patients should be advised that if they miss successive doses of SYNAREL, breakthrough bleeding or ovulation may occur with the potential for conception. If a patient becomes pregnant during treatment, she should discontinue treatment and consult her physician.
4. Those adverse events occurring most frequently in clinical studies with SYNAREL are associated with hypoestrogenism; the most frequently reported are hot flashes, headaches, emotional lability, decreased libido, vaginal dryness, acne, myalgia, and reduction in breast size. Estrogen levels returned to normal after treatment was discontinued. Nasal irritation occurred in about 10% of all patients who used intranasal nafarelin.
5. The induced hypoestrogenic state results in a small loss in bone density over the course of treatment, some of which may not be reversible. During one six-month treatment period, this bone loss should not be important. In patients with major risk factors for decreased bone mineral content such as chronic alcohol and/or tobacco use, strong family history of osteoporosis, or chronic use of drugs that can reduce bone mass such as anticonvulsants or corticosteroids, therapy with SYNAREL may pose an additional risk. In these patients the risks and benefits must be weighed carefully before therapy with SYNAREL is instituted. Repeated courses of treatment with gonadotropin-releasing hormone analogs are not advisable in patients with major risk factors for loss of bone mineral content.
6. Patients with intercurrent rhinitis should consult their physician for the use of a topical nasal decongestant. If the use of a topical nasal decongestant is required during treatment with SYNAREL, the decongestant should not be used until at least 2 hours following dosing with SYNAREL.

   Sneezing during or immediately after dosing with SYNAREL should be avoided, if possible, since this may impair drug absorption.
7. Retreatment cannot be recommended since safety data beyond 6 months are not available.

Drug Interactions

No pharmacokinetic-based drug-drug interaction studies have been conducted with SYNAREL. However, because nafarelin acetate is a peptide that is primarily degraded by peptidase and not by cytochrome P-450 enzymes, and the drug is only about 80% bound to plasma proteins at 4°C, drug interactions would not be expected to occur.

Drug/Laboratory Test Interactions

Administration of SYNAREL in therapeutic doses results in suppression of the pituitary-gonadal system. Normal function is usually restored within 4 to 8 weeks after treatment is discontinued. Therefore, diagnostic tests of pituitary gonadotropic and gonadal functions conducted during treatment and up to 4 to 8 weeks after discontinuation of therapy with SYNAREL may be misleading.

Carcinogenesis, Mutagenesis, Impairment of Fertility

Carcinogenicity studies of nafarelin were conducted in rats (24 months) at doses up to 100 µg/kg/day and mice (18 months) at doses up to 500 µg/kg/day using intramuscular doses (up to 110 times and 560 times the maximum recommended human intranasal dose, respectively). These multiples of the human dose are based on the relative bioavailability of the drug by the two routes of administration. As seen with other GnRH agonists, nafarelin acetate given to laboratory rodents at high doses for prolonged periods induced proliferative responses (hyperplasia and/or neoplasia) of endocrine organs. At 24 months, there was an increase in the incidence of pituitary tumors (adenoma/carcinoma) in high-dose female rats and a dose-related increase in male rats. There was an increase in pancreatic islet cell adenomas in both sexes, and in benign testicular and ovarian tumors in the treated groups. There was a dose-related increase in benign adrenal medullary tumors in treated female rats. In mice, there was a dose-related increase in Harderian gland tumors in males and an increase in pituitary adenomas in high-dose females. No metastases of these tumors were observed. It is known that tumorigenicity in rodents is particularly sensitive to hormonal stimulation.

Mutagenicity studies were performed with nafarelin acetate using bacterial, yeast, and mammalian systems. These studies provided no evidence of mutagenic potential.

Reproduction studies in male and female rats have shown full reversibility of fertility suppression when drug treatment was discontinued after continuous administration for up to 6 months. The effect of treatment of prepubertal rats on the subsequent reproductive performance of mature animals has not been investigated.

Pregnancy, Teratogenic Effects

Pregnancy Category X. See ***'CONTRAINDICATIONS.'*** Intramuscular SYNAREL was administered to rats during the period of organogenesis at 0.4, 1.6, and 6.4 µg/kg/day (about 0.5, 2, and 7 times the maximum recommended human intranasal dose based on the relative bioavailability by the two routes of administration). An increase in major fetal abnormalities was observed in 4/80 fetuses at the highest dose. A similar, repeat study at the same doses in rats and studies in mice and rabbits at doses up to 600 µg/kg/day and 0.18 µg/kg/day, respectively, failed to demonstrate an increase in fetal abnormalities after administration during the period of organogenesis. In rats and rabbits, there was a dose-related increase in fetal mortality and a decrease in fetal weight with the highest dose.

Nursing Mothers

It is not known whether SYNAREL is excreted in human milk. Because many drugs are excreted in human milk, and because the effects of SYNAREL on lactation and/or the breast-fed child have not been determined, SYNAREL should not be used by nursing mothers.

Pediatric Use

Safety and effectiveness of SYNAREL for endometriosis in patients younger than 18 years have not been established.

ADVERSE REACTIONS

In formal clinical trials of 1509 healthy adult patients, symptoms suggestive of drug sensitivity, such as shortness of breath, chest pain, urticaria, rash and pruritus occurred in 3 patients (approximately 0.2%).

As would be expected with a drug which lowers serum estradiol levels, the most frequently reported adverse reactions were those related to hypoestrogenism.

In controlled studies comparing SYNAREL (400 µg/day) and danazol (600 or 800 mg/day), adverse reactions most frequently reported and thought to be drug-related are shown in the figure below.

[See graphic above]

ADVERSE EVENTS DURING 6 MONTHS TREATMENT WITH SYNAREL® 400 µg/day vs DANAZOL 600 OR 800 mg/day

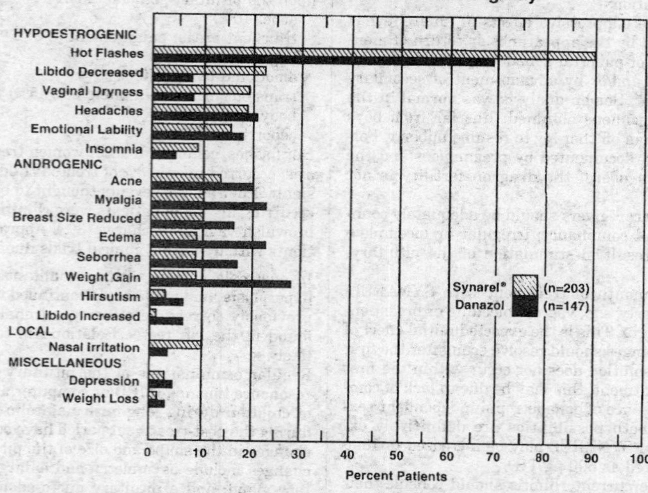

In addition, less than 1% of patients experienced paresthesia, palpitations, chloasma, maculopapular rash, eye pain, asthenia, lactation, breast engorgement, and arthralgia.

Changes in Bone Density

After six months of treatment with SYNAREL, vertebral trabecular bone density and total vertebral bone mass, measured by quantitative computed tomography (QCT), decreased by an average of 8.7% and 4.3%, respectively, compared to pretreatment levels. There was partial recovery of bone density in the post-treatment period; the average trabecular bone density and total bone mass were 4.9% and 3.3% less than the pretreatment levels, respectively. Total vertebral bone mass, measured by dual photon absorptiometry (DPA), decreased by a mean of 5.9% at the end of treatment.

After six months treatment with SYNAREL, bone mass as measured by dual x-ray bone densitometry (DEXA) decreased 3.2%. Mean total vertebral mass, re-examined by DEXA six months after completion of treatment, was 1.4% below pretreatment levels. There was little, if any, decrease in the mineral content in compact bone of the distal radius and second metacarpal. Use of SYNAREL for longer than the recommended six months or in the presence of other known risk factors for decreased bone mineral content may cause additional bone loss.

Changes in Laboratory Values During Treatment

Plasma enzymes. During clinical trials with SYNAREL, regular laboratory monitoring revealed that SGOT and SGPT levels were more than twice the upper limit of normal in only one patient each. There was no other clinical or laboratory evidence of abnormal liver function and levels returned to normal in both patients after treatment was stopped.

Lipids. At enrollment, 9% of the patients in the group taking SYNAREL 400 µg/day and 2% of the patients in the danazol group had total cholesterol values above 250 mg/dL. These patients also had cholesterol values above 250 mg/dL at the end of treatment.

Of those patients whose pretreatment cholesterol values were below 250 mg/dL, 6% in the group treated with SYNAREL and 18% in the danazol group, had post-treatment values above 250 mg/dL.

The mean (± SEM) pretreatment values for total cholesterol from all patients were 191.8 (4.3) mg/dL in the group treated with SYNAREL and 193.1 (4.6) mg/dL in the danazol group. At the end of treatment, the mean values for total cholesterol from all patients were 204.5 (4.8) mg/dL in the group treated with SYNAREL and 207.7 (5.1) mg/dL in the danazol group. These increases from the pretreatment values were statistically significant ($p<0.05$) in both groups.
Triglycerides were increased above the upper limit of 150 mg/dL in 12% of the patients who received SYNAREL and in 7% of the patients who received danazol.
At the end of treatment, no patients receiving SYNAREL had abnormally low HDL cholesterol fractions (less than 30 mg/dL) compared with 43% of patients receiving danazol. None of the patients receiving SYNAREL had abnormally high LDL cholesterol fractions (greater than 190 mg/dL) compared with 15% of those receiving danazol. There was no increase in the LDL/HDL ratio in patients receiving SYNAREL, but there was approximately a 2-fold increase in the LDL/HDL ratio in patients receiving danazol.
Other changes. In comparative studies, the following changes were seen in approximately 10% to 15% of patients. Treatment with SYNAREL was associated with elevations of plasma phosphorus and eosinophil counts, and decreases in serum calcium and WBC counts. Danazol therapy was associated with an increase of hematocrit and WBC.

OVERDOSAGE

In experimental animals, a single subcutaneous administration of up to 60 times the recommended human dose (on a µg/kg basis, not adjusted for bioavailability) had no adverse effects. At present, there is no clinical evidence of adverse effects following overdosage of GnRH analogs.
Based on studies in monkeys, SYNAREL is not absorbed after oral administration.

DOSAGE AND ADMINISTRATION

For the management of endometriosis, the recommended daily dose of SYNAREL is 400 µg. This is achieved by one spray (200 µg) into one nostril in the morning and one spray into the other nostril in the evening. Treatment should be started between days 2 and 4 of the menstrual cycle.
In an occasional patient, the 400 µg daily dose may not produce amenorrhea. For these patients with persistent regular menstruation after 2 months of treatment, the dose of SYNAREL may be increased to 800 µg daily. The 800 µg dose is administered as one spray into each nostril in the morning (a total of two sprays) and again in the evening.
The recommended duration of administration is six months. Retreatment cannot be recommended since safety data for retreatment are not available. If the symptoms of endometriosis recur after a course of therapy, and further treatment with SYNAREL is contemplated, it is recommended that bone density be assessed before retreatment begins to ensure that values are within normal limits.
There appeared to be no significant effect of rhinitis, i.e., nasal congestion, on the systemic bioavailability of SYNAREL; however, if the use of a nasal decongestant for rhinitis is necessary during treatment with SYNAREL, the decongestant should not be used until at least 2 hours following dosing with SYNAREL.
Sneezing during or immediately after dosing with SYNAREL should be avoided, if possible, since this may impair drug absorption.
At 400 µg/day, a bottle of SYNAREL provides a 30-day (about 60 sprays) supply. If the daily dose is increased, increase the supply to the patient to ensure uninterrupted treatment for the recommended duration of therapy.

HOW SUPPLIED

Each 0.5 ounce bottle (NDC 0025-0166-08) contains 8mL SYNAREL (nafarelin acetate) Nasal Solution 2 mg/mL (as nafarelin base), and is supplied with a metered spray pump that delivers 200 µg of nafarelin per spray. A dust cover and a leaflet of patient instructions are also included.
Store upright at 25°C (77°F); excursions permitted to 15–30°C (59–86°F). [See USP Controlled Room Temperature]. Protect from light.
Rx only
U.S. Patent No. 4,234,571.
SEARLE
G.D. Searle & Co.
Chicago IL 60680 USA

10/1/99 • A05579

IDENTIFICATION PROBLEM?
Turn to the **Product Identification Guide,** where you'll find more than 1600 products pictured in actual size and full color.

Serono, Inc.

100 LONGWATER CIRCLE
NORWELL, MA 02061

Direct Inquiries to:
Customer Service, Sales and Ordering
(888) 398-4567
(781) 982-9000

For Medical Information or to report Adverse Drug Experiences Contact:
Product Information and Surveillance
(888) 275-7376
(781) 982-9000 X 5562

Serono, Inc. will be pleased to answer inquiries about the following products:

CETROTIDE™
[*cĕtrō-tīde*]
(cetrorelix acetate for injection)
0.25 mg and 3 mg
FOR SUBCUTANEOUS USE ONLY

DESCRIPTION

Cetrotide™ (cetrorelix acetate for injection) is a synthetic decapeptide with gonadotropin-releasing hormone (GnRH) antagonistic activity. Cetrorelix acetate is an analog of native GnRH with substitutions of amino acids at positions 1, 2, 3, 6, and 10. The molecular formula is Acetyl-*D*-3-(2'-naphtyl)-alanine-*D*-4-chlorophenylalanine-*D*-3-(3'-pyridyl)-alanine-*L*-serine-*L*-tyrosine-*D*-citruline-*L*-leucine-*L*-arginine-*L*-proline-*D*-alanine-amide, and the molecular weight is 1431.06, calculated as the anhydrous free base. The structural formula is as follows:
Cetrorelix acetate
[See graphic below]
Cetrotide™ (cetrorelix acetate for injection) 0.25 mg or 3 mg is a sterile lyophilized powder intended for subcutaneous injection after reconstitution with Sterile Water for Injection, USP (pH 5–8), that comes supplied in either a 1.0 mL (for 0.25 mg vial) or 3.0 mL (for 3 mg vial) pre-filled syringe. Each vial of Cetrotide™ 0.25 mg (multiple dose regimen) contains 0.26–0.27 mg cetrorelix acetate, equivalent to 0.25 mg cetrorelix, and 54.80 mg mannitol. Each vial of Cetrotide™ 3 mg (single dose regimen) contains 3.12–3.24 mg cetrorelix acetate, equivalent to 3 mg cetrorelix, and 164.40 mg mannitol.

CLINICAL PHARMACOLOGY

GnRH induces the production and release of luteinizing hormone (LH) and follicle stimulating hormone (FSH) from the gonadotrophic cells of the anterior pituitary. Due to a positive estradiol (E_2) feedback at midcycle, GnRH liberation is enhanced resulting in an LH-surge. This LH-surge induces the ovulation of the dominant follicle, resumption of oocyte meiosis and subsequently luteinization as indicated by rising progesterone levels.
Cetrotide™ competes with natural GnRH for binding to membrane receptors on pituitary cells and thus controls the release of LH and FSH in a dose-dependent manner. The onset of LH suppression is approximately one hour with the 3 mg dose and two hours with the 0.25 mg dose. This suppression is maintained by continuous treatment and there is a more pronounced effect on LH than on FSH. An initial release of endogenous gonadotropins has not been detected with Cetrotide™, which is consistent with an antagonist effect.
The effects of Cetrotide™ on LH and FSH are reversible after discontinuation of treatment. In women, Cetrotide™ delays the LH-surge, and consequently ovulation, in a dose-dependent fashion. FSH levels are not affected at the doses used during controlled ovarian stimulation. Following a single 3 mg dose of Cetrotide™, duration of action of at least 4 days has been established. A dose of Cetrotide™ 0.25 mg every 24 hours has been shown to maintain the effect.
Pharmacokinetics
The pharmacokinetic parameters of single and multiple doses of Cetrotide™ (cetrorelix acetate for injection) in adult healthy female subjects are summarized in Table 1.
[See table 1 at top of next page]
Absorption
Cetrotide™ is rapidly absorbed following subcutaneous injection, maximal plasma concentrations being achieved approximately one to two hours after administration. The mean absolute bioavailability of Cetrotide™ following subcutaneous administration to healthy female subjects is 85%.
Distribution
The volume of distribution of Cetrotide™ following a single intravenous dose of 3 mg is about 1 1/kg. *In vitro* protein binding to human plasma is 86%.
Cetrotide™ concentrations in follicular fluid and plasma were similar on the day of oocyte pick-up in patients undergoing controlled ovarian stimulation. Following subcutaneous administration of Cetrotide™ 0.25 mg and 3 mg, plasma concentrations of cetrorelix were below or in the range of the lower limit of quantitation on the day of oocyte pick up and embryo transfer.
Metabolism
After subcutaneous administration of 10 mg Cetrotide™ to females and males, Cetrotide™ and small amounts of (1–9), (1–7), (1–6), and (1–4) peptides were found in bile samples over 24 hours.
In *in-vitro* studies, Cetrotide™ was stable against phase I- and phase II-metabolism. Cetrotide™ was transformed by peptidases, and the (1–4) peptide was the predominant metabolite.
Excretion
Following subcutaneous administration of 10 mg cetrorelix to males and females, only unchanged cetrorelix was detected in urine. In 24 hours, cetrorelix and small amounts of the (1–9), (1–7), (1–6), and (1–4) peptides were found in bile samples. 2–4% of the dose was eliminated in the urine as unchanged cetrorelix, while 5–10% was eliminated as cetrorelix and the four metabolites in bile. Therefore, only 7–14% of the total dose was recovered as unchanged cetrorelix and metabolites in urine and bile up to 24 hours. The remaining portion of the dose may not have been recovered since bile and urine were not collected for a longer period of time.
Special Populations
Pharmacokinetic investigations have not been performed either in subjects with impaired renal or liver function, or in the elderly, or in children (see PRECAUTIONS).
Pharmacokinetic differences in different races have not been determined.
There is no evidence of differences in pharmacokinetic parameters for Cetrotide™ between healthy subjects and patients undergoing controlled ovarian stimulation.
Drug-Drug Interactions
No formal drug-drug interaction studies have been performed with Cetrotide™ (see PRECAUTIONS).
Clinical Studies
Seven hundred thirty two (732) patients were treated with Cetrotide™ (cetrorelix acetate for injection) in five (two Phase 2 dose-finding and three Phase 3) clinical trials. The clinical trial population consisted of Caucasians (95.5%) and Black, Asian, Arabian and Others (4.5%). Women were between 19 and 40 years of age (mean: 32). The studies excluded subjects with polycystic ovary syndrome (PCOS), subjects with low or no ovarian reserve, and subjects with stage III-IV endometriosis.
Two dose regimens were investigated in these clinical trials, either a single dose per treatment cycle or multiple dosing. In the Phase 2 studies, a single dose of 3 mg was established as the minimal effective dose for the inhibition of premature LH surges with a protection period of a least 4 days. When Cetrotide™ is administered in a multidose regimen, 0.25 mg was established as the minimal effective dose. The extent and duration of LH-suppression is dose dependent.
In the Phase 3 program, efficacy of the single 3 mg dose regimen of Cetrotide™ and the multiple 0.25 mg dose regimen of Cetrotide™ was established separately in two adequate and well controlled clinical studies utilizing active comparitors. A third non-comparative clinical study evaluated only the multiple 0.25 mg dose regimen of Cetrotide™. The ovarian stimulation treatment with recombinant FSH or human menopausal gonadotropin (hMG) was initiated on day 2 or 3 of a normal menstrual cycle. The dose of gonadotropins was administered according to the individual patient's disposition and response.
In the single dose regimen study, Cetrotide™ 3 mg was administered on the day of controlled ovarian stimulation when adequate estradiol levels (400 pg/ml) were obtained, usually on day 7 (range day 5–12). If hCG was not given within 4 days of the 3 mg dose of Cetrotide™, then 0.25 mg of Cetrotide™ was administered daily beginning 96 hours after the 3 mg injection until and including the day of hCG administration.
In the two multiple dose regimen studies, Cetrotide™ 0.25 mg was started on day 5 or 6 of controlled ovarian stimulation (COS). Both gonadotropins and Cetrotide™ were continued daily (multiple dose regimen) until the injection of human chorionic gonadotropin (hCG).

Continued on next page

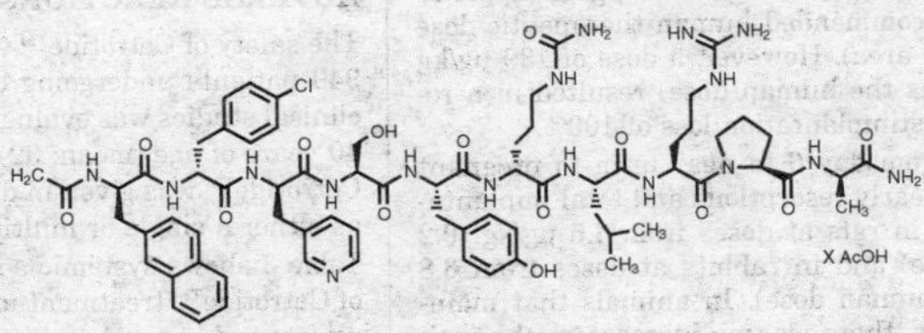

(Ac-*D*-Nal1-*D*-Cpa2-*D*-Pal3-Ser4-Tyr5-*D*-Cit6-Leu7-Arg8-Pro9-*D*-Ala10-NH2)

Cetrotide—Cont.

Oocyte pick-up (OPU) followed by *in vitro* fertilization (IVF) or intracytoplasmic sperm injection (ICSI) as well as embryo transfer (ET) were subsequently performed. The results for Cetrotide™ are summarized below in Table 2.

[See table 2 at right]

In addition to IVF and ICSI, one pregnancy was obtained after intrauterine insemination. In the five Phase 2 and Phase 3 clinical trials, 184 pregnancies have been reported out of a total of 732 patients (including 21 pregnancies following the replacement of frozen-thawed embryos).

In the 3 mg regimen, 9 patients received an additional dose of 0.25 mg of Cetrotide™ and two other patients received two additional doses of 0.25 mg Cetrotide™. The median number of days of Cetrotide™ multiple dose treatment was 5 (range 1–15) in both studies.

No drug related allergic reactions were reported from these clinical studies.

INDICATIONS AND USAGE

Cetrotide™ (cetrorelix acetate for injection) is indicated for the inhibition of premature LH surges in women undergoing controlled ovarian stimulation.

CONTRAINDICATIONS

Cetrotide™ (cetrorelix acetate for injection) is contraindicated under the following conditions:

1. Hypersensitivity to cetrorelix acetate, extrinsic peptide hormones or mannitol.
2. Known hypersensitivity to GnRH or any other GnRH analogs.
3. Known or suspected pregnancy, and lactation (see PRECAUTIONS)

WARNINGS

Cetrotide™ (cetrorelix acetate for injection) should be prescribed by physicians who are experienced in fertility treatment. Before starting treatment with Cetrotide™, pregnancy must be excluded (see CONTRAINDICATIONS and PRECAUTIONS).

PRECAUTIONS

General

Caution is advised in patients with hypersensitivity to GnRH. These patients should be carefully monitored after the first injection. A severe anaphylactic reaction associated with cough, rash and hypotension, was observed in one patient after seven months of treatment with Cetrotide™ (10 mg/day) in a study for an indication unrelated to infertility.

Information for Patients

Prior to therapy with Cetrotide™ (cetrorelix acetate for injection), patients should be informed of the duration of treatment and monitoring procedures that will be required. The risk of possible adverse reactions should be discussed (see ADVERSE REACTIONS). Cetrotide™ should not be prescribed if a patient is pregnant.

If Cetrotide™ is prescribed to patients for self-administration, information for proper use is given in the Patient Leaflet (see below).

Laboratory Tests

After the exclusion of preexisting conditions, enzyme elevations (ALT, AST, GGT, alkaline phosphatase) were found in 1–2% of patients receiving Cetrotide™ during controlled ovarian stimulation. The elevations ranged up to three times the upper limit of normal. The clinical significance of these findings was not determined.

During stimulation with human menopausal gonadotropin, Cetrotide™ had no notable effects on hormone levels aside from inhibition of LH surges.

Drug Interactions

No formal drug interaction studies have been performed with Cetrotide™.

Carcinogenesis, Mutagenesis, Impairment of Fertility

Long-term carcinogenicity studies in animals have not been performed with cetrorelix acetate. Cetrorelix acetate was not genotoxic *in vitro* (Ames test, HPRT test, chromosome aberration test) or *in vivo* (chromosome aberration test, mouse micronucleus test). Cetrorelix acetate induced polyploidy in CHL-Chinese hamster lung fibroblasts, but not in V79-Chinese hamster lung fibroblasts, cultured peripheral human lymphocytes or in an *in-vitro* micronucleus test in the CHL-cell line. Treatment with 0.46 mg/kg cetrorelix acetate for 4 weeks resulted in complete infertility in female rats which was reversed 8 weeks after cessation of treatment.

Pregnancy Category X (see CONTRAINDICATIONS)

Cetrotide™ is contraindicated in pregnant women.

When administered to rats for the first seven days of pregnancy, cetrorelix acetate did not affect the development of the implanted conceptus at doses up to 38 µg/kg (approximately 1 times the recommended human therapeutic dose based on body surface area). However, a dose of 139 µg/kg (approximately 4 times the human dose) resulted in a resorption rate and a postimplantation loss of 100%.

When administered from day 6 to near term to pregnant rats and rabbits, very early resorptions and total implantation losses were seen in rats at doses from 4.6 µg/kg (0.2 times the human dose) and in rabbits at doses from 6.8 µg/kg (0.4 times the human dose). In animals that maintained their pregnancy, there was no increase in the incidence of fetal abnormalities.

Table 1: Pharmacokinetic parameters of Cetrotide™ following 3 mg single or 0.25 mg single and mulitple (daily for 14 days) subcutaneous (sc) administration.

	Single dose 3 mg	Single dose 0.25 mg	Multiple dose 0.25 mg
No. of subjects	12	12	12
t_{max}* [h]	1.5 (0.5–2)	1.0 (0.5–1.5)	1.0 (0.5–2)
$t_{1/2}$* [h]	62.8 (38.2–108)	5.0 (2.4–48.8)	20.6 (4.1–179.3)
C_{max} [ng/ml]	28.5 (22.5–36.2)	4.97 (4.17–5.92)	6.42 (5.18–7.96)
AUC [ng•h/ml]	536 (451–636)	31.4 (23.4–42.0)	44.5 (36.7–54.2)
CL† [ml/min•kg]	1.28[a]		
Vz† [l/kg]	1.16[a]		

Geometric mean (95%CI_{1n}), †arithmetic mean, or *mean (min-max)

t_{max} Time to reach observed maximum plasma concentration

$t_{1/2}$ Elimination half-life

C_{max} Maxinum plasma concentration; multiple dose $C_{ss,\,max}$

AUC Area under the curve; single dose $AUC_{0\text{-}inf}$, multiple dose AUC_{τ}

CL Total plasma clearance

V_z Volume of distribution

[a] Based on iv administration (n=, separate study 0013)

Table 2: Results of Phase 3 Clinical Studies with Cetrotide™ (cetrorelix acetate for injection) 3 mg in a single dose (sd) regimen and 0.25 mg in a multiple dose (md) regimen.

Parameter	Cetrotide™ 3mg (sd, active comparitor study)	Cetrotide™ 0.25 mg (md, active comparitor study)	Cetrotide™ 0.25 mg (md, non-comparative study)
No. of subjects	115	159	303
hCG administered [%]	98.3	96.2	96.0
Oocyte pick-up [%]	98.3	94.3	93.1
LH-surge [%] (LH ≥10 U/L and P[a] ≥ 1 ng/mL)[b]	0.0	1.9	1.0
Serum E_2 [pg/ml] at day hCG[c,d]	1125 (470–2952)	1064 (341–2531)	1185 (311–3676)
Serum LH [U/L] at day hCG[c,d]	1.0 (0.5–2.5)	1.5 (0.5–7.6)	1.1 (0.5–3.5)
No. of follicles ≥11 mm at day hCG[e]	11.2 ± 5.5	10.8 ± 5.2	10.4 ± 4.5
No. of oocytes: IVF[e]	9.2 ± 5.2	7.6 ± 4.3	8.5 ± 5.1
ICSI[e]	10.0 ± 4.2	10.1 ± 5.6	9.3 ± 5.9
Fertilization rate: IVF[e]	0.48 ± 0.33	0.62 ± 0.26	0.60 ± 0.26
ICSI[e]	0.66 ± 0.29	0.63 ± 0.29	0.61 ± 0.25
No. of embroys transferred[e]	2.6 ± 0.9	2.1 ± 0.6	2.7 ± 1.0
Clinical pregnancy rate [%]			
per attempt	22.6	20.8	19.8
per subject with ET	26.3	24.1	23.3

[a] Progesterone
[b] Following initiation of Cetrotide™ therapy
[c] Morning values
[d] Median with 5th–95th percentiles
[e] Mean ± standard deviation

The fetal resorption observed in animals is a logical consequence of the alteration in hormonal levels effected by the antigonadotrophic properties of Cetrotide™, which could result in fetal loss in humans as well. Therefore, this drug should not be used in pregnant women.

Nursing Mothers

It is not known whether Cetrotide™ is excreted in human milk. Because many drugs are excreted in human milk, and because the effects of Cetrotide™ on lactation and/or the breast-fed child have not been determined, Cetrotide™ should not be used by nursing mothers.

Geriatric Use

Cetrotide™ is not intended to be used in subjects aged 65 and over.

ADVERSE REACTIONS

The safety of Cetrotide™ (cetrorelix acetate for injection) in 949 patients undergoing controlled ovarian stimulation in clinical studies was evaluated. Women were between 19 and 40 years of age (mean: 32). 94.0% of them were Caucasian. Cetrotide™ was given in doses ranging from 0.1 mg to 5 mg as either a single or multiple dose.

Table 3 shows systemic adverse events from the beginning of Cetrotide™ treatment until confirmation of pregnancy by ultrasound at an incidence ≥1% in Cetrotide™ treated subjects undergoing COS.

Table 3: Adverse Events in ≥1% (WHO preferred term)	Cetrotide™ N=949 % (n)
Ovarian Hyperstimulation Syndrome#	3.5 (33)
Nausea	1.3 (12)
Headache	1.1 (10)

\# Intensity moderate or severe, or WHO Grade II or III, respectively

Local site reactions (e.g. redness, erythema, bruising, itching, swelling and pruritus) were reported. Usually, they were of a transient nature, mild intensity and short duration.

Two stillbirths were reported in Phase 3 studies of Cetrotide™.

Congenital Anomalies

Clinical follow-up studies of 316 newborns of women administered Cetrotide™ were reviewed. One infant of a set of twin neonates was found to have anencephaly at birth and died after four days. The other twin was normal. Development findings from ongoing baby follow-up included a child with a ventricular septal defect and another child with bilateral congenital glaucoma.

Four pregnancies that resulted in therapeutic abortion in Phase 2 and Phase 3 controlled ovarian stimulation studies had major anomalies (diaphragmatic hernia, trisomy 21, Klinefelter syndrome, polymalformation, and trisomy 18). In three of these four cases, intracytoplasmic sperm injection (ICSI) was the fertilization method employed; in the fourth case, in-vitro fertilization (IVF) was the method employed.

The minor congenital anomalies reported include: supernumerary nipple, bilateral strabismus, imperforate hymen, congenital nevi, hemangiomata, and QT syndrome.

The causal relationship between the reported anomalies and Cetrotide™ is unknown. Multiple factors, genetic and others (including, but not limited to ICSI, IVF, gonadotropins, and progesterone) make causal attribution difficult to study.

OVERDOSAGE

There have been no reports of overdosage with Cetrotide™ 0.25 mg or 3 mg in humans. Single doses up to 120 mg Cetrotide™ have been well tolerated in patients treated for other indications without signs of overdosage.

DOSAGE AND ADMINISTRATION

Ovarian stimulation therapy with gonadotropins (FSH, HMG) is started on cycle Day 2 or 3. The dose of gonadotropins should be adjusted according to individuals response. Cetrotide™ (cetrorelix acetate for injection) may be administered subcutaneously either once daily (0.25 mg dose) or once (3 mg dose) during the early- to mid-follicular phase.

In the single dose regimen, 3 mg of Cetrotide™ is administered when the serum estradiol level is indicative of an appropriate stimulation response, usually on stimulation day 7 (range day 5–9). If hCG has not been administered within four days after injection of Cetrotide™ 3 mg, Cetrotide™ 0.25 mg should be administered once daily until the day of hCG administration.

In the multiple dose regimen, 0.25 mg of Cetrotide™ is administered on either stimulation day 5 (morning or evening) or day 6 (morning) and continued daily until the day of hCG administration.

When assessment by ultrasound shows a sufficient number of follicles of adequate size, hCG is administered to induce ovulation and final maturation of the oocytes. No hCG should be administered if the ovaries show an excessive response to the treatment with gonadotropins to reduce the chance of developing ovarian hyperstimulation syndrome (OHSS).

Administration

Cetrotide™ 0.25 mg and 3 mg can be administered by the patient herself after appropriate instructions by her doctor. Directions for using Cetrotide™ 0.25 mg and 3 mg:

1. Wash hands thoroughly with soap and water.
2. Flip off the plastic cover of the vial and wipe the aluminum ring and the rubber stopper with an alcohol swab.
3. Put the injection needle with the yellow mark (20 gauge) on the pre-filled syringe.
4. Push the needle through the rubber stopper of the vial and slowly inject the solvent into the vial.
5. Leaving the syringe on the vial, gently agitate the vial until the solution is clear and without residues. Avoid forming bubbles.
6. Draw the total contents of the vial into the syringe. If necessary, invert the vial and pull back the needle as far as needed to withdraw the entire contents of the vial.
7. Replace the needle with the yellow mark by the injection needle with the grey mark (27 gauge).
8. Invert the syringe and push the plunger until all air bubbles have been expelled.
9. Choose an injection site at the lower abdominal wall, preferably around the navel. If you are on a multiple dose (0.25 mg) regimen, choose a different injection site each day to minimize local irritation. Use the second alcohol swab to clean the skin at the injection site. Gently pinch up the skin surrounding the site of injection.
10. Insert the needle completely into the skin at an angle of about 45 degrees.
11. Once you have inserted the needle completely, release your grasp of the skin.
12. Gently pull back the plunger of the syringe to check the correct positioning of the needle.
    - If no blood appears, inject the entire solution by slowly pushing the plunger. Thereafter, withdraw the needle and gently press the alcohol swab on the injection site.
    - If blood appears, withdraw the needle with the syringe and gently press the alcohol swab on the injection site. Discard the syringe and the drug vial. Use a new pack and repeat the procedure.
13. Use the syringe and needles only once. Dispose of the syringe and needles properly after use. If available, use a medical waste container for disposal.

HOW SUPPLIED

Cetrotide™ (cetrorelix acetate for injection) 0.25 mg is available in a carton of one packaged tray (NDC 720303122512) or a carton of seven packaged trays (NDC 720303122574). Each packaged tray contains: one glass vial containing 0.26–0.27 mg cetrorelix acetate (corresponding to 0.25 mg cetrorelix), one pre-filled glass syringe with 1 mL of Sterile Water of Injection, USP (pH 5-8), one 20 gauge needle (yellow), one 27 gauge needle (grey), and two alcohol swabs.

Cetrotide™ (cetrorelix acetate for injection) 3 mg is available in a carton of one packaged tray (NDC 720303120310). Each packaged tray contains: one glass vial containing 3.12–3.24 mg cetrorelix acetate (corresponding to 3 mg cetrorelix), one pre-filled glass syringe with 3 mL of Sterile Water for Injection, USP (pH 5-8), one 20 gauge needle (yellow), one 27 gauge needle (grey), and two alcohol swabs.

Storage

Cetrotide™ 3 mg:

Store at 25°C (77°F); excursions permitted to 15–30°C (59–86°F) [see USP Controlled Room Temperature]. Store the packaged tray in the outer carton.

Cetrotide™ 0.25 mg:

Store refrigerated, 2–8°C (36–46°F). Store the packaged tray in the outer carton.

Rx only

Product Information as of August, 2000.

Distributed by: Serono Laboratories, Inc.

Patient Leaflet

Cetrotide™ 0.25 mg and 3 mg

Active ingredient: cetrorelix acetate

Summary

Cetrotide™ blocks the effects of a natural hormone, called gonadotropin-releasing hormone (GnRH). GnRH controls the secretion of another hormone, called luteinizing hormone (LH), which induces ovulation during the menstrual cycle. During hormone treatment for ovarian stimulation, premature ovulation may lead to eggs that are not suitable for fertilization. Cetrotide™ blocks such undesirable premature ovulation.

Uses

Cetrotide™ is used or prevent premature ovulation during controlled ovarian stimulation.

General Cautions

Do not use Cetrotide™ if you

- are allergic to cetrorelix acetate, mannitol or exogenous peptide hormones (medicines similar to Cetrotide™) or
- are pregnant, or think that you might be pregnant, of if you are breast-feeding.

Proper Use

Ovarian stimulation therapy is started on cycle Day 2 or 3. Cetrotide™ is injected under the skin either once daily (0.25 mg dose) or once (3 mg dose), as directed by your physician. When an ultrasound examination shows that you are ready, another drug (hCG) is injected to induce ovulation.

How should you use Cetrotide™?

You may self-inject Cetrotide™ after special instruction from your doctor.

To fully benefit from Cetrotide™, please read carefully and follow the instructions given below, unless your doctor advises you otherwise.

Cetrotide™ is for injection under the skin of the lower abdominal wall, preferably around the belly button. If you are on a multiple dose (0.25 mg) regimen, choose a different injection site each day to minimize local irritation.

Dissolve Cetrotide™ powder only with the water contained in the pre-filled syringe. Do not use a Cetrotide™ solution if it contains particles or if it is not clear.

Before you inject Cetrotide™ yourself, please read the following instructions carefully:

1. Wash your hands well with soap and water.

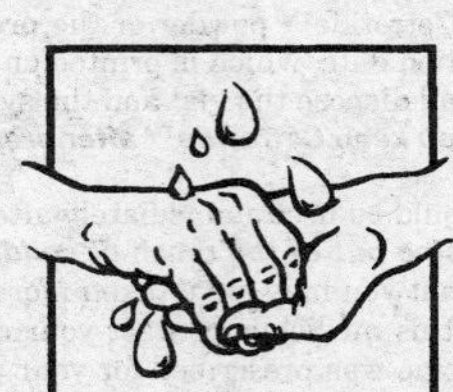

2. On a clean surface, lay out everything you need (one vial, one pre-filled syringe, one injection needle with a yellow mark, one injection needle with a grey mark, and two alcohol wipes).

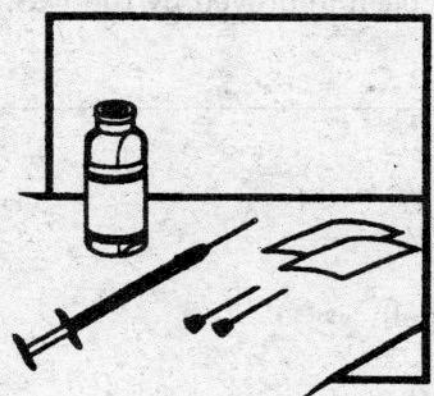

3. Flip off the plastic cover of the vial. Wipe the aluminum ring and the rubber stopper with an alcohol wipe.

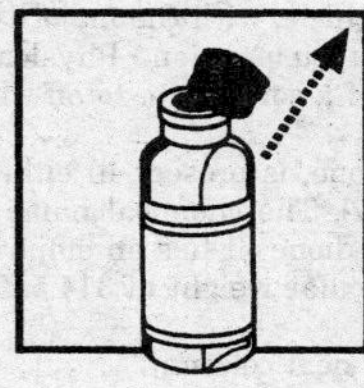

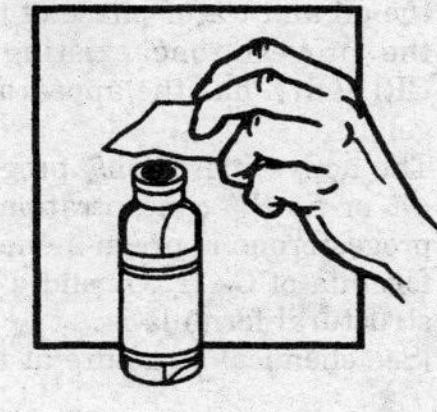

4. Take the injection needle with the yellow mark and remove the wrapping. Take the pre-filled syringe and remove the cover. Put the needle on the syringe and remove the cover of the needle.

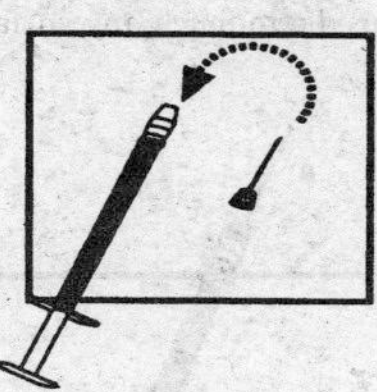

5. Push the needle through the center of the rubber stopper of the vial. Inject the water into the vial by slowly pushing the plunger of the syringe.

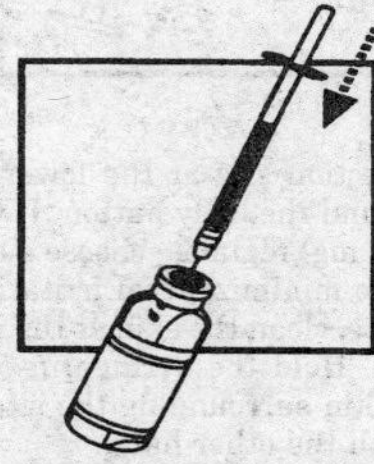

6. Leave the syringe in the vial. Gently shake the vial until the solution is clear and without residue. Avoid forming bubbles during dissolution.

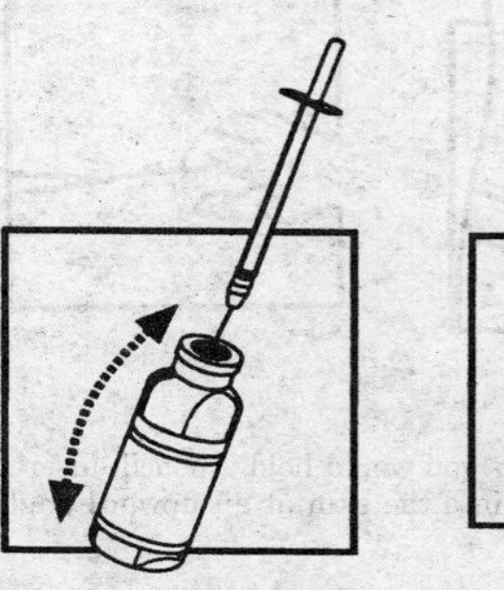

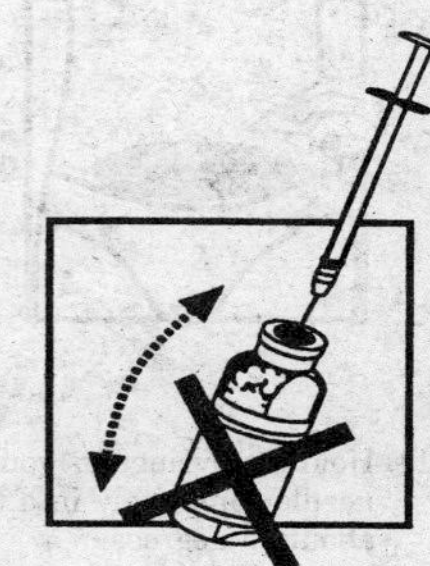

7. Draw the total contents of the vial into the syringe. If liquid is left in the vial, invert the vial, pull back the needle until the opening of the needle is just inside the stopper. If you look from the side through the gap in the stopper. you can control the movement of the needle and the liquid. It is important to withdraw the entire contents of the vial.

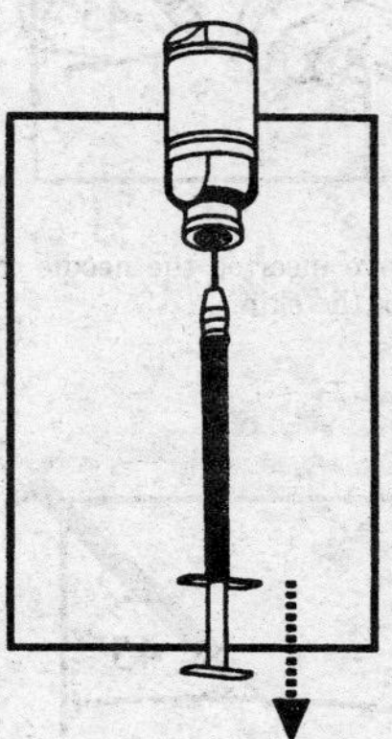

8. Detach the syringe from the needle and lay down the syringe. Take the injection needle with the grey mark and remove its wrapping. Put the needle on the syringe and remove the cover of the needle.

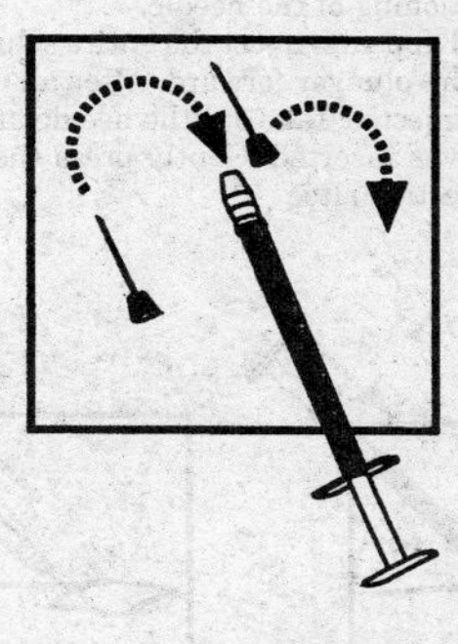

Continued on next page

Cetrotide—Cont.

9. Invert the syringe and push the plunger until all air bubbles have been pushed out. Do not touch the needle or allow the needle to touch any surface.

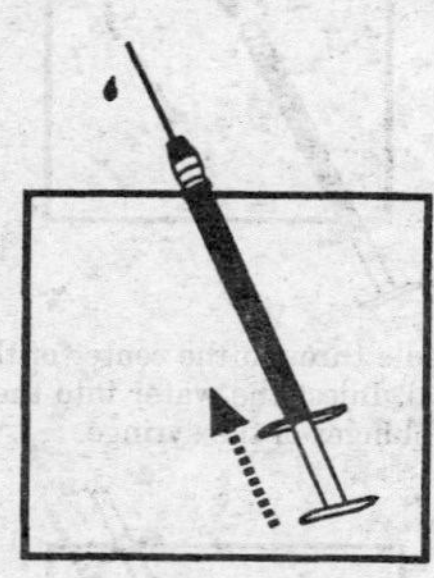

10. Choose an injection site at the lower abdominal wall, preferably around the belly button. If you are on a multiple dose (0.25 mg) regimen, choose a different injection site each day to minimize local irritation. Take the second alcohol wipe, clean the skin at the injection site, and keep the wipe. Hold the syringe in one hand. Gently pinch up the skin surrounding the site of injection and hold firmly with the other hand.

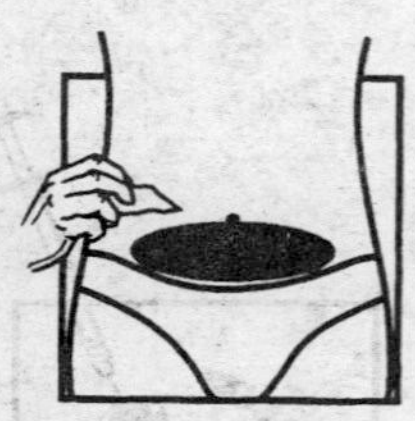

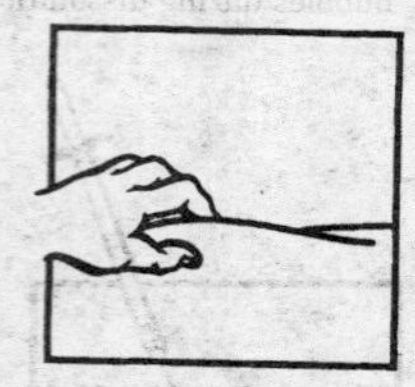

11. Hold the syringe as you would hold a pencil, insert the needle completely into the skin at an upward angle of about 45 degrees.

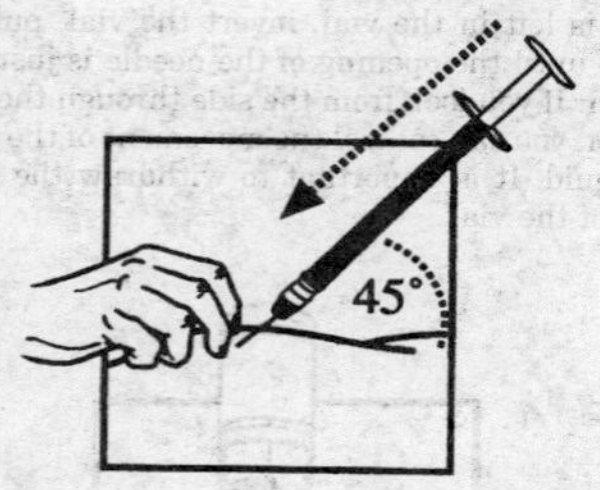

12. Once you have inserted the needle completely, release your grasp of the skin.

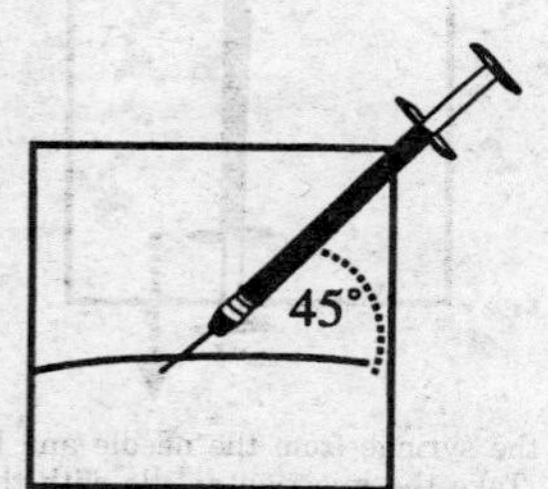

13. Gently pull back the plunger of the syringe to check the correct positioning of the needle.
   - If no blood appears, inject the entire solution by slowly pushing the plunger forward. After all of the solution has been injected, take out the needle at the same angle as it was inserted. Gently press the alcohol wipe on the injection site.

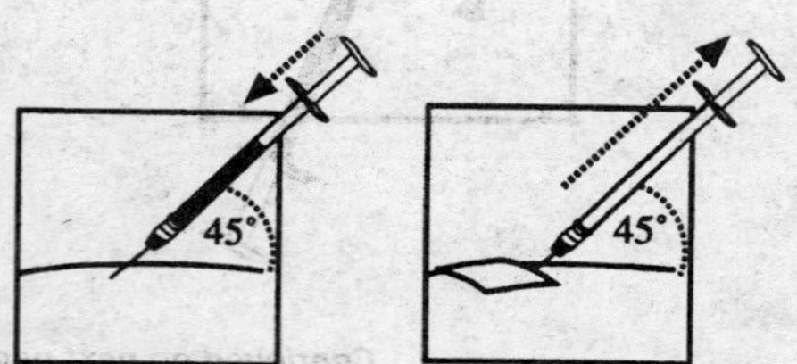

   - If blood appears, withdraw the needle with the syringe and gently press the alcohol wipe on the injection site. Do not use the medicine. Dispose the syringe and the medicine. Use a new packaged tray of Cetrotide™ to repeat the procedure.

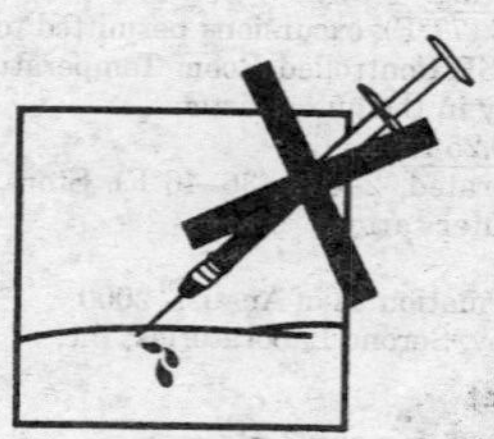

14. Use the syringe and needles only once. Dispose of the syringe and needles immediately after use (put the covers on the needles to avoid injury). If available, a medical waste container should be used for disposal.

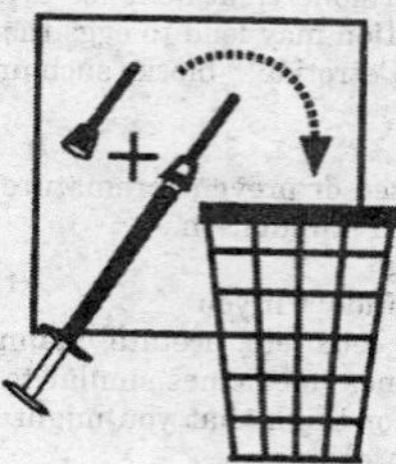

SPECIAL ADVICE

What do you do if you have used too much Cetrotide™?

Contact your doctor in case of overdosage immediately to check whether an adjustment of the further ovarian stimulation procedure is required.

Possible Side Effects

Mild and short lasting reactions may occur at the injection site like reddening, itching, and swelling. Nausea and headache have also been reported.

Call your doctor if you have any side effect not mentioned in this leaflet or if you are unsure about the effect of this medicine.

Storage

How is Cetrotide™ to be stored?

Store Cetrotide™ in a cool dry place protected from excess moisture and heat. Store Cetrotide™ 3 mg at 25°C (77°F). Excursions are permitted to 15–30°C (59–86°F). Store Cetrotide™ 0.25 mg in the refrigerator at 2–8°C (36–46°F). Keep the packaged tray in the outer carton in order to protect it from light.

How long may Cetrotide™ be stored?

Do not use the Cetrotide™ powder or the pre-filled syringe after the expiration date, which is printed on the labels and on the carton, and dispose the vial and the syringe properly.

How long can you keep Cetrotide™ after preparation of the solution?

The solution should be used immediately after preparation.

Store the medicine out of the reach of children.

If you suspect that you may have taken more than the prescribed dose of this medicine, contact your doctor immediately. The medicine was prescribed for your particular condition. Do not use it for another condition or give the drug to others.

This leaflet provides a summary of the information about Cetrotide™. Medicines are sometimes prescribed for uses other than those listed in the Leaflet. If you have any questions or concerns, or want more information about Cetrotide™, contact your doctor or pharmacist.

This Leaflet has been approved by the U.S. Food and Drug Administration.

CRINONE® 4% ℞
CRINONE® 8%

[crĭ ′nōn]

(progesterone gel)

DESCRIPTION

CRINONE® (progesterone gel) is a bioadhesive vaginal gel containing micronized progesterone in an emulsion system, which is contained in single use, one piece polyethylene vaginal applicators. The carrier vehicle is an oil in water emulsion containing the water swellable, but insoluble polymer, polycarbophil. The progesterone is partially soluble in both the oil and water phase of the vehicle, with the majority of the progesterone existing as a suspension. Physically, CRINONE has the appearance of a soft, white to off-white gel.

The active ingredient, progesterone, is present in either a 4% or an 8% concentration (w/w). The chemical name for progesterone is pregn-4-ene-3,20-dione. It has an empirical formula of $C_{21}H_{30}O_2$ and a molecular weight of 314.5. The structural formula is:

[See chemical structure at top of next column]

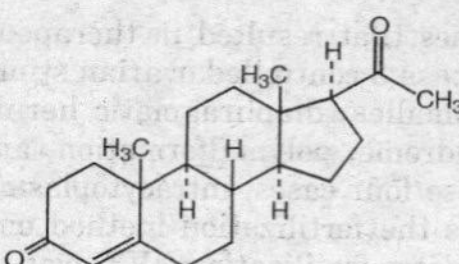

Progesterone exists in two polymorphic forms. Form 1, which is the form used in CRINONE, exists as white orthorhombic prisms with a melting point of 127–131°C.

Each applicator delivers 1.125 grams of CRINONE gel containing either 45 mg (4% gel) or 90 mg (8% gel) of progesterone in a base containing glycerin, mineral oil, polycarbophil, carbomer 934P, hydrogenated palm oil glyceride, sorbic acid, sodium hydroxide and purified water.

CLINICAL PHARMACOLOGY

Progesterone is a naturally occurring steroid that is secreted by the ovary, placenta, and adrenal gland. In the presence of adequate estrogen, progesterone transforms a proliferative endometrium into a secretory endometrium. Progesterone is essential for the development of decidual tissue, and the effect of progesterone on the differentiation of glandular epithelia and stroma has been extensively studied. Progesterone is necessary to increase endometrial receptivity for implantation of an embryo. Once an embryo is implanted, progesterone acts to maintain the pregnancy. Normal or near-normal endometrial responses to oral estradiol and intramuscular progesterone have been noted in functionally agonadal women through the sixth decade of life. Progesterone administration decreases the circulatory levels of gonadotropins.

Pharmacokinetics

Absorption

Due to sustained release properties of CRINONE, progesterone absorption is prolonged with an absorption half-life of approximately 25–50 hours, and an elimination half-life of 5–20 minutes. Therefore, the pharmacokinetics of CRINONE are rate-limited by absorption rather than by elimination.

The bioavailability of progesterone in CRINONE was determined relative to progesterone administered intramuscularly. In a single dose cross-over study, 20 healthy, estrogenized postmenopausal women received 45 mg or 90 mg progesterone vaginally in CRINONE 4% or CRINONE 8%, or 45 mg or 90 mg progesterone intramuscularly. The pharmacokinetic parameters (mean ± standard deviation) are shown in Table 1.

[See table 1 at bottom of next page]

The multiple dose pharmacokinetics of CRINONE 4% and CRINONE 8% administered every other day and CRINONE 8% administered daily or twice daily for 12 days were studied in 10 healthy, estrogenized postmenopausal women in two separate studies. Steady state was achieved within the first 24 hours after initiation of treatment. The pharmacokinetic parameters (mean ± standard deviation) after the last administration of CRINONE 4% or 8% derived from these studies are shown in Table 2.

[See table 2 at bottom of next page]

Distribution

Progesterone is extensively bound to serum proteins (≈ 96–99%), primarily to serum albumin and corticosteroid binding globulin.

Metabolism

The major urinary metabolite of oral progesterone is 5β-pregnan-3α, 20α-diol glucuronide which is present in plasma in the conjugated form only. Plasma metabolites also include 5β-pregnan-3α-ol-20-one (5β-pregnanolone) and 5α-pregnan-3α-ol-20-one (5α-pregnanolone).

Excretion

Progesterone undergoes both biliary and renal elimination. Following an injection of labeled progesterone, 50–60% of the excretion of progesterone metabolites occurs via the kidney; approximately 10% occurs via the bile and feces, the second major excretory pathway. Overall recovery of labeled material accounts for 70% of an administered dose, with the remainder of the dose not characterized with respect to elimination. Only a small portion of unchanged progesterone is excreted in the bile.

Clinical Studies

Assisted Reproductive Technology

In a single-center, open-label study (COL 1620-007US), 99 women (aged 28–47 years) with either partial (n=84) or premature ovarian failure (n=15) who were candidates to receive a donor oocyte transfer as an Assisted Reproductive Technology ("ART") procedure were randomized to receive either CRINONE 8% twice daily (n=68) or intramuscular progesterone 100 mg daily (n=31). The study was divided into three phases (Pilot, Donor Egg and Treatment). The first phase of the study consisted of a test Pilot Cycle to ensure that the administration of transdermal estradiol and progesterone would adequately prime the endometrium to receive the donor egg. The second phase was the Donor Egg Cycle during which a fertilized oocyte was implanted. CRINONE 8% was administered beginning the evening of Day 14 of the Pilot and Donor Egg cycles. Subjects with partial ovarian function also underwent a Pre-Pilot Cycle and a Pre-Donor Egg Cycle during which time they were administered only leuprolide acetate to suppress remaining ovarian function. The Pre-Pilot Cycle, Pilot Cycle, Pre-Donor Egg Cycle, and Donor Egg Cycle each lasted approximately

34 days. The third phase of the study consisted of a 10-week treatment period to maintain a pregnancy until placental autonomy was achieved.

Sixty-one women received CRINONE 8% as part of the Pilot Cycle to determine their endometrial response. Of the 55 evaluable endometrial biopsies in the CRINONE 8% group performed on Day 25–27, all were histologically "in-phase", consistent with luteal phase biopsy specimens of menstruating women at comparable time intervals. Fifty-four women who received CRINONE 8% and had a histologically "in-phase" biopsy received a donor oocyte transfer. Among these 54 CRINONE-treated women, clinical pregnancies (assessed about week 10 after transfer by clinical examination, ultrasound and/or β-hCG levels) occurred in 26 women (48%). In these 54 women, 17 women (31%) delivered a total of 25 newborns, seven women (13%) had a spontaneous abortion and two women (4%) had an elective abortion.

In a second study (COL1620-F01), CRINONE 8% was used in luteal phase support of women with tubal or idiopathic infertility due to endometriosis and normal ovulatory cycles, undergoing *in vitro* fertilization ("IVF") procedures. All women received a GnRH analog to suppress endogenous progesterone, human menopausal gonadotropins, and human chorionic gonadotropin. In this multi-center, open-label study, 139 women (aged 22–38 years) received CRINONE 8% once daily beginning within 24 hours of embryo transfer and continuing through Day 30 post-transfer. Clinical pregnancies assessed at Day 90 post-transfer were seen in 36 (26%) of women. Thirty-two women (23%) delivered newborns and four women (3%) had a spontaneous abortion. (See **PRECAUTIONS**, subsection **Pregnancy**)

Secondary Amenorrhea

In three parallel, open-label studies (COL1620-004US, COL1620-005US, COL1620-009US), 127 women (aged 18–44) with hypothalamic amenorrhea or premature ovarian failure were randomized to receive either CRINONE 4% (n=62) or CRINONE 8% (n=65). All women were treated with either conjugated estrogens 0.625 mg daily (n=100) or transdermal estradiol (delivering 50 mcg/day) twice weekly (n=27).

Estrogen therapy was continuous for the entire three 28-day cycle studies. At Day 15 of the second cycle (six weeks after initiating estrogen replacement), women who demonstrated adequate response to estrogen therapy (by ultrasound) and who continued to be amenorrheic received CRINONE every other day for six doses (Day 15 through Day 25 of the cycle).

In cycle 2, CRINONE 4% induced bleeding in 79% of women and CRINONE 8% induced bleeding in 77% of women. In the third cycle, estrogen was continued and CRINONE was administered every other day beginning on Day 15 for six doses. On Day 24 an endometrial biopsy was performed. In 53 women who received CRINONE 4%, biopsy results were as follows: 7% proliferative, 40% late secretory, 19% mid secretory, 13% early secretory, 7% atrophic, 6% menstrual endometrium, 6% inactive endometrium and 2% negative endometrium. In 54 women who received CRINONE 8%, biopsy results were as follows: 44% late secretory, 19% mid secretory, 11% early secretory, 19% atrophic, 5% menstrual endometrium and 2% "oral contraceptive like" endometrium.

INDICATIONS AND USAGE

Assisted Reproductive Technology

CRINONE 8% is indicated for progesterone supplementation or replacement as part of an Assisted Reproductive Technology ("ART") treatment for infertile women with progesterone deficiency.

Secondary Amenorrhea

CRINONE 4% is indicated for the treatment of secondary amenorrhea.

CRINONE 8% is indicated for use in women who have failed to respond to treatment with CRINONE 4%.

CONTRAINDICATIONS

CRINONE should not be used in individuals with any of the following conditions:

1. Known sensitivity to CRINONE (progesterone or any of the other ingredients)
2. Undiagnosed vaginal bleeding
3. Liver dysfunction or disease
4. Known or suspected malignancy of the breast or genital organs
5. Missed abortion
6. Active thrombophlebitis or thromboembolic disorders, or a history of hormone-associated thrombophlebitis or thromboembolic disorders.

WARNINGS

The physician should be alert to the earliest manifestations of thrombotic disorders (thrombophlebitis, cerebrovascular disorders, pulmonary embolism, and retinal thrombosis). Should any of these occur or be suspected, the drug should be discontinued immediately.

Progesterone and progestins have been used to prevent miscarriage in women with a history of recurrent spontaneous pregnancy losses. No adequate evidence is available to show that they are effective for this purpose.

PRECAUTIONS

General

1. The pretreatment physical examination should include special reference to breast and pelvic organs, as well as Papanicolaou smear.
2. In cases of breakthrough bleeding, as in all cases of irregular vaginal bleeding, nonfunctional causes should be considered. In cases of undiagnosed vaginal bleeding, adequate diagnostic measures should be undertaken.
3. Because progestogens may cause some degree of fluid retention, conditions which might be influenced by this factor (e.g., epilepsy, migraine, asthma, cardiac or renal dysfunction) require careful observation.
4. The pathologist should be advised of progesterone therapy when relevant specimens are submitted.
5. Patients who have a history of psychic depression should be carefully observed and the drug discontinued if the depression recurs to a serious degree.
6. A decrease in glucose tolerance has been observed in a small percentage of patients on estrogen-progestin combination drugs. The mechanism of this decrease is not known. For this reason, diabetic patients should be carefully observed while receiving progestin therapy.

Information for Patients

The product should not be used concurrently with other local intravaginal therapy. If other local intravaginal therapy is to be used concurrently, there should be at least a 6-hour period before or after CRINONE® administration.

Drug Interactions

No drug interactions have been assessed with CRINONE.

Carcinogenesis, Mutagenesis, Impairment of Fertility

Nonclinical toxicity studies to determine the potential of CRINONE to cause carcinogenicity or mutagenicity have not been performed. The effect of CRINONE on fertility has not been evaluated in animals.

Pregnancy (See **CLINICAL PHARMACOLOGY**, subsection **Clinical Studies**)

CRINONE 8% has been used to support embryo implantation and maintain pregnancies through its use as part of ART treatment regimens in two clinical studies (studies COL1620–007US and COL1620-F01). In the first study (COL1620-007US), 54 CRINONE-treated women had donor oocyte transfer procedures, and clinical pregnancies occurred in 26 women (48%). The outcomes of these 26 pregnancies were as follows: one woman had an elective termination of pregnancy at 19 weeks due to congenital malformations (omphalocele) associated with a chromosomal abnormality; one woman pregnant with triplets had an elective termination of her pregnancy; seven women had spontaneous abortions; and 17 women delivered 25 apparently normal newborns.

In the second study (COL1620-F01), CRINONE 8% was used in the luteal phase support of women undergoing *in vitro* fertilization ("IVF") procedures. In this multi-center, open-label study, 139 women received CRINONE 8% once daily beginning within 24 hours of embryo transfer and continuing through Day 30 post-transfer.

Clinical pregnancies assessed at Day 90 post-transfer were seen in 36 (26%) of women. Thirty-two women (23%) delivered newborns and four women (3%) had a spontaneous abortion. Of the 47 newborns delivered, one had a teratoma associated with a cleft palate; one had respiratory distress syndrome; 44 were apparently normal and one was lost to follow-up.

Pediatric Use

Safety and effectiveness in pediatric patients have not been established.

Nursing Mothers

Detectable amounts of progestins have been identified in the milk of mothers receiving them. The effect of this on the nursing infant has not been determined.

ADVERSE REACTIONS

Assisted Reproductive Technology

In a study of 61 women with ovarian failure undergoing a donor oocyte transfer procedure receiving CRINONE 8% twice daily, treatment-emergent adverse events occurring in 5% or more of the women are shown in Table 3.

TABLE 1
Single Dose Relative Bioavailability

	CRINONE 4%	45 mg Intramuscular Progesterone	CRINONE 8%	90 mg Intramuscular Progesterone
C_{max} (ng/mL)	13.15 ± 6.49	39.06 ± 13.68	14.87 ± 6.32	53.76 ± 14.9
$C_{avg\ 0\text{-}24}$ (ng/mL)	6.94 ± 4.24	22.41 ± 4.92	6.98 ± 3.21	28.98 ± 8.75
$AUC_{0\text{-}96}$ (ng•hr/mL)	288.63 ± 273.72	806.26 ± 102.75	296.78 ± 129.90	1378.91 ± 176.39
T_{max} (hr)	5.6 ± 1.84	8.2 ± 6.43	6.8 ± 3.3	9.2 ± 2.7
$t_{1/2}$ (hr)	55.13 ± 28.04	28.05 ± 16.87	34.8 ± 11.3	19.6 ± 6.0
F (%)	27.6		19.8	

C_{max} – maximum progesterone serum concentration
$C_{avg\ 0\text{-}24}$ – average progesterone serum concentration over 24 hours
$AUC_{0\text{-}96}$ – area under the drug concentration versus time curve from 0-96 hours post dose
T_{max} – time to maximum progesterone concentration
$t_{1/2}$ – elimination half-life
F – relative bioavailability

TABLE 2
Multiple Dose Pharmacokinetics

	Assisted Reproductive Technology		Secondary Amenorrhea	
	Daily Dosing 8%	Twice Daily Dosing 8%	Every Other Day Dosing 4%	Every Other Day Dosing 8%
C_{max} (ng/mL)	15.97 ± 5.05	14.57 ± 4.49	13.21 ± 9.46	13.67 ± 3.58
C_{avg} (ng/mL)	8.99 ± 3.53	11.6 ± 3.47	4.05 ± 2.85	6.75 ± 2.83
T_{max} (hr)	5.40 ± 0.97	3.55 ± 2.48	6.67 ± 3.16	7.00 ± 2.88
$AUC_{0\text{-}\tau}$ (ng•hr/mL)	391.98 ± 153.28	138.72 ± 41.58	242.15 ± 167.88	438.36 ± 223.36
$t_{1/2}$ (hr)	45.00 ± 34.70	25.91 ± 6.15	49.87 ± 31.20	39.08 ± 12.88

TABLE 3
Treatment-Emergent Adverse Events
in ≥5% of Women Receiving CRINONE 8%
Twice Daily
Study COL1620-007US (n=61)

Body as a Whole	
Bloating	7%
Cramps NOS	15%
Pain	8%
Central and Peripheral Nervous System	
Dizziness	5%
Headache	13%
Gastro-Intestinal System	
Nausea	7%
Reproductive, Female	
Breast Pain	13%
Moniliasis Genital	5%
Vaginal Discharge	7%

Continued on next page

Crinone—Cont.

Skin and Appendages	
Pruritus Genital	5%

In a second clinical study of 139 women using CRINONE 8% once daily for luteal phase support while undergoing an *in vitro* fertilization procedure, treatment-emergent adverse events reported in ≥5% of the women are shown in Table 4.

TABLE 4
Treatment-Emergent Adverse Events in ≥5% of Women Receiving CRINONE 8% Once Daily
Study COL1620-F01 (n=139)

Body as a Whole	
Abdominal Pain	12%
Perineal Pain Female	17%
Central and Periphal Nervous System	
Headache	17%
Gastro-Intestinal System	
Constipation	27%
Diarrhea	8%
Nausea	22%
Vomiting	5%
Musculo-Skeletal System	
Arthralgia	8%
Psychiatric	
Depression	11%
Libido Decreased	10%
Nervousness	16%
Somnolence	27%
Reproductive, Female	
Breast Enlargement	40%
Dyspareunia	6%
Urinary System	
Nocturia	13%

Secondary Amenorrhea
In three studies, 127 women with secondary amenorrhea received estrogen replacement therapy and CRINONE 4% or 8% every other day for six doses. Treatment emergent adverse events during estrogen and CRINONE treatment that occurred in 5% or more of women are shown in Table 5.

TABLE 5
Treatment Emergent Adverse Events in ≥5% of Women Receiving Estrogen Treatment and CRINONE Every Other Day
Studies COL1620-004US, COL1620-005US, COL1620-009US

	Estrogen +CRINONE 4% n = 62	Estrogen +CRINONE 8% n = 65
Body as a Whole		
Abdominal Pain	3 (5%)	6 (9%)
Appetite Increased	3 (5%)	5 (8%)
Bloating	8 (13%)	8 (12%)
Cramps NOS	12 (19%)	17 (26%)
Fatigue	13 (21%)	14 (22%)
Central and Peripheral Nervous System		
Headache	12 (19%)	10 (15%)
Gastro-Intestinal System		
Nausea	5 (8%)	4 (6%)
Musculo-Skeletal System		
Back Pain	5 (8%)	2 (3%)
Myalgia	5 (8%)	0 (0%)
Psychiatric		
Depression	12 (19%)	10 (15%)
Emotional Lability	14 (23%)	14 (22%)
Sleep Disorder	11 (18%)	12 (18%)
Reproductive, Female		
Vaginal Discharge	7 (11%)	2 (3%)
Resistance Mechanism		
Upper Respiratory Tract Infection	3 (5%)	5 (8%)
Skin and Appendages		
Pruritis genital	1 (2%)	4 (6%)

Additional adverse events reported in women at a frequency <5% in the CRINONE ART and secondary amenorrhea studies and not listed in the tables above include:
Autonomic Nervous System—mouth dry, sweating increased
Body as a Whole—abnormal crying, allergic reaction, allergy, appetite decreased, asthenia, edema, face edema, fever, hot flushes, influenza-like symptoms, water retention, xerophthalmia
Cardiovascular, General—syncope
Central and Peripheral Nervous System—migraine, tremor
Gastro-Intestinal—dyspepsia, eructation, flatulence, gastritis, toothache
Metabolic and Nutritional—thirst
Musculo-Skeletal System—cramps legs, leg pain, skeletal pain
Neoplasm—benign cyst
Platelet, Bleeding & Clotting—purpura
Psychiatric—aggressive reactions, forgetfulness, insomnia
Red Blood Cell—anemia
Reproductive, Female—dysmenorrhea, premenstrual tension, vaginal dryness
Resistance Mechanism—infection, pharyngitis, sinusitis, urinary tract infection
Respiratory System—asthma, dyspnea, hyperventilation, rhinitis
Skin and Appendages—acne, pruritus, rash, seborrhea, skin discoloration, skin disorder, urticaria
Urinary System—cystitis, dysuria, micturition frequency
Vision Disorders—conjunctivitis

OVERDOSAGE
There have been no reports of overdosage with CRINONE. In the case of overdosage, however, discontinue CRINONE, treat the patient symptomatically, and institute supportive measures.
As with all prescription drugs, this medicine should be kept out of the reach of children.

DOSAGE AND ADMINISTRATION
Assisted Reproductive Technology—CRINONE 8% is administered vaginally at a dose of 90 mg once daily in women who require progesterone supplementation. CRINONE 8% is administered vaginally at a dose of 90 mg twice daily in women with partial or complete ovarian failure who require progesterone replacement. If pregnancy occurs, treatment may be continued until placental autonomy is achieved, up to 10–12 weeks.
Secondary Amenorrhea—CRINONE 4% is administered vaginally every other day up to a total of six doses. For women who fail to respond, a trial of CRINONE 8% every other day up to a total of six doses may be instituted. It is important to note that a dosage increase from the 4% gel can only be accomplished by using the 8% gel. Increasing the volume of gel administered does not increase the amount of progesterone absorbed.
SEE CRINONE PATIENT INFORMATION SHEET—HOW TO USE CRINONE. NOTE: The PATIENT INFORMATION SHEET contains special instructions for using the applicator at altitudes above 2500 feet in order to avoid a partial release of CRINONE before vaginal insertion.

HOW SUPPLIED
CRINONE® is available in the following strengths:
4% gel (45 mg) in a single use, one piece, disposable, white polyethylene vaginal applicator with a twist-off top. Each applicator contains 2.6 g of gel and delivers 1.125 g of gel.
NDC – 44087-0804-6 – 6 Single-use prefilled applicators.
8% gel (90 mg) in a single use, one piece, disposable, white polyethylene vaginal applicator with a twist-off top. Each applicator contains 2.6 g of gel and delivers 1.125 g of gel.
NDC – 44087-0808-6 – 6 Single-use prefilled applicators.
NDC – 44087-0818-8 – 18 Single-use prefilled applicators (3 boxes of 6).
Each applicator is wrapped and sealed in a foil overwrap.
Store at controlled room temperature below 25°C (77°F).
Rx Only
U.S. Patent Numbers 4,615,697 and 5,543,150.

Distributed by
Serono Laboratories, Inc.
Randolph, MA 02368
March, 2000

Shown in Product Identification Guide, page 336

FERTINEX® ℞
[fĕr 'tĭn-ĕx]
(urofollitropin for injection, purified)
FOR SUBCUTANEOUS INJECTION

DESCRIPTION
Fertinex® (urofollitropin for injection, purified) is a preparation of highly purified Follicle Stimulating Hormone (FSH) extracted from the urine of post-menopausal women. Purification is by immunoaffinity chromatography using murine monoclonal antibody to human FSH. The purification process results in a consistent FSH isoform profile, significantly enhanced specific activity (8,500–13,500 IU FSH/mg protein), and a highly purified preparation. Each ampule of Fertinex® contains either 75 IU or 150 IU of highly purified FSH and 10 mg lactose in a sterile, lyophilized form. If required, pH is adjusted with 0.1 M hydrochloric acid and/or 0.1 M sodium hydroxide. Fertinex® is administered by subcutaneous injection.
Fertinex® contains an acidic, water soluble glycoprotein biologically standardized for FSH gonadotropin activity in terms of the Second International Reference Preparation for Human Menopausal Gonadotropins established in September, 1964 by the Expert Committee on Biological Standards of the World Health Organization. Negligible amounts (≤0.1 IU LH/1000 IU FSH) of luteinizing hormone (LH) activity are contained in Fertinex®.
Therapeutic Class: Infertility.

CLINICAL PHARMACOLOGY
Fertinex® (urofollitropin for injection, purified) stimulates ovarian follicular growth in women who do not have primary ovarian failure. FSH, the active component of Fertinex®, is the primary hormone responsible for follicular recruitment and development. In order to effect final maturation of the follicle and ovulation in the absence of an endogenous LH surge, human chorionic gonadotropin (hCG) must be given following the administration of Fertinex® when monitoring of the patient indicates that sufficient follicular development has occurred. There may be a degree of interpatient variability in response to FSH administration.
Pharmacokinetics:
In a comparative, single-dose, double-blind, double-dummy, randomized, cross-over study, Fertinex® administered subcutaneously demonstrated a similar pharmacokinetic profile to urofollitropin and Fertinex® administered intramuscularly. No significant differences were found between the treatment groups in AUC/dose and CMAX/dose parameters. A variability in TMAX was observed. Subcutaneous administration of Fertinex® led to a slower absorption rate resulting in a later TMAX (15±7h) than following IM administration of either Fertinex® (10±4h) or urofollitropin (9±4h).
Plasma inhibin levels were measured as a pharmacodynamic marker of FSH activity. The inhibin concentration-time profile of inhibin following Fertinex® administered subcutaneously was found to be similar to that following urofollitropin and Fertinex® administered intramuscularly.
Special Populations: Safety and efficacy of Fertinex® in renal or hepatic insufficiency have not been established.
Drug-Drug Interactions: No clinically significant drug-drug interactions have been reported (see PRECAUTIONS).

Clinical Studies:
1. Ovulation Induction:
The safety and efficacy of Fertinex® administered subcutaneously vs. urofollitropin administered intramuscularly for ovulation induction was assessed in a phase III, open-label, randomized, comparative, multicenter study in oligo-ovulatory infertile women who failed to ovulate or conceive following adequate clomiphene citrate therapy. The purpose of the study was to demonstrate that Fertinex®, a highly purified follicle stimulating hormone (FSH) administered subcutaneously, is clinically not different in terms of safety and efficacy from urofollitropin administered intramuscularly. The principal efficacy parameters recorded were serum estradiol levels, follicular growth, ovulation rate and pregnancy rate. Two hundred eleven patients entered treatment, of whom 108 received Fertinex® and 103 received urofollitropin. Overall, two hundred and four patients (491 cycles) were considered evaluable. There were no differences between the Fertinex® administered subcutaneously and the urofollitropin intramuscular treatment groups in serum estradiol levels and follicular growth (follicle number and size) on the day of human chorionic gonadotropin (hCG) administration, nor were there any differences between the treatment groups in ovulation rates or pregnancy rates per patient.
The results of safety and efficacy with Fertinex® administered subcutaneously for ovulation induction in oligo-ovulatory infertile women are summarized below:
Cumulative Patient Ovulation Rates:
The cumulative patient ovulation rate by cycle is presented for the 102 evaluable patients with documentation of ovulatory status in at least one cycle:

Cycle 1	83%
Cycle 2	97%
Cycle 3	100%

Cumulative Patient Pregnancy Rates:
The cumulative patient pregnancy rate by cycle is presented for 86 evaluable patients who received hCG:

Cycle 1 14%
Cycle 2 21%
Cycle 3 29%

Patients Aborting* 8%
Multiple Births* 21%
Severe Hyperstimulation Syndrome** 0%

* Based upon 25 evaluable clinical pregnancies
** Based upon 108 patients and 266 cycles evaluable for safety

2. Assisted Reproductive Technologies (ART):
The safety and efficacy of Fertinex® administered subcutaneously for Assisted Reproductive Technologies (ART) were assessed in a phase III, multicenter, non-comparative, clinical trial in ovulatory infertile women undergoing stimulation of multiple follicular development for In Vitro Fertilization and Embryo Transfer (IVF/ET) after pituitary downregulation with a GnRH agonist. The initial and maximal doses of Fertinex® were 225 and 450 IU, respectively. The principal parameters recorded were serum estradiol on day of hCG administration, the number and maturity of retrieved oocytes, drug therapy and duration, and clinical pregnancy rate per initiated cycle and per retrieval. One hundred and thirty-nine patients were enrolled in the study; 135 patients were treated with Fertinex® and 122 patients were considered evaluable for efficacy. The results listed below represent mean data of 118 evaluable patients who received hCG in the 10 study centers:

Total number of oocytes recovered 8.4
Mature oocytes recovered 5.9
Maximum serum E2, day hCG (pg/mL) 1682
Total number of ampules (75 IU) 36
Treatment duration (days) 11.5
Clinical pregnancy attempt 23% (0–60)*
Clinical pregnancy transfer 27% (0–60)*
*reflects range across centers

INDICATIONS AND USAGE

Fertinex® (urofollitropin for injection, purified) and hCG given in a sequential manner are indicated for the stimulation of follicular recruitment and development and the induction of ovulation in patients with polycystic ovary syndrome and infertility, who have failed to respond or conceive following adequate clomiphene citrate therapy.
Fertinex® and hCG may also be used to stimulate the development of multiple follicles in ovulatory patients undergoing Assisted Reproductive Technologies (ART) such as in vitro fertilization.

Selection of Patients:
1. Before treatment with Fertinex® (urofollitropin for injection, purified) is instituted, a thorough gynecologic and endocrinologic evaluation must be performed. This should include an assessment of pelvic anatomy. Patients with tubal obstruction should receive Fertinex® only if enrolled in an in vitro fertilization program.
2. Primary ovarian failure should be excluded by the determination of gonadotropin levels.
3. Careful examination should be made to rule out the presence of early pregnancy.
4. Patients in late reproductive life have a greater predisposition to endometrial carcinoma as well as a higher incidence of anovulatory disorders. A thorough diagnostic examination should always be performed before starting Fertinex® therapy in such patients who demonstrate abnormal uterine bleeding or other signs of endometrial abnormalities.
5. Evaluation of the partner's fertility potential should be included in the workup.

CONTRAINDICATIONS

Fertinex® (urofollitropin for injection, purified) is contraindicated in women who exhibit:
1. High levels of FSH indicating primary ovarian failure.
2. Uncontrolled thyroid or adrenal dysfunction.
3. An organic intracranial lesion such as a pituitary tumor.
4. The presence of any cause of infertility other than anovulation, as stated in the "Indications" unless they are candidates for Assisted Reproductive Technologies.
5. Abnormal bleeding of undetermined origin (see "Selection of Patients").
6. Ovarian cysts or enlargement of undetermined origin.
7. Prior hypersensitivity to urofollitropin.

Fertinex® is also contraindicated in women who are pregnant and may cause fetal harm when administered to a pregnant woman. There are limited human data on the effects of Fertinex® when administered during pregnancy.

WARNINGS

Fertinex® (urofollitropin for injection, purified) should only be used by physicians who are thoroughly familiar with infertility problems and their management. It is a potent gonadotropic substance capable of causing mild to severe adverse reactions. Therefore, the lowest dose consistent with the expectation of good results should be used. Gonadotropin therapy requires a certain time commitment by physicians and supportive health professionals, and its use requires the availability of appropriate monitoring facilities (see "Precautions/Laboratory Tests"). Safe and effective use of Fertinex® requires monitoring of ovarian response with serum estradiol and vaginal ultrasound, on a regular basis.
Overstimulation of the Ovary During Fertinex® (urofollitropin for injection, purified) therapy: Ovarian Enlargement: Mild to moderate uncomplicated ovarian enlargement which may be accompanied by abdominal distension and/or abdominal pain occurs in approximately 20% of those treated with urofollitropin and hCG, and generally regresses without treatment within two or three weeks. Careful monitoring of ovarian response can further minimize the risk of overstimulation.
If the ovaries are abnormally enlarged on the last day of Fertinex® therapy, hCG should not be administered in this course of therapy. This will reduce the chances of development of the Ovarian Hyperstimulation Syndrome.
The Ovarian Hyperstimulation Syndrome (OHSS): OHSS is a medical event distinct from uncomplicated ovarian enlargement. Severe OHSS may progress rapidly (within 24 hours to several days) to become a serious medical event. It is characterized by an apparent dramatic increase in vascular permeability which can result in a rapid accumulation of fluid in the peritoneal cavity, thorax, and potentially, the pericardium. The early warning signs of development of OHSS are severe pelvic pain, nausea, vomiting, and weight gain. The following symptomatology has been seen with cases of OHSS: abdominal pain, abdominal distension, gastrointestinal symptoms including nausea, vomiting and diarrhea, severe ovarian enlargement, weight gain, dyspnea, and oliguria. Clinical evaluation may reveal hypovolemia, hemoconcentration, electrolyte imbalances, ascites, hemoperitoneum, pleural effusions, hydrothorax, acute pulmonary distress, and thromboembolic events (see "Pulmonary and Vascular Complications"). Transient liver function test abnormalities suggestive of hepatic dysfunction, which may be accompanied by morphologic changes on liver biopsy, have been reported in association with the Ovarian Hyperstimulation Syndrome (OHSS).
Severe OHSS occurred in approximately 6.0% of patients treated with urofollitropin therapy in the initial clinical trials, in patients treated for anovulation due to polycystic ovarian syndrome. In these studies, prospective monitoring of ovarian response using serum estradiol determination or ultrasonographic visualizations was not routinely employed. In more recent clinical trials in oligo-anovulatory and infertile women in which both estradiol and ultrasound measurements were utilized to monitor follicular development, the incidence of severe OHSS was 0.6%. During studies for in vitro fertilization, four cases of OHSS were reported following 1,586 treatment cycles (0.25%). OHSS may be more severe and more protracted if pregnancy occurs. OHSS develops rapidly; therefore, patients should be followed for at least two weeks after hCG administration. Most often, OHSS occurs after treatment has been discontinued and reaches its maximum at about seven to ten days following treatment. Usually, OHSS resolves spontaneously with the onset of menses. If there is evidence that OHSS may be developing prior to hCG administration (see "Precautions/Laboratory Tests"), the hCG must be withheld. If severe OHSS occurs, treatment must be stopped and the patient should be hospitalized.
A physician experienced in the management of this syndrome, or who is experienced in the management in fluid and electrolyte imbalances should be consulted.
Pulmonary and Vascular Complications: The following paragraph describes serious medical events reported following gonadotropin therapy.
Serious pulmonary conditions (e.g., atelectasis, acute respiratory distress syndrome) have been reported. In addition, thromboembolic events both in association with, and separate from the Ovarian Hyperstimulation Syndrome have been reported. Intravascular thrombosis and embolism can result in reduced blood flow to critical organs or the extremities. Sequelae of such events have included venous thrombophlebitis, pulmonary embolism, pulmonary infarction, cerebral vascular occlusion (stroke), and arterial occlusion resulting in loss of limb. In rare cases, pulmonary complications and/or thromboembolic events have resulted in death.
Multiple Births: Reports of multiple births have been associated with urofollitropin-hCG treatment, including triplet and quintuplet gestations. In clinical studies with Fertinex® 79.2% of the pregnancies following ovulation induction therapy resulted in single births and 20.8% in multiple births. The risk of multiple births in patients undergoing ART procedures is related to the number of embryos replaced. The patient and her partner should be advised of the potential risk of multiple births before starting treatment.

PRECAUTIONS

General: Careful attention should be given to diagnosis in candidates for Fertinex® (urofollitropin for injection, purified) therapy (see "Indications and Usage/Selection of Patients").
Information for Patients: Prior to the therapy with Fertinex®, patients should be informed of the duration of treatment and monitoring of their condition that will be required. Possible adverse reactions (see "Adverse Reactions") and the risk of multiple births should also be discussed.
Laboratory Tests: In most instances, treatment with Fertinex® results only in follicular recruitment and development. In order to effect ovulation in the absence of an endogenous LH surge, hCG must be given following the administration of Fertinex® when monitoring of the patient indicates that sufficient follicular development has occurred. This may be estimated by serum estradiol and vaginal ultrasound. The combination of ultrasound and estradiol is useful for monitoring the development of follicles, timing hCG administration, as well as for detecting ovarian enlargement and minimizing the risk of the Ovarian Hyperstimulation Syndrome and multiple gestation. It is recommended that the number of growing follicles be confirmed using ultrasonography because plasma estrogen alone does not give an indication of the size or number of follicles.
The clinical confirmation of ovulation, with the exception of pregnancy, is obtained by direct and indirect indices of progesterone production. The indices generally used are:
1. A rise in basal body temperature,
2. Increase in serum progesterone, and
3. Menstruation following the shift in basal body temperature.

When used in conjunction with indices of progesterone production, sonographic visualization of the ovaries will assist in determining if ovulation has occurred. Sonographic evidence of ovulation may include the following:
1. Fluid in the cul-de-sac,
2. Ovarian stigmata,
3. Collapsed follicle, and
4. Secretory endometrium.

Accurate interpretation of the indices of follicular development and maturation as well as the determination of ovulation require a physician who is experienced in the interpretation of these tests.
Drug Interactions: No clinically significant drug/drug or drug/food interactions have been reported during Fertinex® therapy.
Carcinogenesis and Mutagenesis: Carcinogenicity and mutagenicity studies have not been performed.
Pregnancy Category X: See "Contraindications".
Nursing Mothers: It is not known whether this drug is excreted in human milk. Because many drugs are excreted in human milk, caution should be exercised if Fertinex® is administered to a nursing woman.

ADVERSE REACTIONS

The following adverse reactions reported during urofollitropin therapy are listed in decreasing order of potential severity:
1. Pulmonary and vascular complications (see "Warnings"),
2. Ovarian Hyperstimulation Syndrome (see "Warnings"),
3. Adnexal torsion (as a complication of ovarian enlargement),
4. Mild to moderate ovarian enlargement,
5. Abdominal pain,
6. Sensitivity to urofollitropin
(Febrile reactions which may be accompanied by chills, musculoskeletal aches, joint pains, malaise, headache, and fatigue have occurred after the administration of urofollitropin. It is not clear whether or not these were pyrogenic responses or possible allergic reactions.)
7. Ovarian cysts,
8. Gastrointestinal symptoms (nausea, vomiting, diarrhea, abdominal cramps, bloating),
9. Pain, rash, swelling, and/or irritation at the site of injection,
10. Breast tenderness,
11. Headache,
12. Dermatological symptoms (dry skin, body rash, hair loss, hives)
13. Hemoperitoneum has been reported during menotropins therapy and, therefore, may also occur during urofollitropin therapy.
14. There have been infrequent reports of ovarian neoplasms, both benign and malignant, in women who have undergone multiple drug regimens for ovulation induction; however, a causal relationship has not been established.

The following medical events have been reported subsequent to pregnancies resulting from urofollitropin therapy:
1. Ectopic Pregnancy
2. Congenital abnormalities
(Three incidents of chromosomal abnormalities and four birth defects have been reported following urofollitropin-hCG or urofollitropin, Pergonal® (menotropins for injection, USP)-hCG therapy in clinical trials for stimulation prior to in vitro fertilization. The aborted pregnancies included one Trisomy 13, one Trisomy 18, and one fetus with multiple congenital anomalies (hydrocephaly, omphalocele, and meningocele). One meningocele, one external ear defect, one dislocated hip and ankle, and one dilated cardiomyopathy in presence of maternal Systemic Lupus Erythematosis were reported. None of these events were thought to be drug-related. The incidence does not exceed that found in the general population).

DRUG ABUSE AND DEPENDENCE

There have been no reports of abuse or dependence with Fertinex® (urofollitropin for injection, purified).

OVERDOSAGE

Aside from possible ovarian hyperstimulation and multiple gestations (see "Warnings"), little is known concerning the consequences of acute overdosage with Fertinex® (urofollitropin for injection, purified).

DOSAGE AND ADMINISTRATION

Dosage:
Polycystic Ovary Syndrome: The dose of Fertinex® (urofollitropin for injection, purified) to stimulate development of the follicle must be individualized for each patient.
The lowest dose consistent with the expectation of good results should be used. Over the course of treatment, doses of Fertinex® may range between 75 IU to 300 IU per day depending on the individual patient response. Fertinex® should be administered until adequate follicular development is indicated by serum estradiol and vaginal ultra-

Continued on next page

Fertinex—Cont.

sonography. A response is generally evident after 5 to 7 days. Subsequent monitoring intervals should be based on individual patient response.

It is recommended that the initial dose of the first cycle be 75 IU of Fertinex® per day, **ADMINISTERED SUBCUTANEOUSLY.** An adjustment in dose may be considered after 5 to 7 days. An additional dose adjustment may also be considered based on individual patient response. The dose should not be increased more than twice in any cycle or by more than one ampule (75 IU) per adjustment. To complete follicular development and effect ovulation in the absence of an endogenous LH surge, hCG, 5,000 U to 10,000 U, should be given 1 day after the last dose of Fertinex®. Human chorionic gonadotropin should be withheld if the serum estradiol is greater than 2,000 pg/mL. If the ovaries are abnormally enlarged or abdominal pain occurs, Fertinex® treatment should be discontinued, hCG should not be administered, and the patient should be advised not to have intercourse; this will reduce the chance of development of the Ovarian Hyperstimulation Syndrome and, should spontaneous ovulation occur, reduce the chance of multiple gestation. A follow-up visit should be conducted in the luteal phase.

The initial dose administered in the subsequent cycles should be individualized for each patient based on her response in the preceding cycle. Doses larger than 300 IU of FSH per day are not routinely recommended. As in the initial cycle, 5,000 U to 10,000 U of hCG must be given 1 day after the last dose of Fertinex® to complete follicular development and induce ovulation. The precautions described above should be followed to minimize the chance of development of the Ovarian Hyperstimulation Syndrome.

The couple should be encouraged to have intercourse daily, beginning on the day prior to the administration of hCG until ovulation becomes apparent from the indices employed for the determination of progestational activity. Care should be taken to ensure insemination. In light of the indices and parameters mentioned, it should become obvious that, unless a physician is willing to devote considerable time to these patients and be familiar with and conduct the necessary laboratory studies, he/she should not use Fertinex®.

Assisted Reproductive Technologies: As in the treatment of patients with polycystic ovary syndrome, the dose of Fertinex® to stimulate development of the follicle must be individualized for each patient. For Assisted Reproductive Technologies, therapy with Fertinex® should be initiated in the early follicular phase (cycle day 2 or 3) at a dose of 150 IU per day, until sufficient follicular development is attained. In most cases, therapy should not exceed ten days.

Administration: Dissolve the contents of one or more ampules of Fertinex® in one-half to one mL of sterile saline (concentration should not exceed 225 IU/0.5 mL) and **ADMINISTER SUBCUTANEOUSLY** immediately. Any unused reconstituted material should be discarded.

Parenteral drug products should be inspected visually, for particulate matter and discoloration prior to administration, whenever solution and container permit.

HOW SUPPLIED

Fertinex® (urofollitropin for injection, purified) is supplied in a sterile, lyophilized form as a white to off-white powder or pellet in ampules containing 75 IU or 150 IU FSH activity. The following package combinations are available:

— 1 ampule 75 IU Fertinex® and 1 ampule 2 mL Sodium Chloride Injection (USP), NDC 44087-7075-1
— 1 ampule 150 IU Fertinex® and 1 ampule 2 mL Sodium Chloride Injection (USP), NDC 44087-7150-1
— 10 ampules 75 IU Fertinex® and 10 ampules 2 mL Sodium Chloride Injection (USP), NDC 44087-7075-3
— 100 ampules 75 IU Fertinex® and 100 ampules 2 mL Sodium Chloride Injection (USP), NDC 44087-7075-4

Lyophilized powder may be stored refrigerated or at room temperature (3°–25°C/37°–77°F). Protect from light. Use immediately after reconstitution. Discard unused material.

Rx Only.

Manufactured for: **SERONO LABORATORIES, INC,**
Randolph, MA 02368 U.S.A.
by: Laboratoires Serono SA, Aubonne, Switzerland

GEREF® ℞
[ge ref]
(sermorelin acetate for injection)
For subcutaneous injection only

DESCRIPTION

Sermorelin acetate is the acetate salt of an amidated synthetic 29-amino acid peptide (GRF 1-29 NH_2) that corresponds to the amino-terminal segment of the naturally occurring human growth hormone-releasing hormone (GHRH or GRF) consisting of 44 amino acid residues. The structural formula for sermorelin acetate is:

Tyr-Ala-Asp-Ala-Ile-Phe-Thr-Asn-Ser-Tyr-
Arg-Lys-Val-Leu-Gly-Gln-Leu-Ser-Ala-Arg-
Lys-Leu-Leu-Gln-Asp-Ile-Met-Ser-Arg-$NH_2 \cdot (C_2H_4O_2)_{3\text{-}6}$

The free base of sermorelin has the empirical formula $C_{149}H_{246}N_{44}O_{42}S$ and a molecular weight of 3,358 daltons.

Geref® is a sterile, non-pyrogenic, lyophilized powder intended for subcutaneous injection after reconstitution with Sodium Chloride Injection, USP. The reconstituted solution has a pH of 5.0 to 5.5.

Geref® is available in vials. The quantitative composition per vial is:

0.5 mg vial: Each vial contains 0.5 mg sermorelin (as the acetate) and 5 mg mannitol. The pH is adjusted with dibasic sodium phosphate and monobasic sodium phosphate buffer.

1.0 mg vial: Each vial contains 1.0 mg sermorelin (as the acetate) and 5 mg mannitol. The pH is adjusted with dibasic sodium phosphate and monobasic sodium phosphate buffer.

CLINICAL PHARMACOLOGY

Geref® (sermorelin acetate for injection) increases plasma growth hormone (GH) concentration by stimulating the pituitary gland to release GH. Geref® is similar to the native hormone (GRF [1-44]-NH_2) in its ability to stimulate GH secretion in humans.

Pharmacokinetics

Absorption

In subcutaneous administration of 2 mg sermorelin to 12 normal volunteers, peak concentrations of sermorelin were reached in 5–20 minutes. The mean absolute bioavailability after SC administration is about 6%.

Distribution

After intravenous administration of 0.25–1.0 mg Geref® to 12 normal volunteers, the mean volume of distribution ranged between 23.7–25.8 liters.

Metabolism

No metabolism studies have been performed in humans.

Elimination

Sermorelin is rapidly cleared from the circulation, with clearance values in adults ranging between 2.4–2.8 L/min. The halflife of Geref® is short, 11–12 minutes after either intravenous or subcutaneous administration.

Special Populations

Gender/Age: No gender data are available in pediatric patients. In normal adults, the clearance of sermorelin in men and women is similar. No age data are available.

Renal/Hepatic Insufficiency: No data are available.

CLINICAL STUDIES

In one multicenter, open-label clinical study in prepubertal children with idiopathic growth hormone deficiency, 110 children were administered Geref® 0.03 mg (30 mcg) per kg per day by subcutaneous injection. Fifty-six patients were evaluable for efficacy at 12 months. Fifty-four patients were considered unevaluable: 24 for eligibility criteria violations; 10 for protocol discontinuation criteria and 20 for failing to satisfy the efficacy criteria at 6 months for continuing in the study. Fifty-six of all 110 patients and 47 of 56 patients in the evaluable patient subset who initiated and continued with Geref® therapy up to 12 months demonstrated an increase of 2 cm/year or more over the baseline height velocity (HV). For the 56 patients in the evaluable patient subset, mean height velocity (± SD) increased from 4.1 ± 1.0 cm/year at baseline to 8.0 ± 1.5 cm/year at 6 months and 7.2 ± 1.3 cm/year at 12 months, an increase of 3.1 ± 1.4 cm/year (p = 0.0001). Mean height standard deviation score (± SD) increased from −3.71 ± 0.92 at baseline to −3.21 ± 0.91 at 12 months, an increase of 0.50 ± 0.23 over the 12 month period (p = 0.0001). Mean changes in bone age at 12 months were proportional to gains in height (1.04 ± 0.58, ΔBA/ΔHA, n=42).

INDICATIONS AND USAGE

Geref® (sermorelin acetate for injection) is indicated for the treatment of idiopathic growth hormone deficiency in children with growth failure. Most of these short, slowly growing children retain pituitary responsiveness to growth hormone releasing hormone.

Selection of Patients and Evaluation of Growth

All children should be pre-pubescent and treatment should be initiated at a bone age of ≤ 7.5 year for females, and ≤ 8 years for males. Prior to initiation of treatment, a growth hormone (GH) stimulation test with Geref® should be performed in all children. Children who do not adequately respond (i.e., peak GH level ≤ 2 ng/mL) should be excluded from Geref® therapy. The relative growth hormone response to the stimulation test with Geref® is not predictive of the growth response to Geref® therapy. Clinical results are better in children with delayed bone age and in whom treatment is initiated as early as possible in the prepubertal period. Height should be assessed at least every six months during treatment. During Geref® therapy, failure to maintain a pattern of growth consistent with a child's age and stage of development requires investigation. Children should be treated with Geref® for an initial period of 6 months and treatment with growth hormone should be initiated for those children with a poor or waning response to Geref®.

CONTRAINDICATIONS

Geref® (sermorelin acetate for injection) should not be used by patients with a known sensitivity to sermorelin or any of the excipients.

WARNINGS

Following reconstitution of Geref® (sermorelin acetate for injection) with the diluent provided, the solution should be administered immediately. Any unused solution should be discarded.

PRECAUTIONS

General: Geref® (sermorelin acetate for injection) therapy should be carried out under the regular guidance of a physician who is experienced in the diagnosis and management of growth disorders.

The growth response of children treated with Geref® should be evaluated on a periodic basis and children with a poor or waning response should be considered for treatment with growth hormone. The effect of Geref® therapy beyond one year and on final adult height remains to be determined.

In clinical studies, the incidence of hypothyroidism during Geref® therapy was 6.5%. In the largest clinical study, 8 of 110 enrolled patients were on thyroid replacement therapy prior to Geref® therapy and an additional 5 after initiating therapy. Untreated hypothyroidism can jeopardize the response to Geref®. Therefore, thyroid hormone determinations should be performed before the initiation and throughout the duration of Geref® therapy. Thyroid hormone replacement therapy should be initiated when indicated.

Bone age should be monitored periodically during Geref® administration, especially in patients who are pubertal and/or receiving concomitant thyroid replacement therapy. Under these circumstances, epiphyseal maturation may progress rapidly.

Patients with growth hormone deficiency secondary to an intracranial lesion were not studied in clinical trials. It is not recommended that such patients be treated with Geref®.

As with the administration of any peptide, local or systemic allergic reactions may occur. Parents/Patients should be informed that such reactions are possible and that prompt medical attention should be sought if allergic reactions occur.

Laboratory Tests: Serum levels of inorganic phosphorus, alkaline phosphatase, GH and IGF-1 may increase with Geref® therapy.

Drug Interaction: Concomitant glucocorticoid therapy may inhibit the response to Geref®. There was no evidence in the controlled studies of Geref®'s interaction with drugs commonly used in the treatment of routine pediatric problems/illnesses. However, formal drug interactions studies have not been conducted.

Carcinogenesis, Mutagenesis, Impairment of Fertility: Long-term animal studies for carcinogenicity and impairment of fertility have not been performed with Geref®. There has been no evidence from studies to date of Geref®-induced genetic toxicity.

Pregnancy: Pregnancy Category C. During teratology studies Geref® produced minor variations in fetuses of rats and rabbits when given at a dose of 0.5 mg/kg/day. This dose is approximately 3 and 6 times the daily human dose calculated on a body surface area (mg/m^2) basis, for rats and rabbits, respectively. There are no adequate and well controlled studies in pregnant women. Geref® should be used during pregnancy only if the potential benefit justifies the potential risk to the fetus.

Nursing Women: It is not known whether Geref® is excreted in human milk. Because many drugs are excreted in human milk, cautions should be exercised when Geref® is administered to a nursing women.

Information For Patients: Patients being treated with Geref® and/or their parents should be informed of the potential benefits and risks associated with treatment. If home use is determined to be desirable by the physician, instructions on appropriate use should be given, including a review of the contents of the Patient Information Insert. This information is intended to aid in the safe and effective administration of the medication. It is not a disclosure of all possible adverse or intended effects.

If home use is prescribed, a puncture resistant container for the disposal of used syringes and needles should be recommended to the patient. Patients and/or parents should be thoroughly instructed in the importance of proper disposal and cautioned against any reuse of needles and syringes (see Patient Information Insert).

Geriatric Use: The safety and effectiveness of Geref® has not been evaluated in clinical studies in patients 65 years old and over. Elderly patients may be more sensitive to the action of Geref®, and may be more prone to develop adverse reactions.

ADVERSE REACTIONS

A large proportion of patients develop anti-GRF antibodies at least once during treatment with Geref® (sermorelin acetate for injection). The significance of these antibodies is not clear and often a positive test at one growth assessment will become negative by the next assessment. The presence of antibodies does not appear to affect growth or appear to be related to a specific adverse reaction profile. No generalized allergic reactions to Geref® have been reported.

The most common treatment-related adverse event (occurring in about 1 patient in 6) is local injection reaction characterized by pain, swelling or redness. Of 350 patients exposed to Geref® in clinical trials, three discontinued therapy due to injection reactions. Other treatment-related adverse events had individual occurrence rates of less than 1% and include: headache, flushing, dysphagia, dizziness, hyperactivity, somnolence and urticaria.

When administered intravenously for diagnostic use, the following adverse reactions have been noted: flushing of the face, injection site pain, redness and/or swelling, nausea, headache, vomiting, dysgeusia, pallor and tightness in the chest.

DRUG ABUSE AND DEPENDENCE

The clinical pharmacology suggests that Geref® is very unlikely to be associated with drug abuse or dependence and there have been no reports of this from clinical trials.

OVERDOSAGE

The recommended dosage of Geref® (sermorelin acetate for injection) should not be exceeded.

DOSAGE AND ADMINISTRATION

A dosage of 0.03 mg (30 mcg) per kg of body weight once daily at bedtime by subcutaneous injection is recommended. It is also recommended that subcutaneous injection sites be periodically rotated.

Treatment with Geref® should be discontinued when the epiphyses are fused. Patients who fail to respond adequately while on Geref® therapy should be evaluated to determine the cause of unresponsiveness.

Height should be assessed at least every six months during treatment. During Geref® therapy, care shoud be taken to ensure that the child continues to grow at a rate consistent with the child's age and stage of development, and treatment with Geref® should be reevaluated if the response is inadequate. Treatment with growth hormone should be considered for children with a poor or waning response to Geref®.

To prevent possible contamination, wipe the rubber vial stopper with an antiseptic solution before puncturing it with the needle. It is recommended that Geref® be administered using sterile, disposable syringes and needles. The syringes should be of small enough volume that the prescribed dose can be drawn from the vial with reasonable accuracy.

After determining the appropriate patient dose, reconstitute each vial of Geref® with 0.5–1.0 mL of Sodium Chloride Injection, USP.

To reconstitute Geref®, inject the diluent into the vial of Geref® aiming the liquid against the glass vial wall. Swirl the vial with a GENTLE rotary motion until contents are dissolved completely. Do not administer Geref® if particles are visible in the reconstituted solution or if the reconstituted solution is cloudy.

HOW SUPPLIED

Before Reconstitution—Vials of Geref® (sermorelin acetate for injection) should be stored refrigerated (2°–8°C/36°–46°F). Expiration dates are stated on the labels.

After Reconstitution—When reconstituted with Sodium Chloride Injection, USP, the reconstituted solution should be administered immediately. Any unused solution should be discarded.

Geref® (sermorelin acetate for injection) is a sterile, nonpyrogenic, lyophilized powder supplied in packages containing:

1 vial 0.5 mg Geref® and 1 vial 2 mL Sodium Chloride Injection, USP NDC 44087-4005-1

1 vial 1.0 mg Geref® and 1 vial 2 mL Sodium Chloride Injection, USP NDC 44087-4010-1

Rx Only

Product information as of August 2000

Manufactured for:
Serono Laboratories, Inc.
Randolph, MA 02368
® Registered trademark of Serono Laboratories, Inc.

GONAL-F® ℞

[gŏn al-ĕf]

(follitropin alfa for injection)
For subcutaneous injection

DESCRIPTION

Gonal-F® (follitropin alfa for injection) is a human follicle stimulating hormone (FSH) preparation of recombinant DNA origin, which consists of two non-covalently linked, non-identical glycoproteins designated as the α- and β-subunits. The α- and β-subunits have 92 and 111 amino acids, respectively, and their primary and tertiary structure are indistinguishable from those of human follicle stimulating hormone. Recombinant FSH production occurs in genetically modified Chinese Hamster Ovary (CHO) cells cultured in bioreactors. Purification by immunochromatography using an antibody specifically binding FSH results in a highly purified preparation with a consistent FSH isoform profile, and a high specific activity. The biological activity of follitropin alfa is determined by measuring the increase in ovary weight in female rats. The in vivo biological activity of follitropin alfa has been calibrated against the second International Reference Preparation for Human Menopausal Gonadotrophins established in September 1964 by the Expert Committee on Biological Standards of the World Health Organization. Gonal-F® contains no luteinizing hormone (LH) activity. Based on available data derived from physico-chemical tests and bioassays, follitropin alfa and follitropin beta, another recombinant follicle stimulating hormone product, are indistinguishable.

Gonal-F® is a sterile, lyophilized powder intended for subcutaneous injection after reconstitution with Sterile Water for Injection, USP. Each ampule of Gonal-F® contains either 37.5 IU, 75 IU, or 150 IU recombinant FSH, 30 mg sucrose, 1.11 mg dibasic sodium phosphate and 0.45 mg monobasic sodium phosphate monohydrate. O-phosphoric acid and/or sodium hydroxide may be used prior to lyophilization for pH adjustment. Under current storage conditions, Gonal-F® may contain up to 15% of oxidized follitropin alfa.

Therapeutic Class: Infertility

Table 1: Pharmacokinetic parameters (mean ± SD) of FSH following administration of Gonal-F®

Population	Female: Healthy female volunteers			IVF/ET patients	Male: Healthy Male Volunteers	
Dose (IU)	Single Dose IM (150)	Single Dose SC (150)	Multiple Dose SC (7× 150)	Multiple Dose SC (5×225)*	Single Dose SC (225 IU)	Multiple Dose SC (7× 225 IU)
AUC - (IU-hr/L)	206 ± 66	176 ± 87	187 ± 61#	—	220 ± 109	186 ±23#
C_{max} (IU/L)	3 ± 1	3 ± 1	9 ± 3	—	2.5 ± 0.8	8.3 ± 0.9
t_{max} (hr)	25 ± 10	16 ± 10	8 ± 6	—	20 ± 14	10.7 ± 6.7
$t_{1/2}$ terminal (hr)	50 ± 27	24 ± 11	24 ± 8	32**	41 ± 14	32 ± 4
CL/F (L/hr)	—	—	—	0.7 ± 0.2	0.86 ± 0.48	0.90 ± 0.12
V_{ss}/F (L)	—	—	—	10 ± 3	—	—
F (%)	76 ± 30	66 ± 39	—	—	—	—

Abbreviations are: IVF/ET: *in vitro* fertilization/embryo transfer; C_{max}: peak concentration (above baseline); t_{max}time of C_{max}; CL/F: apparent clearance; V_{ss}/F: apparent steady-state volume of distribution; $t_{1/2}$: absorption half-life; F: bioavailability compared to IV

\# Steady-state $AUC_{144–168}$ (After the 7th daily SC dose)

* First five days of fixed regimen followed by adjustment of the dose depending on response

** increases with body mass index

CLINICAL PHARMACOLOGY

Gonal-F® (follitropin alfa for injection) stimulates ovarian follicular growth in women who do not have primary ovarian failure. FSH, the active component of Gonal-F® is the primary hormone responsible for follicular recruitment and development. In order to effect final maturation of the follicle and ovulation in the absence of an endogenous LH surge, human chorionic gonadotropin (hCG) must be given following the administration of Gonal-F® when monitoring of the patient indicates that sufficient follicular development has occurred. There is interpatient variability in response to FSH administration. The physico-chemical, immunological, and biological activities of recombinant FSH are comparable to those of pituitary and human menopausal urine-derived FSH. Gonal-F® (follitropin alfa for injection), when administered with hCG, stimulates spermatogenesis in men with hypogonadotropic hypogonadism. FSH, the active component of Gonal-F®, is the primary hormone responsible for spermatogenesis.

Pharmacokinetics

Single dose pharmacokinetics of r-hFSH were determined following intravenous, subcutaneous and intramuscular administration of 150 IU Gonal-F® to 12 healthy, down-regulated female volunteers. Steady-state pharmacokinetics were also determined in 12 healthy down-regulated female volunteers who were administered a single daily dose of 150 IU for seven days. These pharmacokinetics were confirmed in pituitary down-regulated women undergoing *in vitro* fertilization and embryo transfer (IVF/ET), treated with FSH doses of up to 450 IU per day. Additionally, single dose pharmacokinetics of r-hFSH were determined following subcutaneous administration of 225 IU Gonal-F® to 12 healthy adult male volunteers in a cross-over design. Steady state pharmacokinetics were also determined in 6 healthy adult male volunteers who were administered a single daily dose of 225 IU Gonal-F® for 7 days. No significant difference in pharmacokinetics is expected in males versus females when administered Gonal-F® subcutaneously. The pharmacokinetics parameters from these studies are included in Table 1.

[See table above]

Absorption

The absorption rate of Gonal-F® following subcutaneous or intramuscular administration was found to be slower than the elimination rate. Hence the pharmacokinetics of Gonal-F® are absorption rate-limited.

Distribution

Human tissue or organ distribution of FSH has not been determined for Gonal-F®.

After intravenous administration to pituitary down-regulated, healthy female volunteers, the serum profile of FSH appears to be described by a two compartment open model with a distribution half-life of about 2–2.5 hours. Steady-state serum levels were reached after 4 to 5 days of daily administration.

Metabolism/Excretion

FSH metabolism following administration of Gonal-F® has not been studied in humans. Total clearance after IV administration in healthy females was 0.6 L/hr; mean residence time was 17–20 hours. FSH renal clearance was 0.07 L/hr after intravenous administration representing approximately 1/8 of total clearance.

Pharmacodynamics

Following daily subcutaneous administration of 150 IU of Gonal-F® for 7 days in healthy female volunteers, serum inhibin and estradiol, and total follicular volume responded as a function of time, with pronounced inter-individual variability. Pharmacodynamic effect lagged behind FSH serum concentration. Of the three pharmacodynamic parameters, serum inhibin levels responded with the least delay and declined rapidly after discontinuation of Gonal-F®. Follicular growth was most delayed and continued even after discontinuation of Gonal-F® administration, and after serum FSH levels had declined. Maximum follicular volume was better correlated with either inhibin or estradiol peak levels than with FSH concentration. Inhibin rise was an early index of follicular development. In healthy male volunteers, despite high inter-individual variation and the absence of down-regulation, daily administration of 225 IU Gonal-F® was shown to increase the levels of inhibin to reach a plateau during the whole administration period and then return to baseline.

Population pharmacokinetics and pharmacodynamics

To establish the pharmacokinetics and pharmacodynamics of FSH in a target population, measurements performed during a clinical study of *in vitro* fertilization/embryo transfer were used in conjunction with pharmacokinetic data from studies in healthy volunteers. The apparent clearance was comparable to that in healthy volunteers. The absorption rate was found to be influenced by the body mass index (BMI), suggesting that the higher the BMI, the lower the rate of absorption. However, FSH serum levels following fixed (during the first five days) and then adjusted doses of Gonal-F® were found to be poor predictors of follicular growth rate. High pre-treatment serum FSH levels may predict lower follicular growth rates.

Special populations: Safety, efficacy, and pharmacokinetics of Gonal-F® in patients with renal or hepatic insufficiency have not been established.

Drug-Drug Interactions: No drug/drug interaction studies have been conducted (see PRECAUTIONS).

Clinical Studies:

Women:

The safety and efficacy of Gonal-F® have been examined in four clinical studies, two studies for ovulation induction and two studies for assisted reproductive technologies (ART). In these comparative studies, there were no clinically significant differences between treatment groups in study outcomes.

1. Ovulation Induction:

The safety and efficacy of Gonal-F® administered subcutaneously vs. urofollitropin administered intramuscularly were assessed in a phase III, open-label, randomized, comparative, multinational, multicenter study in oligo-anovulatory infertile women who failed to ovulate or conceive following adequate clomiphene citrate therapy (Study 5642). The primary efficacy parameter was the ovulation rate. Two hundred and twenty-two patients entered into the first cycle of treatment, of whom 110 received Gonal-F® and 112 received urofollitropin. Ovulation rates were similar between Gonal-F® and urofollitropin treatment groups. The study results for the 222 patients who received treatment in at least one cycle are summarized in table 2.

Table 2: Cumulative Patient Ovulation and Clinical Pregnancy Rates by Treatment Group in Ovulation Induction

Study 5642	Gonal-F® (n = 110)	urofolitropin (n = 112)
Cumulative Ovulation Rate		
cycle 1	64%	59%
cycle 2	78%	82%
cycle 3	84%	91%
Cumulative Clinical Pregnancy* Rate		
cycle 1	21%	21%
cycle 2	28%	38%
cycle 3	35%	46%

* A clinical pregnancy was defined as a pregnancy during which a fetal sac (with or without heart activity) was visualized by ultrasound on day 34–36 after hCG administration.

For the 90 patients who had a clinical pregnancy (39 in Gonal-F® group; 51 in urofollitropin group), the outcome of the pregnancy was:

Continued on next page

Gonal-F—Cont.

Table 3: Pregnancy Outcome by Treatment Group in Ovulation Induction

Study 5642	Gonal-F® (n = 39)	urofolitropin (n = 51)
Pregnancies not reaching term	20.5%	13.7%
Single births	74.4%	74.5%
Multiple births	5.1%	11.8%

A second randomized, comparative, open-label, multicenter study was conducted in 23 U.S. centers (Study 5727). The primary efficacy parameter was ovulation rate. Ovulation rates were similar between Gonal-F® and urofollitropin treatment groups. Two hundred and thirty-two patients with oligo-anovulatory infertility received treatment with up to three cycles of Gonal-F® administered subcutaneously (118 patients) or urofollitropin administered intramuscularly (114 patients).

The cumulative patient ovulation rate and clinical pregnancy rates by cycle are presented for the 232 patients who received treatment in at least one cycle.

Table 4: Cumulative Patient Ovulation and Clinical Pregnancy Rates by Treatment Group in Ovulation Induction

Study 5727	Gonal-F® (n = 118)	urofolitropin (n = 114)
Cumulative Ovulation Rate		
cycle 1	58%	68%
cycle 2	72%	86%
cycle 3	81%	93%
Cumulative Clinical Pregnancy* Rate		
cycle 1	13%	14%
cycle 2	25%	25%
cycle 3	37%	36%

* A clinical pregnancy was defined as a pregnancy during which a fetal sac (with or without heart activity) was visualized by ultrasound on day 34–36 after hCG administration.

For the 85 patients who had a clinical pregnancy (44 in Gonal-F® group: 41 in urofollitropin group), the outcome of the pregnancy is shown in Table 5.

Table 5: Pregnancy Outcome by Treatment Group in Ovulation Induction

Study 5727	Gonal-F® (n = 44)	urofolitropin (n = 41)
Pregnancies not reaching term	22.7%	22.0%
Single births	63.6%	65.9%
Multiple births	13.7%	12.2%

2. Assisted Reproductive Technologies (ART):
The safety and efficacy of Gonal-F® administered subcutaneously vs. urofollitropin administered intramuscularly were assessed in a phase III, open-label, randomized, comparative, multinational, multicenter study in ovulatory, infertile women undergoing stimulation of multiple follicles for In Vitro Fertilization and Embryo Transfer (IVF/ET) after pituitary down-regulation with a GnRH agonist (Study 5503). The purpose of the study was to demonstrate that Gonal-F®, administered subcutaneously, was clinically not different in terms of safety and efficacy from urofollitropin, administered intramuscularly. The initial and maximal doses of Gonal-F® were 225 and 450 IU, respectively. The primary efficacy parameter was the number of mature preovulatory follicles on the day of hCG administration. One hundred and twenty-three patients were randomized and received either Gonal-F® (60 patients) or urofollitropin (63 patients).

The results summarized in Table 6 are mean data with Gonal-F® and urofollitropin administered to ovulatory infertile women undergoing multiple follicular development for IVF/ET.

Table 6: Treatment Outcomes by Treatment Group in ART

Study 5503	Gonal-F® (n = 60)	urofolitropin (n = 63)
Mean number of follicles ≥ 14 mm in diameter on day of hCG	7.8	9.2
Mean number of oocytes recovered per patient	9.3	10.7
Mean Serum E2 (pg/mL) on day of hCG	1576	2193
Mean treatment duration in days (range)	9.9 (5–20)	9.4 (5–14)
Clinical pregnancy* rate per attempt	20%	16%
Clinical pregnancy* rate per embryo transfer	24%	19%

* A clinical pregnancy was defined as a pregnancy during which a fetal sac (with or without heart activity) was visualized by ultrasound on day 34–36 after hCG administration.

For the 22 patients who had a clinical pregnancy (12 in Gonal-F® group; 10 in urofollitropin group), the outcome of the pregnancy is shown in Table 7.

Table 7: Pregnancy Outcome by Treatment Group in ART

Study 5503	Gonal-F® (n = 12)	urofolitropin (n = 10)
Pregnancies not reaching term	25.0%	20.0%
Single births	41.7%	50.0%
Multiple births	33.3%	30.0%

A second randomized, comparative, open-label, multicenter study was conducted in 7 U.S. centers (Study 5533). One hundred and fourteen patients with ovulatory infertility undergoing IVF/ET were randomized and received either Gonal-F® by subcutaneous administration (56 patients) or urofollitropin by intramuscular administration (58 patients) following pituitary down-regulation with a GnRH agonist. The primary efficacy parameter was the number of mature pre-ovulatory follicles on the day of hCG administration. Results are summarized in table 8.

Table 8: Treatment Outcomes by Treatment Group in ART

Study 5533	Gonal-F® (n = 56)	urofolitropin (n = 58)
Mean number of follicles ≥ 14 mm in diamter on day of hCG	7.2	8.3
Mean number of oocytes recovered per patient	9.3	12.3
Mean Serum E2 (pg/mL) on day of hCG	1236	1513
Mean treatment duration in days (range)	10.0 (5–15)	9.0 (5–12)
Clinical pregnancy* rate per attempt	21%	22%
Clinical pregnancy* rate per embryo transfer	26%	25%

* A clinical pregnancy was defined as a pregnancy during which a fetal sac (with or without heart activity) was visualized by ultrasound on day 34–36 after hCG administration.

For the 25 patients who had a clinical pregnancy (12 in Gonal-F® group; 13 in urofollitropin group), the outcome of the pregnancy is shown in Table 9.

Table 9: Pregnancy Outcome by Treatment Group in ART

Study 5533	Gonal-F® (n = 12)	urofolitropin (n = 13)
Pregnancies not reaching term	33.3%	30.8%
Single births	41.7%	38.5%
Multiple births	25.0%	30.8%

Men:
The safety and efficacy of Gonal-F® administered concomitantly with hCG have been examined in three open-label clinical studies for induction of spermatogenesis in men with primary and secondary hypogonadotropic hypogonadism.

The three multicenter studies involved three to six months of pretreatment with chorionic gonadotropin for injection (Profasi®) to normalize serum testosterone levels, followed by 18 months of treatment with Gonal-F® and hCG. The objective of each study was induction of spermatogenesis (a sperm density of ≥ 1.5 × 10^6/mL).

Study 5844 enrolled 32 patients in six centers in the United Kingdom, France, and Germany. The second trial, Study 6410, was conducted in Australia and enrolled 10 patients in two centers. Study 6793, conducted in 7 centers in the United States, was planned to enroll 32 patients. The interim data for the U.S. study includes 30 of the planned 32 patients. For all 3 studies, a total of 72 patients were enrolled and received hCG and 56 of those patients entered the Gonal-F® treatment phase of the trials.

The populations enrolled in the three studies were similar: Study 5844 studied a naïve population who had had no prior treatment with gonadotropins; mean age was 25.9 (range 16 to 48) years, mean (± SD) testis volume was 2.0 ± 1.2 mL, and 12 of the 32 patients (37.5%) were anosmic. Thirty-one of the patients were Caucasian and one was Asian. In Study 6410, mean age was 36 (range 26 to 48 years), 6 and 1 of the 10 patients had previously been treated with gonadotropins and GnRH, respectively; mean testis volume was 4.5 ± 2.9 mL; and 2 of the 10 patients (20%) were anosmic. Seven patients were Caucasian and three were Asian. In the 30 patients reported in the interim analysis of Study 6793, the mean age was 30.1 (range 22 to 44) years; 4 and 3 of the 30 patients had been treated with gonadotropins and GnRH, respectively, in the past; mean testis volume was 4.4 ± 1.3 mL; and 10 of the 30 patients (33.3%) were anosmic. Twenty-five of the patients were Caucasian, three were Asian, and one each of Moroccan and Indian ancestry.

The primary efficacy endpoint of all three studies was the achievement of a sperm density ≥ 1.5 × 10^6/mL. The study results for the patients treated with Gonal-F® and hCG are summarized in Table 10.

[See table 10 below]

The time to achievement of the primary efficacy endpoint is summarized in Table 11.

[See table 11 at top of next page]

Of the 56 patients who received Gonal-F® in Studies 5844, 6410, and 6793, 12 pregnancies were achieved in 10 partners of the 37 patients who were seeking pregnancy and who currently had a partner during the studies. Thus, pregnancy (clinical and chemical) was documented to have been achieved by 27% of the patients' partners seeking pregnancy during the exposure period to Gonal-F® in the 3 trials. Eight pregnancies continued to term, and 8 healthy babies were born to 7 couples as a result of those studies.

[See table 12 at top of next page]

INDICATIONS AND USAGE

Women:
Gonal-F® (follitropin alfa for injection) is indicated for the induction of ovulation and pregnancy in anovulatory infertile patients in whom the cause of infertility is functional and not due to primary ovarian failure. Gonal-F® is also indicated for the development of multiple follicles in the ovulatory patient participating in an Assisted Reproductive Technology (ART) program.

Selection of Patients:

1. Before treatment with Gonal-F® is instituted, a thorough gynecologic and endocrinologic evaluation must be performed. This should include an assessment of pelvic anatomy. Patients with tubal obstruction should receive Gonal-F® only if enrolled in an *in vitro* fertilization program.
2. Primary ovarian failure should be excluded by the determination of gonadotropin levels.
3. Appropriate evaluation should be performed to exclude pregnancy.
4. Patients in later reproductive life have a greater predisposition to endometrial carcinoma as well as a higher incidence of anovulatory disorders. A thorough diagnostic evaluation should always be performed in patients who demonstrate abnormal uterine bleeding or other signs of endometrial abnormalities before starting Gonal-F® therapy.
5. Evaluation of the partner's fertility potential should be included in the initial evaluation.

Men:
Gonal-F® (follitropin alfa for injection) is indicated for the induction of spermatogenesis in men with primary and secondary hypogonadotropic hypogonadism in whom the cause of infertility is not due to primary testicular failure.

Selection of Patients

1. Before treatment with Gonal-F® is instituted for azoospermia, a thorough medical and endocrinologic evaluation must be performed.
2. Hypogonadotropic hypogonadism should be confirmed, and primary testicular failure should be excluded by the determination of gonadotropin levels.
3. Prior to Gonal-F® therapy for azoospermia in patients with hypogonadotropic hypogonadism, serum testosterone levels should be normalized.

Table 10: Number of Men Receiving Gonal-F® Who Achieved a Sperm Density ≥ 1.5 × 10^6/mL

	Study 5844 (n=26)	Study 6410 (n=8)	Study 6793 (n=22)*
Sperm Concentration ≥ 1.5×10^6/mL			
Yes	12 (46.2%)	5 (62.5%)	14 (63.6%)
No	14 (53.8%)	3 (37.5%)	8 (36.4%)
95% Confidence Interval	(26.6%–66.6%)	(24.5%–91.5%)	(40.7%–82.8%)

* Interim data

CONTRAINDICATIONS

Gonal-F® (follitropin alfa for injection) is contraindicated in women and men who exhibit:

1. Prior hypersensitivity to recombinant FSH preparations or one of their excipients.
2. High levels of FSH indicating primary gonadal failure.
3. Uncontrolled thyroid or adrenal dysfunction.
4. Sex hormone dependent tumors of the reproductive tract and accessory organs.
5. An organic intracranial lesion such as a pituitary tumor.

And in women who exhibit:

6. Abnormal uterine bleeding of undetermined origin (see "Selection of Patients").
7. Ovarian cyst or enlargement of undetermined origin (see "Selection of Patients").
8. Pregnancy.

WARNINGS

Gonal-F® (follitropin alfa for injection) should only be used by physicians who are thoroughly familiar with infertility problems and their management.

Gonal-F® is a potent gonadotropic substance capable of causing Ovarian Hyperstimulation Syndrome (OHSS) in women with or without pulmonary or vascular complications. Gonadotropin therapy requires a certain time commitment by physicians and supportive health professionals, and requires the availability of appropriate monitoring facilities (see "PRECAUTIONS/Laboratory Tests"). Safe and effective use of Gonal-F® in women requires monitoring of ovarian response with serum estradiol and vaginal ultrasound on a regular basis. The lowest effective dose should be used.

Overstimulation of the Ovary During FSH Therapy:

Ovarian Enlargement: Mild to moderate uncomplicated ovarian enlargement which may be accompanied by abdominal distention and/or abdominal pain occurs in approximately 20% of those treated with urofollitropin and hCG, and generally regresses without treatment within two or three weeks. Careful monitoring of ovarian response can further minimize the risk of overstimulation.

If the ovaries are abnormally enlarged on the last day of Gonal-F® therapy, hCG should not be administered in this course of therapy. This will reduce the chances of development of Ovarian Hyperstimulation Syndrome.

Ovarian Hyperstimulation Syndrome (OHSS): OHSS is a medical event distinct from uncomplicated ovarian enlargement. Severe OHSS may progress rapidly (within 24 hours to several days) to become a serious medical event. It is characterized by an apparent dramatic increase in vascular permeability which can result in a rapid accumulation of fluid in the peritoneal cavity, thorax, and potentially, the pericardium. The early warning signs of development of OHSS are severe pelvic pain, nausea, vomiting, and weight gain. The following symptomatology has been seen with cases of OHSS: abdominal pain, abdominal distention, gastrointestinal symptoms including nausea, vomiting and diarrhea, severe ovarian enlargement, weight gain, dyspnea, and oliguria. Clinical evaluation may reveal hypovolemia, hemoconcentration, electrolyte imbalances, ascites, hemoperitoneum, pleural effusions, hydrothorax, acute pulmonary distress, and thromboembolic events (see "Pulmonary and Vascular Complications"). Transient liver function test abnormalities suggestive of hepatic dysfunction, which may be accompanied by morphologic changes on liver biopsy, have been reported in association with Ovarian Hyperstimulation Syndrome (OHSS).

OHSS occurred in 9 of 228 (3.9%) Gonal-F® treated women during ovulation induction clinical trials and of this number, 1 of 228 (0.4%) was classified as severe. In ART clinical studies, OHSS occurred in 0 of 116 (0.0%) Gonal-F® treated women. OHSS may be more severe and more protracted if pregnancy occurs. OHSS develops rapidly: therefore, patients should be followed for at least two weeks after hCG administration. Most often, OHSS occurs after treatment has been discontinued and reaches its maximum at about seven to ten days following treatment. Usually, OHSS resolves spontaneously with the onset of menses. If there is evidence that OHSS may be developing prior to hCG administration (see "PRECAUTIONS/Laboratory Tests"), the hCG must be withheld.

If severe OHSS occurs, treatment must be stopped and the patient should be hospitalized.

A physician experienced in the management of this syndrome, or who is experienced in the management of fluid and electrolyte imbalances should be consulted.

Pulmonary and Vascular Complications:

Serious pulmonary conditions (e.g., atelectasis, acute respiratory distress syndrome and exacerbation of asthma) have been reported. In addition, thromboembolic events both in association with, and separate from Ovarian Hyperstimulation Syndrome have been reported. Intravascular thrombosis and embolism can result in reduced blood flow to critical organs or the extremities. Sequelae of such events have included venous thrombophlebitis, pulmonary embolism, pulmonary infarction, cerebral vascular occlusion (stroke), and arterial occlusion resulting in loss of limb. In rare cases, pulmonary complications and/or thromboembolic events have resulted in death.

Multiple Births: Reports of multiple births have been associated with Gonal-F® treatment. In ovulation induction clinical trials, 12.3% of live births were multiple births in women receiving Gonal-F® and 14.5% of live births were multiple births in women receiving urofollitropin. In IVF/ET clinical trials, 44.0% of live births were multiple births in women receiving Gonal-F® and 41.0% of live births were multiple births in women receiving urofollitropin and is dependent on the number of embryos transferred. The patient should be advised of the potential risk of multiple births before starting treatment.

Table 11: Time to Achievement of Sperm Density ≥ 1.5 × 10⁶/mL in Men Receiving Gonal-F®

		Study 5844 (n=26)	Study 6410 (n=8)	Study 6793 (n=22)*
Number of Men Achieving Sperm Concentration	n	12	5	14
Time (Months) to Sperm Concentration ≥ $1.5{\times}10^6$/mL	Median	12.4	9.1	6.8
	Range	(2.7–18.1)	(8.8–11.7)	(2.8–15.7)

* Interim data

Table 12: Pregnancy Outcome in Partners of Men Desiring Fertility

	Study 5844 (n = 7)	Study 6410 (n = 10)	Study 6793 (n = 20)*
Pregnancy	6 (86%)	3 (30%)	3 (15%)
Pregnancies not reaching term	1 (14%)	1 (10%)	2 (10%)
Single births	5 (71%)	2 (20%)	1 (5%)

* Interim data

PRECAUTIONS

General: Careful attention should be given to the diagnosis of infertility in candidates for Gonal-F® (follitropin alfa for injection) therapy (see "INDICATIONS AND USAGE/ Selection of Patients").

Information for Patients: Prior to therapy with Gonal-F®, patients should be informed of the duration of treatment and monitoring of their condition that will be required. The risks of ovarian hyperstimulation syndrome and multiple births (see **"WARNINGS"**) and other possible adverse reactions (see "ADVERSE REACTIONS") should also be discussed.

Laboratory Tests: In most instances, treatment with Gonal-F® results only in follicular recruitment and development. In the absence of an endogenous LH surge, hCG is given when monitoring of the patient indicates that sufficient follicular development has occurred. This may be estimated by ultrasound alone or in combination with measurement of serum estradiol levels. The combination of both ultrasound and serum estradiol measurement are useful for monitoring the development of follicles, for timing of the ovulatory trigger, as well as for detecting ovarian enlargement and minimizing the risk of the Ovarian Hyperstimulation Syndrome and multiple gestation. It is recommended that the number of growing follicles be confirmed using ultrasonography because plasma estrogens do not give an indication of the size or number of follicles.

The clinical confirmation of ovulation, with the exception of pregnancy, is obtained by direct and indirect indices of progesterone production. The indices most generally used are as follows:

1. A rise in basal body temperature;
2. Increase in serum progesterone; and
3. Menstruation following a shift in basal body temperature.

When used in conjunction with the indices of progesterone production, sonographic visualization of the ovaries will assist in determining if ovulation has occurred. Sonographic evidence of ovulation may include the following:

1. Fluid in the cul-de-sac;
2. Ovarian stigmata;
3. Collapsed follicle; and
4. Secretory endometrium.

Accurate interpretation of the indices of follicle development and maturation require a physician who is experienced in the interpretation of these tests.

Drug Interactions: No drug/drug interaction studies have been performed.

Carcinogenesis, Mutagenesis, Impairment of Fertility: Long-term studies in animals have not been performed to evaluate the carcinogenic potential of Gonal-F®. However, r-hFSH showed no mutagenic activity in a series of tests performed to evaluate its potential genetic toxicity including, bacterial and mammalian cell mutation tests, a chromosomal aberration test, and a micronucleus test.

Impaired fertility has been reported in rats, exposed to pharmacological doses of r-hFSH (≥ 40 IU/kg/day) for extended periods, through reduced fecundity.

Pregnancy: Pregnancy Category X. See "CONTRAINDICATIONS".

Nursing Mothers: It is not known whether this drug is excreted in human milk. Because many drugs are excreted in human milk and because of the potential for serious adverse reactions in the nursing infant from Gonal-F®, a decision should be made whether to discontinue nursing or to discontinue the drug, taking into account the importance of the drug to the mother.

Pediatric Use: Safety and effectiveness in pediatric patients have not been established.

ADVERSE REACTIONS

Women:

The safety of Gonal-F® was examined in four clinical studies that enrolled 691 patients into two studies for ovulation induction (454 patients) and two studies for ART (237 patients).

Adverse events occurring in more than 10% of patients were headache, ovarian cyst, nausea, and upper respiratory tract infection in the U.S. ovulation induction study and headache in the U.S. ART study. Adverse events (without regard to causality assessment) occurring in at least 2% of patients are listed in Table 13 and Table 14.

[See table 13 at top of next page]

Additional adverse events not listed in Table 13 that occurred in 1 to 2% of Gonal-F® treated patients in the U.S. ovulation induction study included the following: leukorrhea, vaginal hemorrhage, migraine, fatigue, asthma, nervousness, somnolence, and hypotension.

[See table 14 at top of next page]

Additional adverse events not listed in Table 14 that occurred in 1 to 2% of Gonal-F® treated patients in the U.S. Assisted Reproductive Technology (ART) study included the following: D&C following delivery or abortion, dysmenorrhea, vaginal hemorrhage, diarrhea, tooth disorder, vomiting, dizziness, paresthesia, abdomen enlarged, chest pain, fatigue, dyspnea, anorexia, anxiety, somnolence, injection site inflammation, injection site reaction, pruritus, pruritus genital, myalgia, thirst, and palpitation.

Two additional clinical studies (for ovulation induction and ART, respectively) were conducted in Europe. The safety profiles from these two studies were comparable to that of the data presented above.

The following medical events have been reported subsequent to pregnancies resulting from Gonal-F® therapy in controlled clinical studies:

1. Spontaneous Abortion
2. Ectopic Pregnancy
3. Premature Labor
4. Postpartum Fever
5. Congenital abnormalities

Two incidents of congenital cardiac malformations have been reported in children born following pregnancies resulting from treatment with Gonal-F® and hCG in Gonal-F® clinical studies 5642 and 5727. In addition, a pregnancy occurring in study 5533 following treatment with Gonal-F® and hCG was complicated by apparent failure of intrauterine growth and terminated for a suspected syndrome of congenital abnormalities. No specific diagnosis was made. The incidence does not exceed that found in the general population.

The following adverse reactions have been previously reported during menotropin therapy:

1. Pulmonary and vascular complications (see "WARNINGS"),
2. Adnexal torsion (as a complication of ovarian enlargement),
3. Mild to moderate ovarian enlargement,
4. Hemoperitoneum

There have been infrequent reports of ovarian neoplasms, both benign and malignant, in women who have undergone multiple drug regimens for ovulation induction; however, a causal relationship has not been established.

Men:

The safety of Gonal-F® was examined in 3 clinical studies that enrolled 72 patients for induction of spermatogenesis fertility of whom 56 patients received Gonal-F®. One hundred twenty-three adverse events, including 7 serious events, were reported in 34 of the 56 patients during Gonal-F® treatment.

In Study 5844, 21 adverse events, including 4 serious adverse events, were reported by 14 of the 26 patients (53.8%) treated with Gonal-F®. Events occurring in more than one patient were varicocele (4) and injection site reactions (4). The 4 serious adverse events were testicular surgery for cryptorchidism, which existed prestudy, hemoptysis, an infected pilonidal cyst, and lymphadenopathy associated with an Epstein-Barr viral infection.

In Study 6410, 3 adverse events were reported in 2 of the 8 patients (24%) treated with Gonal-F®. One serious adverse event was reported, surgery for gynecomastia which existed at baseline.

In the interim analysis of Study 6793, 18 of 22 patients (81.8%) reported a total of 99 adverse events during Gonal-F® treatment. The most common events of possible, probable, or definite relationship to study drug therapy occurring in more than 2 patients were: acne (25 events in 13

Continued on next page

Gonal-F—Cont.

patients; 59% of patients); breast pain (4 events in 3 patients; 13.6% of patients); and fatigue, gynecomastia, and injection site pain (each of which was reported as 2 events by 2 patients; 9.1% of patients). Two serious adverse events (hospitalization for drug abuse and depression) were reported by a single patient in the interim analysis.

A total of 12,026 injections of Gonal-F® were administered by the 56 patients who received Gonal-F® in Studies 5844, 6410, and 6793 combined. The injections were well-tolerated, with no or mild reactions (redness, swelling, bruising and itching) reported by patients for 93.3% of injections. Moderate to severe reactions, consisting primarily of pain, were reported for 4.8% of injections, and no self-assessment was available for 1.9% of injections.

OVERDOSAGE

Aside from possible ovarian hyperstimulation and multiple gestations (see "WARNINGS"), there is no information on the consequences of acute overdosage with Gonal-F® (follitropin alfa for injection).

DOSAGE AND ADMINISTRATION

Dosage:

Infertile Patients with oligo-anovulation: The dose of Gonal-F® (follitropin alfa for injection) to stimulate development of the follicle must be individualized for each patient.

The lowest dose consistent with the expectation of good results should be used. Over the course of treatment, doses of Gonal-F® may range up to 300 IU per day depending on the individual patient response. Gonal-F® should be administered until adequate follicular development is indicated by serum estradiol and vaginal ultrasonography. A response is generally evident after 5 to 7 days. Subsequent monitoring intervals should be based on individual patient response.

It is recommended that the initial dose of the first cycle be 75 IU of Gonal-F® per day, ADMINISTERED SUBCUTANEOUSLY. An incremental adjustment in dose of up to 37.5 IU may be considered after 14 days. Further dose increases of the same magnitude could be made, if necessary, every seven days. Treatment duration should not exceed 35 days unless an E2 rise indicates imminent follicular development. To complete follicular development and effect ovulation in the absence of an endogenous LH surge, chorionic gonadotropin, hCG, (5,000 USP units) should be given 1 day after the last dose of Gonal-F®. Chorionic gonadotropin should be withheld if the serum estradiol is greater than 2,000 pg/mL. If the ovaries are abnormally enlarged or abdominal pain occurs, Gonal-F® treatment should be discontinued, hCG should not be administered, and the patient should be advised not to have intercourse; this may reduce the chance of development of the Ovarian Hyperstimulation Syndrome and, should spontaneous ovulation occur, reduce the chance of multiple gestation. A follow-up visit should be conducted in the luteal phase.

The initial dose administered in the subsequent cycles should be individualized for each patient based on her response in the preceding cycle. Doses larger than 300 IU of FSH per day are not routinely recommended. As in the initial cycle, 5,000 USP units of hCG must be given 1 day after the last dose of Gonal-F® to complete follicular development and induce ovulation. The precautions described above should be followed to minimize the chance of development of the Ovarian Hyperstimulation Syndrome.

The couple should be encouraged to have intercourse daily, beginning on the day prior to the administration of hCG until ovulation becomes apparent from the indices employed for the determination of progestational activity. Care should be taken to ensure insemination. In light of the indices and parameters mentioned, it should become obvious that, unless a physician is willing to devote considerable time to these patients and be familiar with and conduct the necessary laboratory studies, he/she should not use Gonal-F®.

Assisted Reproductive Technologies: As in the treatment of patients with oligo-anovulatory infertility, the dose of Gonal-F® to stimulate development of the follicle must be individualized for each patient. For Assisted Reproductive Technologies, therapy with Gonal-F® should be initiated in the early follicular phase (cycle day 2 or 3) at a dose of 150 IU per day, until sufficient follicular development is attained. In most cases, therapy should not exceed ten days.

In patients undergoing ART, whose endogenous gonadotropin levels are suppressed, Gonal-F® should be initiated at a dose of 225 IU per day. Treatment should be continued until adequate follicular development is indicated as determined by ultrasound in combination with measurement of serum estradiol levels. Adjustments to dose may be considered after five days based on the patient's response; subsequently dosage should be adjusted no more frequently than every 3–5 days and by no more than 75–150 IU additionally at each adjustment. Doses greater than 450 IU per day are not recommended. Once adequate follicular development is evident, hCG (5,000 to 10,000 USP units) should be administered to induce final follicular maturation in preparation for oocyte retrieval. The administration of hCG must be withheld in cases where the ovaries are abnormally enlarged on the last day of therapy. This should reduce the chance of developing OHSS.

Male Patients with Hypogonadotropic Hypogonadism: The dose of Gonal-F® (follitropin alfa for injection) to induce spermatogenesis must be individualized for each patient.

Table 13: US Controlled Trial in Ovulation Induction, Study 5727

Body System Preferred Term	Gonal-F® Patients (%) Experiencing Events Treatment cycles = 288* n = 118	urofollitropin Patients (%) Experiencing Events Treatment cycles = 277 n = 114
Reproductive, Female		
Intermenstrual Bleeding	9.3%	4.4%
Breast Pain Female	4.2%	6.1%
Ovarian Hyperstimulation**	6.8%	3.5%
Dysmenorrhea	2.5%	6.1%
Ovarian Disorder	1.7%	2.6%
Cervix Lesion	2.5%	0.9%
Menstrual Disorder	2.5%	0.9%
Gastro-intestinal System		
Abdominal Pain	9.3%	12.3%
Nausea	13.6%	3.5%
Flatulence	6.8%	8.8%
Diarrhea	7.6%	3.5%
Vomiting	2.5%	2.6%
Dyspepsia	1.7%	3.5%
Central and Peripheral Nervous System		
Headache	22.0%	20.2%
Dizziness	2.5%	0.0%
Neoplasm		
Ovarian Cyst	15.3%	28.9%
Body as a Whole-General		
Pain	5.9%	6.1%
Back Pain	5.1%	1.8%
Influenza-like Symptoms	4.2%	2.6%
Fever	4.2%	1.8%
Respiratory System		
Upper Respiratory Tract Infection	11.9%	7.9%
Sinusitis	5.1%	5.3%
Pharyngitis	2.5%	3.5%
Coughing	1.7%	2.6%
Rhinitis	0.8%	2.6%
Skin and Appendages		
Acne	4.2%	2.6%
Psychiatric		
Emotional Lability	5.1%	2.6%
Urinary System		
Urinary Tract Infection	1.7%	4.4%
Resistance Mechanism		
Moniliasis Genital	2.5%	0.9%
Application Site		
Injection Site Pain	2.5%	0.9%

* up to 3 cycles of therapy
** Severe = 0.8% of 118 patients in Study 5727

Table 14: US Controlled Trial in ART, Study 5533

Body System Preferred Term	Gonal-F® Patients (%) Experiencing Events n = 59	urofollitropin Patients (%) Experiencing Events n = 61
Reproductive, Female		
Intermenstrual Bleeding	3.6%	5.2%
Leukorrhea	1.7%	3.4%
Vaginal Hemorrhage	3.6%	3.4%
Gastro-intestinal System		
Nausea	5.4%	1.7%
Flatulence	3.6%	0.0%
Central and Peripheral Nervous System		
Headache	12.5%	3.4%
Body as a Whole-General		
Abdominal Pain	8.9%	3.4%
Pelvic Pain Female	7.1%	1.7%
Respiratory System		
Upper Respiratory Tract Infection	3.6%	1.7%
Metabolic and Nutritional		
Weight Increase	3.6%	0.0%

Gonal-F® must be given in conjunction with hCG. Prior to concomitant therapy with Gonal-F® and hCG, pretreatment with hCG alone (1,000 to 2,250 USP Units two to three times per week) is required. Treatment should continue for a period sufficient to achieve serum testosterone levels within the normal range. Such pretreatment may require 3 to 6 months and the dose of hCG may need to be increased to achieve normal serum testosterone levels.

After normal serum testosterone levels are reached, the recommended dose of Gonal-F® is 150 IU administered subcutaneously three times a week and the recommended dose of hCG is 1,000 USP Units (or the dose required to maintain serum testosterone levels within the normal range) three times a week. The lowest dose of Gonal-F® which induces spermatogenesis should be utilized. If azoospermia persists, the dose of Gonal-F® may be increased to a maximum dose of 300 IU three times per week. Gonal-F® may need to be administered for up to 18 months to achieve adequate spermatogenesis.

Administration:

Dissolve the contents of one or more ampules of Gonal-F® in one-half to one mL of Sterile Water for Injection, USP (concentration should not exceed 225 IU/0.5 mL) and ADMINISTER SUBCUTANEOUSLY immediately. Any unused reconstituted material should be discarded.

Parenteral drug products should be inspected visually for particulate matter and discoloration prior to administration, whenever solution and container permit.

HOW SUPPLIED

Gonal-F® (follitropin alfa for injection) is supplied in a sterile, lyophilized form in single dose ampules containing 37.5, 75, or 150 IU FSH activity. The following package combinations are available:

— 1 ampule 37.5 IU Gonal-F® and 1 ampule 1 mL Sterile Water for Injection, USP, NDC 44087-9375-1
— 10 ampules 37.5 IU Gonal-F® and 10 ampules 1 mL Sterile Water for Injection, USP, NDC 44087-9375-3
— 100 ampules 37.5 IU Gonal-F® and 100 ampules 1 mL Sterile Water for Injection, USP, NDC 44087-9375-4
— 1 ampule 75 IU Gonal-F® and 1 ampule 1 mL Sterile Water for Injection, USP, NDC 44087-9075-1
— 10 ampules 75 IU Gonal-F® and 10 ampules 1 mL Sterile Water for Injection, USP, NDC 44087-9075-3
— 100 ampules 75 IU Gonal-F® and 100 ampules 1 mL Sterile Water for Injection, USP, NDC 44087-9075-4
— 1 ampule 150 IU Gonal-F® and 1 ampule 1 mL Sterile Water for Injection, USP, NDC 44087-9150-1

Lyophilized ampules may be stored refrigerated or at room temperature (2°–25°C/36°–77°F). Protect from light. Use immediately after reconstitution. Discard unused material.

Rx Only

Distributed by: SERONO LABORATORIES, INC.
Randolph, MA 02368 USA
Revised: June 2000
Code N1900101D 06/00

PERGONAL® ℞

[*per 'go-nal*]
(menotropins for injection, USP)
FOR INTRAMUSCULAR INJECTION

DESCRIPTION

Pergonal® (menotropins for injection, USP) is a purified preparation of gonadotropins extracted from the urine of postmenopausal women. Each ampule of Pergonal® contains 75 IU or 150 IU of follicle-stimulating hormone (FSH) activity and 75 IU or 150 IU of luteinizing hormone (LH) activity, respectively, plus 10 mg lactose in a sterile, lyophilized form. Human Chorionic Gonadotropins (hCG), a naturally occurring hormone in post-menopausal urine, is detected in Pergonal®. Pergonal® is administered by intramuscular injection.

Pergonal® is biologically standardized for FSH and LH (ICSH) gonadotropin activities in terms of the Second International Reference Preparation for Human Menopausal Gonadotropins established in September, 1964 by the Expert Committee on Biological Standards of the World Health Organization.

Both FSH and LH are glycoproteins that are acidic and water soluble.

Therapeutic class: Infertility.

CLINICAL PHARMACOLOGY

Women:

Pergonal® administered for seven to twelve days produces ovarian follicular growth in women who do not have primary ovarian failure. Treatment with Pergonal® in most instances results only in follicular growth and maturation. In order to effect ovulation, human chorionic gonadotropin (hCG) must be given following the administration of Pergonal® when clinical assessment of the patient indicates that sufficient follicular maturation has occurred.

Men:

Pergonal® administered concomitantly with human chorionic gonadotropin (hCG) for at least three months induces spermatogenesis in men with primary or secondary pituitary hypofunction who have achieved adequate masculinization with prior hCG therapy.

INDICATIONS AND USAGE

Women:

Pergonal® and hCG given in a sequential manner are indicated for the induction of ovulation and pregnancy in the anovulatory infertile patient, in whom the cause of anovulation is functional and is not due to primary ovarian failure.

Pergonal® and hCG may also be used to stimulate the development of multiple follicles in ovulatory patients participating in an in vitro fertilization program.

Men:

Pergonal® with concomitant hCG is indicated for the stimulation of spermatogenesis in men who have primary or secondary hypogonadotropic hypogonadism.

Pergonal® with concomitant hCG has proven effective in inducing spermatogenesis in men with primary hypogonadotropic hypogonadism due to a congenital factor or prepubertal hypophysectomy and in men with secondary hypogonadotropic hypogonadism due to hypophysectomy, craniopharyngioma, cerebral aneurysm or chromophobe adenoma.

SELECTION OF PATIENTS

Women:

1. Before treatment with Pergonal® is instituted, a thorough gynecologic and endocrinologic evaluation must be performed. Except for those patients enrolled in an in vitro fertilization program, this should include a hysterosalpingogram (to rule out uterine and tubal pathology) and documentation of anovulation by means of basal body temperature, serial vaginal smears, examination of cervical mucus, determination of serum (or urinary) progesterone, urinary pregnanediol and endometrial biopsy. Patients with tubal pathology should receive Pergonal® only if enrolled in an in vitro fertilization program.
2. Primary ovarian failure should be excluded by the determination of gonadotropin levels.
3. Careful examination should be made to rule out the presence of an early pregnancy.
4. Patients in late reproductive life have a greater predilection to endometrial carcinoma as well as a higher incidence of anovulatory disorders. Cervical dilation and curettage should always be done for diagnosis before starting Pergonal® therapy in such patients who demonstrate abnormal uterine bleeding or other signs of endometrial abnormalities.
5. Evaluation of the husband's fertility potential should be included in the workup.

Men:

Patient selection should be made based on a documented lack of pituitary function. Prior to hormonal therapy, these patients will have low testosterone levels and low or absent gonadotropin levels. Patients with primary hypogonadotropic hypogonadism will have a subnormal development of masculinization, and those with secondary hypogonadotropic hypogonadism will have decreased masculinization.

CONTRAINDICATIONS

Women:

Pergonal® is contraindicated in women who have:

1. A high FSH level indicating primary ovarian failure.
2. Uncontrolled thyroid and adrenal dysfunction.
3. An organic intracranial lesion such as a pituitary tumor.
4. The presence of any cause of infertility other than anovulation, unless they are candidates for in vitro fertilization.
5. Abnormal bleeding of undetermined origin.
6. Ovarian cysts or enlargement not due to polycystic ovary syndrome.
7. Prior hypersensitivity to menotropins.
8. Pergonal® is contraindicated in women who are pregnant and may cause fetal harm when administered to a pregnant woman. There are limited human data on the effects of Pergonal® when administered during pregnancy.

Men:

Pergonal® is contraindicated in men who have:

1. Normal gonadotropin levels indicating normal pituitary function.
2. Elevated gonadotropin levels indicating primary testicular failure.
3. Infertility disorders other than hypogonadotropic hypogonadism.

WARNINGS

Pergonal® is a drug that should only be used by physicians who are thoroughly familiar with infertility problems. It is a potent gonadotropic substance capable of causing mild to severe adverse reactions in women. Gonadotropin therapy requires a certain time commitment by physicians and supportive health professionals, and its use requires the availability of appropriate monitoring facilities (see "Precautions—Laboratory Tests"). In female patients it must be used with a great deal of care.

Overstimulation of the Ovary During Pergonal® Therapy:

Ovarian Enlargement: Mild to moderate uncomplicated ovarian enlargement which may be accompanied by abdominal distension and/or abdominal pain occurs in approximately 20% of those treated with Pergonal® and hCG, and generally regresses without treatment within two or three weeks.

In order to minimize the hazard associated with the occasional abnormal ovarian enlargement which may occur with Pergonal®-hCG therapy, the lowest dose consistent with expectation of good results should be used. Careful monitoring of ovarian response can further minimize the risk of overstimulation.

If the ovaries are abnormally enlarged on the last day of Pergonal® therapy, hCG should not be administered in this course of therapy; this will reduce the chances of development of the Ovarian Hyperstimulation Syndrome.

The Ovarian Hyperstimulation Syndrome (OHSS): OHSS is a medical event distinct from uncomplicated ovarian enlargement. OHSS may progress rapidly to become a serious medical event. It is characterized by an apparent dramatic increase in vascular permeability which can result in a rapid accumulation of fluid in the peritoneal cavity, thorax, and potentially, the pericardium. The early warning signs of development of OHSS are severe pelvic pain, nausea, vomiting, and weight gain. The following symptomatology has been seen with cases of OHSS: abdominal pain, abdominal distension, gastrointestinal symptoms including nausea, vomiting and diarrhea, severe ovarian enlargement, weight gain, dyspnea, and oliguria. Clinical evaluation may reveal hypovolemia, hemoconcentration, electrolyte imbalances, ascites, hemoperitoneum, pleural effusions, hydrothorax, acute pulmonary distress, and thromboembolic events (see "Pulmonary and Vascular Complications" below). Transient liver function test abnormalities suggestive of hepatic dysfunction, which may be accompanied by morphologic changes on liver biopsy, have been reported in association with the Ovarian Hyperstimulation Syndrome (OHSS).

OHSS occurs in approximately 0.4% of patients when the recommended dose is administered and in 1.3% of patients when higher than recommended doses are administered. Cases of OHSS are more common, more severe and more protracted if pregnancy occurs. OHSS develops rapidly; therefore, patients should be followed for at least two weeks after hCG administration. Most often, OHSS occurs after treatment has been discontinued and reaches its maximum at about seven to ten days following treatment. Usually, OHSS resolves spontaneously with the onset of menses. If there is evidence that OHSS may be developing prior to hCG administration (see "Precautions—Laboratory Tests"), the hCG should be withheld.

If OHSS occurs, treatment should be stopped and the patient hospitalized. Treatment is primarily symptomatic, consisting of bed rest, fluid and electrolyte management, and analgesics if needed. The phenomenon of hemoconcentration associated with fluid loss into the peritoneal cavity, pleural cavity, and the pericardial cavity has been seen to occur and should be thoroughly assessed in the following manner: 1) fluid intake and output, 2) weight, 3) hematocrit, 4) serum and urinary electrolytes, 5) urine specific gravity, 6) BUN and creatinine, and 7) abdominal girth. These determinations are to be performed daily or more often if the need arises.

With OHSS there is an increased risk of injury to the ovary. The ascitic, pleural, and pericardial fluid should not be removed unless absolutely necessary to relieve symptoms such as pulmonary distress or cardiac tamponade. Pelvic examination may cause rupture of an ovarian cyst, which may result in hemoperitoneum, and should therefore be avoided. If this does occur, and if bleeding becomes such that surgery is required, the surgical treatment should be designed to control bleeding and to retain as much ovarian tissue as possible. Intercourse should be prohibited in those patients in whom significant ovarian enlargement occurs after ovulation because of the danger of hemoperitoneum resulting from ruptured ovarian cysts.

The management of OHSS may be divided into three phases: the acute, the chronic, and the resolution phases. Because the use of diuretics can accentuate the diminished intravascular volume, diuretics should be avoided except in the late phase of resolution as described below.

Acute Phase: Management during the acute phase should be designed to prevent hemoconcentration due to loss of intravascular volume to the third space and to minimize the risk of thromboembolic phenomena and kidney damage. Treatment is designed to normalize electrolytes while maintaining an acceptable but somewhat reduced intravascular volume. Full correction of the intravascular volume deficit may lead to an unacceptable increase in the amount of third space fluid accumulation. Management includes administration of limited intravenous fluids, electrolytes, and human serum albumin. Monitoring for the development of hyperkalemia is recommended.

Chronic Phase: After stabilizing the patient during the acute phase, excessive fluid accumulation in the third space should be limited by instituting severe potassium, sodium, and fluid restriction.

Resolution Phase: A fall in hematocrit and an increasing urinary output without an increased intake are observed due to the return of third space fluid to the intravascular compartment. Peripheral and/or pulmonary edema may result if the kidneys are unable to excrete third space fluid as rapidly as it is mobilized. Diuretics may be indicated during the resolution phase if necessary to combat pulmonary edema.

Pulmonary and Vascular Complications: Serious pulmonary conditions (e.g., atelectasis, acute respiratory distress syndrome) have been reported. In addition, thromboembolic events both in association with, and separate from, the Ovarian Hyperstimulation Syndrome have been reported following Pergonal® therapy. Intravascular thrombosis and embolism, which may originate in venous or arterial vessels, can result in reduced blood flow to critical organs or the extremities. Sequelae of such events have included venous thrombophlebitis, pulmonary embolism, pulmonary infarction, cerebral vascular occlusion (stroke), and arterial occlusion resulting in loss of limb. In rare cases, pulmonary complications and/or thromboembolic events have resulted in death.

Multiple Births: Data from a clinical trial revealed the following results regarding multiple births: Of the pregnancies following therapy with Pergonal® and hCG, 80% resulted in single births, 15% in twins, and 5% of the total pregnancies resulted in three or more concepti. The patient and her husband should be advised of the frequency and potential hazards of multiple gestation before starting treatment.

Hypersensitivity/Anaphylactic Reactions: Hypersensitivity/anaphylactic reactions associated with Pergonal® administration have been reported in some patients. These reactions presented as generalized urticaria, facial edema, angioneurotic edema, and/or dyspnea suggestive of laryngeal edema. The relationship of these symptoms to uncharacterized urinary proteins is uncertain.

PRECAUTIONS

General: Careful attention should be given to diagnosis in the selection of candidates for Pergonal® therapy (see "Indications and Usage—Selection of Patients").

Information for Patients: Prior to therapy with Pergonal®, patients should be informed of the duration of treatment and the monitoring of their condition that will be required. Possible adverse reactions (see "Adverse Reactions" section) and the risk of multiple births should also be discussed.

Laboratory Tests:

Women:

Treatment for Induction of Ovulation

In most instances, treatment with Pergonal® results only in follicular growth and maturation. In order to effect ovulation, hCG must be given following the administration of Pergonal® when clinical assessment of the patient indicates that sufficient follicular maturation has occurred. This may be directly estimated by measuring serum (or urinary) estrogen levels and sonographic visualization of the ovaries. The combination of both estradiol levels and ultrasonography are useful for monitoring the growth and development of follicles, timing hCG administration, as well as minimizing the risk of the Ovarian Hyperstimulation Syndrome and multiple gestation.

Other clinical parameters which may have potential use for monitoring menotropins therapy include:

a) Changes in the vaginal cytology;
b) Appearance and volume of the cervical mucus;
c) Spinnbarkeit; and
d) Ferning of the cervical mucus.

The above clinical indices provide an indirect estimate of the estrogenic effect upon the target organs, and therefore should only be used adjunctively with more direct estimates of follicular development, i.e., serum estradiol and ultrasonography.

The clinical confirmation of ovulation, with the exception of pregnancy, is obtained by direct and indirect indices of progesterone production. The indices most generally used are as follows:

a) A rise in basal body temperature;
b) Increase in serum progesterone; and

Continued on next page

Pergonal—Cont.

c) Menstruation following the shift in basal body temperature.

When used in conjunction with indices of progesterone production, sonographic visualization of the ovaries will assist in determining if ovulation has occurred. Sonographic evidence of ovulation may include the following:

a) Fluid in the cul-de-sac;
b) Ovarian stigmata; and
c) Collapsed follicle.

Because of the subjectivity of the various tests for the determination of follicular maturation and ovulation, it cannot be overemphasized that the physician should choose tests with which he/she is thoroughly familiar.

Drug Interactions: No clinically significant drug/drug or drug/food adverse interactions have been reported during Pergonal® therapy.

Carcinogenesis and Mutagenesis: Long-term toxicity studies in animals have not been performed to evaluate the carcinogenic potential of Pergonal®.

Pregnancy: Pregnancy Category X. See "Contraindications" section.

Nursing Mothers: It is not known whether this drug is excreted in human milk. Because many drugs are excreted in human milk, caution should be exercised if Pergonal® is administered to a nursing woman.

ADVERSE REACTIONS

Women:

The following adverse reactions, reported during Pergonal® therapy, are listed in decreasing order of potential severity:

1. Pulmonary and vascular complications (see "Warnings")
2. Ovarian Hyperstimulation Syndrome (see "Warnings")
3. Hemoperitoneum
4. Adnexal torsion (as a complication of ovarian enlargement)
5. Mild to moderate ovarian enlargement
6. Ovarian cysts
7. Abdominal pain
8. Sensitivity to Pergonal®
   (Febrile reactions suggestive of allergic response have been reported following the administration of Pergonal®. Reports of flu-like symptoms including fever, chills, musculoskeletal aches, joint pains, nausea, headaches and malaise have also been reported).
9. Gastrointestinal symptoms (nausea, vomiting, diarrhea, abdominal cramps, bloating)
10. Pain, rash, swelling and/or irritation at the site of injection
11. Body rashes
12. Dizziness, tachycardia, dyspnea, tachypnea

The following medical events have been reported subsequent to pregnancies resulting from Pergonal® therapy:

1. Ectopic pregnancy
2. Congenital abnormalities
   From a study of 287 completed pregnancies following Pergonal®-hCG therapy five incidents of birth defects were reported (1.7%). One infant had multiple congenital anomalies consisting of imperforate anus, aplasia of the sigmoid colon, third degree hypospadias, cecovesicle fistula, bifid scrotum, meningocele, bilateral internal tibial torsion, and right metatarsus adductus. Another infant was born with an imperforate anus and possible congenital heart lesions; another had a supernumerary digit; another was born with hypospadias and exstrophy of the bladder; and the fifth child had Down's syndrome. None of the investigators felt that these defects were drug-related. Subsequently one report of an infant death due to hydrocephalus and cardiac anomalies has been received.

There have been infrequent reports of ovarian neoplasms, both benign and malignant, in women who have undergone multiple drug regimens for ovulation induction; however, a causal relationship has not been established.

Men:

1. Gynecomastia may occur occasionally during Pergonal®-hCG therapy. This is a known effect of hCG treatment.
2. Erythrocytosis (hct 50%, hgb 17.8 g%) was recorded in one patient.

DRUG ABUSE AND DEPENDENCE

There have been no reports of abuse or dependence with Pergonal®.

OVERDOSAGE

Aside from possible ovarian hyperstimulation (see "Warnings"), little is known concerning the consequences of acute overdosage with Pergonal®.

DOSAGE AND ADMINISTRATION

Women:

1. Dosage:

The dose of Pergonal® to produce maturation of the follicle must be individualized for each patient. It is recommended that the initial dose to any patient should be 75 IU of FSH/LH per day, **ADMINISTERED INTRAMUSCULARLY**, for seven to twelve days followed by hCG, 5,000 U to 10,000 U, one day after the last dose of Pergonal®. Administration of Pergonal® should not exceed 12 days in a single course of therapy. The patient should be treated until indices of estrogenic activity, as indicated under "Precautions" above, are equivalent to or greater than those of the normal individual. If serum or urinary estradiol determinations or ultrasonographic visualizations are available, they may be useful as a guide to therapy. If the ovaries are abnormally enlarged on the last day of Pergonal® therapy, hCG should not be administered in this course of therapy; this will reduce the chances of development of the Ovarian Hyperstimulation Syndrome. If there is evidence of ovulation but no pregnancy, repeat this dosage regime for at least two more courses before increasing the dose of Pergonal® to 150 IU of FSH/LH per day for seven to twelve days. As before, this dose should be followed by 5,000 U to 10,000 U of hCG one day after the last dose of Pergonal®. A Pergonal® dose of 150 IU of FSH/ LH per day has proven to be the most effective dose especially for in vitro fertilization. If evidence of ovulation is present, but pregnancy does not ensue, repeat the same dose for two more courses. Doses larger than this are not routinely recommended.

During treatment with both Pergonal® and hCG and during a two-week post-treatment period, patients should be examined at least every other day for signs of excessive ovarian stimulation. It is recommended that Pergonal® administration be stopped if the ovaries become abnormally enlarged or abdominal pain occurs. Most of the Ovarian Hyperstimulation Syndrome occurs after treatment has been discontinued and reaches its maximum at about seven to ten days post-ovulation. Patients should be followed for at least two weeks after hCG administration.

The couple should be encouraged to have intercourse daily, beginning on the day prior to the administration of hCG until ovulation becomes apparent from the indices employed for the determination of progestational activity. Care should be taken to insure insemination. In the light of the foregoing indices and parameters mentioned, it should become obvious that, unless a physician is willing to devote considerable time to these patients and be familiar with and conduct the necessary laboratory studies, he/she should not use Pergonal®.

2. Administration:

Dissolve the contents of one ampule of Pergonal® in one to two ml of sterile saline and **ADMINISTER INTRAMUSCULARLY** immediately. Any unused reconstituted material should be discarded. Parenteral drug products should be inspected visually for particulate matter and discoloration prior to administration, whenever solution and container permit.

Men:

1. Dosage:

Prior to concomitant therapy with Pergonal® and hCG, pretreatment with hCG alone (5,000 U three times a week) is required. Treatment should continue for a period sufficient to achieve serum testosterone levels within the normal range and masculinization as judged by the appearance of secondary sex characteristics. Such pretreatment may require four to six months, then the recommended dose of Pergonal® is 75 IU FSH/LH **ADMINISTERED INTRAMUSCULARLY**, three times a week and the recommended dose of hCG is 2,000 U twice a week. Therapy should be carried on for a minimum of four more months to insure detecting spermatozoa in the ejaculate, as it takes 74± 4 days in the human male for germ cells to reach the spermatozoa stage.

If the patient has not responded with evidence of increased spermatogenesis at the end of four months of therapy, treatment may continue with 75 IU FSH/LH three times a week, or the dose can be increased to 150 IU FSH/LH three times a week, with the hCG dose unchanged.

2. Administration:

Dissolve the contents of one ampule of Pergonal® in one to two ml of sterile saline and **ADMINISTER INTRAMUSCULARLY** immediately. Any unused reconstituted material should be discarded. Parenteral drug products should be inspected visually for particulate matter and discoloration prior to administration, whenever solution and container permit.

HOW SUPPLIED

Pergonal® is supplied in a sterile lyophilized form as a white to off-white powder or pellet in ampules containing 75 IU or 150 IU FSH/LH activity. The following package combinations are available:

— 1 ampule 75 IU Pergonal® and 1 ampule 2 ml Sodium Chloride Injection (USP), NDC 44087-0571-7.
— 10 ampules 75 IU Pergonal® and 10 ampules 2 ml Sodium Chloride Injection (USP), NDC 44087-5075-3.
— 1 ampule 150 IU Pergonal® and 1 ampule 2 ml Sodium Chloride Injection (USP), NDC 44087-5150-1.

By biological assay, one IU of LH for the Second International Reference Preparation (2nd-IRP) for hMG is biologically equivalent to approximately $^1/_2$ U of hCG.

Lyophilized powder may be stored refrigerated or at room temperature (3°–25°C/37°–77°F). Protect from light. Use immediately after reconstitution. Discard unused material.

CLINICAL STUDIES

Women:

The results of the clinical experience and effectiveness of the administration of Pergonal® to 1,286 patients in 3,002 courses of therapy are summarized below. The values include patients who were treated with other than the recommended dosage regime. The values for the presently recommended dosage regime are essentially the same.

	%
Patients ovulating	75
Patients pregnant	25
Patients aborting	25*
Multiple pregnancies	20†
Twins	15†
Three or more concepti	5†
Fetal abnormalities	1.7†
Hyperstimulation syndrome	1.3

* Based on total pregnancies
† Based on total deliveries

Results by diagnosis group are summarized below (these values include patients who were treated with other than the present recommended dosage regime):

[See table below]

	% Pts. Ovul.	% Pts. Preg.	% Abort.	% Multi. Preg.	% Twins	% 3 or More Concepti	% Hyperstim. Syndr.
Primary Amenorrhea	62	22	14	25	25	0	0
Secondary Amenorrhea	61	28	24	28	18	10	1.9
Secondary Amen. with Galactorrhea	77	42	21	41	31	10	1.2
Polycystic Ovaries	76	26	39	17	17	0	1.1
Anovulatory Cycles	77	24	15	14	9	5	2.0
Miscellaneous	83	20	36	2	2	0	0.1

Men:

Clinical results of the treatment of men with primary or secondary hypogonadotropic hypogonadism are as follows:

In the Serono Cooperative study, with an adequate treatment period of 3 to 8 months, 60 of 70 men with primary hypogonadotropic hypogonadism and 8 of 11 men with secondary hypogonadotropic hypogonadism responded with mean increases in their sperm counts from less than 5 to 24 million spermatozoa per milliliter of ejaculate. Forty-one wives of 54 men with primary hypogonadotropic hypogonadism desiring offspring and 7 wives of men with secondary hypogonadotropic hypogonadism conceived. Patients treated with Pergonal® and hCG for less than 3 months or with Pergonal® alone did not respond to therapy.

A world-wide data search revealed that of 160 recorded pregnancies as the result of use of Pergonal®-hCG in men, there were 7 spontaneous abortions, one ectopic pregnancy and 3 congenital anomalies at birth (esophageal atresia in a female infant which was later corrected by surgery, unilateral cryptorchidism, inguinal hernia).

Caution: Federal law prohibits dispensing without prescription.

Manufactured for:
SERONO LABORATORIES, INC.
Randolph, MA 02368 USA
by: Laboratoires Serono, SA
Aubonne, Switzerland

Revised: November 1994

PROFASI® ℞

[*pro 'fah-se*]
(chorionic gonadotropin for injection, USP)

FOR INTRAMUSCULAR INJECTION

DESCRIPTION

Human chorionic gonadotropin (HCG), a polypeptide hormone produced by the human placenta, is composed of an alpha and a beta sub-unit. The alpha sub-unit is essentially identical to the alpha sub-units of the human pituitary gonadotropins, luteinizing hormone (LH) and follicle-stimulating hormone (FSH), as well as to the alpha sub-unit of human thyroid-stimulating hormone (TSH). The beta sub-units of these hormones differ in amino acid sequence.

Chorionic Gonadotropin is a water soluble glycoprotein derived from human pregnancy urine. The sterile lyophilized powder is stable. When reconstituted, the solution should be refrigerated and used within 30 days.

Each vial, when reconstituted with provided diluent, will contain:
Chorionic Gonadotropin **2,000, 5,000 or 10,000** USP Units, Mannitol 100 mg, Dibasic Sodium Phosphate 16 mg, Monobasic Sodium Phosphate 4 mg, with Benzyl Alcohol 0.9% as preservative, in Water for Injection.

CLINICAL PHARMACOLOGY

The action of HCG is virtually identical to that of pituitary LH, although HCG appears to have a small degree of FSH activity as well. It stimulates production of gonadal steroid hormones by stimulating the interstitial cells (Leydig cells) of the testis to produce androgens and the corpus luteum of the ovary to produce progesterone. Androgen stimulation in the male leads to the development of secondary sex characteristics and may stimulate testicular descent when no anatomical impediment to descent is present. This descent is usually reversible when HCG is discontinued. During the normal menstrual cycle, LH participates with FSH in the development and maturation of the normal ovarian follicle, and the mid-cycle LH surge triggers ovulation. HCG can substitute for LH in this function.

During a normal pregnancy, HCG secreted by the placenta maintains the corpus luteum after LH secretion decreases, supporting continued secretion of estrogen and progesterone, and preventing menstruation. HCG HAS NO KNOWN EFFECT ON FAT MOBILIZATION, APPETITE OR SENSE OF HUNGER, OR BODY FAT DISTRIBUTION.

INDICATIONS AND USAGE

HCG HAS NOT BEEN DEMONSTRATED TO BE EFFECTIVE ADJUNCTIVE THERAPY IN THE TREATMENT OF OBESITY. THERE IS NO SUBSTANTIAL EVIDENCE THAT IT INCREASES WEIGHT LOSS BEYOND THAT RESULTING FROM CALORIC RESTRICTION, THAT IT CAUSES A MORE ATTRACTIVE OR "NORMAL" DISTRIBUTION OF FAT, OR THAT IT DECREASES THE HUNGER AND DISCOMFORT ASSOCIATED WITH CALORIE-RESTRICTED DIETS.

1. Prepubertal cryptorchidism not due to anatomical obstruction. In general, HCG is thought to induce testicular descent in situations when descent would have occurred at puberty. HCG thus may help to predict whether or not orchiopexy will be needed in the future. Although, in some cases, descent following HCG administration is permanent, in most cases the response is temporary. Therapy is usually instituted between the ages of 4 and 9.
2. Selected cases of hypogonadotropic hypogonadism (hypogonadism secondary to a pituitary deficiency) in males.
3. Induction of ovulation and pregnancy in the anovulatory, infertile woman in whom the cause of anovulation is secondary and not due to primary ovarian failure, and who has been appropriately pretreated with human menotropins.

CONTRAINDICATIONS

Precocious puberty, prostatic carcinoma or other androgen-dependent neoplasm, prior allergic reaction to HCG. HCG may cause fetal harm when administered to a pregnant woman. Combined HCG/PMS (pregnant mare's serum) therapy has been noted to induce high incidences of external congenital anomalies in the offspring of mice, in a dose-dependent manner. The potential extrapolation to humans has not been determined.

WARNINGS

HCG should be used in conjunction with human menopausal gonadotropins only by physicians experienced with infertility problems who are familiar with the criteria for patient selection, contraindications, warnings, precautions, and adverse reactions described in the package insert for menotropins. The principal serious adverse reactions during this use are: (1) Ovarian hyperstimulation, a sydrome of sudden ovarian enlargement, ascites with or without pain, and/or pleural effusion; (2) Enlargement of preexisting ovarian cysts or rupture of ovarian cysts with resultant hemoperitoneum; (3) Multiple births, and (4) Arterial thromboembolism.

The diluent used for reconstitution contains benzyl alcohol. Benzyl alcohol has been reported to be associated with a fatal "Gasping Syndrome" in premature infants.

PRECAUTIONS

General: 1. Induction of androgen secretion by HCG may induce precocious puberty in patients treated for cryptorchidism. Therapy should be discontinued if signs of precocious puberty occur.
2. Since androgens may cause fluid retention, HCG should be used with caution in patients with cardiac or renal disease, epilepsy, migraine, or asthma.

Drug/Laboratory test: HCG can crossreact in the radioimmunoassay of gonadotropins, especially luteinizing hormone. Each individual laboratory should establish the degree of crossreactivity with their gonadotropin assay. Physicians should make the laboratory aware of patients on HCG if gonadotropin levels are requested.

Carcinogenesis, Mutagenesis, Impairment of Fertility: There have been sporadic reports of testicular tumors in otherwise healthy young men receiving HCG for secondary infertility. A causative relationship between HCG and tumor development in these men has not been established. Defects of forelimbs and of the central nervous system, as well as alterations in sex ratio, have been reported in mice on combined gonadotropin and HCG regimens. The dose of gonadotropin used was intended to induce superovulation. No mutagenic effect has been clearly established in humans. Fertility—see "Indications and Usage."

Pregnancy: Teratogenic effects- *-Category X:* See "Contraindications" section. Combined HCG/PMS (pregnant mare's serum) therapy has been noted to induce high incidences of external congenital anomalies in the offspring of mice, in a dose-dependent manner. The potential extrapolation to humans has not been determined.

Nursing Mothers: It is not known whether this drug is excreted in human milk. Because many drugs are excreted in human milk, caution should be exercised when HCG is administered to a nursing woman.

Pediatric Use: Safety and effectiveness in children below the age of 4 have not been established.

ADVERSE REACTIONS (See WARNINGS)

Headache, irritability, restlessness, depression, fatigue, edema, precocious puberty, gynecomastia, pain at the site of injection. Hypersensitivity reactions both localized and systemic in nature, including erythema, urticaria, rash, angioedema, dyspnea and shortness of breath, have been reported. The relationship of these allergic-like events to the polypeptide hormone or the diluent containing benzyl alcohol is not clear.

DOSAGE AND ADMINISTRATION (Intramuscular Use Only):

The dosage regimen employed in any particular case will depend upon the indication for use, the age and weight of the patient, and the physician's preference. The following regimens have been advocated by various authorities.

Prepubertal cryptorchidism not due to anatomical obstruction:
(1) 4,000 USP Units three times weekly for three weeks.
(2) 5,000 USP Units every second day for four injections.
(3) 15 Injections of 500 to 1,000 USP Units over a period of six weeks.
(4) 500 USP Units three times weekly for four to six weeks. If this course of treatment is not successful, another is begun one month later, giving 1,000 USP Units per injection.

Selected cases of hypogonadotropic hypogonadism in males:
(1) 500 to 1,000 USP Units three times a week for three weeks, followed by the same dose twice a week for three weeks.
(2) 4,000 USP Units three times weekly for six to nine months, following which the dosage may be reduced to 2,000 USP Units three times weekly for an additional three months.

Induction of ovulation and pregnancy in the anovulatory, infertile woman in whom the cause of anovulation is secondary and not due to primary ovarian failure and who has been appropriately pre-treated with human menotropins (See prescribing information for menotropins for dosage and administration for that drug product).

5,000 to 10,000 USP Units one day following the last dose of menotropins. (A dosage of 10,000 USP Units is recommended in the labeling for menotropins).

Parenteral drug products should be inspected visually for particulate matter and discoloration prior to administration, whenever solution and container permit.

HOW SUPPLIED

Chorionic gonadotropin for injection, USP, is available in 10 mL lyophilized multiple dose vial sets containing either:
5,000 USP Units per Vial-NDC 44087-8005-3
10,000 USP Units per Vial-NDC 44087-8010-3
with 10 mL vial bacteriostatic water for injection, USP (containing benzyl alcohol 0.9% v/v).

Storage: Store dry product at controlled room temperature 15°–30° C (59°–86° F). AFTER RECONSTITUTION, REFRIGERATE THE PRODUCT AT 2°–8° C (36°–46° F) AND USE WITHIN 30 DAYS.

Rx Only

Manufactured for: SERONO LABORATORIES, INC.
Randolph, MA 02368 USA

Revised January 1999

SAIZEN® ℞

[sī- zen]

[somatropin (rDNA origin) for injection]
For subcutaneous or intramuscular injection

DESCRIPTION

Saizen® [somatropin (rDNA origin) for injection] is a human growth hormone produced by recombinant DNA technology. Saizen® has 191 amino acid residues and a molecular weight of 22,125 daltons. Its amino acid sequence and structure are identical to the dominant form of human pituitary growth hormone. Saizen® is produced by a mammalian cell line (mouse C127) that has been modified by the addition of the human growth hormone gene. Saizen®, with the correct three-dimensional configuration, is secreted directly through the cell membrane into the cell-culture medium for collection and purification.

Saizen® is a highly purified preparation. Biological potency is determined by measuring the increase in body weight induced in hypophysectomized rats.

Saizen® is a sterile, non-pyrogenic, white, lyophilized powder intended for subcutaneous or intramuscular injection after reconstitution with Bacteriostatic Water for Injection, USP (0.9% Benzyl Alcohol). The reconstituted solution has a pH of 6.5 to 8.5.

Saizen® is available in 5 mg and 8.8 mg vials. The quantitative composition per vial is:

5 mg (approximately 15 IU) vial:
Each vial contains 5.0 mg somatropin (approximately 15 IU), 34.2 mg sucrose and 1.165 mg O-phosphoric acid. The pH is adjusted with sodium hydroxide or O-phosphoric acid. The diluent is Bacteriostatic Water for Injection, USP containing 0.9% Benzyl Alcohol added as an antimicrobial preservative.

8.8 mg (approximately 26.4 IU) vial:
Each vial contains 8.8 mg somatropin (approximately 26.4 IU), 60.2 mg sucrose and 2.05 mg O-phosphoric acid. The pH is adjusted with sodium hydroxide or O-phosphoric acid.

CLINICAL PHARMACOLOGY

General

In vitro, preclinical, and clinical testing have demonstrated that Saizen® [somatropin (rDNA origin) for injection] is therapeutically equivalent to pituitary-derived human growth hormone. Clinical studies in normal adults also demonstrated equivalent pharmacokinetics.

Actions that have been demonstrated for Saizen®, somatrem, and/or pituitary-derived human growth hormone include:

A. Tissue Growth–
   1. Skeletal Growth: Saizen® stimulates skeletal growth in prepubertal children with pituitary growth hormone deficiency. Skeletal growth is accomplished at the epiphyseal plates at the ends of long bone. Growth and metabolism of epiphyseal plate cells are directly stimulated by growth hormone and one of its mediators, insulin-like growth factor-I. Serum levels of insulin-like growth factor-I (IGF-I) are low in children and adolescents who are growth hormone deficient, but increase during treatment with Saizen®. Linear growth continues until the growth plates fuse at the end of puberty.
   2. Cell Growth: Treatment with pituitary-derived human growth hormone results in an increase in both the number and the size of skeletal muscle cells.
   3. Organ Growth: Growth hormone of human pituitary origin influences the size and function of internal organs and increases red cell mass. Saizen® has been shown to promote similar organ weight increase to pituitary human growth hormone in an adequate animal model.

B. Protein Metabolism-Linear growth is facilitated in part by growth hormone-stimulated protein synthesis. This is reflected by increased cellular uptake of amino acids and nitrogen retention as demonstrated by a decline in urinary nitrogen excretion and blood urea nitrogen during growth hormone therapy.

C. Carbohydrate Metabolism-Growth hormone is a modulator of carbohydrate metabolism. Children with inadequate secretion of growth hormone sometimes experience fasting hypoglycemia that is improved by treatment with growth hormone. Saizen® therapy may decrease glucose tolerance. Administration of Saizen® to normal adults and patients with growth hormone deficiency resulted in transient increases in mean serum fasting and postprandial insulin levels. However, glucose levels remained in the normal range.

D. Lipid Metabolism-Acute administration of human growth hormone to humans results in lipid mobilization. Nonesterified fatty acids increase in plasma within one hour of Saizen® administration. In growth hormone deficient patients, long-term growth hormone administration often decreases body fat. Mean cholesterol levels decreased in patients treated with Saizen®. The clinical significance of this is unknown.

E. Mineral Metabolism-Growth hormone administration results in the retention of total body potassium, phosphorus, and sodium. Serum calcium levels appear to be unaffected.

F. Connective Tissue/Bone Metabolism-Growth hormone stimulates the synthesis of chondroitin sulfate and collagen as well as the urinary excretion of hydroxyproline.

Pharmacokinetics

Absorption—The absolute bioavailability of recombinant growth hormone (r-hGH) after subcutaneous administration ranges between 70–90%.

Distribution—The mean volume of distribution of r-hGH given to healthy volunteers was estimated to be 12.0 ± 1.08 L.

Metabolism—The metabolic fate of somatropin involves classical protein catabolism in both the liver and kidneys. In renal cells, at least a portion of the breakdown products is returned to the systemic circulation. The mean half-life of intravenous somatropin in normal males is 0.6 hours, whereas subcutaneously and intramuscularly administered somatropin has a half-life of 1.75 and 3.4 hours, respectively. The longer half-life observed after subcutaneous or intramuscular administration is due to slow absorption from the injection site.

Excretion—The mean clearance of intravenously administered r-hGH in six normal male volunteers was 14.6 ± 2.8 L/hr.

SPECIAL POPULATIONS

Pediatric—The pharmacokinetics of r-hGH is similar in children and adults.

Gender—No gender studies have been performed in children. In adults, the clearance of r-hGH in both men and women tends to be similar.

Race—No data are available.

Continued on next page

Saizen—Cont.

Renal Insufficiency—Children and adults with chronic renal failure tend to have decreased clearance of r-hGH as compared to normals.

Hepatic Insufficiency—A reduction in r-hGH clearance has been noted in patients with hepatic dysfunction as compared with normal controls.

INDICATIONS AND USAGE

Saizen® [somatropin (rDNA origin) for injection] is indicated for the long-term treatment of children with growth failure due to inadequate secretion of endogenous growth hormone.

CONTRAINDICATIONS

In general, Saizen® [somatropin (rDNA origin) for injection] is contraindicated in the presence of active neoplasia. Any pre-existing neoplasia should be inactive and its treatment complete prior to instituting therapy with Saizen®. Saizen® should be discontinued if there is evidence of recurrent activity. Since, in rare instances, growth hormone deficiency may be an early sign of the presence of a brain tumor, the presence of such a tumor should be ruled out prior to initiation of treatment. Available information suggests that the rate of tumor recurrence is not increased by growth hormone therapy. Saizen® should not be used for growth promotion in pediatric patients with closed epiphyses.

Saizen® reconstituted with Bacteriostatic Water for Injection, USP (0.9% Benzyl Alcohol) should not be administered to patients with a known sensitivity to Benzyl Alcohol. (See "WARNINGS").

Growth hormone should not be initiated to treat patients with acute critical illness due to complications following open heart or abdominal surgery, multiple accidental trauma or to patients having acute respiratory failure. Two placebo-controlled clinical trials in non-growth hormone deficient adult patients (n=522) with these conditions revealed a significant increase in mortality (41.9% vs. 19.3%) among somatropin treated patients (doses 5.3–8 mg/day) compared to those receiving placebo (see WARNINGS).

WARNINGS

Benzyl Alcohol as a preservative in Bacteriostatic Water for Injection, USP has been associated with toxicity in newborns. If sensitivity to the diluent occurs, Saizen® [somatropin (rDNA origin) for injection] may be reconstituted with Sterile Water for Injection, USP. When Saizen is reconstituted in this manner, the reconstituted solution should be used immediately and any unused solution should be discarded.

See CONTRAINDICATIONS for information on increased mortality in patients with acute critical illnesses in intensive care units due to complications following open heart or abdominal surgery, multiple accidental trauma or with acute respiratory failure. The safety of continuing growth hormone treatment in patients receiving replacement doses for approved indications who concurrently develop these illnesses has not been established. Therefore, the potential benefit of treatment continuation with growth hormone in patients having acute critical illnesses should be weighed against the potential risk.

PRECAUTIONS

General: Saizen® [somatropin (rDNA origin) for injection] therapy should be carried out under the regular guidance of a physician who is experienced in the diagnosis and management of growth disorders.

Because human growth hormone may induce a state of insulin resistance, patients should be observed for evidence of glucose intolerance. Human growth hormone should be used with caution in patients with diabetes mellitus or a family history of diabetes mellitus.

Hypothyroidism may develop during Saizen® therapy. Untreated hypothyroidism will jeopardize the response to growth hormone. Therefore, thyroid hormone determinations should be performed periodically during Saizen® administration and thyroid hormone replacement should be initiated when indicated.

Bone age should be monitored periodically during Saizen® administration especially in patients who are pubertal and/or receiving concomitant thyroid replacement therapy. Under these circumstances, epiphyseal maturation may progress rapidly.

Patients with endocrine disorders, including growth hormone deficiency, may have an increased incidence of slipped capital femoral epiphysis. Any child who develops a limp or complains of hip or knee pain during growth hormone therapy should be evaluated.

Intracranial hypertension (IH) with papilledema, visual changes, headache, nausea and/or vomiting has been reported in a small number of patients treated with growth hormone products and it also has been associated more commonly with IGF-I. Symptoms usually occurred within the first eight weeks of the initiation of growth hormone therapy. In all reported cases, IH-associated signs and symptoms resolved after temporary suspension or termination of therapy. Funduscopic examination of patients is recommended at the initiation and periodically during the course of growth hormone therapy.

When growth hormone is administered subcutaneously at the same site over a long period of time, tissue atrophy may result. This can be avoided by rotating the injection site.

As for any protein, local or systemic allergic reactions may occur. Parents/Patient should be informed that such reactions are possible and that prompt medical attention should be sought if allergic reactions occur.

Laboratory Tests: Serum levels of inorganic phosphorus, alkaline phosphatase, and IGF-I may increase with Saizen® therapy.

Drug Interaction: Concomitant glucocorticoid therapy may inhibit the growth promoting effect of Saizen®. There was no evidence in the controlled studies of Saizen® interaction with drugs commonly used in the treatment of routine pediatric problems/illnesses. However, formal drug interaction studies have not been conducted.

Carcinogenesis, Mutagenesis, Impairment of Fertility: Long-term animal studies for carcinogenicity have not been performed with Saizen®. There is no evidence from animal studies to date of Saizen®-induced mutagenicity or impairment of fertility.

Pregnancy: Teratogenic Effects: Pregnancy Category B. Reproduction studies have been performed in rats and rabbits at doses up to 31 and 62 times, respectively, the human (child) weekly dose based on body surface area. The results have revealed no evidence of impaired fertility or harm to the fetus due to Saizen®. There are, however, no adequate and well controlled studies in pregnant women. Because animal reproduction studies are not always predictive of human response, this drug should be used during pregnancy only if clearly needed.

Nursing Women: It is not known whether Saizen® is excreted in human milk. Because many drugs are excreted in human milk, caution should be exercised when Saizen® is administered to a nursing woman.

Geriatric Use: The safety and effectiveness of Saizen® in patients aged 65 and over have not been evaluated in clinical studies. Elderly patients may be more sensitive to the action of Saizen®, and may be more prone to develop adverse reactions.

Information For Patients: Patients being treated with growth hormone and/or their parents should be informed of the potential benefits and risks associated with treatment. If home use is determined to be desirable by the physician, instructions on appropriate use should be given, including a review of the contents of the Patient Information Insert. This information is intended to aid in the safe and effective administration of the medication. It is not a disclosure of all possible adverse or intended effects.

If home use is prescribed, a puncture resistant container for the disposal of used syringes and needles should be recommended to the patient. Patients and/or parents should be thoroughly instructed in the importance of proper disposal and cautioned against any reuse of needles and syringes (see Patient Information Insert).

ADVERSE REACTIONS

As with all protein pharmaceuticals, a small percentage of patients may develop antibodies to the protein. Anti-growth hormone (GH) antibody capacities below 2 mg/L have not been associated with growth attenuation. In some cases when binding capacity exceeds 2 mg/L, growth attenuation has been described. In clinical studies with Saizen® involving 280 patients (204 naive and 76 transfer patients), one patient at 6 months of therapy developed anti-GH antibodies with binding capacities exceeding 2 mg/L. Despite the high binding capacity, these antibodies were not growth attenuating. The patient was subsequently shown to have a hGH-N gene defect. Thus, genetic analysis should be undertaken in any patient in whom anti-GH antibodies with high binding capacities occur. No antibodies against proteins of the host cells were detected in the sera of patients treated up to five years.

Any patient with well-documented growth hormone deficiency who fails to respond to therapy should be tested for antibodies to human growth hormone and for thyroid status.

In clinical studies in which Saizen® was administered to growth hormone deficient children, the following events were infrequently seen: local reactions at the injection site (such as pain, numbness, redness and swelling), hypothyroidism, hypoglycemia, seizures, exacerbation of pre-existing psoriasis and disturbances in fluid balance.

Leukemia has been reported in a small number of growth hormone deficient patients treated with growth hormone. It is uncertain whether this increased risk is related to the pathology of growth hormone deficiency itself, growth hormone therapy, or other associated treatments such as radiation therapy for intracranial tumors. So far, epidemiological data fail to confirm the hypothesis of a relationship between growth hormone therapy and leukemia.

OVERDOSAGE

Long-term overdosage could result in signs and symptoms of gigantism and/or acromegaly consistent with the known effects of excess human growth hormone.

DOSAGE AND ADMINISTRATION

Saizen® [somatropin (rDNA origin) for injection] dosage and schedule of administration should be individualized for each patient. For the treatment of growth hormone inadequacy, a dosage of 0.06 mg/kg (approximately 0.18 IU/kg) administered 3 times per week by subcutaneous or intramuscular injection is recommended.

Treatment with Saizen® of growth failure due to growth hormone deficiency should be discontinued when the epiphyses are fused. Patients who fail to respond adequately while on Saizen® therapy should be evaluated to determine the cause of unresponsiveness.

To prevent possible contamination, wipe the rubber vial stopper with an antiseptic solution before puncturing it with the needle. It is recommended that Saizen® be administered using sterile, disposable syringes and needles. The syringes should be of small enough volume that the prescribed dose can be drawn from the vial with reasonable accuracy.

After determining the appropriate patient dose, reconstitute each 5 mg vial of Saizen® with 1–3 mL of Bacteriostatic Water for Injection, USP (Benzyl Alcohol preserved). For use in patients sensitive to the diluent see "WARNINGS."

To reconstitute Saizen®, inject the diluent into the vial of Saizen® aiming the liquid against the glass vial wall. Swirl the vial with a **GENTLE** rotary motion until contents are dissolved completely. **DO NOT SHAKE**. Because Saizen® growth hormone is a protein, shaking can result in a cloudy solution. The Saizen® solution should be clear immediately after reconstitution. **DO NOT INJECT** Saizen® if the reconstituted product is cloudy immediately after reconstitution or refrigeration. Occasionally, after refrigeration, small colorless particles may be present in the Saizen® solution. This is not unusual for proteins like Saizen®.

STABILITY AND STORAGE

Before Reconstitution—Saizen® [somatropin (rDNA origin) for injection] should be stored at room temperature (15°–30°C/59°–86°F). Expiration dates are stated on the labels.

After Reconstitution—When reconstituted with the diluent provided, the reconstituted solution should be stored under refrigeration (2°–8°C/36°–46°F) for up to 14 days. Avoid freezing reconstituted vials of Saizen®.

HOW SUPPLIED

Saizen® [somatropin (rDNA origin) for injection] is a sterile, non-pyrogenic, white, lyophilized powder supplied in packages containing:

1 vial of 5 mg (approximately 15 IU) Saizen® and 1 vial of 10 mL Bacteriostatic Water for Injection, USP (0.9% Benzyl Alcohol) NDC 44087-1005-2

1 vial of 8.8 mg (approximately 26.4 IU) Saizen® and 1 vial of 10 mL Bacteriostatic Water for Injection, USP (0.9% Benzyl Alcohol) NDC 44087-1088-1

Rx Only

Product information as of September 2000

Distributed by: Serono Laboratories, Inc., Randolph, MA 02368

®-Registered trademark of Serono Laboratories, Inc., Norwell, MA 02061

SEROPHENE® ℞

[se 'ro-fēn]

(clomiphene citrate tablets, USP)

DESCRIPTION

Each scored white tablet contains: clomiphene citrate, USP 50 mg. Clomiphene citrate is designated chemically as 2-[p-(2-chloro-1,2-diphenylvinyl) phenoxy] triethylamine dihydrogen citrate and is represented structurally as:

$$(C_2H_5)_2NCH_2CH_2O-C_6H_4-C(C_6H_5)=C(Cl)-C_6H_5 \cdot C_6H_8O_7$$

clomiphene citrate, USP (Serophene®)

As shown, one molecule of citric acid is chemically bound with one molecule of the organic base, clomiphene.

Clomiphene citrate is a chemical analog of other triarylethylene compounds such as chlorotrianisene and the cholesterol inhibitor, triparanol.

ACTIONS

Clomiphene citrate, an orally-administered, non-steroidal agent, may induce ovulation in selected anovulatory women. It is a drug of considerable pharmacologic potency. Careful evaluation and selection of the patient and close attention to the timing of the dose is mandatory prior to treatment with clomiphene citrate. Conservative selection and management of the patient contribute to successful therapy of anovulation. Clomiphene citrate induces ovulation in most selected anovulatory patients. The various criteria for ovulation include: an ovulation peak of estrogen excretion followed by a biphasic basal body temperature curve, urinary excretion of pregnanediol at post-ovulatory levels, and endometrial histologic findings characteristic of the luteal phase.

A review of eleven publications appearing between 1964 and 1978 showed that pregnancy occurred in 35% of 5,154 patients with ovulatory dysfunction who received clomiphene citrate.

[See table at bottom of next page]

Clomiphene citrate therapy appears to mediate ovulation through increased output of pituitary gonadotropins. These stimulate the maturation and endocrine activity of the ovarian follicle which is followed by the development and function of the corpus luteum. Increased urinary excretion of gonadotropins and estrogen suggests involvement of the pituitary.

Studies with ^{14}C labeled clomiphene citrate have shown that it is readily absorbed orally in humans and is excreted principally in the feces. An average of 51% of the administered dose was excreted after 5 days. After intravenous administration, 37% was excreted in 5 days. The appearance of ^{14}C in the feces six weeks after administration suggests that the remaining drug and/or metabolites are slowly excreted from a sequestered enterohepatic recirculation pool.

INDICATIONS

Clomiphene citrate is indicated for the treatment of ovulatory failure in patients desiring pregnancy and whose husbands are fertile and potent. Impediments to this goal must be excluded or adequately treated before beginning therapy.
Administration of clomiphene citrate is indicated only in patients with demonstrated ovulatory dysfunction and in whom the following conditions apply:

1. Normal liver function.
2. Physiologic indications of normal endogenous estrogen (as estimated from vaginal smears, endometrial biopsy, assay of serum [or urinary] estrogen, or from bleeding in response to progesterone). Reduced estrogen levels, while less favorable, do not prevent successful therapy.
3. Clomiphene citrate therapy is not effective for those patients with primary pituitary or ovarian failure. It cannot substitute for appropriate therapy of other disturbances leading to ovulatory dysfunction, e.g., diseases of the thyroid or adrenals.
4. Particularly careful evaluation prior to clomiphene citrate therapy should be done in patients with abnormal uterine bleeding. It is most important that neoplastic lesions are detected.

CONTRAINDICATIONS

Pregnancy:
Although no direct effect of clomiphene citrate therapy on the human fetus has been seen established, clomiphene citrate should not be administered in cases of suspected pregnancy as such effects have been reported in animals. To prevent inadvertent clomiphene citrate administration during early pregnancy, the basal body temperature should be recorded throughout all treatment cycles, and therapy should be discontinued if pregnancy is suspected. If the basal body temperature following clomiphene citrate is biphasic and is not followed by menses, the possibility of an ovarian cyst and/or pregnancy should be excluded. Until the correct diagnosis has been determined, the next course of therapy should be delayed.
Clomiphene citrate is also contraindicated in patients who have:

1. Uncontrolled thyroid or adrenal dysfunction.
2. An organic intracranial lesion such as a pituitary tumor.
3. Liver disease or a history of liver dysfunction.
4. Abnormal uterine bleeding of undetermined origin.
5. Ovarian cysts or enlargement not due to polycystic ovarian syndrome.

WARNINGS

Visual Symptoms:
Patients should be warned that blurring and/or other visual symptoms may occur occasionally with clomiphene citrate therapy. These may make activities such as driving or operating machinery more hazardous than usual, particularly under conditions of variable lighting. While their significance is not yet understood (see "Adverse Reactions"), patients having any visual symptoms should discontinue treatment and have a complete ophthalmologic evaluation.
Ovarian Hyperstimulation Syndrome:
The Ovarian Hyperstimulation Syndrome (OHSS) has been reported to occur in patients receiving drug therapy for ovulation induction, including in rare cases patients receiving clomiphene citrate therapy. OHSS is a medical event distinct from uncomplicated ovarian enlargement. OHSS may progress rapidly (within 24 hours to several days) to become a serious medical event. It is characterized by an apparent dramatic increase in vascular permeability which can result in a rapid accumulation of fluid in the peritoneal cavity, thorax, and potentially, the pericardium. The early warning signs of development of OHSS are severe pelvic pain, nausea, vomiting, and weight gain. The following symptomatology has been seen with cases of OHSS: abdominal pain, abdominal distension, gastrointestinal symptoms including nausea, vomiting and diarrhea, severe ovarian enlargement, weight gain, dyspnea, and oliguria. Clinical evaluation may reveal hypovolemia, hemoconcentration, electrolyte imbalances, ascites, hemoperitoneum, pleural effusions, hydrothorax, acute pulmonary distress, and thromboembolic phenomena. Transient liver function test abnormalities, suggestive of hepatic dysfunction, which may be accompanied by morphologic changes on liver biopsy, have been reported in association with the Ovarian Hyperstimulation Syndrome (OHSS).

PRECAUTIONS

Diagnosis Prior to Clomiphene Citrate Therapy:
Careful evaluation should be given to candidates for clomiphene citrate therapy. A complete pelvic examination should be performed prior to treatment and repeated before each subsequent course. Clomiphene citrate should not be given to patients with an ovarian cyst, as further ovarian enlargement may result.
Since the incidence of endometrial carcinoma and of ovulatory disorders increases with age, endometrial biopsy should always exclude the former as causative in such patients. If abnormal uterine bleeding is present, full diagnostic measures are necessary.
Ovarian Overstimulation During Treatment with Clomiphene Citrate:
To minimize the hazard associated with the occasional abnormal ovarian enlargement during clomiphene citrate therapy (see "Adverse Reactions"), the lowest dose producing good results should be chosen. Some patients with polycystic ovarian syndrome are unusually sensitive to gonadotropins and may have an exaggerated response to usual doses of clomiphene citrate. Maximal enlargement of the ovary, whether abnormal or physiologic, does not occur until several days after discontinuation of clomiphene citrate. The patient complaining of pelvic pains after receiving clomiphene citrate should be examined carefully. If enlargement of the ovary occurs, clomiphene citrate therapy should be withheld until the ovaries have returned to pretreatment size, and the dosage or duration of the next course should be reduced. The ovarian enlargement and cyst formation following clomiphene citrate therapy regress spontaneously within a few days or weeks after discontinuing treatment. Therefore, unless a strong indication for laparoscopy (or laparotomy) exists, such cystic enlargement always should be managed conservatively.
Multiple Pregnancy:
In the reviewed publications, the incidence of multiple pregnancies was increased during those cycles in which clomiphene citrate was given. Among the 1,803 pregnancies on which the outcome was reported, 90% were single and 10% twins. Less than 1% of the reported deliveries resulted in triplets or more.
Of these multiple pregnancies, 96-99% resulted in the births of live infants. The patient and her husband should be advised of the frequency and potential hazards of multiple pregnancy before starting treatment.
Additional Precautions:
Prolonged use of clomiphene may increase the risk of a borderline or invasive ovarian tumor.

ADVERSE REACTIONS

At the recommended dosage of clomiphene citrate, side effects occur infrequently and generally do not interfere with treatment. Adverse reactions tend to occur more frequently at higher doses and in the longer treatment courses used in some early studies.
The most frequent adverse reactions to clomiphene citrate include ovarian enlargement (approximately 1 in 7 patients), vasomotor flushes resembling menopausal symptoms which are not usually severe and promptly disappear after treatment is discontinued (approximately 1 in 10 patients), and abdominal discomfort (approximately 1 in 15 patients). Adverse reactions which occur less frequently (approximately 1 in 50 patients or more) include breast tenderness, nausea and vomiting, nervousness, insomnia, and visual disturbances. Other side effects which occur in less than 1 in 100 patients include headache, dizziness and light-headedness, increased urination, depression, fatigue, urticaria and allergic dermatitis, abnormal uterine bleeding, weight gain, ovarian cysts (ovarian enlargement or cysts could, as such, be complicated by adnexal torsion), and reversible hair loss.
Thromboembolic events, such as pulmonary embolism, arterial occlusion, and phlebitis, have been reported rarely in patients treated with clomiphene citrate. It is not clear what, if any, relationship these events have to clomiphene citrate therapy.
When clomiphene citrate is administered at the recommended dose, abnormal ovarian enlargement (see "Precautions") is infrequent, although the usual cyclic variation in ovarian size may be exaggerated. Similarly, mid-cycle ovarian pain (mittelschmerz) may be accentuated.
With prolonged or higher dosage, ovarian enlargement and cyst formation (usually luteal) may occur more often, and the luteal phase of the cycle may be prolonged. Patients with polycystic ovarian syndrome may be unusually sensitive to clomiphene therapy. Rare occurrences of massive ovarian enlargement have been reported, for example, in a patient with polycystic ovarian syndrome whose clomiphene citrate therapy consisted of 100 mg daily for 14 days. Since abnormal ovarian enlargement usually regresses spontaneously, most of these patients should be treated conservatively. The Ovarian Hyperstimulation Syndrome has been reported to occur in rare cases in patients receiving clomiphene citrate therapy (see "Warnings").
The incidence of visual symptoms (see "Warnings" for further recommendations), usually described as "blurring" or spots or flashes (scintillating scotomata), correlates with increasing total dose. Other visual symptoms which may occur include diplopia, phosphenes, photophobia, decreased visual acuity, loss of peripheral vision, and spatial distortion. The symptoms disappear usually within a few days or weeks after clomiphene citrate is discontinued. This may be due to intensification and/or prolongation of after-images. Symptoms often appear first, or are accentuated, upon exposure to a more brightly lit environment.
While measured visual acuity generally has not been affected, in one patient taking 200 mg daily, visual blurring developed on the seventh day of treatment and progressed to severe diminution of visual acuity by the tenth day. No other abnormality was coincident, and the visual acuity was normal by the third day after treatment was stopped. Ophthalmologically definable scotomata and electroretinographic retinal function changes have also been reported.
BSP Laboratory Studies:
Greater than 5% retention of sulfobromophthalein (BSP) has been reported in approximately 10% to 20% of patients in whom it was measured. Retention was usually minimal but was elevated during prolonged clomiphene citrate administration or with apparently unrelated liver disease. In some patients, pre-existing BSP retention decreased even though clomiphene citrate therapy was continued. Other liver function tests were usually normal.
Other Laboratory Studies:
Clomiphene citrate has not been reported to cause a significant abnormality in hematologic or renal tests, in protein bound iodine, or in serum cholesterol levels.
Birth Defects:
The following medical events have been reported subsequent to pregnancies following ovulation induction therapy with clomiphene citrate: ectopic pregnancy and congenital abnormalities such as syndactyly, polydactyly, congenital heart defects, retinal aplasia, hypospadias, ovarian dysplasia, cleft lip/palate, microencephaly and neural tube defects, including anencephaly. Some medical literature reports have implied an increased occurrence of neural tube defects, while others indicate that an increased incidence over that found in the general population does not exist. One case of a congenital abnormality (adactyly) in an infant exposed to clomiphene citrate in utero has been reported.
Of 1,803 births following clomiphene citrate administration, 45 infants with birth defects were reported for a cumulative rate of 2.5%.
Six cases of Down's syndrome, one neonatal death with multiple malformations, and one case of each of the following were reported: club-foot, tibial torsion, blocked tear duct, and hemangioma. The other congenital abnormalities were not described. The investigators did not report that these were presumed to be due to therapy. The cumulative rate of congenital abnormalities does not exceed that reported in the general population.
Ovarian cancer has been reported in a very small number of infertile women who have been treated with clomiphene citrate. A causal relationship between treatment with clomiphene citrate and ovarian cancer has not been established.

DOSAGE AND ADMINISTRATION

General Considerations:
Physicians experienced in managing gynecologic or endocrine disorders should supervise the work-up and treatment of candidate patients for clomiphene citrate therapy. Patients should be chosen for clomiphene citrate therapy only after careful diagnostic evaluation (see "Indications"). The plan of therapy should be outlined in advance. Impediments to achieving the goal of therapy must be excluded or adequately treated before beginning clomiphene citrate.
In determining a starting dose schedule, efficacy must be balanced against potential side effects. For example, the available data so far suggest that ovulation and pregnancy are slightly more attainable with 100 mg/day for 5 days than with 50 mg/day for 5 days. As the dosage is increased, however, ovarian overstimulation and other side effects may be expected to increase. Although the data do not yet establish a relationship between dose level and multiple births, it is reasonable that such a correlation exists on pharmacologic grounds.
For these reasons, treatment of the usual patient should initiate with a 50 mg daily dose for 5 days. The dose may be increased only in those patients who do not respond to the

Continued on next page

PREGNANCIES FOLLOWING CLOMIPHENE CITRATE, USP[a]		(Range)
Number of Patients	= 5,154	
Percent of Patients Ovulating[b]	= 75	(50-94%)
Percent of Ovulatory Cycles	= 53	(33-69%)
Percent of Patients Pregnant	= 35	(11-52%)
Percent Patients Pregnant / Percent Patients Ovulating	= 46	(22-61%)
Percent Live Births	= 86	(74-99.8%)
Percent Abortions	= 14	(0.2-26%)
Percent of Single Births	= 90	(67-100%)
Percent Surviving	= 99	(98.2-100%)
Percent of Multiple Births	= 10	(0-33%)
Percent Surviving	= 96	(82-100%)

a) includes patients receiving other than recommended dosage regimen.
b) average from studies.

Serophene—Cont.

first course (see "Recommended Dosage"). Special treatment with lower dosage over shorter duration is particularly recommended if unusual sensitivity to pituitary gonadotropin is suspected, including patients with polycystic ovarian syndrome (see "Precautions").

Recommended Dosage:
The recommended dosage for the first course of clomiphene citrate is 50 mg (1 tablet) daily for 5 days. Therapy may be started at any time if the patient has had no recent uterine bleeding. If progestin-induced bleeding is intended, or if spontaneous uterine bleeding occurs prior to therapy, the regimen of 50 mg daily for 5 days should be started on or about the fifth day of the cycle. When ovulation occurs at this dosage, there is no advantage to increasing the dose in subsequent cycles of treatment. If ovulation does not appear to have occurred after the first course of therapy, a second course of 100 mg daily (two 50 mg tablets given as a single daily dose) for 5 days may be started. This course may begin as early as 30 days after the previous one. It is recommended that the patient be examined for pregnancy, ovarian enlargement, or cyst formation between each treatment cycle. Increasing the dosage or duration of therapy beyond 100 mg/day for 5 days should not be undertaken.
The majority of patients who respond do so during the first course of therapy, and 3 courses constitute an adequate therapeutic trial. If ovulatory menses do not occur, the diagnosis should be re-evaluated. Treatment beyond this is not recommended in the patient who does not exhibit evidence of ovulation.

Pregnancy:
Properly timed coitus is very important for good results. For regularity of cyclic ovulatory response, it is also important that each course of clomiphene citrate be started on or about the fifth day of the cycle, once ovulation has been established. As with other therapeutic modalities, Serophene® therapy follows the rule of diminishing returns, such that the likelihood of conception diminishes with each succeeding course of therapy. If pregnancy has not been achieved after 3 ovulatory responses to Serophene®, further treatment generally is not recommended. Before starting treatment, patients should be advised of the possibility and potential hazards of multiple pregnancy if conception occurs following clomiphene citrate therapy.

Long-Term Cyclic Therapy —Not Recommended:
Since the relative safety of long-term cyclic therapy has not yet been demonstrated conclusively, and since the majority of patients will ovulate following 3 courses, long-term cyclic therapy is not recommended.

HOW SUPPLIED

Serophene® is available as 50 mg scored white tablets in the following package combinations:
• 1 carton 10 tablets, NDC 44087-8090-6
Each carton contains 2 strips of 5 tablets each.
• 1 carton 30 tablets, NDC 44087-8090-1
Each carton contains 3 strips of 10 tablets, each in a 2 × 5 arrangement.
Protect from light, moisture, and excessive heat. Dispense in well-closed, light resistant container as defined in the USP, with child resistant closure. Store at room temperature (15°–30°C/59°–86°F).
Caution: Federal law prohibits dispensing without prescription.

Manufactured for:
SERONO LABORATORIES, INC.
Randolph, MA 02368 USA
by: TEVA PHARMACEUTICAL INDUSTRIES LTD.
Jerusalem 91010, Israel
Revised: November 1994

SEROSTIM® ℞
[serō-stim]
[somatropin (rDNA origin) for injection]

DESCRIPTION

Serostim® [somatropin (rDNA origin) for injection] is a human growth hormone produced by recombinant DNA technology. Serostim® has 191 amino acid residues and a molecular weight of 22,125 daltons. Its amino acid sequence and structure are identical to the dominant form of human pituitary growth hormone. Serostim® is produced by a mammalian cell line (mouse C127) that has been modified by the addition of the human growth hormone gene. Serostim® is secreted directly through the cell membrane into the cell-culture medium for collection and purification.
Serostim® is a highly purified preparation. Biological potency is determined by measuring the increase in the body weight induced in hypophysectomized rats.
Serostim® is available in 4 mg, 5 mg and 6 mg vials for single dose administration. Each 4 mg vial contains 4.0 mg (approximately 12 IU) somatropin, 27.3 mg sucrose, 0.9 mg phosphoric acid. Each 5 mg vial contains 5.0 mg (approximately 15 IU) somatropin, 34.2 mg sucrose and 1.2 mg phosphoric acid. Each 6 mg vial contains 6.0 mg (approximately 18 IU) somatropin, 41.0 mg sucrose and 1.4 mg phosphoric acid. The pH is adjusted with sodium hydroxide or phosphoric acid to give a pH of 7.4 to 8.5 after reconstitution.

CLINICAL PHARMACOLOGY

Serostim® [somatropin (rDNA origin) for injection] is an anabolic and anticatabolic agent which exerts its influence by interacting with specific receptors on a variety of cell types including myocytes, hepatocytes, adipocytes, lymphocytes, and hematopoietic cells. Some, but not all, of its effects are mediated by another class of hormones known as somatomedins (IGF-1 and IGF-2).
AIDS-associated wasting is a metabolic disorder characterized by abnormalities of intermediary metabolism resulting in weight loss, inappropriate depletion of lean body mass (LBM), and paradoxical preservation of body fat. LBM includes primarily skeletal muscle, organ tissue, blood and blood constituents, and both intracellular and extracellular water. Depletion of LBM results in muscle weakness, organ failure, and death. Unlike nutritional intervention for AIDS-associated wasting, in which supplemental calories are converted predominantly to body fat, Serostim® treatment resulted in an increase in LBM and a decrease in body fat with a significant increase in body weight due to the dominant effect of LBM gain.

Effects on Protein, Lipid, and Carbohydrate Metabolism:
A one-week study in 6 patients with HIV associated wasting has shown that treatment with Serostim® improves nitrogen balance, increases protein-sparing lipid oxidation, and has little effect on overall carbohydrate metabolism.

Lean Body Mass Accrual:
In the same study, treatment with Serostim® resulted in the retention of phosphorous, potassium, nitrogen, and sodium. The ratio of retained potassium and nitrogen during Serostim® therapy was consistent with retention of these elements in lean tissue. In clinical studies (12 weeks), Serostim® significantly increased lean body mass. There was also a proportionate increase in intracellular and extracellular fluid during Serostim® therapy suggesting accretion of normally hydrated lean body tissue.

Physical Performance:
Treadmill performance was examined in a 12-week placebo-controlled study. Work output improved significantly in the Serostim®-treated group after 12 weeks of therapy and was correlated with LBM. No such correlation was seen with body fat. Isometric muscle performance, as measured by grip strength dynamometry, declined, probably as a result of a transient increase in tissue turgor known to occur with r-hGH therapy.

PHARMACOKINETICS

Subcutaneous Absorption: The absolute bioavailability of Serostim® [somatropin (rDNA origin) for injection] after subcutaneous administration of a formulation not equivalent to the marketed formulation was determined to be 70–90%. The $t^1/_2$ (Mean ± SD) after subcutaneous administration is significantly longer than that seen after intravenous administration to normal male volunteers, down-regulated with somatostatin (3.94 ± 3.44 hrs. vs. 0.58 ± 0.08 hrs.), indicating that the subcutaneous absorption of the clinically tested formulation of the compound is slow and rate-limiting.

Distribution: The steady-state volume of distribution (Mean ± SD) following IV administration of Serostim® in healthy volunteers is 12.0 ± 1.08 L.

Metabolism: Although the liver plays a role in the metabolism of growth hormone, GH is primarily cleaved in the kidney. GH undergoes glomerular filtration and after cleavage within the renal cells, the peptides and amino acids are returned to the systemic circulation.

Elimination: The $t^1/_2$ (Mean ± SD) in nine patients with AIDS related wasting with an average weight of 56.7 ± 6.8 kg, given a fixed dose of 6.0 mg r-hGH subcutaneously was 4.28 ± 2.15 hrs. The renal clearance of r-hGH after subcutaneous administration in nine patients with AIDS related wasting was 0.0015 ± 0.0037 L/h. No significant accumulation of r-hGH appears to occur after 6 weeks of dosing as indicated.

Special Populations:

Pediatric: Available evidence suggests that r-hGH clearances are similar in adults and children, but no clinical studies were conducted in children with acquired immune deficiency syndrome or AIDS-related complex.

Gender: Biomedical literature indicates that a gender-related difference in the mean clearance of r-hGH could exist (Clearance of r-hGH in males > Clearance of r-hGH in females). However, no gender-based analysis is available on Serostim® in normal volunteers or patients infected with HIV.

Race: No data are available.

Renal Insufficiency: It has been reported that individuals with chronic renal failure tend to have decreased hGH clearance compared to normals, but there are no data on Serostim® use in the presence of renal insufficiency.

Hepatic Insufficiency: A reduction in r-hGH clearance has been noted in patients with severe liver dysfunction. However, the clinical significance of this in HIV+ patients is unknown.

CLINICAL STUDIES

The clinical efficacy of Serostim® [somatropin (rDNA origin) for injection] was assessed in two placebo-controlled clinical trials. Of the 205 AIDS subjects exposed to GH, only 5 were women. All study subjects received concomitant anti-HIV therapy.

Clinical Trial 1: A multicenter, double-blind, placebo-controlled study compared Serostim® at an average daily dose of 0.1 mg/kg/day administered subcutaneously to placebo in 178 patients with AIDS wasting. The study participants had unintentional weight loss of at least 10% or weighed less than 90% of the lower limit of ideal body weight. In the 140 evaluable patients (those completing a 12-week course of treatment and who were at least 80% compliant with study drug; Serostim® =69, Placebo = 71), the mean difference in weight increase in the Serostim®- treated group was 1.6 kg (3.5 lb). For those patients that had a week two assessment, 76% had weight gain. After 12 weeks of treatment, 74% of the patients treated with Serostim® gained weight while only 48% of the placebo-treated patients gained weight (p=0.002). Mean differences in lean body mass change between the Serostim® treated group and the placebo treated group was 3.1 kg (6.8 lbs) as measured by DEXA. Significant lean body mass gain ($p<0.05$) was achieved in 70% of the patients treated with Serostim® after 12 weeks (see Table 1). No change in LBM was observed in placebo-treated patients. Mean increase in weight and lean body mass and mean decrease in body fat (see Figure 1) were significantly greater in the Serostim® treated group than in the placebo group (p=0.011, $p<0.001$, $p<0.001$, respectively). While depletion of body weight and lean body mass has been associated with increased morbidity and mortality, the clinical significance of treatment-induced weight gain and LBM accrual has yet to be established.
Treatment with Serostim® resulted in a significant increase of physical function as assessed by treadmill exercise testing. The median treadmill work output increased by 13% (p=0.039) at 12 weeks in the group receiving Serostim® (see Figure 2). There was no improvement in the placebo treated group at 12 weeks. Changes in treadmill performance were significantly correlated with changes of lean body mass.
The most common reason for patient drop-out was concurrent medical events including opportunistic infections. There were decreases in serum albumin in both Serostim® and placebo groups. There was up to a 2.7 fold increase in serum IGF-1 levels. No patients developed antibodies to growth hormone.
Patients completing the 12–week placebo-controlled portion of the study were eligible to receive open-label Serostim® therapy, and 96% (n=136) chose to participate. Since this phase of the trial was open-label, and due to limited numbers of evaluable patients, it is difficult to interpret weight and LBM changes. The patients who initially received placebo had significant increases in median weight (1.4 kg, p=0.012) and lean body mass (2.4 kg, $p<0.001$) compared to baseline, during their first 12-weeks on Serostim®. These changes were similar in magnitude to those observed in patients initially treated with Serostim®. For those patients who had initially received Serostim® in the placebo-controlled trials, the median weight change during 12-weeks of open label treatment with Serostim® (-0.2 kg) and LBM change (-0.3 kg) were not significant (p=0.700 and p=0.661, respectively), suggesting that the gains of weight and LBM were not lost.

Figure 1: Trial 1: Mean Changes in Body Composition

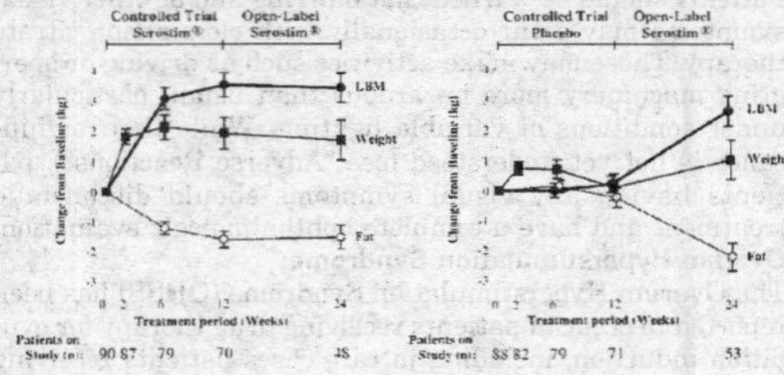

Table 1: Trial 1: Change from Baseline of LBM 12-Week Efficacy Results

	Serostim®		Placebo	
	n	Results	n	Results
Lean Body Mass (kg)	69	+3.1*	69	-0.1
LBM Responders‡	69	70%*	69	12%

‡Major LBM response defined as >4% increase of LBM
*Statistically significantly different from placebo at $p<0.05$
[See figure at top of next column]

Clinical Trial 2: Additional efficacy and safety parameters were evaluated in a second multicenter, double-blind, placebo-controlled study comparing Serostim®, 6 mg/day administered subcutaneously vs. placebo, in AIDS patients with wasting enrolled 177 patients who were randomized in a 2:1 ratio, to receive Serostim® or placebo. In the 78 evaluable patients (those completing a 12-week course of treatment and who were at least 80% compliant with study drug), there was a mean increase in body weight of 1.6 kg, but this change was not significant compared to placebo (p=0.110). The most common reason for patient drop-out was concurrent medical events including opportunistic infections.
Patients were asked to respond to a nine item survey that measured subjective assessments of treatment. Positive findings at 6 and 12 weeks were observed in two of the nine items (change in appearance and overall benefit of treatment). Results of other measures were inconclusive.

Figure 2: Median Treadmill Work Output

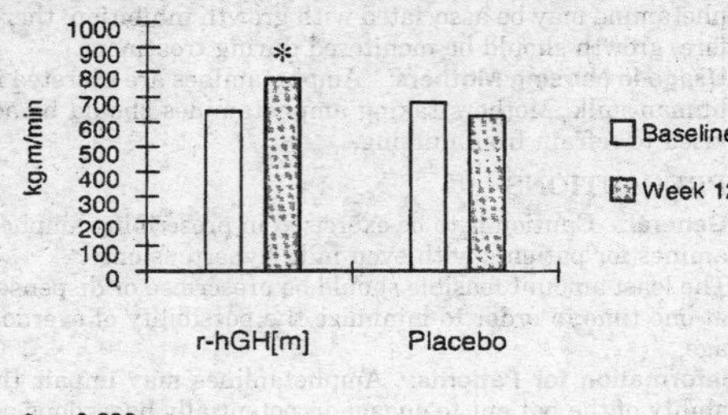

*p = 0.039

Survival Analyses: The two placebo-controlled clinical trials of Serostim® in patients with AIDS wasting up to 12 weeks in length found no difference in survival between groups.

Clinical Trial 3: A third open-label, baseline-controlled, multicenter study conducted in Europe administering Serostim®, 6 mg/day subcutaneously, enrolled 24 patients with AIDS wasting. Twenty patients completed the 12-week treatment regimen and had body composition measurements using bioimpedance analysis. The mean increase over baseline for body weight was 1.6 kg (p=0.137, NS) and for lean body mass was 2.3 kg (p=0.037).

INDICATIONS AND USAGE

Serostim® [somatropin (rDNA origin) for injection] is indicated for the treatment of AIDS wasting or cachexia. This indication is based on analyses of surrogate endpoints in studies of up to 12 weeks in duration. Concomitant antiviral therapy is necessary (see PRECAUTIONS: GENERAL). The continued use of Serostim® treatment should be reevaluated in patients who continue to lose weight in the first two weeks of treatment.

CONTRAINDICATIONS

Growth hormone should not be initiated to treat patients with acute critical illness due to complications following open heart or abdominal surgery, multiple accidental trauma or to patients having acute respiratory failure. Two placebo-controlled clinical trials in non-growth hormone deficient adult patients (n=522) with these conditions revealed a significant increase in mortality (41.9% vs. 19.3%) among somatropin treated patients (doses 5.3–8 mg///day) compared to those receiving placebo (see WARNINGS).

Serostim® [somatropin (rDNA origin) for injection] is contraindicated in patients with a known hypersensitivity to growth hormone.

WARNING

See CONTRAINDICATIONS for information on increased mortality in patients with acute critical illnesses in intensive care units due to complications following open heart or abdominal surgery, multiple accidental trauma or with acute respiratory failure. The safety of continuing growth hormone treatment in patients receiving replacement doses for approved indications who concurrently develop these illnesses has not been established. Therefore, the potential benefit of treatment continuation with growth hormone in patients having acute critical illnesses should be weighed against the potential risk.

PRECAUTIONS

General: Serostim® [somatropin (rDNA origin) for injection] therapy should be carried out under the regular guidance of a physician who is experienced in the diagnosis and management of AIDS. Inadequate nutritional intake, malabsorption and hypogonadism, which are common in individuals with AIDS and which may contribute to catabolism and weight loss, should also be monitored and treated.

HIV and Growth Hormone Considerations: In some experimental systems, recombinant human Growth Hormone (r-hGH) has been shown to potentiate HIV replication in vitro at concentrations ranging from 50–250 ng/ml. There was no increase in virus production when the antiretroviral agents, zidovudine, didanosine or lamivudine were added to the culture medium. Additional in vitro studies have shown that r-hGH does not interfere with the antiviral activity of zalcitabine or stavudine. In the controlled clinical trials, no significant growth hormone-associated increase in viral burden was observed. However, the protocol required all participants to be on concomitant nucleoside analogue therapy for the duration of the study. In view of the potential for acceleration of virus replication, it is recommended that HIV+ patients be maintained on nucleoside analogue therapy for the duration of Serostim® treatment.

Increased tissue turgor (swelling, particularly in the hands and feet) and musculoskeletal discomfort (pain, swelling and/or stiffness) may occur during treatment with Serostim®, but may resolve spontaneously, with analgesic therapy, or after reducing the frequency of dosing (see Dosage and Administration).

Carpal tunnel syndrome may occur during treatment with Serostim®. If the symptoms of carpal tunnel syndrome do not resolve by decreasing the weekly number of doses of Serostim®, it is recommended that treatment be discontinued. Patients should be informed that allergic reactions are possible and that prompt medical attention should be sought if an allergic reaction occurs. None of the 188 study participants with AIDS wasting who were evaluable for antibody assessments and who were treated with Serostim® for the first time developed detectable antibodies to growth hormone (> 4 pg binding). Patients were not rechallenged.

Recombinant Human Growth Hormone (r-hGH) has been associated with acute pancreatitis.

Hyperglycemia may occur in HIV-infected individuals due to a variety of reasons. Serostim® use was associated with a minimal increase of mean blood glucose concentration. Patients with other risk factors for glucose intolerance should be monitored closely during Serostim® therapy.

No cases of intracranial hypertension (IH) have been observed among patients with AIDS wasting treated with Serostim®. The syndrome of IH, with papilledema, visual changes, headache, and nausea and/or vomiting has been reported in a small number of children with growth failure treated with growth hormone products. Nevertheless, funduscopic evaluation of patients is recommended at the initiation and periodically during the course of Serostim® therapy.

Kaposi's sarcoma, lymphoma, and other malignancies are common in HIV+ individuals. There was no increase in the incidence of Kaposi's sarcoma, lymphoma, or in the progression of cutaneous Kaposi's sarcoma in clinical studies of Serostim®. Patients with internal KS lesions were excluded from the studies. Potential effects on other malignancies are unknown.

Information For Patients: Patients being treated with Serostim® should be informed of the potential benefits and risks associated with treatment. Patients should be instructed to contact their physician should they experience any side effects or discomfort during treatment with Serostim®.

It is recommended that Serostim® be administered using sterile, disposable syringes and needles. Patients should be thoroughly instructed in the importance of proper disposal and cautioned against any reuse of needles and syringes. An appropriate container for the disposal of used syringes and needles should be employed.

Patients should be instructed to rotate injection sites to avoid localized tissue atrophy.

Drug Interactions: Formal in vitro drug interaction studies have not been conducted. No data are available on drug interactions between Serostim® and HIV protease inhibitors or the non-nucleoside reverse transcriptase inhibitors.

Carcinogenesis, Mutagenesis, Impairment of Fertility: Long-term animal studies for carcinogenicity have not been performed with Serostim®. There is no evidence from animal studies to date of Serostim®-induced mutagenicity or impairment of fertility.

Pregnancy: Pregnancy Category B. Reproduction studies have been performed in rats and rabbits. Doses up to 5 to 10 times the human dose, based on body surface area, have revealed no evidence of impaired fertility or harm to the fetus due to Serostim®. There are, however, no adequate and well controlled studies in pregnant women. Because animal reproduction studies are not always predictive of human response, this drug should be used during pregnancy only if clearly needed.

Nursing Women: It is not known whether Serostim® is excreted in human milk. Because many drugs are excreted in human milk, caution should be exercised when Serostim® is administered to a nursing woman.

Pediatric Use: In two small studies, 11 children with HIV associated failure to thrive were treated subcutaneously with human growth hormone. In one study, five children (age range, 6 to 17 years) were treated with 0.04 mg/kg/day for 26 weeks. In a second study, six children (age range, 8 to 14 years) were treated with 0.07 mg/kg/day for 4 weeks. Treatment appeared to be well tolerated in both studies. These preliminary data collected on a limited number of patients with HIV associated failure to thrive appear to be consistent with safety observations in growth hormone treated adults with AIDS wasting.

Geriatic Use: Clinical studies with Serostim® did not include sufficient numbers of subjects aged 65 and over to determine whether they respond differently from younger subjects. Elderly patients are more sensitive to growth hormone action, and may be more prone to develop adverse reactions. Thus, dose selection for an elderly patient should be cautious, usually starting at the low end of the dosing range.

ADVERSE REACTIONS

In two placebo-controlled clinical trials in which 205 patients were treated with Serostim® [somatropin (rDNA origin) for injection] the most common adverse reactions judged to be associated with Serostim® were musculoskeletal discomfort and increased tissue turgor (swelling, particularly of the hands or feet) (see PRECAUTIONS: GENERAL). These symptoms were generally rated by investigators as mild to moderate in severity and usually subsided with continued treatment. Discontinuations as a result of these events were rare.

Because of the diverse clinical manifestations of AIDS, and the frequent occurrence of adverse events associated with underlying disease process, it was often difficult to distinguish adverse events possibly associated with the administration of Serostim® from underlying signs or symptoms of AIDS or associated intercurrent illnesses.

Clinical adverse events which occurred during the first 12 weeks of study in at least 10% of those who received Serostim® during the two placebo-controlled trials are listed below by treatment group, without regard to causality assessment.

Table 2: Controlled Trials Adverse Events

Adverse Event	Serostim® (n=205) %	Placebo (n=150) %
Musculoskeletal discomfort	53.7	33.3
Fever	31.2	29.3
Increased tissue turgor	27.3	2.7
Diarrhea	25.9	20.0
Neuropathy	25.9	17.3
Nausea	25.9	16.0
Headache	19.0	20.7
Abdominal pain	17.1	18.7
Fatigue	17.1	16.0
Leukopenia	15.1	24.7
Albuminuria	15.1	9.3
Granulocytopenia	14.1	21.3
Lymphadenopathy	14.1	16.0
Increased sweating	14.1	8.7
Anorexia	12.2	9.3
Anemia	12.2	8.7
Vomiting	11.7	12.0
SGOT increased	11.7	6.0
Insomnia	11.2	9.3
Tachycardia	11.2	6.0
Hyperglycemia	10.2	6.0
SGPT increased	10.2	5.3

Adverse events that occurred in 1% to less than 10% of study participants receiving Serostim® in the two placebo-controlled clinical efficacy studies are listed below by body system. The list of adverse events has been compiled regardless of causal relationship to Serostim®.

Body as a Whole: rigors, flu-like symptoms, back pain, malaise, asthenia, carpal tunnel syndrome (see PRECAUTIONS: GENERAL), chest pain, hot flashes, allergic reaction.

Gastrointestinal System: oral leukoplakia, flatulence, dyspepsia, dry mouth, constipation, ulcerative stomatitis, increased amylase, dysphagia, esophagitis, colitis, pancreatitis, rectal disorder, gastritis, tongue ulceration, gingivitis

Musculoskeletal System: muscle weakness

Central and Peripheral Nervous System: dizziness, convulsions, hypertonia, neuralgia, tremor, encephalopathy, nystagmus, meningism

Respiratory System: dyspnea, coughing, sinusitis, upper respiratory tract infection, pharyngitis, rhinitis, pneumonia, bronchitis, increased sputum, respiratory disorder, bronchospasm, pneumonitis, pleurisy

White Blood Cell and Reticuloendothelial System Disorders: cervical lymphadenopathy, eosinophilia

Skin and appendages: skin disorder, folliculitis, rash, alopecia, photosensitivity reaction, erythematous rash, pruritus, abnormal pigmentation, seborrhea, dermatitis, skin ulceration, acne, skin discoloration, verruca

Psychiatric: depression, anxiety, somnolence, nervousness, appetite increased, amnesia, abnormal thinking

Metabolic and Nutritional: hypertriglyceridemia, increased alkaline phosphatase, dehydration, increased creatine phosphokinase, increased LDH, glycosuria, hypokalemia, cachexia, thirst, acidosis

Immune System Dysfunction: moniliasis, bacterial infection, Pneumocystis carinii infection, viral infection, infection, Herpes simplex, sepsis, abscess, fungal infection, Herpes zoster

Urinary System: hematuria, urinary tract infection, nocturia

Liver and Biliary System: abnormal hepatic function, hepatomegaly, hepatitis

Vision: retinitis, abnormal vision, photophobia

Platelet, Bleeding and Clotting: thrombocytopenia, purpura

Cardiovascular, General: abnormal ECG, heart murmur, hypertension, hypotension

Application Site: injection site pain, injection site reaction

Neoplasms: Kaposi's sarcoma

Male Reproductive: Epididymitis, penis disorder, inguinal hernia

Hearing and Vestibular: earache, ear disorder, decreasing hearing

Endocrine: gynecomastia, male breast pain

The types and incidence of adverse events reported in an open-label, extension trial and in a single, foreign trial, for up to one year, were not different from, or greater in frequency, than those observed in the primary, placebo-controlled, clinical trials.

OVERDOSAGE

Glucose intolerance can occur with overdosage. Long-term overdosage with growth hormone could result in signs and symptoms of acromegaly.

DOSAGE AND ADMINISTRATION

Serostim® [somatropin (rDNA origin) for injection] should be administered subcutaneously daily at bedtime according to the following dosage recommendations.

Continued on next page

Serostim—Cont.

Weight Range	Dose*
>55 kg	6 mg SC daily
45–55 kg	5 mg SC daily
35–45 kg	4 mg SC daily

* Based on an approximate daily dosage of 0.1 mg/kg.

In patients who weigh less than 35 kg, Serostim® should be administered at a dose of 0.1 mg/kg subcutaneously daily at bedtime.
Dose reductions for side effects felt to be related to treatment with Serostim®, which are unresponsive to symptomatic treatment, may be affected by reducing the total daily dose or the number of doses given per week.
In patients who continue to lose weight at week 2, reevaluate for concurrent opportunistic infections or other clinical events.
Injection sites should be rotated.
Safety and effectiveness in pediatric patients with AIDS have not been established.
Each vial of Serostim® 4 mg, 5 mg or 6 mg is reconstituted with 1 mL sterile water for injection.
To reconstitute Serostim®, inject the diluent into the vial of Serostim® aiming the liquid against the glass vial wall. Swirl the vial with a gentle rotary motion until contents are dissolved completely. The Serostim® solution should be clear immediately after reconstitution. **DO NOT INJECT** Serostim® if the reconstituted product is cloudy immediately after reconstitution or refrigeration. Occasionally, after refrigeration, small colorless particles may be present in the Serostim® solution. This is not unusual for proteins like Serostim®.

STABILITY AND STORAGE

Before reconstitution: Serostim® [somatropin (rDNA origin) for injection] should be stored at room temperature, 59°–86°F (15°–30°C). Expiration dates are stated on product labels.
After reconstitution: Use within 24 hours after reconstitution with diluent. The reconstituted solution should be stored under refrigerated conditions (36°–46°F/2°–8°C).
Sterile Diluent, 1 mL (Sterile Water for Injection, USP) should be stored at room temperature, 59°–86°F (15°–30°C).
Avoid freezing vials of Serostim® and Sterile Diluent.

HOW SUPPLIED

Serostim® [somatropin (rDNA origin) for injection] is available in the following forms:

Serostim® vials containing 4 mg (approximately 12 IU) somatropin (mammalian-cell) with Sterile Water for Injection, USP. Package of 7 vials. NDC 44087-0004-7

Serostim® vials containing 5 mg (approximately 15 IU) somatropin (mammalian-cell) with Sterile Water for Injection, USP. Package of 7 vials. NDC 44087-0005-7

Serostim® vials containing 6 mg (approximately 18 IU) somatropin (mammalian-cell) with Sterile Water for Injection, USP. Package of 7 vials. NDC 44087-0006-7

Manufactured for: Serono Laboratories, Inc., Randolph, MA 02368

Rx Only
August 2000

EDUCATIONAL MATERIAL

Access the Serono website www.seronousa.com for product, educational, and service information for practitioners and consumers.
To receive available educational and medical literature about Serono products, or the conditions they treat, phone inquiries can be made by calling the Product Information and Surveillance Group at (888) 275-7376 or (781) 982-9000 X 5562.
To obtain information about scientific, medical, nursing and consumer educational meetings and materials, please contact Serono Symposia USA, Inc., (800) 283-8088, X 2352.

For EMERGENCY telephone numbers, consult the **Manufacturers' Index.**

Shire Richwood Inc.

**7900 TANNERS GATE DRIVE, SUITE 200
FLORENCE, KY 41042**

(For product information see Shire US Inc.)

Shire US Inc.

**7900 TANNERS GATE DRIVE, SUITE 200
FLORENCE, KY 41042**

Direct Inquiries to:
Customer Service
(800) 536-7878
(859) 282-2100
FAX: (859) 282-2118

For Medical Information Contact:
(800) 536-7878

ADDERALL® TABLETS Ⓒ℞

AMPHETAMINES HAVE A HIGH POTENTIAL FOR ABUSE. ADMINISTRATION OF AMPHETAMINES FOR PROLONGED PERIODS OF TIME MAY LEAD TO DRUG DEPENDENCE AND MUST BE AVOIDED. PARTICULAR ATTENTION SHOULD BE PAID TO THE POSSIBILITY OF SUBJECTS OBTAINING AMPHETAMINES FOR NON-THERAPEUTIC USE OR DISTRIBUTION TO OTHERS, AND THE DRUGS SHOULD BE PRESCRIBED OR DISPENSED SPARINGLY.

DESCRIPTION

A single entity amphetamine product combining the neutral sulfate salts of dextroamphetamine and amphetamine, with the dextro isomer of amphetamine saccharate and d, l-amphetamine aspartate.
[See table below]
Inactive ingredients: sucrose, lactose, corn starch, acacia and magnesium stearate.
Colors: ADDERALL 5 mg and 10 mg contain FD & C Blue #1
ADDERALL 20 mg and 30 mg contain FD & C Yellow #6 as a color additive.

CLINICAL PHARMACOLOGY

Amphetamines are non-catecholamine sympathomimetic amines with CNS stimulant activity. Peripheral actions include elevation of systolic and diastolic blood pressures and weak bronchodilator and respiratory stimulant action.
There is neither specific evidence which clearly establishes the mechanism whereby amphetamine produces mental and behavioral effects in children, nor conclusive evidence regarding how these effects relate to the condition of the central nervous system.

INDICATIONS

Attention Deficit Disorder with Hyperactivity: Adderall is indicated as an integral part of a total treatment program which typically includes other remedial measures (psychological, educational, social) for a stabilizing effect in children with behavioral syndrome characterized by the following group of developmentally inappropriate symptoms: moderate to severe distractibility, short attention span, hyperactivity, emotional lability, and impulsivity. The diagnosis of this syndrome should not be made with finality when these symptoms are only of comparatively recent origin. Nonlocalizing (soft) neurological signs, learning disability and abnormal EEG may or may not be present, and a diagnosis of central nervous system dysfunction may or may not be warranted.

In Narcolepsy

CONTRAINDICATIONS

Advanced arteriosclerosis, symptomatic cardiovascular disease, moderate to severe hypertension, hyperthyroidism, known hypersensitivity or idiosyncrasy to the sympathomimetic amines, glaucoma.
Agitated states.
Patients with a history of drug abuse.
During or within 14 days following the administration of monoamine oxidase inhibitors (hypertensive crises may result).

WARNINGS

Clinical experience suggests that in psychotic children, administration of amphetamine may exacerbate symptoms of behavior disturbance and thought disorder. Data are inadequate to determine whether chronic administration of amphetamine may be associated with growth inhibition; therefore, growth should be monitored during treatment.
Usage in Nursing Mothers: Amphetamines are excreted in human milk. Mothers taking amphetamines should be advised to refrain from nursing.

PRECAUTIONS

General: Caution is to be exercised in prescribing amphetamines for patients with even mild hypertension.
The least amount feasible should be prescribed or dispensed at one time in order to minimize the possibility of overdosage.
Information for Patients: Amphetamines may impair the ability of the patient to engage in potentially hazardous activities such as operating machinery or vehicles; the patient should therefore be cautioned accordingly.
Drug Interactions: *Acidifying agents*—Gastrointestinal acidifying agents (guanethidine, reserpine, glutamic acid HCl, ascorbic acid, fruit juices, etc.) lower absorption of amphetamines.
Urinary acidifying agents—(ammonium chloride, sodium acid phosphate, etc.) Increase the concentration of the ionized species of the amphetamine molecule, thereby increasing urinary excretion. Both groups of agents lower blood levels and efficacy of amphetamines.
Adrenergic blockers—Adrenergic blockers are inhibited by amphetamines.
Alkalinizing agents—Gastrointestinal alkalinizing agents (sodium bicarbonate, etc.) increase absorption of amphetamines. Urinary alkalinizing agents (acetazolamide, some thiazides) increase the concentration of the non-ionized species of the amphetamine molecule, thereby decreasing urinary excretion. Both groups of agents increase blood levels and therefore potentiate the actions of amphetamines.
Antidepressants, tricyclic—Amphetamines may enhance the activity of tricyclic or sympathomimetic agents; d-amphetamine with desipramine or protriptyline and possibly other tricyclics cause striking and sustained increases in the concentration of d-amphetamine in the brain; cardiovascular effects can be potentiated.
MAO inhibitors—MAOI antidepressants, as well as a metabolite of furazolidone, slow amphetamine metabolism. This slowing potentiates amphetamines, increasing their effect on the release of norepinephrine and other monoamines from adrenergic nerve endings; this can cause headaches and other signs of hypertensive crisis. A variety of neurological toxic effects and malignant hyperpyrexia can occur, sometimes with fatal results.
Antihistamines—Amphetamines may counteract the sedative effect of antihistamines.
Antihypertensives—Amphetamines may antagonize the hypotensive effects of antihypertensives.
Chlorpromazine—Chlorpromazine blocks dopamine and norepinephrine receptors, thus inhibiting the central stimulant effects of amphetamines, and can be used to treat amphetamine poisoning.
Ethosuximide—Amphetamines may delay intestinal absorption of ethosuximide.
Haloperidol—Haloperidol blocks dopamine receptors, thus inhibiting the central stimulant effects of amphetamines.
Lithium carbonate—The anorectic and stimulatory effects of amphetamines may be inhibited by lithium carbonate.
Meperidine—Amphetamines potentiate the analgesic effect of meperidine.
Methenamine therapy—Urinary excretion of amphetamines is increased, and efficacy is reduced, by acidifying agents used in methenamine therapy.
Norepinephrine—Amphetamines enhance the adrenergic effect of norepinephrine.
Phenobarbital—Amphetamines may delay intestinal absorption of phenobarbital; co-administration of phenobarbital may produce a synergistic anticonvulsant action.
Phenytoin—Amphetamines may delay intestinal absorption of phenytoin; co-administration of phenytoin may produce a synergistic anticonvulsant action.
Propoxyphene—In cases of propoxyphene overdosage, amphetamine CNS stimulation is potentiated and fatal convulsions can occur.
Veratrum alkaloids—Amphetamines inhibit the hypotensive effect of veratrum alkaloids.
Drug/Laboratory Test Interactions:
- Amphetamines can cause a significant elevation in plasma corticosteroid levels. This increase is greatest in the evening.
- Amphetamines may interfere with urinary steroid determinations.

Carcinogenesis/Mutagenesis: Mutagenicity studies and long-term studies in animals to determine the carcinogenic potential of amphetamine, have not been performed.
Pregnancy—Teratogenic Effects: Pregnancy Category C. Amphetamine has been shown to have embryotoxic and teratogenic effects when administered to A/Jax mice and C57BL mice in doses approximately 41 times the maximum human dose. Embryotoxic effects were not seen in New

EACH TABLET CONTAINS:	5 mg	10 mg	20 mg	30 mg
Dextroamphetamine Saccharate	1.25 mg	2.5 mg	5 mg	7.5 mg
Amphetamine Aspartate	1.25 mg	2.5 mg	5 mg	7.5 mg
Dextroamphetamine Sulfate USP	1.25 mg	2.5 mg	5 mg	7.5 mg
Amphetamine Sulfate USP	1.25 mg	2.5 mg	5 mg	7.5 mg
Total amphetamine base equivalence	3.13 mg	6.3 mg	12.6 mg	18.8 mg

Zealand white rabbits given the drug in doses 7 times the human dose nor in rats given 12.5 times the maximum human dose. While there are no adequate and well-controlled studies in pregnant women, there has been one report of severe congenital bony deformity, tracheoesophageal fistula, and anal atresia (vater association) in a baby born to a woman who took dextroamphetamine sulfate with lovastatin during the first trimester of pregnancy. Amphetamines should be used during pregnancy only if the potential benefit justifies the potential risk to the fetus.

Nonteratogenic Effects: Infants born to mothers dependent on amphetamines have an increased risk of premature delivery and low birth weight. Also, these infants may experience symptoms of withdrawal as demonstrated by dysphoria, including agitation, and significant lassitude.

Pediatric Use: Long-term effects of amphetamines in children have not been well established. Amphetamines are not recommended for use in children under 3 years of age with Attention Deficit Disorder with Hyperactivity described under INDICATIONS AND USAGE.

Amphetamines have been reported to exacerbate motor and phonic tics and Tourette's syndrome. Therefore, clinical evaluation for tics and Tourette's syndrome in children and their families should precede use of stimulant medications.

Drug treatment is not indicated in all cases of Attention Deficit Disorder with Hyperactivity and should be considered only in light of the complete history and evaluation of the child. The decision to prescribe amphetamines should depend on the physician's assessment of the chronicity and severity of the child's symptoms and their appropriateness for his/her age. Prescription should not depend solely on the presence of one or more of the behavioral characteristics.

When these symptoms are associated with acute stress reactions, treatment with amphetamines is usually not indicated.

ADVERSE REACTIONS

Cardiovascular: Palpitations, tachycardia, elevation of blood pressure. There have been isolated reports of cardiomyopathy associated with chronic amphetamine use.

Central Nervous System: Psychotic episodes at recommended doses (rare), overstimulation, restlessness, dizziness, insomnia, euphoria, dyskinesia, dysphoria, tremor, headache, exacerbation of motor and phonic tics and Tourette's syndrome.

Gastrointestinal: Dryness of the mouth, unpleasant taste, diarrhea, constipation, other gastrointestinal disturbances. Anorexia and weight loss may occur as undesirable effects when amphetamines are used for other than the anorectic effect.

Allergic: Urticaria.

Endocrine: Impotence, changes in libido.

DRUG ABUSE AND DEPENDENCE

Dextroamphetamine sulfate is a Schedule II controlled substance.

Amphetamines have been extensively abused. Tolerance, extreme psychological dependence, and severe social disability have occurred. There are reports of patients who have increased the dosage to many times that recommended. Abrupt cessation following prolonged high dosage administration results in extreme fatigue and mental depression; changes are also noted on the sleep EEG. Manifestations of chronic intoxication with amphetamines include severe dermatoses, marked insomnia, irritability, hyperactivity, and personality changes. The most severe manifestation of chronic intoxication is psychosis, often clinically indistinguishable from schizophrenia. This is rare with oral amphetamines.

OVERDOSAGE

Individual patient response to amphetamines varies widely. While toxic symptoms occasionally occur as an idiosyncrasy at doses as low as 2 mg, they are rare with doses of less than 15 mg; 30 mg can produce severe reactions, yet doses of 400 to 500 mg are not necessarily fatal.

In rats, the oral LD50 of dextroamphetamine sulfate is 96.8 mg/kg.

Symptoms: Manifestations of acute overdosage with amphetamines include restlessness, tremor, hyperreflexia, rapid respiration, confusion, assaultiveness, hallucinations, panic states, hyperpyrexia and rhabdomyolysis.

Fatigue and depression usually follow the central stimulation.

Cardiovascular effects include arrhythmias, hypertension or hypotension and circulatory collapse.

Gastrointestinal symptoms include nausea, vomiting, diarrhea, and abdominal cramps. Fatal poisoning is usually preceded by convulsions and coma.

Treatment: Consult with a Certified Poison Control Center for up to date guidance and advice. Management of acute amphetamine intoxication is largely symptomatic and includes gastric lavage, administration of activated charcoal, administration of a cathartic and sedation. Experience with hemodialysis or peritoneal dialysis is inadequate to permit recommendation in this regard. Acidification of the urine increases amphetamine excretion, but is believed to increase risk of acute renal failure if myoglobinuria is present. If acute, severe hypertension complicates amphetamine overdosage, administration of intravenous phentolamine has been suggested. However, a gradual drop in blood pressure will usually result when sufficient sedation has been achieved. Chlorpromazine antagonizes the central stimulant effects of amphetamines and can be used to treat amphetamine intoxication.

DOSAGE AND ADMINISTRATION

Regardless of indication, amphetamines should be administered at the lowest effective dosage and dosage should be individually adjusted. Late evening doses should be avoided because of the resulting insomnia.

Attention Deficit Disorder with Hyperactivity: Not recommended for children under 3 years of age. In children from 3 to 5 years of age, start with 2.5 mg daily; daily dosage may be raised in increments of 2.5 mg at weekly intervals until optimal response is obtained.

In children 6 years of age and older, start with 5 mg once or twice daily; daily dosage may be raised in increments of 5 mg at weekly intervals until optimal response is obtained. Only in rare cases will it be necessary to exceed a total of 40 mg per day. Give first dose on awakening; additional doses (1 or 2) at intervals of 4 to 6 hours.

Where possible, drug administration should be interrupted occasionally to determine if there is a recurrence of behavioral symptoms sufficient to require continued therapy.

Narcolepsy: Usual dose 5 mg to 60 mg per day in divided doses, depending on the individual patient response.

Narcolepsy seldom occurs in children under 12 years of age; however, when it does, dextroamphetamine sulfate, may be used. The suggested initial dose for patients aged 6–12 is 5 mg daily; daily dose may be raised in increments of 5 mg at weekly intervals until optimal response is obtained. In patients 12 years of age and older, start with 10 mg daily; daily dosage may be raised in increments of 10 mg at weekly intervals until optimal response is obtained. If bothersome adverse reactions appear (e.g., insomnia or anorexia), dosage should be reduced. Give first dose on awakening; additional doses (1 or 2) at intervals of 4 to 6 hours.

HOW SUPPLIED

ADDERALL® 5 mg: Blue double-scored tablet, debossed "AD" on one side and "5" on the other side (NDC 58521-031-01)

ADDERALL® 10 mg: Blue double-scored tablet, debossed "AD" on one side and "10" on the other side (NDC 58521-032-01)

ADDERALL® 20 mg: Orange double-scored tablet, debossed "AD" on one side and "20" on the other side (NDC 58521-033-01)

ADDERALL® 30 mg: Orange double-scored tablet, debossed "AD" on one side and "30" on the other side (NDC 58521-034-01)

In bottles of 100 tablets.

Dispense in a tight, light-resistant container as defined in the USP.

Store at controlled room temperature 15°–30°C (59°–86°F).

Rx only

Shire Richwood Inc.

Florence, KY 41042

MG #10185 Revised: June 1998

Shown in Product Identification Guide, page 336

AGRYLIN® ℞

(anagrelide hydrochloride)
Capsules
Rx Only

DESCRIPTION

Name: AGRYLIN® (anagrelide hydrochloride)

Dosage Form: 0.5 mg and 1 mg capsules for oral administration

Active Ingredient: AGRYLIN® Capsules contain either 0.5 mg or 1 mg of anagrelide base (as anagrelide hydrochloride).

Inactive Ingredients: Povidone USP, Anhydrous Lactose NF, Lactose Monohydrate NF, Microcrystalline Cellulose NF, Crospovidone NF, Magnesium Stearate NF.

Pharmacological Classification: Platelet-reducing agent.

Chemical Name: 6,7-dichloro-1,5-dihydroimidazo[2,1-b]quinazolin-2(3H)-one monohydrochloride monohydrate.

Molecular formula: $C_{10}H_7Cl_2N_3O \cdot HCl \cdot H_2O$

Molecular weight: 310.55

Structural formula:

Appearance: Off-white powder.

Solubility:

Water	Very slightly soluble
Dimethyl Sulfoxide	Sparingly soluble
Dimethylformamide	Sparingly soluble

CLINICAL PHARMACOLOGY

The mechanism by which anagrelide reduces blood platelet count is still under investigation. Studies in patients support a hypothesis of dose-related reduction in platelet production resulting from a decrease in megakaryocyte hypermaturation. In blood withdrawn from normal volunteers treated with anagrelide, a disruption was found in the postmitotic phase of megakaryocyte development and a reduction in megakaryocyte size and ploidy. At therapeutic doses, anagrelide does not produce significant changes in white cell counts or coagulation parameters, and may have a small, but clinically insignificant effect on red cell parameters. Platelet aggregation is inhibited in people at doses higher than those required to reduce platelet count. Anagrelide inhibits cyclic AMP phosphodiesterase, as well as ADP- and collagen-induced platelet aggregation.

Following oral administration of ^{14}C-anagrelide in people, more than 70% of radioactivity was recovered in urine. Based on limited data, there appears to be a trend toward dose linearity between doses of 0.5 mg and 2.0 mg. At fasting and at a dose of 0.5 mg of anagrelide, the plasma half-life is 1.3 hours. The available plasma concentration time data at steady state in patients showed that anagrelide does not accumulate in plasma after repeated administration. The drug is extensively metabolized; less than 1% is recovered in the urine as anagrelide.

When a 0.5 mg dose of anagrelide was taken after food, its bioavailability (based on AUC values) was modestly reduced by an average of 13.8% and its plasma half-life slightly increased (to 1.8 hours), when compared with drug administered to the same subjects in the fasted state. The peak plasma level was lowered by an average of 45% and delayed by 2 hours.

CLINICAL STUDIES

A total of 942 patients with myeloproliferative disorders including 551 patients with Essential Thrombocythemia (ET), 117 patients with Polycythemia Vera (PV), 178 patients with Chronic Myelogenous Leukemia (CML), and 96 patients with other myeloproliferative disorders (OMPD), were treated with anagrelide in three clinical trials. Patients with OMPD included 87 patients who had Myeloid Metaplasia with Myelofibrosis (MMM), and 9 patients who had unknown myeloproliferative disorders.

Clinical Studies

Patients with ET, PV, CML, or MMM were diagnosed based on the following criteria:

[See table at top of next page]

Patients were enrolled in clinical trials if their platelet count was ≥ 900,000/μL on two occasions or ≥ 650,000/μL on two occasions with documentation of symptoms associated with thrombocythemia. The mean duration of anagrelide therapy for ET, PV, CML, and OMPD patients was 65, 67, 40, and 44 weeks, respectively; 23% of patients received treatment for 2 years. Patients were treated with anagrelide starting at doses of 0.5–2.0 mg every 6 hours. The dose was increased if the platelet count was still high, but to no more than 12 mg each day. Efficacy was defined as reduction of platelet count to or near physiologic levels (150,000-400,000/μL). The criteria for defining subjects as "responders" were reduction in platelets for at least 4 weeks to ≤600,000/μL, or by at least 50% from baseline value. Subjects treated for less than 4 weeks were not considered evaluable. The results are depicted graphically below:

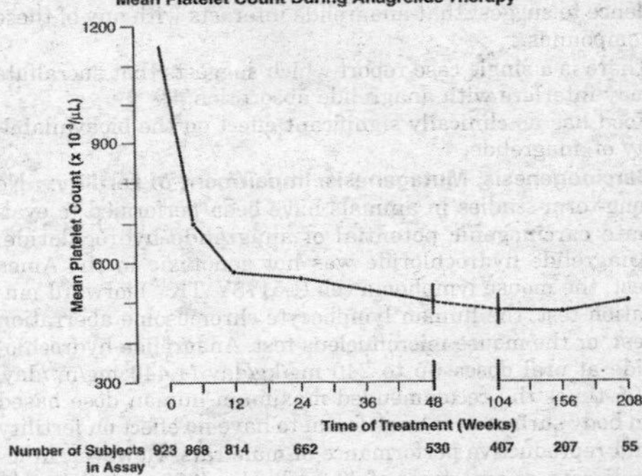

	Time on Treatment							
		Weeks				Years		
	Baseline	4	12	24	48	2	3	4
Mean*	1131	683	575	526	484	460	437	457
N	923†	868	814	662	530	407	207	55

*x 10^3/μL

† Nine hundred and forty-two subjects with myeloproliferative disorders were enrolled in three research studies. Of these, 923 had platelet counts over the duration of the studies.

AGRYLIN® was effective in phlebotomized patients as well as in patients treated with other concomitant therapies including hydroxyurea, aspirin, interferon, radioactive phosphorus, and alkylating agents.

INDICATIONS AND USAGE

AGRYLIN® Capsules are indicated for the treatment of patients with thrombocythemia, secondary to myeloproliferative disorders, to reduce the elevated platelet count and the risk of thrombosis and to ameliorate associated symptoms including thrombo-hemorrhagic events (see CLINICAL STUDIES, DOSAGE and ADMINISTRATION).

WARNINGS

Cardiovascular

Anagrelide should be used with caution in patients with known or suspected heart disease, and only if the potential benefits of therapy outweigh the potential risks. Because of the positive inotropic effects and side-effects of anagrelide, a

Continued on next page

Agrylin—Cont.

ET
- Platelet count ≥900,000/μL on two determinations
- Profound megakaryocytic hyperplasia in bone marrow
- Absence of Philadelphia chromosome
- Normal red cell mass
- Normal serum iron and ferritin and normal marrow iron stores

CML
- Persistent granulocyte count ≥50,000/μL without evidence of infection
- Absolute basophil count ≥ 100/μL
- Evidence for hyperplasia of the granulocytic line in the bone marrow
- Philadelphia chromosome present
- Leucocyte alkaline phophatase ≤ lower limit of the laboratory normal range

PV†
- A1 Increased red cell mass
- A2 Normal arterial oxygen saturation
- A3 Splenomegaly
- B1 Platelet count ≥ 400,000/μL, in absence of iron deficiency or bleeding
- B2 Leucocytosis (≥ 12,000/μL, in the absence of infection)
- B3 Elevated leucocyte alkaline phosphatase
- B4 Elevated Serum B_{12}

† Diagnosis positive if A1, A2, and A3 present; or, if no splenomegaly, diagnosis is positive if A1 and A2 are present with any two of B1, B2, or B3

MMM
- Myelofibrotic (hypocellular, fibrotic) bone marrow
- Prominent megakaryocytic metaplasia in bone marrow
- Splenomegaly
- Moderate to severe normochromic normocytic anemia
- White cell count may be variable; (80,000–100,000/μL)
- Increased platelet count
- Variable red cell mass; teardrop poikilocytes
- Normal to high leucocyte alkaline phosphatase
- Absence of Philadelphia chromosome

pre-treatment cardiovascular examination is recommended along with careful monitoring during treatment. In humans, therapeutic doses of anagrelide may cause cardiovascular effects, including vasodilation, tachycardia, palpitations, and congestive heart failure.

Renal

It is recommended that patients with renal insufficiency (creatinine ≥ 2mg/dL) receive anagrelide when, in the physician's judgment, the potential benefits of therapy outweigh the potential risks. These patients should be monitored closely for signs of renal toxicity while receiving anagrelide (see ADVERSE REACTIONS, Urogenital System).

Hepatic

It is recommended that patients with evidence of hepatic dysfunction (bilirubin, SGOT, or measures of liver function >1.5 times the upper limit of normal) receive anagrelide when, in the physician's judgment, the potential benefits of therapy outweigh the potential risks. These patients should be monitored closely for signs of hepatic toxicity while receiving anagrelide (see ADVERSE REACTIONS, Hepatic System).

PRECAUTIONS

Laboratory Tests: Anagrelide therapy requires close clinical supervision of the patient. While the platelet count is being lowered (usually during the first two weeks of treatment), blood counts (hemoglobin, white blood cells), liver function (SGOT, SGPT) and renal function (serum creatinine, BUN) should be monitored.

In 9 subjects receiving a single 5 mg dose of anagrelide, standing blood pressure fell an average of 22/15 mm Hg, usually accompanied by dizziness. Only minimal changes in blood pressure were observed following a dose of 2 mg.

Cessation of AGRYLIN® Treatment: In general, interruption of anagrelide treatment is followed by an increase in platelet count. After sudden stoppage of anagrelide therapy, the increase in platelet count can be observed within four days.

Drug Interactions: Bioavailability studies evaluating possible interactions between anagrelide and other drugs have not been conducted. The most common medications used concomitantly with anagrelide have been aspirin, acetaminophen, furosemide, iron, ranitidine, hydroxyurea, and allopurinol. The most frequently used concomitant cardiac medication has been digoxin. Although drug-to-drug interaction studies have not been conducted, there is no clinical evidence to suggest that anagrelide interacts with any of these compounds.

There is a single case report which suggests that sucralfate may interfere with anagrelide absorption.

Food has no clinically significant effect on the bioavailability of anagrelide.

Carcinogenesis, Mutagenesis, Impairment of Fertility: No long-term studies in animals have been performed to evaluate carcinogenic potential of anagrelide hydrochloride. Anagrelide hydrochloride was not genotoxic in the Ames test, the mouse lymphoma cell (L5178Y, $TK^{+/-}$) forward mutation test, the human lymphocyte chromosome aberration test, or the mouse micronucleus test. Anagrelide hydrochloride at oral doses up to 240 mg/kg/day (1,440 mg/m^2/day, 195 times the recommended maximum human dose based on body surface area) was found to have no effect on fertility and reproductive performance of male rats. However, in female rats, at oral doses of 60 mg/kg/day (360 mg/m^2/day, 49 times the recommended maximum human dose based on body surface area) or higher, it disrupted implantation when administered in early pregnancy and retarded or blocked parturition when administered in late pregnancy.

Pregnancy: Pregnancy Category C.

(i) Teratogenic Effects

Teratology studies have been performed in pregnant rats at oral doses up to 900 mg/kg/day (5,400 mg/m^2/day, 730 times the recommended maximum human dose based on body surface area) and in pregnant rabbits at oral doses up to 20 mg/kg/day (240 mg/m^2/day, 32 times the recommended maximum human dose based on body surface area) and have revealed no evidence of impaired fertility or harm to the fetus due to anagrelide hydrochloride.

(ii) Nonteratogenic Effects

A fertility and reproductive performance study performed in female rats revealed that anagrelide hydrochloride at oral doses of 60 mg/kg/day (360 mg/m^2/day, 49 times the recommended maximum human dose based on body surface area) or higher disrupted implantation and exerted adverse effect on embryo/fetal survival.

A perinatal and postnatal study performed in female rats revealed that anagrelide hydrochloride at oral doses of 60 mg/kg/day (360 mg/m^2/day, 49 times the recommended maximum human dose based on body surface area) or higher produced delay or blockage of parturition, deaths of nondelivering pregnant dams and their fully developed fetuses, and increased mortality in the pups born.

Five women became pregnant while on anagrelide treatment at doses of 1 to 4 mg/day. Treatment was stopped as soon as it was realized that they were pregnant. All delivered normal, healthy babies. There are no adequate and well-controlled studies in pregnant women. Anagrelide hydrochloride should be used during pregnancy only if the potential benefit justifies the potential risk to the fetus.

Anagrelide is not recommended in women who are or may become pregnant. If this drug is used during pregnancy, or if the patient becomes pregnant while taking this drug, the patient should be apprised of the potential harm to the fetus. Women of child-bearing potential should be instructed that they must not be pregnant and that they should use contraception while taking anagrelide. Anagrelide may cause fetal harm when administered to a pregnant woman.

Nursing Mothers: It is not known whether this drug is excreted in human milk. Because many drugs are excreted in human milk and because of the potential for serious adverse reaction in nursing infants from anagrelide hydrochloride, a decision should be made whether to discontinue nursing or to discontinue the drug, taking into account the importance of the drug to the mother.

Pediatric Use: The safety and efficacy of anagrelide in patients under the age of 16 years have not been established. Myeloproliferative disorders are uncommon in pediatric patients. Anagrelide has been used successfully in 12 pediatric patients (age range 6.8 to 17.4 years; 6 male and 6 female), including 8 patients with ET, 2 patients with CML, 1 patient with PV, and 1 patient with OMPD. Patients were started on therapy with 0.5 mg qid to a maximum daily dose of 10 mg. The median duration of treatment was 18.1 months with a range of 3.1 to 92 months. Three patients received treatment for greater than three years.

ADVERSE REACTIONS

Analysis of the adverse events in a population consisting of 942 patients diagnosed with myeloproliferative diseases of varying etiology (ET: 551; PV: 117; OMPD: 274) has shown that all disease groups have the same adverse event profile. While most reported adverse events during anagrelide therapy have been mild in intensity and have decreased in frequency with continued therapy, serious adverse events were reported in these patients. These include the following: congestive heart failure, myocardial infarction, cardiomyopathy, cardiomegaly, complete heart block, atrial fibrillation, cerebrovascular accident, pericarditis, pulmonary infiltrates, pulmonary fibrosis, pulmonary hypertension, pancreatitis, gastric/duodenal ulceration, and seizure.

Of the 942 patients treated with anagrelide for a mean duration of approximately 65 weeks, 161 (17%) were discontinued from the study because of adverse events or abnormal laboratory test results. The most common adverse events for treatment discontinuation were headache, diarrhea, edema, palpitation, and abdominal pain. Overall, the occurrence rate of all adverse events was 17.9 per 1,000 treatment days. The occurrence rate of adverse events increased at higher dosages of anagrelide.

The most frequently reported adverse reactions to anagrelide (in 5% or greater of 942 patients with myeloproliferative disease) in clinical trials were:

Headache	43.5%
Palpitations	26.1%
Diarrhea	25.7%
Asthenia	23.1%
Edema, other	20.6%
Nausea	17.1%
Abdominal Pain	16.4%
Dizziness	15.4%
Pain, other	15.0%
Dyspnea	11.9%
Flatulence	10.2%
Vomiting	9.7%
Fever	8.9%
Peripheral Edema	8.5%
Rash, including urticaria	8.3%
Chest Pain	7.8%
Anorexia	7.7%
Tachycardia	7.5%
Pharyngitis	6.8%
Malaise	6.4%
Cough	6.3%
Paresthesia	5.9%
Back Pain	5.9%
Pruritus	5.5%
Dyspepsia	5.2%

Adverse events with an incidence of 1% to <5% included:

Body as a Whole System: Flu symptoms, chills, photosensitivity.

Cardiovascular System: Arrhythmia, hemorrhage, cardiovascular disease, angina pectoris, heart failure, postural hypotension, thrombosis, vasodilatation, migraine, syncope.

Digestive System: Constipation, GI distress, GI hemorrhage, gastritis, melena, aphthous stomatitis, eructation.

Hemic & Lymphatic System: Anemia, thrombocytopenia, ecchymosis, lymphadenopathy.

Platelet counts below 100,000/μL occurred in 84 patients (ET: 35; PV: 9; OMPD: 40), reduction below 50,000/μL occurred in 44 patients (ET: 7; PV: 6; OMPD: 31) while on anagrelide therapy. Thrombocytopenia promptly recovered upon discontinuation of anagrelide.

Hepatic System: Elevated liver enzymes were observed in 3 patients (ET: 2; OMPD: 1) during anagrelide therapy.

Musculoskeletal System: Arthralgia, myalgia, leg cramps.

Nervous System: Depression, somnolence, confusion, insomnia, hypertension, nervousness, amnesia.

Nutritional Disorders: Dehydration.

Respiratory System: Rhinitis, epistaxis, respiratory disease, sinusitis, pneumonia, bronchitis, asthma.

Skin and Appendages System: Skin disease, alopecia.

Special Senses: Amblyopia, abnormal vision, tinnitus, visual field abnormality, diplopia.

Urogenital System: Dysuria, Hematuria.

Renal abnormalities occurred in 15 patients (ET: 10; PV: 4; OMPD: 1). Six ET, 4 PV and 1 with OMPD experienced renal failure (approximately 1%) while on anagrelide treatment; in 4 cases, the renal failure was considered to be possibly related to anagrelide treatment. The remaining 11 were found to have pre-existing renal impairment. Doses ranged from 1.5–6.0 mg/day, with exposure periods of 2 to 12 months. No dose adjustment was required because of renal insufficiency.

The adverse event profile for patients in clinical trials on anagrelide therapy (in 5% or greater of 942 patients with myeloproliferative diseases) is shown in the following bar graph:

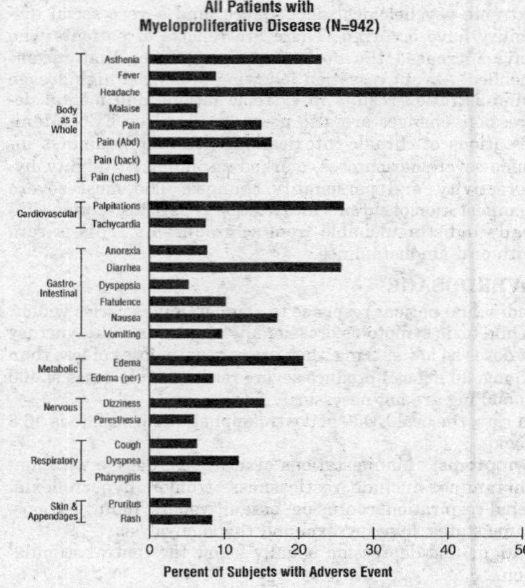

OVERDOSAGE

Acute Toxicity and Symptoms

Single oral doses of anagrelide hydrochloride at 2,500, 1,500 and 200 mg/kg in mice, rats and monkeys, respectively, were not lethal. Symptoms of acute toxicity were: decreased motor activity in mice and rats and softened stools and decreased appetite in monkeys.

There are no reports of overdosage with anagrelide hydrochloride. Platelet reduction from anagrelide therapy is dose-related; therefore, thrombocytopenia, which can potentially cause bleeding, is expected from overdosage. Should overdosage occur, cardiac and central nervous system toxicity can also be expected.

Management and Treatment

In case of overdosage, close clinical supervision of the patient is required; this especially includes monitoring of the platelet count for thrombocytopenia. Dosage should be decreased or stopped, as appropriate, until the platelet count returns to within the normal range.

DOSAGE AND ADMINISTRATION

Treatment with **AGRYLIN®** Capsules should be initiated under close medical supervision. The recommended starting dosage of **AGRYLIN®** is 0.5 mg qid or 1 mg bid, which should be maintained for at least one week. Dosage should then be adjusted to the lowest effective dosage required to reduce and maintain platelet count below 600,000/µL, and ideally to the normal range. The dosage should be increased by not more than 0.5 mg/day in any one week. Dosage should not exceed 10 mg/day or 2.5 mg in a single dose (see PRECAUTIONS). The decision to treat asymptomatic young adults with thrombocythemia secondary to myeloproliferative disorders should be individualized.

To monitor the effect of anagrelide and prevent the occurrence of thrombocytopenia, platelet counts should be performed every two days during the first week of treatment and at least weekly thereafter until the maintenance dosage is reached.

Typically, platelet count begins to respond within 7 to 14 days at the proper dosage. The time to complete response, defined as platelet count ≤ 600,000/µL, ranged from 4 to 12 weeks. Most patients will experience an adequate response at a dose of 1.5 to 3.0 mg/day. Patients with known or suspected heart disease, renal insufficiency, or hepatic dysfunction should be monitored closely.

HOW SUPPLIED

AGRYLIN® is available as:

0.5 mg, opaque, white capsules imprinted "ROBERTS 063" in black ink:

NDC 54092-063-01 = bottle of 100

1 mg, opaque, gray capsules imprinted "ROBERTS 064" in black ink:

NDC 54092-064-01 = bottle of 100

Store from 15° to 25°C (59° to 77°F), in a light-resistant container.

ROBERTS® PHARMACEUTICALS

Manufactured for

Roberts Laboratories Inc., a subsidiary of

ROBERTS PHARMACEUTICAL CORP.

Eatontown, NJ 07724-2274, USA

by MALLINCKRODT INC.

Hobart, NY 13788

Rev. 03/99 063 0117 007

Shown in Product Identification Guide, page 336

CARBATROL® ℞

[*căr-bă 'trōl*]

(carbamazepine extended-release capsules)
200 mg and 300 mg

Prescribing information

> **WARNING**
> APLASTIC ANEMIA AND AGRANULOCYTOSIS HAVE BEEN REPORTED IN ASSOCIATION WITH THE USE OF CARBAMAZEPINE. DATA FROM A POPULATION-BASED CASE-CONTROL STUDY DEMONSTRATE THAT THE RISK OF DEVELOPING THESE REACTIONS IS 5–8 TIMES GREATER THAN IN THE GENERAL POPULATION. HOWEVER, THE OVERALL RISK OF THESE REACTIONS IN THE UNTREATED GENERAL POPULATION IS LOW. APPROXIMATELY SIX PATIENTS PER ONE MILLION POPULATION PER YEAR FOR AGRANULOCYTOSIS AND TWO PATIENTS PER ONE MILLION POPULATION PER YEAR FOR APLASTIC ANEMIA.
> ALTHOUGH REPORTS OF TRANSIENT OR PERSISTENT DECREASED PLATELET OR WHITE BLOOD CELL COUNTS ARE NOT UNCOMMON IN ASSOCIATION WITH THE USE OF CARBAMAZEPINE, DATA ARE NOT AVAILABLE TO ESTIMATE ACCURATELY THEIR INCIDENCE OR OUTCOME. HOWEVER, THE VAST MAJORITY OF THE CASES OF LEUKOPENIA HAVE NOT PROGRESSED TO THE MORE SERIOUS CONDITIONS OF APLASTIC ANEMIA OR AGRANULOCYTOSIS.
> BECAUSE OF THE VERY LOW INCIDENCE OF AGRANULOCYTOSIS AND APLASTIC ANEMIA, THE VAST MAJORITY OF MINOR HEMATOLOGIC CHANGES OBSERVED IN MONITORING OF PATIENTS ON CARBAMAZEPINE ARE UNLIKELY TO SIGNAL THE OCCURRENCE OF EITHER ABNORMALITY. NONETHELESS, COMPLETE PRETREATMENT HEMATOLOGICAL TESTING SHOULD BE OBTAINED AS A BASELINE. IF A PATIENT IN THE COURSE OF TREATMENT EXHIBITS LOW OR DECREASED WHITE BLOOD CELL OR PLATELET COUNTS, THE PATIENT SHOULD BE MONITORED CLOSELY. DISCONTINUATION OF THE DRUG SHOULD BE CONSIDERED IF ANY EVIDENCE OF SIGNIFICANT BONE MARROW DEPRESSION DEVELOPS.

Before prescribing Carbatrol, the physician should be thoroughly familiar with the details of this prescribing information, particularly regarding use with other drugs, especially those which accentuate toxicity potential.

DESCRIPTION

CARBATROL* is an anticonvulsant and specific analgesic for trigeminal neuralgia, available for oral administration as 200 mg and 300 mg extended-release capsules of Carbamazepine, USP. Carbamazepine is a white to off-white powder, practically insoluble in water and soluble in alcohol and in acetone. Its molecular weight is 236.27. Its chemical name is 5H-dibenz[b,f]azepine-5-carboxamide, and its structural formula is:

CARBAMAZEPINE

Carbatrol is a multi-component capsule formulation consisting of three different types of beads: immediate-release beads, extended-release beads, and enteric-release beads. The three bead types are combined in a specific ratio to provide twice daily dosing of Carbatrol.

Inactive ingredients: citric acid, colloidal silicon dioxide, lactose monohydrate, microcrystalline cellulose, polyethylene glycol, povidone, sodium lauryl sulfate, talc, triethyl citrate and other ingredients.

The 200 mg capsule shells contain gelatin-NF, FD&C Red #3, FD&C Yellow #6, Yellow Iron Oxide, FD&C Blue #2, and titanium dioxide, and are imprinted with white ink; and the 300 mg capsule shells contain gelatin-NF, FD&C Blue #2, FD&C Yellow #6, Red Iron Oxide, Yellow Iron Oxide, and titanium dioxide, and are imprinted with white ink.

CLINICAL PHARMACOLOGY

In controlled clinical trials, carbamazepine has been shown to be effective in the treatment of psychomotor and grand mal seizures, as well as trigeminal neuralgia.

Mechanism of Action

Carbamazepine has demonstrated anticonvulsant properties in rats and mice with electrically and chemically induced seizures. It appears to act by reducing polysynaptic responses and blocking the post-tetanic potentiation. Carbamazepine greatly reduces or abolishes pain induced by stimulation of the infraorbital nerve in cats and rats. It depresses thalamic potential and bulbar and polysynaptic reflexes, including the linguomandibular reflex in cats. Carbamazepine is chemically unrelated to other anticonvulsants or other drugs used to control the pain of trigeminal neuralgia. The mechanism of action remains unknown.

The principal metabolite of carbamazepine, carbamazepine-10,11-epoxide, has anticonvulsant activity as demonstrated in several *in vivo* animal models of seizures. Though clinical activity for the epoxide has been postulated, the significance of its activity with respect to the safety and efficacy of carbamazepine has not been established.

Pharmacokinetics

Carbamazepine (CBZ): Taken every 12 hours, carbamazepine extended-release capsules provide steady state plasma levels comparable to immediate-release carbamazepine tablets given every 6 hours, when administered at the same total mg daily dose. Following a single 200 mg oral extended-release dose of carbamazepine, peak plasma concentration was 1.9 ± 0.3 µg/mL and the time to reach the peak was 19 ± 7 hours. Following chronic administration (800 mg every 12 hours), the peak levels were 11.0 ± 2.5 µg/mL and the time to reach the peak was 5.9 ± 1.8 hours. The pharmacokinetics of extended-release carbamazepine is linear over the single dose range of 200–800 mg.

Carbamazepine is 76% bound to plasma proteins. Carbamazepine is primarily metabolized in the liver. Cytochrome P450 3A4 was identified as the major isoform responsible for the formation of carbamazepine-10,11-epoxide. Since carbamazepine induces its own metabolism, the half-life is also variable. Following a single extended-release dose of carbamazepine, the average half-life range from 35–40 hours and 12–17 hours on repeated dosing. The apparent oral clearance following a single dose was 25 ± 5 mL/min and following multiple dosing was 80 ± 30 mL/min.

After oral administration of ^{14}C-carbamazepine, 72% of the administered radioactivity was found in the urine and 28% in the feces. This urinary radioactivity was composed largely of hydroxylated and conjugated metabolites, with only 3% of unchanged carbamazepine.

Carbamazepine-10,11-epoxide (CBZ-E): Carbamazepine-10,11-epoxide is considered to be an active metabolite of carbamazepine. Following a single 200 mg oral extended-release dose of carbamazepine, the peak plasma concentration of carbamazepine-10,11-epoxide was 0.11 ± 0.012 µg/mL and the time to reach the peak was 36 ± 6 hours. Following chronic administration of a extended-release dose of carbamazepine (800 mg every 12 hours), the peak levels of carbamazepine-10,11-epoxide were 2.2 ± 0.9 µg/mL and the time to reach the peak was 14 ± 8 hours. The plasma half-life of carbamazepine-10,11-epoxide following administration of carbamazepine is 34 ± 9 hours. Following a single oral dose of extended-release carbamazepine (200-800 mg) the AUC and C_{max} of carbamazepine-10,11-epoxide were less than 10% of carbamazepine. Following multiple dosing of extended-release carbamazepine (800–1600 mg daily for 14 days), the AUC and C_{max} of carbamazepine-10, 11-epoxide were dose related, ranging from 15.7 µg.hr/mL and 1.5 µg/mL at 800 mg/day to 32.6 µg.hr/mL and 3.2 µg/mL at 1600 mg/day, respectively, and were less than 30% of carbamazepine. Carbamazepine-10,11-epoxide is 50% bound to plasma proteins.

Food Effect: A high fat meal diet increased the rate of absorption of a single 400 mg dose (mean T_{max} was reduced from 24 hours, in the fasting state, to 14 hours and C_{max} increased from 3.2 to 4.3 µg/mL) but not the extent (AUC) of absorption. The elimination half-life remains unchanged between fed and fasting state. The multiple dose study conducted in the fed state showed that the steady-state C_{max} values were within the therapeutic concentration range. The pharmacokinetic profile of extended-release carbamazepine was similar when given by sprinkling the beads over applesauce compared to the intact capsule administered in the fasted state.

* Registered trademark of Shire Richwood Inc.

Special Populations

Hepatic Dysfunction: The effect of hepatic impairment on the pharmacokinetics of carbamazepine is not known. However, given that carbamazepine is primarily metabolized in the liver, it is prudent to proceed with caution in patients with hepatic dysfunction.

Renal Dysfunction: The effect of renal impairment on the pharmacokinetics of carbamazepine is not known.

Gender: No difference in the mean AUC and C_{max} of carbamazepine and carbamazepine-10,11-epoxide was found between males and females.

Age: Carbamazepine is more rapidly metabolized to carbamazepine-10,11-epoxide in young children than adults. In children below the age of 15, there is an inverse relationship between CBZ-E/CBZ ratio and increasing age.

Race: No information is available on the effect of race on the pharmacokinetics of carbamazepine.

INDICATIONS AND USAGE

Epilepsy

Carbatrol is indicated for use as an anticonvulsant drug. Evidence supporting efficacy of carbamazepine as an anticonvulsant was derived from active drug-controlled studies that enrolled patients with the following seizure types:

1. Partial seizures with complex symptomatology (psychomotor, temporal lobe). Patients with these seizures appear to show greater improvements than those with other types.
2. Generalized tonic-clonic seizures (grand mal).
3. Mixed seizure patterns which include the above, or other partial or generalized seizures. Absence seizures (petit mal) do not appear to be controlled by carbamazepine (see PRECAUTIONS, General).

Trigeminal Neuralgia

Carbatrol is indicated in the treatment of the pain associated with true trigeminal neuralgia. Beneficial results have also been reported in glossopharyngeal neuralgia. This drug is not a simple analgesic and should not be used for the relief of trivial aches or pains.

CONTRAINDICATIONS

Carbamazepine should not be used in patients with a history of previous bone marrow depression, hypersensitivity to the drug, or known sensitivity to any of the tricyclic compounds, such as amitriptyline, desipramine, imipramine, protriptyline and nortriptyline. Likewise, on theoretical grounds its use with monoamine oxidase inhibitors is not recommended. Before administration of carbamazepine, MAO inhibitors should be discontinued for a minimum of 14 days, or longer if the clinical situation permits.

WARNINGS

Usage in Pregnancy

Carbamazepine can cause fetal harm when administered to a pregnant women.

Epidemiological data suggest that there may be an association between the use of carbamazepine during pregnancy and congenital malformations, including spina bifida. The prescribing physician will wish to weigh the benefits of therapy against the risks in treating or counseling women of childbearing potential. If this drug is used during pregnancy, or if the patient becomes pregnant while taking this drug, the patient should be apprised of the potential hazard to the fetus.

Retrospective case reviews suggest that, compared with monotherapy, there may be a higher prevalence of teratogenic effects associated with the use of anticonvulsants in combination therapy.

In humans, transplacental passage of carbamazepine is rapid (30–60 minutes), and the drug is accumulated in the fetal tissues, with higher levels found in liver and kidney than in brain and lung.

Carbamazepine has been shown to have adverse effects in reproduction studies in rats when given orally in dosages 10–25 times the maximum human daily dosage (MHDD) of 1200 mg on a mg/kg basis or 1.5–4 times the MHDD on a mg/m^2 basis. In rat teratology studies, 2 of 135 offspring showed kinked ribs at 250 mg/kg and 4 of 119 offspring at 650 mg/kg showed other anomalies (cleft palate, 1; talipes, 1; anophthalmos, 2). In reproduction studies in rats, nursing offspring demonstrated a lack of weight gain and an unkempt appearance at a maternal dosage level of 200 mg/kg.

Antiepileptic drugs should not be discontinued abruptly in patients in whom the drug is administered to prevent major seizures because of the strong possibility of precipitating status epilepticus with attendant hypoxia and threat to

Continued on next page

Carbatrol—Cont.

life. In individual cases where the severity and frequency of the seizure disorder are such that removal of medication does not pose a serious threat to the patient, discontinuation of the drug may be considered prior to and during pregnancy, although it cannot be said with any confidence that even minor seizures do not pose some hazard to the developing embryo or fetus.

Tests to detect defects using current accepted procedures should be considered a part of routine prenatal care in childbearing women receiving carbamazepine.

General

Patients with a history of adverse hematologic reaction to any drug may be particularly at risk.

Severe dermatologic reactions, including toxic epidermal necrolysis (Lyell's syndrome) and Stevens-Johnson syndrome have been reported with carbamazepine. These reactions have been extremely rare. However, a few fatalities have been reported.

Carbamazepine has shown mild anticholinergic activity; therefore, patients with increased intraocular pressure should be closely observed during therapy.

Because of the relationship of the drug to other tricyclic compounds, the possibility of activation of a latent psychosis and, in elderly patients, of confusion or agitation should be considered.

PRECAUTIONS

General

Before initiating therapy, a detailed history and physical examination should be made.

Carbamazepine should be used with caution in patients with a mixed seizure disorder that includes atypical absence seizures, since in these patients carbamazepine has been associated with increased frequency of generalized convulsions (see INDICATIONS AND USAGE).

Therapy should be prescribed only after critical benefit-to-risk appraisal in patients with a history of cardiac, hepatic, or renal damage; adverse hematologic reaction to other drugs; or interrupted courses of therapy with carbamazepine.

Information for Patients

Patients should be made aware of the early toxic signs and symptoms of a potential hematologic problem such as fever, sore throat, rash, ulcers in the mouth, easy bruising, petechial or purpuric hemorrhage, and should be advised to report to the physician immediately if any such signs or symptoms appear.

Since dizziness and drowsiness may occur, patients should be cautioned about the hazards of operating machinery or automobiles or engaging in other potentially dangerous tasks.

If necessary, the Carbatrol capsules can be opened and the contents sprinkled over food, such as a teaspoon of applesauce or other similar food products. Carbatrol capsules or their contents should not be crushed or chewed.

Laboratory Tests

Complete pretreatment blood counts, including platelets and possibly reticulocytes and serum iron, should be obtained as a baseline. If a patient in the course of treatment exhibits low or decreased white blood cell or platelet counts, the patient should be monitored closely. Discontinuation of the drug should be considered if any evidence of significant bone marrow depression develops.

Baseline and periodic evaluations of liver function, particularly in patients with a history of liver disease, must be performed during treatment with this drug since liver damage may occur. The drug should be discontinued immediately in cases of aggravated liver dysfunction or active liver disease.

Baseline and periodic eye examinations, including slit-lamp, funduscopy, and tonometry, are recommended since many phenothiazines and related drugs have been shown to cause eye changes.

Baseline and periodic complete urinalysis and BUN determinations are recommended for patients treated with this agent because of observed renal dysfunction.

Monitoring of blood levels (see CLINICAL PHARMACOLOGY) has increased the efficacy and safety of anticonvulsants. This monitoring may be particularly useful in cases of dramatic increase in seizure frequency and for verification of compliance. In addition, measurement of drug serum levels may aid in determining the cause of toxicity when more than one medication is being used.

Thyroid function tests have been reported to show decreased values with carbamazepine administered alone.

Hyponatremia has been reported in association with carbamazepine use, either alone or in combination with other drugs.

Interference with some pregnancy tests has been reported.

Drug Interactions

Clinically meaningful drug interactions have occurred with concomitant medications and include but are not limited to the following:

Agents that may affect carbamazepine plasma levels:

CYP 3A4 inhibitors inhibit carbamazepine metabolism and can thus increase plasma carbamazepine levels. Drugs that have been shown, or would be expected, to increase plasma carbamazepine levels include:

cimetidine, danazol, diltiazem, macrolides, erythromycin, troleandomycin, clarithromycin, fluoxetine, loratadine, terfenadine, isoniazid, niacinamide, nicotinamide, propoxyphene, ketoconazole, itraconazole, verapamil, valproate.*

CYP 3A4 inducers can increase the rate of carbamazepine metabolism and can thus decrease plasma carbamazepine levels. Drugs that have been shown, or would be expected, to decrease plasma carbamazepine levels include:

cisplatin, doxorubicin HCL, felbamate, rifampin*, phenobarbital, phenytoin, primidone, theophylline.

*increased levels of the active 10, 11-epoxide

Effect of carbamazepine on plasma levels of concomitant agents:

Carbatrol increases levels of clomipramine HCL, phenytoin and primidone.

Carbatrol induces hepatic CYP activity. Carbatrol causes, or would be expected to cause decreased levels of the following:

acetaminophen, alprazolam, clonazepam, clozapine, dicumarol, doxycycline, ethosuximide, haloperidol, methsuximide, oral contraceptives, phensuximide, phenytoin, theophylline, valproate, warfarin.

The doses of these drugs may therefore have to be increased when carbamazepine is added to the therapeutic regimen.

Concomitant administration of carbamazepine and lithium may increase the risk of neurotoxic side effects. Alterations of thyroid function have been reported in combination therapy with other anticonvulsant medications.

Breakthrough bleeding has been reported among patients receiving concomitant oral contraceptives and their reliability may be adversely affected.

Carcinogenesis, Mutagenesis, Impairment of Fertility

Administration of carbamazepine to Sprague-Dawley rats for two years in the diet at doses of 25, 75, and 250 mg/kg/day (low dose approximately 0.2 times the maximum human daily dose of 1200 mg on a mg/m^2 basis), resulted in a dose-related increase in the incidence of hepatocellular tumors in females and of benign interstitial cell adenomas in the testes of males.

Carbamazepine must, therefore, be considered to be carcinogenic in Sprague-Dawley rats. Bacterial and mammalian mutagenicity studies using carbamazepine produced negative results. The significance of these findings relative to the use of carbamazepine in humans is, at present, unknown.

Usage in Pregnancy

Pregnancy Category D (See WARNINGS).

Labor and Delivery

The effect of carbamazepine on human labor and delivery is unknown.

Nursing Mothers

Carbamazepine and its epoxide metabolite are transferred to breast milk and during lactation. The concentrations of carbamazepine and its epoxide metabolite are approximately 50% of the maternal plasma concentration. Because of the potential for serious adverse reactions in nursing infants from carbamazepine, a decision should be made whether to discontinue nursing or to discontinue the drug, taking into account the importance of the drug to the mother.

Pediatric Use

Substantial evidence of carbamazepine effectiveness for use in the management of children with epilepsy (see INDICATIONS for specific seizure types) is derived from clinical investigations performed in adults and from studies in several *in vitro* systems which support the conclusion that (1) the pathogenic mechanisms underlying seizure propagation are essentially identical in adults and children, and (2) the mechanism of action of carbamazepine in treating seizures is essentially identical in adults and children.

Taken as a whole, this information supports a conclusion that the generally acceptable therapeutic range of total carbamazepine in plasma (i.e., 4–12 μg/mL) is the same in children and adults.

The evidence assembled was primarily obtained from short-term use of carbamazepine. The safety of carbamazepine in children has been systematically studied up to 6 months. No longer term data from clinical trials is available.

Geriatric Use

No systematic studies in geriatric patients have been conducted.

ADVERSE REACTIONS

General: If adverse reactions are of such severity that the drug must be discontinued, the physician must be aware that abrupt discontinuation of any anticonvulsant drug in a responsive patient with epilepsy may lead to seizures or even status epilepticus with its life-threatening hazards.

The most severe adverse reactions previously observed with carbamazepine were reported in the hemopoietic system (see BOX WARNING), the skin, and the cardiovascular system.

The most frequently observed adverse reactions, particularly during the initial phases of therapy, are dizziness, drowsiness, unsteadiness, nausea, and vomiting. To minimize the possibility of such reactions, therapy should be initiated at the lowest dosage recommended.

The following additional adverse reactions were previously reported with carbamazepine:

Hemopoietic System: Aplastic anemia, agranulocytosis, pancytopenia, bone marrow depression, thrombocytopenia, leukopenia, leukocytosis, eosinophilia, acute intermittent porphyria.

Skin: Pruritic and erythematous rashes, urticaria, toxic epidermal necrolysis (Lyell's syndrome) (see WARNINGS), Stevens-Johnson syndrome (see WARNINGS), photosensitivity reactions, alterations in skin pigmentation, exfoliative dermatitis, erythema multiforme and nodosum, purpura, aggravation of disseminated lupus erythematosus, alopecia, and diaphoresis. In certain cases, discontinuation of therapy may be necessary. Isolated cases of hirsutism have been reported, but a causal relationship is not clear.

Cardiovascular System: Congestive heart failure, edema, aggravation of hypertension, hypotension, syncope and collapse, aggravation of coronary artery disease, arrhythmias and AV block, thrombophlebitis, thromboembolism, and adenopathy or lymphadenopathy. Some of these cardiovascular complications have resulted in fatalities. Myocardial infarction has been associated with other tricyclic compounds.

Liver: Abnormalities in liver function tests, cholestatic and hepatocellular jaundice, hepatitis.

Respiratory System: Pulmonary hypersensitivity characterized by fever, dyspnea, pneumonitis, or pneumonia.

Genitourinary System: Urinary frequency, acute urinary retention, oliguria with elevated blood pressure, azotemia, renal failure, and impotence. Albuminuria, glycosuria, elevated BUN, and microscopic deposits in the urine have also been reported.

Testicular atrophy occurred in rats receiving carbamazepine orally from 4–52 weeks at dosage levels of 50–400 mg/kg/day. Additionally, rats receiving carbamazepine in the diet for 2 years at dosage levels of 25, 75, and 250 mg/kg/day had a dose-related incidence of testicular atrophy and aspermatogenesis. In dogs, it produced a brownish discoloration, presumably a metabolite, in the urinary bladder at dosage levels of 50 mg/kg/day and higher. Relevance of these findings to humans is unknown.

Nervous System: Dizziness, drowsiness, disturbances of coordination, confusion, headache, fatigue, blurred vision, visual hallucinations, transient diplopia, oculomotor disturbances, nystagmus, speech disturbances, abnormal involuntary movements, peripheral neuritis and paresthesias, depression with agitation, talkativeness, tinnitus, and hyperacusis.

There have been reports of associated paralysis and other symptoms of cerebral arterial insufficiency, but the exact relationship of these reactions to the drug has not been established.

Isolated cases of neuroleptic malignant syndrome have been reported with concomitant use of psychotropic drugs.

Digestive System: Nausea, vomiting, gastric distress and abdominal pain, diarrhea, constipation, anorexia, and dryness of the mouth and pharynx, including glossitis and stomatitis.

Eyes: Scattered punctate cortical lens opacities, as well as conjunctivitis, have been reported. Although a direct causal relationship has not been established, many phenothiazines and related drugs have been shown to cause eye changes.

Musculoskeletal System: Aching joints and muscles, and leg cramps.

Metabolism: Fever and chills, inappropriate antidiuretic hormone (ADH) secretion syndrome has been reported. Cases of frank water intoxication, with decreased serum sodium (hyponatremia) and confusion have been reported in association with carbamazepine use (see PRECAUTIONS, Laboratory Tests). Decreased levels of plasma calcium have been reported.

Other: Isolated cases of a lupus erythematosus-like syndrome have been reported. There have been occasional reports of elevated levels of cholesterol, HDL cholesterol, and triglycerides in patients taking anticonvulsants.

A case of aseptic meningitis, accompanied by myoclonus and peripheral eosinophilia, has been reported in a patient taking carbamazepine in combination with other medications. The patient was successfully dechallenged, and the meningitis reappeared upon rechallenge with carbamazepine.

DRUG ABUSE AND DEPENDENCE

No evidence of abuse potential has been associated with carbamazepine, nor is there evidence of psychological or physical dependence in humans.

OVERDOSAGE

Acute Toxicity

Lowest known lethal dose: adults, >60 g (39-year-old man). Highest known doses survived: adults, 30 g (31-year-old woman): children, 10 g (6-year-old boy); small children, 5 g (3-year-old girl).

Oral LD_{50} in animals (mg/kg): mice, 1100–3750; rats, 3850–4025; rabbits, 1500–2680; guinea pigs, 920.

Signs and Symptoms

The first signs and symptoms appear after 1–3 hours. Neuromuscular disturbances are the most prominent. Cardiovascular disorders are generally milder, and severe cardiac complications occur only when very high doses (>60 g) have been ingested.

Respiration: Irregular breathing, respiratory depression.

Cardiovascular System: Tachycardia, hypotension or hypertension, shock, conduction disorders.

Nervous System and Muscles: Impairment of consciousness ranging in severity to deep coma. Convulsions, especially in small children. Motor restlessness, muscular twitching, tremor, athetoid movements, opisthotonos, ataxia, drowsiness, dizziness, mydriasis, nystagmus, adiadochokinesia, ballism, psychomotor disturbances, dysmetria. Initial hyperreflexia, followed by hyporeflexia.

Gastrointestinal Tract: Nausea, vomiting.

Kidneys and Bladder: Anuria or oliguria, urinary retention.

Laboratory Findings: Isolated instances of overdosage have included leukocytosis, reduced leukocyte count, glycosuria, and acetonuria. EEG may show dysrhythmias.
Combined Poisoning: When alcohol, tricyclic antidepressants, barbiturates, or hydantoins are taken at the same time, the signs and symptoms of acute poisoning with carbamazepine may be aggravated or modified.
Treatment
The prognosis in cases of severe poisoning is critically dependent upon prompt elimination of the drug, which may be achieved by inducing vomiting, irrigating the stomach, and by taking appropriate steps to diminish absorption. If these measures cannot be implemented without risk on the spot, the patient should be transferred at once to a hospital, while ensuring that vital functions are safeguarded. There is no specific antidote.
Elimination of the Drug: Induction of vomiting.
Gastric lavage. Even when more than 4 hours have elapsed following ingestion of the drug, the stomach should be repeatedly irrigated, especially if the patient has also consumed alcohol.
Measures to Reduce Absorption: Activated charcoal, laxatives.
Measures to Accelerate Elimination: Forced diuresis.
Dialysis is indicated only in severe poisoning associated with renal failure. Replacement transfusion is indicated in severe poisoning in small children.
Respiratory Depression: Keep the airways free; resort, if necessary, to endotracheal intubation, artificial respiration, and administration of oxygen.
Hypotension, Shock: Keep the patient's legs raised and administer a plasma expander. If blood pressure fails to rise despite measures taken to increase plasma volume, use of vasoactive substances should be considered.
Convulsions: Diazepam or barbiturates.
Warning: Diazepam or barbiturates may aggravate respiratory depression (especially in children), hypotension, and coma. However, barbiturates should not be used if drugs that inhibit monoamine oxidase have also been taken by the patient either in overdosage or in recent therapy (within 1 week).
Surveillance: Respiration, cardiac function (ECG monitoring), blood pressure, body temperature, pupillary reflexes, and kidney and bladder function should be monitored for several days.
Treatment of Blood Count Abnormalities: If evidence of significant bone marrow depression develops, the following recommendations are suggested: (1) stop the drug, (2) perform daily CBC, platelet, and reticulocyte counts, (3) do a bone marrow aspiration and trephine biopsy immediately and repeat with sufficient frequency to monitor recovery.
Special periodic studies might be helpful as follows: (1) white cell and platelet antibodies, (2) ^{59}Fe-ferrokinetic studies, (3) peripheral blood cell typing, (4) cytogenetic studies on marrow and peripheral blood, (5) bone marrow culture studies for colony-forming units, (6) hemoglobin electrophoresis for A_2 and F hemoglobin, and (7) serum folic acid and B_{12} levels.
A fully developed aplastic anemia will require appropriate, intensive monitoring and therapy, for which specialized consultation should be sought.

DOSAGE AND ADMINISTRATION

Monitoring of blood levels has increased the efficacy and safety of anticonvulsants (see PRECAUTIONS, Laboratory Tests). Dosage should be adjusted to the needs of the individual patients. A low initial daily dosage with gradual increase is advised. As soon as adequate control is achieved, the dosage may be reduced very gradually to the minimum effective level. The Carbatrol capsules may be opened and the beads sprinkled over food, such as a teaspoon of applesauce or other similar food products if this method of administration is preferred. Carbatrol capsules or their contents should not be crushed or chewed. Carbatrol can be taken with or without meals.
Carbatrol is an extended-release formulation for twice a day administration. When converting patients from immediate release carbamazepine to Carbatrol extended-release capsules, the same total daily mg dose of carbamazepine should be administered.
Epilepsy (see INDICATIONS AND USAGE)
Adults and children over 12 years of age. Initial: 200 mg twice daily. Increase at weekly intervals by adding up to 200 mg/day until the optimal response is obtained. Dosage generally should not exceed 1000 mg per day in children 12-15 years of age, and 1200 mg daily in patients above 15 years of age. Doses up to 1600 mg daily have been used in adults.
Maintenance: Adjust dosage to the minimum effective level, usually 800–1200 mg daily.
Children under 12 years of age: Children taking total daily dosages of immediate-release carbamazepine of 400 mg or greater may be converted to the same total daily dosage of Carbatrol extended-release capsules, using a twice daily regimen. Ordinarily, optimal clinical response is achieved at daily doses below 35 mg/kg. If satisfactory clinical response has not been achieved, plasma levels should be measured to determine whether or not they are in the therapeutic range. No recommendation regarding the safety of Carbatrol for use at doses above 35 mg/kg/24 hours can be made.
Combination Therapy: Carbatrol may be used alone or with other anticonvulsants. When added to existing anticonvulsant therapy, the drug should be added gradually while the other anticonvulsants are maintained or gradually decreased, except phenytoin, which may have to be increased (see PRECAUTIONS, Drug Interactions and Pregnancy Category D).
Trigeminal Neuralgia (see INDICATIONS AND USAGE)
Initial: On the first day, start with one 200 mg capsule. This daily dose may be increased by up to 200 mg/day every 12 hours only as needed to achieve freedom from pain. Do not exceed 1200 mg daily.
Maintenance: Control of pain can be maintained in most patients with 400–800 mg daily. However, some patients may be maintained on as little as 200 mg daily, while others may require as much as 1200 mg daily. At least once every 3 months throughout the treatment period, attempts should be made to reduce the dose to the minimum effective level or even to discontinue the drug.

HOW SUPPLIED

Carbatrol (carbamazepine extended-release capsules) is supplied in two dosage strengths.
200 mg-Two-piece hard gelatin capsule (light gray opaque body with bluish green opaque cap) printed with the Shire logo in white ink.
Supplied in bottles of 120 .... NDC 58521-172-12
300 mg-Two-piece hard gelatin capsule (black opaque body with bluish green opaque cap) printed with the Shire logo in white ink.
Supplied in bottles of 120 .... NDC 58521-173-12
Store at controlled room temperature 15–25°C (59–77°F).
Protect from light and moisture. Dispense in tight, light-resistant container as defined in USP.
Rx only.
Manufactured for:
Shire Richwood Inc.
Florence, KY 41042
1-800-536-7878

B5684 Rev. 7/98
Shown in Product Identification Guide, page 336

COLACE® OTC

[*kōlās*]
docusate sodium,
capsules • syrup• liquid (drops)

DESCRIPTION

Colace® (docusate sodium) is a stool softener.
Colace® Capsules, 50 mg, contain the following:
Active Ingredient: contains 50 mg of docusate sodium.
Inactive Ingredients: Polyethylene glycol 400, gelatin, glycerin, sorbitol, propylene glycol, FD&C Red No. 40, D&C Red No. 33.
Colace® Capsules, 100 mg, contain the following:
Active Ingredient: contains 100 mg of docusate sodium.
Inactive Ingredients: Polyethylene glycol 400, gelatin, glycerin, sorbitol, propylene glycol, methylparaben, titanium dioxide, FD&C Red No. 40, D&C Red No. 33, propylparaben, FD&C Yellow No. 6.
Colace® Liquid, 1%, contains the following:
Active Ingredient: each mL contains 10 mg of docusate sodium.
Inactive Ingredients: citric acid, D&C Red No. 33, methylparaben, poloxamer, polyethylene glycol, propylene glycol, propylparaben, sodium citrate, vanillin, and purified water.
Colace® Syrup, 20 mg/5 mL, contains the following:
Active Ingredient: each 5 mL contains 20 mg of docusate sodium.
Inactive Ingredients: alcohol (not more than 1%), citric acid, D&C Red No. 33, FD&C Red No. 40, flavor (natural), menthol, methylparaben, peppermint oil, poloxamer, polyethylene glycol, propylparaben, sodium citrate, sucrose, and purified water.

ACTIONS AND USES

Colace®, a surface-active agent, helps to keep stools soft for easy, natural passage and is not a stimulant laxative, thus, not habit forming. Useful in constipation due to hard stools, in painful anorectal conditions, in cardiac and other conditions in which maximum ease of passage is desirable to avoid difficult or painful defecation, and when peristaltic stimulants are contraindicated.
Note: When peristaltic stimulation is needed due to inadequate bowel motility, see Peri-Colace® (stimulant laxative and stool softener).

CONTRAINDICATIONS

There are no known contraindications to Colace®.

WARNINGS

Do not use when abdominal pain, nausea, or vomiting are present, unless directed by a doctor.
As with any drug, pregnant or nursing women should seek the advice of a health professional before using this product.

SIDE EFFECTS

The incidence of side effects—none of a serious nature—is exceedingly small. Bitter taste, throat irritation, and nausea (primarily associated with the use of the syrup and liquid) are the main side effects reported. Rash has occurred.

ADMINISTRATION AND DOSAGE

Orally —Suggested daily Dosage: *Adults and older children:* 50 to 200 mg *Children 6 to 12:* 40 to 120 mg Liquid.
Infants and children under 3 years of age: As prescribed by physician.
Children 3 to 6 years of age: 2mL one to three times daily
For retention or flushing enemas: Add 5 to 10mL (1 to 2 tsp) of COLACE® liquid to the enema fluid.
The higher doses are recommended for initial therapy. Dosage should be adjusted to individual response. The effect on stools is usually apparent 1 to 3 days after the first dose. Colace® liquid or syrup must be given in a 6 oz. to 8 oz. glass of milk or fruit juice or in infant's formula to prevent throat irritation. *In enemas*—Add 5 to 10 mL Colace® liquid) to a retention or flushing enema.

HOW SUPPLIED

Colace® capsules, 50 mg
NDC 54092-052-30 Bottles of 30
NDC 54092-052-60 Bottles of 60
NDC 54092-052-52 Cartons of 100 single unit packs
NDC 54092-052-11 Blister Pack of 10
Colace® capsules, 100 mg
NDC 54092-053-30 Bottles of 30
NDC 54092-053-60 Bottles of 60
NDC 54092-053-02 Bottles of 250
NDC 54092-053-10 Bottles of 1000
NDC 54092-053-52 Cartons of 100 single unit packs
NDC 54092-053-11 Blister Pack of 10
Note: Colace® capsules should be stored at controlled room temperature (59°–86°F or 15°–30°C)
Colace® liquid, 1% solution; 10 mg/mL (with calibrated dropper)
NDC 54092-414-16 Bottles of 16 fl oz
NDC 54092-414-30 Bottles of 30 mL
Colace® syrup, 20 mg/5-mL teaspoon; contains not more than 1% alcohol
NDC 54092-415-08 Bottles of 8 fl oz
NDC 54092-415-16 Bottles of 16 fl oz
Manufactured for
Roberts Laboratories Inc., a subsidiary of
ROBERTS PHARMACEUTICAL CORPORATION
Eatontown, NJ 07724 USA

DEXTROSTAT® Ⓒ℞

[*deks'trō-stăt*]
Dextroamphetamine Sulfate Tablets, USP
5 mg and 10 mg

> WARNING
> AMPHETAMINES HAVE A HIGH POTENTIAL FOR ABUSE, ADMINISTRATION OF AMPHETAMINES FOR PROLONGED PERIODS OF TIME MAY LEAD TO DRUG DEPENDENCE AND MUST BE AVOIDED. PARTICULAR ATTENTION SHOULD BE PAID TO THE POSSIBILITY OF SUBJECTS OBTAINING AMPHETAMINES FOR NONTHERAPEUTIC USE OR DISTRIBUTION TO OTHERS, AND THE DRUGS SHOULD BE PRESCRIBED OR DISPENSED SPARINGLY.

DESCRIPTION

DextroStat® (dextroamphetamine sulfate) is the dextro isomer of the compound *d,l*-amphetamine sulfate, a sympathomimetic amine of the amphetamine group. Chemically, dextroamphetamine is *d*-alpha-methylphenethylamine, and is present in all forms of DextroStat® as the neutral sulfate. It has a chemical formula of $(C_9H_{13}N)_2 \cdot H_2SO_4$ and a molecular weight of 368.50.
Structural Formula:

CH_2CHNH_2 ; CH_3 ; $]_2 \cdot H_2SO_4$

Each round, yellow, scored tablet contains dextroamphetamine sulfate USP, 5 mg or 10 mg. Each tablet also contains the following inactive ingredients: acacia, corn starch, lactose monohydrate, magnesium stearate, sucrose. 10 mg tablet contains sodium starch glycolate. 5 mg and 10 mg tablets contain FD&C Yellow #5 (tartrazine).

CLINICAL PHARMACOLOGY

Amphetamines are non-catecholamine, sympathomimetic amines with CNS stimulant activity. Peripheral actions include elevations of systolic and diastolic blood pressures and weak bronchodilator and respiratory stimulant action.
There is neither specific evidence which clearly establishes the mechanism whereby amphetamines produce mental and behavioral effects in children, nor conclusive evidence regarding how these effects relate to the condition of the central nervous system.
Pharmacokinetics
The single ingestion of two 5 mg tablets by healthy volunteers produced an average peak dextroamphetamine blood level of 29.2 ng/mL at 2 hours post-administration. The average half-life was 10.25 hours. The average urinary recovery was 45% in 48 hours.

Continued on next page

Dextrostat—Cont.

INDICATIONS AND USAGE

Dextroamphetamine sulfate tablets are indicated:

1. In Narcolepsy.

2. In Attention Deficit Disorder with Hyperactivity, as an integral part of a total treatment program which typically includes other remedial measures (psychological, educational, social) for a stabilizing effect in pediatric patients (ages 3 to 16 years) with a behavioral syndrome characterized by the following group of developmentally inappropriate symptoms: moderate to severe distractibility, short attention span, hyperactivity, emotional lability, and impulsivity. The diagnosis of this syndrome should not be made with finality when these symptoms are only of comparatively recent origin. Nonlocalizing (soft) neurological signs, learning disability and abnormal EEG may or may not be present, and a diagnosis of central nervous system dysfunction may or may not be warranted.

CONTRAINDICATIONS

Advanced arteriosclerosis, symptomatic cardiovascular disease, moderate to severe hypertension, hyperthyroidism, known hypersensitivity or idiosyncrasy to the sympathomimetic amines, glaucoma.

Agitated states.

Patients with a history of drug abuse.

During or within 14 days following the administration of monoamine oxidase inhibitors (hypertensive crises may result).

PRECAUTIONS

General: Caution is to be exercised in prescribing amphetamines for patients with even mild hypertension.

The least amount feasible should be prescribed or dispensed at one time in order to minimize the possibility of overdosage.

These products contain FD&C Yellow No. 5 (tartrazine), which may cause allergic-type reactions (including bronchial asthma) in certain susceptible individuals. Although the overall incidence of FD&C Yellow No. 5 (tartrazine) sensitivity in the general population is low, it is frequently seen in patients who also have aspirin hypersensitivity.

Information for Patients: Amphetamines may impair the ability of the patient to engage in potentially hazardous activities such as operating machinery or vehicles; the patient should therefore be cautioned accordingly.

Drug Interactions:

Acidifying agents—Gastrointestinal acidifying agents (guanethidine, reserpine, glutamic acid HCl, ascorbic acid, fruit juices, etc.) lower absorption of amphetamines. Urinary acidifying agents (ammonium chloride, sodium acid phosphate, etc.) increase the concentration of the ionized species of the amphetamine molecule, thereby increasing urinary excretion. Both groups of agents lower blood levels and efficacy of amphetamines.

Adrenergic blockers—Adrenergic blockers are inhibited by amphetamines.

Alkalinizing agents—Gastrointestinal alkalinizing agents (sodium bicarbonate, etc.) increase absorption of amphetamines. Urinary alkalinizing agents (acetazolamide, some thiazides) increase the concentration of the non-ionized species of the amphetamine molecule, thereby decreasing urinary excretion. Both groups of agents increase blood levels and therefore potentiate the actions of amphetamines.

Antidepressants, tricyclic—Amphetamines may enhance the activity of tricyclic or sympathomimetic agents; *d*-amphetamine with desipramine or protriptyline and possibly other tricyclics cause striking and sustained increases in the concentration of *d*-amphetamine in the brain; cardiovascular effects can be potentiated.

MAO inhibitors—MAOI antidepressants, as well as a metabolite of furazolidone, slow amphetamine metabolism. This slowing potentiates amphetamines, increasing their effect on the release of norepinephrine and other monoamines from adrenergic nerve endings; this can cause headaches and other signs of hypertensive crisis. A variety of neurological toxic effects and malignant hyperpyrexia can occur, sometimes with fatal results.

Antihistamines—Amphetamines may counteract the sedative effect of antihistamines.

Antihypertensives—Amphetamines may antagonize the hypotensive effects of antihypertensives.

Chlorpromazine—Chlorpromazine blocks dopamine and norepinephrine reuptake, thus inhibiting the central stimulant effects of amphetamines, and can be used to treat amphetamine poisoning.

Ethosuximide—Amphetamines may delay intestinal absorption of ethosuximide.

Haloperidol—Haloperidol blocks dopamine and norepinephrine reuptake, thus inhibiting the central stimulant effects of amphetamines.

Lithium carbonate—The stimulatory effects of amphetamines may be inhibited by lithium carbonate.

Meperidine—Amphetamines potentiate the analgesic effect of meperidine.

Methenamine therapy—Urinary excretion of amphetamines is increased, and efficacy is reduced, by acidifying agents used in methenamine therapy.

Norepinephrine—Amphetamines enhance the adrenergic effect of norepinephrine.

Phenobarbital—Amphetamines may delay intestinal absorption of phenobarbital; co-administration of phenobarbital may produce a synergistic anticonvulsant action.

Phenytoin-Amphetamines may delay intestinal absorption of phenytoin; co-administration of phenytoin may produce a synergistic anticonvulsant action.

Propoxyphene—In cases of propoxyphene overdosage, amphetamine CNS stimulation is potentiated and fatal convulsions can occur.

Veratrum alkaloids—Amphetamines inhibit the hypotensive effect of veratrum alkaloids.

Drug/Laboratory Test Interactions:

- Amphetamines can cause a significant elevation in plasma corticosteroid levels. This increase is greatest in the evening.
- Amphetamines may interfere with urinary steroid determinations.

Carcinogenesis/Mutagenesis: Mutagenicity studies and long-term studies in animals to determine the carcinogenic potential of DextroStat® (dextroamphetamine sulfate) have not been performed.

Pregnancy-Teratogenic Effects: Pregnancy Category C. Amphetamine has been shown to have embryotoxic and teratogenic effects when administered to A/Jax mice and C57BL mice in doses approximately 41 times the maximum human dose. Embryotoxic effects were not seen in New Zealand white rabbits given the drug in doses 7 times the human dose nor in rats given 12.5 times the maximum human dose. While there are no adequate and well-controlled studies in pregnant women, there has been one report of severe congenital bony deformity, tracheoesophageal fistula, and anal atresia (Vater association) in a baby born to a woman who took dextroamphetamine sulfate with lovastatin during the first trimester of pregnancy. Amphetamines should be used during pregnancy only if the potential benefit justifies the potential risk to the fetus.

Nonteratogenic Effects: Infants born to mothers dependent on amphetamines have an increased risk of premature delivery and low birth weight. Also, these infants may experience symptoms of withdrawal as demonstrated by dysphoria, including agitation, and significant lassitude.

Nursing Mothers: Amphetamines are excreted in human milk. Mothers taking amphetamines should be advised to refrain from nursing.

Pediatric Use: Long-term effects of amphetamines in pediatric patients have not been well established.

Amphetamines are not recommended for use in pediatric patients under 3 years of age with Attention Deficit Disorder with Hyperactivity described under INDICATIONS AND USAGE.

Clinical experience suggests that in psychotic pediatric patients, administration of amphetamines may exacerbate symptoms of behavior disturbance and thought disorder.

Amphetamines have been reported to exacerbate motor and phonic tics and Tourette's syndrome. Therefore, clinical evaluation for tics and Tourette's syndrome in pediatric patients and their families should precede use of stimulant medications.

Data are inadequate to determine whether chronic administration of amphetamines may be associated with growth inhibition; therefore, growth should be monitored during treatment.

Drug treatment is not indicated in all cases of Attention Deficit Disorder with Hyperactivity and should be considered only in light of the complete history and evaluation of the pediatric patient. The decision to prescribe amphetamines should depend on the physician's assessment of the chronicity and severity of the pediatric patient's symptoms and their appropriateness for his/her age.

Prescription should not depend solely on the presence of one or more of the behavioral characteristics.

When these symptoms are associated with acute stress reactions, treatment with amphetamines is usually not indicated.

ADVERSE REACTIONS

Cardiovascular: Palpitations, tachycardia, elevation of blood pressure. There have been isolated reports of cardiomyopathy associated with chronic amphetamine use.

Central Nervous System:

Psychotic episodes at recommended doses (rare), overstimulation, restlessness, dizziness, insomnia, euphoria, dyskinesia, dysphoria, tremor, headache, exacerbation of motor and phonic tics and Tourette's syndrome.

Gastrointestinal: Dryness of the mouth, unpleasant taste, diarrhea, constipation, other gastrointestinal disturbances. Anorexia and weight loss may occur as undesirable effects.

Allergic: Urticaria.

Endocrine: Impotence, changes in libido.

DRUG ABUSE AND DEPENDENCE

Dextroamphetamine sulfate tablets are a Schedule II controlled substance.

Amphetamines have been extensively abused. Tolerance, extreme psychological dependence and severe social disability have occurred. There are reports of patients who have increased the dosage to many times that recommended. Abrupt cessation following prolonged high dosage administration results in extreme fatigue and mental depression; changes are also noted on the sleep EEG.

Manifestation of chronic intoxication with amphetamines include severe dermatoses, marked insomnia, irritability, hyperactivity and personality changes. The most severe manifestation of chronic intoxication is psychosis, often clinically indistinguishable from schizophrenia. This is rare with oral amphetamines.

OVERDOSAGE

Individual patient response to amphetamines varies widely. While toxic symptoms occasionally occur as an idiosyncrasy at doses as low as 2 mg, they are rare with doses of less than 15 mg; 30 mg can produce severe reactions, yet doses of 400 to 500 mg are not necessarily fatal.

In rats, the oral LD_{50} of dextroamphetamine sulfate is 96.8 mg/kg.

Manifestations of acute overdosage with amphetamines include restlessness, tremor, hyperreflexia, rhabdomyolysis, rapid respiration, hyperpyrexia, confusion, assultiveness, hallucinations, panic states.

Fatigue and depression usually follow the central stimulation.

Cardiovascular effects include arrhythmias, hypertension or hypotension and circulatory collapse. Gastrointestinal symptoms include nausea, vomiting, diarrhea and abdominal cramps. Fatal poisoning is usually preceded by convulsions and coma.

TREATMENT—Consult with a Certified Poison Control Center for up-to-date guidance and advice. Management of acute amphetamine intoxication is largely symptomatic and includes gastric lavage, administration of activated charcoal, administration of a cathartic, and sedation. Experience with hemodialysis or peritoneal dialysis is inadequate to permit recommendation in this regard. Acidification of the urine increases amphetamine excretion, but is believed to increase risk of acute renal failure if myoglobinuria is present. If acute, severe hypertension complicates amphetamine overdosage, administration of intravenous phentolamine has been suggested. However, a gradual drop in blood pressure will usually result when sufficient sedation has been achieved.

DOSAGE AND ADMINISTRATION

Amphetamines should be administered at the lowest effective dosage and dosage should be individually adjusted. Late evening doses should be avoided because of the resulting insomnia.

Narcolepsy: Usual dose 5 to 60 mg per day in divided doses, depending on the individual patient response.

Narcolepsy seldom occurs in pediatric patients under 12 years of age; however, when it does, DextroStat® (dextroamphetamine sulfate) may be used. The suggested initial dose for patients aged 6 to 12 is 5 mg daily; daily dose may be raised in increments of 5 mg at weekly intervals until optimal response is obtained. In patients 12 years of age and older, start with 10 mg daily; daily dosage may be raised in increments of 10 mg at weekly intervals until optimal response is obtained. If bothersome adverse reactions appear (e.g., insomnia or anorexia), dosage should be reduced. Give first dose on awakening; additional doses (1 or 2) at intervals of 4 to 6 hours.

Attention Deficit Disorder with Hyperactivity: Not recommended for pediatric patients under 3 years of age.

In pediatric patients from 3 to 5 years of age, start with 2.5 mg daily; daily dosage may be raised in increments of 2.5 mg at weekly intervals until optimal response is obtained.

In pediatric patients 6 years of age and older, start with 5 mg once or twice daily; daily dosage may be raised in increments of 5 mg at weekly intervals until optimal response is obtained. Only in rare cases will it be necessary to exceed a total of 40 mg per day.

Give first dose on awakening; additional doses (1 or 2) at intervals of 4 to 6 hours.

When possible, drug administration should be interrupted occasionally to determine if there is a recurrence of behavioral symptoms sufficient to require continued therapy.

HOW SUPPLIED

DextroStat®, (dextroamphetamine sulfate) Tablets are available as follows:

5 mg Yellow, Round, Scored Tablet debossed "RP" on one side and "51" on the other side.

NDC #: 58521-451-01 for 100s

10 mg Yellow, Round, Double-Scored Tablet debossed "RP" on one side and "52" on the other side.

NDC #: 58521-452-01 for 100s

Dispense in a tight container as defined in the USP. Store at controlled room temperature 15°–30°C (59°–86°F).

DEA Order Form Required.

Rx only.

Shire Richwood Inc.
Florence, KY 41042
MG #9245 Rev 6/98

Shown in Product Identification Guide, page 336

FARESTON® ℞
(toremifene citrate)
Tablets
PRODUCT INFORMATION

DESCRIPTION

FARESTON (toremifene citrate) Tablets for oral administration each contain 88.5 mg of toremifene citrate, which is equivalent to 60 mg toremifene.

FARESTON is a nonsteroidal antiestrogen. The chemical name of toremifene is: 2-(p-[(Z)-4-chloro-1,2-diphenyl-1-

butenyl]-phenoxy)-N,N-dimethylethylamine citrate (1:1). The structural formula is:

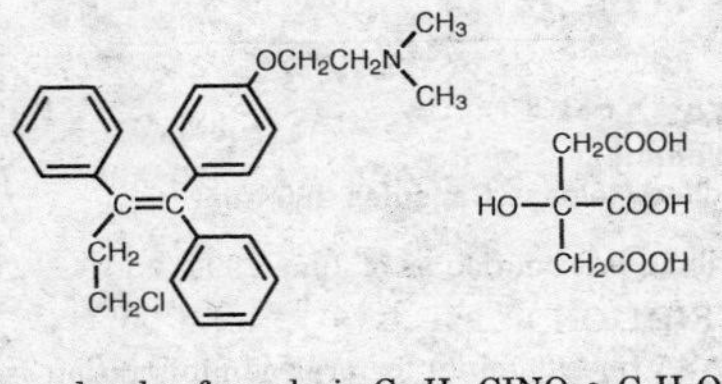

and the molecular formula is $C_{26}H_{28}ClNO \bullet C_6H_8O_7$. The molecular weight of toremifene citrate is 598.10. The pK_a is 8.0. Water solubility at 37°C is 0.63 mg/mL and in 0.02N HCl at 37°C is 0.38 mg/mL.

FARESTON is available only as tablets for oral administration. Inactive ingredients: starch, lactose, povidone, sodium starch glycolate, magnesium stearate, microcrystalline cellulose, and colloidal silicon dioxide.

CLINICAL PHARMACOLOGY

Mechanism of Action: Toremifene is a nonsteroidal triphenylethylene derivative. Toremifene binds to estrogen receptors and may exert estrogenic, antiestrogenic, or both activities, depending upon the duration of treatment, animal species, gender, target organ, or endpoint selected. In general, however, nonsteroidal triphenylethylene derivatives are predominantly antiestrogenic in rats and humans and estrogenic in mice. In rats, toremifene causes regression of established dimethylbenzanthracene (DMBA)-induced mammary tumors. The antitumor effect of toremifene in breast cancer is believed to be mainly due to its antiestrogenic effects, ie, its ability to compete with estrogen for binding sites in the cancer, blocking the growth-stimulating effects of estrogen in the tumor.

Toremifene causes a decrease in the estradiol-induced vaginal cornification index in some postmenopausal women, indicative of its antiestrogenic activity. Toremifene also has estrogenic activity as shown by decreases in serum gonadotropin concentration (FSH and LH).

Pharmacokinetics: The plasma concentration time profile of toremifene declines biexponentially after absorption with a mean distribution half-life of about 4 hours and an elimination half-life of about 5 days. Elimination half-lives of major metabolites, N-demethyltoremifene and (deamino-hydroxy) toremifene were 6 and 4 days, respectively. Mean total clearance of toremifene was approximately 5L/h.

Absorption and Distribution: Toremifene is well absorbed after oral administration and absorption is not influenced by food. Peak plasma concentrations are obtained within 3 hours. Toremifene displays linear pharmacokinetics after single oral doses of 10 to 680 mg. After multiple dosing, dose proportionality was observed for doses of 10 to 400 mg. Steady-state concentrations were reached in about 4–6 weeks. Toremifene has an apparent volume of distribution of 580 L and binds extensively (>99.5%) to serum proteins, mainly to albumin.

Metabolism and Excretion: Toremifene is extensively metabolized, principally by CYP3A4 to N-demethyltoremifene, which is also antiestrogenic but with weak *in vivo* antitumor potency. Serum concentrations of N-demethyltoremifene are 2 to 4 times higher than toremifene at steady state. Toremifene is eliminated as metabolites predominantly in the feces, with about 10% excreted in the urine during a 1-week period. Elimination of toremifene is slow, in part because of enterohepatic circulation.

Special Populations: *Renal insufficiency:* The pharmacokinetics of toremifene and N-demethyltoremifene were similar in normals and in patients with impaired kidney function.

Hepatic insufficiency: The mean elimination half-life of toremifene was increased by less than twofold in 10 patients with hepatic impairment (cirrhosis or fibrosis) compared to subjects with normal hepatic function. The pharmacokinetics of N-demethyltoremifene were unchanged in these patients. Ten patients on anticonvulsants (phenobarbital, clonazepam, phenytoin, and carbamazepine) showed a twofold increase in clearance and a decrease in the elimination half-life of toremifene.

Geriatric patients: The pharmacokinetics of toremifene were studied in 10 healthy young males and 10 elderly females following a single 120 mg dose under fasting conditions. Increases in the elimination half-life (4.2 versus 7.2 days) and the volume of distribution (457 versus 627 L) of toremifene were seen in the elderly females without any change in clearance or AUC.

Race: The pharmacokinetics of toremifene in patients of different races has not been studied.

Drug-drug interactions: No formal drug-drug interaction studies with toremifene have been performed.

CLINICAL STUDIES

Three prospective, randomized, controlled clinical studies (North American, Eastern European, and Nordic) were conducted to evaluate the efficacy of FARESTON for the treatment of breast cancer in postmenopausal women. The patients were randomized to parallel groups receiving FARESTON 60 mg (FAR60) or tamoxifen 20 mg (TAM20) in the North American Study or tamoxifen 40 mg (TAM40) in the Eastern European and Nordic studies. The North American and Eastern European studies also included high-dose toremifene arms of 200 and 240 mg daily, respectively. The studies included postmenopausal patients with estrogen-receptor (ER) positive or estrogen-receptor (ER) unknown metastatic breast cancer. The patients had at least one measurable or evaluable lesion. The primary efficacy variables were response rate (RR) and time to progression (TTP). Survival (S) was also determined. Ninety-five percent confidence intervals (95% CI) were calculated for the difference in RR between FAR60 and TAM groups and the hazard ratio (relative risk for an unfavorable event, such as disease progression or death) between TAM and FAR60 or TTP and S. Two of the 3 studies showed similar results for all effectiveness endpoints. However, the Nordic Study showed a longer time to progression for tamoxifen (see table).

[See table above]

CLINICAL STUDIES

Study	North American		Eastern European		Nordic	
Treatment Group	FAR60	TAM20	FAR60	TAM40	FAR60	TAM40
No. Patients	221	215	157	149	214	201
Responses						
CR[1]+ PR[2]	14+33	11+30	7+25	3+28	19+48	19+56
RR[3](CR + PR)%	21.3	19.1	20.4	20.8	31.3	37.3
Difference in RR	2.2		−0.4		−6.0	
95% CI[4] for Difference in RR	−5.8 to 10.2		−9.5 to 8.6		−15.1 to 3.1	
Time to Progression (TTP)						
Median TTP (mo.)	5.6	5.8	4.9	5.0	7.3	10.2
Hazard Ratio (TAM/FAR)	1.01		1.02		0.80	
95% CI[4] for Hazard Ratio (%)	0.81 to 1.26		0.79 to 1.31		0.64 to 1.00	
Survival (S)						
Median S (mo.)	33.6	34.0	25.4	23.4	33.0	38.7
Hazard Ratio (TAM/FAR)	0.94		0.96		0.94	
95% CI[4] for Hazard Ratio (%)	0.74 to 1.24		0.72 to 1.28		0.73 to 1.22	

[1]CR = complete response; [2]PR = partial response; [3]RR = response rate; [4]CI = confidence interval

The high-dose groups, toremifene 200 mg daily in the North American Study and 240 mg daily in the Eastern European Study, were not superior to the lower toremifene dose groups, with response rates of 22.6% AND 28.7%, median times to progression of 5.6 and 6.1 months, and median survivals of 30.1 and 23.8 months, respectively. The median treatment duration in the three pivotal studies was 5 months (range 4.2–6.3 months).

INDICATION AND USAGE

FARESTON is indicated for the treatment of metastatic breast cancer in postmenopausal women with estrogen-receptor positive or unknown tumors.

CONTRAINDICATIONS

FARESTON is contraindicated in patients with known hypersensitivity to the drug.

WARNINGS

Hypercalcemia and Tumor Flare: As with other antiestrogens, hypercalcemia and tumor flare have been reported in some breast cancer patients with bone metastases during the first weeks of treatment with FARESTON. Tumor flare is a syndrome of diffuse musculoskeletal pain and erythema with increased size of tumor lesions that later regress. It is often accompanied by hypercalcemia. Tumor flare does not imply failure of treatment or represent tumor progression. If hypercalcemia occurs, appropriate measures should be instituted and if hypercalcemia is severe, FARESTON treatment should be discontinued.

Tumorigenicity: Since most toremifene trials have been conducted in patients with metastatic disease, adequate data on the potential endometrial tumorigenicity of long-term treatment with FARESTON are not available. Endometrial hyperplasia has been reported. Some patients treated with FARESTON have developed endometrial cancer, but circumstances (short duration of treatment or prior antiestrogen treatment or premalignant conditions) make it difficult to establish the role of FARESTON.

Endometrial hyperplasia of the uterus was observed in monkeys following 52 weeks of treatment at ≥1 mg/kg and in dogs following 16 weeks of treatment at ≥3 mg/kg with toremifene (about 1/4 and 1.4 times, respectively, the daily maximum recommended human dose on a mg/m^2 basis.

Pregnancy: FARESTON may cause fetal harm when administered to pregnant women. Studies in rats at doses ≥1.0 mg/kg/day (about 1/4 the daily maximum recommended human dose on a mg/m^2 basis) administered during the period of organogenesis, have shown that toremifene is embryotoxic and fetotoxic, as indicated by intrauterine mortality, increased resorption, reduced fetal weight, and fetal anomalies; including malformation of limbs, incomplete ossification, misshapen bones, ribs/spine anomalies, hydroureter, hydronephrosis, testicular displacement, and subcutaneous edema. Fetal anomalies may have been a consequence of maternal toxicity. Toremifene has been shown to cross the placenta and accumulate in the rodent fetus.

In rodent models of fetal reproductive tract development, toremifene produced inhibition of uterine development in female pups similar to diethylstilbestrol (DES) and tamoxifen. The clinical relevance of these changes is not known. Embryotoxicity and fetotoxicity were observed in rabbits at doses ≥1.25 mg/kg/day and 2.5 mg/kg/day, respectively (about 1/3 and 2/3 the daily maximum recommended human dose on a mg/m^2 basis); fetal anomalies included incomplete ossification and anencephaly.

There are no studies in pregnant women. If FARESTON is used during pregnancy, or if the patient becomes pregnant while receiving this drug, the patient should be apprised of the potential hazard to the fetus or potential risk for loss of the pregnancy.

PRECAUTIONS

General: Patients with a history of thromboembolic diseases should generally not be treated with FARESTON. In general, patients with preexisting endometrial hyperplasia should not be given long-term FARESTON treatment. Patients with bone metastases should be monitored closely for hypercalcemia during the first weeks of treatment (see **WARNINGS**). Leukopenia and thrombocytopenia have been reported rarely; leukocyte and platelet counts should be monitored when using FARESTON in patients with leukopenia and thrombocytopenia.

Information for Patients: Vaginal bleeding has been reported in patients using FARESTON. Patients should be informed about this and instructed to contact their physician if such bleeding occurs.

Patients with bone metastases should be informed about the typical signs and symptoms of hypercalcemia and instructed to contact their physician for further assessment if such signs or symptoms occur.

Laboratory Tests: Periodic complete blood counts, calcium levels, and liver function tests should be obtained.

Drug-drug Interactions: Drugs that decrease renal calcium excretion, eg, thiazide diuretics, may increase the risk of hypercalcemia in patients receiving FARESTON. There is a known interaction between antiestrogenic compounds of the triphenylethylene derivative class and coumarin-type anticoagulants (eg, warfarin), leading to an increased prothrombin time. When concomitant use of anticoagulants with FARESTON is necessary, careful monitoring of the prothrombin time is recommended.

Cytochrome P450 3A4 enzyme inducers, such as phenobarbital, phenytoin, and carbamazepine increase the rate of toremifene metabolism, lowering the steady-state concentration in serum. Metabolism of toremifene may be inhibited by drugs known to inhibit the CYP3A4-6 enzymes. Examples of such drugs are ketoconazole and similar antimycotics as well as erythromycin and similar macrolides. This interaction has not been studied and its clinical relevance is uncertain.

Carcinogenesis, Mutagenesis, and Impairment of Fertility: Conventional carcinogenesis studies in rats at doses of 0.12 to 12 mg/kg/day (about 1/100 to 1.5 times the daily maximum recommended human dose on a mg/m^2 basis) for up to 2 years did not show evidence of carcinogenicity. Studies in mice at doses of 1.0 to 30.0 mg/kg/day (about 1/15 to 2 times the daily maximum recommended human dose on a mg/m^2 basis) for up to 2 years revealed increased incidence of ovarian and testicular tumors, and increased incidence of osteoma and osteosarcoma. The significance of the mouse findings is uncertain because of the different role of estrogens in mice and the estrogenic effect of toremifene in mice. An increased incidence of ovarian and testicular tumors in mice has also been observed with other human antiestrogenic agents that have primarily estrogenic activity in mice.

Toremifene has not been shown to be mutagenic in *in vitro* tests (Ames and *E. Coli* bacterial tests). Toremifene is clastogenic *in vitro* (chromosomal aberrations and micronuclei formation in human lymphoblastoid MCL-5 cells) and *in vivo* (chromosomal aberrations in rat hepatocytes). No significant adduct formation could be detected using ^{32}P post-labeling in liver DNA from rats administered toremifene when compared to tamoxifen at similar doses. A study in cultured human lymphocytes indicated that adducting activity of toremifene, detected by ^{32}P post-labeling, was about 1/6 that of tamoxifen at approximately equipotent concentrations. In addition, the DNA adducting activity of toremifene in salmon sperm, using ^{32}P post-labeling, was 1/6 and 1/4 that observed with tamoxifen at equivalent concentrations following activation by rat and human micro-

Continued on next page

Fareston—Cont.

somal systems, respectively. However, toremifene exposure is fourfold the exposure of tamoxifen based on human AUC in serum at recommended clinical doses.

Toremifene produced impairment of fertility and conception in male and female rats at doses ≥25.0 and 0.14 mg/kg/day, respectively (about 3.5 times and 1/50 the daily maximum recommended human dose on a mg/m^2 basis). At these doses, sperm counts, fertility index, and conception rate were reduced in males with atrophy of seminal vesicles and prostate. In females, fertility and reproductive indices were markedly reduced with increased pre- and post-implantation loss. In addition, offspring of treated rats exhibited depressed reproductive indices. Toremifene produced ovarian atrophy in dogs administered doses ≥3 mg/kg/day (about 1.5 times the daily maximum recommended human dose on a mg/m^2 basis) for 16 weeks. Cystic ovaries and reduction in endometrial stromal cellularity were observed in monkeys at doses ≥1 mg/kg/day (about 1/4 the daily maximum recommended human dose on a mg/m^2 basis) for 52 weeks.

Pregnancy: *Pregnancy Category D:* (see **WARNINGS**).

Nursing mothers: Toremifene has been shown to be excreted in the milk of lactating rats. It is not known if this drug is excreted in human milk. (see **WARNINGS** and **PRECAUTIONS**).

Pediatric use: There is no indication for use of FARESTON in pediatric patients.

Geriatric use: The median ages in the three controlled studies ranged from 60 to 66 years. No significant age-related differences in FARESTON effectiveness or safety were noted.

Race: Fourteen percent of patients in the North American Study were non-Caucasian. No significant race-related differences in FARESTON effectiveness or safety were noted.

ADVERSE REACTIONS

Adverse drug reactions are principally due to the antiestrogenic hormonal actions of FARESTON and typically occur at the beginning of treatment.

The incidences of the following eight clinical toxicities were prospectively assessed in the North American Study. The incidence reflects the toxicities that were considered by the investigator to be drug related or possible drug related.

	North American Study	
	FAR60 n = 221	TAM20 n = 215
Hot Flashes	35%	30%
Sweating	20%	17%
Nausea	14%	15%
Vaginal Discharge	13%	16%
Dizziness	9%	7%
Edema	5%	5%
Vomiting	4%	2%
Vaginal Bleeding	2%	4%

Approximately 1% of patients receiving FARESTON (n = 592) in the three controlled studies discontinued treatment as a result of adverse events (nausea and vomiting, fatigue, thrombophlebitis, depression, lethargy, anorexia, ischemic attack, arthritis, pulmonary embolism, and myocardial infarction).

Serious adverse events occurring in patients receiving FARESTON in the three major trials are listed in the table below.

[See table below]

Other adverse events of unclear causal relationship to FARESTON included leukopenia and thrombocytopenia, skin discoloration or dermatitis, constipation, dyspnea, paresis, tremor, vertigo, pruritis, anorexia, reversible corneal opacity (corneal verticulata), asthenia, alopecia, depression, jaundice, and rigors.

In the 200 and 240 mg FARESTON dose arms, the incidence of SGOT elevation and nausea was higher. Approximately 4% of patients were withdrawn for toxicity from the high-dose FARESTON treatment arms. Reasons for withdrawal included hypercalcemia, abnormal liver function tests, and one case of toxic hepatitis, depression, dizziness, incoordination, ataxia, blurry vision, diffuse dermatitis, and a constellation of symptoms consisting of nausea, sweating, and tremor.

OVERDOSAGE

Lethality was observed in rats following single oral doses that were ≥1000 mg/kg (about 150 times the recommended human dose on a mg/m^2 basis) and was associated with gastric atony/dilatation leading to interference with digestion and adrenal enlargement.

Vertigo, headache, and dizziness were observed in healthy volunteer studies at a daily dose of 680 mg for 5 days. The symptoms occurred in two of the five subjects during the third day of the treatment and disappeared within 2 days of discontinuation of the drug. No immediate concomitant changes in any measured clinical chemistry parameters were found. In a study in postmenopausal breast cancer patients, toremifene 400 mg/m^2/day caused dose-limiting nausea, vomiting, and dizziness, as well as reversible hallucinations and ataxia in one patient.

Theoretically, overdose may be manifested as an increase of antiestrogenic effects, such as hot flashes; estrogenic effects, such as vaginal bleeding; or nervous system disorders, such as vertigo, dizziness, ataxia, and nausea. There is no specific antidote and the treatment is symptomatic.

DOSAGE AND ADMINISTRATION

The dosage of FARESTON is 60 mg, once daily, orally. Treatment is generally continued until disease progression is observed.

HOW SUPPLIED

FARESTON Tablets, containing toremifene citrate in an amount equivalent to 60 mg of toremifene, are round, convex, unscored, uncoated, and white, or almost white.

FARESTON Tablets are identified with TO 60 embossed on one side.

FARESTON Tablets are available as:

NDC 54092-170-30 bottles of 30

NDC 54092-170-01 bottles of 100

Store at room temperature, up to 25°C (77°F).

Protect from heat and light.

Manufactured for
Roberts Laboratories Inc., a subsidiary of
ROBERTS PHARMACEUTICAL CORPORATION
Eatontown, NJ 07724, USA
Developed and Manufactured by
Orion Corporation, Espoo, Finland

E702229US-1 170 0117 001 9/99

Shown in Product Identification Guide, page 336

Adverse Events	North American		Eastern European		Nordic	
	FAR60 n=221(%)	TAM20 n=215(%)	FAR60 n=157(%)	TAM40 n=149(%)	FAR60 n=214(%)	TAM40 n=201(%)
Cardiac						
Cardiac Failure	2 (1)	1 (<1)	–	1 (<1)	2 (1)	3 (1.5)
Myocardial Infarction	2 (1)	3 (1.5)	1 (<1)	2 (1)	–	1 (<1)
Arrhythmia	–	–	–	–	3 (1.5)	1 (<1)
Angina Pectoris	–	–	1 (<1)	–	1 (<1)	2 (1)
Ocular*						
Cataracts	22 (10)	16 (7.5)	–	–	–	5 (3)
Dry Eyes	20 (9)	16 (7.5)	–	–	–	–
Abnorma Visual Fields	8 (4)	10 (5)	–	–	–	1 (<1)
Corneal Keratopathy	4 (2)	2 (1)	–	–	–	–
Glaucoma	3 (1.5)	2 (1)	1 (<1)	–	–	1 (<1)
Abnormal Vision/ Diplopia	–	–	–	–	3 (1.5)	–
Thromboembolic						
Pulmonary Embolism	4 (2)	2 (1)	1 (<1)	–	–	1 (<1)
Thrombophlebitis	–	2 (1)	1 (<1)	1 (<1)	4 (2)	3 (1.5)
Thrombosis	–	1 (<1)	1 (<1)	–	3 (1.5)	4 (2)
CVA/TIA	1 (<1)	–	–	1 (<1)	4 (2)	4 (2)
Elevated Liver Tests**						
SGOT	11 (5)	4 (2)	30 (19)	22 (15)	32 (15)	35 (17)
Alkaline Phosphatase	41 (19)	24 (11)	16 (10)	13 (9)	18 (8)	31 (15)
Bilirubin	3 (1.5)	4 (2)	2 (1)	1 (<1)	2 (1)	3 (1.5)
Hypercalcemia	6 (3)	6 (3)	1 (<1)	–	–	–

* Most of the ocular abnormalities were observed in the North American Study in which on-study and biannual ophthalmic examinations were performed. No cases of retinopathy were observed in any arm.

** Elevated defined as follows: North American Study: SGOT >100 IU/L; alkaline phosphatase >200 IU/L; bilirubin >2 mg/dL. Eastern European and Nordic studies: SGOT, alkaline phosphatase, and bilirubin – WHO Grade 1 (1.25 times the upper limit of normal).

PENTASA®

(mesalamine)

Controlled-Release Capsules 250 mg

℞

Prescribing information as of June 1999

DESCRIPTION

PENTASA (mesalamine) for oral administration is a controlled-release formulation of mesalamine, an aminosalicylate anti-inflammatory agent for gastrointestinal use.

Chemically, mesalamine is 5-amino-2-hydroxybenzoic acid. It has a molecular weight of 153.14.

The structural formula is:

Each capsule contains 250 mg of mesalamine. It also contains the following inactive ingredients: acetylated monoglyceride, castor oil, colloidal silicon dioxide, ethylcellulose, hydroxypropyl methylcellulose, starch, stearic acid, sugar, talc, and white wax. The capsule shell contains D&C Yellow #10, FD&C Blue #1, FD&C Green #3, gelatin, titanium dioxide, and other ingredients.

CLINICAL PHARMACOLOGY

Sulfasalazine is split by bacterial action in the colon into sulfapyridine (SP) and mesalamine (5-ASA). It is thought that the mesalamine component is therapeutically active in ulcerative colitis. The usual oral dose of sulfasalazine for active ulcerative colitis in adults is 2 to 4 g per day in divided doses. Four grams of sulfasalazine provide 1.6 g of free mesalamine to the colon.

The mechanism of action of mesalamine (and sulfasalazine) is unknown, but appears to be topical rather than systemic. Mucosal production of arachidonic acid (AA) metabolites, both through the cyclooxygenase pathways, ie, prostanoids, and through the lipoxygenase pathways, ie, leukotrienes (LTs) and hydroxyeicosatetraenoic acids (HETEs), is increased in patients with chronic inflammatory bowel disease, and it is possible that mesalamine diminishes inflammation by blocking cyclooxygenase and inhibiting prostaglandin (PG) production in the colon.

Human Pharmacokinetics and Metabolism

Absorption. PENTASA is an ethylcellulose-coated controlled-release formulation of mesalamine designed to release therapeutic quantities of mesalamine throughout the gastrointestinal tract. Based on urinary excretion data, 20% to 30% of the mesalamine in PENTASA is absorbed. In contrast, when mesalamine is administered orally as an unformulated 1-g aqueous suspension, mesalamine is approximately 80% absorbed.

Plasma mesalamine concentration peaked at approximately 1 µg/mL 3 hours following a 1-g PENTASA dose and declined in a biphasic manner. The literature describes a mean terminal half-life of 42 minutes for mesalamine following intravenous administration. Because of the continuous release and absorption of mesalamine from PENTASA throughout the gastrointestinal tract, the true elimination half-life cannot be determined after oral administration. N-acetylmesalamine, the major metabolite of mesalamine, peaked at approximately 3 hours at 1.8 µg/mL, and its concentration followed a biphasic decline. Pharmacological activities of N-acetylmesalamine are unknown, and other metabolites have not been identified.

Oral mesalamine pharmacokinetics were nonlinear when PENTASA capsules were dosed from 250 mg to 1 g four times daily, with steady-state mesalamine plasma concentrations increasing about nine times, from 0.14 µg/mL to 1.21 µg/mL, suggesting saturable first-pass metabolism. N-acetylmesalamine pharmacokinetics were linear.

Elimination. About 130 mg free mesalamine was recovered in the feces following a single 1-g PENTASA dose, which was comparable to the 140 mg of mesalamine recovered from the molar equivalent sulfasalazine tablet dose of 2.5 g. Elimination of free mesalamine and salicylates in feces increased proportionately with PENTASA dose. N-acetylmesalamine was the primary compound excreted in the urine (19% to 30%) following PENTASA dosing.

CLINICAL TRIALS

In two randomized, double-blind, placebo-controlled, dose-response trials (UC-1 and UC-2) of 625 patients with active mild to moderate ulcerative colitis, PENTASA, at an oral dose of 4 g/day given 1 g four times daily, produced consistent improvement in prospectively identified primary efficacy parameters, PGA, Tx F, and SI as shown in the table below.

The 4-g dose of PENTASA also gave consistent improvement in secondary efficacy parameters, namely the frequency of trips to the toilet, stool consistency, rectal bleeding, abdominal/rectal pain, and urgency. The 4-g dose of PENTASA induced remission as assessed by endoscopic and symptomatic endpoints.

In some patients, the 2-g dose of PENTASA was observed to improve efficacy parameters measured. However, the 2-g dose gave inconsistent results in primary efficacy parameters across the two adequate and well-controlled trials.

[See first table at right]

INDICATIONS AND USAGE

PENTASA is indicated for the induction of remission and for the treatment of patients with mildly to moderately active ulcerative colitis.

CONTRAINDICATIONS

PENTASA is contraindicated in patients who have demonstrated hypersensitivity to mesalamine, any other components of this medication, or salicylates.

PRECAUTIONS

General

Caution should be exercised if PENTASA is administered to patients with impaired hepatic function.

Mesalamine has been associated with an acute intolerance syndrome that may be difficult to distinguish from a flare of inflammatory bowel disease. Although the exact frequency of occurrence cannot be ascertained, it has occurred in 3% of patients in controlled clinical trials of mesalamine or sulfasalazine. Symptoms include cramping, acute abdominal pain and bloody diarrhea, sometimes fever, headache, and rash. If acute intolerance syndrome is suspected, prompt withdrawal is required. If a rechallenge is performed later in order to validate the hypersensitivity, it should be carried out under close medical supervision at reduced dose and only if clearly needed.

Renal

Caution should be exercised if PENTASA is administered to patients with impaired renal function. Single reports of nephrotic syndrome and interstitial nephritis associated with mesalamine therapy have been described in the foreign literature. There have been rare reports of interstitial nephritis in patients receiving PENTASA. In animal studies, a 13-week oral toxicity study in mice and 13-week and 52-week oral toxicity studies in rats and cynomolgus monkeys have shown the kidney to be the major target organ of mesalamine toxicity. Oral daily doses of 2400 mg/kg in mice and 1150 mg/kg in rats produced renal lesions including granular and hyaline casts, tubular degeneration, tubular dilation, renal infarct, papillary necrosis, tubular necrosis, and interstitial nephritis. In cynomolgus monkeys, oral daily doses of 250 mg/kg or higher produced nephrosis, papillary edema, and interstitial fibrosis. Patients with preexisting renal disease, increased BUN or serum creatinine, or proteinuria should be carefully monitored.

Carcinogenesis, Mutagenesis, Impairment of Fertility

In a 104-week dietary carcinogenicity study of mesalamine, CD-1 mice were treated with doses up to 2500 mg/kg/day and it was not tumorigenic. For a 50 kg person of average height (1.46 m^2 body surface area), this represents 2.5 times the recommended human dose on a body surface area basis (2960 mg/m^2/day). In a 104-week dietary carcinogenicity study in Wistar rats, mesalamine up to a dose of 800 mg/kg/day was not tumorigenic. This dose represents 1.5 times the recommended human dose on a body surface area basis.

No evidence of mutagenicity was observed in an in vitro Ames test and an in vivo mouse micronucleus test.

No effects on fertility or reproductive performance were observed in male or female rats at oral doses of mesalamine up to 400 mg/kg/day (0.8 times the recommended human dose based on body surface area).

Semen abnormalities and infertility in men, which have been reported in association with sulfasalazine, have not been seen with PENTASA capsules during controlled clinical trials.

Pregnancy

Category B. Reproduction studies have been performed in rats at doses up to 1000 mg/kg/day (5900 mg/M^2) and rabbits at doses of 800 mg/kg/day (6856 mg/M^2) and have revealed no evidence of teratogenic effects or harm to the fetus due to mesalamine. There are, however, no adequate and well-controlled studies in pregnant women. Because animal reproduction studies are not always predictive of human response, PENTASA should be used during pregnancy only if clearly needed.

Mesalamine is known to cross the placental barrier.

Nursing Mothers

Minute quantities of mesalamine were distributed to breast milk and amniotic fluid of pregnant women following sulfasalazine therapy. When treated with sulfasalazine at a dose equivalent to 1.25 g/day of mesalamine, 0.02 µg/mL to 0.08 µg/mL and trace amounts of mesalamine were measured in amniotic fluid and breast milk, respectively. N-acetylmesalamine, in quantities of 0.07 µg/mL to 0.77 µg/mL and 1.13 µg/mL to 3.44 µg/mL, was identified in the same fluids, respectively.

Caution should be exercised when PENTASA is administered to a nursing woman.

Pediatric Use

Safety and efficacy of PENTASA in pediatric patients have not been established.

ADVERSE REACTIONS

In combined domestic and foreign clinical trials, more than 2100 patients with ulcerative colitis or Crohn's disease received PENTASA therapy. Generally, PENTASA therapy was well tolerated. The most common events (ie, greater than or equal to 1%) were diarrhea (3.4%), headache (2.0%), nausea (1.8%), abdominal pain (1.7%), dyspepsia (1.6%), vomiting (1.5%), and rash (1.0%).

In two domestic placebo-controlled trials involving over 600 ulcerative colitis patients, adverse events were fewer in PENTASA-treated patients than in the placebo group (PENTASA 14% vs placebo 18%) and were not dose-related. Events occurring at 1% or more are shown in the table below. Of these, only nausea and vomiting were more frequent in the PENTASA group. Withdrawal from therapy due to adverse events was more common on placebo than PENTASA (7% vs 4%).

	Clinical Trial UC-1			Clinical Trial UC-2		
		PENTASA			PENTASA	
Parameter Evaluated	PL (n=90)	4 g/day (n=95)	2 g/day (n=97)	PL (n=83)	4 g/day (n=85)	2 g/day (n=83)
PGA	36%	59%*	57%*	31%	55%*	41%
Tx F	22%	9%*	18%	31%	9%*	17%*
SI	−2.5	−5.0*	−4.3*	−1.6	−3.8*	−2.6
Remission†	12%	26%*	24%*	12%	27%*	12%

* $p < 0.05$ vs placebo.

PGA: Physician Global Assessment: proportion of patients with complete or marked improvement.

Tx F: Treatment Failure: proportion of patients developing severe or fulminant UC requiring steroid therapy or hospitalization or worsening of the disease at 7 days of therapy, or lack of significant improvement by 14 days of therapy.

SI: Sigmoidoscopic Index: an objective measure of disease activity rated by a standard (15-point) scale that includes mucosal vascular pattern, erythema, friability, granularity/ulcerations, and mucopus: improvement over baseline.

† Defined as complete resolution of symptoms plus improvement of endoscopic endpoints. To be considered in remission, patients had a "1" score for one of the endoscopic components (mucosal vascular pattern, erythema, granularity, for friability) and "0" for the others.

Table 1. Adverse Events Occurring in More Than 1% of Either Placebo or PENTASA Patients in Domestic Placebo-controlled Ulcerative Colitis Trials. (PENTASA Comparison to Placebo)

Event	PENTASA n=451	Placebo n=173
Diarrhea	16 (3.5%)	13 (7.5%)
Headache	10 (2.2%)	6 (3.5%)
Nausea	14 (3.1%)	—
Abdominal Pain	5 (1.1%)	7 (4.0%)
Melena (Bloody Diarrhea)	4 (0.9%)	6 (3.5%)
Rash	6 (1.3%)	2 (1.2%)
Anorexia	5 (1.1%)	2 (1.2%)
Fever	4 (0.9%)	2 (1.2%)
Rectal Urgency	1 (0.2%)	4 (2.3%)
Nausea and Vomiting	5 (1.1%)	—
Worsening of Ulcerative Colitis	2 (0.4%)	2 (1.2%)
Acne	1 (0.2%)	2 (1.2%)

[See second table above]

Clinical laboratory measurements showed no significant abnormal trends for any test, including measurement of hematologic, liver, and kidney function.

The following adverse events, presented by body system, were reported infrequently (ie, less than 1%) during domestic ulcerative colitis and Crohn's disease trials. In many cases, the relationship to PENTASA has not been established.

Gastrointestinal: abdominal distention, anorexia, constipation, duodenal ulcer, dysphagia, eructation, esophageal ulcer, fecal incontinence, GGTP increase, GI bleeding, increased alkaline phosphatase, LDH increase, mouth ulcer, oral moniliases, pancreatitis, rectal bleeding, SGOT increase, SGPT increase, stool abnormalities (color or texture change), thirst

Dermatological: acne, alopecia, dry skin, eczema, erythema nodosum, nail disorder, photosensitivity, pruritus, sweating, urticaria

Nervous System: depression, dizziness, insomnia, somnolence, paresthesia

Cardiovascular: palpitations, pericarditis, vasodilation

Other: albuminuria, amenorrhea, amylase increase, arthraligia, asthenia, breast pain, conjunctivitis, ecchymosis, edema, fever, hematuria, hypomenorrhea, Kawasaki-like syndrome, leg cramps, lichen planus, lipase increase, malaise, menorrhagia, metrorrhagia, myalgia, pulmonary infiltrates, thrombocythemia, thrombocytopenia, urinary frequency

One week after completion of an 8-week ulcerative colitis study, a 72-year-old male, with no previous history of pulmonary problems, developed dyspnea. The patient was subsequently diagnosed with interstitial pulmonary fibrosis without eosinophilia by one physician and bronchiolitis obliterans with organizing pneumonitis by a second physician. A causal relationship between this event and mesalamine therapy has not been established.

Published case reports and/or spontaneous postmarketing surveillance have described infrequent instances of pericarditis, fatal myocarditis, chest pain and T-wave abnormalities, hypersensitivity pneumonitis, pancreatitis, nephrotic syndrome, interstitial nephritis, hepatitis, aplastic anemia, pancytopenia, leukopenia, agranulocytosis, or anemia while receiving mesalamine therapy. Anemia can be a part of the clinical presentation of inflammatory bowel disease. Allergic reactions, which could involve eosinophilia, can be seen in connection with PENTASA therapy.

Postmarketing Reports

The following events have been identified during post-approval use of products which contain (or are metabolized to) mesalamine in clinical practice. Because they are reported voluntarily from a population of unknown size, estimates of frequency cannot be made. These events have been chosen for inclusion due to a combination of seriousness, frequency of reporting, or potential causal connection to mesalamine:

Gastrointestinal: Reports of hepatotoxicity, including elevated liver function tests (SGOT/AST, SGPT/ALT, GGT, LDH, alkaline phosphatase, bilirubin), jaundice, cholestatic jaundice, cirrhosis, and possible hepatocellular damage including liver necrosis and liver failure. Some of these cases were fatal. One case of Kawasaki-like syndrome which included hepatic function changes was also reported.

OVERDOSAGE

Single oral doses of mesalamine up to 5 g/kg in pigs or a single intravenous dose of mesalamine at 920 mg/kg in rats were not lethal.

There is no clinical experience with PENTASA overdosage. PENTASA is an aminosalicylate, and symptoms of salicylate toxicity may be possible, such as: tinnitus, vertigo, headache, confusion, drowsiness, sweating, hyperventilation, vomiting, and diarrhea. Severe intoxication with salicylates can lead to disruption of electrolyte balance and blood pH, hyperthermia, and dehydration.

Treatment of Overdosage. Since PENTASA is an aminosalicylate, conventional therapy for salicylate toxicity may be beneficial in the event of acute overdosage. This includes prevention of further gastrointestinal tract absorption by emesis and, if necessary, by gastric lavage. Fluid and electrolyte imbalance should be corrected by the administration of appropriate intravenous therapy. Adequate renal function should be maintained.

DOSAGE AND ADMINISTRATION

The recommended dosage for the induction of remission and the symptomatic treatment of mildly to moderately active ulcerative colitis is 1 g (4 PENTASA capsules) four times a day for a total daily dose of 4 g. Treatment duration in controlled trials was up to 8 weeks.

HOW SUPPLIED

PENTASA controlled-release capsules are supplied in bottles of 240 capsules (NDC 54092-189-81); and blister packs of 80 capsules (NDC 54092-189-80). Each green and blue capsule contains 250 mg of mesalamine in controlled-release beads. PENTASA controlled-release capsules are identified with a pentagonal starburst logo and the number 2010 on the green portion and PENTASA 250 mg on the blue portion of the capsules.

Store at controlled room temperature 59° to 86°F (15° to 30°C).

Manufactured for
Roberts Laboratories Inc., a subsidiary of
ROBERTS PHARMACEUTICAL CORPORATION,
Eatontown, NJ 07724, USA

Prescribing Information as of June 1999
Licensed U.S. Patent Nos. B1 4,496,553 and 4,980,173
189 0117 001 50011416

Shown in Product Identification Guide, page 336

Continued on next page

PERI-COLACE® capsules • syrup OTC
(casanthranol and docusate sodium)

DESCRIPTION

Peri-Colace® is a combination of the mild stimulant laxative casanthranol, and the stool-softener Colace® (docusate sodium). Each capsule contains 30 mg of casanthranol and 100 mg of Colace®; the syrup contains 30 mg of casanthranol and 60 mg of Colace® per 15-mL tablespoon (10 mg of casanthranol and 20 mg of Colace® per 5-mL teaspoon) and 10% alcohol.

Peri-Colace® Capsules contain the following inactive ingredients: Polyethylene glycol 400, gelatin, glycerin, sorbitol, propylene glycol, titanium dioxide, methylparaben, FD&C Red No. 40, propylparaben, FD&C Blue No. 1.

Peri-Colace® Syrup contains the following inactive ingredients: alcohol (10% v/v), citric acid, flavors, methyl salicylate, methylparaben, poloxamer, polyethylene glycol, propylparaben, sodium citrate, sorbitol solution, sucrose, and purified water.

ACTION AND USES

Peri-Colace® provides gentle peristaltic stimulation and helps to keep stools soft for easier passage. Bowel movement is induced gently—usually overnight or in 8 to 12 hours. Nausea, griping, abnormally loose stools, and constipation rebound are minimized. Useful in management of chronic or temporary constipation.

Note: To prevent hard stools when laxative stimulation is not needed or undesirable, see Colace® (stool softener).

WARNINGS

Do not use when abdominal pain, nausea, or vomiting are present, unless directed by a doctor. Frequent or prolonged use of this preparation may result in dependence on laxatives.

As with any drug, pregnant or nursing women should seek the advice of a health professional before using this product.

SIDE EFFECTS

The incidence of side effects—none of a serious nature—is exceedingly small. Nausea, abdominal cramping or discomfort, diarrhea, and rash are the main side effects reported.

ADMINISTRATION AND DOSAGE

Adults —1 or 2 capsules, or 1 or 2 tablespoons syrup at bedtime, or as indicated. In severe cases, dosage may be increased to 2 capsules or 2 tablespoons twice daily, or 3 capsules at bedtime. *Children* —1 to 3 teaspoons of syrup at bedtime, or as indicated. Peri-Colace® syrup must be given in a 6 oz. to 8 oz. glass of milk or fruit juice or in infant's formula to prevent throat irritation.

OVERDOSAGE

In addition to symptomatic treatment, gastric lavage, if timely, is recommended in cases of large overdosage.

HOW SUPPLIED

Peri-Colace® Capsules
NDC 54092-054-30 Bottles of 30
NDC 54092-054-60 Bottles of 60
NDC 54092-054-02 Bottles of 250
NDC 54092-054-10 Bottles of 1000
NDC 54092-054-52 Cartons of 100 single unit packs

Note: Peri-Colace® capsules should be stored at controlled room temperatures (59°–86°F or 15°–30°C).

Peri-Colace® Syrup
NDC 54092-418-08 Bottles of 8 fl oz
NDC 54092-418-16 Bottles of 16 fl oz

Peri-Colace®
NDC 54092-054-11 Blister Pack of 10

Manufactured for:
Roberts Laboratories Inc., a subsidiary of
ROBERTS PHARMACEUTICAL CORPORATION
Eatontown, NJ 07724 USA

PROAMATINE® ℞
(midodrine hydrochloride)
Tablets of 2.5 mg and 5 mg

WARNING: Because ProAmatine can cause marked elevation of supine blood pressure, it should be used in patients whose lives are considerably impaired despite standard clinical care. The indication for use of ProAmatine in the treatment of symptomatic orthostatic hypotension is based primarily on a change in a surrogate marker of effectiveness, an increase in systolic blood pressure measured one minute after standing, a surrogate marker considered likely to correspond to a clinical benefit. At present, however, clinical benefits of ProAmatine, principally improved ability to carry out activities of daily living, have not been verified.

DESCRIPTION

Name: ProAmatine® (midodrine hydrochloride) Tablets

Dosage Form: 2.5-mg and 5-mg tablets for oral administration

Active Ingredient: Midodrine hydrochloride, 2.5 mg or 5 mg

Inactive Ingredients: Microcrystalline Cellulose NF, Colloidal Silicone Dioxide NF, Magnesium Stearate NF, Corn Starch NF, Talc USP, FD&C Yellow No. 6 Lake (5-mg tablet)

Pharmacological Classification: Vasopressor/Antihypotensive

Chemical Names (USAN: Midodrine Hydrochloride): (1) Acetamide, 2-amino-*N*-[2-(2,5-dimethoxyphenyl)-2-hydroxyethyl]-monohydrochloride,(±)-; (2) (±) -2-amino-*N*-(β-hydroxy-2,5-dimethoxyphenethyl)acetamide monohydrochloride BAN, INN, JAN: Midodrine

Structural Formula:

HOCHCH₂NHCCH₂NH₂ (C=O) ·HCl, OCH₃, H₃CO

Molecular Formula: $C_{12}H_{18}N_2O_4HCl$; **Molecular Weight:** 290.7

Organoleptic Properties: Odorless, white, crystalline powder

Solubility:	Water:	Soluble
	Methanol:	Sparingly soluble

pKa: 7.8 (0.3% aqueous solution)
pH: 3.5 to 5.5 (5% aqueous solution)
Melting Range: 200 to 203°C

CLINICAL PHARMACOLOGY

Mechanism of Action: ProAmatine forms an active metabolite, desglymidodrine, that is an alpha$_1$-agonist, and exerts its actions via activation of the alpha-adrenergic receptors of the arteriolar and venous vasculature, producing an increase in vascular tone and elevation of blood pressure. Desglymidodrine does not stimulate cardiac beta-adrenergic receptors. Desglymidodrine diffuses poorly across the blood-brain barrier, and is therefore not associated with effects on the central nervous system. Administration of ProAmatine results in a rise in standing, sitting, and supine systolic and diastolic blood pressure in patients with orthostatic hypotension of various etiologies. Standing systolic blood pressure is elevated by approximately 15 to 30 mmHg at 1 hour after a 10-mg dose of midodrine, with some effect persisting for 2 to 3 hours. ProAmatine has no clinically significant effect on standing or supine pulse rates in patients with autonomic failure.

Pharmacokinetics: ProAmatine is a prodrug, i.e., the therapeutic effect of orally administered midodrine is due to the major metabolite desglymidodrine, formed by deglycination of midodrine. After oral administration, ProAmatine is rapidly absorbed. The plasma levels of the prodrug peak after about half an hour, and decline with a half-life of approximately 25 minutes, while the metabolite reaches peak blood concentrations about 1 to 2 hours after a dose of midodrine and has a half-life of about 3 to 4 hours. The absolute bioavailability of midodrine (measured as desglymidodrine) is 93%. The bioavailability of desglymidodrine is not affected by food. Approximately the same amount of desglymidodrine is formed after intravenous and oral administration of midodrine. Neither midodrine nor desglymidodrine is bound to plasma proteins to any significant extent.

Metabolism and Excretion: Thorough metabolic studies have not been conducted, but it appears that deglycination of midodrine to desglymidodrine takes place in many tissues, and both compounds are metabolized in part by the liver. Neither midodrine nor desglymidodrine is a substrate for monoamine oxidase.

Renal elimination of midodrine is insignificant. The renal clearance of desglymidodrine is of the order of 385 mL/minute, most, about 80%, by active renal secretion. The actual mechanism of active secretion has not been studied, but it is possible that it occurs by the base-secreting pathway responsible for the secretion of several other drugs that are bases (see also **Potential for Drug Interactions**).

Clinical Studies

Midodrine has been studied in 3 principal controlled trials, one of 3-weeks duration and 2 of 1 to 2 days duration. All studies were randomized, double-blind and paralled-design trials in patients with orthostatic hypotension of any etiology and supine-to-standing fall of systolic blood pressure of at least 15 mmHg accompanied by at least moderate dizziness/lightheadedness. Patients with pre-existing sustained supine hypertension above 180/110 mmHg were routinely excluded. In a 3-week study in 170 patients, most previously untreated with midodrine, the midodrine-treated patients (10 mg t.i.d., with the last dose not later than 6 P.M.) had significantly higher (by about 20 mmHg) 1-minute standing systolic pressure 1 hour after dosing (blood pressures were not measured at other times) for all 3 weeks. After week 1, midodrine-treated patients had small improvements in dizziness/lightheadedness/unsteadiness scores and global evaluations, but these effects were made difficult to interpret by a high early drop-out rate (about 25% vs 5% on placebo). Supine and sitting blood pressure rose 16/8 and 20/10 mmHg, respectively, on average.

In a 2-day study, after open-label midodrine, known midodrine responders received midodrine 10 mg or placebo at 0, 3, and 6 hours. One-minute standing systolic blood pressures were increased 1 hour after each dose by about 15 mmHg and 3 hours after each dose by about 12 mmHg; 3-minute standing pressures were increased also at 1, but not 3, hours after dosing. There were increases in standing time seen intermittently 1 hour after dosing, but not at 3 hours.

In a 1-day, dose-response trial, single doses of 0, 2.5, 10, and 20 mg of midodrine were given to 25 patients. The 10- and 20-mg doses produced increases in standing 1-minute systolic pressure of about 30 mmHg at 1 hour; the increase was sustained in part for 2 hours after 10 mg and 4 hours after 20 mg. Supine systolic pressure was ≥200 mmHg in 22% of patients on 10 mg and 45% of patients on 20 mg; elevated pressures often lasted 6 hours or more.

INDICATIONS AND USAGE

ProAmatine is indicated for the treatment of symptomatic orthostatic hypotension (OH). Because ProAmatine can cause marked elevation of supine blood pressure (BP > 200 mmHg systolic), it should be used in patients whose lives are considerably impaired despite standard clinical care, including non-pharmacologic treatment (such as support stockings), fluid expansion, and lifestyle alterations. The indication is based on ProAmatine's effect on increases in 1-minute standing systolic blood pressure, a surrogate marker considered likely to correspond to a clinical benefit. At present, however, clinical benefits of ProAmatine, principally improved ability to perform life activities, have not been established. Further clinical trials are underway to verify and describe the clinical benefits of ProAmatine.

After initiation of treatment, ProAmatine should be continued only for patients who report significant symptomatic improvement.

CONTRAINDICATIONS

ProAmatine is contraindicated in patients with severe organic heart disease, acute renal disease, urinary retention, pheochromocytoma or thyrotoxicosis. ProAmatine should not be used in patients with persistent and excessive supine hypertension.

WARNINGS

Supine Hypertension: The most potentially serious adverse reaction associated with ProAmatine therapy is marked elevation of supine arterial blood pressure (supine hypertension). Systolic pressure of about 200 mmHg were seen overall in about 13.4% of patients given 10 mg of ProAmatine. Systolic elevations of this degree were most likely to be observed in patients with relatively elevated pretreatment systolic blood pressures (mean 170 mmHg). There is no experience in patients with initial supine systolic pressure above 180 mmHg, as those patients were excluded from the clinical trials. Use of ProAmatine in such patients is not recommended. Sitting blood pressures were also elevated by ProAmatine therapy. It is essential to monitor supine and sitting blood pressures in patients maintained on ProAmatine.

PRECAUTIONS

General: The potential for supine and sitting hypertension should be evaluated at the beginning of ProAmatine therapy. Supine hypertension can often be controlled by preventing the patient from becoming fully supine, i.e., sleeping with the head of the bed elevated. The patient should be cautioned to report symptoms of supine hypertension immediately. Symptoms may include cardiac awareness, pounding in the ears, headache, blurred vision, etc. The patient should be advised to discontinue the medication immediately if supine hypertension persists. Blood pressure should be monitored carefully when ProAmatine is used concomitantly with other agents that cause vasoconstriction, such as phenylephrine, ephedrine, dihydroergotamine, phenylpropanolamine, or pseudoephedrine.

A slight slowing of the heart rate may occur after administration of ProAmatine, primarily due to vagal reflex. Caution should be exercised when ProAmatine is used concomitantly with cardiac glycosides (such as digitalis), psychopharmacologic agents, beta blockers or other agents that directly or indirectly reduce heart rate. Patients who experience any signs or symptoms suggesting bradycardia (pulse slowing, increased dizziness, syncope, cardiac awareness) should be advised to discontinue ProAmatine and should be re-evaluated.

ProAmatine should be used cautiously in patients with urinary retention problems, as desglymidodrine acts on the alpha-adrenergic receptors of the bladder neck.

ProAmatine should be used with caution in orthostatic hypotensive patients who are also diabetic, as well as those with a history of visual problems who are also taking fludrocortisone acetate, which is known to cause an increase in intraocular pressure and glaucoma.

ProAmatine use has not been studied in patients with renal impairment. Because desglymidodrine is eliminated via the kidneys, and higher blood levels would be expected in such patients. ProAmatine should be used with caution in patients with renal impairment, with a starting dose of 2.5 mg (see **DOSAGE AND ADMINISTRATION**). Renal function should be assessed prior to initial use of ProAmatine.

ProAmatine use has not been studied in patients with hepatic impairment. ProAmatine should be used with caution in patients with hepatic impairment, as the liver has a role in the metabolism of midodrine.

Information for Patients: Patients should be told that certain agents in over-the-counter products, such as cold remedies and diet aids, can elevate blood pressure, and therefore, should be used cautiously with ProAmatine, as they may enhance or potentiate the pressor effects of ProAmatine (see **Drug Interactions**). Patients should also be made aware of the possibility of supine hypertension. They should be told to avoid taking their dose if they are to be supine for any length of time, i.e., they should take their last daily dose of ProAmatine 3 to 4 hours before bedtime to minimize nighttime supine hypertension.

Laboratory Tests: Since desglymidodrine is eliminated by the kidneys and the liver has a role in its metabolism, evaluation of the patient should include assessment of renal and hepatic function prior to initiating therapy and subsequently, as appropriate.

Drug Interactions: When administered concomitantly with ProAmatine, cardiac glycosides may enhance or precipitate bradycardia, A.V. block or arrhythmia.

The use of drugs that stimulate alpha-adrenergic receptors (e.g., phenylephrine, pseudoephedrine, ephedrine, phenylpropanolamine or dihydroergotamine) may enhance or potentiate the pressor effects of ProAmatine. Therefore, caution should be used when ProAmatine is administered concomitantly with agents that cause vasoconstriction.

ProAmatine has been used in patients concomitantly treated with salt-retaining steroid therapy (i.e., fludrocortisone acetate), with or without salt supplementation. The potential for supine hypertension should be carefully monitored in these patients and may be minimized by either reducing the dose of fludrocortisone acetate or decreasing the salt intake prior to initiation of treatment with ProAmatine. Alpha-adrenergic blocking agents, such as prazosin, terazosin, and doxazosin, can antagonize the effects of ProAmatine.

Potential for Drug Interactions: It appears possible, although there is no supporting experimental evidence, that the high renal clearance of desglymidodrine (a base) is due to active tubular secretion by the base-secreting system also responsible for the secretion of such drugs as metformin, cimetidine, ranitidine, procainamide, triamterene, flecainide, and quinidine. Thus there may be a potential for drug-drug interactions with these drugs.

Carcinogenesis, Mutagenesis, Impairment of Fertility: Long-term studies have been conducted in rats and mice at dosages of 3 to 4 times the maximum recommended daily human dose on a mg/m^2 basis, with no indication of carcinogenic effects related to ProAmatine. Studies investigating the mutagenic potential of ProAmatine revealed no evidence of mutagenicity. Other than the dominant lethal assay in male mice, where no impairment of fertility was observed, there have been no studies on the effects of ProAmatine on fertility.

Pregnancy: *Pregnancy Category C.* ProAmatine increased the rate of embryo resorption, reduced fetal body weight in rats and rabbits, and decreased fetal survival in rabbits when given in doses 13 (rat) and 7 (rabbit) times the maximum human dose based on body surface area (mg/m^2). There are no adequate and well-controlled studies in pregnant women. ProAmatine should be used during pregnancy only if the potential benefit justifies the potential risk to the fetus. No teratogenic effects have been observed in studies in rats and rabbits.

Nursing Mothers: It is not known whether this drug is excreted in human milk. Because many drugs are excreted in human milk, caution should be exercised when ProAmatine is administered to a nursing woman.

Pediatric Use: Safety and effectiveness in pediatric patients have not been established.

ADVERSE REACTIONS

The most frequent adverse reactions seen in controlled trials were supine and sitting hypertension; paresthesia and pruritus, mainly of the scalp; goosebumps; chills; urinary urge; urinary retention and urinary frequency.

The frequency of these events in a 3-week placebo-controlled trial is shown in the following table:

Adverse Events

	Placebo n=88		Midodrine n=82	
Event	#of reports	% of patients	#of reports	% of patients
Total # of reports	22		77	
Paresthesia[1]	4	4.5	15	18.3
Piloerection	0	0	11	13.4
Dysuria[2]	0	0	11	13.4
Pruritus[3]	2	2.3	10	12.2
Supine hypertension[4]	0	0	6	7.3
Chills	0	0	4	4.9
Pain[5]	0	0	4	4.9
Rash	1	1.1	2	2.4

1 Includes hyperesthesia and scalp paresthesia
2 Includes dysuria (1), increased urinary frequency (2), impaired urination (1), urinary retention (5), urinary urgency (2)
3 Includes scalp pruritis
4 Includes patients who experienced an increase in supine hypertension
5 Includes abdominal pain and pain increase

Less frequent adverse reactions were headache; feeling of pressure/fullness in the head; vasodilation/flushing face; confusion/thinking abnormality; dry mouth; nervousness/anxiety and rash. Other adverse reactions that occurred rarely were visual field defect; dizziness; skin hyperesthesia; insomnia; somnolence; erythema multiforme; canker sore; dry skin; dysuria; impaired urination; asthenia; backache; pyrosis; nausea; gastrointestinal distress; flatulence and leg cramps.

The most potentially serious adverse reaction associated with ProAmatine therapy is supine hypertension. The feelings of paresthesia, pruritus, piloerection and chills are pilomotor reactions associated with the action of midodrine on the alpha-adrenergic receptors of the hair follicles. Feelings of urinary urgency, retention and frequency are associated with the action of midodrine on the alpha-receptors of the bladder neck.

OVERDOSAGE

Symptoms of overdose could include hypertension, piloerection (goosebumps), a sensation of coldness and urinary retention. There are 2 reported cases of overdosage with ProAmatine, both in young males. One patient ingested ProAmatine drops, 250 mg, experienced systolic blood pressure of greater than 200 mmHg, was treated with an IV injection of 20 mg of phentolamine, and was discharged the same night without any complaints. The other patient ingested 205 mg of ProAmatine (41 5-mg tablets), and was found lethargic and unable to talk, unresponsive to voice but responsive to painful stimuli, hypertensive and bradycardic. Gastric lavage was performed, and the patient recovered fully by the next day without sequelae.

The single doses that would be associated with symptoms of overdose or would be potentially life-threatening are unknown. The oral LD_{50} is approximately 30 to 50 mg/kg in rats, 675 mg/kg in mice, and 125 to 160 mg/kg in dogs.

Desglymidodrine is dialyzable.

Recommended general treatment, based on the pharmacology of the drug, includes induced emesis and administration of alpha-sympatholytic drugs (e.g., phentolamine).

DOSAGE AND ADMINISTRATION

The recommended dose of ProAmatine is 10 mg, 3 times daily. Dosing should take place during the daytime hours when the patient needs to be upright, pursuing the activities of daily life. A suggested dosing schedule of approximately 4-hour intervals is as follows: shortly before or upon arising in the morning, midday, and late afternoon (not later than 6 P.M.). Doses may be given in 3-hour intervals, if required, to control symptoms, but not more frequently. Single doses as high as 20 mg have been given to patients, but severe and persistent systolic supine hypertension occurs at a high rate (about 45%) at this dose. In order to reduce the potential for supine hypertension during sleep, ProAmatine should not be given after the evening meal or less than 4 hours before bedtime. Total daily doses greater than 30 mg have been tolerated by some patients, but their safety and usefulness have not been studied systematically or established. Because of the risk of supine hypertension, ProAmatine should be continued only in patients who appear to attain symptomatic improvement during initial treatment.

The supine and standing blood pressure should be monitored regularly, and the administration of ProAmatine should be stopped if supine blood pressure increases excessively.

Because desglymidodrine is excreted renally, dosing in patients with abnormal renal function should be cautious; although this has not been systematically studied, it is recommended that treatment of these patients be initiated using 2.5-mg doses.

Dosing in children has not been adequately studied.

Blood levels of midodrine and desglymidodrine were similar when comparing levels in patients 65 or older vs. younger than 65 and when comparing males vs. females, suggesting dose modifications for these groups are not necessary.

HOW SUPPLIED

ProAmatine is supplied as 2.5-mg and 5-mg tablets for oral administration. The 2.5-mg tablet is white, round, and biplanar, with a bevelled edge, and is scored on 1 side with "RPC" above and "2.5" below the score, and "003" on the other side. The 5-mg tablet is orange, round, and biplanar, with a bevelled edge, and is scored on 1 side with "RPC" above and "5" below the score, and "004" on the other side.

2.5-milligram
Tablets: NDC 54092-003-01 Bottle of 100
5-milligram
Tablets: NDC 54092-004-01 Bottle of 100

Store from 15°C to 25°C (59°F to 77°F).
Rx only
ROBERTS® PHARMACEUTICALS
Manufactured by NYCOMED Austria GmbH
for Roberts Laboratories Inc.,
a subsidiary of **ROBERTS PHARMACEUTICAL CORPORATION**, Eatontown, NJ 07724-2274, USA

Shown in Product Identification Guide, page 336

SLOW-MAG® OTC
MAGNESIUM CHLORIDE

DESCRIPTION

SLOW-MAG® is enteric coated magnesium chloride available in tablet form in a dosage unit of 64mg magnesium per tablet. Magnesium is an essential mineral of a healthy diet and may help to maintain the functions of the heart, muscles and nervous system.

SLOW-MAG® is a dietary supplement that provides a magnesium chloride formulation that is enteric coated to avoid the stomach upset and diarrhea commonly associated with oral magnesium supplements.

INGREDIENTS

Each tablet contains magnesium chloride hexahydrate, calcium carbonate, povidone, talc, magnesium stearate, cellulose acetate phthalate, diethyl phthalate, titanium dioxide, hydroxypropyl cellulose, FD&C Blue No. 2 Lake.

DIRECTIONS FOR USE

As a dietary supplement, take 2 tablets daily or as directed by a physician. Two 64mg tablets contain 32% of the recommended daily allowance for magnesium.

HOW SUPPLIED

Bottles of 60 tablets.
Do not use if the inner seal or protective band around the cap is broken or missing.
Manufactured for
Roberts Laboratories Inc., a subsidiary of
ROBERTS PHARMACEUTICAL CORPORATION
Eatontown, NJ 07724 USA

Sigma-Tau Pharmaceuticals, Inc.
800 SOUTH FREDERICK AVENUE, SUITE 300
GAITHERSBURG, MARYLAND 20877

Direct Inquiries to:
TEL: (301) 948-1041
800-447-0169
Fax: (301) 948-3194

CARNITOR® ℞
[*căr-nĭ-tor*]
(levocarnitine) Injection
1 g per 5 mL vial and sealed ampoule
FOR INTRAVENOUS USE ONLY.

DESCRIPTION

CARNITOR® (levocarnitine) is a carrier molecule in the transport of long-chain fatty acids across the inner mitochondrial membrane.

The chemical name of levocarnitine is 3-carboxy-2(*R*)-hydroxy-N,N,N-trimethyl-1-propanaminium, inner salt. Levocarnitine is a white crystalline, hygroscopic powder. It is readily soluble in water, hot alcohol, and insoluble in acetone. The specific rotation of levocarnitine is between -29° and -32°. Its chemical structure is:

HO H
C
$(CH_3)_3N^+$—CH_2 CH_2COO^-

Empirical Formula: $C_7H_{15}NO_3$
Molecular Weight: 161.20

CARNITOR® (levocarnitine) Injection is a sterile aqueous solution containing 1 g of levocarnitine per 5 mL vial or sealed ampoule. The pH is adjusted to 6.0-6.5 with hydrochloric acid or sodium hydroxide.

CLINICAL PHARMACOLOGY

CARNITOR® (levocarnitine) is a naturally occurring substance required in mammalian energy metabolism. It has been shown to facilitate long-chain fatty acid entry into cellular mitochondria, thereby delivering substrate for oxidation and subsequent energy production. Fatty acids are utilized as an energy substrate in all tissues except the brain. In skeletal and cardiac muscle, fatty acids are the main substrate for energy production.

Primary systemic carnitine deficiency is characterized by low concentrations of levocarnitine in plasma, RBC, and/or tissues. It has not been possible to determine which symptoms are due to carnitine deficiency and which are due to an underlying organic acidemia, as symptoms of both abnormalities may be expected to improve with CARNITOR®. The literature reports that carnitine can promote the excretion of excess organic or fatty acids in patients with defects in fatty acid metabolism and/or specific organic acidopathies that bioaccumulate acylCoA esters.[1-6]

Secondary carnitine deficiency can be a consequence of inborn errors of metabolism or iatrogenic factors such as hemodialysis. CARNITOR® may alleviate the metabolic abnormalities of patients with inborn errors that result in accumulation of toxic organic acids. Conditions for which this effect has been demonstrated are: glutaric aciduria II, methyl malonic aciduria, propionic acidemia, and medium chain fatty acylCoA dehydrogenase deficiency.[7,8] Autointoxication occurs in these patients due to the accumulations of acylCoA compounds that disrupt intermediary metabolism. The subsequent hydrolysis of the acylCoA compound to its free acid results in acidosis which can be life-threatening.

Continued on next page

Carnitor Injection—Cont.

Levocarnitine clears the acylCoA compound by formation of acylcarnitine, which is quickly excreted. Carnitine deficiency is defined biochemically as abnormally low plasma concentrations of free carnitine, less than 20 µmol/L at one week post term and may be associated with low tissue and/or urine concentrations. Further, this condition may be associated with a plasma concentration ratio of acylcarnitine/levocarnitine greater than 0.4 or abnormally elevated concentrations of acylcarnitine in the urine. In premature infants and newborns, secondary deficiency is defined as plasma levocarnitine concentrations below age-related normal concentrations.

End Stage Renal Disease (ESRD) patients on maintenance hemodialysis may have low plasma carnitine concentrations and an increased ratio of acylcarnitine/carnitine because of reduced intake of meat and dairy products, reduced renal synthesis and dialytic losses. Certain clinical conditions common in hemodialysis patients such as malaise, muscle weakness, cardiomyopathy and cardiac arrhythmias may be related to abnormal carnitine metabolism.

Pharmacokinetic and clinical studies with CARNITOR® have shown that administration of levocarnitine to ESRD patients on hemodialysis results in increased plasma levocarnitine concentrations.

PHARMACOKINETICS

In a relative bioavailability study in 15 healthy adult male volunteers, CARNITOR® Tablets were found to be bio-equivalent to CARNITOR® Oral Solution. Following 4 days of dosing with 6 tablets of CARNITOR® 330 mg b.i.d. or 2 g of CARNITOR® oral solution b.i.d., the maximum plasma concentration (C_{max}) was about 80 µmol/L and the time to maximum plasma concentration (T_{max}) occurred at 3.3 hours.

The plasma concentration profiles of levocarnitine after a slow 3 minute intravenous bolus dose of 20 mg/kg of CARNITOR® were described by a two-compartment model. Following a single i.v. administration, approximately 76% of the levocarnitine dose was excreted in the urine during the 0-24h interval. Using plasma concentrations uncorrected for endogenous levocarnitine, the mean distribution half life was 0.585 hours and the mean apparent terminal elimination half life was 17.4 hours.

The absolute bioavailability of levocarnitine from the two oral formulations of CARNITOR®, calculated after correction for circulating endogenous plasma concentrations of levocarnitine, was 15.1 ± 5.3% for CARNITOR® Tablets and 15.9 ± 4.9% for CARNITOR® Oral Solution.

Total body clearance of levocarnitine (Dose/AUC including endogenous baseline concentrations) was a mean of 4.00 L/h.

Levocarnitine was not bound to plasma protein or albumin when tested at any concentration or with any species including the human.[9]

In a 9-week study, 12 ESRD patients undergoing hemodialysis for at least 6 months received CARNITOR® 20 mg/kg three times per week after dialysis. Prior to initiation of CARNITOR® therapy, mean plasma levocarnitine concentrations were approximately 20 µmol/L pre-dialysis and 6 µmol/L post-dialysis. The table summarizes the pharmacokinetic data (mean ± SD µmol/L) after the first dose of CARNITOR® and after 8 weeks of CARNITOR® therapy.

[See first table above]

After one week of CARNITOR® therapy (3 doses), all patients had trough concentrations between 54 and 180 µmol/L (normal 40–50 µmol/L) and concentrations remained relatively stable or increased over the course of the study.

In a similar study in ESRD patients also receiving 20 mg/kg CARNITOR® 3 times per week after hemodialysis, 12- and 24-week mean pre-dialysis (trough) levocarnitine concentrations were 189 (N=25) and 243 (N=23) µmol/L, respectively.

In a dose-ranging study in ESRD patients undergoing hemodialysis, patients received 10, 20, or 40 mg/kg CARNITOR® 3 times per week following dialysis (N~30 for each dose group). Mean ± SD trough levocarnitine concentrations (µmol/L) by dose after 12 and 24 weeks of therapy are summarized in the table.

	12 weeks	24 weeks
10 mg/kg	116 ± 69	148 ± 50
20 mg/kg	210 ± 58	240 ± 60
40 mg/kg	371 ± 111	456 ± 162

While the efficacy of CARNITOR® to increase carnitine concentrations in patients with ESRD undergoing dialysis has been demonstrated, the effects of supplemental carnitine on the signs and symptoms of carnitine deficiency and on clinical outcomes in this population have not been determined.

METABOLISM AND EXCRETION

In a pharmacokinetic study where five normal adult male volunteers received an oral dose of [^{3}H-methyl]-L-carnitine following 15 days of a high carnitine diet and additional carnitine supplement, 58 to 65% of the administered radioactive dose was recovered in the urine and feces in 5 to 11 days. Maximum concentration of [^{3}H-methyl]-L-carnitine in serum occurred from 2.0 to 4.5 hr after drug administration. Major metabolites found were trimethylamine N-oxide, primarily in urine (8% to 49% of the administered dose) and [^{3}H]-γ-butyrobetaine, primarily in feces (0.44% to 45% of the administered dose). Urinary excretion of levocarnitine was about 4 to 8% of the dose. Fecal excretion of total carnitine was less than 1% of the administered dose.[10]

After attainment of steady state following 4 days of oral administration of CARNITOR® Tablets (1980 mg q12h) or Oral Solution (2000 mg q12h) to 15 healthy male volunteers, the mean urinary excretion of levocarnitine during a single dosing interval (12h) was about 9% of the orally administered dose (uncorrected for endogenous urinary excretion).

N=12	Baseline	Single dose	8 weeks
C_{max}	—	1139 ± 240	1190 ± 270
Trough (pre-dialysis, pre-dose)	21.3 ± 7.7	68.4 ± 26.1	190 ± 55

Adverse Events with a Frequency ≥5% Regardless of Causality by Body System

	Placebo (n=63)	*Levocarnitine 10 mg (n=34)*	*Levocarnitine 20 mg (n=62)*	*Levocarnitine 40 mg (n=34)*	*Levocarnitine 10, 20 & 40 mg (n=130)*
Body as Whole					
Abdominal pain	17	21	5	6	9
Accidental injury	10	12	8	12	10
Allergic reaction	5	6			2
Asthenia	8	9	8	12	9
Back pain	10	9	8	6	8
Chest pain	14	6	15	12	12
Fever	5	6	5	12	7
Flu syndrome	40	15	27	29	25
Headache	16	12	37	3	22
Infection	17	15	10	24	15
Injection site reaction	59	38	27	38	33
Pain	49	21	32	35	30
Cardiovascular					
Arrhythmia	5	3		3	2
Atrial fibrillation			2	6	2
Cardiovascular disorder	6	3	5	6	5
Electrocardiogram abnormal		3		6	2
Hemorrhage	6	9	2	3	4
Hypertension	14	18	21	21	20
Hypotension	19	15	19	3	14
Palpitations		3	8		5
Tachycardia	5	6	5	9	6
Vascular disorder	2		2	6	2
Digestive					
Anorexia	3	3	5	6	5
Constipation	6	3	3	3	3
Diarrhea	19	9	10	35	16
Dyspepsia	10	9	6		5
Gastrointestinal disorder	2	3		6	2
Melena	3	6			2
Nausea	10	9	5	12	8
Stomach atony	5				
Vomiting	16	9	16	21	15
Endocrine System					
Parathyroid disorder	2	6	2	6	4
Hemic/Lymphatic					
Anemia	3	3	5	12	6

(Continued on next page)

INDICATIONS AND USAGE

For the acute and chronic treatment of patients with an inborn error of metabolism which results in secondary carnitine deficiency.

For the prevention and treatment of carnitine deficiency in patients with end stage renal disease who are undergoing dialysis.

CONTRAINDICATIONS

None known.

WARNINGS

None.

PRECAUTIONS

Carcinogenesis, mutagenesis, impairment of fertility

Mutagenicity tests performed in *Salmonella typhimurium*, *Saccharomyces cerevisiae*, and *Schizosaccharomyces pombe* indicate that levocarnitine is not mutagenic. No long-term animal studies have been performed to evaluate the carcinogenic potential of levocarnitine.

Pregnancy

Pregnancy Category B.

Reproductive studies have been performed in rats and rabbits at doses up to 3.8 times the human dose on the basis of surface area and have revealed no evidence of impaired fertility or harm to the fetus due to CARNITOR®. There are, however, no adequate and well controlled studies in pregnant women.

Because animal reproduction studies are not always predictive of human response, this drug should be used during pregnancy only if clearly needed.

Nursing Mothers

Levocarnitine supplementation in nursing mothers has not been specifically studied.

Studies in dairy cows indicate that the concentration of levocarnitine in milk is increased following exogenous administration of levocarnitine. In nursing mothers receiving levocarnitine, any risks to the child of excess carnitine intake need to be weighed against the benefits of levocarnitine supplementation to the mother. Consideration may be given to discontinuation of nursing or of levocarnitine treatment.

Pediatric Use

See Dosage and Administration.

ADVERSE REACTIONS

Transient nausea and vomiting have been observed. Less frequent adverse reactions are body odor, nausea, and gastritis. An incidence for these reactions is difficult to estimate due to the confounding effects of the underlying pathology. Seizures have been reported to occur in patients, with or without pre-existing seizure activity, receiving either oral or intravenous levocarnitine. In patients with pre-existing seizure activity, an increase in seizure frequency and/or severity has been reported.

The table below lists the adverse events that have been reported in two double-blind, placebo-controlled trials in patients on chronic hemodialysis. Events occurring at ≥5% are reported without regard to causality.

[See second table at top of previous page]

Adverse Events with a Frequency ≥5% Regardless of Causality by Body System

	Placebo (n=63)	*Levocarnitine 10 mg (n=34)*	*Levocarnitine 20 mg (n=62)*	*Levocarnitine 40 mg (n=34)*	*Levocarnitine 10, 20 & 40 mg (n=130)*
Metabolic/Nutritional					
Hypercalcemia	3	15	8	6	9
Hyperkalemia	6	6	6	6	6
Hypervolemia	17	3	3	12	5
Peripheral edema	3	6	5	3	5
Weight decrease	3	3	8	3	5
Weight increase	2	3		6	2
Musculo-Skeletal					
Leg cramps	13		8		4
Myalgia	6				
Nervous					
Anxiety	5		2		1
Depression	3	6	5	6	5
Dizziness	11	18	10	15	13
Drug dependence	2	6			2
Hypertonia	5	3			1
Insomnia	6	3	6		4
Paresthesia	3	3	3	12	5
Vertigo		6			2
Respiratory					
Bronchitis			5	3	3
Cough increase	16		10	18	9
Dyspnea	19	3	11	3	7
Pharyngitis	33	24	27	15	23
Respiratory disorder	5				
Rhinitis	10	6	11	6	9
Sinusitis	5		2	3	2
Skin and Appendages					
Pruritus	13		8	3	5
Rash	3		5	3	3
Special Senses					
Amblyopia	2		6		3
Eye disorder	3	6	3		3
Taste perversion			2	9	3
Urogenital					
Urinary tract infect	6	3	3		2
Kidney failure	5	6	6	6	6

OVERDOSAGE

There have been no reports of toxicity from levocarnitine overdosage. Levocarnitine is easily removed from plasma by dialysis. The intravenous LD_{50} of levocarnitine in rats is 5.4 g/kg and the oral LD_{50} of levocarnitine in mice is 19.2 g/kg. Large doses of levocarnitine may cause diarrhea.

DOSAGE AND ADMINISTRATION

CARNITOR® Injection is administered intravenously.

Metabolic Disorders

The recommended dose is 50 mg/kg given as a slow 2-3 minute bolus injection or by infusion. Often a loading dose is given in patients with severe metabolic crisis, followed by an equivalent dose over the following 24 hours. It should be administered q3h or q4h, and never less than q6h either by infusion or by intravenous injection. All subsequent daily doses are recommended to be in the range of 50 mg/kg or as therapy may require. The highest dose administered has been 300 mg/kg.

It is recommended that a plasma carnitine concentration be obtained prior to beginning this parenteral therapy. Weekly and monthly monitoring is recommended as well. This monitoring should include blood chemistries, vital signs, plasma carnitine concentrations (the plasma free carnitine concentration should be between 35 and 60 µmol/L) and overall clinical condition.

ESRD Patients on Hemodialysis

The recommended starting dose is 10-20 mg/kg dry body weight as a slow 2-3 minute bolus injection into the venous return line after each dialysis session. Initiation of therapy may be prompted by trough (pre-dialysis) plasma levocarnitine concentrations that are below normal (40-50 µmol/L). Dose adjustments should be guided by trough (pre-dialysis) levocarnitine concentrations, and downward dose adjustments (e.g. to 5 mg/kg after dialysis) may be made as early as the third or fourth week of therapy.

Parenteral drug products should be inspected visually for particulate matter and discoloration prior to administration, whenever solution and container permit.

COMPATIBILITY AND STABILITY

CARNITOR® Injection is compatible and stable when mixed in parenteral solutions of Sodium Chloride 0.9% or Lactated Ringer's in concentrations ranging from 250 mg/500 mL (0.5 mg/mL) to 4200 mg/500 mL (8.0 mg/mL) and stored at room temperature (25°C) for up to 24 hours in PVC plastic bags.

HOW SUPPLIED

CARNITOR® (levocarnitine) Injection is available in 1 g per 5 mL single dose vials packaged 5 vials per carton (NDC 54482-147-01). CARNITOR® (levocarnitine) Injection 5 mL vial is manufactured for Sigma-Tau Pharmaceuticals, Inc. by Chesapeake Biological Laboratories, Inc. Baltimore, MD 21230-2591.

Store vials at controlled room temperature (25°C). See USP. Discard unused portion of an opened vial, as the formulation does not contain a preservative.

CARNITOR® (levocarnitine) Injection is also available in 1 g per 5 mL single dose ampoules packaged 5 ampoules per carton (NDC 54482-146-09). Made in Italy.

Store ampoules at controlled room temperature (25°C). See USP. Store in carton until their use to protect from light. Discard unused portion of an opened ampoule, as the formulation does not contain a preservative.

CARNITOR® (levocarnitine) is also available in the following dosage forms for oral administration:

CARNITOR® (levocarnitine) Tablets are supplied as 330 mg tablets embossed with "CARNITOR ST" in blister packages, in boxes of 90 tablets (NDC 54482-144-07). Made in Italy.

CARNITOR® (levocarnitine) Oral Solution is supplied in 118 mL (4 FL. OZ.) multiple-unit plastic containers. The multiple-unit containers are packaged 24 per case (NDC 54482-145-08). CARNITOR® (levocarnitine) Oral Solution is manufactured for Sigma-Tau Pharmaceuticals, Inc. by Alpharma USPD, Inc., Baltimore, MD 21244-2654 and/or Hi-Tech Pharmacal Co., Inc., Amityville, NY 11701.

Rx only.

REFERENCES

1. Bohmer, T., Rydning, A. and Solberg, H.E. 1974. Carnitine levels in human serum in health and disease. *Clin. Chim. Acta* 57:55–61.
2. Brooks, H., Goldberg L., Holland, R. *et al.* 1977. Carnitine-induced effects on cardiac and peripheral hemodynamics. *J. Clin. Pharmacol.* 17:561–568.
3. Christiansen, R., Bremer, J. 1976. Active transport of butyrobetaine and carnitine into isolated liver cells. *Biochim. Biophys. Acta* 448:562–577.
4. Lindstedt, S. and Lindstedt, G. 1961. Distribution and excretion of carnitine in the rat. *Acta Chem. Scand.* 15:701–702.
5. Rebouche, C.J. and Engel, A.G. 1983. Carnitine metabolism and deficiency syndromes. *Mayo Clin. Proc.* 58:533–540.

Continued on next page

Carnitor Injection—Cont.

6. Rebouche, C.J. and Paulson, D.J. 1986. Carnitine metabolism and function in humans. *Ann. Rev. Nutr.* 6:41–66.
7. Scriver, C.R., Beaudet, A.L., Sly, W.S. and Valle, D. 1989. *The Metabolic Basis of Inherited Disease*. New York: McGraw-Hill.
8. Schaub, J., Van Hoof, F. and Vis, H.L. 1991. *Inborn Errors of Metabolism*. New York: Raven Press.
9. Marzo, A., Arrigoni Martelli, E., Mancinelli, A., Cardace, G., Corbelletta, C., Bassani, E. and Solbiati, M. 1991. Protein binding of L-carnitine family components. *Eur. J. Drug Met. Pharmacokin.*, Special Issue III: 364–368.
10. Rebouche, C.J. 1991. Quantitative estimation of absorption and degradation of a carnitine supplement by human adults. *Metabolism* 40:1305–1310.

Vials manufactured by: Chesapeake Biological Laboratories, Inc. Baltimore, MD 21230-2591. Ampoules manufactured by: Sigma-Tau S.p.A., Pomezia, Rome, Italy
Sigma-Tau Pharmaceuticals, Inc.
Gaithersburg, MD 20877
PREVIOUS EDITION IS OBSOLETE
STP20182-05/00 Version VIFS-1
533331

CARNITOR® ℞
[car-nĭ-tor]
(Levocarnitine)
Tablets (330 mg)

CARNITOR®
(Levocarnitine)
Oral Solution
(1 g per 10 mL multidose)
For oral use only. Not for parenteral use.

DESCRIPTION

CARNITOR® (Levocarnitine) is (R)-3-carboxy-2-hydroxy-N,N,N-trimethyl-1-propanaminium hydroxide, inner salt. Levocarnitine is a carrier molecule in the transport of long chain fatty acids across the inner mitochondrial membrane. As a bulk drug substance it is a white powder with a melting point of 196-197°C and is readily soluble in water, hot alcohol, and insoluble in acetone. The pH of a solution (1 in 20) is between 6-8 and its pKa value is 3.8. Its chemical structure is:

$$CH_3-\overset{+}{N}(CH_3)_2-CH_2-CH(OH)-CH_2-COO^-$$

Empirical Formula: $C_7H_{15}NO_3$
Molecular Weight: 161.20

Each CARNITOR® (Levocarnitine) Tablet contains 330 mg of levocarnitine and the inactive ingredients magnesium stearate, microcrystalline cellulose and povidone.
Each 118 mL container of the CARNITOR® (Levocarnitine) Oral Solution contains 1 g of levocarnitine/10 mL. Also contains: Artificial Cherry Flavor, D,L-Malic Acid, Purified Water, Sucrose Syrup. Methylparaben NF and Propylparaben NF are added as preservatives. The pH is approximately 5.

CLINICAL PHARMACOLOGY

CARNITOR® (Levocarnitine) is a naturally occurring substance required in mammalian energy metabolism. It has been shown to facilitate long-chain fatty acid entry into cellular mitochondria, therefore delivering substrate for oxidation and subsequent energy production. Fatty acids are utilized as an energy substrate in all tissues except the brain. In skeletal and cardiac muscle they serve as major fuel. Primary systemic carnitine deficiency is characterized by low plasma, RBC, and/or tissue levels. It has not been possible to determine which symptoms are due to carnitine deficiency and which are due to the underlying organic acidemia, as symptoms of both abnormalities may be expected to improve with carnitine. The literature reports that carnitine can promote the excretion of excess organic or fatty acids in patients with defects in fatty acid metabolism and/or specific organic acidopathies that bioaccumulate acyl CoA esters.[1–6]
Secondary levocarnitine deficiency can be a consequence of inborn errors of metabolism. CARNITOR® may alleviate the metabolic abnormalities of patients with inborn errors that result in accumulation of toxic organic acids. Conditions for which this effect was demonstrated are: glutaric aciduria II, methyl malonic aciduria, propionic acidemia, and medium chain fatty acyl CoA dehydrogenase deficiency.[7,8] Autointoxication occurs in these patients due to the accumulations of acyl CoA compounds that disrupt intermediary metabolism. The subsequent hydrolysis of the acyl CoA compound to its free acid results in acidosis that can be life threatening. Levocarnitine clears the acyl CoA compound by formation of acyl carnitine which is quickly excreted.
Levocarnitine deficiency is defined biochemically as abnormally low plasma levels of free carnitine (less than 20 μmol/L at one week post term) and may be associated with low tissue and/or urine levels. Further, this condition may be associated with a ratio of plasma ester/free levocarnitine levels greater than 0.4 or abnormally elevated levels of esterified levocarnitine in the urine. In premature infants and newborns, secondary deficiency is defined as plasma free levocarnitine levels below age related normal levels.

BIOAVAILABILITY/PHARMACOKINETICS
In a relative bioavailability study in 15 healthy adult male volunteers CARNITOR® Tablets were found to be bio-equivalent to CARNITOR® Oral Solution. Following the administration of 1980 mg b.i.d., the maximum plasma concentration level (C_{max}) was 80 nmol/mL and the time to maximum concentration (T_{max}) occurred at 3.3 hours. There were no significant differences for AUC and urinary excretion observed between these two formulations.
In the same bioavailability study of 15 healthy adult males, CARNITOR® (Levocarnitine) Injection administered as a slow 3 minute bolus intravenous injection at a dose of 20 mg/kg showed that free levocarnitine plasma profiles are best fit by a two compartment model. Approximately 76% of free levocarnitine is eliminated in the urine. Using plasma levels uncorrected for endogenous levocarnitine, the mean distribution half life was 0.585 hours and the mean apparent terminal elimination half life was 17.4 hours following a single intravenous dose.
The absolute bioavailability of L-carnitine from CARNITOR® Tablets and Oral Solution was determined compared to the bioavailability of L-carnitine from CARNITOR® Injection Intravenous in 15 healthy male volunteers. After correction for circulating endogenous levels of L-carnitine in the plasma, absolute bioavailability was 15.1% ± 5.3% for L-carnitine from CARNITOR® Tablets and 15.9% ± 4.9% from the Oral Solution.
Total body clearance of L-carnitine (Dose/AUC including endogenous baseline levels) was a mean of 4.00 L/hr. Endogenous baseline levels were not subtracted since total body clearance of L-carnitine does not distinguish between exogenous sources of L-carnitine and endogenously synthesized L-carnitine. Volume of distribution of the intravenously administered dose above baseline endogenous levels was calculated to be a mean of 29.0 L ± 7.1 L (approximately 0.39 L/kg) which is an underestimate of the true volume of distribution since plasma L-carnitine is known to equilibrate slowly with, for instance, muscle L-carnitine.
L-carnitine was not bound to plasma protein or albumin when tested at any concentration or with any species including the human.[9]

METABOLISM AND EXCRETION
Five normal adult male volunteers, administered a dose of [^{3}H-methyl]-L-carnitine following 15 days of a high carnitine diet and additional carnitine supplement, excreted 58 - 65% of administered radioactive dose in 5 to 11 days in the urine and feces. Maximum concentration of [^{3}H-methyl]-L-carnitine in serum occurred from 2.0 to 4.5 hr after drug administration. Major metabolites found were trimethylamine N-oxide, primarily in urine (8% to 49% of the administered dose) and [^{3}H]-γ-butyrobetaine, primarily in feces (0.44% to 45% of the administered dose). Urinary excretion of carnitine was 4% to 8% of the dose. Fecal excretion of total carnitine was less than 1% of total carnitine excretion.[10]
After attainment of steady state following 4 days of oral administration of L-carnitine with CARNITOR® Tablets (1980 mg q12h) or Oral Solution (2000 mg q12h) to 15 healthy male volunteers, urinary excretion of L-carnitine was a mean of 2107 and 2339 μmoles, respectively, equivalent to 8.6% and 9.4%, respectively, of the orally administered doses (uncorrected for endogenous urinary excretion). After a single intravenous dose (20 mg/kg) prior to multiple oral doses, urinary excretion of L-carnitine was 6974 μmoles equivalent to 75.6% of the intravenously administered dose (uncorrected for endogenous urinary excretion).

INDICATIONS AND USAGE

CARNITOR® (Levocarnitine) is indicated in the treatment of primary systemic carnitine deficiency. In the reported cases, the clinical presentation consisted of recurrent episodes of Reye-like encephalopathy, hypoketotic hypoglycemia, and/or cardiomyopathy. Associated symptoms included hypotonia, muscle weakness and failure to thrive. A diagnosis of primary carnitine deficiency requires that serum, red cell and/or tissue carnitine levels be low and that the patient does not have a primary defect in fatty acid or organic acid oxidation (see Clinical Pharmacology). In some patients, particularly those presenting with cardiomyopathy, carnitine supplementation rapidly alleviated signs and symptoms. Treatment should include, in addition to carnitine, supportive and other therapy as indicated by the condition of the patient.
CARNITOR® (Levocarnitine) is also indicated for acute and chronic treatment of patients with an inborn error of metabolism that results in a secondary carnitine deficiency.

CONTRAINDICATIONS

None known.

WARNINGS

None.

PRECAUTIONS

General
CARNITOR® (Levocarnitine) Oral Solution is for oral/internal use only.
Not for parenteral use.
Gastrointestinal reactions may result from too rapid consumption of carnitine. CARNITOR® (Levocarnitine) Oral Solution may be consumed alone, or dissolved in drinks or other liquid foods to reduce taste fatigue. It should be consumed slowly and doses should be spaced evenly throughout the day to maximize tolerance.
Carcinogenesis, mutagenesis, impairment of fertility
Mutagenicity tests performed in *Salmonella typhimurium*, *Saccharomyces cerevisiae*, and *Schizosaccharomyces pombe* indicate that CARNITOR® (Levocarnitine) is not mutagenic. Long-term animal studies have not been conducted to evaluate the carcinogenicity of the compound.
Pregnancy
Pregnancy Category B.
Reproductive studies have been performed in rats and rabbits at doses up to 3.8 times the human dose on the basis of surface area and have revealed no evidence of impaired fertility or harm to the fetus due to CARNITOR®. There are, however, no adequate and well controlled studies in pregnant women. Because animal reproduction studies are not always predictive of human response, this drug should be used during pregnancy only if clearly needed.
Nursing mothers
It is not known whether this drug is excreted in human milk. Because many drugs are excreted in human milk, a decision should be made whether to discontinue nursing or to discontinue the drug, taking into account the importance of the drug to the mother.
Pediatric use
See Dosage and Administration.

ADVERSE REACTIONS

Various mild gastrointestinal complaints have been reported during the long-term administration of oral L- or D,L-carnitine; these include transient nausea and vomiting, abdominal cramps, and diarrhea. Mild myasthenia has been described only in uremic patients receiving D,L-carnitine. Gastrointestinal adverse reactions with CARNITOR® (Levocarnitine) Oral Solution dissolved in liquids might be avoided by a slow consumption of the solution or by a greater dilution. Decreasing the dosage often diminishes or eliminates drug-related patient body odor or gastrointestinal symptoms when present. Tolerance should be monitored very closely during the first week of administration, and after any dosage increases.
Seizures have been reported to occur in patients with or without pre-existing seizure activity receiving either oral or intravenous levocarnitine. In patients with pre-existing seizure activity, an increase in seizure frequency and/or severity has been reported.

OVERDOSAGE

There have been no reports of toxicity from carnitine overdosage. The oral LD_{50} of levocarnitine in mice is 19.2 g/kg. Carnitine may cause diarrhea. Overdosage should be treated with supportive care.

DOSAGE AND ADMINISTRATION

CARNITOR® (Levocarnitine) Tablets.
Adults: The recommended oral dosage for adults is 990 mg two or three times a day using the 330 mg tablets, depending on clinical response.
Infants and children: The recommended oral dosage for infants and children is between 50 and 100 mg/kg/day in divided doses, with a maximum of 3 g/day. Dosage should begin at 50 mg/kg/day. The exact dosage will depend on clinical response.
Monitoring should include periodic blood chemistries, vital signs, plasma carnitine concentrations and overall clinical condition.
CARNITOR® (Levocarnitine) Oral Solution.
For oral use only. **Not for parenteral use.**
Adults: The recommended dosage of levocarnitine is 1 to 3 g/day for a 50 kg subject, which is equivalent to 10 to 30 mL/day of CARNITOR® (Levocarnitine) Oral Solution. Higher doses should be administered only with caution and only where clinical and biochemical considerations make it seem likely that higher doses will be of benefit. Dosage should start at 1 g/day, (10 mL/day), and be increased slowly while assessing tolerance and therapeutic response. Monitoring should include periodic blood chemistries, vital signs, plasma carnitine concentrations, and overall clinical condition.
Infants and children: The recommended dosage of levocarnitine is 50 to 100 mg/kg/day which is equivalent to 0.5 mL/kg/day CARNITOR® (Levocarnitine) Oral Solution. Higher doses should be administered only with caution and only where clinical and biochemical considerations make it seem likely that higher doses will be of benefit. Dosage should start at 50 mg/kg/day, and be increased slowly to a maximum of 3 g/day (30 mL/day) while assessing tolerance and therapeutic response. Monitoring should include periodic blood chemistries, vital signs, plasma carnitine concentrations, and overall clinical condition.
CARNITOR® (Levocarnitine) Oral Solution may be consumed alone or dissolved in drink or other liquid food. Doses should be spaced evenly throughout the day (every three or four hours) preferably during or following meals and should be consumed slowly in order to maximize tolerance.

HOW SUPPLIED

CARNITOR® (Levocarnitine) Tablets are supplied as 330 mg tablets embossed with "CARNITOR ST" in individual blisters, packaged in boxes of 90 (NDC 54482-144-07).
Store at controlled room temperature (25°C). See USP.
CARNITOR® (Levocarnitine) Oral Solution is supplied in 118 mL (4 FL. OZ.) multiple-unit plastic containers. The

multiple-unit containers are packaged 24 per case (NDC 54482-145-08). Store at controlled room temperature (25°C). See USP.
CARNITOR® (Levocarnitine) Oral Solution is manufactured for Sigma-tau Pharmaceuticals, Inc. by: Alpharma USPD, Inc. Baltimore, MD 21244-2654 and/or Hi-Tech Pharmacal Co., Inc. Amityville, NY 11701.
CARNITOR® (Levocarnitine) is also available in the following dosage forms for intravenous injection:
CARNITOR® (levocarnitine) Injection is available in 1 g per 5 mL single dose vials packaged 5 vials per carton (NDC 54482-147-01). CARNITOR® (levocarnitine) Injection 5 mL vial is manufactured for Sigma-Tau Pharmaceuticals, Inc. by Chesapeake Biological Laboratories, Inc. Baltimore, MD 21230-2591.
CARNITOR® (Levocarnitine) Injection is also available in 1 g per 5 mL single dose ampoules packaged 5 ampoules per carton (NDC 54482-146-09). Made in Italy.
Rx only.

REFERENCES

1. Bohmer, T., Rydning, A., Solberg, H.E. 1974. Carnitine levels in human serum in health and disease. *Clin. Chim. Acta* 57:55–61.
2. Brooks, H., Goldberg, L., Holland R. *et al.* 1977. Carnitine-induced effects on cardiac and peripheral hemodynamics. *J. Clin. Pharmacol.* 17:561–568.
3. Christiansen, R., Bremer, J. 1976. Active transport of butyrobetaine and carnitine into isolated liver cells. *Biochim. Biophys. Acta* 448:562–577.
4. Lindstedt, S. and Lindstedt, G. 1961. Distribution and excretion of carnitine in the rat. *Acta Chem. Scand.* 15:701–702.
5. Rebouche, C.J. and Engel, A.G. 1983. Carnitine metabolism and deficiency syndromes. *Mayo Clin. Proc.* 58:533–540.
6. Rebouche, C.J. and Paulson, D.J. 1986. Carnitine metabolism and function in humans. *Ann. Rev. Nutr.* 6:41–66.
7. Scriver, C.R., Beaudet, A.L., Sly, W.S. and Valle, D. 1989. *The Metabolic Basis of Inherited Disease.* New York: McGraw-Hill.
8. Schaub, J., Van Hoof, F. and Vis, H.L. 1991. *Inborn Errors of Metabolism.* New York: Raven Press.
9. Marzo, A., Arrigoni Martelli, E., Mancinelli, A., Cardace, G., Corbelletta, C., Bassani, E. and Solbiati, M. 1991. Protein binding of L-carnitine family components. *Eur. J. Drug Met. Pharmacokin.*, Special Issue III: 364–368.
10. Rebouche, C.J. 1991. Quantitative estimation of absorption and degradation of a carnitine supplement by human adults. *Metabolism* 40:1305–1310.

Sigma-Tau
Pharmaceuticals, Inc.
Gaithersburg, MD 20877

PREVIOUS EDITION IS OBSOLETE
ST-N18-948-05/00 OPI-1

MATULANE® ℞

[*măt'ū-lāne*]
brand of
procarbazine
hydrochloride
CAPSULES

WARNING

It is recommended that MATULANE be given only by or under the supervision of a physician experienced in the use of potent antineoplastic drugs. Adequate clinical and laboratory facilities should be available to patients for proper monitoring of treatment.

DESCRIPTION

Matulane (procarbazine hydrochloride), a hydrazine derivative antineoplastic agent, is available as capsules containing the equivalent of 50 mg procarbazine as the hydrochloride. Each capsule also contains cornstarch, mannitol and talc. Gelatin capsule shells contain parabens (methyl and propyl), potassium sorbate, titanium dioxide, FD&C Yellow No. 6 and D&C Yellow No. 10.
Chemically, procarbazine hydrochloride is *N*-isopropyl-α-(2-methylhydrazino)-*p*-toluamide monohydrochloride. It is a white to pale yellow crystalline powder which is soluble but unstable in water or aqueous solutions. The molecular weight of procarbazine hydrochloride is 257.76 and the structural formula is:

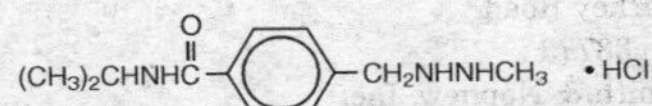

CLINICAL PHARMACOLOGY

The precise mode of cytotoxic action of procarbazine has not been clearly defined. There is evidence that the drug may act by inhibition of protein, RNA and DNA synthesis. Studies have suggested that procarbazine may inhibit transmethylation of methyl groups of methionine into t-RNA. The absence of functional t-RNA could cause the cessation of protein synthesis and consequently DNA and RNA synthesis. In addition, procarbazine may directly damage DNA. Hydrogen peroxide, formed during the auto-oxidation of the drug, may attack protein sulfhydryl groups contained in residual protein which is tightly bound to DNA.
Procarbazine is metabolized primarily in the liver and kidneys. The drug appears to be auto-oxidized to the azo derivative with the release of hydrogen peroxide. The azo derivative isomerizes to the hydrazone, and following hydrolysis splits into a benzyl-aldehyde derivative and methylhydrazine. The methylhydrazine is further degraded to CO_2 and CH_4 and possibly hydrazine, whereas the aldehyde is oxidized to *N*-isopropylterephthalamic acid, which is excreted in the urine.
Procarbazine is rapidly and completely absorbed. Following oral administration of 30 mg of ^{14}C-labeled procarbazine, maximum peak plasma radioactive concentrations were reached within 60 minutes.
After intravenous injection, the plasma half-life of procarbazine is approximately 10 minutes. Approximately 70% of the radioactivity is excreted in the urine as *N*-isopropylterephthalamic acid within 24 hours following both oral and intravenous administration of ^{14}C-labeled procarbazine.
Procarbazine crosses the blood-brain barrier and rapidly equilibrates between plasma and cerebrospinal fluid after oral administration.

INDICATIONS AND USAGE

Matulane is indicated for use in combination with other anticancer drugs for the treatment of Stage III and IV Hodgkin's disease. Matulane is used as part of the MOPP (nitrogen mustard, vincristine, procarbazine, prednisone) regimen.

CONTRAINDICATIONS

Matulane is contraindicated in patients with known hypersensitivity to the drug or inadequate marrow reserve as demonstrated by bone marrow aspiration. Due consideration of this possible state should be given to each patient who has leukopenia, thrombocytopenia or anemia.

WARNINGS

To minimize CNS depression and possible potentiation, barbiturates, antihistamines, narcotics, hypotensive agents or phenothiazines should be used with caution. Ethyl alcohol should not be used since there may be an Antabuse (disulfiram)-like reaction. Because Matulane exhibits some monoamine oxidase inhibitory activity, sympathomimetic drugs, tricyclic antidepressant drugs (eg, amitriptyline HCl, imipramine HCl) and other drugs and foods with known high tyramine content, such as wine, yogurt, ripe cheese and bananas, should be avoided. A further phenomenon of toxicity common to many hydrazine derivatives is hemolysis and the appearance of Heinz-Ehrlich inclusion bodies in erythrocytes.
Pregnancy: *Teratogenic Effects:* Pregnancy Category D. Procarbazine hydrochloride can cause fetal harm when administered to a pregnant woman. While there are no adequate and well-controlled studies with procarbazine hydrochloride in pregnant women, there are case reports of malformations in the offspring of women who were exposed to procarbazine hydrochloride in combination with other antineoplastic agents during pregnancy. Matulane should be used during pregnancy only if the potential benefit justifies the potential risk to the fetus. If this drug is used during pregnancy, or if the patient becomes pregnant while taking this drug, the patient should be apprised of the potential hazard to the fetus. Women of childbearing potential should be advised to avoid becoming pregnant. Procarbazine hydrochloride is teratogenic in the rat when given at doses approximately 4 to 13 times the maximum recommended human therapeutic dose of 6 mg/kg/day.
Nonteratogenic Effects: Procarbazine hydrochloride has not been adequately studied in animals for its effects on peri- and postnatal development. However, neurogenic tumors were noted in the offspring of rats given intravenous injections of 125 mg/kg of procarbazine hydrochloride on day 22 of gestation. Compounds which inhibit DNA, RNA and protein synthesis might be expected to have adverse effects on peri- and post-natal development.
Carcinogenesis, Mutagenesis and Impairment of Fertility:
Carcinogenesis: The carcinogenicity of procarbazine hydrochloride in mice, rats and monkeys has been reported in a considerable number of studies. Instances of a second nonlymphoid malignancy, including acute myelocytic leukemia, have been reported in patients with Hodgkin's disease treated with procarbazine in combination with other chemotherapy and/or radiation. The International Agency for Research on Cancer (IARC) considers that there is "sufficient evidence" for the human carcinogenicity of procarbazine hydrochloride when it is given in intensive regimens which include other antineoplastic agents but that there is inadequate evidence of carcinogenicity in humans given procarbazine hydrochloride alone.
Mutagenesis: Procarbazine hydrochloride has been shown to be mutagenic in a variety of bacterial and mammalian test systems.
Impairment of Fertility: Azoospermia and antifertility effects associated with procarbazine hydrochloride administration in combination with other chemotherapeutic agents for treating Hodgkin's disease have been reported in human clinical studies. Since these patients received multicombination therapy, it is difficult to determine to what extent procarbazine hydrochloride alone was involved in the male germ-cell damage. The usual Segment I fertility/reproduction studies in laboratory animals have not been carried out with procarbazine hydrochloride. However, compounds which inhibit DNA, RNA and/or protein synthesis might be expected to have adverse effects on gametogenesis. Unscheduled DNA synthesis in the testis of rabbits and decreased fertility in male mice treated with procarbazine hydrochloride have been reported.

PRECAUTIONS

General: Undue toxicity may occur if Matulane is used in patients with impairment of renal and/or hepatic function. When appropriate, hospitalization for the initial course of treatment should be considered.
If radiation or a chemotherapeutic agent known to have marrow-depressant activity has been used, an interval of one month or longer without such therapy is recommended before starting treatment with Matulane. The length of this interval may also be determined by evidence of bone marrow recovery based on successive bone marrow studies.
Prompt cessation of therapy is recommended if any one of the following occurs:

Central nervous system signs or symptoms such as paresthesias, neuropathies or confusion.
Leukopenia (white blood count under 4000).
Thrombocytopenia (platelets under 100,000).
Hypersensitivity reaction.
Stomatitis–The first small ulceration or persistent spot soreness around the oral cavity is a signal for cessation of therapy.
Diarrhea–Frequent bowel movements or watery stools.
Hemorrhage or bleeding tendencies.

Bone marrow depression often occurs 2 to 8 weeks after the start of treatment. If leukopenia occurs, hospitalization of the patient may be needed for appropriate treatment to prevent systemic infection.
Information for Patients: Patients should be warned not to drink alcoholic beverages while on Matulane therapy since there may be an Antabuse (disulfiram)-like reaction. They should also be cautioned to avoid foods with known high tyramine content such as wine, yogurt, ripe cheese and bananas. Over-the-counter drug preparations which contain antihistamines or sympathomimetic drugs should also be avoided. Patients taking Matulane should also be warned against the use of prescription drugs without the knowledge and consent of their physician.
Laboratory Tests: Baseline laboratory data should be obtained prior to initiation of therapy. The hematologic status as indicated by hemoglobin, hematocrit, white blood count (WBC), differential, reticulocytes and platelets should be monitored closely–at least every 3 or 4 days.
Hepatic and renal evaluation are indicated prior to beginning therapy. Urinalysis, transaminase, alkaline phosphatase and blood urea nitrogen tests should be repeated at least weekly.
Drug Interactions: See WARNINGS section.
No cross-resistance with other chemotherapeutic agents, radio-therapy or steroids has been demonstrated.
Carcinogenesis, Mutagenesis and Impairment of Fertility: See WARNINGS section.
Pregnancy: Pregnancy Category D. See WARNINGS section.
Nursing Mothers: It is not known whether Matulane is excreted in human milk. Because of the potential for tumorigenicity shown for procarbazine hydrochloride in animal studies, mothers should not nurse while receiving this drug.
Pediatric Use: Undue toxicity, evidenced by tremors, coma and convulsions, has occurred in a few cases. Dosage, therefore, should be individualized (see DOSAGE AND ADMINISTRATION). Very close clinical monitoring is mandatory.

ADVERSE REACTIONS

Leukopenia, anemia and thrombopenia occur frequently. Nausea and vomiting are the most commonly reported side effects.
Other adverse reactions are:
Hematologic: Pancytopenia; eosinophilia; hemolytic anemia; bleeding tendencies such as petechiae, purpura, epistaxis and hemoptysis.
Gastrointestinal: Hepatic dysfunction, jaundice, stomatitis, hematemesis, melena, diarrhea, dysphagia, anorexia, abdominal pain, constipation, dry mouth.
Neurologic: Coma, convulsions, neuropathy, ataxia, paresthesia, nystagmus, diminished reflexes, falling, foot drop, headache, dizziness, unsteadiness.
Cardiovascular: Hypotension, tachycardia, syncope.
Ophthalmic: Retinal hemorrhage, papilledema, photophobia, diplopia, inability to focus.
Respiratory: Pneumonitis, pleural effusion, cough.
Dermatologic: Herpes, dermatitis, pruritus, alopecia, hyperpigmentation, rash, urticaria, flushing.
Allergic: Generalized allergic reactions.
Genitourinary: Hematuria, urinary frequency, nocturia.
Musculoskeletal: Pain, including myalgia and arthralgia; tremors.
Psychiatric: Hallucinations, depression, apprehension, nervousness, confusion, nightmares.
Endocrine: Gynecomastia in prepubertal and early pubertal boys.
Miscellaneous: Intercurrent infections, hearing loss, pyrexia, diaphoresis, lethargy, weakness, fatigue, edema, chills, insomnia, slurred speech, hoarseness, drowsiness.
Second nonlymphoid malignancies, including acute myelocytic leukemia and malignant myelosclerosis, and azoosper-

Continued on next page

Matulane—Cont.

mia have been reported in patients with Hodgkin's disease treated with procarbazine in combination with other chemotherapy and/or radiation.

OVERDOSAGE

The major manifestations of overdosage with Matulane would be anticipated to be nausea, vomiting, enteritis, diarrhea, hypotension, tremors, convulsions and coma. Treatment should consist of either the administration of an emetic or gastric lavage. General supportive measures such as intravenous fluids are advised. Since the major toxicity of procarbazine hydrochloride is hematologic and hepatic, patients should have frequent complete blood counts and liver function tests throughout their period of recovery and for a minimum of two weeks thereafter. Should abnormalities appear in any of these determinations, appropriate measures for correction and stabilization should be immediately undertaken.

The estimated mean lethal dose of procarbazine hydrochloride in laboratory animals varied from approximately 150 mg/kg in rabbits to 1300 mg/kg in mice.

DOSAGE AND ADMINISTRATION

The following doses are for administration of the drug as a single agent. When used in combination with other anticancer drugs, the Matulane dose should be appropriately reduced, eg, in the MOPP regimen, the Matulane dose is 100 mg/m^2 daily for 14 days. All dosages are based on the patient's actual weight. However, the estimated lean body mass (dry weight) is used if the patient is obese or if there has been a spurious weight gain due to edema, ascites or other forms of abnormal fluid retention.

Adults: To minimize the nausea and vomiting experienced by a high percentage of patients beginning Matulane therapy, single or divided doses of 2 to 4 mg/kg/day for the first week are recommended. Daily dosage should then be maintained at 4 to 6 mg/kg/day until maximum response is obtained or until the white blood count falls below 4000/cmm or the platelets fall below 100,000/cmm. When maximum response is obtained, the dose may be maintained at 1 to 2 mg/kg/day. Upon evidence of hematologic or other toxicity (see PRECAUTIONS section), the drug should be discontinued until there has been satisfactory recovery. After toxic side effects have subsided, therapy may then be resumed at the discretion of the physician, based on clinical evaluation and appropriate laboratory studies, at a dosage of 1 to 2 mg/kg/day.

Pediatric Patients: Very close clinical monitoring is mandatory. Undue toxicity, evidenced by tremors, coma and convulsions, has occurred in a few cases. Dosage, therefore, should be individualized. The following dosage schedule is provided as a guideline only.

Fifty (50) mg per square meter of body surface per day is recommended for the first week. Dosage should then be maintained at 100 mg per square meter of body surface per day until maximum response is obtained or until leukopenia or thrombocytopenia occurs. When maximum response is attained, the dose may be maintained at 50 mg per square meter of body surface per day. Upon evidence of hematologic or other toxicity (see PRECAUTIONS section), the drug should be discontinued until there has been satisfactory recovery, based on clinical evaluation and appropriate laboratory tests. After toxic side effects have subsided, therapy may then be resumed.

Procedures for proper handling and disposal of anticancer drugs should be considered. Several guidelines on this subject have been published.[1–6] There is no general agreement that all of the procedures recommended in the guidelines are necessary or appropriate.

HOW SUPPLIED

Capsules, ivory, containing the equivalent of 50 mg procarbazine as the hydrochloride; bottles of 100 (NDC 54482-053-01). Imprint on capsules: MATULANE® sigma-tau.

REFERENCES

1. Recommendations for the safe handling of parenteral antineoplastic drugs. Washington, DC: U.S. Government Printing Office NIH Publication No. 83-2621.
2. AMA Council Report. Guidelines for handling parenteral antineoplastics. *JAMA*. Mar 15, 1985; 253:1590-1592.
3. National Study Commission on Cytotoxic Exposure: Recommendations for handling cytotoxic agents. Available from Louis P. Jeffrey, ScD, Director of Pharmacy Services, Rhode Island Hospital, 593 Eddy Street, Providence, Rhode Island 02902.
4. Clinical Oncological Society of Australia: Guidelines and recommendations for safe handling of antineoplastic agents. *Med J Aust*. Apr 30, 1983; 1:426-428.
5. Jones RB, Frank R, Mass T: Safe handling of chemotherapeutic agents: a report from the Mount Sinai Medical Center. *CA*. Sept-Oct 1983; 33:258-263.
6. ASHP technical assistance bulletin on handling cytotoxic drugs in hospitals. *Am J Hosp Pharm*. Jan 1985; 42:131-137.

Manufactured by
Hoffmann-La Roche Inc
Nutley, NJ 07110
for:
Sigma-Tau Pharmaceuticals, Inc.
800 S. Frederick Avenue
Gaithersburg, MD 20877

Revised: November 1998

25598113-1198

Smith & Nephew, Inc.

11775 STARKEY ROAD
LARGO, FL 33773

Direct Inquiries to:
1-800-3-SANTYL
(1-800-372-6895)
1-800-876-1261
1-727-392-1261

COLLAGENASE SANTYL® OINTMENT ℞

Rx only

DESCRIPTION

Collagenase Santyl® Ointment is a sterile enzymatic debriding ointment which contains 250 collagenase units per gram of white petrolatum USP. The enzyme collagenase is derived from the fermentation by *Clostridium histolyticum*. It possesses the unique ability to digest collagen in necrotic tissue.

CLINICAL PHARMACOLOGY

Since collagen accounts for 75 % of the dry weight of skin tissue, the ability of collagenase to digest collagen in the physiological pH and temperature range makes it particularly effective in the removal of detritus.[1] Collagenase thus contributes towards the formation of granulation tissue and subsequent epithelization of dermal ulcers and severely burned areas.[2, 3, 4, 5, 6] Collagen in healthy tissue or in newly formed granulation tissue is not attacked.[2, 3, 4, 5, 6, 7, 8] There is no information available on collagenase absorption through skin or its concentration in body fluids associated with therapeutic and/or toxic effects, degree of binding to plasma proteins, degree of uptake by a particular organ or in the fetus, and passage across the blood brain barrier.

INDICATIONS AND USAGE

Collagenase Santyl Ointment is indicated for debriding chronic dermal ulcers[2, 3, 4, 5, 6, 8, 9, 10, 11, 12, 13, 14, 15, 16, 17, 18] and severely burned areas.[3, 4, 5, 7, 16, 19, 20, 21]

CONTRAINDICATIONS

Collagenase Santyl Ointment is contraindicated in patients who have shown local or systemic hypersensitivity to collagenase.

PRECAUTIONS

The optimal pH range of collagenase is 6 to 8. Higher or lower pH conditions will decrease the enzyme's activity and appropriate precautions should be taken. The enzymatic activity is also adversely affected by certain detergents, and heavy metal ions such as mercury and silver which are used in some antiseptics. When it is suspected such materials have been used, the site should be carefully cleaned by repeated washing with normal saline before Collagenase Santyl Ointment is applied. Soaks containing metal ions or acidic solutions should be avoided because of the metal ion and low pH. Cleansing materials such as hydrogen peroxide, Dakin's solution, and normal saline are compatible with Collagenase Santyl Ointment.

Debilitated patients should be closely monitored for systemic bacterial infections because of the theoretical possibility that debriding enzymes may increase the risk of bacteremia.

A slight transient erythema has been noted occasionally in the surrounding tissue, particularly when Collagenase Santyl Ointment was not confined to the wound. Therefore, the ointment should be applied carefully within the area of the wound. Safety and effectiveness in pediatric patients have not been established.

ADVERSE REACTIONS

No allergic sensitivity or toxic reactions have been noted in clinical use when used as directed. However, one case of systemic manifestations of hypersensitivity to collagenase in a patient treated for more than one year with a combination of collagenase and cortisone has been reported.

OVERDOSAGE

No systemic or local reaction attributed to overdose has been observed in clinical investigations and clinical use. If deemed necessary the enzyme may be inactivated by washing the area with povidone iodine.

DOSAGE AND ADMINISTRATION

Collagenase Santyl Ointment should be applied once daily (or more frequently if the dressing becomes soiled, as from incontinence). When clinically indicated, crosshatching thick eschar with a #10 blade allows Collagenase Santyl Ointment more surface contact with necrotic debris. It is also desirable to remove, with forceps and scissors, as much loosened detritus as can be done readily. Use Collagenase Santyl Ointment in the following manner:

1— Prior to application the wound should be cleaned of debris and digested material by gently rubbing with a gauze pad saturated with normal saline solution, or with the desired cleansing agent compatible with Collagenase Santyl Ointment (See **PRECAUTIONS**), followed by a normal saline solution rinse.

2— Whenever infection is present, it is desirable to use an appropriate topical antibiotic powder. The antibiotic should be applied to the wound prior to the application of Collagenase Santyl Ointment. Should the infection not respond, therapy with Collagenase Santyl Ointment should be discontinued until remission of the infection.

3— Collagenase Santyl Ointment may be applied to the wound or to a sterile gauze pad which is then applied to the wound and properly secured.

4— Use of Collagenase Santyl Ointment should be terminated when debridement of necrotic tissue is complete and granulation tissue is well established.

HOW SUPPLIED

Collagenase Santyl® Ointment contains 250 units of collagenase enzyme per gram of white petrolatum USP. The potency assay of collagenase is based on the digestion of undenatured collagen (from bovine Archilles tendon) at pH 7.2 and 37°C for 24 hours. The number of peptide bonds cleaved are measured by reaction with ninhydrin. Amino groups released by a trypsin digestion control are subtracted. One net collagenase unit will solubilize ninhydrin reactive material equivalent to 4 micromoles of leucine.

Do not store above 25°C (77°F). Sterility guaranteed until tube is opened.

Collagenase Santyl Ointment is available in 15 gram and 30 gram tubes.

REFERENCES

1— Mandl, I., Adv Enzymol. 23:163, 1961.
2— Boxer, A.M., Gottesman, N., Bernstein, H., & Mandl, I., Geriatrics. 24:75, 1969.
3— Mazurek, I., Med. Welt. 22:150, 1971.
4— Zimmerman, WE., In "Collagenase," Mandl, I., ed., Gordon & Breach, Science Publishers, New York, 1971, p. 131, p. 185.
5— Vetra. H., & Whittaker, D., Geriatrics 30:53, 1975.
6— Rao, D.B., Sane, P.G., & Gerogiev, E.L., J. Am. Geriatrics Soc. 23:22, 1975.
7— Vrabec, R., Moserova, J., Konickova, Z., Behounkova, E., & Blaha, J., J. Hyg. Epidemiol. Microbiol. Immunol. 18:496, 1974.
8— Lippman, H.I., Arch. Phys. Med. Rehabil. 54:588, 1973.
9— German, F.M., In "Collagenase," Mandl, I., ed., Gordon & Breach, Science Publishers, New York, 1971, p. 165.
10— Haimovici, H. & Strauch, B., in "Collagenase," Mandl, I., ed., Gordon & Breach, Science Publishers, New York, 1971, p. 177.
11— Lee, L.K., & Ambrus, J.L., Geriatrics. 30:91, 1975.
12— Locke, R.K., & Heifitz, N.M., J. Am. Pod. Assoc. 65:242, 1975.
13— Varma, A.O., Bugatch, E., & German, F.M., Surg. Gynecol. Obstet. 136:281, 1973.
14— Barrett D., Jr., & Klibanski, A., Am. J. Nurs. 73:849, 1973.
15— Bardfeld, L.A., J. Pod. Ed. 1:41, 1970.
16— Blum, G., Schweiz, Rundschau Med. Praxis 62:820, 1973. Abstr. in Dermatology Digest, Feb. 1974, p. 36.
17— Zaruba, F., Lettl, A. Brozkova, L., Skrdlantova, H., & Krs, V., J. Hyg. Epidemiol. Microbiol. Immunol. 18:499, 1974.
18— Altman, M.I., Goldstein, L., & Horwitz, S., J. Am. Pod. Assoc. 68:11, 1978.
19— Rehn, V.J., Med. Klin. 58:799, 1963.
20— Krauss, H., Koslowski, L., & Zimmermann W.E., Langenbecks Arch. Klin. Chir. 303:23, 1963.
21— Gruenagel, H.H., Med. Klin, 58:442, 1963.

Manufactured by
ADVANCE BIOFACTURES CORPORATION
A Subsidiary of
BIOSPECIFICS TECHNOLOGIES CORP.
35 Wilbur Street
Lynbrook, New York 11563
Distributed by
Smith & Nephew, Inc.
11775 Starkey Road
Largo, FL 33773

Revised: March 2000

0900020-4 PI 06371

Shown in Product Identification Guide, page 336

SmithKline Beecham Consumer Healthcare

Unit of SmithKline Beecham Inc.
POST OFFICE BOX 1467
PITTSBURGH, PA 15230

Direct Inquiries to:
1-800-245-1040 weekdays

DEBROX® Drops **OTC**

[de 'brox]
Ear Wax Removal Aid

(See PDR For Nonprescription Drugs.)

DENAVIR® ℞

brand of
penciclovir cream, 1%
For Dermatologic Use Only

DESCRIPTION

Denavir contains penciclovir, an antiviral agent active against herpes viruses. *Denavir* is available for topical administration as a 1% white cream. Each gram of *Denavir* contains 10 mg of penciclovir and the following inactive ingredients: cetomacrogol 1000 BP, cetostearyl alcohol, mineral oil, propylene glycol, purified water and white petrolatum.
Chemically, penciclovir is known as 9-[4-hydroxy-3-(hydroxymethyl)butyl]guanine. Its molecular formula is $C_{10}H_{15}N_5O_3$; its molecular weight is 253.26. It is a synthetic acyclic guanine derivative and has the following structure:

penciclovir

Penciclovir is a white to pale yellow solid. At 20°C it has a solubility of 0.2 mg/mL in methanol, 1.3 mg/mL in propylene glycol, and 1.7 mg/mL in water. In aqueous buffer (pH 2) the solubility is 10.0 mg/mL. Penciclovir is not hygroscopic. Its partition coefficient in n-octanol/water at pH 7.5 is 0.024 (logP=-1.62).

CLINICAL PHARMACOLOGY

Microbiology

Mechanism of Antiviral Activity: The antiviral compound penciclovir has *in vitro* inhibitory activity against herpes simplex virus types 1 (HSV-1) and 2 (HSV-2). In cells infected with HSV-1 or HSV-2, viral thymidine kinase phosphorylates penciclovir to a monophosphate form which, in turn, is converted to penciclovir triphosphate by cellular kinases. *In vitro* studies demonstrate that penciclovir triphosphate inhibits HSV polymerase competitively with deoxyguanosine triphosphate. Consequently, herpes viral DNA synthesis and, therefore, replication are selectively inhibited.

Antiviral Activity *In Vitro* and *in Vivo*: In cell culture studies, penciclovir has antiviral activity against HSV-1 and HSV-2.
Sensitivity test results, expressed as the concentration of the drug required to inhibit growth of the virus by 50% (IC_{50}) or 99% (IC_{99}) in cell culture, vary depending upon a number of factors, including the assay protocols. See Table 1.
[See table above]

Table 1

Method of Assay	Virus Type	Cell Type	IC_{50} (mcg/mL)	IC_{99} (mcg/mL)
Plaque Reduction	HSV-1 (c.i.)	MRC-5	0.2–0.6	
	HSV-1 (c.i.)	WISH	0.04–0.5	
	HSV-2 (c.i.)	MRC-5	0.9–2.1	
	HSV-2 (c.i.)	WISH	0.1–0.8	
Virus Yield Reduction	HSV-1 (c.i.)	MRC-5		0.4–0.5
	HSV-2 (c.i.)	MRC-5		0.6–0.7
DNA Synthesis Inhibition	HSV-1 (SC16)	MRC-5	0.04	
	HSV-2 (MS)	MRC-5	0.05	

(c.i.) =clinical isolates. The latent state of any herpes virus is not known to respond to any antiviral therapy.

Drug Resistance: Penciclovir-resistant mutants of HSV can result from qualitative changes in viral thymidine kinase or DNA polymerase. The most commonly encountered acyclovir-resistant mutants that are deficient in viral thymidine kinase are also resistant to penciclovir.

Pharmacokinetics

Measurable penciclovir concentrations were not detected in plasma or urine of healthy male volunteers (n=12) following single or repeat application of the 1% cream at a dose of 180 mg penciclovir daily (approximately 67 times the estimated usual clinical dose).

Pediatric Patients: The systemic absorption of penciclovir following topical administration has not been evaluated in patients <18 years of age.

CLINICAL TRIALS

Denavir was studied in two double-blind, placebo (vehicle)-controlled trials for the treatment of recurrent herpes labialis in which otherwise healthy adults were randomized to either *Denavir* or placebo. Therapy was to be initiated by the subjects within 1 hour of noticing signs or symptoms and continued for 4 days, with application of study medication every 2 hours while awake. In both studies, the mean duration of lesions was approximately one-half-day shorter in the subjects treated with *Denavir* (N=1,516) as compared to subjects treated with placebo (N=1,541) (approximately 4.5 days versus 5 days, respectively). The mean duration of lesion pain was also approximately one-half-day shorter in the *Denavir* group compared to the placebo group.

INDICATIONS AND USAGE

Denavir (penciclovir cream) is indicated for the treatment of recurrent herpes labialis (cold sores) in adults.

CONTRAINDICATIONS

Denavir is contraindicated in patients with known hypersensitivity to the product or any of its components.

PRECAUTIONS

General

Denavir should only be used on herpes labialis on the lips and face. Because no data are available, application to human mucous membranes is not recommended. Particular care should be taken to avoid application in or near the eyes since it may cause irritation. The effect of *Denavir* has not been established in immunocompromised patients.

Carcinogenesis, Mutagenesis, Impairment of Fertility

In clinical trials, systemic drug exposure following the topical administration of penciclovir cream was negligible, as the penciclovir content of all plasma and urine samples was below the limit of assay detection (0.1 mcg/mL and 10 mcg/mL, respectively). However, for the purpose of inter-species dose comparisons presented in the following sections, an assumption of 100% absorption of penciclovir from the topically applied product has been used. Based on use of the maximal recommended topical dose of penciclovir of 0.05 mg/kg/day and an assumption of 100% absorption, the maximum theoretical plasma $AUC_{0-24\ hrs}$ for penciclovir is approximately 0.129 mcg.hr/mL.

Carcinogenesis: Two-year carcinogenicity studies were conducted with famciclovir (the oral prodrug of penciclovir) in rats and mice. An increase in the incidence of mammary adenocarcinoma (a common tumor in female rats of the strain used) was seen in female rats receiving 600 mg/kg/day (approximately 395× the maximum theoretical human exposure to penciclovir following application of the topical product, based on area under the plasma concentration curve comparisons [24 hr. AUC]). No increases in tumor incidence were seen among male rats treated at doses up to 240 mg/kg/day (approximately 190× the maximum theoretical human AUC for penciclovir), or in male and female mice at doses up to 600 mg/kg/day (approximately 100× the maximum theoretical human AUC for penciclovir).

Mutagenesis: When tested *in vitro*, penciclovir did not cause an increase in gene mutation in the Ames assay using multiple strains of *S. typhimurium* or *E. coli* (at up to 20,000 mcg/plate), nor did it cause an increase in unscheduled DNA repair in mammalian HeLa S3 cells (at up to 5,000 mcg/mL). However, an increase in clastogenic responses was seen with penciclovir in the L5178Y mouse lymphoma cell assay (at doses ≥1000 mcg/mL) and, in human lymphocytes incubated *in vitro* at doses ≥250 mcg/mL. When tested *in vivo*, penciclovir caused an increase in micronuclei in mouse bone marrow following the intravenous administration of doses ≥500 mg/kg (≥810× the maximum human dose, based on body surface area conversion).

Impairment of Fertility: Testicular toxicity was observed in multiple animal species (rats and dogs) following repeated intravenous administration of penciclovir (160 mg/kg/day and 100 mg/kg/day, respectively, approximately 1155 and 3255× the maximum theoretical human AUC). Testicular changes seen in both species included atrophy of the seminiferous tubules and reductions in epididymal sperm counts and/or an increased incidence of sperm with abnormal morphology or reduced motility. Adverse testicular effects were related to an increasing dose or duration of exposure to penciclovir. No adverse testicular or reproductive effects (fertility and reproductive function) were observed in rats after 10 to 13 weeks dosing at 80 mg/kg/day, or testicular effects in dogs after 13 weeks dosing at 30 mg/kg/day (575 and 845× the maximum theoretical human AUC, respectively). Intravenously administered penciclovir had no effect on fertility or reproductive performance in female rats at doses of up to 80 mg/k/day (260× the maximum human dose [BSA]).
There was no evidence of any clinically significant effects on sperm count, motility or morphology in 2 placebo-controlled clinical trials of Famvir® (famciclovir [the oral prodrug of penciclovir], 250 mg b.i.d.; n=66) in immunocompetent men with recurrent genital herpes, when dosing and follow-up were maintained for 18 and 8 weeks, respectively (approximately 2 and 1 spermatogenic cycles in the human).

Pregnancy

Teratogenic Effects-Pregnancy Category B. No adverse effects on the course and outcome of pregnancy or on fetal development were noted in rats and rabbits following the intravenous administration of penciclovir at doses of 80 and 60 mg/kg/day, respectively (estimated human equivalent doses of 13 and 18 mg/kg/day for the rat and rabbit, respectively, based on body surface area conversion; the body surface area doses being 260 and 355× the maximum recommended dose following topical application of the penciclovir cream). There are, however, no adequate and well-controlled studies in pregnant women. Because animal reproduction studies are not always predictive of human response, penciclovir should be used during pregnancy only if clearly needed.

Nursing Mothers

There is no information on whether penciclovir is excreted in human milk after topical administration. However, following oral administration of famciclovir (the oral prodrug of penciclovir) to lactating rats, penciclovir was excreted in breast milk at concentrations higher than those seen in the plasma. Therefore, a decision should be made whether to discontinue the drug, taking into account the importance of the drug to the mother. There are no data on the safety of penciclovir in newborns.

Pediatric Use

Safety and effectiveness in pediatric patients have not been established.

Geriatic Use

In 74 patients ≥65 years of age, the adverse events profile was comparable to that observed in younger patients.

ADVERSE REACTIONS

In two double-blind, placebo-controlled trials, 1516 patients were treated with Denavir (penciclovir cream) and 1541 with placebo. The most frequently reported adverse event was headache, which occurred in 5.3% of the patients treated with *Denavir* and 5.8% of the placebo-treated patients. The rates of reported local adverse reactions are shown in Table 2 below. One or more local adverse reactions were reported by 2.7% of the patients treated with *Denavir* and 3.9% of placebo-treated patients.

Table 2—Local Adverse Reactions Reported in Phase III Trials

	Penciclovir n=1516 %	Placebo n=1541 %
Application site reaction	1.3	1.8
Hypesthesia/Local anesthesia	0.9	1.4
Taste perversion	0.2	0.3
Pruritus	0.0	0.3
Pain	0.0	0.1
Rash (erythematous)	0.1	0.1
Allergic reaction	0.0	0.1

Two studies, enrolling 108 healthy subjects, were conducted to evaluate the dermal tolerance of 5% penciclovir cream (a 5-fold higher concentration than the commercial formulation) compared to vehicle using repeated occluded patch testing methodology. The 5% penciclovir cream induced mild erythema in approximately one-half of the subjects exposed, an irritancy profile similar to the vehicle control in terms of severity and proportion of subjects with a response. No evidence of sensitization was observed.

OVERDOSAGE

Since penciclovir is poorly absorbed following oral administration, adverse reactions related to penciclovir ingestion are unlikely.
There is no information on overdose.

DOSAGE AND ADMINISTRATION

Denavir should be applied every 2 hours during waking hours for a period of 4 days. Treatment should be started as early as possible (i.e., during the prodrome or when lesions appear).

HOW SUPPLIED

Denavir is supplied in a 1.5 gram tube containing 10 mg of penciclovir per gram.
NDC 00135-315-52
Store at controlled room temperature, 20°–25°C (68°–77°F).

Continued on next page

Denavir—Cont.

CAUTION: Federal law prohibits dispensing without prescription.

Comments or questions? Call toll-free 1-800-320-6022.

Manufactured in Cidra, PR by **SmithKline Beecham Pharmaceuticals,** for **SmithKline Beecham Consumer Healthcare, L.P.,** Pittsburgh, PA 15230

ECOTRIN OTC

Enteric-Coated Aspirin

Antiarthritic, Antiplatelet

COMPREHENSIVE PRESCRIBING INFORMATION

DESCRIPTION

Ecotrin enteric coated aspirin (acetylsalicylic acid) tablets available in 81mg, 325mg and 500 mg tablets for oral administration. The 325 mg and 500 mg tablets contain the following inactive ingredients: Carnuba Wax, Colloidal Silicon Dioxide, FD&C Yellow No. 6, Hydroxypropyl Methylcellulose, Methacrylic Acid Copolymer, Microcrystalline Cellulose, Pregelatinized Starch, Propylene Glycol, Simethicone, Sodium Starch Glycolate, Stearic Acid, Talc, Titanium Dioxide, and Triethyl Citrate. The 81 mg tablets contain Carnuba Wax, Corn Starch, D&C Yellow No. 10, FD&C Yellow No. 6, Hydroxypropyl Methylcellulose, Methacrylic Acid Copolymer, Microcrystalline Cellulose, Propylene Glycol, Simethicone, Stearic Acid, Talc and Triethyl Citrate.

Aspirin is an odorless white, needle-like crystalline or powdery substance. When exposed to moisture, aspirin hydrolyzes into salicylic and acetic acids, and gives off a vinegary-odor. It is highly lipid soluble and slightly soluble in water.

CLINICAL PHARMACOLOGY

Mechanism of Action: Aspirin is a more potent inhibitor of both prostaglandin synthesis and platelet aggregation than other salicylic acid derivatives. The differences in activity between aspirin and salicylic acid are thought to be due to the acetyl group on the aspirin molecule. This acetyl group is responsible for the inactivation of cyclo-oxygenase via acetylation.

PHARMACOKINETICS

Absorption: In general, immediate release aspirin is well and completely absorbed from the gastrointestinal (GI) tract. Following absorption, aspirin is hydrolyzed to salicylic acid with peak plasma levels of salicylic acid occurring within 1–2 hours of dosing (see Pharmacokinetics—Metabolism). The rate of absorption from the GI tract is dependent upon the dosage form, the presence or absence of food, gastric pH (the presence or absence of GI antacids or buffering agents), and other physiologic factors. Enteric coated aspirin products are erratically absorbed from the GI tract.

Distribution: Salicylic acid is widely distibuted to all tissues and fluids in the body including the central nervous system (CNS), breast milk, and fetal tissues. The highest concentrations are found in the plasma, liver, renal cortex, heart, and lungs.

The protein binding of salicylate is concentration-dependent, i.e., non-linear. At low concentrations (< 100 mcg/mL) approximately 90 percent of plasma salicylate is bound to albumin while at higher concentrations (> 400 mcg/mL), only about 75 percent is bound. The early signs of salicylic overdose (salicylism), including tinnitus (ringing in the ears), occur at plasma concentrations approximating 200 mcg/mL. Severe toxic effects are associated with levels > 400 mcg/mL (See Adverse Reactions and Overdosage.)

Metabolism: Aspirin is rapidly hydrolyzed in the plasma to salicylic acid such that plasma levels of aspirin are essentially undetectable 1–2 hours after dosing. Salicylic acid is primarily conjugated in the liver to form salicyluric acid, a phenolic glucuronide, an acyl glucuronide, and a number of minor metabolites. Salicylic acid has a plasma half-life of approximately 6 hours. Salicylate metabolism is saturable and total body clearance decreases at higher serum concentrations due to the limited ability of the liver to form both salicyluric acid and phenolic glucuronide. Following toxic doses (10–20 grams (g)), the plasma half-life may be increased to over 20 hours.

Elimination: The elimination of salicylic acid follows zero order pharmacokinetics; (i.e., the rate of drug elimination is constant in relation to plasma concentration). Renal excretion of unchanged drug depends upon urine pH. As urinary pH rises above 6.5, the renal clearance of free salicylate increases from < 5 percent to > 80 percent. Alkalinization of the urine is a key concept in the management of salicylate overdose. (See Overdosage.) Following therapeutic doses, approximately 10 percent is found excreted in the urine as salicylic acid, 75 percent as salicyluric acid, as the phenolic and acyl glucuronides, respectively.

Pharmacodynamics: Aspirin affects platelet aggregation by irreversibly inhibiting prostaglandin cyclo-oxygenase. This effect lasts for the life of the platelet and prevents the formation of the platelet aggregating factor thromboxane A2. Non-acetylated salicylates do not inhibit this enzyme and have no effect on platelet aggregation. At somewhat higher doses, aspirin reversibly inhibits the formation of prostaglandin I_2 (prostacyclin), which is an arterial vasodilator and inhibits platelet aggregation.

At higher doses aspirin is an effective anti-inflammatory agent, partially due to inhibition of inflammatory mediators via cyclooxygenase inhibition in peripheral tissues. In vitro studies suggest that other mediators of inflammation may also be suppressed by aspirin administration, although the precise mechanism of action has not been elucidated. It is this non-specific suppression of cyclooxygenase activity in peripheral tissues following large doses that leads to its primary side effect of gastric irritation. (See Adverse Reactions.)

CLINICAL STUDIES

Ischemic Stroke and Transient Ischemic Attack (TIA): In clinical trials of subjects with TIA's due to fibrin platelet emboli or ischemic stroke, aspirin has been shown to significantly reduce the risk of the combined endpoint of stroke or death and the combined endpoint of TIA, stroke, or death by about 13–18 percent.

Suspect Acute Myocardial Infarction (MI): In a large, multi-center study of aspirin, streptokinase, and the combination of aspirin and streptokinase in 17,187 patients with suspected acute MI, aspirin treatment produced a 23-percent reduction in the risk of vascular mortality. Aspirin was also shown to have an additional benefit in patients given a thrombolytic agent.

Prevention of Recurrent MI and Unstable Angina Pectoris: These indications are supported by the results of six large, randomized, multi-center, placebo-controlled trials of predominantly male post-MI subjects and one randomized placebo-controlled study of men with unstable angina pectoris. Aspirin therapy in MI subjects was associated with a significant reduction (about 20 percent) in the risk of the combination endpoint of subsequent death and/or nonfatal reinfarction in these patients. In aspirin-treated unstable angina patients the event rate was reduced to 5 percent from the 10 percent rate in the placebo group.

Chronic Stable Angina Pectoris: In a randomized, multi-center, double-blind trial designed to assess the role of aspirin for prevention of MI in patients with chronic stable angina pectoris, aspirin significantly reduced the primary combined endpoint of nonfatal MI, fatal MI, and sudden death by 34 percent. The secondary endpoint for vascular events (first occurrence of MI, stroke, or vascular death) was also significantly reduced (32 percent).

Revascularization Procedures: Most patients who undergo coronary artery revascularization procedures have already had symptomatic coronary artery disease for which aspirin is indicated. Similarly, patients with lesions of the carotid bifurcation sufficient to require carotid endarterectomy are likely to have had a precedent event. Aspirin is recommended for patients who undergo revascularization procedures if there is a preexisting condition for which aspirin is already indicated.

Rheumatologic Diseases: In clinical studies in patients with rheumatoid arthritis, juvenile rheumatoid arthritis, ankylosing spondylitis and osteoarthritis, aspirin has been shown to be effective in controlling various indices of clinical disease activity.

ANIMAL TOXICOLOGY

The acute oral 50 percent lethal dose in rats is about 1.5 g/kg and in mice 1.1 g/kg. Renal papillary necrosis and decreased urinary concentrating ability occur in rodents chronically administered high doses. Dose-dependent gastric mucosal injury occurs in rats and humans. Mammals may develop aspirin toxicosis associated with GI symptoms, circulatory effects, and central nervous system depression. (See Overdosage.)

INDICATIONS AND USAGE

Vascular Indications (Ischemic Stroke, TIA, Acute MI, Prevention of Recurrent MI, Unstable Angina Pectoris, and Chronic Stable Angina Pectoris): Aspirin is indicated to: (1) Reduce the combined risk of death and nonfatal stroke in patients who have had ischemic stroke of transient ischemia of the brain due to fibrin platelet emboli, (2) reduce the risk of vascular mortality in patients with a suspected acute MI, (3) reduce the combined risk of death and nonfatal MI in patients with a previous MI or unstable angina pectoris, and (4) reduce the combined risk of MI and sudden death in patients with chronic stable angina pectoris.

Revascularization Procedures (Coronary Artery Bypass Graft (CABG), Percutaneous Transluminal Coronary Angioplasty (PTCA), and Carotid Endarterectomy): Aspirin is indicated in patients who have undergone revascularization procedures (i.e., CABG, PTCA, or carotid endarterectomy) when there is a preexisting condition for which aspirin is already indicated.

Rheumatologic Disease Indications (Rheumatoid Arthritis, Juvenile Rheumatoid Arthritis, Spondyloarthropathies, Osteoarthritis, and the Arthritis and Pleurisy of Systemic Lupus Erythematosus (SLE)): Aspirin is indicated for the relief of the signs and symptoms of rheumatoid arthritis, juvenile rheumatoid arthritis, osteoarthritis, spondyloarthropathies, and arthritis and pleurisy associated with SLE.

CONTRAINDICATIONS

Allergy: Aspirin is contraindicated in patients with known allergy to nonsteroidal anti-inflammatory drug products and in patients with the syndrome of asthma, rhinitis, and nasal polyps. Aspirin may cause severe urticaria, angioedema, or bronchospasm (asthma).

Reye's Syndrome: Aspirin should not be used in children or teenagers for viral infections, with or without fever, because of the risk of Reye's syndrome with concomitant use of aspirin in certain viral illnesses.

WARNINGS

Alcohol Warning: Patients who consume three or more alcoholic drinks every day should be counseled about the bleeding risks involved with chronic, heavy alcohol use while taking aspirin.

Coagulation Abnormalities: Even low doses of aspirin can inhibit platelet function leading to an increase in bleeding time. This can adversely affect patients with inherited (hemophilia) or acquired (liver disease or vitamin K deficiency) bleeding disorders.

GI Side Effects: GI side effects include stomach pain, heartburn, nausea, vomiting, and gross GI bleeding. Although minor upper GI symptoms, such as dyspepsia, are common and can occur anytime during therapy, physicians should remain alert for signs of ulceration and bleedings, even in the absence of previous GI symptoms. Physicians should inform patients about the signs and symptoms of GI side effects and what steps to take if they occur.

Peptic Ulcer Disease: Patients with a history of active peptic ulcer disease should avoid using aspirin, which can cause gastric mucosal irritation and bleeding.

PRECAUTIONS

General

Renal Failure: Avoid aspirin in patients with severe renal failure (glomerular filtration rate less than 10 mL/minute).

Hepatic Insufficiency: Avoid aspirin in patients with severe hepatic insufficiency.

Sodium Restricted Diets: Patients with sodium-retaining states, such as congestive heart failure or renal failure, should avoid sodium-containing buffered aspirin preparations because of their high sodium content.

Laboratory Tests: Aspirin has been associated with elevated hepatic enzymes, blood urea nitrogen and serum creatinine, hyperkalemia, proteinuria, and prolonged bleeding time.

Drug Interactions

Angiotensin Converting Enzyme (ACE) Inhibitors: The hyponatremic and hypotensive effects of ACE inhibitors may be diminished by the concomitant administration of aspirin due to its direct effect on the renin-angiotensin conversion pathway.

Acetazolamide: Concurrent use of aspirin and acetazolamide can lead to high serum concentrations of acetazolamide (and toxicity) due to competition at the renal tubule for secretion.

Anticoagulant Therapy (Heparin and Warfarin): Patients on anticoagulation therapy are at increased risk for bleeding because of drug-drug interactions and the effect on platelets. Aspirin can displace warfarin from protein binding sites, leading to prolongation of both the prothrombin time and the bleeding time. Aspirin can increase the anticoagulant activity of heparin, increasing bleeding risk.

Anticonvulsants: Salicylate can displace protein-bound phenytoin and valproic acid, leading to a decrease in the total concentration of phenytoin and an increase in serum valproic acid levels.

Beta Blockers: The hypotensive effects of beta blockers may be diminished by the concomitant administration of aspirin due to inhibition of renal prostaglandins, leading to decreased renal blood flow, and salt and fluid retention.

Diuretics: The effectiveness of diuretics in patients with underlying renal or cardiovascular disease may be diminished by the concomitant administration of aspirin due to inhibition of renal prostaglandins, leading to decreased renal blood flow and salt and fluid retention.

Methotrexate: Salicylate can inhibit renal clearance of methotrexate, leading to bone marrow toxicity, especially in the elderly or renal impaired.

Nonsteroidal Anti-inflammatory Drugs (NSAID's): The concurrent use of aspirin with other NSAID's should be avoided because this may increase bleeding or lead to decreased renal function.

Oral Hypoglycemics: Moderate doses of aspirin may increase the effectiveness of oral hypoglycemic drugs, leading to hypoglycemia.

Uricosuric Agents (Probenecid and Sulfinpyrazone): Salicylates antagonize the uricosuric action of uricosuric agents.

Carcinogenesis, Mutagenesis, Impairment of Fertility: Administration of aspirin for 68 weeks at 0.5 percent in the feed of rats was not carcinogenic. In the Ames Salmonella assay, aspirin was not mutagenic; however, aspirin did induce chromosome aberrations in cultured human fibroblasts. Aspirin inhibits ovulation in rats. (See Pregnancy.)

Pregnancy: Pregnant women should only take aspirin if clearly needed. Because of the known effects of NSAID's on the fetal cardiovascular system (closure of the ductus arteriosus), use during the third trimester of pregnancy should be avoided. Salicylate products have also been associated with alterations in maternal and neonatal hemostasis mechanisms, decreased birth weight, and with perinatal mortality.

Labor and Delivery: Aspirin should be avoided 1 week prior to and during labor and delivery because it can result in excessive blood loss at delivery. Prolonged gestation and prolonged labor due to prostaglandin inhibition have been reported.

Nursing Mothers: Nursing mothers should avoid using aspirin because salicylate is excreted in breast milk. Use of high doses may lead to rashes, platelet abnormalities, and bleeding in nursing infants.

Pediatric Use: Pediatric dosing recommendations for juvenile rheumatoid arthritis are based on well-controlled clinical studies. An initial dose of 90–130 mg/kg/day in divided doses, with an increase as needed for anti-inflammatory efficacy (target plasma salicylate levels of 150–300 mcg/mL) are effective. At high doses (i.e., plasma levels of greater than 200 mg/mL), the incidence of toxicity increases.

ADVERSE REACTIONS

Many adverse reactions due to aspirin ingestion are dose-related. The following is a list of adverse reactions that have been reported in the literature. (See Warnings.)

Body as a Whole: Fever, hypothermia, thirst.

Cardiovascular: Dysrhythmias, hypotension, tachycardia.

Central Nervous System: Agitation, cerebral edema, coma, confusion, dizziness, headache, subdural or intracranial hemorrhage, lethargy, seizures.

Fluid and Electrolyte: Dehydration, hyperkalemia, metabolic acidosis, respiratory alkalosis.

Gastrointestinal: Dyspepsia, GI bleeding, ulceration and perforation, nausea, vomiting, transient elevations of hepatic enzymes, hepatitis, Reye's Syndrome, pancreatitis.

Hematologic: Prolongation of the prothrombin time, disseminated intravascular coagulation, coagulopathy, thrombocytopenia.

Hypersensitivity: Acute anaphylaxis, angioedema, asthma, bronchospasm, laryngeal edema, urticaria.

Musculoskeletal: Rhabdomyolysis.

Metabolism: Hypoglycemia (in children), hyperglycemia.

Reproductive: Prolonged pregnancy and labor, stillbirths, lower birth weight infants, antepartum and postpartum bleeding.

Respiratory: Hyperpnea, pulmonary edema, tachypnea.

Special Senses: Hearing loss, tinnitus. Patients with high frequency hearing loss may have difficulty perceiving tinnitus. In these patients, tinnitus cannot be used as a clinical indicator of salicylism.

Urogenital: Interstitial nephritis, papillary necrosis, proteinuria, renal insufficiency and failure.

DRUG ABUSE AND DEPENDENCE

Aspirin is non-narcotic. There is no known potential for addiction associated with the use of aspirin.

OVERDOSAGE

Salicylate toxicity may result from acute ingestion (overdose) or chronic intoxication. The early signs of salicylic overdose (salicylism), including tinnitus (ringing in the ears), occur at plasma concentrations approaching 200 mcg/mL. Plasma concentrations of aspirin above 300 mcg/mL are clearly toxic. Severe toxic effects are associated with levels above 400 mcg/mL. (See Clinical Pharmacology.) A single lethal dose of aspirin in adults is not known with certainty but death may be expected at 30 g. For real or suspected overdose, a Poison Control Center should be contacted immediately. Careful medical management is essential.

Signs and Symptoms: In acute overdose, severe acid-base and electrolyte disturbances may occur and are complicated by hyperthermia and dehydration. Respiratory alkalosis occurs early while hyperventilation is present, but is quickly followed by metabolic acidosis.

Treatment: Treatment consists primarily of supporting vital functions, increasing salicylate elimination, and correcting the acid-base disturbance. Gastric emptying and/or lavage is recommended as soon as possible after ingestion, even if the patient has vomited spontaneously. After lavage and/or emesis, administration of activated charcoal, as a slurry, is beneficial, if less than 3 hours have passed since ingestion. Charcoal adsorption should not be employed prior to emesis and lavage.

Severity of aspirin intoxication is determined by measuring the blood salicylate level. Acid-base status should be closely followed with serial blood gas and serum pH measurements. Fluid and electrolyte balance should be maintained.

In severe cases, hyperthermia and hypovolemia are the major immediate threats to life. Children should be sponged with tepid water. Replacement fluid should be administered intravenously and augmented with correction of acidosis. Plasma electrolytes and pH should be monitored to promote alkaline diuresis of salicylate if renal function is normal. Infusion of glucose may be required to control hypoglycemia. Hemodialysis and peritoneal dialysis can be performed to reduce the body drug content. In patients with renal insufficiency or in cases of life-threatening intoxication, dialysis is usually required. Exchange transfusion may be indicated in infants and young children.

DOSAGE AND ADMINISTRATION

Each dose of aspirin should be taken with a full glass of water unless patient is fluid restricted. Anti-inflammatory and analgesic dosages should be individualized. When aspirin is used in high doses, the development of tinnitus may be used as a clinical sign of elevated plasma salicylate levels except in patients with high frequency hearing loss.

Ischemic Stroke and TIA: 50–325 mg once a day. Continue therapy indefinitely.

Suspected Acute MI: The initial dose of 160–162.5 mg is administered as soon as an MI is suspected. The maintenance dose of 160–162.5 mg a day is continued for 30 days post infarction. After 30 days, consider further therapy based on dosage and administration for prevention of recurrent MI.

Prevention of Recurrent MI: 75–325 mg once a day. Continue therapy indefinitely.

Unstable Angina Pectoris: 75–325 mg once a day. Continue therapy indefinitely.

Chronic Stable Angina Pectoris: 75–325 mg once a day. Continue therapy indefinitely.

CABG: 325 mg daily starting 6 hours post-procedure. Continue therapy for 1 year post-procedure.

PTCA: The initial dose of 325 mg should be given 2 hours pre-surgery. Maintenance dose is 160–325 mg daily. Continue therapy indefinitely.

Carotid Endarterectomy: Doses of 80 mg once daily to 650 mg twice daily, started presurgery, are recommended. Continue therapy indefinitely.

Rheumatoid Arthritis: The initial dose is 3 g a day in divided doses. Increase as needed for anti-inflammatory efficacy with target plasma salicylate levels of 150–300 mcg/mL. At high doses (i.e., plasma levels of greater than 200 mg/mL), the incidence of toxicity increases.

Juvenile Rheumatoid Arthritis: Initial dose is 90–130 mg/kg/day in divided doses. Increase as needed for anti-inflammatory efficacy with target plasma salicylate levels of 150–300 mcg/mL. At high doses (i.e., plasma levels of greater than 200 mg/mL), the incidence of toxicity increases.

Spondyloarthropathies: Up to 4 g per day in divided doses.

Osteoarthritis: Up to 3 g per day in divided doses.

Arthritis and Pleurisy of SLE: The initial dose is 3 g a day in divided doses. Increase as needed for anti-inflammatory efficacy with target plasma salicylate levels of 150–300 mcg/mL. At high doses (i.e., plasma levels of greater than 200 mg/mL), the incidence of toxicity increases.

HOW SUPPLIED

81 mg convex orange film coated tablet with ECOTRIN LOW printed in black ink on one side of the tablet. Available as follows

NDC 0108-0117-82 Bottle of 36 tablets

NDC 0108-0117-83 Bottle of 120 tablets

325 mg convex orange film coated tablet with ECOTRIN REG printed in black ink on one side of the tablet. Available as follows:

NDC 0108-0014-26 Bottle of 100 tablets

NDC 0108-0014-29 Bottle of 250 tablets

500 mg convex orange film coated tablet with ECOTRIN MAX printed in black ink on one side of the tablet. Available as follows:

NDC 0108-0016-23 Bottle of 60 tablets

NDC 0108-0016-27 Bottle of 150 tablets

Store in a tight container at 25°C (77° F); excursions permitted to 15–30° C (59–86° F).

FEOSOL®Caplets OTC

Hematinic
Iron Supplement

DESCRIPTION

FEOSOL Caplets contain pure iron micro particles called carbonyl iron. Replacing FEOSOL Capsules, this advanced formula is specially designed to be well absorbed, gentle on the stomach and offers enhanced safety in the event of an accidental overdose. Each FEOSOL carbonyl iron caplet delivers 45 mg of pure elemental iron, the same amount of elemental iron contained in the 225 mg ferrous sulfate capsule. At equivalent doses, carbonyl iron and ferrous sulfate were shown to be equally efficacious in correcting hemoglobin, hematocrit and serum iron levels in iron-deficient patients[1].

SAFETY

According to the American Association of Poison Control Centers, iron containing supplements are the leading cause of pediatric poisoning deaths for children under six in the United States[2]. Widely used as a food additive, carbonyl iron must be gastrically solubilized before it can be absorbed, giving it lower toxicity and enhancing its safety versus any of the ferrous salts[3]. As a result, carbonyl iron presents less chance of harm from accidental overdose. In addition, at equivalent doses, carbonyl iron side effects are no greater than those experienced with ferrous sulfate[4].

WARNINGS

Do not exceed recommended dosage. The treatment of any anemic condition should be under the advice and supervision of a physician. Since oral iron products interfere with absorption of oral tetracycline antibiotics, these products should not be taken within two hours of each other. Occasional gastrointestinal discomfort (such as nausea) may be minimized by taking with meals. Iron containing medication may occasionally cause constipation or diarrhea.

If you are pregnant or nursing a baby, seek the advice of a health professional before using this product.

WARNING: Accidental overdose of iron-containing products is a leading cause of fatal poisoning in children under 6. Keep this product out of reach of children. In case of accidental overdose, call a doctor or poison control center immediately.

SUPPLEMENT FACTS

Serving Size: 1 Caplet

Amount per Caplet	% Daily Value
Iron 45 mg	250%

INGREDIENTS

Lactose, Sorbitol, Carbonyl Iron, Hydroxypropyl Methylcellulose. Contains 1% or less of the following ingredients: Carnauba Wax, Crospovidone, FD&C Blue #2 Al Lake, FD&C Red #40 Al Lake, FD&C Yellow #6 Al Lake, Magnesium Stearate, Polydextrose, Polyethylene Glycol, Polyethylene Glycol 8000 (Powder), Stearic Acid, Titanium Dioxide, Triacetin.

DIRECTIONS

Adults—one caplet daily or as directed by a physician. Children under 12 years: Consult a physician.

TAMPER-EVIDENT FEATURE

Each caplet is encased in a plastic cell with a foil back; do not use if cell or foil is broken.

REFERENCES

[1]Devasthali SD, Gordeuk VR, Brittenham GM, et al, "Bioavailability of Carbonyl Iron: A randomized, double-blind study." Eur J Haematology, 1991; 46:272–278.

[2]FDA Consumer; March 1996:7

[3]Heubers, JA, Brittenham GM, Csiba E and Finch CA. "Absorption of carbonyl iron." J Lab Clin Med 1986; 108:473–78.

[4]Devasthali SD, Gordeuk VR, Brittenham GM, et al, "Bioavailability of a Carbonyl Iron: A randomized, double-blind study." Eur J Haematology, 1991; 46:272–278.

Store at room temperature, avoid excessive heat (greater than 100°F) or humidity.

HOW SUPPLIED

Boxes of 30 and 60 caplets in blisters. Also available in single unit packages of 100 caplets intended for institutional use

Also Available: Feosol Tablets and Feosol Elixir.

Comments or Questions? Call Toll-Free 1-800-245-1040 Weekdays.

SmithKline Beecham Consumer Healthcare, L.P.
Pittsburgh, PA 15230 Made in USA

FEOSOL® TABLETS OTC

Hematinic
Iron Supplement

DESCRIPTION

Feosol tablets provide the body with ferrous sulfate—an iron supplement for iron deficiency and iron deficiency anemia when the need for such therapy has been determined by a physician.

Supplement Facts

Serving Size: 1 Tablet

Amount per Tablet	**% Daily Value**
Iron 65 mg	360%

INGREDIENTS

Dried ferrous sulfate 200 mg (65 mg of elemental iron) equivalent to 325 mg of ferrous sulfate, USP per tablet, Lactose, Sorbitol, Cospovidone, Magnesium Stearate, Carnauba Wax. Contains 2% or less of the following ingredients: FD&C Blue #1, FD&C Yellow #6, Hydroxypropyl Methylcellulose, Polydextrose, Polyethylene Glycol, Titanium Dioxide, Triacetin.

DIRECTIONS

Adults and children 12 years and over—One tablet daily or as directed by a physician. Children under 12 years—Consult a physician.

TAMPER-EVIDENT FEATURES:

Each tablet is encased in a plastic cell with a foil back; do not use if cell or foil is broken.

Comments or Questions?
Call toll-free 800-245-1040 weekdays.

WARNINGS

Do not exceed recommended dosage. The treatment of any anemic condition should be under the advice and supervision of a physician. Since oral iron products interfere with absorption of oral tetracycline antibiotics, these products should not be taken within two hours of each other. Occassional gastrointestinal discomfort (such as nausea) may be minimized by taking with meals. Iron containing medication may occassionally cause constipation or diarrhea.

If you are pregnant or nursing a baby, seek the advice of a health professional before using this product.

WARNING: Accidental overdose of iron-contraining products is a leading cause of fatal poisoning in children under 6. Keep this product out of reach of children. In case of accidental overdose, call a doctor, or poison control center immediately.

Store at room temperature (59–86 F).

Not USP for dissolution.

HOW SUPPLIED

Cartons of 100 tablets in child-resistant blisters.

Previously packaged in bottles.

Also available in caplets and elixir.

Comments or Questions?

Call Toll-Free 1-800-245-1040 Weekdays

SmithKline Beecham Consumer Healthcare, L.P.
Pittsburgh, PA 15230
Made in USA

Continued on next page

GAVISCON® REGULAR AND EXTRA STRENGTH TABLETS **OTC**
Antacid Tablets
GAVISCON® REGULAR AND EXTRA STRENGTH LIQUID ANTACID
[*gav 'is-kon*]

(See PDR For Nonprescription Drugs.)

GLY–OXIDE® Liquid **OTC**
[*gli 'ok-sīd*]

(See PDR For Nonprescription Drugs.)

MASSENGILL® Douches, Towelettes and Cleansing Wash **OTC**
[*mas 'sen-gil*]

(See PDR for Nonprescription Drugs)

NICODERM® CQ® **OTC**
Nicotine Transdermal System/Stop Smoking Aid

Formerly available only by prescription
Available as:
Step 1 - 21 mg/24 hours
Step 2 - 14 mg/24 hours
Step 3 - 7 mg/24 hours

If you smoke:
More than 10 cigarettes per Day: Start with Step 1
10 Cigarettes a Day or Less: Start with Step 2

WHAT IS THE NICODERM CQ PATCH AND HOW IS IT USED?
NicoDerm CQ is a small, nicotine containing patch. When you put on a NicoDerm CQ patch, nicotine passes through the skin and into your body. NicoDerm CQ is very thin and uses special material to control how fast nicotine passes through the skin. Unlike the sudden jolts of nicotine delivered by cigarettes, the amount of nicotine you receive remains relatively smooth throughout the 24 or 16 hours period you wear the NicoDerm CQ patch. This helps to reduce cravings you may have for nicotine.

Active Ingredient: Nicotine

Purpose: Stop Smoking Aid

Use: reduces withdrawal symptoms, including nicotine craving, associated with quitting smoking

Directions
- **if you are under 18 years of age, ask a doctor before use**
- before using this product, read the enclosed user's guide for complete directions and other information
- stop smoking completely when you begin using the patch
- **if you smoke more than 10 cigarettes per day,** use according to the following 10 week schedule:

STEP 1 (21 mg)	STEP 2 (14 mg)	STEP 3 (7 mg)
Initial Treatment Period Weeks 1–6	Step Down Treatment Period	Step Down Treatment Period
	Weeks 7–8	Weeks 9–10

- if you smoke **10 or less cigarettes per day,** do not use **STEP 1 (21 mg).** Start with **STEP 2 (14 mg)** for 6 weeks, then
- **STEP 3 (7 mg)** for two weeks and then stop.
- steps 2 and 3 allow you to gradually reduce your level of nicotine. Completing the full program will increase your chances of quitting successfully.
- apply one new patch every 24 hours on skin that is dry, clean and hairless
- remove backing from patch and immediately press onto skin. Hold for 10 seconds.
- wash hands after applying or removing patch. Throw away the patch in the enclosed disposal tray. See enclosed user's guide for safety and handling.
- you may wear the patch for 16 or 24 hours
- if you crave cigarettes when you wake up, wear the patch for 24 hours
- if you have vivid dreams or other sleep disturbances, you may remove the patch at bedtime and apply a new one in the morning
- the used patch should be removed and a new one applied to a different skin site at the same time each day
- do not wear more than one patch at a time
- do not cut patch in half or into smaller pieces
- do not leave patch on for more than 24 hours because it may irritate your skin and loses strength after 24 hours
- stop using the patch at the end of 10 weeks. If you started with **STEP 2,** stop using the patch at the end of 8 weeks. If you still feel the need to use the patch talk to your doctor.

Warnings
Do Not Use
- if you continue to smoke, chew tobacco, use snuff, or use a nicotine gum or other nicotine containing products

Ask a doctor before use if you have
- heart disease, recent heart attack, or irregular heartbeat. Nicotine can increase your heart rate.
- high blood pressure not controlled with medication. Nicotine can increase your blood pressure.
- an allergy to adhesive tape or skin problems because you are more likely to get rashes

Ask a doctor or pharmacist before use if you are
- using a non-nicotine stop smoking drug
- taking a prescription medication for depression or asthma. Your prescription dose may need to be adjusted.

Stop use and ask a doctor if
- skin redness caused by the patch does not go away after four days, or if skin swells, or you get a rash
- irregular heartbeat or palpitations occur
- you get symptoms of nicotine overdose such as nausea, vomiting, dizziness, weakness and rapid heartbeat

If pregnant or breast feeding, ask a health professional before use. Nicotine can increase your baby's heart rate. First try to stop without the nicotine patch.

Keep out of reach of children and pets. Used patches have enough nicotine to poison children and pets. If swallowed, get medical help or contact a Poison Control Center right away. Dispose of the used patches by folding sticky ends together and inserting in disposal tray in this box.

When using this product
- do not smoke even when not wearing the patch. The nicotine in your skin will still be entering your blood stream for several hours after you take off the patch.
- if you have vivid dreams or other sleep disturbances remove this patch at bedtime

READ THE LABEL
Read the carton and the User's Guide before using this product. Keep the carton and User's Guide. They contain important information.

Inactive Ingredients: Ethylene vinyl acetate-copolymer, polyisobutylene and high density polyethylene between pigmented and clear polyester backings.

Store at 20–25°C (68–77°F)

TO INCREASE YOUR SUCCESS IN QUITTING:
1. You must be motivated to quit.
2. Complete the full treatment program, applying a new patch every day.
3. Use with a support program as described in the Users Guide.

NicoDerm CQ User's Guide
KEYS TO SUCCESS
1) You must really want to quit smoking for **NicoDerm® CQ®** to help you.
2) Complete the full program, applying a new patch every day.
3) **NicoDerm CQ** works best when used together with a support program: See page 3 for details.
4) If you have trouble using **NicoDerm CQ**, ask your doctor or pharmacist or call SmithKline Beecham at 1-800-834-5895 weekdays (10:00 am 4:30 pm EST).

SO, YOU'VE DECIDED TO QUIT.
Congratulations. Your decision to stop smoking is one of the most important things you can do to improve your health. Quitting smoking is a two-part process that involves:
1) overcoming your physical need for nicotine, and
2) breaking your smoking habit.
NicoDerm CQ helps smokers quit by reducing nicotine withdrawal symptoms.
Many NicoDerm CQ users will be able to stop smoking for a few days but often will start smoking again. Most smokers have to try to quit several times before they completely stop. Your own chances of quitting smoking depend on how strongly you are addicted to nicotine, how much you want to quit, and how closely you follow a quitting plan like the one that comes with NicoDerm CQ.

QUITTING SMOKING IS HARD!
If you find you cannot stop or if you start smoking again after using NicoDerm CQ please talk to a health care professional who can help you find a program that may work better for you. Breaking this addiction doesn't happen overnight.
Because NicoDerm CQ provides some nicotine, the NicoDerm CQ patch will help you stop smoking by reducing nicotine withdrawal symptoms such as nicotine craving, nervousness and irritability.
This User's Guide will give you support as you become a non-smoker. It will answer common questions about NicoDerm CQ and give tips to help you stop smoking, and should be referred to often.

WHERE TO GET HELP.
You are more likely to stop smoking by using NicoDerm CQ with a support program that helps you break your smoking habit. There may be support groups in your area for people trying to quit. Call your local chapter of the American Lung Association, American Cancer Society or American Heart Association for further information. Toll free phone numbers are printed on the wallet card on the back cover of this User's Guide.
If you find you cannot stop smoking or if you start smoking again after using NicoDerm CQ, remember breaking this addiction doesn't happen overnight. You may want to talk to a health care professional who can help you improve your chances of quitting the next time you try NicoDerm CQ or another method.

LET'S GET ORGANIZED.
Your reason for quitting may be a combination of concerns about health, the effect of smoking on your appearance, and pressure from your family and friends to stop smoking. Or maybe you're concerned about the dangerous effect of second-hand smoke on the people you care about.
All of these are good reasons. You probably have others. Decide your most important reasons, and write them down on the wallet card inside the back cover of this User's Guide. Carry this card with you. In difficult moments, when you want to smoke, the card will remind you why you are quitting.

WHAT YOU'RE UP AGAINST.
Smoking is addictive in two ways. Your need for nicotine has become both physical and mental. You must overcome both addictions to stop smoking. So while NicoDerm CQ will lessen your body's craving for nicotine, you've got to want to quit smoking to overcome the mental dependence on cigarettes. Once you've decided that you're going to quit, it's time to get started. But first, there are some important cautions you should consider.

SOME IMPORTANT WARNINGS.
This product is only for those who want to stop smoking.

Do not use
- if you continue to smoke, chew tobacco, use snuff or use a nicotine gum or other nicotine products.

Ask a doctor before use if you have
- heart disease, recent heart attack, or irregular heartbeat. Nicotine can increase your heart rate.
- high blood pressure not controlled with medication. Nicotine can increase your blood pressure.
- an allergy to adhesive tape or have skin problems because you are more likely to get rashes.

Ask a doctor or pharmacist before use if you are
- using a non-nicotine stop smoking drug
- taking a prescription medication for asthma or depression. Your prescription dose may need to be adjusted.

When using this product
- do not smoke even when not wearing the patch. The nicotine in your skin will still be entering your bloodstream for several hours after you take off the patch.
- you have vivid dreams or other sleep disturbances remove this patch at bedtime.

Stop use and ask a doctor if
- skin redness caused by the patch does not go away after four days, or if your skin swells or you get a rash.
- irregular heartbeat or palpitations occur
- you get symptoms of nicotine overdose, such as nausea, vomiting, dizziness, weakness and rapid heartbeat.

If pregnant or breast-feeding, ask a health professional before use. Nicotine can increase your baby's heart rate. First try to stop smoking without the nicotine patch.

Keep out of reach of children and pets. Used patches have enough nicotine to poison children and pets. If swallowed, get medical help or contact a Poison Control Center right away. Dispose of the used patches by folding sticky ends together and inserting in the disposal tray in this box.

LET'S GET STARTED.
If you are under 18 years of age, ask a doctor before use.
Becoming a non-smoker starts today. Your first step is to read through this entire User's Guide carefully.

First, check that you bought the right starting dose.
If you smoke more than 10 cigarettes a day, begin with Step 1 (21 mg). As the carton indicates, people who smoke 10 or less cigarettes per day should not use Step 1 (21 mg). They should start with Step 2 (14 mg). Throughout this User's Guide we will give specific instructions for people who smoke 10 or less cigarettes per day.

Next, set your personalized quitting schedule.
Take out a calendar that you can use to track your progress. Pick a quit date, and mark this on your calendar using the stickers in the middle of this User's Guide, as described below.

DIRECTIONS: FOR PEOPLE WHO SMOKE MORE THAN 10 CIGARETTES PER DAY

STEP 1. (Weeks 1–6). Your quit date (and the day you'll start using NicoDerm CQ patch).
Choose your quit date (it should be soon).
This is the day you will quit smoking cigarettes entirely and begin using NicoDerm CQ to reduce your cravings for nicotine. Place the Step 1 sticker on this date. For the first six weeks, you'll use the highest-strength (21 mg) NicoDerm CQ patches. Be sure to follow the directions on page 10.
Completing the full program will increase your chances of quitting successfully. This is done by changing over to the Step 1 (14mg) patch for 2 weeks followed by a final 2 weeks with the Step 3 (7mg) patch. The Step 2 and Step 3 treatment periods allow you to gradually reduce the amount of nicotine you get, rather than stopping suddenly, and will increase your chances of quitting.

STEP 2. (Weeks 7–8). The day you'll start reducing your use of NicoDerm CQ patch.
Switching to Step 2 (14mg) patches after 6 weeks begins to gradually reduce your nicotine usage. Place the Step 2 sticker on this date (the first day of week seven). Use the 14mg patches for two weeks.

STEP 3. (Weeks 9–10). The day you'll further start reducing your use of NicoDerm CQ patch.
After eight weeks, nicotine intake is further reduced by moving down to Step 3 (7mg) patches. Place the Step 3 sticker on this date (the first day of week nine). Use the 7 mg patches for two weeks.

THE NICODERM CQ PROGRAM

STEP 1	STEP 2	STEP 3
Use one 21 mg patch/day	Use one 14 mg patch/day	Use one 7 mg patch/day
Weeks 1–6	Weeks 7–8	Weeks 9–10

STOP USING NICODERM CQ AT THE END OF WEEK 10. If you still feel the need to use the patch after Week 10, talk with your doctor or health professional.

DIRECTIONS: FOR PEOPLE WHO SMOKE 10 OR LESS CIGARETTES PER DAY

Do not use Step 1 (21 mg).

Begin with STEP 2 – Initial Treatment Period (Weeks 1–6): 14mg patches.

Choose our quit date (it should be soon). This is the Day you will quit smoking cigarettes entirely and begin using NicoDerm CQ to reduce your cravings for nicotine. Place the Step 2 sticker on this date. For the first six weeks, you'll use the Step 2 (14mg) NicoDerm CQ patches. Be sure to follow the directions on page 10.

Continue with STEP 3 – Step Down Treatment Period (Weeks 7–8): 7mg patches.

Completing the full program will increase your chances of quitting successfully. This is done by changing over to the Step 3 (7mg) patches for 2 weeks. The two week step down treatment period allows you to gradually reduce the amount of nicotine you get, rather than stopping suddenly, and will increase your chances of quitting. Place the Step 3 sticker on the first day of week seven. Use the 7mg patches for two weeks. People who smoke 10 or less cigarettes per day should not use NicoDerm CQ for longer than 8 weeks. If you still feel the need to use NicoDerm CQ after 8 weeks, talk with your doctor.

PLAN AHEAD.

Because smoking is an addiction, it is not easy to stop. After you've given up nicotine, you may still have a strong urge to smoke. Plan ahead NOW for these times, so you're not tempted to start smoking again in a moment of weakness. The following tips may help:

- Keep the phone numbers of supportive friends and family members handy.
- Keep a record of your quitting process. Track whether you feel a craving for cigarettes. In the event that you slip, immediately stop smoking and resume your quit attempt with the NicoDerm CQ patch. If you smoke at all, write down what you think caused the slip.
- Put together an Emergency Kit that includes items that will help take your mind off occasional urges to smoke. You might include cinnamon gum or lemon drops to suck on, a relaxing cassette tape, and something for your hands to play with, like a smooth rock, rubber band or small metal balls.
- Set aside some small rewards, like a new magazine or a gift certificate from your favorite store, which you'll "give" yourself after passing difficult hurdles.
- Think now about the times when you most often want a cigarette, and then plan what else you might do instead of smoking. For instance, you might plan to take your coffee break in a new location, or take a walk right after dinner, so you won't be tempted to smoke.

HOW NICODERM CQ WORKS.

NicoDerm CQ patches provide nicotine to your system. They work as a temporary aid to help you quit smoking by reducing nicotine withdrawal symptoms, including nicotine craving. NicoDerm CQ provides a lower level of nicotine to your blood than cigarettes, and allows you to gradually do away with your body's need for nicotine.

Because NicoDerm CQ does not contain the tar or carbon monoxide of cigarette smoke, it does not have the same health dangers as tobacco. However, it still delivers nicotine, the addictive part of cigarette smoke. Nicotine can cause side effects such as headache, nausea, upset stomach, and dizziness.

HOW TO USE NICODERM CQ PATCHES.

Read all the following instructions, and the instructions on the outer carton, before using NicoDerm CQ. Refer to them often to make sure you're using NicoDerm CQ correctly. Please refer to the audio tape for additional help.

1) Stop smoking completely before you start using NicoDerm CQ.

2) To reduce nicotine craving and other withdrawal symptoms, use NicoDerm CQ according to the directions on pages 6–8.

3) Insert used NicoDerm CQ patches in the child resistant disposal tray provided in the box – safely away from children and pets.

When to apply and remove NicoDerm CQ patches.

Each day apply a new patch to a different place on skin that is dry, clean and hairless. **You can wear a NicoDerm CQ patch for either 16 or 24 hours.** If you crave cigarettes when you wake up, wear the patch for 24 hours. If you begin to have vivid dreams or other disruptions of your sleep while wearing the patch 24 hours, try taking the patch off at bedtime (after about 16 hours) and putting on a new one when you get up the next day.

PLACE THESE STICKERS ON YOUR CALENDAR

STEP 1	**STEP 2**
A new 21 mg patch every day AT THE BEGINNING OF WEEK #1 (QUIT DAY)	A new 14 mg patch every day AT THE BEGINNING OF WEEK #7

For people who smoke 10 or less cigarettes per day: Do not use STEP 1 (21 mg). Use STEP 2 (14 mg) at the beginning of week #1 and STEP 3 (7 mg) at the beginning of week #7.

PLACE THESE STICKERS ON YOUR CALENDAR

STEP 3	**EX-SMOKER**
A new 7 mg patch every day AT THE BEGINNING OF WEEK #9	WHEN YOU HAVE COMPLETED YOUR QUITTING PROGRAM

Do not smoke even when you are not wearing the patch. Remove the used patch and put on a new patch at the same time every day. Applying the patch at about the same time each day (first thing in the morning, for instance) will help you remember when to put on a new patch. Do not leave the same NicoDerm CQ patch on for more than 24 hours because it may irritate your skin and because it loses strength after 24 hours.

Do not use NicoDerm CQ continuously for more than 10 weeks (8 weeks for people who smoke 10 or less cigarettes per day).

How to apply a NicoDerm CQ patch.

1. Do not remove the NicoDerm CQ patch from its sealed protective pouch until you are ready to use it. NicoDerm CQ patches will lose nicotine to the air if you store them out of the pouch.

2. Choose a non-hairy, clean, dry area of skin. Do not put a NicoDerm CQ patch on skin that is burned, broken out, cut, or irritated in any way. Make sure your skin is free of lotion and soap before applying a patch.

3. A clear, protective liner covers the sticky back side of the NicoDerm CQ patch—the side that will be put on your skin. The liner has a slit down the middle to help you remove it from the patch. With the sticky back side facing you, pull half the liner away from the NicoDerm CQ patch starting at the middle slit, as shown in the illustration above. Hold the NicoDerm CQ patch at one of the outside edges (touch the sticky side as little as possible), and pull off the other half of the protective liner.

Place this liner in the slot in the disposable tray provided in the NicoDerm CQ package where it will be out of reach of children and pets.

4. Immediately apply the sticky side of the NicoDerm CQ patch to your skin. **Press the patch firmly on your skin with the heel of your hand for at least 10 seconds.** Make sure it sticks well to your skin, especially around the edges.

5. Wash your hands when you have finished applying the NicoDerm CQ patch. Nicotine on your hands could get into your eyes and nose, and cause stinging, redness, or more serious problems.

6. After 24 or 16 hours, remove the patch you have been wearing. Fold the used NicoDerm CQ patch in half with the sticky side together. Carefully dispose of the used patch in the slot of the disposal tray provided in the NicoDerm CQ package where it will be out of the reach of children and pets. Even used patches have enough nicotine to poison children and pets. Wash your hands.

7. Chose a different place on your skin to apply the next NicoDerm CQ patch and repeat Steps 1 to 6. Do not apply a new patch to a previously used skin site for at least one week.

If your NicoDerm CQ patch gets wet during wearing.

Water will not harm the NicoDerm CQ patch you are wearing if applied properly. You can bathe, swim, or shower for short periods while you are wearing the NicoDerm CQ patch.

If your NicoDerm CQ patch comes off while wearing.

NicoDerm CQ patches generally stick well to most people's skin. However, a patch may occasionally come off. If your NicoDerm CQ patch falls off during the day, put on a new patch, making sure you select a non-hairy, non-irritated area of the skin that is clean and dry.

If the soap you use has lanolin or moisturizers, the patch may not stick well. Using a different soap may help. Body creams, lotions and sunscreens can also cause problems with keeping your patch on. Do not apply creams or lotions to the place on your skin where you will put the patch.

If you have followed the directions and the patch still does not stick to you, try using medical adhesive tape over the patch.

Disposing of NicoDerm CQ patches.

Fold the used patch in half with the sticky side together. Carefully dispose of the patch in the disposal slot of the tray provided in the NicoDerm CQ package where it will be out of the reach of children and pets. Small amounts of nicotine, even from a used patch, can poison children and pets. **Keep all nicotine patches away from children and pets.** Wash your hands after disposing of the patch.

If your skin reacts to the NicoDerm CQ patch.

When you first put on a NicoDerm CQ patch, mild itching, burning, or tingling is normal and should go away within an hour. After you remove a NicoDerm CQ patch, the skin under the patch might be somewhat red. Your skin should not stay red for more than a day after removing the patch. **Stop use and ask a doctor if skin redness caused by the patch does not go away after four days, or if your skin swells, or you get a rash. Do not put on a new patch.**

Storage Instructions

Keep each NicoDerm CQ patch in its protective pouch, unopened, until you are ready to use it, because the patch will lose nicotine to the air if it's outside the pouch.

Store NicoDerm CQ patches at 20–25 C (68–77 F) because they are sensitive to heat. Remember, the inside of your car can reach temperatures much higher than this. A slight yellowing of the sticky side of the patch is normal. Do not use NicoDerm CQ patches stored in pouches that are open or torn.

TIPS TO MAKE QUITTING EASIER.

Within the first few weeks of giving up smoking, you may be tempted to smoke for pleasure, particularly after completing a difficult task, or at a party or bar. Hear are some tips to help get you through the important first stages of becoming a nonsmoker:

On Your Quit Date:

Ask your family, friends and co-workers to support you in your efforts to stop smoking.

- Throw away all your cigarettes, matches, lighters, ashtrays, etc.
- Keep busy on your quit day. Exercise. Go to a movie. Take a walk. Get together with friends.
- Figure out how much money you'll save by not smoking. Most ex-smokers can save more than $1,000 a year on the price of cigarettes alone.
- Write down what you will do with the money you save.
- Know your high risk situations and plan ahead how you will deal with them.
- Visit your dentist and have your teeth cleaned to get rid of the tobacco stains.

Right after Quitting:

- During the first few days after you've stopped smoking, spend as much time as possible at places where smoking is not allowed.
- Drink large quantities of water and fruit juices.
- Try to avoid alcohol, coffee and other beverages you associate with smoking.
- Remember that temporary urges to smoke will pass, even if you don't smoke a cigarette.
- Keep your hands busy with something like a pencil or a paper clip.
- Find other activities that help you relax without cigarettes. Swim, jog, take a walk, play basketball.

Don't worry too much about gaining weight. Watch what you eat, take time for daily exercise, and change your eating habits if you need to.

- Laughter helps. Watch or read something funny

WHAT TO EXPECT.

The First Few Days.

Your body is now coming back into balance. During the first few days after you stop smoking, you might feel edgy and nervous and have trouble concentrating. You might get headaches, feel dizzy and a little out of sorts, feel sweaty or have stomach upsets. You might even have trouble sleeping at first. These are typical nicotine withdrawal symptoms that will go away with time. Your smoker's cough will get worse before it gets better. But don't worry, that's a good sign. Coughing helps clear the tar deposits out of your lungs.

After A Week Or Two.

By now you should be feeling more confident that you can handle those smoking urges. Many of your nicotine withdrawal symptoms have left by now, and you should be noticing some positive signs: less coughing, better breathing and an improved sense of taste and smell, to name a few.

After A Month.

You probably have the urge to smoke much less often now. But urges may still occur, and when they do, they are likely to be powerful ones that come out of nowhere. Don't let them catch you off guard. Plan ahead for these difficult times.

Concentrate on the ways non-smokers are more attractive than smokers. Their skin is less likely to wrinkle. Their teeth are whiter, cleaner. Their breath is fresher.

Their hair and clothes smell better. That cough that seems to make even a laugh sound more like a rattle is a thing of the past. Their children and others around them are healthier, too.

What To Do About Relapse.

What should you do if you slip and start smoking again? The answer is simple. A lapse of one or two or even a few cigarettes should not spoil your efforts! Throw away your cigarettes, forgive yourself and continue with the program. Listen to the Audio Tape again and re-read the User's Guide to ensure that you're using NicoDerm CQ correctly and following the other important tips for dealing with the mental and social dependence on nicotine. Your doctor, pharmacist or other health professional can also provide useful counseling on the importance of stopping smoking. You should consider them partners in your quit attempt.

What To Do About Relapse After a Successful Quit Attempt.

If you have taken up regular smoking again, don't be discouraged. Research shows that the best thing you can do is try again, since several quitting attempts may be needed before you're successful. And your chances of quitting successfully increase with each quit attempt.

The important thing is to learn from your last attempt.

- Admit that you've slipped, but don't treat yourself as a failure.
- Try to identify the "trigger" that caused you to slip, and prepare a better plan for dealing with this problem next time.
- Talk positively to yourself – tell yourself that you have learned something from this experience.

Continued on next page

Nicoderm CQ—Cont.

- Make sure you used NicoDerm CQ patches correctly
- Remember that it takes practice to do anything, and quitting smoking is no exception.

WHEN THE STRUGGLE IS OVER.
Once you've stopped smoking, take a second and pat yourself on your back. Now do it again. You deserve it. Remember now why you decided to stop smoking in the first place. Look at your list of reasons. Read them again. And smile. Now think about all the money you are saving and what you'll do with it. All the non-smoking places you can go, and what you might do there. All those years you may have added to your life, and what you'll do with them. Remember that temptation may not be gone forever. However, the hard part is behind you so look forward with a positive attitude, and enjoy your new life as a non-smoker.

QUESTIONS & ANSWERS

1. How will I feel when I stop smoking and start using NicoDerm CQ?
You'll need to prepare yourself for some nicotine withdrawal symptoms. These begin almost immediately after you stop smoking, and are usually at their worst during the first three or four days. Understand that any of the following is possible:
- craving for nicotine
- anxiety, irritability, restlessness, mood changes, nervousness
- disruptions of your sleep
- drowsiness
- trouble concentrating
- increased appetite and weight gain headaches, muscular pain, constipation, fatigue.

NicoDerm CQ reduces nicotine withdrawal symptoms such as irritability and nervousness, as well as the craving for nicotine you used to satisfy by having a cigarette.

2. Is NicoDerm CQ just substituting one form of nicotine for another?
NicoDerm CQ does contain nicotine. The purpose of NicoDerm CQ is to provide you with enough nicotine to reduce the physical withdrawal symptoms so you can deal with the mental aspects of quitting.

3. Can I be hurt by using NicoDerm CQ?
For most adults, the amount of nicotine delivered from the patch is less than from smoking. If you believe you may be sensitive to even this amount of nicotine, you should not use this product without advice from your doctor. There are also some important warnings in this User's Guide (See page 4).

4. Will I gain weight?
Many people do tend to gain a few pounds the first 8–10 weeks after they stop smoking. This is a very small price to pay for the enormous gains that you will make in your overall health and attractiveness. If you continue to gain weight after the first two months, try to analyze what you're doing differently. Reduce your fat intake, choose healthy snacks, and increase your physical activity to burn off the extra calories. Drink lots of water. This is good for your body and skin, and also helps to reduce the amount you eat.

5. Is NicoDerm CQ more expensive than smoking?
The total cost of NicoDerm CQ program is similar to what a person who smokes one and a half packs of cigarettes a day would spend on cigarettes for the same period of time. Also, use of NicoDerm CQ is only a short-term cost, while the cost of smoking is a long-term cost, including the health problems smoking causes.

6. What if I slip up?
Discard your cigarettes, forgive yourself and then get back on track. Don't consider yourself a failure or punish yourself. In fact, people who have already tried to quit are more likely to be successful the next time.

GOOD LUCK!

WALLET CARD
My most important reasons to quit smoking are:

WALLET CARD
Where to call for Help:

American Lung Association	American Cancer Society	American Heart Association
800-586-4872	800-227-2345	800-242-8721

For people who smoke more than 10 cigarettes per day:

STEP 1	STEP 2	STEP 3
Use one 21 mg patch/day	Use one 14 mg patch/day	Use one 7 mg patch/day
Weeks 1–6	Weeks 7–8	Weeks 9–10

People who smoke 10 or less cigarettes per day. Do not use STEP 1 (21 mg). Use STEP 2 (14 mg) for six weeks and STEP 3 (7 mg) for two weeks and then stop.

For your family's protection, NicoDerm CQ patches are supplied in child resistant pouches. Do not use if individual pouch is open or torn.

Manufactured by ALZA Corporation, Mountain View, CA 94043 for SmithKline Beecham Consumer Healthcare, L.P. Comments or Questions? Call 1–800–834–5895 Weekdays. (10 a.m.–4:30 p.m. EST).

- **Not for sale to those under 18 years of age.**
- **Proof of age required.**
- **Not for sale in vending machines or from any source where proof of age cannot be verified.**

Available as
NicoDerm CQ Step 1 (21 mg/24 hours)–7 Patches*
NicoDerm CQ Step 1 (21 mg/24 hours)–14 Patches*
NicoDerm CQ Step 2 (14 mg/24 hours)–7 Patches*
NicoDerm CQ Step 2 (14 mg/24 hours)–14 Patches
NicoDerm CQ Step 3 (7 mg/24 hours)–7 Patches**
NicoDerm CQ Step 3 (7 mg/24 hours)–14 Patches
* User's Guide, Audio Tape & Child Resistant Disposal Tray
** User's Guide, & Child Resistant Disposal Tray

NICORETTE® OTC

Nicotine Polacrilex Gum/Stop Smoking Aid
Available in Original 2mg and 4mg Strength and Mint 2mg and 4mg Strength

If you smoke:
UNDER 25 CIGARETTES A DAY: Use 2 mg
OVER 24 CIGARETTES A DAY: Use 4 mg

Action: Stop Smoking Aid

Use:
- To reduce withdrawal symptoms, including nicotine craving, associated with quitting smoking.

Directions:
- Stop smoking completely when you begin using Nicorette.
- Read the enclosed User's Guide before using Nicorette.
- Use properly as directed in the User's Guide.
- Don't eat or drink for 15 minutes before using Nicorette or while chewing a piece.
- Use according to the following 12 week schedule:

Weeks 1 to 6	Weeks 7 to 9	Weeks 10 to 12
1 piece every 1 to 2 hours	1 piece every 2 to 4 hours	1 piece every 4 to 8 hours

- Do not exceed 24 pieces a day.
- Stop using Nicorette at the end of week 12. If you still feel the need for Nicorette, talk with your doctor.

Warnings:
- Keep this and all drugs out of the reach of children and pets. In case of accidental overdose, seek professional assistance or contact a poison control center immediately.
- Nicotine can increase your baby's heart rate; if you are pregnant or nursing a baby, seek the advice of a health professional before using this product.

DO NOT USE IF YOU
- Continue to smoke, chew tobacco, use snuff, or use a nicotine patch or other nicotine containing products.

ASK YOUR DOCTOR BEFORE USE IF YOU
- Are under 18 years of age.
- Have heart disease, recent heart attack, or irregular heartbeat. Nicotine can increase your heart rate.
- Have high blood pressure not controlled with medication. Nicotine can increase blood pressure.
- Have stomach ulcer or take insulin for diabetes.
- Take prescription medicine for depression or asthma. Your prescription dose may need to be adjusted.

STOP USE AND SEE YOUR DOCTOR IF YOU HAVE
- Mouth, teeth or jaw problems.
- Irregular heartbeat, palpitations.
- Symptoms of nicotine overdose such as nausea, vomiting, dizziness, weakness and rapid heartbeat.

READ THE LABEL
Read the carton and the User's Guide before taking this product. Do not discard carton or User's Guide. They contain important information.

Original [2 mg] Inactive Ingredients: Flavors, glycerin, gum base, sodium carbonate, sorbitol, sodium bicarbonate.
Original [4 mg] Inactive Ingredients: Flavors, glycerin, gum base, sodium carbonate, sorbitol, D&C Yellow 10.
Mint 2 mg Inactive Ingredients: Gum base, magnesium oxide, menthol, peppermint oil, sodium bicarbonate, sodium carbonate, xylitol.
Mint 4 mg Inactive Ingredients: Gum base, magnesium oxide, menthol, peppermint oil, sodium carbonate, xylitol, D&C yellow #10.
Do not store above 86°F (30°C). Protect from light.

TO INCREASE YOUR SUCCESS IN QUITTING:
1. **You must be motivated to quit.**
2. **Use Enough** —**Chew at least 9 pieces** of Nicorette per day during the first six weeks.
3. **Use long enough** —Use Nicorette for the full 12 weeks.
4. **Use with a support program** as described in the enclosed User's Guide.

USER'S GUIDE:

HOW TO USE NICORETTE TO HELP YOU QUIT SMOKING
KEYS TO SUCCESS
1) You must really want to quit smoking for Nicorette to help you.
2) You can greatly increase your chances for success by using at least 9 to 12 pieces every day when you start using Nicorette.
3) You should continue to use Nicorette as explained in the User's Guide for 12 full weeks.
4) Nicorette works best when used together with a support program.
5) If you have trouble using Nicorette, ask your doctor or pharmacist or call SmithKline Beecham at 1-800-419-4766 weekdays (10:00am–4:30pm EST).

SO YOU DECIDED TO QUIT
Congratulations. Your decision to stop smoking is an important one. That's why you've made the right choice in choosing Nicorette gum. Your own chances of quitting smoking depend on how much you want to quit, how strongly you are addicted to tobacco, and how closely you follow a quitting program like the one that comes with Nicorette.

QUITTING SMOKING IS HARD!
If you've tried to quit before and haven't succeeded, don't be discouraged! Quitting isn't easy. It takes time, and most people try a few times before they are successful. The important thing is to try again until you succeed. This User's Guide will give you support as you become a non-smoker. It will answer common questions about Nicorette and give tips to help you stop smoking, and should be referred to often.

WHERE TO GET HELP
You are more likely to stop smoking by using Nicorette with a support program that helps you break your smoking habit. There may be support groups in your area for people trying to quit. Call your local chapter of the American Lung Association (1-800-586-4872), American Cancer Society (1-800-227-2345) or American Heart Association (1-800-242-8721) for further information. If you find you cannot stop smoking or if you start smoking again after using Nicorette, remember breaking this addiction doesn't happen overnight. You may want to talk to a health care professional who can help you improve your chances of quitting the next time you try Nicorette or another method.

LET'S GET ORGANIZED
Your reason for quitting may be a combination of concerns about health, the effect of smoking on your appearance, and pressure from your family and friends to stop smoking. Or maybe you're concerned about the dangerous effect of second-hand smoke on the people you care about. All of these are good reasons. You probably have others. Decide your most important reasons, and write them down on the wallet card inside the back cover of the User's Guide. Carry this card with you. In difficult moments, when you want to smoke, the card will remind you why you are quitting.

WHAT YOU'RE UP AGAINST
Smoking is addictive in two ways. Your need for nicotine has become both physical and mental. You must overcome both addictions to stop smoking. So while Nicorette will lessen your body's physical addition to nicotine, you've got to want to quit smoking to overcome the mental dependence on cigarettes. Once you've decided that you're going to quit, it's time to get started. But first, there are some important cautions you should consider.

SOME IMPORTANT CAUTIONS
This product is only for those who want to stop smoking. Do not smoke, chew tobacco, use snuff or nicotine patches while using Nicorette. If you have heart disease, a recent heart attack, irregular heartbeats, palpitations, high blood pressure not controlled with medication, stomach ulcer, or take insulin for diabetes, ask your doctor whether you should use Nicorette. As with any drug, if you are pregnant or nursing a baby, seek the advice of a health professional before using this product. If you take a prescription medication for asthma or depression, be sure your doctor knows you are quitting smoking. Your prescription medication dose may need to be adjusted. Those under 18 should use this product under a doctor's care. Symptoms of nicotine overdose may include vomiting and diarrhea. Young children are more likely to have additional symptoms, including weakness. Also, seizures have been seen in children who swallowed cigarettes. Keep this and all drugs out of the reach of children. In case of accidental overdose, seek professional assistance or contact a poison control center immediately.

LET'S GET STARTED
Becoming a non-smoker starts today. Your first step is to read through the entire User's Guide carefully. **Next, set your personalized quitting schedule.** Take out a calendar that you can use to track your progress, and identify four dates, using the stickers in the User's Guide.

STEP 1: Your quit date (and the day you'll start using Nicorette gum). Choose your quit date (it should be soon). This is the day you will quit smoking cigarettes entirely and begin using Nicorette to satisfy your craving for nicotine. For the first six weeks, you'll use a piece of Nicorette every hour or two. Be sure to follow the directions on pages 8 and 11 of the User's Guide. Place the Step 1 sticker on this date.

STEP 2: The day you'll start reducing your use of Nicorette. After six weeks, you'll begin gradually reducing your Nicorette usage to one piece every two to four hours. Place the Step 2 sticker on this date (the first day of week seven).

STEP 3: The day you'll further reduce your use of Nicorette. Nine weeks after you begin using Nicorette, you will further reduce your nicotine intake by using one piece every four to eight hours. Place the Step 3 sticker on this date (the first day of week ten). For the next three weeks, you'll use a piece of Nicorette every four to eight hours. **End of treatment: The day you'll complete Nicorette therapy. Nicorette** should not be used for longer than twelve weeks. Identify the date thirteen weeks after the date you chose in Step 1 and place the "EX-Smoker" sticker on your calendar.

PLAN AHEAD
Because smoking is an addiction, it is not easy to stop. After you've given up cigarettes, you will still have a strong urge to smoke. Plan ahead NOW for these times, so you're not defeated in a moment of weakness. The following tips may help:
- Keep the phone numbers of supportive friends and family members handy.

- Keep a record of your quitting process. Track the number of Nicorette pieces you use each day, and whether you feel a craving for cigarettes. If you smoke at all, write down what you think caused the slip.
- Put together an Emergency Kit that includes items that will help take your mind off occasional urges to smoke. Include cinnamon gum or lemon drops to suck on, a relaxing cassette tape and something for your hands to play with, like a smooth rock, rubber band or small metal balls.
- Set aside some small rewards, like a new magazine or a gift certificate from your favorite store, which you'll 'give' yourself after passing difficult hurdles.
- Think now about the times when you most often want a cigarette, and then plan what else you might do instead of smoking. For instance, you might plan to take your coffee break in a new location, or take a walk right after dinner, so you won't be tempted to smoke.

HOW NICORETTE GUM WORKS

Nicorette's sugar-free chewing pieces provide nicotine to your system—they work as a temporary aid to help you quit smoking by reducing nicotine withdrawal symptoms. Nicorette provides a lower level of nicotine to your blood than cigarettes, and allows you to gradually do away with your body's need for nicotine. Because Nicorette does not contain the tar or carbon monoxide of cigarette smoke, it does not have the same health dangers as tobacco. However, it still delivers nicotine, the addictive part of cigarette smoke. Nicotine can cause side effects such as headache, nausea, upset stomach and dizziness.

HOW TO USE NICORETTE GUM

Before you can use Nicorette correctly, you have to practice! That sounds silly, but it isn't.

Nicorette isn't like ordinary chewing gum. It's a medicine, and must be chewed a certain way to work right. Chewed like ordinary gum, Nicorette won't work well and can cause side effects. An overdose can occur if you chew more than one piece of Nicorette at the same time, or if you chew many pieces one after another. Read all the following instructions before using Nicorette. Refer to them often to make sure you're using Nicorette gum correctly. If you chew too fast, or do not chew correctly, you may get hiccups, heartburn, or other stomach problems.

1. Stop smoking completely before you start using Nicorette.
2. To reduce craving and other withdrawal symptoms, use Nicorette according to the dosage schedule on page 11 of the User's Guide.
3. Chew each Nicorette piece very slowly several times.
4. Stop chewing when you notice a peppery taste, or a slight tingling in your mouth. (This usually happens after about 15 chews, but may vary from person to person.)
5. "PARK" the Nicorette piece between your cheek and gum and leave it there.
6. When the peppery taste or tingle is almost gone (in about a minute), start to chew a few times slowly again. When the taste or tingle returns, stop again.
7. Park the Nicorette piece again (in a different place in your mouth).
8. Repeat steps 3 to 7 (chew, chew, park) until most of the nicotine is gone from the Nicorette piece (usually happens in about half an hour; the peppery taste or tingle won't return).
9. Throw away the used Nicorette piece, safely away from children and pets.

See the chart in the **"DIRECTIONS"** section above for the recommended usage schedule for Nicorette.

To improve your chances of quitting, use at least 9 pieces of Nicorette a day. Heavier smokers may need more pieces to reduce their cravings. Don't eat or drink for 15 minutes before using Nicorette or while chewing a piece. The effectiveness of Nicorette may be reduced by some foods and drinks, such as coffee, juices, wine or soft drinks.

HOW TO REDUCE YOUR NICORETTE USAGE

The goal of using Nicorette is to slowly reduce your dependence on nicotine. The schedule for using Nicorette will help you reduce your nicotine craving gradually. Here are some tips to help you cut back during each step:

- After a while, start chewing each Nicorette piece for only 10 to 15 minutes, instead of half an hour. Then gradually begin to reduce the number of pieces used.
- Or, try chewing each piece for longer than half an hour, but reduce the number of pieces you use each day.
- Substitute ordinary chewing gum for some of the Nicorette pieces you would normally use. Increase the number of pieces of ordinary gum as you cut back on the Nicorette pieces.

STOP USING NICORETTE AT THE END OF WEEK 12. If you still feel the need to use Nicorette after Week 12, talk with your doctor.

TIPS TO MAKE QUITTING EASIER

Within the first few weeks of giving up smoking, you may be tempted to smoke for pleasure, particularly after completing a difficult task, or at a party or bar. Here are some tips to help get you through the important first stages of becoming a non-smoker:

On your Quit Date:

- Ask your family, friends, and co-workers to support you in your efforts to stop smoking.
- Throw away all your cigarettes, matches, lighters, ashtrays, etc.
- Keep busy on your quit day. Exercise. Go to a movie. Take a walk. Get together with friends.
- Figure out how much money you'll save by not smoking. Most ex-smokers can save more than $1,000 a year.
- Write down what you will do with the money you save.
- Know your high risk situations and plan ahead how you will deal with them.
- Keep Nicorette gum near your bed, so you'll be prepared for any nicotine cravings when you wake up in the morning.
- Visit your dentist and have your teeth cleaned to get rid of the tobacco stains.

Right after Quitting:

- During the first few days after you've stopped smoking, spend as much time as possible at places where smoking is not allowed.
- Drink large quantities of water and fruit juices.
- Try to avoid alcohol, coffee and other beverages you associate with smoking.
- Remember that temporary urges to smoke will pass, even if you don't smoke a cigarette.
- Keep your hands busy with something like a pencil or a paper clip.
- Find other activities which help you relax without cigarettes. Swim, jog, take a walk, play basketball.
- Don't worry too much about gaining weight. Watch what you eat, take time for daily exercise, and change your eating habits if you need to.
- Laughter helps. Watch or read something funny.

WHAT TO EXPECT

Your body is now coming back into balance. During the first few days after you stop smoking, you might feel edgy and nervous and have trouble concentrating. You might get headaches, feel dizzy and a little out of sorts, feel sweaty or have stomach upsets. You might even have trouble sleeping at first. These are typical withdrawal symptoms that will go away with time. Your smoker's cough will get worse before it gets better. But don't worry, that's a good sign. Coughing helps clear the tar deposits out of your lungs.

After a Week or Two.

By now you should be feeling more confident that you can handle those smoking urges. Many of your withdrawal symptoms have left by now, and you should be noticing some positive signs: less coughing, better breathing and an improved sense of taste and smell, to name a few.

After a Month.

You probably have the urge to smoke much less often now. But urges may still occur, and when they do, they are likely to be powerful ones that come out of nowhere. Don't let them catch you off guard. Plan ahead for these difficult times. Concentrate on the ways non-smokers are more attractive than smokers. Their skin is less likely to wrinkle. Their teeth are whiter, cleaner. Their breath is fresher. Their hair and clothes smell better. That cough seems to make even a laugh sound more like a rattle is a thing of the past. Their children and others around them are healthier, too.

What To Do About Relapse.

What should you do if you slip and start smoking again? The answer is simple. A lapse of one or two or even a few cigarettes has not spoiled your efforts! Discard your cigarettes, forgive yourself and try again. If you start smoking again, keep your box of Nicorette for your next quit attempt. If you have taken up regular smoking again, don't be discouraged. Research shows that the best thing you can do is to try again. The important thing is to learn from your last attempt.

- Admit that you've slipped, but don't treat yourself as a failure.
- Try to identify the 'trigger' that caused you to slip, and prepare a better plan for dealing with this problem next time.
- Talk positively to yourself—tell yourself that you have learned something from this experience.
- Make sure you used Nicorette gum correctly over the full 12 weeks to reduce your craving for nicotine.
- Remember that it takes practice to do anything, and quitting smoking is no exception.

WHEN THE STRUGGLE IS OVER

Once you've stopped smoking, take a second and pat yourself on the back. Now do it again. You deserve it. Remember now why you decided to stop smoking in the first place. Look at your list of reasons. Read them again. And smile. Now think about all the money you are saving and what you'll do with it. All the non-smoking places you can go, and what you might do there. All those years you may have added to your life, and what you'll do with them. Remember that temptation may not be gone forever. However, the hard part is behind you, so look forward with a positive attitude and enjoy your new life as a non-smoker.

QUESTIONS & ANSWERS

1. How will I feel when I stop smoking and start using Nicorette? You'll need to prepare yourself for some nicotine withdrawal symptoms. These begin almost immediately after you stop smoking, and are usually at their worst during the first three to four days. Understand that any of the following is possible:

- craving for cigarettes
- anxiety, irritability, restlessness, mood changes, nervousness
- drowsiness
- trouble concentrating
- increased appetite and weight gain
- headaches, muscular pain, constipation, fatigue.

Nicorette can help provide relief from withdrawal symptoms such as irritability and nervousness, as well as the craving for nicotine you used to satisfy by having a cigarette.

2. Is Nicorette just substuting one form of nicotine for another? Nicorette does contain nicotine. The purpose of Nicorette is to provide you with enough nicotine to help control the physical withdrawal symptoms so you can deal with the mental aspects of quitting. During the 12 week program, you will gradually reduce your nicotine intake by switching to fewer pieces each day. Remember, don't use Nicorette together with nicotine patches or other nicotine containing products.

3. Can I be hurt by using Nicorette? For most adults, the amount of nicotine in the gum is less than from smoking. Some people will be sensitive to even this amount of nicotine and should not use this product without advice from their doctor. Because Nicorette is a gum-based product, chewing it can cause dental fillings to loosen and aggravate other mouth, tooth and jaw problems. Nicorette can also cause hiccups, heartburn and other stomach problems especially if chewed too quickly or not chewed correctly.

4. Will I gain weight? Many people do tend to gain a few pounds in the first 8–10 weeks after they stop smoking. This is a very small price to pay for the enormous gains that you will make in your overall health and attractiveness. If you continue to gain weight after the first two months, try to analyze what you're doing differently. Reduce your fat intake, choose healthy snacks, and increase your physical activity to burn off the extra calories.

5. Is Nicorette more expensive than smoking? The total cost of Nicorette for the twelve week program is about equal to what a person who smokes one and a half packs of cigarettes a day would spend on cigarettes for the same period of time. Also use of Nicorette is only a short-term cost, while the cost of smoking is a long-term cost, because of the health problems smoking causes.

6. What if I slip up? Discard your cigarettes, forgive yourself and then get back on track. Don't consider yourself a failure or punish yourself. In fact, people who have already tried to quit are more likely to be successful the next time. **GOOD LUCK!**

[End User's Guide]

To remove the gum, tear off a single unit.
Peel off backing starting at corner with loose edge.
Push gum through foil.

Blister packaged for your protection. Do not use if individual seals are broken.

Manufactured by Pharmacia & Upjohn AB, Stockholm, Sweden for SmithKline Beecham Consumer Healthcare, LP Pittsburgh, PA 15230

Comments or Questions? Call 1-800-419-4766 weekdays. (10 a.m.–4:30 p.m. EST).

- **Not for sale to those under 18 years of age.**
- **Proof of age required.**
- **Not for sale in vending machines or from any source where proof of age cannot be verified.**

Nicorette Original and Mint are available in:
2 mg or 4 mg Starter kit*—108 pieces
2 mg or 4 mg Refill—48 pieces
*User's Guide and Audio Tape included in kit

OS-CAL® 250+D, 500+D **OTC**
calcium & vitamin D supplement
OS-CAL® 500 and 500 Chewable Tablets
calcium supplement
[*ahs 'kal*]

(See PDR For Dietary Supplements.)

SINGLET® **OTC**
[*sĭn 'glĕt*]
Pain Reliever-Fever Reducer/
Nasal Decongestant/Antihistamine

(See PDR For Nonprescription Drugs.)

TAGAMET HB 200® **OTC**
Cimetidine Tablets 200 mg/Acid Reducer
TAGAMET HB 200 **OTC**
Cimetidine Suspension 200 mg/Acid Reducer

(See PDR For Nonprescription Drugs)

TUMS® REGULAR, TUMS E-X®, & TUMS ULTRA® **OTC**
Antacid/Calcium Supplement Tablets

(See PDR For Nonprescription Drugs.)

SmithKline Beecham Pharmaceuticals

ONE FRANKLIN PLAZA
P.O. BOX 7929
PHILADELPHIA, PA 19101

For Medical Information Contact:
Medical Department
800-366-8900, ext. 5231

Questions should be directed to Product Information, 1-800-366-8900, ext. 5231.

PRODUCT CODE INDEX

Code	Product, Form and Strength
A30	*Albenza* Tablets 200 mg
189	*Augmentin* 125 mg Chewable Tablets
190	*Augmentin* 250 mg Chewable Tablets
A58	*Avandia* 2 mg Tablets
A59	*Avandia* 4 mg Tablets
A60	*Avandia* 8 mg Tablets
B27	*Bactroban* Cream
C44	*Compazine* Spansule Capsules 10 mg
C46	*Compazine* Spansule Capsules 15 mg
C60	*Compazine* Suppositories 2½ mg
C61	*Compazine* Suppositories 5 mg
C62	*Compazine* Suppositories 25 mg
C66	*Compazine* Tablets 5 mg
C67	*Compazine* Tablets 10 mg
V39	*Coreg* Tablets 3.125 mg
V40	*Coreg* Tablets 6.25 mg
V41	*Coreg* Tablets 12.5 mg
V42	*Coreg* Tablets 25 mg
E12	*Dexedrine* Spansule Capsules 5 mg
E13	*Dexedrine* Spansule Capsules 10 mg
E14	*Dexedrine* Spansule Capsules 15 mg
E19	*Dexedrine* Tablets 5 mg
J10	*Eskalith* Controlled Release Tablets 450 mg
H01	*Hycamtin* Injection 4 mg/5 mL
P15	*Paxil* Oral Suspension
P10	*Paxil* 10 mg Tablets
P11	*Paxil* 20 mg Tablets
P12	*Paxil* 30 mg Tablets
P13	*Paxil* 40 mg Tablets
R90	*Requip* Tablets 0.25 mg
R91	*Requip* Tablets 0.5 mg
R92	*Requip* Tablets 1 mg
R93	*Requip* Tablets 2 mg
R96	*Requip* Tablets 4 mg
R94	*Requip* Tablets 5 mg
S03	*Stelazine* Tablets 1 mg
S04	*Stelazine* Tablets 2 mg
S06	*Stelazine* Tablets 5 mg
S07	*Stelazine* Tablets 10 mg
T63	*Thorazine* Spansule Capsules 30 mg
T64	*Thorazine* Spansule Capsules 75 mg
T66	*Thorazine* Spansule Capsules 150 mg
T70	*Thorazine* Suppositories 25 mg
T71	*Thorazine* Suppositories 100 mg
T73	*Thorazine* Tablets 10 mg
T74	*Thorazine* Tablets 25 mg
T76	*Thorazine* Tablets 50 mg
T77	*Thorazine* Tablets 100 mg
T79	*Thorazine* Tablets 200 mg

ALBENZA™ ℞

[al-ben´-za]
brand of albendazole Tablets

DESCRIPTION

Albenza (albendazole) is an orally administered broad-spectrum anthelmintic. Chemically it is Methyl 5-(propylthio)-2-benzimidazolecarbamate. Its molecular formula is $C_{12}H_{15}N_3O_2S$. Its molecular weight is 265.34. It has the following chemical structure:

albendazole

Albendazole is a white to off-white powder. It is soluble in dimethylsulfoxide, strong acids and strong bases. It is slightly soluble in methanol, chloroform, ethyl acetate and acetonitrile. Albendazole is practically insoluble in water. Each white to off-white, film-coated tablet contains 200 mg of albendazole.

Inactive ingredients consist of: carnauba wax, hydroxypropyl methylcellulose, lactose monohydrate, magnesium stearate, microcrystalline cellulose, povidone, sodium lauryl sulfate, sodium saccharin, sodium starch glycolate, and starch.

CLINICAL PHARMACOLOGY

Pharmacokinetics

Absorption and Metabolism

Albendazole is poorly absorbed from the gastrointestinal tract due to its low aqueous solubility. Albendazole concentrations are negligible or undetectable in plasma as it is rapidly converted to the sulfoxide metabolite prior to reaching the systemic circulation. The systemic anthelmintic activity has been attributed to the primary metabolite, albendazole sulfoxide. Oral bioavailability appears to be enhanced when albendazole is coadministered with a fatty meal (estimated fat content 40 g) as evidenced by higher (up to 5-fold on average) plasma concentrations of albendazole sulfoxide as compared to the fasted state.

Maximal plasma concentrations of albendazole sulfoxide are typically achieved 2 to 5 hours after dosing and are on average 1.31 mcg/mL (range 0.46 to 1.58 mcg/mL) following oral doses of albendazole (400 mg) in six hydatid disease patients, when administered with a fatty meal. Plasma concentrations of albendazole sulfoxide increase in a dose-proportional manner over the therapeutic dose range following ingestion of a fatty meal (fat content 43.1 g). The mean apparent terminal elimination half-life of albendazole sulfoxide typically ranges from 8 to 12 hours in twenty-five normal subjects, as well as in fourteen hydatid and eight neurocysticercosis patients.

Following 4 weeks of treatment with albendazole (200 mg three times daily), twelve patients' plasma concentrations of albendazole sulfoxide were approximately 20% lower than those observed during the first half of the treatment period, suggesting that albendazole may induce its own metabolism.

Distribution

Albendazole sulfoxide is 70% bound to plasma protein and is widely distributed throughout the body; it has been detected in urine, bile, liver, cyst wall, cyst fluid, and cerebral spinal fluid (CSF). Concentrations in plasma were 3- to 10-fold and 2- to 4-fold higher than those simultaneously determined in cyst fluid and CSF, respectively. Limited *in vitro* and clinical data suggest that albendazole sulfoxide may be eliminated from cysts at a slower rate than observed in plasma.

Metabolism and Excretion

Albendazole is rapidly converted in the liver to the primary metabolite, albendazole sulfoxide, which is further metabolized to albendazole sulfone and other primary oxidative metabolites that have been identified in human urine. Following oral administration, albendazole has not been detected in human urine. Urinary excretion of albendazole sulfoxide is a minor elimination pathway with less than 1% of the dose recovered in the urine. Biliary elimination presumably accounts for a portion of the elimination as evidenced by biliary concentrations of albendazole sulfoxide similar to those achieved in plasma.

Special Populations

Patients with Impaired Renal Function: The pharmacokinetics of albendazole in patients with impaired renal function has not been studied. However, since renal elimination of albendazole and its primary metabolite, albendazole sulfoxide, is negligible, it is unlikely that clearance of these compounds would be altered in these patients.

Biliary Effects: In patients with evidence of extrahepatic obstruction (n=5), the systemic availability of albendazole sulfoxide was increased, as indicated by a 2-fold increase in maximum serum concentration and a 7-fold increase in area under the curve. The rate of absorption/conversion and elimination of albendazole sulfoxide appeared to be prolonged with mean T_{max} and serum elimination half-life values of 10 hours and 31.7 hours, respectively. Plasma concentrations of parent albendazole were measurable in only one of five patients.

Pediatrics: Following single-dose administration of 200 mg to 300 mg (approximately 10 mg/kg) albendazole to three fasted and two fed pediatric patients with hydatid cyst disease (age range 6 to 13 years), albendazole sulfoxide pharmacokinetics were similar to those observed in fed adults.

Elderly Patients: Although no studies have investigated the effect of age on albendazole sulfoxide pharmacokinetics, data in twenty-six hydatid cyst patients (up to 79 years) suggest pharmacokinetics similar to those in young healthy subjects.

Microbiology

The principal mode of action for albendazole is by its inhibitory effect on tubulin polymerization which results in the loss of cytoplasmic microtubules.

In the specified treatment indications albendazole appears to be active against the larval forms of the following organisms:

Echinococcus granulosus
Taenia solium

INDICATIONS AND USAGE

Albenza (albendazole) is indicated for the treatment of the following infections:

Neurocysticercosis. *Albenza* is indicated for the treatment of parenchymal neurocysticercosis due to active lesions caused by larval forms of the pork tapeworm, *Taenia solium.*

Lesions considered responsive to albendazole therapy appear as nonenhancing cysts with no surrounding edema on contrast-enhanced computerized tomography. Clinical studies in patients with lesions of this type demonstrate a 74% to 88% reduction in number of cysts; 40% to 70% of albendazole-treated patients showed resolution of all active cysts.

Hydatid disease. *Albenza* is indicated for the treatment of cystic hydatid disease of the liver, lung, and peritoneum, caused by the larval form of the dog tapeworm, *Echinococcus granulosus.*

This indication is based on combined clinical studies which demonstrated non-infectious cyst contents in approximately 80–90% of patients given *Albenza* for 3 cycles of therapy of 28 days each. (See **DOSAGE AND ADMINISTRATION.**) Clinical cure (disappearance of cysts) was seen in approximately 30% of these patients, and improvement (reduction in cyst diameter of ≥25%) was seen in an additional 40%.

NOTE: When medically feasible, surgery is considered the treatment of choice for hydatid disease. When administering *Albenza* in the pre- or post-surgical setting, optimal killing of cyst contents is achieved when three courses of therapy have been given.

NOTE: The efficacy of albendazole in the therapy of alveolar hydatid disease caused by *Echinococcus multilocularis* has not been clearly demonstrated in clinical studies.

CONTRAINDICATIONS

Albenza (albendazole) is contraindicated in patients with known hypersensitivity to the benzimidazole class of compounds or any components of *Albenza.*

WARNINGS

Rare fatalities associated with the use of *Albenza* have been reported due to granulocytopenia or pancytopenia. (See **PRECAUTIONS.**) Blood counts should be monitored at the beginning of each 28-day cycle of therapy, and every 2 weeks while on therapy with albendazole. Albendazole may be continued if the total white blood cell count and absolute neutrophil count decrease appear modest and do not progress. Albendazole should not be used in pregnant women except in clinical circumstances where no alternative management is appropriate. Patients should not become pregnant for at least 1 month following cessation of albendazole therapy. If a patient becomes pregnant while taking this drug, albendazole should be discontinued immediately. If pregnancy occurs while taking this drug, the patient should be apprised of the potential hazard to the fetus.

PRECAUTIONS

General: Patients being treated for neurocysticercosis should receive appropriate steroid and anticonvulsant therapy as required. Oral or intravenous corticosteroids should be considered to prevent cerebral hypertensive episodes during the first week of anticysticeral therapy.

Cysticercosis may, in rare cases, involve the retina. Before initiating therapy for neurocysticercosis, the patient should be examined for the presence of retinal lesions. If such lesions are visualized, the need for anticysticeral therapy should be weighed against the possibility of retinal damage caused by albendazole-induced changes to the retinal lesion.

Information for Patients

Patients should be advised that:

- Albendazole may cause fetal harm, therefore, women of childbearing age should begin treatment after a negative pregnancy test.
- Women of childbearing age should be cautioned against becoming pregnant while on albendazole or within 1 month of completing treatment.
- During albendazole therapy, because of the possibility of harm to the liver or bone marrow, routine (every 2 weeks) monitoring of blood counts and liver function tests should take place.
- Albendazole should be taken with food.

Laboratory Tests

White Blood Cell Count: Albendazole has been shown to cause occasional (less than 1% of treated patients) reversible reductions in total white blood cell count. Rarely, more significant reductions may be encountered including granulocytopenia, agranulocytosis, or pancytopenia. Blood counts should be performed at the start of each 28-day treatment cycle and every 2 weeks during each 28-day cycle. Albendazole may be continued if the total white blood cell count decrease appears modest and does not progress.

Liver Function: In clinical trials, treatment with albendazole has been associated with mild to moderate elevations of hepatic enzymes in approximately 16% of patients. These have returned to normal upon discontinuation of therapy.

Liver function tests (transaminases) should be performed before the start of each treatment cycle and at least every 2 weeks during treatment. If enzymes are significantly increased, albendazole therapy should be discontinued. Therapy can be reinstituted when liver enzymes have returned to pretreatment levels, but laboratory tests should be performed frequently during repeat therapy.

Patients with abnormal liver function test results prior to commencing albendazole therapy should be carefully evaluated, since the drug is metabolized by the liver and has been associated with hepatotoxicity in a few patients.

Theophylline: Although single doses of albendazole have been shown not to inhibit theophylline metabolism (see **Drug Interactions**), albendazole does induce cytochrome P450 1A in human hepatoma cells. Therefore, it is recommended that plasma concentrations of theophylline be monitored during and after treatment with Albenza (albendazole).

Indication	Patient Weight	Dose	Duration
Hydatid Disease	60 kg or greater	400 mg b.i.d., with meals	28-day cycle followed by a 14-day albendazole-free interval, for a total of 3 cycles
	less than 60 kg	15 mg/kg/day given in divided doses b.i.d. with meals (maximum total daily dose 800 mg)	
	NOTE: When administering *Albenza* in the pre- or post-surgical setting, optimal killing of cyst contents is achieved when three courses of therapy have been given.		
Neurocysticercosis	60 kg or greater	400 mg b.i.d., with meals	8–30 days
	less than 60 kg	15 mg/kg/day given in divided doses b.i.d. with meals (maximum total daily dose 800 mg)	

Drug Interactions
Dexamethasone: Steady-state trough concentrations of albendazole sulfoxide were about 56% higher when 8 mg dexamethasone was coadministered with each dose of albendazole (15 mg/kg/day) in eight neurocysticercosis patients.
Praziquantel: In the fed state, praziquantel (40 mg/kg) increased mean maximum plasma concentration and area under the curve of albendazole sulfoxide by about 50% in healthy subjects (n=10) compared with a separate group of subjects (n=6) given albendazole alone. Mean T_{max} and mean plasma elimination half-life of albendazole sulfoxide were unchanged. The pharmacokinetics of praziquantel were unchanged following coadministration with albendazole (400 mg).
Cimetidine: Albendazole sulfoxide concentrations in bile and cystic fluid were increased (about 2-fold) in hydatid cyst patients treated with cimetidine (10 mg/kg/day) (n=7) compared with albendazole (20 mg/kg/day) alone (n=12). Albendazole sulfoxide plasma concentrations were unchanged 4 hours after dosing.
Theophylline: The pharmacokinetics of theophylline (aminophylline 5.8 mg/kg infused over 20 minutes) were unchanged following a single oral dose of albendazole (400 mg) in 6 healthy subjects.
Carcinogenesis, Mutagenesis, Impairment of Fertility
Long-term carcinogenicity studies were conducted in mice and rats. In the mouse study, albendazole was administered in the diet at doses of 25, 100 and 400 mg/kg/day (0.1, 0.5, and 2 times the recommended human dose based on body surface area in mg/m^2, respectively) for 108 weeks. In the rat study, albendazole was administered in the diet at doses of 3.5, 7, and 20 mg/kg/day (0.04, 0.08, and 0.21 times the recommended human dose based on body surface area in mg/m^2, respectively) for 117 weeks. There was no evidence of increased incidence of tumors in the treated mice and rats when compared to the control group.
In genotoxicity tests, albendazole was found negative in an Ames Salmonella/Microsome Plate mutation assay with and without metabolic activation or with and without pre-incubation, cell-mediated Chinese Hamster Ovary chromosomal aberration test and *in vivo* mouse micronucleus test. In the *in vitro* BALB/3T3 cells transformation assay, albendazole produced weak activity in the presence of metabolic activation while no activity was found in the absence of metabolic activation.
Albendazole did not adversely affect male or female fertility in the rat at an oral dose of 30 mg/kg/day (0.32 times the recommended human dose based on body surface area in mg/m^2).
Pregnancy
Teratogenic Effects—Pregnancy Category C: Albendazole has been shown to be teratogenic (to cause embryotoxicity and skeletal malformations) in pregnant rats and rabbits. The teratogenic response in the rat was shown at oral doses of 10 and 30 mg/kg/day (0.10 times and 0.32 times the recommended human dose based on body surface area in mg/m^2, respectively) during gestation days 6 to 15 and in pregnant rabbits at oral doses of 30 mg/kg/day (0.60 times the recommended human dose based on body surface area in mg/m^2) administered during gestation days 7 to 19. In the rabbit study, maternal toxicity (33% mortality) was noted at 30 mg/kg/day. In mice, no teratogenic effects were observed at oral doses up to 30 mg/kg/day (0.16 times the recommended human dose based on body surface area in mg/m^2), administered during gestation days 6 to 15.
There are no adequate and well-controlled studies of albendazole administration in pregnant women. Albendazole should be used during pregnancy only if the potential benefit justifies the potential risk to the fetus. (See **WARNINGS**.)
Nursing Mothers: Albendazole is excreted in animal milk. It is not known whether it is excreted in human milk. Because many drugs are excreted in human milk, caution should be exercised when albendazole is administered to a nursing woman.
Pediatric Use: Experience in children under the age of 6 years is limited. In hydatid disease, infection in infants and young children is uncommon, but no problems have been encountered in those who have been treated. In neurocysticercosis, infection is more frequently encountered. In five published studies involving pediatric patients as young as 1 year, no significant problems were encountered, and the efficacy appeared similar to the adult population.
Geriatric Use: Experience in patients 65 years of age or older is limited. The number of patients treated for either hydatid disease or neurocysticercosis is limited, but no problems associated with an older population have been observed.

ADVERSE REACTIONS

The adverse event profile of albendazole differs between hydatid disease and neurocysticercosis. Adverse events occurring with a frequency of ≥1% in either disease are described in the table below.
These symptoms were usually mild and resolved without treatment. Treatment discontinuations were predominantly due to leukopenia (0.7%) or hepatic abnormalities (3.8% in hydatid disease). The following incidence reflects events that were reported by investigators to be at least possibly or probably related to albendazole.

Adverse Event Incidence ≥1% in Hydatid Disease and Neurocysticercosis

Adverse Event	Hydatid Disease	Neurocysticercosis
Abnormal Liver Function Tests	15.6	<1.0
Abdominal Pain	6.0	0
Nausea/Vomiting	3.7	6.2
Headache	1.3	11.0
Dizziness/Vertigo	1.2	<1.0
Raised Intracranial Pressure	0	1.5
Meningeal Signs	0	1.0
Reversible Alopecia	1.6	<1.0
Fever	1.0	0

The following adverse events were observed at an incidence of <1%:
Hematologic: Leukopenia. There have been rare reports of granulocytopenia, pancytopenia, agranulocytosis, or thrombocytopenia. (See **WARNINGS.**)
Dermatologic: Rash, urticaria.
Hypersensitivity: Allergic reactions.
Renal: Acute renal failure related to albendazole therapy has been observed.

OVERDOSAGE

Significant toxicity and mortality were shown in male and female mice at doses exceeding 5,000 mg/kg; in rats, at estimated doses between 1,300 and 2,400 mg/kg; in hamsters, at doses exceeding 10,000 mg/kg; and in rabbits, at estimated doses between 500 and 1,250 mg/kg. In the animals, symptoms were demonstrated in a dose-response relationship and included diarrhea, vomiting, tachycardia, and respiratory distress.
One overdosage has been reported with Albenza (albendazole) in a patient who took at least 16 grams over 12 hours. No untoward effects were reported. In case of overdosage, symptomatic therapy (e.g., gastric lavage and activated charcoal) and general supportive measures are recommended.

DOSAGE AND ADMINISTRATION

Dosing of *Albenza* will vary, depending upon which of the following parasitic infections is being treated.
[See table at top of page]
Patients being treated for neurocysticercosis should receive appropriate steroid and anticonvulsant therapy as required. Oral or intravenous corticosteroids should be considered to prevent cerebral hypertensive episodes during the first week of treatment.

HOW SUPPLIED

Albenza (albendazole) is supplied as 200 mg, white to off-white, circular, biconvex, bevel-edged, film-coated Tiltab® tablets in bottles of 112.
NDC 0007-5500-40 .... Bottles of 112
Store between 20° and 25°C (68° and 77°F).
AL:L1
Shown in Product Identification Guide, page 336

AMOXIL® ℞

[ă-mŏx-ĭl]
brand of amoxicillin capsules, tablets, chewable tablets, and powder for oral suspension

DESCRIPTION

Amoxil formulations contain amoxicillin, a semisynthetic antibiotic, an analog of ampicillin, with a broad spectrum of bactericidal activity against many gram-positive and gram-negative microorganisms. Chemically it is (2*S*,5*R*,6*R*)-6-[(*R*)-(-)-2-amino-2-(*p*-hydroxyphenyl)acetamido]-3,3-dimethyl-7-oxo-4-thia-1-azabicyclo[3.2.0]heptane-2-carboxylic acid trihydrate. It may be represented structurally as:

The amoxicillin molecular formula is $C_{16}H_{19}N_3O_5S \cdot 3H_2O$, and the molecular weight is 419.45.
Amoxil capsules, tablets, and powder for oral suspension are intended for oral administration.
Capsules: Each *Amoxil* capsule, with royal blue opaque cap and pink opaque body, contains 250 mg or 500 mg amoxicillin as the trihydrate. The cap and body of the 250-mg capsule are imprinted with the product name AMOXIL and 250; the cap and body of the 500-mg capsule are imprinted with AMOXIL and 500. Inactive ingredients: D&C Red No. 28, FD&C Blue No. 1, FD&C Red No. 40, gelatin, magnesium stearate, and titanium dioxide.
Tablets: Each tablet contains 500 mg or 875 mg amoxicillin as the trihydrate. Each film-coated, capsule-shaped, pink tablet is debossed with AMOXIL centered over 500 or 875, respectively. The 875-mg tablet is scored on the reverse side. Inactive ingredients: colloidal silicon dioxide, crospovidone, FD&C Red No. 30 aluminum lake, hydroxypropyl methylcellulose, magnesium stearate, microcrystalline cellulose, polyethylene glycol, sodium starch glycolate, and titanium dioxide.
Chewable Tablets: Each cherry-banana-peppermint-flavored tablet contains 125 mg, 200 mg, 250 mg or 400 mg amoxicillin as the trihydrate. The 125-mg and 250-mg pink, oval tablets are imprinted with the product name AMOXIL on one side and 125 or 250 on the other side. Inactive ingredients: citric acid, corn starch, FD&C Red No. 40, flavorings, glycine, mannitol, magnesium stearate, saccharin sodium, silica gel, and sucrose. Each 125-mg chewable tablet contains 0.0019 mEq (0.044 mg) of sodium; the 250-mg chewable tablet contains 0.0037 mEq (0.085 mg) of sodium. Each 200-mg chewable tablet contains 0.0005 mEq (0.0107 mg) of sodium; the 400-mg chewable tablet contains 0.0009 mEq (0.0215 mg) of sodium. The 200-mg and 400-mg pale pink round tablets are imprinted with the product name AMOXIL and 200 or 400 along the edge of one side. Inactive ingredients: aspartame•, crospovidone NF, FD&C Red No. 40 aluminum lake, flavorings, magnesium stearate and mannitol.
•See **PRECAUTIONS.**
Powder for Oral Suspension: Each 5 mL of reconstituted suspension contains 125 mg, 200 mg, 250 mg or 400 mg amoxicillin as the trihydrate. Each 5 mL of the 125-mg reconstituted suspension contains 0.11 mEq (2.51 mg) of sodium; each 5 mL of the 250-mg reconstituted suspension contains 0.15 mEq (3.36 mg) of sodium. Each 5 mL of the 200-mg reconstituted suspension contains 0.15 mEq (3.39 mg) of sodium; each 5 mL of the 400-mg reconstituted suspension contains 0.19 mEq (4.33 mg) of sodium.
Pediatric Drops for Oral Suspension: Each mL of reconstituted suspension contains 50 mg amoxicillin as the trihydrate and 0.03 mEq (0.69 mg) of sodium.
Amoxicillin trihydrate for oral suspension 125 mg/5 mL (reconstituted) is a strawberry-flavored pink suspension; the 200 mg/5 mL, 250 mg/5 mL (or 50 mg/mL), and 400 mg/5 mL are bubble-gum-flavored pink suspensions. Inactive ingredients: FD&C Red No. 3, flavorings, silica gel, sodium benzoate, sodium citrate, sucrose, and xanthan gum.

CLINICAL PHARMACOLOGY

Amoxicillin is stable in the presence of gastric acid and is rapidly absorbed after oral administration. The effect of food

Continued on next page

Information on the SmithKline Beecham Pharmaceuticals products appearing here is based on the labeling in effect on June 15, 2000. Further information on these and other products may be obtained from the Medical Department, SmithKline Beecham Pharmaceuticals, One Franklin Plaza, Philadelphia, PA 19101.

Amoxil—Cont.

on the absorption of amoxicillin from *Amoxil* tablets and *Amoxil* suspension has been partially investigated. The 400-mg and 875-mg formulations have been studied only when administered at the start of a light meal. However, food effect studies have not been performed with the 200-mg and 500-mg formulations. Amoxicillin diffuses readily into most body tissues and fluids, with the exception of brain and spinal fluid, except when meninges are inflamed. The half-life of amoxicillin is 61.3 minutes. Most of the amoxicillin is excreted unchanged in the urine; its excretion can be delayed by concurrent administration of probenecid. In blood serum, amoxicillin is approximately 20% protein-bound.

Orally administered doses of 250 mg and 500 mg amoxicillin capsules result in average peak blood levels 1 to 2 hours after administration in the range of 3.5 µg/mL to 5.0 µg/mL and 5.5 µg/mL to 7.5 µg/mL, respectively.

Mean amoxicillin pharmacokinetic parameters from an open, two-part, single-dose crossover bioequivalence study in 27 adults comparing 875 mg of Amoxil (amoxicillin) with 875 mg of Augmentin® (amoxicillin/clavulanate potassium) showed that the 875-mg tablet of *Amoxil* produces an $AUC_{0-\infty}$ of 35.4 ± 8.1 µg.hr./mL and a C_{max} of 13.8 ± 4.1 µg/mL. Dosing was at the start of a light meal following an overnight fast.

Amoxicillin chewable tablets, 125 mg and 250 mg, produced blood levels similar to those achieved with the corresponding doses of amoxicillin oral suspensions. Orally administered doses of amoxicillin suspension, 125 mg/5 mL and 250 mg/5 mL, result in average peak blood levels 1 to 2 hours after administration in the range of 1.5 µg/mL to 3.0 µg/mL and 3.5 µg/mL to 5.0 µg/mL, respectively.

Oral administration of single doses of 400-mg *Amoxil* chewable tablets and 400-mg/5 mL suspension to 24 adult volunteers yielded comparable pharmacokinetic data:

Dose†	$AUC_{0-\infty}$ (ug.hr./mL)	C_{max} (ug/mL)‡
amoxicillin	amoxicillin (±S.D.)	amoxicillin (±S.D.)
400 mg (5 mL of suspension)	17.1 (3.1)	5.92 (1.62)
400 mg (one chewable tablet)	17.9 (2.4)	5.18 (1.64)

† Administered at the start of a light meal.
‡ Mean values of 24 normal volunteers. Peak concentrations occurred approximately 1 hour after the dose.

Detectable serum levels are observed up to 8 hours after an orally administered dose of amoxicillin. Following a 1-gram dose and utilizing a special skin window technique to determine levels of the antibiotic, it was noted that therapeutic levels were found in the interstitial fluid. Approximately 60% of an orally administered dose of amoxicillin is excreted in the urine within 6 to 8 hours.

Microbiology

Amoxicillin is similar to ampicillin in its bactericidal action against susceptible organisms during the stage of active multiplication. It acts through the inhibition of biosynthesis of cell wall mucopeptide. Amoxicillin has been shown to be active against most strains of the following microorganisms, both *in vitro* and in clinical infections as described in the **INDICATIONS AND USAGE** section.

Aerobic gram-positive microorganisms:

Enterococcus faecalis
Staphylococcus spp.† (β-lactamase-negative strains only)
Streptococcus pneumoniae
Streptococcus spp. (α- and β-hemolytic strains only)

† Staphylococci which are susceptible to amoxicillin but resistant to methicillin/oxacillin should be considered as resistant to amoxicillin.

Aerobic gram-negative microorganisms:

Escherichia coli (β-lactamase-negative strains only)
Haemophilus influenzae (β-lactamase-negative strains only)
Neisseria gonorrhoeae (β-lactamase-negative strains only)
Proteus mirabilis (β-lactamase-negative strains only)

Helicobacter:

Helicobacter pylori

Susceptibility tests

Dilution techniques: Quantitative methods are used to determine antimicrobial minimum inhibitory concentrations (MICs). These MICs provide estimates of the susceptibility of bacteria to antimicrobial compounds. The MICs should be determined using a standardized procedure. Standardized procedures are based on a dilution method[1] (broth or agar) or equivalent with standardized inoculum concentrations and standardized concentrations of **ampicillin** powder. Ampicillin is sometimes used to predict susceptibility of *Streptococcus pneumoniae* to amoxicillin; however, some intermediate strains have been shown to be susceptible to amoxicillin. Therefore, *Streptococcus pneumoniae* susceptibility should be tested using amoxicillin powder. The MIC values should be interpreted according to the following criteria:

For gram-positive aerobes:

Enterococcus

MIC (µg/mL)	Interpretation
≤8	Susceptible (S)
≥16	Resistant (R)

Staphylococcus[a]

MIC (µg/mL)	Interpretation
≤ 0.25	Susceptible (S)
≥0.5	Resistant (R)

Streptococcus (except *S. pneumoniae*)

MIC (µg/mL)	Interpretation
≤0.25	Susceptible (S)
0.5 to 4	Intermediate (I)
≥8	Resistant (R)

S. pneumoniae[b]
(**Amoxicillin** powder should be used to determine susceptibility.)

MIC (µg/mL)	Interpretation
≤0.5	Susceptible (S)
1	Intermediate (I)
≥2	Resistant (R)

For gram-negative aerobes:

Enterobacteriaceae

MIC (µg/mL)	Interpretation
≤8	Susceptible (S)
16	Intermediate (I)
≥32	Resistant (R)

H. influenzae[c]

MIC (µg/mL)	Interpretation
≤1	Susceptible (S)
2	Intermediate (I)
≥4	Resistant (R)

a. Staphylococci which are susceptible to amoxicillin but resistant to methicillin/oxacillin should be considered as resistant to amoxicillin.
b. These interpretive standards are applicable only to broth microdilution susceptibility tests using cation-adjusted Mueller-Hinton broth with 2–5% lysed horse blood.
c. These interpretive standards are applicable only to broth microdilution test with *Haemophilus influenzae* using *Haemophilus* Test Medium (HTM).[1]

A report of "Susceptible" indicates that the pathogen is likely to be inhibited if the antimicrobial compound in the blood reaches the concentrations usually achievable. A report of "Intermediate" indicates that the result should be considered equivocal, and, if the microorganism is not fully susceptible to alternative, clinically feasible drugs, the test should be repeated. This category implies possible clinical applicability in body sites where the drug is physiologically concentrated or in situations where high dosage of drug can be used. This category also provides a buffer zone which prevents small uncontrolled technical factors from causing major discrepancies in interpretation. A report of "Resistant" indicates that the pathogen is not likely to be inhibited if the antimicrobial compound in the blood reaches the concentrations usually achievable; other therapy should be selected.

Standardized susceptibility test procedures require the use of laboratory control microorganisms to control the technical aspects of the laboratory procedures. Standard **ampicillin** powder should provide the following MIC values:

Microorganism	MIC (µg/mL)
E. coli ATCC 25922	2 to 8
E. faecalis ATCC 29212	0.5 to 2
H. influenzae ATCC 49247[d]	2 to 8
S. aureus ATCC 29213	0.25 to 1

Using **amoxicillin** to determine susceptibility:

Microorganism	MIC Range (µg/mL)
S. pneumoniae ATCC 49619[e]	0.03 to 0.12

d. This quality control range is applicable to only *H. influenzae* ATCC 49247 tested by a broth microdilution procedure using HTM.[1]
e. This quality control range is applicable to only *S. pneumoniae* ATCC 49619 tested by the broth microdilution procedure using cation-adjusted Mueller-Hinton broth with 2–5% lysed horse blood.

Diffusion techniques: Quantitative methods that require measurement of zone diameters also provide reproducible estimates of the susceptibility of bacteria to antimicrobial compounds. One such standardized procedure[2] requires the use of standardized inoculum concentrations. This procedure uses paper disks impregnated with 10 µg ampicillin to test the susceptibility of microorganisms, except *S. pneumoniae*, to amoxicillin. Interpretation involves correlation of the diameter obtained in the disk test with the MIC for **ampicillin**.

Reports from the laboratory providing results of the standard single-disk susceptibility test with a 10-µg ampicillin disk should be interpreted according to the following criteria:

For gram-positive aerobes:

Enterococcus

Zone Diameter (mm)	Interpretation
≥17	Susceptible (S)
≤16	Resistant (R)

Staphylococcus[f]

Zone Diameter (mm)	Interpretation
≥29	Susceptible (S)
≤28	Resistant (R)

β-hemolytic streptococci

Zone Diameter (mm)	Interpretation
≥26	Susceptible (S)
19 to 25	Intermediate (I)
≤18	Resistant (R)

NOTE: For streptococci (other than β-hemolytic streptococci and *S. pneumoniae*), an ampicillin MIC should be determined.

S. pneumoniae
S. pneumoniae should be tested using a 1-µg oxacillin disk. Isolates with oxacillin zone sizes of ≥20 mm are susceptible to amoxicillin. An amoxicillin MIC should be determined on isolates of *S. pneumoniae* with oxacillin zone sizes of ≤19 mm.

For gram-negative aerobes:

Enterobacteriaceae

Zone Diameter (mm)	Interpretation
≥17	Susceptible (S)
14 to 16	Intermediate (I)
≤13	Resistant (R)

H. influenzae[g]

Zone Diameter (mm)	Interpretation
≥22	Susceptible (S)
19 to 21	Intermediate (I)
≤18	Resistant (R)

f. Staphylococci which are susceptible to amoxicillin but resistant to methicillin/oxacillin should be considered as resistant to amoxicillin.
g. These interpretive standards are applicable only to disk diffusion susceptibility tests with *H. influenzae* using *Haemophilus* Test Medium (HTM).[2]

Interpretation should be as stated above for results using dilution techniques.

As with standard dilution techniques, disk diffusion susceptibility test procedures require the use of laboratory control microorganisms. The 10-µg **ampicillin** disk should provide the following zone diameters in these laboratory test quality control strains:

Microorganism	Zone diameter (mm)
E. coli ATCC 25922	16 to 22
H. influenzae ATCC 49247[h]	13 to 21
S. aureus ATCC 25923	27 to 35

Using 1-µg **oxacillin** disk:

Microorganism	Zone diameter (mm)
S. pneumoniae ATCC 49619[i]	8 to 12

h. This quality control range is applicable to only *H. influenzae* ATCC 49247 tested by a disk diffusion procedure using HTM.[2]
i. This quality control range is applicable to only *S. pneumoniae* ATCC 49619 tested by a disk diffusion procedure using Mueller-Hinton agar supplemented with 5% sheep blood and incubated in 5% CO_2.

Susceptibility testing for *Helicobacter pylori*

In vitro susceptibility testing methods and diagnostic products currently available for determining minimum inhibitory concentrations (MICs) and zone sizes have not been standardized, validated, or approved for testing *H. pylori* microorganisms.

Culture and susceptibility testing should be obtained in patients who fail triple therapy. If clarithromycin resistance is found, a non-clarithromycin-containing regimen should be used.

INDICATIONS AND USAGE

Amoxil (amoxicillin) is indicated in the treatment of infections due to susceptible (ONLY β-lactamase-negative) strains of the designated microorganisms in the conditions listed below:

Infections of the ear, nose, and throat due to *Streptococcus* spp. (α- and β-hemolytic strains only), *Streptococcus pneumoniae, Staphylococcus* spp., or *H. influenzae*

Infections of the genitourinary tract due to *E. coli, P. mirabilis*, or *E. faecalis*

Infections of the skin and skin structure due to *Streptococcus* spp. (α- and β-hemolytic strains only), *Staphylococcus* spp., or *E. coli*

Infections of the lower respiratory tract due to *Streptococcus* spp. (α- and β-hemolytic strains only), *Streptococcus pneumoniae, Staphylococcus* spp., or *H. influenzae*

Gonorrhea, acute uncomplicated (ano-genital and urethral infections) due to *N. gonorrhoeae* (males and females)

Therapy may be instituted prior to obtaining results from bacteriological and susceptibility studies to determine the causative organisms and their susceptibility to amoxicillin. Indicated surgical procedures should be performed.

H. pylori eradication to reduce the risk of duodenal ulcer recurrence

Triple therapy: *Amoxil*/clarithromycin/lansoprazole

Amoxil, in combination with clarithromycin plus lansoprazole as triple therapy, is indicated for the treatment of patients with *H. pylori* infection and duodenal ulcer disease (active or one-year history of a duodenal ulcer) to eradicate *H. pylori*. Eradication of *H. pylori* has been shown to reduce the risk of duodenal ulcer recurrence. (See **CLINICAL STUDIES** and **DOSAGE AND ADMINISTRATION**.)

Dual therapy: *Amoxil*/lansoprazole
Amoxil (amoxicillin), in combination with lansoprazole delayed-release capsules as dual therapy, is indicated for the treatment of patients with *H. pylori* infection and duodenal ulcer disease (active or one-year history of a duodenal ulcer) **who are either allergic or intolerant to clarithromycin or in whom resistance to clarithromycin is known or suspected.** (See the clarithromycin package insert, **MICROBIOLOGY.**) Eradication of *H. pylori* has been shown to reduce the risk of duodenal ulcer recurrence. (See **CLINICAL STUDIES** and **DOSAGE AND ADMINISTRATION.**)

CONTRAINDICATIONS

A history of allergic reaction to any of the penicillins is a contraindication.

WARNINGS

SERIOUS AND OCCASIONALLY FATAL HYPERSENSITIVITY (ANAPHYLACTIC) REACTIONS HAVE BEEN REPORTED IN PATIENTS ON PENICILLIN THERAPY. ALTHOUGH ANAPHYLAXIS IS MORE FREQUENT FOLLOWING PARENTERAL THERAPY, IT HAS OCCURRED IN PATIENTS ON ORAL PENICILLINS. THESE REACTIONS ARE MORE LIKELY TO OCCUR IN INDIVIDUALS WITH A HISTORY OF PENICILLIN HYPERSENSITIVITY AND/OR A HISTORY OF SENSITIVITY TO MULTIPLE ALLERGENS. THERE HAVE BEEN REPORTS OF INDIVIDUALS WITH A HISTORY OF PENICILLIN HYPERSENSITIVITY WHO HAVE EXPERIENCED SEVERE REACTIONS WHEN TREATED WITH CEPHALOSPORINS. BEFORE INITIATING THERAPY WITH *AMOXIL*, CAREFUL INQUIRY SHOULD BE MADE CONCERNING PREVIOUS HYPERSENSITIVITY REACTIONS TO PENICILLINS, CEPHALOSPORINS, OR OTHER ALLERGENS. IF AN ALLERGIC REACTION OCCURS, *AMOXIL* SHOULD BE DISCONTINUED AND APPROPRIATE THERAPY INSTITUTED. **SERIOUS ANAPHYLACTIC REACTIONS REQUIRE IMMEDIATE EMERGENCY TREATMENT WITH EPINEPHRINE. OXYGEN, INTRAVENOUS STEROIDS, AND AIRWAY MANAGEMENT, INCLUDING INTUBATION, SHOULD ALSO BE ADMINISTERED AS INDICATED.**
Pseudomembranous colitis has been reported with nearly all antibacterial agents, including amoxicillin, and may range in severity from mild to life-threatening. Therefore, it is important to consider this diagnosis in patients who present with diarrhea subsequent to the administration of antibacterial agents.
Treatment with antibacterial agents alters the normal flora of the colon and may permit overgrowth of clostridia. Studies indicate that a toxin produced by *Clostridium difficile* is a primary cause of "antibiotic-associated colitis."
After the diagnosis of pseudomembranous colitis has been established, appropriate therapeutic measures should be initiated. Mild cases of pseudomembranous colitis usually respond to drug discontinuation alone. In moderate to severe cases, consideration should be given to management with fluids and electrolytes, protein supplementation, and treatment with an antibacterial drug clinically effective against *Clostridium difficile* colitis.

PRECAUTIONS

General: The possibility of superinfections with mycotic or bacterial pathogens should be kept in mind during therapy. If superinfections occur, amoxicillin should be discontinued and appropriate therapy instituted.
Phenylketonurics: Each 200 mg *Amoxil* chewable tablet contains 1.82 mg phenylalanine; each 400 mg chewable tablet contains 3.64 mg phenylalanine. The *Amoxil* suspensions do not contain phenylalanine and can be used by phenylketonurics.
Laboratory Tests: As with any potent drug, periodic assessment of renal, hepatic, and hematopoietic function should be made during prolonged therapy.
All patients with gonorrhea should have a serologic test for syphilis at the time of diagnosis. Patients treated with amoxicillin should have a follow-up serologic test for syphilis after 3 months.
Drug Interactions: Probenecid decreases the renal tubular secretion of amoxicillin. Concurrent use of amoxicillin and probenecid may result in increased and prolonged blood levels of amoxicillin.
Chloramphenicol, macrolides, sulfonamides, and tetracyclines may interfere with the bactericidal effects of penicillin. This has been demonstrated *in vitro*; however, the clinical significance of this interaction is not well documented.
Drug/Laboratory Test Interactions: High urine concentrations of ampicillin may result in false-positive reactions when testing for the presence of glucose in urine using Clinitest®, Benedict's Solution or Fehling's Solution. Since this effect may also occur with amoxicillin, it is recommended that glucose tests based on enzymatic glucose oxidase reactions (such as Clinistix® or Tes-Tape®) be used.
Following administration of ampicillin to pregnant women, a transient decrease in plasma concentration of total conjugated estriol, estriol-glucuronide, conjugated estrone, and estradiol has been noted. This effect may also occur with amoxicillin.
Carcinogenesis, Mutagenesis, Impairment of Fertility: Long-term studies in animals have not been performed to evaluate carcinogenic potential. Studies to detect mutagenic potential of amoxicillin alone have not been conducted; however, the following information is available from tests on a 4:1 mixture of amoxicillin and potassium clavulanate (*Augmentin*). *Augmentin* was non-mutagenic in the Ames bacterial mutation assay, and the yeast gene conversion assay. *Augmentin* was weakly positive in the mouse lymphoma assay, but the trend toward increased mutation frequencies in this assay occurred at doses that were also associated with decreased cell survival. *Augmentin* was negative in the mouse micronucleus test, and in the dominant lethal assay in mice. Potassium clavulanate alone was tested in the Ames bacterial mutation assay and in the mouse micronucleus test, and was negative in each of these assays. In a multi-generation reproduction study in rats, no impairment of fertility or other adverse reproductive effects were seen at doses up to 500 mg/kg (approximately 3 times the human dose in mg/m^2).
Pregnancy: *Teratogenic Effects. Pregnancy Category B.* Reproduction studies have been performed in mice and rats at doses up to ten (10) times the human dose and have revealed no evidence of impaired fertility or harm to the fetus due to amoxicillin. There are, however, no adequate and well-controlled studies in pregnant women. Because animal reproduction studies are not always predictive of human response, this drug should be used during pregnancy only if clearly needed.
Labor and Delivery: Oral ampicillin-class antibiotics are poorly absorbed during labor. Studies in guinea pigs showed that intravenous administration of ampicillin slightly decreased the uterine tone and frequency of contractions but moderately increased the height and duration of contractions. However, it is not known whether use of amoxicillin in humans during labor or delivery has immediate or delayed adverse effects on the fetus, prolongs the duration of labor, or increases the likelihood that forceps delivery or other obstetrical intervention or resuscitation of the newborn will be necessary.
Nursing Mothers: Penicillins have been shown to be excreted in human milk. Amoxicillin use by nursing mothers may lead to sensitization of infants. Caution should be exercised when amoxicillin is administered to a nursing woman.
Pediatric Use: Because of incompletely developed renal function in neonates and young infants, the elimination of amoxicillin may be delayed. Dosing of Amoxil (amoxicillin) should be modified in pediatric patients 12 weeks or younger (≤3 months). (See **DOSAGE AND ADMINISTRATION**-Neonates and infants.)

ADVERSE REACTIONS

As with other penicillins, it may be expected that untoward reactions will be essentially limited to sensitivity phenomena. They are more likely to occur in individuals who have previously demonstrated hypersensitivity to penicillins and in those with a history of allergy, asthma, hay fever, or urticaria. The following adverse reactions have been reported as associated with the use of penicillins:
Gastrointestinal: nausea, vomiting, diarrhea, and hemorrhagic/pseudomembranous colitis.
Onset of pseudomembranous colitis symptoms may occur during or after antibiotic treatment. (See **WARNINGS**.)
Hypersensitivity Reactions: Serum sickness like reactions, erythematous maculopapular rashes, erythema multiforme, Stevens-Johnson Syndrome, exfoliative dermatitis, toxic epidermal necrolysis, hypersensitivity vasculitis and urticaria have been reported.
NOTE: These hypersensitivity reactions may be controlled with antihistamines and, if necessary, systemic corticosteroids. Whenever such reactions occur, amoxicillin should be discontinued unless, in the opinion of the physician, the condition being treated is life-threatening and amenable only to amoxicillin therapy.
Liver: A moderate rise in AST (SGOT) and/or ALT (SGPT) has been noted, but the significance of this finding is unknown. Hepatic dysfunction including cholestatic jaundice, hepatic cholestasis and acute cytolytic hepatitis have been reported.
Hemic and Lymphatic Systems: Anemia, including hemolytic anemia, thrombocytopenia, thrombocytopenic purpura, eosinophilia, leukopenia, and agranulocytosis have been reported during therapy with penicillins. These reactions are usually reversible on discontinuation of therapy and are believed to be hypersensitivity phenomena.
Central Nervous System: Reversible hyperactivity, agitation, anxiety, insomnia, confusion, convulsions, behavioral changes, and/or dizziness have been reported rarely.
Combination therapy with clarithromycin and lansoprazole
In clinical trials using combination therapy with amoxicillin plus clarithromycin and lansoprazole, and amoxicillin plus lansoprazole, no adverse reactions peculiar to these drug combinations were observed. Adverse reactions that have occurred have been limited to those that had been previously reported with amoxicillin, clarithromycin, or lansoprazole.
Triple therapy: amoxicillin/clarithromycin/lansoprazole
The most frequently reported adverse events for patients who received triple therapy were diarrhea (7%), headache (6%), and taste perversion (5%). No treatment-emergent adverse events were observed at significantly higher rates with triple therapy than with any dual therapy regimen.
Dual therapy: amoxicillin/lansoprazole
The most frequently reported adverse events for patients who received amoxicillin t.i.d. plus lansoprazole t.i.d. dual therapy were diarrhea (8%) and headache (7%). No treatment-emergent adverse events were observed at significantly higher rates with amoxicillin t.i.d. plus lansoprazole t.i.d. dual therapy than with lansoprazole alone.
For more information on adverse reactions with clarithromycin or lansoprazole, refer to their package inserts, **ADVERSE REACTIONS.**

OVERDOSAGE

In case of overdosage, discontinue medication, treat symptomatically, and institute supportive measures as required. If the overdosage is very recent and there is no contraindication, an attempt at emesis or other means of removal of drug from the stomach may be performed. A prospective study of 51 pediatric patients at a poison-control center suggested that overdosages of less than 250 mg/kg of amoxicillin are not associated with significant clinical symptoms and do not require gastric emptying.[3]
Interstitial nephritis resulting in oliguric renal failure has been reported in a small number of patients after overdosage with amoxicillin. Renal impairment appears to be reversible with cessation of drug administration. High blood levels may occur more readily in patients with impaired renal function because of decreased renal clearance of amoxicillin. Amoxicillin may be removed from circulation by hemodialysis.

DOSAGE AND ADMINISTRATION

Amoxil capsules, chewable tablets and oral suspensions may be given without regard to meals. The 400-mg suspension, 400-mg chewable tablet and the 875-mg tablet have been studied only when administered at the start of a light meal. However, food effect studies have not been performed with the 200-mg and 500-mg formulations.
Neonates and infants aged ≤12 weeks (≤3 months)
Due to incompletely developed renal function affecting elimination of amoxicillin in this age group, the recommended upper dose of Amoxil (amoxicillin) is 30 mg/kg/day divided q12h.
[See table at top of next page]
After reconstitution, the required amount of suspension should be placed directly on the child's tongue for swallowing. Alternate means of administration are to add the required amount of suspension to formula, milk, fruit juice, water, ginger ale, or cold drinks. These preparations should then be taken immediately. To be certain the child is receiving full dosage, such preparations should be consumed in entirety.
All patients with gonorrhea should be evaluated for syphilis. (See **PRECAUTIONS** - Laboratory Tests.)
Larger doses may be required for stubborn or severe infections.
General: It should be recognized that in the treatment of chronic urinary tract infections, frequent bacteriological and clinical appraisals are necessary. Smaller doses than those recommended above should not be used. Even higher doses may be needed at times. In stubborn infections, therapy may be required for several weeks. It may be necessary to continue clinical and/or bacteriological follow-up for several months after cessation of therapy. Except for gonorrhea, treatment should be continued for a minimum of 48 to 72 hours beyond the time that the patient becomes asymptomatic or evidence of bacterial eradication has been obtained. It is recommended that there be at least 10 days' treatment for any infection caused by *Streptococcus pyogenes* to prevent the occurrence of acute rheumatic fever.
H. pylori eradication to reduce the risk of duodenal ulcer recurrence
Triple therapy: Amoxil/*clarithromycin/lansoprazole*
The recommended adult oral dose is 1 gram *Amoxil*, 500 mg clarithromycin, and 30 mg lansoprazole, all given twice daily (q12h) for 14 days. (See **INDICATIONS AND USAGE.**)
Dual therapy: Amoxil/*lansoprazole*
The recommended adult oral dose is 1 gram Amoxil (amoxicillin) and 30 mg lansoprazole, each given three times daily (q8h) for 14 days. (See **INDICATIONS AND USAGE.**)
Please refer to clarithromycin and lansoprazole full prescribing information for **CONTRAINDICATIONS** and **WARNINGS**, and for information regarding dosing in elderly and renally impaired patients.
Dosing recommendations for adults with impaired renal function:
Patients with impaired renal function do not generally require a reduction in dose unless the impairment is severe. Severely impaired patients with a glomerular filtration rate of <30 mL/minute should not receive the 875-mg tablet. Patients with a glomerular filtration rate of 10 to 30 mL/minute should receive 500 mg or 250 mg every 12 hours, depending on the severity of the infection. Patients with a

Continued on next page

Information on the SmithKline Beecham Pharmaceuticals products appearing here is based on the labeling in effect on June 15, 2000. Further information on these and other products may be obtained from the Medical Department, SmithKline Beecham Pharmaceuticals, One Franklin Plaza, Philadelphia, PA 19101.

Amoxil—Cont.

less than 10 mL/minute glomerular filtration rate should receive 500 mg or 250 mg every 24 hours, depending on severity of the infection.

Hemodialysis patients should receive 500 mg or 250 mg every 24 hours, depending on severity of the infection. They should receive an additional dose both during and at the end of dialysis.

There are currently no dosing recommendations for pediatric patients with impaired renal function.

Directions For Mixing Oral Suspension

Prepare suspension at time of dispensing as follows: Tap bottle until all powder flows freely. Add approximately 1/3 of the total amount of water for reconstitution (see table below) and shake vigorously to wet powder. Add remainder of the water and again shake vigorously.

125 mg/5 mL

Bottle Size	Amount of Water Required for Reconstitution
80 mL	62 mL
100 mL	78 mL
150 mL	116 mL

Each teaspoonful (5 mL) will contain 125 mg amoxicillin.

200 mg/5 mL

Bottle Size	Amount of Water Required for Reconstitution
5 mL	5 mL
50 mL	39 mL
75 mL	57 mL
100 mL	76 mL

Each teaspoonful (5 mL) will contain 200 mg amoxicillin.

250 mg/5 mL

Bottle Size	Amount of Water Required for Reconstitution
80 mL	59 mL
100 mL	74 mL
150 mL	111 mL

Each teaspoonful (5 mL) will contain 250 mg amoxicillin.

400 mg/5 mL

Bottle Size	Amount of Water Required for Reconstitution
5 mL	5 mL
50 mL	36 mL
75 mL	54 mL
100 mL	71 mL

Each teaspoonful (5 mL) will contain 400 mg amoxicillin.

Directions For Mixing Pediatric Drops

Prepare pediatric drops at time of dispensing as follows: Add the required amount of water (see table below) to the bottle and shake vigorously. Each mL of suspension will then contain amoxicillin trihydrate equivalent to 50 mg amoxicillin.

Bottle Size	Amount of Water Required for Reconstitution
15 mL	12 mL
30 mL	23 mL

NOTE: SHAKE BOTH ORAL SUSPENSION AND PEDIATRIC DROPS WELL BEFORE USING. Keep bottle tightly closed. Any unused portion of the reconstituted suspension must be discarded after 14 days. Refrigeration preferable, but not required.

HOW SUPPLIED

Amoxil (amoxicillin) Capsules. Each capsule contains 250 mg or 500 mg amoxicillin as the trihydrate.

250-mg Capsule

NDC 0029-6006-30	bottles of 100
NDC 0029-6006-32	bottles of 500

500-mg Capsule

NDC 0029-6007-30	bottles of 100
NDC 0029-6007-32	bottles of 500

Amoxil (amoxicillin) Tablets. Each tablet contains 500 mg or 875 mg amoxicillin as the trihydrate.

500-mg Tablet

NDC 0029-6046-12	bottles of 20
NDC 0029-6046-20	bottles of 100
NDC 0029-6046-25	bottles of 500

875-mg Tablet

NDC 0029-6047-12	bottles of 20
NDC 0029-6047-20	bottles of 100
NDC 0029-6047-25	bottles of 500

Amoxil (amoxicillin) Chewable Tablets. Each cherry-banana-peppermint-flavored tablet contains 125 mg, 200 mg, 250 mg or 400 mg amoxicillin as the trihydrate.

125-mg Tablet

NDC 0029-6004-39	bottles of 60

200-mg Tablet

NDC 0029-6044-12	bottles of 20
NDC 0029-6044-20	bottles of 100

250-mg Tablet

NDC 0029-6005-13	bottles of 30
NDC 0029-6005-30	bottles of 100

400-mg Tablet

NDC 0029-6045-12	bottles of 20
NDC 0029-6045-20	bottles of 100

Amoxil (amoxicillin) for Oral Suspension. Each 5 mL of reconstituted strawberry-flavored suspension contains 125

Adults and pediatric patients >3 months

Infection	Severity‡	Usual Adult Dose	Usual Dose for Children >3 months§ ‖
Ear/nose/throat	Mild/Moderate	500 mg every 12 hours or 250 mg every 8 hours	25 mg/kg/day in divided doses every 12 hours **or** 20 mg/kg/day in divided doses every 8 hours
	Severe	875 mg every 12 hours or 500 mg every 8 hours	45 mg/kg/day in divided doses every 12 hours **or** 40 mg/kg/day in divided doses every 8 hours
Lower respiratory tract	Mild/Moderate or Severe	875 mg every 12 hours or 500 mg every 8 hours	45 mg/kg/day in divided doses every 12 hours **or** 40 mg/kg/day in divided doses every 8 hours
Skin/skin structure	Mild/Moderate	500 mg every 12 hours or 250 mg every 8 hours	25 mg/kg/day in divided doses every 12 hours **or** 20 mg/kg/day in divided doses every 8 hours
	Severe	875 mg every 12 hours or 500 mg every 8 hours	45 mg/kg/day in divided doses every 12 hours **or** 40 mg/kg/day in divided doses every 8 hours
Genitourinary tract	Mild/Moderate	500 mg every 12 hours or 250 mg every 8 hours	25 mg/kg/day in divided doses every 12 hours **or** 20 mg/kg/day in divided doses every 8 hours
	Severe	875 mg every 12 hours or 500 mg every 8 hours	45 mg/kg/day in divided doses every 12 hours **or** 40 mg/kg/day in divided doses every 8 hours
Gonorrhea Acute, uncomplicated ano-genital and urethral infections in males and females		3 grams as single oral dose	<u>Prepubertal</u> children: 50 mg/kg *Amoxil,* combined with 25 mg/kg probenecid as a single dose. **NOTE: SINCE PROBENECID IS CONTRAINDICATED IN CHILDREN UNDER 2 YEARS, DO NOT USE THIS REGIMEN IN THESE CASES.**

‡ Dosing for infections caused by less susceptible organisms should follow the recommendations for severe infections.

§ The children's dosage is intended for individuals whose weight is less than 40 kg. Children weighing 40 kg or more should be dosed according to the adult recommendations.

‖ Each strength of *Amoxil* suspension is available as a chewable tablet for use by older children.

mg amoxicillin as the trihydrate. Each 5 mL of reconstituted bubble-gum-flavored suspension contains 200, 250, or 400 mg amoxicillin as the trihydrate.

125 mg/5 mL

NDC 0029-6008-21	80-mL bottle
NDC 0029-6008-23	100-mL bottle
NDC 0029-6008-22	150-mL bottle

200 mg/5 mL

NDC 0029-6048-54	50-mL bottle
NDC 0029-6048-55	75-mL bottle
NDC 0029-6048-59	100-mL bottle

250 mg/5 mL

NDC 0029-6009-21	80-mL bottle
NDC 0029-6009-23	100-mL bottle
NDC 0029-6009-22	150-mL bottle

400 mg/5 mL

NDC 0029-6049-54	50-mL bottle
NDC 0029-6049-55	75-mL bottle
NDC 0029-6049-59	100-mL bottle

NDC 0029-6048-18	**200-mg unit dose bottle**
NDC 0029-6049-18	**400-mg unit dose bottle**

Amoxil (amoxicillin) Pediatric Drops for Oral Suspension. Each mL of bubble-gum-flavored reconstituted suspension contains 50 mg amoxicillin as the trihydrate.

NDC 0029-6035-20	15-mL bottle
NDC 0029-6038-39	30-mL bottle

Store capsules, unreconstituted powder, and 125-mg and 250-mg chewable tablets at or below 20° C (68° F). The 200-mg and 400-mg chewable tablets may be stored at or below 25° C (77° F). Store 500-mg and 875-mg tablets at or below 25° C (77° F). Dispense in a tight container.

CLINICAL STUDIES

<u>*H. pylori* eradication to reduce the risk of duodenal ulcer recurrence</u>

Randomized, double-blind clinical studies performed in the U.S. in patients with *H. pylori* and duodenal ulcer disease (defined as an active ulcer or history of an ulcer within one year) evaluated the efficacy of lansoprazole in combination with amoxicillin capsules and clarithromycin tablets as triple 14-day therapy, or in combination with amoxicillin capsules as dual 14-day therapy, for the eradication of *H. pylori.* Based on the results of these studies, the safety and efficacy of two different eradication regimens were established:

Triple therapy: amoxicillin 1 gram b.i.d./clarithromycin 500 mg b.i.d./lansoprazole 30 mg b.i.d.

Dual therapy: amoxicillin 1 gram t.i.d./lansoprazole 30 mg t.i.d.

All treatments were for 14 days. *H. pylori* eradication was defined as two negative tests (culture and histology) at 4 to 6 weeks following the end of treatment.

Triple therapy was shown to be more effective than all possible dual therapy combinations. Dual therapy was shown to be more effective than both monotherapies. Eradication of *H. pylori* has been shown to reduce the risk of duodenal ulcer recurrence.

H. pylori Eradication Rates - Triple Therapy (amoxicillin/clarithromycin/lansoprazole) Percent of Patients Cured [95% Confidence Interval] (Number of Patients)		
	Triple Therapy	Triple Therapy
Study	Evaluable Analysis†	Intent-to-Treat Analysis‡
Study 1	92§ [80.0–97.7] (n=48)	86§ [73.3–93.5] (n=55)
Study 2	86 ‖ [75.7–93.6] (n=66)	83 ‖ [72.0–90.8] (n=70)

† This analysis was based on evaluable patients with confirmed duodenal ulcer (active or within one year) and *H. pylori* infection at baseline defined as at least two of three positive endoscopic tests from CLOtest®, (Delta West Ltd., Bentley, Australia), histology and/or culture. Patients were included in the analysis if they completed the study. Additionally, if patients dropped out of the study due to an adverse event related to the study drug, they were included in the analysis as failures of therapy.

‡ Patients were included in the analysis if they had documented *H. pylori* infection at baseline as defined above and had a confirmed duodenal ulcer (active or within one year). All dropouts were included as failures of therapy.

§ ($p<0.05$) versus lansoprazole/amoxicillin and lansoprazole/clarithromycin dual therapy.

‖ ($p<0.05$) versus clarithromycin/amoxicillin dual therapy.

H. pylori Eradication Rates - Dual Therapy (amoxicillin/lansoprazole) Percent of Patients Cured [95% Confidence Interval] (Number of Patients)		
	Dual Therapy	Dual Therapy
Study	Evaluable Analysis¶	Intent-to-Treat Analysis††
Study 1	77‡‡ [62.5–87.2] (n=51)	70‡‡ [56.8–81.2] (n=60)
Study 2	66§§ [51.9–77.5] (n=58)	61§§ [48.5–72.9] (n=67)

¶ This analysis was based on evaluable patients with confirmed duodenal ulcer (active or within one year) and *H. pylori* infection at baseline defined as at least two of three positive endoscopic tests from CLOtest®, histology and/or culture. Patients were included in the analysis if they completed the study. Additionally, if patients dropped out of the study due to an adverse event related to the study drug, they were included in the analysis as failures of therapy.

†† Patients were included in the analysis if they had documented *H. pylori* infection at baseline as defined above and had a confirmed duodenal ulcer (active or within one year). All dropouts were included as failures of therapy.

‡‡ ($p<0.05$) versus lansoprazole alone.

§§ ($p<0.05$) versus lansoprazole alone or amoxicillin alone.

REFERENCES

1. National Committee for Clinical Laboratory Standards. Methods for Dilution Antimicrobial Susceptibility Tests for Bacteria that Grow Aerobically - Fourth Edition; Approved Standard. NCCLS Document M7-A4, Vol. 17, No. 2. NCCLS, Wayne, PA, January 1997.
2. National Committee for Clinical Laboratory Standards. Performance Standards for Antimicrobial Disk Susceptibility Tests - Sixth Edition; Approved Standard. NCCLS Document M2-A6, Vol. 17, No. 1. NCCLS, Wayne, PA, January 1997.
3. Swanson-Biearman B, Dean BS, Lopez G, Krenzelok EP. The effects of penicillin and cephalosporin ingestions in children less than six years of age. *Vet Hum Toxicol* 1988;30:66-67.

Rx only

SmithKline Beecham Pharmaceuticals
Philadelphia, PA 19101
AM:L19

Shown in Product Identification Guide, page 336

ANCEF® ℞

[an-sef']

(brand of sterile cefazolin for injection and cefazolin injection)

DESCRIPTION

Ancef (cefazolin for injection) is a semi-synthetic cephalosporin for parenteral administration. It is the sodium salt of 3-{[(5-methyl-1, 3, 4-thiadiazol-2-yl) thio]-methyl}-8-oxo-7-[2-(1H-tetrazol-1-yl) acetamido] -5- thia-1-azabicyclo [4.2.0] oct-2-ene-2-carboxylic acid.

The sodium content is 48 mg per gram of cefazolin.

Ancef in lyophilized form is supplied in vials equivalent to 500 mg or 1 gram of cefazolin; in "Piggyback" Vials for intravenous admixture equivalent to 1 gram of cefazolin; and in Pharmacy Bulk Vials equivalent to 10 grams of cefazolin.

Ancef is also supplied as a frozen, sterile, nonpyrogenic solution of cefazolin sodium in an iso-osmotic diluent in plastic containers. After thawing, the solution is intended for intravenous use.

The plastic container is fabricated from a specially designed multilayer plastic, PL 2040. Solutions are in contact with the polyethylene layer of this container and can leach out certain of the chemical components of the plastic in very small amounts within the expiration period. However, the suitability of the plastic has been confirmed in tests in animals according to the USP biological tests for plastic containers as well as by tissue culture toxicity studies.

CLINICAL PHARMACOLOGY

Human Pharmacology: After intramuscular administration of *Ancef* to normal volunteers, the mean serum concentrations were 37 mcg/mL at 1 hour and 3 mcg/mL at 8 hours following a 500 mg dose, and 64 mcg/mL at 1 hour and 7 mcg/mL at 8 hours following a 1 gram dose.

Studies have shown that following intravenous administration of *Ancef* to normal volunteers, mean serum concentrations peaked at approximately 185 mcg/mL and were approximately 4 mcg/mL at 8 hours for a 1 gram dose.

The serum half-life for *Ancef* is approximately 1.8 hours following I.V. administration and approximately 2.0 hours following I.M. administration.

In a study (using normal volunteers) of constant intravenous infusion with dosages of 3.5 mg/kg for 1 hour (approximately 250 mg) and 1.5 mg/kg the next 2 hours (approximately 100 mg), *Ancef* produced a steady serum level at the third hour of approximately 28 mcg/mL.

Studies in patients hospitalized with infections indicate that Ancef (cefazolin for injection) produces mean peak serum levels approximately equivalent to those seen in normal volunteers.

Bile levels in patients without obstructive biliary disease can reach or exceed serum levels by up to five times; however, in patients with obstructive biliary disease, bile levels of *Ancef* are considerably lower than serum levels (< 1.0 mcg/mL).

In synovial fluid, the *Ancef* level becomes comparable to that reached in serum at about 4 hours after drug administration.

Studies of cord blood show prompt transfer of *Ancef* across the placenta. *Ancef* is present in very low concentrations in the milk of nursing mothers.

Ancef is excreted unchanged in the urine. In the first 6 hours approximately 60% of the drug is excreted in the urine and this increases to 70% to 80% within 24 hours. *Ancef* achieves peak urine concentrations of approximately 2400 mcg/mL and 4000 mcg/mL respectively following 500 mg and 1 gram intramuscular doses.

In patients undergoing peritoneal dialysis (2 l/hr.), *Ancef* produced mean serum levels of approximately 10 and 30 mcg/mL after 24 hours' instillation of a dialyzing solution containing 50 mg/l and 150 mg/l, respectively. Mean peak levels were 29 mcg/mL (range 13–44 mcg/mL) with 50 mg/l (three patients), and 72 mcg/mL (range 26–142 mcg/mL) with 150 mg/l (six patients). Intraperitoneal administration of *Ancef* is usually well tolerated.

Controlled studies on adult normal volunteers, receiving 1 gram 4 times a day for 10 days, monitoring CBC, SGOT, SGPT, bilirubin, alkaline phosphatase, BUN, creatinine and urinalysis, indicated no clinically significant changes attributed to *Ancef.*

Microbiology: *In vitro* tests demonstrate that the bactericidal action of cephalosporins results from inhibition of cell wall synthesis. Ancef (cefazolin for injection) is active against the following organisms *in vitro* and in clinical infections:

Staphylococcus aureus (including penicillinase-producing strains)
Staphylococcus epidermidis
Methicillin-resistant staphylococci are uniformly resistant to cefazolin
Group A beta-hemolytic streptococci and other strains of streptococci (many strains of enterococci are resistant)
Streptococcus pneumoniae
Escherichia coli
Proteus mirabilis
Klebsiella species
Enterobacter aerogenes
Haemophilus influenzae

Most strains of indole positive Proteus (*Proteus vulgaris*), *Enterobacter cloacae, Morganella morganii* and *Providencia rettgeri* are resistant. *Serratia, Pseudomonas, Mima, Herellea* species are almost uniformly resistant to cefazolin.

Disk Susceptibility Tests

Disk diffusion technique—Quantitative methods that require measurement of zone diameters give the most precise estimates of antibiotic susceptibility. One such procedure[1] has been recommended for use with disks to test susceptibility to cefazolin.

Reports from a laboratory using the standardized single-disk susceptibility test[1] with a 30 mcg cefazolin disk should be interpreted according to the following criteria:

Susceptible organisms produce zones of 18 mm or greater, indicating that the tested organism is likely to respond to therapy.

Organisms of intermediate susceptibility produce zones 15 to 17 mm, indicating that the tested organism would be susceptible if high dosage is used or if the infection is confined to tissues and fluids (e.g., urine), in which high antibiotic levels are attained.

Resistant organisms produce zones of 14 mm or less, indicating that other therapy should be selected.

1 Bauer, A.W.; Kirby, W.M.M.; Sherris, J.C., and Turck, M.: Antibiotic Testing by a Standardized Single Disc Method, Am. J. Clin. Path. 45:493, 1966. Standardized Disc Susceptibility Test, Federal Register 39:19182-19184, 1974.

For gram-positive isolates, a zone of 18 mm is indicative of a cefazolin-susceptible organism when tested with either the cephalosporin-class disk (30 mcg cephalothin) or the cefazolin disk (30 mcg cefazolin).

Gram-negative organisms should be tested with the cefazolin disk (using the above criteria), since cefazolin has been shown by *in vitro* tests to have activity against certain strains of *Enterobacteriaceae* found resistant when tested with the cephalothin disk. Gram-negative organisms having zones of less than 18 mm around the cephalothin disk may be susceptible to cefazolin.

Standardized procedures require use of control organisms. The 30 mcg cefazolin disk should give zone diameter between 23 and 29 mm for *E. coli* ATCC 25922 and between 29 and 35 mm for *S. aureus* ATCC 25923.

The cefazolin disk should not be used for testing susceptibility to other cephalosporins.

Dilution techniques—A bacterial isolate may be considered susceptible if the minimal inhibitory concentration (MIC) for cefazolin is not more than 16 mcg per mL. Organisms are considered resistant if the MIC is equal to or greater than 64 mcg per mL.

The range of MIC's for the control strains are as follows:
S. aureus ATCC 25923, 0.25 to 1.0 mcg/mL
E. coli ATCC 25922, 1.0 to 4.0 mcg/mL

INDICATIONS AND USAGE

Ancef (cefazolin for injection) is indicated in the treatment of the following serious infections due to susceptible organisms:

RESPIRATORY TRACT INFECTIONS due to *Streptococcus pneumoniae, Klebsiella* species, *Haemophilus influenzae, Staphylococcus aureus* (penicillin-sensitive and penicillin-resistant) and group A beta-hemolytic streptococci.

Injectable benzathine penicillin is considered to be the drug of choice in treatment and prevention of streptococcal infections, including the prophylaxis of rheumatic fever.

Ancef is effective in the eradication of streptococci from the nasopharynx; however, data establishing the efficacy of *Ancef* in the subsequent prevention of rheumatic fever are not available at present.

URINARY TRACT INFECTIONS due to *Escherichia coli, Proteus mirabilis, Klebsiella* species and some strains of enterobacter and enterococci.

SKIN AND SKIN STRUCTURE INFECTIONS due to *Staphylococcus aureus* (penicillin-sensitive and penicillin-resistant), group A beta-hemolytic streptococci and other strains of streptococci.

BILIARY TRACT INFECTIONS due to *Escherichia coli,* various strains of streptococci, *Proteus mirabilis, Klebsiella* species and *Staphylococcus aureus.*

BONE AND JOINT INFECTIONS due to *Staphylococcus aureus.*

GENITAL INFECTIONS (i.e., prostatitis, epididymitis) due to *Escherichia coli, Proteus mirabilis, Klebsiella* species and some strains of enterococci.

SEPTICEMIA due to *Streptococcus pneumoniae, Staphylococcus aureus* (penicillin-sensitive and penicillin-resistant), *Proteus mirabilis, Escherichia coli* and *Klebsiella* species.

ENDOCARDITIS due to *Staphylococcus aureus* (penicillin-sensitive and penicillin-resistant) and group A beta-hemolytic streptococci.

Appropriate culture and susceptibility studies should be performed to determine susceptibility of the causative organism to *Ancef.*

PERIOPERATIVE PROPHYLAXIS: The prophylactic administration of *Ancef* preoperatively, intraoperatively and postoperatively may reduce the incidence of certain postoperative infections in patients undergoing surgical procedures which are classified as contaminated or potentially contaminated (e.g., vaginal hysterectomy, and cholecystectomy in high-risk patients such as those over 70 years of age, with acute cholecystitis, obstructive jaundice or common duct bile stones).

The perioperative use of *Ancef* may also be effective in surgical patients in whom infection at the operative site would present a serious risk (e.g., during open-heart surgery and prosthetic arthroplasty).

Continued on next page

Information on the SmithKline Beecham Pharmaceuticals products appearing here is based on the labeling in effect on June 15, 2000. Further information on these and other products may be obtained from the Medical Department, SmithKline Beecham Pharmaceuticals, One Franklin Plaza, Philadelphia, PA 19101.

Ancef—Cont.

The prophylactic administration of *Ancef* should usually be discontinued within a 24-hour period after the surgical procedure. In surgery where the occurrence of infection may be particularly devastating (e.g., open-heart surgery and prosthetic arthroplasty), the prophylactic administration of *Ancef* may be continued for 3 to 5 days following the completion of surgery.
If there are signs of infection, specimens for cultures should be obtained for the identification of the causative organism so that appropriate therapy may be instituted.
(See DOSAGE AND ADMINISTRATION.)

CONTRAINDICATIONS

ANCEF (CEFAZOLIN FOR INJECTION) IS CONTRAINDICATED IN PATIENTS WITH KNOWN ALLERGY TO THE CEPHALOSPORIN GROUP OF ANTIBIOTICS.

WARNINGS

BEFORE THERAPY WITH *ANCEF* IS INSTITUTED, CAREFUL INQUIRY SHOULD BE MADE TO DETERMINE WHETHER THE PATIENT HAS HAD PREVIOUS HYPERSENSITIVITY REACTIONS TO CEFAZOLIN, CEPHALOSPORINS, PENICILLINS, OR OTHER DRUGS. IF THIS PRODUCT IS GIVEN TO PENICILLIN-SENSITIVE PATIENTS, CAUTION SHOULD BE EXERCISED BECAUSE CROSS-HYPERSENSITIVITY AMONG BETA-LACTAM ANTIBIOTICS HAS BEEN CLEARLY DOCUMENTED AND MAY OCCUR IN UP TO 10% OF PATIENTS WITH A HISTORY OF PENICILLIN ALLERGY. IF AN ALLERGIC REACTION TO *ANCEF* OCCURS, DISCONTINUE TREATMENT WITH THE DRUG. SERIOUS ACUTE HYPERSENSITIVITY REACTIONS MAY REQUIRE TREATMENT WITH EPINEPHRINE AND OTHER EMERGENCY MEASURES, INCLUDING OXYGEN, IV FLUIDS, IV ANTIHISTAMINES, CORTICOSTEROIDS, PRESSOR AMINES AND AIRWAY MANAGEMENT, AS CLINICALLY INDICATED.

Pseudomembranous colitis has been reported with nearly all antibacterial agents, including cefazolin, and may range in severity from mild to life-threatening. Therefore, it is important to consider this diagnosis in patients who present with diarrhea subsequent to the administration of antibacterial agents.

Treatment with antibacterial agents alters the normal flora of the colon and may permit overgrowth of clostridia. Studies indicate that a toxin produced by *Clostridium difficile* is a primary cause of "antibiotic-associated colitis."

After the diagnosis of pseudomembranous colitis has been established, therapeutic measures should be initiated. Mild cases of pseudomembranous colitis usually respond to drug discontinuation alone. In moderate to severe cases, consideration should be given to management with fluids and electrolytes, protein supplementation and treatment with an oral antibacterial drug clinically effective against *C. difficile* colitis.

PRECAUTIONS

General—Prolonged use of Ancef (cefazolin for injection) may result in the overgrowth of nonsusceptible organisms. Careful clinical observation of the patient is essential.

When *Ancef* is administered to patients with low urinary output because of impaired renal function, lower daily dosage is required (see DOSAGE AND ADMINISTRATION).

As with other beta-lactam antibiotics, seizures may occur if inappropriately high doses are administered to patients with impaired renal function (see DOSAGE AND ADMINISTRATION).

Ancef, as with all cephalosporins, should be prescribed with caution in individuals with a history of gastrointestinal disease, particularly colitis.

Drug Interactions—Probenecid may decrease renal tubular secretion of cephalosporins when used concurrently, resulting in increased and more prolonged cephalosporin blood levels.

Drug/Laboratory Test Interactions—A false positive reaction for glucose in the urine may occur with Benedict's solution, Fehling's solution or with Clinitest® tablets, but not with enzyme-based tests such as Clinistix® and Tes-Tape®.

Positive direct and indirect antiglobulin (Coombs) tests have occurred; these may also occur in neonates whose mothers received cephalosporins before delivery.

Carcinogenesis/Mutagenesis — Mutagenicity studies and long-term studies in animals to determine the carcinogenic potential of Ancef (cefazolin for injection) have not been performed.

Pregnancy — Teratogenic Effects — Pregnancy Category B. Reproduction studies have been performed in rats, mice and rabbits at doses up to 25 times the human dose and have revealed no evidence of impaired fertility or harm to the fetus due to *Ancef*. There are, however, no adequate and well-controlled studies in pregnant women. Because animal reproduction studies are not always predictive of human response, this drug should be used during pregnancy only if clearly needed.

Labor and Delivery—When cefazolin has been administered prior to caesarean section, drug levels in cord blood have been approximately one quarter to one third of maternal drug levels. The drug appears to have no adverse effect on the fetus.

Nursing Mothers—Ancef (cefazolin for injection) is present in very low concentrations in the milk of nursing mothers. Caution should be exercised when *Ancef* is administered to a nursing woman.

Pediatric Use—Safety and effectiveness for use in premature infants and neonates have not been established. See DOSAGE AND ADMINISTRATION for recommended dosage in pediatric patients over 1 month.

The potential for the toxic effect in pediatric patients from chemicals that may leach from the single-dose I.V. preparation in plastic has not been determined.

ADVERSE REACTIONS

The following reactions have been reported:

Gastrointestinal: Diarrhea, oral candidiasis (oral thrush), vomiting, nausea, stomach cramps, anorexia and pseudomembranous colitis. Onset of pseudomembranous colitis symptoms may occur during or after antibiotic treatment (see WARNINGS). Nausea and vomiting have been reported rarely.

Allergic: Anaphylaxis, eosinophilia, itching, drug fever, skin rash, Stevens-Johnson syndrome.

Hematologic: Neutropenia, leukopenia, thrombocytopenia, thrombocythemia.

Hepatic and Renal: Transient rise in SGOT, SGPT, BUN and alkaline phosphatase levels has been observed without clinical evidence of renal or hepatic impairment.

Local Reactions: Rare instances of phlebitis have been reported at site of injection. Pain at the site of injection after intramuscular administration has occurred infrequently. Some induration has occurred.

Other Reactions: Genital and anal pruritus (including vulvar pruritus, genital moniliasis and vaginitis).

DOSAGE AND ADMINISTRATION

Usual Adult Dosage

Type of Infection	Dose	Frequency
Moderate to severe infections	500 mg to 1 gram	every 6 to 8 hrs.
Mild infections caused by susceptible gram + cocci	250 mg to 500 mg	every 8 hours
Acute, uncomplicated urinary tract infections	1 gram	every 12 hours
Pneumococcal pneumonia	500 mg	every 12 hours
Severe, life-threatening infections (e.g., endocarditis, septicemia)*	1 gram to 1.5 grams	every 6 hours

* In rare instances, doses of up to 12 grams of *Ancef* per day have been used.

Perioperative Prophylactic Use

To prevent postoperative infection in contaminated or potentially contaminated surgery, recommended doses are:

a. 1 gram I.V. or I.M. administered 1/2 hour to 1 hour prior to the start of surgery.
b. For lengthy operative procedures (e.g., 2 hours or more), 500 mg to 1 gram I.V. or I.M. during surgery (administration modified depending on the duration of the operative procedure).
c. 500 mg to 1 gram I.V. or I.M. every 6 to 8 hours for 24 hours postoperatively.

It is important that (1) the preoperative dose be given just (1/2 to 1 hour) prior to the start of surgery so that adequate antibiotic levels are present in the serum and tissues at the time of initial surgical incision; and (2) *Ancef* be administered, if necessary, at appropriate intervals during surgery to provide sufficient levels of the antibiotic at the anticipated moments of greatest exposure to infective organisms.

In surgery where the occurrence of infection may be particularly devastating (e.g., open-heart surgery and prosthetic arthroplasty), the prophylactic administration of Ancef (cefazolin for injection) may be continued for 3 to 5 days following the completion of surgery.

Dosage Adjustment for Patients with Reduced Renal Function

Ancef may be used in patients with reduced renal function with the following dosage adjustments: Patients with a creatinine clearance of 55 mL/min. or greater or a serum creatinine of 1.5 mg % or less can be given full doses. Patients with creatinine clearance rates of 35 to 54 mL/min. or serum creatinine of 1.6 to 3.0 mg % can also be given full doses but dosage should be restricted to at least 8 hour intervals. Patients with creatinine clearance rates of 11 to 34 mL/min. or serum creatinine of 3.1 to 4.5 mg % should be given 1/2 the usual dose every 12 hours. Patients with creatinine clearance rates of 10 mL/min. or less or serum creatinine of 4.6 mg % or greater should be given 1/2 the usual dose every 18 to 24 hours. All reduced dosage recommendations apply after an initial loading dose appropriate to the severity of the infection. Patients undergoing peritoneal dialysis: See Human Pharmacology.

Pediatric Dosage

In pediatric patients, a total daily dosage of 25 to 50 mg per kg (approximately 10 to 20 mg per pound) of body weight, divided into three or four equal doses, is effective for most mild to moderately severe infections. Total daily dosage may be increased to 100 mg per kg (45 mg per pound) of body weight for severe infections. Since safety for use in premature infants and in neonates has not been established, the use of Ancef (cefazolin for injection) in these patients is not recommended.

Pediatric Dosage Guide

Weight		25 mg/kg/Day Divided into 3 Doses		25 mg/kg/Day Divided into 4 Doses	
Lbs	Kg	Approximate Single Dose mg/q8h	Vol. (mL) needed with dilution of 125 mg/mL	Approximate Single Dose mg/q6h	Vol. (mL) needed with dilution of 125 mg/mL
10	4.5	40 mg	0.35 mL	30 mg	0.25 mL
20	9.0	75 mg	0.60 mL	55 mg	0.45 mL
30	13.6	115 mg	0.90 mL	85 mg	0.70 mL
40	18.1	150 mg	1.20 mL	115 mg	0.90 mL
50	22.7	190 mg	1.50 mL	140 mg	1.10 mL

Weight		50 mg/kg/Day Divided into 3 Doses		50 mg/kg/Day Divided into 4 Doses	
Lbs	Kg	Approximate Single Dose mg/q8h	Vol. (mL) needed with dilution of 225 mg/mL	Approximate Single Dose mg/q6h	Vol. (mL) needed with dilution of 225 mg/mL
10	4.5	75 mg	0.35 mL	55 mg	0.25 mL
20	9.0	150 mg	0.70 mL	110 mg	0.50 mL
30	13.6	225 mg	1.00 mL	170 mg	0.75 mL
40	18.1	300 mg	1.35 mL	225 mg	1.00 mL
50	22.7	375 mg	1.70 mL	285 mg	1.25 mL

In pediatric patients with mild to moderate renal impairment (creatinine clearance of 70 to 40 mL/min.), 60 percent of the normal daily dose given in equally divided doses every 12 hours should be sufficient. In patients with moderate impairment (creatinine clearance of 40 to 20 mL/min.), 25 percent of the normal daily dose given in equally divided doses every 12 hours should be adequate. Pediatric patients with severe renal impairment (creatinine clearance of 20 to 5 mL/min.) may be given 10 percent of the normal daily dose every 24 hours. All dosage recommendations apply after an initial loading dose.

RECONSTITUTION

Preparation of Parenteral Solution

Parenteral drug products should be SHAKEN WELL when reconstituted, and inspected visually for particulate matter prior to administration. If particulate matter is evident in reconstituted fluids, the drug solutions should be discarded. When reconstituted or diluted according to the instructions below, Ancef (cefazolin for injection) is stable for 24 hours at room temperature or for 10 days if stored under refrigeration (5°C or 41°F). Reconstituted solutions may range in color from pale yellow to yellow without a change in potency.

Single-Dose Vials

For I.M. injection, I.V. direct (bolus) injection or I.V. infusion, reconstitute with Sterile Water for Injection according to the following table. SHAKE WELL.

Vial Size	Amount of Diluent	Approximate Concentration	Approximate Available Volume
500 mg	2.0 mL	225 mg/mL	2.2 mL
1 gram	2.5 mL	330 mg/mL	3.0 mL

Pharmacy Bulk Vials

Add Sterile Water for Injection, Bacteriostatic Water for Injection or Sodium Chloride Injection according to the table below. SHAKE WELL.

Vial Size	Amount of Diluent	Approximate Concentration	Approximate Available Volume
10 grams	45 mL	1 gram/5 mL	51 mL
	96 mL	1 gram/10 mL	102 mL

"Piggyback" Vials

Reconstitute with 50 to 100 mL of Sodium Chloride Injection or other I.V. solution listed under ADMINISTRATION. When adding diluent to vial, allow air to escape by using a small vent needle or by pumping the syringe. SHAKE WELL. Administer with primary I.V. fluids, as a single dose.

ADMINISTRATION

Intramuscular Administration—Reconstitute vials with Sterile Water for Injection according to the dilution table above. Shake well until dissolved. *Ancef* should be injected into a large muscle mass. Pain on injection is infrequent with *Ancef*.

Intravenous Administration—Direct (bolus) injection: Following reconstitution according to the above table, further

dilute vials with approximately 5 mL Sterile Water for Injection. Inject the solution slowly over 3 to 5 minutes, directly or through tubing for patients receiving parenteral fluids (see list below).
Intermittent or continuous infusion: Dilute reconstituted *Ancef* in 50 to 100 mL of one of the following solutions:
- Sodium Chloride Injection, USP
- 5% or 10% Dextrose Injection, USP
- 5% Dextrose in Lactated Ringer's Injection, USP
- 5% Dextrose and 0.9% Sodium Chloride Injection, USP
- 5% Dextrose and 0.45% Sodium Chloride Injection, USP
- 5% Dextrose and 0.2% Sodium Chloride Injection, USP
- Lactated Ringer's Injection, USP
- Invert Sugar 5% or 10% in Sterile Water for Injection
- Ringer's Injection, USP
- 5% Sodium Bicarbonate Injection, USP

DIRECTIONS FOR USE OF ANCEF (CEFAZOLIN INJECTION) GALAXY® CONTAINER (PL 2040 PLASTIC)
Ancef in Galaxy® Container (PL 2040 Plastic) is to be administered either as a continuous or intermittent infusion using sterile equipment.
Storage
Store in a freezer capable of maintaining a temperature of −20°C.X(−4°F).
Thawing of Plastic Container
Thaw frozen container at 25°C or 77°F or under refrigeration (5°C or 41°F). (DO NOT FORCE THAW BY IMMERSION IN WATER BATHS OR BY MICROWAVE IRRADIATION.)
Check for minute leaks by squeezing container firmly. If leaks are detected, discard solution as sterility may be impaired.
Do not add supplementary medication.
The container should be visually inspected. Components of the solution may precipitate in the frozen state and will dissolve upon reaching room temperature with little or no agitation. Potency is not affected. Agitate after solution has reached room temperature. If after visual inspection the solution remains cloudy or if an insoluble precipitate is noted or if any seals or outlet ports are not intact, the container should be discarded.
The thawed solution is stable for 30 days under refrigeration (5°C or 41°F) and 48 hours at 25°C or 77°F. Do not refreeze thawed antibiotics.
Use sterile equipment. It is recommended that the intravenous administration apparatus be replaced at least once every 48 hours.
CAUTION: Do not use plastic containers in series connections. Such use could result in air embolism due to residual air being drawn from the primary container before administration of the fluid from the secondary container is complete.
Preparation for administration:
1. Suspend container from eyelet support.
2. Remove plastic protector from outlet port at bottom of container.
3. Attach administration set. Refer to complete directions accompanying set.

HOW SUPPLIED

Ancef (cefazolin for injection)—supplied in vials equivalent to 500 mg or 1 gram of cefazolin; in "Piggyback" Vials for intravenous admixture equivalent to 1 gram of cefazolin; and in Pharmacy Bulk Vials equivalent to 10 grams of cefazolin.
Ancef (cefazolin injection) as a frozen, iso-osmotic, sterile, nonpyrogenic solution in plastic containers—supplied in 50 mL single-dose containers equivalent to 500 mg or 1 gram of cefazolin. Dextrose Hydrous, USP, has been added to the above dosages to adjust osmolality (approximately 2.4 grams and 2 grams, respectively). Store at or below −20°C (−4°F). (See DIRECTIONS FOR USE OF ANCEF [CEFAZOLIN INJECTION] GALAXY® CONTAINER [PL 2040 PLASTIC].)
As with other cephalosporins, *Ancef* tends to darken depending on storage conditions; within the stated recommendations, however, product potency is not adversely affected. Before reconstitution protect from light and store at Controlled Room Temperature 20° to 25°C (68° to 77°F).
Ancef supplied as a frozen, iso-osmotic, sterile, nonpyrogenic solution in plastic containers is manufactured for SmithKline Beecham Pharmaceuticals by Baxter Healthcare Corporation, Deerfield, IL 60015.
Galaxy is a registered trademark of Baxter International Inc.

Rx only

AF:L52
Shown in Product Identification Guide, page 336

AUGMENTIN® ℞
[*og 'men-tin*]
amoxicillin/clavulanate potassium
Powder for Oral Suspension and Chewable Tablets

DESCRIPTION

Augmentin is an oral antibacterial combination consisting of the semisynthetic antibiotic amoxicillin and the β-lactamase inhibitor, clavulanate potassium (the potassium salt of clavulanic acid). Amoxicillin is an analog of ampicillin, derived from the basic penicillin nucleus, 6-aminopenicillanic acid. The amoxicillin molecular formula is $C_{16}H_{19}N_3O_5S \bullet 3H_2O$ and the molecular weight is 419.46. Chemically, amoxicillin is (*2S,5R,6R*)-6-[(*R*)-(-)-2-Amino-2-(*p* -hydroxyphenyl)acetamido] -3,3-dimethyl-7-oxo-4-thia-1-azabicyclo[3.2.0]heptane-2- carboxylic acid trihydrate and may be represented structurally as:

Clavulanic acid is produced by the fermentation of *Streptomyces clavuligerus*. It is a β-lactam structurally related to the penicillins and possesses the ability to inactivate a wide variety of β-lactamases by blocking the active sites of these enzymes. Clavulanic acid is particularly active against the clinically important plasmid mediated β-lactamases frequently responsible for transferred drug resistance to penicillins and cephalosporins. The clavulanate potassium molecular formula is $C_8H_8KNO_5$ and the molecular weight is 237.25. Chemically clavulanate potassium is potassium (Z)-(*2R,5R*)-3-(2-hydroxyethylidene) -7-oxo-4-oxa-1-azabicyclo [3.2.0]-heptane-2-carboxylate and may be represented structurally as:

Inactive Ingredients: Powder for Oral Suspension—Colloidal silicon dioxide, flavorings (See HOW SUPPLIED), succinic acid, xanthan gum, and one or more of the following: aspartame•, hydroxypropyl methylcellulose, mannitol, silica gel, silicon dioxide and sodium saccharin. Chewable Tablets—Colloidal silicon dioxide, flavorings (See HOW SUPPLIED), magnesium stearate, mannitol and one or more of the following: aspartame•, D&C Yellow No. 10, FD&C Red No. 40, glycine, sodium saccharin and succinic acid.
•See PRECAUTIONS—Information for Patients.
Each 125 mg chewable tablet and each 5 mL of reconstituted *Augmentin* 125 mg/5 mL oral suspension contains 0.16 mEq potassium. Each 250 mg chewable tablet and each 5 mL of reconstituted *Augmentin* 250 mg/5 mL oral suspension contains 0.32 mEq potassium. Each 200 mg chewable tablet and each 5 mL of reconstituted *Augmentin* 200 mg/5 mL oral suspension contains 0.14 mEq potassium. Each 400 mg chewable tablet and each 5 mL of reconstituted *Augmentin* 400 mg/5 mL oral suspension contains 0.29 mEq of potassium.

CLINICAL PHARMACOLOGY

Amoxicillin and clavulanate potassium are well absorbed from the gastrointestinal tract after oral administration of *Augmentin*. Dosing in the fasted or fed state has minimal effect on the pharmacokinetics of amoxicillin. While *Augmentin* can be given without regard to meals, absorption of clavulanate potassium when taken with food is greater relative to the fasted state. In one study, the relative bioavailability of clavulanate was reduced when *Augmentin* was dosed at 30 and 150 minutes after the start of a high fat breakfast. The safety and efficacy of *Augmentin* have been established in clinical trials where *Augmentin* was taken without regard to meals.
Oral administration of single doses of 400 mg *Augmentin* chewable tablets and 400 mg/5 mL suspension to 28 adult volunteers yielded comparable pharmacokinetic data:
[See table above]

Dose† (amoxicillin/clavulanate potassium)	AUC $_{0-\infty}$ (μg.hr./mL) amoxicillin (±S.D.)	AUC $_{0-\infty}$ (μg.hr./mL) clavulanate potassium (±S.D.)	C_{max} (μg/mL)‡ amoxicillin (±S.D.)	C_{max} (μg/mL)‡ clavulanate potassium (±S.D.)
400/57 mg (5 mL of suspension)	17.29 ±2.28	2.34 ±0.94	6.94 ±1.24	1.10 ±0.42
400/57 mg (one chewable tablet)	17.24 ±2.64	2.17 ±0.73	6.67 ±1.37	1.03 ±0.33

† Administered at the start of a light meal.
‡ Mean values of 28 normal volunteers. Peak concentrations occurred approximately 1 hour after the dose.

Oral administration of 5 mL of *Augmentin* 250 mg/5 mL suspension or the equivalent dose of 10 mL *Augmentin* 125 mg/5 mL suspension provides average peak serum concentrations approximately 1 hour after dosing of 6.9 μg/mL for amoxicillin and 1.6 μg/mL for clavulanic acid. The areas under the serum concentration curves obtained during the first 4 hours after dosing were 12.6 μg.hr./mL for amoxicillin and 2.9 μg.hr./mL for clavulanic acid when 5 mL of *Augmentin* 250 mg/5 mL suspension or equivalent dose of 10 mL of *Augmentin* 125 mg/5 mL suspension was administered to adult volunteers. One *Augmentin* 250 mg chewable tablet or 2 *Augmentin* 125 mg chewable tablets are equivalent to 5 mL of *Augmentin* 250 mg/5 mL suspension and provide similar serum levels of amoxicillin and clavulanic acid.
Amoxicillin serum concentrations achieved with *Augmentin* are similar to those produced by the oral administration of equivalent doses of amoxicillin alone. The half-life of amoxicillin after the oral administration of *Augmentin* is 1.3 hours and that of clavulanic acid is 1.0 hour. Time above the minimum inhibitory concentration of 1.0 μg/mL for amoxicillin has been shown to be similar after corresponding q12h and q8h dosing regimens of *Augmentin* in adults and children.
Approximately 50% to 70% of the amoxicillin and approximately 25% to 40% of the clavulanic acid are excreted unchanged in urine during the first 6 hours after administration of 10 mL of *Augmentin* 250 mg/5 mL suspension.
Concurrent administration of probenecid delays amoxicillin excretion but does not delay renal excretion of clavulanic acid.
Neither component in *Augmentin* is highly protein-bound; clavulanic acid has been found to be approximately 25% bound to human serum and amoxicillin approximately 18% bound.
Amoxicillin diffuses readily into most body tissues and fluids with the exception of the brain and spinal fluid. The results of experiments involving the administration of clavulanic acid to animals suggest that this compound, like amoxicillin, is well distributed in body tissues.
Two hours after oral administration of a single 35 mg/kg dose of *Augmentin* suspension to fasting children, average concentrations of 3.0 μg/mL of amoxicillin and 0.5 μg/mL of clavulanic acid were detected in middle ear effusions.
Microbiology: Amoxicillin is a semisynthetic antibiotic with a broad spectrum of bactericidal activity against many gram-positive and gram-negative microorganisms. Amoxicillin is, however, susceptible to degradation by β-lactamases and, therefore, the spectrum of activity does not include organisms which produce these enzymes. Clavulanic acid is a β-lactam, structurally related to the penicillins, which possesses the ability to inactivate a wide range of β-lactamase enzymes commonly found in microorganisms resistant to penicillins and cephalosporins. In particular, it has good activity against the clinically important plasmid mediated β-lactamases frequently responsible for transferred drug resistance.
The formulation of amoxicillin and clavulanic acid in *Augmentin* protects amoxicillin from degradation by β-lactamase enzymes and effectively extends the antibiotic spectrum of amoxicillin to include many bacteria normally resistant to amoxicillin and other β-lactam antibiotics. Thus, *Augmentin* possesses the distinctive properties of a broad-spectrum antibiotic and a β-lactamase inhibitor.
Amoxicillin/clavulanic acid has been shown to be active against most strains of the following microorganisms, both *in vitro* and in clinical infections as described in the INDICATIONS AND USAGE section.
GRAM-POSITIVE AEROBES
Staphylococcus aureus (β-lactamase and non-β-lactamase producing)§
§Staphylococci which are resistant to methicillin/oxacillin must be considered resistant to amoxicillin/clavulanic acid.
GRAM-NEGATIVE AEROBES
Enterobacter species (Although most strains of *Enterobacter* species are resistant *in vitro,* clinical efficacy has been demonstrated with *Augmentin* in urinary tract infections caused by these organisms.)
Escherichia coli (β-lactamase and non-β-lactamase producing)
Haemophilus influenzae (β-lactamase and non-β-lactamase producing)
Klebsiella species (All known strains are β-lactamase producing.)
Moraxella catarrhalis (β-lactamase and non-β-lactamase producing)
The following *in vitro* data are available, **but their clinical significance is unknown.**
Amoxicillin/clavulanic acid exhibits *in vitro* minimal inhibitory concentrations (MICs) of 0.5 μg/mL or less against most (≥90%) strains of *Streptococcus pneumoniae* [II]; MICs of 0.06 μg/mL or less against most (≥90%) strains of *Neisseria gonorrhoeae;* MICs of 4 μg/mL or less against most (≥90%) strains of staphylococci and anaerobic bacteria; and MICs of 8 μg/mL or less against most (≥90%) strains of other listed organisms. However, with the exception of organisms shown to respond to amoxicillin alone, the safety and effectiveness of amoxicillin/clavulanic acid in treating clinical infections due to these microorganisms have not been established in adequate and well-controlled clinical trials.

Continued on next page

Information on the SmithKline Beecham Pharmaceuticals products appearing here is based on the labeling in effect on June 15, 2000. Further information on these and other products may be obtained from the Medical Department, SmithKline Beecham Pharmaceuticals, One Franklin Plaza, Philadelphia, PA 19101.

Augmentin Powder/Chewable—Cont.

¶Because amoxicillin has greater *in vitro* activity against *Streptococcus pneumoniae* than does ampicillin or penicillin, the majority of *S. pneumoniae* strains with intermediate susceptibility to ampicillin or penicillin are fully susceptible to amoxicillin.

GRAM-POSITIVE AEROBES

Enterococcus faecalis ¶

Staphylococcus epidermidis (β-lactamase and non-β-lactamase producing)

Staphylococcus saprophyticus (β-lactamase and non-β-lactamase producing)

Streptococcus pneumoniae ¶**

Streptococcus pyogenes ¶**

viridans group *Streptococcus* ¶**

GRAM-NEGATIVE AEROBES

Eikenella corrodens (β-lactamase and non-β-lactamase producing)

Neisseria gonorrhoeae ¶ (β-lactamase and non-β-lactamase producing)

Proteus mirabilis ¶ (β-lactamase and non-β-lactamase producing)

ANAEROBIC BACTERIA

Bacteroides species, including *Bacteroides fragilis* (β-lactamase and non-β-lactamase producing)

Fusobacterium species (β-lactamase and non-β-lactamase producing)

Peptostreptococcus species**

¶ Adequate and well-controlled clinical trials have established the effectiveness of amoxicillin alone in treating certain clinical infections due to these organisms.

** These are non-β-lactamase-producing organisms and, therefore, are susceptible to amoxicillin alone.

SUSCEPTIBILITY TESTING

Dilution Techniques: Quantitative methods are used to determine antimicrobial minimal inhibitory concentrations (MICs). These MICs provide estimates of the susceptibility of bacteria to antimicrobial compounds. The MICs should be determined using a standardized procedure. Standardized procedures are based on a dilution method[1] (broth or agar) or equivalent with standardized inoculum concentrations and standardized concentrations of amoxicillin/clavulanate potassium powder.

The recommended dilution pattern utilizes a constant amoxicillin/clavulanate potassium ratio of 2 to 1 in all tubes with varying amounts of amoxicillin. MICs are expressed in terms of the amoxicillin concentration in the presence of clavulanic acid at a constant 2 parts amoxicillin to 1 part clavulanic acid. The MIC values should be interpreted according to the following criteria:

RECOMMENDED RANGES FOR AMOXICILLIN/CLAVULANIC ACID SUSCEPTIBILITY TESTING

For gram-negative enteric aerobes:

MIC (μg/mL)	Interpretation
≤8/4	Susceptible (S)
16/8	Intermediate (I)
≥32/16	Resistant (R)

For *Staphylococcus* †† and *Haemophilus* species:

MIC (μg/mL)	Interpretation
≤4/2	Susceptible (S)
≥8/4	Resistant (R)

†† Staphylococci which are susceptible to amoxicillin/clavulanic acid but resistant to methicillin/oxacillin must be considered as resistant.

For *Streptococcus pneumoniae:* Isolates should be tested using amoxicillin/clavulanic acid and the following criteria should be used:

MIC (μg/mL)	Interpretation
≤0.5/0.25	Susceptible (S)
1/0.5	Intermediate (I)
≥2/1	Resistant (R)

A report of "Susceptible" indicates that the pathogen is likely to be inhibited if the antimicrobial compound in the blood reaches the concentration usually achievable. A report of "Intermediate" indicates that the result should be considered equivocal, and, if the microorganism is not fully susceptible to alternative, clinically feasible drugs, the test should be repeated. This category implies possible clinical applicability in body sites where the drug is physiologically concentrated or in situations where high dosage of drug can be used. This category also provides a buffer zone that prevents small uncontrolled technical factors from causing major discrepancies in interpretation. A report of "Resistant" indicates that the pathogen is not likely to be inhibited if the antimicrobial compound in the blood reaches the concentrations usually achievable; other therapy should be selected.

Standardized susceptibility test procedures require the use of laboratory control microorganisms to control the technical aspects of the laboratory procedures. Standard amoxicillin/clavulanate potassium powder should provide the following MIC values:

Microorganism	MIC Range (μg/mL)‡‡
Escherichia coli ATCC 25922	2 to 8
Escherichia coli ATCC 35218	4 to 16
Enterococcus faecalis ATCC 29212	0.25 to 1.0
Haemophilus influenzae ATCC 49247	2 to 16
Staphylococcus aureus ATCC 29213	0.12 to 0.5
Streptococcus pneumoniae ATCC 49619	0.03 to 0.12

‡‡ Expressed as concentration of amoxicillin in the presence of clavulanic acid at a constant 2 parts amoxicillin to 1 part clavulanic acid.

Diffusion Techniques: Quantitative methods that require measurement of zone diameters also provide reproducible estimates of the susceptibility of bacteria to antimicrobial compounds. One such standardized procedure[2] requires the use of standardized inoculum concentrations. This procedure uses paper disks impregnated with 30 μg of amoxicillin/clavulanate potassium (20 μg amoxicillin plus 10 μg clavulanate potassium) to test the susceptibility of microorganisms to amoxicillin/clavulanic acid.

Reports from the laboratory providing results of the standard single-disk susceptibility test with a 30 μg amoxicillin/clavulanate potassium (20 μg amoxicillin plus 10 μg clavulanate potassium) disk should be interpreted according to the following criteria:

RECOMMENDED RANGES FOR AMOXICILLIN/CLAVULANIC ACID SUSCEPTIBILITY TESTING

For *Staphylococcus* §§ species and *H. influenzae*[a]:

Zone Diameter (mm)	Interpretation
≥20	Susceptible (S)
≤19	Resistant (R)

For other organisms except *S. pneumoniae*[b] and *N. gonorrhoeae*[c]:

Zone Diameter (mm)	Interpretation
≥18	Susceptible (S)
14 to 17	Intermediate (I)
≤13	Resistant (R)

§§ Staphylococci which are resistant to methicillin/oxacillin must be considered as resistant to amoxicillin/clavulanic acid.

[a] A broth microdilution method should be used for testing *H. influenzae.* Beta-lactamase negative, ampicillin-resistant strains must be considered resistant to amoxicillin/clavulanic acid.

[b] Susceptibility of *S. pneumoniae* should be determined using a 1 μg oxacillin disk. Isolates with oxacillin zone sizes of ≥20 mm are susceptible to amoxicillin/clavulanic acid. An amoxicillin/clavulanic acid MIC should be determined on isolates of *S. pneumoniae* with oxacillin zone sizes of ≤19 mm.

[c] A broth microdilution method should be used for testing *N. gonorrhoeae* and interpreted according to penicillin breakpoints.

Interpretation should be as stated above for results using dilution techniques. Interpretation involves correlation of the diameter obtained in the disk test with the MIC for amoxicillin/clavulanic acid.

As with standardized dilution techniques, diffusion methods require the use of laboratory control microorganisms that are used to control the technical aspects of the laboratory procedures. For the diffusion technique, the 30 μg amoxicillin/clavulanate potassium (20 μg amoxicillin plus 10 μg clavulanate potassium) disk should provide the following zone diameters in these laboratory quality control strains:

Microorganism	Zone Diameter (mm)
Escherichia coli ATCC 25922	19 to 25 mm
Escherichia coli ATCC 35218	18 to 22 mm
Staphylococcus aureus ATCC 25923	28 to 36 mm

INDICATIONS AND USAGE

Augmentin is indicated in the treatment of infections caused by susceptible strains of the designated organisms in the conditions listed below:

Lower Respiratory Tract Infections—caused by β-lactamase-producing strains of *Haemophilus influenzae* and *Moraxella (Branhamella) catarrhalis.*

Otitis Media—caused by β-lactamase-producing strains of *Haemophilus influenzae* and *Moraxella (Branhamella) catarrhalis.*

Sinusitis—caused by β-lactamase-producing strains of *Haemophilus influenzae* and *Moraxella (Branhamella) catarrhalis.*

Skin and Skin Structure Infections—caused by β-lactamase-producing strains of *Staphylococcus aureus, Escherichia coli* and *Klebsiella* spp.

Urinary Tract Infections—caused by β-lactamase-producing strains of *Escherichia coli, Klebsiella* spp. and *Enterobacter* spp.

While *Augmentin* is indicated only for the conditions listed above, infections caused by ampicillin-susceptible organisms are also amenable to *Augmentin* treatment due to its amoxicillin content. Therefore, mixed infections caused by ampicillin-susceptible organisms and β-lactamase-producing organisms susceptible to *Augmentin* should not require the addition of another antibiotic. Because amoxicillin has greater *in vitro* activity against *Streptococcus pneumoniae* than does ampicillin or penicillin, the majority of *S. pneumoniae* strains with intermediate susceptibility to ampicillin or penicillin are fully susceptible to amoxicillin and *Augmentin.* (See Microbiology subsection.)

Bacteriological studies, to determine the causative organisms and their susceptibility to *Augmentin,* should be performed together with any indicated surgical procedures.

Therapy may be instituted prior to obtaining the results from bacteriological and susceptibility studies to determine the causative organisms and their susceptibility to *Augmentin* when there is reason to believe the infection may involve any of the β-lactamase-producing organisms listed above. Once the results are known, therapy should be adjusted, if appropriate.

CONTRAINDICATIONS

Augmentin is contraindicated in patients with a history of allergic reactions to any penicillin. It is also contraindicated in patients with a previous history of *Augmentin*-associated cholestatic jaundice/hepatic dysfunction.

WARNINGS

SERIOUS AND OCCASIONALLY FATAL HYPERSENSITIVITY (ANAPHYLACTIC) REACTIONS HAVE BEEN REPORTED IN PATIENTS ON PENICILLIN THERAPY. THESE REACTIONS ARE MORE LIKELY TO OCCUR IN INDIVIDUALS WITH A HISTORY OF PENICILLIN HYPERSENSITIVITY AND/OR A HISTORY OF SENSITIVITY TO MULTIPLE ALLERGENS. THERE HAVE BEEN REPORTS OF INDIVIDUALS WITH A HISTORY OF PENICILLIN HYPERSENSITIVITY WHO HAVE EXPERIENCED SEVERE REACTIONS WHEN TREATED WITH CEPHALOSPORINS. BEFORE INITIATING THERAPY WITH *AUGMENTIN,* CAREFUL INQUIRY SHOULD BE MADE CONCERNING PREVIOUS HYPERSENSITIVITY REACTIONS TO PENICILLINS, CEPHALOSPORINS OR OTHER ALLERGENS. IF AN ALLERGIC REACTION OCCURS, *AUGMENTIN* SHOULD BE DISCONTINUED AND THE APPROPRIATE THERAPY INSTITUTED. **SERIOUS ANAPHYLACTIC REACTIONS REQUIRE IMMEDIATE EMERGENCY TREATMENT WITH EPINEPHRINE. OXYGEN, INTRAVENOUS STEROIDS AND AIRWAY MANAGEMENT, INCLUDING INTUBATION, SHOULD ALSO BE ADMINISTERED AS INDICATED.**

Pseudomembranous colitis has been reported with nearly all antibacterial agents, including *Augmentin,* and has ranged in severity from mild to life-threatening. Therefore, it is important to consider this diagnosis in patients who present with diarrhea subsequent to the administration of antibacterial agents.

Treatment with antibacterial agents alters the normal flora of the colon and may permit overgrowth of clostridia. Studies indicate that a toxin produced by *Clostridium difficile* is one primary cause of "antibiotic associated colitis."

After the diagnosis of pseudomembranous colitis has been established, appropriate therapeutic measures should be initiated. Mild cases of pseudomembranous colitis usually respond to drug discontinuation alone. In moderate to severe cases, consideration should be given to management with fluids and electrolytes, protein supplementation and treatment with an antibacterial drug clinically effective against *Clostridium difficile* colitis.

Augmentin should be used with caution in patients with evidence of hepatic dysfunction. Hepatic toxicity associated with the use of *Augmentin* is usually reversible. On rare occasions, deaths have been reported (less than 1 death reported per estimated 4 million prescriptions worldwide). These have generally been cases associated with serious underlying diseases or concomitant medications. (See CONTRAINDICATIONS and ADVERSE REACTIONS—*Liver.*)

PRECAUTIONS

General: While *Augmentin* possesses the characteristic low toxicity of the penicillin group of antibiotics, periodic assessment of organ system functions, including renal, hepatic and hematopoietic function, is advisable during prolonged therapy. A high percentage of patients with mononucleosis who receive ampicillin develop an erythematous skin rash. Thus, ampicillin class antibiotics should not be administered to patients with mononucleosis.

The possibility of superinfections with mycotic or bacterial pathogens should be kept in mind during therapy. If superinfections occur (usually involving *Pseudomonas* or *Candida*), the drug should be discontinued and/or appropriate therapy instituted.

Information for the Patient: Augmentin may be taken every 8 hours or every 12 hours, depending on the strength of the product prescribed. Each dose should be taken with a meal or snack to reduce the possibility of gastrointestinal upset. Many antibiotics can cause diarrhea. If diarrhea is severe or lasts more than 2 or 3 days, call your doctor.

Make sure your child completes the entire prescribed course of treatment, even if he/she begins to feel better after a few days. Keep suspension refrigerated. Shake well before using. When dosing a child with *Augmentin* suspension (liquid), use a dosing spoon or medicine dropper. Be sure to rinse the spoon or dropper after each use. Bottles of *Augmentin* suspension may contain more liquid than required. Follow your doctor's instructions about the amount to use and the days of treatment your child requires. Discard any unused medicine.

Phenylketonurics: Each 200 mg *Augmentin* chewable tablet contains 2.1 mg phenylalanine; each 400 mg chewable tablet contains 4.2 mg phenylalanine; each 5 mL of either the 200 mg/5 mL or 400 mg/5 mL oral suspension contains 7 mg phenylalanine. The other *Augmentin* products do not contain phenylalanine and can be used by phenylketonurics. Contact your physician or pharmacist.

Drug Interactions: Probenecid decreases the renal tubular secretion of amoxicillin. Concurrent use with *Augmentin* may result in increased and prolonged blood levels of amoxicillin. Co-administration of probenecid cannot be recommended.

The concurrent administration of allopurinol and ampicillin increases substantially the incidence of rashes in patients receiving both drugs as compared to patients receiving ampicillin alone. It is not known whether this potentiation of ampicillin rashes is due to allopurinol or the hyperuricemia present in these patients. There are no data with *Augmentin* and allopurinol administered concurrently.

In common with other broad-spectrum antibiotics, *Augmentin* may reduce the efficacy of oral contraceptives.

Drug/Laboratory Test Interactions: Oral administration of *Augmentin* will result in high urine concentrations of amoxicillin. High urine concentrations of ampicillin may result in false-positive reactions when testing for the presence of glucose in urine using Clinitest®, Benedict's Solution or Fehling's Solution. Since this effect may also occur with amoxicillin and therefore *Augmentin*, it is recommended that glucose tests based on enzymatic glucose oxidase reactions (such as Clinistix® or Tes-Tape®) be used.

Following administration of ampicillin to pregnant women a transient decrease in plasma concentration of total conjugated estriol, estriol-glucuronide, conjugated estrone and estradiol has been noted. This effect may also occur with amoxicillin and therefore *Augmentin*.

Carcinogenesis, Mutagenesis, Impairment of Fertility: Long-term studies in animals have not been performed to evaluate carcinogenic potential.

Mutagenesis: The mutagenic potential of *Augmentin* was investigated *in vitro* with an Ames test, a human lymphocyte cytogenetic assay, a yeast test and a mouse lymphoma forward mutation assay, and *in vivo* with mouse micronucleus tests and a dominant lethal test. All were negative apart from the *in vitro* mouse lymphoma assay where weak activity was found at very high, cytotoxic concentrations.

Impairment of Fertility: Augmentin at oral doses of up to 1200 mg/kg/day (5.7 times the maximum human dose, 1480 mg/m^2/day, based on body surface area) was found to have no effect on fertility and reproductive performance in rats, dosed with a 2:1 ratio formulation of amoxicillin:clavulanate.

Teratogenic effects. Pregnancy (Category B): Reproduction studies performed in pregnant rats and mice given *Augmentin* at oral dosages up to 1200 mg/kg/day, equivalent to 7200 and 4080 mg/m^2/day, respectively (4.9 and 2.8 times the maximum human oral dose based on body surface area), revealed no evidence of harm to the fetus due to *Augmentin*. There are, however, no adequate and well-controlled studies in pregnant women. Because animal reproduction studies are not always predictive of human response, this drug should be used during pregnancy only if clearly needed.

Labor and Delivery: Oral ampicillin class antibiotics are generally poorly absorbed during labor. Studies in guinea pigs have shown that intravenous administration of ampicillin decreased the uterine tone, frequency of contractions, height of contractions and duration of contractions. However, it is not known whether the use of *Augmentin* in humans during labor or delivery has immediate or delayed adverse effects on the fetus, prolongs the duration of labor, or increases the likelihood that forceps delivery or other obstetrical intervention or resuscitation of the newborn will be necessary.

Nursing Mothers: Ampicillin class antibiotics are excreted in the milk; therefore, caution should be exercised when *Augmentin* is administered to a nursing woman.

Pediatric Use: Because of incompletely developed renal function in neonates and young infants, the elimination of amoxicillin may be delayed. Dosing of *Augmentin* should be modified in pediatric patients younger than 12 weeks (3 months). (See DOSAGE AND ADMINISTRATION–Pediatric.)

ADVERSE REACTIONS

Augmentin is generally well tolerated. The majority of side effects observed in clinical trials were of a mild and transient nature and less than 3% of patients discontinued therapy because of drug-related side effects. From the original premarketing studies, where both pediatric and adult patients were enrolled, the most frequently reported adverse effects were diarrhea/loose stools (9%), nausea (3%), skin rashes and urticaria (3%), vomiting (1%) and vaginitis (1%). The overall incidence of side effects, and in particular diarrhea, increased with the higher recommended dose. Other less frequently reported reactions include: abdominal discomfort, flatulence and headache.

In pediatric patients (aged 2 months to 12 years), one U.S./Canadian clinical trial was conducted which compared *Augmentin* 45/6.4 mg/kg/day (divided q12h) for 10 days versus *Augmentin* 40/10 mg/kg/day (divided q8h) for 10 days in the treatment of acute otitis media. A total of 575 patients were enrolled, and only the suspension formulations were used in this trial. Overall, the adverse event profile seen was comparable to that noted above. However, there were differences in the rates of diarrhea, skin rashes/urticaria, and diaper area rashes. (See CLINICAL STUDIES.)

The following adverse reactions have been reported for ampicillin class antibiotics:

Gastrointestinal: Diarrhea, nausea, vomiting, indigestion, gastritis, stomatitis, glossitis, black "hairy" tongue, mucocutaneous candidiasis, enterocolitis, and hemorrhagic/pseudomembranous colitis. Onset of pseudomembranous colitis symptoms may occur during or after antibiotic treatment. (See WARNINGS.)

Hypersensitivity Reactions: Skin rashes, pruritus, urticaria, angioedema, serum sickness-like reactions (urticaria or skin rash accompanied by arthritis, arthralgia, myalgia and frequently fever), erythema multiforme (rarely Stevens-Johnson Syndrome) and an occasional case of exfoliative dermatitis (including toxic epidermal necrolysis) have been reported. These reactions may be controlled with antihistamines and, if necessary, systemic corticosteroids. Whenever such reactions occur, the drug should be discontinued, unless the opinion of the physician dictates otherwise. Serious and occasional fatal hypersensitivity (anaphylactic) reactions can occur with oral penicillin. (See WARNINGS.)

Liver: A moderate rise in AST (SGOT) and/or ALT (SGPT) has been noted in patients treated with ampicillin class antibiotics but the significance of these findings is unknown. Hepatic dysfunction, including increases in serum transaminases (AST and/or ALT), serum bilirubin and/or alkaline phosphatase, has been infrequently reported with *Augmentin*. It has been reported more commonly in the elderly, in males, or in patients on prolonged treatment. The histologic findings on liver biopsy have consisted of predominantly cholestatic, hepatocellular, or mixed cholestatic-hepatocellular changes. The onset of signs/symptoms of hepatic dysfunction may occur during or several weeks after therapy has been discontinued. The hepatic dysfunction, which may be severe, is usually reversible. On rare occasions, deaths have been reported (less than 1 death reported per estimated 4 million prescriptions worldwide). These have generally been cases associated with serious underlying diseases or concomitant medications.

Renal: Interstitial nephritis and hematuria have been reported rarely.

Hemic and Lymphatic Systems: Anemia, including hemolytic anemia, thrombocytopenia, thrombocytopenic purpura, eosinophilia, leukopenia and agranulocytosis have been reported during therapy with penicillins. These reactions are usually reversible on discontinuation of therapy and are believed to be hypersensitivity phenomena. A slight thrombocytosis was noted in less than 1% of the patients treated with *Augmentin*. There have been reports of increased prothrombin time in patients receiving *Augmentin* and anticoagulant therapy concomitantly.

Central Nervous System: Agitation, anxiety, behavioral changes, confusion, convulsions, dizziness, insomnia, and reversible hyperactivity have been reported rarely.

OVERDOSAGE

Most patients have been asymptomatic following overdosage or have experienced primarily gastrointestinal symptoms including stomach and abdominal pain, vomiting, and diarrhea. Rash, hyperactivity, or drowsiness have also been observed in a small number of patients.

In the case of overdosage, discontinue *Augmentin*, treat symptomatically, and institute supportive measures as required. If the overdosage is very recent and there is no contraindication, an attempt at emesis or other means of removal of drug from the stomach may be performed. A prospective study of 51 pediatric patients at a poison center suggested that overdosages of less than 250 mg/kg of amoxicillin are not associated with significant clinical symptoms and do not require gastric emptying.[3]

Interstitial nephritis resulting in oliguric renal failure has been reported in a small number of patients after overdosage with amoxicillin. Renal impairment appears to be reversible with cessation of drug administration. High blood levels may occur more readily in patients with impaired renal function because of decreased renal clearance of both amoxicillin and clavulanate. Both amoxicillin and clavulanate are removed from the circulation by hemodialysis.

DOSAGE AND ADMINISTRATION

Dosage:

Pediatric Patients: Based on the amoxicillin component, *Augmentin* should be dosed as follows:

Neonates and infants aged < 12 weeks (3 months)

Due to incompletely developed renal function affecting elimination of amoxicillin in this age group, the recommended dose of *Augmentin* is 30 mg/kg/day divided q12h, based on the amoxicillin component. Clavulanate elimination is unaltered in this age group. Experience with the 200 mg/5 mL formulation in this age group is limited and, thus, use of the 125 mg/5 mL oral suspension is recommended.

Patients aged 12 weeks (3 months) and older

INFECTIONS	DOSING REGIMEN	
	q12h‖	q8h
	200 mg/5 mL or 400 mg/5 mL oral suspension¶¶	125 mg/5 mL or 250 mg/5 mL oral suspension¶¶
Otitis media***, sinusitis, lower respiratory tract infections, and more severe infections	45 mg/kg/day q12h	40 mg/kg/day q8h
Less severe infections	25 mg/kg/day q12h	20 mg/kg/day q8h

‖ The q12h regimen is recommended as it is associated with significantly less diarrhea. (See CLINICAL STUDIES.) However, the q12h formulations (200 mg and 400 mg) contain aspartame and should not be used by phenylketonurics.

¶¶ Each strength of *Augmentin* suspension is available as a chewable tablet for use by older children.

*** Duration of therapy studied and recommended for acute otitis media is 10 days.

Pediatric patients weighing 40 kg and more should be dosed according to the following adult recommendations: The usual adult dose is 1 *Augmentin* 500 mg tablet every 12 hours or 1 *Augmentin* 250 mg tablet every 8 hours. For more severe infections and infections of the respiratory tract, the dose should be 1 *Augmentin* 875 mg tablet every 12 hours or 1 *Augmentin* 500 mg tablet every 8 hours. Among adults treated with 875 mg every 12 hours, significantly fewer experienced severe diarrhea or withdrawals with diarrhea vs. adults treated with 500 mg every 8 hours. For detailed adult dosage recommendations, please see complete prescribing information for *Augmentin* Tablets.

Hepatically impaired patients should be dosed with caution and hepatic function monitored at regular intervals. (See WARNINGS.)

Adults: Adults who have difficulty swallowing may be given the 125 mg/5 mL or 250 mg/5 mL suspension in place of the 500 mg tablet. The 200 mg/5 mL suspension or the 400 mg/5 mL suspension may be used in place of the 875 mg tablet. See dosage recommendations above for children weighing 40 kg or more.

The *Augmentin* 250 mg tablet and the 250 mg chewable tablet do *not* contain the same amount of clavulanic acid (as the potassium salt). The *Augmentin* 250 mg tablet contains 125 mg of clavulanic acid, whereas the 250 mg chewable tablet contains 62.5 mg of clavulanic acid. Therefore, the *Augmentin* 250 mg tablet and the 250 mg chewable tablet should *not* be substituted for each other, as they are not interchangeable.

Due to the different amoxicillin to clavulanic acid ratios in the *Augmentin* 250 mg tablet (250/125) versus the *Augmentin* 250 mg chewable tablet (250/62.5), the *Augmentin* 250 mg tablet should not be used until the child weighs at least 40 kg and more.

DIRECTIONS FOR MIXING ORAL SUSPENSION

Prepare a suspension at time of dispensing as follows: Tap bottle until all the powder flows freely. Add approximately 2/3 of the total amount of water for reconstitution (see table below) and shake vigorously to suspend powder. Add remainder of the water and again shake vigorously.

***Augmentin* 125 mg/5 mL Suspension**

Bottle Size	Amount of Water Required for Reconstitution
75 mL	67 mL
100 mL	90 mL
150 mL	134 mL

Each teaspoonful (5 mL) will contain 125 mg amoxicillin and 31.25 mg of clavulanic acid as the potassium salt.

***Augmentin* 200 mg/5 mL Suspension**

Bottle Size	Amount of Water Required for Suspension
50 mL	47 mL
75 mL	69 mL
100 mL	91 mL

Each teaspoonful (5 mL) will contain 200 mg amoxicillin and 28.5 mg of clavulanic acid as the potassium salt.

***Augmentin* 250 mg/5 mL Suspension**

Bottle Size	Amount of Water Required for Reconstitution
75 mL	65 mL
100 mL	87 mL
150 mL	130 mL

Each teaspoonful (5 mL) will contain 250 mg amoxicillin and 62.5 mg of clavulanic acid as the potassium salt.

***Augmentin* 400 mg/5 mL Suspension**

Bottle Size	Amount of Water Required for Suspension
50 mL	44 mL
75 mL	66 mL
100 mL	87 mL

Each teaspoonful (5 mL) will contain 400 mg amoxicillin and 57.0 mg of clavulanic acid as the potassium salt.

Continued on next page

Information on the SmithKline Beecham Pharmaceuticals products appearing here is based on the labeling in effect on June 15, 2000. Further information on these and other products may be obtained from the Medical Department, SmithKline Beecham Pharmaceuticals, One Franklin Plaza, Philadelphia, PA 19101.

Augmentin Powder/Chewable—Cont.

Note: SHAKE ORAL SUSPENSION WELL BEFORE USING.

Reconstituted suspension must be stored under refrigeration and discarded after 10 days.

Administration: *Augmentin* may be taken without regard to meals; however, absorption of clavulanate potassium is enhanced when *Augmentin* is administered at the start of a meal. To minimize the potential for gastrointestinal intolerance, *Augmentin* should be taken at the start of a meal.

HOW SUPPLIED

***AUGMENTIN* 125 MG/5 ML FOR ORAL SUSPENSION:** Each 5 mL of reconstituted banana-flavored suspension contains 125 mg amoxicillin and 31.25 mg clavulanic acid as the potassium salt.

NDC 0029-6085-39 .... 75 mL bottle
NDC 0029-6085-23 .... 100 mL bottle
NDC 0029-6085-22 .... 150 mL bottle

***AUGMENTIN* 200 MG/5 ML FOR ORAL SUSPENSION:** Each 5 mL of reconstituted orange-raspberry-flavored suspension contains 200 mg amoxicillin and 28.5 mg clavulanic acid as the potassium salt.

NDC 0029-6087-29 .... 50 mL bottle
NDC 0029-6087-39 .... 75 mL bottle
NDC 0029-6087-51 .... 100 mL bottle

***AUGMENTIN* 250 MG/5 ML FOR ORAL SUSPENSION:** Each 5 mL of reconstituted orange-flavored suspension contains 250 mg amoxicillin and 62.5 mg clavulanic acid as the potassium salt.

NDC 0029-6090-39 .... 75 mL bottle
NDC 0029-6090-23 .... 100 mL bottle
NDC 0029-6090-22 .... 150 mL bottle

***AUGMENTIN* 400 MG/5 ML FOR ORAL SUSPENSION:** Each 5 mL of reconstituted orange-raspberry-flavored suspension contains 400 mg amoxicillin and 57 mg clavulanic acid as the potassium salt.

NDC 0029-6092-29 .... 50 mL bottle
NDC 0029-6092-39 .... 75 mL bottle
NDC 0029-6092-51 .... 100 mL bottle

***AUGMENTIN* 125 MG CHEWABLE TABLETS:** Each mottled yellow, round, lemon-lime-flavored tablet, debossed with BMP 189, contains 125 mg amoxicillin as the trihydrate and 31.25 mg clavulanic acid as the potassium salt.

NDC 0029-6073-47 .... carton of 30 tablets

***AUGMENTIN* 200 MG CHEWABLE TABLETS:** Each mottled pink, round, biconvex, cherry-banana-flavored tablet contains 200 mg amoxicillin as the trihydrate and 28.5 mg clavulanic acid as the potassium salt.

NDC 0029-6071-12 .... carton of 20 tablets

***AUGMENTIN* 250 MG CHEWABLE TABLETS:** Each mottled yellow, round, lemon-lime-flavored tablet, debossed with BMP 190, contains 250 mg amoxicillin as the trihydrate and 62.5 mg clavulanic acid as the potassium salt.

NDC 0029-6074-47 .... carton of 30 tablets

***AUGMENTIN* 400 MG CHEWABLE TABLETS:** Each mottled pink, round, biconvex, cherry-banana-flavored tablet contains 400 mg amoxicillin as the trihydrate and 57.0 mg clavulanic acid as the potassium salt.

NDC 0029-6072-12 .... carton of 20 tablets

***AUGMENTIN* is also supplied as:**

***AUGMENTIN* 250 MG TABLETS** (250 mg amoxicillin/125 mg clavulanic acid):

NDC 0029-6075-27 .... bottles of 30
NDC 0029-6075-31 .... 100 Unit Dose tablets

***AUGMENTIN* 500 MG TABLETS** (500 mg amoxicillin/125 mg clavulanic acid):

NDC 0029-6080-12 .... bottles of 20
NDC 0029-6080-31 .... 100 Unit Dose tablets

***AUGMENTIN* 875 MG TABLETS** (875 mg amoxicillin/125 mg clavulanic acid):

NDC 0029-6086-12 .... bottles of 20
NDC 0029-6086-21 .... 100 Unit Dose tablets

Store tablets and dry powder at or below 25°C (77°F). Dispense in original container. Store reconstituted suspension under refrigeration. Discard unused suspension after 10 days.

CLINICAL STUDIES

In pediatric patients (aged 2 months to 12 years), one U.S./Canadian clinical trial was conducted which compared *Augmentin* 45/6.4 mg/kg/day (divided q12h) for 10 days versus *Augmentin* 40/10 mg/kg/day (divided q8h) for 10 days in the treatment of acute otitis media. Only the suspension formulations were used in this trial. A total of 575 patients were enrolled, with an even distribution among the two treatment groups and a comparable number of patients were evaluable (i.e., ≥84%) per treatment group. Strict otitis media-specific criteria were required for eligibility and a strong correlation was found at the end of therapy and follow-up between these criteria and physician assessment of clinical response. The clinical efficacy rates at the end of therapy visit (defined as 2–4 days after the completion of therapy) and at the follow-up visit (defined as 22–28 days post-completion of therapy) were comparable for the two treatment groups, with the following cure rates obtained for the evaluable patients: At end of therapy, 87.2% (n=265) and 82.3% (n=260) for 45 mg/kg/day q12h and 40 mg/kg/day q8h, respectively. At follow-up, 67.1% (n=249) and 68.7% (n=243) for 45 mg/kg/day q12h and 40 mg/kg/day q8h, respectively.

The incidence of diarrhea††† was significantly lower in patients in the q12h treatment group compared to patients who received the q8h regimen (14.3% and 34.3%, respectively). In addition, the number of patients with either severe diarrhea or who were withdrawn with diarrhea was significantly lower in the q12h treatment group (3.1% and 7.6% for the q12h/10 day and q8h/10 day, respectively). In the q12h treatment group, 3 patients (1.0%) were withdrawn with an allergic reaction, while 1 patient (0.3%) in the q8h group was withdrawn for this reason. The number of patients with a candidal infection of the diaper area was 3.8% and 6.2% for the q12h and q8h groups, respectively.

It is not known if the finding of a statistically significant reduction in diarrhea with the oral suspensions dosed q12h, versus suspensions dosed q8h, can be extrapolated to the chewable tablets. The presence of mannitol in the chewable tablets may contribute to a different diarrhea profile. The q12h oral suspensions are sweetened with aspartame only.

††† Diarrhea was defined as either: (a) three or more watery or four or more loose/watery stools in one day; OR (b) two watery stools per day or three loose/watery stools per day for two consecutive days.

REFERENCES

1. National Committee for Clinical Laboratory Standards. Methods for Dilution Antimicrobial Susceptibility Tests for Bacteria That Grow Aerobically — Third Edition. Approved Standard NCCLS Document M7-A3, Vol. 13, No. 25. NCCLS, Villanova, PA, Dec. 1993.
2. National Committee for Clinical Laboratory Standards. Performance Standard for Antimicrobial Disk Susceptibility Tests — Fifth Edition. Approved Standard NCCLS Document M2-A5, Vol. 13, No. 24. NCCLS, Villanova, PA, Dec. 1993.
3. Swanson-Biearman B, Dean BS, Lopez G, Krenzelok EP. The effects of penicillin and cephalosporin ingestions in children less than six years of age. *Vet Hum Toxicol* 1988; 30:66–67.

Rx only
AG:PL6A

Shown in Product Identification Guide, page 336

AUGMENTIN® ℞

[og' men-tin]
amoxicillin/clavulanate potassium Tablets

DESCRIPTION

Augmentin is an oral antibacterial combination consisting of the semisynthetic antibiotic amoxicillin and the β-lactamase inhibitor, clavulanate potassium (the potassium salt of clavulanic acid). Amoxicillin is an analog of ampicillin, derived from the basic penicillin nucleus, 6-aminopenicillanic acid. The amoxicillin molecular formula is $C_{16}H_{19}N_3O_5S{\cdot}3H_2O$ and the molecular weight is 419.46. Chemically, amoxicillin is (2*S*,5*R*,6*R*)-6-[(*R*)-(-)-2-Amino-2-(*p*-hydroxyphenyl)acetamido] -3,3- dimethyl -7-oxo-4-thia -1- azabicyclo[3.2.0]heptane-2-carboxylic acid trihydrate and may be represented structurally as:

HO–C₆H₄–CH(NH₂)–CO–NH– [bicyclic structure] CH₃, CH₃, COOH 3H₂O

Clavulanic acid is produced by the fermentation of *Streptomyces clavuligerus*. It is a β-lactam structurally related to the penicillins and possesses the ability to inactivate a wide variety of β-lactamases by blocking the active sites of these enzymes. Clavulanic acid is particularly active against the clinically important plasmid mediated β-lactamases frequently responsible for transferred drug resistance to penicillins and cephalosporins. The clavulanate potassium molecular formula is $C_8H_8KNO_5$ and the molecular weight is 237.25. Chemically clavulanate potassium is potassium (*Z*)-(2*R*, 5*R*)-3-(2-hydroxyethylidene)-7-oxo-4-oxa-1-azabicyclo[3.2.0]-heptane-2-carboxylate, and may be represented structurally as:

[structure: CH₂OH, H, COOK]

Inactive Ingredients: Colloidal silicon dioxide, hydroxypropyl methylcellulose, magnesium stearate, microcrystalline cellulose, polyethylene glycol, sodium starch glycolate and titanium dioxide.

Each *Augmentin* tablet contains 0.63 mEq potassium.

CLINICAL PHARMACOLOGY

Amoxicillin and clavulanate potassium are well absorbed from the gastrointestinal tract after oral administration of *Augmentin*. Dosing in the fasted or fed state has minimal effect on the pharmacokinetics of amoxicillin. While *Augmentin* can be given without regard to meals, absorption of clavulanate potassium when taken with food is greater relative to the fasted state. In one study, the relative bioavailability of clavulanate was reduced when *Augmentin* was dosed at 30 and 150 minutes after the start of a high fat breakfast. The safety and efficacy of *Augmentin* have been established in clinical trials where *Augmentin* was taken without regard to meals.

Mean* amoxicillin and clavulanate potassium pharmacokinetic parameters are shown in the table below:

[See table below]

Dose† and regimen	AUC$_{0-24}$ (µg.hr/mL)		C$_{max}$ (µg/mL)	
amoxicillin/ clavulanate potassium	amoxicillin (±S.D.)	clavulanate potassium (±S.D.)	amoxicillin (±S.D.)	clavulanate potassium (±S.D.)
250/125 mg q8h	26.7 ± 4.56	12.6 ± 3.25	3.3 ± 1.12	1.5 ± 0.70
500/125 mg q12h	33.4 ± 6.76	8.6 ± 1.95	6.5 ± 1.41	1.8 ± 0.61
500/125 mg q8h	53.4 ± 8.87	15.7 ± 3.86	7.2 ± 2.26	2.4 ± 0.83
875/125 mg q12h	53.5 ± 12.31	10.2 ± 3.04	11.6 ± 2.78	2.2 ± 0.99

* Mean values of 14 normal volunteers (n=15 for clavulanate potassium in the low-dose regimens). Peak concentrations occurred approximately 1.5 hours after the dose.
† Administered at the start of a light meal.

Amoxicillin serum concentrations achieved with *Augmentin* are similar to those produced by the oral administration of equivalent doses of amoxicillin alone. The half-life of amoxicillin after the oral administration of *Augmentin* is 1.3 hours and that of clavulanic acid is 1.0 hour.

Approximately 50% to 70% of the amoxicillin and approximately 25% to 40% of the clavulanic acid are excreted unchanged in urine during the first 6 hours after administration of a single *Augmentin* 250 mg or 500 mg tablet.

Concurrent administration of probenecid delays amoxicillin excretion but does not delay renal excretion of clavulanic acid.

Neither component in *Augmentin* is highly protein-bound; clavulanic acid has been found to be approximately 25% bound to human serum and amoxicillin approximately 18% bound.

Amoxicillin diffuses readily into most body tissues and fluids with the exception of the brain and spinal fluid. The results of experiments involving the administration of clavulanic acid to animals suggest that this compound, like amoxicillin, is well distributed in body tissues.

Microbiology: Amoxicillin is a semisynthetic antibiotic with a broad spectrum of bactericidal activity against many gram-positive and gram-negative microorganisms. Amoxicillin is, however, susceptible to degradation by β-lactamases and, therefore, the spectrum of activity does not include organisms which produce these enzymes. Clavulanic acid is a β-lactam, structurally related to the penicillins, which possesses the ability to inactivate a wide range of β-lactamase enzymes commonly found in microorganisms resistant to penicillins and cephalosporins. In particular, it has good activity against the clinically important plasmid mediated β-lactamases frequently responsible for transferred drug resistance.

The formulation of amoxicillin and clavulanic acid in *Augmentin* protects amoxicillin from degradation by β-lactamase enzymes and effectively extends the antibiotic spectrum of amoxicillin to include many bacteria normally resistant to amoxicillin and other β-lactam antibiotics. Thus, *Augmentin* possesses the properties of a broad-spectrum antibiotic and a β-lactamase inhibitor.

Amoxicillin/clavulanic acid has been shown to be active against most strains of the following microorganisms, both *in vitro* and in clinical infections as described in the INDICATIONS AND USAGE section.

GRAM-POSITIVE AEROBES

Staphylococcus aureus (β-lactamase and non-β-lactamase producing)‡

‡Staphylococci which are resistant to methicillin/oxacillin must be considered resistant to amoxicillin/clavulanic acid.

GRAM-NEGATIVE AEROBES

Enterobacter species (Although most strains of *Enterobacter* species are resistant *in vitro*, clinical efficacy has been demonstrated with *Augmentin* in urinary tract infections caused by these organisms.)

Escherichia coli (β-lactamase and non-β-lactamase producing)

Haemophilus influenzae (β-lactamase and non-β-lactamase producing)

Klebsiella species (All known strains are β-lactamase producing.)

Moraxella catarrhalis (β-lactamase and non-β-lactamase producing)

The following *in vitro* data are available, **but their clinical significance is unknown.**

Amoxicillin/clavulanic acid exhibits *in vitro* minimal inhibitory concentrations (MICs) of 0.5 µg/mL or less against most (≥90%) strains of *Streptococcus pneumoniae*§; MICs of 0.06 µg/mL or less against most (≥90%) strains of *Neisseria gonorrhoeae*; MICs of 4 µg/mL or less against most (≥90%) strains of staphylococci and anaerobic bacteria; and MICs of 8 µg/mL or less against most (≥90%) strains of other listed organisms. However, with the exception of organisms shown to respond to amoxicillin alone, the safety and effectiveness of amoxicillin/clavulanic acid in treating clinical infections due to these microorganisms have not been established in adequate and well-controlled clinical trials.

§Because amoxicillin has greater *in vitro* activity against *Streptococcus pneumoniae* than does ampicillin or penicillin, the majority of *S. pneumoniae* strains with intermediate susceptibility to amipicillin or penicillin are fully susceptible to amoxicillin.

GRAM-POSITIVE AEROBES

Enterococcus faecalis[II]
Staphylococcus epidermidis (β-lactamase and non-β-lactamase producing)
Staphylococcus saprophyticus (β-lactamase and non-β-lactamase producing)
Streptococcus pneumoniae[II ¶]
Streptococcus pyogenes[II ¶]
viridans group *Streptococcus*[II ¶]

GRAM-NEGATIVE AEROBES

Eikenella corrodens (β-lactamase and non-β-lactamase producing)
Neisseria gonorrhoeae[II] (β-lactamase and non-β-lactamase producing)
Proteus mirabilis[II] (β-lactamase and non-β-lactamase producing)

ANAEROBIC BACTERIA

Bacteroides species, including *Bacteroides fragilis* (β-lactamase and non-β-lactamase producing)
Fusobacterium species (β-lactamase and non-β-lactamase producing)
Peptostreptococcus species¶

[II]Adequate and well-controlled clinical trials have established the effectiveness of amoxicillin alone in treating certain clinical infections due to these organisms.

¶These are non-β-lactamase-producing organisms and, therefore, are susceptible to amoxicillin alone.

SUSCEPTIBILITY TESTING

Dilution Techniques: Quantitative methods are used to determine antimicrobial minimal inhibitory concentrations (MICs). These MICs provide estimates of the susceptibility of bacteria to antimicrobial compounds. The MICs should be determined using a standardized procedure. Standardized procedures are based on a dilution method[1] (broth or agar) or equivalent with standardized inoculum concentrations and standardized concentrations of amoxicillin/clavulanate potassium powder.

The recommended dilution pattern utilizes a constant amoxicillin/clavulanate potassium ratio of 2 to 1 in all tubes with varying amounts of amoxicillin. MICs are expressed in terms of the amoxicillin concentration in the presence of clavulanic acid at a constant 2 parts amoxicillin to 1 part clavulanic acid. The MIC values should be interpreted according to the following criteria:

RECOMMENDED RANGES FOR AMOXICILLIN/CLAVULANIC ACID SUSCEPTIBILITY TESTING

For gram-negative enteric aerobes:

MIC (μg/mL)	Interpretation
≤8/4	Susceptible (S)
16/8	Intermediate (I)
≥32/16	Resistant (R)

For *Staphylococcus*** and *Haemophilus* species:

MIC (μg/mL)	Interpretation
≤4/2	Susceptible (S)
≥8/4	Resistant (R)

** Staphylococci which are susceptible to amoxicillin/clavulanic acid but resistant to methicillin/oxacillin must be considered as resistant.

For *Streptococcus pneumoniae*: Isolates should be tested using amoxicillin/clavulanic acid and the following criteria should be used:

MIC (μg/mL)	Interpretation
≤0.5/0.25	Susceptible (S)
1/0.5	Intermediate (I)
≥2/1	Resistant (R)

A report of "Susceptible" indicates that the pathogen is likely to be inhibited if the antimicrobial compound in the blood reaches the concentration usually achievable. A report of "Intermediate" indicates that the result should be considered equivocal, and, if the microorganism is not fully susceptible to alternative, clinically feasible drugs, the test should be repeated. This category implies possible clinical applicability in body sites where the drug is physiologically concentrated or in situations where high dosage of drug can be used. This category also provides a buffer zone which prevents small uncontrolled technical factors from causing major discrepancies in interpretation. A report of "Resistant" indicates that the pathogen is not likely to be inhibited if the antimicrobial compound in the blood reaches the concentrations usually achievable; other therapy should be selected.

Standardized susceptibility test procedures require the use of laboratory control microorganisms to control the technical aspects of the laboratory procedures. Standard amoxicillin/clavulanate potassium powder should provide the following MIC values:

Microorganism	MIC Range (μg/mL) ††
Escherichia coli ATCC 25922	2 to 8
Escherichia coli ATCC 35218	4 to 16
Enterococcus faecalis ATCC 29212	0.25 to 1.0
Haemophilus influenzae ATCC 49247	2 to 16
Staphylococcus aureus ATCC 29213	0.12 to 0.5
Streptococcus pneumoniae ATCC 49619	0.03 to 0.12

†† Expressed as concentration of amoxicillin in the presence of clavulanic acid at a constant 2 parts amoxicillin to 1 part clavulanic acid.

Diffusion Techniques: Quantitative methods that require measurement of zone diameters also provide reproducible estimates of the susceptibility of bacteria to antimicrobial compounds. One such standardized procedure[2] requires the use of standardized inoculum concentrations. This procedure uses paper disks impregnated with 30 μg of amoxicillin/clavulanate potassium (20 μg amoxicillin plus 10 μg clavulanate potassium) to test the susceptibility of microorganisms to amoxicillin/clavulanic acid.

Reports from the laboratory providing results of the standard single-disk susceptibility test with a 30 μg amoxicillin/clavulanate acid (20 μg amoxicillin plus 10 μg clavulanate potassium) disk should be interpreted according to the following criteria:

RECOMMENDED RANGES FOR AMOXICILLIN/CLAVULANIC ACID SUSCEPTIBILITY TESTING

For *Staphylococcus*‡‡ species and *H. influenzae*[a]:

Zone Diameter (mm)	Interpretation
≥20	Susceptible (S)
≤19	Resistant (R)

For other organisms except *S. pneumoniae*[b] and *N. gonorrhoeae*[c]:

Zone Diameter (mm)	Interpretation
≥18	Susceptible (S)
14 to 17	Intermediate (I)
≤13	Resistant (R)

‡‡ Staphylococci which are resistant to methicillin/oxacillin must be considered as resistant to amoxicillin/clavulanic acid.

[a] A broth microdilution method should be used for testing *H. influenzae.* Beta-lactamase negative, ampicillin-resistant strains must be considered resistant to amoxicillin/clavulanic acid.

[b] Susceptibility of *S. pneumoniae* should be determined using a 1 μg oxacillin disk. Isolates with oxacillin zone sizes of ≥20 mm are susceptible to amoxicillin/clavulanic acid. An amoxicillin/clavulanic acid MIC should be determined on isolates of *S. pneumoniae* with oxacillin zone sizes of ≤19 mm.

[c] A broth microdilution method should be used for testing *N. gonorrhoeae* and interpreted according to penicillin breakpoints.

Interpretation should be as stated above for results using dilution techniques. Interpretation involves correlation of the diameter obtained in the disk test with the MIC for amoxicillin/clavulanic acid.

As with standardized dilution techniques, diffusion methods require the use of laboratory control microorganisms that are used to control the technical aspects of the laboratory procedures. For the diffusion technique, the 30 μg amoxicillin/clavulanate potassium (20 μg amoxicillin plus 10 μg clavulanate potassium) disk should provide the following zone diameters in these laboratory quality control strains:

Microorganism	Zone Diameter (mm)
Escherichia coli ATCC 25922	19 to 25
Escherichia coli ATCC 35218	18 to 22
Staphylococcus aureus ATCC 25923	28 to 36

INDICATIONS AND USAGE

Augmentin is indicated in the treatment of infections caused by susceptible strains of the designated organisms in the conditions listed below:

Lower Respiratory Tract Infections—caused by β-lactamase-producing strains of *Haemophilus influenzae* and *Moraxella (Branhamella) catarrhalis.*

Otitis Media—caused by β-lactamase-producing strains of *Haemophilus influenzae* and *Moraxella (Branhamella) catarrhalis.*

Sinusitis—caused by β-lactamase-producing strains of *Haemophilus influenzae* and *Moraxella (Branhamella) catarrhalis.*

Skin and Skin Structure Infections—caused by β-lactamase-producing strains of *Staphylococcus aureus, Escherichia coli* and *Klebsiella* spp.

Urinary Tract Infections—caused by β-lactamase-producing strains of *Escherichia coli, Klebsiella* spp. and *Enterobacter* spp.

While *Augmentin* is indicated only for the conditions listed above, infections caused by ampicillin-susceptible organisms are also amenable to *Augmentin* treatment due to its amoxicillin content. Therefore, mixed infections caused by ampicillin-susceptible organisms and β-lactamase-producing organisms susceptible to *Augmentin* should not require the addition of another antibiotic. Because amoxicillin has greater *in vitro* activity against *Streptococcus pneumoniae* than does ampicillin or penicillin, the majority of *S. pneumoniae* strains with intermediate susceptibility to ampicillin or penicillin are fully susceptible to amoxicillin and *Augmentin.* (See Microbiology subsection.)

Bacteriological studies, to determine the causative organisms and their susceptibility to *Augmentin,* should be performed together with any indicated surgical procedures.

Therapy may be instituted prior to obtaining the results from bacteriological and susceptibility studies to determine the causative organisms and their susceptibility to *Augmentin* when there is reason to believe the infection may involve any of the β-lactamase-producing organisms listed above. Once the results are known, therapy should be adjusted, if appropriate.

CONTRAINDICATIONS

Augmentin is contraindicated in patients with a history of allergic reactions to any penicillin. It is also contraindicated in patients with a previous history of *Augmentin*-associated cholestatic jaundice/hepatic dysfunction.

WARNINGS

SERIOUS AND OCCASIONALLY FATAL HYPERSENSITIVITY (ANAPHYLACTIC) REACTIONS HAVE BEEN REPORTED IN PATIENTS ON PENICILLIN THERAPY. THESE REACTIONS ARE MORE LIKELY TO OCCUR IN INDIVIDUALS WITH A HISTORY OF PENICILLIN HYPERSENSITIVITY AND/OR A HISTORY OF SENSITIVITY TO MULTIPLE ALLERGENS. THERE HAVE BEEN REPORTS OF INDIVIDUALS WITH A HISTORY OF PENICILLIN HYPERSENSITIVITY WHO HAVE EXPERIENCED SEVERE REACTIONS WHEN TREATED WITH CEPHALOSPORINS. BEFORE INITIATING THERAPY WITH *AUGMENTIN,* CAREFUL INQUIRY SHOULD BE MADE CONCERNING PREVIOUS HYPERSENSITIVITY REACTIONS TO PENICILLINS, CEPHALOSPORINS OR OTHER ALLERGENS. IF AN ALLERGIC REACTION OCCURS, *AUGMENTIN* SHOULD BE DISCONTINUED AND THE APPROPRIATE THERAPY INSTITUTED. **SERIOUS ANAPHYLACTIC REACTIONS REQUIRE IMMEDIATE EMERGENCY TREATMENT WITH EPINEPHRINE. OXYGEN, INTRAVENOUS STEROIDS AND AIRWAY MANAGEMENT, INCLUDING INTUBATION, SHOULD ALSO BE ADMINISTERED AS INDICATED.**

Pseudomembranous colitis has been reported with nearly all antibacterial agents, including *Augmentin,* and has ranged in severity from mild to life-threatening. Therefore, it is important to consider this diagnosis in patients who present with diarrhea subsequent to the administration of antibacterial agents.

Treatment with antibacterial agents alters the normal flora of the colon and may permit overgrowth of clostridia. Studies indicate that a toxin produced by *Clostridium difficile* is one primary cause of "antibiotic associated colitis."

After the diagnosis of pseudomembranous colitis has been established, appropriate therapeutic measures should be initiated. Mild cases of pseudomembranous colitis usually respond to drug discontinuation alone. In moderate to severe cases, consideration should be given to management with fluids and electrolytes, protein supplementation and treatment with an antibacterial drug clinically effective against *Clostridium difficile* colitis.

Augmentin should be used with caution in patients with evidence of hepatic dysfunction. Hepatic toxicity associated with the use of *Augmentin* is usually reversible. On rare occasions, deaths have been reported (less than 1 death reported per estimated 4 million prescriptions worldwide). These have generally been cases associated with serious underlying diseases or concomitant medications. (See CONTRAINDICATIONS and ADVERSE REACTIONS—*Liver.*)

PRECAUTIONS

General: While *Augmentin* possesses the characteristic low toxicity of the penicillin group of antibiotics, periodic assessment of organ system functions, including renal, hepatic and hematopoietic function, is advisable during prolonged therapy.

A high percentage of patients with mononucleosis who receive ampicillin develop an erythematous skin rash. Thus, ampicillin class antibiotics should not be administered to patients with mononucleosis.

The possibility of superinfections with mycotic or bacterial pathogens should be kept in mind during therapy. If superinfections occur (usually involving *Pseudomonas* or *Candida*), the drug should be discontinued and/or appropriate therapy instituted.

Drug Interactions: Probenecid decreases the renal tubular secretion of amoxicillin. Concurrent use with *Augmentin* may result in increased and prolonged blood levels of amoxicillin. Co-administration of probenecid cannot be recommended.

The concurrent administration of allopurinol and ampicillin increases substantially the incidence of rashes in patients receiving both drugs as compared to patients receiving ampicillin alone. It is not known whether this potentiation of

Continued on next page

Information on the SmithKline Beecham Pharmaceuticals products appearing here is based on the labeling in effect on June 15, 2000. Further information on these and other products may be obtained from the Medical Department, SmithKline Beecham Pharmaceuticals, One Franklin Plaza, Philadelphia, PA 19101.

Augmentin Tablets—Cont.

ampicillin rashes is due to allopurinol or the hyperuricemia present in these patients. There are no data with *Augmentin* and allopurinol administered concurrently.
In common with other broad-spectrum antibiotics, *Augmentin* may reduce the efficacy of oral contraceptives.
Drug/Laboratory Test Interactions: Oral administration of *Augmentin* will result in high urine concentrations of amoxicillin. High urine concentrations of ampicillin may result in false-positive reactions when testing for the presence of glucose in urine using Clinitest®, Benedict's Solution or Fehling's Solution. Since this effect may also occur with amoxicillin and therefore *Augmentin*, it is recommended that glucose tests based on enzymatic glucose oxidase reactions (such as Clinistix® or Tes-Tape®) be used.
Following administration of ampicillin to pregnant women a transient decrease in plasma concentration of total conjugated estriol, estriol-glucuronide, conjugated estrone and estradiol has been noted. This effect may also occur with amoxicillin and therefore *Augmentin*.
Carcinogenesis, Mutagenesis, Impairment of Fertility: Long-term studies in animals have not been performed to evaluate carcinogenic potential.
Mutagenesis: The mutagenic potential of *Augmentin* was investigated *in vitro* with an Ames test, a human lymphocyte cytogenetic assay, a yeast test and a mouse lymphoma forward mutation assay, and *in vivo* with mouse micronucleus tests and a dominant lethal test. All were negative apart from the *in vitro* mouse lymphoma assay where weak activity was found at very high, cytotoxic concentrations.
Impairment of Fertility: *Augmentin* at oral doses of up to 1200 mg/kg/day (5.7 times the maximum human dose, 1480 mg/m^2/day, based on body surface area) was found to have no effect on fertility and reproductive performance in rats, dosed with a 2:1 ratio formulation of amoxicillin:clavulanate.
Teratogenic effects. Pregnancy (Category B): Reproduction studies performed in pregnant rats and mice given *Augmentin* at oral dosages up to 1200 mg/kg/day, equivalent to 7200 and 4080 mg/m^2/day, respectively (4.9 and 2.8 times the maximum human oral dose based on body surface area), revealed no evidence of harm to the fetus due to *Augmentin*. There are, however, no adequate and well-controlled studies in pregnant women. Because animal reproduction studies are not always predictive of human response, this drug should be used during pregnancy only if clearly needed.
Labor and Delivery: Oral ampicillin class antibiotics are generally poorly absorbed during labor. Studies in guinea pigs have shown that intravenous administration of ampicillin decreased the uterine tone, frequency of contractions, height of contractions and duration of contractions. However, it is not known whether the use of *Augmentin* in humans during labor or delivery has immediate or delayed adverse effects on the fetus, prolongs the duration of labor, or increases the likelihood that forceps delivery or other obstetrical intervention or resuscitation of the newborn will be necessary.
Nursing Mothers: Ampicillin class antibiotics are excreted in the milk; therefore, caution should be exercised when *Augmentin* is administered to a nursing woman.

ADVERSE REACTIONS

Augmentin is generally well tolerated. The majority of side effects observed in clinical trials were of a mild and transient nature and less than 3% of patients discontinued therapy because of drug-related side effects. The most frequently reported adverse effects were diarrhea/loose stools (9%), nausea (3%), skin rashes and urticaria (3%), vomiting (1%) and vaginitis (1%). The overall incidence of side effects, and in particular diarrhea, increased with the higher recommended dose. Other less frequently reported reactions include: abdominal discomfort, flatulence and headache.
The following adverse reactions have been reported for ampicillin class antibiotics:
Gastrointestinal: Diarrhea, nausea, vomiting, indigestion, gastritis, stomatitis, glossitis, black "hairy" tongue, mucocutaneous candidiasis, enterocolitis, and hemorrhagic/pseudomembranous colitis. Onset of pseudomembranous colitis symptoms may occur during or after antibiotic treatment. (See WARNINGS.)
Hypersensitivity Reactions: Skin rashes, pruritus, urticaria, angioedema, serum sickness-like reactions (urticaria or skin rash accompanied by arthritis, arthralgia, myalgia and frequently fever), erythema multiforme (rarely Stevens-Johnson Syndrome) and an occasional case of exfoliative dermatitis (including toxic epidermal necrolysis) have been reported. These reactions may be controlled with antihistamines and, if necessary, systemic corticosteroids. Whenever such reactions occur, the drug should be discontinued, unless the opinion of the physician dictates otherwise. Serious and occasional fatal hypersensitivity (anaphylactic) reactions can occur with oral penicillin. (See WARNINGS.)
Liver: A moderate rise in AST (SGOT) and/or ALT (SGPT) has been noted in patients treated with ampicillin class antibiotics but the significance of these findings is unknown. Hepatic dysfunction, including increases in serum transaminases (AST and/or ALT), serum bilirubin and/or alkaline phosphatase, has been infrequently reported with *Augmentin*. It has been reported more commonly in the elderly, in males, or in patients on prolonged treatment. The histologic findings on liver biopsy have consisted of predominantly cholestatic, hepatocellular, or mixed cholestatic-hepatocellular changes. The onset of signs/symptoms of hepatic dysfunction may occur during or several weeks after therapy has been discontinued. The hepatic dysfunction, which may be severe, is usually reversible. On rare occasions, deaths have been reported (less than 1 death reported per estimated 4 million prescriptions worldwide). These have generally been cases associated with serious underlying diseases or concomitant medications.
Renal: Interstitial nephritis and hematuria have been reported rarely.
Hemic and Lymphatic Systems: Anemia, including hemolytic anemia, thrombocytopenia, thrombocytopenic purpura, eosinophilia, leukopenia and agranulocytosis have been reported during therapy with penicillins. These reactions are usually reversible on discontinuation of therapy and are believed to be hypersensitivity phenomena. A slight thrombocytosis was noted in less than 1% of the patients treated with *Augmentin*. There have been reports of increased prothrombin time in patients receiving *Augmentin* and anticoagulant therapy concomitantly.
Central Nervous System: Agitation, anxiety, behavioral changes, confusion, convulsions, dizziness, insomnia, and reversible hyperactivity have been reported rarely.

OVERDOSAGE

Most patients have been asymptomatic following overdosage or have experienced primarily gastrointestinal symptoms including stomach and abdominal pain, vomiting, and diarrhea. Rash, hyperactivity, or drowsiness have also been observed in a small number of patients.
In the case of overdosage, discontinue *Augmentin*, treat symptomatically, and institute supportive measures as required. If the overdosage is very recent and there is no contraindication, an attempt at emesis or other means of removal of drug from the stomach may be performed. A prospective study of 51 pediatric patients at a poison center suggested that overdosages of less than 250 mg/kg of amoxicillin are not associated with significant clinical symptoms and do not require gastric emptying.[3]
Interstitial nephritis resulting in oliguric renal failure has been reported in a small number of patients after overdosage with amoxicillin. Renal impairment appears to be reversible with cessation of drug administration. High blood levels may occur more readily in patients with impaired renal function because of decreased renal clearance of both amoxicillin and clavulanate. Both amoxicillin and clavulanate are removed from the circulation by hemodialysis. (See DOSAGE AND ADMINISTRATION for recommended dosing for patients with impaired renal function.)

DOSAGE AND ADMINISTRATION

Since both the *Augmentin* 250 mg and 500 mg tablets contain the same amount of clavulanic acid (125 mg, as the potassium salt), 2 *Augmentin* 250 mg tablets are not equivalent to 1 *Augmentin* 500 mg tablet. Therefore, 2 *Augmentin* 250 mg tablets should not be substituted for 1 *Augmentin* 500 mg tablet.
Dosage:
Adults: The usual adult dose is 1 *Augmentin* 500 mg tablet every 12 hours or 1 *Augmentin* 250 mg tablet every 8 hours. For more severe infections and infections of the respiratory tract, the dose should be 1 *Augmentin* 875 mg tablet every 12 hours or 1 *Augmentin* 500 mg tablet every 8 hours.
Patients with impaired renal function do not generally require a reduction in dose unless the impairment is severe. Severely impaired patients with a glomerular filtration rate of <30 mL/minute should not receive the 875 mg tablet. Patients with a glomerular filtration rate of 10 to 30 mL/minute should receive 500 mg or 250 mg every 12 hours, depending on the severity of the infection. Patients with a less than 10 mL/minute glomerular filtration rate should receive 500 mg or 250 mg every 24 hours, depending on severity of the infection.
Hemodialysis patients should receive 500 mg or 250 mg every 24 hours, depending on severity of the infection. They should receive an additional dose both during and at the end of dialysis.
Hepatically impaired patients should be dosed with caution and hepatic function monitored at regular intervals. (See WARNINGS.)
Pediatric Patients: Pediatric patients weighing 40 kg or more should be dosed according to the adult recommendations.
Due to the different amoxicillin to clavulanic acid ratios in the *Augmentin* 250 mg tablet (250/125) versus the *Augmentin* 250 mg chewable tablet (250/62.5), the *Augmentin* 250 mg tablet should not be used until the pediatric patient weighs at least 40 kg or more.
Administration: *Augmentin* may be taken without regard to meals; however, absorption of clavulanate potassium is enhanced when *Augmentin* is administered at the start of a meal. To minimize the potential for gastrointestinal intolerance, *Augmentin* should be taken at the start of a meal.

HOW SUPPLIED

***AUGMENTIN* 250 MG TABLETS:** Each white oval film-coated tablet, debossed with AUGMENTIN on 1 side and 250/125 on the other side, contains 250 mg amoxicillin as the trihydrate and 125 mg clavulanic acid as the potassium salt.
NDC 0029-6075-27 .... bottles of 30
NDC 0029-6075-31 .... Unit Dose (10×10) 100 tablets
***AUGMENTIN* 500 MG TABLETS:** Each white oval film-coated tablet, debossed with AUGMENTIN on 1 side and 500/125 on the other side, contains 500 mg amoxicillin as the trihydrate and 125 mg clavulanic acid as the potassium salt.
NDC 0029-6080-12 .... bottles of 20
NDC 0029-6080-31 .... Unit Dose (10×10) 100 tablets
***AUGMENTIN* 875 MG TABLETS:** Each scored white capsule-shaped tablet, debossed with AUGMENTIN 875 on 1 side and scored on the other side, contains 875 mg amoxicillin as the trihydrate and 125 mg clavulanic acid as the potassium salt.
NDC 0029-6086-12 .... bottles of 20
NDC 0029-6086-21 .... Unit Dose (10×10) 100 tablets
***AUGMENTIN* is also supplied as:**
AUGMENTIN 125 MG/5 ML (125 mg amoxicillin/31.25 mg clavulanic acid) FOR ORAL SUSPENSION:
NDC 0029-6085-39 .... 75 mL bottle
NDC 0029-6085-23 .... 100 mL bottle
NDC 0029-6085-22 .... 150 mL bottle
AUGMENTIN 200 MG/5 ML (200 mg amoxicillin/28.5 mg clavulanic acid) FOR ORAL SUSPENSION:
NDC 0029-6087-29 .... 50 mL bottle
NDC 0029-6087-39 .... 75 mL bottle
NDC 0029-6087-51 .... 100 mL bottle
AUGMENTIN 250 MG/5 ML (250 mg amoxicillin/62.5 mg clavulanic acid) FOR ORAL SUSPENSION:
NDC 0029-6090-39 .... 75 mL bottles
NDC 0029-6090-23 .... 100 mL bottle
NDC 0029-6090-22 .... 150 mL bottle
AUGMENTIN 400 MG/5 ML (400 mg amoxicillin/57 mg clavulanic acid) FOR ORAL SUSPENSION:
NDC 0029-6092-29 .... 50 mL bottle
NDC 0029-6092-39 .... 75 mL bottles
NDC 0029-6092-51 .... 100 mL bottle
AUGMENTIN 125 MG (125 mg amoxicillin/31.25 mg clavulanic acid) CHEWABLE TABLETS:
NDC 0029-6073-47 .... carton of 30 (5×6) tablets
AUGMENTIN 200 MG (200 mg amoxicillin/28.5 mg clavulanic acid) CHEWABLE TABLETS:
NDC 0029-6071-12 .... carton of 20 tablets
AUGMENTIN 250 MG (250 mg amoxicillin/62.5 mg clavulanic acid) CHEWABLE TABLETS:
NDC 0029-6074-47 .... carton of 30 (5×6) tablets
AUGMENTIN 400 MG (400 mg amoxicillin/57.0 mg clavulanic acid) CHEWABLE TABLETS:
NDC 0029-6072-12 .... carton of 20 tablets
Store tablets and dry powder at or below 25°C (77°F). Dispense in original container.

CLINICAL STUDIES

Data from two pivotal studies in 1,191 patients treated for either lower respiratory tract infections or complicated urinary tract infections compared a regimen of 875 mg *Augmentin* tablets q12h to 500 mg *Augmentin* tablets dosed q8h (584 and 607 patients, respectively). Comparable efficacy was demonstrated between the q12h and q8h dosing regimens. There was no significant difference in the percentage of adverse events in each group. The most frequently reported adverse event was diarrhea; incidence rates were similar for the 875 mg q12h and 500 mg q8h dosing regimens (14.9% and 14.3%, respectively). However, there was a statistically significant difference ($p<0.05$) in rates of severe diarrhea or withdrawals with diarrhea between the regimens: 1.0% for 875 mg q12h dosing versus 2.5% for the 500 mg q8h dosing.
In one of these pivotal studies, 629 patients with either pyelonephritis or a complicated urinary tract infection (i.e., patients with abnormalities of the urinary tract that predispose to relapse of bacteriuria following eradication) were randomized to receive either 875 mg *Augmentin* tablets q12h or 500 mg *Augmentin* tablets q8h in the following distribution:

	875 mg q12h	500 mg q8h
Pyelonephritis	173 patients	188 patients
Complicated UTI	135 patients	133 patients
Total patients	308	321

The number of bacteriologically evaluable patients was comparable between the two dosing regimens. *Augmentin* produced comparable bacteriological success rates in patients assessed 2 to 4 days immediately following end of therapy. The bacteriologic efficacy rates were comparable at one of the follow-up visits (5 to 9 days post-therapy) and at a late post-therapy visit (in the majority of cases, this was 2 to 4 weeks post-therapy), as seen in the table below:

	875 mg q12h	500 mg q8h
2 to 4 days	81%, n=58	80%, n=54
5 to 9 days	58.5%, n=41	51.9%, n=52
2 to 4 weeks	52.5%, n=101	54.8%, n=104

As noted before, though there was no significant difference in the percentage of adverse events in each group, there was a statistically significant difference in rates of severe diarrhea or withdrawals with diarrhea between the regimens.

REFERENCES

1. National Committee for Clinical Laboratory Standards. Methods for Dilution Antimicrobial Susceptibility Tests for Bacteria that Grow Aerobically—Third Edition. Approved Standard NCCLS Document M7-A3, Vol. 13, No. 25. NCCLS, Villanova, PA, December 1993.
2. National Committee for Clinical Laboratory Standards. Performance Standards for Antimicrobial Disk Susceptibility Tests—Fifth Edition. Approved Standard NCCLS Document M2-A5, Vol. 13, No. 24. NCCLS, Villanova, PA, December 1993.

3. Swanson-Bierman B, Dean BS, Lopez G, Krenzelok EP. The effects of penicillin and cephalosporin ingestions in children less than six years of age. *Vet Hum Toxicol* 1988; 30:66–67.

Rx only
AG:AL6

Shown in Product Identification Guide, page 336

AVANDIA® ℞

[ă-vaṅ-dee-ă]
brand of rosiglitazone maleate tablets

DESCRIPTION

Avandia (rosiglitazone maleate) is an oral antidiabetic agent which acts primarily by increasing insulin sensitivity. *Avandia* is used in the management of type 2 diabetes mellitus (also known as non-insulin-dependent diabetes mellitus [NIDDM] or adult-onset diabetes). *Avandia* improves glycemic control while reducing circulating insulin levels. Pharmacological studies in animal models indicate that rosiglitazone improves sensitivity to insulin in muscle and adipose tissue and inhibits hepatic gluconeogenesis. Rosiglitazone maleate is not chemically or functionally related to the sulfonylureas, the biguanides, or the alpha-glucosidase inhibitors.

Chemically, rosiglitazone maleate is (±)-5-[[4-[2-(methyl-2-pyridinylamino)ethoxy]phenyl]methyl]-2,4-thiazolidinedione, (*Z*)-2-butenedioate (1:1) with a molecular weight of 473.52 (357.44 free base). The molecule has a single chiral center and is present as a racemate. Due to rapid interconversion, the enantiomers are functionally indistinguishable. The structural formula is:

rosiglitazone maleate

The molecular formula is $C_{18}H_{19}N_3O_3S{\bullet}C_4H_4O_4$. Rosiglitazone maleate is a white to off-white solid with a melting point range of 122° to 123° C. The pKa values of rosiglitazone maleate are 6.8 and 6.1. It is readily soluble in ethanol and a buffered aqueous solution with pH of 2.3; solubility decreases with increasing pH in the physiological range.

Each pentagonal film-coated Tiltab® tablet contains rosiglitazone maleate equivalent to rosiglitazone, 2 mg, 4 mg, or 8 mg, for oral administration. Inactive ingredients are: hydroxypropyl methylcellulose, lactose monohydrate, magnesium stearate, microcrystalline cellulose, polyethylene glycol 3000, sodium starch glycolate, titanium dioxide, triacetin, and one or more of the following: synthetic red and yellow iron oxides and talc.

CLINICAL PHARMACOLOGY

Mechanism of Action

Rosiglitazone, a member of the thiazolidinedione class of antidiabetic agents, improves glycemic control by improving insulin sensitivity. Rosiglitazone is a highly selective and potent agonist for the peroxisome proliferator-activated receptor-gamma (PPARγ). In humans, PPAR receptors are found in key target tissues for insulin action such as adipose tissue, skeletal muscle, and liver. Activation of PPARγ nuclear receptors regulates the transcription of insulin-responsive genes involved in the control of glucose production, transport, and utilization. In addition, PPARγ-responsive genes also participate in the regulation of fatty acid metabolism.

Insulin resistance is a common feature characterizing the pathogenesis of type 2 diabetes. The antidiabetic activity of rosiglitazone has been demonstrated in animal models of type 2 diabetes in which hyperglycemia and/or impaired glucose tolerance is a consequence of insulin resistance in target tissues. Rosiglitazone reduces blood glucose concentrations and reduces hyperinsulinemia in the ob/ob obese mouse, db/db diabetic mouse, and fa/fa fatty Zucker rat. Rosiglitazone also prevents the development of overt diabetes in both the db/db mouse and Zucker fa/fa Diabetic Fatty rat models.

In animal models, rosiglitazone's antidiabetic activity was shown to be mediated by increased sensitivity to insulin's action in the liver, muscle, and adipose tissues. The expression of the insulin-regulated glucose transporter GLUT-4 was increased in adipose tissue. Rosiglitazone did not induce hypoglycemia in animal models of type 2 diabetes and/or impaired glucose tolerance.

Pharmacokinetics and Drug Metabolism

Maximum plasma concentration (C_{max}) and the area under the curve (AUC) of rosiglitazone increase in a dose-proportional manner over the therapeutic dose range (Table 1). The elimination half-life is 3 to 4 hours and is independent of dose.

[See table 1 above]

Absorption

The absolute bioavailability of rosiglitazone is 99%. Peak plasma concentrations are observed about 1 hour after dosing. Administration of rosiglitazone with food resulted in no change in overall exposure (AUC), but there was an approximately 28% decrease in C_{max} and a delay in T_{max} (1.75 hours). These changes are not likely to be clinically significant; therefore, Avandia (rosiglitazone maleate) may be administered with or without food.

Table 1. Mean (SD) Pharmacokinetic Parameters for Rosiglitazone Following Single Oral Doses (N=32)

Parameter	1 mg Fasting	2 mg Fasting	8 mg Fasting	8 mg Fed
$AUC_{0\text{-}inf}$ [ng.hr./mL]	358 (112)	733 (184)	2971 (730)	2890 (795)
C_{max} [ng/mL]	76 (13)	156 (42)	598 (117)	432 (92)
Half-life [hr.]	3.16 (0.72)	3.15 (0.39)	3.37 (0.63)	3.59 (0.70)
CL/F* [L/hr.]	3.03 (0.87)	2.89 (0.71)	2.85 (0.69)	2.97 (0.81)

* CL/F = Oral Clearance.

Table 2. Summary of Mean Lipid Changes in 26-Week Placebo-Controlled and 52-Week Glyburide-Controlled Monotherapy Studies

	Placebo-controlled Studies Week 26			Glyburide-controlled Study Week 26 and Week 52			
		Avandia		Glyburide titration		*Avandia* 8 mg	
	Placebo	4 mg daily*	8 mg daily*	Wk 26	Wk 52	Wk 26	Wk 52
Free Fatty Acids							
N	207	428	436	181	168	166	145
Baseline (mean)	18.1	17.5	17.9	26.4	26.4	26.9	26.6
% Change from baseline (mean)	+0.2%	−7.8%	−14.7%	−2.4%	−4.7%	−20.8%	−21.5%
LDL							
N	190	400	374	175	160	161	133
Baseline (mean)	123.7	126.8	125.3	142.7	141.9	142.1	142.1
% Change from baseline (mean)	+4.8%	+14.1%	+18.6%	−0.9%	−0.5%	+11.9%	+12.1%
HDL							
N	208	429	436	184	170	170	145
Baseline (mean)	44.1	44.4	43.0	47.2	47.7	48.4	48.3
% Change from baseline (mean)	+8.0%	+11.4%	+14.2%	+4.3%	+8.7%	+14.0%	+18.5%

*Once daily and twice daily dosing groups were combined.

Distribution

The mean (CV%) oral volume of distribution (Vss/F) of rosiglitazone is approximately 17.6 (30%) liters, based on a population pharmacokinetic analysis. Rosiglitazone is approximately 99.8% bound to plasma proteins, primarily albumin.

Metabolism

Rosiglizatone is extensively metabolized with no unchanged drug excreted in the urine. The major routes of metabolism were N-demethylation and hydroxylation, followed by conjugation with sulfate and glucuronic acid. All the circulating metabolites are considerably less potent than parent and, therefore, are not expected to contribute to the insulin-sensitizing activity of rosiglitazone.

In vitro data demonstrate that rosiglitazone is predominantly metabolized by Cytochrome P_{450} (CYP) isoenzyme 2C8, with CYP2C9 contributing as a minor pathway.

Excretion

Following oral or intravenous administration of [^{14}C]rosiglitazone maleate, approximately 64% and 23% of the dose was eliminated in the urine and in the feces, respectively. The plasma half-life of [^{14}C]related material ranged from 103 to 158 hours.

Population Pharmacokinetics in Patients with Type 2 Diabetes

Population pharmacokinetic analyses from three large clinical trials including 642 men and 405 women with type 2 diabetes (aged 35 to 80 years) showed that the pharmacokinetics of rosiglitazone are not influenced by age, race, smoking, or alcohol consumption. Both oral clearance (CL/F) and oral steady-state volume of distribution (Vss/F) were shown to increase with increases in body weight. Over the weight range observed in these analyses (50 to 150 kg), the range of predicted CL/F and Vss/F values varied by <1.7-fold and <2.3-fold, respectively. Additionally, rosiglitazone CL/F was shown to be influenced by both weight and gender, being lower (about 15%) in female patients.

Special Populations

Age: Results of the population pharmacokinetic analysis (n=716 <65 years; n=331 ≥65 years) showed that age does not significantly affect the pharmacokinetics of rosiglitazone.

Gender: Results of the population pharmacokinetics analysis showed that the mean oral clearance of rosiglitazone in female patients (n=405) was approximately 6% lower compared to male patients of the same body weight (n=642).

As monotherapy and in combination with metformin, *Avandia* improved glycemic control in both males and females. In metformin combination studies, efficacy was demonstrated with no gender differences in glycemic response.

In monotherapy studies, a greater therapeutic response was observed in females; however, in more obese patients, gender differences were less evident. For a given body mass index (BMI), females tend to have a greater fat mass than males. Since the molecular target PPARγ is expressed in adipose tissues, this differentiating characteristic may account, at least in part, for the greater response to *Avandia* in females. Since therapy should be individualized, no dose adjustments are necessary based on gender alone.

Hepatic Impairment: Unbound oral clearance of rosiglitazone was significantly lower in patients with moderate to severe liver disease (Child-Pugh Class B/C) compared to healthy subjects. As a result, unbound C_{max} and $AUC_{0\text{-}inf}$ were increased 2- and 3-fold, respectively. Elimination half-life for rosiglitazone was about 2 hours longer in patients with liver disease, compared to healthy subjects.

Therapy with Avandia (rosiglitazone maleate) should not be initiated if the patient exhibits clinical evidence of active liver disease or increased serum transaminase levels (ALT >2.5X upper limit of normal) at baseline (see PRECAUTIONS, *Hepatic Effects*).

Renal Impairment: There are no clinically relevant differences in the pharmacokinetics of rosiglitazone in patients with mild to severe renal impairment or in hemodialysis-dependent patients compared to subjects with normal renal function. No dosage adjustment is therefore required in such patients receiving *Avandia*. Since metformin is contraindicated in patients with renal impairment, co-administration of metformin with *Avandia* is contraindicated in these patients.

Race: Results of a population pharmacokinetic analysis including subjects of Caucasian, black, and other ethnic origins indicate that race has no influence on the pharmacokinetics of rosiglitazone.

Pediatric Use: The safety and effectiveness of *Avandia* in pediatric patients have not been established.

Pharmacodynamics and Clinical Effects

In clinical studies, treatment with *Avandia* resulted in an improvement in glycemic control, as measured by fasting

Continued on next page

Information on the SmithKline Beecham Pharmaceuticals products appearing here is based on the labeling in effect on June 15, 2000. Further information on these and other products may be obtained from the Medical Department, SmithKline Beecham Pharmaceuticals, One Franklin Plaza, Philadelphia, PA 19101.

Avandia—Cont.

plasma glucose (FPG) and hemoglobin A1c (HbA1c), with a concurrent reduction in insulin and C-peptide. Postprandial glucose and insulin were also reduced. This is consistent with the mechanism of action of *Avandia* as an insulin sensitizer. The improvement in glycemic control was durable, with maintenance of effect for 52 weeks. The maximum recommended daily dose is 8 mg. Dose-ranging studies suggested that no additional benefit was obtained with a total daily dose of 12 mg.

The addition of *Avandia* to either metformin or a sulfonylurea resulted in significant reductions in hyperglycemia compared to any of these agents alone. These results are consistent with an additive effect on glycemic control when *Avandia* is used as combination therapy.

Reduction in hyperglycemia was associated with increases in weight. In the 26-week clinical trials, the mean weight gain in patients treated with *Avandia* was 1.2 kg (4 mg daily) to 3.5 kg (8 mg daily) when administered as monotherapy, 0.7 kg (4 mg daily) and 2.3 kg (8 mg daily) when administered in combination with metformin, and 1.8 kg (4 mg daily) when administered in combination with a sulfonylurea. A mean weight loss of about 1 kg was seen for both placebo and metformin alone in these studies. The mean change in weight was negligible for patients treated with a sulfonylurea alone in these studies. In the 52-week glyburide-controlled study, there was a mean weight gain of 1.75 kg and 2.95 kg for patients treated with 4 mg and 8 mg of *Avandia* daily, respectively, versus 1.9 kg in glyburide-treated patients.

Patients with lipid abnormalities were not excluded from clinical trials of *Avandia*. In all 26-week controlled trials, across the recommended dose range, *Avandia* as monotherapy was associated with increases in total cholesterol, LDL, and HDL and decreases in free fatty acids. These changes were statistically significantly different from placebo or glyburide controls (Table 2).

Increases in LDL occurred primarily during the first 1 to 2 months of therapy with *Avandia* and LDL levels remained elevated above baseline throughout the trials. In contrast, HDL continued to rise over time. As a result, the LDL/HDL ratio peaked after 2 months of therapy and then appeared to decrease over time. Because of the temporal nature of lipid changes, the 52-week glyburide-controlled study is most pertinent to assess long-term effects on lipids. At baseline, week 26, and week 52, mean LDL/HDL ratios were 3.1, 3.2, and 3.0, respectively, for *Avandia* 4 mg twice daily. The corresponding values for glyburide were 3.2, 3.1, and 2.9. The differences in change from baseline between *Avandia* and glyburide at week 52 were statistically significant.

The pattern of LDL and HDL changes following therapy with *Avandia* in combination with a sulfonylurea or metformin were generally similar to those seen with *Avandia* in monotherapy.

The changes in triglycerides during therapy with Avandia (rosiglitazone maleate) were variable and were generally not statistically different from placebo or glyburide controls.

[See table 2 at top of previous page]

Clinical Studies

Monotherapy

A total of 2315 patients with type 2 diabetes, previously treated with diet alone or antidiabetic medication(s), were treated with *Avandia* as monotherapy in six double-blind studies, which included two 26-week placebo-controlled studies, one 52-week glyburide-controlled study, and three placebo-controlled dose-ranging studies of 8 to 12 weeks duration. Previous antidiabetic medication(s) were withdrawn and patients entered a 2 to 4 week placebo run-in period prior to randomization.

Two 26-week, double-blind, placebo-controlled trials, in patients with type 2 diabetes with inadequate glycemic control (mean baseline FPG approximately 228 mg/dL and mean baseline HbA1c 8.9%), were conducted. Treatment with *Avandia* produced statistically significant improvements in FPG and HbA1c compared to baseline and relative to placebo (Table 3).

[See table 3 below]

When administered at the same total daily dose, *Avandia* was generally more effective in reducing FPG and HbA1c when administered in divided doses twice daily compared to once daily doses. However, for HbA1c, the difference between the 4 mg once daily and 2 mg twice daily doses was not statistically significant.

Long-term maintenance of effect was evaluated in a 52-week, double-blind, glyburide-controlled trial in patients with type 2 diabetes. Patients were randomized to treatment with Avandia (rosiglitazone maleate) 2 mg twice daily (N=195) or *Avandia* 4 mg twice daily (N=189) or glyburide (N=202) for 52 weeks. Patients receiving glyburide were given an initial dosage of either 2.5 mg/day or 5.0 mg/day. The dosage was then titrated in 2.5 mg/day increments over the next 12 weeks, to a maximum dosage of 15.0 mg/day in order to optimize glycemic control. Thereafter the glyburide dose was kept constant.

The median titrated dose of glyburide was 7.5 mg. All treatments resulted in a statistically significant improvement in glycemic control from baseline (Figures 1 and 2). At the end of week 52, the reduction from baseline in FPG and HbA1c was −40.8 mg/dL and −0.53% with *Avandia* 4 mg twice daily; −25.4 mg/dL and −0.27% with *Avandia* 2 mg twice daily; and −30.0 mg/dL and −0.72% with glyburide. For HbA1c, the difference between *Avandia* 4 mg twice daily and glyburide was not statistically significant at week 52. The initial fall in FPG with glyburide was greater than with *Avandia*; however, this effect was less durable over time. The improvement in glycemic control seen with *Avandia* 4 mg twice daily at week 26 was maintained through week 52 of the study.

Figure 1. Mean FPG Over Time in a 52-Week Glyburide-Controlled Study

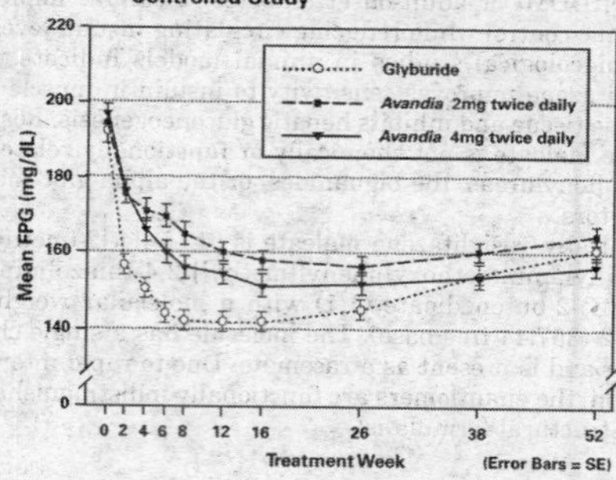

Figure 2. Mean HbA1c Over Time in a 52-Week Glyburide-Controlled Study

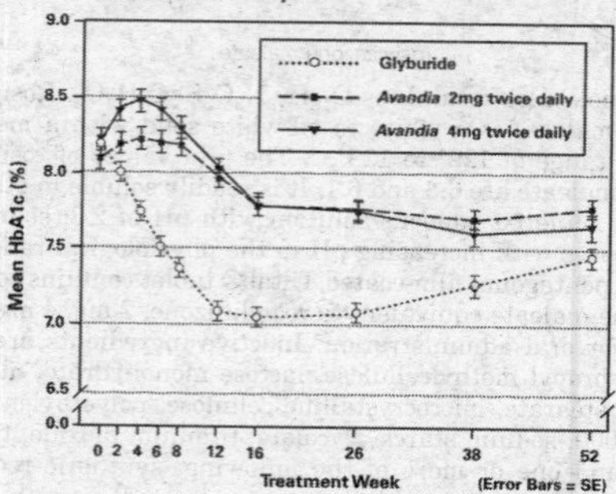

Hypoglycemia was reported in 12.1% of glyburide-treated patients versus 0.5% (2 mg twice daily) and 1.6% (4 mg twice daily) of patients treated with *Avandia*. The improvements in glycemic control were associated with a mean weight gain of 1.75 kg and 2.95 kg for patients treated with 2 mg and 4 mg twice daily of *Avandia*, respectively, versus 1.9 kg in glyburide-treated patients. In patients treated with *Avandia*, C-peptide, insulin, pro-insulin, and pro-insulin split products were significantly reduced in a dose-ordered fashion, compared to an increase in the glyburide-treated patients.

Combination with Metformin

A total of 670 patients with type 2 diabetes participated in two 26-week, randomized, double-blind, placebo/active-controlled studies designed to assess the efficacy of Avandia (rosiglitazone maleate) in combination with metformin. *Avandia*, administered in either once daily or twice daily dosing regimens, was added to the therapy of patients who were inadequately controlled on a maximum dose (2.5 grams/day) of metformin.

In one study, patients inadequately controlled on 2.5 grams/day of metformin (mean baseline FPG 216 mg/dL and mean baseline HbA1c 8.8%) were randomized to receive *Avandia* 4 mg once daily, *Avandia* 8 mg once daily, or placebo in addition to metformin. A statistically significant improvement in FPG and HbA1c was observed in patients treated with the combinations of metformin and *Avandia* 4 mg once daily and *Avandia* 8 mg once daily, versus patients continued on metformin alone (Table 4).

[See table 4 at top of next page]

In a second 26-week study, patients with type 2 diabetes inadequately controlled on 2.5 grams/day of metformin who were randomized to receive the combination of *Avandia* 4 mg twice daily and metformin (N=105) showed a statistically significant improvement in glycemic control with a mean treatment effect for FPG of −56 mg/dL and a mean treatment effect for HbA1c of −0.8% over metformin alone. The combination of metformin and *Avandia* resulted in lower levels of FPG and HbA1c than either agent alone.

Patients who were inadequately controlled on a maximum dose (2.5 grams/day) of metformin and who were switched to monotherapy with Avandia (rosiglitazone maleate) demonstrated loss of glycemic control, as evidenced by increases in FPG and HbA1c. In this group, increases in LDL and VLDL were also seen.

Combination with a Sulfonylurea

A total of 1216 patients with type 2 diabetes participated in three 26-week randomized, double-blind, placebo/active-

Table 3. Glycemic Parameters in Two 26-Week Placebo-Controlled Trials

	Placebo	*Avandia* 2 mg twice daily	*Avandia* 4 mg twice daily
STUDY A			
N	158	166	169
FPG (mg/dL)			
Baseline (mean)	229	227	220
Change from baseline (mean)	19	−38	−54
Difference from placebo (adjusted mean)		−58*	−76*
Responders (≥30 mg/dL decrease from baseline)	16%	54%	64%
HbA1c(%)			
Baseline (mean)	9.0	9.0	8.8
Change from baseline (mean)	0.9	−0.3	−0.6
Difference from placebo (adjusted mean)		−1.2*	−1.5*
Responders (≥0.7% decrease from baseline)	6%	40%	42%

	Placebo	*Avandia* 4 mg once daily	*Avandia* 2 mg twice daily	*Avandia* 8 mg once daily	*Avandia* 4 mg twice daily
STUDY B					
N	173	180	186	181	187
FPG (mg/dL)					
Baseline (mean)	225	229	225	228	228
Change from baseline (mean)	8	−25	−35	−42	−55
Difference from placebo (adjusted mean)		−31*	−43*	−49*	−62*
Responders (≥30 mg/dL decrease from baseline)	19%	45%	54%	58%	70%
HbA1c (%)					
Baseline (mean)	8.9	8.9	8.9	8.9	9.0
Change from baseline (mean)	0.8	0.0	−0.1	−0.3	−0.7
Difference from placebo (adjusted mean)	—	−0.8*	−0.9*	−1.1*	−1.5*
Responders (≥0.7% decrease from baseline)	9%	28%	29%	39%	54%

* <0.0001 compared to placebo.

controlled studies designed to assess the efficacy and safety of *Avandia* in combination with a sulfonylurea. *Avandia* 2 mg or 4 mg daily, was administered either once daily or in divided doses twice daily, to patients inadequately controlled on a sulfonylurea.

In the two placebo-controlled studies, patients inadequately controlled on sulfonylureas that were randomized to single dose or divided doses of *Avandia* 4 mg daily plus a sulfonylurea showed significantly reduced FPG and HbA1c compared to sulfonylurea plus placebo (Table 5).

[See table 5 in next column]

In the third study, including patients on prior single or multiple therapies, in patients inadequately controlled on the maximal dose of glyburide (20 mg daily), *Avandia* 2 mg twice daily plus sulfonylurea significantly reduced FPG (n=98, mean change from baseline of −31 mg/dL) and HbA1c (mean change from baseline of −0.5%) compared to sulfonylurea plus placebo (n=99, mean change from baseline of FPG of +24 mg/dL and of HbA1c of +0.9%). The combination of sulfonylurea and *Avandia* resulted in lower levels of FPG and HbA1c than either agent alone. Patients who were switched from maximal dose of glyburide to 2 mg twice daily *Avandia* monotherapy demonstrated loss of glycemic control, as evidenced by increases in FPG and HbA1c.

INDICATIONS AND USAGE

Avandia is indicated as an adjunct to diet and exercise to improve glycemic control in patients with type 2 diabetes mellitus. *Avandia* is indicated as monotherapy.

Avandia is also indicated for use in combination with a sulfonylurea or metformin when diet, exercise and *Avandia* alone or diet, exercise plus the single agent do not result in adequate glycemic control. For patients inadequately controlled with a maximum dose of a sulfonylurea or metformin, *Avandia* should be added to, rather than substituted for, a sulfonylurea or metformin.

Management of type 2 diabetes should include diet control. Caloric restriction, weight loss, and exercise are essential for the proper treatment of the diabetic patient because they help improve insulin sensitivity. This is important not only in the primary treatment of type 2 diabetes, but also in maintaining the efficacy of drug therapy. Prior to initiation of therapy with Avandia (rosiglitazone maleate), secondary causes of poor glycemic control, e.g., infection, should be investigated and treated.

CONTRAINDICATIONS

Avandia is contraindicated in patients with known hypersensitivity to this product or any of its components.

PRECAUTIONS

General

Due to its mechanism of action, *Avandia* is active only in the presence of insulin. Therefore, *Avandia* should not be used in patients with type 1 diabetes or for the treatment of diabetic ketoacidosis.

Patients receiving *Avandia* in combination with other oral hypoglycemic agents may be at risk for hypoglycemia, and a reduction in the dose of the concomitant agent may be necessary.

Ovulation: Therapy with *Avandia*, like other thiazolidinediones, may result in ovulation in some premenopausal anovulatory women. As a result, these patients may be at an increased risk for pregnancy while taking *Avandia*. (See PRECAUTIONS, Pregnancy, Pregnancy Category C.) Thus, adequate contraception in premenopausal women should be recommended. This possible effect has not been specifically investigated in clinical studies so the frequency of this occurrence is not known.

Although hormonal imbalance has been seen in preclinical studies (see Carcinogenesis, Mutagenesis, Impairment of Fertility), the clinical significance of this finding is not known. If unexpected menstrual dysfunction occurs, the benefits of continued therapy with *Avandia* should be reviewed.

Hematologic: Across all controlled clinical studies, decreases in hemoglobin and hematocrit (mean decreases in individual studies ≤1.0 gram/dL and ≤3.3%, respectively) were observed for both *Avandia* alone and in combination with a sulfonylurea or metformin. The changes occurred primarily during the first 4 to 8 weeks of therapy and remained relatively constant thereafter. White blood cell counts also decreased slightly in patients treated with *Avandia*. The observed changes may be related to the increased plasma volume observed with treatment with *Avandia* and have not been associated with any significant hematologic clinical effects (see ADVERSE REACTIONS, Laboratory Abnormalities).

Edema: *Avandia* should be used with caution in patients with edema. In a clinical study in healthy volunteers who received *Avandia* 8 mg once daily for 8 weeks, there was a small, statistically significant increase in median plasma volume (1.8 mL/kg) compared to placebo.

In controlled clinical trials of patients with type 2 diabetes, mild to moderate edema was reported in patients treated with *Avandia* (See ADVERSE REACTIONS).

Since thiazolidinediones can cause fluid retention, which can exacerbate congestive heart failure, patients at risk for heart failure (particularly those on insulin) should be monitored for signs and symptoms of heart failure (See PRECAUTIONS, *Use in Patients with Heart Failure*).

Use in Patients with Heart Failure: In preclinical studies, thiazolidinediones, including rosiglitazone, caused plasma volume expansion and pre-load-induced cardiac hypertrophy. Two ongoing echocardiography studies in patients with type 2 diabetes (a 52-week study with *Avandia* 4 mg twice daily [n=86] and a 26-week study with 8 mg once daily [n=90]), have shown no deleterious alteration in cardiac structure or function. These studies were designed to detect a change in left ventricular mass of 10% or more.

Patients with New York Heart Association (NYHA) Class 3 and 4 cardiac status were not studied during the clinical trials. *Avandia* is not indicated in patients with NYHA Class 3 and 4 cardiac status unless the expected benefit is judged to outweigh the potential risk.

Hepatic Effects: Another drug of the thiazolidinedione class, troglitazone, has been associated with idiosyncratic hepatotoxicity, and very rare cases of liver failure, liver transplants, and death have been reported during postmarketing clinical use. In pre-approval controlled clinical trials in patients with type 2 diabetes, troglitazone was more frequently associated with clinically significant elevations in liver enzymes (ALT>3X upper limit of normal) compared to placebo, and very rare cases of reversible jaundice were reported.

In clinical studies in 4598 patients treated with *Avandia*, encompassing approximately 3600 patient years of exposure, there was no evidence of drug-induced hepatotoxicity or elevation of ALT levels.

In controlled trials, 0.2% of patients treated with *Avandia* had elevations in ALT >3X the upper limit of normal compared to 0.2% on placebo and 0.5% on active comparators. The ALT elevations in patients treated with *Avandia* were reversible and were not clearly causally related to therapy with Avandia (rosiglitazone maleate).

Although available clinical data show no evidence of *Avandia*-induced hepatotoxicity or ALT elevations, rosiglitazone is structurally related to troglitazone, which has been associated with idiosyncratic hepatotoxicity and rare cases of liver failure, liver transplants, and death. Pending the availability of the results of additional large, long-term controlled clinical trials and postmarketing safety data following wide clinical use of *Avandia* to more fully define its hepatic safety profile, it is recommended that patients treated with *Avandia* undergo periodic monitoring of liver enzymes. Liver enzymes should be checked prior to the initiation of therapy with *Avandia* in all patients. Therapy with *Avandia* should not be initiated in patients with increased baseline liver enzyme levels (ALT>2.5X upper limit of normal). In patients with normal baseline liver enzymes, following initiation of therapy with *Avandia*, it is recommended that liver enzymes be monitored every 2 months for the first 12 months, and periodically thereafter. Patients with mildly elevated liver enzymes (ALT levels one to 2.5X upper limit of normal) at baseline or during therapy with *Avandia* should be evaluated to determine the cause of the liver enzyme elevation. Initiation of, or continuation of, therapy with *Avandia* in patients with mild liver enzyme elevations should proceed with caution and include close clinical follow-up, including more frequent liver enzyme monitoring, to determine if the liver enzyme elevations resolve or worsen. If at

Continued on next page

Table 4. Glycemic Parameters in a 26-Week Combination Study

	Metformin	*Avandia* 4 mg once daily + metformin	*Avandia* 8 mg once daily + metformin
N	113	116	110
FPG (mg/dL)			
Baseline (mean)	214	215	220
Change from baseline (mean)	6	−33	−48
Difference from placebo (adjusted mean)		−40*	−53*
Responders (≥30 mg/dL decrease from baseline)	20%	45%	61%
HbA1c (%)			
Baseline (mean)	8.6	8.9	8.9
Change from baseline (mean)	0.5	−0.6	−0.8
Difference from placebo (adjusted mean)		−1.0*	−1.2*
Responders (≥0.7% decrease from baseline)	11%	45%	52%

* <0.0001 compared to metformin.

Table 5. Glycemic Parameters in Two 26-Week Combination Studies

Study C (patients on prior sulfonylurea monotherapy)	**Sulfonylurea**	***Avandia* 2 mg twice daily + sulfonylurea**
N	192	183
FPG (mg/dL)		
Baseline (mean)	207	205
Change from baseline (mean)	+6	−38
Difference from placebo (adjusted mean)	–	−44*
Responders (≥30 mg/dL decrease from baseline)	21%	56%
HbA1c (%)		
Baseline (mean)	9.2	9.2
Change from baseline (mean)	+0.2	−0.9
Difference from placebo (adjusted mean)		−1.0*
Study D (patients on prior single or multiple therapies)	**Sulfonylurea**	***Avandia* 4 mg once daily + sulfonylurea**
N	115	116
FPG (mg/dL)		
Baseline (mean)	209	214
Change from baseline (mean)	+23	−25
Difference from placebo (adjusted mean)	–	−47*
Responders (≥30 mg/dL decrease from baseline)	13%	46%
HbA1c (%)		
Baseline (mean)	8.9	9.1
Change from baseline (mean)	+0.6	−0.3
Difference from placebo (adjusted mean)	–	−0.9*

* ≤0.0001 compared to sulfonylurea plus placebo.

Information on the SmithKline Beecham Pharmaceuticals products appearing here is based on the labeling in effect on June 15, 2000. Further information on these and other products may be obtained from the Medical Department, SmithKline Beecham Pharmaceuticals, One Franklin Plaza, Philadelphia, PA 19101.

Avandia—Cont.

any time ALT levels increase to >3X upper limit of normal in patients on therapy with *Avandia*, liver enzyme levels should be rechecked as soon as possible. If ALT levels remain >3X the upper limit of normal, therapy with *Avandia* should be discontinued.

There are no data available to evaluate the safety of *Avandia* in patients who experience liver abnormalities, hepatic dysfunction, or jaundice while on troglitazone. Avandia (rosiglitazone maleate) should not be used in patients who experienced jaundice while taking troglitazone. For patients with normal hepatic enzymes who are switched from troglitazone to *Avandia*, a 1-week washout is recommended before starting therapy with *Avandia*.

If any patient develops symptoms suggesting hepatic dysfunction, which may include unexplained nausea, vomiting, abdominal pain, fatigue, anorexia and/or dark urine, liver enzymes should be checked. The decision whether to continue the patient on therapy with *Avandia* should be guided by clinical judgment pending laboratory evaluations. If jaundice is observed, drug therapy should be discontinued.

Laboratory Tests

Periodic fasting blood glucose and HbA1c measurements should be performed to monitor therapeutic response.

Liver enzyme monitoring is recommended prior to initiation of therapy with *Avandia* in all patients and periodically thereafter (See PRECAUTIONS, *Hepatic Effects* and ADVERSE REACTIONS, Serum Transaminase Levels).

Information for Patients

Patients should be informed of the following:

Management of type 2 diabetes should include diet control. Caloric restriction, weight loss, and exercise are essential for the proper treatment of the diabetic patient because they help improve insulin sensitivity. This is important not only in the primary treatment of type 2 diabetes, but in maintaining the efficacy of drug therapy.

It is important to adhere to dietary instructions and to regularly have blood glucose and glycosylated hemoglobin tested. Patients should be advised that it can take 2 weeks to see a reduction in blood glucose and 2 to 3 months to see full effect. Patients should be informed that blood will be drawn to check their liver function prior to the start of therapy and every 2 months for the first 12 months, and periodically thereafter. Patients with unexplained symptoms of nausea, vomiting, abdominal pain, fatigue, anorexia, or dark urine should immediately report these symptoms to their physician.

Avandia can be taken with or without meals.

When using *Avandia* in combination with other oral hypoglycemic agents, the risk of hypoglycemia, its symptoms and treatment, and conditions that predispose to its development should be explained to patients and their family members.

Therapy with *Avandia*, like other thiazolidinediones, may result in ovulation in some premenopausal anovulatory women. As a result, these patients may be at an increased risk for pregnancy while taking *Avandia*. (See PRECAUTIONS, Pregnancy, Pregnancy Category C.) Thus, adequate contraception in premenopausal women should be recommended. This possible effect has not been specifically investigated in clinical studies so the frequency of this occurrence is not known.

Drug Interactions

Drugs Metabolized by Cytochrome P_{450}

In vitro drug metabolism studies suggest that rosiglitazone does not inhibit any of the major P_{450} enzymes at clinically relevant concentrations. *In vitro* data demonstrate that rosiglitazone is predominantly metabolized by CYP2C8, and to a lesser extent, 2C9.

Avandia (4 mg twice daily) was shown to have no clinically relevant effect on the pharmacokinetics of nifedipine and oral contraceptives (ethinylestradiol and norethindrone), which are predominantly metabolized by CYP3A4.

Glyburide: Avandia (2 mg twice daily) taken concomitantly with glyburide (3.75 to 10 mg/day) for 7 days did not alter the mean steady-state 24-hour plasma glucose concentrations in diabetic patients stabilized on glyburide therapy.

Metformin: Concurrent administration of *Avandia* (2 mg twice daily) and metformin (500 mg twice daily) in healthy volunteers for 4 days had no effect on the steady-state pharmacokinetics of either metformin or rosiglitazone.

Acarbose: Coadministration of acarbose (100 mg three times daily) for 7 days in healthy volunteers had no clinically relevant effect on the pharmacokinetics of a single oral dose of *Avandia*.

Digoxin: Repeat oral dosing of *Avandia* (8 mg once daily) for 14 days did not alter the steady-state pharmacokinetics of digoxin (0.375 mg once daily) in healthy volunteers.

Warfarin: Repeat dosing with *Avandia* had no clinically relevant effect on the steady-state pharmacokinetics of warfarin enantiomers.

Ethanol: A single administration of a moderate amount of alcohol did not increase the risk of acute hypoglycemia in type 2 diabetes mellitus patients treated with Avandia (rosiglitazone maleate).

Ranitidine: Pretreatment with ranitidine (150 mg twice daily for 4 days) did not alter the pharmacokinetics of either single oral or intravenous doses of rosiglitazone in healthy volunteers. These results suggest that the absorption of oral rosiglitazone is not altered in conditions accompanied by increases in gastrointestinal pH.

Table 6. Adverse Events (≥5% in Any Treatment Group) Reported by Patients in Double-blind Clinical Trials with *Avandia* as Monotherapy

Preferred Term	*Avandia* Monotherapy N = 2526 %	Placebo N = 601 %	Metformin N = 225 %	Sulfonylureas* N = 626 %
Upper respiratory tract infection	9.9	8.7	8.9	7.3
Injury	7.6	4.3	7.6	6.1
Headache	5.9	5.0	8.9	5.4
Back pain	4.0	3.8	4.0	5.0
Hyperglycemia	3.9	5.7	4.4	8.1
Fatigue	3.6	5.0	4.0	1.9
Sinusitis	3.2	4.5	5.3	3.0
Diarrhea	2.3	3.3	15.6	3.0
Hypoglycemia	0.6	0.2	1.3	5.9

*Includes patients receiving glyburide (N=514), gliclazide (N=91) or glipizide (N=21).

Carcinogenesis, Mutagenesis, Impairment of Fertility

Carcinogenesis: A 2-year carcinogenicity study was conducted in Charles River CD-1 mice at doses of 0.4, 1.5, and 6 mg/kg/day in the diet (highest dose equivalent to approximately 12 times human AUC at the maximum recommended human daily dose). Sprague-Dawley rats were dosed for 2 years by oral gavage at doses of 0.05, 0.3, and 2 mg/kg/day (highest dose equivalent to approximately 10 and 20 times human AUC at the maximum recommended human daily dose for male and female rats, respectively).

Rosiglitazone was not carcinogenic in the mouse. There was an increase in incidence of adipose hyperplasia in the mouse at doses ≥1.5 mg/kg/day (approximately 2 times human AUC at the maximum recommended human daily dose). In rats, there was a significant increase in the incidence of benign adipose tissue tumors (lipomas) at doses ≥0.3 mg/kg/day (approximately 2 times human AUC at the maximum recommended human daily dose). These proliferative changes in both species are considered due to the persistent pharmacological overstimulation of adipose tissue.

Mutagenesis: Rosiglitazone was not mutagenic or clastogenic in the *in vitro* bacterial assays for gene mutation, the *in vitro* chromosome aberration test in human lymphocytes, the *in vivo* mouse micronucleus test, and the *in vivo/in vitro* rat UDS assay. There was a small (about 2-fold) increase in mutation in the *in vitro* mouse lymphoma assay in the presence of metabolic activation.

Impairment of Fertility: Rosiglitazone had no effects on mating or fertility of male rats given up to 40 mg/kg/day (approximately 116 times human AUC at the maximum recommended human daily dose). Rosiglitazone altered estrous cyclicity (2 mg/kg/day) and reduced fertility (40 mg/kg/day) of female rats in association with lower plasma levels of progesterone and estradiol (approximately 20 and 200 times human AUC at the maximum recommended human daily dose, respectively). No such effects were noted at 0.2 mg/kg/day (approximately 3 times human AUC at the maximum recommended human daily dose). In monkeys, rosiglitazone (0.6 and 4.6 mg/kg/day; approximately 3 and 15 times human AUC at the maximum recommended human daily dose, respectively) diminished the follicular phase rise in serum estradiol with consequential reduction in the luteinizing hormone surge, lower luteal phase progesterone levels, and amenorrhea. The mechanism for these effects appears to be direct inhibition of ovarian steroidogenesis.

Animal Toxicology

Heart weights were increased in mice (3 mg/kg/day), rats (5 mg/kg/day), and dogs (2 mg/kg/day) with rosiglitazone treatments (approximately 5, 22, and 2 times human AUC at the maximum recommended human daily dose, respectively). Morphometric measurement indicated that there was hypertrophy in cardiac ventricular tissues, which may be due to increased heart work as a result of plasma volume expansion.

Pregnancy

Pregnancy Category C

There was no effect on implantation or the embryo with rosiglitazone treatment during early pregnancy in rats, but treatment during mid-late gestation was associated with fetal death and growth retardation in both rats and rabbits. Teratogenicity was not observed at doses up to 3 mg/kg in rats and 100 mg/kg in rabbits (approximately 20 and 75 times human AUC at the maximum recommended human daily dose, respectively). Rosiglitazone caused placental pathology in rats (3 mg/kg/day). Treatment of rats during gestation through lactation reduced litter size, neonatal viability, and postnatal growth, with growth retardation reversible after puberty. For effects on the placenta, embryo/fetus, and offspring, the no-effect dose was 0.2 mg/kg/day in rats and 15 mg/kg/day in rabbits. These no-effect levels are approximately 4 times human AUC at the maximum recommended human daily dose.

There are no adequate and well-controlled studies in pregnant women. Avandia (rosiglitazone maleate) should not be used during pregnancy unless the potential benefit justifies the potential risk to the fetus.

Because current information strongly suggests that abnormal blood glucose levels during pregnancy are associated with a higher incidence of congenital anomalies as well as increased neonatal morbidity and mortality, most experts recommend that insulin monotherapy be used during pregnancy to maintain blood glucose levels as close to normal as possible.

Labor and Delivery

The effect of rosiglitazone on labor and delivery in humans is not known.

Nursing Mothers

Drug related material was detected in milk from lactating rats. It is not known whether *Avandia* is excreted in human milk. Because many drugs are excreted in human milk, *Avandia* should not be administered to a nursing woman.

ADVERSE REACTIONS

In clinical trials, approximately 4600 patients with type 2 diabetes have been treated with *Avandia*; 3300 patients were treated for 6 months or longer and 2000 patients were treated for 12 months or longer.

***Avandia* Monotherapy and Oral Combination Therapy Studies**

The incidence and types of adverse events reported in clinical trials of *Avandia* as monotherapy are shown in Table 6. [See table 6 above]

There were a small number of patients treated with *Avandia* who had adverse events of anemia and edema. Overall, these events were generally mild to moderate in severity and usually did not require discontinuation of treatment with *Avandia*.

In double-blind studies, anemia was reported in 1.9% of patients receiving *Avandia* compared to 0.7% on placebo, 0.6% on sulfonylureas and 2.2% on metformin. Edema was reported in 4.8% of patients receiving *Avandia* compared to 1.3% on placebo, 1.0% on sulfonylureas, and 2.2% on metformin. Overall, the types of adverse experiences reported when *Avandia* was used in combination with a sulfonylurea or metformin were similar to those during monotherapy with *Avandia*. Reports of anemia (7.1%) were greater in patients treated with a combination of *Avandia* and metformin compared to monotherapy with *Avandia* or in combination with a sulfonylurea.

Lower pre-treatment hemoglobin/hematocrit levels in patients enrolled in the metformin combination clinical trials may have contributed to the higher reporting rate of anemia in these studies (see Laboratory Abnormalities, Hematologic).

Laboratory Abnormalities

Hematologic: Decreases in mean hemoglobin and hematocrit occurred in a dose-related fashion in patients treated with *Avandia* (mean decreases in individual studies up to 1.0 gram/dL hemoglobin and up to 3.3% hematocrit). The time course and magnitude of decreases were similar in patients treated with a combination of *Avandia* and a sulfonylurea or metformin, or *Avandia* monotherapy. Pre-treatment levels of hemoglobin and hematocrit were lower in patients in metformin combination studies and may have contributed to the higher reporting rate of anemia. White blood cell counts also decreased slightly in patients treated with *Avandia*. Decreases in hematologic parameters may be related to increased plasma volume observed with treatment with *Avandia*.

Lipids: Changes in serum lipids have been observed following treatment with *Avandia* (see CLINICAL PHARMACOLOGY, Pharmacodynamics and Clinical Effects).

Serum Transaminase Levels: In clinical studies in 4598 patients treated with Avandia (rosiglitazone maleate) encompassing approximately 3600 patient years of exposure, there was no evidence of drug-induced hepatotoxicity or elevated ALT levels.

In controlled trials, 0.2% of patients treated with *Avandia* had reversible elevations in ALT >3X the upper limit of normal compared to 0.2% on placebo and 0.5% on active comparators. Hyperbilirubinemia was found in 0.3% of patients treated with *Avandia* compared with 0.9% treated with placebo and 1% in patients treated with active comparators.

In the clinical program including long-term, open-label experience, the rate per 100 patient years exposure of ALT increase to >3X the upper limit of normal was 0.35 for patients treated with *Avandia*, 0.59 for placebo-treated patients, and 0.78 for patients treated with active comparator agents.

In pre-approval clinical trials, there were no cases of idiosyncratic drug reactions leading to hepatic failure (See PRECAUTIONS, *Hepatic Effects*).

DOSAGE AND ADMINISTRATION

The management of antidiabetic therapy should be individualized. *Avandia* may be administered either at a starting dose of 4 mg as a single daily dose or divided and administered in the morning and evening. For patients who respond inadequately following 8 to 12 weeks of treatment, as determined by reduction in FPG, the dose may be increased to 8 mg daily as indicated below. Reductions in glycemic parameters by dose and regimen are described under CLINICAL PHARMACOLOGY, Clinical Studies. *Avandia* may be taken with or without food.

Monotherapy

The usual starting dose of *Avandia* is 4 mg administered either as a single dose once daily or in divided doses twice daily. In clinical trials, the 4 mg twice daily regimen resulted in the greatest reduction in FPG and HbA1c.

Combination Therapy with a Sulfonylurea or Metformin

When *Avandia* is added to existing therapy, the current dose of sulfonylurea or metformin can be continued upon initiation of *Avandia* therapy.

Sulfonylurea:

When used in combination with sulfonylurea, the recommended dose of *Avandia* is 4 mg administered as either a single dose once daily or in divided doses twice daily. If patients report hypoglycemia, the dose of the sulfonylurea should be decreased.

Metformin:

The usual starting dose of *Avandia* in combination with metformin is 4 mg administered as either a single dose once daily or in divided doses twice daily. It is unlikely that the dose of metformin will require adjustment due to hypoglycemia during combination therapy with *Avandia*.

Maximum Recommended Dose:

The dose of *Avandia* should not exceed 8 mg daily, as a single dose or divided twice daily. The 8 mg daily dose has been shown to be safe and effective in clinical studies as monotherapy and in combination with metformin. Doses of *Avandia* greater than 4 mg daily in combination with a sulfonylurea have not been studied in adequate and well-controlled clinical trials. In clinical trials, the 8 mg daily regimen resulted in the greatest reduction in FPG and HbA1c.

Avandia may be taken with or without food.

No dosage adjustments are required for the elderly.

No dosage adjustment is necessary when *Avandia* is used as monotherapy in patients with renal impairment. Since metformin is contraindicated in such patients, concomitant administration of metformin and *Avandia* is also contraindicated in patients with renal impairment.

Therapy with *Avandia* should not be initiated if the patient exhibits clinical evidence of active liver disease or increased serum transaminase levels (ALT >2.5X the upper limit of normal at start of therapy) (See PRECAUTIONS, *Hepatic Effects* and CLINICAL PHARMACOLOGY, Hepatic Impairment). Liver enzyme monitoring is recommended in all patients prior to initiation of therapy with *Avandia* and periodically thereafter (See PRECAUTIONS, *Hepatic Effects*).

There are no data on the use of *Avandia* in patients under 18 years of age; therefore, use of *Avandia* in pediatric patients is not recommended.

OVERDOSAGE

Limited data are available with regard to overdosage in humans. In clinical studies in volunteers, Avandia (rosiglitazone maleate) has been administered at single oral doses of up to 20 mg and was well-tolerated. In the event of an overdose, appropriate supportive treatment should be initiated as dictated by the patient's clinical status.

HOW SUPPLIED

Tablets: Each pentagonal film-coated Tiltab® tablet contains rosiglitazone as the maleate as follows: 2 mg—pink, debossed with SB on one side and 2 on the other; 4 mg—orange, debossed with SB on one side and 4 on the other; 8 mg—red-brown, debossed with SB on one side and 8 on the other.

2 mg bottles of 30: NDC 0029-3158-13
2 mg bottles of 60: NDC 0029-3158-18
2 mg bottles of 100: NDC 0029-3158-20
2 mg bottles of 500: NDC 0029-3158-25
2 mg SUP 100s: NDC 0029-3158-21

4 mg bottles of 30: NDC 0029-3159-13
4 mg bottles of 60: NDC 0029-3159-18
4 mg bottles of 100: NDC 0029-3159-20
4 mg bottles of 500: NDC 0029-3159-25
4 mg SUP 100s: NDC 0029-3159-21

8 mg bottles of 30: NDC 0029-3160-13
8 mg bottles of 100: NDC 0029-3160-20
8 mg bottles of 500: NDC 0029-3160-25
8 mg SUP 100s: NDC 0029-3160-21

STORAGE

Store at 25° C (77° F); excursions 15°–30° C (59°–86° F). Dispense in a tight, light-resistant container.

Rx only

AV:L3

Shown in Product Identification Guide, page 336

BACTROBAN® OINTMENT ℞

[*back 'tro-ban*]
(mupirocin ointment), 2%
For Dermatologic Use

DESCRIPTION

Each gram of Bactroban Ointment (mupirocin ointment), 2% contains 20 mg mupirocin in a bland water miscible ointment base (polyethylene glycol ointment, N.F.) consisting of polyethylene glycol 400 and polyethylene glycol 3350.

Mupirocin is a naturally occurring antibiotic. The chemical name is (*E*)-(2*S*,3*R*,4*R*,5*S*)-5-[(2*S*,3*S*,4*S*,5*S*)-2,3-Epoxy-5-hydroxy-4-methylhexyl]tetrahydro-3,4-dihydroxy-β-methyl-2*H*-pyran-2-crotonic acid, ester with 9-hydroxynonanoic acid. The molecular formula of mupirocin is $C_{26}H_{44}O_9$ and the molecular weight is 500.63. The chemical structure is:

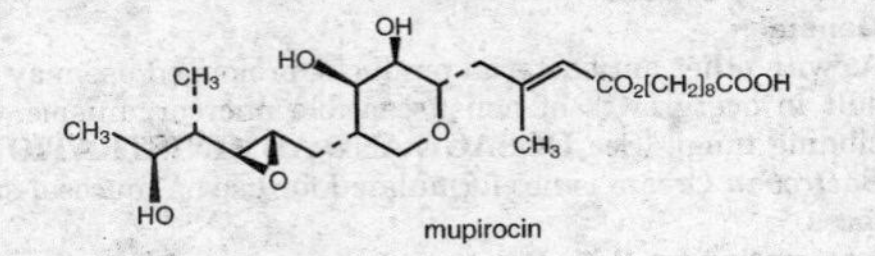

mupirocin

CLINICAL PHARMACOLOGY

Application of ^{14}C-labeled mupirocin ointment to the lower arm of normal male subjects followed by occlusion for 24 hours showed no measurable systemic absorption (<1.1 nanogram mupirocin per milliliter of whole blood). Measurable radioactivity was present in the stratum corneum of these subjects 72 hours after application.

Following intravenous or oral administration, mupirocin is rapidly metabolized. The principal metabolite, monic acid, is eliminated by renal excretion, and demonstrates no antibacterial activity. In a study conducted in seven healthy adult male subjects, the elimination half-life after intravenous administration of mupirocin was 20 to 40 minutes for mupirocin and 30 to 80 minutes for monic acid. The pharmacokinetics of mupirocin has not been studied in individuals with renal insufficiency.

Microbiology: Mupirocin is an antibacterial agent produced by fermentation using the organism *Pseudomonas fluorescens*. It is active against a wide range of gram-positive bacteria including methicillin-resistant *Staphylococcus aureus* (MRSA). It is also active against certain gram-negative bacteria. Mupirocin inhibits bacterial protein synthesis by reversibly and specifically binding to bacterial isoleucyl transfer-RNA synthetase. Due to this unique mode of action, mupirocin demonstrates no *in vitro* cross-resistance with other classes of antimicrobial agents.

Resistance occurs rarely. However, when mupirocin resistance does occur, it appears to result from the production of a modified isoleucyl-tRNA synthetase. High-level plasmid-mediated resistance (MIC >1024 mcg/mL) has been reported in some strains of *S. aureus* and coagulase-negative staphylococci.

Mupirocin is bactericidal at concentrations achieved by topical administration. However, the minimum bactericidal concentration (MBC) against relevant pathogens is generally eight-fold to thirty-fold higher than the minimum inhibitory concentration (MIC). In addition, mupirocin is highly protein bound (>97%), and the effect of wound secretions on the MICs of mupirocin has not been determined.

Mupirocin has been shown to be active against most strains of *Staphylococcus aureus* and *Streptococcus pyogenes*, both *in vitro* and in clinical studies. (See **INDICATIONS AND USAGE.**) The following *in vitro* data are available, BUT THEIR CLINICAL SIGNIFICANCE IS UNKNOWN. Mupirocin is active against most strains of *Staphylococcus epidermidis* and *Staphylococcus saprophyticus*.

INDICATIONS AND USAGE

Bactroban Ointment (mupirocin ointment), 2% is indicated for the topical treatment of impetigo due to: *Staphylococcus aureus* and *Streptococcus pyogenes*.

CONTRAINDICATIONS

This drug is contraindicated in individuals with a history of sensitivity reactions to any of its components.

WARNINGS

Bactroban Ointment is not for ophthalmic use.

PRECAUTIONS

If a reaction suggesting sensitivity or chemical irritation should occur with the use of Bactroban Ointment (mupirocin ointment) 2%, treatment should be discontinued and appropriate alternative therapy for the infection instituted.

As with other antibacterial products, prolonged use may result in overgrowth of nonsusceptible organisms, including fungi.

Bactroban Ointment is not formulated for use on mucosal surfaces. Intranasal use has been associated with isolated reports of stinging and drying. A paraffin-based formulation—Bactroban® Nasal (mupirocin calcium ointment)—is available for intranasal use.

Polyethylene glycol can be absorbed from open wounds and damaged skin and is excreted by the kidneys. In common with other polyethylene glycol-based ointments, *Bactroban* Ointment should not be used in conditions where absorption of large quantities of polyethylene glycol is possible, especially if there is evidence of moderate or severe renal impairment.

Information for Patients: Use this medication only as directed by your healthcare provider. It is for external use only. Avoid contact with the eyes. The medication should be stopped and your healthcare practitioner contacted if irritation, severe itching, or rash occurs.

If impetigo has not improved in 3 to 5 days, contact your healthcare practitioner.

Drug Interactions: The effect of the concurrent application of *Bactroban* Ointment and other drug products has not been studied.

Carcinogenesis, Mutagenesis, Impairment of Fertility: Long-term studies in animals to evaluate carcinogenic potential of mupirocin have not been conducted.

Results of the following studies performed with mupirocin calcium or mupirocin sodium *in vitro* and *in vivo* did not indicate a potential for genotoxicity: rat primary hepatocyte unscheduled DNA synthesis, sediment analysis for DNA strand breaks, *Salmonella* reversion test (Ames), *Escherichia coli* mutation assay, metaphase analysis of human lymphocytes, mouse lymphoma assay, and bone marrow micronuclei assay in mice.

Reproduction studies were performed in male and female rats with mupirocin administered subcutaneously at doses up to 14 times a human topical dose (approximately 60 mg mupirocin per day) on a mg/m² basis and revealed no evidence of impaired fertility and reproductive performance from mupirocin.

Pregnancy

Teratogenic Effects.

Pregnancy Category B: Reproduction studies have been performed in rats and rabbits with mupirocin administered subcutaneously at doses up to 22 and 43 times, respectively, the human topical dose (approximately 60 mg mupirocin per day) on a mg/m² basis and revealed no evidence of harm to the fetus due to mupirocin. There are, however, no adequate and well-controlled studies in pregnant women. Because animal studies are not always predictive of human response, this drug should be used during pregnancy only if clearly needed.

Nursing Mothers: It is not known whether this drug is excreted in human milk. Because many drugs are excreted in human milk, caution should be exercised when *Bactroban* Ointment is administered to a nursing woman.

Pediatric Use: The safety and effectiveness of *Bactroban* Ointment have been established in the age range of 2 months to 16 years. Use of *Bactroban* Ointment in these age groups is supported by evidence from adequate and well-controlled studies of *Bactroban* Ointment in impetigo in pediatric patients studied as a part of the pivotal clinical trials. (See **CLINICAL STUDIES.**)

ADVERSE REACTIONS

The following local adverse reactions have been reported in connection with the use of *Bactroban* Ointment: burning, stinging, or pain in 1.5% of patients; itching in 1% of patients; rash, nausea, erythema, dry skin, tenderness, swelling, contact dermatitis, and increased exudate in less than 1% of patients.

DOSAGE AND ADMINISTRATION

A small amount of *Bactroban* Ointment should be applied to the affected area three times daily. The area treated may be covered with a gauze dressing if desired. Patients not showing a clinical response within 3 to 5 days should be re-evaluated.

CLINICAL STUDIES

The efficacy of topical *Bactroban* Ointment in impetigo was tested in two studies. In the first, patients with impetigo were randomized to receive either *Bactroban* Ointment or vehicle placebo t.i.d. for 8 to 12 days. Clinical efficacy rates at end of therapy in the evaluable populations (adults and pediatric patients included) were 71% for *Bactroban* Ointment (n=49) and 35% for vehicle placebo (n=51). Pathogen eradication rates in the evaluable populations were 94% for *Bactroban* Ointment and 62% for vehicle placebo. There were no side effects reported in the group receiving *Bactroban* Ointment.

In the second study, patients with impetigo were randomized to receive either *Bactroban* Ointment t.i.d. or 30 to 40 mg/kg oral erythromycin ethylsuccinate per day (this was an unblinded study) for 8 days. There was a follow-up visit 1 week after treatment ended. Clinical efficacy rates at the follow-up visit in the evaluable populations (adults and pediatric patients included) were 93% for *Bactroban* Ointment (n=29) and 78.5% for erythromycin (n=28). Pathogen eradication rates in the evaluable patient populations were 100% for both test groups. There were no side effects reported in the *Bactroban* Ointment group.

Pediatrics

There were 91 pediatric patients aged 2 months to 15 years in the first study described above. Clinical efficacy rates at end of therapy in the evaluable populations were 78% for *Bactroban* Ointment (n=42) and 36% for vehicle placebo (n=49). In the second study described above, all patients were pediatric except two adults in the group receiving *Bactroban* Ointment. The age range of the pediatric patients was 7 months to 13 years. The clinical efficacy rate for *Bactroban* Ointment (n=27) was 96%, and for erythromycin it was unchanged (78.5%).

HOW SUPPLIED

Bactroban Ointment (mupirocin ointment), 2% is supplied in 15 gram, 22 gram and 30 gram tubes.

NDC 0029-1525-22 (15 gram tube)
NDC 0029-1525-44 (22 gram tube)
NDC 0029-1525-25 (30 gram tube)

Continued on next page

Information on the SmithKline Beecham Pharmaceuticals products appearing here is based on the labeling in effect on June 15, 2000. Further information on these and other products may be obtained from the Medical Department, SmithKline Beecham Pharmaceuticals, One Franklin Plaza, Philadelphia, PA 19101.

Bactroban Ointment—Cont.

Store at controlled room temperature 20° to 25°C (68° to 77°F).

℞ only

BC:L10C

BACTROBAN® CREAM ℞

[*back- 'trō-ban*]
brand of
mupirocin calcium cream, 2%
For Dermatologic Use

DESCRIPTION

Bactroban Cream (mupirocin calcium cream), 2% contains the dihydrate crystalline calcium hemi-salt of the antibiotic mupirocin. Chemically, it is (α*E*,2*S*,3*R*,4*R*,5*S*)-5-[(2*S*,3*S*,4*S*,5*S*)-2,3-Epoxy-5-hydroxy-4-methylhexyl]tetrahydro-3,4-dihydroxy-β-methyl-2*H*-pyran-2-crotonic acid, ester with 9-hydroxynonanoic acid, calcium salt (2:1), dihydrate.

The molecular formula of mupirocin calcium is $(C_{26}H_{43}O_9)_2Ca \bullet 2H_2O$, and the molecular weight is 1075.3. The molecular weight of mupirocin free acid is 500.6. The structural formula of mupirocin calcium is:

Bactroban Cream is a white cream that contains 2.15% w/w mupirocin calcium (equivalent to 2.0% mupirocin free acid) in an oil and water-based emulsion. The inactive ingredients are benzyl alcohol, cetomacrogol 1000, cetyl alcohol, mineral oil, phenoxyethanol, purified water, stearyl alcohol and xanthan gum.

CLINICAL PHARMACOLOGY

Pharmacokinetics

Systemic absorption of mupirocin through intact human skin is minimal. The systemic absorption of mupirocin was studied following application of *Bactroban* Cream three times a day for 5 days to various skin lesions (greater than 10 cm in length or 100 cm^2 in area) in 16 adults (aged 29 to 60 years) and 10 children (aged 3 to 12 years). Some systemic absorption was observed as evidenced by the detection of the metabolite, monic acid, in urine. Data from this study indicated more frequent occurrence of percutaneous absorption in children (90% of patients) compared to adults (44% of patients). However, the observed urinary concentrations in children (0.07 – 1.3 μg/mL [1 pediatric patient had no detectable level]) are within the observed range (0.08 – 10.03 μg/mL [9 adults had no detectable level]) in the adult population. In general, the degree of percutaneous absorption following multiple dosing appears to be minimal in adults and children. Any mupirocin reaching the systemic circulation is rapidly metabolized, predominantly to inactive monic acid, which is eliminated by renal excretion.

Microbiology

Mupirocin is an antibacterial agent produced by fermentation using the organism *Pseudomonas fluorescens*. It is active against a wide range of gram-positive bacteria including methicillin-resistant *Staphylococcus aureus* (MRSA). It is also active against certain gram-negative bacteria. Mupirocin inhibits bacterial protein synthesis by reversibly and specifically binding to bacterial isoleucyl transfer-RNA synthetase. Due to this unique mode of action, mupirocin demonstrates no *in vitro* cross-resistance with other classes of antimicrobial agents.

Resistance occurs rarely. However, when mupirocin resistance does occur, it appears to result from the production of a modified isoleucyl-tRNA synthetase. High-level plasmid-mediated resistance (MIC >1024 mcg/mL) has been reported in some strains of *S. aureus* and coagulase-negative staphylococci.

Mupirocin is bactericidal at concentrations achieved by topical application. However, the minimum bactericidal concentration (MBC) against relevant pathogens is generally eight-fold to thirty-fold higher than the minimum inhibitory concentration (MIC). In addition, mupirocin is highly protein bound (>97%), and the effect of wound secretions on the MICs of mupirocin has not been determined.

Mupirocin has been shown to be active against most strains of *Staphylococcus aureus* and *Streptococcus pyogenes*, both *in vitro* and in clinical studies. (See **INDICATIONS AND USAGE** section.) The following *in vitro* data are available, BUT THEIR CLINICAL SIGNIFICANCE IS UNKNOWN. Mupirocin is active against most strains of *Staphylococcus epidermidis* and *Staphylococcus saprophyticus*.

INDICATIONS AND USAGE

Bactroban Cream (mupirocin calcium cream), 2% is indicated for the treatment of secondarily infected traumatic skin lesions (up to 10 cm in length or 100 cm^2 in area) due to susceptible strains of *Staphylococcus aureus* and *Streptococcus pyogenes*.

CONTRAINDICATIONS

Bactroban Cream is contraindicated in patients with known hypersensitivity to any of the constituents of the product.

WARNINGS

Avoid contact with the eyes.

In the event of a sensitization or severe local irritation from *Bactroban* Cream, usage should be discontinued, and appropriate alternative therapy for the infection instituted.

PRECAUTIONS

General

As with other antibacterial products, prolonged use may result in overgrowth of nonsusceptible microorganisms, including fungi. (See **DOSAGE AND ADMINISTRATION**.) *Bactroban* Cream is not formulated for use on mucosal surfaces.

Information for Patients

- Use this medication only as directed by your healthcare provider. It is for external use only. Avoid contact with the eyes.
- The treated area may be covered by gauze dressing if desired.
- Report to your healthcare provider any signs of local adverse reactions. The medication should be stopped and your healthcare provider contacted if irritation, severe itching or rash occurs.
- If no improvement is seen in 3 to 5 days, contact your healthcare provider.

Drug Interactions

The effect of the concurrent application of topical mupirocin calcium cream and other topical products has not been studied.

Carcinogenesis, Mutagenesis, Impairment of Fertility

Long-term studies in animals to evaluate carcinogenic potential of mupirocin calcium have not been conducted.

Results of the following studies performed with mupirocin calcium or mupirocin sodium *in vitro* and *in vivo* did not indicate a potential for mutagenicity: rat primary hepatocyte unscheduled DNA synthesis, sediment analysis for DNA strand breaks, *Salmonella* reversion test (Ames), *Escherichia coli* mutation assay, metaphase analysis of human lymphocytes, mouse lymphoma assay, and bone marrow micronuclei assay in mice.

Fertility studies were performed in rats with mupirocin administered subcutaneously at doses up to 49 times a human topical dose of 1 gram/day (approximately 20 mg mupirocin per day) on a mg/m^2 basis and revealed no evidence of impaired fertility from mupirocin sodium.

Pregnancy

Teratogenic Effects. Pregnancy Category B. Teratology studies have been performed in rats and rabbits with mupirocin administered subcutaneously at doses up to 78 and 154 times, respectively, a human topical dose of 1 gram/day (approximately 20 mg mupirocin per day) on a mg/m^2 basis and revealed no evidence of harm to the fetus due to mupirocin. There are, however, no adequate and well-controlled studies in pregnant women. Because animal reproduction studies are not always predictive of human response, this drug should be used during pregnancy only if clearly needed.

Nursing Mothers

It is not known whether this drug is excreted in human milk. Because many drugs are excreted in human milk, caution should be exercised when *Bactroban* Cream is administered to a nursing woman.

Pediatric Use

The safety and effectiveness of *Bactroban* Cream have been established in the age groups 3 months to 16 years. Use of *Bactroban* Cream in these age groups is supported by evidence from adequate and well-controlled studies of *Bactroban* Cream in adults with additional data from 93 pediatric patients studied as part of the pivotal trials in adults. (See **CLINICAL STUDIES** section.)

Geriatric Use

In two well-controlled studies, 30 patients over 65 years old were treated with *Bactroban* Cream. No overall difference in the efficacy or safety of *Bactroban* Cream was observed in this patient population when compared to that observed in younger patients.

ADVERSE REACTIONS

In two randomized, double-blind, double-dummy trials, 339 patients were treated with topical *Bactroban* Cream plus oral placebo. Adverse events thought to be possibly or probably drug-related occurred in 28 (8.3%) patients. The incidence of those events that were reported in at least 1% of patients enrolled in these trials were: headache (1.7%), rash and nausea (1.1% each).

Other adverse events thought to be possibly or probably drug-related which occurred in less than 1% of patients were: abdominal pain, burning at application site, cellulitis, dermatitis, dizziness, pruritus, secondary wound infection, and ulcerative stomatitis.

In a supportive study in the treatment of secondarily infected eczema, 82 patients were treated with *Bactroban* Cream. The incidence of adverse events thought to be possibly or probably drug-related was as follows: nausea (4.9%), headache and burning at application site (3.6% each), pruritus (2.4%) and one report each of abdominal pain, bleeding secondary to eczema, pain secondary to eczema, hives, dry skin and rash.

OVERDOSAGE

Intravenous infusions of 252 mg, as well as single oral doses of 500 mg of mupirocin, have been well tolerated in healthy adult subjects. There is no information regarding overdose of *Bactroban* Cream.

DOSAGE AND ADMINISTRATION

A small amount of *Bactroban* Cream should be applied to the affected area three times daily for 10 days. The area treated may be covered with gauze dressing if desired. Patients not showing a clinical response within 3 to 5 days should be re-evaluated.

CLINICAL STUDIES

The efficacy of topical *Bactroban* Cream for the treatment of secondarily infected traumatic skin lesions (e.g., lacerations, sutured wounds and abrasions not more than 10 cm in length or 100 cm^2 in total area) was compared to that of oral cephalexin in two randomized, double-blind, double-dummy clinical trials. Clinical efficacy rates at follow-up in the per protocol populations (adults and pediatric patients included) were 96.1% for *Bactroban* Cream (n=231) and 93.1% for oral cephalexin (n=219). Pathogen eradication rates at follow-up in the per protocol populations were 100% for both *Bactroban* Cream and oral cephalexin.

Pediatrics

There were 93 pediatric patients aged 2 weeks to 16 years enrolled per protocol in the secondarily infected skin lesion studies, although only 3 were less than 2 years of age in the *Bactroban* Cream treated population. Patients were randomized to either 10 days of topical *Bactroban* Cream t.i.d. or 10 days of oral cephalexin (250 mg q.i.d. for patients >40 kg or 25 mg/kg/day oral suspension in four divided doses for patients ≤40 kg). Clinical efficacy at follow-up (7 to 12 days post-therapy) in the per protocol populations was 97.7% (43/44) for *Bactroban* Cream and 93.9% (46/49) for cephalexin. Only one adverse event (headache) was thought to be possibly or probably related to drug therapy in the *Bactroban* Cream intent-to-treat pediatric population of 70 children (1.4%).

HOW SUPPLIED

Bactroban Cream (mupirocin calcium cream), 2% is supplied in 15 gram and 30 gram tubes.

NDC 0029-1527-22 (15 gram tube)
NDC 0029-1527-25 (30 gram tube)
Store at or below 25°C (77°F). Do not freeze.

Manufactured by **DPT Laboratories**
San Antonio, TX 78215

Distributed by
SmithKline Beecham Pharmaceuticals
Philadelphia, PA 19101
BB:L2

BACTROBAN® NASAL ℞

[*back 'tro-ban*]
brand of mupirocin calcium ointment, 2%
for intranasal use only

DESCRIPTION

Bactroban Nasal (mupirocin calcium ointment), 2% contains the dihydrate crystalline calcium hemi-salt of the antibiotic mupirocin. Chemically, it is (α *E*,2*S*,3*R*,4*R*,5*S*)-5-[(2*S*,3*S*,4*S*,5*S*)-2,3-Epoxy-5-hydroxy-4-methylhexyl] tetrahydro-3,4-dihydroxy-β-methyl-2*H*-pyran-2-crotonic acid, ester with 9-hydroxynonanoic acid, calcium salt (2:1), dihydrate.

The molecular formula of mupirocin calcium is $(C_{26}H_{43}O_9)_2Ca \cdot 2H_2O$, and the molecular weight is 1075.3. The molecular weight of mupirocin free acid is 500.6. The structural formula of mupirocin calcium is:

Bactroban Nasal is a white to off-white ointment that contains 2.15% w/w mupirocin calcium (equivalent to 2.0% pure mupirocin free acid) in a soft white ointment base. The inactive ingredients are paraffin and a mixture of glycerin esters (Softisan® 649).

CLINICAL PHARMACOLOGY

Pharmacokinetics

Following single or repeated intranasal applications of 0.2 gram of *Bactroban* Nasal t.i.d. for 3 days to five healthy **adult** male subjects, no evidence of systemic absorption of mupirocin was demonstrated. The dosage regimen used in this study was for pharmacokinetic characterization only. (See **DOSAGE AND ADMINISTRATION** for proper clinical dosing information.)

In this study, the concentrations of mupirocin in urine and of monic acid in urine and serum were below the limit of determination of the assay for up to 72 hours after the applications. The lowest levels of determination of the assay used were 50 ng/mL of mupirocin in urine, 75 ng/mL of monic acid in urine, and 10 ng/mL of monic acid in serum. Based on the detectable limit of the urine assay for monic acid, one can extrapolate that a mean of 3.3% (range: 1.2–5.1%) of the applied dose could be systemically absorbed from the nasal mucosa of **adults**.

Data from a report of a pharmacokinetic study in neonates and premature infants indicate that, unlike in adults, significant systemic absorption occurred following intranasal administration of *Bactroban* Nasal in this population. **At this time, the pharmacokinetic properties of mupirocin following intranasal application of *Bactroban* Nasal have not been adequately characterized in neonates or other children less than 12 years of age, and in addition, the safety of the product in children less than 12 years of age has not been established.**

The effect of the concurrent application of intranasal mupirocin calcium ointment, 2% with other intranasal products has not been studied. (See **PRECAUTIONS, Drug Interactions.**)

Following intravenous or oral administration, mupirocin is rapidly metabolized. The principal metabolite, monic acid, demonstrates no antibacterial activity. In a study conducted in seven healthy adult male subjects, the elimination half-life after intravenous administration of mupirocin was 20 to 40 minutes for mupirocin and 30 to 80 minutes for monic acid. Monic acid is predominantly eliminated by renal excretion. The pharmacokinetics of mupirocin has not been studied in individuals with renal insufficiency.

Microbiology

Mupirocin is an antibacterial agent produced by fermentation using the organism *Pseudomonas fluorescens.* Mupirocin inhibits bacterial protein synthesis by reversibly and specifically binding to bacterial isoleucyl transfer-RNA synthetase. Due to this mode of action, mupirocin demonstrates no *in vitro* cross-resistance with other classes of antimicrobial agents.

When mupirocin resistance does occur, it appears to result from the production of a modified isoleucyl-tRNA synthetase. High-level plasmid-mediated resistance (MIC >1024 mcg/mL) has been reported in some strains of *S. aureus* and coagulase-negative staphylococci.

Mupirocin is bactericidal at concentrations achieved topically by intranasal administration. However, the minimum bactericidal concentration (MBC) against relevant intranasal pathogens is generally eight-fold to thirty-fold higher than the minimum inhibitory concentration (MIC). In addition, mupirocin is highly protein bound (>97%), and the effect of nasal secretions on the MIC's of intranasally applied mupirocin has not been determined.

Mupirocin has been shown to be active against most strains of methicillin-resistant *S. aureus,* both *in vitro* and in clinical studies of the eradication of nasal colonization. *Bactroban* Nasal only has established clinical utility in nasal eradication as part of a comprehensive program to curtail institutional outbreaks of infections with methicillin-resistant *S. aureus.* (See **INDICATIONS AND USAGE.**)

The following *in vitro* data are available, **but their clinical significance is unknown.** Mupirocin exhibits *in vitro* MIC's of 1 mcg/mL or less against most (>90%) strains of methicillin-susceptible *S. aureus*; however, the safety and effectiveness of mupirocin calcium in eradicating nasal colonization of and preventing subsequent infections due to methicillin-susceptible *S. aureus* have not been established.

INDICATIONS AND USAGE

Bactroban Nasal (mupirocin calcium ointment), 2% is indicated for the eradication of nasal colonization with methicillin-resistant *Staphylococcus aureus* in adult patients and health care workers as part of a comprehensive infection control program to reduce the risk of infection among patients at high risk of methicillin-resistant *S. aureus* infection during institutional outbreaks of infections with this pathogen.

NOTE:

(1) There are insufficient data at this time to establish that this product is safe and effective as part of an intervention program to prevent autoinfection of high-risk patients from their own nasal colonization with *S. aureus.*

(2) There are insufficient data at this time to recommend use of *Bactroban* Nasal for general prophylaxis of any infection in any patient population.

(3) Greater than 90% of subjects/patients in clinical trials had eradication of nasal colonization 2 to 4 days after therapy was completed. Approximately 30% recolonization was reported in one domestic study within 4 weeks after completion of therapy. These eradication rates were clinically and statistically superior to those reported in subjects/patients in the vehicle-treated arms of the adequate and well-controlled studies. Those treated with vehicle had eradication rates of 5% to 30% at 2 to 4 days post-therapy with 85% to 100% recolonization within 4 weeks.

All adequate and well-controlled trials of this product were vehicle-controlled; therefore, no data from direct, head-to-head comparisons with other products are available at this time.

CONTRAINDICATIONS

Bactroban Nasal is contraindicated in patients with known hypersensitivity to any of the constituents of the product.

WARNINGS

AVOID CONTACT WITH THE EYES. Application of *Bactroban* Nasal to the eye under testing conditions has caused severe symptoms such as burning and tearing. These symptoms resolved within days to weeks after discontinuation of the ointment.

In the event of a sensitization or severe local irritation from *Bactroban* Nasal, usage should be discontinued.

PRECAUTIONS

General

As with other antibacterial products, prolonged use may result in overgrowth of nonsusceptible microorganisms, including fungi. (See **DOSAGE AND ADMINISTRATION.**)

Information for Patients

Patients should be given the following instructions:

— Apply approximately one-half of the ointment from the single-use tube directly into one nostril and the other half into the other nostril;
— Avoid contact of the medication with the eyes;
— Discard the tube after using, do not re-use;
— Press the sides of the nose together and gently massage after application to spread the ointment throughout the inside of the nostrils; and
— Discontinue usage of the medication and call your health care practitioner if sensitization or severe local irritation occurs.

Drug Interactions

The effect of the concurrent application of intranasal mupirocin calcium and other intranasal products has not been studied. Until further information is known, mupirocin calcium ointment, 2% should not be applied concurrently with any other intranasal products.

Carcinogenesis, Mutagenesis, Impairment of Fertility

Long-term studies in animals to evaluate carcinogenic potential of mupirocin calcium have not been conducted.

Results of the following studies performed with mupirocin calcium or mupirocin sodium *in vitro* and *in vivo* did not indicate a potential for mutagenicity: rat primary hepatocyte unscheduled DNA synthesis, sediment analysis for DNA strand breaks, *Salmonella* reversion test (Ames), *Escherichia coli* mutation assay, metaphase analysis of human lymphocytes, mouse lymphoma assay, and bone marrow micronuclei assay in mice.

Reproduction studies were performed in rats with mupirocin administered subcutaneously at doses up to **40** times the human intranasal dose (approximately 20 mg mupirocin per day) on a mg/m^2 basis and revealed no evidence of impaired fertility from mupirocin sodium.

Pregnancy

Teratogenic Effects. Pregnancy Category B. Reproduction studies have been performed in rats and rabbits with mupirocin administered subcutaneously at doses up to 65 and 130 times, respectively, the human intranasal dose (approximately 20 mg mupirocin per day) on a mg/m^2 basis and revealed no evidence of harm to the fetus due to mupirocin. There are, however, no adequate and well-controlled studies in pregnant women. Because animal reproduction studies are not always predictive of human response, this drug should be used during pregnancy only if clearly needed.

Nursing Mothers

It is not known whether this drug is excreted in human milk. Because many drugs are excreted in human milk, caution should be exercised when *Bactroban* Nasal is administered to a nursing woman.

Pediatric Use

Safety in children under the age of 12 years has not been established. (See **CLINICAL PHARMACOLOGY.**)

ADVERSE REACTIONS

Clinical Trials

In clinical trials, 210 domestic and 2,130 foreign adult subjects/patients received *Bactroban* Nasal ointment. Less than 1% of domestic or foreign subjects and patients in clinical trials were withdrawn due to adverse events.

The most frequently reported adverse events in foreign clinical trials were as follows: rhinitis (1.0%), taste perversion (0.8%), pharyngitis (0.5%).

In domestic clinical trials, 17% (36/210) of adults treated with *Bactroban* Nasal ointment reported adverse events thought to be at least possibly drug-related. The incidence of adverse events that were reported in at least 1% of adults enrolled in domestic clinical trials were as follows:

ADVERSE EVENTS (≥1% INCIDENCE)- ADULTS IN U.S. TRIALS

	% of Subjects/Patients Experiencing Event *Bactroban* Nasal 2% (n=210)
Headache	9%
Rhinitis	6%
Respiratory disorder, including upper respiratory tract congestion	5%
Pharyngitis	4%
Taste perversion	3%
Burning/Stinging	2%
Cough	2%
Pruritus	1%

The following events thought possibly drug-related were reported in less than 1% of adults enrolled in domestic clinical trials: blepharitis, diarrhea, dry mouth, ear pain, epistaxis, nausea and rash.

All adequate and well-controlled clinical trials have been performed using *Bactroban* Nasal ointment, 2% in one arm and the vehicle ointment in the other arm of the study. No adequate and well-controlled safety data are available from direct, head-to-head comparative studies of this product and other products for this indication.

OVERDOSAGE

Following single or repeated intranasal applications of *Bactroban* Nasal to adults, no evidence for systemic absorption of mupirocin was obtained. Intravenous infusions of 252 mg, as well as single oral doses of 500 mg of mupirocin, have been well tolerated in healthy adult subjects. There is no information regarding local overdose of *Bactroban* Nasal or regarding oral ingestion of the nasal ointment formulation.

DOSAGE AND ADMINISTRATION

(See **INDICATIONS AND USAGE.**)

Adults (12 years of age and older): Approximately one-half of the ointment from the single-use tube should be applied into one nostril and the other half into the other nostril twice daily (morning and evening) for 5 days.

After application, the nostrils should be closed by pressing together and releasing the sides of the nose repetitively for approximately 1 minute. This will spread the ointment throughout the nares.

The single-use 1.0 gram tube will deliver a total of approximately 0.5 grams of the ointment (approximately 0.25 grams/nostril).

The tube should be discarded after usage; it should not be re-used.

The safety and effectiveness of applications of this medication for greater than 5 days have not been established. There are no human clinical or pre-clinical animal data to support the use of this product in a chronic manner or in manners other than those described in this package insert. Until further information is known, *Bactroban* Nasal should not be applied concurrently with any other intranasal products.

HOW SUPPLIED

Bactroban Nasal (mupirocin calcium ointment), 2% is supplied in 1.0 gram tubes packaged in cartons of 10.

NDC 0029-1526-11 (1.0 gram tubes in packages of 10).

Store at or below 25°C (77°F).

REFERENCE

1. National Committee for Clinical Laboratory Standards. Methods for Dilution Antimicrobial Susceptibility Tests for Bacteria That Grow Aerobically—Third Edition; Approved Standard NCCLS Document M7-A3. Vol. 12, No. 25, NCCLS, Villanova, PA, December 1993.

Manufactured by **DPT Laboratories**
San Antonio, TX 78215
Distributed by **SmithKline Beecham Pharmaceuticals**
Philadelphia, PA 19101
BN:L3

COMPAZINE® ℞

[*komp 'ah-zeen*]
brand of prochlorperazine
antiemetic • tranquilizer

DESCRIPTION

Compazine (prochlorperazine) is a phenothiazine derivative, present in *Compazine* tablets and *Spansule* sustained release capsules as the maleate. Its chemical name is 2-chloro-10-[3-(4-methyl-1-piperazinyl)propyl]-10*H*-phenothiazine(*Z*)-2-butenedioate (1:2).

prochlorperazine maleate

Compazine vials and syrup contain prochlorperazine as the edisylate salt and *Compazine* suppositories contain prochlorperazine base. Empirical formulas (and molecular weights) are: prochlorperazine maleate—$C_{20}H_{24}ClN_3S \bullet 2C_4H_4O_4$ (606.10); prochlorperazine edisylate—$C_{20}H_{24}ClN_3S \bullet C_2H_6O_6S_2$ (564.14); and prochlorperazine base—$C_{20}H_{24}ClN_3S$ (373.95).

Tablets—Each round, yellow-green, coated tablet contains prochlorperazine maleate equivalent to prochlorperazine as follows: 5 mg imprinted SKF and C66; 10 mg imprinted SKF and C67.

5 mg and 10 mg Tablets—Inactive ingredients consist of cellulose, lactose, magnesium stearate, polyethylene glycol, sodium croscarmellose, titanium dioxide, D&C Yellow No. 10, FD&C Blue No. 2, FD&C Yellow No. 6, FD&C Red No. 40, iron oxide, starch, stearic acid and trace amounts of other inactive ingredients, including aluminum lake dyes.

Continued on next page

Information on the SmithKline Beecham Pharmaceuticals products appearing here is based on the labeling in effect on June 15, 2000. Further information on these and other products may be obtained from the Medical Department, SmithKline Beecham Pharmaceuticals, One Franklin Plaza, Philadelphia, PA 19101.

Compazine—Cont.

Spansule® sustained release capsules—Each Compazine® *Spansule* capsule is so prepared that an initial dose is released promptly and the remaining medication is released gradually over a prolonged period. Food slows absorption of prochlorperazine and decreases C_{max} by 23% and AUC by 13%.

Each capsule, with black cap and natural body, contains prochlorperazine maleate equivalent to prochlorperazine. The 10 mg capsule is imprinted 10 mg and 3344 on the black cap and is imprinted 10 mg and SB on the natural body. The 15 mg capsule is imprinted 15 mg and 3346 on the black cap and is imprinted 15 mg and SB on the natural body. Inactive ingredients consist of ammonio methacrylate co-polymer, D&C Green No. 5, D&C Yellow No. 10, FD&C Blue No. 1, FD&C Blue No. 1 aluminum lake, FD&C Red No. 40, FD&C Yellow No. 6, gelatin, hyroxypropyl methylcellulose, propylene glycol, silicon dioxide, simethicone emulsion, sodium lauryl sulfate, sorbic acid, sugar spheres, talc, triethyl citrate, and trace amounts of other inactive ingredients.

Vials, 2 mL (5 mg/mL) and 10 mL (5 mg/mL)—Each mL contains, in aqueous solution, 5 mg prochlorperazine as the edisylate, 5 mg sodium biphosphate, 12 mg sodium tartrate, 0.9 mg sodium saccharin and 0.75% benzyl alcohol as preservative.

Suppositories—Each suppository contains $2^1/_2$ mg, 5 mg or 25 mg of prochlorperazine; with glycerin, glyceryl monopalmitate, glyceryl monostearate, hydrogenated cocoanut oil fatty acids and hydrogenated palm kernel oil fatty acids.

Syrup—Each 5 mL (1 teaspoonful) of clear, yellow-orange, fruit-flavored liquid contains 5 mg of prochlorperazine as the edisylate. Inactive ingredients consist of FD&C Yellow No. 6, flavors, polyoxyethylene polyoxypropylene glycol, sodium benzoate, sodium citrate, sucrose and water.

INDICATIONS

For control of severe nausea and vomiting.

For management of the manifestations of psychotic disorders.

Compazine (prochlorperazine) is effective for the short-term treatment of generalized non-psychotic anxiety. However, *Compazine* is not the first drug to be used in therapy for most patients with non-psychotic anxiety, because certain risks associated with its use are not shared by common alternative treatments (e.g., benzodiazepines).

When used in the treatment of non-psychotic anxiety, *Compazine* should not be administered at doses of more than 20 mg per day or for longer than 12 weeks, because the use of *Compazine* at higher doses or for longer intervals may cause persistent tardive dyskinesia that may prove irreversible (see WARNINGS).

The effectiveness of *Compazine* as treatment for non-psychotic anxiety was established in 4-week clinical studies of outpatients with generalized anxiety disorder. This evidence does not predict that *Compazine* will be useful in patients with other non-psychotic conditions in which anxiety, or signs that mimic anxiety, are found (e.g., physical illness, organic mental conditions, agitated depression, character pathologies, etc.).

Compazine has not been shown effective in the management of behavioral complications in patients with mental retardation.

CONTRAINDICATIONS

Do not use in patients with known hypersensitivity to phenothiazines.

Do not use in comatose states or in the presence of large amounts of central nervous system depressants (alcohol, barbiturates, narcotics, etc.).

Do not use in pediatric surgery.

Do not use in pediatric patients under 2 years of age or under 20 lbs. Do not use in children for conditions for which dosage has not been established.

WARNINGS

The extrapyramidal symptoms which can occur secondary to Compazine (prochlorperazine) may be confused with the central nervous system signs of an undiagnosed primary disease responsible for the vomiting, e.g., Reye's syndrome or other encephalopathy. The use of Compazine (prochlorperazine) and other potential hepatotoxins should be avoided in children and adolescents whose signs and symptoms suggest Reye's syndrome.

Tardive Dyskinesia: Tardive dyskinesia, a syndrome consisting of potentially irreversible, involuntary, dyskinetic movements, may develop in patients treated with neuroleptic (antipsychotic) drugs. Although the prevalence of the syndrome appears to be highest among the elderly, especially elderly women, it is impossible to rely upon prevalence estimates to predict, at the inception of neuroleptic treatment, which patients are likely to develop the syndrome. Whether neuroleptic drug products differ in their potential to cause tardive dyskinesia is unknown.

Both the risk of developing the syndrome and the likelihood that it will become irreversible are believed to increase as the duration of treatment and the total cumulative dose of neuroleptic drugs administered to the patient increase. However, the syndrome can develop, although much less commonly, after relatively brief treatment periods at low doses.

There is no known treatment for established cases of tardive dyskinesia, although the syndrome may remit, partially or completely, if neuroleptic treatment is withdrawn. Neuroleptic treatment itself, however, may suppress (or partially suppress) the signs and symptoms of the syndrome and thereby may possibly mask the underlying disease process.

The effect that symptomatic suppression has upon the long-term course of the syndrome is unknown.

Given these considerations, neuroleptics should be prescribed in a manner that is most likely to minimize the occurrence of tardive dyskinesia. Chronic neuroleptic treatment should generally be reserved for patients who suffer from a chronic illness that, 1) is known to respond to neuroleptic drugs, and 2) for whom alternative, equally effective, but potentially less harmful treatments are *not* available or appropriate. In patients who do require chronic treatment, the smallest dose and the shortest duration of treatment producing a satisfactory clinical response should be sought. The need for continued treatment should be reassessed periodically.

If signs and symptoms of tardive dyskinesia appear in a patient on neuroleptics, drug discontinuation should be considered. However, some patients may require treatment despite the presence of the syndrome.

For further information about the description of tardive dyskinesia and its clinical detection, please refer to the sections on PRECAUTIONS and ADVERSE REACTIONS.

Neuroleptic Malignant Syndrome (NMS): A potentially fatal symptom complex sometimes referred to as Neuroleptic Malignant Syndrome (NMS) has been reported in association with antipsychotic drugs. Clinical manifestations of NMS are hyperpyrexia, muscle rigidity, altered mental status and evidence of autonomic instability (irregular pulse or blood pressure, tachycardia, diaphoresis and cardiac dysrhythmias).

The diagnostic evaluation of patients with this syndrome is complicated. In arriving at a diagnosis, it is important to identify cases where the clinical presentation includes both serious medical illness (e.g., pneumonia, systemic infection, etc.) and untreated or inadequately treated extrapyramidal signs and symptoms (EPS). Other important considerations in the differential diagnosis include central anticholinergic toxicity, heat stroke, drug fever and primary central nervous system (CNS) pathology.

The management of NMS should include 1) immediate discontinuation of antipsychotic drugs and other drugs not essential to concurrent therapy, 2) intensive symptomatic treatment and medical monitoring, and 3) treatment of any concomitant serious medical problems for which specific treatments are available. There is no general agreement about specific pharmacological treatment regimens for uncomplicated NMS.

If a patient requires antipsychotic drug treatment after recovery from NMS, the potential reintroduction of drug therapy should be carefully considered. The patient should be carefully monitored, since recurrences of NMS have been reported.

An encephalopathic syndrome (characterized by weakness, lethargy, fever, tremulousness and confusion, extrapyramidal symptoms, leukocytosis, elevated serum enzymes, BUN and FBS) has occurred in a few patients treated with lithium plus a neuroleptic. In some instances, the syndrome was followed by irreversible brain damage. Because of a possible causal relationship between these events and the concomitant administration of lithium and neuroleptics, patients receiving such combined therapy should be monitored closely for early evidence of neurologic toxicity and treatment discontinued promptly if such signs appear. This encephalopathic syndrome may be similar to or the same as neuroleptic malignant syndrome (NMS).

Patients with bone marrow depression or who have previously demonstrated a hypersensitivity reaction (e.g., blood dyscrasias, jaundice) with a phenothiazine should not receive any phenothiazine, including *Compazine*, unless in the judgment of the physician the potential benefits of treatment outweigh the possible hazards.

Compazine (prochlorperazine) may impair mental and/or physical abilities, especially during the first few days of therapy. Therefore, caution patients about activities requiring alertness (e.g., operating vehicles or machinery).

Phenothiazines may intensify or prolong the action of central nervous system depressants (e.g., alcohol, anesthetics, narcotics).

Usage in Pregnancy: Safety for the use of *Compazine* during pregnancy has not been established. Therefore, *Compazine* is not recommended for use in pregnant patients except in cases of severe nausea and vomiting that are so serious and intractable that, in the judgment of the physician, drug intervention is required and potential benefits outweigh possible hazards.

There have been reported instances of prolonged jaundice, extrapyramidal signs, hyperreflexia or hyporeflexia in newborn infants whose mothers received phenothiazines.

Nursing Mothers: There is evidence that phenothiazines are excreted in the breast milk of nursing mothers. Caution should be exercised when *Compazine* is administered to a nursing woman.

PRECAUTIONS

The antiemetic action of Compazine (prochlorperazine) may mask the signs and symptoms of overdosage of other drugs and may obscure the diagnosis and treatment of other conditions such as intestinal obstruction, brain tumor and Reye's syndrome (see WARNINGS).

When *Compazine* is used with cancer chemotherapeutic drugs, vomiting as a sign of the toxicity of these agents may be obscured by the antiemetic effect of *Compazine*.

Because hypotension may occur, large doses and parenteral administration should be used cautiously in patients with impaired cardiovascular systems. To minimize the occurrence of hypotension after injection, keep patient lying down and observe for at least $^1/_2$ hour. If hypotension occurs after parenteral or oral dosing, place patient in head-low position with legs raised. If a vasoconstrictor is required, Levophed®* and Neo-Synephrine®† are suitable. Other pressor agents, including epinephrine, should not be used because they may cause a paradoxical further lowering of blood pressure.

Aspiration of vomitus has occurred in a few post-surgical patients who have received Compazine (prochlorperazine) as an antiemetic. Although no causal relationship has been established, this possibility should be borne in mind during surgical aftercare.

Deep sleep, from which patients can be aroused, and coma have been reported, usually with overdosage.

Neuroleptic drugs elevate prolactin levels; the elevation persists during chronic administration. Tissue culture experiments indicate that approximately one third of human breast cancers are prolactin-dependent *in vitro*, a factor of potential importance if the prescribing of these drugs is contemplated in a patient with a previously detected breast cancer. Although disturbances such as galactorrhea, amenorrhea, gynecomastia and impotence have been reported, the clinical significance of elevated serum prolactin levels is unknown for most patients. An increase in mammary neoplasms has been found in rodents after chronic administration of neuroleptic drugs. Neither clinical nor epidemiologic studies conducted to date, however, have shown an association between chronic administration of these drugs and mammary tumorigenesis; the available evidence is considered too limited to be conclusive at this time.

Chromosomal aberrations in spermatocytes and abnormal sperm have been demonstrated in rodents treated with certain neuroleptics.

As with all drugs which exert an anticholinergic effect, and/or cause mydriasis, prochlorperazine should be used with caution in patients with glaucoma.

Because phenothiazines may interfere with thermoregulatory mechanisms, use with caution in persons who will be exposed to extreme heat.

Phenothiazines can diminish the effect of oral anticoagulants.

Phenothiazines can produce alpha-adrenergic blockade.

Thiazide diuretics may accentuate the orthostatic hypotension that may occur with phenothiazines.

Antihypertensive effects of guanethidine and related compounds may be counteracted when phenothiazines are used concomitantly.

Concomitant administration of propranolol with phenothiazines results in increased plasma levels of both drugs.

Phenothiazines may lower the convulsive threshold; dosage adjustments of anticonvulsants may be necessary. Potentiation of anticonvulsant effects does not occur. However, it has been reported that phenothiazines may interfere with the metabolism of Dilantin®‡ and thus precipitate *Dilantin* toxicity.

The presence of phenothiazines may produce false-positive phenylketonuria (PKU) test results.

Long-Term Therapy: Given the likelihood that some patients exposed chronically to neuroleptics will develop tardive dyskinesia, it is advised that all patients in whom chronic use is contemplated be given, if possible, full information about this risk. The decision to inform patients and/or their guardians must obviously take into account the clinical circumstances and the competency of the patient to understand the information provided.

To lessen the likelihood of adverse reactions related to cumulative drug effect, patients with a history of long-term therapy with Compazine (prochlorperazine) and/or other neuroleptics should be evaluated periodically to decide whether the maintenance dosage could be lowered or drug therapy discontinued.

Children with acute illnesses (e.g., chickenpox, CNS infections, measles, gastroenteritis) or dehydration seem to be much more susceptible to neuromuscular reactions, particularly dystonias, than are adults. In such patients, the drug should be used only under close supervision.

Drugs which lower the seizure threshold, including phenothiazine derivatives, should not be used with Amipaque®§.

As with other phenothiazine derivatives, Compazine (prochlorperazine) should be discontinued at least 48 hours before myelography, should not be resumed for at least 24 hours postprocedure, and should not be used for the control of nausea and vomiting occurring either prior to myelography with *Amipaque*, or postprocedure.

ADVERSE REACTIONS

Drowsiness, dizziness, amenorrhea, blurred vision, skin reactions and hypotension may occur. Neuroleptic Malignant Syndrome (NMS) has been reported in association with antipsychotic drugs (see WARNINGS).

Cholestatic jaundice has occurred. If fever with grippe-like symptoms occurs, appropriate liver studies should be conducted. If tests indicate an abnormality, stop treatment. There have been a few observations of fatty changes in the livers of patients who have died while receiving the drug. No causal relationship has been established.

Leukopenia and agranulocytosis have occurred. Warn patients to report the sudden appearance of sore throat or other signs of infection. If white blood cell and differential counts indicate leukocyte depression, stop treatment and start antibiotic and other suitable therapy.

Neuromuscular (Extrapyramidal) Reactions

These symptoms are seen in a significant number of hospitalized mental patients. They may be characterized by motor restlessness, be of the dystonic type, or they may resemble parkinsonism.

Depending on the severity of symptoms, dosage should be reduced or discontinued. If therapy is reinstituted, it should be at a lower dosage. Should these symptoms occur in children or pregnant patients, the drug should be stopped and not reinstituted. In most cases barbiturates by suitable route of administration will suffice. (Or, injectable Benadryl®[‡] may be useful.) In more severe cases, the administration of an anti-parkinsonism agent, except levodopa, usually produces rapid reversal of symptoms. Suitable supportive measures such as maintaining a clear airway and adequate hydration should be employed.

Motor Restlessness: Symptoms may include agitation or jitteriness and sometimes insomnia. These symptoms often disappear spontaneously. At times these symptoms may be similar to the original neurotic or psychotic symptoms. Dosage should not be increased until these side effects have subsided.

If these symptoms become too troublesome, they can usually be controlled by a reduction of dosage or change of drug. Treatment with anti-parkinsonian agents, benzodiazepines or propranolol may be helpful.

Dystonias: Symptoms may include: spasm of the neck muscles, sometimes progressing to torticollis; extensor rigidity of back muscles, sometimes progressing to opisthotonos; carpopedal spasm, trismus, swallowing difficulty, oculogyric crisis and protrusion of the tongue.

These usually subside within a few hours, and almost always within 24 to 48 hours, after the drug has been discontinued.

In mild cases, reassurance or a barbiturate is often sufficient. *In moderate cases,* barbiturates will usually bring rapid relief. *In more severe adult cases,* the administration of an anti-parkinsonism agent, except levodopa, usually produces rapid reversal of symptoms. *In children,* reassurance and barbiturates will usually control symptoms. (Or, injectable *Benadryl* may be useful. Note: See *Benadryl* prescribing information for appropriate *children's* dosage.) If appropriate treatment with anti-parkinsonism agents or *Benadryl* fails to reverse the signs and symptoms, the diagnosis should be reevaluated.

Pseudo-parkinsonism: Symptoms may include: mask-like facies; drooling; tremors; pillrolling motion; cogwheel rigidity; and shuffling gait. Reassurance and sedation are important. In most cases these symptoms are readily controlled when an anti-parkinsonism agent is administered concomitantly. Anti-parkinsonism agents should be used only when required. Generally, therapy of a few weeks to 2 or 3 months will suffice. After this time patients should be evaluated to determine their need for continued treatment. (Note: Levodopa has not been found effective in pseudo-parkinsonism.) Occasionally it is necessary to lower the dosage of Compazine (prochlorperazine) or to discontinue the drug.

Tardive Dyskinesia: As with all antipsychotic agents, tardive dyskinesia may appear in some patients on long-term therapy or may appear after drug therapy has been discontinued. The syndrome can also develop, although much less frequently, after relatively brief treatment periods at low doses. This syndrome appears in all age groups. Although its prevalence appears to be highest among elderly patients, especially elderly women, it is impossible to rely upon prevalence estimates to predict at the inception of neuroleptic treatment which patients are likely to develop the syndrome. The symptoms are persistent and in some patients appear to be irreversible. The syndrome is characterized by rhythmical involuntary movements of the tongue, face, mouth or jaw (e.g., protrusion of tongue, puffing of cheeks, puckering of mouth, chewing movements). Sometimes these may be accompanied by involuntary movements of extremities. In rare instances, these involuntary movements of the extremities are the only manifestations of tardive dyskinesia. A variant of tardive dyskinesia, tardive dystonia, has also been described.

There is no known effective treatment for tardive dyskinesia; anti-parkinsonism agents do not alleviate the symptoms of this syndrome. It is suggested that all antipsychotic agents be discontinued if these symptoms appear.

Should it be necessary to reinstitute treatment, or increase the dosage of the agent, or switch to a different antipsychotic agent, the syndrome may be masked.

It has been reported that fine vermicular movements of the tongue may be an early sign of the syndrome and if the medication is stopped at that time the syndrome may not develop.

Contact Dermatitis: Avoid getting the Injection solution on hands or clothing because of the possibility of contact dermatitis.

Adverse Reactions Reported with Compazine (prochlorperazine) or Other Phenothiazine Derivatives: Adverse reactions with different phenothiazines vary in type, frequency and mechanism of occurrence, i.e., some are dose-related, while others involve individual patient sensitivity. Some adverse reactions may be more likely to occur, or occur with greater intensity, in patients with special medical problems, e.g., patients with mitral insufficiency or pheochromocytoma have experienced severe hypotension following recommended doses of certain phenothiazines.

Not all of the following adverse reactions have been observed with every phenothiazine derivative, but they have been reported with 1 or more and should be borne in mind when drugs of this class are administered: extrapyramidal symptoms (opisthotonos, oculogyric crisis, hyperreflexia, dystonia, akathisia, dyskinesia, parkinsonism) some of which have lasted months and even years—particularly in elderly patients with previous brain damage; grand mal and petit mal convulsions, particularly in patients with EEG abnormalities or history of such disorders; altered cerebrospinal fluid proteins; cerebral edema; intensification and prolongation of the action of central nervous system depressants (opiates, analgesics, antihistamines, barbiturates, alcohol), atropine, heat, organophosphorus insecticides; autonomic reactions (dryness of mouth, nasal congestion, headache, nausea, constipation, obstipation, adynamic ileus, ejaculatory disorders/impotence, priapism, atonic colon, urinary retention, miosis and mydriasis); reactivation of psychotic processes, catatonic-like states; hypotension (sometimes fatal); cardiac arrest; blood dyscrasias (pancytopenia, thrombocytopenic purpura, leukopenia, agranulocytosis, eosinophilia, hemolytic anemia, aplastic anemia); liver damage (jaundice, biliary stasis); endocrine disturbances (hyperglycemia, hypoglycemia, glycosuria, lactation, galactorrhea, gynecomastia, menstrual irregularities, false-positive pregnancy tests); skin disorders (photosensitivity, itching, erythema, urticaria, eczema up to exfoliative dermatitis); other allergic reactions (asthma, laryngeal edema, angioneurotic edema, anaphylactoid reactions); peripheral edema; reversed epinephrine effect; hyperpyrexia; mild fever after large I.M. doses; increased appetite; increased weight; a systemic lupus erythematosus-like syndrome; pigmentary retinopathy; with prolonged administration of substantial doses, skin pigmentation, epithelial keratopathy, and lenticular and corneal deposits.

EKG changes—particularly nonspecific, usually reversible Q and T wave distortions—have been observed in some patients receiving phenothiazine tranquilizers.

Although phenothiazines cause neither psychic nor physical dependence, sudden discontinuance in long-term psychiatric patients may cause temporary symptoms, e.g., nausea and vomiting, dizziness, tremulousness.

Note: There have been occasional reports of sudden death in patients receiving phenothiazines. In some cases, the cause appeared to be cardiac arrest or asphyxia due to failure of the cough reflex.

DOSAGE AND ADMINISTRATION

Notes on Injection: *Stability*—This solution should be protected from light. This is a clear, colorless to pale yellow solution; a slight yellowish discoloration will not alter potency. If markedly discolored, solution should be discarded.

Compatibility—It is recommended that Compazine (prochlorperazine) Injection not be mixed with other agents in the syringe.

DOSAGE AND ADMINISTRATION—ADULTS

(For children's dosage and administration, see below.) Dosage should be increased more gradually in debilitated or emaciated patients.

Elderly Patients: In general, dosages in the lower range are sufficient for most elderly patients. Since they appear to be more susceptible to hypotension and neuromuscular reactions, such patients should be observed closely. Dosage should be tailored to the individual, response carefully monitored and dosage adjusted accordingly. Dosage should be increased more gradually in elderly patients.

1. To Control Severe Nausea and Vomiting: Adjust dosage to the response of the individual. Begin with the lowest recommended dosage.

Oral Dosage—Tablets: Usually one 5 mg or 10 mg tablet 3 or 4 times daily. Daily dosages above 40 mg should be used only in resistant cases.

***Spansule* capsules:** Initially, usually one 15 mg capsule on arising or one 10 mg capsule q12h. Daily doses above 40 mg should be used only in resistant cases.

Rectal Dosage: 25 mg twice daily.

I.M. Dosage: Initially 5 to 10 mg (1 to 2 mL) injected *deeply* into the upper outer quadrant of the buttock. If necessary, repeat every 3 or 4 hours. Total I.M. dosage should not exceed 40 mg per day.

I.V. Dosage: $2\frac{1}{2}$ to 10 mg ($\frac{1}{2}$ to 2 mL) by slow I.V. injection or infusion at a rate not to exceed 5 mg per minute. *Compazine* Injection may be administered either undiluted or diluted in isotonic solution. A single dose of the drug should not exceed 10 mg; total I.V. dosage should not exceed 40 mg per day. When administered I.V., do not use bolus injection. Hypotension is a possibility if the drug is given by I.V. injection or infusion.

Subcutaneous administration is not advisable because of local irritation.

2. Adult Surgery (for severe nausea and vomiting): Total parenteral dosage should not exceed 40 mg per day. Hypotension is a possibility if the drug is given by I.V. injection or infusion.

I.M. Dosage: 5 to 10 mg (1 to 2 mL) 1 to 2 hours before induction of anesthesia (repeat once in 30 minutes, if necessary), or to control acute symptoms during and after surgery (repeat once if necessary).

I.V. Dosage: 5 to 10 mg (1 to 2 mL) as a slow I.V. injection or infusion 15 to 30 minutes before induction of anesthesia, or to control acute symptoms during or after surgery. Repeat once if necessary. Compazine (prochlorperazine) may be administered either undiluted or diluted in isotonic solution, but a single dose of the drug should not exceed 10 mg. The rate of administration should not exceed 5 mg per minute. When administered I.V., do not use bolus injection.

3. In Adult Psychiatric Disorders: Adjust dosage to the response of the individual and according to the severity of the condition. Begin with the lowest recommended dose. Although response ordinarily is seen within a day or 2, longer treatment is usually required before maximal improvement is seen.

Oral Dosage: *Non-Psychotic Anxiety*—Usual dosage is 5 mg 3 or 4 times daily; by *Spansule* capsule, usually one 15 mg capsule on arising or one 10 mg capsule q12h. Do not administer in doses of more than 20 mg per day or for longer than 12 weeks.

Psychotic Disorders—*In relatively mild conditions,* as seen in private psychiatric practice or in outpatient clinics, dosage is 5 or 10 mg 3 or 4 times daily.

In moderate to severe conditions, for hospitalized or adequately supervised patients, usual starting dosage is 10 mg 3 or 4 times daily. Increase dosage gradually until symptoms are controlled or side effects become bothersome. When dosage is increased by small increments every 2 or 3 days, side effects either do not occur or are easily controlled. Some patients respond satisfactorily on 50 to 75 mg daily.

In more severe disturbances, optimum dosage is usually 100 to 150 mg daily.

I.M. Dosage: For immediate control of severely disturbed adults, inject an initial dose of 10 to 20 mg (2 to 4 mL) *deeply* into the upper outer quadrant of the buttock. Many patients respond shortly after the first injection. If necessary, however, repeat the initial dose every 2 to 4 hours (or, in resistant cases, every hour) to gain control of the patient. More than three or four doses are seldom necessary. After control is achieved, switch patient to an oral form of the drug at the same dosage level or higher. If, in rare cases, parenteral therapy is needed for a prolonged period, give 10 to 20 mg (2 to 4 mL) every 4 to 6 hours. Pain and irritation at the site of injection have seldom occurred.

Subcutaneous administration is not advisable because of local irritation.

DOSAGE AND ADMINISTRATION—CHILDREN

Do not use in pediatric surgery.

Children seem more prone to develop extrapyramidal reactions, even on moderate doses. Therefore, use lowest effective dosage. Tell parents not to exceed prescribed dosage, since the possibility of adverse reactions increases as dosage rises.

Occasionally the patient may react to the drug with signs of restlessness and excitement; if this occurs, do not administer additional doses. Take particular precaution in administering the drug to children with acute illnesses or dehydration (see under Dystonias).

When writing a prescription for the $2\frac{1}{2}$ mg size suppository, write "$2\frac{1}{2}$," not "2.5"; this will help avoid confusion with the 25 mg adult size.

1. Severe Nausea and Vomiting in Children: Compazine (prochlorperazine) should not be used in pediatric patients under 20 pounds in weight or 2 years of age. It should not be used in conditions for which children's dosages have not been established. Dosage and frequency of administration should be adjusted according to the severity of the symptoms and the response of the patient. The duration of activity following intramuscular administration may last up to 12 hours. Subsequent doses may be given by the same route if necessary.

Oral or Rectal Dosage: More than 1 day's therapy is seldom necessary.

Weight	Usual Dosage	Not to Exceed
under 20 lbs not recommended		
20 to 29 lbs	$2\frac{1}{2}$ mg 1 or 2 times a day	7.5 mg per day
30 to 39 lbs	$2\frac{1}{2}$ mg 2 or 3 times a day	10 mg per day
40 to 85 lbs	$2\frac{1}{2}$ mg 3 times a day or 5 mg 2 times a day	15 mg per day

I.M. Dosage: Calculate each dose on the basis of 0.06 mg of the drug per lb of body weight; give by deep I.M. injection. Control is usually obtained with one dose.

2. In Psychotic Children:

Oral or Rectal Dosage: For children 2 to 12 years, starting dosage is $2\frac{1}{2}$ mg 2 or 3 times daily. Do not give more than 10 mg the first day. Then increase dosage according to patient's response.

Continued on next page

Information on the SmithKline Beecham Pharmaceuticals products appearing here is based on the labeling in effect on June 15, 2000. Further information on these and other products may be obtained from the Medical Department, SmithKline Beecham Pharmaceuticals, One Franklin Plaza, Philadelphia, PA 19101.

Compazine—Cont.

FOR AGES 2 to 5, total daily dosage usually does not exceed 20 mg.
FOR AGES 6 to 12, total daily dosage usually does not exceed 25 mg.
I.M. Dosage: For ages under 12, calculate each dose on the basis of 0.06 mg of Compazine (prochlorperazine) per lb of body weight; give by deep I.M. injection. Control is usually obtained with one dose. After control is achieved, switch the patient to an oral form of the drug at the same dosage level or higher.

OVERDOSAGE

(See also ADVERSE REACTIONS.)
SYMPTOMS—Primarily involvement of the extrapyramidal mechanism producing some of the dystonic reactions described above.
Symptoms of central nervous system depression to the point of somnolence or coma. Agitation and restlessness may also occur. Other possible manifestations include convulsions, EKG changes and cardiac arrhythmias, fever and autonomic reactions such as hypotension, dry mouth and ileus.
TREATMENT—It is important to determine other medications taken by the patient since multiple-dose therapy is common in overdosage situations. Treatment is essentially symptomatic and supportive. Early gastric lavage is helpful. Keep patient under observation and maintain an open airway, since involvement of the extrapyramidal mechanism may produce dysphagia and respiratory difficulty in severe overdosage. **Do not attempt to induce emesis because a dystonic reaction of the head or neck may develop that could result in aspiration of vomitus.** Extrapyramidal symptoms may be treated with anti-parkinsonism drugs, barbiturates or *Benadryl*. See prescribing information for these products. Care should be taken to avoid increasing respiratory depression.
If administration of a stimulant is desirable, amphetamine, dextroamphetamine or caffeine with sodium benzoate is recommended.
Stimulants that may cause convulsions (e.g., picrotoxin or pentylenetetrazol) should be avoided.
If hypotension occurs, the standard measures for managing circulatory shock should be initiated. If it is desirable to administer a vasoconstrictor, *Levophed* and *Neo-Synephrine* are most suitable. Other pressor agents, including epinephrine, are not recommended because phenothiazine derivatives may reverse the usual elevating action of these agents and cause a further lowering of blood pressure.
Limited experience indicates that phenothiazines are *not* dialyzable.
Special note on Spansule *capsules*—Since much of the *Spansule* capsule medication is coated for gradual release, therapy directed at reversing the effects of the ingested drug and at supporting the patient should be continued for as long as overdosage symptoms remain. Saline cathartics are useful for hastening evacuation of pellets that have not already released medication.

HOW SUPPLIED

Tablets—5 and 10 mg, in bottles of 100; in Single Unit Packages of 100 (intended for institutional use only).
5 mg 100's: NDC 0007-3366-20
5 mg SUP 100's: NDC 0007-3366-21
10 mg 100's: NDC 0007-3367-20
10 mg SUP 100's: NDC 0007-3367-21
***Spansule* capsules**—10 and 15 mg, in bottles of 50.
10 mg 50's: NDC 0007-3344-15
15 mg 50's: NDC 0007-3346-15
Vials—2 mL (5 mg/mL), in boxes of 25 and 10 mL (5 mg/mL), in boxes of 1.
2 mL (5 mg/mL), in boxes of 25: NDC 0007-3352-16
10 mL (5 mg/mL), in boxes of 1: NDC 0007-3343-01
Suppositories—2½ mg (for young children), 5 mg (for older children) and 25 mg (for adults), in boxes of 12.
2½ mg, in boxes of 12: NDC 0007-3360-03
5 mg, in boxes of 12: NDC 0007-3361-03
25 mg, in boxes of 12: NDC 0007-3362-03
Syrup—5 mg/5 mL (1 teaspoonful) in 4 fl oz bottles.
5 mg/5 mL, 4 fl oz: NDC 0007-3363-44

Store Compazine (prochlorperazine) vials below 30°C (86°F). Do not freeze. Other dosage forms can be stored between 15° and 30°C (59° and 86°F). Protect from light.
* norepinephrine bitartrate, Sanofi Pharmaceuticals.
† phenylephrine hydrochloride, Sanofi Pharmaceuticals.
‡ phenytoin, Parke-Davis.
§ metrizamide, Sanofi Pharmaceuticals.
‖ diphenhydramine hydrochloride, Parke-Davis.

℞ only

CZ:L92

Shown in Product Identification Guide, page 337

COREG® ℞

[kō-reg]
brand of carvedilol Tablets

DESCRIPTION

Carvedilol is a nonselective β-adrenergic blocking agent with α_1-blocking activity. It is (±)-1-(Carbazol-4-yloxy)-3-[[2-(o-methoxyphenoxy)ethyl]amino]-2-propanol. It is a racemic mixture with the following structure:

carvedilol

Tablets for Oral Administration:
Coreg (carvedilol) is a white, oval, film-coated tablet containing 3.125 mg, 6.25 mg, 12.5 mg or 25 mg of carvedilol. The 6.25 mg, 12.5 mg and 25 mg tablets are Tiltab® tablets. Inactive ingredients consist of colloidal silicon dioxide, crospovidone, hydroxypropyl methylcellulose, lactose, magnesium stearate, polyethylene glycol, polysorbate 80, povidone, sucrose and titanium dioxide.
Carvedilol is a white to off-white powder with a molecular weight of 406.5 and a molecular formula of $C_{24}H_{26}N_2O_4$. It is freely soluble in dimethylsulfoxide; soluble in methylene chloride and methanol; sparingly soluble in 95% ethanol and isopropanol; slightly soluble in ethyl ether; and practically insoluble in water, gastric fluid (simulated, TS, pH 1.1) and intestinal fluid (simulated, TS without pancreatin, pH 7.5).

CLINICAL PHARMACOLOGY

Coreg is a racemic mixture in which nonselective β-adrenoreceptor blocking activity is present in the S(-) enantiomer and α-adrenergic blocking activity is present in both R(+) and S(-) enantiomers at equal potency. *Coreg* has no intrinsic sympathomimetic activity.

Pharmacokinetics
Coreg is rapidly and extensively absorbed following oral administration, with absolute bioavailability of approximately 25% to 35% due to a significant degree of first-pass metabolism. Following oral administration, the apparent mean terminal elimination half-life of carvedilol generally ranges from 7 to 10 hours. Plasma concentrations achieved are proportional to the oral dose administered. When administered with food, the rate of absorption is slowed, as evidenced by a delay in the time to reach peak plasma levels, with no significant difference in extent of bioavailability. Taking *Coreg* with food should minimize the risk of orthostatic hypotension.
Carvedilol is extensively metabolized. Following oral administration of radiolabelled carvedilol to healthy volunteers, carvedilol accounted for only about 7% of the total radioactivity in plasma as measured by area under the curve (AUC). Less than 2% of the dose was excreted unchanged in the urine. Carvedilol is metabolized primarily by aromatic ring oxidation and glucuronidation. The oxidative metabolites are further metabolized by conjugation via glucuronidation and sulfation. The metabolites of carvedilol are excreted primarily via the bile into the feces. Demethylation and hydroxylation at the phenol ring produce three active metabolites with β-receptor blocking activity. Based on preclinical studies, the 4′-hydroxyphenyl metabolite is approximately 13 times more potent than carvedilol for β-blockade.
Compared to carvedilol, the three active metabolites exhibit weak vasodilating activity. Plasma concentrations of the active metabolites are about one-tenth of those observed for carvedilol and have pharmacokinetics similar to the parent.
Carvedilol undergoes stereoselective first-pass metabolism with plasma levels of R(+)-carvedilol approximately 2 to 3 times higher than S(-)-carvedilol following oral administration in healthy subjects. The mean apparent terminal elimination half-lives for R(+)-carvedilol range from 5 to 9 hours compared with 7 to 11 hours for the S(-)-enantiomer.
The primary P450 enzymes responsible for the metabolism of both R(+) and S(-)-carvedilol in human liver microsomes were CYP2D6 and CYP2C9 and to a lesser extent CYP3A4, 2C19, 1A2, and 2E1. CYP2D6 is thought to be the major enzyme in the 4′- and 5′-hydroxylation of carvedilol, with a potential contribution from 3A4. CYP2C9 is thought to be of primary importance in the O-methylation pathway of S(-)-carvedilol.
Carvedilol is subject to the effects of genetic polymorphism with poor metabolizers of debrisoquin (a marker for cytochrome P450 2D6) exhibiting 2- to 3-fold higher plasma concentrations of R(+)-carvedilol compared to extensive metabolizers. In contrast, plasma levels of S(-)- carvedilol are increased only about 20% to 25% in poor metabolizers, indicating this enantiomer is metabolized to a lesser extent by cytochrome P450 2D6 than R(+)-carvedilol. The pharmacokinetics of carvedilol do not appear to be different in poor metabolizers of S-mephenytoin (patients deficient in cytochrome P450 2C19).
Carvedilol is more than 98% bound to plasma proteins, primarily with albumin. The plasma-protein binding is independent of concentration over the therapeutic range. Carvedilol is a basic, lipophilic compound with a steady-state volume of distribution of approximately 115 L, indicating substantial distribution into extravascular tissues. Plasma clearance ranges from 500 to 700 mL/min.
Congestive Heart Failure: Steady-state plasma concentrations of carvedilol and its enantiomers increased proportionally over the 6.25 to 50 mg dose range in patients with congestive heart failure. Compared to healthy subjects, congestive heart failure patients had increased mean AUC and C_{max} values for carvedilol and its enantiomers, with up to 50% to 100% higher values observed in 6 patients with NYHA class IV heart failure. The mean apparent terminal elimination half-life for carvedilol was similar to that observed in healthy subjects.
Pharmacokinetic Drug-Drug Interactions: Since carvedilol undergoes substantial oxidative metabolism, the metabolism and pharmacokinetics of carvedilol may be affected by induction or inhibition of cytochrome P450 enzymes.
Rifampin: In a pharmacokinetic study conducted in 8 healthy male subjects, rifampin (600 mg daily for 12 days) decreased the AUC and C_{max} of carvedilol by about 70%.
Cimetidine: In a pharmacokinetic study conducted in 10 healthy male subjects, cimetidine (1000 mg/day) increased the steady-state AUC of carvedilol by 30% with no change in C_{max}.
Glyburide: In 12 healthy subjects, combined administration of carvedilol (25 mg once daily) and a single dose of glyburide did not result in a clinically relevant pharmacokinetic interaction for either compound.
Hydrochlorothiazide: A single oral dose of carvedilol 25 mg did not alter the pharmacokinetics of a single oral dose of hydrochlorothiazide 25 mg in 12 patients with hypertension. Likewise, hydrochlorothiazide had no effect on the pharmacokinetics of carvedilol.
Digoxin: Following concomitant administration of carvedilol (25 mg once daily) and digoxin (0.25 mg once daily) for 14 days, steady-state AUC and trough concentrations of digoxin were increased by 14% and 16%, respectively, in 12 hypertensive patients.
Torsemide: In a study of 12 healthy subjects, combined oral administration of carvedilol 25 mg once daily and torsemide 5 mg once daily for 5 days did not result in any significant differences in their pharmacokinetics compared with administration of the drugs alone.
Warfarin: Carvedilol (12.5 mg twice daily) did not have an effect on the steady-state prothrombin time ratios and did not alter the pharmacokinetics of R(+)- and S(-)-warfarin following concomitant administration with warfarin in 9 healthy volunteers.

Special Populations
Elderly: Plasma levels of carvedilol average about 50% higher in the elderly compared to young subjects.
Hepatic Impairment: Compared to healthy subjects, patients with cirrhotic liver disease exhibit significantly higher concentrations of carvedilol (approximately 4- to 7-fold) following single-dose therapy (see WARNINGS, Hepatic Injury).
Renal Insufficiency: Although carvedilol is metabolized primarily by the liver, plasma concentrations of carvedilol have been reported to be increased in patients with renal impairment. Based on mean AUC data, approximately 40% to 50% higher plasma concentrations of carvedilol were observed in hypertensive patients with moderate to severe renal impairment compared to a control group of hypertensive patients with normal renal function. However, the ranges of AUC values were similar for both groups. Changes in mean peak plasma levels were less pronounced, approximately 12% to 26% higher in patients with impaired renal function.
Consistent with its high degree of plasma protein-binding, carvedilol does not appear to be cleared significantly by hemodialysis.

Pharmacodynamics and Clinical Trials
Congestive Heart Failure
Pharmacodynamics
The basis for the beneficial effects of Coreg (carvedilol) in congestive heart failure is not established.
Two placebo-controlled studies compared the acute hemodynamic effects of *Coreg* to baseline measurements in 59 and 49 patients with NYHA class II-IV heart failure receiving diuretics, ACE inhibitors, and digitalis. There were significant reductions in systemic blood pressure, pulmonary artery pressure, pulmonary capillary wedge pressure, and heart rate. Initial effects on cardiac output, stroke volume index, and systemic vascular resistance were small and variable.
These studies measured hemodynamic effects again at 12 to 14 weeks. *Coreg* significantly reduced systemic blood pressure, pulmonary artery pressure, right atrial pressure, systemic vascular resistance, and heart rate, while stroke volume index was increased.
Among 839 patients with NYHA class II-III heart failure treated for 26 to 52 weeks in 4 U.S. placebo-controlled trials, average left ventricular ejection fraction (EF) measured by radionuclide ventriculography increased by 8 EF units (%) in *Coreg* patients and by 2 EF units in placebo patients (between-group difference of 6 EF units). This treatment effect was nominally statistically significant in each trial.

Hypertension
Pharmacodynamics
The mechanism by which β-blockade produces an antihypertensive effect has not been established.
β-adrenoreceptor blocking activity has been demonstrated in animal and human studies showing that carvedilol (1) reduces cardiac output in normal subjects; (2) reduces exercise- and/or isoproterenol-induced tachycardia and (3) reduces reflex orthostatic tachycardia. Significant β-adrenoreceptor blocking effect is usually seen within 1 hour of drug administration.
α_1-adrenoreceptor blocking activity has been demonstrated in human and animal studies, showing that carvedilol (1) attenuates the pressor effects of phenylephrine; (2) causes vasodilation and (3) reduces peripheral vascular resistance.

These effects contribute to the reduction of blood pressure and usually are seen within 30 minutes of drug administration.

Due to the α_1-receptor blocking activity of carvedilol, blood pressure is lowered more in the standing than in the supine position, and symptoms of postural hypotension (1.8%), including rare instances of syncope, can occur. Following oral administration, when postural hypotension has occurred, it has been transient and is uncommon when Coreg (carvedilol) is administered with food at the recommended starting dose and titration increments are closely followed (see DOSAGE AND ADMINISTRATION).

In hypertensive patients with normal renal function, therapeutic doses of *Coreg* decreased renal vascular resistance with no change in glomerular filtration rate or renal plasma flow. Changes in excretion of sodium, potassium, uric acid and phosphorus in hypertensive patients with normal renal function were similar after *Coreg* and placebo.

Coreg has little effect on plasma catecholamines, plasma aldosterone or electrolyte levels, but it does significantly reduce plasma renin activity when given for at least 4 weeks. It also increases levels of atrial natriuretic peptide.

CLINICAL TRIALS

Congestive Heart Failure

Four U.S. multicenter, double-blind, placebo-controlled studies enrolled 1094 patients (696 randomized to carvedilol) with NYHA class II-III heart failure and ejection fraction <0.35. The vast majority were on digitalis, diuretics, and an ACE inhibitor at study entry. Patients were assigned to the studies based upon exercise ability. An Australia-New Zealand double-blind, placebo-controlled study enrolled 415 patients (half randomized to carvedilol) with less severe heart failure. All protocols excluded patients expected to undergo cardiac surgery during the 6 to 12 months of double-blind follow-up. All randomized patients had tolerated a 2-week course on carvedilol 6.25 mg b.i.d.

In each study, there was a primary end-point, either progression of heart failure (one U.S. study) or exercise tolerance (2 U.S. studies meeting enrollment goals and the Australia-New Zealand study). There were many secondary end-points specified in these studies, including NYHA classification, patient and physician global assessments, and cardiovascular hospitalization. Death was not a specified end-point in any study, but it was analyzed in all studies. Other analyses not prospectively planned included the sum of deaths and total cardiovascular hospitalizations. In situations where the primary end-points of a trial do not show a significant benefit of treatment, assignment of significance values to the other results is complex, and such values need to be interpreted cautiously.

The results of the U.S. and Australia-New Zealand trials were as follows:

Slowing Progression of Heart Failure: One U.S. multicenter study (366 subjects) had as its primary end-point the sum of cardiovascular mortality, cardiovascular hospitalization, and sustained increase in heart failure medications. Heart failure progression was reduced, during an average follow-up of 7 months, by 48% (p=0.008).

In the Australia-New Zealand study, death and total hospitalizations were reduced by about 25% over 18 to 24 months. In the three largest U.S. studies, death and total hospitalizations were reduced by 19%, 39% and 49%, nominally statistically significant in the last two studies. The Australia-New Zealand results were statistically borderline.

Functional Measures: None of the multicenter studies had NYHA classification as a primary end-point, but all such studies had it as a secondary end-point. There was at least a trend toward improvement in NYHA class in all studies. Exercise tolerance was the primary end-point in 3 studies; in none was a statistically significant effect found.

Subjective Measures: Quality of life, as measured with a standard questionnaire (a primary end-point in one study), was unaffected by carvedilol. However, patients' and investigators' global assessments showed significant improvement in most studies.

Mortality: Mortality was not a planned end-point in any study. Overall, in the U.S. trials, mortality was reduced, nominally significantly so in 2 studies, but the actual effect size and statistical significance of this observation are difficult to define.

Hypertension

Coreg was studied in two placebo-controlled trials that utilized twice-daily dosing, at total daily doses of 12.5 to 50 mg. In these and other studies, the starting dose did not exceed 12.5 mg. At 50 mg per day, *Coreg* reduced sitting trough (12-hour) blood pressure by about 9/5.5 mm Hg; at 25 mg/day the effect was about 7.5/3.5 mm Hg. Comparisons of trough to peak blood pressure showed a trough to peak ratio for blood pressure response of about 65%. Heart rate fell by about 7.5 beats per minute at 50 mg/day. In general, as is true for other β-blockers, responses were smaller in black than non-black patients. There were no age- or gender-related differences in response.

The peak antihypertensive effect occurred 1 to 2 hours after a dose. The dose-related blood pressure response was accompanied by a dose-related increase in adverse effects (see ADVERSE REACTIONS).

INDICATIONS AND USAGE

Congestive Heart Failure

Coreg is indicated for the treatment of mild or moderate (NYHA class II or III) heart failure of ischemic or cardiomyopathic origin, in conjunction with digitalis, diuretics, and ACE inhibitor, to reduce the progression of disease as evidenced by cardiovascular death, cardiovascular hospitalization, or the need to adjust other heart failure medications.

Coreg may be used in patients unable to tolerate an ACE inhibitor. *Coreg* may be used in patients who are or are not receiving digitalis, hydralazine or nitrate therapy.

Hypertension

Coreg (carvedilol) is also indicated for the management of essential hypertension. It can be used alone or in combination with other antihypertensive agents, especially thiazide-type diuretics (see PRECAUTIONS, Drug Interactions).

CONTRAINDICATIONS

Coreg is contraindicated in patients with NYHA class IV decompensated cardiac failure requiring intravenous inotropic therapy, bronchial asthma (two cases of death from status asthmaticus have been reported in patients receiving single doses of *Coreg*) or related bronchospastic conditions, second- or third-degree AV block, sick sinus syndrome (unless a permanent pacemaker is in place), cardiogenic shock or severe bradycardia.

Use of *Coreg* in patients with clinically manifest hepatic impairment is not recommended.

Coreg is contraindicated in patients with hypersensitivity to the drug.

WARNINGS

Hepatic Injury: Mild hepatocellular injury, confirmed by rechallenge, has occurred rarely with *Coreg* therapy. In controlled studies of hypertensive patients, the incidence of liver function abnormalities reported as adverse experiences was 1.1% (13 of 1,142 patients) in patients receiving *Coreg* and 0.9% (4 of 462 patients) in those receiving placebo. One patient receiving carvedilol in a placebo-controlled trial withdrew for abnormal hepatic function.

In controlled studies of congestive heart failure, the incidence of liver function abnormalities reported as adverse experiences was 5.0% (38 of 765 patients) in patients receiving *Coreg* and 4.6% (20 of 437 patients) in those receiving placebo. Three patients receiving carvedilol (0.4%) and two patients receiving placebo (0.5%) in placebo-controlled trials withdrew for abnormal hepatic function.

Hepatic injury has been reversible and has occurred after short- and/or long-term therapy with minimal clinical symptomatology. No deaths due to liver function abnormalities have been reported.

At the first symptom/sign of liver dysfunction (e.g., pruritus, dark urine, persistent anorexia, jaundice, right upper quadrant tenderness or unexplained "flu-like" symptoms), laboratory testing should be performed. If the patient has laboratory evidence of liver injury or jaundice, carvedilol should be stopped and not restarted.

Peripheral Vascular Disease: β-blockers can precipitate or aggravate symptoms of arterial insufficiency in patients with peripheral vascular disease. Caution should be exercised in such individuals.

Anesthesia and Major Surgery: If *Coreg* treatment is to be continued perioperatively, particular care should be taken when anesthetic agents which depress myocardial function, such as ether, cyclopropane and trichloroethylene, are used. See OVERDOSAGE for information on treatment of bradycardia and hypertension.

Diabetes and Hypoglycemia: β-blockers may mask some of the manifestations of hypoglycemia, particularly tachycardia. Nonselective β-blockers may potentiate insulin-induced hypoglycemia and delay recovery of serum glucose levels. Patients subject to spontaneous hypoglycemia, or diabetic patients receiving insulin or oral hypoglycemic agents, should be cautioned about these possibilities and carvedilol should be used with caution. In congestive heart failure patients, there is a risk of worsening hyperglycemia (see PRECAUTIONS).

Thyrotoxicosis: β-adrenergic blockade may mask clinical signs of hyperthyroidism, such as tachycardia. Abrupt withdrawal of β-blockade may be followed by an exacerbation of the symptoms of hyperthyroidism or may precipitate thyroid storm.

PRECAUTIONS

General

Since Coreg (carvedilol) has β-blocking activity, it should not be discontinued abruptly, particularly in patients with ischemic heart disease. Instead, it should be discontinued over 1 to 2 weeks.

In clinical trials, *Coreg* caused bradycardia in about 2% of hypertensive patients and 9% of congestive heart failure patients. If pulse rate drops below 55 beats/min., the dosage should be reduced.

Hypotension and postural hypotension occurred in 9.7% and syncope in 3.4% of congestive heart failure patients receiving carvedilol compared to 3.6% and 2.5% of placebo patients, respectively. The risk for these events was highest during the first 30 days of dosing, corresponding to the up-titration period and was a cause for discontinuation of therapy in 0.7% of carvedilol patients, compared to 0.4% of placebo patients.

Postural hypotension occurred in 1.8% and syncope in 0.1% of hypertensive patients, primarily following the initial dose or at the time of dose increase and was a cause for discontinuation of therapy in 1% of patients.

To decrease the likelihood of syncope or excessive hypotension, treatment should be initiated with 3.125 mg b.i.d. for congestive heart failure patients and 6.25 mg b.i.d. for hypertensive patients. Dosage should then be increased slowly, according to recommendations in the DOSAGE AND ADMINISTRATION section, and the drug should be taken with food. During initiation of therapy, the patient should be cautioned to avoid situations such as driving or hazardous tasks, where injury could result should syncope occur.

Rarely, use of carvedilol in patients with congestive heart failure has resulted in deterioration of renal function. Patients at risk appear to be those with low blood pressure (systolic BP<100 mm Hg), ischemic heart disease and diffuse vascular disease, and/or underlying renal insufficiency. Renal function has returned to baseline when carvedilol was stopped. In patients with these risk factors it is recommended that renal function be monitored during up-titration of carvedilol and the drug discontinued or dosage reduced if worsening of renal function occurs.

Worsening cardiac failure or fluid retention may occur during up-titration of carvedilol. If such symptoms occur, diuretics should be increased and the carvedilol dose should not be advanced until clinical stability resumes (see DOSAGE AND ADMINISTRATION). Occasionally it is necessary to lower the carvedilol dose or temporarily discontinue it. Such episodes do not preclude subsequent successful titration of carvedilol.

In patients with pheochromocytoma, an α-blocking agent should be initiated prior to the use of any β-blocking agent. Although carvedilol has both α- and β-blocking pharmacologic activities, there has been no experience with its use in this condition. Therefore, caution should be taken in the administration of carvedilol to patients suspected of having pheochromocytoma.

Agents with non-selective β-blocking activity may provoke chest pain in patients with Prinzmetal's variant angina. There has been no clinical experience with carvedilol in these patients although the α-blocking activity may prevent such symptoms. However, caution should be taken in the administration of carvedilol to patients suspected of having Prinzmetal's variant angina.

Risk of Anaphylactic Reaction

While taking β-blockers, patients with a history of severe anaphylactic reaction to a variety of allergens may be more reactive to repeated challenge, either accidental, diagnostic or therapeutic. Such patients may be unresponsive to the usual doses of epinephrine used to treat allergic reaction.

Nonallergic Bronchospasm (e.g., chronic bronchitis and emphysema)

Patients with bronchospastic disease should, in general, not receive β-blockers. *Coreg* may be used with caution, however, in patients who do not respond to, or cannot tolerate, other antihypertensive agents. It is prudent, if Coreg (carvedilol) is used, to use the smallest effective dose, so that inhibition of endogenous or exogenous β-agonists is minimized.

In clinical trials of patients with congestive heart failure, patients with bronchospastic disease were enrolled if they did not require oral or inhaled medication to treat their bronchospastic disease. In such patients, it is recommended that carvedilol be used with caution. The dosing recommendations should be followed closely and the dose should be lowered if any evidence of bronchospasm is observed during up-titration.

Hypertensive Patients with Left Ventricular Failure: In hypertensive patients who have congestive heart failure controlled with digitalis, diuretics and/or an angiotensin-converting enzyme inhibitor, Coreg (carvedilol) may be used. However, since it is likely that such patients are dependent, in part, on sympathetic stimulation for circulatory support, it is recommended that dosing follow the instructions for patients with congestive heart failure.

In congestive heart failure patients with diabetes, carvedilol therapy may lead to worsening hyperglycemia, which responds to intensification of hypoglycemic therapy. It is recommended that blood glucose be monitored when carvedilol dosing is initiated, adjusted, or discontinued.

Information for Patients

Patients taking *Coreg* should be advised of the following:

— they should not interrupt or discontinue using *Coreg* without a physician's advice.

— congestive heart failure patients should consult their physician if they experience signs or symptoms of worsening heart failure such as weight gain or increasing shortness of breath.

— they may experience a drop in blood pressure when standing, resulting in dizziness and, rarely, fainting. Patients should sit or lie down when these symptoms of lowered blood pressure occur.

— if patients experience dizziness or fatigue, they should avoid driving or hazardous tasks.

— they should consult a physician if they experience dizziness or faintness, in case the dosage should be adjusted.

— they should take *Coreg* with food.

— diabetic patients should report any changes in blood sugar levels to their physician.

— contact lens wearers may experience decreased lacrimation.

Continued on next page

Information on the SmithKline Beecham Pharmaceuticals products appearing here is based on the labeling in effect on June 15, 2000. Further information on these and other products may be obtained from the Medical Department, SmithKline Beecham Pharmaceuticals, One Franklin Plaza, Philadelphia, PA 19101.

Coreg—Cont.

Drug Interactions
(Also see CLINICAL PHARMACOLOGY, Pharmacokinetic Drug-Drug Interactions.)
Inhibitors of CYP2D6; poor metabolizers of debrisoquin: Interactions of carvedilol with strong inhibitors of CYP2D6 (such as quinidine, fluoxetine, paroxetine, and propafenone) have not been studied, but these drugs would be expected to increase blood levels of the R(+) enantiomer of carvedilol (see CLINICAL PHARMACOLOGY). Retrospective analysis of side effects in clinical trials showed that poor 2D6 metabolizers had a higher rate of dizziness during up-titration, presumably resulting from vasodilating effects of the higher concentrations of the α-blocking R(+) enantiomer.
Catecholamine-depleting agents: Patients taking both agents with β-blocking properties and a drug that can deplete catecholamines (e.g., reserpine and monoamine oxidase inhibitors) should be observed closely for signs of hypotension and/or severe bradycardia.
Clonidine: Concomitant administration of clonidine with agents with β-blocking properties may potentiate blood-pressure- and heart-rate-lowering effects. When concomitant treatment with agents with β-blocking properties and clonidine is to be terminated, the β-blocking agent should be discontinued first. Clonidine therapy can then be discontinued several days later by gradually decreasing the dosage.
Cyclosporin: Modest increases in mean trough cyclosporin concentrations were observed following initiation of carvedilol treatment in 21 renal transplant patients suffering from chronic vascular rejection. In about 30% of patients, the dose of cyclosporin had to be reduced in order to maintain cyclosporin concentrations within the therapeutic range, while in the remainder no adjustment was needed. On the average for the group, the dose of cyclosporin was reduced about 20% in these patients. Due to wide inter-individual variability in the dose adjustment required, it is recommended that cyclosporin concentrations be monitored closely after initiation of carvedilol therapy and that the dose of cyclosporin be adjusted as appropriate.
Digoxin: Digoxin concentrations are increased by about 15% when digoxin and carvedilol are administered concomitantly. Both digoxin and *Coreg* slow AV conduction. Therefore, increased monitoring of digoxin is recommended when initiating, adjusting or discontinuing *Coreg*.
Inducers and inhibitors of hepatic metabolism: Rifampin reduced plasma concentrations of carvedilol by about 70%. Cimetidine increased AUC by about 30% but caused no change in C_{max}.
Calcium channel blockers: Isolated cases of conduction disturbance (rarely with hemodynamic compromise) have been observed when *Coreg* is co-administered with diltiazem. As with other agents with β-blocking properties, if Coreg (carvedilol) is to be administered orally with calcium channel blockers of the verapamil or diltiazem type, it is recommended that ECG and blood pressure be monitored.
Insulin or oral hypoglycemics: Agents with β-blocking properties may enhance the blood-sugar-reducing effect of insulin and oral hypoglycemics. Therefore, in patients taking insulin or oral hypoglycemics, regular monitoring of blood glucose is recommended.

Carcinogenesis, Mutagenesis, Impairment of Fertility
In 2-year studies conducted in rats given carvedilol at doses up to 75 mg/kg/day (12 times the maximum recommended human dose [MRHD] when compared on a mg/m^2 basis) or in mice given up to 200 mg/kg/day (16 times the MRHD on a mg/m^2 basis), carvedilol had no carcinogenic effect.
Carvedilol was negative when tested in a battery of genotoxicity assays, including the Ames and the CHO/HGPRT assays for mutagenicity and the *in vitro* hamster micronucleus and *in vivo* human lymphocyte cell tests for clastogenicity.
At doses ≥200 mg/kg/day (≥32 times the MRHD as mg/m^2) carvedilol was toxic to adult rats (sedation, reduced weight gain) and was associated with a reduced number of successful matings, prolonged mating time, significantly fewer corpora lutea and implants per dam and complete resorption of 18% of the litters. The no-observed-effect dose level for overt toxicity and impairment of fertility was 60 mg/kg/day (10 times the MRHD as mg/m^2).

Pregnancy: Teratogenic Effects. Pregnancy Category C.
Studies performed in pregnant rats and rabbits given carvedilol revealed increased post-implantation loss in rats at doses of 300 mg/kg/day (50 times the MRHD as mg/m^2) and in rabbits at doses of 75 mg/kg/day (25 times the MRHD as mg/m^2). In the rats, there was also a decrease in fetal body weight at the maternally toxic dose of 300 mg/kg/day (50 times the MRHD as mg/m^2), which was accompanied by an elevation in the frequency of fetuses with delayed skeletal development (missing or stunted 13th rib). In rats the no-observed-effect level for developmental toxicity was 60 mg/kg/day (10 times the MRHD as mg/m^2); in rabbits it was 15 mg/kg/day (5 times the MRHD as mg/m^2). There are no adequate and well-controlled studies in pregnant women. *Coreg* should be used during pregnancy only if the potential benefit justifies the potential risk to the fetus.

Nursing Mothers
It is not known whether this drug is excreted in human milk. Studies in rats have shown that carvedilol and/or its metabolites (as well as other β-blockers) cross the placental barrier and are excreted in breast milk. There was increased mortality at one week post-partum in neonates from rats treated with 60 mg/kg/day (10 times the MRHD as mg/m^2) and above during the last trimester through day 22 of lactation. Because many drugs are excreted in human milk and because of the potential for serious adverse reactions in nursing infants from β-blockers, especially bradycardia, a decision should be made whether to discontinue nursing or to discontinue the drug, taking into account the importance of the drug to the mother. The effects of other α- and β-blocking agents have included perinatal and neonatal distress.

Pediatric Use
Safety and efficacy in patients younger than 18 years of age have not been established.

Geriatric Use
Of the 765 patients with congestive heart failure randomized to *Coreg* in U.S. clinical trials, 31% (235) were 65 years of age or older. Of 1,869 patients receiving *Coreg* in congestive heart failure trials worldwide, 39% were 65 years of age or older. There were no notable differences in efficacy or the incidence of adverse events between older and younger patients.
Of the 2,065 hypertensive patients in U.S. clinical trials of efficacy or safety who were treated with Coreg (carvedilol), 21% (436) were 65 years of age or older. Of 3,722 patients receiving *Coreg* in hypertension clinical trials conducted worldwide, 24% were 65 years of age or older. There were no notable differences in efficacy or the incidence of adverse events between older and younger patients. With the exception of dizziness (incidence 8.8% in the elderly vs. 6% in younger patients), there were no events for which the incidence in the elderly exceeded that in the younger population by greater than 2.0%.
Similar results were observed in a postmarketing surveillance study of 3,328 *Coreg* patients, of whom approximately 20% were 65 years of age or older.

ADVERSE REACTIONS

Congestive Heart Failure
Coreg has been evaluated for safety in congestive heart failure in more than 1,900 patients worldwide of whom 1,300 participated in U.S. clinical trials. Approximately 54% of the total treated population received *Coreg* for at least 6 months and 20% received *Coreg* for at least 12 months. The adverse experience profile of *Coreg* in congestive heart failure patients was consistent with the pharmacology of the drug and the health status of the patients. In U.S. clinical trials comparing *Coreg* in daily doses up to 100 mg (n=765) to placebo (n=437), 5.4% of *Coreg* patients discontinued for adverse experiences vs. 8.0% of placebo patients.
Table 1 shows adverse events in U.S. placebo-controlled clinical trials of congestive heart failure patients that occurred with an incidence of greater than 2% regardless of causality and were more frequent in drug-treated patients than placebo-treated patients. Median study medication exposure was 6.33 months for both Coreg (carvedilol) and placebo patients.
[See table 1 below]

Table 1 **Adverse Events in U.S. Placebo-Controlled Congestive Heart Failure Trials Incidence >2%, Regardless of Causality; Withdrawal Rates due to Adverse Events**

	Adverse Reactions		Withdrawals	
	Coreg **(n=765)** % occurrence	**Placebo (n=437)** % occurrence	***Coreg*** **(n=765)** % withdrawals	**Placebo (n=437)** % withdrawals
Autonomic Nervous System				
Sweating increased	2.9	2.1	—	—
Body as a Whole				
Fatigue	23.9	22.4	0.7	0.7
Chest pain	14.4	14.2	0.1	—
Pain	8.6	7.6	—	0.2
Injury	5.9	5.5	—	—
Drug level increased	5.1	3.7	—	0.2
Edema generalized	5.1	2.5	—	—
Edema dependent	3.7	1.8	—	—
Fever	3.1	2.3	—	—
Edema legs	2.2	0.2	0.1	0.2
Cardiovascular				
Bradycardia	8.8	0.9	0.8	—
Hypotension	8.5	3.4	0.4	0.2
Syncope	3.4	2.5	0.3	0.2
Hypertension	2.9	2.5	0.1	—
AV block	2.9	0.5	—	—
Angina pectoris aggravated	2.0	1.1	—	—
Central Nervous System				
Dizziness	32.4	19.2	0.4	—
Headache	8.1	7.1	0.3	—
Paresthesia	2.0	1.8	0.1	—
Gastrointestinal				
Diarrhea	11.8	5.9	0.3	—
Nausea	8.5	4.8	—	—
Abdominal Pain	7.2	7.1	0.3	—
Vomiting	6.3	4.3	0.1	—
Hematologic				
Thrombocytopenia	2.0	0.5	0.1	—
Metabolic				
Hyperglycemia	12.2	7.8	0.1	—
Weight increase	9.7	6.9	0.1	0.5
Gout	6.3	6.2	—	—
BUN increased	6.0	4.6	0.3	0.2
NPN increased	5.8	4.6	0.3	0.2
Hypercholesterolemia	4.1	2.5	—	—
Dehydration	2.1	1.6	—	—
Hypervolemia	2.0	0.9	—	—
Musculoskeletal				
Back pain	6.9	6.6	—	—
Arthralgia	6.4	4.8	0.1	0.2
Myalgia	3.4	2.7	—	—
Resistance Mechanism				
Upper respiratory tract infection	18.3	17.6	—	—
Infection	2.2	0.9	—	—
Respiratory				
Sinusitis	5.4	4.3	—	—
Bronchitis	5.4	3.4	—	0.2
Pharyngitis	3.1	2.7	—	—
Urinary/Renal				
Urinary tract infection	3.1	2.7	—	—
Hematuria	2.9	2.1	—	—
Vision				
Vision abnormal	5.0	1.8	0.1	—

Incidence >2%, Regardless of Causality; Withdrawal Rates due to Adverse Events
In addition to the events in Table 1, asthenia, cardiac failure, flatulence, anorexia, dyspepsia, palpitation, extrasystoles, hyperkalemia, arthritis, angina pectoris, insomnia, depression, anemia, viral infection, dyspnea, coughing, respiratory disorder, rhinitis, rash, and leg cramps were also reported, but rates were equal to, or more common in, placebo-treated patients.
The following adverse events were reported more frequently with *Coreg* in U.S. placebo-controlled trials in patients with congestive heart failure:
Incidence >1% to <2%
Body as a Whole: Peripheral edema, allergy, sudden death, malaise, hypovolemia.

Cardiovascular: Fluid overload, postural hypotension.
Central and Peripheral Nervous System: Hypesthesia, vertigo.
Gastrointestinal: Melena, periodontitis.
Liver and Biliary System: SGPT increased, SGOT increased.
Metabolic and Nutritional: Hyperuricemia, hypoglycemia, hyponatremia, increased alkaline phosphatase, glycosuria.
Platelet, Bleeding and Clotting: Prothrombin decreased, purpura.
Psychiatric: Somnolence.
Reproductive, male: Impotence.
Urinary System: Abnormal renal function, albuminuria.

POSTMARKETING EXPERIENCE

The following adverse reaction has been reported in postmarketing experience: reports of aplastic anemia have been rare and received only when carvedilol was administered concomitantly with other medications associated with the event.

Hypertension

Coreg (carvedilol) has been evaluated for safety in hypertension in more than 2,193 patients in U.S. clinical trials and in 2,976 patients in international clinical trials. Approximately 36% of the total treated population received *Coreg* for at least 6 months. In general, *Coreg* was well tolerated at doses up to 50 mg daily. Most adverse events reported during *Coreg* therapy were of mild to moderate severity. In U.S. controlled clinical trials directly comparing *Coreg* monotherapy in doses up to 50 mg (n=1,142) to placebo (n=462), 4.9% of *Coreg* patients discontinued for adverse events vs. 5.2% of placebo patients. Although there was no overall difference in discontinuation rates, discontinuations were more common in the carvedilol group for postural hypotension (1% vs. 0). The overall incidence of adverse events in U.S. placebo-controlled trials was found to increase with increasing dose of *Coreg*. For individual adverse events this could only be distinguished for dizziness, which increased in frequency from 2% to 5% as total daily dose increased from 6.25 mg to 50 mg.

Table 2 shows adverse events in U.S. placebo-controlled clinical trials for hypertension that occurred with an incidence of greater than 1% regardless of causality, and that were more frequent in drug-treated patients than placebo-treated patients.

[See table above]

Table 2 **Adverse Events in U.S. Placebo-Controlled Hypertension Trials Incidence ≥1%, Regardless of Causality; Withdrawal Rates due to Adverse Events**

	Adverse Reactions		Withdrawals	
	Coreg **(n=1,142)** % occurrence	**Placebo (n=462)** % occurrence	***Coreg*** **(n=1,142)** % withdrawals	**Placebo (n=462)** % withdrawals
Body as a Whole				
Fatigue	4.3	3.9	0.3	0.2
Injury	2.9	2.6	0.1	—
Cardiovascular				
Bradycardia	2.1	0.2	0.4	—
Postural hypotension	1.8	—	1.0	—
Dependent edema	1.7	1.5	0.1	0.4
Peripheral edema	1.4	0.4	0.2	—
Central Nervous System				
Dizziness	6.2	5.4	0.4	1.3
Insomnia	1.6	0.6	—	0.2
Somnolence	1.8	1.5	—	—
Gastrointestinal				
Abdominal pain	1.4	1.3	0.1	—
Diarrhea	2.2	1.3	0.1	—
Hematologic				
Thrombocytopenia	1.1	0.2	—	—
Metabolic				
Hypertriglyceridemia	1.2	0.2		—
Musculoskeletal				
Back pain	2.3	1.5	0.1	—
Resistance Mechanism				
Viral infection	1.8	1.3	—	—
Respiratory				
Rhinitis	2.1	1.9	—	—
Pharyngitis	1.5	0.6	—	—
Dyspnea	1.4	0.9	0.4	0.2
Urinary/Renal				
Urinary tract infection	1.8	0.6	—	—

In addition to the events in Table 2, chest pain, dyspepsia, headache, nausea, pain, sinusitis and upper respiratory tract infection were also reported, but rates were at least as great in placebo-treated patients.

The following adverse events were reported as possibly or probably related in worldwide open or controlled trials with Coreg (carvedilol) in patients with hypertension or congestive heart failure.

Incidence >0.1% to ≤1%

Cardiovascular: Peripheral ischemia, tachycardia.
Central and Peripheral Nervous System: Hypokinesia.
Gastrointestinal: Bilirubinemia, increased hepatic enzymes (0.2% of hypertension patients and 0.4% of congestive heart failure patients were discontinued from therapy because of increases in hepatic enzymes; see WARNINGS, Hepatic Injury).
General: Substernal chest pain, edema.
Psychiatric: Nervousness, sleep disorder, aggravated depression, impaired concentration, abnormal thinking, paroniria, emotional lability.
Respiratory System: Asthma (see CONTRAINDICATIONS).
Reproductive: Male: decreased libido.
Skin and Appendages: Pruritus, rash erythematous, rash maculopapular, rash psoriaform, photosensitivity reaction.
Special Senses: Tinnitus.
Urinary System: Micturition frequency.
Autonomic Nervous System: Dry mouth, sweating increased.
Metabolic and Nutritional: Hypokalemia, diabetes mellitus, hypertriglyceridemia.
Hematologic: Anemia, leukopenia.

The following events were reported in ≤0.1% of patients and are potentially important: complete AV block, bundle branch block, myocardial ischemia, cerebrovascular disorder, convulsions, migraine, neuralgia, paresis, anaphylactoid reaction, alopecia, exfoliative dermatitis, amnesia, GI hemorrhage, bronchospasm, pulmonary edema, decreased hearing, respiratory alkalosis, increased BUN, decreased HDL, pancytopenia and atypical lymphocytes.

Other adverse events occurred sporadically in single patients and cannot be distinguished from concurrent disease states or medications.

Coreg therapy has not been associated with clinically significant changes in routine laboratory tests in hypertensive patients. No clinically relevant changes were noted in serum potassium, fasting serum glucose, total triglycerides, total cholesterol, HDL cholesterol, uric acid, blood urea nitrogen or creatinine.

OVERDOSAGE

The acute oral LD_{50} doses in male and female mice and male and female rats are over 8000 mg/kg.

Overdosage may cause severe hypotension, bradycardia, cardiac insufficiency, cardiogenic shock and cardiac arrest. Respiratory problems, bronchospasms, vomiting, lapses of consciousness and generalized seizures may also occur.

The patient should be placed in a supine position and, where necessary, kept under observation and treated under intensive-care conditions. Gastric lavage or pharmacologically induced emesis may be used shortly after ingestion. The following agents may be administered:

for excessive bradycardia: atropine, 2 mg IV.

to support cardiovascular function: glucagon, 5 to 10 mg IV rapidly over 30 seconds, followed by a continuous infusion of 5 mg/hour; sympathomimetics (dobutamine, isoprenaline, adrenaline) at doses according to body weight and effect.

If peripheral vasodilation dominates, it may be necessary to administer adrenaline or noradrenaline with continuous monitoring of circulatory conditions. For therapy-resistant bradycardia, pacemaker therapy should be performed. For bronchospasm, β-sympathomimetics (as aerosol or IV) or aminophylline IV should be given. In the event of seizures, slow IV injection of diazepam or clonazepam is recommended.

NOTE: In the event of severe intoxication where there are symptoms of shock, treatment with antidotes must be continued for a sufficiently long period of time consistent with the 7- to 10-hour half-life of carvedilol.

Cases of overdosage with *Coreg* alone or in combination with other drugs have been reported. Quantities ingested in some cases exceeded 1000 milligrams. Symptoms experienced included low blood pressure and heart rate. Standard supportive treatment was provided and individuals recovered.

DOSAGE AND ADMINISTRATION

Congestive Heart Failure

DOSAGE MUST BE INDIVIDUALIZED AND CLOSELY MONITORED BY A PHYSICIAN DURING UP-TITRATION. Prior to initiation of *Coreg*, the dosing of digitalis, diuretics and ACE inhibitors (if used) should be stabilized. The recommended starting dose of *Coreg* is 3.125 mg twice daily for two weeks. If this dose is tolerated, it can then be increased to 6.25 mg twice daily. Dosing should then be doubled every 2 weeks to the highest level tolerated by the patient. At initiation of each new dose, patients should be observed for signs of dizziness or light-headedness for one hour. The maximum recommended dose is 25 mg twice daily in patients weighing less than 85 kg (187 lbs) and 50 mg twice daily in patients weighing more than 85 kg. Coreg (carvedilol) should be taken with food to slow the rate of absorption and reduce the incidence of orthostatic effects.

Before each dose increase the patient should be seen in the office and evaluated for symptoms of worsening heart failure, vasodilation (dizziness, light-headedness, symptomatic hypotension) or bradycardia, in order to determine tolerability of *Coreg*. Transient worsening of heart failure may be treated with increased doses of diuretics although occasionally it is necessary to lower the dose of *Coreg* or temporarily discontinue it. Symptoms of vasodilation often respond to a reduction in the dose of diuretics or ACE inhibitor. If these changes do not relieve symptoms, the dose of *Coreg* may be decreased. The dose of *Coreg* should not be increased until symptoms of worsening heart failure or vasodilation have been stabilized. Initial difficulty with titration should not preclude later attempts to introduce *Coreg*. If congestive heart failure patients experience bradycardia (pulse rate below 55 beats/min.), the dose of *Coreg* should be reduced.

Hypertension

DOSAGE MUST BE INDIVIDUALIZED. The recommended starting dose of *Coreg* is 6.25 mg twice daily. If this dose is tolerated, using standing systolic pressure measured about 1 hour after dosing as a guide, the dose should be maintained for 7 to 14 days, and then increased to 12.5 mg twice daily if needed, based on trough blood pressure, again using standing systolic pressure one hour after dosing as a guide for tolerance. This dose should also be maintained for 7 to 14 days and can then be adjusted upward to 25 mg twice daily if tolerated and needed. The full antihypertensive effect of *Coreg* is seen within 7 to 14 days. Total daily dose should not exceed 50 mg. *Coreg* should be taken with food to slow the rate of absorption and reduce the incidence of orthostatic effects.

Addition of a diuretic to *Coreg*, or *Coreg* to a diuretic can be expected to produce additive effects and exaggerate the orthostatic component of *Coreg* action.

Coreg (carvedilol) should not be given to patients with severe hepatic impairment (see CONTRAINDICATIONS).

HOW SUPPLIED

Tablets: White, oval, film-coated tablets: 3.125 mg-engraved with 39 and SB, in bottles of 100; 6.25 mg-engraved with 4140 and SB, in bottles of 100; 12.5 mg-engraved with 4141 and SB, in bottles of 100; 25 mg-engraved with 4142 and SB, in bottles of 100. The 6.25 mg, 12.5 mg and 25 mg tablets are Tiltab® tablets.

Store below 30°C (86°F). Protect from moisture. Dispense in a tight, light-resistant container.

3.125 mg 100's: NDC 0007-4139-20
6.25 mg 100's: NDC 0007-4140-20
12.5 mg 100's: NDC 0007-4141-20
25 mg 100's: NDC 0007-4142-20

Coreg is a registered trademark.

Coreg is copromoted by SmithKline Beecham Pharmaceuticals and Roche Laboratories Inc.

Rx only

Manufactured and distributed by
SmithKline Beecham Pharmaceuticals
Philadelphia, PA 19101
CO:L5A

Shown in Product Identification Guide, page 337

DEXEDRINE®

[dex 'eh-dreen]

brand of dextroamphetamine sulfate

SPANSULE® CAPSULES

brand of sustained release capsules and TABLETS

ⒸⅡ

WARNING

AMPHETAMINES HAVE A HIGH POTENTIAL FOR ABUSE. ADMINISTRATION OF AMPHETAMINES FOR PROLONGED PERIODS OF TIME MAY LEAD TO DRUG DEPENDENCE AND MUST BE AVOIDED.

Continued on next page

Information on the SmithKline Beecham Pharmaceuticals products appearing here is based on the labeling in effect on June 15, 2000. Further information on these and other products may be obtained from the Medical Department, SmithKline Beecham Pharmaceuticals, One Franklin Plaza, Philadelphia, PA 19101.

Dexedrine Spansule—Cont.

PARTICULAR ATTENTION SHOULD BE PAID TO THE POSSIBILITY OF SUBJECTS OBTAINING AMPHETAMINES FOR NON-THERAPEUTIC USE OR DISTRIBUTION TO OTHERS, AND THE DRUGS SHOULD BE PRESCRIBED OR DISPENSED SPARINGLY.

DESCRIPTION

Dexedrine (dextroamphetamine sulfate) is the dextro isomer of the compound *d,l*-amphetamine sulfate, a sympathomimetic amine of the amphetamine group. Chemically, dextroamphetamine is *d*-alpha-methylphenethylamine, and is present in all forms of *Dexedrine* as the neutral sulfate.

Spansule® capsules

Each *Spansule* sustained release capsule is so prepared that an initial dose is released promptly and the remaining medication is released gradually over a prolonged period.

Each capsule, with brown cap and clear body, contains dextroamphetamine sulfate. The 5 mg capsule is imprinted 5 mg and 3512 on the brown cap and is imprinted 5 mg and SB on the clear body. The 10 mg capsule is imprinted 10 mg—3513—on the brown cap and is imprinted 10 mg—SB—on the clear body. The 15 mg capsule is imprinted 15 mg and 3514 on the brown cap and is imprinted 15 mg and SB on the clear body. A narrow bar appears above and below 15 mg and 3514. Product reformulation in 1996 has caused a minor change in the color of the time-released pellets within each capsule. Inactive ingredients now consist of cetyl alcohol, D&C Yellow No. 10, dibutyl sebacate, ethylcellulose, FD&C Blue No. 1, FD&C Blue No. 1 aluminum lake, FD&C Red No. 40, FD&C Yellow No. 6, gelatin, hydroxypropyl methylcellulose, propylene glycol, povidone, silicon dioxide, sodium lauryl sulfate, sugar spheres and trace amounts of other inactive ingredients.

Tablets

Each triangular, orange, scored tablet is debossed SKF and E19 and contains dextroamphetamine sulfate, 5 mg. Inactive ingredients consist of calcium sulfate, FD&C Yellow No. 5 (tartrazine), FD&C Yellow No. 6, gelatin, lactose, mineral oil, starch, stearic acid, sucrose, talc and trace amounts of other inactive ingredients.

CLINICAL PHARMACOLOGY

Amphetamines are non-catecholamine, sympathomimetic amines with CNS stimulant activity. Peripheral actions include elevations of systolic and diastolic blood pressures and weak bronchodilator and respiratory stimulant action.

There is neither specific evidence which clearly establishes the mechanism whereby amphetamines produce mental and behavioral effects in children, nor conclusive evidence regarding how these effects relate to the condition of the central nervous system.

Dexedrine (dextroamphetamine sulfate) *Spansule* capsules are formulated to release the active drug substance *in vivo* in a more gradual fashion than the standard formulation, as demonstrated by blood levels. The formulation has not been shown superior in effectiveness over the same dosage of the standard, noncontrolled-release formulations given in divided doses.

Pharmacokinetics

The pharmacokinetics of the tablet and sustained release capsule were compared in 12 healthy subjects. The extent of bioavailability of the sustained release capsule was similar compared to the immediate release tablet. Following administration of three 5 mg tablets, average maximal dextroamphetamine plasma concentrations (C_{max}) of 36.6 ng/mL were achieved at approximately 3 hours. Following administration of one 15 mg sustained release capsule, maximal dextroamphetamine plasma concentrations were obtained approximately 8 hours after dosing. The average C_{max} was 23.5 ng/mL. The average plasma $T^1/_2$ was similar for both the tablet and sustained release capsule and was approximately 12 hours.

In 12 healthy subjects, the rate and extent of dextroamphetamine absorption were similar following administration of the sustained released capsule formulation in the fed (58 to 75 gm fat) and fasted state.

INDICATIONS AND USAGE

Dexedrine (dextroamphetamine sulfate) is indicated:

1. In Narcolepsy.

2. In Attention Deficit Disorder with Hyperactivity, as an integral part of a total treatment program which typically includes other remedial measures (psychological, educational, social) for a stabilizing effect in pediatric patients (ages 3 years to 16 years) with a behavioral syndrome characterized by the following group of developmentally inappropriate symptoms: moderate to severe distractibility, short attention span, hyperactivity, emotional lability, and impulsivity. The diagnosis of this syndrome should not be made with finality when these symptoms are only of comparatively recent origin. Nonlocalizing (soft) neurological signs, learning disability, and abnormal EEG may or may not be present, and a diagnosis of central nervous system dysfunction may or may not be warranted.

CONTRAINDICATIONS

Advanced arteriosclerosis, symptomatic cardiovascular disease, moderate to severe hypertension, hyperthyroidism, known hypersensitivity or idiosyncrasy to the sympathomimetic amines, glaucoma.

Agitated states.

Patients with a history of drug abuse.

During or within 14 days following the administration of monoamine oxidase inhibitors (hypertensive crises may result).

PRECAUTIONS

General: Caution is to be exercised in prescribing amphetamines for patients with even mild hypertension.

The least amount feasible should be prescribed or dispensed at one time in order to minimize the possibility of overdosage.

The tablets contain FD&C Yellow No. 5 (tartrazine), which may cause allergic-type reactions (including bronchial asthma) in certain susceptible individuals. Although the overall incidence of FD&C Yellow No. 5 (tartrazine) sensitivity in the general population is low, it is frequently seen in patients who also have aspirin hypersensitivity.

Information for Patients: Amphetamines may impair the ability of the patient to engage in potentially hazardous activities such as operating machinery or vehicles; the patient should therefore be cautioned accordingly.

Drug Interactions

Acidifying agents—Gastrointestinal acidifying agents (guanethidine, reserpine, glutamic acid HCl, ascorbic acid, fruit juices, etc.) lower absorption of amphetamines. Urinary acidifying agents (ammonium chloride, sodium acid phosphate, etc.) increase the concentration of the ionized species of the amphetamine molecule, thereby increasing urinary excretion. Both groups of agents lower blood levels and efficacy of amphetamines.

Adrenergic blockers—Adrenergic blockers are inhibited by amphetamines.

Alkalinizing agents—Gastrointestinal alkalinizing agents (sodium bicarbonate, etc.) increase absorption of amphetamines. Urinary alkalinizing agents (acetazolamide, some thiazides) increase the concentration of the non-ionized species of the amphetamine molecule, thereby decreasing urinary excretion. Both groups of agents increase blood levels and therefore potentiate the actions of amphetamines.

Antidepressants, tricyclic—Amphetamines may enhance the activity of tricyclic or sympathomimetic agents; d-amphetamine with desipramine or protriptyline and possibly other tricyclics cause striking and sustained increases in the concentration of d-amphetamine in the brain; cardiovascular effects can be potentiated.

MAO inhibitors—MAOI antidepressants, as well as a metabolite of furazolidone, slow amphetamine metabolism. This slowing potentiates amphetamines, increasing their effect on the release of norepinephrine and other monoamines from adrenergic nerve endings; this can cause headaches and other signs of hypertensive crisis. A variety of neurological toxic effects and malignant hyperpyrexia can occur, sometimes with fatal results.

Antihistamines—Amphetamines may counteract the sedative effect of antihistamines.

Antihypertensives—Amphetamines may antagonize the hypotensive effects of antihypertensives.

Chlorpromazine—Chlorpromazine blocks dopamine and norepinephrine reuptake, thus inhibiting the central stimulant effects of amphetamines, and can be used to treat amphetamine poisoning.

Ethosuximide—Amphetamines may delay intestinal absorption of ethosuximide.

Haloperidol—Haloperidol blocks dopamine and norepinephrine reuptake, thus inhibiting the central stimulant effects of amphetamines.

Lithium carbonate—The stimulatory effects of amphetamines may be inhibited by lithium carbonate.

Meperidine—Amphetamines potentiate the analgesic effect of meperidine.

Methenamine therapy—Urinary excretion of amphetamines is increased, and efficacy is reduced, by acidifying agents used in methenamine therapy.

Norepinephrine—Amphetamines enhance the adrenergic effect of norepinephrine.

Phenobarbital—Amphetamines may delay intestinal absorption of phenobarbital; co-administration of phenobarbital may produce a synergistic anticonvulsant action.

Phenytoin—Amphetamines may delay intestinal absorption of phenytoin; co-administration of phenytoin may produce a synergistic anticonvulsant action.

Propoxyphene—In cases of propoxyphene overdosage, amphetamine CNS stimulation is potentiated and fatal convulsions can occur.

Veratrum alkaloids—Amphetamines inhibit the hypotensive effect of veratrum alkaloids.

Drug/Laboratory Test Interactions

- Amphetamines can cause a significant elevation in plasma corticosteroid levels. This increase is greatest in the evening.
- Amphetamines may interfere with urinary steroid determinations.

Carcinogenesis/Mutagenesis: Mutagenicity studies and long-term studies in animals to determine the carcinogenic potential of Dexedrine (dextroamphetamine sulfate) have not been performed.

Pregnancy—Teratogenic Effects: Pregnancy Category C. *Dexedrine* has been shown to have embryotoxic and teratogenic effects when administered to A/Jax mice and C57BL mice in doses approximately 41 times the maximum human dose. Embryotoxic effects were not seen in New Zealand white rabbits given the drug in doses 7 times the human dose nor in rats given 12.5 times the maximum human dose.

While there are no adequate and well-controlled studies in pregnant women, there has been one report of severe congenital bony deformity, tracheoesophageal fistula, and anal atresia (Vater association) in a baby born to a woman who took dextroamphetamine sulfate with lovastatin during the first trimester of pregnancy. *Dexedrine* should be used during pregnancy only if the potential benefit justifies the potential risk to the fetus.

Nonteratogenic Effects: Infants born to mothers dependent on amphetamines have an increased risk of premature delivery and low birth weight. Also, these infants may experience symptoms of withdrawal as demonstrated by dysphoria, including agitation, and significant lassitude.

Nursing Mothers: Amphetamines are excreted in human milk. Mothers taking amphetamines should be advised to refrain from nursing.

Pediatric Use: Long-term effects of amphetamines in pediatric patients have not been well established.

Amphetamines are not recommended for use in pediatric patients under 3 years of age with Attention Deficit Disorder with Hyperactivity described under INDICATIONS AND USAGE.

Clinical experience suggests that in psychotic children, administration of amphetamines may exacerbate symptoms of behavior disturbance and thought disorder.

Amphetamines have been reported to exacerbate motor and phonic tics and Tourette's syndrome. Therefore, clinical evaluation for tics and Tourette's syndrome in children and their families should precede use of stimulant medications.

Data are inadequate to determine whether chronic administration of amphetamines may be associated with growth inhibition; therefore, growth should be monitored during treatment.

Drug treatment is not indicated in all cases of Attention Deficit Disorder with Hyperactivity and should be considered only in light of the complete history and evaluation of the child. The decision to prescribe amphetamines should depend on the physician's assessment of the chronicity and severity of the child's symptoms and their appropriateness for his/her age. Prescription should not depend solely on the presence of one or more of the behavioral characteristics.

When these symptoms are associated with acute stress reactions, treatment with amphetamines is usually not indicated.

ADVERSE REACTIONS

Cardiovascular: Palpitations, tachycardia, elevation of blood pressure. There have been isolated reports of cardiomyopathy associated with chronic amphetamine use.

Central Nervous System: Psychotic episodes at recommended doses (rare), overstimulation, restlessness, dizziness, insomnia, euphoria, dyskinesia, dysphoria, tremor, headache, exacerbation of motor and phonic tics and Tourette's syndrome.

Gastrointestinal: Dryness of the mouth, unpleasant taste, diarrhea, constipation, other gastrointestinal disturbances. Anorexia and weight loss may occur as undesirable effects.

Allergic: Urticaria.

Endocrine: Impotence, changes in libido.

DRUG ABUSE AND DEPENDENCE

Dextroamphetamine sulfate is a Schedule II controlled substance.

Amphetamines have been extensively abused. Tolerance, extreme psychological dependence and severe social disability have occurred. There are reports of patients who have increased the dosage to many times that recommended. Abrupt cessation following prolonged high dosage administration results in extreme fatigue and mental depression; changes are also noted on the sleep EEG.

Manifestations of chronic intoxication with amphetamines include severe dermatoses, marked insomnia, irritability, hyperactivity and personality changes. The most severe manifestation of chronic intoxication is psychosis, often clinically indistinguishable from schizophrenia. This is rare with oral amphetamines.

OVERDOSAGE

Individual patient response to amphetamines varies widely. While toxic symptoms occasionally occur as an idiosyncrasy at doses as low as 2 mg, they are rare with doses of less than 15 mg; 30 mg can produce severe reactions, yet doses of 400 to 500 mg are not necessarily fatal.

In rats, the oral LD_{50} of dextroamphetamine sulfate is 96.8 mg/kg.

Manifestations of acute overdosage with amphetamines include restlessness, tremor, hyperreflexia, rhabdomyolysis, rapid respiration, hyperpyrexia, confusion, assaultiveness, hallucinations, panic states.

Fatigue and depression usually follow the central stimulation.

Cardiovascular effects include arrhythmias, hypertension or hypotension and circulatory collapse. Gastrointestinal symptoms include nausea, vomiting, diarrhea and abdominal cramps. Fatal poisoning is usually preceded by convulsions and coma.

TREATMENT—Consult with a Certified Poison Control Center for up-to-date guidance and advice. Management of acute amphetamine intoxication is largely symptomatic and includes gastric lavage, administration of activated charcoal, administration of a cathartic, and sedation. Experience with hemodialysis or peritoneal dialysis is inadequate to permit recommendation in this regard. Acidification of the urine increases amphetamine excretion, but is believed to increase risk of acute renal failure if myoglobinuria is

present. If acute, severe hypertension complicates amphetamine overdosage, administration of intravenous phentolamine (Regitine®, CIBA) has been suggested. However, a gradual drop in blood pressure will usually result when sufficient sedation has been achieved.
Chlorpromazine antagonizes the central stimulant effects of amphetamines and can be used to treat amphetamine intoxication.
Since much of the *Spansule* capsule medication is coated for gradual release, therapy directed at reversing the effects of the ingested drug and at supporting the patient should be continued for as long as overdosage symptoms remain. Saline cathartics are useful for hastening the evacuation of pellets that have not already released medication.

DOSAGE AND ADMINISTRATION

Amphetamines should be administered at the lowest effective dosage and dosage should be individually adjusted. Late evening doses—particularly with the *Spansule* capsule form—should be avoided because of the resulting insomnia.
Narcolepsy: Usual dose 5 to 60 mg per day in divided doses, depending on the individual patient response.
Narcolepsy seldom occurs in children under 12 years of age; however, when it does, Dexedrine (dextroamphetamine sulfate) may be used. The suggested initial dose for patients aged 6 to 12 is 5 mg daily; daily dose may be raised in increments of 5 mg at weekly intervals until optimal response is obtained. In patients 12 years of age and older, start with 10 mg daily; daily dosage may be raised in increments of 10 mg at weekly intervals until optimal response is obtained. If bothersome adverse reactions appear (e.g., insomnia or anorexia), dosage should be reduced. *Spansule* capsules may be used for once-a-day dosage wherever appropriate. With tablets, give first dose on awakening; additional doses (1 or 2) at intervals of 4 to 6 hours.
Attention Deficit Disorder with Hyperactivity: Not recommended for pediatric patients under 3 years of age.
In pediatric patients from 3 to 5 years of age, start with 2.5 mg daily, by tablet; daily dosage may be raised in increments of 2.5 mg at weekly intervals until optimal response is obtained.
In pediatric patients 6 years of age and older, start with 5 mg once or twice daily; daily dosage may be raised in increments of 5 mg at weekly intervals until optimal response is obtained. Only in rare cases will it be necessary to exceed a total of 40 mg per day.
Spansule capsules may be used for once-a-day dosage wherever appropriate.
With tablets, give first dose on awakening; additional doses (1 or 2) at intervals of 4 to 6 hours.
Where possible, drug administration should be interrupted occasionally to determine if there is a recurrence of behavioral symptoms sufficient to require continued therapy.

HOW SUPPLIED

***Dexedrine* Spansule capsules:** Each capsule, with brown cap and clear body, contains dextroamphetamine sulfate. The 5 mg capsule is imprinted 5 mg and 3512 on the brown cap and is imprinted 5 mg and SB on the clear body. The 10 mg capsule is imprinted 10 mg—3513—on the brown cap and is imprinted 10 mg—SB—on the clear body. The 15 mg capsule is imprinted 15 mg and 3514 on the brown cap and is imprinted 15 mg and SB on the clear body. A narrow bar appears above and below 15 mg and 3514. Available: 5 mg, 10 mg, and 15 mg in bottles of 100.
Store at controlled room temperature between 20° and 25°C (68° and 77°F) [see USP]. Dispense in a tight, light-resistant container.
5 mg 100's: NDC 0007-3512-20
10 mg 100's: NDC 0007-3513-20
15 mg 100's: NDC 0007-3514-20
Dexedrine Spansule capsules are manufactured by **International Processing Corporation,** Winchester, KY 40391.
Dexedrine (dextroamphetamine sulfate) Tablets: Triangular, orange, scored, debossed SKF and E19. Available: 5 mg in bottles of 100.
Store between 15° and 30°C (59° and 86°F). Dispense in a tight, light-resistant container.
5 mg 100's: NDC 0007-3519-20
SmithKline Beecham Pharmaceuticals
Philadelphia, PA 19101
Comarketed with **Mallinckrodt, Inc.** St. Louis, MO 63134
DX:L49A **Rx only**

Shown in Product Identification Guide, page 337

DYAZIDE® ℞

[dye-uh-zide ']
capsules
diuretic • antihypertensive

DESCRIPTION

Each *Dyazide* capsule for oral use, with opaque red cap and opaque white body, contains hydrochlorothiazide 25 mg and triamterene 37.5 mg, and is imprinted with the product name DYAZIDE and SB. Hydrochlorothiazide is a diuretic/antihypertensive agent and triamterene is an antikaliuretic agent.
Hydrochlorothiazide is slightly soluble in water. It is soluble in dilute ammonia, dilute aqueous sodium hydroxide and dimethylformamide. It is sparingly soluble in methanol.
Hydrochlorothiazide is 6-chloro-3,4-dihydro-2H -1,2,4-benzothiadiazine-7-sulfonamide 1,1-dioxide and its structural formula is:

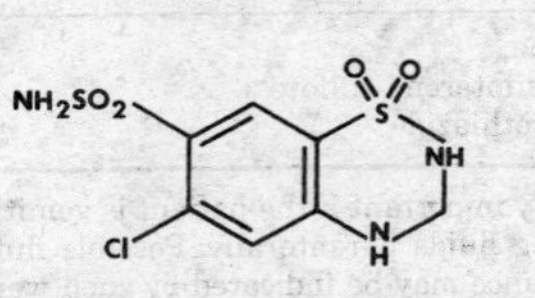

At 50°C, triamterene is practically insoluble in water (less than 0.1%). It is soluble in formic acid, sparingly soluble in methoxyethanol and very slightly soluble in alcohol.
Triamterene is 2,4,7-triamino-6-phenylpteridine and its structural formula is:

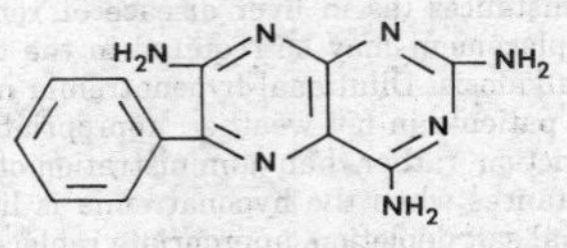

Inactive ingredients consist of benzyl alcohol, cetylpyridinium chloride, D&C Red No. 33, FD&C Yellow No. 6, gelatin, glycine, lactose, magnesium stearate, microcrystalline cellulose, povidone, polysorbate 80, sodium starch glycolate, titanium dioxide and trace amounts of other inactive ingredients.
Dyazide capsules meet Drug Release Test 3 as published in the USP 23 monograph for Triamterene and Hydrochlorothiazide Capsules.

CLINICAL PHARMACOLOGY

Dyazide is a diuretic/antihypertensive drug product that combines natriuretic and antikaliuretic effects. Each component complements the action of the other. The hydrochlorothiazide component blocks the reabsorption of sodium and chloride ions, and thereby increases the quantity of sodium traversing the distal tubule and the volume of water excreted. A portion of the additional sodium presented to the distal tubule is exchanged there for potassium and hydrogen ions. With continued use of hydrochlorothiazide and depletion of sodium, compensatory mechanisms tend to increase this exchange and may produce excessive loss of potassium, hydrogen and chloride ions. Hydrochlorothiazide also decreases the excretion of calcium and uric acid, may increase the excretion of iodide and may reduce glomerular filtration rate. The exact mechanism of the antihypertensive effect of hydrochlorothiazide is not known.
The triamterene component of *Dyazide* exerts its diuretic effect on the distal renal tubule to inhibit the reabsorption of sodium in exchange for potassium and hydrogen ions. Its natriuretic activity is limited by the amount of sodium reaching its site of action. Although it blocks the increase in this exchange that is stimulated by mineralocorticoids (chiefly aldosterone) it is not a competitive antagonist of aldosterone and its activity can be demonstrated in adrenalectomized rats and patients with Addison's disease. As a result, the dose of triamterene required is not proportionally related to the level of mineralocorticoid activity, but is dictated by the response of the individual patients, and the kaliuretic effect of concomitantly administered drugs. By inhibiting the distal tubular exchange mechanism, triamterene maintains or increases the sodium excretion and reduces the excess loss of potassium, hydrogen and chloride ions induced by hydrochlorothiazide. As with hydrochlorothiazide, triamterene may reduce glomerular filtration and renal plasma flow. Via this mechanism it may reduce uric acid excretion although it has no tubular effect on uric acid reabsorption or secretion. Triamterene does not affect calcium excretion. No predictable antihypertensive effect has been demonstrated for triamterene.
Duration of diuretic activity and effective dosage range of the hydrochlorothiazide and triamterene components of *Dyazide* are similar. Onset of diuresis with *Dyazide* takes place within 1 hour, peaks at 2 to 3 hours and tapers off during the subsequent 7 to 9 hours.
Dyazide capsule is well absorbed.
Upon administration of a single oral dose to fasted normal male volunteers, the following mean pharmacokinetic parameters were determined:
[See table at top of next page]
where AUC(0–48), Cmax, Tmax and Ae represent area under the plasma concentration versus time plot, maximum plasma concentration, time to reach Cmax and amount excreted in urine over 48 hours.
Dyazide capsule is bioequivalent to a single-entity 25 mg hydrochlorothiazide tablet and 37.5 mg triamterene capsule used in the double-blind clinical trial below. (See Clinical Trials.)
In a limited study involving 12 subjects, coadministration of *Dyazide* with a high-fat meal resulted in: (1) an increase in the mean bioavailability of triamterene by about 67% (90% confidence interval = 0.99, 1.90), p-hydroxytriamterene sulfate by about 50% (90% confidence interval = 1.06, 1.77), hydrochlorothiazide by about 17% (90% confidence interval = 0.90, 1.34); (2) increases in the peak concentrations of triamterene and p-hydroxytriamterene; and (3) a delay of up to 2 hours in the absorption of the active constituents.
Clinical Trials
A placebo-controlled, double-blind trial was conducted to evaluate the efficacy of *Dyazide* capsules. This trial demonstrated that *Dyazide* (25 mg hydrochlorothiazide/37.5 mg triamterene) was effective in controlling blood pressure while reducing the incidence of hydrochlorothiazide-induced hypokalemia. This trial involved 636 patients with mild to moderate hypertension controlled by hydrochlorothiazide 25 mg daily and who had hypokalemia (serum potassium <3.5 mEq/L) secondary to the hydrochlorothiazide. Patients were randomly assigned to 4 weeks' treatment with once-daily regimens of 25 mg hydrochlorothiazide plus placebo, or 25 mg hydrochlorothiazide combined with one of the following doses of triamterene: 25 mg, 37.5 mg, 50 mg or 75 mg.
Blood pressure and serum potassium were monitored at baseline and throughout the trial. All five treatment groups had similar mean blood pressure and serum potassium concentrations at baseline (mean systolic blood pressure range: 137±14 mmHg to 140±16 mmHg; mean diastolic blood pressure range: 86±9 mmHg to 88±8 mmHg; mean serum potassium range: 2.3 to 3.4 mEq/L with the majority of patients having values between 3.1 and 3.4 mEq/L).
While all triamterene regimens reversed hypokalemia, at week 4 the 37.5 mg regimen proved optimal compared with the other tested regimens. On this regimen, 81% of the patients had a significant ($p<0.05$) reversal of hypokalemia vs. 59% of patients on the placebo/hydrochlorothiazide regimen. The mean serum potassium concentration on 37.5 mg triamterene went from 3.2±0.2 mEq/L at baseline to 3.7±0.3 mEq/L at week 4, a significantly greater ($p<0.05$) improvement than that achieved with placebo/hydrochlorothiazide (i.e., 3.2±0.2 mEq/L at baseline and 3.5±0.4 mEq/L at week 4). Also, 51% of patients in the 37.5 mg triamterene group had an increase in serum potassium of ≥0.5 mEq/L at week 4 vs. 33% in the placebo group. The 37.5 mg triamterene/25 mg hydrochlorothiazide regimen also maintained control of blood pressure; mean supine systolic blood pressure at week 4 was 138±21 mmHg while mean supine diastolic blood pressure was 87±13 mmHg.

INDICATIONS AND USAGE

This fixed combination drug is not indicated for the initial therapy of edema or hypertension except in individuals in whom the development of hypokalemia cannot be risked.
Dyazide is indicated for the treatment of hypertension or edema in patients who develop hypokalemia on hydrochlorothiazide alone.
Dyazide is also indicated for those patients who require a thiazide diuretic and in whom the development of hypokalemia cannot be risked.
Dyazide may be used alone or as an adjunct to other antihypertensive drugs, such as beta-blockers. Since *Dyazide* may enhance the action of these agents, dosage adjustments may be necessary.
Usage in Pregnancy: The routine use of diuretics in an otherwise healthy woman is inappropriate and exposes mother and fetus to unnecessary hazard. Diuretics do not prevent development of toxemia of pregnancy, and there is no satisfactory evidence that they are useful in the treatment of developed toxemia.
Edema during pregnancy may arise from pathological causes or from the physiologic and mechanical consequences of pregnancy. Diuretics are indicated in pregnancy when edema is due to pathologic causes, just as they are in the absence of pregnancy. Dependent edema in pregnancy resulting from restriction of venous return by the expanded uterus is properly treated through elevation of the lower extremities and use of support hose; use of diuretics to lower intravascular volume in this case is illogical and unnecessary. There is hypervolemia during normal pregnancy which is harmful to neither the fetus nor the mother (in the absence of cardiovascular disease), but which is associated with edema, including generalized edema in the majority of pregnant women. If this edema produces discomfort, increased recumbency will often provide relief. In rare instances this edema may cause extreme discomfort which is not relieved by rest. In these cases a short course of diuretics may provide relief and may be appropriate.

CONTRAINDICATIONS

Antikaliuretic Therapy and Potassium Supplementation
Dyazide should not be given to patients receiving other potassium-sparing agents such as spironolactone, amiloride or other formulations containing triamterene. Concomitant potassium-containing salt substitutes should also not be used.
Potassium supplementation should not be used with *Dyazide* except in severe cases of hypokalemia. Such concomitant therapy can be associated with rapid increases in serum potassium levels. If potassium supplementation is used, careful monitoring of the serum potassium level is necessary.
Impaired Renal Function
Dyazide is contraindicated in patients with anuria, acute and chronic renal insufficiency or significant renal impairment.

Continued on next page

Information on the SmithKline Beecham Pharmaceuticals products appearing here is based on the labeling in effect on June 15, 2000. Further information on these and other products may be obtained from the Medical Department, SmithKline Beecham Pharmaceuticals, One Franklin Plaza, Philadelphia, PA 19101.

	AUC(0–48) ng*hrs/mL (±SD)	Cmax ng/mL (±SD)	Median Tmax hrs	Ae mg (±SD)
triamterene	148.7 (87.9)	46.4 (29.4)	1.1	2.7 (1.4)
hydroxytriamterene sulfate	1865 (471)	720 (364)	1.3	19.7 (6.1)
hydrochlorothiazide	834 (177)	135.1 (35.7)	2.0	14.3 (3.8)

Dyazide—Cont.

Hypersensitivity
Hypersensitivity to either drug in the preparation or to other sulfonamide-derived drugs is a contraindication.

Hyperkalemia
Dyazide should not be used in patients with preexisting elevated serum potassium.

WARNINGS: Hyperkalemia

Abnormal elevation of serum potassium levels (greater than or equal to 5.5 mEq/liter) can occur with all potassium-sparing diuretic combinations, including *Dyazide*. Hyperkalemia is more likely to occur in patients with renal impairment and diabetes (even without evidence of renal impairment), and in the elderly or severely ill. Since uncorrected hyperkalemia may be fatal, serum potassium levels must be monitored at frequent intervals especially in patients first receiving *Dyazide*, when dosages are changed or with any illness that may influence renal function.

If hyperkalemia is suspected (warning signs include paresthesias, muscular weakness, fatigue, flaccid paralysis of the extremities, bradycardia and shock), an electrocardiogram (ECG) should be obtained. However, it is important to monitor serum potassium levels because hyperkalemia may not be associated with ECG changes.

If hyperkalemia is present, *Dyazide* should be discontinued immediately and a thiazide alone should be substituted. If the serum potassium exceeds 6.5 mEq/liter more vigorous therapy is required. The clinical situation dictates the procedures to be employed. These include the intravenous administration of calcium chloride solution, sodium bicarbonate solution and/or the oral or parenteral administration of glucose with a rapid-acting insulin preparation. Cationic exchange resins such as sodium polystyrene sulfonate may be orally or rectally administered. Persistent hyperkalemia may require dialysis.

The development of hyperkalemia associated with potassium-sparing diuretics is accentuated in the presence of renal impairment (see CONTRAINDICATIONS section). Patients with mild renal functional impairment should not receive this drug without frequent and continuing monitoring of serum electrolytes. Cumulative drug effects may be observed in patients with impaired renal function. The renal clearances of hydrochlorothiazide and the pharmacologically active metabolite of triamterene, the sulfate ester of hydroxytriamterene, have been shown to be reduced and the plasma levels increased following *Dyazide* administration to elderly patients and patients with impaired renal function.

Hyperkalemia has been reported in diabetic patients with the use of potassium-sparing agents even in the absence of apparent renal impairment. Accordingly, serum electrolytes must be frequently monitored if *Dyazide* is used in diabetic patients.

Metabolic or Respiratory Acidosis
Potassium-sparing therapy should also be avoided in severely ill patients in whom respiratory or metabolic acidosis may occur. Acidosis may be associated with rapid elevations in serum potassium levels. If *Dyazide* is employed, frequent evaluations of acid/base balance and serum electrolytes are necessary.

PRECAUTIONS

Diabetes
Caution should be exercised when administering *Dyazide* to patients with diabetes, since thiazides may cause hyperglycemia, glycosuria and alter insulin requirements in diabetes. Also, diabetes mellitus may become manifest during thiazide administration.

Impaired Hepatic Function
Thiazides should be used with caution in patients with impaired hepatic function. They can precipitate hepatic coma in patients with severe liver disease. Potassium depletion induced by the thiazide may be important in this connection. Administer *Dyazide* cautiously and be alert for such early signs of impending coma as confusion, drowsiness and tremor; if mental confusion increases discontinue *Dyazide* for a few days. Attention must be given to other factors that may precipitate hepatic coma, such as blood in the gastrointestinal tract or preexisting potassium depletion.

Hypokalemia
Hypokalemia is uncommon with *Dyazide*; but, should it develop, corrective measures should be taken such as potassium supplementation or increased intake of potassium-rich foods. Institute such measures cautiously with frequent determinations of serum potassium levels, especially in patients receiving digitalis or with a history of cardiac arrhythmias. If serious hypokalemia (serum potassium less than 3.0 mEq/L) is demonstrated by repeat serum potassium determinations, *Dyazide* should be discontinued and potassium chloride supplementation initiated. Less serious hypokalemia should be evaluated with regard to other coexisting conditions and treated accordingly.

Electrolyte Imbalance
Electrolyte imbalance, often encountered in such conditions as heart failure, renal disease or cirrhosis of the liver, may also be aggravated by diuretics and should be considered during *Dyazide* therapy when using high doses for prolonged periods or in patients on a salt-restricted diet. Serum determinations of electrolytes should be performed, and are particularly important if the patient is vomiting excessively or receiving fluids parenterally. Possible fluid and electrolyte imbalance may be indicated by such warning signs as: dry mouth, thirst, weakness, lethargy, drowsiness, restlessness, muscle pain or cramps, muscular fatigue, hypotension, oliguria, tachycardia and gastrointestinal symptoms.

Hypochloremia
Although any chloride deficit is generally mild and usually does not require specific treatment except under extraordinary circumstances (as in liver disease or renal disease), chloride replacement may be required in the treatment of metabolic alkalosis. Dilutional hyponatremia may occur in edematous patients in hot weather; appropriate therapy is water restriction, rather than administration of salt, except in rare instances when the hyponatremia is life threatening. In actual salt depletion, appropriate replacement is the therapy of choice.

Renal Stones
Triamterene has been found in renal stones in association with the other usual calculus components. *Dyazide* should be used with caution in patients with a history of renal stones.

Laboratory Tests
Serum Potassium: The normal adult range of serum potassium is 3.5 to 5.0 mEq per liter with 4.5 mEq often being used for a reference point. If hypokalemia should develop, corrective measures should be taken such as potassium supplementation or increased dietary intake of potassium-rich foods.

Institute such measures cautiously with frequent determinations of serum potassium levels. Potassium levels persistently above 6 mEq per liter require careful observation and treatment. Serum potassium levels do not necessarily indicate true body potassium concentration. A rise in plasma pH may cause a decrease in plasma potassium concentration and an increase in the intracellular potassium concentration. Discontinue corrective measures for hypokalemia immediately if laboratory determinations reveal an abnormal elevation of serum potassium. Discontinue *Dyazide* and substitute a thiazide diuretic alone until potassium levels return to normal.

Serum Creatinine and BUN: *Dyazide* may produce an elevated blood urea nitrogen level, creatinine level or both. This apparently is secondary to a reversible reduction of glomerular filtration rate or a depletion of intravascular fluid volume (prerenal azotemia) rather than renal toxicity; levels usually return to normal when *Dyazide* is discontinued. If azotemia increases, discontinue *Dyazide*. Periodic BUN or serum creatinine determinations should be made, especially in elderly patients and in patients with suspected or confirmed renal insufficiency.

Serum PBI: Thiazide may decrease serum PBI levels without sign of thyroid disturbance.

Parathyroid Function: Thiazides should be discontinued before carrying out tests for parathyroid function. Calcium excretion is decreased by thiazides. Pathologic changes in the parathyroid glands with hypercalcemia and hypophosphatemia have been observed in a few patients on prolonged thiazide therapy. The common complications of hyperparathyroidism such as bone resorption and peptic ulceration have not been seen.

Drug Interactions
Angiotensin-converting enzyme inhibitors: Potassium-sparing agents should be used with caution in conjunction with angiotensin-converting enzyme (ACE) inhibitors due to an increased risk of hyperkalemia.

Oral hypoglycemic drugs: Concurrent use with chlorpropamide may increase the risk of severe hyponatremia.

Nonsteroidal anti-inflammatory drugs: A possible interaction resulting in acute renal failure has been reported in a few patients on *Dyazide* when treated with indomethacin, a nonsteroidal anti-inflammatory agent. Caution is advised in administering nonsteroidal anti-inflammatory agents with *Dyazide*.

Lithium: Lithium generally should not be given with diuretics because they reduce its renal clearance and increase the risk of lithium toxicity. Read circulars for lithium preparations before use of such concomitant therapy with *Dyazide*.

Surgical considerations: Thiazides have been shown to decrease arterial responsiveness to norepinephrine (an effect attributed to loss of sodium). This diminution is not sufficient to preclude effectiveness of the pressor agent for therapeutic use. Thiazides have also been shown to increase the paralyzing effect of nondepolarizing muscle relaxants such as tubocurarine (an effect attributed to potassium loss); consequently caution should be observed in patients undergoing surgery.

Other Considerations: Concurrent use of hydrochlorothiazide with amphotericin B or corticosteroids or corticotropin (ACTH) may intensify electrolyte imbalance, particularly hypokalemia, although the presence of triamterene minimizes the hypokalemic effect.

Thiazides may add to or potentiate the action of other antihypertensive drugs. See INDICATIONS AND USAGE for concomitant use with other antihypertensive drugs.

The effect of oral anticoagulants may be decreased when used concurrently with hydrochlorothiazide; dosage adjustments may be necessary.

Dyazide may raise the level of blood uric acid; dosage adjustments of antigout medication may be necessary to control hyperuricemia and gout.

The following agents given together with triamterene may promote serum potassium accumulation and possibly result in hyperkalemia because of the potassium-sparing nature of triamterene, especially in patients with renal insufficiency: blood from blood bank (may contain up to 30 mEq of potassium per liter of plasma or up to 65 mEq per liter of whole blood when stored for more than 10 days); low-salt milk (may contain up to 60 mEq of potassium per liter); potassium-containing medications (such as parenteral penicillin G potassium); salt substitutes (most contain substantial amounts of potassium).

Exchange resins, such as sodium polystyrene sulfonate, whether administered orally or rectally, reduce serum potassium levels by sodium replacement of the potassium; fluid retention may occur in some patients because of the increased sodium intake.

Chronic or overuse of laxatives may reduce serum potassium levels by promoting excessive potassium loss from the intestinal tract; laxatives may interfere with the potassium-retaining effects of triamterene.

The effectiveness of methenamine may be decreased when used concurrently with hydrochlorothiazide because of alkalinization of the urine.

Drug/Laboratory Test Interactions
Triamterene and quinidine have similar fluorescence spectra; thus, *Dyazide* will interfere with the fluorescent measurement of quinidine.

Carcinogenesis, Mutagenesis, Impairment of Fertility

Carcinogenesis
Long-term studies have not been conducted with *Dyazide* (the triamterene/hydrochlorothiazide combination), or with triamterene alone.

Hydrochlorothiazide: Two-year feeding studies in mice and rats, conducted under the auspices of the National Toxicology Program (NTP), treated mice and rats with doses of hydrochlorothiazide up to 600 and 100 mg/kg/day, respectively. On a body-weight basis, these doses are 600 times (in mice) and 100 times (in rats) the Maximum Recommended Human Dose (MRHD) for the hydrochlorothiazide component of *Dyazide* at 50 mg/day (or 1.0 mg/kg/day based on 50 kg individuals). On the basis of body-surface area, these doses are 56 times (in mice) and 21 times (in rats) the MRHD. These studies uncovered no evidence of carcinogenic potential of hydrochlorothiazide in rats or female mice, but there was equivocal evidence of hepatocarcinogenicity in male mice.

Mutagenesis
Studies of the mutagenic potential of *Dyazide* (the triamterene/hydrochlorothiazide combination), or of triamterene alone have not been performed.

Hydrochlorothiazide: Hydrochlorothiazide was not genotoxic in *in vitro* assays using strains TA 98, TA 100, TA 1535, TA 1537 and TA 1538 of *Salmonella typhimurium* (the Ames test); in the Chinese Hamster Ovary (CHO) test for chromosomal aberrations; or in *in vivo* assays using mouse germinal cell chromosomes, Chinese hamster bone marrow chromosomes, and the *Drosophila* sex-linked recessive lethal trait gene. Positive test results were obtained in the *in vitro* CHO Sister Chromatid Exchange (clastogenicity) test, and in the mouse Lymphoma Cell (mutagenicity) assays, using concentrations of hydrochlorothiazide of 43 to 1300 mcg/mL. Positive test results were also obtained in the *Aspergillus nidulans* nondisjunction assay, using an unspecified concentration of hydrochlorothiazide.

Impairment of Fertility
Studies of the effects of *Dyazide* (the triamterene/hydrochlorothiazide combination), or of triamterene alone on animal reproductive function have not been conducted.

Hydrochlorothiazide: Hydrochlorothiazide had no adverse effects on the fertility of mice and rats of either sex in studies wherein these species were exposed, via their diet, to doses of up to 100 and 4 mg/kg/day, respectively, prior to mating and throughout gestation. Corresponding multiples of the MRHD are 100 (mice) and 4 (rats) on the basis of body-weight and 9.4 (mice) and 0.8 (rats) on the basis of body-surface area.

Pregnancy: Category C
Teratogenic Effects
Dyazide: Animal reproduction studies to determine the potential for fetal harm by *Dyazide* have not been conducted. However, a One Generation Study in the rat approximated *Dyazide* composition by using a 1:1 ratio of triamterene to hydrochlorothiazide (30:30 mg/kg/day); there was no evidence of teratogenicity at those doses which were, on a body-weight basis, 15 and 30 times, respectively, the MRHD, and on the basis of body-surface area, 3.1 and 6.2 times, respectively, the MRHD.

The safe use of *Dyazide* in pregnancy has not been established since there are no adequate and well-controlled studies with *Dyazide* in pregnant women. *Dyazide* should be used during pregnancy only if the potential benefit justifies the risk to the fetus.

Triamterene: Reproduction studies have been performed in rats at doses as high as 20 times the MRHD on the basis of body-weight, and 6 times the human dose on the basis of body-surface area without evidence of harm to the fetus due to triamterene.

Because animal reproduction studies are not always predictive of human response, this drug should be used during pregnancy only if clearly needed.

Hydrochlorothiazide: Hydrochlorothiazide was orally administered to pregnant mice and rats during respective periods of major organogenesis at doses up to 3000 and 1000 mg/kg/day, respectively. At these doses, which are multiples of the MRHD equal to 3000 for mice and 1000 for rats, based on body-weight, and equal to 282 for mice and 206 for rats, based on body-surface area, there was no evidence of harm to the fetus.

There are, however, no adequate and well-controlled studies in pregnant women. Because animal reproduction studies are not always predictive of human response, this drug should be used during pregnancy only if clearly needed.

Nonteratogenic Effects—Thiazides and triamterene have been shown to cross the placental barrier and appear in cord blood. The use of thiazides and triamterene in pregnant women requires that the anticipated benefit be weighed against possible hazards to the fetus. These hazards include fetal or neonatal jaundice, pancreatitis, thrombocytopenia and possible other adverse reactions which have occurred in the adult.

Nursing Mothers—Thiazides and triamterene in combination have not been studied in nursing mothers. Triamterene appears in animal milk; this may occur in humans. Thiazides are excreted in human breast milk. If use of the combination drug product is deemed essential, the patient should stop nursing.

Pediatric Use—Safety and effectiveness in children have not been established.

ADVERSE REACTIONS

Adverse effects are listed in decreasing order of frequency; however, the most serious adverse effects are listed first regardless of frequency. The serious adverse effects associated with *Dyazide* have commonly occurred in less than 0.1% of patients treated with this product.

Hypersensitivity: anaphylaxis, rash, urticaria, photosensitivity.

Cardiovascular: arrhythmia, postural hypotension.

Metabolic: diabetes mellitus, hyperkalemia, hyperglycemia, glycosuria, hyperuricemia, hypokalemia, hyponatremia, acidosis, hypochloremia.

Gastrointestinal: jaundice and/or liver enzyme abnormalities, pancreatitis, nausea and vomiting, diarrhea, constipation, abdominal pain.

Renal: acute renal failure (one case of irreversible renal failure has been reported), interstitial nephritis, renal stones composed primarily of triamterene, elevated BUN and serum creatinine, abnormal urinary sediment.

Hematologic: leukopenia, thrombocytopenia and purpura, megaloblastic anemia.

Musculoskeletal: muscle cramps.

Central Nervous System: weakness, fatigue, dizziness, headache, dry mouth.

Miscellaneous: impotence, sialadenitis.

Thiazides alone have been shown to cause the following additional adverse reactions:

Central Nervous System: paresthesias, vertigo.

Ophthalmic: xanthopsia, transient blurred vision.

Respiratory: allergic pneumonitis, pulmonary edema, respiratory distress.

Other: necrotizing vasculitis, exacerbation of lupus.

Hematologic: aplastic anemia, agranulocytosis, hemolytic anemia.

Neonate and infancy: thrombocytopenia and pancreatitis—rarely, in newborns whose mothers have received thiazides during pregnancy.

DOSAGE AND ADMINISTRATION

The usual dose of *Dyazide* is one or two capsules given once daily, with appropriate monitoring of serum potassium and of the clinical effect. (See WARNINGS, Hyperkalemia.)

OVERDOSAGE

Electrolyte imbalance is the major concern (see WARNINGS section). Symptoms reported include: polyuria, nausea, vomiting, weakness, lassitude, fever, flushed face and hyperactive deep tendon reflexes. If hypotension occurs, it may be treated with pressor agents such as levarterenol to maintain blood pressure. Carefully evaluate the electrolyte pattern and fluid balance. Induce immediate evacuation of the stomach through emesis or gastric lavage. There is no specific antidote.

Reversible acute renal failure following ingestion of 50 tablets of a product containing a combination of 50 mg triamterene and 25 mg hydrochlorothiazide has been reported. Although triamterene is largely protein-bound (approximately 67%), there may be some benefit to dialysis in cases of overdosage.

HOW SUPPLIED

Capsules containing 25 mg hydrochlorothiazide and 37.5 mg triamterene, in bottles of 1000 capsules; in Single Unit Packages (unit-dose) of 100 (intended for institutional use only); in Patient-Pak™ unit-of-use bottles of 100.

They are supplied as follows:

NDC 0007-3650-21—Single Unit Packages (unit-dose) of 100 (intended for institutional use only).

NDC 0007-3650-22—in Patient-Pak™ unit-of-use bottles of 100.

NDC 0007-3650-30—bottles of 1000.

Store at controlled room temperature 20° to 25°C (68° to 77°F). Protect from light. Dispense in a tight, light-resistant container.

Rx only

DZ: L67A

Shown in Product Identification Guide, page 337

ENGERIX-B® ℞

[en 'jur-ix bee]

Hepatitis B Vaccine (Recombinant)

DESCRIPTION

Engerix-B [Hepatitis B Vaccine (Recombinant)] is a noninfectious recombinant DNA hepatitis B vaccine developed and manufactured by SmithKline Beecham Biologicals. It contains purified surface antigen of the virus obtained by culturing genetically engineered *Saccharomyces cerevisiae* cells, which carry the surface antigen gene of the hepatitis B virus. The surface antigen expressed in *Saccharomyces cerevisiae* cells is purified by several physicochemical steps and formulated as a suspension of the antigen adsorbed on aluminum hydroxide. The procedures used to manufacture *Engerix-B* result in a product that contains no more than 5% yeast protein. No substances of human origin are used in its manufacture.

Engerix-B is supplied as a sterile suspension for intramuscular administration. The vaccine is ready for use without reconstitution; it must be shaken before administration since a fine white deposit with a clear colorless supernatant may form on storage.

Pediatric/Adolescent

Each 0.5 mL of vaccine consists of 10 mcg of hepatitis B surface antigen adsorbed on 0.25 mg aluminum hydroxide. The pediatric/adolescent vaccine is formulated without preservatives. The pediatric formulation contains a trace amount of thimerosal (<0.5 mcg mercury) from the manufacturing process, sodium chloride (9 mg/mL) and phosphate buffers (disodium phosphate dihydrate, 0.98 mg/mL; sodium dihydrogen phosphate dihydrate, 0.71 mg/mL).

Adult

Each 1 mL adult dose consists of 20 mcg of hepatitis B surface antigen adsorbed on 0.5 mg aluminum as aluminum hydroxide. The adult vaccine is formulated with a preservative. The adult formulation contains thimerosal (25 mcg mercury), sodium chloride (9 mg/mL) and phosphate buffers (disodium phosphate dihydrate, 0.98 mg/mL; sodium dihydrogen phosphate dihydrate, 0.71 mg/mL).

CLINICAL PHARMACOLOGY

Several hepatitis viruses are known to cause a systemic infection resulting in major pathologic changes in the liver (e.g., A, B, C, D, E). The estimated lifetime risk of HBV infection in the United States varies from almost 100% for the highest-risk groups to approximately 5% for the population as a whole.[1] Hepatitis B infection can have serious consequences including acute massive hepatic necrosis, chronic active hepatitis and cirrhosis of the liver. Sixty to 80% of neonates and 6 to 10% of adults who are infected in the United States will become hepatitis B virus carriers.[1] It has been estimated that more than 170 million people in the world today are persistently infected with hepatitis B virus.[2] The Centers for Disease Control (CDC) estimates that there are approximately 0.75 to 1.0 million chronic carriers of hepatitis B virus in the United States.[1] Those patients who become chronic carriers can infect others and are at increased risk of developing primary hepatocellular carcinoma. Among other factors, infection with hepatitis B may be the single most important factor for development of this carcinoma.[1,3]

Reduced Risk of Hepatocellular Carcinoma: According to the CDC, the hepatitis B vaccine is recognized as the first anti-cancer vaccine because it can prevent primary liver cancer.[4]

A clear link has been demonstrated between chronic hepatitis B infection and the occurrence of hepatocellular carcinoma. In a Taiwanese study, the institution of universal childhood immunization against hepatitis B virus has been shown to decrease the incidence of hepatocellular carcinoma among children.[5] In a Korean study in adult males, vaccination against hepatitis B virus has been shown to decrease the incidence of, and risk of, developing hepatocellular carcinoma in adults.[6]

Considering the serious consequences of infection, immunization should be considered for all persons at potential risk of exposure to the hepatitis B virus. Mothers infected with hepatitis B virus can infect their infants at, or shortly after, birth if they are carriers of the HBsAg antigen or develop an active infection during the third trimester of pregnancy. Infected infants usually become chronic carriers. Therefore, screening of pregnant women for hepatitis B is recommended.[1] Because a vaccination strategy limited to high-risk individuals has failed to substantially lower the overall incidence of hepatitis B infection, the Advisory Committee on Immunization Practices (ACIP) recommends vaccination of all persons from birth to age 18.[7] The Committee on Infectious Diseases of the American Academy of Pediatrics (AAP) has also endorsed universal infant immunization as part of a comprehensive strategy for the control of hepatitis B infection.[8] The AAP, American Academy of Family Physicians (AAFP) and American Medical Association (AMA) also recommend routine vaccination of adolescents 11 to 12 years of age who have not been vaccinated previously.[9] The AAP further recommends that providers administer hepatitis B vaccine to all previously unvaccinated adolescents.[10] (See INDICATIONS AND USAGE.) There is no specific treatment for acute hepatitis B infection. However, those who develop anti-HBs antibodies after active infection are usually protected against subsequent infection. Antibody titers $\geq$10 mIU/mL against HBsAg are recognized as conferring protection against hepatitis B.[11] Seroconversion is defined as antibody titers $\geq$1 mIU/mL.

Reduced Risk of Hepatocellular Carcinoma: According to the CDC, the hepatitis B vaccine is recognized as the first anti-cancer vaccine because it can prevent primary liver cancer.[4]

A clear link has been demonstrated between chronic hepatitis B infection and the occurrence of hepatocellular carcinoma. In a Taiwanese study, the institution of universal childhood immunization against hepatitis B virus has been shown to decrease the incidence of heptocellular carcinoma among children.[5] In a Korean study in adult males, vaccination against hepatitis B virus has been shown to decrease the incidence of, and risk of, developing hepatocellular carcinoma in adults.[6]

Considering the serious consequences of infection, immunization should be considered for all persons at potential risk of exposure to the hepatitis B virus. Mothers infected with hepatitis B virus can infect their infants at, or shortly after, birth if they are carriers of the HBsAg antigen or develop an active infection during the third trimester of pregnancy. Infected infants usually become chronic carriers. Therefore, screening of pregnant women for hepatitis B is recommended.[1] Because of vaccination strategy limited to high-risk individuals has failed to substantially lower the overall incidence of hepatitis B infection, the Advisory Committee on Immunization Practices (ACIP) recommends vaccination of all persons from birth to age 18.[7] The Committee on Infectious Diseases of the American Academy of Pediatrics (AAP) has also endorsed universal infant immunization as part of a comprehensive strategy for the control of hepatitis B infection.[8] The AAP, American Academy of Family Physicians (AAFP) and American Medical Association (AMA) also recommend routine vaccination of adolescents 11 to 12 years of age who have not been vaccinated previously.[9] The AAP further recommends that providers administer hepatitis B vaccine to all previously unvaccinated adolescents.[10] (See INDICATIONS AND USAGE.) There is no specific treatment for acute hepatitis B infection. However, those who develop anti-HBs antibodies after active infection are usually protected against subsequent infection. Antibody titers $\geq$10 mIU/mL against HBsAg are recognized as conferring protection against hepatitis B.[11] Seroconversion is defined as antibody titers $\geq$1 mIU/mL.

Immunogenicity in Healthy Adults and Adolescents: Clinical trials in healthy adult and adolescent subjects have shown that following a course of three doses of 20 mcg Engerix-B [Hepatitis B Vaccine (Recombinant)] given according to the ACIP recommended schedule of injections at months 0, 1 and 6, the seroprotection (antibody titers $\geq$10 mIU/mL) rate for all individuals was 79% at month 6 and 96% at month 7; the geometric mean antibody titer (GMT) for seroconverters at month 7 was 2,204 mIU/mL. On an alternate schedule (injections at months 0, 1 and 2) designed for certain populations (e.g., neonates born of hepatitis B infected mothers, individuals who have or might have been recently exposed to the virus, and certain travelers to high-risk areas. See INDICATIONS AND USAGE.), 99% of all individuals were seroprotected at month 3 and remained protected through month 12. On the alternate schedule, an additional dose at 12 months produced a GMT for seroconverters at month 13 of 9,163 mIU/mL.

Immunogenicity in Adolescents: In clinical trials with healthy adolescent subjects 11 through 19 years of age, immunization with 10 mcg using a 0, 1, 6-month schedule produced a seroprotection rate of 97% at month 8 (N=119) with a GMT of 1,989 mIU/mL (N=118, 95% confidence intervals=1,318–3,020). Immunization with 20 mcg using a 0, 1, 6-month schedule produced a seroprotection rate of 99% at month 8 (N=122) with a GMT of 7,672 mIU/mL (N=122, 95% confidence intervals=5,248–10,965).

Immunogenicity in Neonates: Immunization with 10 mcg at 0, 1 and 2 months of age produced a seroprotection rate of 96% in infants by month 4, with a GMT among seroconverters of 210 mIU/mL (N=311); an additional dose at month 12 produced a GMT among seroconverters of 2,941 mIU/mL at month 13 (N=126).

Immunization with 10 mcg at 0, 1 and 6 months of age produced seroconversion in 100% of infants by month 7 with a GMT of 713 mIU/mL (N=52), and the seroprotection rate was 97%.

Continued on next page

Information on the SmithKline Beecham Pharmaceuticals products appearing here is based on the labeling in effect on June 15, 2000. Further information on these and other products may be obtained from the Medical Department, SmithKline Beecham Pharmaceuticals, One Franklin Plaza, Philadelphia, PA 19101.

Engerix-B—Cont.

Clinical trials indicate that administration of hepatitis B immune globulin at birth does not alter the response to Engerix-B [Hepatitis B Vaccine (Recombinant)].

Immunogenicity in Pediatric Patients: In clinical trials with 242 children ages 6 months to, and including, 10 years given 10 mcg at months 0, 1 and 6, the seroprotection rate was 98% 1 to 2 months after the third dose; the GMT of seroconverters was 4,023 mIU/mL.

Immunogenicity in Older Subjects: Among older subjects given 20 mcg at months 0, 1 and 6, the seroprotection rate 1 month after the third dose was 88%. However, as with other hepatitis B vaccines, in adults over 40 years of age, *Engerix-B* vaccine produced anti-HBs titers that were lower than those in younger adults (GMT among seroconverters 1 month after the third 20 mcg dose with a 0, 1, 6-month schedule: 610 mIU/mL for individuals over 40 years of age, N=50).

In a separate clinical trial including both children and adolescents aged 5 to 16 years, 10 mcg of *Engerix-B* was administered at 0, 1, and 6 months (N=181) or 0, 12, and 24 months (N=161). Immediately before the third dose of vaccine, seroprotection was achieved in 92.3% of subjects vaccinated on the 0, 1, 6-month schedule and 88.8% of subjects on the 0, 12, 24-month schedule (117.9 mIU/mL vs. 162.1 mIU/mL, respectively, p=0.18). One month following the third dose, seroprotection was achieved in 99.5% of children vaccinated on the 0, 1, 6-month schedule compared to 98.1% of those on the 0, 12, 24-month schedule. GMTs were higher (p=0.02) for children receiving vaccine on the 0, 1, 6-month schedule compared to those on the 0, 12, 24-month schedule (5687.4 mIU/mL vs. 3158.7 mIU/mL, respectively). The clinical relevance of this finding is unknown.

Immunogenicity in Subjects with Chronic Hepatitis C: In a clinical trial of subjects with chronic hepatitis C, 31 subjects received *Engerix-B* on the usual 0, 1, 6-month schedule. All subjects responded with seroprotective titers. The GMT of anti-HBs was 1,260 mIU/mL (95% Cl:709-2237).

Hemodialysis Patients: Hemodialysis patients given hepatitis B vaccines respond with lower titers,[12] which remain at protective levels for shorter durations than in normal subjects. In a study in which patients on chronic hemodialysis (mean time on dialysis was 24 months; N=562) received 40 mcg of the plasma-derived vaccine at months 0, 1 and 6, approximately 50% of patients achieved antibody titers ≥10 mIU/mL.[12] Since a fourth dose of *Engerix-B* given to healthy adults at month 12 following the 0, 1, 2-month schedule resulted in a substantial increase in the GMT (see above), a four-dose regimen was studied in hemodialysis patients. In a clinical trial of adults who had been on hemodialysis for a mean of 56 months (N=43), 67% of patients were seroprotected 2 months after the last dose of 40 mcg of *Engerix-B* (two × 20 mcg) given on a 0, 1, 2, 6-month schedule; the GMT among seroconverters was 93 mIU/mL.

Protective Efficacy: Protective efficacy with Engerix-B [Hepatitis B Vaccine (Recombinant)] has been demonstrated in a clinical trial in neonates at high risk of hepatitis B infection.[13,14] Fifty-eight neonates born of mothers who were both HBsAg and HBeAg positive were given *Engerix-B* (10 mcg at 0, 1 and 2 months) without concomitant hepatitis B immune globulin. Two infants became chronic carriers in the 12-month follow-up period after initial inoculation. Assuming an expected carrier rate of 70%,[1] the protective efficacy rate against the chronic carrier state during the first 12 months of life was 95%.

Other Clinical Studies: In one study,[15] four of 244 (1.6%) adults (homosexual men) at high risk of contracting hepatitis B virus became infected during the period prior to completion of three doses of *Engerix-B* (20 mcg at 0, 1, 6 months). No additional patients became infected during the 18-month follow-up period after completion of the immunization course.

Interchangeability with Other Hepatitis B Vaccines: Recombinant DNA vaccines are produced in yeast by expression of a hepatitis B virus gene sequence that codes for the hepatitis B surface antigen. Like plasma-derived vaccine, the yeast-derived vaccines are protein particles visible by electron microscopy and have hepatitis B surface antigen epitopes as determined by monoclonal antibody analyses. Yeast-derived vaccines have been shown by *in vitro* analyses to induce antibodies (anti-HBs) which are immunologically comparable by epitope specificity and binding affinity to antibodies induced by plasma-derived vaccine.[16] In cross absorption studies, no differences were detected in the spectra of antibodies induced in man to plasma-derived or to yeast-derived hepatitis B vaccines.[16]

Additionally, patients immunized approximately 3 years previously with plasma-derived vaccine and whose antibody titers were <100 mIU/mL (GMT: 35 mIU/mL; range: 9–94) were given a 20 mcg dose of Engerix-B [Hepatitis B Vaccine (Recombinant)]. All patients, including two who had not responded to the plasma-derived vaccine, showed a response to *Engerix-B* (GMT: 5,069 mIU/mL; range: 624 –15,019). There have been no clinical studies in which a three-dose vaccine series was initiated with a plasma-derived hepatitis B vaccine and completed with *Engerix-B*, or vice versa. However, because the *in vitro* and *in vivo* studies described above indicate the comparability of the antibody produced in response to plasma-derived vaccine and *Engerix-B*, it should be possible to interchange the use of *Engerix-B* and plasma-derived vaccines (but see CONTRAINDICATIONS).

A controlled study (N=48) demonstrated that completion of a course of immunization with one dose of *Engerix-B* (20 mcg, month 6) following two doses of Recombivax HB®* (10 mcg, months 0 and 1) produced a similar GMT (4,077 mIU/mL) to immunization with three doses of *Recombivax HB* (10 mcg, months 0, 1 and 6; 2,654 mIU/mL). Thus, *Engerix-B* can be used to complete a vaccination course initiated with *Recombivax HB*.

INDICATIONS AND USAGE

Engerix-B is indicated for immunization against infection caused by all known subtypes of hepatitis B virus. As hepatitis D (caused by the delta virus) does not occur in the absence of hepatitis B infection, it can be expected that hepatitis D will also be prevented by *Engerix-B* vaccination.

Engerix-B will not prevent hepatitis caused by other agents, such as hepatitis A, C and E viruses, or other pathogens known to infect the liver.

Immunization is recommended in persons of all ages, especially those who are, or will be, at increased risk of exposure to hepatitis B virus,[1] for example:

Health Care Personnel: Dentists and oral surgeons. Dental, medical and nursing students. Physicians, surgeons and podiatrists. Nurses. Paramedical and ambulance personnel and custodial staff who may be exposed to the virus via blood or other patient specimens. Dental hygienists and dental nurses. Laboratory and blood-bank personnel handling blood, blood products, and other patient specimens. Hospital cleaning staff who handle waste.

Selected Patients and Patient Contacts: Patients and staff in hemodialysis units and hematology/oncology units. Patients requiring frequent and/or large volume blood transfusions or clotting factor concentrates (e.g., persons with hemophilia, thalassemia, sickle-cell anemia, cirrhosis). Clients (residents) and staff of institutions for the mentally handicapped. Classroom contacts of deinstitutionalized mentally handicapped persons who have persistent hepatitis B surface antigenemia and who show aggressive behavior. Household and other intimate contacts of persons with persistent hepatitis B surface antigenemia.

Infants, Including Those Born of HBsAG-Positive Mothers Whether HBeAg Positive or Negative (See DOSAGE AND ADMINISTRATION.)

Adolescents (See CLINICAL PHARMACOLOGY.)

Subpopulations with a Known High Incidence of the Disease, such as: Alaskan Eskimos. Pacific Islanders. Indochinese immigrants. Haitian immigrants. Refugees from other HBV endemic areas. All infants of women born in areas where the infection is highly endemic.

Individuals with Chronic Hepatitis C: Risk factors for hepatitis C are similar to those for hepatitis B. Consequently, immunization with hepatitis B vaccine is recommended for individuals with chronic hepatitis C.

Persons Who May Be Exposed to the Hepatitis B Virus by Travel to High-Risk Areas (See ACIP Guidelines, 1990.)

Military Personnel Identified as Being at Increased Risk

Morticians and Embalmers

Persons at Increased Risk of the Disease Due to Their Sexual Practices,[17] such as: Persons with more than one sexual partner in a 6-month period. Persons who have contracted a sexually transmitted disease. Homosexually active males. Female prostitutes.

Prisoners

Users of Illicit Injectable Drugs

Others: Police and fire department personnel who render first aid or medical assistance, and any others who, through their work or personal life-style, may be exposed to the hepatitis B virus. Adoptees from countries of high HBV endemicity.

Use with Other Vaccines: The Immunization Practices Advisory Committee states that, in general, simultaneous administration of certain live and inactivated pediatric vaccines has not resulted in impaired antibody responses or increased rates of adverse reactions.[18] Separate sites and syringes should be used for simultaneous administration of injectable vaccines.

CONTRAINDICATIONS

Hypersensitivity to yeast or any other component of the vaccine is a contraindication for use of the vaccine. Patients experiencing hypersensitivity after an Engerix-B [Hepatitis B Vaccine (Recombinant)] injection should not receive further injections of *Engerix-B*.

WARNINGS

Hepatitis B has a long incubation period. Hepatitis B vaccination may not prevent hepatitis B infection in individuals who had an unrecognized hepatitis B infection at the time of vaccine administration. Additionally, it may not prevent infection in individuals who do not achieve protective antibody titers.

PRECAUTIONS

General As with other vaccines, although a moderate or severe febrile illness is sufficient reason to postpone vaccination, minor illnesses such as mild upper respiratory infections with or without low-grade fever are not contraindications.[18]

Prior to immunization, the patient's medical history should be reviewed. The physician should review the patient's immunization history for possible vaccine sensitivity, previous vaccination-related adverse reactions and occurrence of any adverse-event-related symptoms and/or signs, in order to determine the existence of any contraindication to immunization with *Engerix-B* and to allow an assessment of benefits and risks. Epinephrine injection (1:1000) and other appropriate agents used for the control of immediate allergic reactions must be immediately available should an acute anaphylactic reaction occur.

A separate sterile syringe and needle or a sterile disposable unit should be used for each individual patient to prevent transmission of hepatitis or other infectious agents from one person to another. Needles should be disposed of properly and should not be recapped.

Special care should be taken to prevent injection into a blood vessel.

As with any vaccine administered to immunosuppressed persons or persons receiving immunosuppressive therapy, the expected immune response may not be obtained. For individuals receiving immunosuppressive therapy, deferral of vaccination for at least 3 months after therapy may be considered.[18]

Multiple Sclerosis: Although no causal relationship has been established, rare instances of exacerbation of multiple sclerosis have been reported following administration of hepatitis B vaccines and other vaccines. In persons with multiple sclerosis, the benefit of immunization for prevention of hepatitis B infection and sequelae must be weighed against the risk of exacerbation of the disease.

Information for the Patient

Patients, parents or guardians should be informed of the potential benefits and risks of the vaccine, and of the importance of completing the immunization series. As with any vaccine, it is important when a subject returns for the next dose in a series that he/she be questioned concerning occurrence of any symptoms and/or signs of an adverse reaction after a previous dose of the same vaccine. Patients, parents or guardians should be told to report severe or unusual adverse reactions to their healthcare provider.

The parent or guardian should be given the Vaccine Information Materials, which are required by the National Childhood Vaccine Injury Act of 1986 to be given prior to immunization.

Drug Interactions

For information regarding simultaneous administration with other vaccines, refer to INDICATIONS AND USAGE.

Carcinogenesis, Mutagenesis, Impairment of Fertility

Engerix-B [Hepatitis B Vaccine (Recombinant)] has not been evaluated for carcinogenic or mutagenic potential, or for impairment of fertility.

Pregnancy Pregnancy Category C: Animal reproduction studies have not been conducted with *Engerix-B*. It is also not known whether *Engerix-B* can cause fetal harm when administered to a pregnant woman or can affect reproduction capacity. *Engerix-B* should be given to a pregnant woman only if clearly needed.

Nursing Mothers It is not known whether *Engerix-B* is excreted in human milk. Because many drugs are excreted in human milk, caution should be exercised when *Engerix-B* is administered to a nursing woman.

Pediatric Use *Engerix-B* has been shown to be well tolerated and highly immunogenic in infants and children of all ages. Newborns also respond well; maternally transferred antibodies do not interfere with the active immune response to the vaccine. (See CLINICAL PHARMACOLOGY for seroconversion rates and titers in neonates and children. See DOSAGE AND ADMINISTRATION for recommended pediatric dosage and for recommended dosage for infants born of HBsAg-positive mothers.)

ADVERSE REACTIONS

Engerix-B [Hepatitis B Vaccine (Recombinant)] is generally well tolerated. As with any vaccine, however, it is possible that expanded commercial use of the vaccine could reveal rare adverse reactions.

Ten double-blind studies involving 2,252 subjects showed no significant difference in the frequency or severity of adverse experiences between *Engerix-B* and plasma-derived vaccines. In 36 clinical studies a total of 13,495 doses of *Engerix-B* were administered to 5,071 healthy adults and children who were initially seronegative for hepatitis B markers, and healthy neonates. All subjects were monitored for 4 days post-administration. Frequency of adverse experiences tended to decrease with successive doses of *Engerix-B*. Using a symptom checklist,† the most frequently reported adverse reactions were injection site soreness (22%) and fatigue† (14%). Other reactions are listed below.

Incidence 1% to 10% of Injections

Local reactions at injection site: Induration; erythema; swelling.

Body as a whole: Fever (>37.5°C).

Nervous system: Headache†; dizziness.†

† Parent or guardian completed forms for children and neonates. Neonatal checklist did not include headache, fatigue or dizziness.

Incidence <1% of Injections

Local reactions at injection site: Pain; pruritus; ecchymosis.

Body as a whole: Sweating; malaise; chills; weakness; flushing; tingling.

Cardiovascular system: Hypotension.

Respiratory system: Influenza-like symptoms; upper respiratory tract illnesses.

Gastrointestinal system: Nausea; anorexia; abdominal pain/cramps; vomiting; constipation; diarrhea.

Lymphatic system: Lymphadenopathy.

Musculoskeletal system: Pain/stiffness in arm, shoulder or neck; arthralgia; myalgia; back pain.

Skin and appendages: Rash; urticaria; petechiae; pruritus; erythema.
Nervous system: Somnolence; insomnia; irritability; agitation.

Additional adverse experiences have been reported with the commercial use of *Engerix-B*. Those listed below are to serve as alerting information to physicians.

Hypersensitivity: Anaphylaxis; erythema multiforme including Stevens-Johnson syndrome; angioedema; arthritis. An apparent hypersensitivity syndrome (serum-sickness-like) of delayed onset has been reported days to weeks after vaccination, including: arthralgia/arthritis (usually transient), fever and dermatologic reactions such as urticaria, erythema multiforme, ecchymoses and erythema nodosum (see CONTRAINDICATIONS).
Cardiovascular system: Tachycardia/palpitations.
Respiratory system: Bronchospasm including asthma-like symptoms.
Gastrointestinal system: Abnormal liver function tests; dyspepsia.
Nervous system: Migraine; syncope; paresis; neuropathy including hypoesthesia, paresthesia, Guillain-Barré syndrome and Bell's palsy, transverse myelitis; optic neuritis; multiple sclerosis; seizures.
Hematologic: Thrombocytopenia.
Skin and appendages: Eczema; purpura; herpes zoster; erythema nodosum; alopecia.
Special senses: Conjunctivitis; keratitis; visual disturbances; vertigo; tinnitus; earache.

Reporting Adverse Events

The National Childhood Vaccine Injury Act requires that the manufacturer and lot number of the vaccine administered be recorded by the healthcare provider in the vaccine recipient's permanent medical record, along with the date of administration of the vaccine and the name, address and title of the person administering the vaccine.[18] The Act further requires the healthcare provider to report to the U.S. Department of Health and Human Services via VAERS the occurrences following immunization of any event set forth in the Vaccine Injury Table including: anaphylaxis or anaphylactic shock within 4 hours, encephalopathy or encephalitis within 72 hours, or any sequelae thereof (including death).[19,20] In addition, any event considered a contraindication to further doses should be reported. The VAERS toll-free number is 1-800-822-7967.

DOSAGE AND ADMINISTRATION

Injection: Engerix-B [Hepatitis B Vaccine (Recombinant)] should be administered by intramuscular injection. *Do not inject intravenously or intradermally.* In adults, the injection should be given in the deltoid region but it may be preferable to inject in the anterolateral thigh in neonates and infants, who have smaller deltoid muscles. *Engerix-B* should not be administered in the gluteal region; such injections may result in suboptimal response. The attending physician should determine final selection of the injection site and needle size, depending upon the patient's age and the size of the target muscle. A 1–inch 23–gauge needle is sufficient to penetrate the anterolateral thigh in infants younger than 12 months of age. A $^5/_8$–inch 25–gauge needle may be used to administer the vaccine in the deltoid region of toddlers and children up to, and including, 10 years of age. The 1–inch 23–gauge needle is appropriate for use in older children and adults.[18]

Engerix-B may be administered subcutaneously to persons at risk of hemorrhage (e.g., hemophiliacs). However, hepatitis B vaccines administered subcutaneously are known to result in lower GMTs. Additionally, when other aluminum-adsorbed vaccines have been administered subcutaneously, an increased incidence of local reactions including subcutaneous nodules has been observed. Therefore, subcutaneous administration should be used only in persons who are at risk of hemorrhage with intramuscular injections.

Preparation for Administration: Shake well before withdrawal and use. Parenteral drug products should be inspected visually for particulate matter or discoloration prior to administration. With thorough agitation, Engerix-B [Hepatitis B Vaccine (Recombinant)] is a slightly turbid white suspension. Discard if it appears otherwise. The vaccine should be used as supplied; no dilution is necessary. The full recommended dose of the vaccine should be used. Any vaccine remaining in a single-dose vial should be discarded.

Dosing Schedules: The usual immunization regimen (see Table 1) consists of three doses of vaccine given according to the following schedule: 1st dose: at elected date; 2nd dose: 1 month later; 3rd dose: 6 months after first dose.

[See table 1 above]

Table 1. Recommended dosage and administration schedule

Group	Dose	Schedule
Infants born of:		
HBsAg-negative mothers	10 mcg/0.5 mL	0, 1, 6 months
HBsAg-positive mothers	10 mcg/0.5 mL	0, 1, 6 months
Children:		
Birth through 10 years of age	10 mcg/0.5 mL	0, 1, 6 months
Adolescents:		
11 through 19 years of age	10 mcg/0.5 mL	0, 1, 6 months
Adults (>19 years)	20 mcg/1.0 mL	0, 1, 6 months
Adult hemodialysis	40 mcg/2.0 mL[a]	0, 1, 2, 6 months

[a] Two × 20 mcg in one or two injections.

For hemodialysis patients, in whom vaccine-induced protection is less complete and may persist only as long as antibody levels remain above 10 mIU/mL, the need for booster doses should be assessed by annual antibody testing. 40 mcg (two × 20 mcg) booster doses with *Engerix-B* should be given when antibody levels decline below 10 mIU/mL.[1] Data show individuals given a booster with *Engerix-B* achieve high antibody titers. (See CLINICAL PHARMACOLOGY.)

There are alternate dosing and administration schedules which may be used for specific populations (see Table 2 and accompanying explanations).

[See table 2 above]

Table 2. Alternate dosage and administration schedules

Group	Dose	Schedules
Infants born of:		
HBsAg-negative mothers	10 mcg/0.5 mL	0, 1, 2, 12 months[b]
Children:		
Birth through 10 years of age	10 mcg/0.5 mL	0, 1, 2, 12 months[b]
5 through 10 years of age	10 mcg/0.5 mL	0, 12, 24 months[c]
Adolescents:		
11 through 16 years of age	10 mcg/0.5 mL	0, 12, 24 months[c]
11 through 19 years of age	20 mcg/1.0 mL	0, 1, 6 months
11 through 19 years of age	20 mcg/1.0 mL	0, 1, 2, 12 months[b]
Adults (>19 years)	20 mcg/1.0 mL	0, 1, 2, 12 months[b]

[b] This schedule is designed for certain populations (e.g., neonates born of hepatitis B infected mothers, others who have or might have been recently exposed to the virus, certain travelers to high-risk areas. See INDICATIONS AND USAGE). On this alternate schedule, an additional dose at 12 months is recommended for prolonged maintenance of protective titers.
[c] For children and adolescents for whom an extended administration schedule is acceptable based on risk of exposure.

booster vaccinations: Whenever administration of a booster dose is appropriate, the dose of *Engerix-B* is 10 mcg for children 10 years of age and under; 20 mcg for adolescents 11 through 19 years of age and 20 mcg for adults. Studies have demonstrated a substantial increase in antibody titers after Engerix-B [Hepatitis B Vaccine (Recombinant)] booster vaccination following an initial course with both plasma- and yeast-derived vaccines. (See CLINICAL PHARMACOLOGY.)

See previous section for discussion on booster vaccination for adult hemodialysis patients.

Known or presumed exposure to hepatitis B virus: Unprotected individuals with known or presumed exposure to the hepatitis B virus (e.g., neonates born of infected mothers, others experiencing percutaneous or permucosal exposure) should be given hepatitis B immune globulin (HBIG) in addition to Engerix-B [Hepatitis B Vaccine (Recombinant)] in accordance with ACIP recommendations[1] and with the package insert for HBIG. Engerix-B [Hepatitis B Vaccine (Recombinant)] can be given on either dosing schedule (see above).

STORAGE

Store between 2° and 8°C (36° and 46°F). *Do not freeze;* discard if product has been frozen. Do not dilute to administer.

HOW SUPPLIED

Adult Dose

20 mcg/mL in Single-Dose Vials in packages of 1 and 25 vials.
NDC 58160-860-01 (package of 1)
NDC 58160-860-16 (package of 25)
20 mcg/mL in Single-Dose Prefilled Disposable Syringes.
NDC 58160-861-05 (package of 5)
20 mcg/mL in Single-Dose Prefilled Disposable Tip-Lok® Syringes with 1-inch 23-gauge needles.
NDC 58160-861-35 (package of 5)
NDC 58160-861-26 (package of 25)

Pediatric/Adolescent Doses

10 mcg/0.5 mL in Single-Dose Vials in packages of 1 and 10 vials.
NDC 58160-856-01 (package of 1)
NDC 58160-856-11 (package of 10)
10 mcg/0.5 mL in Single-Dose Prefilled Disposable Tip-Lok® Syringes with 1-inch 23-gauge needles.
NDC 58160-856-35 (package of 5)
NDC 58160-856-26 (package of 25)
10 mcg/0.5 mL in Single-Dose Prefilled Disposable Tip-Lok® Syringes with $^5/_8$-inch 25-gauge needles.
NDC 58160-856-36 (package of 5)
NDC 58160-856-27 (package of 25)

REFERENCES

1. Centers for Disease Control: Protection against viral hepatitis: recommendations of the Immunization Practices Advisory Committee (ACIP). *MMWR.* 39(No. RR-2), 1990. 2. Robinson, W.S.: Hepatitis B virus and the delta virus. In Mandell, G.L., Douglas, R.G., Bennett, J.E. (eds): *Principles and practice of infectious diseases,* vol. 3, New York, John Wiley & Sons, 1990, pp. 1204-1231. 3. Beasley, R.P., et al.: Efficacy of hepatitis B immune globulin for prevention of perinatal transmission of hepatitis B virus carrier state: final report of a randomized double-blind, placebo-controlled trial. *Hepatology* 3:135-141, 1983. 4. Centers for Disease Control and Prevention. *Federal Register,* Feb. 23, 1999,64(35):9044–9045. 5. Chang M.H., Chen C.J., Lai M.S. Universal hepatitis B vaccination in Taiwan and the incidence of hepatocellular carcinoma in children. *N. Engl. J. Med.* 1997;336(26): 1855–1859. 6. Lee M.S., Kim D.H., et al. Hepatitis B vaccination and reduced risk of primary liver cancer among male adults: A cohort study in Korea. *Int. J. Epidemiol.* 1998;27:316–319. 7. Centers for Disease Control and Prevention: Effectiveness of a Seventh Grade School Entry Vaccination Requirement—Statewide and Orange County, Florida. 1997–1998. *MMWR.* 1998; 47(34):714. 8. Committee on Infectious Diseases: Universal hepatitis B immunization. *Pediatrics.* 89(4):795-800, 1992. 9. Centers for Disease Control: Immunization of adolescents: recommendations of the Advisory Committee on Immunization Practices, the American Academy of Pediatrics, the American Academy of Family Physicians, and the American Medical Association. *MMWR.* 45(No. RR-13), 1996. 10. American Academy of Pediatrics: Immunization in special clinical circumstances: adolescents and college populations and hepatitis vaccines. In Peter, G. (ed): *1994 Redbook: Report of the Committee on Infectious Diseases.* 23rd ed. Elk Grove Village, IL, American Academy of Pediatrics, 1994, pp 64–65, 224–237. 11. Ambrosch, F.: Persistence of vaccine-induced antibodies to hepatitis B surface antigen–the need for booster vaccination in adult subjects. *Postgrad. Med. J.* 63(Suppl. 2):129-135, 1987. 12. Stevens, C.E., et al.: Hepatitis B vaccine in patients receiving hemodialysis. *N. Engl. J. Med.* 311:496-501, 1984. 13. Andre, F.E., and Safary, A.: Clinical experience with a yeast-derived hepatitis B vaccine. In Zuckerman, A.J.(ed): *Viral hepatitis and liver disease,* Alan R. Liss, Inc., 1988, pp. 1025-1030. 14. Poovorawan, Y., et al.: Protective efficacy of a recombinant DNA hepatitis B vaccine in neonates of HBe antigen-positive mothers. *JAMA.* 261(22):3278-3281, June 9, 1989. 15. Goilav, C., et al.: Immunization of homosexual men with a recombinant DNA vaccine against hepatitis B: immunogenicity and protection. In Zuckerman, A.J. (ed): *Viral hepatitis and liver disease,* Alan R. Liss, Inc., 1988, pp. 1057-1058. 16. Hauser, P., et al.: Immunological properties of recombinant HBsAg produced in yeast. *Postgrad. Med. J.* 63(Suppl. 2):83-91, 1987. 17. Centers for Disease Control and Prevention. 1998 Guidelines for treatment of sexually transmitted diseases. *MMWR.* 1998;47 (RR-1):102. 18. Centers for Disease Control and Prevention: General Recommendations on Immunization: Recommendations of the Advisory Committee on Immunization Practices (ACIP). *MMWR.* 1994;43(RR-1):1–38. 19. Centers for Disease Control. National Childhood Vaccine Injury Act: Requirements for permanent vaccination records and for reporting of selected events after vaccination. *MMWR.* 1988;Vol.37 (No. 13):197–200. 20. National Vaccine Injury Compensation Program: Revision of the vaccine injury table. *Federal Register.* Wednesday, February 8, 1995;Vol. 60 (No. 26): 7694.

* yeast-derived, Hepatitis B Vaccine, MSD.

Continued on next page

Information on the SmithKline Beecham Pharmaceuticals products appearing here is based on the labeling in effect on June 15, 2000. Further information on these and other products may be obtained from the Medical Department, SmithKline Beecham Pharmaceuticals, One Franklin Plaza, Philadelphia, PA 19101.

Engerix-B—Cont.

U.S. License No. 1090

Manufactured by **SmithKline Beecham Biologicals**
Rixensart, Belgium
Distributed by **SmithKline Beecham Pharmaceuticals**
Philadelphia, PA 19101
Engerix-B and *Tip-Lok* are registered trademarks of SmithKline Beecham.
Rx only

EB:L30

Shown in Product Identification Guide, page 337

ESKALITH® ℞

[*ess-kah 'lith*]
(brand of lithium carbonate)
Capsules, 300 mg

ESKALITH CR® ℞

(brand of lithium carbonate)
Controlled Release Tablets, 450 mg

WARNING

Lithium toxicity is closely related to serum lithium levels, and can occur at doses close to therapeutic levels. Facilities for prompt and accurate serum lithium determinations should be available before initiating therapy (see DOSAGE AND ADMINISTRATION).

DESCRIPTION

Eskalith contains lithium carbonate, a white, light alkaline powder with molecular formula Li_2CO_3 and molecular weight 73.89. Lithium is an element of the alkali-metal group with atomic number 3, atomic weight 6.94 and an emission line at 671 nm on the flame photometer.

***Eskalith* Capsules:** Each capsule, with opaque gray cap and opaque yellow body, is imprinted with the product name ESKALITH and SB and contains lithium carbonate, 300 mg. Inactive ingredients consist of benzyl alcohol, cetylpyridinium chloride, D&C Yellow No. 10, FD&C Green No. 3, FD&C Red No. 40, FD&C Yellow No. 6, gelatin, lactose, magnesium stearate, povidone, sodium lauryl sulfate, titanium dioxide and trace amounts of other inactive ingredients.

***Eskalith CR* Controlled Release Tablets:** Each round, yellow, biconvex tablet, debossed with SKF and J10 on one side and scored on the other side, contains lithium carbonate, 450 mg. Inactive ingredients consist of alginic acid, gelatin, iron oxide, magnesium stearate and sodium starch glycolate.

Eskalith CR tablets 450 mg are designed to release a portion of the dose initially and the remainder gradually; the release pattern of the controlled release tablets reduces the variability in lithium blood levels seen with the immediate release dosage forms.

ACTIONS

Preclinical studies have shown that lithium alters sodium transport in nerve and muscle cells and effects a shift toward intraneuronal metabolism of catecholamines, but the specific biochemical mechanism of lithium action in mania is unknown.

INDICATIONS

Eskalith (lithium carbonate) is indicated in the treatment of manic episodes of manic-depressive illness. Maintenance therapy prevents or diminishes the intensity of subsequent episodes in those manic-depressive patients with a history of mania.

Typical symptoms of mania include pressure of speech, motor hyperactivity, reduced need for sleep, flight of ideas, grandiosity, elation, poor judgment, aggressiveness and possibly hostility. When given to a patient experiencing a manic episode, *Eskalith* may produce a normalization of symptomatology within 1 to 3 weeks.

WARNINGS

Lithium should generally not be given to patients with significant renal or cardiovascular disease, severe debilitation or dehydration, or sodium depletion, since the risk of lithium toxicity is very high in such patients. If the psychiatric indication is life-threatening, and if such a patient fails to respond to other measures, lithium treatment may be undertaken with extreme caution, including daily serum lithium determinations and adjustment to the usually low doses ordinarily tolerated by these individuals. In such instances, hospitalization is a necessity.

Chronic lithium therapy may be associated with diminution of renal concentrating ability, occasionally presenting as nephrogenic diabetes insipidus, with polyuria and polydipsia. Such patients should be carefully managed to avoid dehydration with resulting lithium retention and toxicity. This condition is usually reversible when lithium is discontinued.

Morphologic changes with glomerular and interstitial fibrosis and nephron atrophy have been reported in patients on chronic lithium therapy. Morphologic changes have also been seen in manic-depressive patients never exposed to lithium. The relationship between renal functional and morphologic changes and their association with lithium therapy have not been established.

When kidney function is assessed, for baseline data prior to starting lithium therapy or thereafter, routine urinalysis and other tests may be used to evaluate tubular function (e.g., urine specific gravity or osmolality following a period of water deprivation, or 24-hour urine volume) and glomerular function (e.g., serum creatinine or creatinine clearance). During lithium therapy, progressive or sudden changes in renal function, even within the normal range, indicate the need for reevaluation of treatment.

An encephalopathic syndrome (characterized by weakness, lethargy, fever, tremulousness and confusion, extrapyramidal symptoms, leukocytosis, elevated serum enzymes, BUN and FBS) has occurred in a few patients treated with lithium plus a neuroleptic. In some instances, the syndrome was followed by irreversible brain damage. Because of a possible causal relationship between these events and the concomitant administration of lithium and neuroleptics, patients receiving such combined therapy should be monitored closely for early evidence of neurologic toxicity and treatment discontinued promptly if such signs appear. This encephalopathic syndrome may be similar to or the same as neuroleptic malignant syndrome (NMS).

Lithium toxicity is closely related to serum lithium levels, and can occur at doses close to therapeutic levels (see DOSAGE AND ADMINISTRATION).

Outpatients and their families should be warned that the patient must discontinue lithium carbonate therapy and contact his physician if such clinical signs of lithium toxicity as diarrhea, vomiting, tremor, mild ataxia, drowsiness or muscular weakness occur.

Lithium carbonate may impair mental and/or physical abilities. Caution patients about activities requiring alertness (e.g., operating vehicles or machinery).

Lithium may prolong the effects of neuromuscular blocking agents. Therefore, neuromuscular blocking agents should be given with caution to patients receiving lithium.

Usage in Pregnancy: Adverse effects on implantation in rats, embryo viability in mice and metabolism *in vitro* of rat testes and human spermatozoa have been attributed to lithium, as have teratogenicity in submammalian species and cleft palates in mice.

In humans, lithium carbonate may cause fetal harm when administered to a pregnant woman. Data from lithium birth registries suggest an increase in cardiac and other anomalies, especially Ebstein's anomaly. If this drug is used in women of childbearing potential, or during pregnancy, or if a patient becomes pregnant while taking this drug, the patient should be apprised of the potential hazard to the fetus.

Usage in Nursing Mothers: Lithium is excreted in human milk. Nursing should not be undertaken during lithium therapy except in rare and unusual circumstances where, in the view of the physician, the potential benefits to the mother outweigh possible hazards to the child.

Usage in Pediatric Patients: Since information regarding the safety and effectiveness of lithium carbonate in children under 12 years of age is not available, its use in such patients is not recommended.

There has been a report of a transient syndrome of acute dystonia and hyperreflexia occurring in a 15 kg child who ingested 300 mg of lithium carbonate.

Usage in the Elderly: Elderly patients often require lower lithium dosages to achieve therapeutic serum levels. They may also exhibit adverse reactions at serum levels ordinarily tolerated by younger patients.

PRECAUTIONS

The ability to tolerate lithium is greater during the acute manic phase and decreases when manic symptoms subside (see DOSAGE AND ADMINISTRATION).

Caution should be used when lithium and diuretics are used concomitantly because diuretic-induced sodium loss may reduce the renal clearance of lithium and increase serum lithium levels with risk of lithium toxicity. Patients receiving such combined therapy should have serum lithium levels monitored closely and the lithium dosage adjusted if necessary.

The distribution space of lithium approximates that of total body water. Lithium is primarily excreted in urine with insignificant excretion in feces. Renal excretion of lithium is proportional to its plasma concentration. The half-life of elimination of lithium is approximately 24 hours. Lithium decreases sodium reabsorption by the renal tubules which could lead to sodium depletion. Therefore, it is essential for the patient to maintain a normal diet, including salt, and an adequate fluid intake (2500 to 3000 mL) at least during the initial stabilization period. Decreased tolerance to lithium has been reported to ensue from protracted sweating or diarrhea and, if such occur, supplemental fluid and salt should be administered under careful medical supervision and lithium intake reduced or suspended until the condition is resolved.

In addition to sweating and diarrhea, concomitant infection with elevated temperatures may also necessitate a temporary reduction or cessation of medication.

Previously existing underlying thyroid disorders do not necessarily constitute a contraindication to lithium treatment; where hypothyroidism exists, careful monitoring of thyroid function during lithium stabilization and maintenance allows for correction of changing thyroid parameters, if any; where hypothyroidism occurs during lithium stabilization and maintenance, supplemental thyroid treatment may be used.

Indomethacin and piroxicam have been reported to increase significantly, steady-state plasma lithium levels. In some cases, lithium toxicity has resulted from such interactions. There is also some evidence that other nonsteroidal anti-inflammatory agents may have a similar effect. When such combinations are used, increased plasma lithium level monitoring is recommended. Concurrent use of metronidazole with lithium may provoke lithium toxicity due to reduced renal clearance. Patients receiving such combined therapy should be monitored closely.

There is evidence that angiotensin-converting enzyme inhibitors, such as enalapril and captopril, may substantially increase steady-state plasma lithium levels, sometimes resulting in lithium toxicity. When such combinations are used, lithium dosage may need to be decreased, and plasma lithium levels should be measured more often.

Concurrent use of calcium channel blocking agents with lithium may increase the risk of neurotoxicity in the form of ataxia, tremors, nausea, vomiting, diarrhea and/or tinnitus. Caution is recommended.

The concomitant administration of lithium with selective serotonin reuptake inhibitors should be undertaken with caution as this combination has been reported to result in symptoms such as diarrhea, confusion, tremor, dizziness and agitation.

The following drugs can lower serum lithium concentrations by increasing urinary lithium excretion: acetazolamide, urea, xanthine preparations and alkalinizing agents such as sodium bicarbonate.

The following have also been shown to interact with lithium: methyldopa, phenytoin and carbamazepine.

ADVERSE REACTIONS

The occurrence and severity of adverse reactions are generally directly related to serum lithium concentrations as well as to individual patient sensitivity to lithium, and generally occur more frequently and with greater severity at higher concentrations.

Adverse reactions may be encountered at serum lithium levels below 1.5 mEq/L. Mild to moderate adverse reactions may occur at levels from 1.5 to 2.5 mEq/L, and moderate to severe reactions may be seen at levels of 2.0 mEq/L and above.

Fine hand tremor, polyuria and mild thirst may occur during initial therapy for the acute manic phase, and may persist throughout treatment. Transient and mild nausea and general discomfort may also appear during the first few days of lithium administration.

These side effects usually subside with continued treatment or a temporary reduction or cessation of dosage. If persistent, cessation of lithium therapy may be required.

Diarrhea, vomiting, drowsiness, muscular weakness and lack of coordination may be early signs of lithium intoxication, and can occur at lithium levels below 2.0 mEq/L. At higher levels, ataxia, giddiness, tinnitus, blurred vision and a large output of dilute urine may be seen. Serum lithium levels above 3.0 mEq/L may produce a complex clinical picture, involving multiple organs and organ systems. Serum lithium levels should not be permitted to exceed 2.0 mEq/L during the acute treatment phase.

The following reactions have been reported and appear to be related to serum lithium levels, including levels within the therapeutic range: **Neuromuscular/Central Nervous System**—tremor, muscle hyperirritability (fasciculations, twitching, clonic movements of whole limbs), hypertonicity, ataxia, choreo-athetotic movements, hyperactive deep tendon reflex, extrapyramidal symptoms including acute dystonia, cogwheel rigidity, blackout spells, epileptiform seizures, slurred speech, dizziness, vertigo, downbeat nystagmus, incontinence of urine or feces, somnolence, psychomotor retardation, restlessness, confusion, stupor, coma, tongue movements, tics, tinnitus, hallucinations, poor memory, slowed intellectual functioning, startled response, worsening of organic brain syndromes, myasthenia gravis (rarely); **Cardiovascular**—cardiac arrhythmia, hypotension, peripheral circulatory collapse, bradycardia, sinus node dysfunction with severe bradycardia (which may result in syncope); **Gastrointestinal**—anorexia, nausea, vomiting, diarrhea, gastritis, salivary gland swelling, abdominal pain, excessive salivation, flatulence, indigestion; **Genitourinary**—glycosuria, decreased creatinine clearance, albuminuria, oliguria, and symptoms of nephrogenic diabetes insipidus including polyuria, thirst and polydipsia; **Dermatologic**—drying and thinning of hair, alopecia, anesthesia of skin, acne, chronic folliculitis, xerosis cutis, psoriasis or its exacerbation, generalized pruritus with or without rash, cutaneous ulcers, angioedema; **Autonomic**—blurred vision, dry mouth, impotence/sexual dysfunction; **Thyroid Abnormalities**—euthyroid goiter and/or hypothyroidism (including myxedema) accompanied by lower T_3 and T_4. I^{131} uptake may be elevated. (See PRECAUTIONS.) Paradoxically, rare cases of hyperthyroidism have been reported; **EEG Changes**—diffuse slowing, widening of the frequency spectrum, potentiation and disorganization of background rhythm; **EKG Changes**—reversible flattening, isoelectricity or inversion of T-waves; **Miscellaneous**—fatigue, lethargy, transient scotomata, exophthalmos, dehydration, weight loss, leukocytosis, headache, transient hyperglycemia, hypercalcemia, hyperparathyroidism, excessive weight gain, edematous swelling of ankles or wrists, metallic taste, dysgeusia/taste distortion, salty taste, thirst, swollen lips, tightness in chest, swollen and/or painful joints, fever, polyarthralgia, dental caries.

Some reports of nephrogenic diabetes insipidus, hyperparathyroidism and hypothyroidism which persist after lithium discontinuation have been received.

A few reports have been received of the development of painful discoloration of fingers and toes and coldness of the extremities within one day of the starting of treatment with

lithium. The mechanism through which these symptoms (resembling Raynaud's syndrome) developed is not known. Recovery followed discontinuance.
Cases of pseudotumor cerebri (increased intracranial pressure and papilledema) have been reported with lithium use. If undetected, this condition may result in enlargement of the blind spot, constriction of visual fields and eventual blindness due to optic atrophy.
Lithium should be discontinued, if clinically possible, if this syndrome occurs.

DOSAGE AND ADMINISTRATION

Immediate release capsules are usually given t.i.d. or q.i.d. Doses of controlled release tablets are usually given b.i.d. (approximately 12-hour intervals). When initiating therapy with immediate release or controlled release lithium, dosage must be individualized according to serum levels and clinical response.
When switching a patient from immediate release capsules to the Eskalith CR (lithium carbonate) Controlled Release Tablets, give the same total daily dose when possible. Most patients on maintenance therapy are stabilized on 900 mg daily, e.g., 450 mg *Eskalith CR* b.i.d. When the previous dosage of immediate release lithium is not a multiple of 450 mg, for example, 1500 mg, initiate *Eskalith CR* dosage at the multiple of 450 mg nearest to, but *below,* the original daily dose, i.e., 1350 mg. When the two doses are unequal, give the larger dose in the evening. In the above example, with a total daily dosage of 1350 mg, generally 450 mg *Eskalith CR* should be given in the morning and 900 mg *Eskalith CR* in the evening. If desired, the total daily dosage of 1350 mg can be given in three equal 450 mg *Eskalith CR* doses. These patients should be monitored at 1 to 2 week intervals, and dosage adjusted if necessary, until stable and satisfactory serum levels and clinical state are achieved.
When patients require closer titration than that available with *Eskalith CR* doses in increments of 450 mg, immediate release capsules should be used.
Acute Mania—Optimal patient response to Eskalith (lithium carbonate) can usually be established and maintained with 1800 mg per day in divided doses. Such doses will normally produce the desired serum lithium level ranging between 1.0 and 1.5 mEq/L.
Dosage must be individualized according to serum levels and clinical response. Regular monitoring of the patient's clinical state and serum lithium levels is necessary. Serum levels should be determined twice per week during the acute phase, and until the serum level and clinical condition of the patient have been stabilized.
Long-Term Control—The desirable serum lithium levels are 0.6 to 1.2 mEq/L. Dosage will vary from one individual to another, but usually 900 mg to 1200 mg per day in divided doses will maintain this level. Serum lithium levels in uncomplicated cases receiving maintenance therapy during remission should be monitored at least every two months.
Patients unusually sensitive to lithium may exhibit toxic signs at serum levels below 1.0 mEq/L.
N.B.: Blood samples for serum lithium determinations should be drawn immediately prior to the next dose when lithium concentrations are relatively stable (i.e., 8 to 12 hours after the previous dose). Total reliance must not be placed on serum levels alone. Accurate patient evaluation requires both clinical and laboratory analysis.
Elderly patients often respond to reduced dosage, and may exhibit signs of toxicity at serum levels ordinarily tolerated by younger patients.

OVERDOSAGE

The toxic levels for lithium are close to the therapeutic levels. It is therefore important that patients and their families be cautioned to watch for early toxic symptoms and to discontinue the drug and inform the physician should they occur. Toxic symptoms are listed in detail under ADVERSE REACTIONS.

Treatment

No specific antidote for lithium poisoning is known. Early symptoms of lithium toxicity can usually be treated by reduction or cessation of dosage of the drug and resumption of the treatment at a lower dose after 24 to 48 hours. In severe cases of lithium poisoning, the first and foremost goal of treatment consists of elimination of this ion from the patient. Treatment is essentially the same as that used in barbiturate poisoning: 1) gastric lavage, 2) correction of fluid and electrolyte imbalance, and 3) regulation of kidney function. Urea, mannitol and aminophylline all produce significant increases in lithium excretion. Hemodialysis is an effective and rapid means of removing the ion from the severely toxic patient. Infection prophylaxis, regular chest X-rays and preservation of adequate respiration are essential.

HOW SUPPLIED

Capsules: gray and yellow, imprinted with the product name ESKALITH and SB, in bottles of 100.
300 mg 100's: NDC 0007-4007-20
Controlled Release Tablets: round, yellow, biconvex, debossed with SKF and J10 on one side and scored on the other side, in bottles of 100.
450 mg 100's: NDC 0007-4010-20
STORAGE CONDITIONS: Store between 15° and 30°C (59° and 86°F).

Rx only

EL:L46

Shown in Product Identification Guide, page 337

FAMVIR®

[fam'-vir]
(brand of famciclovir)
Tablets

℞

DESCRIPTION

Famvir contains famciclovir, an orally administered prodrug of the antiviral agent penciclovir. Chemically, famciclovir is known as 2-[2-(2-amino-9*H*-purin-9-yl)ethyl]-1,3-propanediol diacetate. Its molecular formula is $C_{14}H_{19}N_5O_4$; its molecular weight is 321.3. It is a synthetic acyclic guanine derivative and has the following structure:

famciclovir

Famciclovir is a white to pale yellow solid. It is freely soluble in acetone and methanol, and sparingly soluble in ethanol and isopropanol. At 25° C famciclovir is freely soluble (>25% w/v) in water initially, but rapidly precipitates as the sparingly soluble (2–3% w/v) monohydrate. Famciclovir is not hygroscopic below 85% relative humidity. Partition coefficients are: octanol/water (pH 4.8) *P*=1.09 and octanol/phosphate buffer (pH 7.4) *P*=2.08.
Tablets for Oral Administration: Each white, film-coated tablet contains famciclovir. The 125 mg and 250 mg tablets are round; the 500 mg tablets are oval. Inactive ingredients consist of hydroxypropyl cellulose, hydroxypropyl methylcellulose, lactose, magnesium stearate, polyethylene glycols, sodium starch glycolate and titanium dioxide.

MICROBIOLOGY

Mechanism of Antiviral Activity: Famciclovir undergoes rapid biotransformation to the active antiviral compound penciclovir, which has inhibitory activity against herpes simplex virus types 1 (HSV-1) and 2 (HSV-2) and varicella zoster virus (VZV). In cells infected with HSV-1, HSV-2 or VZV, viral thymidine kinase phosphorylates penciclovir to a monophosphate form that, in turn, is converted to penciclovir triphosphate by cellular kinases. *In vitro* studies demonstrate that penciclovir triphosphate inhibits HSV-2 DNA polymerase competitively with deoxyguanosine triphosphate. Consequently, herpes viral DNA synthesis and, therefore, replication are selectively inhibited.
Penciclovir triphosphate has an intracellular half-life of 10 hours in HSV-1-, 20 hours in HSV-2- and 7 hours in VZV-infected cells cultured *in vitro*; however, the clinical significance is unknown.
Antiviral Activity *In Vitro* and *In Vivo*: In cell culture studies, penciclovir has antiviral activity against the following herpesviruses (listed in decreasing order of potency): HSV-1, HSV-2 and VZV. Sensitivity test results, expressed as the concentration of the drug required to inhibit the growth of the virus by 50% (IC_{50}) or 99% (IC_{99}) in cell culture, vary greatly depending upon a number of factors, including the assay protocols, and in particular the cell type used. See Table 1.
[See table 1 at top of next page]
Drug Resistance: Penciclovir-resistant mutants of HSV and VZV can result from complete loss of viral thymidine kinase activity (TK negative), reduced TK activity (TK altered) or DNA polymerase mutations. The most commonly encountered acyclovir-resistant mutants that are TK negative are also resistant to penciclovir. The possibility of viral resistance to penciclovir should be considered in patients who fail to respond or experience recurrent viral infections during therapy.

CLINICAL PHARMACOLOGY

Pharmacokinetics

Absorption and Bioavailability: Famciclovir is the diacetyl 6-deoxy analog of the active antiviral compound penciclovir. Following oral administration, little or no famciclovir is detected in plasma or urine.
The absolute bioavailability of famciclovir is 77±8% as determined following the administration of a 500 mg famciclovir oral dose and a 400 mg penciclovir intravenous dose to 12 healthy male subjects.
Penciclovir concentrations increased in proportion to dose over a famciclovir dose range of 125 mg to 750 mg administered as a single dose. Single oral dose administration of 125 mg, 250 mg or 500 mg famciclovir to healthy male volunteers across 17 studies gave the following pharmacokinetic parameters:

Table 2

Dose	AUC (0–inf)† (mcg.hr./mL)	C_{max}‡ (mcg/mL)	T_{max}§ (h)
125 mg	2.24	0.8	0.9
250 mg	4.48	1.6	0.9
500 mg	8.95	3.3	0.9

† AUC (0–inf) (mcg.hr./mL)=area under the plasma concentration-time profile extrapolated to infinity.
‡ C_{max} (mcg/mL)=maximum observed plasma concentration.
§ T_{max} (h)=time to C_{max}.

Following single oral-dose administration of 500 mg famciclovir to seven patients with herpes zoster, the mean ± SD AUC, C_{max}, and T_{max} were 12.1±1.7 mcg.hr./mL, 4.0±0.7 mcg/mL, and 0.7±0.2 hours, respectively. The AUC of penciclovir was approximately 35% greater in patients with herpes zoster as compared to healthy volunteers. Some of this difference may be due to differences in renal function between the two groups.
There is no accumulation of penciclovir after the administration of 500 mg famciclovir t.i.d. for 7 days.
Penciclovir C_{max} decreased approximately 50% and T_{max} was delayed by 1.5 hours when a capsule formulation of famciclovir was administered with food (nutritional content was approximately 910 Kcal and 26% fat). There was no effect on the extent of availability (AUC) of penciclovir. There was an 18% decrease in C_{max} and a delay in T_{max} of about 1 hour when famciclovir was given 2 hours after a meal as compared to its administration 2 hours before a meal. Because there was no effect on the extent of systemic availability of penciclovir, it appears that *Famvir* can be taken without regard to meals.
Distribution: The volume of distribution (Vd_β) was 1.08±0.17 L/kg in 12 healthy male subjects following a single intravenous dose of penciclovir at 400 mg administered as a 1-hour intravenous infusion.
Penciclovir is <20% bound to plasma proteins over the concentration range of 0.1 to 20 mcg/mL. The blood/plasma ratio of penciclovir is approximately 1.
Metabolism: Following oral administration, famciclovir is deacetylated and oxidized to form penciclovir. Metabolites that are inactive include 6-deoxy penciclovir, monoacetylated penciclovir, and 6-deoxy monoacetylated penciclovir (5%, <0.5% and <0.5% of the dose in the urine, respectively). Little or no famciclovir is detected in plasma or urine. An *in vitro* study using human liver microsomes demonstrated that cytochrome P450 does not play an important role in famciclovir metabolism. The conversion of 6-deoxy penciclovir to penciclovir is catalyzed by aldehyde oxidase.
Elimination: Approximately 94% of administered radioactivity was recovered in urine over 24 hours (83% of the dose was excreted in the first 6 hours) after the administration of 5 mg/kg radiolabeled penciclovir as a 1-hour infusion to three healthy male volunteers. Penciclovir accounted for 91% of the radioactivity excreted in the urine.
Following the oral administration of a single 500 mg dose of radiolabeled famciclovir to three healthy male volunteers, 73% and 27% of administered radioactivity were recovered in urine and feces over 72 hours, respectively. Penciclovir accounted for 82% and 6-deoxy penciclovir accounted for 7% of the radioactivity excreted in the urine. Approximately 60% of the administered radiolabeled dose was collected in urine in the first 6 hours.
After intravenous administration of penciclovir in 48 healthy male volunteers, mean ± S.D. total plasma clearance of penciclovir was 36.6±6.3 L/hr (0.48±0.09 L/hr/kg). Penciclovir renal clearance accounted for 74.5±8.8% of total plasma clearance.
Renal clearance of penciclovir following the oral administration of a single 500 mg dose of famciclovir to 109 healthy male volunteers was 27.7±7.6 L/hr.
The plasma elimination half-life of penciclovir was 2.0±0.3 hours after intravenous administration of penciclovir to 48 healthy male volunteers and 2.3±0.4 hours after oral administration of 500 mg famciclovir to 124 healthy male volunteers. The half-life in seven patients with herpes zoster was 3.0±1.1 hours.
HIV-Infected Patients: Following oral administration of a single dose of 500 mg famciclovir (the oral prodrug of penciclovir) to HIV-positive patients, the pharmacokinetic parameters of penciclovir were comparable to those observed in healthy subjects.
Renal Insufficiency: Apparent plasma clearance, renal clearance, and the plasma-elimination rate constant of penciclovir decreased linearly with reductions in renal function. After the administration of a single 500 mg famciclovir oral dose (n=27) to healthy volunteers and to volunteers with varying degrees of renal insufficiency (CL_{CR} ranged from 6.4 to 138.8 mL/min.), the following results were obtained (Table 3):
[See table 3 at top of next page]
In a multiple dose study of famciclovir conducted in subjects with varying degrees of renal impairment (n=18), the pharmacokinetics of penciclovir were comparable to those after single doses.
A dosage adjustment is recommended for patients with renal insufficiency (see DOSAGE AND ADMINISTRATION).
Hepatic Insufficiency: Well-compensated chronic liver disease (chronic hepatitis [n=6], chronic ethanol abuse [n=8], or primary biliary cirrhosis [n=1]) had no effect on the extent of availability (AUC) of penciclovir following a single dose of 500 mg famciclovir. However, there was a 44% decrease in penciclovir mean maximum plasma concentration and the time to maximum plasma concentration was in-

Continued on next page

Information on the SmithKline Beecham Pharmaceuticals products appearing here is based on the labeling in effect on June 15, 2000. Further information on these and other products may be obtained from the Medical Department, SmithKline Beecham Pharmaceuticals, One Franklin Plaza, Philadelphia, PA 19101.

Famvir—Cont.

creased by 0.75 hours in patients with hepatic insufficiency compared to normal volunteers. No dosage adjustment is recommended for patients with well-compensated hepatic impairment. The pharmacokinetics of penciclovir have not been evaluated in patients with severe uncompensated hepatic impairment.

Elderly Subjects: Based on cross-study comparisons, mean penciclovir AUC was 40% larger and penciclovir renal clearance was 22% lower after the oral administration of famciclovir in elderly volunteers (n=18, age 65 to 79 years) compared to younger volunteers. Some of this difference may be due to differences in renal function between the two groups.

Gender: The pharmacokinetics of penciclovir were evaluated in 18 healthy male and 18 healthy female volunteers after single-dose oral administration of 500 mg famciclovir. AUC of penciclovir was 9.3±1.9 mcg.hr./mL and 11.1±2.1 mcg.hr./mL in males and females, respectively. Penciclovir renal clearance was 28.5±8.9 L/hr and 21.8±4.3 L/hr, respectively. These differences were attributed to differences in renal function between the two groups. No famciclovir dosage adjustment based on gender is recommended.

Pediatric Patients: The pharmacokinetics of famciclovir or penciclovir have not been evaluated in patients <18 years of age.

Race: The pharmacokinetics of famciclovir or penciclovir with respect to race have not been evaluated.

Drug Interactions

Effects on penciclovir

No clinically significant alterations in penciclovir pharmacokinetics were observed following single-dose administration of 500 mg famciclovir after pre-treatment with multiple doses of allopurinol, cimetidine, theophylline, or zidovudine. No clinically significant effect on penciclovir pharmacokinetics was observed following multiple-dose (t.i.d.) administration of famciclovir (500 mg) with multiple doses of digoxin.

Effects of famciclovir on co-administered drugs

The steady-state pharmacokinetics of digoxin were not altered by concomitant administration of multiple doses of famciclovir (500 mg t.i.d.). No clinically significant effect on the pharmacokinetics of zidovudine or zidovudine glucuronide was observed following a single oral dose of 500 mg famciclovir.

CLINICAL TRIALS

Herpes Zoster

Famvir (famciclovir) was studied in a placebo-controlled, double-blind trial of 419 immunocompetent adults with uncomplicated herpes zoster. Comparisons included *Famvir* 500 mg t.i.d., *Famvir* 750 mg t.i.d., or placebo. Treatment was begun within 72 hours of initial lesion appearance and therapy was continued for 7 days.

The median time to full crusting in *Famvir*-treated patients was 5 days compared to 7 days in placebo-treated patients. The times to full crusting, loss of vesicles, loss of ulcers, and loss of crusts were shorter for *Famvir* 500 mg-treated patients than for placebo-treated patients in the overall study population. The effects of *Famvir* were greater when therapy was initiated within 48 hours of rash onset; it was also more pronounced in patients 50 years of age or older. Among the 65.2% of patients with at least one positive viral culture, *Famvir*-treated patients had a shorter median duration of viral shedding than placebo-treated patients (1 day and 2 days, respectively).

There were no overall differences in the duration of pain before rash healing between *Famvir* and placebo-treated groups. In addition, there was no difference in the incidence of pain after rash healing (postherpetic neuralgia) between the treatment groups. In the 186 patients (44.4% of total study population) who did develop postherpetic neuralgia, the median duration of postherpetic neuralgia was shorter in patients treated with *Famvir* 500 mg than in those treated with placebo (63 days and 119 days, respectively). No additional efficacy was demonstrated with higher doses of *Famvir*.

A double-blind controlled trial in 545 immunocompetent adults with uncomplicated herpes zoster treated within 72 hours of initial lesion appearance compared three doses of *Famvir* to acyclovir 800 mg 5 times per day. Times to full lesion crusting and times to loss of acute pain were comparable for all groups and there were no statistically significant differences in the time to loss of postherpetic neuralgia between *Famvir* and acyclovir-treated groups.

Herpes Simplex Infections

Recurrent Genital Herpes: In two placebo-controlled trials, 626 immunocompetent adults with a recurrence of genital herpes were treated with *Famvir* 125 mg b.i.d. (n=160), *Famvir* 250 mg b.i.d. (n=169), *Famvir* 500 mg b.i.d. (n=154) or placebo (n=143) for 5 days. Treatment was initiated within 6 hours of either symptom onset or lesion appearance. In the two studies combined, the median time to healing in *Famvir* 125 mg-treated patients was 4 days compared to 5 days in placebo-treated patients and the median time to cessation of viral shedding was 1.8 vs. 3.4 days in *Famvir* 125 mg and placebo recipients, respectively. The median time to loss of all symptoms was 3.2 days in *Famvir* 125 mg-treated patients vs. 3.8 days in placebo-treated patients. No additional efficacy was demonstrated with higher doses of *Famvir*.

Suppression of Recurrent Genital Herpes: 934 immunocompetent adults with a history of 6 or more recurrences per year were randomized into two double-blind, 1-year, placebo-controlled trials. Comparisons included *Famvir* 125 mg t.i.d., 250 mg b.i.d., 250 mg t.i.d. and placebo. At one-year, 60% to 65% of patients were still receiving *Famvir* and 25% were receiving placebo treatment. Patient reported recurrence rates for the 250 mg b.i.d. dose at 6 and 12 months are shown in Table 4.

[See table 4 above]

Famvir-treated patients had approximately 1/5 the median number of recurrences as compared to placebo-treated patients.

Higher doses of *Famvir* were not associated with an increase in efficacy.

Recurrent Mucocutaneous Herpes Simplex Infection in HIV-Infected Patients

A randomized, double-blind, multicenter study compared famciclovir 500 mg twice daily for 7 days (n=150) with oral acyclovir 400 mg 5 times daily for 7 days (n=143) in HIV-infected patients with recurrent mucocutaneous HSV infection treated within 48 hours of lesion onset. Approximately 40% of patients had a CD_4 count below 200 cells/mm^3, 54% of patients had anogenital lesions and 35% had orolabial lesions. Famciclovir therapy was comparable to oral acyclovir in reducing new lesion formation and in time to complete healing.

INDICATIONS AND USAGE

Herpes Zoster: Famvir (famciclovir) is indicated for the treatment of acute herpes zoster (shingles).

Herpes Simplex Infections: *Famvir* is indicated for:
- treatment or suppression of recurrent genital herpes in immunocompetent patients
- treatment of recurrent mucocutaneous herpes simplex infections in HIV-infected patients.

CONTRAINDICATIONS

Famvir (famciclovir) is contraindicated in patients with known hypersensitivity to the product, its components, and Denavir® (penciclovir cream).

PRECAUTIONS

General

The efficacy of *Famvir* has not been established for initial episode genital herpes infection, ophthalmic zoster, disseminated zoster or in immunocompromised patients with herpes zoster.

Table 1

Method of Assay	Virus Type	Cell Type	IC_{50} (mcg/mL)	IC_{99}
Plaque Reduction	VZV (c.i.)	MRC-5	5.0 ± 3.0	
	VZV (c.i.)	Hs68	0.9 ± 0.4	
	HSV-1 (c.i.)	MRC-5	0.2 – 0.6	
	HSV-1 (c.i.)	WISH	0.04 – 0.5	
	HSV-2 (c.i.)	MRC-5	0.9 – 2.1	
	HSV-2 (c.i.)	WISH	0.1 – 0.8	
Virus Yield Reduction	HSV-1 (c.i.)	MRC-5		0.4 – 0.5
	HSV-2 (c.i.)	MRC-5		0.6 – 0.7
DNA Synthesis Inhibition	VZV (Ellen)	MRC-5	0.1	
	HSV-1 (SC16)	MRC-5	0.04	
	HSV-2 (MS)	MRC-5	0.05	

(c.i.) = clinical isolates.

Table 3

Parameter (mean ± S.D.)	CL_{CR}† ≥60 (mL/min.)	CL_{CR} 40–59 (mL/min.)	CL_{CR} 20–39 (mL/min.)	CL_{CR} <20 (mL/min.)
CL_{CR} (mL/min)	88.1 ± 20.6	49.3 ± 5.9	26.5 ± 5.3	12.7 ± 5.9
CL_R (L/hr)	30.1 ± 10.6	13.0 ± 1.3‡	4.2 ± 0.9	1.6 ± 1.0
CL/F§ (L/hr)	66.9 ± 27.5	27.3 ± 2.8	12.8 ± 1.3	5.8 ± 2.8
Half-life (hr)	2.3 ± 0.5	3.4 ± 0.7	6.2 ± 1.6	13.4 ± 10.2
n	15	5	4	3

† CL_{CR} is measured creatinine clearance.
‡ n=4.
§ CL/F consists of bioavailability factor and famciclovir to penciclovir conversion factor.

Table 4

	Recurrence Rates at 6 Months: Famvir 250 mg b.i.d.	Recurrence Rates at 6 Months: Placebo	Recurrence Rates at 12 Months: Famvir 250 mg b.i.d.	Recurrence Rates at 12 Months: Placebo
n	236	233	236	233
Recurrence-free	39%	10%	29%	6%
Recurrences†	47%	74%	53%	78%
Lost to Follow-up‡	14%	16%	17%	16%

† Based on patient reported data; not necessarily confirmed by a physician.
‡ Patients recurrence-free at time of last contact prior to withdrawal.

Table 5
Selected Adverse Events Reported by ≥2% of Patients in Placebo-controlled Famvir (famciclovir) Trials*

	Incidence					
	Herpes Zoster		Recurrent Genital Herpes		Genital Herpes-Suppression	
Event	*Famvir* (n=273) %	Placebo (n=146) %	*Famvir* (n=640) %	Placebo (n=225) %	*Famvir* (n=458) %	Placebo (n=63) %
Nervous System						
Headache	22.7	17.8	23.6	16.4	39.3	42.9
Paresthesia	2.6	0.0	1.3	0.0	0.9	0.0
Migraine	0.7	0.7	1.3	0.4	3.1	0.0
Gastrointestinal						
Nausea	12.5	11.6	10.0	8.0	7.2	9.5
Diarrhea	7.7	4.8	4.5	7.6	9.0	9.5
Vomiting	4.8	3.4	1.3	0.9	3.1	1.6
Flatulence	1.5	0.7	1.9	2.2	4.8	1.6
Abdominal Pain	1.1	3.4	3.9	5.8	7.9	7.9
Body as a Whole						
Fatigue	4.4	3.4	6.3	4.4	4.8	3.2
Skin and Appendages						
Pruritus	3.7	2.7	0.9	0.0	2.2	0.0
Rash	0.4	0.7	0.6	0.4	3.3	1.6
Reproductive Female						
Dysmenorrhea	0.0	0.7	2.2	1.3	7.6	6.3

*Patients may have entered into more than one clinical trial.

Dosage adjustment is recommended when administering *Famvir* to patients with creatinine clearance values <60 mL/min. (see DOSAGE AND ADMINISTRATION). In patients with underlying renal disease who have received inappropriately high doses of *Famvir* for their level of renal function, acute renal failure has been reported.

Information for Patients

Patients should be informed that *Famvir* is not a cure for genital herpes. There are no data evaluating whether *Famvir* will prevent transmission of infection to others. As genital herpes is a sexually transmitted disease, patients should avoid contact with lesions or intercourse when lesions and/or symptoms are present to avoid infecting partners. Genital herpes can also be transmitted in the absence of symptoms through asymptomatic viral shedding. If medical management of recurrent episodes is indicated, patients should be advised to initiate therapy at the first sign or symptom.

Drug Interactions

Concurrent use with probenecid or other drugs significantly eliminated by active renal tubular secretion may result in increased plasma concentrations of penciclovir.

The conversion of 6-deoxy penciclovir to penciclovir is catalyzed by aldehyde oxidase. Interactions with other drugs metabolized by this enzyme could potentially occur.

Carcinogenesis, Mutagenesis, Impairment of Fertility

Famciclovir was administered orally unless otherwise stated.

Carcinogenesis: Two-year dietary carcinogenicity studies with famciclovir were conducted in rats and mice. An increase in the incidence of mammary adenocarcinoma (a common tumor in animals of this strain) was seen in female rats receiving the high dose of 600 mg/kg/day (1.5 to 9.0x the human systemic exposure at the recommended daily oral doses of 500 mg t.i.d., 250 mg b.i.d., or 125 mg b.i.d. based on area under the plasma concentration curve comparisons [24 hr AUC] for penciclovir). No increases in tumor incidence were reported in male rats treated at doses up to 240 mg/kg/day (0.9 to 5.4x the human AUC), or in male and female mice at doses up to 600 mg/kg/day (0.4 to 2.4x the human AUC).

Mutagenesis: Famciclovir and penciclovir (the active metabolite of famciclovir) were tested for genotoxic potential in a battery of *in vitro* and *in vivo* assays. Famciclovir and penciclovir were negative in *in vitro* tests for gene mutations in bacteria (*S. typhimurium* and *E. coli*) and unscheduled DNA synthesis in mammalian HeLa 83 cells (at doses up to 10,000 and 5000 mcg/plate, respectively). Famciclovir was also negative in the L5178Y mouse lymphoma assay (5000 mcg/mL), the *in vivo* mouse micronucleus test (4800 mg/kg), and rat dominant lethal study (5000 mg/kg). Famciclovir induced increases in polyploidy in human lymphocytes *in vitro* in the absence of chromosomal damage (1200 mcg/mL). Penciclovir was positive in the L5178Y mouse lymphoma assay for gene mutation/chromosomal aberrations, with and without metabolic activation (1000 mcg/mL). In human lymphocytes, penciclovir caused chromosomal aberrations in the absence of metabolic activation (250 mcg/mL). Penciclovir caused an increased incidence of micronuclei in mouse bone marrow *in vivo* when administered intravenously at doses highly toxic to bone marrow (500 mg/kg), but not when administered orally.

Impairment of Fertility: Testicular toxicity was observed in rats, mice, and dogs following repeated administration of famciclovir or penciclovir. Testicular changes included atrophy of the seminiferous tubules, reduction in sperm count, and/or increased incidence of sperm with abnormal morphology or reduced motility. The degree of toxicity to male reproduction was related to dose and duration of exposure. In male rats, decreased fertility was observed after 10 weeks of dosing at 500 mg/kg/day (1.9 to 11.4x the human AUC). The no observable effect level for sperm and testicular toxicity in rats following chronic administration (26 weeks) was 50 mg/kg/day (0.2 to 1.2x the human systemic exposure based on AUC comparisons). Testicular toxicity was observed following chronic administration to mice (104 weeks) and dogs (26 weeks) at doses of 600 mg/kg/day (0.4 to 2.4x the human AUC) and 150 mg/kg/day (1.7 to 10.2x the human AUC), respectively.

Famciclovir had no effect on general reproductive performance or fertility in female rats at doses up to 1000 mg/kg/day (3.6 to 21.6x the human AUC).

Two placebo-controlled studies in a total of 130 otherwise healthy men with a normal sperm profile over an 8-week baseline period and recurrent genital herpes receiving oral *Famvir* (250 mg b.i.d.) (n=66) or placebo (n=64) therapy for 18 weeks showed no evidence of significant effects on sperm count, motility or morphology during treatment or during an 8-week follow-up.

Pregnancy

Teratogenic Effects—Pregnancy Category B. Famciclovir was tested for effects on embryo-fetal development in rats and rabbits at oral doses up to 1000 mg/kg/day (approximately 3.6 to 21.6x and 1.8 to 10.8x the human systemic exposure to penciclovir based on AUC comparisons for the rat and rabbit, respectively) and intravenous doses of 360 mg/kg/day in rats (2 to 12x the human dose based on body surface area [BSA] comparisons) or 120 mg/kg/day in rabbits (1.5 to 9.0x the human dose [BSA]). No adverse effects were observed on embryo-fetal development. Similarly, no adverse effects were observed following intravenous administration of penciclovir to rats (80 mg/kg/day, 0.4 to 2.6x the human dose [BSA]) or rabbits (60 mg/kg/day, 0.7 to 4.2x the human dose [BSA]). There are, however, no adequate and well-controlled studies in pregnant women. Because animal reproduction studies are not always predictive of human response, famciclovir should be used during pregnancy only if the benefit to the patient clearly exceeds the potential risk to the fetus.

Table 6
Selected Laboratory Abnormalities in Genital Herpes Suppression Studies*

Parameter	*Famvir* (n = 660)† %	Placebo (n = 210)† %
Anemia (<0.8 × NRL)	0.1	0.0
Leukopenia (<0.75 × NRL)	1.3	0.9
Neutropenia (<0.8 × NRL)	3.2	1.5
AST (SGOT) (>2 × NRH)	2.3	1.2
ALT (SGPT) (>2 × NRH)	3.2	1.5
Total Bilirubin (>1.5 × NRH)	1.9	1.2
Serum Creatinine (>1.5 × NRH)	0.2	0.3
Amylase (>1.5 × NRH)	1.5	1.9
Lipase (>1.5 × NRH)	4.9	4.7

*Percentage of patients with laboratory abnormalities that were increased or decreased from baseline and were outside of specified ranges.
†n values represent the minimum number of patients assessed for each laboratory parameter.
NRH = Normal Range High.
NRL = Normal Range Low.

Table 7

Indication and Normal Dosage Regimen	Creatinine Clearance (mL/min.)	Adjusted Dosage Regimen Dose (mg)	Dosing Interval
Herpes Zoster 500 mg every 8 hours	>60	500	every 8 hours
	40–59	500	every 12 hours
	20–39	500	every 24 hours
	<20	250	every 24 hours
	HD*	250	following each dialysis
Recurrent Genital Herpes 125 mg every 12 hours	≥40	125	every 12 hours
	20–39	125	every 24 hours
	<20	125	every 24 hours
	HD*	125	following each dialysis
Suppression of Recurrent Genital Herpes 250 mg every 12 hours	≥40	250	every 12 hours
	20–39	125	every 12 hours
	<20	125	every 24 hours
	HD*	125	following each dialysis
Recurrent Orolabial and Genital Herpes Simplex Infection in HIV-Infected Patients 500 mg every 12 hours	≥40	500	every 12 hours
	20–39	500	every 24 hours
	<20	250	every 24 hours
	HD*	250	following each dialysis

* Hemodialysis

Pregnancy Exposure Registry: To monitor maternal-fetal outcomes of pregnant women exposed to *Famvir*, SmithKline Beecham maintains a *Famvir* Pregnancy Registry. Physicians are encouraged to register their patients by calling (800) 366-8900, ext. 5231.

Nursing Mothers

Following oral administration of famciclovir to lactating rats, penciclovir was excreted in breast milk at concentrations higher than those seen in the plasma. It is not known whether it is excreted in human milk. There are no data on the safety of *Famvir* in infants.

Usage in Children

Safety and efficacy in children under the age of 18 years have not been established.

Geriatric Use

Of 816 patients with herpes zoster in clinical studies who were treated with *Famvir*, 248 (30.4%) were ≥65 years of age and 103 (13%) were ≥75 years of age. No overall differences were observed in the incidence or types of adverse events between younger and older patients.

ADVERSE REACTIONS

Immunocompetent Patients

The safety of *Famvir* has been evaluated in clinical studies involving 816 *Famvir*-treated patients with herpes zoster (*Famvir*, 250 mg t.i.d. to 750 mg t.i.d.); 528 *Famvir*-treated patients with recurrent genital herpes (*Famvir*, 125 mg b.i.d. to 500 mg t.i.d.); and 1,197 patients with recurrent genital herpes treated with *Famvir* as suppressive therapy (125 mg q.d. to 250 mg t.i.d.) of which 570 patients received *Famvir* (open-labeled and/or double-blind) for at least 10 months. Table 5 lists selected adverse events.

[See table 5 at top of previous page]

The following adverse events have been reported during post-approval use of *Famvir:* urticaria, hallucinations and confusion (including delirium, disorientation, confusional state, occurring predominantly in the elderly). Because these adverse events are reported voluntarily from a population of unknown size, estimates of frequency cannot be made.

Table 6 lists selected laboratory abnormalities in genital herpes suppression trials.

[See table 6 above]

HIV-Infected Patients

In HIV-infected patients, the most frequently reported adverse events for famciclovir (500 mg twice daily; n=150) and acyclovir (400 mg, 5x/day; n=143), respectively, were headache (16.0 vs 15.4%), nausea (10.7 vs 12.6%), diarrhea (6.7 vs 10.5%), vomiting (4.7 vs 3.5%), fatigue (4.0 vs 2.1%), and abdominal pain (3.3 vs 5.6%).

OVERDOSAGE

Appropriate symptomatic and supportive therapy should be given. Penciclovir is removed by hemodialysis (see PRECAUTIONS, General).

DOSAGE AND ADMINISTRATION

Herpes Zoster

The recommended dosage is 500 mg every 8 hours for 7 days. Therapy should be initiated promptly as soon as herpes zoster is diagnosed. No data are available on efficacy of treatment started greater than 72 hours after rash onset.

Herpes Simplex Infections

Recurrent genital herpes: The recommended dosage is 125 mg twice daily for 5 days. Initiate therapy at the first sign or symptom if medical management of a genital herpes recurrence is indicated. The efficacy of *Famvir* has not been established when treatment is initiated more than 6 hours after onset of symptoms or lesions.

Suppression of recurrent genital herpes: The recommended dosage is 250 mg twice daily for up to 1 year. The safety and efficacy of *Famvir* therapy beyond 1 year of treatment have not been established.

HIV-Infected Patients

For recurrent orolabial or genital herpes simplex infection, the recommended dosage is 500 mg twice daily for 7 days.

Continued on next page

Information on the SmithKline Beecham Pharmaceuticals products appearing here is based on the labeling in effect on June 15, 2000. Further information on these and other products may be obtained from the Medical Department, SmithKline Beecham Pharmaceuticals, One Franklin Plaza, Philadelphia, PA 19101.

Famvir—Cont.

In patients with reduced renal function, dosage reduction is recommended (see PRECAUTIONS, General).
[See table 7 at top of previous page]

Administration with Food

When famciclovir was administered with food, penciclovir C_{max} decreased approximately 50%. Because the systemic availability of penciclovir (AUC) was not altered, it appears that *Famvir* may be taken without regard to meals.

HOW SUPPLIED

Famvir is supplied as film-coated tablets as follows: 125 mg in bottles of 30; 250 mg in bottles of 30; and 500 mg in bottles of 30 and Single Unit Packages of 50 (intended for institutional use only).

Famvir 125 mg tablets are white, round, debossed with FAMVIR on one side and 125 on the other.
125 mg 30's: NDC 0007-4115-13

Famvir 250 mg tablets are white, round, debossed with FAMVIR on one side and 250 on the other.
250 mg 30's: NDC 0007-4116-13

Famvir 500 mg tablets are white, oval, debossed with FAMVIR on one side and 500 on the other.
500 mg 30's: NDC 0007-4117-13
500 mg SUP 50's: NDC 0007-4117-19
Store between 15° and 30° C (59° and 86° F).

Rx only

Manufactured in Crawley, UK
by **SmithKline Beecham Pharmaceuticals**
for **SmithKline Beecham Pharmaceuticals**
Philadelphia, PA 19101
FV:L16A

Shown in Product Identification Guide, page 337

HEPATITIS A VACCINE, INACTIVATED ℞
HAVRIX®
[have 'rix]

DESCRIPTION

Havrix (Hepatitis A Vaccine, Inactivated) is a noninfectious hepatitis A vaccine developed and manufactured by SmithKline Beecham Biologicals. The virus (strain HM175) is propagated in MRC_5 human diploid cells. After removal of the cell culture medium, the cells are lysed to form a suspension. This suspension is purified through ultrafiltration and gel permeation chromatography procedures. Treatment of this lysate with formalin ensures viral inactivation. *Havrix* contains a sterile suspension of inactivated virus; viral antigen activity is referenced to a standard using an enzyme linked immunosorbent assay (ELISA), and is therefore expressed in terms of ELISA Units (EL.U.).

Havrix is supplied as a sterile suspension for intramuscular administration. The vaccine is ready for use without reconstitution; it must be shaken before administration to assure a uniform suspension. After shaking, the vaccine is a homogenous white turbid suspension.

Each 1 mL adult dose of vaccine consists of not less than 1440 EL.U. of viral antigen, adsorbed on 0.5 mg of aluminum, as aluminum hydroxide.

There are two pediatric dose formulations, each with its own dosing schedule (see DOSAGE AND ADMINISTRATION). The formulations are: not less than 360 EL.U. of viral antigen/0.5 mL; not less than 720 EL.U. of viral antigen/ 0.5 mL. Each dose is adsorbed onto 0.25 mg of aluminum, as aluminum hydroxide.

The vaccine preparations also contain 0.5% (w/v) of 2-phenoxyethanol as a preservative. Other excipients are: amino acid supplement (0.3% w/v) in a phosphate-buffered saline solution and polysorbate 20 (0.05 mg/mL). Residual MRC_5 cellular proteins (not more than 5 mcg/adult dose) and traces of formalin (not more than 0.1 mg/mL) are present.

CLINICAL PHARMACOLOGY

The hepatitis A virus (HAV) belongs to the picornavirus family. Only one serotype of HAV has been described.[1]

Hepatitis A is highly contagious with the predominant mode of transmission being person-to-person via the fecal-oral route. Infection has been shown to be spread (1) by contaminated water or food; (2) by infected food handlers[2]; (3) after breakdown in usual sanitary conditions or after floods or natural disasters; (4) by ingestion of raw or undercooked shellfish (oysters, clams, mussels) from contaminated waters[3]; (5) during travel to areas of the world with poor hygienic conditions[4,5]; (6) among institutionalized children and adults[6]; (7) in day-care centers where children have not been toilet trained[7]; (8) by parenteral transmission, either blood transfusions or sharing needles with infected people.[1]

The level of economic development influences the prevalence of hepatitis A and the age at which it is most likely to occur. In developing countries with poor hygiene and sanitation, about 90% of children are infected by age 5 years.[1] As conditions improve, the prevalence decreases and the age at which infection occurs increases. Hence it is more likely to occur in adulthood, when disease is generally more severe and more likely to be fatal.[1] In the United States, attack rates for hepatitis A infection are cyclical and vary by population. The rates have increased gradually from 9.2 per 100,000 in 1983 to 14.6 per 100,000 in 1989.[8]

The incubation period for hepatitis A averages 28 days (range: 15 to 50 days).[9] The course of hepatitis A infection is extremely variable, ranging from asymptomatic infection to icteric hepatitis. However, most adults (76% to 97%)[10] become symptomatic. Symptoms range from mild and transient to severe and prolonged and may include fever, nausea, vomiting and diarrhea in the prodromal phase, followed by jaundice in up to 88% of adults, as well as hepatomegaly and biochemical evidence of hepatocellular damage.[10] Recovery is generally complete and followed by protection against HAV infection. However, illness may be prolonged, and relapse of clinical illness and viral shedding have been described.[11]

Hepatitis A infection is often asymptomatic in children under 2 years of age, who nonetheless excrete the virus in their stool and thereby serve as a source of infection.[10] In older patients and persons with underlying liver disease,[1] it is generally much more severe. This is reflected in mortality rates. While an overall case fatality rate of 0.6% has been reported, a case fatality rate of 2.7% has been reported in patients ≥49 years of age.[1] Indeed, while 67% of cases occur in children, over 70% of deaths occur in those over the age of 49 years.[1]

There is no chronic carrier state. The virus replicates in the liver and is excreted in bile. The highest concentrations of HAV are found in stools of infected persons during the 2-week period immediately before the onset of jaundice and decline after jaundice appears.[12] Children and infants may shed HAV for longer periods than adults, possibly lasting as long as several weeks after the onset of clinical illness.[13] Chronic shedding of HAV in feces has not been demonstrated, but relapses of hepatitis A can occur in as many as 20% of patients[1,14] and fecal shedding of HAV may recur at this time.[11]

The presence of antibodies to HAV (anti-HAV) confers protection against hepatitis A infection. However, the lowest titer needed to confer protection has not been determined.

In a chimpanzee challenge study, the quality of protection afforded by immune globulin (IG) prepared from initially seronegative human volunteers vaccinated with *Havrix* was comparable to that afforded by commercial IG. In this experiment chimpanzees immunized with either preparation developed passive-active immunity, when challenged with wild-type HAV. No animal in either group developed clinical illness.

In vitro studies in a randomly selected subset of human subjects (n=80) showed anti-HAV induced by *Havrix* to have functional activity. This was demonstrated by a neutralization assay and a competitive inhibition assay using a panel of monoclonal antibodies known to have neutralizing activity.

Immunogenicity in Adults: In three clinical studies involving over 400 healthy adult volunteers given a single 1440 EL.U. dose of *Havrix*, specific humoral antibodies against HAV were elicited in more than 96% of subjects when measured 1 month after vaccination. By day 15, 80% to 98% of vaccinees had already seroconverted (anti-HAV ≥20 mIU/mL [the lower limit of antibody measurement by current assay]). Geometric mean titers (GMTs) of seroconverters ranged from 264 to 339 mIU/mL at day 15 and increased to a range of 335 to 637 mIU/mL by 1 month following vaccination.[15]

The GMTs obtained following a single dose of *Havrix* are at least several times higher than that expected following receipt of IG.

In a clinical study using 2.5 to 5 times the standard dose of IG (standard dose=0.02 to 0.06 mL/kg), the GMT in recipients was 146 mIU/mL at 5 days post-administration, 77 mIU/mL at month 1 and 63 mIU/mL at month 2.[15]

In two clinical trials in which a booster dose of 1440 EL.U. was given 6 months following the initial dose, 100% of vaccinees (n=269) were seropositive 1 month after the booster dose, with GMTs ranging from 3318 mIU/mL to 5925 mIU/ mL. The titers obtained from this additional dose approximate those observed several years after natural infection.

In a subset of vaccinees (n=89), a single dose of *Havrix* 1440 EL.U. elicited specific anti-HAV neutralizing antibodies in more than 94% of vaccinees when measured 1 month after vaccination. These neutralizing antibodies persisted until month 6. One hundred percent of vaccinees had neutralizing antibodies when measured 1 month after a booster dose given at month 6.

Immunogenicity of *Havrix* was studied in subjects with chronic liver disease of various etiologies. 189 healthy adults and 220 adults with either chronic hepatitis B (n=46), chronic hepatitis C (n=104) or moderate chronic liver disease of other etiology (n=70) were vaccinated with *Havrix* 1440 EL.U. on a 0, 6 month schedule. The last group consisted of alcoholic cirrhosis (n=17), autoimmune hepatitis (n=10), chronic hepatitis/cryptogenic cirrhosis (n=9), hemochromatosis (n=2), primary biliary cirrhosis (n=15), primary sclerosing cholangitis (n=4) and unspecified (n=13). At each time point, GMTs were lower for subjects with chronic liver disease than for healthy subjects. At month 7, the GMTs ranged from 478 mIU/mL (chronic hepatitis C) to 1245 mIU/mL (healthy), as determined by a commercial ELISA. The relevance of these data to the duration of protection afforded by *Havrix* is unknown. One month after the first dose, seroconversion rates in adults with chronic liver disease were lower than in healthy adults. However, 1 month after the booster dose at month 6, seroconversion rates were similar in all groups; rates ranged from 94.7% to 98.1%.

Immunogenicity in Children and Adolescents: In six clinical studies involving pediatric vaccinees (n=762) ranging from 1 to 18 years of age, the GMT following two doses of *Havrix* 360 EL.U. given 1 month apart ranged from 197 to 660 mIU/mL. Ninety-nine percent of subjects seroconverted following two doses. When a booster (third) dose of *Havrix* 360 EL.U. was administered 6 months following the initial dose, all subjects were seropositive 1 month following the booster dose with GMTs rising to a range of 3388 to 4643 mIU/mL. In one study in which children were followed for an additional 6 months, all subjects remained seropositive. Solicited adverse effects were similar in frequency and nature to those seen following administration of Engerix-B® [Hepatitis B Vaccine (Recombinant)].

In four clinical studies, children and adolescents (n=314), ranging from 2 to 19 years of age, were immunized with two doses of *Havrix* 720 EL.U./0.5 mL given six months apart. One month after the first dose, seroconversion ranged from 96.8% to 100%, with GMTs of 194 mIU/mL to 305 mIU/mL. In studies in which sera were obtained 2 weeks following the initial dose, seroconversion ranged from 91.6% to 96.1%. One month following a booster dose at month 6, all subjects were seropositive with GMTs ranging from 2495 mIU/mL to 3644 mIU/mL.[15]

In one additional study in which the booster dose was delayed until 1 year following the initial dose, 95.2% of the subjects were seropositive just prior to administration of the booster dose. One month later, all subjects were seropositive with a GMT of 2657 mIU/mL.[15]

Also, *Havrix* has been found to be highly efficacious in a clinical study of children at high risk of HAV infection (see below).

At present, the duration of protection afforded by *Havrix* has not been established. Therefore it is unknown if the protection provided to immunized children will last until adulthood.

Protective Efficacy: Protective efficacy with *Havrix* has been demonstrated in a double-blind, randomized controlled study in school children (age 1 to 16 years) in Thailand who were at high risk of HAV infection. A total of 40,119 children were randomized to be vaccinated with either *Havrix* 360 EL.U. or *Engerix-B* at 0, 1, 12 months. 19,037 children received a primary course (0, 1 months) of *Havrix* and 19,120 children received a primary course (0, 1 months) of *Engerix-B*. 38,157 children entered surveillance at day 138 and were observed for an additional 8 months. Using the protocol-defined endpoint (≥2 days absence from school, ALT level >45 U/mL, and a positive result in the HAVAB-M test), 32 cases of clinical hepatitis A occurred in the control group; in the *Havrix* group, two cases were identified. These two cases were mild both in terms of biochemical and clinical indices of hepatitis A disease. Thus the calculated efficacy rate for prevention of clinical hepatitis A was 94% (95% confidence intervals 74% to 98%).[16]

In outbreak investigations occurring in the trial, 26 clinical cases of hepatitis A (of a total of 34 occurring in the trial) occurred. No cases occurred in *Havrix* vaccinees.

Using additional virological and serological analyses post hoc, the efficacy of *Havrix* was confirmed. Up to three additional cases of very mild clinical illness may have occurred in vaccinees. Using available testing, these illnesses could neither be proven nor disproven to have been caused by HAV. By including these as cases, the calculated efficacy rate for prevention of clinical hepatitis A would be 84% (95% confidence intervals 60% to 94%).

In a study designed to interrupt an epidemic of hepatitis A among Native Americans in Alaska, vaccination with a single dose of *Havrix* (1440 EL.U./mL in adults, 720 EL.U./0.5 mL in children and adolescents), appeared to be efficacious.[15]

INDICATIONS AND USAGE

Havrix is indicated for active immunization of persons ≥2 years of age against disease caused by hepatitis A virus (HAV).

Havrix will not prevent hepatitis caused by other agents such as hepatitis B virus, hepatitis C virus, hepatitis E virus or other pathogens known to infect the liver.

Immunization with *Havrix* is indicated for those people desiring protection against hepatitis A. Primary immunization should be completed at least 2 weeks prior to expected exposure to HAV. Individuals who are, or will be, at increased risk of infection by HAV include:

Travelers.

Persons traveling to areas of higher endemicity for hepatitis A. These areas include, but are not limited to, Africa, Asia (except Japan), the Mediterranean basin, eastern Europe, the Middle East, Central and South America, Mexico, and parts of the Caribbean. Current CDC advisories should be consulted with regard to specific locales.

Military personnel.

People living in, or relocating to, areas of high endemicity.

Certain ethnic and geographic populations that experience cyclic hepatitis A epidemics such as:

Native peoples of Alaska and the Americas.

People with chronic liver disease, including:

—Alcoholic cirrhosis
—Chronic hepatitis B
—Chronic hepatitis C
—Autoimmune hepatitis
—Primary biliary cirrhosis

Others.

—Persons engaging in high-risk sexual activity (such as men having sex with men)[17]
—Residents of a community experiencing an outbreak of hepatitis A
—Users of illicit injectable drugs

—Persons who have clotting-factor disorders (hemophiliacs and other recipients of therapeutic blood products)
Hepatitis A transmission has been documented in persons with clotting disorders. Susceptible persons in this category, especially those who receive solvent-detergent-treated clotting-factor concentrates, should be vaccinated against hepatitis A[18] (see PRECAUTIONS and DOSAGE AND ADMINISTRATION).
Although the epidemiology of hepatitis A does not permit the identification of other specific populations at high risk of disease, outbreaks of hepatitis A or exposure to hepatitis A virus have been described in a variety of populations in which *Havrix* may be useful:
—Certain institutional workers (e.g., caretakers for the developmentally challenged)
—Employees of child day-care centers
—Laboratory workers who handle live hepatitis A virus
—Handlers of primate animals that may be harboring HAV

People exposed to hepatitis A.
For those requiring both immediate and long-term protection, *Havrix* may be administered concomitantly with IG.
The ACIP has issued the following recommendations regarding food handlers: "Persons who work as food handlers can contract hepatitis A and transmit HAV to others. To decrease the frequency of evaluations of food handlers with hepatitis A and the need for postexposure prophylaxis of patrons, vaccination may be considered where state or local health authorities or private employers determine that such vaccination is cost-effective."[18]

CONTRAINDICATIONS

Havrix is contraindicated in people with known hypersensitivity to any component of the vaccine.

WARNINGS

There have been rare reports of anaphylaxis/anaphylactoid reactions following commercial use of the vaccine in other countries. Patients experiencing hypersensitivity reactions after a *Havrix* injection should not receive further *Havrix* injections. (See CONTRAINDICATIONS.)
Hepatitis A has a relatively long incubation period (15 to 50 days). Hepatitis A vaccine may not prevent hepatitis A infection in individuals who have an unrecognized hepatitis A infection at the time of vaccination. Additionally, it may not prevent infection in individuals who do not achieve protective antibody titers (although the lowest titer needed to confer protection has not been determined).

PRECAUTIONS

General

As with any parenteral vaccine, epinephrine should be available for use in case of anaphylaxis or anaphylactoid reaction.
As with any vaccine, administration of *Havrix* should be delayed, if possible, in people with any febrile illness, except when, in the opinion of the physician, withholding vaccine entails the greater risk.
Havrix should be administered with caution to people with thrombocytopenia or a bleeding disorder since bleeding may occur following an intramuscular administration to these subjects.
As with any vaccine, if administered to immunosuppressed persons or persons receiving immunosuppressive therapy, the expected immune response may not be obtained.[19]
Care is to be taken by the health-care provider for the safe and effective use of *Havrix*.
Prior to an injection of any vaccine, all known precautions should be taken to prevent adverse reactions. This includes a review of the patient's history with respect to possible hypersensitivity to the vaccine or similar vaccines.
A separate sterile syringe and needle (for single-dose vial) or a sterile disposable unit (prefilled syringe) must be used for each patient to prevent the transmission of infectious agents from person to person. Needles should not be recapped and should be properly disposed.
Special care should be taken to ensure that *Havrix* is not injected into a blood vessel.

Information for Patients

Patients, parents or guardians should be fully informed of the benefits and risks of immunization with *Havrix*.
Havrix is indicated in a variety of situations (see INDICATIONS AND USAGE). For persons traveling to endemic or epidemic areas, current CDC advisories should be consulted with regard to specific locales.
Travelers should take all necessary precautions to avoid contact with or ingestion of contaminated food or water.
The duration of immunity following a complete schedule of immunization with *Havrix* has not been established.

Drug Interactions

Preliminary results suggest that the concomitant administration of a wide variety of other vaccines is unlikely to interfere with the immune response to *Havrix*.
As with other intramuscular injections, *Havrix* should be given with caution to individuals on anticoagulant therapy.
When concomitant administration of other vaccines or IG is required, they should be given with different syringes and at different injection sites.

Carcinogenesis, Mutagenesis, Impairment of Fertility

Havrix has not been evaluated for its carcinogenic potential, mutagenic potential or potential for impairment of fertility.

Pregnancy: Pregnancy Category C.

Animal reproduction studies have not been conducted with *Havrix*. It is also not known whether *Havrix* can cause fetal harm when administered to a pregnant woman or can affect reproduction capacity. *Havrix* should be given to a pregnant woman only if clearly needed.

Nursing Mothers

It is not known whether *Havrix* is excreted in human milk. Because many drugs are excreted in human milk, caution should be exercised when *Havrix* is administered to a nursing woman.

Pediatric Use

Havrix is well tolerated and highly immunogenic and effective in children ≥2 years of age. (See CLINICAL PHARMACOLOGY for immunogenicity and efficacy data. See DOSAGE AND ADMINISTRATION for recommended dosage.)

ADVERSE REACTIONS

During clinical trials involving more than 31,000 individuals receiving doses ranging from 360 EL.U. to 1440 EL.U. and during extensive postmarketing experience in Europe, Havrix (Hepatitis A Vaccine, Inactivated) has been generally well tolerated. As with all pharmaceuticals, however, it is possible that expanded commercial use of the vaccine could reveal rare adverse events not observed in clinical studies.
The frequency of solicited adverse events tended to decrease with successive doses of *Havrix*. Most events reported were considered by the subjects as mild and did not last for more than 24 hours.
Of solicited adverse events in clinical trials, the most frequently reported by volunteers was injection-site soreness (56% of adults and 21% of children); however, less than 0.5% of soreness was reported as severe. Headache was reported by 14% of adults and less than 9% of children. Other solicited and unsolicited events occurring during clinical trials are listed below:

Incidence 1% to 10% of Injections

Local reactions at injection site: induration, redness, swelling.
Body as a whole: fatigue, fever (>37.5°C), malaise.
Gastrointestinal: anorexia, nausea.

Incidence <1% of Injections

Local reaction at injection site: hematoma.
Dermatologic: pruritus, rash, urticaria.
Respiratory: pharyngitis, other upper respiratory tract infections.
Gastrointestinal: abdominal pain, diarrhea, dysgeusia, vomiting.
Musculoskeletal: arthralgia, elevation of creatine phosphokinase, myalgia.
Hematologic: lymphadenopathy.
Central nervous system: hypertonic episode, insomnia, photophobia, vertigo.

Additional Safety Data

Safety data were obtained from two additional sources in which large populations were vaccinated. In an outbreak setting in which 4,930 individuals were immunized with a single dose of either 720 EL.U. or 1440 EL.U. of *Havrix*, the vaccine was well-tolerated and no serious adverse events due to vaccination were reported. Overall, less than 10% of vaccinees reported solicited general adverse events following the vaccine. The most common solicited local adverse event was pain at the injection site, reported in 22.3% of subjects at 24 hours and decreasing to 2.4% by 72 hours.
In a field efficacy trial, 19,037 children received the 360 EL.U. dose of *Havrix*. The most commonly reported adverse events following administration of *Havrix* were injection-site pain (9.5%) and tenderness (8.1%), which were reported following first doses of *Havrix*. Other adverse events were infrequent and comparable to the control vaccine *Engerix-B*. Additionally, no serious adverse events due to the vaccine were reported. The large trial further allowed for analysis of rare adverse events, including hospitalization and death. No significant differences were found between the cohorts.
In subjects with chronic liver disease, *Havrix* was safe and well-tolerated. Local injection site reactions were similar among all four groups and no serious adverse reactions attributed to the vaccine were reported in subjects with chronic liver disease.

Postmarketing Reports

Rare voluntary reports of adverse events in people receiving *Havrix* that have been reported since market introduction of the vaccine include the following:
Local: localized edema.
While no causal relationship has been established, the following rare events have been reported:
Body as a whole: anaphylaxis/anaphylactoid reactions, somnolence.
Cardiovascular: syncope.
Hepatobiliary: jaundice, hepatitis.
Dermatologic: erythema multiforme, hyperhydrosis, angioedema.
Respiratory: dyspnea.
Hematologic: lymphadenopathy.
Central nervous system: convulsions, encephalopathy, dizziness, neuropathy, myelitis, paresthesia, Guillain-Barré syndrome, multiple sclerosis.
Other: congenital abnormality.

Reporting of Adverse Events

The U.S. Department of Health and Human Services has established the Vaccine Adverse Events Reporting System (VAERS) to accept reports of suspected adverse events after the administration of any vaccine, including, but not limited to, the reporting of events required by the National Childhood Vaccine Injury Act of 1986. The toll-free number for VAERS forms and information is 1-800-822-7967.[20]

DOSAGE AND ADMINISTRATION

Havrix should be administered by intramuscular injection. *Do not inject intravenously, intradermally or subcutaneously.* In adults, the injection should be given in the deltoid region. *Havrix* should not be administered in the gluteal region; such injections may result in suboptimal response.
Havrix may be administered concomitantly with IG, although the ultimate antibody titer obtained is likely to be lower than when the vaccine is given alone. *Havrix* has been administered simultaneously with *Engerix-B* without interference with their respective immune responses.
For individuals with clotting-factor disorders who are at risk of hemorrhage following intramuscular injection, the ACIP recommends that when any intramuscular vaccine is indicated for such patients, "...it should be administered intramuscularly if, in the opinion of a physician familiar with the patient's bleeding risk, the vaccine can be administered with reasonable safety by this route. If the patient receives antihemophilia or other similar therapy, intramuscular vaccination can be scheduled shortly after such therapy is administered. A fine needle (≤23 gauge) can be used for the vaccination and firm pressure applied to the site (without rubbing) for at least two minutes. The patient or family should be instructed concerning the risk of hematoma from the injection."[21]
When concomitant administration of other vaccines or IG is required, they should be given with different syringes and at different injection sites.
Preparation for Administration: Shake vial or syringe well before withdrawal and use. Parenteral drug products should be inspected visually for particulate matter or discoloration prior to administration. With thorough agitation, *Havrix* is a turbid white suspension. Discard if it appears otherwise.
The vaccine should be used as supplied; no dilution or reconstitution is necessary. The full recommended dose of the vaccine should be used. After removal of the appropriate volume from a single-dose vial, any vaccine remaining in the vial should be discarded.
Primary immunization for adults consists of a single dose of 1440 EL.U. in 1 mL. Primary immunization for children and adolescents (2 through 18 years of age) may follow either of these two schedules:

Group	Dose	Schedule
Children and adolescents (2 through 18 years of age)	Primary course: 360 EL.U./0.5 mL	two doses, given 1 month apart (month 0 and month 1)
	Booster: 360 EL.U./0.5 mL	6 to 12 months after primary course
	OR	
	Primary course: 720 EL.U./0.5 mL	one dose (month 0)
	Booster: 720 EL.U./0.5 mL	6 to 12 months after primary course

Individuals should not be alternated between the 360 EL.U. and 720 EL.U. doses. Those who receive an initial 360 EL.U. dose should continue on the 360 EL.U. dosing schedule. Likewise, those individuals who receive a single 720 EL.U. primary dose should receive a 720 EL.U. booster dose.
For all age groups, a booster dose is recommended anytime between 6 and 12 months after the initiation of the primary dose in order to ensure the highest antibody titers.
In those with an impaired immune system, adequate anti-HAV response may not be obtained after the primary immunization course. Such patients may therefore require administration of additional doses of vaccine.

STORAGE

Store between 2° and 8°C (36° and 46°F). Do not freeze; discard if product has been frozen. Do not dilute to administer.

HOW SUPPLIED

360 EL.U./0.5 mL in Single-Dose Vials
NDC 58160-836-01 Package of 1
720 EL.U./0.5 mL in Single-Dose Vials and Prefilled Syringes
NDC 58160-837-01 Package of 1 Single-Dose Vial
NDC 58160-837-02 Package of 1 Prefilled Syringe
NDC 58160-837-05 Package of 5 Prefilled Syringes with 5/8-inch 25-gauge needles
NDC 58160-837-11 Package of 10 Single-Dose Vials
NDC 58160-837-26 Package of 25 Prefilled Disposable Tip-Lok® Syringes with 5/8-inch 25-gauge needles

Continued on next page

Information on the SmithKline Beecham Pharmaceuticals products appearing here is based on the labeling in effect on June 15, 2000. Further information on these and other products may be obtained from the Medical Department, SmithKline Beecham Pharmaceuticals, One Franklin Plaza, Philadelphia, PA 19101.

Havrix—Cont.

NDC 58160-837-35 Package of 5 Prefilled Disposable Tip-Lok® Syringes with 5/8-inch 25-gauge needles
1440 EL.U./mL in Single-Dose Vials, Prefilled Syringes and Multi-Dose Vials
NDC 58160-835-01 Package of 1 Single-Dose Vial
NDC 58160-835-05 Package of 5 Prefilled Syringes with 1-inch 23-gauge needles
NDC 58160-835-07 Package of 1 Multi-Dose Vial, containing 10 doses
NDC 58160-835-32 Package of 1 Prefilled Disposable Tip-Lok® Syringe with 1-inch 23-gauge needle
NDC 58160-835-35 Package of 5 Prefilled Disposable Tip-Lok® Syringes with 1-inch 23-gauge needles

REFERENCES

1. Hadler SC: Global impact of hepatitis A virus infection changing patterns. In Hollinger FB, Lemon SM, Margolis H (eds): *Viral Hepatitis and Liver Disease.* Baltimore, Williams & Wilkins, 1991, pp. 14-20. **2.** Dienstag JL, Routenberg JA, Purcell RH, et al: Foodhandler-associated outbreak of hepatitis type A. An immune electron microscopic study. *Ann Intern Med.* 1975;83:647. **3.** Mackowiak PA, Caraway CT, Portnoy BL: Oyster-associated hepatitis. Lessons from the Louisiana experience. *Am J Epidemiol.* 1976;103:181. **4.** Woodson RD, Clinton JJ: Hepatitis prophylaxis abroad. Effectiveness of immune serum globulin in protecting Peace Corps volunteers. *JAMA.* 1969;1009:1053. **5.** Krugman S, Giles JP: Viral hepatitis. New light on an old disease. *JAMA.* 1970;212:1019. **6.** Mosley JW: Hepatitis types B and non-B. Epidemiologic background. *JAMA.* 1975;233:967. **7.** Hadler SC, Erben JJ, Francis DP, et al: Risk factors for hepatitis A in daycare centers. *J Infect Dis.* 1982;145:255. **8.** Shapiro CN, Shaw SE, Mandel EJ, Hadler SC: Epidemiology of hepatitis A in the United States. In Hollinger FB, Lemon SM, Margolis H (eds): *Viral Hepatitis and Liver Disease.* Baltimore, Williams & Wilkins, 1991, pp. 71-76. **9.** Centers for Disease Control: Protection against viral hepatitis: Recommendations of the Immunization Practices Advisory Committee (ACIP). *MMWR.* 1990;39(No. RR-2):1-26. **10.** Lemon SM: Type A viral hepatitis: new developments in an old disease. *N Engl J Med.* Oct. 24, 1985;313(17):1059-1067. **11.** Sjogren MH, Tanno H, Fay O, et al: Hepatitis A virus in stool during clinical relapse. *Ann Intern Med.* 1987;106:221-226. **12.** Hollinger FB, Ticehurst J: Hepatitis A Virus. In Hollinger FB, Robinson WS, Purcell RH, et al (eds): *Viral Hepatitis.* New York, Raven Press, 1990, pp. 1-37. **13.** Tassopoulos NC, Papaevangelou GJ, Ticehurst JR, et al: Fecal excretion of Greek strains of hepatitis A virus in patients with hepatitis A and in experimentally infected chimpanzees. *J Infect Dis.* 1986; 154:231-237. **14.** Chiriaco P, Gaudalupi C, Armigliato MK, et al: Polyphasic course of hepatitis type A in children. *J Infect Dis.* 1986; 153:378. **15.** Data on file, SmithKline Beecham Pharmaceuticals. **16.** Innis BL, Snitbhan R, Kunasol P, et al: Protection against hepatitis A by an inactivated vaccine. *JAMA.* 1994;271(17):1328-1364. **17.** Centers for Disease Control and Prevention: 1998 Guidelines for treatment of sexually transmitted diseases. *MMWR* 1998; 47 (No. RR-1): 100. **18.** Centers for Disease Control and Prevention: Prevention of hepatitis A through active or passive immunization. Recommendations of the Advisory Committee on Immunization Practices (ACIP). *MMWR.* 1996; 45(No. RR-15): 21–23. **19.** ACIP: Use of vaccines and immune globulins in persons with altered immunocompetence. *MMWR.* 1993;42 (No. RR-4). **20.** Centers for Disease Control: Vaccine Adverse Event Reporting System—United States. *MMWR.* 1990;39:730–733. **21.** Centers for Disease Control and Prevention: General recommendations on immunization. Recommendations of the Advisory Committee on Immunization Practices (ACIP). *MMWR.* 1994;43(No. RR-1):23.

U.S. License No. 1090
Manufactured by **SmithKline Beecham Biologicals**
Rixensart, Belgium
Distributed by **SmithKline Beecham Pharmaceuticals**
Philadelphia, PA 19101
Havrix and *Tip-Lok* are registered trademarks of SmithKline Beecham.
Rx only
HA:L13

Shown in Product Identification Guide, page 337

HYCAMTIN® ℞

[hī-kam-tin]
brand of topotecan hydrochloride for Injection (for intravenous use)

WARNING

Hycamtin (topotecan hydrochloride) for Injection should be administered under the supervision of a physician experienced in the use of cancer chemotherapeutic agents. Appropriate management of complications is possible only when adequate diagnostic and treatment facilities are readily available.
Therapy with *Hycamtin* should not be given to patients with baseline neutrophil counts of less than 1500 cells/mm^3. In order to monitor the occurrence of bone marrow suppression, primarily neutropenia, which may be severe and result in infection and death, frequent peripheral blood cell counts should be performed on all patients receiving *Hycamtin.*

Table 1. Efficacy of Hycamtin (topotecan hydrochloride) vs. Paclitaxel in Ovarian Cancer

Parameter	*Hycamtin* (n=112)		Paclitaxel (n=114)
Complete Response Rate	5%		3%
Partial Response Rate	16%		11%
Overall Response Rate	21%		14%
95% Confidence Interval	13 to 28%		8 to 20%
(p-value)		(0.20)	
Response Duration (weeks)	n=23		n=16
Median	25.9		21.6
95% Confidence Interval	22.1 to 32.9		16.0 to 34.0
hazard-ratio (*Hycamtin:* paclitaxel)		0.78	
(p-value)		(0.48)	
Time to Progression (weeks)			
Median	18.9		14.7
95% Confidence Interval	12.1 to 23.6		11.9 to 18.3
hazard-ratio (*Hycamtin:* paclitaxel)		0.76	
(p-value)		(0.07)	
Survival (weeks)			
Median	63.0		53.0
95% Confidence Interval	46.6 to 71.9		42.3 to 68.7
hazard-ratio (*Hycamtin:* paclitaxel)		0.97	
(p-value)		(0.87)	

The calculation for duration of response was based on the interval between first response and time to progression.

Table 2. Efficacy of Hycamtin (topotecan hydrochloride) vs CAV (cyclophosphamide-doxorubicin-vincristine) in Small Cell Lung Cancer Patients Sensitive to First-Line Chemotherapy

Parameter	*Hycamtin* (n=107)		CAV (n=104)
Complete Response Rate	0%		1%
Partial Response Rate	24%		17%
Overall Response Rate	24%		18%
Difference in Overall Response Rates		6%	
95% Confidence Interval of the Difference		(−6 to 18%)	
Response Duration (weeks)	n=26		n=19
Median	14.4		15.3
95% Confidence Interval	13.1 to 18.0		13.1 to 23.1
hazard-ratio (*Hycamtin*:CAV)		1.42 (0.73 to 2.76)	
(p-value)		(0.30)	
Time to Progression (weeks)			
Median	13.3		12.3
95% Confidence Interval	11.4 to 16.4		11.0 to 14.1
hazard-ratio (*Hycamtin*:CAV)		0.92 (0.69 to 1.22)	
(p-value)		(0.55)	
Survival (weeks)			
Median	25.0		24.7
95% Confidence Interval	20.6 to 29.6		21.7 to 30.3
hazard-ratio (*Hycamtin*:CAV)		1.04 (0.78 to 1.39)	
(p-value)		(0.80)	

The calculation for duration of response was based on the interval between first response and time to progression.

DESCRIPTION

Hycamtin (topotecan hydrochloride) is a semi-synthetic derivative of camptothecin and is an anti-tumor drug with topoisomerase I-inhibitory activity.
Hycamtin (topotecan hydrochloride) for Injection is supplied as a sterile lyophilized, buffered, light yellow to greenish powder available in single-dose vials. Each vial contains topotecan hydrochloride equivalent to 4 mg of topotecan as free base. The reconstituted solution ranges in color from yellow to yellow-green and is intended for administration by intravenous infusion.
Inactive ingredients are mannitol, 48 mg, and tartaric acid, 20 mg. Hydrochloric acid and sodium hydroxide may be used to adjust the pH. The solution pH ranges from 2.5 to 3.5.
The chemical name for topotecan hydrochloride is (*S*)-10-[(dimethylamino)methyl]-4-ethyl-4,9-dihydroxy-1*H*-pyrano [3′,4′:6,7] indolizino [1,2-*b*]quinoline-3,14-(4*H*,12*H*)-dione monohydrochloride. It has the molecular formula $C_{23}H_{23}N_3O_5 \bullet HCl$ and a molecular weight of 457.9.
Topotecan hydrochloride has the following structural formula:
[See chemical structure at top of next column]
It is soluble in water and melts with decomposition at 213° to 218°C.

CLINICAL PHARMACOLOGY

Mechanism of Action

Topoisomerase I relieves torsional strain in DNA by inducing reversible single strand breaks. Topotecan binds to the topoisomerase I-DNA complex and prevents religation of these single strand breaks. The cytotoxicity of topotecan is thought to be due to double strand DNA damage produced during DNA synthesis when replication enzymes interact with the ternary complex formed by topotecan, topoisomerase I and DNA. Mammalian cells cannot efficiently repair these double strand breaks.

Pharmacokinetics

The pharmacokinetics of topotecan have been evaluated in cancer patients following doses of 0.5 to 1.5 mg/m^2 administered as a 30-minute infusion. Topotecan exhibits multiexponential pharmacokinetics with a terminal half-life of 2 to

3 hours. Total exposure (AUC) is approximately dose-proportional. Binding of topotecan to plasma proteins is about 35%.

Metabolism and Elimination: Topotecan undergoes a reversible pH dependent hydrolysis of its lactone moiety; it is the lactone form that is pharmacologically active. At pH≤4 the lactone is exclusively present whereas the ring-opened hydroxy-acid form predominates at physiologic pH. *In vitro* studies in human liver microsomes indicate that metabolism of topotecan to a N-demethylated metabolite represents a minor metabolic pathway.

In humans, about 30% of the dose is excreted in the urine and renal clearance is an important determinant of topotecan elimination (see Special Populations).

Special Populations

Gender: The overall mean topotecan plasma clearance in male patients was approximately 24% higher than in female patients, largely reflecting difference in body size.

Geriatrics: Topotecan pharmacokinetics have not been specifically studied in an elderly population, but population pharmacokinetic analysis in female patients did not identify age as a significant factor. Decreased renal clearance, common in the elderly, is a more important determinant of topotecan clearance.

Race: The effect of race on topotecan pharmacokinetics has not been studied.

Renal Impairment: In patients with mild renal impairment (creatinine clearance of 40 to 60 mL/min.), topotecan plasma clearance was decreased to about 67% of the value in patients with normal renal function. In patients with moderate renal impairment (Cl_{cr} of 20 to 39 mL/min.), topotecan plasma clearance was reduced to about 34% of the value in control patients, with an increase in half-life. Mean half-life, estimated in three renally impaired patients, was about 5.0 hours. Dosage adjustment is recommended for these patients (see DOSAGE AND ADMINISTRATION).

Hepatic Impairment: Plasma clearance in patients with hepatic impairment (serum bilirubin levels between 1.7 and 15.0 mg/dL) was decreased to about 67% of the value in patients without hepatic impairment. Topotecan half-life increased slightly, from 2.0 hours to 2.5 hours, but these hepatically impaired patients tolerated the usual recommended topotecan dosage regimen (see DOSAGE AND ADMINISTRATION).

Drug Interactions: Pharmacokinetic studies of the interaction of topotecan with concomitantly administered medications have not been formally investigated. *In vitro* inhibition studies using marker substrates known to be metabolized by human P450 CYP1A2, CYP2A6, CYP2C8/9, CYP2C19, CYP2D6, CYP2E, CYP3A, or CYP4A or dihydropyrimidine dehydrogenase indicate that the activities of these enzymes were not altered by topotecan. Enzyme inhibition by topotecan has not been evaluated *in vivo*.

Pharmacodynamics: The dose-limiting toxicity of topotecan is leukopenia. White blood cell count decreases with increasing topotecan dose or topotecan AUC. When topotecan is administered at a dose of 1.5 mg/m²/day for 5 days, an 80% to 90% decrease in white blood cell count at nadir is typically observed after the first cycle of therapy.

CLINICAL STUDIES

Ovarian Cancer

Hycamtin (topotecan hydrochloride) was studied in two clinical trials of 223 patients given topotecan with metastatic ovarian carcinoma. All patients had disease that had recurred on, or was unresponsive to, a platinum-containing regimen. Patients in these two studies received an initial dose of 1.5 mg/m² given by intravenous infusion over 30 minutes for 5 consecutive days, starting on day 1 of a 21-day course.

One study was a randomized trial of 112 patients treated with *Hycamtin* (1.5 mg/m²/day × 5 days starting on day 1 of a 21-day course) and 114 patients treated with paclitaxel (175 mg/m² over 3 hours on day 1 of a 21-day course). All patients had recurrent ovarian cancer after a platinum-containing regimen or had not responded to at least one prior platinum-containing regimen. Patients who did not respond to the study therapy, or who progressed, could be given the alternative treatment.

Response rates, response duration and time to progression are shown in Table 1.

[See table 1 at top of previous page]

The median time to response was 7.6 weeks (range 3.1 to 21.7) with *Hycamtin* compared to 6.0 weeks (range 2.4 to 18.1) with paclitaxel. Consequently, the efficacy of *Hycamtin* may not be achieved if patients are withdrawn from treatment prematurely.

In the crossover phase, 8 of 61 (13%) patients who received *Hycamtin* after paclitaxel had a partial response and 5 of 49 (10%) patients who received paclitaxel after *Hycamtin* had a response (two complete responses).

Hycamtin was active in ovarian cancer patients who had developed resistance to platinum-containing therapy, defined as tumor progression while on, or tumor relapse within 6 months after completion of, a platinum-containing regimen. One complete and six partial responses were seen in 60 patients, for a response rate of 12%. In the same study, there were no complete responders and four partial responders on the paclitaxel arm, for a response rate of 7%.

Hycamtin was also studied in an open-label, non-comparative trial in 111 patients with recurrent ovarian cancer after treatment with a platinum-containing regimen, or who had not responded to one prior platinum-containing regimen. The response rate was 14% (95% CI=7% to 20%). The median duration of response was 22 weeks (range 4.6 to 41.9 weeks). The time to progression was 11.3 weeks (range 0.7 to 72.1 weeks). The median survival was 67.9 weeks (range 1.4 to 112.9 weeks).

Small Cell Lung Cancer

Hycamtin (topotecan hydrochloride) was studied in 426 patients with recurrent or progressive small cell lung cancer in one randomized, comparative study and in three single arm studies.

Randomized Comparative Study

In a randomized, comparative, Phase 3 trial, 107 patients were treated with *Hycamtin* (1.5 mg/m²/day × 5 days starting on day 1 of a 21-day course) and 104 patients were treated with CAV (1000 mg/m² cyclophosphamide, 45 mg/m² doxorubicin, 2 mg vincristine administered sequentially on day 1 of a 21-day course). All patients were considered sensitive to first-line chemotherapy (responders who then subsequently progressed ≥60 days after completion of first-line therapy). A total of 77% of patients treated with *Hycamtin* and 79% of patients treated with CAV received platinum/etoposide with or without other agents as first-line chemotherapy.

Response rates, response duration, time to progression, and survival are shown in Table 2.

[See table 2 at top of previous page]

Table 3. Percentage of Patients with Symptom Improvement*: *Hycamtin* versus CAV in Patients with Small Cell Lung Cancer

Symptom	*Hycamtin* (n=107) n**	(%)	CAV (n=104) n**	(%)
Shortness of Breath	68	(28)	61	(7)
Interference with Daily Activity	67	(27)	63	(11)
Fatigue	70	(23)	65	(9)
Hoarseness	40	(33)	38	(13)
Cough	69	(25)	61	(15)
Insomnia	57	(33)	53	(19)
Anorexia	56	(32)	57	(16)
Chest Pain	44	(25)	41	(17)
Hemoptysis	15	(27)	12	(33)

* Defined as improvement sustained over at least two courses compared to baseline.
**Number of patients with baseline and at least one post-baseline assessment.

Table 4. Summary of Hematologic Adverse Events in Patients Receiving *Hycamtin*

Hematologic Adverse Events	Patients n = 879 % Incidence	Courses n = 4124 % Incidence
Neutropenia		
<1,500 cells/mm³	97	81
<500 cells/mm³	78	39
Leukopenia		
<3,000 cells/mm³	97	80
<1,000 cells/mm³	32	11
Thrombocytopenia		
<75,000 cells/mm³	69	42
<25,000 cells/mm³	27	9
Anemia		
<10 g/dL	89	71
<8 g/dL	37	14
Sepsis or fever/infection with grade 4 neutropenia	23	7
Platelet transfusions	15	4
RBC transfusions	52	22

Table 5. Summary of Non-hematologic Adverse Events in Patients Receiving Hycamtin (topotecan hydrochloride)

Non-hematologic Adverse Events	All Grades % Incidence		Grade 3 % Incidence		Grade 4 % Incidence	
	n = 879 Patients	n = 4124 Courses	n = 879 Patients	n = 4124 Courses	n = 879 Patients	n = 4124 Courses
Gastrointestinal						
Nausea	64	42	7	2	1	<1
Vomiting	45	22	4	1	1	<1
Diarrhea	32	14	3	1	1	<1
Constipation	29	15	2	1	1	<1
Abdominal Pain	22	10	2	1	2	<1
Stomatitis	18	8	1	<1	<1	<1
Anorexia	19	9	2	1	<1	<1
Body as a Whole						
Fatigue	29	22	5	2	0	0
Fever	28	11	1	<1	<1	<1
Pain*	23	11	2	1	1	<1
Asthenia	25	13	4	1	2	<1
Skin/Appendages						
Alopecia	49	54	NA	NA	NA	NA
Rash**	16	6	1	<1	0	0
Respiratory System						
Dyspnea	22	11	5	2	3	1
Coughing	15	7	1	<1	0	0
CNS/Peripheral Nervous System						
Headache	18	7	1	<1	<1	0

* Pain includes body pain, back pain and skeletal pain.
**Rash also includes pruritus, rash erythematous, urticaria, dermatitis, bullous eruption and rash maculopapular.

Continued on next page

Information on the SmithKline Beecham Pharmaceuticals products appearing here is based on the labeling in effect on June 15, 2000. Further information on these and other products may be obtained from the Medical Department, SmithKline Beecham Pharmaceuticals, One Franklin Plaza, Philadelphia, PA 19101.

Hycamtin—Cont.

The time to response was similar in both arms: *Hycamtin* median of 6 weeks (range 2.4 to 15.7) versus CAV median 6 weeks (range 5.1 to 18.1).
Changes on a disease-related symptom scale in patients who received *Hycamtin* or who received CAV are presented in Table 3. It should be noted that not all patients had all symptoms nor did all patients respond to all questions. Each symptom was rated on a four category scale with an improvement defined as a change in one category from baseline sustained over two courses. Limitations in interpretation of the rating scale and responses preclude formal statistical analysis.
[See table 3 at top of previous page]

Single Arm Studies
Hycamtin (topotecan hydrochloride) was also studied in three open-label, non-comparative trials in a total of 319 patients with recurrent or progressive small cell lung cancer after treatment with first-line chemotherapy. In all three studies, patients were stratified as either sensitive (responders who then subsequently progressed ≥90 days after completion of first-line therapy) or refractory (no response to first-line chemotherapy or who responded to first-line therapy and then progressed within 90 days of completing first-line therapy). Response rates ranged from 11% to 31% for sensitive patients and 2% to 7% for refractory patients. Median time to progression and median survival were similar in all three studies and the comparative study.

INDICATIONS AND USAGE

Hycamtin is indicated for the treatment of:
- metastatic carcinoma of the ovary after failure of initial or subsequent chemotherapy.
- small cell lung cancer sensitive disease after failure of first-line chemotherapy. In clinical studies submitted to support approval, sensitive disease was defined as disease responding to chemotherapy but subsequently progressing at least 60 days (in the Phase 3 study) or at least 90 days (in the Phase 2 studies) after chemotherapy (See Clinical Studies Section).

CONTRAINDICATIONS

Hycamtin is contraindicated in patients who have a history of hypersensitivity reactions to topotecan or to any of its ingredients. *Hycamtin* should not be used in patients who are pregnant or breast-feeding, or those with severe bone marrow depression.

WARNINGS

Bone marrow suppression (primarily neutropenia) is the dose-limiting toxicity of topotecan. Neutropenia is not cumulative over time. The following data on myelosuppression with topotecan is based on the combined experience of 879 patients with metastatic ovarian cancer or small cell lung cancer.
Neutropenia: Grade 4 neutropenia (<500 cells/mm^3) was most common during course 1 of treatment (60% of patients) and occurred in 39% of all courses, with a median duration of 7 days. The nadir neutrophil count occurred at a median of 12 days. Therapy-related sepsis or febrile neutropenia occurred in 23% of patients and sepsis was fatal in 1%.
Thrombocytopenia: Grade 4 thrombocytopenia (<25,000/mm^3) occurred in 27% of patients and in 9% of courses, with a median duration of 5 days and platelet nadir at a median of 15 days. Platelet transfusions were given to 15% of patients in 4% of courses.
Anemia: Grade 3/4 anemia (<8 g/dL) occurred in 37% of patients and in 14% of courses. Median nadir was at day 15. Transfusions were needed in 52% of patients in 22% of courses.
In ovarian cancer, the overall treatment-related death rate was 1%. In the comparative study in small cell lung cancer, however, the treatment-related death rates were 5% for *Hycamtin* and 4% for CAV.
Monitoring of Bone Marrow Function: *Hycamtin* should only be administered in patients with adequate bone marrow reserves, including baseline neutrophil count of at least 1,500 cells/mm^3 and platelet count at least 100,000/mm^3. Frequent monitoring of peripheral blood cell counts should be instituted during treatment with *Hycamtin*. Patients should not be treated with subsequent courses of *Hycamtin* until neutrophils recover to >1,000 cells/mm^3, platelets recover to >100,000 cells/mm^3 and hemoglobin levels recover to 9.0 g/dL (with transfusion if necessary). Severe myelotoxicity has been reported when *Hycamtin* is used in combination with cisplatin (see Drug Interactions).
Pregnancy: *Hycamtin* may cause fetal harm when administered to a pregnant woman. The effects of topotecan on pregnant women have not been studied. If topotecan is used during a patient's pregnancy, or if a patient becomes pregnant while taking topotecan, she should be warned of the potential hazard to the fetus. Fecund women should be warned to avoid becoming pregnant. In rabbits, a dose of 0.10 mg/kg/day (about equal to the clinical dose on a mg/m^2 basis) given on days 6 through 20 of gestation caused maternal toxicity, embryolethality, and reduced fetal body weight. In the rat, a dose of 0.23 mg/kg/day (about equal to the clinical dose on a mg/m^2 basis) given for 14 days before mating through gestation day 6 caused fetal resorption, microphthalmia, pre-implant loss, and mild maternal toxicity. A dose of 0.10 mg/kg/day (about half the clinical dose on a mg/m^2 basis) given to rats on days 6 through 17 of gestation caused an increase in post-implantation mortality. This dose also caused an increase in total fetal malformations. The most frequent malformations were of the eye (microphthalmia, anophthalmia, rosette formation of the retina, coloboma of the retina, ectopic orbit), brain (dilated lateral and third ventricles), skull and vertebrae.

Table 6. Comparative Toxicity Profiles for Ovarian Cancer Patients Randomized to Receive *Hycamtin* or Paclitaxel

Adverse Event	Hycamtin		Paclitaxel	
	Pts	Courses	Pts	Courses
	n=112	n=597	n=114	n=589
Hematologic Grade 3/4	%	%	%	%
Grade 4 Neutropenia (<500 cells/mL)	80	36	21	9
Grade 3/4 Anemia (Hgb < 8 g/dL)	41	16	6	2
Grade 4 Thrombocytopenia (<25,000 plts/mL)	27	10	3	<1
Fever/Grade 4 Neutropenia	23	6	4	1
Documented Sepsis	5	1	2	<1
Death related to Sepsis	2	NA	0	NA
Non-hematologic Grade 3/4				
Gastrointestinal				
Abdominal Pain	5	1	4	1
Constipation	5	1	0	0
Diarrhea	6	2	1	<1
Intestinal Obstruction	5	1	4	1
Nausea	10	3	2	<1
Stomatitis	1	<1	1	<1
Vomiting	10	2	3	<1
Constitutional				
Anorexia	4	1	0	0
Dyspnea	6	2	5	1
Fatigue	7	2	6	2
Malaise	2	<1	2	<1
Neuromuscular				
Arthralgia	1	<1	3	<1
Asthenia	5	2	3	1
Chest Pain	2	<1	1	<1
Headache	1	<1	2	1
Myalgia	0	0	3	2
Pain*	5	1	7	2
Skin/Appendages				
Rash**	0	0	1	<1
Liver/Biliary				
Increased Hepatic Enzymes†	1	<1	1	<1

* Pain includes body pain, skeletal pain and back pain.
** Rash also includes pruritus, rash erythematous, urticaria, dermatitis, bullous eruption and rash maculopapular.
† Increased hepatic enzymes includes increased SGOT/AST, increased SGPT/ALT and increased hepatic enzymes.

PRECAUTIONS

General: Inadvertent extravasation with Hycamtin (topotecan hydrochloride) has been associated only with mild local reactions such as erythema and bruising.
Hematology: Monitoring of bone marrow function is essential (see WARNINGS and DOSAGE AND ADMINISTRATION).
Carcinogenesis, Mutagenesis, Impairment of Fertility: Carcinogenicity testing of topotecan has not been performed. Topotecan, however, is known to be genotoxic to mammalian cells and is a probable carcinogen. Topotecan was mutagenic to L5178Y mouse lymphoma cells and clastogenic to cultured human lymphocytes with and without metabolic activation. It was also clastogenic to mouse bone marrow. Topotecan did not cause mutations in bacterial cells.
Drug Interactions: Concomitant administration of G-CSF can prolong the duration of neutropenia, so if G-CSF is to be used, it should not be initiated until day 6 of the course of therapy, 24 hours after completion of treatment with *Hycamtin*.[1]
Myelosuppression was more severe when *Hycamtin* was given in combination with cisplatin in Phase I studies. In a reported study on concomitant administration of cisplatin 50 mg/m^2 and *Hycamtin* at a dose of 1.25 mg/m^2/day × 5 days, one of three patients had severe neutropenia for 12 days and a second patient died with neutropenic sepsis. There are no adequate data to define a safe and effective regimen for *Hycamtin* and cisplatin in combination.
Pregnancy: Pregnancy Category D. (See WARNINGS.)
Nursing Mothers: It is not known whether the drug is excreted in human milk. Breast-feeding should be discontinued when women are receiving *Hycamtin* (see CONTRAINDICATIONS).
Pediatric Use: Safety and effectiveness in pediatric patients have not been established.

ADVERSE REACTIONS

Data in the following section are based on the combined experience of 453 patients with metastatic ovarian carcinoma, and 426 patients with small cell lung cancer treated with *Hycamtin*. Table 4 lists the principal hematologic toxicities and Table 5 lists non-hematologic toxicities occurring in at least 15% of patients.
[See table 4 at top of previous page]
[See table 5 at top of previous page]
Premedications were not routinely used in these clinical studies.
Hematologic: (See WARNINGS.)
Gastrointestinal: The incidence of nausea was 64% (8% grade 3/4) and vomiting occurred in 45% (6% grade 3/4) of patients (see Table 5). The prophylactic use of antiemetics

was not routine in patients treated with *Hycamtin*. Thirty-two percent of patients had diarrhea (4% grade 3/4), 29% constipation (2% grade 3/4) and 22% had abdominal pain (4% grade 3/4). Grade 3/4 abdominal pain was 6% in ovarian cancer patients and 2% in small cell lung cancer patients.

Skin/Appendages: Total alopecia (grade 2) occurred in 31% of patients.

Central and Peripheral Nervous System: Headache (18% of patients) was the most frequently reported neurologic toxicity. Paresthesia occurred in 7% of patients but was generally grade 1.

Liver/Biliary: Grade 1 transient elevations in hepatic enzymes occurred in 8% of patients. Greater elevations, grade 3/4, occurred in 4%. Grade 3/4 elevated bilirubin occurred in <2% of patients.

Respiratory: The incidence of grade 3/4 dyspnea was 4% in ovarian cancer patients and 12% in small cell lung cancer patients.

Table 6 shows the grade 3/4 hematologic and major non-hematologic adverse events in the topotecan/paclitaxel comparator trial in ovarian cancer.

[See table 6 at top of previous page]

Premedications were not routinely used in patients randomized to *Hycamtin*, while patients receiving paclitaxel received routine pretreatment with corticosteroids, diphenhydramine, and histamine receptor type 2 blockers.

Table 7 shows the grade 3/4 hematologic and major non-hematologic adverse events in the topotecan/CAV comparator trial in small cell lung cancer.

[See table 7 above]

Premedications were not routinely used in patients randomized to *Hycamtin*, while patients receiving CAV received routine pretreatment with corticosteroids, diphenhydramine, and histamine receptor type 2 blockers.

Postmarketing Reports of Adverse Events. Reports of adverse events in patients taking Hycamtin (topotecan hydrochloride) received after market introduction, which are not listed above, include the following:

Hematologic: *Rare* — severe bleeding (in association with thrombocytopenia).

Skin/Appendages: *Rare* — severe dermatitis, severe pruritus.

Body as a Whole: *Infrequent* — allergic manifestations; *rare* — anaphylactoid reactions, angioedema.

OVERDOSAGE

There is no known antidote for overdosage with *Hycamtin*. The primary anticipated complication of overdosage would consist of bone marrow suppression.

One patient on a single-dose regimen of 17.5 mg/m^2 given on day 1 of a 21-day cycle had received a single dose of 35 mg/m^2. This patient experienced severe neutropenia (nadir of 320/mm^3) 14 days later but recovered without incident.

The LD_{10} in mice receiving single intravenous infusions of *Hycamtin* was 75 mg/m^2 (CI 95%: 47 to 97).

DOSAGE AND ADMINISTRATION

Prior to administration of the first course of *Hycamtin*, patients must have a baseline neutrophil count of >1500 cells/mm^3 and a platelet count of >100,000 cells/mm^3. The recommended dose of Hycamtin (topotecan hydrochloride) is 1.5 mg/m^2 by intravenous infusion over 30 minutes daily for 5 consecutive days, starting on day 1 of a 21-day course. In the absence of tumor progression, a minimum of four courses is recommended because tumor response may be delayed. The median time to response in three ovarian clinical trials was 9 to 12 weeks and median time to response in four small cell lung cancer trials was 5 to 7 weeks. In the event of severe neutropenia during any course, the dose should be reduced by 0.25 mg/m^2 for subsequent courses. Alternatively, in the event of severe neutropenia, G-CSF may be administered following the subsequent course (before resorting to dose reduction) starting from day 6 of the course (24 hours after completion of topotecan administration).

Adjustment of Dose in Special Populations

Hepatic Impairment: No dosage adjustment appears to be required for treating patients with impaired hepatic function (plasma bilirubin >1.5 to <10 mg/dL).

Renal Functional Impairment: No dosage adjustment appears to be required for treating patients with mild renal impairment (Cl_{cr} 40 to 60 mL/min.). Dosage adjustment to 0.75 mg/m^2 is recommended for patients with moderate renal impairment (20 to 39 mL/min.). Insufficient data are available in patients with severe renal impairment to provide a dosage recommendation.

Elderly Patients: No dosage adjustment appears to be needed in the elderly, other than adjustments related to renal function.

PREPARATION FOR ADMINISTRATION

Precautions: *Hycamtin* is a cytotoxic anticancer drug. As with other potentially toxic compounds, *Hycamtin* should be prepared under a vertical laminar flow hood while wearing gloves and protective clothing. If *Hycamtin* solution contacts the skin, wash the skin immediately and thoroughly with soap and water. If *Hycamtin* contacts mucous membranes, flush thoroughly with water.

Preparation for Intravenous Administration: Each *Hycamtin* 4 mg vial is reconstituted with 4 mL Sterile Water for Injection. Then the appropriate volume of the reconstituted solution is diluted in either 0.9% Sodium Chloride Intravenous Infusion or 5% Dextrose Intravenous Infusion prior to administration.

Table 7. Comparative Toxicity Profiles for Small Cell Lung Cancer Patients Randomized to Receive Hycamtin (topotecan hydrochloride) or CAV

	Hycamtin		CAV	
Adverse Event	**Pts n=107**	**Courses n=446**	**Pts n=104**	**Courses n=359**
Hematologic Grade 3/4	%	%	%	%
Grade 4 Neutropenia (<500 cells/mL)	70	38	72	51
Grade 3/4 Anemia (Hgb < 8 g/dL)	42	18	20	7
Grade 4 Thrombocytopenia (<25,000 plts/mL)	29	10	5	1
Fever/Grade 4 Neutropenia	28	9	26	13
Documented Sepsis	5	1	5	1
Death related to Sepsis	3	NA	1	NA
Non-hematologic Grade 3/4				
Gastrointestinal				
Abdominal Pain	6	1	4	2
Constipation	1	<1	0	0
Diarrhea	1	<1	0	0
Nausea	8	2	6	2
Stomatitis	2	<1	1	<1
Vomiting	3	<1	3	1
Constitutional				
Anorexia	3	1	4	2
Dyspnea	9	5	14	7
Fatigue	6	4	10	3
Neuromuscular				
Asthenia	9	4	7	2
Headache	0	0	2	<1
Pain*	5	2	7	4
Respiratory System				
Coughing	2	1	0	0
Pneumonia	8	2	6	2
Skin/Appendages				
Rash**	1	<1	1	<1
Liver/Biliary				
Increased Hepatic Enzymes†	1	<1	0	0

* Pain includes body pain, skeletal pain and back pain.
** Rash also includes pruritus, rash erythematous, urticaria, dermatitis, bullous eruption and rash maculopapular.
† Increased hepatic enzymes includes increased SGOT/AST, increased SGPT/ALT and increased hepatic enzymes.

Because the lyophilized dosage form contains no antibacterial preservative, the reconstituted product should be used immediately.

STABILITY

Unopened vials of Hycamtin (topotecan hydrochloride) are stable until the date indicated on the package when stored between 20° and 25° C (68° and 77° F) [see USP] and protected from light in the original package. Because the vials contain no preservative, contents should be used immediately after reconstitution.

Reconstituted vials of *Hycamtin* diluted for infusion are stable at approximately 20° to 25° C (68° to 77° F) and ambient lighting conditions for 24 hours.

HOW SUPPLIED

Hycamtin (topotecan hydrochloride) for Injection is supplied in 4 mg (free base) single-dose vials.
NDC 0007-4201-01 (package of 1)
NDC 0007-4201-05 (package of 5)

Storage: Store the vials protected from light in the original cartons at controlled room temperature between 20° and 25° C (68° and 77° F) [see USP].

Handling and Disposal: Procedures for proper handling and disposal of anticancer drugs should be used. Several guidelines on this subject have been published.[1-7] There is no general agreement that all of the procedures recommended in the guidelines are necessary or appropriate.

REFERENCES

1. Recommendations for the safe handling of parenteral antineoplastic drugs. NIH Publication No. 83-2621. For sale by the Superintendent of Documents, US Government Printing Office, Washington, DC 20402.
2. AMA Council Report. Guidelines for handling parenteral antineoplastics. *JAMA*. 1985;253(11):1590–1592.
3. National Study Commission on Cytotoxic Exposure-recommendations for handling cytotoxic agents. Available from Louis P. Jeffry, Chairman, National Study Commission on Cytotoxic Exposure. Massachusetts College of Pharmacy and Allied Health Sciences, 179 Longwood Avenue, Boston, Massachusetts 02115.
4. Clinical Oncological Society of Australia. Guidelines and recommendations for safe handling of antineoplastic agents. *Med J Austr.* 1983;1:426–428.
5. Jones RB, et al. Safe handling of chemotherapeutic agents: A report from the Mount Sinai Medical Center. *CA-A Cancer Journal for Clinicians*. 1983;Sept./Oct.:258–263.

Continued on next page

Information on the SmithKline Beecham Pharmaceuticals products appearing here is based on the labeling in effect on June 15, 2000. Further information on these and other products may be obtained from the Medical Department, SmithKline Beecham Pharmaceuticals, One Franklin Plaza, Philadelphia, PA 19101.

Hycamtin—Cont.

6. American Society of Hospital Pharmacists Technical Assistance Bulletin on Handling Cytotoxic and Hazardous Drugs. *Am J Hosp Pharm.* 1990;47:1033–1049.
7. Controlling Occupational Exposure to Hazardous Drugs. (OSHA Work-Practice Guidelines), *Am J Health-Syst Pharm.* 1996;53:1669–1685.

Rx only

SmithKline Beecham Pharmaceuticals
Philadelphia, PA 19101
HY:L10

Shown in Product Identification Guide, page 337

INFANRIX® Diphtheria and Tetanus Toxoids and Acellular Pertussis Vaccine Adsorbed

℞

DESCRIPTION

Infanrix (Diphtheria and Tetanus Toxoids and Acellular Pertussis Vaccine Adsorbed) is a sterile combination of diphtheria and tetanus toxoids and three pertussis antigens [inactivated pertussis toxin (PT), filamentous hemagglutinin (FHA) and pertactin (69 kiloDalton outer membrane protein)] adsorbed onto aluminum hydroxide. *Infanrix* is intended for intramuscular injection only. After shaking, the vaccine is a homogeneous white turbid suspension.

Three acellular pertussis antigens (pertussis toxin [PT], filamentous hemagglutinin [FHA] and pertactin) are isolated from phase 1 *Bordetella pertussis* culture grown in modified Stainer-Scholte liquid medium. PT and FHA are extracted from the fermentation broth by adsorption on hydroxyapatite gel; pertactin is extracted from the cells by heat treatment and flocculation using barium chloride. These antigens are purified in successive chromatographic steps: PT and FHA by hydrophobic, affinity and size exclusion; pertactin by ion exchange, hydrophobic and size exclusion processes. PT is detoxified using formaldehyde and glutaraldehyde. FHA and pertactin are treated with formaldehyde.

Diphtheria toxin is produced by growing *Corynebacterium diphtheriae* in Linggoud and Fenton medium containing a bovine extract. Tetanus toxin is produced by growing *Clostridium tetani* in a modified Latham medium. Both toxins are detoxified with formaldehyde, concentrated by ultrafiltration, and purified by precipitation, sterile filtration and dialysis.

Each antigen is individually adsorbed onto aluminum hydroxide. Each 0.5 mL dose contains, by assay, not more than 0.625 mg aluminum. Each 0.5 mL dose is formulated to contain 25 Lf diphtheria toxoid, 10 Lf tetanus toxoid (both toxoids induce at least 2 antitoxin units/mL of serum in the guinea pig potency test), 25 mcg PT, 25 mcg FHA and 8 mcg pertactin. The potency of the pertussis component is evaluated by measurement of the antibody response to PT, FHA and pertactin in immunized mice using an ELISA.

Each 0.5 mL dose also contains 2.5 mg 2-phenoxyethanol as a preservative, 4.5 mg sodium chloride, water for injection and not more than 0.02% (w/v) residual formaldehyde. The vaccine contains polysorbate 80 (Tween 80) which is used in the production of the pertussis concentrate. The inactivated acellular pertussis components contribute less than 5 endotoxin units (EU) per 0.5 mL dose.

Diphtheria and Tetanus Toxoids adsorbed bulk concentrates for further manufacturing use are produced by Chiron Behring GmbH & Co, Marburg, Germany. The acellular pertussis antigens are manufactured by SmithKline Beecham Biologicals S.A., Rixensart, Belgium. Formulation, filling, testing, packaging and release of the vaccine are conducted by SmithKline Beecham Biologicals S.A.

CLINICAL PHARMACOLOGY

Simultaneous immunization against diphtheria, tetanus and pertussis during infancy and childhood using a conventional whole-cell DTP vaccine has been a routine practice in the United States since the late 1940s. It has played a major role in markedly reducing the incidence of, and deaths from, each of these diseases.

Diphtheria

Diphtheria is primarily a localized and generalized intoxication caused by diphtheria toxin, an extracellular protein metabolite of toxigenic strains of *Corynebacterium diphtheriae.* While the incidence of diphtheria in the United States has decreased from over 200,000 cases reported in 1921,[1] before the general use of diphtheria toxoid, to only 30 cases of respiratory diphtheria reported from 1983 to 1993,[2] the ratio of fatalities to attack rate has remained constant at about 5% to 10%. The highest case fatality rates are in the very young and in the elderly. Diphtheria remains a serious disease in some areas of the world as evidenced by the recent outbreak in the former Soviet Union.[3] Protection against disease is due to the development of neutralizing antibodies to the diphtheria toxin. Following adequate immunization with diphtheria toxoid, it is thought that protection lasts for at least 10 years.[1] Serum antitoxin levels of at least 0.01 antitoxin units per mL are generally regarded as protective.[4] This significantly reduces both the risk of developing diphtheria and the severity of clinical illness. Immunization with diphtheria toxoid does not, however, eliminate carriage of *C. diphtheriae* in the pharynx or nose or on the skin.[1] Efficacy of the diphtheria toxoid used in Infanrix (Diphtheria and Tetanus Toxoids and Acellular Pertussis Vaccine Adsorbed) was determined on the basis of immunogenicity studies, with a comparison to a serological correlate of protection (0.01 antitoxin units/mL) established by the Panel on Review of Bacterial Vaccines and Toxoids.[4] A Vero cell toxin neutralizing test confirmed the ability of infant sera (N=45), obtained 1 month after the primary course, to neutralize diphtheria toxin. Protective titers (≥0.01 antitoxin units/mL of serum) were achieved in 100% of the sera tested.

Tetanus

Tetanus is an intoxication manifested primarily by neuromuscular dysfunction caused by a potent exotoxin released by *Clostridium tetani.* The incidence of tetanus in the United States has dropped dramatically with the routine use of tetanus toxoid to a record low of 45 cases in 1992.[2] Tetanus in the U.S. is primarily a disease of older adults. Of 99 tetanus patients with complete information reported to the Centers for Disease Control and Prevention during 1987 and 1988, 68% were ≥50 years of age, while only 6 were <20 years of age. No cases of neonatal tetanus were reported. Overall, the case-fatality rate was 21%. The disease continues to occur almost exclusively among persons who are unvaccinated or inadequately vaccinated or whose vaccination histories are unknown or uncertain.[5]

Spores of *C. tetani* are ubiquitous. Serological tests indicate that naturally acquired immunity to tetanus toxin does not occur in the U.S. Thus, universal primary immunization with tetanus toxoid, with subsequent maintenance of adequate antitoxin levels by means of timed boosters, is necessary to protect all age groups.[1] Protection against disease is due to the development of neutralizing antibodies to the tetanus toxin. Tetanus toxoid is a highly effective antigen and a completed primary series generally induces serum antitoxin levels of at least 0.01 antitoxin units per mL, a level which has been reported to be protective.[4] It is thought that protection persists for at least 10 years.[1] Efficacy of the tetanus toxoid used in *Infanrix* was determined on the basis of immunogenicity studies with a comparison to a serological correlate of protection (0.01 antitoxin units per mL) established by the Panel on Review of Bacterial Vaccines and Toxoids.[4] An *in vivo* mouse toxin neutralizing test confirmed the ability of infant sera (N=45), obtained 1 month after the primary course, to neutralize tetanus toxin. Protective titers (≥0.01 antitoxin units/mL of serum) were achieved in 100% of the sera tested.

Pertussis

Pertussis (whooping cough) is a disease of the respiratory tract caused by *Bordetella pertussis.* Pertussis is highly communicable (attack rates in unimmunized household contacts of up to 90% have been reported[6]) and can cause severe disease, particularly among the very young.[1] Since immunization against pertussis became widespread, the number of reported cases and associated mortality in the United States have declined from an average annual incidence and mortality of 150 cases and 6 deaths per 100,000 population, respectively, in the early 1940s, to annual reported incidences of 1.6, 2.6 and 1.8 cases per 100,000 population in 1992, 1993 and 1994, respectively.[2,7] Precise epidemiologic data do not exist, since bacteriological confirmation of pertussis can be obtained in less than half of the suspected cases. Most reported illness from *B. pertussis* occurs in infants and young children in whom complications can be severe. From 1980 to 1989, of 10,749 pertussis cases reported nationally in infants less than 1 year of age, 69% were hospitalized, 22% had pneumonia, 3.0% had seizures, 0.9% had encephalopathy and 0.6% died.[8] Older children and adults, in whom classic signs are often absent, may go undiagnosed and may serve as reservoirs of disease.[9]

Routine vaccination with whole-cell DTP vaccine has significantly reduced pertussis-related morbidity and mortality. However, concerns regarding reactogenicity of whole-cell DTP vaccine have spurred development of safer pertussis vaccines with high efficacy. The role of the different components produced by *B. pertussis* in either the pathogenesis of, or the immunity to, pertussis is not well understood.

Antigenic components of *B. pertussis* believed to contribute to protective immunity include: pertussis toxin; filamentous hemagglutinin; and pertactin.[10,11] Although the role of these antigens in providing protective immunity in humans is not well understood, clinical trials which evaluated candidate acellular DTP vaccines manufactured by SmithKline Beecham Biologicals supported the efficacy of three-component *Infanrix.*[12-14]

Infanrix, which contains three pertussis antigens (PT, FHA and pertactin), has been shown to be effective in preventing WHO-defined pertussis in two published clinical trials when administered as a primary series.[13,14]

A double-blind, randomized, placebo-controlled (DT) trial conducted in Italy, sponsored by the National Institutes of Health (NIH), assessed the absolute protective efficacy of *Infanrix* when administered at 2, 4 and 6 months of age.[13] A total of 15,601 infants were immunized with one of two tricomponent acellular DTP vaccines (containing inactivated PT, FHA and pertactin), or with a U.S.-licensed whole-cell DTP vaccine manufactured by Connaught Laboratories, Inc., or with DT vaccine alone. The mean length of follow-up was 17 months, beginning 30 days after the third dose of vaccine. The population used in the primary analysis of vaccine efficacy included 4,481 *Infanrix* vaccinees, 4,348 whole-cell DTP vaccinees and 1,470 DT vaccinees. After three doses, the protective efficacy of *Infanrix* against WHO-defined typical pertussis (21 days or more of paroxysmal cough with infection confirmed by culture and/or serologic testing) was 84% (95% CI: 76% to 89%) while the efficacy of the whole-cell DTP vaccine was 36% (95% CI: 14% to 52%). When the definition of pertussis was expanded to include clinically milder disease with respect to type and duration of cough, with infection confirmed by culture and/or serologic testing, the efficacy of *Infanrix* was calculated to be 71% (95% CI: 60% to 78%) against >7 days of any cough and 73% (95% CI: 63% to 80%) against ≥14 days of any cough. A longer follow-up of the Italian trial showed that after three doses, the absolute efficacy of *Infanrix* remained high against WHO-defined pertussis at 78% (95% CI: 62% to 87%) in children whose average age was then 33 months (20-39 months).[15]

A prospective, blinded efficacy trial was also conducted in Germany employing a household contact study design.[14] In preparation for this study, three doses of Infanrix (Diphtheria and Tetanus Toxoids and Acellular Pertussis Vaccine Adsorbed) were administered at 3, 4 and 5 months of age to more than 22,000 children living in six areas of Germany in a large safety and immunogenicity trial. Infants who did not participate in this trial could have received whole-cell DTP vaccine (manufactured by Behringwerke A.G., Germany) or DT vaccine. Pediatricians were asked to monitor households with a first potential case (index case) of typical pertussis which was identified by spontaneous presentation to a physician. Households were enrolled in the study if there was at least one other household member (a household contact) 6 to 47 months of age. Prospective follow-up of household contacts of index cases for the incidence and progression of pertussis was performed by a separate physician who was blinded to the vaccination status of the household. Calculation of vaccine efficacy was based on attack rates of pertussis in household contacts classified by vaccination status. Of the 173 unvaccinated household contacts, 96 developed WHO-defined pertussis (21 days or more of paroxysmal cough with infection confirmed by culture and/or serologic testing), as compared to 7 of 112 contacts vaccinated with *Infanrix* and 1 of 75 contacts vaccinated with whole-cell DTP vaccine. The protective efficacy of *Infanrix* was calculated to be 89% (95% CI: 77% to 95%), with no indication of waning of protection up until the time of the booster. The protective efficacy of the whole-cell DTP vaccine was calculated to be 98% (95% CI: 83% to 100%). The average age of *Infanrix* vaccinees at the time of follow-up in this trial was 13 months (range 6-25 months). When the definition of pertussis was expanded to include clinically milder disease, with infection confirmed by culture and/or serologic testing, the efficacy of *Infanrix* against ≥7 days of any cough was 67% (95% CI: 52% to 78%) and against ≥7 days of paroxysmal cough was 81% (95% CI: 68% to 89%). The corresponding efficacy rates of *Infanrix* against ≥14 days of any cough or paroxysmal cough were 73% (95% CI: 59% to 82%) and 84% (95% CI: 71% to 91%), respectively.

Immune Response to Infanrix *Administered as a Three-Dose Primary Series*

The immune responses to each of the three pertussis antigens contained in *Infanrix* were evaluated in sera obtained 1 month after the third dose of vaccine in each of three studies (schedule of administration: 2, 4 and 6 months of age in the Italian efficacy study and one U.S. study; 3, 4 and 5 months of age in the German efficacy study). One month after the third dose of *Infanrix,* the response rates to each pertussis antigen were similar in all three studies. Thus, although a serologic correlate of protection for pertussis has not been established, the antibody responses to these three pertussis antigens (PT, FHA and pertactin) in a U.S. population were similar to those achieved in two populations in which efficacy of *Infanrix* was demonstrated.

Immune Response to Simultaneously Administered Vaccines

In a small clinical trial in the United States, *Infanrix* was given simultaneously, at separate sites, with hepatitis B vaccine, *Haemophilus influenzae* type b vaccine (Hib) and poliovirus vaccine live oral (OPV), at 2, 4 and 6 months of age. One month after the third dose of hepatitis B vaccine given simultaneously with *Infanrix,* 100% of infants demonstrated anti-HBs antibodies ≥10 mIU/mL (N=64). Ninety percent of infants who received Hib simultaneously with *Infanrix* achieved anti-PRP antibodies ≥1 mcg/mL (N=72), and 96% to 100% of infants who received OPV simultaneously with *Infanrix* showed protective neutralizing antibody to poliovirus types 1, 2 and 3 (N=60–61).[16]

In the Italian efficacy trial, 92% of infants received hepatitis B vaccine with the first and second dose of *Infanrix.* Ninety-four percent of infants received OPV with the first and second dose of *Infanrix.*[13]

INDICATIONS AND USAGE

Infanrix is indicated for active immunization against diphtheria, tetanus and pertussis (whooping cough) in infants and children 6 weeks to 7 years of age (prior to seventh birthday). Because of the substantial risks of complications from pertussis disease, completion of a primary series of vaccine early in life is strongly recommended.[1]

Individuals 7 years of age or older should not receive this vaccine. In such individuals, Tetanus and Diphtheria Toxoids Adsorbed For Adult Use (Td) is preferable to use of either tetanus or diphtheria vaccines alone.

Children who have recovered from culture-confirmed pertussis need not receive further doses of a pertussis-containing vaccine, but should receive additional doses of Diphtheria and Tetanus Toxoids Adsorbed (DT) for pediatric use to complete the series in accordance with ACIP recommendations.[1]

In instances where the pertussis vaccine component is contraindicated, Diphtheria and Tetanus Toxoids Adsorbed (DT) for pediatric use may be substituted for each of the remaining doses[1] (see CONTRAINDICATIONS).

The decision to administer or delay vaccination because of a current or recent febrile illness depends on the severity of symptoms and on the etiology of the disease. All vaccines can be administered to persons with minor illness such as diarrhea, mild upper respiratory infections with or without low-grade fever or other low-grade febrile illness.[17,18]

Where passive protection is required, Tetanus Immune Globulin and/or Diphtheria Antitoxin may also be administered at separate sites.[1,17]

As with any vaccine, *Infanrix* may not protect 100% of individuals receiving the vaccine.

This product is not recommended for treatment of actual infections.

CONTRAINDICATIONS

Hypersensitivity to any component of the vaccine is a contraindication (see DESCRIPTION).

It is a contraindication to use this vaccine after an immediate anaphylactic reaction temporally associated with a previous dose. Because of the uncertainty as to which component of the vaccine might be responsible, no further vaccination with diphtheria, tetanus or pertussis should be given. Alternatively, because of the importance of tetanus vaccination, such individuals may be referred to an allergist for evaluation.[1]

Immunization should be deferred during the course of a moderate or severe febrile illness or acute infection (see PRECAUTIONS).[1,17,18]

Elective immunization should be deferred during an outbreak of poliomyelitis.[19]

Safety data on the use of Infanrix (Diphtheria and Tetanus Toxoids and Acellular Pertussis Vaccine Adsorbed) in children for whom whole-cell pertussis vaccine is contraindicated are not available. Until such data are available, it would be prudent to consider Advisory Committee on Immunization Practices (ACIP) and American Academy of Pediatrics (AAP) contraindications to whole-cell DTP vaccine as contraindications to *Infanrix*.[1,18,20]

The ACIP states that "if any of the following events occur in temporal relationship to the administration of DTP, further vaccination with DTP is contraindicated":

1. An immediate anaphylactic reaction.
2. Encephalopathy (not due to another identifiable cause). This is defined as an acute, severe central nervous system disorder occurring within 7 days following vaccination (with whole-cell DTP or acellular DTP), and generally consisting of major alterations in consciousness, unresponsiveness, generalized or focal seizures that persist more than a few hours, with failure to recover within 24 hours. Even though causation by DTP vaccine cannot be established, no subsequent doses of pertussis vaccine should be given.

WARNINGS

If any of the following events occur in temporal relation to receipt of whole-cell DTP or acellular DTP vaccine, the decision to give subsequent doses of vaccine containing the pertussis component should be carefully considered. There may be circumstances, such as high incidence of pertussis, in which the potential benefits outweigh possible risks, particularly since these events have not been proven to cause permanent sequelae.[1,18] The following events were previously considered contraindications and are now considered precautions by the ACIP:

- **Temperature of ≥40.5°C (105°F) within 48 hours not due to another identifiable cause**
- **Collapse or shock-like state (hypotonic-hyporesponsive episode) within 48 hours**
- **Persistent, inconsolable crying lasting ≥3 hours, occurring within 48 hours**
- **Convulsions with or without fever occurring within 3 days**

In the Italian efficacy trial, the incidence of temperature ≥104°F, crying for 3 hours or more and seizures within 48 hours of vaccination was less than that following administration of whole-cell DTP vaccine manufactured by Connaught Laboratories, Inc. No hypotonic-hyporesponsive episodes were reported after administration of *Infanrix* in this trial[13] (see ADVERSE EVENTS–Table 7).

A committee of the Institute of Medicine (IOM) has concluded that evidence is consistent with a causal relationship between whole-cell DTP vaccine and acute neurologic illness, and under special circumstances, between whole-cell DTP vaccine and chronic neurologic disease in the context of the National Childhood Encephalopathy Study (NCES) report.[21,22] However, the IOM committee concluded that the evidence was insufficient to indicate whether or not whole-cell DTP vaccine increased the overall risk of chronic neurologic disease.[22] While acute encephalopathy and permanent neurologic damage have not been reported in temporal association after administration of *Infanrix*, the data at this time are insufficient to rule this out.

The ACIP and the AAP recognize certain circumstances in which children with stable central nervous system disorders, such as well-controlled seizures or satisfactorily explained single seizures, may receive pertussis vaccine. The decision to administer a pertussis-containing vaccine to such children must be made by the physician on an individual basis, with consideration of all relevant factors, and assessment of potential risks and benefits for that individual.

Table 1.[13] Adverse Events (%) Occurring Within the 3 Days Following Vaccination of Italian Infants with Either *Infanrix* or Whole-Cell DTP at 2, 4 and 6 Months of Age

	Infanrix			Whole-Cell DTP Vaccine		
	Dose 1	**Dose 2**	**Dose 3**	**Dose 1**	**Dose 2**	**Dose 3**
No. of infants	4,696	4,560	4,505	4,678	4,474	4,368
Local						
Redness	4.8	8.6	16.0	27.1	24.2	28.0
Redness ≥2.4 cm	1.0	1.3	3.5	12.4	7.3	7.7
Swelling	5.2	8.2	14.5	28.9	23.5	25.8
Swelling ≥2.4 cm	0.7	1.2	2.9	13.1	7.4	8.0
Tenderness	4.7	4.0	5.2	36.0	26.8	25.9
Systemic						
Fever ≥100.4°F*	7.1	7.9	9.0	46.8	36.1	39.8
Irritability	36.3	34.9	28.8	57.2	50.1	47.2
Drowsiness	34.9	18.8	11.4	54.0	34.1	23.0
Loss of Appetite	16.5	13.9	11.5	31.2	22.8	19.1
Vomiting	5.8†	4.1†	3.3	6.7	4.7	4.8
Crying ≥1 Hour	3.9	3.3	2.2	17.3	11.1	8.2

*Rectal temperatures.
†For the comparison of *Infanrix* and whole-cell DTP vaccine, all adverse events reached statistical significance ($p<0.001$) at all doses except vomiting at doses 1 and 2, which was not statistically significant at $p<0.05$.

ACIP and AAP have issued guidelines for such children.[1,18,20] The parent or guardian should be advised of the potential increased risk involved (see Information for the Patient).

Studies suggest that, when given whole-cell DTP vaccine, infants and children with a history of convulsions in first-degree family members (i.e., siblings and parents) have a 2.4-fold increased risk for neurologic events compared with those without such histories.[23] However, the ACIP has concluded that a history of convulsions or other central nervous system disorders in parents or siblings is not a contraindication to pertussis vaccine and that children with such family histories should receive pertussis vaccine according to the recommended schedule.[1,17,18,24]

For children at higher risk for seizures than the general population, it may be prudent to extend the ACIP and AAP recommendations for whole-cell DTP vaccine to *Infanrix:* that acetaminophen be administered at age-appropriate doses at the time of DTP vaccination and every 4 to 6 hours for 24 hours.[1,18,20]

Infanrix should not be given to infants or children with any coagulation disorder, including thrombocytopenia, that would contraindicate intramuscular injection unless the potential benefit clearly outweighs the risk of administration.

PRECAUTIONS

Although a moderate or severe febrile illness is sufficient reason to postpone vaccination, minor illnesses such as mild upper respiratory infections with or without low-grade fever are not contraindications.[1,18]

Before the injection of any biological, the physician should take all reasonable precautions to prevent allergic or other adverse reactions, including understanding the use of the biological concerned, and the nature of the side effects and adverse reactions that may follow its use.

Prior to immunization, the patient's medical history should be reviewed. The physician should review the patient's immunization history for possible vaccine sensitivity, previous vaccination-related adverse reactions and occurrence of any adverse-event-related symptoms and/or signs, in order to determine the existence of any contraindication to immunization with *Infanrix* and to allow an assessment of benefits and risks. Epinephrine injection (1:1000) and other appropriate agents used for the control of immediate allergic reactions must be immediately available should an acute anaphylactic reaction occur.

A separate sterile syringe and needle or a sterile disposable unit should be used for each individual patient to prevent transmission of hepatitis or other infectious agents from one person to another. Needles should be disposed of properly and should not be recapped.

Special care should be taken to prevent injection into a blood vessel.

Infanrix (Diphtheria and Tetanus Toxoids and Acellular Pertussis Vaccine Adsorbed) is not contraindicated for use in individuals with HIV infection.[17,25]

As with any vaccine, if administered to immunosuppressed persons, including individuals receiving immunosuppressive therapy, the expected immune response may not be obtained.[25]

Information for the Patient

Parents or guardians should be informed of the potential benefits and risks of the vaccine, and of the importance of completing the immunization series. It is important when a child returns for the next dose in a series that the parent/guardian be questioned concerning occurrence of any symptoms and/or signs of an adverse reaction after a previous dose of the same vaccine. The physician should inform the parents or guardians about the potential for adverse reactions that have been temporally associated with administration of *Infanrix* or other pertussis-containing vaccines. The parents or guardians of infants and children with a family history of convulsions should be advised of the potential increased risk of seizures following DTP vaccination. In particular, they should be told, before the child is vaccinated, to seek immediate medical evaluation in the unlikely event of a seizure.[24] The adult accompanying the recipient should be told to report severe or unusual adverse reactions to the physician or clinic where the vaccine was administered.

The parent or guardian should be given the Vaccine Information Materials, which are required by the National Childhood Vaccine Injury Act of 1986 to be given prior to immunization.

The U.S. Department of Health and Human Services has established a Vaccine Adverse Event Reporting System (VAERS) to accept all reports of suspected adverse events after the administration of any vaccine, including but not limited to the reporting of events required by the National Childhood Vaccine Injury Act of 1986.[26] The VAERS toll-free number is 1-800-822-7967.

Drug Interactions

For information regarding simultaneous administration with other vaccines, refer to DOSAGE AND ADMINISTRATION and CLINICAL PHARMACOLOGY.

As with other intramuscular injections, *Infanrix* should not be given to infants or children on anticoagulant therapy unless the potential benefit clearly outweighs the risk of administration (see WARNINGS).

Immunosuppressive therapies, including irradiation, antimetabolites, alkylating agents, cytotoxic drugs and corticosteroids (used in greater than physiologic doses), may reduce the immune response to vaccines. Although no specific data from studies with pertussis vaccine under these conditions are available, if immunosuppressive therapy will be discontinued shortly, it would be reasonable to defer immunization until the patient has been off therapy for 1 month; otherwise, the patient should be vaccinated while still on therapy (see PRECAUTIONS).[1] If *Infanrix* is administered to a person receiving immunosuppressive therapy, or a recent injection of immune globulin, or who has an immunodeficiency disorder, an adequate immunologic response may not be obtained.

Tetanus Immune Globulin or Diphtheria Antitoxin, if used, should be given at a separate site, with a separate needle and syringe.

Carcinogenesis, Mutagenesis, Impairment of Fertility

Infanrix has not been evaluated for carcinogenic or mutagenic potential, or for impairment of fertility.

Pregnancy: Pregnancy Category C

Animal reproduction studies have not been conducted with *Infanrix*. It is not known whether *Infanrix* can cause fetal harm when administered to a pregnant woman or if *Infanrix* can affect reproductive capacity. *Infanrix* is not recommended for use in a pregnant woman. *Infanrix* is not recommended for persons 7 years of age or older.

Pediatric Use

Safety and effectiveness of *Infanrix* in infants below the age of 6 weeks have not been established (see DOSAGE AND ADMINISTRATION). *Infanrix* is not recommended for individuals 7 years of age or older. Tetanus and Diphtheria Adsorbed For Adult Use (Td) is to be used in individuals 7 years of age or older.

ADVERSE REACTIONS

A total of 92,502 doses of *Infanrix* has been administered in clinical studies. In these studies, 28,749 infants have received *Infanrix* as a three-dose primary series, 5,830 children have received *Infanrix* as a fourth dose following three doses of *Infanrix*, and 22 children have received *Infanrix* as a fifth dose following four doses of *Infanrix*. In addition, 439 children and 169 children have received *Infanrix* as a fourth or fifth dose following three or four doses of whole-cell DTP

Continued on next page

Information on the SmithKline Beecham Pharmaceuticals products appearing here is based on the labeling in effect on June 15, 2000. Further information on these and other products may be obtained from the Medical Department, SmithKline Beecham Pharmaceuticals, One Franklin Plaza, Philadelphia, PA 19101.

Infanrix—Cont.

vaccine, respectively. In comparative studies, *Infanrix* has been shown to be followed by fewer of the local and systemic adverse reactions commonly associated with whole-cell DTP vaccination. However, studies have shown that the rate of erythema, swelling and fever increased with successive doses of *Infanrix*.

In the double-blind, randomized comparative trial in Italy, safety data in a three-dose primary series are available for 4,696 infants who received at least one dose of *Infanrix* and 4,678 infants who received at least one dose of U.S.-licensed whole-cell DTP vaccine manufactured by Connaught Laboratories, Inc.[13,15] Data were actively collected by parents using standardized diaries for eight consecutive evenings after each vaccine dose with follow-up telephone calls made by nurses after the eighth day. Table 1 lists adverse events reported during the three days after each dose. All common solicited adverse events were less frequent following vaccination with *Infanrix* as compared to whole-cell DTP after each one of the three doses.

[See table 1 at top of previous page]

A similar reduction in adverse events was seen in a randomized, double-blind, comparative trial conducted in the U.S. when Infanrix (Diphtheria and Tetanus Toxoids and Acellular Pertussis Vaccine Adsorbed) was compared to two U.S.-licensed whole-cell DTP vaccines. Adverse events were actively solicited using standardized diaries with follow-up telephone calls made at days 1, 4 and 8 by blinded study personnel. Table 2 summarizes the frequency of adverse events within 3 days of the three primary immunizing doses. The incidence of redness, swelling, pain, fever (rectal temperature >101°F), fussiness, drowsiness and poor appetite, were lower following *Infanrix* than following either whole-cell DTP vaccine.

[See table 2 above]

The frequencies of adverse reactions following each dose in children who received *Infanrix* at 2, 4 and 6 months of age in a U.S. NIH-sponsored trial are shown in Table 3. Of the 120 infants who received the three-dose primary series, a subset of 76 received a fourth dose of *Infanrix* at 15 to 20 months of age. Adverse events were actively solicited using standardized diaries with follow-up telephone calls made at day 3 by blinded study personnel.

[See table 3 above]

Of 22,505 children who had previously received three doses of *Infanrix* at 3, 4 and 5 months of age in the large German safety study, 5,361 received a fourth dose at 10 to 36 (mean 20) months of age. Standardized diaries were available on 2,457 children receiving the primary series and 1,809 children receiving the fourth dose. Local and systemic reaction rates within 3 days of vaccination for each dose are reported in Table 4. In this study, the rate of erythema, swelling, pain and fever increased with successive doses of *Infanrix*.

[See table 4 above]

In another study conducted in Germany, which was double-blinded and randomized, additional safety data are available from 13- to 27-month-old children who received Infanrix (Diphtheria and Tetanus Toxoids and Acellular Pertussis Vaccine Adsorbed) or whole-cell DTP vaccine, manufactured by Behringwerke, A.G., as a fourth dose. These children had previously received three doses of the same vaccine. The rates of adverse events, which were actively solicited using standardized diaries, are presented in Table 5. The incidence of redness, swelling, severe swelling (greater than 2 cm), pain, fever, severe fever (rectal temperature >103.1°F), restlessness, loss of appetite, vomiting, drowsiness and unusual crying was lower following vaccination with *Infanrix* compared to whole-cell DTP vaccine.

[See table 5 at bottom of next page]

Cases of edematous swelling, generally beginning within 48 hours of vaccination and resolving spontaneously over an average of 4 days without sequelae, have been reported with *Infanrix*.[15] In the German study in which 5,361 children received a fourth dose of *Infanrix* after three doses of the same vaccine, swelling of the injected thigh was reported spontaneously in 62 vaccinees (1.2%). This swelling was associated with pain upon digital pressure in 53% of cases, with rectal temperature ≥100.4°F in 45% of cases, and with injection site redness in 71% of cases (redness of the entire thigh was reported in 17% of such cases). The mean difference in the circumference of the thighs in those subjects in whom this was measured (N=17) was 2.2 cm (range: 0.5 to 5 cm). In 1,809 children for whom standardized diaries were available, edematous swelling was observed in 2.5% of vaccinees. In clinical studies of *Infanrix* to date, edematous swelling has been seen only with *Infanrix* as a fourth dose in *Infanrix*-primed individuals. In other countries where *Infanrix* has been licensed, limb swelling has been reported rarely following administration of *Infanrix* at any dose, including the primary series. Edematous swelling has also been reported following administration of other acellular DTP vaccines,[29] acellular pertussis vaccine alone (without DT),[30] whole-cell DTP vaccine[31] and other vaccines.[32]

Table 6 lists the frequency of adverse events in U.S. children who received *Infanrix* (N=110) or U.S.-licensed whole-cell DTP vaccine (N=55) manufactured by Lederle Laboratories at 15 to 20 months of age[33] and in U.S. children who received *Infanrix* (N=115) or U.S.-licensed whole-cell DTP vaccine (N=57) manufactured by Lederle Laboratories at 4 to 6 years of age.[34] All children had previously received three or four doses of whole-cell DTP vaccine at approximately 2, 4, 6 and 15–18 months of age. Adverse events

Table 2.[27] Adverse Events (%) Occurring Within the 3 Days Following Vaccination of U.S. Infants with Either *Infanrix* or Whole-Cell DTP at 2, 4 and 6 Months of Age

	Infanrix			Whole-Cell DTP Vaccine-Lederle			Whole-Cell DTP Vaccine-Connaught		
	Dose 1	Dose 2	Dose 3	Dose 1	Dose 2	Dose 3	Dose 1	Dose 2	Dose 3
No. of infants	407	402	395	74	73	73	76	75	74
Local									
Redness*	10.6	19.4	25.8	28.4	42.5	39.7	35.5	50.7	50.0
Swelling	7.4†¶	12.2†¶	17.5¶	23.0†	26.0†	27.4	30.3¶	37.3¶	31.1¶
Pain*‡	2.7	2.0	1.5	17.6	15.1	9.6	38.2	17.3	14.9
Systemic									
Fever >101°F§	0.5†¶	0.7†¶	5.1	12.2†	8.2†	6.8	14.5¶	18.7¶	8.1
Fussiness**	3.9†¶	3.5†¶	4.1	25.7†	13.7†	6.8	21.1¶	16.0¶	8.1
Drowsiness	26.3†¶	16.4†¶	12.9†	51.4†	34.2†	23.3†	52.6¶	28.0¶	18.9
Poor Appetite	8.1†¶	7.7	6.6	31.1†	15.1	9.6	19.7¶	14.7	9.5
Vomiting	6.6	3.7	3.8	8.1	4.1	2.7	7.9	2.7	2.7

‡ Moderate or severe = cried or protested to touch or cried when leg moved.
** Moderate or severe = prolonged crying and refusal to play or persistent crying that could not be comforted.
§ Rectal temperatures.
* p<0.05 for the comparison of *Infanrix* and both whole-cell DTP vaccines.
† p<0.05 for the comparison of *Infanrix* and whole-cell DTP vaccine-Lederle.
¶ p<0.05 for the comparison of *Infanrix* and whole-cell DTP vaccine-Connaught.

Table 3.[15,28] Adverse Events (%) Occurring Within the 3 Days Following Vaccination with *Infanrix* in U.S. Infants and Children in Which All Doses Were *Infanrix*

	Primary (N = 120 infants)			Booster (N = 76 children)
Event	Dose 1 (2 months)	Dose 2 (4 months)	Dose 3 (6 months)	Dose 4 (15 to 20 months)
Local				
Redness	16.6	15.4	26.3	39.5
Swelling	12.5	15.4	21.0	32.9
Pain*	5.0	5.1	0.9	10.5
Systemic				
Fever (>101°F)†	0.0	0.9	3.5	6.6
Anorexia	7.5	6.0	9.6	11.8
Vomiting	5.8	6.8	3.5	2.6
Drowsiness	37.5	19.7	13.2	6.6
Fussiness‡	3.3	7.7	8.8	9.2

* Moderate or severe = cried or protested to touch or cried when limb moved.
† Rectal temperatures for primary series; oral temperatures for booster.
‡ Moderate or severe = prolonged crying and refusal to play or persistent crying that could not be comforted.

Table 4.[15] Adverse Events (%) Occurring Within the 3 Days Following Vaccination with *Infanrix* in German Infants and Children in Which All Doses Were *Infanrix*

	Primary (N=2,457 infants)			Booster (N=1,809 children)*
Event	Dose 1 (3 months)	Dose 2 (4 months)	Dose 3 (5 months)	Dose 4 (10 to 36 months†)
Local				
Redness	8.9	23.6	26.6	45.9
Redness >2 cm	0.0	0.5	1.3	13.8
Swelling	3.9	14.1	18.5	35.4
Swelling >2 cm	0.0	0.3	1.3	11.4
Pain	2.0	2.6	3.7	26.3
Systemic				
Fever (≥100.4°F)‡	6.3	8.3	13.3	26.4
Fever (>103.1°F)‡	0.0	0.1	0.1	1.1
Loss of Appetite	8.0	7.4	6.5	11.6
Vomiting	4.3	3.9	3.4	2.9
Restlessness	10.3	9.5	8.6	15.9
Unusual Crying	3.9	4.3	4.1	6.4
Diarrhea	6.0	4.9	4.0	11.0

* May not be same children as in primary series.
† Mean = 20 months.
‡ Rectal temperatures.

were actively solicited using standardized diaries with follow-up telephone calls made at days 1, 4 and 8 by blinded study personnel. Significantly fewer solicited local and general adverse events were reported following *Infanrix* than following whole-cell DTP vaccine when administered as the fourth or fifth dose in those previously primed with three or four doses of whole-cell DTP vaccine.

[See table 6 at bottom of next page]

Severe adverse events reported from the double-blind, randomized comparative Italian study involving 4,696 children administered Infanrix (Diphtheria and Tetanus Toxoids and Acellular Pertussis Vaccine Adsorbed) or 4,678 children administered whole-cell DTP vaccine (manufactured by Connaught Laboratories, Inc.) as a three-dose primary series are shown in Table 7. The incidence of rectal temperature ≥104°F, hypotonic-hyporesponsive episodes and persistent crying ≥3 hours following administration of *Infanrix* was significantly less than that following administration of whole-cell DTP vaccine.[13] Hospitalization rates and death rates within 7 days of vaccination were similar between *Infanrix* and DT vaccine recipients.[15]

[See table 7 at bottom of next page]

In the large German safety trial that enrolled 22,505 infants (66,867 doses of *Infanrix* administered as a three-dose primary series), all subjects were monitored for unsolicited adverse events that occurred within 28 days following vaccination using report cards. In a subset of subjects (N=2,457), these cards were standardized diaries which solicited specific adverse events that occurred within 8 days of each vaccination in addition to unsolicited adverse events which occurred throughout the course of the entire trial (from study enrollment until approximately 30 days following the third vaccination). Cards from the whole cohort were returned at subsequent visits and were supplemented by spontaneous reporting by parents and a medical history after the first and second doses of vaccine. In the subset of

2,457, adverse events following the third dose of vaccine were reported via standardized diaries and spontaneous reporting at a follow-up visit. Adverse events in the remainder of the cohort were reported via report cards which were returned by mail approximately 28 days after the third dose of vaccine. Adverse events (rates per 1,000 doses) occurring within 7 days including those events deemed by investigators as related as well as those felt to be unrelated to vaccination included: unusual crying (0.09), febrile seizure (0.0), afebrile seizure (0.13) and hypotonic-hyporesponsive episodes (0.01).

Rates of serious adverse experiences that are less common than those reported in the German safety trial are not known at this time.

In clinical trials involving more than 29,000 infants and children, 14 deaths in Infanrix (Diphtheria and Tetanus Toxoids and Acellular Pertussis Vaccine Adsorbed) recipients were reported. Causes of deaths included nine cases of Sudden Infant Death Syndrome (SIDS) and one of each of the following: meal aspiration, hepatoblastoma, neuroblastoma, invasive bacterial infection and sudden death in a child greater than 1 year of age. None of these events was determined to be vaccine-related. The rate of SIDS observed in the large German safety study was 0.3/1000 vaccinated infants. The rate of SIDS in the Italian efficacy trial was 0.4/1000 *Infanrix*-vaccinated infants. The reported rate of SIDS in the U.S. from 1985 to 1991 was 1.5/1000 live births.[35] By chance alone, some cases of SIDS can be expected to follow receipt of whole-cell DTP or acellular DTP vaccine.[18]

Rarely, an anaphylactic reaction (i.e., hives, swelling of the mouth, difficulty breathing, hypotension, shock) has been reported after receiving preparations containing diphtheria, tetanus and/or pertussis antigens.[1,18] Arthus-type hypersensitivity reactions, characterized by severe local reactions, may follow receipt of tetanus toxoid. A few cases of peripheral mono-neuropathy have been reported following tetanus toxoid administration, although the IOM concluded that the evidence was inadequate to accept or reject a causal relationship.[36]

A review by the IOM found evidence for a causal relationship between receipt of tetanus toxoid and both brachial neuritis and Guillain-Barré Syndrome.[36]

Additional Adverse Reactions Evaluated in Conjunction with Whole-Cell DTP Vaccination

Whole-cell DTP vaccine has been associated with acute encephalopathy.[21] In the National Childhood Encephalopathy Study (NCES), a large, case-control study in England, children 2 to 35 months of age with serious, acute neurologic disorders, such as encephalopathy or complicated convulsion(s), were more likely to have received DTP vaccine in the 7 days preceding onset than their age-matched controls. Among children presumed to be neurologically normal before entering the study, the relative risk (estimated by odds ratio) of a neurologic illness occurring within the 7-day period following receipt of DTP dose, compared to children not receiving DTP vaccine in the 7-day period before onset of their illness, was 3.3 (p<0.001). The attributable risk for all neurologic events was estimated to be 1:140,000 doses of DTP vaccine administered. In this study, a causal relationship between receipt of DTP vaccine and permanent neurologic injury was suggested.[1,37–40]

A 10-year follow-up to the NCES demonstrated that children who experience a serious acute neurologic illness following whole-cell DTP vaccine are at increased risk for chronic nervous system dysfunction or death.[41] However, the IOM concluded that the results were insufficient to determine whether DTP vaccine increases the overall risk for chronic nervous system dysfunction in children.[18,22]

Subsequent studies have failed to provide evidence in support of a causal relationship between DTP vaccination and either serious acute neurologic illness or permanent neurologic injury.[42–45] The ACIP and AAP continue to recommend the use of DTP vaccine.

Among a subset of children who were participating in the NCES and who had infantile spasms, both DTP and DT vaccination appeared either to precipitate early manifestations of the condition or to lead to its identification by parents.[46] IOM reviewed this and other studies and concluded that neither vaccine causes the illness.[18,21,45,47] The incidence of onset of infantile spasms increases at 3 to 9 months of age, the time period in which the second and third doses of DTP vaccine are generally given. Therefore, some cases of infantile spasms can be expected to be temporally associated with receipt of whole-cell DTP or acellular DTP vaccine by chance alone.

SIDS has occurred in infants following administration of whole-cell DTP and acellular DTP vaccine. Large case-control studies of SIDS in the United States have shown that SIDS was not causally related to receipt of DTP vaccine.[48,49] It should be recognized that the first three primary immunizing doses of DTP vaccine are usually administered to infants 2 to 6 months old and that approximately 85% of SIDS cases occur between the ages of 1 and 6 months, with the peak incidence occurring at 6 weeks to 4 months of age. By chance alone, some cases of SIDS can be expected to be temporally related to recent receipt of whole-cell DTP or acellular DTP vaccine. A review by the committee of the IOM concluded that available evidence did not indicate a causal relation between DTP vaccine and SIDS.[18,21]

A bulging fontanelle associated with increased intracranial pressure, which occurred within 24 hours following DTP immunization, has been reported, although a causal relationship has not been established.[50–52]

As with any vaccine, there is the possibility that broad use of Infanrix (Diphtheria and Tetanus Toxoids and Acellular Pertussis Vaccine Adsorbed) could reveal adverse reactions not observed in clinical trials.

Reporting Adverse Events

The National Childhood Vaccine Injury Act requires that the manufacturer and lot number of the vaccine administered be recorded by the healthcare provider in the vaccine recipient's permanent medical record, along with the date of administration of the vaccine and the name, address and title of the person administering the vaccine.[53] The Act further requires the healthcare provider to report to the U.S. Department of Health and Human Services via VAERS the occurrence following immunization of any event set forth in the Vaccine Injury Table including: anaphylaxis or anaphylactic shock within 4 hours, encephalopathy or encephalitis within 72 hours, or any sequelae thereof (including death).[53,54] In addition, any event considered a contraindication to further doses should be reported.

DOSAGE AND ADMINISTRATION

Preparation for Administration

Shake the vial well before withdrawal and use. The vaccine is ready to use without reconstitution. Parenteral drug products should be inspected visually for particulate matter or discoloration prior to administration, whenever solution and container permit. With thorough agitation, *Infanrix* is a homogeneous white turbid suspension. Discard if it appears otherwise. Since this product is a suspension containing an adjuvant, shake vigorously to obtain a uniform suspension prior to withdrawal from the vial. DO NOT USE IF RESUSPENSION DOES NOT OCCUR WITH VIGOROUS SHAKING. After removal of the 0.5 mL dose, any vaccine remaining in the vial should be discarded.

Infanrix should be administered by intramuscular injection. The preferred sites are the anterolateral aspects of the thigh or the deltoid muscle of the upper arm. The vaccine should not be injected in the gluteal area or areas where there may be a major nerve trunk. Before injection, the skin at the injection site should be cleaned and prepared with a

Continued on next page

Table 5.[15] Adverse Events (%) Occurring Within the 3 Days Following Vaccination with *Infanrix* or Whole-Cell DTP (Fourth Dose) in German Children Who Had Received Three Previous Doses of the Same Vaccine

Event	*Infanrix* After *Infanrix* Primary (N=268)	Whole-Cell DTP Vaccine After Whole-Cell DTP Vaccine Primary (N=92)
Local		
Redness	32.8	43.5
Redness >2 cm	4.5	3.3
Swelling	22.4	31.5
Swelling >2 cm	3.0	7.6
Pain*	15.7	55.4
Systemic		
Fever (≥100.4°F)*†	26.9	64.1
Fever (>103.1°F)†‡	0.4	4.3
Restlessness*	12.3	32.6
Loss of Appetite*	10.8	43.5
Vomiting	3.4	7.6
Drowsiness*	10.4	31.5
Unusual Crying*	7.8	33.7

* p<0.0001.
† Rectal temperatures.
‡ p<0.05.

Table 6.[33,34] Adverse Events (%) Occurring Within the 3 Days Following Vaccination with *Infanrix* Administered at 15 to 20 Months and 4 to 6 Years of Age in U.S. Children Who Had Previously Received Three or Four Doses of Whole-Cell DTP Vaccine

	15 to 20 months Three Previous Doses of Whole-Cell DTP Vaccine		4 to 6 years Four Previous Doses of Whole-Cell DTP Vaccine	
Event	*Infanrix* (N=110)	Whole-Cell DTP Vaccine (N=55)	*Infanrix* (N=115)	Whole-Cell DTP Vaccine (N=57)
Local				
Redness*	23	45	19	40
Redness† >10 mm	5	31	7	26
Swelling	14	24	15*	33*
Swelling >10 mm	7	15	8	18
Pain†§	5	38	12	40
Systemic				
Fever* ≥99.4°F‡	25	42	23	47
Fever† >100.5°F‡	2	20	1	12
Fussiness	34†	69†	20	30
Drowsiness	9*	24*	11	18
Poor Appetite*	9	20	6	16
Vomiting	2	0	1	4

* p<0.05.
† p<0.0001.
‡ Oral temperatures.
§ Moderate or severe = cried or protested to touch or cried when arm moved.

Table 7.[13] Severe Adverse Events Occurring Within 48 Hours Following Vaccination with *Infanrix* or Whole-Cell DTP in Italian Infants at 2, 4 or 6 Months of Age

	Infanrix (N=13,761 doses)		Whole-Cell DTP Vaccine (N=13,520 Doses)	
Event	Number	Rate/ 1,000 Doses	Number	Rate/ 1,000 Doses
Fever ≥104°F*†	5	0.36	32	2.4
Hypotonic-Hyporesponsive Episode‡	0	0	9	0.67
Persistent crying ≥3 hours*	6	0.44	54	4.0
Seizures**	1§	0.07	3¶	0.22

* p <0.001.
† Rectal temperatures.
‡ p = 0.002.
§ Maximum rectal temperature within 72 hours of vaccination = 103.1°F.
¶ Maximum rectal temperature within 72 hours of vaccination = 99.5°F, 101.3°F and 102.2°F.
** Not statistically significant at p<0.05.

Information on the SmithKline Beecham Pharmaceuticals products appearing here is based on the labeling in effect on June 15, 2000. Further information on these and other products may be obtained from the Medical Department, SmithKline Beecham Pharmaceuticals, One Franklin Plaza, Philadelphia, PA 19101.

Infanrix—Cont.

suitable germicide. After insertion of the needle, aspirate to ensure that the needle has not entered a blood vessel.
Do not administer this product subcutaneously.

Primary Immunization

The primary immunization course for children less than 7 years of age is three doses of 0.5 mL, given intramuscularly, at 4- to 8-week intervals (preferably 8 weeks). The customary age for the first dose is 2 months of age, but it may be given starting at 6 weeks of age and up to the seventh birthday. It is recommended that *Infanrix* be given for all three doses since no interchangeability data on acellular DTP vaccines exist for the primary series. *Infanrix* may be used to complete the primary series in infants who have received one or two doses of whole-cell DTP vaccine. However, the safety and efficacy of *Infanrix* in such infants have not been evaluated.

Booster Immunization

When *Infanrix* is given for the primary series, a fourth dose is recommended at 15 to 20 months of age. The interval between the third and fourth dose should be at least 6 months. At this time, data are insufficient to establish the frequency of adverse events following a fifth dose of *Infanrix* in children who have previously received four doses of *Infanrix*.

If a child has received whole-cell DTP vaccine for one or more doses, *Infanrix* may be given to complete the five-dose series. A fourth dose is recommended at 15 to 20 months of age. The interval between the third and fourth dose should be at least 6 months. Children 4 to 6 years of age (up to the seventh birthday) who received all four doses by the fourth birthday, including one or more doses of whole-cell DTP vaccine, should receive a single dose of *Infanrix* before entering kindergarten or elementary school. This dose is not needed if the fourth dose was given on or after the fourth birthday.

Additional Dosing Information

If any recommended dose of pertussis vaccine cannot be given, DT (For Pediatric Use) should be given as needed to complete the series.

Interruption of the recommended schedule with a delay between doses should not interfere with the final immunity achieved with *Infanrix*. There is no need to start the series over again, regardless of the time elapsed between doses.

The use of reduced volume (fractional doses) is not recommended. The effect of such practices on the frequency of serious adverse events and on protection against disease has not been determined.[17]

Preterm infants should be vaccinated according to their chronological age from birth.[17]

For persons 7 years of age or older, Tetanus and Diphtheria Toxoids (Td) for adult use should be given for routine booster immunization against tetanus and diphtheria.

Simultaneous Vaccine Administration

In clinical trials, *Infanrix* was routinely administered, at separate sites, concomitantly with one or more of the following vaccines: poliovirus vaccine live oral (OPV), hepatitis B vaccine, and *Haemophilus influenzae* type b vaccine (Hib) (see CLINICAL PHARMACOLOGY).

No data are available on the simultaneous administration of measles, mumps and rubella vaccine (MMR), varicella vaccine or inactivated polio virus (IPV) with *Infanrix*.

When concomitant administration of other vaccines is required, they should be given with different syringes and at different injection sites.

The ACIP encourages routine simultaneous administration of acellular DTP, OPV (or IPV), Hib, MMR and hepatitis B vaccine for children who are at the recommended age to receive these vaccines and for whom no specific contraindications exist at the time of the visit, unless, in the judgment of the provider, complete vaccination of the child will not be compromised by administering vaccines at different visits. Simultaneous administration is particularly important if the child might not return for subsequent vaccinations.[17]

STORAGE

Store *Infanrix* between 2°and 8°C (36°and 46°F). **Do not freeze.** Discard if the vaccine has been frozen. Do not use after expiration date shown on the label.

HOW SUPPLIED

Infanrix (Diphtheria and Tetanus Toxoids and Acellular Pertussis Vaccine Adsorbed) is supplied as a turbid white suspension in vials containing a 0.5 mL single dose, in packages of 10 vials.

NDC 58160-840-11 (package of 10)

References

1. Centers for Disease Control. Diphtheria, tetanus and pertussis: Recommendations for vaccine use and other preventive measures. Recommendations of the Immunization Practices Advisory Committee (ACIP). *MMWR.* 1991;Vol. 40 (No. RR-10):1–28.
2. Centers for Disease Control and Prevention. Summary of Notifiable Diseases, United States, 1993. *MMWR.* 1994;Vol. 42 (No. 53):1–28.
3. Centers for Disease Control and Prevention. Diphtheria Epidemic-New independent states of the former Soviet Union, 1990-1994. *MMWR.* 1995;44 (No.10):177–181.
4. Biological products; bacterial vaccines and toxoids; implementation of efficacy review. *Federal Register.* Friday, December 13, 1985; Vol. 50 (No. 240):51002–51117.
5. Centers for Disease Control. Tetanus—United States, 1987 and 1988. *MMWR.* 1990;Vol. 39 (No. 3):37–44.
6. Kendrick PL. Secondary familial attack rates from pertussis in vaccinated and unvaccinated children. *Am J Hygiene.* 1940;32:89–91.
7. Centers for Disease Control. Pertussis—United States, January 1992-June 1995. *MMWR.* 1995; Vol. 44 (No. 28):525–529.
8. Farizo KM, et al. Epidemiologic features of pertussis in the United States, 1980-1989. *Clin Infect Dis.* 1992;14: 708–719.
9. Nennig ME, et al. Prevalence and incidence of adult pertussis in an urban population. *JAMA.* 1996; Vol. 275 (No. 21):1672–1674.
10. Cowell JL, et al. Prospective protective antigens and animal models for pertussis. In: Leive L and Schlessinger D, eds. *Microbiology-1984.* Washington, DC: American Society for Microbiology, 1984, pp. 172–175.
11. Shahin RD, et al. Characterization of the protective capacity and immunogenicity of the 69-kD outer membrane protein of *Bordetella pertussis. J Exper Med.* 1990;171(1):63–73.
12. Gustafsson L, et al. A controlled trial of a two-component acellular, a five-component acellular, and a whole-cell pertussis vaccine. *N Engl J Med.* 1996;334(6):349–355.
13. Greco D, et al. A controlled trial of two acellular vaccines and one whole-cell vaccine against pertussis. *N Engl J Med.* 1996;334(6):341–348.
14. Schmitt H-J, et al. Efficacy of acellular pertussis vaccine in early childhood after household exposure. *JAMA.* 1996;275(1):37–41.
15. Data on file, SmithKline Beecham Pharmaceuticals, Philadelphia, PA.
16. Blatter M, et al. Immunogenicity of diphtheria-tetanus-acellular pertussis (DT-tricomponent Pa), hepatitis B (HB) and *Haemophilus influenzae* type b (Hib) vaccines administered concomitantly at separate sites along with oral poliovirus vaccine (OPV) in infants. Abstract G102, Interscience Conference on Antimicrobial Agents and Chemotherapy, 1996.
17. Centers for Disease Control and Prevention. General recommendations on immunization. Recommendations of the Advisory Committee on Immunization Practices (ACIP). *MMWR.* 1994; Vol. 43 (No. RR-1):1–38.
18. Centers for Disease Control and Prevention. Update: Vaccine side effects, adverse reactions, contraindications, and precautions—recommendations of the Advisory Committee on Immunization Practices (ACIP). *MMWR.* 1996;Vol. 45 (No. RR-12):1–35.
19. Wilson GS. The hazards of immunization. Provocation poliomyelitis. 1967, pp. 270–274.
20. American Academy of Pediatrics. Pertussis. *Report of the Committee on Infectious Diseases.* 23rd ed. Elk Grove Village, IL: American Academy of Pediatrics, 1994.
21. Howson CP, et al. Adverse effects of pertussis and rubella vaccines. Institute of Medicine (IOM). Washington, DC: National Academy Press, 1991.
22. Stratton KR, et al. DPT vaccine and chronic nervous system dysfunction: a new analysis. Institute of Medicine (IOM). Washington, DC: National Academy Press, 1994 (Supplement).
23. Livengood JR, et al. Family history of convulsions and use of pertussis vaccine. *J Pediatr.* 1989;115(4):527–531.
24. Centers for Disease Control. Pertussis immunization: family history of convulsions and use of antipyretics-supplementary ACIP statement. Recommendations of the Immunization Practices Advisory Committee (ACIP). *MMWR.* 1987;Vol. 36 (No. 18):281–282.
25. Centers for Disease Control and Prevention. Use of vaccines and immune globulins for persons with altered immunocompetence. Recommendations of the Advisory Committee on Immunization Practices (ACIP). *MMWR.* 1993;Vol. 42 (No. RR-4):1–3.
26. Centers for Disease Control. Vaccine Adverse Event Reporting System-United States. *MMWR.* 1990;Vol. 39 (No. 41):730–733.
27. Bernstein HH, et al. Reactogenicity and immunogenicity of a three-component acellular pertussis vaccine administered as the primary series to 2, 4 and 6 month-old infants in the United States. *Vaccine.* 1995;Vol. 13(17): 1631–1635.
28. Decker MD, et al. Comparison of 13 acellular pertussis vaccines: adverse reactions. *Pediatrics.* 1995;96:557–566.
29. Noble GR, et al. Acellular and whole-cell pertussis vaccines in Japan. Report of a visit by US scientists. *JAMA.* 1987;257(10):1351–1356.
30. Blennow M, et al. Adverse reactions and serologic response to a booster dose of acellular pertussis vaccine in children immunized with acellular or whole-cell vaccine as infants. *Pediatrics.* 1989;84(1):62–67.
31. Pim C, et al. Local reactions to kindergarten DPT boosters—Cranbrook. *Dis Surveill.* 1988; 9:230–239.
32. Gold R, et al. Safety and immunogenicity of *Haemophilus influenzae* vaccine (tetanus toxoid conjugate) administered concurrently or combined with diphtheria and tetanus toxoids, pertussis vaccine and inactivated poliomyelitis vaccine to healthy infants at two, four and six months of age. *Pediatr Infect Dis J.* 1994;13:348–355.
33. Bernstein HH, et al. Comparison of a three-component acellular pertussis vaccine with a whole-cell pertussis vaccine in 15- through 20-month-old infants. *Pediatrics.* 1994;93(4):656–659.
34. Annunziato PW, et al. Comparison of a three-component acellular pertussis vaccine with a whole-cell pertussis vaccine in 4- through 6-year-old children. *Arch Pediatr Adolesc Med.* 1994;148:503–507.
35. Willinger M, et al. Infant sleep position and risk for Sudden Infant Death Syndrome: Report of meeting held January 13 and 14, 1994, National Institutes of Health, Bethesda, MD. *Pediatrics.* 1994;93:814–819.
36. Stratton KR, et al. Adverse events associated with childhood vaccines. Evidence bearing on causality. Institute of Medicine (IOM). Washington, DC: National Academy Press, 1994.
37. Miller D, et al. Pertussis vaccine and whooping cough as risk factors for acute neurological illness and death in young children. *Dev Biol Stand.* 1985;61:389–394.
38. Miller DL, et al. Pertussis immunization and serious acute neurological illness in children. *Br Med J.* 1981;282:1595–1599.
39. Ross E, et al. Risk and pertussis vaccine (letter). *Arch Dis Child.* 1986;61:98–99.
40. Miller D, et al. Severe neurological illness: further analyses of the British National Childhood Encephalopathy Study. *Tokai J Exp Clin Med.* 1988;13(suppl):145–155.
41. Miller DL, et al. Pertussis immunization and serious acute neurological illnesses in children. *Br Med J.* 1993;307:1171–1176.
42. Pollock TM, et al. A 7-year survey of disorders attributed to vaccination in North West Thames region. *Lancet.* 1983;1:753–757.
43. Walker AM, et al. Neurologic events following diphtheria-tetanus-pertussis immunization. *Pediatrics.* 1988;81(3):345–349.
44. Griffin MR, et al. Risk of seizures and encephalopathy after immunization with the diphtheria-tetanus-pertussis vaccine. *JAMA.* 1990;263(12):1641–1645.
45. Shields WD, et al. Relationship of pertussis immunization to the onset of neurologic disorders: a retrospective epidemiologic study. *J Pediatr.* 1988;113:801–805.
46. Bellman MH, et al. Infantile spasms and pertussis immunization. *Lancet.* 1983;(1):1031–1034.
47. Melchior JC. Infantile spasms and early immunization against whooping cough: Danish survey from 1970 to 1975. *Arch Dis Child.* 1977;52:134–137.
48. Griffin MR, et al. Risk of Sudden Infant Death Syndrome after immunization with the diphtheria-tetanus-pertussis vaccine. *N Engl J Med.* 1988; Vol. 319 (10): 618–623.
49. Hoffman HJ, et al. Diphtheria-tetanus-pertussis immunization and sudden infant death: Results of the National Institute of Child Health and Human Development Cooperative Epidemiological Study of Sudden Infant Death Syndrome Risk Factors. *Pediatrics.* 1987; 79(4):598–611.
50. Jacob J, et al. Increased intracranial pressure after diphtheria, tetanus and pertussis immunization. *Am J Dis Child.* 1979;133(2):217–218.
51. Mathur R, et al. Bulging fontanel following triple vaccine. *Indian Pediatr.* 1981;18(6):417–418.
52. Shendurnikar N, et al. Bulging fontanel following DPT vaccine. *Indian Pediatr.* 1986; 23(11):960.
53. Centers for Disease Control. National Childhood Vaccine Injury Act: Requirements for permanent vaccination records and for reporting of selected events after vaccination. *MMWR.* 1988;Vol. 37 (No. 13):197–200.
54. National Vaccine Injury Compensation Program: Revision of the vaccine injury table. *Federal Register.* Wednesday, February 8, 1995; Vol. 60 (No. 26):7694.

Manufactured by **SmithKline Beecham Biologicals**
Rixensart, Belgium, U.S. License 1090, and
Chiron Behring GmbH & Co
Marburg, Germany, U.S. License 0097
Distributed by **SmithKline Beecham Pharmaceuticals**
Philadelphia, PA 19101
Rx only
Infanrix is a registered trademark of SmithKline Beecham.
Veterans Administration/Military/PHS—0.5 mL Single-Dose Vial, 10's, 6505-01-442-6262.
IN:L3

Shown in Product Identification Guide, page 337

KYTRIL® ℞

[*kī ′-tril*]
granisetron hydrochloride Injection

DESCRIPTION

Kytril (granisetron hydrochloride) Injection is an antinauseant and antiemetic agent. Chemically it is *endo*-N-(9-methyl-9-azabicyclo [3.3.1] non-3-yl)-1-methyl-1H-indazole-3-carboxamide hydrochloride with a molecular weight of 348.9 (312.4 free base). Its empirical formula is $C_{18}H_{24}N_4O \cdot HCl$ while its chemical structure is:

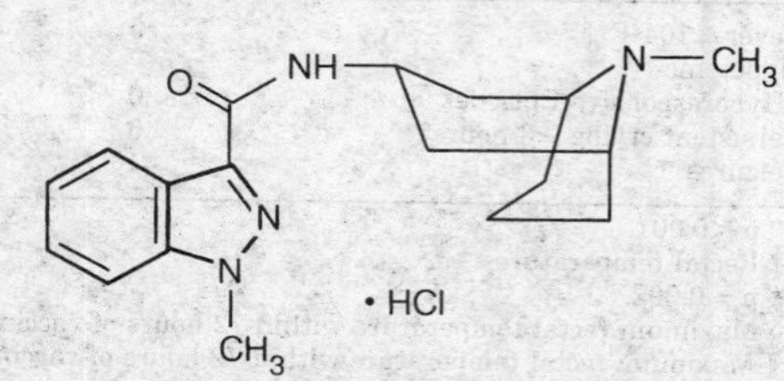

granisetron hydrochloride

Granisetron hydrochloride is a white to off-white solid that is readily soluble in water and normal saline at 20°C. *Kytril* Injection is a clear, colorless, sterile, nonpyrogenic, aqueous solution for intravenous administration.

Kytril is available in 1 mL single-dose and 4 mL multi-dose vials.

Single-Dose Vials: Each 1 mL of preservative-free aqueous solution contains 1.12 mg granisetron hydrochloride equivalent to granisetron, 1.0 mg and sodium chloride, 9.0 mg. The solution's pH ranges from 4.7 to 7.3.

Multi-Dose Vials: Each 1 mL contains 1.12 mg granisetron hydrochloride equivalent to granisetron, 1.0 mg; sodium chloride, 9 mg; citric acid, 2 mg; benzyl alcohol, 10 mg, as a preservative. The solution's pH ranges from 4.0 to 6.0.

CLINICAL PHARMACOLOGY

Granisetron is a selective 5-hydroxytryptamine$_3$ (5-HT$_3$) receptor antagonist with little or no affinity for other serotonin receptors, including 5-HT$_1$; 5-HT$_{1A}$; 5-HT$_{1B/C}$; 5-HT$_2$; for alpha$_1$-, alpha$_2$- or beta-adrenoreceptors; for dopamine-D$_2$; or for histamine-H$_1$; benzodiazepine; picrotoxin, or opioid receptors.

Serotonin receptors of the 5-HT$_3$ type are located peripherally on vagal nerve terminals and centrally in the chemoreceptor trigger zone of the area postrema. During chemotherapy-induced vomiting, mucosal enterochromaffin cells release serotonin, which stimulates 5-HT$_3$ receptors. This evokes vagal afferent discharge, inducing vomiting. Animal studies demonstrate that, in binding to 5-HT$_3$ receptors, granisetron blocks serotonin stimulation and subsequent vomiting after emetogenic stimuli such as cisplatin. In the ferret animal model, a single granisetron injection prevented vomiting due to high-dose cisplatin or arrested vomiting within 5 to 30 seconds.

In most human studies, granisetron has had little effect on blood pressure, heart rate or ECG. No evidence of an effect on plasma prolactin or aldosterone concentrations has been found in other studies.

Kytril Injection exhibited no effect on oro-cecal transit time in normal volunteers given a single intravenous infusion of 50 mcg/kg or 200 mcg/kg. Single and multiple oral doses slowed colonic transit in normal volunteers.

Pharmacokinetics

In adult cancer patients undergoing chemotherapy and in volunteers, infusion of a single 40 mcg/kg dose of *Kytril* Injection produced the following mean pharmacokinetic data:

[See table 1 above]

There was high inter and intrasubject variability noted in these studies. No difference in mean AUC was found between males and females, although males had a higher C_{max} generally.

Granisetron metabolism involves N-demethylation and aromatic ring oxidation followed by conjugation. Animal studies suggest that some of the metabolites may also have 5-HT$_3$ receptor antagonist activity.

Clearance is predominantly by hepatic metabolism. In normal volunteers, approximately 12% of the administered dose is eliminated unchanged in the urine in 48 hours. The remainder of the dose is excreted as metabolites, 49% in the urine and 34% in the feces.

In vitro liver microsomal studies show that granisetron's major route of metabolism is inhibited by ketoconazole, suggestive of metabolism mediated by the cytochrome P-450 3A subfamily.

Plasma protein binding is approximately 65% and granisetron distributes freely between plasma and red blood cells.

Elderly: The ranges of the pharmacokinetic parameters in elderly volunteers (mean age 71 years), given a single 40 mcg/kg intravenous dose of *Kytril* Injection, were generally similar to those in younger healthy volunteers; mean values were lower for clearance and longer for half-life in the elderly (see Table 1).

Pediatric Patients: A pharmacokinetic study in pediatric cancer patients (2 to 16 years of age), given a single 40 mcg/kg intravenous dose of *Kytril* Injection, showed that volume of distribution and total clearance increased with age. No relationship with age was observed for peak plasma concentration or terminal phase plasma half-life. When volume of distribution and total clearance are adjusted for body weight, the pharmacokinetics of granisetron are similar in pediatric and adult cancer patients.

Renal Failure Patients: Total clearance of granisetron was not affected in patients with severe renal failure who received a single 40 mcg/kg intravenous dose of *Kytril* Injection.

Hepatically Impaired Patients: A pharmacokinetic study in patients with hepatic impairment due to neoplastic liver involvement showed that total clearance was approximately halved compared to patients without hepatic impairment. Given the wide variability in pharmacokinetic parameters noted in patients and the good tolerance of doses well above the recommended 10 mcg/kg dose, dosage adjustment in patients with possible hepatic functional impairment is not necessary.

CLINICAL TRIALS

Kytril Injection has been shown to prevent nausea and vomiting associated with single-day and repeat cycle cancer chemotherapy.

Single-Day Chemotherapy

Cisplatin-Based Chemotherapy: In a double-blind, placebo-controlled study in 28 cancer patients, *Kytril* Injection, administered as a single intravenous infusion of 40 mcg/kg,

Table 1. Pharmacokinetic Parameters in Adult Cancer Patients Undergoing Chemotherapy and in Volunteers, Following a Single Intravenous 40 mcg/kg Dose of Kytril (granisetron hydrochloride) Injection

	Peak Plasma Concentration (ng/mL)	Terminal Phase Plasma Half-Life (h)	Total Clearance (L/h/kg)	Volume of Distribution (L/kg)
Cancer Patients				
Mean	63.8*	8.95*	0.38*	3.07*
Range	18.0 to 176	0.90 to 31.1	0.14 to 1.54	0.85 to 10.4
Volunteers				
21 to 42 years				
Mean	64.3†	4.91†	0.79†	3.04†
Range	11.2 to 182	0.88 to 15.2	0.20 to 2.56	1.68 to 6.13
65 to 81 years				
Mean	57.0†	7.69†	0.44†	3.97†
Range	14.6 to 153	2.65 to 17.7	0.17 to 1.06	1.75 to 7.01

* 5-minute infusion.
† 3-minute infusion.

Table 3. Prevention of Chemotherapy-Induced Nausea and Vomiting—Single-Day High-Dose Cisplatin Therapy [1]

	Kytril Injection (mcg/kg)			*P*-Value (vs. 2 mcg/kg)	
	2	10	40	10	40
Number of Patients	52	52	53		
Response Over 24 Hours					
Complete Response[2]	31%	62%	68%	<0.002	<0.001
No Vomiting	38%	65%	74%	<0.001	<0.001
No More Than Mild Nausea	58%	75%	79%	NS	0.007

1. Cisplatin administration began within 10 minutes of *Kytril* Injection infusion and continued for 2.6 hours (mean). Mean cisplatin doses were 96 to 99 mg/m^2.
2. No vomiting and no moderate or severe nausea.

Table 4. Prevention of Chemotherapy-Induced Nausea and Vomiting—Single-Day High-Dose and Low-Dose Cisplatin Therapy[1]

	Kytril Injection (mcg/kg)				*P*-Value (vs. 5 mcg/kg)		
	5	10	20	40	10	20	40
High-Dose Cisplatin							
Number of Patients	40	49	48	47			
Response Over 24 Hours							
Complete Response[2]	18%	41%	40%	47%	0.018	0.025	0.004
No Vomiting	28%	47%	44%	53%	NS	NS	0.016
No Nausea	15%	35%	38%	43%	0.036	0.019	0.005
Low-Dose Cisplatin							
Number of Patients	42	41	40	46			
Response Over 24 Hours							
Complete Response[2]	29%	56%	58%	41%	0.012	0.009	NS
No Vomiting	36%	63%	65%	43%	0.012	0.008	NS
No Nausea	29%	56%	38%	33%	0.012	NS	NS

1. Cisplatin administration began within 10 minutes of *Kytril* Injection infusion and continued for 2 hours (mean). Mean cisplatin doses were 64 and 98 mg/m^2 for low and high strata.
2. No vomiting and no use of rescue antiemetic.

was significantly more effective than placebo in preventing nausea and vomiting induced by cisplatin chemotherapy. See Table 2.

Table 2. Prevention of Chemotherapy-Induced Nausea and Vomiting—Single-Day Cisplatin Therapy [1]

	Kytril Injection	Placebo	*P*-Value
Number of Patients	14	14	
Response Over 24 Hours			
Complete Response[2]	93%	7%	<0.001
No Vomiting	93%	14%	<0.001
No More Than Mild Nausea	93%	7%	<0.001

1. Cisplatin administration began within 10 minutes of *Kytril* Injection infusion and continued for 1.5 to 3.0 hours. Mean cisplatin dose was 86 mg/m^2 in the *Kytril* Injection group and 80 mg/m^2 in the placebo group.
2. No vomiting and no moderate or severe nausea.

Kytril Injection was also evaluated in a randomized dose response study of cancer patients receiving cisplatin ≥75 mg/m^2. Additional chemotherapeutic agents included: anthracyclines, carboplatin, cytostatic antibiotics, folic acid derivatives, methylhydrazine, nitrogen mustard analogs, podophyllotoxin derivatives, pyrimidine analogs and vinca alkaloids. *Kytril* Injection doses of 10 and 40 mcg/kg were superior to 2 mcg/kg in preventing cisplatin-induced nausea and vomiting, but 40 mcg/kg was not significantly superior to 10 mcg/kg. See Table 3.

[See table 3 above]

Kytril (granisetron hydrochloride) Injection was also evaluated in a double-blind, randomized dose response study of 353 patients stratified for high (≥80 to 120 mg/m^2) or low (50 to 79 mg/m^2) cisplatin dose. Response rates of patients for both cisplatin strata are given in Table 4.

[See table 4 above]

For both the low and high cisplatin strata, the 10, 20 and 40 mcg/kg doses were more effective than the 5 mcg/kg dose in preventing nausea and vomiting within 24 hours of chemotherapy administration. The 10 mcg/kg dose was at least as effective as the higher doses.

Moderately Emetogenic Chemotherapy: *Kytril* Injection, 40 mcg/kg, was compared with the combination of chlorpromazine (50 to 200 mg/24 hours) and dexamethasone (12 mg) in patients treated with moderately emetogenic chemotherapy, including primarily carboplatin >300 mg/m^2, cisplatin 20 to 50 mg/m^2 and cyclophosphamide >600 mg/m^2. *Kytril* Injection was superior to the chlorpromazine regimen in preventing nausea and vomiting. See Table 5.

Table 5. Prevention of Chemotherapy-Induced Nausea and Vomiting—Single-Day Moderately Emetogenic Chemotherapy

	Kytril Injection	Chlorpromazine[1]	*P*-Value
Number of Patients	133	133	
Response Over 24 Hours			
Complete Response[2]	68%	47%	<0.001
No Vomiting	73%	53%	<0.001
No More Than Mild Nausea	77%	59%	<0.001

1. Patients also received dexamethasone, 12 mg.
2. No vomiting and no moderate or severe nausea.

In other studies of moderately emetogenic chemotherapy, no significant difference in efficacy was found between *Kytril* doses of 40 mcg/kg and 160 mcg/kg doses.

Repeat-Cycle Chemotherapy

In an uncontrolled trial, 512 cancer patients received *Kytril* Injection, 40 mcg/kg, prophylactically, for two cycles of chemotherapy, 224 patients received it for at least four cycles and 108 patients received it for at least six cycles.

Continued on next page

Information on the SmithKline Beecham Pharmaceuticals products appearing here is based on the labeling in effect on June 15, 2000. Further information on these and other products may be obtained from the Medical Department, SmithKline Beecham Pharmaceuticals, One Franklin Plaza, Philadelphia, PA 19101.

Kytril Injection—Cont.

Kytril Injection efficacy remained relatively constant over the first six repeat cycles, with complete response rates (no vomiting and no moderate or severe nausea in 24 hours) of 60% to 69%. No patients were studied for more than 15 cycles.

Pediatric Studies

A randomized double-blind study evaluated the 24-hour response of 80 pediatric cancer patients (age 2 to 16 years) to *Kytril* Injection 10, 20 or 40 mcg/kg. Patients were treated with cisplatin ≥60 mg/m^2, cytarabine ≥3 g/m^2, cyclophosphamide ≥1 g/m^2 or nitrogen mustard ≥6 mg/m^2. See Table 6.

Table 6. Prevention of Chemotherapy-Induced Nausea and Vomiting in Pediatric Patients

	Kytril Injection Dose (mcg/kg)		
	10	20	40
Number of Patients	29	26	25
Median Number of Vomiting Episodes	2	3	1
Complete Response Over 24 Hours[1]	21%	31%	32%

1. No vomiting and no moderate or severe nausea.

A second pediatric study compared *Kytril* Injection 20 mcg/kg to chlorpromazine plus dexamethasone in 88 patients treated with ifosfamide ≥3 g/m^2/day for two or three days. *Kytril* Injection was administered on each day of ifosfamide treatment. At 24 hours, 22% of *Kytril* Injection patients achieved complete response (no vomiting and no moderate or severe nausea in 24 hours) compared with 10% on the chlorpromazine regimen. The median number of vomiting episodes with *Kytril* Injection was 1.5; with chlorpromazine it was 7.0.

INDICATIONS AND USAGE

Kytril (granisetron hydrochloride) Injection is indicated for the prevention of nausea and vomiting associated with initial and repeat courses of emetogenic cancer therapy, including high-dose cisplatin.

CONTRAINDICATIONS

Kytril Injection is contraindicated in patients with known hypersensitivity to the drug or to any of its components.

PRECAUTIONS

Drug Interactions

Granisetron does not induce or inhibit the cytochrome P-450 drug-metabolizing enzyme system. There have been no definitive drug-drug interaction studies to examine pharmacokinetic or pharmacodynamic interaction with other drugs, but in humans, *Kytril* Injection has been safely administered with drugs representing benzodiazepines, neuroleptics and anti-ulcer medications commonly prescribed with antiemetic treatments. *Kytril* Injection also does not appear to interact with emetogenic cancer chemotherapies. Because granisetron is metabolized by hepatic cytochrome P-450 drug-metabolizing enzymes, inducers or inhibitors of these enzymes may change the clearance and, hence, the half-life of granisetron.

Carcinogenesis, Mutagenesis, Impairment of Fertility

In a 24-month carcinogenicity study, rats were treated orally with granisetron 1, 5 or 50 mg/kg/day (6, 30 or 300 mg/m^2/day). The 50 mg/kg/day dose was reduced to 25 mg/kg/day (150 mg/m^2/day) during week 59 due to toxicity. For a 50 kg person of average height (1.46m^2 body surface area), these doses represent 16, 81 and 405 times the recommended clinical dose (0.37 mg/m^2, i.v.) on a body surface area basis. There was a statistically significant increase in the incidence of hepatocellular carcinomas and adenomas in males treated with 5 mg/kg/day (30 mg/m^2/day, 81 times the recommended human dose based on body surface area) and above, and in females treated with 25 mg/kg/day (150 mg/m^2/day, 405 times the recommended human dose based on body surface area). No increase in liver tumors was observed at a dose of 1 mg/kg/day (6 mg/m^2/day, 16 times the recommended human dose based on body surface area) in males and 5 mg/kg/day (30 mg/m^2/day, 81 times the recommended human dose based on body surface area) in females. In a 12-month oral toxicity study, treatment with granisetron 100 mg/kg/day (600 mg/m^2/day, 1622 times the recommended human dose based on body surface area) produced hepatocellular adenomas in male and female rats while no such tumors were found in the control rats. A 24-month mouse carcinogenicity study of granisetron did not show a statistically significant increase in tumor incidence, but the study was not conclusive.

Because of the tumor findings in rat studies, Kytril (granisetron hydrochloride) Injection should be prescribed only at the dose and for the indication recommended (see INDICATIONS AND USAGE, and DOSAGE AND ADMINISTRATION).

Granisetron was not mutagenic in *in vitro* Ames test and mouse lymphoma cell forward mutation assay, and *in vivo* mouse micronucleus test and *in vitro* and *ex vivo* rat hepatocyte UDS assays. It, however, produced a significant increase in UDS in HeLa cells *in vitro* and a significant increased incidence of cells with polyploidy in an *in vitro* human lymphocyte chromosomal aberration test.

Granisetron at subcutaneous doses up to 6 mg/kg/day (36 mg/m^2/day, 97 times the recommended human dose based on body surface area) was found to have no effect on fertility and reproductive performance of male and female rats.

Pregnancy

Teratogenic Effects. Pregnancy Category B. Reproduction studies have been performed in pregnant rats at intravenous doses up to 9 mg/kg/day (54 mg/m^2/day, 146 times the recommended human dose based on body surface area) and pregnant rabbits at intravenous doses up to 3 mg/kg/day (35.4 mg/m^2/day, 96 times the recommended human dose based on body surface area) and have revealed no evidence of impaired fertility or harm to the fetus due to granisetron. There are, however, no adequate and well-controlled studies in pregnant women. Because animal reproduction studies are not always predictive of human response, this drug should be used during pregnancy only if clearly needed.

Nursing Mothers

It is not known whether granisetron is excreted in human milk. Because many drugs are excreted in human milk, caution should be exercised when *Kytril* Injection is administered to a nursing woman.

Pediatric Use

See DOSAGE AND ADMINISTRATION for use in children 2 to 16 years of age. Safety and effectiveness in children under 2 years of age have not been established.

Geriatric Use

During clinical trials, 713 patients 65 years of age or older received Kytril (granisetron HCl) Injection. Effectiveness and safety were similar in patients of various ages.

ADVERSE REACTIONS

The following have been reported during controlled clinical trials or in the routine management of patients. The percentage figures are based on clinical trial experience only. Table 7 gives the comparative frequencies of the five most commonly reported adverse events (≥3%) in patients receiving *Kytril* Injection, in single-day chemotherapy trials. These patients received chemotherapy, primarily cisplatin, and intravenous fluids during the 24-hour period following *Kytril* Injection administration. Events were generally recorded over seven days post-*Kytril* Injection administration. In the absence of a placebo group, there is uncertainty as to how many of these events should be attributed to *Kytril*, except for headache, which was clearly more frequent than in comparison groups.

Table 7. Principal Adverse Events in Clinical Trials—Single-Day Chemotherapy

	Percent of Patients with Event	
	Kytril Injection 40 mcg/kg (n=1,268)	Comparator[1] (n=422)
Headache	14%	6%
Asthenia	5%	6%
Somnolence	4%	15%
Diarrhea	4%	6%
Constipation	3%	3%

1. Metoclopramide/dexamethasone and phenothiazines/dexamethasone.

In over 3,000 patients receiving *Kytril* Injection (2 to 160 mcg/kg) in single-day and multiple-day clinical trials with emetogenic cancer therapies, adverse events, other than those in Table 7, were observed; attribution of many of these events to *Kytril* is uncertain.

Hepatic: In comparative trials, mainly with cisplatin regimens, elevations of AST and ALT (>2 times the upper limit of normal) following administration of *Kytril* Injection occurred in 2.8% and 3.3% of patients, respectively. These frequencies were not significantly different from those seen with comparators (AST: 2.1%; ALT: 2.4%).

Cardiovascular: Hypertension (2%); hypotension, arrhythmias such as sinus bradycardia, atrial fibrillation, varying degrees of A-V block, ventricular ectopy including non-sustained tachycardia, and ECG abnormalities have been observed rarely.

Central Nervous System: Agitation, anxiety, CNS stimulation and insomnia were seen in less than 2% of patients. Extrapyramidal syndrome occurred rarely and only in the presence of other drugs associated with this syndrome.

Hypersensitivity: Rare cases of hypersensitivity reactions, sometimes severe (e.g., anaphylaxis, shortness of breath, hypotension, urticaria) have been reported.

Other: Fever (3%), taste disorder (2%), skin rashes (1%). In multiple-day comparative studies, fever occurred more frequently with *Kytril* Injection (8.6%) than with comparative drugs (3.4%, $P < 0.014$), which usually included dexamethasone.

OVERDOSAGE

There is no specific antidote for Kytril (granisetron hydrochloride) Injection overdosage. In case of overdosage, symptomatic treatment should be given. Overdosage of up to 38.5 mg of granisetron hydrochloride injection has been reported without symptoms or only the occurrence of a slight headache.

DOSAGE AND ADMINISTRATION

The recommended dosage for *Kytril* Injection is 10 mcg/kg administered intravenously within 30 minutes before initiation of chemotherapy, and only on the day(s) chemotherapy is given. *Kytril* Injection may be administered intravenously either undiluted over 30 seconds, or diluted with 0.9% Sodium Chloride or 5% Dextrose and infused over 5 minutes.

Pediatric Use: The recommended dose in children 2 to 16 years of age is 10 mcg/kg (see CLINICAL TRIALS). Children under 2 years of age have not been studied.

Use in the Elderly, Renal Failure Patients or Hepatically Impaired Patients: No dosage adjustment is recommended. (See CLINICAL PHARMACOLOGY, Pharmacokinetics.)

Infusion Preparation

Kytril Injection, administered as a 5–minute infusion, should be diluted in 0.9% Sodium Chloride or 5% Dextrose to a total volume of 20 to 50 mL.

Stability

Intravenous infusion of *Kytril* Injection should be prepared at the time of administration. However, *Kytril* Injection has been shown to be stable for at least 24 hours when diluted in 0.9% Sodium Chloride or 5% Dextrose and stored at room temperature under normal lighting conditions.

As a general precaution, *Kytril* Injection should not be mixed in solution with other drugs. Parenteral drug products should be inspected visually for particulate matter and discoloration before administration whenever solution and container permit.

HOW SUPPLIED

Kytril (granisetron hydrochloride) Injection, 1 mg/mL (free base), is supplied in 1 mL Single-Use Vials and 4 mL Multi-Dose Vials.

NDC 0029-4149-01 (package of 1 Single-Dose Vial)

NDC 0029-4152-01 (package of 1 Multi-Dose Vial)

Store single-dose vials and multi-dose vials at 25°C (77°F); excursions permitted to 15–30°C (59–86°F).

Once the multi-dose vial is penetrated, its contents should be used within 30 days.

Do not freeze. Protect from light. Rx only

KY:L11A

Shown in Product Identification Guide, page 337

KYTRIL® ℞

[kī '-tril]

granisetron hydrochloride

Tablets

DESCRIPTION

Kytril Tablets contain granisetron hydrochloride, an antinauseant and antiemetic agent. Chemically it is *endo*-N-(9-methyl-9-azabicyclo [3.3.1] non-3-yl)-1-methyl-1H-indazole-3-carboxamide hydrochloride with a molecular weight of 348.9 (312.4 free base). Its empirical formula is $C_{18}H_{24}N_4O \bullet HCl$, while its chemical structure is:

granisetron hydrochloride

Granisetron hydrochloride is a white to off-white solid that is readily soluble in water and normal saline at 20°C.

Tablets for Oral Administration: Each white, triangular, biconvex, film-coated *Kytril* Tablet contains 1.12 mg granisetron hydrochloride equivalent to granisetron, 1 mg. Inactive ingredients are: hydroxypropyl methylcellulose, lactose, magnesium stearate, microcrystalline cellulose, polyethylene glycol, polysorbate 80, sodium starch glycolate and titanium dioxide.

CLINICAL PHARMACOLOGY

Granisetron is a selective 5-hydroxytryptamine$_3$ (5-HT$_3$) receptor antagonist with little or no affinity for other serotonin receptors, including 5-HT$_1$; 5-HT$_{1A}$; 5-HT$_{1B/C}$; 5-HT$_2$; for alpha$_1$-, alpha$_2$-, or beta-adrenoreceptors; for dopamine-D$_2$; or for histamine-H$_1$; benzodiazepine; picrotoxin, or opioid receptors.

Serotonin receptors of the 5-HT$_3$ type are located peripherally on vagal nerve terminals and centrally in the chemoreceptor trigger zone of the area postrema. During chemotherapy that induces vomiting, mucosal enterochromaffin cells release serotonin, which stimulates 5-HT$_3$ receptors. This evokes vagal afferent discharge, inducing vomiting. Animal studies demonstrate that, in binding to 5-HT$_3$ receptors, granisetron blocks serotonin stimulation and subsequent vomiting after emetogenic stimuli such as cisplatin. In the ferret animal model, a single granisetron injection prevented vomiting due to high-dose cisplatin or arrested vomiting within 5 to 30 seconds.

In most human studies, granisetron has had little effect on blood pressure, heart rate or ECG. No evidence of an effect on plasma prolactin or aldosterone concentrations has been found in other studies.

Following single and multiple oral doses, *Kytril* slowed colonic transit in normal volunteers. However, *Kytril* had no effect on oro-cecal transit time in normal volunteers when given as a single intravenous (IV) infusion of 50 mcg/kg or 200 mcg/kg.

Pharmacokinetics

In healthy volunteers and adult cancer patients undergoing chemotherapy, administration of oral *Kytril* produced the following mean pharmacokinetic data:

[See table 1 in next column]

The effects of gender on the pharmacokinetics of oral *Kytril* have not been studied. However, after intravenous infusion of *Kytril,* no difference in mean AUC was found between males and females, although males had a higher C_{max} generally.

When oral *Kytril* was administered with food, AUC was decreased by 5% and C_{max} increased by 30% in non-fasted healthy volunteers who received a single dose of 10 mg.

Granisetron metabolism involves N-demethylation and aromatic ring oxidation followed by conjugation. Animal studies suggest that some of the metabolites may also have 5-HT_3 receptor antagonist activity.

Clearance is predominantly by hepatic metabolism. In normal volunteers, approximately 11% of the orally administered dose is eliminated unchanged in the urine in 48 hours. The remainder of the dose is excreted as metabolites, 48% in the urine and 38% in the feces.

In vitro liver microsomal studies show that granisetron's major route of metabolism is inhibited by ketoconazole, suggestive of metabolism mediated by the cytochrome P-450 3A subfamily.

Plasma protein binding is approximately 65% and granisetron distributes freely between plasma and red blood cells.

In elderly and pediatric patients and in patients with renal failure or hepatic impairment, the pharmacokinetics of granisetron was determined following administration of intravenous *Kytril:*

Elderly: The ranges of the pharmacokinetic parameters in elderly volunteers (mean age 71 years), given a single 40 mcg/kg intravenous dose of *Kytril* Injection, were generally similar to those in younger healthy volunteers; mean values were lower for clearance and longer for half-life in the elderly.

Renal Failure Patients: Total clearance of granisetron was not affected in patients with severe renal failure who received a single 40 mcg/kg intravenous dose of *Kytril* Injection.

Hepatically Impaired Patients: A pharmacokinetic study with intravenous *Kytril* in patients with hepatic impairment due to neoplastic liver involvement showed that total clearance was approximately halved compared to patients without hepatic impairment. Given the wide variability in pharmacokinetic parameters noted in patients and the good tolerance of doses well above the recommended dose, dosage adjustment in patients with possible hepatic functional impairment is not necessary.

Pediatric Patients: A pharmacokinetic study in pediatric cancer patients (2 to 16 years of age), given a single 40 mcg/kg intravenous dose of *Kytril* Injection, showed that volume of distribution and total clearance increased with age. No relationship with age was observed for peak plasma concentration or terminal phase plasma half-life. When volume of distribution and total clearance are adjusted for body weight, the pharmacokinetics of granisetron are similar in pediatric and adult cancer patients.

Table 1. Pharmacokinetic Parameters (Median [range]) Following Oral Kytril (granisetron hydrochloride)

	Peak Plasma Concentration (ng/mL)	Terminal Phase Plasma Half-Life (h)	Volume of Distribution (L/kg)	Total Clearance (L/h/kg)
Cancer Patients 1.0 mg b.i.d., 7 days (n=27)	5.99 [0.63 to 30.9]	N.D.*	N.D.	0.52 [0.09 to 7.37]
Volunteers single 1.0 mg dose (n=39)	3.63 [0.27 to 9.14]	6.23 [0.96 to 19.9]	3.94 [1.89 to 39.4]	0.41 [0.11 to 24.6]

* Not determined after oral administration; following a single intravenous dose of 40 mcg/kg, terminal phase half-life was determined to be 8.95 hours.

N.D. Not determined

Table 2. Prevention of Nausea and Vomiting 24 Hours Post-Chemotherapy[1]

	Percentages of Patients Oral *Kytril* Dose			
Efficacy Measures	**0.25 mg b.i.d. (n=229) %**	**0.5 mg b.i.d. (n=235) %**	**1.0 mg b.i.d. (n=233) %**	**2.0 mg b.i.d. (n=233) %**
Complete Response[2]	61	70*	81*†	72*
No Vomiting	66	77*	88*	79*
No Nausea	48	57	63*	54

1. Chemotherapy included oral and injectable cyclophosphamide, carboplatin, cisplatin (20 mg/m² to 50 mg/m²), dacarbazine, doxorubicin, epirubicin.
2. No vomiting, no moderate or severe nausea, no rescue medication.

* Statistically significant ($P<0.01$) vs. 0.25 mg b.i.d.

† Statistically significant ($P<0.01$) vs. 0.5 mg b.i.d.

Table 3. Prevention of Nausea and Vomiting 24 Hours Post-Chemotherapy[1]

	Percentages of Patients		
Efficacy Measures	**Oral *Kytril* 1.0 mg b.i.d. (n=354) %**	**Oral *Kytril* 2.0 mg q.d. (n=343) %**	**Prochlorperazine[2] 10.0 mg b.i.d. (n=111) %**
Complete Response[3]	69*	64*	41
No Vomiting	82*	77*	48
No Nausea	51*	53*	35
Total Control[4]	51*	50*	33

1. Moderately emetogenic chemotherapeutic agents included cisplatin (20 mg/m² to 50 mg/m²), oral and intravenous cyclophosphamide, carboplatin, dacarbazine, doxorubicin.
2. Historical control from a previous double-blind *Kytril* trial.
3. No vomiting, no moderate or severe nausea, no rescue medication.
4. No vomiting, no nausea, no rescue medication.

* Statistically significant ($P<0.05$) vs. prochlorperazine historical control.

CLINICAL TRIALS

Chemotherapy-induced Nausea and Vomiting

Oral *Kytril* prevents nausea and vomiting associated with initial and repeat courses of emetogenic cancer therapy, as shown by 24-hour efficacy data from studies using both moderately- and highly-emetogenic chemotherapy.

Moderately Emetogenic Chemotherapy: The first trial compared oral *Kytril* doses of 0.25 to 2.0 mg b.i.d., in 930 cancer patients receiving, principally, cyclophosphamide, carboplatin and cisplatin (20 mg/m² to 50 mg/m²). Efficacy was based on: complete response (i.e., no vomiting, no moderate or severe nausea, no rescue medication), no vomiting and no nausea. Table 2 summarizes the results of this study.

[See table 2 above]

Results from a second double-blind, randomized trial evaluating *Kytril* 2.0 mg q.d. and *Kytril* 1.0 mg b.i.d. were compared to prochlorperazine 10 mg b.i.d. derived from a historical control. At 24 hours, there was no statistically significant difference in efficacy between the two oral *Kytril* regimens. Both regimens were statistically superior to the prochlorperazine control regimen (See Table 3).

[See table 3 above]

Results from a *Kytril* 2.0 mg q.d. alone treatment arm in a third double-blind, randomized trial, were compared to prochlorperazine (PCPZ), 10 mg b.i.d., derived from a historical control. The 24-hour results for *Kytril* 2.0 mg q.d. were statistically superior to PCPZ for all efficacy parameters: complete response (58%), no vomiting (79%), no nausea (51%), total control (49%). The PCPZ rates are shown in Table 3.

Cisplatin-based Chemotherapy: The first double-blind trial compared oral *Kytril* 1.0 mg b.i.d., relative to placebo (historical control), in 119 cancer patients receiving high-dose cisplatin (mean dose 80 mg/m²). At 24 hours, oral *Kytril* 1.0 mg b.i.d. was significantly ($P<0.001$) superior to placebo (historical control) in all efficacy parameters: complete response (52%), no vomiting (56%) and no nausea (45%). The placebo rates were 7%, 14% and 7%, respectively, for the three efficacy parameters.

Results from a *Kytril* 2.0 mg q.d. alone treatment arm in a second double-blind, randomized trial, were compared to both *Kytril* 1.0 mg b.i.d. and placebo historical controls. The 24-hour results for *Kytril* 2.0 mg q.d. were: complete response (44%), no vomiting (58%), no nausea (46%), total control (40%). The efficacy of *Kytril* 2.0 mg q.d. was comparable to *Kytril* 1.0 mg b.i.d. and statistically superior to placebo. The placebo rates were 7%, 14%, 7%, 7%, respectively, for the four parameters.

No controlled study comparing granisetron injection with the oral formulation to prevent chemotherapy-induced nausea and vomiting has been performed.

Radiation-induced Nausea and Vomiting

Total Body Irradiation: In a double-blind randomized study, 18 patients receiving *Kytril* Tablets, 2.0 mg daily, experienced significantly greater antiemetic protection compared to patients in a historical negative control group who received conventional (non-5-HT_3 antagonist) antiemetics. Total body irradiation consisted of 11 fractions of 120 cGy administered over 4 days, with three fractions on each of the first 3 days, and two fractions on the fourth day. *Kytril* Tablets were given one hour before the first radiation fraction of each day.

Twenty-two percent (22%) of patients treated with *Kytril* Tablets did not experience vomiting or receive rescue antiemetics over the entire 4-day dosing period, compared to 0% of patients in the historical negative control group ($P<0.01$). In addition, patients who received *Kytril* Tablets also experienced significantly fewer emetic episodes during the first day of radiation and over the 4-day treatment period, compared to patients in the historical negative control group. The median time to the first emetic episode was 36 hours for patients who received *Kytril* Tablets.

Fractionated Abdominal Radiation: The efficacy of *Kytril,* 2 mg daily, was evaluated in a double-blind, placebo-controlled randomized trial of 260 patients. *Kytril* Tablets were given 1 hour before radiation, composed of up to 20 daily fractions of 180 to 300 cGy each. The exceptions were patients with seminoma or those receiving whole abdomen irradiation who initially received 150 cGy per fraction. Radiation was administered to the upper abdomen with a field size of at least 100 cm².

The proportion of patients without emesis and those without nausea for *Kytril* Tablets, compared to placebo, were statistically significant ($P<0.0001$) at 24 hours after radiation, irrespective of the radiation dose. *Kytril* was superior to placebo in patients receiving up to 10 daily fractions of radiation, but was not superior to placebo in patients receiving 20 fractions.

Patients treated with *Kytril* Tablets (n=134) had a significantly longer time to the first episode of vomiting (35 vs. 9 days, $P<0.001$) relative to those patients who received placebo (n=126), and a significantly longer time to the first episode of nausea (11 vs. 1 day, $P<0.001$). *Kytril* provided significantly greater protection from nausea and vomiting than placebo.

INDICATIONS AND USAGE

Kytril (granisetron hydrochloride) is indicated for the prevention of:

1) nausea and vomiting associated with initial and repeat courses of emetogenic cancer therapy, including high-dose cisplatin.
2) nausea and vomiting associated with radiation, including total body irradiation and fractionated abdominal radiation.

CONTRAINDICATIONS

Kytril is contraindicated in patients with known hypersensitivity to the drug or any of its components.

PRECAUTIONS

Drug Interactions

Granisetron does not induce or inhibit the cytochrome P-450 drug-metabolizing enzyme system. There have been no definitive drug-drug interaction studies to examine pharmacokinetic or pharmacodynamic interaction with other drugs but, in humans, *Kytril* Injection has been safely administered with drugs representing benzodiazepines, neuroleptics and anti-ulcer medications commonly prescribed with antiemetic treatments. *Kytril* Injection also does not appear to interact with emetogenic cancer chemotherapies. Because granisetron is metabolized by hepatic cytochrome P-450 drug-metabolizing enzymes, inducers or inhibitors of these enzymes may change the clearance and, hence, the half-life of granisetron.

Carcinogenesis, Mutagenesis, Impairment of Fertility

In a 24-month carcinogenicity study, rats were treated orally with granisetron 1, 5 or 50 mg/kg/day (6, 30 or 300 mg/m²/day). The 50 mg/kg/day dose was reduced to 25 mg/kg/day (150 mg/m²/day) during week 59 due to toxicity. For a 50 kg person of average height (1.46m² body surface area),

Continued on next page

Information on the SmithKline Beecham Pharmaceuticals products appearing here is based on the labeling in effect on June 15, 2000. Further information on these and other products may be obtained from the Medical Department, SmithKline Beecham Pharmaceuticals, One Franklin Plaza, Philadelphia, PA 19101.

Kytril Tablets—Cont.

these doses represent 4, 20 and 101 times the recommended clinical dose (1.48 mg/m^2, oral) on a body surface area basis. There was a statistically significant increase in the incidence of hepatocellular carcinomas and adenomas in males treated with 5 mg/kg/day (30 mg/m^2/day, 20 times the recommended human dose based on body surface area) and above, and in females treated with 25 mg/kg/day (150 mg/m^2/day, 101 times the recommended human dose based on body surface area). No increase in liver tumors was observed at a dose of 1 mg/kg/day (6 mg/m^2/day, 4 times the recommended human dose based on body surface area) in males and 5 mg/kg/day (30 mg/m^2/day, 20 times the recommended human dose based on body surface area) in females. In a 12-month oral toxicity study, treatment with granisetron 100 mg/kg/day (600 mg/m^2/day, 405 times the recommended human dose based on body surface area) produced hepatocellular adenomas in male and female rats while no such tumors were found in the control rats. A 24-month mouse carcinogenicity study of granisetron did not show a statistically significant increase in tumor incidence, but the study was not conclusive.

Because of the tumor findings in rat studies, Kytril (granisetron hydrochloride) Tablets should be prescribed only at the dose and for the indication recommended (see INDICATIONS AND USAGE, and DOSAGE AND ADMINISTRATION).

Granisetron was not mutagenic in *in vitro* Ames test and mouse lymphoma cell forward mutation assay, and *in vivo* mouse micronucleus test and *in vitro* and *ex vivo* rat hepatocyte UDS assays. It, however, produced a significant increase in UDS in HeLa cells *in vitro* and a significant increased incidence of cells with polyploidy in an *in vitro* human lymphocyte chromosomal aberration test.

Granisetron at oral doses up to 100 mg/kg/day (600 mg/m^2/day, 405 times the recommended human dose based on body surface area) was found to have no effect on fertility and reproductive performance of male and female rats.

Pregnancy

Teratogenic Effects. Pregnancy Category B. Reproduction studies have been performed in pregnant rats at oral doses up to 125 mg/kg/day (750 mg/m^2/day, 507 times the recommended human dose based on body surface area) and pregnant rabbits at oral doses up to 32 mg/kg/day (378 mg/m^2/day, 255 times the recommended human dose based on body surface area) and have revealed no evidence of impaired fertility or harm to the fetus due to granisetron. There are, however, no adequate and well-controlled studies in pregnant women. Because animal reproduction studies are not always predictive of human response, this drug should be used during pregnancy only if clearly needed.

Nursing Mothers

It is not known whether granisetron is excreted in human milk. Because many drugs are excreted in human milk, caution should be exercised when *Kytril* is administered to a nursing woman.

Pediatric Use

Safety and effectiveness in children have not been established.

Geriatric Use

During clinical trials, 325 patients 65 years of age or older received oral *Kytril*; 298 were 65 to 74 years of age and 27 were 75 years of age or older. Efficacy and safety were maintained with increasing age.

ADVERSE REACTIONS

Chemotherapy-induced Nausea and Vomiting

Over 3,700 patients have received oral *Kytril* in clinical trials with emetogenic cancer therapies consisting primarily of cyclophosphamide or cisplatin regimens.

In patients receiving oral *Kytril* 1.0 mg b.i.d. for 1, 7 or 14 days, 2.0 mg q.d. for 1 day, the following table lists adverse experiences reported in more than 5% of the patients with comparator and placebo incidences.

[See table 4 below]

Other adverse events reported in clinical trials were:

Gastrointestinal: In single-day dosing studies in which adverse events were collected for 7 days, nausea (20%) and vomiting (12%) were recorded as adverse events after the 24-hour efficacy assessment period.

Hepatic: In comparative trials, elevation of AST and ALT (>2 times the upper limit of normal) following the administration of oral *Kytril* occurred in 5% and 6% of patients, respectively. These frequencies were not significantly different from those seen with comparators (AST: 2%; ALT: 9%).

Cardiovascular: Hypertension (1%); hypotension, angina pectoris, atrial fibrillation and syncope have been observed rarely.

Central Nervous System: Dizziness (5%), insomnia (5%), anxiety (2%), somnolence (1%). One case compatible with but not diagnostic of extrapyramidal symptoms has been reported in a patient treated with oral *Kytril*.

Hypersensitivity: Rare cases of hypersensitivity reactions, sometimes severe (e.g., anaphylaxis, shortness of breath, hypotension, urticaria) have been reported.

Other: Fever (5%). Events often associated with chemotherapy also have been reported: leukopenia (9%), decreased appetite (6%), anemia (4%), alopecia (3%), thrombocytopenia (2%).

Over 5,000 patients have received injectable *Kytril* in clinical trials.

Table 5 gives the comparative frequencies of the five commonly reported adverse events (≥3%) in patients receiving *Kytril* Injection, 40 mcg/kg, in single-day chemotherapy trials. These patients received chemotherapy, primarily cisplatin, and intravenous fluids during the 24-hour period following *Kytril* Injection administration.

Table 5. Principal Adverse Events in Clinical Trials—Single-Day Chemotherapy

	Percent of Patients with Event	
	Kytril Injection[1] 40 mcg/kg (n=1,268)	Comparator[2] (n=422)
Headache	14%	6%
Asthenia	5%	6%
Somnolence	4%	15%
Diarrhea	4%	6%
Constipation	3%	3%

1. Adverse events were generally recorded over 7 days post-*Kytril* Injection administration.
2. Metoclopramide/dexamethasone and phenothiazines/dexamethasone.

In the absence of a placebo group, there is uncertainty as to how many of these events should be attributed to *Kytril*, except for headache, which was clearly more frequent than in comparison groups.

Radiation-induced Nausea and Vomiting

In controlled clinical trials, the adverse events reported by patients receiving *Kytril* tablets and concurrent radiation were similar to those reported by patients receiving *Kytril* tablets prior to chemotherapy. The most frequently reported adverse events were diarrhea, asthenia and constipation. Headache, however, was less prevalent in this patient population.

OVERDOSAGE

There is no specific treatment for granisetron hydrochloride overdosage. In case of overdosage, symptomatic treatment should be given. Overdosage of up to 38.5 mg of granisetron hydrochloride injection has been reported without symptoms or only the occurrence of a slight headache.

DOSAGE AND ADMINISTRATION

Emetogenic Chemotherapy

The recommended adult dosage of oral Kytril (granisetron hydrochloride) is 2 mg once daily or 1 mg twice daily. In the 2 mg once-daily regimen, two 1 mg tablets are given up to 1 hour before chemotherapy. In the 1 mg twice-daily regimen, the first 1 mg tablet is given up to 1 hour before chemotherapy, and the second tablet, 12 hours after the first. Either regimen is administered only on the day(s) chemotherapy is given. Continued treatment, while not on chemotherapy, has not been found to be useful.

Use in the Elderly, Pediatric Patients, Renal Failure Patients or Hepatically Impaired Patients: No dosage adjustment is recommended. (See CLINICAL PHARMACOLOGY, Pharmacokinetics.)

Radiation (either Total Body Irradiation or Fractionated Abdominal Radiation): The recommended adult dosage of oral *Kytril* is 2 mg once daily. Two 1 mg tablets are taken within 1 hour of radiation.

Pediatric Use: There is no experience with oral *Kytril* in the prevention of radiation-induced nausea and vomiting in pediatric patients.

Use in the Elderly: No dosage adjustment is recommended.

HOW SUPPLIED

Tablets: White, triangular, biconvex, film-coated tablets; tablets are debossed K1 on one face.

1 mg Unit of Use 2's: NDC 0029-4151-39

1 mg SUP 20's: NDC 0029-4151-05 (intended for institutional use only)

Store between 15° and 30°C (59° and 86°F). Protect from light.

Rx only

Manufactured in Crawley, UK by
SmithKline Beecham Pharmaceuticals, for
SmithKline Beecham Pharmaceuticals,
Philadelphia, PA 19101
KY:L6T-A

Shown in Product Identification Guide, page 337

Table 4. Principal Adverse Events in Clinical Trials

	Percent of Patients with Event			
	Oral *Kytril*[1] 1.0 mg b.i.d. (n=978)	Oral *Kytril*[1] 2.0 mg q.d. (n=1450)	Comparator[2] (n=599)	Placebo (n=185)
Headache[3]	21%	20%	13%	12%
Constipation	18%	14%	16%	8%
Asthenia	14%	18%	10%	4%
Diarrhea	8%	9%	10%	4%
Abdominal pain	6%	4%	6%	3%
Dyspepsia	4%	6%	5%	4%

1. Adverse events were recorded for 7 days when oral *Kytril* was given on a single day and for up to 28 days when oral *Kytril* was administered for 7 or 14 days.
2. Metoclopramide/dexamethasone; phenothiazines/dexamethasone; dexamethasone alone; prochlorperazine.
3. Usually mild to moderate in severity.

LYMErix® ℞

Lyme Disease Vaccine (Recombinant OspA)

DESCRIPTION

LYMErix [Lyme Disease Vaccine (Recombinant OspA)] is a noninfectious recombinant vaccine developed and manufactured by SmithKline Beecham Biologicals. The causative agent of Lyme disease is *Borrelia burgdorferi;* in North America, all Lyme disease is due to *Borrelia burgdorferi sensu stricto*. The vaccine contains lipoprotein OspA, an outer surface protein of *Borrelia burgdorferi sensu stricto* ZS7, as expressed by *Escherichia coli*. Lipoprotein OspA is a single polypeptide chain of 257 amino acids with lipids covalently bonded to the N terminus. No substance of animal origin is used in the commercial manufacturing process. Fermentation media consist primarily of inorganic salts, and vitamins, with small quantities of antifoam (contains silicon), kanamycin sulfate (an aminoglycoside antibiotic), and yeast extract. Silicon and kanamycin are removed to levels below detection (<7 ppm and <10 ppb, respectively). The vaccine is adsorbed onto aluminum hydroxide.

LYMErix is supplied as a sterile suspension in single-dose vials and prefilled syringes for intramuscular administration. The vaccine is ready for use without reconstitution; it must be shaken before administration to ensure a uniform turbid white suspension.

Each 0.5 mL dose of vaccine consists of 30 mcg of lipoprotein OspA adsorbed onto 0.5 mg aluminum as aluminum hydroxide adjuvant. Each dose of the vaccine preparation contains 10 mM phosphate buffered saline and 2.5 mg of 2-phenoxyethanol, a bacteriostatic agent.

The potency of the vaccine is evaluated by immunizing mice with LYMErix® [Lyme Disease Vaccine (Recombinant OspA)] and measuring their serum antibody response to OspA by ELISA.

CLINICAL PHARMACOLOGY

Microbiology

Lyme disease is a multisystem disease caused by infection with the bacterial spirochete, *B. burgdorferi,* which is transmitted by *Ixodes* ticks. The enzootic life cycle of *B. burgdorferi* is dependent upon its transmission between a vector, the *Ixodes* tick, and a reservoir host, most commonly the white-footed mouse. Tick larvae usually feed in the late summer and acquire *B. burgdorferi* from an infected animal host. Nymphal ticks feed in the late spring and summer, and serve as the most common source of human infection. Adult ticks feed in the fall, winter and early spring, with the white-tailed deer being the preferred host. Adult ticks can also transmit *B. burgdorferi* to humans.[1] Both deer and rodent hosts are necessary to maintain the enzootic cycle of *B. burgdorferi*.

Epidemiology

Lyme disease is the most commonly diagnosed vector-borne disease in the United States, with over 99,000 cases reported to the Centers for Disease Control and Prevention (CDC) from 1982 to 1996. During that time, the incidence of reported cases increased by at least 32-fold. Although most cases have been reported in the Northeast, upper Midwest and Pacific coastal areas of the United States, infections have been reported in almost all states.[2] The incidence rates vary considerably from state to state and even within states at the county level.[2]

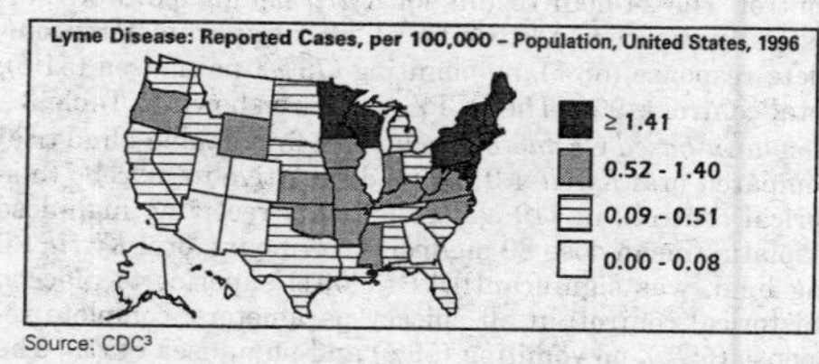

Source: CDC[3]

The trend of an increasing incidence in some established endemic areas continues, along with the geographic spread of the causative organism to new areas.[1,2,4,5]

Lyme disease has a bimodal age distribution, with the highest number of cases occurring in children 2 to 15 years of age and adults 30 to 55 years of age.[4]

[See figure at top of next column]

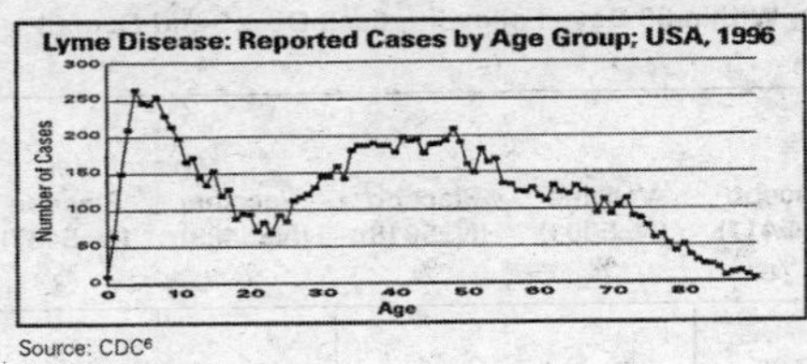

Source: CDC[6]

The primary risk factor for Lyme disease is exposure to wooded or grassy areas inhabited by *B. burgdorferi*-infected ticks. Such areas may include woodlands, meadows, or residential yards in endemic areas.[5] Cases have been reported in people whose only exposure to *B. burgdorferi* has been while on vacation in an endemic area.[1]

Lyme disease has been reported to occur throughout the year.[7,8] Peak incidence of Lyme disease varies by region and may vary annually based on fluctuations in local climatic conditions.[1,5,7,8] For example, the peak occurs in the late spring and summer in the Northeast United States, coincident with the feeding of nymphal ticks, the most common source of human infection. Transmission can occur also in the fall, winter, and early spring when adult ticks are feeding.[1]

Clinical Manifestations: Lyme disease has a variable incubation period.[5] Lyme disease is a multisystem disease, which has been described as having early and late stages. The early stage is usually characterized by a rash (erythema migrans) and may be accompanied by fever, fatigue, myalgias and/or arthralgias. Erythema migrans represents a localized cutaneous infection and is the presenting symptom in 60% to 80% of cases. Early disseminated manifestations include secondary skin lesions, neurologic involvement (meningitis, facial palsy, other cranial neuritides, radiculoneuritis), cardiac involvement (atrioventricular block, myocarditis), and musculoskeletal symptoms usually consisting of migratory pain in joints and the surrounding soft tissue structures.[9]

Late stage disease (persistent infection) occurs months to years after initial infection and may be manifested as chronic arthritis, chronic neurologic abnormalities or acrodermatitis chronica atrophicans. Not all patients with Lyme disease have this characteristic progression of symptoms. Late stage disease usually requires more intensive therapy and may result in permanent sequelae. In particular, late neurologic involvement is associated with chronic, slowly progressive disease.[10]

The rate of asymptomatic infection has not been well studied in adults. In the LYMErix [Lyme Disease Vaccine (Recombinant OspA)] study, the rate of asymptomatic infection (for definition, see *Clinical Efficacy*, Asymptomatic *B. burgdorferi* infection) was approximately 0.25% per year with one case of asymptomatic infection occurring for every four cases of erythema migrans.

Late stage disease may result from early disease that is either unrecognized or fails to respond to treatment, or from asymptomatic infection. The relative importance of these conditions in predisposing to the development of late stage disease is unknown.

Diagnosis: Diagnosis is based on clinical manifestations, epidemiologic information and laboratory evaluation. Confirming the diagnosis may be difficult in some cases.

At a consensus meeting of the CDC and ASTPHLD (Association of State, Territorial and Public Health Laboratory Directors), a two-step approach was recommended if serologic evaluation of Lyme disease is required.[11] A sensitive screening test such as an enzyme-linked immunosorbent assay (ELISA) or immunofluorescent assay (IFA) is recommended as the initial laboratory test and, if positive or equivocal, immunoblot (Western blot) testing should be performed to confirm the results (see Laboratory Test Interactions).

LYMErix *Mechanism of Action:* *LYMErix* stimulates specific antibodies directed against *B. burgdorferi*. The organism contains several outer surface proteins, with lipoprotein OspA being immunodominant.[12] Administration of lipoprotein OspA to mice resulted in the formation of specific IgG anti-OspA antibodies, including those directed against a specific epitope, LA-2 (designated LA-2 equivalent antibodies). These antibodies have demonstrated bactericidal activity. Studies have shown that mice immunized with recombinant lipoprotein OspA are protected against disease after tick challenge with *B. burgdorferi*.[13] LA-2 equivalent antibody titers have been shown to correlate with protection against infection in laboratory animals.[14]

B. burgdorferi express OspA while residing in the midgut of the infected tick, but OspA is downregulated after tick attachment and is usually undetectable or absent when *B. burgdorferi* is inoculated into the human host.[15] Thus, a novel hypothesis has been proposed to explain the effectiveness of lipoprotein OspA vaccination: when infected ticks bite humans who have been vaccinated with *LYMErix*, the vaccine-induced antibodies are taken up by the tick and interact with the *B. burgdorferi* in the midgut of the tick, thereby preventing transmission of the organism to the host. This mechanism has been suggested by a pre-clinical study in which *B. burgdorferi* were detected by immunofluorescence assay in none of the ticks that fed on OspA-immunized mice, compared with 72% of ticks that fed on control-immunized mice.[13]

Clinical Efficacy

A randomized, double-blind, multicentered, placebo-controlled trial has shown that *LYMErix* confers protection against Lyme disease.[16] This trial was conducted in highly endemic areas of the United States, primarily in the Northeast, and enrolled 10,936 subjects (5,469 vaccinees; 5,467 placebo recipients) ages 15 to 70 years. Subjects with a history of previous Lyme disease were not excluded from this trial.

Subjects vaccinated with three doses of *LYMErix* or placebo at months 0, 1 and 12 were observed for 20 months after the first injection (January 1995 through November 1996). The primary endpoint of the trial was the incidence of definite Lyme disease after two doses of vaccine. Each subject was actively followed for symptomatic disease during the entire observation period and was assessed for possible asymptomatic infection (as evidenced by IgG Western blot seroconversion) at months 12 and 20.

Definite Lyme disease

In the pivotal efficacy trial, definite Lyme disease was defined as clinical manifestations (erythema migrans, neurologic, musculoskeletal or cardiovascular involvement) with laboratory confirmation (positive culture for *B. burgdorferi* from skin biopsy; positive polymerase chain reaction [PCR] result for *B. burgdorferi* from skin biopsy, synovial fluid, or CSF; or IgM or IgG Western blot seroconversion) as defined by CDC/ASTPHLD criteria.[11]

Post-second dose efficacy was measured beginning at 4 weeks following the second dose through to month 12. Post-third dose efficacy was measured from the third dose through to month 20.

Prevention of Definite Lyme Disease: Vaccine efficacy against definite Lyme disease was 78% (95% CI: 59% to 88%) after three doses of vaccine administered according to protocol (13 cases among 4,765 subjects in the vaccine group; 58 cases among 4,784 subjects in the placebo group). Vaccine efficacy against definite Lyme disease was 50% (95% CI: 14% to 71%) after two doses of vaccine administered according to protocol (20 cases among 5,148 subjects in the vaccine group; 40 cases among 5,166 subjects in the placebo group).

Asymptomatic *B. burgdorferi* infection

In the pivotal efficacy trial, subjects were defined as having asymptomatic infection when, in the absence of recognizable clinical symptoms, IgG Western blot seroconversion occurred either between months 2 and 12 of the first year, or between months 12 and 20 of the second year.

Prevention of Asymptomatic Infection: Vaccine efficacy against asymptomatic *B. burgdorferi* was 100% (95% CI: 30% to 100%) after three doses of vaccine administered according to protocol (0 cases among 4,765 subjects in the vaccine group; 13 cases among 4,784 subjects in the placebo group). Vaccine efficacy against asymptomatic *B. burgdorferi* was 83% (95% CI: 25% to 96%) after two doses of vaccine administered according to protocol (two cases among 5,148 subjects in the vaccine group; 12 cases among 5,166 subjects in the placebo group).

Possible Lyme disease

In the pivotal efficacy trial, possible Lyme disease was defined as a flu-like illness (fever, chills, fatigue, headache, joint or muscle aches) with IgM or IgG Western blot seroconversion, or physician-diagnosed erythema migrans with negative laboratory results.

Prevention of Possible Lyme Disease: Following the three-dose course of vaccine administered according to protocol, efficacy was 48% (95% CI: 1% to 73%) against possible Lyme disease. Fourteen of the subjects in the vaccine group developed a possible case of Lyme disease, compared to 27 placebo recipients. Following two doses of vaccine administered according to protocol, the vaccine efficacy against possible Lyme disease was 21% (95% CI: −45% to 56%). Nineteen subjects who received two doses of vaccine developed possible Lyme disease, compared to 24 placebo recipients.

The data regarding flu-like illnesses due to possible Lyme disease may be confounded by possible cross-reactivity and/or co-infection with *Ehrlichia*, which may cause a flu-like illness and false-positive IgM Western blot for *B. burgdorferi*.[17]

Lyme Disease Manifestations and Laboratory Diagnosis in the Efficacy Trial: The clinical presentation of the 131 cases of definite Lyme disease was as follows: erythema migrans, 128 (32 vaccine, 96 placebo); arthritis, 1 (vaccine); trigeminal neuralgia, 1 (placebo); and facial palsy, 1 (placebo). Of the 128 cases with erythema migrans, additional presenting clinical manifestations included: facial palsy, 3 (1 vaccine, 2 placebo) and trigeminal neuralgia, 1 (placebo). The duration of erythema migrans was similar for both vaccine and placebo recipients.

Subjects were treated at either acute presentation of Lyme disease symptoms, following laboratory confirmation of symptoms, or following laboratory confirmation of asymptomatic infection. Active surveillance and prompt treatment of identified cases may have accounted for the low incidence of late Lyme disease manifestations.

A similar proportion of definite Lyme disease cases in both vaccine and placebo groups were confirmed by positive culture, PCR analysis, or Western blot seroconversion.

Immunogenicity in Persons 15 to 70 Years of Age: In the pivotal efficacy trial, immunogenicity of LYMErix [Lyme Disease Vaccine (Recombinant OspA)] was assessed by measuring IgG anti-OspA antibodies and LA-2 equivalent antibodies in a subset of subjects 15 to 70 years of age enrolled at one study center.

Table 1 shows the seropositivity rates and geometric mean titers (GMTs) following the second and third doses of *LYMErix*.

[See table above]

Table 1. Immunogenicity in Vaccines

Antibody	Sampling Time	Seropositivity* % (n/N)	GMT-EL.U./mL (95% CI)
Total IgG Anti-OspA	1 mo. after dose 2	99% (260/264)	1227 (1029, 1463)
	Pre-dose 3†	83% (201/241)	116 (96, 139)
	1 mo. after dose 3	100% (267/267)	6006 (5180, 6963)
	8 mos. after dose 3	98% (262/267)	1991 (1686, 2351)
			GMT-ng/mL (95% CI)
LA-2 Equivalent	1 mo. after dose 2	96% (236/245)	909 (773, 1067)
	Pre-dose 3†	58% (150/258)	132 (118, 149)
	1 mo. after dose 3	99% (220/222)	4402 (3686, 5257)
	8 mos. after dose 3	97% (217/223)	1935 (1628, 2300)

*Seropositivity defined as an IgG OspA antibody titer ≥20 EL.U./mL or a LA-2 equivalent antibody titer ≥100 ng/mL.
†At month 12.
n/N = number of seropositive subjects/total subjects tested.
% = percentage of seropositive subjects.

Subjects in the placebo group did not develop detectable anti-OspA seropositivity at the sampling time points indicated in the above table.

INDICATION AND USAGE

LYMErix is indicated for active immunization against Lyme disease in individuals 15 to 70 years of age.

Individuals most at risk may be those who live or work in *B. burgdorferi*-infected tick-infested grassy or wooded areas (e.g., landscaping, brush clearing, forestry, and wildlife and parks management),[4,18–21] as well as those who plan travel to or pursue recreational activities (e.g., hiking, camping, fishing and hunting) in such areas. Most cases of Lyme disease in the United States are thought to be acquired in the peri-residential environment, through routine activities of property maintenance, recreation, and/or exercise of pets.[19,22]

Previous infection with *B. burgdorferi* may not confer protective immunity.[23] Therefore people with a prior history of Lyme disease may benefit from vaccination with *LYMErix*.

Safety and efficacy for this vaccine are based on administration of the second and third doses several weeks prior to the onset of the *Borrelia* transmission season in the local geographic area (see DOSAGE AND ADMINISTRATION).

LYMErix is not a treatment for Lyme disease.

As with any vaccine, *LYMErix* may not protect 100% of individuals. The vaccine should not be administered to persons outside of the indicated age range.

CONTRAINDICATIONS

LYMErix is contraindicated in people with known hypersensitivity to any component of the vaccine.

PRECAUTIONS

General

LYMErix will not prevent disease in those who have unrecognized infection at the time of vaccination. *LYMErix* will not provide protection against other tick-borne diseases such as babesiosis or ehrlichiosis.

Treatment-resistant Lyme arthritis (antibiotic refractory), a rare complication of *B. burgdorferi* infection, has been associated with immune reactivity to OspA of *B. burgdorferi*.[24] Since the underlying etiology is not clearly understood, it is recommended that *LYMErix* not be administered to such patients.

As with other vaccines, although a moderate or severe febrile illness is sufficient reason to postpone vaccination, minor illnesses such as mild upper respiratory infections with or without low-grade fever are not contraindications.[25]

Before the injection of any biological, the physician should take all reasonable precautions to prevent allergic or other

Continued on next page

Information on the SmithKline Beecham Pharmaceuticals products appearing here is based on the labeling in effect on June 15, 2000. Further information on these and other products may be obtained from the Medical Department, SmithKline Beecham Pharmaceuticals, One Franklin Plaza, Philadelphia, PA 19101.

LYMErix—Cont.

adverse reactions, including understanding the use of the product concerned, and the nature of the side effects and adverse reactions that may follow its use.

Prior to immunization with any vaccine, the patient's history should be reviewed. The physician should review the patient's immunization history for possible vaccine sensitivity, previous vaccination-related adverse reactions and occurrence of any adverse-event-related symptoms and/or signs, in order to determine the existence of any contraindication to immunization and to allow an assessment of benefits and risks. Epinephrine injection (1:1000) and other appropriate agents used for the control of immediate allergic reactions must be immediately available should an acute anaphylactic reaction occur.

Packaging for the *LYMErix* Tip-Lok™ syringe contains dry natural rubber, which may cause allergic reactions; packaging for the vial does not contain natural rubber.

A separate sterile syringe and needle or a sterile disposable unit must be used for each patient to prevent the transmission of infectious agents from person to person. Needles should be disposed of properly and should not be recapped.

As with any vaccine administered to immunosuppressed persons or persons receiving immunosuppressive therapy, the expected immune response may not be obtained. For individuals receiving immunosuppressive therapy, deferral of vaccination for three months after therapy may be considered.[26]

Information for Patients

In addition to vaccination with LYMErix [Lyme Disease Vaccine (Recombinant OspA)], people can further decrease their risk of acquiring tick-borne infections by taking standard preventive measures (e.g., wearing long-sleeved shirts, long pants rather than shorts, tucking pants into socks, treating clothing with tick repellent, and checking for and removing attached ticks).[2]

Patients, parents or guardians should be informed of the benefits and risks of immunization with *LYMErix*, and of the importance of completing the immunization series. As with any vaccine, it is important when a subject returns for the next dose in a series that he/she be questioned concerning the occurrence of any symptoms and/or signs after a previous dose of the same vaccine and adverse events be reported. The U.S. Department of Health and Human Services has established a Vaccine Adverse Events Reporting System (VAERS) to accept all reports of suspected adverse events after the administration of any vaccine. The VAERS toll-free number is 1-800-822-7967.

The duration of immunity following a complete schedule of immunization with *LYMErix* has not been established.

It is important to note that subjects with a prior history of *B. burgdorferi* infection may not have protection against subsequent disease[23] or asymptomatic infection.

Individuals should be informed that vaccination with *LYMErix* may induce a false-positive ELISA result for *B. burgdorferi* infection (see Laboratory Test Interactions). Patients should be advised to inform health care professionals that they have been immunized with *LYMErix*, since it may affect laboratory testing for diagnosing Lyme disease.

Laboratory Test Interactions

LYMErix immunization results in the generation of anti-OspA antibodies, which can be detected by an enzyme-linked immunosorbent assay (ELISA) for *B. burgdorferi*. The incidence of positive IgG ELISA tests is dependent on the sensitivity and specificity of the ELISA assay and the titer of anti-OspA antibody. In general, there is an association between anti-OspA titer and IgG ELISA index or Optical Density (OD) ratio; the higher the titer of anti-OspA achieved, the higher the IgG ELISA index or OD ratio. Therefore, because vaccination may result in a positive IgG ELISA in the absence of infection, it is important to perform Western blot testing if the ELISA test is positive or equivocal in vaccinated individuals who are being evaluated for suspected Lyme disease.

Following vaccination, the appearance of a 31kD OspA band, possibly accompanied by other lower molecular weight bands on an immunoblot (Western blot), should not interfere with the determination of positivity when assessed by CDC/ ASTPHLD criteria.[11]

Drug Interactions

No data are available on the immune response to *LYMErix* when administered concurrently with other vaccines. As with other intramuscular injections, *LYMErix* should not be given to individuals on anticoagulant therapy, unless the potential benefit clearly outweighs the risk of administration.

Carcinogenesis, Mutagenesis, Impairment of Fertility

LYMErix has not been evaluated for carcinogenic or mutagenic potential, or for impairment of fertility.

Pregnancy

Teratogenic Effects: Pregnancy Category C. Animal reproductive studies have not been conducted with *LYMErix*. It is also not known whether *LYMErix* can cause fetal harm when administered to a pregnant woman or can affect reproductive capacity. *LYMErix* should be given to a pregnant woman only if clearly needed.

Health care providers are encouraged to register pregnant women who receive LYMErix [Lyme Disease Vaccine (Recombinant OspA)] in the SmithKline Beecham Pharmaceuticals vaccination pregnancy registry by calling 1-800-366-8900, ext. 5231.

Nursing Mothers

It is not known whether *LYMErix* is excreted in human milk. Because many drugs are excreted in human milk, caution should be exercised when *LYMErix* is administered to a nursing woman.

Table 2. Incidence (≥1%) of Unsolicited Adverse Events Occurring Within 30 Days Following Each Dose* and Overall (after Doses 1, 2 or 3)

	Dose 1		Dose 2		Dose 3		Overall	
Events	**Vaccine (N=5469) %**	**Placebo (N=5467) %**	**Vaccine (N=5397) %**	**Placebo (N=5417) %**	**Vaccine (N=5001) %**	**Placebo (N=5018) %**	**Vaccine (N=5469) %**	**Placebo (N=5467) %**
Local								
Injection site pain	17.96[c]	4.90	8.76[c]	2.95			21.87[c]	6.91
Injection site reaction							1.54[b]	0.91
General Body as a Whole								
Achiness	1.57	1.19	1.22	0.90			2.78	2.25
Chills/Rigors							2.05[c]	0.73
Fatigue	2.03	1.96	1.72	1.42			3.86	3.42
Fever	1.35[a]	0.91					2.58[c]	1.61
Infection viral	1.88	1.66					2.83	2.45
Influenza-like symptoms	1.44[a]	0.93					2.54[c]	1.66
Nausea							1.12	1.04
Musculoskeletal System								
Arthralgia	3.22	2.67	3.11	2.60	1.24	1.16	6.78	6.05
Back pain							1.90	1.55
Myalgia	2.69[c]	1.72	1.52[a]	0.98			4.83[c]	2.94
Stiffness							0.95	1.21
Nervous System								
Dizziness							1.01	1.08
Headache	3.51	2.96	2.39	2.33			5.61	5.09
Respiratory System								
Bronchitis							1.10	1.28
Coughing							1.50	1.46
Pharyngitis	1.39	1.12	1.15	1.20			2.52	2.45
Rhinitis	1.50	1.46					2.41	2.47
Sinusitis	1.74	1.57	1.26	1.27			3.16	2.93
Upper respiratory tract infection	2.63	3.22	1.65	1.75			4.35	4.98
Skin/Appendages								
Rash							1.37	1.08

*Includes events obtained through spontaneous reports following each dose and events reported 1 month after doses 1 and 2 (when all subjects were queried regarding the occurrence of any adverse event since the previous vaccination).

a. p-value <0.05. b. p-value <0.01. c. p-value <0.001.

Pediatric Use

Safety and efficacy in pediatric subjects younger than 15 years of age have not been evaluated. Therefore, the vaccine is not indicated for this age group at this time.

ADVERSE REACTIONS

During clinical trials involving 6,478 individuals receiving a total of 18,047 doses, *LYMErix* has been generally well tolerated.

Subjects with the following conditions: chronic joint or neurologic illness related to Lyme disease; diseases associated with joint swelling (including rheumatoid arthritis) or diffuse musculoskeletal pain; second- or third-degree atrioventricular block or a pacemaker were excluded from the efficacy trial because such conditions could interfere with the assessment of Lyme disease in the trial. Therefore, data are limited regarding the safety of the vaccine in subjects with these conditions (see below).

Unsolicited Adverse Events

The most frequently reported (≥1%) unsolicited adverse events within 30 days of vaccination for all subjects receiving at least one dose (n=10,936) in the double-blind, placebo-controlled efficacy trial are shown in Table 2.

[See table 2 above]

The most frequently reported (≥1%) unsolicited adverse events occurring more than 30 days following vaccination for all subjects (n=10,936) in the double-blind, placebo-controlled efficacy trial are shown in Table 3.

[See table 3 at bottom of next page]

Separate post hoc analyses were conducted to assess two subsets of musculoskeletal events which occurred either early (≤30 days) or late (>30 days) post-vaccination. There were no significant differences, either early or late, between the vaccine and placebo recipients with regard to experiencing arthritis, aggravated arthritis, arthropathy or arthrosis. However, vaccine recipients were significantly more likely than placebo recipients to experience early events of arthralgia or myalgia after each dose [for dose 1: odds ratio (OR), (95% CI) = 1.35 (1.13, 1.61); dose 2: OR = 1.28 (1.05, 1.56); dose 3: OR = 1.59 (1.18, 2.16)]. With regard to late events of arthralgia or myalgia, there were no significant differences between vaccine and placebo recipients.

There was no significant difference in the rates of cardiac adverse events between vaccine and placebo recipients. Neurologic adverse events which occurred at a rate <1% in the vaccine group and were noted to occur with a similar frequency in placebo recipients included: carpal tunnel syndrome, migraine, paralysis, tremor, coma, dysphonia, ataxia, multiple sclerosis, myasthenia gravis, meningitis, trigeminal neuralgia, nystagmus, neuritis, neuralgia, nerve root lesion, neuropathy, hyperesthesia, hyperkinesia, and intracranial hypertension.

Overall, approximately 18% of subjects enrolled in the study had a prior history of some musculoskeletal condition (19% vaccinees, 18% placebo recipients). In a post hoc subgroup analysis, there was no significant difference between vaccine and placebo recipients with regard to development of musculoskeletal events (defined as arthritis, arthropathy, arthrosis, synovitis, tendinitis, polymyalgia rheumatica, bursitis or rheumatoid arthritis and lasting more than 30 days) in those with a prior history of musculoskeletal conditions. However, both vaccine and placebo recipients with a prior history of musculoskeletal conditions were more likely to experience musculoskeletal events than subjects without such prior history.

Solicited Adverse Events

The frequency of solicited local and systemic adverse events was evaluated in a subset of subjects (n=938) who comprised the total enrollment at one study center in the efficacy trial. Of these 938 subjects, 800 completed a 4-day diary card following each of three doses, and were evaluable according to protocol. Table 4 shows the percentage of subjects reporting a solicited symptom following any one of the three doses and overall. The majority of the solicited events were mild to moderate in severity and limited in duration.

[See table 4 at bottom of next page]

Subjects with Previous Lyme Disease

Subjects with previous Lyme disease were assessed using two definitions: subjects whose baseline sera were evaluated for Western blot (WB) positivity and subjects who at study entry self-reported a previous history of Lyme disease.

Study participants did not routinely have baseline sera tested by WB for Lyme disease. WB at baseline was performed for subjects who were noted to have a positive or equivocal WB during a visit for suspected Lyme disease or when tested at months 12 or 20. Baseline serology was thus found to be positive in 250 subjects out of 628 tested. The nature and incidence of adverse events (either early or late) did not differ between vaccinees determined to have been WB-positive at baseline (n=124) compared to vaccinees determined to have been WB-negative at baseline (n=151).

There were 1,206 subjects enrolled in the study who self-reported a previous history of Lyme disease (610 vaccinees, 596 placebo recipients). For adverse events occurring within the first 30 days, there was an increased incidence of musculoskeletal symptoms in vaccinees with a history of Lyme disease compared to vaccinees with no history of Lyme disease (20% vs. 13%, p<0.001). No such difference was observed in the placebo group (13% vs. 11%, p=0.24). Subjects with a previous history of Lyme disease had an increased incidence of late (>30 days post-vaccination) musculoskeletal symptoms compared to subjects without a history of Lyme disease in both the vaccine and placebo groups. There was no significant difference in late musculoskeletal adverse events between vaccine and placebo recipients with a history of Lyme disease (33% vs. 35%, p=0.51).

Subjects with a self-reported prior history of Lyme disease had a greater incidence of psychiatric disorders (early and late); central, peripheral and autonomic nervous system disorders (late); and gastrointestinal disorders (late) than subjects with no prior history of Lyme disease. However, there was no significant difference in the incidence of any of these disorders between vaccine and placebo recipients with a prior history of Lyme disease.

Among the 10,936 subjects enrolled in the efficacy trial and followed for 20 months, a total of 15 deaths occurred (10 vaccine, 5 placebo). None of these deaths were judged to be treatment-related by investigators. In the vaccine group, causes of death included: cancer (5), myocardial infarction (3), sudden death (1), cardiac arrest (1). In the placebo group, causes of death included: cancer (1), sudden cardiac death (1), cardiac arrest (1), septic shock (1), homicide (1). As with all pharmaceuticals, it is possible that expanded commercial use of the vaccine could reveal rare adverse events not observed in clinical studies.

Table 3. Incidence (≥1%) of Unsolicited Adverse Events Occurring More Than 30 Days Following Doses 2 and 3* and Overall (after Doses 1, 2 or 3)

	Dose					
	2		3		Overall	
Events	Vaccine (N=5397) %	Placebo (N=5417) %	Vaccine (N=5001) %	Placebo (N=5018) %	Vaccine (N=5469) %	Placebo (N=5467) %
Body as a Whole						
Achiness	1.50	1.38			2.30	2.18
Chills/Rigors	1.30	1.05			1.74	1.76
Fatigue	3.24	3.43	1.86	1.81	5.01	4.98
Fever	2.28	2.60	1.34	1.30	3.58	3.82
Infection viral	1.43	1.74			2.19	2.34
Influenza-like symptoms	2.33	2.10			2.87	2.76
Cardiovascular System						
Hypertension					0.93	1.24
Gastrointestinal System						
Diarrhea					1.01	1.19
Musculoskeletal System						
Arthralgia	9.93	10.04	4.72	4.46	13.64	13.55
Arthritis	1.98	1.74	1.04	1.12	2.91	2.84
Arthrosis	1.22	1.09			1.66	1.50
Back pain	2.69	2.73			3.58	3.46
Myalgia	2.78	2.22	1.14	1.28	4.02	3.40
Stiffness	1.82	1.59			2.47	2.40
Tendinitis	1.45	1.05			1.92	1.63
Nervous System						
Depression					1.02	1.10
Dizziness					1.02	1.26
Headache	3.56	3.05	1.36	1.49	5.06	4.72
Hypesthesia	2.20	2.66			2.96	3.60
Paresthesia	2.69	2.20	1.06	0.98	3.60	2.98
Respiratory System						
Bronchitis					1.32	1.39
Pharyngitis	1.70	1.68			2.19	2.12
Rhinitis	0.94	1.07			1.41	1.37
Sinusitis	2.33	2.53			3.07	3.11
Upper respiratory tract infection	2.02	2.29			2.80	3.00
Skin/Appendages						
Contact dermatitis	1.50	1.75			1.68	1.94
Rash	2.39	1.99			3.07	2.71

*Data for adverse events occurring more than 30 days after dose 1 are not provided because most subjects received dose 2 approximately 30 days after dose 1.

Note: No significant differences in adverse events were noted between treatment groups after any dose and overall.

Table 4. The Incidence of Local and General Solicited Adverse Events (including Severe Events) Reported After Each Dose and Overall

	Dose							
	1		2		3		Overall	
Events	Vaccine (N=402) %	Placebo (N=398) %	Vaccine (N=402) %	Placebo (N=398) %	Vaccine (N=402) %	Placebo (N=398) %	Vaccine (N=402) %	Placebo (N=398) %
Local Symptoms								
Redness, any	21.64[c]	8.29	16.67[c]	7.04	25.12[c]	11.81	41.79[c]	20.85
Redness, severe*	2.2[b]	0.0	1.0	0.0	2.5[b]	0.0	4.2[c]	0.0
Soreness, any	81.59[c]	36.68	76.37[c]	30.90	82.59[c]	52.26	93.53[c]	68.09
Soreness, severe†	1.2	0.0	1.0	0.3	3.0[b]	0.3	5.0[c]	0.0
Swelling, any	14.43[c]	4.27	11.44[c]	3.27	19.15[c]	6.78	29.85[c]	11.31
Swelling, severe*	0.0	0.0	0.0	0.0	0.5	0.0	0.5	0.0
General Symptoms								
Arthralgia, any	11.94[c]	4.52	10.70	8.29	13.43[b]	7.54	25.62[b]	16.33
Arthralgia, severe†	0.7	0.0	0.2	0.3	0.0	0.3	1.0	0.5
Fatigue, any	20.90	16.83	20.15[c]	11.81	21.89[a]	16.33	40.80[a]	32.91
Fatigue, severe†	0.5	0.05	1.5	1.3	1.0	1.0	3.0	2.3
Headache, any	20.65	19.10	14.43	12.31	19.90	18.34	38.56	37.19
Headache, severe†	0.5	0.05	1.2	0.5	1.2	1.8	3.0	2.8
Rash, any	4.23[a]	1.51	4.98[a]	2.01	5.47[b]	1.76	11.69[b]	5.28
Rash, severe*	0.0	0.0	0.0	0.0	0.2	0.0	0.2	0.0
Fever ≥99.5°F	1.49	0.75	1.00	0.50	1.00	1.01	3.48	2.26
Fever >102.2°F	0.0	0.0	0.0	0.0	0.0	0.0	0.0	0.0

*Severe = measuring >3.0 cm and persisting longer than 24 hours.

†Severe = preventing everyday normal activity.

a. p-value <0.05. b. p-value <0.01. c. p-value <0.001.

DOSAGE AND ADMINISTRATION

Primary immunization against Lyme disease consists of a 30 mcg/0.5 mL dose of *LYMErix* given at 0, 1 and 12 months.

Vaccination with all three doses is required to achieve optimal protection.

Safety and efficacy for this vaccine are based on administration of the second and third doses several weeks prior to the onset of the *Borrelia* transmission season in the local geographic area (see INDICATION AND USAGE). For example, in the pivotal efficacy trial performed primarily in the Northeast United States (see *Clinical Efficacy*), individuals were vaccinated between January and April in both years of the trial.

LYMErix [Lyme Disease Vaccine (Recombinant OspA)] should be administered by intramuscular injection in the deltoid region. *Do not inject intravenously, intradermally or subcutaneously.*

Preparation for Administration: Shake well before withdrawal and use. Parenteral drug products should be inspected visually for particulate matter or discoloration prior to administration. With thorough agitation, *LYMErix* is a turbid white suspension. Discard if it appears otherwise. Any vaccine remaining in a single-dose vial should be discarded.

The vaccine should be used as supplied; no dilution or reconstitution is necessary. The full recommended dose of the vaccine should be used.

As with other intramuscular injections, *LYMErix* should not be given to individuals on anticoagulant therapy or with clotting disorders, unless the potential benefit clearly outweighs the risk of administration.

No data are available on the immune response to *LYMErix* when administered concurrently with other vaccines. When concomitant administration of other vaccines is required, they should be given with different syringes and at different injection sites (see Drug Interactions).

STORAGE

Store between 2° and 8°C (36° and 46°F). Do not freeze; discard if product has been frozen.

HOW SUPPLIED

LYMErix [Lyme Disease Vaccine (Recombinant OspA)] is supplied in Single-Dose (30 mcg/0.5 mL) Vials and Prefilled Syringes

NDC 58160-845-11 Package of 10 Single-Dose Vials

NDC 58160-845-32 Package of 1 Prefilled Disposable Tip-Lok® Syringe with 1-inch 23-gauge needle

NDC 58160-845-35 Package of 5 Prefilled Disposable Tip-Lok® Syringes with 1-inch 23-gauge needles

REFERENCES

1. Dennis DT. Epidemiology. In: Coyle P (ed). *Lyme Disease*. Mosby Year Book, Inc. 1993:27–36.
2. Centers for Disease Control and Prevention. Lyme Disease—United States, 1996. *MMWR*. June 13, 1997; Vol. 46:23;533–534.
3. Centers for Disease Control and Prevention. Lyme Disease—United States, 1996. *MMWR*. October 31, 1997;Vol. 45:53;41.
4. Goldstein MD, Schwartz BS, Friedmann C, et al. Lyme disease in New Jersey outdoor workers: a statewide survey of seroprevalence and tick exposure. *Am J Public Health*. 1990;80:1225–1229.
5. Dennis DT. Lyme disease. *Dermatol Clin*. 1995;13(3): 537–551.
6. Data on file from Centers for Disease Control and Prevention (LYR198), SmithKline Beecham Pharmaceuticals.
7. Data on file from Centers for Disease Control and Prevention (LYR598:12 monthly incidence tables for Lyme Disease. *MMWR*. 1997;46:Nos. 5, 8, 13, 17, 22, 23, 31, 35, 39, 44, 47, 51), SmithKline Beecham Pharmaceuticals.
8. Fish D. Environmental risk and prevention of Lyme disease. *Am J Med*. 1995;98 (suppl 4A):4A2S–4A9S.
9. Steere AC. *Borrelia burgdorferi* (Lyme Disease, Lyme Borreliosis). In: Mandell, Bennett, Dolin (eds). *Mandell, Douglas and Bennett's Principles and Practices of Infectious Disease*. 4th ed. 1995:chapter 219:2143–2155.
10. Nocton JJ, Steere AC. Lyme Disease. In: *Advances in Internal Medicine*. Mosby Year Book, Inc. 1995;40:69–115.
11. Centers for Disease Control and Prevention. Recommendations for test performance and interpretation from the Second National Conference on Serologic Diagnosis of Lyme Disease. *MMWR*. 1995;44:590–591.
12. Fikrig E, Barthold SW, Marcantonio N, et al. Roles of OspA, OspB, and flagellin in protective immunity to Lyme borreliosis in the laboratory mouse. *Infect Immun*. 1992;60:657–661.
13. Fikrig E, Telford SR, Barthold SW, et al. Elimination of *Borrelia burgdorferi* from vector ticks feeding on OspA-immunized mice. *Proc Natl Acad Sci* (USA). 1992;89: 5418–5421.

Continued on next page

Information on the SmithKline Beecham Pharmaceuticals products appearing here is based on the labeling in effect on June 15, 2000. Further information on these and other products may be obtained from the Medical Department, SmithKline Beecham Pharmaceuticals, One Franklin Plaza, Philadelphia, PA 19101.

LYMErix—Cont.

14. Golde WT, Piesman J, Dolan MC, et al. Reactivity with a specific epitope of outer surface protein A predicts protection from infection with the Lyme disease spirochete, *Borrelia burgdorferi*. *Infect Immun*. 1997;65:882–889.
15. Schwan TG, Piesman J, Golde WT, et al. Induction of an outer surface protein on *Borrelia burgdorferi* during tick feeding. *Proc Natl Acad Sci* (USA). 1995;92:2909–2913.
16. Data on file (LYR 1098), SmithKline Beecham Pharmaceuticals.
17. Wormser GP, Horowitz HW, Nowakowski J, et al. Positive Lyme disease serology in patients with clinical and laboratory evidence of human granulocytic ehrlichiosis. *Am J Clin Pathol*. 1997;107:142–147.
18. Bowen GS, Schulze TL, Hayne C, et al. A focus of Lyme disease in Monmouth County, New Jersey. *Am J Epidemiol*. 1984;120:387–394.
19. Smith PF, Benach JL, White DJ, et al. Occupational risk of Lyme disease in endemic areas of New York State. *Ann NY Acad Sci*. 1988;539:289–301.
20. Schwartz BS, Goldstein MC, Childs JE. Longitudinal study of *Borrelia burgdorferi* infection in New Jersey outdoor workers, 1988–1991. *Am J Epidemiol*. 1994; 139(5):504–512.
21. Schwartz BS, Goldstein MD. Lyme disease in outdoor workers: risk factors, preventive measures, and tick removal methods. *Am J Epidemiol*. 1990; 131(5):877–885.
22. Steere AC, Broderick TF, Malawista SE. Erythema chronicum migrans and Lyme arthritis: epidemiologic evidence for a tick vector. *Am J Epidemiol*. 1978; 108(4): 312–321.
23. Nowakowski J, Schwartz I, Nadelman RB, et al. Culture-confirmed infection and reinfection with *Borrelia burgdorferi*. *Ann Intern Med*. 1997;127:130–132.
24. Gross DM, Forsthuber T, Tary-Lehmann M, et al: Identification of LFA-1 as a candidate autoantigen in treatment-resistant Lyme arthritis. *Science*. 1998;281:703–706.
25. Centers for Disease Control and Prevention. Update: Vaccine side effects, adverse reactions, contraindications and precautions—recommendations of the Advisory Committee on Immunization Practices (ACIP). *MMWR*. 1996;Vol. 45(RR-12): 1–35.
26. Centers for Disease Control and Prevention. General recommendations on immunization recommendations of the Advisory Committee on Immunization Practices (ACIP). *MMWR*. 1994;Vol. 43 (RR-1):1–38.

U.S. License No. 1090
Manufactured by
SmithKline Beecham Biologicals
Rixensart, Belgium
Distributed by
SmithKline Beecham Pharmaceuticals
Philadelphia, PA 19101

Rx only

LYMErix and *Tip-Lok* are registered trademarks of SmithKline Beecham.
LY:L3B

Shown in Product Identification Guide, page 337

ORNADE® SPANSULE® CAPSULES ℞

[*or 'naid*]
brand of sustained release capsules

DESCRIPTION

Ornade is a combination of an oral nasal decongestant and an antihistamine.

Each *Ornade* Spansule capsule contains phenylpropanolamine hydrochloride, 75 mg and chlorpheniramine maleate, 12 mg. Inactive ingredients consist of benzyl alcohol, cetylpyridinium chloride, FD&C Blue No. 1, FD&C Red No. 3, FD&C Yellow No. 6, D&C Red No. 27, D&C Red No. 30, gelatin, glyceryl distearate, iron oxide, polyethylene glycol, povidone, silicon dioxide, sodium lauryl sulfate, starch, sucrose, titanium dioxide, wax and trace amounts of other inactive ingredients.

Each *Ornade* Spansule capsule is so prepared that an initial dose is released promptly and the remaining medication is released gradually over a prolonged period.

CLINICAL PHARMACOLOGY

Phenylpropanolamine Hydrochloride

Phenylpropanolamine hydrochloride is a sympathomimetic agent which is closely related to ephedrine in chemical structure and pharmacologic action, but produces less central nervous system stimulation than ephedrine. It is a vasoconstrictor with decongestant action on nasal and upper respiratory tract mucosal membranes.

Chlorpheniramine Maleate

Chlorpheniramine maleate is an antihistamine with anticholinergic (drying) and sedative side effects. Antihistamines appear to compete with histamine for H_1 cell receptor sites on effector cells.

Pharmacokinetics

A single *Ornade* Spansule capsule produces blood levels comparable to those produced by administration of three 25 mg doses of phenylpropanolamine hydrochloride and three 4 mg doses of chlorpheniramine maleate in conventional release form given at 4-hour intervals. At steady-state conditions, the following peak levels are reached after the oral administration of an *Ornade* Spansule capsule: 21 ng/mL chlorpheniramine maleate in 7.7 hours; 173 ng/mL phenylpropanolamine hydrochloride in 6.1 hours; under these circumstances, the half-lives are approximately 21 and 7 hours, respectively.

INDICATIONS AND USAGE

For the treatment of the symptoms of seasonal and perennial allergic rhinitis and vasomotor rhinitis, including nasal obstruction (congestion); also for the treatment of runny nose, sneezing and nasal congestion associated with the common cold.

CONTRAINDICATIONS

Hypersensitivity to either phenylpropanolamine hydrochloride or chlorpheniramine maleate and other antihistamines of similar chemical structure; severe hypertension; coronary artery disease.

This drug should NOT be used in newborn or premature infants.

Because of the higher risk of antihistamines for infants generally, and for newborns and prematures in particular, antihistamine therapy is contraindicated in nursing mothers.

As with any product containing a sympathomimetic, *Ornade* Spansule capsules should NOT be used in patients taking monoamine oxidase (MAO) inhibitors.

WARNINGS

Ornade Spansule capsules may potentiate the effects of alcohol and other CNS depressants. Also, this product should not be taken simultaneously with other products containing phenylpropanolamine hydrochloride or amphetamines.

Ornade Spansule capsules should be used with considerable caution in patients with narrow-angle glaucoma, stenosing peptic ulcer, pyloroduodenal obstruction, symptomatic prostatic hypertrophy, or bladder neck obstruction.

Use in Children: In infants and children, especially, antihistamines in *overdosage* may cause hallucinations, convulsions, or death. As in adults, antihistamines may diminish mental alertness in children. In the young child, particularly, they may produce excitation.

Use in the Elderly (approximately 60 years or older): Antihistamines are more likely to cause dizziness, sedation and hypotension in elderly patients.

PRECAUTIONS

General: Use with caution in patients with lower respiratory disease including asthma, hypertension, cardiovascular disease, hyperthyroidism, increased intraocular pressure, or diabetes.

Information for Patients: Caution patients about activities requiring alertness (e.g., operating vehicles or machinery). Also caution patients about the possible additive effects of alcohol and other CNS depressants (hypnotics, sedatives, tranquilizers, etc.), and not to take simultaneously other products containing phenylpropanolamine hydrochloride or amphetamines. Patients should not take *Ornade* Spansule capsules in conjunction with a monoamine oxidase inhibitor or an oral anticoagulant.

Drug Interactions: *Ornade* Spansule capsules may interact with alcohol and other CNS depressants to potentiate their effects.

This product may have additive effects when taken simultaneously with other products containing phenylpropanolamine hydrochloride or amphetamines.

MAO inhibitors prolong and intensify the anticholinergic (drying) effects of antihistamines and potentiate the pressor effects of sympathomimetics such as phenylpropanolamine hydrochloride (see CONTRAINDICATIONS).

Phenylpropanolamine hydrochloride should not be used with ganglionic blocking drugs—such as mecamylamine—which potentiate reactions of sympathomimetics. It also should not be used with adrenergic blocking drugs, such as guanethidine sulfate or bethanidine, since it antagonizes the hypotensive action of these drugs.

The action of oral anticoagulants may be inhibited by antihistamines.

The CNS depressant and atropine-like effects of anticholinergics may be potentiated by concomitant administration of antihistamines. Concomitant administration of anticholinergics such as trihexyphenidyl, and other drugs with anticholinergic action (such as imipramine), with antihistamines may result in xerostomia.

β-adrenergic blockers may be antagonized by antihistamines.

Concomitant administration of corticosteroids and antihistamines may decrease the effects of the corticosteroids by enzyme induction.

Antihistamines inhibit norepinephrine reuptake by tissues and therefore potentiate the cardiovascular effects of norepinephrine.

Concomitant use of antihistamines with phenothiazines may produce an additive CNS depressant effect; concomitant use also may cause urinary retention or glaucoma.

Carcinogenesis, Mutagenesis, Impairment of Fertility: A long-term oncogenic study in rats with the chlorpheniramine maleate component of *Ornade* Spansule capsules did not produce an increase in the incidence of tumors in the drug-treated groups, as compared with the controls. No evidence of mutagenicity was found when chlorpheniramine maleate was evaluated in a battery of mutagenic studies, including the Ames test.

In an early study in rats with chlorpheniramine maleate a reduction in fertility was observed in female rats at doses approximately 67 times the human dose. More recent studies in rabbits and rats, using more appropriate methodology and doses up to approximately 50 and 85 times the human dose, showed no reduction in fertility.

There are no studies available which indicate whether phenylpropanolamine hydrochloride has carcinogenic or mutagenic effects or impairs fertility.

Pregnancy, Teratogenic Effects, Pregnancy Category B: Reproduction studies have been performed with the components of *Ornade* Spansule capsules. Studies with chlorpheniramine maleate in rabbits and rats at doses up to 50 times and 85 times the human dose, respectively, revealed no evidence of harm to the fetus. A study with phenylpropanolamine hydrochloride in rats at doses up to 7 times the human dose revealed no evidence of harm to the fetus. There are, however, no adequate and well-controlled studies in pregnant women. Because animal reproduction studies are not always predictive of human response, *Ornade* Spansule capsules should be used during pregnancy only if clearly needed.

Nonteratogenic Effects: Studies of chlorpheniramine maleate in rats showed a decrease in the postnatal survival rate of offspring of animals dosed with 33 and 67 times the human dose.

Nursing Mothers: Small amounts of antihistamines are excreted in breast milk. Because of the higher risk with antihistamines in infants generally, and for newborns and prematures in particular, *Ornade* Spansule capsules should not be administered to a nursing mother (see CONTRAINDICATIONS).

Pediatric Use: The safety and effectiveness of *Ornade* Spansule capsules in children under 12 years of age have not been established.

In infants and children, especially, antihistamines in *overdosage* may cause hallucinations, convulsions, or death.

As in adults, antihistamines may diminish mental alertness in children. In the young child, particularly, they may produce excitation. (See WARNINGS.)

ADVERSE REACTIONS

The following adverse reactions have been reported following the use of antihistamines and/or sympathomimetic amines:

General: Anaphylactic shock; chills; drug rash; excessive dryness of mouth, nose and throat; increased intraocular pressure; excessive perspiration; photosensitivity; urticaria; weakness.

Cardiovascular System: Angina pain; extrasystoles; headache; hypertension; hypotension; palpitations; tachycardia.

Hematologic: Agranulocytosis; hemolytic anemia; leukopenia; thrombocytopenia.

Nervous System: Blurred vision; confusion; convulsions; diplopia; disturbed coordination; dizziness; drowsiness; euphoria; excitation; fatigue; hysteria; insomnia; irritability; acute labyrinthitis; nervousness; neuritis; paresthesia; restlessness; sedation; tinnitus; tremor; vertigo.

GI System: Abdominal pain; anorexia; constipation; diarrhea; epigastric distress; nausea; vomiting.

GU System: Dysuria; early menses; urinary frequency; urinary retention.

Respiratory System: Thickening of bronchial secretions; tightness of chest and wheezing; nasal stuffiness.

OVERDOSAGE

In the event of overdosage, emergency treatment should be started immediately.

Symptoms: Effects of antihistamine overdosage may vary from central nervous system depression (sedation, apnea, diminished mental alertness, cardiovascular collapse) to stimulation (insomnia, hallucinations, tremors, or convulsions) to death.

Other signs and symptoms may be dizziness, tinnitus, ataxia, blurred vision and hypotension. Stimulation is particularly likely in children, as are atropine-like signs and symptoms (dry mouth; fixed, dilated pupils; flushing; hyperthermia; and gastrointestinal symptoms). In large doses, sympathomimetics may cause giddiness, headache, nausea, vomiting, sweating, thirst, tachycardia, precordial pain, palpitations, difficulty in micturition, muscular weakness and tenseness, anxiety, restlessness and insomnia. Many patients can present a toxic psychosis with delusions and hallucinations. Some may develop cardiac arrhythmias, circulatory collapse, convulsions, coma and respiratory failure.

Toxicity: In acute oral toxicity tests in rats, the LD_{50} for the ratio of 75 mg phenylpropanolamine hydrochloride and 12 mg chlorpheniramine maleate was 774.2 mg/kg; in mice, the LD_{50} for the formulation was 757.4 mg/kg.

Treatment: The patient should be induced to vomit even if emesis has occurred spontaneously. Pharmacologically induced vomiting by the administration of ipecac syrup is a preferred method. But vomiting should not be induced in patients with impaired consciousness. The action of ipecac is facilitated by physical activity and by the administration of 8 to 12 fluid ounces of water. If emesis does not occur within 15 minutes, the dose of ipecac should be repeated. Precautions against aspiration must be taken, especially in infants and children.

Following emesis, any drug remaining in the stomach may be adsorbed by activated charcoal administered as a slurry with water. If vomiting is unsuccessful or contraindicated, gastric lavage should be performed. Isotonic and one-half isotonic saline are the lavage solutions of choice. Since much of the *Spansule* capsule medication is coated for gradual release, saline cathartics should be administered to hasten evacuation of pellets that have not already released medication. Saline cathartics, such as milk of magnesia, draw water into the bowel by osmosis and therefore may be valuable for their action in rapid dilution of bowel content. Dialysis has not been reported to be effective in the treatment of phenylpropanolamine hydrochloride and chlorpheniramine maleate overdosage. After emergency treatment, the patient should continue to be medically monitored.

Treatment of the signs and symptoms of overdosage is symptomatic and supportive. *Stimulants* (analeptic agents) should *not* be used. Vasopressors may be used to treat hypotension. Short-acting barbiturates, diazepam, or paraldehyde may be administered to control seizures. Hyperpyrexia, especially in children, may require treatment with tepid water sponge baths or a hypothermic blanket. Apnea is treated with ventilatory support.

DOSAGE AND ADMINISTRATION

Adults and children 12 years of age and over—one capsule every 12 hours.

Ornade Spansule capsules are not recommended in children under 12.

HOW SUPPLIED

In gelatin capsules with opaque red cap and natural body. Each capsule is imprinted with the product name ORNADE and SB, and filled with small red, white and gray pellets; in bottles of 50 and 500 capsules, and in Single Unit Packages of 100 capsules (intended for institutional use only). Each capsule contains 75 mg phenylpropanolamine hydrochloride and 12 mg chlorpheniramine maleate. Capsules should be stored between 15° and 30°C (59° and 86°F).

NDC 0007-4421-15 50's

NDC 0007-4421-25 500's

WARNING: Manufactured with carbon tetrachloride and methyl chloroform, substances which harm public health and environment by destroying ozone in the upper atmosphere.

OR:L42

Shown in Product Identification Guide, page 337

PARNATE® ℞

[*pahr 'naight*]

brand of tranylcypromine sulfate

tablets 10 mg

Before prescribing, the physician should be familiar with the entire contents of this prescribing information.

DESCRIPTION

Chemically, tranylcypromine sulfate is (±)-*trans* -2-phenylcyclopropylamine sulfate (2:1).

Each round, rose-red, film-coated tablet is imprinted with the product name PARNATE and SKF and contains tranylcypromine sulfate equivalent to 10 mg of tranylcypromine. Inactive ingredients consist of cellulose, citric acid, croscarmellose sodium, D&C Red No. 7, FD&C Blue No. 2, FD&C Red No. 40, FD&C Yellow No. 6, gelatin, iron oxide, lactose, magnesium stearate, talc, titanium dioxide and trace amounts of other inactive ingredients.

NOTE: Parnate (tranylcypromine sulfate) tablets have been changed from rose-red sugar-coated tablets to rose-red film-coated tablets. The film-coated tablets differ in size from the sugar-coated tablets, but the drug content remains unchanged.

ACTION

Tranylcypromine is a non-hydrazine monoamine oxidase inhibitor with a rapid onset of activity. It increases the concentration of epinephrine, norepinephrine, and serotonin in storage sites throughout the nervous system and, in theory, this increased concentration of monoamines in the brain stem is the basis for its antidepressant activity. When tranylcypromine is withdrawn, monoamine oxidase activity is recovered in 3 to 5 days, although the drug is excreted in 24 hours.

INDICATIONS

For the treatment of Major Depressive Episode Without Melancholia.

Parnate (tranylcypromine sulfate) should be used in adult patients who can be closely supervised. It should rarely be the first antidepressant drug given. Rather, the drug is suited for patients who have failed to respond to the drugs more commonly administered for depression.

The effectiveness of *Parnate* has been established in adult outpatients, most of whom had a depressive illness which would correspond to a diagnosis of Major Depressive Episode Without Melancholia. As described in the American Psychiatric Association's Diagnostic and Statistical Manual, third edition (DSM III), Major Depressive Episode implies a prominent and relatively persistent (nearly every day for at least 2 weeks) depressed or dysphoric mood that usually interferes with daily functioning and includes at least 4 of the following 8 symptoms: change in appetite, change in sleep, psychomotor agitation or retardation, loss of interest in usual activities or decrease in sexual drive, increased fatigability, feelings of guilt or worthlessness, slowed thinking or impaired concentration and suicidal ideation or attempts.

The effectiveness of *Parnate* in patients who meet the criteria for Major Depressive Episode with Melancholia (endogenous features) has not been established.

SUMMARY OF CONTRAINDICATIONS

Parnate (tranylcypromine sulfate) should not be administered in combination with any of the following: MAO inhibitors or dibenzazepine derivatives; sympathomimetics (including amphetamines); some central nervous system depressants (including narcotics and alcohol); antihypertensive, diuretic, antihistaminic, sedative or anesthetic drugs; bupropion HCl; buspirone HCl; dextromethorphan; cheese or other foods with a high tyramine content; or excessive quantities of caffeine.

Parnate (tranylcypromine sulfate) should not be administered to any patient with a confirmed or suspected cerebrovascular defect or to any patient with cardiovascular disease, hypertension or history of headache.

(For complete discussion of contraindications and warnings, see below.)

CONTRAINDICATIONS

Parnate (tranylcypromine sulfate) is contraindicated:

1. In patients with cerebrovascular defects or cardiovascular disorders

Parnate should not be administered to any patient with a confirmed or suspected cerebrovascular defect or to any patient with cardiovascular disease or hypertension.

2. In the presence of pheochromocytoma

Parnate should not be used in the presence of pheochromocytoma since such tumors secrete pressor substances.

3. In combination with MAO inhibitors or with dibenzazepine-related entities

Parnate (tranylcypromine sulfate) should not be administered together or in rapid succession with other MAO inhibitors or with dibenzazepine-related entities. Hypertensive crises or severe convulsive seizures may occur in patients receiving such combinations.

In patients being transferred to *Parnate* from another MAO inhibitor or from a dibenzazepine-related entity, allow a medication-free interval of at least a week, then initiate *Parnate* using half the normal starting dosage for at least the first week of therapy. Similarly, at least a week should elapse between the discontinuance of *Parnate* and the administration of another MAO inhibitor or a dibenzazepine-related entity, or the readministration of *Parnate*.

The following list includes some other MAO inhibitors, dibenzazepine-related entities and tricyclic antidepressants, and the companies which market them.

Other MAO Inhibitors

Generic Name	Trademark
Furazolidone	Furoxone® (Roberts Laboratories)
Isocarboxazid	Marplan® (Roche Laboratories)
Pargyline HCl	Eutonyl® (Abbott Laboratories)
Pargyline HCl and methyclothiazide	Eutron® (Abbott Laboratories)
Phenelzine sulfate	Nardil® (Parke-Davis)
Procarbazine HCl	Matulane® (Roche Laboratories)

Dibenzazepine-Related and Other Tricyclics

Generic Name	Trademark
Amitriptyline HCl	Elavil® (Zeneca)
	Endep® (Roche Products)
Perphenazine and amitriptyline HCl	Etrafon® (Schering)
	Triavil® (Merck and Co.)
Clomipramine hydrochloride	Anafranil® (CibaGeneva)
Desipramine HCl	Norpramin® (Marion Merrell Dow)
	Pertofrane® (Rhône-Poulenc Rorer Pharmaceuticals)
Imipramine HCl	Janimine™ (Abbott Laboratories)
	Tofranil® (CibaGeneva)
Nortriptyline HCl	Aventyl® (Eli Lilly & Co.)
	Pamelor® (Sandoz)
Protriptyline HCl	Vivactil® (Merck and Co.)
Doxepin HCl	Adapin® (Fisons)
	Sinequan® (Roerig)
Carbamazepine	Tegretol® (CibaGeneva)
Cyclobenzaprine HCl	Flexeril® (Merck and Co.)
Amoxapine	Asendin™ (Lederle)
Maprotiline HCl	Ludiomil® (CibaGeneva)
Trimipramine maleate	Surmontil® (Wyeth-Ayerst Laboratories)

4. In combination with bupropion

The concurrent administration of a MAO inhibitor and bupropion hydrochloride (Wellbutrin®, Burroughs Wellcome) is contraindicated. At least 14 days should elapse between discontinuation of a MAO inhibitor and initiation of treatment with bupropion hydrochloride.

5. In combination with dexfenfluramine hydrochloride

Because Redux (dexfenfluramine hydrochloride, Wyeth) is a serotonin releaser and reuptake inhibitor, it should not be used concomitantly with Parnate (tranylcypromine sulfate).

6. In combination with selective serotonin reuptake inhibitors (SSRIs)

As a general rule, *Parnate* should not be administered in combination with any SSRI. There have been reports of serious, sometimes fatal, reactions (including hyperthermia, rigidity, myoclonus, autonomic instability with possible rapid fluctuations of vital signs, and mental status changes that include extreme agitation progressing to delirium and coma) in patients receiving fluoxetine (Prozac®, Lilly) in combination with a monoamine oxidase inhibitor (MAOI), and in patients who have recently discontinued fluoxetine and are then started on a MAOI. Some cases presented with features resembling neuroleptic malignant syndrome. Therefore, fluoxetine and other SSRIs should not be used in combination with a MAOI, or within 14 days of discontinuing therapy with a MAOI. Since fluoxetine and its major metabolite have very long elimination half-lives, at least 5 weeks should be allowed after stopping fluoxetine before starting a MAOI.

At least 2 weeks should be allowed after stopping sertraline (Zoloft®, Roerig) or paroxetine (Paxil®, SmithKline Beecham Pharmaceuticals) before starting a MAOI.

7. In combination with buspirone

Parnate (tranylcypromine sulfate) should not be used in combination with buspirone HCl (BuSpar®, Bristol-Myers Squibb), since several cases of elevated blood pressure have been reported in patients taking MAO inhibitors who were then given buspirone HCl. At least 10 days should elapse between the discontinuation of *Parnate* and the institution of buspirone HCl.

8. In combination with sympathomimetics

Parnate (tranylcypromine sulfate) should not be administered in combination with sympathomimetics, including amphetamines, and over-the-counter drugs such as cold, hay fever or weight-reducing preparations that contain vasoconstrictors.

During *Parnate* therapy, it appears that certain patients are particularly vulnerable to the effects of sympathomimetics when the activity of certain enzymes is inhibited. Use of sympathomimetics and compounds such as guanethidine, methyldopa, reserpine, dopamine, levodopa and tryptophan with *Parnate* may precipitate hypertension, headache and related symptoms. In addition, use with tryptophan may precipitate disorientation, memory impairment and other neurologic and behavioral signs.

9. In combination with meperidine

Do not use meperidine concomitantly with MAO inhibitors or within 2 or 3 weeks following MAOI therapy. Serious reactions have been precipitated with concomitant use, including coma, severe hypertension or hypotension, severe respiratory depression, convulsions, malignant hyperpyrexia, excitation, peripheral vascular collapse and death. It is thought that these reactions may be mediated by accumulation of 5-HT (serotonin) consequent to MAO inhibition.

10. In combination with dextromethorphan

The combination of MAO inhibitors and dextromethorphan has been reported to cause brief episodes of psychosis or bizarre behavior.

11. In combination with cheese or other foods with a high tyramine content

Hypertensive crises have sometimes occurred during *Parnate* therapy after ingestion of foods with a high tyramine content. In general, the patient should avoid protein foods in which aging or protein breakdown is used to increase flavor. In particular, patients should be instructed not to take foods such as cheese (particularly strong or aged varieties), sour cream, Chianti wine, sherry, beer (including nonalcoholic beer), liqueurs, pickled herring, anchovies, caviar, liver, canned figs, dried fruits (raisins, prunes, etc.) bananas, raspberries, avocados, overripe fruit, chocolate, soy sauce, sauerkraut, the pods of broad beans (fava beans), yeast extracts, yogurt, meat extracts or meat prepared with tenderizers.

12. In patients undergoing elective surgery

Patients taking *Parnate* should not undergo elective surgery requiring general anesthesia. Also, they should not be given cocaine or local anesthesia containing sympathomimetic vasoconstrictors. The possible combined hypotensive effects of *Parnate* and spinal anesthesia should be kept in mind. *Parnate* should be discontinued at least 10 days prior to elective surgery.

ADDITIONAL CONTRAINDICATIONS

In general, the physician should bear in mind the possibility of a lowered margin of safety when Parnate (tranylcypromine sulfate) is administered in combination with potent drugs.

1. *Parnate* should not be used in combination with some central nervous system depressants such as narcotics and alcohol, or with hypotensive agents. A marked potentiating effect on these classes of drugs has been reported.

Continued on next page

Information on the SmithKline Beecham Pharmaceuticals products appearing here is based on the labeling in effect on June 15, 2000. Further information on these and other products may be obtained from the Medical Department, SmithKline Beecham Pharmaceuticals, One Franklin Plaza, Philadelphia, PA 19101.

Parnate—Cont.

2. Anti-parkinsonism drugs should be used with caution in patients receiving *Parnate* since severe reactions have been reported.
3. *Parnate* should not be used in patients with a history of liver disease or in those with abnormal liver function tests.
4. Excessive use of caffeine in any form should be avoided in patients receiving *Parnate*.

WARNING TO PHYSICIANS

Parnate (tranylcypromine sulfate) is a potent agent with the capability of producing serious side effects. *Parnate* is not recommended in those depressive reactions where other antidepressant drugs may be effective. **It should be reserved for patients who can be closely supervised and who have not responded satisfactorily to the drugs more commonly administered for depression.**

Before prescribing, the physician should be completely familiar with the full material on dosage, side effects and contraindications on these pages, with the principles of MAO inhibitor therapy and the side effects of this class of drugs. Also, the physician should be familiar with the symptomatology of mental depressions and alternate methods of treatment to aid in the careful selection of patients for *Parnate* therapy. In depressed patients, the possibility of suicide should always be considered and adequate precautions taken.

Pregnancy Warning: Use of any drug in pregnancy, during lactation or in women of childbearing age requires that the potential benefits of the drug be weighed against its possible hazards to mother and child.

Animal reproductive studies show that *Parnate* passes through the placental barrier into the fetus of the rat, and into the milk of the lactating dog. The absence of a harmful action of *Parnate* on fertility or on postnatal development by either prenatal treatment or from the milk of treated animals has not been demonstrated. Tranylcypromine is excreted in human milk.

WARNING TO THE PATIENT

Patients should be instructed to report promptly the occurrence of headache or other unusual symptoms, i.e., palpitation and/or tachycardia, a sense of constriction in the throat or chest, sweating, dizziness, neck stiffness, nausea or vomiting.

Patients should be warned against eating the foods listed in Section 11 under Contraindications while on Parnate (tranylcypromine sulfate) therapy. Also, they should be told not to drink alcoholic beverages. The patient should also be warned about the possibility of hypotension and faintness, as well as drowsiness sufficient to impair performance of potentially hazardous tasks such as driving a car or operating machinery.

Patients should also be cautioned not to take concomitant medications, whether prescription or over-the-counter drugs such as cold, hay fever or weight-reducing preparations, without the advice of a physician. They should be advised not to consume excessive amounts of caffeine in any form. Likewise, they should inform other physicians, and their dentist, about their use of *Parnate*.

WARNINGS

HYPERTENSIVE CRISES: The most important reaction associated with Parnate (tranylcypromine sulfate) is the occurrence of hypertensive crises which have sometimes been fatal.

These crises are characterized by some or all of the following symptoms: occipital headache which may radiate frontally, palpitation, neck stiffness or soreness, nausea or vomiting, sweating (sometimes with fever and sometimes with cold, clammy skin) and photophobia. Either tachycardia or bradycardia may be present, and associated constricting chest pain and dilated pupils may occur. **Intracranial bleeding, sometimes fatal in outcome, has been reported in association with the paradoxical increase in blood pressure.**

In all patients taking *Parnate* blood pressure should be followed closely to detect evidence of any pressor response. It is emphasized that full reliance should not be placed on blood pressure readings, but that the patient should also be observed frequently.

Therapy should be discontinued immediately upon the occurrence of palpitation or frequent headaches during *Parnate* therapy. These signs may be prodromal of a hypertensive crisis.

**Important:
Recommended treatment in
hypertensive crises**

If a hypertensive crisis occurs, Parnate (tranylcypromine sulfate) should be discontinued and therapy to lower blood pressure should be instituted immediately. Headache tends to abate as blood pressure is lowered. On the basis of present evidence, phentolamine (available as Regitine®*) is recommended. (The dosage reported for phentolamine is 5 mg I.V.) Care should be taken to administer this drug slowly in order to avoid producing an excessive hypotensive effect. Fever should be managed by means of external cooling. Other symptomatic and supportive measures may be desirable in particular cases. Do not use parenteral reserpine.

PRECAUTIONS

Hypotension

Hypotension has been observed during Parnate (tranylcypromine sulfate) therapy. Symptoms of postural hypotension are seen most commonly but not exclusively in patients with pre-existent hypertension; blood pressure usually returns rapidly to pretreatment levels upon discontinuation of the drug. At doses above 30 mg daily, postural hypotension is a major side effect and may result in syncope. Dosage increases should be made more gradually in patients showing a tendency toward hypotension at the beginning of therapy. Postural hypotension may be relieved by having the patient lie down until blood pressure returns to normal.

Also, when *Parnate* is combined with those phenothiazine derivatives or other compounds known to cause hypotension, the possibility of additive hypotensive effects should be considered.

OTHER PRECAUTIONS

There have been reports of drug dependency in patients using doses of tranylcypromine significantly in excess of the therapeutic range. Some of these patients had a history of previous substance abuse. The following withdrawal symptoms have been reported: restlessness, anxiety, depression, confusion, hallucinations, headache, weakness and diarrhea.

Drugs which lower the seizure threshold, including MAO inhibitors, should not be used with Amipaque®†. As with other MAO inhibitors, Parnate (tranylcypromine sulfate) should be discontinued at least 48 hours before myelography and should not be resumed for at least 24 hours post-procedure.

In depressed patients, the possibility of suicide should always be considered and adequate precautions taken. Exclusive reliance on drug therapy to prevent suicidal attempts is unwarranted, as there may be a delay in the onset of therapeutic effect or an increase in anxiety and agitation. Also, some patients fail to respond to drug therapy or may respond only temporarily.

MAO inhibitors may have the capacity to suppress anginal pain that would otherwise serve as a warning of myocardial ischemia.

The usual precautions should be observed in patients with impaired renal function since there is a possibility of cumulative effects in such patients.

Older patients may suffer more morbidity than younger patients during and following an episode of hypertension or malignant hyperthermia. Older patients have less compensatory reserve to cope with any serious adverse reaction. Therefore, *Parnate* should be used with caution in the elderly population.

Although excretion of *Parnate* is rapid, inhibition of MAO may persist up to 10 days following discontinuation.

Because the influence of *Parnate* on the convulsive threshold is variable in animal experiments, suitable precautions should be taken if epileptic patients are treated.

Some MAO inhibitors have contributed to hypoglycemic episodes in diabetic patients receiving insulin or oral hypoglycemic agents. Therefore, *Parnate* should be used with caution in diabetics using these drugs.

Parnate may aggravate coexisting symptoms in depression, such as anxiety and agitation.

Use Parnate (tranylcypromine sulfate) with caution in hyperthyroid patients because of their increased sensitivity to pressor amines.

Parnate should be administered with caution to patients receiving Antabuse®‡. In a single study, rats given high intraperitoneal doses of *d* or *l* isomers of tranylcypromine sulfate plus disulfiram experienced severe toxicity including convulsions and death. Additional studies in rats given high oral doses of racemic tranylcypromine sulfate (*Parnate*) and disulfiram produced no adverse interaction.

ADVERSE REACTIONS

Overstimulation which may include increased anxiety, agitation and manic symptoms is usually evidence of excessive therapeutic action. Dosage should be reduced, or a phenothiazine tranquilizer should be administered concomitantly.

Patients may experience restlessness or insomnia; may notice some weakness, drowsiness, episodes of dizziness or dry mouth; or may report nausea, diarrhea, abdominal pain or constipation. Most of these effects can be relieved by lowering the dosage or by giving suitable concomitant medication.

Tachycardia, significant anorexia, edema, palpitation, blurred vision, chills and impotence have each been reported.

Headaches without blood pressure elevation have occurred.

Rare instances of hepatitis and skin rash have been reported.

Impaired water excretion compatible with the syndrome of inappropriate secretion of antidiuretic hormone (SIADH) has been reported.

Tinnitus, muscle spasm, tremors, myoclonic jerks, numbness, paresthesia, urinary retention and retarded ejaculation have been reported.

Hematologic disorders including anemia, leukopenia, agranulocytosis and thrombocytopenia have been reported.

Post-Introduction Reports

The following are spontaneously reported adverse events temporally associated with *Parnate* therapy. No clear relationship between *Parnate* and these events has been established. Localized scleroderma, flare-up of cystic acne, ataxia, confusion, disorientation, memory loss, urinary frequency, urinary incontinence, urticaria, fissuring in corner of mouth, akinesia.

DOSAGE AND ADMINISTRATION

Dosage should be adjusted to the requirements of the individual patient. Improvement should be seen within 48 hours to 3 weeks after starting therapy.

The usual effective dosage is 30 mg per day, usually given in divided doses. If there are no signs of improvement after a reasonable period (up to 2 weeks), then the dosage may be increased in 10 mg per day increments at intervals of 1 to 3 weeks; the dosage range may be extended to a maximum of 60 mg per day from the usual 30 mg per day.

OVERDOSAGE

SYMPTOMS: The characteristic symptoms that may be caused by overdosage are usually those described above. However, an intensification of these symptoms and sometimes severe additional manifestations may be seen, depending on the degree of overdosage and on individual susceptibility. Some patients exhibit insomnia, restlessness and anxiety, progressing in severe cases to agitation, mental confusion and incoherence. Hypotension, dizziness, weakness and drowsiness may occur, progressing in severe cases to extreme dizziness and shock. A few patients have displayed hypertension with severe headache and other symptoms. Rare instances have been reported in which hypertension was accompanied by twitching or myoclonic fibrillation of skeletal muscles with hyperpyrexia, sometimes progressing to generalized rigidity and coma.

TREATMENT: Gastric lavage is helpful if performed early. Treatment should normally consist of general supportive measures, close observation of vital signs and steps to counteract specific symptoms as they occur, since MAO inhibition may persist. The management of hypertensive crises is described under WARNINGS in the HYPERTENSIVE CRISES section.

External cooling is recommended if hyperpyrexia occurs. Barbiturates have been reported to help relieve myoclonic reactions, but frequency of administration should be controlled carefully because Parnate (tranylcypromine sulfate) may prolong barbiturate activity. When hypotension requires treatment, the standard measures for managing circulatory shock should be initiated. If pressor agents are used, the rate of infusion should be regulated by careful observation of the patient because an exaggerated pressor response sometimes occurs in the presence of MAO inhibition. Remember that the toxic effect of *Parnate* may be delayed or prolonged following the last dose of the drug. Therefore, the patient should be closely observed for at least a week. It is not known if tranylcypromine is dialyzable.

HOW SUPPLIED

Parnate is supplied as round, rose-red, film-coated tablets imprinted with the product name PARNATE and SKF and contains tranylcypromine sulfate equivalent to 10 mg of tranylcypromine, in bottles of 100 with a desiccant.

10 mg 100's: NDC 0007-4471-20

Store between 15° and 30°C (59° and 86°F).

---

*phentolamine mesylate USP, CibaGeneva.
†metrizamide, Sanofi Winthrop Pharmaceuticals.
‡disulfiram, Wyeth-Ayerst Laboratories.
PT:L64

Shown in Product Identification Guide, page 337

PAXIL® ℞

[packs 'ill]
**brand of
paroxetine
hydrochloride
tablets and oral suspension**

DESCRIPTION

Paxil (paroxetine hydrochloride) is an orally administered antidepressant with a chemical structure unrelated to other selective serotonin reuptake inhibitors or to tricyclic, tetracyclic or other available antidepressant agents. It is the hydrochloride salt of a phenylpiperidine compound identified chemically as (-)-*trans*-4*R*-(4'-fluorophenyl)-3*S*-[(3',4'-methylenedioxyphenoxy) methyl] piperidine hydrochloride hemihydrate and has the empirical formula of $C_{19}H_{20}FNO_3 \cdot HCl \cdot 1/2H_2O$. The molecular weight is 374.8 (329.4 as free base). The structural formula is:

paroxetine hydrochloride

Paroxetine hydrochloride is an odorless, off-white powder, having a melting point range of 120° to 138° C and a solubility of 5.4 mg/mL in water.

Tablets

Each film-coated tablet contains paroxetine hydrochloride equivalent to paroxetine as follows: 10 mg-yellow; 20 mg-pink (scored); 30 mg-blue, 40 mg-green. Inactive ingredients consist of dibasic calcium phosphate dihydrate, hydroxypropyl methylcellulose, magnesium stearate, polyethylene glycols, polysorbate 80, sodium starch glycolate, titanium dioxide and one or more of the following: D&C Red No. 30, D&C Yellow No. 10, FD&C Blue No. 2, FD&C Yellow No. 6.

Suspension for Oral Administration
Each 5 mL of orange-colored, orange-flavored liquid contains paroxetine hydrochloride equivalent to paroxetine, 10 mg. Inactive ingredients consist of polacrilin potassium, microcrystalline cellulose, propylene glycol, glycerin, sorbitol, methyl paraben, propyl paraben, sodium citrate dihydrate, citric acid anhydrate, sodium saccharin, flavorings, FD&C Yellow No. 6 and simethicone emulsion, USP.

CLINICAL PHARMACOLOGY

Pharmacodynamics
The antidepressant action of paroxetine and its efficacy in the treatment of social anxiety disorder, obsessive compulsive disorder (OCD) and panic disorder (PD) is presumed to be linked to potentiation of serotonergic activity in the central nervous system resulting from inhibition of neuronal reuptake of serotonin (5-hydroxy-tryptamine, 5-HT). Studies at clinically relevant doses in humans have demonstrated that paroxetine blocks the uptake of serotonin into human platelets. *In vitro* studies in animals also suggest that paroxetine is a potent and highly selective inhibitor of neuronal serotonin reuptake and has only very weak effects on norepinephrine and dopamine neuronal reuptake. *In vitro* radioligand binding studies indicate that paroxetine has little affinity for muscarinic, alpha$_1$-, alpha$_2$-, beta-adrenergic-, dopamine (D_2)-, 5-HT_1-, 5-HT_2- and histamine (H_1)-receptors; antagonism of muscarinic, histaminergic and alpha$_1$-adrenergic receptors has been associated with various anticholinergic, sedative and cardiovascular effects for other psychotropic drugs.
Because the relative potencies of paroxetine's major metabolites are at most 1/50 of the parent compound, they are essentially inactive.

Pharmacokinetics
Paroxetine is equally bioavailable from oral suspension and tablet.
Paroxetine hydrochloride is completely absorbed after oral dosing of a solution of the hydrochloride salt. In a study in which normal male subjects (n=15) received 30 mg tablets daily for 30 days, steady-state paroxetine concentrations were achieved by approximately 10 days for most subjects, although it may take substantially longer in an occasional patient. At steady state, mean values of C_{max}, T_{max}, C_{min} and $T_{1/2}$ were 61.7 ng/mL (CV 45%), 5.2 hr. (CV 10%), 30.7 ng/mL (CV 67%) and 21.0 hr. (CV 32%), respectively. The steady-state C_{max} and C_{min} values were about 6 and 14 times what would be predicted from single-dose studies. Steady-state drug exposure based on AUC_{0-24} was about 8 times greater than would have been predicted from single-dose data in these subjects. The excess accumulation is a consequence of the fact that one of the enzymes that metabolizes paroxetine is readily saturable.
In steady-state dose proportionality studies involving elderly and nonelderly patients, at doses of 20 to 40 mg daily for the elderly and 20 to 50 mg daily for the nonelderly, some nonlinearity was observed in both populations, again reflecting a saturable metabolic pathway. In comparison to C_{min} values after 20 mg daily, values after 40 mg daily were only about 2 to 3 times greater than doubled.
The effects of food on the bioavailability of paroxetine were studied in subjects administered a single dose with and without food. AUC was only slightly increased (6%) when drug was administered with food but the C_{max} was 29% greater, while the time to reach peak plasma concentration decreased from 6.4 hours post-dosing to 4.9 hours.
Paroxetine is extensively metabolized after oral administration. The principal metabolites are polar and conjugated products of oxidation and methylation, which are readily cleared. Conjugates with glucuronic acid and sulfate predominate, and major metabolites have been isolated and identified. Data indicate that the metabolites have no more than 1/50 the potency of the parent compound at inhibiting serotonin uptake. The metabolism of paroxetine is accomplished in part by cytochrome $P_{450}IID_6$. Saturation of this enzyme at clinical doses appears to account for the nonlinearity of paroxetine kinetics with increasing dose and increasing duration of treatment. The role of this enzyme in paroxetine metabolism also suggests potential drug-drug interactions (see PRECAUTIONS).
Approximately 64% of a 30 mg oral solution dose of paroxetine was excreted in the urine with 2% as the parent compound and 62% as metabolites over a 10-day post-dosing period. About 36% was excreted in the feces (probably via the bile), mostly as metabolites and less than 1% as the parent compound over the 10-day post-dosing period.
Distribution: Paroxetine distributes throughout the body, including the CNS, with only 1% remaining in the plasma.
Protein Binding: Approximately 95% and 93% of paroxetine is bound to plasma protein at 100 ng/mL and 400 ng/mL, respectively. Under clinical conditions, paroxetine concentrations would normally be less than 400 ng/mL. Paroxetine does not alter the *in vitro* protein binding of phenytoin or warfarin.
Renal and Liver Disease: Increased plasma concentrations of paroxetine occur in subjects with renal and hepatic impairment. The mean plasma concentrations in patients with creatinine clearance below 30 mL/min. was approximately 4 times greater than seen in normal volunteers. Patients with creatinine clearance of 30 to 60 mL/min. and patients with hepatic functional impairment had about a 2-fold increase in plasma concentrations (AUC, C_{max}).
The initial dosage should therefore be reduced in patients with severe renal or hepatic impairment, and upward titration, if necessary, should be at increased intervals (see DOSAGE AND ADMINISTRATION).
Elderly Patients: In a multiple-dose study in the elderly at daily paroxetine doses of 20, 30 and 40 mg, C_{min} concentrations were about 70% to 80% greater than the respective C_{min} concentrations in nonelderly subjects. Therefore the initial dosage in the elderly should be reduced (see DOSAGE AND ADMINISTRATION).

Clinical Trials

Depression
The efficacy of Paxil (paroxetine hydrochloride) as a treatment for depression has been established in 6 placebo-controlled studies of patients with depression (ages 18 to 73). In these studies *Paxil* was shown to be significantly more effective than placebo in treating depression by at least 2 of the following measures: Hamilton Depression Rating Scale (HDRS), the Hamilton depressed mood item, and the Clinical Global Impression (CGI)-Severity of Illness. Paxil (paroxetine hydrochloride) was significantly better than placebo in improvement of the HDRS sub-factor scores, including the depressed mood item, sleep disturbance factor and anxiety factor.
A study of depressed outpatients who had responded to *Paxil* (HDRS total score <8) during an initial 8-week open-treatment phase and were then randomized to continuation on *Paxil* or placebo for 1 year demonstrated a significantly lower relapse rate for patients taking *Paxil* (15%) compared to those on placebo (39%). Effectiveness was similar for male and female patients.

Obsessive Compulsive Disorder
The effectiveness of *Paxil* in the treatment of obsessive compulsive disorder (OCD) was demonstrated in two 12-week multicenter placebo-controlled studies of adult outpatients (Studies 1 and 2). Patients in all studies had moderate to severe OCD (DSM-IIIR) with mean baseline ratings on the Yale Brown Obsessive Compulsive Scale (YBOCS) total score ranging from 23 to 26. Study 1, a dose-range finding study where patients were treated with fixed doses of 20, 40 or 60 mg of paroxetine/day demonstrated that daily doses of paroxetine 40 and 60 mg are effective in the treatment of OCD. Patients receiving doses of 40 and 60 mg paroxetine experienced a mean reduction of approximately 6 and 7 points, respectively, on the YBOCS total score which was significantly greater than the approximate 4 point reduction at 20 mg and a 3 point reduction in the placebo-treated patients. Study 2 was a flexible dose study comparing paroxetine (20 to 60 mg daily) with clomipramine (25 to 250 mg daily). In this study, patients receiving paroxetine experienced a mean reduction of approximately 7 points on the YBOCS total score which was significantly greater than the mean reduction of approximately 4 points in placebo-treated patients.
The following table provides the outcome classification by treatment group on Global Improvement items of the Clinical Global Impressions (CGI) scale for Study 1.

Outcome Classification (%) on CGI-Global Improvement Item for Completers in Study 1

Outcome Classification	Placebo (n=74)	*Paxil* 20 mg (n=75)	*Paxil* 40 mg (n=66)	*Paxil* 60 mg (n=66)
Worse	14%	7%	7%	3%
No Change	44%	35%	22%	19%
Minimally Improved	24%	33%	29%	34%
Much Improved	11%	18%	22%	24%
Very Much Improved	7%	7%	20%	20%

Subgroup analyses did not indicate that there were any differences in treatment outcomes as a function of age or gender.
The long-term maintenance effects of *Paxil* in OCD were demonstrated in a long-term extension to Study 1. Patients who were responders on paroxetine during the 3-month double-blind phase and a 6-month extension on open-label paroxetine (20 to 60 mg/day) were randomized to either paroxetine or placebo in a 6-month double-blind relapse prevention phase. Patients randomized to paroxetine were significantly less likely to relapse than comparably treated patients who were randomized to placebo.

Panic Disorder
The effectiveness of Paxil (paroxetine hydrochloride) in the treatment of panic disorder was demonstrated in three 10- to 12-week multicenter, placebo-controlled studies of adult outpatients (Studies 1–3). Patients in all studies had panic disorder (DSM-IIIR), with or without agoraphobia. In these studies, *Paxil* was shown to be significantly more effective than placebo in treating panic disorder by at least 2 out of 3 measures of panic attack frequency and on the Clinical Global Impression Severity of Illness score.
Study 1 was a 10-week dose-range finding study; patients were treated with fixed paroxetine doses of 10, 20, or 40 mg/day or placebo. A significant difference from placebo was observed only for the 40 mg/day group. At endpoint, 76% of patients receiving paroxetine 40 mg/day were free of panic attacks, compared to 44% of placebo-treated patients.
Study 2 was a 12-week flexible-dose study comparing paroxetine (10 to 60 mg daily) and placebo. At endpoint, 51% of paroxetine patients were free of panic attacks compared to 32% of placebo-treated patients.
Study 3 was a 12-week flexible-dose study comparing paroxetine (10 to 60 mg daily) to placebo in patients concurrently receiving standardized cognitive behavioral therapy. At endpoint, 33% of the paroxetine-treated patients showed a reduction to 0 or 1 panic attacks compared to 14% of placebo patients.
In both Studies 2 and 3, the mean paroxetine dose for completers at endpoint was approximately 40 mg/day of paroxetine.
Long-term maintenance effects of *Paxil* in panic disorder were demonstrated in an extension to Study 1. Patients who were responders during the 10-week double-blind phase and during a 3-month double-blind extension phase were randomized to either paroxetine (10, 20, or 40 mg/day) or placebo in a 3-month double-blind relapse prevention phase. Patients randomized to paroxetine were significantly less likely to relapse than comparably treated patients who were randomized to placebo.
Subgroup analyses did not indicate that there were any differences in treatment outcomes as a function of age or gender.

Social Anxiety Disorder
The effectiveness of *Paxil* in the treatment of social anxiety disorder was demonstrated in three 12-week, multicenter, placebo-controlled studies (Studies 1–3) of adult outpatients with social anxiety disorder (DSM-IV). In these studies, the effectiveness of *Paxil* compared to placebo was evaluated on the basis of (1) the proportion of responders, as defined by a Clinical Global Impressions (CGI) Improvement score of 1 (very much improved) or 2 (much improved), and (2) change from baseline in the Liebowitz Social Anxiety Scale (LSAS).
Studies 1 and 2 were flexible-dose studies comparing paroxetine (20 to 50 mg daily) and placebo. Paroxetine demonstrated statistically significant superiority over placebo on both the CGI Improvement responder criterion and the Liebowitz Social Anxiety Scale (LSAS). In Study 1, for patients who completed to week 12, 69% of paroxetine-treated patients compared to 29% of placebo-treated patients were CGI Improvement responders. In Study 2, CGI Improvement responders were 77% and 42% for the paroxetine- and placebo-treated patients, respectively.
Study 3 was a 12-week study comparing fixed paroxetine doses of 20, 40 or 60 mg/day with placebo. Paroxetine 20 mg was demonstrated to be significantly superior to placebo on both the LSAS Total Score and the CGI Improvement responder criterion; there were trends for superiority over placebo for the 40 and 60 mg/day dose groups. There was no indication in this study of any additional benefit for doses higher than 20 mg/day.
Subgroup analyses did not indicate differences in treatment outcomes as a function of age, race, or gender.

INDICATIONS AND USAGE

Depression
Paxil (paroxetine hydrochloride) is indicated for the treatment of depression.
The efficacy of *Paxil* in the treatment of a major depressive episode was established in 6-week controlled trials of outpatients whose diagnoses corresponded most closely to the DSM-III category of major depressive disorder (see CLINICAL PHARMACOLOGY). A major depressive episode implies a prominent and relatively persistent depressed or dysphoric mood that usually interferes with daily functioning (nearly every day for at least 2 weeks); it should include at least 4 of the following 8 symptoms: change in appetite, change in sleep, psychomotor agitation or retardation, loss of interest in usual activities or decrease in sexual drive, increased fatigue, feelings of guilt or worthlessness, slowed thinking or impaired concentration, and a suicide attempt or suicidal ideation.
The antidepressant action of *Paxil* in hospitalized depressed patients has not been adequately studied.
The efficacy of *Paxil* in maintaining an antidepressant response for up to 1 year was demonstrated in a placebo-controlled trial (see CLINICAL PHARMACOLOGY). Nevertheless, the physician who elects to use *Paxil* for extended periods should periodically re-evaluate the long-term usefulness of the drug for the individual patient.

Obsessive Compulsive Disorder
Paxil is indicated for the treatment of obsessions and compulsions in patients with obsessive compulsive disorder (OCD) as defined in the DSM-IV. The obsessions or compulsions cause marked distress, are time-consuming, or significantly interfere with social or occupational functioning.
The efficacy of *Paxil* was established in two 12-week trials with obsessive compulsive outpatients whose diagnoses corresponded most closely to the DSM-IIIR category of obsessive compulsive disorder (see CLINICAL PHARMACOLOGY—Clinical Trials).
Obsessive compulsive disorder is characterized by recurrent and persistent ideas, thoughts, impulses or images (obsessions) that are ego-dystonic and/or repetitive, purposeful and intentional behaviors (compulsions) that are recognized by the person as excessive or unreasonable.
Long-term maintenance of efficacy was demonstrated in a 6-month relapse prevention trial. In this trial, patients as-

Continued on next page

Information on the SmithKline Beecham Pharmaceuticals products appearing here is based on the labeling in effect on June 15, 2000. Further information on these and other products may be obtained from the Medical Department, SmithKline Beecham Pharmaceuticals, One Franklin Plaza, Philadelphia, PA 19101.

Paxil—Cont.

signed to paroxetine showed a lower relapse rate compared to patients on placebo (see CLINICAL PHARMACOLOGY). Nevertheless, the physician who elects to use *Paxil* for extended periods should periodically re-evaluate the long-term usefulness of the drug for the individual patient (see DOSAGE AND ADMINISTRATION).

Panic Disorder

Paxil is indicated for the treatment of panic disorder, with or without agoraphobia, as defined in DSM-IV. Panic disorder is characterized by the occurrence of unexpected panic attacks and associated concern about having additional attacks, worry about the implications or consequences of the attacks, and/or a significant change in behavior related to the attacks.

The efficacy of Paxil (paroxetine hydrochloride) was established in three 10- to 12-week trials in panic disorder patients whose diagnoses corresponded to the DSM-IIIR category of panic disorder (see CLINICAL PHARMACOLOGY—Clinical Trials).

Panic disorder (DSM-IV) is characterized by recurrent unexpected panic attacks, i.e., a discrete period of intense fear or discomfort in which four (or more) of the following symptoms develop abruptly and reach a peak within 10 minutes: (1) palpitations, pounding heart, or accelerated heart rate; (2) sweating; (3) trembling or shaking; (4) sensations of shortness of breath or smothering; (5) feeling of choking; (6) chest pain or discomfort; (7) nausea or abdominal distress; (8) feeling dizzy, unsteady, lightheaded, or faint; (9) derealization (feelings of unreality) or depersonalization (being detached from oneself); (10) fear of losing control; (11) fear of dying; (12) paresthesias (numbness or tingling sensations); (13) chills or hot flushes.

Long-term maintenance of efficacy was demonstrated in a 3-month relapse prevention trial. In this trial, patients with panic disorder assigned to paroxetine demonstrated a lower relapse rate compared to patients on placebo (see CLINICAL PHARMACOLOGY). Nevertheless, the physician who prescribes *Paxil* for extended periods should periodically re-evaluate the long-term usefulness of the drug for the individual patient.

Social Anxiety Disorder

Paxil is indicated for the treatment of social anxiety disorder, also known as social phobia, as defined in DSM-IV (300.23). Social anxiety disorder is characterized by a marked and persistent fear of one or more social or performance situations in which the person is exposed to unfamiliar people or to possible scrutiny by others. Exposure to the feared situation almost invariably provokes anxiety, which may approach the intensity of a panic attack. The feared situations are avoided or endured with intense anxiety or distress. The avoidance, anxious anticipation, or distress in the feared situation(s) interferes significantly with the person's normal routine, occupational or academic functioning, or social activities or relationships, or there is marked distress about having the phobias. Lesser degrees of performance anxiety or shyness generally do not require psychopharmacological treatment.

The efficacy of Paxil (paroxetine hydrochloride) was established in three 12-week trials in adult patients with social anxiety disorder (DSM-IV). *Paxil* has not been studied in children or adolescents with social phobia (see CLINICAL PHARMACOLOGY—Clinical Trials).

The effectiveness of *Paxil* in long-term treatment of social anxiety disorder, i.e., for more than 12 weeks, has not been systematically evaluated in adequate and well-controlled trials. Therefore, the physician who elects to prescribe *Paxil* for extended periods should periodically re-evaluate the long-term usefulness of the drug for the individual patient (see DOSAGE AND ADMINISTRATION).

CONTRAINDICATIONS

Concomitant use in patients taking monoamine oxidase inhibitors (MAOIs) is contraindicated (see WARNINGS and PRECAUTIONS).

Paxil is contraindicated in patients with a hypersensitivity to paroxetine or any of the inactive ingredients in *Paxil*.

WARNINGS

Potential for Interaction with Monoamine Oxidase Inhibitors

In patients receiving another serotonin reuptake inhibitor drug in combination with a monoamine oxidase inhibitor (MAOI), there have been reports of serious, sometimes fatal, reactions including hyperthermia, rigidity, myoclonus, autonomic instability with possible rapid fluctuations of vital signs, and mental status changes that include extreme agitation progressing to delirium and coma. These reactions have also been reported in patients who have recently discontinued that drug and have been started on a MAOI. Some cases presented with features resembling neuroleptic malignant syndrome. While there are no human data showing such an interaction with *Paxil*, limited animal data on the effects of combined use of paroxetine and MAOIs suggest that these drugs may act synergistically to elevate blood pressure and evoke behavioral excitation. Therefore, it is recommended that Paxil (paroxetine hydrochloride) not be used in combination with a MAOI, or within 14 days of discontinuing treatment with a MAOI. At least 2 weeks should be allowed after stopping *Paxil* before starting a MAOI.

PRECAUTIONS

General

Activation of Mania/Hypomania: During premarketing testing, hypomania or mania occurred in approximately 1.0% of *Paxil*-treated unipolar patients compared to 1.1% of active-control and 0.3% of placebo-treated unipolar patients. In a subset of patients classified as bipolar, the rate of manic episodes was 2.2% for *Paxil* and 11.6% for the combined active-control groups. As with all antidepressants, *Paxil* should be used cautiously in patients with a history of mania.

Seizures: During premarketing testing, seizures occurred in 0.1% of *Paxil*-treated patients, a rate similar to that associated with other antidepressants. *Paxil* should be used cautiously in patients with a history of seizures. It should be discontinued in any patient who develops seizures.

Suicide: The possibility of a suicide attempt is inherent in depression and may persist until significant remission occurs. Close supervision of high-risk patients should accompany initial drug therapy. Prescriptions for *Paxil* should be written for the smallest quantity of tablets consistent with good patient management, in order to reduce the risk of overdose.

Hyponatremia: Several cases of hyponatremia have been reported. The hyponatremia appeared to be reversible when *Paxil* was discontinued. The majority of these occurrences have been in elderly individuals, some in patients taking diuretics or who were otherwise volume depleted.

Abnormal Bleeding: There have been several reports of abnormal bleeding (mostly ecchymosis and purpura) associated with paroxetine treatment, including a report of impaired platelet aggregation. While a causal relationship to paroxetine is unclear, impaired platelet aggregation may result from platelet serotonin depletion and contribute to such occurrences.

Use in Patients with Concomitant Illness: Clinical experience with *Paxil* in patients with certain concomitant systemic illness is limited. Caution is advisable in using *Paxil* in patients with diseases or conditions that could affect metabolism or hemodynamic responses.

Paxil has not been evaluated or used to any appreciable extent in patients with a recent history of myocardial infarction or unstable heart disease. Patients with these diagnoses were excluded from clinical studies during the product's premarket testing. Evaluation of electrocardiograms of 682 patients who received *Paxil* in double-blind, placebo-controlled trials, however, did not indicate that *Paxil* is associated with the development of significant ECG abnormalities. Similarly, Paxil (paroxetine hydrochloride) does not cause any clinically important changes in heart rate or blood pressure.

Increased plasma concentrations of paroxetine occur in patients with severe renal impairment (creatinine clearance <30 mL/min.) or severe hepatic impairment. A lower starting dose should be used in such patients (see DOSAGE AND ADMINISTRATION).

Information for Patients

Physicians are advised to discuss the following issues with patients for whom they prescribe *Paxil:*

Interference with Cognitive and Motor Performance: Any psychoactive drug may impair judgment, thinking or motor skills. Although in controlled studies *Paxil* has not been shown to impair psychomotor performance, patients should be cautioned about operating hazardous machinery, including automobiles, until they are reasonably certain that *Paxil* therapy does not affect their ability to engage in such activities.

Completing Course of Therapy: While patients may notice improvement with *Paxil* therapy in 1 to 4 weeks, they should be advised to continue therapy as directed.

Concomitant Medication: Patients should be advised to inform their physician if they are taking, or plan to take, any prescription or over-the-counter drugs, since there is a potential for interactions.

Alcohol: Although *Paxil* has not been shown to increase the impairment of mental and motor skills caused by alcohol, patients should be advised to avoid alcohol while taking *Paxil*.

Pregnancy: Patients should be advised to notify their physician if they become pregnant or intend to become pregnant during therapy.

Nursing: Patients should be advised to notify their physician if they are breast-feeding an infant (see PRECAUTIONS—Nursing Mothers).

Laboratory Tests

There are no specific laboratory tests recommended.

Drug Interactions

Tryptophan: As with other serotonin reuptake inhibitors, an interaction between paroxetine and tryptophan may occur when they are co-administered. Adverse experiences, consisting primarily of headache, nausea, sweating and dizziness, have been reported when tryptophan was administered to patients taking Paxil (paroxetine hydrochloride). Consequently, concomitant use of *Paxil* with tryptophan is not recommended.

Monoamine Oxidase Inhibitors: See CONTRAINDICATIONS and WARNINGS.

Warfarin: Preliminary data suggest that there may be a pharmacodynamic interaction (that causes an increased bleeding diathesis in the face of unaltered prothrombin time) between paroxetine and warfarin. Since there is little clinical experience, the concomitant administration of *Paxil* and warfarin should be undertaken with caution.

Sumatriptan: There have been rare postmarketing reports describing patients with weakness, hyperreflexia, and incoordination following the use of a selective serotonin reuptake inhibitor (SSRI) and sumatriptan. If concomitant treatment with sumatriptan and an SSRI (e.g., fluoxetine, fluvoxamine, paroxetine, sertraline) is clinically warranted, appropriate observation of the patient is advised.

Drugs Affecting Hepatic Metabolism: The metabolism and pharmacokinetics of paroxetine may be affected by the induction or inhibition of drug-metabolizing enzymes.

Cimetidine–Cimetidine inhibits many cytochrome P_{450} (oxidative) enzymes. In a study where *Paxil* (30 mg q.d.) was dosed orally for 4 weeks, steady-state plasma concentrations of paroxetine were increased by approximately 50% during co-administration with oral cimetidine (300 mg t.i.d.) for the final week. Therefore, when these drugs are administered concurrently, dosage adjustment of Paxil (paroxetine hydrochloride) after the 20 mg starting dose should be guided by clinical effect. The effect of paroxetine on cimetidine's pharmacokinetics was not studied.

Phenobarbital–Phenobarbital induces many cytochrome P_{450} (oxidative) enzymes. When a single oral 30 mg dose of *Paxil* was administered at phenobarbital steady state (100 mg q.d. for 14 days), paroxetine AUC and $T_{1/2}$ were reduced (by an average of 25% and 38%, respectively) compared to paroxetine administered alone. The effect of paroxetine on phenobarbital pharmacokinetics was not studied. Since *Paxil* exhibits nonlinear pharmacokinetics, the results of this study may not address the case where the 2 drugs are both being chronically dosed. No initial *Paxil* dosage adjustment is considered necessary when co-administered with phenobarbital; any subsequent adjustment should be guided by clinical effect.

Phenytoin—When a single oral 30 mg dose of *Paxil* was administered at phenytoin steady state (300 mg q.d. for 14 days), paroxetine AUC and $T_{1/2}$ were reduced (by an average of 50% and 35%, respectively) compared to *Paxil* administered alone. In a separate study, when a single oral 300 mg dose of phenytoin was administered at paroxetine steady state (30 mg q.d. for 14 days), phenytoin AUC was slightly reduced (12% on average) compared to phenytoin administered alone. Since both drugs exhibit nonlinear pharmacokinetics, the above studies may not address the case where the two drugs are both being chronically dosed. No initial dosage adjustments are considered necessary when these drugs are co-administered; any subsequent adjustments should be guided by clinical effect (see ADVERSE REACTIONS—Postmarketing Reports).

Drugs Metabolized by Cytochrome $P_{450}IID_6$: Many drugs, including most antidepressants (paroxetine, other SSRIs and many tricyclics), are metabolized by the cytochrome P_{450} isozyme $P_{450}IID_6$. Like other agents that are metabolized by $P_{450}IID_6$, paroxetine may significantly inhibit the activity of this isozyme. In most patients (>90%), this $P_{450}IID_6$ isozyme is saturated early during *Paxil* dosing. In one study, daily dosing of *Paxil* (20 mg q.d.) under steady-state conditions increased single dose desipramine (100 mg) C_{max}, AUC and $T_{1/2}$ by an average of approximately two-, five- and three-fold, respectively. Concomitant use of *Paxil* with other drugs metabolized by cytochrome $P_{450}IID_6$ has not been formally studied but may require lower doses than usually prescribed for either *Paxil* or the other drug.

Therefore, co-administration of *Paxil* with other drugs that are metabolized by this isozyme, including certain antidepressants (e.g., nortriptyline, amitriptyline, imipramine, desipramine and fluoxetine), phenothiazines (e.g., thioridazine) and Type 1C antiarrhythmics (e.g., propafenone, flecainide and encainide), or that inhibit this enzyme (e.g., quinidine), should be approached with caution.

At steady state, when the $P_{450}IID_6$ pathway is essentially saturated, paroxetine clearance is governed by alternative P_{450} isozymes which, unlike $P_{450}IID_6$, show no evidence of saturation (see PRECAUTIONS—Tricyclic Antidepressants).

Drugs Metabolized by Cytochrome $P_{450}IIIA_4$: An *in vivo* interaction study involving the co-administration under steady-state conditions of paroxetine and terfenadine, a substrate for cytochrome $P_{450}IIIA_4$, revealed no effect of paroxetine on terfenadine pharmacokinetics. In addition, *in vitro* studies have shown ketoconazole, a potent inhibitor of $P_{450}IIIA_4$ activity, to be at least 100 times more potent than paroxetine as an inhibitor of the metabolism of several substrates for this enzyme, including terfenadine, astemizole, cisapride, triazolam, and cyclosporin. Based on the assumption that the relationship between paroxetine's *in vitro* Ki and its lack of effect on terfenadine's *in vivo* clearance predicts its effect on other $IIIA_4$ substrates, paroxetine's extent of inhibition of $IIIA_4$ activity is not likely to be of clinical significance.

Tricyclic Antidepressants (TCA): Caution is indicated in the co-administration of tricyclic antidepressants (TCAs) with *Paxil*, because paroxetine may inhibit TCA metabolism. Plasma TCA concentrations may need to be monitored, and the dose of TCA may need to be reduced, if a TCA is co-administered with *Paxil* (see PRECAUTIONS—Drugs Metabolized by Cytochrome $P_{450}IID_6$).

Drugs Highly Bound to Plasma Protein: Because paroxetine is highly bound to plasma protein, administration of *Paxil* to a patient taking another drug that is highly protein bound may cause increased free concentrations of the other drug, potentially resulting in adverse events. Conversely, adverse effects could result from displacement of paroxetine by other highly bound drugs.

Alcohol: Although *Paxil* does not increase the impairment of mental and motor skills caused by alcohol, patients should be advised to avoid alcohol while taking Paxil (paroxetine hydrochloride).

Lithium: A multiple-dose study has shown that there is no pharmacokinetic interaction between *Paxil* and lithium carbonate. However, since there is little clinical experience, the concurrent administration of paroxetine and lithium should be undertaken with caution.

Digoxin: The steady-state pharmacokinetics of paroxetine was not altered when administered with digoxin at steady state. Mean digoxin AUC at steady state decreased by 15% in the presence of paroxetine. Since there is little clinical experience, the concurrent administration of paroxetine and digoxin should be undertaken with caution.

Diazepam: Under steady-state conditions, diazepam does not appear to affect paroxetine kinetics. The effects of paroxetine on diazepam were not evaluated.

Procyclidine: Daily oral dosing of *Paxil* (30 mg q.d.) increased steady-state AUC_{0-24}, C_{max} and C_{min} values of procyclidine (5 mg oral q.d.) by 35%, 37% and 67%, respectively, compared to procyclidine alone at steady state. If anticholinergic effects are seen, the dose of procyclidine should be reduced.

Beta-Blockers: In a study where propranolol (80 mg b.i.d.) was dosed orally for 18 days, the established steady-state plasma concentrations of propranolol were unaltered during co-administration with *Paxil* (30 mg q.d.) for the final 10 days. The effects of propranolol on paroxetine have not been evaluated (see ADVERSE REACTIONS—Postmarketing Reports).

Theophylline: Reports of elevated theophylline levels associated with *Paxil* treatment have been reported. While this interaction has not been formally studied, it is recommended that theophylline levels be monitored when these drugs are concurrently administered.

Electroconvulsive Therapy (ECT): There are no clinical studies of the combined use of ECT and *Paxil*.

Carcinogenesis, Mutagenesis, Impairment of Fertility

Carcinogenesis: Two-year carcinogenicity studies were conducted in rodents given paroxetine in the diet at 1, 5, and 25 mg/kg/day (mice) and 1, 5, and 20 mg/kg/day (rats). These doses are up to 2.4 (mouse) and 3.9 (rat) times the maximum recommended human dose (MRHD) for depression and social anxiety disorder on a mg/m^2 basis. Because the MRHD for depression is slightly less than that for OCD (50 mg vs. 60 mg), the doses used in these carcinogenicity studies were only 2.0 (mouse) and 3.2 (rat) times the MRHD for OCD. There was a significantly greater number of male rats in the high-dose group with reticulum cell sarcomas (1/100, 0/50, 0/50 and 4/50 for control, low-, middle- and high-dose groups, respectively) and a significantly increased linear trend across dose groups for the occurrence of lymphoreticular tumors in male rats. Female rats were not affected. Although there was a dose-related increase in the number of tumors in mice, there was no drug-related increase in the number of mice with tumors. The relevance of these findings to humans is unknown.

Mutagenesis: Paroxetine produced no genotoxic effects in a battery of 5 *in vitro* and 2 *in vivo* assays that included the following: bacterial mutation assay, mouse lymphoma mutation assay, unscheduled DNA synthesis assay, and tests for cytogenetic aberrations *in vivo* in mouse bone marrow and *in vitro* in human lymphocytes and in a dominant lethal test in rats.

Impairment of Fertility: A reduced pregnancy rate was found in reproduction studies in rats at a dose of paroxetine of 15 mg/kg/day which is 2.9 times the MRHD for depression and social anxiety disorder or 2.4 times the MRHD for OCD on a mg/m^2 basis. Irreversible lesions occurred in the reproductive tract of male rats after dosing in toxicity studies for 2 to 52 weeks. These lesions consisted of vacuolation of epididymal tubular epithelium at 50 mg/kg/day and atrophic changes in the seminiferous tubules of the testes with arrested spermatogenesis at 25 mg/kg/day (9.8 and 4.9 times the MRHD for depression and social anxiety disorder; 8.2 and 4.1 times the MRHD for OCD and PD on a mg/m^2 basis).

Pregnancy

Teratogenic Effects—Pregnancy Category C

Reproduction studies were performed at doses up to 50 mg/kg/day in rats and 6 mg/kg/day in rabbits administered during organogenesis. These doses are equivalent to 9.7 (rat) and 2.2 (rabbit) times the maximum recommended human dose (MRHD) for depression and social anxiety disorder (50 mg) and 8.1 (rat) and 1.9 (rabbit) times the MRHD for OCD, on a mg/m^2 basis. These studies have revealed no evidence of teratogenic effects. However, in rats, there was an increase in pup deaths during the first 4 days of lactation when dosing occurred during the last trimester of gestation and continued throughout lactation. This effect occurred at a dose of 1 mg/kg/day or 0.19 times (mg/m^2) the MRHD for depression and social anxiety disorder and at 0.16 times (mg/m^2) the MRHD for OCD. The no-effect dose for rat pup mortality was not determined. The cause of these deaths is not known. There are no adequate and well-controlled studies in pregnant women. Because animal reproduction studies are not always predictive of human response, this drug should be used during pregnancy only if the potential benefit justifies the potential risk to the fetus.

Labor and Delivery

The effect of paroxetine on labor and delivery in humans is unknown.

	Depression		OCD		Panic Disorder		Social Anxiety Disorder	
	Paxil	Placebo	*Paxil*	Placebo	*Paxil*	Placebo	*Paxil*	Placebo
CNS								
Somnolence	2.3%	0.7%	—		1.9%	0.3%	3.4%	0.3%
Insomnia	—	—	1.7%	0%	1.3%	0.3%	3.1%	0%
Agitation	1.1%	0.5%	—					
Tremor	1.1%	0.3%	—				1.7%	0%
Anxiety	—	—	—				1.1%	0%
Dizziness	—	—	1.5%	0%			1.9%	0%
Gastro-intestinal								
Constipation	—		1.1%	0%				
Nausea	3.2%	1.1%	1.9%	0%	3.2%	1.2%	4.0%	0.3%
Diarrhea	1.0%	0.3%	—					
Dry mouth	1.0%	0.3%	—					
Vomiting	1.0%	0.3%	—				1.0%	0%
Flatulence							1.0%	0.3%
Other								
Asthenia	1.6%	0.4%	1.9%	0.4%			2.5%	0.6%
Abnormal ejaculation[1]	1.6%	0%	2.1%	0%			4.9%	0.6%
Sweating	1.0%	0.3%	—				1.1%	0%
Impotence[1]	—		1.5%	0%				
Libido Decreased							1.0%	0%

Where numbers are not provided the incidence of the adverse events in Paxil (paroxetine hydrochloride) patients was not >1% or was not greater than or equal to two times the incidence of placebo.

1. Incidence corrected for gender.

Table 1. Treatment-Emergent Adverse Experience Incidence in Placebo-Controlled Clinical Trials for Depression[1]

Body System	Preferred Term	*Paxil* (n=421)	Placebo (n=421)
Body as a Whole	Headache	18%	17%
	Asthenia	15%	6%
Cardiovascular	Palpitation	3%	1%
	Vasodilation	3%	1%
Dermatologic	Sweating	11%	2%
	Rash	2%	1%
Gastrointestinal	Nausea	26%	9%
	Dry Mouth	18%	12%
	Constipation	14%	9%
	Diarrhea	12%	8%
	Decreased Appetite	6%	2%
	Flatulence	4%	2%
	Oropharynx Disorder[2]	2%	0%
	Dyspepsia	2%	1%
Musculoskeletal	Myopathy	2%	1%
	Myalgia	2%	1%
	Myasthenia	1%	0%
Nervous System	Somnolence	23%	9%
	Dizziness	13%	6%
	Insomnia	13%	6%
	Tremor	8%	2%
	Nervousness	5%	3%
	Anxiety	5%	3%
	Paresthesia	4%	2%
	Libido Decreased	3%	0%
	Drugged Feeling	2%	1%
	Confusion	1%	0%
Respiration	Yawn	4%	0%
Special Senses	Blurred Vision	4%	1%
	Taste Perversion	2%	0%
Urogenital System	Ejaculatory Disturbance[3,4]	13%	0%
	Other Male Genital Disorders[3,5]	10%	0%
	Urinary Frequency	3%	1%
	Urination Disorder[6]	3%	0%
	Female Genital Disorders[3,7]	2%	0%

1. Events reported by at least 1% of patients treated with Paxil (paroxetine hydrochloride) are included, except the following events which had an incidence on placebo ≥ *Paxil:* abdominal pain, agitation, back pain, chest pain, CNS stimulation, fever, increased appetite, myoclonus, pharyngitis, postural hypotension, respiratory disorder (includes mostly "cold symptoms" or "URI"), trauma and vomiting.
2. Includes mostly "lump in throat" and "tightness in throat."
3. Percentage corrected for gender.
4. Mostly "ejaculatory delay."
5. Includes "anorgasmia," "erectile difficulties," "delayed ejaculation/orgasm," and "sexual dysfunction," and "impotence."
6. Includes mostly "difficulty with micturition" and "urinary hesitancy."
7. Includes mostly "anorgasmia" and "difficulty reaching climax/orgasm."

Nursing Mothers

Like many other drugs, paroxetine is secreted in human milk, and caution should be exercised when Paxil (paroxetine hydrochloride) is administered to a nursing woman.

Pediatric Use

Safety and effectiveness in the pediatric population have not been established.

Geriatric Use

In worldwide premarketing *Paxil* clinical trials, 17% of *Paxil*-treated patients (approximately 700) were 65 years of age or older. Pharmacokinetic studies revealed a decreased clearance in the elderly, and a lower starting dose is recommended; there were, however, no overall differences in the adverse event profile between elderly and younger patients, and effectiveness was similar in younger and older patients (see CLINICAL PHARMACOLOGY and DOSAGE AND ADMINISTRATION).

Continued on next page

Information on the SmithKline Beecham Pharmaceuticals products appearing here is based on the labeling in effect on June 15, 2000. Further information on these and other products may be obtained from the Medical Department, SmithKline Beecham Pharmaceuticals, One Franklin Plaza, Philadelphia, PA 19101.

Paxil—Cont.

ADVERSE REACTIONS

Associated with Discontinuation of Treatment

Twenty percent (1,199/6,145) of *Paxil* patients in worldwide clinical trials in depression and 16.1% (84/522), 11.8% (64/542) and 9.4% (44/469) of *Paxil* patients in worldwide trials in social anxiety disorder, OCD and panic disorder, respectively, discontinued treatment due to an adverse event. The most common events (≥1%) associated with discontinuation and considered to be drug related (i.e., those events associated with dropout at a rate approximately twice or greater for *Paxil* compared to placebo) included the following:

[See first table at top of previous page]

Commonly Observed Adverse Events

Depression

The most commonly observed adverse events associated with the use of paroxetine (incidence of 5% or greater and incidence for *Paxil* at least twice that for placebo, derived from Table 1 below) were: asthenia, sweating, nausea, decreased appetite, somnolence, dizziness, insomnia, tremor, nervousness, ejaculatory disturbance and other male genital disorders.

Obsessive Compulsive Disorder

The most commonly observed adverse events associated with the use of paroxetine (incidence of 5% or greater and incidence for *Paxil* at least twice that of placebo, derived from Table 2 below) were: nausea, dry mouth, decreased appetite, constipation, dizziness, somnolence, tremor, sweating, impotence and abnormal ejaculation.

Panic Disorder

The most commonly observed adverse events associated with the use of paroxetine (incidence of 5% or greater and incidence for *Paxil* at least twice that for placebo, derived from Table 2 below) were: asthenia, sweating, decreased appetite, libido decreased, tremor, abnormal ejaculation, female genital disorders and impotence.

Social Anxiety Disorder

The most commonly observed adverse events associated with the use of paroxetine (incidence of 5% or greater and incidence for *Paxil* at least twice that for placebo, derived from Table 2 below) were: sweating, nausea, dry mouth, constipation, decreased appetite, somnolence, tremor, libido decreased, yawn, abnormal ejaculation, female genital disorders and impotence.

Incidence in Controlled Clinical Trials

The prescriber should be aware that the figures in the tables following cannot be used to predict the incidence of side effects in the course of usual medical practice where patient characteristics and other factors differ from those which prevailed in the clinical trials. Similarly, the cited frequencies cannot be compared with figures obtained from other clinical investigations involving different treatments, uses and investigators. The cited figures, however, do provide the prescribing physician with some basis for estimating the relative contribution of drug and nondrug factors to the side effect incidence rate in the populations studied.

Depression

Table 1 enumerates adverse events that occurred at an incidence of 1% or more among paroxetine-treated patients who participated in short-term (6-week) placebo-controlled trials in which patients were dosed in a range of 20 to 50 mg/day. Reported adverse events were classified using a standard COSTART-based Dictionary terminology.

[See second table at top of previous page]

Obsessive Compulsive Disorder, Panic Disorder and Social Anxiety Disorder

Table 2 enumerates adverse events that occurred at a frequency of 2% or more among OCD patients on *Paxil* who participated in placebo-controlled trials of 12-weeks duration in which patients were dosed in a range of 20 to 60 mg/day or among patients with panic disorder on *Paxil* who participated in placebo-controlled trials of 10- to 12-weeks duration in which patients were dosed in a range of 10 to 60 mg/day or among patients with social anxiety disorder on Paxil (paroxetine hydrochloride) who participated in placebo-controlled trials of 12-weeks duration in which patients were dosed in a range of 20 to 50 mg/day.

[See table 2 above]

Dose Dependency of Adverse Events: A comparison of adverse event rates in a fixed-dose study comparing *Paxil* 10, 20, 30 and 40 mg/day with placebo in the treatment of depression revealed a clear dose dependency for some of the more common adverse events associated with *Paxil* use, as shown in the following table:

[See table 3 at bottom of next page]

In a fixed-dose study comparing placebo and *Paxil* 20, 40 and 60 mg in the treatment of OCD, there was no clear relationship between adverse events and the dose of Paxil (paroxetine hydrochloride) to which patients were assigned. No new adverse events were observed in the *Paxil* 60 mg dose group compared to any of the other treatment groups.

In a fixed-dose study comparing placebo and *Paxil* 10, 20 and 40 mg in the treatment of panic disorder, there was no clear relationship between adverse events and the dose of *Paxil* to which patients were assigned, except for asthenia, dry mouth, anxiety, libido decreased, tremor and abnormal ejaculation. In flexible dose studies, no new adverse events were observed in patients receiving *Paxil* 60 mg compared to any of the other treatment groups.

In a fixed-dose study comparing placebo and *Paxil* 20, 40 and 60 mg in the treatment of social anxiety disorder, for most of the adverse events, there was no clear relationship between adverse events and the dose of Paxil (paroxetine hydrochloride) to which patients were assigned.

Adaptation to Certain Adverse Events: Over a 4- to 6-week period, there was evidence of adaptation to some adverse events with continued therapy (e.g., nausea and dizziness), but less to other effects (e.g., dry mouth, somnolence and asthenia).

Male and Female Sexual Dysfunction with SSRIs: Although changes in sexual desire, sexual performance and sexual satisfaction often occur as manifestations of a psychiatric disorder, they may also be a consequence of pharmacologic treatment. In particular, some evidence suggests that selective serotonin reuptake inhibitors (SSRIs) can cause such untoward sexual experiences.

Reliable estimates of the incidence and severity of untoward experiences involving sexual desire, performance and satisfaction are difficult to obtain, however, in part because patients and physicians may be reluctant to discuss them. Accordingly, estimates of the incidence of untoward sexual experience and performance cited in product labeling, are likely to underestimate their actual incidence.

In placebo-controlled clinical trials involving more than 1,800 patients, the ranges for the reported incidence of sexual side effects in males and females with depression, OCD, panic disorder, and social anxiety disorder are displayed in Table 4 below.

[See table 4 at bottom of next page]

There are no adequate and well-controlled studies examining sexual dysfunction with paroxetine treatment.

Paroxetine treatment has been associated with several cases of priapism. In those cases with a known outcome, patients recovered without sequelae.

While it is difficult to know the precise risk of sexual dysfunction associated with the use of SSRIs, physicians should routinely inquire about such possible side effects.

Weight and Vital Sign Changes: Significant weight loss may be an undesirable result of treatment with *Paxil* for

Table 2. Treatment-Emergent Adverse Experience Incidence in Placebo-Controlled Clinical Trials for Obsessive Compulsive Disorder, Panic Disorder and Social Anxiety Disorder[1]

		Obsessive Compulsive Disorder		Panic Disorder		Social Anxiety Disorder	
Body System	Preferred Term	*Paxil* (n=542)	Placebo (n=265)	*Paxil* (n=469)	Placebo (n=324)	*Paxil* (n=425)	Placebo (n=339)
Body as a Whole	Asthenia	22%	14%	14%	5%	22%	14%
	Abdominal Pain	—	—	4%	3%	—	—
	Chest Pain	3%	2%	—	—	—	—
	Back Pain	—	—	3%	2%	—	—
	Chills	2%	1%	2%	1%	—	—
	Trauma	—	—	—	—	3%	1%
Cardio-vascular	Vasodilation	4%	1%	—	—	—	—
	Palpitation	2%	0%	—	—	—	—
Derma-tologic	Sweating	9%	3%	14%	6%	9%	2%
	Rash	3%	2%	—	—	—	—
Gastro-intestinal	Nausea	23%	10%	23%	17%	25%	7%
	Dry Mouth	18%	9%	18%	11%	9%	3%
	Constipation	16%	6%	8%	5%	5%	2%
	Diarrhea	10%	10%	12%	7%	9%	6%
	Decreased Appetite	9%	3%	7%	3%	8%	2%
	Dyspepsia	—	—	—	—	4%	2%
	Flatulence	—	—	—	—	4%	2%
	Increased Appetite	4%	3%	2%	1%	—	—
	Vomiting	—	—	—	—	2%	1%
Musculo-skeletal	Myalgia	—	—	—	—	4%	3%
Nervous System	Insomnia	24%	13%	18%	10%	21%	16%
	Somnolence	24%	7%	19%	11%	22%	5%
	Dizziness	12%	6%	14%	10%	11%	7%
	Tremor	11%	1%	9%	1%	9%	1%
	Nervousness	9%	8%	—	—	8%	7%
	Libido Decreased	7%	4%	9%	1%	12%	1%
	Agitation	—	—	5%	4%	3%	1%
	Anxiety	—	—	5%	4%	5%	4%
	Abnormal Dreams	4%	1%	—	—	—	—
	Concentration Impaired	3%	2%	—	—	4%	1%
	Depersonali-zation	3%	0%	—	—	—	—
	Myoclonus	3%	0%	3%	2%	2%	1%
	Amnesia	2%	1%	—	—	—	—
Respiratory System	Rhinitis	—	—	3%	0%	—	—
	Pharyngitis	—	—	—	—	4%	2%
	Yawn	—	—	—	—	5%	1%
Special Senses	Abnormal Vision	4%	2%	—	—	4%	1%
	Taste Perversion	2%	0%	—	—	—	—
Urogenital System	Abnormal Ejaculation[2]	23%	1%	21%	1%	28%	1%
	Dysmenorrhea	—	—	—	—	5%	4%
	Female Genital Disorder[2]	3%	0%	9%	1%	9%	1%
	Impotence[2]	8%	1%	5%	0%	5%	1%
	Urinary Frequency	3%	1%	2%	0%	—	—
	Urination Impaired	3%	0%	—	—	—	—
	Urinary Tract Infection	2%	1%	2%	1%	—	—

1. Events reported by at least 2% of OCD, panic disorder, and social anxiety disorder *Paxil*-treated patients are included, except the following events which had an incidence on placebo ≥*Paxil*: [OCD]: abdominal pain, agitation, anxiety, back pain, cough increased, depression, headache, hyperkinesia, infection, paresthesia, pharyngitis, respiratory disorder, rhinitis and sinusitis. [panic disorder]: abnormal dreams, abnormal vision, chest pain, cough increased, depersonalization, depression, dysmenorrhea, dyspepsia, flu syndrome, headache, infection, myalgia, nervousness, palpitation, paresthesia, pharyngitis, rash, respiratory disorder, sinusitis, taste perversion, trauma, urination impaired and vasodilation. [social anxiety disorder]: abdominal pain, depression, headache, infection, respiratory disorder and sinusitis.
2. Percentage corrected for gender.

some patients but, on average, patients in controlled trials had minimal (about 1 pound) weight loss vs. smaller changes on placebo and active control. No significant changes in vital signs (systolic and diastolic blood pressure, pulse and temperature) were observed in patients treated with *Paxil* in controlled clinical trials.

ECG Changes: In an analysis of ECGs obtained in 682 patients treated with *Paxil* and 415 patients treated with placebo in controlled clinical trials, no clinically significant changes were seen in the ECGs of either group.

Liver Function Tests: In placebo-controlled clinical trials, patients treated with *Paxil* exhibited abnormal values on liver function tests at no greater rate than that seen in placebo-treated patients. In particular, the *Paxil*-vs.-placebo comparisons for alkaline phosphatase, SGOT, SGPT and bilirubin revealed no differences in the percentage of patients with marked abnormalities.

Other Events Observed During the Premarketing Evaluation of Paxil (paroxetine hydrochloride)

During its premarketing assessment in depression, multiple doses of *Paxil* were administered to 6,145 patients in phase 2 and 3 studies. The conditions and duration of exposure to *Paxil* varied greatly and included (in overlapping categories) open and double-blind studies, uncontrolled and controlled studies, inpatient and outpatient studies, and fixed-dose and titration studies. During premarketing clinical trials in OCD, panic disorder, and social anxiety disorder, 542, 469, and 522 patients, respectively, received multiple doses of *Paxil*. Untoward events associated with this exposure were recorded by clinical investigators using terminology of their own choosing. Consequently, it is not possible to provide a meaningful estimate of the proportion of individuals experiencing adverse events without first grouping similar types of untoward events into a smaller number of standardized event categories.

In the tabulations that follow, reported adverse events were classified using a standard COSTART-based Dictionary terminology. The frequencies presented, therefore, represent the proportion of the 7,678 patients exposed to multiple doses of Paxil (paroxetine hydrochloride) who experienced an event of the type cited on at least one occasion while receiving *Paxil*. All reported events are included except those already listed in Tables 1 and 2, those reported in terms so general as to be uninformative and those events where a drug cause was remote. It is important to emphasize that although the events reported occurred during treatment with paroxetine, they were not necessarily caused by it.

Events are further categorized by body system and listed in order of decreasing frequency according to the following definitions: frequent adverse events are those occurring on one or more occasions in at least 1/100 patients (only those not already listed in the tabulated results from placebo-controlled trials appear in this listing); infrequent adverse events are those occurring in 1/100 to 1/1000 patients; rare events are those occurring in fewer than 1/1000 patients. Events of major clinical importance are also described in the PRECAUTIONS section.

Body as a Whole: *frequent*: chills, malaise; *infrequent*: allergic reaction, face edema, neck pain; *rare*: adrenergic syndrome, cellulitis, moniliasis, neck rigidity, pelvic pain, peritonitis, ulcer.

Cardiovascular System: *frequent:* hypertension, syncope, tachycardia; *infrequent:* bradycardia, hematoma, hypotension, migraine; *rare:* angina pectoris, arrhythmia nodal, atrial fibrillation, bundle branch block, cerebral ischemia, cerebrovascular accident, congestive heart failure, heart block, low cardiac output, myocardial infarct, myocardial ischemia, pallor, phlebitis, pulmonary embolus, supraventricular extrasystoles, thrombophlebitis, thrombosis, varicose vein, vascular headache, ventricular extrasystoles.

Digestive System: *infrequent:* bruxism, colitis, dysphagia, eructation, gastritis, gastroenteritis, gingivitis, glossitis, increased salivation, liver function tests abnormal, rectal hemorrhage, ulcerative stomatitis; *rare:* aphthous stomatitis, bloody diarrhea, bulimia, cholelithiasis, duodenitis, enteritis, esophagitis, fecal impactions, fecal incontinence, gum hemorrhage, hematemesis, hepatitis, ileus, intestinal obstruction, jaundice, melena, mouth ulceration, peptic ulcer, salivary gland enlargement, stomach ulcer, stomatitis, tongue discoloration, tongue edema, tooth caries.

Endocrine System: *rare:* diabetes mellitus, hyperthyroidism, hypothyroidism, thyroiditis.

Hemic and Lymphatic Systems: *infrequent:* anemia, eosinophilia, leukocytosis, leukopenia, lymphadenopathy, purpura; *rare:* abnormal erythrocytes, basophilia, hypochromic anemia, iron deficiency anemia, lymphedema, abnormal lymphocytes, lymphocytosis, microcytic anemia, monocytosis, normocytic anemia, thrombocythemia, thrombocytopenia.

Metabolic and Nutritional: *frequent:* weight gain, weight loss; *infrequent:* alkaline phosphatase increased, edema, peripheral edema, SGOT increased, SGPT increased, thirst; *rare:* bilirubinemia, BUN increased, creatinine phosphokinase increased, dehydration, gamma globulins increased, gout, hypercalcemia, hypercholesteremia, hyperglycemia, hyperkalemia, hyperphosphatemia, hypocalcemia, hypoglycemia, hypokalemia, hyponatremia, ketosis, lactic dehydrogenase increased.

Musculoskeletal System: *frequent:* arthralgia; *infrequent:* arthritis; *rare:* arthrosis, bursitis, myositis, osteoporosis, generalized spasm, tenosynovitis, tetany.

Nervous System: *frequent:* amnesia, CNS stimulation, concentration impaired, depression, emotional lability, vertigo; *infrequent:* abnormal thinking, alcohol abuse, ataxia, delirium, depersonalization, dystonia, dyskinesia, euphoria, hallucinations, hostility, hyperkinesia, hypertonia, hypesthesia, hypokinesia, incoordination, lack of emotion, libido increased, manic reaction, neurosis, paralysis, paranoid reaction, psychosis; *rare:* abnormal gait, akinesia, antisocial reaction, aphasia, choreoathetosis, circumoral paresthesias, convulsion, delusions, diplopia, drug dependence, dysarthria, extrapyramidal syndrome, fasciculations, grand mal convulsion, hyperalgesia, hysteria, manic-depressive reaction, meningitis, myelitis, neuralgia, neuropathy, nystagmus, peripheral neuritis, psychotic depression, reflexes decreased, reflexes increased, stupor, trismus, withdrawal syndrome.

Respiratory System: *frequent:* cough increased, rhinitis, sinusitis; *infrequent:* asthma, bronchitis, dyspnea, epistaxis, hyperventilation, pneumonia, respiratory flu; *rare:* emphysema, hemoptysis, hiccups, lung fibrosis, pulmonary edema, sputum increased, voice alteration.

Skin and Appendages: *frequent:* pruritus; *infrequent:* acne, alopecia, contact dermatitis, dry skin, ecchymosis, eczema, herpes simplex, maculopapular rash, photosensitivity, urticaria; *rare:* angioedema, erythema nodosum, erythema multiforme, fungal dermatitis, furunculosis, herpes zoster, hirsutism, seborrhea, skin discoloration, skin hypertrophy, skin ulcer, vesiculobullous rash.

Special Senses: *infrequent:* abnormality of accommodation, conjunctivitis, ear pain, eye pain, mydriasis, otitis media, photophobia, tinnitus; *rare:* amblyopia, anisocoria, blepharitis, cataract, conjunctival edema, corneal ulcer, deafness, exophthalmos, eye hemorrhage, glaucoma, hyperacusis, keratoconjunctivitis, night blindness, otitis externa, parosmia, ptosis, retinal hemorrhage, taste loss, visual field defect.

Urogenital System: *infrequent:* abortion, amenorrhea, breast pain, cystitis, dysuria, hematuria, menorrhagia, nocturia, polyuria, urinary incontinence, urinary retention, urinary urgency, vaginal moniliasis, vaginitis; *rare:* breast atrophy, breast enlargement, epididymitis, female lactation, fibrocystic breast, kidney calculus, kidney pain, leukorrhea, mastitis, metrorrhagia, nephritis, oliguria, pyuria, urethritis, uterine spasm, urolith, vaginal hemorrhage.

Postmarketing Reports

Voluntary reports of adverse events in patients taking Paxil (paroxetine hydrochloride) that have been received since market introduction and not listed above that may have no causal relationship with the drug include acute pancreatitis, elevated liver function tests (the most severe cases were deaths due to liver necrosis, and grossly elevated transaminases associated with severe liver dysfunction), Guillain-Barré syndrome, toxic epidermal necrolysis, priapism, thrombocytopenia, syndrome of inappropriate ADH secretion, symptoms suggestive of prolactinemia and galactorrhea, neuroleptic malignant syndrome-like events; extrapyramidal symptoms which have included akathisia, bradykinesia, cogwheel rigidity, dystonia, hypertonia, oculogyric crisis which has been associated with concomitant use of pimozide, tremor and trismus; and serotonin syndrome, associated in some cases with concomitant use of serotonergic drugs and with drugs which may have impaired *Paxil* metabolism (symptoms have included agitation, confusion, diaphoresis, hallucinations, hyperreflexia, myoclonus, shivering, tachycardia and tremor). There have been spontaneous reports that abrupt discontinuation may lead to symptoms such as dizziness, sensory disturbances, agitation or anxiety, nausea and sweating; these events are generally self-limiting. There has been a case report of an elevated phenytoin level after 4 weeks of *Paxil* and phenytoin co-administration. There has been a case report of severe hypotension when *Paxil* was added to chronic metoprolol treatment.

DRUG ABUSE AND DEPENDENCE

Controlled Substance Class: Paxil (paroxetine hydrochloride) is not a controlled substance.

Physical and Psychologic Dependence: *Paxil* has not been systematically studied in animals or humans for its potential for abuse, tolerance or physical dependence. While the clinical trials did not reveal any tendency for any drug-seeking behavior, these observations were not systematic and it is not possible to predict on the basis of this limited experience the extent to which a CNS-active drug will be misused, diverted and/or abused once marketed. Consequently, patients should be evaluated carefully for history of drug abuse, and such patients should be observed closely for signs of *Paxil* misuse or abuse (e.g., development of tolerance, incrementations of dose, drug-seeking behavior).

OVERDOSAGE

Human Experience: Overdose with *Paxil* (up to 2000 mg) alone and in combination with other drugs has been reported. Signs and symptoms of overdose with *Paxil* include nausea, vomiting, sedation, dizziness, sweating, and facial flush. There are no reports of coma or convulsions following overdosage with *Paxil* alone. A fatal outcome has been reported rarely when *Paxil* was taken in combination with other agents, or when taken alone.

Overdosage Management: Treatment should consist of those general measures employed in the management of overdosage with any antidepressant.

Continued on next page

Table 3. Treatment-Emergent Adverse Experience Incidence in a Depression Dose-Comparison Trial*

Body System/ Preferred Term	Placebo n=51	Paxil 10 mg n=102	20 mg n=104	30 mg n=101	40 mg n=102
Body as a Whole					
Asthenia	0.0%	2.9%	10.6%	13.9%	12.7%
Dermatology					
Sweating	2.0%	1.0%	6.7%	8.9%	11.8%
Gastrointestinal					
Constipation	5.9%	4.9%	7.7%	9.9%	12.7%
Decreased Appetite	2.0%	2.0%	5.8%	4.0%	4.9%
Diarrhea	7.8%	9.8%	19.2%	7.9%	14.7%
Dry Mouth	2.0%	10.8%	18.3%	15.8%	20.6%
Nausea	13.7%	14.7%	26.9%	34.7%	36.3%
Nervous System					
Anxiety	0.0%	2.0%	5.8%	5.9%	5.9%
Dizziness	3.9%	6.9%	6.7%	8.9%	12.7%
Nervousness	0.0%	5.9%	5.8%	4.0%	2.9%
Paresthesia	0.0%	2.9%	1.0%	5.0%	5.9%
Somnolence	7.8%	12.7%	18.3%	20.8%	21.6%
Tremor	0.0%	0.0%	7.7%	7.9%	14.7%
Special Senses					
Blurred Vision	2.0%	2.9%	2.9%	2.0%	7.8%
Urogenital System					
Abnormal Ejaculation	0.0%	5.8%	6.5%	10.6%	13.0%
Impotence	0.0%	1.9%	4.3%	6.4%	1.9%
Male Genital Disorders	0.0%	3.8%	8.7%	6.4%	3.7%

*Rule for including adverse events in table: incidence at least 5% for one of paroxetine groups and ≥ twice the placebo incidence for at least one paroxetine group.

Table 4. Incidence of Sexual Adverse Events in Controlled Clinical Trials

	Paxil	Placebo
n (males)	925	655
Decreased libido	6%–14%	0%–5%
Ejaculatory disturbance	13%–28%	0%–1%
Impotence	2%–8%	0%–1%
n (females)	932	694
Decreased libido	1%–9%	0%–2%
Orgasmic disturbance	2%–9%	0%–1%

Information on the SmithKline Beecham Pharmaceuticals products appearing here is based on the labeling in effect on June 15, 2000. Further information on these and other products may be obtained from the Medical Department, SmithKline Beecham Pharmaceuticals, One Franklin Plaza, Philadelphia, PA 19101.

Paxil—Cont.

Ensure an adequate airway, oxygenation, and ventilation. Monitor cardiac rhythm and vital signs. General supportive and symptomatic measures are also recommended. Induction of emesis is not recommended. Gastric lavage with a large-bore orogastric tube with appropriate airway protection, if needed, may be indicated if performed soon after ingestion, or in symptomatic patients.

Activated charcoal should be administered. Due to the large volume of distribution of this drug, forced diuresis, dialysis, hemoperfusion and exchange transfusion are unlikely to be of benefit. No specific antidotes for paroxetine are known.

A specific caution involves patients who are taking or have recently taken paroxetine who might ingest excessive quantities of a tricyclic antidepressant. In such a case, accumulation of the parent tricyclic and/or an active metabolite may increase the possibility of clinically significant sequelae and extend the time needed for close medical observation (see Drugs Metabolized by Cytochrome $P_{450}IID_6$ under PRECAUTIONS).

In managing overdosage, consider the possibility of multiple drug involvement. The physician should consider contacting a poison control center for additional information on the treatment of any overdose. Telephone numbers for certified poison control centers are listed in the *Physicians' Desk Reference* (PDR).

DOSAGE AND ADMINISTRATION

Depression

Usual Initial Dosage: Paxil (paroxetine hydrochloride) should be administered as a single daily dose with or without food, usually in the morning. The recommended initial dose is 20 mg/day. Patients were dosed in a range of 20 to 50 mg/day in the clinical trials demonstrating the antidepressant effectiveness of *Paxil*. As with all antidepressants, the full antidepressant effect may be delayed. Some patients not responding to a 20 mg dose may benefit from dose increases, in 10 mg/day increments, up to a maximum of 50 mg/day. Dose changes should occur at intervals of at least 1 week.

Maintenance Therapy: There is no body of evidence available to answer the question of how long the patient treated with *Paxil* should remain on it. It is generally agreed that acute episodes of depression require several months or longer of sustained pharmacologic therapy. Whether the dose of an antidepressant needed to induce remission is identical to the dose needed to maintain and/or sustain euthymia is unknown.

Systematic evaluation of the efficacy of Paxil (paroxetine hydrochloride) has shown that efficacy is maintained for periods of up to 1 year with doses that averaged about 30 mg.

Obsessive Compulsive Disorder

Usual Initial Dosage: Paxil (paroxetine hydrochloride) should be administered as a single daily dose with or without food, usually in the morning. The recommended dose of *Paxil* in the treatment of OCD is 40 mg daily. Patients should be started on 20 mg/day and the dose can be increased in 10 mg/day increments. Dose changes should occur at intervals of at least 1 week. Patients were dosed in a range of 20 to 60 mg/day in the clinical trials demonstrating the effectiveness of *Paxil* in the treatment of OCD. The maximum dosage should not exceed 60 mg/day.

Maintenance Therapy: Long-term maintenance of efficacy was demonstrated in a 6-month relapse prevention trial. In this trial, patients with OCD assigned to paroxetine demonstrated a lower relapse rate compared to patients on placebo (see CLINICAL PHARMACOLOGY). OCD is a chronic condition, and it is reasonable to consider continuation for a responding patient. Dosage adjustments should be made to maintain the patient on the lowest effective dosage, and patients should be periodically reassessed to determine the need for continued treatment.

Panic Disorder

Usual Initial Dosage: *Paxil* should be administered as a single daily dose with or without food, usually in the morning. The target dose of *Paxil* in the treatment of panic disorder is 40 mg/day. Patients should be started on 10 mg/day. Dose changes should occur in 10 mg/day increments and at intervals of at least 1 week. Patients were dosed in a range of 10 to 60 mg/day in the clinical trials demonstrating the effectiveness of *Paxil*. The maximum dosage should not exceed 60 mg/day.

Maintenance Therapy: Long-term maintenance of efficacy was demonstrated in a 3-month relapse prevention trial. In this trial, patients with panic disorder assigned to paroxetine demonstrated a lower relapse rate compared to patients on placebo (see CLINICAL PHARMACOLOGY). Panic disorder is a chronic condition, and it is reasonable to consider continuation for a responding patient. Dosage adjustments should be made to maintain the patient on the lowest effective dosage, and patients should be periodically reassessed to determine the need for continued treatment.

Social Anxiety Disorder

Usual Initial Dosage: *Paxil* should be administered as a single daily dose with or without food, usually in the morning. The recommended and initial dosage is 20 mg/day. In clinical trials the effectiveness of *Paxil* was demonstrated in patients dosed in a range of 20 to 60 mg/day. While the safety of *Paxil* has been evaluated in patients with social anxiety disorder at doses up to 60 mg/day, available information does not suggest any additional benefit for doses above 20 mg/day. (See CLINICAL PHARMACOLOGY).

Maintenance Therapy: There is no body of evidence available to answer the question of how long the patient treated with *Paxil* should remain on it. Although the efficacy of *Paxil* beyond 12 weeks of dosing has not been demonstrated in controlled clinical trials, social anxiety disorder is recognized as a chronic condition, and it is reasonable to consider continuation of treatment for a responding patient. Dosage adjustments should be made to maintain the patient on the lowest effective dosage, and patients should be periodically reassessed to determine the need for continued treatment.

Dosage for Elderly or Debilitated, and Patients with Severe Renal or Hepatic Impairment: The recommended initial dose is 10 mg/day for elderly patients, debilitated patients, and/or patients with severe renal or hepatic impairment. Increases may be made if indicated. Dosage should not exceed 40 mg/day.

Switching Patients to or from a Monoamine Oxidase Inhibitor: At least 14 days should elapse between discontinuation of a MAOI and initiation of *Paxil* therapy. Similarly, at least 14 days should be allowed after stopping Paxil (paroxetine hydrochloride) before starting a MAOI.

NOTE: SHAKE SUSPENSION WELL BEFORE USING.

HOW SUPPLIED

Tablets: Film-coated, modified-oval as follows:

10 mg yellow tablets engraved on the front with PAXIL and on the back with 10.

NDC 0029-3210-13 Bottles of 30

20 mg pink, scored tablets engraved on the front with PAXIL and on the back with 20.

NDC 0029-3211-13 Bottles of 30
NDC 0029-3211-20 Bottles of 100
NDC 0029-3211-21 SUP 100's (intended for institutional use only)

30 mg blue tablets engraved on the front with PAXIL and on the back with 30.

NDC 0029-3212-13 Bottles of 30

40 mg green tablets engraved on the front with PAXIL and on the back with 40.

NDC 0029-3213-13 Bottles of 30

Store tablets between 15° and 30° C (59° and 86° F).

Oral Suspension: Orange-colored, orange-flavored, 10 mg/5 mL, in 250 mL white bottles. Manufactured in Crawley, UK, by SmithKline Beecham Pharmaceuticals.

NDC 0029-3215-48

Store suspension at or below 25° C (77° F).

SmithKline Beecham Pharmaceuticals **Rx only**
Philadelphia, PA 19101
PX:L16A

Shown in Product Identification Guide, page 337

RELAFEN® ℞

[rel 'ah-fen]
brand of nabumetone tablets

DESCRIPTION

Relafen (nabumetone) is a naphthylalkanone designated chemically as 4-(6-methoxy-2-naphthalenyl)-2-butanone. It has the following structure:

nabumetone

Nabumetone is a white to off-white crystalline substance with a molecular weight of 228.3. It is nonacidic and practically insoluble in water, but soluble in alcohol and most organic solvents. It has an n-octanol:phosphate buffer partition coefficient of 2400 at pH 7.4.

Tablets for Oral Administration: Each oval-shaped, film-coated tablet contains 500 mg or 750 mg of nabumetone. Inactive ingredients consist of hydroxypropyl methylcellulose, microcrystalline cellulose, polyethylene glycol, polysorbate 80, sodium lauryl sulfate, sodium starch glycolate and titanium dioxide. The 750 mg tablets also contain iron oxides.

CLINICAL PHARMACOLOGY

Relafen is a nonsteroidal anti-inflammatory drug (NSAID) that exhibits anti-inflammatory, analgesic and antipyretic properties in pharmacologic studies. As with other nonsteroidal anti-inflammatory agents, its mode of action is not known. However, the ability to inhibit prostaglandin synthesis may be involved in the anti-inflammatory effect.

The parent compound is a prodrug, which undergoes hepatic biotransformation to the active component, 6-methoxy-2-naphthylacetic acid (6MNA), that is a potent inhibitor of prostaglandin synthesis.

6-methoxy-2-naphthylacetic acid (6MNA)

It is acidic and has an n-octanol:phosphate buffer partition coefficient of 0.5 at pH 7.4.

Pharmacokinetics

After oral administration, approximately 80% of a radiolabelled dose of nabumetone is found in the urine, indicating that nabumetone is well absorbed from the gastrointestinal tract. Nabumetone itself is not detected in the plasma because, after absorption, it undergoes rapid biotransformation to the principal active metabolite, 6-methoxy-2-naphthylacetic acid (6MNA). Approximately 35% of a 1000 mg oral dose of nabumetone is converted to 6MNA and 50% is converted into unidentified metabolites which are subsequently excreted in the urine. Following oral administration of *Relafen,* 6MNA exhibits pharmacokinetic characteristics that generally follow a one-compartment model with first order input and first order elimination.

6MNA is more than 99% bound to plasma proteins. The free fraction is dependent on total concentration of 6MNA and is proportional to dose over the range of 1000 mg to 2000 mg. It is 0.2% to 0.3% at concentrations typically achieved following administration of *Relafen* 1000 mg and is approximately 0.6% to 0.8% of the total concentrations at steady state following daily administration of 2000 mg.

Steady-state plasma concentrations of 6MNA are slightly lower than predicted from single-dose data. This may result from the higher fraction of unbound 6MNA which undergoes greater hepatic clearance.

Coadministration of food increases the rate of absorption and subsequent appearance of 6MNA in the plasma but does not affect the extent of conversion of nabumetone into 6MNA. Peak plasma concentrations of 6MNA are increased by approximately one third.

Coadministration with an aluminum-containing antacid had no significant effect on the bioavailability of 6MNA.

[See table below]

The simulated curves in the graph below illustrate the range of active metabolite plasma concentrations that would be expected from 95% of patients following 1000 mg to 2000 mg doses to steady state. The cross-hatched area represents the expected overlap in plasma concentrations due to intersubject variation following oral administration of 1000 mg to 2000 mg of *Relafen.*

Nabumetone Active Metabolite (6MNA) Plasma Concentrations at Steady State Following Once-Daily Dosing of Nabumetone
1000 mg (n=31) 2000 mg (n=12)

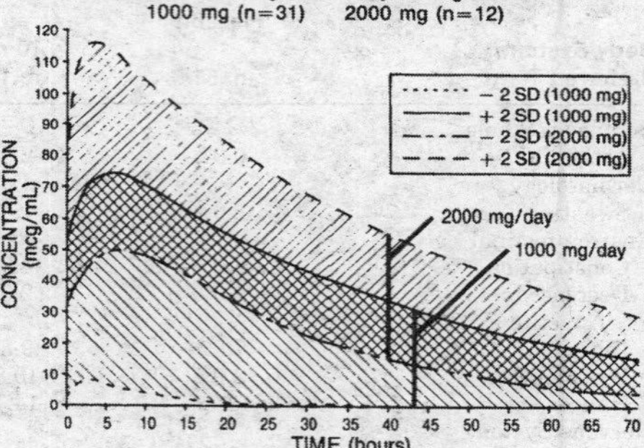

6MNA undergoes biotransformation in the liver, producing inactive metabolites that are eliminated as both free metabolites and conjugates. None of the known metabolites of 6MNA has been detected in plasma. Preliminary *in vivo* and *in vitro* studies suggest that unlike other NSAIDs, there is no evidence of enterohepatic recirculation of the active metabolite. Approximately 75% of a radiolabelled dose was recovered in urine in 48 hours. Approximately 80% was recovered in 168 hours. A further 9% appeared in the feces. In the first 48 hours, metabolites consisted of:

—nabumetone, unchanged	not detectable
—6-methoxy-2-naphthylacetic acid (6MNA), unchanged	<1%
—6MNA, conjugated	11%

Table 1. Mean pharmacokinetic parameters of nabumetone active metabolite (6MNA) at steady state following oral administration of 1000 mg or 2000 mg doses of Relafen (nabumetone)

Abbreviation (units)	Young Adults Mean ± SD 1000 mg n=31	Young Adults Mean ± SD 2000 mg n=12	Elderly Mean ± SD 1000 mg n=27
t_{max} (hours)	3.0 (1.0 to 12.0)	2.5 (1.0 to 8.0)	4.0 (1.0 to 10.0)
$t^1/_2$ (hours)	22.5 ± 3.7	26.2 ± 3.7	29.8 ± 8.1
CL_{SS}/F (mL/min.)	26.1 ± 17.3	21.0 ± 4.0	18.6 ± 13.4
Vd_{SS}/F (L)	55.4 ± 26.4	53.4 ± 11.3	50.2 ± 25.3

—6-hydroxy-2-naphthylacetic acid (6HNA), unchanged 5%
—6HNA, conjugated 7%
—4-(6-hydroxy-2-naphthyl)-butan-2-ol, conjugated 9%
—*O*-desmethyl-nabumetone, conjugated 7%
—unidentified minor metabolites 34%
Total % Dose: 73%

Following oral administration of dosages of 1000 mg to 2000 mg to steady state, the mean plasma clearance of 6MNA is 20 to 30 mL/min. and the elimination half-life is approximately 24 hours.

Elderly Patients: Steady-state plasma concentrations in elderly patients were generally higher than in young healthy subjects. (See Table 1 for summary of pharmacokinetic parameters.)

Renal Insufficiency: In studies of patients with renal insufficiency, the mean terminal half-life of 6MNA was increased in patients with severe renal dysfunction (creatinine clearance <30 mL/min./1.73 m^2). In patients undergoing hemodialysis, steady-state plasma concentrations of the active metabolite were similar to those observed in healthy subjects. Due to extensive protein-binding, 6MNA is not dialyzable.

Hepatic Impairment: Data in patients with severe hepatic impairment are limited. Biotransformation of nabumetone to 6MNA and the further metabolism of 6MNA to inactive metabolites is dependent on hepatic function and could be reduced in patients with severe hepatic impairment (history of or biopsy-proven cirrhosis).

Special Studies

Gastrointestinal: Relafen (nabumetone) was compared to aspirin in inducing gastrointestinal blood loss. Food intake was not monitored. Studies utilizing ^{51}Cr-tagged red blood cells in healthy males showed no difference in fecal blood loss after 3 or 4 weeks' administration of *Relafen* 1000 mg or 2000 mg daily when compared to either placebo-treated or nontreated subjects. In contrast, aspirin 3600 mg daily produced an increase in fecal blood loss when compared to the *Relafen*-treated, placebo-treated or nontreated subjects. The clinical relevance of the data is unknown.

The following endoscopy trials entered patients who had been previously treated with NSAIDs. These patients had varying baseline scores and different courses of treatment. The trials were not designed to correlate symptoms and endoscopy scores. The clinical relevance of these endoscopy trials, i.e., either G.I. symptoms or serious G.I. events, is not known.

Ten endoscopy studies were conducted in 488 patients who had baseline and post-treatment endoscopy. In 5 clinical trials that compared a total of 194 patients on *Relafen* 1000 mg daily or naproxen 250 mg or 500 mg twice daily for 3 to 12 weeks, *Relafen* treatment resulted in fewer patients with endoscopically detected lesions (>3 mm). In 2 trials a total of 101 patients on *Relafen* 1000 mg or 2000 mg daily or piroxicam 10 mg to 20 mg for 7 to 10 days, there were fewer *Relafen* patients with endoscopically detected lesions. In 3 trials of a total of 47 patients on *Relafen* 1000 mg daily or indomethacin 100 mg to 150 mg daily for 3 to 4 weeks, the endoscopy scores were higher with indomethacin. Another 12-week trial in a total of 171 patients compared the results of treatment with *Relafen* 1000 mg/day to ibuprofen 2400 mg/day and ibuprofen 2400 mg/day plus misoprostol 800 mcg/day. The results showed that patients treated with *Relafen* had a lower number of endoscopically detected lesions (>5 mm) than patients treated with ibuprofen alone but comparable to the combination of ibuprofen plus misoprostol. The results did not correlate with abdominal pain.

Other: In 1-week repeat-dose studies in healthy volunteers, *Relafen* 1000 mg daily had little effect on collagen-induced platelet aggregation and no effect on bleeding time. In comparison, naproxen 500 mg daily suppressed collagen-induced platelet aggregation and significantly increased bleeding time.

CLINICAL TRIALS

Osteoarthritis: The use of *Relafen* in relieving the signs and symptoms of osteoarthritis was assessed in double-blind controlled trials in which 1,047 patients were treated for 6 weeks to 6 months. In these trials, *Relafen* in a dose of 1000 mg/day administered at night was comparable to naproxen 500 mg/day and to aspirin 3600 mg/day.

Rheumatoid Arthritis: The use of *Relafen* in relieving the signs and symptoms of rheumatoid arthritis was assessed in double-blind, randomized, controlled trials in which 770 patients were treated for 3 weeks to 6 months. *Relafen,* in a dose of 1000 mg/day administered at night was comparable to naproxen 500 mg/day and to aspirin 3600 mg/day.

In controlled clinical trials of rheumatoid arthritis patients, *Relafen* has been used in combination with gold, d-penicillamine and corticosteroids.

INDIVIDUALIZATION OF DOSING

There is considerable interpatient variation in response to *Relafen.* Therapy is usually initiated at a *Relafen* dose of 1000 mg daily, then adjusted, if needed, based on clinical response.

In clinical trials with osteoarthritis and rheumatoid arthritis patients, most patients responded to *Relafen* in doses of 1000 mg/day administered nightly; total daily dosages up to 2000 mg were used. In open-labelled studies, 1,490 patients were permitted dosage increases and were followed for approximately 1 year (mode). Twenty percent of patients (n=294) were withdrawn for lack of effectiveness during the first year of these open-labelled studies. The following table provides patient-exposure to doses used in the U.S. clinical trials:

Table 2. Clinical double-blind and open-labelled trials of Relafen (nabumetone) in osteoarthritis and rheumatoid arthritis

Relafen Dose	Number of Patients		Mean/Mode Duration of Treatment (yrs.)	
	OA	RA	OA	RA
500 mg	17	6	0.4/–	0.2/–
1000 mg	917	701	1.2/1	1.4/1
1500 mg	645	224	2.3/1	1.7/1
2000 mg	15	100	0.6/1	1.3/1

As with other NSAIDs, the lowest dose should be sought for each patient. Patients weighing under 50 kg may be less likely to require dosages beyond 1000 mg. Therefore, after observing the response to initial therapy, the dose should be adjusted to meet individual patients' requirements.

INDICATIONS AND USAGE

Relafen is indicated for acute and chronic treatment of signs and symptoms of osteoarthritis and rheumatoid arthritis.

CONTRAINDICATIONS

Relafen is contraindicated in patients who have previously exhibited hypersensitivity to it.

Relafen is contraindicated in patients in whom *Relafen,* aspirin or other NSAIDs induce asthma, urticaria or other allergic-type reactions. Fatal asthmatic reactions have been reported in such patients receiving NSAIDs.

WARNINGS

Risk of G.I. Ulceration, Bleeding and Perforation with NSAID Therapy: Serious gastrointestinal toxicity such as bleeding, ulceration and perforation can occur at any time, with or without warning symptoms, in patients treated chronically with NSAID therapy. Although minor upper gastrointestinal problems, such as dyspepsia, are common, usually developing early in therapy, physicians should remain alert for ulceration and bleeding in patients treated chronically with NSAIDs even in the absence of previous G.I. tract symptoms.

In controlled clinical trials involving 1,677 patients treated with *Relafen* (1,140 followed for 1 year and 927 for 2 years), the cumulative incidence of peptic ulcers was 0.3% (95% Cl; 0%, 0.6%) at 3 to 6 months, 0.5% (95% Cl; 0.1%, 0.9%) at 1 year and 0.8% (95% Cl; 0.3%, 1.3%) at 2 years. Physicians should inform patients about the signs and symptoms of serious G.I. toxicity and what steps to take if they occur. In patients with active peptic ulcer, physicians must weigh the benefits of Relafen (nabumetone) therapy against possible hazards, institute an appropriate ulcer treatment regimen and monitor the patients' progress carefully.

Studies to date have not identified any subset of patients not at risk of developing peptic ulceration and bleeding. Except for a prior history of serious G.I. events and other risk factors known to be associated with peptic ulcer disease, such as alcoholism, smoking, etc., no risk factors (e.g., age, sex) have been associated with increased risk. Elderly or debilitated patients seem to tolerate ulceration or bleeding less well than other individuals and most spontaneous reports of fatal G.I. events are in this population.

High doses of any NSAID probably carry a greater risk of these reactions, although controlled clinical trials showing this do not exist in most cases. In considering the use of relatively large doses (within the recommended dosage range), sufficient benefit should be anticipated to offset the potential increased risk of G.I. toxicity.

PRECAUTIONS

General

Renal Effects: As a class, NSAIDs have been associated with renal papillary necrosis and other abnormal renal pathology during long-term administration to animals.

A second form of renal toxicity often associated with NSAIDs is seen in patients with conditions leading to a reduction in renal blood flow or blood volume, where renal prostaglandins have a supportive role in the maintenance of renal perfusion. In these patients, administration of an NSAID results in a dose-dependent decrease in prostaglandin synthesis and, secondarily, in a reduction of renal blood flow, which may precipitate overt renal decompensation. Patients at greatest risk of this reaction are those with impaired renal function, heart failure, liver dysfunction, those taking diuretics, and the elderly. Discontinuation of NSAID therapy is typically followed by recovery to the pretreatment state.

Because nabumetone undergoes extensive hepatic metabolism, no adjustment of *Relafen* dosage is generally necessary in patients with renal insufficiency. However, as with all NSAIDs, patients with impaired renal function should be monitored more closely than patients with normal renal function (see CLINICAL PHARMACOLOGY, Special Studies). The oxidized and conjugated metabolites of 6MNA are eliminated primarily by the kidneys. The extent to which these largely inactive metabolites may accumulate in patients with renal failure has not been studied. As with other drugs whose metabolites are excreted by the kidneys, the possibility that adverse reactions (not listed in ADVERSE REACTIONS) may be attributable to these metabolites should be considered.

Hepatic Function: As with other NSAIDs, borderline elevations of one or more liver function tests may occur in up to 15% of patients. These abnormalities may progress, may remain essentially unchanged, or may return to normal with continued therapy. The ALT (SGPT) test is probably the most sensitive indicator of liver dysfunction. Meaningful (3 times the upper limit of normal) elevations of ALT (SGPT) or AST (SGOT) have occurred in controlled clinical trials of Relafen (nabumetone) in less than 1% of patients. A patient with symptoms and/or signs suggesting liver dysfunction, or in whom an abnormal liver test has occurred, should be evaluated for evidence of the development of a more severe hepatic reaction while on *Relafen* therapy. Severe hepatic reactions, including jaundice and fatal hepatitis, have been reported with other NSAIDs. Although such reactions are rare, if abnormal liver tests persist or worsen, if clinical signs and symptoms consistent with liver disease develop, or if systemic manifestations occur (e.g., eosinophilia, rash, etc.), *Relafen* should be discontinued. Because nabumetone's biotransformation to 6MNA is dependent upon hepatic function, the biotransformation could be decreased in patients with severe hepatic dysfunction. Therefore, *Relafen* should be used with caution in patients with severe hepatic impairment (see Pharmacokinetics, *Hepatic Impairment*).

Fluid Retention and Edema: Fluid retention and edema have been observed in some patients taking *Relafen.* Therefore, as with other NSAIDs, *Relafen* should be used cautiously in patients with a history of congestive heart failure, hypertension or other conditions predisposing to fluid retention.

Photosensitivity: Based on U.V. light photosensitivity testing, *Relafen* may be associated with more reactions to sun exposure than might be expected based on skin tanning types.

Information for Patients: *Relafen,* like other drugs of its class, is not free of side effects. The side effects of these drugs can cause discomfort and, rarely, there are more serious side effects, such as gastrointestinal bleeding, which may result in hospitalization and even fatal outcome.

NSAIDs are often essential agents in the management of arthritis, but they also may be commonly employed for conditions which are less serious. Physicians may wish to discuss with their patients the potential risks (see WARNINGS, PRECAUTIONS and ADVERSE REACTIONS) and likely benefits of NSAID treatment, particularly when the drugs are used for less serious conditions where treatment without NSAIDs may represent an acceptable alternative to both the patient and the physician.

Laboratory Tests: Because severe G.I. tract ulceration and bleeding can occur without warning symptoms, physicians should follow chronically treated patients for signs and symptoms of ulceration and bleeding, and should inform them of the importance of this follow-up (see WARNINGS, Risk of G.I. Ulceration, Bleeding and Perforation with NSAID Therapy).

Drug Interactions: *In vitro* studies have shown that, because of its affinity for protein, 6MNA may displace other protein-bound drugs from their binding site. Caution should be exercised when administering *Relafen* with warfarin since interactions have been seen with other NSAIDs.

Concomitant administration of an aluminum-containing antacid had no significant effect on the bioavailability of 6MNA. When administered with food or milk, there is more rapid absorption; however, the total amount of 6MNA in the plasma is unchanged (see Pharmacokinetics).

Carcinogenesis, Mutagenesis: In two-year studies conducted in mice and rats, nabumetone had no statistically significant tumorigenic effect. Nabumetone did not show mutagenic potential in the Ames test and mouse micronucleus test *in vivo.* However, nabumetone- and 6MNA-treated lymphocytes in culture showed chromosomal aberrations at 80 mcg/mL and higher concentrations (equal to the average human exposure to *Relafen* at the maximum recommended dose).

Impairment of Fertility: Nabumetone did not impair fertility of male or female rats treated orally at doses of 320 mg/kg/day (1888 mg/m^2) before mating.

Pregnancy: Teratogenic Effects. Pregnancy Category C. Nabumetone did not cause any teratogenic effect in rats given up to 400 mg/kg (2360 mg/m^2) and in rabbits up to 300 mg/kg (3540 mg/m^2) orally. However, increased post-implantation loss was observed in rats at 100 mg/kg (590 mg/m^2) orally and at higher doses (equal to the average human exposure to 6MNA at the maximum recommended human dose). There are no adequate, well-controlled studies in pregnant women. This drug should be used during pregnancy only if clearly needed.

Because of the known effect of prostaglandin-synthesis-inhibiting drugs on the human fetal cardiovascular system

Continued on next page

Information on the SmithKline Beecham Pharmaceuticals products appearing here is based on the labeling in effect on June 15, 2000. Further information on these and other products may be obtained from the Medical Department, SmithKline Beecham Pharmaceuticals, One Franklin Plaza, Philadelphia, PA 19101.

Relafen—Cont.

(closure of ductus arteriosus), use of Relafen (nabumetone) during the third trimester of pregnancy is not recommended.

Labor and Delivery: The effects of *Relafen* on labor and delivery in women are not known. As with other drugs known to inhibit prostaglandin synthesis, an increased incidence of dystocia and delayed parturition occurred in rats treated throughout pregnancy.

Nursing Mothers: *Relafen* is not recommended for use in nursing mothers because of the possible adverse effects of prostaglandin-synthesis-inhibiting drugs on neonates. It is not known whether nabumetone or its metabolites are excreted in human milk; however, 6MNA is excreted in the milk of lactating rats.

Pediatric Use: Safety and effectiveness in pediatric patients have not been established.

Geriatric Use: Of the 1,677 patients in U.S. clinical studies who were treated with *Relafen*, 411 patients (24%) were 65 years of age or older; 22 patients (1%) were 75 years of age or older. No overall differences in efficacy or safety were observed between these older patients and younger ones. Similar results were observed in a 1-year, non-U.S. postmarketing surveillance study of 10,800 *Relafen* patients, of whom 4,577 patients (42%) were 65 years of age or older.

ADVERSE REACTIONS

Adverse reaction information was derived from blinded-controlled and open-labelled clinical trials and from worldwide marketing experience. In the description below, rates of the more common events (greater than 1%) and many of the less common events (less than 1%) represent results of U.S. clinical studies.

Of the 1,677 patients who received *Relafen* during U.S. clinical trials, 1,524 were treated for at least 1 month, 1,327 for at least 3 months, 929 for at least a year and 750 for at least 2 years. Over 300 patients have been treated for 5 years or longer.

The most frequently reported adverse reactions were related to the gastrointestinal tract. They were diarrhea, dyspepsia and abdominal pain.

Incidence ≥1% — Probably Causally Related

Gastrointestinal: Diarrhea (14%), dyspepsia (13%), abdominal pain (12%), constipation*, flatulence*, nausea*, positive stool guaiac*, dry mouth, gastritis, stomatitis, vomiting.

Central Nervous System: Dizziness*, headache*, fatigue, increased sweating, insomnia, nervousness, somnolence.

Dermatologic: Pruritus*, rash*.

Special Senses: Tinnitus*.

Miscellaneous: Edema*.

*Incidence of reported reaction between 3% and 9%. Reactions occurring in 1% to 3% of the patients are unmarked.

Incidence <1% — Probably Causally Related†

Gastrointestinal: Anorexia, cholestatic jaundice, duodenal ulcer, dysphagia, gastric ulcer, gastroenteritis, gastrointestinal bleeding, increased appetite, liver function abnormalities, melena.

Central Nervous System: Asthenia, agitation, anxiety, confusion, depression, malaise, paresthesia, tremor, vertigo.

Dermatologic: Bullous eruptions, photosensitivity, urticaria, pseudoporphyria cutanea tarda, *toxic epidermal necrolysis.*

Cardiovascular: Vasculitis.

Metabolic: Weight gain.

Respiratory: Dyspnea, *eosinophilic pneumonia, hypersensitivity pneumonitis.*

Genitourinary: Albuminuria, azotemia, *hyperuricemia, interstitial nephritis, nephrotic syndrome, vaginal bleeding.*

Special Senses: Abnormal vision.

Hypersensitivity: *Anaphylactoid reaction, anaphylaxis,* angioneurotic edema.

† Adverse reactions reported only in worldwide postmarketing experience or in the literature, not seen in clinical trials, are considered rarer and are italicized.

Incidence <1% — Causal Relationship Unknown‡

Gastrointestinal: Bilirubinuria, duodenitis, eructation, gallstones, gingivitis, glossitis, pancreatitis, rectal bleeding.

Central Nervous System: Nightmares.

Dermatologic: Acne, alopecia, *erythema multiforme, Stevens-Johnson Syndrome.*

Cardiovascular: Angina, arrhythmia, hypertension, myocardial infarction, palpitations, syncope, thrombophlebitis.

Respiratory: Asthma, cough.

Genitourinary: Dysuria, hematuria, impotence, renal stones.

Special Senses: Taste disorder.

Body as a Whole: Fever, chills.

Hematologic/Lymphatic: Anemia, leukopenia, granulocytopenia, thrombocytopenia.

Metabolic/Nutritional: Hyperglycemia, hypokalemia, weight loss.

‡ Adverse reactions reported only in worldwide postmarketing experience or in the literature, not seen in clinical trials, are considered rarer and are italicized.

OVERDOSAGE

Since only 1 case of Relafen (nabumetone) overdose has been reported, the experience is limited. If acute overdose occurs, it is recommended that the stomach be emptied by vomiting or lavage and general supportive measures be instituted, as necessary. In addition, the use of activated charcoal, up to 60 grams, may effectively reduce nabumetone absorption. Coadministration of nabumetone with charcoal to man has resulted in an 80% decrease in maximum plasma concentrations of the active metabolite.

The 1 overdose occurred in a 17-year-old female patient who had a history of abdominal pain and was hospitalized for increased abdominal pain following ingestion of 30 *Relafen* tablets (15 grams total). Stools were negative for occult blood and there was no fall in serum hemoglobin concentration. The patient had no other symptoms. She was given an H_2-receptor antagonist and discharged from the hospital without sequelae.

DOSAGE AND ADMINISTRATION

Osteoarthritis and Rheumatoid Arthritis

The recommended starting dose is 1000 mg taken as a single dose with or without food. Some patients may obtain more symptomatic relief from 1500 mg to 2000 mg per day. Relafen (nabumetone) can be given in either a single or twice-daily dose. Dosages over 2000 mg per day have not been studied. The lowest effective dose should be used for chronic treatment.

HOW SUPPLIED

Tablets: Oval-shaped, film-coated: 500 mg—white, imprinted with the product name RELAFEN and 500, in bottles of 100, and in Single Unit Packages of 100 (intended for institutional use only). 750 mg—beige, imprinted with the product name RELAFEN and 750, in bottles of 100, and in Single Unit Packages of 100 (intended for institutional use only).

Store at 25°C (77°F); excursions permitted to 15–30°C (59–86°F) in well-closed container; dispense in light-resistant container.

500 mg 100's: NDC 0029-4851-20
500 mg SUP 100's: NDC 0029-4851-21

750 mg 100's: NDC 0029-4852-20
750 mg SUP 100's: NDC 0029-4852-21

Rx only

RL:L9

Shown in Product Identification Guide, page 337

REQUIP® ℞

[ri-'kwip]
brand of
ropinirole hydrochloride
Tablets

DESCRIPTION

Requip (ropinirole hydrochloride), an orally administered anti-Parkinsonian drug, is a non-ergoline dopamine agonist. It is the hydrochloride salt of 4-[2-(dipropylamino)-ethyl]-1,3-dihydro-2H-indol-2-one monohydrochloride and has an empirical formula of $C_{16}H_{24}N_2O{\bullet}HCl$. The molecular weight is 296.84 (260.38 as the free base).

The structural formula is:

$N(CH_2CH_2CH_3)_2{\bullet}HCl$

ropinirole hydrochloride

Ropinirole hydrochloride is a white to pale greenish-yellow powder with a melting range of 243° to 250°C and a solubility of 133 mg/mL in water.

Each pentagonal film-coated Tiltab® tablet with beveled edges contains ropinirole hydrochloride equivalent to ropinirole, 0.25 mg, 0.5 mg, 1 mg, 2 mg, 4 mg or 5 mg. Inactive ingredients consist of: croscarmellose sodium, hydrous lactose, magnesium stearate, microcrystalline cellulose, and one or more of the following: FD&C Blue No. 2 aluminum lake, FD&C Yellow No. 6 aluminum lake, hydroxypropyl methylcellulose, iron oxides, polyethylene glycol, polysorbate 80, titanium dioxide.

CLINICAL PHARMACOLOGY

Mechanism of Action

Requip is a non-ergoline dopamine agonist with high relative *in vitro* specificity and full intrinsic activity at the D_2 and D_3 dopamine receptor subtypes, binding with higher affinity to D_3 than to D_2 or D_4 receptor subtypes. The relevance of D_3 receptor binding in Parkinson's disease is unknown.

Ropinirole has moderate *in vitro* affinity for opioid receptors. Ropinirole and its metabolites have negligible *in vitro* affinity for dopamine D_1, 5-HT_1, 5-HT_2, benzodiazepine, GABA, muscarinic, alpha$_1$-, alpha$_2$-, and beta-adrenoreceptors.

The precise mechanism of action of *Requip* as a treatment for Parkinson's disease is unknown, although it is believed to be due to stimulation of post-synaptic dopamine D_2-type receptors within the caudate-putamen in the brain. This conclusion is supported by studies that show that ropinirole improves motor function in various animal models of Parkinson's disease. In particular, ropinirole attenuates the motor deficits induced by lesioning the ascending nigrostriatal dopaminergic pathway with the neurotoxin 1-methyl-4-phenyl-1,2,3,6-tetrahydropyridine (MPTP) in primates.

Clinical Pharmacology Studies

In healthy normotensive subjects, single oral doses of *Requip* in the range 0.01 to 2.5 mg had little or no effect on supine blood pressure and pulse rates. Upon standing, *Requip* caused decreases in systolic and diastolic blood pressure at doses above 0.25 mg. In some subjects, these changes were associated with the emergence of orthostatic symptoms, bradycardia and, in one case, transient sinus arrest with syncope. The effect of repeat dosing and slow titration of *Requip* was not studied in healthy volunteers.

The mechanism of *Requip*-induced postural hypotension is presumed to be due to a D_2-mediated blunting of the noradrenergic response to standing and subsequent decrease in peripheral vascular resistance. Nausea is a common concomitant of orthostatic signs and symptoms.

At oral doses as low as 0.2 mg, *Requip* suppressed serum prolactin concentrations in healthy male volunteers.

Requip had no dose-related effect on ECG wave form and rhythm in young healthy male volunteers in the range of 0.01 to 2.5 mg.

Pharmacokinetics

Absorption, Distribution, Metabolism and Elimination

Ropinirole is rapidly absorbed after oral administration, reaching peak concentration in approximately 1-2 hours. In clinical studies, over 88% of a radiolabeled dose was recovered in urine and the absolute bioavailability was 55%, indicating a first pass effect. Relative bioavailability from a tablet compared to an oral solution is 85%. Food does not affect the extent of absorption of ropinirole, although its T_{max} is increased by 2.5 hours when the drug is taken with a meal. The clearance of ropinirole after oral administration to patients is 47 L/hr (cv=45%) and its elimination half-life is approximately 6 hours. Ropinirole is extensively metabolized by the liver to inactive metabolites and displays linear kinetics over the therapeutic dosing range of 1 mg to 8 mg t.i.d. Steady-state concentrations are expected to be achieved within 2 days of dosing. Accumulation upon multiple dosing is predictive from single dosing.

Ropinirole is widely distributed throughout the body, with an apparent volume of distribution of 7.5 L/kg (cv=32%). It is up to 40% bound to plasma proteins and has a blood-to-plasma ratio of 1:1.

The major metabolic pathways are N-despropylation and hydroxylation to form the inactive N-despropyl and hydroxy metabolites. *In vitro* studies indicate that the major cytochrome P_{450} isozyme involved in the metabolism of ropinirole is CYP1A2, an enzyme known to be stimulated by smoking and omeprazole, and inhibited by, for example, fluvoxamine, mexiletine, and the older fluoroquinolones, such as ciprofloxacin and norfloxacin. The N-despropyl metabolite is converted to carbamyl glucuronide, carboxylic acid, and N-despropyl hydroxy metabolites. The hydroxy metabolite of ropinirole is rapidly glucuronidated. Less than 10% of the administered dose is excreted as unchanged drug in urine. N-despropyl ropinirole is the predominant metabolite found in urine (40%), followed by the carboxylic acid metabolite (10%), and the glucuronide of the hydroxy metabolite (10%).

P_{450} Interaction: *In vitro* metabolism studies showed that CYP1A2 was the major enzyme responsible for the metabolism of ropinirole. There is thus the potential for inhibitors or substrates of this enzyme to alter its clearance when coadministered with ropinirole. Therefore, if therapy with a drug known to be a potent inhibitor of CYP1A2 is stopped or started during treatment with *Requip*, adjustment of the *Requip* dose may be required.

Population Subgroups

Because therapy with *Requip* is initiated at a subtherapeutic dosage and gradually titrated upward according to clinical tolerability to obtain the optimum therapeutic effect, adjustment of the initial dose based on gender, weight or age is not necessary.

Age: Oral clearance of ropinirole is reduced by 30% in patients above 65 years of age compared to younger patients. Dosage adjustment is not necessary in the elderly (above 65 years) as the dose of ropinirole is to be individually titrated to clinical response.

Gender: Female and male patients showed similar oral clearance.

Race: The influence of race on the pharmacokinetics of ropinirole has not been evaluated.

Cigarette Smoking: The effect of smoking on the oral clearance of ropinirole has not been evaluated. Smoking is expected to increase the clearance of ropinirole since CYP1A2 is known to be induced by smoking.

Renal Impairment: Based on population pharmacokinetic analysis, no difference was observed in the pharmacokinetics of ropinirole in patients with moderate renal impairment (creatinine clearance between 30 to 50 mL/min.) compared to an age-matched population with creatinine clearance above 50 mL/min. Therefore, no dosage adjustment is necessary in moderately renally impaired patients. The use of Requip (ropinirole hydrochloride) in patients with severe renal impairment has not been studied.

The effect of hemodialysis on drug removal is not known, but because of the relatively high apparent volume of distribution of ropinirole (525 L), the removal of the drug by hemodialysis is unlikely.

Hepatic Impairment: The pharmacokinetics of ropinirole have not been studied in hepatically impaired patients. These patients may have higher plasma levels and lower clearance of the drug than patients with normal hepatic function. The drug should be titrated with caution in this population.

Other Diseases: Population pharmacokinetic analysis revealed no change in the oral clearance of ropinirole in patients with concomitant diseases, such as hypertension, depression, osteoporosis/arthritis, and insomnia, compared to patients with Parkinson's disease only.

Clinical Trials

The effectiveness of *Requip* in the treatment of Parkinson's disease was evaluated in a multi-national drug development program consisting of 11 randomized, controlled trials. Four were conducted in patients with early Parkinson's disease and no concomitant L-dopa and 7 were conducted in patients with advanced Parkinson's disease with concomitant L-dopa.

Among these 11 studies, three placebo-controlled studies provide the most persuasive evidence of ropinirole's effectiveness in the management of patients with Parkinson's disease who were and were not receiving concomitant L-dopa. Two of these three trials enrolled patients with early Parkinson's disease (without L-dopa) and one enrolled patients receiving L-dopa.

In these studies a variety of measures were used to assess the effects of treatment (e.g., the Unified Parkinson's Disease Rating Scale [UPDRS], Clinical Global Impression scores, patient diaries recording time "on" and "off," and tolerability of L-dopa dose reductions).

In both studies of early Parkinson's disease (without L-dopa) patients, the motor component (Part III) of the UPDRS was the primary outcome assessment. The UPDRS is a four-part multi-item rating scale intended to evaluate mentation (Part I), activities of daily living (Part II), motor performance (Part III), and complications of therapy (Part IV). Part III of the UPDRS contains 14 items designed to assess the severity of the cardinal motor findings in patients with Parkinson's disease (e.g., tremor, rigidity, bradykinesia, postural instability, etc.) scored for different body regions and has a maximum (worst) score of 108. Responders were defined as patients with at least a 30% reduction in the Part III score.

In the study of advanced Parkinson's disease (with L-dopa) patients, both reduction in percent awake time spent "off" and the ability to reduce the daily use of L-dopa were assessed as a combined endpoint and individually.

Studies in Patients with Early Parkinson's Disease (without L-dopa)

One early therapy study was a 12-week multicenter study in which 63 patients (41 on *Requip*) with idiopathic Parkinson's disease receiving concomitant anti-Parkinson medication (but not L-dopa) were randomized to either *Requip* or placebo. Patients had a mean disease duration of approximately 2 years. Patients were eligible for enrollment if they presented with bradykinesia and at least tremor, rigidity, or postural instability. In addition, they must have been classified as Hoehn & Yahr Stage I-IV. This scale, ranging from I=unilateral involvement with minimal impairment to V=confined to wheelchair or bed, is a standard instrument used for staging patients with Parkinson's disease. The primary outcome measure in this trial was the proportion of patients experiencing a decrease (compared to baseline) of at least 30% in the UPDRS motor score.

Patients were titrated for up to 10 weeks, starting at 0.5 mg b.i.d., with weekly increments of 0.5 mg b.i.d. to a maximum of 5 mg b.i.d. Once patients reached their maximally tolerated dose (or 5 mg b.i.d.), they were maintained on that dose through 12 weeks. The mean dose achieved by patients at study endpoint was 7.4 mg/day. At the end of 12 weeks, 71% of *Requip*-treated patients were responders, compared with 41% of patients in the placebo group (p=0.021).

Statistically significant differences between the percentage of responders on *Requip* compared to placebo were seen after 8 weeks of treatment.

In addition, the mean percentage improvement from baseline in the Total Motor Score was 43% in *Requip*-treated patients compared with 21% in placebo-treated patients (p=0.018).

Statistically significant differences in UPDRS motor score between *Requip* and placebo were seen after 2 weeks of treatment.

The median daily dose at which a 30% reduction in UPDRS motor score was sustained was 4 mg.

The second trial in early Parkinson's disease (without L-dopa) patients was a double-blind, randomized, placebo-controlled 6-month study. Patients were essentially similar to those in the study described above; concomitant use of selegiline was allowed, but patients were not permitted to use anticholinergics or amantadine during the study. Patients had a mean disease duration of 2 years and limited (not more than a 6-week period) or no prior exposure to L-dopa. The starting dose of *Requip* in this trial was 0.25 mg t.i.d. The dose was titrated at weekly intervals by increments of 0.25 mg t.i.d. to a dose of 1.0 mg t.i.d. Further titrations at weekly intervals were at increments of 0.5 mg t.i.d. up to a dose of 3.0 mg t.i.d and then weekly at increments of 1.0 mg t.i.d. Patients were to be titrated to a dose of at least 1.5 mg t.i.d. and then to their maximally tolerated dose, up to a maximum of 8.0 mg t.i.d. The mean dose attained in patients at study endpoint was 15.7 mg/day.

The primary measure of effectiveness was the mean percent reduction (improvement) from baseline in the UPDRS Motor Score. In this study 241 patients were enrolled. At the end of the 6-month study, *Requip*-treated patients had 22% improvement in motor score, compared with a 4% worsening in the placebo group ($p<0.001$).

Table 1: Treatment-Emergent Adverse Event[1] Incidence in Double-blind, Placebo-controlled Early Parkinson's Disease (without L-dopa) Trials (Events ≥2% of Patients Treated with *Requip* and Numerically More Frequent than the Placebo Group)

	Requip N = 157 (%)	Placebo N = 147 (%)
Autonomic Nervous System		
Flushing	3	1
Dry Mouth	5	3
Increased Sweating	6	4
Body as a Whole		
Asthenia	6	1
Chest Pain	4	2
Dependent Edema	6	3
Leg Edema	7	1
Fatigue	11	4
Malaise	3	1
Pain	8	4
Cardiovascular General		
Hypertension	5	3
Hypotension	2	0
Orthostatic Symptoms	6	5
Syncope	12	1
Central/Peripheral Nervous System		
Dizziness	40	22
Hyperkinesia	2	1
Hypesthesia	4	2
Vertigo	2	0
Gastrointestinal System		
Abdominal Pain	6	3
Anorexia	4	1
Dyspepsia	10	5
Flatulence	3	1
Nausea	60	22
Vomiting	12	7
Heart Rate/Rhythm		
Extrasystoles	2	1
Atrial Fibrillation	2	0
Palpitation	3	2
Tachycardia	2	0

Statistically significant differences in UPDRS motor score improvement between *Requip* and placebo were seen after 12 weeks of treatment.

Study in Patients with Advanced Parkinson's Disease (with L-dopa)

This double-blind, randomized, placebo-controlled 6-month trial evaluated 148 patients (Hoehn & Yahr II-IV) who were not adequately controlled on L-dopa. Patients in this study had a mean disease duration of approximately 9 years, had been exposed to L-dopa for approximately 7 years, and had experienced "on-off" periods with L-dopa therapy. Patients previously receiving stable doses of selegiline, amantadine and/or anticholinergic agents could continue on these agents during the study. Patients were started at a *Requip* dose of 0.25 mg t.i.d. and titrated upward by weekly intervals until an optimal therapeutic response was achieved. The maximum dose of study medication was 8 mg t.i.d. All patients had to be titrated to at least a dose of 2.5 mg t.i.d. Patients could then be maintained on this dose level or higher for the remainder of the study. Once a dose of 2.5 mg t.i.d. was achieved, patients underwent a mandatory reduction in their L-dopa dose, to be followed by additional mandatory reductions with continued escalation of the *Requip* dose. Reductions in the dosage of L-dopa were also allowed if patients experienced adverse events that the investigator considered related to dopaminergic therapy. The mean dose attained at study endpoint was 16.3 mg/day. The primary outcome was the proportion of responders, defined as patients who were able both to achieve a decrease (compared to baseline) of at least 20% in their L-dopa dose and a decrease of at least 20% in the proportion of the time awake in the "off" condition (a period of time during the day when patients are particularly immobile), as determined by patient diary. In addition, the mean percent change from baseline in daily L-dopa dose was examined.

At the end of 6 months, 28% of *Requip*-treated patients were classified as responders (based on combined endpoint) while 11% of placebo-treated patients were responders (p=0.02). Based on the protocol-mandated reductions in L-dopa dosage with escalating *Requip* doses, *Requip*-treated patients had a 19.4% mean reduction in L-dopa dose while placebo-treated patients had a 3% reduction ($p<0.001$). L-dopa dosage reduction was also allowed during the study if dyskinesias or other dopaminergic effects occurred. Overall, reduction of L-dopa dose was sustained in 87% of *Requip*-treated

Continued on next page

Information on the SmithKline Beecham Pharmaceuticals products appearing here is based on the labeling in effect on June 15, 2000. Further information on these and other products may be obtained from the Medical Department, SmithKline Beecham Pharmaceuticals, One Franklin Plaza, Philadelphia, PA 19101.

Requip—Cont.

patients and in 57% of patients on placebo. On average, the L-dopa dose was reduced by 31% in *Requip*-treated patients. The mean number of "off" hours per day during baseline was 6.4 hours for *Requip*-treated patients and 7.3 hours for patients treated with placebo. At the end of the 6-month study, patients treated with *Requip* had a mean of 4.9 hours per day of "off" time, while placebo-treated patients had a mean of 6.4 hours per day of "off" time.

INDICATIONS AND USAGE

Requip (ropinirole hydrochloride) is indicated for the treatment of the signs and symptoms of idiopathic Parkinson's disease.

The effectiveness of *Requip* was demonstrated in randomized, controlled trials in patients with early Parkinson's disease who were not receiving concomitant L-dopa therapy as well as in patients with advanced disease on concomitant L-dopa (see CLINICAL PHARMACOLOGY, Clinical Trials).

CONTRAINDICATIONS

Requip is contraindicated for patients known to have hypersensitivity to the product.

WARNINGS

Falling Asleep During Activities of Daily Living:

Patients treated with *Requip* have reported falling asleep while engaged in activities of daily living, including the operation of motor vehicles which sometimes resulted in accidents. Although many of these patients reported somnolence while on *Requip*, some perceived that they had no warning signs such as excessive drowsiness, and believed that they were alert prior to the event. Some of these events have been reported as late as one year after initiation of treatment.

Somnolence is a common occurrence in patients receiving *Requip*. Many clinical experts believe that falling asleep while engaged in activities of daily living always occurs in a setting of pre-existing somnolence although patients may not give such a history. For this reason, prescribers should continually reassess patients for drowsiness or sleepiness especially since some of the events occur well after the start of treatment. Prescribers should also be aware that patients may not acknowledge drowsiness or sleepiness until directly questioned about drowsiness or sleepiness during specific activities.

Before initiating treatment with *Requip*, patients should be advised of the potential to develop drowsiness and specifically asked about factors that may increase the risk with *Requip* such as concomitant sedating medications, the presence of sleep disorders, and concomitant medications that increase ropinirole plasma levels (e.g., ciprofloxacin—see PRECAUTIONS, Drug Interactions). If a patient develops significant daytime sleepiness or episodes of falling asleep during activities that require active participation (e.g., conversations, eating, etc.), *Requip* should ordinarily be discontinued. [See DOSAGE AND ADMINISTRATION for guidance in discontinuing *Requip*.] If a decision is made to continue *Requip*, patients should be advised to not drive and to avoid other potentially dangerous activities. There is insufficient information to establish that dose reduction will eliminate episodes of falling asleep while engaged in activities of daily living.

Syncope

Syncope, sometimes associated with bradycardia, was observed in association with ropinirole in both early Parkinson's disease (without L-dopa) patients and advanced Parkinson's disease (with L-dopa) patients. In the two double-blind placebo-controlled studies of *Requip* in patients with Parkinson's disease who were not being treated with L-dopa, 11.5% (18 of 157) of patients on *Requip* had syncope compared to 1.4% (2 of 147) of patients on placebo. Most of these cases occurred more than 4 weeks after initiation of therapy with *Requip*, and were usually associated with a recent increase in dose.

Of 208 patients being treated with both L-dopa and *Requip*, in placebo-controlled advanced Parkinson's disease trials, there were reports of syncope in 6 (2.9%) compared to 2 of 120 (1.7%) of placebo/L-dopa patients.

Because the studies of *Requip* excluded patients with significant cardiovascular disease, it is not known to what extent the estimated incidence figures apply to Parkinson's disease patients as a whole. Therefore, patients with severe cardiovascular disease should be treated with caution.

Two of 47 Parkinson's disease patient volunteers enrolled in phase 1 studies had syncope following a 1 mg dose. In phase 1 studies including 110 healthy volunteers, one patient developed hypotension, bradycardia, and sinus arrest of 26 seconds accompanied by syncope; the patient recovered spontaneously without intervention. One other healthy volunteer reported syncope.

Symptomatic Hypotension

Dopamine agonists, in clinical studies and clinical experience, appear to impair the systemic regulation of blood pressure, with resulting postural hypotension, especially during dose escalation. Parkinson's disease patients, in addition, appear to have an impaired capacity to respond to a postural challenge. For these reasons, Parkinson's patients being treated with dopaminergic agonists ordinarily (1) require careful monitoring for signs and symptoms of postural hypotension, especially during dose escalation, and (2) should be informed of this risk (see PRECAUTIONS, Information for Patients).

Table 1: Treatment-Emergent Adverse Event[1] Incidence in Double-blind, Placebo-controlled Early Parkinson's Disease (without L-dopa) Trials (Events ≥2% of Patients Treated with *Requip* and Numerically More Frequent than the Placebo Group)

	Requip N = 157 (%)	Placebo N = 147 (%)
Metabolic/Nutritional		
Increased Alkaline Phosphatase	3	1
Psychiatric		
Amnesia	3	1
Impaired Concentration	2	0
Confusion	5	1
Hallucination	5	1
Somnolence	40	6
Yawning	3	0
Reproductive Male		
Impotence	3	1
Resistance Mechanism		
Viral Infection	11	3
Respiratory System		
Bronchitis	3	1
Dyspnea	3	0
Pharyngitis	6	4
Rhinitis	4	3
Sinusitis	4	3
Urinary System		
Urinary Tract Infection	5	4
Vascular Extracardiac		
Peripheral Ischemia	3	0
Vision		
Eye Abnormality	3	1
Abnormal Vision	6	3
Xerophthalmia	2	0

1. Patients may have reported multiple adverse experiences during the study or at discontinuation; thus, patients may be included in more than one category.

Although the clinical trials were not designed to systematically monitor blood pressure, there were individual reported cases of postural hypotension in early Parkinson's disease (without L-dopa) *Requip*-treated patients. Most of these cases occurred more than 4 weeks after initiation of therapy with *Requip*, and were usually associated with a recent increase in dose.

In phase 1 studies of *Requip* that included 110 healthy volunteers, nine subjects had documented symptomatic postural hypotension. These episodes appeared mainly at doses above 0.8 mg and these doses are higher than the starting doses recommended for Parkinson's disease patients. In eight of these nine individuals, the hypotension was accompanied by bradycardia, but did not develop into syncope. (See Syncope above.) None of these events resulted in death or hospitalization.

One of 47 Parkinson's disease patient volunteers enrolled in phase 1 studies had documented hypotension following a 2 mg dose on two occasions.

Hallucinations

In double-blind, placebo-controlled, early therapy studies in patients with Parkinson's disease who were not treated with L-dopa, 5.2% (8 of 157) of patients treated with *Requip* reported hallucinations, compared to 1.4% of patients on placebo (2 of 147). Among those patients receiving both *Requip* and L-dopa, in advanced Parkinson's disease (with L-dopa) studies, 10.1% (21 of 208) were reported to experience hallucinations, compared to 4.2% (5 of 120) of patients treated with placebo and L-dopa.

Hallucinations were of sufficient severity to cause discontinuation of treatment in 1.3% of the early Parkinson's disease (without L-dopa) patients and 1.9% of the advanced Parkinson's disease (with L-dopa) patients compared to 0% and 1.7% of placebo patients, respectively.

PRECAUTIONS

General

Dyskinesia: *Requip* may potentiate the dopaminergic side effects of L-dopa and may cause and/or exacerbate pre-existing dyskinesia. Decreasing the dose of L-dopa may ameliorate this side effect.

Renal and Hepatic: No dosage adjustment is needed in patients with mild to moderate renal impairment (creatinine clearance of 30 to 50 mL/min.). Because the use of *Requip* in patients with severe renal or hepatic impairment has not been studied, administration of *Requip* to such patients should be carried out with caution.

Events Reported with Dopaminergic Therapy:

Withdrawal Emergent Hyperpyrexia and Confusion: Although not reported with *Requip*, a symptom complex resembling the neuroleptic malignant syndrome (characterized by elevated temperature, muscular rigidity, altered consciousness, and autonomic instability), with no other obvious etiology, has been reported in association with rapid dose reduction, withdrawal of, or changes in anti-Parkinsonian therapy.

Fibrotic Complications: Cases of retroperitoneal fibrosis, pulmonary infiltrates, pleural effusion, and pleural thickening have been reported in some patients treated with ergot-derived dopaminergic agents. While these complications may resolve when the drug is discontinued, complete resolution does not always occur.

Although these adverse events are believed to be related to the ergoline structure of these compounds, whether other, nonergot derived dopamine agonists can cause them is unknown.

In the *Requip* development program, a 69-year-old man with obstructive lung disease was treated with *Requip* for 16 months and developed pleural thickening and effusion accompanied by lower extremity edema, cardiomegaly, pleuritic pain, and shortness of breath. Pleural biopsy demonstrated chronic inflammation and sclerosis. The effusion resolved after medical therapy and discontinuation of *Requip*. The patient was lost to follow-up. The relationship of these events to Requip (ropinirole hydrochloride) cannot be established.

Retinal pathology in albino rats: Retinal degeneration was observed in albino rats in the 2-year carcinogenicity study at all doses tested (equivalent to 0.6 to 20 times the maximum recommended human dose on a mg/m^2 basis), but was statistically significant at the highest dose (50 mg/kg/

day). Additional studies to further evaluate the specific pathology (e.g., loss of photoreceptor cells) have not been performed. Similar changes were not observed in a 2-year carcinogenicity study in albino mice or in rats or monkeys treated for 1 year.
The potential significance of this effect in humans has not been established, but cannot be disregarded because disruption of a mechanism that is universally present in vertebrates (e.g., disk shedding) may be involved.
Binding to melanin: *Requip* binds to melanin-containing tissues (i.e., eyes, skin) in pigmented rats. After a single dose, long-term retention of drug was demonstrated, with a half-life in the eye of 20 days. It is not known if *Requip* accumulates in these tissues over time.

Information for Patients

Patients should be instructed to take *Requip* only as prescribed.
Requip can be taken with or without food. Since ingestion with food reduces the maximum concentration (C_{max}) of *Requip*, patients should be advised that taking *Requip* with food may reduce the occurrence of nausea. However, this has not been established in controlled clinical trials.
Patients should be informed that hallucinations can occur, and that the elderly are at a higher risk than younger patients with Parkinson's disease.
Patients should be advised that they may develop postural (orthostatic) hypotension with or without symptoms such as dizziness, nausea, syncope, and sometimes sweating. Hypotension and/or orthostatic symptoms may occur more frequently during initial therapy or with an increase in dose at any time (cases have been seen after weeks of treatment). Accordingly, patients should be cautioned against rising rapidly after sitting or lying down, especially if they have been doing so for prolonged periods, and especially at the initiation of treatment with *Requip*.
Patients should be alerted to the potential sedating effects associated with *Requip* including somnolence and the possibility of falling asleep while engaged in activities of daily living. Since somnolence is a frequent adverse event with potentially serious consequences, patients should neither drive a car nor engage in other potentially dangerous activities until they have gained sufficient experience with *Requip* to gauge whether or not it affects their mental and/or motor performance adversely. Patients should be advised that if increased somnolence or episodes of falling asleep during activities of daily living (e.g., watching television, passenger in a car, etc.) are experienced at any time during treatment, they should not drive or participate in potentially dangerous activities until they have contacted their physician. Because of possible additive effects, caution should be advised when patients are taking other sedating medications or alcohol in combination with *Requip* and when taking concomitant medications that increase plasma levels of ropinirole (e.g., ciprofloxacin).
Because of the possible additive sedative effects, caution should also be used when patients are taking alcohol or other CNS depressants (e.g., benzodiazepines, antipsychotics, antidepressants, etc.) in combination with *Requip*.
Because of the possibility that ropinirole may be excreted in breast milk, patients should be advised to notify their physicians if they intend to breast-feed or are breast-feeding an infant.
Because ropinirole has been shown to have adverse effects on embryo-fetal development, including teratogenic effects, in animals, and because experience in humans is limited, patients should be advised to notify their physician if they become pregnant or intend to become pregnant during therapy (see PRECAUTIONS, Pregnancy).

Drug Interactions

P_{450} Interaction: *In vitro* metabolism studies showed that CYP1A2 was the major enzyme responsible for the metabolism of ropinirole. There is thus the potential for substrates or inhibitors of this enzyme when coadministered with ropinirole to alter its clearance. Therefore, if therapy with a drug known to be a potent inhibitor of CYP1A2 is stopped or started during treatment with *Requip*, adjustment of the *Requip* dose may be required.
L-dopa: Co-administration of carbidopa + L-dopa (Sinemet® 10/100 mg b.i.d.) with ropinirole (2.0 mg t.i.d.) had no effect on the steady-state pharmacokinetics of ropinirole (n=28 patients). Oral administration of *Requip* 2.0 mg t.i.d. increased mean steady state C_{max} of L-dopa by 20% but its AUC was unaffected (n=23 patients).
Digoxin: Co-administration of *Requip* (2.0 mg t.i.d.) with digoxin (0.125–0.25 mg q.d.) did not alter the steady-state pharmacokinetics of digoxin in 10 patients.
Theophylline: Administration of theophylline (300 mg b.i.d., a substrate of CYP1A2) did not alter the steady-state pharmacokinetics of ropinirole (2 mg t.i.d.) in 12 patients with Parkinson's disease. Ropinirole (2 mg t.i.d.) did not alter the pharmacokinetics of theophylline (5 mg/kg i.v.) in 12 patients with Parkinson's disease.
Ciprofloxacin: Co-administration of ciprofloxacin (500 mg b.i.d.), an inhibitor of CYP1A2, with ropinirole (2 mg t.i.d.) increased ropinirole AUC by 84% on average, and C_{max} by 60% (n=12 patients).
Estrogens: Population pharmacokinetic analysis revealed that estrogens (mainly ethinylestradiol: intake 0.6–3 mg over 4-month to 23-year period) reduced the oral clearance of ropinirole by 36% in 16 patients. Dosage adjustment may not be needed for *Requip* in patients on estrogen therapy because patients must be carefully titrated with ropinirole to tolerance or adequate effect. However, if estrogen therapy is stopped or started during treatment with *Requip*, then adjustment of the Requip (ropinirole hydrochloride) dose may be required.
Dopamine Antagonists: Since ropinirole is a dopamine agonist, it is possible that dopamine antagonists, such as neuroleptics (phenothiazines, butyrophenones, thioxanthenes) or metoclopramide, may diminish the effectiveness of *Requip*. Patients with major psychotic disorders, treated with neuroleptics, should only be treated with dopamine agonists if the potential benefits outweigh the risks.
Population analysis showed that commonly administered drugs, e.g., selegiline, amantadine, tricyclic antidepressants, benzodiazepines, ibuprofen, thiazides, antihistamines, and anticholinergics did not affect the oral clearance of ropinirole.

Carcinogenesis, Mutagenesis, Impairment of Fertility

Two-year carcinogenicity studies were conducted in Charles River CD-1 mice at doses of 5, 15, and 50 mg/kg/day and in Sprague-Dawley rats at doses of 1.5, 15, and 50 mg/kg/day (top doses equivalent to 10 times and 20 times, respectively, the maximum recommended human dose of 24 mg/day on a mg/m² basis). In the male rat, there was a significant increase in testicular Leydig cell adenomas at all doses tested, i.e., ≥1.5 mg/kg (0.6 times the maximum recommended human dose on a mg/m² basis). This finding is of questionable significance because the endocrine mechanisms believed to be involved in the production of Leydig cell hyperplasia and

Continued on next page

Table 2: Treatment-Emergent Adverse Event[1] Incidence in Double-blind, Placebo-controlled Advanced Parkinson's Disease (with L-dopa) Trials (Events ≥2% of Patients Treated with *Requip* and Numerically More Frequent than the Placebo Group)

	Requip N = 208 (%)	Placebo N = 120 (%)
Autonomic Nervous System		
Dry Mouth	5	1
Increased Sweating	7	2
Body as a Whole		
Increased Drug Level	7	3
Pain	5	3
Cardiovascular General		
Hypotension	2	1
Syncope	3	2
Central/Peripheral Nervous System		
Dizziness	26	16
Dyskinesia	34	13
Falls	10	7
Headache	17	12
Hypokinesia	5	4
Paresis	3	0
Paresthesia	5	3
Tremor	6	3
Gastrointestinal System		
Abdominal Pain	9	8
Constipation	6	3
Diarrhea	5	3
Dysphagia	2	1
Flatulence	2	1
Nausea	30	18
Increased Saliva	2	1
Vomiting	7	4
Metabolic/Nutritional		
Weight Decrease	2	1
Musculoskeletal System		
Arthralgia	7	5
Arthritis	3	1
Psychiatric		
Amnesia	5	1
Anxiety	6	3
Confusion	9	2
Abnormal Dreaming	3	2
Hallucination	10	4
Nervousness	5	3
Somnolence	20	8

Information on the SmithKline Beecham Pharmaceuticals products appearing here is based on the labeling in effect on June 15, 2000. Further information on these and other products may be obtained from the Medical Department, SmithKline Beecham Pharmaceuticals, One Franklin Plaza, Philadelphia, PA 19101.

Requip—Cont.

adenomas in rats are not relevant to humans. In the female mouse, there was an increase in benign uterine endometrial polyps at a dose of 50 mg/kg/day (10 times the maximum recommended human dose on a mg/m^2 basis).

Ropinirole was not mutagenic or clastogenic in the *in vitro* Ames test, the *in vitro* chromosome aberration test in human lymphocytes, the *in vitro* mouse lymphoma (L1578Y cells) assay, and the *in vivo* mouse micronucleus test.

When administered to female rats prior to and during mating and throughout pregnancy, ropinirole caused disruption of implantation at doses of 20 mg/kg/day (8 times the maximum recommended human dose on a mg/m^2 basis) or greater. This effect is thought to be due to the prolactin-lowering effect of ropinirole. In humans, chorionic gonadotropin, not prolactin, is essential for implantation. In rat studies using low doses (5 mg/kg) during the prolactin-dependent phase of early pregnancy (gestation days 0–8), ropinirole did not affect female fertility at dosages up to 100 mg/kg/day (40 times the maximum recommended human dose on a mg/m^2 basis). No effect on male fertility was observed in rats at dosages up to 125 mg/kg/day (50 times the maximum recommended human dose on a mg/m^2 basis).

Pregnancy

Pregnancy Category C: In animal reproduction studies, ropinirole has been shown to have adverse effects on embryo-fetal development, including teratogenic effects. Ropinirole given to pregnant rats during organogenesis (20 mg/kg on gestation days 6 and 7 followed by 20, 60, 90, 120 or 150 mg/kg on gestation days 8 through 15) resulted in decreased fetal body weight at 60 mg/kg/day, increased fetal death at 90 mg/kg/day, and digital malformations at 150 mg/kg/day (24, 36 and 60 times the maximum recommended clinical dose on a mg/m^2 basis, respectively). The combined administration of ropinirole (10 mg/kg/day; 8 times the maximum recommended human dose on a mg/m^2 basis) and L-dopa (250 mg/kg/day) to pregnant rabbits during organogenesis produced a greater incidence and severity of fetal malformations (primarily digit defects) than were seen in the offspring of rabbits treated with L-dopa alone. No indication of an effect on development of the conceptus was observed in rabbits when a maternally toxic dose of ropinirole was administered alone (20 mg/kg/day: 16 times the maximum recommended human dose on a mg/m^2 basis). In a perinatal-postnatal study in rats, 10 mg/kg/day (4 times the maximum recommended human dose on a mg/m^2 basis) of ropinirole impaired growth and development of nursing offspring and altered neurological development of female offspring.

There are no adequate and well-controlled studies using *Requip* in pregnant women. *Requip* should be used during pregnancy only if the potential benefit outweighs the potential risk to the fetus.

Nursing Mothers

Requip inhibits prolactin secretion in humans and could potentially inhibit lactation.

Studies in rats have shown that *Requip* and/or its metabolite(s) is excreted in breast milk. It is not known whether this drug is excreted in human milk. Because many drugs are excreted in human milk and because of the potential for serious adverse reactions in nursing infants from *Requip*, a decision should be made whether to discontinue nursing or to discontinue the drug, taking into account the importance of the drug to the mother.

Pediatric Use

Safety and effectiveness in the pediatric population have not been established.

ADVERSE REACTIONS

During the pre-marketing development of *Requip*, patients received *Requip* either without L-dopa (early Parkinson's disease studies) or as concomitant therapy with L-dopa (advanced Parkinson's disease studies). Because these 2 populations may have differential risks for various adverse events, this section will, in general, present adverse event data for these 2 populations separately.

Early Parkinson's Disease (without L-dopa)

The most commonly observed adverse events (>5%) in the double-blind, placebo-controlled early Parkinson's disease trials associated with the use of *Requip* (n=157) not seen at an equivalent frequency among the placebo-treated patients (n=147) were, in order of decreasing incidence: nausea, dizziness, somnolence, headache, vomiting, syncope, fatigue, dyspepsia, viral infection, constipation, pain, increased sweating, asthenia, dependent/leg edema, orthostatic symptoms, abdominal pain, pharyngitis, confusion, hallucinations, urinary tract infections, and abnormal vision.

Approximately 24% of 157 *Requip*-treated patients who participated in the double-blind, placebo-controlled early Parkinson's disease (without L-dopa) trials discontinued treatment due to adverse events compared to 13% of 147 patients who received placebo. The adverse events most commonly causing discontinuation of treatment by *Requip*-treated patients were: nausea (6.4%), dizziness (3.8%), aggravated Parkinson's disease (1.3%), hallucinations (1.3%), somnolence (1.3%), vomiting (1.3%) and headache (1.3%). Of these, hallucinations appear to be dose-related. While other adverse events leading to discontinuation may be dose-related, the titration design utilized in these trials precluded an adequate assessment of the dose response. For example, in the larger of the 2 trials described in CLINICAL PHARMACOLOGY, Clinical Trials, the difference in the rate of discontinuations emerged only after 10 weeks of treatment, suggesting, although not proving, that the effect could be related to dose.

Adverse Event Incidence in Controlled Clinical Studies

Table 1 lists treatment-emergent adverse events that occurred in ≥2% of patients with early Parkinson's disease (without L-dopa) treated with *Requip* participating in the double-blind, placebo-controlled studies and were numerically more common in the *Requip* group. In these studies, either Requip (ropinirole hydrochloride) or placebo was used as early therapy (i.e., without L-dopa).

The prescriber should be aware that these figures cannot be used to predict the incidence of adverse events in the course of usual medical practice where patient characteristics and other factors differ from those that prevailed in the clinical studies. Similarly, the cited frequencies cannot be compared with figures obtained from other clinical investigations involving different treatments, uses and investigators. However, the cited figures do provide the prescribing physician with some basis for estimating the relative contribution of drug and non-drug factors to the adverse-events incidence rate in the population studied.

[See table 1 on pages 3123 and 3124]

Other events reported by 1% or more of early Parkinson's disease (without L-dopa) patients treated with *Requip*, but that were equally or more frequent in the placebo group were: headache, upper respiratory infection, insomnia, arthralgia, tremor, back pain, anxiety, dyskinesias, aggravated Parkinsonism, depression, falls, myalgia, leg cramps, paresthesias, nervousness, diarrhea, arthritis, hot flushes, weight loss, rash, cough, hyperglycemia, muscle spasm, arthrosis, abnormal dreams, dystonia, increased salivation, bradycardia, gout, basal cell carcinoma, gingivitis, hematuria, and rigors.

Table 2: Treatment-Emergent Adverse Event[1] Incidence in Double-blind, Placebo-controlled Advanced Parkinson's Disease (with L-dopa) Trials (Events ≥2% of Patients Treated with *Requip* and Numerically More Frequent than the Placebo Group)

	Requip N = 208 (%)	Placebo N = 120 (%)
Red Blood Cell		
Anemia	2	0
Resistance Mechanism		
Upper Repiratory Tract Infection	9	8
Respiratory System		
Dyspnea	3	2
Urinary System		
Pyuria	2	1
Urinary Incontinence	2	1
Urinary Tract Infection	6	3
Vision		
Diplopia	2	1

1. Patients may have reported multiple adverse experiences during the study or at discontinuation; thus, patients may be included in more than one category.

Among the treatment-emergent adverse events in patients treated with *Requip*, hallucinations appear to be dose-related.

The incidence of adverse events was not materially different between women and men.

Advanced Parkinson's Disease (with L-dopa)

The most commonly observed adverse events (>5%), in the double-blind, placebo-controlled advanced Parkinson's disease (with L-dopa) trials associated with the use of *Requip* (n = 208) as an adjunct to L-dopa not seen at an equivalent frequency among the placebo-treated patients (n = 120) were, in order of decreasing incidence: dyskinesias, nausea, dizziness, aggravated Parkinsonism, somnolence, headache, insomnia, injury, hallucinations, falls, abdominal pain, upper respiratory infection, confusion, increased sweating, vomiting, viral infection, increased drug level, arthralgia, tremor, anxiety, urinary tract infection, constipation, dry mouth, pain, hypokinesia, and paresthesia.

Approximately 24% of 208 patients who received Requip (ropinirole hydrochloride) in the double-blind, placebo-controlled advanced Parkinson's disease (with L-dopa) trials discontinued treatment due to adverse events compared to 18% of 120 patients who received placebo. The events most commonly (≥1%) causing discontinuation of treatment by *Requip*-treated patients were: dizziness (2.9%), dyskinesias (2.4%), vomiting (2.4%), confusion (2.4%), nausea (1.9%), hallucinations (1.9%), anxiety (1.9%), and increased sweating (1.4%). Of these, hallucinations and dyskinesias appear to be dose-related.

Adverse Event Incidence in Controlled Clinical Studies

Table 2 lists treatment-emergent adverse events that occurred in ≥2% of patients with advanced Parkinson's disease (with L-dopa) treated with *Requip* who participated in the double-blind, placebo-controlled studies and were numerically more common in the *Requip* group. In these studies, either *Requip* or placebo was used as an adjunct to L-dopa. Adverse events were usually mild or moderate in intensity.

The prescriber should be aware that these figures cannot be used to predict the incidence of adverse events in the course of usual medical practice where patient characteristics and other factors differ from those that prevailed in the clinical studies. Similarly, the cited frequencies cannot be compared with figures obtained from other clinical investigations involving different treatments, uses, and investigators. However, the cited figures do provide the prescribing physician with some basis for estimating the relative contribution of drug and non-drug factors to the adverse-events incidence rate in the population studied.

[See table 2 on previous page and below]

Other events reported by 1% or more of patients treated with both *Requip* and L-dopa, but equally or more frequent in the placebo/L-dopa group were: myocardial infarction, orthostatic symptoms, virus infections, asthenia, dyspepsia, myalgia, back pain, depression, leg cramps, fatigue, rhinitis, chest pain, hematuria, vertigo, tinnitus, leg edema, hot flushes, abnormal gait, hyperkinesia, and pharyngitis.

Among the treatment-emergent adverse events in patients treated with *Requip*, hallucinations and dyskinesias appear to be dose-related.

Other Adverse Events Observed During All Phase 2/3 Clinical Trials: *Requip* has been administered to 1,599 individuals in clinical trials. During these trials, all adverse events were recorded by the clinical investigators using terminology of their own choosing. To provide a meaningful estimate of the proportion of individuals having adverse events, similar types of events were grouped into a smaller number of standardized categories using modified WHOART dictionary terminology. These categories are used in the listing below. The frequencies presented represent the proportion of the 1,599 individuals exposed to *Requip* who experienced events of the type cited on at least one occasion while receiving *Requip*. All reported events that occurred at least twice (or once for serious or potentially serious events), except those already listed above, trivial events, and terms too vague to be meaningful are included, without regard to determination of a causal relationship to Requip (ropinirole hydrochloride), except that events very unlikely to be drug-related have been deleted.

Events are further classified within body system categories and enumerated in order of decreasing frequency using the following definitions: frequent adverse events are defined as those occurring in at least 1/100 patients and infrequent adverse events are those occurring in 1/100 to 1/1000 patients and rare events are those occurring in fewer than 1/1000 patients.

Body as a Whole: *infrequent* — cellulitis, peripheral edema, fever, influenza-like symptoms, enlarged abdomen, precordial chest pain, and generalized edema; *rare* — ascites.

Cardiovascular: *infrequent* — cardiac failure, bradycardia, tachycardia, supraventricular tachycardia, angina pectoris, bundle branch block, cardiac arrest, cardiomegaly, aneurysm, mitral insufficiency; *rare* — ventricular tachycardia.

Central/Peripheral Nervous System: *frequent* — neuralgia; *infrequent* — involuntary muscle contractions, hypertonia, dysphonia, abnormal coordination, extrapyramidal disorder, migraine, choreoathetosis, coma, stupor, aphasia, convulsions, hypotonia, peripheral neuropathy, paralysis; *rare* — grand mal convulsions, hemiparesis, hemiplegia.

Endocrine: *infrequent* — hypothyroidism, gynecomastia, hyperthyroidism; *rare* — goiter, SIADH.

Gastrointestinal: *infrequent* — increased hepatic enzymes, bilirubinemia, cholecystitis, cholelithiasis colitis, dysphagia, periodontitis, fecal incontinence, gastroesophageal reflux, hemorrhoids, toothache, eructation, gastritis, esophagitis, hiccups, diverticulitis, duodenal ulcer, gastric ulcer, melena, duodenitis, gastrointestinal hemorrhage, glossitis, rectal hemorrhage, pancreatitis, stomatitis and ulcerative stomatitis, tongue edema; *rare* — biliary pain, hemorrhagic gastritis, hematemesis, salivary duct obstruction.

Hematologic: *infrequent* — purpura, thrombocytopenia, hematoma, Vitamin B12 deficiency, hypochromic anemia, eosinophilia, leukocytosis, leukopenia, lymphocytosis, lymphopenia, lymphedema.

Metabolic/Nutritional: *frequent* — increased BUN; *infrequent* — hypoglycemia, increased alkaline phosphatase, increased LDH, weight increase, hyperphosphatemia, hyperuricemia, diabetes mellitus, glycosuria, hypokalemia, hypercholesterolemia, hyperkalemia, acidosis, hyponatremia, thirst, increased CPK, dehydration; *rare* — hypochloremia.

Musculoskeletal: *infrequent* — aggravated arthritis, tendinitis, osteoporosis, bursitis, polymyalgia rheumatica, muscle weakness, skeletal pain, torticollis; *rare* — Dupuytren's contracture requiring surgery.

Neoplasm: *infrequent* — malignant breast neoplasm; *rare* — bladder carcinoma, benign brain neoplasm, esophageal carcinoma, malignant laryngeal neoplasm, lipoma, rectal carcinoma, uterine neoplasm.

Psychiatric: *infrequent* — increased libido, agitation, apathy, impaired concentration, depersonalization, paranoid reaction, personality disorder, euphoria, delirium, dementia, delusion, emotional lability, decreased libido, manic reaction, somnambulism, aggressive reaction, neurosis; *rare* — suicide attempt.

Genito-urinary: *infrequent* — amenorrhea, vaginal hemorrhage, penile disorder, prostatic disorder, balanoposthitis, epididymitis, perineal pain, dysuria, micturition frequency, albuminuria, nocturia, polyuria, renal calculus; *rare* — breast enlargement, mastitis, uterine hemorrhage, ejaculation disorder, Peyronie's Disease, pyelonephritis, acute renal failure, uremia.

Resistance Mechanism: *infrequent* — herpes zoster, otitis media, sepsis, abscess, herpes simplex, fungal infection, genital moniliasis.

Respiratory: *infrequent* — asthma, epistaxis, laryngitis, pleurisy, pulmonary edema.

Skin/Appendage: *infrequent* — pruritis, dermatitis, eczema, skin ulceration, alopecia, skin hypertrophy, skin discoloration, urticaria, fungal dermatitis, furunculosis, hyperkeratosis, photosensitivity reaction, psoriasis, maculopapular rash, psoriaform rash, seborrhea.

Special Senses: *infrequent* — tinnitus, earache, decreased hearing, abnormal lacrimation, conjunctivitis, blepharitis, glaucoma, abnormal accommodation, blepharospasm, eye pain, photophobia; *rare* — scotoma.

Vascular Extracardiac: *infrequent* — varicose veins, phlebitis, peripheral gangrene; *rare* — limb embolism, pulmonary embolism, gangrene, subarachnoid hemorrhage, deep thrombophlebitis, leg thrombophlebitis, thrombosis.

Falling Asleep During Activities of Daily Living: Patients treated with *Requip* have reported falling asleep while engaged in activities of daily living, including operation of a motor vehicle which sometimes resulted in accidents (see bolded **WARNING**).

DRUG ABUSE AND DEPENDENCE

Controlled Substance Class

Requip is not a controlled substance.

Physical and Psychological Dependence

Animal studies and human clinical trials with Requip (ropinirole hydrochloride) did not reveal any potential for drug-seeking behavior or physical dependence.

OVERDOSAGE

There were no reports of intentional overdose of *Requip* in the premarketing clinical trials. A total of 27 patients accidentally took more than their prescribed dose of *Requip*, with 10 patients ingesting more than 24 mg/day. The largest overdose reported in premarketing clinical trials was 435 mg taken over a 7-day period (62.1 mg/day). Of patients who received a dose greater than 24 mg/day, one experienced mild oro-facial dyskinesia, another patient experienced intermittent nausea. Other symptoms reported with accidental overdoses were: agitation, increased dyskinesia, grogginess, sedation, orthostatic hypotension, chest pain, confusion, vomiting and nausea.

Overdose Management

It is anticipated that the symptoms of *Requip* overdose will be related to its dopaminergic activity. General supportive measures are recommended. Vital signs should be maintained, if necessary. Removal of any unabsorbed material (e.g., by gastric lavage) should be considered.

DOSAGE AND ADMINISTRATION

In all clinical studies, dosage was initiated at a subtherapeutic level and gradually titrated to therapeutic response. The dosage should be increased to achieve a maximum therapeutic effect, balanced against the principal side effects of nausea, dizziness, somnolence and dyskinesia.

Requip should be taken three times daily. *Requip* can be taken with or without food. Since ingestion with food reduces the maximum concentration (C_{max}) of *Requip*, patients should be advised that taking *Requip* with food may reduce the occurrence of nausea. However, this has not been established in controlled clinical trials.

The recommended starting dose is 0.25 mg three times daily. Based on individual patient response, dosage should then be titrated with weekly increments as described in the table below. After week 4, if necessary, daily dosage may be increased by 1.5 mg per day on a weekly basis up to a dose of 9 mg per day, and then by up to 3 mg per day weekly to a total dose of 24 mg per day.

Ascending-Dose Schedule of *Requip*

Week	Dosage	Total Daily Dose
1	0.25 mg three times daily	0.75 mg
2	0.5 mg three times daily	1.5 mg
3	0.75 mg three times daily	2.25 mg
4	1.0 mg three times daily	3.0 mg

Doses greater than 24 mg/day have not been tested in clinical trials.

When *Requip* is administered as adjunct therapy to L-dopa, the concurrent dose of L-dopa may be decreased gradually as tolerated. L-dopa dosage reduction was allowed during the advanced Parkinson's disease (with L-dopa) study if dyskinesias or other dopaminergic effects occurred. Overall, reduction of L-dopa dose was sustained in 87% of *Requip*-treated patients and in 57% of patients on placebo. On average the L-dopa dose was reduced by 31% in *Requip*-treated patients.

Requip should be discontinued gradually over a 7-day period. The frequency of administration should be reduced from three times daily to twice daily for 4 days. For the remaining 3 days, the frequency should be reduced to once daily prior to complete withdrawal of Requip (ropinirole hydrochloride).

HOW SUPPLIED

Tablets: Each pentagonal film-coated Tiltab® tablet with beveled edges contains ropinirole hydrochloride as follows: 0.25 mg–white imprinted with SB and 4890; 0.5 mg–yellow imprinted with SB and 4891; 1.0 mg–green imprinted with SB and 4892; 2.0 mg–pale yellowish pink imprinted with SB and 4893; 4.0 mg–pale brown imprinted with SB and 4896; 5.0 mg–blue imprinted with SB and 4894.

0.25 mg SUP 30's: NDC 0007-4890-14
0.25 mg bottles of 100: NDC 0007-4890-20
0.5 mg SUP 30's: NDC 0007-4891-14
0.5 mg bottles of 100: NDC 0007-4891-20
1 mg SUP 30's: NDC 0007-4892-14
1 mg bottles of 100: NDC 0007-4892-20
2 mg SUP 30's: NDC 0007-4893-14
2 mg bottles of 100: NDC 0007-4893-20
4 mg bottles of 100: NDC 0007-4896-20
5 mg SUP 30's: NDC 0007-4894-14
5 mg bottles of 100: NDC 0007-4894-20

STORAGE

Protect from light and moisture. Close container tightly after each use.

Store at controlled room temperature 20°–25°C (68°–77°F) [see USP].

Manufactured in Crawley, UK by **SmithKline Beecham Pharmaceuticals**, for

SmithKline Beecham Pharmaceuticals, Philadelphia, PA 19101

RQ:L8 Rx only

Shown in Product Identification Guide, page 337

STELAZINE® ℞

[stel 'ah-zeen]

brand of trifluoperazine hydrochloride

Antianxiety/Antipsychotic

DESCRIPTION

Tablets: Each round, blue, film-coated tablet contains trifluoperazine hydrochloride equivalent to trifluoperazine as follows: 1 mg imprinted SKF and S03; 2 mg imprinted SKF and S04; 5 mg imprinted SKF and S06; 10 mg imprinted SKF and S07. Inactive ingredients consist of cellulose, croscarmellose sodium, FD&C Blue No. 2, FD&C Yellow No. 6, FD&C Red No. 40, gelatin, iron oxide, lactose, magnesium stearate, talc, titanium dioxide and trace amounts of other inactive ingredients.

Multi-Dose Vials, 10 mL (2 mg/mL)—Each mL contains, in aqueous solution, trifluoperazine, 2 mg, as the hydrochloride; sodium tartrate, 4.75 mg; sodium biphosphate, 11.6 mg; sodium saccharin, 0.3 mg; benzyl alcohol, 0.75%, as preservative.

Concentrate—Each mL of clear, yellow, banana-vanilla-flavored liquid contains 10 mg of trifluoperazine as the hydrochloride. Inactive ingredients consist of D&C Yellow No. 10, FD&C Yellow No. 6, flavor, sodium benzoate, sodium bisulfite, sucrose and water.

N.B.: The Concentrate is for use in severe neuropsychiatric conditions when oral medication is preferred and other oral forms are considered impractical.

INDICATIONS

For the management of the manifestations of psychotic disorders.

Stelazine (trifluoperazine HCl) is effective for the short-term treatment of generalized non-psychotic anxiety. However, *Stelazine* is not the first drug to be used in therapy for most patients with non-psychotic anxiety because certain risks associated with its use are not shared by common alternative treatments (i.e., benzodiazepines).

When used in the treatment of non-psychotic anxiety, *Stelazine* should not be administered at doses of more than 6 mg per day or for longer than 12 weeks because the use of *Stelazine* at higher doses or for longer intervals may cause persistent tardive dyskinesia that may prove irreversible (see WARNINGS).

The effectiveness of *Stelazine* as a treatment for non-psychotic anxiety was established in a 4-week clinical multicenter study of outpatients with generalized anxiety disorder (DSM-III). This evidence does not predict that *Stelazine* will be useful in patients with other non-psychotic conditions in which anxiety, or signs that mimic anxiety, are found (i.e., physical illness, organic mental conditions, agitated depression, character pathologies, etc.).

Stelazine (trifluoperazine HCl) has not been shown effective in the management of behavioral complications in patients with mental retardation.

CONTRAINDICATIONS

A known hypersensitivity to phenothiazines, comatose or greatly depressed states due to central nervous system depressants and, in cases of existing blood dyscrasias, bone marrow depression and pre-existing liver damage.

WARNINGS

Tardive Dyskinesia: Tardive dyskinesia, a syndrome consisting of potentially irreversible, involuntary, dyskinetic movements, may develop in patients treated with neuroleptic (antipsychotic) drugs. Although the prevalence of the syndrome appears to be highest among the elderly, especially elderly women, it is impossible to rely upon prevalence estimates to predict, at the inception of neuroleptic treatment, which patients are likely to develop the syndrome. Whether neuroleptic drug products differ in their potential to cause tardive dyskinesia is unknown.

Both the risk of developing the syndrome and the likelihood that it will become irreversible are believed to increase as the duration of treatment and the total cumulative dose of neuroleptic drugs administered to the patient increase. However, the syndrome can develop, although much less commonly, after relatively brief treatment periods at low doses.

There is no known treatment for established cases of tardive dyskinesia, although the syndrome may remit, partially or completely, if neuroleptic treatment is withdrawn. Neuroleptic treatment itself, however, may suppress (or partially suppress) the signs and symptoms of the syndrome and thereby may possibly mask the underlying disease process. The effect that symptomatic suppression has upon the long-term course of the syndrome is unknown.

Given these considerations, neuroleptics should be prescribed in a manner that is most likely to minimize the occurrence of tardive dyskinesia. Chronic neuroleptic treatment should generally be reserved for patients who suffer from a chronic illness that 1) is known to respond to neuroleptic drugs, and, 2) for whom alternative, equally effective, but potentially less harmful treatments are *not* available or appropriate. In patients who do require chronic treatment, the smallest dose and the shortest duration of treatment producing a satisfactory clinical response should be sought. The need for continued treatment should be reassessed periodically.

If signs and symptoms of tardive dyskinesia appear in a patient on neuroleptics, drug discontinuation should be considered. However, some patients may require treatment despite the presence of the syndrome.

For further information about the description of tardive dyskinesia and its clinical detection, please refer to the sections on PRECAUTIONS and ADVERSE REACTIONS.

Neuroleptic Malignant Syndrome (NMS)

A potentially fatal symptom complex sometimes referred to as Neuroleptic Malignant Syndrome (NMS) has been reported in association with antipsychotic drugs. Clinical manifestations of NMS are hyperpyrexia, muscle rigidity, altered mental status and evidence of autonomic instability (irregular pulse or blood pressure, tachycardia, diaphoresis, and cardiac dysrhythmias).

The diagnostic evaluation of patients with this syndrome is complicated. In arriving at a diagnosis, it is important to identify cases where the clinical presentation includes both serious medical illness (e.g., pneumonia, systemic infection, etc.) and untreated or inadequately treated extrapyramidal signs and symptoms (EPS). Other important considerations in the differential diagnosis include central anticholinergic toxicity, heat stroke, drug fever and primary central nervous system (CNS) pathology.

The management of NMS should include 1) immediate discontinuation of antipsychotic drugs and other drugs not essential to concurrent therapy, 2) intensive symptomatic treatment and medical monitoring, and 3) treatment of any concomitant serious medical problems for which specific treatments are available. There is no general agreement about specific pharmacological treatment regimens for uncomplicated NMS.

If a patient requires antipsychotic drug treatment after recovery from NMS, the potential reintroduction of drug ther-

Continued on next page

Information on the SmithKline Beecham Pharmaceuticals products appearing here is based on the labeling in effect on June 15, 2000. Further information on these and other products may be obtained from the Medical Department, SmithKline Beecham Pharmaceuticals, One Franklin Plaza, Philadelphia, PA 19101.

Stelazine—Cont.

apy should be carefully considered. The patient should be carefully monitored, since recurrences of NMS have been reported.

An encephalopathic syndrome (characterized by weakness, lethargy, fever, tremulousness and confusion, extrapyramidal symptoms, leukocytosis, elevated serum enzymes, BUN and FBS) has occurred in a few patients treated with lithium plus a neuroleptic. In some instances, the syndrome was followed by irreversible brain damage. Because of a possible causal relationship between these events and the concomitant administration of lithium and neuroleptics, patients receiving such combined therapy should be monitored closely for early evidence of neurologic toxicity and treatment discontinued promptly if such signs appear. This encephalopathic syndrome may be similar to or the same as neuroleptic malignant syndrome (NMS).

Patients who have demonstrated a hypersensitivity reaction (e.g., blood dyscrasias, jaundice) with a phenothiazine should not be re-exposed to any phenothiazine, including Stelazine (trifluoperazine HCl), unless in the judgment of the physician the potential benefits of treatment outweigh the possible hazard.

Stelazine Concentrate contains sodium bisulfite, a sulfite that may cause allergic-type reactions including anaphylactic symptoms and life-threatening or less severe asthmatic episodes in certain susceptible people. The overall prevalence of sulfite sensitivity in the general population is unknown and probably low. Sulfite sensitivity is seen more frequently in asthmatic than in non-asthmatic people.

Stelazine (trifluoperazine HCl) may impair mental and/or physical abilities, especially during the first few days of therapy. Therefore, caution patients about activities requiring alertness (e.g., operating vehicles or machinery).

If agents such as sedatives, narcotics, anesthetics, tranquilizers or alcohol are used either simultaneously or successively with the drug, the possibility of an undesirable additive depressant effect should be considered.

Usage in Pregnancy: Safety for the use of *Stelazine* during pregnancy has not been established. Therefore, it is not recommended that the drug be given to pregnant patients except when, in the judgment of the physician, it is essential. The potential benefits should clearly outweigh possible hazards. There are reported instances of prolonged jaundice, extrapyramidal signs, hyperreflexia or hyporeflexia in newborn infants whose mothers received phenothiazines.

Reproductive studies in rats given over 600 times the human dose showed an increased incidence of malformations above controls and reduced litter size and weight linked to maternal toxicity. These effects were not observed at half this dosage. No adverse effect on fetal development was observed in rabbits given 700 times the human dose nor in monkeys given 25 times the human dose.

Nursing Mothers: There is evidence that phenothiazines are excreted in the breast milk of nursing mothers. Because of the potential for serious adverse reactions in nursing infants from trifluoperazine, a decision should be made whether to discontinue nursing or to discontinue the drug, taking into account the importance of the drug to the mother.

PRECAUTIONS

General

Given the likelihood that some patients exposed chronically to neuroleptics will develop tardive dyskinesia, it is advised that all patients in whom chronic use is contemplated be given, if possible, full information about this risk. The decision to inform patients and/or their guardians must obviously take into account the clinical circumstances and the competency of the patient to understand the information provided.

Thrombocytopenia and anemia have been reported in patients receiving the drug. Agranulocytosis and pancytopenia have also been reported—warn patients to report the sudden appearance of sore throat or other signs of infection. If white blood cell and differential counts indicate cellular depression, stop treatment and start antibiotic and other suitable therapy.

Jaundice of the cholestatic type of hepatitis or liver damage has been reported. If fever with grippe-like symptoms occurs, appropriate liver studies should be conducted. If tests indicate an abnormality, stop treatment.

One result of therapy may be an increase in mental and physical activity. For example, a few patients with angina pectoris have complained of increased pain while taking the drug. Therefore, angina patients should be observed carefully and, if an unfavorable response is noted, the drug should be withdrawn.

Because hypotension has occurred, large doses and parenteral administration should be avoided in patients with impaired cardiovascular systems. To minimize the occurrence of hypotension after injection, keep patient lying down and observe for at least $^1/_2$ hour. If hypotension occurs from parenteral or oral dosing, place patient in head-low position with legs raised. If a vasoconstrictor is required, Levophed®* and Neo-Synephrine®† are suitable. Other pressor agents, including epinephrine, should not be used as they may cause a paradoxical further lowering of blood pressure.

Since certain phenothiazines have been reported to produce retinopathy, the drug should be discontinued if ophthalmoscopic examination or visual field studies should demonstrate retinal changes.

An antiemetic action of Stelazine (trifluoperazine HCl) may mask the signs and symptoms of toxicity or overdosage of other drugs and may obscure the diagnosis and treatment of other conditions such as intestinal obstruction, brain tumor and Reye's syndrome.

With prolonged administration at high dosages, the possibility of cumulative effects, with sudden onset of severe central nervous system or vasomotor symptoms, should be kept in mind.

Neuroleptic drugs elevate prolactin levels; the elevation persists during chronic administration. Tissue culture experiments indicate that approximately $^1/_3$ of human breast cancers are prolactin-dependent in vitro, a factor of potential importance if the prescribing of these drugs is contemplated in a patient with a previously detected breast cancer. Although disturbances such as galactorrhea, amenorrhea, gynecomastia and impotence have been reported, the clinical significance of elevated serum prolactin levels is unknown for most patients. An increase in mammary neoplasms has been found in rodents after chronic administration of neuroleptic drugs. Neither clinical nor epidemiologic studies conducted to date, however, have shown an association between chronic administration of these drugs and mammary tumorigenesis; the available evidence is considered too limited to be conclusive at this time.

Chromosomal aberrations in spermatocytes and abnormal sperm have been demonstrated in rodents treated with certain neuroleptics.

Because phenothiazines may interfere with thermoregulatory mechanisms, use with caution in persons who will be exposed to extreme heat.

As with all drugs which exert an anticholinergic effect, and/or cause mydriasis, trifluoperazine should be used with caution in patients with glaucoma.

Phenothiazines may diminish the effect of oral anticoagulants.

Phenothiazines can produce alpha-adrenergic blockade.

Concomitant administration of propranolol with phenothiazines results in increased plasma levels of both drugs.

Antihypertensive effects of guanethidine and related compounds may be counteracted when phenothiazines are used concurrently.

Thiazide diuretics may accentuate the orthostatic hypotension that may occur with phenothiazines.

Phenothiazines may lower the convulsive threshold; dosage adjustments of anticonvulsants may be necessary. Potentiation of anticonvulsant effects does not occur. However, it has been reported that phenothiazines may interfere with the metabolism of Dilantin®‡ and thus precipitate *Dilantin* toxicity.

Drugs which lower the seizure threshold, including phenothiazine derivatives, should not be used with Amipaque®§. As with other phenothiazine derivatives, *Stelazine* should be discontinued at least 48 hours before myelography, should not be resumed for at least 24 hours postprocedure and should not be used for the control of nausea and vomiting occurring either prior to myelography or postprocedure with *Amipaque.*

The presence of phenothiazines may produce false-positive phenylketonuria (PKU) test results.

Long-Term Therapy: To lessen the likelihood of adverse reactions related to cumulative drug effect, patients with a history of long-term therapy with Stelazine (trifluoperazine HCl) and/or other neuroleptics should be evaluated periodically to decide whether the maintenance dosage could be lowered or drug therapy discontinued.

ADVERSE REACTIONS

Drowsiness, dizziness, skin reactions, rash, dry mouth, insomnia, amenorrhea, fatigue, muscular weakness, anorexia, lactation, blurred vision and neuromuscular (extrapyramidal) reactions.

Neuromuscular (Extrapyramidal) Reactions

These symptoms are seen in a significant number of hospitalized mental patients. They may be characterized by motor restlessness, be of the dystonic type, or they may resemble parkinsonism.

Depending on the severity of symptoms, dosage should be reduced or discontinued. If therapy is reinstituted, it should be at a lower dosage. Should these symptoms occur in children or pregnant patients, the drug should be stopped and not reinstituted. In most cases barbiturates by suitable route of administration will suffice. (Or, injectable Benadryl®‖ may be useful.) In more severe cases, the administration of an anti-parkinsonism agent, except levodopa, usually produces rapid reversal of symptoms. Suitable supportive measures such as maintaining a clear airway and adequate hydration should be employed.

Motor Restlessness: Symptoms may include agitation or jitteriness and sometimes insomnia. These symptoms often disappear spontaneously. At times these symptoms may be similar to the original neurotic or psychotic symptoms. Dosage should not be increased until these side effects have subsided.

If this phase becomes too troublesome, the symptoms can usually be controlled by a reduction of dosage or change of drug. Treatment with anti-parkinsonian agents, benzodiazepines or propranolol may be helpful.

Dystonias: Symptoms may include: spasm of the neck muscles, sometimes progressing to torticollis; extensor rigidity of back muscles, sometimes progressing to opisthotonos; carpopedal spasm, trismus, swallowing difficulty, oculogyric crisis and protrusion of the tongue.

These usually subside within a few hours, and almost always within 24 to 48 hours, after the drug has been discontinued.

In mild cases, reassurance or a barbiturate is often sufficient. *In moderate cases,* barbiturates will usually bring rapid relief. *In more severe adult cases,* the administration of an anti-parkinsonism agent, except levodopa, usually produces rapid reversal of symptoms. Also, intravenous caffeine with sodium benzoate seems to be effective. *In children,* reassurance and barbiturates will usually control symptoms. (Or, injectable *Benadryl* may be useful.) Note: See *Benadryl* prescribing information for appropriate children's dosage. If appropriate treatment with anti-parkinsonism agents or *Benadryl* fails to reverse the signs and symptoms, the diagnosis should be reevaluated.

Pseudo-parkinsonism: Symptoms may include: mask-like facies; drooling; tremors; pill-rolling motion; cogwheel rigidity; and shuffling gait. Reassurance and sedation are important. In most cases these symptoms are readily controlled when an anti-parkinsonism agent is administered concomitantly. Anti-parkinsonism agents should be used only when required. Generally, therapy of a few weeks to 2 to 3 months will suffice. After this time patients should be evaluated to determine their need for continued treatment. (Note: Levodopa has not been found effective in pseudo-parkinsonism.) Occasionally it is necessary to lower the dosage of Stelazine (trifluoperazine HCl) or to discontinue the drug.

Tardive Dyskinesia: As with all antipsychotic agents, tardive dyskinesia may appear in some patients on long-term therapy or may appear after drug therapy has been discontinued. The syndrome can also develop, although much less frequently, after relatively brief treatment periods at low doses. This syndrome appears in all age groups. Although its prevalence appears to be highest among elderly patients, especially elderly women, it is impossible to rely upon prevalence estimates to predict at the inception of neuroleptic treatment which patients are likely to develop the syndrome. The symptoms are persistent and in some patients appear to be irreversible. The syndrome is characterized by rhythmical involuntary movements of the tongue, face, mouth or jaw (e.g., protrusion of tongue, puffing of cheeks, puckering of mouth, chewing movements). Sometimes these may be accompanied by involuntary movements of extremities. In rare instances, these involuntary movements of the extremities are the only manifestations of tardive dyskinesia. A variant of tardive dyskinesia, tardive dystonia, has also been described.

There is no known effective treatment for tardive dyskinesia; anti-parkinsonism agents do not alleviate the symptoms of this syndrome. If clinically feasible, it is suggested that all antipsychotic agents be discontinued if these symptoms appear. Should it be necessary to reinstitute treatment, or increase the dosage of the agent, or switch to a different antipsychotic agent, the syndrome may be masked.

It has been reported that fine vermicular movements of the tongue may be an early sign of the syndrome and if the medication is stopped at that time the syndrome may not develop.

Adverse Reactions Reported with Stelazine (trifluoperazine HCl) or Other Phenothiazine Derivatives: Adverse effects with different phenothiazines vary in type, frequency, and mechanism of occurrence, i.e., some are dose-related, while others involve individual patient sensitivity. Some adverse effects may be more likely to occur, or occur with greater intensity, in patients with special medical problems, e.g., patients with mitral insufficiency or pheochromocytoma have experienced severe hypotension following recommended doses of certain phenothiazines.

Neuroleptic Malignant Syndrome (NMS) has been reported in association with antipsychotic drugs. (See WARNINGS.)

Not all of the following adverse reactions have been observed with every phenothiazine derivative, but they have been reported with one or more and should be borne in mind when drugs of this class are administered: extrapyramidal symptoms (opisthotonos, oculogyric crisis, hyperreflexia, dystonia, akathisia, dyskinesia, parkinsonism) some of which have lasted months and even years—particularly in elderly patients with previous brain damage; grand mal and petit mal convulsions, particularly in patients with EEG abnormalities or history of such disorders; altered cerebrospinal fluid proteins; cerebral edema; intensification and prolongation of the action of central nervous system depressants (opiates, analgesics, antihistamines, barbiturates, alcohol), atropine, heat, organophosphorus insecticides; autonomic reactions (dryness of mouth, nasal congestion, headache, nausea, constipation, obstipation, adynamic ileus, ejaculatory disorders/impotence, priapism, atonic colon, urinary retention, miosis and mydriasis); reactivation of psychotic processes, catatonic-like states; hypotension (sometimes fatal); cardiac arrest; blood dyscrasias (pancytopenia, thrombocytopenic purpura, leukopenia, agranulocytosis, eosinophilia, hemolytic anemia, aplastic anemia); liver damage (jaundice, biliary stasis); endocrine disturbances (hyperglycemia, hypoglycemia, glycosuria, lactation, galactorrhea, gynecomastia, menstrual irregularities, false-positive pregnancy tests); skin disorders (photosensitivity, itching, erythema, urticaria, eczema up to exfoliative dermatitis); other allergic reactions (asthma, laryngeal edema, angioneurotic edema, anaphylactoid reactions); peripheral edema; reversed epinephrine effect; hyperpyrexia; mild fever after large I.M. doses; increased appetite; increased weight; a systemic lupus erythematosus-like syndrome; pigmentary retinopathy; with prolonged administration of substantial doses, skin pigmentation, epithelial keratopathy, and lenticular and corneal deposits.

EKG changes—particularly nonspecific, usually reversible Q and T wave distortions—have been observed in some patients receiving phenothiazine tranquilizers. Although phenothiazines cause neither psychic nor physical dependence, sudden discontinuance in long-term psychiatric patients may cause temporary symptoms, e.g., nausea and vomiting, dizziness, tremulousness.

Note: There have been occasional reports of sudden death in patients receiving phenothiazines. In some cases, the cause appeared to be cardiac arrest or asphyxia due to failure of the cough reflex.

DOSAGE AND ADMINISTRATION—ADULTS

Dosage should be adjusted to the needs of the individual. The lowest effective dosage should always be used. Dosage should be increased more gradually in debilitated or emaciated patients. When maximum response is achieved, dosage may be reduced gradually to a maintenance level. Because of the inherent long action of the drug, patients may be controlled on convenient b.i.d. administration; some patients may be maintained on once-a-day administration.

When Stelazine (trifluoperazine HCl) is administered by intramuscular injection, equivalent oral dosage may be substituted once symptoms have been controlled.

Note: Although there is little likelihood of contact dermatitis due to the drug, persons with known sensitivity to phenothiazine drugs should avoid direct contact.

Elderly Patients: In general, dosages in the lower range are sufficient for most elderly patients. Since they appear to be more susceptible to hypotension and neuromuscular reactions, such patients should be observed closely. Dosage should be tailored to the individual, response carefully monitored, and dosage adjusted accordingly. Dosage should be increased more gradually in elderly patients.

Non-psychotic Anxiety

Usual dosage is 1 or 2 mg twice daily. Do not administer at doses of more than 6 mg per day or for longer than 12 weeks.

Psychotic Disorders

Oral: Usual starting dosage is 2 mg to 5 mg b.i.d. (Small or emaciated patients should always be started on the lower dosage.)

Most patients will show optimum response on 15 mg or 20 mg daily, although a few may require 40 mg a day or more. Optimum therapeutic dosage levels should be reached within 2 or 3 weeks.

When the Concentrate dosage form is to be used, it should be added to 60 mL (2 fl oz) or more of diluent *just prior to administration* to insure palatability and stability. Vehicles suggested for dilution are: tomato or fruit juice, milk, simple syrup, orange syrup, carbonated beverages, coffee, tea or water. Semisolid foods (soup, puddings, etc.) may also be used.

Intramuscular (for prompt control of severe symptoms): Usual dosage is 1 mg to 2 mg ($^1/_2$ to 1 mL) by deep intramuscular injection q4 to 6h, p.r.n. More than 6 mg within 24 hours is rarely necessary.

Only in very exceptional cases should intramuscular dosage exceed 10 mg within 24 hours. Injections should not be given at intervals of less than 4 hours because of a possible cumulative effect.

Note: Stelazine (trifluoperazine HCl) Injection has been usually well tolerated and there is little, if any, pain and irritation at the site of injection.

This solution should be protected from light. This is a clear, colorless to pale yellow solution; a slight yellowish discoloration will not alter potency. If markedly discolored, solution should be discarded.

DOSAGE AND ADMINISTRATION—PSYCHOTIC CHILDREN

Dosage should be adjusted to the weight of the child and severity of the symptoms. These dosages are for children, ages 6 to 12, who are hospitalized or under close supervision.

Oral: The starting dosage is 1 mg administered once a day or b.i.d. Dosage may be increased gradually until symptoms are controlled or until side effects become troublesome.

While it is usually not necessary to exceed dosages of 15 mg daily, some older children with severe symptoms may require higher dosages.

Intramuscular: There has been little experience with the use of Stelazine (trifluoperazine HCl) Injection in children. However, if it is necessary to achieve rapid control of severe symptoms, 1 mg ($^1/_2$ mL) of the drug may be administered intramuscularly once or twice a day.

OVERDOSAGE

(See also under ADVERSE REACTIONS.) SYMPTOMS—Primarily involvement of the extrapyramidal mechanism producing some of the dystonic reactions described above. Symptoms of central nervous system depression to the point of somnolence or coma. Agitation and restlessness may also occur. Other possible manifestations include convulsions, EKG changes and cardiac arrhythmias, fever and autonomic reactions such as hypotension, dry mouth and ileus.

TREATMENT—It is important to determine other medications taken by the patient since multiple dose therapy is common in overdosage situations. Treatment is essentially symptomatic and supportive. Early gastric lavage is helpful. Keep patient under observation and maintain an open airway, since involvement of the extrapyramidal mechanism may produce dysphagia and respiratory difficulty in severe overdosage. **Do not attempt to induce emesis because a dystonic reaction of the head or neck may develop that could result in aspiration of vomitus.** Extrapyramidal symptoms may be treated with anti-parkinsonism drugs, barbiturates, or *Benadryl.* See prescribing information for these products. Care should be taken to avoid increasing respiratory depression. If administration of a stimulant is desirable, amphetamine, dextroamphetamine or caffeine with sodium benzoate is recommended. Stimulants that may cause convulsions (e.g., picrotoxin or pentylenetetrazol) should be avoided.

If hypotension occurs, the standard measures for managing circulatory shock should be initiated. If it is desirable to administer a vasoconstrictor, *Levophed* and *Neo-Synephrine* are most suitable. Other pressor agents, including epinephrine, are not recommended because phenothiazine derivatives may reverse the usual elevating action of these agents and cause a further lowering of blood pressure.

Limited experience indicates that phenothiazines are *not* dialyzable.

HOW SUPPLIED

Tablets, 1 mg, 2 mg, 5 mg and 10 mg in bottles of 100.

1 mg 100's: NDC 0108-4903-20
2 mg 100's: NDC 0108-4904-20
5 mg 100's: NDC 0108-4906-20
10 mg 100's: NDC 0108-4907-20

Multi-Dose Vials, 10 mL (2 mg/mL), in 1's:
NDC 0108-4902-01

Concentrate (for institutional use), 10 mg/mL, in 2 fl oz bottles and in cartons of 12 bottles.

The Concentrate form is light-sensitive. For this reason, it should be protected from light and dispensed in amber bottles. *Refrigeration is not required.*

10 mg/mL 2 fl oz (carton of 12): NDC 0108-4901-42

Store all Stelazine (trifluoperazine HCl) formulations between 15° and 30°C (59° and 86°F).

---

* norepinephrine bitartrate, Sanofi Winthrop Pharmaceuticals.
† phenylephrine hydrochloride, Sanofi Winthrop Pharmaceuticals.
‡ phenytoin, Parke-Davis.
§ metrizamide, Sanofi Winthrop Pharmaceuticals.
‖ diphenhydramine hydrochloride, Parke-Davis.

Rx only

SZ:L71

Shown in Product Identification Guide, page 337

TAGAMET® ℞

[tag 'ah-met]
brand of cimetidine tablets
cimetidine hydrochloride liquid and
cimetidine hydrochloride injection

DESCRIPTION

Tagamet (cimetidine) is a histamine H_2-receptor antagonist. Chemically it is *N* "-cyano- *N* -methyl-*N* '-[2-[[(5-methyl-1 *H*-imidazol-4-yl) methyl] thio]-ethyl]-guanidine.

The empirical formula for cimetidine is $C_{10}H_{16}N_6S$ and for cimetidine hydrochloride, $C_{10}H_{16}N_6SHCl$; these represent molecular weights of 252.34 and 288.80, respectively.

CH_3 $CH_2SCH_2CH_2NHCNHCH_3$
N—C≡N
HN N

Cimetidine

Cimetidine contains an imidazole ring, and is chemically related to histamine.

(The liquid and injection dosage forms contain cimetidine as the hydrochloride.)

Cimetidine has a bitter taste and characteristic odor.

Solubility Characteristics: Cimetidine is soluble in alcohol, slightly soluble in water, very slightly soluble in chloroform and insoluble in ether. Cimetidine hydrochloride is freely soluble in water, soluble in alcohol, very slightly soluble in chloroform and practically insoluble in ether.

Tablets for Oral Administration: Each light green, film-coated tablet contains cimetidine as follows: 200 mg—round, imprinted with the product name TAGAMET, SKF and 200; 300 mg—round, debossed with the product name TAGAMET, SB and 300; 400 mg—oval Tiltab® tablets, debossed with the product name TAGAMET, SB and 400; 800 mg—oval Tiltab® tablets, debossed with the product name TAGAMET, SB and 800. Inactive ingredients consist of cellulose, D&C Yellow No. 10, FD&C Blue No. 2, FD&C Red No. 40, FD&C Yellow No. 6, hydroxypropyl methylcellulose, iron oxides, magnesium stearate, povidone, propylene glycol, sodium lauryl sulfate, sodium starch glycolate, starch, titanium dioxide and trace amounts of other inactive ingredients.

Liquid for Oral Administration: Each 5 mL (1 teaspoonful) of clear, light orange, mint-peach flavored liquid contains cimetidine hydrochloride equivalent to cimetidine, 300 mg; alcohol, 2.8%. Inactive ingredients consist of FD&C Yellow No. 6, flavors, methylparaben, polyoxyethylene polyoxypropylene glycol, propylene glycol, propylparaben, saccharin sodium, sodium chloride, sodium phosphate, sorbitol and water.

Injection:

Single-Dose Vials for Intramuscular or Intravenous Administration: Each 2 mL contains, in sterile aqueous solution (pH range 3.8 to 6), cimetidine hydrochloride equivalent to cimetidine, 300 mg; phenol, 10 mg.

Multi-Dose Vials for Intramuscular or Intravenous Administration: 8 mL (300 mg/2 mL): Each 2 mL contains, in sterile aqueous solution (pH range 3.8 to 6), cimetidine hydrochloride equivalent to cimetidine, 300 mg; phenol, 10 mg.

Single-Dose Premixed Plastic Containers for Intravenous Administration: Each 50 mL of sterile aqueous solution (pH range 5 to 7) contains cimetidine hydrochloride equivalent to 300 mg cimetidine and 0.45 grams sodium chloride. No preservative has been added.

The plastic container is fabricated from specially formulated polyvinyl chloride. The amount of water that can permeate from inside the container into the overwrap is insufficient to affect the solution significantly. Solutions in contact with the plastic container can leach out certain of its chemical components in very small amounts within the expiration period, e.g., di 2-ethylhexyl phthalate (DEHP), up to 5 parts per million. However, the safety of the plastic has been confirmed in tests in animals according to the USP biological tests for plastic containers as well as by tissue culture toxicity studies.

ADD-Vantage®* Vials for Intravenous Administration: Each 2 mL contains, in sterile aqueous solution (pH range 3.8 to 6), cimetidine hydrochloride equivalent to cimetidine, 300 mg; phenol, 10 mg.

All of the above injection formulations are pyrogen free, and sodium hydroxide N.F. is used as an ingredient to adjust the pH.

CLINICAL PHARMACOLOGY

Tagamet (cimetidine) competitively inhibits the action of histamine at the histamine H_2 receptors of the parietal cells and thus is a histamine H_2-receptor antagonist.

Tagamet is not an anticholinergic agent. Studies have shown that *Tagamet* inhibits both daytime and nocturnal basal gastric acid secretion. *Tagamet* also inhibits gastric acid secretion stimulated by food, histamine, pentagastrin, caffeine and insulin.

Antisecretory Activity

1) **Acid Secretion:** *Nocturnal: Tagamet* 800 mg orally at bedtime reduces mean hourly H^+ activity by greater than 85% over an 8-hour period in duodenal ulcer patients, with no effect on daytime acid secretion. *Tagamet* 1600 mg orally h.s. produces 100% inhibition of mean hourly H^+ activity over an 8-hour period in duodenal ulcer patients, but also reduces H^+ activity by 35% for an additional 5 hours into the following morning. *Tagamet* 400 mg b.i.d. and 300 mg q.i.d. decrease nocturnal acid secretion in a dose-related manner, i.e., 47% to 83% over a 6- to 8-hour period and 54% over a 9-hour period, respectively.

Food Stimulated: During the first hour after a standard experimental meal, oral *Tagamet* 300 mg inhibited gastric acid secretion in duodenal ulcer patients by at least 50%. During the subsequent 2 hours *Tagamet* inhibited gastric acid secretion by at least 75%.

The effect of a 300 mg breakfast dose of *Tagamet* continued for at least 4 hours and there was partial suppression of the rise in gastric acid secretion following the luncheon meal in duodenal ulcer patients. This suppression of gastric acid output was enhanced and could be maintained by another 300 mg dose of *Tagamet* given with lunch.

In another study, *Tagamet* 300 mg given with the meal increased gastric pH as compared with placebo.

	Mean Gastric pH	
	Tagamet	**Placebo**
1 hour	3.5	2.6
2 hours	3.1	1.6
3 hours	3.8	1.9
4 hours	6.1	2.2

24-Hour Mean H^+ Activity: *Tagamet* 800 mg h.s., 400 mg b.i.d. and 300 mg q.i.d. all provide a similar, moderate (less than 60%) level of 24-hour acid suppression. However, the 800 mg h.s. regimen exerts its entire effect on nocturnal acid, and does not affect daytime gastric physiology.

Chemically Stimulated: Oral Tagamet (cimetidine) significantly inhibited gastric acid secretion stimulated by betazole (an isomer of histamine), pentagastrin, caffeine and insulin as follows:

Stimulant	Stimulant Dose	*Tagamet*	% Inhibition
Betazole	1.5mg/kg (sc)	300mg (po)	85% at $2^1/_2$ hours
Pentagastrin	6mcg/kg/ hr (iv)	100mg/hr (iv)	60% at 1 hour

Continued on next page

Information on the SmithKline Beecham Pharmaceuticals products appearing here is based on the labeling in effect on June 15, 2000. Further information on these and other products may be obtained from the Medical Department, SmithKline Beecham Pharmaceuticals, One Franklin Plaza, Philadelphia, PA 19101.

Tagamet—Cont.

Caffeine	5mg/kg/hr (iv)	300mg (po)	100% at 1 hour
Insulin	0.03 units/kg/hr (iv)	100mg/hr (iv)	82% at 1 hour

When food and betazole were used to stimulate secretion, inhibition of hydrogen ion concentration usually ranged from 45% to 75% and the inhibition of volume ranged from 30% to 65%.

Parenteral administration also significantly inhibits gastric acid secretion. In a crossover study involving patients with active or healed duodenal or gastric ulcers, either continuous I.V. infusion of *Tagamet* 37.5 mg/hour (900 mg/day) or intermittent injection of *Tagamet* 300 mg q6h (1200 mg/day) maintained gastric pH above 4.0 for more than 50% of the time under steady-state conditions.

2) **Pepsin:** Oral *Tagamet* 300 mg reduced total pepsin output as a result of the decrease in volume of gastric juice.

3) **Intrinsic Factor:** Intrinsic factor secretion was studied with betazole as a stimulant. Oral *Tagamet* 300 mg inhibited the rise in intrinsic factor concentration produced by betazole, but some intrinsic factor was secreted at all times.

*ADD-Vantage® is a trademark of Abbott Laboratories.

Other

Lower Esophageal Sphincter Pressure and Gastric Emptying

Tagamet has no effect on lower esophageal sphincter (LES) pressure or the rate of gastric emptying.

Pharmacokinetics

Tagamet is rapidly absorbed after oral administration and peak levels occur in 45 to 90 minutes. The half-life of *Tagamet* is approximately 2 hours. Both oral and parenteral (I.V. or I.M.) administration provide comparable periods of therapeutically effective blood levels; blood concentrations remain above that required to provide 80% inhibition of basal gastric acid secretion for 4 to 5 hours following a dose of 300 mg.

Steady-state blood concentrations of cimetidine with continuous infusion of *Tagamet* are determined by the infusion rate and clearance of the drug in the individual patient. In a study of peptic ulcer patients with normal renal function, an infusion rate of 37.5 mg/hour produced average steady-state plasma cimetidine concentrations of about 0.9 mcg/mL. Blood levels with other infusion rates will vary in direct proportion to the infusion rate.

The principal route of excretion of *Tagamet* is the urine. Following parenteral administration, most of the drug is excreted as the parent compound; following oral administration, the drug is more extensively metabolized, the sulfoxide being the major metabolite. Following a single oral dose, 48% of the drug is recovered from the urine after 24 hours as the parent compound. Following I.V. or I.M. administration, approximately 75% of the drug is recovered from the urine after 24 hours as the parent compound.

CLINICAL TRIALS

Duodenal Ulcer

Tagamet (cimetidine) has been shown to be effective in the treatment of active duodenal ulcer and, at reduced dosage, in maintenance therapy following healing of active ulcers.

Active Duodenal Ulcer: *Tagamet* accelerates the rate of duodenal ulcer healing. Healing rates reported in U.S. and foreign controlled trials with *Tagamet* are summarized below, beginning with the regimen providing the lowest nocturnal dose.

Duodenal Ulcer Healing Rates with Various *Tagamet* Dosage Regimens*

Regimen	300 mg q.i.d.	400 mg b.i.d.	800 mg h.s.	1600 mg h.s.
week 4	68%	73%	80%	86%
week 6	80%	80%	89%	—
week 8	—	92%	94%	—

* Averages from controlled clinical trials.

A U.S., double-blind, placebo-controlled, dose-ranging study demonstrated that all once-daily at bedtime (h.s.) *Tagamet* regimens were superior to placebo in ulcer healing and that *Tagamet* 800 mg h.s. healed 75% of patients at 4 weeks. The healing rate with 800 mg h.s. was significantly superior to 400 mg h.s. (66%) and not significantly different from 1600 mg h.s. (81%).

In the U.S. dose-ranging trial, over 80% of patients receiving *Tagamet* 800 mg h.s. experienced nocturnal pain relief after 1 day. Relief from daytime pain was reported in approximately 70% of patients after 2 days. As with ulcer healing, the 800 mg h.s. dose was superior to 400 mg h.s. and not different from 1600 mg h.s.

In foreign, double-blind studies with *Tagamet* 800 mg h.s., 79% to 85% of patients were healed at 4 weeks.

While short-term treatment with Tagamet (cimetidine) can result in complete healing of the duodenal ulcer, acute therapy will not prevent ulcer recurrence after *Tagamet* has been discontinued. Some follow-up studies have reported that the rate of recurrence once therapy was discontinued was slightly higher for patients healed on *Tagamet* than for patients healed on other forms of therapy; however, the *Tagamet*-treated patients generally had more severe disease.

Maintenance Therapy in Duodenal Ulcer: Treatment with a reduced dose of *Tagamet* has been proven effective as maintenance therapy following healing of active duodenal ulcers.

In numerous placebo-controlled studies conducted worldwide, the percent of patients with observed ulcers at the end of 1 year's therapy with *Tagamet* 400 mg h.s. was significantly lower (10% to 45%) than in patients receiving placebo (44% to 70%). Thus, from 55% to 90% of patients were maintained free of observed ulcers at the end of 1 year with *Tagamet* 400 mg h.s.

Factors such as smoking, duration and severity of disease, gender, and genetic traits may contribute to variations in actual percentages.

Trials of other anti-ulcer therapy, whether placebo-controlled, positive-controlled or open, have demonstrated a range of results similar to that seen with *Tagamet.*

Active Benign Gastric Ulcer

Tagamet has been shown to be effective in the short-term treatment of active benign gastric ulcer.

In a multicenter, double-blind U.S. study, patients with endoscopically confirmed benign gastric ulcer were treated with *Tagamet* 300 mg four times a day or with placebo for 6 weeks. Patients were limited to those with ulcers ranging from 0.5 to 2.5 cm in size. Endoscopically confirmed healing at 6 weeks was seen in significantly* more *Tagamet*-treated patients than in patients receiving placebo, as shown below:

	Tagamet	Placebo
week 2	14/63 (22%)	7/63 (11%)
total at week 6	43/65 (66%) *	30/67 (45%)

*p<0.05

In a similar multicenter U.S. study of the 800 mg h.s. oral regimen, the endoscopically confirmed healing rates were:

	Tagamet	Placebo
total at week 6	63/83 (76%) *	44/80 (55%)

*p = 0.005

Similarly, in worldwide double-blind clinical studies, endoscopically evaluated benign gastric ulcer healing rates were consistently higher with *Tagamet* than with placebo.

Gastroesophageal Reflux Disease

In two multicenter, double-blind, placebo-controlled studies in patients with gastroesophageal reflux disease (GERD) and endoscopically proven erosions and/or ulcers, *Tagamet* was significantly more effective than placebo in healing lesions. The endoscopically confirmed healing rates were:

Trial		*Tagamet* (800 mg b.i.d.)	*Tagamet* (400 mg q.i.d.)	Placebo	p-Value (800 mg b.i.d. vs. placebo)
1	Week 6	45%	52%	26%	0.02
	Week 12	60%	66%	42%	0.02
2	Week 6	50%		20%	<0.01
	Week 12	67%		36%	<0.01

In these trials *Tagamet* was superior to placebo by most measures in improving symptoms of day- and night-time heartburn, with many of the differences statistically significant. The q.i.d. regimen was generally somewhat better than the b.i.d. regimen where these were compared.

Prevention of Upper Gastrointestinal Bleeding in Critically Ill Patients

A double-blind, placebo-controlled randomized study of continuous infusion cimetidine was performed in 131 critically ill patients (mean APACHE II score = 15.99) to compare the incidence of upper gastrointestinal bleeding, manifested as hematemesis or bright red blood which did not clear after adjustment of the nasogastric tube and a 5 to 10 minute lavage, persistent Gastroccult® positive coffee grounds for 8 consecutive hours which did not clear with 100 cc lavage and/or which were accompanied by a drop in hematocrit of 5 percentage points, or melena, with an endoscopically documented upper gastrointestinal source of bleed. 14% (9/65) of patients treated with cimetidine continuous infusion developed bleeding compared to 33% (22/66) of the placebo group. Coffee grounds was the manifestation of bleeding that accounted for the difference between groups. Another randomized, double-blind placebo-controlled study confirmed these results for an end point of upper gastrointestinal bleeding with a confirmed upper gastrointestinal source noted on endoscopy, and by post hoc analyses of bleeding episodes between groups.

Pathological Hypersecretory Conditions
(such as Zollinger-Ellison Syndrome)

Tagamet significantly inhibited gastric acid secretion and reduced occurrence of diarrhea, anorexia and pain in patients with pathological hypersecretion associated with Zollinger-Ellison Syndrome, systemic mastocytosis and multiple endocrine adenomas. Use of *Tagamet* was also followed by healing of intractable ulcers.

INDICATIONS AND USAGE

Tagamet (cimetidine) is indicated in:

(1) Short-term treatment of active duodenal ulcer. Most patients heal within 4 weeks and there is rarely reason to use *Tagamet* at full dosage for longer than 6 to 8 weeks (see Dosage and Administration–Duodenal Ulcer). Concomitant antacids should be given as needed for relief of pain. However, simultaneous administration of *Tagamet* and antacids is not recommended, since antacids have been reported to interfere with the absorption of *Tagamet.*

(2) Maintenance therapy for duodenal ulcer patients at reduced dosage after healing of active ulcer. Patients have been maintained on continued treatment with *Tagamet* 400 mg h.s. for periods of up to 5 years.

(3) Short-term treatment of active benign gastric ulcer. There is no information concerning usefulness of treatment periods of longer than 8 weeks.

(4) Erosive gastroesophageal reflux disease (GERD). Erosive esophagitis diagnosed by endoscopy. Treatment is indicated for 12 weeks for healing of lesions and control of symptoms. The use of *Tagamet* beyond 12 weeks has not been established (see Dosage and Administration—GERD).

(5) Prevention of upper gastrointestinal bleeding in critically ill patients.

(6) The treatment of pathological hypersecretory conditions (i.e., Zollinger-Ellison Syndrome, systemic mastocytosis, multiple endocrine adenomas).

CONTRAINDICATIONS

Tagamet is contraindicated for patients known to have hypersensitivity to the product.

PRECAUTIONS

General: Rare instances of cardiac arrhythmias and hypotension have been reported following the rapid administration of Tagamet (cimetidine hydrochloride) Injection by intravenous bolus.

Symptomatic response to *Tagamet* therapy does not preclude the presence of a gastric malignancy. There have been rare reports of transient healing of gastric ulcers despite subsequently documented malignancy.

Reversible confusional states (see Adverse Reactions) have been observed on occasion, predominantly, but not exclusively, in severely ill patients. Advancing age (50 or more years) and preexisting liver and/or renal disease appear to be contributing factors. In some patients these confusional states have been mild and have not required discontinuation of *Tagamet* therapy. In cases where discontinuation was judged necessary, the condition usually cleared within 3 to 4 days of drug withdrawal.

Drug Interactions: *Tagamet,* apparently through an effect on certain microsomal enzyme systems, has been reported to reduce the hepatic metabolism of warfarin-type anticoagulants, phenytoin, propranolol, nifedipine, chlordiazepoxide, diazepam, certain tricyclic antidepressants, lidocaine, theophylline and metronidazole, thereby delaying elimination and increasing blood levels of these drugs.

Clinically significant effects have been reported with the warfarin anticoagulants; therefore, close monitoring of prothrombin time is recommended, and adjustment of the anticoagulant dose may be necessary when *Tagamet* is administered concomitantly. Interaction with phenytoin, lidocaine and theophylline has also been reported to produce adverse clinical effects.

However, a crossover study in healthy subjects receiving either *Tagamet* 300 mg q.i.d. or 800 mg h.s. concomitantly with a 300 mg b.i.d. dosage of theophylline (Theo-Dur®, Key Pharmaceuticals, Inc.) demonstrated less alteration in steady-state theophylline peak serum levels with the 800 mg h.s. regimen, particularly in subjects aged 54 years and older. Data beyond 10 days are not available. (Note: All patients receiving theophylline should be monitored appropriately, regardless of concomitant drug therapy.)

Dosage of the drugs mentioned above and other similarly metabolized drugs, particularly those of low therapeutic ratio or in patients with renal and/or hepatic impairment, may require adjustment when starting or stopping concomitantly administered *Tagamet* to maintain optimum therapeutic blood levels.

Alteration of pH may affect absorption of certain drugs (e.g., ketoconazole). If these products are needed, they should be given at least 2 hours before cimetidine administration.

Additional clinical experience may reveal other drugs affected by the concomitant administration of *Tagamet.*

Carcinogenesis, Mutagenesis, Impairment of Fertility: In a 24-month toxicity study conducted in rats, at dose levels of 150, 378 and 950 mg/kg/day (approximately 8 to 48 times the recommended human dose), there was a small increase in the incidence of benign Leydig cell tumors in each dose group; when the combined drug-treated groups and control groups were compared, this increase reached statistical significance. In a subsequent 24-month study, there were no differences between the rats receiving 150 mg/kg/day and the untreated controls. However, a statistically significant increase in benign Leydig cell tumor incidence was seen in the rats that received 378 and 950 mg/kg/day. These tumors were common in control groups as well as treated groups and the difference became apparent only in aged rats.

Tagamet (cimetidine) has demonstrated a weak antiandrogenic effect. In animal studies this was manifested as reduced prostate and seminal vesicle weights. However, there was no impairment of mating performance or fertility, nor any harm to the fetus in these animals at doses 8 to 48 times the full therapeutic dose of *Tagamet,* as compared with controls. The cases of gynecomastia seen in patients treated for 1 month or longer may be related to this effect. In human studies, *Tagamet* has been shown to have no effect on spermatogenesis, sperm count, motility, morphology or *in vitro* fertilizing capacity.

Pregnancy: Teratogenic Effects. Pregnancy Category B: Reproduction studies have been performed in rats, rabbits and mice at doses up to 40 times the normal human dose and have revealed no evidence of impaired fertility or harm to the fetus due to *Tagamet.* There are, however, no adequate and well-controlled studies in pregnant women. Because animal reproductive studies are not always predictive of human response, this drug should be used during pregnancy only if clearly needed.

Nursing Mothers: Cimetidine is secreted in human milk and, as a general rule, nursing should not be undertaken while a patient is on a drug.

Pediatric Use: Clinical experience in children is limited. Therefore, *Tagamet* therapy cannot be recommended for children under 16, unless, in the judgment of the physician, anticipated benefits outweigh the potential risks. In very limited experience, doses of 20 to 40 mg/kg per day have been used.

Immunocompromised Patients: In immunocompromised patients, decreased gastric acidity, including that produced by acid-suppressing agents such as cimetidine, may increase the possibility of a hyperinfection of strongyloidiasis.

ADVERSE REACTIONS

Adverse effects reported in patients taking *Tagamet* are described below by body system. Incidence figures of 1 in 100 and greater are generally derived from controlled clinical studies.

Gastrointestinal: Diarrhea (usually mild) has been reported in approximately 1 in 100 patients.

CNS: Headaches, ranging from mild to severe, have been reported in 3.5% of 924 patients taking 1600 mg/day, 2.1% of 2,225 patients taking 800 mg/day and 2.3% of 1,897 patients taking placebo. Dizziness and somnolence (usually mild) have been reported in approximately 1 in 100 patients on either 1600 mg/day or 800 mg/day.

Reversible confusional states, e.g., mental confusion, agitation, psychosis, depression, anxiety, hallucinations, disorientation, have been reported predominantly, but not exclusively, in severely ill patients. They have usually developed within 2 to 3 days of initiation of *Tagamet* therapy and have cleared within 3 to 4 days of discontinuation of the drug.

Endocrine: Gynecomastia has been reported in patients treated for 1 month or longer. In patients being treated for pathological hypersecretory states, this occurred in about 4% of cases while in all others the incidence was 0.3% to 1% in various studies. No evidence of induced endocrine dysfunction was found, and the condition remained unchanged or returned toward normal with continuing Tagamet (cimetidine) treatment.

Reversible impotence has been reported in patients with pathological hypersecretory disorders, e.g., Zollinger-Ellison Syndrome, receiving *Tagamet,* particularly in high doses, for at least 12 months (range 12 to 79 months, mean 38 months). However, in large-scale surveillance studies at regular dosage, the incidence has not exceeded that commonly reported in the general population.

Hematologic: Decreased white blood cell counts in *Tagamet*-treated patients (approximately 1 per 100,000 patients), including agranulocytosis (approximately 3 per million patients), have been reported, including a few reports of recurrence on rechallenge. Most of these reports were in patients who had serious concomitant illnesses and received drugs and/or treatment known to produce neutropenia. Thrombocytopenia (approximately 3 per million patients) and, very rarely, cases of pancytopenia or aplastic anemia have also been reported. As with some other H_2-receptor antagonists, there have been extremely rare reports of immune hemolytic anemia.

Hepatobiliary: Dose-related increases in serum transaminase have been reported. In most cases they did not progress with continued therapy and returned to normal at the end of therapy. There have been rare reports of cholestatic or mixed cholestatic-hepatocellular effects. These were usually reversible. Because of the predominance of cholestatic features, severe parenchymal injury is considered highly unlikely. However, as in the occasional liver injury with other H_2-receptor antagonists, in exceedingly rare circumstances fatal outcomes have been reported.

There has been reported a single case of biopsy-proven periportal hepatic fibrosis in a patient receiving *Tagamet.*

Rare cases of pancreatitis, which cleared on withdrawal of the drug, have been reported.

Hypersensitivity: Rare cases of fever and allergic reactions including anaphylaxis and hypersensitivity vasculitis, which cleared on withdrawal of the drug, have been reported.

Renal: Small, possibly dose-related increases in plasma creatinine, presumably due to competition for renal tubular secretion, are not uncommon and do not signify deteriorating renal function. Rare cases of interstitial nephritis and urinary retention, which cleared on withdrawal of the drug, have been reported.

Cardiovascular: Rare cases of bradycardia, tachycardia and A-V heart block have been reported with H_2-receptor antagonists.

Musculoskeletal: There have been rare reports of reversible arthralgia and myalgia; exacerbation of joint symptoms in patients with preexisting arthritis has also been reported. Such symptoms have usually been alleviated by a reduction in Tagamet (cimetidine) dosage. Rare cases of polymyositis have been reported, but no causal relationship has been established.

Integumental: Mild rash and, very rarely, cases of severe generalized skin reactions including Stevens-Johnson syndrome, epidermal necrolysis, erythema multiforme, exfoliative dermatitis and generalized exfoliative erythroderma have been reported with H_2-receptor antagonists. Reversible alopecia has been reported very rarely.

Immune Function: There have been extremely rare reports of strongyloidiasis hyperinfection in immunocompromised patients.

OVERDOSAGE

Studies in animals indicate that toxic doses are associated with respiratory failure and tachycardia that may be controlled by assisted respiration and the administration of a beta-blocker.

Reported acute ingestions orally of up to 20 grams have been associated with transient adverse effects similar to those encountered in normal clinical experience. The usual measures to remove unabsorbed material from the gastrointestinal tract, clinical monitoring and supportive therapy should be employed.

There have been reports of severe CNS symptoms, including unresponsiveness, following ingestion of between 20 and 40 grams of cimetidine, and extremely rare reports following concomitant use of multiple CNS-active medications and ingestion of cimetidine at doses less than 20 grams. An elderly, terminally ill dehydrated patient with organic brain syndrome receiving concomitant antipsychotic agents and *Tagamet* 4800 mg intravenously over a 24-hour period experienced mental deterioration with reversal on *Tagamet* discontinuation.

There have been two deaths in adults who were reported to have ingested over 40 grams orally on a single occasion.

DOSAGE AND ADMINISTRATION

Duodenal Ulcer

Active Duodenal Ulcer: Clinical studies have indicated that suppression of nocturnal acid is the most important factor in duodenal ulcer healing (see Clinical Pharmacology—Acid Secretion). This is supported by recent clinical trials (see Clinical Trials—Active Duodenal Ulcer). Therefore, there is no apparent rationale, except for familiarity with use, for treating with anything other than a once-daily at bedtime dosage regimen (h.s.).

In a U.S. dose-ranging study of 400 mg h.s., 800 mg h.s. and 1600 mg h.s., a continuous dose response relationship for ulcer healing was demonstrated.

However, 800 mg h.s. is the dose of choice for most patients, as it provides a high healing rate (the difference between 800 mg h.s. and 1600 mg h.s. being small), maximal pain relief, a decreased potential for drug interactions (see Precautions—Drug Interactions) and maximal patient convenience. Patients unhealed at 4 weeks, or those with persistent symptoms, have been shown to benefit from 2 to 4 weeks of continued therapy.

It has been shown that patients who both have an endoscopically demonstrated ulcer larger than 1.0 cm and are also heavy smokers (i.e., smoke one pack of cigarettes or more per day) are more difficult to heal. There is some evidence which suggests that more rapid healing can be achieved in this subpopulation with *Tagamet* 1600 mg at bedtime. While early pain relief with either 800 mg h.s. or 1600 mg h.s. is equivalent in all patients, 1600 mg h.s. provides an appropriate alternative when it is important to ensure healing within 4 weeks for this subpopulation. Alternatively, approximately 94% of all patients will also heal in 8 weeks with *Tagamet* 800 mg h.s.

Other *Tagamet* regimens in the U.S. which have been shown to be effective are: 300 mg four times daily, with meals and at bedtime, the original regimen with which U.S. physicians have the most experience, and 400 mg twice daily, in the morning and at bedtime (see Clinical Trials—Active Duodenal Ulcer).

Concomitant antacids should be given as needed for relief of pain. However, simultaneous administration of *Tagamet* and antacids is not recommended, since antacids have been reported to interfere with the absorption of Tagamet (cimetidine).

While healing with *Tagamet* often occurs during the first week or two, treatment should be continued for 4 to 6 weeks unless healing has been demonstrated by endoscopic examination.

Maintenance Therapy for Duodenal Ulcer: In those patients requiring maintenance therapy, the recommended adult oral dose is 400 mg at bedtime.

Active Benign Gastric Ulcer

The recommended adult oral dosage for short-term treatment of active benign gastric ulcer is 800 mg h.s., or 300 mg four times a day with meals and at bedtime. Controlled clinical studies were limited to 6 weeks of treatment (see Clinical Trials). 800 mg h.s. is the preferred regimen for most patients based upon convenience and reduced potential for drug interactions. Symptomatic response to *Tagamet* does not preclude the presence of a gastric malignancy. It is important to follow gastric ulcer patients to assure rapid progress to complete healing.

Erosive Gastroesophageal Reflux Disease (GERD)

The recommended adult oral dosage for the treatment of erosive esophagitis that has been diagnosed by endoscopy is 1600 mg daily in divided doses (800 mg b.i.d. or 400 mg q.i.d.) for 12 weeks. The use of *Tagamet* beyond 12 weeks has not been established.

Prevention of Upper Gastrointestinal Bleeding

The recommended adult dosing regimen is continuous I.V. infusion of 50 mg/hour. Patients with creatinine clearance less than 30 cc/min. should receive half the recommended dose. Treatment beyond 7 days has not been studied.

Pathological Hypersecretory Conditions
(such as Zollinger-Ellison Syndrome)

Recommended adult oral dosage: 300 mg four times a day with meals and at bedtime. In some patients it may be necessary to administer higher doses more frequently. Doses should be adjusted to individual patient needs, but should not usually exceed 2400 mg per day and should continue as long as clinically indicated.

Parenteral Administration

In hospitalized patients with pathological hypersecretory conditions or intractable ulcers, or in patients who are unable to take oral medication, *Tagamet* may be administered parenterally.

The doses and regimen for parenteral administration in patients with GERD have not been established.

All parenteral drug products should be inspected visually for particulate matter and discoloration prior to administration.

Recommendations for parenteral administration:

Intramuscular injection: 300 mg q 6 to 8 hours (no dilution necessary). Transient pain at the site of injection has been reported.

Intravenous injection: 300 mg q 6 to 8 hours. In some patients it may be necessary to increase dosage. When this is necessary, the increases should be made by more frequent administration of a 300 mg dose, but should not exceed 2400 mg per day. Dilute Tagamet (cimetidine hydrochloride) Injection, 300 mg, in Sodium Chloride Injection (0.9%) or another compatible I.V. solution (see Stability of *Tagamet* Injection) to a total volume of 20 mL and inject over a period of not less than 5 minutes (see Precautions).

Intermittent intravenous infusion: 300 mg q 6 to 8 hours, infused over 15 to 20 minutes. In some patients it may be necessary to increase dosage. When this is necessary, the increases should be made by more frequent administration of a 300 mg dose, but should not exceed 2400 mg per day. **Vials:** Dilute *Tagamet* Injection, 300 mg, in at least 50 mL of 5% Dextrose Injection, or another compatible I.V. solution (see Stability of *Tagamet* Injection). **Plastic containers:** Use premixed *Tagamet* Injection, 300 mg, in 0.9% Sodium Chloride in 50 mL plastic containers. **ADD-Vantage® Vials:** Dilute contents of one vial in an ADD-Vantage® Diluent Container, available in 50 mL and 100 mL sizes of 0.9% Sodium Chloride Injection, and 5% Dextrose Injection.

Continuous intravenous infusion: 37.5 mg/hour (900 mg/day). For patients requiring a more rapid elevation of gastric pH, continuous infusion may be preceded by a 150 mg loading dose administered by I.V. infusion as described above. Dilute 900 mg *Tagamet* Injection in a compatible I.V. fluid (see Stability of *Tagamet* Injection) for constant rate infusion over a 24-hour period. Note: *Tagamet* may be diluted in 100 to 1000 mL; however, a volumetric pump is recommended if the volume for 24-hour infusion is less than 250 mL. In one study in patients with pathological hypersecretory states, the mean infused dose of cimetidine was 160 mg/hour with a range of 40 to 600 mg/hour. These doses maintained the intragastric acid secretory rate at 10 mEq/hour or less. The infusion rate should be adjusted to individual patient requirements.

DIRECTIONS FOR USE OF TAGAMET (cimetidine hydrochloride) INJECTION IN PLASTIC CONTAINERS

To open: Tear overwrap down side at slit and remove solution containers.

Some opacity of the plastic due to moisture absorption during the sterilization process may be observed. This is normal and does not affect solution quality or safety. The opacity will diminish gradually.

Do not add other drugs to premixed *Tagamet* Injection in plastic containers.

CAUTION: Check for minute leaks by squeezing inner bag firmly. If leaks are found, discard solution as sterility may be impaired. Additives should not be introduced into this solution. Do not use if the solution is cloudy or precipitated or if the seal is not intact.

Do not use plastic containers in series connections. Such use could result in air embolism due to residual air being drawn from the primary container before administration of the fluid from the secondary container is complete.

Continued on next page

Information on the SmithKline Beecham Pharmaceuticals products appearing here is based on the labeling in effect on June 15, 2000. Further information on these and other products may be obtained from the Medical Department, SmithKline Beecham Pharmaceuticals, One Franklin Plaza, Philadelphia, PA 19101.

Tagamet—Cont.

Use sterile equipment.

Preparation for administration:

1. Suspend container from eyelet support.
2. Remove plastic protector from outlet port at bottom of container.
3. Attach administration set. Refer to complete directions accompanying set.

DIRECTIONS FOR USE OF TAGAMET® INJECTION IN ADD-VANTAGE® VIALS are enclosed in ADD-Vantage® Vial packaging.

Stability of *Tagamet* Injection

When added to or diluted with most commonly used intravenous solutions, e.g., Sodium Chloride Injection (0.9%), Dextrose Injection (5% or 10%), Lactated Ringer's Solution, 5% Sodium Bicarbonate Injection, Tagamet (cimetidine hydrochloride) Injection should not be used after more than 48 hours of storage at room temperature.

Tagamet Injection premixed in plastic containers is stable through the labeled expiration date when stored under the recommended conditions.

Dosage Adjustment for Patients with Impaired Renal Function

Patients with severely impaired renal function have been treated with *Tagamet.* However, such usage has been very limited. On the basis of this experience the recommended dosage is 300 mg q 12 hours orally or by intravenous injection. Should the patient's condition require, the frequency of dosing may be increased to q 8 hours or even further with caution. In severe renal failure, accumulation may occur and the lowest frequency of dosing compatible with an adequate patient response should be used. When liver impairment is also present, further reductions in dosage may be necessary. Hemodialysis reduces the level of circulating *Tagamet.* Ideally, the dosage schedule should be adjusted so that the timing of a scheduled dose coincides with the end of hemodialysis.

Patients with creatinine clearance less than 30 cc/min. who are being treated for prevention of upper gastrointestinal bleeding should receive half the recommended dose.

HOW SUPPLIED

Tablets: Light green, film-coated as follows: 200 mg—round, imprinted with the product name TAGAMET, SKF and 200—tablets in bottles of 100; 300 mg—round, debossed with the product name TAGAMET, SB and 300—tablets in bottles of 100 and Single Unit Packages of 100 (intended for institutional use only); 400 mg—oval-shaped Tiltab®, debossed with the product name TAGAMET, SB and 400—tablets in bottles of 60 and Single Unit Packages of 100 (intended for institutional use only); 800 mg—oval-shaped Tiltab®, debossed with the product name TAGAMET, SB and 800—tablets in bottles of 30 and Single Unit Packages of 100 (intended for institutional use only).

Store between 15° and 30°C (59° and 86°F); dispense in a tight light-resistant container.

200 mg 100's: NDC 0108-5012-20
300 mg 100's: NDC 0108-5013-20
300 mg SUP 100's: NDC 0108-5013-21
400 mg 60's: NDC 0108-5026-18
400 mg SUP 100's: NDC 0108-5026-21
800 mg 30's: NDC 0108-5027-13
800 mg SUP 100's: NDC 0108-5027-21

Liquid: Clear, light orange, mint-peach flavored, as follows: 300 mg/5 mL in 8 fl oz (237 mL) amber glass bottles; 300 mg/5 mL in single-dose units in packages of 10 (intended for institutional use only).

Store between 15° and 30°C (59° and 86°F); dispense in a tight light-resistant container.

300 mg/5 mL 8 fl oz: NDC 0108-5014-48
300 mg/5 mL SUP 10's: NDC 0108-5014-10

Injection:

Vials: 300 mg/2 mL in single-dose vials, in packages of 25, and in 8 mL multi-dose vials, in packages of 10 and 25.

Store between 15° and 30°C (59° and 86°F); do not refrigerate.

300 mg/2 mL Single-Dose Vials: NDC 0108-5017-16 (package of 25 vials)

300 mg/2 mL in 8 mL Multi-Dose Vials:
NDC 0108-5022-11 (package of 10 vials)
NDC 0108-5022-16 (package of 25 vials)

Single-Dose Premixed Plastic Containers: 300 mg in 50 mL of 0.9% Sodium Chloride in single-dose plastic containers, in packages of 4 units. No preservative has been added.

Exposure of the premixed product to excessive heat should be avoided. It is recommended the product be stored between 15° and 30°C (59° and 86°F). Brief exposure up to 40°C does not adversely affect the premixed product.

300 mg/50 mL SUP's: NDC 0108-5029-04

ADD-Vantage® Vials: 300 mg/2 mL in single-dose ADD-Vantage® Vials, in packages of 25.

Store between 15° and 30°C (59° and 86°F); do not refrigerate.

300 mg/2 mL: NDC 0108-5031-16 (package of 25 vials)

Tagamet (cimetidine hydrochloride) Injection premixed in single-dose plastic containers is manufactured for SmithKline Beecham Pharmaceuticals by Baxter Healthcare Corporation, Deerfield, IL 60015.

TG:L92A

Shown in Product Identification Guide, page 337

TAZICEF® ℞

[taz ′i-sef]

brand of ceftazidime for injection
for intravenous or intramuscular use

DESCRIPTION

Ceftazidime is a semisynthetic, broad-spectrum, beta-lactam antibiotic for parenteral administration. It is the pentahydrate of pyridinium, 1-[[7-[[(2-amino-4-thiazolyl)[(1-carboxy-1-methylethoxy) imino]acetyl]amino]-2-carboxy-8-oxo-5-thia-1-azabicyclo (4.2.0.)oct-2-en-3-yl] methyl]-, hydroxide,inner salt, [6R-[6α,7β(Z)]]. It has the following structure:

The empirical formula is $C_{22}H_{32}N_6O_{12}S_2$, representing a molecular weight of 636.6.

Tazicef (ceftazidime for injection) is a sterile, dry, powdered mixture of ceftazidime pentahydrate and sodium carbonate. The sodium carbonate at a concentration of 118 mg/gram of ceftazidime activity has been admixed to facilitate dissolution. The total sodium content of the mixture is approximately 54 mg (2.3 mEq)/gram of ceftazidime activity.

Tazicef in sterile crystalline form is supplied in vials equivalent to 1 gram or 2 grams of anhydrous ceftazidime, in piggyback vials equivalent to 1 gram or 2 grams of anhydrous ceftazidime and in ADD-Vantage® vials equivalent to 1 gram or 2 grams of anhydrous ceftazidime. Solutions of *Tazicef* range in color from light yellow to amber, depending on the diluent and volume used. The pH of freshly reconstituted solutions usually ranges from 5 to 8.

CLINICAL PHARMACOLOGY

After IV administration of 500-mg and 1-gram doses of ceftazidime over 5 minutes to normal adult male volunteers, mean peak serum concentrations of 45 mcg/mL and 90 mcg/mL, respectively, were achieved. After IV infusion of 500-mg, 1-gram and 2-gram doses of ceftazidime over 20 to 30 minutes to normal adult male volunteers, mean peak serum concentrations of 42 mcg/mL, 69 mcg/mL and 170 mcg/mL, respectively, were achieved. The average serum concentrations following IV infusion of 500-mg, 1-gram and 2-gram doses to these volunteers over an 8-hour interval are given in Table 1.

Table 1

Ceftazidime IV Dosage	Serum Concentrations (mcg/mL)				
	0.5 hr.	1 hr.	2 hr.	4 hr.	8 hr.
500 mg	42	25	12	6	2
1 gram	60	39	23	11	3
2 grams	129	75	42	13	5

The absorption and elimination of ceftazidime were directly proportional to the size of the dose. The half-life following IV administration was approximately 1.9 hours. Less than 10% of ceftazidime was protein bound. The degree of protein binding was independent of concentration. There was no evidence of accumulation of ceftazidime in the serum in individuals with normal renal function following multiple IV doses of 1 gram and 2 grams every 8 hours for 10 days.

Following IM administration of 500-mg and 1-gram doses of ceftazidime to normal adult volunteers, the mean peak serum concentrations were 17 mcg/mL and 39 mcg/mL, respectively, at approximately 1 hour. Serum concentrations remained above 4 mcg/mL for 6 and 8 hours after the IM administration of 500-mg and 1-gram doses, respectively. The half-life of ceftazidime in these volunteers was approximately 2 hours.

The presence of hepatic dysfunction had no effect on the pharmacokinetics of ceftazidime in individuals administered 2 grams intravenously every 8 hours for 5 days. Therefore, a dosage adjustment from the normal recommended dosage is not required for patients with hepatic dysfunction, provided renal function is not impaired.

Approximately 80% to 90% of an IM or IV dose of ceftazidime is excreted unchanged by the kidneys over a 24-hour period. After the IV administration of single 500-mg or 1-gram doses, approximately 50% of the dose appeared in the urine in the first 2 hours. An additional 20% was excreted between 2 and 4 hours after dosing, and approximately another 12% of the dose appeared in the urine between 4 and 8 hours later. The elimination of ceftazidime by the kidneys resulted in high therapeutic concentrations in the urine.

The mean renal clearance of ceftazidime was approximately 100 mL/min. The calculated plasma clearance of approximately 115 mL/min. indicated nearly complete elimination of ceftazidime by the renal route. Administration of probenecid before dosing had no effect on the elimination kinetics of ceftazidime. This suggested that ceftazidime is eliminated by glomerular filtration and is not actively secreted by renal tubular mechanisms.

Since ceftazidime is eliminated almost solely by the kidneys, its serum half-life is significantly prolonged in patients with impaired renal function. Consequently, dosage adjustments in such patients as described in the DOSAGE AND ADMINISTRATION section are suggested.

Therapeutic concentrations of ceftazidime are achieved in the following body tissues and fluids.

[See table below]

Microbiology: Ceftazidime is bactericidal in action, exerting its effect by inhibition of enzymes responsible for cell-wall synthesis. A wide range of gram-negative organisms is susceptible to ceftazidime *in vitro,* including strains resistant to gentamicin and other aminoglycosides. In addition, ceftazidime has been shown to be active against gram-positive organisms. It is highly stable to most clinically important beta-lactamases, plasmid or chromosomal, which are produced by both gram-negative and gram-positive organisms and, consequently, is active against many strains resistant to ampicillin and other cephalosporins.

Ceftazidime has been shown to be active against the following organisms both *in vitro* and in clinical infections (see INDICATIONS AND USAGE).

Aerobes, Gram-Negative: *Citrobacter* spp. (including *Citrobacter freundii* and *Citrobacter diversus*); *Enterobacter* spp. (including *Enterobacter cloacae* and *Enterobacter aerogenes*); *Escherichia coli; Haemophilus influenzae,* including ampicillin-resistant strains; *Klebsiella* spp. (including *Klebsiella pneumoniae*); *Neisseria meningitidis; Proteus mirabilis; Proteus vulgaris; Pseudomonas* spp. (including *Pseudomonas aeruginosa*); and *Serratia* spp.

Aerobes, Gram-Positive: *Staphylococcus aureus,* including penicillinase- and non-penicillinase-producing strains; *Streptococcus agalactiae* (group B streptococci); *Streptococcus pneumoniae;* and *Streptococcus pyogenes* (group A beta-hemolytic streptococci).

Anaerobes: *Bacteroides* spp. (NOTE: Many strains of *Bacteroides fragilis* are resistant).

Ceftazidime has been shown to be active *in vitro* against most strains of the following organisms; however, the clinical significance of these data is unknown: *Acinetobacter* spp.; *Clostridium* spp. (not including *Clostridium difficile*); *Haemophilus parainfluenzae; Morganella morganii* (formerly *Proteus morganii*); *Neisseria gonorrhoeae; Peptococcus* spp.; *Peptostreptococcus* spp.; *Providencia* spp. (including *Providencia rettgeri,* formerly *Proteus rettgeri*); *Salmonella* spp.; *Shigella* spp.; *Staphylococcus epidermidis;* and *Yersinia enterocolitica.*

Ceftazidime and the aminoglycosides have been shown to be synergistic *in vitro* against *Pseudomonas aeruginosa* and

Table 2. Ceftazidime Concentrations in Body Tissues and Fluids

Tissue or Fluid	Dose/Route	No. Patients	Time of Sample Post-Dose	Average Tissue or Fluid Level (mcg/mL or mcg/g)
Urine	500 mg IM	6	0 to 2 hours	2,100.0
	2 grams IV	6	0 to 2 hours	12,000.0
Bile	2 grams IV	3	90 min.	36.4
Synovial fluid	2 grams IV	13	2 hours	25.6
Peritoneal fluid	2 grams IV	8	2 hours	48.6
Sputum	1 gram IV	8	1 hour	9.0
Cerebrospinal fluid (inflamed	2 grams q8h IV	5	120 min.	9.8
meninges)	2 grams q8h IV	6	180 min.	9.4
Aqueous humor	2 grams IV	13	1 to 3 hours	11.0
Blister fluid	1 gram IV	7	2 to 3 hours	19.7
Lymphatic fluid	1 gram IV	7	2 to 3 hours	23.4
Bone	2 grams IV	8	0.67 hour	31.1
Heart muscle	2 grams IV	35	30 to 280 min.	12.7
Skin	2 grams IV	22	30 to 180 min.	6.6
Skeletal muscle	2 grams IV	35	30 to 280 min.	9.4
Myometrium	2 grams IV	31	1 to 2 hours	18.7

the enterobacteriaceae. Ceftazidime and carbenicillin have also been shown to be synergistic *in vitro* against *Pseudomonas aeruginosa.*

Ceftazidime is not active *in vitro* against: methicillin-resistant staphylococci, *Streptococcus faecalis* and many other enterococci, *Listeria monocytogenes, Campylobacter* spp., or *Clostridium difficile.*

Susceptibility Tests: ***Diffusion Techniques:*** Quantitative methods that require measurement of zone diameters give an estimate of antibiotic susceptibility. One such procedure [1–3] has been recommended for use with disks to test susceptibility to ceftazidime.

Reports from the laboratory giving results of the standard single-disk susceptibility test with a 30 mcg ceftazidime disk should be interpreted according to the following criteria:

Susceptible organisms produce zones of 18 mm or greater, indicating that the test organism is likely to respond to therapy.

Organisms that produce zones of 15 mm to 17 mm are expected to be susceptible if high dosage is used or if the infection is confined to tissues and fluids (e.g., urine) in which high antibiotic levels are attained.

Resistant organisms produce zones of 14 mm or less, indicating that other therapy should be selected.

Organisms should be tested with the ceftazidime disk, since ceftazidime has been shown by *in vitro* tests to be active against certain strains found resistant when other betalactam disks are used.

Standardized procedures require the use of laboratory control organisms. The 30 mcg ceftazidime disk should give zone diameters between 25 mm and 32 mm for *Escherichia coli* ATCC 25922. For *Pseudomonas aeruginosa* ATCC 27853, the zone diameters should be between 22 mm and 29 mm. For *Staphylococcus aureus* ATCC 25923, the zone diameters should be between 16 mm and 20 mm.

Dilution Techniques: In other susceptibility testing procedures, e.g., ICS agar dilution or the equivalent, a bacterial isolate may be considered susceptible if the minimum inhibitory concentration (MIC) value for ceftazidime is not more than 16 mcg/mL. Organisms are considered resistant to ceftazidime if the MIC is ≥64 mcg/mL. Organisms having an MIC value of <64 mcg/mL but >16 mcg/mL are expected to be susceptible if high dosage is used or if the infection is confined to tissues and fluids (e.g., urine) in which high antibiotic levels are attained.

As with standard diffusion methods, dilution procedures require the use of laboratory control organisms. Standard ceftazidime powder should give MIC values in the range of 4 mcg/mL to 16 mcg/mL for *Staphylococcus aureus* ATCC 25923. For *Escherichia coli* ATCC 25922, the MIC range should be between 0.125 mcg/mL and 0.5 mcg/mL. For *Pseudomonas aeruginosa* ATCC 27853, the MIC range should be between 0.5 mcg/mL and 2 mcg/mL.

INDICATIONS AND USAGE

Tazicef (ceftazidime for injection) is indicated for the treatment of patients with infections caused by susceptible strains of the designated organisms in the following diseases:

1. Lower Respiratory Tract Infections, including pneumonia, caused by *Pseudomonas aeruginosa* and other *Pseudomonas* spp.; *Haemophilus influenzae,* including ampicillin-resistant strains; *Klebsiella* spp.; *Enterobacter* spp.; *Proteus mirabilis; Escherichia coli; Serratia* spp.; *Citrobacter* spp.; *Streptococcus pneumoniae;* and *Staphylococcus aureus* (methicillin-susceptible strains).

2. Skin and Skin-Structure Infections caused by *Pseudomonas aeruginosa; Klebsiella* spp.; *Escherichia coli; Proteus* spp., including *Proteus mirabilis* and indole-positive *Proteus; Enterobacter* spp.; *Serratia* spp.; *Staphylococcus aureus* (methicillin-susceptible strains); and *Streptococcus pyogenes* (group A beta-hemolytic streptococci).

3. Urinary Tract Infections, both complicated and uncomplicated, caused by *Pseudomonas aeruginosa; Enterobacter* spp.; *Proteus* spp., including *Proteus mirabilis* and indole-positive *Proteus; Klebsiella* spp.; and *Escherichia coli.*

4. Bacterial Septicemia caused by *Pseudomonas aeruginosa, Klebsiella* spp., *Haemophilus influenzae, Escherichia coli, Serratia* spp., *Streptococcus pneumoniae,* and *Staphylococcus aureus* (methicillin-susceptible strains).

5. Bone and Joint Infections caused by *Pseudomonas aeruginosa; Klebsiella* spp.; *Enterobacter* spp., and *Staphylococcus aureus* (methicillin-susceptible strains).

6. Gynecologic Infections, including endometritis, pelvic cellulitis, and other infections of the female genital tract caused by *Escherichia coli.*

7. Intra-abdominal Infections, including peritonitis caused by *Escherichia coli, Klebsiella* spp., and *Staphylococcus aureus* (methicillin-susceptible strains) and polymicrobial infections caused by aerobic and anaerobic organisms and *Bacteroides* spp. (many strains of *Bacteroides fragilis* are resistant).

8. Central Nervous System Infections, including meningitis, caused by *Haemophilus influenzae* and *Neisseria meningitidis.* Ceftazidime has also been used successfully in a limited number of cases of meningitis due to *Pseudomonas aeruginosa* and *Streptococcus pneumoniae.*

Specimens for bacterial cultures should be obtained before therapy in order to isolate and identify causative organisms and to determine their susceptibility to ceftazidime. Therapy may be instituted before results of susceptibility studies are known; however, once these results become available, the antibiotic treatment should be adjusted accordingly.

Tazicef (ceftazidime for injection) may be used alone in cases of confirmed or suspected sepsis. Ceftazidime has been used successfully in clinical trials as empiric therapy in cases where various concomitant therapies with other antibiotics have been used.

Tazicef may also be used concomitantly with other antibiotics, such as aminoglycosides, vancomycin and clindamycin, in severe and life-threatening infections and in the immunocompromised patient. When such concomitant treatment is appropriate, prescribing information in the labeling for the other antibiotics should be followed. The dose depends on the severity of the infection and the patient's condition.

CONTRAINDICATIONS

Tazicef is contraindicated in patients who have shown hypersensitivity to ceftazidime or the cephalosporin group of antibiotics.

WARNINGS

BEFORE THERAPY WITH *TAZICEF* IS INSTITUTED, CAREFUL INQUIRY SHOULD BE MADE TO DETERMINE WHETHER THE PATIENT HAS HAD PREVIOUS HYPERSENSITIVITY REACTIONS TO CEFTAZIDIME, CEPHALOSPORINS, PENICILLINS, OR OTHER DRUGS. IF THIS PRODUCT IS TO BE GIVEN TO PENICILLIN-SENSITIVE PATIENTS, CAUTION SHOULD BE EXERCISED BECAUSE CROSS-HYPERSENSITIVITY AMONG BETA-LACTAM ANTIBIOTICS HAS BEEN CLEARLY DOCUMENTED AND MAY OCCUR IN UP TO 10% OF PATIENTS WITH A HISTORY OF PENICILLIN ALLERGY. IF AN ALLERGIC REACTION TO *TAZICEF* OCCURS, DISCONTINUE TREATMENT WITH THE DRUG. SERIOUS ACUTE HYPERSENSITIVITY REACTIONS MAY REQUIRE TREATMENT WITH EPINEPHRINE AND OTHER EMERGENCY MEASURES, INCLUDING OXYGEN, IV FLUIDS, IV ANTIHISTAMINES, CORTICOSTEROIDS, PRESSOR AMINES AND AIRWAY MANAGEMENT, AS CLINICALLY INDICATED.

Pseudomembranous colitis has been reported with nearly all antibacterial agents, including ceftazidime, and may range in severity from mild to life-threatening. Therefore, it is important to consider this diagnosis in patients who present with diarrhea subsequent to the administration of antibacterial agents.

Treatment with antibacterial agents alters the normal flora of the colon and may permit overgrowth of clostridia. Studies indicate that a toxin produced by *Clostridium difficile* is a primary cause of "antibiotic-associated colitis."

After the diagnosis of pseudomembranous colitis has been established, appropriate therapeutic measures should be initiated. Mild cases of pseudomembranous colitis usually respond to drug discontinuation alone. In moderate to severe cases, consideration should be given to management with fluids and electrolytes, protein supplementation and treatment with an oral antibacterial drug clinically effective against *Clostridium difficile* colitis.

Elevated levels of ceftazidime in patients with renal insufficiency can lead to seizures, encephalopathy, asterixis and neuromuscular excitability (see PRECAUTIONS).

PRECAUTIONS

General: Ceftazidime has not been shown to be nephrotoxic; however, high and prolonged serum antibiotic concentrations can occur from usual dosages in patients with transient or persistent reduction of urinary output because of renal insufficiency. The total daily dosage should be reduced when ceftazidime is administered to patients with renal insufficiency (see DOSAGE AND ADMINISTRATION). Elevated levels of ceftazidime in these patients can lead to seizures, encephalopathy, asterixis and neuromuscular excitability. Continued dosage should be determined by degree of renal impairment, severity of infection and susceptibility of the causative organisms.

As with other antibiotics, prolonged use of Tazicef (ceftazidime for injection) may result in overgrowth of nonsusceptible organisms. Repeated evaluation of the patient's condition is essential. If superinfection occurs during therapy, appropriate measures should be taken.

Inducible type-1 beta-lactamase resistance has been noted with some organisms (e.g., *Enterobacter* spp., *Pseudomonas* spp., and *Serratia* spp.). As with other extended-spectrum beta-lactam antibiotics, resistance can develop during therapy, leading to clinical failure in some cases. When treating infections caused by these organisms, periodic susceptibility testing should be performed when clinically appropriate. If patients fail to respond to monotherapy, an aminoglycoside or similar agent should be considered.

Cephalosporins may be associated with a fall in prothrombin activity. Those at risk include patients with renal or hepatic impairment, or poor nutritional state, as well as patients receiving a protracted course of antimicrobial therapy. Prothrombin time should be monitored in patients at risk and exogenous vitamin K administered as indicated.

Tazicef should be prescribed with caution in individuals with a history of gastrointestinal disease, particularly colitis.

Distal necrosis can occur after inadvertent intra-arterial administration of ceftazidime.

Drug Interactions: Nephrotoxicity has been reported following concomitant administration of cephalosporins with aminoglycoside antibiotics or potent diuretics, such as furosemide. Renal function should be carefully monitored, especially if higher dosages of the aminoglycosides are to be administered or if therapy is prolonged, because of the potential nephrotoxicity and ototoxicity of aminoglycoside antibiotics. Nephrotoxicity and ototoxicity were not noted when ceftazidime was given alone in clinical trials.

Chloramphenicol has been shown to be antagonistic to beta-lactam antibiotics, including ceftazidime, based on *in vitro* studies and time kill curves with enteric gram-negative bacilli. Due to the possibility of antagonism *in vivo*, particularly when bactericidal activity is desired, this drug combination should be avoided.

Drug/Laboratory Test Interactions: The administration of ceftazidime may result in a false-positive reaction for glucose in the urine when using Clinitest® tablets, Benedict's solution or Fehling's solution. It is recommended that glucose tests based on enzymatic glucose oxidase reactions (such as Clinistix® or Tes-Tape®) be used.

Carcinogenesis, Mutagenesis, Impairment of Fertility: Long-term studies in animals have not been performed to evaluate carcinogenic potential. However, a mouse micronucleus test and an Ames test were both negative for mutagenic effects.

Pregnancy: ***Teratogenic Effects:*** Pregnancy Category B. Reproduction studies have been performed in mice and rats at doses up to 40 times the human dose and have revealed no evidence of impaired fertility or harm to the fetus due to *Tazicef.* There are, however, no adequate and well-controlled studies in pregnant women. Because animal reproduction studies are not always predictive of human response, this drug should be used during pregnancy only if clearly needed.

Nursing Mothers: Ceftazidime is excreted in human milk in low concentrations. Caution should be exercised when *Tazicef* is administered to a nursing woman.

Pediatric Use: (See DOSAGE AND ADMINISTRATION).

ADVERSE REACTIONS

Ceftazidime is generally well-tolerated. The incidence of adverse reactions associated with the administration of ceftazidime was low in clinical trials. The most common were local reactions following IV injection and allergic and gastrointestinal reactions. Other adverse reactions were encountered infrequently. No disulfiram-like reactions were reported.

The following adverse effects from clinical trials were considered to be either related to ceftazidime therapy or were of uncertain etiology:

Local Effects, reported in fewer than 2% of patients, were phlebitis and inflammation at the site of injection (1 in 69 patients).

Hypersensitivity Reactions, reported in 2% of patients, were pruritus, rash and fever. Toxic epidermal necrolysis, Stevens-Johnson syndrome, and erythema multiforme have also been reported with cephalosporin antibiotics, including ceftazidime. Immediate reactions, generally manifested by rash and/or pruritus, occurred in 1 in 285 patients. Angioedema and anaphylaxis (bronchospasm and/or hypotension) have been reported very rarely.

Gastrointestinal Symptoms, reported in fewer than 2% of patients, were diarrhea (1 in 78), nausea (1 in 156), vomiting (1 in 500) and abdominal pain (1 in 416). The onset of pseudomembranous colitis symptoms may occur during or after treatment (see WARNINGS).

Central Nervous System Reactions (fewer than 1%) include headache, dizziness and paresthesia. Seizures have been reported with several cephalosporins, including ceftazidime. In addition, encephalopathy, asterixis and neuromuscular excitability have been reported in renally impaired patients treated with unadjusted dosage regimens of ceftazidime (see PRECAUTIONS: General).

Less Frequent Adverse Events (fewer than 1%) were candidiasis (including oral thrush) and vaginitis.

Hematologic: Rare cases of hemolytic anemia have been reported.

Laboratory Test Changes noted during Tazicef (ceftazidime for injection) clinical trials were transient and included: eosinophilia (1 in 13), positive Coombs' test without hemolysis (1 in 23), thrombocytosis (1 in 45), and slight elevations in one or more of the hepatic enzymes, aspartate aminotransferase (AST,SGOT) (1 in 16), alanine aminotransferase (ALT, SGPT) (1 in 15), LDH (1 in 18), GGT (1 in 19) and alkaline phosphatase (1 in 23). As with some other cephalosporins, transient elevations of blood urea, blood urea nitrogen and/or serum creatinine were observed occasionally. Transient leukopenia, neutropenia, agranulocytosis, thrombocytopenia and lymphocytosis were seen very rarely.

Observed During Clinical Practice: In addition to the adverse events reported from clinical trials, the following events have been identified during post-approval use of ceftazidime. Because they are reported voluntarily from a population of unknown size, estimates of frequency cannot be made. These events have been chosen for inclusion due to a combination of their seriousness, frequency of reporting, or potential causal connection to ceftazidime.

General: Anaphylactic or anaphylactoid reactions, which, in rare instances, were severe (e.g., cardiopulmonary ar-

Continued on next page

Information on the SmithKline Beecham Pharmaceuticals products appearing here is based on the labeling in effect on June 15, 2000. Further information on these and other products may be obtained from the Medical Department, SmithKline Beecham Pharmaceuticals, One Franklin Plaza, Philadelphia, PA 19101.

Tazicef—Cont.

rest), including laryngeal edema, stridor, and urticaria; pain at injection site.

Hepatobiliary Tract and Pancreas: Hyperbilirubinemia.

Renal and Genitourinary: Renal impairment.

Cephalosporin-Class Adverse Reactions: In addition to the adverse reactions listed above that have been observed in patients treated with ceftazidime, the following adverse reactions and altered laboratory tests have been reported for cephalosporin-class antibiotics:

Adverse Reactions: Urticaria, colitis, renal dysfunction, toxic nephropathy, hepatic dysfunction including cholestasis, aplastic anemia, hemorrhage.

Altered Laboratory Tests: Prolonged prothrombin time, false-positive test for urinary glucose, elevated bilirubin, pancytopenia.

OVERDOSAGE

Ceftazidime overdosage has occurred in patients with renal failure. Reactions have included seizure activity, encephalopathy, asterixis and neuromuscular excitability. Patients who receive an acute overdosage should be carefully observed and given supportive treatment. In the presence of renal insufficiency, hemodialysis or peritoneal dialysis may aid in the removal of ceftazidime from the body.

DOSAGE AND ADMINISTRATION

Dosage: The usual adult dosage is 1 gram administered intravenously or intramuscularly every 8 or 12 hours. The dosage and route should be determined by the susceptibility of the causative organisms, the severity of infection and the condition and renal function of the patient.

The guidelines for dosage of Tazicef (ceftazidime for injection) are listed in Table 3. The following dosage schedule is recommended.

Table 3. Recommended Dosage Schedule

	Dose	Frequency
Adults		
Usual recommended dose	**1 gram IV or IM**	**q8 or 12h**
Uncomplicated urinary tract infections	250 mg IV or IM	q12h
Bone and joint infections	2 grams IV	q12h
Complicated urinary tract infections	500 mg IV or IM	q8 or 12h
Uncomplicated pneumonia; mild skin and skin structure infections	500 mg to 1 gram IV or IM	q8h
Serious gynecological and intra-abdominal infections	2 grams IV	q8h
Meningitis	2 grams IV	q8h
Very severe life-threatening infections, especially in immunocompromised patients	2 grams IV	q8h
Lung infections caused by *Pseudomonas* spp. in patients with cystic fibrosis with normal renal function*	30 to 50 mg/kg IV to a maximum of 6 grams/day	q8h
Neonates (0 – 4 weeks)	30 mg/kg IV	q12h
Infants and children (1 month – 12 years)	30 to 50 mg/kg IV to a maximum of 6 grams/day†	q8h

*Although clinical improvement has been shown, bacteriological cures cannot be expected in patients with chronic respiratory disease and cystic fibrosis.

†The higher dose should be reserved for immunocompromised pediatric patients or pediatric patients with cystic fibrosis or meningitis.

Impaired Hepatic Function: No adjustment in dosage is required for patients with hepatic dysfunction.

Impaired Renal Function: Ceftazidime is excreted by the kidneys, almost exclusively by glomerular filtration. Therefore, in patients with impaired renal function (glomerular filtration rate [GFR] <50 mL/min.), it is recommended that the dosage of ceftazidime be reduced to compensate for its slower excretion. In patients with suspected renal insufficiency, an initial loading dose of 1 gram of ceftazidime may be given. An estimate of GFR should be made to determine the appropriate maintenance dose. The recommended dosage is presented in Table 4.

Table 4. Recommended Maintenance Doses of Tazicef (ceftazidime for injection) in Renal Insufficiency

NOTE: IF THE DOSE RECOMMENDED IN TABLE 3 ABOVE IS LOWER THAN THAT RECOMMENDED FOR PATIENTS WITH RENAL INSUFFICIENCY AS OUTLINED IN TABLE 4, THE LOWER DOSE SHOULD BE USED.

Creatinine Clearance (mL/min.)	Recommended Unit Dose of *Tazicef*	Frequency of Dosing
50 – 31	1 gram	q12h
30 – 16	1 gram	q24h
15 – 6	500 mg	q24h
<5	500 mg	q48h

When only serum creatinine is available, the following formula (Cockcroft's equation)[4] may be used to estimate creatinine clearance. The serum creatinine should represent a steady state of renal function:

Males:

$$\text{Creatinine clearance (mL/min.)} = \frac{\text{Weight (kg)} \times (140 - \text{age})}{72 \times \text{serum creatinine (mg/dL)}}$$

Females:
$0.85 \times$ male value

In patients with severe infections who would normally receive 6 grams of *Tazicef* daily were it not for renal insufficiency, the unit dose given in the table above may be increased by 50% or the dosing frequency increased appropriately. Further dosing should be determined by therapeutic monitoring, severity of the infection and susceptibility of the causative organism.

In pediatric patients as for adults, the creatinine clearance should be adjusted for body surface area or lean body mass and the dosing frequency reduced in cases of renal insufficiency.

In patients undergoing hemodialysis, a loading dose of 1 gram is recommended, followed by 1 gram after each hemodialysis period.

Tazicef (ceftazidime for injection) can also be used in patients undergoing intra-peritoneal dialysis and continuous ambulatory peritoneal dialysis. In such patients, a loading dose of 1 gram of *Tazicef* may be given, followed by 500 mg every 24 hours. In addition to IV use, *Tazicef* can be incorporated in the dialysis fluid at a concentration of 250 mg for 2 liters of dialysis fluid.

Note: Generally *Tazicef* should be continued for 2 days after the signs and symptoms of infection have disappeared, but in complicated infections longer therapy may be required.

Administration: *Tazicef* may be given intravenously or by deep IM injection into a large muscle mass such as the upper outer quadrant of the gluteus maximus or lateral part of the thigh. Intra-arterial administration should be avoided (see PRECAUTIONS).

Note: *Tazicef* in ADD-Vantage® vials is not intended for direct IV or IM injection.

Intramuscular Administration: For IM administration, *Tazicef* should be reconstituted with Sterile Water for Injection. Refer to Table 5.

Intravenous Administration: The IV route is preferable for patients with bacterial septicemia, bacterial meningitis, peritonitis, or other severe or life-threatening infections, or for patients who may be poor risks because of lowered resistance resulting from such debilitating conditions as malnutrition, trauma, surgery, diabetes, heart failure or malignancy, particularly if shock is present or pending.

For direct intermittent IV administration, reconstitute *Tazicef* as directed in Table 5 with Sterile Water for Injection. Slowly inject directly into the vein over a period of 3 to 5 minutes or give through the tubing of an administration set while the patient is also receiving one of the compatible IV fluids (see COMPATIBILITY AND STABILITY).

For IV infusion, reconstitute the 1- or 2-gram piggyback vial with 100 mL of Sodium Chloride Injection or one of the compatible IV fluids listed under the COMPATIBILITY AND STABILITY section. Alternatively, reconstitute the 1-gram or 2-gram vial and add an appropriate quantity of the resulting solution to an IV container with one of the compatible IV fluids.

Intermittent intravenous infusion with a Y-type administration set can be accomplished with compatible solutions. However, during infusion of a solution containing ceftazidime it is desirable to discontinue the other solution.

All vials of *Tazicef* as supplied are under reduced pressure. When *Tazicef* is dissolved, carbon dioxide is released and a positive pressure develops. See RECONSTITUTION.

Solutions of *Tazicef*, like those of most beta-lactam antibiotics, should not be added to solutions of aminoglycoside antibiotics because of potential interaction.

However, if concurrent therapy with *Tazicef* and an aminoglycoside is indicated, each of these antibiotics can be administered separately to the same patient.

***TAZICEF* INJECTION IN ADD-VANTAGE® VIALS**

Note: Tazicef (ceftazidime for injection) in the ADD-Vantage® vial is intended to be administered as a single-dose intravenous infusion with the ADD-Vantage® flexible diluent container.

Tazicef in single-dose ADD-Vantage® vials should be prepared as directed (see RECONSTITUTION, for ADD-Vantage® Vials) with either 0.9% Sodium Chloride Injection in the 50 mL or 100 mL flexible diluent containers, 0.45% Sodium Chloride Injection in the 50 mL container or 5% Dextrose Injection in the 50 mL or 100 mL containers.

RECONSTITUTION

Single-Dose Vials:

For IM injection, IV direct (bolus) injection or IV infusion, reconstitute with Sterile Water for Injection according to the following table. The vacuum may assist entry of the diluent. SHAKE WELL.

Table 5

Vial Size	Amount of Diluent to Be Added	Approx. Avail. Volume	Approximate Ceftazidime Concentration
Intramuscular or Intravenous Direct (bolus) Injection			
1 gram	3.0 mL	3.6 mL	280 mg/mL
Intravenous Infusion			
1 gram	10 mL	10.6 mL	95 mg/mL
2 gram	10 mL	11.2 mL	180 mg/mL

Withdraw the total volume of solution into the syringe (the pressure in the vial may aid withdrawal). The withdrawn solution may contain some bubbles of carbon dioxide.

Note: As with the administration of all parenteral products, accumulated gases should be expressed from the syringe immediately before injection of *Tazicef*.

These solutions of *Tazicef* are stable for 24 hours at room temperature or 7 days if refrigerated (5°C). Slight yellowing does not affect potency.

For IV infusion, dilute reconstituted solution in 50 to 100 mL of one of the parenteral fluids listed under COMPATIBILITY AND STABILITY.

"Piggyback" Vials:

For IV infusion, reconstitute with 10 mL of Sodium Chloride Injection according to the following table. The vacuum may assist entry of the diluent. SHAKE WELL.

Table 6

Vial Size	Diluent to Be Added	Approx. Avail. Volume	Approx. Avg. Concentration
1 gram	100 mL*	100 mL	10 mg/mL
2 gram	100 mL*	100 mL	20 mg/mL

*Addition should be in two stages.

Insert a gas relief needle through the vial closure to relieve the internal pressure. With the gas relief needle in position, add the remaining 90 mL of Sodium Chloride Injection. Remove the gas relief needle and syringe needle; shake the vial and set up for infusion in the normal way.

Note: To preserve product sterility, it is important that a gas relief needle is not inserted through the vial closure before the product has dissolved.

These solutions of Tazicef (ceftazidime for injection) are stable for 24 hours at room temperature or 7 days if refrigerated (5°C). Slight yellowing does not affect potency.

ADD-Vantage® Vials: ADD-Vantage® vials of Tazicef (ceftazidime for injection) are to be reconstituted only with 0.9% Sodium Chloride Injection or 5% Dextrose Injection in the 50 mL or 100 mL flexible diluent containers, or with 0.45% Sodium Chloride Injection in the 50 mL container.

DIRECTIONS FOR USE OF TAZICEF® (CEFTAZIDIME FOR INJECTION) IN ADD-VANTAGE® VIALS

To Open Diluent Container:

Peel overwrap at corner and remove solution container. Some opacity of the plastic due to moisture absorption during the sterilization process may be observed. This is normal and does not affect the solution quality or safety. The opacity will diminish gradually.

To Assemble Vial and Flexible Diluent Container:
(Use Aseptic Technique)

1. Remove the protective covers from the top of the vial and the vial port on the diluent container as follows:
   a. To remove the breakaway vial cap, swing the pull ring over the top of the vial and pull down far enough to start the opening (SEE FIGURE 1), then pull straight up to remove the cap. (SEE FIGURE 2.)
   Note: Do not access vial with syringe.

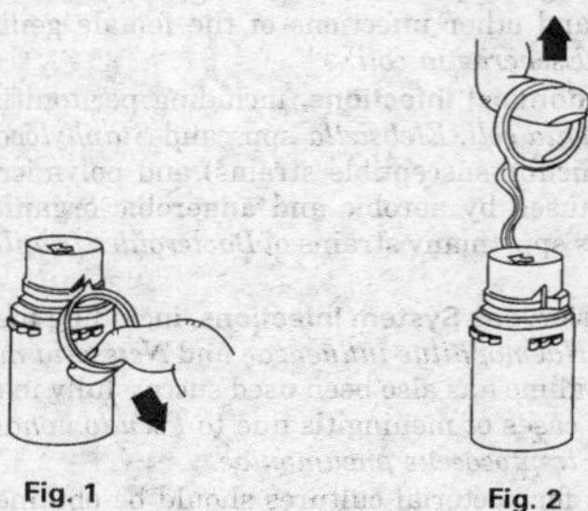

Fig. 1 **Fig. 2**

   b. To remove the vial port cover, grasp the tab on the pull ring, pull up to break the three tie strings, then pull back to remove the cover. (SEE FIGURE 3.)

2. Screw the vial into the vial port until it will go no further. THE VIAL MUST BE SCREWED IN TIGHTLY TO ASSURE A SEAL. This occurs approximately 1/2 turn (180°) after the first audible click. (SEE FIGURE 4.) The clicking sound does not assure a seal; the vial must be turned as far as it will go.
Note: Once vial is sealed, do not attempt to remove. (SEE FIGURE 4.)
3. Recheck the vial to assure that it is tight by trying to turn it further in the direction of assembly.
4. Label appropriately.

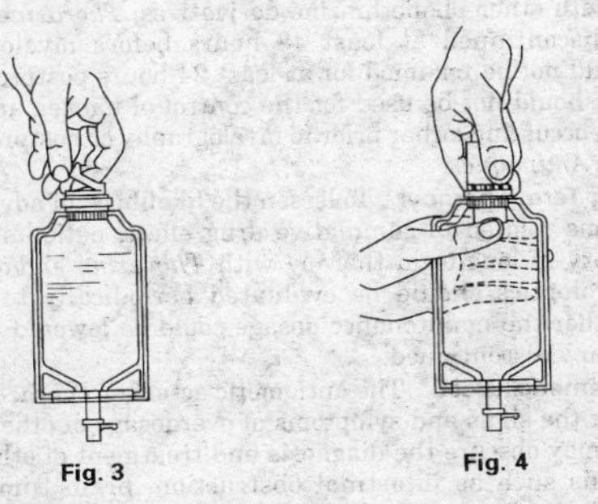
Fig. 3 Fig. 4

To Reconstitute the Drug:
1. Squeeze the bottom of the diluent container gently to inflate the portion of the container surrounding the end of the drug vial.
2. With the other hand, push the drug vial down into the container telescoping the walls of the container. Grasp the inner cap of the vial through the walls of the container. (SEE FIGURE 5.)
3. Pull the inner cap from the drug vial. (SEE FIGURE 6.) Verify that the rubber stopper has been pulled out, allowing the drug and diluent to mix.
4. Mix container contents thoroughly and use within the specified time.

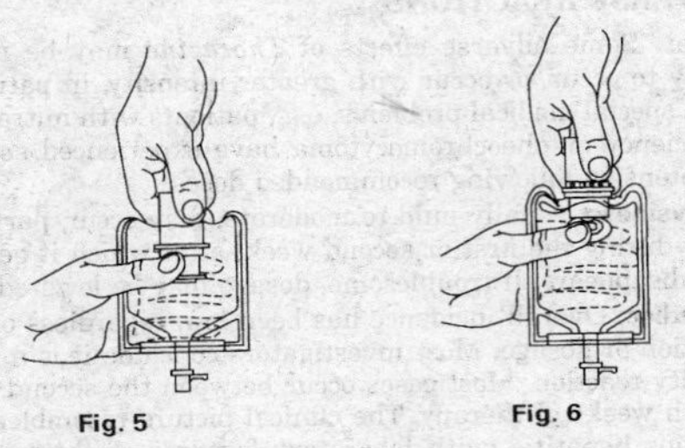
Fig. 5 Fig. 6

Preparation for Administration:
(Use Aseptic Technique)
1. Confirm the activation and admixture of vial contents.
2. Check for leaks by squeezing container firmly. If leaks are found discard unit as sterility may be impaired.
3. Close flow control clamp of administration set.
4. Remove cover from outlet port at bottom of container.
5. Insert piercing pin of administration set into port with a twisting motion until the pin is firmly seated. **Note:** See full directions on administration set carton.
6. Lift the free end of the hanger loop on the bottom of the vial, breaking the two tie strings. Bend the loop outward to lock it in the upright position, then suspend container from hanger.
7. Squeeze and release drip chamber to establish proper fluid level in chamber.
8. Open flow control clamp and clear air from set. Close clamp.
9. Attach set to venipuncture device. If device is not in dwelling, prime and make venipuncture.
10. Regulate rate of administration with flow control clamp.

WARNING: Do not use flexible container in series connections.

COMPATIBILITY AND STABILITY

Intramuscular: Tazicef (ceftazidime for injection) when reconstituted as directed with Sterile Water for Injection, maintains satisfactory potency for 24 hours at room temperature or for 7 days under refrigeration (5°C). Solutions in Sterile Water for Injection that are frozen immediately after reconstitution in the original container are stable for 3 months when stored at −20°C. Once thawed, solutions should not be refrozen. Thawed solutions may be stored for up to 8 hours at room temperature or for 4 days in a refrigerator (5°C).

Intravenous: Tazicef (ceftazidime for injection) when reconstituted as directed with Sterile Water for Injection, maintains satisfactory potency for 24 hours at room temperature or for 7 days under refrigeration. Solutions in Sterile Water for Injection in the original container or in 0.9% Sodium Chloride Injection in Viaflex® small volume containers that are frozen immediately after reconstitution are stable for 3 months when stored at −20°C. For larger volumes where it may be necessary to warm the frozen product (to a maximum of 40°C), care should be taken to avoid heating after thawing is complete. Do not force thaw by immersion in water baths or by microwave irradiation. Once thawed, solutions should not be refrozen. Thawed solutions may be stored for up to 8 hours at room temperature or for 4 days in a refrigerator (5°C).

Tazicef is compatible with the more commonly used IV infusion fluids. Solutions at concentrations between 1 mg/mL and 40 mg/mL in the following infusion fluids may be stored for up to 24 hours at room temperature or 7 days if refrigerated: 0.9% Sodium Chloride Injection; Ringer's Injection USP; Lactated Ringer's Injection USP; 5% Dextrose Injection; 5% Dextrose and 0.225% Sodium Chloride Injection; 5% Dextrose and 0.45% Sodium Chloride Injection; 5% Dextrose and 0.9% Sodium Chloride Injection; 10% Dextrose Injection.

Tazicef is less stable in Sodium Bicarbonate Injection than in other IV fluids. It is not recommended as a diluent. Solutions of *Tazicef* in 5% Dextrose and 0.9% Sodium Chloride Injection are stable for at least 6 hours at room temperature in plastic tubing, drip chambers and volume control devices of common IV infusion sets.

Ceftazidime at a concentration of 20 mg/mL has been found physically compatible for 24 hours at room temperature or 7 days under refrigeration in Sterile Water for Injection when admixed with: cefazolin sodium 330 mg/mL; heparin 1000 units/mL; and cimetidine HCl 150 mg/mL.

Ceftazidime at a concentration of 20 mg/mL has been found physically compatible for 24 hours at room temperature or 7 days under refrigeration in 5% Dextrose Injection when admixed with potassium chloride 40 mEq/L.

Vancomycin solution exhibits a physical incompatibility when mixed with a number of drugs, including ceftazidime. The likelihood of precipitation with ceftazidime is dependent on the concentrations of vancomycin and ceftazidime present. It is therefore recommended, when both drugs are to be administered by intermittent IV infusion, that they be given separately, flushing the IV lines (with one of the compatible IV fluids) between the administration of these two agents.

ADD-Vantage® Vials: Ordinarily, ADD-Vantage® vials should be reconstituted only when it is certain that the patient is ready to receive the drug. However, *Tazicef* in ADD-Vantage® vials is stable for 24 hours at room temperature when reconstituted as directed (see RECONSTITUTION, ADD-Vantage® Vials and DIRECTIONS FOR USE OF TAZICEF® INJECTION IN ADD-VANTAGE® VIALS).

Note: Parenteral drug products should be inspected visually for particulate matter prior to administration whenever solution and container permit.

As with other cephalosporins, *Tazicef* powder, as well as solutions, tends to darken depending on storage conditions; within the stated recommendations, however, product potency is not adversely affected.

HOW SUPPLIED

Tazicef in the dry state should be stored at Controlled Room Temperature 20° to 25°C (68° to 77°F) and protected from light. Tazicef (ceftazidime for injection) is a dry, white to off-white powder supplied in vials as follows:
Vials: equivalent to 1 gram and 2 grams of ceftazidime.
1 gram (tray of 25): NDC 0007-5082-16
2 gram (tray of 10): NDC 0007-5084-11
"Piggyback" Vials for IV admixture: equivalent to 1 gram and 2 grams of ceftazidime.
1 gram (tray of 10): NDC 0007-5083-11
2 gram (tray of 10): NDC 0007-5085-11
ADD-Vantage® Vials: equivalent to 1 gram and 2 grams of ceftazidime.
1 gram: NDC 0007-5090-16
2 gram: NDC 0007-5091-11
Also available as:
Pharmacy Bulk Vials: equivalent to 6 grams of ceftazidime.
6 gram (tray of 10): NDC 0007-5086-11
Galaxy® Containers (PL 2040 Plastic): equivalent to 1 gram and 2 grams of ceftazidime.
1 gram 1's: NDC 0007-5088-04
2 gram 1's: NDC 0007-5089-04
ADD-Vantage® is a registered trademark of Abbott Laboratories.
Galaxy is a registered trademark of Baxter International Inc.

REFERENCES

1. Bauer AW, Kirby WMM, Sherris JC, Turck M. Antibiotic susceptibility testing by a standardized single disk method. *Am J Clin Pathol.* 1966;45:493-496.
2. National Committee for Clinical Laboratory Standards. *Approved Standard: Performance Standards for Antimicrobial Disc Susceptibility Tests.* (M2-A3), December, 1984.
3. Certification procedure for antibiotic sensitivity discs (21 CFR 460.1). *Federal Register.* May 30, 1974;39:19182-19184.
4. Cockcroft DW, Gault MH. Prediction of creatinine clearance from serum creatinine. *Nephron.* 1976;16:31-41.

℞ only

Jointly manufactured by
SmithKline Beecham Pharmaceuticals
Philadelphia, PA 19101 and
Bristol-Myers Squibb Co.
New York, NY 10154
TF:L18

THORAZINE® ℞

[*thor 'ah-zeen*]
brand of chlorpromazine
tranquilizer · antiemetic

DESCRIPTION

Thorazine (chlorpromazine) is 10-(3-dimethylaminopropyl)-2-chlorphenothiazine, a dimethylamine derivative of phenothiazine. It is present in oral and injectable forms as the hydrochloride salt, and in the suppositories as the base.

Tablets—Each round, orange, coated tablet contains chlorpromazine hydrochloride as follows: 10 mg imprinted SKF and T73; 25 mg imprinted SKF and T74; 50 mg imprinted SKF and T76; 100 mg imprinted SKF and T77; 200 mg imprinted SKF and T79. Inactive ingredients consist of benzoic acid, croscarmellose sodium, D&C Yellow No. 10, FD&C Blue No. 2, FD&C Yellow No. 6, gelatin, hydroxypropyl methylcellulose, lactose, magnesium stearate, methylparaben, polyethylene glycol, propylparaben, talc, titanium dioxide and trace amounts of other inactive ingredients.

Spansule® sustained release capsules—Each *Thorazine* Spansule® capsule is so prepared that an initial dose is released promptly and the remaining medication is released gradually over a prolonged period.

Each capsule, with opaque orange cap and natural body, contains chlorpromazine hydrochloride as follows: 30 mg imprinted SKF and T63; 75 mg imprinted SKF and T64; 150 mg imprinted SKF and T66. Inactive ingredients consist of benzyl alcohol, calcium sulfate, cetylpyridinium chloride, FD&C Yellow No. 6, gelatin, glyceryl distearate, glyceryl monostearate, iron oxide, povidone, silicon dioxide, sodium lauryl sulfate, starch, sucrose, titanium dioxide, wax and trace amounts of other inactive ingredients.

Ampuls—Each mL contains, in aqueous solution, chlorpromazine hydrochloride, 25 mg; ascorbic acid, 2 mg; sodium bisulfite, 1 mg; sodium chloride, 6 mg; sodium sulfite, 1 mg.

Multi-Dose Vials—Each mL contains, in aqueous solution, chlorpromazine hydrochloride, 25 mg; ascorbic acid, 2 mg; sodium bisulfite, 1 mg; sodium chloride, 1 mg; sodium sulfite, 1 mg; benzyl alcohol, 2%, as a preservative.

Syrup—Each 5 mL (1 teaspoonful) of clear, orange-custard flavored liquid contains chlorpromazine hydrochloride, 10 mg. Inactive ingredients consist of citric acid, flavors, sodium benzoate, sodium citrate, sucrose and water.

Suppositories—Each suppository contains chlorpromazine, 25 or 100 mg, glycerin, glyceryl monopalmitate, glyceryl monostearate, hydrogenated coconut oil fatty acids and hydrogenated palm kernel oil fatty acids.

ACTIONS

The precise mechanism whereby the therapeutic effects of chlorpromazine are produced is not known. The principal pharmacological actions are psychotropic. It also exerts sedative and antiemetic activity. Chlorpromazine has actions at all levels of the central nervous system—primarily at subcortical levels—as well as on multiple organ systems. Chlorpromazine has strong antiadrenergic and weaker peripheral anticholinergic activity; ganglionic blocking action is relatively slight. It also possesses slight antihistaminic and antiserotonin activity.

INDICATIONS

For the management of manifestations of psychotic disorders.
To control nausea and vomiting.
For relief of restlessness and apprehension before surgery.
For acute intermittent porphyria.
As an adjunct in the treatment of tetanus.
To control the manifestations of the manic type of manic-depressive illness.
For relief of intractable hiccups.
For the treatment of severe behavioral problems in children (1 to 12 years of age) marked by combativeness and/or explosive hyperexcitable behavior (out of proportion to immediate provocations), and in the short-term treatment of hyperactive children who show excessive motor activity with accompanying conduct disorders consisting of some or all of the following symptoms: impulsivity, difficulty sustaining attention, aggressivity, mood lability and poor frustration tolerance.

CONTRAINDICATIONS

Do not use in patients with known hypersensitivity to phenothiazines.
Do not use in comatose states or in the presence of large amounts of central nervous system depressants (alcohol, barbiturates, narcotics, etc.).

WARNINGS

The extrapyramidal symptoms which can occur secondary to Thorazine (chlorpromazine) may be confused with the central nervous system signs of an undiagnosed primary disease responsible for the vomiting, e.g., Reye's syndrome or other encephalopathy. The use of *Thorazine* and other

Continued on next page

Information on the SmithKline Beecham Pharmaceuticals products appearing here is based on the labeling in effect on June 15, 2000. Further information on these and other products may be obtained from the Medical Department, SmithKline Beecham Pharmaceuticals, One Franklin Plaza, Philadelphia, PA 19101.

Thorazine—Cont.

potential hepatotoxins should be avoided in children and adolescents whose signs and symptoms suggest Reye's syndrome.

Tardive Dyskinesia: Tardive dyskinesia, a syndrome consisting of potentially irreversible, involuntary, dyskinetic movements, may develop in patients treated with neuroleptic (antipsychotic) drugs. Although the prevalence of the syndrome appears to be highest among the elderly, especially elderly women, it is impossible to rely upon prevalence estimates to predict, at the inception of neuroleptic treatment, which patients are likely to develop the syndrome. Whether neuroleptic drug products differ in their potential to cause tardive dyskinesia is unknown.

Both the risk of developing the syndrome and the likelihood that it will become irreversible are believed to increase as the duration of treatment and the total cumulative dose of neuroleptic drugs administered to the patient increase. However, the syndrome can develop, although much less commonly, after relatively brief treatment periods at low doses.

There is no known treatment for established cases of tardive dyskinesia, although the syndrome may remit, partially or completely, if neuroleptic treatment is withdrawn. Neuroleptic treatment itself, however, may suppress (or partially suppress) the signs and symptoms of the syndrome and thereby may possibly mask the underlying disease process. The effect that symptomatic suppression has upon the long-term course of the syndrome is unknown.

Given these considerations, neuroleptics should be prescribed in a manner that is most likely to minimize the occurrence of tardive dyskinesia. Chronic neuroleptic treatment should generally be reserved for patients who suffer from a chronic illness that, 1) is known to respond to neuroleptic drugs, and, 2) for whom alternative, equally effective, but potentially less harmful treatments are *not* available or appropriate. In patients who do require chronic treatment, the smallest dose and the shortest duration of treatment producing a satisfactory clinical response should be sought. The need for continued treatment should be reassessed periodically.

If signs and symptoms of tardive dyskinesia appear in a patient on neuroleptics, drug discontinuation should be considered. However, some patients may require treatment despite the presence of the syndrome.

For further information about the description of tardive dyskinesia and its clinical detection, please refer to the sections on PRECAUTIONS and ADVERSE REACTIONS.

Neuroleptic Malignant Syndrome (NMS): A potentially fatal symptom complex sometimes referred to as Neuroleptic Malignant Syndrome (NMS) has been reported in association with antipsychotic drugs. Clinical manifestations of NMS are hyperpyrexia, muscle rigidity, altered mental status and evidence of autonomic instability (irregular pulse or blood pressure, tachycardia, diaphoresis and cardiac dysrhythmias).

The diagnostic evaluation of patients with this syndrome is complicated. In arriving at a diagnosis, it is important to identify cases where the clinical presentation includes both serious medical illness (e.g., pneumonia, systemic infection, etc.) and untreated or inadequately treated extrapyramidal signs and symptoms (EPS). Other important considerations in the differential diagnosis include central anticholinergic toxicity, heat stroke, drug fever and primary central nervous system (CNS) pathology.

The management of NMS should include 1) immediate discontinuation of antipsychotic drugs and other drugs not essential to concurrent therapy, 2) intensive symptomatic treatment and medical monitoring, and 3) treatment of any concomitant serious medical problems for which specific treatments are available. There is no general agreement about specific pharmacological treatment regimens for uncomplicated NMS.

If a patient requires antipsychotic drug treatment after recovery from NMS, the potential reintroduction of drug therapy should be carefully considered. The patient should be carefully monitored, since recurrences of NMS have been reported.

An encephalopathic syndrome (characterized by weakness, lethargy, fever, tremulousness and confusion, extrapyramidal symptoms, leukocytosis, elevated serum enzymes, BUN and FBS) has occurred in a few patients treated with lithium plus a neuroleptic. In some instances, the syndrome was followed by irreversible brain damage. Because of a possible causal relationship between these events and the concomitant administration of lithium and neuroleptics, patients receiving such combined therapy should be monitored closely for early evidence of neurologic toxicity and treatment discontinued promptly if such signs appear. This encephalopathic syndrome may be similar to or the same as neuroleptic malignant syndrome (NMS).

Thorazine (chlorpromazine) ampuls and multi-dose vials contain sodium bisulfite and sodium sulfite, sulfites that may cause allergic-type reactions including anaphylactic symptoms and life-threatening or less severe asthmatic episodes in certain susceptible people. The overall prevalence of sulfite sensitivity in the general population is unknown and probably low. Sulfite sensitivity is seen more frequently in asthmatic than in nonasthmatic people.

Patients with bone marrow depression or who have previously demonstrated a hypersensitivity reaction (e.g., blood dyscrasias, jaundice) with a phenothiazine should not receive any phenothiazine, including *Thorazine,* unless in the judgment of the physician the potential benefits of treatment outweigh the possible hazard.

Thorazine may impair mental and/or physical abilities, especially during the first few days of therapy. Therefore, caution patients about activities requiring alertness (e.g., operating vehicles or machinery).

The use of alcohol with this drug should be avoided due to possible additive effects and hypotension.

Thorazine may counteract the antihypertensive effect of guanethidine and related compounds.

Usage in Pregnancy: Safety for the use of Thorazine (chlorpromazine) during pregnancy has not been established. Therefore, it is not recommended that the drug be given to pregnant patients except when, in the judgment of the physician, it is essential. The potential benefits should clearly outweigh possible hazards. There are reported instances of prolonged jaundice, extrapyramidal signs, hyperreflexia or hyporeflexia in newborn infants whose mothers received phenothiazines.

Reproductive studies in rodents have demonstrated potential for embryotoxicity, increased neonatal mortality and nursing transfer of the drug. Tests in the offspring of the drug-treated rodents demonstrate decreased performance. The possibility of permanent neurological damage cannot be excluded.

Nursing Mothers: There is evidence that chlorpromazine is excreted in the breast milk of nursing mothers. Because of the potential for serious adverse reactions in nursing infants from chlorpromazine, a decision should be made whether to discontinue nursing or to discontinue the drug, taking into account the importance of the drug to the mother.

PRECAUTIONS

General

Given the likelihood that some patients exposed chronically to neuroleptics will develop tardive dyskinesia, it is advised that all patients in whom chronic use is contemplated be given, if possible, full information about this risk. The decision to inform patients and/or their guardians must obviously take into account the clinical circumstances and the competency of the patient to understand the information provided.

Thorazine (chlorpromazine) should be administered cautiously to persons with cardiovascular, liver or renal disease. There is evidence that patients with a history of hepatic encephalopathy due to cirrhosis have increased sensitivity to the CNS effects of *Thorazine* (i.e., impaired cerebration and abnormal slowing of the EEG).

Because of its CNS depressant effect, *Thorazine* should be used with caution in patients with chronic respiratory disorders such as severe asthma, emphysema and acute respiratory infections, particularly in children (1 to 12 years of age).

Because *Thorazine* can suppress the cough reflex, aspiration of vomitus is possible.

Thorazine (chlorpromazine) prolongs and intensifies the action of CNS depressants such as anesthetics, barbiturates and narcotics. When *Thorazine* is administered concomitantly, about $^1/_4$ to $^1/_2$ the usual dosage of such agents is required. When *Thorazine* is not being administered to reduce requirements of CNS depressants, it is best to stop such depressants before starting *Thorazine* treatment. These agents may subsequently be reinstated at low doses and increased as needed.

Note: *Thorazine* does *not* intensify the anticonvulsant action of barbiturates. Therefore, dosage of anticonvulsants, including barbiturates, should *not* be reduced if *Thorazine* is started. Instead, start *Thorazine* at low doses and increase as needed.

Use with caution in persons who will be exposed to extreme heat, organophosphorus insecticides, and in persons receiving atropine or related drugs.

Neuroleptic drugs elevate prolactin levels; the elevation persists during chronic administration. Tissue culture experiments indicate that approximately $^1/_3$ of human breast cancers are prolactin-dependent *in vitro,* a factor of potential importance if the prescribing of these drugs is contemplated in a patient with a previously detected breast cancer. Although disturbances such as galactorrhea, amenorrhea, gynecomastia and impotence have been reported, the clinical significance of elevated serum prolactin levels is unknown for most patients. An increase in mammary neoplasms has been found in rodents after chronic administration of neuroleptic drugs. Neither clinical nor epidemiologic studies conducted to date, however, have shown an association between chronic administration of these drugs and mammary tumorigenesis; the available evidence is considered too limited to be conclusive at this time.

Chromosomal aberrations in spermatocytes and abnormal sperm have been demonstrated in rodents treated with certain neuroleptics.

As with all drugs which exert an anticholinergic effect, and/or cause mydriasis, chlorpromazine should be used with caution in patients with glaucoma.

Chlorpromazine diminishes the effect of oral anticoagulants.

Phenothiazines can produce alpha-adrenergic blockade.

Chlorpromazine may lower the convulsive threshold; dosage adjustments of anticonvulsants may be necessary. Potentiation of anticonvulsant effects does not occur. However, it has been reported that chlorpromazine may interfere with the metabolism of Dilantin®* and thus precipitate *Dilantin* toxicity.

Concomitant administration with propranolol results in increased plasma levels of both drugs.

Thiazide diuretics may accentuate the orthostatic hypotension that may occur with phenothiazines.

The presence of phenothiazines may produce false-positive phenylketonuria (PKU) test results.

Drugs which lower the seizure threshold, including phenothiazine derivatives, should not be used with Amipaque®†. As with other phenothiazine derivatives, *Thorazine* should be discontinued at least 48 hours before myelography, should not be resumed for at least 24 hours postprocedure, and should not be used for the control of nausea and vomiting occurring either prior to myelography or postprocedure with *Amipaque*.

Long-Term Therapy: To lessen the likelihood of adverse reactions related to cumulative drug effect, patients with a history of long-term therapy with *Thorazine* and/or other neuroleptics should be evaluated periodically to decide whether the maintenance dosage could be lowered or drug therapy discontinued.

Antiemetic Effect: The antiemetic action of *Thorazine* may mask the signs and symptoms of overdosage of other drugs and may obscure the diagnosis and treatment of other conditions such as intestinal obstruction, brain tumor and Reye's syndrome. (See WARNINGS.)

When *Thorazine* is used with cancer chemotherapeutic drugs, vomiting as a sign of the toxicity of these agents may be obscured by the antiemetic effect of *Thorazine*.

Abrupt Withdrawal: Like other phenothiazines, Thorazine (chlorpromazine) is not known to cause psychic dependence and does not produce tolerance or addiction. There may be, however, following abrupt withdrawal of high-dose therapy, some symptoms resembling those of physical dependence such as gastritis, nausea and vomiting, dizziness and tremulousness. These symptoms can usually be avoided or reduced by gradual reduction of the dosage or by continuing concomitant anti-parkinsonism agents for several weeks after *Thorazine* is withdrawn.

ADVERSE REACTIONS

Note: Some adverse effects of *Thorazine* may be more likely to occur, or occur with greater intensity, in patients with special medical problems, e.g., patients with mitral insufficiency or pheochromocytoma have experienced severe hypotension following recommended doses.

Drowsiness, usually mild to moderate, may occur, particularly during the first or second week, after which it generally disappears. If troublesome, dosage may be lowered.

Jaundice: Overall incidence has been low, regardless of indication or dosage. Most investigators conclude it is a sensitivity reaction. Most cases occur between the second and fourth weeks of therapy. The clinical picture resembles infectious hepatitis, with laboratory features of obstructive jaundice, rather than those of parenchymal damage. It is usually promptly reversible on withdrawal of the medication; however, chronic jaundice has been reported.

There is no conclusive evidence that preexisting liver disease makes patients more susceptible to jaundice. Alcoholics with cirrhosis have been successfully treated with Thorazine (chlorpromazine) without complications. Nevertheless, the medication should be used cautiously in patients with liver disease. Patients who have experienced jaundice with a phenothiazine should not, if possible, be reexposed to *Thorazine* or other phenothiazines.

If fever with grippe-like symptoms occurs, appropriate liver studies should be conducted. If tests indicate an abnormality, stop treatment.

Liver function tests in jaundice induced by the drug may mimic extrahepatic obstruction; withhold exploratory laparotomy until extrahepatic obstruction is confirmed.

Hematological Disorders, including agranulocytosis, eosinophilia, leukopenia, hemolytic anemia, aplastic anemia, thrombocytopenic purpura and pancytopenia have been reported.

Agranulocytosis—Warn patients to report the sudden appearance of sore throat or other signs of infection. If white blood cell and differential counts indicate cellular depression, stop treatment and start antibiotic and other suitable therapy.

Most cases have occurred between the fourth and tenth weeks of therapy; patients should be watched closely during that period.

Moderate suppression of white blood cells is not an indication for stopping treatment unless accompanied by the symptoms described above.

Cardiovascular:

Hypotensive Effects—Postural hypotension, simple tachycardia, momentary fainting and dizziness may occur after the first injection; occasionally after subsequent injections; rarely, after the first oral dose. Usually recovery is spontaneous and symptoms disappear within $^1/_2$ to 2 hours. Occasionally, these effects may be more severe and prolonged, producing a shock-like condition.

To minimize hypotension after injection, keep patient lying down and observe for at least $^1/_2$ hour. To control hypotension, place patient in head-low position with legs raised. If a vasoconstrictor is required, Levophed®‡ and Neo-Synephrine®§ are the most suitable. Other pressor agents, including epinephrine, should not be used as they may cause a paradoxical further lowering of blood pressure.

EKG Changes—particularly nonspecific, usually reversible Q and T wave distortions—have been observed in some patients receiving phenothiazine tranquilizers, including Thorazine (chlorpromazine).

Note: Sudden death, apparently due to cardiac arrest, has been reported.

CNS Reactions:

Neuromuscular (Extrapyramidal) Reactions—Neuromuscular reactions include dystonias, motor restlessness, pseudo-parkinsonism and tardive dyskinesia, and appear to be dose-related. They are discussed in the following paragraphs:

Dystonias: Symptoms may include spasm of the neck muscles, sometimes progressing to acute, reversible torticollis; extensor rigidity of back muscles, sometimes progressing to opisthotonos; carpopedal spasm, trismus, swallowing difficulty, oculogyric crisis and protrusion of the tongue. These usually subside within a few hours, and almost always within 24 to 48 hours after the drug has been discontinued.

In mild cases, reassurance or a barbiturate is often sufficient. *In moderate cases,* barbiturates will usually bring rapid relief. *In more severe adult cases,* the administration of an anti-parkinsonism agent, except levodopa, usually produces rapid reversal of symptoms. *In children (1 to 12 years of age),* reassurance and barbiturates will usually control symptoms. (Or, parenteral Benadryl®[ll] may be useful. See *Benadryl* prescribing information for appropriate children's dosage.) If appropriate treatment with anti-parkinsonism agents or *Benadryl* fails to reverse the signs and symptoms, the diagnosis should be reevaluated.

Suitable supportive measures such as maintaining a clear airway and adequate hydration should be employed when needed. If therapy is reinstituted, it should be at a lower dosage. Should these symptoms occur in children or pregnant patients, the drug should not be reinstituted.

Motor Restlessness: Symptoms may include agitation or jitteriness and sometimes insomnia. These symptoms often disappear spontaneously. At times these symptoms may be similar to the original neurotic or psychotic symptoms. Dosage should not be increased until these side effects have subsided.

If these symptoms become too troublesome, they can usually be controlled by a reduction of dosage or change of drug. Treatment with anti-parkinsonian agents, benzodiazepines or propranolol may be helpful.

Pseudo-parkinsonism: Symptoms may include: mask-like facies, drooling, tremors, pillrolling motion, cogwheel rigidity and shuffling gait. In most cases these symptoms are readily controlled when an anti-parkinsonism agent is administered concomitantly. Anti-parkinsonism agents should be used only when required. Generally, therapy of a few weeks to 2 or 3 months will suffice. After this time patients should be evaluated to determine their need for continued treatment. (Note: Levodopa has not been found effective in neuroleptic-induced pseudo-parkinsonism.) Occasionally it is necessary to lower the dosage of Thorazine (chlorpromazine) or to discontinue the drug.

Tardive Dyskinesia: As with all antipsychotic agents, tardive dyskinesia may appear in some patients on long-term therapy or may appear after drug therapy has been discontinued. The syndrome can also develop, although much less frequently, after relatively brief treatment periods at low doses. This syndrome appears in all age groups. Although its prevalence appears to be highest among elderly patients, especially elderly women, it is impossible to rely upon prevalence estimates to predict at the inception of neuroleptic treatment which patients are likely to develop the syndrome. The symptoms are persistent and in some patients appear to be irreversible. The syndrome is characterized by rhythmical involuntary movements of the tongue, face, mouth or jaw (e.g., protrusion of tongue, puffing of cheeks, puckering of mouth, chewing movements). Sometimes these may be accompanied by involuntary movements of extremities. In rare instances, these involuntary movements of the extremities are the only manifestations of tardive dyskinesia. A variant of tardive dyskinesia, tardive dystonia, has also been described.

There is no known effective treatment for tardive dyskinesia; anti-parkinsonism agents do not alleviate the symptoms of this syndrome. If clinically feasible, it is suggested that all antipsychotic agents be discontinued if these symptoms appear. Should it be necessary to reinstitute treatment, or increase the dosage of the agent, or switch to a different antipsychotic agent, the syndrome may be masked.

It has been reported that fine vermicular movements of the tongue may be an early sign of the syndrome and if the medication is stopped at that time the syndrome may not develop.

Adverse Behavioral Effects—Psychotic symptoms and catatonic-like states have been reported rarely.

Other CNS Effects—Neuroleptic Malignant Syndrome (NMS) has been reported in association with antipsychotic drugs. (See WARNINGS.)

Cerebral edema has been reported.

Convulsive seizures *(petit mal* and *grand mal)* have been reported, particularly in patients with EEG abnormalities or history of such disorders.

Abnormality of the cerebrospinal fluid proteins has also been reported.

Allergic Reactions of a mild urticarial type or photosensitivity are seen. Avoid undue exposure to sun. More severe reactions, including exfoliative dermatitis, have been reported occasionally.

Contact dermatitis has been reported in nursing personnel; accordingly, the use of rubber gloves when administering *Thorazine* liquid or injectable is recommended.

In addition, asthma, laryngeal edema, angioneurotic edema and anaphylactoid reactions have been reported.

Endocrine Disorders: Lactation and moderate breast engorgement may occur in females on large doses. If persistent, lower dosage or withdraw drug. False-positive pregnancy tests have been reported, but are less likely to occur when a serum test is used. Amenorrhea and gynecomastia have also been reported. Hyperglycemia, hypoglycemia and glycosuria have been reported.

Autonomic Reactions: Occasional dry mouth; nasal congestion; nausea; obstipation; constipation; adynamic ileus; urinary retention; priapism; miosis and mydriasis, atonic colon, ejaculatory disorders/impotence.

Special Considerations in Long-Term Therapy: Skin pigmentation and ocular changes have occurred in some patients taking substantial doses of Thorazine (chlorpromazine) for prolonged periods.

Skin Pigmentation—Rare instances of skin pigmentation have been observed in hospitalized mental patients, primarily females who have received the drug usually for 3 years or more in dosages ranging from 500 mg to 1500 mg daily. The pigmentary changes, restricted to exposed areas of the body, range from an almost imperceptible darkening of the skin to a slate gray color, sometimes with a violet hue. Histological examination reveals a pigment, chiefly in the dermis, which is probably a melanin-like complex. The pigmentation may fade following discontinuance of the drug.

Ocular Changes—Ocular changes have occurred more frequently than skin pigmentation and have been observed both in pigmented and nonpigmented patients receiving Thorazine (chlorpromazine) usually for 2 years or more in dosages of 300 mg daily and higher. Eye changes are characterized by deposition of fine particulate matter in the lens and cornea. In more advanced cases, star-shaped opacities have also been observed in the anterior portion of the lens. The nature of the eye deposits has not yet been determined. A small number of patients with more severe ocular changes have had some visual impairment. In addition to these corneal and lenticular changes, epithelial keratopathy and pigmentary retinopathy have been reported. Reports suggest that the eye lesions may regress after withdrawal of the drug.

Since the occurrence of eye changes seems to be related to dosage levels and/or duration of therapy, it is suggested that long-term patients on moderate to high dosage levels have periodic ocular examinations.

Etiology—The etiology of both of these reactions is not clear, but exposure to light, along with dosage/duration of therapy, appears to be the most significant factor. If either of these reactions is observed, the physician should weigh the benefits of continued therapy against the possible risks and, on the merits of the individual case, determine whether or not to continue present therapy, lower the dosage, or withdraw the drug.

Other Adverse Reactions: Mild fever may occur after large I.M. doses. Hyperpyrexia has been reported. Increases in appetite and weight sometimes occur. Peripheral edema and a systemic lupus erythematosus-like syndrome have been reported.

Note: There have been occasional reports of sudden death in patients receiving phenothiazines. In some cases, the cause appeared to be cardiac arrest or asphyxia due to failure of the cough reflex.

DOSAGE AND ADMINISTRATION—ADULTS

Adjust dosage to individual and the severity of his condition, recognizing that the milligram for milligram potency relationship among all dosage forms has not been precisely established clinically. It is important to increase dosage until symptoms are controlled. Dosage should be increased more gradually in debilitated or emaciated patients. In continued therapy, gradually reduce dosage to the lowest effective maintenance level, after symptoms have been controlled for a reasonable period.

In general, dosage recommendations for other oral forms of the drug may be applied to Spansule® brand sustained release capsules on the basis of total daily dosage in milligrams.

The 100 mg and 200 mg tablets are for use in severe neuropsychiatric conditions.

Increase parenteral dosage only if hypotension has not occurred. Before using I.M., see IMPORTANT NOTES ON INJECTION.

Elderly Patients—In general, dosages in the lower range are sufficient for most elderly patients. Since they appear to be more susceptible to hypotension and neuromuscular reactions, such patients should be observed closely. Dosage should be tailored to the individual, response carefully monitored, and dosage adjusted accordingly. Dosage should be increased more gradually in elderly patients.

Psychotic Disorders—Increase dosage gradually until symptoms are controlled. Maximum improvement may not be seen for weeks or even months. Continue optimum dosage for 2 weeks; then gradually reduce dosage to the lowest effective maintenance level. Daily dosage of 200 mg is not unusual. Some patients require higher dosages (e.g., 800 mg daily is not uncommon in discharged mental patients).

HOSPITALIZED PATIENTS: ACUTELY DISTURBED OR MANIC—*I.M.:* 25 mg (1 mL). If necessary, give additional 25 to 50 mg injection in 1 hour. Increase subsequent I.M. doses gradually over several days—up to 400 mg q4 to 6h in exceptionally severe cases—until patient is controlled. Usually patient becomes quiet and cooperative within 24 to 48 hours and oral doses may be substituted and increased until the patient is calm. 500 mg a day is generally sufficient. While gradual increases to 2,000 mg a day or more may be necessary, there is usually little therapeutic gain to be achieved by exceeding 1,000 mg a day for extended periods. In general, dosage levels should be lower in the elderly, the emaciated and the debilitated. LESS ACUTELY DISTURBED—*Oral:* 25 mg t.i.d. Increase gradually until effective dose is reached—usually 400 mg daily. OUTPATIENTS—*Oral:* 10 mg t.i.d. or q.i.d., or 25 mg b.i.d. or t.i.d. MORE SEVERE CASES—*Oral:* 25 mg t.i.d. After 1 or 2 days, daily dosage may be increased by 20 to 50 mg at semiweekly intervals until patient becomes calm and cooperative. PROMPT CONTROL OF SEVERE SYMPTOMS—*I.M.:* 25 mg (1 mL). If necessary, repeat in 1 hour. Subsequent doses should be oral, 25 to 50 mg t.i.d.

Nausea and Vomiting—*Oral:* 10 to 25 mg q4 to 6h, p.r.n., increased, if necessary. *I.M.:* 25 mg (1 mL). If no hypotension occurs, give 25 to 50 mg q3 to 4h, p.r.n., until vomiting stops. Then switch to oral dosage. *Rectal:* One 100 mg suppository q6 to 8h, p.r.n. In some patients, half this dose will do.

DURING SURGERY—*I.M.:* 12.5 mg (0.5 mL). Repeat in $^1/_2$ hour if necessary and if no hypotension occurs. *I.V.:* 2 mg per fractional injection, at 2-minute intervals. Do not exceed 25 mg. Dilute to 1 mg/mL, i.e., 1 mL (25 mg) mixed with 24 mL of saline.

Presurgical Apprehension—*Oral:* 25 to 50 mg, 2 to 3 hours before the operation. *I.M.:* 12.5 to 25 mg (0.5 to 1 mL), 1 to 2 hours before operation.

Intractable Hiccups—*Oral:* 25 to 50 mg t.i.d. or q.i.d. If symptoms persist for 2 to 3 days, give 25 to 50 mg (1 to 2 mL) I.M. Should symptoms persist, use *slow* I.V. infusion with patient flat in bed: 25 to 50 mg (1 to 2 mL) in 500 to 1,000 mL of saline. Follow blood pressure closely.

Acute Intermittent Porphyria—*Oral:* 25 to 50 mg t.i.d. or q.i.d. Can usually be discontinued after several weeks, but maintenance therapy may be necessary for some patients. *I.M.:* 25 mg (1 mL) t.i.d. or q.i.d. until patient can take oral therapy.

Tetanus—*I.M.:* 25 to 50 mg (1 to 2 mL) given 3 or 4 times daily, usually in conjunction with barbiturates. Total doses and frequency of administration must be determined by the patient's response, starting with low doses and increasing gradually. *I.V.:* 25 to 50 mg (1 to 2 mL). Dilute to at least 1 mg per mL and administer at a rate of 1 mg per minute.

DOSAGE AND ADMINISTRATION—PEDIATRIC PATIENTS (6 months to 12 years of age)

Thorazine (chlorpromazine) should generally not be used in pediatric patients under 6 months of age except where potentially lifesaving. It should not be used in conditions for which specific pediatric dosages have not been established.

Severe Behavioral Problems—OUTPATIENTS—Select route of administration according to severity of patient's condition and increase dosage gradually as required. *Oral:* $^1/_4$ mg/lb body weight q4 to 6h, p.r.n. (e.g., for 40 lb child—10 mg q4 to 6h). *Rectal:* $^1/_2$ mg/lb body weight q6 to 8h, p.r.n. (e.g., for 20 to 30 lb child—half a 25 mg suppository q6 to 8h). *I.M.:* $^1/_4$ mg/lb body weight q6 to 8h, p.r.n.

HOSPITALIZED PATIENTS—As with outpatients, start with low doses and increase dosage gradually. In severe behavior disorders or psychotic conditions, higher dosages (50 to 100 mg daily, and in older children, 200 mg daily or more) may be necessary. There is little evidence that behavior improvement in severely disturbed mentally retarded patients is further enhanced by doses beyond 500 mg per day. *Maximum I.M. Dosage:* Children up to 5 years (or 50 lbs), not over 40 mg/day; 5 to 12 years (or 50 to 100 lbs), not over 75 mg/day except in unmanageable cases.

Nausea and Vomiting—Dosage and frequency of administration should be adjusted according to the severity of the symptoms and response of the patient. The duration of activity following intramuscular administration may last up to 12 hours. Subsequent doses may be given by the same route if necessary. *Oral:* $^1/_4$ mg/lb body weight (e.g., 40 lb child—10 mg q4 to 6h). *Rectal:* $^1/_2$ mg/lb body weight q6 to 8h, p.r.n. (e.g., 20 to 30 lb child—half of a 25 mg suppository q6 to 8h). *I.M.:* $^1/_4$ mg/lb body weight q6 to 8h, p.r.n. *Maximum I.M. Dosage:* Pediatric patients 6 months to 5 yrs. (or 50 lbs), not over 40 mg/day; 5 to 12 yrs. (or 50 to 100 lbs), not over 75 mg/day except in severe cases. DURING SURGERY—*I.M.:* $^1/_8$ mg/lb body weight. Repeat in $^1/_2$ hour if necessary and if no hypotension occurs. *I.V.:* 1 mg per fractional injection at 2-minute intervals and not exceeding recommended I.M. dosage. Always dilute to 1 mg/ mL, i.e., 1 mL (25 mg) mixed with 24 mL of saline.

Presurgical Apprehension—$^1/_4$ mg/lb body weight, either *orally* 2 to 3 hours before operation, or *I.M.* 1 to 2 hours before.

Tetanus—*I.M.* or *I.V.:* $^1/_4$ mg/lb body weight q6 to 8h. When given I.V., dilute to at least 1 mg/mL and administer at rate

Continued on next page

Information on the SmithKline Beecham Pharmaceuticals products appearing here is based on the labeling in effect on June 15, 2000. Further information on these and other products may be obtained from the Medical Department, SmithKline Beecham Pharmaceuticals, One Franklin Plaza, Philadelphia, PA 19101.

Thorazine—Cont.

of 1 mg per 2 minutes. In patients up to 50 lbs, do not exceed 40 mg daily; 50 to 100 lbs, do not exceed 75 mg, except in severe cases.

IMPORTANT NOTES ON INJECTION

Inject slowly, deep into upper outer quadrant of buttock. Because of possible hypotensive effects, reserve parenteral administration for bedfast patients or for acute ambulatory cases, and keep patient lying down for at least 1/2 hour after injection. If irritation is a problem, dilute Injection with saline or 2% procaine; mixing with other agents in the syringe is not recommended. Subcutaneous injection is not advised. Avoid injecting undiluted Thorazine (chlorpromazine) into vein. I.V. route is only for severe hiccups, surgery and tetanus.

Because of the possibility of contact dermatitis, avoid getting solution on hands or clothing. This solution should be protected from light. This is a clear, colorless to pale yellow solution; a slight yellowish discoloration will not alter potency. If markedly discolored, solution should be discarded. For information on sulfite sensitivity, see the WARNINGS section of this labeling.

Note on Concentrate: When the Concentrate is to be used, add the desired dosage of Concentrate to 60 mL (2 fl oz) or more of diluent *just prior to administration*. This will insure palatability and stability. Vehicles suggested for dilution are: tomato or fruit juice, milk, simple syrup, orange syrup, carbonated beverages, coffee, tea or water. Semisolid foods (soups, puddings, etc.) may also be used. The Concentrate is light sensitive; it should be protected from light and dispensed in amber glass bottles. *Refrigeration is not required.*

OVERDOSAGE

(See also ADVERSE REACTIONS.)

SYMPTOMS—Primarily symptoms of central nervous system depression to the point of somnolence or coma. Hypotension and extrapyramidal symptoms.

Other possible manifestations include agitation and restlessness, convulsions, fever, autonomic reactions such as dry mouth and ileus, EKG changes and cardiac arrhythmias.

TREATMENT—It is important to determine other medications taken by the patient since multiple drug therapy is common in overdosage situations. Treatment is essentially symptomatic and supportive. Early gastric lavage is helpful. Keep patient under observation and maintain an open airway, since involvement of the extrapyramidal mechanism may produce dysphagia and respiratory difficulty in severe overdosage. **Do not attempt to induce emesis because a dystonic reaction of the head or neck may develop that could result in aspiration of vomitus.** Extrapyramidal symptoms may be treated with anti-parkinsonism drugs, barbiturates, or *Benadryl*. See prescribing information for these products. Care should be taken to avoid increasing respiratory depression.

If administration of a stimulant is desirable, amphetamine, dextroamphetamine, or caffeine with sodium benzoate is recommended. Stimulants that may cause convulsions (e.g., picrotoxin or pentylenetetrazol) should be avoided.

If hypotension occurs, the standard measures for managing circulatory shock should be initiated. If it is desirable to administer a vasoconstrictor, *Levophed* and *Neo-Synephrine* are most suitable. Other pressor agents, including epinephrine, are not recommended because phenothiazine derivatives may reverse the usual elevating action of these agents and cause a further lowering of blood pressure.

Limited experience indicates that phenothiazines are *not* dialyzable.

Special note on Spansule® capsules—Since much of the *Spansule* capsule medication is coated for gradual release, therapy directed at reversing the effects of the ingested drug and at supporting the patient should be continued for as long as overdosage symptoms remain. Saline cathartics are useful for hastening evacuation of pellets that have not already released medication.

HOW SUPPLIED

Tablets: 10 mg, in bottles of 100; 25 mg or 50 mg, in bottles of 100 and 1000. For use in severe neuropsychiatric conditions, 100 mg and 200 mg, in bottles of 100 and 1000.

NDC 0007-5073-20 10 mg 100's
NDC 0007-5074-20 25 mg 100's
NDC 0007-5074-30 25 mg 1000's
NDC 0007-5076-20 50 mg 100's
NDC 0007-5076-30 50 mg 1000's
NDC 0007-5077-20 100 mg 100's
NDC 0007-5077-30 100 mg 1000's
NDC 0007-5079-20 200 mg 100's
NDC 0007-5079-30 200 mg 1000's

Spansule® brand of sustained release capsules: 30 mg, 75 mg or 150 mg, in bottles of 50.

NDC 0007-5063-15 30 mg 50's
NDC 0007-5064-15 75 mg 50's
NDC 0007-5066-15 150 mg 50's

Ampuls: 1 mL and 2 mL (25 mg/mL), in boxes of 10.

NDC 0007-5060-11 25 mg/mL in 1 mL Ampuls (box of 10)
NDC 0007-5061-11 25 mg/mL in 2 mL Ampuls (box of 10)

Multi-Dose Vials: 10 mL (25 mg/mL), in boxes of 1.

NDC 0007-5062-01 25 mg/mL in 10 mL Multi-Dose Vials (box of 1)

Syrup: 10 mg/5 mL, in 4 fl oz bottles.

NDC 0007-5072-44 10 mg/5 mL 4 fl oz

Suppositories: 25 mg or 100 mg, in boxes of 12.

NDC 0007-5070-03 25 mg (box of 12)
NDC 0007-5071-03 100 mg (box of 12)

All dosage forms except Syrup should be stored between 15° and 30°C (59° and 86°F). Syrup should be stored below 25°C (77°F).

* phenytoin, Parke-Davis.
† metrizamide, Sanofi Winthrop Pharmaceuticals.
‡ norepinephrine bitartrate, Sanofi Winthrop Pharmaceuticals.
§ phenylephrine hydrochloride, Sanofi Winthrop Pharmaceuticals.
‖ diphenhydramine hydrochloride, Parke-Davis.

WARNING: Thorazine® *Spansule* capsules are manufactured with carbon tetrachloride and methyl chloroform, substances which harm public health and environment by destroying ozone in the upper atmosphere.

TZ:L83

Shown in Product Identification Guide, page 338

TIMENTIN® ℞

[*tī 'mĕn-tĭn*]

brand of sterile ticarcillin disodium and clavulanate potassium for Intravenous Administration

DESCRIPTION

Timentin is a sterile injectable antibacterial combination consisting of the semisynthetic antibiotic, ticarcillin disodium, and the β-lactamase inhibitor, clavulanate potassium (the potassium salt of clavulanic acid), for intravenous administration. Ticarcillin is derived from the basic penicillin nucleus, 6-amino-penicillanic acid.

Chemically, ticarcillin disodium is *N*-(2-Carboxy-3,3-dimethyl -7-oxo-4-thia-1-azabicyclo[3.2.0] hept-6-yl)-3-thiophenemalonamic acid disodium salt and may be represented as:

Clavulanic acid is produced by the fermentation of *Streptomyces clavuligerus*. It is a β-lactam structurally related to the penicillins and possesses the ability to inactivate a wide variety of β-lactamases by blocking the active sites of these enzymes. Clavulanic acid is particularly active against the clinically important plasmid-mediated β-lactamases frequently responsible for transferred drug resistance to penicillins and cephalosporins.

Chemically, clavulanate potassium is potassium (Z)-(2*R*,5*R*)-3-(2-hydroxyethylidene)-7-oxo-4-oxa-1-azabicyclo [3.2.0]heptane-2-carboxylate and may be represented structurally as:

Timentin is supplied as a white to pale yellow powder for reconstitution. *Timentin* is very soluble in water, its solubility being greater than 600 mg/mL. The reconstituted solution is clear, colorless or pale yellow, having a pH of 5.5 to 7.5.

For the *Timentin* 3.1 gram and 3.2 gram dosages, the theoretical sodium content is 4.75 mEq (109 mg) per gram of *Timentin*. The theoretical potassium content is 0.15 mEq (6 mg) and 0.3 mEq (11.9 mg) per gram of *Timentin* for the 3.1 gram and 3.2 gram dosages, respectively.

CLINICAL PHARMACOLOGY

After an intravenous infusion (30 min.) of 3.1 grams or 3.2 grams *Timentin*, peak serum concentrations of both ticarcillin and clavulanic acid are attained immediately after completion of infusion. Ticarcillin serum levels are similar to those produced by the administration of equivalent amounts of ticarcillin alone with a mean peak serum level of 330 µg/mL for the 3.1 gram and 3.2 gram formulations. The corresponding mean peak serum levels for clavulanic acid were 8 µg/mL and 16 µg/mL for the 3.1 gram and 3.2 gram formulations, respectively. (See following table.)

[See table below]

The mean area under the serum concentration curves for ticarcillin was 485 µg.hr./mL for the *Timentin* 3.1 gram and 3.2 gram formulations. The corresponding areas under the serum concentration curves for clavulanic acid were 8.2 µg.hr./mL and 15.6 µg.hr./mL for the *Timentin* 3.1 gram and 3.2 gram formulations, respectively.

The mean serum half-lives of ticarcillin and clavulanic acid in healthy volunteers are 1.1 hours and 1.1 hours, respectively, following administration of 3.1 grams or 3.2 grams of *Timentin*.

In pediatric patients receiving approximately 50 mg/kg *Timentin* (30:1 ratio ticarcillin to clavulanate), mean ticarcillin serum half-lives were 4.4 hours in neonates (n=18) and 1.0 hour in infants and children (n=41). The corresponding clavulanate serum half-lives averaged 1.9 hours in neonates (n=14) and 0.9 hour in infants and children (n=40). Area under the serum concentration time curves averaged 339 µg.hr./mL in infants and children (n=41), whereas the corresponding mean clavulanate area under the serum concentration time curves was approximately 7 µg.hr./mL in the same population (n=40).

Approximately 60% to 70% of ticarcillin and approximately 35% to 45% of clavulanic acid are excreted unchanged in urine during the first 6 hours after administration of a single dose of *Timentin* to normal volunteers with normal renal function. Two hours after an intravenous injection of 3.1 grams or 3.2 grams *Timentin*, concentrations of ticarcillin in urine generally exceed 1500 µg/mL. The corresponding concentrations of clavulanic acid in urine generally exceed 40 µg/mL and 70 µg/mL following administration of the 3.1 gram and 3.2 gram doses, respectively. By 4 to 6 hours after injection, the urine concentrations of ticarcillin and clavulanic acid usually decline to approximately 190 µg/mL and 2 µg/mL, respectively, for both doses. Neither component of *Timentin* is highly protein bound; ticarcillin has been found to be approximately 45% bound to human serum protein and clavulanic acid approximately 9% bound.

Somewhat higher and more prolonged serum levels of ticarcillin can be achieved with the concurrent administration of probenecid; however, probenecid does not enhance the serum levels of clavulanic acid.

Ticarcillin can be detected in tissues and interstitial fluid following parenteral administration.

Penetration of ticarcillin into bile and pleural fluid has been demonstrated. The results of experiments involving the administration of clavulanic acid to animals suggest that this compound, like ticarcillin, is well distributed in body tissues.

An inverse relationship exists between the serum half-life of ticarcillin and creatinine clearance. The dosage of *Timentin* need only be adjusted in cases of severe renal impairment. (See **DOSAGE AND ADMINISTRATION.)**

Ticarcillin may be removed from patients undergoing dialysis; the actual amount removed depends on the duration and type of dialysis.

MICROBIOLOGY: Ticarcillin is a semisynthetic antibiotic with a broad spectrum of bactericidal activity against many gram-positive and gram-negative aerobic and anaerobic bacteria.

Ticarcillin is, however, susceptible to degradation by β-lactamases and, therefore, the spectrum of activity does not normally include organisms which produce these enzymes. Clavulanic acid is a β-lactam, structurally related to the penicillins, which possesses the ability to inactivate a wide range of β-lactamase enzymes commonly found in microorganisms resistant to penicillins and cephalosporins. In particular, it has good activity against the clinically important plasmid-mediated β-lactamases frequently responsible for transferred drug resistance.

The formulation of ticarcillin with clavulanic acid in *Timentin* protects ticarcillin from degradation by β-lactamase enzymes and effectively extends the antibiotic spectrum of ticarcillin to include many bacteria normally resistant to ticarcillin and other β-lactam antibiotics. Thus *Timentin* possesses the distinctive properties of a broad-spectrum antibiotic and a β-lactamase inhibitor.

While *in vitro* studies have demonstrated the susceptibility of most strains of the following organisms, clinical efficacy for infections other than those included in the INDICATIONS AND USAGE section has not been documented:

<u>GRAM-NEGATIVE BACTERIA:</u> *Pseudomonas aeruginosa* (β-lactamase and non-β-lactamase producing), *Pseudomonas* species including *P. maltophilia* (β-lactamase and non-β-lactamase producing), *Escherichia coli* (β-lactamase and non-β-lactamase producing), *Proteus mirabilis* (β-lactamase and non-β-lactamase producing), *Proteus vulgaris* (β-lacta-

SERUM LEVELS IN ADULTS
AFTER A 30-MINUTE I.V. INFUSION OF TIMENTIN®

TICARCILLIN SERUM LEVELS (µg/mL)

Dose	0	15 min.	30 min.	1 hr.	1.5 hr.	3.5 hr.	5.5 hr.
3.1 gram	324 (293 to 388)	223 (184 to 293)	176 (135 to 235)	131 (102 to 195)	90 (65 to 119)	27 (19 to 37)	6 (5 to 7)
3.2 gram	336 (301 to 386)	214 (180 to 258)	186 (160 to 218)	122 (108 to 136)	78 (33 to 113)	29 (19 to 44)	10 (5 to 15)

CLAVULANIC ACID SERUM LEVELS (µg/mL)

Dose	0	15 min.	30 min.	1 hr.	1.5 hr.	3.5 hr.	5.5 hr.
3.1 gram	8.0 (5.3 to 10.3)	4.6 (3.0 to 7.6)	2.6 (1.8 to 3.4)	1.8 (1.6 to 2.2)	1.2 (0.8 to 1.6)	0.3 (0.2 to 0.3)	0
3.2 gram	15.8 (11.7 to 21.0)	8.3 (6.4 to 10.0)	5.2 (3.5 to 6.3)	3.4 (1.9 to 4.0)	2.5 (1.3 to 3.4)	0.5 (0.2 to 0.8)	0

mase and non-β-lactamase producing), *Providencia rettgeri* (formerly *Proteus rettgeri*) (β-lactamase and non-β-lactamase producing), *Providencia stuartii* (β-lactamase and non-β-lactamase producing), *Morganella morganii* (formerly *Proteus morganii*) (β-lactamase and non-β-lactamase producing), *Enterobacter* species (Although most strains of *Enterobacter* species are resistant *in vitro*, clinical efficacy has been demonstrated with *Timentin* in urinary tract infections caused by these organisms.), *Acinetobacter* species (β-lactamase and non-β-lactamase producing), *Hemophilus influenzae* (β-lactamase and non-β-lactamase producing), *Branhamella catarrhalis* (β-lactamase and non-β-lactamase producing), *Serratia* species including *S. marcescens* (β-lactamase and non-β-lactamase producing), *Neisseria gonorrhoeae* (β-lactamase and non-β-lactamase producing), *Neisseria meningitidis**, *Salmonella* species (β-lactamase and non-β-lactamase producing), *Klebsiella* species including *K. pneumoniae* (β-lactamase and non-β-lactamase producing), *Citrobacter* species including *C. freundii, C. diversus* and *C. amalonaticus* (β-lactamase and non-β-lactamase producing).

GRAM-POSITIVE BACTERIA: *Staphylococcus aureus* (β-lactamase and non-β-lactamase producing), *Staphylococcus saprophyticus, Staphylococcus epidermidis* (coagulase-negative staphylococci) (β-lactamase and non-β-lactamase producing), *Streptococcus pneumoniae** (*D. pneumoniae*), *Streptococcus bovis**, *Streptococcus agalactiae** (Group B), *Streptococcus faecalis** (*Enterococcus*), *Streptococcus pyogenes** (Group A, β-hemolytic), Viridans group streptococci*.

ANAEROBIC BACTERIA: *Bacteroides* species, including *B. fragilis* group (*B. fragilis, B. vulgatus*) (β-lactamase and non-β-lactamase producing), non-*B. fragilis* (*B. melaninogenicus*) (β-lactamase and non-β-lactamase producing), *B. thetaiotaomicron, B. ovatus, B. distasonis* (β-lactamase and non-β-lactamase-producing), *Clostridium* species including *C. perfringens, C. difficile, C. sporogenes, C. ramosum* and *C. bifermentans**, *Eubacterium* species, *Fusobacterium* species including *F. nucleatum* and *F. necrophorum**, *Peptococcus* species*, *Peptostreptococcus* species*, *Veillonella* species.

*These are non-β-lactamase-producing strains and therefore are susceptible to ticarcillin alone. Some of the β-lactamase-producing strains are also susceptible to ticarcillin alone.

In vitro synergism between *Timentin* and gentamicin, tobramycin or amikacin against multiresistant strains of *Pseudomonas aeruginosa* has been demonstrated.

SUSCEPTIBILITY TESTING:

Diffusion Technique: An 85 mcg *Timentin* (75 mcg ticarcillin plus 10 mcg clavulanic acid) diffusion disk is available for use with the Kirby-Bauer method. Based on the zone sizes given below, a report of "Susceptible" indicates that the infecting organism is likely to respond to *Timentin* therapy, while a report of "Resistant" indicates that the organism is not likely to respond to therapy with this antibiotic. A report of "Intermediate" susceptibility indicates that the organism would be susceptible to *Timentin* at a higher dosage or if the infection is confined to tissues or fluids (e.g., urine) in which high antibiotic levels are attained.

Dilution Technique: Broth or agar dilution methods may be used to determine the minimal inhibitory concentration (MIC) values for bacterial isolates to *Timentin*. Tubes should be inoculated with the test culture containing 10^4 to 10^5 CFU/mL or plates spotted with a test solution containing 10^3 to 10^4 CFU/mL.

The recommended dilution pattern utilizes a constant level of clavulanic acid, 2 mcg/mL, in all tubes together with varying amounts of ticarcillin. MICs are expressed in terms of the ticarcillin concentration in the presence of 2 mcg/mL clavulanic acid.

[See table above]

RECOMMENDED RANGES FOR *TIMENTIN* SUSCEPTIBILITY TESTING[1–3]

Diffusion Method Disk Zone Size, mm			Dilution Method MIC Correlates[4], mcg/mL	
Res.	Inter.	Susc.	Res.	Susc.
≤11	12 to 14	≥15	≥128	≤64

[1] The non-β-lactamase-producing organisms which are normally susceptible to ticarcillin will have similar zone sizes as for ticarcillin.

[2] Staphylococci which are susceptible to *Timentin* but resistant to methicillin, oxacillin or nafcillin must be considered as resistant.

[3] The quality control cultures should have the following assigned daily ranges for *Timentin*:

		Disks	MIC Range (mcg/mL)
E. coli	(ATCC 25922)	24 to 30 mm	2/2 to 8/2
S. aureus	(ATCC 25923)	32 to 40 mm	—
Ps. aeruginosa	(ATCC 27853)	20 to 28 mm	8/2 to 32/2
E. coli	(ATCC 35218)	21 to 25 mm	4/2 to 16/2
S. aureus	(ATCC 29213)	—	0.5/2 to 2/2

[4] Expressed as concentration of ticarcillin in the presence of a constant 2.0 mcg/mL concentration of clavulanic acid.

INDICATIONS AND USAGE

Timentin is indicated in the treatment of infections caused by susceptible strains of the designated microorganisms in the conditions listed below:

Septicemia, including bacteremia, caused by β-lactamase-producing strains of *Klebsiella* spp.*, *E. coli**, *Staphylococcus aureus**, or *Pseudomonas aeruginosa** (or other *Pseudomonas* species*)

Lower Respiratory Infections caused by β-lactamase-producing strains of *Staphylococcus aureus, Hemophilus influenzae**, or *Klebsiella* spp.*

Bone and Joint Infections caused by β-lactamase-producing strains of *Staphylococcus aureus*

Skin and Skin Structure Infections caused by β-lactamase-producing strains of *Staphylococcus aureus, Klebsiella* spp.*, or *E. coli**

Urinary Tract Infections (complicated and uncomplicated) caused by β-lactamase-producing strains of *E. coli, Klebsiella* spp., *Pseudomonas aeruginosa** (or other *Pseudomonas* spp.*), *Citrobacter* spp.*, *Enterobacter cloacae**, *Serratia marcescens**, or *Staphylococcus aureus**

Gynecologic Infections endometritis caused by β-lactamase-producing strains of *B. melaninogenicus**, *Enterobacter* spp. (including *E. cloacae**), *Escherichia coli, Klebsiella pneumoniae**, *Staphylococcus aureus*, or *Staphylococcus epidermidis*

Intra-abdominal Infections peritonitis caused by β-lactamase-producing strains of *Escherichia coli, Klebsiella pneumoniae*, or *Bacteroides fragilis** group

*Efficacy for this organism in this organ system was studied in fewer than 10 infections.

NOTE: For information on use in pediatric patients (≥3 months of age) see PRECAUTIONS–Pediatric Use and CLINICAL STUDIES sections. There are insufficient data to support the use of *Timentin* in pediatric patients under 3 months of age or for the treatment of septicemia and/or infections in the pediatric population where the suspected or proven pathogen is *Haemophilus influenzae* type b.

While *Timentin* is indicated only for the conditions listed above, infections caused by ticarcillin-susceptible organisms are also amenable to *Timentin* treatment due to its ticarcillin content. Therefore, mixed infections caused by ticarcillin-susceptible organisms and β-lactamase-producing organisms susceptible to ticarcillin/clavulanic acid should not require the addition of another antibiotic.

Appropriate culture and susceptibility tests should be performed before treatment in order to isolate and identify organisms causing infection and to determine their susceptibility to ticarcillin/clavulanic acid. Because of its broad spectrum of bactericidal activity against gram-positive and gram-negative bacteria, *Timentin* is particularly useful for the treatment of mixed infections and for presumptive therapy prior to the identification of the causative organisms. *Timentin* has been shown to be effective as single drug therapy in the treatment of some serious infections where normally combination antibiotic therapy might be employed.

Therapy with *Timentin* may be initiated before results of such tests are known when there is reason to believe the infection may involve any of the β-lactamase-producing organisms listed above; however, once these results become available, appropriate therapy should be continued.

Based on the *in vitro* synergism between ticarcillin/clavulanic acid and aminoglycosides against certain strains of *Pseudomonas aeruginosa*, combined therapy has been successful, especially in patients with impaired host defenses. Both drugs should be used in full therapeutic doses. As soon as results of culture and susceptibility tests become available, antimicrobial therapy should be adjusted as indicated.

CONTRAINDICATIONS

Timentin is contraindicated in patients with a history of hypersensitivity reactions to any of the penicillins.

WARNINGS

SERIOUS AND OCCASIONALLY FATAL HYPERSENSITIVITY (ANAPHYLACTIC) REACTIONS HAVE BEEN REPORTED IN PATIENTS ON PENICILLIN THERAPY. THESE REACTIONS ARE MORE LIKELY TO OCCUR IN INDIVIDUALS WITH A HISTORY OF PENICILLIN HYPERSENSITIVITY AND/OR A HISTORY OF SENSITIVITY TO MULTIPLE ALLERGENS. THERE HAVE BEEN REPORTS OF INDIVIDUALS WITH A HISTORY OF PENICILLIN HYPERSENSITIVITY WHO HAVE EXPERIENCED SEVERE REACTIONS WHEN TREATED WITH CEPHALOSPORINS. BEFORE INITIATING THERAPY WITH *TIMENTIN*, CAREFUL INQUIRY SHOULD BE MADE CONCERNING PREVIOUS HYPERSENSITIVITY REACTIONS TO PENICILLINS, CEPHALOSPORINS, OR OTHER ALLERGENS. IF AN ALLERGIC REACTION OCCURS, *TIMENTIN* SHOULD BE DISCONTINUED AND THE APPROPRIATE THERAPY INSTITUTED. **SERIOUS ANAPHYLACTIC REACTIONS REQUIRE IMMEDIATE EMERGENCY TREATMENT WITH EPINEPHRINE. OXYGEN, INTRAVENOUS STEROIDS AND AIRWAY MANAGEMENT, INCLUDING INTUBATION, SHOULD ALSO BE PROVIDED AS INDICATED.**

Pseudomembranous colitis has been reported with nearly all antibacterial agents, including *Timentin*, and may range in severity from mild to life-threatening. Therefore, it is important to consider this diagnosis in patients who present with diarrhea subsequent to the administration of antibacterial agents.

Treatment with antibacterial agents alters the normal flora of the colon and may permit overgrowth of clostridia. Studies indicate that a toxin produced by *Clostridium difficile* is a primary cause of "antibiotic-associated colitis."

After the diagnosis of pseudomembranous colitis has been established, appropriate therapeutic measures should be initiated. Mild cases of pseudomembranous colitis usually respond to drug discontinuation alone. In moderate to severe cases, consideration should be given to management with fluids and electrolytes, protein supplementation and treatment with an antibacterial drug clinically effective against *Clostridium difficile* colitis.

When very high doses of *Timentin* are administered, especially in the presence of impaired renal function, patients may experience convulsions. (See **ADVERSE REACTIONS** and **OVERDOSAGE**.)

PRECAUTIONS

General: While *Timentin* possesses the characteristic low toxicity of the penicillin group of antibiotics, periodic assessment of organ system functions, including renal, hepatic, and hematopoietic function, is advisable during prolonged therapy.

Bleeding manifestations have occurred in some patients receiving β-lactam antibiotics. These reactions have been associated with abnormalities of coagulation tests such as clotting time, platelet aggregation, and prothrombin time and are more likely to occur in patients with renal impairment.

If bleeding manifestations appear, *Timentin* treatment should be discontinued and appropriate therapy instituted.

Timentin has only rarely been reported to cause hypokalemia; however, the possibility of this occurring should be kept in mind particularly when treating patients with fluid and electrolyte imbalance. Periodic monitoring of serum potassium may be advisable in patients receiving prolonged therapy.

The theoretical sodium content is 4.75 mEq (109 mg) per gram of *Timentin*. This should be considered when treating patients requiring restricted salt intake.

As with any penicillin, an allergic reaction, including anaphylaxis, may occur during *Timentin* administration, particularly in a hypersensitive individual.

The possibility of superinfections with mycotic or bacterial pathogens should be kept in mind, particularly during prolonged treatment. If superinfections occur, appropriate measures should be taken.

Drug/Laboratory Test Interactions: As with other penicillins, the mixing of *Timentin* with an aminoglycoside in solutions for parenteral administration can result in substantial inactivation of the aminoglycoside.

Probenecid interferes with the renal tubular secretion of ticarcillin, thereby increasing serum concentrations and prolonging serum half-life of the antibiotic.

High urine concentrations of ticarcillin may produce false-positive protein reactions (pseudoproteinuria) with the following methods: sulfosalicylic acid and boiling test, acetic acid test, biuret reaction and nitric acid test. The bromphenol blue (Multi-stix®) reagent strip test has been reported to be reliable.

The presence of clavulanic acid in *Timentin* may cause a nonspecific binding of IgG and albumin by red cell membranes leading to a false-positive Coombs test.

Carcinogenesis, Mutagenesis, Impairment of Fertility: Long-term studies in animals have not been performed to evaluate carcinogenic potential. However, results from assays for gene mutation *in vitro* using bacteria (Ames tests) and yeast, and for chromosomal effects *in vitro* in human lymphocytes, and *in vivo* in mouse bone marrow (micronucleus test) indicate that *Timentin* is without any mutagenic potential.

Pregnancy (Category B): Reproduction studies have been performed in rats given doses up to 1050 mg/kg/day and have revealed no evidence of impaired fertility or harm to the fetus due to *Timentin*. There are, however, no adequate and well-controlled studies in pregnant women. Because animal reproduction studies are not always predictive of human response, this drug should be used during pregnancy only if clearly needed.

Nursing Mothers: It is not known whether this drug is excreted in human milk. Because many drugs are excreted in human milk, caution should be exercised when *Timentin* is administered to a nursing woman.

Pediatric Use: The safety and effectiveness of *Timentin* have been established in the age group of 3 months to 16 years. Use of *Timentin* in these age groups is supported by evidence from adequate and well-controlled studies of *Timentin* in adults with additional efficacy, safety, and pharmacokinetic data from both comparative and non-comparative studies in pediatric patients. There are insufficient data to support the use of *Timentin* in pediatric patients under 3 months of age or for the treatment of septicemia and/or in-

Continued on next page

Information on the SmithKline Beecham Pharmaceuticals products appearing here is based on the labeling in effect on June 15, 2000. Further information on these and other products may be obtained from the Medical Department, SmithKline Beecham Pharmaceuticals, One Franklin Plaza, Philadelphia, PA 19101.

Timentin—Cont.

fections in the pediatric population where the suspected or proven pathogen is *Haemophilus influenzae* type b.
In those patients in whom meningeal seeding from a distant infection site or in whom meningitis is suspected or documented, or in patients who require prophylaxis against central nervous system infection, an alternate agent with demonstrated clinical efficacy in this setting should be used.

ADVERSE REACTIONS

As with other penicillins, the following adverse reactions may occur:
Hypersensitivity reactions: skin rash, pruritus, urticaria, arthralgia, myalgia, drug fever, chills, chest discomfort, and anaphylactic reactions
Central nervous system: headache, giddiness, neuromuscular hyperirritability, or convulsive seizures
Gastrointestinal disturbances: disturbances of taste and smell, stomatitis, flatulence, nausea, vomiting and diarrhea, epigastric pain, and pseudomembranous colitis have been reported. Onset of pseudomembranous colitis symptoms may occur during or after antibiotic treatment. (See **WARNINGS**.)
Hemic and lymphatic systems: thrombocytopenia, leukopenia, neutropenia, eosinophilia, reduction of hemoglobin or hematocrit, and prolongation of prothrombin time and bleeding time
Abnormalities of hepatic and renal function tests: elevation of serum aspartate aminotransferase (SGOT), serum alanine aminotransferase (SGPT), serum alkaline phosphatase, serum LDH, serum bilirubin. There have been reports of transient hepatitis and cholestatic jaundice—as with some other penicillins and some cephalosporins. Elevation of serum creatinine and/or BUN, hypernatremia, reduction in serum potassium and uric acid
Local reactions: pain, burning, swelling, and induration at the injection site and thrombophlebitis with intravenous administration
Available safety data for pediatric patients treated with *Timentin* demonstrate a similar adverse event profile to that observed in adult patients.

DRUG ABUSE AND DEPENDENCE

Neither *Timentin* abuse nor *Timentin* dependence has been reported.

OVERDOSAGE

As with other penicillins, neurotoxic reactions may arise when very high doses of *Timentin* are administered, especially in patients with impaired renal function. (See **WARNINGS** and **ADVERSE REACTIONS**—*Central nervous system.*)
In case of overdosage, discontinue *Timentin*, treat symptomatically, and institute supportive measures as required. Ticarcillin may be removed from circulation by hemodialysis. The molecular weight, degree of protein binding, and pharmacokinetic profile of clavulanic acid together with information from a single patient with renal insufficiency all suggest that this compound may also be removed by hemodialysis.

DOSAGE AND ADMINISTRATION

Timentin should be administered by intravenous infusion (30 min.).
Adults: The usual recommended dosage for systemic and urinary tract infections for average (60 kg) adults is 3.1 grams *Timentin* (3.1 gram vial containing 3 grams ticarcillin and 100 mg clavulanic acid) given every 4 to 6 hours. For gynecologic infections, *Timentin* should be administered as follows: Moderate infections 200 mg/kg/day in divided doses every 6 hours and for severe infections 300 mg/kg/day in divided doses every 4 hours. For patients weighing less than 60 kg, the recommended dosage is 200 to 300 mg/kg/day, based on ticarcillin content, given in divided doses every 4 to 6 hours.
In urinary tract infections, a dosage of 3.2 grams *Timentin* (3.2 gram vial containing 3 grams ticarcillin and 200 mg clavulanic acid) given every 8 hours is adequate.
Pediatric Patients (≥3 months):
For patients <60 kg:
In patients <60 kg, *Timentin* is dosed at 50 mg/kg/dose based on the ticarcillin component. *Timentin* should be administered as follows: Mild to moderate infections 200 mg/kg/day in divided doses every 6 hours; for severe infections, 300 mg/kg/day in divided doses every 4 hours.
For patients ≥60 kg:
For mild to moderate infections, 3.1 grams *Timentin* (3 grams of ticarcillin and 100 mg of clavulanic acid) administered every 6 hours; for severe infections, 3.1 grams every 4 hours.
Renal impairment:
For infections complicated by renal insufficiency†, an initial loading dose of 3.1 grams should be followed by doses based on creatinine clearance and type of dialysis as indicated below:
[See first table above]
Dosage for any individual patient must take into consideration the site and severity of infection, the susceptibility of the organisms causing infection, and the status of the patient's host defense mechanisms.
The duration of therapy depends upon the severity of infection. Generally, *Timentin* should be continued for at least 2 days after the signs and symptoms of infection have disappeared. The usual duration is 10 to 14 days; however, in difficult and complicated infections, more prolonged therapy may be required.

Creatinine clearance mL/min.	Dosage
over 60	3.1 grams every 4 hrs.
30 to 60	2 grams every 4 hrs.
10 to 30	2 grams every 8 hrs.
less than 10	2 grams every 12 hrs.
less than 10 with hepatic dysfunction	2 grams every 24 hrs.
patients on peritoneal dialysis	3.1 grams every 12 hrs.
patients on hemodialysis	2 grams every 12 hrs. supplemented with 3.1 grams after each dialysis

To calculate creatinine clearance‡ from a serum creatinine value use the following formula.

$$C_{cr} = \frac{(140-\text{Age})\ (\text{wt. in kg})}{72 \times S_{cr}\ (\text{mg}/100\ \text{mL})}$$

This is the calculated creatinine clearance for adult males; for females it is 15% less.

‡Cockcroft, D.W., et al: Prediction of Creatinine Clearance from Serum Creatinine. Nephron 16:31–41, 1976.

†The half-life of ticarcillin in patients with renal failure is approximately 13 hours.

STABILITY PERIOD
(3.1 gram and 3.2 gram Vials and Piggyback Bottles)

Intravenous Solution (ticarcillin concentrations of 10 mg/mL to 100 mg/mL)	Room Temperature 21° to 24°C (70° to 75°F)	Refrigerated 4°C (40°F)
Dextrose Injection 5%, USP	24 hours	3 days
Sodium Chloride Injection, USP	24 hours	7 days
Lactated Ringer's Injection, USP	24 hours	7 days

Frequent bacteriologic and clinical appraisals are necessary during therapy of chronic urinary tract infection and may be required for several months after therapy has been completed; persistent infections may require treatment for several weeks, and doses smaller than those indicated above should not be used.
In certain infections, involving abscess formation, appropriate surgical drainage should be performed in conjunction with antimicrobial therapy.

INTRAVENOUS ADMINISTRATION
DIRECTIONS FOR USE
3.1 gram and 3.2 gram Vials and Piggyback Bottles

The 3.1 gram or 3.2 gram vial should be reconstituted by adding approximately 13 mL of Sterile Water for Injection, USP, or Sodium Chloride Injection, USP, and shaking well. When dissolved, the concentration of ticarcillin will be approximately 200 mg/mL with corresponding concentrations of 6.7 mg/mL and 13.4 mg/mL clavulanic acid for the 3.1 gram and 3.2 gram respective doses. Conversely, each 5.0 mL of the 3.1 gram dose reconstituted with approximately 13 mL of diluent will contain approximately 1 gram of ticarcillin and 33 mg of clavulanic acid. For the 3.2 gram dose reconstituted with 13 mL of diluent, each 5.0 mL will contain 1 gram of ticarcillin and 66 mg of clavulanic acid.
INTRAVENOUS INFUSION: The dissolved drug should be further diluted to desired volume using the recommended solution listed in the COMPATIBILITY AND STABILITY Section (STABILITY PERIOD) to a concentration between 10 mg/mL to 100 mg/mL. The solution of reconstituted drug may then be administered over a period of 30 minutes by direct infusion or through a Y-type intravenous infusion set. If this method or the "piggyback" method of administration is used, it is advisable to discontinue temporarily the administration of any other solutions during the infusion of *Timentin*.
Stability—For I.V. solutions, see STABILITY PERIOD below.
When *Timentin* is given in combination with another antimicrobial, such as an aminoglycoside, each drug should be given separately in accordance with the recommended dosage and routes of administration for each drug.
After reconstitution and prior to administration, *Timentin*, as with other parenteral drugs, should be inspected visually for particulate matter. If this condition is evident, the solution should be discarded.
The color of reconstituted solutions of *Timentin* normally ranges from light to dark yellow depending on concentration, duration and temperature of storage while maintaining label claim characteristics.

COMPATIBILITY AND STABILITY
3.1 gram and 3.2 gram Vials and Piggyback Bottles
(Dilutions derived from a stock solution of 200 mg/mL)

The concentrated stock solution at 200 mg/mL is stable for up to 6 hours at room temperature 21° to 24°C (70° to 75°F) or up to 72 hours under refrigeration 4°C (40°F).
If the concentrated stock solution (200 mg/mL) is held for up to 6 hours at room temperature 21° to 24°C (70° to 75°F) or up to 72 hours under refrigeration 4°C (40°F) and further diluted to a concentration between 10 mg/mL and 100 mg/mL with any of the diluents listed below, then the following stability periods apply.
[See second table above]
If the concentrated stock solution (200 mg/mL) is stored for up to 6 hours at room temperature and then further diluted to a concentration between 10 mg/mL and 100 mg/mL, solutions of Sodium Chloride Injection, USP, and Lactated Ringer's Injection, USP, may be stored frozen −18°C (0°F) for up to 30 days. Solutions prepared with Dextrose Injection 5%, USP, may be stored frozen −18°C (0°F) for up to 7 days. All thawed solutions should be used within 8 hours or discarded. Once thawed, solutions should not be refrozen.
NOTE: *Timentin* is incompatible with Sodium Bicarbonate.
Unused solutions must be discarded after the time periods listed above.

HOW SUPPLIED

Timentin (sterile ticarcillin disodium and clavulanate potassium).
Each 3.1 gram vial contains sterile ticarcillin disodium equivalent to 3 grams ticarcillin and sterile clavulanate potassium equivalent to 0.1 gram clavulanic acid.
NDC 0029-6571-26 .... 3.1 gram Vial
NDC 0029-6571-21 .... 3.1 gram Piggyback Bottle
Timentin is also supplied as:
NDC 0029-6571-40 .... 3.1 gram ADD-Vantage®§ Antibiotic Vial
Each 31 gram Pharmacy Bulk Package contains sterile ticarcillin disodium equivalent to 30 grams ticarcillin and sterile clavulanate potassium equivalent to 1 gram clavulanic acid.
NDC 0029-6579-21 .... 31 gram Pharmacy Bulk Package
Timentin vials should be stored at or below 24°C (75°F).
NDC 0029-6571-31 ...... *Timentin* as an iso-osmotic, sterile, nonpyrogenic, frozen solution in Galaxy®[II] (PL 2040) Plastic Containers—supplied in 100 mL single-dose containers equivalent to 3 grams ticarcillin and clavulanate potassium equivalent to 0.1 gram clavulanic acid.

CLINICAL STUDIES

Timentin has been studied in a total of 296 pediatric patients (excluding neonates and infants less than 3 months) in six controlled clinical trials. The majority of patients studied had intra-abdominal infections, and the primary comparator was clindamycin and gentamicin with or without ampicillin. At the end-of-therapy visit, comparable efficacy was reported in the *Timentin* and appropriate comparator arms.
Timentin was also evaluated in an additional 408 pediatric patients (excluding neonates and infants less than 3 months) in three uncontrolled U.S. clinical trials. Patients were treated across a broad range of presenting diagnoses including: infections in bone and joint, skin and skin structure, lower respiratory tract, urinary tract, as well as intra-abdominal and gynecologic infections. Patients received *Timentin* either 300 mg/kg/day (based on the ticarcillin component) divided q4h for severe infection or 200 mg/kg/day (based on the ticarcillin component) divided q6h for mild to moderate infections. The efficacy rates were comparable to those obtained in the controlled trials.
The adverse event profile in these 704 *Timentin*-treated pediatric patients was comparable to that seen in adult patients.
§ADD-Vantage® is a trademark of Abbott Laboratories.
[II]Galaxy® is a trademark of Baxter International Inc.
Rx only
TI:L8IV

Shown in Product Identification Guide, page 338

For information on over-the-counter drugs, consult **PDR For Nonprescription Drugs**.

Solvay Pharmaceuticals, Inc.
901 SAWYER ROAD
MARIETTA, GA 30062

For Medical Information Contact:
Generally:
Medical Information Department
(800) 241-1643
In Emergencies:
(770) 429-7110

Sales and Ordering:
Orders may be placed by calling this toll free number:
(800) 241-1643
Mail orders should be sent to:
Solvay Pharmaceuticals
Order Entry Department
901 Sawyer Road
Marietta, GA 30062

ACEON® ℞

[ā-sē-ŏn]
(perindopril erbumine) Tablets

USE IN PREGNANCY
When used in pregnancy during the second and third trimesters, ACE inhibitors can cause injury and even death to the developing fetus. When pregnancy is detected, ACEON® should be discontinued as soon as possible. See **WARNINGS: Fetal/Neonatal Morbidity and Mortality.**

DESCRIPTION

ACEON® (perindopril erbumine) is the tert-butylamine salt of perindopril, the ethyl ester of a non-sulfhydryl angiotensin converting enzyme (ACE) inhibitor. Perindopril erbumine is chemically described as (2S,3aS,7aS)-1-[(S)-N-[(S)-1-Carboxybutyl]alanyl]hexahydro-2-indolinecarboxylic acid, 1-ethyl ester, compound with tert-butylamine (1:1). Its molecular formula is $C_{19}H_{32}N_2O_5C_4H_{11}N$. Its structural formula is:

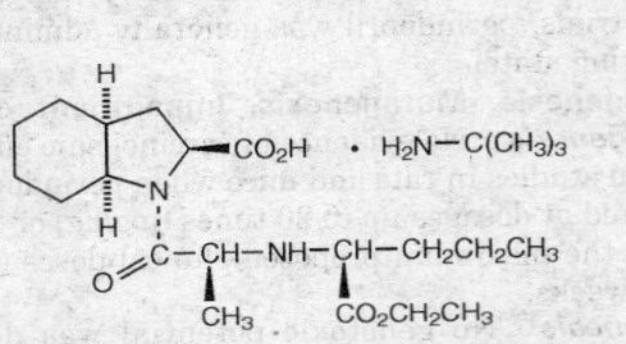

Perindopril erbumine is a white, crystalline powder with a molecular weight of 368.47 (free acid) or 441.61 (salt form). It is freely soluble in water (60% w/w), alcohol and chloroform.

Perindopril is the free acid form of perindopril erbumine, is a pro-drug and metabolized *in vivo* by hydrolysis of the ester group to form perindoprilat, the biologically active metabolite.

ACEON® Tablets are available in 2 mg, 4 mg and 8 mg strengths for oral administration. In addition to perindopril erbumine, each tablet contains the following inactive ingredients: colloidal silica (hydrophobic), lactose, magnesium stearate and microcrystalline cellulose. The 4 and 8 mg tablets also contain iron oxide.

CLINICAL PHARMACOLOGY

Mechanism of Action: ACEON® (perindopril erbumine) is a pro-drug for perindoprilat, which inhibits ACE in human subjects and animals. The mechanism through which perindoprilat lowers blood pressure is believed to be primarily inhibition of ACE activity. ACE is a peptidyl dipeptidase that catalyzes conversion of the inactive decapeptide, angiotensin I, to the vasoconstrictor, angiotensin II. Angiotensin II is a potent peripheral vasoconstrictor, which stimulates aldosterone secretion by the adrenal cortex, and provides negative feedback on renin secretion. Inhibition of ACE results in decreased plasma angiotensin II, leading to decreased vasoconstriction, increased plasma renin activity and decreased aldosterone secretion. The latter results in diuresis and natriuresis and may be associated with a small increase of serum potassium.

ACE is identical to kininase II, an enzyme that degrades bradykinin. Whether increased levels of bradykinin, a potent vasodepressor peptide, play a role in the therapeutic effects of ACEON® remains to be elucidated.

While the principal mechanism of perindopril in blood pressure reduction is believed to be through the renin-angiotensin-aldosterone system, ACE inhibitors have some effect even in apparent low-renin hypertension. Perindopril has been studied in relatively few black patients, usually a low-renin population, and the average response of diastolic blood pressure to perindopril was about half the response seen in nonblacks, a finding consistent with previous experience of other ACE inhibitors.

After administration of perindopril, ACE is inhibited in a dose- and blood concentration-related fashion, with the maximal inhibition of 80 to 90% attained by 8 mg persisting for 10 to 12 hours. Twenty-four hour ACE inhibition is about 60% after these doses. The degree of ACE inhibition achieved by a given dose appears to diminish over time (the ID_{50} increases). The pressor response to an angiotensin I infusion is reduced by perindopril, but this effect is not as persistent as the effect on ACE; there is about 35% inhibition at 24 hours after a 12 mg dose.

Pharmacokinetics: Oral administration of ACEON® (perindopril erbumine) results in its rapid absorption with peak plasma concentrations occurring at approximately 1 hour. The absolute oral bioavailability of perindopril is about 75%. Following absorption, approximately 30 to 50% of systemically available perindopril is hydrolyzed to its active metabolite, perindoprilat, which has a mean bioavailability of about 25%. Peak plasma concentrations of perindoprilat are attained 3 to 7 hours after perindopril administration. The presence of food in the gastrointestinal tract does not affect the rate or extent of absorption of perindopril but reduces bioavailability of perindoprilat by about 35%. (See **PRECAUTIONS: Food Interactions.**)

With 4, 8 and 16 mg doses of ACEON®, C_{max} and AUC of perindopril and perindoprilat increase in a linear and dose-proportional manner following both single oral dosing and at steady state during a once-a-day multiple dosing regimen.

Perindopril exhibits multiexponential pharmacokinetics following oral administration. The mean half-life of perindopril associated with most of its elimination is approximately 0.8 to 1.0 hours. At very low plasma concentrations of perindopril (<3 ng/mL), there is a prolonged terminal elimination half-life, similar to that seen with other ACE inhibitors, that results from slow dissociation of perindopril from plasma/tissue ACE binding sites. Perindopril does not accumulate with a once-a-day multiple dosing regimen. Mean total body clearance of perindopril is 219 to 362 mL/min and its mean renal clearance is 23.3 to 28.6 mL/min.

Perindopril is extensively metabolized following oral administration, with only 4 to 12% of the dose recovered unchanged in the urine. Six metabolites resulting from hydrolysis, glucuronidation and cyclization via dehydration have been identified. These include the active ACE inhibitor, perindoprilat (hydrolyzed perindopril), perindopril and perindoprilat glucuronides, dehydrated perindopril and the diastereoisomers of dehydrated perindoprilat. In humans, hepatic esterase appears to be responsible for the hydrolysis of perindopril.

The active metabolite, perindoprilat, also exhibits multiexponential pharmacokinetics following the oral administration of ACEON®. Formation of perindoprilat is gradual with peak plasma concentrations occurring between 3 and 7 hours. The subsequent decline in plasma concentration shows an apparent mean half-life of 3 to 10 hours for the majority of the elimination, with a prolonged terminal elimination half-life of 30 to 120 hours resulting from slow dissociation of perindoprilat from plasma/tissue ACE binding sites. During repeated oral once-daily dosing with perindopril, perindoprilat accumulates about 1.5 to 2.0 fold and attains steady state plasma levels in 3 to 6 days. The clearance of perindoprilat and its metabolites is almost exclusively renal.

Approximately 60% of circulating perindopril is bound to plasma proteins, and only 10 to 20% of perindoprilat is bound. Therefore, drug interactions mediated through effects on protein binding are not anticipated.

At usual antihypertensive dosages, little radioactivity (<5% of the dose) was distributed to the brain after administration of ^{14}C-perindopril to rats.

Radioactivity was detectable in fetuses and in milk after administration of ^{14}C-perindopril to pregnant and lactating rats.

Elderly Patients: Plasma concentrations of both perindopril and perindoprilat in elderly patients (>70 yrs) are approximately twice those observed in younger patients, reflecting both increased conversion of perindopril to perindoprilat and decreased renal excretion of perindoprilat. (See **PRECAUTIONS: Geriatric Use.**)

Heart Failure Patients: Perindoprilat clearance is reduced in congestive heart failure patients, resulting in a 40% higher dose interval AUC. (See **DOSAGE AND ADMINISTRATION.**)

Patients with Renal Insufficiency: With perindopril erbumine doses of 2 to 4 mg, perindoprilat AUC increases with decreasing renal function. At creatinine clearances of 30 to 80 mL/min, AUC is about double that of 100 mL/min. When creatinine clearance drops below 30 mL/min, AUC increases more markedly.

In a limited number of patients studied, perindopril dialysis clearance ranged from 41.7 to 76.7 mL/min (mean 52.0 mL/min). Perindoprilat dialysis clearance ranged from 37.4 to 91.0 mL/min (mean 67.2 mL/min). (See **DOSAGE AND ADMINISTRATION.**)

Patients with Hepatic Insufficiency. The bioavailability of perindoprilat is increased in patients with impaired hepatic function. Plasma concentrations of perindoprilat in patients with impaired liver function were about 50% higher than those observed in healthy subjects or hypertensive patients with normal liver function.

Pharmacodynamics: In placebo-controlled studies of perindopril monotherapy (2 to 16 mg q.d.) in patients with a mean blood pressure of about 150/100 mm Hg, 2 mg had little effect, but doses of 4 to 16 mg lowered blood pressure. The 8 and 16 mg doses were indistinguishable, and both had a greater effect than the 4 mg dose. The magnitude of the blood pressure effect was similar in the standing and supine positions, generally about 1 mm Hg greater on standing. In these studies, doses of 8 and 16 mg per day gave supine, trough blood pressure reductions of 9 to 15/5 to 6 mm Hg. When once-daily and twice-daily dosing were compared, the B.I.D. regimen was generally slightly superior, but by not more than about 0.5 to 1 mm Hg. After 2 to 16 mg doses of perindopril, the trough mean systolic and diastolic blood pressure effects were approximately equal to the peak effects (measured 3 to 7 hours after dosing.). Trough effects were about 75 to 100% of peak effects. When perindopril was given to patients receiving 25 mg HCTZ, it had an added effect similar in magnitude to its effect as monotherapy, but 2 to 8 mg doses were approximately equal in effectiveness. In general, the effect of perindopril occurred promptly, with effects increasing slightly over several weeks.

In hemodynamic studies carried out in animal models of hypertension, blood pressure reduction after perindopril administration was accompanied by a reduction in peripheral arterial resistance and improved arterial wall compliance.

In studies carried out in patients with essential hypertension, the reduction in blood pressure was accompanied by a reduction in peripheral resistance with no significant changes in heart rate or glomerular filtration rate. An increase in the compliance of large arteries was also observed, suggesting a direct effect on arterial smooth muscle, consistent with the results of animal studies.

Formal interaction studies of ACEON® have not been carried out with antihypertensive agents other than thiazides. Limited experience in controlled and uncontrolled trials coadministering ACEON® with a calcium channel blocker, a loop diuretic or triple therapy (beta-blocker, vasodilator and a diuretic) do not suggest any unexpected interactions. In general, ACE inhibitors have less than additive effects when given with beta-adrenergic blockers, presumably because both work in part through the renin angiotension system. A controlled pharmacokinetic study has shown no effect on plasma digoxin concentrations when coadministered with ACEON®. (See **PRECAUTIONS: Drug Interactions.**)

In uncontrolled studies in patients with insulin-dependent diabetes, perindopril did not appear to affect glycemic control. In long-term use, no effect on urinary protein excretion was seen in these patients.

The effectiveness of ACEON® was not influenced by sex and it was less effective in blacks than in nonblacks. In elderly patients (≥60 years), the mean blood pressure effect was somewhat smaller than in younger patients, although the difference was not significant.

INDICATIONS AND USAGE

ACEON® (perindopril erbumine) is indicated for the treatment of patients with essential hypertension. ACEON® may be used alone or given with other classes of antihypertensives, especially thiazide diuretics.

When using ACEON®, consideration should be given to the fact that another angiotensin converting enzyme inhibitor (captopril) has caused agranulocytosis, particularly in patients with renal impairment or collagen vascular disease. Available data are insufficient to determine whether ACEON® has a similar potential. (See **WARNINGS.**)

In considering use of ACEON®, it should be noted that in controlled trials ACE inhibitors have an effect on blood pressure that is less in black patients than in nonblacks. In addition, it should be noted that black patients receiving ACE inhibitor monotherapy have been reported to have a higher incidence of angioedema compared to nonblacks. (See **WARNINGS: Angioedema.**)

CONTRAINDICATIONS

ACEON® (perindopril erbumine) is contraindicated in patients known to be hypersensitive to this product or to any other ACE inhibitor. ACEON® is also contraindicated in patients with a history of angioedema related to previous treatment with an ACE inhibitor.

WARNINGS

Anaphylactoid and Possibly Related Reactions: Presumably because angiotensin-converting enzyme inhibitors affect the metabolism of eicosanoids and polypeptides, including endogenous bradykinin, patients receiving ACE inhibitors (including ACEON®) may be subject to a variety of adverse reactions, some of them serious.

Angioedema: Angioedema involving the face, extremities, lips, tongue, glottis and/or larynx has been reported in patients treated with ACE inhibitors, including ACEON® (perindopril erbumine) (0.1% of patients treated with ACEON® in U.S. clinical trials). In such cases, ACEON® should be promptly discontinued and the patient carefully observed until the swelling disappears. In instances where swelling has been confined to the face and lips, the condition has generally resolved without treatment, although antihistamines have been useful in relieving symptoms. Angioedema associated with involvement of the tongue, glottis or larynx may be fatal due to airway obstruction. Appropriate therapy, such as subcutaneous epinephrine solution 1:1000 (0.3 to 0.5 mL), should be promptly administered. Patients with a history of angioedema unrelated to ACE inhibitor therapy may be at increased risk of angioedema while receiving an ACE inhibitor.

Anaphylactoid Reactions During Desensitization: Two patients undergoing desensitizing treatment with hymenoptera venom while receiving ACE inhibitors sustained life-threatening anaphylactoid reactions. In the same patients, these reactions were avoided when ACE inhibitors were

Continued on next page

Aceon—Cont.

temporarily withheld, but they reappeared upon inadvertent rechallenge.

Anaphylactoid Reactions During Membrane Exposure: Anaphylactoid reactions have been reported in patients dialyzed with high-flux membranes and treated concomitantly with an ACE inhibitor. Anaphylactoid reactions have also been reported in patients undergoing low-density lipoprotein apheresis with dextran sulfate absorption.

Hypotension: Like other ACE inhibitors, ACEON® can cause symptomatic hypotension. ACEON® has been associated with hypotension in 0.3% of uncomplicated hypertensive patients in U.S. placebo-controlled trials. Symptoms related to orthostatic hypotension were reported in another 0.8% of patients.

Symptomatic hypotension associated with the use of ACE inhibitors is more likely to occur in patients who have been volume and/or salt-depleted, as a result of prolonged diuretic therapy, dietary salt restriction, dialysis, diarrhea or vomiting. Volume and/or salt depletion should be corrected before initiating therapy with ACEON®. (See **DOSAGE AND ADMINISTRATION.**)

In patients with congestive heart failure, with or without associated renal insufficiency, ACE inhibitors may cause excessive hypotension, and may be associated with oliguria or azotemia, and rarely with acute renal failure and death. In patients with ischemic heart disease or cerebrovascular disease such an excessive fall in blood pressure could result in a myocardial infarction or a cerebrovascular accident.

In patients at risk of excessive hypotension, ACEON® therapy should be started under very close medical supervision. Patients should be followed closely for the first two weeks of treatment and whenever the dose of ACEON® and/or diuretic is increased.

If excessive hypotension occurs, the patient should be placed immediately in a supine position and, if necessary, treated with an intravenous infusion of physiological saline. ACEON® treatment can usually be continued following restoration of volume and blood pressure.

Neutropenia/Agranulocytosis: Another ACE inhibitor, captopril, has been shown to cause agranulocytosis and bone marrow depression, rarely in uncomplicated patients but more frequently in patients with renal impairment, especially patients with a collagen vascular disease such as systemic lupus erythematosus or scleroderma. Available data from clinical trials of ACEON® are insufficient to show whether ACEON® causes agranulocytosis at similar rates.

Fetal/Neonatal Morbidity and Mortality: ACE inhibitors can cause fetal and neonatal morbidity and death when administered to pregnant women. Several dozen cases have been reported in the world literature. When pregnancy is detected, ACE inhibitors should be discontinued as soon as possible.

The use of ACE inhibitors during the second and third trimesters of pregnancy has been associated with fetal and neonatal injury, including hypotension, neonatal skull hypoplasia, anuria, reversible or irreversible renal failure and death. Oligohydramnios has also been reported, presumably resulting from decreased fetal renal function; oligohydramnios in this setting has been associated with fetal limb contractures, craniofacial deformation and hypoplastic lung development. Prematurity, intrauterine growth retardation and patent ductus arteriosus have also been reported, although it is not clear whether these occurrences were due to the ACE-inhibitor exposure.

These adverse effects do not appear to have resulted from intrauterine ACE-inhibitor exposure that has been limited to the first trimester. Mothers whose embryos and fetuses are exposed to ACE inhibitors only during the first trimester should be so informed. Nonetheless, when patients become pregnant, physicians should make every effort to discontinue the use of ACEON® as soon as possible.

Rarely (probably less often than once in every thousand pregnancies), no alternative to ACE inhibitors will be found. In these rare cases, the mothers should be apprised of the potential hazards to their fetuses, and serial ultrasound examinations should be performed to assess the intra-amniotic environment.

If oligohydramnios is observed, ACEON® should be discontinued unless it is considered life-saving for the mother. Contraction stress testing (CST), a non-stress test (NST) or biophysical profiling (BPP) may be appropriate, depending upon the week of pregnancy. Patients and physicians should be aware, however, that oligohydramnios may not appear until after the fetus has sustained irreversible injury.

Infants with histories of *in utero* exposure to ACE inhibitors should be closely observed for hypotension, oliguria and hyperkalemia. If oliguria occurs, attention should be directed toward support of blood pressure and renal perfusion. Exchange transfusion or dialysis may be required as means of reversing hypotension and/or substituting for disordered renal function. Perindopril, which crosses the placenta, can theoretically be removed from the neonatal circulation by these means, but limited experience has not shown that such removal is central to the treatment of these infants.

No teratogenic effects of perindopril were seen in studies of pregnant rats, mice, rabbits and cynomologous monkeys. On a mg/m^2 basis, the doses used in these studies were 6 times (in mice), 670 times (in rats), 50 times (in rabbits) and 17 times (in monkeys) the maximum recommended human dose (assuming a 50 kg adult). On a mg/kg basis, these multiples are 60 times (in mice), 3,750 times (in rats), 150 times (in rabbits) and 50 times (in monkeys) the maximum recommended human dose.

Hepatic Failure: Rarely, ACE inhibitors have been associated with a syndrome that starts with cholestatic jaundice and progresses to fulminant hepatic necrosis and (sometimes) death. The mechanism of this syndrome is not understood. Patients receiving ACE inhibitors who develop jaundice or marked elevations of hepatic enzymes should discontinue the ACE inhibitor and receive appropriate medical follow-up.

PRECAUTIONS

General: ***Impaired Renal Function:*** As a consequence of inhibiting the renin-angiotensin-aldosterone system, changes in renal function may be anticipated in susceptible individuals.

Hypertensive Patients with Congestive Heart Failure: In patients with severe congestive heart failure, where renal function may depend on the activity of the renin-angiotensin-aldosterone system, treatment with ACE inhibitors, including ACEON®, may be associated with oliguria and/or progressive azotemia, and rarely with acute renal failure and/or death.

Hypertensive Patients with Renal Artery Stenosis: In hypertensive patients with unilateral or bilateral renal artery stenosis, increases in blood urea nitrogen and serum creatinine may occur. Experience with ACE inhibitors suggests that these increases are usually reversible upon discontinuation of the drug. In such patients, renal function should be monitored during the first few weeks of therapy.

Some hypertensive patients without apparent pre-existing renal vascular disease have developed increases in blood urea nitrogen and serum creatinine, usually minor and transient. These increases are more likely to occur in patients treated concomitantly with a diuretic and in patients with pre-existing renal impairment. Reduction of dosages of ACEON®, the diuretic or both may be required. In some cases, discontinuation of either or both drugs may be necessary.

Evaluation of hypertensive patients should always include an assessment of renal function. (See **DOSAGE AND ADMINISTRATION.**)

Hyperkalemia: Elevations of serum potassium have been observed in some patients treated with ACE inhibitors, including ACEON®. In U.S. controlled clinical trials, 1.4% of the patients receiving ACEON® and 2.3% of patients receiving placebo showed increased serum potassium levels to greater than 5.7 mEq/L. Most cases were isolated single values that did not appear clinically relevant and were rarely a cause for withdrawal. Risk factors for the development of hyperkalemia include renal insufficiency, diabetes mellitus and the concomitant use of agents such as potassium-sparing diuretics, potassium supplements and/or potassium-containing salt substitutes. Drugs associated with increases in serum potassium should be used cautiously, if at all, with ACEON®. (See **Drug Interactions.**)

Cough: Presumably due to the inhibition of the degradation of endogenous bradykinin, persistent nonproductive cough has been reported with all ACE inhibitors, always resolving after discontinuation of therapy. ACE inhibitor-induced cough should be considered in the differential diagnosis of cough. In controlled trials with perindopril, cough was present in 12% of perindopril patients and 4.5% of patients given placebo.

Surgery/Anesthesia: In patients undergoing surgery or during anesthesia with agents that produce hypotension, ACEON® may block angiotensin II formation that would otherwise occur secondary to compensatory renin release. Hypotension attributable to this mechanism can be corrected by volume expansion.

Information for Patients: ***Angioedema:*** Angioedema, including laryngeal edema, can occur with ACE inhibitor therapy, especially following the first dose. Patients should be told to report immediately signs or symptoms suggesting angioedema (swelling of face, extremities, eyes, lips, tongue, hoarseness or difficulty in swallowing or breathing) and to take no more drug before consulting a physician.

Symptomatic Hypotension: As with any antihypertensive therapy, patients should be cautioned that lightheadedness can occur, especially during the first few days of therapy and that it should be reported promptly. Patients should be told that if fainting occurs, ACEON® should be discontinued and a physician consulted.

All patients should be cautioned that inadequate fluid intake or excessive perspiration, diarrhea or vomiting can lead to an excessive fall in blood pressure in association with ACE inhibitor therapy.

Hyperkalemia: Patients should be advised not to use potassium supplements or salt substitutes containing potassium without a physician's advice.

Neutropenia: Patients should be told to report promptly any indication of infection (*e.g.,* sore throat, fever) which could be a sign of neutropenia.

Pregnancy: Female patients of childbearing age should be told about the consequences of second and third trimester exposure to ACE inhibitors, and they should also be told that these consequences do not appear to have resulted from intrauterine ACE-inhibitor exposure that has been limited to the first trimester. These patients should be asked to report pregnancies to their physicians as soon as possible.

Drug Interactions: ***Diuretics:*** Patients on diuretics, and especially those started recently, may occasionally experience an excessive reduction of blood pressure after initiation of ACEON® therapy. The possibility of hypotensive effects can be minimized by either discontinuing the diuretic or increasing the salt intake prior to initiation of treatment with perindopril. If diuretics cannot be interrupted, close medical supervision should be provided with the first dose of ACEON®, for at least two hours and until blood pressure has stabilized for another hour. (See **WARNINGS** and **DOSAGE AND ADMINISTRATION.**)

The rate and extent of perindopril absorption and elimination are not affected by concomitant diuretics. The bioavailability of perindoprilat was reduced by diuretics, however, and this was associated with a decrease in plasma ACE inhibition.

Potassium Supplements and Potassium-Sparing Diuretics: ACEON® may increase serum potassium because of its potential to decrease aldosterone production. Use of potassium-sparing diuretics (spironolactone, amiloride, triamterene and others), potassium supplements or other drugs capable of increasing serum potassium (indomethacin, heparin, cyclosporine and others) can increase the risk of hyperkalemia. Therefore, if concomitant use of such agents is indicated, they should be given with caution and the patient's serum potassium should be monitored frequently.

Lithium: Increased serum lithium and symptoms of lithium toxicity have been reported in patients receiving concomitant lithium and ACE inhibitor therapy. These drugs should be coadministered with caution and frequent monitoring of serum lithium concentration is recommended. Use of a diuretic may further increase the risk of lithium toxicity.

Digoxin: A controlled pharmacokinetic study has shown no effect on plasma digoxin concentrations when coadministered with ACEON®, but an effect of digoxin on the plasma concentration of perindopril/perindoprilat has not been excluded.

Gentamicin: Animal data have suggested the possibility of interaction between perindopril and gentamicin. However, this has not been investigated in human studies. Coadministration of both drugs should proceed with caution.

Food Interaction: Oral administration of ACEON® with food does not significantly lower the rate or extent of perindopril absorption relative to the fasted state. However, the extent of biotransformation of perindopril to the active metabolite, perindoprilat, is reduced approximately 43%, resulting in a reduction in the plasma ACE inhibition curve of approximately 20%, probably clinically insignificant. In clinical trials, perindopril was generally administered in a non-fasting state.

Carcinogenesis, Mutagenesis, Impairment of Fertility: ***Carcinogenesis:*** No evidence of carcinogenic effect was observed in studies in rats and mice when perindopril was administered at dosages up to 20 times (mg/kg) or 2 to 4 times (mg/m^2) the maximum proposed clinical doses (16 mg/day) for 104 weeks.

Mutagenesis: No genotoxic potential was detected for ACEON®, perindoprilat and other metabolites in various *in vitro* and *in vivo* investigations, including the Ames test, the *Saccharomyces cerevisiae* D4 test, cultured human lymphocytes, TK ± mouse lymphoma assay, mouse and rat micronucleus tests and Chinese hamster bone marrow assay.

Impairment of Fertility: There was no meaningful effect on reproductive performance or fertility in the rat given up to 30 times (mg/kg) or 6 times (mg/m^2) the proposed maximum clinical dosage of ACEON® during the period of spermatogenesis in males or oogenesis and gestation in females.

Pregnancy: Pregnancy Categories C (first trimester) and D (second and third trimesters). (See **WARNINGS: Fetal/Neonatal Morbidity and Mortality.**)

Nursing Mothers: Milk of lactating rats contained radioactivity following administration ^{14}C-perindopril. It is not known whether perindopril is secreted in human milk. Because many drugs are secreted in human milk, caution should be exercised when ACEON® is given to nursing mothers.

Pediatric Use: Safety and effectiveness of ACEON® in pediatric patients have not been established.

Geriatric Use: The mean blood pressure effect of perindopril was somewhat smaller in patients over 60 than in younger patients, although the difference was not significant. Plasma concentrations of both perindopril and perindoprilat were increased in elderly patients compared to concentrations in younger patients. No adverse effects were clearly increased in older patients with the exception of dizziness and possibly rash. Experience with ACEON® in elderly patients at daily doses exceeding 8 mg is limited.

ADVERSE REACTIONS

ACEON® (perindopril erbumine) has been evaluated for safety in approximately 3,400 patients with hypertension in U.S. and foreign clinical trials. ACEON® was in general well-tolerated in the patient populations studied, the side effects were usually mild and transient. Although dizziness was reported more frequently in placebo patients (8.5%) than in perindopril patients (8.2%), the incidence appeared to increase with an increase in perindopril dose.

The data presented here are based on results from the 1,417 ACEON®-treated patients who participated in the U.S. clinical trials. Over 220 of these patients were treated with ACEON® for at least one year.

In placebo-controlled U.S. clinical trials, the incidence of premature discontinuation of therapy due to adverse events was 6.5% in patients treated with ACEON® and 6.7% in patients treated with placebo. The most common causes were cough, headache, asthenia and dizziness.

Among 1,012 patients in placebo-controlled U.S. trials, the overall frequency of reported adverse events was similar in patients treated with ACEON® and in those treated with placebo (approximately 75% in each group). Adverse events that occurred in 1% or greater of the patients and that were more common for perindopril than placebo by at least 1% (regardless of whether they were felt to be related to study drug) are shown in the first two columns below. Of these adverse events, those considered possibly or probably related to study drug are shown in the last two columns.
[See table above]

FREQUENCY OF ADVERSE EVENTS (%)

	All Adverse Events		Possibly—or Probably—Related Adverse Events	
	Perindopril n=789	Placebo n=223	Perindopril n=789	Placebo n=223
Cough	12.0	4.5	6.0	1.8
Back Pain	5.8	3.1	0.0	0.0
Sinusitis	5.2	3.6	0.6	0.0
Viral Infection	3.4	1.6	0.3	0.0
Upper Extremity Pain	2.8	1.4	0.2	0.0
Hypertonia	2.7	1.4	0.2	0.0
Dyspepsia	1.9	0.9	0.3	0.0
Fever	1.5	0.5	0.3	0.0
Proteinuria	1.5	0.5	1.0	0.5
Ear Infection	1.3	0.0	0.0	0.0
Palpitation	1.1	0.0	0.9	0.0

Of these, cough was the reason for withdrawal in 1.3% of perindopril and 0.4% of placebo patients. While dizziness was not reported more frequently in the perindopril group (8.2%) than in the placebo group (8.5%), it was clearly increased with dose, suggesting a causal relationship with perindopril. Other commonly reported complaints (1% or greater), regardless of causality, include: headache (23.8%), upper respiratory infection (8.6%), asthenia (7.9%), rhinitis (4.8%), low extremity pain (4.7%), diarrhea (4.3%), edema (3.9%), pharyngitis (3.3%), urinary tract infection (2.8%), abdominal pain (2.7%), sleep disorder (2.5%), chest pain (2.4%), injury, paresthesia, nausea, rash (each 2.3%), seasonal allergy, depression (each 2.0%), abnormal ECG (1.8%), ALT increase (1.7%), tinnitus, vomiting (each 1.5%), neck pain, male sexual dysfunction (each 1.4%), triglyceride increase, somnolence (each 1.3%), joint pain, nervousness, myalgia, menstrual disorder (each 1.1%), flatulence and arthritis (each 1.0%), but none of those was more frequent by at least 1% on perindopril than on placebo. Depending on the specific adverse event, approximately 30 to 70% of the common complaints were considered possibly or probably related to treatment.

Below is a list (by body system) of adverse experiences reported in 0.3 to 1% of patients in U.S. placebo-controlled studies without regard to attribution to therapy. Less frequent but medically important adverse events are also included; the incidence of these events is given in parentheses.

Body as a Whole: malaise, pain, cold/hot sensation, chills, fluid retention, orthostatic symptoms, anaphylactic reaction, facial edema, angioedema (0.1%).

Gastrointestinal: constipation, dry mouth, dry mucous membrane, appetite increased, gastroenteritis.

Respiratory: posterior nasal drip, bronchitis, rhinorrhea, throat disorder, dyspnea, sneezing, epistaxis, hoarseness, pulmonary fibrosis (<0.1%).

Urogenital: vaginitis, kidney stone, flank pain, urinary frequency, urinary retention.

Cardiovascular: hypotension, ventricular extrasystole, myocardial infarction, vasodilation, syncope, abnormal conduction, heart murmur, orthostatic hypotension.

Endocrine: gout.

Hematology: hematoma, ecchymosis.

Musculoskeletal: arthralgia, myalgia.

CNS: migraine, amnesia, vertigo, cerebral vascular accident (0.2%).

Psychiatric: anxiety, psychosexual disorder.

Dermatology: sweating, skin infection, tinea, pruritus, dry skin, erythema, fever blisters, purpura (0.1%).

Special Senses: conjunctivitis, earache.

Laboratory: potassium decrease, uric acid increase, alkaline phosphatase increase, cholesterol increase, AST increase, creatinine increase, hematuria, glucose increase.

When ACEON® was given concomitantly with thiazide diuretics, adverse events were generally reported at the same rate as those for ACEON® alone, except for a higher incidence of abnormal laboratory findings known to be related to treatment with thiazide diuretics alone (*e.g.*, increases in serum uric acid, triglycerides and cholesterol and decreases in serum potassium).

Potential Adverse Effects Reported with ACE Inhibitors: Other medically important adverse effects reported with other available ACE inhibitors include: cardiac arrest, eosinophilic pneumonitis, neutropenia/agranulocytosis, pancytopenia, anemia (including hemolytic and aplastic), thrombocytopenia, acute renal failure, nephritis, hepatic failure, jaundice (hepatocellular or cholestatic), symptomatic hyponatremia, bullous pemphigus, exfoliative dermatitis and a syndrome which may include: arthralgia/arthritis, vasculitis, serositis, myalgia, fever, rash or other dermatologic manifestations, a positive ANA, leukocytosis, eosinophilia or an elevated ESR. Many of these adverse effects have also been reported for perindopril.

Fetal/Neonatal Morbidity and Mortality: See **WARNINGS: Fetal/Neonatal Morbidity and Mortality.**

Clinical Laboratory Test Findings: Hematology, clinical chemistry and urinalysis parameters have been evaluated in U.S. placebo-controlled trials. In general, there were no clinically significant trends in laboratory test findings.

Hyperkalemia: In clinical trials, 1.4% of the patients receiving ACEON® and 2.3% of the patients receiving placebo showed serum potassium levels greater than 5.7 mEq/L. (See **PRECAUTIONS.**)

BUN/Serum Creatinine Elevations: Elevations, usually transient and minor, of BUN and serum creatinine have been observed. In placebo-controlled clinical trials, the proportion of patients experiencing increases in serum creatinine were similar in the ACEON® and placebo treatment groups. Rapid reduction of long-standing or markedly elevated blood pressure by any antihypertensive therapy can result in decreases in the glomerular filtration rate and, in turn, lead to increases in BUN or serum creatinine. (See **PRECAUTIONS.**)

Hematology: Small decreases in hemoglobin and hematocrit occur frequently in hypertensive patients treated with ACEON®, but are rarely of clinical importance. In controlled clinical trials, no patient was discontinued from therapy due to the development of anemia. Leukopenia (including neutropenia) was observed in 0.1% of patients in U.S. clinical trials (See **WARNINGS.**)

Liver Function Tests: Elevations in ALT (1.6% ACEON® vs 0.9% placebo) and AST (0.5% ACEON® vs 0.4% placebo) have been observed in U.S. placebo-controlled clinical trials. The elevations were generally mild and transient and resolved after discontinuation of therapy.

OVERDOSAGE

In animals, doses of perindopril up to 2500 mg/kg in mice, 3000 mg/kg in rats and 1600 mg/kg in dogs were non-lethal. Past experiences were scant but suggested that overdosage with other ACE inhibitors was also fairly well tolerated by humans. The most likely manifestation is hypotension, and treatment should be symptomatic and supportive. Therapy with the ACE inhibitor should be discontinued, and the patient should be observed. Dehydration, electrolyte imbalance and hypotension should be treated by established procedures.

However, of the reported cases of perindopril overdosage, one (dosage unknown) required assisted ventilation and the other developed hypothermia, circulatory arrest and died following ingestion of up to 180 mg of perindopril. The intervention for perindopril overdose may require vigorous support (see below).

Laboratory determinations of serum levels of perindopril and its metabolites are not widely available, and such determinations have, in any event, no established role in the management of perindopril overdose.

No data are available to suggest physiological maneuvers (*e.g.*, maneuvers to change the pH of the urine) that might accelerate elimination of perindopril and its metabolites. Perindopril can be removed by hemodialysis, with clearance of 52 mL/min for perindopril and 67 mL/min for perindoprilat.

Angiotensin II could presumably serve as a specific antagonist-antidote in the settling of perindopril overdose, but angiotensin II is essentially unavailable outside of scattered research facilities. Because the hypotensive effect of perindopril is achieved through vasodilation and effective hypovolemia, it is reasonable to treat perindopril overdose by infusion of normal saline solution.

DOSAGE AND ADMINISTRATION

Use in Uncomplicated Hypertensive Patients: In patients with essential hypertension, the recommended initial dose is 4 mg once a day. The dosage may be titrated upward until blood pressure, when measured just before the next dose, is controlled or to a maximum of 16 mg per day. The usual maintenance dose range is 4 to 8 mg administered as a single daily dose. ACEON® may also be administered in two divided doses. When once-daily dosing was compared to twice-daily dosing in clinical studies, the B.I.D. regimen was generally slightly superior, but not by more than about 0.5 to 1.0 mm Hg.

Use in the Elderly Patients: As in younger patients, the recommended initial dosages of ACEON® for the elderly (>65 years) is 4 mg daily in one or in two divided doses. The daily dosage may be titrated upward until blood pressure, when measured just before the next dose, is controlled, but experience with ACEON® is limited in the elderly at doses exceeding 8 mg. Dosages above 8 mg should be administered with caution and under close medical supervision. (See **PRECAUTIONS: Geriatric Use.**)

Use in Concomitant Diuretics: If blood pressure is not adequately controlled with perindopril alone, a diuretic may be added. In patients currently being treated with a diuretic, symptomatic hypotension occasionally can occur following the initial dose of perindopril. To reduce likelihood of such reaction, the diuretic should, if possible, be discontinued 2 to 3 days prior to beginning of ACEON® therapy. (See **WARNINGS.**) Then, if blood pressure is not controlled with ACEON® alone, the diuretic should be resumed.

If the diuretic cannot be discontinued, an initial dose of 2 to 4 mg daily in one or in two divided doses should be used with careful medical supervision for several hours and until blood pressure has stabilized. The dosage should then be titrated as described above. (See **WARNINGS** and **PRECAUTIONS: Drug Interactions.**)

Use in Patients with Impaired Renal Function: Kinetic data indicate that perindoprilat elimination is decreased in renally impaired patients, with a marked increase in accumulation when creatinine clearance drops below 30 mL/min. In such patients (creatinine clearance <30 mL/min), safety and efficacy of ACEON® have not been established. For patients with lesser degrees of impairment (creatinine clearance above 30 mL/min), the initial dosage should be 2 mg/day and dosage should not exceed 8 mg/day due to limited clinical experience. During dialysis, perindopril is removed with the same clearance as in patients with normal renal function.

HOW SUPPLIED

Tablets 2 mg: Scored one side, white, oblong (debossed "ACEON 2" on one side and debossed with "SLV" on both sides of score on the other side)

Bottles of 100 .... NDC 0032-1101-01

Tablets 4 mg: Scored one side, pink, oblong (debossed "ACEON 4" on one side and debossed with "SLV" on both sides of score on the other side)

Bottles of 100 .... NDC 0032-1102-01

Tablets 8 mg: Scored one side, salmon-colored, oblong (debossed "ACEON 8" on one side and debossed with "SLV" on both sides of score on the other side)

Bottles of 100 .... NDC 0032-1103-01

Storage Conditions: Store at controlled room temperature 20 to 25°C (68 to 77°F) [see USP]. Protect from moisture.

Rx only

Keep out of the reach of children.

Manufactured by:
RHÔNE-POULENC RORER PHARMACEUTICALS INC.
Manati, Puerto Rico 00674

Marketed by:
Solvay Pharmaceuticals, Inc.
Marietta, GA 30062

9605/9594 2E Rev 7/99

Shown in Product Identification Guide, page 338

CORTENEMA® ℞

(Hydrocortisone Retention Enema)
100 mg/60 mL
Disposable Unit for Rectal Use Only

DESCRIPTION

Each disposable unit (60 mL) contains:
Hydrocortisone, 100 mg in an aqueous solution containing carbomer 934P, polysorbate 80, purified water, sodium hydroxide and methylparaben, 0.18% as a preservative.

CORTENEMA® is a convenient disposable single-dose hydrocortisone enema designed for ease of self-administration. Hydrocortisone is a naturally occurring glucocorticoid (adrenal corticosteroid), similar to its acetate and sodium hemisuccinate derivatives, is partially absorbed following rectal administration. Absorption studies in ulcerative colitis patients have shown up to 50% absorption of hydrocortisone administered as CORTENEMA® and up to 30% of hydrocortisone acetate administered in an identical vehicle.

ACTIONS

CORTENEMA® provides the potent anti-inflammatory effect of hydrocortisone. Because this drug is absorbed from the colon, it acts both topically and systemically. Although rectal hydrocortisone, used as recommended for CORTENEMA®, has a low incidence of reported adverse reactions, prolonged use presumably may cause systemic reactions associated with oral dosage forms.

INDICATIONS AND USAGE

CORTENEMA® is indicated as adjunctive therapy in the treatment of ulcerative colitis, especially distal forms, including ulcerative proctitis, ulcerative proctosigmoiditis, and left-sided ulcerative colitis. It has proved useful also in some cases involving the transverse and ascending colons.

CONTRAINDICATIONS

Systemic fungal infections; and ileocolostomy during the immediate or early post-operative period.

WARNINGS

In severe ulcerative colitis, it is hazardous to delay needed surgery while awaiting response to medical treatment.

Continued on next page

Cortenema—Cont.

Damage to the rectal wall can result from careless or improper insertion of an enema tip.
In patients on corticosteroid therapy subjected to unusual stress, increased dosage of rapidly acting corticosteroids before, during, and after the stressful situation is indicated.
Corticosteroids may mask some signs of infection, and new infections may appear during their use. There may be decreased resistance and inability to localize infection when corticosteroids are used.
Prolonged use of corticosteroids may produce posterior subcapsular cataracts, glaucoma with possible damage to the optic nerves, and may enhance the establishment of secondary ocular infections due to fungi or viruses.
Usage in pregnancy: Since adequate human reproduction studies have not been done with corticosteroids, the use of these drugs in pregnancy, nursing mothers or women of childbearing potential requires that the possible benefits of the drug be weighed against the potential hazards to the mother and embryo or fetus. Neonates born of mothers who have received substantial doses of corticosteroids during pregnancy should be carefully observed for signs of hypoadrenalism.
Average and large doses of hydrocortisone or cortisone can cause elevation of blood pressure, salt and water retention, and increased excretion of potassium. These effects are less likely to occur with the synthetic derivatives except when used in large doses. Dietary salt restriction and potassium supplementation may be necessary. All corticosteroids increase calcium excretion.
While on corticosteroid therapy patients should not be vaccinated against smallpox. Other immunization procedures should not be undertaken in patients who are on corticosteroids, especially on high dose, because of possible hazards of neurological complications and a lack of antibody response.
If corticosteroids are indicated in patients with latent tuberculosis or tuberculin reactivity, close observation is necessary as reactivation of the disease may occur. During prolonged corticosteroid therapy, these patients should receive chemoprophylaxis.

PRECAUTIONS

CORTENEMA® hydrocortisone retention enema should be used with caution where there is a probability of impending perforation, abscess or other pyogenic infection; fresh intestinal anastomoses; obstruction; or extensive fistulas and sinus tracts. Use with caution in presence of active or latent peptic ulcer; diverticulitis; renal insufficiency; hypertension; osteoporosis; and myasthenia gravis.
Steroid therapy might impair prognosis in surgery by increasing the hazard of infection. If infection is suspected, appropriate antibiotic therapy must be administered, usually in larger than ordinary doses.
Drug-induced secondary adrenocortical insufficiency may occur with prolonged CORTENEMA® therapy. This is minimized by gradual reduction of dosage. This type of relative insufficiency may persist for months after discontinuation of therapy; therefore, in any situation of stress occurring during that period, hormone therapy should be reinstituted. Since mineralocorticoid secretion may be impaired, salt and/or a mineralocorticoid should be administered concurrently.
There is an enhanced effect of corticosteroids on patients with hypothyroidism and in those with cirrhosis.
Corticosteroid should be used cautiously in patients with ocular herpes simplex because of possible corneal perforation.
The lowest possible dose of corticosteroid should be used to control the conditions under treatment, and when reduction in dosage is possible, the reduction should be gradual.
Psychic derangement may appear when corticosteroids are used, ranging from euphoria, insomnia, mood swings, personality changes, and severe depression, to frank psychotic manifestations. Also, existing emotional instability or psychotic tendencies may be aggravated by corticosteroids.
Aspirin should be used cautiously in conjunction with corticosteroids in hypoprothrombinemia.
Pediatric Use
Safety and effectiveness in pediatric patients have not been established.
Growth and development of pediatric patients on prolonged corticosteroid therapy should be carefully observed.

ADVERSE REACTIONS

Local pain or burning, and rectal bleeding attributed to CORTENEMA® have been reported rarely. Apparent exacerbations or sensitivity reactions also occur rarely. The following adverse reactions should be kept in mind whenever corticosteroids are given by rectal administration.
Fluid and Electrolyte Disturbances: Sodium retention; fluid retention; congestive heart failure in susceptible patients; potassium loss; hypokalemic alkalosis; hypertension. **Musculoskeletal:** Muscle weakness; steroid myopathy; loss of muscle mass; osteoporosis; vertebral compression fractures; asceptic necrosis of femoral and humeral heads; pathologic fracture of long bones. **Gastrointestinal:** Peptic ulcer with possible perforation and hemorrhage; pancreatitis; abdominal distention; ulcerative esophagitis. **Dermatologic:** Impaired wound healing; thin fragile skin; petechiae and ecchymoses; facial erythema; increased sweating; may suppress reactions to skin tests. **Neurological:** Convulsions; increased intracranial pressure with papilledema (pseudotumor cerebri) usually after treatment; vertigo; headache. **Endocrine:** Menstrual irregularities; development of Cushingoid state; suppression of growth in pediatric patients; secondary adrenocortical and pituitary unresponsiveness, particularly in times of stress, as in trauma, surgery or illness; decreased carbohydrate tolerance; manifestations of latent diabetes requirements for insulin or oral hypoglycemic agents in diabetics. **Ophthalmic:** Posterior subcapsular cataracts; increased intraocular pressure; glaucoma; exophthalmos. **Metabolic:** Negative nitrogen balance due to protein catabolism.

DOSAGE AND ADMINISTRATION

The use of CORTENEMA® hydrocortisone retention enema is predicated upon the concomitant use of modern supportive measures such as rational dietary control, sedatives, antidiarrheal agents, antibacterial therapy, blood replacement if necessary, etc.
The usual course of therapy is one CORTENEMA® nightly for 21 days, or until the patient comes into remission both clinically and proctologically. Clinical symptoms usually subside promptly within 3 to 5 days. Improvement in the appearance of the mucosa, as seen by sigmoidoscopic examination, may lag somewhat behind clinical improvement. Difficult cases may require as long as 2 or 3 months of CORTENEMA® treatment. Where the course of therapy extends beyond 21 days, CORTENEMA® should be discontinued gradually by reducing administration to every other night for 2 or 3 weeks.
If clinical or proctologic improvement fails to occur within 2 or 3 weeks after starting CORTENEMA®, discontinue its use.
Symptomatic improvement, evidenced by decreased diarrhea and bleeding; weight gain; improved appetite; lessened fever; and decreased leukocytosis, may be misleading and should not be used as the sole criterion in judging efficacy. Sigmoidoscopic examination and X-ray visualization are essential for adequate monitoring of ulcerative colitis. Biopsy is useful for differential diagnosis.
Patient instructions for administering CORTENEMA® are enclosed in each box of seven units. We recommend that the patient lie on his left side during administration and for 30 minutes thereafter, so that the fluid will distribute throughout the left colon. Every effort should be made to retain the enema for at least an hour and preferably, all night. This may be facilitated by prior sedation and/or antidiarrheal medication, especially early in therapy, when the urge to evacuate is great.

HOW SUPPLIED

CORTENEMA®, hydrocortisone 100 mg retention enema, is supplied as disposable single-dose bottles with lubricated rectal applicator tips, in boxes of seven × 60 mL (NDC 0032-1904-82) and boxes of one × 60 mL (NDC 0032-1904-73).
Store at controlled room temperature, 15°–30°C (59°–86°F).
Rx Only

0638
7E Rev 2/98

Solvay Pharmaceuticals
Marietta, GA 30062

CREON® 5 ℞
CREON® 10
CREON® 20
MINIMICROSPHERES®
(Pancrelipase Delayed-release Capsules, USP)

PRESCRIBING INFORMATION

DESCRIPTION

CREON® 5, CREON® 10, and CREON® 20 Capsules are orally administered and contain delayed-release MINIMICROSPHERES® of pancrelipase, which is of porcine pancreatic origin. Each CREON 5 Capsule contains lipase 5,000 USP Units, protease 18,750 USP Units and amylase 16,600 USP Units. Each CREON 10 Capsule contains lipase 10,000 USP Units, protease 37,500 USP Units and amylase 33,200 USP Units. Each CREON 20 Capsule contains lipase 20,000 USP Units, protease 75,000 USP Units and amylase 66,400 USP Units.
Inactive ingredients include dibutyl phthalate, dimethicone, hydroxypropylmethylcellulose phthalate, light mineral oil and polyethylene glycol. The capsule shells contain gelatin, red iron oxide, titanium dioxide, yellow iron oxide. The CREON 5 capsule shell contains FD & C blue No. 2. In addition, the CREON 10 capsule shell contains black iron oxide and the CREON® 5, CREON 10, and CREON 20 Capsules imprinting ink contains dimethicone, 2-ethoxyethanol, shellac, soya lecithin and titanium dioxide.

CLINICAL PHARMACOLOGY

The pancreatic enzymes in CREON 5, CREON 10, and CREON 20 Capsules are enteric-coated to resist gastric destruction or inactivation. The pancreatic enzymes catalyze the hydrolysis of fats to glycerol and fatty acids, protein into proteoses and derived substances and starch into dextrins and short chain sugars.

INDICATIONS

CREON 5, CREON 10, and CREON 20 Capsules are indicated for patients with pancreatic exocrine insufficiency as is often associated with:
- cystic fibrosis
- chronic pancreatitis
- post-pancreatectomy
- post-gastrointestinal bypass surgery (e.g., Billroth II gastroenterostomy)
- ductal obstruction from neoplasm (e.g., of the pancreas or common bile duct)

CONTRAINDICATIONS

CREON 5, CREON 10, and CREON 20 Capsules are contraindicated in the early stages of acute pancreatitis or in patients who are known to be hypersensitive to pork protein.

WARNINGS

Should symptoms of hypersensitivity appear, discontinue medication and initiate symptomatic and supportive therapy if necessary.
Strictures in the ileo-cecal region and/or ascending colon have been reported in cystic fibrosis patients treated with high doses of high-potency pancreatic enzyme supplements containing 20,000 or greater USP units of lipase per capsule. The underlying mechanism is unknown, but caution should be exercised when doses in excess of 6,000 USP units per kg per meal fail to resolve symptoms, especially in patients with a history of intestinal complications such as meconium ileus equivalent, short bowel syndrome, surgery or Crohn's disease. If symptoms suggestive of gastrointestinal obstruction occur, the possibility of bowel stricture should be investigated including evaluation of pancreatic enzyme therapy.

PRECAUTIONS

CREON 5, CREON 10, and CREON 20 Capsules MINIMICROSPHERES® SHOULD NOT BE CRUSHED OR CHEWED or placed on foods having a pH greater than 5.5. These can dissolve the protective enteric coating resulting in early release of enzymes, irritation of oral mucosa, and/or loss of enzyme activity.
Information for Patients: CREON 5, CREON 10, and CREON 20 Capsules are a pancreatic enzyme product prescribed to promote improved digestion of foods, especially fat. The prescribed dosage should be taken with each meal and snack or as directed by the physician. The capsules can be swallowed whole, or the contents poured on soft, bland food. Care should be taken to avoid chewing or crushing of the capsule contents, which can result in early release of enzymes, irritation of oral mucosa, and/or loss of enzyme activity. Patients should maintain adequate fluid intake. The prescribed dose range should not be exceeded without calling your doctor.
The most common adverse reactions involve the stomach and intestine including diarrhea, nausea, vomiting, bloating, constipation, stomach cramps or pain. If these symptoms are persistent, contact your doctor.
Carcinogenesis, Mutagenesis, Impairment of Fertility: Long-term studies in animals have not been performed to evaluate carcinogenic potential.
Pregnancy, Category C: Animal reproduction studies have not been conducted with pancrelipase. It is also not known whether pancrelipase can cause fetal harm when administered to a pregnant woman or can affect reproduction capacity. CREON 5, CREON 10, and CREON 20 Capsules should be given to a pregnant woman only if clearly needed.
Nursing Mothers: It is not known whether this drug is excreted in human milk. Because many drugs are excreted in human milk, caution should be exercised when CREON 5, CREON 10, and CREON 20 Capsules are administered to a nursing mother.

ADVERSE REACTIONS

The most frequently reported adverse reactions to pancreatic enzyme-containing products are gastrointestinal in nature which may include nausea, vomiting, bloating, cramping, constipation or diarrhea. Less frequently, allergic-type reactions have also been observed. Very high doses of pancreatin have been associated with hyperuricosuria and hyperuricemia.

DOSAGE AND ADMINISTRATION

Clinical experience should dictate initial starting dose. Doses should be taken during meals or snacks, not before or after. Do not take without food.
Adults and Children Over 6 Years Old:
CREON 5: Usual initial starting dosage is two to four CREON 5 Capsules per meal or snack.
CREON 10: Usual initial starting dosage is one to two CREON 10 Capsules per meal or snack.
CREON 20: Usual initial starting dosage is one CREON 20 capsule per meal or snack.
Children Under 6 Years Old:
CREON 5: The exact dosage of CREON 5 Capsules should be selected based on clinical experience for this age group. Patients can be started on one to two capsules per meal or snack.
CREON 10: Usual initial starting dosage is up to one CREON 10 Capsule per meal or snack.
CREON 20: The exact dosage of CREON 20 Capsules should be selected based on clinical experience for this age group.
For cystic fibrosis patients typical doses are 1,500–3,000 USP lipase units/kg/meal.
Dosage should be adjusted according to the severity of the disease, control of steatorrhea and maintenance of good nutritional status. Doses in excess of 6,000 USP lipase units/kg/meal are not recommended.
Dose increases, if required, should occur with careful monitoring of body weight and stool fat content. When changing strengths of pancreatic enzyme products, care should be

taken to maintain equivalent lipase units for each divided dosage.

It is important to ensure adequate hydration of patients at all times while taking pancreatic enzymes.

Where swallowing of capsules is difficult, the capsules may be carefully opened and the MINIMICROSPHERES® added to a small amount of soft food, with a pH less than 5.5. The soft food should be swallowed immediately without chewing and followed with a glass of water or juice to insure swallowing.

HOW SUPPLIED

CREON® 5 MINIMICROSPHERES® (Pancrelipase Delayed-release Capsules, USP) are available in a two-piece gelatin capsule (orange opaque top half, blue opaque bottom half) imprinted in white with "SOLVAY" and "1205". Each capsule contains tan-colored delayed-release MINIMICROSPHERES® of pancrelipase supplied in bottles of:

100 .... NDC 0032-1205-01
250 .... NDC 0032-1205-07

CREON® 10 MINIMICROSPHERES® (Pancrelipase Delayed-release Capsules, USP) are available in a two-piece gelatin capsule (brown opaque top half, natural transparent bottom half) imprinted in white with "SOLVAY" and "1210". Each capsule contains tan-colored delayed-release MINIMICROSPHERES® of pancrelipase supplied in bottles of:

100 .... NDC 0032-1210-01
250 .... NDC 0032-1210-07

CREON® 20 MINIMICROSPHERES® (Pancrelipase Delayed-release Capsules, USP) are available in a two-piece gelatin capsule (orange opaque top half, natural transparent bottom half) imprinted in white with "SOLVAY" and "1220". Each capsule contains tan-colored delayed release MINIMICROSPHERES® of pancrelipase supplied in bottles of:

100 .... NDC 0032-1220-01
250 .... NDC 0032-1220-07

CREON 5, CREON 10, and CREON 20 Capsules must be stored at 25°C (77°F); excursions permitted to 15°–30°C (59°–86°F). [see USP Controlled Room Temperature.] PROTECT FROM MOISTURE. DO NOT REFRIGERATE. Dispense in tight, light-resistant containers. For human consumption only.

Rx only

Manufactured By:
Solvay Pharmaceuticals GmbH
Hannover, Germany

Marketed by:
SOLVAY PHARMACEUTICALS, Inc.
Marietta, GA 30062
Rev 6/98

Shown in Product Identification Guide, page 338

ESTRATAB® ℞

(Esterified Estrogens Tablets, USP)
0.3 mg, 0.625 mg, 2.5 mg
Physician Labeling

1. **ESTROGENS HAVE BEEN REPORTED TO INCREASE THE RISK OF ENDOMETRIAL CARCINOMA IN POSTMENOPAUSAL WOMEN.**
   Close clinical surveillance of all women taking estrogens is important. Adequate diagnostic measures, including endometrial sampling when indicated, should be undertaken to rule out malignancy in all cases of undiagnosed persistent or recurring abnormal vaginal bleeding. There is no evidence that "natural" estrogens are more or less hazardous than "synthetic" estrogens at equi-estrogenic doses.
2. **ESTROGENS SHOULD NOT BE USED DURING PREGNANCY.**
   There is no indication for estrogen therapy during pregnancy or during the immediate postpartum period. Estrogens are ineffective for the prevention or treatment of threatened or habitual abortion. Estrogens are not indicated for the prevention of postpartum breast engorgement.
   Estrogen therapy during pregnancy is associated with an increased risk of congenital defects in the reproductive organs of the fetus, and possibly other birth defects. Studies of women who received diethylstilbestrol (DES) during pregnancy have shown that female offspring have an increased risk of vaginal adenosis, squamous-cell dysplasia of the uterine cervix, and clear cell vaginal cancer later in life; male offspring have an increased risk of urogenital abnormalities and possibly testicular cancer later in life. The 1985 DES Task Force concluded that use of DES during pregnancy is associated with a subsequent increased risk of breast cancer in the mothers, although a causal relationship is still unproven and the observed level of excess risk is similar to that for a number of other breast cancer risk factors.

DESCRIPTION

ESTRATAB® (Esterified Estrogens Tablets, USP)

Each blue, sugarcoated tablet contains 0.3 mg. Each yellow, sugarcoated tablet contains 0.625 mg. Each light purple, sugarcoated tablet contains 2.5 mg.

Table 1. Mean Percent Change From Baseline in Lumbar Spine (L1-L4) BMD

	Mean Percent Change in Lumbar Spine BMD 6 Mos.	12 Mos.	18 Mos.	24 Mos.
Placebo	-0.25	-1.04[a]	-1.65[a]	-1.97[a]
ESTRATAB® 0.3 mg	0.81[a,b]	1.32[a,b]	1.47[a,b]	1.42[a,b]
ESTRATAB® 0.625 mg	1.32[a,b]	2.17[a,b]	2.13[a,b]	2.29[a,b]
ESTRATAB® 1.25 mg	2.98[a,b]	3.69[a,b]	4.11[a,b]	4.36[a,b]

[a] $p < 0.05$ compared to baseline
[b] $p < 0.05$ compared to placebo

Table 2. Mean Percent Change From Baseline in Hip BMD

	Mean Percent Change in Hip BMD 6 Mos.	12 Mos.	18 Mos.	24 Mos.
Placebo	-0.06	-0.48	-0.48	-0.82
ESTRATAB® 0.3 mg	1.09[a,b]	1.21[a,b]	1.71[a,b]	1.59[a,b]
ESTRATAB® 0.625 mg	0.73	1.71[a,b]	2.25[a,b]	2.28[a,b]
ESTRATAB® 1.25 mg	1.46[a,b]	1.55[a,b]	1.72[a,b]	2.06[a,b]

[a] $p < 0.05$ compared to baseline
[b] $p < 0.05$ compared to placebo

ESTRATAB® Tablets for oral administration is a mixture of the sodium salts of the sulfate esters of the estrogenic substances, principally estrone, that are prepared synthetically from plant sterol precursors. Esterified Estrogens, USP contain not less than 75.0 percent and not more than 85.0 percent of sodium estrone sulfate, and not less than 6.0 percent and not more than 15.0 percent of sodium equilin sulfate, in such proportion that the total of these two components is not less than 90.0 percent.

Inactive Ingredients: Acacia, calcium carbonate, carnauba wax, carboxymethylcellulose sodium, citric acid, colloidal silicon dioxide, diacetylated monoglyceride, gelatin, anhydrous lactose, magnesium stearate, methylparaben, microcrystalline cellulose, pharmaceutical glaze, povidone, propylparaben, shellac, sodium benzoate, sodium bicarbonate, sorbic acid, sucrose, corn starch, talc, titanium dioxide and tribasic calcium phosphate. The 0.3 mg tablet coating contains FD&C Blue #1 Lake; the 0.625 mg tablet coating contains D&C Yellow #10 Lake, FD&C Yellow #6 Lake and FD&C Blue #2 Lake; and the 2.5 mg tablet coating contains FD&C Red #40 Lake and FD&C Blue #2 Lake. In addition, the tablet imprinting ink for the 0.3 mg and 0.625 mg tablets contains black iron oxide, FD&C Blue #2 Lake, FD&C Red #40 Lake and FD&C Yellow #6 Lake. The 2.5 mg imprinting ink contains Soya lecithin, dimethyl polysiloxane, pharmaceutical shellac and titanium dioxide.

ACTIONS/CLINICAL PHARMACOLOGY

Estrogen drug products act by regulating the transcription of a limited number of genes. Estrogens diffuse through cell membranes, distribute themselves throughout the cell, and bind to and activate the nuclear estrogen receptor, a DNA-binding protein which is found in estrogen-responsive tissues. The activated estrogen receptor binds to specific DNA sequences, or hormone response elements, which enhance the transcription of adjacent genes and in turn lead to the observed effects. Estrogen receptors have been identified in tissues of the reproductive tract, breast, pituitary, hypothalamus, liver, and bone of women.

Estrogens are important in the development and maintenance of the female reproductive system and secondary sex characteristics. By direct action, they cause growth and development of the uterus, Fallopian tubes, and vagina. With other hormones, such as pituitary hormones and progesterone, they cause enlargement of the breasts through promotion of ductal growth, stromal development, and the accretion of fat. Estrogens are intricately involved with other hormones, especially progesterone, in the processes of the ovulatory menstrual cycle and pregnancy, and affect the release of pituitary gonadotropins. They also contribute to the shaping of the skeleton, maintenance of tone and elasticity of urogenital structures, changes in epiphyses of the long bones that allow for the pubertal growth spurt and its termination, and pigmentation of the nipples and genitals.

Estrogens occur naturally in several forms. The primary source of estrogen in normally cycling adult women is the ovarian follicle, which secretes 70 to 500 micrograms of estradiol daily, depending on the phase of the menstrual cycle. This is converted primarily to estrone, which circulates in roughly equal proportion to estradiol, and to small amounts of estriol. After menopause, most endogenous estrogen is produced by conversion of androstenedione, secreted by the adrenal cortex, to estrone by peripheral tissues. Thus, estrone – – especially in its sulfate ester form – – is the most abundant circulating estrogen in postmenopausal women. Although circulating estrogens exist in a dynamic equilibrium of metabolic interconversions, estradiol is the principle intracellular human estrogen and is substantially more potent than estrone or estriol at the receptor.

Estrogens used in therapy are well absorbed through the skin, mucous membranes, and gastrointestinal tract. When applied for a local action, absorption is usually sufficient to cause systemic effects. When conjugated with aryl and alkyl groups for parenteral administration, the rate of absorption of oily preparations is slowed with a prolonged duration of action, such that a single intramuscular injection of estradiol valerate or estradiol cypionate is absorbed over several weeks.

Administered estrogens and their esters are handled within the body essentially the same as the endogenous hormones. Metabolic conversion of estrogens occurs primarily in the liver (first pass effect), but also at local target tissue sites. Complex metabolic processes result in a dynamic equilibrium of circulating conjugated and unconjugated estrogenic forms which are continually interconverted, especially between estrone and estradiol and between esterified and non-esterified forms. Although naturally-occurring estrogens circulate in the blood largely bound to sex hormone-binding globulin and albumin, only unbound estrogens enter target tissue cells. A significant proportion of the circulating estrogen exists as sulfate conjugates, especially estrone sulfate, which serves as a circulating reservoir for the formation of more active estrogenic species. A certain proportion of the estrogen is excreted into the bile and then reabsorbed from the intestine. During this enterohepatic recirculation, estrogens are desulfated and resulfated and undergo degradation through conversion to less active estrogens (estriol and other estrogens), oxidation to nonestrogenic substances (catecholestrogens, which interact with catecholamine metabolism, especially in the central nervous system), and conjugation with glucuronic acids (which are then rapidly excreted in the urine).

When given orally, naturally-occurring estrogens and their esters are extensively metabolized (first pass effect) and circulate primarily as estrone sulfate, with smaller amounts of other conjugated and unconjugated estrogenic species. This results in limited oral potency. By contrast, synthetic estrogens, such as ethinyl estradiol and the nonsteroidal estrogens, are degraded very slowly in the liver and other tissues, which results in their high intrinsic potency. Estrogen drug products administered by non-oral routes are not subject to first-pass metabolism, but also undergo significant hepatic uptake, metabolism, and enterohepatic recycling.

Clinical Studies

A two-year, double-blind, placebo-controlled, randomized study was conducted in 406 postmenopausal women to determine the efficacy of continuously administered ESTRATAB® Tablets (0.3 mg, 0.625 mg, and 1.25 mg), unopposed by a progestin, on the prevention of postmenopausal osteoporosis. Efficacy was evaluated by semi-annual determination of lumbar spine (L1-L4) BMD and hip BMD changes (DXA). The results (see Tables 1, 2 and Figures 1,2) of this study demonstrate that ESTRATAB® Tablets, at doses of 0.3 mg, 0.625 mg, and 1.25 mg, is effective in the prevention of postmenopausal osteoporosis. Compared to placebo, patients treated with ESTRATAB® Tablets had significant increases in lumbar BMD and hip BMD.

[See table 1 above]
[See table 2 above]
[See figure 2 at top of next column]

Figure 1. Percent Change From Baseline in Lumbar Spine (L1-L4) BMD Over 24 Months

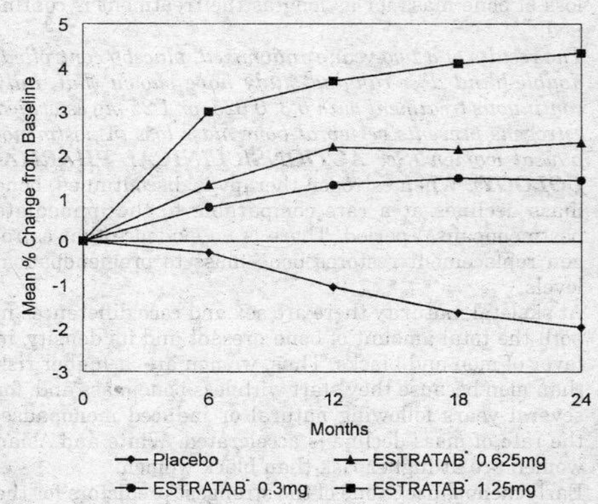

Continued on next page

Estratab—Cont.

Figure 2. Percent Change From Baseline in Hip BMD Over 24 Months

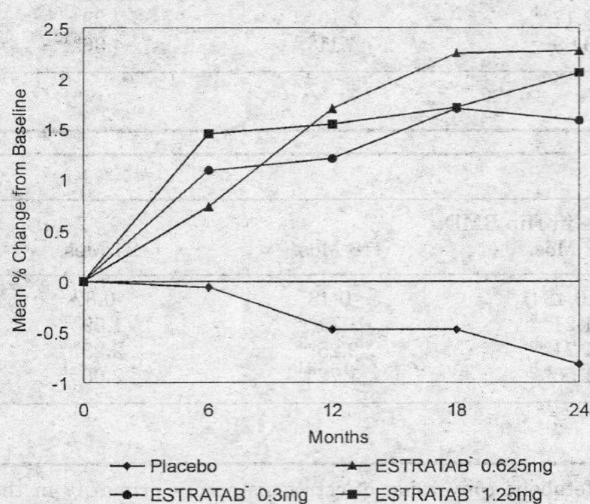

INFORMATION REGARDING ENDOMETRIAL EFFECTS. As shown in Table 3, only one case of endometrial hyperplasia occurred in the groups treated with placebo or unopposed 0.3-mg ESTRATAB® Tablets. The incidence of endometrial hyperplasia was significantly greater with unopposed ESTRATAB® Tablets in doses of 0.625 mg and 1.25 mg.
[See table above]

INFORMATION REGARDING LIPID EFFECTS. As shown in Table 4, ESTRATAB® Tablets increase HDL-Cholesterol and decrease LDL-Cholesterol. The following table summarizes mean percent changes from baseline values after 2 years of treatment.
[See table above]

Table 3. Incidence of Endometrial Hyperplasia After 1 and 2 Years

	Incidence of Hyperplasia				
		1 Year		2 Years	
	No. Pat.	N	%	N	%
Placebo	60	1	1.67	1	1.67
ESTRATAB® 0.3 mg	59	1	1.69	1	1.69
ESTRATAB® 0.625 mg	59	12	20.3[a,b]	17	28.8[a,b]
ESTRATAB® 1.25 mg	60	26	43.3[a,b]	32	53.3[a,b]

[a] $p < 0.05$ compared to baseline
[b] $p < 0.05$ compared to ESTRATAB® 0.3 mg

Table 4. Mean Percent Change From Baseline in Lipid Parameters After Two Years

	Lipid Parameters			
	HDL Cholesterol	LDL Cholesterol	Triglycerides	Total Cholesterol
Placebo	2.64	1.22	17.34[a]	1.98
ESTRATAB® 0.3 mg	5.59[a]	-4.62[a,b]	15.02[a]	-1.89
ESTRATAB® 0.625 mg	10.54[a,b]	-3.71	16.03[a]	0.09
ESTRATAB® 1.25 mg	12.31[a,b]	-14.71[a,b]	28.77[a]	-5.15[a,b]

[a] $p < 0.05$ compared to baseline
[b] $p < 0.05$ compared to placebo

INDICATIONS AND USAGE

ESTRATAB® Tablets are indicated in the:

1. Treatment of moderate to severe vasomotor symptoms associated with the menopause. (There is no adequate evidence that estrogens are effective for nervous symptoms or depression which might occur during menopause, and they should not be used to treat these conditions).
2. Treatment of vulval and vaginal atrophy.
3. Treatment of hypoestrogenism due to hypogonadism, castration, or primary ovarian failure.
4. Treatment of breast cancer (for palliation only) in appropriately selected women and men with metastatic disease.
5. Treatment of advanced androgen - dependent carcinoma of the prostate (for palliation only).
6. Prevention of osteoporosis.

Since estrogen administration is associated with risk as well as benefit, selection of patients should ideally be based on prospective identification of risk factors for developing osteoporosis. Unfortunately, there is no certain way to identify those women who will develop osteoporotic fractures. Most prospective studies of efficacy for this indication have been carried out in white menopausal women, without stratification by other risk factors, and tend to show a universally salutary effect on bone. Thus, patient selection must be individualized based on the balance of risks and benefits. A more favorable risk/benefit ratio exists in a hysterectomized woman because she has no risk of endometrial cancer (see Boxed Warning).

Estrogen replacement therapy reduces bone resorption and retards or halts postmenopausal bone loss. Case-control studies have shown an approximately 60 percent reduction in hip and wrist fractures in women whose estrogen replacement was begun within a few years of menopause. Studies also suggest that estrogen reduces the rate of vertebral fractures. Even when started as late as 6 years after menopause, estrogen prevents further loss of bone mass for as long as the treatment is continued.

The results of a two-year, randomized, placebo-controlled, double-blind dose-ranging study have shown that daily continuous treatment with 0.3, 0.625, or 1.25 mg esterified estrogens prevents vertebral bone mass loss in postmenopausal women (See ***ACTIONS/CLINICAL PHARMACOLOGY****).* When estrogen therapy is discontinued, bone mass declines at a rate comparable to the immediate postmenopausal period. There is no evidence that estrogen replacement restores bone mass to premenopausal levels.

At skeletal maturity there are sex and race differences in both the total amount of bone present and its density, in favor of men and blacks. Thus, women are at higher risk than men because they start with less bone mass and, for several years following natural or induced menopause, the rate of mass decline is accelerated. White and Asian women are at higher risk than black women.

Early menopause is one of the strongest predictors for the development of osteoporosis. In addition, other factors affecting the skeleton which are associated with osteoporosis include genetic factors (small build, family history), endocrine factors (nulliparity, thyrotoxicosis, hyperparathyroidism, Cushing's syndrome, hyperprolactinemia, Type I diabetes), lifestyle (cigarette smoking, alcohol abuse, sedentary exercise habits) and nutrition (below average body weight, dietary calcium intake).

The mainstays of prevention and management of osteoporosis are estrogen, an adequate lifetime calcium intake, and exercise. Postmenopausal women absorb dietary calcium less efficiently than premenopausal women and require an average of 1500 mg/day of elemental calcium to remain in neutral calcium balance. By comparison, premenopausal women require about 1000 mg/day and the average calcium intake in the USA is 400–600 mg/day. Therefore, when not contraindicated, calcium supplementation may be helpful.

Weight-bearing exercise and nutrition may be important adjuncts to the prevention and management of osteoporosis. Immobilization and prolonged bed rest produce rapid bone loss, while weight-bearing exercise has been shown both to reduce bone loss and to increase bone mass. The optimal type and amount of physical activity that would prevent osteoporosis have not been established. However, in two studies, an hour of walking and running exercises twice or three times weekly significantly increased lumbar spine bone mass.

CONTRAINDICATIONS

Estrogens should not be used in individuals with any of the following conditions:

1. Known or suspected pregnancy (See Boxed Warning). Estrogens may cause fetal harm when administered to a pregnant woman.
2. Known or suspected cancer of the breast except in appropriately selected patients being treated for metastatic disease.
3. Known or suspected estrogen-dependent neoplasia.
4. Undiagnosed abnormal genital bleeding.
5. Active thrombophlebitis or thromboembolic disorders.

WARNINGS

1. **Induction of malignant neoplasms**

Endometrial Cancer: The reported endometrial cancer risk among unopposed estrogen users is about 2- to 12-fold greater than in non-users, and appears dependent on duration of treatment and on estrogen dose. Most studies show no significant increased risk associated with use of estrogens for less than one year. The greatest risk appears associated with prolonged use – – with increased risks of 15- to 24-fold for five to ten years or more. In three studies, persistence of risk was demonstrated for 8 to over 15 years after cessation of estrogen treatment. In one study a significant decrease in the incidence of endometrial cancer occurred six months after estrogen withdrawal. Concurrent progestin therapy may offset this risk but the overall health impact in postmenopausal women is not known (see **PRECAUTIONS**).

Breast Cancer: While the majority of studies have not shown an increased risk of breast cancer in women who have ever used estrogen replacement therapy, some have reported a moderately increased risk (relative risks of 1.3–2.0) in those taking higher doses or those taking lower doses for prolonged periods of time, especially in excess of 10 years. Other studies have not shown this relationship.

Congenital lesions with malignant potential: Estrogen therapy during pregnancy is associated with an increased risk of fetal congenital reproductive tract disorders, and possibly other birth defects. Studies of women who received DES during pregnancy have shown that female offspring have an increased risk of vaginal adenosis, squamous cell dysplasia of the uterine cervix, and clear cell vaginal cancer later in life; male offspring have an increased risk of urogenital abnormalities and possibly testicular cancer later in life. Although some of these changes are benign, others are precursors of malignancy.

2. **Gallbladder disease**

Two studies have reported a 2- to 4-fold increase in the risk of gallbladder disease requiring surgery in women receiving postmenopausal estrogens.

3. **Cardiovascular disease**

Large doses of estrogen (5 mg conjugated estrogens per day), comparable to those used to treat cancer of the prostate and breast, have been shown in a large prospective clinical trial in men to increase the risks of nonfatal myocardial infarction, pulmonary embolism, and thrombophlebitis. These risks cannot necessarily be extrapolated from men to women. However, to avoid the theoretical cardiovascular risk caused by high estrogen doses, the dose for estrogen replacement therapy should not exceed the lowest effective dose.

4. **Elevated Blood Pressure**

Occasional blood pressure increases during estrogen replacement therapy have been attributed to idiosyncratic reactions to estrogens. More often, blood pressure has remained the same or has dropped. One study showed that postmenopausal estrogen users have higher blood pressure than nonusers. Two other studies showed slightly lower blood pressure among estrogen users compared to nonusers. Postmenopausal estrogen use does not increase the risk of stroke. Nonetheless, blood pressure should be monitored at regular intervals with estrogen use.

5. **Hypercalcemia**

Administration of estrogens may lead to severe hypercalcemia in patients with breast cancer and bone metastases. If this occurs, the drug should be stopped and appropriate measures taken to reduce the serum calcium level.

PRECAUTIONS

General

1. ***Addition of a progestin:*** Studies of the addition of a progestin for ten or more days of a cycle of estrogen administration have reported a lowered incidence of endometrial hyperplasia than would be induced by estrogen treatment alone. Morphological and biochemical studies of endometria suggest that 10 to 14 days of progestin are needed to provide maximal maturation of the endometrium and to reduce the likelihood of hyperplastic changes.

There are, however, possible risks which may be associated with the use of progestins in estrogen replacement regimens. These include:

(a) adverse effects on lipoprotein metabolism (lowering HDL and raising LDL) which could diminish the purported cardioprotective effects of estrogen therapy (see **PRECAUTIONS** below);
(b) impairment of glucose tolerance; and
(c) possible enhancement of mitotic activity in breast epithelial tissue, although few epidemiological data are available to address this point (see **PRECAUTIONS** below).

The choice of progestin, its dose, and its regimen may be important in minimizing these adverse effects, but these issues will require further study before they are clarified.

2. ***Cardiovascular risk:*** **A causal relationship between estrogen replacement therapy and reduction of cardiovascular disease in postmenopausal women has not been proven. Furthermore, the effect of added progestins on this putative benefit is not yet known.**

In recent years many published studies have suggested that there may be a cause-effect relationship between postmenopausal oral estrogen replacement therapy **without added progestins** and a decrease in cardiovascular disease in women. Although most of the observational studies which assessed this statistical association have reported a 20% to 50% reduction in coronary heart disease risk and associated mortality in estrogen takers, the following should be considered when interpreting these reports:

(a) Because only one of these studies was randomized and it was too small to yield statistically significant results, all relevant studies were subject to selection bias. Thus, the apparently reduced risk of coronary artery disease cannot be attributed with certainty to estrogen replacement therapy. It may instead have been caused by life-style and medical characteristics of the women studied with the result that healthier women were selected for estrogen therapy. In general, treated women were of higher socioeconomic and educational status, more slender, more physically active, more likely to have undergone surgical menopause, and less likely to have diabetes than the untreated women. Although some studies attempted to control for these selection factors, it is common for properly designed randomized trials to fail to confirm benefits suggested by less rigorous study designs. Thus, ongoing and future large-scale randomized trials may fail to confirm this apparent benefit.

(b) Current medical practice often includes the use of concomitant progestin therapy in women with intact uteri (see **PRECAUTIONS** and **WARNINGS**). While the effects of added progestins on the risk of ischemic heart disease are not known, all available progestins reverse at least some of the favorable effects of estrogens on HDL and LDL levels.

(c) While the effects of added progestins on the risk of breast cancer are also unknown, available epidemiological evidence suggests that progestins do not reduce, and may enhance, the moderately increased breast cancer incidence that has been reported with prolonged estrogen replacement therapy (see **WARNINGS** above).

Because relatively long-term use of estrogens by a woman with a uterus has been shown to induce endometrial cancer, physicians often recommend that women who are deemed candidates for hormone replacement should take progestins as well as estrogens. When considering prescribing concomitant estrogens and progestins for hormone replacement therapy, physicians and patients are advised to carefully weigh the potential benefits and risks of the added progestin. Large-scale randomized, placebo-controlled, prospective clinical trials are required to clarify these issues.

3. ***Physical Examination:*** A complete medical and family history should be taken prior to the initiation of any estrogen therapy. The pretreatment and periodic physical examinations should include special reference to blood pressure, breasts, abdomen, and pelvic organs, and should include a Papanicolaou smear. As a general rule, estrogen should not be prescribed for longer than one year without reexamining the patient.
4. ***Hypercoagulability:*** Some studies have shown that women taking estrogen replacement therapy have hypercoagulability, primarily related to decreased antithrombin activity. This effect appears dose- and duration-dependent and is less pronounced than that associated with oral contraceptive use. Also, postmenopausal women tend to have increased coagulation parameters at baseline compared to premenopausal women. There is some suggestion that low dose postmenopausal mestranol may increase the risk of thromboembolism, although the majority of studies (of primarily conjugated estrogen users) reports no such increase. There is insufficient information on hypercoagulability in women who have had previous thromboembolic disease.
5. ***Familial hyperlipoproteinemia:*** Estrogen therapy may be associated with massive elevations of plasma triglycerides leading to pancreatitis and other complications in patients with familial defects of lipoprotein metabolism.
6. ***Fluid retention:*** Because estrogen may cause some degree of fluid retention, conditions which might be exacerbated by this factor such as asthma, epilepsy, migraine, and cardiac or renal dysfunction, require careful observation.
7. ***Uterine bleeding and mastodynia:*** Certain patients may develop undesirable manifestations of estrogenic stimulation, such as abnormal uterine bleeding, and mastodynia.
8. ***Impaired liver function:*** Estrogens may be poorly metabolized in patients with impaired liver function and should be administered with caution.

Information for the Patient

See text of Patient Package Insert below which appears after the **HOW SUPPLIED** section.

Laboratory Tests

Estrogen administration should generally be guided by clinical response at the smallest dose, rather than laboratory monitoring, for relief of symptoms for those indications in which symptoms are observable. For prevention of osteoporosis, however, see **DOSAGE AND ADMINISTRATION** section.

Drug/Laboratory Test Interactions

1. Accelerated prothrombin time, partial thromboplastin time, and platelet aggregation time; increased platelet count; increased factors II, VII antigen, VIII antigen, VIII coagulant activity, IX, X, XII, VII-X complex, II-VII-X complex, and beta-thromboglobulin; decreased levels of anti-factor Xa and antithrombin III, decreased antithrombin III activity; increased levels of fibrinogen and fibrinogen activity; increased plasminogen antigen and activity.
2. Increased thyroid-binding globulin (TBG) leading to increased circulating total thyroid hormone, as measured by protein-bound iodine (PBI), T4 levels (by column or by radioimmunoassay) or T3 levels by radioimmunoassay. T3 resin uptake is decreased, reflecting the elevated TBG. Free T4 and T3 concentrations are unaltered.
3. Other binding proteins may be elevated in serum, i.e., corticosteroid binding globulin (CBG), sex hormone-binding globulin (SHBG), leading to increased circulating corticosteroids and sex steroids respectively. Free or biologically active hormone concentrations are unchanged. Other plasma proteins may be increased (angiotensinogen/renin substrate, alpha-1-antitrypsin, ceruloplasmin).
4. Increased plasma HDL and HDL-2 subfraction concentrations, reduced LDL cholesterol concentration, increased triglyceride levels.
5. Impaired glucose tolerance.
6. Reduced response to metyrapone test.
7. Reduced serum folate concentration.

Carcinogenesis, Mutagenesis, Impairment of Fertility

Long-term, continuous administration of natural and synthetic estrogens in certain animal species increases the frequency of carcinomas of the breast, uterus, cervix, vagina, testis and liver. See **CONTRAINDICATIONS** and **WARNINGS**.

Pregnancy Category X

Estrogens should not be used during pregnancy. See **CONTRAINDICATIONS** and Boxed Warning.

Nursing Mothers

As a general principle, the administration of any drug to nursing mothers should be done only when clearly necessary since many drugs are excreted in human milk. In addition, estrogen administration to nursing mothers has been shown to decrease the quantity and quality of the milk.

ADVERSE REACTIONS

The following additional adverse reactions have been reported with estrogen therapy (See **WARNINGS** regarding induction of neoplasia, adverse effects on the fetus, increased incidence of gallbladder disease, cardiovascular disease, elevated blood pressure, and hypercalcemia.)

1. **Genitourinary system:**
   Changes in vaginal bleeding pattern and abnormal withdrawal bleeding or flow.
   Breakthrough bleeding, spotting.
   Increase in size of uterine leiomyomata.
   Vaginal candidiasis.
   Change in amount of cervical secretion.
2. **Breasts:**
   Tenderness, enlargement.
3. **Gastrointestinal:**
   Nausea, vomiting.
   Abdominal cramps, bloating.
   Cholestatic jaundice.
   Increased incidence of gallbladder disease.
4. **Skin:**
   Chloasma or melasma which may persist when drug is discontinued.
   Erythema multiforme.
   Erythema nodosum.
   Hemorrhagic eruption.
   Loss of scalp hair.
   Hirsutism.
5. **Eyes:**
   Steepening of corneal curvature.
   Intolerance to contact lenses.
6. **CNS:**
   Headache, migraine, dizziness.
   Mental depression.
   Chorea
7. **Miscellaneous:**
   Increase or decrease in weight.
   Reduced carbohydrate tolerance.
   Aggravation of porphyria.
   Edema.
   Changes in libido.

OVERDOSAGE

Serious ill effects have not been reported following acute ingestion of large doses of estrogen-containing oral contraceptives by young children. Overdosage of estrogen may cause nausea and vomiting, and withdrawal bleeding may occur in females.

DOSAGE AND ADMINISTRATION

1. **Given cyclically for short term use only:**
   For treatment of moderate to severe *vasomotor* symptoms, atrophic vaginitis, or kraurosis vulvae associated with the menopause. The lowest dose that will control symptoms should be chosen and medication should be discontinued as promptly as possible. Administration should be cyclic (e.g., three weeks on and one week off). Attempts to discontinue or taper medication should be made at three to six month intervals.
   Usual dosage ranges:
   Vasomotor symptoms – 1.25 mg daily. If the patient has not menstruated within the last two months or more, cyclic administration is started arbitrarily. If the patient is menstruating, cyclic administration is started on day 5 of bleeding.
   Atrophic vaginitis and kraurosis vulvae – 0.3 mg to 1.25 mg or more daily, depending upon the tissue response of the individual patient. Administer cyclically.
2. **Given cyclically:** Female hypogonadism; female castration; primary ovarian failure.
   Usual dosage ranges:
   Female hypogonadism – 2.5 to 7.5 mg daily, in divided doses for 20 days, followed by a rest period of 10 days' duration. If bleeding does not occur by the end of this period, the same dosage schedule is repeated. The number of courses of estrogen therapy necessary to produce bleeding may vary depending on the responsiveness of the endometrium.
   If bleeding occurs before the end of the 10 day period, begin a 20 day estrogen-progestin cyclic regimen with ESTRATAB® (Esterified Estrogens Tablets, USP), 2.5 to 7.5 mg daily in divided doses, for 20 days. During the last five days of estrogen therapy, give an oral progestin. If bleeding occurs before this regimen is concluded, therapy is discontinued and may be resumed on the fifth day of bleeding.
   Female castration, and primary ovarian failure – 1.25 mg daily, cyclically. Adjust dosage upward or downward according to severity of symptoms and response of the patient. For maintenance, adjust dosage to lowest level that will provide effective control.
3. **Given chronically:** Inoperable progressing prostatic cancer – 1.25 to 2.5 mg three times daily. The effectiveness of therapy can be judged by phosphatase determinations as well as by symptomatic improvement of the patient. Inoperable progressing breast cancer in appropriately selected men and postmenopausal women. (See **INDICATIONS**) – – Suggested dosage is 10 mg three times daily for a period of at least three months.
4. **For prevention of osteoporosis** – – therapy with ESTRATAB® Tablets to prevent postmenopausal bone loss should be initiated as soon as possible after menopause. Therapy should be initiated at a daily dose of 0.3 mg and may be increased to a maximum daily dose of 1.25 mg if necessary to control concurrent menopausal symptoms.
   Discontinuation of estrogen replacement therapy may reestablish the natural rate of bone loss.
   Treated patients with an intact uterus should be monitored closely for signs of endometrial cancer, and appropriate diagnostic measures should be taken to rule out malignancy in the event of persistent or recurring abnormal vaginal bleeding.

HOW SUPPLIED

ESTRATAB® (Esterified Estrogens Tablets, USP) are available in the following strengths and package sizes:

— Each blue tablet with black imprint "SOLVAY 1014" contains 0.3 mg, in bottles of 100 (NDC 0032-1014-01).
— Each yellow tablet with black imprint "SOLVAY 1022" contains 0.625 mg, in bottles of 100 (NDC 0032-1022-01) and 1000 (NDC 0032-1022-10).
— Each light purple tablet with white imprint "SOLVAY 1025" contains 2.5 mg, in bottles of 100 (NDC 0032-1025-01).

Storage

Store and dispense in tight, light-resistant containers as defined in the USP. Store below 30°C (86°F). Protect from moisture.

℞ only

Manufactured by:

Solvay
Pharmaceuticals, Inc.
Marietta, GA 30062

INFORMATION FOR THE PATIENT

This leaflet describes when and how to use estrogens and the risks of estrogen treatment.

Estrogens have important benefits but also some risks. You must decide, with your doctor, whether the risks to you of estrogen use are acceptable because of their benefits. If you use estrogens, check with your doctor to make sure you are using the lowest possible dose that works, and that you don't use them for longer than necessary. How long you need to use estrogens will depend on the reason for use.

1. **ESTROGENS INCREASE THE RISK OF CANCER OF THE UTERUS IN WOMEN WHO HAVE HAD THEIR MENOPAUSE ("CHANGE OF LIFE")**
   If you use any estrogen-containing drug, it is important to visit your doctor regularly and report any unusual vaginal bleeding right away. Vaginal bleeding after menopause may be a warning sign of uterine cancer. Your doctor should evaluate any unusual vaginal bleeding to find out the cause.
2. **ESTROGENS SHOULD NOT BE USED DURING PREGNANCY.**
   Estrogens do not prevent miscarriage (spontaneous abortion) and are not needed in the days following childbirth. If you take estrogens during pregnancy, your unborn child has a greater than usual chance of having birth defects. The risk of developing these defects is small, but clearly larger than the risk in children whose mothers did not take estrogen during pregnancy. These birth defects may affect the baby's urinary system and sex organs. Daughters born to mothers who took DES (an estrogen drug) have a higher than usual chance of developing cancer of the vagina or cervix when they become teenagers or young adults. Sons may have a higher than usual chance of developing cancer of the testicles when they become teenagers or young adults.

USES OF ESTROGEN

(NOT EVERY ESTROGEN DRUG IS APPROVED FOR EVERY USE LISTED IN THIS SECTION). If you want to know which of these possible uses are approved for the medicine prescribed for you, ask your doctor or pharmacist to show you the professional labeling.

You can also look up the specific estrogen product in a book called the "Physicians' Desk Reference", which is available

Continued on next page

Estratab—Cont.

in many book stores and public libraries. (Generic drugs carry virtually the same labeling information as their brand name versions).

To reduce moderate or severe menopausal symptoms. Estrogens are hormones made by the ovaries of normal women. Between ages 45 and 55, the ovaries normally stop making estrogens. This leads to a drop in body estrogen levels which causes the "change of life" or menopause (the end of monthly menstrual periods). If both ovaries are removed during an operation before natural menopause takes place, the sudden drop in estrogen levels causes "surgical menopause".

When the estrogen levels begin dropping, some women develop very uncomfortable symptoms, such as feelings of warmth in the face, neck, and chest, or sudden intense episodes of heat and sweating ("hot flashes" or "hot flushes"). Using estrogen drugs can help the body adjust to lower estrogen levels and reduce these symptoms. Most women have only mild menopausal symptoms or none at all and do not need to use estrogen drugs for these symptoms. Others may need to take estrogens for a few months while their bodies adjust to lower estrogen levels. The majority of women do not need estrogen replacement for longer than six months for these symptoms.

To treat vulval and vaginal atrophy (itching, burning, dryness in or around the vagina, difficulty or burning on urination) associated with menopause.

To treat certain conditions in which a young woman's ovaries do not produce enough estrogen naturally.

To treat certain types of abnormal vaginal bleeding due to hormonal imbalance when your doctor has found no serious cause of the bleeding.

To treat certain cancers in special situations, in men and women.

To prevent thinning of bones. Osteoporosis is a thinning of the bones that makes them weaker and allows them to break more easily. The bones of the spine, wrists and hips break most often in osteoporosis. Both men and women start to lose bone mass after about age 40, but women lose bone mass faster after the menopause. Using estrogens after the menopause slows down bone thinning and may prevent bones from breaking. Lifelong adequate calcium intake, either in the diet (such as dairy products) or by calcium supplements (to reach a total daily intake of 1000 milligrams per day before menopause or 1500 milligrams per day after menopause), may help to prevent osteoporosis. Regular weight-bearing exercise (like walking and running for an hour, two or three times a week) may also help to prevent osteoporosis. Before you change your calcium intake or exercise habits, it is important to discuss these lifestyle changes with your doctor to find out if they are safe for you.

Since estrogen use has some risks, only women who are likely to develop osteoporosis should use estrogens for prevention. Women who are likely to develop osteoporosis often have the following characteristics: white or Asian race, slim, cigarette smokers, and a family history of osteoporosis in a mother, sister, or aunt. Women who have relatively early menopause, often because their ovaries were removed during an operation ("surgical menopause"), are more likely to develop osteoporosis than women whose menopause happens at the average age.

WHO SHOULD NOT USE ESTROGENS

Estrogens should not be used:

During pregnancy (see Boxed Warning). If you think you may be pregnant, do not use any form of estrogen-containing drug. Using estrogens while you are pregnant may cause your unborn child to have birth defects. Estrogens do not prevent miscarriage.

If you have unusual vaginal bleeding which has not been evaluated by your doctor (see Boxed Warning). Unusual vaginal bleeding can be a warning sign of cancer of the uterus, especially if it happens after menopause. Your doctor must find out the cause of the bleeding so that he or she can recommend the proper treatment. Taking estrogens without visiting your doctor can cause you serious harm if your vaginal bleeding is caused by cancer of the uterus.

If you have had cancer. Since estrogens increase the risk of certain types of cancers, you should not use estrogens if you have ever had cancer of the breast or uterus, unless your doctor recommends that the drug may help in the cancer treatment. (For certain patients with breast or prostate cancer, estrogens may help.)

If you have any circulation problems. Estrogen drugs should not be used except in unusually special situations in which your doctor judges that you need estrogen therapy so much that the risks are acceptable. Men and women with abnormal blood clotting conditions should avoid estrogen use (see **DANGERS OF ESTROGENS**, below).

When they do not work. During menopause, some women develop nervous symptoms or depression. Estrogens do not relieve these symptoms. You may have heard that taking estrogens for years after menopause will keep your skin soft and supple and keep you feeling young. There is no evidence for these claims and such long-term estrogen use may have serious risks.

After childbirth or when breastfeeding a baby. Estrogens should not be used to try to stop the breasts from filling with milk after a baby is born. Such treatment may increase the risk of developing blood clots (see **DANGERS OF ESTROGENS**, below).

If you are breastfeeding, you should avoid using any drugs because many drugs pass through to the baby in the milk. While nursing a baby, you should take drugs only on the advice of your health care provider.

DANGERS OF ESTROGENS

Cancer of the uterus. Your risk of developing cancer of the uterus gets higher the longer you use estrogens and the larger doses you use. One study showed that after women stop taking estrogens, this higher cancer risk quickly returns to the usual level of risk (as if you had never used estrogen therapy). Three other studies showed that the cancer risk stayed high for 8 to more than 15 years after stopping estrogen treatment. **Because of this risk, IT IS IMPORTANT TO TAKE THE LOWEST DOSE THAT WORKS AND TO TAKE IT ONLY AS LONG AS YOU NEED IT.**

Using progestin therapy together with estrogen therapy may reduce the higher risk of uterine cancer related to estrogen use (but see **OTHER INFORMATION**, below).

If you have had your uterus removed (total hysterectomy), there is no danger of developing cancer of the uterus.

Cancer of the breast. Most studies have not shown a higher risk of breast cancer in women who have ever used estrogens. However, some studies have reported that breast cancer developed more often (up to twice the usual rate) in women who used estrogens for long periods of time (especially more than 10 years), or who used higher doses for shorter time periods.

Regular breast examinations by a health professional and monthly self-examination are recommended for all women.

Gallbladder disease. Women who use estrogens after menopause are more likely to develop gallbladder disease needing surgery than women who do not use estrogens.

Abnormal blood clotting. Taking estrogens may cause changes in your blood clotting system. These changes allow the blood to clot more easily, possibly allowing clots to form in your bloodstream. If blood clots do form in your bloodstream, they can cut off the blood supply to vital organs, causing serious problems. These problems may include a stroke (by cutting off blood to the brain), a heart attack (by cutting off blood to the heart), a pulmonary embolus (by cutting off blood to the lungs), or other problems. Any of these conditions may cause death or serious long term disability. However, most studies of low dose estrogen usage by women do not show an increased risk of these complications.

SIDE EFFECTS

In addition to the risks listed above, the following side effects have been reported with estrogen use:

- Nausea, vomiting
- Breast tenderness or enlargement.
- Enlargement of benign tumors ("fibroids") of the uterus.
- Retention of excess fluid. This may make some conditions worsen, such as asthma, epilepsy, migraine, heart disease, or kidney disease.
- A spotty darkening of the skin, particularly on the face.

REDUCING RISK OF ESTROGEN USE

If you use estrogens, you can reduce your risks by doing these things:

See your doctor regularly. While you are using estrogens, it is important to visit your doctor at least once a year for a check-up. If you develop vaginal bleeding while taking estrogens, you may need further evaluation. If members of your family have had breast cancer or if you have ever had breast lumps or an abnormal mammogram (breast x-ray), you may need to have more frequent breast examinations.

Reassess your need for estrogens. You and your doctor should reevaluate whether or not you still need estrogens at least every six months.

Be alert for signs of trouble. If any of these warning signals (or any other unusual symptoms) happen while you are using estrogens, call your doctor immediately:

- Abnormal bleeding from the vagina (possible uterine cancer).
- Pains in the calves or chest, sudden shortness of breath, or coughing blood (possible clot in the legs, heart, or lungs).
- Severe headache or vomiting, dizziness, faintness, changes in vision or speech, weakness or numbness of an arm or leg (possible clots in the brain or eye).
- Breast lumps (possible breast cancer; ask your doctor or health professional to show you how to examine your breasts monthly).
- Yellowing of the skin or eyes (possible liver problem).
- Pain, swelling, or tenderness in the abdomen (possible gallbladder problem).

OTHER INFORMATION

Estrogens increase the risk of developing a condition (endometrial hyperplasia) that may lead to cancer of the lining of the uterus. Taking progestins, another hormone drug, with estrogens lowers the risk of developing this condition. Therefore, if your uterus has not been removed, your doctor may prescribe a progestin for you to take together with the estrogen.

You should know, however, that taking estrogens with progestins may have additional risks. These include:

— unhealthy effects on blood fats (especially the lowering of HDL blood cholesterol, the "good" blood fat which protects against heart disease);

— unhealthy effects on blood sugar (which might make a diabetic condition worse); and

— a possible further increase in breast cancer risk which may be associated with long-term estrogen use.

Some research had shown that estrogens taken **without** progestins may protect women against developing heart disease. However, this is not certain. The protection shown may have been caused by the characteristics of the estrogen-treated women, and not by the estrogen treatment itself. In general, treated women were slimmer, more physically active, and were less likely to have diabetes than the untreated women. These characteristics are known to protect against heart disease.

You are cautioned to discuss very carefully with your doctor or health care provider all the possible risks and benefits of long-term estrogen and progestin treatment as they affect you personally.

Your doctor has prescribed this drug for you and you alone. Do not give the drug to anyone else.

If you will be taking calcium supplements as part of the treatment to help prevent osteoporosis, check with your doctor about how much to take.

Keep this and all drugs out of the reach of children. In case of overdose, call your doctor, hospital, or poison control center immediately.

This leaflet provides a summary of the most important information about estrogens. If you want more information, ask your doctor or pharmacist to show you the professional labeling. The professional labeling is also published in a book called the "Physicians' Desk Reference," which is available in book stores and public libraries. Generic drugs carry virtually the same labeling information as their brand name versions.

HOW SUPPLIED

ESTRATAB® (Esterified Estrogens Tablets, USP) for oral administration.

Each blue tablet contains 0.3 mg.

Each yellow tablet contains 0.625 mg.

Each light purple tablet contains 2.5 mg.

℞ only

The appearance of ESTRATAB® Tablets is a trademark of Solvay Pharmaceuticals, Inc.

1222
7E Rev 2/98

Solvay
Pharmaceuticals, Inc.
Marietta, GA 30062

Shown in Product Identification Guide, page 338

ESTRATEST® ℞

[es 'trah-test]

ESTRATEST® H.S. ℞

(Esterified Estrogens and Methyltestosterone) Tablets

WARNINGS

1. ESTROGENS HAVE BEEN REPORTED TO INCREASE THE RISK OF ENDOMETRIAL CARCINOMA.

Three independent case control studies have reported an increased risk of endometrial cancer in postmenopausal women exposed to exogenous estrogens for prolonged periods.[1–3] This risk was independent of the other known risk factors for endometrial cancer. These studies are further supported by the finding that incidence rates of endometrial cancer have increased sharply since 1969 in eight different areas of the United States with population-based cancer reporting systems, an increase which may be related to the rapidly expanding use of estrogens during the last decade.[4]

The three case control studies reported that the risk of endometrial cancer in estrogen users was about 4.5 to 13.9 times greater than in nonusers. The risk appears to depend on both duration of treatment[1] and on estrogen dose.[3] In view of these findings, when estrogens are used for the treatment of menopausal symptoms, the lowest dose that will control symptoms should be utilized and medication should be discontinued as soon as possible. When prolonged treatment is medically indicated, the patient should be reassessed on at least a semiannual basis to determine the need for continued therapy. Although the evidence must be considered preliminary, one study suggests that cyclic administration of low doses of estrogen may carry less risk than continuous administration;[3] it therefore appears prudent to utilize such a regimen.

Close clinical surveillance of all women taking estrogens is important. In all cases of undiagnosed persistent or recurring abnormal vaginal bleeding, adequate diagnostic measures should be undertaken to rule out malignancy.

There is no evidence at present that "natural" estrogens are more or less hazardous than "synthetic" estrogens at equiestrogenic doses.

2. ESTROGENS SHOULD NOT BE USED DURING PREGNANCY.

The use of female sex hormones, both estrogens and progestogens, during early pregnancy may seriously damage the offspring. It has been shown that females exposed in utero to diethylstilbestrol, a non-steroidal estrogen, have an increased risk of developing in later life a form of vaginal or cervical cancer that is ordinarily extremely rare.[5,6] This risk has been estimated as not greater than 4 per 1000 exposures.[7] Furthermore, a high percentage of such exposed women (from 30 to 90 percent) have been found to have vaginal adenosis,[8–12] epithelial changes of the vagina and cervix. Although these changes are histologically benign, it is not known whether they are precursors of malignancy. Although similar data are not available with the use of other estrogens, it cannot be presumed they would not induce similar changes.

Several reports suggest an association between intrauterine exposure to female sex hormones and congenital anomalies, including congenital heart defects and limb reduction defects.[13–16] One case control study[16] estimated a 4.7 fold increased risk of limb reduction defects in infants exposed in utero to sex hormones (oral contraceptives, hormone withdrawal tests for pregnancy, or attempted treatment for threatened abortion). Some of these exposures were very short and involved only a few days of treatment. The data suggest that the risk of limb reduction defects in exposed fetuses is somewhat less than 1 per 1000.

In the past, female sex hormones have been used during pregnancy in an attempt to treat threatened or habitual abortion. There is considerable evidence that estrogens are ineffective for these indications, and there is no evidence from well controlled studies that progestogens are effective for these uses.

If ESTRATEST® or ESTRATEST® H.S. is used during pregnancy, or if the patient becomes pregnant while taking this drug, she should be apprised of the potential risks to the fetus, and the advisability of pregnancy continuation.

DESCRIPTION

ESTRATEST®: Each dark green, capsule shaped, sugar-coated oral tablet contains: 1.25 mg of Esterified Estrogens, USP and 2.5 mg of Methyltestosterone.

ESTRATEST® H.S. (Half-Strength): Each light green, capsule shaped, sugar-coated oral tablet contains: 0.625 mg of Esterified Estrogens, USP and 1.25 mg of Methyltestosterone.

Esterified Estrogens

Esterified Estrogens, USP is a mixture of the sodium salts of the sulfate esters of the estrogenic substances, principally estrone, that are of the type excreted by pregnant mares. Esterified Estrogens contain not less than 75.0 percent and not more than 85.0 percent of sodium estrone sulfate, and not less than 6.0 percent and not more than 15.0 percent of sodium equilin sulfate, in such proportion that the total of these two components is not less than 90.0 percent.

Category: Estrogens

Methyltestosterone

Methyltestosterone is an androgen. Androgens are derivatives of cyclopentano-perhydrophenanthrene. Endogenous androgens are C-19 steroids with a side chain at C-17, and with two angular methyl groups. Testosterone is the primary endogenous androgen. Fluoxymesterone and methyltestosterone are synthetic derivatives of testosterone.

Methyltestosterone is a white to light yellow crystalline substance that is virtually insoluble in water but soluble in organic solvents. It is stable in air but decomposes in light.

Methyltestosterone structural formula:

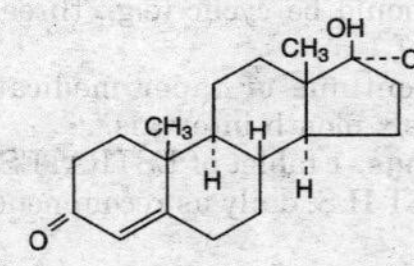

$C_{20}H_{30}O_2$, 302.46

Androst-4-en-3-one, 17-hydroxy-17-methyl-, (17B)-

Category: Androgen.

ESTRATEST® and ESTRATEST® H.S. Tablets contain the following inactive ingredients: acacia, calcium carbonate, citric acid, gelatin, lactose (anhydrous), magnesium stearate, methylparaben, microcrystalline cellulose, pharmaceutical glaze, povidone, propylparaben, sodium benzoate, sodium bicarbonate, sodium carboxymethylcellulose, sorbic acid, sucrose, starch (corn), talc, titanium dioxide, tribasic calcium phosphate, and other minor ingredients.

ESTRATEST® Tablets also contain: FD&C Blue No. 1 Lake, FD&C Yellow No. 6 Lake, and FD&C Yellow No. 10 Lake.

ESTRATEST® H.S. Tablets also contain: FD&C Yellow No. 10 Lake, FD&C Blue No. 1 Lake, and FD&C Blue No. 2 Lake.

CLINICAL PHARMACOLOGY

Estrogens: Estrogens are important in the development and maintenance of the female reproductive system and secondary sex characteristics. They promote growth and development of the vagina, uterus, and fallopian tubes, and enlargement of the breasts. Indirectly, they contribute to the shaping of the skeleton, maintenance of tone and elasticity of urogenital structures, changes in the epiphyses of the long bones that allow for the pubertal growth spurt and its termination, growth of axillary and pubic hair, and pigmentation of the nipples and genitals. Decline of estrogenic activity at the end of the menstrual cycle can bring on menstruation, although the cessation of progesterone secretion is the most important factor in the mature ovulatory cycle. However, in the preovulatory or nonovulatory cycle, estrogen is the primary determinant in the onset of menstruation. Estrogens also affect the release of pituitary gonadotropins.

The pharmacologic effects of esterified estrogens are similar to those of endogenous estrogens. They are soluble in water and are well absorbed from the gastrointestinal tract.

In responsive tissues (female genital organs, breasts, hypothalamus, pituitary) estrogens enter the cell and are transported into the nucleus. As a result of estrogen action, specific RNA and protein synthesis occurs.

Estrogen Pharmacokinetics

Metabolism and inactivation occur primarily in the liver. Some estrogens are excreted into the bile; however they are reabsorbed from the intestine and returned to the liver through the portal venous system. Water soluble esterified estrogens are strongly acidic and are ionized in body fluids, which favor excretion through the kidneys since tubular reabsorption is minimal.

Androgens: Endogenous androgens are responsible for the normal growth and development of the male sex organs and for maintenance of secondary sex characteristics. These effects include the growth and maturation of prostate, seminal vesicles, penis, and scrotum; the development of male hair distribution, such as beard, pubic, chest, and axillary hair, laryngeal enlargement, vocal cord thickening, alterations in body musculature, and fat distribution. Drugs in this class also cause retention of nitrogen, sodium, potassium, phosphorus, and decreased urinary excretion of calcium. Androgens have been reported to increase protein anabolism and decrease protein catabolism. Nitrogen balance is improved only when there is sufficient intake of calories and protein. Androgens are responsible for the growth spurt of adolescence and for the eventual termination of linear growth which is brought about by fusion of the epiphyseal growth centers. In children, exogenous androgens accelerate linear growth rates, but may cause a disproportionate advancement in bone maturation. Use over long periods may result in fusion of the epiphyseal growth centers and termination of growth process. Androgens have been reported to stimulate the production of red blood cells by enhancing the production of erythropoietic stimulating factor.

Androgen Pharmacokinetics

Testosterone given orally is metabolized by the gut and 44 percent is cleared by the liver in the first pass. Oral doses as high as 400 mg per day are needed to achieve clinically effective blood levels for full replacement therapy. The synthetic androgens (methyltestosterone and fluoxymesterone) are less extensively metabolized by the liver and have longer half-lives. They are more suitable than testosterone for oral administration.

Testosterone in plasma is 98 percent bound to a specific testosterone-estradiol binding globulin, and about 2 percent is free. Generally, the amount of this sex-hormone binding globulin in the plasma will determine the distribution of testosterone between free and bound forms, and the free testosterone concentration will determine its half-life.

About 90 percent of a dose of testosterone is excreted in the urine as glucuronic and sulfuric acid conjugates of testosterone and its metabolites; about 6 percent of a dose is excreted in the feces, mostly in the unconjugated form. Inactivation of testosterone occurs primarily in the liver. Testosterone is metabolized to various 17-keto steroids through two different pathways. There are considerable variations of the half-life of testosterone as reported in the literature, ranging from 10 to 100 minutes.

In many tissues the activity of testosterone appears to depend on reduction to dihydrotestosterone, which binds to cytosol receptor proteins. The steroid-receptor complex is transported to the nucleus where it initiates transcription events and cellular changes related to androgen action.

INDICATIONS AND USAGE

ESTRATEST® and ESTRATEST® H.S. are indicated in the treatment of:

Moderate to severe *vasomotor* symptoms associated with the menopause in those patients not improved by estrogens alone. (There is no evidence that estrogens are effective for nervous symptoms or depression without associated vasomotor symptoms, and they should not be used to treat such conditions.)

ESTRATEST® AND ESTRATEST® H.S. HAVE NOT BEEN SHOWN TO BE EFFECTIVE FOR ANY PURPOSE DURING PREGNANCY AND ITS USE MAY CAUSE SEVERE HARM TO THE FETUS (SEE BOXED WARNING).

CONTRAINDICATIONS

Estrogens should not be used in women with any of the following conditions:

1. Known or suspected cancer of the breast except in appropriately selected patients being treated for metastatic disease.
2. Known or suspected estrogen-dependent neoplasia.
3. Known or suspected pregnancy (See Boxed Warning).
4. Undiagnosed abnormal genital bleeding.
5. Active thrombophlebitis or thromboembolic disorders.
6. A past history of thrombophlebitis, thrombosis, or thromboembolic disorders associated with previous estrogen use (except when used in treatment of breast malignancy).

Methyltestosterone should not be used in:

1. The presence of severe liver damage.
2. Pregnancy and in breast-feeding mothers because of the possibility of masculinization of the female fetus or breast-fed infant.

WARNINGS

Associated with Estrogens

1. *Induction of malignant neoplasms.* Long term continuous administration of natural and synthetic estrogens in certain animal species increases the frequency of carcinomas of the breast, cervix, vagina, and liver. There is now evidence that estrogens increase the risk of carcinoma of the endometrium in humans (See Boxed Warning).

   At the present time there is no satisfactory evidence that estrogens given to postmenopausal women increase the risk of cancer of the breast,[18] although a recent long-term follow-up of a single physician's practice has raised this possibility.[18a] Because of the animal data, there is a need for caution in prescribing estrogens for women with a strong family history of breast cancer or who have breast nodules, fibrocystic disease, or abnormal mammograms.
2. *Gallbladder disease.* A recent study has reported a 2 to 3-fold increase in the risk of surgically confirmed gallbladder disease in women receiving postmenopausal estrogens,[18] similar to the 2-fold increase previously noted in users of oral contraceptives.[19–24a] In the case of oral contraceptives the increased risk appeared after two years of use.[24]
3. *Effects similar to those caused by estrogen-progestogen oral contraceptives.* There are several serious adverse effects of oral contraceptives, most of which have not, up to now, been documented as consequences of postmenopausal estrogen therapy. This may reflect the comparatively low doses of estrogen used in postmenopausal women. It would be expected that the larger doses of estrogen used to treat prostatic or breast cancer or postpartum breast engorgement are more likely to result in these adverse effects, and, in fact, it has been shown that there is an increased risk of thrombosis in men receiving estrogens for prostatic cancer and women for postpartum breast engorgement.[20–23]
   a. Thromboembolic disease. It is now well established that users of oral contraceptives have an increased risk of various thromboembolic and thrombotic vascular diseases, such as thrombophlebitis, pulmonary embolism, stroke, and myocardial infarction.[24–31] Cases of retinal thrombosis, mesenteric thrombosis, and optic neuritis have been reported in oral contraceptive users. There is evidence that the risk of several of these adverse reactions is related to the dose of the drug.[32,33]

      An increased risk of postsurgery thromboembolic complications has also been reported in users of oral contraceptives.[34,35] If feasible, estrogen should be discontinued at least 4 weeks before surgery of the type associated with an increased risk of thromboembolism, or during periods of prolonged immobilization.

      While an increased rate of thromboembolic and thrombotic disease in postmenopausal users of estrogens has not been found,[18–36] this does not rule out the possibility that such an increase may be present or that subgroups of women who have underlying risk factors or who are receiving relatively large doses of estrogens may have increased risk. Therefore estrogens should not be used in persons with active thrombophlebitis or thromboembolic disorders, and they should not be used (except in treatment of malignancy) in persons with a history of such disorders in association with estrogen use. They should be used with caution in patients with cerebral vascular or coronary artery disease and only for those in whom estrogens are clearly needed.

      Large doses of estrogen (5 mg esterified estrogens per day), comparable to those used to treat cancer of the prostate and breast, have been shown in a large prospective clinical trial in men[37] to increase the risk of nonfatal myocardial infarction, pulmonary embolism and thrombophlebitis. When estrogen doses of this size are used, any of the thromboembolic and thrombotic adverse effects associated with oral contraceptive use should be considered a clear risk.

   b. Hepatic adenoma. Benign hepatic adenomas appear to be associated with the use of oral contraceptives.[38–40] Although benign and rare, these may rupture and may cause death through intra-abdominal hemorrhage. Such lesions have not yet been reported in association with other estrogen or progestogen preparations but should be considered in estrogen users having abdominal pain and tenderness, abdominal mass, or hypovolemic shock. Hepatocellular carcinoma has also been reported in women taking estrogen-containing oral contraceptives.[39] The relationship of this malignancy to these drugs is not known at this time.
   c. Elevated blood pressure. Increased blood pressure is not uncommon in women using oral contraceptives. There is now a report that this may occur with use of estrogens in the menopause[41] and blood pressure should be monitored with estrogen use, especially if high doses are used.
   d. Glucose tolerance. A worsening of glucose tolerance has been observed in a significant percentage of patients on estrogen-containing oral contraceptives. For this reason, diabetic patients should be carefully observed while receiving estrogens.
4. *Hypercalcemia.* Administration of estrogens may lead to severe hypercalcemia in patients with breast cancer and bone metastases. If this occurs, the drug should be stopped and appropriate measures taken to reduce the serum calcium level.

Associated with Methyltestosterone

In patients with breast cancer, androgen therapy may cause hypercalcemia by stimulating osteolysis. In this case, the drug should be discontinued.

Continued on next page

Estratest/Estratest H.S.—Cont.

Prolonged use of high doses of androgens has been associated with the development of peliosis hepatis and hepatic neoplasms including hepatocellular carcinoma. (See PRECAUTIONS—*Carcinogenesis*). Peliosis hepatis can be a life-threatening or fatal complication.
Cholestatic hepatitis and jaundice occur with 17-alpha-alkylandrogens at a relatively low dose. If cholestatic hepatitis with jaundice appears or if liver function tests become abnormal, the androgen should be discontinued and the etiology should be determined. Drug-induced jaundice is reversible when the medication is discontinued.
Edema with or without heart failure may be a serious complication in patients with preexisting cardiac, renal, or hepatic disease. In addition to discontinuation of the drug, diuretic therapy may be required.

PRECAUTIONS

Associated with Estrogens

A. General Precautions.

1. A complete medical and family history should be taken prior to the initiation of any estrogen therapy. The pretreatment and periodic physical examinations should include special reference to blood pressure, breasts, abdomen, and pelvic organs, and should include a Papanicolaou smear. As a general rule, estrogen should not be prescribed for longer than one year without another physical examination being performed.
2. Fluid retention—Because estrogens may cause some degree of fluid retention, conditions which might be influenced by this factor such as asthma, epilepsy, migraine, and cardiac or renal dysfunction, require careful observation.
3. Certain patients may develop undesirable manifestations of excessive estrogenic stimulation, such as abnormal or excessive uterine bleeding, mastodynia, etc.
4. Oral contraceptives appear to be associated with an increased incidence of mental depression.[24] Although it is not clear whether this is due to the estrogenic or progestogenic component of the contraceptive, patients with a history of depression should be carefully observed.
5. Preexisting uterine leiomyomata may increase in size during estrogen use.
6. The pathologist should be advised of estrogen therapy when relevant specimens are submitted.
7. Patients with a past history of jaundice during pregnancy have an increased risk of recurrence of jaundice while receiving estrogen-containing oral contraceptive therapy. If jaundice develops in any patient receiving estrogen, the medication should be discontinued while the cause is investigated.
8. Estrogens may be poorly metabolized in patients with impaired liver function and they should be administered with caution in such patients.
9. Because estrogens influence the metabolism of calcium and phosphorus, they should be used with caution in patients with metabolic bone diseases that are associated with hypercalcemia or in patients with renal insufficiency.
10. Because of the effects of estrogens on epiphyseal closure, they should be used judiciously in young patients in whom bone growth is not complete.
11. Certain endocrine and liver function tests may be affected by estrogen-containing oral contraceptives. The following similar changes may be expected with larger doses of estrogen:

a. Increased sulfobromophthalein retention.
b. Increased prothrombin and factors VII, VIII, IX and X; decreased antithrombin 3; increased norepinephrine-induced platelet aggregability.
c. Increased thyroid binding globulin (TBG) leading to increased circulating total thyroid hormone, as measured by PBI, T4 by column, or T4 by radioimmunoassay. Free T3 resin uptake is decreased, reflecting the elevated TBG; free T4 concentration is unaltered.
d. Impaired glucose tolerance.
e. Decreased pregnanediol excretion.
f. Reduced response to metyrapone test.
g. Reduced serum folate concentration.
h. Increased serum triglyceride and phospholipid concentration.

B. Information for the Patient. See text of Patient Package Insert which appears after the REFERENCES.

C. Pregnancy Category X. See CONTRAINDICATIONS and Boxed WARNING.

D. Nursing Mothers. As a general principle, the administration of any drug to nursing mothers should be done only when clearly necessary since many drugs are excreted in human milk.

Associated with Methyltestosterone

A. General Precautions.

1. Women should be observed for signs of virilization (deepening of the voice, hirsutism, acne, clitoromegaly, and menstrual irregularities). Discontinuation of drug therapy at the time of evidence of mild virilism is necessary to prevent irreversible virilization. Such virilization is usual following androgen use at high doses.
2. Prolonged dosage of androgen may result in sodium and fluid retention. This may present a problem, especially in patients with compromised cardiac reserve or renal disease.
3. Hypersensitivity may occur rarely.
4. PBI may be decreased in patients taking androgens.
5. Hypercalcemia may occur. If this does occur, the drug should be discontinued.

B. Information for the Patient.
The physician should instruct patients to report any of the following side effects of androgens:
Women: Hoarseness, acne, changes in menstrual periods, or more hair on the face.
All Patients: Any nausea, vomiting, changes in skin color or ankle swelling.

C. Laboratory tests.
1. Women with disseminated breast carcinoma should have frequent determination of urine and serum calcium levels during the course of androgen therapy (See WARNINGS).
2. Because of the hepatotoxicity associated with the use of 17-alpha-alkylated androgens, liver function tests should be obtained periodically.
3. Hemoglobin and hematocrit should be checked periodically for polycythemia in patients who are receiving high doses of androgens.

D. Drug Interactions.
1. *Anticoagulants* C-17 substituted derivatives of testosterone, such as methandrostenolone, have been reported to decrease the anticoagulant requirements of patients receiving oral anticoagulants. Patients receiving oral anticoagulant therapy require close monitoring, especially when androgens are started or stopped.
2. *Oxyphenbutazone.* Concurrent administration of oxyphenbutazone and androgens may result in elevated serum levels of oxyphenbutazone.
3. *Insulin.* In diabetic patients the metabolic effects of androgens may decrease blood glucose and insulin requirements.

E. Drug/Laboratory Test Interferences.
Androgens may decrease levels of thyroxine-binding globulin, resulting in decreased T_4 serum levels and increased resin uptake of T_3 and T_4. Free thyroid hormone levels remain unchanged, however, and there is no clinical evidence of thyroid dysfunction.

F. Carcinogenesis.
Animal Data. Testosterone has been tested by subcutaneous injection and implantation in mice and rats. The implant induced cervical-uterine tumors in mice, which metastasized in some cases. There is suggestive evidence that injection of testosterone into some strains of female mice increases their susceptibility to hepatoma. Testosterone is also known to increase the number of tumors and decrease the degree of differentiation of chemically induced carcinomas of the liver in rats.
Human Data. There are rare reports of hepatocellular carcinoma in patients receiving long-term therapy with androgens in high doses. Withdrawal of the drugs did not lead to regression of the tumors in all cases.
Geriatric patients treated with androgens may be at an increased risk for the development of prostatic hypertrophy and prostatic carcinoma.

G. Pregnancy.
Teratogenic Effects. Pregnancy Category X (see CONTRAINDICATIONS).

H. Nursing Mothers.
It is not known whether androgens are excreted in human milk. Because many drugs are excreted in human milk and because of the potential for serious adverse reactions in nursing infants from androgens, a decision should be made whether to discontinue nursing or to discontinue the drug, taking into account the importance of the drug to the mother.

ADVERSE REACTIONS

Associated with Estrogens (See Warnings regarding induction of neoplasia, adverse effects on the fetus, increased incidence of gallbladder disease, and adverse effects similar to those of oral contraceptives, including thromboembolism).
The following additional adverse reactions have been reported with estrogenic therapy, including oral contraceptives:

1. Genitourinary system.
Breakthrough bleeding, spotting, change in menstrual flow.
Dysmenorrhea.
Premenstrual-like syndrome.
Amenorrhea during and after treatment.
Increase in size of uterine fibromyomata.
Vaginal candidiasis.
Change in cervical erosion and in degree of cervical secretion.
Cystitis-like syndrome.

2. Breasts.
Tenderness, enlargement, secretion.

3. Gastrointestinal.
Nausea, vomiting.
Abdominal cramps, bloating.
Cholestatic jaundice.

4. Skin.
Chloasma or melasma which may persist when drug is discontinued.
Erythema multiforme.
Erythema nodosum.
Hemorrhagic eruption.
Loss of scalp hair.
Hirsutism.

5. Eyes.
Steepening of corneal curvature.
Intolerance to contact lenses.

6. CNS.
Headache, migraine, dizziness.
Mental depression.
Chorea.

7. Miscellaneous.
Increase or decrease in weight.
Reduced carbohydrate tolerance.
Aggravation of porphyria.
Edema.
Changes in libido.

Associated with Methyltestosterone

A. Endocrine and Urogenital.
1. *Female:* The most common side effects of androgen therapy are amenorrhea and other menstrual irregularities, inhibition of gonadotropin secretion, and virilization, including deepening of the voice and clitoral enlargement. The latter usually is not reversible after androgens are discontinued. When administered to a pregnant woman androgens cause virilization of external genitalia of the female fetus.
2. *Skin and Appendages:* Hirsutism, male pattern of baldness, and acne.
3. *Fluid and Electrolyte Disturbances:* Retention of sodium, chloride, water, potassium, calcium, and inorganic phosphates.
4. *Gastrointestinal:* Nausea, cholestatic jaundice, alterations in liver function test, rarely hepatocellular neoplasms, and peliosis hepatis (see WARNINGS).
5. *Hematologic:* Suppression of clotting factors II, V, VII, and X, bleeding in patients on concomitant anticoagulant therapy, and polycythemia.
6. *Nervous System:* Increased or decreased libido, headache, anxiety, depression, and generalized paresthesia.
7. *Metabolic:* Increased serum cholesterol.
8. *Miscellaneous:* Inflammation and pain at the site of intramuscular injection or subcutaneous implantation of testosterone containing pellets, stomatitis with buccal preparations, and rarely anaphylactoid reactions.

OVERDOSAGE

Numerous reports of ingestion of large doses of estrogen-containing oral contraceptives by young children indicate that serious ill effects do not occur. Overdosage of estrogen may cause nausea, and withdrawal bleeding may occur in females.
There have been no reports of acute overdosage with the androgens.

DOSAGE AND ADMINISTRATION

1. *Given cyclically for short-term use only:*
For treatment of moderate to severe *vasomotor* symptoms associated with the menopause in patients not improved by estrogen alone.
The lowest dose that will control symptoms should be chosen and medication should be discontinued as promptly as possible.
Administration should be cyclic (e.g., three weeks on and one week off).
Attempts to discontinue or taper medication should be made at three to six month intervals.
Usual Dosage Range: 1 tablet of ESTRATEST or 1 to 2 tablets of ESTRATEST H.S. daily as recommended by the physician.
Treated patients with an intact uterus should be monitored closely for signs of endometrial cancer and appropriate diagnostic measures should be taken to rule out malignancy in the event of persistent or recurring abnormal vaginal bleeding.

HOW SUPPLIED

ESTRATEST® (Imprinted "SOLVAY 1026") in bottles of 100—NDC 0032-1026-01 and 1000—NDC 0032-1026-10.
ESTRATEST® (Dark green, capsule shaped, sugar-coated oral tablets) contains: 1.25 mg of Esterified Estrogens, USP and 2.5 mg of Methyltestosterone, USP.
ESTRATEST® H.S. (Imprinted "SOLVAY 1023") in bottles of 100—NDC 0032-1023-01.
ESTRATEST® H.S. "Half-Strength" (Light green, capsule shaped, sugar-coated oral tablets) contains: 0.625 mg of Esterified Estrogens, USP and 1.25 mg of Methyltestosterone, USP.
Store at controlled room temperature, 15°–30°C (59°–86°F).
Rx only

REFERENCES

1. Ziel, H.K., *et al.:* N. Engl. J. Med. *293* :1167–1170, 1975.
2. Smith, D.C., *et al.:* N. Engl. J. Med. *293* :1164–1167, 1975.
3. Mack, T.M., *et al.:* N. Engl. J. Med. *294* :1262–1267, 1976.
4. Weiss, N.S., *et al.:* N. Engl. J. Med. *294* :1259–1262, 1976.
5. Herbst, A.L., *et al.:* N. Engl. J. Med. *284* :878–881, 1971.
6. Greenwald, P., *et al.:* N. Engl. J. Med. *285* :390–392, 1971.
7. Lanier, A., *et al.:* Mayo Clin. Proc. *48* :793–799, 1973.
8. Herbst, A., *et al.:* Obstet. Gynecol. *40* :287–298, 1972.
9. Herbst, A., *et al.:* Am. J. Obstet. Gynecol. *118* :607–615, 1974.

10. Herbst, A., *et al.*: N. Engl. J. Med. *292* :334–339, 1975.
11. Stafl, A., *et al.*: Obstet. Gynecol. *43* :118–128, 1974.
12. Sherman, A.I., *et al.*: Obstet. Gynecol. *44* :531–545, 1974.
13. Gal, I., *et al.*: Nature *216* :83, 1967.
14. Levy, E.P., *et al.*: Lancet *1* :611, 1973.
15. Nora, J., *et al.*: Lancet *1* :941–942, 1973.
16. Janerich, D.T., *et al.*: N. Engl. J. Med. *291* :697–700, 1974.
17. Estrogens for Oral or Parenteral Use: Federal Register *40* :8212, 1975.
18. Boston Collaborative Drug Surveillance Program: N. Engl. J. Med. *290* :15–19, 1974.
18a. Hoover, R., *et al.*: N. Engl. J. Med. *295* :401–405, 1976.
19. Boston Collaborative Drug Surveillance Program: Lancet *1* :1399–1404, 1973.
20. Daniel, D.G., *et al.*: Lancet *2* :287–289, 1967.
21. The Veterans Administration Cooperative Urological Research Group: J. Urol. *98* :516–522, 1967.
22. Bailar, J. C.: Lancet *2* :560, 1967.
23. Blackard, C., *et al.*: Cancer *26* :249–256, 1970.
24. Royal College of General Practitioners: J.R. Coll, Gen. Pract. *13* :267–279, 1967.
25. Inman, W.H.W., *et al.*: Br. Med. J. *2* :193–199, 1968.
26. Vessey, M.P., *et al.*: Br. Med. J. *2* :651–657, 1969.
27. Sartwell, P.E., *et al.*: Am. J. Epidemiol, *90* :365–380, 1969.
28. Collaborative Group for the Study of Stroke in Young Women: N. Engl. J. Med. *288* :871–878, 1973.
29. Collaborative Group for the Study of Stroke in Young Women: J.A.M.A. *231* :718–722, 1975.
30. Mann, J.I., *et al.*: Br. Med. J. *2* :245–248, 1975.
31. Mann, J.I., *et al.*: Br. Med. J. *2* :241–245, 1975.
32. Inman, W.H.W., *et al.*: Br. Med. J. *2* :203–209, 1970.
33. Stolley, P.D., *et al.*: Am. J. Epidemiol, *102* :197–208, 1975.
34. Vessey, M.P., *et al.*: Br. Med. J. *3* :123–126, 1970.
35. Greene, G.R., *et al.*: Am. J. Public Health *62* :680–685, 1972.
36. Rosenberg, L., *et al.*: N. Engl. J. Med. *294* :1256–1259, 1976.
37. Coronary Drug Project Research Group: J.A.M.A. *214* : 1303–1313, 1970.
38. Baum, J., *et al.*: Lancet *2* :926–928, 1973.
39. Mays, E.T., *et al.*: J.A.M.A. *235* :730–732, 1976.
40. Edmondson, H.A., *et al.*: N. Engl. J. Med. *294* :470–472, 1976.
41. Pfeffer, R.I., *et al.*: Am. J. Epidemiol, *103* :445–456, 1976.

INFORMATION FOR THE PATIENT

WHAT YOU SHOULD KNOW ABOUT ESTROGENS

Estrogens are female hormones produced by the ovaries. The ovaries make several different kinds of estrogens. In addition, scientists have been able to make a variety of synthetic estrogens. As far as we know, all these estrogens have similar properties and therefore much the same usefulness, side effects, and risks. This leaflet is intended to help you understand what estrogens are used for, the risks involved in their use, and how to use them as safely as possible.
This leaflet includes the most important information about estrogens, but not all the information. If you want to know more, you can ask your doctor or pharmacist to let you read the package insert prepared for the doctor.

USES OF ESTROGEN

Estrogens are prescribed by doctors for a number of purposes, including:
1. To provide estrogen during a period of adjustment when a woman's ovaries no longer produce it, in order to prevent certain uncomfortable symptoms of estrogen deficiency. (All women normally stop producing estrogens, generally between the ages of 45 and 55; this is called the menopause).
2. To prevent symptoms of estrogen deficiency when a woman's ovaries have been removed surgically before the natural menopause.
3. To prevent pregnancy. (Estrogens are given along with a progestogen, another female hormone; these combinations are called oral contraceptives or birth controll pills. Patient labeling is available to women taking oral contraceptives and they will not be discussed in this leaflet).
4. To treat certain cancers in women and men.

THERE IS NO PROPER USE OF ESTROGENS IN A PREGNANT WOMAN.

ESTROGENS IN THE MENOPAUSE

In the natural course of their lives, all women eventually experience a decrease in estrogen production. This usually occurs between ages 45 and 55 but may occur earlier or later. Sometimes the ovaries may need to be removed before natural menopause by an operation, producing a "surgical menopause."
When the amount of estrogen in the blood begins to decrease, many women may develop typical symptoms: Feelings of warmth in the face, neck, and chest or sudden intense episodes of heat and sweating throughout the body (called "hot flashes" or "hot flushes"). These symptoms are sometimes very uncomfortable. A few women eventually develop changes in the vagina (called "atrophic vaginitis") which cause discomfort, especially during and after intercourse.
Estrogens can be prescribed to treat these symptoms of the menopause. It is estimated that considerably more than half of all women undergoing the menopause have only mild symptoms or no symptoms at all and therefore do not need estrogens. Other women may need estrogens for a few months, while their bodies adjust to lower estrogen levels. Sometimes the need will be for periods longer than six months. In an attempt to avoid overstimulation of the uterus (womb), estrogens are usually given cyclically during each month of use, that is three weeks of pills followed by one week without pills.
Sometimes women experience nervous symptoms or depression during menopause. There is no evidence that estrogens are effective for such symptoms and they should not be used to treat them, although other treatment may be needed.
You may have heard that taking estrogens for long periods (years) after the menopause will keep your skin soft and supple and keep you feeling young. There is no evidence that this is so, however, and such long-term treatment carries important risks.

THE DANGERS OF ESTROGENS

1. **Cancer of the uterus.** If estrogens are used in the postmenopausal period for more than a year, there is an increased risk of **endometrial cancer** (cancer of the uterus). Women taking estrogens have roughly 5 to 10 times as great a chance of getting this cancer as women who take no estrogens. To put this another way, while a postmenopausal woman not taking estrogens has 1 chance in 1,000 each year of getting cancer of the uterus, a woman taking estrogens has 5 to 10 chances in 1,000 each year. For this reason **it is important to take estrogens only when you really need them.**
   The risk of this cancer is greater the longer estrogens are used and also seems to be greater when larger doses are taken. For this reason, **It is important to take the lowest dose of estrogen that will control symptoms and to take it only as long as it is needed.** If estrogens are needed for longer periods of time, your doctor will want to reevaluate your need for estrogens at least every six months.
   Women using estrogens should report any irregular vaginal bleeding to their doctors; such bleeding may be of no importance, but it can be an early warning of cancer of the uterus. If you have undiagnosed vaginal bleeding, you should not use estrogens until a diagnosis is made and you are certain there is no cancer of the uterus.
2. **Other possible cancers.** Estrogens can cause development of other tumors in animals, such as tumors of the breast, cervix, vagina, or liver, when given for a long time. At present there is no good evidence that women using estrogen in the menopause have an increased risk of such tumors, but there is no way yet to be sure they do not; and one study raises the possibility that use of estrogens in the menopause may increase the risk of breast cancer many years later. This is a further reason to use estrogens only when clearly needed. While you are taking estrogens, it is important that you go to your doctor at least once a year for a physical examination. Also, if members of your family have had breast cancer or if you have had breast nodules or abnormal mammograms (breast x-rays), your doctor may wish to carry out more frequent examinations of your breasts.
3. **Gallbladder disease.** Women who use estrogens after menopause are more likely to develop gallbladder disease needing surgery as women who do not use estrogens. Birth control pills have a similar effect.
4. **Abnormal blood clotting.** Oral contraceptives increase the risk of blood clotting in various parts of the body. This can result in a stroke (if the clot is in the brain), a heart attack (clot in a blood vessel of the heart), or pulmonary embolus (a clot which forms in the legs or pelvis, then breaks off and travels to the lungs). Any of these can be fatal. At this time use of estrogens in the menopause is not known to cause such blood clotting, but this has not been fully studied and there could still prove to be such a risk. It is recommended that if you have had clotting in the legs or lungs or a heart attack or stroke while you were using estrogens or birth control pills, you should not use estrogens (unless they are being used to treat cancer of the breast or prostate). If you have had a stroke or heart attack or if you have angina pectoris, estrogens should be used with great caution and only if clearly needed (for example, if you have severe symptoms of the menopause).
   The larger doses of estrogen used to prevent swelling of the breasts after pregnancy have been reported to cause clotting in the legs and lungs.

SPECIAL WARNING ABOUT PREGNANCY

You should not receive estrogen if you are pregnant. If this should occur, there is a greater than usual chance that the developing child will be born with a birth defect, although the possibility remains fairly small. A female child may have an increased risk of developing cancer of the vagina or cervix later in life (in the teens or twenties). Every possible effort should be made to avoid exposure to estrogens during pregnancy. If exposure occurs, see your doctor.

OTHER EFFECTS OF ESTROGENS

In addition to the serious known risks of estrogens described above, estrogens have the following side effects and potential risks:
1. **Nausea and vomiting.** The most common side effect of estrogen therapy is nausea. Vomiting is less common.
2. **Effects on breasts.** Estrogens may cause breast tenderness or enlargement and may cause the breasts to secrete a liquid. These effects are not dangerous.
3. **Effects on the uterus.** Estrogens may cause benign fibroid tumors of the uterus to get larger.
   Some women will have menstrual bleeding when estrogens are stopped. But if the bleeding occurs on days you are still taking estrogens you should report this to your doctor.
4. **Effect on liver.** Women taking oral contraceptives develop on rare occasions a benign tumor of the liver which can rupture and bleed into the abdomen. So far, these tumors have not been reported in women using estrogens in the menopause, but you should report any swelling or unusual pain or tenderness in the abdomen to your doctor immediately.
   Women with a past history of jaundice (yellowing of the skin and white parts of the eyes) may get jaundice again during estrogen use. If this occurs, stop taking estrogens and see your doctor.
5. **Other effects.** Estrogens may cause excess fluid to be retained in the body. This may make some conditions worse, such as epilepsy, migraine, heart disease, or kidney disease.

SUMMARY

Estrogens have important uses, but they have serious risks as well. You must decide, with your doctor, whether the risks are acceptable to you in view of the benefits of treatment. Except where your doctor has prescribed estrogens for use in special cases of cancer of the breast or prostate, you should not use estrogens if you have cancer of the breast or uterus, are pregnant, have undiagnosed abnormal vaginal bleeding, or have had a stroke, heart attack or angina, or clotting in the legs or lungs in the past while you were taking estrogens.
You can use estrogens as safely as possible by understanding that your doctor will require regular physical examinations while you are taking them and will try to discontinue the drug as soon as possible and use the smallest dose possible. Be alert for signs of trouble including:
1. Abnormal bleeding from the vagina.
2. Pains in the calves or chest or sudden shortness of breath, or coughing blood (indicating possible clots in the legs, heart, or lungs).
3. Severe headaches, dizziness, faintness, or changes in vision (indicating possible developing clots in the brain or eye).
4. Breast lumps (you should ask your doctor how to examine your own breasts).
5. Jaundice (yellowing of the skin).
6. Mental depression.

Based on his or her assessment of your medical needs, your doctor has prescribed this drug for you. Do not give the drug to anyone else.

HOW SUPPLIED

ESTRATEST® H.S. a combination of Esterified Estrogens and Methyltestosterone. Each capsule-shaped light green, sugar coated Tablet contains: 0.625 mg of Esterified Estrogens, USP and 1.25 mg of Methyltestosterone, USP.
ESTRATEST® a combination of Esterified Estrogens and Methyltestosterone. Each capsule-shaped dark green sugar-coated Tablet contains: 1.25 mg of Esterified Estrogens, USP and 2.5 mg of Methyltestosterone, USP.
Rx only

Solvay Pharmaceuticals, Inc.
Marietta, GA 30062 0978 8E Rev 6/98

Shown in Product Identification Guide, page 338

LITHOBID® ℞

[lĭth' ō-bĭd"]
(Lithium Carbonate, USP)
Slow-Release Tablets
300 mg

> **WARNING**
> Lithium toxicity is closely related to serum lithium levels, and can occur at doses close to therapeutic levels. Facilities for prompt and accurate serum lithium determinations should be available before initiating therapy (see **DOSAGE AND ADMINISTRATION**).

DESCRIPTION

LITHOBID® Tablets contain lithium carbonate, a white, odorless alkaline powder with molecular formula Li_2CO_3 and molecular weight 73.89. Lithium is an element of the alkali-metal group with atomic number 3, atomic weight 6.94 and an emission line at 671 nm on the flame photometer.
Each peach-colored, film-coated, slow-release tablet contains 300 mg of lithium carbonate. This slowly dissolving, film-coated tablet is designed to give lower serum lithium peak concentrations than obtained with conventional oral lithium dosage forms. Inactive ingredients consist of calcium stearate, carnauba wax, cellulose compounds, FD&C Blue No. 2 Aluminum Lake, FD&C Red No. 40 Aluminum Lake, FD&C Yellow No. 6 Aluminum Lake, povidone, propylene glycol, sodium chloride, sodium lauryl sulfate, sodium starch glycolate, sorbitol and titanium dioxide. Product meets USP Drug Release Test 1.

Continued on next page

Lithobid—Cont.

ACTIONS

Preclinical studies have shown that lithium alters sodium transport in nerve and muscle cells and effects a shift toward intraneuronal metabolism of catecholamines, but the specific biochemical mechanism of lithium action in mania is unknown.

INDICATIONS

Lithium is indicated in the treatment of manic episodes of manic-depressive illness. Maintenance therapy prevents or diminishes the intensity of subsequent episodes in those manic-depressive patients with a history of mania.

Typical symptoms: of mania include pressure of speech, motor hyperactivity, reduced need for sleep, flight of ideas, grandiosity, elation, poor judgment, aggressiveness, and possibly hostility. When given to a patient experiencing a manic episode, lithium may produce a normalization of symptomatology within 1 to 3 weeks.

WARNINGS

Lithium should generally not be given to patients with significant renal or cardiovascular disease, severe debilitation, dehydration, sodium depletion, and to patients receiving diuretics, or angiotensin converting enzyme (ACE) inhibitors, since the risk of lithium toxicity is very high in such patients. If the psychiatric indication is life threatening, and if such a patient fails to respond to other measures, lithium treatment may be undertaken with extreme caution, including daily serum lithium determinations and adjustment to the usually low doses ordinarily tolerated by these individuals. In such instances, hospitalization is a necessity.

Chronic lithium therapy may be associated with diminution of renal concentrating ability, occasionally presenting as nephrogenic diabetes insipidus, with polyuria and polydipsia. Such patients should be carefully managed to avoid dehydration with resulting lithium retention and toxicity. This condition is usually reversible when lithium is discontinued.

Morphologic changes with glomerular and interstitial fibrosis and nephron atrophy have been reported in patients on chronic lithium therapy. Morphologic changes have also been seen in manic-depressive patients never exposed to lithium. The relationship between renal function and morphologic changes and their association with lithium therapy have not been established.

Kidney function should be assessed prior to and during lithium therapy. Routine urinalysis and other tests may be used to evaluate tubular function (e.g., urine specific gravity or osmolality following a period of water deprivation, or 24-hour urine volume) and glomerular function (e.g., serum creatinine or creatinine clearance). During lithium therapy, progressive or sudden changes in renal function, even within the normal range, indicate the need for re-evaluation of treatment.

An encephalopathic syndrome (characterized by weakness, lethargy, fever, tremulousness and confusion, extrapyramidal symptoms, leukocytosis, elevated serum enzymes, BUN and FBS) has occurred in a few patients treated with lithium plus a neuroleptic, most notably haloperidol. In some instances, the syndrome was followed by irreversible brain damage. Because of possible causal relationship between these events and the concomitant administration of lithium and neuroleptic drugs, patients receiving such combined therapy or patients with organic brain syndrome or other CNS impairment should be monitored closely for early evidence of neurologic toxicity and treatment discontinued promptly if such signs appear. This encephalopathic syndrome may be similar to or the same as Neuroleptic Malignant Syndrome (NMS).

Lithium toxicity is closely related to serum lithium concentrations and can occur at doses close to the therapeutic concentrations (see **DOSAGE AND ADMINISTRATION**).

Outpatients and their families should be warned that the patient must discontinue lithium therapy and contact his physician if such clinical signs of lithium toxicity as diarrhea, vomiting, tremor, mild ataxia, drowsiness, or muscular weakness occur.

Lithium may prolong the effects of neuromuscular blocking agents. Therefore, neuromuscular blocking agents should be given with caution to patients receiving lithium.

Usage in Pregnancy

Adverse effects on nidation in rats, embryo viability in mice, and metabolism in vitro of rat testis and human spermatozoa have been attributed to lithium, as have teratogenicity in submammalian species and cleft palate in mice.

In humans, lithium may cause fetal harm when administered to a pregnant woman. Data from lithium birth registries suggest an increase in cardiac and other anomalies especially Ebstein's anomaly. If this drug is used in women of childbearing potential, or during pregnancy, or if a patient becomes pregnant while taking this drug, the patient should be apprised by their physician of the potential hazard to the fetus.

Usage in Nursing Mothers

Lithium is excreted in human milk. Nursing should not be undertaken during lithium therapy except in rare and unusual circumstances where, in the view of the physician, the potential benefits to the mother outweigh possible hazard to the infant or neonate. Signs and symptoms of lithium toxicity such as hypertonia, hypothermia, cyanosis and ECG changes have been reported in some infants and neonates.

Pediatric Use

Safety and effectiveness in pediatric patients under 12 years of age have not been determined; its use in these patients is not recommended.

There has been a report of transient syndrome of acute dystonia and hyperreflexia occurring in a 15 kg pediatric patient who ingested 300 mg of lithium carbonate.

PRECAUTIONS

The ability to tolerate lithium is greater during the acute manic phase and decreases when manic symptoms subside (see **DOSAGE AND ADMINISTRATION**).

The distribution space of lithium approximates that of total body water. Lithium is primarily excreted in urine with insignificant excretion in feces. Renal excretion of lithium is proportional to its plasma concentration. The elimination half-life of lithium is approximately 24 hours. Lithium decreases sodium reabsorption by the renal tubules which could lead to sodium depletion. Therefore, it is essential for the patient to maintain a normal diet, including salt, and an adequate fluid intake (2500–3500 mL) at least during the initial stabilization period. Decreased tolerance to lithium has been reported to ensue from protracted sweating or diarrhea and, if such occur, supplemental fluid and salt should be administered under careful medical supervision and lithium intake reduced or suspended until the condition is resolved.

In addition to sweating and diarrhea, concomitant infection with elevated temperatures may also necessitate a temporary reduction or cessation of medication.

Previously existing thyroid disorders do not necessarily constitute a contraindication to lithium treatment. Where hypothyroidism preexists, careful monitoring of thyroid function during lithium stabilization and maintenance allows for correction of changing thyroid parameters and/or adjustment of lithium doses, if any. If hypothyroidism occurs during lithium stabilization and maintenance, supplemental thyroid treatment may be used.

In general, the concomitant use of diuretics or angiotensin converting enzyme (ACE) inhibitors with lithium carbonate should be avoided. In those cases where concomitant use is necessary extreme caution is advised since sodium loss from these drugs may reduce the renal clearance of lithium resulting in increased serum lithium concentrations with the risk of lithium toxicity. When such combinations are used, the lithium dosage may need to be decreased, and more frequent monitoring of lithium serum concentrations is recommended. See **WARNINGS** for additional caution information.

Concomitant administration of carbamazepine and lithium may increase the risk of neurotoxic side effects.

The following drugs can lower serum lithium concentrations by increasing urinary lithium excretion: acetazolamide, urea, xanthine preparations and alkalinizing agents such as sodium bicarbonate.

Concomitant extended use of iodide preparations, especially potassium iodide, with lithium may produce hypothyroidism. Indomethacin and piroxicam have been reported to significantly increase steady state serum lithium concentrations. In some cases lithium toxicity has resulted from such interactions. There is also some evidence that other nonsteroidal, anti-inflammatory agents may have a similar effect. When such combinations are used, increased serum lithium concentrations monitoring is recommended.

Concurrent use of calcium channel blocking agents with lithium may increase the risk of neurotoxicity in the form of ataxia, tremors, nausea, vomiting, diarrhea and/or tinnitus.

Concurrent use of metronidazole with lithium may provoke lithium toxicity due to reduced renal clearance. Patients receiving such combined therapy should be monitored closely.

Concurrent use of fluoxetine with lithium has resulted in both increased and decreased serum lithium concentrations. Patients receiving such combined therapy should be monitored closely.

Lithium may impair mental and/or physical abilities. Patients should be cautioned about activities requiring alertness (e.g., operating vehicles or machinery).

Usage in Pregnancy

Pregnancy Category D. (see **WARNINGS**).

Usage in Nursing Mothers

Because of the potential for serious adverse reactions in nursing infants and neonates from lithium, a decision should be made whether to discontinue nursing or to discontinue the drug, taking into account the importance of the drug to the mother (see **WARNINGS**).

Pediatric Use

Safety and effectiveness in pediatric patients below the age of 12 have not been established (see **WARNINGS**).

Usage in the Elderly

Elderly patients often require lower lithium dosages to achieve therapeutic serum concentrations. They may also exhibit adverse reactions at serum concentrations ordinarily tolerated by younger patients. Additionally, patients with renal impairment may also require lower lithium doses (see **WARNINGS**).

ADVERSE REACTIONS

The occurrence and severity of adverse reactions are generally directly related to serum lithium concentrations and to individual patient sensitivity to lithium. They generally occur more frequently and with greater severity at higher concentrations.

Adverse reactions may be encountered at serum lithium concentrations below 1.5 mEq/L. Mild to moderate adverse reactions may occur at concentrations from 1.5–2.5 mEq/L, and moderate to severe reactions may be seen at concentrations from 2.0 mEq/L and above.

Fine hand tremor, polyuria and mild thirst may occur during initial therapy for the acute manic phase and may persist throughout treatment. Transient and mild nausea and general discomfort may also appear during the first few days of lithium administration.

These side effects usually subside with continued treatment or with a temporary reduction or cessation of dosage. If persistent, a cessation of lithium therapy may be required. Diarrhea, vomiting, drowsiness, muscular weakness and lack of coordination may be early signs of lithium intoxication, and can occur at lithium concentrations below 2.0 mEq/L. At higher concentrations giddiness, ataxia, blurred vision, tinnitus and a large output of dilute urine may be seen. Serum lithium concentrations above 3.0 mEq/L may produce a complex clinical picture involving multiple organs and organ systems. Serum lithium concentrations should not be permitted to exceed 2.0 mEq/L during the acute treatment phase.

The following reactions have been reported and appear to be related to serum lithium concentrations, including concentrations within the therapeutic range:

Central Nervous System: tremor, muscle hyperirritability (fasiculations, twitching, clonic movements of whole limbs), hypertonicity, ataxia, choreoathetotic movements, hyperactive deep tendon reflex, extrapyramidal symptoms including acute dystonia, cogwheel rigidity, blackout spells, epileptiform seizures, slurred speech, dizziness, vertigo, downbeat nystagmus, incontinence of urine or feces, somnolence, psychomotor retardation, restlessness, confusion, stupor, coma, tongue movements, tics, tinnitus, hallucinations, poor memory, slowed intellectual functioning, startled response, worsening of organic brain syndromes. Cases of Pseudotumor Cerebri (increased intracranial pressure and papilledema) have been reported with lithium use. If undetected, this condition may result in enlargement of the blind spot, constriction of visual fields and eventual blindness due to optic atrophy. Lithium should be discontinued, if clinically possible, if this syndrome occurs. **Cardiovascular**: cardiac arrhythmia, hypotension, peripheral circulatory collapse, bradycardia, sinus node dysfunction with severe bradycardia (which may result in syncope); **Gastrointestinal**: anorexia, nausea, vomiting, diarrhea, gastritis, salivary gland swelling, abdominal pain, excessive salivation, flatulence, indigestion; **Genitourinary**: glycosuria, decreased creatinine clearance, albuminuria, oliguria, and symptoms of nephrogenic diabetes insipidus including polyuria, thirst and polydipsia; **Dermatologic**: drying and thinning of hair, alopecia, anesthesia of skin, acne, chronic folliculitis, xerosis cutis, psoriasis or its exacerbation, generalized pruritus with or without rash, cutaneous ulcers, angioedema; **Autonomic Nervous System**: blurred vision, dry mouth, impotence/sexual dysfunction; **Thyroid Abnormalities**: euthyroid goiter and/or hypothyroidism (including myxedema) accompanied by lower T_3 and T_4. ^{131}Iodine uptake may be elevated (see **PRECAUTIONS**). Paradoxically, rare cases of hyperthyroidism have been reported. **EEG Changes**: diffuse slowing, widening of frequency spectrum, potentiation and disorganization of background rhythm. **EKG Changes**: reversible flattening, isoelectricity or inversion of T-waves. **Miscellaneous**: Fatigue, lethargy, transient scotomata, exophthalmos, dehydration, weight loss, leucocytosis, headache, transient hyperglycemia, hypercalcemia, hyperparathyroidism, albuminuria, excessive weight gain, edematous swelling of ankles or wrists, metallic taste, dysgeusia/taste distortion, salty taste, thirst, swollen lips, tightness in chest, swollen and/or painful joints, fever, polyarthralgia, and dental caries.

Some reports of nephrogenic diabetes insipidus, hyperparathyroidism and hypothyroidism which persist after lithium discontinuation have been received.

A few reports have been received of the development of painful discoloration of fingers and toes and coldness of the extremities within one day of starting lithium treatment. The mechanism through which these symptoms (resembling Raynaud's Syndrome) developed is not known. Recovery followed discontinuance.

DOSAGE AND ADMINISTRATION

Acute Mania

Optimal patient response can usually be established with 1800 mg/day in the following dosages:

ACUTE MANIA

	Morning	Afternoon	Nighttime
LITHOBID® Slow-Release Tablets[1]	3 tabs (900 mg)		3 tabs (900 mg)

[1] Can also be administered on 600 mg t.i.d. recommended dosing interval.

Such doses will normally produce an effective serum lithium concentration ranging between 1.0 and 1.5 mEq/L. Dosage must be individualized according to serum concentrations and clinical response. Regular monitoring of the patient's clinical state and of serum lithium concentrations is necessary. Serum concentrations should be determined twice per week during the acute phase, and until the serum concentrations and clinical condition of the patient have been stabilized.

Long-Term Control
Desirable serum lithium concentrations are 0.6 to 1.2 mEq/L which can usually be achieved with 900–1200 mg/day. Dosage will vary from one individual to another, but generally the following dosages will maintain this concentration.

LONG TERM			
	Morning	Afternoon	Nighttime
LITHOBID® Slow-Release Tablets[1]	2 tabs (600 mg)		2 tabs (600 mg)

[1] Can be administered on t.i.d. recommended dosing interval up to 1200 mg/day.

Serum lithium concentrations in uncomplicated cases receiving maintenance therapy during remission should be monitored at least every two months. Patients abnormally sensitive to lithium may exhibit toxic signs at serum concentrations of 1.0 to 1.5 mEq/L. Elderly patients often respond to reduced dosage, and may exhibit signs of toxicity at serum concentrations ordinarily tolerated by other patients.

N.B.: Blood samples for serum lithium determinations should be drawn immediately prior to the next dose when lithium concentrations are relatively stable (i.e., 8–12 hours after previous dose). Total reliance must not be placed on serum concentrations alone. Accurate patient evaluation requires both clinical and laboratory analysis. LITHOBID® Slow-Release Tablets must be swallowed whole and never chewed or crushed.

OVERDOSAGE

The toxic concentrations for lithium (≥1.5 mEq/L) are close to the therapeutic concentrations (0.6–1.2 mEq/L). It is therefore important that patients and their families be cautioned to watch for early toxic symptoms and to discontinue the drug and inform the physician should they occur. (Toxic symptoms are listed in detail under **ADVERSE REACTIONS**.)

Treatment
No specific antidote for lithium poisoning is known. Treatment is supportive. Early symptoms of lithium toxicity can usually be treated by reduction or cessation of dosage of the drug and resumption of the treatment at a lower dose after 24 to 48 hours. In severe cases of lithium poisoning, the first and foremost goal of treatment consists of elimination of this ion from the patient.
Treatment is essentially the same as that used in barbiturate poisoning: 1) gastric lavage, 2) correction of fluid and electrolyte imbalance and, 3) regulation of kidney functioning. Urea, mannitol, and aminophylline all produce significant increases in lithium excretion. Hemodialysis is an effective and rapid means of removing the ion from the severely toxic patient. However, patient recovery may be slow. Infection prophylaxis, regular chest X-rays, and preservation of adequate respiration are essential.

HOW SUPPLIED

LITHOBID® (Lithium Carbonate, USP) Slow-Release Tablets, 300 mg, peach-colored imprinted "SOLVAY 4492"
Bottles of 100
NDC 0032-4492-01
Bottles of 1000
NDC 0032-4492-10
Store between 59°–86°F (15°–30°C). Protect from moisture. Dispense in tight, child-resistant container (USP).
℞ only
Solvay Pharmaceuticals, Inc.
Marietta, GA 30062
0990
7E Rev 7/99

Shown in Product Identification Guide, page 338

LUVOX® ℞
[lū-vŏx]
(Fluvoxamine Maleate) Tablets
25 mg, 50 mg and 100 mg

DESCRIPTION

Fluvoxamine maleate is a selective serotonin (5-HT) reuptake inhibitor (SSRI) belonging to a new chemical series, the 2-aminoethyl oxime ethers of aralkylketones. It is chemically unrelated to other SSRIs and clomipramine. It is chemically designated as 5-methoxy-4′-(trifluoromethyl)valerophenone-(E)-O-(2-aminoethyl)oxime maleate (1:1) and has the empirical formula $C_{15}H_{21}O_2N_2F_3 \bullet C_4H_4O_4$. Its molecular weight is 434.4.
The structural formula is:

F_3C-[benzene ring]-C(=N-O-CH_2-CH_2-NH_2)-CH_2-CH_2-CH_2-CH_2-O-CH_3 • HCCOOH ‖ HCCOOH

Fluvoxamine maleate is a white or off white, odorless, crystalline powder which is sparingly soluble in water, freely soluble in ethanol and chloroform and practically insoluble in diethyl ether.
LUVOX® (Fluvoxamine Maleate) Tablets are available in 25 mg, 50 mg and 100 mg strengths for oral administration. In addition to the active ingredient, fluvoxamine maleate, each tablet contains the following inactive ingredients: carnauba wax, hydroxypropyl methylcellulose, mannitol, polyethylene glycol, polysorbate 80, pregelatinized starch (potato), silicon dioxide, sodium stearyl fumarate, starch (corn), and titanium dioxide. The 50 mg and 100 mg tablets also contain synthetic iron oxides.

CLINICAL PHARMACOLOGY

Pharmacodynamics
The mechanism of action of fluvoxamine maleate in Obsessive Compulsive Disorder is presumed to be linked to its specific serotonin reuptake inhibition in brain neurons. In preclinical studies, it was found that fluvoxamine inhibited neuronal uptake of serotonin.
In *in vitro* studies fluvoxamine maleate had no significant affinity for histaminergic, alpha or beta adrenergic, muscarinic, or dopaminergic receptors. Antagonism of some of these receptors is thought to be associated with various sedative, cardiovascular, anticholinergic, and extrapyramidal effects of some psychotropic drugs.

Pharmacokinetics
Bioavailability: The absolute bioavailability of fluvoxamine maleate is 53%. Oral bioavailability is not significantly affected by food.
In a dose proportionality study involving fluvoxamine maleate at 100, 200 and 300 mg/day for 10 consecutive days in 30 normal volunteers, steady state was achieved after about a week of dosing. Maximum plasma concentrations at steady state occurred within 3–8 hours of dosing and reached concentrations averaging 88, 283 and 546 ng/mL, respectively. Thus, fluvoxamine had nonlinear pharmacokinetics over this dose range, i.e., higher doses of fluvoxamine maleate produced disproportionately higher concentrations than predicted from the lower dose.
Distribution/Protein Binding: The mean apparent volume of distribution for fluvoxamine is approximately 25 L/kg, suggesting extensive tissue distribution.
Approximately 80% of fluvoxamine is bound to plasma protein, mostly albumin, over a concentration range of 20 to 2000 ng/mL.
Metabolism: Fluvoxamine maleate is extensively metabolized by the liver; the main metabolic routes are oxidative demethylation and deamination. Nine metabolites were identified following a 5 mg radiolabelled dose of fluvoxamine maleate, constituting approximately 85% of the urinary excretion products of fluvoxamine. The main human metabolite was fluvoxamine acid which, together with its N-acetylated analog, accounted for about 60% of the urinary excretion products. A third metabolite, fluvoxethanol, formed by oxidative deamination, accounted for about 10%. Fluvoxamine acid and fluvoxethanol were tested in an *in vitro* assay of serotonin and norepinephrine reuptake inhibition in rats; they were inactive except for a weak effect of the former metabolite on inhibition of serotonin uptake (1–2 orders of magnitude less potent than the parent compound). Approximately 2% of fluvoxamine was excreted in urine unchanged. (See **PRECAUTIONS—Drug Interactions**)
Elimination: Following a ^{14}C-labelled oral dose of fluvoxamine maleate (5 mg), an average of 94% of drug-related products was recovered in the urine within 71 hours.
The mean plasma half-life of fluvoxamine at steady state after multiple oral doses of 100 mg/day in healthy, young volunteers was 15.6 hours.
Elderly Subjects: In a study of LUVOX® Tablets at 50 and 100 mg comparing elderly (ages 66–73) and young subjects (ages 19–35), mean maximum plasma concentrations in the elderly were 40% higher. The multiple dose elimination half-life of fluvoxamine was 17.4 and 25.9 hours in the elderly compared to 13.6 and 15.6 hours in the young subjects at steady state for 50 and 100 mg doses, respectively.
In elderly patients, the clearance of fluvoxamine was reduced by about 50% and, therefore, LUVOX® Tablets should be slowly titrated during initiation of therapy.
Hepatic and Renal Disease: A cross study comparison (healthy subjects vs. patients with hepatic dysfunction) suggested a 30% decrease in fluvoxamine clearance in association with hepatic dysfunction. The mean minimum plasma concentrations in renally impaired patients (creatinine clearance of 5 to 45 mL/min) after 4 and 6 weeks of treatment (50 mg bid, N=13) were comparable to each other, suggesting no accumulation of fluvoxamine in these patients. (See **PRECAUTIONS—*Use in Patients with Concomitant Illness***)

Clinical Trials
Adult OCD Studies: The effectiveness of LUVOX® Tablets for the treatment of Obsessive Compulsive Disorder (OCD) was demonstrated in two 10-week multicenter, parallel group studies of adult outpatients. Patients in these trials were titrated to a total daily fluvoxamine maleate dose of 150 mg/day over the first two weeks of the trial, following which the dose was adjusted within a range of 100–300 mg/day (on a bid schedule), on the basis of response and tolerance. Patients in these studies had moderate to severe OCD (DSM-III-R), with mean baseline ratings on the Yale-Brown Obsessive Compulsive Scale (Y-BOCS), total score of 23. Patients receiving fluvoxamine maleate experienced mean reductions of approximately 4 to 5 units on the Y-BOCS total score, compared to a 2 unit reduction for placebo patients.
The following table provides the outcome classification by treatment group on the Global Improvement item of the Clinical Global Impressions (CGI) scale for both studies combined.

OUTCOME CLASSIFICATION (%) ON CGI-GLOBAL IMPROVEMENT ITEM FOR COMPLETERS IN POOL OF TWO ADULT OCD STUDIES

Outcome Classification	Fluvoxamine (N = 120)	Placebo (N = 134)
Very Much Improved	13%	2%
Much Improved	30%	10%
Minimally Improved	22%	32%
No Change	31%	51%
Worse	4%	6%

Exploratory analyses for age and gender effects on outcomes did not suggest any differential responsiveness on the basis of age or sex.
Pediatric OCD Study: The effectiveness of LUVOX® Tablets for the treatment of OCD was also demonstrated in a 10-week multicenter, parallel group study in a pediatric outpatient population (children and adolescents, ages 8–17). Patients in this study were titrated to a total daily fluvoxamine dose of approximately 100 mg/day over the first two weeks of the trial, following which the dose was adjusted within a range of 50–200 mg/day (on a bid schedule) on the basis of response and tolerance. Patients in these studies had moderate to severe OCD (DSM-III-R) with mean baseline ratings on the Children's Yale-Brown Obsessive Compulsive Scale (CY-BOCS), total score of 24. Patients receiving fluvoxamine maleate experienced mean reductions of approximately 6 units on the CY-BOCS total score, compared to a 3 unit reduction for placebo patients.
The following table provides the outcome classification by treatment group on the Global Improvement item of the Clinical Global Impression (CGI) scale for the pediatric study.

OUTCOME CLASSIFICATION (%) ON CGI-GLOBAL IMPROVEMENT ITEM FOR COMPLETERS IN PEDIATRIC STUDY

Outcome Classification	Fluvoxamine (N = 38)	Placebo (N = 36)
Very Much Improved	21%	11%
Much Improved	18%	17%
Minimally Improved	37%	22%
No Change	16%	44%
Worse	8%	6%

Post hoc exploratory analyses for gender effects on outcomes did not suggest any differential responsiveness on the basis of gender. Further exploratory analyses revealed a prominent treatment effect in the 8–11 age group and essentially no effect in the 12–17 age group. The significance of these results is not known at this time.

INDICATIONS AND USAGE

LUVOX® Tablets are indicated for the treatment of obsessions and compulsions in patients with Obsessive Compulsive Disorder (OCD), as defined in the DSM-III-R. The obsessions or compulsions cause marked distress, are time-consuming, or significantly interfere with social or occupational functioning.
The efficacy of LUVOX® Tablets was established in three 10-week trials with obsessive compulsive outpatients with the diagnosis of Obsessive Compulsive Disorder as defined in DSM-III-R. (See **Clinical Trials** under **CLINICAL PHARMACOLOGY.**)
Obsessive Compulsive Disorder is characterized by recurrent and persistent ideas, thoughts, impulses or images (obsessions) that are ego-dystonic and/or repetitive, purposeful, and intentional behaviors (compulsions) that are recognized by the person as excessive or unreasonable.
The effectiveness of LUVOX® Tablets for long-term use, i.e., for more than 10 weeks, has not been systematically evaluated in placebo-controlled trials. Therefore, the physician who elects to use LUVOX® Tablets for extended periods should periodically re-evaluate the long-term usefulness of the drug for the individual patient. (See **DOSAGE AND ADMINISTRATION**)

CONTRAINDICATIONS

Co-administration of terfenadine, astemizole, cisapride, or pimozide with LUVOX® Tablets is contraindicated (see **WARNINGS** and **PRECAUTIONS**).
LUVOX® Tablets are contraindicated in patients with a history of hypersensitivity to fluvoxamine maleate.

Continued on next page

Luvox—Cont.

WARNINGS

Potential for Interaction with Monoamine Oxidase Inhibitors

In patients receiving another serotonin reuptake inhibitor drug in combination with monoamine oxidase inhibitors (MAOI), there have been reports of serious, sometimes fatal, reactions including hyperthermia, rigidity, myoclonus, autonomic instability with possible rapid fluctuations of vital signs, and mental status changes that include extreme agitation progressing to delirium and coma. These reactions have also been reported in patients who have discontinued that drug and have been started on a MAOI. Some cases presented with features resembling neuroleptic malignant syndrome. Therefore, it is recommended that LUVOX® Tablets not be used in combination with a MAOI, or within 14 days of discontinuing treatment with a MAOI. After stopping LUVOX® Tablets, at least 2 weeks should be allowed before starting a MAOI.

Potential Terfenadine, Astemizole, Cisapride, and Pimozide Interactions

Terfenadine, astemizole, cisapride, and pimozide are all metabolized by the cytochrome P450IIIA4 isozyme, and it has been demonstrated that ketoconazole, a potent inhibitor of IIIA4, blocks the metabolism of these drugs, resulting in increased plasma concentrations of parent drug. Increased plasma concentrations of terfenadine, astemizole, cisapride, and pimozide cause QT prolongation and have been associated with torsades de pointes-type ventricular tachycardia, sometimes fatal. As noted below, a substantial pharmacokinetic interaction has been observed for fluvoxamine in combination with alprazolam, a drug that is known to be metabolized by the IIIA4 isozyme. Although it has not been definitively demonstrated that fluvoxamine is a potent IIIA4 inhibitor, it is likely to be, given the substantial interaction of fluvoxamine with alprazolam. Consequently, it is recommended that fluvoxamine not be used in combination with either terfenadine, astemizole, cisapride, or pimozide (see CONTRAINDICATIONS and PRECAUTIONS).

Other Potentially Important Drug Interactions

(Also see **PRECAUTIONS—Drug Interactions**)

Benzodiazepines: Benzodiazepines metabolized by hepatic oxidation (e.g., alprazolam, midazolam, triazolam, etc.) should be used with caution because the clearance of these drugs is likely to be reduced by fluvoxamine. The clearance of benzodiazepines metabolized by glucuronidation (e.g., lorazepam, oxazepam, temazepam) is unlikely to be affected by fluvoxamine.

Alprazolam—When fluvoxamine maleate (100 mg qd) and alprazolam (1 mg qid) were co-administered to steady state, plasma concentrations and other pharmacokinetic parameters (AUC, C_{max}, $T_{½}$) of alprazolam were approximately twice those observed when alprazolam was administered alone; oral clearance was reduced by about 50%. The elevated plasma alprazolam concentrations resulted in decreased psychomotor performance and memory. This interaction, which has not been investigated using higher doses of fluvoxamine, may be more pronounced if a 300 mg daily dose is co-administered, particularly since fluvoxamine exhibits non-linear pharmacokinetics over the dosage range 100–300 mg. If alprazolam is co-administered with LUVOX® Tablets, the initial alprazolam dosage should be at least halved and titration to the lowest effective dose is recommended. No dosage adjustment is required for LUVOX® Tablets.

Diazepam—The co-administration of LUVOX® Tablets and diazepam is generally not advisable. Because fluvoxamine reduces the clearance of both diazepam and its active metabolite, N-desmethyldiazepam, there is a strong likelihood of substantial accumulation of both species during chronic co-administration.

Evidence supporting the conclusion that it is inadvisable to co-administer fluvoxamine and diazepam is derived from a study in which healthy volunteers taking 150 mg/day of fluvoxamine were administered a single oral dose of 10 mg of diazepam. In these subjects (N=8), the clearance of diazepam was reduced by 65% and that of N-desmethyldiazepam to a level that was too low to measure over the course of the 2 week long study.

It is likely that this experience significantly underestimates the degree of accumulation that might occur with repeated diazepam administration. Moreover, as noted with alprazolam, the effect of fluvoxamine may even be more pronounced when it is administered at higher doses.

Accordingly, diazepam and fluvoxamine should not ordinarily be co-administered.

Theophylline: The effect of steady-state fluvoxamine (50 mg bid) on the pharmacokinetics of a single dose of theophylline (375 mg as 442 mg aminophylline) was evaluated in 12 healthy non-smoking, male volunteers. The clearance of theophylline was decreased approximately three-fold. Therefore, if theophylline is co-administered with fluvoxamine maleate, its dose should be reduced to one third of the usual daily maintenance dose and plasma concentrations of theophylline should be monitored. No dosage adjustment is required for LUVOX® Tablets.

Warfarin: When fluvoxamine maleate (50 mg tid) was administered concomitantly with warfarin for two weeks, warfarin plasma concentrations increased by 98% and prothrombin times were prolonged. Thus patients receiving oral anticoagulants and LUVOX® Tablets should have their prothrombin time monitored and their anticoagulant dose adjusted accordingly. No dosage adjustment is required for LUVOX® Tablets.

PRECAUTIONS

General

Activation of Mania/Hypomania: During premarketing studies involving primarily depressed patients, hypomania or mania occurred in approximately 1% of patients treated with fluvoxamine. In a ten week pediatric OCD study, 2 out of 57 patients (4%) treated with fluvoxamine experienced manic reactions, compared to none of 63 placebo patients. Activation of mania/hypomania has also been reported in a small proportion of patients with major affective disorder who were treated with other marketed antidepressants. As with all antidepressants, LUVOX® Tablets should be used cautiously in patients with a history of mania.

Seizures: During premarketing studies, seizures were reported in 0.2% of fluvoxamine-treated patients. LUVOX® Tablets should be used cautiously in patients with a history of seizures. It should be discontinued in any patient who develops seizures.

Suicide: The possibility of a suicide attempt is inherent in patients with depressive symptoms, whether these occur in primary depression or in association with another primary disorder such as OCD. Close supervision of high risk patients should accompany initial drug therapy. Prescriptions for LUVOX® Tablets should be written for the smallest quantity of tablets consistent with good patient management in order to reduce the risk of overdose.

Hyponatremia: Several cases of hyponatremia have been reported. In cases where the outcome was known, the hyponatremia appeared to be reversible when fluvoxamine was discontinued. The majority of these occurrences have been in elderly individuals, some in patients taking diuretics or with concomitant conditions that might cause hyponatremia. In patients receiving LUVOX® Tablets and suffering from Syndrome of Inappropriate Secretion of Antidiuretic Hormone (SIADH), displacement syndromes, edematous states, adrenal disease or conditions of fluid loss, it is recommended that serum electrolytes, especially sodium as well as BUN and plasma creatinine, be monitored regularly.

Use in Patients with Concomitant Illness: Closely monitored clinical experience with LUVOX® Tablets in patients with concomitant systemic illness is limited. Caution is advised in administering LUVOX® Tablets to patients with diseases or conditions that could affect hemodynamic responses or metabolism.

LUVOX® Tablets have not been evaluated or used to any appreciable extent in patients with a recent history of myocardial infarction or unstable heart disease. Patients with these diagnoses were systematically excluded from many clinical studies during the product's premarketing testing. Evaluation of the electrocardiograms for patients with depression or OCD who participated in premarketing studies revealed no differences between fluvoxamine and placebo in the emergence of clinically important ECG changes.

In patients with liver dysfunction, fluvoxamine clearance was decreased by approximately 30%. LUVOX® Tablets should be slowly titrated in patients with liver dysfunction during the initiation of treatment.

Information for Patients

Physicians are advised to discuss the following issues with patients for whom they prescribe LUVOX® Tablets:

Interference with Cognitive or Motor Performance: Since any psychoactive drug may impair judgement, thinking, or motor skills, patients should be cautioned about operating hazardous machinery, including automobiles, until they are certain that LUVOX® Tablets therapy does not adversely affect their ability to engage in such activities.

Pregnancy: Patients should be advised to notify their physicians if they become pregnant or intend to become pregnant during therapy with LUVOX® Tablets.

Nursing: Patients receiving LUVOX® Tablets should be advised to notify their physicians if they are breast feeding an infant. (See **PRECAUTIONS—Nursing Mothers**)

Concomitant Medication: Patients should be advised to notify their physicians if they are taking, or plan to take, any prescription or over-the-counter drugs, since there is a potential for clinically important interactions with LUVOX® Tablets.

Alcohol: As with other psychotropic medications, patients should be advised to avoid alcohol while taking LUVOX® Tablets.

Allergic Reactions: Patients should be advised to notify their physicians if they develop a rash, hives, or a related allergic phenomenon during therapy with LUVOX® Tablets.

Laboratory Tests

There are no specific laboratory tests recommended.

Drug Interactions

Potential Interactions with Drugs that Inhibit or are Metabolized by Cytochrome P450 Isozymes: Multiple hepatic cytochrome P450 (CYP450) enzymes are involved in the oxidative biotransformation of a large number of structurally different drugs and endogenous compounds. The available knowledge concerning the relationship of fluvoxamine and the CYP450 enzyme system has been obtained mostly from pharmacokinetic interaction studies conducted in healthy volunteers, but some preliminary *in vitro* data are also available. Based on a finding of substantial interactions of fluvoxamine with certain of these drugs (see later parts of this section and also **WARNINGS** for details) and limited *in vitro* data for the IIIA4 isozyme, it appears that fluvoxamine inhibits the following isozymes that are known to be involved in the metabolism of the listed drugs:

IA2	IIC9	IIIA4
Warfarin	Warfarin	Alprazolam
Theophylline		
Propranolol		

In vitro data suggest that fluvoxamine is a relatively weak inhibitor of the IID6 isozyme.

Approximately 7% of the normal population has a genetic defect that leads to reduced levels of activity of cytochrome P450IID6 isozyme. Such individuals have been referred to as "poor metabolizers" (PM) of drugs such as debrisoquin, dextromethorphan, and tricyclic antidepressants. While none of the drugs studied for drug interactions significantly affected the pharmacokinetics of fluvoxamine, an *in vivo* study of fluvoxamine single-dose pharmacokinetics in 13 PM subjects demonstrated altered pharmacokinetic properties compared to 16 "extensive metabolizers" (EM): mean Cmax, AUC, and half-life were increased by 52%, 200%, and 62%, respectively, in the PM compared to the EM group. This suggests that fluvoxamine is metabolized, at least in part, by IID6 isozyme. Caution is indicated in patients known to have reduced levels of P450IID6 activity and those receiving concomitant drugs known to inhibit this isozyme (e.g. quinidine).

The metabolism of fluvoxamine has not been fully characterized and the effects of potent P450 isozyme inhibition, such as the ketoconazole inhibition of IIIA4, on fluvoxamine metabolism have not been studied.

A clinically significant fluvoxamine interaction is possible with drugs having a narrow therapeutic ratio such as terfenadine, astemizole, cisapride, or pimozide, warfarin, theophylline, certain benzodiazepines and phenytoin. If LUVOX® Tablets are to be administered together with a drug that is eliminated via oxidative metabolism and has a narrow therapeutic window, plasma levels and/or pharmacodynamic effects of the latter drug should be monitored closely, at least until steady-state conditions are reached (See **CONTRAINDICATIONS** and **WARNINGS**).

CNS Active Drugs:

Monoamine Oxidase Inhibitors: See **WARNINGS**

Alprazolam: See **WARNINGS**

Diazepam: See **WARNINGS**

Alcohol: Studies involving single 40 g doses of ethanol (oral administration in one study and intravenous in the other) and multiple dosing with fluvoxamine maleate (50 mg bid) revealed no effect of either drug on the pharmacokinetics or pharmacodynamics of the other.

Carbamazepine: Elevated carbamazepine levels and symptoms of toxicity have been reported with the co-administration of fluvoxamine maleate and carbamazepine.

Clozapine: Elevated serum levels of clozapine have been reported in patients taking fluvoxamine maleate and clozapine. Since clozapine related seizures and orthostatic hypotension appear to be dose related, the risk of these adverse events may be higher when fluvoxamine and clozapine are co-administered. Patients should be closely monitored when fluvoxamine maleate and clozapine are used concurrently.

Lithium: As with other serotonergic drugs, lithium may enhance the serotonergic effects of fluvoxamine and, therefore, the combination should be used with caution. Seizures have been reported with the co-administration of fluvoxamine maleate and lithium.

Lorazepam: A study of multiple doses of fluvoxamine maleate (50 mg bid) in healthy male volunteers (N=12) and a single dose of lorazepam (4 mg single dose) indicated no significant pharmacokinetic interaction. On average, both lorazepam alone and lorazepam with fluvoxamine produced substantial decrements in cognitive functioning; however, the co-administration of fluvoxamine and lorazepam did not produce larger mean decrements compared to lorazepam alone.

Methadone: Significantly increased methadone (plasma level:dose) ratios have been reported when fluvoxamine maleate was administered to patients receiving maintenance methadone treatment, with symptoms of opioid intoxication in one patient. Opioid withdrawal symptoms were reported following fluvoxamine maleate discontinuation in another patient.

Sumatriptan: There have been rare postmarketing reports describing patients with weakness, hyperreflexia, and incoordination following the use of a selective serotonin reuptake inhibitor (SSRI) and sumatriptan. If concomitant treatment with sumatriptan and an SSRI (e.g., fluoxetine, fluvoxamine, paroxetine, sertraline) is clinically warranted, appropriate observation of the patient is advised.

Tacrine: In a study of 13 healthy, male volunteers, a single 40 mg dose of tacrine added to fluvoxamine 100 mg/day administered at steady-state was associated with five- and eight-fold increases in tacrine Cmax and AUC, respectively, compared to the administration of tacrine alone. Five subjects experienced nausea, vomiting, sweating, and diarrhea following co-administration, consistent with the cholinergic effects of tacrine.

Tricyclic Antidepressants (TCAs): Significantly increased plasma TCA levels have been reported with the co-administration of fluvoxamine maleate and amitriptyline, clomipramine or imipramine. Caution is indicated with the coadministration of LUVOX® Tablets and TCAs; plasma TCA concentrations may need to be monitored, and the dose of TCA may need to be reduced.

Tryptophan: Tryptophan may enhance the serotonergic effects of fluvoxamine, and the combination should, therefore, be used with caution. Severe vomiting has been reported with the co-administration of fluvoxamine maleate and tryptophan.

Other Drugs:

Theophylline: See **WARNINGS**

Warfarin: See **WARNINGS**

Digoxin: Administration of fluvoxamine maleate 100 mg daily for 18 days (N=8) did not significantly affect the pharmacokinetics of a 1.25 mg single intravenous dose of digoxin.

Diltiazem: Bradycardia has been reported with the co-administration of fluvoxamine maleate and diltiazem.

Propranolol and Other Beta-Blockers: Co-administration of fluvoxamine maleate 100 mg per day and propranolol 160 mg per day in normal volunteers resulted in a mean five-fold increase (range 2 to 17) in minimum propranolol plasma concentrations. In this study, there was a slight potentiation of the propranolol-induced reduction in heart rate and reduction in the exercise diastolic pressure.

One case of bradycardia and hypotension and a second case of orthostatic hypotension have been reported with the co-administration of fluvoxamine maleate and metoprolol.

If propranolol or metoprolol is co-administered with LUVOX® Tablets, a reduction in the initial beta-blocker dose and more cautious dose titration are recommended. No dosage adjustment is required for LUVOX® Tablets.

Co-administration of fluvoxamine maleate 100 mg per day with atenolol 100 mg per day (N=6) did not affect the plasma concentrations of atenolol. Unlike propranolol and metoprolol which undergo hepatic metabolism, atenolol is eliminated primarily by renal excretion.

Effects of Smoking on Fluvoxamine Metabolism: Smokers had a 25% increase in the metabolism of fluvoxamine compared to nonsmokers.

Electroconvulsive Therapy (ECT): There are no clinical studies establishing the benefits or risks of combined use of ECT and fluvoxamine maleate.

Carcinogenesis, Mutagenesis, Impairment of Fertility

Carcinogenesis: There is no evidence of carcinogenicity, mutagenicity or impairment of fertility with fluvoxamine maleate.

There was no evidence of carcinogenicity in rats treated orally with fluvoxamine maleate for 30 months or hamsters treated orally with fluvoxamine maleate for 20 (females) or 26 (males) months. The daily doses in the high dose groups in these studies were increased over the course of the study from a minimum of 160 mg/kg to a maximum of 240 mg/kg in rats, and from a minimum of 135 mg/kg to a maximum of 240 mg/kg in hamsters. The maximum dose of 240 mg/kg is approximately 6 times the maximum human daily dose on a mg/m^2 basis.

Mutagenesis: No evidence of mutagenic potential was observed in a mouse micronucleus test, an *in vitro* chromosome aberration test, or the Ames microbial mutagen test with or without metabolic activation.

Impairment of Fertility: In fertility studies of male and female rats, up to 80 mg/kg/day orally of fluvoxamine maleate (approximately 2 times the maximum human daily dose on a mg/m^2 basis) had no effect on mating performance, duration of gestation, or pregnancy rate.

Pregnancy

Teratogenic Effects—Pregnancy Category C: In teratology studies in rats and rabbits, daily oral doses of fluvoxamine maleate of up to 80 and 40 mg/kg, respectively (approximately 2 times the maximum human daily dose on a mg/m^2 basis) caused no fetal malformations. However, in other reproduction studies in which pregnant rats were dosed through weaning there was (1) an increase in pup mortality at birth (seen at 80 mg/kg and above but not at 20 mg/kg), and (2) decreases in postnatal pup weights (seen at 160 but not at 80 mg/kg) and survival (seen at all doses; lowest dose tested = 5 mg/kg). (Doses of 5, 20, 80, and 160 mg/kg are approximately 0.1, 0.5, 2, and 4 times the maximum human daily dose on a mg/m^2 basis.) While the results of a cross-fostering study implied that at least some of these results likely occurred secondarily to maternal toxicity, the role of a direct drug effect on the fetuses or pups could not be ruled out. There are no adequate and well-controlled studies in pregnant women. Fluvoxamine maleate should be used during pregnancy only if the potential benefit justifies the potential risk to the fetus.

Labor and Delivery

The effect of fluvoxamine on labor and delivery in humans is unknown.

Nursing Mothers

As for many other drugs, fluvoxamine is secreted in human breast milk. The decision of whether to discontinue nursing or to discontinue the drug should take into account the potential for serious adverse effects from exposure to fluvoxamine in the nursing infant as well as the potential benefits of LUVOX® (Fluvoxamine Maleate) Tablets therapy to the mother.

Pediatric Use

The efficacy of fluvoxamine maleate for the treatment of Obsessive Compulsive Disorder was demonstrated in a 10-week multicenter placebo controlled study with 120 outpatients ages 8–17. The adverse event profile observed in that study was generally similar to that observed in adult studies with fluvoxamine (see **ADVERSE REACTIONS** and **DOSAGE AND ADMINISTRATION**).

Decreased appetite and weight loss have been observed in association with the use of fluvoxamine as well as other SSRIs. Consequently, regular monitoring of weight and growth is recommended if treatment of a child with an SSRI is to be continued long term.

The risks, if any, that may be associated with fluvoxamine's extended use in children and adolescents with OCD have not been systematically assessed. The prescriber should be mindful that the evidence relied upon to conclude that fluvoxamine is safe for use in children and adolescents derives from relatively short term clinical studies and from extrapolation of experience gained with adult patients. In particular, there are no studies that directly evaluate the effects of long term fluvoxamine use on the growth, development, and maturation of children and adolescents. Although there is no affirmative finding to suggest that fluvoxamine possesses a capacity to adversely affect growth, development or maturation, the absence of such findings is not compelling evidence of the absence of the potential of fluvoxamine to have adverse effects in chronic use.

Geriatric Use

Approximately 230 patients participating in controlled premarketing studies with LUVOX® Tablets were 65 years of age or over. No overall differences in safety were observed between these patients and younger patients. Other reported clinical experience has not identified differences in response between the elderly and younger patients. However, fluvoxamine has been associated with several cases of clinically significant hyponatremia in elderly patients (see **PRECAUTIONS, General**). Furthermore, the clearance of fluvoxamine is decreased by about 50% in elderly compared to younger patients (see **Pharmacokinetics** under **CLINICAL PHARMACOLOGY**), and greater sensitivity of some older individuals also cannot be ruled out. Consequently, LUVOX® Tablets should be slowly titrated during initiation of therapy.

ADVERSE REACTIONS

Associated with Discontinuation of Treatment

Of the 1087 OCD and depressed patients treated with fluvoxamine maleate in controlled clinical trials conducted in North America, 22% discontinued treatment due to an adverse event. The most common events (≥1%) associated with discontinuation and considered to be drug related (i.e., those events associated with dropout at a rate at least twice that of placebo) included:

Table 1
ADVERSE EVENTS ASSOCIATED WITH DISCONTINUATION OF TREATMENT IN OCD AND DEPRESSION POPULATIONS

BODY SYSTEM/ ADVERSE EVENT	PERCENTAGE OF PATIENTS FLUVOXAMINE	PLACEBO
BODY AS A WHOLE		
Headache	3%	1%
Asthenia	2%	<1%
Abdominal Pain	1%	0%
DIGESTIVE		
Nausea	9%	1%
Diarrhea	1%	<1%
Vomiting	2%	<1%
Anorexia	1%	<1%
Dyspepsia	1%	<1%
NERVOUS SYSTEM		
Insomnia	4%	1%
Somnolence	4%	<1%
Nervousness	2%	<1%
Agitation	2%	<1%
Dizziness	2%	<1%
Anxiety	1%	<1%
Dry Mouth	1%	<1%

Incidence in Controlled Trials

Commonly Observed Adverse Events in Controlled Clinical Trials:

LUVOX® Tablets have been studied in controlled trials of OCD (N=320) and depression (N=1350). In general, adverse event rates were similar in the two data sets as well as in the pediatric OCD study. The most commonly observed adverse events associated with the use of LUVOX® Tablets and likely to be drug-related (incidence of 5% or greater and at least twice that for placebo) derived from Table 2 were: *somnolence, insomnia, nervousness, tremor, nausea, dyspepsia, anorexia, vomiting, abnormal ejaculation, asthenia, and sweating.* In a pool of two studies involving only patients with OCD, the following additional events were identified using the above rule: *dry mouth, decreased libido, urinary frequency, anorgasmia, rhinitis and taste perversion.* In a study of pediatric patients with OCD, the following additional events were identified using the above rule: *agitation, depression, dysmenorrhea, flatulence, hyperkinesia, and rash.*

Adverse Events Occurring at an Incidence of 1%: Table 2 enumerates adverse events that occurred in adults at a frequency of 1% or more, and were more frequent than in the placebo group, among patients treated with LUVOX® Tablets in two short-term placebo controlled OCD trials (10 week) and depression trials (6 week) in which patients were dosed in a range of generally 100 to 300 mg/day. This table shows the percentage of patients in each group who had at least one occurrence of an event at some time during their treatment. Reported adverse events were classified using a standard COSTART-based Dictionary terminology.

The prescriber should be aware that these figures cannot be used to predict the incidence of side effects in the course of usual medical practice where patient characteristics and other factors may differ from those that prevailed in the clinical trials. Similarly, the cited frequencies cannot be compared with figures obtained from other clinical investigations involving different treatments, uses, and investigators. The cited figures, however, do provide the prescribing physician with some basis for estimating the relative contribution of drug and non-drug factors to the side-effect incidence rate in the population studied.

Table 2
TREATMENT-EMERGENT ADVERSE EVENT INCIDENCE RATES BY BODY SYSTEM IN ADULT OCD AND DEPRESSION POPULATIONS COMBINED[1]

BODY SYSTEM/ ADVERSE EVENT	Percentage of Patients Reporting Event FLUVOXAMINE N=892	PLACEBO N=778
BODY AS WHOLE		
Headache	22	20
Asthenia	14	6
Flu Syndrome	3	2
Chills	2	1
CARDIOVASCULAR		
Palpitations	3	2
DIGESTIVE SYSTEM		
Nausea	40	14
Diarrhea	11	7
Constipation	10	8
Dyspepsia	10	5
Anorexia	6	2
Vomiting	5	2
Flatulence	4	3
Tooth Disorder[2]	3	1
Dysphagia	2	1
NERVOUS SYSTEM		
Somnolence	22	8
Insomnia	21	10
Dry Mouth	14	10
Nervousness	12	5
Dizziness	11	6
Tremor	5	1
Anxiety	5	3
Vasodilation[3]	3	1
Hypertonia	2	1
Agitation	2	1
Decreased Libido	2	1
Depression	2	1
CNS Stimulation	2	1
RESPIRATORY SYSTEM		
Upper Respiratory Infection	9	5
Dyspnea	2	1
Yawn	2	0
SKIN		
Sweating	7	3
SPECIAL SENSES		
Taste Perversion	3	1
Amblyopia[4]	3	2
UROGENITAL		
Abnormal Ejaculation[5,6]	8	1
Urinary Frequency	3	2
Impotence[6]	2	1
Anorgasmia	2	0
Urinary Retention	1	0

1 Events for which fluvoxamine maleate incidence was equal or less than placebo are not listed in the table above, but include the following: abdominal pain, abnormal dreams, appetite increase, back pain, chest pain, confusion, dysmenorrhea, fever, infection, leg cramps, migraine, myalgia, pain, paresthesia, pharyngitis, postural hypotension, pruritus, rash, rhinitis, thirst and tinnitus.

2 Includes "toothache", "tooth extraction and abscess," and "caries."

3 Mostly feeling warm, hot, or flushed.

4 Mostly "blurred vision."

5 Mostly "delayed ejaculation."

6 Incidence based on number of male patients.

Adverse Events in OCD Placebo Controlled Studies Which are Markedly Different (defined as at least a two-fold difference) in Rate from the Pooled Event Rates in OCD and Depression Placebo Controlled Studies: The events in OCD studies with a two-fold decrease in rate compared to event rates in OCD and depression studies were dysphagia and amblyopia (mostly blurred vision). Additionally, there was an approximate 25% decrease in nausea.

The events in OCD studies with a two-fold increase in rate compared to event rates in OCD and depression studies were: *asthenia, abnormal ejaculation (mostly delayed ejaculation), anxiety, infection, rhinitis, anorgasmia (in males), depression, libido decreased, pharyngitis, agitation, impo-*

Continued on next page

Luvox—Cont.

tence, myoclonus/twitch, thirst, weight loss, leg cramps, myalgia and urinary retention. These events are listed in order of decreasing rates in the OCD trials.

Other Adverse Events in OCD Pediatric Population

In pediatric patients (N=57) treated with LUVOX® Tablets, the overall profile of adverse events was generally similar to that seen in adult studies, as shown in Table 2. However, the following adverse events, not appearing in Table 2, were reported in two or more of the pediatric patients and were more frequent with LUVOX® Tablets than with placebo: abnormal thinking, cough increase, dysmenorrhea, ecchymosis, emotional lability, epistaxis, hyperkinesia, infection, manic reaction, rash, sinusitis, and weight decrease.

Vital Sign Changes

Comparisons of fluvoxamine maleate and placebo groups in separate pools of short-term OCD and depression trials on (1) median change from baseline on various vital signs variables and on (2) incidence of patients meeting criteria for potentially important changes from baseline on various vital signs variables revealed no important differences between fluvoxamine maleate and placebo.

Laboratory Changes

Comparisons of fluvoxamine maleate and placebo groups in separate pools of short-term OCD and depression trials on (1) median change from baseline on various serum chemistry, hematology, and urinalysis variables and on (2) incidence of patients meeting criteria for potentially important changes from baseline on various serum chemistry, hematology, and urinalysis variables revealed no important differences between fluvoxamine maleate and placebo.

ECG Changes

Comparisons of fluvoxamine maleate and placebo groups in separate pools of short-term OCD and depression trials on (1) mean change from baseline on various ECG variables and on (2) incidence of patients meeting criteria for potentially important changes from baseline on various ECG variables revealed no important differences between fluvoxamine maleate and placebo.

Other Events Observed During the Premarketing Evaluation of LUVOX® Tablets

During premarketing clinical trials conducted in North America and Europe, multiple doses of fluvoxamine maleate were administered for a combined total of 2737 patient exposures in patients suffering OCD or Major Depressive Disorder. Untoward events associated with this exposure were recorded by clinical investigators using descriptive terminology of their own choosing. Consequently, it is not possible to provide a meaningful estimate of the proportion of individuals experiencing adverse events without first grouping similar types of untoward events into a limited (i.e., reduced) number of standard event categories.

In the tabulations which follow, a standard COSTART-based Dictionary terminology has been used to classify reported adverse events. If the COSTART term for an event was so general as to be uninformative, it was replaced with a more informative term. The frequencies presented, therefore, represent the proportion of the 2737 patient exposures to multiple doses of fluvoxamine maleate who experienced an event of the type cited on at least one occasion while receiving fluvoxamine maleate. All reported events are included in the list below, with the following exceptions: 1) those events already listed in Table 2, which tabulates incidence rates of common adverse experiences in placebo-controlled OCD and depression clinical trials, are excluded; 2) those events for which a drug cause was considered remote (i.e., neoplasia, gastrointestinal carcinoma, herpes simplex, herpes zoster, application site reaction, and unintended pregnancy) are omitted; and 3) events which were reported in only one patient and judged to not be potentially serious are not included. It is important to emphasize that, although the events reported did occur during treatment with fluvoxamine maleate, a causal relationship to fluvoxamine maleate has not been established.

Events are further classified within body system categories and enumerated in order of decreasing frequency using the following definitions: frequent adverse events are defined as those occurring on one or more occasions in at least 1/100 patients; infrequent adverse events are those occurring between 1/100 and 1/1000 patients; and rare adverse events are those occurring in less than 1/1000 patients.

Body as a Whole: *Frequent:* accidental injury, malaise; *Infrequent:* allergic reaction, neck pain, neck rigidity, overdose, photosensitivity reaction, suicide attempt; *Rare:* cyst, pelvic pain, sudden death.

Cardiovascular System: *Frequent:* hypertension, hypotension, syncope, tachycardia; *Infrequent:* angina pectoris, bradycardia, cardiomyopathy, cardiovascular disease, cold extremities, conduction delay, heart failure, myocardial infarction, pallor, pulse irregular, ST segment changes; *Rare:* AV block, cerebrovascular accident, coronary artery disease, embolus, pericarditis, phlebitis, pulmonary infarction, supraventricular extrasystoles.

Digestive System: *Frequent:* elevated liver transaminases; *Infrequent:* colitis, eructation, esophagitis, gastritis, gastroenteritis, gastrointestinal hemorrhage, gastrointestinal ulcer, gingivitis, glossitis, hemorrhoids, melena, rectal hemorrhage, stomatitis; *Rare:* biliary pain, cholecystitis, cholelithiasis, fecal incontinence, hematemesis, intestinal obstruction, jaundice.

Endocrine System: *Infrequent:* hypothyroidism; *Rare:* goiter.

Hemic and Lymphatic Systems: *Infrequent:* anemia, ecchymosis, leukocytosis, lymphadenopathy, thrombocytopenia; *Rare:* leukopenia, purpura.

Metabolic and Nutritional Systems: *Frequent:* edema, weight gain, weight loss; *Infrequent:* dehydration, hypercholesterolemia; *Rare:* diabetes mellitus, hyperglycemia, hyperlipidemia, hypoglycemia, hypokalemia, lactate dehydrogenase increased.

Musculoskeletal System: *Infrequent:* arthralgia, arthritis, bursitis, generalized muscle spasm, myasthenia, tendinous contracture, tenosynovitis; *Rare:* arthrosis, myopathy, pathological fracture.

Nervous System: *Frequent:* amnesia, apathy, hyperkinesia, hypokinesia, manic reaction, myoclonus, psychotic reaction; *Infrequent:* agoraphobia, akathisia, ataxia, CNS depression, convulsion, delirium, delusion, depersonalization, drug dependence, dyskinesia, dystonia, emotional lability, euphoria, extrapyramidal syndrome, gait unsteady, hallucinations, hemiplegia, hostility, hypersomnia, hypochondriasis, hypotonia, hysteria, incoordination, increased salivation, increased libido, neuralgia, paralysis, paranoid reaction, phobia, psychosis, sleep disorder, stupor, twitching, vertigo; *Rare:* akinesia, coma, fibrillations, mutism, obsessions, reflexes decreased, slurred speech, tardive dyskinesia, torticollis, trismus, withdrawal syndrome.

Respiratory System: *Frequent:* cough increased, sinusitis; *Infrequent:* asthma, bronchitis, epistaxis, hoarseness, hyperventilation; *Rare:* apnea, congestion of upper airway, hemoptysis, hiccups, laryngismus, obstructive pulmonary disease, pneumonia.

Skin: *Infrequent:* acne, alopecia, dry skin, eczema, exfoliative dermatitis, furunculosis, seborrhea, skin discoloration, urticaria.

Special Senses: *Infrequent:* accommodation abnormal, conjunctivitis, deafness, diplopia, dry eyes, ear pain, eye pain, mydriasis, otitis media, parosmia, photophobia, taste loss, visual field defect; *Rare:* corneal ulcer, retinal detachment.

Urogenital System: *Infrequent:* anuria, breast pain, cystitis, delayed menstruation[1], dysuria, female lactation[1], hematuria, menopause[1], menorrhagia[1], metrorrhagia[1], nocturia, polyuria, premenstrual syndrome[1], urinary incontinence, urinary tract infection, urinary urgency, urination impaired, vaginal hemorrhage[1], vaginitis[1]; *Rare:* kidney calculus, hematospermia[2], oliguria.

[1]Based on the number of females.

[2]Based on the number of males.

Non-US Postmarketing Reports

Voluntary reports of adverse events in patients taking LUVOX® Tablets that have been received since market introduction and are of unknown causal relationship to LUVOX® Tablets use include: toxic epidermal necrolysis, Stevens-Johnson syndrome, Henoch-Schoenlein purpura, bullous eruption, priapism, agranulocytosis, neuropathy, aplastic anemia, anaphylactic reaction, hyponatremia, acute renal failure, hepatitis, and severe akinesia with fever when fluvoxamine was co-administered with antipsychotic medication.

DRUG ABUSE AND DEPENDENCE

Controlled Substance Class

LUVOX® Tablets are not controlled substances.

Physical and Psychological Dependence

The potential for abuse, tolerance and physical dependence with fluvoxamine maleate has been studied in a nonhuman primate model. No evidence of dependency phenomena was found. The discontinuation effects of LUVOX® Tablets were not systematically evaluated in controlled clinical trials. LUVOX® Tablets were not systematically studied in clinical trials for potential for abuse, but there was no indication of drug-seeking behavior in clinical trials. It should be noted, however, that patients at risk for drug dependency were systematically excluded from investigational studies of fluvoxamine maleate. Generally, it is not possible to predict on the basis of preclinical or premarketing clinical experience the extent to which a CNS active drug will be misused, diverted, and/or abused once marketed. Consequently, physicians should carefully evaluate patients for a history of drug abuse and follow such patients closely, observing them for signs of fluvoxamine maleate misuse or abuse (i.e., development of tolerance, incrementation of dose, drug-seeking behavior).

OVERDOSAGE

Human Experience

Worldwide exposure to fluvoxamine maleate includes over 37,000 patients treated in clinical trials and an estimated exposure of 4,500,000 patients treated during foreign marketing experience (circa 1992). Of the 354 cases of deliberate or accidental overdose involving fluvoxamine maleate reported from this population, there were 19 deaths. Of the 19 deaths, 2 were in patients taking fluvoxamine maleate alone and the remaining 17 were in patients taking fluvoxamine maleate along with other drugs. In the remaining 335 patients, 309 had complete recovery after gastric lavage or symptomatic treatment. One patient had persistent mydriasis after the event, and a second patient had a bowel infarction requiring a hemicolectomy. In the remaining 24 patients the outcome was unknown. The highest reported overdose of fluvoxamine maleate involved a non-lethal ingestion of 10,000 mg (equivalent of 1–3 months' dosage). The patient fully recovered with no sequelae.

Commonly observed adverse events associated with fluvoxamine maleate overdose included drowsiness, vomiting, diarrhea, and dizziness. Other notable signs and symptoms seen with fluvoxamine maleate overdose (single or mixed drugs) included coma, tachycardia, bradycardia, hypotension, ECG abnormalities, liver function abnormalities, convulsions, and symptoms such as aspiration pneumonitis, respiratory difficulties or hypokalemia that may occur secondary to loss of consciousness or vomiting.

Management of Overdose

Treatment should consist of those general measures employed in the management of overdosage with any antidepressant.

Ensure an adequate airway, oxygenation, and ventilation. Monitor cardiac rhythm and vital signs. General supportive and symptomatic measures are also recommended. Induction of emesis is not recommended. Gastric lavage with a large-bore orogastric tube with appropriate airway protection, if needed, may be indicated if performed soon after ingestion, or in symptomatic patients.

Activated charcoal should be administered. Due to the large volume of distribution of this drug, forced diuresis, dialysis, hemoperfusion and exchange transfusion are unlikely to be of benefit. No specific antidotes for fluvoxamine are known.

A specific caution involves patients taking, or recently having taken, fluvoxamine who might ingest excessive quantities of a tricyclic antidepressant. In such a case, accumulation of the parent tricyclic and/or an active metabolite may increase the possibility of clinically significant sequelae and extend the time needed for close medical observation (see Tricyclic Antidepressants (TCAs) under **PRECAUTIONS**).

In managing overdosage, consider the possibility of multiple drug involvement. The physician should consider contacting a poison control center for additional information on the treatment of any overdose. Telephone numbers for certified poison control centers are listed in the *Physicians' Desk Reference* (PDR).

DOSAGE AND ADMINISTRATION

Dosage for Adults

The recommended starting dose for LUVOX® Tablets in adult patients is 50 mg, administered as a single daily dose at bedtime. In the controlled clinical trials establishing the effectiveness of LUVOX® Tablets in OCD, patients were titrated within a dose range of 100 to 300 mg/day. Consequently, the dose should be increased in 50 mg increments every 4 to 7 days, as tolerated, until maximum therapeutic benefit is achieved, not to exceed 300 mg per day. It is advisable that a total daily dose of more than 100 mg should be given in two divided doses. If the doses are not equal, the larger dose should be given at bedtime.

Dosage for Pediatric Population (children and adolescents)

The recommended starting dose for LUVOX® Tablets in pediatric populations (ages 8–17 years) is 25 mg, administered as a single daily dose at bedtime. In a controlled clinical trial establishing the effectiveness of LUVOX® Tablets in OCD, pediatric patients (ages 8–17) were titrated within a dose range of 50 to 200 mg/day. The dose should be increased in 25 mg increments every 4 to 7 days, as tolerated, until maximum therapeutic benefit is achieved, not to exceed 200 mg per day. It is advisable that a total daily dose of more then 50 mg should be given in two divided doses. If the two divided doses are not equal, the larger dose should be given at bedtime.

Dosage for Elderly or Hepatically Impaired Patients

Elderly patients and those with hepatic impairment have been observed to have a decreased clearance of fluvoxamine maleate. Consequently, it may be appropriate to modify the initial dose and the subsequent dose titration for these patient groups.

Maintenance/Continuation Extended Treatment

Although the efficacy of LUVOX® Tablets beyond 10 weeks of dosing for OCD has not been documented in controlled trials, OCD is a chronic condition, and it is reasonable to consider continuation for a responding patient. Dosage adjustments should be made to maintain the patient on the lowest effective dosage, and patients should be periodically reassessed to determine the need for continued treatment.

HOW SUPPLIED

Tablets 25 mg: unscored, white, elliptical, film-coated (debossed "SOLVAY" and "4202" on one side)

Bottles of 100 .... NDC 0032-4202-01
Unit dose pack of 100 .... NDC 0032-4202-11

Tablets 50 mg: scored, yellow, elliptical, film-coated (debossed "SOLVAY" and "4205" on one side and scored on the other)

Bottles of 100 .... NDC 0032-4205-01
Bottles of 1000 .... NDC 0032-4205-10
Unit dose pack of 100 .... NDC 0032-4205-11

Tablets 100 mg: scored, beige, elliptical, film-coated (debossed "SOLVAY" and "4210" on one side and scored on the other)

Bottles of 100 .... NDC 0032-4210-01
Bottles of 1000 .... NDC 0032-4210-10
Unit dose pack of 100 .... NDC 0032-4210-11

LUVOX® Tablets should be protected from high humidity and stored at controlled room temperature, 15°–30°C (59°–86°F).

Dispense in tight containers.

Rx only

Solvay Pharmaceuticals
Marietta, GA 30062
1280/1285
15E Rev 5/99

Shown in Product Identification Guide, page 338

PROMETRIUM® ℞

[prō mē' trium]
(progesterone, USP)
Capsules 100 mg
Capsules 200 mg

DESCRIPTION

PROMETRIUM® (progesterone, USP) Capsules contain micronized progesterone for oral administration. Progesterone has a molecular weight of 314.47 and an empirical formula of $C_{21}H_{30}O_2$. Progesterone (pregn-4-ene-3, 20-dione) is a white or creamy white, odorless, crystalline powder practically insoluble in water, soluble in alcohol, acetone and dioxane and sparingly soluble in vegetable oils, stable in air, melting between 126° and 131°C. The structural formula is:

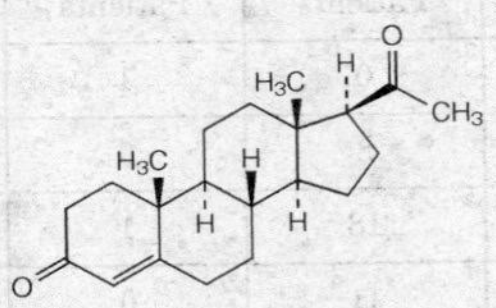

Progesterone is synthesized from a starting material from a plant source and is chemically identical to progesterone of human ovarian origin. PROMETRIUM Capsules are available in multiple strengths to afford dosage flexibility for optimum management. PROMETRIUM Capsules contain 100 mg or 200 mg micronized progesterone.

The inactive ingredients for PROMETRIUM Capsules 100 mg include: peanut oil NF, gelatin NF, glycerin USP, lecithin NF, titanium dioxide USP, D&C Yellow No. 10, and FD&C Red No. 40.

The inactive ingredients for PROMETRIUM Capsules 200 mg include: peanut oil NF, gelatin NF, glycerin USP, lecithin NF, titanium dioxide USP, D&C Yellow No. 10, and FD&C Yellow No. 6.

CLINICAL PHARMACOLOGY

PROMETRIUM Capsules are an oral dosage form of micronized progesterone which is chemically identical to progesterone of ovarian origin. The oral bioavailability of progesterone is increased through micronization.

Pharmacokinetics

Absorption

After oral administration of progesterone as a micronized soft gelatin capsule formulation, maximum serum concentrations were attained within 3 hours. The absolute bioavailability of micronized progesterone is not known. Table 1 summarizes the mean pharmacokinetic parameters in postmenopausal women after five oral daily doses of PROMETRIUM Capsules 100 mg as a micronized soft-gelatin capsule formulation.

[See table 1 above]

Serum progesterone concentrations appeared linear and dose proportional following multiple dose administration of PROMETRIUM Capsules 100 mg over the dose range 100 mg/day to 300 mg/day in postmenopausal women. Although doses greater than 300 mg/day were not studied in females, serum concentrations from a study in male volunteers appeared linear and dose proportional between 100 mg/day and 400 mg/day. The pharmacokinetic parameters in male volunteers were generally consistent with those seen in postmenopausal women.

Distribution

Progesterone is approximately 96%–99% bound to serum proteins, primarily to serum albumin (50%–54%) and transcortin (43%–48%).

Metabolism

Progesterone is metabolized primarily by the liver largely to pregnanediols and pregnanolones. Pregnanediols and pregnanolones are conjugated in the liver to glucuronide and sulfate metabolites. Progesterone metabolites which are excreted in the bile may be deconjugated and may be further metabolized in the gut via reduction, dehydroxylation, and epimerization.

Excretion

The glucuronide and sulfate conjugates of pregnanediol and pregnanolone are excreted in the bile and urine. Progesterone metabolites which are excreted in the bile may undergo enterohepatic recycling or may be excreted in the feces.

Special Populations

The pharmacokinetics of PROMETRIUM Capsules have not been assessed in low body weight or obese patients.

Race:
There is insufficient information available from trials conducted with PROMETRIUM Capsules to compare progesterone pharmacokinetics in different racial groups.

Hepatic Insufficiency:
No formal studies have evaluated the effect of hepatic disease on the disposition of progesterone. However, since progesterone is metabolized by the liver, use in patients with severe liver dysfunction or disease is contraindicated (see **CONTRAINDICATIONS**). If treatment with progesterone is indicated in patients with mild to moderate hepatic dysfunction, these patients should be monitored carefully.

Renal Insufficiency:
No formal studies have evaluated the effect of renal disease on the disposition of progesterone. Since progesterone metabolites are eliminated mainly by the kidneys, PROMETRIUM Capsules should be used with caution and only with careful monitoring in patients with renal dysfunction. (see **PRECAUTIONS**)

Table 1

Parameter	PROMETRIUM Capsules Dose QD		
	100 mg	200 mg	300 mg
Cmax (ng/ml)	17.3 ± 21.9[a]	38.1 ± 37.8	60.6 ± 72.5
Tmax (hr)	1.5 ± 0.8	2.3 ± 1.4	1.7 ± 0.6
AUC (0–10) (ng•hr/ml)	43.3 ± 30.8	101.2 ± 66.0	175.7 ± 170.3

[a] Mean ± S.D.

Table 2

Mean (±S.D.) Pharmacokinetic Parameters for Estradiol, Estrone and Equilin Following Coadministration of Conjugated Estrogens 0.625 mg and PROMETRIUM Capsules 200 mg for 12 Days to Postmenopausal Women

	Conjugated Estrogens			Conjugated Estrogens plus PROMETRIUM Capsules		
Drug	Cmax (ng/mL)	Tmax (hr)	AUC (0–24h) (ng•h/mL)	Cmax (ng/mL)	Tmax (hr)	AUC (0–24h) (ng•h/mL)
Estradiol	0.037 ±0.048	12.7 ±9.1	0.676 ±0.737	0.030 ±0.032	17.32 ±1.21	0.561 ±0.572
Estrone Total[a]	3.68 ±1.55	10.6 ±6.8	61.3 ±26.36	4.93 ±2.07	7.5 ±3.8	85.9 ±41.2
Equilin Total[a]	2.27 ±0.95	6.0 ±4.0	28.8 ±13.0	3.22 ±1.13	5.3 ±2.6	38.1 ±20.2

[a] Total estrogens is the sum of conjugated and unconjugated estrogen.

Table 3

Incidence of Endometrial Hyperplasia in Women Receiving 3 Years of Treatment

Endometrial Diagnosis	Treatment Group					
	Conjugated Estrogens 0.625 mg + PROMETRIUM Capsules 200 mg (cyclical)		Conjugated Estrogens 0.625 mg (only)		Placebo	
	Number of Patients	% of Patients	Number of Patients	% of Patients	Number of Patients	% of Patients
	N=117		N=115		N=116	
Hyperplasia[a]	7	6	74	64	3	3
Adenocarcinoma	0	0	0	0	1	1
Atypical hyperplasia	1	1	14	12	0	0
Complex hyperplasia	0	0	27	23	1	1
Simple hyperplasia	6	5	33	29	1	1

[a] Most advanced result to least advanced result:
Adenocarcinoma > atypical hyperplasia > complex hyperplasia > simple hyperplasia

Food-Drug Interaction:

Concomitant food ingestion increased the bioavailability of PROMETRIUM Capsules relative to a fasting state when administered to postmenopausal women at a dose of 200 mg.

Drug-Drug Interaction:

The metabolism of progesterone by human liver microsomes was inhibited by ketoconazole (IC_{50} <0.1 μM). Ketoconazole is a known inhibitor of cytochrome P450 3A4, hence these data suggest that ketoconazole or other known inhibitors of this enzyme may increase the bioavailability of progesterone. The clinical relevance of the *in vitro* findings is unknown.

Coadministration of conjugated estrogens and PROMETRIUM Capsules to 29 postmenopausal women over a 12 day period resulted in an increase in total estrone concentrations (Cmax 3.68 ng/ml to 4.93 ng/ml) and total equilin concentrations (Cmax 2.27 ng/ml to 3.22 ng/ml) and a decrease in circulating 17β estradiol concentrations (Cmax 0.037 ng/ml to 0.030 ng/ml). The half-life of the conjugated estrogens was similar with coadministration of PROMETRIUM Capsules. Table 2 summarizes the pharmacokinetic parameters.

[See table 2 above]

Clinical Studies

Endometrial Protection

In a randomized double-blind clinical trial, 358 postmenopausal women, each with an intact uterus, received treatment for up to 36 months. The treatment groups were: PROMETRIUM Capsules at the dose of 200 mg/day for 12 days per 28 day cycle in combination with conjugated estrogens 0.625 mg/day (n=120); conjugated estrogens 0.625 mg/day only (n=119); or placebo (n=119). The subjects in all three treatment groups were primarily Caucasian women (87% or more of each group). The results for the incidence of endometrial hyperplasia in women receiving up to 3 years of treatment are shown in Table 3. A comparison of the PROMETRIUM Capsules plus conjugated estrogens treatment group to the conjugated estrogens only group showed a significantly lower rate of hyperplasia (6% combination product vs. 64% estrogen alone) in the PROMETRIUM Capsules plus conjugated estrogens treatment group throughout 36 months of treatment.

[See table 3 above]

The times to diagnosis of endometrial hyperplasia over 36 months of treatment are shown in Figure 1. This figure illustrates graphically that the proportion of patients with hyperplasia was significantly greater for the conjugated estrogens group (64%) compared to the conjugated estrogens plus PROMETRIUM Capsules group (6%).

[See figure 1 at top of next column]

The discontinuation rates due to hyperplasia over the 36 months of treatment are as shown in Table 4. For any degree of hyperplasia, the discontinuation rate for patients who received conjugated estrogens plus PROMETRIUM Capsules was similar to that of the placebo only group, while the discontinuation rate for patients who received conjugated estrogens alone was significantly higher. Women who permanently discontinued treatment due to hyperplasia were similar in demographics to the overall study population.

[See table 4 at top of next page]

In the same three year clinical trial, postmenopausal women were treated with PROMETRIUM Capsules in combination with conjugated estrogens, conjugated estrogens only, or placebo. There was no statistically significant differ-

Continued on next page

Prometrium—Cont.

Figure 1

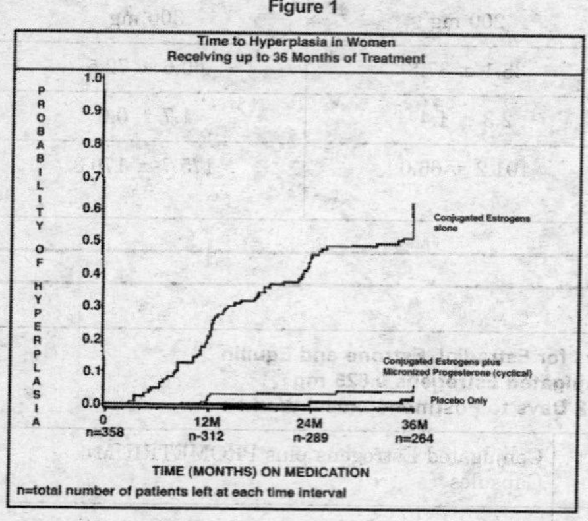

ence between the PROMETRIUM Capsules plus conjugated estrogens group and the conjugated estrogens only group in increases of HDL-C and triglycerides, or in decreases of LDL-C. The changes observed in lipid profiles are shown in Table 5.

[See table 5 above]

Secondary Amenorrhea

In a single-center, randomized, double-blind clinical study that included premenopausal women with secondary amenorrhea for at least 90 days, administration of 10 days of PROMETRIUM Capsules therapy resulted in 80% of women experiencing withdrawal bleeding within 7 days of the last dose of PROMETRIUM Capsules, 300 mg/day (n=20), compared to 10% of women experiencing withdrawal bleeding in the placebo group (n=21).

The rate of secretory transformation was evaluated in a multicenter, randomized, double-blind clinical study in estrogen-primed postmenopausal women. PROMETRIUM Capsules administered orally for 10 days at 400 mg/day (n=22) induced complete secretory changes in the endometrium in 45% of women compared to 0% in the placebo group (n=23).

INDICATIONS AND USAGE

PROMETRIUM Capsules are indicated for use in the prevention of endometrial hyperplasia in non-hysterectomized postmenopausal women who are receiving conjugated estrogens tablets. They are also indicated for use in secondary amenorrhea.

CONTRAINDICATIONS

1. **Known sensitivity to PROMETRIUM Capsules or its ingredients. PROMETRIUM Capsules contain peanut oil and should never be used by patients allergic to peanuts.**
2. Known or suspected pregnancy.
3. Thrombophlebitis, thromboembolic disorders, cerebral apoplexy, or patients with a past history of these conditions.
4. Severe liver dysfunction or disease.
5. Known or suspected malignancy of breast or genital organs.
6. Undiagnosed vaginal bleeding.
7. Missed abortion.
8. As a diagnostic test for pregnancy.

WARNINGS

1. The physician should be alert to the earliest manifestations of thrombotic disorders (thrombophlebitis, cerebrovascular disorders, pulmonary embolism, and retinal thrombosis). Should any of these occur or be suspected, the drug should be discontinued immediately.
2. Discontinue medication pending examination if there is sudden partial or complete loss of vision, or if there is a sudden onset of proptosis, diplopia or migraine. If examination reveals papilledema or retinal vascular lesions, medication should be withdrawn.
3. The administration of any drug to nursing mothers should be done only when clearly necessary since many drugs are excreted in human milk. Detectable amounts of progestin have been identified in the milk of mothers receiving progestins. The effect of this on the nursing infant has not been determined.
4. Retrospective studies of morbidity and mortality in Great Britain and studies of morbidity in the United States have shown a statistically significant association between thrombophlebitis, pulmonary embolism, cerebral thrombosis and embolism, and the use of oral contraceptives. The estimate of the relative risk of thromboembolism in the study by Vessey and Doll was about seven fold, while Sartwell and associates in the United States found a relative risk of 4.4, meaning that the users are several times as likely to undergo thromboembolic disease without evident cause as nonusers. The American study also indicated that the risk did not persist after discontinuation of administration, and that it was not enhanced by long-continued administration. The American study was not designed to evaluate a difference between products.

Table 4

Discontinuation Rate Due to Hyperplasia Over 36 Months of Treatment

Most Advanced Biopsy Result Through 36 Months of Treatment	Treatment Group					
	Conjugated Estrogens + PROMETRIUM Capsules (cyclical)		Conjugated Estrogens (only)		Placebo	
	N = 120		N = 119		N = 119	
	Number of Patients	% of Patients	Number of Patients	% of Patients	Number of Patients	% of Patients
Adenocarcinoma	0	0	0	0	1	1
Atypical hyperplasia	1	1	10	8	0	0
Complex hyperplasia	0	0	21	18	1	1
Simple hyperplasia	1	1	13	11	0	0

Table 5

Mean Changes from Baseline in Lipid Profiles After 36 Months of Treatment

Parameter	Treatment Group Mean (Mean % Change)					
	Conjugated Estrogens 0.625 mg + PROMETRIUM Capsules 200 mg (cyclical)[a] N = 176 to 177[b]		Conjugated Estrogens 0.625 mg (only) N = 171 to 173[b]		Placebo N = 171	
	Mean change	Mean % change	Mean change	mean % change	Mean change	mean % change
LIPID PROFILE						
HDL-C (mmol/L)	0.07	5.1	0.10	7.2	−0.05	−2
LDL-C (mmol/L)	−0.43	−11.8	−0.36	−9.5	−0.14	−2.9
Cholesterol (mmol/L)	−0.26	−4.0	−0.22	−3.6	−0.15	−1.8
Triglyceride (mmol/L)[c]	0.20	17.8	0.15	13.7	0.01	0.6

a: There are no significant changes ($p<0.05$) from conjugated estrogens values.
b: Number of subjects (N) varies by parameter.
c: Computed from log transformed data.

Table 6

Mean Changes from Baseline in Insulin and Glucose Levels After 36 Months of Treatment

Parameter		Treatment Group Mean (Mean % Change)					
		Conjugated Estrogens 0.625 mg + PROMETRIUM Capsules 200 mg (cyclical)[a] N = 173 to 176[b]		Conjugated Estrogens 0.625 mg (only) N = 170 to 172[b]		Placebo N = 171	
		mean	mean % change	mean	mean % change	mean	mean % change
OGTT							
Insulin (pmol/L)	fasting	−2.2	−6.2	−1.1	−3.2	5.1	14.2
	2 hour	−45.2	−14.5	−23.9	−7.9	−29.7	−9.1
Glucose (mg/dL)	fasting	−3.0	−2.9	−2.7	−2.7	−1.0	−0.9
	2 hour	3.6	5.2	5.0	7.8	2.1	3.9

a: There are no significant changes ($p<0.05$) from conjugated estrogens values
b: Number of subjects (N) varies by parameter

PRECAUTIONS

General

1. The pretreatment physical examination should include special reference to breast and pelvic organs, as well as Papanicolaou smear.
2. Because progesterone may cause some degree of fluid retention, conditions which might be influenced by this factor, such as epilepsy, migraine, asthma, cardiac or renal dysfunction, require careful observation.
3. In cases of breakthrough bleeding, as in any cases of irregular bleeding per vaginum, nonfunctional causes should be borne in mind. In cases of undiagnosed vaginal bleeding, adequate diagnostic measures are indicated.
4. Patients who have a history of psychic depression should be carefully observed and the drug discontinued if the depression recurs to a serious degree.
5. Any possible influence of prolonged progestin therapy on pituitary, ovarian, adrenal, hepatic or uterine functions awaits further study.
6. Although concomitant use of conjugated estrogens and PROMETRIUM Capsules did not result in a decrease in glucose tolerance, diabetic patients should be carefully observed while receiving estrogen-progestin therapy.
7. The pathologist should be advised of progestin therapy when relevant specimens are submitted.
8. Because of the occurrence of thrombotic disorders (thrombophlebitis, pulmonary embolism, retinal thrombosis, and cerebrovascular disorders) in patients taking estrogen-progestin combinations, the physician should be alert to the earliest manifestation of these disorders.
9. Transient dizziness may occur in some patients. Use caution when driving a motor vehicle or operating machinery. A small percentage of women may experience extreme dizziness and/or drowsiness during initial therapy. For these women, bedtime dosing is advised.

Information for the Patient

See accompanying Patient Insert.

General: This product contains peanut oil and should not be used if you are allergic to peanuts.

Drug Lab Test Interactions

The following laboratory results may be altered by the use of estrogen-progestin combination drugs:

Increased sulfobromophthalein retention and other hepatic function tests.
Coagulation tests: increase in prothrombin factors VII, VIII, IX and X.
Metyrapone test.
Pregnanediol determination.
Thyroid function: increase in PBI, and butanol extractable protein bound iodine
and decrease in T3 uptake values.

Fasting and 2-hour plasma insulin and glucose levels following an oral glucose tolerance test (OGTT) and fibrinogen levels were measured in patients receiving PROMETRIUM Capsules at a dose of 200 mg/day for 12 days per 28 day cycle in combination with conjugated estrogens 0.625 mg/day (n=120). Table 6 summarizes this data. Plasma insulin levels 2 hours post-OGTT were decreased from baseline. The fasting plasma glucose and fasting plasma insulin levels were also decreased from baseline. Glucose levels 2 hours post-OGTT were increased slightly. There was no effect on fibrinogen levels.
For information on changes in lipid profile, see the Clinical Studies subsection, Table 5.
[See table 6 at top of previous page]

Carcinogenesis, Mutagenesis, Impairment of Fertility
Progesterone has not been tested for carcinogenicity in animals by the oral route of administration. When implanted into female mice, progesterone produced mammary carcinomas, ovarian granulosa cell tumors and endometrial stromal sarcomas (1). In dogs, long-term intramuscular injections produced nodular hyperplasia and benign and malignant mammary tumors (2). Subcutaneous or intramuscular injections of progesterone decreased the latency period and increased the incidence of mammary tumors in rats previously treated with a chemical carcinogen (3).
Progesterone did not show evidence of genotoxicity in *in vitro* studies for point mutations or for chromosomal damage. *In vivo* studies for chromosome damage have yielded positive results in mice at oral doses of 1000 mg/kg and 2000 mg/kg (4). Exogenously administered progesterone has been shown to inhibit ovulation in a number of species and it is expected that high doses given for an extended duration would impair fertility until the cessation of treatment.

Pregnancy Category B
Reproductive studies have been performed in mice at doses up to 9 times the human oral dose (5, 6), in rats at doses up to 44 times the human oral dose (7, 8), in rabbits at a dose of 10 µg/day delivered locally within the uterus by an implanted device (9), in guinea pigs at doses of approximately one-half the human oral dose (10) and in rhesus monkeys (11) at doses approximately the human dose, all based on body surface area, and have revealed little or no evidence of impaired fertility or harm to the fetus due to progesterone. Several studies in women exposed to progesterone have not demonstrated any significant increase in fetal malformations (12). A single case of cleft palate was observed in the child of a woman using PROMETRIUM Capsules in early pregnancy, although definitive causality has not been established. Rare instances of fetal death have been reported in pregnant women prescribed PROMETRIUM Capsules for unapproved indications. Because the studies in humans cannot rule out the possibility of harm, PROMETRIUM Capsules should be used during pregnancy only if indicated (see **CONTRAINDICATIONS**).

Nursing Mothers
The administration of any drug to nursing mothers should be done only when clearly necessary since many drugs are excreted in human milk. Detectable amounts of progestin have been identified in the milk of nursing mothers receiving progestins. The effect of this on the nursing infant has not been determined.

Pediatric Use
The safety and effectiveness of PROMETRIUM Capsules in pediatric patients have not been established.

ADVERSE REACTIONS

Endometrial Protection
Table 7 lists adverse experiences which were reported in ≥2% of patients (regardless of relationship to treatment) who received cyclic PROMETRIUM Capsules, 200 mg daily (12 days per calendar month cycle) with daily 0.625 mg conjugated estrogen, in a multicenter, randomized, double-blind, placebo-controlled clinical trial in 875 postmenopausal women.
[See table 7 above]

Secondary Amenorrhea
Table 8 lists adverse experiences which were reported in ≥5% of patients receiving PROMETRIUM Capsules, 400 mg/day, in a multicenter, randomized, double-blind, placebo-controlled clinical trial in estrogen-primed (6 weeks) postmenopausal women receiving conjugated estrogens 0.625 mg/day and cyclic (10 days per calendar month cycle) PROMETRIUM Capsules at a dose of 400 mg/day, for three cycles.
[See table 8 above]
The most common adverse experiences reported in ≥5% of patients in all PROMETRIUM Capsules dosage groups studied in this trial (100 mg/day to 400 mg/day) were: dizziness (16%), breast pain (11%), headache (10%), abdominal pain (10%), fatigue (9%), viral infection (7%), abdominal distention (6%), musculoskeletal pain (6%), emotional lability (6%), irritability (5%), and upper respiratory tract infection (5%).
Other adverse events reported in <5% of patients taking PROMETRIUM Capsules include:

Table 7

Adverse Experiences (≥2%) Reported in an 875 Patient Placebo-Controlled Trial in Postmenopausal Women over a 3-Year Period (Percentage (%) of Patients Reporting)

	PROMETRIUM Capsules 200 mg with Conjugated Estrogens 0.625 mg (N=178)	Conjugated Estrogens 0.625 mg (only) (N=175)	Placebo (N=174)
Headache	31	30	27
Breast Tenderness	27	16	6
Joint Pain	20	22	29
Depression	19	18	12
Dizziness	15	5	9
Abdominal Bloating	12	10	5
Hot Flashes	11	14	35
Urinary Problems	11	10	9
Abdominal Pain	10	13	10
Vaginal Discharge	10	10	3
Nausea/Vomiting	8	6	7
Worry	8	5	4
Chest Pain	7	4	5
Diarrhea	7	7	4
Night Sweats	7	5	17
Breast Pain	6	6	2
Swelling of Hands and Feet	6	9	9
Vaginal Dryness	6	8	10
Constipation	3	3	2
Breast Carcinoma	2	<1	<1
Breast Excisional Biopsy	2	1	<1
Cholecystectomy	2	<1	<1

Table 8

Adverse Experiences (≥5%) Reported in Patients Using 400 mg/day in a Placebo-Controlled Trial in Estrogen-Primed Postmenopausal Women

Adverse Experience	PROMETRIUM Capsules 400 mg N=25	Placebo N=24
	Percentage (%) of Patients	
Fatigue	8	4
Headache	16	8
Dizziness	24	4
Abdominal Distention (Bloating)	8	8
Abdominal Pain (Cramping)	20	13
Diarrhea	8	4
Nausea	8	0
Back Pain	8	8
Musculoskeletal Pain	12	4
Irritability	8	4
Breast Pain	16	8
Infection Viral	12	0
Coughing	8	0

Autonomic Nervous System Disorders: dry mouth
Body As A Whole: accidental injury, chest pain, fever
Cardiovascular System Disorders: hypertension
Central and Peripheral Nervous System Disorders: confusion, somnolence, speech disorder
Gastrointestinal System Disorders: constipation, dyspepsia, gastroenteritis, hemorrhagic rectum, hiatus hernia, vomiting
Hearing and Vestibular Disorders: earache
Heart Rate and Rhythm Disorders: palpitation
Metabolic and Nutritional Disorders: edema, edema peripheral
Musculoskeletal System Disorders: arthritis, leg cramps, hypertonia, muscle disorder, myalgia
Myo/Endo/Pericardial and Valve Disorders: angina pectoris
Psychiatric Disorders: anxiety, impaired concentration, insomnia, personality disorder
Reproductive System Disorders: leukorrhea, uterine fibroid, vaginal dryness, fungal vaginitis, vaginitis
Resistance Mechanism Disorders: abscess, herpes simplex
Respiratory System Disorders: bronchitis, nasal congestion, pharyngitis, pneumonitis, sinusitis

Continued on next page

Prometrium—Cont.

Skin and Appendages Disorders: acne, verruca, wound debridement
Urinary System Disorders: urinary tract infection
Vision Disorders: abnormal vision
White Cell and Resistance Disorders: lymphadenopathy
The following adverse experiences have been reported with PROMETRIUM Capsules in other U.S. clinical trials: increased sweating, asthenia, tooth disorder, anorexia, increased appetite, nervousness, and breast enlargement.
The following spontaneous adverse events have been reported during the foreign marketing of PROMETRIUM Capsules: reversible cases of hepatitis and elevated transaminases. These events occurred mainly in patients receiving high doses of up to 1200 mg.
The following additional adverse experiences have been observed in women taking progestins in general: breakthrough bleeding, spotting, change in menstrual flow, amenorrhea, changes in weight (increase or decrease), changes in the cervical squamo-columnar junction and cervical secretions, cholestatic jaundice, anaphylactoid reactions and anaphylaxis, rash (allergic) with and without pruritus, melasma or chloasma, pyrexia, and insomnia.

OVERDOSAGE

No studies on overdosage have been conducted in humans. In the case of overdosage, PROMETRIUM Capsules should be discontinued, and the patient should be treated symptomatically.

DOSAGE AND ADMINISTRATION

Prevention of endometrial hyperplasia—PROMETRIUM Capsules should be given as a single daily dose in the evening, 200 mg orally for 12 days sequentially per 28 day cycle, to postmenopausal women with a uterus who are receiving daily conjugated estrogens tablets.
Secondary Amenorrhea—PROMETRIUM Capsules may be given as a single daily dose of 400 mg in the evening for 10 days.

HOW SUPPLIED

PROMETRIUM® (progesterone, USP) Capsules 100 mg are round, peach-colored capsules branded with black imprint "SV", available in bottles of 100 capsules (NDC0032-1708-01).
PROMETRIUM® (progesterone, USP) Capsules 200 mg are oval, pale yellow- colored capsules branded with black imprint "SV2", available in bottles of 100 capsules (NDC0032-1711-01).
Store at 25°C (77°F). Excursions permitted to 15–30°C (59–86°F).
Dispense in tight, light-resistant container as defined in USP/NF, accompanied by a Patient Insert.
Protect from excessive moisture.
Rx only

References:

1. International Agency for Research on Cancer (IARC) V.6, 1974; IARC V.21, 1979.
2. K.S. Larrson and D. Machin, Safety requirements for contraceptive steroids. F. Michal (ed.) Cambridge University Press, Cambridge. pp. 30–269, 1989.
3. Sixth Annual Report on Carcinogens V.2, pp 693–696, 1991.
4. Med. Sci. Res. 1987; 15:703–704.
5. Johnstone, E.E. and Franklin, R.R. (1964). Assay of progestins for fetal virilizing properties using the mouse. *Obstet Gynecol.* 23:359–62.
6. Seegmiller, R.E., Nelson, G.W. and Johnson, C.K. (1983) Evaluation of the teratogenic potential of Delalutin (17-hydroxyprogesterone caproate) in mice. *Teratology* 28: 201–8.
7. Suchowsky, G.K. and Junkmann, K. (1961). A study of the virilizing effects of progesterone on the female rat fetus. *Endocrinolgy* 68:341–9.
8. Scholer, H.F.L. and de Wachter, A.M. (1961). Evaluation of androgenic properties of progestational compounds in the rat by the female foetal masculinization test. *Acta. Endocrinol.* 38:128–36.
9. Hudson, R., Pharriss, B.B., Tillson, S.A. and Reno, F. (1978). Preclinical evaluation of intrauterine progesterone as a contraceptive agent. III. Embryology and toxicology. *Contraception* 17:489–97.
10. Foote, W.D., Foote, W.C., and Foote, L.H. (1968). Influence of certain natural and synthetic steroids on genital development in guinea pigs. *Fertil. Steril.* 19:606–15.
11. Wharton, L.R. Jr. and Scott, R.B. (1964). Experimental production of genital lesions with norethindrone. *Am J. Obstet. Gynecol.* 89:701–15
12. Scialli, A.R. (1988). Developmental effects of progesterone and its derivatives. *Reproductive Toxicol.* 2:3–11.

Manufactured by: R. P. Scherer North America, St. Petersburg, FL 33716
Marketed by: Solvay Pharmaceuticals, Inc., Marietta, GA 30062.

9563 3E Rev 9/99
Shown in Product Identification Guide, page 338

ROWASA® ℞

[*rō-ā'sǎ*]
(Mesalamine)
Rectal Suspension Enema
4.0 grams/unit (60 mL)

DESCRIPTION

The active ingredient in ROWASA® Rectal Suspension Enema, a disposable (60 mL) unit, is mesalamine, also known as 5-aminosalicylic acid (5-ASA). Chemically, mesalamine is 5-amino-2-hydroxybenzoic acid.
The empirical formula is $C_7H_7NO_3$, representing a molecular weight of 153.14. The structural formula is:

COOH, OH, H_2N

Each rectal suspension enema unit contains 4 grams of mesalamine. In addition to mesalamine the preparation contains the inactive ingredients carbomer 934P, edetate disodium, potassium acetate, potassium metabisulfite, purified water and xanthan gum. Sodium benzoate is added as a preservative. The disposable unit consists of an applicator tip protected by a polyethylene cover and lubricated with USP white petrolatum. The unit has a one-way valve to prevent back flow of the dispensed product.

CLINICAL PHARMACOLOGY

Sulfasalazine is split by bacterial action in the colon into sulfapyridine (SP) and mesalamine (5-ASA). It is thought that the mesalamine component is therapeutically active in ulcerative colitis [A.K. Azad Khan *et al*, **Lancet** 2:892–895 (1977)]. The usual oral dose of sulfasalazine for active ulcerative colitis in adults is two to four grams per day in divided doses. Four grams of sulfasalazine provide 1.6 g of free mesalamine to the colon. Each ROWASA® suspension enema delivers up to 4 g of mesalamine to the left side of the colon. The mechanism of action of mesalamine (and sulfasalazine) is unknown, but appears to be topical rather than systemic. Mucosal production of arachidonic acid (AA) metabolites, both through the cyclooxygenase pathways, i.e., prostanoids, and through the lipoxygenase pathways, i.e., leukotrienes (LTs) and hydroxyeicosatetraenoic acids (HETEs) is increased in patients with chronic inflammatory bowel disease, and it is possible that mesalamine diminishes inflammation by blocking cyclooxygenase and inhibiting prostaglandin (PG) production in the colon.

Preclinical Toxicology
Preclinical studies have shown the kidney to be the major target organ for mesalamine toxicity. Adverse renal function changes were observed in rats after a single 600 mg/kg oral dose, but not after a 200 mg/kg dose. Gross kidney lesions, including papillary necrosis, were observed after a single oral >900 mg/kg dose, and after i.v. doses of >214 mg/kg. Mice responded similarly. In a 13-week oral (gavage) dose study in rats, the high dose of 640 mg/kg/day mesalamine caused deaths, probably due to renal failure, and dose-related renal lesions (papillary necrosis and/or multifocal tubular injury) were seen in most rats given the high dose (males and females) as well as in males receiving lower doses 160 mg/kg/day. Renal lesions were not observed in the 160 mg/kg/day female rats. Minimal tubular epithelial damage was seen in the 40 mg/kg/day males and was reversible. In a six-month oral study in dogs, the no-observable dose level of mesalamine was 40 mg/kg/day and doses of 80 mg/kg/day and higher caused renal pathology similar to that described for the rat. In a combined 52-week toxicity and 127-week carcinogenicity study in rats, degeneration in kidneys was observed at doses of 100 mg/kg/day and above admixed with diet for 52 weeks, and at 127 weeks increased incidence of kidney degeneration and hyalinization of basement membranes and Bowman's capsule were seen at 100 mg/kg/day and above. In the 12 month eye toxicity study in dogs, Keratoconjunctivitis Sicca (KCS) occurred at oral doses of 40 mg/kg/day and above. The oral preclinical studies were done with a highly bioavailable suspension where absorption throughout the gastrointestinal tract occurred. The human dose of 4 grams represents approximately 80 mg/kg but when mesalamine is given rectally as a suspension, absorption is poor and limited to the distal colon (see **Pharmacokinetics**). Overt renal toxicity has not been observed (see **ADVERSE REACTIONS** and **PRECAUTIONS**), but the potential must be considered.

Pharmacokinetics
Mesalamine administered rectally as ROWASA® Rectal Suspension Enema is poorly absorbed from the colon and is excreted principally in the feces during subsequent bowel movements. The extent of absorption is dependent upon the retention time of the drug product, and there is considerable individual variation. At steady state, approximately 10 to 30% of the daily 4-gram dose can be recovered in cumulative 24-hour urine collections. Other than the kidney, the organ distribution and other bioavailability characteristics of absorbed mesalamine in man are not known. It is known that the compound undergoes acetylation but whether this process takes place at colonic or systemic sites has not been elucidated.
Whatever the metabolic site, most of the absorbed mesalamine is excreted in the urine as the N-acetyl-5-ASA metabolite. The poor colonic absorption of rectally administered mesalamine is substantiated by the low serum concentration of 5-ASA and N-acetyl-5-ASA seen in ulcerative colitis patients after dosage with mesalamine. Under clinical conditions patients demonstrated plasma levels 10 to 12 hours post mesalamine administration of 2 µg/mL, about two-thirds of which was the N-acetyl metabolite. While the elimination half-life of mesalamine is short (0.5 to 1.5 h), the acetylated metabolite exhibits a half-life of 5 to 10 hours [U. Klotz, **Clin. Pharmacokin.** 10:285–302 (1985)]. In addition, steady state plasma levels demonstrated a lack of accumulation of either free or metabolized drug during repeated daily administrations.

Efficacy
In a placebo-controlled, international, multicenter trial of 153 patients with active distal ulcerative colitis, proctosigmoiditis or proctitis, ROWASA® Rectal Suspension Enema reduced the overall disease activity index (DAI) and individual components as follows:
[See table below]
Differences between ROWASA® and placebo were also statistically different in subgroups of patients on concurrent sulfasalazine and in those having an upper disease boundary between 5 and 20 or 20 and 40 cm. Significant differences between ROWASA® and placebo were not achieved in those subgroups of patients on concurrent prednisone or with an upper disease boundary between 40 and 50 cm.

INDICATIONS AND USAGE

ROWASA® Rectal Suspension Enema is indicated for the treatment of active mild to moderate distal ulcerative colitis, proctosigmoiditis or proctitis.

CONTRAINDICATIONS

ROWASA® Rectal Suspension Enema is contraindicated for patients known to have hypersensitivity to the drug or any component of this medication.

WARNINGS

ROWASA® Rectal Suspension Enema contains potassium metabisulfite, a sulfite that may cause allergic-type reactions including anaphylactic symptoms and life-threatening or less severe asthmatic episodes in certain susceptible people. The overall prevalence of sulfite sensitivity in the gen-

EFFECT OF TREATMENT ON SEVERITY OF DISEASE
DATA FROM U.S.-CANADA TRIAL
COMBINED RESULTS OF EIGHT CENTERS
Activity Indices, mean

		N	Baseline	Day 22	End-Point	Change Baseline to End-Point†
Overall DAI	ROWASA®	76	7.42	4.05**	3.37***	-55.07%***
	Placebo	77	7.40	6.03	5.83	-21.58%
Stool Frequency	ROWASA®		1.58	1.11*	1.01**	-0.57*
	Placebo		1.92	1.47	1.50	-0.41
Rectal Bleeding	ROWASA®		1.82	0.59***	0.51***	-1.30***
	Placebo		1.73	1.21	1.11	-0.61
Mucosal Inflammation	ROWASA®		2.17	1.22**	0.96***	-1.21**
	Placebo		2.18	1.74	1.61	-0.56
Physician's Assessment of Disease Severity	ROWASA®		1.86	1.13***	0.88***	-0.97***
	Placebo		1.87	1.62	1.55	-0.30

Each parameter has a 4-point scale with a numerical rating:
0=normal, 1=mild, 2=moderate, 3=severe. The four parameters are added together to produce a maximum overall DAI of 12.
† Percent change for overall DAI only (calculated by taking the average of the change for each individual patient).
* Significant ROWASA®/placebo difference. $p<0.05$
** Significant ROWASA®/placebo difference. $p<0.01$
*** Significant ROWASA®/placebo difference. $p<0.001$

eral population is unknown but probably low. Sulfite sensitivity is seen more frequently in asthmatic or in atopic nonasthmatic persons. Epinephrine is the preferred treatment for serious allergic or emergency situations even though epinephrine injection contains sodium or potassium metabisulfite with the above-mentioned potential liabilities. The alternatives to using epinephrine in a life-threatening situation may not be satisfactory. The presence of a sulfite(s) in epinephrine injection should not deter the administration of the drug for treatment of serious allergic or other emergency situations.

PRECAUTIONS

Mesalamine has been implicated in the production of an acute intolerance syndrome characterized by cramping, acute abdominal pain and bloody diarrhea, sometimes fever, headache and a rash; in such cases prompt withdrawal is required. The patient's history of sulfasalazine intolerance, if any, should be re-evaluated. If a rechallenge is performed later in order to validate the hypersensitivity it should be carried out under close supervision and only if clearly needed, giving consideration to reduced dosage. In the literature one patient previously sensitive to sulfasalazine was rechallenged with 400 mg oral mesalamine; within eight hours she experienced headache, fever, intensive abdominal colic, profuse diarrhea and was readmitted as an emergency. She responded poorly to steroid therapy and two weeks later a pancolectomy was required.

Although renal abnormalities were not noted in the clinical trials with ROWASA® Rectal Suspension Enema, the possibility of increased absorption of mesalamine and concomitant renal tubular damage as noted in the preclinical studies must be kept in mind. Patients on ROWASA® Rectal Suspension Enema, especially those on concurrent oral products which liberate mesalamine and those with preexisting renal disease, should be carefully monitored with urinalysis, BUN and creatinine studies.

In a clinical trial most patients who were hypersensitive to sulfasalazine were able to take mesalamine enemas without evidence of any allergic reaction. Nevertheless, caution should be exercised when mesalamine is initially used in patients known to be allergic to sulfasalazine. These patients should be instructed to discontinue therapy if signs of rash or fever become apparent.

While using ROWASA® Rectal Suspension Enema some patients have developed pancolitis. However, extension of upper disease boundary and/or flare-ups occurred less often in the ROWASA® suspension enema treated group than in the placebo-treated group.

Rare instances of pericarditis have been reported with mesalamine containing products including sulfasalazine. Cases of pericarditis have also been reported as manifestations of inflammatory bowel disease. In the cases reported with ROWASA® Rectal Suspension Enema there have been positive rechallenges with mesalamine or mesalamine containing products. In one of these cases, however, a second rechallenge with sulfasalazine was negative throughout a 2 month follow-up. Chest pain or dyspnea in patients treated with ROWASA® Rectal Suspension Enema should be investigated with this information in mind.

Discontinuation of ROWASA® Rectal Suspension Enema may be warranted in some cases, but rechallenge with mesalamine can be performed under careful clinical observation should the continued therapeutic need for mesalamine be present.

Carcinogenesis, Mutagenesis, Impairment of Fertility

Mesalamine caused no increase in the incidence of neoplastic lesions over controls in a two-year study of Wistar rats fed up to 320 mg/kg/day of mesalamine admixed with diet. Mesalamine is not mutagenic to Salmonella typhimurium tester strains TA98, TA100, TA1535, TA1537, TA1538. There were no reverse mutations in an assay using E. coli strain WP2UVRA. There were no effects in an *in vivo* mouse micronucleus assay at 600 mg/kg and in an *in vivo* sister chromatid exchange at doses up to 610 mg/kg. No effects on fertility were observed in rats receiving up to 320 mg/kg/day. The oligospermia and infertility in men associated with sulfasalazine have not been reported with mesalamine.

Pregnancy (Category B)

Teratologic studies have been performed in rats and rabbits at oral doses up to five and eight times respectively, the maximum recommended human dose, and have revealed no evidence of harm to the embryo or the fetus. There are, however, no adequate and well controlled studies in pregnant women for either sulfasalazine or 5-ASA. Because animal reproduction studies are not always predictive of human response, 5-ASA should be used during pregnancy only if clearly needed.

Nursing Mothers

It is not known whether mesalamine or its metabolite(s) are excreted in human milk. As a general rule, nursing should not be undertaken while a patient is on a drug since many drugs are excreted in human milk.

Pediatric Use

Safety and effectiveness in pediatric patients have not been established.

ADVERSE REACTIONS

Clinical Adverse Experience

ROWASA® Rectal Suspension Enema is usually well tolerated. Most adverse effects have been mild and transient.

[See table above]

In addition, the following adverse events have been associated with ROWASA® Rectal Suspension Enema and other mesalamine containing products: nephrotoxicity, pancreatitis, fibrosing alveolitis and elevated liver enzymes. Cases of pancreatitis and fibrosing alveolitis have been reported as manifestations of inflammatory bowel disease as well.

ADVERSE REACTIONS OCCURRING IN MORE THAN 0.1% OF ROWASA® RECTAL SUSPENSION ENEMA TREATED PATIENTS (COMPARISON TO PLACEBO)

SYMPTOM	ROWASA® N=815 N	%	PLACEBO N=128 N	%
Abdominal Pain/Cramps/Discomfort	66	8.10	10	7.81
Headache	53	6.50	16	12.50
Gas/Flatulence	50	6.13	5	3.91
Nausea	47	5.77	12	9.38
Flu	43	5.28	1	0.78
Tired/Weak/Malaise/Fatigue	28	3.44	8	6.25
Fever	26	3.19	0	0.00
Rash/Spots	23	2.82	4	3.12
Cold/Sore Throat	19	2.33	9	7.03
Diarrhea	17	2.09	5	3.91
Leg/Joint Pain	17	2.09	1	0.78
Dizziness	15	1.84	3	2.34
Bloating	12	1.47	2	1.56
Back Pain	11	1.35	1	0.78
Pain on Insertion of Enema Tip	11	1.35	1	0.78
Hemorrhoids	11	1.35	0	0.00
Itching	10	1.23	1	0.78
Rectal Pain	10	1.23	0	0.00
Constipation	8	0.98	4	3.12
Hair Loss	7	0.86	0	0.00
Peripheral Edema	5	0.61	11	8.59
UTI/Urinary Burning	5	0.61	4	3.12
Rectal Pain/Soreness/Burning	5	0.61	3	2.34
Asthenia	1	0.12	4	3.12
Insomnia	1	0.12	3	2.34

Hair Loss

Mild hair loss characterized by "more hair in the comb" but no withdrawal from clinical trials has been observed in seven of 815 mesalamine patients but none of the placebo-treated patients. In the literature there are at least six additional patients with mild hair loss who received either mesalamine or sulfasalazine. Retreatment is not always associated with repeated hair loss.

OVERDOSAGE

There have been no documented reports of serious toxicity in man resulting from massive overdosing with mesalamine. Under ordinary circumstances, mesalamine absorption from the colon is limited.

DOSAGE AND ADMINISTRATION

The usual dosage of ROWASA® (mesalamine) Rectal Suspension Enema in 60 mL units is one rectal instillation (4 grams) once a day, preferably at bedtime, and retained for approximately eight hours. While the effect of ROWASA® (mesalamine) may be seen within three to twenty-one days, the usual course of therapy would be from three to six weeks depending on symptoms and sigmoidoscopic findings. Studies available to date have not assessed if ROWASA® Rectal Suspension Enema will modify relapse rates after the 6-week short-term treatment.

Patients should be instructed to shake the bottle well to make sure the suspension is homogeneous. The patient should remove the protective sheath from the applicator tip. Holding the bottle at the neck will not cause any of the medication to be discharged. The position most often used is obtained by lying on the left side (to facilitate migration into the sigmoid colon); with the lower leg extended and the upper right leg flexed forward for balance. An alternative is the knee-chest position. The applicator tip should be gently inserted in the rectum pointing toward the umbilicus. A steady squeezing of the bottle will discharge most of the preparation. The preparation should be taken at bedtime with the objective of retaining it all night. Patient instructions are included with every seven units.

HOW SUPPLIED

ROWASA® suspension for rectal administration is an off-white to tan colored suspension. Each disposable enema bottle contains 4.0 grams of mesalamine in 60 mL aqueous suspension. Enema bottles are supplied in boxed, foil-wrapped trays of seven (NDC 0032-1924-82). ROWASA® enemas are for rectal use only.

Rx only

Patient instructions are included.

Store at controlled room temperature 15° to 30°C (59° to 86°F). Once the foil-wrapped unit of seven bottles is opened, all enemas should be used promptly as directed by your physician. **Contents of enemas removed from the foil pouch may darken with time. Slight darkening will not affect potency, however, enemas with dark brown contents should be discarded.**

NOTE: ROWASA® Rectal Suspension Enema will cause staining of direct contact surfaces, including but not limited to fabrics, flooring, painted surfaces, marble, granite, vinyl, and enamel. Take care in choosing a suitable location for administration of this product.

0645
11E Rev 6/98

U.S. Pat. Nos. 4657900 and RE33239

Solvay Pharmaceuticals, Inc.
Marietta, GA 30062

PATIENT INSTRUCTIONS

How to Use this Medication.

Best results are achieved if the bowel is emptied immediately before the medication is given.

NOTE: ROWASA® Rectal Suspension Enema will cause staining of direct contact surfaces, including but not limited to fabrics, flooring, painted surfaces, marble, granite, vinyl, and enamel. Take care in choosing a suitable location for administration of this product.

1. Remove the Bottles

a. Remove the bottles from the protective foil pouch by tearing or by using scissors as shown, being careful not to squeeze or puncture bottles. ROWASA® rectal suspension is an off-white to tan colored suspension. Once the foil-wrapped unit of seven bottles is opened, all enemas should be used promptly as directed by your physician. **Contents of enemas removed from the foil pouch may darken with time. Slight darkening will not affect potency, however, enemas with dark brown contents should be discarded.**

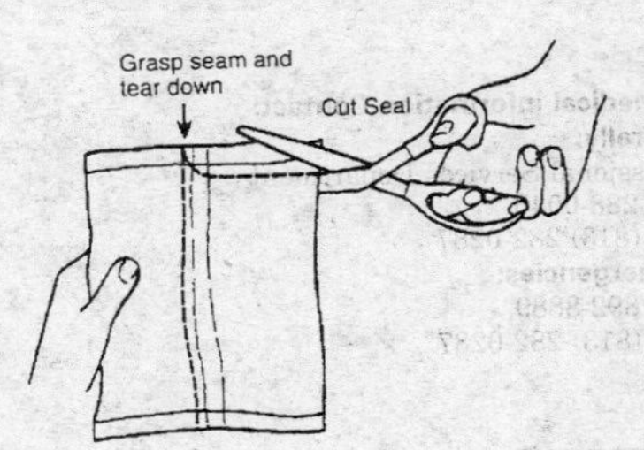

2. Prepare the Medication for Administration

a. Shake the bottle well to make sure that the medication is thoroughly mixed.

b. Remove the protective sheath from the applicator tip. Hold the bottle at the neck so as not to cause any of the medication to be discharged.

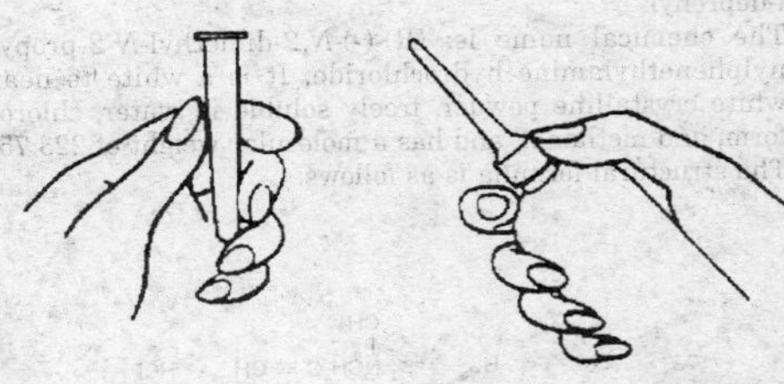

3. Assume the Correct Body Position

a. Best results are obtained by lying on the left side with the left leg extended and the right leg flexed forward for balance.

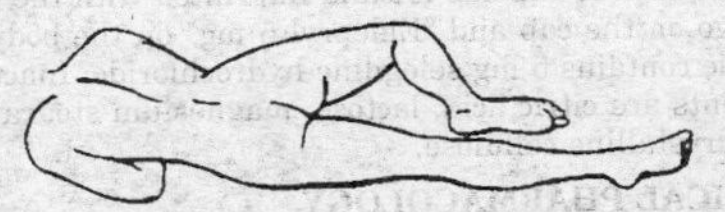

Continued on next page

Rowasa—Cont.

b. An alternative to lying on the left side is the "knee-chest" position as shown here.

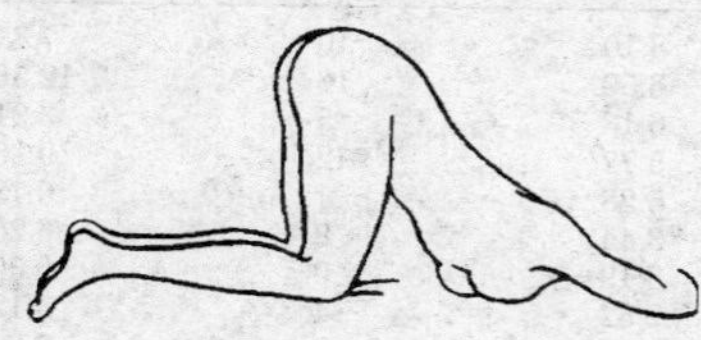

4. Administer the Medication

a. Gently insert the lubricated applicator tip into the rectum to prevent damage to the rectal wall, pointed slightly toward the navel.

b. Grasp the bottle firmly, then tilt slightly so that the nozzle is aimed toward the back, squeeze slowly to instill the medication. Steady hand pressure will discharge most of the medication. After administering, withdraw and discard the bottle.

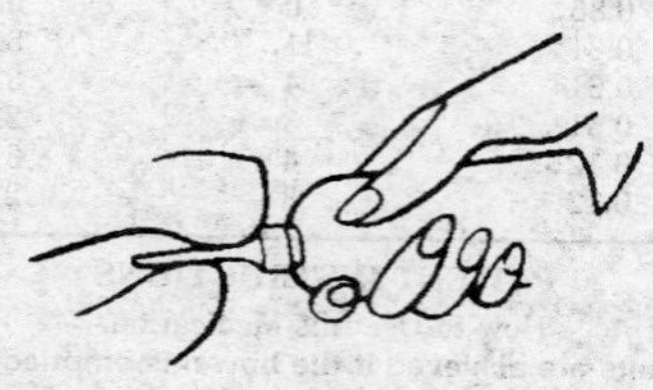

c. Remain in position for at least 30 minutes to allow thorough distribution of the medication internally. Retain the medication all night, if possible.

0645 11E
Rev 6/98
Solvay
Pharmaceuticals, Inc.
Marietta, GA 30062

Shown in Product Identification Guide, page 338

Somerset Pharmaceuticals, Inc.

2202 NORTH WESTSHORE BOULEVARD
SUITE 450
TAMPA, FLORIDA 33607

For Medical Information Contact:
Generally:
Professional Services Department
(813) 288-0040
FAX: (813) 282-0287
In Emergencies:
(800) 892-8889
FAX: (813) 282-0287

ELDEPRYL® ℞
(SELEGILINE HYDROCHLORIDE)
CAPSULES

DESCRIPTION

ELDEPRYL (selegiline hydrochloride) is a levorotatory acetylenic derivative of phenethylamine. It is commonly referred to in the clinical and pharmacological literature as l-deprenyl.

The chemical name is: (R)-(-)-*N*,2-dimethyl-*N*-2-propynylphenethylamine hydrochloride. It is a white to near white crystalline powder, freely soluble in water, chloroform, and methanol, and has a molecular weight of 223.75. The structural formula is as follows:

$$C_6H_5-CH_2-C(H)(CH_3)-N(CH_3)CH_2C\equiv CH \cdot HCl$$

Each aqua blue capsule is band imprinted with the Somerset logo on the cap and "Eldepryl 5 mg" on the body. Each capsule contains 5 mg selegiline hydrochloride. Inactive ingredients are citric acid, lactose, magnesium stearate, and microcrystalline cellulose.

CLINICAL PHARMACOLOGY

The mechanisms accounting for selegiline's beneficial adjunctive action in the treatment of Parkinson's disease are not fully understood. Inhibition of monoamine oxidase, type B, activity is generally considered to be of primary importance; in addition, there is evidence that selegiline may act through other mechanisms to increase dopaminergic activity.

Selegiline is best known as an irreversible inhibitor of monoamine oxidase (MAO), an intracellular enzyme associated with the outer membrane of mitochondria. Selegiline inhibits MAO by acting as a 'suicide' substrate for the enzyme; that is, it is converted by MAO to an active moiety which combines irreversibly with the active site and/or the enzyme's essential FAD cofactor. Because selegiline has greater affinity for type B rather than for type A active sites, it can serve as a selective inhibitor of MAO type B if it is administered at the recommended dose.

MAOs are widely distributed throughout the body; their concentration is especially high in liver, kidney, stomach, intestinal wall, and brain. MAOs are currently subclassified into two types, A and B, which differ in their substrate specificity and tissue distribution. In humans, intestinal MAO is predominantly type A, while most of that in brain is type B.

In CNS neurons, MAO plays an important role in the catabolism of catecholamines (dopamine, norepinephrine and epinephrine) and serotonin. MAOs are also important in the catabolism of various exogenous amines found in a variety of foods and drugs. MAO in the GI tract and liver (primarily type A), for example, is thought to provide vital protection from exogenous amines (e.g., tyramine) that have the capacity, if absorbed intact, to cause a 'hypertensive crisis,' the so-called 'cheese reaction.' (If large amounts of certain exogenous amines gain access to the systemic circulation - e.g., from fermented cheese, red wine, herring, over-the-counter cough/cold medications, etc. - they are taken up by adrenergic neurons and displace norepinephrine from storage sites within membrane bound vesicles. Subsequent release of the displaced norepinephrine causes the rise in systemic blood pressure, etc.)

In theory, since MAO A of the gut is not inhibited, patients treated with selegiline at a dose of 10 mg a day should be able to take medications containing pharmacologically active amines and consume tyramine-containing foods without risk of uncontrolled hypertension. Although rare, a few reports of hypertensive reactions have occurred in patients receiving Eldepryl at the recommended dose, with tyramine-containing foods. In addition, one case of hypertensive crisis has been reported in a patient taking the recommended dose of selegiline and a sympathomimetic medication, ephedrine. The pathophysiology of the 'cheese reaction' is complicated and, in addition to its ability to inhibit MAO B selectively, selegiline's relative freedom from this reaction has been attributed to an ability to prevent tyramine and other indirect acting sympathomimetics from displacing norepinephrine from adrenergic neurons. However, until the pathophysiology of the cheese reaction is more completely understood, it seems prudent to assume that selegiline can ordinarily only be used safely without dietary restrictions at doses where it presumably selectively inhibits MAO B (e.g., 10 mg/day).

In short, attention to the dose dependent nature of selegiline's selectivity is critical if it is to be used without elaborate restrictions being placed on diet and concomitant drug use although, as noted above, a few cases of hypertensive reactions have been reported at the recommended dose. (See WARNINGS and PRECAUTIONS.)

It is important to be aware that selegiline may have pharmacological effects unrelated to MAO B inhibition. As noted above, there is some evidence that it may increase dopaminergic activity by other mechanisms, including interfering with dopamine re-uptake at the synapse. Effects resulting from selegiline administration may also be mediated through its metabolites. Two of its three principal metabolites, amphetamine and methamphetamine, have pharmacological actions of their own; they interfere with neuronal uptake and enhance release of several neurotransmitters (e.g., norepinephrine, dopamine, serotonin). However, the extent to which these metabolites contribute to the effects of selegiline are unknown.

Rationale for the Use of a Selective Monoamine Oxidase Type B Inhibitor in Parkinson's Disease: Many of the prominent symptoms of Parkinson's disease are due to a deficiency of striatal dopamine that is the consequence of a progressive degeneration and loss of a population of dopaminergic neurons which originate in the substantia nigra of the midbrain and project to the basal ganglia or striatum. Early in the course of Parkinson's Disease, the deficit in the capacity of these neurons to synthesize dopamine can be overcome by administration of exogenous levodopa, usually given in combination with a peripheral decarboxylase inhibitor (carbidopa).

With the passage of time, due to the progression of the disease and/or the effect of sustained treatment, the efficacy and quality of the therapeutic response to levodopa diminishes. Thus, after several years of levodopa treatment, the response, for a given dose of levodopa, is shorter, has less predictable onset and offset (i.e., there is 'wearing off'), and is often accompanied by side effects (e.g., dyskinesia, akinesias, on-off phenomena, freezing, etc.).

This deteriorating response is currently interpreted as a manifestation of the inability of the ever decreasing population of intact nigrostriatal neurons to synthesize and release adequate amounts of dopamine.

MAO B inhibition may be useful in this setting because, by blocking the catabolism of dopamine, it would increase the net amount of dopamine available (i.e., it would increase the pool of dopamine). Whether or not this mechanism or an alternative one actually accounts for the observed beneficial effects of adjunctive selegiline is unknown.

Selegiline's benefit in Parkinson's disease has only been documented as an adjunct to levodopa/carbidopa. Whether or not it might be effective as a sole treatment is unknown, but past attempts to treat Parkinson's disease with non-selective MAOI monotherapy are reported to have been unsuccessful. It is important to note that attempts to treat Parkinsonian patients with combinations of levodopa and currently marketed non-selective MAO inhibitors were abandoned because of multiple side effects including hypertension, increase in involuntary movement, and toxic delirium.

Pharmacokinetic Information (Absorption, Distribution, Metabolism and Elimination—ADME):

The absolute bioavailability of selegiline following oral dosing is not known; however, selegiline undergoes extensive metabolism (presumably attributable to presystemic clearance in gut and liver). The major plasma metabolites are N-desmethylselegiline, L-amphetamine and L-methamphetamine. Only N-desmethylselegiline has MAO-B inhibiting activity. The peak plasma levels of these metabolites following a single oral dose of 10 mg are from 4 to almost 20 times greater than that of the maximum plasma concentration of selegiline [1 ng/mL]. The maximum concentrations of amphetamine and methamphetamine, however, are far below those ordinarily expected to produce clinically important effects.

Single oral dose studies do not predict multiple dose kinetics, however. At steady state the peak plasma level of selegiline is 4 fold that obtained following a single dose. Metabolite concentrations increase to a lesser extent, averaging 2 fold that seen after a single dose.

The bioavailability of selegiline is increased 3 to 4 fold when it is taken with food.

The extent of systemic exposure to selegiline at a given dose varies considerably among individuals. Estimates of systemic clearance of selegiline are not available. Following a single oral dose, the mean elimination half-life of selegiline is two hours. Under steady state conditions the elimination half-life increases to ten hours.

Because selegiline's inhibition of MAO-B is irreversible, it is impossible to predict the extent of MAO-B inhibition from steady state plasma levels. For the same reason, it is not possible to predict the rate of recovery of MAO-B activity as a function of plasma levels. The recovery of MAO-B activity is a function of de novo protein synthesis; however, information about the rate of de novo protein synthesis is not yet available. Although platelet MAO-B activity returns to the normal range within 5 to 7 days of selegiline discontinuation, the linkage between platelet and brain MAO-B inhibition is not fully understood nor is the relationship of MAO-B inhibition to the clinical effect established (see Clinical Pharmacology).

Special Populations:

Renal Impairment:

No pharmacokinetic information is available on selegiline or its metabolites in renally impaired subjects.

Hepatic Impairment:

No pharmacokinetic information is available on selegiline or its metabolites in hepatically impaired subjects.

Age:

Although a general conclusion about the effects of age on the pharmacokinetics of selegiline is not warranted because of the size of the sample evaluated (12 subjects greater than 60 years of age, 12 subjects between the ages of 18 to 30), systemic exposure was about twice as great in older as compared to a younger population given a single oral dose of 10 mg.

Gender:

No information is available on the effects of gender on the pharmacokinetics of selegiline.

INDICATIONS AND USAGE

ELDEPRYL is indicated as an adjunct in the management of Parkinsonian patients being treated with levodopa/carbidopa who exhibit deterioration in the quality of their response to this therapy. There is no evidence from controlled studies that selegiline has any beneficial effect in the absence of concurrent levodopa therapy.

Evidence supporting this claim was obtained in randomized controlled clinical investigations that compared the effects of added selegiline or placebo in patients receiving levodopa/carbidopa. Selegiline was significantly superior to placebo on all three principal outcome measures employed: change from baseline in daily levodopa/carbidopa dose, the amount of 'off' time, and patient self-rating of treatment success. Beneficial effects were also observed on other measures of treatment success (e.g., measures of reduced end of dose akinesia, decreased tremor and sialorrhea, improved speech and dressing ability and improved overall disability as assessed by walking and comparison to previous state).

CONTRAINDICATIONS

ELDEPRYL is contraindicated in patients with a known hypersensitivity to this drug.

ELDEPRYL is contraindicated for use with meperidine (DEMEROL & other trade names). This contraindication is often extended to other opioids. (See Drug Interactions.)

WARNINGS

Selegiline should not be used at daily doses exceeding those recommended (10 mg/day) because of the risks associated with nonselective inhibition of MAO. (See CLINICAL PHARMACOLOGY.)

The selectivity of selegiline for MAO B may not be absolute even at the recommended daily dose of 10 mg a day. Rare cases of hypertensive reactions associated with ingestion of tyramine-containing foods have been reported in patients taking the recommended daily dose of selegiline. The selectivity is further diminished with increasing daily doses. The precise dose at which selegiline becomes a non-selective inhibitor of all MAO is unknown, but may be in the range of 30 to 40 mg a day.

Severe CNS toxicity associated with hyperpyrexia and death have been reported with the combination of tricyclic antidepressants and nonselective MAOIs (NARDIL, PARNATE). A similar reaction has been reported for a patient on amitriptyline and ELDEPRYL. Another patient receiving protriptyline and ELDEPRYL developed tremors, agitation, and restlessness followed by unresponsiveness and death two weeks after ELDEPRYL was added. Related adverse events including hypertension, syncope, asystole, diaphoresis, seizures, changes in behavioral and mental status, and muscular rigidity have also been reported in some patients receiving ELDEPRYL and various tricyclic antidepressants.

Serious, sometimes fatal, reactions with signs and symptoms that may include hyperthermia, rigidity, myoclonus, autonomic instability with rapid fluctuations of the vital signs, and mental status changes that include extreme agitation progressing to delirium and coma have been reported with patients receiving a combination of fluoxetine hydrochloride (PROZAC) and non-selective MAOIs. Similar signs have been reported in some patients on the combination of ELDEPRYL (10 mg a day) and selective serotonin reuptake inhibitors including fluoxetine, sertraline and paroxetine.

Since the mechanisms of these reactions are not fully understood, it seems prudent, in general, to avoid this combination of ELDEPRYL and tricyclic antidepressants as well as ELDEPRYL and selective serotonin reuptake inhibitors. At least 14 days should elapse between discontinuation of ELDEPRYL and initiation of treatment with a tricyclic antidepressant or selective serotonin reuptake inhibitors. Because of the long half-lives of fluoxetine and its active metabolite, at least five weeks (perhaps longer, especially if fluoxetine has been prescribed chronically and/or at higher doses) should elapse between discontinuation of fluoxetine and initiation of treatment with ELDEPRYL.

PRECAUTIONS

General:

Some patients given selegiline may experience an exacerbation of levodopa associated side effects, presumably due to the increased amounts of dopamine reaction with super sensitive, post-synaptic receptors. These effects may often be mitigated by reducing the dose of levodopa/carbidopa by approximately 10 to 30%.

The decision to prescribe selegiline should take into consideration that the MAO system of enzymes is complex and incompletely understood and there is only a limited amount of carefully documented clinical experience with selegiline. Consequently, the full spectrum of possible responses to selegiline may not have been observed in pre-marketing evaluation of the drug. It is advisable, therefore, to observe patients closely for atypical responses.

Information for Patients:

Patients should be advised of the possible need to reduce levodopa dosage after the initiation of ELDEPRYL therapy.

Patients (or their families if the patient is incompetent) should be advised not to exceed the daily recommended dose of 10 mg. The risk of using higher daily doses of selegiline should be explained, and a brief description of the 'cheese reaction' provided. Rare hypertensive reactions with selegiline at recommended doses associated with dietary influences have been reported.

Consequently, it may be useful to inform patients (or their families) about the signs and symptoms associated with MAOI induced hypertensive reactions. In particular, patients should be urged to report, immediately, any severe headache or other atypical or unusual symptoms not previously experienced.

Laboratory Tests:

No specific laboratory tests are deemed essential for the management of patients on ELDEPRYL. Periodic routine evaluation of all patients, however, is appropriate.

Drug Interactions:

The occurrence of stupor, muscular rigidity, severe agitation, and elevated temperature has been reported in some patients receiving the combination of selegiline and meperidine. Symptoms usually resolve over days when the combination is discontinued. This is typical of the interaction of meperidine and MAOIs. Other serious reactions (including severe agitation, hallucinations, and death) have been reported in patients receiving this combination (see **CONTRAINDICATIONS**). Severe toxicity has also been reported in patients receiving the combination of tricyclic antidepressants and ELDEPRYL and selective serotonin reuptake inhibitors and ELDEPRYL. (See **WARNINGS** for details). One case of hypertensive crisis has been reported in a patient taking the recommended doses of selegiline and a sympathomimetic medication (ephedrine).

Carcinogenesis, Mutagenesis, and Impairment of Fertility:

Assessment of the carcinogenic potential of selegiline in mice and rats is ongoing.

Selegiline did not induce mutations or chromosomal damage when tested in the bacterial mutation assay in Salmonella typhimurium and in an *in vivo* chromosomal aberration assay. While these studies provide some reassurance that selegiline is not mutagenic or clastogenic, they are not definitive because of methodological limitations. No definitive *in vitro* chromosomal aberration or *in vitro* mammalian gene mutation assays have been performed.

The effect of selegiline on fertility has not been adequately assessed.

Pregnancy:

Pregnancy Category C: No teratogenic effects were observed in a study of embryo-fetal development in Sprague-Dawley rats at oral doses of 4, 12, and 36 mg/kg or 4, 12 and 35 times the human therapeutic dose on a mg/m^2 basis. No teratogenic effects were observed in a study of embryo-fetal development in New Zealand White rabbits at oral doses of 5, 25, and 50 mg/kg or 10, 48, and 95 times the human therapeutic dose on a mg/m^2 basis; however, in this study, the number of litters produced at the two higher doses was less than recommended for assessing teratogenic potential. In the rat study, there was a decrease in fetal body weight at the highest dose tested. In the rabbit study, increases in total resorptions and % post-implantation loss, and a decrease in the number of live fetuses per dam occurred at the highest dose tested. In a peri- and postnatal development study in Sprague-Dawley rats (oral doses of 4, 16, and 64 mg/kg or 4, 15, and 62 times the human therapeutic dose on a mg/m^2 basis), an increase in the number of stillbirths and decreases in the number of pups per dam, pup survival, and pup body weight (at birth and throughout the lactation period) were observed at the two highest doses. At the highest dose tested, no pups born alive survived to Day 4 postpartum. Postnatal development at the highest dose tested in dams could not be evaluated because of the lack of surviving pups. The reproductive performance of the untreated offspring was not assessed.

There are no adequate and well-controlled studies in pregnant women. Selegiline should be used during pregnancy only if the potential benefit justifies the potential risk to the fetus.

Nursing Mothers:

It is not known whether selegiline hydrochloride is excreted in human milk. Because many drugs are excreted in human milk, consideration should be given to discontinuing the use of all but absolutely essential drug treatments in nursing women.

Pediatric Use:

The effects of selegiline hydrochloride in children have not been evaluated.

ADVERSE REACTIONS

Introduction:

The number of patients who received selegiline in prospectively monitored pre-marketing studies is limited. While other sources of information about the use of selegiline are available (e.g., literature reports, foreign post-marketing reports, etc.) they do not provide the kind of information necessary to estimate the incidence of adverse events. Thus, overall incidence figures for adverse reactions associated with the use of selegiline cannot be provided. Many of the adverse reactions seen have also been reported as symptoms of dopamine excess.

Moreover, the importance and severity of various reactions reported often cannot be ascertained. One index of relative importance, however, is whether or not a reaction caused treatment discontinuation. In prospective pre-marketing studies, the following events led, in decreasing order of frequency, to discontinuation of treatment with selegiline: nausea, hallucinations, confusion, depression, loss of balance, insomnia, orthostatic hypotension, increased akinetic involuntary movements, agitation, arrhythmia, bradykinesia, chorea, delusions, hypertension, new or increased angina pectoris, and syncope. Events reported only once as a cause of discontinuation are ankle edema, anxiety, burning lips/mouth, constipation, drowsiness/lethargy, dystonia, excess perspiration, increased freezing, gastrointestinal bleeding, hair loss, increased tremor, nervousness, weakness, and weight loss.

Experience with ELDEPRYL obtained in parallel, placebo controlled, randomized studies provides only a limited basis for estimates of adverse reaction rates. The following reactions that occurred with greater frequency among the 49 patients assigned to selegiline as compared to the 50 patients assigned to placebo in the only parallel, placebo controlled trial performed in patients with Parkinson's disease are shown in the following Table. None of these adverse reactions led to a discontinuation of treatment.

INCIDENCE OF TREATMENT-EMERGENT ADVERSE EXPERIENCES IN THE PLACEBO-CONTROLLED CLINICAL TRIAL

Adverse Event	Number of Patients Reporting Events	
	selegiline hydrochloride N=49	placebo N=50
Nausea	10	3
Dizziness/Lightheaded/Fainting	7	1
Abdominal Pain	4	2
Confusion	3	0
Hallucinations	3	1
Dry mouth	3	1
Vivid Dreams	2	0
Dyskinesias	2	5
Headache	2	1

The following events were reported once in either or both groups:

Ache, generalized	1	0
Anxiety/Tension	1	1
Anemia	0	1
Diarrhea	1	0
Hair Loss	0	1
Insomnia	1	1
Lethargy	1	0
Leg pain	1	0
Low back pain	1	0
Malaise	0	1
Palpitations	1	0
Urinary Retention	1	0
Weight Loss	1	0

In all prospectively monitored clinical investigations, enrolling approximately 920 patients, the following adverse events, classified by body system, were reported.

Central Nervous System:

Motor/Coordination/Extrapyramidal:

increased tremor, chorea, loss of balance, restlessness, blepharospasm, increased bradykinesia, facial grimace, falling down, heavy leg, muscle twitch*, myoclonic jerks*, stiff neck, tardive dyskinesia, dystonic symptoms, dyskinesia, involuntary movements, freezing, festination, increased apraxia, muscle cramps.

Mental Status/Behavioral/Psychiatric:

hallucinations, dizziness, confusion, anxiety, depression, drowsiness, behavior/mood change, dreams/nightmares, tiredness, delusions, disorientation, lightheadedness, impaired memory*, increased energy*, transient high*, hollow feeling, lethargy/malaise, apathy, overstimulation, vertigo, personality change, sleep disturbance, restlessness, weakness, transient irritability.

Pain/Altered Sensation:

headache, back pain, leg pain, tinnitus, migraine, supraorbital pain, throat burning, generalized ache, chills, numbness of toes/fingers, taste disturbance.

Autonomic Nervous System:

dry mouth, blurred vision, sexual dysfunction.

Cardiovascular:

orthostatic hypotension, hypertension, arrhythmia, palpitations, new or increased angina pectoris, hypotension, tachycardia, peripheral edema, sinus bradycardia, syncope.

Gastrointestinal:

nausea/vomiting, constipation, weight loss, anorexia, poor appetite, dysphagia, diarrhea, heartburn, rectal bleeding, bruxism*, gastrointestinal bleeding (exacerbation of preexisting ulcer disease).

Genitourinary/Gynecologic/Endocrine:

slow urination, transient anorgasmia*, nocturia, prostatic hypertrophy, urinary hesitancy, urinary retention, decreased penile sensation*, urinary frequency.

Skin and Appendages:

increased sweating, diaphoresis, facial hair, hair loss, hematoma, rash, photosensitivity.

Miscellaneous:

asthma, diplopia, shortness of breath, speech affected.

Postmarketing Reports:

The following experiences were described in spontaneous post-marketing reports. These reports do not provide sufficient information to establish a clear causal relationship with the use of ELDEPRYL.

CNS:

Seizure in dialyzed chronic renal failure patient on concomitant medications.

*indicates events reported only at doses greater than 10 mg/day.

OVERDOSAGE

Selegiline:

No specific information is available about clinically significant overdoses with ELDEPRYL. However, experience gained during selegiline's development reveals that some individuals exposed to doses of 600 mg of d,l-selegiline suffered severe hypotension and psychomotor agitation.

Since the selective inhibition of MAO B by selegiline hydrochloride is achieved only at doses in the range recommended for the treatment of Parkinson's disease (e.g., 10 mg/day), overdoses are likely to cause significant inhibition of both MAO A and MAO B. Consequently, the signs and symptoms of overdose may resemble those observed with marketed non-selective MAO inhibitors [e.g., tranylcypromine (PARNATE), isocarboxazide (MARPLAN), and phenelzine (NARDIL)].

Overdose with Non-Selective MAO Inhibition:

NOTE:

This section is provided for reference; it does not describe events that have actually been observed with selegiline in overdose.

Characteristically, signs and symptoms of non-selective MAOI overdose may not appear immediately. Delays of up to 12 hours between ingestion of drug and the appearance of signs may occur. Importantly, the peak intensity of the syndrome may not be reached for upwards of a day following the overdose. Death has been reported following overdosage. Therefore, immediate hospitalization, with continuous patient observation and monitoring for a period of at least two days following the ingestion of such drugs in overdose, is strongly recommended.

Continued on next page

Eldepryl—Cont.

The clinical picture of MAOI overdose varies considerably; its severity may be a function of the amount of drug consumed. The central nervous and cardiovascular systems are prominently involved.

Signs and symptoms of overdosage may include, alone or in combination, any of the following: drowsiness, dizziness, faintness, irritability, hyperactivity, agitation, severe headache, hallucinations, trismus, opisthotonos, convulsions, and coma; rapid and irregular pulse, hypertension, hypotension and vascular collapse; precordial pain, respiratory depression and failure, hyperpyrexia, diaphoresis, and cool, clammy skin.

Treatment Suggestions For Overdose:

NOTE:

Because there is no recorded experience with selegiline overdose, the following suggestions are offered based upon the assumption that selegiline overdose may be modeled by non-selective MAOI poisoning. In any case, up-to-date information about the treatment of overdose can often be obtained from a certified Regional Poison Control Center. Telephone numbers of certified Poison Control Centers are listed in the Physicians' Desk Reference (PDR).

Treatment of overdose with non-selective MAOIs is symptomatic and supportive. Induction of emesis or gastric lavage with instillation of charcoal slurry may be helpful in early poisoning, provided the airway has been protected against aspiration. Signs and symptoms of central nervous system stimulation, including convulsions, should be treated with diazepam, given slowly intravenously. Phenothiazine derivatives and central nervous system stimulants should be avoided. Hypotension and vascular collapse should be treated with intravenous fluids and, if necessary, blood pressure titration with an intravenous infusion of a dilute pressor agent. It should be noted that adrenergic agents may produce a markedly increased pressor response.

Respiration should be supported by appropriate measures, including management of the airway, use of supplemental oxygen, and mechanical ventilatory assistance, as required.

Body temperature should be monitored closely. Intensive management of hyperpyrexia may be required. Maintenance of fluid and electrolyte balance is essential.

DOSAGE AND ADMINISTRATION

ELDEPRYL is intended for administration to Parkinsonian patients receiving levodopa/carbidopa therapy who demonstrate a deteriorating response to this treatment. The recommended regimen for the administration of ELDEPRYL is 10 mg per day administered as divided doses of 5 mg each taken at breakfast and lunch. There is no evidence that additional benefit will be obtained from the administration of higher doses. Moreover, higher doses should ordinarily be avoided because of the increased risk of side effects.

After two to three days of selegiline treatment, an attempt may be made to reduce the dose of levodopa/carbidopa. A reduction of 10 to 30% was achieved with the typical participant in the domestic placebo controlled trials who was assigned to selegiline treatment. Further reductions of levodopa/carbidopa may be possible during continued selegiline therapy.

HOW SUPPLIED

ELDEPRYL capsules are available containing 5 mg of selegiline hydrochloride. Each aqua blue capsule is band imprinted with the Somerset logo on the cap and "Eldepryl 5 mg" on the body.

They are available as:

NDC 39506-022-60 bottles of 60 capsules.
NDC 39506-022-30 bottles of 300 capsules.

Store at controlled room temperature, 59° to 86°F (15° to 30°C).

Rx only

SOMERSET
PHARMACEUTICALS, INC.
Tampa, FL 33607
Literature issued July 1998
ELD:R16

Shown in Product Identification Guide, page 338

Star Pharmaceuticals, Inc.

1990 N.W. 44TH STREET
POMPANO BEACH, FL 33064-8712

Direct Inquiries to:
Scott L. Davidson, President
(954) 971-9704
For Medical Information Contact:
Scott L. Davidson
(800) 845-7827
Sales and Ordering:
(800) 845-7827
FAX: (954) 971-7718
http://www.starpharm.com

APHRODYNE® ℞

[af"ro-din']
brand of yohimbine hydrochloride

DESCRIPTION

Yohimbine is a 3a-15a-20β-17a- hydroxy Yohimbine-16a-carboxylic acid methyl ester. The alkaloid is found in Rubaceae and related trees and is also found in Rauwolfia Serpentina (L) Benth.

Yohimbine is an indolalkylamine alkaloid with chemical similarity to reserpine. It is a crystalline powder, odorless. Each compressed caplet contains 5.4 mg (1/12 gr.) of Yohimbine Hydrochloride.

ACTION

Yohimbine blocks presynaptic alpha-2 adrenergic receptors. Its action on peripheral blood vessels resembles that of reserpine, though it is weaker and of short duration. Yohimbine's peripheral autonomic nervous system effect is to increase parasympathetic (cholinergic) and decrease sympathetic (adrenergic) activity. It is to be noted that in male sexual performance, erection is linked to cholinergic activity and to alpha-2 adrenergic blockade which may theoretically result in increased penile inflow, decreased penile outflow or both.

Yohimbine exerts a stimulating action on the mood and may increase anxiety. Such actions have not been adequately studied or related to dosage although they appear to require high doses of the drug. Yohimbine has a mild anti-diuretic action, probably via stimulation of hypothalmic center and release of posterior pituitary hormone.

Reportedly Yohimbine exerts no significant influence on cardiac stimulation and other effects mediated by β-adrenergic receptors. Its effect on blood pressure, if any, would be to lower it; however, no adequate studies are at hand to quantitate this effect in terms of Yohimbine dosage.

INDICATIONS

APHRODYNE® is indicated as a sympatholytic and mydriatic. Impotence has been successfully treated with yohimbine in male patients with vascular or diabetic origins and psychogenic origins (18 mg/day).

CONTRAINDICATIONS

Renal diseases, and patients sensitive to the drug. In view of the limited and inadequate information at hand, no precise tabulation can be offered of additional contraindications.

WARNING

Generally, this drug is not proposed for use in females and certainly must not be used during pregnancy. Neither is this drug proposed for use in pediatric, geriatric or cardio-renal patients with gastric or duodenal ulcer history. Nor should it be used in conjunction with mood-modifying drugs such as antidepressants or in psychiatric patients in general.

ADVERSE REACTIONS

Yohimbine readily penetrates the CNS and produces a complex pattern of responses in lower doses than required to produce peripheral α-adrenergic blockage. These include anti-diuresis, a general picture of central excitation including elevated blood pressure and heart rate, increased motor activity, irritability and tremor. Sweating, nausea and vomiting are common after parenteral administration of the drug.[1,2] Also dizziness, headache, and skin flushing have been reported.[1,3]

DOSAGE AND ADMINISTRATION

Experimental dosage reported in treatment of erectile impotence:[1,3,4] 1 caplet (5.4mg) 3 times a day, to adult males taken orally. Occasional side effects reported with this dosage are nausea, dizziness or nervousness. In the event of side effects dosage is to be reduced to 1/2 caplet 3 times a day, followed by gradual increases to 1 caplet 3 times a day. Reported therapy not more than 10 weeks.[3]

HOW SUPPLIED

APHRODYNE® scored caplets are aqua, debossed with APHRO DYNE. They are available in bottles of 100 NDC 0076-0401-03) and 1000 (NDC 0076-0401-04).

MANUFACTURED FOR:
Star Pharmaceuticals, Inc.,

Revised February 1991

PROSED®/DS ℞

[prō-sĕd DS]

DESCRIPTION

PROSED®/DS is a dark blue, round, sugar-coated compressed tablet for oral administration imprinted with **PROSED®/DS.**

Methenamine	81.6 mg
Phenyl Salicylate	36.2 mg
Methylene Blue	10.8 mg
Benzoic Acid	9.0 mg
Atropine Sulfate	0.06 mg
Hyoscyamine Sulfate	0.06 mg

METHENAMINE (Hexamethylenetetramine) exists as colorless, lustrous crystals or white crystalline powder. Its solutions are alkaline to litmus. Freely soluble in water; soluble in alcohol and in chloroform.

PHENYL SALICYLATE (2-hydroxybenzoic acid phenyl ester) exists as white crystals with a melting point of 40–43°C. It is very slightly soluble in water and freely soluble in alcohol.

METHYLENE BLUE (methylthionine chloride) exists as dark green crystals. It is soluble in water and in chloroform; sparingly soluble in alcohol.

BENZOIC ACID (benzenecarboxylic acid) exists as white crystals, scales or needles. It has a slight odor and is slightly soluble in water; freely soluble in alcohol, in chloroform and in ether.

ATROPINE SULFATE (d/tropyl tropate) is an alkaloid of belladonna. It exists as a odorless, white crystalline powder that is slowly affected by light. It is very soluble in water and freely soluble in alcohol.

HYOSCYAMINE SULFATE (*l*-tropyl tropate) is an alkaloid of belladonna. It exists as a white crystalline powder. Its solutions are alkaline to litmus and affected by light. It is slightly soluble in water; freely soluble in alcohol; sparingly soluble in ether.

PROSED®/DS tablets contain the inactive ingredients calcium sulfate, dicalcium phosphate anhydrous, talc, kaolin, polyvinylpyrollidone, magnesium stearate, methylparaben, propylparaben, FD&C Blue #1 Aluminum Lake, FD&C Blue #2 Aluminum Lake, titanium dioxide, sodium benzoate, acacia, gelatin, sugar, white beeswax, carnauba, polyvinyl acetate phthalate, triethyl citrate, stearic acid.

CLINICAL PHARMACOLOGY

METHENAMINE degrades in an acidic urine environment releasing formaldehyde which provides bactericidal or bacteriostatic action. It is well absorbed from the gastrointestinal tract. 70 to 90% reaches the urine unchanged at which point it is hydrolyzed if the urine is acidic. Within 24 hours it is almost completely (90%) excreted; of this amount at pH 5, approximately 20% is formaldehyde. Protein binding—some formaldehyde is bound to substances in the urine and surrounding tissues. Methenamine is freely distributed to body tissue and fluids but is not clinically significant as it does not hydrolyze at a pH greater than 6.8.

PHENYL SALICYLATE releases salicylate, a mild analgesic for pain.

METHYLENE BLUE possesses weak antiseptic properties. It is well absorbed by the gastrointestinal tract and is rapidly reduced to leukomethylene blue which is stabilized in some combination form in the urine. 75% is excreted unchanged.

BENZOIC ACID has mild antibacterial and antifungal action. It also helps maintain an acid pH in the urine necessary for the degradation of methenamine.

ATROPINE SULFATE AND HYOSCYAMINE SULFATE are parasympatholytic drugs which relax smooth muscles. Protein binding for both atropine sulfate and hyoscyamine sulfate is moderate. Biotransformation for both atropine sulfate and hyoscyamine sulfate is hepatic. They are well absorbed from the gastrointestinal tract. Atropine sulfate is excreted 30 to 50% unchanged and the majority of hyoscyamine sulfate is excreted unchanged.

INDICATIONS AND USAGE

PROSED®/DS is indicated for the relief of discomfort of the lower urinary tract caused by hypermotility resulting from inflammation or diagnostic procedures and in the treatment of cystitis, urethritis and trigonitis when caused by organisms which maintain or produce an acid urine and are susceptible to formaldehyde.

CONTRAINDICATIONS

Risk-benefit should be considered when the following medical problems exist: glaucoma, urinary bladder neck obstruction, pyloric or duodenal obstruction or cardiospasm. Hypersensitivity to any of the ingredients.

WARNINGS

Do not exceed recommended dosage. If rapid pulse, dizziness, or blurring of vision occurs, discontinue use immediately.

PRECAUTIONS

Cross sensitivity and/or related problems: patients intolerant of other belladonna alkaloids or other salicylates may be intolerant of this medication also. Delay in gastric emptying could complicate the management of gastric ulcers.

Pregnancy/Reproduction (FDA Pregnancy Category C): Atropine, hyoscyamine and methenamine cross the placenta. Studies have not been done in either animals or humans. It is not known whether **PROSED®/DS** tablets can cause fetal harm when administered to a pregnant woman or can affect reproduction capacity. **PROSED®/DS** tablets should be given to a pregnant woman only if clearly needed.

Nursing mothers: Methenamine and traces of atropine and hyoscyamine are excreted in breast milk. Caution should be exercised when **PROSED®/DS** tablets are administered to a nursing mother.

Prolonged use: There have been no studies to establish the safety of prolonged use in humans. No known long-term animal studies have been performed to evaluate carcinogenic potential.

Pediatric: Infants and young children are especially susceptible to the toxic effect of the belladonna alkaloids.

Geriatric: Use with caution in elderly patients as they may respond to the usual doses of the belladonna alkaloids with excitement, agitation, drowsiness, or confusion.

Drug Interactions: As a result of atropine's and hyoscamine's effects on gastrointestinal motility and gastric emptying, absorption of other oral medications may be decreased during concurrent use with this combination medication.

Urinary alkalizers and thiazide diuretics: May cause the urine to become alkaline reducing the effectiveness of methenamine by inhibiting its conversion to formaldehyde.

Antimuscarinics: Concurrent use may intensify antimuscarinic effects of atropine and hyoscyamine because of secondary antimuscarinic activities of these medications.

Antacids/antidiarrheals: Concurrent use may reduce absorption of atropine and hyoscyamine resulting in decreased therapeutic effectiveness. Concurrent use with antacids may cause urine to become alkaline reducing the effectiveness of methenamine by inhibiting its conversion to formaldehyde. Doses of these medications should be spaced 1 hour apart from doses of atropine and hyoscyamine.

Antimyasthenics: Concurrent use with atropine and hyoscyamine may further reduce intestinal motility, therefore, caution is recommended.

Ketoconazole-atropine and hyoscyamine may cause increased gastrointestinal pH. Concurrent administration with atropine and hyoscyamine may result in marked reduction in the absorption of ketoconazole. Patients should be advised to take this combination at least 2 hours after ketoconazole.

Monoamine oxidase (MAO) inhibitors: Concurrent use with atropine and hyoscyamine may intensify antimuscarinic side effects.

Opioid (narcotic) analgesics may result in increased risk of severe constipation.

Sulfonamides: These drugs may precipitate with formaldehyde in the urine increasing the danger of crystalluria.

Patients should be advised that the urine and/or stools may become blue to blue-green as a result of the excretion of methylene blue.

ADVERSE REACTIONS

Cardiovascular—rapid pulse, flushing
Central Nervous System—blurred vision, dizziness
Respiratory—shortness of breath or troubled breathing
Genitourinary—difficult micturition, acute urinary retention
Gastrointestinal—dry mouth, nausea/vomiting.

DRUG ABUSE AND DEPENDENCE

A dependence on the use of **PROSED®/DS** has not been reported and due to the nature of its ingredients, abuse of **PROSED®/DS** is not expected.

OVERDOSAGE

Emesis or gastric lavage. Slow intravenous administration of physostigmine in doses of 1 to 4 mg (0.5 to 1 mg in children) repeated as needed in one to two hours to reverse severe antimuscarinic symptoms. Administration of small doses of diazepam to control excitement and seizures. Artificial respiration with oxygen if needed for respiratory depression. Adequate hydration. Symptomatic treatment as necessary.

DOSAGE AND ADMINISTRATION

Adults: One tablet orally 4 times per day followed by liberal fluid intake.
Older children: Dosage must be individualized by physician.
Not recommended for use in children up to 12 years of age.

HOW SUPPLIED

Round, deep blue, sugar-coated tablets imprinted with **"PROSED®/DS"**. Bottles of 100 (NDC 0076-0108-03), and 1000 (NDC 0076-0108-04) tablets.
NDC 0076-0108-03

STORAGE

Store in a dry place between 15° and 30°C (59° to 86°F).
Keep container tightly closed.

Code#STA108-031 **Rev. 3/97**

Manufactured For:
STAR PHARMACEUTICALS, INC.
Pompano Beach, FL 33064

URO-KP-NEUTRAL® Caplet ℞

[*ū 'ro-kp-nū 'tral*]

DESCRIPTION

Each light peach caplet contains 258 mg phosphorous, 49.4 mg potassium and 262.4 mg sodium derived from sodium phosphate monobasic anhydrous, dipotassium phosphate anhydrous, and disodium phosphate anhydrous.

INDICATIONS

URO-KP-NEUTRAL® increases urinary phosphate and pyrophosphate. As a phosphorus supplement, each caplet supplies 25% of the U. S. Recommended Daily Allowance (U. S. RDA) of phosphorus for adults.

CONTRAINDICATIONS

This product is contraindicated in patients with infected phosphate stones, in patients with severely impaired renal function (less than 30% of normal) and in the presence of hyperphosphatemia.

PRECAUTIONS

General: This product contains potassium and sodium and should be used with caution if regulation of these elements is desired. Occasionally, some individuals may experience a mild laxative effect during the first few days of phosphate therapy. If laxation persists to an unpleasant degree, reduce the daily dosage until this effect subsides or, if necessary, discontinue the use of this product.

Caution should be exercised when prescribing this product in the following conditions: Cardiac disease (particularly in digitalized patients); severe adrenal insufficiency (Addison's disease); acute dehydration; severe renal insufficiency; renal function impairment or chronic renal disease; extensive tissue breakdown (such as severe burns); myotonia congenita; cardiac failure; cirrhosis of the liver or severe hepatic disease; peripheral or pulmonary edema; hypernatremia; hypertension; toxemia of pregnancy; hypoparathyroidism; and acute pancreatitis. Rickets may benefit from phosphate therapy, but caution should be exercised. High serum phosphate may increase the incidence of extraskeletal calcification.

Information for Patients: Patients with kidney stones may pass old stones when phosphate therapy is started and should be warned of this possibility. Patients should be advised to avoid the use of antacids containing aluminum, magnesium or calcium which may prevent the absorption of phosphate.

Laboratory Tests: Careful monitoring of renal function and serum electrolytes (calcium, phosphorus, potassium, sodium) may be required at periodic intervals during phosphate therapy. Other tests may be warranted in some patients, depending on conditions.

Drug Interactions: The use of antacids containing magnesium, aluminum or calcium in conjunction with phosphate preparations may bind the phosphate and prevent its absorption. Concurrent use of antihypertensives, especially diazoxide, guanethidine, hydralazine, methyldopa, or rauwolfia alkaloids; or corticosteroids, especially mineralcorticoids or corticotropin, with sodium phosphate may result in hypernatremia. Calcium-containing preparations and/or vitamin D may antagonize the effects of phosphates in the treatment of hypercalcemia. Potassium-containing medications or potassium-sparing diuretics may cause hyperkalemia. Patients should have serum potassium level determinations at periodic intervals.

Carcinogenesis, Mutagenesis, Impairment of Fertility: There have been no studies in animals or humans to evalute the carcinogenesis, mutagenesis, or impairment of fertility for this product.

Pregnancy: Pregnancy Category C. Animal reproduction studies have not been conducted with this product. It is also not known whether this product can cause fetal harm when administered to a pregnant woman or can affect reproduction capacity. This product should be given to a pregnant woman only if clearly needed.

Nursing Mothers: It is not known whether this drug is excreted in human milk. Because many drugs are excreted in human milk, caution should be exercised when this product is administered to a nursing woman.

ADVERSE REACTIONS

Gastrointestinal upset (diarrhea, nausea, stomach pain, and vomiting) may occur with phosphate therapy. Also, bone and joint pain (possible phosphate-induced osteomalacia) could occur. The following adverse effects may be observed (primarily from sodium or potassium): headaches; dizziness; mental confusion; seizures; weakness or heaviness of legs; unusual tiredness or weakness; muscle cramps; numbness, tingling, pain, or weakness of hands or feet; numbness or tingling around lips; fast or irregular heartbeat; shortness of breath or troubled breathing; swelling of feet or lower legs; unusual weight gain; low urine output; unusual thirst.

DOSAGE

Adults: One or two tablets four times a day with a full glass of water.

HOW SUPPLIED

Light peach, film coated caplet with the Star logo and number 109 debossed on each caplet. Bottles of 100 caplets (NDC 0076-0109-03).

CAUTION

Federal law prohibits dispensing without a prescription.
Manufactured for:
Star Pharmaceuticals, Inc.

Rev. 7/92

UROLENE BLUE® ℞

[*ū 'ro-lene blue*]
Methylene Blue Tablets

Each blue coated tablet contains Methylene blue USP 65 mg.

HOW SUPPLIED

Bottles of 100 and 1000.
NDC 0076-0501-03 & 04

VIRILON® Ⓒ℞

[*vir 'i-lon*]
Methyltestosterone Macro-Beads Capsules
Oral Androgen Macro-Beads

Each capsule contains Methyltestosterone ..... USP 10 mg. In a special base. Look for the grey and white seeds in the black and transparent capsule, available only from Star Pharmaceuticals.

HOW SUPPLIED

Bottles of 100 and 1000.
NDC 0076-0301-03 & 04

VIRILON® IM Ⓒ℞

brand of testosterone cypionate
injection sterile solution
200 mg/ml
For Intramuscular Use Only

HOW SUPPLIED

Multiple dose vials of 10 ml containing 200 mg/ml.
NDC 0076-0302-10

Write for complete prescribing information for all Star products.

Stiefel Laboratories, Inc.

255 ALHAMBRA CIRCLE
CORAL GABLES, FL 33134

Direct Inquiries to:
Professional Services Department
(305) 443-3800

BREVOXYL®-4 ℞

[*brĕv-ăhx-il*]
(benzoyl peroxide 4%)

BREVOXYL®-8 ℞

(benzoyl peroxide 8%)

DESCRIPTION

Brevoxyl-4 and Brevoxyl-8 are topical preparations containing benzoyl peroxide 4% and 8%, respectively, as the active ingredient in a gel vehicle containing purified water, cetyl alcohol, dimethyl isosorbide, fragrance, simethicone, stearyl alcohol and ceteareth-20. The structural formula of benzoyl peroxide is:

CLINICAL PHARMACOLOGY

The exact method of action of benzoyl peroxide in acne vulgaris is not known. Benzoyl peroxide is an antibacterial agent with demonstrated activity against *Propionibacterium acnes.* This action, combined with the mild keratolytic effect of benzoyl peroxide is believed to be responsible for its usefulness in acne.

Benzoyl peroxide is absorbed by the skin where it is metabolized to benzoic acid and excreted as benzoate in the urine.

INDICATIONS AND USAGE

Brevoxyl-4 and Brevoxyl-8 are indicated for use in the topical treatment of mild to moderate acne vulgaris. Brevoxyl may be used as an adjunct in acne treatment regimens including antibiotics, retinoic acid products, and sulfur/salicylic acid containing preparations.

CONTRAINDICATIONS

Brevoxyl-4 and Brevoxyl-8 should not be used in patients who have shown hypersensitivity to benzoyl peroxide or to any of the other ingredients in the product.

PRECAUTIONS

General—For external use only. Avoid contact with eyes and mucous membranes. **AVOID CONTACT WITH HAIR, FABRICS OR CARPETING AS BENZOYL PEROXIDE WILL CAUSE BLEACHING.**

Carcinogenesis, Mutagenesis, Impairment of Fertility—Based upon all available evidence, benzoyl peroxide is not considered to be a carcinogen. However, data from a study using mice known to be highly susceptible to cancer suggest that benzoyl peroxide acts as a tumor promoter. The clinical significance of the findings is not known.

Continued on next page

Brevoxyl-4/Brevoxyl-8—Cont.

Pregnancy: Category C—Animal reproduction studies have not been conducted with benzoyl peroxide. It is also not known whether benzoyl peroxide can cause fetal harm when administered to a pregnant woman or can affect reproduction capacity. Benzoyl peroxide should be used by a pregnant woman only if clearly needed.

Nursing Mothers—It is not known whether this drug is excreted in human milk. Because many drugs are excreted in human milk, caution should be exercised when benzoyl peroxide is administered to a nursing woman.

Pediatric Use—Safety and effectiveness in children below the age of 12 have not been established.

ADVERSE REACTIONS

Contact sensitization reactions are associated with the use of topical benzoyl peroxide products and may be expected to occur in 10 to 25 of 1000 patients. The most frequent adverse reactions associated with benzoyl peroxide use are excessive erythema and peeling which may be expected to occur in 5 of 100 patients. Excessive erythema and peeling most frequently appear during the initial phase of drug use and may normally be controlled by reducing frequency of use.

DOSAGE AND ADMINISTRATION

Therapy may be initiated with either Brevoxyl-4 or Brevoxyl-8. The medication should be applied once or twice daily to affected areas. Frequency of use should be adjusted to obtain the desired clinical response. Gentle cleansing of the affected areas prior to application of Brevoxyl-4 or Brevoxyl-8 may be beneficial. Clinically visible improvement will normally occur by the third week of therapy. Maximum lesion reduction may be expected after approximately eight to twelve weeks of drug use. Continuing use of the drug is normally required to maintain a satisfactory clinical response.

HOW SUPPLIED

Brevoxyl-4 and Brevoxyl-8 are supplied in 42.5 g (1.5 oz) and 90 g (3.1 oz) tubes.
Brevoxyl-4
42.5 g tube NDC 0145-2374-06
90 g tube NDC 0145-2374-08
Brevoxyl-8
42.5 g tube NDC 0145-2384-06
90 g tube NDC 0145-2384-08
Store at controlled room temperature 15°–30°C (59°–86°F).
U.S. Patent No. 4,923,900

BREVOXYL®-4 Cleansing Lotion ℞
[*brev-ăhx-il*]
(benzoyl peroxide 4%)
BREVOXYL-8 Cleansing Lotion ℞
(benzoyl peroxide 8%)

DESCRIPTION

Brevoxyl-4 and Brevoxyl-8 Cleansing Lotions are topical preparations containing benzoyl peroxide as the active ingredient.

Brevoxyl-4 and Brevoxyl-8 Cleansing Lotions contain benzoyl peroxide 4% and 8%, respectively, in a lathering vehicle containing purified water, cetyl alcohol, citric acid, dimethyl isosorbide, docusate sodium, hydroxypropyl methylcellulose, laureth-12, magnesium aluminum silicate, propylene glycol, sodium hydroxide, sodium lauryl sulfoacetate, and sodium octoxynol-2 ethane sulfonate.

The structural formula of benzoyl peroxide is:

CLINICAL PHARMACOLOGY

The exact method of action of benzoyl peroxide in acne vulgaris is not known. Benzoyl peroxide is an antibacterial agent with demonstrated activity against *Propionibacterium acnes.* This action, combined with the mild keratolytic effect of benzoyl peroxide is believed to be responsible for its usefulness in acne.

Benzoyl peroxide is absorbed by the skin where it is metabolized to benzoic acid and excreted as benzoate in the urine.

INDICATIONS AND USAGE

Brevoxyl-4 and Brevoxyl-8 Cleansing Lotions are indicated for use in the topical treatment of mild to moderate acne vulgaris. Brevoxyl-4 or Brevoxyl-8 Cleansing Lotion may be used as an adjunct in acne treatment regimens including antibiotics, retinoic acid products, and sulfur/salicylic acid containing preparations.

CONTRAINDICATIONS

Brevoxyl-4 and Brevoxyl-8 Cleansing Lotions should not be used in patients who have shown hypersensitivity to benzoyl peroxide or to any of the other ingredients in the product.

PRECAUTIONS

General—For external use only. Avoid contact with eyes and mucous membranes. **AVOID CONTACT WITH HAIR, FABRICS OR CARPETING AS BENZOYL PEROXIDE WILL CAUSE BLEACHING.**

Carcinogenesis, Mutagenesis, Impairment of Fertility—Based upon all available evidence, benzoyl peroxide is not considered to be a carcinogen. However, data from a study using mice known to be highly susceptible to cancer suggest that benzoyl peroxide acts as a tumor promoter. The clinical significance of the findings is not known.

Pregnancy: Category C—Animal reproduction studies have not been conducted with benzoyl peroxide. It is also not known whether benzoyl peroxide can cause fetal harm when administered to a pregnant woman or can affect reproduction capacity. Benzoyl peroxide should be used by a pregnant woman only if clearly needed.

Nursing Mothers—It is not known whether this drug is excreted in human milk. Because many drugs are excreted in human milk, caution should be exercised when benzoyl peroxide is administered to a nursing woman.

Pediatric Use—Safety and effectiveness in children below the age of 12 have not been established.

ADVERSE REACTIONS

Contact sensitization reactions are associated with the use of topical benzoyl peroxide products and may be expected to occur in 10 to 25 of 1000 patients. The most frequent adverse reactions associated with benzoyl peroxide use are excessive erythema and peeling which may be expected to occur in 5 of 100 patients. Excessive erythema and peeling most frequently appear during the initial phase of drug use and may normally be controlled by reducing frequency of use.

DOSAGE AND ADMINISTRATION

Shake well before using. Wash the affected areas once a day during the first week, and twice a day thereafter as tolerated. Wet skin areas to be treated; apply Brevoxyl-4 or Brevoxyl-8 Cleansing Lotion, work to a full lather, rinse thoroughly and pat dry. Frequency of use should be adjusted to obtain the desired clinical response. Clinically visible improvement will normally occur by the third week of therapy. Maximum lesion reduction may be expected after approximately eight to twelve weeks of drug use. Continuing use of the drug is normally required to maintain a satisfactory clinical response.

HOW SUPPLIED

Brevoxyl-4 Cleansing Lotion is supplied in 297 g (10.5 oz) plastic bottles NDC 0145-2310-05.
Brevoxyl-8 Cleansing Lotion is supplied in 297 g (10.5 oz) plastic bottles NDC 0145-2410-05.
Store at controlled room temperature 15°–30°C (59°–86°F).

BREVOXYL®-4 ℞
[*brev 'ăhx-il*]
Creamy Wash
(benzoyl peroxide 4%)
BREVOXYL®-8 ℞
Creamy Wash
(benzoyl peroxide 8%)
ACNE WASH FOR TOPICAL USE

DESCRIPTION

Brevoxyl-4 Creamy Wash and Brevoxyl-8 Creamy Wash are topical preparations containing benzoyl peroxide as the active ingredient. Brevoxyl-4 Creamy Wash and Brevoxyl-8 Creamy Wash contain: 4% and 8% Benzoyl Peroxide, respectively, in a lathering cream vehicle containing Cetostearyl Alcohol, Cocamidopropyl Betaine, Corn Starch, Dimethyl Isosorbide, Glycerin, Glycolic Acid, Hydrogenated Castor Oil, Imidurea, Methylparaben, Mineral Oil, PEG-14M, Purified Water, Sodium Hydroxide, Sodium PCA, Sodium Potassium Lauryl Sulfate, Titanium Dioxide.

The structural formula of benzoyl peroxide is:

CLINICAL PHARMACOLOGY

The exact method of action of benzoyl peroxide in acne vulgaris is not known. Benzoyl peroxide is an antibacterial agent with demonstrated activity against *Propionibacterium acnes.* This action, combined with the mild keratolytic effect of benzoyl peroxide is believed to be responsible for its usefulness in acne.

Benzoyl peroxide is absorbed by the skin where it is metabolized to benzoic acid and excreted as benzoate in the urine.

INDICATIONS AND USAGE

Brevoxyl-4 Creamy Wash and Brevoxyl-8 Creamy Wash are indicated for use in the topical treatment of mild to moderate acne vulgaris. Brevoxyl-4 Creamy Wash and Brevoxyl-8 Creamy Wash may be used as an adjunct in acne treatment regimens including antibiotics, retinoic acid products, and sulfur/salicylic acid containing preparations.

CONTRAINDICATIONS

Brevoxyl-4 Creamy Wash and Brevoxyl-8 Creamy Wash should not be used in patients who have shown hypersensitivity to benzoyl peroxide or to any of the other ingredients in the product.

PRECAUTIONS

General—For external use only. Avoid contact with eyes and mucous membranes. **AVOID CONTACT WITH HAIR, FABRICS OR CARPETING AS BENZOYL PEROXIDE WILL CAUSE BLEACHING.**

Carcinogenesis, Mutagenesis, Impairment of Fertility—Based upon all available evidence, benzoyl peroxide is not considered to be a carcinogen. However, data from a study using mice known to be highly susceptible to cancer suggest that benzoyl peroxide acts as a tumor promoter. The clinical significance of the findings is not known.

Pregnancy: Category C—Animal reproduction studies have not been conducted with benzoyl peroxide. It is also not known whether benzoyl peroxide can cause fetal harm when administered to a pregnant woman or can affect reproduction capacity. Benzoyl peroxide should be used by a pregnant woman only if clearly needed.

Nursing Mothers—It is not known whether this drug is excreted in human milk. Because many drugs are excreted in human milk, caution should be exercised when benzoyl peroxide is administered to a nursing woman.

Pediatric Use—Safety and effectiveness in children below the age of 12 have not been established.

ADVERSE REACTIONS

Contact sensitization reactions are associated with the use of topical benzoyl peroxide products and may be expected to occur in 10 to 25 of 1000 patients. The most frequent adverse reactions associated with benzoyl peroxide use are excessive erythema and peeling which may be expected to occur in 5 of 100 patients. Excessive erythema and peeling most frequently appear during the initial phase of drug use and may normally be controlled by reducing frequency of use.

DOSAGE AND ADMINISTRATION

Shake well before using. Wash the affected areas once a day during the first week, and twice a day thereafter as tolerated. Wet skin areas to be treated; apply Brevoxyl-4 Creamy Wash or Brevoxyl-8 Creamy Wash, work to a full lather, rinse thoroughly and pat dry. Frequency of use should be adjusted to obtain the desired clinical response. Clinically visible improvement will normally occur by the third week of therapy. Maximum lesion reduction may be expected after approximately eight to twelve weeks of drug use. Continuing use of the drug is normally required to maintain a satisfactory clinical response.

HOW SUPPLIED

Brevoxyl-4 Creamy Wash is supplied in 170.1 g (6.0 oz) tubes NDC 0145-2474-06.
Brevoxyl-8 Creamy Wash is supplied in 170.1 g (6.0 oz) tubes NDC 0145-2484-06.
Store at controlled room temperature, 15°–30°C (59°–86°F).

CLINDETS® ℞
[*klĭn-dĕtz'*]
(Clindamycin Phosphate Pledgets)
1%*
***equivalent to 1% clindamycin**
(10 mg/mL)
FOR EXTERNAL USE ONLY

DESCRIPTION

Clindets® (Clindamycin Phosphate Pledgets) contain clindamycin phosphate, USP at a concentration equivalent to 10 mg clindamycin per milliliter in a vehicle of isopropyl alcohol 52% v/v, propylene glycol and water. Each Clindets® pledget applicator contains approximately 1 mL of Clindamycin Phosphate Topical Solution. Clindamycin Phosphate Topical Solution has a pH range between 4.0 and 7.0.

Clindamycin phosphate is a water soluble ester of the semi-synthetic antibiotic produced by a 7(S)-chloro-substitution of the 7(R)-hydroxyl group of the parent antibiotic lincomycin. It occurs as a white to off-white, hygroscopic, crystalline powder. It is freely soluble in water, slightly soluble in dehydrated alcohol, very slightly soluble in acetone and practically insoluble in chloroform, benzene, and ether. Clindamycin phosphate is odorless or practically odorless, and has a bitter taste.

Chemically, clindamycin phosphate is $C_{18}H_{34}ClN_2O_8PS$. It has the following structural formula:

The chemical name for clindamycin phosphate is Methyl 7-chloro-6,7,8-trideoxy-6-(1-methyl-*trans*-4-propyl-L-2-pyrrolidinecarboxamido)-1-thio-L-*threo*-α-D-*galacto*-octopyranoside 2-(dihydrogen phosphate). (MW=504.97)

CLINICAL PHARMACOLOGY

Although clindamycin phosphate is inactive *in vitro,* rapid *in vivo* hydrolysis converts this compound to the antibacterially active clindamycin.

Cross resistance has been demonstrated between clindamycin and lincomycin.

Treatment Emergent Adverse Event	Number of patients reporting events Solution n=553 (%)	Gel n=148 (%)	Lotion n=160 (%)
Burning	62 (11)	15 (10)	17 (11)
Itching	36 (7)	15 (10)	17 (11)
Burning/Itching	60 (11)	# (-)	# (-)
Dryness	105 (19)	34 (23)	29 (18)
Erythema	86 (16)	10 (7)	22 (14)
Oiliness/Oily Skin	8 (1)	26 (18)	12* (10)
Peeling	61 (11)	# (-)	11 (7)

\# not recorded   * of 126 subjects

Antagonism has been demonstrated between clindamycin and erythromycin.

Following multiple topical applications of clindamycin phosphate at a concentration equivalent to 10 mg clindamycin per mL in an isopropyl alcohol and water solution, very low levels of clindamycin are present in the serum (0-3 ng/mL) and less than 0.2% of the dose is recovered in urine as clindamycin.

Clindamycin activity has been demonstrated in comedones from acne patients. The mean concentration of antibiotic activity in extracted comedones after application of a Clindamycin Phosphate Pledget for 4 weeks was 597 mcg/g of comedonal material (range 0-1490). Clindamycin *in vitro* inhibits all *Propionibacterium acnes* cultures tested (MICs 0.4 mcg/mL). Free fatty acids on the skin surface have been decreased from approximately 14% to 2% following application of clindamycin.

INDICATIONS AND USAGE

Clindets are indicated in the treatment of acne vulgaris. In view of the potential for diarrhea, bloody diarrhea and pseudomembranous colitis, the physician should consider whether other agents are more appropriate. (See CONTRAINDICATIONS, WARNINGS, and ADVERSE REACTIONS.)

CONTRAINDICATIONS

Clindets are contraindicated in individuals with a history of hypersensitivity to preparations containing clindamycin or lincomycin, a history of regional enteritis or ulcerative colitis, or a history of antibiotic-associated colitis.

WARNINGS

Orally and parenterally administered clindamycin has been associated with severe colitis which may result in patient death. Use of the topical formulation of clindamycin results in absorption of the antibiotic from the skin surface. Diarrhea, bloody diarrhea, and colitis (including pseudomembranous colitis) have been reported with the use of topical and systemic clindamycin.

Studies indicate a toxin(s) produced by *clostridia* is one primary cause of antibiotic-associated colitis. The colitis is usually characterized by severe persistent diarrhea and severe abdominal cramps and may be associated with the passage of blood and mucus. Endoscopic examination may reveal pseudomembranous colitis. Stool culture for *Clostridium difficile* and stool assay for *C. difficile* toxin may be helpful diagnostically.

When significant diarrhea occurs, the drug should be discontinued. Large bowel endoscopy should be considered to establish a definitive diagnosis in cases of severe diarrhea.

Antiperistatic agents such as opiates and diphenoxylate with atropine may prolong and/or worsen the condition.

Vancomycin has been found to be effective in the treatment of antibiotic-associated pseudomembranous colitis produced by *Clostridium difficile.* The usual adult dosage is 500 milligrams to 2 grams of vancomycin orally per day in three to four divided doses administered for 7 to 10 days. Cholestyramine or colestipol resins bind to vancomycin *in vitro.* If both a resin and vancomycin are to be administered concurrently, it may be advisable to separate the time of administration of each drug.

Diarrhea, colitis, and pseudomembranous colitis have been observed to begin up to several weeks following cessation of oral and parenteral therapy with clindamycin.

PRECAUTIONS

General

Clindets contain an alcohol base which will cause burning and irritation of the eyes. In the event of accidental contact with sensitive surfaces (eye, abraded skin, mucuous membranes), bathe with copious amounts of cool tap water. The solution has an unpleasant taste and caution should be exercised when applying medication around the mouth.

Clindets should be prescribed with caution in atopic individuals.

Drug Interactions

Clindamycin has been shown to have neuromuscular blocking properties that may enhance the action of other neuromuscular blocking agents. Therefore, it should be used with caution in patients receiving such agents.

Pregnancy: Teratogenic effects-Pregnancy Category B

Reproduction studies have been performed in rats and mice using subcutaneous and oral doses of clindamycin ranging from 100 to 600 mg/kg/day and have revealed no evidence of impaired fertility or harm to the fetus due to clindamycin. There are, however, no adequate and well-controlled studies in pregnant women. Because animal reproduction studies are not always predictive of human response, this drug should be used during pregnancy only if clearly needed.

Nursing Mothers

It is not known whether clindamycin is excreted in human milk following use of Clindets. However, orally and parenterally administered clindamycin has been reported to appear in breast milk. Because of the potential for serious adverse reactions in nursing infants, a decision should be made whether to discontinue nursing or to discontinue the drug, taking into account the importance of the drug to the mother.

Pediatric Use

Safety and effectiveness in the pediatric population under the age of 12 has not been established.

ADVERSE REACTIONS

In 18 clinical studies of various topical formulations of clindamycin phosphate using placebo vehicle and/or active comparator drugs as controls, patients experienced a number of treatment emergent adverse dermatological events (see table below).

[See table above]

OVERDOSAGE

Topically applied Clindamycin Phosphate formulations can be absorbed in sufficient amounts to produce systemic effects. (See WARNINGS.)

DOSAGE AND ADMINISTRATION

Apply a thin film using a Clindets applicator for the application of Clindamycin Phosphate Topical Solution twice daily to affected area. More than one pledget may be used. Each pledget should be used only once and then discarded. Remove pledget from foil just before use. Do not use if the seal is broken.

Discard after single use.

HOW SUPPLIED

Clindets® (Clindamycin Phosphate Pledgets) 1%* * equivalent to 1% clindamycin (10 mg/mL) is available in the following size:

60 pledget container — NDC 0145-2472-60

Store at controlled room temperature, 15°–30°C (59°–86°F).

CLOBEVATE® ℞

[klō' bə-vāt]

(Clobetasol Propionate Gel)

0.05%*

***potency expressed as clobetasol propionate**

FOR TOPICAL DERMATOLOGIC USE ONLY— NOT FOR OPHTHALMIC, ORAL, OR INTRAVAGINAL USE

DESCRIPTION

Clobevate® (Clobetasol Propionate Gel) contains the active compound clobetasol propionate, a synthetic corticosteroid, for topical dermatologic use. Clobetasol, an analog of prednisolone, has a high degree of glucocorticoid activity and a slight degree of mineralocorticoid activity.

Chemically, clobetasol propionate is 21-Chloro-9-fluoro-11β,17-dihydroxy-16β-methylpregna-1,4-diene-3,20-dione 17-propionate, and it has the following structural formula:

Clobetasol propionate has the molecular formula $C_{25}H_{32}ClFO_5$ and a molecular weight of 466.98. It is a white to cream-colored crystalline powder insoluble in water.

Each gram, for topical administration, contains clobetasol propionate 0.5 mg in a base of propylene glycol, carbomer 934P, sodium hydroxide, and purified water.

CLINICAL PHARMACOLOGY

Like other topical corticosteroids, clobetasol propionate has anti-inflammatory, antipruritic, and vasoconstrictive properties. The mechanism of the anti-inflammatory activity of the topical steroids, in general, is unclear. However, corticosteroids are thought to act by the induction of phospholipase A_2 inhibitory proteins, collectively called lipocortins. It is postulated that these proteins control the biosynthesis of potent mediators of inflammation such as prostaglandins and leukotrienes by inhibiting the release of their common precursor, arachidonic acid. Arachidonic acid is released from membrane phospholipids by phospholipase A_2.

Pharmacokinetics: The extent of percutaneous absorption of topical corticosteroids is determined by many factors, including the vehicle and the integrity of the epidermal barrier. Occlusive dressing with hydrocortisone for up to 24 hours has not been demonstrated to increase penetration; however, occlusion of hydrocortisone for 96 hours markedly enhances penetration. Topical corticosteroids can be absorbed from normal intact skin, while inflammation and/or other disease processes in the skin may increase percutaneous absorption. Greater absorption was observed for the clobetasol propionate gel formulation as compared to the cream formulation in *in vitro* human skin penetration studies.

Studies performed with Clobevate indicate that it is in the super-high range of potency as compared with other topical corticosteroids.

INDICATIONS AND USAGE

Clobevate is a super-high potency corticosteroid formulation indicated for the relief of the inflammatory and pruritic manifestations of corticosteroid-responsive dermatoses.

Treatment beyond 2 consecutive weeks is not recommended, and the total dosage should not exceed 50 g per week because of the potential for the drug to suppress the hypothalamic-pituitary-adrenal (HPA) axis. Use in children under 12 years of age is not recommended.

CONTRAINDICATIONS

Clobevate is contraindicated in those patients with a history of hypersensitivity to any of the components of the preparation.

PRECAUTIONS

General: Clobetasol propionate is a highly potent topical corticosteroid that has been shown to suppress the HPA axis at doses as low as 2 g per day.

Systemic absorption of topical corticosteroids can produce reversible HPA axis suppression with the potential for glucocorticosteroid insufficiency after withdrawal from treatment. Manifestations of Cushing's syndrome, hyperglycemia, and glucosuria can also be produced in some patients by systemic absorption of topical corticosteroids while on therapy.

Patients receiving a large dose applied to a large surface area should be evaluated periodically for evidence of HPA axis suppression. This may be done by using the ACTH stimulation, a.m. plasma cortisol, and urinary free cortisol tests. Patients receiving super-potent corticosteroids should not be treated for more than 2 weeks at a time, and only small areas should be treated at any one time due to the increased risk of HPA suppression.

If HPA axis suppression is noted, an attempt should be made to withdraw the drug, to reduce the frequency of application, or to substitute a less potent corticosteroid. Recovery of HPA axis function is generally prompt and complete upon discontinuation of topical corticosteroids. Infrequently, signs and symptoms of glucocorticosteroid insufficiency may occur that require supplemental systemic corticosteroids. For information on systemic supplementation, see prescribing information for those products.

Children may be more susceptible to systemic toxicity from equivalent doses due to their larger skin surface to body mass ratios (see PRECAUTIONS: Pediatric Use).

If irritation develops, Clobevate should be discontinued and appropriate therapy instituted. Allergic contact dermatitis with corticosteroids is usually diagnosed by observing *failure to heal* rather than noting a clinical exacerbation as with most topical products not containing corticosteroids. Such an observation should be corroborated with appropriate diagnostic patch testing.

If concomitant skin infections are present or develop, an appropriate antifungal or antibacterial agent should be used. If a favorable response does not occur promptly, use of Clobevate should be discontinued until the infection has been adequately controlled.

Clobevate should not be used in the treatment of rosacea or perioral dermatitis, and should not be used on the face, groin, or axillae.

Information for Patients: Patients using topical corticosteroids should receive the following information and instructions:

1. This medication is to be used as directed by the physician. It is for external use only. Avoid contact with the eyes.
2. This medication should not be used for any disorder other than that for which it was prescribed.
3. The treated skin area should not be bandaged or otherwise covered or wrapped so as to be occlusive unless directed by the physician.
4. Patients should report any signs of local adverse reactions to the physician.
5. Patients should inform their physicians that they are using Clobevate if surgery is contemplated.

Laboratory Tests: The following tests may be helpful in evaluating patients for HPA axis suppression:

ACTH stimulation test
A.M. plasma cortisol test
Urinary free cortisol test

Carcinogenesis, Mutagenesis, Impairment of Fertility: Long-term animal studies have not been performed to evaluate the carcinogenic potential of clobetasol propionate.

Continued on next page

Clobevate—Cont.

Studies in the rat following oral administration at dosage levels up to 50 mg/kg per day revealed no significant effect on the males. The females exhibited an increase in the number of resorbed embryos and a decrease in the number of living fetuses at the highest dose.
Clobetasol propionate was nonmutagenic in three different test systems: the Ames test, the *Saccharomyces cerevisiae* gene conversion assay, and the *E. coli* B WP2 fluctuation test.
Pregnancy: ***Teratogenic Effects: Pregnancy Category C:*** Corticosteroids have been shown to be teratogenic in laboratory animals when administered systemically at relatively low dosage levels. Some corticosteroids have been shown to be teratogenic after dermal application to laboratory animals.
Clobetasol propionate has not been tested for teratogenicity by this route; however, it is absorbed percutaneously, and when administered subcutaneously it was a significant teratogen in both the rabbit and mouse. Clobetasol propionate has greater teratogenic potential than steroids that are less potent.
Teratogenicity studies in mice using the subcutaneous routes resulted in fetotoxicity at the highest dose tested (1 mg/kg) and teratogenicity at all dose levels tested down to 0.03 mg/kg. These doses are approximately 0.33 and 0.01 times, respectively, the human topical dose of Clobevate. Abnormalities seen included cleft palate and skeletal abnormalities.
In rabbits, clobetasol propionate given by the same route was teratogenic at doses of 3 and 10 mcg/kg. These doses are approximately 0.001 and 0.003 times, respectively, the human topical dose of Clobevate. Abnormalities seen included cleft palate, cranioschisis, and other skeletal abnormalities.
There are no adequate and well-controlled studies of the teratogenic potential of clobetasol propionate in pregnant women. Clobevate should be used during pregnancy only if the potential benefit justifies the potential risk to the fetus.
Nursing Mothers: Systemically administered corticosteroids appear in human milk and could suppress growth, interfere with endogenous corticosteroid production, or cause other untoward effects. It is not known whether topical administration of corticosteroids could result in sufficient systemic absorption to produce detectable quantities in human milk. Because many drugs are excreted in human milk, caution should be exercised when Clobevate is administered to a nursing woman.
Pediatric Use: Safety and effectiveness of Clobevate in children and infants have not been established; therefore, use in children under 12 years of age is not recommended. Because of a higher ratio of skin surface area to body mass, children are at a greater risk than adults of HPA axis suppression when they are treated with topical corticosteroids. They are therefore also at greater risk of glucocorticosteroid insufficiency after withdrawal of treatment and of Cushing's syndrome while on treatment. Adverse effects including striae have been reported with inappropriate use of topical corticosteroids in infants and children (see PRECAUTIONS).
HPA axis suppression, Cushing's syndrome, and intracranial hypertension have been reported in children receiving topical corticosteroids. Manifestations of adrenal suppression in children include linear growth retardation, delayed weight gain, low plasma cortisol levels, and absence of response to ACTH stimulation. Manifestations of intracranial hypertension include bulging fontanelles, headaches, and bilateral papilledema.

ADVERSE REACTIONS

In a controlled trial with Clobevate, the only reported adverse reaction that was considered to be drug related was a report of burning sensation (1.8% of treated patients).
In larger controlled clinical trials with other clobetasol propionate formulations, the most frequently reported adverse reactions have included burning, stinging, irritation, pruritus, erythema, folliculitis, cracking and fissuring of the skin, numbness of the fingers, skin atrophy, and telangiectasia (all less than 2%).
Cushing's syndrome has been reported in infants and adults as a result of prolonged use of topical clobetasol propionate formulations.
The following additional local adverse reactions are reported infrequently with topical corticosteroids, but may occur more frequently with super-high potency corticosteroids such as Clobevate. These reactions are listed in approximate decreasing order of occurrence: dryness, hypertrichosis, acneiform eruptions, hypopigmentation, perioral dermatitis, allergic contact dermatitis, secondary infection, irritation, striae, and miliaria.

OVERDOSAGE

Topically applied Clobevate can be absorbed in sufficient amounts to produce systemic effects (see PRECAUTIONS).

DOSAGE AND ADMINISTRATION

Apply a thin layer of Clobevate to the affected areas twice daily and rub in gently and completely (see INDICATIONS AND USAGE).
Clobevate is a super-high potency topical corticosteroid; therefore, **treatment should be limited to 2 consecutive weeks, and amounts greater than 50 g per week should not be used.**
As with other highly active corticosteroids, therapy should be discontinued when control has been achieved. If no improvement is seen within 2 weeks, reassessment of diagnosis may be necessary.
Clobevate should not be used with occlusive dressings.

HOW SUPPLIED

Clobevate (Clobetasol Propionate Gel) 0.05% is supplied in 45-g (NDC 0145-2790-04) tubes.
Store between 15° and 30°C (59° and 86°F). Clobevate should not be refrigerated.

LACTICARE®–HC Lotion 1%, 2½% ℞
[lăk 'tĭ-kār ″]
(hydrocortisone lotion, USP)

CONTAINS

Each mL of LactiCare-HC Lotion 1% and 2½% (hydrocortisone lotion, USP) contains 10 mg and 25 mg respectively of hydrocortisone in a vehicle consisting of carbomer 940, sodium PCA, lactic acid, sodium hydroxide, stearyl alcohol (and) ceteareth-20, glyceryl stearate (and) PEG-100 stearate, cetyl alcohol, isopropyl palmitate, light mineral oil, myristyl lactate, DMDM hydantoin, dehydroacetic acid, fragrance and purified water.

HOW SUPPLIED

Lacticare®-HC Lotion 1% (hydrocortisone lotion, USP) is available in the following size:
118 mL (4 fl oz) bottle NDC 0145-2537-04
Lacticare®-HC Lotion 2½% (hydrocortisone lotion, USP) is available in the following sizes:
59 mL (2 fl oz) bottle NDC 0145-2538-02
118 mL (4 fl oz) bottle NDC 0145-2538-04

PANOXYL® 5 ℞
[pan 'ăhx-il]
(benzoyl peroxide 5%)

PANOXYL® 10 ℞
(benzoyl peroxide 10%)

HOW SUPPLIED

PanOxyl 5 and PanOxyl 10 are supplied in 56.7 gram and 113.4 gram tubes.

PanOxyl 5
56.7 g (2.0 oz) tube NDC 0145-2372-06
113.4 g (4.0 oz) tube NDC 0145-2372-08
PanOxyl 10
56.7 g (2.0 oz) tube NDC 0145-2373-06
113.4 g (4.0 oz) tube NDC 0145-2373-08
U.S. Patent 4056611

PANOXYL® AQ 2½ ℞
[pan 'ăhx-il]
(benzoyl peroxide 2½%)

PANOXYL® AQ 5 ℞
(benzoyl peroxide 5%)

PANOXYL® AQ 10 ℞
(benzoyl peroxide 10%)

HOW SUPPLIED

PanOxyl AQ 2½, PanOxyl AQ 5, and PanOxyl AQ 10 are supplied in 56.7 gram and 113.4 gram tubes.

PanOxyl AQ 2½
56.7 g (2.0 oz) tube NDC 0145-2375-06
113.4 g (4.0 oz) tube NDC 0145-2375-08
PanOxyl AQ 5
56.7 g (2.0 oz) tube NDC 0145-2376-06
113.4 g (4.0 oz) tube NDC 0145-2376-08
PanOxyl AQ 10
56.7 g (2.0 oz) tube NDC 0145-2377-06
113.4 g (4.0 oz) tube NDC 0145-2377-08

SULFOXYL® Lotion Regular ℞
SULFOXYL® Lotion Strong ℞
[sul 'fox-ul]

HOW SUPPLIED

Sulfoxyl Lotion Regular and Sulfoxyl Lotion Strong are supplied in 59 milliliter (2 fluid ounce) plastic bottles.

Sulfoxyl Lotion Regular	**Sulfoxyl Lotion Strong**
NDC 0145-3518-07	NDC 0145-3519-07

For EMERGENCY telephone numbers, consult the **Manufacturers' Index**.

SuperGen, Inc.

1059 SERPENTINE LANE
PLEASANTON, CA 94566

For Customer Service and Placing Orders Contact:
Nipent: 800-222-6883
Mitomycin: 800-905-5474
For Medical or Drug Information Contact:
Professional Services:
888-43-SUPER
888-437-8737
In Emergencies:
415-487-8441
For Corporate Headquarters:
800-353-1075

MITOMYCIN ℞
FOR INJECTION, USP

DESCRIPTION

Mitomycin (also known as mitomycin-C) is an antibiotic isolated from the broth of *Streptomyces caespitosus* which has been shown to have antitumor activity. The compound is heat stable, has a high melting point, and is freely soluble in organic solvents.
Mitomycin for Injection is a sterile dry mixture of mitomycin and mannitol, which when reconstituted with Sterile Water for Injection provides a solution for intravenous administration. Mitomycin for Injection is supplied in vials containing 5 mg and 20 mg of mitomycin. Each 5 mg vial of Mitomycin for Injection contains mitomycin 5 mg and mannitol 10 mg. Each 20 mg vial of Mitomycin for Injection contains mitomycin 20 mg and mannitol 40 mg.
Mitomycin is a blue-violet crystalline powder with the molecular formula of $C_{15}H_{18}N_4O_5$ and a molecular weight of 334.33. Its chemical name is 7-amino-9α-methoxymitosane.

HOW SUPPLIED

Mitomycin for Injection, USP
NDC **62701-010-01**–5 mg mitomycin in an amber vial, individually packaged in single cartons.
NDC **62701-011-01**–20 mg mitomycin in an amber vial, individually packaged in single cartons.
Storage: Store dry powder at controlled room temperatures 15° to 30°C (59° to 86°F), protected from light. Protect reconstituted solution from light. Store solution under refrigeration 2° to 8°C (36° to 46°F), discard after 14 days. If unrefrigerated, discard after 7 days.
Rx Only

NIPENT® ℞
(pentostatin for injection)

> **WARNING**
>
> NIPENT should be administered under the supervision of a physician qualified and experienced in the use of cancer chemotherapeutic agents. The use of higher doses than those specified (see **DOSAGE AND ADMINISTRATION**) is not recommended. Dose-limiting severe renal, liver, pulmonary, and CNS toxicities occurred in Phase 1 studies that used NIPENT at higher doses (20–50 mg/m^2 in divided doses over 5 days) than recommended.
> In a clinical investigation in patients with refractory chronic lymphocytic leukemia using NIPENT at the recommended dose in combination with fludarabine phosphate, 4 of 6 patients entered in the study had severe or fatal pulmonary toxicity. The use of NIPENT in combination with fludarabine phosphate is not recommended.

DESCRIPTION

NIPENT® (pentostatin for injection) is supplied as a sterile, apyrogenic, lyophilized powder in single-dose vials for intravenous administration. Each vial contains 10 mg of pentostain and 50 mg of Mannitol, USP. The pH of the final product is maintained between 7.0 and 8.5 by addition of sodium hydroxide or hydrochloric acid.
Pentostatin, also known as 2′-deoxycoformycin (DCF), is a potent inhibitor of the enzyme adenosine deaminase and is isolated from fermentation cultures of *Streptomyces antibioticus*. Pentostatin is known chemically as (R)-3-(2–deoxy-β-D-*erythro* -pentofuranosyl)-3,6,7,8-tetrahydroimidazo[4,5-*d*] [1,3]diazepin-8-ol with a molecular formula of $C_{11}H_{16}N_4O_4$ and a molecular weight of 268.27.
Pentostain is a white to off-white solid, freely soluble in distilled water.
The molecular structure of pentostatin is:
[See chemical structure at top of next column]

CLINICAL PHARMACOLOGY

Mechanism of Action

Pentostatin is a potent transition state inhibitor of the enzyme adenosine deaminase (ADA). The greatest activity of ADA is found in cells of the lymphoid system with T-cells having higher activity than B-cells and T-cell malignancies higher ADA activity than B-cell malignancies. Pentostatin

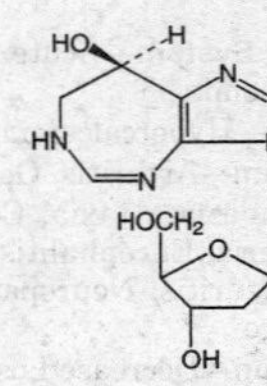

inhibition of ADA, particularly in the presence of adenosine or deoxyadenosine, leads to cytotoxicity, and this is believed to be due to elevated intracellular levels of dATP which can block DNA synthesis through inhibition of ribonucleotide reductase. Pentostatin can also inhibit RNA synthesis as well as cause increased DNA damage. In addition to elevated dATP, these mechanisms may also contribute to the overall cytotoxic effect of pentostatin. The precise mechanism of pentostain's antitumor effect, however, in hairy cell leukemia is not known.

Pharmacokinetics/Drug Metabolism

A tissue distribution and whole-body autoradiography study in the rat revealed that radioactivity concentrations were highest in the kidneys with very little central nervous system penetration.

In man, following a single dose of 4 mg/m^2 of pentostain infused over 5 minutes, the distribution half-life was 11 minutes, the mean terminal half-life was 5.7 hours, the mean plasma clearance was 68 mL/min/m^2, and approximately 90% of the dose was excreted in the urine as unchanged pentostatin and/or metabolites as measured by adenosine deaminase inhibitory activity. The plasma protein binding of pentostatin is low, approximately 4%.

A positive correlation was observed between pentostatin clearance and creatinine clearance (CrCl) in patients with creatinine clearance values ranging from 60 mL/min to 130 mL/min.[1] Pentostatin half-life in patients with renal impairment (CrCl <50 mL/min, n=2) was 18 hours, which was much longer than that observed in patients with normal renal function (CrCl >60 mL/min, n=14), about 6 hours.

CLINICAL STUDIES

The following table provides efficacy results for 4 groups (columns) of patients with hairy cell leukemia: patients who initially received NIPENT, patients who initially received alpha-interferon (IFN), and 2 different groups of patients who received NIPENT after proving to be refractory to, or intolerant of IFN therapy. The first 2 groups represent treatment results from the SWOG 8691 study, a large multicenter study comparing NIPENT and IFN in untreated (frontline) patients with confirmed hairy cell leukemia. The third group represents evaluable patients from the SWOG study who crossed over to NIPENT after initially receiving IFN. The fourth group, labeled NCI Phase 2 studies, displays pooled results of 2 noncomparative studies (MD Anderson and CALGB), in which NIPENT was used to treat patients with confirmed IFN-refractory disease.

In the SWOG 8691 study, NIPENT was administered at a dose of 4 mg/m^2 every 2 weeks. After 6 months of treatment, patients were evaluated for response. If a complete response was achieved, 2 additional doses of NIPENT were administered and then discontinued. If a partial response was achieved. NIPENT was continued for up to an additional 6 months. NIPENT was discontinued for stable disease after 6 months or progressive disease after 2 months of therapy. IFN was administered 3 million units subcutaneously 3 times per week. Patients who achieved a complete or partial response after 6 months of treatment continued on IFN for another 6 months. IFN was discontinued if patients did not achieve a complete or partial response after 6 months of initial treatment or progressed after 2 months. This study allowed crossover of patients intolerant of, or refractory to, initial treatment.

Interferon-refractory patients enrolled into the MD Anderson study received NIPENT at a dose of 4 mg/m^2 every other week for 3 months and responding patients received 3 additional months. CALGB patients received 4 mg/m^2 of NIPENT every other week for 3 months and responding patients were treated monthly for up to 9 additional months. Almost all patients had a PS of 0 to 2 in the Phase 2 and 3 studies.

For each study, a complete response (CR) required clearing of the peripheral blood and bone marrow of all hairy cells, normalization of organomegaly and lymphadenopathy by physical examination, and recovery of hemoglobin to at least 12 g/dL, platelet count to at least 100,000/mm^3, and granulocyte count to at least 1500/mm^3. A partial response (PR) required that the percentage of hairy cells in the blood and bone marrow decrease by more than 50%, enlarged organs and lymph nodes decrease by more than 50% by physical examination, and hematologic parameters had to meet the same criteria as for complete response. The table below reports the response rate for 2 groups of patients: (1) Evaluable, ie, patients who could be evaluated for response and (2) Intent-to-Treat, ie, patients diagnosed with hairy cell leukemia.

[See table above]

Parameter		FRONTLINE		IFN-REFRACTORY[a]	
		Evaluable NIPENT N=138	Evaluable IFN N=130	SWOG 8691[b] Crossover N=79	NCI Phase 2 Studies N=44
Response Rates (%)					
Evaluable	CR	84	18	85	58
	PR	6	24	4	28
Intent-to-Treat		*N=170*	*N=170*		
	CR	*68*	*14*		
	PR	*5*	*18*		
Median Time to Response (months)					
	CR	6.6	11.5	6.0	4.2
	PR	4.0	6.2	5.8	—
Median Duration of Response (months)					
	CR	NR	8.3	NR	>7.7[c] (CALGB) >15.2[c] (MDA)
	PR	NR	15.2	NR	—
% Estimated to be in Response After 24 Months					
	CR	76	16	85	—
	PR	50	21	—	—
Median Time to Recovery (days)					
ANC (1500/mm^3)		70	106	—	—
Platelets (100,000/mm^3)		22	36	—	—

NR = Not reached by Kaplan-Meier method; ANC = Absolute neutrophil count.
[a]Evaluable patients
[b]Patients either refractory to, or intolerant of, IFN
[c]Kaplan-Meier estimate

The results show that frontline patients treated with NIPENT achieved a significantly higher rate of response than those treated with IFN. The time to recovery of neutrophil and platelet counts was shorter with NIPENT treatment and the estimated duration of response was longer. The response rate in IFN-refractory patients treated with NIPENT was similar to that in NIPENT-treated frontline patients. At a median follow-up duration of 46 months, there was no statistically significant difference in survival between hairy cell leukemia patients initially treated with NIPENT and those initially treated with IFN. However, no definite conclusions regarding survival can be made from these results because they are complicated by the fact that the majority of IFN patients crossed over to NIPENT treatment.

In the Phase 3 SWOG study, 25 patients with hairy cell leukemia died during treatment or follow-up: 18 patients had last received NIPENT (3 of whom had crossed over from IFN), and 7 patients had last received IFN (1 of whom crossed over from NIPENT). Eleven of the 25 deaths occurred within 60 days of the last dose of treatment. Of these, hairy cell leukemia was cited by the investigators as a contributory cause for 1 death in the NIPENT group and 3 deaths in the IFN group. Additionally, infection contributed to the deaths of 3 patients in the NIPENT group and 2 patients in the IFN group. Approximately 4% of hairy cell leukemia patients, in each arm, died more than 60 days after the last dose of either treatment and there was no outstanding cause of death among these patients.

INDICATIONS AND USAGE

NIPENT is indicated as single-agent treatment for both untreated and alpha-interferon-refractory hairy cell leukemia patients with active disease as defined by clinically significant anemia, neutropenia, thrombocytopenia, or disease-related symptoms.

CONTRAINDICATIONS

NIPENT is contraindicated in patients who have demonstrated hypersensitivity to NIPENT.

WARNINGS

See **Boxed Warning**.

Patients with hairy cell leukemia may experience myelosuppression primarily during the first few courses of treatment. Patients with infections prior to NIPENT treatment have in some cases developed worsening of their condition leading to death, whereas others have achieved complete response. Patients with infection should be treated only when the potential benefit of treatment justifies the potential risk to the patient. Efforts should be made to control the infection before treatment is initiated or resumed.

In patients with progressive hairy cell leukemia, the initial courses of NIPENT treatment were associated with worsening of neutropenia. Therefore, frequent monitoring of complete blood counts during this time is necessary. If severe neutropenia continues beyond the initial cycles, patients should be evaluated for disease status, including a bone marrow examination.

Elevations in liver function tests occurred during treatment with NIPENT and were generally reversible.

Renal toxicity was observed at higher doses in early studies; however, in patients treated at the recommended dose, elevations in serum creatinine were usually minor and reversible. There were some patients who began treatment with normal renal function who had evidence of mild to moderate toxicity at a final assessment. (See **DOSAGE AND ADMINISTRATION**.)

Rashes, occasionally severe, were commonly reported and may worsen with continued treatment. Withholding of treatment may be required (See **DOSAGE AND ADMINISTRATION**.)

Acute pulmonary edema and hypotension, leading to death, have been reported in the literature in patients treated with pentostatin in combination with carmustine, etoposide and high dose cyclophosphamide as part of the ablative regimen for bone marrow transplant.

Pregnancy Category D

Pentostatin can cause fetal harm when administered to a pregnant woman. Pentostatin was administered intravenously at doses of 0, 0.01, 0.1, or 0.75 mg/kg/day (0, 0.06, 0.6, and 4.5 mg/m^2) to pregnant rats on days 6 through 15 of gestation. Drug-related maternal toxicity occurred at doses of 0.1 and 0.75 mg/kg/day (0.6 and 4.5 mg/m^2). Teratogenic effects were observed at 0.75 mg/kg/day (4.5 mg/m^2) manifested by increased incidence of various skeletal malformations. In a dose range-finding study, pentostatin was administered intravenously to rats at doses of 0, 0.05, 0.1, 0.5, 0.75, or 1 mg/kg/day (0, 0.3, 0.6, 3, 4.5, 6 mg/m^2) on days 6 through 15 of gestation. Fetal malformations that were observed were an omphalocele at 0.05 mg/kg (0.3 mg/m^2), gastroschisis at 0.75 mg/kg and 1 mg/kg (4.5 and 6 mg/m^2), and a flexure defect of the hindlimbs at 0.75 mg/kg (4.5 mg/m^2). Pentostatin was also shown to be teratogenic in mice when administered as a single 2 mg/kg (6 mg/m^2) intraperitoneal injection on day 7 of gestation. Pentostatin was not teratogenic in rabbits when administered intravenously on days 6 through 18 of gestation at doses of 0, 0.005, 0.01, or 0.02 mg/kg/day (0, 0.015, 0.03, or 0.06 mg/m^2); however, maternal toxicity, abortions, early deliveries, and deaths occurred in all drug-treated groups. There are no adequate and well-controlled studies in pregnant women. If NIPENT is used during pregnancy, or if the patient becomes pregnant while taking (receiving) this drug, the patient should be apprised of the potential hazard to the fetus. Women of childbearing potential receiving NIPENT should be advised to avoid becoming pregnant.

PRECAUTIONS

General

Therapy with NIPENT requires regular patient observation and monitoring of hematologic parameters and blood chemistry values. If severe adverse reactions occur, the drug should be withheld (see **DOSAGE AND ADMINISTRATION**), and appropriate corrective measures should be taken according to the clinical judgment of the physician.

NIPENT treatment should be withheld or discontinued in patients showing evidence of nervous system toxicity.

Information for Patients

Patients should be advised of the signs and symptoms of adverse events associated with NIPENT therapy. (See **ADVERSE REACTIONS**.)

Laboratory Tests

Prior to initiating therapy witn NIPENT, renal function should be assessed with a serum creatinine and/or a creatinine clearance assay. (See **CLINICAL PHARMACOLOGY** and **DOSAGE AND ADMINISTRATION**.) Complete blood counts and serum creatinine should be performed before each dose of NIPENT and at other appropriate periods during therapy (see **DOSAGE AND ADMINISTRATION**). Severe neutropenia has been observed following the early courses of treatment with NIPENT and therefore frequent monitoring of complete blood counts is recommended during this time. If hematologic parameters do not improve with subsequent courses, patients should be evaluated for disease status, including a bone marrow examination. Periodic monitoring of the peripheral blood for hairy cells should be performed to assess the response to treatment.

In addition, bone marrow aspirates and biopsies may be required at 2 to 3 month intervals to assess the response to treatment.

Drug Interactions

Allopurinol and NIPENT are both associated with skin rashes. Based on clinical studies in 25 refractory patients who received both NIPENT and allopurinol, the combined use of NIPENT and allopurinol did not appear to produce a higher incidence of skin rashes than observed with NIPENT

Continued on next page

Nipent—Cont.

alone. There has been a report of one patient who received both drugs and experienced a hypersensitivity vasculitis that resulted in death. It was unclear whether this adverse event and subsequent death resulted from the drug combination.

Biochemical studies have demonstrated that pentostatin enhances the effects of vidarabine, a purine nucleoside with antiviral activity. The combined use of vidarabine and NIPENT may result in an increase in adverse reactions associated with each drug. The therapeutic benefit of the drug combination has not been established.

The combined use of NIPENT and fludarabine phosphate is not recommended because it may be associated with an increased risk of fatal pulmonary toxicity (see **WARNINGS**).

Acute pulmonary edema and hypotension, leading to death, have been reported in the literature in patients treated with pentostatin in combination with carmustine, etoposide and high dose cyclophosphamide as part of the ablative regimen for bone marrow transplant.

Carcinogenesis, Mutagenesis, Impairment of Fertility

Carcinogenesis: No animal carcinogenicity studies have been conducted with pentostatin.

Mutagenesis: Pentostatin was nonmutagenic when tested in *Salmonella typhimurium* strains TA-98, TA-1535, TA-1537, and TA-1538. When tested with strain TA-100, a repeatable statistically significant response trend was observed with and without metabolic activation. The response was 2.1 to 2.2 fold higher than the background at 10 mg/plate, the maximum possible drug concentration. Formulated pentostatin was clastogenic in the *in vivo* mouse bone marrow micronucleus assay at 20, 120, and 240 mg/kg. Pentostatin was not mutagenic to V79 Chinese hamster lung cells at the HGPRT locus exposed 3 hours to concentrations of 1 to 3 mg/mL, with or without metabolic activation. Pentostatin did not significantly increase chromosomal aberrations in V79 Chinese hamster lung cells exposed 3 hours to 1 to 3 mg/mL in the presence or absence of metabolic activation.

Impairment of Fertility: No fertility studies have been conducted in animals; however, in a 5-day intravenous toxicity study in dogs, mild seminiferous tubular degeneration was observed with doses of 1 and 4 mg/kg. The possible adverse effects on fertility in humans have not been determined.

Pregnancy

Pregnancy Category D: (See **WARNINGS**)

Nursing Mothers

It is not known whether NIPENT is excreted in human milk. Because many drugs are excreted in human milk, and because of the potential for serious adverse reactions in nursing infants from pentostatin, a decision should be made whether to discontinue nursing or discontinue the drug, taking into account the importance of NIPENT to the mother.

Pediatric Use

Safety and effectiveness in children or adolescents have not been established.

ADVERSE REACTIONS

Most patients treated for hairy cell leukemia in the five NCI-sponsored Phase 2 and the Phase 3 SWOG study experienced an adverse event. The following table lists the most frequently occurring adverse events in patients treated with NIPENT (both frontline and IFN-refractory patients) compared with IFN (frontline only), regardless of drug association. The drug association of some adverse events is uncertain as they may be associated with the disease itself (eg, infection, hematologic suppression), but other events, such as the gastrointestinal symptoms, rashes, and abnormal liver function tests, can in many cases be attributed to the drug. Most adverse events that were asssessed for severity were either mild or moderate, and diminished in frequency with continued therapy.

	Percent of Patients		
All Adverse Events[a]	Frontline, Treated With NIPENT N=180	Frontline, Treated With IFN N=176	IFN-Refractory Treated With NIPENT N=197
Nausea and/or Vomiting	63	22	53[b]
Fever	46	59	42
Rash	43	30	26
Fatigue	42	55	29
Leukopenia	22	15	60
Pruritus	21	6	10
Coughing/Increased Cough	20	15	17
Myalgia	19	36	11
Chills	19	34	11
Headache	17	29	13
Diarrhea	17	17	15
Abdominal Pain	16	15	4
Anorexia	13	10	16
Upper Respiratory Infection	13	8	16
Asthenia	12	13	10
Stomatitis	12	7	5
Rhinitis	11	15	10
Dyspnea	11	13	8
Anemia	8	5	35
Pain	8	19	20
Pharyngitis	8	11	10
Sweating Increased/Sweating	8	21	10
Viral Infection	8	17	NR
Infection	7[c]	2[c]	36
Arthralgia	6	14	3
Thrombocytopenia	6	6	32
Skin Disorder	4	5	17
Allergic Reaction	2	1	11
Hepatic Disorder/Elevated Liver Function Tests[d]	2	2	19
Neurologic Disorder, CNS/CNS Toxicity	1	NR	11
Lung Disorder/Disease	NR	1	12
Nausea	NR	NR	22
Genitourinary Disorder	NR	NR	15

NR = Not Reported

[a] Occurring in more than 10% of patients, in any group, regardless of drug association

[b] Includes only nausea with vomiting

[c] These figures represent only unspecified infections. Refer to infection table.

[d] Elevated liver enzymes and liver disorder for SWOG

The total incidence for all types of infections is considerably higher for both treatment groups in the SWOG 8691 study than is listed in the table above. An intent-to-treat analysis of infections found that 38% of patients treated with NIPENT and 34% of patients treated with IFN averaged 2.4 and 1.9 documented infections during treatment, respectively. The following table lists the different types of infections that were reported as adverse events during the initial phase of the SWOG study. There were no apparent differences in the types of infection between the 2 treatment groups, with the possible exception of herpes zoster which was reported more frequently for NIPENT (8%) than for IFN (1%).

	Percent of Patients	
Type of Infection	Frontline, Treated With NIPENT N=180	Frontline, Treated With IFN N=176
Upper Respiratory Infection	13	8
Rhinitis	11	15
Herpes Zoster	8	1
Pharyngitis	8	11
Viral Infection	8	17
Infection (Unspecified)	7	2
Sinusitis	6	4
Cellulitis	6	3
Bacterial Infection	5	4
Pneumonia	5	7
Conjunctivitis	4	2
Furunculosis	4	<1
Herpes Simplex	4	1
Bronchitis	3	2
Sepsis	3	2
Urinary Tract Infection	3	3
Abscess, Skin	2	4
Moniliasis, Oral	2	<1
Mycotic Infection, Skin	<1	3
Osteomyelitis	1	0

The drug relatedness of the adverse events listed below cannot be excluded. The following adverse events occurred in 3% to 10% of NIPENT-treated patients in the initial phase of the SWOG study:

Body as a Whole—Chest Pain, Death, Face Edema, Peripheral Edema

Cardiovascular System—Hemorrhage, Hypotension

Digestive System—Dental Abnormalities, Dyspepsia, Flatulence, Gingivitis

Hemic and Lymphatic System—Agranulocytosis

Laboratory Deviations—Elevated Creatinine

Musculoskeletal System—Arthralgia

Nervous System—Confusion, Dizziness, Insomnia, Paresthesia, Somnolence

Psychobiologic Function—Anxiety, Depression, Nervousness

Respiratory System—Asthma

Skin & Appendages—Skin Dry, Urticaria

The remaining adverse events which occurred in less than 3% of NIPENT-treated patients during the initial phase of the SWOG study:

Body as a Whole—Flu-like Symptoms, Hangover Effect, Neoplasm

Cardiovascular System—Angina Pectoris, Arrhythmia, A-V Block, Bradycardia, Extrasystoles Ventricular, Heart Arrest, Heart Failure, Hypertension, Pericardial Effusion, Phlebitis, Pulmonary Embolus, Sinus Arrest, Tachycardia, Thrombophlebitis Deep, Vasculitis

Digestive System—Constipation, Dysphagia, Glossitis, Ileus

Hemic and Lymphatic System—Acute Leukemia, Anemia-Hemolytic, Aplastic Anemia

Laboratory Deviations—Hypercalcemia, Hyponatremia

Musculoskeletal System—Arthritis, Gout

Nervous System—Amnesia, Ataxia, Convulsions, Dreaming Abnormal, Dysarthria, Encephalitis, Hyperkinesia, Meningism, Neuralgia, Neuritis, Neuropathy, Paralysis, Syncope, Twitching, Vertigo

Psychobiologic Function—Decrease/Loss Libido, Emotional Liability, Hallucination, Hostility, Neurosis, Thinking Abnormal

Respiratory System—Bronchospasm, Larynx Edema

Skin and Appendages—Acne, Alopecia, Eczema, Petechial Rash, Photosensitivity Reaction

Special Senses—Amblyopia, Deafness, Earache, Eyes Dry, Labyrinthitis, Lacrimation Disorder, Nonreactive Eye, Photophobia, Retinopathy, Tinnitus, Unusual Taste, Vision Abnormal, Watery Eyes

Urogenital System—Amenorrhea, Breast Lump, Impotence, Kidney Function Abnormal, Nephropathy, Renal Failure, Renal Insufficiency, Renal Stone

One patient with hairy cell leukemia treated with NIPENT during another clinical study developed unilateral uveitis with vision loss.

Nineteen (5%) patients withdrew from the Phase 3 SWOG 8691 study because of adverse events; 9 during initial NIPENT treatment, 4 during NIPENT crossover, 5 during initial IFN treatment, and 1 during both initial IFN treatment and NIPENT crossover. In the Phase 2 studies in IFN-refractory hairy cell leukemia, 11% of patients withdrew from treatment with NIPENT due to an adverse event.

OVERDOSAGE

No specific antidote for NIPENT overdose is known. NIPENT administered at higher doses (20 to 50 mg/m^2 in divided doses over 5 days) than recommended was associated with deaths due to severe renal, hepatic, pulmonary, and CNS toxicity. In case of overdose, management would include general supportive measures through any period of toxicity that occurs.

DOSAGE AND ADMINISTRATION

It is recommended that patients receive hydration with 500 to 1,000 mL of 5% Dextrose in 0.5 Normal Saline or equivalent before NIPENT administration. An additional 500 mL of 5% Dextrose or equivalent should be administered after NIPENT is given.

The recommended dosage of NIPENT for the treatment of hairy cell leukemia is 4 mg/m^2 every other week. NIPENT may be administered intravenously by bolus injection or diluted in a larger volume and given over 20 to 30 minutes. (See **Preparation of Intravenous Solution**.)

Higher doses are not recommended.

No extravasation injuries were reported in clinical studies.

The optimal duration of treatment has not been determined. In the absence of major toxicity and with observed continuing improvement, the patient should be treated until a complete response has been achieved. Although not established as required, the administration of two additional doses has been recommended following the achievement of a complete response.

All patients receiving NIPENT at 6 months should be assessed for response to treatment. If the patient has not achieved a complete or partial response, treatment with NIPENT should be discontinued.

If the patient has achieved a partial response, NIPENT treatment should be continued in an effort to achieve a complete response. At any time thereafter that a complete response is achieved, two additional doses of NIPENT are recommended. NIPENT treatment should then be stopped. If the best response to treatment at the end of 12 months is a partial response, it is recommended that treatment with NIPENT be stopped.

Withholding or discontinuation of individual doses may be needed when severe adverse reactions occur. Drug treatment should be withheld in patients with severe rash, and withheld or discontinued in patients showing evidence of nervous system toxicity.

NIPENT treatment should be withheld in patients with active infection occurring during the treatment but may be resumed when the infection is controlled.

Patients who have elevated serum creatinine should have their dose withheld and a creatinine clearance determined. There are insufficient data to recommend a starting or a subsequent dose for patients with impaired renal function (creatinine clearance <60 mL/min).

Patients with impaired renal function should be treated only when the potential benefit justifies the potential risk. Two patients with impaired renal function (creatinine clearances 50 to 60 mL/min) achieved complete response without unusual adverse events when treated with 2 mg/m^2.

No dosage reduction is recommended at the start of therapy with NIPENT in patients with anemia, neutropenia, or thrombocytopenia. In addition, dosage reductions are not recommended during treatment in patients with anemia and thrombocytopenia if patients can be otherwise supported hematologically. NIPENT should be temporarily withheld if the absolute neutrophil count falls during treatment below 200 cells/mm^3 in a patient who had an initial neutrophil count greater than 500 cells/mm^3 and may be resumed when the count returns to predose levels.

Preparation of Intravenous Solution

1. Procedures for proper handling and disposal of anticancer drugs should be followed. Several guidelines on this subject have been published.[2–7] There is no general agreement that all of the procedures recommended in the guidelines are necessary or appropriate. Spills and wastes should be treated with a 5% sodium hypochlorite solution prior to disposal.
2. Protective clothing including polyethylene gloves must be worn.
3. Transfer 5 mL of Sterile Water for Injection, USP to the vial containing NIPENT and mix thoroughly to obtain complete dissolution of a solution yielding 2 mg/mL. Parenteral drug products should be inspected visually for particulate matter and discoloration prior to administration.
4. NIPENT may be given intravenously by bolus injection or diluted in a larger volume (25 to 50 mL) with 5% Dextrose Injection, USP or 0.9% Sodium Chloride Injection, USP. Dilution of the entire contents of a reconstituted vial with 25 mL or 50 mL provides a pentostatin concentration of 0.33 mg/mL or 0.18 mg/mL, respectively, for the diluted solutions.
5. NIPENT solution when diluted for infusion with 5% Dextrose Injection, USP or 0.9% Sodium Chloride Injection, USP does not interact with PVC infusion containers or administration sets at concentrations of 0.18 mg/mL to 0.33 mg/mL.

Stability

NIPENT vials are stable at refrigerated storage temperature 2° to 8°C (36° to 46°F) for the period stated on the package. Vials reconstituted or reconstituted and further diluted as directed may be stored at room temperature and ambient light but should be used within 8 hours because NIPENT contains no preservatives.

HOW SUPPLIED

NIPENT (pentostatin for injection) is supplied as a sterile lyophilized white to off-white powder in single-dose vials containing 10 mg of pentostatin. The vials are packed in individual cartons. **NDC 62701-800-01**

Storage: Store NIPENT vials under refrigerated storage conditions 2° to 8°C (36° to 46°F).

Rx Only

REFERENCES

1. Malspeis L, et al. Clinical Pharmacokinetics of 2'-Deoxycoformycin. Cancer Treatment Symposia 2:7–15, 1984.
2. Recommendations for the safe handling of parenteral antineoplastic drugs. NIH publication 83-2621. For sale by the Superintendent of Documents, US Government Printing Office, Washington, NC 20402.
3. AMA council report. Guidelines for handling parenteral antineoplastics. JAMA 253:1590–2, 1985.
4. National Study Commission on Cytotoxic Exposure–Recommendations for handling cytotoxic agents. Available from Louis P. Jeffery, Sc.D., Chairman, National Study Commission on Cytotoxic Exposure, Massachusetts College of Pharmacy and Allied Health Sciences, 179 Longwood Ave, Boston, Massachusetts 02115.
5. Clinical Oncology Society of Australia: Guidelines and recommendations for safe handling of antineoplastic agents. Med J Australia 1:426–8, 1983.
6. Jones RB, et al. Safe handling of chemotherapeutic agents: A report from the Mount Sinai Medical Center. CA: A Cancer Journal for Clinicians 33:258–63, 1983.
7. American Society of Hospital Pharmacists technical assistance bulletin on handling cytotoxic and hazardous drugs. Am J Hosp Pharm 47:1033–49, 1990.

800P1 Rev. April, 1998

Swiss Bioceutical International, Ltd.

2533 NORTH CARSON STREET
SUITE 3573
CARSON CITY, NV 89706

Direct Inquiries to:

Executive Director
(775) 841-7020
FAX: (775) 883-2384
www.imuplus.com

IMUPlus™ OTC

[*ĭm-ū-plus*]
Bioactive Non-Denatured
Whey Protein Isolate Formula

IMU*Plus*™ is a pharmaceutical grade (>99.0%) non-denatured whey protein isolate formula: a functional food naturally providing bioactive precursors for the intracellular production of glutathione, a critical constituent for the immune system and a vital antioxidant and detoxifying agent. IMUPlus non-denatured proteins are important contributors to the following body processes:

- REPAIR OF RNA AND DNA
- PRODUCTION OF ANTIOXIDANTS AND HORMONES
- REMOVAL OF TOXIC METALS
- WOUND HEALING
- CREATION OF NEW MUSCLE MASS, INHIBITION OF HARMFUL BACTERIA AND VIRUSES IN THE GASTROINTESTINAL TRACT
- PRODUCTION OF HEMOGLOBIN, ENZYMES, HORMONES, ANTIBODIES

Nutritional Facts
Serving Size 1 pouch (10g)
Servings per Container 60

Amount per Serving

Calories 40	
	% Daily Value*
Total Fat 0g	0%
Sodium 25mg	1%
Total Carbohydrates 0g	0%
Protein 9g	
Calcium 6%	Iron 4%

Not a significant source of calories from fat, saturated fat, cholesterol, dietary fiber, sugars, vitamin A and vitamin C

* Percent Daily Values are based on a 2,000 calorie diet.

These statements have not been evaluated by the FDA. This product is not intended to diagnose, cure, prevent or treat any diseases.

NUTRITIONAL CONTENT

	1 POUCH 10 gm	100 gm	1 CARTON 60 POUCHES
TOTAL FAT	0.01 gm	0.13 gm	0.78 gm
SATURATED FAT	0.01 gm	0.08 gm	0.48 gm
POLY-UNSATURATED FAT	0	0.01 gm	0.06 gm
MONO-UNSATURATED FAT	0	0.04 gm	0.24 gm
CHOLESTEROL	0.04 mg	0.37 mg	2.22 mg
SODIUM	25 mg	250 mg	1500 mg
POTASSIUM	30 mg	300 mg	1800 mg
TOTAL CARBOHYDRATE	0.10 gm	1.0 gm	6 gm
DIETARY FIBER	0	0	0
SUGARS	0.15 gm	1.5 gm	9 gm
PROTEIN	9 gm	90 gm	540 gm
VITAMIN A	<1 gm	<10 gm	<60 gm
VITAMIN C	0	0	0
CALCIUM	60 mg	600 mg	3600 mg
MAGNESIUM	9 mg	90 mg	540 mg
CHLORIDE	0.5 mg	5 mg	30 mg
IRON	0.93 mg	9.3 mg	55.80 mg
THIAMIN	0	0	0
RIBOFLAVIN	0	0	0
NIACIN	0	0	0
PHOSPHORUS	21 mg	210 mg	1260 mg
CALORIES	40	400	2400
CALORIES FROM FAT	0.1	1.0	3

DOSAGE: 2 Pouches per day for Immune Maintenance
3–5 Pouches for all Major immune diseases.

DIRECTIONS

Fill a large glass with 6 ounces of distilled water -Or- combine * compatible protein with the distilled water. Empty a pouch of IMUPlus™ into the liquid. Using a fork, stir until mixture thickens. Let stand 5–10 minutes. Stir again and drink.
2. For easy mixing use our Portable Mixer designed to preserve the non-denatured quality of IMUPlus™.

BEST RESULTS

At least 30 minutes before eating in the morning, take pouch #1. Take pouch #2 between 3–4 p.m. or as directed by your healthcare professional.

CAUTION

Store in a cool dry place or refrigerate. Never mix in an electric blender. This will 'denature' the IMUPlus™ bioactive benefits.

HOW SUPPLIED

60 pouch Carton (600 gm)
1 pouch (10 gm)

INGREDIENT

Whey Protein Isolate Formula

Distributed by: SWISS BIOCEUTICAL INTERNATIONAL, LTD
2533 North Carson Street,
Suite 3573
Carson City, Nevada 89706
Note* Not an MLM Company
Telephone: (775) 841-7020
Fax: (775) 883-2384
Web: www.IMUPlus.com
Product of U.S.A. K-kosher seal
Packaged in U.S.A.
Patent Pending

Takeda Pharmaceuticals America, Inc.

475 HALF DAY ROAD, SUITE 500
LINCOLNSHIRE, IL 60069

Direct Inquiries to:

Sales and Ordering:
Customer Service
(877) 5 TAKEDA
(877) 582-5332

For Medical Information Contact:

Generally:
(877) TAKEDA 7
(877) 825-3327

Adverse Drug Experiences:
(877) TAKEDA 7
(877) 825-3327

ACTOS® ℞

[*act-ōs*]
(pioglitazone hydrochloride) Tablets

DESCRIPTION

ACTOS (pioglitazone hydrochloride) is an oral antidiabetic agent that acts primarily by decreasing insulin resistance. ACTOS is used in the management of type 2 diabetes mellitus (also known as non-insulin-dependent diabetes mellitus [NIDDM] or adult-onset diabetes). Pharmacological studies indicate that ACTOS improves sensitivity to insulin in muscle and adipose tissue and inhibits hepatic gluconeogenesis. ACTOS improves glycemic control while reducing circulating insulin levels.

Pioglitazone [(±)-5-[[4-[2-(5-ethyl-2-pyridinyl)ethoxy]phenyl]methyl]-2,4-] thiazolidinedione monohydrochloride belongs to a different chemical class and has a different pharmacological action than the sulfonylureas, metformin, or the α-glucosidase inhibitors. The molecule contains one asymmetric carbon, and the compound is synthesized and used as the racemic mixture. The two enantiomers of pioglitazone inter-convert in vivo. No differences were found in the pharmacologic activity between the two enantiomers. The structural formula is as shown:

CH3 N O S O NH O • HCl

Pioglitazone hydrochloride is an odorless white crystalline powder that has a molecular formula of $C_{19}H_{20}N_2O_3S \cdot HCl$ and a molecular weight of 392.90 daltons. It is soluble in N,N-dimethylformamide, slightly soluble in anhydrous ethanol, very slightly soluble in acetone and acetonitrile, practically insoluble in water, and insoluble in ether.

ACTOS is available as a tablet for oral administration containing 15 mg, 30 mg, or 45 mg of pioglitazone (as the base) formulated with the following excipients: lactose monohydrate NF, hydroxypropylcellulose NF, carboxymethylcellulose calcium NF, and magnesium stearate NF.

CLINICAL PHARMACOLOGY

Mechanism of Action

ACTOS is a thiazolidinedione antidiabetic agent that depends on the presence of insulin for its mechanism of action. ACTOS decreases insulin resistance in the periphery and in the liver resulting in increased insulin-dependent glucose disposal and decreased hepatic glucose output. Unlike sulfonylureas, pioglitazone is not an insulin secretagogue. Pi-

Continued on next page

Actos—Cont.

oglitazone is a potent and highly selective agonist for peroxisome proliferator-activated receptor-gamma (PPARγ). PPAR receptors are found in tissues important for insulin action such as adipose tissue, skeletal muscle, and liver. Activation of PPARγ nuclear receptors modulates the transcription of a number of insulin responsive genes involved in the control of glucose and lipid metabolism.

In animal models of diabetes, pioglitazone reduces the hyperglycemia, hyperinsulinemia, and hypertriglyceridemia characteristic of insulin-resistant states such as type 2 diabetes. The metabolic changes produced by pioglitazone result in increased responsiveness of insulin-dependent tissues and are observed in numerous animal models of insulin resistance.

Since pioglitazone enhances the effects of circulating insulin (by decreasing insulin resistance), it does not lower blood glucose in animal models that lack endogenous insulin.

Pharmacokinetics and Drug Metabolism

Serum concentrations of total pioglitazone (pioglitazone plus active metabolites) remain elevated 24 hours after once daily dosing. Steady-state serum concentrations of both pioglitazone and total pioglitazone are achieved within 7 days. At steady-state, two of the pharmacologically active metabolites of pioglitazone, Metabolites III (M-III) and IV (M-IV), reach serum concentrations equal to or greater than pioglitazone. In both healthy volunteers and in patients with type 2 diabetes, pioglitazone comprises approximately 30% to 50% of the peak total pioglitazone serum concentrations and 20% to 25% of the total area under the serum concentration-time curve (AUC).

Maximum serum concentration (C_{max}), AUC, and trough serum concentrations (C_{min}) for both pioglitazone and total pioglitazone increase proportionally at doses of 15 mg and 30 mg per day. There is a slightly less than proportional increase for pioglitazone and total pioglitazone at a dose of 60 mg per day.

Absorption: Following oral administration, in the fasting state, pioglitazone is first measurable in serum within 30 minutes, with peak concentrations observed within 2 hours. Food slightly delays the time to peak serum concentration to 3 to 4 hours, but does not alter the extent of absorption.

Distribution: The mean apparent volume of distribution (Vd/F) of pioglitazone following single-dose administration is 0.63 ± 0.41 (mean ± SD) L/kg of body weight. Pioglitazone is extensively protein bound (> 99%) in human serum, principally to serum albumin. Pioglitazone also binds to other serum proteins, but with lower affinity. Metabolites M-III and M-IV also are extensively bound (> 98%) to serum albumin.

Metabolism: Pioglitazone is extensively metabolized by hydroxylation and oxidation; the metabolites also partly convert to glucuronide or sulfate conjugates. Metabolites M-II and M-IV (hydroxy derivatives of pioglitazone) and M-III (keto derivative of pioglitazone) are pharmacologically active in animal models of type 2 diabetes. In addition to pioglitazone, M-III and M-IV are the principal drug-related species found in human serum following multiple dosing. At steady-state, in both healthy volunteers and in patients with type 2 diabetes, pioglitazone comprises approximately 30% to 50% of the total peak serum concentrations and 20% to 25% of the total AUC.

Pioglitazone incubated with expressed human P450 or human liver microsomes results in the formation of M-IV and to a much lesser degree, M-II. The major cytochrome P450 isoforms involved in the hepatic metabolism of pioglitazone are CYP2C8 and CYP3A4 with contributions from a variety of other isoforms including the mainly extrahepatic CYP1A1. Ketoconazole inhibited up to 85% of hepatic pioglitazone metabolism in vitro at a concentration equal molar to pioglitazone. Pioglitazone did not inhibit P450 activity when incubated with human P450 liver microsomes. In vivo human studies have not been performed to investigate any induction of CYP3A4 by pioglitazone.

Excretion and Elimination: Following oral administration, approximately 15% to 30% of the pioglitazone dose is recovered in the urine. Renal elimination of pioglitazone is negligible, and the drug is excreted primarily as metabolites and their conjugates. It is presumed that most of the oral dose is excreted into the bile either unchanged or as metabolites and eliminated in the feces.

The mean serum half-life of pioglitazone and total pioglitazone ranges from 3 to 7 hours and 16 to 24 hours, respectively. Pioglitazone has an apparent clearance, CL/F, calculated to be 5 to 7 L/hr.

Special Populations

Renal Insufficiency: The serum elimination half-life of pioglitazone, M-III, and M-IV remains unchanged in patients with moderate (creatinine clearance 30 to 60 mL/min) to severe (creatinine clearance < 30 mL/min) renal impairment when compared to normal subjects. No dose adjustment in patients with renal dysfunction is recommended (see DOSAGE AND ADMINISTRATION).

Hepatic Insufficiency: Compared with normal controls, subjects with impaired hepatic function (Child-Pugh Grade B/C) have an approximate 45% reduction in pioglitazone and total pioglitazone mean peak concentrations but no change in the mean AUC values.

ACTOS therapy should not be initiated if the patient exhibits clinical evidence of active liver disease or serum transaminase levels (ALT) exceed 2.5 times the upper limit of normal (see PRECAUTIONS, Hepatic Effects).

Table 1 Lipids in a 26-Week Placebo-Controlled Dose-Ranging Study

	Placebo	ACTOS 15 mg Once Daily	ACTOS 30 mg Once Daily	ACTOS 45 mg Once Daily
Triglycerides (mg/dL)	N=79	N=79	N=84	N=77
Baseline (mean)	262.8	283.8	261.1	259.7
Percent change from baseline (mean)	4.8%	-9.0%	-9.6%	-9.3%
HDL Cholesterol (mg/dL)	N=79	N=79	N=83	N=77
Baseline (mean)	41.7	40.4	40.8	40.7
Percent change from baseline (mean)	8.1%	14.1%	12.2%	19.1%
LDL Cholesterol (mg/dL)	N=65	N=63	N=74	N=62
Baseline (mean)	138.8	131.9	135.6	126.8
Percent change from baseline (mean)	4.8%	7.2%	5.2%	6.0%
Total Cholesterol (mg/dL)	N=79	N=79	N=84	N=77
Baseline (mean)	224.6	220.0	222.7	213.7
Percent change from baseline (mean)	4.4%	4.6%	3.3%	6.4%

Figure 1 Mean Change from Baseline for FBG and HbA_{1c} in a 26-Week Placebo-Controlled Dose-Ranging Study

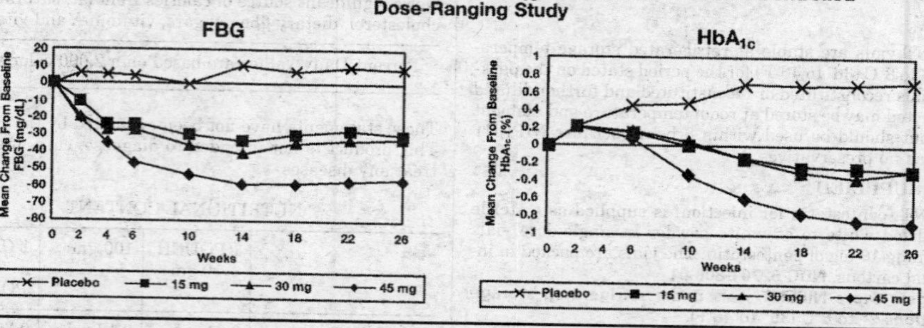

Table 2 Glycemic Parameters in a 26-Week Placebo-Controlled Dose-Ranging Study

	Placebo	ACTOS 15 mg Once Daily	ACTOS 30 mg Once Daily	ACTOS 45 mg Once Daily
Total Population				
HbA_{1c} (%)	N=79	N=79	N=85	N=76
Baseline (mean)	10.4	10.2	10.2	10.3
Change from baseline (adjusted mean⁺)	0.7	-0.3	-0.3	-0.9
Difference from placebo (adjusted mean⁺)		1.0*	-1.0*	-1.6*
FBG (mg/dL)	N=79	N=79	N=84	N=77
Baseline (mean)	268	267	269	276
Change from baseline (adjusted mean⁺)	9	-30	-32	-56
Difference from placebo (adjusted mean⁺)		-39*	-41*	-65*

⁺ Adjusted for baseline, pooled center, and pooled center by treatment interaction
* $p \leq 0.050$ vs. placebo

Elderly: In healthy elderly subjects, peak serum concentrations of pioglitazone and total pioglitazone are not significantly different, but AUC values are slightly higher and the terminal half-life values slightly longer than for younger subjects. These changes were not of a magnitude that would be considered clinically relevant.

Pediatrics: Pharmacokinetic data in the pediatric population are not available.

Gender: The mean C_{max} and AUC values were increased 20% to 60% in females. As monotherapy and in combination with sulfonylurea, metformin, or insulin, ACTOS improved glycemic control in both males and females. In controlled clinical trials, hemoglobin A_{1c} (HbA_{1c}) decreases from baseline were generally greater for females than for males (average mean difference in HbA_{1c} 0.5%). Since therapy should be individualized for each patient to achieve glycemic control, no dose adjustment is recommended based on gender alone.

Ethnicity: Pharmacokinetic data among various ethnic groups are not available.

Pharmacodynamics and Clinical Effects

Clinical studies demonstrate that ACTOS improves insulin sensitivity in insulin-resistant patients. ACTOS enhances cellular responsiveness to insulin, increases insulin-dependent glucose disposal, improves hepatic sensitivity to insulin, and improves dysfunctional glucose homeostasis. In patients with type 2 diabetes, the decreased insulin resistance produced by ACTOS results in lower blood glucose concentrations, lower plasma insulin levels, and lower HbA_{1c} values. Based on results from an open-label extension study, the glucose lowering effects of ACTOS appear to persist for at least one year. In controlled clinical trials, ACTOS in combination with sulfonylurea, metformin, or insulin had an additive effect on glycemic control.

Patients with lipid abnormalities were included in clinical trials with ACTOS. Overall, patients treated with ACTOS had mean decreases in triglycerides, mean increases in HDL cholesterol, and no consistent mean changes in LDL and total cholesterol.

In a 26-week, placebo-controlled, dose-ranging study, mean triglyceride levels decreased in the 15 mg, 30 mg, and 45 mg ACTOS dose groups compared to a mean increase in the placebo group. Mean HDL levels increased to a greater extent in patients treated with ACTOS than in the placebo-treated patients. There were no consistent differences for LDL and total cholesterol in patients treated with ACTOS compared to placebo (Table 1).

[See table 1 above]

In the two other monotherapy studies (24 weeks and 16 weeks) and in combination therapy studies with sulfonylurea (16 weeks) and metformin (16 weeks), the results were generally consistent with the data above. For patients treated with ACTOS, the placebo-corrected mean changes from baseline decreased 5% to 26% for triglycerides and increased 6% to 13% for HDL cholesterol.

In the combination therapy study with insulin (16 weeks), the placebo-corrected mean percent change from baseline in triglyceride values for patients treated with ACTOS was also decreased. A placebo-corrected mean change from baseline in LDL cholesterol of 7% was observed for the 15 mg dose group. Similar results to those noted above for HDL and total cholesterol were observed.

In all clinical trials, a reduction in HbA_{1c} was accompanied by increased body weight in patients treated with ACTOS in a dose-related manner. The change in average weight in U.S. placebo-controlled monotherapy trials ranged from 0.5 kg to 2.8 kg for patients treated with ACTOS and -1.3 kg to -1.9 kg for placebo-treated patients. In combination with sulfonylurea, the change in average weight was 1.9 kg and 2.9 kg for 15 mg and 30 mg of ACTOS, respectively, and -0.8 kg for placebo. In combination with insulin, the change in average weight was 2.3 kg and 3.7 kg for 15 mg and 30 mg of ACTOS, respectively, and 0 kg for placebo. In combination with metformin, the change in average weight was 1.0 kg for 30 mg of ACTOS and -1.4 kg for placebo.

Clinical Studies

Monotherapy

In the U.S., three randomized, double-blind, placebo-controlled trials with durations from 16 to 26 weeks were con-

ducted to evaluate the use of ACTOS as monotherapy in patients with type 2 diabetes. These studies examined ACTOS at doses up to 45 mg or placebo once daily in 865 patients.
In a 26-week dose-ranging study, 408 patients with type 2 diabetes were randomized to receive 7.5 mg, 15 mg, 30 mg, or 45 mg of ACTOS, or placebo once daily. Therapy with any previous antidiabetic agent was discontinued 8 weeks prior to the double-blind period. Treatment with 15 mg, 30 mg, and 45 mg of ACTOS produced statistically significant improvements in HbA_{1c} and fasting blood glucose (FBG) at endpoint compared to placebo (see Figure 1, Table 2).
Figure 1 shows the time course for changes in FBG and HbA_{1c} for the entire study population in this 26-week study.
[See figure 1 at top of previous page]
Table 2 shows HbA_{1c} and FBG values for the entire study population.
[See table 2 at top of previous page]
The study population included patients not previously treated with antidiabetic medication (naïve; 31%) and patients who were receiving antidiabetic medication at the time of study enrollment (previously treated; 69%). The data for the naïve and previously treated patient subsets are shown in Table 3. All patients entered an 8 week washout/run-in period prior to double-blind treatment. This run-in period was associated with little change in HbA_{1c} and FBG values from screening to baseline for the naïve patients; however, for the previously-treated group, washout from previous antidiabetic medication resulted in deterioration of glycemic control and increases in HbA_{1c} and FBG. Although most patients in the previously-treated group had a decrease from baseline in HbA_{1c} and FBG with ACTOS, in many cases the values did not return to screening levels by the end of the study. The study design did not permit the evaluation of patients who switched directly to ACTOS from another antidiabetic agent.
[See table 3 above]
In a 24-week study, 260 patients with type 2 diabetes were randomized to one of two forced-titration ACTOS treatment groups or a mock titration placebo group. Therapy with any previous antidiabetic agent was discontinued 6 weeks prior to the double-blind period. In one ACTOS treatment group, patients received an initial dose of 7.5 mg once daily. After four weeks, the dose was increased to 15 mg once daily and after another four weeks, the dose was increased to 30 mg once daily for the remainder of the study (16 weeks). In the second ACTOS treatment group, patients received an initial dose of 15 mg once daily and were titrated to 30 mg once daily and 45 mg once daily in a similar manner. Treatment with ACTOS, as described, produced statistically significant improvements in HbA_{1c} and FBG at endpoint compared to placebo (see Table 4).
[See table 4 above]
For patients who had not been previously treated with antidiabetic medication (24%), mean values at screening were 10.1% for HbA_{1c} and 238 mg/dL for FBG. At baseline, mean HbA_{1c} was 10.2% and mean FBG was 243 mg/dL. Compared with placebo, treatment with ACTOS titrated to a final dose of 30 mg and 45 mg resulted in reductions from baseline in mean HbA_{1c} of 2.3% and 2.6% and mean FBG of 63 mg/dL and 95 mg/dL, respectively. For patients who had been previously treated with antidiabetic medication (76%), this medication was discontinued at screening. Mean values at screening were 9.4% for HbA_{1c} and 216 mg/dL for FBG. At baseline, mean HbA_{1c} was 10.7% and mean FBG was 290 mg/dL. Compared with placebo, treatment with ACTOS titrated to a final dose of 30 mg and 45 mg resulted in reductions from baseline in mean HbA_{1c} of 1.3% and 1.4% and mean FBG of 55 mg/dL and 60 mg/dL, respectively. For many previously-treated patients, HbA_{1c} and FBG had not returned to screening levels by the end of the study.
In a 16-week study, 197 patients with type 2 diabetes were randomized to treatment with 30 mg of ACTOS or placebo once daily. Therapy with any previous antidiabetic agent was discontinued 6 weeks prior to the double-blind period. Treatment with 30 mg of ACTOS produced statistically significant improvements in HbA_{1c} and FBG at endpoint compared to placebo (see Table 5).
[See table 5 above]
For patients who had not been previously treated with antidiabetic medication (40%), mean values at screening were 10.3% for HbA_{1c} and 240 mg/dL for FBG. At baseline, mean HbA_{1c} was 10.4% and mean FBG was 254 mg/dL. Compared with placebo, treatment with ACTOS 30 mg resulted in reductions from baseline in mean HbA_{1c} of 1.0% and mean FBG of 62 mg/dL. For patients who had been previously treated with antidiabetic medication (60%), this medication was discontinued at screening. Mean values at screening were 9.4% for HbA_{1c} and 216 mg/dL for FBG. At baseline, mean HbA_{1c} was 10.6% and mean FBG was 287 mg/dL. Compared with placebo, treatment with ACTOS 30 mg resulted in reductions from baseline in mean HbA_{1c} of 1.3% and mean FBG of 46 mg/dL. For many previously-treated patients, HbA_{1c} and FBG had not returned to screening levels by the end of the study.

Combination Therapy

Three 16-week, randomized, double-blind, placebo-controlled clinical studies were conducted to evaluate the effects of ACTOS on glycemic control in patients with type 2 diabetes who were inadequately controlled ($HbA_{1c} \geq 8\%$) despite current therapy with a sulfonylurea, metformin, or insulin. Previous diabetes treatment may have been monotherapy or combination therapy.
In one combination study, 560 patients with type 2 diabetes on a sulfonylurea, either alone or combined with another antidiabetic agent, were randomized to receive 15 mg or 30 mg of ACTOS or placebo once daily in addition to their current sulfonylurea regimen. Any other antidiabetic agent was withdrawn. Compared with placebo, the addition of ACTOS to the sulfonylurea significantly reduced the mean HbA_{1c} by 0.9% and 1.3% for the 15 mg and 30 mg doses, respectively. Compared with placebo, mean FBG decreased by 39 mg/dL (15 mg dose) and 58 mg/dL (30 mg dose). The therapeutic effect of ACTOS in combination with sulfonylurea was observed in patients regardless of whether the patients were receiving low, medium, or high doses of sulfonylurea (< 50%, 50%, or > 50% of the recommended maximum daily dose).
In a second combination study, 328 patients with type 2 diabetes on metformin either alone or combined with another antidiabetic agent, were randomized to receive either 30 mg of ACTOS or placebo once daily in addition to their metformin. Any other antidiabetic agent was withdrawn. Compared to placebo, the addition of ACTOS to metformin significantly reduced the mean HbA_{1c} by 0.8% and decreased the mean FBG by 38 mg/dL. The therapeutic effect of ACTOS in combination with metformin was observed in patients regardless of whether the patients were receiving lower or higher doses of metformin (< 2000 mg per day or ≥ 2000 mg per day).
In a third combination study, 566 patients with type 2 diabetes receiving a median of 60.5 units per day of insulin, either alone or combined with another antidiabetic agent, were randomized to receive either 15 mg or 30 mg of ACTOS or placebo once daily in addition to their insulin. Any other antidiabetic agent was discontinued. Compared to placebo, treatment with ACTOS in addition to insulin significantly reduced both HbA_{1c} (0.7% for the 15 mg dose and 1.0% for the 30 mg dose) and FBG (35 mg/dL for the 15 mg dose and 49 mg/dL for the 30 mg dose). The therapeutic effect of ACTOS in combination with insulin was observed in patients regardless of whether the patients were receiving lower or higher doses of insulin (< 60.5 units per day or ≥ 60.5 units per day).

Table 3 Glycemic Parameters in a 26-Week Placebo-Controlled Dose-Ranging Study

	Placebo	ACTOS 15 mg Once Daily	ACTOS 30 mg Once Daily	ACTOS 45 mg Once Daily
Naïve to Therapy				
HbA_{1c} (%)	N=25	N=26	N=26	N=21
Screening (mean)	9.3	10.0	9.5	9.8
Baseline (mean)	9.0	9.9	9.3	10.0
Change from baseline (adjusted mean*)	0.6	-0.8	-0.6	-1.9
Difference from placebo (adjusted mean*)		-1.4	-1.3	-2.6
FBG (mg/dL)	N=25	N=26	N=26	N=21
Screening (mean)	223	245	239	239
Baseline (mean)	229	251	225	235
Change from baseline (adjusted mean*)	16	-37	-41	-64
Difference from placebo (adjusted mean*)		-52	-56	-80
Previously Treated				
HbA_{1c} (%)	N=54	N=53	N=59	N=55
Screening (mean)	9.3	9.0	9.1	9.0
Baseline (mean)	10.9	10.4	10.4	10.6
Change from baseline (adjusted mean*)	0.8	-0.1	-0.0	-0.6
Difference from placebo (adjusted mean*)		-1.0	-0.9	-1.4
FBG (mg/dL)	N=54	N=53	N=58	N=56
Screening (mean)	222	209	230	215
Baseline (mean)	285	275	286	292
Change from baseline (adjusted mean*)	4	-32	-27	-55
Difference from placebo (adjusted mean*)		-36	-31	-59

* Adjusted for baseline and pooled center

Table 4 Glycemic Parameters in a 24-Week Placebo-Controlled Forced-Titration Study

	Placebo	ACTOS 30 mg⁺ Once Daily	ACTOS 45 mg⁺ Once Daily
Total Population			
HbA_{1c} (%)	N=83	N=85	N=85
Baseline (mean)	10.8	10.3	10.8
Change from baseline (adjusted mean⁺⁺)	0.9	-0.6	-0.6
Difference from placebo (adjusted mean⁺⁺)		-1.5*	-1.5*
FBG (mg/dL)	N=78	N=82	N=85
Baseline (mean)	279	268	281
Change from baseline (adjusted mean⁺⁺)	18	-44	-50
Difference from placebo (adjusted mean⁺⁺)		-62*	-68*

⁺ Final dose in forced titration
⁺⁺ Adjusted for baseline, pooled center, and pooled center by treatment interaction
* p ≤ 0.050 vs. placebo

Table 5 Glycemic Parameters in a 16-Week Placebo-Controlled Study

	Placebo	ACTOS 30 mg Once Daily
Total Population		
HbA_{1c} (%)	N=93	N=100
Baseline (mean)	10.3	10.5
Change from baseline (adjusted mean⁺)	0.8	-0.6
Difference from placebo (adjusted mean⁺)		-1.4*
FBG (mg/dL)	N=91	N=99
Baseline (mean)	270	273
Change from baseline (adjusted mean⁺)	8	-50
Difference from placebo (adjusted mean⁺)		-58*

⁺ Adjusted for baseline, pooled center, and pooled center by treatment interaction
* p ≤ 0.050 vs. placebo

INDICATIONS AND USAGE

ACTOS is indicated as an adjunct to diet and exercise to improve glycemic control in patients with type 2 diabetes (non-insulin-dependent diabetes mellitus, NIDDM). ACTOS is indicated for monotherapy. ACTOS is also indicated for use in combination with a sulfonylurea, metformin, or insulin when diet and exercise plus the single agent does not result in adequate glycemic control.
Management of type 2 diabetes should also include nutritional counseling, weight reduction as needed, and exercise. These efforts are important not only in the primary treatment of type 2 diabetes, but also to maintain the efficacy of drug therapy.

Continued on next page

Actos—Cont.

CONTRAINDICATIONS

ACTOS is contraindicated in patients with known hypersensitivity to this product or any of its components.

PRECAUTIONS

General

ACTOS exerts its antihyperglycemic effect only in the presence of insulin. Therefore, ACTOS should not be used in patients with type 1 diabetes or for the treatment of diabetic ketoacidosis.

Hypoglycemia: Patients receiving ACTOS in combination with insulin or oral hypoglycemic agents may be at risk for hypoglycemia, and a reduction in the dose of the concomitant agent may be necessary.

Ovulation: Therapy with ACTOS, like other thiazolidinediones, may result in ovulation in some premenopausal anovulatory women. As a result, these patients may be at an increased risk for pregnancy while taking ACTOS. Thus, adequate contraception in premenopausal women should be recommended. This possible effect has not been investigated in clinical studies so the frequency of this occurrence is not known.

Hematologic: ACTOS may cause decreases in hemoglobin and hematocrit. Across all clinical studies, mean hemoglobin values declined by 2% to 4% in patients treated with ACTOS. These changes primarily occurred within the first 4 to 12 weeks of therapy and remained relatively constant thereafter. These changes may be related to increased plasma volume and have not been associated with any significant hematologic clinical effects (see ADVERSE REACTIONS, Laboratory Abnormalities).

Edema: ACTOS should be used with caution in patients with edema. In double-blind clinical trials of patients with type 2 diabetes, mild to moderate edema was reported in patients treated with ACTOS (see ADVERSE REACTIONS).

Cardiac: In preclinical studies, thiazolidinediones, including pioglitazone, cause plasma volume expansion and preload-induced cardiac hypertrophy (see PRECAUTIONS, Animal Toxicology). In a six-month placebo-controlled study of 334 patients with type 2 diabetes and a long-term (one year or more) open-label study of more than 350 patients with type 2 diabetes, echocardiographic evaluation revealed no significant increase in mean left ventricular mass index or significant decrease in mean cardiac index in patients treated with ACTOS.

In clinical trials that excluded patients with New York Heart Association (NYHA) Class III and IV cardiac status, no increased incidence of serious cardiac adverse events potentially related to volume expansion (e.g., congestive heart failure) was observed. Patients with NYHA Class III and IV cardiac status were not studied in ACTOS clinical trials. ACTOS is not indicated in patients with NYHA Class III or IV cardiac status.

Hepatic Effects: Another drug of the thiazolidinedione class, troglitazone, has been associated with idiosyncratic hepatotoxicity, and very rare cases of liver failure, liver transplants, and death have been reported during postmarketing clinical use. In pre-approval controlled clinical trials in patients with type 2 diabetes, troglitazone was more frequently associated with clinically significant elevations of hepatic enzymes (ALT > 3 times the upper limit of normal) compared to placebo, and very rare cases of reversible jaundice were reported.

In clinical studies worldwide, over 4500 subjects have been treated with ACTOS. In U.S. clinical studies, over 2500 patients with type 2 diabetes received ACTOS. There was no evidence of drug-induced hepatotoxicity or elevation of ALT levels.

During placebo-controlled clinical trials in the U.S., a total of 4 of 1526 (0.26%) patients treated with ACTOS and 2 of 793 (0.25%) placebo-treated patients had ALT values ≥ 3 times the upper limit of normal. The ALT elevations in patients treated with ACTOS were reversible and were not clearly related to therapy with ACTOS.

Although available clinical data show no evidence of ACTOS-induced hepatotoxicity or ALT elevations, pioglitazone is structurally related to troglitazone, which has been associated with idiosyncratic hepatotoxicity and rare cases of liver failure, liver transplants, and death. Pending the availability of additional large, long-term controlled clinical trials and postmarketing safety data following wide clinical use of ACTOS to more fully define its hepatic safety profile, it is recommended that patients treated with ACTOS undergo periodic monitoring of liver enzymes. Serum ALT (alanine transaminase) levels should be evaluated prior to the initiation of therapy with ACTOS in all patients, every two months for the first year of therapy, and periodically thereafter. Liver function tests should also be obtained for patients if symptoms suggestive of hepatic dysfunction occur, e.g., nausea, vomiting, abdominal pain, fatigue, anorexia, dark urine. The decision whether to continue the patient on therapy with ACTOS should be guided by clinical judgement pending laboratory evaluations. If jaundice is observed, drug therapy should be discontinued.

Therapy with ACTOS should not be initiated if the patient exhibits clinical evidence of active liver disease or the ALT levels exceed 2.5 times the upper limit of normal. Patients with mildly elevated liver enzymes (ALT levels at 1 to 2.5 times the upper limit of normal) at baseline or any time during therapy with ACTOS should be evaluated to determine the cause of the liver enzyme elevation. Initiation of, or continuation of, therapy with ACTOS in patients with mildly elevated liver enzymes should proceed with caution and include the appropriate clinical follow-up which may include more frequent liver enzyme monitoring. If serum transaminase levels are increased (ALT > 2.5 times the upper limit of normal), liver function tests should be evaluated more frequently until the levels return to normal or pretreatment values. If ALT levels exceed 3 times the upper limit of normal, the test should be repeated as soon as possible. If ALT levels remain > 3 times the upper limit of normal or if the patient is jaundiced, ACTOS therapy should be discontinued.

There are no data available to evaluate the safety of ACTOS in patients who experienced liver abnormalities, hepatic dysfunction, or jaundice while on troglitazone. ACTOS should not be used in patients who experienced jaundice while taking troglitazone. For patients with normal hepatic enzymes who are switched from troglitazone to ACTOS, a one-week washout is recommended before starting therapy with ACTOS.

Laboratory Tests

FBG and HbA_{1c} measurements should be performed periodically to monitor glycemic control and the therapeutic response to ACTOS.

Liver enzyme monitoring is recommended prior to initiation of therapy with ACTOS in all patients and periodically thereafter (see PRECAUTIONS, General, Hepatic Effects and ADVERSE REACTIONS, Serum Transaminase Levels).

Information for Patients

It is important to instruct patients to adhere to dietary instructions and to have blood glucose and glycosylated hemoglobin tested regularly. During periods of stress such as fever, trauma, infection, or surgery, medication requirements may change and patients should be reminded to seek medical advice promptly.

Patients should be told that blood tests for liver function will be performed prior to the start of therapy, every two months for the first year, and periodically thereafter. Patients should be told to seek immediate medical advice for unexplained nausea, vomiting, abdominal pain, fatigue, anorexia, or dark urine.

Patients should be told to take ACTOS once daily. ACTOS can be taken with or without meals. If a dose is missed on one day, the dose should not be doubled the following day.

When using combination therapy with insulin or oral hypoglycemic agents, the risks of hypoglycemia, its symptoms and treatment, and conditions that predispose to its development should be explained to patients and their family members.

Therapy with ACTOS, like other thiazolidinediones, may result in ovulation in some premenopausal anovulatory women. As a result, these patients may be at an increased risk for pregnancy while taking ACTOS. Thus, adequate contraception in premenopausal women should be recommended. This possible effect has not been investigated in clinical studies so the frequency of this occurrence is not known.

Drug Interactions

Oral Contraceptives: Administration of another thiazolidinedione with an oral contraceptive containing ethinyl estradiol and norethindrone reduced the plasma concentrations of both hormones by approximately 30%, which could result in loss of contraception. The pharmacokinetics of coadministration of ACTOS and oral contraceptives have not been evaluated in patients receiving ACTOS and an oral contraceptive. Therefore, additional caution regarding contraception should be exercised in patients receiving ACTOS and an oral contraceptive.

Glipizide: In healthy volunteers, coadministration of ACTOS (45 mg once daily) and glipizide (5.0 mg once daily) for seven days did not alter the steady-state pharmacokinetics of glipizide.

Digoxin: In healthy volunteers, coadministration of ACTOS (45 mg once daily) with digoxin (0.25 mg once daily) for seven days did not alter the steady-state pharmacokinetics of digoxin.

Warfarin: In healthy volunteers, coadministration of ACTOS (45 mg once daily) for seven days with warfarin did not alter the steady-state pharmacokinetics of warfarin. In addition, ACTOS has no clinically significant effect on prothrombin time when administered to patients receiving chronic warfarin therapy.

Metformin: In healthy volunteers, coadministration of metformin (1000 mg) and ACTOS (45 mg) after seven days of ACTOS (45 mg once daily) did not alter the pharmacokinetics of the single dose of metformin.

The cytochrome P450 isoform CYP3A4 is partially responsible for the metabolism of pioglitazone. Specific formal pharmacokinetic interaction studies have not been conducted with ACTOS and other drugs metabolized by this enzyme such as: erythromycin, astemizole, calcium channel blockers, cisapride, corticosteroids, cyclosporine, HMG-CoA reductase inhibitors, tacrolimus, triazolam, and trimetrexate, as well as inhibitory drugs such as ketoconazole and itraconazole. In vitro, ketoconazole appears to significantly inhibit the metabolism of pioglitazone (see CLINICAL PHARMACOLOGY, Metabolism). Pending the availability of additional data, patients receiving ketoconazole concomitantly with ACTOS should be evaluated more frequently with respect to glycemic control.

Carcinogenesis, Mutagenesis, Impairment of Fertility

A two-year carcinogenicity study was conducted in male and female rats at oral doses up to 63 mg/kg (approximately 14 times the maximum recommended human oral dose of 45 mg based on mg/m^2). Drug-induced tumors were not observed in any organ except for the urinary bladder. Benign and/or malignant transitional cell neoplasms were observed in male rats at 4 mg/kg/day and above (approximately equal to the maximum recommended human oral dose based on mg/m^2). The relationship of these findings in male rats to humans is unclear. A two-year carcinogenicity study was conducted in male and female mice at oral doses up to 100 mg/kg/day (approximately 11 times the maximum recommended human oral dose based on mg/m^2). No drug-induced tumors were observed in any organ.

During prospective evaluation of urinary cytology involving more than 1800 patients receiving ACTOS in clinical trials up to one year in duration, no new cases of bladder tumors were identified. Occasionally, abnormal urinary cytology results indicating possible malignancy were observed in both patients treated with ACTOS (0.72%) and patients treated with placebo (0.88%).

Pioglitazone HCl was not mutagenic in a battery of genetic toxicology studies, including the Ames bacterial assay, a mammalian cell forward gene mutation assay (CHO/HPRT and AS52/XPRT), an in vitro cytogenetics assay using CHL cells, an unscheduled DNA synthesis assay, and an in vivo micronucleus assay.

No adverse effects upon fertility were observed in male and female rats at oral doses up to 40 mg/kg pioglitazone HCl daily prior to and throughout mating and gestation (approximately 9 times the maximum recommended human oral dose based on mg/m^2).

Animal Toxicology

Heart enlargement has been observed in mice (100 mg/kg), rats (4 mg/kg and above) and dogs (3 mg/kg) treated orally with pioglitazone HCl (approximately 11, 1, and 2 times the maximum recommended human oral dose for mice, rats, and dogs, respectively, based on mg/m^2). In a one-year rat study, drug-related early death due to apparent heart dysfunction occurred at an oral dose of 160 mg/kg/day (approximately 35 times the maximum recommended human oral dose based on mg/m^2). Heart enlargement was seen in a 13-week study in monkeys at oral doses of 8.9 mg/kg and above (approximately 4 times the maximum recommended human oral dose based on mg/m^2), but not in a 52-week study at oral doses up to 32 mg/kg (approximately 13 times the maximum recommended human oral dose based on mg/m^2).

Pregnancy

Pregnancy Category C. Pioglitazone was not teratogenic in rats at oral doses up to 80 mg/kg or in rabbits given up to 160 mg/kg during organogenesis (approximately 17 and 40 times the maximum recommended human oral dose based on mg/m^2, respectively). Delayed parturition and embryotoxicity (as evidenced by increased postimplantation losses, delayed development and reduced fetal weights) were observed in rats at oral doses of 40 mg/kg/day and above (approximately 10 times the maximum recommended human oral dose based on mg/m^2). No functional or behavioral toxicity was observed in offspring of rats. In rabbits, embryotoxicity was observed at an oral dose of 160 mg/kg (approximately 40 times the maximum recommended human oral dose based on mg/m^2). Delayed postnatal development, attributed to decreased body weight, was observed in offspring of rats at oral doses of 10 mg/kg and above during late gestation and lactation periods (approximately 2 times the maximum recommended human oral dose based on mg/m^2).

There are no adequate and well-controlled studies in pregnant women. ACTOS should be used during pregnancy only if the potential benefit justifies the potential risk to the fetus.

Because current information strongly suggests that abnormal blood glucose levels during pregnancy are associated with a higher incidence of congenital anomalies, as well as increased neonatal morbidity and mortality, most experts recommend that insulin be used during pregnancy to maintain blood glucose levels as close to normal as possible.

Nursing Mothers

Pioglitazone is secreted in the milk of lactating rats. It is not known whether ACTOS is secreted in human milk. Because many drugs are excreted in human milk, ACTOS should not be administered to a breast-feeding woman.

Pediatric Use

Safety and effectiveness of ACTOS in pediatric patients have not been established.

Elderly Use

Approximately 500 patients in placebo-controlled clinical trials of ACTOS were 65 and over. No significant differences in effectiveness and safety were observed between these patients and younger patients.

ADVERSE REACTIONS

In worldwide clinical trials, over 3700 patients with type 2 diabetes have been treated with ACTOS. In U.S. clinical trials, over 2500 patients have received ACTOS, over 1100 patients have been treated for 6 months or longer, and over 450 patients for one year or longer.

The overall incidence and types of adverse events reported in placebo-controlled clinical trials of ACTOS monotherapy at doses of 7.5 mg, 15 mg, 30 mg, or 45 mg once daily are shown in Table 6.

Table 6 Placebo-Controlled Clinical Studies of ACTOS Monotherapy: Adverse Events Reported at a Frequency ≥ 5% of Patients Treated with ACTOS

(% of Patients)

	Placebo N=259	ACTOS N=606
Upper Respiratory Tract Infection	8.5	13.2
Headache	6.9	9.1
Sinusitis	4.6	6.3
Myalgia	2.7	5.4
Tooth Disorder	2.3	5.3
Diabetes Mellitus Aggravated	8.1	5.1
Pharyngitis	0.8	5.1

The types of clinical adverse events reported when ACTOS was used in combination with sulfonylureas (N=373), metformin (N=168), or insulin (N=379) were generally similar to those reported during ACTOS monotherapy with the exception of an increase in the occurrence of edema in the insulin combination study (pioglitazone 15% and placebo 7%). The incidence of withdrawals from clinical trials due to an adverse event other than hyperglycemia was similar for patients treated with placebo (2.8%) or ACTOS (3.3%).
Mild to moderate hypoglycemia was reported during combination therapy with sulfonylurea or insulin. Hypoglycemia was reported for 1% of placebo-treated patients and 2% of patients when ACTOS was used in combination with a sulfonylurea. In combination with insulin, hypoglycemia was reported for 5% of placebo-treated patients, 8% for patients treated with 15 mg of ACTOS, and 15% for patients treated with 30 mg of ACTOS (see PRECAUTIONS, General, Hypoglycemia).
In U.S. double-blind studies, anemia was reported for 1.0% of patients treated with ACTOS and 0.0% of placebo-treated patients in monotherapy studies. Anemia was reported for 1.6% of patients treated with ACTOS and 1.6% of placebo-treated patients in combination with insulin. Anemia was reported for 0.3% of patients treated with ACTOS and 1.6% of placebo-treated patients in combination with sulfonylurea. Anemia was reported for 1.2% of patients treated with ACTOS and 0.0% of placebo-treated patients in combination with metformin.
In all U.S. clinical trials, edema was reported more frequently in patients treated with ACTOS than placebo-treated patients. In monotherapy studies, edema was reported for 4.8% of patients treated with ACTOS versus 1.2% of placebo-treated patients. Edema was reported most frequently in the insulin combination study (15.3% for patients treated with ACTOS versus 7.0% for placebo-treated patients). All events were considered mild or moderate in intensity (see PRECAUTIONS, General, Edema).

Laboratory Abnormalities

Hematologic: ACTOS may cause decreases in hemoglobin and hematocrit. Across all clinical studies, mean hemoglobin values declined by 2% to 4% in patients treated with ACTOS. These changes generally occurred within the first 4 to 12 weeks of therapy and remained relatively stable thereafter. These changes may be related to increased plasma volume associated with ACTOS therapy and have not been associated with any significant hematologic clinical effects.
Serum Transaminase Levels: During placebo-controlled clinical trials in the U.S., a total of 4 of 1526 (0.26%) patients treated with ACTOS and 2 of 793 (0.25%) placebo-treated patients had ALT values ≥ 3 times the upper limit of normal. During all clinical studies in the U.S., 11 of 2561 (0.43%) patients treated with ACTOS had ALT values ≥ 3 times the upper limit of normal. All patients with follow-up values had reversible elevations in ALT. In the population of patients treated with ACTOS, mean values for bilirubin, AST, ALT, alkaline phosphatase, and GGT were decreased at the final visit compared with baseline. Fewer than 0.12% of patients treated with ACTOS were withdrawn from clinical trials in the U.S. due to abnormal liver function tests. In pre-approval clinical trials, there were no cases of idiosyncratic drug reactions leading to hepatic failure (see PRECAUTIONS, Hepatic Effects).
CPK Levels: During required laboratory testing in clinical trials, sporadic, transient elevations in creatine phosphokinase levels (CPK) were observed. A single, isolated elevation to greater than 10 times the upper limit of normal (values of 2150 to 8610) was noted in 7 patients. Five of these patients continued to receive ACTOS and the other two patients had completed receiving study medication at the time of the elevated value. These elevations resolved without any apparent clinical sequelae. The relationship of these events to ACTOS therapy is unknown.

OVERDOSAGE

During controlled clinical trials, one case of overdose with ACTOS was reported. A male patient took 120 mg per day for four days, then 180 mg per day for seven days. The patient denied any clinical symptoms during this period.
In the event of overdosage, appropriate supportive treatment should be initiated according to patient's clinical signs and symptoms.

DOSAGE AND ADMINISTRATION

ACTOS should be taken once daily without regard to meals. The management of antidiabetic therapy should be individualized. Ideally, the response to therapy should be evaluated using HbA_{1c} which is a better indicator of long-term glycemic control than FBG alone. HbA_{1c} reflects glycemia over the past two to three months. In clinical use, it is recommended that patients be treated with ACTOS for a period of time adequate to evaluate change in HbA_{1c} (three months) unless glycemic control deteriorates.

Monotherapy

ACTOS monotherapy in patients not adequately controlled with diet and exercise may be initiated at 15 mg or 30 mg once daily. For patients who respond inadequately to the initial dose of ACTOS, the dose can be increased in increments up to 45 mg once daily. For patients not responding adequately to monotherapy, combination therapy should be considered.

Combination Therapy

Sulfonylureas: ACTOS in combination with a sulfonylurea may be initiated at 15 mg or 30 mg once daily. The current sulfonylurea dose can be continued upon initiation of ACTOS therapy. If patients report hypoglycemia, the dose of the sulfonylurea should be decreased.
Metformin: ACTOS in combination with metformin may be initiated at 15 mg or 30 mg once daily. The current metformin dose can be continued upon initiation of ACTOS therapy. It is unlikely that the dose of metformin will require adjustment due to hypoglycemia during combination therapy with ACTOS.
Insulin: ACTOS in combination with insulin may be initiated at 15 mg or 30 mg once daily. The current insulin dose can be continued upon initiation of ACTOS therapy. In patients receiving ACTOS and insulin, the insulin dose can be decreased by 10% to 25% if the patient reports hypoglycemia or if plasma glucose concentrations decrease to less than 100 mg/dL. Further adjustments should be individualized based on glucose-lowering response.

Maximum Recommended Dose

The dose of ACTOS should not exceed 45 mg once daily since doses higher than 45 mg once daily have not been studied in placebo-controlled clinical studies. No placebo-controlled clinical studies of more than 30 mg once daily have been conducted in combination therapy.
Dose adjustment in patients with renal insufficiency is not recommended (see CLINICAL PHARMACOLOGY, Pharmacokinetics and Drug Metabolism).
Therapy with ACTOS should not be initiated if the patient exhibits clinical evidence of active liver disease or increased serum transaminase levels (ALT greater than 2.5 times the upper limit of normal) at start of therapy (see PRECAUTIONS, General, Hepatic Effects and CLINICAL PHARMACOLOGY, Special Populations, Hepatic Insufficiency). Liver enzyme monitoring is recommended in all patients prior to initiation of therapy with ACTOS and periodically thereafter (see PRECAUTIONS, General, Hepatic Effects).
There are no data on the use of ACTOS in patients under 18 years of age; therefore, use of ACTOS in pediatric patients is not recommended.
No data are available on the use of ACTOS in combination with another thiazolidinedione.

HOW SUPPLIED

ACTOS is available in 15 mg, 30 mg, and 45 mg tablets as follows:
15 mg Tablet: white to off-white, round, convex, non-scored tablet with "ACTOS" on one side, and "15" on the other, available in:
NDC 64764-151-04 Bottle of 30
NDC 64764-151-05 Bottle of 90
NDC 64764-151-06 Bottle of 500
30 mg Tablet: white to off-white, round, flat, non-scored tablet with "ACTOS" on one side and "30" on the other, available in:
NDC 64764-301-14 Bottle of 30
NDC 64764-301-15 Bottle of 90
NDC 64764-301-16 Bottle of 500
45 mg Tablet: white to off-white, round, flat, non-scored tablet with "ACTOS" on one side, and "45" on the other, available in:
NDC 64764-451-24 Bottle of 30
NDC 64764-451-25 Bottle of 90
NDC 64764-451-26 Bottle of 500

STORAGE

Store at 25°C (77°F); excursions permitted to 15–30°C (59–86°F) [see USP Controlled Room Temperature]. Keep container tightly closed, and protect from moisture and humidity.

Rx only

Manufactured by:
Takeda Chemical Industries, Ltd.
Osaka, Japan
Marketed by:
Takeda Pharmaceuticals America, Inc.
475 Half Day Road, Suite 500
Lincolnshire, IL 60069
and
Eli Lilly and Company
Lilly Corporate Center
Indianapolis, IN 46285

ACTOS® is a registered trademark of Takeda Chemical Industries, Ltd.
5012100-02 Revised: February 2000
Shown in Product Identification Guide, page 338

TAP Pharmaceuticals Inc.
LAKE FOREST, IL 60045

For Medical Information Contact:
Medical Department
(800) 622-2011 (LUPRON)
(800) 478-9526 (PREVACID)
In Emergencies:
(800) 622-2011 (LUPRON)
(800) 478-9526 (PREVACID)

LUPRON® ℞
(leuprolide acetate) Injection

DESCRIPTION

LUPRON (leuprolide acetate) Injection is a synthetic nonapeptide analog of naturally occurring gonadotropin releasing hormone (GnRH or LH-RH). The analog possesses greater potency than the natural hormone. The chemical name is 5-Oxo-L-prolyl-L-histidyl-L-tryptophyl-L-seryl-L-tyrosyl-D-leucyl-L-leucyl-L-arginyl-N-ethyl-L-prolinamide acetate (salt) with the following structural formula:
[See chemical structure at top of next page]
LUPRON is a sterile, aqueous solution intended for subcutaneous injection. It is available in a 2.8 mL multiple-dose vial containing 5 mg/mL of leuprolide acetate, sodium chloride for tonicity adjustment, 9 mg/mL of benzyl alcohol as a preservative and water for injection. The pH may have been adjusted with sodium hydroxide and/or acetic acid.

CLINICAL PHARMACOLOGY

Leuprolide acetate, an LH-RH agonist, acts as a potent inhibitor of gonadotropin secretion when given continuously and in therapeutic doses. Animal and human studies indicate that following an initial stimulation, chronic administration of leuprolide acetate results in suppression of ovarian and testicular steroidogenesis. This effect is reversible upon discontinuation of drug therapy. Administration of leuprolide acetate has resulted in inhibition of the growth of certain hormone dependent tumors (prostatic tumors in Noble and Dunning male rats and DMBA-induced mammary tumors in female rats) as well as atrophy of the reproductive organs.
In humans, subcutaneous administration of single daily doses of leuprolide acetate results in an initial increase in circulation levels of luteinizing hormone (LH) and follicle stimulating hormone (FSH), leading to a transient increase in levels of the gonadal steroids (testosterone and dihydrotestosterone in males, and estrone and estradiol in pre-menopausal females). However, continuous daily administration of leuprolide acetate results in decreased levels of LH and FSH in all patients. In males, testosterone is reduced to castrate levels. In pre-menopausal females, estrogens are reduced to post-menopausal levels. These decreases occur within two to four weeks after initiation of treatment, and castrate levels of testosterone in prostatic cancer patients have been demonstrated for periods of up to five years.
Leuprolide acetate is not active when given orally. Bioavailability by subcutaneous administration is comparable to that by intravenous administration. Leuprolide acetate has a plasma half-life of approximately three hours. The metabolism, distribution and excretion of leuprolide acetate in man have not been determined.

INDICATIONS AND USAGE

LUPRON (leuprolide acetate) Injection is indicated in the palliative treatment of advanced prostatic cancer. It offers an alternative treatment of prostatic cancer when orchiectomy or estrogen administration are either not indicated or unacceptable to the patient. In a controlled study comparing LUPRON 1 mg/day given subcutaneously to DES (diethylstilbestrol), 3 mg/day, the survival rate for the two groups was comparable after two years treatment. The objective response to treatment was also similar for the two groups.

CONTRAINDICATIONS

A report of an anaphylactic reaction to synthetic GnRH (Factrel) has been reported in the medical literature.[1]
LUPRON is contraindicated in women who are or may become pregnant while receiving the drug. When administered on day 6 of pregnancy at test dosages of 0.00024, 0.0024, and 0.024 mg/kg (1/600 to 1/6 the human dose) to rabbits, LUPRON produced a dose-related increase in major fetal abnormalities. Similar studies in rats failed to demonstrate an increase in fetal malformations. There was increased fetal mortality and decreased fetal weights with the two higher doses of LUPRON in rabbits and with the highest dose in rats. The effects on fetal mortality are logical consequences of the alterations in hormonal levels brought

Continued on next page

Lupron—Cont.

about by this drug. Therefore, the possibility exists that spontaneous abortion may occur if the drug is administered during pregnancy.

WARNINGS

Isolated cases of worsening of signs and symptoms during the first weeks of treatment have been reported. Worsening of symptoms may contribute to paralysis with or without fatal complications.

PRECAUTIONS

Patients with metastatic vertebral lesions and/or with urinary tract obstruction should be closely observed during the first few weeks of therapy (see "**ADVERSE REACTIONS**" section).

Patients with known allergies to benzyl alcohol, an ingredient of the drug's vehicle, may present symptoms of hypersensitivity, usually local, in the form of erythema and induration at the injection site.

Information for Patients: See Information for Patients which appears after the "**HOW SUPPLIED**" section.

Laboratory Tests: Response to leuprolide acetate should be monitored by measuring serum levels of testosterone and acid phosphatase. In the majority of patients, testosterone levels increased above baseline during the first week, declining thereafter to baseline levels or below by the end of the second week of treatment. Castrate levels were reached within two to four weeks and once attained were maintained for as long as drug administration continued. Transient increases in acid phosphatase levels occurred sometimes early in treatment. However, by the fourth week, the elevated levels usually decreased to values at or near baseline.

Drug Interactions: None have been reported.

Carcinogenesis, Mutagenesis, Impairment of Fertility: Two-year carcinogenicity studies were conducted in rats and mice. In rats, a dose-related increase of benign pituitary hyperplasia and benign pituitary adenomas was noted at 24 months when the drug was administered subcutaneously at high daily doses (0.6 to 4 mg/kg). In mice no pituitary abnormalities were observed at a dose as high as 60 mg/kg for two years. Patients have been treated with leuprolide acetate for up to three years with doses as high as 10 mg/day and for two years with doses as high as 20 mg/day without demonstrable pituitary abnormalities.

Mutagenicity studies have been performed with leuprolide acetate using bacterial and mammalian systems. These studies provided no evidence of a mutagenic potential.

Clinical and pharmacologic studies with leuprolide acetate and similar analogs have shown full reversibility of fertility suppression when the drug is discontinued after continuous administration for periods of up to 24 weeks. However, no clinical studies have been conducted with leuprolide acetate to assess the reversibility of fertility suppression.

Pregnancy Category X. See "**CONTRAINDICATIONS**" section.

ADVERSE REACTIONS

In the majority of patients testosterone levels increased above baseline during the first week, declining thereafter to baseline levels or below by the end of the second week of treatment. This transient increase was occasionally associated with a temporary worsening of signs and symptoms, usually manifested by an increase in bone pain (See "**WARNINGS**" section). In a few cases a temporary worsening of existing hematuria and urinary tract obstruction occurred during the first week. Temporary weakness and paresthesia of the lower limbs have been reported in a few cases.

Potential exacerbations of signs and symptoms during the first few weeks of treatment is a concern in patients with vertebral metastases and/or urinary obstruction which, if aggravated, may lead to neurological problems or increase the obstruction.

In a comparative trial of LUPRON (leuprolide acetate) Injection versus DES, in 5% or more of the patients receiving either drug, the following adverse reactions were reported to have a possible or probable relationship to drug as ascribed by the treating physician. Often, causality is difficult to assess in patients with metastatic prostate cancer. Reactions considered not drug related are excluded.

	LUPRON (N=98)	DES (N=101)
	Number of Reports	
Cardiovascular System		
Congestive heart failure	1	5
ECG changes/ischemia	19	22
High blood pressure	8	5
Murmur	3	8
Peripheral edema	12	30
Plebitis/thrombosis	2	10
Gastrointestinal System		
Anorexia	6	5
Constipation	7	9
Nausea/vomiting	5	17
Endocrine System		
*Decreased testicular size	7	11
*Gynecomastia/breast tenderness or pain	7	63
*Hot flashes	55	12
*Impotence	4	12
Hemic and Lymphatic System		
Anemia	5	5
Musculoskeletal System		
Bone pain	5	2
Myalgia	3	9
Central/Peripheral Nervous System		
Dizziness/lightheadedness	5	7
General pain	13	13
Headache	7	4
Insomnia/sleep disorders	7	5
Respiratory System		
Dyspnea	2	8
Sinus congestion	5	6
Integumentary System		
Dermatitis	5	8
Urogenital System		
Frequency/urgency	6	8
Hematuria	6	4
Urinary tract infection	3	7
Miscellaneous		
Asthenia	10	10

*Physiologic effect of decreased testosterone.

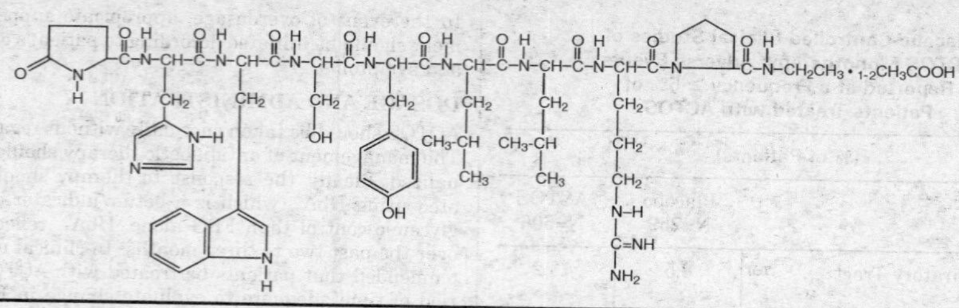

In this same study, the following adverse reactions were reported in less than 5% of the patients on LUPRON.

Cardiovascular System—Angina, Cardiac arrhythmias, Myocardial infarction, Pulmonary emboli; *Gastrointestinal System*—Diarrhea, Dysphagia, Gastrointestinal bleeding, Gastrointestinal disturbance, Peptic ulcer, Rectal polyps; *Endocrine System*—Libido decrease, Thyroid enlargement; *Musculoskeletal System*—Joint pain; *Central/Peripheral Nervous System*—Anxiety, Blurred vision, Lethargy, Memory disorder, Mood swings, Nervousness, Numbness, Paresthesia, Peripheral neuropathy, Syncope/blackouts, Taste disorders; *Respiratory System*—Cough, Pleural rub, Pneumonia, Pulmonary fibrosis; *Integumentary System*—Carcinoma of skin/ear, Dry skin, Ecchymosis, Hair loss, Itching, Local skin reactions, Pigmentation, Skin lesions; *Urogenital System*—Bladder spasms, Dysuria, Incontinence, Testicular pain, Urinary obstruction; *Miscellaneous*—Depression, Diabetes, Fatigue, Fever/chills, Hypoglycemia, Increased BUN, Increased calcium, Increased creatinine, Infection/inflammation, Ophthalmologic disorders, Swelling (temporal bone).

The following additional adverse reactions have been reported with LUPRON or LUPRON DEPOT (leuprolide acetate for depot suspension) during other clinical trials and/or during postmarketing surveillance. Reactions considered as nondrug related by the treating physician are excluded.

Cardiovascular System—Hypotension, Transient ischemic attack/stroke; *Gastrointestinal System*—Hepatic dysfunction; *Endocrine System*—Libido increase; *Hemic and Lymphatic System*—Decreased WBC, Hemoptysis; *Musculoskeletal System*—Ankylosing spondylosis, Pelvic fibrosis; *Central/Peripheral Nervous System*—Hearing disorder, Peripheral neuropathy, Spinal fracture/paralysis; *Respiratory System*—Pulmonary infiltrate, Respiratory disorders; *Integumentary System*—Hair growth; *Urogenital System*—Penile swelling, Prostate pain; *Miscellaneous*—Hypoproteinemia, Hard nodule in throat, Weight gain, Increased uric acid.

OVERDOSAGE

In rats subcutaneous administration of 250 to 500 times the recommended human dose, expressed on a per body weight basis, resulted in dyspnea, decreased activity, and local irritation at the injection site. There is no evidence at present that there is a clinical counterpart of this phenomenon. In early clinical trials with leuprolide acetate doses as high as 20 mg/day for up to two years caused no adverse effects differing from those observed with the 1 mg/day dose.

DOSAGE AND ADMINISTRATION

The recommended dose is 1 mg (0.2 mL or 20 unit mark) administered as a single daily subcutaneous injection. As with other drugs administered chronically by subcutaneous injection, the injection site should be varied periodically.

NOTE: As with all parenteral products, inspect container's solution for discoloration and particulate matter before each use.

HOW SUPPLIED

LUPRON (leuprolide acetate) Injection is a sterile solution supplied in a 2.8 mL multiple-dose vial, NDC 0300-3612-28. Store below 77° F (25° C). Do not freeze. Protect from light—store vial in carton until use.

Each 0.2 mL contains 1 mg of leuprolide acetate, sodium chloride for tonicity adjustment, 1.8 mg of benzyl alcohol as preservative and water for injection. The pH may have been adjusted with sodium hydroxide and/or acetic acid.

Rx ONLY

U.S. Patent Nos. 4,005,063 and 4,005,194.

REFERENCE

1. MacLeod TL, Eisen A, Sussman GL, et al: Anaphylactic reaction to synthetic luteinizing hormone-releasing hormone. *Fertil Steril* 1987 Sept;48(3):500-502.

INFORMATION FOR PATIENTS

NOTE: Be sure to consult your physician with any questions you may have or for information about LUPRON (leuprolide acetate) Injection and its use.

WHAT IS LUPRON?

LUPRON (leuprolide acetate) Injection is chemically similar to gonadotropin releasing hormone (GnRH or LH-RH) a hormone which occurs naturally in your body.

Normally, your body releases small amounts of LH-RH and this leads to events which stimulate the production of sex hormones.

However, when you inject LUPRON (leuprolide acetate) Injection, the normal events that lead to sex hormone production are interrupted and testosterone is no longer produced by the testes.

LUPRON must be injected because, like insulin which is injected by diabetics, LUPRON is inactive when taken by mouth.

If you were to discontinue the drug for any reason, your body would begin making testosterone again.

DIRECTIONS FOR USING LUPRON

1. Wash hands thoroughly with soap and water.
2. If using a new bottle for the first time, flip off the plastic cover to expose the gray rubber stopper. Wipe metal ring and rubber stopper with an alcohol wipe each time you use LUPRON. Check the liquid in the container. If it is not clear or has particles in it, DO NOT USE IT. Exchange it at your pharmacy for another container.
3. Remove outer wrapping from one syringe. Pull plunger back until the tip of the plunger is at the 0.2 mL or 20 unit mark.
4. Take cover off needle. Push the needle through the center of the rubber stopper on the LUPRON bottle.
5. Push the plunger all the way in to inject air into the bottle.
6. Keep the needle in the bottle and turn the bottle upside down. Check to make sure the tip of the needle is in the liquid. Slowly pull back on the plunger, until the syringe fills to the 0.2 mL or 20 unit mark.
7. Toward the end of a two-week period, the amount of LUPRON left in the bottle will be small. Take special care to hold the bottle straight and to keep the needle tip in liquid while pulling back on the plunger.
8. Keeping the needle in the bottle and the bottle upside down, check for air bubbles in the syringe. If you see any, push the plunger *slowly* in to push the air bubble back into the bottle. Keep the tip of the needle in the liquid and pull the plunger back again to fill to the 0.2 mL or 20 unit mark.
9. Do this again if necessary to eliminate air bubbles. Remove needle from bottle and lay syringe down. DO NOT TOUCH THE NEEDLE OR ALLOW THE NEEDLE TO TOUCH ANY SURFACE.
10. To protect your skin, inject each daily dose at a different body spot.
11. Choose an injection spot. Cleanse the injection spot with another alcohol wipe.
12. Hold the syringe in one hand. Hold the skin taut, or pull up a little flesh with the other hand, as you were instructed.
13. Holding the syringe as you would a pencil, thrust the needle all the way into the skin at a 90° angle.
14. Hold an alcohol wipe down on your skin where the needle is inserted and withdraw the needle at the same angle it was inserted.
15. Use the disposable syringe only once and dispose of it properly as you were instructed. Needles thrown into a garbage bag could accidentally stick someone. NEVER LEAVE SYRINGES, NEEDLES OR DRUGS WHERE CHILDREN CAN REACH THEM.

SOME SPECIAL ADVICE

- You may experience hot flashes when using LUPRON (leuprolide acetate) Injection. During the first few weeks of treatment you may experience increased bone pain, increased difficulty in urinating, and less commonly but most importantly, you may experience the onset or aggravation of nerve symptoms. In any of these events, discuss the symptoms with your doctor.
- You may experience some irritation at the injection site, such as burning, itching or swelling. These reactions are usually mild and go away. If they do not, tell your doctor.
- Do not stop taking your injections because you feel better. You need an injection every day to make sure LUPRON keeps working for you.

- If you need to use an alternate to the syringe supplied with LUPRON, insulin syringes should be utilized.
- When the drug level gets low, take special care to hold the bottle straight up and down and to keep the needle tip in liquid while pulling back on the plunger.
- Do not try to get every last drop out of the bottle. This will increase the possibility of drawing air into the syringe and getting an incomplete dose. Some extra drug has been provided so that you can withdraw the recommended number of doses.
- Tell your pharmacist when you will need LUPRON so it will be at the pharmacy when you need it.
- Store below 77° F (25° C). Do not store near a radiator or other very warm place. Do not freeze.
  Protect from light—store vial in carton until use.
- Do not leave your drug or hypodermic syringes where anyone can pick them up.
- Keep this and all other medications out of reach of children.

TAP Pharmaceuticals Inc.
Deerfield, IL 60015, U.S.A.
Lupron Injection manufactured by Abbott Laboratories, North Chicago, IL 60064
®—Registered
Ref. 03-4881-R1 Revised: July, 1998

Shown in Product Identification Guide, page 338

For Pediatric Use
LUPRON® ℞
(leuprolide acetate) Injection

DESCRIPTION

Leuprolide acetate is a synthetic nonapeptide analog of naturally occurring gonadotropin releasing hormone (GnRH or LH-RH). The analog possesses greater potency than the natural hormone. The chemical name is 5-Oxo-L-prolyl-L-histidyl-L-tryptophyl-L-seryl-L-tyrosyl-D-leucyl-L-leucyl-L-arginyl-N-ethyl-L-prolinamide acetate (salt) with the following structural formula:

[See chemical structure above]

LUPRON Injection is a sterile, aqueous solution intended for daily subcutaneous injection.

- A 2.8 mL multiple dose vial contains leuprolide acetate (5 mg/mL), sodium chloride (6.3 mg/mL) for tonicity adjustment, benzyl alcohol as a preservative (9 mg/mL), and water for injection. The pH may have been adjusted with sodium hydroxide and/or acetic acid.

CLINICAL PHARMACOLOGY

Leuprolide acetate, a GnRH agonist, acts as a potent inhibitor of gonadotropin secretion when given continuously and in therapeutic doses. Human studies indicate that following an initial stimulation of gonadotropins, chronic stimulation with leuprolide acetate results in suppression or "downregulation" of these hormones and consequent suppression of ovarian and testicular steroidogenesis. These effects are reversible on discontinuation of drug therapy.

Leuprolide acetate is not active when given orally. In adults, bioavailability by subcutaneous administration is comparable to that by intravenous administration; and leuprolide acetate has a plasma half-life of approximately three hours. The metabolism, distribution and excretion of leuprolide acetate in humans have not been determined. A pharmacokinetic study of leuprolide acetate in children has not been performed.

In children with central precocious puberty (CPP), stimulated and basal gonadotropins are reduced to prepubertal levels. Testosterone and estradiol are reduced to prepubertal levels in males and females respectively. Reduction of gonadotropins will allow for normal physical and psychological growth and development. Natural maturation occurs when gonadotropins return to pubertal levels following discontinuation of leuprolide acetate.

The following physiologic effects have been noted with the chronic administration of leuprolide acetate in this patient population.

1. **Skeletal Growth.** A measurable increase in body length can be noted since the epiphyseal plates will not close prematurely.
2. **Organ growth.** Reproductive organs will return to a prepubertal state.
3. **Menses.** Menses, if present, will cease.

INDICATIONS AND USAGE

LUPRON Injection is indicated in the treatment of children with central precocious puberty. Children should be selected using the following criteria:

1. Clinical diagnosis of CPP (idiopathic or neurogenic) with onset of secondary sexual characteristics earlier than 8 years in females and 9 years in males.
2. Clinical diagnosis should be confirmed prior to initiation of therapy:
   - Confirmation of diagnosis by a pubertal response to a GnRH stimulation test. The sensitivity and methodology of this assay must be understood.
   - Bone age advanced one year beyond the chronological age.
3. Baseline evaluation should also include:
   - Height and weight measurements.
   - Sex steroid levels.
   - Adrenal steroid level to exclude congenital adrenal hyperplasia. 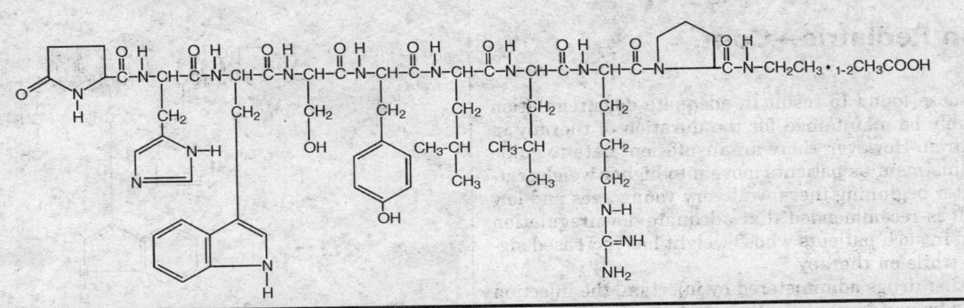
   - Beta human chorionic gonadotropin level to rule out a chorionic gonadotropin secreting tumor.
   - Pelvic/adrenal/testicular ultrasound to rule out a steroid secreting tumor.
   - Computerized tomography of the head to rule out intracranial tumor.

CONTRAINDICATIONS

LUPRON Injection is contraindicated in women who are or may become pregnant while receiving the drug. When administered on day 6 of pregnancy at test dosages of 0.00024, 0.0024, and 0.024 mg/kg (1/1200 to 1/12 the human pediatric dose) to rabbits, LUPRON produced a dose-related increase in major fetal abnormalities. Similar studies in rats failed to demonstrate an increase in fetal malformations. There was increased fetal mortality and decreased fetal weights with the two higher doses of LUPRON in rabbits and with the highest dose in rats. The effects on fetal mortality are logical consequences of the alterations in hormonal levels brought about by this drug. Therefore, the possibility exists that spontaneous abortion may occur if the drug is administered during pregnancy.

Leuprolide acetate is contraindicated in children demonstrating hypersensitivity to GnRH, GnRH agonist analogs, or any of the excipients.

A report of an anaphylactic reaction to synthetic GnRH (Factrel) has been reported in the medical literature.[1]

WARNINGS

During the early phase of therapy, gonadotropins and sex steroids rise above baseline because of the natural stimulatory effect of the drug. Therefore, an increase in clinical signs and symptoms may be observed (see "**CLINICAL PHARMACOLOGY**" section).

Noncompliance with drug regimen or inadequate dosing may result in inadequate control of the pubertal process. The consequences of poor control include the return of pubertal signs such as menses, breast development, and testicular growth. The long-term consequences of inadequate control of gonadal steroid secretion are unknown, but may include a further compromise of adult stature.

PRECAUTIONS

Patients with known allergies to benzyl alcohol, an ingredient of the vehicle of Lupron Injection, may present symptoms of hypersensitivity, usually local, in the form of erythema and induration at the injection site.

Laboratory Tests: Response to leuprolide acetate should be monitored 1–2 months after the start of therapy with a GnRH stimulation test and sex steroid levels. Measurement of bone age for advancement should be done every 6–12 months.

Sex steroids may increase or rise above prepubertal levels if the dose is inadequate (see "**WARNINGS**" section). Once a therapeutic dose has been established, gonadotropin and sex steroid levels will decline to prepubertal levels.

Drug Interactions: No pharmacokinetic-based drug-drug interaction studies have been conducted. However, because leuprolide acetate is a peptide that is primarily degraded by peptidase and not by cytochrome P-450 enzymes as noted in specific studies, and the drug is only about 46% bound to plasma proteins, drug interactions would not be expected to occur.

Drug/Laboratory Test Interactions: Administration of leuprolide acetate in therapeutic doses results in suppression of the pituitary-gonadal system. Normal function is usually restored within 4 to 12 weeks after treatment is discontinued.

Information for Parents: Prior to starting therapy with LUPRON Injection, the parent or guardian must be aware of the importance of continuous therapy. Adherence to daily drug administration schedules must be accepted if therapy is to be successful.

- During the first 2 months of therapy, a female may experience menses or spotting. If bleeding continues beyond the second month, notify the physician.
- Any irritation at the injection site should be reported to the physician immediately.
- Report any unusual signs or symptoms to the physician.

Carcinogenesis, Mutagenesis, Impairment of Fertility: A two-year carcinogenicity study was conducted in rats and mice. In rats, a dose-related increase of benign pituitary hyperplasia and benign pituitary adenomas was noted at 24 months when the drug was administered subcutaneously at high daily doses (0.6 to 4 mg/kg). There was a significant but not dose-related increase of pancreatic islet-cell adenomas in females and of testes interstitial cell adenomas in males (highest incidence in the low dose group). In mice, no leuprolide acetate-induced tumors or pituitary abnormalities were observed at a dose as high as 60 mg/kg for two years. Adult patients have been treated with leuprolide acetate for up to three years with doses as high as 10 mg/day and for two years with doses as high as 20 mg/day without demonstrable pituitary abnormalities.

Although no clinical studies have been completed in children to assess the full reversibility of fertility suppression, animal studies (prepubertal and adult rats and monkeys) with leuprolide acetate and other GnRH analogs have shown functional recovery. However, following a study with leuprolide acetate, immature male rats demonstrated tubular degeneration in the testes even after a recovery period. In spite of the failure to recover histologically, the treated males proved to be as fertile as the controls. Also, no histologic changes were observed in the female rats following the same protocol. In both sexes, the offspring of the treated animals appeared normal. The effect of the treatment of the parents on the reproductive performance of the F1 generation was not tested. The clinical significance of these findings is unknown.

Pregnancy Category X. See "**CONTRAINDICATIONS**" section.

Nursing Mothers: It is not known whether leuprolide acetate is excreted in human milk. LUPRON should not be used by nursing mothers.

ADVERSE REACTIONS

Potential exacerbation of signs and symptoms during the first few weeks of treatment (See "**PRECAUTIONS**" section) is a concern in patients with rapidly advancing central precocious puberty.

In two studies of children with central precocious puberty, in 2% or more of the patients receiving the drug, the following adverse reactions were reported to have a possible or probable relationship to drug as ascribed by the treating physician. Reactions considered not drug related are excluded.

	Number of Patients N = 395	(Percent)
Body as a Whole		
General Pain	7	(2)
Integumentary System		
Acne/Seborrhea	7	(2)
Injection Site Reactions		
Including Abscess	21	(5)
Rash Including		
Erythema Multiforme	8	(2)
Urogenital System		
Vaginitis/Bleeding/ Discharge	7	(2)

In those same studies, the following adverse reactions were reported in less than 2% of the patients.

Body as a Whole—Body Odor, Fever, Headache, Infection; *Cardiovascular System*—Syncope, Vasodilation; *Digestive System*—Dysphagia, Gingivitis, Nausea/Vomiting; *Endocrine System*—Accelerated Sexual Maturity; *Metabolic and Nutritional Disorders*—Peripheral Edema, Weight Gain; *Nervous System*—Nervousness, Personality Disorder, Somnolence, Emotional Lability; *Respiratory System*—Epistaxis; *Integumentary System*—Alopecia, Skin Striae; *Urogenital System*—Cervix Disorder, Gynecomastia/Breast Disorders, Urinary Incontinence.

See other package inserts for adverse events reported in other patient populations.

OVERDOSAGE

In rats, subcutaneous administration of 125 to 250 times the recommended human pediatric dose, expressed on a per body weight basis, resulted in dyspnea, decreased activity, and local irritation at the injection site. There is no evidence at present that there is a clinical counterpart of this phenomenon. In early clinical trials using leuprolide acetate in adult patients, doses as high as 20 mg/day for up to two years caused no adverse effects differing from those observed with the 1 mg/day dose.

DOSAGE AND ADMINISTRATION

LUPRON INJECTION can be administered by a patient/parent or health care professional.

The dose of LUPRON Injection must be individualized for each child. The dose is based on a mg/kg ratio of drug to body weight. Younger children require higher doses on a mg/kg ratio.

For either dosage form, after 1–2 months of initiating therapy or changing doses, the child must be monitored with a GnRH stimulation test, sex steroids, and Tanner staging to confirm downregulation. Measurements of bone age for advancement should be monitored every 6–12 months. The dose should be titrated upward until no progression of the condition is noted either clinically and/or by laboratory parameters.

Continued on next page

Lupron Pediatric—Cont.

The first dose found to result in adequate downregulation can probably be maintained for the duration of therapy in most children. However, there are insufficient data to guide dosage adjustment as patients move into higher weight categories after beginning therapy at very young ages and low dosages. It is recommended that adequate downregulation be verified in such patients whose weight has increased significantly while on therapy.
As with other drugs administered by injection, the injection site should be varied periodically.
Discontinuation of LUPRON Injection should be considered before age 11 for females and age 12 for males.
The recommended starting dose is 50 mcg/kg/day administered as a single subcutaneous injection. If total downregulation is not achieved, the dose should be titrated upward by 10 mcg/kg/day. This dose will be considered the maintenance dose.
NOTE: As with other parenteral products, inspect container's solution for discoloration and particulate matter before each use.

HOW SUPPLIED

LUPRON (leuprolide acetate) Injection is a sterile solution.

- A 2.8 mL multiple dose vial (NDC 0300-3612-28) contains leuprolide acetate (5 mg/mL), sodium chloride (6.3 mg/mL) for tonicity adjustment, benzyl alcohol as a preservative (9 mg/mL), and water for injection. The pH may have been adjusted with sodium hydroxide and/or acetic acid.
- Store below 77°F (25°C). Do not freeze. Protect from light—store vial in carton until use.
- Use the syringes supplied with LUPRON Injection. Insulin syringes may be substituted for use with Lupron Injection. The volume of drug for the dose will vary depending on the syringe used and the concentration of drug.

Rx ONLY

U.S. Patent Nos. 4,005,063; 4,005,194.

REFERENCE

1. MacLeod TL, et al. Anaphylactic reaction to synthetic luteinizing hormone-releasing hormone. *Fertil Steril* 1987 Sept;48(3):500-502.

TAP Pharmaceuticals Inc.
Deerfield, IL 60015, U.S.A.
Lupron Injection manufactured by Abbott Laboratories, North Chicago, IL 60064
®–Registered
Ref. 03-4881-R1 Revised: July, 1998

This is combined labeling. Examples of different fonts appear below.

- General information
- Information on endometriosis
- **Information on uterine fibroids**

LUPRON DEPOT® 3.75 mg ℞
(leuprolide acetate for depot suspension)

DESCRIPTION

Leuprolide acetate is a synthetic nonapeptide analog of naturally occurring gonadotropin-releasing hormone (GnRH or LH-RH). The analog possesses greater potency than the natural hormone. The chemical name is 5-oxo-L-prolyl-L-histidyl-L-tryptophyl-L-seryl-L-tyrosyl-D-leucyl-L-leucyl-L-arginyl-N-ethyl-L-prolinamide acetate (salt) with the following structural formula:
[See chemical structure above]
LUPRON DEPOT is available in a prefilled dual-chamber syringe containing sterile lyophilized microspheres which, when mixed with diluent, become a suspension intended as a monthly intramuscular injection.
The front chamber of LUPRON DEPOT 3.75 mg prefilled dual-chamber syringe contains leuprolide acetate (3.75 mg), purified gelatin (0.65 mg), DL-lactic and glycolic acids copolymer (33.1 mg), and D-mannitol (6.6 mg). The second chamber of diluent contains carboxymethylcellulose sodium (5 mg), D-mannitol (50 mg), polysorbate 80 (1 mg), water for injection, USP, and glacial acetic acid, USP to control pH.
During the manufacture of LUPRON DEPOT 3.75 mg, acetic acid is lost, leaving the peptide.

CLINICAL PHARMACOLOGY

Leuprolide acetate is a long-acting GnRH analog. A single monthly injection of LUPRON DEPOT 3.75 mg results in an initial stimulation followed by a prolonged suppression of pituitary gonadotropins. Repeated dosing at monthly intervals results in decreased secretion of gonadal steroids; consequently, tissues and functions that depend on gonadal steroids for their maintenance become quiescent. This effect is reversible on discontinuation of drug therapy.
Leuprolide acetate is not active when given orally. Intramuscular injection of the depot formulation provides plasma concentrations of leuprolide over a period of one month.

Pharmacokinetics

Absorption A single dose of LUPRON DEPOT 3.75 mg was administered by intramuscular injection to healthy female volunteers. The absorption of leuprolide was characterized by an initial increase in plasma concentration, with peak concentration ranging from 4.6 to 10.2 ng/mL at four

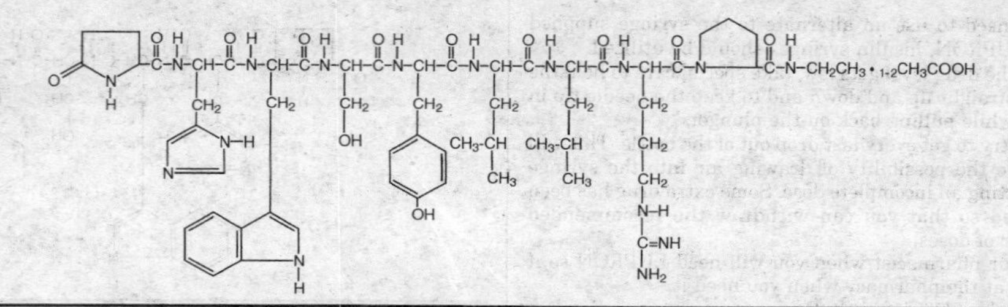

FIGURE 1-PERCENT OF PATIENTS WITH SIGNS/SYMPTOMS AT BASELINE, FINAL TREATMENT VISIT, AND AFTER 6 AND 12 MONTHS OF FOLLOW-UP

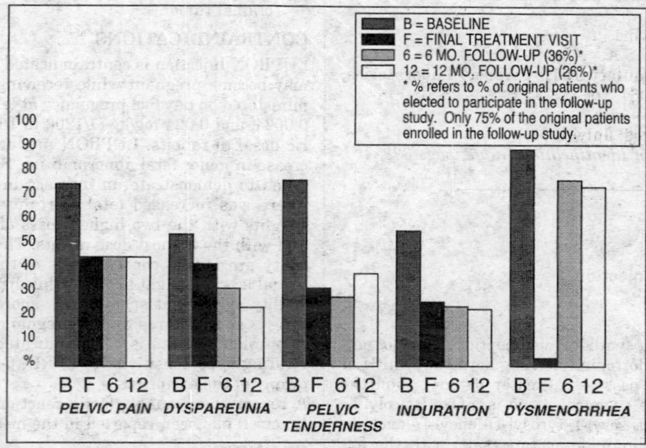

hours postdosing. However, intact leuprolide and an inactive metabolite could not be distinguished by the assay used in the study. Following the initial rise, leuprolide concentrations started to plateau within two days after dosing and remained relatively stable for about four to five weeks with plasma concentrations of about 0.30 ng/mL.

Distribution The mean steady-state volume of distribution of leuprolide following intravenous bolus administration to healthy male volunteers was 27 L. *In vitro* binding to human plasma proteins ranged from 43% to 49%.

Metabolism In healthy male volunteers, a 1 mg bolus of leuprolide administered intravenously revealed that the mean systemic clearance was 7.6 L/h, with a terminal elimination half-life of approximately 3 hours based on a two compartment model.
In rats and dogs, administration of ^{14}C-labeled leuprolide was shown to be metabolized to smaller inactive peptides, a pentapeptide (Metabolite I), tripeptides (Metabolites II and III) and a dipeptide (Metabolite IV). These fragments may be further catabolized.
The major metabolite (M-I) plasma concentrations measured in 5 prostate cancer patients reached maximum concentration 2 to 6 hours after dosing and were approximately 6% of the peak parent drug concentration. One week after dosing, mean plasma M-I concentrations were approximately 20% of mean leuprolide concentrations.

Excretion Following administration of LUPRON DEPOT 3.75 mg to 3 patients, less than 5% of the dose was recovered as parent and M-I metabolite in the urine.

Special Populations The pharmacokinetics of the drug in hepatically and renally impaired patients have not been determined.

CLINICAL STUDIES

Endometriosis: In controlled clinical studies, LUPRON DEPOT 3.75 mg monthly for six months was shown to be comparable to danazol 800 mg/day in relieving the clinical sign/symptoms of endometriosis (pelvic pain, dysmenorrhea, dyspareunia, pelvic tenderness, and induration) and in reducing the size of endometrial implants as evidenced by laparoscopy. The clinical significance of a decrease in endometriotic lesions is not known at this time, and in addition laparoscopic staging of endometriosis does not necessarily correlate with the severity of symptoms.
LUPRON DEPOT 3.75 mg monthly induced amenorrhea in 74% and 98% of the patients after the first and second treatment months respectively. Most of the remaining patients reported episodes of only light bleeding or spotting. In the first, second and third post-treatment months, normal menstrual cycles resumed in 7%, 71% and 95% respectively, of those patients who did not become pregnant.
Figure 1 illustrates the percent of patients with symptoms at baseline, final treatment visit and sustained relief at 6 and 12 months following discontinuation of treatment for the various symptoms evaluated during the study. This included all patients at end of treatment and those who elected to participate in the follow-up periods. This might provide a slight bias in the results at follow-up as 75% of the original patients entered the follow-up study, and 36% were evaluated at 6 months and 26% at 12 months respectively.
[See figure 1 above]
Hormonal replacement therapy: Clinical studies suggest that the addition of hormonal replacement therapy (estrogen and/or progestin) to LUPRON is effective in reducing loss of bone mineral density which occurs with LUPRON, without compromising the efficacy of LUPRON in relieving symptoms of endometriosis. The optimal drug/dose is not established.

Uterine Leiomyomata (Fibroids): **In controlled clinical trials, administration of LUPRON DEPOT 3.75 mg for a period of three or six months was shown to decrease uterine and fibroid volume, thus allowing for relief of clinical symptoms (abdominal bloating, pelvic pain, and pressure). Excessive vaginal bleeding (menorrhagia and menometrorrhagia) decreased, resulting in improvement in hematologic parameters.**
In three clinical trials, enrollment was not based on hematologic status. Mean uterine volume decreased by 41% and myoma volume decreased by 37% at final visit as evidenced by ultrasound or MRI. These patients also experienced a decrease in symptoms including excessive vaginal bleeding and pelvic discomfort. Benefit occurred by three months of therapy, but additional gain was observed with an additional three months of LUPRON DEPOT 3.75 mg. Ninety-five percent of these patients became amenorrheic with 61%, 25%, and 4% experiencing amenorrhea during the first, second, and third treatment months respectively.
Post-treatment follow-up was carried out for a small percentage of LUPRON DEPOT 3.75 mg patients among the 77% who demonstrated a ≥ 25% decrease in uterine volume while on therapy. Menses usually returned within two months of cessation of therapy. Mean time to return to pretreatment uterine size was 8.3 months. Regrowth did not appear to be related to pretreatment uterine volume.
In another controlled clinical study, enrollment was based on hematocrit ≤ 30% and/or hemoglobin ≤ 10.2 g/dL. Administration of LUPRON DEPOT 3.75 mg, concomitantly with iron, produced an increase of ≥ 6% hematocrit and ≥ 2 g/dL hemoglobin in 77% of patients at three months of therapy. The mean change in hematocrit was 10.1% and the mean change in hemoglobin was 4.2 g/dL. Clinical response was judged to be a hematocrit of ≥ 36% and hemoglobin of ≥ 12 g/dL, thus allowing for autologous blood donation prior to surgery. At three months, 75% of patients met this criterion.
At three months, 80% of patients experienced relief from either menorrhagia or menometrorrhagia. As with the previous studies, episodes of spotting and menstrual-like bleeding were noted in some patients.
In this same study, a decrease of ≥ 25% was seen in uterine and myoma volumes in 60% and 54% of patients respectively. LUPRON DEPOT 3.75 mg was found to relieve symptoms of bloating, pelvic pain, and pressure.
There is no evidence that pregnancy rates are enhanced or adversely affected by the use of LUPRON DEPOT 3.75 mg.

INDICATIONS AND USAGE

Endometriosis:
LUPRON DEPOT 3.75 mg is indicated for management of endometriosis, including pain relief and reduction of endometriotic lesions. Experience with LUPRON DEPOT 3.75 mg in females has been limited to women 18 years of age and older treated for 6 months.

Uterine Leiomyomata (Fibroids):
LUPRON DEPOT 3.75 mg concomitantly with iron therapy is indicated for the preoperative hematologic improvement of patients with anemia caused by uterine leiomyomata. The clinician may wish to consider a one-month trial period on iron alone inasmuch as some of the patients will respond to iron alone. (See clinical trial results below.) LUPRON may be added if the response to iron

alone is considered inadequate. Recommended duration of therapy with LUPRON DEPOT 3.75 mg is *up to* three months.
Experience with LUPRON DEPOT in females has been limited to women 18 years of age and older.

PERCENT OF PATIENTS ACHIEVING HEMOGLOBIN ≥ 12 GM/DL

Treatment Group	Week 4	Week 8	Week 12
LUPRON DEPOT 3.75 mg with Iron	41*	71**	79*
Iron Alone	17	40	56

* P-Value < 0.01
**P-Value < 0.001

CONTRAINDICATIONS

1. Hypersensitivity to GnRH, GnRH agonist analogs or any of the excipients in LUPRON DEPOT.
2. Undiagnosed abnormal vaginal bleeding.
3. LUPRON DEPOT is contraindicated in women who are or may become pregnant while receiving the drug. LUPRON DEPOT may cause fetal harm when administered to a pregnant woman. Major fetal abnormalities were observed in rabbits but not in rats after administration of LUPRON DEPOT throughout gestation. There was increased fetal mortality and decreased fetal weights in rats and rabbits. (See **Pregnancy** section.) The effects on fetal mortality are expected consequences of the alterations in hormonal levels brought about by the drug. If this drug is used during pregnancy, or if the patient becomes pregnant while taking this drug, the patient should be apprised of the potential hazard to the fetus.
4. Use in women who are breast-feeding. (See **Nursing Mothers** section.)
5. A report of an anaphylactic reaction to synthetic GnRH (Factrel) has been reported in the medical literature.[1]

WARNINGS

Safe use of leuprolide acetate in pregnancy has not been established clinically. Before starting treatment with LUPRON DEPOT, pregnancy must be excluded.

When used monthly at the recommended dose, LUPRON DEPOT usually inhibits ovulation and stops menstruation. Contraception is not insured, however, by taking LUPRON DEPOT. Therefore, patients should use non-hormonal methods of contraception. Patients should be advised to see their physician if they believe they may be pregnant. If a patient becomes pregnant during treatment, the drug must be discontinued and the patient must be apprised of the potential risk to the fetus.

During the early phase of therapy, sex steroids temporarily rise above baseline because of the physiologic effect of the drug. Therefore, an increase in clinical signs and symptoms may be observed during the initial days of therapy, but these will dissipate with continued therapy.

PRECAUTIONS

Information for Patients An information pamphlet for patients is included with the product. Patients should be aware of the following information:

1. Since menstruation should stop with effective doses of LUPRON DEPOT, the patient should notify her physician if regular menstruation persists. Patients missing successive doses of LUPRON DEPOT may experience breakthrough bleeding.
2. Patients should not use LUPRON DEPOT if they are pregnant, breast feeding, have undiagnosed abnormal vaginal bleeding, or are allergic to any of the ingredients in LUPRON DEPOT.
3. Safe use of the drug in pregnancy has not been established clinically. Therefore, a non-hormonal method of contraception should be used during treatment. Patients should be advised that if they miss successive doses of LUPRON DEPOT, breakthrough bleeding or ovulation may occur with the potential for conception. If a patient becomes pregnant during treatment, she should discontinue treatment and consult her physician.
4. Adverse events occurring in clinical studies with LUPRON DEPOT that are associated with hypoestrogenism include: hot flashes, headaches, emotional lability, decreased libido, acne, myalgia, reduction in breast size, and vaginal dryness. Estrogen levels returned to normal after treatment was discontinued.
5. The induced hypoestrogenic state **also** results in a small loss in bone density over the course of treatment, some of which may not be reversible. For a period up to six months, this bone loss should not be important. In patients with major risk factors for decreased bone mineral content such as chronic alcohol and/or tobacco use, strong family history of osteoporosis, or chronic use of drugs that can reduce bone mass such as anticonvulsants or corticosteroids, LUPRON DEPOT therapy may pose an additional risk. In these patients, the risks and benefits must be weighed carefully before therapy with LUPRON DEPOT is instituted. Repeated courses of therapy with gonadotropin-releasing hormone analogs beyond six months are not advisable in patients with major risk factors for loss of bone mineral content. Clinical studies suggest that the addition of hormonal replacement therapy (estrogen and/or progestin) to LUPRON is effective in reducing loss of bone mineral density which occurs with LUPRON, without compromising the efficacy of LUPRON in relieving symptoms of endometriosis. The optimal drug/dose is not established.
6. Retreatment cannot be recommended since safety data beyond six months are not available.

FIGURE 2–ADVERSE EVENTS REPORTED DURING 6 MONTHS OF TREATMENT WITH LUPRON DEPOT 3.75 MG

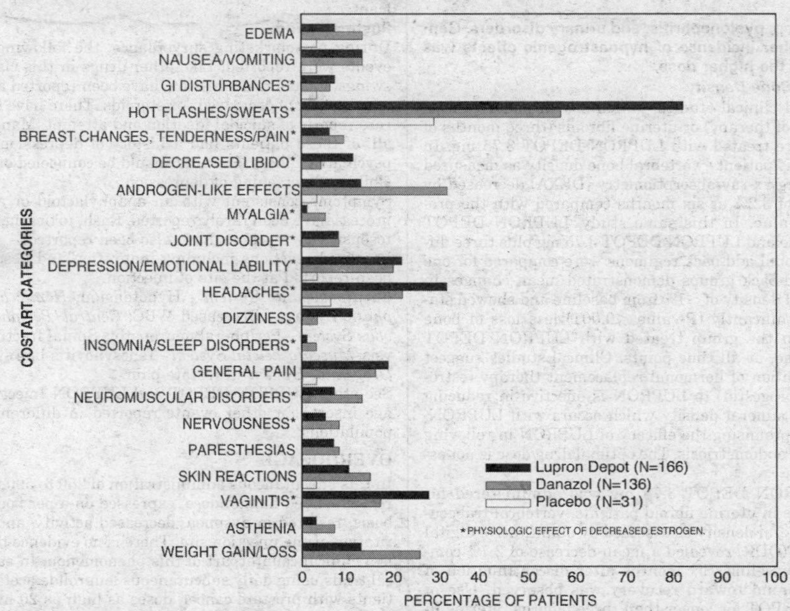

Laboratory Tests See **ADVERSE REACTIONS** section.

Drug Interactions No pharmacokinetic-based drug-drug interaction studies have been conducted with LUPRON DEPOT. However, because leuprolide acetate is a peptide that is primarily degraded by peptidase and not by cytochrome P-450 enzymes as noted in specific studies, and the drug is only about 46% bound to plasma proteins, drug interactions would not be expected to occur.

Drug/Laboratory Test Interactions Administration of LUPRON DEPOT in therapeutic doses results in suppression of the pituitary-gonadal system. Normal function is usually restored within three months after treatment is discontinued. Therefore, diagnostic tests of pituitary gonadotropic and gonadal functions conducted during treatment and for up to three months after discontinuation of LUPRON DEPOT may be misleading.

Carcinogenesis, Mutagenesis, Impairment of Fertility A two-year carcinogenicity study was conducted in rats and mice. In rats, a dose-related increase of benign pituitary hyperplasia and benign pituitary adenomas was noted at 24 months when the drug was administered subcutaneously at high daily doses (0.6 to 4 mg/kg). There was a significant but not dose-related increase of pancreatic islet-cell adenomas in females and of testicular interstitial cell adenomas in males (highest incidence in the low dose group). In mice, no leuprolide acetate-induced tumors or pituitary abnormalities were observed at a dose as high as 60 mg/kg for two years. Patients have been treated with leuprolide acetate for up to three years with doses as high as 10 mg/day and for two years with doses as high as 20 mg/day without demonstrable pituitary abnormalities.

Mutagenicity studies have been performed with leuprolide acetate using bacterial and mammalian systems. These studies provided no evidence of a mutagenic potential.

Clinical and pharmacologic studies in adults (>18 years) with leuprolide acetate and similar analogs have shown reversibility of fertility suppression when the drug is discontinued after continuous administration for periods of up to 24 weeks. Although no clinical studies have been completed in children to assess the full reversibility of fertility suppression, animal studies (prepubertal and adult rats and monkeys) with leuprolide acetate and other GnRH analogs have shown functional recovery.

Pregnancy, Teratogenic Effects Pregnancy Category X. (See **CONTRAINDICATIONS** section.) When administered on day 6 of pregnancy at test dosages of 0.00024, 0.0024, and 0.024 mg/kg (1/300 to 1/3 of the human dose) to rabbits, LUPRON DEPOT produced a dose-related increase in major fetal abnormalities. Similar studies in rats failed to demonstrate an increase in fetal malformations. There was increased fetal mortality and decreased fetal weights with the two higher doses of LUPRON DEPOT in rabbits and with the highest dose (0.024 mg/kg) in rats.

Nursing Mothers It is not known whether LUPRON DEPOT is excreted in human milk. Because many drugs are excreted in human milk, and because the effects of LUPRON DEPOT on lactation and/or the breast-fed child have not been determined, LUPRON DEPOT should not be used by nursing mothers.

Pediatric Use See LUPRON DEPOT-PED® (leuprolide acetate for depot suspension) labeling for the safety and effectiveness in children with central precocious puberty.

ADVERSE REACTIONS

Clinical Trials

Estradiol levels may increase during the first weeks following the initial injection, but then decline to menopausal levels. This transient increase in estradiol can be associated with a temporary worsening of signs and symptoms. (See **WARNINGS** section.)

As would be expected with a drug that lowers serum estradiol levels, the most frequently reported adverse reactions were those related to hypoestrogenism.

Endometriosis: In controlled studies comparing LUPRON DEPOT 3.75 mg monthly and danazol (800 mg/day) or placebo, adverse reactions most frequently reported and thought to be possibly or probably drug-related are shown in Figure 2.

[See figure 2 above]

Cardiovascular System - Palpitations, Syncope, Tachycardia; *Gastrointestinal System* - Appetite changes, Dry mouth, Thirst; *Central/Peripheral Nervous System* - Anxiety,* Delusions, Memory Disorder, Personality disorder; *Integumentary System* - Alopecia, Ecchymosis, Hair disorder; *Urogenital System* - Dysuria,* Lactation; *Miscellaneous* - Lymphadenopathy, Ophthalmologic disorders.*

Uterine Leiomyomata (Fibroids): **In controlled clinical trials comparing LUPRON DEPOT 3.75 mg and placebo, adverse events reported in >5% of patients and thought to be potentially related to drug are noted in the following table.**

	Lupron Depot 3.75 mg N=166 (%)	Placebo N=163 (%)
Body as a Whole		
Asthenia	14 (8.4)	8 (4.9)
General pain	14 (8.4)	10 (6.1)
Headache*	43 (25.9)	29 (17.8)
Cardiovascular System		
Hot flashes/sweats*	121 (72.9)	29 (17.8)
Metabolic and Nutritional Disorders		
Edema	9 (5.4)	2 (1.2)
Musculoskeletal System		
Joint disorder*	13 (7.8)	5 (3.1)
Nervous System		
Depression/emotional lability*	18 (10.8)	7 (4.3)
Urogenital System		
Vaginitis*	19 (11.4)	3 (1.8)

Symptoms reported in < 5% of patients included: *Body as Whole* - Body odor, Flu syndrome, Injection site reactions; *Cardiovascular System* - Tachycardia; *Digestive System* - Appetite changes, Dry mouth, GI disturbances, Nausea/vomiting; *Metabolic and Nutritional Disorders* - Weight changes; *Musculoskeletal System* - Myalgia; *Nervous System* - Anxiety, Decreased libido,* Dizziness, Insomnia, Nervousness,* Neuromuscular disorders,* Paresthesias; *Respiratory System* - Rhinitis; *Integumentary System* - Androgen-like effects, Nail disorder, Skin reactions; *Special Senses* - Conjunctivitis, Taste perversion; *Urogenital System* - Breast changes,* Menstrual disorders.

*** = Physiologic effect of the drug.**

In one controlled clinical trial, patients received a higher dose (7.5 mg) of LUPRON DEPOT. Events seen with this dose that were thought to be potentially related to drug and were not seen at the lower dose included palpitations, syncope, glossitis, ecchymosis, hypesthesia, confu-

Continued on next page

Lupron Depot 3.75 mg—Cont.

sion, lactation, pyelonephritis, and urinary disorders. Generally, a higher incidence of hypoestrogenic effects was observed at the higher dose.

Changes in Bone Density

In controlled clinical studies, patients with endometriosis (six months of therapy) or uterine fibroids (three months of therapy) were treated with LUPRON DEPOT 3.75 mg. In endometriosis patients, vertebral bone density as measured by dual energy x-ray absorptiometry (DEXA) decreased by an average of 3.2% at six months compared with the pretreatment value. In this same study, LUPRON DEPOT 3.75 mg alone and LUPRON DEPOT 3.75 mg plus three different hormonal add-back regimens were compared for one year. All add-back groups demonstrated mean changes in bone mineral density of ≤1% from baseline and showed statistically significantly (P-value <0.001) less loss of bone density than the group treated with LUPRON DEPOT 3.75 mg alone, at all time points. Clinical studies suggest that the addition of hormonal replacement therapy (estrogen and/or progestin) to LUPRON is effective in reducing loss of bone mineral density which occurs with LUPRON, without compromising the efficacy of LUPRON in relieving symptoms of endometriosis. The optimal drug/dose is not established.

When LUPRON DEPOT 3.75 mg was administered for three months in uterine fibroid patients, vertebral trabecular bone mineral density as assessed by quantitative digital radiography (QDR) revealed a mean decrease of 2.7% compared with baseline. Six months after discontinuation of therapy, a trend toward recovery was observed. Use of LUPRON DEPOT for longer than three months (uterine fibroids) or six months (endometriosis) or in the presence of other known risk factors for decreased bone mineral content may cause additional bone loss **and is not recommended.**

Changes in Laboratory Values During Treatment

Plasma Enzymes

Endometriosis: During clinical trials with LUPRON DEPOT 3.75 mg, regular laboratory monitoring revealed that AST levels were more than twice the upper limit of normal in only one patient. There was no clinical or other laboratory evidence of abnormal liver function.

Uterine Leiomyomata (Fibroids): **In clinical trials with LUPRON DEPOT 3.75 mg, five (3%) patients had a post-treatment transaminase value that was at least twice the baseline value and above the upper limit of the normal range. None of the laboratory increases were associated with clinical symptoms.**

Lipids

Endometriosis: At enrollment, 4% of the LUPRON DEPOT 3.75 mg patients and 1% of the danazol patients had total cholesterol values above the normal range. These patients also had cholesterol values above the normal range at the end of treatment.

Of those patients whose pretreatment cholesterol values were in the normal range, 7% of the LUPRON DEPOT 3.75 mg patients and 9% of the danazol patients had post-treatment values above the normal range.

The mean (±SEM) pretreatment values for total cholesterol from all patients were 178.8 (2.9) mg/dL in the LUPRON DEPOT 3.75 mg groups and 175.3 (3.0) mg/dL in the danazol group. At the end of treatment, the mean values for total cholesterol from all patients were 193.3 mg/dL in the LUPRON DEPOT 3.75 mg group and 194.4 mg/dL in the danazol group. These increases from the pretreatment values were statistically significant (p<0.03) in both groups.

Triglycerides were increased above the upper limit of normal in 12% of the patients who received LUPRON DEPOT 3.75 mg and in 6% of the patients who received danazol.

At the end of treatment, HDL cholesterol fractions decreased below the lower limit of the normal range in 2% of the LUPRON DEPOT 3.75 mg patients compared with 54% of those receiving danazol. LDL cholesterol fractions increased above the upper limit of the normal range in 6% of the patients receiving LUPRON DEPOT 3.75 mg compared with 23% of those receiving danazol. There was no increase in the LDL/HDL ratio in patients receiving LUPRON DEPOT 3.75 mg but there was approximately a two-fold increase in the LDL/HDL ratio in patients receiving danazol.

Uterine Leiomyomata (Fibroids): **In patients receiving LUPRON DEPOT 3.75 mg, mean changes in cholesterol (+11 mg/dL to +29 mg/dL), LDL cholesterol (+8 mg/dL to +22 mg/dL), HDL cholesterol (0 to +6 mg/dL), and the LDL/HDL ratio (-0.1 to +0.5) were observed across studies. In the one study in which triglycerides were determined, the mean increase from baseline was 32 mg/dL.**

Other Changes

Endometriosis: In comparative studies, the following changes were seen in approximately 5% to 8% of patients. LUPRON DEPOT 3.75 mg was associated with elevations of LDH and phosphorus, and decreases in WBC counts. Danazol therapy was associated with increases in hematocrit, platelet count, and LDH.

Uterine Leiomyomata (Fibroids):

Hematology: (See CLINICAL STUDIES section.) In LUPRON DEPOT 3.75 mg treated patients, although there were statistically significant mean decreases in platelet counts from baseline to final visit, the last mean platelet counts were within the normal range. Decreases in total WBC count and neutrophils were observed, but were not clinically significant.

Chemistry: Slight to moderate mean increases were noted for glucose, uric acid, BUN, creatinine, total protein, albumin, bilirubin, alkaline phosphatase, LDH, calcium, and phosphorus. None of these increases were clinically significant.

Postmarketing

During postmarketing surveillance, the following adverse events were reported. Like other drugs in this class, mood swings, including depression, have been reported as a physiologic effect of decreased sex steroids. There have been very rare reports of suicidal ideation and attempt. Many, but not all, of these patients had a history of depression or other psychiatric illness. Patients should be counseled on the possibility of worsening of depression.

Symptoms consistent with an anaphylactoid or asthmatic process have been rarely reported. Rash, urticaria, and photosensitivity reactions have also been reported.

Localized reactions including induration and abscess have been reported at the site of injection.

Cardiovascular System - Hypotension; *Hemic and Lymphatic System* - Decreased WBC; *Central/Peripheral Nervous System* - Peripheral neuropathy, Spinal fracture/paralysis; *Musculoskeletal System* - Tenosynovitis-like symptoms; *Urogenital System* - Prostate pain.

See other LUPRON DEPOT and LUPRON Injection package inserts for other events reported in different patient populations.

OVERDOSAGE

In rats subcutaneous administration of 250 to 500 times the recommended human dose, expressed on a per body weight basis, resulted in dyspnea, decreased activity, and local irritation at the injection site. There is no evidence that there is a clinical counterpart of this phenomenon. In early clinical trials using daily subcutaneous leuprolide acetate in patients with prostate cancer, doses as high as 20 mg/day for up to two years caused no adverse effects differing from those observed with the 1 mg/day dose.

DOSAGE AND ADMINISTRATION

LUPRON DEPOT Must Be Administered Under The Supervision Of A Physician.

The recommended dose of LUPRON DEPOT is 3.75 mg, incorporated in a depot formulation. The lyophilized microspheres are to be reconstituted and administered monthly as a single intramuscular injection, in accord with the following directions:

1. To prepare for injection, screw the white plunger into the end stopper until the stopper begins to turn.
2. Remove and discard the tab around the base of the needle.
3. Holding the syringe upright, release the diluent by SLOWLY PUSHING the plunger until the first stopper is at the blue line in the middle of the barrel.
4. Gently shake the syringe to thoroughly mix the particles to form a uniform suspension. The suspension will appear milky.
5. If the microspheres (particles) adhere to the stopper, tap the syringe against your finger.
6. Then remove the needle guard and advance the plunger to expel the air from the syringe.
7. At the time of reconstitution, inject the entire contents of the syringe intramuscularly as you would for a normal injection. The suspension settles very quickly following reconstitution; therefore it is preferable that LUPRON DEPOT 3.75 mg be mixed and used immediately. Reshake suspension if settling occurs.

Since the product does not contain a preservative, the suspension should be discarded if not used immediately.

Endometriosis: The recommended duration of administration is six months. Retreatment cannot be recommended since safety data for retreatment are not available. If the symptoms of endometriosis recur after a course of therapy, and further treatment with LUPRON DEPOT 3.75 mg is contemplated, it is recommended that bone density be assessed before retreatment begins to ensure that values are within normal limits.

Uterine Leiomyomata (Fibroids): **Recommended duration of therapy with LUPRON DEPOT 3.75 mg is *up to* 3 months. The symptoms associated with uterine leiomyomata will recur following discontinuation of therapy. If additional treatment with LUPRON DEPOT 3.75 mg is contemplated, bone density should be assessed prior to initiation of therapy to ensure that values are within normal limits.**

As with other drugs administered by injection, the injection site should be varied periodically.

HOW SUPPLIED

LUPRON DEPOT 3.75 mg is packaged as follows:

Kit with prefilled dual-chamber syringe NDC 0300-3641-01

Each syringe contains sterile lyophilized microspheres which is leuprolide incorporated in a biodegradable copolymer of lactic and glycolic acids. When mixed with diluent, LUPRON DEPOT 3.75 mg is administered as a single monthly IM injection.

Store at 25°C (77°F); excursions permitted to 15–30°C (59–86°F) [See USP Controlled Room Temperature]

Rx only

REFERENCE

1. MacLeod TL, *et al.* Anaphylactic reaction to synthetic luteinizing hormone-releasing hormone. *Fertil Steril* 1987 Sept;48(3):500-502.

U.S. Patent Nos. 4,652,441; 4,677,191; 4,728,721; 4,849,228; 4,917,893; 4,954,298; 5,330,767; 5,476,663; 5,575,987; 5,631,020; 5,631,021; and 5,716,640.

Manufactured for
TAP Pharmaceuticals Inc.
Lake Forest, IL 60045, U.S.A.
by Takeda Chemical Industries, Ltd. Osaka, JAPAN 541

®-Registered Trademark

(No. 3641)
03-5043-R12; Revised: April 2000

Shown in Product Identification Guide, page 338

LUPRON DEPOT® 7.5 mg ℞
(leuprolide acetate for depot suspension)

DESCRIPTION

Leuprolide acetate is a synthetic nonapeptide analog of naturally occurring gonadotropin-releasing hormone (GnRH or LH-RH). The analog possesses greater potency than the natural hormone. The chemical name is 5-oxo-L-prolyl-L-histidyl-L-tryptophyl-L-seryl-L-tyrosyl-D-leucyl-L-leucyl-L-arginyl-N-ethyl-L-prolinamide acetate (salt) with the following structural formula:

[See chemical structure at bottom of next page]

LUPRON DEPOT is available in a prefilled dual-chamber syringe containing sterile lyophilized microspheres which, when mixed with diluent, become a suspension intended as a monthly intramuscular injection.

The front chamber of LUPRON DEPOT 7.5 mg prefilled dual-chamber syringe contains leuprolide acetate (7.5 mg), purified gelatin (1.3 mg), DL-lactic and glycolic acids copolymer (66.2 mg), and D-mannitol (13.2 mg). The second chamber of diluent contains carboxymethylcellulose sodium (5 mg), D-mannitol (50 mg), polysorbate 80 (1 mg), water for injection, USP, and glacial acetic acid, USP to control pH.

During the manufacture of LUPRON DEPOT 7.5 mg, acetic acid is lost, leaving the peptide.

CLINICAL PHARMACOLOGY

Leuprolide acetate, an LH-RH agonist, acts as a potent inhibitor of gonadotropin secretion when given continuously and in therapeutic doses. Animal and human studies indicate that following an initial stimulation, chronic administration of leuprolide acetate results in suppression of ovarian and testicular steroidogenesis. This effect is reversible upon discontinuation of drug therapy. Administration of leuprolide acetate has resulted in inhibition of the growth of certain hormone dependent tumors (prostatic tumors in Noble and Dunning male rats and DMBA-induced mammary tumors in female rats) as well as atrophy of the reproductive organs.

In humans, administration of leuprolide acetate results in an initial increase in circulating levels of luteinizing hormone (LH) and follicle stimulating hormone (FSH), leading to a transient increase in levels of the gonadal steroids (testosterone and dihydrotestosterone in males, and estrone and estradiol in premenopausal females). However, continuous administration of leuprolide acetate results in decreased levels of LH and FSH. In males, testosterone is reduced to castrate levels. In premenopausal females, estrogens are reduced to postmenopausal levels. These decreases occur within two to four weeks after initiation of treatment. Castrate levels of testosterone in prostatic cancer patients have been demonstrated for up to 10 years.

Leuprolide acetate is not active when given orally.

Pharmacokinetics

Absorption Following a single injection of LUPRON DEPOT 7.5 mg to patients, mean plasma leuprolide concentration was almost 20 ng/mL at 4 hours and 0.36 ng/mL at 4 weeks. However, intact leuprolide and an inactive major metabolite could not be distinguished by the assay which was employed in the study. Nondetectable leuprolide plasma concentrations have been observed during chronic LUPRON DEPOT 7.5 mg administration, but testosterone levels appear to be maintained at castrate levels.

Distribution The mean steady-state volume of distribution of leuprolide following intravenous bolus administration to healthy male volunteers was 27 L. *In vitro* binding to human plasma proteins ranged from 43% to 49%.

Metabolism In healthy male volunteers, a 1 mg bolus of leuprolide administered intravenously revealed that the mean systemic clearance was 7.6 L/h, with a terminal elimination half-life of approximately 3 hours based on a two compartment model.

In rats and dogs, administration of ^{14}C-labeled leuprolide was shown to be metabolized to smaller inactive peptides, a pentapeptide (Metabolite I), tripeptides (Metabolites II and III) and a dipeptide (Metabolite IV). These fragments may be further catabolized.

The major metabolite (M-I) plasma concentrations measured in 5 prostate cancer patients reached maximum concentration 2 to 6 hours after dosing and were approximately 6% of the peak parent drug concentration. One week after dosing, mean plasma M-I concentrations were approximately 20% of mean leuprolide concentrations.

Excretion Following administration of LUPRON DEPOT 3.75 mg to 3 patients, less than 5% of the dose was recovered as parent and M-I metabolite in the urine.

Special Populations The pharmacokinetics of the drug in hepatically and renally impaired patients have not been determined.

Drug Interactions No pharmacokinetic-based drug-drug interaction studies have been conducted with LUPRON DEPOT. However, because leuprolide acetate is a peptide that is primarily degraded by peptidase and the drug is only about 46% bound to plasma proteins, drug interactions would not be expected to occur.

CLINICAL STUDIES

In an open-label, non-comparative, multicenter clinical study of LUPRON DEPOT 7.5 mg, 56 patients with stage D_2 prostatic adenocarcinoma and no prior systemic treatment were enrolled. The objectives were to determine if a 7.5 mg depot formulation of leuprolide injected once every 4 weeks would reduce and maintain serum testosterone to castrate range (≤50 ng/dL), to evaluate objective clinical response, and to assess the safety of the formulation. During the initial 24 weeks, serum testosterone was measured weekly, biweekly, or every four weeks and objective tumor response assessments were performed at Weeks 12 and 24. Once the patient completed the initial 24-week treatment phase, treatment continued at the investigator's discretion. Data from the initial 24-week treatment phase are summarized in this section.

In the majority of patients, serum testosterone increased by 50% or more above baseline during the first week of treatment. Serum testosterone suppressed to the castrate range within 30 days of the initial depot injection in 94% (51/54) of patients for whom testosterone suppression was achieved (2 patients withdrew prior to onset of suppression) and within 66 days in all 54 patients. Mean serum testosterone suppressed to castrate level by Week 3. The median dosing interval between injections was 28 days. One escape from suppression (2 consecutive testosterone values >50 ng/dL after achieving castrate level) was noted at Week 18, associated with a substantial dosing delay. In this patient, serum testosterone returned to the castrate range at the next monthly measurement. Serum testosterone was minimally above the castrate range on a single occasion for 4 other patients. No clinical significance was attributed to these rises in testosterone.

Secondary efficacy endpoints evaluated included objective tumor response, assessed by clinical evaluations of tumor burden (complete response, partial response, objectively stable, and progression), as well as changes in local disease status, assessed by digital rectal examination, and changes in prostatic acid phosphatase (PAP). These evaluations were performed at Weeks 12 and 24. The objective tumor response analysis showed a "no progression" (ie. complete or partial response, or stable disease) in 77% (40/52) of patients at Week 12, and in 84% (42/50) of patients at Week 24. Local disease improved or remained stable in all (42) patients evaluated at Week 12 and in 98% (41/42) of patients elevated at Week 24. PAP normalized or decreased at Week 12 and/or 24 in the majority of patients with elevated baseline PAP.

Periodic monitoring of serum testosterone and PSA levels is recommended, especially if the anticipated clinical or biochemical response to treatment has not been achieved. It should be noted that results of testosterone determinations are dependent on assay methodology. It is advisable to be aware of the type and precision of the assay methodology to make appropriate clinical and therapeutic decisions.

INDICATIONS AND USAGE

LUPRON DEPOT 7.5 mg is indicated in the palliative treatment of advanced prostatic cancer.

CONTRAINDICATIONS

1. Hypersensitivity to GnRH, GNRH agonist analogs or any of the excipients in LUPRON DEPOT.
   Reports of an anaphylactic reaction to synthetic GnRH (Factrel) or GnRH agonist analogs have been reported in the medical literature.[1]
2. All formulations of LUPRON DEPOT are contraindicated in women who are or may become pregnant while receiving the drug. LUPRON DEPOT may cause fetal harm when administered to a pregnant woman. Major fetal abnormalities were observed in rabbits but not in rats after administration of LUPRON DEPOT throughout gestation. There was increased fetal mortality and decreased fetal weights in rats and rabbits. The effects on fetal mortality are expected consequences of the alterations in hormonal levels brought about by this drug. Therefore, the possibility exists that spontaneous abortion may occur. If this drug is administered during pregnancy or if the patient becomes pregnant while taking any formulation of LUPRON DEPOT, the patient should be apprised of the potential Hazard to the fetus.

WARNINGS

Initially, LUPRON DEPOT, like other LH-RH agonists, causes increases in serum levels of testosterone to approximately 50% above baseline during the first week of treatment. Transient worsening of symptoms, or the occurrence of additional signs and symptoms of prostate cancer, may occasionally develop during the first few weeks of LUPRON DEPOT treatment. A small number of patients may experience a temporary increase in bone pain, which can be managed symptomatically. As with other LH-RH agonists, isolated cases of ureteral obstruction and spinal cord compression have been observed, which may contribute to paralysis with or without fatal complications.

For patients at risk, initiation of therapy with daily LUPRON® (leuprolide acetate) Injection (See **DOSAGE AND ADMINISTRATION** section of the LUPRON Injection labeling.) for the first two weeks to facilitate withdrawal of treatment may be considered. If spinal cord compression or renal impairment develops, standard treatment of these complications should be instituted.

PRECAUTIONS

Information for Patients An information pamphlet for patients is included with the product.

General Patients with metastatic vertebral lesions and/or with urinary tract obstruction should be closely observed during the first few weeks of therapy. (See **WARNINGS** section.)

Laboratory Tests Response to LUPRON DEPOT 7.5 mg should be monitored by measuring serum levels of testosterone as well as prostate-specific antigen. In the majority of patients, testosterone levels increased above baseline during the first week, declining thereafter to baseline levels or below by the end of the second week. Castrate levels were reached within two to four weeks and once achieved were maintained for the duration of treatment in all 54 patients. Minimal and transient increases to above the castrate level occurred in eight patients. (See **CLINICAL STUDIES** section.)

Drug Interactions (See **Pharmacokinetics**.)

Drug/Laboratory Test Interactions Administration of LUPRON DEPOT in therapeutic doses results in suppression of the pituitary-gonadal system. Normal function is usually restored within three months after treatment is discontinued. Due to the supression of the pituitary-gonadal system by LUPRON DEPOT, diagnostic tests of pituitary gonadotropic and gonadal functions conducted during treatment and for up to three months after discontinuation of LUPRON DEPOT may be affected.

Carcinogenesis, Mutagenesis, Impairment of Fertility Two-year carcinogenicity studies were conducted in rats and mice. In rats, a dose-related increase of benign pituitary hyperplasia and benign pituitary adenomas was noted at 24 months when the drug was administered subcutaneously at high daily doses (0.6 to 4 mg/kg). There was a significant but not dose-related increase of pancreatic islet-cell adenomas in females and of testicular interstitial cell adenomas in males (highest incidence in the low dose group). In mice, no leuprolide acetate-induced tumors or pituitary abnormalities were observed at a dose as high as 60 mg/kg for two years. Patients have been treated with leuprolide acetate for up to three years with doses as high as 10 mg/day and for two years with doses as high as 20 mg/day without demonstrable pituitary abnormalities.

Mutagenicity studies have been performed with leuprolide acetate using bacterial and mammalian systems. These studies provided no evidence of a mutagenic potential.

Clinical and pharmacologic studies in adults (≥ 18 years) with leuprolide acetate and similar analogs have shown reversibility of fertility suppression when the drug is discontinued after continuous administration for periods of up to 24 weeks.

Pregnancy Category X. (See **CONTRAINDICATIONS** section.)

Pediatric Use See LUPRON DEPOT-PED® (leuprolide acetate for depot suspension) labeling for the safety and effectiveness of the monthly formulation in children with central precocious puberty.

ADVERSE REACTIONS

Clinical Trials

In the majority of patients testosterone levels increased above baseline during the first week, declining thereafter to baseline levels or below by the end of the second week of treatment.

Potential exacerbations of signs and symptoms during the first few weeks of treatment is a concern in patients with vertebral metastases and/or urinary obstruction or hematuria which, if aggravated, may lead to neurological problems such as temporary weakness and/or paresthesia of the lower limbs or worsening of urinary symptoms. (See **WARNINGS** section.)

In a clinical trial of LUPRON DEPOT 7.5 mg, the following adverse reactions were reported in 5% or more of the patients during the initial 24-week treatment period regardless of causality.

LUPRON DEPOT 7.5 mg (N=56)

	N	(%)
Body as a Whole		
General pain	13	(23.2)
Infection	3	(5.4)
Cardiovascular System		
Hot flashes/sweats*	32	(57.1)
Digestive System		
GI disorders	8	(14.3)
Metabolic and Nutritional Disorders		
Edema	8	(14.3)
Nervous System		
Libido decreased*	3	(5.4)
Respiratory System		
Respiratory disorder	6	(10.7)
Urogenital System		
Urinary disorder	7	(12.5)
Impotence*	3	(5.4)
Testicular atrophy*	3	(5.4)

*Due to the expected physiologic effect of decreased testosterone levels.

In this same study, the following adverse reactions were reported in less than 5% of the patients on LUPRON DEPOT 7.5 mg.

Body as a Whole—Asthenia, Cellulitis, Fever, Headache, Injection site reaction, Neoplasm; *Cardiovascular System*—Angina, Congestive heart failure; *Digestive System*—Anorexia, Dysphagia, Eructation, Peptic ulcer; *Hemic and Lymphatic System*—Ecchymosis; *Musculoskeletal System*—Myalgia; *Nervous System*—Agitation, Insomnia/sleep disorders, Neuromuscular disorders; *Respiratory System*—Emphysema, Hemoptysis, Lung edema, Sputum increased; *Skin and Appendages*—Hair disorder, Skin reaction; *Urogenital System*—Balanitis, Breast enlargement, Urinary tract infection.

Laboratory: Abnormalities of certain parameters were observed, but their relationship to drug treatment are difficult to assess in this population. The following were recorded in ≥5% of patients at final visit: Decreased albumin, decreased hemoglobin/hematocrit, decreased prostatic acid phosphatase, decreased total protein, decreased urine specific gravity, hyperglycemia, hyperuricemia, increased BUN, increased creatinine, increased liver function tests (AST, LDH), increased phosphorus, increased platelets, increased prostatic acid phosphatase, increased total cholesterol, increased urine specific gravity, leukopenia.

Postmarketing

During postmarketing surveillance which includes other dosage forms and other patient populations, the following adverse events were reported.

Symptoms consistent with an anaphylactoid or asthmatic process have been rarely (incidence rate of about 0.002%) reported. Rash, urticaria, and photosensitivity reactions have also been reported.

Localized reactions including induration and abscess have been reported at the site of injection.

Symptoms consistent with a fibromyalgia (eg, joint and muscle pain, headaches, sleep disorders, gastrointestinal distress, and shortness of breath) have been reported individually and collectively.

Cardiovascular System—Hypotension, Pulmonary embolism; *Hemic and Lymphatic System*—Decreased WBC; *Central/Peripheral Nervous System*—Peripheral neuropathy, Spinal fracture/paralysis; *Musculoskeletal System*—Tenosynovitis-like symptoms; *Urogenital System*—Prostate pain.

Changes in Bone Density: Decreased bone density has been reported in the medical literature in men who have had orchiectomy or who have been treated with an LH-RH agonist analog. In a clinical trial, 25 men with prostate cancer, 12 of whom had been treated previously with leuprolide acetate for at least six months, underwent bone density studies as a result of pain. The leuprolide-treated group had lower bone density scores than the nontreated control group. It can be anticipated that long periods of medical castration in men will have effects on bone density.

See other LUPRON DEPOT and LUPRON Injection package inserts for other events reported in women and pediatric populations.

OVERDOSAGE

In clinical trials using daily subcutaneous leuprolide acetate in patients with prostate cancer, doses as high as 20 mg/day for up to two years caused no adverse effects differing from those observed with the 1 mg/day dose.

DOSAGE AND ADMINISTRATION

LUPRON DEPOT Must Be Administered Under The Supervision Of A Physician.

The recommended dose of LUPRON DEPOT is 7.5 mg, incorporated in a depot formulation. The lyophilized microspheres are to be reconstituted and administered monthly as a single intramuscular injection, in accord with the following directions:

1. To prepare for injection, screw the white plunger into the end stopper until the stopper begins to turn.
2. Remove and discard the tab around the base of the needle.
3. Holding the syringe upright, release the diluent by SLOWLY PUSHING the plunger until the first stopper is at the blue line in the middle of the barrel.

Continued on next page

Lupron Depot 7.5 mg—Cont.

4. Gently shake the syringe to thoroughly mix the particles to form a uniform suspension. The suspension will appear milky.
5. If the microspheres (particles) adhere to the stopper, tap the syringe against your finger.
6. Then remove the needle guard and advance the plunger to expel the air from the syringe.
7. At the time of reconstitution, inject the entire contents of the syringe intramuscularly as you would for a normal injection. The suspension settles very quickly following reconstitution; therefore, it is preferable that LUPRON DEPOT 7.5 mg be mixed and used immediately. Reshake suspension if settling occurs.

Since the product does not contain a preservative, the suspension should be discarded if not used immediately.
As with other drugs administered by injection, the injection site should be varied periodically.

HOW SUPPLIED

LUPRON DEPOT 7.5 mg is packaged as follows:

Kit with prefilled dual-chamber syringe NDC 0300-3642-01

Each syringe contains sterile lyophilized microspheres which is leuprolide incorporated in a biodegradable copolymer of lactic and glycolic acids. When mixed with diluent, LUPRON DEPOT 7.5 mg is administered as a single monthly IM injection.
An information pamphlet for patients is included with the kit.

Store at 25°C (77°F); excursions permitted to 15–30°C (59–86°F). [See USP Controlled Room Temperature.]

Rx only

REFERENCE

1. MacLeod TL, *et al.* Anaphylactic reaction to synthetic luteinizing hormone-releasing hormone. *Fertil Steril* 1987 Sept; 48(3):500-502.
2. U.S. Patent Nos. 4,652,441; 4,677,191; 4,728,721; 4,849,228; 4,917,893; 4,954,298; 5,330,767; 5,476,663; 5,575,987; 5,631,020; 5,631,021; and 5,716,640.

Manufactured for
TAP Pharmaceuticals Inc.
Lake Forest, IL 60045, U.S.A.
by Takeda Chemical Industries, Ltd. Osaka, JAPAN 541

®-Registered Trademark

(No. 3642)
03-5046-R10; Revised: April 2000

Shown in Product Identification Guide, page 338

This is combined labeling. Examples of different fonts appear below.
- General information
- Information on endometriosis
- **Information on uterine fibroids**

LUPRON DEPOT®–3 Month 11.25 mg ℞
(leuprolide acetate for depot suspension)

3-MONTH FORMULATION

DESCRIPTION

Leuprolide acetate is a synthetic nonapeptide analog of naturally occurring gonadotropin-releasing hormone (GnRH or LH-RH). The analog possesses greater potency than the natural hormone. The chemical name is 5-oxo-L-prolyl-L-histidyl-L-tryptophyl-L-seryl-L-tyrosyl-D-leucyl-L-leucyl-L-arginyl-N-ethyl-L-prolinamide acetate (salt) with the following structural formula:

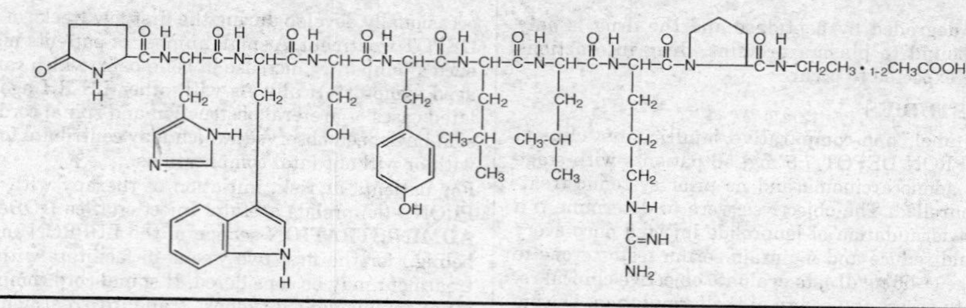

[See chemical structure above]

LUPRON DEPOT–3 Month 11.25 mg is available in a prefilled dual-chamber syringe containing sterile lyophilized microspheres which, when mixed with diluent become a suspension intended as an intramuscular injection to be given **ONCE EVERY THREE MONTHS.**

The front chamber of LUPRON DEPOT–3 Month 11.25 mg prefilled dual-chamber syringe contains leuprolide acetate (11.25 mg), polylactic acid (99.3 mg) and D-mannitol (19.45 mg). The second chamber of diluent contains carboxymethylcellulose sodium (7.5 mg), D-mannitol (75.0 mg), polysorbate 80 (1.5 mg), water for injection, USP, and glacial acetic acid, USP to control pH.

During the manufacture of LUPRON DEPOT–3 Month 11.25 mg, acetic acid is lost, leaving the peptide.

CLINICAL PHARMACOLOGY

Leuprolide acetate is a long-acting GnRH analog. A single injection of LUPRON DEPOT–3 Month 11.25 mg will result in an initial stimulation followed by a prolonged suppression of pituitary gonadotropins. Repeated dosing at quarterly (LUPRON DEPOT–3 Month 11.25 mg) intervals results in decreased secretion of gonadal steroids; consequently, tissues and functions that depend on gonadal steroids for their maintenance become quiescent. This effect is reversible on discontinuation of drug therapy.

Leuprolide acetate is not active when given orally.

Pharmacokinetics

Absorption Following a single injection of the three month formulation of LUPRON DEPOT–3 Month 11.25 mg in female subjects, a mean plasma leuprolide concentration of 36.3 ng/mL was observed at 4 hours. Leuprolide appeared to be released at a constant rate following the onset of steady-state levels during the third week after dosing and mean levels then declined gradually to near the lower limit of detection by 12 weeks. The mean (± standard deviation) leuprolide concentration from 3 to 12 weeks was 0.23 ± 0.09 ng/mL. However, intact leuprolide and an inactive major metabolite could not be distinguished by the assay which was employed in the study. The initial burst, followed by the rapid decline to a steady-state level, was similar to the release pattern seen with the monthly formulation.

Distribution The mean steady-state volume of distribution of leuprolide following intravenous bolus administration to healthy male volunteers was 27 L. *In vitro* binding to human plasma proteins ranged from 43% to 49%.

Metabolism In healthy male volunteers, a 1 mg bolus of leuprolide administered intravenously revealed that the mean systemic clearance was 7.6 L/h, with a terminal elimination half-life of approximately 3 hours based on a two compartment model.

In rats and dogs, administration of ^{14}C-labeled leuprolide was shown to be metabolized to smaller inactive peptides, a pentapeptide (Metabolite I), tripeptides (Metabolites II and III) and a dipeptide (Metabolite IV). These fragments may be further catabolized.

In a pharmacokinetic/pharmacodynamic study of endometriosis patients, intramuscular 11.25 mg LUPRON DEPOT (n=19) every 12 weeks or intramuscular 3.75 mg LUPRON DEPOT (n=15) every 4 weeks was administered for 24 weeks. There was no statistically significant difference between the 2 treatment groups in trough plasma concentrations of leuprolide or M-I collected from weeks 4 through 24. No accumulation of plasma leuprolide or M-I concentrations was observed with multiple dosing of either treatment group. There was also no statistically significant difference in changes of serum estradiol concentration from baseline between the 2 treatment groups.

M-I Plasma concentrations measured in 5 prostate cancer patients reached maximum concentration 2 to 6 hours after dosing and were approximately 6% of the peak parent drug concentration. One week after dosing, mean plasma M-I concentrations were approximately 20% of mean leuprolide concentrations.

Excretion Following administration of LUPRON DEPOT 3.75 mg to 3 patients, less than 5% of the dose was recovered as parent and M-I metabolite in the urine.

Special Populations The pharmacokinetics of the drug in hepatically and renally impaired patients have not been determined.

Drug Interactions No pharmacokinetic-based drug-drug interaction studies have been conducted with LUPRON DEPOT. However, because leuprolide acetate is a peptide that is primarily degraded by peptidase and not by cytochrome P-450 enzymes as noted in specific studies, and the drug is only about 46% bound to plasma proteins, drug interactions would not be expected to occur.

CLINICAL STUDIES

In a pharmacokinetic/pharmacodynamic study of healthy female subjects (N=20), the onset of estradiol suppression was observed for individual subjects between day 4 and week 4 after dosing. By the third week following the injection, the mean estradiol concentration (8 pg/mL) was in the menopausal range. Throughout the remainder of the dosing period, mean serum estradiol levels ranged from the menopausal to the early follicular range.

Serum estradiol was suppressed to ≤20 pg/mL in all subjects within four weeks and remained suppressed (≤40 pg/mL) in 80% of subjects until the end of the 12-week dosing interval, at which time two of these subjects had a value between 40 and 50 pg/mL. Four additional subjects had at least two consecutive elevations of estradiol (range 43–240 pg/mL) levels during the 12-week dosing interval, but there was no indication of luteal function for any of the subjects during this period.

LUPRON DEPOT–3 Month 11.25 mg induced amenorrhea in 85% (N=17) of subjects during the initial month and 100% during the second month following the injection. All subjects remained amenorrheic through the remainder of the 12-week dosing interval. Episodes of light bleeding and spotting were reported by a majority of subjects during the first month after the injection and in a few subjects at later time-points. Menses resumed on average 12 weeks (range 2.9 to 20.4 weeks) following the end of the 12-week dosing interval.

LUPRON DEPOT–3 Month 11.25 mg produced similar pharmacodynamic effects in terms of hormonal and menstrual suppression to those achieved with monthly injections of LUPRON DEPOT 3.75 mg during the controlled clinical trials for the management of endometriosis and the anemia caused by uterine fibroids.

Endometriosis: In a Phase IV pharmacokinetic/pharmacodynamic study of patients, LUPRON DEPOT-3 Month 11.25 mg (N=21) was shown to be comparable to monthly LUPRON DEPOT 3.75 mg (N=20) in relieving the clinical signs/symptoms of endometriosis (dysmenorrhea, non-menstrual pelvic pain, pelvic tenderness and pelvic induration). In both treatment groups, suppression of menses was achieved in 100% of the patients who remained in the study for at least 60 days. Suppression is defined as no new menses for at least 60 consecutive days.

In controlled clinical studies, LUPRON DEPOT 3.75 mg monthly for six months was shown to be comparable to danazol 800 mg/day in relieving the clinical sign/symptoms of endometriosis (pelvic pain, dysmenorrhea, dyspareunia, pelvic tenderness, and induration) and in reducing the size of endometrial implants as evidenced by laparoscopy.

The clinical significance of a decrease in endometriotic lesions is not known at this time, and in addition laparoscopic staging of endometriosis does not necessarily correlate with the severity of symptoms.

LUPRON DEPOT 3.75 mg monthly induced amenorrhea in 74% and 98% of the patients after the first and second treatment months respectively. Most of the remaining patients reported episodes of only light bleeding or spotting. In the first, second and third post-treatment months, normal menstrual cycles resumed in 7%, 71% and 95% respectively, of those patients who did not become pregnant.

Figure 1 illustrates the percent of patients with symptoms at baseline, final treatment visit and sustained relief at 6 and 12 months following discontinuation of treatment for the various symptoms evaluated during the two controlled clinical studies. A total of 166 patients received LUPRON DEPOT 3.75 mg. Seventy-five percent (N=125) of these elected to participate in the follow-up periods. Of these patients, 36% and 24% are included in the 6 month and 12 month follow-up analysis, respectively. All the patients who had a pain evaluation at baseline and at a minimum of one treatment visit, are included in the Baseline (B) and final treatment visit (F) analysis.

[See figure 1 above]

FIGURE 1 - PERCENT OF PATIENTS WITH SIGN/SYMPTOMS OF ENDOMETRIOSIS AT BASELINE, FINAL TREATMENT VISIT, AND AFTER 6 AND 12 MONTHS OF FOLLOW-UP

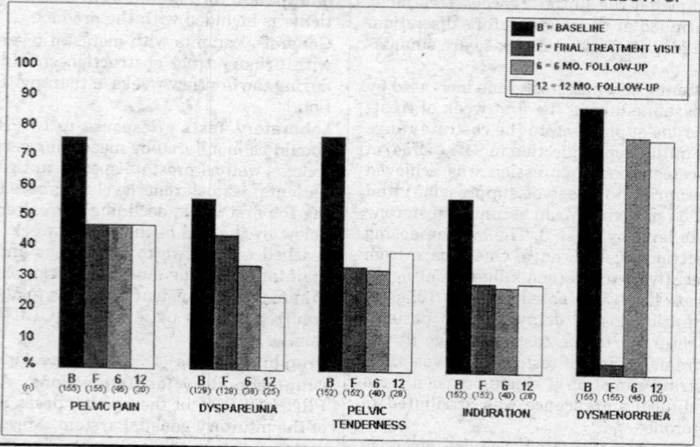

Hormonal replacement therapy: Clinical studies suggest that the addition of hormonal replacement therapy (estrogen and/or progestin) to LUPRON is effective in reducing loss of bone mineral density which occurs with LUPRON, without compromising the efficacy of LUPRON in relieving symptoms of endometriosis. The optimal drug/dose is not established.

Uterine Leiomyomata (Fibroids): **LUPRON DEPOT 3.75 mg for a period of three to six months was studied in four controlled clinical trials.**

In one of these clinical studies, enrollment was based on hematocrit ≤ 30% and/or hemoglobin ≤ 10.2 g/dL. Administration of LUPRON DEPOT 3.75 mg, concomitantly with iron, produced an increase of ≥ 6% hematocrit and ≥ 2 g/dL hemoglobin in 77% of patients at three months of therapy. The mean change in hematocrit was 10.1% and the mean change in hemoglobin was 4.2 g/dL. Clinical response was judged to be a hematocrit of ≥ 36% and hemoglobin of ≥ 12 g/dL, thus allowing for autologous blood donation prior to surgery. At two and three months respectively, 71% and 75% of patients met this criterion (Table 1). These data suggest however, that some patients may benefit from iron alone or 1 to 2 months of LUPRON DEPOT 3.75 mg.

Table 1:
PERCENT OF PATIENTS ACHIEVING
HEMATOCRIT ≥ 36% AND HEMOGLOBIN ≥ 12 GM/DL

Treatment Group	Week 4	Week 8	Week 12
LUPRON DEPOT 3.75 mg with Iron (N=104)	40*	71**	75*
Iron Alone (N=98)	17	39	49

* P-Value <0.01
**P-Value <0.001

Excessive vaginal bleeding (menorrhagia or menometrorrhagia) decreased in 80% of patients at three months. Episodes of spotting and menstrual-like bleeding were noted in 16% of patients at final visit.

In this same study, a decrease of ≥ 25% was seen in uterine and myoma volumes in 60% and 54% of patients respectively. The mean fibroid diameter was 6.3 cm at pretreatment and decreased to 5.6 cm at the end of treatment. LUPRON DEPOT 3.75 mg was found to relieve symptoms of bloating, pelvic pain, and pressure.

In three other controlled clinical trials, enrollment was not based on hematologic status. Mean uterine volume decreased by 41% and myoma volume decreased by 37% at final visit as evidenced by ultrasound or MRI. The mean fibroid diameter was 5.6 cm at pretreatment and decreased to 4.7 cm at the end of treatment. These patients also experienced a decrease in symptoms including excessive vaginal bleeding and pelvic discomfort. Ninety-five percent of these patients became amenorrheic with 61%, 25%, and 4% experiencing amenorrhea during the first, second, and third treatment months respectively.

In addition, posttreatment follow-up was carried out in one clinical trial for a small percentage of LUPRON DEPOT 3.75 mg patients (N=46) among the 77% who demonstrated a ≥ 25% decrease in uterine volume while on therapy. Menses usually returned within two months of cessation of therapy. Mean time to return to pretreatment uterine size was 8.3 months. Regrowth did not appear to be related to pretreatment uterine volume.

There is no evidence that pregnancy rates are enhanced or adversely affected by the use of LUPRON DEPOT.

INDICATIONS AND USAGE

Endometriosis:

LUPRON DEPOT–3 Month 11.25 mg is indicated for management of endometriosis, including pain relief and reduction of endometriotic lesions.

Experience with LUPRON DEPOT in females has been limited to women 18 years of age and older treated for no more than 6 months.

Uterine Leiomyomata (Fibroids):

LUPRON DEPOT–3 Month 11.25 mg concomitantly with iron therapy is indicated for the preoperative hematologic improvement of patients with anemia caused by uterine leiomyomata. The clinician may wish to consider a one-month trial period on iron alone inasmuch as some of the patients will respond to iron alone. (See Table 1, CLINICAL STUDIES section.) LUPRON may be added if the response to iron alone is considered inadequate. Recommended therapy is a single injection of LUPRON DEPOT–3 Month 11.25 mg. This dosage form is indicated only for women for whom three months of hormonal suppression is deemed necessary.

Experience with LUPRON DEPOT in females has been limited to women 18 years of age and older treated for no more than 6 months.

CONTRAINDICATIONS

1. Hypersensitivity to GnRH, GnRH agonist analogs or any of the excipients in LUPRON DEPOT. A report of an anaphylactic reaction to synthetic GnRH (Factrel) has been reported in the medical literature.[1]
2. LUPRON DEPOT is contraindicated in women who are or may become pregnant while receiving the drug. LUPRON DEPOT may cause fetal harm when administered to a pregnant woman. Major fetal abnormalities were observed in rabbits but not in rats after administration of LUPRON DEPOT throughout gestation. There was increased fetal mortality and decreased fetal weights in rats and rabbits. (See **Pregnancy** section.) The effects on fetal mortality are expected consequences of the alterations in hormonal levels brought about by the drug. If this drug is used during pregnancy or if the patient becomes pregnant while taking this drug, the patient should be apprised of the potential hazard to the fetus.
3. Use in women who are breast-feeding. (See **Nursing Mothers** section.)
4. Undiagnosed abnormal vaginal bleeding.

Table 2:
Adverse Events Reported to be Causally Related to Drug in ≥ 5% of Patients

	Endometriosis (2 Studies)			**Uterine Fibroids (4 Studies)**	
	LUPRON DEPOT 3.75 mg N=166 N (%)	Danazol N=136 N (%)	Placebo N=31 N (%)	**LUPRON DEPOT 3.75 mg N=166 N (%)**	**Placebo N=163 N (%)**
Body as a Whole					
Asthenia	5 (3)	9 (7)	0 (0)	**14 (8.4)**	**8 (4.9)**
General pain	31 (19)	22 (16)	1 (3)	**14 (8.4)**	**10 (6.1)**
Headache*	53 (32)	30 (22)	2 (6)	**43 (25.9)**	**29 (17.8)**
Cardiovascular System					
Hot flashes/sweats*	139 (84)	77 (57)	9 (29)	**121 (72.9)**	**29 (17.8)**
Gastrointestinal System					
Nausea/vomiting	21 (13)	17 (13)	1 (3)	**8 (4.8)**	**6 (3.7)**
GI disturbances*	11 (7)	8 (6)	1 (3)	**5 (3.0)**	**2 (1.2)**
Metabolic and Nutritional Disorders					
Edema	12 (7)	17 (13)	1 (3)	**9 (5.4)**	**2 (1.2)**
Weight gain/loss	22 (13)	36 (26)	0 (0)	**5 (3.0)**	**2 (1.2)**
Endocrine System					
Acne	17 (10)	27 (20)	0 (0)	**0 (0)**	**0 (0)**
Hirsutism	2 (1)	9 (7)	1 (3)	**1 (0.6)**	**0 (0)**
Musculoskeletal System					
Joint disorder*	14 (8)	11 (8)	0 (0)	**13 (7.8)**	**5 (3.1)**
Myalgia*	1 (1)	7 (5)	0 (0)	**1 (0.6)**	**0 (0)**
Nervous System					
Decreased libido*	19 (11)	6 (4)	0 (0)	**3 (1.8)**	**0 (0)**
Depression/emotional lability*	36 (22)	27 (20)	1 (3)	**18 (10.8)**	**7 (4.3)**
Dizziness	19 (11)	4 (3)	0 (0)	**3 (1.8)**	**6 (3.7)**
Nervousness*	8 (5)	11 (8)	0 (0)	**8 (4.8)**	**1 (0.6)**
Neuromuscular disorders*	11 (7)	17 (13)	0 (0)	**3 (1.8)**	**0 (0)**
Paresthesias	12 (7)	11 (8)	0 (0)	**2 (1.2)**	**1 (0.6)**
Skin and Appendages					
Skin reactions	17 (10)	20 (15)	1 (3)	**5 (3.0)**	**2 (1.2)**
Urogenital System					
Breast changes/tenderness/pain*	10 (6)	12 (9)	0 (0)	**3 (1.8)**	**7 (4.3)**
Vaginitis*	46 (28)	23 (17)	0 (0)	**19 (11.4)**	**3 (1.8)**

WARNINGS

1. As the effects of LUPRON DEPOT–3 Month 11.25 mg are present throughout the course of therapy, the drug should only be used in patients who require hormonal suppression for at least three months.
2. Experience with LUPRON DEPOT in females has been limited to six months; therefore, exposure should be limited to six months of therapy.
3. When used at the recommended dose and dosing interval, LUPRON DEPOT usually inhibits ovulation and stops menstruation. Contraception is not insured, however, by taking LUPRON DEPOT. Therefore, patients should use non-hormonal methods of contraception. Patients should be advised to see their physician if they believe they may be pregnant. If a patient becomes pregnant during treatment, the drug must be discontinued and the patient must be apprised of the potential risk to the fetus. (See **CONTRAINDICATIONS** section.)
4. During the early phase of therapy, sex steroids temporarily rise above baseline because of the physiologic effect of the drug. Therefore, an increase in clinical signs and symptoms may be observed during the initial days of therapy, but these will dissipate with continued therapy.

PRECAUTIONS

Information for Patients An information pamphlet for patients is included with the product. Patients should be aware of the following information:

1. Since menstruation should stop with effective doses of LUPRON DEPOT, the patient should notify her physician if regular menstruation persists. Patients missing successive doses of LUPRON DEPOT may experience breakthrough bleeding.
2. Patients should not use LUPRON DEPOT if they are pregnant, breast feeding, have undiagnosed abnormal vaginal bleeding, or are allergic to any of the ingredients in LUPRON DEPOT.
3. LUPRON DEPOT is contraindicated for use during pregnancy. Therefore, a non-hormonal method of contraception should be used during treatment. Patients should be advised that if they miss successive doses of LUPRON DEPOT, breakthrough bleeding or ovulation may occur with the potential for conception. If a patient becomes pregnant during treatment, she should discontinue treatment and consult her physician.
4. Adverse events occurring in clinical studies with LUPRON DEPOT that are associated with hypoestrogenism include: hot flashes, headaches, emotional lability, decreased libido, acne, myalgia, reduction in breast size, and vaginal dryness. Estrogen levels returned to normal after treatment was discontinued.
5. The induced hypoestrogenic state **also** results in a small loss in bone density over the course of treatment, which may not be fully reversible. In patients with major risk factors for decreased bone mineral content such as chronic alcohol and/or tobacco use, strong family history of osteoporosis, or chronic use of drugs that can reduce bone mass such as anticonvulsants or corticosteroids, LUPRON DEPOT therapy may pose an additional risk. In these patients, the risks and benefits must be weighed carefully before therapy with LUPRON DEPOT is instituted. Clinical studies suggest that the addition of hormonal replacement therapy (estrogen and/or progestin) to LUPRON is effective in reducing loss of bone mineral density which occurs with LUPRON, without compromising the efficacy of LUPRON in relieving symptoms of endometriosis. The optimal drug/dose is not established.
6. Treatment for more than six months cannot be recommended since safety data beyond six months are not available.

Laboratory Tests See **ADVERSE REACTIONS** section.

Drug/Laboratory Test Interactions See **ADVERSE REACTIONS** section. Administration of LUPRON DEPOT in therapeutic doses results in suppression of the pituitary-gonadal system. Normal function is usually restored within three months after treatment is discontinued. Due to the suppression of the pituitary-gonadal system by LUPRON DEPOT, diagnostic tests of pituitary gonadotropic and gonadal functions conducted during treatment and for up to three months after discontinuation of LUPRON DEPOT may be affected.

Carcinogenesis, Mutagenesis, Impairment of Fertility A two-year carcinogenicity study was conducted in rats and mice. In rats, a dose-related increase of benign pituitary hyperplasia and benign pituitary adenomas was noted at 24 months when the drug was administered subcutaneously at high daily doses (0.6 to 4 mg/kg). There was a significant but not dose-related increase of pancreatic islet-cell adenomas in females and of testicular interstitial cell adenomas in males (highest incidence in the low dose group). In mice, no leuprolide acetate-induced tumors or pituitary abnormalities were observed at a dose as high as 60 mg/kg for two years. Patients have been treated with leuprolide acetate for up to three years with doses as high as 10 mg/day and for two years with doses as high as 20 mg/day without demonstrable pituitary abnormalities.

Mutagenicity studies have been performed with leuprolide acetate using bacterial and mammalian systems. These studies provided no evidence of a mutagenic potential.

Clinical and pharmacologic studies in adults (> 18 years) with leuprolide acetate and similar analogs have shown reversibility of fertility suppression when the drug is discontinued after continuous administration for periods of up to 24 weeks.

Pregnancy, Teratogenic Effects Pregnancy Category X. (See **CONTRAINDICATIONS** section.) When administered on day 6 of pregnancy at test dosages of 0.00024, 0.0024, and 0.024 mg/kg (1/300 to 1/3 of the human dose) to rabbits, LUPRON DEPOT produced a dose-related increase in major fetal abnormalities. Similar studies in rats failed to demonstrate an increase in fetal malformations. There was increased fetal mortality and decreased fetal weights with the two higher doses of LUPRON DEPOT in rabbits and with the highest dose (0.024 mg/kg) in rats.

Nursing Mothers It is not known whether LUPRON DEPOT is excreted in human milk. Because many drugs are excreted in human milk, and because the effects of LUPRON DEPOT on lactation and/or the breast-fed child have

Continued on next page

Lupron Depot-3 mo. 11.25 mg—Cont.

not been determined, LUPRON DEPOT should not be used by nursing mothers.

Pediatric Use Safety and effectiveness of LUPRON DEPOT–3 Month 11.25 mg have not been established in pediatric patients. See LUPRON DEPOT-PED® (leuprolide acetate for depot suspension) labeling for the safety and effectiveness in children with central precocious puberty.

ADVERSE REACTIONS

Clinical Trials

The **monthly formulation of LUPRON DEPOT 3.75 mg** was utilized in controlled clinical trials that studied the drug in 166 endometriosis and 166 uterine fibroids patients. Adverse events reported in ≥ 5% of patients in either of these populations and thought to be potentially related to drug are noted in Table 2.

[See table 2 at top of previous page]

In these same studies, symptoms reported in < 5% of patients included: *Body as a Whole*—Body odor, Flu syndrome, Injection site reactions; *Cardiovascular System*—Palpitations, Syncope, Tachycardia; *Digestive System*—Appetite changes, Dry mouth, Thirst; *Endocrine System*—Androgen-like effects; *Hemic and Lymphatic System*—Ecchymosis, Lymphadenopathy; *Nervous System*—Anxiety,* Insomnia/Sleep disorders,* Delusions, Memory disorder, Personality disorder; *Respiratory System*—Rhinitis; *Skin and Appendages*—Alopecia, Hair disorder, Nail disorder; *Special Senses*—Conjunctivitis, Ophthalmologic disorders,* Taste perversion; *Urogenital System*—Dysuria,* Lactation, Menstrual disorders.

* = Physiologic effect of the drug.

In one controlled clinical trial utilizing the monthly formulation of LUPRON DEPOT, patients diagnosed with uterine fibroids received a higher dose (7.5 mg) of LUPRON DEPOT. Events seen with this dose that were thought to be potentially related to drug and were not seen at the lower dose included glossitis, hypesthesia, lactation, pyelonephritis, and urinary disorders. Generally, a higher incidence of hypoestrogenic effects was observed at the higher dose.

In a pharmacokinetic trial involving 20 healthy female subjects receiving LUPRON DEPOT–3 Month 11.25 mg, a few adverse events were reported with this formulation that were not reported previously. These included face edema, agitation, laryngitis, and ear pain.

In a Phase IV study involving endometriosis patients receiving LUPRON DEPOT 3.75 mg (N=20) or LUPRON DEPOT-3 Month 11.25 mg (N=21), similar adverse events were reported by the two groups of patients. In general the safety profiles of the two formulations were comparable in this study.

Changes in Bone Density

In controlled clinical studies, patients with endometriosis (six months of therapy) or uterine fibroids (three months of therapy) were treated with LUPRON DEPOT 3.75 mg. In endometriosis patients, vertebral bone density as measured by dual energy x-ray absorptiometry (DEXA) decreased by an average of 3.2% at six months compared with the pretreatment value. In this same study, LUPRON DEPOT 3.75 mg alone and LUPRON DEPOT 3.75 mg plus three different hormonal add-back regimens were compared for one year. All add-back groups demonstrated mean changes in bone mineral density of ≤1% from baseline and showed statistically significantly (P-value <0.001) less loss of bone density than the group treated with LUPRON DEPOT 3.75 mg alone, at all time points. Clinical studies suggest that the addition of hormonal replacement therapy (estrogen and/or progestin) to LUPRON is effective in reducing loss of bone mineral density which occurs with LUPRON, without compromising the efficacy of LUPRON in relieving symptoms of endometriosis. The optimal drug/dose is not established. In the Phase IV, six-month pharmacokinetic/pharmacodynamic study in endometriosis patients who were treated with LUPRON DEPOT 3.75 mg or LUPRON DEPOT-3 Month 11.25 mg, vertebral bone density measured by DEXA decreased compared with baseline by an average of 3.0% and 2.8% at six months for the two groups, respectively.

When LUPRON DEPOT 3.75 mg was administered for three months in uterine fibroid patients, vertebral trabecular bone mineral density as assessed by quantitative digital radiography (QDR) revealed a mean decrease of 2.7% compared with baseline. Six months after discontinuation of therapy, a trend toward recovery was observed. Use of LUPRON DEPOT for longer than three months (uterine fibroids) or six months (endometriosis) or in the presence of other known risk factors for decreased bone mineral content may cause additional bone loss **and is not recommended.**

Changes in Laboratory Values During Treatment

Liver Enzymes

Three percent of uterine fibroid patients treated with LUPRON DEPOT 3.75 mg, manifested posttreatment transaminase values that were at least twice the baseline value and above the upper limit of the normal range. None of the laboratory increases were associated with clinical symptoms.

Lipids

Triglycerides were increased above the upper limit of normal in 12% of the endometriosis patients who received LUPRON DEPOT 3.75 mg and in 32% of the subjects receiving LUPRON DEPOT–3 Month 11.25 mg.

Of those endometriosis and uterine fibroid patients whose pretreatment cholesterol values were in the normal range, mean change following therapy was +16 mg/dL to +17 mg/dL in endometriosis patients and +11 mg/dL to +29 mg/dL in uterine fibroid patients. In the endometriosis treated patients, increases from the pretreatment values were statistically significant (p<0.03). There was essentially no increase in the LDL/HDL ratio in patients from either population receiving LUPRON DEPOT 3.75 mg.

Chemistry

Slight to moderate mean increases were noted for glucose, uric acid, BUN, creatinine, total protein, albumin, bilirubin, alkaline phosphatase, LDH, calcium, and phosphorus. None of these increases were clinically significant.

Postmarketing

During postmarketing surveillance with other dosage forms and in the same and/or different populations, the following adverse events were reported. Like other drugs in this class, mood swings, including depression, have been reported as a physiologic effect of decreased sex steroids. There have been very rare reports of suicidal ideation and attempt. Many, but not all, of these patients had a history of depression or other psychiatric illness. Patients should be counseled on the possibility of worsening of depression.

Symptoms consistent with an anaphylactoid or asthmatic process have been reported. Rash, urticaria, and photosensitivity reactions have also been reported.

Localized reactions including induration and abscess have been reported at the site of injection.

Symptoms consistent with fibromyalgia (eg: joint and muscle pain, headaches, sleep disorders, gastrointestinal distress, and shortness of breath) have been reported individually and collectively.

Cardiovascular System—Hypotension, Pulmonary embolism; *Hemic and Lymphatic System*—Decreased WBC; *Central/Peripheral Nervous System*—Peripheral neuropathy, Spinal fracture/paralysis; *Musculoskeletal System*—Tenosynovitis-like symptoms; *Urogenital System*—Prostate pain.

See other LUPRON DEPOT and LUPRON Injection package inserts for other events reported in the same and different patient populations.

OVERDOSAGE

In clinical trials using daily subcutaneous leuprolide acetate in patients with prostate cancer, doses as high as 20 mg/day for up to two years caused no adverse effects differing from those observed with the 1 mg/day dose.

DOSAGE AND ADMINISTRATION

LUPRON DEPOT Must Be Administered Under the Supervision of a Physician.

Endometriosis: The recommended dose of LUPRON DEPOT–3 Month 11.25 mg is one injection every three months, for a maximum recommended duration of six months. Retreatment cannot be recommended since safety data for retreatment are not available. If the symptoms of endometriosis recur after a course of therapy, and further treatment with LUPRON DEPOT–3 Month 11.25 mg is contemplated, it is recommended that bone density be assessed before retreatment begins to ensure that values are within normal limits.

Uterine Leiomyomata (Fibroids): **The recommended dose of LUPRON DEPOT–3 Month 11.25 mg is one injection. The symptoms associated with uterine leiomyomata will recur following discontinuation of therapy. If additional treatment with LUPRON DEPOT–3 Month 11.25 mg is contemplated, bone density should be assessed prior to initiation of therapy to ensure that values are within normal limits.**

Due to different release characteristics, a fractional dose of the 3-month depot formulation is not equivalent to the same dose of the monthly formulation and should not be given.

Incorporated in a depot formulation, the lyophilized microspheres are to be reconstituted and administered as a single intramuscular injection, in accord with the following directions:

1. To prepare for injection, screw the white plunger into the end stopper until the stopper begins to turn.
2. Remove and discard the tab around the base of the needle.
3. Holding the syringe upright, release the diluent by SLOWLY PUSHING the plunger until the first stopper is at the blue line in the middle of the barrel.
4. Gently shake the syringe to thoroughly mix the particles to form a uniform suspension. The suspension will appear milky.
5. If the microspheres (particles) adhere to the stopper, tap the syringe against your finger.
6. Then remove the needle guard and advance the plunger to expel the air from the syringe.
7. At the time of reconstitution, inject the entire contents of the syringe intramuscularly as you would for a normal injection. The suspension settles very quickly following reconstitution; therefore, it is preferable that LUPRON DEPOT–3 Month 11.25 mg be mixed and used immediately. Reshake suspension if settling occurs.

Since the product does not contain a preservative, the suspension should be discarded if not used immediately.

As with other drugs administered by injection, the injection site should be varied periodically.

HOW SUPPLIED

LUPRON DEPOT–3 Month 11.25 mg is packaged as follows:

Kit with prefilled
dual-chamber syringe NDC 0300-3663-01

Each syringe contains sterile lyophilized microspheres which are leuprolide acetate incorporated in a biodegradable polymer of polylactic acid. When mixed with 1.5 mL of diluent, LUPRON DEPOT–3 Month 11.25 mg is administered as a single IM injection **EVERY THREE MONTHS.**

Store at 25°C (77°F); excursions permitted to 15–30°C (59–86°F) [See USP Controlled Room Temperature]

Rx only

REFERENCE

1. MacLeod TL, *et al.* Anaphylactic reaction to synthetic luteinizing hormone-releasing hormone. *Fertil Steril* 1987 Sept;48(3):500–502.

U.S. Patent Nos. 4,652,441; 4,728,721; 4,849,228; 4,917,893; 4,954,298; 5,330,767; 5,476,663; 5,480,656; 5,575,987; 5,631,020; 5,631,021; 5,643,607; and 5,716,640.

Manufactured for
TAP Pharmaceuticals Inc.
Lake Forest, IL 60045, U.S.A.
by Takeda Chemical Industries, Ltd. Osaka, JAPAN 541
®—Registered Trademark

(No. 3663)

03-5052-R7; Revised: April 2000

Shown in Product Identification Guide, page 338

LUPRON DEPOT®-3 Month 22.5 mg ℞
(leuprolide acetate for depot suspension)

3-MONTH FORMULATION

DESCRIPTION

Leuprolide acetate is a synthetic nonapeptide analog of naturally occurring gonadotropin-releasing hormone (GnRH or LH-RH). The analog possesses greater potency than the natural hormone. The chemical name is 5-oxo-L-prolyl-L-histidyl-L-tryptophyl-L-seryl-L-tyrosyl-D-leucyl-L-leucyl-L-arginyl-N-ethyl-L-prolinamide acetate (salt) with the following structural formula:

[See chemical structure at top of next page]

LUPRON DEPOT-3 Month 22.5 mg is available in a prefilled dual-chamber syringe containing sterile lyophilized microspheres which, when mixed with diluent, become a suspension intended as an intramuscular injection to be given **ONCE EVERY THREE MONTHS (84 days).**

The front chamber of LUPRON DEPOT-3 Month 22.5 mg prefilled dual-chamber syringe contains leuprolide acetate (22.5 mg), polylactic acid (198.6 mg) and D-mannitol (38.9 mg). The second chamber of diluent contains carboxymethylcellulose sodium (7.5 mg), D-mannitol (75.0 mg), polysorbate 80 (1.5 mg), water for injection, USP, and glacial acetic acid, USP to control pH.

During the manufacture of LUPRON DEPOT-3 Month 22.5 mg, acetic acid is lost, leaving the peptide.

CLINICAL PHARMACOLOGY

Leuprolide acetate, an LH-RH agonist, acts as a potent inhibitor of gonadotropin secretion when given continuously and in therapeutic doses. Animal and human studies indicate that following an initial stimulation, chronic administration of leuprolide acetate results in suppression of ovarian and testicular steroidogenesis. This effect is reversible upon discontinuation of drug therapy. Administration of leuprolide acetate has resulted in inhibition of the growth of certain hormone dependent tumors (prostatic tumors in Noble and Dunning male rats and DMBA-induced mammary tumors in female rats) as well as atrophy of the reproductive organs.

In humans, administration of leuprolide acetate results in an initial increase in circulating levels of luteinizing hormone (LH) and follicle stimulating hormone (FSH), leading to a transient increase in levels of the gonadal steroids (testosterone and dihydrotestosterone in males, and estrone and estradiol in premenopausal females). However, continuous administration of leuprolide acetate results in decreased levels of LH and FSH. In males, testosterone is reduced to castrate levels. In premenopausal females, estrogens are reduced to postmenopausal levels. These decreases occur within two to four weeks after initiation of treatment, and castrate levels of testosterone in prostatic cancer patients have been demonstrated for more than five years. Leuprolide acetate is not active when given orally.

Pharmacokinetics

Absorption Following a single injection of the three month formulation of LUPRON DEPOT-3 Month 22.5 mg in patients, mean peak plasma leuprolide concentration of 48.9 ng/mL was observed at 4 hours and then declined to 0.67 ng/mL at 12 weeks. Leuprolide appeared to be released at a constant rate following the onset of steady-state levels during the third week after dosing, providing steady plasma concentrations through the 12-week dosing interval. However, intact leuprolide and an inactive major metabolite could not be distinguished by the assay which was employed in the study. Detectable levels of leuprolide were present at all measurement points in all patients. The initial burst, followed by the rapid decline to a steady-state level, was similar to the release pattern seen with the monthly formulation.

Distribution The mean steady-state volume of distribution of leuprolide following intravenous bolus administration to healthy male volunteers was 27 L. *In vitro* binding to human plasma proteins ranged from 43% to 49%.

Metabolism In healthy male volunteers, a 1 mg bolus of leuprolide administered intravenously revealed that the mean systemic clearance was 7.6 L/h, with a terminal elimination half-life of approximately 3 hours based on a two compartment model.

In rats and dogs, administration of ^{14}C-labeled leuprolide was shown to be metabolized to smaller inactive peptides, a pentapeptide (Metabolite I), tripeptides (Metabolites II and III) and a dipeptide (Metabolite IV). These fragments may be further catabolized.

The major metabolite (M-I) plasma concentrations measured in 5 prostate cancer patients reached maximum concentration 2 to 6 hours after dosing and were approximately 6% of the peak parent drug concentration. One week after dosing, mean plasma M-I concentrations were approximately 20% of mean leuprolide concentrations.

Excretion Following administration of LUPRON DEPOT 3.75 mg to 3 patients, less than 5% of the dose was recovered as parent and M-I metabolite in the urine.

Special Populations The pharmacokinetics of the drug in hepatically and renally impaired patients have not been determined.

CLINICAL STUDIES

In clinical studies, serum testosterone was suppressed to castrate within 30 days in 87 of 92 (95%) patients and within an additional two weeks in three patients. Two patients did not suppress for 15 and 28 weeks, respectively. Suppression was maintained in all of these patients with the exception of transient minimal testosterone elevations in one of them, and in another an increase in serum testosterone to above the castrate range was recorded during the 12 hour observation period after a subsequent injection. This represents stimulation of gonadotropin secretion.

An 85% rate of "no progression" was achieved during the initial 24 weeks of treatment. A decrease from baseline in serum PSA of ≥90% was reported in 71% of the patients and a change to within the normal range (≤3.99 ng/mL) in 63% of the patients.

Periodic monitoring of serum testosterone and PSA levels is recommended, especially if the anticipated clinical or biochemical response to treatment has not been achieved. It should be noted that results of testosterone determinations are dependent on assay methodology. It is advisable to be aware of the type and precision of the assay methodology to make appropriate clinical and therapeutic decisions.

INDICATIONS AND USAGE

LUPRON DEPOT-3 Month 22.5 mg is indicated in the palliative treatment of advanced prostatic cancer. It offers an alternative treatment of prostatic cancer when orchiectomy or estrogen administration are either not indicated or unacceptable to the patient. In clinical trials, the safety and efficacy of LUPRON DEPOT-3 Month 22.5 mg were similar to that of the original daily subcutaneous injection and the monthly depot formulation.

CONTRAINDICATIONS

A report of an anaphylactic reaction to synthetic GnRH (Factrel) has been reported in the medical literature.[1]

LUPRON DEPOT is contraindicated in women who are or may become pregnant while receiving the drug. When administered on day 6 of pregnancy at test dosages of 0.00024, 0.0024, and 0.024 mg/kg (1/600 to 1/6 of the human dose) to rabbits, the monthly formulation of LUPRON DEPOT produced a dose-related increase in major fetal abnormalities. Similar studies in rats failed to demonstrate an increase in fetal malformations. There was increased fetal mortality and decreased fetal weights with the two higher doses of the monthly formulation of LUPRON DEPOT in rabbits and with the highest dose in rats. The effects on fetal mortality are logical consequences of the alterations in hormonal levels brought about by this drug. Therefore, the possibility exists that spontaneous abortion may occur if the drug is administered during pregnancy.

WARNINGS

Isolated cases of worsening of signs and symptoms during the first weeks of treatment have been reported with LH-RH analogs. Worsening of symptoms may contribute to paralysis with or without fatal complications. For patients at risk, the physician may consider initiating therapy with daily LUPRON® (leuprolide acetate) Injection for the first two weeks to facilitate withdrawal of treatment if that is considered necessary.

PRECAUTIONS

General Patients with metastatic vertebral lesions and/or with urinary tract obstruction should be closely observed during the first few weeks of therapy. (See **WARNINGS** section.)

Laboratory Tests Response to LUPRON DEPOT-3 Month 22.5 mg should be monitored by measuring serum levels of testosterone, as well as prostate-specific antigen and prostatic acid phosphatase. In the majority of patients, testosterone levels increased above baseline during the first week, declining thereafter to baseline levels or below by the end of the second week. Castrate levels were reached within two to four weeks and once achieved were maintained for as long as the patients received their injections.

Drug Interactions No pharmacokinetic-based drug-drug interaction studies have been conducted with LUPRON DEPOT. However, because leuprolide acetate is a peptide that is primarily degraded by peptidase and not by cytochrome P-450 enzymes as noted in specific studies, and the drug is only about 46% bound to plasma proteins, drug interactions would not be expected to occur.

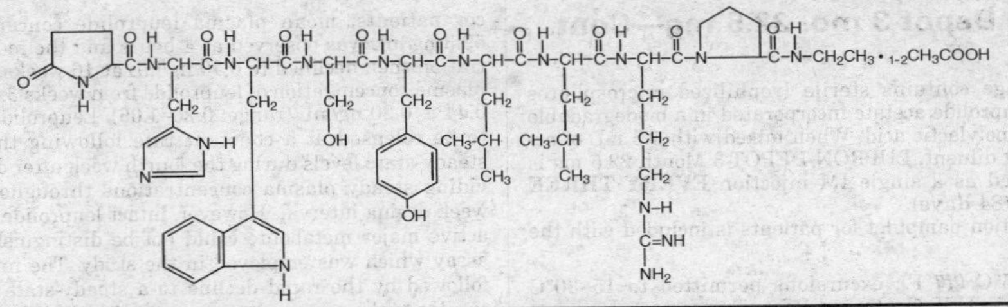

Drug/Laboratory Test Interactions Administration of LUPRON DEPOT 3.75 mg in women results in suppression of the pituitary-gonadal system. Normal function is usually restored within one to three months after treatment is discontinued. Therefore, diagnostic tests of pituitary gonadotropic and gonadal functions conducted during treatment and up to three months after discontinuation of LUPRON DEPOT 3.75 mg therapy may be misleading.

Carcinogenesis, Mutagenesis, Impairment of Fertility Two-year carcinogenicity studies were conducted in rats and mice. In rats, a dose-related increase of benign pituitary hyperplasia and benign pituitary adenomas was noted at 24 months when the drug was administered subcutaneously at high daily doses (0.6 to 4 mg/kg). There was a significant but not dose-related increase of pancreatic islet-cell adenomas in females and of testicular interstitial cell adenomas in males (highest incidence in the low dose group). In mice no pituitary abnormalities were observed at a dose as high as 60 mg/kg for two years. Patients have been treated with leuprolide acetate for up to three years with doses as high as 10 mg/day and for two years with doses as high as 20 mg/day without demonstrable pituitary abnormalities.

Mutagenicity studies have been performed with leuprolide acetate using bacterial and mammalian systems. These studies provided no evidence of a mutagenic potential.

Clinical and pharmacologic studies in adults (≥18 years) with leuprolide acetate and similar analogs have shown reversibility of fertility suppression when the drug is discontinued after continuous administration for periods of up to 24 weeks.

Pregnancy, Teratogenic Effects

Pregnancy Category X. (See **CONTRAINDICATIONS** section.)

Pediatric Use See LUPRON DEPOT-PED® (leuprolide acetate for depot suspension) labeling for the safety and effectiveness of the monthly formulation in children with central precocious puberty.

ADVERSE REACTIONS

Clinical Trials

In the majority of patients testosterone levels increased above baseline during the first week, declining thereafter to baseline levels or below by the end of the second week of treatment.

Potential exacerbations of signs and symptoms during the first few weeks of treatment is a concern in patients with vertebral metastases and/or urinary obstruction or hematuria which, if aggravated, may lead to neurological problems such as temporary weakness and/or paresthesia of the lower limbs or worsening of urinary symptoms. (See **WARNINGS** section.)

In two clinical trials of LUPRON DEPOT-3 Month 22.5 mg, the following adverse reactions were reported to have a possible or probable relationship to drug as ascribed by the treating physician in 5% or more of the patients receiving the drug. **Often, causality is difficult to assess in patients with metastatic prostate cancer.** Reactions considered not drug-related are excluded.

	LUPRON DEPOT-3 Month 22.5 mg N=94	(%)
Body as a Whole		
Asthenia	7	(7.4)
General Pain	25	(26.6)
Headache	6	(6.4)
Injection Site Reaction	13	(13.8)
Cardiovascular System		
Hot flashes/Sweats*	55	(58.5)
Digestive System		
GI Disorders	15	(16.0)
Musculoskeletal System		
Joint Disorders	11	(11.7)
Central/Peripheral Nervous System		
Dizziness/Vertigo	6	(6.4)
Insomnia/Sleep Disorders	8	(8.5)
Neuromuscular Disorders	9	(9.6)
Respiratory System		
Respiratory Disorders	6	(6.4)
Skin and Appendages		
Skin Reaction	8	(8.5)
Urogenital System		
Testicular Atrophy*	19	(20.2)
Urinary Disorders	14	(14.9)

In these same studies, the following adverse reactions were reported in less than 5% of the patients on LUPRON DEPOT-3 Month 22.5 mg.

Body As A Whole—Enlarged abdomen, Fever; *Cardiovascular System*—Arrhythmia, Bradycardia, Heart failure, Hypertension, Hypotension, Varicose vein; *Digestive System*—Anorexia, Duodenal ulcer, Increased appetite, Thirst/dry mouth; *Hemic and Lymphatic System*—Anemia, Lymphedema; *Metabolic and Nutritional Disorders*—Dehydration, Edema; *Central/Peripheral Nervous System*—Anxiety, Delusions, Depression, Hypesthesia, Libido decreased*, Nervousness, Paresthesia; *Respiratory System*—Epistaxis, Pharyngitis, Pleural effusion, Pneumonia; *Special Senses*—Abnormal vision, Amblyopia, Dry eyes, Tinnitus; *Urogenital System*—Gynecomastia, Impotence*, Penis disorders, Testis disorders.

Laboratory: Abnormalities of certain parameters were observed, but are difficult to assess in this population. The following were recorded in ≥ 5% of patients: Increased BUN, Hyperglycemia, Hyperlipidemia (total cholesterol, LDL-cholesterol, triglycerides), Hyperphosphatemia, Abnormal liver function tests, Increased PT, Increased PTT. Additional laboratory abnormalities reported were: Decreased platelets, Decreased potassium and Increased WBC.

*Physiologic effect of decreased testosterone.

Postmarketing

During postmarketing surveillance, which includes other dosage forms, the following adverse events were reported. Symptoms consistent with an anaphylactoid or asthmatic process have been rarely reported. Rash, urticaria, and photosensitivity reactions have also been reported.

Localized reactions including induration and abscess have been reported at the site of injection.

Hemic and Lymphatic System—Decreased WBC; *Central/Peripheral Nervous System*—Peripheral neuropathy, Spinal fracture/paralysis; *Musculoskeletal System*—Tenosynovitis-like symptoms; *Urogenital System*— Prostate pain.

See other LUPRON DEPOT and LUPRON Injection package inserts for other events reported in different patient populations.

OVERDOSAGE

In rats subcutaneous administration of 250 to 500 times the recommended human dose, expressed on a per body weight basis, resulted in dyspnea, decreased activity, and local irritation at the injection site. There is no evidence at present that there is a clinical counterpart of this phenomenon. In early clinical trials with daily subcutaneous leuprolide acetate, doses as high as 20 mg/day for up to two years caused no adverse effects differing from those observed with the 1 mg/day dose.

DOSAGE AND ADMINISTRATION

LUPRON DEPOT Must Be Administered Under The Supervision Of A Physician.

The recommended dose of LUPRON DEPOT-3 Month 22.5 mg to be administered is one injection every three months (84 days). Due to different release characteristics, a fractional dose of this 3-month depot formulation is not equivalent to the same dose of the monthly formulation and should not be given.

Incorporated in a depot formulation, the lyophilized microspheres are to be reconstituted and administered every three months as a single intramuscular injection, in accord with the following directions:

1. To prepare for injection, screw the white plunger into the end stopper until the stopper begins to turn.
2. Remove and discard the tab around the base of the needle.
3. Holding the syringe upright, release the diluent by SLOWLY PUSHING the plunger until the first stopper is at the blue line in the middle of the barrel.
4. Gently shake the syringe to thoroughly mix the particles to form a uniform suspension. The suspension will appear milky.
5. If the microspheres (particles) adhere to the stopper, tap the syringe against your finger.
6. Then remove the needle guard and advance the plunger to expel the air from the syringe.
7. Inject the entire contents of the syringe intramuscularly as you would for a normal injection.

Although the potency of the reconstituted suspension has been shown to be stable for 24 hours, since the product does not contain a preservative, the suspension should be discarded if not used immediately.

As with other drugs administered by injection, the injection site should be varied periodically.

HOW SUPPLIED

LUPRON DEPOT-3 Month 22.5 mg is packaged as follows:

Kit with prefilled dual-chamber syringe (NDC 0300-3346-01)

Continued on next page

Lupron Depot-3 mo. 22.5 mg—Cont.

Each syringe contains sterile lyophilized microspheres which is leuprolide acetate incorporated in a biodegradable polymer of polylactic acid. When mixed with 1.5 mL of accompanying diluent, LUPRON DEPOT-3 Month 22.5 mg is administered as a single IM injection **EVERY THREE MONTHS (84 days).**
An information pamphlet for patients is included with the kit.

Store at 25°C (77°F); excursions permitted to 15–30°C (59–86°F) [see USP Controlled Room Temperature]

Rx only

REFERENCE

1. MacLeod TL, *et al.* Anaphylactic reaction to synthetic luteinizing hormone-releasing hormone. *Fertil Steril* 1987 Sept; 48(3):500–502.

U.S. Patent Nos. 4,652,441; 4,728,721; 4,849,228; 4,917,893; 4,954,298; 5,330,767; 5,476,663; 5,480,656; 5,575,987; 5,631,020; 5,631,021; 5,643,607; and 5,716,640.

Manufactured for
TAP Pharmaceuticals Inc.
Lake Forest, IL 60045, U.S.A.
by Takeda Chemical Industries, Ltd. Osaka, JAPAN 541

®—Registered trademark

(No. 3346)
03-5028-R5; Revised: March 2000

Shown in Product Identification Guide, page 338

LUPRON DEPOT®-4 Month 30 mg ℞
(leuprolide acetate for depot suspension)

4-MONTH FORMULATION

DESCRIPTION

Leuprolide acetate is a synthetic nonapeptide analog of naturally occurring gonadotropin-releasing hormone (GnRH or LH-RH). The analog possesses greater potency than the natural hormone. The chemical name is 5-oxo-L-prolyl-L-histidyl-L-tryptophyl-L-seryl-L-tyrosyl-D-leucyl-L-leucyl-L-arginyl-N-ethyl-L-prolinamide acetate (salt) with the following structural formula:
[See chemical structure below]
LUPRON DEPOT-4 Month 30 mg is available in a prefilled dual-chamber syringe containing sterile lyophilized microspheres which, when mixed with diluent, become a suspension intended as an intramuscular injection to be given **ONCE EVERY FOUR MONTHS (16 weeks).**
The front chamber of LUPRON DEPOT-4 Month 30 mg prefilled dual-chamber syringe contains leuprolide acetate (30 mg), polylactic acid (264.8 mg) and D-mannitol (51.9 mg). The second chamber of diluent contains carboxymethylcellulose sodium (7.5 mg), D-mannitol (75.0 mg), polysorbate 80 (1.5 mg), water for injection, USP, and glacial acetic acid, USP to control pH.
During the manufacture of LUPRON DEPOT-4 Month 30 mg, acetic acid is lost, leaving the peptide.

CLINICAL PHARMACOLOGY

Leuprolide acetate, an LH-RH agonist, acts as a potent inhibitor of gonadotropin secretion when given continuously and in therapeutic doses. Animal and human studies indicate that following an initial stimulation, chronic administration of leuprolide acetate results in suppression of ovarian and testicular steroidogenesis. This effect is reversible upon discontinuation of drug therapy. Administration of leuprolide acetate has resulted in inhibition of the growth of certain hormone dependent tumors (prostatic tumors in Noble and Dunning male rats and DMBA-induced mammary tumors in female rats) as well as atrophy of the reproductive organs.
In humans, administration of leuprolide acetate results in an initial increase in circulating levels of luteinizing hormone (LH) and follicle stimulating hormone (FSH), leading to a transient increase in levels of the gonadal steroids (testosterone and dihydrotestosterone in males, and estrone and estradiol in premenopausal females). However, continuous administration of leuprolide acetate results in decreased levels of LH and FSH. In males, testosterone is reduced to castrate levels. In premenopausal females, estrogens are reduced to postmenopausal levels. These decreases occur within two to four weeks after initiation of treatment. Castrate levels of testosterone in prostatic cancer patients have been demonstrated for more than five years.
Leuprolide acetate is not active when given orally.

Pharmacokinetics

Absorption Following a single injection of LUPRON DEPOT-4 Month 30 mg in sixteen orchiectomized prostate cancer patients, mean plasma leuprolide concentration of 59.3 ng/mL was observed at 4 hours and the mean concentration then declined to 0.30 ng/mL at 16 weeks. The mean plasma concentration of leuprolide from weeks 3.5 to 16 was 0.44 ± 0.20 ng/mL (range: 0.20–1.06). Leuprolide appeared to be released at a constant rate following the onset of steady-state levels during the fourth week after dosing, providing steady plasma concentrations throughout the 16-week dosing interval. However, intact leuprolide and an inactive major metabolite could not be distinguished by the assay which was employed in the study. The initial burst, followed by the rapid decline to a steady-state level, was similar to the release pattern seen with the other depot formulations.

Distribution The mean steady-state volume of distribution of leuprolide following intravenous bolus administration to healthy male volunteers was 27 L. *In vitro* binding to human plasma proteins ranged from 43% to 49%.

Metabolism In healthy male volunteers, a 1 mg bolus of leuprolide administered intravenously revealed that the mean systemic clearance was 7.6 L/h, with a terminal elimination half-life of approximately 3 hours based on a two compartment model.
In rats and dogs, administration of ^{14}C-labeled leuprolide was shown to be metabolized to smaller inactive peptides, a pentapeptide (Metabolite I), tripeptides (Metabolites II and III) and a dipeptide (Metabolite IV). These fragments may be further catabolized.
The major metabolite (M-I) plasma concentrations measured in 5 prostate cancer patients reached maximum concentration 2 to 6 hours after dosing and were approximately 6% of the peak parent drug concentration. One week after dosing, mean plasma M-I concentrations were approximately 20% of mean leuprolide concentrations.

Excretion Following administration of LUPRON DEPOT 3.75 mg to 3 patients, less than 5% of the dose was recovered as parent and M-I metabolite in the urine.

Special Populations The pharmacokinetics of the drug in hepatically and renally impaired patients have not been determined.

Drug Interactions No pharmacokinetic-based drug-drug interaction studies have been conducted with LUPRON DEPOT. However, because leuprolide acetate is a peptide that is primarily degraded by peptidase and the drug is only about 46% bound to plasma proteins, drug interactions would not be expected to occur.

CLINICAL STUDIES

In an open-label, noncomparative, multicenter clinical study of LUPRON DEPOT-4 Month 30 mg, 49 patients with stage D2 prostatic adenocarcinoma (with no prior treatment) were enrolled. The objectives were to determine whether a 30 mg depot formulation of leuprolide injected once every 16 weeks would reduce and maintain serum testosterone levels at castrate levels (≤ 50 ng/dL), and to assess the safety of the formulation. The study was divided into an initial 32-week treatment phase and a long-term treatment phase. Serum testosterone levels were determined biweekly or weekly during the first 32 weeks of treatment. Once the patient completed the initial 32-week treatment period, treatment continued at the investigator's discretion with serum testosterone levels being done every 4 months prior to the injection.
In the majority of patients, testosterone levels increased 50% or more above the baseline during the first week of treatment. Mean serum testosterone subsequently suppressed to castrate levels within 30 days of the first injection in 94% of patients and within 43 days in all 49 patients during the initial 32-week treatment period. The median dosing interval between injections was 112 days. One escape from suppression (two consecutive testosterone values > 50 ng/dL after castrate levels achieved) was noted at Week 16. In this patient, serum testosterone increased to above the castrate range following the second depot injection (Week 16) but returned to the castrate level by Week 18. No adverse events were associated with this rise in serum testosterone. A second patient had a rise in testosterone at Week 17, then returned to the castrate level by Week 18 and remained there through Week 32. In the long-term treatment phase two patients experienced testosterone elevations, both at Week 48. Testosterone for one patient returned to the castrate range at Week 52, and one patient discontinued the study at Week 48 due to disease progression.
Secondary efficacy endpoints evaluated in the study were the objective tumor response as assessed by clinical evaluations of tumor burden (complete response, partial response, objectively stable and progression) and evaluations of changes in prostatic involvement and prostate-specific antigen (PSA). These evaluations were performed at Weeks 16 and 32 of the treatment phase. The long-term treatment phase monitored PSA at each visit (every 16 weeks). The objective tumor response analysis showed "no progression" (i.e. complete or partial response, or stable disease) in 86% (37/43) of patients at Week 16, and in 77% (37/48) of patients at Week 32. Local disease improved or remained stable in all patients evaluated at Week 16 and/or 32. For patients with elevated baseline PSA, 50% (23/46) had a normal PSA (< 4.0 ng/mL) at Week 16, and 51% (19/37) had a normal PSA at Week 32.
Periodic monitoring of serum testosterone and PSA levels is recommended, especially if the anticipated clinical or biochemical response to treatment has not been achieved. It should be noted that results of testosterone determinations are dependent on assay methodology. It is advisable to be aware of the type and precision of the assay methodology to make appropriate clinical and therapeutic decisions.
Using historical comparisons, the safety and efficacy of LUPRON DEPOT-4 Month 30 mg appear similar to the other LUPRON DEPOT formulations.

INDICATIONS AND USAGE

LUPRON DEPOT-4 Month 30 mg is indicated in the palliative treatment of advanced prostatic cancer.

CONTRAINDICATIONS

1. Hypersensitivity to GnRH, GnRH agonist analogs or any of the excipients in LUPRON DEPOT. Reports of anaphylactic reactions to synthetic GnRH (Factrel) or GnRH agonist analogs have been reported in the medical literature.
2. This formulation is not indicated for use in women (See LUPRON DEPOT 3.75 mg and LUPRON DEPOT-3 Month 11.25 mg package inserts.)
3. All formulations of LUPRON DEPOT are contraindicated in women who are or may become pregnant while receiving the drug. LUPRON DEPOT may cause fetal harm when administered to a pregnant woman. Major fetal abnormalities were observed in rabbits but not in rats after administration of LUPRON DEPOT throughout gestation. There was increased fetal mortality and decreased fetal weights in rats and rabbits. The effects on fetal mortality are expected consequences of the alterations in hormonal levels brought about by this drug. Therefore, the possibility exists that spontaneous abortion may occur. If this drug is used during pregnancy, or if the patient becomes pregnant while taking any formulation of LUPRON DEPOT, the patient should be apprised of the potential hazard to the fetus.

WARNINGS

Initially, LUPRON DEPOT, like other LH-RH agonists, causes increases in serum levels of testosterone to approximately 50% above baseline during the first week of treatment. Transient worsening of symptoms, or the occurrence of additional signs and symptoms of prostate cancer, may occasionally develop during the first few weeks of LUPRON DEPOT treatment. A small number of patients may experience a temporary increase in bone pain, which can be managed symptomatically. As with other LH-RH agonists, isolated cases of ureteral obstruction and spinal cord compression have been observed, which may contribute to paralysis with or without fatal complications.
For patients at risk, initiation of therapy with daily LUPRON® (leuprolide acetate) Injection (See **DOSAGE AND ADMINISTRATION** section in the LUPRON Injection labeling.) for the first two weeks to facilitate withdrawal of treatment may be considered. If spinal cord compression or renal impairment develops, standard treatment of these complications should be instituted.

PRECAUTIONS

Information for Patients An information pamphlet for patients is included with the product.

General Patients with metastatic vertebral lesions and/or with urinary tract obstruction should be closely observed during the first few weeks of therapy. (See **WARNINGS** section.)

Laboratory Tests Response to LUPRON DEPOT-4 Month 30 mg should be monitored by measuring serum levels of testosterone as well as prostate-specific antigen. In the majority of patients, testosterone levels increased above baseline during the first week, declining thereafter to baseline levels or below by the end of the second week. Castrate levels were reached within two to four weeks and once achieved were maintained in most (45/49) patients for as long as the patients received their injections (See **CLINICAL STUDIES** and **ADVERSE REACTIONS** section.)

Drug Interactions See **CLINICAL PHARMACOLOGY, Pharmacokinetics** section.

Drug/Laboratory Test Interactions Administration of LUPRON DEPOT in therapeutic doses results in suppression of the pituitary-gonadal system. Normal function is usually restored within three months after treatment is discontinued. Due to the suppression of the pituitary-gonadal system by LUPRON DEPOT, diagnostic tests of pituitary gonadotropic and gonadal functions conducted during treatment and for up to three months after discontinuation of LUPRON DEPOT may be affected.

Carcinogenesis, Mutagenesis, Impairment of Fertility Two-year carcinogenicity studies were conducted in rats and mice. In rats, a dose-related increase of benign pituitary hyperplasia and benign pituitary adenomas was noted at 24 months when the drug was administered subcutaneously at high daily doses (0.6 to 4 mg/kg). There was a significant but not dose-related increase of pancreatic islet-cell adenomas in females and of testicular interstitial cell ad-

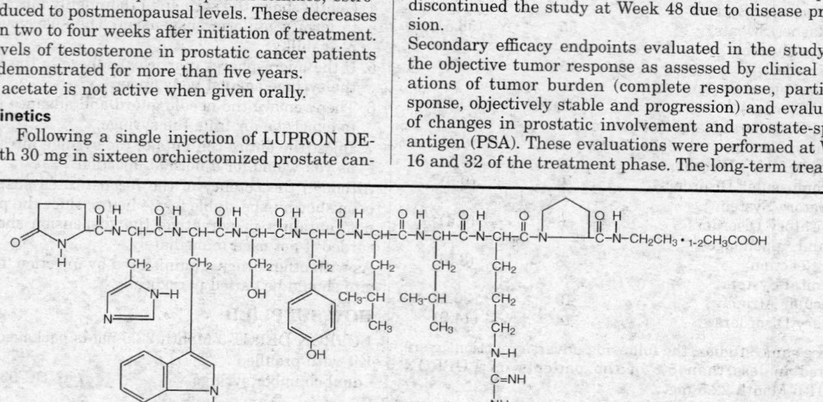

enomas in males (highest incidence in the low dose group). In mice no pituitary abnormalities were observed at a dose as high as 60 mg/kg for two years. Patients have been treated with leuprolide acetate for up to three years with doses as high as 10 mg/day and for two years with doses as high as 20 mg/day without demonstrable pituitary abnormalities.
Mutagenicity studies have been performed with leuprolide acetate using bacterial and mammalian systems. These studies provided no evidence of a mutagenic potential.
Clinical and pharmacologic studies in adults (≥18 years) with leuprolide acetate and similar analogs have shown reversibility of fertility suppression when the drug is discontinued after continuous administration for periods of up to 24 weeks.

Pregnancy, Teratogenic Effects. Pregnancy Category X. (See **CONTRAINDICATIONS** section.)

Pediatric Use Safety and effectiveness of LUPRON DEPOT-4 Month 30 mg have not been established in pediatric patients. See LUPRON DEPOT-PED® (leuprolide acetate for depot suspension) labeling for the safety and effectiveness of the monthly formulation in children with central precocious puberty.

ADVERSE REACTIONS

Clinical Trials

The 4-month formulation of LUPRON DEPOT 30 mg was utilized in clinical trials that studied the drug in 49 nonorchiectomized prostate cancer patients for 32 weeks or longer and in 24 orchiectomized prostate cancer patients for 20 weeks.
In the majority of nonorchiectomized patients, testosterone levels increased 50% or more above baseline during the first week of treatment with LUPRON DEPOT, declining thereafter to baseline levels or below by the end of the second week of treatment. Therefore, potential exacerbations of signs and symptoms during the first few weeks of treatment are of concern in patients with vertebral metastases and/or urinary obstruction or hematuria which, if aggravated, may lead to neurological problems such as temporary weakness and/or paresthesia of the lower limbs or worsening of urinary symptoms. (See **WARNINGS** section.)
In the above described clinical trials, the following adverse reactions were reported in ≥ 5% of the patients during the treatment period regardless of causality.
[See table above]
In these same studies, the following adverse reactions were reported in less than 5% of the patients on LUPRON DEPOT-4 Month 30 mg.
Body As a Whole—Abscess, Accidental injury, Allergic reaction, Cyst, Fever, Generalized edema, Hernia, Neck pain, Neoplasm; *Cardiovascular System*—Atrial fibrillation, Deep thrombophlebitis, Hypertension; *Digestive System*—Anorexia, Eructation, Gastrointestinal hemorrhage, Gingivitis, Gum hemorrhage, Hepatomegaly, Increased appetite, Intestinal obstruction, Peridontal abscess; *Hemic and Lymphatic System*—Lymphadenopathy; *Metabolic and Nutritional Disorders*—Healing abnormal, Hypoxia, Weight loss; *Musculoskeletal System*—Leg cramps, Pathological fracture, Ptosis; *Nervous System*—Abnormal thinking, Amnesia, Confusion, Convulsion, Dementia, Depression, Insomnia/sleep disorders, Libido decreased*, Neuropathy, Paralysis; *Respiratory System*—Asthma, Bronchitis, Hiccup, Lung disorder, Sinusitis, Voice alteration; *Skin and Appendages*—Herpes zoster, Melanosis; *Urogenital System*—Bladder carcinoma, Epididymitis, Impotence*, Prostate disorder, Testicular atrophy*, Urinary incontinence, Urinary tract infection.

* Due to the expected physiologic effects of decreased testosterone levels.

Laboratory: Abnormalities of certain parameters were observed, but their relationship to drug treatment is difficult to assess in this population. The following were recorded in ≥ 5% of patients: Decreased bicarbonate, Decreased hemoglobin/hematocrit/RBC, Hyperlipidemia (total cholesterol, LDL-cholesterol, triglycerides), Decreased HDL-cholesterol, Eosinophilia, Increased glucose, Increased liver function tests (ALT, AST, GGTP, LDH), Increased phosphorus. Additional laboratory abnormalities were reported: Increased BUN and PT, Leukopenia, Thrombocytopenia, Uricaciduria.

Postmarketing

During postmarketing surveillance, which includes other dosage forms and other patient populations, the following adverse events were reported. Symptoms consistent with an anaphylactoid or asthmatic process have been reported. Rash, urticaria, and photosensitivity reactions have also been reported. Localized reactions including induration and abscess have been reported at the site of injection.
Cardiovascular System—Hypotension; *Hemic and Lymphatic System*—Decreased WBC; *Central/Peripheral Nervous System*—Peripheral neuropathy, Spinal fracture/paralysis; *Musculoskeletal System*—Tenosynovitis-like symptoms; *Urogenital System*—Prostate pain.
Changes in Bone Density: Decreased bone density has been reported in the medical literature in men who have had orchiectomy or who have been treated with an LH-RH agonist analog. In a clinical trial, 25 men with prostate cancer, 12 of whom had been treated previously with leuprolide acetate for at least six months, underwent bone density studies as a result of pain. The leuprolide-treated group had lower bone density scores than the nontreated control group. It can be anticipated that long periods of medical castration in men will have effects on bone density.

Adverse Events Reported in ≥5% of Patients Regardless of Causality

	LUPRON DEPOT-4 Month 30 mg Nonorchiectomized, N=49 Study 013		Orchiectomized, N=24 Study 012	
	N	(%)	N	(%)
Body As a Whole				
Asthenia	6	(12.2)	1	(4.2)
Flu Syndrome	6	(12.2)	0	(0.0)
General Pain	16	(32.7)	1	(4.2)
Headache	5	(10.2)	1	(4.2)
Injection Site Reaction	4	(8.2)	9	(37.5)
Cardiovascular System				
Hot flashes/Sweats*	23	(46.9)	2	(8.3)
Digestive System				
GI Disorders	5	(10.2)	3	(12.5)
Metabolic and Nutritional Disorders				
Dehydration	4	(8.2)	0	(0.0)
Edema	4	(8.2)	5	(20.8)
Musculoskeletal System				
Joint Disorder	8	(16.3)	1	(4.2)
Myalgia	4	(8.2)	0	(0.0)
Nervous System				
Dizziness/Vertigo	3	(6.1)	2	(8.3)
Neuromuscular Disorders	3	(6.1)	1	(4.2)
Paresthesia	4	(8.2)	1	(4.2)
Respiratory System				
Respiratory Disorder	4	(8.2)	1	(4.2)
Skin and Appendages				
Skin Reaction	6	(12.2)	0	(0.0)
Urogenital System				
Urinary Disorders	5	(10.2)	4	(16.7)

See other LUPRON DEPOT and LUPRON Injection package inserts for other events reported in women and pediatric populations.

OVERDOSAGE

In clinical trials using daily subcutaneous leuprolide acetate in patients with prostate cancer, doses as high as 20 mg/day for up to two years caused no adverse effects differing from those observed with the 1 mg/day dose.

DOSAGE AND ADMINISTRATION

LUPRON DEPOT Must Be Administered Under The Supervision Of A Physician.
The recommended dose of LUPRON DEPOT-4 Month 30 mg to be administered is one injection **EVERY FOUR MONTHS (16 weeks).** Due to different release characteristics, a fractional dose of this 4-month depot formulation is not equivalent to the same dose of the monthly formulation and should not be given.
Incorporated in a depot formulation, the lyophilized microspheres are to be reconstituted and administered **EVERY FOUR MONTHS (16 weeks)** as a single intramuscular injection, in accord with the following directions:

1. To prepare for injection, screw the white plunger into the end stopper until the stopper begins to turn.
2. Remove and discard the tab around the base of the needle.
3. Holding the syringe upright, release the diluent by SLOWLY PUSHING the plunger until the first stopper is at the blue line in the middle of the barrel.
4. Gently shake the syringe to thoroughly mix the particles to form a uniform suspension. The suspension will appear milky.
5. If the microspheres (particles) adhere to the stopper, tap the syringe against your finger.
6. Then remove the needle guard and advance the plunger to expel the air from the syringe.
7. At the time of reconstitution, inject the entire contents of the syringe intramuscularly as you would for a normal injection. The suspension settles very quickly following reconstitution; therefore, it is preferable that LUPRON DEPOT-4 Month 30 mg be mixed and used immediately. Reshake suspension if settling occurs.

Since the product does not contain a preservative, the suspension should be discarded if not used immediately.
As with other drugs administered by injection, the injection site should be varied periodically.

HOW SUPPLIED

LUPRON DEPOT-4 Month 30 mg is packaged as follows:
Kit with prefilled dual-chamber syringe NDC 0300-3683-01
Each syringe contains sterile lyophilized microspheres which is leuprolide acetate incorporated in a biodegradable polymer of polylactic acid. When mixed with 1.5 mL of accompanying diluent, LUPRON DEPOT-4 Month 30 mg is administered as a single IM injection **EVERY FOUR MONTHS (16 weeks).**
Store at 25°C (77°F); excursions permitted to 15–30°C (59–86°F) [See USP Controlled Room Temperature]

Rx only

U.S. Patent Nos. 4,652,441; 4,728,721; 4,849,228; 4,917,893; 4,954,298; 5,330,767; 5,476,663; 5,480,656; 5,575,987; 5,631,020; 5,631,021; 5,643,607; and 5,716,640.

Manufactured for
TAP Pharmaceuticals Inc.
Lake Forest, IL 60045, U.S.A.
by Takeda Chemical Industries, Ltd. Osaka, JAPAN 541

® - Registered trademark
(No. 3683)
03-5055-R3; Revised: April 2000

Shown in Product Identification Guide, page 338

LUPRON DEPOT-PED® ℞

(leuprolide acetate for depot suspension)
7.5 mg, 11.25 mg and 15 mg

DESCRIPTION

Leuprolide acetate is a synthetic nonapeptide analog of naturally occurring gonadotropin-releasing hormone (GnRH or LH-RH). The analog possesses greater potency than the natural hormone. The chemical name is 5-oxo-L-prolyl-L-histidyl -L- tryptophyl-L-seryl-L-tyrosyl-D-leucyl-L-leucyl-L-arginyl-N-ethyl-L-prolinamide acetate (salt) with the following structural formula:
[See chemical structure at top of next page]
LUPRON DEPOT-PED is available in a prefilled dual-chamber syringe containing sterile lyophilized microspheres which, when mixed with diluent, become a suspension intended as a single intramuscular injection.
The front chamber of LUPRON DEPOT-PED 7.5 mg, 11.25 mg, and 15 mg prefilled dual-chamber syringe contains leuprolide acetate (7.5/11.25/15 mg), purified gelatin (1.3/1.95/2.6 mg), DL-lactic and glycolic acids copolymer (66.2/99.3/132.4 mg), and D-mannitol (13.2/19.8/26.4 mg). The second chamber of diluent contains carboxymethylcellulose sodium (5 mg), D-mannitol (50 mg), polysorbate 80 (1mg), water for injection, USP, and glacial acetic acid, USP to control pH.
During the manufacture of LUPRON DEPOT-PED, acetic acid is lost, leaving the peptide.

CLINICAL PHARMACOLOGY

Leuprolide acetate, a GnRH agonist, acts as a potent inhibitor of gonadotropin secretion when given continuously and in therapeutic doses. Human studies indicate that following an initial stimulation of gonadotropins, chronic stimulation with leuprolide acetate results in suppression or "downregulation" of these hormones and consequent suppression of ovarian and testicular steroidogenesis. These effects are reversible on discontinuation of drug therapy.
Leuprolide acetate is not active when given orally.

Pharmacokinetics

Absorption Following a single LUPRON DEPOT 7.5 mg injection to adult patients, mean peak leuprolide plasma concentration was almost 20 ng/mL at 4 hours and then declined to 0.36 ng/mL at 4 weeks. However, intact leuprolide and an inactive major metabolite could not be distinguished by the assay which was employed in the study. Nondetectable leuprolide plasma concentrations have been observed during chronic LUPRON DEPOT 7.5 mg administration, but testosterone levels appear to be maintained at castrate levels.

Distribution The mean steady-state volume of distribution of leuprolide following intravenous bolus administration to healthy male volunteers was 27 L. *In vitro* binding to human plasma proteins ranged from 43% to 49%.

Metabolism In healthy male volunteers, a 1 mg bolus of leuprolide administered intravenously revealed that the

Continued on next page

Lupron Depot-PED—Cont.

mean systemic clearance was 7.6 L/h, with a terminal elimination half-life of approximately 3 hours based on a two compartment model.

In rats and dogs, administration of ^{14}C-labeled leuprolide was shown to be metabolized to smaller inactive peptides, a pentapeptide (Metabolite I), tripeptides (Metabolites II and III) and a dipeptide (Metabolite IV). These fragments may be further catabolized.

The major metabolite (M-I) plasma concentrations measured in 5 prostate cancer patients reached maximum concentration 2 to 6 hours after dosing and were approximately 6% of the peak parent drug concentration. One week after dosing, mean plasma M-I concentrations were approximately 20% of mean leuprolide concentrations.

Excretion Following administration of LUPRON DEPOT 3.75 mg to 3 patients, less than 5% of the dose was recovered as parent and M-I metabolite in the urine.

Special Populations The pharmacokinetics of the drug in hepatically and renally impaired patients have not been determined.

CLINICAL STUDIES

In children with central precocious puberty (CPP), stimulated and basal gonadotropins are reduced to prepubertal levels. Testosterone and estradiol are reduced to prepubertal levels in males and females respectively. Reduction of gonadotropins will allow for normal physical and psychological growth and development. Natural maturation occurs when gonadotropins return to pubertal levels following discontinuation of leuprolide acetate.

The following physiologic effects have been noted with the chronic administration of leuprolide acetate in this patient population.

1. ***Skeletal Growth.*** A measurable increase in body length can be noted since the epiphyseal plates will not close prematurely.
2. ***Organ Growth.*** Reproductive organs will return to a prepubertal state.
3. ***Menses.*** Menses, if present, will cease.

In a study of 22 children with central precocious puberty, doses of LUPRON DEPOT were given every 4 weeks and plasma levels were determined according to weight categories as summarized below:

[See table above]

INDICATIONS AND USAGE

LUPRON DEPOT-PED is indicated in the treatment of children with central precocious puberty. Children should be selected using the following criteria:

1. Clinical diagnosis of CPP (idiopathic or neurogenic) with onset of secondary sexual characteristics earlier than 8 years in females and 9 years in males.
2. Clinical diagnosis should be confirmed prior to initiation of therapy:
   - Confirmation of diagnosis by a pubertal response to a GnRH stimulation test. The sensitivity and methodology of this assay must be understood.
   - Bone age advanced one year beyond the chronological age.
3. Baseline evaluation should also include:
   - Height and weight measurements.
   - Sex steroid levels.
   - Adrenal steroid level to exclude congenital adrenal hyperplasia.
   - Beta human chorionic gonadotropin level to rule out a chorionic gonadotropin-secreting tumor.
   - Pelvic/adrenal/testicular ultrasound to rule out a steroid secreting tumor.
   - Computerized tomography of the head to rule out intracranial tumor.

CONTRAINDICATIONS

LUPRON DEPOT-PED is contraindicated in women who are or may become pregnant while receiving the drug. When administered on day 6 of pregnancy at test dosages of 0.00024, 0.0024, and 0.024 mg/kg (1/1200 to 1/12 of the human pediatric dose) to rabbits, LUPRON DEPOT produced a dose-related increase in major fetal abnormalities. Similar studies in rats failed to demonstrate an increase in fetal malformations. There was increased fetal mortality and decreased fetal weights with the two higher doses of LUPRON DEPOT in rabbits and with the highest dose in rats. The effects on fetal mortality are logical consequences of the alterations in hormonal levels brought about by this drug. Therefore, the possibility exists that spontaneous abortion may occur if the drug is administered during pregnancy.

Leuprolide acetate is contraindicated in children demonstrating hypersensitivity to GnRH, GnRH agonist analogs, or any of the excipients.

A report of an anaphylactic reaction to synthetic GnRH (Factrel) has been reported in the medical literature.[1]

WARNINGS

During the early phase of therapy, gonadotropins and sex steroids rise above baseline because of the natural stimulatory effect of the drug. Therefore, an increase in clinical signs and symptoms may be observed. (See **CLINICAL PHARMACOLOGY** section.)

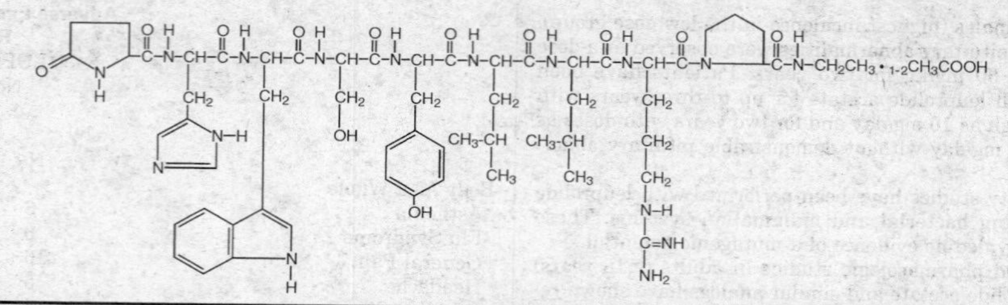

Patient Weight Range (kg)	Group Weight Average (kg)	Dose (mg)	Trough Plasma Leuprolide Level Mean ± SD (ng/mL)*
20.2–27.0	22.7	7.5	0.77±0.033
28.4–36.8	32.5	11.25	1.25±1.06
39.3–57.5	44.2	15.0	1.59±0.65

* Group average values determined at Week 4 immediately prior to leuprolide injection. Drug levels at 12 and 24 weeks were similar to respective 4 week levels.

Noncompliance with drug regimen or inadequate dosing may result in inadequate control of the pubertal process. The consequences of poor control include the return of pubertal signs such as menses, breast development, and testicular growth. The long-term consequences of inadequate control of gonadal steroid secretion are unknown, but may include a further compromise of adult stature.

PRECAUTIONS

Laboratory Tests Response to LUPRON DEPOT-PED should be monitored 1–2 months after the start of therapy with a GnRH stimulation test and sex steroid levels. Measurement of bone age for advancement should be done every 6–12 months.

Sex steroids may increase or rise above prepubertal levels if the dose is inadequate. (See **WARNINGS** section.) Once a therapeutic dose has been established, gonadotropin and sex steroid levels will decline to prepubertal levels.

Drug Interactions No pharmacokinetic-based drug-drug interaction studies have been conducted. However, because leuprolide acetate is a peptide that is primarily degraded by peptidase and not by cytochrome P-450 enzymes as noted in specific studies, and the drug is only about 46% bound to plasma proteins, drug interactions would not be expected to occur.

Drug/Laboratory Test Interactions Administration of LUPRON DEPOT 3.75 mg in women results in suppression of the pituitary-gonadal system. Normal function is usually restored within three months after treatment is discontinued. Therefore, diagnostic tests of pituitary gonadotropic and gonadal functions conducted during treatment and for up to three months after discontinuation of LUPRON DEPOT therapy may be misleading.

Information for Parents Prior to starting therapy with LUPRON DEPOT-PED, the parent or guardian must be aware of the importance of continuous therapy. Adherence to 4 week drug administration schedules must be accepted if therapy is to be successful.

- During the first 2 months of therapy, a female may experience menses or spotting. If bleeding continues beyond the second month, notify the physician.
- Any irritation at the injection site should be reported to the physician immediately.
- Report any unusual signs or symptoms to the physician.

Carcinogenesis, Mutagenesis, Impairment of Fertility A two-year carcinogenicity study was conducted in rats and mice. In rats, a dose-related increase of benign pituitary hyperplasia and benign pituitary adenomas was noted at 24 months when the drug was administered subcutaneously at high daily doses (0.6 to 4 mg/kg). There was a significant but not dose-related increase of pancreatic islet-cell adenomas in females and of testicular interstitial cell adenomas in males (highest incidence in the low dose group). In mice, no leuprolide acetate-induced tumors or pituitary abnormalities were observed at a dose as high as 60 mg/kg for two years. Adult patients have been treated with leuprolide acetate for up to three years with doses as high as 10 mg/day and for two years with doses as high as 20 mg/day without demonstrable pituitary abnormalities.

Although no clinical studies have been completed in children to assess the full reversibility of fertility suppression, animal studies (prepubertal and adult rats and monkeys) with leuprolide acetate and other GnRH analogs have shown functional recovery. However, following a study with leuprolide acetate, immature male rats demonstrated tubular degeneration in the testes even after a recovery period. In spite of the failure to recover histologically, the treated males proved to be as fertile as the controls. Also, no histologic changes were observed in the female rats following the same protocol. In both sexes, the offspring of the treated animals appeared normal. The effect of the treatment of the parents on the reproductive performance of the F1 generation was not tested. The clinical significance of these findings is unknown.

Pregnancy, Teratogenic Effects Pregnancy Category X. See **CONTRAINDICATIONS** section.

Nursing Mothers It is not known whether leuprolide acetate is excreted in human milk. LUPRON should not be used by nursing mothers.

ADVERSE REACTIONS

Clinical Trials

Potential exacerbation of signs and symptoms during the first few weeks of treatment. (See **PRECAUTIONS** section.) is a concern in patients with rapidly advancing central precocious puberty.

In two studies of children with central precocious puberty, in 2% or more of the patients receiving the drug, the following adverse reactions were reported to have a possible or probable relationship to drug as ascribed by the treating physician. Reactions which are not considered drug-related are excluded.

	Number of Patients N=395	(%)
Body as a Whole		
General Pain	7	(2)
Integumentary System		
Acne/Seborrhea	7	(2)
Injection Site Reactions Including Abscess	21	(5)
Rash Including Erythema Multiforme	8	(2)
Urogenital System		
Vaginitis/Bleeding/ Discharge	7	(2)

In those same studies, the following adverse reactions were reported in less than 2% of the patients.

Body as a Whole—Body Odor, Fever, Headache, Infection; *Cardiovascular System*—Syncope, Vasodilation; *Digestive System*—Dysphagia, Gingivitis, Nausea/Vomiting; *Endocrine System*—Accelerated Sexual Maturity; *Metabolic and Nutritional Disorders*—Peripheral Edema, Weight Gain; *Nervous System*—Emotional Lability, Nervousness, Personality Disorder, Somnolence; *Respiratory System*—Epistaxis; *Integumentary System*—Alopecia, Skin Striae; *Urogenital System*—Cervix Disorder, Gynecomastia/Breast Disorders, Urinary Incontinence.

Postmarketing

During postmarketing surveillance, which includes other dosage forms, the following adverse events were reported. Symptoms consistent with an anaphylactoid or asthmatic process have been rarely reported. Rash, urticaria, and photosensitivity reactions have also been reported.

Localized reactions including induration and abscess have been reported at the site of injection.

Cardiovascular System—Hypotension; *Hemic and Lymphatic System*—Decreased WBC; *Central/Peripheral Nervous System*—Peripheral neuropathy, Spinal fracture/paralysis; *Musculoskeletal System*—Tenosynovitis-like symptoms; *Urogenital System*—Prostate pain.

See other LUPRON DEPOT and LUPRON Injection package inserts for other events reported in different patient populations.

OVERDOSAGE

In rats, subcutaneous administration of 125 to 250 times the recommended human pediatric dose, expressed on a per body weight basis, resulted in dyspnea, decreased activity, and local irritation at the injection site. There is no evidence at present that there is a clinical counterpart of this phenomenon. In early clinical trials using leuprolide acetate in adult patients, doses as high as 20 mg/day for up to two years caused no adverse effects differing from those observed with the 1 mg/day dose.

DOSAGE AND ADMINISTRATION

LUPRON DEPOT-PED must be administered under the supervision of a physician.

The dose of LUPRON DEPOT-PED must be individualized for each child. The dose is based on a mg/kg ratio of drug to body weight. Younger children require higher doses on a mg/kg ratio.

For each dosage form, after 1-2 months of initiating therapy or changing doses, the child must be monitored with a

GnRH stimulation test, sex steroids, and Tanner staging to confirm downregulation. Measurements of bone age for advancement should be monitored every 6-12 months. The dose should be titrated upward until no progression of the condition is noted either clinically and/or by laboratory parameters.
The first dose found to result in adequate downregulation can probably be maintained for the duration of therapy in most children. However, there are insufficient data to guide dosage adjustment as patients move into higher weight categories after beginning therapy at very young ages and low dosages. It is recommended that adequate downregulation be verified in such patients whose weight has increased significantly while on therapy.
Discontinuation of LUPRON DEPOT-PED should be considered before age 11 for females and age 12 for males.
The recommended starting dose is 0.3 mg/kg/4 weeks (minimum 7.5 mg) administered as a single intramuscular injection. The starting dose will be dictated by the child's weight.

≤ 25 kg	7.5 mg
> 25–37.5 kg	11.25 mg
> 37.5 kg	15 mg

If total downregulation is not achieved, the dose should be titrated upward in increments of 3.75 mg every 4 weeks. This dose will be considered the maintenance dose.
The lyophilized microspheres are to be reconstituted and administered as a single intramuscular injection, in accord with the following directions:

1. To prepare for injection, screw the white plunger into the end stopper until the stopper begins to turn.
2. Remove and discard the tab around the base of the needle.
3. Holding the syringe upright, release the diluent by SLOWLY PUSHING the plunger until the first stopper is at the blue line in the middle of the barrel.
4. Gently shake the syringe to thoroughly mix the particles to form a uniform suspension. The suspension will appear milky.
5. If the microspheres (particles) adhere to the stopper, tap the syringe against your finger.
6. Then remove the needle guard and advance the plunger to expel the air from the syringe.
7. Inject the entire contents of the syringe intramuscularly as you would for a normal injection.

Although the potency of the reconstituted suspension has been shown to be stable for 24 hours, since the product does not contain a preservative, the suspension should be discarded if not used immediately.
As with other drugs administered by injection, the injection site should be varied periodically.

HOW SUPPLIED

LUPRON DEPOT-PED is packaged as follows:
Kit with prefilled dual-chamber syringe
7.5 mg NDC 0300-2108-01
Kit with prefilled dual-chamber syringe
11.25 mg NDC 0300-2282-01
Kit with prefilled dual-chamber syringe
15 mg NDC 0300-2440-01
Each syringe contains sterile lyophilized microspheres which is leuprolide incorporated in a biodegradable copolymer of lactic and glycolic acids. When mixed with diluent, LUPRON DEPOT-PED is administered as a single IM injection.
An information pamphlet for parents is included with the kit.
Store at 25°C (77°F); excursions permitted to 15–30°C (59–86°F) [See USP Controlled Room Temperature]

Rx only

REFERENCE

1. MacLeod TL, *et al.* Anaphylactic reaction to synthetic luteinizing hormone-releasing hormone. *Fertil Steril* 1987 Sept;48(3):500–502.

U.S. Patent Nos. 4,652,441; 4,677,191; 4,728,721; 4,849,228; 4,917,893; 4,954,298; 5,330,767; and 5,476,663.

Manufactured for
TAP Pharmaceuticals Inc.
Lake Forest, IL 60045, U.S.A.
Takeda Chemical Industries, Ltd.
Osaka, JAPAN 541
®—Registered Trademark
(Nos. 2108, 2282, 2440)
03-5010-R8; Revised: April 2000

PREVACID® ℞
[prē′-va-sĭd]
(lansoprazole)
Delayed-Release Capsules

DESCRIPTION

The active ingredient in PREVACID (lansoprazole) Delayed-Release Capsules is a substituted benzimidazole, 2-[[[3-methyl-4-(2,2,2-trifluoroethoxy)-2-pyridyl] methyl] sulfinyl] benzimidazole, a compound that inhibits gastric acid secretion. Its empirical formula is $C_{16}H_{14}F_3N_3O_2S$ with a molecular weight of 369.37. The structural formula is:
[See chemical structure at top of next column]

Table 1
Mean Antisecretory Effects after Single and Multiple Daily Dosing

Parameter	Baseline Value	PREVACID 15 mg Day 1	PREVACID 15 mg Day 5	PREVACID 30 mg Day 1	PREVACID 30 mg Day 5	Omeprazole 20 mg Day 1	Omeprazole 20 mg Day 5
Mean 24-Hour pH	2.1	2.7⁺	4.0⁺	3.6*	4.9*	2.5	4.2⁺
Mean Nighttime pH	1.9	2.4	3.0⁺	2.6	3.8*	2.2	3.0⁺
% Time Gastric pH>3	18	33⁺	59⁺	51*	72*	30⁺	61⁺
% Time Gastric pH>4	12	22⁺	49⁺	41*	66*	19	51⁺

NOTE: An intragastric pH of >4 reflects a reduction in gastric acid by 99%.
*(p<0.05) versus baseline, lansoprazole 15 mg and omeprazole 20 mg.
⁺(p<0.05) versus baseline only.

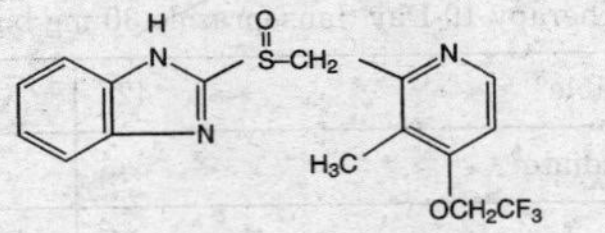

Lansoprazole is a white to brownish-white odorless crystalline powder which melts with decomposition at approximately 166°C. Lansoprazole is freely soluble in dimethylformamide; soluble in methanol; sparingly soluble in ethanol; slightly soluble in ethyl acetate, dichloromethane and acetonitrile; very slightly soluble in ether; and practically insoluble in hexane and water.
Lansoprazole is stable when exposed to light for up to two months. The compound degrades in aqueous solution, the rate of degradation increasing with decreasing pH. At 25°C the $t_{½}$ is approximately 0.5 hour at pH 5.0 and approximately 18 hours at pH 7.0.
PREVACID is supplied in delayed-release capsules for oral administration. The delayed-release capsules contain the active ingredient, lansoprazole, in the form of enteric-coated granules and are available in two dosage strengths: 15 mg and 30 mg of lansoprazole per capsule. Each delayed-release capsule contains enteric-coated granules consisting of lansoprazole, hydroxypropyl cellulose, low substituted hydroxypropyl cellulose, colloidal silicon dioxide, magnesium carbonate, methacrylic acid copolymer, starch, talc, sugar sphere, sucrose, polyethylene glycol, polysorbate 80, and titanium dioxide. Components of the gelatin capsule include gelatin, titanium dioxide, D&C Red No. 28, FD&C Blue No. 1, FD&C Green No. 3*, and FD&C Red No. 40.
* PREVACID 15-mg capsules only.

CLINICAL PHARMACOLOGY

Pharmacokinetics and Metabolism

PREVACID Delayed-Release Capsules contain an enteric-coated granule formulation of lansoprazole. Absorption of lansoprazole begins only after the granules leave the stomach. Absorption is rapid, with mean peak plasma levels of lansoprazole occurring after approximately 1.7 hours. Peak plasma concentrations of lansoprazole (C_{max}) and the area under the plasma concentration curve (AUC) of lansoprazole are approximately proportional in doses from 15 mg to 60 mg after single-oral administration. Lansoprazole does not accumulate and its pharmacokinetics are unaltered by multiple dosing.

Absorption

The absorption of lansoprazole is rapid, with mean C_{max} occurring approximately 1.7 hours after oral dosing, and relatively complete with absolute bioavailability over 80%. In healthy subjects, the mean (± SD) plasma half-life was 1.5 (± 1.0) hours. Both C_{max} and AUC are diminished by about 50% if the drug is given 30 minutes after food as opposed to the fasting condition. There is no significant food effect if the drug is given before meals.

Distribution

Lansoprazole is 97% bound to plasma proteins. Plasma protein binding is constant over the concentration range of 0.05 to 5.0 µg/mL.

Metabolism

Lansoprazole is extensively metabolized in the liver. Two metabolites have been identified in measurable quantities in plasma (the hydroxylated sulfinyl and sulfone derivatives of lansoprazole). These metabolites have very little or no antisecretory activity. Lansoprazole is thought to be transformed into two active species which inhibit acid secretion by (H^+,K^+)-ATPase within the parietal cell canaliculus, but are not present in the systemic circulation. The plasma elimination half-life of lansoprazole does not reflect its duration of suppression of gastric acid secretion. Thus, the plasma elimination half-life is less than two hours, while the acid inhibitory effect lasts more than 24 hours.

Elimination

Following single-dose oral administration of lansoprazole, virtually no unchanged lansoprazole was excreted in the urine. In one study, after a single oral dose of ^{14}C-lansoprazole, approximately one-third of the administered radiation was excreted in the urine and two-thirds was recovered in the feces. This implies a significant biliary excretion of the metabolites of lansoprazole.

Special Populations

Geriatric
The clearance of lansoprazole is decreased in the elderly, with elimination half-life increased approximately 50% to 100%. Because the mean half-life in the elderly remains between 1.9 to 2.9 hours, repeated once daily dosing does not result in accumulation of lansoprazole. Peak plasma levels were not increased in the elderly.
Pediatric
The pharmacokinetics of lansoprazole has not been investigated in patients <18 years of age.
Gender
In a study comparing 12 male and 6 female human subjects, no gender differences were found in pharmacokinetics and intragastric pH results. (Also see **Use in Women.**)
Renal Insufficiency
In patients with severe renal insufficiency, plasma protein binding decreased by 1.0%–1.5% after administration of 60 mg of lansoprazole. Patients with renal insufficiency had a shortened elimination half-life and decreased total AUC (free and bound). AUC for free lansoprazole in plasma, however, was not related to the degree of renal impairment, and C_{max} and T_{max} were not different from subjects with healthy kidneys.
Hepatic Insufficiency
In patients with various degrees of chronic hepatic disease, the mean plasma half-life of the drug was prolonged from 1.5 hours to 3.2–7.2 hours. An increase in mean AUC of up to 500% was observed at steady state in hepatically-impaired patients compared to healthy subjects. Dose reduction in patients with severe hepatic disease should be considered.
Race
The pooled mean pharmacokinetic parameters of lansoprazole from twelve U.S. Phase 1 studies (N=513) were compared to the mean pharmacokinetic parameters from two Asian studies (N=20). The mean AUCs of lansoprazole in Asian subjects were approximately twice those seen in pooled U.S. data; however, the inter-individual variability was high. The C_{max} values were comparable.

Pharmacodynamics

Mechanism of action

Lansoprazole belongs to a class of antisecretory compounds, the substituted benzimidazoles, that do not exhibit anticholinergic or histamine H_2-receptor antagonist properties, but that suppress gastric acid secretion by specific inhibition of the (H^+,K^+)-ATPase enzyme system at the secretory surface of the gastric parietal cell. Because this enzyme system is regarded as the acid (proton) pump within the parietal cell, lansoprazole has been characterized as a gastric acid-pump inhibitor, in that it blocks the final step of acid production. This effect is dose-related and leads to inhibition of both basal and stimulated gastric acid secretion irrespective of the stimulus.

Antisecretory activity

After oral administration, lansoprazole was shown to significantly decrease the basal acid output and significantly increase the mean gastric pH and percent of time the gastric pH was >3 and >4. Lansoprazole also significantly reduced meal-stimulated gastric acid output and secretion volume, as well as pentagastrin-stimulated acid output. In patients with hypersecretion of acid, lansoprazole significantly reduced basal and pentagastrin-stimulated gastric acid secretion. Lansoprazole inhibited the normal increases in secretion volume, acidity and acid output induced by insulin.
In a crossover study comparing lansoprazole 15 and 30 mg with omeprazole 20 mg for five days, the following effects on intragastric pH were noted. See Table 1.
[See table above]
After the initial dose in this study, increased gastric pH was seen within 1–2 hours with lansoprazole 30 mg, 2–3 hours with lansoprazole 15 mg, and 3–4 hours with omeprazole 20 mg. After multiple daily dosing, increased gastric pH was seen within the first hour postdosing with lansoprazole 30 mg and within 1–2 hours postdosing with lansoprazole 15 mg and omeprazole 20 mg.
Acid suppression may enhance the effect of antimicrobials in eradicating *Helicobacter pylori (H. pylori)*. The percentage of time gastric pH was elevated above 5 and 6 was evaluated in a crossover study of PREVACID given q.d., b.i.d. and t.i.d. See Table 2.

Continued on next page

Prevacid—Cont.

Table 2
Mean Antisecretory Effects After 5 Days of b.i.d. and t.i.d. Dosing

	PREVACID			
Parameter	30 mg q.d.	15 mg b.i.d.	30 mg b.i.d.	30 mg t.i.d.
% Time Gastric pH>5	43	47	59⁺	77*
% Time Gastric pH>6	20	23	28	45*

⁺ ($p<0.05$) versus PREVACID 30 mg q.d.
* ($p<0.05$) versus PREVACID 30 mg q.d., 15 mg b.i.d. and 30 mg b.i.d.

The inhibition of gastric acid secretion as measured by intragastric pH returns gradually to normal over two to four days after multiple doses. There is no indication of rebound gastric acidity.

Enterochromaffin-like (ECL) cell effects

During lifetime exposure of rats with up to 150 mg/kg/day of lansoprazole dosed seven days per week, marked hypergastrinemia was observed followed by ECL cell proliferation and formation of carcinoid tumors, especially in female rats. (See **PRECAUTIONS, Carcinogenesis, Mutagenesis, Impairment of Fertility.**)

Gastric biopsy specimens from the body of the stomach from approximately 150 patients treated continuously with lansoprazole for at least one year did not show evidence of ECL cell effects similar to those seen in rat studies. Longer term data are needed to rule out the possibility of an increased risk of the development of gastric tumors in patients receiving long-term therapy with lansoprazole.

Other gastric effects in humans

Lansoprazole did not significantly affect mucosal blood flow in the fundus of the stomach. Due to the normal physiologic effect caused by the inhibition of gastric acid secretion, a decrease of about 17% in blood flow in the antrum, pylorus, and duodenal bulb was seen. Lansoprazole significantly slowed the gastric emptying of digestible solids. Lansoprazole increased serum pepsinogen levels and decreased pepsin activity under basal conditions and in response to meal stimulation or insulin injection. As with other agents that elevate intragastric pH, increases in gastric pH were associated with increases in nitrate-reducing bacteria and elevation of nitrite concentration in gastric juice in patients with gastric ulcer. No significant increase in nitrosamine concentrations was observed.

Serum gastrin effects

In over 2100 patients, median fasting serum gastrin levels increased 50% to 100% from baseline but remained within normal range after treatment with lansoprazole given orally in doses of 15 mg to 60 mg. These elevations reached a plateau within two months of therapy and returned to pretreatment levels within four weeks after discontinuation of therapy.

Endocrine effects

Human studies for up to one year have not detected any clinically significant effects on the endocrine system. Hormones studied include testosterone, luteinizing hormone (LH), follicle stimulating hormone (FSH), sex hormone binding globulin (SHBG), dehydroepiandrosterone sulfate (DHEA-S), prolactin, cortisol, estradiol, insulin, aldosterone, parathormone, glucagon, thyroid stimulating hormone (TSH), triiodothyronine (T_3), thyroxine (T_4), and somatotropic hormone (STH). Lansoprazole in oral doses of 15 to 60 mg for up to one year had no clinically significant effect on sexual function. In addition, lansoprazole in oral doses of 15 to 60 mg for two to eight weeks had no clinically significant effect on thyroid function.

In 24-month carcinogenicity studies in Sprague-Dawley rats with daily dosages up to 150 mg/kg, proliferative changes in the Leydig cells of the testes, including benign neoplasm, were increased compared to control rates.

Other effects

No systemic effects of lansoprazole on the central nervous system, lymphoid, hematopoietic, renal, hepatic, cardiovascular or respiratory systems have been found in humans. No visual toxicity was observed among 56 patients who had extensive baseline eye evaluations, were treated with up to 180 mg/day of lansoprazole and were observed for up to 58 months. Other rat-specific findings after lifetime exposure included focal pancreatic atrophy, diffuse lymphoid hyperplasia in the thymus, and spontaneous retinal atrophy.

CLINICAL PHARMACOLOGY

Microbiology

Lansoprazole, clarithromycin and/or amoxicillin have been shown to be active against most strains of *Helicobacter pylori in vitro* and in clinical infections as described in the **INDICATIONS AND USAGE** section.

Table 3
Clarithromycin Susceptibility Test Results and Clinical/Bacteriological Outcomes[a]

Clarithromycin Pretreatment Results		Clarithromycin Post-treatment Results				
		H. pylori negative-eradicated	*H. pylori* positive-not eradicated			
			Post-treatment susceptibility results			
			S[b]	I[b]	R[b]	No MIC
Triple Therapy 14-Day (lansoprazole 30 mg b.i.d./amoxicillin 1 gm b.i.d./clarithromycin 500 mg b.i.d.) (M95-399, M93-131, M95-392)						
Susceptible[b]	112	105				7
Intermediate[b]	3	3				
Resistant[b]	17	6			7	4
Triple Therapy 10-Day (lansoprazole 30 mg b.i.d./amoxicillin 1 gm b.i.d./clarithromycin 500 mg b.i.d.) (M95-399)						
Susceptible[b]	42	40	1		1	
Intermediate[b]						
Resistant[b]	4	1			3	

[a] Includes only patients with pretreatment clarithromycin susceptibility test results
[b] Susceptibility (S) MIC ≤ 0.25 μg/mL, Intermediate (I) MIC 0.5–1.0 μg/mL, Resistant (R) MIC ≥ 2 μg/mL

Table 4
Duodenal Ulcer Healing Rates

	PREVACID			Placebo
Week	15 mg q.d. (N=68)	30 mg q.d. (N=74)	60 mg q.d. (N=70)	(N=72)
2	42.4%*	35.6%*	39.1%*	11.3%
4	89.4%*	91.7%*	89.9%*	46.1%

*($p\leq0.001$) versus placebo.

Helicobacter

Helicobacter pylori

Pretreatment Resistance

Clarithromycin pretreatment resistance (≥ 2.0 μg/mL) was 9.5% (91/960) by E-test and 11.3% (12/106) by agar dilution in the dual and triple therapy clinical trials (M93-125, M93-130, M93-131, M95-392, and M95-399).

Amoxicillin pretreatment susceptible isolates (≤ 0.25 μg/mL) occurred in 97.8% (936/957) and 98.0% (98/100) of the patients in the dual and triple therapy clinical trials by E-test and agar dilution, respectively. Twenty-one of 957 patients (2.2%) by E-test and 2 of 100 patients (2.0%) by agar dilution had amoxicillin pretreatment MICs of > 0.25 μg/mL. One patient on the 14-day triple therapy regimen had an unconfirmed pretreatment amoxicillin minimum inhibitory concentration (MIC) of > 256 μg/mL by E-test and the patient was eradicated of *H. pylori*. See Table 3.

[See table 3 above]

Patients not eradicated of *H. pylori* following lansoprazole/amoxicillin/clarithromycin triple therapy will likely have clarithromycin resistant *H. pylori*. Therefore, for those patients who fail therapy, clarithromycin susceptibility testing should be done when possible. Patients with clarithromycin resistant *H. pylori* should not be treated with lansoprazole/amoxicillin/clarithromycin triple therapy or with regimens which include clarithromycin as the sole antimicrobial agent.

<u>Amoxicillin Susceptibility Test Results and Clinical/Bacteriological Outcomes</u>

In the dual and triple therapy clinical trials, 82.6% (195/236) of the patients that had pretreatment amoxicillin susceptible MICs (≤ 0.25 μg/mL) were eradicated of H. pylori. Of those with pretreatment amoxicillin MICs of > 0.25 μg/mL, three of six had the H. pylori eradicated. A total of 30% (21/70) of the patients failed lansoprazole 30 mg t.i.d./amoxicillin 1 gm t.i.d. dual therapy and a total of 12.8% (22/172) of the patients failed the 10- and 14-day triple therapy regimens. Post-treatment susceptibility results were not obtained on 11 of the patients who failed therapy. Nine of the 11 patients with amoxicillin post-treatment MICs that failed the triple therapy regimen also had clarithromycin resistant H. pylori isolates.

<u>Susceptibility Test for *Helicobacter pylori*</u>

The reference methodology for susceptibility testing of *H. pylori* is agar dilution MICs.[1] One to three microliters of an inoculum equivalent to a No. 2 McFarland standard (1×10^7 - 1×10^8 CFU/mL for *H. pylori*) are inoculated directly onto freshly prepared antimicrobial containing Mueller-Hinton agar plates with 5% aged defibrinated sheep blood (≥ 2 weeks old). The agar dilution plates are incubated at 35°C in a microaerobic environment produced by a gas generating system suitable for campylobacters. After 3 days of incubation, the MICs are recorded as the lowest concentration of antimicrobial agent required to inhibit growth of the organism. The clarithromycin and amoxicillin MIC values should be interpreted according to the following criteria:

Clarithromycin MIC (μg/mL)[a]	Interpretation
≤ 0.25	Susceptible (S)
0.5–1.0	Intermediate (I)
≥ 2.0	Resistant (R)
Amoxicillin MIC (μg/mL)[b]	Interpretation
≤ 0.25	Susceptible (S)

[a] These are tentative breakpoints for the agar dilution methodology and they should not be used to interpret results obtained using alternative methods.
[b] There were not enough organisms with MICs > 0.25 μg/mL to determine a resistance breakpoint.

Standardized susceptibility test procedures require the use of laboratory control microorganisms to control the technical aspects of the laboratory procedures. Standard clarithromycin and amoxicillin powders should provide the following MIC values:

Microorganism	Antimicrobial Agent	MIC (μg/mL)[a]
H. pylori ATCC 43504	Clarithromycin	0.015–0.12 mcg/mL
H. pylori ATCC 43504	Amoxicillin	0.015–0.12 mcg/mL

[a] These are quality control ranges for the agar dilution methodology and they should not be used to control test results obtained using alternative methods.

Reference

1. National Committee for Clinical Laboratory Standards. Summary Minutes, Subcommittee on Antimicrobial Susceptibility Testing, Tampa, FL, January 11–13, 1998.

CLINICAL STUDIES

Duodenal Ulcer

In a U.S. multicenter, double-blind, placebo-controlled, dose-response (15, 30, and 60 mg of PREVACID once daily) study of 284 patients with endoscopically documented duodenal ulcer, the percentage of patients healed after two and four weeks was significantly higher with all doses of PREVACID than with placebo. There was no evidence of a greater or earlier response with the two higher doses compared with PREVACID 15 mg. Based on this study and the second study described below, the recommended dose of PREVACID in duodenal ulcer is 15 mg per day. See Table 4.

[See table 4 above]

PREVACID 15 mg was significantly more effective than placebo in relieving day and nighttime abdominal pain and in decreasing the amount of antacid taken per day.

In a second U.S. multicenter study, also double-blind, placebo-controlled, dose-comparison (15 and 30 mg of PREVACID once daily), and including a comparison with ranitidine, in 280 patients with endoscopically documented duodenal ulcer, the percentage of patients healed after four weeks was significantly higher with both doses of PREVACID than

Table 5
Duodenal Ulcer Healing Rates

Week	PREVACID 15 mg q.d. (N=80)	PREVACID 30 mg q.d. (N=77)	Ranitidine 300 mg h.s. (N=82)	Placebo (N=41)
2	35.0%	44.2%	30.5%	34.2%
4	92.3%**	80.3%*	70.5%*	47.5%

*(p≤0.05) versus placebo.
**(p≤0.05) versus placebo and ranitidine.

Table 6
***H. pylori* Eradication Rates—Triple Therapy**
(PREVACID/amoxicillin/clarithromycin)
Percent of Patients Cured
[95% Confidence Interval]
(Number of Patients)

Study	Duration	Triple Therapy Evaluable Analysis*	Triple Therapy Intent-to-Treat Analysis#
M93-131	14 days	92† [80.0–97.7] (N=48)	86† [73.3–93.5] (N=55)
M95-392	14 days	86‡ [75.7–93.6] (N=66)	83‡ [72.0–90.8] (N=70)
M95-399+	14 days	85 [77.0–91.0] (N=113)	82 [73.9–88.1] (N=126)
	10 days	84 [76.0–89.8] (N=123)	81 [73.9–87.6] (N=135)

* Based on evaluable patients with confirmed duodenal ulcer (active or within one year) and *H. pylori* infection at baseline defined as at least two of three positive endoscopic tests from CLOtest® (Delta West Ltd., Bentley, Australia), histology and/or culture. Patients were included in the analysis if they completed the study. Additionally, if patients dropped out of the study due to an adverse event related to the study drug, they were included in the evaluable analysis as failures of therapy.
\# Patients were included in the analysis if they had documented *H. pylori* infection at baseline as defined above and had a confirmed duodenal ulcer (active or within one year). All dropouts were included as failures of therapy.
† (p<0.05) versus PREVACID/amoxicillin and PREVACID/clarithromycin dual therapy
‡ (p<0.05) versus clarithromcyin/amoxicillin dual therapy
\+ The 95% confidence interval for the difference in eradication rates, 10-day minus 14-day is (-10.5, 8.1) in the evaluable analysis and (-9.7, 9.1) in the intent-to-treat analysis.

Table 7
***H. pylori* Eradication Rates—14-Day Dual Therapy**
PREVACID/amoxicillin)
Percent of Patients Cured
[95% Confidence Interval]
(Number of Patients)

Study	Dual Therapy Evaluable Analysis*	Dual Therapy Intent-to-Treat Analysis#
M93-131	77† [62.5–87.2] (N=51)	70† [56.8–81.2] (N=60)
M93-125	66‡ [51.9–77.5] (N=58)	61‡ [48.5–72.9] (N=67)

* Based on evaluable patients with confirmed duodenal ulcer (active or within one year) and *H. pylori* infection at baseline defined as at least two of three positive endoscopic tests from CLOtest®, histology and/or culture. Patients were included in the analysis if they completed the study. Additionally, if patients dropped out of the study due to an adverse event related to the study drug, they were included in the analysis as failures of therapy.
\# Patients were included in the analysis if they had documented *H. pylori* infection at baseline as defined above and had a confirmed duodenal ulcer (active or within one year). All dropouts were included as failures of therapy.
† (p<0.05) versus PREVACID alone.
‡ (p<0.05) versus PREVACID alone or amoxicillin alone.

Table 8
Endoscopic Remission Rates

Trial	Drug	No. of Pts.	Percent in Endoscopic Remission 0–3 mo.	0–6 mo.	0–12 mo.
#1	PREVACID 15 mg q.d.	86	90%*	87%*	84%*
	Placebo	83	49%	41%	39%
#2	PREVACID 30 mg q.d.	18	94%	94%*	85%*
	PREVACID 15 mg q.d.	15	87%*	79%*	70%*
	Placebo	15	33%	0%	0%

%=Life Table Estimate
*(p≤0.001) versus placebo.

with placebo. There was no evidence of a greater or earlier response with the higher dose of PREVACID. Although the 15 mg dose of PREVACID was superior to ranitidine at 4 weeks, the lack of significant difference at 2 weeks and the absence of a difference between 30 mg of PREVACID and ranitidine leaves the comparative effectiveness of the two agents undetermined. See Table 5.
[See table 5 above]

***H. pylori* Eradication to Reduce the Risk of Duodenal Ulcer Recurrence**
Randomized, double-blind clinical studies performed in the U.S. in patients with *H. pylori* and duodenal ulcer disease (defined as an active ulcer or history of an ulcer within one year) evaluated the efficacy of PREVACID in combination with amoxicillin capsules and clarithromycin tablets as triple 14-day therapy or in combination with amoxicillin capsules as dual 14-day therapy for the eradication of *H. pylori*. Based on the results of these studies, the safety and efficacy of two different eradication regimens were established:

Triple therapy: PREVACID 30 mg b.i.d./amoxicillin 1 gm b.i.d./clarithromycin 500 mg b.i.d.
Dual therapy: PREVACID 30 mg t.i.d./amoxicillin 1 gm t.i.d.

All treatments were for 14 days. *H. pylori* eradication was defined as two negative tests (culture and histology) at 4–6 weeks following the end of treatment.
Triple therapy was shown to be more effective than all possible dual therapy combinations. Dual therapy was shown to be more effective than both monotherapies. Eradication of *H. pylori* has been shown to reduce the risk of duodenal ulcer recurrence.
A randomized, double-blind clinical study performed in the U.S. in patients with *H. pylori* and duodenal ulcer disease (defined as an active ulcer or history of an ulcer within one year) compared the efficacy of PREVACID triple therapy for 10 and 14 days. This study established that the 10-day triple therapy was equivalent to the 14-day triple therapy in eradicating *H. pylori.* See Tables 6 and 7.
[See table 6 at left]
[See table 7 below]

Long-Term Maintenance Treatment of Duodenal Ulcers
PREVACID has been shown to prevent the recurrence of duodenal ulcers. Two independent, double-blind, multicenter, controlled trials were conducted in patients with endoscopically confirmed healed duodenal ulcers. Patients remained healed significantly longer and the number of recurrences of duodenal ulcers was significantly less in patients treated with PREVACID than in patients treated with placebo over a 12-month period. In trial #2, no significant difference was noted between PREVACID 15 mg and 30 mg in maintaining remission. See Table 8.
[See table 8 below]

Gastric Ulcer
In a U.S. multicenter, double-blind, placebo-controlled study of 253 patients with endoscopically documented gastric ulcer, the percentage of patients healed at four and eight weeks was significantly higher with PREVACID 15 mg and 30 mg once a day than with placebo.
Patients treated with any PREVACID dose reported significantly less day and night abdominal pain along with fewer days of antacid use and fewer antacid tablets used per day than the placebo group.
Independent substantiation of the effectiveness of PREVACID 30 mg was provided by a meta-analysis of published and unpublished data. See Table 9.
[See table 9 at top of next page]

Gastroesophageal Reflux Disease (GERD)
Symptomatic GERD
In a U.S. multicenter, double-blind, placebo-controlled study of 214 patients with frequent GERD symptoms, but no esophageal erosions by endoscopy, significantly greater relief of heartburn associated with GERD was observed with the administration of lansoprazole 15 mg once daily up to 8 weeks than with placebo. No significant additional benefit from lansoprazole 30 mg once daily was observed.
The intent-to-treat analyses demonstrated significant reduction in frequency and severity of day and night heartburn. Data for frequency and severity for the 8-week treatment period are shown in Table 10 and Figures 1 and 2.
[See table 10 at top of next page]

Figure 1
Mean Severity of Day Heartburn By Study Day For Evaluable Patients (3=Severe, 2=Moderate, 1=Mild, 0=None)

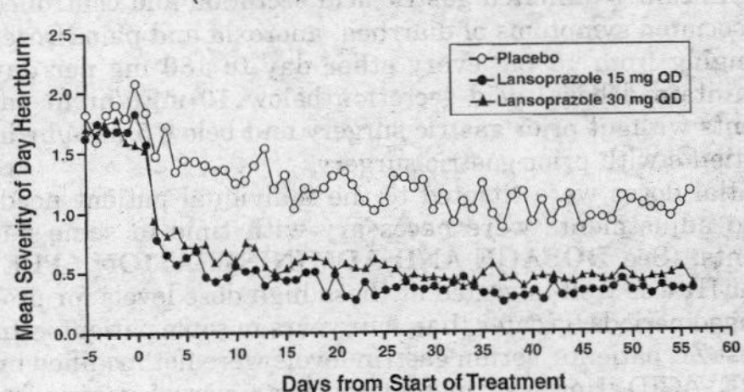

Figure 2
Mean Severity of Night Heartburn By Study Day For Evaluable Patients (3=Severe, 2=Moderate, 1=Mild, 0=None)

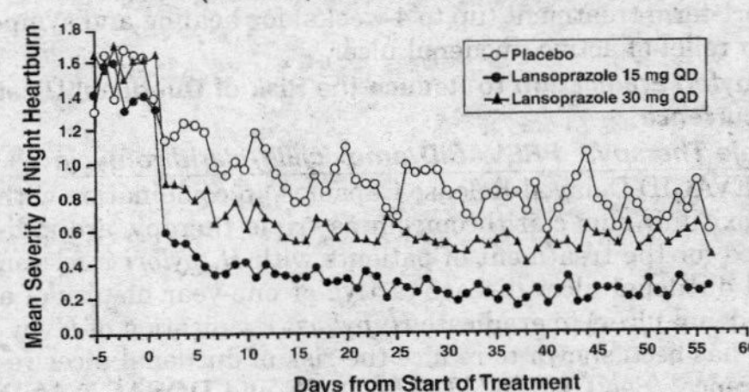

Erosive Esophagitis
In a U.S. multicenter, double-blind, placebo-controlled study of 269 patients entering with an endoscopic diagnosis of

Continued on next page

Prevacid—Cont.

esophagitis with mucosal grading of 2 or more and grades 3 and 4 signifying erosive disease, the percentages of patients with healing were as shown in Table 11.
[See table 11 at right]
In this study, all PREVACID groups reported significantly greater relief of heartburn and less day and night abdominal pain along with fewer days of antacid use and fewer antacid tablets taken per day than the placebo group.
Although all doses were effective, the earlier healing in the higher two doses suggests 30 mg q.d. as the recommended dose.
PREVACID was also compared in a U.S. multicenter, double-blind study to a low dose of ranitidine in 242 patients with erosive reflux esophagitis. PREVACID at a dose of 30 mg was significantly more effective than ranitidine 150 mg b.i.d. as shown in Table 12.
[See table 12 below]
In addition, patients treated with PREVACID reported less day and nighttime heartburn and took less antacid tablets for fewer days than patients taking ranitidine 150 mg b.i.d.
Although this study demonstrates effectiveness of PREVACID in healing erosive esophagitis, it does not represent an adequate comparison with ranitidine because the recommended ranitidine dose for esophagitis is 150 mg q.i.d., twice the dose used in this study.
In the two trials described and in several smaller studies involving patients with moderate to severe erosive esophagitis, PREVACID produced healing rates similar to those shown above.
In a U.S. multicenter, double-blind, active-controlled study, 30 mg of PREVACID was compared with ranitidine 150 mg b.i.d. in 151 patients with erosive reflux esophagitis that was poorly responsive to a minimum of 12 weeks of treatment with at least one H_2-receptor antagonist given at the dose indicated for symptom relief or greater, namely, cimetidine 800 mg/day, ranitidine 300 mg/day, famotidine 40 mg/day or nizatidine 300 mg/day. PREVACID 30 mg was more effective than ranitidine 150 mg b.i.d. in healing reflux esophagitis, and the percentage of patients with healing were as shown in Table 13. This study does not constitute a comparison of the effectiveness of histamine H_2-receptor antagonists with PREVACID, as all patients had demonstrated unresponsiveness to the histamine H_2-receptor antagonist mode of treatment. It does indicate, however, that PREVACID may be useful in patients failing on a histamine H_2-receptor antagonist.
[See table 13 below]

Long-Term Maintenance Treatment of Erosive Esophagitis
Two independent, double-blind, multicenter, controlled trials were conducted in patients with endoscopically confirmed healed esophagitis. Patients remained in remission significantly longer and the number of recurrences of erosive esophagitis was significantly less in patients treated with PREVACID than in patients treated with placebo over a 12-month period. See Table 14.
[See table 14 below]
Regardless of initial grade of erosive esophagitis, PREVACID 15 mg and 30 mg were similar in maintaining remission.

Pathological Hypersecretory Conditions Including Zollinger-Ellison Syndrome
In open studies of 57 patients with pathological hypersecretory conditions, such as Zollinger-Ellison (ZE) syndrome with or without multiple endocrine adenomas, PREVACID significantly inhibited gastric acid secretion and controlled associated symptoms of diarrhea, anorexia and pain. Doses ranging from 15 mg every other day to 180 mg per day maintained basal acid secretion below 10 mEq/hr in patients without prior gastric surgery and below 5 mEq/hr in patients with prior gastric surgery.
Initial doses were titrated to the individual patient need, and adjustments were necessary with time in some patients. (See **DOSAGE AND ADMINISTRATION**.) PREVACID was well tolerated at these high dose levels for prolonged periods (greater than four years in some patients). In most ZE patients, serum gastrin levels were not modified by PREVACID. However, in some patients, serum gastrin increased to levels greater than those present prior to initiation of lansoprazole therapy.

Table 9
Gastric Ulcer Healing Rates

Week	PREVACID 15 mg q.d. (N=65)	PREVACID 30 mg q.d. (N=63)	PREVACID 60 mg q.d. (N=61)	Placebo (N=64)
4	64.6%*	58.1%*	53.3%*	37.5%
8	92.2%*	96.8%*	93.2%*	76.7%

*(p≤0.05) versus placebo.

Table 10
Frequency of Heartburn

Variable	Placebo (n=43)	PREVACID 15 mg (n=80)	PREVACID 30 mg (n=86)
		Median	
% of Days without Hearburn			
Week 1	0%	71%*	46%*
Week 4	11%	81%*	76%*
Week 8	13%	84%*	82%*
% of Nights without Heartburn			
Week 1	17%	86%*	57%*
Week 4	25%	89%*	73%*
Week 8	36%	92%*	80%*

*(p<0.01) versus placebo.

Table 11
Erosive Esophagitis Healing Rates

Week	PREVACID 15 mg q.d. (N=69)	PREVACID 30 mg q.d. (N=65)	PREVACID 60 mg q.d. (N=72)	Placebo (N=63)
4	67.6%*	81.3%**	80.6%**	32.8%
6	87.7%*	95.4%*	94.3%*	52.5%
8	90.0%*	95.4%*	94.4%*	52.5%

*(p≤0.001) versus placebo.
**(p≤0.05) versus PREVACID 15 mg and placebo.

Table 12
Erosive Esophagitis Healing Rates

Week	PREVACID 30 mg q.d. (N=115)	Ranitidine 150 mg b.i.d. (N=127)
2	66.7%*	38.7%
4	82.5%*	52.0%
6	93.0%*	67.8%
8	92.1%*	69.9%

*(p≤0.001) versus ranitidine.

Table 13
Reflux Esophagitis Healing Rates in Patients Poorly Responsive to Histamine H_2-Receptor Antagonist Therapy

Week	PREVACID 30 mg q.d. (N=100)	Ranitidine 150 mg b.i.d. (N=51)
4	74.7%*	42.6%
8	83.7%*	32.0%

*(p≤0.001) versus ranitidine.

Table 14
Endoscopic Remission Rates

Trial	Drug	No. of Pts.	Percent in Endoscopic Remission 0–3 mo.	0–6 mo.	0–12 mo.
#1	PREVACID 15 mg q.d.	59	83%*	81%*	79%*
	PREVACID 30 mg q.d.	56	93%*	93%*	90%*
	Placebo	55	31%	27%	24%
#2	PREVACID 15 mg q.d.	50	74%*	72%*	67%*
	PREVACID 30 mg q.d.	49	75%*	72%*	55%*
	Placebo	47	16%	13%	13%

%=Life Table Estimate
*(p≤0.001) versus placebo.

INDICATIONS AND USAGE

Short-Term Treatment of Active Duodenal Ulcer
PREVACID Delayed-Release Capsules are indicated for short-term treatment (up to 4 weeks) for healing and symptom relief of active duodenal ulcer.

***H. pylori* Eradication to Reduce the Risk of Duodenal Ulcer Recurrence**

Triple Therapy: PREVACID/amoxicillin/clarithromycin
PREVACID Delayed-Release Capsules, in combination with amoxicillin plus clarithromycin as triple therapy, are indicated for the treatment of patients with *H. pylori* infection and duodenal ulcer disease (active or one-year history of a duodenal ulcer) to eradicate *H. pylori*. Eradication of *H. pylori* has been shown to reduce the risk of duodenal ulcer recurrence. (See **CLINICAL STUDIES** and **DOSAGE AND ADMINISTRATION**.)

Dual Therapy: PREVACID/amoxicillin
PREVACID Delayed-Release Capsules, in combination with amoxicillin as dual therapy, are indicated for the treatment of patients with *H. pylori* infection and duodenal ulcer disease (active or one-year history of a duodenal ulcer) **who are either allergic or intolerant to clarithromycin or in whom resistance to clarithromycin is known or suspected.** (See the clarithromycin package insert, **MICROBIOLOGY** section.) Eradication of *H. pylori* has been shown to reduce the risk of duodenal ulcer recurrence. (See **CLINICAL STUDIES** and **DOSAGE AND ADMINISTRATION**.)

Maintenance of Healed Duodenal Ulcers
PREVACID Delayed-Release Capsules are indicated to maintain healing of duodenal ulcers. Controlled studies do not extend beyond 12 months.

Short-Term Treatment of Active Benign Gastric Ulcer
PREVACID Delayed-Release Capsules are indicated for short-term treatment (up to 8 weeks) for healing and symptom relief of active benign gastric ulcer.

Gastroesophageal Reflux Disease (GERD)

Short-Term Treatment of Symptomatic GERD
PREVACID Delayed-Release Capsules are indicated for the treatment of heartburn and other symptoms associated with GERD.

Short-Term Treatment of Erosive Esophagitis
PREVACID Delayed-Release Capsules are indicated for short-term treatment (up to 8 weeks) for healing and symptom relief of all grades of erosive esophagitis.
For patients who do not heal with PREVACID for 8 weeks (5-10%), it may be helpful to give an additional 8 weeks of treatment.
If there is a recurrence of erosive esophagitis an additional 8-week course of PREVACID may be considered.

Maintenance of Healing of Erosive Esophagitis
PREVACID Delayed-Release Capsules are indicated to maintain healing of erosive esophagitis. Controlled studies did not extend beyond 12 months.

Pathological Hypersecretory Conditions Including Zollinger-Ellison Syndrome
PREVACID Delayed-Release Capsules are indicated for the long-term treatment of pathological hypersecretory conditions, including Zollinger-Ellison syndrome.

CONTRAINDICATIONS

PREVACID Delayed-Release Capsules are contraindicated in patients with known hypersensitivity to any component of the formulation.
Amoxicillin is contraindicated in patients with a known hypersensitivity to any penicillin. (Please refer to full prescribing information for amoxicillin before prescribing.)
Clarithromycin is contraindicated in patients with a known hypersensitivity to any macrolide antibiotic, and in patients receiving terfenadine therapy who have preexisting cardiac abnormalities or electrolyte disturbances. (Please refer to full prescribing information for clarithromycin before prescribing.)

WARNINGS

CLARITHROMYCIN SHOULD NOT BE USED IN PREGNANT WOMEN EXCEPT IN CLINICAL CIRCUMSTANCES WHERE NO ALTERNATIVE THERAPY IS APPROPRIATE. IF PREGNANCY OCCURS WHILE TAKING CLARITHROMYCIN, THE PATIENT SHOULD BE APPRISED OF THE POTENTIAL HAZARD TO THE FETUS. (SEE **WARNINGS** IN PRESCRIBING INFORMATION FOR CLARITHROMYCIN.)
Pseudomembranous colitis has been reported with nearly all antibacterial agents, including clarithromycin and amoxicillin, and may range in severity from mild to life threatening. Therefore, it is important to consider this diagnosis in patients who present with diarrhea subsequent to the administration of antibacterial agents.
Treatment with antibacterial agents alters the normal flora of the colon and may permit overgrowth of clostridia. Studies indicate that a toxin produced by *Clostridium difficile* is a primary cause of "antibiotic-associated colitis".
After the diagnosis of pseudomembranous colitis has been established, therapeutic measures should be initiated. Mild cases of pseudomembranous colitis usually respond to discontinuation of the drug alone. In moderate to severe cases, consideration should be given to management with fluids and electrolytes, protein supplementation, and treatment with an antibacterial drug clinically effective against *Clostridium difficile* colitis.
Serious and occasionally fatal hypersensitivity (anaphylactic) reactions have been reported in patients on penicillin therapy. These reactions are more apt to occur in individuals with a history of penicillin hypersensitivity and/or a history of sensitivity to multiple allergens.
There have been well documented reports of individuals with a history of penicillin hypersensitivity reactions who have experienced severe hypersensitivity reactions when treated with a cephalosporin. Before initiating therapy with any penicillin, careful inquiry should be made concerning previous hypersensitivity reactions to penicillins, cephalosporins, and other allergens. If an allergic reaction occurs, amoxicillin should be discontinued and the appropriate therapy instituted.
SERIOUS ANAPHYLACTIC REACTIONS REQUIRE IMMEDIATE EMERGENCY TREATMENT WITH EPINEPHRINE. OXYGEN, INTRAVENOUS STEROIDS, AND AIRWAY MANAGEMENT, INCLUDING INTUBATION, SHOULD ALSO BE ADMINISTERED AS INDICATED.

PRECAUTIONS

General
Symptomatic response to therapy with lansoprazole does not preclude the presence of gastric malignancy.
Information for Patients
PREVACID Delayed-Release Capsules should be taken before eating.
Alternative Administration Options
For patients who have difficulty swallowing capsules, PREVACID Delayed-Release Capsules can be opened, and the intact granules contained within can be sprinkled on one tablespoon of either applesauce, ENSURE® pudding, cottage cheese, yogurt, or strained pears and swallowed immediately. The granules should not be chewed or crushed. Alternatively, PREVACID Delayed-Release Capsules may be emptied into a small volume of either orange juice or tomato juice (60 mL – approximately 2 ounces), mixed briefly and swallowed immediately. To insure complete delivery of the dose, the glass should be rinsed with two or more volumes of juice and the contents swallowed immediately. The granules have also been shown *in vitro* to remain intact when exposed to apple, cranberry, grape, orange, pineapple, prune, tomato, and V-8® vegetable juice and stored for up to 30 minutes.
For patients who have a nasogastric tube in place, PREVACID Delayed-Release Capsules can be opened and the intact granules mixed in 40 mL of apple juice and injected through the nasogastric tube into the stomach. After administering the granules, the nasogastric tube should be flushed with additional apple juice to clear the tube.
Drug Interactions
Lansoprazole is metabolized through the cytochrome P_{450} system, specifically through the CYP3A and CYP2C19 isozymes. Studies have shown that lansoprazole does not have clinically significant interactions with other drugs metabolized by the cytochrome P_{450} system, such as warfarin, antipyrine, indomethacin, ibuprofen, phenytoin, propranolol, prednisone, diazepam, clarithromycin, or terfenadine in healthy subjects. These compounds are metabolized through various cytochrome P_{450} isozymes including CYP1A2, CYP2C9, CYP2C19, CYP2D6, and CYP3A. When lansoprazole was administered concomitantly with theophylline (CYP1A2, CYP3A), a minor increase (10%) in the clearance of theophylline was seen. Because of the small magnitude and the direction of the effect on theophylline clearance, this interaction is unlikely to be of clinical concern. Nonetheless, individual patients may require additional titration of their theophylline dosage when lansoprazole is started or stopped to ensure clinically effective blood levels.
Lansoprazole has also been shown to have no clinically significant interaction with amoxicillin.
In a single-dose crossover study examining lansoprazole 30 mg and omeprazole 20 mg each administered alone and concomitantly with sucralfate 1 gram, absorption of the proton pump inhibitors was delayed and their bioavailability was reduced by 17% and 16%, respectively, when administered concomitantly with sucralfate. Therefore, proton pump inhibitors should be taken at least 30 minutes prior to sucralfate. In clinical trials, antacids were administered concomitantly with PREVACID Delayed-Release Capsules; this did not interfere with its effect.
Lansoprazole causes a profound and long-lasting inhibition of gastric acid secretion; therefore, it is theoretically possible that lansoprazole may interfere with the absorption of drugs where gastric pH is an important determinant of bioavailability (eg, ketoconazole, ampicillin esters, iron salts, digoxin).
Carcinogenesis, Mutagenesis, Impairment of Fertility
In two 24-month carcinogenicity studies, Sprague-Dawley rats were treated orally with doses of 5 to 150 mg/kg/day, about 1 to 40 times the exposure on a body surface (mg/m^2) basis, of a 50-kg person of average height (1.46 m^2 body surface area) given the recommended human dose of 30 mg/day (22.2 mg/m^2). Lansoprazole produced dose-related gastric enterochromaffin-like (ECL) cell hyperplasia and ECL cell carcinoids in both male and female rats. It also increased the incidence of intestinal metaplasia of the gastric epithelium in both sexes. In male rats, lansoprazole produced a dose-related increase of testicular interstitial cell adenomas. The incidence of these adenomas in rats receiving doses of 15 to 150 mg/kg/day (4 to 40 times the recommended human dose based on body surface area) exceeded the low background incidence (range = 1.4 to 10%) for this strain of rat. Testicular interstitial cell adenoma also occurred in 1 of 30 rats treated with 50 mg/kg/day (13 times the recommended human dose based on body surface area) in a 1-year toxicity study.
In a 24-month carcinogenicity study, CD-1 mice were treated orally with doses of 15 to 600 mg/kg/day, 2 to 80 times the recommended human dose based on body surface area. Lansoprazole produced a dose-related increased incidence of gastric ECL cell hyperplasia. It also produced an increased incidence of liver tumors (hepatocellular adenoma plus carcinoma). The tumor incidences in male mice treated with 300 and 600 mg/kg/day (40 to 80 times the recommended human dose based on body surface area) and female mice treated with 150 to 600 mg/kg/day (20 to 80 times the recommended human dose based on body surface area) exceeded the ranges of background incidences in historical controls for this strain of mice. Lansoprazole treatment produced adenoma of rete testis in male mice receiving 75 to 600 mg/kg/day (10 to 80 times the recommended human dose based on body surface area).
Lansoprazole was not genotoxic in the Ames test, the *ex vivo* rat hepatocyte unscheduled DNA synthesis (UDS) test, the *in vivo* mouse micronucleus test or the rat bone marrow cell chromosomal aberration test. It was positive in *in vitro* human lymphocyte chromosomal aberration assays.
Lansoprazole at oral doses up to 150 mg/kg/day (40 times the recommended human dose based on body surface area) was found to have no effect on fertility and reproductive performance of male and female rats.
Pregnancy: Teratogenic Effects.
Pregnancy Category B
Lansoprazole
Teratology studies have been performed in pregnant rats at oral doses up to 150 mg/kg/day (40 times the recommended human dose based on body surface area) and pregnant rabbits at oral doses up to 30 mg/kg/day (16 times the recommended human dose based on body surface area) and have revealed no evidence of impaired fertility or harm to the fetus due to lansoprazole.
There are, however, no adequate or well-controlled studies in pregnant women. Because animal reproduction studies are not always predictive of human response, this drug should be used during pregnancy only if clearly needed.
Pregnancy Category C
Clarithromycin
See **WARNINGS** (above) and full prescribing information for clarithromycin before using in pregnant women.
Nursing Mothers
Lansoprazole or its metabolites are excreted in the milk of rats. It is not known whether lansoprazole is excreted in human milk. Because many drugs are excreted in human milk, because of the potential for serious adverse reactions in nursing infants from lansoprazole, and because of the potential for tumorigenicity shown for lansoprazole in rat carcinogenicity studies, a decision should be made whether to discontinue nursing or to discontinue the drug, taking into account the importance of the drug to the mother.
Pediatric Use
Safety and effectiveness in pediatric patients have not been established.
Use in Women
Over 800 women were treated with lansoprazole. Ulcer healing rates in females were similar to those in males. The incidence rates of adverse events were also similar to those seen in males.
Use in Geriatric Patients
Ulcer healing rates in elderly patients are similar to those in a younger age group. The incidence rates of adverse events and laboratory test abnormalities are also similar to those seen in younger patients. For elderly patients, dosage and administration of lansoprazole need not be altered for a particular indication.

ADVERSE REACTIONS

Clinical
Worldwide, over 6100 patients have been treated with lansoprazole in Phase 2–3 clinical trials involving various dosages and durations of treatment. In general, lansoprazole treatment has been well tolerated in both short-term and long-term trials.
The following adverse events shown in Table 15, were reported by the treating physician to have a possible or probable relationship to drug in 1% or more of PREVACID-treated patients and occurred at a greater rate in PREVACID-treated patients than placebo-treated patients:
[See table 15 above]

Table 15
Incidence of Possibly or Probably Treatment-Related Adverse Events in Short-term, Placebo-Controlled Studies

Body System/Adverse Event	PREVACID (N=1457) %	Placebo (N=467) %
Body as a Whole		
Abdominal Pain	1.8	1.3
Digestive System		
Diarrhea	3.6	2.6
Nausea	1.4	1.3

Headache was also seen at greater than 1% incidence but was more common on placebo. The incidence of diarrhea was similar between patients who received placebo and patients who received lansoprazole 15 mg and 30 mg, but higher in the patients who received lansoprazole 60 mg (2.9%, 1.4%, 4.2%, and 7.4%, respectively).
The most commonly reported possibly or probably treatment-related adverse event during maintenance therapy was diarrhea.
Additional adverse experiences occurring in <1% of patients or subjects in domestic trials are shown below. Refer to **Postmarketing** for adverse reactions occurring since the drug was marketed.
Body as a Whole—asthenia, candidiasis, chest pain (not otherwise specified), edema, fever, flu syndrome, halitosis, infection (not otherwise specified), malaise; *Cardiovascular System*—angina, cerebrovascular accident, hypertension/hypotension, myocardial infarction, palpitations, shock (circulatory failure), vasodilation; *Digestive System*—anorexia, bezoar, cardiospasm, cholelithiasis, constipation, dry mouth/thirst, dyspepsia, dysphagia, eructation, esophageal stenosis, esophageal ulcer, esophagitis, fecal discoloration, flatulence, gastric nodules/fundic gland polyps, gastroenteritis, gastrointestinal hemorrhage, hematemesis, increased appetite, increased salivation, melena, rectal hemorrhage, stomatitis, tenesmus, ulcerative colitis; *Endocrine System*—diabetes mellitus, goiter, hyperglycemia/hypoglycemia; *Hemic and Lymphatic System*—anemia, hemolysis; *Metabolic and Nutritional Disorders*—gout, weight gain/loss; *Musculoskeletal System*—arthritis/arthralgia, musculoskeletal pain, myalgia; *Nervous System*—agitation, amnesia, anxiety, apathy, confusion, depression, dizziness/syncope, hallucinations, hemiplegia, hostility aggravated, libido decreased, nervousness, paresthesia, thinking abnormality; *Respiratory System*—asthma, bronchitis, cough increased, dyspnea, epistaxis, hemoptysis, hiccup, pneumonia, upper respiratory inflammation/infection; *Skin and Appendages*—acne, alopecia, pruritus, rash, urticaria; *Special Senses*—blurred vision, deafness, eye pain, otitis media, taste perversion, tinnitus, visual field defect; *Urogenital System*—abnormal menses, albuminuria, breast enlargement/gynecomastia, breast tenderness, glycosuria, hematuria, impotence, kidney calculus.

Postmarketing
On-going Safety Surveillance: Additional adverse experiences have been reported since lansoprazole has been mar-

Continued on next page

Prevacid—Cont.

keted. The majority of these cases are foreign-sourced and a relationship to lansoprazole has not been established. Because these events were reported voluntarily from a population of unknown size, estimates of frequency cannot be made. These events are listed below by COSTART body system.

Body as a Whole—anaphylactoid-like reaction; *Digestive System*—hepatotoxicity, vomiting; *Hemic and Lymphatic System*—agranulocytosis, aplastic anemia, hemolytic anemia, leukopenia, neutropenia, pancytopenia, thrombocytopenia, and thrombotic thrombocytopenic purpura; *Special Senses*—speech disorder; *Urogenital System*—urinary retention.

Combination Therapy with Amoxicillin and Clarithromycin

In clinical trials using combination therapy with PREVACID plus amoxicillin and clarithromycin, and PREVACID plus amoxicillin, no adverse reactions peculiar to these drug combinations were observed. Adverse reactions that have occurred have been limited to those that had been previously reported with PREVACID, amoxicillin, or clarithromycin.

Triple Therapy: PREVACID/amoxicillin/clarithromycin

The most frequently reported adverse events for patients who received triple therapy for 14 days were diarrhea (7%), headache (6%), and taste perversion (5%). There were no statistically significant differences in the frequency of reported adverse events between the 10- and 14-day triple therapy regimens. No treatment-emergent adverse events were observed at significantly higher rates with triple therapy than with any dual therapy regimen.

Dual Therapy: PREVACID/amoxicillin

The most frequently reported adverse events for patients who received PREVACID t.i.d. plus amoxicillin t.i.d. dual therapy were diarrhea (8%) and headache (7%). No treatment-emergent adverse events were observed at significantly higher rates with PREVACID t.i.d. plus amoxicillin t.i.d. dual therapy than with PREVACID alone.

For more information on adverse reactions with amoxicillin or clarithromycin, refer to their package inserts, **ADVERSE REACTIONS** sections.

Laboratory Values

The following changes in laboratory parameters for lansoprazole were reported as adverse events:

Abnormal liver function tests, increased SGOT (AST), increased SGPT (ALT), increased creatinine, increased alkaline phosphatase, increased globulins, increased GGTP, increased/decreased/abnormal WBC, abnormal AG ratio, abnormal RBC, bilirubinemia, eosinophilia, hyperlipemia, increased/decreased electrolytes, increased/decreased cholesterol, increased glucocorticoids, increased LDH, increased/decreased/abnormal platelets, and increased gastrin levels. Additional isolated laboratory abnormalities were reported.

In the placebo controlled studies, when SGOT (AST) and SGPT (ALT) were evaluated, 0.4% (1/250) placebo patients and 0.3% (2/795) lansoprazole patients had enzyme elevations greater than three times the upper limit of normal range at the final treatment visit. None of these patients reported jaundice at any time during the study.

In clinical trials using combination therapy with PREVACID plus amoxicillin and clarithromycin, and PREVACID plus amoxicillin, no increased laboratory abnormalities particular to these drug combinations were observed.

For more information on laboratory value changes with amoxicillin or clarithromycin, refer to their package inserts, **ADVERSE REACTIONS** section.

OVERDOSAGE

Oral doses up to 5000 mg/kg in rats (approximately 1300 times the recommended human dose based on body surface area) and mice (about 675.7 times the recommended human dose based on body surface area) did not produce deaths or any clinical signs.

Lansoprazole is not removed from the circulation by hemodialysis. In one reported case of overdose, the patient consumed 600 mg of lansoprazole with no adverse reaction.

DOSAGE AND ADMINISTRATION

Short-Term Treatment of Duodenal Ulcer

The recommended adult oral dose is 15 mg once daily for 4 weeks. (See **INDICATIONS AND USAGE.**)

***H. pylori* Eradication to Reduce the Risk of Duodenal Ulcer Recurrence**

Triple Therapy: PREVACID/amoxicillin/clarithromycin

The recommended adult oral dose is 30 mg PREVACID, 1 gram amoxicillin, and 500 mg clarithromycin, all given twice daily (q 12h) for 10 or 14 days. (See **INDICATIONS AND USAGE.**)

Dual Therapy: PREVACID/amoxicillin

The recommended adult oral dose is 30 mg PREVACID and 1 gram amoxicillin, each given three times daily (q 8h) for 14 days. (See **INDICATIONS AND USAGE.**)

Please refer to amoxicillin and clarithromycin full prescribing information for **CONTRAINDICATIONS** and **WARNINGS**, and for information regarding dosing in elderly and renally-impaired patients.

Maintenance of Healed Duodenal Ulcers

The recommended adult oral dose is 15 mg once daily. (See **CLINICAL STUDIES.**)

Short-Term Treatment of Gastric Ulcer

The recommended adult oral dose is 30 mg once daily for up to eight weeks. (See **CLINICAL STUDIES.**)

Gastroesophageal Reflux Disease (GERD)

Short-Term Treatment of Symptomatic GERD

The recommended adult oral dose is 15 mg once daily for up to 8 weeks.

Short-Term Treatment of Erosive Esophagitis

The recommended adult oral dose is 30 mg once daily for up to 8 weeks. For patients who do not heal with PREVACID for 8 weeks (5-10%), it may be helpful to give an additional 8 weeks of treatment. (See **INDICATIONS AND USAGE.**)

If there is a recurrence of erosive esophagitis, an additional 8-week course of PREVACID may be considered.

Maintenance of Healing of Erosive Esophagitis

The recommended adult oral dose is 15 mg once daily. (See **CLINICAL STUDIES.**)

Pathological Hypersecretory Conditions Including Zollinger-Ellison Syndrome

The dosage of PREVACID in patients with pathologic hypersecretory conditions varies with the individual patient. The recommended adult oral starting dose is 60 mg once a day. Doses should be adjusted to individual patient needs and should continue for as long as clinically indicated. Dosages up to 90 mg b.i.d. have been administered. Daily dosages of greater than 120 mg should be administered in divided doses. Some patients with Zollinger-Ellison syndrome have been treated continuously with PREVACID for more than four years.

No dosage adjustment is necessary in patients with renal insufficiency or the elderly. For patients with severe liver disease, dosage adjustment should be considered.

PREVACID Delayed-Release Capsules should be taken before eating. In the clinical trials, antacids were used concomitantly with PREVACID.

Alternative Administration Options

For patients who have difficulty swallowing capsules, PREVACID Delayed-Release Capsules can be opened, and the intact granules contained within can be sprinkled on one tablespoon of either applesauce, ENSURE® pudding, cottage cheese, yogurt, or strained pears and swallowed immediately. The granules should not be chewed or crushed. Alternatively, PREVACID Delayed-Release Capsules may be emptied into a small volume of either orange juice or tomato juice (60 mL – approximately 2 ounces), mixed briefly and swallowed immediately. To insure complete delivery of the dose, the glass should be rinsed with two or more volumes of juice and the contents swallowed immediately. The granules have also been shown *in vitro* to remain intact when exposed to apple, cranberry, grape, orange, pineapple, prune, tomato, and V-8® vegetable juice and stored for up to 30 minutes.

For patients who have a nasogastric tube in place, PREVACID Delayed-Release Capsules can be opened and the intact granules mixed in 40 mL of apple juice and injected through the nasogastric tube into the stomach. After administering the granules, the nasogastric tube should be flushed with additional apple juice to clear the tube.

HOW SUPPLIED

PREVACID Delayed-Release Capsules, 15 mg, are opaque, hard gelatin, colored pink and green with the TAP logo and "PREVACID 15" imprinted on the capsules. The 30 mg are opaque, hard gelatin, colored pink and black with the TAP logo and "PREVACID 30" imprinted on the capsules. They are available as follows:

NDC 0300-1541-30
Unit of use bottles of 30: 15-mg capsules
NDC 0300-1541-13
Bottles of 100: 15-mg capsules
NDC 0300-1541-19
Bottles of 1000: 15-mg capsules
NDC 0300-1541-11
Unit dose package of 100: 15-mg capsules
NDC 0300-3046-13
Bottles of 100: 30-mg capsules
NDC 0300-3046-19
Bottles of 1000: 30-mg capsules
NDC 0300-3046-11
Unit dose package of 100: 30-mg capsules

Storage: PREVACID capsules should be stored in a tight container protected from moisture.

Store between 15°C and 30°C (59°F and 86°F).

Rx only

U.S. Patent Nos. 4,628,098; 4,689,333; 5,013,743; 5,026,560 and 5,045,321.

Manufactured for TAP Pharmaceuticals Inc. Lake Forest, Illinois 60045, U.S.A. by Takeda Chemical Industries Limited, Osaka, Japan 541

ENSURE® is a registered trademark of Abbott Laboratories. V-8® is a registered trademark of the Campbell Soup Company.

03-5036-R14-Rev. March 2000

Shown in Product Identification Guide, page 338

PREVPAC® ℞

(lansoprazole 30-mg capsules, amoxicillin 500-mg capsules, USP, and clarithromycin 500-mg tablets)

THESE PRODUCTS ARE INTENDED ONLY FOR USE AS DESCRIBED. The individual products contained in this package should not be used alone or in combination for other purposes. The information described in this labeling concerns only the use of these products as indicated in this daily administration pack. For information on use of the individual components when dispensed as individual medications outside this combined use for treating *Helicobacter pylori (H. pylori)*, please see the package inserts for each individual product.

DESCRIPTION

PREVPAC consists of a daily administration pack containing two PREVACID 30-mg capsules, four amoxicillin 500-mg capsules, USP, and two clarithromycin 500-mg tablets, for oral administration.

PREVACID® (lansoprazole) Delayed-Release Capsules

The active ingredient in PREVACID capsules is a substituted benzimidazole, 2-[[[3-methyl-4-(2,2,2-trifluoroethoxy)-2-pyridyl] methyl]sulfinyl] benzimidazole, a compound that inhibits gastric acid secretion. Its empirical formula is $C_{16}H_{14}F_3N_3O_2S$ with a molecular weight of 369.37. The structural formula is:

Lansoprazole is a white to brownish-white odorless crystalline powder which melts with decomposition at approximately 166°C. Lansoprazole is freely soluble in dimethylformamide; soluble in methanol; sparingly soluble in ethanol; slightly soluble in ethyl acetate, dichloromethane and acetonitrile; very slightly soluble in ether; and practically insoluble in hexane and water.

Each delayed-release capsule contains enteric-coated granules consisting of lansoprazole (30 mg), hydroxypropyl cellulose, low substituted hydroxypropyl cellulose, colloidal silicon dioxide, magnesium carbonate, methacrylic acid copolymer, starch, talc, sugar sphere, sucrose, polyethylene glycol, polysorbate 80, and titanium dioxide. Components of the gelatin capsule include gelatin, titanium dioxide, D&C Red No. 28, FD&C Blue No. 1, and FD&C Red No. 40.

TRIMOX® (amoxicillin, USP)

Amoxicillin, USP, (2*S*,5*R*,6*R*)-6-[(*R*)-(–)-2-Amino-2-(*p*-hydroxyphenyl)acetamido]-3,3-dimethyl-7-oxo-4-thia-1-azabicyclo[3.2.0]heptane-2-carboxylic acid trihydrate, is a semisynthetic penicillin, an analogue of ampicillin. It has the following chemical structure:

The empirical formula is $C_{16}H_{18}N_3O_5S \cdot 3H_2O$, and the molecular weight is 419.45.

The maroon and light-pink capsules contain amoxicillin trihydrate equivalent to 500 mg of amoxicillin. The inactive ingredient in the capsules is magnesium stearate.

BIAXIN® Filmtab® (clarithromycin tablets)

Clarithromycin is a semi-synthetic macrolide antibiotic. Chemically, it is 6-*0*-methylerythromycin. The molecular formula is $C_{38}H_{69}NO_{13}$, and the molecular weight is 747.96. The structural formula is:

Clarithromycin is a white to off-white crystalline powder. It is soluble in acetone, slightly soluble in methanol, ethanol, and acetonitrile, and practically insoluble in water.

Each yellow oval film-coated tablet contains 500 mg of clarithromycin and the following inactive ingredients: cellulosic polymers, croscarmellose sodium, D&C Yellow No. 10, FD&C Blue No. 1, magnesium stearate, povidone, propylene glycol, silicon dioxide, sorbic acid, sorbitan monooleate, stearic acid, talc, titanium dioxide, and vanillin.

CLINICAL PHARMACOLOGY

Pharmacokinetics

Pharmacokinetics when all three of the PREVPAC components (PREVACID capsules, amoxicillin capsules, clarithromycin tablets) were coadministered has not been studied. Studies have shown no clinically significant interactions of PREVACID and amoxicillin or PREVACID and clarithromycin when administered together. There is no information about the gastric mucosal concentrations of PREVACID, amoxicillin and clarithromycin after administration of these agents concomitantly. The systemic pharmacokinetic information presented below is based on studies in which each product was administered alone.

PREVACID:

PREVACID capsules contain an enteric-coated granule formulation of lansoprazole. Absorption of lansoprazole begins only after the granules leave the stomach. Absorption is rapid, with mean peak plasma levels of lansoprazole occurring after approximately 1.7 hours. Peak plasma concentrations of lansoprazole (C_{max}) and the area under the plasma concentration curve (AUC) of lansoprazole are approximately proportional in doses from 15 mg to 60 mg after single-oral administration. Lansoprazole does not accumulate and its pharmacokinetics are unaltered by multiple dosing. The absorption of lansoprazole is rapid, with mean C_{max} occurring approximately 1.7 hours after oral dosing, and relatively complete with absolute bioavailability over 80%. In healthy subjects, the mean (± SD) plasma half-life was 1.5 (± 1.0) hours. Both C_{max} and AUC are diminished by about 50% if the drug is given 30 minutes after food as opposed to the fasting condition. There is no significant food effect if the drug is given before meals.

Lansoprazole is 97% bound to plasma proteins. Plasma protein binding is consistent over the concentration range of 0.05 to 5.0 mcg/mL.

Lansoprazole is extensively metabolized in the liver. Two metabolites have been identified in measurable quantities in plasma (the hydroxylated sulfinyl and sulfone derivatives of lansoprazole). These metabolites have very little or no antisecretory activity. Lansoprazole is thought to be transformed into two active species which inhibit acid secretion by (H^+,K^+)-ATPase within the parietal cell canaliculus, but are not present in the systemic circulation. The plasma elimination half-life of lansoprazole does not reflect its duration of suppression of gastric acid secretion. Thus, the plasma elimination half-life is less than two hours while the acid inhibitory effect lasts more than 24 hours.

Following single-dose oral administration of PREVACID, virtually no unchanged lansoprazole was excreted in the urine. In one study, after a single oral dose of ^{14}C-lansoprazole, approximately one-third of the administered radiation was excreted in the urine and two-thirds was recovered in the feces. This implies a significant biliary excretion of the metabolites of lansoprazole.

The clearance of lansoprazole is decreased in the elderly, with elimination half-life increased approximately 50% to 100%. Because the mean half-life in the elderly remains between 1.9 to 2.9 hours, repeated once daily dosing does not result in accumulation of lansoprazole. Peak plasma levels were not increased in the elderly.

In patients with severe renal insufficiency, plasma protein binding decreased by 1.0%–1.5% after administration of 60 mg of lansoprazole. Patients with renal insufficiency had a shortened elimination half-life and decreased total AUC (free and bound). AUC for free lansoprazole in plasma, however, was not related to the degree of renal impairment, and C_{max} and T_{max} were not different from subjects with healthy kidneys.

In patients with various degrees of chronic hepatic disease, the mean plasma half-life of the drug was prolonged from 1.5 hours to 3.2–7.2 hours. An increase in mean AUC of up to 500% was observed at steady state in hepatically-impaired patients compared to healthy subjects. Dose reduction in patients with severe hepatic disease should be considered.

The pooled pharmacokinetic parameters of PREVACID from twelve U.S. Phase I studies (N=513) were compared to the mean pharmacokinetic parameters from two Asian studies (N=20). The mean AUCs of PREVACID in Asian subjects are approximately twice that seen in pooled U.S. data; however, the inter-individual variability is high. The C_{max} values are comparable.

Amoxicillin:

Amoxicillin is stable in the presence of gastric acid and is well absorbed from the gastrointestinal tract and may be given with no regard to food. It diffuses readily into most body tissues and fluids, with the exception of brain and spinal fluid, except when meninges are inflamed. The half-life of amoxicillin is 61.3 minutes. Most of the amoxicillin is excreted unchanged in the urine; its excretion can be delayed by concurrent administration of probenecid. Amoxicillin is not highly protein-bound. In blood serum, amoxicillin is approximately 20% protein-bound as compared to 60% for penicillin G.

Orally administered doses of 500-mg amoxicillin capsules result in average peak blood levels 1 to 2 hours after administration in the range of 5.5 to 7.5 μg/mL.

Detectable serum levels are observed up to eight hours after an orally administered dose of amoxicillin. Approximately 60% of an orally administered dose of amoxicillin is excreted in the urine within 6 to 8 hours.

Clarithromycin:

Clarithromycin is rapidly absorbed from the gastrointestinal tract after oral administration. The absolute bioavailability of 250 mg clarithromycin tablets was approximately 50%. Food slightly delays both the onset of clarithromycin absorption and the formation of the antimicrobially active metabolite, 14-OH clarithromycin, but does not affect the extent of bioavailability. Therefore, clarithromycin tablets may be given without regard to food.

In fasting healthy human subjects, peak serum concentrations were attained within two hours after oral dosing. Steady-state peak serum clarithromycin concentrations were attained in two to three days and were approximately 2 to 3 μg/mL with a 500-mg dose administered every 12 hours. The elimination half-life of clarithromycin was 5 to 7 hours with 500 mg administered every 8 to 12 hours. The nonlinearity of clarithromycin pharmacokinetics is slight at the recommended dose of 500 mg administered every 12 hours. With a 500-mg dose every 8 to 12 hours, the peak steady-state concentration of 14-OH clarithromycin, the principal metabolite, is up to 1 μg/mL and its elimination

Clarithromycin Susceptibility Test Results and Clinical/Bacteriological Outcomes[a]

Clarithromycin Pretreatment Results		Clarithromycin Post-treatment Results				
		H. pylori negative-eradicated	*H. pylori* positive- not eradicated Post-treatment susceptibility results S[b]	I[b]	R[b]	No MIC
Triple Therapy 14-Day (lansoprazole 30 mg b.i.d./amoxicillin 1 gm b.i.d./clarithromycin 500 mg b.i.d.) (M95-399, M93-131, M95-392)						
Susceptible[b]	112	105				7
Intermediate[b]	3	3				
Resistant[b]	17	6			7	4
Triple Therapy 10-Day (lansoprazole 30 mg b.i.d./amoxicillin 1 gm b.i.d./clarithromycin 500 mg b.i.d.) (M95-399)						
Susceptible[b]	42	40	1		1	
Intermediate[b]						
Resistant[b]	4	1			3	

[a] Includes only patients with pretreatment clarithromycin susceptibility test results

[b] Susceptible (S) MIC ≤ 0.25 μg/mL, Intermediate (I) MIC 0.5–1.0 μg/mL, Resistant (R) MIC ≥ 2 μg/mL

half-life is about 7 to 9 hours. The steady-state concentration of this metabolite is generally attained within 2 to 3 days.

After a 500-mg tablet every 12 hours, the urinary excretion of clarithromycin is approximately 30%. The renal clearance of clarithromycin approximates the normal glomerular filtration rate. The major metabolite found in urine is 14-OH clarithromycin, which accounts for an additional 10% to 15% of the dose with a 500-mg tablet administered every 12 hours.

The steady-state concentrations of clarithromycin in subjects with impaired hepatic function did not differ from those in normal subjects; however, the 14-OH clarithromycin concentrations were lower in the hepatically impaired subjects. The decreased formation of 14-OH clarithromycin was at least partially offset by an increase in renal clearance of clarithromycin in the subjects with impaired hepatic function when compared to healthy subjects.

The pharmacokinetics of clarithromycin was also altered in subjects with impaired renal function. (See **PRECAUTIONS** and **DOSAGE AND ADMINISTRATION.**)

Pharmacodynamics

MICROBIOLOGY

Lansoprazole, clarithromycin and/or amoxicillin have been shown to be active against most strains of *Helicobacter pylori in vitro* and in clinical infections as described in the **INDICATIONS AND USAGE** section.

Helicobacter

Helicobacter pylori

Pretreatment Resistance

Clarithromycin pretreatment resistance (≥ 2.0 μg/mL) was 9.5% (91/960) by E-test and 11.3% (12/106) by agar dilution in the dual and triple therapy clinical trials (M93-125, M93-130, M93-131, M95-392, and M95-399).

Amoxicillin pretreatment susceptible isolates (≤ 0.25 μg/mL) occurred in 97.8% (936/957) and 98.0% (98/100) of the patients in the dual and triple therapy clinical trials by E-test and agar dilution, respectively. Twenty-one of 957 patients (2.2%) by E-test and 2 of 100 patients (2.0%) by agar dilution had amoxicillin pretreatment MICs of > 0.25 μg/mL. One patient on the 14-day triple therapy regimen had an unconfirmed pretreatment amoxicillin minimum inhibitory concentration (MIC) of > 256 μg/mL by E-test and the patient was eradicated of *H. pylori*.

[See table above]

Patients not eradicated of *H. pylori* following lansoprazole/amoxicillin/clarithromycin triple therapy will likely have clarithromycin resistant *H. pylori*. Therefore, for those patients who fail therapy, clarithromycin susceptibility testing should be done when possible. Patients with clarithromycin resistant *H. pylori* should not be treated with lansoprazole/amoxicillin/clarithromycin triple therapy or with regimens which include clarithromycin as the sole antimicrobial agent.

Amoxicillin Susceptibility Test Results and Clinical/Bacteriological Outcomes

In the dual and triple therapy clinical trials, 82.6% (195/236) of the patients that had pretreatment amoxicillin susceptible MICs (≤ 0.25 μg/mL) were eradicated of *H. pylori*. Of those with pretreatment amoxicillin MICs of > 0.25 μg/mL, three of six had the *H. pylori* eradicated. A total of 30% (21/70) of the patients failed lansoprazole 30 mg t.i.d./amoxicillin 1 gm t.i.d. dual therapy and a total of 12.8% (22/172) of the patients failed the 10- and 14-day triple therapy regimens. Post-treatment susceptibility results were not obtained on 11 of the patients who failed therapy. Nine of the 11 patients with amoxicillin post-treatment MICs that failed the triple therapy regimen also had clarithromycin resistant *H. pylori* isolates.

Susceptibility Test for *Helicobacter pylori*

The reference methodology for susceptibility testing of *H. pylori* is agar dilution MICs.[1] One to three microliters of an inoculum equivalent to a No. 2 McFarland standard ($1 \times 10^7 - 1 \times 10^8$ CFU/mL for *H. pylori*) are inoculated directly onto freshly prepared antimicrobial containing Mueller-Hinton agar plates with 5% aged defibrinated sheep blood (≥ 2 weeks old). The agar dilution plates are incubated at 35°C in a microaerobic environment produced by a gas generating system suitable for campylobacters. After 3 days of incubation, the MICs are recorded as the lowest concentration of antimicrobial agent required to inhibit growth of the organism. The clarithromycin and amoxicillin MIC values should be interpreted according to the following criteria:

Clarithromycin MIC (μg/mL)[a]	Interpretation
≤ 0.25	Susceptible (S)
0.5–1.0	Intermediate (I)
≥ 2.0	Resistant (R)

Amoxicillin MIC (μg/mL)[b]	Interpretation
≤ 0.25	Susceptible (S)

[a] These are tentative breakpoints for the agar dilution methodology and they should not be used to interpret results obtained using alternative methods.

[b] There were not enough organisms with MICs > 0.25 μg/mL to determine a resistance breakpoint.

Standardized susceptibility test procedures require the use of laboratory control microorganisms to control the technical aspects of the laboratory procedures. Standard clarithromycin and amoxicillin powders should provide the following MIC values:

Microorganisms	Antimicrobial Agent	MIC (μg/mL)[a]
H. pylori ATCC 43504	Clarithromycin	0.015–0.12 mcg/mL
H. pylori ATCC 43504	Amoxicillin	0.015–0.12 mcg/mL

[a] These are quality control ranges for the agar dilution methodology and they should not be used to control test results obtained using alternative methods.

Reference

1. National Committee for Clinical Laboratory Standards. Summary Minutes, Subcommittee on Antimicrobial Susceptibility Testing, Tampa, FL, January 11–13, 1998.

Antisecretory activity

After oral administration, lansoprazole was shown to significantly decrease the basal acid output and significantly increase the mean gastric pH and percent of time the gastric pH was >3 and >4. Lansoprazole also significantly reduced meal-stimulated gastric acid output and secretion volume, as well as pentagastrin-stimulated acid output. In patients with hypersecretion of acid, lansoprazole significantly reduced basal and pentagastrin-stimulated gastric acid secretion. Lansoprazole inhibited the normal increases in secretion volume, acidity and acid output induced by insulin.

In a crossover study comparing lansoprazole 15 and 30 mg with omeprazole 20 mg for five days, the following effects on intragastric pH were noted:

[See first table at top of next page]

After the initial dose in this study, increased gastric pH was seen within 1–2 hours with lansoprazole 30 mg, 2–3 hours with lansoprazole 15 mg, and 3–4 hours with omeprazole 20 mg. After multiple daily dosing, increased gastric pH was seen within the first hour postdosing with lansoprazole 30 mg and within 1–2 hours postdosing with lansoprazole 15 mg and omeprazole 20 mg.

The percentage of time gastric pH was elevated above 5 and 6 was evaluated in a crossover study of PREVACID given q.d., b.i.d. and t.i.d.

[See second table at top of next page]

The inhibition of gastric acid secretion as measured by intragastric pH returns gradually to normal over two to four days after multiple doses. There is no indication of rebound gastric acidity.

CLINICAL STUDIES

***H. pylori* Eradication to Reduce the Risk of Duodenal Ulcer Recurrence**

Randomized, double-blind clinical studies performed in the U.S. in patients with *H. pylori* and duodenal ulcer disease

Continued on next page

Prevpac—Cont.

(defined as an active ulcer or history of an ulcer within one year) evaluated the efficacy of PREVPAC as triple 14-day therapy for the eradication of *H. pylori*. The triple therapy regimen (PREVACID 30 mg BID plus amoxicillin 1 gm BID plus clarithromycin 500 mg BID) produced statistically significantly higher eradication rates than PREVACID plus amoxicillin, PREVACID plus clarithromycin, and amoxicillin plus clarithromycin dual therapies.

H. pylori eradication was defined as two negative tests (culture and histology) at 4 to 6 weeks following the end of treatment.

Triple therapy was shown to be more effective than all possible dual therapy combinations. The combination of PREVACID plus amoxicillin and clarithromycin as triple therapy was effective in eradicating *H. pylori*. Eradication of *H. pylori* has been shown to reduce the risk of duodenal ulcer recurrence.

A randomized, double-blind clinical study performed in the U.S. in patients with *H. pylori* and duodenal ulcer disease (defined as an active ulcer or history of an ulcer within one year) compared the efficacy of PREVACID triple therapy for 10 and 14 days. This study established that the 10-day triple therapy was equivalent to the 14-day triple therapy in eradicating *H. pylori*.

[See third table at right]

INDICATIONS AND USAGE

***H. pylori* Eradication to Reduce the Risk of Duodenal Ulcer Recurrence**

The components in PREVPAC (PREVACID, amoxicillin, and clarithromycin) are indicated for the treatment of patients with *H. pylori* infection and duodenal ulcer disease (active or one-year history of a duodenal ulcer) to eradicate *H. pylori*. Eradication of *H. pylori* has been shown to reduce the risk of duodenal ulcer recurrence (See **CLINICAL STUDIES** and **DOSAGE AND ADMINISTRATION**).

CONTRAINDICATIONS

PREVPAC is contraindicated in patients with known hypersensitivity to any component of the formulation of PREVACID, any macrolide antibiotic, or any penicillin.

Concomitant administration of PREVPAC with cisapride, pimozide, or terfenadine is contraindicated. There have been postmarketing reports of drug interactions when clarithromycin and/or erythromycin are co-administered with cisapride, pimozide, or terfenadine resulting in cardiac arrhythmias (QT prolongation, ventricular tachycardia, ventricular fibrillation, and torsades de pointes) most likely due to inhibition of hepatic metabolism of these drugs by erythromycin and clarithromycin. Fatalities have been reported.

WARNINGS

Amoxicillin:

Serious and occasionally fatal hypersensitivity (anaphylactoid) reactions have been reported in patients on penicillin therapy. Although anaphylaxis is more frequent following parenteral therapy, it has occurred in patients on oral penicillins. These reactions are more apt to occur in individuals with a history of penicillin hypersensitivity and/or a history of sensitivity to multiple allergens.

There have been well documented reports of individuals with a history of penicillin hypersensitivity reactions who have experienced severe hypersensitivity reactions when treated with a cephalosporin. Before initiating therapy with any penicillin, careful inquiry should be made concerning previous hypersensitivity reactions to penicillins, cephalosporins, and other allergens. If an allergic reaction occurs, amoxicillin should be discontinued and the appropriate therapy instituted.

SERIOUS ANAPHYLACTOID REACTIONS REQUIRE IMMEDIATE EMERGENCY TREATMENT WITH EPINEPHRINE. OXYGEN, INTRAVENOUS STEROIDS, AND AIRWAY MANAGEMENT, INCLUDING INTUBATION, SHOULD ALSO BE ADMINISTERED AS INDICATED.

Clarithromycin:

CLARITHROMYCIN SHOULD NOT BE USED IN PREGNANT WOMEN EXCEPT IN CLINICAL CIRCUMSTANCES WHERE NO ALTERNATIVE THERAPY IS APPROPRIATE. IF PREGNANCY OCCURS WHILE TAKING CLARITHROMYCIN, THE PATIENT SHOULD BE APPRISED OF THE POTENTIAL HAZARD TO THE FETUS. CLARITHROMYCIN HAS DEMONSTRATED ADVERSE EFFECTS OF PREGNANCY OUTCOME AND/OR EMBRYO-FETAL DEVELOPMENT IN MONKEYS, RATS, MICE, AND RABBITS AT DOSES THAT PRODUCED PLASMA LEVELS 2 TO 17 TIMES THE SERUM LEVELS ACHIEVED IN HUMANS TREATED AT THE MAXIMUM RECOMMENDED HUMAN DOSES. (See PRECAUTIONS - *Pregnancy.*)

Pseudomembranous colitis has been reported with nearly all antibacterial agents, including clarithromycin, and may range in severity from mild to life threatening. Therefore, it is important to consider this diagnosis in patients who present with diarrhea subsequent to the administration of antibacterial agents.

Treatment with antibacterial agents alters the normal flora of the colon and may permit overgrowth of clostridia. Studies indicate that a toxin produced by *Clostridium difficile* is a primary cause of "antibiotic-associated colitis."

After the diagnosis of pseudomembranous colitis has been established, therapeutic measures should be initiated. Mild cases of pseudomembranous colitis usually respond to discontinuation of the drug alone. In moderate to severe cases, consideration should be given to management with fluids and electrolytes, protein supplementation, and treatment with an antibacterial drug clinically effective against *Clostridium difficile* colitis.

Mean Antisecretory Effects after Single and Multiple Daily Dosing

Parameter	Baseline Value	PREVACID 15 mg Day 1	PREVACID 15 mg Day 5	PREVACID 30 mg Day 1	PREVACID 30 mg Day 5	Omeprazole 20 mg Day 1	Omeprazole 20 mg Day 5
Mean 24-Hour pH	2.1	2.7+	4.0+	3.6*	4.9*	2.5	4.2+
Mean Nighttime pH	1.9	2.4	3.0+	2.6	3.8*	2.2	3.0+
% Time Gastric pH>3	18	33+	59+	51*	72*	30+	61+
% Time Gastric pH>4	12	22+	49+	41*	66*	19	51+

NOTE: An intragastric pH of >4 reflects a reduction in gastric acid by 99%.
*(p<0.05) versus baseline, lansoprazole 15 mg and omeprazole 20 mg.
+(p<0.05) versus baseline only.

Mean Antisecretory Effects After 5 Days of b.i.d. and t.i.d. Dosing

Parameter	PREVACID 30 mg q.d.	PREVACID 15 mg b.i.d.	PREVACID 30 mg b.i.d.	PREVACID 30 mg t.i.d.
% Time Gastric pH>5	43	47	59+	77*
% Time Gastric pH>6	20	23	28	45*

+(p<0.05) versus PREVACID 30 mg q.d.
*(p<0.05) versus PREVACID 30 mg q.d., 15 mg b.i.d. and 30 mg b.i.d.

***H. pylori* Eradication Rates—Triple Therapy**
(PREVACID/amoxicillin/clarithromycin)
Percent of Patients Cured
[95% Confidence Interval]
(Number of patients)

Study	Duration	Triple Therapy Evaluable Analysis*	Triple Therapy Intent-to-Treat Analysis#
M93-131	14 days	92† [80.0–97.7] (N=48)	86† [73.3–93.5] (N=55)
M95-392	14 days	86‡ [75.7–93.6] (N=66)	83‡ [72.0–90.8] (N=70)
M95-399+	14 days	85 [77.0–91.0] (N=113)	82 [73.9–88.1] (N=126)
	10 days	84 [76.0–89.8] (N=123)	81 [73.9–87.6] (N=135)

* Based on evaluable patients with confirmed duodenal ulcer (active or within one year) and *H. pylori* infection at baseline defined as at least two of three positive endoscopic tests from CLOtest® (Delta West Ltd., Bentley, Australia), histology and/or culture. Patients were included in the analysis if they completed the study. Additionally, if patients dropped out of the study due to an adverse event related to the study drug, they were included in the evaluable analysis as failures of therapy.
\# Patients were included in the analysis if they had documented *H. pylori* infection at baseline as defined above and had a confirmed duodenal ulcer (active or within one year). All dropouts were included as failures of therapy.
† (p<0.05) versus PREVACID/amoxicillin and PREVACID/clarithromycin dual therapy
‡ (p<0.05) versus clarithromycin/amoxicillin dual therapy
\+ The 95% confidence interval for the difference in eradication rates, 10-day minus 14-day is (-10.5, 8.1) in the evaluable analysis and (-9.7, 9.1) in the intent-to-treat analysis.

PRECAUTIONS

Clarithromycin is principally excreted via the liver and kidney. Clarithromycin may be administered without dosage adjustment to patients with hepatic impairment and normal renal function. However, in the presence of severe renal impairment with or without coexisting hepatic impairment, decreased dosage or prolonged dosing intervals may be appropriate.

The possibility of superinfections with mycotic organisms or bacterial pathogens should be kept in mind during therapy. In such cases, discontinue PREVPAC and substitute appropriate treatment.

Symptomatic response to therapy with PREVACID does not preclude the presence of gastric malignancy.

Information for Patients: Each dose of PREVPAC contains four pills: one pink and black capsule (PREVACID), two maroon and light-pink capsules (amoxicillin) and one yellow tablet (clarithromycin). Each dose should be taken twice per day before eating. Patients should be instructed to swallow each pill whole.

Drug Interactions

PREVACID:

PREVACID is metabolized through the cytochrome P_{450} system, specifically through the CYP3A and CYP2C19 isozymes. Studies have shown that PREVACID does not have clinically significant interactions with other drugs metabolized by the cytochrome P_{450} system, such as warfarin, antipyrine, indomethacin, ibuprofen, phenytoin, propranolol, prednisone, diazepam, clarithromycin, or terfenadine in healthy subjects. These compounds are metabolized through various cytochrome P_{450} isozymes including CYP1A2, CYP2C9, CYP2C19, CYP2D6, and CYP3A. When PREVACID was administered concomitantly with theophylline (CYP1A2, CYP3A), a minor increase (10%) in the clearance of theophylline was seen. Because of the small magnitude and the direction of the effect on theophylline clearance, this interaction is unlikely to be of clinical concern. Nonetheless, individual patients may require additional titration of their theophylline dosage when PREVACID is started or stopped to ensure clinically effective blood levels.

PREVACID has also been shown to have no clinically significant interaction with amoxicillin.

In a single-dose crossover study examining PREVACID 30 mg and omeprazole 20 mg each administered alone and concomitantly with sucralfate 1 gram, absorption of the proton pump inhibitors was delayed and their bioavailability was reduced by 17% and 16%, respectively, when administered concomitantly with sucralfate. Therefore, proton pump inhibitors should be taken at least 30 minutes prior to sucralfate. In clinical trials, antacids were administered concomitantly with PREVACID Delayed-Release Capsules; this did not interfere with its effect.

PREVACID causes a profound and long-lasting inhibition of gastric acid secretion; therefore, it is theoretically possible that PREVACID may interfere with the absorption of drugs where gastric pH is an important determinant of bioavailability (eg, ketoconazole, ampicillin esters, iron salts, digoxin).

Clarithromycin:

Clarithromycin use in patients who are receiving theophylline may be associated with an increase of serum theophylline concentrations. Monitoring of serum theophylline concentrations should be considered for patients receiving high doses of theophylline or with baseline concentrations in the upper therapeutic range. In two studies in which theophylline was administered with clarithromycin (a theophylline sustained-release formulation was dosed at either 6.5 mg/kg or 12 mg/kg together with 250 or 500 mg q12h clarithromycin), the steady-state levels of C_{max}, C_{min}, and the area under the serum concentration time curve (AUC) of theophylline increased about 20%.

Concomitant administration of single doses of clarithromycin and carbamazepine has been shown to result in increased plasma concentrations of carbamazepine. Blood level monitoring of carbamazepine may be considered.

When clarithromycin and terfenadine were coadministered, plasma concentrations of the active acid metabolite of terfenadine were threefold higher, on average, than the values observed when terfenadine was administered alone. The pharmacokinetics of clarithromycin and the 14-hydroxy-clarithromycin were not significantly affected by coadministration of terfenadine once clarithromycin reached steady-state conditions. Concomitant administration of clarithromycin with terfenadine is contraindicated. (See **CONTRAINDICATIONS**.)

Spontaneous reports in the postmarketing period suggest that concomitant administration of clarithromycin and oral anticoagulants may potentiate the effects of the oral anticoagulants. Prothrombin times should be carefully monitored while patients are receiving clarithromycin and oral anticoagulants simultaneously.

Elevated digoxin serum concentrations in patients receiving clarithromycin and digoxin concomitantly have also been reported in postmarketing surveillance. Some patients have shown clinical signs consistent with digoxin toxicity, including potentially fatal arrhythmias. Serum digoxin levels should be carefully monitored while patients are receiving digoxin and clarithromycin simultaneously.

For information on interactions between clarithromycin in combination with other drugs which may be administered to HIV-infected patients, see the BIAXIN package insert, Drug Interactions, under the **PRECAUTIONS** section.

The following drug interactions, other than increased serum concentrations of carbamazepine and active acid metabolite of terfenadine, have not been reported in clinical trials with clarithromycin; however, they have been observed with erythromycin products and/or with clarithromycin in postmarketing experience.

Concurrent use of erythromycin or clarithromycin and ergotamine or dihydroergotamine has been associated in some patients with acute ergot toxicity characterized by severe peripheral vasospasm and dysesthesia.

Erythromycin has been reported to decrease the clearance of triazolam and, thus, may increase the pharmacologic effect of triazolam. There have been postmarketing reports of drug interactions and CNS effects (e.g., somnolence and confusion) with the concomitant use of clarithromycin and triazolam.

There have been reports of an interaction between erythromycin and astemizole resulting in QT prolongation and torsades de pointes. Concomitant administration of erythromycin and astemizole is contraindicated. Because clarithromycin is also metabolized by cytochrome P_{450}, concomitant administration of clarithromycin with astemizole is not recommended.

As with other macrolides, clarithromycin has been reported to increase concentrations of HMG-CoA reductase inhibitors (e.g., lovastatin and simvastatin), through inhibition of cytochrome P_{450} metabolism of these drugs. Rare reports of rhabdomyolysis have been reported in patients taking these drugs concomitantly.

The use of erythromycin and clarithromycin in patients concurrently taking drugs metabolized by the cytochrome P_{450} system may be associated with elevations in serum levels of these other drugs. There have been reports of interactions of erythromycin and/or clarithromycin with carbamazepine, cyclosporine, tacrolimus, hexobarbital, phenytoin, alfentanil, disopyramide, lovastatin, bromocriptine, valproate, terfenadine, cisapride, pimozide, rifabutin, and astemizole. Serum concentrations of drugs metabolized by the cytochrome P_{450} system should be monitored closely in patients concurrently receiving these drugs.

Carcinogenesis, Mutagenesis, Impairment of Fertility

PREVACID:

In two 24-month carcinogenicity studies, Sprague-Dawley rats were treated orally with doses of 5 to 150 mg/kg/day, about 1 to 40 times the exposure on a body surface (mg/m^2) basis, of a 50-kg person of average height (1.46 m^2 body surface area) given the recommended human dose of 30 mg/day (22.2 mg/m^2). Lansoprazole produced dose-related gastric enterochromaffin-like (ECL) cell hyperplasia and ECL cell carcinoids in both male and female rats. It also increased the incidence of intestinal metaplasia of the gastric epithelium in both sexes. In male rats, lansoprazole produced a dose-related increase of testicular interstitial cell adenomas. The incidence of these adenomas in rats receiving doses of 15 to 150 mg/kg/day (4 to 40 times the recommended human dose based on body surface area) exceeded the low background incidence (range = 1.4 to 10%) for this strain of rat. Testicular interstitial cell adenoma also occurred in 1 of 30 rats treated with 50 mg/kg/day (13 times the recommended human dose based on body surface area) in a 1-year toxicity study.

In a 24-month carcinogenicity study, CD-1 mice were treated orally with doses of 15 to 600 mg/kg/day, 2 to 80 times the recommended human dose based on body surface area. Lansoprazole produced a dose-related increased incidence of gastric ECL cell hyperplasia. It also produced an increased incidence of liver tumors (hepatocellular adenoma plus carcinoma). The tumor incidences in male mice treated with 300 and 600 mg/kg/day (40 to 80 times the recommended human dose based on body surface area) and female mice treated with 150 to 600 mg/kg/day (20 to 80 times the recommended human dose based on body surface area) exceeded the ranges of background incidences in historical controls for this strain of mice. Lansoprazole treatment produced adenoma of rete testis in male mice receiving 75 to 600 mg/kg/day (10 to 80 times the recommended human dose based on body surface area).

Lansoprazole was not genotoxic in the Ames test, the *ex vivo* rat hepatocyte unscheduled DNA synthesis (UDS) test, the *in vivo* mouse micronucleus test or the rat bone marrow cell chromosomal aberration test. It was positive in *in vitro* human lymphocyte chromosomal aberration assays.

Lansoprazole at oral doses up to 150 mg/kg/day (40 times the recommended human dose based on body surface area) was found to have no effect on fertility and reproductive performance of male and female rats.

Amoxicillin:

Long-term studies in animals have not been performed with amoxicillin.

Clarithromycin:

The following *in vitro* mutagenicity tests have been conducted with clarithromycin:

Salmonella/Mammalian Microsomes Test
Bacterial Induced Mutation Frequency Test
In Vitro Chromosome Aberration Test
Rat Hepatocyte DNA Synthesis Assay
Mouse Lymphoma Assay
Mouse Dominant Lethal Study
Mouse Micronucleus Test

All tests had negative results except the *In Vitro* Chromosome Aberration Test which was weakly positive in one test and negative in another.

In addition, a Bacterial Reverse-Mutation Test (Ames Test) has been performed on clarithromycin metabolites with negative results.

Fertility and reproduction studies have shown that daily doses of up to 160 mg/kg/day (1.3 times the recommended maximum human dose based on mg/m^2) to male and female rats caused no adverse effects on the estrous cycle, fertility, parturition, or number and viability of offspring. Plasma levels in rats after 150 mg/kg/day were 2 times the human serum levels.

In the 150 mg/kg/day monkey studies, plasma levels were 3 times the human serum levels. When given orally at 150 mg/kg/day (2.4 times the recommended maximum human dose based on mg/m^2), clarithromycin was shown to produce embryonic loss in monkeys. This effect has been attributed to marked maternal toxicity of the drug at this high dose.

In rabbits, *in utero* fetal loss occurred at an intravenous dose of 33 mg/m^2, which is 17 times less than the maximum proposed human oral daily dose of 618 mg/m^2.

Long-term studies in animals have not been performed to evaluate the carcinogenic potential of clarithromycin.

Pregnancy

Teratogenic Effects. Pregnancy Category C

Category C is based on the pregnancy category for clarithromycin.

Four teratogenicity studies in rats (three with oral doses and one with intravenous doses up to 160 mg/kg/day administered during the period of major organogenesis) and two in rabbits at oral doses up to 125 mg/kg/day (approximately 2 times the recommended maximum human dose based on mg/m^2) or intravenous doses of 30 mg/kg/day administered during gestation days 6 to 18 failed to demonstrate any teratogenicity from clarithromycin. Two additional oral studies in a different rat strain at similar doses and similar conditions demonstrated a low incidence of cardiovascular anomalies at doses of 150 mg/kg/day administered during gestation days 6 to 15. Plasma levels after 150 mg/kg/day were 2 times the human serum levels. Four studies in mice revealed a variable incidence of cleft palate following oral doses of 1000 mg/kg/day (2 and 4 times the recommended maximum human dose based on mg/m^2, respectively) during gestation days 6 to 15. Cleft palate was also seen at 500 mg/kg/day. The 1000 mg/kg/day exposure resulted in plasma levels 17 times the human serum levels. In monkeys, an oral dose of 70 mg/kg/day (an approximate equidose of the recommended maximum human dose based on mg/m^2) produced fetal growth retardation at plasma levels that were 2 times the human serum levels.

There were no adequate and well-controlled studies of PREVPAC in pregnant women. PREVPAC should be used during pregnancy only if the potential benefit justifies the potential risk to the fetus. (See **WARNINGS**.)

Labor and Delivery

Oral ampicillin-class antibiotics are poorly absorbed during labor. Studies in guinea pigs showed that intravenous administration of ampicillin slightly decreased the uterine tone and frequency of contractions, but moderately increased the height and duration of contractions. However, it is not known whether use of these drugs in humans during labor or delivery has immediate or delayed adverse effects on the fetus, prolongs the duration of labor, or increases the likelihood that forceps delivery or other obstetrical intervention or resuscitation of the newborn will be necessary.

Nursing Mothers

Amoxicillin is excreted in human milk in very small amounts. Because of the potential for serious adverse reactions in nursing infants from PREVPAC, a decision should be made whether to discontinue nursing or to discontinue the drug therapy, taking into account the importance of the therapy to the mother.

Pediatric Use

Safety and effectiveness of PREVPAC in pediatric patients infected with *H. pylori* have not been established (See **CONTRAINDICATIONS** and **WARNINGS**).

Geriatric Use

Elderly patients may suffer from asymptomatic renal and hepatic dysfunction. Care should be taken when administering PREVPAC to this patient population.

ADVERSE REACTIONS

The most common adverse reactions (≥ 3%) reported in clinical trials when all three components of this therapy were given concomitantly for 14 days are listed in the table below.

Adverse Reactions Most Frequently Reported in Clinical Trials (≥3%)

Adverse Reaction	Triple Therapy n=138 (%)
Diarrhea	7.0
Headache	6.0
Taste Perversion	5.0

The additional adverse reactions which were reported as possibly or probably related to treatment (< 3%) in clinical trials when all three components of this therapy were given concomitantly are listed below and divided by body system: *Body as a Whole*—abdominal pain; *Digestive System*—dark stools, dry mouth/thirst, glossitis, rectal itching, nausea, oral moniliasis, stomatitis, tongue discoloration, tongue disorder, vomiting; *Musculoskeletal System*—myalgia; *Nervous System*—confusion, dizziness; *Respiratory System*—respiratory disorders; *Skin and Appendages*—skin reactions; *Urogenital System*—vaginitis, vaginal moniliasis. There were no statistically significant differences in the frequency of reported adverse events between the 10- and 14-day triple therapy regimens.

PREVACID:

The following adverse reactions from the labeling for lansoprazole are provided for information.

Worldwide, over 6100 patients have been treated with lansoprazole in Phase II-III clinical trials involving various dosages and duration of treatment. In general, lansoprazole treatment has been well tolerated in both short-term and long-term trials.

Incidence in Clinical Trials

The following adverse events were reported by the treating physician to have a possible or probable relationship to drug in 1% or more of patients treated with PREVACID capsules and occurred at a greater rate in patients treated with PREVACID capsules than placebo-treated patients:

Incidence of Possibly or Probably Treatment-Related Adverse Events in Short-term, Placebo-Controlled Studies

Body System/Adverse Event	PREVACID (N=1457) %	Placebo (N=467) %
Body as a Whole		
Abdominal Pain	1.8	1.3
Digestive System		
Diarrhea	3.6	2.6
Nausea	1.4	1.3

Headache was also seen at greater than 1% incidence but was more common on placebo. The incidence of diarrhea is similar between placebo and lansoprazole 15 mg and 30 mg patients, but higher in the lansoprazole 60 mg patients (2.9%, 1.4%, 4.2%, and 7.4%, respectively).

The most commonly reported possibly or probably treatment-related adverse event during maintenance therapy was diarrhea.

Additional adverse experiences occurring in <1% of patients or subjects in domestic and/or international trials, or occurring since the drug was marketed, are shown below within each body system.

In short-term and long-term studies, the following adverse events were reported in <1% of the lansoprazole-treated patients:

Body as a Whole—anaphylactoid-like reaction, asthenia, candidiasis, chest pain (not otherwise specified), edema, fever, flu syndrome, halitosis, infection (not otherwise specified), malaise; *Cardiovascular System*—angina, cerebrovascular accident, hypertension/hypotension, myocardial infarction, palpitations, shock (circulatory failure), vasodilation; *Digestive System*—melena, anorexia, bezoar, cardiospasm, cholelithiasis, constipation, dry mouth/thirst, dyspepsia, dysphagia, eructation, esophageal stenosis, esophageal ulcer, esophagitis, fecal discoloration, flatulence, gastric nodules/fundic gland polyps, gastroenteritis, gastrointestinal hemorrhage, hematemesis, increased appetite, increased salivation, rectal hemorrhage, stomatitis, tenesmus, ulcerative colitis, vomiting; *Endocrine System*—diabetes mellitus, goiter, hyperglycemia/hypoglycemia; *Hematologic and Lymphatic System**—agranulocytosis, anemia, aplastic anemia, hemolysis, hemolytic anemia, leukopenia, neutropenia, pancytopenia, thrombocytopenia, and thrombotic thrombocytopenic purpura; *Metabolic and Nutritional Disorders*—gout, weight gain/loss; *Musculoskeletal System*—arthritis/arthralgia, musculoskeletal pain, myalgia; *Nervous System*—agitation, amnesia, anxiety, apathy, confusion, depression, dizziness/syncope, hallucinations, hemiplegia, hostility aggravated, libido decreased, nervousness, paresthesia, thinking abnormality; *Respiratory System*—asthma, bronchitis, cough increased, dyspnea, epistaxis, hemoptysis, hiccup, pneumonia, upper respiratory inflammation/infection; *Skin and Appendages*—acne, alopecia, pruri-

Continued on next page

Prevpac—Cont.

tus, rash, urticaria; *Special Senses*—blurred vision, deafness, eye pain, visual field defect, otitis media, taste perversion, tinnitus; *Urogenital System*—abnormal menses, albuminuria, breast enlargement/gynecomastia, breast tenderness, glycosuria, hematuria, impotence, kidney calculus.
*The majority of hematologic cases received were foreign-sourced and their relationship to lansoprazole was unclear.

Laboratory Values

The following changes in laboratory parameters were reported as adverse events.

Abnormal liver function tests, increased SGOT (AST), increased SGPT (ALT), increased creatinine, increased alkaline phosphatase, increased globulins, increased GGTP, increased/decreased/abnormal WBC, abnormal AG ratio, abnormal RBC, bilirubinemia, eosinophilia, hyperlipemia, increased/decreased electrolytes, increased/decreased cholesterol, increased glucocorticoids, increased LDH, increased/decreased/abnormal platelets, and increased gastrin levels. Additional isolated laboratory abnormalities were reported.

In the placebo-controlled studies, when SGOT (AST) and SGPT (ALT) were evaluated, 0.4% (1/250) placebo patients and 0.3% (2/795) lansoprazole patients had enzyme elevations greater than three times the upper limit of normal range at the final treatment visit. None of these patients reported jaundice at any time during the study.

Amoxicillin:

The following adverse reactions from the labeling for amoxicillin are provided for information.

As with other penicillins, it may be expected that untoward reactions will be essentially limited to sensitivity phenomena. They are more likely to occur in individuals who have previously demonstrated hypersensitivity to penicillins and in those with a history of allergy, asthma, hay fever, or urticaria. Glossitis, stomatitis, black "hairy" tongue, nausea, vomiting, and diarrhea have been reported as associated with the use of penicillin. (These reactions are usually associated with oral dosage forms.)

Hypersensitivity Reactions—Skin rashes and urticaria have been reported frequently. A few cases of exfoliative dermatitis and erythema multiforme have been reported. Anaphylaxis is the most serious reaction experienced and has usually been associated with the parenteral dosage form. Urticaria, other skin rashes, and serum sickness-like reactions may be controlled with antihistamines and, if necessary, systemic corticosteroids. Whenever such reactions occur, penicillin should be discontinued unless, in the opinion of the physician, the condition being treated is life threatening and amenable only to penicillin therapy. Serious anaphylactic reactions require the immediate use of epinephrine, oxygen, and intravenous steroids.

Liver—A moderate rise in serum glutamic oxaloacetic transaminase (SGOT) has been noted, particularly in infants, but the significance of this finding is unknown.

Hemic and Lymphatic Systems—Anemia, thrombocytopenia, thrombocytopenic purpura, eosinophilia, leukopenia, and agranulocytosis have been reported during therapy with the penicillins. These reactions are usually reversible on discontinuation of therapy and are believed to be hypersensitivity phenomena.

Clarithromycin:

The following adverse reactions from the labeling for clarithromycin are provided for information.

The majority of side effects observed in clinical trials were of a mild and transient nature. Fewer than 3% of adult patients without mycobacterial infections discontinued therapy because of drug-related side effects.

The most frequently reported events in adults were diarrhea (3%), nausea (3%), abnormal taste (3%), dyspepsia (2%), abdominal pain/discomfort (2%), and headache (2%). Most of these events were described as mild or moderate in severity. Of the reported adverse events, only 1% was described as severe.

Postmarketing Experience:

Allergic reactions ranging from urticaria and mild skin eruptions to rare cases of anaphylaxis and Stevens-Johnson syndrome have occurred. Other spontaneously reported adverse events include glossitis, stomatitis, oral moniliasis, vomiting, tongue discoloration, thrombocytopenia, leukopenia, neutropenia, and dizziness. There have been reports of tooth discoloration in patients treated with clarithromycin. Tooth discoloration is usually reversible with professional dental cleaning. There have been isolated reports of hearing loss, which is usually reversible, occurring chiefly in elderly women. Reports of alterations of the sense of smell, usually in conjunction with taste perversion or taste loss have also been reported.

Transient CNS events including anxiety, behavioral changes, confusional states, depersonalization, disorientation, hallucinations, insomnia, manic behavior, nightmares, psychosis, tinnitus, tremor, and vertigo have been reported during postmarketing surveillance. Events usually resolve with discontinuation of the drug.

Hepatic dysfunction, including increased liver enzymes and hepatocellular and/or cholestatic hepatitis, with or without jaundice, has been infrequently reported with clarithromycin. This hepatic dysfunction may be severe and is usually reversible. In very rare instances, hepatic failure with fatal outcome has been reported and generally has been associated with serious underlying diseases and/or concomitant medications.

There have been rare reports of hypoglycemia, some of which have occurred in patients taking oral hypoglycemic agents or insulin.

Rarely, erythromycin and clarithromycin have been associated with ventricular arrhythmias, including ventricular tachycardia and torsades de pointes in individuals with prolonged QT_C intervals.

Changes in Laboratory Values: Changes in laboratory values with possible clinical significance were as follows: *Hepatic*—elevated SGPT (ALT) <1%, SGOT (AST) <1%, GGT <1%, alkaline phosphatase <1%, LDH <1%, total bilirubin <1%; *Hematologic*—decreased WBC <1%, elevated prothrombin time 1%; *Renal*—elevated BUN 4%, elevated serum creatinine <1%. GGT, alkaline phosphatase, and prothrombin time are from adult studies only.

OVERDOSAGE

In case of an overdose, patients should contact a physician, poison control center, or emergency room. There is neither a pharmacologic basis nor data suggesting an increased toxicity of the combination compared to individual components.

Lansoprazole:

Oral doses up to 5000 mg/kg in rats (approximately 1300 times the 30 mg human dose based on body surface area) and mice (about 675.7 times the 30 mg human dose based on body surface area) did not produce deaths or any clinical signs.

Lansoprazole is not removed from the circulation by hemodialysis. In one reported case of overdose, the patient consumed 600 mg of lansoprazole with no adverse reaction.

Amoxicillin:

In case of overdosage, discontinue medication, treat symptomatically and institute supportive measures as required. Amoxicillin can be removed from circulation by hemodialysis.

DOSAGE AND ADMINISTRATION

***H. pylori* Eradication to Reduce the Risk of Duodenal Ulcer Recurrence**

The recommended adult oral dose is 30 mg PREVACID, 1 g amoxicillin, and 500 mg clarithromycin administered together twice daily (morning and evening) for 10 or 14 days. (See **INDICATIONS AND USAGE**.)

PREVPAC is not recommended in patients with creatinine clearance less than 30mL/min.

HOW SUPPLIED

PREVPAC is supplied as an individual daily administration pack, each containing:

PREVACID:

– two opaque, hard gelatin, black and pink PREVACID 30-mg capsules, with the TAP logo and "PREVACID 30" imprinted on the capsules.

TRIMOX:

– four maroon and light-pink amoxicillin 500-mg capsules, USP, with "BRISTOL 7279" imprinted on the capsules.

BIAXIN Filmtab:

– two yellow oval film-coated clarithromycin 500-mg tablets with the Abbott logo and "KL" imprinted in blue on one side of the tablets.

NDC 0300-3702-01 Daily administration pack
NDC 0300-3702-11 Daily administration card

Storage: Protect from light and moisture.
Store at a controlled room temperature between 59°F and 86°F (15°C and 30°C).
Rx only
U.S. Patent No. 5,013,743
PREVPAC is distributed by TAP Pharmaceuticals Inc.
PREVACID® (lansoprazole) Delayed-Release Capsules
Manufactured for TAP Pharmaceuticals Inc.
Deerfield, Illinois 60015-1595, U.S.A.
by Takeda Chemical Industries, Limited,
Osaka, Japan 541
Distributed by TAP Pharmaceuticals Inc.
TRIMOX® (amoxicillin, USP)
Manufactured by APOTHECON® A Bristol-Myers Squibb Company Princeton, NJ 08540, U.S.A.
BIAXIN® Filmtab® (clarithromycin tablets)
Manufactured by Abbott Laboratories North Chicago, IL 60064, U.S.A.
Ref. 03-4943-R2; Revised: January, 1999

Shown in Product Identification Guide, page 338

NOTICE
Before prescribing or administering
any product described in
PHYSICIANS' DESK REFERENCE
check the **PDR Supplements**
for revised information.

TevaMarion Partners

10450 B HICKMAN MILLS DR
KANSAS CITY, MO 64137

For Direct Inquiries Contact:
(816) 966-3977

COPAXONE® ℞
(glatiramer acetate for injection)

DESCRIPTION

COPAXONE® is the brand name for glatiramer acetate (formerly known as copolymer-1). Glatiramer acetate, the active ingredient of COPAXONE®, consists of the acetate salts of synthetic polypeptides, containing four naturally occurring amino acids: L-glutamic acid, L-alanine, L-tyrosine, and L-lysine with an average molar fraction of 0.141, 0.427, 0.095, and 0.338, respectively. The average molecular weight of glatiramer acetate is 4,700–11,000 daltons.

Chemically, glatiramer acetate is designated L-glutamic acid polymer with L-alanine, L-lysine and L-tyrosine, acetate (salt). Its structural formula is:

$$(\text{Glu, Ala, Lys, Tyr})_\chi \cdot \chi CH_3COOH$$
$$(C_5H_9NO_4 \cdot C_3H_7NO_2 \cdot C_6H_{14}N_2O_2 \cdot C_9H_{11}NO_3)_\chi \cdot \chi C_2H_4O_2$$

CAS - 147245-92-9

COPAXONE® is a white to off-white, sterile, lyophilized powder containing 20 mg of glatiramer acetate and 40 mg of mannitol. It is supplied in single-use vials for subcutaneous administration after reconstitution with the diluent supplied (Sterile Water for Injection).

CLINICAL PHARMACOLOGY

Mechanism of Action

The mechanism(s) by which glatiramer acetate exerts its effects in patients with Multiple Sclerosis (MS) is (are) unknown. However, it is thought to act by modifying immune processes that are currently believed to be responsible for the pathogenesis of MS. This view of glatiramer acetate derives from knowledge that it reduces the incidence and severity of experimental allergic encephalomyelitis, a condition induced in several animal species through immunization against central nervous system derived material containing myelin and often used as an experimental animal model of MS.

Because glatiramer acetate can modify immune function, concerns exist about its potential to alter naturally occurring immune responses. Results of a limited battery of tests designed to evaluate the risk produced no finding of concern; nevertheless, there is no logical way to absolutely exclude this possibility (see **PRECAUTIONS**).

Pharmacokinetics

Pharmacokinetics studies in humans have not been performed. It is assumed, however, based in part on the results of animal studies, that a substantial fraction of a subcutaneous injection of glatiramer acetate is hydrolyzed locally. Some fraction of injected material is presumed to enter the lymphatic circulation, enabling it to reach regional lymph nodes, and some may enter the systemic circulation intact.

Clinical Trials

Evidence supporting the effectiveness of glatiramer acetate in decreasing the frequency of relapses in patients with Relapsing-Remitting Multiple Sclerosis (RR MS) derives from two placebo-controlled trials, both of which used a glatiramer acetate dose of 20 mg/day. (No other dose has been studied in placebo-controlled trials of RR MS.)

One trial was performed at a single center. It enrolled 50 patients (glatiramer acetate, 25; placebo, 25) who were randomized to receive daily doses of either glatiramer acetate, 20 mg subcutaneously, or placebo. Patients were diagnosed with RR MS by standard criteria, and had had at least 2 exacerbations during the 2 years immediately preceding enrollment. Patients were ambulatory, as evidenced by a score of no more than 6 on the Kurtzke Expanded Disability Scale Score (DSS), a standard scale ranging from 0-Normal to 10-Death due to MS. A score of 6 is defined as one at which a patient is still ambulatory with assistance; a score of 7 means the patient must use a wheelchair.

Patients were examined every 3 months for 2 years, as well as within several days of a presumed exacerbation. To confirm an exacerbation, a blinded neurologist had to document objective neurologic signs, as well as document the existence of other criteria (e.g., the persistence of the lesion for at least 48 hours).

The protocol-specified primary outcome measure was the proportion of patients in each treatment group who remained exacerbation free for the 2 years of the trial, but two other important outcomes were also specified as endpoints: 1) the frequency of attacks during the trial, and 2) the change in the number of attacks compared with the number which occurred during the previous 2 years.

The following table presents the values of the three outcomes described above, as well as several protocol-specified secondary measures. These values are based on the intent-to-treat population (i.e., all patients who received at least 1 dose of treatment and who had at least 1 on-treatment assessment):

[See first table at top of next page]

The second trial was a multicenter trial of similar design to the first study, and was performed in 11 US centers. A total of 251 patients (glatiramer acetate 125; placebo, 126) were enrolled. The primary outcome measure was the Mean 2 Year Relapse Rate. The table below presents the values of this outcome for the intent-to-treat population, as well as several secondary measures:

[See second table at right]

In both studies glatiramer acetate exhibited a clear beneficial effect on relapse rate, and it is based on this evidence that glatiramer acetate is considered effective.

INDICATIONS AND USAGE

COPAXONE® is indicated for reduction of the frequency of relapses in patients with Relapsing-Remitting Multiple Sclerosis.

CONTRAINDICATIONS

COPAXONE® is contraindicated in patients with known hypersensitivity to glatiramer acetate or mannitol.

WARNINGS

The only recommended route of administration of COPAXONE® injection is the subcutaneous route. COPAXONE® should not be administered by the intravenous route.

PRECAUTIONS

General

Patients should be instructed in self-injection techniques to assure the safe administration of COPAXONE® (see **PRECAUTIONS: Information for Patients** and the **COPAXONE® PATIENT INFORMATION** Booklet). Current data indicate that no special caution is required for patients operating an automobile or using complex machinery.

Considerations Regarding the Use of a Product Capable of Modifying Immune Response

Because glatiramer acetate can modify immune response, it could possibly interfere with useful immune function. For example, treatment with glatiramer acetate might, in theory, interfere with the recognition of foreign antigens in a way that would undermine the body's tumor surveillance and its defenses against infection. There is no evidence that glatiramer acetate does this, but there has as yet been no systematic evaluation of the risk. Also, while glatiramer acetate is intended to minimize the autoimmune response to myelin, the possibility exists that continued alteration of cellular immunity from chronic treatment with glatiramer acetate might result in untoward effects. Because glatiramer acetate is an antigenic material it is possible that its use may lead to the induction of host responses that are untoward.

Although there is no evidence that use of glatiramer acetate induces untoward host responses in humans, systematic surveillance for these effects has not been undertaken. Studies in both the rat and monkey, however, have suggested that immune complexes are deposited in the renal glomeruli. Furthermore, in a controlled trial of 125 RR MS patients given glatiramer acetate, 20 mg, subcutaneously every day for 2 years, serum IgG levels reached approximately 3 times baseline values in 80% of patients within 3 to 6 months of initiation of treatment. These values returned to about 50% greater than baseline during the remainder of treatment.

Although glatiramer acetate is intended to minimize the autoimmune response to myelin, there is the possibility that continued alteration of cellular immunity due to chronic treatment with glatiramer acetate might result in untoward effects. Anaphylaxis can be associated with the administration of almost any foreign substance. Based on the protein nature of glatiramer acetate, the risk of anaphylaxis cannot be excluded. Of the approximately 900 patients treated in premarketing trials, none experienced anaphylactic shock.

Information for Patients

To assure safe and effective use of COPAXONE®, the following information and instructions should be given to patients:

1. Inform your physician if you are pregnant, if you are planning to have a child, or if you become pregnant while taking this medication.
2. Inform your physician if you are nursing.
3. Do not change the dose or dosing schedule without consulting your physician.
4. Do not stop taking the drug without consulting your physician.

Patients should be instructed in the use of aseptic techniques when administering COPAXONE®. Appropriate instructions for COPAXONE® reconstitution and self-injection should be given, including a careful review of the **COPAXONE® PATIENT INFORMATION** Booklet. The first injection should be performed under the supervision of an appropriately qualified health care professional. Patient understanding and use of aseptic self-injection techniques and procedures should be periodically reevaluated. Patients should be cautioned against the reuse of needles or syringes and instructed in safe disposal procedures. They should use a puncture-resistant container for disposal of used needles and syringes. Patients should be instructed on the safe disposal of full containers.

Awareness of Adverse Reactions: Physicians are advised to counsel patients about adverse reactions associated with the use of COPAXONE® (see **ADVERSE REACTIONS** section). In addition, patients should be advised to read the **COPAXONE® PATIENT INFORMATION** Booklet and resolve any questions regarding it prior to beginning COPAXONE® therapy.

Outcome	Glatiramer Acetate (N=25)	Placebo (N=25)	P-Value
% Relapse Free	14/25 (56%)	7/25 (28%)	0.085
Mean Relapse Frequency	0.6/2 years	2.4/2 years	0.005
Change in Relapse Rate	3.2	1.6	0.025
Median Time to First Relapse (days)	>700	150	0.03
% of Patients Progression Free*	20/25 (80%)	13/25 (52%)	0.07

*Progression is defined as an increase of at least 1 point on the DSS, persisting for at least 3 consecutive months.

Outcome	Glatiramer Acetate	Placebo	P-Value
Mean Relapse Rate	1.19/2 years	1.68/2 years	0.055
% Relapse Free	42/125 (34%)	34/126 (27%)	0.25
Median Time to First Relapse (days)	287	198	0.23
% of Patients Progression Free	98/125 (78%)	95/126 (75%)	0.48
Mean Change in DSS	-0.05	+0.21	0.023

Laboratory Tests

Data collected during premarketing development do not suggest the need for routine laboratory monitoring.

Drug Interactions

Interactions between COPAXONE® and other drugs have not been fully evaluated. Results from existing clinical trials do not suggest any significant interactions of COPAXONE® with therapies commonly used in MS patients, including the concurrent use of corticosteroids for up to 28 days. COPAXONE® has not been formally evaluated in combination with Interferon beta. However, 10 patients who switched from therapy with Interferon beta to COPAXONE® did not report any serious and unexpected adverse reactions thought to be related to treatment.

Drug/Laboratory Test Interactions

None are known.

Carcinogenesis, Mutagenesis, Impairment of Fertility

Carcinogenesis

Results of tests to assess the carcinogenic potential of glatiramer acetate in mice and rats are unavailable; these studies are in progress.

Mutagenesis

Glatiramer acetate was not mutagenic in four strains of *Salmonella typhimurium* and two strains of *Escherichia coli* (Ames test) or in the *in vitro* mouse lymphoma assay in L5178Y cells. Glatiramer acetate was clastogenic in two separate *in vitro* chromosomal aberration assays in cultured human lymphocytes; it was not clastogenic in an *in vivo* mouse bone marrow micronucleus assay.

Impairment of Fertility

In a multigeneration reproduction and fertility study in rats, glatiramer acetate at subcutaneous doses of up to 36 mg/kg (18 times the recommended human daily dose of 20 mg on a mg/m^2 basis) had no adverse effects on reproductive parameters.

Pregnancy: Pregnancy Category B. No adverse effects on embryofetal development occurred in reproduction studies in rats and rabbits receiving subcutaneous doses of up to 37.5 mg/kg of glatiramer acetate during the period of organogenesis (18 and 36 times the human dose of 20 mg on a mg/m^2 basis respectively). In a prenatal and postnatal study in which rats received subcutaneous glatiramer acetate at doses of up to 36 mg/kg from day 15 of pregnancy throughout lactation, no significant effects on delivery or on offspring growth and development were observed.

There are no adequate and well-controlled studies in pregnant women. Because animal reproduction studies are not always predictive of human response, glatiramer acetate should be used during pregnancy only if clearly needed.

Labor and Delivery

In a prenatal and postnatal study, in which rats received subcutaneous glatiramer acetate at doses of up to 36 mg/kg from day 15 of pregnancy throughout lactation, no significant effects on delivery or on offspring growth and development were observed. The relevance of these findings to humans is unknown.

Nursing Mothers

It is not known whether glatiramer acetate is excreted in human milk. Because many drugs are excreted in human milk, caution should be exercised when COPAXONE® is administered to a nursing woman.

Pediatric Use

The safety and efficacy of COPAXONE® have not been established in individuals under 18 years of age.

Use in the Elderly

COPAXONE® has not been studied specifically in elderly patients.

Use in Patients with Impaired Renal Function

The pharmacokinetics of glatiramer acetate in patients with impaired renal function have not been determined.

ADVERSE REACTIONS

During premarketing clinical trials approximately 850 MS patients and 50 patients in clinical pharmacology trials received at least one dose of glatiramer acetate.

In controlled clinical trials the most commonly observed adverse experiences associated with the use of glatiramer acetate and not seen at an equivalent frequency among placebo-treated patients were: injection site reactions, vasodilatation, chest pain, asthenia, infection, pain, nausea, arthralgia, anxiety, and hypertonia.

Approximately 8% of the 893 subjects receiving glatiramer acetate discontinued treatment because of an adverse reaction. The adverse reactions most commonly associated with discontinuation were: injection site reaction (6.5%), vasodilatation, unintended pregnancy, depression, dyspnea, urticaria, tachycardia, dizziness, and tremor.

Immediate Post-Injection Reaction

Approximately 10% of MS patients exposed to glatiramer acetate in premarketing studies experienced a constellation of symptoms immediately after injection that included flushing, chest pain, palpitations, anxiety, dyspnea, constriction of the throat, and urticaria. In clinical trials, the symptoms were generally transient and self-limited and did not require specific treatment. In general, these symptoms have their onset several months after the initiation of treatment, although they may occur earlier, and a given patient may experience one or several episodes of these symptoms. Whether or not any of these symptoms actually represent a specific syndrome is uncertain. During the postmarketing period, there have been reports of patients with similar symptoms who received emergency medical care.

Whether an immunologic or non-immunologic mechanism mediates these episodes, or whether several similar episodes seen in a given patient have identical mechanisms is unknown.

Chest Pain

Approximately 26% of glatiramer acetate patients in the multicenter controlled trial (compared to 10% of placebo patients) experienced at least one episode of what was described as transient chest pain. While some of these episodes occurred in the context of the Immediate Post-Injection Reaction described above, many did not. The temporal relationship of this chest pain to an injection of glatiramer acetate was not always known. The pain was transient (usually lasting only a few minutes), often unassociated with other symptoms, and appeared to have no important clinical sequelae. EKG monitoring was not performed during any of these episodes. Some patients experienced more than one such episode, and episodes usually began at least 1 month after the initiation of treatment. The pathogenesis of this symptom is unknown.

Incidence in Controlled Clinical Studies: The following table lists treatment-emergent signs and symptoms that occurred in at least 2% of MS patients treated with glatiramer acetate in placebo-controlled trials. These signs and symptoms were numerically more common in patients treated with glatiramer acetate than in patients treated with placebo. These trials include the two controlled trials in RR MS patients and a controlled trial in patients with Chronic Progressive MS. Adverse reactions were usually mild in intensity.

The prescriber should be aware that these figures cannot be used to predict the frequency of adverse experiences in the course of usual medical practice where patient characteristics and other factors may differ from those prevailing during clinical studies. Similarly, the cited frequencies cannot be directly compared with figures obtained from other clinical investigations involving different treatments, uses, or investigators. An inspection of these frequencies, however, does provide the prescriber with one basis on which to estimate the relative contribution of drug and nondrug factors to the adverse reaction incidences in the population studied.

[See table at top of next page]

Other events which occurred in at least 2% of glatiramer acetate patients but were present at equal or greater rates in the placebo group included:

Continued on next page

Copaxone—Cont.

Body as a Whole: Headache, injection site ecchymosis, accidental injury, abdominal pain, allergic rhinitis, neck rigidity, and malaise.
Digestive System: Dyspepsia, constipation, dysphagia, fecal incontinence, flatulence, nausea and vomiting, gastritis, gingivitis, periodontal abscess, and dry mouth.
Musculoskeletal: Myasthenia and myalgia.
Nervous System: Dizziness, hypesthesia, paresthesia, insomnia, depression, dysesthesia, incoordination, somnolence, abnormal gait, amnesia, emotional lability, Lhermitte's sign, abnormal thinking, twitching, euphoria, and sleep disorder.
Respiratory System: Pharyngitis, sinusitis, increased cough and laryngitis.
Skin and Appendages: Acne, alopecia, and nail disorder.
Special Senses: Abnormal vision, diplopia, amblyopia, eye pain, conjunctivitis, tinnitus, taste perversion, and deafness.
Urogenital System: Urinary tract infection, urinary frequency, urinary incontinence, urinary retention, dysuria, cystitis, metrorrhagia, breast pain, and vaginitis.

Data on adverse reactions occurring in the controlled clinical trials were analyzed to evaluate differences based on sex. No clinically significant differences were identified. Ninety-two percent of patients in these clinical trials were Caucasian. This percentage reflects the racial composition of the MS population. In addition, the vast majority of patients treated with COPAXONE® were between the ages of 18 and 45. Consequently, data are inadequate to perform an analysis of the adverse reaction incidence related to clinically relevant age subgroups.

Laboratory analyses were performed on all patients participating in the clinical program for glatiramer acetate. Clinically significant laboratory values for hematology, chemistry, and urinalysis were similar for both glatiramer acetate and placebo groups in blinded clinical trials. No patient receiving glatiramer acetate withdrew from any trial because of abnormal laboratory findings.

Other Adverse Events Observed During Clinical Trials

Glatiramer acetate was administered to approximately 900 individuals during premarketing clinical trials, only some of which were placebo-controlled. During these trials, all adverse events were recorded by the clinical investigators, using terminology of their own choosing. To provide a meaningful estimate of the proportion of individuals having adverse events, similar types of events were grouped into standardized categories using COSTART dictionary terminology. The frequencies given represent the proportion of the 979 individuals exposed to glatiramer acetate who had data available for this determination. All reported events occurring at least twice and potentially important events occurring once are included except those already listed in the previous table, those too general to be informative, trivial events, and those not reasonably related to the drug. Additional adverse reactions reported during the postmarketing period are included.

Events are further classified within body system categories and listed in order of decreasing frequency using the following definitions: *Frequent* adverse events are defined as those occurring in at least 1/100 patients; *Infrequent* adverse events are those occurring in 1/100 to 1/1000 patients; *Rare* adverse events are those occurring in less than 1/1000 patients.

Body as a Whole:
- ◆ *Frequent:* Injection site edema, injection site atrophy, abscess, injection site hypersensitivity.
- ◆ *Infrequent:* Injection site hematoma, injection site fibrosis, moon face, cellulitis, generalized edema, hernia, injection site abscess, serum sickness, suicide attempt, injection site hypertrophy, injection site melanosis, lipoma, and photosensitivity reaction.

Cardiovascular:
- ◆ *Frequent:* Hypertension.
- ◆ *Infrequent:* Hypotension, midsystolic click, systolic murmur, atrial fibrillation, bradycardia, fourth heart sound, postural hypotension, and varicose veins.

Digestive:
- ◆ *Infrequent:* Dry mouth, stomatitis, burning sensation on tongue, cholecystitis, colitis, esophageal ulcer, esophagitis, gastrointestinal carcinoma, gum hemorrhage, hepatomegaly, increased appetite, melena, mouth ulceration, pancreas disorder, pancreatitis, rectal hemorrhage, tenesmus, tongue discoloration, and duodenal ulcer.

Endocrine:
- ◆ *Infrequent:* Goiter, hyperthyroidism, and hypothyroidism.

Gastrointestinal:
- ◆ *Frequent:* Bowel urgency, oral moniliasis, salivary gland enlargement, tooth caries, and ulcerative stomatitis.

Hemic and Lymphatic:
- ◆ *Infrequent:* Leukopenia, anemia, cyanosis, eosinophilia, hematemesis, lymphedema, pancytopenia, and splenomegaly.

Metabolic and Nutritional:
- ◆ *Infrequent:* Weight loss, alcohol intolerance, Cushing's syndrome, gout, abnormal healing, and xanthoma.

Musculoskeletal:
- ◆ *Infrequent:* Arthritis, muscle atrophy, bone pain, bursitis, kidney pain, muscle disorder, myopathy, osteomyelitis, tendon pain, and tenosynovitis.

Controlled Trials in Patients with Multiple Sclerosis: Incidence of Glatiramer Acetate Adverse Reactions ≥2% and More Frequent than Placebo

Preferred Term	Glatiramer Acetate (N = 201) N	Glatiramer Acetate (N = 201) %	Placebo (N = 206) N	Placebo (N = 206) %
Body as a Whole				
Asthenia	83	41	78	38
Back Pain	33	16	30	15
Bacterial Infection	11	5	9	4
Chest Pain	43	21	22	11
Chills	8	4	2	1
Cyst	5	2	1	0
Face Edema	12	6	2	1
Fever	17	8	15	7
Flu Syndrome	38	19	35	17
Infection	101	50	99	48
Injection Site Erythema	132	66	40	19
Injection Site Hemorrhage	11	5	6	3
Injection Site Induration	26	13	1	0
Injection Site Inflammation	98	49	22	11
Injection Site Mass	54	27	21	10
Injection Site Pain	147	73	78	38
Injection Site Pruritus	80	40	12	6
Injection Site Urticaria	10	5	0	0
Injection Site Welt	22	11	5	2
Neck Pain	16	8	9	4
Pain	56	28	52	25
Cardiovascular System				
Migraine	10	5	5	2
Palpitations	35	17	16	8
Syncope	10	5	5	2
Tachycardia	11	5	8	4
Vasodilatation	55	27	21	10
Digestive System				
Anorexia	17	8	15	7
Diarrhea	25	12	23	11
Gastroenteritis	6	3	2	1
Gastrointestinal Disorder	10	5	8	4
Nausea	44	22	34	17
Vomiting	13	6	8	4
Hemic and Lymphatic System				
Ecchymosis	16	8	13	6
Lymphadenopathy	25	12	12	6
Metabolic and Nutritional				
Edema	5	3	1	0
Peripheral Edema	14	7	8	4
Weight Gain	7	3	0	0
Musculoskeletal System				
Arthralgia	49	24	39	19
Nervous System				
Agitation	8	4	4	2
Anxiety	46	23	40	19
Confusion	5	2	1	0
Foot Drop	6	3	4	2
Hypertonia	44	22	37	18
Nervousness	4	2	2	1
Nystagmus	5	2	2	1
Speech Disorder	5	2	3	1
Tremor	14	7	7	3
Vertigo	12	6	11	5
Respiratory System				
Bronchitis	18	9	12	6
Dyspnea	38	19	15	7
Laryngismus	10	5	7	3
Rhinitis	29	14	27	13
Skin and Appendages				
Erythema	8	4	4	2
Herpes Simplex	8	4	6	3
Pruritus	36	18	26	13
Rash	37	18	30	15
Skin Nodule	4	2	1	0
Sweating	31	15	21	10
Urticaria	9	4	5	2
Special Senses				
Ear Pain	15	7	12	6
Eye Disorder	8	4	1	0
Urogenital System				
Dysmenorrhea	12	6	10	5
Urinary Urgency	20	10	17	8
Vaginal Moniliasis	16	8	9	4

Nervous:
- ◆ *Frequent:* Abnormal dreams, emotional lability, and stupor.
- ◆ *Infrequent:* Aphasia, ataxia, convulsion, circumoral paresthesia, depersonalization, hallucinations, hostility, hypokinesia, coma, concentration disorder, facial paralysis, decreased libido, manic reaction, memory impairment, myoclonus, neuralgia, paranoid reaction, paraplegia, psychotic depression, and transient stupor.

Respiratory:
- ◆ *Frequent:* Hyperventilation, hay-fever.
- ◆ *Infrequent:* Asthma, pneumonia, epistaxis, hypoventilation, and voice alteration.

Skin and Appendages:
- ◆ *Frequent:* Eczema, herpes zoster, pustular rash, skin atrophy, and warts.
- ◆ *Infrequent:* Dry skin, skin hypertrophy, dermatitis, furunculosis, psoriasis, angioedema, contact dermatitis, erythema nodosum, fungal dermatitis, maculopapular rash, pigmentation, benign skin neoplasm, skin carcinoma, skin striae, and vesiculobullous rash.

Special Senses:
- ◆ *Frequent:* Visual field defect.
- ◆ *Infrequent:* Dry eyes, otitis externa, ptosis, cataract, corneal ulcer, mydriasis, optic neuritis, photophobia, and taste loss.

Urogenital:
- ◆ *Frequent:* Amenorrhea, hematuria, impotence, menorrhagia, suspicious papanicolaou smear, urinary frequency and vaginal hemorrhage.
- ◆ *Infrequent:* Vaginitis, flank pain (kidney), abortion, breast engorgement, breast enlargement, carcinoma *in situ* cervix, fibrocystic breast, kidney calculus, nocturia, ovarian cyst, priapism, pyelonephritis, abnormal sexual function, and urethritis.

Postmarketing Clinical Experience

Postmarketing experience has shown an adverse event profile similar to that presented above. Reports of adverse reactions occuring under treatment with COPAXONE® (glatiramer acetate) not mentioned, above that have been received since market introduction and that may have or not have causal relationship to the drug include the following:

Body as a Whole: sepsis; LE syndrome; hydrocephalus; enlarged abdomen; injection site hypersensitivity; allergic reaction; anaphylactoid reaction
Cardiovascular System: thrombosis; peripheral vascular disease; pericardial effusion; myocardial infarct; deep thrombophlebitis; coronary occlusion; congestive heart failure; cardiomyopathy cardiomegaly; arrythmia; angina pectoris
Digestive System: tongue edema; stomach ulcer hemorrhage; liver function abnormality; liver damage; hepatitis; eructation; cirrhosis of the liver; cholelithiasis
Hemic and Lymphatic System: thrombocytopenia; lymphoma-like reaction; acute leukemia
Metabolic and Nutritional Disorders: hypercholesterolemia
Musculoskeleton System: rheumatoid arthritis; generalized spasm
Nervous System: myelitis; meningitis; CNS neoplasm; cerebrovascular accident; brain edema; abnormal dreams; aphasia; convulsion; neuralgia
Respiratory System: pulmonary embolus; pleural effusion; carcinoma of lung; hay fever
Special Senses: glaucoma; blindness; visual field defect
Urogenital System: urogenital neoplasm; urine abnormality; ovarian carcinoma; nephrosis; kidney failure; breast carcinoma; bladder carcinoma; urinary frequency

DRUG ABUSE AND DEPENDENCE

No evidence or experience suggests that abuse or dependence occurs with COPAXONE® therapy; however, the risk of dependence has not been systematically evaluated.

DOSAGE AND ADMINISTRATION

The recommended dose of COPAXONE® for the treatment of RR MS is 20 mg/day injected subcutaneously.

Instructions for Use

To reconstitute lyophilized COPAXONE® for injection, use a sterile syringe and Mixject Vial Adapter to transfer the diluent supplied, Sterile Water for Injection, into the COPAXONE® vial. Gently swirl the vial of COPAXONE® and let stand at room temperature until the solid material is completely dissolved. Inspect the reconstituted product visually and discard or return the product to the pharmacist before use if it contains particulate matter.
Soon after reconstitution, withdraw the solution into the syringe. Replace the Mixject Vial Adapter with a 27 gauge, ½″ needle and inject the solution subcutaneously. Sites for self-injection include arms, abdomen, hips, and thighs. A vial is suitable for single use only; unused portions should be discarded. (See the **COPAXONE® PATIENT INFORMATION** Booklet for **INSTRUCTIONS FOR INJECTING COPAXONE®**.)

HOW SUPPLIED

COPAXONE® is supplied as a sterile, lyophilized material containing 20 mg of glatiramer acetate and 40 mg of mannitol, USP. The drug is packaged in a USP Type 1 amber glass, single-use 2 mL vial. A separate vial, containing 1.1 mL of diluent (Sterile Water for Injection) is included for each vial of drug.
The recommended storage condition for the unreconstituted product is refrigeration (2°C to 8°C / 36°F to 46°F). However, excursions from recommended storage conditions to room temperature conditions (15° to 30°C / 59° to 86°F) for up to one week have been shown to have no adverse impact on the product. Exposure to higher temperatures or intense light should be avoided.
The diluent may be stored at room temperature.
COPAXONE® contains no preservative. It should be used immediately after reconstitution.
COPAXONE® is available in packs of 32 amber vials of sterile, lyophilized material for subcutaneous injection (NDC 0088-1150-03). The diluent for COPAXONE® is supplied in packs of 32 clear vials.

℞ **only.**

COPAXONE® (glatiramer acetate for injection) PATIENT INFORMATION

This booklet tells patients about COPAXONE® [coe PAX own] (glatiramer acetate for injection, formerly known as copolymer-1) and how to use COPAXONE® with the Mixject Vial Adapter. COPAXONE® treats Relapsing-Remitting Multiple Sclerosis.

- Before you begin using COPAXONE®, make sure you understand all the information in this booklet about its possible benefits and risks. If you do not understand some of the information in this booklet, contact your doctor for help.
- COPAXONE® is not recommended for use in pregnancy. Therefore, tell your doctor if you are pregnant, if you are planning to have a child, or if you become pregnant while you are taking this medicine.
- Tell your doctor if you are nursing. We do not know if COPAXONE® is passed through the milk to the baby.
- Do not change the dose or dosing schedule without talking with your doctor.
- Do not stop taking the drug without talking with your doctor.
- The most common side effects of COPAXONE® are redness, pain, swelling, itching, or a lump at the site of injection. These reactions are usually mild and seldom require professional treatment. Be sure to tell your doctor about any side effects.
- Some patients report a short-term reaction right after injecting COPAXONE®. This reaction can involve flushing (feeling of warmth and/or redness), chest tightness or pain with heart palpitations, anxiety, and trouble breathing. These symptoms generally appear within minutes of an injection, last about 15 minutes, and go away by themselves without further problems.
- After you inject COPAXONE®, call your doctor right away if you develop hives, skin rash with irritation, dizziness, sweating, chest pain, trouble breathing, severe pain at the injection site or other uncomfortable changes in your general health. Make no more injections until your doctor tells you to begin again.
- If symptoms become severe, call 911 or the appropriate emergency phone number in your area. Make no more injections until your physician tells you to begin again.
- Your prescription includes two types of vials (small bottles): brown vials containing COPAXONE® and clear vials of sterile water (diluent).
- Store the brown vials of COPAXONE® in the refrigerator as soon as you bring them home.
- Store the clear vials labeled "Sterile Water for Injection" (diluent) at room temperature.
- Keep COPAXONE® out of the reach of children.

INSTRUCTIONS FOR MIXING (RECONSTITUTING) AND INJECTING COPAXONE®

Read all of the following instructions before you reconstitute and inject COPAXONE®.

Are you left-handed?

Drawings in this leaflet show patients who are right-handed. If you are left-handed, do what comes naturally. You will probably find it most comfortable to hold the syringe in your left hand, and hold the vial between thumb and forefinger of your right hand.

Safety Tips:

- Use only the supplies provided with your COPAXONE® kit.
- Wash your hands well before beginning. Do not touch your hair or skin after washing.
- Keep the items sterile. Do not touch the needle, the piercing spike of the vial adapter, or the tops of the cleaned vials.
- Make sure none of the items in your kit have been opened.
- Never mix COPAXONE® with tap water.
- Do not reuse opened materials. Throw away unused portion of the COPAXONE® and sterile water (diluent).
- Throw away used syringes in a proper container. Ask your doctor if you do not know how to do this.
- Contact your doctor if you have questions.

There are 4 basic steps for injecting COPAXONE®:
1. Gathering the materials.
2. Mixing COPAXONE® and sterile water (reconstitution). This involves adding sterile water to the dry COPAXONE®.
3. Preparing the injection syringe.
4. Giving yourself the injection.

STEP 1. Gathering the Materials

1) Put the items you will need on a clean flat surface in a well-lighted area. The items and where you will find them are listed in the table below.

[See table above]

The item	Supplied in
• 1 brown vial of COPAXONE®	COPAXONE® drug product package
• 1 clear vial of Sterile Water For Injection, USP (diluent) • 1 syringe (3cc)* • 1 injection needle (27 gauge, ½″) • 1 Mixject Vial Adapter • 3 alcohol wipes (preps or swabs)	Self Injection Administration Package
• 1 Dry cotton ball	Not supplied

**One cubic centimeter (cc) represents the same amount as one-milliliter (mL). Use the scale that is on the syringe.*

2) To prevent infection, wash and dry your hands. Do not touch your hair or skin after washing.
3) Remove the 3-cc syringe from its protective wrapper by peeling back the paper label.
4) Place the syringe on the clean surface.
5) Remove the injection needle from its protective wrapper by peeling back the paper label. Place the injection needle on the clean surface. Do not remove the plastic needle shield yet.

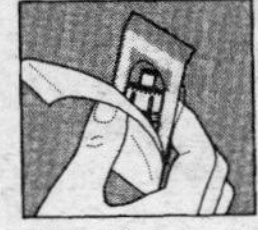
Figure 1

6) Open the Mixject Vial Adapter package by peeling back the paper and the plastic. Peel back only half-way. Do not open the package completely. Hold the wide side of the Mixject Vial Adapter through the package so you will not get germs on the Mixject Vial Adapter (Figure 1).

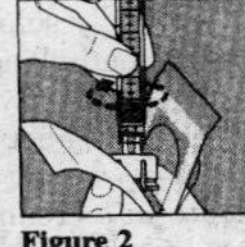
Figure 2

7) Remove the plastic tip cap from the 3-cc syringe. Without removing the Mixject Vial Adapter from its package, connect the syringe to the Mixject Vial Adapter by twisting the syringe (rotation). Make sure that the syringe is tightly attached to the Mixject Vial Adapter (Figure 2).
8) Place the package containing the Mixject Vial Adapter with the attached syringe on the clean surface.
9) Remove the plastic cover from the clear sterile water (diluent) vial. Use an alcohol wipe to clean the rubber top. Do the same for the brown COPAXONE® vial with a fresh alcohol wipe. **Do not touch the rubber tops after they are cleaned.** Let both rubber tops dry for a few seconds.

Important:
- **To avoid spreading germs, do not touch any of the following:**
  the needle
  the piercing spike of the Mixject Vial Adapter
  the top of either vial
- Use only the Sterile Water for Injection, USP (diluent) from the Self Injection Administration Package when mixing (reconstituting) COPAXONE®.
- If you have questions, contact your doctor or nurse before going further in reconstituting and injecting COPAXONE®. You may also contact **Shared Solutions™** by calling 1-800-887-8100.

STEP 2. Mixing COPAXONE® and Diluent (Reconstitution)

1) Hold the syringe with one hand. Remove the Mixject Vial Adapter from its paper wrapper. Do not touch the Mixject Vial Adapter. Pull the plunger back to the 1.1 cc line to draw air into the syringe (see insert, Figure 5).
2) With 2 fingers of one hand, hold the clear diluent vial on a stable surface like a table or kitchen counter. Hold the connection between the Mixject Vial Adapter and the syringe with the other hand. Insert the piercing spike of the Mixject Vial Adapter all the way in through the rubber top of the clear sterile water vial, using a rotating and pushing movement. (Figure 3)

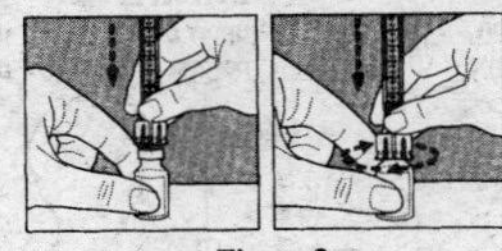
Figure 3

3) Push the plunger of the syringe all the way in.
4) Turn the connected syringe and vial upside down and pull the plunger out until all the diluent is drawn into the syringe. If there are air bubbles inside the syringe, tap the side of the syringe to make them float to the top (Figure 4). Push the plunger in until the top of the black plunger ring is in line with the bottom of the 1.1 cc line on the syringe (as shown by the arrow in Figure 5).

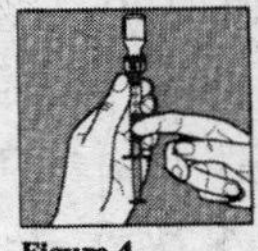
Figure 4

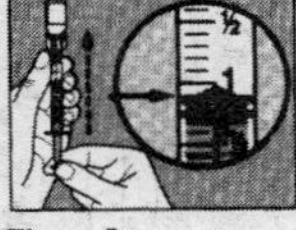
Figure 5

5) Holding the syringe containing the sterile water (diluent) and the Mixject Vial Adapter, remove the clear vial. Throw it away by putting it in a safe hard-walled container, such as an empty liquid laundry detergent container.

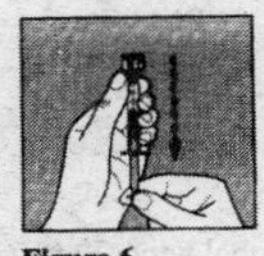
Figure 6

6) Take the 3 cc syringe containing the sterile water (diluent) and pull the plunger back to the 2.0 cc line to draw air into the syringe (Figure 6).
7) Hold the brown COPAXONE® vial on a stable surface with 2 fingers of one hand. Hold the connected Mixject Vial Adapter and the syringe with the other hand. Insert the piercing spike of the Mixject Vial Adapter all the way in through the rubber top of the COPAXONE® vial, using a rotating and pushing movement.

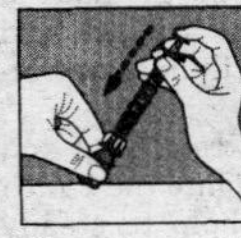
Figure 7

8) Slowly inject all the sterile water and air into the vial by pressing the plunger all the way in. To avoid bubbles, do not inject the sterile water directly onto the COPAXONE®. Instead, inject the sterile water so it runs down the inside of the vial glass. You can do this if you keep the vial tilted while injecting (Figure 7).
9) **Do not shake the vial.** Gently swirl the vial until all the medicine dissolves and the solution looks clear. The

Continued on next page

Copaxone—Cont.

COPAXONE® is now mixed (reconstituted). Keeping the vial, adapter, and syringe connected, let them rest and warm up for about 5 minutes.

10) Look for particles in the solution. Do not use the solution if there are any particles in it.

STEP 3. Preparing the Injection Syringe

1) Hold the syringe with one hand and make sure that the plunger is pressed all the way in. Turn the vial upside down. To give the full dose of COPAXONE®, withdraw all of the solution into the syringe and Mixject Vial Adapter by slowly pulling the plunger out. This amount will be about 1.1 cc. Again, if there are air bubbles inside the syringe, tap the side of the syringe to make them float to the top. Inject any air back into the vial by pushing the plunger in gently.

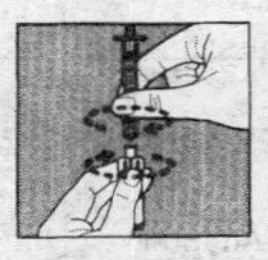
Figure 8

2) Keep the brown vial of COPAXONE® and the Mixject Vial Adapter connected to each other. Disconnect them from the syringe by turning them together (rotation) (Figure 8). Throw away the COPAXONE® vial and the Mixject Vial Adapter by putting them in a safe hard-walled container.

3) When you connect the injection needle (27 gauge, $^1/_2$") to the syringe, keep the plastic cover on the needle. Make sure that the needle is tightly placed in its proper position. The syringe is now ready to use.

4) Place the ready-to-use syringe on the clean surface.

STEP 4. Giving Yourself the Injection

Before you begin the procedure to self-inject the COPAXONE®:

- **Decide where you will inject yourself.** There are seven injection sites on your body, and **you should not use any site more than once each week.** Marking a calendar each day will help you keep track of the sites you have used (Figure 9).
- **Be consistent.** Give yourself the injection at the same time each day. Choose a time when you feel strongest.
- **Have a friend or relative with you if you need help.** You may have had a friend attend the injection training session as your assistant. Especially when you first start giving yourself injections, your assistant should be with you.

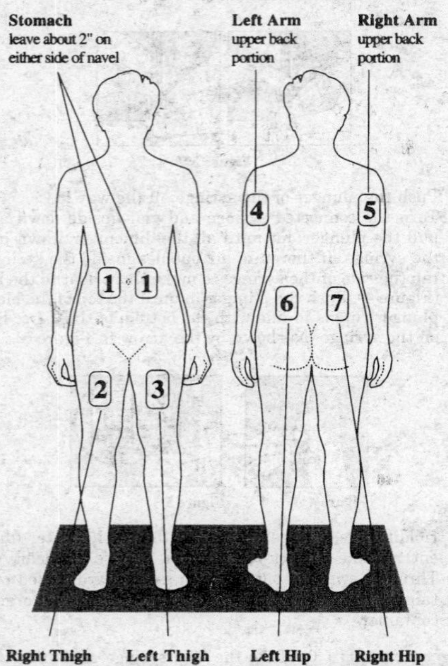

Figure 9

1) Clean the injection site with a fresh alcohol wipe. Let the site dry.
2) Pick up the 3-cc syringe you already filled with COPAXONE® as you would pick up a pencil, using the hand you write with. Remove the plastic cover from the needle.

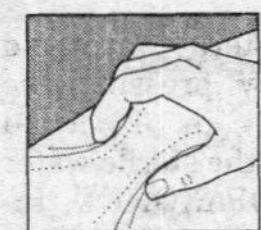
Figure 10

3) For sites that are **not** on the back of your arms, pinch about a 2-inch fold of skin between your thumb and index finger (Figure 10).
4) Holding the syringe straight up and down insert the needle into the 2-inch fold of skin. It may help to steady your hand by resting the heel of your hand against your body.

> **How do I reach the upper back of my arms?**
> For the 2 injection sites on the upper back of the arms, it is not possible to pinch 2 inches of skin with one hand and inject yourself with the other hand. Ask your nurse for instruction on how to use these sites.

5) When the needle is all the way in, release the fold of skin.
6) Inject the medicine by holding the syringe steady while pushing down on the plunger. The injection should take just a few seconds (Figure 11).

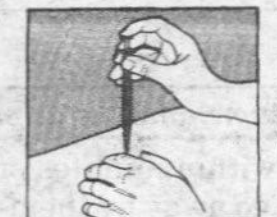
Figure 11

7) Pull the needle straight out.
8) Press a dry cotton ball on the injection site for a few seconds. Do not rub or massage the site.
9) Put the plastic cover back on the needle.
10) Throw away the needle, syringe, Mixject Vial Adapter, and the used vials in a safe, hard-walled container, according to your physician's instructions and the laws of your state.

What is the proper use of needles and syringes?
Needles, syringes, and vials should be used for only one injection each. Place all used syringes, needles, and vials in a hard-walled plastic container, such as an empty liquid laundry detergent container. Keep the cover of this container tight and out of the reach of children. When the container is full, check with your doctor or nurse about proper disposal, as laws vary from state to state.

How should COPAXONE® and the sterile water (diluent) be stored?
Store the brown vials of sterile, lyophilized material for subcutaneous injection COPAXONE® in a refrigerator (36–46°F/2–8°C). If you cannot have refrigerator storage, COPAXONE® can be stored at room temperature (59–86°F/15–30°C) for up to one week. Do not store COPAXONE® at room temperature for longer than one week. Avoid exposure to higher temperatures or very bright light.
The clear vials of sterile water (diluent) may be stored at room temperature.

What is the shelf-life of COPAXONE®?
Do not use COPAXONE® after the expiration date (EXP) printed on the vial label.
COPAXONE® does not contain preservatives. Therefore, it should be used right away after you reconstitute (mix) it. If you cannot use it right away after reconstitution, throw it away.

Manufactured For:
TEVA Marion Partners
Kansas City, MO 64134
Manufactured By:
Ben Venue Laboratories
Bedford, OH 44146
or
TEVA Pharmaceutical Industries, Ltd.
Kfar-Saba, 44102, Israel

I20162
Rev. R 5/2000

Shown in Product Identification Guide, page 338

Ther-Rx Corporation

13622 LAKEFRONT DRIVE
ST. LOUIS, MISSOURI 63045

For direct inquiries contact:
(314) 209-1517 phone
(314) 770-0371 fax

GYNAZOLE-1™ ℞

(Butoconazole Nitrate)
Vaginal Cream, 2%
Rx Only

DESCRIPTION

GYNAZOLE•1™ (butoconazole nitrate) vaginal cream, 2% contains butoconazole nitrate 2%, an imidazole derivative with antifungal activity. Its chemical name is (±)-1-[4-(p-chlorophenyl)-2-[(2,6-dichlorophenyl)thio]butyl] imidazole mononitrate, and it has the following chemical structure:

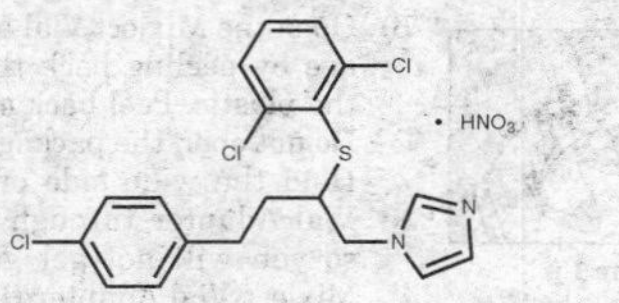

Butoconazole nitrate is a white to off-white crystalline powder with a molecular weight of 474.79. It is sparingly soluble in methanol; slightly soluble in chloroform, methylene chloride, acetone, and ethanol; very slightly soluble in ethyl acetate; and practically insoluble in water. It melts at about 159°C with decomposition.
GYNAZOLE•1™ contains 2% butoconazole nitrate in a cream of edetate disodium, glyceryl monoisostearate, methylparaben, mineral oil, polyglyceryl-3 oleate, propylene glycol, propylparaben, colloidal silicon dioxide, sorbitol solution, purified water, and microcrystalline wax.

CLINICAL PHARMACOLOGY

Following vaginal administration of butoconazole nitrate vaginal cream, 2% to 3 women, 1.7% (range 1.3–2.2%) of the dose was absorbed on average. Peak plasma levels (13.6–18.6 ng radioequivalents/mL of plasma) of the drug and its metabolites are attained between 12 and 24 hours after vaginal administration.

Microbiology
The exact mechanism of the antifungal action of butoconazole nitrate is unknown; however, it is presumed to function as other imidazole derivatives via inhibition of steroid synthesis.
Imidazoles generally inhibit the conversion of lanosterol to ergosterol, resulting in a change in fungal cell membrane lipid composition. This structural change alters cell permeability and, ultimately, results in the osmotic disruption or growth inhibition of the fungal cell.
Butoconazole nitrate is an imidazole derivative that has fungicidal activity *in vitro* and is clinically effective against vaginal infections due to *Candida albicans*.

INDICATIONS AND USAGE

GYNAZOLE•1™ (butoconazole nitrate) vaginal cream, 2% is indicated for the local treatment of vulvovaginal infections caused by *Candida albicans*. The diagnosis should be confirmed by KOH smears and/or cultures.
Note: GYNAZOLE•1™ is safe and effective in non-pregnant women; however, the safety and effectiveness of this product in pregnant women has not been established. (See PRECAUTIONS: Pregnancy.)

CONTRAINDICATIONS

GYNAZOLE•1™ is contraindicated in patients with a history of hypersensitivity to any of the components of the product.

WARNINGS

This cream contains mineral oil. Mineral oil may weaken latex or rubber products such as condoms or vaginal contraceptive diaphragms; therefore, use of such products within 72 hours following treatment with GYNAZOLE•1™ is not recommended.
Recurrent vaginal yeast infections, especially those that are difficult to eradicate, can be an early sign of infection with the human immunodeficiency virus (HIV) in women who are considered at risk for HIV infection.

PRECAUTIONS

General
If clinical symptoms persist, tests should be repeated to rule out other pathogens, to confirm the original diagnosis, and rule out other conditions that may predispose a patient to recurrent vaginal fungal infections.

Carcinogenesis, Mutagenesis, Impairment of Fertility
Carcinogenesis: Long term studies in animals have not been performed to evaluate the carcinogenic potential of this drug.
Mutagenicity: Butoconazole nitrate was not mutagenic when tested in the Ames bacterial test, yeast, chromosomal aberration assay in CHO cells, CHO/HGPRT point mutation assay, mouse micronucleus, and rat dominant lethal assays.
Impairment of Fertility: No impairment of fertility was seen in rabbits or rats administered butoconazole nitrate in oral doses up to 30 mg/kg/day (5 times the human dose based on mg/M^2) or 100 mg/kg/day (10 times the human dose based on mg/M^2), respectively.

Pregnancy
Pregnancy Category C.
In pregnant rats administered 6 mg/kg/day of butoconazole nitrate intravaginally during the period of organogenesis, there was an increase in resorption rate and decrease in litter size; however, no teratogenicity was noted. This dose represents a 130- to 353-fold margin of safety based on serum levels achieved in rats following intravaginal administration compared to the serum levels achieved in humans following intravaginal administration of the recommended therapeutic dose of butoconazole nitrate.
Butoconazole nitrate has no apparent adverse effect when administered orally to pregnant rats throughout organogenesis at dose levels up to 50 mg/kg/day (5 times the human dose based on mg/M^2). Daily oral doses of 100, 300 or 750 mg/kg/day (10, 30 or 75 times the human dose based on mg/M^2 respectively) resulted in fetal malformations (abdominal wall defects, cleft palate), but maternal stress was also evident at these higher dose levels. There were, however, no adverse effects on litters of rabbits who received butoconazole nitrate orally, even at maternally stressful dose levels (e.g., 150 mg/kg, 24 times the human dose based on mg/M^2).
Butoconazole nitrate, like other azole anti-fungal agents, causes dystocia in rats when treatment is extended through parturition. However, this effect was not apparent in rabbits treated with as much as 100 mg/kg/day orally (16 times the human dose based on mg/M^2).
There are, however, no adequate and well-controlled studies in pregnant women. GYNAZOLE•1™ should be used during pregnancy only if the potential benefit justifies the potential risk to the fetus.

Nursing Mothers
It is not known whether this drug is excreted in human milk. Because many drugs are excreted in human milk, caution should be exercised when butoconazole nitrate is administered to a nursing woman.

Pediatric Use
Safety and effectiveness in children have not been established.

ADVERSE REACTIONS

Of the 314 patients treated with GYNAZOLE•1™ for 1 day in controlled clinical trials, 18 patients (5.7%) reported complaints such as vulvar/vaginal burning, itching, soreness and swelling, pelvic or abdominal pain or cramping, or a combination of two or more of these symptoms. In 3 patients (1%) these complaints were considered treatment-related. Five of the 18 patients reporting adverse events discontinued the study because of them.

D0SAGE AND ADMINISTRATION

The recommended dose of GYNAZOLE•1™ is one applicatorful of cream (approximately 5 grams of the cream) intravaginally. This amount of cream contains approximately 100 mg of butoconazole nitrate.

HOW SUPPLIED

GYNAZOLE•1™ (butoconazole nitrate) vaginal cream, 2% is available in cartons containing one single-dose prefilled disposable applicator (NDC 64011-001-08).
Store at 25°C (77°F): excursions permitted to 15°–30°C (59°–86°F). (See USP Controlled Room Temperature). Avoid heat above 30°C (86°F).
U.S. Patent Nos. 4,078,071, 4,551,148, 4,636,202 and 5,266,329
Manufactured for Ther-Rx Corporation by KV Pharmaceutical Co.
St. Louis, MO 63144

Shown in Product Identification Guide, page 338

MICRO-K® EXTENCAPS® ℞
MICRO-K® 10 EXTENCAPS®
(Potassium Chloride Extended-Release Capsules, USP)

DESCRIPTION

Micro-K Extencaps capsules and Micro-K 10 Extencaps capsules are oral dosage forms of microencapsulated potassium chloride containing 600 and 750 mg, respectively, of potassium chloride USP equivalent to 8 and 10 mEq of potassium.
Dispersibility of potassium chloride (KCl) is accomplished by microencapsulation and a dispersing agent. The resultant flow characteristics of the KCl microcapsules and the controlled release of K ions by the microcapsular membrane are intended to avoid the possibility that excessive amounts of KCl can be localized at any point on the mucosa of the gastrointestinal tract.
Each crystal of KCl is microencapsulated by a patented process with an insoluble polymeric coating which functions as a semi-permeable membrane; it allows for the controlled release of potassium and chloride ions over an eight- to ten-hour period. Fluids pass through the membrane and gradually dissolve the potassium chloride within the microcapsules. The resulting potassium chloride solution slowly diffuses outward through the membrane. Micro-K and Micro-K 10 are electrolyte replenishers. The chemical name of the active ingredient is potassium chloride and the structural formula is KCl. Potassium chloride USP occurs as a white, granular powder or as colorless crystals. It is odorless and has a saline taste. Its solutions are neutral to litmus. It is freely soluble in water and insoluble in alcohol.
The inactive ingredients present are edible ink, ethylcellulose, FD&C Blue 2 Aluminum Lake, FD&C Yellow 6, gelatin, magnesium stearate, sodium lauryl sulfate, titanium dioxide. May contain FD&C Red 40 and Yellow 6 Aluminum Lakes.

CLINICAL PHARMACOLOGY

Potassium ion is the principal intracellular cation of most body tissues. Potassium ions participate in a number of essential physiological processes, including the maintenance of intracellular tonicity, the transmission of nerve impulses, the contraction of cardiac, skeletal, and smooth muscle and the maintenance of normal renal function.
Potassium depletion may occur whenever the rate of potassium loss through renal excretion and/or loss from the gastrointestinal tract exceeds the rate of potassium intake. Such depletion usually develops slowly as a consequence of prolonged therapy with oral diuretics, primary or secondary hyperaldosteronism, diabetic ketoacidosis, severe diarrhea, or inadequate replacement of potassium in patients on prolonged parenteral nutrition. Potassium depletion due to these causes is usually accompanied by a concomitant deficiency of chloride and is manifested by hypokalemia and metabolic alkalosis. Potassium depletion may produce weakness, fatigue, disturbances of cardiac rhythm (primarily ectopic beats), prominent U-waves in the electrocardiogram, and in advanced cases, flaccid paralysis and/or impaired ability to concentrate urine.
Potassium depletion associated with metabolic alkalosis is managed by correcting the fundamental causes of the deficiency whenever possible and administering supplemental potassium chloride, in the form of high potassium food or potassium chloride solution, capsules or tablets. In rare circumstances (e.g., patients with renal tubular acidosis) potassium depletion may be associated with metabolic acidosis and hyperchloremia. In such patients potassium replacement should be accomplished with potassium salts other than the chloride, such as potassium bicarbonate, potassium citrate, or potassium acetate.

INDICATIONS AND USAGE

BECAUSE OF REPORTS OF INTESTINAL AND GASTRIC ULCERATION AND BLEEDING WITH SLOW-RELEASE POTASSIUM CHLORIDE PREPARATIONS, THESE DRUGS SHOULD BE RESERVED FOR THOSE PATIENTS WHO CANNOT TOLERATE OR REFUSE TO TAKE LIQUID OR EFFERVESCENT POTASSIUM PREPARATIONS OR FOR PATIENTS IN WHOM THERE IS A PROBLEM OF COMPLIANCE WITH THESE PREPARATIONS.

1. **For therapeutic use** in patients with hypokalemia with or without metabolic alkalosis; in digitalis intoxication and in patients with hypokalemic familial periodic paralysis.
2. **For prevention** of potassium depletion when the dietary intake of potassium is inadequate in the following conditions: patients receiving digitalis and diuretics for congestive heart failure; hepatic cirrhosis with ascites; states of aldosterone excess with normal renal function; potassium-losing nephropathy, and certain diarrheal states.
3. **The use of potassium salts** in patients receiving diuretics for uncomplicated essential hypertension is often unnecessary when such patients have a normal dietary pattern. Serum potassium should be checked periodically, however, and, if hypokalemia occurs, dietary supplementation with potassium-containing foods may be adequate to control milder cases. In more severe cases, supplementation with potassium salts may be indicated.

CONTRAINDICATIONS

Potassium supplements are contraindicated in patients with hyperkalemia since a further increase in serum potassium concentration in such patients can produce cardiac arrest.
Hyperkalemia may complicate any of the following conditions: chronic renal failure, systemic acidosis, such as diabetic acidosis, acute dehydration, extensive tissue breakdown as in severe burns, adrenal insufficiency, or the administration of a potassium-sparing diuretic (e.g., spironolactone, triamterene, amiloride) (see **OVERDOSAGE**).
Controlled-release formulations of potassium chloride have produced esophageal ulceration in certain cardiac patients with esophageal compression due to an enlarged left atrium. Potassium supplementation, when indicated in such patients, should be given as a liquid preparation.
All solid oral dosage forms of potassium chloride are contraindicated in any patient in whom there is structural, pathological (e.g., diabetic gastroparesis), or pharmacologic (use of anticholinergic agents or other agents with anticholinergic properties at sufficient doses to exert anticholinergic effects) cause for arrest or delay in capsule passage through the gastrointestinal tract.

WARNINGS

Hyperkalemia (see **OVERDOSAGE**)
In patients with impaired mechanisms for excreting potassium, the administration of potassium salts can produce hyperkalemia and cardiac arrest. This occurs most commonly in patients given potassium by the intravenous route but may also occur in patients given potassium orally. Potentially fatal hyperkalemia can develop rapidly and be asymptomatic.
The use of potassium salts in patients with chronic renal disease, or any other condition which impairs potassium excretion, requires particularly careful monitoring of the serum potassium concentration and appropriate dosage adjustments.
Interaction with Potassium-Sparing Diuretics
Hypokalemia should not be treated by the concomitant administration of potassium salts and a potassium-sparing diuretic (e.g., spironolactone or triamterene), since the simultaneous administration of these agents can produce severe hyperkalemia.
Interaction with Angiotensin Converting Enzyme Inhibitors
Angiotensin converting enzyme (ACE) inhibitors (e.g., captopril, enalapril) will produce some potassium retention by inhibiting aldosterone production. Potassium supplements should be given to patients receiving ACE inhibitors only with close monitoring.
Gastrointestinal Lesions
Potassium chloride tablets have produced stenotic and/or ulcerative lesions of the small bowel and deaths, in addition to upper gastrointestinal bleeding. These lesions are caused by a high localized concentration of potassium ion in the region of a rapidly dissolving tablet which injures the bowel wall and thereby produces obstruction, hemorrhage, or perforation.
Micro-K® Extencaps® contain microcapsules which disperse upon dissolution of the hard gelatin capsule. The microcapsules are formulated to provide a controlled release of potassium chloride. The dispersibility of the microcapsules and the controlled release of ions from the microcapsules are intended to minimize the possibility of a high local concentration near the gastrointestinal mucosa and the ability of the KCl to cause stenosis or ulceration. Other means of accomplishing this (e.g., incorporation of KCl into a wax matrix) have reduced the frequency of such lesions to less than one per 100,000 patient years (compared with 40 to 50 per 100,000 patient years with enteric-coated KCl), but have not eliminated them. The frequency of GI lesions with Micro-K® Extencaps® is, at present, unknown. Micro-K® Extencaps® should be discontinued immediately and the possibility of bowel obstruction or perforation considered if severe vomiting, abdominal pain, distention, or gastrointestinal bleeding occurs.
Metabolic Acidosis
Hypokalemia in patients with metabolic acidosis should be treated with an alkalinizing potassium salt, such as potassium bicarbonate, potassium citrate, or potassium acetate.

PRECAUTIONS

General The diagnosis of potassium depletion is ordinarily made by demonstrating hypokalemia in a patient with a clinical history suggesting some cause for potassium depletion. In interpreting the serum potassium level, the physician should bear in mind that acute alkalosis *per se* can produce hypokalemia in the absence of a deficit in total body potassium, while acute acidosis *per se* can increase the serum potassium concentration into the normal range even in the presence of a reduced total body potassium. The treatment of potassium depletion, particularly in the presence of cardiac disease, renal disease, or acidosis, requires careful attention to acid-base balance and appropriate monitoring of serum electrolytes, the electrocardiogram, and the clinical status of the patient.
Information for Patients
Physicians should consider reminding the patient of the following: To take each dose with meals and with water or other suitable liquid. To take this medicine following the frequency and amount prescribed by the physician. This is especially important if the patient is also taking diuretics and/or digitalis preparations. To check with the physician if there is trouble swallowing capsules or if the capsules seem to stick in the throat. To check with the physician at once if tarry stools or other evidence of gastrointestinal bleeding is noticed. To take each dose without crushing, chewing, or sucking the capsule.
Laboratory Test Regular serum potassium determinations are recommended, especially in patients with renal insufficiency or diabetic nephropathy. When blood is drawn for analysis of plasma potassium it is important to recognize that artifactual elevations can occur after improper venipuncture technique or as a result of in vitro hemolysis of the sample.
Drug Interactions Potassium-sparing diuretic, angiotensin converting enzyme inhibitors (see **WARNINGS**).
Carcinogenesis, Mutagenesis, Impairment of Fertility Carcinogenicity, mutagenicity and fertility studies in animals have not been performed. Potassium is a normal dietary constituent.
Pregnancy, Teratogenic Effects – Category C Animal reproduction stuides have not been conducted with Micro-K®. It is unlikely that potassium supplementation that does not lead to hyperkalemia would have an adverse effect on the fetus or would affect reproductive capacity.
Nursing Mothers The normal potassium ion content of human milk is about 13 mEq per liter. Since oral potassium becomes part of the body potassium pool, so long as body potassium is not excessive, the contribution of potassium chloride supplementation should have little or no effect on the level in human milk.
Pediatric Use Safety and effectiveness in pediatric patients have not been established.
Geriatric Use Clinical studies of Micro-K® Extencaps® did not include sufficient numbers of subjects aged 65 and over to determine whether they respond differently from younger subjects. Other reported clinical experience has not identified differences in responses between the elderly and younger patients. In general, dose selection for an elderly patient should be cautious, usually starting at the low end of the dosing range, reflecting the greater frequency of decreased hepatic, renal, or cardiac function, and of concomitant disease or other drug therapy.
This drug is known to be substantially excreted by the kidney, and the risk of toxic reactions to this drug may be greater in patients with impaired renal function. Because elderly patients are more likely to have decreased renal function, care should be taken in dose selection, and it may be useful to monitor renal function.

ADVERSE REACTIONS

One of the most severe adverse effects is hyperkalemia (see **CONTRAINDICATIONS, WARNINGS** and **OVERDOSAGE**). Gastrointestinal bleeding and ulceration have been reported in patients treated with Micro-K® Extencaps® (see **WARNINGS**). In addition to gastrointestinal bleeding and ulceration, perforation and obstruction have been reported in patients treated with other solid KCl dosage forms, and may occur with Micro-K® Extencaps®.
The most common adverse reactions to the oral potassium salts are nausea, vomiting, abdominal pain/discomfort, and diarrhea. These symptoms are due to irritation of the gastrointestinal tract and are best managed by taking the dose with meals, or reducing the amount taken at one time.

OVERDOSAGE

The administration of oral potassium salts to persons with normal excretory mechanisms for potassium rarely causes serious hyperkalemia. However, if excretory mechanisms are impaired or if potassium is administered too rapidly intravenously, potentially fatal hyperkalemia can result (see **CONTRAINDICATIONS** and **WARNINGS**). It is important to recognize that hyperkalemia is usually asymptomatic and may be manifested only by an increased serum po-

Continued on next page

Micro-K—Cont.

tassium concentration and characteristic electrocardiogram changes (peaking of T-waves, loss of P-wave, depression of S-T segment, and prolongation of the QT interval). Late manifestations include muscle paralysis and cardiovascular collapse from cardiac arrest.
Treatment measures for hyperkalemia include the following: (1) elimination of foods and medications containing potassium and of potassium-sparing diuretics; (2) intravenous administration of 300 to 500 mL/hr of 10% dextrose solution containing 10 to 20 units of insulin per 1,000 mL; (3) correction of acidosis, if present, with intravenous sodium bicarbonate; (4) use of exchange resins, hemodialysis, or peritoneal dialysis.
In treating hyperkalemia, it should be recalled that in patients who have been stabilized on digitalis, too rapid a lowering of the serum potassium concentration can produce digitalis toxicity.

DOSAGE AND ADMINISTRATION

The usual dietary intake of potassium by the average adult is 50 to 100 mEq per day. Potassium depletion sufficient to cause hypokalemia usually requires the loss of 200 or more mEq of potassium from the total body store.
Dosage must be adjusted to the individual needs of each patient. The dose for the prevention of hypokalemia is typically in the range of 20 mEq per day. Doses of 40 to 100 mEq per day or more are used for the treatment of potassium depletion. Dosage should be divided if more than 20 mEq per day is given such that no more than 20 mEq is given in a single dose.
Because of the potential for gastric irritation (see **WARNINGS**), Micro-K Extencaps should be taken with meals and with a full glass of water or other liquid.
Patients who have difficulty swallowing capsules may sprinkle the contents of the capsule onto a spoonful of soft food. The soft food, such as applesauce or pudding, should be swallowed immediately without chewing and followed with a glass of cool water or juice to ensure complete swallowing of the microcapsules. The food used should not be hot and should be soft enough to be swallowed without chewing. Any microcapsule/food mixture should be used immediately and not stored for future use.

HOW SUPPLIED

Micro-K® Extencaps® are pale orange capsules, monogrammed Micro-K® and Ther-Rx/010, each containing 600 mg microencapsulated potassium chloride (equivalent to 8 mEq K) in bottles of 100 (NDC 64011-010-04), 500 (NDC 64011-010-08) and Dis-Co® unit dose packs of 100 (NDC 64011-010-11).
Micro-K® Extencaps® are pale orange and opaque white capsules, monogrammed Micro-K® 10 and Ther-Rx/009, each containing 750 mg microencapsulated potassium chloride (equivalent to 10 mEq K) in bottles of 100 (NDC 64011-009-04), 100 Unit-of-Use (NDC 64011-009-21), bottles of 500 (NDC 64011-009-08), and DisCo® unit dose packs of 100 (NDC 64011-009-11).
Store at controlled room temperature, between 20° C and 25° C (68° F–77° F).
Dispense in tight container.
Manufactured by
Pharmaceutical Division
A.H. Robins Company
Richmond, VA 23220
for Ther-Rx Corporation
St. Louis, MO 63045

Rev. 6/00

Shown in Product Identification Guide, page 338

PRECARE® Chewables ℞
Flavored Prenatal Multivitamin/Mineral Tablet

Rx Only

DESCRIPTION

Each orange-colored tablet contains:
Vitamin C (as Ester-C®[1])* .... 50 mg
Calcium (as calcium carbonate) .... 250 mg
Iron (as MicroMask™ ferrous fumarate) .... 40 mg
Vitamin D_3 (cholecalciferol) .... 6 mcg
Vitamin E (as dl-α-tocopheryl acetate) .... 3.5 mg
Vitamin B_6 (as pyridoxine HCl) .... 2 mg
Folic Acid, USP .... 1 mg
Magnesium (as magnesium oxide, USP) .... 50 mg
Zinc (as zinc oxide, USP) .... 15 mg
Copper (as cupric oxide) .... 2 mg
Inactive Ingredients: Citric acid, FD&C yellow No. 6 lake, flow agents, natural non-nutritive and nutritive sweetening agents, natural and artificial flavors.
KEEP THIS AND ALL DRUGS OUT OF THE REACH OF CHILDREN

[1] Ester-C as a patented pharmaceutical grade material consisting of calcium ascorbate and calcium theronate.
*Logo and Ester-C® is a registered trademark of Inter-Cal Corporation.

WARNING: Accidental overdose of iron-containing products is a leading cause of fatal poisoning in children under 6. Keep this product out of the reach of children. In case of accidental overdose, call a doctor or poison control center immediately.

INDICATIONS

PreCare® Chewable is indicated to provide vitamin and mineral supplementation throughout pregnancy and during the postnatal period—for both lactating and non-lactating mothers. They are also useful for improving nutritional status prior to conception.

CONTRAINDICATIONS

This product is contraindicated in patients with a known hypersensitivity to any of the ingredients.

WARNINGS

Folic acid alone is improper therapy in the treatment of pernicious anemia and other megaloblastic anemias where Vitamin B_{12} is deficient.

PRECAUTIONS

Folic acid in doses above 0.1 mg daily may obscure pernicious anemia, in that hematologic remission can occur while neurological manifestations remain progressive.

PEDIATRIC USE

Safety and effectiveness in pediatric patients has not been established.

GERIATRIC USE

Clinical studies on this product have not been performed to determine whether elderly subjects respond differently from younger subjects. In general, dose selection for an elderly patient should be cautious, usually starting at the low end of the dosing range, reflecting the greater frequency of decreased hepatic, renal, or cardiac function, and of concomitant disease or other drug therapy.

ADVERSE REACTIONS

Allergic sensitization has been reported following both oral and parenteral administration of folic acid.

DOSAGE AND ADMINISTRATION

Usual dosage is one tablet daily, or as prescribed by a physician.

HOW SUPPLIED

PreCare® Chewable tablets for oral administration are supplied as orange-colored, flavored tablets, debossed "Thx" on one side and "024" on the other side in child-resistant, unit dose packages of 100 tablets (10×10 Unit Dose Packs) (NDC 64011-024-11). Store at controlled room temperature, 15°–30°C (59°–86°F).
NOTICE: Contact with moisture may produce surface discoloration or erosion of the tablet.
U.S. Patents No. 4,822,816, 5,070,085 and 5,494,681
Other U.S. Patents Pending Rev. 6/00

Shown in Product Identification Guide, page 338

PRECARE® CONCEIVE™ ℞
Preconception/Prenatal Multivitamin/Mineral Tablet

Rx only

DESCRIPTION

Each diamond shaped, film coated yellow tablet contains:
Vitamin C (as Ester-C®[1])* .... 60 mg
Calcium (as Calcium Carbonate) .... 200 mg
Iron (as Ferrous Fumarate and Carbonyl Iron) .... 30 mg
Vitamin E (as dl-Alpha-Tocopheryl Acetate) .... 30 IU
Thiamine (as Thiamine Mononitrate) .... 3 mg
Riboflavin (as Riboflavin, USP) .... 3.4 mg
Niacin (as Niacinamide, USP) .... 20 mg
Pyridoxine (as Pyridoxine HCl, USP) .... 50 mg
Folic Acid, USP .... 1 mg
Magnesium (as Magnesium Oxide) .... 100 mg
Cyanocobalamin .... 12 mcg
Zinc (as Zinc Oxide) .... 15 mg
Copper (as Cupric Oxide) .... 2 mg
Inactive Ingredients: Cellulose polymers, flow agents, pigment, natural wax, D&C yellow #10 aluminum lake, FD&C yellow #6 aluminum lake, lactose and other ingredients.

[1] Ester-C® is a patented pharmaceutical grade material consisting of calcium ascorbate and calcium threonate.
Ester-C® is a registered trademark of Inter-Cal Corporation.
*Logo and Ester-C are licensed trademarks of Inter-Cal Corporation.

WARNING: Accidental overdose of iron-containing products is a leading cause of fatal poisoning in children under 6. Keep this product out of the reach of children. In case of accidental overdose, call a doctor or poison control center immediately.

INDICATIONS

PreCare® Conceive™ tablets are indicated to provide vitamin and mineral supplementation which is useful to improve nutritional status prior to conception and throughout pregnancy.

CONTRAINDICATIONS

This product is contraindicated in patients with a known hypersensitivity to any of the ingredients.

WARNING

Folic acid alone is improper therapy in the treatment of pernicious anemia and other megaloblastic anemias where Vitamin B_{12} is deficient.

PRECAUTIONS

Folic acid in doses above 0.1 mg daily may obscure pernicious anemia, in that hematologic remission can occur while neurological manifestations remain progressive.
PEDIATRIC USE: Safety and effectiveness in pediatric patients has not been established.

GERIATRIC USE: Clinical studies on this product have not been performed to determine whether elderly subjects respond differently from younger subjects. In general, dose selection for elderly patients should be cautious, usually starting at the low end of the dosing range, reflecting the greater frequency of decreased hepatic, renal, or cardiac function, and of concomitant disease or other drug therapy.

ADVERSE REACTIONS

Allergic sensitization has been reported following both oral and parenteral administration of folic acid.

DOSAGE AND ADMINISTRATION

Usual dosage is one tablet daily, or as prescribed by a physician.

HOW SUPPLIED

PreCare® Conceive™ tablets for oral administration are supplied as diamond shaped, film coated yellow tablets, debossed "Ther-Rx" on one side and "014" on the other side in child-resistant, unit dose packages of 100 tablets (10 × 10 Unit Dose Packs) (NDC 64011-014-11).
Store at controlled room temperature 15°–30°C (59°–86°F).
Manufactured by
KV Pharmaceutical Co. for
Ther-Rx Corporation
St. Louis, MO 63045
U.S. Patents No. 4,822,816, 5,070,085, 5,494,681
Other U.S. Patent Pending

Rev. 6/00

Shown in Product Identification Guide, page 338

PRECARE® PRENATAL ℞
Multivitamin/Mineral Film Coated Caplet

DESCRIPTION

Each peach film coated caplet contains:
Vitamin C (as Ester-C®[1])* .... 50 mg
Calcium (as Calcium Carbonate) .... 250 mg
Iron (as Ferrous Fumarate and Carbonyl Iron) .... 40 mg
Vitamin E (as dl-Alpha-Tocopheryl Acetate) .... 3.5 mg
Vitamin D_3 (Cholecalciferol) .... 6 mcg
Thiamine (as Thiamine Mononitrate, USP) .... 3.0 mg
Riboflavin, USP .... 3.4 mg
Niacin (as Niacinamide, USP) .... 20 mg
Pyridoxine (as Pyridoxine HCl, USP) .... 20 mg
Folic Acid, USP .... 1 mg
Cyanocobalamin .... 12 mcg
Magnesium (as Magnesium Oxide, USP) .... 50 mg
Zinc (as Zinc Sulfate, USP) .... 15 mg
Copper (as Cupric Sulfate) .... 2 mg
Inactive Ingredients: Natural oils, natural wax, cellulose polymers, flow agents, FD&C yellow No. 6 aluminum lake, and other ingredients.

[1] Ester-C® is a patented pharmaceutical grade material consisting of calcium ascorbate and calcium threonate.
*Logo and Ester-C® are licensed trademarks of Inter-Cal Corporation.

WARNING: Accidental overdose of iron-containing products is a leading cause of fatal poisoning in children under 6. Keep this product out of the reach of children. In case of accidental overdose, call a doctor or poison control center immediately.

INDICATIONS

PreCare® Prenatal caplets are indicated to provide vitamin and mineral supplementation throughout pregnancy and during the postnatal period—for both lactating and non-lactating mothers. It is also useful for improving nutritional status prior to conception.

CONTRAINDICATIONS

This product is contraindicated in patients with a known hypersensitivity to any of the ingredients.

WARNING

Folic acid alone is improper therapy in the treatment of pernicious anemia and other megaloblastic anemias where Vitamin B_{12} is deficient.

PRECAUTIONS

Folic acid in doses above 0.1 mg daily may obscure pernicious anemia, in that hematologic remission can occur while neurological manifestations remain progressive.

PEDIATRIC USE

Safety and effectiveness in pediatric patients has not been established.

GERIATRIC USE

Clinical studies on this product have not been performed to determine whether elderly subjects respond differently from younger subjects. In general, dose selection for elderly patients should be cautious, usually starting at the low end of the dosing range, reflecting the greater frequency of decreased hepatic, renal, or cardiac function, and of concomitant disease or other drug therapy.

ADVERSE REACTIONS

Allergic sensitization has been reported following both oral and parenteral administration of folic acid.

DOSAGE AND ADMINISTRATION

Usual dosage is one caplet daily, or as prescribed by a physician.

HOW SUPPLIED

PreCare® Prenatal Multivitamin/Mineral Caplets for oral administration are supplied as peach, film coated tablets, debossed "Ther-Rx" on one side and "025" with partial bisect on the other side in child-resistant, unit dose packages of 100 caplets (10×10 Unit Dose Packs) (NDC 64011-025-11).
Store at controlled room temperature 15°–30°C (59°–86°F)
U.S. Patents No. 4,822,816, 5,070,085, 5,494,681
Manufactured by
KV Pharmaceutical Company for
Ther-Rx Corporation
St. Louis, MO 63045
7/00

Shown in Product Identification Guide, page 338

PREMESISRx™ ℞

Prescription Multivitamin/Mineral Tablet with Controlled-Release Vitamin B_6

DESCRIPTION

Each blue tablet contains:

Vitamin B_6 (as pyridoxine HCl)	75 mg
Vitamin B_{12} (cyanocobalamin)	12 mcg
Folic Acid, USP	1 mg
Calcium (as calcium carbonate)	200 mg

Inactive Ingredients: Natural waxes, cellulose polymers, FD&C blue No. 1 aluminum lake, D&C yellow No. 10 aluminum lake, flow agents and other ingredients.

INDICATIONS

PremesisRx™ tablets are indicated to provide vitamin and mineral supplementation during pregnancy and may be used in conjunction with a physician-prescribed regimen to minimize pregnancy related nausea.

CONTRAINDICATIONS

This product is contraindicated in patients with a known hypersensitivity to any of the ingredients.

WARNINGS

Folic acid alone is improper therapy in the treatment of pernicious anemia and other megaloblastic anemias where Vitamin B_{12} is deficient.

PRECAUTIONS

Folic acid in doses above 0.1 mg daily may obscure pernicious anemia, in that hematologic remission can occur while neurological manifestations remain progressive.

PEDIATRIC USE

Safety and effectiveness in pediatric patients has not been established.

GERIATRIC USE

Clinical studies on this product have not been performed to determine whether elderly subjects respond differently from younger subjects. In general, dose selection for elderly patients should be cautious, usually starting at the low end of the dosing range, reflecting the greater frequency of decreased hepatic, renal, or cardiac function, and of concomitant disease or other drug therapy.

ADVERSE REACTIONS

Allergic sensitization has been reported following both oral and parenteral administration of folic acid.

DOSAGE AND ADMINISTRATION

Usual dosage is one tablet daily, or as prescribed by a physician.

HOW SUPPLIED

PremesisRx™ tablets for oral administration are supplied as blue, oval tablets, debossed "Ther-Rx" on one side and "019" on the other side in bottles of 100 tablets (NDC 64011-019-04). Store at controlled room temperature, 15°–30°C (59°–86°F).
U.S. Patents Pending
Manufactured by
KV Pharmaceutical Company for
Ther-Rx Corporation
St. Louis, MO 63045
04-017 © Ther-Rx Corporation 7/00

Shown in Product Identification Guide, page 338

UCB Pharma, Inc.

1950 LAKE PARK DRIVE
SMYRNA, GA 30080

Direct Inquiries to:
UCB Pharma, Inc.
1950 Lake Park Drive
Smyrna, GA 30080
(800) 477–7877

For Medical Information Contact:
Medical Affairs Department
24 hours a day, seven days a week:
(800) 477–7877

DURATUSS™ Tablets ℞

120 mg pseudoephedrine hydrochloride and 600 mg guaifenesin

DESCRIPTION

Each long-acting, film-coated, dye-free Duratuss Tablet contains:

Pseudoephedrine Hydrochloride	120 mg
Guaifenesin	600 mg

Also contains ethylcellulose, hydrogenated vegetable oil (type 1), magnesium stearate, microcrystalline cellulose, and talc. Film coating composed of hydroxypropyl methylcellulose, polyethylene glycol, polysorbate 80, titanium dioxide, and artificial flavoring.

HOW SUPPLIED

Duratuss™ Tablets (120 mg pseudoephedrine hydrochloride and 600 mg guaifenesin) are supplied as white, film-coated, dye-free, oval-shaped tablets debossed "ucb" on one side and scored and debossed "612" on the other side in bottles of 100 (NDC 50474-612-01), 500 tablets (NCD 50474-612-50), and 1000 tablets (NDC 50474-612-70).
Store at controlled room temperature 25°C(77°F); excursions permitted to 15–30°C(59–86°F). [See USP Controlled Room Temperature]
Protect from light and moisture.

Manufactured for
UCB Pharma, Inc.,
Smyrna, GA 30080
by **Schwarz Pharma**
Manufacturing, Inc.
Seymour, IN 47274

Rev. 7/00

Shown in Product Identification Guide, page 338

DURATUSS™ G TABLETS ℞

guaifenesin 1200 mg

DESCRIPTION

Each long-acting, film-coated, dye-free Duratuss G Tablet contains:

Guaifenesin	1200 mg

The inactive ingredients for Duratuss G Tablets are as follows: ethylcellulose, hydrogenated vegetable oil (type 1) and magnesium stearate. Film coating composed of hydrolyzed gelatin, hydroxypropyl methylcellulose and polyethylene glycol.

HOW SUPPLIED

Duratuss™ G Tablets (guaifenesin 1200 mg) are supplied as scored, white, film-coated, dye-free, capsule-shaped tablets debossed 'ucb/620' on one side, in bottles of 100 tablets (NDC 50474-620-01), 500 tablets (NDC 50474-620-50) and 1000 tablets (NDC 50474-620-70).
Store at 25°C (77°F); excursions permitted to 15°–30°C (59°–86°F). [see USP Controlled Room Temperature] Protect from light and moisture.

Manufactured for
UCB Pharma, Inc.
Smyrna, GA 30080
by **Schwarz Pharma**
Manufacturing, Inc.
Seymour, IN 47274

Rev. 3/00

Shown in Product Identification Guide, page 338

DURATUSS™ GP Tablets ℞

(1200 mg guaifenesin and 120 mg pseudoephedrine hydrochloride)

DESCRIPTION

Each long-acting, film-coated, dye-free, DURATUSS™ GP tablet for oral administration contains:

Guaifenesin	1200 mg
Pseudoephedrine hydrochloride	120 mg

Also contains microcrystalline cellulose, magnesium stearate and other ingredients. Film coating composed of hydroxypropyl methylcellulose and polyethylene glycol.
Guaifenesin is an expectorant with the chemical name 1,2-propanediol, 3-(2-methoxyphenoxy)-, (±)-. The molecular weight is 198.22. The molecular formula is $C_{10}H_{14}O_4$. Guaifenesin occurs as white to slightly gray crystalline substance, which may have a slight characteristic odor. It is soluble in water, in alcohol, in chloroform, and in propylene glycol and sparingly soluble in glycerin. The chemical structure is shown below:

Pseudoephedrine hydrochloride, is an adrenergic (vasoconstrictor) agent with the chemical name benzenemethanol, α-[1-(methylamino)etyl]-, [S-(R*,R*)]-, hydrochloride. The molecular weight is 201.69. The molecular formula is $C_{10}H_{15}NO \cdot HCl$. Pseudoephedrine hydrochloride occurs as fine, white to off-white crystals or powder, having a faint characteristic odor. It is very soluble in water, freely soluble in alcohol and sparingly soluble in chloroform. The chemical structure is shown below:

CLINICAL PHARMACOLOGY

Overview: Guaifenesin is an expectorant, which increases respiratory tract fluid secretions and helps loosen phlegm and bronchial secretions. By reducing the viscosity of secretions, guaifenesin increases the efficiency of the mucociliary mechanism in removing accumulated secretions from the upper and lower airway. As a result, sinus and bronchial drainage is improved and nonproductive coughs become more productive and less frequent.
Pseudoephedrine hydrochloride is an orally effective nasal decongestant that acts on alpha-adrenergic receptors in the mucosa of the respiratory tract producing vasoconstriction. Pseudoephedrine shrinks swollen nasal mucus membranes, reduces tissue hyperemia, edema and nasal congestion and increases nasal airway patency. Drainage of sinus secretions is increased and obstructed eustachian ostia may be opened. Pseudoephedrine produces little if any rebound congestion. Pseudoephedrine produces peripheral effects similar to those of ephedrine and central effects similar to, but less intense than, amphetamines. It has potential for excitatory side effects.
Pharmacokinetics: Guaifenesin is readily absorbed from the gastrointestinal tract and is rapidly metabolized and excreted in the urine. Guaifenesin has a plasma half-life of one hour. The major urinary metabolite is β-(2-methoxyphenoxy) lactic acid.
Pseudoephedrine has been shown to have a mean elimination half-life of 4–6 hours, which is dependent on urine pH. The elimination half-life is decreased at urine pH lower than 6 and may be increased at urine pH higher than 8.
Special Populations:
Pediatric Patients: DURATUSS GP contains a fixed dose of pseudoephedrine hydrochloride 120 mg in an extended release formulation. This product is not recommended for pediatric patients under 12 years of age.
Renal Impairment: About 55–75% of an administered dose of pseudoephedrine hydrochloride is excreted unchanged in the urine; the remainder is apparently metabolized in the liver. Therefore, pseudoephedrine may accumulate in patients with renal insufficiency.
Dosing adjustment may be necessary in patients with moderate or severe renal impairment and in patients on dialysis.
Hepatic Impairment: The effect of hepatic impairment on pseudoephedrine pharmacokinetics is unknown.

INDICATIONS

DURATUSS GP tablets are indicated for the relief of nasal congestion due to the common cold, hay fever or other upper respiratory allergies and nasal congestion associated with sinusitis. To promote nasal or sinus drainage; for the relief of eustachian tube congestion; for adjunctive therapy in serous otitis media; for the symptomatic relief of respiratory conditions characterized by dry, nonproductive cough and in the presence of tenacious mucus and/or mucus plugs in the respiratory tract.

CONTRAINDICATIONS

DURATUSS GP is contraindicated in those patients with a known hypersensitivity to it or any of its ingredients.
Due to its pseudoephedrine component, DURATUSS GP is contraindicated in patients with narrow-angle glaucoma or urinary retention, and in patients receiving monoamine oxidase (MAO) inhibitor therapy or within fourteen (14) days of stopping such treatment (see Drug/Drug Interactions). It is also contraindicated in patients with severe hypertension, or severe coronary artery disease, and in those who have shown hypersensitivity, or idiosyncrasy to its components, to adrenergic agents, or to other drugs of similar chemical structures. Manifestations of patient idiosyncrasy to adrenergic agents include: insomnia, dizziness, weakness, tremor, or arrhythmias.

WARNINGS

Sympathomimetic amines should be used judiciously and sparingly in patients with hypertension, peripheral vascu-

Continued on next page

Duratuss GP—Cont.

lar disease, diabetes mellitus, ischemic heart disease, increased intraocular pressure, hyperthyroidism, renal impairment, or prostatic hypertrophy (see CONTRAINDICATIONS). Sympathomimetic amines may produce central nervous system stimulation with convulsions or cardiovascular collapse with accompanying hypotension. The elderly are more likely to have adverse reactions to sympathomimetic amines.

PRECAUTIONS

Information for Patients: Patients taking DURATUSS GP should receive the following information: Patients should be instructed to take DURATUSS GP only as prescribed. **Do not exceed the recommended dose.** If nervousness, dizziness, or sleeplessness occur, discontinue use and consult physician.

Patients who are hypersensitive to it or any of its ingredients should not use this product. Due to its pseudoephedrine component, this product should not be used by patients with narrow-angle glaucoma, urinary retention, or patients receiving a monoamine oxidase (MAO) inhibitor or within 14 days of stopping use of a MAO inhibitor. Patients with severe hypertension or severe coronary artery disease also should not use it.

As with other sympathomimetic drugs, DURATUSS GP should be used cautiously in the presence of hypertension, peripheral vascular disease, diabetes mellitus, ischemic heart disease, increased intraocular pressure, hyperthyroidism, renal impairment, or prostatic hypertrophy. Sympathomimetic amines may produce central nervous system stimulation with convulsions or cardiovascular collapse with accompanying hypotension. The elderly are more likely to have adverse reactions to sympathomimetic amines.

Patients should consult their physician if they are or wish to become pregnant.

Do not crush or chew DURATUSS GP tablets before ingestion to preserve the long-acting effect.

Drug/Drug Interactions: Due to the pseudoephedrine component, DURATUSS GP is contraindicated in patients taking monoamine oxidase (MAO) inhibitors and for fourteen (14) days after stopping use of a MAO inhibitor. Concomitant use with antihypertensive drugs which interfere with sympathetic activity (e.g. methyldopa, mecamylamine, and reserpine) may reduce their antihypertensive effects. Increased ectopic pacemaker activity can occur when pseudoephedrine is used concomitantly with digitalis. Care should be taken in the administration of DURATUSS GP concomitantly with other sympathomimetic amines because combined effects on the cardiovascular system may be harmful to the patient (See CONTRAINDICATIONS and WARNINGS).

Drug/Laboratory Test Interactions: Guaifenesin interferes with the colorimetric determination of 5-hydroxy-indolacetic acid (5-HIAA) and vanillylmandelic acid (VMA).

Carcinogenesis, Mutagenesis, Impairment of Fertility: There are no animal or *in vitro* studies on the combination product guaifenesin and pseudoephedrine hydrochloride to evaluate carcinogenesis, mutagenesis, and impairment of fertility.

Two-year feeding studies in rats and mice conducted under the auspices of National Toxicology Program (NTP) demonstrated no evidence of carcinogenic potential with ephedrine sulfate, a structurally related drug with pharmacological properties similar to pseudoephedrine, at doses up to 10 and 27 mg/kg, respectively (approximately 16 and 100% of the maximum recommended daily dose of pseudoephedrine hydrochloride in adults on a mg/m^2 basis).

Pregnancy Category C: There are no adequate and well-controlled studies with guaifenesin and/or pseudoephedrine hydrochloride in pregnant women. DURATUSS GP should be used in pregnant women only if the potential benefit justifies the potential risk to the fetus.

Nursing Mothers: It is not known if guaifenesin is excreted in human milk.

Pseudoephedrine hydrochloride administered alone distributes into breast milk of lactating human females.

Because of the potential for serious adverse reactions in nursing infants from sympathomimetic amines, a decision should be made whether to discontinue nursing or to discontinue the drug, taking into account the importance of the drug to the mother.

Pediatric Use: DURATUSS GP contains a fixed dose of pseudoephedrine hydrochloride 120 mg in an extended release formulation. This product is not recommended for pediatric patients under 12 years of age. The safety and effectiveness of DURATUSS GP in pediatric patients under the age of 12 years have not been established.

Geriatric Use: The elderly are more likely to have adverse reactions to sympathomimetic amines. In general, dose selection for an elderly patient should be cautious reflecting the greater frequency of decreased hepatic, renal, or cardiac function, and of concomitant disease or other drug therapy. The pseudoephedrine component of DURATUSS GP is known to be substantially excreted by the kidney, and the risk of toxic reactions to this drug may be greater in patients with impaired renal function. Because elderly patients are more likely to have decreased renal function, care should be taken in dose selection, and it may be useful to monitor renal function.

Use in Patients with Impaired Renal Function: Dose should be adjusted in patients with decreased renal function. Patients should be given a lower total daily dose because they have reduced elimination of pseudoephedrine.

ADVERSE REACTIONS

Guaifenesin: Guaifenesin is well tolerated. Side effects are generally mild and infrequent. Nausea and vomiting are the most frequently occurring side effects. Dizziness, headache, and rash (including urticaria) have been reported rarely.

Pseudoephedrine hydrochloride: Pseudoephedrine hydrochloride may cause mild CNS stimulation in hypersensitivity patients. Nervousness, excitability, dizziness, weakness, or insomnia may occur. Headache, nausea, drowsiness, tachycardia, palpitation, pressor activity, and cardiac arrhythmias have been reported. Sympathomimetic drugs have also been associated with other untoward effects such as fear, anxiety, tenseness, tremor, hallucinations, seizures, pallor, respiratory difficulty, dysuria, and cardiovascular collapse.

DRUG ABUSE AND DEPENDENCE

There is no information to indicate that abuse or dependency occurs with guaifenesin or with the combination of guaifenesin and pseudoephedrine.

However, like other central nervous system stimulants, pseudoephedrine has been abused. At high doses, subjects commonly experience an elevation of mood; a sense of increased energy and alertness and decreased appetite. Some individuals become anxious, irritable, and loquacious. In addition to the marked euphoria, the user experiences a sense of markedly enhanced physical strength and mental capacity. With continued use, tolerance develops, the user increases the dose, and toxic signs and symptoms appear. Depression may follow rapid withdrawal.

OVERDOSAGE

Since the effects of DURATUSS GP may last up to 12 hours, treatment of overdosage should be directed towards supporting the patient and reversing the effects of the drug for at least that length of time.

In large doses, sympathomimetics may give rise to giddiness, headache, nausea, vomiting, sweating, thirst, tachycardia, precordial pain, palpitations, difficulty in micturition, muscular weakness and tenseness, anxiety, restlessness, and insomnia. Many patients can present a toxic psychosis with delusions and hallucinations. Some may develop cardiac arrhythmias, circulatory collapse, convulsions, coma and respiratory failure.

DOSAGE AND ADMINISTRATION

Adults and pediatric patients 12 years of age and older: The recommended dose of DURATUSS GP is one tablet every 12 hours, not to exceed 2 tablets in 24 hours.

Dosing adjustments may be necessary in patients with moderate or severe renal impairment and in patients on dialysis.

Do not crush or chew DURATUSS GP tablets before ingestion to preserve the long-acting effect.

HOW SUPPLIED

DURATUSS™ GP (1200 mg guaifenesin and 120 mg pseudoephedrine hydrochloride) is supplied as scored, white, film-coated, dye-free, oval-shaped tablets, debossed "ucb/640" on one side, in bottles of 100 tablets, NDC 50474-640-01.

STORAGE

Store at controlled room temperature 25°C (77°F); excursions permitted to 15–30°C (59–86°F). [See USP Controlled Room Temperature]

Protect from light and moisture.

Manufactured for
UCB Pharma, Inc.
Smyrna, GA 30080
Manufactured by
Mikart, Inc.
Atlanta, GA 30318
Rev. 5/00
P/N: 1003322
Code 0870A00

Shown in Product Identification Guide, page 338

DURATUSS™ DM Elixir ℞

20 mg dextromethorphan hydrobromide and 200 mg guaifenesin per 5 mL

DESCRIPTION

Each 5 mL (one teaspoonful) of Duratuss DM Elixir contains:

Dextromethorphan hydrobromide .... 20 mg
Guaifenesin .... 200 mg
Alcohol 5%

Also contains citric acid, high fructose corn syrup, propylene glycol, purified water, saccharin sodium, sodium benzoate, FD&C Red No. 40, FD&C Red No. 3, FD&C Blue No. 1, and artificial flavoring.

HOW SUPPLIED

Duratuss™ DM Elixir is a purple-colored, fruit-flavored liquid containing 20 mg dextromethorphan hydrobromide and 200 mg guaifenesin per 5 mL with 5% alcohol. It is supplied in containers of 1 pint (473 mL), NDC 50474-630-16 and 1 gallon (3785 mL), NDC 50474-630-28.

Store at 25°C (77°F); excursions permitted to 15–30°C (59–86°F) [see USP Controlled Room Temperature]

Dispense in a tight, light-resistant container with a child-resistant closure.

Manufactured for
UCB Pharma, Inc.
Smyrna, GA 30080
by **Vintage Pharmaceuticals, Inc.**
Huntsville, AL 35811
Rev. 4/00

Shown in Product Identification Guide, page 338

DURATUSS™ HD Elixir Ⓒ III

2.5 mg hydrocodone bitartrate
30 mg pseudoephedrine hydrochloride, and 100 mg guaifenesin per 5 mL
Rx only

DESCRIPTION

Each 5 mL (one teaspoonful) of Duratuss HD Elixir contains:

Hydrocodon Bitartrate .... 2.5 mg
Pseudoephedrine Hydrochloride .... 30 mg
Guaifenesin .... 100 mg
Alcohol 5%

Also contains citric acid anhydrous, glucose liquid, methylparaben, propylene glycol, propylparaben, purified water, saccharin sodium, sorbitol solution, sucrose, FD&C Red #40, natural and artificial flavoring.

HOW SUPPLIED

Duratuss™ HD Elixir is a red-colored, fruit punch-flavored liquid containing 2.5 mg hydrocodone bitartrate, 30 mg pseudoephedrine hydrochloride, and 100 mg guaifenesin per 5 mL, with 5% alcohol. It is supplied in containers of 1 pint (473 mL), NDC 50474-610-16, and 1 gallon (3785 mL), NDC 50474-610-28.

Store at 25°C (77°F); excursions permitted to 15–30°C (59–86°F) [see USP Controlled Room Temperature]

Dispense in a tight, light-resistant container with a child-resistant closure.

Manufactured for
UCB Pharma, Inc.,
Smyrna, GA 30080
by Mikart, Inc.,
Atlanta, GA 30318
Rev. 7/00

Shown in Product Identification Guide, page 338

KEPPRA™ ℞

[*kĕp-ră*]

levetiracetam
250•500•750 mg tablets
PRESCRIBING INFORMATION

℞ only

DESCRIPTION

Keppra™ (levetiracetam) is an antiepileptic drug available as 250 mg (blue), 500 mg (yellow) and 750 mg (orange) tablets for oral administration.

The chemical name of levetiracetam, a single enantiomer, is (-)-(S)-α-ethyl-2-oxo-1-pyrrolidine acetamide, its molecular formula is $C_8H_{14}N_2O_2$ and its molecular weight is 170.21.

Levetiracetam is chemically unrelated to existing antiepileptic drugs (AEDs). It has the following structural formula:

N O CH₃CH₂ H CONH₂

Levetiracetam is a white to off-white crystalline powder with a faint odor and a bitter taste. It is very soluble in water (104.0 g/100 mL). It is freely soluble in chloroform (65.3g/100 mL) and in methanol (53.6 g/100 mL), soluble in ethanol (16.5 g/100 mL), sparingly soluble in acetonitrile (5.7 g/100 mL) and practically insoluble in n-hexane.

Keppra tablets contain the labeled amount of levetiracetam. Inactive ingredients: colloidal silicon dioxide, corn starch, hydroxypropyl methylcellulose, magnesium stearate, polyethylene glycol 4000, povidone, talc, titanium dioxide and coloring agents.

The individual tablets contain the following coloring agents:
250 mg tablets: FD&C Blue No. 2,
500 mg tablets: FD&C Blue No. 2 and yellow iron oxide,
750 mg tablets: FD&C Blue No. 2, FD&C Yellow No. 6 and red iron oxide.

CLINICAL PHARMACOLOGY

Mechanism of Action The precise mechanism(s) by which levetiracetam exerts its antiepileptic effect is unknown and does not appear to derive from any interaction with known mechanisms involved in inhibitory and excitatory neurotransmission. The antiepileptic activity of levetiracetam was assessed in a number of animal models of epileptic seizures. Levetiracetam did not inhibit single seizures induced by maximal stimulation with electrical current or different chemoconvulsants and showed only minimal activity in submaximal stimulation and in threshold tests. Protection was observed, however, against secondarily generalized activity from focal seizures induced by pilocarpine and kainic acid, two chemoconvulsants that induce seizures that mimic some features of human complex partial seizures with secondary generalization. Levetiracetam also displayed inhibitory properties in the kindling model in rats, another model of human complex partial seizures, both during kindling development and in the fully kindled state. The predictive value of these animal models for specific types of human epilepsy is uncertain.

In vitro studies show that levetiracetam, up to 1700 µg/L, did not result in significant ligand displacement at known receptor binding sites. Second messenger systems, ion channel proteins, glutamate receptor-mediated neurotransmission, muscimol-induced chloride flux and gamma-aminobutyric acid-transaminase and glutamate decarboxylase activities were unaffected by levetiracetam. Benzodiazepine receptor antagonists had no effect on levetiracetam's protection against seizures. In contrast, a stereoselective binding site for the drug has been demonstrated to exist exclusively in synaptic plasma membranes in the CNS, and not in peripheral tissue.

In vitro and *in vivo* recordings of epileptiform activity from the hippocampus have shown that levetiracetam inhibits burst firing without affecting normal neuronal excitability, suggesting that levetiracetam may selectively prevent hypersynchronization of epileptiform burst firing and propagation of seizure activity.

Pharmacokinetics The pharmacokinetics of levetiracetam have been studied in healthy adult subjects, adults and pediatric patients with epilepsy, elderly subjects and subjects with renal and hepatic impairment.

Overview Levetiracetam is rapidly and almost completely absorbed after oral administration. The pharmacokinetics are linear and time-invariant, with low intra- and intersubject variability. The extent of bioavailability of levetiracetam is not affected by food. Levetiracetam is not protein-bound (<10% bound) and its volume of distribution is close to the volume of intracellular and extracellular water. Sixty-six percent (66%) of the dose is renally excreted unchanged. The major metabolic pathway of levetiracetam (24% of dose) is an enzymatic hydrolysis of the acetamide group. It is not liver cytochrome P450 dependent. The metabolites have no known pharmacological activity and are renally excreted. Plasma half-life of levetiracetam across studies is approximately 6–8 hours. It is increased in the elderly (primarily due to impaired renal clearance) and in subjects with renal impairment.

Absorption and Distribution Absorption of levetiracetam is rapid, with peak plasma concentrations occurring in about an hour following oral administration in fasted subjects. The oral bioavailability of levetiracetam tablets is 100%. Food does not affect the extent of absorption of levetiracetam but it decreases C_{max} by 20% and delays T_{max} by 1.5 hours. The pharmacokinetics of levetiracetam are linear over the dose range of 500–5000 mg. Steady state is achieved after 2 days of multiple twice-daily dosing. Levetiracetam and its major metabolite are less than 10% bound to plasma proteins; clinically significant interactions with other drugs through competition for protein binding sites are therefore unlikely.

Metabolism Levetiracetam is not extensively metabolized in humans. The major metabolic pathway is the enzymatic hydrolysis of the acetamide group, which produces the carboxylic acid metabolite, ucb L057 (24%) and is not dependent on any liver cytochrome P450 isoenzymes. The major metabolite is inactive in animal seizure models. Two minor metabolites were identified as the product of hydroxylation of the 2-oxo-pyrrolidine ring (2% of dose) and opening of the 2-oxo-pyrrolidine ring in position 5 (1% of dose). There is no enantiomeric interconversion of levetiracetam or its major metabolite.

Elimination Levetiracetam plasma half-life in adults is 7 ± 1 hour and is unaffected by either dose or repeated administration. Levetiracetam is eliminated from the systemic circulation by renal excretion as unchanged drug which represents 66% of administered dose. The total body clearance is 0.96 mL/min/kg and the renal clearance is 0.6 mL/min/kg. The mechanism of excretion is glomerular filtration with subsequent partial tubular reabsorption. The metabolite ucb L057 is excreted by glomerular filtration and active tubular secretion with a renal clearance of 4 mL/min/kg. Levetiracetam elimination is correlated to creatinine clearance. Levetiracetam clearance is reduced in patients with impaired renal function (see Special Populations, Renal Impairment and DOSAGE AND ADMINISTRATION, Patients with Impaired Renal Function).

Pharmacokinetic Interactions *In vitro* data on metabolic interactions indicate that levetiracetam is unlikely to produce, or be subject to, pharmacokinetic interactions. Levetiracetam and its major metabolite, at concentrations well above C_{max} levels achieved within the therapeutic dose range, are neither inhibitors of, nor high affinity substrates for, human liver cytochrome P450 isoforms, epoxide hydrolase, or UDP-glucuronidation enzymes. In addition, levetiracetam does not affect the *in vitro* glucuronidation of valproic acid.

Potential pharmacokinetic interactions were assessed in clinical pharmacokinetic studies (phenytoin, warfarin, digoxin, oral contraceptives) and through pharmacokinetic screening in the placebo-controlled clinical studies in epilepsy patients (see PRECAUTIONS, Drug Interactions).

Special Populations Elderly Pharmacokinetics of levetiracetam were evaluated in 16 elderly subjects (age 61–88 years) with creatinine clearance ranging from 30 to 74 mL/min. Following oral administration of twice daily dosing for 10 days, total body clearance decreased by 38% and the half-life was 2.5 hours longer in the elderly compared to healthy adults. This is most likely due to the decrease in renal function in these subjects.

Pediatric Patients Pharmacokinetics of levetiracetam were evaluated in 24 pediatric patients (age 6–12 years) after single dose (20 mg/kg). The apparent clearance of levetiracetam was approximately 40% higher than in adults.

Gender Levetiracetam C_{max} and AUC were 20% higher in women (N=11) compared to men (N=12). However, clearances adjusted for body weight were comparable.

Race Formal pharmacokinetic studies of the effects of race have not been conducted. Cross study comparisons involving Caucasians (N=12) and Asians (N=12), however, show that pharmacokinetics of levetiracetam were comparable between the two races. Because levetiracetam is primarily renally excreted and there are no important racial differences in creatinine clearance, pharmacokinetic differences due to race are not expected.

Renal Impairment The disposition of levetiracetam was studied in subjects with varying degrees of renal function. Total body clearance of levetiracetam is reduced in patients with impaired renal function by 40% in the mild group (CLcr = 50–80 mL/min), 50% in the moderate group (CLcr = 30–50 mL/min) and 60% in the severe renal impairment group (CLcr <30 mL/min). Clearance of levetiracetam is correlated with creatinine clearance.

In anuric (end stage renal disease) patients, the total body clearance decreased 70% compared to normal subjects (CLcr >80 mL/min). Approximately 50% of the pool of levetiracetam in the body is removed during a standard 4-hour hemodialysis procedure.

Dosage should be reduced in patients with impaired renal function receiving levetiracetam, and supplemental doses should be given to patients after dialysis (see PRECAUTIONS and DOSAGE AND ADMINISTRATION, Patients with Impaired Renal Function).

Hepatic Impairment In subjects with mild (Child-Pugh A) to moderate (Child-Pugh B) hepatic impairment, the pharmacokinetics of levetiracetam were unchanged. In patients with severe hepatic impairment (Child-Pugh C), total body clearance was 50% that of normal subjects, but decreased renal clearance accounted for most of the decrease. No dose adjustment is needed for patients with hepatic impairment.

CLINICAL STUDIES

Effectiveness in Partial Onset Seizures The effectiveness of Keppra as adjunctive therapy (added to other antiepileptic drugs) in adults was established in three multicenter, randomized, double-blind, placebo-controlled clinical studies in patients who had refractory partial onset seizures with or without secondary generalization. In these studies, 904 patients were randomized to placebo, 1000 mg, 2000 mg, or 3000 mg/day. Patients enrolled in Study 1 or Study 2 had refractory partial onset seizures for at least 2 years and had taken two or more classical AEDs. At the time of the study, patients were taking a stable dose regimen of at least one and could take a maximum of two AEDs. During the baseline period, patients had to have experienced at least four partial onset seizures during each 4-week period.

Study 1 Study 1 was a double-blind, placebo-controlled, parallel-group study conducted at 41 sites in the United States comparing Keppra 1000 mg/day (N=97), Keppra 3000 mg/day (N=101) and placebo (N=95) given in equally divided doses twice daily. After a prospective baseline period of 12 weeks, patients were randomized to one of the three treatment groups described above. The 18-week treatment period consisted of a 6-week titration period, followed by a 12-week fixed dose evaluation period, during which concomitant AED regimens were held constant. The primary measure of effectiveness was a between group comparison of the percent reduction in weekly partial seizure frequency relative to placebo over the entire randomized treatment period (titration + evaluation period). Secondary outcome variables included the responder rate (incidence of patients with ≥50% reduction from baseline in partial onset seizure frequency). The results of the analysis of Study 1 are displayed in Table 1.

Table 1: Reduction in Weekly Frequency of Partial Onset Seizures in Study 1

	Placebo (N=95)	Keppra 1000 mg/day (N=97)	Keppra 3000 mg/day (N=101)
Percent reduction in partial seizure frequency over placebo	—	26.1% $P<0.001$	30.1% $P<0.001$

The percentage of patients (y-axis) who achieved ≥50% reduction in weekly seizure rates from baseline in partial onset seizure frequency over the entire randomized treatment period (titration + evaluation period) within the three treatment groups (x-axis) is presented in Figure 1.

[See figure 1 at top of next column]

Figure 1: Responder Rate (≥50% Reduction From Baseline) in Study 1

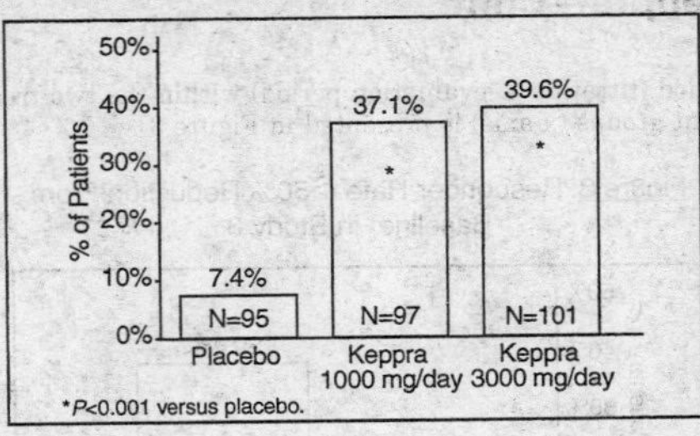

Study 2 Study 2 was a double-blind, placebo-controlled, crossover study conducted at 62 centers in Europe comparing Keppra 1000 mg/day (N=106), Keppra 2000 mg/day (N=105) and placebo (N=111) given in equally divided doses twice daily.

The first period of the study (Period A) was designed to be analyzed as a parallel-group study. After a prospective baseline period of up to 12 weeks, patients were randomized to one of the three treatment groups described above. The 16-week treatment period consisted of the 4-week titration period followed by a 12-week fixed dose evaluation period, during which concomitant AED regimens were held constant. The primary measure of effectiveness was a between group comparison of the percent reduction in weekly partial seizure frequency relative to placebo over the entire randomized treatment period (titration + evaluation period). Secondary outcome variables included the responder rate (incidence of patients with ≥50% reduction from baseline in partial onset seizure frequency). The results of the analysis of Period A are displayed in Table 2.

Table 2: Reduction in Weekly Frequency of Partial Onset Seizures in Study 2—Period A

	Placebo (N=111)	Keppra 1000 mg/day (N=106)	Keppra 2000 mg/day (N=105)
Percent reduction in partial seizure frequency over placebo	—	17.1% $P\leq0.001$	21.4% $P\leq0.001$

The percentage of patients (y-axis) who achieved ≥50% reduction in weekly seizure rates from baseline in partial onset seizure frequency over the entire randomized treatment period (titration + evaluation period) within the three treatment groups (x-axis) is presented in Figure 2.

Figure 2: Responder Rate (≥50% Reduction From Baseline) in Study 2 – Period A

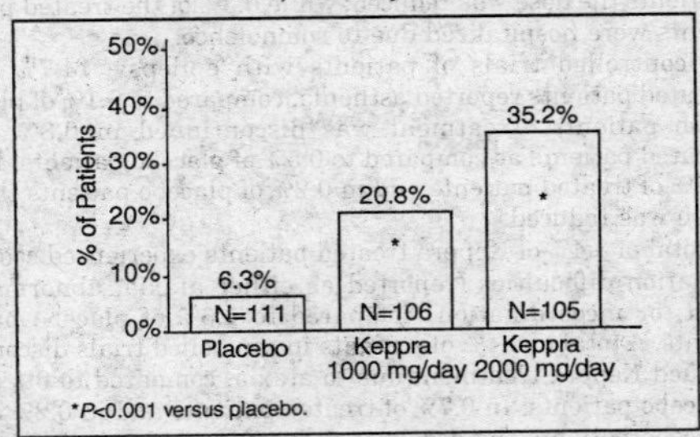

The comparison of Keppra 2000 mg/kg to Keppra 1000 mg/day for responder rate was statistically significant ($P=0.02$). Analysis of the trial as a crossover yielded similar results.

Study 3 Study 3 was a double-blind, placebo-controlled, parallel-group study conducted at 47 centers in Europe comparing Keppra 3000 mg/day (N=180) and placebo (N=104) in patients with refractory partial onset seizures, with or without secondary generalization, receiving only one concomitant AED. Study drug was given in two divided doses. After a prospective baseline period of 12 weeks, patients were randomized to one of two treatment groups described above. The 16-week treatment period consisted of a 4-week titration period, followed by a 12-week fixed dose evaluation period, during which concomitant AED doses were held constant. The primary measure of effectiveness was a between group comparison of the percent reduction in weekly seizure frequency relative to placebo over the entire randomized treatment period (titration + evaluation period). Secondary outcome variables included the responder rate (incidence of patients with ≥50% reduction from baseline in partial onset seizure frequency). Table 3 displays the results of the analysis of Study 3.

Table 3: Reduction in Weekly Frequency of Partial Onset Seizures in Study 3

	Placebo (N=104)	Keppra 3000 mg/day (N=180)
Percent reduction in partial seizure frequency over placebo	—	23.0% $P<0.001$

The percentage of patients (y-axis) who achieved ≥50% reduction in weekly seizure rates from baseline in partial onset seizure frequency over the entire randomized treatment

Continued on next page

Keppra—Cont.

period (titration + evaluation period) within the two treatment groups (x-axis) is presented in Figure 3.

Figure 3: Responder Rate (≥50% Reduction From Baseline) in Study 3

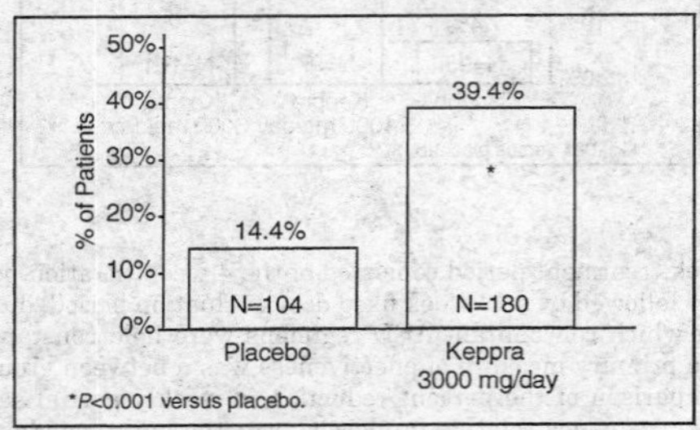

INDICATIONS AND USAGE

Keppra (levetiracetam) is indicated as adjunctive therapy in the treatment of partial onset seizures in adults with epilepsy.

CONTRAINDICATIONS

This product should not be administered to patients who have previously exhibited hypersensitivity to levetiracetam or any of the inactive ingredients in Keppra tablets.

WARNINGS

Neuropsychiatric Adverse Events Keppra use is associated with the occurrence of central nervous system adverse events that can be classified into the following categories: 1) somnolence and fatigue, 2) coordination difficulties, and 3) behavioral abnormalities.

In controlled trials of patients with epilepsy, 14.8% of Keppra treated patients reported somnolence, compared to 8.4% of placebo patients. There was no clear dose response up to 3000 mg/day. In a study where there was no titration, about 45% of patients receiving 4000 mg/day reported somnolence. The somnolence was considered serious in 0.3% of the treated patients, compared to 0% in the placebo group. About 3% of Keppra treated patients discontinued treatment due to somnolence, compared to 0.7% of placebo patients. In 1.4% of treated patients and in 0.9% of placebo patients the dose was reduced, while 0.3% of the treated patients were hospitalized due to somnolence.

In controlled trials of patients with epilepsy, 14.7% of treated patients reported asthenia, compared to 9.1% of placebo patients. Treatment was discontinued in 0.8% of treated patients as compared to 0.5% of placebo patients. In 0.5% of treated patients and in 0.2% of placebo patients the dose was reduced.

A total of 3.4% of Keppra treated patients experienced coordination difficulties (reported as either ataxia, abnormal gait, or incoordination) compared to 1.6% of placebo patients. A total of 0.4% of patients in controlled trials discontinued Keppra treatment due to ataxia, compared to 0% of placebo patients. In 0.7% of treated patients and in 0.2% of placebo patients the dose was reduced due to coordination difficulties while one of the treated patients was hospitalized due to worsening of preexisting ataxia.

Somnolence, asthenia and coordination difficulties occurred most frequently within the first 4 weeks of treatment.

In controlled trials of patients with epilepsy, 5 (0.7%) of Keppra treated patients experienced psychotic symptoms compared to 1 (0.2%) placebo patient. Two (0.3%) Keppra treated patients were hospitalized and their treatment was discontinued. Both events, reported as psychosis, developed within the first week of treatment and resolved within 1 to 2 weeks following treatment discontinuation. Two other events, reported as hallucinations, occurred after 1–5 months and resolved within 2–7 days while the patients remained on treatment. In one patient experiencing psychotic depression occurring within a month, symptoms resolved within 45 days while the patient continued treatment. A total of 13.3% of Keppra patients experienced other behavioral symptoms (reported as agitation, hostility, anxiety, apathy, emotional lability, depersonalization, depression, etc.) compared to 6.2% of placebo patients.

Approximately half of these patients reported these events within the first 4 weeks. A total of 1.7% of treated patients discontinued treatment due to these events, compared to 0.2% of placebo patients. The treatment dose was reduced in 0.8% of treated patients and in 0.5% of placebo patients. A total of 0.8% of treated patients had a serious behavioral event (compared to 0.2% of placebo patients) and were hospitalized.

In addition, 4 (0.5%) of treated patients attempted suicide compared to 0% of placebo patients. One of these patients successfully committed suicide. In the other 3 patients, the events did not lead to discontinuation or dose reduction. The events occurred after patients had been treated for between 4 weeks and 6 months.

Withdrawal Seizures Antiepileptic drugs, including Keppra, should be withdrawn gradually to minimize the potential of increased seizure frequency.

PRECAUTIONS

Hematologic Abnormalities Minor, but statistically significant, decreases compared to placebo in total mean RBC count (0.03×10^6/mm^2), mean hemoglobin (0.09 g/dL), and mean hematocrit (0.38%) were seen in Keppra treated patients in controlled trials.

A total of 3.2% of treated and 1.8% of placebo patients had at least one possibly significant ($\leq 2.8 \times 10^9$/L) decreased WBC, and 2.4% of treated and 1.4% of placebo patients had at least one possibly significant ($\leq 1.0 \times 10^9$/L) decreased neutrophil count. Of the treated patients with a low neutrophil count, all but one rose towards or to baseline with continued treatment. No patient was discontinued secondary to low neutrophil counts.

Hepatic Abnormalities There were no meaningful changes in mean liver function tests (LFT) in controlled trials; lesser LFT abnormalities were similar in drug and placebo treated patients in controlled trials (1.4%). No patients were discontinued from controlled trials for LFT abnormalities except for 1 (0.07%) epilepsy patient receiving open treatment.

Information For Patients Patients should be instructed to take Keppra only as prescribed.

Patients should be advised to notify their physician if they become pregnant or intend to become pregnant during therapy.

Patients should be advised that Keppra may cause dizziness and somnolence. Accordingly, patients should be advised not to drive or operate machinery or engage in other hazardous activities until they have gained sufficient experience on Keppra to gauge whether it adversely affects their performance of these activities.

Laboratory Tests Although most laboratory tests are not systematically altered with Keppra treatment, there have been relatively infrequent abnormalities seen in hematologic parameters and liver function tests.

Use in Patients With Impaired Renal Function Caution should be taken in dosing patients with moderate and severe renal impairment and patients undergoing hemodialysis. Dosage should be reduced in patients with impaired renal function receiving Keppra and supplemental doses should be given to patients after dialysis (see CLINICAL PHARMACOLOGY and DOSAGE AND ADMINISTRATION, Patients with Impaired Renal Function).

Drug Interactions *In vitro* data on metabolic interactions indicate that Keppra is unlikely to produce, or be subject to, pharmacokinetic interactions. Levetiracetam and its major metabolite, at concentrations well above C_{max} levels achieved within the therapeutic dose range, are neither inhibitors of nor high affinity substrates for human liver cytochrome P450 isoforms, epoxide hydrolase or UDP-glucuronidation enzymes. In addition, levetiracetam does not affect the *in vitro* glucuronidation of valproic acid.

Levetiracetam circulates largely unbound (<10% bound) to plasma proteins; clinically significant interactions with other drugs through competition for protein binding sites are therefore unlikely.

Potential pharmacokinetic interactions were assessed in clinical pharmacokinetic studies (phenytoin, warfarin, digoxin, oral contraceptive) and through pharmacokinetic screening in the placebo-controlled clinical studies in epilepsy patients.

Drug-Drug Interactions Between Keppra and Existing Antiepileptic Drugs (AEDs) Potential drug interactions between Keppra and existing AEDs (phenytoin, carbamazepine, valproic acid, phenobarbital, lamotrigine, gabapentin and primidone) were assessed by evaluating the serum concentrations of levetiracetam and these AEDs during placebo-controlled clinical studies. These data indicate that levetiracetam does not influence the plasma concentration of existing AEDs and that these AEDs do not influence the pharmacokinetics of levetiracetam.

Other Drug Interactions Oral Contraceptives Keppra (500 mg twice daily) did not influence the pharmacokinetics of an oral contraceptive containing 0.03 mg ethinyl estradiol and 0.15 mg levonorgestrel, or of the luteinizing hormone and progesterone levels, indicating that impairment of contraceptive efficacy is unlikely. Coadministration of this oral contraceptive did not influence the pharmacokinetics of levetiracetam.

Digoxin Keppra (1000 mg twice daily) did not influence the pharmacokinetics and pharmacodynamics (ECG) of digoxin given as a 0.25 mg dose every day. Coadministration of digoxin did not influence the pharmacokinetics of levetiracetam.

Warfarin Keppra (1000 mg twice daily) did not influence the pharmacokinetics of R and S warfarin. Prothrombin time was not affected by levetiracetam. Coadministration of warfarin did not affect the pharmacokinetics of levetiracetam.

Probenecid Probenecid, a renal tubular secretion blocking agent, administered at a dose of 500 mg four times a day, did not change the pharmacokinetics of levetiracetam 1000 mg twice daily. C^{ss}_{max} of the metabolite, ucb L057, was approximately doubled in the presence of probenecid while the fraction of drug excreted unchanged in the urine remained the same. Renal clearance of ucb L057 in the presence of probenecid decreased 60%, probably related to competitive inhibition of tubular secretion of ucb L057. The effect of Keppra on probenecid was not studied.

Carcinogenesis, Mutagenesis, Impairment of Fertility

Carcinogenesis Rats were dosed with levetiracetam in the diet for 104 weeks at doses of 50, 300 and 1800 mg/kg/day. The highest dose corresponds to 6 times the maximum recommended daily human dose (MRHD) of 3000 mg on a mg/m^2 basis and it also provided systemic exposure (AUC) approximately 6 times that achieved in humans receiving the MRHD. There was no evidence of carcinogenicity. A study was conducted in which mice received levetiracetam in the diet for 80 weeks at doses of 60, 240 and 960 mg/kg/day (high dose is equivalent to 2 times the MRHD on a mg/m^2 or exposure basis). Although no evidence for carcinogenicity was seen, the potential for a carcinogenic response has not been fully evaluated in that species because adequate doses have not been studied.

Mutagenesis Levetiracetam was not mutagenic in the Ames test or in mammalian cells *in vitro* in the Chinese hamster ovary/HGPRT locus assay. It was not clastogenic in an *in vitro* analysis of metaphase chromosomes obtained from Chinese hamster ovary cells or in an *in vivo* mouse micronucleus assay. The hydrolysis product and major human metabolite of levetiracetam (ucb L057) was not mutagenic in the Ames test or the *in vitro* mouse lymphoma assay.

Impairment of Fertility No adverse effects on male or female fertility or reproductive performance were observed in rats at doses up to 1800 mg/kg/day (approximately 6 times the maximum recommended human dose on a mg/m^2 or exposure basis).

Pregnancy

Pregnancy Category C In animal studies, levetiracetam produced evidence of developmental toxicity at doses similar to or greater than human therapeutic doses.

Administration to female rats throughout pregnancy and lactation was associated with increased incidences of minor fetal skeletal abnormalities and retarded offspring growth pre- and/or postnatally at doses ≥350 mg/kg/day (approximately equivalent to the maximum recommended human dose of 3000 mg [MRHD] on a mg/m^2 basis) and with increased pup mortality and offspring behavioral alterations at a dose of 1800 mg/kg/day (6 times the MRHD on a mg/m^2 basis). The developmental no effect dose was 70 mg/kg/day (0.2 times the MRHD on a mg/m^2 basis). There was no overt maternal toxicity at the doses used in this study.

Treatment of pregnant rabbits during the period of organogenesis resulted in increased embryofetal mortality and increased incidences of minor fetal skeletal abnormalities at doses ≥600 mg/kg/day (approximately 4 times MRHD on a mg/m^2 basis) and in decreased fetal weights and increased incidences of fetal malformations at a dose of 1800 mg/kg/day (12 times the MRHD on a mg/m^2 basis). The developmental no effect dose was 200 mg/kg/day (1.3 times the MRHD on a mg/m^2 basis). Maternal toxicity was also observed at 1800 mg/kg/day.

When pregnant rats were treated during the period of organogenesis, fetal weights were decreased and the incidence of fetal skeletal variations was increased at a dose of 3600 mg/kg/day (12 times the MRHD). 1200 mg/kg/day (4 times the MRHD) was a developmental no effect dose. There was no evidence of maternal toxicity in this study.

Treatment of rats during the last third of gestation and throughout lactation produced no adverse developmental or maternal effects at doses of up to 1800 mg/kg/day (6 times the MRHD on a mg/m^2 basis).

There are no adequate and well-controlled studies in pregnant women. Keppra should be used during pregnancy only if the potential benefit justifies the potential risk to the fetus.

Pregnancy Exposure Registry To facilitate monitoring fetal outcomes of pregnant women exposed to Keppra physicians are encouraged to register patients, before fetal outcome is known (e.g., ultrasound, results of aminocentesis, etc.), in the Antiepileptic Drug Pregnancy Registry by calling (888) 233-2334 (toll free).

Labor and Delivery The effect of Keppra on labor and delivery in humans is unknown.

Nursing Mothers It is not known whether this drug is excreted in human milk. Because many drugs are excreted in human milk, caution should be exercised when Keppra is administered to a nursing woman.

Pediatric Use Safety and effectiveness in patients below the age of 16 have not been established.

Geriatric Use Of the total number of subjects in clinical studies of levetiracetam, 347 were 65 and over. No overall differences in safety were observed between these subjects and younger subjects. There were insufficient numbers of elderly subjects in controlled trials of epilepsy to adequately assess the effectiveness of Keppra in these patients.

A study in 16 elderly subjects (age 61–88 years) with oral administration of single dose and multiple twice-daily doses for 10 days showed no pharmacokinetic differences related to age alone.

Levetiracetam is known to be substantially excreted by the kidney, and the risk of adverse reactions to this drug may be greater in patients with impaired renal function. Because elderly patients are more likely to have decreased renal function, care should be taken in dose selection, and it may be useful to monitor renal function.

Use in Patients With Impaired Renal Function Clearance of levetiracetam is decreased in patients with renal impairment and is correlated with creatinine clearance. The dosage should be reduced in patients with impaired renal function receiving Keppra and supplemental doses should be given to patients after dialysis (see DOSAGE AND ADMINISTRATION, Patients with Impaired Renal Function).

ADVERSE REACTIONS

In well-controlled clinical studies, the most frequently reported adverse events associated with the use of Keppra in combination with other AEDs, not seen at an equivalent frequency among placebo-treated patients, were somnolence, asthenia, infection and dizziness.

Table 4 lists treatment-emergent adverse events that occurred in at least 1% of patients with epilepsy treated with Keppra participating in placebo-controlled studies and were numerically more common in patients treated with Keppra than placebo. In these studies, either Keppra or placebo was added to concurrent AED therapy. Adverse events were usually mild to moderate in intensity.

The prescriber should be aware that these figures, obtained when Keppra was added to concurrent AED therapy, cannot be used to predict the frequency of adverse experiences in the course of usual medical practice where patient characteristics and other factors may differ from those prevailing during clinical studies. Similarly, the cited frequencies cannot be directly compared with figures obtained from other clinical investigations involving different treatments, uses, or investigators. An inspection of these frequencies, however, does provide the prescriber with one basis to estimate the relative contribution of drug and non-drug factors to the adverse event incidences in the population studied.

Table 4: Incidence (%) of Treatment-emergent Adverse Events in Placebo-controlled, Add-on Studies by Body System (Adverse Events Occurred in at Least 1% of Keppra-treated Patients and Occurred More Frequently than Placebo-treated Patients)

Body System/ Adverse Event	Keppra (N=769) %	Placebo (N=439) %
Body as a Whole		
Asthenia	15	9
Headache	14	13
Infection	13	8
Pain	7	6
Digestive System		
Anorexia	3	2
Nervous System		
Amnesia	2	1
Anxiety	2	1
Ataxia	3	1
Depression	4	2
Dizziness	9	4
Emotional Lability	2	0
Hostility	2	1
Nervousness	4	2
Paresthesia	2	1
Somnolence	15	8
Vertigo	3	1
Respiratory System		
Cough Increased	2	1
Pharyngitis	6	4
Rhinitis	4	3
Sinusitis	2	1
Special Senses		
Diplopia	2	1

Other events reported by 1% or more of patients treated with Keppra but as or more frequent in the placebo group were: abdominal pain, accidental injury, amblyopia, arthralgia, back pain, bronchitis, chest pain, confusion, constipation, convulsion, diarrhea, drug level increased, dyspepsia, ecchymosis, fever, flu syndrome, fungal infection, gastroenteritis, gingivitis, grand mal convulsion, insomnia, nausea, otitis media, rash, thinking abnormal, tremor, urinary tract infection, vomiting and weight gain.

Time Course of Onset of Adverse Events Of the most frequently reported adverse events, asthenia, somnolence and dizziness appeared to occur predominantly during the first 4 weeks of treatment with Keppra.

Discontinuation or Dose Reduction in Well-Controlled Clinical Studies In well-controlled clinical studies, 15.0% of patients receiving Keppra and 11.6% receiving placebo either discontinued or had a dose reduction as a result of an adverse event. The adverse events most commonly associated (>1%) with discontinuation or dose reduction in either treatment group are presented in Table 5.

$$CLcr = \frac{[140\text{-age (years)}] \times \text{weight (kg)}}{72 \times \text{serum creatinine (mg/dL)}} \quad (\times 0.85 \text{ for female patients})$$

Dosing Adjustment Regimen for Patients With Impaired Renal Function

Group	Creatinine Clearance (mL/min)	Dosage (mg)	Frequency
Normal	>80	500 to 1,500	Every 12 h
Mild	50 – 80	500 to 1,000	Every 12 h
Moderate	30 – 50	250 to 750	Every 12 h
Severe	< 30	250 to 500	Every 12 h
ESRD patients using dialysis	—	500 to 1,000	[1]Every 24 h

[1]Following dialysis, a 250 to 500 mg supplemental dose is recommended.

Table 5: Adverse Events Most Commonly Associated With Discontinuation or Dose Reduction in Placebo-controlled Studies in Patients With Epilepsy

	Number (%)	
	Keppra (N=769)	Placebo (N=439)
Asthenia	10 (1.3%)	3 (0.7%)
Convulsion	23 (3.0%)	15 (3.4%)
Dizziness	11 (1.4%)	0
Somnolence	34 (4.4%)	7 (1.6%)
Rash	0	5 (1.1%)

Comparison of Gender, Age and Race The overall adverse experience profile of Keppra was similar between females and males. There are insufficient data to support a statement regarding the distribution of adverse experience reports by age and race.

DRUG ABUSE AND DEPENDENCE

The abuse and dependence potential of Keppra has not been evaluated in human studies.

OVERDOSAGE

Signs, Symptoms and Laboratory Findings of Acute Overdosage in Humans The highest known dose of Keppra received in the clinical development program was 6000 mg/day. Other than drowsiness, there were no adverse events in the few known cases of overdose.

Treatment or Management of Overdose There is no specific antidote for overdose with Keppra. If indicated, elimination of unabsorbed drug should be attempted by emesis or gastric lavage; usual precautions should be observed to maintain airway. General supportive care of the patient is indicated including monitoring of vital signs and observation of the clinical status of patient. A Certified Poison Control Center should be contacted for up to date information on the management of overdose with Keppra.

Hemodialysis Standard hemodialysis procedures result in significant clearance of levetiracetam (approximately 50% in 4 hours) and should be considered in cases of overdose. Although hemodialysis has not been performed in the few known cases of overdose, it may be indicated by the patient's clinical state or in patients with significant renal impairment.

DOSAGE AND ADMINISTRATION

Keppra is indicated as adjunctive treatment of partial onset seizures in adults with epilepsy.

In clinical trials, daily doses of 1000 mg, 2000 mg and 3000 mg, given as twice a day dosing, were shown to be effective. Although in some studies there was a tendency toward greater response with higher dose (see CLINICAL STUDIES), a consistent increase in response with increased dose has not been shown.

Treatment should be initiated with a daily dose of 1000 mg/day, given as twice daily dosing (500 mg BID). Additional dosing increments may be given (1000 mg/day additional evey 2 weeks) to a maximum recommended daily dose of 3000 mg. Long term experience at doses greater than 3000 mg/day is relatively minimal, and there is no evidence that doses greater than 3000 mg/day confer additional benefit.

Keppra is given orally with or without food.

Patients With Impaired Renal Function Keppra dosing must be individualized according to the patient's renal function status. Recommended doses and adjustment for dose are shown in the Table below. To use this dosing table, an estimate of the patient's creatinine clearance (CLcr) in mL/min is needed. CLcr in mL/min may be estimated from serum creatinine (mg/dL) determination using the following formula:

[See first table above]

[See second table above]

HOW SUPPLIED

Keppra™ (levetiracetam) tablets, 250 mg are blue, oblong-shaped, scored, film-coated tablets debossed with "ucb" and "250" on one side. They are supplied in containers of 120 tablets (NDC 50474-591-40).

Keppra™ (levetiracetam) tablets, 500 mg are yellow, oblong-shaped, scored, film-coated tablets debossed with "ucb" and "500" on one side. They are supplied in containers of 120 tablets (NDC 50474-592-40).

Keppra™ (levetiracetam) tablets, 750 mg are orange, oblong-shaped, scored, film-coated tablets debossed with "ucb" and "750" on one side. They are supplied in containers of 120 tablets (NDC 50474-593-40.

Storage

Store at 25°C (77°F); excursions permitted to 15–30°C (59–86°F).

[see USP Controlled Room Temperature]

FOR MEDICAL INFORMATION

Contact: Medical Affairs Department
Phone: (800) 447-7877
Fax: (770) 803-2174
UCB Pharma, Inc.
Smyrna, GA 30080
Rev. 12/99

Shown in Product Identification Guide, page 339

LORTAB® 2.5/500 Tablets Ⓒ III
Hydrocodone Bitartrate and Acetaminophen Tablets, USP
2.5 mg/500 mg
Rev. 8/98

LORTAB® 5/500 Tablets Ⓒ III
Hydrocodone Bitartrate and Acetaminophen Tablets, USP
5 mg/500 mg
Rev. 2/99

LORTAB® 7.5/500 Tablets Ⓒ III
Hydrocodone Bitartrate and Acetaminophen Tablets, USP
7.5 mg/500 mg
Rev. 7/98

LORTAB® 10/500 Tablets Ⓒ III
Hydrocodone Bitartrate and Acetaminophen Tablets, USP
10 mg/500 mg
Rev. 1/99

LORTAB® Elixir Ⓒ III
Hydrocodone Bitartrate and Acetaminophen Elixir, 7.5 mg/500 mg per 15 mL
Rx only
Rev. 6/98

DESCRIPTION

Hydrocodone bitartrate and acetaminophen is supplied in tablet and liquid forms for oral administration.

WARNING: May be habit forming (see PRECAUTIONS, Information for Patients, and DRUG ABUSE AND DEPENDENCE).

Hydrocodone bitartrate is an opioid analgesic and antitussive and occurs as fine, white crystals or as a crystalline powder. It is affected by light. The chemical name is 4,5α-epoxy-3-methoxy-17-methylmorphinan-6-one tartrate (1:1) hydrate (2:5). It has the following structural formula:

$C_{18}H_{21}NO_3 \cdot C_4H_6O_6 \cdot 2\frac{1}{2}H_2O$ MW=494.50

Acetaminophen, 4'-hydroxyacetanilide, a slightly bitter, white, odorless, crystalline powder, is a non-opiate, non-salicylate analgesic and antipyretic. It has the following structural formula:

CH_3CONH–⟨benzene ring⟩–OH

$C_8H_9NO_2$ MW=151.17

Continued on next page

Lortab—Cont.

Each Lortab 2.5/500 contains:

Hydrocodone Bitartrate	2.5 mg
Acetaminophen	500 mg

In addition, each tablet contains the following inactive ingredients: colloidal silicon dioxide, croscarmellose sodium, crospovidone, microcrystalline cellulose, povidone, pregelatinized starch, stearic acid and sugar spheres which are composed of starch derived from corn, sucrose, and FD&C Red #3.

Each Lortab 5/500 contains:

Hydrocodone Bitartrate	5 mg
Acetaminophen	500 mg

In addition, each tablet contains the following inactive ingredients: corn starch, FD&C Blue #1 Lake, gelatin, magnesium stearate, microcrystalline cellulose, povidone, pregelatinized starch, sodium starch glycolate, and sugar spheres.

Each Lortab 7.5/500 contains:

Hydrocodone Bitartrate	7.5 mg
Acetaminophen	500 mg

In addition, each tablet contains the following inactive ingredients: colloidal silicon dioxide, croscarmellose sodium, crospovidone, microcrystalline cellulose, povidone, pregelatinized starch, stearic acid, and sugar spheres which are composed of starch derived from corn, sucrose, FD&C Blue #1 and D&C Yellow #10.

Each Lortab 10/500 tablet contains:

Hydrocodone Bitartrate	10 mg
Acetaminophen	500 mg

In addition, each tablet contains the following inactive ingredients: D&C Red No. 27 Aluminum Lake, D&C Red No. 30 Aluminum Lake, colloidal silicon dioxide, croscarmellose sodium, crospovidone, microcrystalline cellulose, povidone, pregelatinized starch, starch (corn), and stearic acid.

Lortab Elixir contains:	Per 5 mL	Per 15 mL
Hydrocodone Bitartrate	2.5 mg	7.5 mg
Acetaminophen	167 mg	500 mg
Alcohol	7%	7%

In addition, the liquid contains the following inactive ingredients: citric acid anhydrous, ethyl maltol, glycerin, methyl paraben, propylene glycol, propylparaben, purified water, saccharin sodium, sorbitol solution, sucrose, with D&C Yellow #10 and FD&C Yellow #6 as coloring and natural and artificial flavoring.

CLINICAL PHARMACOLOGY

Hydrocodone is a semisynthetic narcotic analgesic and antitussive with multiple actions qualitatively similar to those of codeine. Most of these involve the central nervous system and smooth muscle. The precise mechanism of action of hydrocodone and other opiates is not known, although it is believed to relate to the existence of opiate receptors in the central nervous system. In addition to analgesia, narcotics may produce drowsiness, changes in mood and mental clouding.

The analgesic action of acetaminophen involves peripheral influences, but the specific mechanism is as yet undetermined. Antipyretic activity is mediated through hypothalamic heat regulating centers. Acetaminophen inhibits prostaglandin synthetase. Therapeutic doses of acetaminophen have negligible effects on the cardiovascular or respiratory systems; however, toxic doses may cause circulatory failure and rapid, shallow breathing.

Pharmacokinetics: The behavior of the individual components is described below.

Hydrocodone: Following a 10 mg oral dose of hydrocodone administered to five adult male subjects, the mean peak concentration was 23.6 ± 5.2 ng/mL. Maximum serum levels were achieved at 1.3 ± 0.3 hours and the half-life was determined to be 3.8 ± 0.3 hours. Hydrocodone exhibits a complex pattern of metabolism including O-demethylation, N-demethylation and 6-keto reduction to the corresponding 6-α- and 6-β- hydroxymetabolites.

See OVERDOSAGE for toxicity information.

Acetaminophen: Acetaminophen is rapidly absorbed from the gastrointestinal tract and is distributed throughout most body tissues. The plasma half-life is 1.25 to 3 hours, but may be increased by liver damage and following overdosage. Elimination of acetaminophen is principally by liver metabolism (conjugation) and subsequent renal execretion of metabolites. Approximately 85% of an oral dose appears in the urine within 24 hours of administration, most as the glucuronide conjugate, with small amounts of other conjugates and unchanged drug.

See OVERDOSAGE for toxicity information.

INDICATIONS AND USAGE

Lortab Tablets & Elixir are indicated for the relief of moderate to moderately severe pain.

CONTRAINDICATIONS

This product should not be administered to patients who have previously exhibited hypersensitivity to hydrocodone or acetaminophen.

WARNINGS

Respiratory Depression: At high doses or in sensitive patients, hydrocodone may produce dose-related respiratory depression by acting directly on the brain stem respiratory center. Hydrocodone also affects the center that controls respiratory rhythm, and may produce irregular and periodic breathing.

Head Injury and Increased Intracranial Pressure: The respiratory depressant effects of narcotics and their capacity to elevate cerebrospinal fluid pressure may be markedly exaggerated in the presence of head injury, other intracranial lesions or a preexisting increase in intracranial pressure. Furthermore, narcotics produce adverse reactions which may obscure the clinical course of patients with head injuries.

Acute Abdominal Conditions: The administration of narcotics may obscure the diagnosis or clinical course of patients with acute abdominal conditions.

PRECAUTIONS

General: Special Risk Patients: As with any narcotic analgesic agent, Lortab Tablets & Elixir should be used with caution in elderly or debilitated patients, and those with severe impairment of hepatic or renal function, hypothyroidism, Addison's disease, prostatic hypertrophy or urethral stricture. The usual precautions should be observed and the possibility of respiratory depression should be kept in mind.

Cough Reflex: Hydrocodone suppresses the cough reflex; as with all narcotics, caution should be exercised when Lortab Tablets or Elixir are used postoperatively and in patients with pulmonary disease.

Information for Patients: Hydrocodone, like all narcotics, may impair the mental and/or physical abilities required for the performance of potentially hazardous tasks such as driving a car or operating machinery; patients should be cautioned accordingly.

Alcohol and other CNS depressants may produce an additive CNS depression, when taken with this combination product, and should be avoided.

Hydrocodone may be habit-forming. Patients should take the drug only for as long as it is prescribed, in the amounts prescribed, and no more frequently than prescribed.

Laboratory Tests: In patients with severe hepatic or renal disease, effects of therapy should be monitored with serial liver and/or renal function tests.

Drug Interactions: Patients receiving narcotics, antihistamines, antipsychotics, antianxiety agents, or other CNS depressants (including alcohol) concomitantly with hydrocodone bitartrate and acetaminophen tablets or elixir may exhibit an additive CNS depression. When combined therapy is contemplated, the dose of one or both agents should be reduced.

The use of MAO inhibitors or tricyclic antidepressants with hydrocodone preparations may increase the effect of either the antidepressant or hydrocodone.

Drug/Laboratory Test Interactions: Acetaminophen may produce false-positive test results for urinary 5-hydroxyindoleacetic acid.

Carcinogenesis, Mutagenesis, Impairment of Fertility: No adequate studies have been conducted in animals to determine whether hydrocodone or acetaminophen have a potential for carcinogenesis, mutagenesis, or impairment of fertility.

Pregnancy:

Teratogenic Effects: Pregnancy Category C: There are no adequate and well-controlled studies in pregnant women. Lortab Tablets or Elixir should be used during pregnancy only if the potential benefit justifies the potential risk to the fetus.

Nonteratogenic Effects: Babies born to mothers who have been taking opioids regularly prior to delivery will be physically dependent. The withdrawal signs include irritability and excessive crying, tremors, hyperactive reflexes, increased respiratory rate, increased stools, sneezing, yawning, vomiting, and fever. The intensity of the syndrome does not always correlate with the duration of maternal opioid use or dose. There is no consensus on the best method of managing withdrawal.

Labor and Delivery: As with all narcotics, administration of this product to the mother shortly before delivery may result in some degree of respiratory depression in the newborn, especially if higher doses are used.

Nursing Mothers: Acetaminophen is excreted in breast milk in small amounts, but the significance of its effects on nursing infants is not known. It is not known whether hydrocodone is excreted in human milk. Because many drugs are excreted in human milk and because of the potential for serious adverse reactions in nursing infants from hydrocodone and acetaminophen, a decision should be made whether to discontinue nursing or to discontinue the drug, taking into account the importance of the drug to the mother.

Pediatric Use: Safety and effectiveness in the pediatric population have not been established.

ADVERSE REACTIONS

The most frequently reported adverse reactions are lightheadedness, dizziness, sedation, nausea and vomiting. These effects seem to be more prominent in ambulatory than in non-ambulatory patients, and some of these adverse reactions may be alleviated if the patient lies down.

Other adverse reactions include:

Central Nervous System: Drowsiness, mental clouding, lethargy, impairment of mental and physical performance, anxiety, fear, dysphoria, psychic dependence, mood changes.

Gastrointestinal System: Prolonged administration of Lortab Tablets or Elixir may produce constipation.

Genitourinary System: Ureteral spasm, spasm of vesical sphincters and urinary retention have been reported with opiates.

Respiratory Depression: Hydrocodone bitartrate may produce dose-related respiratory depression by acting directly on brain stem respiratory centers (see OVERDOSAGE).

Dermatological: Skin rash, pruritus.

The following adverse drug events may be borne in mind as potential effects of acetaminophen: allergic reactions, rash, thrombocytopenia, agranulocytosis.

Potential effects of high dosage are listed in the OVERDOSAGE section.

DRUG ABUSE AND DEPENDENCE

Controlled Substance: Lortab Tablets & Elixir are classified as Schedule III controlled substances.

Abuse and Dependence: Psychic dependence, physical dependence, and tolerance may develop upon repeated administration of narcotics; therefore, this product should be prescribed and administered with caution. However, psychic dependence is unlikely to develop when hydrocodone bitartrate and acetaminophen tablets or elixir are used for a short time for the treatment of pain.

Physical dependence, the condition in which continued administration of the drug is required to prevent the appearance of a withdrawal syndrome, assumes clinically significant proportions only after several weeks of continued narcotic use, although some mild degree of physical dependence may develop after a few days of narcotic therapy. Tolerance, in which increasingly large doses are required in order to produce the same degree of analgesia, is manifested initially by a shortened duration of analgesic effect, and subsequently by decreases in the intensity of analgesia. The rate of development of tolerance varies among patients.

OVERDOSAGE

Following an acute overdosage, toxicity may result from hydrocodone or acetaminophen.

Signs and Symptoms:

Hydrocodone: Serious overdose with hydrocodone is characterized by respiratory depression (a decrease in respiratory rate and/or tidal volume, Cheyne-Stokes respiration, cyanosis), extreme somnolence progressing to stupor or coma, skeletal muscle flaccidity, cold and clammy skin, and sometimes bradycardia and hypotension. In severe overdosage, apnea, circulatory collapse, cardiac arrest and death may occur.

Acetaminophen: In acetaminophen overdosage: dose-dependent, potentially fatal hepatic necrosis is the most serious adverse effect. Renal tubular necrosis, hypoglycemic coma, and thrombocytopenia may also occur.

Early symptoms following a potentially hepatotoxic overdose may include: nausea, vomiting, diaphoresis and general malaise. Clinical and laboratory evidence of hepatic toxicity may not be apparent until 48 to 72 hours post-ingestion.

In adults, hepatic toxicity has rarely been reported with acute overdoses of less than 10 grams or fatalities with less than 15 grams.

Treatment: A single or multiple overdose with hydrocodone and acetaminophen is a potentially lethal polydrug overdose, and consultation with a regional poison control center is recommended.

Immediate treatment includes support of cardiorespiratory function and measures to reduce drug absorption. Vomiting should be induced mechanically, or with syrup of ipecac, if the patient is alert (adequate pharyngeal and laryngeal reflexes). Oral activated charcoal (1 g/kg) should follow gastric emptying. The first dose should be accompanied by an appropriate cathartic. If repeated doses are used, the cathartic might be included with alternate doses as required. Hypotension is usually hypovolemic and should respond to fluids. Vasopressors and other supportive measures should be employed as indicated. A cuffed endo-tracheal tube should be inserted before gastric lavage of the unconscious patient and, when necessary, to provide assisted respiration.

Meticulous attention should be given to maintaining adequate pulmonary ventilation. In severe cases of intoxication, peritoneal dialysis, or preferably hemodialysis may be considered. If hypoprothrombinemia occurs due to acetaminophen overdose, vitamin K should be administered intravenously.

Naloxone, a narcotic antagonist, can reverse respiratory depression and coma associated with opioid overdose. Naloxone hydrochloride 0.4 mg to 2 mg is given parenterally. Since the duration of action of hydrocodone may exceed that of the naloxone, the patient should be kept under continuous surveillance and repeated doses of the antagonist should be administered as needed to maintain adequate respiration. A narcotic antagonist should not be administered in the absence of clinically significant respiratory or cardiovascular depression.

If the dose of acetaminophen may have exceeded 140 mg/kg, acetylcysteine should be administered as early as possible. Serum acetaminophen levels should be obtained, since levels four or more hours following ingestion help predict acetaminophen toxicity. Do not await acetaminophen assay results before initiating treatment. Hepatic enzymes should be obtained initially, and repeated at 24-hour intervals.

Methemoglobinemia over 30% should be treated with methylene blue by slow intravenous administration.

The toxic dose for adults for acetaminophen is 10 g.

DOSAGE AND ADMINISTRATION

Dosage should be adjusted according to severity of pain and response of the patient. However, it should be kept in mind that tolerance to hydrocodone can develop with continued use and that the incidence of untoward effects is dose related.

The usual adult dosage for LORTAB® 2.5/500 tablets is one or two tablets every four to six hours as needed for pain. The total daily dosage should not exceed 8 tablets.

The usual adult dosage for LORTAB® 5/500 tablets is one or two tablets every four to six hours as needed for pain. The total daily dosage should not exceed 8 tablets.

The usual adult dosage for LORTAB® 7.5/500 tablets is one tablet every four to six hours as needed for pain. The total daily dosage should not exceed 6 tablets.

The usual adult dosage for LORTAB® 10/500 tablets is one tablet every four to six hours as needed for pain. The total daily dosage should not exceed 6 tablets.

The usual adult dosage for LORTAB® ELIXIR is one tablespoonful (15 mL) every four to six hours as needed for pain. The total daily dosage should not exceed 6 tablespoonfuls.

HOW SUPPLIED

LORTAB® 2.5/500 (Hydrocodone Bitartrate and Acetaminophen Tablets, USP 2.5 mg/500 mg) contain hydrocodone bitartrate 2.5 mg and acetaminophen 500 mg. They are supplied as white with pink specks, capsule-shaped, bisected tablets, debossed "ucb" on one side and "901" on the other side, in containers of 100 tablets NDC 50474-925-01.

LORTAB® 5/500 (Hydrocodone Bitartrate and Acetaminophen Tablets, USP 5 mg/500 mg) contain hydrocodone bitartrate 5 mg and acetaminophen 500 mg. They are supplied as white with blue specks, capsule-shaped, bisected tablets, debossed "ucb" on one side and "902" on the other side, in containers of 100 tablets NDC 50474-902-01, in containers of 500 tablets NDC 50474-902-50, and in hospital unit-dose packages of 100 tablets [4×25] NDC 50474-902-60.

LORTAB® 7.5/500 (Hydrocodone Bitartrate and Acetaminophen Tablets, USP 7.5 mg/500 mg) contain hydrocodone bitartrate 7.5 mg and acetaminophen 500 mg. They are supplied as white with green specks, capsule-shaped, bisected tablets, debossed "ucb" on one side and "903" on the other side, in containers of 100 tablets NDC 50474-907-01, in containers of 500 tablets NDC 50474-907-50, and in hospital unit-dose packages of 100 tablets [4×25] NDC 50474-907-60.

Lortab® 10/500 (Hydrocodone Bitartrate and Acetaminophen Tablets, USP 10 mg/500 mg) contain hydrocodone bitartrate 10 mg and acetaminophen 500 mg. They are supplied as pink, capsule-shaped, bisected tablets, debossed "ucb" one one side and "910" on the other side, in containers of 100 tablets NDC 50474-910-01, 500 tablets NDC 50474-910-50, and in hospital unit-dose packages of 100 tablets [4×25] NDC 50474-910-60.

LORTAB® Elixir (Hydrocodone Bitartrate and Acetaminophen Elixir, 7.5mg/500 mg per 15 mL) is a yellow-colored, tropical fruit punch flavored liquid containing hydrocodone bitartrate 7.5 mg and acetaminophen 500 mg per 15 mL, with 7% alcohol. It is supplied in containers of 1 pint (473 mL) NDC 50474-909-16.

Storage: Store at controlled room temperature, 15°–30°C (59°–86°F).

Dispense in a tight, light-resistant container with a child-resistant closure.

A Schedule CIII Narcotic

Manufactured for:
UCB PHARMA, INC.
Smyrna, GA 30080
Lortab® 2.5/500, Lortab® 7.5/500, Lortab® Elixir
Manufactured by:
Mikart, Inc.
Atlanta, GA 30318
Lortab® 5/500, Lortab® 10/500
Manufactured by:
Mallinckrodt Inc
Hobart, NY 13788

8/00

Shown in Product Identification Guide, page 339

THEO-24® ℞

(theophylline anhydrous)
Extended-release capsules 100, 200, 300, & 400 mg

DESCRIPTION

Theophylline

Theophylline is structurally classified as a methylxanthine. It occurs as a white, odorless, crystalline powder with a bitter taste. Anhydrous theophylline has the chemical name 1H-Purine-2,6-dione,3,7-dihydro-1,3-dimethyl-, and is represented by the following structural formula:

CH3, O, H, N, N, O, N, N, CH3

The molecular formula of anhydrous theophylline is $C_7H_8N_4O_2$ with a molecular weight of 180.17.

Theo-24® is available as capsules intended for oral administration, containing 100 mg, 200 mg, 300 mg, or 400 mg of anhydrous theophylline per capsule, in an extended-release formulation which allows a 24-hour dosing interval for appropriate patients.

Inactive ingredients are edible ink (which contains synthetic black iron oxide, FD&C Blue No. 1, FD&C Blue No. 2, FD&C Yellow No. 6, D&C Yellow No. 10, FD&C Red No. 40), ethylcellulose, gelatin, pharmaceutical glaze, colloidal silicon dioxide, starch, sucrose, talc, titanium dioxide, and coloring agents: 100 mg—includes FD&C Yellow No. 6; 200 mg—FD&C Red No. 3 and D&C Yellow No. 10; 300 mg—FD&C Blue No.1 and FD&C Red No. 40; 400 mg—FD&C Red No. 40 and D&C Red No. 28.

Theo-24 Extended-release capsules meet Drug Release Test 6 as published in the USP 23 monograph for Theophylline Extended-release Capsules.

CLINICAL PHARMACOLOGY

Mechanism of Action;

Theophylline has two distinct actions in the airways of patients with reversible obstruction: smooth muscle relaxation (i.e., bronchodilation) and suppression of the response of the airways to stimuli (i.e., non-bronchodilator prophylactic effects). While the mechanisms of action of theophylline are not known with certainty, studies in animals suggest that bronchodilation is mediated by the inhibition of two isozymes of phosphodiesterase (PDE III and, to a lesser extent, PDE IV) while non-bronchodilator prophylactic actions are probably mediated through one or more different molecular mechanisms that do not involve inhibition of PDE III or antagonism of adenosine receptors. Some of the adverse effects associated with theophylline appear to be mediated by inhibition of PDE III (e.g., hypotension, tachycardia, headache, and emesis) and adenosine receptor antagonism (e.g., alterations in cerebral blood flow).

Theophylline increases the force of contraction of diaphragmatic muscles. This action appears to be due to enhancement of calcium uptake through an adenosine-mediated channel.

Serum Concentration-Effect Relationship:

Bronchodilation occurs over the serum theophylline concentration range of 5–20 mcg/mL. Clinically important improvement in symptom control has been found in most studies to require peak serum theophylline concentrations >10 mcg/mL, but patients with mild disease may benefit from lower concentrations. At serum theophylline concentrations >20 mcg/mL, both the frequency and severity of adverse reactions increase. In general, maintaining peak serum theophylline concentrations between 10 and 15 mcg/mL will achieve most of the drug's potential therapeutic benefit while minimizing the risk of serious adverse events.

Pharmacokinetics:

Overview Theophylline is rapidly and completely absorbed after oral administration in solution or immediate-release solid oral dose form. Theophylline does not undergo any appreciable pre-systemic elimination, distributes freely into fat-free tissues and is extensively metabolized in the liver.

The pharmacokinetics of theophylline vary widely among similar patients and cannot be predicted by age, sex, body weight or other demographic characteristics. In addition, certain concurrent illnesses and alterations in normal physiology (see Table I) and co-administration of other drugs (see Table II) can significantly alter the pharmacokinetic characteristics of theophylline. Within-subject variability in metabolism has also been reported in some studies, especially in acutely ill patients. It is, therefore, recommended that serum theophylline concentrations be measured frequently in acutely ill patients (e.g., at 24-hr intervals) and periodically in patients receiving long-term therapy, e.g., at 6–12 month intervals. More frequent measurements should be made in the presence of any condition that may significantly alter theophylline clearance (see PRECAUTIONS, Laboratory Tests).

[See table above]

Table I. Mean and range of total body clearance and half-life of theophylline related to age and altered physiological states.¶

Population characteristics		Total body clearance* mean (range)†† (mL/kg/min)	Half-life mean (range)††, (hr)
Age			
Premature neonates			
postnatal age 3–15 days		0.29 (0.09–0.49)	30 (17–43)
postnatal age 25–57 days		0.64 (0.04–1.2)	20 (9.4–30.6)
Term infants			
postnatal age 1–2 days		NR†	25.7 (25–26.5)
postnatal age 3–30 weeks		NR†	11 (6–29)
Children			
1–4 years		1.7 (0.5–2.9)	3.4 (1.2–5.6)
4–12 years		1.6 (0.8–2.4)	NR†
13–15 years		0.9 (0.48–1.3)	NR†
6–17 years		1.4 (0.2–2.6)	3.7 (1.5–5.9)
Adults (16–60 years)			
otherwise healthy non-smoking asthmatics		0.65 (0.27–1.03)	8.7 (6.1–12.8)
Elderly (>60 years)			
non-smokers with normal cardiac, liver, and renal function		0.41 (0.21–0.61)	9.8 (1.6–18)
Concurrent illness or altered physiological state			
Acute pulmonary edema		0.33** (0.07–2.45)	19** (3.1–82)
COPD>60 years, stable non-smoker >1 year		0.54 (0.44–0.64)	11 (9.4–12.6)
COPD with cor-pulmonale		0.48 (0.08–0.88)	NR†
Cystic fibrosis (14–28 years)		1.25 (0.31–2.2)	6.0 (1.8–10.2)
Fever associated with acute viral respiratory illness (children 9–15 years)		NR†	7.0 (1.0–13)
Liver disease -	cirrhosis	0.31** (0.1–0.7)	32** (10–56)
	acute hepatitis	0.35 (0.25–0.45)	19.2 (16.6–21.8)
	cholestasis	0.65 (0.25–1.45)	14.4 (5.7–31.8)
Pregnancy -	1st trimester	NR†	8.5 (3.1–13.9)
	2nd trimester	NR†	8.8 (3.8–13.8)
	3rd trimester	NR†	13.0 (8.4–17.6)
Sepsis with multi-organ failure		0.47 (0.19–1.9)	18.8 (6.3–24.1)
Thyroid disease -	hypothyroid	0.38 (0.13–0.57)	11.6 (8.2–25)
	hyperthyroid	0.8 (0.68–0.97)	4.5 (3.7–5.6)

¶ For various North American patient populations from literature reports. Different rates of elimination and consequent dosage requirements have been observed among other peoples.
* Clearance represents the volume of blood completely cleared of theophylline by the liver in one minute. Values listed were generally determined at serum theophylline concentrations <20 mcg/mL; clearance may decrease and half-life may increase at higher serum concentrations due to non-linear pharmacokinetics.
†† Reported range or estimated range (mean ± 2 SD) where actual range not reported.
† NR = not reported or not reported in a comparable format.
** Median

Note: In addition to the factors listed above, theophylline clearance is increased and half-life decreased by low carbohydrate/high protein diets, parenteral nutrition, and daily consumption of charcoal-broiled beef. A high carbohydrate/low protein diet can decrease the clearance and prolong the half-life of theophylline.

Absorption Theophylline is rapidly and completely absorbed after oral administration in solution or immediate-release solid oral dosage form. After a single immediate-release dose of 5 mg/kg in adults, a mean peak serum concentration of about 10 mcg/mL (range 5–15 mcg/mL) can be expected 1–2 hr after dose. Co-administration of theophylline with food or antacids does not cause clinically significant changes in the absorption of theophylline from immediate-release dosage forms.

Theo-24 capsules contain hundreds of coated beads of theophylline. Each bead is an individual extended-release delivery system. After dissolution of the capsules these beads are released and distributed in the gastrointestinal tract, thus minimizing the probability of high local concentrations of theophylline at any particular site.

In a 6-day multiple-dose study involving 18 subjects (with theophylline clearance rates between 0.57 and 1.02 mL/kg/min) who had fasted overnight and 2 hours after morning

Continued on next page

Theo-24—Cont.

dosing, Theo-24 given once daily in a dose of 1500 mg produced serum theophylline levels that ranged between 5.7 mcg/mL and 22 mcg/mL. The mean minimum and maximum values were 11.6 mcg/mL and 18.1 mcg/mL, respectively, with an average peak-trough difference of 6.5 mcg/mL. The mean percent fluctuation $[(C_{max}-C_{min}/C_{min})\times100]$ equals 80%. A 24-hour single-dose study demonstrated an approximately proportional increase in serum levels as the dose was increased from 600 to 1500 mg.

Taking Theo-24 with a high-fat-content meal may result in a significant increase in the peak serum level and in the extent of absorption of theophylline as compared to administration in the fasted state (see PRECAUTIONS, Drug/Food Interactions).

Following the single-dose administration (8 mg/kg) of Theo-24 to 20 normal subjects who had fasted overnight and 2 hours after morning dosing, peak serum theophylline concentrations of 4.8 ± 1.5 (SD) mcg/mL were obtained at 13.3 ± 4.7 (SD) hours. The amount of the dose absorbed was approximately 13% at 3 hours, 31% at 6 hours, 55% at 12 hours, 70% at 16 hours, and 88% at 24 hours. The extent of theophylline bioavailability from Theo-24 was comparable to the most widely used 12-hour extended-release product when both products were administered every 12 hours.

Distribution Once theophylline enters the systemic circulation, about 40% is bound to plasma protein, primarily albumin. Unbound theophylline distributes throughout body water, but distributes poorly into body fat. The apparent volume of distribution of theophylline is approximately 0.45 L/kg (range 0.3–0.7 L/kg) based on ideal body weight. Theophylline passes freely across the placenta, into breast milk and into the cerebrospinal fluid (CSF). Saliva theophylline concentrations approximate unbound serum concentrations, but are not reliable for routine or therapeutic monitoring unless special techniques are used. An increase in the volume of distribution of theophylline, primarily due to reduction in plasma protein binding, occurs in premature neonates, patients with hepatic cirrhosis, uncorrected acidemia, the elderly and in women during the third trimester of pregnancy. In such cases, the patient may show signs of toxicity at total (bound + unbound) serum concentrations of theophylline in the therapeutic range (10–20 mcg/mL) due to elevated concentrations of the pharmacologically active unbound drug. Similarly, a patient with decreased theophylline binding may have a sub-therapeutic total drug concentration while the pharmacologically active unbound concentration is in the therapeutic range. If only total serum theophylline concentration is measured, this may lead to an unnecessary and potentially dangerous dose increase. In patients with reduced protein binding, measurement of unbound serum theophylline concentration provides a more reliable means of dosage adjustment than measurement of total serum theophylline concentration. Generally, concentrations of unbound theophylline should be maintained in the range of 6–12 mcg/mL.

Metabolism Following oral dosing, theophylline does not undergo any measurable first-pass elimination. In adults and children beyond one year of age, approximately 90% of the dose is metabolized in the liver. Biotransformation takes place through demethylation to 1-methylxanthine and 3-methylxanthine and hydroxylation to 1,3-dimethyluric acid. 1-methylxanthine is further hydroxylated, by xanthine oxidase, to 1-methyluric acid. About 6% of a theophylline dose is N-methylated to caffeine. Theophylline demethylation to 3-methylxanthine is catalyzed by cytochrome P-450 1A2, while cytochromes P-450 2E1 and P-450 3A3 catalyze the hydroxylation to 1,3-dimethyluric acid. Demethylation to 1-methylxanthine appears to be catalyzed either by cytochrome P-450 1A2 or a closely related cytochrome. In neonates, the N-demethylation pathway is absent while the function of the hydroxylation pathway is markedly deficient. The activity of these pathways slowly increases to maximal levels by one year of age.

Caffeine and 3-methylxanthine are the only theophylline metabolites with pharmacologic activity. 3–methylxanthine has approximately one tenth the pharmacologic activity of theophylline and serum concentrations in adults with normal renal function are <1 mcg/mL. In patients with end-stage renal disease, 3-methylxanthine may accumulate to concentrations that approximate the unmetabolized theophylline concentration. Caffeine concentrations are usually undetectable in adults regardless of renal function. In neonates, caffeine may accumulate to concentrations that approximate the unmetabolized theophylline concentration and thus, exert a pharmacologic effect.

Both the N-demethylation and hydroxylation pathways of theophylline biotransformation are capacity-limited. Due to the wide intersubject variability of the rate of theophylline metabolism, non-linearity of elimination may begin in some patients at serum theophylline concentrations <10 mcg/mL. Since this non-linearity results in more than proportional changes in serum theophylline concentrations with changes in dose, it is advisable to make increases or decreases in dose in small increments in order to achieve desired changes in serum theophylline concentrations (see DOSAGE AND ADMINISTRATION, Table VI). Accurate prediction of dose-dependency of theophylline metabolism in patients *a priori* is not possible, but patients with very high initial clearance rates (i.e., low steady state serum theophylline concentrations at above average doses) have the greatest likelihood of experiencing large changes in serum theophylline concentration in response to dosage changes.

Excretion In neonates, approximately 50% of the theophylline dose is excreted unchanged in the urine. Beyond the first three months of life, approximately 10% of the theophylline dose is excreted unchanged in the urine. The remainder is excreted in the urine mainly as 1,3-dimethyluric acid (35-40%), 1-methyluric acid (20-25%) and 3-methylxanthine (15-20%). Since little theophylline is excreted unchanged in the urine and since active metabolites of theophylline (i.e., caffeine, 3-methylxanthine) do not accumulate to clinically significant levels even in the face of end-stage renal disease, no dosage adjustment for renal insufficiency is necessary in adults and children >3 months of age. In contrast, the large fraction of the theophylline dose excreted in the urine as unchanged theophylline and caffeine in neonates requires careful attention to dose reduction and frequent monitoring of serum theophylline concentrations in neonates with reduced renal function (See WARNINGS).

Serum concentrations at Steady State After multiple doses of theophylline, steady state is reached in 30–65 hours (average 40 hours) in adults. At steady state, on a dosage regimen with 6-hour intervals, the expected mean trough concentration is approximately 60% of the mean peak concentration, assuming a mean theophylline half-life of 8 hours. The difference between peak and trough concentrations is larger in patients with more rapid theophylline clearance. In patients with high theophylline clearance and half-lives of about 4–5 hours, such as children age 1 to 9 years, the trough serum theophylline concentration may be only 30% of peak with a 6-hour dosing interval. In these patients a slow release formulation would allow a longer dosing interval (8–12 hours) with a smaller peak/trough difference.

Special Populations (See Table I for mean clearance and half-life values)

Geriatric The clearance of theophylline is decreased by an average of 30% in healthy elderly adults (>60 years) compared to healthy young adults. Careful attention to dose reduction and frequent monitoring of serum theophylline concentrations are required in elderly patients (see WARNINGS).

Pediatrics The clearance of theophylline is very low in neonates (see WARNINGS). Theophylline clearance reaches maximal values by one year of age, remains relatively constant until about 9 years of age and then slowly decreases by approximately 50% to adult values at about age 16. Renal excretion of unchanged theophylline in neonates amounts to about 50% of the dose, compared to about 10% in children older than three months and in adults. Careful attention to dosage selection and monitoring of serum theophylline concentrations are required in pediatric patients (see WARNINGS and DOSAGE AND ADMINISTRATION).

Gender Gender differences in theophylline clearance are relatively small and unlikely to be of clinical significance. Significant reduction in theophylline clearance, however, has been reported in women on the 20th day of the menstrual cycle and during the third trimester of pregnancy.

Race Pharmacokinetic differences in theophylline clearance due to race have not been studied.

Renal Insufficiency Only a small fraction, e.g., about 10% of the administered theophylline dose is excreted unchanged in the urine of children greater than three months of age and adults. Since little theophylline is excreted unchanged in the urine and since active metabolites of theophylline (i.e., caffeine, 3-methylxanthine) do not accumulate to clinically significant levels even in the face of end-stage renal disease, no dosage adjustment for renal insufficiency is necessary in adults and children >3 months of age. In contrast, approximately 50% of the administered theophylline dose is excreted unchanged in the urine in neonates. Careful attention to dose reduction and frequent monitoring of serum theophylline concentrations are required in neonates with decreased renal function (see WARNINGS).

Hepatic Insufficiency Theophylline clearance is decreased by 50% or more in patients with hepatic insufficiency (e.g., cirrhosis, acute hepatitis, cholestasis). Careful attention to dose reduction and frequent monitoring of serum theophylline concentrations are required in patients with reduced hepatic function (see WARNINGS).

Congestive Heart Failure (CHF) Theophylline clearance is decreased by 50% or more in patients with CHF. The extent of reduction in theophylline clearance in patients with CHF appears to be directly correlated to the severity of the cardiac disease. Since theophylline clearance is independent of liver blood flow, the reduction in clearance appears to be due to impaired hepatocyte function rather than reduced perfusion. Careful attention to dose reduction and frequent monitoring of serum theophylline concentrations are required in patients with CHF (see WARNINGS).

Smokers Tobacco and marijuana smoking appears to increase the clearance of theophylline by induction of metabolic pathways. Theophylline clearance has been shown to increase by approximately 50% in young adult tobacco smokers and by approximately 80% in elderly tobacco smokers compared to non-smoking subjects. Passive smoke exposure has also been shown to increase theophylline clearance by up to 50%. Abstinence from tobacco smoking for one week causes a reduction of approximately 40% in theophylline clearance. Careful attention to dose reduction and frequent monitoring of serum theophylline concentrations are required in patients who stop smoking (see WARNINGS). Use of nicotine gum has been shown to have no effect on theophylline clearance.

Fever Fever, regardless of its underlying cause, can decrease the clearance of theophylline. The magnitude and duration of the fever appear to be directly correlated to the degree of decrease of theophylline clearance. Precise data are lacking, but a temperature of 39°C (102°F) for at least 24 hours is probably required to produce a clinically significant increase in serum theophylline concentrations. Children with rapid rates of theophylline clearance (i.e., those who require a dose that is substantially larger than average [e.g., >22 mg/kg/day] to achieve a therapeutic peak serum theophylline concentration when afebrile) may be at greater risk of toxic effects from decreased clearance during sustained fever. Careful attention to dose reduction and frequent monitoring of serum theophylline concentrations are required in patients with sustained fever (see WARNINGS).

Miscellaneous

Other factors associated with decreased theophylline clearance include the third trimester of pregnancy, sepsis with multiple organ failure, and hypothyroidism. Careful attention to dose reduction and frequent monitoring of serum theophylline concentrations are required in patients with any of these conditions (see WARNINGS). Other factors associated with increased theophylline clearance include hyperthyroidism and cystic fibrosis.

Clinical Studies:

In patients with chronic asthma, including patients with severe asthma requiring inhaled corticosteroids or alternate-day oral corticosteroids, many clinical studies have shown that theophylline decreases the frequency and severity of symptoms, including nocturnal exacerbations, and decreases the "as needed" use of inhaled $beta_2$ agonists. Theophylline has also been shown to reduce the need for short courses of daily oral prednisone to relieve exacerbations of airway obstruction that are unresponsive to bronchodilators in asthmatics.

In patients with chronic obstructive pulmonary disease (COPD), clinical studies have shown that theophylline decreases dyspnea, air trapping, the work of breathing, and improves contractility of diaphragmatic muscles with little or no improvement in pulmonary function measurements.

INDICATIONS AND USAGE

Theophylline is indicated for the treatment of the symptoms and reversible airflow obstruction associated with chronic asthma and other chronic lung diseases, e.g., emphysema and chronic bronchitis.

CONTRAINDICATIONS

Theo-24 is contraindicated in patients with a history of hypersensitivity to theophylline or other components in the product.

WARNINGS

Concurrent Illness:

Theophylline should be used with extreme caution in patients with the following clinical conditions due to the increased risk of exacerbation of the concurrent condition:

Active peptic ulcer disease
Seizure disorders
Cardiac arrhythmias (not including bradyarrhythmias)

Conditions That Reduce Theophylline Clearance:

There are several readily indentifiable causes of reduced theophylline clearance. ***If the total daily dose is not appropriately reduced in the presence of these risk factors, severe and potentially fatal theophylline toxicity can occur.*** Careful consideration must be given to the benefits and risks of theophylline use and the need for more intensive monitoring of serum theophylline concentrations in patients with the following risk factors:

Age

Neonates (term and premature)
Children <1 year
Elderly (>60 years)

Concurrent Diseases

Acute pulmonary edema
Congestive heart failure
Cor-pulmonale
Fever; ≥102°F for 24 hours or more; or lesser temperature elevations for longer periods
Hypothyroidism
Liver disease; cirrhosis, acute hepatitis
Reduced renal function in infants <3 months of age
Sepsis with multi-organ failure
Shock

Cessation of Smoking

Drug Interactions Adding a drug that inhibits theophylline metabolism (e.g., cimetidine, erythromycin, tacrine) or stopping a concurrently administered drug that enhances theophylline metabolism (e.g., carbamazepine, rifampin). (see PRECAUTIONS, Drug Interactions, Table II).

When Signs or Symptoms of Theophylline Toxicity Are Present:

Whenever a patient receiving theophylline develops nausea or vomiting, particularly repetitive vomiting, or other signs or symptoms consistent with theophylline toxicity (even if another cause may be suspected), additional doses of theophylline should be withheld and a serum theophylline concentration measured immediately. Patients should be instructed not to continue any dosage that causes adverse effects and to withhold subsequent doses until the symptoms have resolved, at which time the clinician may instruct the patient to resume the drug at a lower dosage (see DOSAGE AND ADMINISTRATION, Dosing Guidelines, Table VI).

Table II. Clinically significant drug interactions with theophylline*.

Drug	Type of Interaction	Effect**
Adenosine	Theophylline blocks adenosine receptors.	Higher doses of adenosine may be required to achieve desired effect.
Alcohol	A single large dose of alcohol (3 mL/kg of whiskey) decreases theophylline clearance for up to 24 hours.	30% increase
Allopurinol	Decreases theophylline clearance at allopurinol doses ≥600 mg/day.	25% increase
Aminoglutethimide	Increases theophylline clearance by induction of microsomal enzyme activity.	25% decrease
Carbamazepine	Similar to aminoglutethimide.	30% decrease
Cimetidine	Decreases theophylline clearance by inhibiting cytochrome P450 1A2.	70% increase
Ciprofloxacin	Similar to cimetidine.	40% increase
Clarithomycin	Similar to erythromycin.	25% increase
Diazepam	Benzodiazepines increase CNS concentrations of adenosine, a potent CNS depressant, while theophylline blocks adenosine receptors.	Larger diazepam doses may be required to produce desired level of sedation. Discontinuation of theophylline without reduction of diazepam dose may result in respiratory depression.
Disulfiram	Decreases theophylline clearance by inhibiting hydroxylation and demethylation.	50% increase
Enoxacin	Similar to cimetidine.	300% increase
Ephedrine	Synergistic CNS effects	Increased frequency of nausea, nervousness, and insomnia.
Erythromycin	Erythromycin metabolite decreases theophylline clearance by inhibiting cytochrome P450 3A3.	35% increase. Erythromycin steady-state serum concentrations decrease by a similar amount.
Estrogen	Estrogen containing oral contraceptives decrease theophylline clearance in a dose-dependent fashion. The effect of progesterone on theophylline clearance is unknown.	30% increase
Flurazepam	Similar to diazepam.	Similar to diazepam.
Fluvoxamine	Similar to cimetidine	Similar to cimetidine
Halothane	Halothane sensitizes the myocardium to catecholamines, theophylline increases release of endogenous catecholamines.	Increased risk of ventricular arrhythmias.
Interferon, human recombinant alpha-A	Decreases theophylline clearance.	100% increase
Isoproterenol (IV)	Increases theophylline clearance.	20% decrease

(Continued on next page)

Dosage Increases:
Increases in the dose of theophylline should not be made in response to an acute exacerbation of symptoms of chronic lung disease since theophylline provides little added benefit to inhaled beta$_2$-selective agonists and systemically administered corticosteroids in this circumstance and increases the risk of adverse effects. A peak steady-state serum theophylline concentration should be measured before increasing the dose in response to persistent chronic symptoms to ascertain whether an increase in dose is safe. Before increasing the theophylline dose on the basis of a low serum concentration, the clinician should consider whether the blood sample was obtained at an appropriate time in relationship to the dose and whether the patient has adhered to the prescribed regimen (see PRECAUTIONS, Laboratory Tests).
As the rate of theophylline clearance may be dose-dependent (i.e., steady-state serum concentrations may increase disproportionately to the increase in dose), an increase in dose based upon a sub-therapeutic serum concentration measurement should be conservative. In general, limiting dose increases to about 25% of the previous total daily dose will reduce the risk of unintended excessive increases in serum theophylline concentration (see DOSAGE AND ADMINISTRATION, Table VI).

PRECAUTIONS

General:
Careful consideration of the various interacting drugs and physiologic conditions that can alter theophylline clearance and require dosage adjustment should occur prior to initiation of theophylline therapy, prior to increases in theophylline dose, and during follow up (see WARNINGS). The dose of theophylline selected for initiation of therapy should be low and, ***if tolerated***, increased slowly over a period of a week or longer with the final dose guided by monitoring serum theophylline concentrations and the patient's clinical response (see DOSAGE AND ADMINISTRATION, Table V).
Monitoring Serum Theophylline Concentrations:
Serum theophylline concentration measurements are readily available and should be used to determine whether the dosage is appropriate. Specifically, the serum theophylline concentration should be measured as follows:

1. When initiating therapy to guide final dosage adjustment after titration.
2. Before making a dose increase to determine whether the serum concentration is sub-therapeutic in a patient who continues to be symptomatic.
3. Whenever signs or symptoms of theophylline toxicity are present.
4. Whenever there is a new illness, worsening of a chronic illness or a change in the patient's treatment regimen that may alter theophylline clearance (e.g., fever >102°F sustained for ≥24 hours, hepatitis, or drugs listed in Table II are added or discontinued).

To guide a dose increase, the blood sample should be obtained at the time of the expected peak serum theophylline concentration; 12 hours after a dose at steady-state (expected peak serum theophylline concentration range is between 5–15 mcg/mL). For most patients, steady-state will be reached after 3 days of dosing when no doses have been missed, no extra doses have been added, and none of the doses have been taken at unequal intervals. A trough concentration (i.e., at the end of the dosing interval) provides no additional useful information and may lead to an inappropriate dose increase since the peak serum theophylline concentration can be two or more times greater than the trough concentration with an extended-release formulation. If the serum sample is drawn more or less than twelve (12) hours after the dose, the results must be interpreted with caution since the concentration may not be reflective of the peak concentration. In contrast, when signs or symptoms of theophylline toxicity are present, the serum sample should be obtained as soon as possible, analyzed immediately, and the result reported to the clinician without delay. In patients in whom decreased serum protein binding is suspected (e.g., cirrhosis, women during the third trimester of pregnancy), the concentration of unbound theophylline should be measured and the dosage adjusted to achieve an unbound concentration of 6-12 mcg/mL.
Saliva concentrations of theophylline cannot be used reliably to adjust dosage without special techniques.
Effects on Laboratory Tests:
As a result of its pharmacological effects, theophylline at serum concentrations within the 10–20 mcg/mL range modestly increases plasma glucose (from a mean of 88 mg% to 98 mg%), uric acid (from a mean of 4 mg/dL to 6 mg/dL), free fatty acids (from a mean of 451 µEq/L to 800 µEq/L, total cholesterol (from a mean of 140 vs 160 mg/dL), HDL (from a mean of 36 to 50 mg/dL), HDL/LDL ratio (from a mean of 0.5 to 0.7), and urinary free cortisol excretion (from a mean of 44 to 63 mcg/24 hr). Theophylline at serum concentrations within the 10–20 mcg/mL range may also transiently decrease serum concentrations of triiodothyronine (144 before, 131 after one week and 142 ng/dL after 4 weeks of theophylline). The clinical importance of these changes should be weighed against the potential therapeutic benefit of theophylline in individual patients.
Information for Patients:
The patient (or parent/care giver) should be instructed to seek medical advice whenever nausea, vomiting, persistent headache, insomnia or rapid heart beat occurs during treatment with theophylline, even if another cause is suspected. The patient should be instructed to contact their clinician if they develop a new illness, especially if accompanied by a persistent fever, if they experience worsening of a chronic illness, if they start or stop smoking cigarettes or marijuana, or if another clinician adds a new medication or discontinues a previously prescribed medication. Patients should be instructed to inform all clinicians involved in their care that they are taking theophylline, especially when a medication is being added or deleted from their treatment. Patients should be instructed to not alter the dose, timing of the dose, or frequency of administration without first consulting their clinician. If a dose is missed, the patient should be instructed to take the next dose at the usually scheduled time and to not attempt to make up for the missed dose.
Patients should be instructed to take this medication each morning at approximately the same time and not to exceed the prescribed dose.
Patients who require a relatively high dose of theophylline should be informed of important considerations relating to time of drug administration and meal content (see PRECAUTIONS, Drug/Food Interactions, and DOSAGE AND ADMINISTRATION).
Drug Interactions:
Drug/Drug Interactions Theophylline interacts with a wide variety of drugs. The interaction may be pharmacodynamic, i.e., alterations in the therapeutic response to theophylline or another drug or occurrence of adverse effects without a change in serum theophylline concentration. More frequently, however, the interaction is pharmacokinetic, i.e., the rate of theophylline clearance is altered by another drug resulting in increased or decreased serum theophylline concentrations. Theophylline only rarely alters the pharmacokinetics of other drugs.
The drugs listed in Table II have the potential to produce clinically significant pharmacodynamic or pharmacokinetic interactions with theophylline. The information in the "Effect" column of Table II assumes that the interacting drug is being added to a steady-state theophylline regimen. If theophylline is being initiated in a patient who is already taking a drug that inhibits theophylline clearance (e.g., cimetidine, erythromycin), the dose of theophylline required to achieve a therapeutic serum theophylline concentration will be smaller. Conversely, if theophylline is being initiated in a patient who is already taking a drug that enhances theophylline clearance (e.g., rifampin), the dose of theophylline required to achieve a therapeutic serum theophylline concentration will be larger. Discontinuation of a concomitant drug that increases theophylline clearance will result in accumulation of theophylline to potentially toxic levels, unless the theophylline dose is appropriately reduced. Discontinuation of a concomitant drug that inhibits theophylline clearance will result in decreased serum theophylline concentrations, unless the theophylline dose is appropriately increased.
The drugs listed in Table III have either been documented not to interact with theophylline or do not produce a clinically significant interaction (i.e., <15% change in theophylline clearance).
The listing of drugs in Tables II and III are current as of January 2, 1996. New interactions are continuously being reported for theophylline, especially with new chemical entities. **The clinician should not assume that a drug does not interact with theophylline if it is not listed in Table II.** Before addition of a newly available drug in a patient receiving theophylline, the package insert of the new drug and/or the medical literature should be consulted to determine if an interaction between the new drug and theophylline has been reported.
[See table above]
[See table at top of next page]

Table III. Drugs that have been documented not to interact with theophylline or drugs that produce no clinically significant interaction with theophylline.*

albuterol,
 systemic and inhaled
amoxicillin
ampicillin,
 with or without sulbactam
atenolol
azithromycin
caffeine,
 dietary ingestion
cefaclor
co-trimoxazole
 (trimethoprim and sulfamethoxazole)
diltiazem
dirithomycin
enflurane
famotidine
felodipine
finasteride
hydrocortisone
lomefloxacin
mebendazole
medroxyprogesterone
methylprednisolone
metronidazole
metoprolol
nadolol
nifedipine
nizatidine
norfloxacin
ofloxacin
omeprazole
prednisone, prednisolone
ranitidine
rifabutin
roxithromycin
sorbitol
 (purgative doses do not inhibit theophylline absorption)

Continued on next page

Theo-24—Cont.

isoflurane	sucralfate
isoniazid	terbutaline, systemic
isradipine	terfenadine
influenza vaccine	tetracycline
ketoconazole	tocainide

* **Refer to PRECAUTIONS, Drug Interactions for information regarding table.**

Drug/Food Interactions Taking Theo-24 less than one hour before a high-fat-content meal, such as 8 oz whole milk, 2 fried eggs, 2 bacon strips, 2 oz hashed brown potatoes, and 2 slices of buttered toast (about 985 calories, including approximately 71 g of fat) may result in a significant increase in peak serum level and in the extent of absorption of theophylline as compared to administration in the fasted state. In some cases (especially with doses of 900 mg or more taken less than one hour before a high-fat-content meal) serum theophylline levels may exceed the 20 mcg/mL level, above which theophylline toxicity is more likely to occur.

The Effect of Other Drugs on Theophylline Serum Concentration Measurements:
Most serum theophylline assays in clinical use are immunoassays which are specific for theophylline. Other xanthines such as caffeine, dyphylline, and pentoxifylline are not detected by these assays. Some drugs (e.g., cefazolin, cephalothin), however, may interfere with certain HPLC techniques. Caffeine and xanthine metabolites in neonates or patients with renal dysfunction may cause the reading from some dry reagent office methods to be higher than the actual serum theophylline concentration.

Carcinogenesis, Mutagenesis, and Impairment of Fertility:
Long term carcinogenicity studies have been carried out in mice (oral doses 30–150 mg/kg) and rats (oral doses 5–75 mg/kg). Results are pending.
Theophylline has been studied in Ames salmonella, *in vivo* and *in vitro* cytogenetics, micronucleus and Chinese hamster ovary test systems and has not been shown to be genotoxic.
In a 14 week continuous breeding study, theophylline, administered to mating pairs of B6C3F$_1$ mice at oral doses of 120, 270 and 500 mg/kg (approximately 1.0–3.0 times the human dose on a mg/m^2 basis) impaired fertility, as evidenced by decreases in the number of live pups per litter, decreases in the mean number of litters per fertile pair, and increases in the gestation period at the high dose as well as decreases in the proportion of pups born alive at the mid and high dose. In 13 week toxicity studies, theophylline was administered to F344 rats and B6C3F$_1$ mice at oral doses of 40–300 mg/kg (approximately 2.0 times the human dose on a mg/m^2 basis). At the high dose, systemic toxicity was observed in both species including decreases in testicular weight.

Pregnancy:
CATEGORY C: There are no adequate and well controlled studies in pregnant women. Additionally, there are no teratogenicity studies in non-rodents (e.g., rabbits). Theophylline was not shown to be teratogenic in CD-1 mice at oral doses up to 400 mg/kg, approximately 2.0 times the human dose on a mg/m^2 basis or in CD-1 rats at oral doses up to 260 mg/kg, approximately 3.0 times the recommended human dose on a mg/m^2 basis. At a dose of 220 mg/kg, embryotoxicity was observed in rats in the absence of maternal toxicity.

Nursing Mothers:
Theophylline is excreted into breast milk and may cause irritability or other signs of mild toxicity in nursing human infants. The concentration of theophylline in breast milk is about equivalent to the maternal serum concentration. An infant ingesting a liter of breast milk containing 10–20 mcg/mL of theophylline a day is likely to receive 10–20 mg of theophylline per day. Serious adverse effects in the infant are unlikely unless the mother has toxic serum theophylline concentrations.

Pediatric Use:
Theophylline is safe and effective for the approved indications in pediatric patients (See, INDICATIONS AND USAGE). The maintenance dose of theophylline must be selected with caution in pediatric patients since the rate of theophylline clearance is highly variable across the age range of neonates to adolescents (see CLINICAL PHARMACOLOGY, Table I, WARNINGS, and DOSAGE AND ADMINISTRATION, Table V). Due to the immaturity of theophylline metabolic pathways in infants under the age of one year, particular attention to dosage selection and frequent monitoring of serum theophylline concentrations are required when theophylline is prescribed to pediatric patients in this group.

Geriatric Use:
Elderly patients are at significantly greater risk of experiencing serious toxicity from theophylline than younger patients due to pharmacokinetic and pharmacodynamic changes associated with aging. Theophylline clearance is reduced in patients greater than 60 years of age, resulting in increased serum theophylline concentrations in response to a given theophylline dose. Protein binding may be decreased in the elderly resulting in a larger proportion of the total serum theophylline concentration in the pharmacologically active unbound form. Elderly patients also appear to be more sensitive to the toxic effects of theophylline after chronic overdosage than younger patients. For these reasons, the maximum daily dose of theophylline in patients greater than 60 years of age ordinarily should not exceed 400 mg/day unless the patient continues to be symptomatic and the peak steady state serum theophylline concentration is <10 mcg/mL (see DOSAGE AND ADMINISTRATION). Theophylline doses greater than 400 mg/day should be prescribed with caution in elderly patients.

Table II. Clinically significant drug interactions with theophylline*. (Continued)

Drug	Type of Interaction	Effect**
Ketamine	Pharmacologic	May lower theophylline seizure threshold.
Lithium	Theophylline increases renal lithium clearance.	Lithium dose required to achieve a therapeutic serum concentration increased an average of 60%.
Lorazepam	Similar to diazepam.	Similar to diazepam.
Methotrexate (MTX)	Decreases theophylline clearance.	20% increase after low dose MTX, higher dose MTX may have a greater effect.
Mexiletine	Similar to disulfiram.	80% increase
Midazolam	Similar to diazepam.	Similar to diazepam.
Moricizine	Increases theophylline clearance.	25% decrease
Pancuronium	Theophylline may antagonize non-depolarizing neuromuscular blocking effects; possibly due to phosphodiesterase inhibition.	Larger dose of pancuronium may be required to achieve neuromuscular blockade.
Pentoxifylline	Decreases theophylline clearance.	30% increase
Phenobarbital (PB)	Similar to aminoglutethimide.	25% decrease after two weeks of concurrent PB.
Phenytoin	Phenytoin increases theophylline clearance by increasing microsomal enzyme activity. Theophylline decreases phenytoin absorption.	Serum theophylline and phenytoin concentrations decrease about 40%.
Propafenone	Decreases theophylline clearance and pharmacologic interaction.	40% increase. Beta$_2$ blocking effect may decrease efficacy of theophylline.
Propranolol	Similar to cimetidine and pharmacologic interaction.	100% increase. Beta$_2$ blocking effect may decrease efficacy of theophylline.
Rifampin	Increases theophylline clearance by increasing cytochrome P450 1A2 and 3A3 activity.	20–40% decrease
Sulfinpyrazone	Increases theophylline clearance by increasing demethylation and hydroxylation. Decreases renal clearance of theophylline.	20% decrease
Tacrine	Similar to cimetidine, also increases renal clearance of theophylline.	90% increase
Thiabendazole	Decreases theophylline clearance.	190% increase
Ticlopidine	Decreases theophylline clearance.	60% increase
Troleandomycin	Similar to erythromycin.	33–100% increase depending on troleandomycin dose.
Verapamil	Similar to disulfiram.	20% increase

* **Refer to PRECAUTIONS, Drug Interactions for further information regarding table.**
** **Average effect on steady-state theophylline concentration or other clinical effect for pharmacologic interactions. Individual patients may experience larger changes in serum theophylline concentration than the value listed.**

ADVERSE REACTIONS

Adverse reactions associated with theophylline are generally mild when peak serum theophylline concentrations are <20 mcg/mL and mainly consist of transient caffeine-like adverse effects such as nausea, vomiting, headache, and insomnia. When peak serum theophylline concentrations exceed 20 mcg/mL, however, theophylline produces a wide range of adverse reactions including persistent vomiting, cardiac arrhythmias, and intractable seizures which can be lethal (see OVERDOSE). The transient caffeine-like adverse reactions occur in about 50% of patients when theophylline therapy is initiated at doses higher than recommended initial doses (e.g., >300 mg/day in adults and >12 mg/kg/day in children beyond 1 year of age). During the initiation of theophylline therapy, caffeine-like adverse effects may transiently alter patient behavior, especially in school age children, but this response rarely persists. Initiation of theophylline therapy at a low dose with subsequent slow titration to a predetermined age-related maximum dose will significantly reduce the frequency of these transient adverse effects (see DOSAGE AND ADMINISTRATION, Table V). In a small percentage of patients (<3% of children and <10% of adults) the caffeine-like adverse effects persist during maintenance therapy, even at peak serum theophylline concentrations within the therapeutic range (i.e., 10–20 mcg/mL). Dosage reduction may alleviate the caffeine-like adverse effects in these patients, however, persistent adverse effects should result in a reevaluation of the need for continued theophylline therapy and the potential therapeutic benefit of alternative treatment.
Other adverse reactions that have been reported at serum theophylline concentrations <20 mcg/mL include diarrhea, irritability, restlessness, fine skeletal muscle tremors, and transient diuresis. In patients with hypoxia secondary to COPD, multifocal atrial tachycardia and flutter have been reported at serum theophylline concentrations ≥15 mcg/mL. There have been a few isolated reports of seizures at serum theophylline concentrations <20 mcg/mL in patients with an underlying neurological disease or in elderly patients. The occurrence of seizures in elderly patients with serum theophylline concentrations <20 mcg/mL may be secondary to decreased protein binding resulting in a larger proportion of the total serum theophylline concentration in the pharmacologically active unbound form. The clinical characteristics of the seizures reported in patients with serum theophylline concentrations <20 mcg/mL have generally been milder than seizures associated with excessive serum theophylline concentrations resulting from an overdose (i.e., they have generally been transient, often stopped without anticonvulsant therapy, and did not result in neurological residua).

Table IV. Manifestations of theophylline toxicity.*

	Percentage of patients reported with sign or symptom			
	Acute Overdose (Large Single Ingestion)		Chronic Overdosage (Multiple Excessive Doses)	
Sign/Symptom	Study 1 (n=157)	Study 2 (n=14)	Study 1 (n=92)	Study 2 (n=102)
Asymptomatic	NR**	0	NR**	6
Gastrointestinal				
Vomiting	73	93	30	61
Abdominal Pain	NR**	21	NR**	12
Diarrhea	NR**	0	NR**	14
Hematemesis	NR**	0	NR**	2
Metabolic/Other				
Hypokalemia	85	79	44	43
Hyperglycemia	98	NR**	18	NR**
Acid/base disturbance	34	21	9	5
Rhabdomyolysis	NR**	7	NR**	0
Cardiovascular				
Sinus tachycardia	100	86	100	62
Other supraventricular tachycardias	2	21	12	14
Ventricular premature beats	3	21	10	19
Atrial fibrillation or flutter	1	NR**	12	NR**
Multifocal atrial tachycardia	0	NR**	2	NR**

Ventricular arrythmias with hemodynamic instability	7	14	40	0
Hypotension/shock	NR**	21	NR**	8
Neurologic				
Nervousness	NR**	64	NR**	21
Tremors	38	29	16	14
Disorientation	NR**	7	NR**	11
Seizures	5	14	14	5
Death	3	21	10	4

* These data are derived from two studies in patients with serum theophylline concentrations >30 mcg/mL. In the first study (Study #1—Shanon, Ann Intern Med 1993; 119:1161–67), data were prospectively collected from 249 consecutive cases of theophylline toxicity referred to a regional poison center for consultation. In the second study (Study #2—Sessler, Am J Med 1990;88:567–76), data were retrospectively collected from 116 cases with serum theophylline concentrations >30 mcg/mL among 6000 blood samples obtained for measurement of serum theophylline concentrations in three emergency departments. Differences in the incidence of manifestations of theophylline toxicity between the two studies may reflect sample selection as a result of study design (e.g., in Study #1, 48% of the patients had acute intoxications versus only 10% in Study #2) and different methods of reporting results.

** NR = Not reported in a comparable manner.

OVERDOSAGE

General:

The chronicity and pattern of theophylline overdosage significantly influences clinical manifestations of toxicity, management and outcome. There are two common presentations: *(1) acute overdose*, i.e., ingestion of a single large excessive dose (>10 mg/kg) as occurs in the context of an attempted suicide or isolated medication error, and *(2) chronic overdosage*, i.e., ingestion of repeated doses that are excessive for the patient's rate of theophylline clearance. The most common causes of chronic theophylline overdosage include patient or care giver error in dosing, clinician prescribing of an excessive dose or a normal dose in the presence of factors known to decrease the rate of theophylline clearance, and increasing the dose in response to an exacerbation of symptoms without first measuring the serum theophylline concentration to determine whether a dose increase is safe.

Severe toxicity from theophylline overdose is a relatively rare event. In one health maintenance organization, the frequency of hospital admissions for chronic overdosage of theophylline was about 1 per 1000 person-years exposure. In another study, among 6000 blood samples obtained for measurement of serum theophylline concentration, for any reason, from patients treated in an emergency department, 7% were in the 20-30 mcg/mL range and 3% were >30 mcg/mL. Approximately two-thirds of the patients with serum theophylline concentrations in the 20-30 mcg/mL range had one or more manifestations of toxicity while >90% of patients with serum theophylline concentrations >30 mcg/mL were clinically intoxicated. Similarly, in other reports, serious toxicity from theophylline is seen principally at serum concentrations >30 mcg/mL.

Several studies have described the clinical manifestations of theophylline overdose and attempted to determine the factors that predict life-threatening toxicity. In general, patients who experience an acute overdose are less likely to experience seizures than patients who have experienced a chronic overdosage, unless the peak serum theophylline concentration is >100 mcg/mL. After a chronic overdosage, generalized seizures, life-threatening cardiac arrhythmias, and death may occur at serum theophylline concentrations >30 mcg/mL. The severity of toxicity after chronic overdosage is more strongly correlated with the patient's age than the peak serum theophylline concentration; patients >60 years are at the greatest risk for severe toxicity and mortality after a chronic overdosage. Pre-existing or concurrent disease may also significantly increase the susceptibility of a patient to a particular toxic manifestation, e.g., patients with neurologic disorders have an increased risk of seizures and patients with cardiac disease have an increased risk of cardiac arrhythmias for a given serum theophylline concentration compared to patients without the underlying disease.

The frequency of various reported manifestations of theophylline overdose according to the mode of overdose are listed in Table IV.

Other manifestations of theophylline toxicity include increases in serum calcium, creatine kinase, myoglobin and leukocyte count, decreases in serum phosphate and magnesium, acute myocardial infarction, and urinary retention in men with obstructive uropathy.

Seizures associated with serum theophylline concentrations >30 mcg/mL are often resistant to anticonvulsant therapy and may result in irreversible brain injury if not rapidly controlled. Death from theophylline toxicity is most often secondary to cardiorespiratory arrest and/or hypoxic encephalopathy following prolonged generalized seizures or intractable cardiac arrhythmias causing hemodynamic compromise.

Overdose Management:

General Recommendations for Patients with Symptoms of Theophylline Overdose or Serum Theophylline Concentrations >30 mcg/mL (Note: Serum theophylline concentrations may continue to increase after presentation of the patient for medical care.

1. While simultaneously instituting treatment, contact a regional poison center to obtain updated information and advice on individualizing the recommendations that follow.
2. Institute supportive care, including establishment of intravenous access, maintenance of the airway, and electrocardiographic monitoring.
3. Treatment of seizures Because of the high morbidity and mortality associated with theophylline-induced seizures, treatment should be rapid and aggressive. Anticonvulsant therapy should be initiated with an intravenous benzodiazepine, e.g., diazepam, in increments of 0.1-0.2 mg/kg every 1-3 minutes until seizures are terminated. Repetitive seizures should be treated with a loading dose of phenobarbital (20 mg/kg infused over 30-60 minutes). Case reports of theophylline overdose in humans and animal studies suggest that phenytoin is ineffective in terminating theophylline-induced seizures. The doses of benzodiazepines and phenobarbital required to terminate theophylline-induced seizures are close to the doses that may cause severe respiratory depression or respiratory arrest; the clinician should therefore be prepared to provide assisted ventilation. Elderly patients and patients with COPD may be more susceptible to the respiratory depressant effects of anticonvulsants. Barbiturate-induced coma or administration of general anesthesia may be required to terminate repetitive seizures or status epilepticus. General anesthesia should be used with caution in patients with theophylline overdose because fluorinated volatile anesthetics may sensitize the myocardium to endogenous catecholamines released by theophylline. Enflurane appears less likely to be associated with this effect than halothane and may, therefore, be safer. Neuromuscular blocking agents alone should not be used to terminate seizures since they abolish the musculoskeletal manifestations without terminating seizure activity in the brain.
4. Anticipate need for anticonvulsants In patients with theophylline overdose who are at a high risk for theophylline-induced seizures, e.g., patients with acute overdoses and serum theophylline concentrations >100 mcg/mL or chronic overdosage in patients >60 years of age with serum theophylline concentrations >30 mcg/mL, the need for anticonvulsant therapy should be anticipated. A benzodiazepine such as diazepam should be drawn into a syringe and kept at the patient's bedside and medical personnel qualified to treat seizures should be immediately available. In selected patients at high risk for theophylline-induced seizures, consideration should be given to the administration of prophylactic anticonvulsant therapy. Situations where prophylactic anticonvulsant therapy should be considered in high risk patients include anticipated delays in instituting methods for extracorporeal removal of theophylline (e.g., transfer of a high risk patient from one health care facility to another for extracorporeal removal) and clinical circumstances that significantly interfere with efforts to enhance theophylline clearance (e.g., a neonate where dialysis may not be technically feasible or a patient with vomiting unresponsive to antiemetics who is unable to tolerate multiple-dose oral activated charcoal). In animal studies, prophylactic administration of phenobarbital, but not phenytoin, has been shown to delay the onset of theophylline-induced generalized seizures and to increase the dose of theophylline required to induce seizures (i.e., markedly increases the LD_{50}). Although there are no controlled studies in humans, a loading dose of intravenous phenobarbital (20 mg/kg infused over 60 minutes) may delay or prevent life-threatening seizures in high risk patients while efforts to enhance theophylline clearance are continued. Phenobarbital may cause respiratory depression, particularly in elderly patients and patients with COPD.
5. Treatment of cardiac arrhythmias Sinus tachycardia and simple ventricular premature beats are not harbingers of life-threatening arrhythmias, they do not require treatment in the absence of hemodynamic compromise, and they resolve with declining serum theophylline concentrations. Other arrhythmias, especially those associated with hemodynamic compromise, should be treated with antiarrhythmic therapy appropriate for the type of arrhythmia.
6. Gastrointestinal decontamination Oral activated charcoal (0.5 g/kg up to 20 g and repeat at least once 1-2 hours after the first dose) is extremely effective in blocking the absorption of theophylline throughout the gastrointestinal tract, even when administered several hours after ingestion. If the patient is vomiting, the charcoal should be administered through a nasogastric tube or after administration of an antiemetic. Phenothiazine antiemetics such as prochlorperazine or perphenazine should be avoided since they can lower the seizure threshold and frequently cause dystonic reactions. A single dose of sorbitol may be used to promote stooling to facilitate removal of theophylline bound to charcoal from the gastrointestinal tract. Sorbitol, however, should be dosed with caution since it is a potent purgative which can cause profound fluid and electrolyte abnormalities, particularly after multiple doses. Commercially available fixed combinations of liquid charcoal and sorbitol should be avoided in young children and after the first dose in adolescents and adults since they do not allow for individualization of charcoal and sorbitol dosing. Ipecac syrup should be avoided in theophylline overdoses. Although ipecac induces emesis, it does not reduce the absorption of theophylline unless administered within 5 minutes of ingestion and even then is less effective than oral activated charcoal. Moreover, ipecac-induced emesis may persist for several hours after a single dose and significantly decrease the retention and the effectiveness of oral activated charcoal.
7. Serum theophylline concentration monitoring The serum theophylline concentration should be measured immediately upon presentation, 2-4 hours later, and then at sufficient intervals, e.g., every 4 hours, to guide treatment decisions and to assess the effectiveness of therapy. Serum theophylline concentrations may continue to increase after presentation of the patient for medical care as a result of continued absorption of theophylline from the gastrointestinal tract. Serial monitoring of serum theophylline concentrations should be continued until it is clear that the concentration is no longer rising and has returned to non-toxic levels.
8. General monitoring procedures Electrocardiographic monitoring should be initiated on presentation and continued until the serum theophylline level has returned to a non-toxic level. Serum electrolytes and glucose should be measured on presentation and at appropriate intervals indicated by clinical circumstances. Fluid and electrolyte abnormalities should be promptly corrected. **Monitoring and treatment should be continued until the serum concentration decreases below 20 mcg/mL.**
9. Enhance clearance of theophylline Multiple-dose oral activated charcoal (e.g., 0.5 g/kg up to 20 g, every two hours) increases the clearance of theophylline at least twofold by adsorption of theophylline secreted into gastrointestinal fluids. Charcoal must be retained in, and pass through, the gastrointestinal tract to be effective; emesis should therefore be controlled by administration of appropriate antiemetics. Alternatively, the charcoal can be administered continuously through a nasogastric tube in conjunction with appropriate antiemetics. A single dose of sorbitol may be administered with the activated charcoal to promote stooling to facilitate clearance of the adsorbed theophylline from the gastrointestinal tract. Sorbitol alone does not enhance clearance of theophylline and should be dosed with caution to prevent excessive stooling which can result in severe fluid and electrolyte imbalances. Commercially available fixed combinations of liquid charcoal and sorbitol should be avoided in young children and after the first dose in adolescents and adults since they do not allow for individualization of charcoal and sorbitol dosing. In patients with intractable vomiting, extracorporeal methods of theophylline removal should be instituted (see OVERDOSAGE, Extracorporeal Removal).

Specific Recommendations:

Acute Overdose

A. Serum Concentration >20 <30 mcg/mL
   1. Administer a single dose of oral activated charcoal.
   2. Monitor the patient and obtain a serum theophylline concentration in 2-4 hours to insure that the concentration is not increasing.

B. Serum Concentration >30 <100 mcg/mL
   1. Administer multiple dose oral activated charcoal and measures to control emesis.
   2. Monitor the patient and obtain serial theophylline concentrations every 2-4 hours to gauge the effectiveness of therapy and to guide further treatment decisions.
   3. Institute extracorporeal removal if emesis, seizures, or cardiac arrhythmias cannot be adequately controlled (see OVERDOSAGE, Extracorporeal Removal).

C. Serum Concentration >100 mcg/mL
   1. Consider prophylactic anticonvulsant therapy.
   2. Administer multiple-dose oral activated charcoal and measures to control emesis.
   3. Consider extracorporeal removal, even if the patient has not experienced a seizure (see OVERDOSAGE, Extracorporeal Removal).
   4. Monitor the patient and obtain serial theophylline concentrations every 2-4 hours to gauge the effectiveness of therapy and to guide further treatment decisions.

Chronic Overdosage

A. Serum Concentration >20<30 mcg/mL (with manifestations of theophylline toxicity)
   1. Administer a single dose of oral activated charcoal.
   2. Monitor the patient and obtain a serum theophylline concentration in 2–4 hours to insure that the concentration is not increasing.

B. Serum Concentration >30 mcg/mL in patients <60 years of age
   1. Administer multiple-dose oral activated charcoal and measures to control emesis.
   2. Monitor the patient and obtain serial theophylline concentrations every 2–4 hours to gauge the effectiveness of therapy and to guide further treatment decisions.
   3. Institute extracorporeal removal if emesis, seizures, or cardiac arrhythmias cannot be adequately controlled (see OVERDOSAGE, Extracorporeal Removal).

C. Serum Concentration >30 mcg/mL in patients ≥60 years of age.
   1. Consider prophylactic anticonvulsant therapy.
   2. Administer multiple-dose oral activated charcoal and measures to control emesis.

Continued on next page

Theo-24—Cont.

3. Consider extracorporeal removal even if the patient has not experienced a seizure (see OVERDOSAGE, Extracorporeal Removal).

4. Monitor the patient and obtain serial theophylline concentrations every 2–4 hours to gauge the effectiveness of therapy and to guide further treatment decisions.

Extracorporeal Removal:
Increasing the rate of theophylline clearance by extracorporeal methods may rapidly decrease serum concentrations, but the risks of the procedure must be weighed against the potential benefit. Charcoal hemoperfusion is the most effective method of extracorporeal removal, increasing theophylline clearance up to six fold, but serious complications, including hypotension, hypocalcemia, platelet consumption and bleeding diatheses may occur. Hemodialysis is about as efficient as multiple-dose oral activated charcoal and has a lower risk of serious complications than charcoal hemoperfusion. Hemodialysis should be considered as an alternative when charcoal hemoperfusion is not feasible and multiple-dose oral charcoal is ineffective because of intractable emesis. Serum theophylline concentrations may rebound 5–10 mcg/mL after discontinuation of charcoal hemoperfusion or hemodialysis due to redistribution of theophylline from the tissue compartment. Peritoneal dialysis is ineffective for theophylline removal; exchange transfusions in neonates have been minimally effective.

DOSAGE AND ADMINISTRATION

General Considerations:
Theo-24, like other extended-release theophylline products, is intended for patients with relatively continuous or recurring symptoms who have a need to maintain therapeutic serum levels of theophylline. It is not intended for patients experiencing an acute episode of bronchospasm (associated with asthma, chronic bronchitis, or emphysema). Such patients require rapid relief of symptoms and should be treated with an immediate-release or intravenous theophylline preparation (or other bronchodilators) and not with extended-release products.

Patients who metabolize theophylline at a normal or slow rate are reasonable candidates for once-daily dosing with Theo-24. Patients who metabolize theophylline rapidly (e.g, the young, smokers, and some nonsmoking adults) and who have symptoms repeatedly at the end of a dosing interval, will require either increased doses given once a day or preferably, are likely to be better controlled by a schedule of twice-daily dosing. Those patients who require increased daily doses are more likely to experience relatively wide peak-trough differences and may be candidates for twice-a-day dosing with Theo-24.

Patients should be instructed to take this medication each morning at approximately the same time and not to exceed the prescribed dose.

Recent studies suggest that dosing of extended-release theophylline products at night (after the evening meal) results in serum concentrations of theophylline which are not identical to those recorded during waking hours and may be characterized by early trough and delayed peak levels. This appears to occur whether the drug is given as an immediate-release, extended-release, or intravenous product. To avoid this phenomenon when two doses per day are prescribed, it is recommended that the second dose be given 10 to 12 hours after the morning dose and before the evening meal.

Food and posture, along with changes associated with circadian rhythm, may influence the rate of absorption and/or clearance rates of theophylline from extended-release dosage forms administered at night. The exact relationship of these and other factors to nighttime serum concentrations and the clinical significance of such findings require additional study. Therefore, it is not recommended that Theo-24 (when used as a once-a-day product) be administered at night.

Patients who require a relatively high dose of theophylline (i.e., a dose equal to or greater than 900 mg or 13 mg/kg, whichever is less) should not take Theo-24 less than 1 hour before a high-fat-content meal since this may result in a significant increase in peak serum level and in the extent of absorption of theophylline as compared to administration in the fasted state (see PRECAUTIONS, Drug/Food Interactions).

The steady-state peak serum theophylline concentration is a function of the dose, the dosing interval, and the rate of theophylline absorption and clearance in the individual patient. Because of marked individual differences in the rate of theophylline clearance, the dose required to achieve a peak serum theophylline concentration in the 10–20 mcg/mL range varies fourfold among otherwise similar patients in the absence of factors known to alter theophylline clearance (e.g., 400–1600 mg/day in adults <60 years old and 10–36 mg/kg/day in children 1–9 years old). For a given population there is no single theophylline dose that will provide both safe and effective serum concentrations for all patients. Administration of the median theophylline dose required to achieve a therapeutic serum theophylline concentration in a given population may result in either sub-therapeutic or potentially toxic serum theophylline concentrations in individual patients. For example, at a dose of 900 mg/day in adults <60 years or 22 mg/kg/day in children 1–9 years, the steady-state peak serum theophylline concentration will be <10 mcg/mL in about 30% of patients, 10–20 mcg/mL in about 50% and 20–30 mcg/mL in about 20% of patients. **The dose of theophylline must be individualized on the basis of peak serum theophylline concentration measurements in order to achieve a dose that will provide maximum potential benefit with minimal risk of adverse effects.**

Transient caffeine-like adverse effects and excessive serum concentrations in slow metabolizers can be avoided in most patients by starting with a sufficiently low dose and slowly increasing the dose, if judged to be clinically indicated, in small increments (See Table V). Dose increases should only be made if the previous dosage is well tolerated and at intervals of no less than 3 days to allow serum theophylline concentrations to reach the new steady state. Dosage adjustment should be guided by serum theophylline concentration measurement (see PRECAUTIONS, Laboratory Tests and DOSAGE AND ADMINISTRATION, Table VI). Health care providers should instruct patients and care givers to discontinue any dosage that causes adverse effects, to withhold the medication until these symptoms are gone and to then resume therapy at a lower, previously tolerated dosage (see WARNINGS).

If the patient's symptoms are well controlled, there are no apparent adverse effects, and no intervening factors that might alter dosage requirements (see WARNINGS and PRECAUTIONS), serum theophylline concentrations should be monitored at 6 month intervals for rapidly growing children and at yearly intervals for all others. In acutely ill patients, serum theophylline concentrations should be monitored at frequent intervals, e.g., every 24 hours.

Theophylline distributes poorly into body fat, therefore, mg/kg dose should be calculated on the basis of ideal body weight.

Table V contains theophylline dosing titration schema recommended for patients in various age groups and clinical circumstances. Table VI contains recommendations for theophylline dosage adjustment based upon serum theophylline concentrations. **Application of these general dosing recommendations to individual patients must take into account the unique clinical characteristics of each patient. In general, these recommendations should serve as the upper limit for dosage adjustments in order to decrease the risk of potentially serious adverse events associated with unexpected large increases in serum theophylline concentration.**

Table V. Dosing initiation and titration (as anhydrous theophylline).*

A. Children (12–15 years) and adults (16–60 years) without risk factors for impaired clearance.

Titration Step	*Children <45 kg*	*Children >45 kg and adults*
1. Starting Dosage	12–14 mg/kg/day up to a maximum of 300 mg/day divided Q 24 hrs*	300–400 mg/day[1] divided Q 24 hrs*
2. After 3 days, *if tolerated,* increase dose to:	16 mg/kg/day up to a maximum of 400 mg/day divided Q 24 hrs*	400–600 mg/day[1] divided Q 24 hrs *
3. After 3 more days, *if tolerated* and *if needed,* increase dose to:	20 mg/kg/day up to a maximum of 600 mg/day divided Q 24 hrs*	As with all theophylline products, doses greater than 600 mg should be titrated according to blood level (see Table VI)

[1] If caffeine-like effects occur, then consideration should be given to a lower dose and titrating the dose more slowly (see ADVERSE REACTIONS).

B. Patients with risk factors for impaired clearance, the elderly (>60 years), and those in whom it is not feasible to monitor serum theophylline concentrations: In children 12–15 years of age, the final theophylline dose should not exceed 16 mg/kg/day up to a maximum of 400 mg/day in the presence of risk factors for reduced theophylline clearance (see WARNINGS) or if it is not feasible to monitor serum theophylline concentrations. In adolescents ≥16 years and adults, including the elderly, the final theophylline dose should not exceed 400 mg/day in the presence of risk factors for reduced theophylline clearance (see WARNINGS) or if it is not feasible to monitor serum theophylline concentrations.

* Patients with more rapid metabolism, clinically identified by higher than average dose requirements, should receive a smaller dose more frequently to prevent breakthrough symptoms resulting from low trough concentrations before the next dose. A reliably absorbed slow-release formulation will decrease fluctuations and permit longer dosing intervals.

Table VI. Dosage adjustment guided by serum theophylline concentration.

Peak Serum Concentration	**Dosage Adjustment**
<9.9 mcg/mL	If symptoms are not controlled and current dosage is tolerated, increase dose about 25%. Recheck serum concentration after three days for further dosage adjustment.
10–14.9 mcg/mL	If symptoms are controlled and current dosage is tolerated, maintain dose and recheck serum concentration at 6–12 month intervals.¶ If symptoms are not controlled and current dosage is tolerated consider adding additional medication(s) to treatment regimen.
15–19.9 mcg/mL	Consider 10% decrease in dose to provide greater margin of safety even if current dosage is tolerated.¶
20–24.9 mcg/mL	Decrease dose by 25% even if no adverse effects are present. Recheck serum concentration after 3 days to guide further dosage adjustment.
25–30 mcg/mL	Skip next dose and decrease subsequent doses at least 25% even if no adverse effects are present. Recheck serum concentration after 3 days to guide further dosage adjustment. If symptomatic, consider whether overdose treatment is indicated (see recommendations for chronic overdosage).
>30 mcg/mL	Treat overdose as indicated (see recommendations for chronic overdosage). If theophylline is subsequently resumed, decrease dose by at least 50% and recheck serum concentration after 3 days to guide further dosage adjustment.

¶ Dose reduction and/or serum theophylline concentration measurement is indicated whenever adverse effects are present, physiologic abnormalities that can reduce theophylline clearance occur (e.g., sustained fever), or a drug that interacts with theophylline is added or discontinued (see WARNINGS).

HOW SUPPLIED

Theo-24® (theophylline anhydrous) is supplied in extended-release capsules containing 100, 200, 300 or 400 mg of anhydrous theophylline.

Theo-24 100 mg capsules are yellow-orange and clear, with markings Theo-24, 100 mg, ucb, and 2832, supplied as:

NDC Number	Size
50474-100-01	bottle of 100

Theo-24 200 mg capsules are red-orange and clear, with markings Theo-24, 200 mg, ucb, and 2842, supplied as:

NDC Number	Size
50474-200-01	bottle of 100
50474-200-50	bottle of 500
50474-200-60	carton of 100 unit dose

Theo-24 300 mg capsules are red and clear, with markings Theo-24, 300 mg, ucb, and 2852, supplied as:

NDC Number	Size
50474-300-01	bottle of 100
50474-300-50	bottle of 500
50474-300-60	carton of 100 unit dose

Theo-24 400 mg capsules are pink and clear, with markings Theo-24, 400 mg, ucb, and 2902, supplied as:

NDC Number	Size
50474-400-01	bottle of 100
50474-400-50	bottle of 500

Store below 77°F (25°C).

Manufactured for **UCB Pharma, Inc.** Smyrna, GA 30080 by **G. D. Searle & Co.,** Chicago, IL 60680 — Revised: 3/98

Shown in Product Identification Guide, page 339

TRINSICON® ℞

[tren 'sa-kon]

Hematinic Concentrate With Intrinsic Factor

DESCRIPTION

Each TRINSICON capsule contains:

Special liver-stomach concentrate (containing intrinsic factor)	240 mg
Vitamin B_{12} (activity equivalent)	15 mcg
Iron, elemental (as ferrous fumarate)	110 mg
Ascorbic acid (vitamin C)	75 mg
Folic acid	0.5 mg

with other factors of vitamin B complex present in the liver-stomach concentrate.

Each capsule also contains FD&C Blue No. 1, D&C Red No. 28, FD&C Red No. 40, D&C Yellow No. 10, gelatin, silicon dioxide, corn starch, edible ink, silicone fluid, sodium lauryl sulfate and titanium dioxide.

HOW SUPPLIED

Dark pink and dark red capsules imprinted "ucb/364" in child-resistant, unit-dose packages of 60 capsules [6 × 10] (NDC 50474-364-23), and of 100 capsules [10 × 10] (NDC 50474-364-28).

Manufactured for
UCB Pharma, Inc.
Smyrna, GA 30080
By **Mallinckrodt Inc**
Hobart, NY 13788

Revised 5/98

Shown in Product Identification Guide, page 339

VICON FORTE® Capsules ℞

[*vī 'kon for 'tā*]

Therapeutic Vitamins-Minerals

DESCRIPTION

Each black and orange VICON FORTE capsule for oral administration contains:

Vitamin A	8,000 IU
Vitamin E	50 IU
Ascorbic acid	150 mg
Zinc sulfate, USP*	80 mg
Magnesium sulfate, USP†	70 mg
Niacinamide	25 mg
Thiamine mononitrate	10 mg
d-Calcium pantothenate	10 mg
Riboflavin	5 mg
Manganese chloride	4 mg
Pyridoxine hydrochloride	2 mg
Folic acid	1 mg
Vitamin B_{12} (Cyanocobalamin)	10 mcg

* As 50 mg dried zinc sulfate.
† As 50 mg dried magnesium sulfate.

Each capsule also contains edible ink, FD&C Blue No. 1, FD&C Red No. 40, FD&C Yellow No. 6, gelatin, lactose, magnesium stearate, silicon dioxide, sodium lauryl sulfate, and titanium dioxide.

HOW SUPPLIED

Orange and black capsules imprinted with "ucb" and "316" in bottles of 60 (NDC 50474-316-22) and 500 (NDC 50474-316-24) and unit-dose packs of 100 (NDC 50474-316-27).

Dispense in tight, light-resistant container with a child resistant closure.

Manufactured for
UCB Pharma, Inc.,
Smyrna, GA 30080
by Mallinckrodt Inc.
Hobart, NY 13788

Revised 4/98

Shown in Product Identification Guide, page 339

Unimed Pharmaceuticals, Inc.

A Solvay Pharmaceuticals, Inc. Company
FOUR PARKWAY NORTH, SUITE 200
DEERFIELD, ILLINOIS 60015-2544

Direct Inquiries to:
(847) 282-5400

ANADROL®-50 Ⓒ ℞

(oxymetholone)
50 mg Tablets

DESCRIPTION

ANADROL (oxymetholone) tablets for oral administration each contain 50 mg of the steroid oxymetholone, a potent anabolic and androgenic drug.

The chemical name for oxymetholone is 17β-hydroxy-2-(hydroxymethylene)-17-methyl-5α-androstan-3-one. The structural formula is:

Inactive Ingredients— lactose, magnesium stearate, povidone, starch

CLINICAL PHARMACOLOGY

Anabolic steroids are synthetic derivatives of testosterone. Nitrogen balance is improved with anabolic agents but only when there is sufficient intake of calories and protein. Whether this positive nitrogen balance is of primary benefit in the utilization of protein-building dietary substances has not been established. Oxymetholone enhances the production and urinary excretion of erythropoietin in patients with anemias due to bone marrow failure and often stimulates erythropoiesis in anemias due to deficient red cell production.

Certain clinical effects and adverse reactions demonstrate the androgenic properties of this class of drugs. Complete dissociation of anabolic and androgenic effects has not been achieved. The actions of anabolic steroids are therefore similar to those of male sex hormones with the possibility of causing serious disturbances of growth and sexual development if given to young children. They suppress the gonadotropic functions of the pituitary and may exert a direct effect upon the testes.

INDICATIONS AND USAGE

ANADROL-50 is indicated in the treatment of anemias caused by deficient red cell production. Acquired aplastic anemia, congenital aplastic anemia, myelofibrosis and the hypoplastic anemias due to the administration of myelotoxic drugs often respond. ANADROL-50 should not replace other supportive measures such as transfusion, correction of iron, folic acid, vitamin B_{12} or pyridoxine deficiency, antibacterial therapy and the appropriate use of corticosteroids.

CONTRAINDICATIONS

1. Carcinoma of the prostate or breast in male patients.
2. Carcinoma of the breast in females with hypercalcemia; androgenic anabolic steroids may stimulate osteolytic resorption of bones.
3. Oxymetholone can cause fetal harm when administered to pregnant women. It is contraindicated in women who are or may become pregnant. If the patient becomes pregnant while taking the drug, she should be apprised of the potential hazard to the fetus.
4. Nephrosis or the nephrotic phase of nephritis.
5. Hypersensitivity to the drug.
6. Severe hepatic dysfunction.

WARNINGS

The following conditions have been reported in patients receiving androgenic anabolic steroids as a general class of drugs:

> Peliosis hepatis, a condition in which liver and sometimes splenic tissue is replaced with blood-filled cysts, has been reported in patients receiving androgenic anabolic steroid therapy. These cysts are sometimes present with minimal hepatic dysfunction, but at other times they have been associated with liver failure. They are often not recognized until life-threatening liver failure or intra-abdominal hemorrhage develops. Withdrawal of drug usually results in complete disappearance of lesions.
>
> Liver cell tumors are also reported. Most often these tumors are benign and androgen-dependent, but fatal malignant tumors have been reported. Withdrawal of drug often results in regression or cessation of progression of the tumor. However, hepatic tumors associated with androgens or anabolic steroids are much more vascular than other hepatic tumors and may be silent until life-threatening intra-abdominal hemorrhage develops.
>
> Blood lipid changes that are known to be associated with increased risk of atherosclerosis are seen in patients treated with androgens and anabolic steroids. These changes include decreased high density lipoprotein and sometimes increased low density lipoprotein. The changes may be very marked and could have a serious impact on the risk of atherosclerosis and coronary artery disease.

Cholestatic hepatitis and jaundice occur with 17-alpha-alkylated androgens at relatively low doses. Clinical jaundice may be painless, with or without pruritus. It may also be associated with acute hepatic enlargement and right upper-quadrant pain, which has been mistaken for acute (surgical) obstruction of the bile duct. Drug-induced jaundice is usually reversible when the medication is discontinued. Continued therapy has been associated with hepatic coma and death. Because of the hepatoxicity associated with oxymetholone administration, periodic liver function tests are recommended.

In patients with breast cancer, anabolic steroid therapy may cause hypercalcemia by stimulating osteolysis. In this case, the drug should be discontinued.

Edema with or without congestive heart failure may be a serious complication in patients with pre-existing cardiac, renal or hepatic disease. Concomitant administration with adrenal steroids or ACTH may add to the edema. This is generally controllable with appropriate diuretic and/or digitalis therapy.

Geriatric male patients treated with androgenic anabolic steroids may be at an increased risk for the development of prostate hypertrophy and prostatic carcinoma.

Anabolic steroids have not been shown to enhance athletic ability.

PRECAUTIONS

General:

Women should be observed for signs of virilization (deepening of the voice, hirsutism, acne and clitoromegaly). To prevent irreversible change, drug therapy must be discontinued when mild virilism is first detected. Such virilization is usual following androgenic anabolic steroid use at high doses. Some virilizing changes in women are irreversible even after prompt discontinuance of therapy and are not prevented by concomitant use of estrogens. Menstrual irregularities, including amenorrhea, may also occur.

The insulin or oral hypoglycemic dosage may need adjustment in diabetic patients who receive anabolic steroids.

Anabolic steroids may cause suppression of clotting factors II, V, VII and X, and an increase in prothrombin time.

Information for the patient:

The physician should instruct patients to report any of the following side effects of androgens.

Adult or Adolescent Males: Too frequent or persistent erections of the penis, appearance or aggravation of acne.

Women: Hoarseness, acne, changes in menstrual periods or more hair on the face.

All Patients: Any nausea, vomiting, changes in skin color or ankle swelling.

Laboratory Tests:

Women with disseminated breast carcinoma should have frequent determination of urine and serum calcium levels during the course of androgenic anabolic steroid therapy (see WARNINGS).

Because of the hepatoxicity associated with the use of 17-alpha-alkylated androgens, liver function tests should be obtained periodically.

Periodic (every 6 months) x-ray examinations of bone age should be made during treatment of prepubertal patients to determine the rate of bone maturation and the effects of androgenic anabolic steroid therapy on the epiphyseal centers.

Anabolic steroids have been reported to lower the level of high-density lipoproteins and raise the level of low-density lipoproteins. These changes usually revert to normal on discontinuation of treatment. Increased low-density lipoproteins and decreased high-density lipoproteins are considered cardiovascular risk factors. Serum lipids and high-density lipoprotein cholesterol should be determined periodically.

Hemoglobin and hematocrit should be checked periodically for polycythemia in patients who are receiving high doses of anabolics.

Because iron deficiency anemia has been observed in some patients treated with oxymetholone, periodic determination of the serum iron and iron binding capacity is recommended. If iron deficiency is detected, it should be appropriately treated with supplementary iron.

Oxymetholone has been shown to decrease 17-ketosteroid excretion.

Drug Interaction:

Anabolic steroids may increase sensitivity to anticoagulants; therefore, dosage of an anticoagulant may have to be decreased in order to maintain the prothrombin time at the desired therapeutic level.

Drug/Laboratory Test Interferences:

Therapy with androgenic anabolic steroids may decrease levels of thyroxine-binding globulin resulting in decreased total T_4 serum levels and increased resin uptake of T_3 and T_4. Free thyroid hormone levels remain unchanged and there is no clinical evidence of thyroid dysfunction. Altered tests usually persist for 2 to 3 weeks after stopping anabolic therapy.

Anabolic steroids may cause an increase in prothrombin time.

Anabolic steroids have been shown to alter fasting blood sugar and glucose tolerance tests.

Carcinogenesis, Mutagenesis, Impairment of Fertility:

Animal data: Testosterone has been tested by subcutaneous injection and implantation in mice and rats. The implant induced cervical-uterine tumors in mice, which metastasized in some cases. There is suggestive evidence that injection of testosterone into some strains of female mice increases their susceptibility to hepatoma. Testosterone is also known to increase the number of tumors and decrease the degree of differentiation of chemically induced carcinomas of the liver in rats.

Human data: There are rare reports of hepatocellular carcinoma in patients receiving long-term therapy with androgens in high doses. Withdrawal of the drugs did not lead to regression of the tumors in all cases.

Geriatric patients treated with androgens may be at an increased risk of developing prostatic hypertrophy and prostatic carcinoma although conclusive evidence to support this concept is lacking.

This compound has not been tested for mutagenic potential. However, as noted above, carcinogenic effects have been attributed to treatment with androgenic hormones. The potential carcinogenic effects likely occur through a hormonal mechanism rather than by a direct chemical interaction mechanism.

Impairment of fertility was not tested directly in animal species. However, as noted below under ADVERSE REACTIONS, oligospermia in males and amenorrhea in females are potential adverse effects of treatment with ANADROL® Tablets. Therefore, impairment of fertility is a possible outcome of treatment with ANADROL.

Pregnancy:

Pregnancy category X. See CONTRAINDICATIONS.

Nursing Mothers:

It is not known whether anabolics are excreted in human milk. Because of the potential for serious adverse reactions in nursed infants from anabolics, women who take oxymetholone should not nurse.

Continued on next page

Anadrol-50—Cont.

Pediatric Use:
Anabolic/androgenic steroids should be used very cautiously in children and only by specialists who are aware of their effects on bone maturation.
Anabolic agents may accelerate epiphyseal maturation more rapidly than linear growth in children, and the effect may continue for 6 months after the drug has been stopped. Therefore, therapy should be monitored by x-ray studies at 6-month intervals in order to avoid the risk of compromising the adult height.

ADVERSE REACTIONS

Hepatic:
Cholestatic jaundice with, rarely, hepatic necrosis and death. Hepatocellular neoplasms and peliosis hepatis have been reported in association with long-term androgenic anabolic steroid therapy (see WARNINGS).
Genitourinary System:
In Men:
Prepubertal: Phallic enlargement and increased frequency of erections.
Postpubertal: Inhibition of testicular function, testicular atrophy and oligospermia, impotence, chronic priapism, epididymitis, bladder irritability and decrease in seminal volume.
In Women:
Clitoral enlargement, menstrual irregularities.
In Both Sexes:
Increased or decreased libido.
CNS: Excitation, insomnia.
Gastrointestinal: Nausea, vomiting, diarrhea.
Hematologic: Bleeding in patients on concomitant anticoagulant therapy, iron-deficiency anemia.
Leukemia has been observed in patients with aplastic anemia treated with oxymetholone. The role, if any, of oxymetholone is unclear because malignant transformation has been seen in blood dyscrasias and leukemia has been reported in patients with aplastic anemia who have not been treated with oxymetholone.
Breast: Gynecomastia.
Larynx: Deepening of the voice in women.
Hair: Hirsutism and male-pattern baldness in women, male-pattern of hair loss in postpubertal males.
Skin: Acne (especially in women and prepubertal boys).
Skeletal: Premature closure of epiphyses in children (see PRECAUTIONS, Pediatric Use), muscle cramps.
Body as a Whole: Chills.
Fluid and Electrolytes: Edema, retention of serum electrolytes (sodium, chloride, potassium, phosphate, calcium).
Metabolic/Endocrine: Decreased glucose tolerance (see PRECAUTIONS), increased serum levels of low-density lipoproteins and decreased levels of high-density lipoproteins (see PRECAUTIONS, Laboratory Tests), increased creatine and creatinine excretion, increased serum levels of creatinine phosphokinase (CPK). Reversible changes in liver function tests also occur, including increased bromsulphalein (BSP) retention and increases in serum bilirubin, glutamic oxaloacetic transaminase (SGOT), and alkaline phosphatase.

DRUG ABUSE AND DEPENDENCE

Controlled Substance:
ANADROL-50 is considered to be a controlled substance and is listed in Schedule III.

OVERDOSAGE

There have been no reports of acute overdosage with anabolics.

DOSAGE AND ADMINISTRATION

The recommended daily dose in children and adults is 1–5 mg/kg body weight per day. The usual effective dose is 1–2 mg/kg/day but higher doses may be required, and the dose should be individualized. Response is not often immediate, and a minimum trial of three to six months should be given. Following remission, some patients may be maintained without the drug; others may be maintained on an established lower daily dosage. A continued maintenance dose is usually necessary in patients with congenital aplastic anemia.

HOW SUPPLIED

ANADROL-50 (oxymetholone) is supplied in bottles of 100 white scored tablets imprinted with 8633 and UNIMED (NDC 0051-8633-33).

Store at 15° to 30°C (59° to 86°F).

CAUTION: Federal law prohibits dispensing without prescription.

6/17/97

Manufactured for
Unimed Pharmaceuticals, Inc.
Buffalo Grove IL 60089
by Oread, Inc.
Palo Alto, CA 94304
Shown in Product Identification Guide, page 339

ANDROGEL™ 1%

Ⓒ℞

(testosterone gel)
A.09.063.0030563

Issued 3/00

DESCRIPTION

AndroGel™ (testosterone gel) is a clear, colorless hydroalcoholic gel containing 1% testosterone. AndroGel™ provides continuous transdermal delivery of testosterone, the primary circulating endogenous androgen, for 24 hours following a single application to intact, clean, dry skin of the shoulders, upper arms and/or abdomen.
A daily application of AndroGel™ 5 G, 7.5 G, or 10 G delivers 50 mg, 75 mg, or 100 mg of testosterone, respectively, per day, to the skin's surface. Approximately 10% of the applied testosterone dose is absorbed across skin of average permeability during a 24-hour period.
The active pharmacologic ingredient in AndroGel™ is testosterone. Testosterone USP is a white to practically white crystalline powder chemically described as 17-beta hydroxyandrost-4-en-3-one.

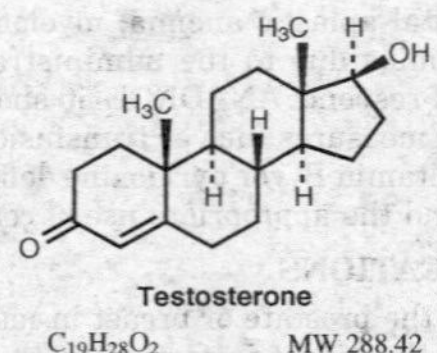

Testosterone

$C_{19}H_{28}O_2$ MW 288.42

Inactive ingredients in AndroGel™ are ethanol 68.9%, purified water, sodium hydroxide, Carbomer 940 and isopropyl myristate; these ingredients are not pharmacologically active.

CLINICAL PHARMACOLOGY

AndroGel™ (testosterone gel) delivers physiologic amounts of testosterone, producing circulating testosterone concentrations that approximate normal levels (298–1043 ng/dL) seen in healthy men.
Testosterone—General Androgen Effects:
Endogenous androgens, including testosterone and dihydrotestosterone (DHT), are responsible for the normal growth and development of the male sex organs and for maintenance of secondary sex characteristics. These effects include the growth and maturation of prostate, seminal vesicles, penis, and scrotum; the development of male hair distribution, such as facial, pubic, chest, and axillary hair; laryngeal enlargement, vocal cord thickening, alterations in body musculature, and fat distribution. Testosterone and DHT are necessary for the normal development of secondary sex characteristics. Male hypogonadism results from insufficient secretion of testosterone and is characterized by low serum testosterone concentrations. Symptoms associated with male hypogonadism include impotence and decreased sexual desire, fatigue and loss of energy, mood depression, regression of secondary sexual characteristics and osteoporosis. Hypogonadism is a risk factor for osteoporosis in men.
Drugs in the androgen class also promote retention of nitrogen, sodium, potassium, phosphorus, and decreased urinary excretion of calcium. Androgens have been reported to increase protein anabolism and decrease protein catabolism. Nitrogen balance is improved only when there is sufficient intake of calories and protein.
Androgens are responsible for the growth spurt of adolescence and for the eventual termination of linear growth brought about by fusion of the epiphyseal growth centers. In children, exogenous androgens accelerate linear growth rates but may cause a disproportionate advancement in bone maturation. Use over long periods may result in fusion of the epiphyseal growth centers and termination of the growth process. Androgens have been reported to stimulate the production of red blood cells by enhancing erythropoietin production.
During exogenous administration of androgens, endogenous testosterone release may be inhibited through feedback inhibition of pituitary luteinizing hormone (LH). At large doses of exogenous androgens, spermatogenesis may also be suppressed through feedback inhibition of pituitary follicle-stimulating hormone (FSH).
There is a lack of substantial evidence that androgens are effective in accelerating fracture healing or in shortening post-surgical convalescence.

Pharmacokinetics

Absorption
AndroGel™ is a hydroalcoholic formulation that dries quickly when applied to the skin surface. The skin serves as a reservoir for the sustained release of testosterone into the systemic circulation. In a study with the 10 G dose (to deliver 100 mg testosterone), all patients showed an increase in serum testosterone within 30 minutes, and eight of nine patients had a serum testosterone concentration within the normal range by 4 hours after the initial application. Absorption of testosterone into the blood continues for the entire 24-hour dosing interval. Serum concentrations approximate the steady state level by the end of the first 24 hours and are at steady state by the second or third day of dosing.
With single daily applications of AndroGel™, follow-up measurements 30, 90 and 180 days after starting treatment have confirmed that serum testosterone concentrations are generally maintained within the eugonadal range. Figure 1 summarizes the 24-hour pharmacokinetic profiles of testosterone for patients maintained on 5 G or 10 G of AndroGel™ (to deliver 50 or 100 mg of testosterone, respectively) for 30 days. The average (±SD) daily testosterone concentration produced by AndroGel™ 10 G on Day 30 was 792 (±294) ng/dL and by AndroGel™ 5 G 566 (±262) ng/dL.

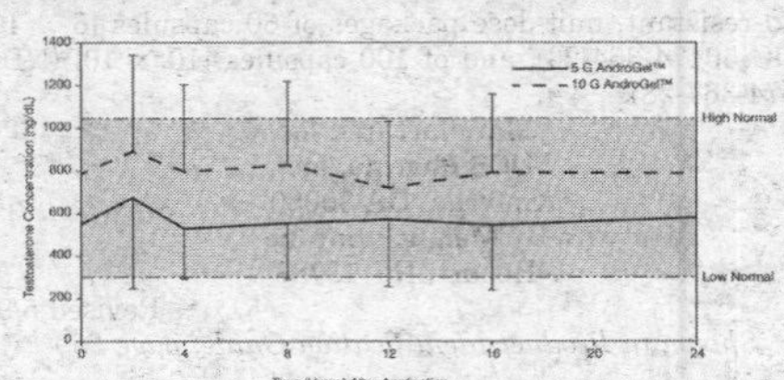

Figure 1. Mean (±SD) Steady-State Serum Testosterone Concentrations on Day 30 in Patients Applying AndroGel™ Once Daily

When AndroGel™ treatment is discontinued after achieving steady state, serum testosterone levels remain in the normal range for 24 to 48 hours but return to their pretreatment levels by the fifth day after the last application.

Distribution
Circulating testosterone is chiefly bound in the serum to sex hormone-binding globulin (SHBG) and albumin. The albumin-bound fraction of testosterone easily dissociates from albumin and is presumed to be bioactive. The portion of testosterone bound to SHBG is not considered biologically active. The amount of SHBG in the serum and the total testosterone level will determine the distribution of bioactive and nonbioactive androgen. SHBG-binding capacity is high in prepubertal children, declines during puberty and adulthood, and increases again during the later decades of life. Approximately 40% of testosterone in plasma is bound to SHBG, 2% remains unbound (free) and the rest is bound to albumin and other proteins.

Metabolism
There is considerable variation in the half-life of testosterone as reported in the literature, ranging from ten to 100 minutes. Testosterone is metabolized to various 17-ketosteroids through two different pathways. The major active metabolites of testosterone are estradiol and DHT. DHT binds with greater affinity to SHBG than does testosterone. In many tissues, the activity of testosterone depends on its reduction to DHT, which binds to cytosol receptor proteins. The steroid-receptor complex is transported to the nucleus where it initiates transcription and cellular changes related to androgen action. In reproductive tissues, DHT is further metabolized to 3-α and 3-β androstanediol.
DHT concentrations increased in parallel with testosterone concentrations during AndroGel™ treatment. After 180 days of treatment, mean DHT concentrations were within the normal range with 5 G AndroGel™ and were about 7% above the normal range after a 10 G dose. The mean steady state DHT/T ratio during 180 days of AndroGel™ treatment remained within normal limits (as determined by the analytical laboratory involved with this clinical trial) and ranged from 0.23 to 0.29 (5 G/day) and from 0.27 to 0.33 (10 G/day).

Excretion
About 90% of a dose of testosterone given intramuscularly is excreted in the urine as glucuronic and sulfuric acid conjugates of testosterone and its metabolites; about 6% of a dose is excreted in the feces, mostly in the unconjugated form. Inactivation of testosterone occurs primarily in the liver.

Special Populations

In patients treated with AndroGel™, there are no observed differences in the average daily serum testosterone concentration at steady-state based on age, cause of hypogonadism or body mass index. No formal studies were conducted involving patients with renal or hepatic insufficiencies.

CLINICAL STUDIES

AndroGel™ 1% was evaluated in a multicenter, randomized, parallel-group, active-controlled, 180-day trial in 227 hypogonadal men. The study was conducted in 2 phases. During the Initial Treatment Period (Days 1–90), 73 patients were randomized to AndroGel™ 5 G daily (to deliver 50 mg testosterone), 78 patients to AndroGel™ 10 G daily (to deliver 100 mg testosterone), and 76 patients to a non-scrotal testosterone transdermal system (5 mg daily). The study was double-blind for dose of AndroGel™ but open-label for active control. Patients who were originally randomized to AndroGel™ and who had single-sample serum testosterone levels above or below the normal range on Day 60 were titrated to 7.5 G daily (to deliver 75 mg testosterone) on Day 91. During the Extended Treatment Period (Days 91–180), 51 patients continued on AndroGel™ 5 G daily, 52 patients continued on AndroGel™ 10 G daily, 41 patients continued on a non-scrotal testosterone transdermal system (5 mg daily), and 40 patients received AndroGel™ 7.5 G daily.
Mean peak, trough and average serum testosterone concentrations within the normal range (298–1043 ng/dL) were achieved on the first day of treatment with doses of 5 G and 10 G. In patients continuing on AndroGel™ 5 G and 10 G, these mean testosterone levels were maintained within the normal range for the 180-day duration of the study. Figure 2 summarizes the 24-hour pharmacokinetic profiles of testosterone administered as AndroGel™ for 30, 90 and 180 days. Testosterone concentrations were maintained as long as the patient continued to properly apply the prescribed AndroGel™ treatment.
[See figure 2 at top of next column]
Table 1 summarizes the mean testosterone concentrations on Treatment Day 180 for patients receiving 5 G, 7.5 G, or

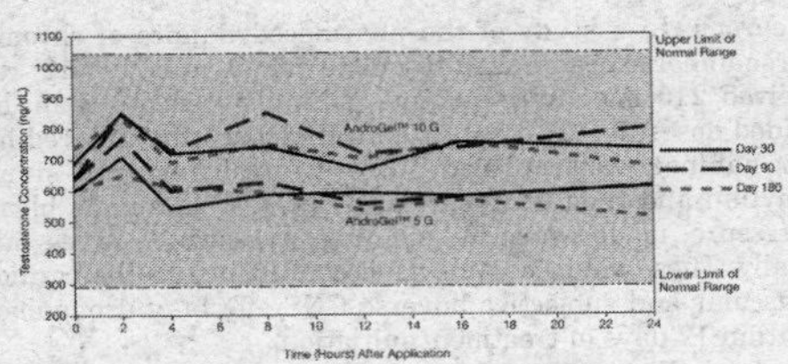

Figure 2. Mean Steady-State Testosterone Concentrations in Patients with Once-Daily AndroGel™ Therapy

10 G of AndroGel™. The 7.5 G dose produced mean concentrations intermediate to those produced by 5 G and 10 G of AndroGel™.

Table 1: Mean (± SD) Steady-State Serum Testosterone Concentrations During Therapy (Day 180)

	5 G N = 44	7.5 G N = 37	10 G N = 48
C_{avg}	555 ± 225	601 ± 309	713 ± 209
C_{max}	830 ± 347	901 ± 471	1083 ± 434
C_{min}	371 ± 165	406 ± 220	485 ± 156

Of 129 hypogonadal men who were appropriately titrated with AndroGel™ and who had sufficient data for analysis, 87% achieved an average serum testosterone level within the normal range on Treatment Day 180.

AndroGel™ 5 G/day and 10 G/day resulted in significant increases over time in total body mass and total body lean mass, while total body fat mass and the percent body fat decreased significantly. These changes were maintained for 180 days of treatment. Changes in the 7.5 G dose group were similar. Bone mineral density in both hip and spine increased significantly from Baseline to Day 180 with 10 G AndroGel.™

AndroGel™ treatment at 5 G/day and 10 G/day for 90 days produced significant improvement in libido (measured by sexual motivation, sexual activity and enjoyment of sexual activity as assessed by patient responses to a questionnaire). The degree of penile erection as subjectively estimated by the patients, increased with AndroGel™ treatment, as did the subjective score for "satisfactory duration of erection." AndroGel™ treatment at 5 G/day and 10 G/day produced positive effects on mood and fatigue. Similar changes were seen after 180 days of treatment and in the group treated with the 7.5 G dose.

DHT concentrations increased in parallel with testosterone concentrations at AndroGel™ doses of 5 G/day and 10 G/day, but the DHT/T ratio stayed within the normal range, indicating enhanced availability of the major physiologically active androgen. Serum estradiol (E2) concentrations increased significantly within 30 days of starting treatment with AndroGel™ 5 or 10 G/day and remained elevated throughout the treatment period but remained within the normal range for eugonadal men. Serum levels of SHBG decreased very slightly (1 to 11%) during AndroGel™ treatment. In men with hypergonadotropic hypogonadism, serum levels of LH and FSH fell in a dose- and time-dependent manner during treatment with AndroGel.™

Potential for testosterone transfer:

The potential for dermal testosterone transfer following AndroGel™ use was evaluated in a clinical study between males dosed with AndroGel™ and their untreated female partners. Two to 12 hours after AndroGel™ (10 G) application by the male subjects, the couples (N=38 couples) engaged in daily, 15-minute sessions of vigorous skin-to-skin contact so that the female partners gained maximum exposure to the AndroGel™ application sites. Under these study conditions, all unprotected female partners had a serum testosterone concentration >2 times the baseline value at some time during the study. When a shirt covered the application site(s), the transfer of testosterone from the males to the female partners was completely prevented.

Table 2. Adverse Events Possibly, Probably or Definitely Related to Use of AndroGel™ in the Controlled Clinical Trial

Adverse Event	5 G	7.5 G	10 G
Acne	1%	3%	8%
Alopecia	1%	0%	1%
Application Site Reaction	5%	3%	4%
Asthenia	0%	3%	1%
Depression	1%	0%	1%
Emotional Lability	0%	3%	3%
Gynecomastia	1%	0%	3%
Headache	4%	3%	0%
Hypertension	3%	0%	3%
Lab Test Abnormal*	6%	5%	3%
Libido Decreased	0%	3%	1%
Nervousness	0%	3%	1%
Pain Breast	1%	3%	1%
Prostate Disorder**	3%	3%	5%
Testis Disorder	3%	0%	0%

* *Lab test abnormal* occurred in nine patients with one or more of the following events: elevated hemoglobin or hematocrit, hyperlipidemia, elevated triglycerides, hypokalemia, decreased HDL, elevated glucose, elevated creatinine, or elevated total bilirubin.

** *Prostate disorders* included five patients with enlarged prostate, one patient with BPH, and one patient with elevated PSA results.

Table 3. Incidence of Adverse Events Possibly, Probably or Definitely Related to the Use of AndroGel™ in the Long-Term, Follow-up Study

	Dose of AndroGel™		
Adverse Event	**5 G**	**7.5 G**	**10 G**
Lab Test Abnormal*	4.2%	0.0%	6.3%
Peripheral Edema	1.4%	0.0%	3.1%
Acne	2.8%	0.0%	12.5%
Application Site Reaction	9.7%	10.0%	3.1%
Prostate Disorder**	2.8%	5.0%	18.8%
Urination Impaired	2.8%	0.0%	0.0%

* *Lab test abnormal* included one patient each with elevated GGTP, elevated hematocrit and hemoglobin, increased total bilirubin, worsened hyperlipidemia, decreased HDL, and hypokalemia.

** *Prostate disorders* included enlarged prostate, elevated PSA results, and in one patient, a new diagnosis of prostate cancer; three patients (one taking 7.5 G daily and two taking 10 G daily) discontinued AndroGel™ treatment during the long-term study because of such disorders.

INDICATIONS AND USAGE

AndroGel™ is indicated for replacement therapy in males for conditions associated with a deficiency or absence of endogenous testosterone:

1. Primary hypogonadism (congenital or acquired)—testicular failure due to cryptorchidism, bilateral torsion, orchitis, vanishing testis syndrome, orchiectomy, Klinefelter's syndrome, chemotherapy, or toxic damage from alcohol or heavy metals. These men usually have low serum testosterone levels and gonadotropins (FSH, LH) above the normal range.
2. Hypogonadotropic hypogonadism (congenital or acquired)—idiopathic gonadotropin or luteinizing hormone-releasing hormone (LHRH) deficiency or pituitary-hypothalamic injury from tumors, trauma, or radiation. These men have low testosterone serum levels but have gonadotropins in the normal or low range.

AndroGel™ has not been clinically evaluated in males under 18 years of age.

CONTRAINDICATIONS

Androgens are contraindicated in men with carcinoma of the breast or known or suspected carcinoma of the prostate.

AndroGel™ is not indicated for use in women, has not been evaluated in women, and must not be used in women.

Pregnant women should avoid skin contact with AndroGel™ application sites in men. Testosterone may cause fetal harm. In the event that unwashed or unclothed skin to which AndroGel™ has been applied does come in direct contact with the skin of a pregnant woman, the general area of contact on the woman should be washed with soap and water as soon as possible. *In vitro* studies show that residual testosterone is removed from the skin surface by washing with soap and water.

AndroGel™ should not be used in patients with known hypersensitivity to any of its ingredients.

WARNINGS

1. Prolonged use of high doses of orally active 17-alpha-alkyl androgens (e.g., methyltestosterone) has been associated with serious hepatic adverse effects (peliosis hepatitis, hepatic neoplasms, cholestatic hepatitis, and jaundice). Peliosis hepatitis can be a life-threatening or fatal complication. Long-term therapy with testosterone enanthate, which elevates blood levels for prolonged periods, has produced multiple hepatic adenomas. Testosterone is not known to produce these adverse effects.
2. Geriatric patients treated with androgens may be at an increased risk for the development of prostatic hyperplasia and prostatic carcinoma.
3. Geriatric patients and other patients with clinical or demographic characteristics that are recognized to be associated with an increased risk of prostate cancer should be evaluated for the presence of prostate cancer prior to initiation of testosterone replacement therapy. In men receiving testosterone replacement therapy, surveillance for prostate cancer should be consistent with current practices for eugonadal men (see PRECAUTIONS: Carcinogenesis, Mutagenesis, Impairment of Fertility and Laboratory Tests).
4. Edema with or without congestive heart failure may be a serious complication in patients with preexisting cardiac, renal, or hepatic disease. In addition to discontinuation of the drug, diuretic therapy may be required.
5. Gynecomastia frequently develops and occasionally persists in patients being treated for hypogonadism.
6. The treatment of hypogonadal men with testosterone esters may potentiate sleep apnea in some patients, especially those with risk factors such as obesity or chronic lung diseases.

PRECAUTIONS

Transfer of testosterone to another person can occur when vigorous skin-to-skin contact is made with the application site (see Clinical Studies). The following precautions are recommended to minimize potential transfer of testosterone from AndroGel™-treated skin to another person:

- Patients should wash their hands immediately with soap and water after application of AndroGel.™
- Patients should cover the application site(s) with clothing after the gel has dried (e.g. a shirt).
- In the event that unwashed or unclothed skin to which AndroGel™ has been applied does come in direct contact with the skin of another person, the general area of contact on the other person should be washed with soap and water as soon as possible. *In vitro* studies show that residual testosterone is removed from the skin surface by washing with soap and water.

Changes in body hair distribution, significant increase in acne, or other signs of virilization of the female partner should be brought to the attention of a physician.

General

The physician should instruct patients to report any of the following:

- Too frequent or persistent erections of the penis.
- Any nausea, vomiting, changes in skin color, or ankle swelling.
- Breathing disturbances, including those associated with sleep.

Information for Patients

Advise patients to carefully read the information brochure that accompanies each carton of 30 AndroGel™ single-use packets.

Advise patients of the following:

- AndroGel™ should not be applied to the scrotum.
- AndroGel™ should be applied once daily to clean dry skin.
- After application of AndroGel™, it is currently unknown for how long showering or swimming should be delayed. For optimal absorption of testosterone, it appears reasonable to wait at least 5–6 hours after application prior to showering or swimming. Nevertheless, showering or swimming after just 1 hour should have a minimal effect on the amount of AndroGel™ absorbed if done very infrequently.

Laboratory Tests

1. Hemoglobin and hematocrit levels should be checked periodically (to detect polycythemia) in patients on long-term androgen therapy.
2. Liver function, prostatic specific antigen, cholesterol, and high-density lipoprotein should be checked periodically.
3. To ensure proper dosing, serum testosterone concentrations should be measured (see DOSAGE AND ADMINISTRATION).

Drug Interactions

Oxyphenbutazone: Concurrent administration of oxyphenbutazone and androgens may result in elevated serum levels of oxyphenbutazone.

Insulin: In diabetic patients, the metabolic effects of androgens may decrease blood glucose and, therefore, insulin requirements.

Propranolol: In a published pharmacokinetic study of an injectable testosterone product, administration of testosterone cypionate led to an increased clearance of propranolol in the majority of men tested.

Corticosteroids: The concurrent administration of testosterone with ACTH or corticosteroids may enhance edema formation; thus these drugs should be administered cautiously, particularly in patients with cardiac or hepatic disease.

Continued on next page

Androgel—Cont.

Drug/Laboratory Test Interactions
Androgens may decrease levels of thyroxin-binding globulin, resulting in decreased total T4 serum levels and increased resin uptake of T3 and T4. Free thyroid hormone levels remain unchanged, however, and there is no clinical evidence of thyroid dysfunction.
Carcinogenesis, Mutagenesis, Impairment of Fertility
Animal Data: Testosterone has been tested by subcutaneous injection and implantation in mice and rats. In mice, the implant induced cervical-uterine tumors, which metastasized in some cases. There is suggestive evidence that injection of testosterone into some strains of female mice increases their susceptibility to hepatoma. Testosterone is also known to increase the number of tumors and decrease the degree of differentiation of chemically induced carcinomas of the liver in rats.
Human Data: There are rare reports of hepatocellular carcinoma in patients receiving long-term oral therapy with androgens in high doses. Withdrawal of the drugs did not lead to regression of the tumors in all cases.
Geriatric patients treated with androgens may be at an increased risk for the development of prostatic hyperplasia and prostatic carcinoma.
Geriatric patients and other patients with clinical or demographic characteristics that are recognized to be associated with an increased risk of prostate cancer should be evaluated for the presence of prostate cancer prior to initiation of testosterone replacement therapy.
In men receiving testosterone replacement therapy, surveillance for prostate cancer should be consistent with current practices for eugonadal men.
Pregnancy Category X (see Contraindications)—Teratogenic Effects: AndroGel™ is not indicated for women and must not be used in women.
Nursing Mothers: AndroGel™ is not indicated for women and must not be used in women.
Pediatric Use: Safety and efficacy of AndroGel™ in pediatric patients have not been established.

ADVERSE REACTIONS

In a controlled clinical study, 154 patients were treated with AndroGel™ for up to 6 months (see Clinical Studies). Adverse Events possibly, probably or definitely related to the use of AndroGel™ and reported by ≥1% of the patients are listed in Table 2.
[See table 2 at top of previous page]
The following adverse events possibly related to the use of AndroGel™ occurred in fewer than 1% of patients: amnesia, anxiety, discolored hair, dizziness, dry skin, hirsutism, hostility, impaired urination, paresthesia, penis disorder, peripheral edema, sweating, and vasodilation.
In this clinical trial of AndroGel™, skin reactions at the site of application were occasionally reported with AndroGel™, but none was severe enough to require treatment or discontinuation of drug.
Six (4%) patients in this trial had adverse events that led to discontinuation of AndroGel™. These events included the following: cerebral hemorrhage, convulsion (neither of which were considered related to AndroGel™ administration), depression, sadness, memory loss, elevated prostate specific antigen and hypertension. No AndroGel™ patients discontinued due to skin reactions.
In an uncontrolled pharmacokinetic study of 10 patients, two had adverse events associated with AndroGel™; these were asthenia and depression in one patient and increased libido and hyperkinesia in the other. Among 17 patients in foreign clinical studies there was 1 instance each of acne, erythema and benign prostate adenoma associated with a 2.5% testosterone gel formulation applied dermally.
One hundred six (106) patients have received AndroGel™ for up to 12 months in a long-term follow-up study for patients who completed the controlled clinical trial. The preliminary safety results from this study are consistent with those reported for the controlled clinical trial. Table 3 summarizes those adverse events possibly, probably or definitely related to the use of AndroGel™ and reported by at least 1% of the total number of patients during long-term exposure to AndroGel.™
[See table 3 at top of previous page]

DRUG ABUSE AND DEPENDENCE

AndroGel™ contains testosterone, a Schedule III controlled substance as defined by the Anabolic Steroids Control Act. Oral ingestion of AndroGel™ will not result in clinically significant testosterone concentrations due to extensive first-pass metabolism.

OVERDOSAGE

There is one report of acute overdosage by injection of testosterone enanthate: testosterone levels of up to 11,400 ng/dL were implicated in a cerebrovascular accident.

DOSAGE AND ADMINISTRATION

The recommended starting dose of AndroGel™ 1% is 5 G (to deliver 50 mg of testosterone) applied once daily (preferably in the morning) to clean, dry, intact skin of the shoulders, and upper arms and/or abdomen. Upon opening the packet(s), the entire contents should be squeezed into the palm of the hand and immediately applied to the application sites. Application sites should be allowed to dry for a few minutes prior to dressing. Hands should be washed with soap and water after AndroGel™ has been applied.
Do not apply AndroGel™ to the genitals.
Serum testosterone levels should be measured approximately 14 days after initiation of therapy to ensure proper dosing. If the serum testosterone concentration is below the normal range, or if the desired clinical response is not achieved, the daily AndroGel™ 1% dose may be increased from 5 G to 7.5 G and from 7.5 G to 10 G as instructed by the physician.

HOW SUPPLIED

AndroGel™ contains testosterone, a Schedule III controlled substance as defined by the Anabolic Steroids Control Act. AndroGel™ is supplied in unit-dose aluminum foil packets in cartons of 30. Each packet contains 2.5 G or 5.0 G of gel to deliver 25 mg or 50 mg of testosterone, respectively, and is supplied as follows:

NDC Number	Strength	Package Size
0051-8425-30	1% (25 mg)	30 packets: 2.5 G per packet
0051-8450-30	1% (50 mg)	30 packets: 5 G per packet

Storage
Store at controlled room temperature 20–25°C (68–77°F) [see USP].
Disposal
Used AndroGel™ packets should be discarded in household trash in a manner that prevents accidental application or ingestion by children or pets.
Rx ONLY
Manufactured by Laboratoires Besins Iscovesco
Montrouge, France
For:
Unimed Pharmaceuticals, Inc.
Buffalo Grove, IL 60089-1864, USA
UNIMED PHARMACEUTICALS, INC.
A Solvay Pharmaceuticals, Inc. Company
AG01-032700-01
A.09.063.0030563
Issued 3/00
Shown in Product Identification Guide, page 339

MARINOL® Ⓒ℞
(dronabinol)
Capsules
℞ only.

Dronabinol is a cannabinoid designated chemically as (6a*R*-*trans*)-6a,7,8,10a-tetrahydro-6,6,9-trimethyl-3-pentyl-6*H*-dibenzo[*b*,*d*]pyran-1-ol. Dronabinol has the following empirical and structural formulas:

$C_{21}H_{30}O_2$ (molecular weight = 314.47)

Dronabinol, the active ingredient in Marinol, is synthetic delta-9-tetrahydrocannabinol (delta-9-THC). Delta-9-tetrahydrocannabinol is also a naturally occurring component of *Cannabis sativa L.* (Marijuana).
Dronabinol is a light yellow resinous oil that is sticky at room temperature and hardens upon refrigeration. Dronabinol is insoluble in water and is formulated in sesame oil. It has a pK_a of 10.6 and an octanol-water partition coefficient: 6,000:1 at pH 7.
Capsules for oral administration: Marinol is supplied as round, soft gelatin capsules containing either 2.5 mg, 5 mg, or 10 mg dronabinol. Each Marinol capsule is formulated with the following inactive ingredients: FD&C Blue No. 1 (5 mg), FD&C Red No. 40 (5 mg), FD&C Yellow No. 6 (5 mg and 10 mg), gelatin, glycerin, methylparaben, propylparaben, sesame oil, and titanium dioxide.

CLINICAL PHARMACOLOGY

Dronabinol is an orally active cannabinoid which, like other cannabinoids, has complex effects on the central nervous system (CNS), including central sympathomimetic activity. Cannabinoid receptors have been discovered in neural tissues. These receptors may play a role in mediating the effects of dronabinol and other cannabinoids.
Pharmacodynamics: Dronabinol-induced sympathomimetic activity may result in tachycardia and/or conjunctival injection. Its effects on blood pressure are inconsistent, but occasional subjects have experienced orthostatic hypotension and/or syncope upon abrupt standing.
Dronabinol also demonstrates reversible effects on appetite, mood, cognition, memory, and perception. These phenomena appear to be dose-related, increasing in frequency with higher dosages, and subject to great interpatient variability.
After oral administration, dronabinol has an onset of action of approximately 0.5 to 1 hours and peak effect at 2 to 4 hours. Duration of action for psychoactive effects is 4 to 6 hours, but the appetite stimulant effect of dronabinol may continue for 24 hours or longer after administration.
Tachyphylaxis and tolerance develop to some of the pharmacologic effects of dronabinol and other cannabinoids with chronic use, suggesting an indirect effect on sympathetic neurons. In a study of the pharmacodynamics of chronic dronabinol exposure, healthy male volunteers (N = 12) received 210 mg/day dronabinol, administered orally in divided doses, for 16 days. An initial tachycardia induced by dronabinol was replaced successively by normal sinus rhythm and then bradycardia. A decrease in supine blood pressure, made worse by standing, was also observed initially. These volunteers developed tolerance to the cardiovascular and subjective adverse CNS effects of dronabinol within 12 days of treatment initiation.
Tachyphylaxis and tolerance do not, however, appear to develop to the appetite stimulant effect of Marinol. In studies involving patients with Acquired Immune Deficiency Syndrome (AIDS), the appetite stimulant effect of Marinol has been sustained for up to five months in clinical trials, at dosages ranging from 2.5 mg/day to 20 mg/day.
Pharmacokinetics:
Absorption and Distribution: Marinol (dronabinol) is almost completely absorbed (90 to 95%) after single oral doses. Due to the combined effects of first pass hepatic metabolism and high lipid solubility, only 10 to 20% of the administered dose reaches the systemic circulation. Dronabinol has a large apparent volume of distribution, approximately 10 L/kg, because of its lipid solubility. The plasma protein binding of dronabinol and its metabolites is approximately 97%.
The elimination phase of dronabinol can be described using a two compartment model with an initial (alpha) half-life of about 4 hours and a terminal (beta) half-life of 25 to 36 hours. Because of its large volume of distribution, dronabinol and its metabolites may be excreted at low levels for prolonged periods of time.
Metabolism: Dronabinol undergoes extensive first-pass hepatic metabolism, primarily by microsomal hydroxylation, yielding both active and inactive metabolites. Dronabinol and its principal active metabolite, 11-OH-delta-9-THC, are present in approximately equal concentrations in plasma. Concentrations of both parent drug and metabolite peak at approximately 2 to 4 hours after oral dosing and decline over several days. Values for clearance average about 0.2 L/kg-hr, but are highly variable due to the complexity of cannabinoid distribution.
Elimination: Dronabinol and its biotransformation products are excreted in both feces and urine. Biliary excretion is the major route of elimination with about half of a radio-labeled oral dose being recovered from the feces within 72 hours as contrasted with 10 to 15% recovered from urine. Less than 5% of an oral dose is recovered unchanged in the feces.
Following single dose administration, low levels of dronabinol metabolites have been detected for more than 5 weeks in the urine and feces.
In a study of Marinol involving AIDS patients, urinary cannabinoid/creatinine concentration ratios were studied biweekly over a six week period. The urinary cannabinoid/creatinine ratio was closely correlated with dose. No increase in the cannabinoid/creatinine ratio was observed after the first two weeks of treatment, indicating that steady-state cannabinoid levels had been reached. This conclusion is consistent with predictions based on the observed terminal half-life of dronabinol.
Special Populations: The pharmacokinetic profile of Marinol has not been investigated in either pediatric or geriatric patients.

CLINICAL TRIALS

Appetite Stimulation: The appetite stimulant effect of Marinol (dronabinol) in the treatment of AIDS-related anorexia associated with weight loss was studied in a randomized, double-blind, placebo-controlled study involving 139 patients. The initial dosage of Marinol in all patients was 5 mg/day, administered in doses of 2.5 mg one hour before lunch and one hour before supper. In pilot studies, early morning administration of Marinol appeared to have been associated with an increased frequency of adverse experiences, as compared to dosing later in the day. The effect of Marinol on appetite, weight, mood, and nausea was measured at scheduled intervals during the six-week treatment period. Side effects (feeling high, dizziness, confusion, somnolence) occurred in 13 of 72 patients (18%) at this dosage level and the dosage was reduced to 2.5 mg/day, administered as a single dose at supper or bedtime.
As compared to placebo, Marinol treatment resulted in a statistically significant improvement in appetite as measured by visual analog scale (see figure). Trends toward improved body weight and mood, and decreases in nausea were also seen.
After completing the 6-week study, patients were allowed to continue treatment with Marinol in an open-label study, in which there was a sustained improvement in appetite.
[See figure at top of next column]
Antiemetic: Marinol (dronabinol) treatment of chemotherapy-induced emesis was evaluated in 454 patients with cancer, who received a total of 750 courses of treatment of various malignancies. The antiemetic efficacy of Marinol was greatest in patients receiving cytotoxic therapy with MOPP for Hodgkin's and non-Hodgkin's lymphomas. Marinol dosages ranged from 2.5 mg/day to 40 mg/day, administered in equally divided doses every four to six hours (four times daily). As indicated in the following table, escalating the Marinol dose above 7 mg/m^2 increased the frequency of adverse experiences, with no additional antiemetic benefit.
[See table at top of next page]

Appetite Change from Baseline

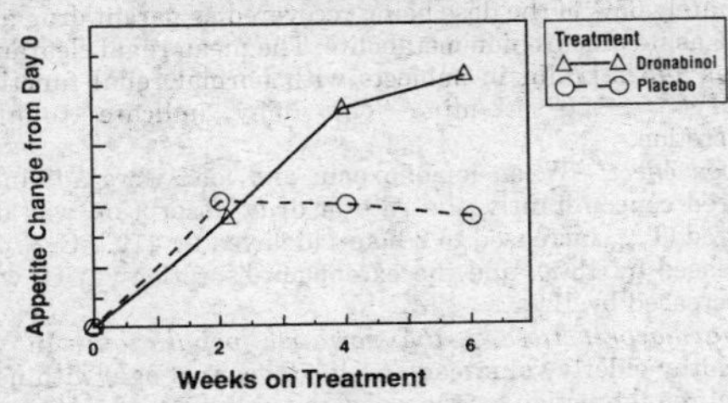

Combination antiemetic therapy with Marinol and a phenothiazine (prochlorperazine) may result in synergistic or additive antiemetic effects and attenuate the toxicities associated with each of the agents.

INDIVIDUALIZATION OF DOSAGES

The pharmacologic effects of Marinol (dronabinol) are dose-related and subject to considerable interpatient variability. Therefore, dosage individualization is critical in achieving the maximum benefit of Marinol treatment.

Appetite Stimulation: In the clinical trials, the majority of patients were treated with 5 mg/day Marinol, although the dosages ranged from 2.5 to 20 mg/day. For an adult:

1. Begin with 2.5 mg before lunch and 2.5 mg before supper.
   If CNS symptoms (feeling high, dizziness, confusion, somnolence) do occur, they usually resolve in 1 to 3 days with continued dosage.
2. If CNS symptoms are severe or persistant, reduce the dose to 2.5 mg before supper. If symptoms continue to be a problem, taking the single dose in the evening or at bedtime may reduce their severity.
3. When adverse effects are absent or minimal and further therapeutic effect is desired, increase the dose to 2.5 mg before lunch and 5 mg before supper or 5 and 5 mg. Although most patients respond to 2.5 mg twice daily, 10 mg twice daily has been tolerated in about half of the patients in appetite stimulation studies.

The pharmacologic effects of Marinol are reversible upon treatment cessation.

Antiemetic: Most patients respond to 5 mg three or four times daily. Dosage may be escalated during a chemotherapy cycle or at subsequent cycles, based upon initial results. Therapy should be initiated at the lowest recommended dosage and titrated to clinical response. Administration of Marinol with phenothiazines, such as prochlorperazine, has resulted in improved efficacy as compared to either drug alone, without additional toxicity.

Pediatrics: Marinol is not recommended for AIDS-related anorexia in pediatric patients because it has not been studied in this population. The pediatric dosage for the treatment of chemotherapy-induced emesis is the same as in adults. Caution is recommended in prescribing Marinol for children because of the psychoactive effects.

Geriatrics: Caution is advised in prescribing Marinol in elderly patients because they are generally more sensitive to the psychoactive effects of drugs. In antiemetic studies, no difference in tolerance or efficacy was apparent in patients > 55 years old.

INDICATIONS AND USAGE

Marinol (dronabinol) is indicated for the treatment of:

1. anorexia associated with weight loss in patients with AIDS; and
2. nausea and vomiting associated with cancer chemotherapy in patients who have failed to respond adequately to conventional antiemetic treatments.

CONTRAINDICATIONS

Marinol (dronabinol) is contraindicated in any patient who has a history of hypersensitivity to any cannabinoid or sesame oil.

WARNINGS

Patients receiving treatment with Marinol should be specifically warned not to drive, operate machinery, or engage in any hazardous activity until it is established that they are able to tolerate the drug and to perform such tasks safely.

PRECAUTIONS

General: The risk/benefit ratio of Marinol (dronabinol) use should be carefully evaluated in patients with the following medical conditions because of individual variation in response and tolerance to the effects of Marinol.

Marinol should be used with caution in patients with cardiac disorders because of occasional hypotension, possible hypertension, syncope, or tachycardia (see CLINICAL PHARMACOLOGY).

Marinol should be used with caution in patients with a history of substance abuse, including alcohol abuse or dependence, because they may be more prone to abuse Marinol as well. Multiple substance abuse is common and marijuana, which contains the same active compound, is a frequently abused substance.

Marinol should be used with caution and careful psychiatric monitoring in patients with mania, depression, or schizophrenia because Marinol may exacerbate these illnesses.

Marinol should be used with caution in patients receiving concomitant therapy with sedatives, hypnotics or other psychoactive drugs because of the potential for additive or synergistic CNS effects.

Marinol Dose: Response Frequency and Adverse Experiences*
(N = 750 treatment courses)

	Response Frequency (%)			Adverse Events Frequency (%)		
Marinol Dose	Complete	Partial	Poor	None	Nondysphoric	Dysphoric
< 7 mg/m^2	36	32	32	23	65	12
> 7 mg/m^2	33	31	36	13	58	28

*Nondysphoric events consisted of drowsiness, tachycardia, etc.

Marinol should be used with caution in pregnant patients, nursing mothers, or pediatric patients because it has not been studied in these patient populations.

Marinol should be used with caution for treatment of anorexia and weight loss in elderly patients with AIDS because they may be more sensitive to the psychoactive effects and because its use in these patients has not been studied.

Information for Patients: Patients receiving treatment with Marinol (dronabinol) should be alerted to the potential for additive central nervous system depression if Marinol is used concomitantly with alcohol or other CNS depressants such as benzodiazepines and barbiturates.

Patients receiving treatment with Marinol should be specifically warned not to drive, operate machinery, or engage in any hazardous activity until it is established that they are able to tolerate the drug and to perform such tasks safely.

Patients using Marinol should be advised of possible changes in mood and other adverse behavioral effects of the drug so as to avoid panic in the event of such manifestations. Patients should remain under the supervision of a responsible adult during initial use of Marinol and following dosage adjustments.

Drug Interactions: In studies involving patients with AIDS and/or cancer, Marinol (dronabinol) has been coadministered with a variety of medications (e.g., cytotoxic agents, anti-infective agents, sedatives, or opioid analgesics) without resulting in any clinically significant drug/drug interactions. Although no drug/drug interactions were discovered during the clinical trials of Marinol, cannabinoids may interact with other medications through both metabolic and pharmacodynamic mechanisms. Dronabinol is highly protein bound to plasma proteins, and therefore, might displace other protein-bound drugs. Although this displacement has not been confirmed *in vivo*, practitioners should monitor patients for a change in dosage requirements when administering dronabinol to patients receiving other highly protein-bound drugs. Published reports of drug/drug interactions involving cannabinoids are summarized in the following table.

CONCOMITANT DRUG	CLINICAL EFFECT(S)
Amphetamines, cocaine, other sympathomimetic agents	Additive hypertension, tachycardia, possibly cardiotoxicity
Atropine, scopolamine, antihistamines, other anticholinergic agents	Additive or super-additive tachycardia, drowsiness
Amitriptyline, amoxapine, desipramine, other tricyclic antidepressants	Additive tachycardia, hypertension, drowsiness
Barbiturates, benzodiazepines, ethanol, lithium, opioids, buspirone, antihistamines, muscle relaxants, other CNS depressants	Additive drowsiness and CNS depression
Disulfiram	A reversible hypomanic reaction was reported in a 28 y/o man who smoked marijuana; confirmed by dechallenge and rechallenge
Fluoxetine	A 21 y/o female with depression and bulimia receiving 20 mg/day fluoxetine × 4 wks became hypomanic after smoking marijuana; symptoms resolved after 4 days
Antipyrine, barbiturates	Decreased clearance of these agents, presumably via competitive inhibition of metabolism
Theophylline	Increased theophylline metabolism reported with smoking of marijuana; effect similar to that following smoking tobacco

Carcinogenesis, Mutagenesis, Impairment of Fertility: Carcinogenicity studies have not been performed with dronabinol. Mutagenicity testing of dronabinol was negative in an Ames test. In a long-term study (77 days) in rats, oral administration of dronabinol at doses of 30 to 150 mg/m^2, equivalent to 0.3 to 1.5 times maximum recommended human dose (MRHD) of 90 mg/m^2/day in cancer patients or 2 to 10 times MRHD of 15 mg/m^2/day in AIDS patients, reduced ventral prostate, seminal vesicle and epididymal weights and caused a decrease in seminal fluid volume. Decreases in spermatogenesis, number of developing germ cells, and number of Leydig cells in the testis were also observed. However, sperm count, mating success and testosterone levels were not affected. The significance of these animal findings in humans is not known.

Pregnancy: Pregnancy Category C. Reproduction studies with dronabinol have been performed in mice at 15 to 450 mg/m^2, equivalent to 0.2 to 5 times maximum recommended human dose (MRHD) of 90 mg/m^2/day in cancer patients or 1 to 30 times MRHD of 15 mg/m^2/day in AIDS patients, and in rats at 74 to 295 mg/m^2 (equivalent to 0.8 to 3 times MRHD of 90 mg/m^2 in cancer patients or 5 to 20 times MRHD of 15 mg/m^2/day in AIDS patients). These studies have revealed no evidence of teratogenicity due to dronabinol. At these dosages in mice and rats, dronabinol decreased maternal weight gain and number of viable pups and increased fetal mortality and early resorptions. Such effects were dose dependent and less apparent at lower doses which produced less maternal toxicity. There are no adequate and well-controlled studies in pregnant women. Dronabinol should be used only if the potential benefit justifies the potential risk to the fetus.

Nursing Mothers: Use of Marinol is not recommended in nursing mothers since, in addition to the secretion of HIV virus in breast milk, dronabinol is concentrated in and secreted in human breast milk and is absorbed by the nursing baby.

ADVERSE REACTIONS

Adverse experiences information summarized in the tables below was derived from well-controlled clinical trials conducted in the US and US territories involving 474 patients exposed to Marinol (dronabinol). Studies of AIDS-related weight loss included 157 patients receiving dronabinol at a dose of 2.5 mg twice daily and 67 receiving placebo. Studies of different durations were combined by considering the first occurrence of events during the first 28 days. Studies of nausea and vomiting related to cancer chemotherapy included 317 patients receiving dronabinol and 68 receiving placebo.

A cannabinoid dose-related "high" (easy laughing, elation and heightened awareness) has been reported by patients receiving Marinol in both the antiemetic (24%) and the lower dose appetite stimulant clinical trials (8%) (see CLINICAL TRIALS).

The most frequently reported adverse experiences in patients with AIDS during placebo-controlled clinical trials involved the CNS and were reported by 33% of patients receiving Marinol. About 25% of patients reported a minor CNS adverse event during the first 2 weeks and about 4% reported such an event each week for the next 6 weeks thereafter.

PROBABLY CAUSALLY RELATED: Incidence greater than 1%.

Rates derived from clinical trials in AIDS-related anorexia (N=157) and chemotherapy-related nausea (N=317). Rates were generally higher in the anti-emetic use (given in parentheses).

Body as a whole: Asthenia.
Cardiovascular: Palpitations, tachycardia, vasodilation/facial flush.
Digestive: Abdominal pain*, nausea*, vomiting*.
Nervous system: (Amnesia), anxiety/nervousness, (ataxia), confusion, depersonalization, dizziness*, euphoria*, (hallucination), paranoid reaction*, somnolence*, thinking abnormal*.

*Incidence of events 3% to 10%

PROBABLY CAUSALLY RELATED: Incidence less than 1%.

Event rates derived from clinical trials in AIDS-related anorexia (N=157) and chemotherapy-related nausea (N=317).

Cardiovascular: Conjunctivitis*, hypotension*.
Digestive: Diarrhea*, fecal incontinence.
Musculoskeletal: Myalgias.
Nervous system: Depression, nightmares, speech difficulties, tinnitus.
Skin and Appendages: Flushing*.
Special senses: Vision difficulties.

*Incidence of events 0.3% to 1%.

CAUSAL RELATIONSHIP UNKNOWN: Incidence less than 1%.

The clinical significance of the association of these events with Marinol treatment is unknown, but they are reported as alerting information for the clinician.

Body as a whole: Chills, headache, malaise.
Digestive: Anorexia, hepatic enzyme elevation.
Respiratory: Cough, rhinitis, sinusitis.
Skin and Appendages: Sweating.

Continued on next page

Marinol—Cont.

DRUG ABUSE AND DEPENDENCE

Marinol (dronabinol) is one of the psychoactive compounds present in cannabis, and is abusable and controlled [Schedule III (CIII)] under the Controlled Substances Act. Both psychological and physiological dependence have been noted in healthy individuals receiving dronabinol, but addiction is uncommon and has only been seen after prolonged high dose administration.

Chronic abuse of cannabis has been associated with decrements in motivation, cognition, judgment, and perception. The etiology of these impairments is unknown, but may be associated with the complex process of addiction rather than an isolated effect of the drug. No such decrements in psychological, social or neurological status have been associated with the administration of Marinol for therapeutic purposes.

In an open-label study in patients with AIDS who received Marinol for up to five months, no abuse, diversion or systematic change in personality or social functioning were observed despite the inclusion of a substantial number of patients with a past history of drug abuse.

An abstinence syndrome has been reported after the abrupt discontinuation of dronabinol in volunteers receiving dosages of 210 mg/day for 12 to 16 consecutive days. Within 12 hours after discontinuation, these volunteers manifested symptoms such as irritability, insomnia, and restlessness. By approximately 24 hours post-dronabinol discontinuation, withdrawal symptoms intensified to include "hot flashes", sweating, rhinorrhea, loose stools, hiccoughs and anorexia. These withdrawal symptoms gradually dissipated over the next 48 hours. Electroencephalographic changes consistent with the effects of drug withdrawal (hyperexcitation) were recorded in patients after abrupt dechallenge. Patients also complained of disturbed sleep for several weeks after discontinuing therapy with high dosages of dronabinol.

OVERDOSAGE

Signs and symptoms following MILD Marinol (dronabinol) intoxication include drowsiness, euphoria, heightened sensory awareness, altered time perception, reddened conjunctiva, dry mouth and tachycardia; following MODERATE intoxication include memory impairment, depersonalization, mood alteration, urinary retention, and reduced bowel motility; and following SEVERE intoxication include decreased motor coordination, lethargy, slurred speech, and postural hypotension. Apprehensive patients may experience panic reactions and seizures may occur in patients with existing seizure disorders.

The estimated lethal human dose of intravenous dronabinol is 30 mg/kg (2100 mg/70kg). Significant CNS symptoms in antiemetic studies followed oral dose of 0.4 mg/kg (28 mg/70 kg) of Marinol.

Management: A potentially serious oral ingestion, if recent, should be managed with gut decontamination. In unconscious patients with a secure airway, instill activated charcoal (30 to 100 g in adults, 1 to 2 g/kg in infants) via a nasogastric tube. A saline cathartic or sorbitol may be added to the first dose of activated charcoal. Patients experiencing depressive, hallucinatory or psychotic reactions should be placed in a quiet area and offered reassurance. Benzodiazepines (5 to 10 mg diazepam *po*) may be used for treatment of extreme agitation. Hypotension usually responds to Trendelenburg position and IV fluids. Pressors are rarely required.

DOSAGE AND ADMINISTRATION

Appetite stimulation: Initially, 2.5 mg Marinol (dronabinol) should be administered orally twice daily (b.i.d.), before lunch and supper. For patients unable to tolerate this 5 mg/day dosage of Marinol, the dosage can be reduced to 2.5 mg/day, administered as a single dose in the evening or at bedtime. If clinically indicated and in the absence of significant adverse effects, the dosage may be gradually increased to a maximum of 20 mg/day Marinol, administered in divided oral doses. Caution should be exercised in escalating the dosage of Marinol because of the increased frequency of dose-related adverse experiences at higher dosages (see PRECAUTIONS).

Antiemetic: Marinol is best administered at an initial dose of 5 mg/m^2, given 1 to 3 hours prior to the administration of chemotherapy, then every 2 to 4 hours after chemotherapy is given, for a total of 4 to 6 doses/day. Should the 5 mg/m^2 dose prove to be ineffective, and in the absence of significant side effects, the dose may be escalated by 2.5 mg/m^2 increments to a maximum of 15 mg/m^2 per dose. Caution should be exercised in dose escalation, however, as the incidence of disturbing psychiatric symptoms increases significantly at maximum dose (see PRECAUTIONS).

STORAGE CONDITIONS

Marinol (dronabinol) should be packaged in a well-closed container and stored in a cool environment between 8° and 15°C (46° and 59°F) and alternatively could be stored in a refrigerator. Protect from freezing.

HOW SUPPLIED

MARINOL® CAPSULES (dronabinol solution in sesame oil in soft gelatin capsules)

2.5 mg white capsules (Identified RL).

NDC 0054-2601-11: Bottles of 25 capsules.
NDC 0054-2601-21: Bottles of 60 capsules.
NDC 0054-2601-25: Bottles of 100 capsules.

5 mg dark brown capsules (Identified RL).

NDC 0054-2602-11: Bottles of 25 capsules.
NDC 0054-2602-25: Bottles of 100 capsules.

10 mg orange capsules (Identified RL).

NDC 0054-2603-11: Bottles of 25 capsules.
NDC 0054-2603-21: Bottles of 60 capsules.

MARINOL® is a registered trademark of Unimed Pharmaceuticals, Inc. and is
marketed by Roxane Laboratories, Inc.
under license from Unimed Pharmaceuticals, Inc.
Manufactured by Banner Pharmacaps, Inc.
Chatsworth CA 91311

4056020 **Revised October 1999**
109 © RLI, 1999

Roxane Laboratories, Inc.
Columbus, Ohio 43216

Shown in Product Identification Guide, page 339

MAXAQUIN® ℞

[*măx 'ah-kwĭn*]
(lomefloxacin hydrochloride)
Film-coated Tablets

DESCRIPTION

Maxaquin (lomefloxacin HCl) is a synthetic broad-spectrum antimicrobial agent for oral administration. Lomefloxacin HCl, a difluoroquinolone, is the monohydrochloride salt of (±)-1-ethyl-6,8-difluoro-1,4-dihydro-7-(3-methyl-1-piperazinyl)-4-oxo-3-quinolinecarboxylic acid. Its empirical formula is $C_{17}H_{19}F_2N_3O_3 \cdot HCl$, and its structural formula is:

[structural formula: F, O, O, OH, N, HN, F, N, CH_2CH_3, •HCl, CH_3]

Lomefloxacin HCl is a white to pale yellow powder with a molecular weight of 387.8. It is slightly soluble in water and practically insoluble in alcohol. Lomefloxacin HCl is stable to heat and moisture but is sensitive to light in dilute aqueous solution.

Maxaquin is available as a film-coated tablet formulation containing 400 mg of lomefloxacin base, present as the hydrochloride salt. The base content of the hydrochloride salt is 90.6%. The inactive ingredients are carboxymethylcellulose calcium, hydroxypropyl cellulose, hydroxypropyl methylcellulose, lactose, magnesium stearate, polyethylene glycol, polyoxyl 40 stearate, and titanium dioxide.

CLINICAL PHARMACOLOGY

Pharmacokinetics in healthy volunteers: In 6 fasting healthy male volunteers, approximately 95% to 98% of a single oral dose of lomefloxacin was absorbed. Absorption was rapid following single doses of 200 and 400 mg (T_{max} 0.8 to 1.4 hours). Mean plasma concentration increased proportionally between 100 and 400 mg as shown below:

Dose (mg)	Mean Peak Plasma Concentration (μg/mL)	Area Under Curve (AUC) (μg•h/mL)
100	0.8	5.6
200	1.4	10.9
400	3.2	26.1

In 6 healthy male volunteers administered 400 mg of lomefloxacin on an empty stomach qd for 7 days, the following mean pharmacokinetic parameter values were obtained:

C_{max}	2.8 μg/mL
C_{min}	0.27 μg/mL
$AUC_{0-24\ h}$	25.9 μg•h/mL
T_{max}	1.5 h
$t_{1/2}$	7.75 h

The elimination half-life in 8 subjects with normal renal function was approximately 8 hours. At 24 hours postdose, subjects with normal renal function receiving single doses of 200 or 400 mg had mean plasma lomefloxacin concentrations of 0.10 and 0.24 μg/mL, respectively. Steady-state concentrations were achieved within 48 hours of initiating therapy with one-a-day dosing. There was no drug accumulation with single-daily dosing in patients with normal renal function.

Approximately 65% of an orally administered dose was excreted in the urine as unchanged drug in patients with normal renal function. Following a 400-mg dose of lomefloxacin administered qd for 7 days, the mean urine concentration 4 hours postdose was in excess of 300 μg/mL. The mean urine concentration exceeded 35 μg/mL for at least 24 hours after dosing.

Following a single 400-mg dose, the solubility of lomefloxacin in urine usually exceeded its peak urinary concentration 2- to 6-fold. In this study, urine pH affected the solubility of lomefloxacin with solubilities ranging from 7.8 mg/mL at pH 5.2, to 2.4 mg/mL at pH 6.5, and 3.03 mg/mL at pH 8.12.

The urinary excretion of lomefloxacin was virtually complete within 72 hours after cessation of dosing, with approximately 65% of the dose being recovered as parent drug and 9% as its glucuronide metabolite. The mean renal clearance was 145 mL/min in subjects with normal renal function (GFR = 120 mL/min). This may indicate tubular secretion.

Food effect: When lomefloxacin and food were administered concomitantly, the rate of drug absorption was delayed (T_{max} increased to 2 hours [delayed by 41%], C_{max} decreased by 18%), and the extent of absorption (AUC) was decreased by 12%.

Pharmacokinetics in the geriatric population: In 16 healthy elderly volunteers (61 to 76 years of age) with normal renal function for their age, the half-life of lomefloxacin (mean of 8 hours) and its peak plasma concentration (mean of 4.2 μg/mL) following a single 400-mg dose were similar to those in 8 younger subjects dosed with a single 400-mg dose. Thus, drug absorption appears unaffected in the elderly. Plasma clearance was, however, reduced in this elderly population by approximately 25%, and the AUC was increased by approximately 33%. This slower elimination most likely reflects the decreased renal function normally observed in the geriatric population.

Pharmacokinetics in renally impaired patients: In 8 patients with creatinine clearance (Cl_{Cr}) between 10 and 40 mL/min/1.73 m^2, the mean AUC after a single 400-mg dose of lomefloxacin increased 335% over the AUC demonstrated in patients with a Cl_{Cr} > 80 mL/min/1.73 m^2. Also, in these patients, the mean $t_{1/2}$ increased to 21 hours. In 8 patients with Cl_{Cr} < 10 mL/min/1.73 m^2, the mean AUC after a single 400-mg dose of lomefloxacin increased 700% over the AUC demonstrated in patients with a Cl_{Cr} > 80 mL/min/1.73 m^2. In these patients with Cl_{Cr} < 10 mL/min/1.73 m^2, the mean $t_{1/2}$ increased to 45 hours. The plasma clearance of lomefloxacin was closely correlated with creatinine clearance, ranging from 31 mL/min/1.73 m^2 when creatinine clearance was zero to 271 mL/min/1.73 m^2 at a normal creatinine clearance of 110 mL/min/1.73 m^2. Peak lomefloxacin concentrations were not affected by the degree of renal function when single doses of lomefloxacin were administered. Adjustment of dosage schedules for patients with such decreases in renal function is warranted. (See **Dosage and Administration**.)

Pharmacokinetics in patients with cirrhosis: In 12 patients with histologically confirmed cirrhosis, no significant changes in rate or extent of lomefloxacin exposure (C_{max}, T_{max}, $t_{1/2}$, or AUC) were observed when they were administered 400 mg of lomefloxacin as a single dose. No data are available in cirrhotic patients treated with multiple doses of lomefloxacin. Cirrhosis does not appear to reduce the nonrenal clearance of lomefloxacin. There does not appear to be a need for a dosage reduction in cirrhotic patients, provided adequate renal function is present.

Metabolism and pharmacodynamics of lomefloxacin: Lomefloxacin is minimally metabolized although 5 metabolites have been identified in human urine. The glucuronide metabolite is found in the highest concentration and accounts for approximately 9% of the administered dose. The other 4 metabolites together account for < 0.5% of the dose.

Approximately 10% of an oral dose was recovered as unchanged drug in the feces.

Serum protein binding of lomefloxacin is approximately 10%.

The following are mean tissue- or fluid-to-plasma ratios of lomefloxacin following oral administration. Studies have not been conducted to assess the penetration of lomefloxacin into human cerebrospinal fluid.

Tissue or Body Fluid	Mean Tissue- or Fluid-to-Plasma Ratio
Bronchial mucosa	2.1
Bronchial secretions	0.6
Prostatic tissue	2.0
Sputum	1.3
Urine	140.0

In two studies including 74 healthy volunteers, the minimal dose of UVA light needed to cause erythema (MED-UVA) was inversely proportional to plasma lomefloxacin concentration. The MED-UVA values (16 hours and 12 hours postdose) were significantly higher than the MED-UVA values 2 hours postdose at steady state. Increasing the interval between lomefloxacin dosing and exposure to UVA light increased the amount of light energy needed for photoreaction. In a study of 27 healthy volunteers, the steady state AUC values and C_{min} values were equivalent whether the drug was administered in the morning or in the evening.

Microbiology: Lomefloxacin is a bactericidal agent with in vitro activity against a wide range of gram-negative and gram-positive organisms. The bactericidal action of lomefloxacin results from interference with the activity of the bacterial enzyme DNA gyrase, which is needed for the transcription and replication of bacterial DNA. The minimum bactericidal concentration (MBC) generally does not exceed the minimum inhibitory concentration (MIC) by more than a factor of 2, except for staphylococci, which usually have MBCs 2 to 4 times the MIC.

Lomefloxacin has been shown to be active against most strains of the following organisms both in vitro and in clinical infections: (See **Indications and Usage**.)

Gram-positive aerobes

Staphylococcus saprophyticus

Gram-negative aerobes
Citrobacter diversus
Enterobacter cloacae
Escherichia coli
Haemophilus influenzae
Klebsiella pneumoniae
Moraxella catarrhalis
Proteus mirabilis
Pseudomonas aeruginosa (urinary tract only—See **Indications and Usage** and **Warnings**)

The following in vitro data are available; however, their clinical significance is unknown.

Lomefloxacin exhibits in vitro MICs of 2 μg/mL or less against most strains of the following organisms; however, the safety and effectiveness of lomefloxacin in treating clinical infections due to these organisms have not been established in adequate and well-controlled trials:

Gram-positive aerobes
Staphylococcus aureus (including methicillin-resistant strains)
Staphylococcus epidermidis (including methicillin-resistant strains)

Gram-negative aerobes
Aeromonas hydrophila
Citrobacter freundii
Enterobacter aerogenes
Enterobacter agglomerans
Haemophilus parainfluenzae
Hafnia alvei
Klebsiella oxytoca
Klebsiella ozaenae
Morganella morganii
Proteus vulgaris
Providencia alcalifaciens
Providencia rettgeri
Serratia liquefaciens
Serratia marcescens

Other organisms:
Legionella pneumophila

Beta-lactamase production should have no effect on the in vitro activity of lomefloxacin.

Most group A, B, D, and G streptococci, *Streptococcus pneumoniae, Pseudomonas cepacia, Ureaplasma urealyticum, Mycoplasma hominis,* and anaerobic bacteria are resistant to lomefloxacin.

Lomefloxacin appears slightly less active in vitro when tested at acidic pH. An increase in inoculum size has little effect on the in vitro activity of lomefloxacin. In vitro resistance to lomefloxacin develops slowly (multiple-step mutation). Rapid one-step development of resistance occurs only rarely ($<10^{-9}$) in vitro.

Cross-resistance between lomefloxacin and other quinolone-class antimicrobial agents has been reported; however, cross-resistance between lomefloxacin and members of other classes of antimicrobial agents, such as aminoglycosides, penicillins, tetracyclines, cephalosporins, or sulfonamides has not yet been reported. Lomefloxacin is active in vitro against some strains of cephalosporin- and aminoglycoside-resistant gram-negative bacteria.

Susceptibility tests

Diffusion techniques: Quantitative methods that require measurement of zone diameters give the most precise estimate of the susceptibility of bacteria to antimicrobial agents. One such standardized procedure[1] that has been recommended for use with disks to test the susceptibility of organisms to lomefloxacin uses the 10-μg lomefloxacin disk. Interpretation involves correlation of the diameter obtained in the disk test with the MIC for lomefloxacin.

Reports from the laboratory giving results of the standard single-disk susceptibility test with a 10-μg lomefloxacin disk should be interpreted according to the following criteria:

Zone Diameter (mm)	Interpretation
≥22	Susceptible (S)
19–21	Intermediate (I)
≤18	Resistant (R)

A report of "susceptible" indicates that the pathogen is likely to be inhibited by generally achievable drug concentrations. A report of "intermediate" indicates that the result should be considered equivocal, and, if the organism is not fully susceptible to alternative clinically feasible drugs, the test should be repeated. This category provides a buffer zone that prevents small uncontrolled technical factors from causing major discrepancies in interpretation. A report of "resistant" indicates that achievable drug concentrations are unlikely to be inhibitory, and other therapy should be selected.

Standardized susceptibility test procedures require the use of laboratory control organisms. The 10-μg lomefloxacin disk should give the following zone diameters:

Organism	Zone Diameter (mm)
S aureus (ATCC 25923)	23–29
E coli (ATCC 25922)	27–33
P aeruginosa (ATCC 27853)	22–28

Dilution techniques: Use a standardized dilution method[2] (broth, agar, or microdilution) or equivalent with lomefloxacin powder. The MIC values obtained should be interpreted according to the following criteria:

MIC (μg/mL)	Interpretation
≤2	Susceptible (S)
4	Intermediate (I)
≥8	Resistant (R)

As with standard diffusion techniques, dilution methods require the use of laboratory control organisms. Standard lomefloxacin powder should provide the following MIC values:

Organism	MIC (μg/mL)
S aureus (ATCC 29213)	0.25–2.0
E coli (ATCC 25922)	0.03–0.12
P aeruginosa (ATCC 27853)	1.0–4.0

INDICATIONS AND USAGE

Treatment:

Maxaquin (lomefloxacin HCl) film-coated tablets are indicated for the treatment of adults with mild to moderate infections caused by susceptible strains of the designated microorganisms in the conditions listed below: (See **Dosage and Administration** for specific dosing recommendations.)

LOWER RESPIRATORY TRACT

Acute Bacterial Exacerbation of Chronic Bronchitis caused by *Haemophilus influenzae* or *Moraxella catarrhalis.**

NOTE: MAXAQUIN IS NOT INDICATED FOR THE EMPIRIC TREATMENT OF ACUTE BACTERIAL EXACERBATION OF CHRONIC BRONCHITIS WHEN IT IS PROBABLE THAT *S PNEUMONIAE* IS A CAUSATIVE PATHOGEN. *S PNEUMONIAE* EXHIBITS IN VITRO RESISTANCE TO LOMEFLOXACIN, AND THE SAFETY AND EFFICACY OF LOMEFLOXACIN IN THE TREATMENT OF PATIENTS WITH ACUTE BACTERIAL EXACERBATION OF CHRONIC BRONCHITIS CAUSED BY *S PNEUMONIAE* HAVE NOT BEEN DEMONSTRATED. IF LOMEFLOXACIN IS TO BE PRESCRIBED FOR GRAM-STAIN-GUIDED EMPIRIC THERAPY OF ACUTE BACTERIAL EXACERBATION OF CHRONIC BRONCHITIS, IT SHOULD BE USED ONLY IF SPUTUM GRAM STAIN DEMONSTRATES AN ADEQUATE QUALITY OF SPECIMEN (>25 PMNs/LPF) AND THERE IS BOTH A PREDOMINANCE OF GRAM-NEGATIVE MICROORGANISMS AND NOT A PREDOMINANCE OF GRAM-POSITIVE MICROORGANISMS.

URINARY TRACT

Uncomplicated Urinary Tract Infections (cystitis) caused by *Escherichia coli, Klebsiella pneumoniae, Proteus mirabilis,* or *Staphylococcus saprophyticus.* (See **DOSAGE AND ADMINISTRATION** and **CLINICAL STUDIES—UNCOMPLICATED CYSTITIS**.)

Complicated Urinary Tract Infections caused by *Escherichia coli, Klebsiella pneumoniae, Proteus mirabilis, Pseudomonas aeruginosa, Citrobacter diversus,** or *Enterobacter cloacae.**

NOTE: In clinical trials with patients experiencing complicated urinary tract infections (UTIs) due to *P aeruginosa*, 12 of 16 patients had the microorganism eradicated from the urine after therapy with lomefloxacin. None of the patients had concomitant bacteremia. Serum levels of lomefloxacin do not reliably exceed the MIC of *Pseudomonas* isolates. THE SAFETY AND EFFICACY OF LOMEFLOXACIN IN TREATING PATIENTS WITH *PSEUDOMONAS* BACTEREMIA HAVE NOT BEEN ESTABLISHED.

*Although treatment of infections due to this microorganism in this organ system demonstrated a clinically acceptable overall outcome, efficacy was studied in fewer than 10 infections.

Appropriate culture and susceptibility tests should be performed before antimicrobial treatment in order to isolate and identify microorganisms causing infection and to determine their susceptibility to lomefloxacin. In patients with UTIs, therapy with Maxaquin film-coated tablets may be initiated before results of these tests are known; once these results become available, appropriate therapy should be continued. In patients with an acute bacterial exacerbation of chronic bronchitis, therapy should not be started empirically with lomefloxacin when there is a probability the causative pathogen is *S pneumoniae.*

Beta-lactamase production should have no effect on lomefloxacin activity.

Prevention/prophylaxis:

Maxaquin is indicated preoperatively for the prevention of infection in the following situations:

- Transrectal prostate biopsy: to reduce the incidence of urinary tract infection, in the early and late postoperative periods (3–5 days and 3–4 weeks postsurgery).
- Transurethral surgical procedures: to reduce the incidence of urinary tract infection in the early postoperative period (3–5 days postsurgery).

Efficacy in decreasing the incidence of infections other than urinary tract infection has not been established. Maxaquin, like all drugs for prophylaxis of transurethral surgical procedures, usually should not be used in minor urologic procedures for which prophylaxis is not indicated (eg, simple cystoscopy or retrograde pyelography). (See **Dosage and Administration.**)

CONTRAINDICATIONS

Maxaquin (lomefloxacin HCl) is contraindicated in persons with a history of hypersensitivity to lomefloxacin or any member of the quinolone group of antimicrobial agents.

WARNINGS

MODERATE TO SEVERE PHOTOTOXIC REACTIONS HAVE OCCURRED IN PATIENTS EXPOSED TO DIRECT OR INDIRECT SUNLIGHT OR TO ARTIFICAL ULTRAVIOLET LIGHT (eg, sunlamps) DURING OR FOLLOWING TREATMENT WITH LOMEFLOXACIN. THESE REACTIONS HAVE ALSO OCCURRED IN PATIENTS EXPOSED TO SHADED OR DIFFUSE LIGHT, INCLUDING EXPOSURE THROUGH GLASS. PATIENTS SHOULD BE ADVISED TO DISCONTINUE LOMEFLOXACIN THERAPY AT THE FIRST SIGNS OR SYMPTOMS OF A PHOTOTOXICITY REACTION SUCH AS A SENSATION OF SKIN BURNING, REDNESS, SWELLING, BLISTERS, RASH, ITCHING, OR DERMATITIS.

These phototoxic reactions have occurred with and without the use of sunscreens or sunblocks. Single doses of lomefloxacin have been associated with these types of reactions. In a few cases, recovery was prolonged for several weeks. As with some other types of phototoxicity, there is the potential for exacerbation of the reaction on re-exposure to sunlight or artificial ultraviolet light prior to complete recovery from the reaction. In rare cases, reactions have recurred up to several weeks after stopping lomefloxacin therapy.

EXPOSURE TO DIRECT OR INDIRECT SUNLIGHT (EVEN WHEN USING SUNSCREENS OR SUNBLOCKS) SHOULD BE AVOIDED WHILE TAKING LOMEFLOXACIN AND FOR SEVERAL DAYS FOLLOWING THERAPY. LOMEFLOXACIN THERAPY SHOULD BE DISCONTINUED IMMEDIATELY AT THE FIRST SIGNS OR SYMPTOMS OF PHOTOTOXICITY. RISK OF PHOTOTOXICITY MAY BE REDUCED BY TAKING LOMEFLOXACIN IN THE EVENING (See **Dosage and Administration**).

THE SAFETY AND EFFICACY OF LOMEFLOXACIN IN PEDIATRIC PATIENTS AND ADOLESCENTS (UNDER THE AGE OF 18 YEARS), PREGNANT WOMEN, AND LACTATING WOMEN HAVE NOT BEEN ESTABLISHED. (See **PRECAUTIONS—*Pediatric Use, Pregnancy,*** and ***Nursing Mothers*** subsections). The oral administration of multiple doses of lomefloxacin to juvenile dogs at 0.3 times and to rats at 5.4 times the recommended adult human dose based on mg/m^2 (0.6 and 34 times the recommended adult human dose based on mg/kg, respectively) caused arthropathy and lameness. Histopathologic examination of the weight-bearing joints of these animals revealed permanent lesions of the cartilage. Other quinolones also produce erosions of cartilage of weight-bearing joints and other signs of arthropathy in juvenile animals of various species. (See **Animal Pharmacology.**)

Convulsions have been reported in patients receiving lomefloxacin. Whether the convulsions were directly related to lomefloxacin administration has not yet been established. However, convulsions, increased intracranial pressure, and toxic psychoses have been reported in patients receiving other quinolones. Nevertheless, lomefloxacin has been associated with a possible increased risk of seizures compared to other quinolones. Some of these may occur with a relative absence of predisposing factors. Quinolones may also cause central nervous system (CNS) stimulation, which may lead to tremors, restlessness, lightheadedness, confusion, and hallucinations. If any of these reactions occurs in patients receiving lomefloxacin, the drug should be discontinued and appropriate measures instituted. However, until more information becomes available, lomefloxacin, like all other quinolones, should be used with caution in patients with known or suspected CNS disorders, such as severe cerebral arteriosclerosis, epilepsy, or other factors that predispose to seizures. (See **Adverse Reactions.**) Psychiatric disturbances, agitation, anxiety, and sleep disorders may be more common with lomefloxacin than other products in the quinolone class.

The safety and efficacy of lomefloxacin in the treatment of acute bacterial exacerbation of chronic bronchitis due to *S pneumoniae* have not been demonstrated. This product should not be used empirically in the treatment of acute bacterial exacerbation of chronic bronchitis when it is probable that *S pneumoniae* is a causative pathogen.

In clinical trials of complicated UTIs due to *P aeruginosa*, 12 of 16 patients had the microorganism eradicated from the urine after therapy with lomefloxacin. No patients had concomitant bacteremia. Serum levels of lomefloxacin do not reliably exceed the MIC of *Pseudomonas* isolates. THE SAFETY AND EFFICACY OF LOMEFLOXACIN IN TREATING PATIENTS WITH *PSEUDOMONAS* BACTEREMIA HAVE NOT BEEN ESTABLISHED.

Serious and occasionally fatal hypersensitivity (anaphylactoid or anaphylactic) reactions, some following the first dose, have been reported in patients receiving quinolone therapy. Some reactions were accompanied by cardiovascular collapse, loss of consciousness, tingling, pharyngeal or facial edema, dyspnea, urticaria, or itching. Only a few of these patients had a history of previous hypersensitivity reactions. Serious hypersensitivity reactions have also been reported following treatment with lomefloxacin. If an allergic reaction to lomefloxacin occurs, discontinue the drug. Serious acute hypersensitivity reactions may require immediate emergency treatment with epinephrine. Oxygen, in-

Continued on next page

Maxaquin—Cont.

travenous fluids, antihistamines, corticosteroids, pressor amines, and airway management, including intubation, should be administered as indicated.

Pseudomembranous colitis has been reported with nearly all antibacterial agents, including lomefloxacin, and may range from mild to life-threatening in severity. Therefore, it is important to consider this diagnosis in patients who present with diarrhea subsequent to the administration of antibacterial agents. Treatment with antimicrobial agents alters the normal flora of the colon and may permit overgrowth of clostridia. Studies indicate that a toxin produced by *Clostridium difficile* is a primary cause of "antibiotic-associated colitis." After the diagnosis of pseudomembranous colitis has been established, therapeutic measures should be initiated. Mild cases of pseudomembranous colitis usually respond to discontinuation of drug alone. In moderate to severe cases, consideration should be given to management with fluids and electrolytes, protein supplementation, and treatment with an antibacterial drug clinically effective against *C difficile* colitis.

Ruptures of the shoulder, hand, and Achilles tendons that required surgical repair or resulted in prolonged disability have been reported with lomefloxacin. Lomefloxacin should be discontinued if the patient experiences pain, inflammation, or rupture of a tendon. Patients should rest and refrain from exercise until the diagnosis of tendinitis or tendon rupture has been confidently excluded. Tendon rupture can occur at any time during or after therapy with lomefloxacin.

PRECAUTIONS

General:

Alteration of the dosage regimen is recommended for patients with impairment of renal function ($Cl_{Cr} < 40$ mL/min/1.73 m^2). (See **Dosage and Administration**.)

Information for patients:

Patients should be advised

- to avoid to the maximum extent possible direct or indirect sunlight (including exposure through glass and exposure through sunscreens and sunblocks) and artificial ultraviolet light (eg, sunlamps) during treatment with lomefloxacin and for several days after therapy;
- that they may reduce the risk of developing phototoxicity from sunlight by taking the daily dose of lomefloxacin at least 12 hours before exposure to the sun (eg, in the evening);
- to discontinue lomefloxacin therapy at the first signs or symptoms of phototoxicity reaction such as a sensation of skin burning, redness, swelling, blisters, rash, itching, or dermatitis;
- that a patient who has experienced a phototoxic reaction should avoid re-exposure to sunlight and artificial ultraviolet light until he has completely recovered from the reaction. In rare cases, reactions have recurred up to several weeks after stopping lomefloxacin therapy.
- to drink fluid liberally;
- that lomefloxacin can be taken without regard to meals;
- that mineral supplements or vitamins with iron or minerals should not be taken within the 2-hour period before or after taking lomefloxacin (see **Drug Interactions**);
- that sucralfate and antacids containing magnesium or aluminum, or Videx® (didanosine), chewable/buffered tablets or the pediatric powder for oral solution should not be taken within 4 hours before or 2 hours after taking lomefloxacin (see **PRECAUTIONS—Drug Interactions**);
- that lomefloxacin can cause dizziness and lightheadedness and, therefore, patients should know how they react to lomefloxacin before they operate an automobile or machinery or engage in activities requiring mental alertness and coordination;
- to discontinue treatment and inform their physician if they experience pain, inflammation, or rupture of a tendon, and to rest and refrain from exercise until the diagnosis of tendinitis or tendon rupture has been confidently excluded;
- that lomefloxacin may be associated with hypersensitivity reactions, even following the first dose, and to discontinue the drug at the first sign of a skin rash or other allergic reaction;
- that convulsions have been reported in patients taking quinolones, including lomefloxacin, and to notify their physician before taking this drug if there is a history of this condition.

Drug interactions:

Theophylline: In three pharmacokinetic studies including 46 normal, healthy subjects, theophylline clearance and concentration were not significantly altered by the addition of lomefloxacin. In clinical studies where patients were on chronic theophylline therapy, lomefloxacin had no measurable effect on the mean distribution of theophylline concentrations or the mean estimates of theophylline clearance. Though individual theophylline levels fluctuated, there were no clinically significant symptoms of drug interaction.

Antacids and sucralfate: Sucralfate and antacids containing magnesium or aluminum, as well as formulations containing divalent and trivalent cations such as Videx® (didanosine), chewable/buffered tablets or the pediatric powder for oral solution can form chelation complexes with lomefloxacin and interfere with its bioavailability. Sucralfate administered 2 hours before lomefloxacin resulted in a slower absorption (mean C_{max} decreased by 30% and mean T_{max} increased by 1 hour) and a lesser extent of absorption (mean AUC decreased by approximately 25%). Magnesium- and aluminum-containing antacids, administered concomitantly with lomefloxacin, significantly decreased the bioavailability (48%) of lomefloxacin. Separating the doses of antacid and lomefloxacin minimizes this decrease in bioavailability; therefore, administration of these agents should precede lomefloxacin dosing by 4 hours or follow lomefloxacin dosing by at least 2 hours.

Caffeine: Two hundred mg of caffeine (equivalent to 1 to 3 cups of American coffee) was administered to 16 normal, healthy volunteers who had achieved steady-state blood concentrations of lomefloxacin after being dosed at 400 mg qd. This did not result in any statistically or clinically relevant changes in the pharmacokinetic parameters of either caffeine or its major metabolite, paraxanthine. No data are available on potential interactions in individuals who consume greater than 200 mg of caffeine per day or in those, such as the geriatric population, who are generally believed to be more susceptible to the development of drug-induced CNS-related adverse effects. Other quinolones have demonstrated moderate to marked interference with the metabolism of caffeine, resulting in a reduced clearance, a prolongation of plasma half-life, and an increase in symptoms that accompany high levels of caffeine.

Cimetidine: Cimetidine has been demonstrated to interfere with the elimination of other quinolones. This interference has resulted in significant increases in half-life and AUC. The interaction between lomefloxacin and cimetidine has not been studied.

Cyclosporine: Elevated serum levels of cyclosporine have been reported with concomitant use of cyclosporine with other members of the quinolone class. Interaction between lomefloxacin and cyclosporine has not been studied.

Omeprazole: No clinically significant changes in lomefloxacin pharmacokinetics (AUC, C_{max}, or T_{max}) were observed when a single dose of lomefloxacin 400 mg was given after multiple doses of omeprazole (20 mg qd) in 13 healthy volunteers. Changes in omeprazole pharmacokinetics were not studied.

Phenytoin: No significant differences were observed in mean phenytoin AUC, C_{max}, C_{min} or T_{max} (although C_{max} increased by 11%) when extended phenytoin sodium capsules (100 mg tid) were coadministered with lomefloxacin (400 mg qd) for five days in 15 healthy males. Lomefloxacin is unlikely to have a significant effect on phenytoin metabolism.

Probenecid: Probenecid slows the renal elimination of lomefloxacin. An increase of 63% in the mean AUC and increases of 50% and 4%, respectively, in the mean T_{max} and mean C_{max} were noted in 1 study of 6 individuals.

Terfenadine: No clinically significant changes occurred in heart rate or corrected QT intervals, or in terfenadine metabolite or lomefloxacin pharmacokinetics, during concurrent administration of lomefloxacin and terfenadine at steady-state in 28 healthy males.

Warfarin: Quinolones may enhance the effects of the oral anticoagulant, warfarin, or its derivatives. When these products are administered concomitantly, prothrombin or other suitable coagulation tests should be monitored closely. However, no clinically or statistically significant differences in prothrombin time ratio or warfarin enantiomer pharmacokinetics were observed in a small study of 7 healthy males who received both warfarin and lomefloxacin under steady-state conditions.

Carcinogenesis, mutagenesis, impairment of fertility:

Carcinogenesis: Hairless (Skh-1) mice were exposed to UVA light for 3.5 hours five times every two weeks for up to 52 weeks while concurrently being administered lomefloxacin. The lomefloxacin doses used in this study caused a phototoxic response. In mice treated with both UVA and lomefloxacin concomitantly, the time to development of skin tumors was 16 weeks. In mice treated concomitantly in this model with both UVA and other quinolones, the times to development of skin tumors ranged from 28 to 52 weeks.

Ninety-two percent (92%) of the mice treated concomitantly with both UVA and lomefloxacin developed well-differentiated squamous cell carcinomas of the skin. These squamous cell carcinomas were nonmetastatic and were endophytic in character. Two-thirds of these squamous cell carcinomas contained large central keratinous inclusion masses and were thought to arise from the vestigial hair follicles in these hairless animals.

In this model, mice treated with lomefloxacin alone did not develop skin or systemic tumors.

There are no data from similar models using pigmented mice and/or fully haired mice.

The clinical significance of these findings to humans is unknown.

Mutagenesis: One in vitro mutagenicity test (CHO/HGPRT assay) was weakly positive at lomefloxacin concentrations ≥226 μg/mL and negative at concentrations <226 μg/mL. Two other in vitro mutagenicity tests (chromosomal aberrations in Chinese hamster ovary cells, chromosomal aberrations in human lymphocytes) and two in vivo mouse micronucleus mutagenicity tests were all negative.

Impairment of fertility: Lomefloxacin did not affect the fertility of male and female rats at oral doses up to 8 times the recommended human dose based on mg/m^2 (34 times the recommended human dose based on mg/kg).

Pregnancy: Teratogenic effects. Pregnancy Category C.

Reproductive function studies have been performed in rats at doses up to 8 times the recommended human dose based on mg/m^2 (34 times the recommended human dose based on mg/kg), and no impaired fertility or harm to the fetus was reported due to lomefloxacin. Increased incidence of fetal loss in monkeys has been observed at approximately 3 to 6 times the recommended human dose based on mg/m^2 (6 to 12 times the recommended human dose based on mg/kg). No teratogenicity has been observed in rats and monkeys at up to 16 times the recommended human dose exposure. In the rabbit, maternal toxicity and associated fetotoxicity, decreased placental weight, and variations of the coccygeal vertebrae occurred at doses 2 times the recommended human exposure based on mg/m^2. There are, however, no adequate and well-controlled studies in pregnant women. Lomefloxacin should be used during pregnancy only if the potential benefit justifies the potential risk to the fetus.

Nursing mothers:

It is not known whether lomefloxacin is excreted in human milk. However, it is known that other drugs of this class are excreted in human milk and that lomefloxacin is excreted in the milk of lactating rats. Because of the potential for serious adverse reactions from lomefloxacin in nursing infants, a decision should be made whether to discontinue nursing or to discontinue the drug, taking into account the importance of the drug to the mother.

Pediatric use:

The safety and effectiveness of lomefloxacin in pediatric patients and adolescents less than 18 years of age have not been established. Lomefloxacin causes arthropathy in juvenile animals of several species. (See **Warnings** and **Animal Pharmacology**.)

Geriatric use:

Of the total number of subjects in clinical studies of lomefloxacin, 25% were ≥65 years and 9% were ≥75 years. No overall differences in safety or effectiveness were observed between these subjects and younger subjects, and other reported clinical experience has not identified differences in responses between the elderly and younger patients, but greater sensitivity of some older individuals cannot be ruled out.

This drug is known to be substantially excreted by the kidney, and the risk of toxic reactions to this drug may be greater in patients with impaired renal function. Because elderly patients are more likely to have decreased renal function, care should be taken in dose selection, and it may be useful to monitor renal function. (See **Clinical Pharmacology**—*Pharmacokinetics in the geriatric population.*)

ADVERSE REACTIONS

In clinical trials, most of the adverse events reported were mild to moderate in severity and transient in nature. During these clinical investigations, 5,623 patients received Maxaquin. In 2.2% of the patients, lomefloxacin was discontinued because of adverse events, primarily involving the gastrointestinal system (0.7%), skin (0.7%), or CNS (0.5%).

Adverse clinical events:

The events with the highest incidence (≥1%) in patients, regardless of relationship to drug, were headache (3.6%), nausea (3.5%), photosensitivity (2.3%) [see **Warnings**], dizziness (2.1%), diarrhea (1.4%), and abdominal pain (1.2%).

Additional clinical events reported in <1% of patients treated with Maxaquin, regardless of relationship to drug, are listed below:

Autonomic: increased sweating, dry mouth, flushing, syncope.

Body as a whole: fatigue, back pain, malaise, asthenia, chest pain, face edema, hot flashes, influenza-like symptoms, edema, chills, allergic reaction, anaphylactoid reaction, decreased heat tolerance.

Cardiovascular: tachycardia, hypertension, hypotension, myocardial infarction, angina pectoris, cardiac failure, bradycardia, arrhythmia, phlebitis, pulmonary embolism, extrasystoles, cerebrovascular disorder, cyanosis, cardiomyopathy.

Central and peripheral nervous system: tremor, vertigo, paresthesias, twitching, hypertonia, convulsions, hyperkinesia, coma.

Gastrointestinal: dyspepsia, vomiting, flatulence, constipation, gastrointestinal bleeding, dysphagia, stomatitis, tongue discoloration, gastrointestinal inflammation.

Hearing: earache, tinnitus.

Hematologic: purpura, lymphadenopathy, thrombocythemia, anemia, thrombocytopenia, increased fibrinolysis.

Hepatic: abnormal liver function.

Metabolic: thirst, hyperglycemia, hypoglycemia, gout.

Musculoskeletal: arthralgia, myalgia, leg cramps.

Ophthalmologic: abnormal vision, conjunctivitis, photophobia, eye pain, abnormal lacrimation.

Psychiatric: insomnia, nervousness, somnolence, anorexia, depression, confusion, agitation, increased appetite, depersonalization, paranoid reaction, anxiety, paroniria, abnormal thinking, concentration impairment.

Reproductive system: Female: vaginal moniliasis, vaginitis, leukorrhea, menstrual disorder, perineal pain, intermenstrual bleeding. Male: epididymitis, orchitis.

Resistance mechanism: viral infection, moniliasis, fungal infection.

Respiratory: respiratory infection, rhinitis, pharyngitis, dyspnea, cough, epistaxis, bronchospasm, respiratory disorder, increased sputum, stridor, respiratory depression.

Skin/Allergic: pruritus, rash, urticaria, skin exfoliation, bullous eruption, eczema, skin disorder, acne, skin discoloration, skin ulceration, angiodema. (See also *Body as a whole.*)

Special senses: taste perversion.

Urinary: hematuria, micturition disorder, dysuria, strangury, anuria.

Adverse laboratory events:

Changes in laboratory parameters, listed as adverse events, without regard to drug relationship include:

Hematologic: monocytosis (0.2%), eosinophilia (0.1%), leukopenia (0.1%), leukocytosis (0.1%).

Renal: elevated BUN (0.1%), decreased potassium (0.1%), increased creatinine (0.1%).

Hepatic: elevations of ALT (SGPT) (0.4%), AST (SGOT) (0.3%), bilirubin (0.1%), alkaline phosphatase (0.1%).

Additional laboratory changes occurring in <0.1% in the clinical studies included: elevation of serum gamma glutamyl transferase, decrease in total protein or albumin, prolongation of prothrombin time, anemia, decrease in hemoglobin, thrombocythemia, thrombocytopenia, abnormalities of urine specific gravity or serum electrolytes, increased albumin, elevated ESR, albuminuria, macrocytosis.

Quinolone-class adverse events:

Post-marketing adverse events: Adverse events reported from worldwide marketing experience with lomefloxacin are: anaphylaxis, cardiopulmonary arrest, laryngeal or pulmonary edema, ataxia, cerebral thrombosis, hallucinations, painful oral mucosa, pseudomembranous colitis, hemolytic anemia, hepatitis, tendinitis, diplopia, photophobia, phobia, exfoliative dermatitis, hyperpigmentation, Stevens-Johnson syndrome, toxic epidermal necrolysis, dysgeusia, interstitial nephritis, polyuria, renal failure, urinary retention, and vasculitis.

Quinolone-class adverse events: Additional quinolone-class adverse events include: erythema nodosum, hepatic necrosis, possible exacerbation of myasthenia gravis, dysphasia, nystagmus, intestinal perforation, manic reaction, renal calculi, acidosis and hiccough.

Laboratory adverse events include: agranulocytosis, elevation of serum triglycerides, elevation of serum cholesterol, elevation of blood glucose, elevation of serum potassium, albuminuria, candiduria, and crystalluria.

OVERDOSAGE

Information on overdosage in humans is limited. In the event of acute overdosage, the stomach should be emptied by inducing vomiting or by gastric lavage, and the patient should be carefully observed and given supportive treatment. Adequate hydration must be maintained. Hemodialysis or peritoneal dialysis is unlikely to aid in the removal of lomefloxacin as < 3% is removed by these modalities.

Clinical signs of acute toxicity in rodents progressed from salivation to tremors, decreased activity, dyspnea, and clonic convulsions prior to death. These signs were noted in rats and mice as lomefloxacin doses were increased.

DOSAGE AND ADMINISTRATION

Maxaquin (lomefloxacin HCl) may be taken without regard to meals. Sucralfate and antacids containing magnesium or aluminum, or Videx® (didanosine), chewable/buffered tablets or the pediatric powder for oral solution should not be taken within 4 hours before or 2 hours after taking lomefloxacin. Risk of reaction to solar UVA light may be reduced by taking Maxaquin at least 12 hours before exposure to the sun (eg, in the evening). (See **Clinical Pharmacology**.)

See **Indications and Usage** for information on appropriate pathogens and patient populations.

Treatment:

Patients with normal renal function: The recommended daily dose of Maxaquin is described in the following chart:

[See first table above]

Elderly patients: No dosage adjustment is needed for elderly patients with normal renal function ($Cl_{Cr} \geq 40$ mL/min/1.73 m^2).

Patients with impaired renal function: Lomefloxacin is primarily eliminated by renal excretion. (See **Clinical Pharmacology.**) Modification of dosage is recommended in patients with renal dysfunction. In patients with a creatinine clearance > 10 mL/min/1.73 m^2 but < 40 mL/min/1.73 m^2, the recommended dosage is an initial loading dose of 400 mg followed by daily maintenance doses of 200 mg (1/2 tablet) once daily for the duration of treatment. It is suggested that serial determinations of lomefloxacin levels be performed to determine any necessary alteration in the appropriate next dosing interval.

If only the serum creatinine is known, the following formula may be used to estimate creatinine clearance.

$$\text{Men: } \frac{(\text{weight in kg}) \times (140 - \text{age})}{(72) \times \text{serum creatinine (mg/dL)}}$$

$$\text{Women: } (0.85) \times (\text{calculated value for men})$$

Dialysis patients: Hemodialysis removes only a negligible amount of lomefloxacin (3% in 4 hours). Hemodialysis patients should receive an initial loading dose of 400 mg followed by daily maintenance doses of 200 mg (1/2 tablet) once daily for the duration of treatment.

Patients with cirrhosis: Cirrhosis does not reduce the nonrenal clearance of lomefloxacin. The need for a dosage reduction in this population should be based on the degree of renal function of the patient and on the plasma concentrations. (See **Clinical Pharmacology** and **Dosage and Administration**–*Patients with impaired renal function.*)

Prevention/prophylaxis:

The recommended dose of Maxaquin is described in the following chart:

Infection	Unit Dose	Frequency	Duration	Daily Dose
Acute bacterial exacerbation of chronic bronchitis	400 mg	qd	10 days	400 mg
Uncomplicated cystitis in females caused by *E. coli*	400 mg	qd	3 days	400 mg
(see **CLINICAL STUDIES—UNCOMPLICATED CYSTITIS.**)				
Uncomplicated cystitis caused by *K pneumoniae, P mirabilis,* or *S saprophyticus*	400 mg	qd	10 days	400 mg
Complicated UTI	400 mg	qd	14 days	400 mg

STUDIES 1, 2, AND 3

U.S. AND CANADIAN STUDIES

	Lomefloxacin 3-Day Treatment	**Norfloxacin 3-Day Treatment**	**Ofloxacin 3-Day Treatment**	**Trimethoprim/ sulfamethoxazole 10-Day Treatment**
E coli	133/135 (99%)	36/39 (92%)	65/67 (97%)	33/34 (97%)
K pneumoniae	7/7 (100%)	2/2 (100%)	4/4 (100%)	2/2 (100%)
P mirabilis	8/8 (100%)	1/1 (100%)	2/2 (100%)	1/1 (100%)
S saprophyticus	11/11 (100%)	3/3 (100%)	1/1 (100%)	0/0

SWEDISH STUDY

	Lomefloxacin 3-Day Treatment	**Lomefloxacin 7-Day Treatment**	**Norfloxacin 7-Day Treatment**
E coli	101/109 (93%)	102/104 (98%)	108/110 (98%)
K pneumoniae	2/2 (100%)	5/5 (100%)	1/1 (100%)
P mirabilis	0/0	6/6 (100%)	4/4 (100%)
S saprophyticus	11/17 (65%)	23/23 (100%)	16/16 (100%)

Procedure	Dose	Oral Administration
Transrectal prostate biopsy	400 mg single dose	1–6 hours prior to procedure
Transurethral surgical procedures*	400 mg single dose	2–6 hours prior to procedure

* When preoperative prophylaxis is considered appropriate.

HOW SUPPLIED

Maxaquin (lomefloxacin HCl) is supplied as a scored, film-coated tablet containing the equivalent of 400 mg of lomefloxacin base present as the hydrochloride. The tablet is oval, white, and film-coated with "MAXAQUIN 400" debossed on one side and scored on the other side and is supplied in:

NDC Number	Size
0051-1651-02	bottle of 20
0051-1651-32	carton of 100 unit dose

Store at 59° to 77°F (15° to 25°C).

CLINICAL STUDIES—UNCOMPLICATED CYSTITIS

In three controlled clinical studies of uncomplicated cystitis in females, two performed in the United States and one in Canada, lomefloxacin was compared to other oral antimicrobial agents. In these studies, using very strict evaluability criteria and microbiological criteria at 5–9 days post-therapy follow-up, the following bacterial eradication outcomes were obtained:

[See second table above]

STUDY 4

In a controlled clinical study of uncomplicated cystitis performed in Sweden, lomefloxacin 3-day treatment was compared with lomefloxacin 7-day treatment and norfloxacin 7-day treatment. In this study, using very strict evaluability criteria and microbiological criteria at 5–9 days post-therapy follow-up, the following bacterial eradication outcomes were obtained:

[See third table above]

ANIMAL PHARMACOLOGY

Lomefloxacin and other quinolones have been shown to cause arthropathy in juvenile animals. Arthropathy, involving multiple diarthrodial joints, was observed in juvenile dogs administered lomefloxacin at doses as low as 4.5 mg/kg for 7 to 8 days (0.3 times the recommended human dose based on mg/m^2 or 0.6 times the recommended human dose based on mg/kg). In juvenile rats, no changes were observed in the joints with doses up to 91 mg/kg for 7 days (2 times the recommended human dose based on mg/m^2 or 11 times the recommended human dose based on mg/kg). (See **Warnings.**)

In a 13-week oral rat study, gamma globulin decreased when lomefloxacin was administered at less than the recommended human exposure. Beta globulin decreased when lomefloxacin was administered at 0.6 to 2 times the recommended human dose based on mg/m^2. The A/G ratio increased when lomefloxacin was administered at 6 to 20 times the human dose. Following a 4-week recovery period, beta globulins in the females and A/G ratios in the females returned to control values. Gamma globulin values in the females and beta and gamma globulins and A/G ratios in the males were still statistically significantly different from control values. No effects on globulins were seen in oral studies in dogs or monkeys in the limited number of specimens collected.

Twenty-seven NSAIDs, administered concomitantly with lomefloxacin, were tested for seizure induction in mice at approximately 2 times the recommended human dose based on mg/m^2. At a dose of lomefloxacin equivalent to the recommended human exposure based on mg/m^2 (10 times the human dose based on mg/kg), only fenbufen, when coadministered, produced an increase in seizures.

Crystalluria and ocular toxicity, seen with some related quinolones, were not observed in any lomefloxacin-treated animals, either in studies designed to look for these effects specifically or in subchronic and chronic toxicity studies in rats, dogs, and monkeys.

Long-term, high-dose systemic use of other quinolones in experimental animals has caused lenticular opacities; however, this finding was not observed with lomefloxacin.

REFERENCES

1. National Committee for Clinical Laboratory Standards, *Performance Standards for Antimicrobial Disk Susceptibility Tests*–4th ed. Approved Standard NCCLS Document M2–A4, vol 10, No. 7, NCCLS, Villanova, Pa, 1990. **2.** National Committee for Clinical Laboratory Standards. *Methods for Dilution Antimicrobial Susceptibility Tests for Bacteria that Grow Aerobically*–2nd ed. Approved Standard NCCLS Document M7–A2, vol 10, No. 8 NCCLS, Villanova, PA, 1990.

Revised: May 26, 1999

A05229-2

Manufactured for
Unimed Pharmaceuticals, Inc.
Buffalo Grove IL 60089
by Searle & Co.
San Juan PR 00936

Maxaquin is a registered trademark of G.D. Searle & Co.

Shown in Product Identification Guide, page 339

TEVETEN® ℞

brand of eprosartan mesylate tablets

400 mg and 600 mg

USE IN PREGNANCY

When used in pregnancy during the second and third trimesters, drugs that act directly on the renin-angiotensin system can cause injury and even death to the developing fetus. When pregnancy is detected,

Continued on next page

Teveten—Cont.

TEVETEN® Tablets should be discontinued as soon as possible. See WARNINGS: Fetal/Neonatal Morbidity and Mortality.

DESCRIPTION

TEVETEN® (eprosartan mesylate) Tablet is a non-biphenyl non-tetrazole angiotensin II receptor (AT_1) antagonist. A selective non-peptide molecule, TEVETEN® Tablets are chemically described as the monomethanesulfonate of (*E*)-2-butyl-1-(*p*-carboxybenzyl)-α-2-thienylmethylimidazole-5-acrylic acid.

Its empirical formula is $C_{23}H_{24}N_2O_4S \bullet CH_4O_3S$ and molecular weight is 520.625. Its structural formula is

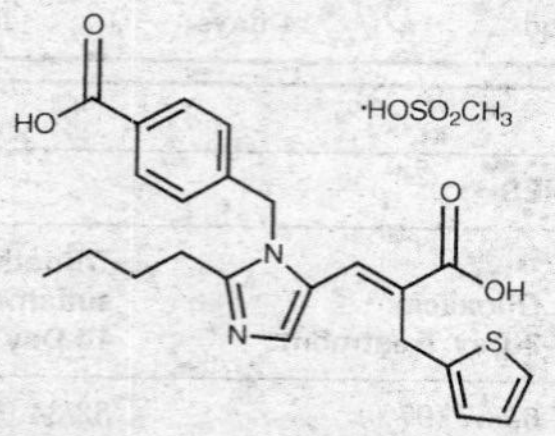

Eprosartan mesylate is a white to off-white free-flowing crystalline powder that is insoluble in water, freely soluble in ethanol, and melts between 248°C and 250°C.

TEVETEN® Tablets are available as aqueous film-coated tablets containing eprosartan mesylate equivalent to 400 mg or 600 mg eprosartan zwitterion (pink, oval, scored Tiltab® or white, non-scored, capsule-shaped tablets, respectively). **Inactive ingredients:** The 400 mg tablet contains the following: croscarmellose sodium, hydroxypropyl methylcellulose, iron oxide red, iron oxide yellow, lactose monohydrate, magnesium stearate, microcrystalline cellulose, polyethylene glycol, polysorbate 80, pregelatinized starch, titanium dioxide. The 600 mg tablet contains crospovidone, hydroxypropyl methylcellulose, lactose monohydrate, magnesium stearate, microcrystalline cellulose, polyethylene glycol, polysorbate 80, pregelatinized starch, titanium dioxide.

CLINICAL PHARMACOLOGY

Mechanism of Action

Angiotensin II (formed from angiotensin I in a reaction catalyzed by angiotensin-converting enzyme [kininase II]), a potent vasoconstrictor, is the principal pressor agent of the renin-angiotensin system. Angiotensin II also stimulates aldosterone synthesis and secretion by the adrenal cortex, cardiac contraction, renin resorption of sodium, activity of the sympathetic nervous system, and smooth muscle cell growth. Eprosartan blocks the vasoconstrictor and aldosterone-secreting effects of angiotensin II by selectively blocking the binding of angiotensin II to the AT_1 receptor found in many tissues (e.g., vascular smooth muscle, adrenal gland). There is also an AT_2 receptor found in many tissues but it is not known to be associated with cardiovascular homeostasis. Eprosartan does not exhibit any partial agonist activity at the AT_1 receptor. Its affinity for the AT_1 receptor is 1,000 times greater than for the AT_2 receptor. *In vitro* binding studies indicate that eprosartan is a reversible, competitive inhibitor of the AT_1 receptor.

Blockade of the AT_1 receptor removes the negative feedback of angiotensin II on renin secretion, but the resulting increased plasma renin activity and circulating angiotensin II do not overcome the effect of eprosartan on blood pressure.

TEVETEN® (eprosartan mesylate) Tablets do not inhibit kininase II, the enzyme that converts angiotensin I to angiotensin II and degrades bradykinin; whether this has clinical relevance is not known. It does not bind to or block other hormone receptors or ion channels known to be important in cardiovascular regulation.

Pharmacokinetics

General

Absolute bioavailability following a single 300 mg oral dose of eprosartan is approximately 13%. Eprosartan plasma concentrations peak at 1 to 2 hours after an oral dose in the fasted state. Administering eprosartan with food delays absorption, and causes variable changes (<25%) in C_{max} and AUC values which do not appear clinically important.

Plasma concentrations of eprosartan increase in a slightly less than dose-proportional manner over the 100 mg to 800 mg dose range. The terminal elimination half-life of eprosartan following oral administration is typically 5 to 9 hours. Eprosartan does not significantly accumulate with chronic use.

Metabolism and Excretion

Eprosartan is eliminated by biliary and renal excretion, primarily as unchanged compound. Less than 2% of an oral dose is excreted in the urine as a glucuronide. There are no active metabolites following oral and intravenous dosing with [^{14}C] eprosartan in human subjects. Eprosartan was the only drug-related compound found in the plasma and feces. Following intravenous [^{14}C] eprosartan, about 61% of the material is recovered in the feces and about 37% in the urine. Following an oral dose of [^{14}C] eprosartan, about 90% is recovered in the feces and about 7% in the urine. Approximately 20% of the radioactivity excreted in the urine was an acyl glucuronide of eprosartan with the remaining 80% being unchanged eprosartan.

Distribution

Plasma protein binding of eprosartan is high (approximately 98%) and constant over the concentration range achieved with therapeutic doses.

The pooled population pharmacokinetic analysis from two Phase 3 trials of 299 men and 172 women with mild to moderate hypertension (aged 20 to 93 years) showed that eprosartan exhibited a population mean oral clearance (CL/F) for an average 60-year-old patient of 48.5 L/hr. The population mean steady-state volume of distribution (Vss/F) was 308 liters. Eprosartan pharmacokinetics were not influenced by weight, race, gender or severity of hypertension at baseline. Oral clearance was shown to be a linear function of age with CL/F decreasing 0.62 L/hr. for every year increase.

Special Populations

Pediatric: Eprosartan pharmacokinetics have not been investigated in patients younger than 18 years of age.

Geriatric: Following single oral dose administration of eprosartan to healthy elderly men (aged 68 to 78 years), AUC, C_{max}, and T_{max} eprosartan values increased, on average by approximately twofold, compared to healthy young men (aged 20 to 39 years) who received the same dose. The extent of plasma protein binding was not influenced by age.

Gender: There was no difference in the pharmacokinetics and plasma protein binding between men and women following single oral dose administration of eprosartan.

Race: A pooled population pharmacokinetic analysis of 442 Caucasian and 29 non-Caucasian hypertensive patients showed that oral clearance and steady-state volume of distribution were not influenced by race.

Renal Insufficiency: Following administration of eprosartan 200 mg b.i.d. for 7 days, patients with mild renal impairment (CL_{cr} 60 to 80 mL/min.) showed mean eprosartan C_{max} and AUC values similar to subjects with normal renal function. Compared to patients with normal renal function, mean AUC and C_{max} values were approximately 30% higher in patients with moderate renal impairment (CL_{cr} 30 to 59 mL/min.) and 50% higher in patients with severe renal impairment (CL_{cr} 5 to 29 mL/min.). The unbound eprosartan fraction was not influenced by mild to moderate renal impairment but increased approximately twofold in a few patients with severe renal impairment. No dosage adjustment is necessary for patients with renal impairment. Eprosartan was poorly removed by hemodialysis (CL_{HD} <1 L/hr.) (see DOSAGE AND ADMINISTRATION).

Hepatic Insufficiency: Eprosartan AUC (but not C_{max}) values increased, on average, by approximately 40% in men with decreased hepatic function compared to healthy men after a single 100 mg oral dose of eprosartan. Hepatic disease was defined as a documented clinical history of chronic hepatic abnormality diagnosed by liver biopsy, liver/spleen scan or clinical laboratory tests. The extent of eprosartan plasma protein binding was not influenced by hepatic dysfunction. No dosage adjustment is necessary for patients with hepatic impairment (see DOSAGE AND ADMINISTRATION).

Drug Interactions

Concomitant administration of eprosartan and digoxin had no effect on single oral-dose digoxin pharmacokinetics. Concomitant administration of eprosartan and warfarin had no effect on steady-state prothrombin time ratios (INR) in healthy volunteers. Concomitant administration of eprosartan and glyburide in diabetic patients did not affect 24-hour plasma glucose profiles. Eprosartan pharmacokinetics were not affected by concomitant administration of ranitidine. Eprosartan did not inhibit human cytochrome P450 enzymes CYP1A, 2A6, 2C9/8, 2C19, 2D6, 2E and 3A *in vitro*. Eprosartan is not metabolized by the cytochrome P450 system; eprosartan steady-state concentrations were not affected by concomitant administration of ketoconazole or fluconazole, potent inhibitors of CYP3A and 2C9, respectively.

Pharmacodynamics and Clinical Effects

Eprosartan inhibits the pharmacologic effects of angiotensin II infusions in healthy adult men. Single oral doses of eprosartan from 10 mg to 400 mg have been shown to inhibit the vasopressor, renal vasoconstrictive and aldosterone secretory effects of infused angiotensin II with complete inhibition evident at doses of 350 mg and above. Eprosartan inhibits the pressor effects of angiotensin II infusions. A single oral dose of 350 mg of eprosartan inhibits pressor effects by approximately 100% at peak, with approximately 30% inhibition persisting for 24 hours. The absence of angiotensin II AT_1 agonist activity has been demonstrated in healthy adult men. In hypertensive patients treated chronically with eprosartan, there was a twofold rise in angiotensin II plasma concentration and a twofold rise in plasma renin activity, while plasma aldosterone levels remained unchanged. Serum potassium levels also remained unchanged in these patients.

Achievement of maximal blood pressure response to a given dose in most patients may take 2 to 3 weeks of treatment. Onset of blood pressure reduction is seen within 1 to 2 hours of dosing with few instances of orthostatic hypotension. Blood pressure control is maintained with once- or twice-daily dosing over a 24-hour period. Discontinuing treatment with eprosartan does not lead to a rapid rebound increase in blood pressure.

There was no change in mean heart rate in patients treated with eprosartan in controlled clinical trials.

Eprosartan increases mean effective renal plasma flow (ERPF) in salt-replete and salt-restricted normal subjects. A dose-related increase in ERPF of 25% to 30% occurred in salt-restricted normal subjects, with the effect plateauing between 200 mg and 400 mg doses. There was no change in ERPF in hypertensive patients and patients with renal insufficiency on normal salt diets. Eprosartan did not reduce glomerular filtration rate in patients with renal insufficiency or in patients with hypertension, after 7 days and 28 days of dosing, respectively. In hypertensive patients and patients with chronic renal insufficiency, eprosartan did not change fractional excretion of sodium and potassium.

Eprosartan (1200 mg once daily for 7 days or 300 mg twice daily for 28 days) had no effect on the excretion of uric acid in healthy men, patients with essential hypertension or those with varying degrees of renal insufficiency.

There were no effects on mean levels of fasting triglycerides, total cholesterol, HDL cholesterol, LDL cholesterol or fasting glucose.

Clinical Trials

The safety and efficacy of TEVETEN® (eprosartan mesylate) Tablets have been evaluated in controlled clinical trials worldwide that enrolled predominantly hypertensive patients with sitting DBP ranging from 95 mmHg to ≤115 mmHg. There is also some experience with use of eprosartan together with other antihypertensive drugs in more severe hypertension.

The antihypertensive effects of TEVETEN® Tablets were demonstrated principally in five placebo-controlled trials (4 to 13 weeks' duration) including dosages of 400 mg to 1200 mg given once daily (two studies), 25 mg to 400 mg twice daily (two studies), and one study comparing total daily doses of 400 mg to 800 mg given once daily or twice daily. The five studies included 1,111 patients randomized to eprosartan and 395 patients randomized to placebo. The studies showed dose-related antihypertensive responses.

At study endpoint, patients treated with TEVETEN® Tablets at doses of 600 mg to 1200 mg given once daily experienced significant decreases in sitting systolic and diastolic blood pressure at trough, with differences from placebo of approximately 5–10/3–6 mmHg. Limited experience is available with the dose of 1200 mg administered once daily. In a direct comparison of 200 mg to 400 mg b.i.d. with 400 mg to 800 mg q.d. of TEVETEN® Tablets, effects at trough were similar. Patients treated with TEVETEN® Tablets at doses of 200 mg to 400 mg given twice daily experienced significant decreases in sitting systolic and diastolic blood pressure at trough, with differences from placebo of approximately 7–10/4–6 mmHg.

Peak (1 to 3 hours) effects were uniformly, but moderately, larger than trough effects with b.i.d. dosing, with the trough-to-peak ratio for diastolic blood pressure 65% to 80%. In the once-daily dose-response study, trough-to-peak response of ≤50% were observed at some doses (including 1200 mg), suggesting attenuation of effect at the end of the dosing interval.

The antihypertensive effect of TEVETEN® Tablets was similar in men and women, but was somewhat smaller in patients over 65. There were too few black subjects to determine whether their response was similar to Caucasians. In general, blacks (usually a low renin population) have had smaller responses to ACE inhibitors and angiotensin II inhibitors than Caucasian populations.

Angiotensin-converting enzyme (ACE) inhibitor-induced cough (a dry, persistent cough) can lead to discontinuation of ACE inhibitor therapy. In one study, patients who had previously coughed while taking an ACE inhibitor were treated with eprosartan, an ACE inhibitor (enalapril) or placebo for six weeks. The incidence of dry, persistent cough was 2.2% on eprosartan, 4.4% on placebo, and 20.5% on the ACE inhibitor; P=0.008 for the comparison of eprosartan with enalapril. In a second study comparing the incidence of cough in 259 patients treated with eprosartan to 261 patients treated with the ACE inhibitor enalapril, the incidence of dry, persistent cough in eprosartan-treated patients (1.5%) was significantly lower (P=0.018) than that observed in patients treated with the ACE inhibitor (5.4%). In addition, analysis of overall data from six double-blind clinical trials involving 1,554 patients showed an incidence of spontaneously reported cough in patients treated with eprosartan of 3.5%, similar to placebo (2.6%).

INDICATIONS AND USAGE

TEVETEN® Tablets are indicated for the treatment of hypertension. It may be used alone or in combination with other antihypertensives such as diuretics and calcium channel blockers.

CONTRAINDICATIONS

TEVETEN® Tablets are contraindicated in patients who are hypersensitive to this product or any of its components.

WARNINGS

Fetal/Neonatal Morbidity and Mortality

Drugs that act directly on the renin-angiotensin system can cause fetal and neonatal morbidity and death when administered to pregnant women. Several dozen cases have been reported in the world literature in patients who were taking angiotensin-converting enzyme inhibitors. When pregnancy is detected, TEVETEN® (eprosartan mesylate) Tablets should be discontinued as soon as possible.

The use of drugs that act directly on the renin-angiotensin system during the second and third trimesters of pregnancy has been associated with fetal and neonatal injury, including hypotension, neonatal skull hypoplasia, anuria, reversible or irreversible renal failure, and death. Oligohydramnios has also been reported, presumably resulting from decreased fetal renal function; oligohydramnios in this setting has been associated with fetal limb contractures, craniofacial deformation, and hypoplastic lung development. Prematurity, intrauterine growth retardation, and patent ductus arteriosus have also been reported, although it is not clear whether these occurrences were due to exposure to the drug.

These adverse effects do not appear to have resulted from intrauterine drug exposure that has been limited to the first trimester. Mothers whose embryos and fetuses are exposed to an angiotensin II receptor antagonist only during the first trimester should be so informed. Nonetheless, when patients become pregnant, physicians should advise the patient to discontinue the use of eprosartan as soon as possible.

Rarely (probably less often than once in every thousand pregnancies), no alternative to a drug acting on the renin-angiotensin system will be found. In these rare cases, the mothers should be apprised of the potential hazards to their fetuses, and serial ultrasound examinations should be performed to assess the intra-amniotic environment.

If oligohydramnios is observed, TEVETEN® Tablets should be discontinued unless it is considered life-saving for the mother. Contraction stress testing (CST), a nonstress test (NST) or biophysical profiling (BPP) may be appropriate, depending upon the week of pregnancy. Patients and physicians should be aware, however, that oligohydramnios may not appear until after the fetus has sustained irreversible injury.

Infants with histories of *in utero* exposure to an angiotensin II receptor antagonist should be closely observed for hypotension, oliguria, and hyperkalemia. If oliguria occurs, attention should be directed toward support of blood pressure and renal perfusion. Exchange transfusion or dialysis may be required as means of reversing hypotension and/or substituting for disordered renal function.

Eprosartan mesylate has been shown to produce maternal and fetal toxicities (maternal and fetal mortality, low maternal body weight and food consumption, resorptions, abortions and litter loss) in pregnant rabbits given oral doses as low as 10 mg eprosartan/kg/day. No maternal or fetal adverse effects were observed at 3 mg/kg/day; this oral dose yielded a systemic exposure (AUC) to unbound eprosartan 0.8 times that achieved in humans given 400 mg b.i.d. No adverse effects on *in utero* or postnatal development and maturation of offspring were observed when eprosartan mesylate was administered to pregnant rats at oral doses up to 1000 mg eprosartan/kg/day (the 1000 mg eprosartan/kg/day dose in non-pregnant rats yielded systemic exposure to unbound eprosartan approximately 0.6 times the exposure achieved in humans given 400 mg b.i.d.).

Hypotension in Volume- and/or Salt-Depleted Patients

In patients with an activated renin-angiotensin system, such as volume- and/or salt-depleted patients (e.g., those being treated with diuretics), symptomatic hypotension may occur. These conditions should be corrected prior to administration of TEVETEN® Tablets, or the treatment should start under close medical supervision. If hypotension occurs, the patient should be placed in the supine position and, if necessary, given an intravenous infusion of normal saline. A transient hypotensive response is not a contraindication to further treatment, which usually can be continued without difficulty once the blood pressure has stabilized.

PRECAUTIONS

Risk of Renal Impairment

As a consequence of inhibiting the renin-angiotensin-aldosterone system, changes in renal function have been reported in susceptible individuals treated with angiotensin II antagonists; in some patients, these changes in renal function were reversible upon discontinuation of therapy. In patients whose renal function may depend on the activity of the renin-angiotensin-aldosterone system (e.g., patients with severe congestive heart failure), treatment with angiotensin-converting enzyme inhibitors and angiotensin II receptor antagonists has been associated with oliguria and/or progressive azotemia and (rarely) with acute renal failure and/or death. TEVETEN® (eprosartan mesylate) Tablets would be expected to behave similarly.

In studies of ACE inhibitors in patients with unilateral or bilateral renal artery stenosis, increases in serum creatinine or BUN have been reported. Similar effects have been reported in angiotensin II antagonists; in some patients, these effects were reversible upon discontinuation of therapy.

Information for Patients

Pregnancy: Female patients of childbearing age should be told about the consequences of second- and third-trimester exposure to drugs that act on the renin-angiotensin system, and they should also be told that these consequences do not appear to have resulted from intrauterine drug exposure that has been limited to the first trimester. These patients should be asked to report pregnancies to their physicians as soon as possible so that treatment may be discontinued under medical supervision.

Drug Interactions

Eprosartan has been shown to have no effect on the pharmacokinetics of digoxin and the pharmacodynamics of warfarin and glyburide. Thus, no dosing adjustments are necessary during concomitant use with these agents. Because eprosartan is not metabolized by the cytochrome P450 system, inhibitors of CYP450 enzyme would not be expected to affect its metabolism, and ketoconazole and fluconazole, potent inhibitors of CYP3A and 2C9, respectively, have been shown to have no effect on eprosartan pharmacokinetics. Ranitidine also has no effect on eprosartan pharmacokinetics.

Eprosartan (up to 400 mg b.i.d. or 800 mg q.d.) doses have been safely used concomitantly with a thiazide diuretic (hydrochlorothiazide). Eprosartan doses of up to 300 mg b.i.d. have been safely used concomitantly with sustained-release calcium channel blockers (sustained-release nifedipine) with no clinically significant adverse interactions.

Carcinogenesis, Mutagenesis, Impairment of Fertility

Eprosartan mesylate was not carcinogenic in dietary restricted rats or *ad libitum* fed mice dosed at 600 mg and 2000 mg eprosartan/kg/day, respectively, for up to 2 years. In male and female rats, the systemic exposure (AUC) to unbound eprosartan at the dose evaluated was only approximately 20% of the exposure achieved in humans given 400 mg b.i.d. In mice, the systemic exposure (AUC) to unbound eprosartan was approximately 25 times the exposure achieved in humans given 400 mg b.i.d.

Eprosartan mesylate was not mutagenic *in vitro* in bacteria or mammalian cells (mouse lymphoma assay). Eprosartan mesylate also did not cause structural chromosomal damage *in vivo* (mouse micronucleus assay). In human peripheral lymphocytes *in vitro*, eprosartan mesylate was equivocal for clastogenicity with metabolic activation, and was negative without metabolic activation. In the same assay, eprosartan mesylate was positive for polyploidy with metabolic activation and equivocal for polyploidy without metabolic activation.

Eprosartan mesylate had no adverse effects on the reproductive performance of male or female rats at oral doses up to 1000 mg eprosartan/kg/day. This dose provided systemic exposure (AUC) to unbound eprosartan approximately 0.6 times the exposure achieved in humans given 400 mg b.i.d.

Pregnancy

Pregnancy Category C (first trimester) and D (second and third trimesters): See WARNINGS: Fetal/Neonatal Morbidity and Mortality.

Nursing Mothers

Eprosartan is excreted in animal milk; it is not known whether eprosartan is excreted in human milk. Because many drugs are excreted in human milk and because of the potential for serious adverse reactions in nursing infants from eprosartan, a decision should be made whether to discontinue nursing or to discontinue the drug, taking into account the importance of the drug to the mother.

Pediatric Use

Safety and effectiveness in pediatric patients have not been established.

Geriatric Use

Of the total number of patients receiving TEVETEN® Tablets in clinical studies, 29% (681 of 2,334) were 65 years and over, while 5% (124 of 2,334) were 75 years and over. Based on the pooled data from randomized trials, the decrease in diastolic blood pressure and systolic blood pressure with TEVETEN® Tablets was slightly less in patients ≥65 years of age compared to younger patients. In a study of only patients over the age of 65, TEVETEN® Tablets at 200 mg twice daily (and increased optionally up to 300 mg twice daily) decreased diastolic blood pressure on average by 3 mmHg (placebo corrected). Adverse experiences were similar in younger and older patients.

ADVERSE REACTIONS

TEVETEN® Tablets have been evaluated for safety in more than 3,300 healthy volunteers and patients worldwide, including more than 1,460 patients treated for more than 6 months, and more than 980 patients treated for 1 year or longer. TEVETEN® Tablets were well tolerated at doses up to 1200 mg daily. Most adverse events were of mild or moderate severity and did not require discontinuation of therapy. The overall incidence of adverse experiences and the incidences of specific adverse events reported with eprosartan were similar to placebo.

Adverse experiences were similar in patients regardless of age, gender, or race. Adverse experiences were not dose-related.

In placebo-controlled clinical trials, about 4% of 1,202 of patients treated with TEVETEN® Tablets discontinued therapy due to clinical adverse experiences, compared to 6.5% of 352 patients given placebo.

Adverse Events Occurring at an Incidence of 1% or More Among Eprosartan-treated Patients: The following table lists adverse events that occurred at an incidence of 1% or more among eprosartan-treated patients who participated in placebo-controlled trials of 8 to 13 weeks' duration, using doses of 25 mg to 400 mg twice daily, and 400 mg to 1200 mg once daily. The overall incidence of adverse events reported with TEVETEN® Tablets (54.4%) was similar to placebo (52.8%).

Table 1. Adverse Events Reported by ≥1% of Patients Receiving TEVETEN® (eprosartan mesylate) Tablets and Were More Frequent on Eprosartan than Placebo

Event	Incidence Eprosartan (n=1,202) %	Placebo (n=352) %
Body as a Whole		
Infection viral	2	1
Injury	2	1
Fatigue	2	1
Gastrointestinal		
Abdominal pain	2	1
Metabolic and Nutritional		
Hypertriglyceridemia	1	0
Musculoskeletal		
Arthralgia	2	1
Nervous System		
Depression	1	0
Respiratory		
Upper respiratory tract infection	8	5
Rhinitis	4	3
Pharyngitis	4	3
Coughing	4	3
Urogenital		
Urinary tract infection	1	0

The following adverse events were also reported at a rate of 1% or greater in patients treated with eprosartan, but were as, or more, frequent in the placebo group: headache, myalgia, dizziness, sinusitis, diarrhea, bronchitis, dependent edema, dyspepsia, chest pain.

Facial edema was reported in 5 patients receiving eprosartan. Angioedema has been reported with other angiotensin II antagonists.

In addition to the adverse events above, potentially important events that occurred in at least two patients/subjects exposed to eprosartan or other adverse events that occurred in <1% of patients in clinical studies are listed below. It cannot be determined whether events were causally related to eprosartan:

Body as a Whole: alcohol intolerance, asthenia, substernal chest pain, peripheral edema, fatigue, fever, hot flushes, influenza-like symptoms, malaise, rigors, pain;
Cardiovascular: angina pectoris, bradycardia, abnormal ECG, specific abnormal ECG, extrasystoles, atrial fibrillation, hypotension, tachycardia, palpitations;
Gastrointestinal: anorexia, constipation, dry mouth, esophagitis, flatulence, gastritis, gastroenteritis, gingivitis, nausea, periodontitis, toothache, vomiting;
Hematologic: anemia purpura;
Liver and Biliary: increased SGOT, increased SGPT;
Metabolic and Nutritional: increased creatine phosphokinase, diabetes mellitus, glycosuria, gout, hypercholesterolemia, hyperglycemia, hyperkalemia, hypokalemia, hyponatremia;
Musculoskeletal: arthritis, aggravated arthritis, arthrosis, skeletal pain, tendinitis, back pain;
Nervous System/Psychiatric: anxiety, ataxia, insomnia, migraine, neuritis, nervousness, paresthesia, somnolence, tremor, vertigo;
Resistance Mechanism: herpes simplex, otitis externa, otitis media, upper respiratory tract infection;
Respiratory: asthma, epistaxis;
Skin and Appendages: eczema, furunculosis, pruritus, rash, maculopapular rash, increased sweating;
Special Senses: conjunctivitis, abnormal vision, xerophthalmia, tinnitus;
Urinary: albuminuria, cystitis, hematuria, micturition frequency, polyuria, renal calculus, urinary incontinence;
Vascular: leg cramps, peripheral ischemia.

Laboratory Test Findings: In placebo-controlled studies, clinically important changes in standard laboratory parameters were rarely associated with administration of TEVETEN® (eprosartan mesylate) Tablets. Patients were rarely withdrawn from TEVETEN® Tablets because of laboratory test results.

Creatinine, Blood Urea Nitrogen: Minor elevations in creatinine and in BUN occurred in 0.6% and 1.3%, respectively, of patients taking TEVETEN® Tablets and 0.9% and 0.3%, respectively, of patients given placebo in controlled clinical trials. Two patients were withdrawn from clinical trials for elevations in serum creatinine and BUN, and three additional patients were withdrawn for increases in serum creatinine.

Liver Function Tests: Minor elevations of ALAT, ASAT, and alkaline phosphatase occurred for comparable percentages of patients taking TEVETEN® (eprosartan mesylate) Tablets or placebo in controlled clinical trials. An elevated ALAT of >3.5 × ULN occurred in 0.1% of patients taking TEVETEN® Tablets (one patient) and in no patient given placebo in controlled clinical trials. Four patients were withdrawn from clinical trials for an elevation in liver function tests.

Hemoglobin: A greater than 20% decrease in hemoglobin was observed in 0.1% of patients taking TEVETEN® Tablets (one patient) and in no patient given placebo in controlled clinical trials. Two patients were withdrawn from clinical trials for anemia.

Leukopenia: A WBC count of $\leq 3.0 \times 10^3/mm^3$ occurred in 0.3% of patients taking TEVETEN® Tablets and in 0.3% of patients given placebo in controlled clinical trials. One patient was withdrawn from clinical trials for leukopenia.

Neutropenia: A neutrophil count of $\leq 1.5 \times 10^3/mm^3$ occurred in 1.3% of patients taking TEVETEN® Tablets and in 1.4% of patients given placebo in controlled clinical trials. No patient was withdrawn from any clinical trials for neutropenia.

Thrombocytopenia: A platelet count of $\leq 100 \times 10^9/L$ occurred in 0.3% of patients taking TEVETEN® Tablets (one patient) and in no patient given placebo in controlled clinical trials. Four patients receiving TEVETEN® Tablets in clinical trials were withdrawn for thrombocytopenia. In one

Continued on next page

Teveten—Cont.

case, thrombocytopenia was present prior to dosing with TEVETEN® Tablets.

Serum Potassium: A potassium value of ≥5.6 mmol/L occurred in 0.9% of patients taking TEVETEN® Tablets and 0.3% of patients given placebo in controlled clinical trials. One patient was withdrawn from clinical trials for hyperkalemia and three for hypokalemia.

OVERDOSAGE

Limited data are available regarding overdosage. Appropriate symptomatic and supportive therapy should be given if overdosage should occur. There was no mortality in rats and mice receiving oral doses of up to 3000 mg eprosartan/kg and in dogs receiving oral doses of up to 1000 mg eprosartan/kg.

DOSAGE AND ADMINISTRATION

The usual recommended starting dose of TEVETEN® Tablets is 600 mg once daily when used as monotherapy in patients who are not volume-depleted (see WARNINGS, Hypotension in Volume- and/or Salt-Depleted Patients). TEVETEN® Tablets can be administered once or twice daily and total daily doses ranging from 400 mg to 800 mg. There is limited experience with doses beyond 800 mg/day.

If the antihypertensive effect measured at trough using once-daily dosing is inadequate, a twice-a-day regimen at the same total daily dose or an increase in dose may give a more satisfactory response. Achievement of maximum blood pressure reduction in most patients may take 2 to 3 weeks.

TEVETEN® Tablets may be used in combination with other antihypertensive agents such as thiazide diuretics or calcium channel blockers if additional blood-pressure-lowering effect is required. Discontinuation of treatment with eprosartan does not lead to a rapid rebound increase in blood pressure.

Elderly, Hepatically Impaired or Renally Impaired Patients: No initial dosing adjustment is generally necessary for elderly or hepatically impaired patients or those with renal impairment.

TEVETEN® Tablets may be taken with or without food.

HOW SUPPLIED

TEVETEN® (eprosartan mesylate) Tablets are available as aqueous film-coated tablets as follows:

400 mg pink, scored Tiltab®, oval tablets debossed with 5044 on both sides of the tablet.

NDC 0051-5044-01 (bottles of 100)

NDC 0051-5044-42 (unit dose box of 50)

600 mg white, non-scored, capsule-shaped tablets, debossed with "SOLVAY" on one side and 5046 on the other.

NDC 0051-5046-01 (bottles of 100)

NDC 0051-5046-42 (unit dose box of 50)

STORAGE

Store at controlled room temperature 20° to 25°C (68° to 77°F) [see USP].

Rx only

Manufactured by:
SmithKline Beecham Pharmaceuticals
Crawley, UK

Marketed by:
UNIMED Pharmaceuticals, Inc.,
A Solvay Pharmaceuticals, Inc. Company,
Buffalo Grove, IL 60089-1862

2E Rev 11/99
Printed in U.S.A.
50186US3

Shown in Product Identification Guide, page 339

Upsher-Smith Laboratories, Inc.

14905 23RD AVE. NORTH
MINNEAPOLIS, MN 55447

For Medical Information Contact:
Write: Professional Services Department
or call: (800) 654-2299
(during business hours-8:00 am to 5:00 pm CST)

ALTINAC™ Cream ℞

[*ăll-tĭn-ăc*]

(Tretinoin Cream, USP)

DESCRIPTION

Altinac™ Cream (Tretinoin Cream, USP) is used for the topical treatment of acne vulgaris. Each gram of Altinac™ Cream contains tretinoin in either of three strengths, 0.1% (1 mg), 0.05% (0.5 mg), or 0.025% (0.25 mg) in a hydrophilic cream vehicle which includes the following inactive ingredients: stearic acid, isopropyl myristate, polyoxyl 40 stearate, stearyl alcohol, xanthan gum, sorbic acid, butylated hydroxytoluene, and purified water. Chemically, tretinoin is *all-trans*-retinoic acid.

HOW SUPPLIED

Altinac™ Cream (Tretinoin Cream, USP) is supplied as (NDC 0245-9045-22) 0.025%, 20g; (NDC 0245-9045-19) 0.025%, 45g; (NDC 0245-9047-22) 0.05%, 20g; (NDC 0245-9047-19) 0.05%, 45g; (NDC 0245-9049-22) 0.1%, 20g; (NDC 0245-9049-19) 0.1%, 45g.

FOLGARD™ Tablets OTC

[*fōl'-gärd*]

Folic Acid, Vitamin B-6, Vitamin B-12 Combination Dietary Supplement

DESCRIPTION

Folgard™ is a unique formulation of 800 mcg folic acid, 10 mg vitamin B-6 and 115 mcg vitamin B-12. Taking a folic acid supplement can mask a B-vitamin deficiency. Folgard™ includes vitamin B-6 and B-12 to help ensure that this does not occur.

HOW SUPPLIED

Bottles of 60 tablets: List No. 0245-0017-60

KLOR-CON® POWDER ℞

[*klōr 'kon*]

Potassium Chloride for Oral Solution, USP
20 mEq (1.5 g) per packet

DESCRIPTION

Each packet contains 1.5 g potassium chloride providing potassium 20 mEq and chloride 20 mEq. Fruit-flavored with artificial color and sweetener (saccharin) added.

HOW SUPPLIED

KLOR-CON® Powder 20 mEq: Cartons of 30 and 100 packets.

30's NDC 0245-0035-30, 100's NDC 0245-0035-01

KLOR-CON®/25 POWDER ℞

[*klōr 'kon*]

Potassium Chloride for Oral Solution, USP
25 mEq (1.875 g) per packet

DESCRIPTION

Each packet contains 1.875 g potassium chloride providing potassium 25 mEq and chloride 25 mEq. Fruit-flavored with artificial color and sweetener (saccharin) added.

HOW SUPPLIED

KLOR-CON®/25 Powder 25 mEq:
Cartons of 30, 100 and 250 packets.
30's NDC 0245-0037-30, 100's NDC 0245-0037-01

KLOR-CON® 8/KLOR-CON® 10 ℞

[*klōr 'kon*]

Potassium Chloride
Extended-release Tablets, USP
8 mEq and 10 mEq

DESCRIPTION

KLOR-CON® Extended-release Tablets, USP are a solid oral dosage form of potassium chloride. Each contains 600 mg or 750 mg of potassium chloride equivalent to 8 mEq or 10 mEq of potassium in a wax matrix tablet. This formulation is intended to slow the release of potassium so that the likelihood of a high localized concentration of potassium chloride within the gastrointestinal tract is reduced.

HOW SUPPLIED

Film coated, Klor-Con® 8 (blue), Klor-Con® 10 (yellow), imprinted round tablets containing:

600 mg potassium chloride (equivalent to 8 mEq) in bottles of 100 (NDC 0245-0040-11), bottles of 500 (NDC 0245-0040-15), unit-dose packages of 100 (NDC 0245-0040-01) and bulk packs of 5,000 for repack only (NDC 0245-0040-55).

750 mg potassium chloride (equivalent to 10 mEq) in bottles of 100 (NDC 0245-0041-11), bottles of 500 (NDC 0245-0041-15), unit-dose packages of 100 (NDC 0245-0041-01) and bulk packs of 5,000 for repack only (NDC 0245-0041-55).

Shown in Product Identification Guide, page 339

KLOR-CON®/EF 25mEq ℞

[*klōr 'kon*]

Potassium Bicarbonate Effervescent Tablets for Oral Solution, USP

DESCRIPTION

Each effervescent tablet in solution provides 25 mEq (978 mg) potassium as bicarbonate and citrate. Fruit-flavored with artificial color and sweetener (saccharin) added.

HOW SUPPLIED

KLOR-CON®/EF 25 mEq effervescent tablets in cartons of 30 and 100 individually wrapped tablets.

30's NDC 0245-0039-30, 100's NDC 0245-0039-01

NIACOR® ℞

[*nī 'ă-kōr*]

NIACIN TABLETS, USP
500 mg

DESCRIPTION

Niacin or nicotinic acid, a water-soluble B-complex vitamin and antihyperlipidemic agent, is 3-pyridinecarboxylic acid. Each NIACOR® tablet, for oral administration, contains 500 mg of nicotinic acid.

HOW SUPPLIED

NIACOR® is available in bottles of 100 tablets (NDC 0245-0067-11).

PACERONE® ℞

[*pă-sĕ-rōn*]

(Amiodarone HCl)
Tablets, 200 mg

DESCRIPTION

Pacerone® (Amiodarone HCl) Tablets are a member of a new class of antiarrhythmic drugs with predominantly Class III (Vaughan Williams' classification) effects, available for oral administration as pink, scored tablets containing 200 mg of amiodarone hydrochloride. The inactive ingredients present are lactose monohydrate, magnesium stearate, povidone, pregelatinized corn starch, sodium starch glycolate, stearic acid, FD&C Red 40 and FD&C Yellow 6.

Amiodarone hydrochloride, the active ingredient in Pacerone®, is a benzofuran derivative: 2-butyl-3-benzofuranyl 4-[2-(diethylamino)-ethoxy]-3,5-diiodophenyl ketone hydrochloride. It is not chemically related to any other available antiarrhythmic drug.

The structural formula is as follows:

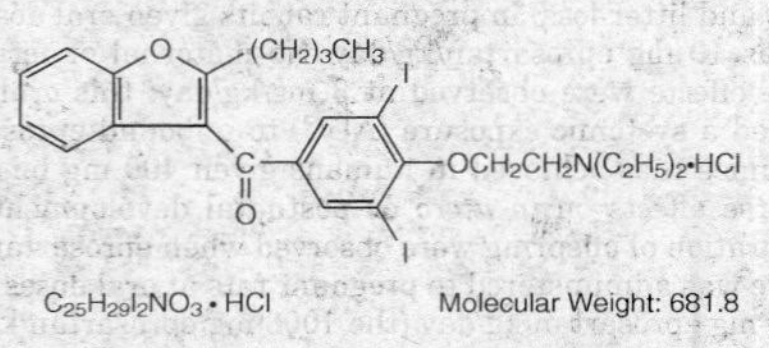

$(CH_2)_3CH_3$; $-OCH_2CH_2N(C_2H_5)_2 \cdot HCl$

$C_{25}H_{29}I_2NO_3 \cdot HCl$ Molecular Weight: 681.8

Amiodarone HCl is a white to cream-colored crystalline powder. It is slightly soluble in water, soluble in alcohol and freely soluble in chloroform. It contains 37.3% iodine by weight.

CLINICAL PHARMACOLOGY

Electrophysiology/Mechanisms of Action

In animals, amiodarone HCl is effective in the prevention or suppression of experimentally-induced arrhythmias. The antiarrhythmic effect of amiodarone may be due to at least two major properties; 1) a prolongation of the myocardial cell-action potential duration and refractory period and 2) non-competitive alpha- and beta-adrenergic inhibition.

Amiodarone prolongs the duration of the action potential of all cardiac fibers while causing minimal reduction of dV/dt (maximal upstroke velocity of the action potential). The refractory period is prolonged in all cardiac tissues. Amiodarone increases the cardiac refractory period without influencing resting membrane potential, except in automatic cells where the slope of the prepotential is reduced, generally reducing automaticity. These electrophysiologic effects are reflected in a decreased sinus rate of 15 to 20%, increased PR and QT intervals of about 10%, the development of U-waves and changes in T-wave contour. These changes should not require discontinuation of Pacerone® as they are evidence of its pharmacological action, although amiodarone can cause marked sinus bradycardia or sinus arrest and heart block. On rare occasions, QT prolongation has been associated with worsening of arrhythmia (see "**WARNINGS**").

Hemodynamics

In animal studies and after intravenous administration in man, amiodarone relaxes vascular smooth muscle, reduces peripheral vascular resistance (afterload) and slightly increases cardiac index. After oral dosing, however, amiodarone produces no significant change in left ventricular ejection fraction (LVEF), even in patients with depressed LVEF. After acute intravenous dosing in man, amiodarone may have a mild negative inotropic effect.

Pharmacodynamics

Following oral administration in man, amiodarone is slowly and variably absorbed. The bioavailability of amiodarone is approximately 50%, but has varied between 35 and 65% in various studies. Maximum plasma concentrations are attained 3 to 7 hours after a single dose. Despite this, the onset of action may occur in 2 to 3 days, but more commonly takes 1 to 3 weeks, even with loading doses. Plasma concentrations with chronic dosing at 100 to 600 mg/day are approximately dose proportional, with a mean 0.5 mg/L increase for each 100 mg/day. These means, however, include considerable individual variability. Food increases the rate and extent of absorption of amiodarone. The effects of food upon the bioavailability of amiodarone have been studied in 30 healthy subjects who received a single 600 mg dose immediately after consuming a high fat meal and following an overnight fast. The area under the plasma concentration-time curve (AUC) and the peak plasma concentration (C_{max}) of amiodarone increased by 2.3 (range 1.7 to 3.6) and 3.8

(range 2.7 to 4.4) times, respectively, in the presence of food. Food also increased the rate of absorption of amiodarone, decreasing the time to peak plasma concentration (T_{max}) by 37%. The mean AUC and mean C_{max} of desethylamiodarone increased by 55% (range 58 to 101%) and 32% (range 4 to 84%), respectively, but there was no change in the T_{max} in the presence of food.
Amiodarone has a very large but variable volume of distribution, averaging about 60 L/kg, because of extensive accumulation in various sites, especially adipose tissue and highly perfused organs, such as the liver, lung and spleen. One major metabolite of amiodarone, desethylamiodarone (DEA), has been identified in man; it accumulates to an even greater extent in almost all tissues. No data are available on the activity of DEA in humans, but in animals, it has significant electrophysiologic and antiarrhythmic effects generally similar to amiodarone itself. DEA's precise role and contribution to the antiarrhythmic activity of oral amiodarone are not certain. The development of maximal ventricular Class III effects after oral amiodarone administration in humans correlates more closely with DEA accumulation over time than with amiodarone accumulation.
Amiodarone is eliminated primarily by hepatic metabolism and biliary excretion and there is negligible excretion of amiodarone or DEA in urine. Neither amiodarone nor DEA is dialyzable.
In clinical studies of 2 to 7 days, clearance of amiodarone after intravenous administration in patients with VT and VP ranged between 220 and 440 mL/hr/kg. Age, sex, renal disease and hepatic disease (cirrhosis) do not have marked effects on the disposition of amiodarone or DEA. Renal impairment does not influence the pharmacokinetics of amiodarone. After a single dose of intravenous amiodarone in cirrhotic patients, significantly lower C_{max} and average concentration values are seen for DEA, but mean amiodarone levels are unchanged. Normal subjects over 65 years of age show lower concentrations (about 100 mL/hr/kg) than younger subjects (about 150 mL/hr/kg) and an increase in $t_{1/2}$ from about 20 to 47 days.
In patients with severe left ventricular disposition, the pharmacokinetics of amiodarone are not significantly altered but the terminal disposition $t_{1/2}$ of DEA is prolonged. Although no dosage adjustment for patients with renal, hepatic or cardiac abnormalities has been defined during chronic treatment with amiodarone, close clinical monitoring is prudent for elderly patients and those with severe left ventricular dysfunction.
In patients, following discontinuation of chronic oral therapy, amiodarone has been shown to have a biphasic elimination with an initial one-half reduction of plasma levels after 2.5 to 10 days. A much slower terminal plasma-elimination phase shows a half-life of the parent compound ranging from 26 to 107 days, with a mean of approximately 53 days and most patients in the 40- to 55-day range. In the absence of a loading-dose period, steady-state plasma concentrations, at constant oral dosing, would therefore be reached between 130 and 535 days, with an average of 265 days. For the metabolite, the mean plasma-elimination half-life was approximately 61 days. These data probably reflect an initial elimination of drug from well-perfused tissue (the 2.5- to 10-day half-life phase), followed by a terminal phase representing extremely slow elimination from poorly perfused tissue compartments such as fat.
Following single dose administration in 12 healthy subjects, amiodarone exhibited multi-compartmental pharmacokinetics with a mean apparent plasma terminal elimination half-life of 58 days (range 15 to 142 days) for amiodarone and 36 days (range 14 to 75 days) for the active metabolite (DEA). The considerable intersubject variation in both phases of elimination, as well as uncertainty as to what compartment is critical to drug effect, requires attention to individual responses once arrhythmia control is achieved with loading doses because the correct maintenance dose is determined, in part, by the elimination rates. Daily maintenance doses of Pacerone® should be based on individual patient requirements (see "**DOSAGE AND ADMINISTRATION**").
Amiodarone and its metabolite have a limited transplacental transfer of approximately 10 to 50%. The parent drug and its metabolite have been detected in breast milk.
Amiodarone is highly protein-bound (approximately 96%).
Although electrophysiologic effects, such as prolongation QTc, can be seen within hours after a parenteral dose of amiodarone, effects on abnormal rhythms are not seen before 2 to 3 days and usually require 1 to 3 weeks, even when a loading dose is used. There may be a continued increase in effect for longer periods still. There is evidence that the time to effect is shorter when a loading-dose regimen is used.
Consistent with the slow rate of elimination, antiarrhythmic effects persist for weeks or months after Pacerone® is discontinued, but the time of recurrence is variable and unpredictable. In general, when the drug is resumed after recurrence of the arrhythmia, control is established relatively rapidly compared to the initial response, presumably because tissue stores were not wholly depleted at the time of recurrence.

Pharmacodynamics

There is no well-established relationship of plasma concentration to effectiveness, but it does appear that concentrations much below 1 mg/L are often ineffective and that levels above 2.5 mg/L are generally not needed. Within individuals, dose reductions and ensuing decreased plasma concentrations can result in loss of arrhythmia control. Plasma-concentration measurements can be used to identify patients whose levels are unusually low, and who might benefit from a dose increase, or unusually high, and who might have dosage reduction in the hope of minimizing side effects. Some observations have suggested a plasma concentration, dose or dose/duration relationship for side effects such as pulmonary fibrosis, liver-enzyme elevations, corneal deposits and facial pigmentation, peripheral neuropathy, gastrointestinal and central nervous system effects.

Monitoring Effectiveness

Predicting the effectiveness of any antiarrhythmic agent in long-term prevention of recurrent ventricular tachycardia and ventricular fibrillation is difficult and controversial, with highly qualified investigators recommending use of ambulatory monitoring, programmed electrical stimulation with various stimulation regimens, or a combination of these, to assess response. There is no present consensus on many aspects of how best to assess effectiveness, but there is a reasonable consensus on some aspects.
1. If a patient with a history of cardiac arrest does not manifest a hemodynamically unstable arrhythmia during electrocardiographic monitoring prior to treatment, assessment of the effectiveness of amiodarone requires some provocative approach, either exercise or programmed electrical stimulation (PES).
2. Whether provocation is also needed in patients who do manifest their life-threatening arrhythmias spontaneously is not settled, but there are reasons to consider PES or other provocation in such patients. In the fraction of patients whose PES-inducible arrhythmia can be made noninducible by amiodarone (a fraction that has varied widely in various series from less than 10% to almost 40%, perhaps due to different stimulation criteria), the prognosis has been almost uniformly excellent, with very low recurrence (ventricular tachycardia or sudden death) rates. More controversial is the meaning of continued inducibility. There has been an impression that continued inducibility in amiodarone patients may not fortell a poor prognosis but, in fact, many observers have found greater recurrence rates in patients who remain inducible than in those who do not. A number of criteria have been proposed, however, for identifying patients who remain inducible but who seem likely nonetheless to do well on Pacerone®. These criteria include increased difficulty of induction (more stimuli or more rapid stimuli), which has been reported to predict a lower rate of recurrence, and ability to tolerate the induced ventricular tachycardia without severe symptoms, a finding that has been reported to correlate with better survival but not with lower recurrence rates. While these criteria require confirmation and further study in general, *easier* inducibility or *poorer* tolerance of the induced arrhythmia should suggest consideration of a need to revise treatment.
Several predictors of success not based on PES have also been suggested, including complete elimination of all nonsustained ventricular tachycardia on ambulatory monitoring and very low premature ventricular-beat rates (less than 1 VPB/1,000 normal beats).
While these tissues remain unsettled for amiodarone, as for other agents, the prescriber of Pacerone® should have access to (direct or through referral), and familiarity with, the full range of evaluatory procedures used in the care of patients with life-threatening arrhythmias.
It is difficult to describe the effectiveness rates of Pacerone®, as these depend on the specific arrhythmia treated, the success criteria used, the underlying cardiac disease of the patient, the number of drugs tried before resorting to Pacerone®, the duration of follow-up, the dose of amiodarone HCl, the use of additional antiarrhythmic agents and many other factors. As amiodarone has been studied principally in patients with refractory life-threatening ventricular arrhythmias, in whom drug therapy must be selected on the basis of response and cannot be assigned arbitrarily, randomized comparisons with other agents or placebo have not been possible. Reports of series of treated patients with a history of cardiac arrest and mean follow-up of one year or more have given mortality (due to arrhythmia) rates that were highly variable, ranging from less than 5% to over 30%, with most series in the range of 10 to 15%. Overall arrhythmia-recurrence rates (fatal and nonfatal) also were highly variable (and, as noted above, depended on response to PES and other measures), and depend on whether patients who do not seem to respond initially are included. In most cases, considering only patients who seemed to respond well enough to be placed on long-term treatment, recurrence rates have ranged from 20 to 40% in series with a mean follow-up of a year or more.

INDICATIONS AND USAGE

Because of its life-threatening side effects and the substantial management difficulties associated with amiodarone use (see "**WARNINGS**" below), Pacerone® (Amiodarone HCl) Tablets are indicated only for the treatment of the following documented, life-threatening recurrent ventricular arrhythmias when these have not responded to documented adequate doses of other available antiarrhythmics or when alternative agents could not be tolerated.
1. Recurrent ventricular fibrillation.
2. Recurrent hemodynamically unstable ventricular tachycardia.
As is the case for other antiarrhythmic agents, there is no evidence from controlled trials that the use of amiodarone HCl favorably affects survival.
Pacerone® (Amiodarone HCl) Tablets should be used only by physicians familiar with and with access to (directly or through referral) the use of all available modalities for treating recurrent life-threatening ventricular arrhythmias, and who have access to appropriate monitoring facilities, including in-hospital and ambulatory continuous electrocardiographic monitoring and electrophysiologic techniques. Because of the life-threatening nature of the arrhythmias treated, potential interactions with prior therapy and potential exacerbation of the arrhythmia, initiation of therapy with Pacerone® should be carried out in the hospital.

CONTRAINDICATIONS

Pacerone® is contraindicated in severe sinus-node dysfunction, causing marked sinus bradycardia; second- and third-degree atrioventricular block; and when episodes of bradycardia have caused syncope (except when used in conjunction with a pacemaker).
Pacerone® is contraindicated in patients with a known hypersensitivity to the drug.

WARNINGS

Pacerone® is intended for use only in patients with the indicated life-threatening arrhythmias because amiodarone use is accompanied by substantial toxicity.
Amiodarone has several potentially fatal toxicities, the most important of which is pulmonary toxicity (hypersensitivity pneumonitis or interstitial/alveolar pneumonitis) that has resulted in clinically manifest disease at rates as high as 10 to 17% in some series of patients with ventricular arrhythmias given doses around 400 mg/day, and as abnormal diffusion capacity without symptoms in a much higher percentage of patients. Pulmonary toxicity has been fatal about 10% of the time. Liver injury is common with amiodarone, but is usually mild and evidenced only by abnormal liver enzymes. Overt liver disease can occur, however, and has been fatal in a few cases. Like other antiarrhythmics, amiodarone can exacerbate the arrhythmia, e.g., by making the arrhythmia less well tolerated or more difficult to reverse. This has occurred in 2 to 5% of patients in various series, and significant heart block or sinus bradycardia has been seen in 2 to 5%. All of these events should be manageable in the proper clinical setting in most cases. Although the frequency of such proarrhythmic events does not appear greater with amiodarone than with many other agents used in this population, the effects are prolonged when they occur. Even in patients at high risk of arrhythmic death, in whom the toxicity of amiodarone is an acceptable risk, Pacerone® poses major management problems that could be life-threatening in a population at risk of sudden death, so that every effort should be made to utilize alternative agents first.
The difficulty of using Pacerone® effectively and safely itself poses a significant risk to patients. Patients with the indicated arrhythmias must be hospitalized while the loading dose of Pacerone® is given, and a response generally requires at least one week, usually two or more. Because absorption and elimination are variable, maintenance-dose selection is difficult, and it is not unusual to require dosage decrease of discontinuation of treatment. In a retrospective survey of 192 patients with ventricular tachyarrhythmias, 84 required dose reduction and 18 required at least temporary discontinuation because of adverse effects, and several series have reported 15 to 20% overall frequencies of discontinuation due to adverse reactions. The time at which a previously controlled life-threatening arrhythmia will recur after discontinuation or dose adjustment is unpredictable, ranging from weeks to months. The patient is obviously at great risk during this time and may need prolonged hospitalization. Attempts to substitute other antiarrhythmic agents when Pacerone® must be stopped will be made difficult by the gradually, but unpredictably, changing amiodarone body burden. A similar problem exists when amiodarone is not effective; it still poses the risk of an interaction with whatever subsequent treatment is tried.

Mortality

In the National Heart, Lung and Blood Institute's Cardiac Arrhythmia Suppression Trial (CAST), a long-term, multi-centered, randomized, double-blind study in patients with asymptomatic non-life-threatening ventricular arrhythmias who had had myocardial infarctions more than six days but less than two years previously, an excessive mortality or nonfatal cardiac arrest rate was seen in patients treated with encainide or flecainide (56/730) compared with that seen in patients assigned to matched placebo-treated groups (22/725). The average duration of treatment with encainide or flecainide in this study was ten months.
Amiodarone therapy was evaluated in two multi-centered, randomized, double-blind, placebo-controlled trials involving 1202 (Canadian Amiodarone Myocardial Infarction Arrhythmia Trial; CAMIAT) and 1486 (European Myocardial Infarction Amiodarone Trial; EMIAT) post-MI patients followed for up to 2 years. Patients in CAMIAT qualified with ventricular arrhythmias, and those randomized to amiodarone received weight- and response-adjusted doses of 200 to 400 mg/day. Patients in EMIAT qualified with ejection fraction <40%, and those randomized to amiodarone received fixed doses of 200 mg/day. Both studies had weeks-long loading dose schedules. Intent-to-treat all-cause mortality results were as follows:
[See table at bottom of next page]

Continued on next page

Pacerone—Cont.

These data are consistent with the results of a pooled analysis of smaller, controlled studies involving patients with structural heart disease (including myocardial infarction).

Pulmonary Toxicity

Amiodarone may cause a clinical syndrome of cough and progressive dyspnea accompanied by functional, radiographic, gallium scan, and pathological data consistent with pulmonary toxicity, the frequency of which varies from 2 to 7% in most published reports, but is as high as 10 to 17% in some reports. Therefore, when Pacerone® therapy is initiated, a baseline chest X-ray and pulmonary-function tests, including diffusion capacity, should be performed. The patient should return for a history, physical exam and chest X-rays every 3 to 6 months.

Preexisting pulmonary disease does not appear to increase the risk of developing pulmonary toxicity; however, these patients have a poorer prognosis if pulmonary toxicity does develop.

Pulmonary toxicity secondary to amiodarone seems to result from either indirect or direct toxicity as represented by hypersensitivity pneumonitis or interstitial/alveolar pneumonitis, respectively.

Hypersensitivity pneumonitis usually appears earlier in the course of therapy and rechallenging these patients with Pacerone® results in a more rapid recurrence of greater severity. Bronchoalveolar lavage is the procedure of choice to confirm this diagnosis, which can be made when a T suppressor/cytotoxic (CD8-positive) lymphocytosis is noted. Steroid therapy should be instituted and Pacerone® therapy discontinued in these patients.

Interstitial/alveolar pneumonitis may result from the release of oxygen radicals and/or phospholipidosis and is characterized by findings of diffuse alveolar damage, interstitial pneumonitis or fibrosis in lung biopsy specimens. Phospholipidosis (foamy cells, foamy macrophages), due to inhibition of phospholipase, will be present in most cases of amiodarone-induced pulmonary toxicity; however, these changes also are present in approximately 50% of all patients on amiodarone therapy. These cells should be used as markers of therapy, but not as evidence of toxicity. A diagnosis of amiodarone-induced interstitial/alveolar pneumonitis should lead, at a minimum, to dose reduction or, preferably, to withdrawal of Pacerone® to establish reversibility, especially if other acceptable antiarrhythmic therapies are available. Where these measures have been instituted, a reduction in symptoms of amiodarone-induced pulmonary toxicity was usually noted within the first week, and a clinical improvement was greatest in the first two to three weeks. Chest X-ray changes usually resolve within two to four months. According to some experts, steroids may prove beneficial. Prednisone in doses of 40 to 60 mg/day or equivalent doses of other steroids have been given and tapered over the course of several weeks depending upon the condition of the patient. In some cases rechallenge with amiodarone at a lower dose has not resulted in return to toxicity. Recent reports suggest that the use of lower loading and maintenance doses of amiodarone are associated with a decreased incidence of amiodarone-induced pulmonary toxicity.

In a patient receiving Pacerone®, any new respiratory symptoms should suggest the possibility of pulmonary toxicity, and the history, physical exam, chest X-ray and pulmonary function tests (with diffusion capacity) should be repeated and evaluated. A 15% decrease in diffusion capacity has a high sensitivity but only a moderate specificity for pulmonary toxicity; as the decrease in diffusion capacity approaches 30%, the sensitivity decreases but the specificity increases. A gallium scan also may be performed as part of the diagnostic workup.

Fatalities, secondary to pulmonary toxicity, have occurred in approximately 10% of cases. However, in patients with life-threatening arrhythmias, discontinuation of Pacerone® therapy due to suspected drug-induced pulmonary toxicity should be undertaken with caution, as the most common cause of death in these patients is sudden cardiac death. Therefore, every effort should be made to rule out other causes of respiratory impairment (i.e., congestive heart failure with Swan-Ganz catherization if necessary, respiratory infection, pulmonary embolism, malignancy, etc.) before discontinuing Pacerone® in these patients. In addition, bronchoalveolar lavage, trans-bronchial lung biopsy and/or open lung biopsy may be necessary to confirm the diagnosis, especially in those cases where no acceptable alternative therapy is available.

If a diagnosis of amiodarone-induced hypersensitivity pneumonitis is made, Pacerone® should be discontinued, and treatment with steroids should be instituted. If a diagnosis of amiodarone-induced interstitial/alveolar pneumonitis is made, steroid therapy should be and, preferably, Pacerone® discontinued or, at a minimum, reduced in dosage. Some cases of amiodarone-induced interstitial/alveolar pneumonitis may resolve following a reduction in Pacerone® dosage in conjunction with the administration of steroids. In some patients, rechallenge at a lower dose has not resulted in return of interstitial/alveolar pneumonitis; however, in some patients (perhaps because of severe alveolar damage) the pulmonary lesions have not been reversible.

Worsened Arrhythmia

Amiodarone, like other antiarrhythmics, can cause serious exacerbation of the presenting arrhythmia, a risk that may be enhanced by the presence of concomitant antiarrhythmics. Exacerbation has been reported in about 2 to 5% in most series, and has included new ventricular fibrillation, incessant ventricular tachycardia, increased resistance to cardioversion and polymorphic ventricular tachycardia associated with QT prolongation (Torsade de Pointes). In addition, amiodarone has caused symptomatic bradycardia or sinus arrest with suppression of escape foci in 2 to 4% of patients.

Liver Injury

Elevations of hepatic enzyme levels are seen frequently in patients exposed to amiodarone and in most cases are asymptomatic. If the increase exceeds three times normal, or doubles in a patient with an elevated baseline, discontinuation of Pacerone® or dosage reduction should be considered. In a few cases in which biopsy has been done, the histology has resembled that of alcoholic hepatitis or cirrhosis. Hepatic failure has been a rare cause of death in patients treated with amiodarone.

Loss of Vision

Cases of optic neuropathy and/or optic neuritis, usually resulting in visual impairment, have been reported in patients treated with amiodarone. In some cases, visual impairment has progressed to permanent blindness. Optic neuropathy and/or neuritis may occur at any time following initiation of therapy. A causal relationship to the drug has not been clearly established. If symptoms of visual impairment appear, such as changes in visual acuity and decreases in peripheral vision, prompt opthalmic examination is recommended. Appearance of optic neuropathy and/or neuritis calls for re-evaluation of Pacerone® therapy. The risks and complications of antiarrhythmic therapy with Pacerone® must be weighed against its benefits in patients whose lives are threatened by cardiac arrhythmias. Regular ophthalmic examination, including fundoscopy and slit-lamp examination, is recommended during administration of Pacerone®. (See "**ADVERSE REACTIONS**").

Neonatal Hypo- or Hyperthyroidism

Amiodarone can cause fetal harm when administered to a pregnant woman. Although amiodarone use during pregnancy is uncommon, there have been a small number of published reports of congenital goiter/hypothyroidism and hyperthyroidism. If Pacerone® (Amiodarone HCl) tablets are used during pregnancy, or if the patients becomes pregnant while taking Pacerone®, the patient should be apprised of the potential hazard to the fetus.

In general, Pacerone® should be used during pregnancy only if the potential benefit to the mother justifies the unknown risk to the fetus.

In pregnant rats and rabbits, amiodarone HCl in doses of 25 mg/kg/day (approximately 0.4 and 0.9 times, respectively, the maximum recommended human maintenance dose*) had no adverse effects on the fetus. In the rabbit, 75 mg/kg/day (approximately 2.7 times the maximum recommended human maintenance dose*) caused abortions in greater than 90% of the animals. In the rat, doses of 50 mg/kg/day or more were associated with slight displacement of the testes and an increased incidence of incomplete ossification of some skull and digital bones; at 100 mg/kg/day or more, fetal body weights were reduced; at 200 mg/kg/day, there was an increased incidence of fetal resorption. (These doses in the rat are approximately 0.8, 1.6 and 3.2 times the maximum recommended human maintenance dose.*) Adverse events on fetal growth and survival also were noted in one of two strains of mice at a dose of 5 mg/kg/day (approximately 0.04 times the maximum recommended human maintenance dose*).

*600 mg in a 50 kg patient (doses compared on a body surface area basis)

PRECAUTIONS

Impairment of Vision

Optic Neuropathy and/or Neuritis

Cases of optic neuropathy and optic neuritis have been reported (see "**WARNINGS**").

Corneal Microdeposits

Corneal microdeposits appear in the majority of adults treated with amiodarone. They are usually discernible only by slit-lamp examination, but give rise to symptoms such as visual halos or blurred vision in as many as 10% of patients. Corneal microdeposits are reversible upon reduction of dose or termination of treatment. Asymptomatic microdeposits alone are not a reason to reduce dose or discontinue treatment (see "**ADVERSE REACTIONS**").

Neurologic

Chronic administration of oral amiodarone in rare instances may lead to the development of peripheral neuropathy that may resolve when amiodarone is discontinued, but this resolution has been slow and incomplete.

Photosensitivity

Amiodarone has induced photosensitization in about 10% of patients; some protection may be afforded by the use of sun-barrier creams or protective clothing. During long-term treatment, a blue-gray discoloration of the exposed skin may occur. The risk may be increased in patients of fair complexion or those with excessive sun exposure, and may be related to cumulative dose and duration of therapy.

Thyroid Abnormalities

Amiodarone inhibits peripheral conversion of thyroxine (T_4) to triiodothyronine (T_3) and may cause increased thyroxine levels, decreased T_3 levels and increased levels of inactive reverse T_3 (rT_3) in clinically euthyroid patients. It is also a potential source of large amounts of inorganic iodine. Because of its release of inorganic iodine, or perhaps for other reasons, amiodarone can cause either hypothyroidism or hyperthyroidism. Thyroid function should be monitored prior to treatment and periodically thereafter, particularly in elderly patients, and in any patient with a history of thyroid nodules, goiter or other thyroid dysfunction. Because of the slow elimination of amiodarone and its metabolites, high plasma iodide levels, altered thyroid function and abnormal thyroid-function tests may persist for several weeks or even months following Pacerone® (Amiodarone HCl) Tablets withdrawal.

Hypothyroidism has been reported in 2 to 4% of patients in most series, but in 8 to 10% in some series. This condition may be identified by relevant clinical symptoms and particularly by elevated serum TSH levels. In some clinically hypothyroid amiodarone-treated patients, free thyroxine index values may be normal. Hypothyroidism is best managed by Pacerone® dose reduction and/or thyroid hormone supplement. However, therapy must be individualized, and it may be necessary to discontinue Pacerone® in some patients.

Hyperthyroidism occurs in about 2% of patients receiving amiodarone, but the incidence may be higher among patients with prior inadequate dietary iodine intake. Amiodarone-induced hyperthyroidism usually poses a greater hazard to the patient than hypothyroidism because of the possibility of arrhythmia breakthrough or aggravation. In fact, IF ANY NEW SIGNS OF ARRHYTHMIA APPEAR, THE POSSIBILITY OF HYPERTHYROIDISM SHOULD BE CONSIDERED. Hyperthyroidism is best identified by relevant clinical symptoms and signs, accompanied usually by abnormally elevated levels of serum T_3 RIA, and further elevations of serum T_4, and a subnormal serum TSH level (using a sufficiently sensitive TSH assay). The finding of a flat TSH response to TRH is confirmatory of hyperthyroidism and may be sought in equivocal cases. Since arrhythmia breakthroughs may accompany amiodarone-induced hyperthyroidism, aggressive medical treatment is indicated, including, if possible, dose reduction or withdrawal of Pacerone®. The institution of antithyroid drugs, beta-adrenergic blockers and/or temporary corticosteroid therapy may be necessary. The action of antithyroid drugs may be especially delayed in amiodarone-induced thyrotoxicosis because of substantial quantities of preformed thyroid hormones stored in the gland. Radioactive iodine therapy is contraindicated because of the low radioiodine uptake associated with amiodarone-induced hyperthyroidism. Experience with thyroid surgery in this setting is extremely limited, and this form of therapy runs the theoretical risk of inducing thyroid storm. Amiodarone-induced hyperthyroidism may be followed by a transient period of hypothyroidism.

Surgery

Volatile Anesthetic Agents: Close perioperative monitoring is recommended in patients undergoing general anesthesia who are on amiodarone therapy as they may be more sensitive to the myocardial depressant and conduction effects of halogenated inhalational anesthetics.

Hypotension Postbypass: Rare occurrences of hypotension upon discontinuation of cardiopulmonary bypass during open-heart surgery in patients receiving amiodarone have been reported. The relationship of this event to Pacerone® therapy is unknown.

Adult Respiratory Distress Syndrome (ARDS): Postoperatively, rare occurrences of ARDS have been reported in patients receiving amiodarone therapy who have undergone either cardiac or noncardiac surgery. Although patients usually respond well to vigorous respiratory therapy, in rare instances the outcome has been fatal. Until further studies have been performed, it is recommended that FiO_2 and the determinants of oxygen therapy delivery to the tissues (e.g., SaO_2, PaO_2) be closely monitored in patients on amiodarone.

Laboratory Tests

Elevations in liver enzymes (SGOT and SGPT) can occur. Liver enzymes in patients on relatively high maintenance doses should be monitored on a regular basis. Persistent significant elevations in the liver enzymes or hepatomegaly should alert the physician to consider reducing the maintenance dose of Pacerone® or discontinuing therapy.

Amiodarone alters the results of thyroid-function tests, causing an increase in serum T_4 and serum reverse T_3, and a decline in serum T_3 levels. Despite these biochemical changes, most patients remain clinically euthyroid.

Drug Interactions

Although only a small number of drug-drug interactions with amiodarone have been explored formally, most of these have shown such an interaction. The potential for other interactions should be anticipated, particularly for drugs with potentially serious toxicity, such as other antiarrhythmics.

	Placebo		Amiodarone		Relative Risk	
	N	Deaths	N	Deaths		95% CI
EMIAT	743	102	743	103	0.99	0.76–1.31
CAMIAT	596	68	606	57	0.88	0.58–1.16

If such drugs are needed, their dose should be reassessed and, where appropriate, plasma concentration measured.
In view of the long and variable half-life of amiodarone, potential for drug interactions exists not only with concomitant medication but also with drugs administered after discontinuation of Pacerone®.

Cyclosporine
Concomitant use of amiodarone and cyclosporine has been reported to produce persistently elevated plasma concentrations of cyclosporine resulting in elevated creatinine, despite reduction in dose of cyclosporine.

Digitalis
Administration of amiodarone to patients receiving digoxin therapy regularly results in an increase in the serum digoxin concentration that may reach toxic levels with resultant clinical toxicity. **On initiation of Pacerone®, the need for digitalis therapy should be reviewed and the dose reduced by approximately 50% of discontinued.** If digitalis treatment is continued, serum levels should be closely monitored and patients observed for clinical evidence of toxicity. These precautions probably should apply to digitoxin administration as well.

Anticoagulants
Potentiation of warfarin-type anticoagulant response is almost always seen in patients receiving amiodarone and can result in serious or fatal bleeding. **The dose of the anticoagulant should be reduced by one-third to one-half, and prothrombin times should be monitored closely.**

Antiarrhythmic Agents
Other antiarrhythmic drugs, such as quinidine, procainamide, disopyramide and phenytoin, have been used concurrently with amiodarone.
There have been case reports of increased steady-state levels of quinidine, procainamide and phenytoin during concomitant therapy with amiodarone. In general, any added antiarrhythmic drug should be initiated at a lower than usual dose with careful monitoring.
In general, combination of Pacerone® (Amidarone HCl) Tablets with other antiarrhythmic therapy should be reversed for patients with life-threatening ventricular arrhythmias who are incompletely responsive to a single agent or incompletely responsive to amiodarone. During transfer to Pacerone®, the dose levels of previously administered agents should be reduced by 30 to 50% several days after the addition of Pacerone®, when arrhythmia suppression should be beginning. The continued need for the other antiarrhythmic agent should be reviewed after the effects of amiodarone have been established, and discontinuation ordinarily should be attempted. If the treatment is continued, these patients should be particularly carefully monitored for adverse effects, especially conduction disturbances and exacerbation of tachyarrhythmias, as Pacerone® is continued. In Pacerone® treated patients who require additional antiarrhythmic therapy, the initial dose of such agents should be approximately half of the usual recommended dose.
Pacerone should be used with caution in patients receiving beta-blocking agents or calcium antagonists because of the possible potentiation of bradycardia, sinus arrest and AV block; if necessary, Pacerone® can continue to be used after insertion of a pacemaker in patients with severe bradycardia or sinus arrest.
Volatile Anesthetic Agents (see "**PRECAUTIONS**, **Surgery**, *Volatile Anesthetic Agents*").
[See first table above]

SUMMARY OF DRUG INTERACTIONS WITH PACERONE®

Concomitant Drug	Interaction: Onset (days)	Interaction: Magnitude	Recommended Dose Reduction of Concomitant Drug
Warfarin	3 to 4	Increases prothrombin time by 100%	↓ 1/3 to 1/2
Digoxin	1	Increases serum concentration by 70%	↓ 1/2
Quinidine	2	Increases serum concentration by 33%	↓ 1/3 to 1/2 (or discontinue)
Procainamide	<7	Increases plasma concentration by 55%; NAPA*concentration by 33%	↓ 1/3 (or discontinue)

*NAPA = n-acetyl procainamide.

	Loading Dose (Daily)	Adjustment and Maintenance Dose (Daily)	
Ventricular Arrhythmias	1 to 3 weeks	~1 month	usual maintenance
	800 to 1,600 mg	600 to 800 mg	400 mg

Electrolyte Disturbances
Since antiarrhythmic drugs may be ineffective or may be arrhythmogenic in patients with hypokalemia, any potassium or magnesium deficiency should be corrected before instituting Pacerone® therapy.

Carcinogenesis, Mutagenesis, Impairment of Fertility
Amiodarone HCl was associated with a statistically significant, dose-related increase in the incidence of thyroid tumors (follicular adenoma and/or carcinoma) in rats. The incidence of thyroid tumors was greater than control even at the lowest dose level tested, i.e., 5 mg/kg/day (approximately 0.08 times the maximum recommended human maintenance dose*).
Mutagenicity studies (Ames, micronucleus and lysogenic tests) with amiodarone were negative. In a study in which amiodarone HCl was administered to male and female rats, beginning 9 weeks prior to mating, reduced fertility was observed at a dose level of 90 mg/kg/day (approximately 1.4 times the maximum recommended human maintenance dose*).

*600 mg in a 50 kg patient (dose compared on a body surface area basis)

Pregnancy: Pregnancy Category D
See "**WARNINGS, Neonatal Hypo- or Hyperthyroidism**".

Labor and Delivery
It is not known whether the use of Pacerone® (Amiodarone HCl) Tablets during labor or delivery has any immediate or delayed adverse effects. Preclinical studies in rodents have not shown any effect of amiodarone on the duration of gestation or on parturition.

Nursing Mothers
Amiodarone is excreted in human milk, suggesting that breast-feeding could expose the nursing infant to a significant dose of the drug. Nursing offspring of lactating rats administered amiodarone have been shown to be less viable and have reduced body-weight gains. Therefore, when Pacerone® therapy is indicated, the mother should be advised to discontinue nursing.

Pediatric Use
The safety and effectiveness of Pacerone® in pediatric patients have not been established.

Geriatric Use
Clinical studies of amiodarone tablets did not include sufficient numbers of subjects aged 65 and over to determine whether they respond differently from younger subjects. Other reported clinical experience has not identified differences in responses between the elderly and younger patients. In general, dose selection for an elderly patient should be cautious, usually starting at the low end of the dosing range, reflecting the greater frequency of decreased hepatic, renal or cardiac function, and of concomitant disease or other drug therapy.

ADVERSE REACTIONS

Adverse reactions have been very common in virtually all series of patients treated with amiodarone HCl for ventricular arrhythmias with relatively large doses of drug (400 mg/day and above), occurring in about three-fourths of all patients and causing discontinuation in 7 to 18%. The most serious reactions are pulmonary toxicity, exacerbation of arrhythmia and rare serious liver injury (see "**WARNINGS**"), but other adverse effects constitute important problems. They are often reversible with dose reduction or cessation of amiodarone treatment. Most of the adverse effects appear to become more frequent with continued treatment beyond six months, although rates appear to remain relatively constant beyond one year. The time and dose relationships of adverse effects are under continued study.
Neurologic problems are extremely common, occurring in 20 to 40% of patients and including malaise and fatigue, tremor and involuntary movements, poor coordination and gait, and peripheral neuropathy; they are rarely a reason to stop therapy and may respond to dose reductions or discontinuation (see "**PRECAUTIONS**").
Gastrointestinal complaints, most commonly nausea, vomiting, constipation and anorexia, occur in about 25% of patients but rarely require discontinuation of drug. These commonly occur during high-dose administration (i.e, loading dose) and usually respond to dose reduction or divided doses.
Ophthalmic abnormalities including optic neuropathy and/or optic neuritis, in some cases progressing to permanent blindness, papilledema, corneal degeneration, photosensitivity, eye discomfort, scotoma, lens opacities and macular degeneration, have been reported. (See "**WARNINGS**".)
Asymptomatic corneal microdeposits are present in virtually all adult patients who have been on drug for more than 6 months. Some patients develop eye symptoms of halos, photophobia and dry eyes. Vision is rarely affected and drug discontinuation is rarely needed.
Dermatological adverse reactions occur in about 15% of patients, with photosensitivity being most common (about 10%). Sunscreen and protection from sun exposure may be helpful, and drug discontinuation is not usually necessary. Prolonged exposure to amiodarone occasionally results in blue-gray pigmentation. This is slowly and occasionally incompletely reversible on discontinuation of drug but is of cosmetic importance only.
Cardiovascular adverse reactions, other than exacerbation of the arrhythmias, include the uncommon occurrence of congestive heart failure (3%) and bradycardia. Bradycardia usually responds to dosage reduction but may require a pacemaker for control. CHF rarely requires drug discontinuation. Cardiac conduction abnormalities occur infrequently and are reversible on discontinuation of drug.
Hepatitis, cholestatic hepatitis, cirrhosis, epididymitis, vasculitis, pseudotumor cerebri, thrombocytopenia, angioedema, bronchiolitis obliterans organizing pneumonia (possibly fatal), pleuritis, pancreatitis, toxic epidermal necrolysis, pancytopenia and neutropenia also have been reported in patients receiving amiodarone.
The following side-effect rates are based on a retrospective study of 241 patients treated for 2 to 1,515 days (mean 441.3 days).

The following side effects were each reported in 10 to 33% of patients:
Gastrointestinal: Nausea and vomiting.

The following side effects were each reported in 4 to 9% of patients:
Dermatologic: Solar dermatitis/photosensitivity.
Neurologic: Malaise and fatigue, tremor/abnormal involuntary movements, lack of coordination, abnormal gait/ataxia, dizziness, paresthesias.
Gastrointestinal: Constipation, anorexia.
Ophthalmologic: Visual disturbances.
Hepatic: Abnormal liver-function tests.
Respiratory: Pulmonary inflammation or fibrosis.

The following side effects were each reported in 1 to 3% of patients:
Thyroid: Hypothyroidism, hyperthyroidism.
Neurologic: Decreased libido, insomnia, headache, sleep disturbances.
Cardiovascular: Congestive heart failure, cardiac arrhythmias, SA node dysfunction.
Gastrointestinal: Abdominal pain.
Hepatic: Nonspecific hepatic disorders.
Other: Flushing, abnormal taste and smell, edema, abnormal salivation, coagulation abnormalities.

The following side effects were each reported in less than 1% of patients:
Blue skin discoloration, rash, spontaneous ecchymosis, alopecia, hypotension and cardiac conduction abnormalities.
In surveys of almost 5,000 patients treated in open U.S. studies and in published reports of treatment with amiodarone HCl, the adverse reactions most frequently requiring discontinuation of drug included pulmonary infiltrates or fibrosis, paroxysmal ventricular tachycardia, congestive heart failure and elevation of liver enzymes. Other symptoms causing discontinuations less often included visual disturbances, solar dermatitis, blue skin discoloration, hyperthyroidism and hypothyroidism.

OVERDOSAGE

There have been a few reported cases of amiodarone HCl overdose in which 3 to 8 grams were taken. There were no deaths or permanent sequelae. The acute oral LD_{50} of amiodarone HCl in mice and rats is greater than 3,000 mg/kg.
In addition to general supportive measures, the patient's cardiac rhythm and blood pressure should be monitored, and if bradycardia ensues, a β-adrenergic agonist or a pacemaker may be used. Hypotension with inadequate tissue perfusion should be treated with positive inotropic and/or vasopressor agents. Neither amiodarone nor its metabolite is dialyzable.

DOSAGE AND ADMINISTRATION

BECAUSE OF THE UNIQUE PHARMACOKINETIC PROPERTIES, DIFFICULT DOSING SCHEDULE AND SEVERITY OF SIDE EFFECTS IF PATIENTS ARE IMPROPERLY MONITORED, PACERONE® SHOULD BE ADMINISTERED ONLY BY PHYSICIANS WHO ARE EXPERIENCED IN THE TREATMENT OF LIFE-THREATENING ARRHYTHMIAS WHO ARE THOROUGHLY FAMILIAR WITH THE RISKS AND BENEFITS OF AMIODARONE THERAPY, AND WHO HAVE ACCESS TO LABORATORY FACILITIES CAPABLE OF ADEQUATELY MONITORING THE EFFECTIVENESS AND SIDE EFFECTS OF TREATMENT.
In order to insure that an antiarrhythmic effect will be observed without waiting several months, loading doses are required. A uniform, optimal dosage schedule for administration of Pacerone® has not been determined. Because of the food effect on absorption, Pacerone® should be administered consistently with regard to meals (see "**CLINICAL PHARMACOLOGY**"). Individual patient titration is suggested according to the following guidelines.
For life-threatening ventricular arrhythmias, such as ventricular fibrillation or hemodynamically unstable ventricular tachycardia: Close monitoring of the patients is indi-

Continued on next page

Pacerone—Cont.

cated during the loading phase, particularly until risk of recurrent ventricular tachycardia or fibrillation has abated. Because of the serious nature of the arrhythmia and the lack of predictable time course of effect, loading should be performed in a hospital setting. Loading doses of 800 to 1,600 mg/day are required for 1 to 3 weeks (occasionally longer) until initial response occurs. (Administration of Pacerone® in divided doses with meals is suggested for total daily doses of 1,000 mg or higher, or when gastrointestinal intolerance occurs.) If side effects become excessive, the dose should be reduced. Elimination of recurrence of ventricular fibrillation and tachycardia usually occurs within 1 to 3 weeks, along with reduction in complex and total ventricular ectopic beats.

Upon starting Pacerone® therapy, an attempt should be made to gradually discontinue prior antiarrhythmic drugs (see section on "**Drug Interactions**"). When adequate arrhythmia control is achieved, or if side effects become prominent, Pacerone® dose should be reduced to 600 to 800 mg/day for one month and then to the maintenance dose, usually 400 mg/day (see "**CLINICAL PHARMACOLOGY, Monitoring Effectiveness**"). Some patients may require larger maintenance doses, up to 600 mg/day, and some can be controlled on lower doses. Pacerone® may be administered as a single daily dose, or in patients with severe gastrointestinal intolerance, as a b.i.d. dose. In each patient, the chronic maintenance dose should be determined according to antiarrhythmic effect as assessed by symptoms, Holter recordings and/or programmed electrical stimulation, and by patient tolerance. Plasma concentrations may be helpful in evaluating nonresponsiveness or unexpectedly severe toxicity (see "**CLINICAL PHARMACOLOGY**").

The lowest effective dose should be used to prevent the occurrence of side effects. In all instances, the physician must be guided by the severity of the individual patient's arrhythmia and response to therapy.

When dosage adjustments are necessary, the patient should be closely monitored for an extended period of time because of the long and variable half-life of amiodarone and the difficulty in predicting the time required to attain a new steady-state level of drug. Dosage suggestions are summarized below:

[See second table at top of previous page]

HOW SUPPLIED

Pacerone® (Amiodarone HCl) Tablets, 200 mg, are available in bottles of 60 tablets (NDC 0245-0147-60), bottles of 90 tablets (NDC 0245-0147-90), bottles of 500 tablets (NDC 0245-0147-15) and in unit dose cartons of 100 tablets (10 cards containing 10 tablets each) (NDC 0245-0147-01).

Pacerone® Tablets are pink, round, flat-faced, scored, uncoated tablets, debossed with "P_{200}" on the unscored side, and "U-S" above and "0147" below the score on the reverse side.

Store at room temperature, approximately 25°C (77°F). Protect from light and moisture.

Dispense in a tight, light-resistant container with a child-resistant closure.

Manufactured by
UPSHER-SMITH LABORATORIES, INC.
Minneapolis, MN 55447
US Patent 5,785,995
Rev. 0200 PCPI.0200

Shown in Product Identification Guide, page 339

PENTOXIL® ℞

[pen-tox-il]
(Pentoxifylline Extended-release Tablets, 400 mg)

DESCRIPTION

Pentoxil® (Pentoxifylline Extended-release Tablets) for oral administration contain 400 mg of the active drug and the following inactive ingredients: D&C Red No. 27 Aluminum Lake, FD&C Blue No.1 Aluminum Lake, hydroxypropyl methylcellulose USP, magnesium stearate NF, polyethylene glycol NF, polysorbate 80 NF, povidone USP, silicon dioxide NF, and titanium dioxide USP, in an extended-release formulation.

HOW SUPPLIED

Pentoxil® (Pentoxifylline Extended-release Tablets) is available for oral administration as 400 mg light-pink, unscored, film-coated, capsule-shaped tablets imprinted U-S 027; supplied in bottles of 100 (NDC 0245-0027-11); bottles of 500 (NDC 0245-0027-15); bottles of 5000 (NDC 0245-0027-55), and Unit Dose Packs of 100 (NDC 0245-0027-01).

PREVALITE® ℞

[prē 'vă līt]
(Cholestyramine for Oral Suspension, USP)

DESCRIPTION

Prevalite® (Cholestyramine for Oral Suspension, USP), the chloride salt of a basic anion exchange resin, a cholesterol-lowering agent, is intended for oral administration.

HOW SUPPLIED

Available in cartons of forty-two and sixty single-dose packets and in cans containing 231 grams. 5.5 grams of Prevalite® contain 4 grams of anhydrous cholestyramine resin.
NDC 0245-0036-42 Cartons of 42, 5.5 g packets
NDC 0245-0036-60 Cartons of 60, 5.5 g packets
NDC 0245-0036-23 Cans, 231 g (42 doses)

RMS® Suppositories ℂ ℞

(Rectal Morphine Sulfate)

DESCRIPTION

Suppositories contain 5, 10, 20, or 30 mg of morphine sulfate. Morphine sulfate suppositories are prepared from a hydrogenated vegetable oil base and other ingredients (contains BHA and BHT as preservatives), and are suitable for rectal administration.

HOW SUPPLIED

RMS® Suppositories are individually sealed in color-coded wrappers to aid in identification. 5 mg suppositories (white wrapper/blue print), NDC 0245-0160-12, 12 per carton. 10 mg suppositories (white wrapper/green print), NDC 0245-0161-12, 12 per carton. 20 mg suppositories (white wrapper/red print), NDC 0245-0162-12, 12 per carton. 30 mg suppositories (white wrapper/gold print), NDC 0245-0163-12, 12 per carton.

DEA ORDER FORM REQUIRED

SSKI® ℞

Potassium Iodide Oral Solution, USP (Saturated) 1 g/ml

DESCRIPTION

SSKI® (Potassium Iodide Oral Solution, USP) is a saturated solution of potassium iodide containing 1 g of potassium iodide per ml.

HOW SUPPLIED

SSKI® (Potassium Iodide Oral Solution, USP) is supplied in 1 fluid ounce (30 ml) bottles (NDC 0245-0003-31) with a calibrated dropper marked to deliver 0.3 ml (300 mg) and 0.6 ml (600 mg); and 8 fluid ounce (237 ml) bottles (NDC 0245-0003-08).

Notice: When exposed to cold temperatures, crystallization may occur, but on warming and shaking, the crystals will redissolve. If the solution turns brownish yellow in color, it should be discarded.

SLO–NIACIN® Tablets OTC

(polygel® controlled-release niacin)
Dietary Supplement

DESCRIPTION

Slo-Niacin® Tablets are manufactured utilizing a unique, patented polygel® controlled-release delivery system. This exclusive technology assures the gradual and measured release of niacin (nicotinic acid) and is designed to reduce the incidence of flushing and itching commonly associated with niacin use. Slo-Niacin® Tablets are available in 250 mg, 500 mg, and 750 mg strengths.

HOW SUPPLIED

250 mg tablets in bottles of 100: List No. 0245–0062–11
500 mg tablets in bottles of 100: List No. 0245–0063–11
750 mg tablets in bottles of 100: List No. 0245–0064–11
U.S. Patent No. 5,126,145 and 5,268,181

Shown in Product Identification Guide, page 339

U.S. Pharmaceutical Corporation

2401-C MELLON COURT
DECATUR, GA 30035

Direct Inquiries to:
Peter J. Krebs, Ph.D.
CEO Management Unit
(800) 330-3040,
or
Clayton W. Bishop
National Sales Manager
(877) 775-2418
or
(800) 330-3040

CENOGEN-OB™ ℞

(Prenatal-Vitamin-Mineral Capsules)

DESCRIPTION

Each blue and pink **Cenogen-OB™** capsule contains:

Ferrous Fumarate (anhydrous)	324 mg
(Equivalent to about 106 mg of Elemental Iron)	
Sodium Ascorbate (Vit. C)	200 mg
Vit. B-1, Thiamine Mononitrate	10 mg
Vit. B-2, Riboflavin	6 mg
Vit. B-6, Pyridoxine HCl	5 mg
Vit. B-12, Cyanocobalamin Concentrate	15 mg
Folic Acid	1 mg
Niacinamide	30 mg
Pantothenic Acid (as calcium pantothenate)	10 mg
Zinc (as Zinc Sulfate)	8.2 mg
Magnesium (as Magnesium Sulfate)	6.9 mg
Manganese (as Manganese Sulfate)	1.3 mg
Copper (as Copper Sulfate)	0.8 mg

Dosage Adults, 1 capsule daily, between meals or at bedtime, orally

HOW SUPPLIED

Child resistant 10 x 10 blister packs in containers of 100 capsules, NDC 52747-130-70.

Dispense in a tight, light resistant container as defined in the USP/NF with a child resistant closure. Store at controlled room temperature 15°–30°C (59°–86°F).

Keep in Cool Dry Place. Capsules are non-USP.

CAUTION: RX only 5/2000

HEMOCYTE™ Tablets OTC

(ferrous fumarate 324 mg.)

HOW SUPPLIED

Boxes of 100 child-proof tablets NDC 52747-307-70
Boxes of 30 child-proof tablets NDC 52747-307-30

HEMOCYTE PLUS™ Tabules ℞

Iron-Vitamin-Mineral Complex

DESCRIPTION

Each tabule contains:

Ferrous Fumarate (anhydrous)	324 mg.
[Equivalent to about 106 mg. of Elemental Iron]	
Sodium Ascorbate (Vit. C)	200 mg.
Vit. B-1—Thiamine Mononitrate	10 mg.
Vit. B-2—Riboflavin	6 mg.
Vit. B-6—Pyridoxine HCl	5 mg.
Vit. B-12—Cyanocobalamin Concentrate	5mcg.
Folic Acid	1 mg.
Niacinamide	30 mg.
Calcium Pantothenate	10 mg.
Zinc (as Zinc Sulfate)	18.2 mg.
Magnesium (as Magnesium Sulfate)	6.9 mg.
Manganese (as Manganese Sulfate)	1.3 mg.
Copper (as Copper Sulfate)	0.8 mg.

HOW SUPPLIED

Boxes of 100 child-proof tablets NDC 52747-308-70
Boxes of 30 child-proof tablets NDC 52747-308-30

HEMOCYTE-F ELIXIR ℞

Iron, Folic Acid, and Vitamin B12 Complex

DESCRIPTION

Each Teaspoon Contains:

Elemental Iron	100 mg
(As a polysaccharide-iron complex)	
Folic Acid	1 mg
Vitamin B12	25 mcg
Alcohol	10%
(Sugar Free)	

HOW SUPPLIED

Bottles of 16 oz. NDC 52747-404-90

HEMOCYTE–F TABLETS ℞

DESCRIPTION

Each tablet contains:

Ferrous Fumarate (anhydrous)	324 mg.
Folic Acid	1 mg.

HOW SUPPLIED

Boxes of 100 child proof tablets NDC 52747-306-70
Boxes of 30 child proof tablets NDC 52747-306-30

MAGSAL™ TABLETS ℞

DESCRIPTION

Each tablet contains:

Magnesium Salicylate	600 mg.
Phenyltoloxamine Dihydrogen Citrate	25 mg.

HOW SUPPLIED

Bottles of 100 NDC 52747-321-60

MEDIGESIC® Capsules ℞

DESCRIPTION

Each capsule or tablet contains:

Butalbital*	50 mg
*WARNING: May be habit forming.	
Acetaminophen	325 mg
Caffeine	40 mg

HOW SUPPLIED

Capsules: Bottles of 100 NDC 52747-600-60

MEDIPLEX ULTRA OTC
(Vitamin-Mineral Complex)

DESCRIPTION

Each tabule contains:

Vitamin E - dl-alpha Tocopheryl Acetate	100 I.U.
Vitamin C-Ascorbic Acid	300 mg.
Vitamin B12 - Cyanocabalmin Concentrate	25 mcg
Vitamin B1 - Thiamine	25 mg.
Niacinamide	100 mg.
Folic Acid	0.4 mg.
Vitamin B6 - Pyridoxine	10 mg.
Vitamin B2 - Riboflavin	10 mg.
Calcium Pantothenate	25 mg.
Zinc (as Zinc Sulfate)	18 mg.
Magnesium (as Magnesium Sulfate)	7 mg.
Manganese (as Manganese Sulfate)	1.3 mg.
Copper (as Cupric Sulfate)	0.8 mg.

HOW SUPPLIED

Bottles of 100 NDC 52747-305-70

NOREL DM™ OTC
Antihistamine
Nasal Decongestant
Cough Suppressant
Alcohol Free • Sugar Free • Dye Free

DESCRIPTION

Each teaspoonful (5ml) contains:

Dextromethorphan hydrobromide	15 mg
Chlorpheniramine maleate	4 mg
Phenylephrine hydrochloride	10 mg

HOW SUPPLIED

Bottles of 1 pint (16 fluid ounces)
NDC# 52747-410-90

NOREL PLUS ℞
Decongestant–Analgesic–Antihistaminic

DESCRIPTION

Each yellow and white capsule for oral administration contains:

Acetaminophen	325 mg
Phenyltoloxamine Dihydrogen Citrate	25 mg
Phenylpropanolamine Hydrochloride	25 mg
Chlorpheniramine Maleate	4 mg

HOW SUPPLIED

Bottles of 100 NDC 52747-128-60

USANA, Incorporated

3838 WEST PARKWAY BOULEVARD
SALT LAKE CITY, UTAH 84120-6336

Direct Inquiries to:
Ph: (801) 954 7860
Fax: (801) 954 7658

Active Calcium OTC

COMPOSITION

Each Active Calcium tablet contains the following minerals:

Calcium (as citrate)	135 mg
Magnesium (as aminoate*)	90 mg
Silicon (as aminoate*)	2.25 mg
Boron (as aminoate*)	330 mcg
Vitamin D_3	40 IU

*Amino acid chelate from rice protein

ADVANTAGES

Each tablet contains a balanced blend of calcium, magnesium, vitamin D, boron and silicon; five nutrients required for bone development, bone remodeling and skeletal health. This non-prescription product meets USP guidelines for potency (as applicable), uniformity and disintegration, and is manufactured according to pharmaceutical cGMP standards.

RECOMMENDED USE

Take 4–8 tablets by mouth daily.

SUPPLIED

Capsule-shaped tablet, mottled greenish-white color, with clear film coating, and with USANA imprint. In bottle of 240 tablets.

Shown in Product Identification Guide, page 339

CHELATED MINERAL OTC
[*chē'-latĕd mineral*]

COMPOSITION

Each Chelated Mineral contains the following minerals:

Calcium (as citrate)	90 mg
Magnesium (as aminoate*)	100 mg
Zinc (as citrate)	6.7 mg
Manganese (as aminoate*)	1.7 mg
Boron (as aminoate*)	1 mg
Copper (as aminoate*)	1 mg
Chromium (as picolinate)	100 mcg
Iodine (as potassium iodide)	75 mcg
Selenium (as aminoate*)	66.7 mcg
Molybdenum (as aminoate*)	16 mcg
Trace minerals	33 mg

*amino acid chelate from rice protein.

ADVANTAGES

Each tablet contains a complete and balanced blend of essential minerals in bioavailable forms. The Chelated Mineral is designed to be taken with USANA's Mega Antioxidant to provide the full complement of essential nutrients required for health. This non-prescription product meets USP guidelines for potency (as applicable), uniformity and disintegration, and is manufactured according to pharmaceutical cGMP standards.

RECOMMENDED USE

Take 3 tablets by mouth daily, spread evenly throughout the day, or as is convenient.

SUPPLIED

Oblong shaped tablet, off-white color, with clear film coating and with USANA imprint. In bottle of 90 tablets.

Shown in Product Identification Guide, page 339

COQUINONE™ OTC
[*cokwinōn*]

COMPOSITION

Each CoQuinone™ contains the following:

Coenzyme Q_{10}	10 mg
Alpha Lipoic Acid	12.5 mg

ADVANTAGES

CoQuinone™ contains a hydrosoluble form of Coenzyme Q_{10} (CoQ_{10}) that is 2.5 times more bioavailable than material supplied in dry tablet/capsule formulas. The higher blood levels of CoQ_{10} supplied enhance mitochondrial production of ATP. CoQ_{10} is a rate-limiting factor in the electron transport chain involved in mitochondrial production of ATP. It is also involved in neutralizing free radicals generated during ATP production. As such, CoQ_{10} helps the body maintain healthy skeletal and cardiac muscle. Alpha lipoic acid is included in the formula as a lipid-soluble antioxidant to recycle CoQ_{10} from the prooxidant form to the antioxidant form. This non-prescription product meets USP guidelines for uniformity and disintegration and is manufactured according to cGMP standards.

RECOMMENDED USE

Take 2 or 3 capsules by mouth daily.

SUPPLIED

Oval shaped, soft gelatin capsule, orange-colored, opaque, imprinted with USANA in white edible ink. Capsules contain an orange colored liquid. In bottle of 60 soft-gel capsules.

Shown in Product Identification Guide, page 339

MEGA ANTIOXIDANT OTC
[*mēga aenti-óksid'nt*]

COMPOSITION

Each Mega Antioxidant contains the following vitamins and antioxidants:

Beta carotene	5,670 IU
Vitamin C (as Poly C, a blend of calcium, zinc, potassium and magnesium ascorbates)	433 mg
Vitamin D_3	67 IU
Vitamin E	150 IU
Vitamin K	20 mcg
Vitamin B1 (Thiamine HCl)	9 mg
Vitamin B2 (Riboflavin)	9 mg
Niacin and Niacinamide	13.3 mg
Vitamin B6 (Pyridoxine HCl)	9 mg
Folate	333 mcg
Vitamin B12 (Cyanocobalamin)	20 mcg
Biotin	16.7 mcg
Pantothenic Acid	30 mg
Bioflavonoid Complex (Rutin, Quercetin, Hesperidin, Green Tea Extract, Bilberry Extract)	69.4 mg
Inositol	50 mg
Choline Bitartrate	33.3 mg
Cruciferrous Extract	33.3 mg
N-Acetyl-L-Cysteine	21.7 mg
Para-Aminobenzoic Acid	16.7 mg
Bromelain	16.7 mg
Alpha-Lipoic Acid	5 mg
Coenzyme Q10	4 mg
Reduced Glutathione	3.3 mg
Broccoli Concentrate	3.3 mg
Mixed Carotenoids (Lutein and Zeaxanthin)	67 mcg

ADVANTAGES

A comprehensive and balanced formula containing the essential vitamins and antioxidants at levels substantially higher than RDA amounts. In addition to the traditionally recognized essential nutrients, the formula contains a unique blend of dietary antioxidants including mixed carotenoids, a bioflavonoid complex, cruciferous extracts and a glutathione complex to provide full-spectrum antioxidant protection. This formula is designed to be taken with USANA's Chelated Mineral to provide the full compliment of essential nutrients required for health. This non-prescription product meets USP guidelines for potency (as applicable), uniformity and disintegration, and is manufactured according to pharmaceutical cGMP standards.

RECOMMENDED USE

Three tablets by mouth daily, spread evenly throughout the day, or as is convenient.

SUPPLIED

Oblong shaped tablets, mottled orange-brown color, with clear film coating and with USANA imprint. In bottle of 90 tablets.

Shown in Product Identification Guide, page 339

PROFLAVANOL® OTC
[*prou fléivənol*]

COMPOSITION

Each Proflavanol contains the following:

Vitamin C (Poly C)	100 mg
Grape seed extract	30 mg
Ascorbyl palmitate	12 mg

ADVANTAGES

A potent antioxidant formula combining the proanthocyanidins (bioflavonoids) from standardized grape seed extract with vitamin C in the form of ascorbate salts and ascorbyl palmitate. Proflavanol is designed to be taken as a standalone antioxidant, or preferably in combination with USANA's Mega Antioxidant and Chelated Mineral to provide additional antioxidant protection. This non-prescription product meets USP guidelines for uniformity and disintegration and is manufactured according to pharmaceutical cGMP standards.

RECOMMENDED USE

Take 2–4 tablets by mouth daily.

SUPPLIED

Round, buff colored tablet, with clear film coating, without imprint or distinguishing marks. In bottle of 90 tablets.

Shown in Product Identification Guide, page 339

IDENTIFICATION PROBLEM?
Turn to the **Product Identification Guide**, where you'll find more than 1600 products pictured in actual size and full color.

Vitaline Corporation

385 WILLIAMSON WAY
ASHLAND, OR 97520

Direct Inquiries to:
Jed D. Meese, Technical Director
(800) 648-4755
(541) 482-9231
FAX: (541) 482-9112
E-Mail: jmeese@vitaline.com

L-CARNITINE USP OTC

250mg Tablets, 500mg Scored Caplets and 500mg Chewable Wafers

L-CARNITINE

500mg Capsules
(from 736mg L-Carnitine Tartrate)

DESCRIPTION

Carnitine is a naturally occurring substance, which is essential for fatty acid oxidation and energy production. Without it, long-chain fatty acids cannot cross from cellular cytoplasma into the mitochondria and out again, resulting in loss of energy and toxic accumulations of free fatty acids. Ninety-five percent of the body's carnitine is found in cardiac and skeletal tissue; these muscles rely upon fatty acid oxidation for most of their energy.

INDICATIONS

Dietary supplementation of L-Carnitine for individuals who may benefit from supplementation of this essential nutrient. Renal dialysis patients and individuals with immune system deficiencies may benefit from L-Carnitine supplementation.

ADVERSE REACTIONS

None reported.

SUGGESTED USE

As a dietary supplement: Adults, one gram daily or as directed by physician, registered dietician or nutritionist. Children, as directed by physician.

HOW SUPPLIED

250mg tablets in bottles of 90 NDC 54022-2100-1
500mg scored caplets in bottles of 30 NDC 54022-2120-1
500mg chewable wafers in bottles of 30 NDC 54022-2700-1
500mg capsules in bottles of 30 NDC 54022-2800-1

REFERENCES

1) Effects of L-Carnitine Supplementation on Muscular Symptoms in Hemodialyzed Patients. Y. Saskurauchi, Y. Matsumoto, T. Shinzato, I. Takai, Y. Nakamura, M. Sato, S. Nakai, M. Miwa, H. Morita, T. Miwa, I. Amano, K. Maeda, *American Journal of Kidney Diseases,* 32(2)258–264, August 1998
2) Anemia and Carnitine Supplementation in Hemodialyzed Patients. Kletzmajr, J., et al., *Kidney International,* 55(Suppl 69):S93–S106, March 1999
3) Carnitine and its Derivatives in Cardiovascular Disease. Arsenian, M.A., *Progress in Cardiovascular Diseases,* 40(3): 265–286, Nov.-Dec. 1997

COENZYME Q_{10} OTC

(Ubiquinone)
200mg, 100mg & 60mg Chewable Wafers
200mg, 60mg & 25mg Tablets, and
60mg Lipospheres Softgels

DESCRIPTION

Coenzyme Q_{10} (CoQ_{10}) is an essential nutrient that is a cofactor in the mitochondrial electron transport chain, the biochemical pathway in cellular respiration from which ATP and metabolic energy are derived. Since nearly all cellular functions are dependent on energy, CoQ_{10} is essential for the health of all human tissues and organs. The involvement of CoQ_{10} as a redox carrier of the respiratory chain is well established on the basis of both reconstitution studies and kinetic evidence.

In addition to CoQ_{10}'s vital role in cellular energy production, it also functions as a powerful, highly effective antioxidant. These functions of CoQ_{10} support normal heart function. Studies show that CoQ_{10} also enhances vitamin E's ability to destroy free radicals.

SUGGESTED USE

As a dietary supplement: Adults, 60mg–200mg daily or as directed by physician or registered dietician. Children, as directed by physician.

ADVERSE REACTIONS

None reported.

HOW SUPPLIED

Bottles of 30, 60, 500 and 1000.
200mg with 400 I.U. Vitamin E chewable wafers, NDC 54022-2091, 100mg with 300 I.U. Vitamin E chewable wafers, NDC 54022-2090, 60mg chewable wafers, NDC 54022-2085, 200mg tablets, NDC 54022-8002, 60mg tablets, NDC 54022-2081, 25mg tablets, NDC 54022-2055, 60mg Liposphere softgels 54022-2075

REFERENCES

1) Coenzyme Q_{10} Administration Increases Brain Mitochondrial Concentrations and Exerts Neuroprotective Effects. Matthews, R.T., Beal, M.F., et al. *Proceedings of the National Academy of Sciences of the United States of America,* 95(15):8892-7, July 21, 1998
2) Overview of the Use of CoQ_{10} in Cardiovascular Disease. Langsjoen, P., *The First Conference of the International Co-Enzyme Q_{10} Association,* Boston, MA, May 21–24, 1998 (reprint available)
3) Plasma Coenzyme Q_{10} Concentrations in Breast Cancer: Prognosis and Therapeutic Consequences. P. Jolliet, et al., *International Journal of Clinical Pharmacology and Therapeutics,* 36(9):506-9, 1998
4) Absorption, Tolerability, and Effects on Mitochondrial Activity of Oral Coenzyme Q10 in Parkinsonian Patients. Shultz C.W., et al. *Neurology,* 50:793-795, March 1998
5) Introduction to Coenzyme Q_{10}. Langsjoen, Peter H., M.D., F.A.C.C., Tyler, TX 75701, 1996

VIVUS, Inc.

1172 CASTRO STREET
MOUNTAIN VIEW, CA 94040

Direct Inquiries to:
(888) 345-6873

For Medical Information or Emergencies Contact:
Medical Services Department @ VIVUS:
(650) 934-5200
FAX: (650) 934-5389

MUSE® ℞

(alprostadil)
urethral suppository

DESCRIPTION

MUSE® (alprostadil) is a single-use, medicated transurethral system for the delivery of alprostadil to the male urethra. Alprostadil is suspended in polyethylene glycol 1450 (as excipient) and is formed into a medicated pellet (microsuppository measuring 1.4 mm in diameter by 3 mm or 6 mm in length) that resides in the tip of a translucent hollow applicator. MUSE is administered by inserting the applicator stem into the urethra after urination. The pellet containing alprostadil is delivered by depressing the applicator button (**see Figure 1**). The components of the delivery system are constructed of medical grade polypropylene. Each MUSE system is packaged in an individual foil pouch.

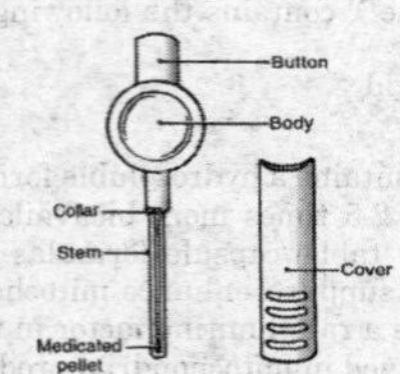

Figure 1: Diagram of the MUSE Transurethral System

The active ingredient in MUSE is alprostadil, which is chemically identical to the naturally occurring eicosanoid, prostaglandin E_1 (PGE_1). The chemical name for alprostadil is prost-13-en-1-oic acid, 11,15-dihydroxy-9-oxo-(11α, 13E, 15S)-(1R,2R,3R)-3-hydroxy-2-[(E)-(3S)-3-hydroxy-1-octenyl]-5-oxo-cyclopentane heptanoic acid, and the molecular weight is 354.49. The empirical formula is $C_{20}H_{34}O_5$. The structural formula of alprostadil is represented below:

Alprostadil is a white to off-white crystalline powder with a melting point between 115° and 116°C. Its solubility at 35°C is 8000 mcg per 100 mL double-distilled water. The inactive ingredient in MUSE is polyethylene glycol 1450, USP. There are no other active agents or excipients in MUSE.

MUSE is available in 4 dosage strengths: 125 mcg, 250 mcg, 500 mcg, and 1000 mcg.

CLINICAL PHARMACOLOGY

Mechanism of Action: Prostaglandin E_1 is a naturally occurring acidic lipid that is synthesized from fatty acid precursors by most mammalian tissues and has a variety of pharmacologic effects. Human seminal fluid is a rich source of prostaglandins, including PGE_1 and PGE_2, and the total concentration of prostaglandins in ejaculate has been estimated to be approximately 100–200 mcg/mL. In vitro, alprostadil (PGE_1) has been shown to cause dose-dependent smooth muscle relaxation in isolated corpus cavernosum and corpus spongiosum preparations. Additionally, vasodilation has been demonstrated in isolated cavernosal artery segments that were pre-contracted with either norepinephrine or prostaglandin $F_{2\alpha}$. When alprostadil was injected into the corpus cavernosum of pigtail monkeys in vivo, dose-dependent increases in cavernosal artery blood flow were observed.

In human studies using Doppler duplex ultrasonography, intraurethral administration of 500 mcg of MUSE resulted in an increase in cavernosal artery diameter and a 5- to 10-fold increase in peak systolic flow velocities. These results suggest that intraurethral alprostadil is absorbed from the urethra, transported throughout the erectile bodies by communicating vessels between the corpus spongiosum and corpora cavernosa, and able to induce vasodilation of the targeted vascular beds.

The vasodilatory effects of alprostadil on the cavernosal arteries and the trabecular smooth muscle of the corpora cavernosa result in rapid arterial inflow and expansion of the lacunar spaces within the corpora. As the expanded corporal sinusoids are compressed against the tunica albuginea, venous outflow through subtunical vessels is impeded and penile rigidity develops. This process is referred to as the corporal veno-occlusive mechanism.

The most notable systemic effects of alprostadil are vasodilation, inhibition of platelet aggregation, and stimulation of intestinal and uterine smooth muscle. Intravenous doses of 1 to 10 micrograms per kilogram of body weight lower blood pressure in mammals by decreasing peripheral resistance. Reflex increases in cardiac output and heart rate may accompany these effects.

Pharmacokinetics: About 80% of alprostadil administered by MUSE is absorbed within 10 minutes and is rapidly cleared from the systemic circulation by the lungs, leaving barely detectable systemic blood levels.

Absorption: MUSE is designed to deliver alprostadil directly to the urethral lining for transfer via the corpus spongiosum to the corpora cavernosa. Intraurethral administration of MUSE is preceded by urination, and the residual urine disperses the medicated pellet, permitting alprostadil to be absorbed by the urethral mucosa. The transurethral absorption of alprostadil after MUSE administration is biphasic. Initial absorption is rapid, with approximately 80% of an administered dose absorbed within 10 minutes. The mean time to the maximum plasma PGE_1 concentration after a 1000 mcg intraurethral dose of MUSE is approximately 16 minutes.

In 10 normal human volunteers, endogenous PGE_1 levels in the ejaculate averaged 31 mcg (range 0–161 mcg). In these same volunteers, an average of 123 mcg of additional PGE_1 (range 30–369 mcg) was present in the ejaculate obtained 10 minutes after the highest dose (1000 mcg) of MUSE. The mean total endogenous PGE content (PGE_1, PGE_2, 19-OH-PGE_1, and 19-OH-PGE_2) of the ejaculate in these subjects was 444 mcg (range 0–1423 mcg).

Distribution: Following MUSE administration, alprostadil is absorbed from the urethral mucosa into the corpus spongiosum. A portion of the administered dose is transported to the corpora cavernosa through collateral vessels, while the remainder passes into the pelvic venous circulation through veins draining the corpus spongiosum. The half-life of alprostadil in humans is short, varying between 30 seconds and 10 minutes, depending on the body compartment in which it is measured and the physiological status of the subject. Nearly all of the alprostadil entering the central venous circulation is removed in a single pass through the lungs; thus peripheral venous plasma levels of PGE_1 are low or undetectable ($<$2 picograms/mL) after MUSE administration. The mean maximum plasma PGE_1 concentration following intraurethral administration of the highest dose of MUSE (1000 mcg) was barely detectable (11.4 picograms/mL). In a study of 14 subjects, the plasma PGE_1 level was shown to be undetectable within 60 minutes of MUSE administration in most subjects.

Metabolism: Alprostadil is rapidly metabolized locally by enzymatic oxidation of the 15-hydroxyl group to 15-keto-PGE_1. The enzyme catalyzing this process has been isolated from many tissues in the lower genitourinary tract including the urethra, prostate, and corpus cavernosum. 15-keto-PGE_1 retains little (1–2%) of the biological activity of PGE_1. 15-keto-PGE_1 is rapidly reduced at the C_{13}–C_{14} position to form the most abundant metabolite in plasma, 13, 14-dihydro, 15-keto PGE_1 (DHK-PGE_1), which is biologically inactive. The majority of DHK-PGE_1 is further metabolized to smaller prostaglandin remnants that are cleared primarily by the kidney and liver. Between 60% and 90% of PGE_1 has been shown to be metabolized after 1 pass through the pulmonary capillary beds.

Excretion: After intravenous administration of tritium-labeled alprostadil in man, labeled drug disappears rapidly from the blood in the first 10 minutes, and by 1 hour radioactivity in the blood reaches a low level. The metabolites of alprostadil are excreted primarily by the kidney, with approximately 90% of an administered intravenous dose excreted in the urine within 24 hours of dosing. The remainder is excreted in the feces. There is no evidence of tissue retention of alprostadil or its metabolites following intravenous administration.

Pharmacokinetics in Special Populations:

Pulmonary Disease: The near-complete pulmonary first-pass metabolism of PGE_1 is the primary factor influencing the systemic pharmacokinetics of MUSE and is a reason that peripheral venous plasma levels of PGE_1 are low or undetectable (<2 picograms/mL) following MUSE administration. Patients with pulmonary disease therefore may have a reduced capacity to clear the drug. In patients with the adult respiratory distress syndrome (ARDS), pulmonary extraction of intravascularly administered alprostadil was reduced by approximately 15% compared to a control group of patients with normal respiratory function (66±3.2% vs. 78±2.4%).

Geriatrics: The effects of age on the pharmacokinetics of alprostadil have not been evaluated.

CLINICAL TRIALS

The MUSE system was evaluated in 7 placebo-controlled trials of various design in over 2500 patients with a history of erectile dysfunction of various etiologies. These trials assessed erectile function in the clinic and sexual intercourse in outpatient settings. In studies of sexual performance, patients were screened in the clinic, generally using doses of 125 mcg to 1000 mcg, for a satisfactory erectile response, then sent home with the selected dose or placebo for evaluation of sexual performance. Not all patients beginning titration had a successful dose and some patients could not tolerate MUSE, principally because of penile pain, so that the success rates in the studies described below must be understood to represent response rates only in patients who were successfully titrated.

In 2 identical multicenter, double-blind, placebo-controlled, parallel-group studies, 1511 monogamous and heterosexual patients with a mean 4-year history of erectile dysfunction and at least a 3-month history of no erections adequate for sexual intercourse without medical assistance, were enrolled and began dose titration in the clinic with doses between 125 mcg and 1000 mcg. 996 patients (66%) completed dose titration, achieved an erection sufficient for intercourse, and were randomized equally to placebo or active treatment and followed during at-home treatment for up to 3 months. 874 patients and partners completed 3 months of follow-up. About 10%, 20%, 30%, and 40% of patients were titrated to 125 mcg, 250 mcg, 500 mcg, and 1000 mcg, respectively. Couples on active therapy were more likely to have at least 1 successful sexual intercourse (65% vs. 19%) than were couples on placebo. Among patients who reported successful intercourse at least once with active treatment, approximately 7 of 10 MUSE systems resulted in successful sexual intercourse. Results were similar in patients with erectile dysfunction stemming from surgery or trauma, diabetes, vascular disease, or other etiologies, and were similar in Caucasians and non-Caucasians. In administrations resulting in sexual intercourse, the duration of erections sufficient for penetration was 6 minutes on placebo and 16 minutes on active drug. Successful therapy with MUSE was associated with improvement in the quality of life measures of "emotional well-being" for patients and "relationship with partner" for both patients and their female partners.

INDICATIONS AND USAGE

MUSE is indicated for the treatment of erectile dysfunction. Studies that established benefit demonstrated improvements in success rates for sexual intercourse compared with similarly administered placebo.

CONTRAINDICATIONS

MUSE is contraindicated in men with any of the following:

1. Known hypersensitivity to alprostadil.
2. Abnormal penile anatomy: MUSE is contraindicated in patients with urethral stricture, balanitis (inflammation/infection of the glans of the penis), severe hypospadias and curvature, and in patients with acute or chronic urethritis.
3. Sickle cell anemia or trait, thrombocythemia, polycythemia, multiple myeloma: MUSE is contraindicated in patients who are prone to venous thrombosis or who have a hyperviscosity syndrome and are therefore at increased risk of priapism (rigid erection lasting 6 or more hours).
4. MUSE should not be used in men for whom sexual activity is inadvisable (see General Precautions).
5. MUSE should not be used for sexual intercourse with a pregnant woman unless the couple uses a condom barrier.

WARNINGS

Because of the potential for symptomatic hypotension and syncope, which occurred in 3% and 0.4%, respectively, of patients during in-clinic dosing, MUSE titration should be carried out under medical supervision. During post-marketing surveillance syncope occurring within one hour of administration has been reported. Patients should be cautioned to avoid activities, such as driving or hazardous tasks, where injury could result if hypotension or syncope were to occur after MUSE administration.

PRECAUTIONS

General Precautions:

1. A complete medical history and physical examination should be undertaken to exclude reversible causes of erectile dysfunction prior to the initiation of MUSE therapy. In addition, underlying disorders that might preclude the use of MUSE (see CONTRAINDICATIONS) should be sought.
2. *Cardiovascular effects:* During in-clinic dosing, patients should be monitored for symptoms of hypotension, and the lowest effective dose of MUSE should be prescribed.
3. *Hematologic effects:* Patients administering MUSE improperly may be at risk of urethral abrasion resulting in minor bleeding or spotting. Patients on anticoagulant therapy or with bleeding disorders may be at higher risk of bleeding. Patients on anticoagulant therapy have been safely treated with MUSE; however, the risk/benefit ratio in these patients should be considered prior to prescribing MUSE.
4. *Resumption of sexual activity:* Sexual intercourse is considered a vigorous physical activity, and it increases heart rate as well as cardiac work. Physicians may want to examine the cardiac fitness of patients prior to treating erectile dysfunction.
5. *Priapism and prolonged erection:* In clinical trials of MUSE, priapism (rigid erection lasting ≥6 hours) and prolonged erection (rigid erection lasting 4 hours and <6 hours) were reported infrequently (<0.1% and 0.3% of patients, respectively). Nevertheless, these events are a potential risk of pharmacologic therapy and can cause penile injury. Physicians should lower the dose or consider discontinuing MUSE treatment in any patient who develops priapism or prolonged erection.
6. *Drug-Drug Interactions:* Because there are low or undetectable (<2 picograms/mL) amounts of alprostadil found in the peripheral venous circulation following MUSE administration, systemic drug-drug interactions with MUSE are unlikely. Although formal studies have not been conducted, the concomitant use of MUSE and antihypertensive medications may increase the risk of hypotension. It is therefore advised that caution be used in the administration of MUSE to individuals on anti-hypertensive medications. In addition, the presence of medications in the circulation that attenuate erectile function may influence the response to MUSE.
7. *Drug-Device Interactions:* Use of MUSE in patients with penile implants has not been studied.
8. *Sexual Preference:* There is no experience in homosexual men and no experience with other than vaginal intercourse.

Information for Patients: Patients should be informed that MUSE offers no protection from the transmission of sexually transmitted diseases. Patients and partners who use MUSE need to be counseled about the protective measures that are necessary to guard against the spread of sexually transmitted agents, including the human immunodeficiency virus (HIV).

Although unreported in clinical trials, there is the possibility that an overdosage of MUSE can cause priapism, a painful erection of the penis sustained for hours and unrelieved by sexual intercourse or masturbation. This condition is serious and, if untreated, it can lead to permanent inability to have an erection. Patients who experience a prolonged erection should seek prompt medical attention.

Patients should be instructed how to administer MUSE. A patient package insert must be given to each patient at the initiation of MUSE therapy.

Information for Partners: Partners of patients using MUSE should be informed that MUSE offers no protection from the transmission of sexually transmitted diseases. Patients and partners who use MUSE should be counseled about the protective measures that are necessary to guard against the spread of sexually transmitted agents, including the human immunodeficiency virus (HIV). Human semen contains PGE_1, but additional amounts may be present from MUSE administration (see CLINICAL PHARMACOLOGY). Partners who have experienced an extended period of sexual abstinence should be encouraged to seek advice from a health care professional prior to resuming sexual intercourse. The use of a water-based lubricant may facilitate vaginal penetration.

It is recommended that couples using MUSE employ adequate contraception if the female partner is of childbearing potential. There is no information on the effects on early pregnancy of PGE_1 at the levels received by female partners. MUSE has no contraceptive properties. MUSE should not be used if the female partner is pregnant, unless the couple uses a condom barrier.

Carcinogenesis, Mutagenesis, Impairment of Fertility: Long-term carcinogenicity studies of alprostadil have not been conducted. Alprostadil showed no evidence of mutagenicity in vitro in the Ames bacterial reverse mutation test, the unscheduled DNA synthesis assay in rat hepatocytes, or the Chinese hamster ovary forward gene mutation assay; nor was there evidence of mutagenicity in vivo in the mouse micronucleus assay. Alprostadil concentrations increased chromosomal aberrations above control incidence in the in vitro Chinese hamster ovary chromosomal aberration assay. In dogs, sperm concentration, morphology, and motility were unaffected by daily intraurethral administration of up to 3000 mcg MUSE (alprostadil) for 13 weeks (200 mcg/kg/day or about 3.5 times the maximum recommended daily dose adjusted for body surface area). Alprostadil concentrations of 400 mcg/mL had no effect on human sperm motility or viability in vitro.

Pregnancy: Pregnancy Category C: Alprostadil has been shown to be embryotoxic (decreased fetal weight) when administered as a subcutaneous bolus to pregnant rats at doses as low as 500 mcg/kg/day. Doses of 2000 mcg/kg/day resulted in increased resorptions, reduced numbers of live fetuses, increased incidences of visceral and skeletal variations (primarily left umbilical artery and generalized reduction in ossification of the entire skeleton) and gross visceral and skeletal malformations (primarily edema, hydrocephaly, anophthalmia/microphthalmia, and skeletal anomalies). The latter dose produced maternal toxicity (ataxia, lethargy, diarrhea, and retarded body weight gain). When administered by continuous intravenous infusion, evidence of embryotoxicity (decreased fetal weight gain and increased incidence of hydroureter) was observed at 2000 mcg/kg/day, a dose that was also associated with a decrease in maternal weight gain. Intravaginal administration of up to 4000 mcg/day of MUSE (alprostadil) to pregnant rabbits (1100 mcg/kg/day or about 12.5 times the maximum recommended daily dose adjusted for body surface area) resulted in no evidence of harm to the fetus. MUSE should not be used for sexual intercourse with a pregnant woman unless the couple uses a condom barrier.

Nursing Mothers and Pediatric Use: MUSE is not indicated for use in newborns, children, or women.

ADVERSE REACTIONS

In-Clinic Titration: In the 2 largest double-blind, parallel, placebo-controlled trials, 1511 patients received MUSE at least 1 time in the clinic setting. The most frequently reported drug-related side effects during in-clinic titration included pain in the penis (36%), urethra (13%), or testes (5%). These discomforts were most commonly reported as mild and transient, but about 7% of patients withdrew at this stage because of adverse events. Urethral bleeding/spotting and other minor abrasions to the urethra were reported in approximately 3% of patients. Symptomatic lowering of blood pressure (hypotension) occurred in 3% of patients; in addition, some lowering of blood pressure may occur without symptoms. Dizziness was reported in 4% of patients. Syncope (fainting) was reported by 0.4% of patients. (See **WARNINGS**).

Home Treatment: 996 patients (66% of those who began titration) were studied during the home treatment portion of 2 Phase III placebo-controlled studies. Fewer than 2% of patients discontinued from these studies primarily because of adverse events. The following table summarizes the frequency of adverse events reported by patients using MUSE or placebo.

Adverse Events Reported by ≥2% of Patients Treated with MUSE and More Common than on Placebo At Home in Phase III Placebo-Controlled Clinical Studies for up to 3 Months

Event	MUSE n = 486	Placebo n = 511
UROGENITAL SYSTEM		
Penile Pain	32%	3%
Urethral Burning	12%	4%
Minor Urethral Bleeding/Spotting	5%	1%
Testicular Pain	5%	1%
NERVOUS SYSTEM		
Dizziness	2%	<1%
BODY AS A WHOLE		
Flu Symptoms	4%	2%
Headache	3%	2%
Pain	3%	1%
Accidental Injury	3%	2%
Back Pain	2%	1%
Pelvic Pain	2%	<1%
RESPIRATORY		
Rhinitis	2%	<1%
Infection	3%	2%

Other drug-related side effects observed during in-clinic titration and home treatment include swelling of leg veins, leg pain, perineal pain, and rapid pulse, each occurring in <2% of patients.

Female Partner Adverse Events: The most common drug-related adverse event reported by female partners during placebo-controlled clinical studies was vaginal burning/itching, reported by 5.8% of partners of patients on active vs. 0.8% of partners of patients on placebo. It is unknown whether this adverse event experienced by female partners was a result of the medication or a result of resuming sexual intercourse, which occurred much more frequently in partners of patients on active medication.

OVERDOSAGE

Overdosage has not been reported with MUSE. Overdosage with MUSE may result in hypotension, persistent penile pain, and possibly priapism (rigid erection lasting ≥6h). Priapism can result in permanent worsening of erectile function. Patients suspected of overdosage who develop these symptoms should be kept under medical supervision until systemic or local symptoms have resolved.

DOSAGE AND ADMINISTRATION

MUSE is a transurethral delivery system available in 4 dosage strengths: 125 mcg, 250 mcg, 500 mcg, and 1000 mcg. MUSE should be administered as needed to achieve an erection. The onset of effect is within 5–10 minutes after administration. The duration of effect is approximately 30–60 minutes. However, the actual duration will vary from patient to patient. Each patient should be instructed by a medical professional on proper technique for administering MUSE prior to self-administration. The maximum frequency of use is no more than 2 systems per 24-hour period.

Initiation of Therapy: Dose titration should be administered under the supervision of a physician to test a patient's responsiveness to MUSE, to demonstrate proper administration technique (see detailed instructions for MUSE administration in patient package insert), and to monitor for evidence of hypotension (see **WARNINGS**). Patients should

Continued on next page

MUSE—Cont.

be individually titrated to the lowest dose that is sufficient for sexual intercourse. The lower doses of MUSE (125 mcg or 250 mcg) are recommended for initial dosing. If necessary, the dose should be increased (or decreased) on separate occasions in a stepwise manner until the patient achieves an erection that is sufficient for sexual intercouse.

Home Treatment Regimen: MUSE should be used as needed to achieve an erection. The maximum frequency of use is 2 administrations per 24-hour period. Each MUSE is for single use only and should be properly discarded after use.

HOW SUPPLIED

MUSE is supplied in individual foil pouches containing one (1) system per pouch. MUSE is available in unit cartons containing six (6) systems. MUSE is available in the following 4 dosage strengths:

Dosage Strength	NDC Numbers Carton	Pouch	Identifying Package Color
125 mcg	62541-110-06	62541-110-01	Tan
250 mcg	62541-120-06	62541-120-01	Green
500 mcg	62541-130-06	62541-130-01	Blue
1000 mcg	62541-140-06	62541-140-01	Burgundy

STORAGE AND HANDLING

Store unopened foil pouches in a refrigerator at 2°–8°C (36°–46°F). Do not expose MUSE to temperatures above 30°C (86°F). MUSE may be kept by the patient at room temperature (below 30°C or 86°F) for up to 14 days prior to use.

Caution: Federal law prohibits dispensing without prescription.

Medical information line at VIVUS 1-888-345-MUSE (1-888-345-6873).

Revised February 1998

PATIENT INFORMATION

Please read this pamphlet before using MUSE® (alprostadil). This pamphlet is a quick reference source on important information about MUSE for you and your partner. **Before administering MUSE, please review the patient video and education booklet. These materials provide visual instruction and more detailed information as well as practical tips on how to use MUSE.**

WHAT IS MUSE?

MUSE represents a unique approach for the treatment of erectile dysfunction, commonly called impotence. It is based on the discovery that the urethra (the normal pathway for urine) can absorb certain medications into the surrounding erectile tissues thereby creating an erection. There are 4 dose strengths available: 125, 250, 500, and 1000 micrograms. The MUSE applicator (Fig. 1) contained in each foil pouch is intended for 1 administration only. Your dose of MUSE will be determined by you and your physician. After administration, the erection process will begin within 5–10 minutes, and may last 30–60 minutes. However, the actual duration will vary from patient to patient.

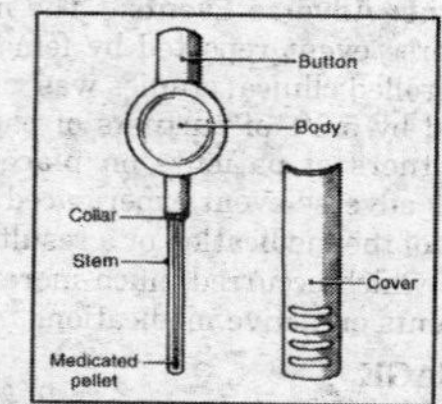

Figure 1.

WHAT IS MUSE USED FOR?

MUSE is indicated for the treatment of erectile dsyfunction. Erectile dysfunction is the inability to attain or maintain an erection sufficient for sexual intercourse.

WHO SHOULD NOT USE MUSE?

You should not use MUSE if you have any of the following:

- Known hypersensitivity to alprostadil (the active medication in MUSE)
- An abnormally formed penis
- Have been advised not to undertake sexual activity
- Conditions that might result in long-lasting erections, such as sickle cell anemia or trait, leukemia, or tumor of the bone marrow (multiple myeloma)
- MUSE should not be used for sexual intercourse with a pregnant woman unless the couple uses a condom barrier.

WHAT ARE THE POSSIBLE SIDE EFFECTS OF MUSE?

The most common side effects that have been observed using MUSE follow:

- Aching in the penis, testicles, legs, and in the perineum (area between the penis and rectum)
- Warmth or burning sensation in the urethra
- Redness of the penis due to increased blood flow
- Minor urethral bleeding or spotting due to improper administration.

Side effects reported less frequently:

- Prolonged erection— PLEASE NOTE: IF YOUR ERECTION IS RIGID FOR MORE THAN 4 HOURS, CALL YOUR DOCTOR PROMPTLY.
- Swelling of leg veins
- Light-headedness/Dizziness
- Fainting— PLEASE NOTE: AFTER USING MUSE, YOU SHOULD AVOID ACTIVITIES, SUCH AS DRIVING OR HAZARDOUS TASKS, WHERE INJURY COULD RESULT IF DIZZINESS OR FAINTING WERE TO OCCUR. IN PATIENTS EXPERIENCING THESE SYMPTOMS, THE SYMPTOMS HAVE USUALLY OCCURRED DURING INITIATION OF THERAPY AND WITHIN ONE HOUR OF MUSE ADMINISTRATION.
- Rapid pulse.

If you have a history of fainting be sure to discuss this with your doctor prior to using MUSE. If you do experience dizziness or feel faint, this may be due to the lowering of your blood pressure. Lie down immediately and raise your legs. If symptoms persist, call your doctor promptly. Because of the potential for these side effects, MUSE titration should be carried out under medical supervision.

Changing Your Dosage

It is assumed that you and your doctor have determined the proper dose of MUSE. If you suspect that your dose needs to be increased or decreased to achieve the response that works best for you, please call your doctor to determine if your dose needs to be reevaluated. Do not use MUSE more than twice in a 24-hour period.

WHAT ARE THE POSSIBLE SIDE EFFECTS OF MUSE FOR YOUR PARTNER?

The most common reported side effects observed in women whose partners use MUSE are mild vaginal itching or burning. Using a water-based lubricant can help to make vaginal penetration easier. Your partner may want to consult her health care provider if she has not had sexual intercourse for an extended period of time.

IMPORTANT INFORMATION FOR YOU AND YOUR PARTNER

Pregnancy

MUSE has no contraceptive properties.

Because MUSE has not been tested during human pregnancy, it is recommended that couples use adequate contraception if the female partner is of childbearing potential. MUSE should not be used for sexual intercourse with a pregnant woman unless the couple uses a condom barrier.

Sexually Transmitted Diseases

MUSE will not protect you or your partner from sexually transmitted diseases like chlamydia, gonorrhea, herpes simplex virus, viral hepatitis, human immunodeficiency virus (HIV—the virus that causes AIDS), human papilloma virus (genital warts), and syphilis. Latex condoms can protect against these sexually transmitted diseases.

HOW SHOULD I STORE MUSE?

It is recommended that MUSE be stored in a refrigerator. MUSE may be kept at room temperature (less than 30°C/86°F) for up to 14 days prior to use. It is very important that MUSE not be exposed to temperatures above 30°C/86°F since this will make MUSE ineffective. MUSE should not be exposed to high temperatures or placed in direct sunlight.

Storage when traveling

When traveling, store MUSE in a portable ice pack or cooler. Do not store in the trunk of a car or in baggage storage areas where MUSE may be exposed to extremes in temperature.

HOW TO ADMINISTER MUSE:

1. Immediately prior to administration, urinate and gently shake the penis several times to remove excess urine. A moist urethra makes administration of MUSE easier. The medicated pellet has been specially developed to dissolve in the small quantity of urine that remains in the urethra after urination.
2. Open the foil pouch by tearing fully across the notched edge (Fig. 2). Let the MUSE slide out of the pouch. Save the pouch for discarding the MUSE applicator later.

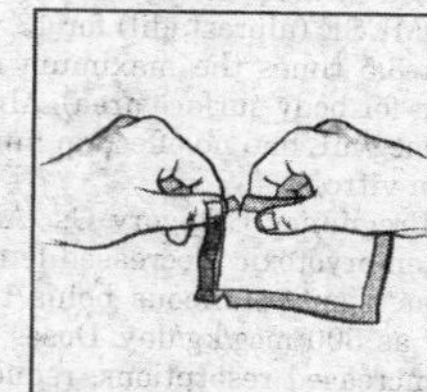
Figure 2.

3. To remove the protective cover from the applicator stem (Fig. 3), hold the body of the applicator with your thumb and forefinger. Twist the body and pull out the applicator from the cover, being careful not to push in or pull out the applicator button. Avoid touching the applicator stem and tip. Save the cover for discarding the MUSE applicator later.

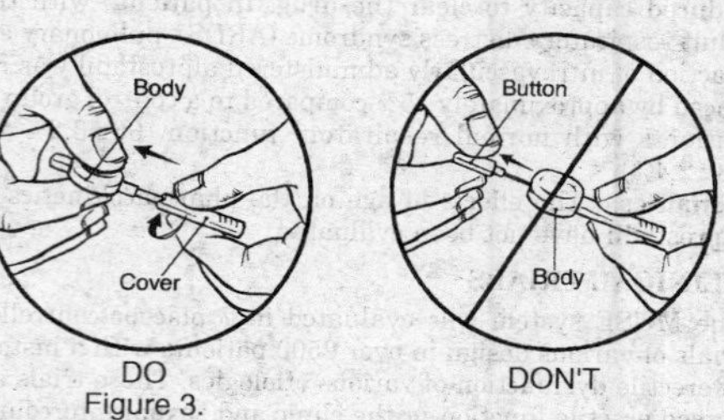

Figure 3.

4. Visually inspect the MUSE. The MUSE system is see-through, and you will be able to see the medicated pellet at the end of the stem. Make sure that the pellet is present before insertion (Fig. 4).

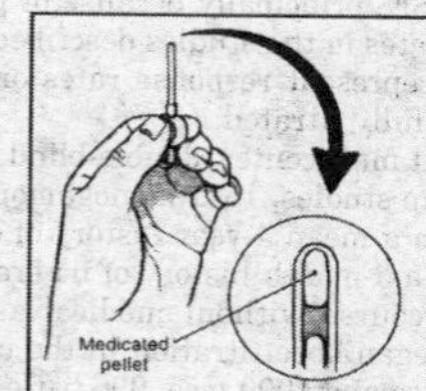

Figure 4.

5. Hold the applicator in a way which is the most comfortable for you (Fig. 5A and 5B).

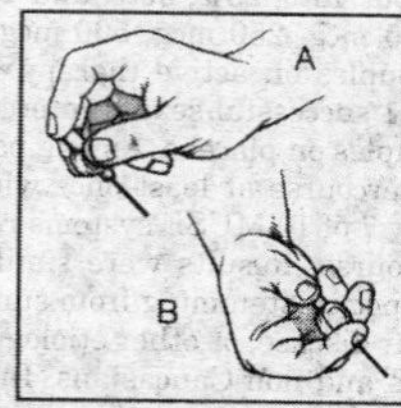

Figure 5.

6. Please review Figure 6A, the anatomy of the penis.

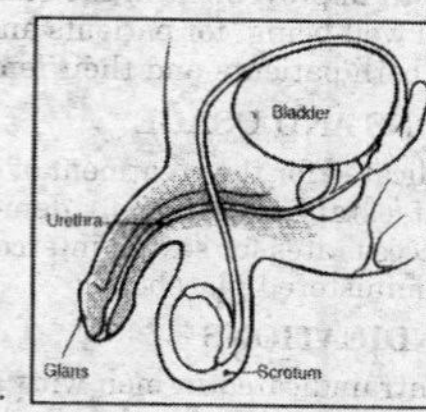

Figure 6A.

While sitting or standing, whichever is more comfortable for you, take several seconds to gently and slowly stretch the penis upward to its full length, with gentle compression from top to bottom of the glans (Fig. 6B). This straightens and opens the urethra. Slowly insert the MUSE stem into the urethra up to the collar (Fig. 6C). If you feel any discomfort or a pulling sensation, withdraw the applicator slightly and then gently reinsert.

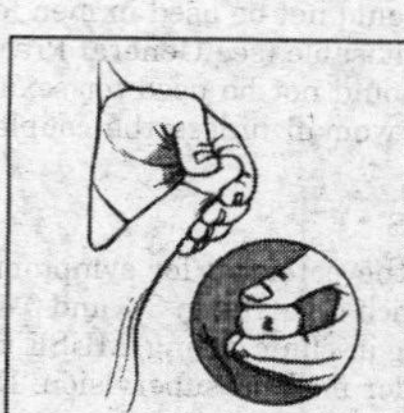
Figure 6B.

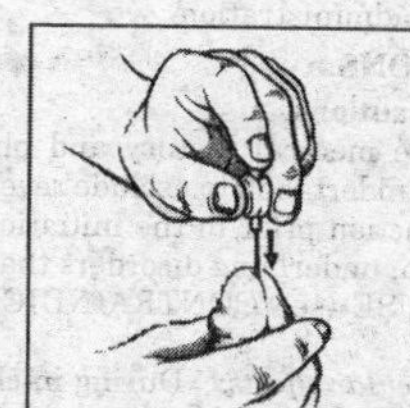
Figure 6C.

7. Gently and completely push down (Fig. 7) the button at the top of the applicator until it stops. It is important to do this to ensure that the medicated pellet is completely

released. Hold the applicator in this position for 5 seconds.

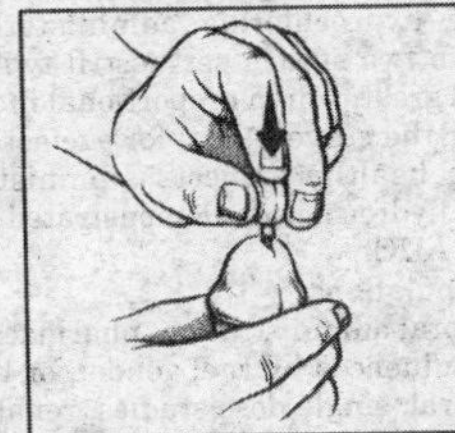

Figure 7.

8. Gently rock the applicator from side to side. This will separate the medicated pellet from the applicator tip (Fig. 8). If you apply too much pressure you may scratch the lining of the urethra causing it to bleed.

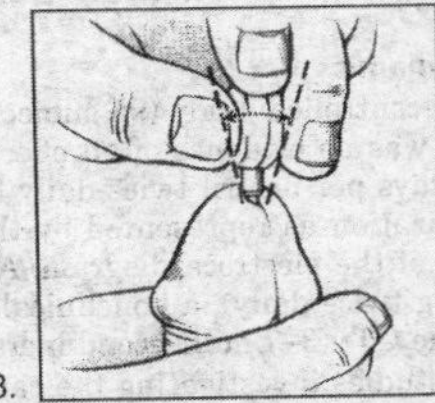

Figure 8.

9. Remove the applicator while keeping the penis upright.
10. Visually inspect the applicator tip to see that the medication is no longer in the applicator. Do not touch the stem. If you notice some residual medication in the end of the applicator, gently reinsert into the urethra and repeat steps 7, 8, and 9.
11. Holding the penis upright and stretched to its full length, roll the penis firmly between your hands for at least 10 seconds. This will ensure that the medication is adequately distributed along the walls of the urethra (Fig. 9). If you feel a burning sensation, it may help to continue to roll the penis for an additional 30–60 seconds or until the burning subsides.

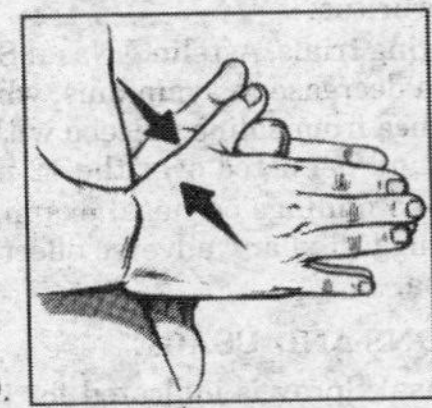

Figure 9.

12. Remember, each MUSE is good for a single administration only. Replace the cover on the MUSE applicator, place in the opened foil pouch, fold, and discard as normal household waste.

After you have administered MUSE, it is important to sit, or preferably stand or walk about for 10 minutes while the erection is developing. This increases blood flow to the penis and will enhance your erection.

ADDITIONAL INFORMATION AND PRACTICAL TIPS

Factors Which May Enhance Your Erection:
- Being well rested and relaxed
- Sexual foreplay with your partner or self-stimulation while sitting or standing
- Pelvic exercises (for example, Kegel exercises)—these consist of tightening and releasing your pelvic and buttock muscles. These are the muscles you use to stop urination
- Various positions that may favor blood flow into the penis. Please refer to the patient starter booklet and video for illustrative examples.

Factors Which May Reduce Your Erection:
- Anxiety, fatigue, tension, and too much alcohol
- Lying on your back too soon after administration of MUSE may decrease blood flow to the penis and result in loss of erection
- Urination or dribbling immediately following administration may result in loss of medication from the urethra
- Using medications that contain decongestants, such as over-the-counter cold remedies, allergy, sinus medications, and appetite suppressants, may block the effect of MUSE.

COMMONLY ASKED QUESTIONS ABOUT MUSE

Will insertion of MUSE hurt?
At first, you may feel some minor discomfort from insertion. Urinating prior to administration will reduce the chance of discomfort or abrasions and is important for dissolving the medicated pellet. Be sure to straighten your penis to its full length when inserting the MUSE applicator. With repeated use, administration will become much easier.

What are the side effects associated with MUSE?
Most of the side effects reported in men are relatively minor and include burning and aching in the penis and groin. Rarely noted are prolonged erection, light-headedness, dizziness, fainting, rapid pulse, and swelling of the leg veins. If you feel dizzy, light-headed, faint, or experience rapid pulse, lie down immediately and raise your legs. If symptoms persist, call your doctor promptly. Because of the potential for these side effects, MUSE titration should be carried out under medical supervision.
(See also: **"WHAT ARE THE POSSIBLE SIDE EFFECTS OF MUSE?"**)
In women, mild vaginal itching and burning have been observed.

After I administer MUSE, can we immediately lie down and begin sexual activity?
You can begin sexual activity, but having the man lie down, especially on his back shortly after administration, is not recommended. This will reduce blood flow to the penis and may reduce the erection. It is important to sit, stand or walk about for 10 minutes after administration. Many couples have used this time to incorporate various types of foreplay. After this initial period, you can assume different positions leading to sexual intercourse. Some couples have noticed that the erection is better maintained in positions that favor blood flow into the penis during intercourse.
Please review the video and patient starter booklet available from your doctor which illustrates various positions that will enhance your erection.

How long will the effect of MUSE last?
An erection should begin within 5–10 minutes after administering MUSE. The duration of effect is approximately 30–60 minutes. However, the actual duration will vary from patient to patient.

What will the erection be like? How will it compare to the erections I had when I was younger?
An effective dose of MUSE should produce an erection sufficient for sexual intercourse. MUSE may not create an erection such as those you experienced when you were younger. Some patients may experience some mild pain and aching in the penis or groin area. Also, your erection may continue after orgasm.

How do I know if I have the correct dose of MUSE?
You and your physician will determine the appropriate dose of MUSE. If your erection cannot be maintained for the time needed to have foreplay and sexual intercourse, you may need to have your dose increased. Similarly, an erection that lasts longer than desired may require a dose decrease. Call your doctor if you suspect you may require a dosing adjustment.

After my erection is over, will my penis feel sensitive?
Your penis may feel full, warm, and somewhat sensitive to the touch. These effects are normal and may last a few hours.

Can I reuse MUSE?
No. MUSE is intended for single-dose application only.

How do I dispose of the MUSE applicator?
After you have administered MUSE, replace the cap on the applicator, place in the opened foil pouch, fold, and discard as normal household waste.

If my erection lasts longer than desired, what should I do?
Note: Call your doctor promptly if you have a rigid erection that lasts more than 4 hours.
An application of ice packs to the inner thigh may shorten the duration of the erection, since the cold will restrict blood flow to the penis. If used, ice packs should be applied alternately to each inner thigh for a period not exceeding 10 minutes.

How often can I safely use MUSE?
MUSE should not be used more than twice per day.

If you have any additional questions about MUSE, please call the toll free patient information line at VIVUS 1-888-367-MUSE (1-888-367-6873).

MUSE® IS A REGISTERED TRADEMARK OF VIVUS, INC. IN THE U.S. AND OTHER COUNTRIES.
VIVUS, Inc.
Mountain View, CA 94043 February 1998

Shown in Product Identification Guide, page 339

Wakefield Pharmaceuticals, Inc.

310 MAXWELL ROAD, SUITE 100
ALPHARETTA, GA 30004

Direct Inquiries to:
(770) 664-1661
FAX: (770) 664-1126

Products Described:

Biohist® LA Tablets
Muco-fen® 800 Tablets
Muco-fen® 800 DM Tablets
Profen Forte DM® Tablets
Profen Forte® Tablets
Profen II DM® Liquid
Profen II DM® Tablets
Profen II® Tablets

Other Products Available:

Muco-fen® 1200 Tablets
Muco-fen® DM Tablets
Muco-fen® LA Tablets
Profen LA® Tablets

BIOHIST® LA TABLETS ℞
[*bīō-hĭst*]
Chlorpheniramine Maleate/Pseudoephedrine HCl

DESCRIPTION
Each time-released, dye free, scored tablet contains:
Chlorpheniramine Maleate .... 12 mg
Pseudoephedrine Hydrochloride .... 120 mg

DOSAGE
Adults and children over 12 years of age: ½–1 tablet every 12 hours
Children 6–12 years of age: ½ tablet every 12 hours

HOW SUPPLIED
Bottles of 100 tablets (NDC 59310-112-10)

MUCO-FEN® 800 DM TABLETS ℞
[*mū-co-fin*]
Guaifenesin/Dextromehorphan HBr

DESCRIPTION
Each time-released, dye free, scored tablet contains:
Guaifenesin .... 800 mg
Dextromethorphan Hydrobromide .... 60 mg

DOSAGE
Adults and children over 12 years of age: 1 tablet every 12 hours not to exceed 2 tablets in 24 hours
Children 6–12 years of age: ½ tablet every 12 hours not to exceed 1 tablet in 24 hours

HOW SUPPLIED
Bottles of 100 tablets (NDC 59310-114-10)

MUCO-FEN® 800 Tablets ℞
[*mū-co-fin*]
Guaifenesin

DESCRIPTION
Each time-released, dye free, scored tablet contains:
Guaifenesin .... 800 mg

DOSAGE
Adults and children over 12 years of age: 1–1½ tablets every 12 hours not to exceed 3 tablets (2400 mg) in 24 hours
Children 6–12 years of age: ½ tablet every 12 hours not to exceed 1200 mg in 24 hours

HOW SUPPLIED
Bottles of 100 tablets (NDC 59310-109-10)

PROFEN II® TABLETS ℞
[*prō'-fin*]
Phenylpropanolamine HCl/Guaifenesin

DESCRIPTION
Each time-released, dye free, scored tablet contains:
Phenylpropanolamine Hydrochloride .... 37.5 mg
Guaifenesin .... 600 mg

DOSAGE
Adults and children over 12 years of age: 1–2 tablets every 12 hours not to exceed 4 tablets in 24 hours
Children 6–12 years of age: 1 tablet every 12 hours not to exceed 2 tablets in 24 hours

HOW SUPPLIED
Bottles of 100 tablets (NDC 59310-107-10)

PROFEN II DM® Liquid ℞
[*prō'-fin*]
Dextromethorphan HBr/Phenylpropanolamine HCl/Guaifenesin

DESCRIPTION
Each 5 mL (one teaspoonful) contains:
Dextromethorphan Hydrobromide .... 10 mg
Phenylpropanolamine Hydrochloride .... 12.5 mg
Guaifenesin .... 200 mg
In a sugar free, dye free and alcohol free base.

DOSAGE
Adults and children 12 years or older: 1–2 teaspoonfuls every 4 hours not to exceed 12 teaspoonfuls in 24 hours. Children 6–12 years of age: $^1/_2$–1 teaspoonful every 4 hours not to exceed 6 teaspoonfuls in 24 hours. Children 2–6 years of age: $^1/_4$–$^1/_2$ teaspoonful not to exceed 3 teaspoonfuls in 24 hours. Children under 2 years: As directed by physician.

HOW SUPPLIED
PROFEN II DM® LIQUID is available as a sugar, alcohol and dye-free clear liquid having a cherry odor and flavor.
Pint Bottles: NDC 59310-201-16.

Continued on next page

PROFEN II DM® TABLETS ℞
[*prō ′-fin*]
Dextromethorphan HBr/Phenylpropanolamine HCl/Guaifenesin

DESCRIPTION

Each time-released, dye free, scored tablet contains:
Dextromethorphan Hydrobromide .... 30 mg
Phenylpropanolamine Hydrochloride .... 37.5 mg
Guaifenesin .... 600 mg

DOSAGE

Adults and children over 12 years of age: 1–2 tablets every 12 hours not to exceed 4 tablets in 24 hours
Children 6–12 years of age: 1 tablet every 12 hours not to exceed 2 tablets in 24 hours

HOW SUPPLIED

Bottles of 100 tablets (NDC 59310-110-10)

PROFEN FORTE® TABLETS ℞
[*prō′-fin*]
Phenylpropanolamine HCl/Guaifenesin

DESCRIPTION

Each time-released, dye free, scored tablet contains:
Phenylpropanolamine Hydrochloride .... 75 mg
Guaifenesin .... 800 mg

DOSAGE

Adults and children over 12 years of age: 1 tablet every 12 hours not to exceed 2 tablets in 24 hours
Children 6–12 years of age: ½ tablet every 12 hours not to exceed 1 tablet in 24 hours

HOW SUPPLIED

Bottles of 100 tablets (NDC 59310-115-10)

PROFEN FORTE DM® TABLETS ℞
[*prō ′-fin*]
Dextromethorphan HBr/Phenylpropanolamine HCl/Guaifenesin

DESCRIPTION

Each time-released, dye free, scored tablet contains:
Dextromethorphan Hydrobromide .... 60 mg
Phenylpropanolamine Hydrochloride .... 75 mg
Guaifenesin .... 800 mg

DOSAGE

Adults and children over 12 years of age: 1 tablet every 12 hours not to exceed 2 tablets in 24 hours
Children 6–12 years of age: ½ tablet every 12 hours not to exceed 1 tablet in 24 hours

HOW SUPPLIED

Bottles of 100 tablets (NDC 59310-116-10)

Wakunaga Consumer Products

**23501 MADERO
MISSION VIEJO, CA 92691**

Direct Inquiries to:
(800) 527-5200

KYOLIC®
Odor Modified Garlic Supplement

Active Ingredient: Each caplet contains 600 mg Aged Garlic Extract™.

Suggested Use: As a dietary supplement, take 1 or more caplets daily with food to promote healthy circulation.

How Supplied: Boxes of 30 Caplets.
Shown in Product Identification Guide, page 343

PROBIATA®
Probiotic Dietary Supplement

Active Ingredient: L. acidophilus

Suggested Use: Take one tablet, twice daily with meals. Replenishes healthy intestinal flora to avoid disorders such as diarrhea, constipation and yeast discomfort caused by antibiotic usage.

How Supplied: Bottles of 30 tablets.
Shown in Product Identification Guide, page 343

Wallace Laboratories

**P.O. BOX 1001
CRANBURY, NJ 08512**

For Medical Information, Contact:
Generally:
Professional Services
800-526-3840
After Hours and Weekend Emergencies:
(609) 655-6474
Wallace Laboratories
Sales and Ordering:
Div. of Carter-Wallace, Inc
P.O. Box 1001
Cranbury, NJ 08512

AQUATENSEN® ℞
(methyclothiazide tablets, USP, 5 mg)
Tablets

ASTELIN® ℞
(azelastine hydrochloride)
Nasal Spray, 137 mcg
For Intranasal Use Only

DESCRIPTION

Astelin® (azelastine hydrochloride) Nasal Spray, 137 micrograms (mcg), is an antihistamine formulated as a metered-spray solution for intranasal administration. Azelastine hydrochloride occurs as a white, almost odorless, crystalline powder with a bitter taste. It has a molecular weight of 418.37. It is sparingly soluble in water, methanol, and propylene glycol and slightly soluble in ethanol, octanol, and glycerine. It has a melting point of about 225°C and the pH of a saturated solution is between 5.0 and 5.4. Its chemical name is (±)-1-(2H)-phthalazinone,4-[(4-chlorophenyl) methyl]-2-(hexahydro-1-methyl-1H-azepin-4-yl)-, monohydrochloride. Its molecular formula is $C_{22}H_{24}ClN_3O \bullet HCl$ with the following chemical structure:

Astelin® Nasal Spray contains 0.1% azelastine hydrochloride in an aqueous solution at pH 6.8 ± 0.3. It also contains benzalkonium chloride (125 mcg/mL), edetate disodium, hydroxypropyl methyl cellulose, citric acid, dibasic sodium phosphate, sodium chloride, and purified water.
After priming, each metered spray delivers a 0.137 mL mean volume containing 137 mcg of azelastine hydrochloride (equivalent to 125 mcg of azelastine base). Each bottle can deliver 100 metered sprays.

CLINICAL PHARMACOLOGY

Azelastine hydrochloride, a phthalazinone derivative, exhibits histamine H_1-receptor antagonist activity in isolated tissues, animal models, and humans. Astelin® Nasal Spray is administered as a racemic mixture with no difference in pharmacologic activity noted between the enantiomers in *in vitro* studies. The major metabolite, desmethylazelastine, also possesses H_1-receptor antagonist activity.

Pharmacokinetics and Metabolism
After intranasal administration, the systemic bioavailability of azelastine hydrochloride is approximately 40%. Maximum plasma concentrations (Cmax) are achieved in 2–3 hours. Based on intravenous and oral administration, the elimination half-life, steady-state volume of distribution, and plasma clearance are 22 hours, 14.5 L/kg, and 0.5 L/h/kg, respectively. Approximately 75% of an oral dose of radiolabeled azelastine hydrochloride was excreted in the feces with less than 10% as unchanged azelastine. Azelastine is oxidatively metabolized to the principal active metabolite, desmethylazelastine, by the cytochrome P450 enzyme system. The specific P450 isoforms responsible for the biotransformation of azelastine have not been identified; however, clinical interaction studies with the known CYP3A4 inhibitor erythromycin failed to demonstrate a pharmacokinetic interaction. In a multiple-dose, steady-state drug interaction study in normal volunteers, cimetidine (400 mg twice daily), a nonspecific P450 inhibitor, raised orally administered azelastine (4 mg twice daily) concentrations by approximately 65%.
The major active metabolite, desmethylazelastine, was not measurable (below assay limits) after single-dose intranasal administration of azelastine hydrochloride. After intranasal dosing of azelastine hydrochloride to steady-state, plasma concentrations of desmethylazelastine range from 20–50% of azelastine concentrations. When azelastine hydrochloride is administered orally, desmethylazelastine has an elimination half-life of 54 hours. Limited data indicate that the metabolite profile is similar when azelastine hydrochloride is administered via the intranasal or oral route.
In vitro studies with human plasma indicate that the plasma protein binding of azelastine and desmethylazelastine are approximately 88% and 97%, respectively.
Azelastine hydrochloride administered intranasally at doses above two sprays per nostril twice daily for 29 days resulted in greater than proportional increases in Cmax and area under the curve (AUC) for azelastine.
Studies in healthy subjects administered oral doses of azelastine hydrochloride demonstrated linear responses in Cmax and AUC.

Special Populations
Following oral administration, pharmacokinetic parameters were not influenced by age, gender, or hepatic impairment. Based on oral, single-dose studies, renal insufficiency (creatine clearance <50 mL/min) resulted in a 70–75% higher Cmax and AUC compared to normal subjects. Time to maximum concentration was unchanged.
Oral azelastine has been safely administered to over 1400 asthmatic subjects, supporting the safety of administering Astelin® Nasal Spray to allergic rhinitis patients with asthma.

Pharmacodynamics
In a placebo-controlled study (95 subjects with allergic rhinitis), there was no evidence of an effect of Astelin® Nasal Spray (2 sprays per nostril twice daily for 56 days) on cardiac repolarization as represented by the corrected QT interval (QTc) of the electrocardiogram. At higher oral exposures (≥4 mg twice daily), a nonclinically significant mean change on the QTc (3–7 millisecond increase) was observed.
Interaction studies investigating the cardiac repolarization effects of concomitantly administered oral azelastine hydrochloride and erythromycin or ketoconazole were conducted. Oral erythromycin had no effect on azelastine pharmacokinetics or QTc based on analysis of serial electrocardiograms. Ketoconazole interfered with the measurement of azelastine plasma levels; however, no effects on QTc were observed (see PRECAUTIONS, Drug Interactions).

Clinical Trials
U.S. placebo-controlled clinical trials of Astelin® Nasal Spray included 322 patients with seasonal allergic rhinitis who received two sprays per nostril twice a day for up to 4 weeks. These trials included 55 pediatric patients ages 12 to 16 years. Astelin® Nasal Spray significantly improved a complex of symptoms, which included rhinorrhea, sneezing, and nasal pruritus.
In dose-ranging trials, Astelin® Nasal Spray administration resulted in a decrease in symptoms, which reached statistical significance from saline placebo within 3 hours after initial dosing and persisted over the 12-hour dosing interval.
There were no findings on nasal examination in an 8-week study that suggested any adverse effect of azelastine on the nasal mucosa.

INDICATIONS AND USAGE

Astelin® Nasal Spray is indicated for the treatment of the symptoms of seasonal allergic rhinitis such as rhinorrhea, sneezing, and nasal pruritus in adults and children 5 years and older.

CONTRAINDICATIONS

Astelin® Nasal Spray is contraindicated in patients with a known hypersensitivity to azelastine hydrochloride or any of its components.

PRECAUTIONS

Activities Requiring Mental Alertness: In clinical trials, the occurrence of somnolence has been reported in some patients taking Astelin® Nasal Spray; due caution should therefore be exercised when driving a car or operating potentially dangerous machinery. Concurrent use of Astelin® Nasal Spray with alcohol or other CNS depressants should be avoided because additional reductions in alertness and additional impairment of CNS performance may occur.
Information for Patients: Patients should be instructed to use Astelin® Nasal Spray only as prescribed. For the proper use of the nasal spray and to attain maximum improvement, the patient should read and follow carefully the accompanying patient instructions. Patients should be instructed to prime the delivery system before initial use and after storage for 3 or more days (see PATIENT INSTRUCTIONS FOR USE). Patients should also be instructed to store the bottle upright at room temperature with the pump tightly closed and out of the reach of children. In case of accidental ingestion by a young child, seek professional assistance or contact a poison control center immediately.
Patients should be advised against the concurrent use of Astelin® Nasal Spray with other antihistamines without consulting a physician. Patients who are, or may become, pregnant should be told that this product should be used in pregnancy or during lactation only if the potential benefit justifies the potential risks to the fetus or nursing infant. Patients should be advised to assess their individual responses to Astelin® Nasal Spray before engaging in any activity requiring mental alertness, such as driving a car or operating machinery. Patients should be advised that the concurrent use of Astelin® Nasal Spray with alcohol or other CNS depressants may lead to additional reductions in alertness and impairment of CNS performance and should be avoided (see Drug Interactions).
Drug Interactions:
Concurrent use of Astelin® Nasal Spray with alcohol or other CNS depressants should be avoided because additional reductions in alertness and additional impairment of CNS performance may occur.

Cimetidine (400 mg twice daily) increased the mean Cmax and AUC of orally administered azelastine hydrochloride (4 mg twice daily) by approximately 65%. Ranitidine hydrochloride (150 mg twice daily) had no effect on azelastine pharmacokinetics.
Interaction studies investigating the cardiac effects, as measured by the corrected QT interval (QTc), of concomitantly administered oral azelastine hydrochloride and erythromycin or ketoconazole were conducted. Oral erythromycin (500 mg three times daily for seven days) had no effect on azelastine pharmacokinetics or QTc based on analyses of serial electrocardiograms. Ketoconazole (200 mg twice daily for seven days) interfered with the measurement of azelastine plasma concentrations; however, no effects on QTc were observed.
No significant pharmacokinetic interaction was observed with the coadministration of an oral 4 mg dose of azelastine hydrochloride twice daily and theophylline 300 mg or 400 mg twice daily.
Carcinogenesis, Mutagenesis, Impairment of Fertility: In 2 year carcinogenicity studies in rats and mice azelastine hydrochloride did not show evidence of carcinogenicity at oral doses up to 30 mg/kg and 25 mg/kg, respectively (approximately 240 and 100 times the maximum recommended daily intranasal dose in adults and children on a mg/m^2 basis).
Azelastine hydrochloride showed no genotoxic effects in the Ames test, DNA repair test, mouse lymphoma forward mutation assay, mouse micronucleus test, or chromosomal aberration test in rat bone marrow.
Reproduction and fertility studies in rats showed no effects on male or female fertility at oral doses up to 30 mg/kg (approximately 240 times the maximum recommended daily intranasal dose in adults on a mg/m^2 basis). At 68.6 mg/kg (approximately 560 times the maximum recommended daily intranasal dose in adults on a mg/m^2 basis), the duration of estrous cycles was prolonged and copulatory activity and the number of pregnancies were decreased. The numbers of corpora lutea and implantations were decreased; however, pre-implantation loss was not increased.
Pregnancy Category C: Azelastine hydrochloride has been shown to cause developmental toxicity. Treatment of mice with an oral dose of 68.6 mg/kg (approximately 280 times the maximum recommended daily intranasal dose in adults on a mg/m^2 basis) caused embryo-fetal death, malformations (cleft palate; short or absent tail; fused, absent or branched ribs), delayed ossification and decreased fetal weight. This dose also caused maternal toxicity as evidenced by decreased body weight. Neither fetal nor maternal effects occurred at a dose of 3 mg/kg (approximately 10 times the maximum recommended daily intranasal dose in adults on a mg/m^2 basis).
In rats, an oral dose of 30 mg/kg (approximately 240 times the maximum recommended daily intranasal dose in adults on a mg/m^2 basis) caused malformations (oligo-and brachydactylia), delayed ossification and skeletal variations, in the absence of maternal toxicity. At 68.6 mg/kg (approximately 560 times the maximum recommended daily intranasal dose in adults on a mg/m^2 basis) azelastine hydrochloride also caused embryo-fetal death and decreased fetal weight; however, the 68.6 mg/kg dose caused severe maternal toxicity. Neither fetal nor maternal effects occurred at a dose of 3 mg/kg (approximately 25 times the maximum recommended daily intranasal dose in adults on a mg/m^2 basis).
In rabbits, oral doses of 30 mg/kg and greater (approximately 500 times the maximum recommended daily intranasal dose in adults on a mg/m^2 basis) caused abortion, delayed ossification and decreased fetal weight; however, these doses also resulted in severe maternal toxicity. Neither fetal nor maternal effects occurred at a dose of 0.3 mg/kg (approximately 5 times the maximum recommended daily intranasal dose in adults on a mg/m^2 basis).
There are no adequate and well-controlled clinical studies in pregnant women. Astelin® Nasal Spray should be used during pregnancy only if the potential benefit justifies the potential risk to the fetus.
Nursing Mothers:
It is not known whether azelastine hydrochloride is excreted in human milk. Because many drugs are excreted in human milk, caution should be exercised when Astelin® Nasal Spray is administered to a nursing woman.
Pediatric Use: The safety and effectiveness of Astelin® Nasal Spray at a dose of 1 spray per nostril twice daily has been established for patients 5 through 11 years of age for the treatment of symptoms of seasonal allergic rhinitis. The safety of this dosage of Astelin® Nasal Spray was established in well-controlled studies of this dose in 176 patients 5 to 12 years of age treated for up to 6 weeks. The effectiveness of Astelin® Nasal Spray at this dose is based on an extrapolation of the finding of efficacy in adults, on the likelihood that the disease course, pathophysiology and response to treatment are substantially similar in children compared to adults, and on supportive data from controlled clinical trials in patients 5 to 12 years of age at the dose of 1 spray per nostril twice daily. The safety and effectiveness of Astelin® Nasal Spray in patients below the age of 5 years have not been established.
Geriatric Use: U.S. placebo-controlled clinical trials included 11 patients above the age of 60 years who were treated with Astelin® Nasal Spray. While this number is very small and no substantial conclusions can be drawn, the adverse events in this group were similar to patients under age 60 years.

ADVERSE REACTIONS

Adverse experience information for Astelin® Nasal Spray is derived from six well-controlled, 2-day to 8-week clinical studies which included 391 patients who received Astelin® Nasal Spray at a dose of 2 sprays per nostril twice daily. In placebo-controlled efficacy trials, the incidence of discontinuation due to adverse reactions in patients receiving Astelin® Nasal Spray was not significantly different from vehicle placebo (2.2% vs 2.8%, respectively).
In these clinical studies, adverse events that occurred statistically significantly more often in patients treated with Astelin® Nasal Spray versus vehicle placebo included bitter taste (19.7% vs 0.6%), somnolence (11.5% vs 5.4%), weight increase (2.0% vs 0%), and myalgia (1.5% vs 0%).
The following adverse events were reported with frequencies ≥2% in the Astelin® Nasal Spray treatment group and more frequently than placebo in short-term (≤2 days) and long-term (2–8 weeks) clinical trials.

ADVERSE EVENT	Astelin® Nasal Spray n = 391	Vehicle Placebo n = 353
Bitter Taste*	19.7	0.6
Headache	14.8	12.7
Somnolence*	11.5	5.4
Nasal Burning	4.1	1.7
Pharyngitis	3.8	2.8
Dry Mouth	2.8	1.7
Paroxysmal Sneezing	3.1	1.1
Nausea	2.8	1.1
Rhinitis	2.3	1.4
Fatigue	2.3	1.4
Dizziness	2.0	1.4
Epistaxis	2.0	1.4
Weight Increase*	2.0	0.0

*P<0.05, Fisher's Exact Test (two-tailed)

A total of 176 patients 5 to 12 years of age were exposed to Astelin® Nasal Spray at a dose of 1 spray each nostril twice daily in 3 placebo-controlled studies. In these studies, adverse events that occurred more frequently in patients treated with Astelin® Nasal Spray than with placebo, and that were not represented in the adult adverse event table above include rhinitis/cold symptoms (17.0% vs 9.5%), cough (11.4% vs 8.3%), conjunctivitis (5.1% vs 1.8%), and asthma (4.5% vs 4.1%).
The following events were observed infrequently (<2% and exceeding placebo incidence) in patients who received Astelin® Nasal Spray (2 sprays/nostril twice daily) in U.S. clinical trials.
Cardiovascular: flushing, hypertension, tachycardia.
Dermatological: contact dermatitis, eczema, hair and follicle infection, furunculosis.
Digestive: constipation, gastroenteritis, glossitis, ulcerative stomatitis, vomiting, increased SGPT, aphthous stomatitis.
Metabolic and Nutritional: increased appetite.
Musculoskeletal: myalgia, temporomandibular dislocation.
Neurological: hyperkinesia, hypoesthesia, vertigo.
Psychological: anxiety, depersonalization, depression, nervousness, sleep disorder, thinking abnormal.
Respiratory: bronchospasm, coughing, throat burning, laryngitis.
Special Senses: conjunctivitis, eye abnormality, eye pain, watery eyes, taste loss.
Urogenital: albuminuria, amenorrhea, breast pain, hematuria, increased urinary frequency.
Whole Body: allergic reaction, back pain, herpes simplex, viral infection, malaise, pain in extremities, abdominal pain.
In controlled trials involving nasal and oral azelastine hydrochloride formulations, there were infrequent occurrences of hepatic transaminase elevations. The clinical relevance of these reports has not been established.
In addition, the following spontaneous adverse events have been reported during the marketing of Astelin® Nasal Spray and causal relationship with the drug is unknown: anaphylactoid reaction, application site irritation, chest pain, nasal congestion, confusion, diarrhea, dyspnea, facial edema, involuntary muscle contractions, paresthesia, parosmia, pruritus, rash, tolerance, urinary retention, vision abnormal and xerophthalmia.

OVERDOSAGE

There have been no reported overdosages with Astelin® Nasal Spray. Acute overdosage by adults with this dosage form is unlikely to result in clinically significant adverse events, other than increased somnolence, since one bottle of Astelin® Nasal Spray contains 17 mg of azelastine hydrochloride. Clinical studies in adults with single doses of the oral formulation of azelastine hydrochloride (up to 16 mg) have not resulted in increased incidence of serious adverse events. General supportive measures should be employed if overdose occurs. There is no known antidote to Astelin® Nasal Spray. Oral ingestion of antihistamines has the potential to cause serious adverse effects in young children. Accordingly, Astelin® Nasal Spray should be kept out of the reach of children. Oral doses of 120 mg/kg and greater (approximately 460 times the maximum recommended daily intranasal dose in adults and children on a mg/m^2 basis) were lethal in mice. Responses seen prior to death were tremor, convulsions, decreased muscle tone, and salivation. In dogs, single oral doses as high as 10 mg/kg (approximately 260 times the maximum recommended daily intranasal dose in adults and children on a mg/m^2 basis) were well tolerated, but single oral doses of 20 mg/kg were lethal.

DOSAGE AND ADMINISTRATION

The recommended dose of Astelin® Nasal Spray in adults and children 12 years and older is two sprays per nostril twice daily. In children 5 years to 11 years of age, the recommended dose of Astelin® Nasal Spray is one spray per nostril twice daily. Before initial use, the screw cap on the bottle should be replaced with the pump unit and the delivery system should be primed with 4 sprays or until a fine mist appears. When 3 or more days have elapsed since the last use, the pump should be reprimed with 2 sprays or until a fine mist appears.
CAUTION: Avoid spraying in the eyes.
Directions for Use: Illustrated patient instructions for proper use accompany each package of Astelin® Nasal Spray.

HOW SUPPLIED

Astelin® (azelastine hydrochloride) Nasal Spray, 137 mcg, (NDC 0037-0241-10) is supplied as a package containing a total of 200 metered sprays in two high-density polyethylene (HDPE) bottles fitted with screw caps. A separate metered-dose spray pump unit and a leaflet of patient instructions are also provided. The spray pump unit is packaged in a polyethylene wrapper and consists of a nasal spray pump fitted with a blue safety clip and a blue plastic dust cover. Each Astelin® (azelastine hydrochloride) Nasal Spray, 137 mcg, bottle contains 17 mg (1mg/mL) of azelastine hydrochloride to be used with the supplied metered-dose spray pump unit. Each bottle can deliver 100 metered sprays. Each spray delivers a mean of 0.137 mL solution containing 137 mcg of azelastine hydrochloride.
ATTENTION: The imprinted expiration date applies to the product in the bottles with screw caps. After the spray pump is inserted into the first bottle of the dispensing package, both bottles of product should be discarded after 3 months, not to exceed the expiration date imprinted on the label.
Storage: Store at controlled room temperature 20°–25°C (68°–77°F). Protect from freezing.

Manufactured by
Wallace Laboratories
Division of Carter-Wallace, Inc.
Cranbury, NJ 08512-0181 for
Wallace Laboratories/ASTA Medica LLC

IN-023S3-10 Rev.4/00

Shown in Product Identification Guide, page 339

DEPEN® ℞
(penicillamine tablets, USP)
Titratable Tablets

> Physicians planning to use penicillamine should thoroughly familiarize themselves with its toxicity, special dosage considerations, and therapeutic benefits. Penicillamine should never be used casually. Each patient should remain constantly under the close supervision of the physician. Patients should be warned to report promptly any symptoms suggesting toxicity.

DESCRIPTION

Penicillamine is 3-mercapto-D-valine, a disease modifying antirheumatic drug. It is a white or practically white, crystalline powder, freely soluble in water, slightly soluble in alcohol, and insoluble in ether, acetone, benzene, and carbon tetrachloride. Although its configuration is D, it is levorotatory as usually measured:

$$[\alpha]^{25°}_{D} = -62.5° \pm 2.0° \ (C = 1, 1N\,NaOH)$$

The empirical formula is $C_5H_{11}NO_2S$, giving it a molecular weight of 149.21. The structural formula is:

```
     CH3 H
      |  |
HS—C——C—COOH
      |  |
     CH3 NH2
```

It reacts readily with formaldehyde or acetone to form a thiazolidine-carboxylic acid.
Depen® (penicillamine tablets, USP) Titratable Tablets for oral administration contain 250 mg of penicillamine.
Other ingredients (inactive): edetate disodium, hydroxypropyl methylcellulose, lactose, magnesium stearate, magnesium trisilicate, polyethylene glycol, povidone, simethicone emulsion, starch, and stearic acid.

CLINICAL PHARMACOLOGY

Penicillamine is a chelating agent recommended for the removal of excess copper in patients with Wilson's disease. From *in vitro* studies which indicate that one atom of copper

Continued on next page

Depen—Cont.

combines with two molecules of penicillamine, it would appear that one gram of penicillamine should be followed by the excretion of about 200 milligrams of copper; however, the actual amount excreted is about one percent of this.
Penicillamine also reduces excess cystine excretion in cystinuria. This is done, at least in part, by disulfide interchange between penicillamine and cystine, resulting in formation of penicillamine-cysteine disulfide, a substance that is much more soluble than cystine and is excreted readily.
Penicillamine interferes with the formation of cross-links between tropocollagen molecules and cleaves them when newly formed.
The mechanism of action of penicillamine in rheumatoid arthritis is unknown, although it appears to suppress disease activity. Unlike cytotoxic immunosuppressants, penicillamine markedly lowers IgM rheumatoid factor but produces no significant depression in absolute levels of serum immunoglobulins. Also unlike cytotoxic immunosuppressants, which act on both, penicillamine *in vitro* depresses T-cell activity but not B-cell activity.
In vitro, penicillamine dissociates macroglobulins (rheumatoid factor) although the relationship of the activity to its effect in rheumatoid arthritis is not known.
In rheumatoid arthritis, the onset of therapeutic response to DEPEN may not be seen for two or three months. In those patients who respond, however, the first evidence of suppression of symptoms such as pain, tenderness, and swelling usually is generally apparent within three months. The optimum duration of therapy has not been determined. If remissions occur, they may last from months to years but usually require continued treatment (see DOSAGE AND ADMINISTRATION).
In all patients receiving penicillamine, it is important that DEPEN be given on an empty stomach, at least one hour before meals or two hours after meals, and at least one hour apart from any other drug, food or milk. This permits maximum absorption and reduces the likelihood of inactivation by metal binding in the gastrointestinal tract.
Methodology for determining the bioavailability of penicillamine is not available; however, penicillamine is known to be a very soluble substance.

INDICATIONS

DEPEN is indicated in the treatment of Wilson's disease, cystinuria, and in patients with severe, active rheumatoid arthritis who have failed to respond to an adequate trial of conventional therapy. Available evidence suggests that DEPEN is not of value in ankylosing spondylitis.
Wilson's Disease—Wilson's disease (hepatolenticular degeneration) results from the interaction of an inherited defect and an abnormality in copper metabolism. The metabolic defect, which is the consequence of the autosomal inheritance of one abnormal gene from each parent, manifests itself in a greater positive copper balance than normal. As a result, copper is deposited in several organs and appears eventually to produce pathologic effects most prominently seen in the brain, where degeneration is widespread; in the liver, where fatty infiltration, inflammation, and hepatocellular damage progress to postnecrotic cirrhosis; in the kidney, where tubular and glomerular dysfunction results; and in the eye, where characteristic corneal copper deposits are known as Kayser-Fleischer rings.
Two types of patients require treatment for Wilson's disease: (1) the symptomatic, and (2) the asymptomatic in whom it can be assumed the disease will develop in the future if the patient is not treated.
Diagnosis, suspected on the basis of family or individual history, physical examination, or a low serum concentration of ceruloplasmin*, is confirmed by the demonstration of Kayser-Fleischer rings or, particularly in the asymptomatic patient, by the quantitative demonstration in a liver biopsy specimen of a concentration of copper in excess of 250 mcg/g dry weight.
Treatment has two objectives:
(1) to minimize dietary intake and absorption of copper.
(2) to promote excretion of copper deposited in tissues.
The first objective is attained by a daily diet that contains no more than one or two milligrams of copper. Such a diet should exclude, most importantly, chocolate, nuts, shellfish, mushrooms, liver, molasses, broccoli, and cereals enriched with copper, and be composed to as great an extent as possible of foods with a low copper content. Distilled or demineralized water should be used if the patient's drinking water contains more than 0.1 mg of copper per liter.
For the second objective, a copper chelating agent is used. In symptomatic patients, this treatment usually produces marked neurologic improvement, fading of Kayser-Fleischer rings, and gradual amelioration of hepatic dysfunction and psychic disturbances.
Clinical experience to date suggests that life is prolonged with the above regimen.
Noticeable improvement may not occur for one to three months. Occasionally, neurologic symptoms become worse during initiation of therapy with DEPEN. Despite this, the drug should not be discontinued permanently. Although temporary interruption may result in clinical improvement of the neurological symptoms, it carries an increased risk of developing a sensitivity reaction upon resumption of therapy (See WARNINGS).

* For quantitative test for serum ceruloplasmin see: Morell, A.G.; Windsor, J.; Sternlieb, I; Scheinberg, I.H.: Measurement of the concentration of ceruloplasmin in serum by determination of its oxidase activity, in "Laboratory Diagnosis of Liver Disease," F.W. Sunderman; F.W. Sunderman, Jr., (eds.), St. Louis, Warren H. Green, Inc., 1968, pp. 193–195.

Treatment of asymptomatic patients has been carried out for over ten years. Symptoms and signs of the disease appear to be prevented indefinitely if daily treatment with DEPEN can be continued.
Cystinuria—Cystinuria is characterized by excessive urinary excretion of the dibasic amino acids, arginine, lysine, ornithine, and cystine, and the mixed disulfide of cysteine and homocysteine. The metabolic defect that leads to cystinuria is inherited as an autosomal, recessive trait. Metabolism of the affected amino acids is influenced by at least two abnormal factors: (1) defective gastrointestinal absorption and (2) renal tubular dysfunction.
Arginine, lysine, ornithine, and cysteine are soluble substances, readily excreted. There is no apparent pathology connected with their excretion in excessive quantities.
Cystine, however, is so slightly soluble at the usual range of urinary pH that it is not excreted readily, and so crystallizes and forms stones in the urinary tract. Stone formation is the only known pathology in cystinuria. Normal daily output of cystine is 40 to 80 mg. In cystinuria, output is greatly increased and may exceed 1 g/day. At 500 to 600 mg/day, stone formation is almost certain. When it is more than 300 mg/day, treatment is indicated.
Conventional treatment is directed at keeping urinary cystine diluted enough to prevent stone formation, keeping the urine alkaline enough to dissolve as much cystine as possible, and minimizing cystine production by a diet low in methionine (the major dietary precursor of cystine). Patients must drink enough fluid to keep urine specific gravity below 1.010, take enough alkali to keep urinary pH at 7.5 to 8, and maintain a diet low in methionine. This diet is not recommended in growing children and probably is contraindicated in pregnancy because of its low protein content (see PRECAUTIONS).
When these measures are inadequate to control recurrent stone formation, DEPEN may be used as additional therapy. When patients refuse to adhere to conventional treatment, DEPEN may be a useful substitute. It is capable of keeping cystine excretion to near normal values, thereby hindering stone formation and the serious consequences of pyelonephritis and impaired renal function that develop in some patients.
Bartter and colleagues depict the process by which penicillamine interacts with cystine to form penicillamine-cysteine mixed disulfide as:

CSSC + PS′ ⇄ CS′ + CSSP
PSSP + CS′ ⇄ PS′ + CSSP
CSSC + PSSP ⇄ 2 CSSP
CSSC = cystine
CS′ = deprotonated cysteine
PSSP = penicillamine
PS′ = deprotonated penicillamine sulfhydryl
CSSP = penicillamine-cysteine mixed disulfide

In this process, it is assumed that the deprotonated form of penicillamine, PS′, is the active factor in bringing about the disulfide interchange.
Rheumatoid Arthritis—Because DEPEN can cause severe adverse reactions, its use in rheumatoid arthritis should be restricted to patients who have severe, active disease and who have failed to respond to an adequate trial of conventional therapy. Even then, benefit-to-risk ratio should be carefully considered. Other measures, such as rest, physiotherapy, salicylates, and corticosteroids should be used, when indicated, in conjunction with DEPEN (see PRECAUTIONS).

CONTRAINDICATIONS

Except for treatment of Wilson's disease or certain cases of cystinuria, use of penicillamine during pregnancy is contraindicated (see WARNINGS).
Although breast milk studies have not been reported in animals or humans, mothers on therapy with penicillamine should not nurse their infants.
Patients with a history of penicillamine-related aplastic anemia or agranulocytosis should not be restarted on penicillamine (see WARNINGS and ADVERSE REACTIONS).
Because of its potential for causing renal damage, penicillamine should not be administered to rheumatoid arthritis patients with a history or other evidence of renal insufficiency.

WARNINGS

The use of penicillamine has been associated with fatalities due to certain diseases, such as aplastic anemia, agranulocytosis, thrombocytopenia, Goodpasture's syndrome, and myasthenia gravis.
Because of the potential for serious hematological and renal adverse reactions to occur at any time, routine urinalysis, white and differential blood cell count, hemoglobin determination, and direct platelet count must be done every two weeks for at least the first six months of penicillamine therapy and monthly thereafter. Patients should be instructed to report promptly the development of signs and symptoms of granulocytopenia and/or thrombocytopenia such as fever, sore throat, chills, bruising, or bleeding. The above laboratory studies should then be promptly repeated.
Leukopenia and thrombocytopenia have been reported to occur in up to five percent of patients during penicillamine therapy. Leukopenia is of the granulocytic series and may or may not be associated with an increase in eosinophils. A confirmed reduction in WBC below 3500 per cubic mL mandates discontinuance of penicillamine therapy. Thrombocytopenia may be on an idiosyncratic basis with decreased or absent megakaryocytes in the marrow, when it is part of an aplastic anemia. In other cases the thrombocytopenia is presumably on an immune basis since the number of megakaryocytes in the marrow has been reported to be normal or sometimes increased. The development of a platelet count below 100,000 per cubic mL, even in the absence of clinical bleeding, requires at least temporary cessation of penicillamine therapy. A progressive fall in either platelet count or WBC in three successive determinations, even though values are still within the normal range, likewise requires at least temporary cessation.
Proteinuria and/or hematuria may develop during therapy and may be warning signs of membranous glomerulopathy which can progress to a nephrotic syndrome. Close observation of these patients is essential. In some patients the proteinuria disappears with continued therapy; in others penicillamine must be discontinued. When a patient develops proteinuria or hematuria the physician must ascertain whether it is a sign of drug-induced glomerulopathy or is unrelated to penicillamine.
Rheumatoid arthritis patients who develop moderate degrees of proteinuria may be continued cautiously on penicillamine therapy, provided that quantitative 24-hour urinary protein determinations are obtained at intervals of one to two weeks. Penicillamine dosage should not be increased under these circumstances. Proteinuria which exceeds 1 g/24 hours, or proteinuria which is progressively increasing requires either discontinuance of the drug or a reduction in the dosage. In some patients, proteinuria has been reported to clear following reduction in dosage.
In rheumatoid arthritis patients, penicillamine should be discontinued if unexplained gross hematuria or persistent microscopic hematuria develops.
In patients with Wilson's disease or cystinuria the risks of continued penicillamine therapy in patients manifesting potentially serious urinary abnormalities must be weighed against the expected therapeutic benefits.
When penicillamine is used in cystinuria, an annual x-ray for renal stones is advised. Cystine stones form rapidly, sometimes in six months.
Up to one year or more may be required for any urinary abnormalities to disappear after penicillamine has been discontinued.
Because of rare reports of intrahepatic cholestasis and toxic hepatitis, liver function tests are recommended every six months for the duration of therapy.
Goodpasture's syndrome has occurred rarely. The development of abnormal urinary findings associated with hemoptysis and pulmonary infiltrates on x-ray requires immediate cessation of penicillamine.
Obliterative bronchiolitis has been reported rarely. The patient should be cautioned to report immediately pulmonary symptoms such as exertional dyspnea, unexplained cough, or wheezing. Pulmonary function studies should be considered at that time.
Myasthenic syndrome sometimes progressing to myasthenia gravis has been reported. Ptosis and diplopia, with weakness of the extraocular muscles, are often early signs of myasthenia. In the majority of cases, symptoms of myasthenia have receded after withdrawal of penicillamine.
Most of the various forms of pemphigus have occurred during treatment with penicillamine. Pemphigus vulgaris and pemphigus foliaceus are reported most frequently, usually as a late complication of therapy. The seborrhea-like characteristics of pemphigus foliaceus may obscure an early diagnosis. When pemphigus is suspected, DEPEN should be discontinued. Treatment has consisted of high doses of corticosteroids alone or, in some cases, concomitantly with an immunosuppressant. Treatment may be required for only a few weeks or months, but may need to be continued for more than a year.
Once instituted for Wilson's disease or cystinuria, treatment with penicillamine should, as a rule, be continued on a daily basis. Interruptions for even a few days have been followed by sensitivity reactions after reinstitution of therapy.
Use in Pregnancy—Penicillamine has been shown to be teratogenic in rats when given in doses 6 times higher than the highest dose recommended for human use (based on a standard weight of 50 kg). Skeletal defects, cleft palates, and fetal toxicity (resorptions) have been reported.
There are no controlled studies on the use of penicillamine in pregnant women. Although normal outcomes have been reported, characteristic congenital cutis laxa and associated birth defects have been reported in infants born of mothers who received therapy with penicillamine during pregnancy. Penicillamine should be used in women of childbearing potential only when the expected benefits outweigh the possible hazards. Women on therapy with penicillamine who are of childbearing potential should be apprised of this risk, advised to report promptly any missed menstrual periods or other indications of possible pregnancy, and followed closely for early recognition of pregnancy.
Wilson's Disease—Reported experience* shows that continued treatment with penicillamine throughout pregnancy protects the mother against relapse of the Wilson's disease, and that discontinuation of penicillamine has deleterious effects on the mother.
If penicillamine is administered during pregnancy to patients with Wilson's disease, it is recommended that the daily dosage be limited to 1 g. If cesarean section is planned, the daily dosage should be limited to 250 mg during the last

six weeks of pregnancy and postoperatively until wound healing is complete.

Cystinuria—If possible, penicillamine should not be given during pregnancy to women with cystinuria (see CONTRAINDICATIONS). There are reports of women with cystinuria on therapy with penicillamine who gave birth to infants with generalized connective tissue defects who died following abdominal surgery. If stones continue to form in these patients, the benefits of therapy to the mother must be evaluated against the risk to the fetus.

Rheumatoid Arthritis—Penicillamine should not be administered to rheumatoid arthritis patients who are pregnant (see CONTRAINDICATIONS) and should be discontinued promptly in patients in whom pregnancy is suspected or diagnosed.

There is a report that a woman with rheumatoid arthritis treated with less than one gram a day of penicillamine during pregnancy gave birth (cesarean delivery) to an infant with growth retardation, flattened face with broad nasal bridge, low set ears, short neck with loose skin folds, and unusually lax body skin.

* Scheinberg, I.H., Sternlieb, I.: *N Engl J Med 293:* 1300–1302, December 18, 1975.

PRECAUTIONS

Some patients may experience drug fever, a marked febrile response to penicillamine, usually in the second or third week following initiation of therapy. Drug fever may sometimes be accompanied by a macular cutaneous eruption.

In the case of drug fever in patients with Wilson's disease or cystinuria, penicillamine should be temporarily discontinued until the reaction subsides. Then penicillamine should be reinstituted with a small dose that is gradually increased until the desired dosage is attained. Systemic steroid therapy may be necessary, and is usually helpful, in such patients in whom toxic reactions develop a second or third time.

In the case of drug fever in rheumatoid arthritis patients, because other treatments are available, penicillamine should be discontinued and another therapeutic alternative tried, since experience indicates that the febrile reaction will recur in a very high percentage of patients upon readministration of penicillamine.

The skin and mucous membranes should be observed for allergic reactions. Early and late rashes have occurred. Early rash occurs during the first few months of treatment and is more common. It is usually a generalized pruritic, erythematous, maculopapular, or morbilliform rash and resembles the allergic rash seen with other drugs. Early rash usually disappears within days after stopping penicillamine and seldom recurs when the drug is restarted at a lower dosage. Pruritus and early rash may often be controlled by the concomitant administration of antihistamines. Less commonly, a late rash may be seen, usually after six months or more of treatment, and requires discontinuation of penicillamine. It is usually on the trunk, is accompanied by intense pruritus, and is usually unresponsive to topical corticosteroid therapy. Late rash may take weeks to disappear after penicillamine is stopped and usually recurs if the drug is restarted.

The appearance of a drug eruption accompanied by fever, arthralgia, lymphadenopathy, or other allergic manifestations usually requires discontinuation of penicillamine. Certain patients will develop a positive antinuclear antibody (ANA) test and some of these may show a lupus erythematosus-like syndrome similar to drug-induced lupus associated with other drugs. The lupus erythematosus-like syndrome is not associated with hypocomplementemia and may be present without nephropathy. The development of a positive ANA test does not mandate discontinuance of the drug; however, the physician should be alerted to the possibility that a lupus erythematosus-like syndrome may develop in the future.

Some patients may develop oral ulcerations which in some cases have the appearance of aphthous stomatitis. The stomatitis usually recurs on rechallenge but often clears on a lower dosage. Although rare, cheilosis, glossitis, and gingivostomatitis have also been reported. These oral lesions are frequently dose-related and may preclude further increase in penicillamine dosage or require discontinuation of the drug.

Hypogeusia (a blunting or diminution in taste perception) has occurred in some patients. This may last two to three months or more and may develop into a total loss of taste; however, it is usually self-limited, despite continued penicillamine treatment. Such taste impairment is rare in patients with Wilson's disease.

Penicillamine should not be used in patients who are receiving concurrently gold therapy, antimalarial or cytotoxic drugs, oxyphenbutazone, or phenylbutazone because these drugs are also associated with similar serious hematologic and renal adverse reactions. Patients who have had gold salt therapy discontinued due to a major toxic reaction may be at greater risk of serious adverse reactions with penicillamine, but not necessarily of the same type.

Patients who are allergic to penicillin may theoretically have cross-sensitivity to penicillamine. The possibility of reactions from contamination of penicillamine by trace amounts of penicillin has been eliminated now that penicillamine is being produced synthetically rather than as a degradation product of penicillin.

Because of their dietary restrictions, patients with Wilson's disease and cystinuria should be given 25 mg/day of pyridoxine during therapy, since penicillamine increases the requirement for this vitamin. Patients also may receive benefit from a multivitamin preparation, although there is no evidence that deficiency of any vitamin other than pyridoxine is associated with penicillamine. In Wilson's disease, multi-vitamin preparations must be copper-free.

Rheumatoid arthritis patients whose nutrition is impaired should also be given a daily supplement of pyridoxine. Mineral supplements should not be given, since they may block the response to penicillamine.

Iron deficiency may develop, especially in children and in menstruating women. In Wilson's disease, this may be a result of adding the effects of the low copper diet, which is probably also low in iron, and the penicillamine to the effects of blood loss or growth. In cystinuria, a low methionine diet may contribute to iron deficiency, since it is necessarily low in protein. If necessary, iron may be given in short courses, but a period of two hours should elapse between administration of penicillamine and iron, since orally administered iron has been shown to reduce the effects of penicillamine.

Penicillamine causes an increase in the amount of soluble collagen. In the rat this results in inhibition of normal healing and also a decrease in tensile strength of intact skin. In man this may be the cause of increased skin friability at sites especially subject to pressure or trauma, such as shoulders, elbows, knees, toes, and buttocks. Extravasations of blood may occur and may appear as purpuric areas, with external bleeding if the skin is broken, or as vesicles containing dark blood. Neither type is progressive. There is no apparent association with bleeding elsewhere in the body and no associated coagulation defect has been found. Therapy with penicillamine may be continued in the presence of these lesions. They may not recur if dosage is reduced. Other reported effects probably due to the action of penicillamine on collagen are excessive wrinkling of the skin and development of small, white papules at venipuncture and surgical sites.

The effects of penicillamine on collagen and elastin make it advisable to consider a reduction in dosage to 250 mg/day when surgery is contemplated. Reinstitution of full therapy should be delayed until wound healing is complete.

Carcinogenesis—Long-term animal carcinogenicity studies have not been done with penicillamine. There is a report that five of ten autoimmune disease-prone NZB hybrid mice developed lymphocytic leukemia after 6 months' intraperitoneal treatment with a dose of 400 mg/kg penicillamine 5 days per week.

Nursing Mothers—See CONTRAINDICATIONS.

Pediatric Use—The efficacy of DEPEN in pediatric patients with juvenile rheumatoid arthritis has not been established.

ADVERSE REACTIONS

Penicillamine is a drug with a high incidence of untoward reactions, some of which are potentially fatal. Therefore, it is mandatory that patients receiving penicillamine therapy remain under close medical supervision throughout the period of drug administration (see WARNINGS and PRECAUTIONS).

Reported incidences (%) for the most commonly occurring adverse reactions in rheumatoid arthritis patients are noted, based on 17 representative clinical trials reported in the literature (1270 patients).

Allergic—Generalized pruritus, early and late rashes (5%), pemphigus (see WARNINGS), and drug eruptions which may be accompanied by fever, arthralgia, or lymphadenopathy have occurred (see WARNINGS and PRECAUTIONS). Some patients may show a lupus erythematosus-like syndrome similar to drug-induced lupus produced by other pharmacological agents (see PRECAUTIONS).

Urticaria and exfoliative dermatitis have occurred.

Thyroiditis has been reported; hypoglycemia in association with anti-insulin antibodies has been reported. These reactions are extremely rare.

Some patients may develop a migratory polyarthralgia, often with objective synovitis (see DOSAGE AND ADMINISTRATION).

Gastrointestinal—Anorexia, epigastric pain, nausea, vomiting, or occasional diarrhea may occur (17%).

Isolated cases of reactivated peptic ulcer have occurred, as have hepatic dysfunction and pancreatitis. Intrahepatic cholestasis and toxic hepatitis have been reported rarely. There have been a few reports of increased serum alkaline phosphatase, lactic dehydrogenase, and positive cephalin flocculation and thymol turbidity tests.

Some patients may report a blunting, diminution, or total loss of taste perception (12%); or may develop oral ulcerations. Although rare, cheilosis, glossitis, and gingivo-stomatitis have been reported (see PRECAUTIONS).

Gastrointestinal side effects are usually reversible following cessation of therapy.

Hematological—Penicillamine can cause bone marrow depression (see WARNINGS). Leukopenia (2%) and thrombocytopenia (4%) have occurred. Fatalities have been reported as a result of thrombocytopenia, agranulocytosis, aplastic anemia, and sideroblastic anemia.

Thrombotic thrombocytopenic purpura, hemolytic anemia, red cell aplasia, monocytosis, leukocytosis, eosinophilia, and thrombocytosis have also been reported.

Renal—Patients on penicillamine therapy may develop proteinuria (6%) and/or hematuria which, in some, may progress to the development of the nephrotic syndrome as a result of an immune complex membranous glomerulopathy (see WARNINGS).

Central Nervous System—Tinnitus, optic neuritis, and peripheral sensory and motor neuropathies (including polyradiculoneuropathy, i.e., Guillain-Barre Syndrome) have been reported. Muscular weakness may or may not occur with the peripheral neuropathies.

Neuromuscular—Myasthenia gravis (see WARNINGS).

Other—Adverse reactions that have been reported rarely include thrombophlebitis; hyperpyrexia (see PRECAUTIONS); falling hair or alopecia; lichen planus; polymyositis; dermatomyositis; mammary hyperplasia; elastosis perforans serpiginosa; toxic epidermal necrolysis; anetoderma (cutaneous macular atrophy); and Goodpasture's syndrome, a severe and ultimately fatal glomerulonephritis associated with intra-alveolar hemorrhage (see WARNINGS). Fatal renal vasculitis has also been reported. Allergic alveolitis, obliterative bronchiolitis, interstitial pneumonitis, and pulmonary fibrosis have been reported in patients with severe rheumatoid arthritis, some of whom were receiving penicillamine. Bronchial asthma also has been reported.

Increased skin friability, excessive wrinkling of skin, and development of small, white papules at venipuncture and surgical sites have been reported (see PRECAUTIONS).

The chelating action of the drug may cause increased excretion of other heavy metals such as zinc, mercury, and lead.

There have been reports associating penicillamine with leukemia. However, circumstances involved in these reports are such that a cause and effect relationship to the drug has not been established.

DOSAGE AND ADMINISTRATION

In all patients receiving penicillamine, it is important that DEPEN be given on an empty stomach, at least one hour before meals or two hours after meals, and at least one hour apart from any other drug, food, or milk. Because penicillamine increases the requirement for pyridoxine, patients may require a daily supplement of pyridoxine (see PRECAUTIONS).

Wilson's Disease—Optimal dosage can be determined by measurement of urinary copper excretion and the determination of free copper in the serum. The urine must be collected in copper-free glassware, and should be quantitatively analyzed for copper before and soon after initiation of therapy with DEPEN.

Determination of 24-hour urinary copper excretions is of greatest value in the first week of therapy with penicillamine. In the absence of any drug reaction, a dose between 0.75 and 1.5 g that results in an initial 24-hour cupriuresis of over 2 mg should be continued for about three months, by which time the most reliable method of monitoring maintenance treatment is the determination of free copper in the serum. This equals the difference between quantitatively determined total copper and ceruloplasmin-copper. Adequately treated patients will usually have less than 10 mcg free copper/dL of serum. It is seldom necessary to exceed a dosage of 2 g/day. If the patient is intolerant to therapy with DEPEN, alternative treatment is trientine hydrochloride.

In patients who cannot tolerate as much as 1 g/day initially, initiating dosage with 250 mg/day, and increasing gradually to the requisite amount, gives closer control of the effects of the drug and may help to reduce the incidence of adverse reactions.

Cystinuria—It is recommended that DEPEN be used along with conventional therapy. By reducing urinary cystine, it decreases crystalluria and stone formation. In some instances, it has been reported to decrease the size of, and even to dissolve, stones already formed.

The usual dosage of DEPEN in the treatment of cystinuria is 2 g/day for adults, with a range of 1 to 4 g/day. For pediatric patients, dosage can be based on 30 mg/kg/day. The total daily amount should be divided into four doses. If four equal doses are not feasible, give the larger portion at bedtime. If adverse reactions necessitate a reduction in dosage, it is important to retain the bedtime dose.

Initiating dosage with 250 mg/day, and increasing gradually to the requisite amount, gives closer control of the effects of the drug and may help to reduce the incidence of adverse reactions.

In addition to taking DEPEN, patients should drink copiously. It is especially important to drink about a pint of fluid at bedtime and another pint once during the night when urine is more concentrated and more acid than during the day. The greater the fluid intake, the lower the required dosage of DEPEN.

Dosage must be individualized to an amount that limits cystine excretion to 100–200 mg/day in those with no history of stones, and below 100 mg/day in those who have had stone formation and/or pain. Thus, in determining dosage, the inherent tubular defect, the patient's size, age, and rate of growth, and his diet and water intake all must be taken into consideration.

The standard nitroprusside cyanide test has been reported useful as a qualitative measure of the effective dose*: Add 2 mL of freshly prepared 5 percent sodium cyanide to 5 mL of a 24-hour aliquot of protein-free urine and let stand ten minutes. Add 5 drops of freshly prepared 5 percent sodium nitroprusside and mix. Cystine will turn the mixture magenta. If the result is negative, it can be assumed that cystine excretion is less than 100 mg/g creatinine.

* Lotz, M., Potts, J.T. and Bartter, F.C.: *BritMed J 2:* 521, August 28, 1965 (in Medical Memoranda).

Although penicillamine is rarely excreted unchanged, it also will turn the mixture magenta. If there is any question as to

Continued on next page

Depen—Cont.

which substance is causing the reaction, a ferric chloride test can be done to eliminate doubt: Add 3 percent ferric chloride dropwise to the urine. Penicillamine will turn the urine an immediate and quickly fading blue. Cystine will not produce any change in appearance.

Rheumatoid Arthritis—The principal rule of treatment with DEPEN in rheumatoid arthritis is patience. The onset of therapeutic response is typically delayed. Two or three months may be required before the first evidence of a clinical response is noted (see CLINICAL PHARMACOLOGY). When treatment with DEPEN has been interrupted because of adverse reactions or other reasons, the drug should be reintroduced cautiously by starting with a lower dosage and increasing slowly.

Initial Therapy—The currently recommended dosage regimen in rheumatoid arthritis begins with a single daily dose of 125 mg or 250 mg which is thereafter increased at one to three month intervals, by 125 mg or 250 mg/day, as patient response and tolerance indicate. If a satisfactory remission of symptoms is achieved, the dose associated with the remission should be continued (see Maintenance Therapy). If there is no improvement and there are no signs of potentially serious toxicity after two to three months of treatment with doses of 500–750 mg/day, increases of 250 mg/day at two to three month intervals may be continued until a satisfactory remission occurs (see Maintenance Therapy) or signs of toxicity develop (see WARNINGS and PRECAUTIONS). If there is no discernible improvement after three to four months of treatment with 1000 to 1500 mg of penicillamine/day, it may be assumed the patient will not respond and DEPEN should be discontinued.

Maintenance Therapy—The maintenance dosage of DEPEN must be individualized, and may require adjustment during the course of treatment. Many patients respond satisfactorily to a dosage within the 500–750 mg/day range. Some need less.

Changes in maintenance dosage levels may not be reflected clinically or in the erythrocyte sedimentation rate for two to three months after each dosage adjustment.

Some patients will subsequently require an increase in the maintenance dosage to achieve maximal disease suppression. In those patients who do respond, but who evidence incomplete suppression of their disease after the first six to nine months of treatment, the daily dosage of DEPEN may be increased by 125 mg or 250 mg/day at three-month intervals. It is unusual in current practice to employ a dosage in excess of 1 g/day, but up to 1.5 g/day has sometimes been required.

Management of Exacerbations—During the course of treatment some patients may experience an exacerbation of disease activity following an initial good response.

These may be self-limited and can subside within twelve weeks. They are usually controlled by the addition of nonsteroidal anti-inflammatory drugs, and only if the patient has demonstrated a true "escape" phenomenon (as evidenced by failure of the flare to subside within this time period) should an increase in the maintenance dose ordinarily be considered.

In the rheumatoid patient, migratory polyarthralgia due to penicillamine is extremely difficult to differentiate from an exacerbation of the rheumatoid arthritis. Discontinuance or a substantial reduction in the dosage of DEPEN for up to several weeks will usually determine which of these processes is responsible for the arthralgia.

Duration of Therapy—The optimum duration of DEPEN therapy in rheumatoid arthritis has not been determined. If the patient has been in remission for six months or more, a gradual, stepwise dosage reduction in decrements of 125 mg or 250 mg/day at approximately three month intervals may be attempted.

Concomitant Drug Therapy—DEPEN should not be used in patients who are receiving gold therapy, antimalarial or cytotoxic drugs, oxyphenbutazone, or phenylbutazone (see PRECAUTIONS). Other measures, such as salicylates, other nonsteroidal anti-inflammatory drugs or systemic corticosteroids may be continued when DEPEN is initiated. After improvement commences, analgesic and anti-inflammatory drugs may be slowly discontinued as symptoms permit. Steroid withdrawal must be done gradually, and many months of DEPEN treatment may be required before steroids can be completely eliminated.

Dosage Frequency—Based on clinical experience, dosages up to 500 mg/day can be given as a single daily dose. Dosages in excess of 500 mg/day should be administered in divided doses.

HOW SUPPLIED

Depen® (penicillamine tablets, USP) Titratable Tablets: 250 mg scored, oval, white tablets coded with 37-4401 and Wallace; available in bottles of 100 (NDC 0037-4401-01).

Storage: Store at controlled room temperature 20°–25°C (68°–77°F). Protect from moisture.

Dispense in a tight container.

Manufactured by
Wallace Laboratories
Division of Carter-Wallace, Inc.
Cranbury, NJ 08512-0181 for
Wallace Laboratories/ASTA Medica LLC

IN-030F2-11 Rev. 10/98

DIUTENSEN®-R ℞
(methyclothiazide and reserpine)
Tablets

FELBATOL® ℞
(felbamate)
Tablets 400 mg and 600 mg,
Oral Suspension 600 mg/5 mL

Before Prescribing Felbatol® (felbamate), the physician should be thoroughly familiar with the details of this prescribing information.

FELBATOL® SHOULD NOT BE USED BY PATIENTS UNTIL THERE HAS BEEN A COMPLETE DISCUSSION OF THE RISKS AND THE PATIENT, PARENT, OR GUARDIAN HAS PROVIDED WRITTEN INFORMED CONSENT (SEE PATIENT INFORMATION/CONSENT SECTION).

WARNING

1. APLASTIC ANEMIA

THE USE OF FELBATOL® (felbamate) IS ASSOCIATED WITH A MARKED INCREASE IN THE INCIDENCE OF APLASTIC ANEMIA. ACCORDINGLY, FELBATOL® SHOULD ONLY BE USED IN PATIENTS WHOSE EPILEPSY IS SO SEVERE THAT THE RISK OF APLASTIC ANEMIA IS DEEMED ACCEPTABLE IN LIGHT OF THE BENEFITS CONFERRED BY ITS USE (SEE **INDICATIONS**). ORDINARILY, A PATIENT SHOULD NOT BE PLACED ON AND/OR CONTINUED ON FELBATOL® WITHOUT CONSIDERATION OF APPROPRIATE EXPERT HEMATOLOGIC CONSULTATION.

AMONG FELBATOL® TREATED PATIENTS, APLASTIC ANEMIA (PANCYTOPENIA IN THE PRESENCE OF A BONE MARROW LARGELY DEPLETED OF HEMATOPOIETIC PRECURSORS) OCCURS AT AN INCIDENCE THAT MAY BE MORE THAN A 100 FOLD GREATER THAN THAT SEEN IN THE UNTREATED POPULATION (I.E., 2 TO 5 PER MILLION PERSONS PER YEAR). THE RISK OF DEATH IN PATIENTS WITH APLASTIC ANEMIA GENERALLY VARIES AS A FUNCTION OF ITS SEVERITY AND ETIOLOGY; CURRENT ESTIMATES OF THE OVERALL CASE FATALITY RATE ARE IN THE RANGE OF 20 TO 30%, BUT RATES AS HIGH AS 70% HAVE BEEN REPORTED IN THE PAST.

THERE ARE TOO FEW FELBATOL® ASSOCIATED CASES, AND TOO LITTLE KNOWN ABOUT THEM TO PROVIDE A RELIABLE ESTIMATE OF THE SYNDROME'S INCIDENCE OR ITS CASE FATALITY RATE OR TO IDENTIFY THE FACTORS, IF ANY, THAT MIGHT CONCEIVABLY BE USED TO PREDICT WHO IS AT GREATER OR LESSER RISK.

IN MANAGING PATIENTS ON FELBATOL®, IT SHOULD BE BORNE IN MIND THAT THE CLINICAL MANIFESTATION OF APLASTIC ANEMIA MAY NOT BE SEEN UNTIL AFTER A PATIENT HAS BEEN ON FELBATOL® FOR SEVERAL MONTHS. (E.G., ONSET OF APLASTIC ANEMIA AMONG FELBATOL® EXPOSED PATIENTS FOR WHOM DATA ARE AVAILABLE HAS RANGED FROM 5 TO 30 WEEKS). HOWEVER, THE INJURY TO BONE MARROW STEM CELLS THAT IS HELD TO BE ULTIMATELY RESPONSIBLE FOR THE ANEMIA MAY OCCUR WEEKS TO MONTHS EARLIER. ACCORDINGLY, PATIENTS WHO ARE DISCONTINUED FROM FELBATOL® REMAIN AT RISK FOR DEVELOPING ANEMIA FOR A VARIABLE, AND UNKNOWN, PERIOD AFTERWARDS.

IT IS NOT KNOWN WHETHER OR NOT THE RISK OF DEVELOPING APLASTIC ANEMIA CHANGES WITH DURATION OF EXPOSURE. CONSEQUENTLY, IT IS NOT SAFE TO ASSUME THAT A PATIENT WHO HAS BEEN ON FELBATOL® WITHOUT SIGNS OF HEMATOLOGIC ABNORMALITY FOR LONG PERIODS OF TIME IS WITHOUT RISK.

IT IS NOT KNOWN WHETHER OR NOT THE DOSE OF FELBATOL® AFFECTS THE INCIDENCE OF APLASTIC ANEMIA.

IT IS NOT KNOWN WHETHER OR NOT CONCOMITANT USE OF ANTIEPILEPTIC DRUGS AND/OR OTHER DRUGS AFFECTS THE INCIDENCE OF APLASTIC ANEMIA.

APLASTIC ANEMIA TYPICALLY DEVELOPS WITHOUT PREMONITORY CLINICAL OR LABORATORY SIGNS, THE FULL BLOWN SYNDROME PRESENTING WITH SIGNS OF INFECTION, BLEEDING, OR ANEMIA. ACCORDINGLY, ROUTINE BLOOD TESTING CANNOT BE RELIABLY USED TO REDUCE THE INCIDENCE OF APLASTIC ANEMIA, BUT, IT WILL, IN SOME CASES, ALLOW THE DETECTION OF THE HEMATOLOGIC CHANGES BEFORE THE SYNDROME DECLARES ITSELF CLINICALLY. FELBATOL® SHOULD BE DISCONTINUED IF ANY EVIDENCE OF BONE MARROW DEPRESSION OCCURS.

2. HEPATIC FAILURE

HEPATIC FAILURE RESULTING IN FATALITIES HAS BEEN REPORTED WITH A MARKED INCREASE IN THE FREQUENCY IN PATIENTS RECEIVING FELBATOL® (felbamate). ACCORDINGLY, FELBATOL® SHOULD ONLY BE USED IN PATIENTS WHOSE EPILEPSY IS SO SEVERE THAT THE RISK OF LIVER FAILURE IS OUTWEIGHED BY THE POTENTIAL BENEFITS OF SEIZURE CONTROL.

ALTHOUGH FULL INFORMATION IS NOT YET AVAILABLE, THE NUMBER OF CASES REPORTED GREATLY EXCEEDS THE NUMBER THAT IS EXPECTED BASED ON THE ANNUAL INCIDENCE OF ACUTE LIVER FAILURE IN THE UNITED STATES (I.E., ABOUT 2,000 CASES PER YEAR).

THERE ARE TOO FEW FELBATOL® ASSOCIATED CASES OF HEPATIC FAILURE AND TOO LITTLE KNOWN ABOUT THEM TO PROVIDE EITHER A RELIABLE ESTIMATE OF ITS INCIDENCE OR TO IDENTIFY THE FACTORS, IF ANY, THAT MIGHT BE USED TO PREDICT WHICH PATIENT IS AT GREATER OR LESSER RISK.

IT IS NOT KNOWN WHETHER OR NOT THE RISK OF DEVELOPING HEPATIC FAILURE CHANGES WITH DURATION OF EXPOSURE.

IT IS NOT KNOWN WHETHER OR NOT THE DOSAGE OF FELBATOL® AFFECTS THE INCIDENCE OF HEPATIC FAILURE.

IT IS NOT KNOWN WHETHER CONCOMITANT USE OF OTHER ANTIEPILEPTIC DRUGS AND/OR OTHER DRUGS AFFECTS THE INCIDENCE OF HEPATIC FAILURE.

FELBATOL® SHOULD NOT BE PRESCRIBED FOR ANYONE WITH A HISTORY OF HEPATIC DYSFUNCTION.

PATIENTS PRESCRIBED FELBATOL® SHOULD HAVE LIVER FUNCTION TESTS (AST, ALT, BILIRUBIN) PERFORMED BEFORE INITIATING FELBATOL® AND AT 1- TO 2-WEEK INTERVALS WHILE TREATMENT CONTINUES. A PATIENT WHO DEVELOPS ABNORMAL LIVER FUNCTION TESTS SHOULD BE IMMEDIATELY WITHDRAWN FROM FELBATOL® TREATMENT.

DESCRIPTION

Felbatol® (felbamate) is an antiepileptic available as 400 mg and 600 mg tablets and as a 600 mg/5 mL suspension for oral administration. Its chemical name is 2-phenyl-1,3-propanediol dicarbamate.

Felbamate is a white to off-white crystalline powder with a characteristic odor. It is very slightly soluble in water, slightly soluble in ethanol, sparingly soluble in methanol, and freely soluble in dimethyl sulfoxide. The molecular weight is 238.24; felbamate's molecular formula is $C_{11}H_{14}N_2O_4$; its structural formula is:

$CH_2-O-C(=O)-NH_2$
C_6H_5-CH
$CH_2-O-C(=O)-NH_2$

The inactive ingredients for Felbatol® (felbamate) tablets 400 mg and 600 mg are starch, microcrystalline cellulose, croscarmellose sodium, lactose, magnesium stearate, FD&C Yellow No. 6, D&C Yellow No. 10, and FD&C Red No. 40 (600 mg tablets only). The inactive ingredients for Felbatol® (felbamate) suspension 600 mg/5mL are sorbitol, glycerin, microcrystalline cellulose, carboxymethylcellulose sodium, simethicone, polysorbate 80, methylparaben, saccharin sodium, propylparaben, FD&C Yellow No. 6, FD&C Red No. 40, flavorings, and purified water.

CLINICAL PHARMACOLOGY

Mechanism of Action:

The mechanism by which felbamate exerts its anticonvulsant activity is unknown, but in animal test systems designed to detect anticonvulsant activity, felbamate has properties in common with other marketed anticonvulsants. Felbamate is effective in mice and rats in the maximal electroshock test, the subcutaneous pentylenetetrazol seizure test, and the subcutaneous picrotoxin seizure test. Felbamate also exhibits anticonvulsant activity against seizures induced by intracerebroventricular administration of glutamate in rats and N-methyl-D,L-aspartic acid in mice. Protection against maximal electroshock-induced seizures suggests that felbamate may reduce seizure spread, an effect possibly predictive of efficacy in generalized tonic-clonic or partial seizures. Protection against pentylenetetrazol-induced seizures suggests that felbamate may increase seizure threshold, an effect considered to be predictive of potential efficacy in absence seizures.

Receptor-binding studies *in vitro* indicate that felbamate has weak inhibitory effects on GABA-receptor binding, benzodiazepine receptor binding, and is devoid of activity at the MK-801 receptor binding site of the NMDA receptor-ionophore complex. However, felbamate does interact as an antagonist at the strychnine-insensitive glycine recognition site of the NMDA receptor-ionophore complex. Felbamate is not effective in protecting chick embryo retina tissue against the neurotoxic effects of the excitatory amino acid agonists NMDA, kainate, or quisqualate *in vitro*.

The monocarbamate, p-hydroxy, and 2-hydroxy metabolites were inactive in the maximal electroshock-induced seizure test in mice. The monocarbamate and p-hydroxy metabolites had only weak (0.2 to 0.6) activity compared with felbamate in the subcutaneous pentylenetetrazol seizure test. These metabolites did not contribute significantly to the anticonvulsant action of felbamate.

Pharmacokinetics:

The numbers in the pharmacokinetic section are mean ± standard deviation.

Felbamate is well-absorbed after oral administration. Over 90% of the radioactivity after a dose of 1000 mg ^{14}C felbamate was found in the urine. Absolute bioavailability (oral vs. parenteral) has not been measured. The tablet and suspension were each shown to be bioequivalent to the capsule used in clinical trials, and pharmacokinetic parameters of the tablet and suspension are similar. There was no effect of food on absorption of the tablet; the effect of food on absorption of the suspension has not been evaluated.

Following oral administration, felbamate is the predominant plasma species (about 90% of plasma radioactivity). About 40–50% of absorbed dose appears unchanged in urine, and an additional 40% is present as unidentified metabolites and conjugates. About 15% is present as parahydroxyfelbamate, 2-hydroxyfelbamate, and felbamate monocarbamate, none of which have significant anticonvulsant activity.

Binding of felbamate to human plasma protein was independent of felbamate concentrations between 10 and 310 micrograms/mL. Binding ranged from 22% to 25%, mostly to albumin, and was dependent on the albumin concentration.

Felbamate is excreted with a terminal half-life of 20–23 hours, which is unaltered after multiple doses. Clearance after a single 1200 mg dose is 26±3 mL/hr/kg, and after multiple daily doses of 3600 mg is 30±8 mL/hr/kg. The apparent volume of distribution was 756±82 mL/kg after a 1200 mg dose. Felbamate Cmax and AUC are proportionate to dose after single and multiple doses over a range of 100–800 mg single doses and 1200–3600 mg daily doses. Cmin (trough) blood levels are also dose proportional. Multiple daily doses of 1200, 2400, and 3600 mg gave Cmin values of 30±5, 55±8, and 83±21 micrograms/mL (N=10 patients). Linear and dose proportional pharmacokinetics were also observed at doses above 3600 mg/day up to the maximum dose studied of 6000 mg/day. Felbamate gave dose proportional steady-state peak plasma concentrations in children age 4–12 over a range of 15, 30, and 45 mg/kg/day with peak concentrations of 17, 32, and 49 micrograms/mL.

The effects of race and gender on felbamate pharmacokinetics have not been systematically evaluated, but plasma concentrations in males (N=5) and females (N=4) given felbamate have been similar. The effects of felbamate kinetics on hepatic functional impairment have not been evaluated.

Renal Impairment: Felbamate's single dose monotherapy pharmacokinetic parameters were evaluated in 12 otherwise healthy individuals with renal impairment. Reduced felbamate clearance and a longer half-life were associated with diminishing renal function.

Pharmacodynamics:

Typical Physiologic Responses:

1. Cardiovascular:

In adults, there is no effect of felbamate on blood pressure. Small but statistically significant mean increases in heart rate were seen during adjunctive therapy and monotherapy; however, these mean increases of up to 5 bpm were not clinically significant. In children, no clinically relevant changes in blood pressure or heart rate were seen during adjunctive therapy or monotherapy with felbamate.

2. Other Physiologic Effects:

The only other change in vital signs was a mean decrease of approximately 1 respiration per minute in respiratory rate during adjunctive therapy in children. In adults, statistically significant mean reductions in body weight were observed during felbamate monotherapy and adjunctive therapy. In children, there were mean decreases in body weight during adjunctive therapy and monotherapy; however, these mean changes were not statistically significant. These mean reductions in adults and children were approximately 5% of the mean weights at baseline.

CLINICAL STUDIES

The results of controlled clinical trials established the efficacy of Felbatol® (felbamate) as monotherapy and adjunctive therapy in adults with partial-onset seizures with or without secondary generalization and in partial and generalized seizures associated with Lennox-Gastaut syndrome in children.

Felbatol® Monotherapy Trials in Adults

Felbatol® (3600 mg/day given QID) and low-dose valproate (15 mg/kg/day) were compared as monotherapy during a 112-day treatment period in a multicenter and a single-center double-blind efficacy trial. Both trials were conducted according to an identical study design. During a 56-day baseline period, all patients had at least four partial-onset seizures per 28 days and were receiving one antiepileptic drug at a therapeutic level, the most common being carbamazepine. In the multicenter trial, baseline seizure frequencies were 12.4 per 28 days in the Felbatol® group and 21.3 per 28 days in the low-dose valproate group. In the single-center trial, baseline seizure frequencies were 18.1 per 28 days in the Felbatol® group and 15.9 per 28 days in the low-dose valproate group. Patients were converted to monotherapy with Felbatol® or low-dose valproic acid during the first 28 days of the 112-day treatment period. Study endpoints were completion of 112 study days or fulfilling an escape criterion. Criteria for escape relative to baseline were: (1) twofold increase in monthly seizure frequency, (2) twofold increase in highest 2-day seizure frequency, (3) single generalized tonic-clonic seizure (GTC) if none occurred during baseline, or (4) significant prolongation of GTCs. The primary efficacy variable was the number of patients in each treatment group who met escape criteria.

In the multicenter trial, the percentage of patients who met escape criteria was 40% (18/45) in the Felbatol® group and 78% (39/50) in the low-dose valproate group. In the single-center trial, the percentage of patients who met escape criteria was 14% (3/21) in the Felbatol® group and 90% (19/21) in the low-dose valproate group. In both trials, the difference in the percentage of patients meeting escape criteria was statistically significant (P<.001) in favor of Felbatol®. These two studies by design were intended to demonstrate the effectiveness of Felbatol® monotherapy. The studies were not designed or intended to demonstrate comparative efficacy of the two drugs. For example, valproate was not used at the maximally effective dose.

Felbatol® Adjunctive Therapy Trials in Adults

A double-blind, placebo-controlled crossover trial consisted of two 10-week outpatient treatment periods. Patients with refractory partial-onset seizures who were receiving phenytoin and carbamazepine at therapeutic levels were administered Felbatol® (felbamate) as add-on therapy at a starting dosage of 1400 mg/day in three divided doses, which was increased to 2600 mg/day in three divided doses. Among the 56 patients who completed the study, the baseline seizure frequency was 20 per month. Patients treated with Felbatol® had fewer seizures than patients treated with placebo for each treatment sequence. There was a 23% (P=.018) difference in percentage seizure frequency reduction in favor of Felbatol®.

Felbatol® 3600 mg/day given QID and placebo were compared in a 28-day double-blind add-on trial in patients who had their standard antiepileptic drugs reduced while undergoing evaluations for surgery of intractable epilepsy. All patients had confirmed partial-onset seizures with or without generalization, seizure frequency during surgical evaluation not exceeding an average of four partial seizures per day or more than one generalized seizure per day, and a minimum average of one partial or generalized tonic-clonic seizure per day for the last 3 days of the surgical evaluation. The primary efficacy variable was time to fourth seizure after randomization to treatment with Felbatol® or placebo. Thirteen (46%) of 28 patients in the Felbatol® group versus 29 (88%) of 33 patients in the placebo group experienced a fourth seizure. The median times to fourth seizure were greater than 28 days in the Felbatol® group and 5 days in the placebo group. The difference between Felbatol® and placebo in time to fourth seizure was statistically significant (P=.002) in favor of Felbatol®.

Felbatol® Adjunctive Therapy Trial in Children with Lennox-Gastaut Syndrome

In a 70-day double-blind, placebo-controlled add-on trial in the Lennox-Gastaut syndrome, Felbatol® 45 mg/kg/day given QID was superior to placebo in controlling the multiple seizure types associated with this condition. Patients had at least 90 atonic and/or atypical absence seizures per month while receiving therapeutic dosages of one or two other antiepileptic drugs. Patients had a past history of using an average of eight antiepileptic drugs. The most commonly used antiepileptic drug during the baseline period was valproic acid. The frequency of all types of seizures during the baseline period was 1617 per month in the Felbatol® group and 716 per month in the placebo group. Statistically significant differences in the effect on seizure frequency favored Felbatol® over placebo for total seizures (26% reduction vs 5% increase, P<.001), atonic seizures (44% reduction vs 7% reduction, P=.002), and generalized tonic-clonic seizures (40% reduction vs 12% increase, P=.017). Parent/guardian global evaluations based on impressions of quality of life with respect to alertness, verbal responsiveness, general well-being, and seizure control significantly (P<.001) favored Felbatol® over placebo.

When efficacy was analyzed by gender in four well-controlled trials of felbamate as adjunctive and monotherapy for partial-onset seizures and Lennox-Gastaut syndrome, a similar response was seen in 122 males and 142 females.

INDICATIONS AND USAGE

Felbatol® is not indicated as a first line antiepileptic treatment (see **Warnings**). Felbatol® is recommended for use only in those patients who respond inadequately to alternative treatments and whose epilepsy is so severe that a substantial risk of aplastic anemia and/or liver failure is deemed acceptable in light of the benefits conferred by its use.

If these criteria are met and the patient has been fully advised of the risk and has provided written, informed consent, Felbatol® can be considered for either monotherapy or adjunctive therapy in the treatment of partial seizures, with and without generalization, in adults with epilepsy and as adjunctive therapy in the treatment of partial and generalized seizures associated with Lennox-Gastaut syndrome in children.

CONTRAINDICATIONS

Felbatol® is contraindicated in patients with known hypersensitivity to Felbatol®, its ingredients, or known sensitivity to other carbamates. It should not be used in patients with a history of any blood dyscrasia or hepatic dysfunction.

WARNINGS

See Boxed Warning regarding aplastic anemia and hepatic failure.

Antiepileptic drugs should not be suddenly discontinued because of the possibility of increasing seizure frequency.

PRECAUTIONS

A study in otherwise healthy individuals with renal dysfunction indicated that prolonged half-life and reduced clearance of felbamate are associated with diminishing renal function. Felbamate should be used with caution in patients with renal dysfunction (see **DOSAGE AND ADMINISTRATION**).

Information for Patients: Patients should be informed that the use of Felbatol® is associated with aplastic anemia and hepatic failure, potentially fatal conditions acutely or over a long term.

The physician should obtain written, informed consent prior to initiation of Felbatol® therapy (see **PATIENT INFORMATION/CONSENT** section).

Aplastic anemia in the general population is relatively rare. The absolute risk for the individual patient is not known with any degree of reliability, but patients on Felbatol® may be at more than a 100 fold greater risk for developing the syndrome than the general population.

The long term outlook for patients with aplastic anemia is variable. Although many patients are apparently cured, others require repeated transfusions and other treatments for relapses, and some, although surviving for years, ultimately develop serious complications that sometimes prove fatal (e.g., leukemia).

At present there is no way to predict who is likely to get aplastic anemia, nor is there a documented effective means to monitor the patient so as to avoid and/or reduce the risk. Patients with a history of any blood dyscrasia should not receive Felbatol®.

Patients should be advised to be alert for signs of infection, bleeding, easy bruising, or signs of anemia (fatigue, weakness, lassitude, etc.) and should be advised to report to the physician immediately if any such signs or symptoms appear.

Hepatic failure in the general population is relatively rare. The absolute risk for an individual patient is not known with any degree of reliability but patients on Felbatol® are at a greater risk for developing hepatic failure than the general population.

At present, there is no way to predict who is likely to develop hepatic failure, however, patients with a history of hepatic dysfunction should not be started on Felbatol®.

Patients should be advised to follow their physician's directives for liver function testing both before starting Felbatol® (felbamate) and at frequent intervals while taking Felbatol®.

Laboratory Tests: Full hematologic evaluations should be performed before Felbatol® therapy, frequently during therapy, and for a significant period of time after discontinuation of Felbatol® therapy. While it might appear prudent to perform frequent CBCs in patients continuing on Felbatol®, there is no evidence that such monitoring will allow early detection of marrow suppression before aplastic anemia occurs. (See **Boxed Warnings**.) Complete pretreatment blood counts, including platelets and reticulocytes should be obtained as a baseline. If any hematologic abnormalities are detected during the course of treatment, immediate consultation with a hematologist is advised. Felbatol® should be discontinued if any evidence of bone marrow depression occurs.

Liver function testing (AST, ALT, bilirubin) should be done before Felbatol® is started and at 1- to 2-week intervals while the patient is taking Felbatol®. If any liver abnormalities are detected during the course of treatment, Felbatol® should be discontinued immediately. (see **PATIENT INFORMATION/CONSENT**).

Drug Interactions:

The drug interaction data described in this section were obtained from controlled clinical trials and studies involving otherwise healthy adults with epilepsy.

Use in Conjunction with Other Antiepileptic Drugs (See DOSAGE AND ADMINISTRATION):

The addition of Felbatol® to antiepileptic drugs (AEDs) affects the steady-state plasma concentrations of AEDs. The net effect of these interactions is summarized in the following table:

AED Coadministered	AED Concentration	Felbatol® Concentration
Phenytoin	↑	↓
Valproate	↑	↔**
Carbamazepine (CBZ) *CBZ epoxide	↓ ↑	↓
Phenobarbital	↑	↓

*Not administered, but an active metabolite of carbamazepine.

**No significant effect.

Specific Effects of Felbatol® on Other Antiepileptic Drugs:

Phenytoin: Felbatol® causes an increase in steady-state phenytoin plasma concentrations. In 10 otherwise healthy

Continued on next page

Felbatol—Cont.

subjects with epilepsy ingesting phenytoin, the steady-state trough (Cmin) phenytoin plasma concentration was 17±5 micrograms/mL. The steady-state Cmin increased to 21±5 micrograms/mL when 1200 mg/day of felbamate was coadministered. Increasing the felbamate dose to 1800 mg/day in six of these subjects increased the steady-state phenytoin Cmin to 25±7 micrograms/mL. In order to maintain phenytoin levels, limit adverse experiences, and achieve the felbamate dose of 3600 mg/day, a phenytoin dose reduction of approximately 40% was necessary for eight of these 10 subjects.

In a controlled clinical trial, a 20% reduction of the phenytoin dose at the initiation of Felbatol® therapy resulted in phenytoin levels comparable to those prior to Felbatol® administration.

Carbamazepine: Felbatol® causes a decrease in the steady-state carbamazepine plasma concentrations and an increase in the steady-state carbamazepine epoxide plasma concentration. In nine otherwise healthy subjects with epilepsy ingesting carbamazepine, the steady-state trough (Cmin) carbamazepine concentration was 8±2 micrograms/mL. The carbamazepine steady-state Cmin decreased 31% to 5±1 micrograms/mL when felbamate (3000 mg/day, divided into three doses) was coadministered. Carbamazepine epoxide steady-state Cmin concentrations increased 57% from 1.0±0.3 to 1.6±0.4 micrograms/mL with the addition of felbamate.

In clinical trials, similar changes in carbamazepine and carbamazepine epoxide were seen.

Valproate: Felbatol® causes an increase in steady-state valproate concentrations. In four subjects with epilepsy ingesting valproate, the steady-state trough (Cmin) valproate plasma concentration was 63±16 micrograms/mL. The steady-state Cmin increased to 78±14 micrograms/mL when 1200 mg/day of felbamate was coadministered. Increasing the felbamate dose to 2400 mg/day increased the steady-state valproate Cmin to 96±25 micrograms/mL. Corresponding values for free valproate Cmin concentrations were 7±3, 9±4, and 11±6 micrograms/mL for 0, 1200, and 2400 mg/day Felbatol®, respectively. The ratios of the AUCs of unbound valproate to the AUCs of the total valproate were 11.1%, 13.0%, and 11.5%, with coadministration of 0, 1200, and 2400 mg/day of Felbatol®, respectively. This indicates that the protein binding of valproate did not change appreciably with increasing doses of Felbatol®.

Phenobarbital: Coadministration of felbamate with phenobarbital causes an increase in phenobarbital plasma concentrations. In 12 otherwise healthy male volunteers ingesting phenobarbital, the steady-state trough (Cmin) phenobarbital concentration was 14.2 micrograms/mL. The steady-state Cmin concentration increased to 17.8 micrograms/mL when 2400 mg/day of felbamate was coadministered for one week.

Effects of Other Antiepileptic Drugs on Felbatol®:

Phenytoin: Phenytoin causes an approximate doubling of the clearance of Felbatol® (felbamate) at steady state and, therefore, the addition of phenytoin causes an approximate 45% decrease in the steady-state trough concentrations of Felbatol® as compared to the same dose of Felbatol® given as monotherapy.

Carbamazepine: Carbamazepine causes an approximate 50% increase in the clearance of Felbatol® at steady state and, therefore, the addition of carbamazepine results in an approximate 40% decrease in the steady-state trough concentrations of Felbatol® as compared to the same dose of Felbatol® given as monotherapy.

Valproate: Available data suggest that there is no significant effect of valproate on the clearance of Felbatol® at steady state. Therefore, the addition of valproate is not expected to cause a clinically important effect on Felbatol® (felbamate) plasma concentrations.

Phenobarbital: It appears that phenobarbital may reduce plasma felbamate concentrations. Steady-state plasma felbamate concentrations were found to be 29% lower than the mean concentrations of a group of newly diagnosed subjects with epilepsy also receiving 2400 mg of felbamate a day.

Effects of Antacids on Felbatol®:

The rate and extent of absorption of a 2400 mg dose of Felbatol® as monotherapy given as tablets was not affected when coadministered with antacids.

Effects of Erythromycin on Felbatol®:

The coadministration of erythromycin (1000 mg/day) for 10 days did not alter the pharmacokinetic parameters of Cmax, Cmin, AUC, Cl/kg or tmax at felbamate daily doses of 3000 or 3600 mg/day in 10 otherwise healthy subjects with epilepsy.

Effects of Felbatol® on Low-Dose Combination Oral Contraceptives:

A group of 24 nonsmoking, healthy white female volunteers established on an oral contraceptive regimen containing 30 µg ethinyl estradiol and 75 µg gestodene for at least 3 months received 2400 mg/day of felbamate from midcycle (day 15) to midcycle (day 14) of two consecutive oral contraceptive cycles. Felbamate treatment resulted in a 42% decrease in the gestodene AUC 0–24, but no clinically relevant effect was observed on the pharmacokinetic parameters of ethinyl estradiol. No volunteer showed hormonal evidence of ovulation, but one volunteer reported intermenstrual bleeding during felbamate treatment.

Drug/Laboratory Test Interactions: There are no known interactions of Felbatol® with commonly used laboratory tests.

Carcinogenesis, Mutagenesis, Impairment of Fertility:

Carcinogenicity studies were conducted in mice and rats. Mice received felbamate as a feed admixture for 92 weeks at doses of 300, 600, and 1200 mg/kg and rats were also dosed by feed admixture for 104 weeks at doses of 30, 100, and 300 (males) or 10, 30, and 100 (females) mg/kg. The maximum doses in these studies produced steady-state plasma concentrations that were equal to or less than the steady-state plasma concentrations in epileptic patients receiving 3600 mg/day. There was a statistically significant increase in hepatic cell adenomas in high-dose male and female mice and in high-dose female rats. Hepatic hypertrophy was significantly increased in a dose-related manner in mice, primarily males, but also in females. Hepatic hypertrophy was not found in female rats. The relationship between the occurrence of benign hepatocellular adenomas and the finding of liver hypertrophy resulting from liver enzyme induction has not been examined. There was a statistically significant increase in benign interstitial cell tumors of the testes in high-dose male rats receiving felbamate. The relevance of these findings to humans is unknown.

As a result of the synthesis process, felbamate could contain small amounts of two known animal carcinogens, the genotoxic compound ethyl carbamate (urethane) and the nongenotoxic compound methyl carbamate. It is theoretically possible that a 50 kg patient receiving 3600 mg of felbamate could be exposed to up to 0.72 micrograms of urethane and 1800 micrograms of methyl carbamate. These daily doses are approximately 1/35,000 (urethane) and 1/5,500 (methyl carbamate) on a mg/kg basis, and 1/10,000 (urethane) and 1/1,600 (methyl carbamate) on a mg/m^2 basis, of the dose levels shown to be carcinogenic in rodents. Any presence of these two compounds in felbamate used in the lifetime carcinogenicity studies was inadequate to cause tumors.

Microbial and mammalian cell assays revealed no evidence of mutagenesis in the Ames *Salmonella*/microsome plate test, CHO/HGPRT mammalian cell forward gene mutation assay, sister chromatid exchange assay in CHO cells, and bone marrow cytogenetics assay.

Reproduction and fertility studies in rats showed no effects on male or female fertility at oral doses of up to 13.9 times the human total daily dose of 3600 mg on a mg/kg basis, or up to 3 times the human total daily dose on a mg/m^2 basis.

Pregnancy: Pregnancy Category C. The incidence of malformations was not increased compared to control in offspring of rats or rabbits given doses up to 13.9 times (rat) and 4.2 times (rabbit) the human daily dose on a mg/kg basis, or 3 times (rat) and less than 2 times (rabbit) the human daily dose on a mg/m^2 basis. However, in rats, there was a decrease in pup weight and an increase in pup deaths during lactation. The cause for these deaths is not known. The no effect dose for rat pup mortality was 6.9 times the human dose on a mg/kg basis or 1.5 times the human dose on a mg/m^2 basis.

Placental transfer of felbamate occurs in rat pups. There are, however, no studies in pregnant women. Because animal reproduction studies are not always predictive of human response, this drug should be used during pregnancy only if clearly needed.

Labor and Delivery: The effect of felbamate on labor and delivery in humans is unknown.

Nursing Mothers: Felbamate has been detected in human milk. The effect on the nursing infant is unknown (see **Pregnancy** section).

Pediatric Use: The safety and effectiveness of Felbatol® in children other than those with Lennox-Gastaut syndrome has not been established.

Geriatric Use: No systematic studies in geriatric patients have been conducted. Clinical studies of Felbatol® did not include sufficient numbers of patients aged 65 and over to determine whether they respond differently from younger patients. Other reported clinical experience has not identified differences in responses between the elderly and younger patients. In general, dosage selection for an elderly patient should be cautious, usually starting at the low end of the dosing range, reflecting the greater frequency of decreased hepatic, renal, or cardiac function, and of concomitant disease or other drug therapy.

ADVERSE REACTIONS

The most common adverse reactions seen in association with Felbatol® (felbamate) in adults during monotherapy are anorexia, vomiting, insomnia, nausea, and headache. The most common adverse reactions seen in association with Felbatol® in adults during adjunctive therapy are anorexia, vomiting, insomnia, nausea, dizziness, somnolence, and headache.

The most common adverse reactions seen in association with Felbatol® in children during adjunctive therapy are anorexia, vomiting, insomnia, headache, and somnolence.

The dropout rate because of adverse experiences or intercurrent illnesses among adult felbamate patients was 12 percent (120/977). The dropout rate because of adverse experiences or intercurrent illnesses among pediatric felbamate patients was six percent (22/357). In adults, the body systems associated with causing these withdrawals in order of frequency were: digestive (4.3%), psychological (2.2%), whole body (1.7%), neurological (1.5%), and dermatological (1.5%). In children, the body systems associated with causing these withdrawals in order of frequency were: digestive (1.7%), neurological (1.4%), dermatological (1.4%), psychological (1.1%), and whole body (1.0%). In adults, specific events with an incidence of 1% or greater associated with causing these withdrawals, in order of frequency were: anorexia (1.6%), nausea (1.4%), rash (1.2%), and weight decrease (1.1%). In children, specific events with an incidence of 1% or greater associated with causing these withdrawals, in order of frequency was rash (1.1%).

Incidence in Clinical Trials:

The prescriber should be aware that the figures cited in the following table cannot be used to predict the incidence of side effects in the course of usual medical practice where patient characteristics and other factors differ from those which prevailed in the clinical trials. Similarly, the cited frequencies cannot be compared with figures obtained from other clinical investigations involving different investigators, treatments, and uses including the use of Felbatol® (felbamate) as adjunctive therapy where the incidence of adverse events may be higher due to drug interactions. The cited figures, however, do provide the prescribing physician with some basis for estimating the relative contribution of drug and nondrug factors to the side effect incidence rate in the population studied.

Adults

Incidence in Controlled Clinical Trials — Monotherapy Studies in Adults:

The table that follows enumerates adverse events that occurred at an incidence of 2% or more among 58 adult patients who received Felbatol® monotherapy at dosages of 3600 mg/day in double-blind controlled trials. Reported adverse events were classified using standard WHO-based dictionary terminology.

Adults
Treatment-Emergent Adverse Event
Incidence in Controlled Monotherapy Trials

Body System/Event	Felbatol®* (N=58) %	Low Dose Valproate** (N=50) %
Body as a Whole		
Fatigue	6.9	4.0
Weight Decrease	3.4	0
Face Edema	3.4	0
Central Nervous System		
Insomnia	8.6	4.0
Headache	6.9	18.0
Anxiety	5.2	2.0
Dermatological		
Acne	3.4	0
Rash	3.4	0
Digestive		
Dyspepsia	8.6	2.0
Vomiting	8.6	2.0
Constipation	6.9	2.0
Diarrhea	5.2	0
SGPT Increased	5.2	2.0
Metabolic/Nutritional		
Hypophosphatemia	3.4	0
Respiratory		
Upper Respiratory Tract Infection	8.6	4.0
Rhinitis	6.9	0
Special Senses		
Diplopia	3.4	4.0
Otitis Media	3.4	0
Urogenital		
Intramenstrual Bleeding	3.4	0
Urinary Tract Infection	3.4	2.0

*3600 mg/day;
**15 mg/kg/day

Incidence in Controlled Add-On Clinical Studies in Adults:

The table that follows enumerates adverse events that occurred at an incidence of 2% or more among 114 adult patients who received Felbatol® adjunctive therapy in add-on controlled trials at dosages up to 3600 mg/day. Reported adverse events were classified using standard WHO-based dictionary terminology.

Many adverse experiences that occurred during adjunctive therapy may be a result of drug interactions. Adverse experiences during adjunctive therapy typically resolved with conversion to monotherapy, or with adjustment of the dosage of other antiepileptic drugs.

Adults
Treatment-Emergent Adverse Event
Incidence in Controlled Add-On Trials

Body System/Event	Felbatol® (N=114) %	Placebo (N=43) %
Body as a Whole		
Fatigue	16.8	7.0
Fever	2.6	4.7
Chest Pain	2.6	0
Central Nervous System		
Headache	36.8	9.3
Somnolence	19.3	7.0
Dizziness	18.4	14.0
Insomnia	17.5	7.0
Nervousness	7.0	2.3
Tremor	6.1	2.3

Anxiety	5.3	4.7
Gait Abnormal	5.3	0
Depression	5.3	0
Paraesthesia	3.5	2.3
Ataxia	3.5	0
Mouth Dry	2.6	0
Stupor	2.6	0
Dermatological		
Rash	3.5	4.7
Digestive		
Nausea	34.2	2.3
Anorexia	19.3	2.3
Vomiting	16.7	4.7
Dyspepsia	12.3	7.0
Constipation	11.4	2.3
Diarrhea	5.3	2.3
Abdominal Pain	5.3	0
SGPT Increased	3.5	0
Musculoskeletal		
Myalgia	2.6	0
Respiratory		
Upper Respiratory Tract Infection	5.3	7.0
Sinusitis	3.5	0
Pharyngitis	2.6	0
Special Senses		
Diplopia	6.1	0
Taste Perversion	6.1	0
Vision Abnormal	5.3	2.3

Children

Incidence in a Controlled Add-On Trial in Children with Lennox-Gastaut Syndrome:

The table that follows enumerates adverse events that occurred more than once among 31 pediatric patients who received Felbatol® up to 45 mg/kg/day or a maximum of 3600 mg/day. Reported adverse events were classified using standard WHO-based dictionary terminology.

Children
Treatment-Emergent Adverse Event
Incidence in a Controlled Add-On Lennox-Gastaut Trial

Body System/Event	Felbatol® (N=31) %	Placebo (N=27) %
Body as a Whole		
Fever	22.6	11.1
Fatigue	9.7	3.7
Weight Decrease	6.5	0
Pain	6.5	0
Central Nervous System		
Somnolence	48.4	11.1
Insomnia	16.1	14.8
Nervousness	16.1	18.5
Gait Abnormal	9.7	0
Headache	6.5	18.5
Thinking Abnormal	6.5	3.7
Ataxia	6.5	3.7
Urinary Incontinence	6.5	7.4
Emotional Lability	6.5	0
Miosis	6.5	0
Dermatological		
Rash	9.7	7.4
Digestive		
Anorexia	54.8	14.8
Vomiting	38.7	14.8
Constipation	12.9	0
Hiccup	9.7	3.7
Nausea	6.5	0
Dyspepsia	6.5	3.7
Hematologic		
Purpura	12.9	7.4
Leukopenia	6.5	0
Respiratory		
Upper Respiratory Tract Infection	45.2	25.9
Pharyngitis	9.7	3.7
Coughing	6.5	0
Special Senses		
Otitis Media	9.7	0

Other Events Observed in Association with the Administration of Felbatol® (felbamate):

In the paragraphs that follow, the adverse clinical events, other than those in the preceding tables, that occurred in a total of 977 adults and 357 children exposed to Felbatol® (felbamate) and that are reasonably associated with its use are presented. They are listed in order of decreasing frequency. Because the reports cite events observed in open-label and uncontrolled studies, the role of Felbatol® in their causation cannot be reliably determined.

Events are classified within body system categories and enumerated in order of decreasing frequency using the following definitions: frequent adverse events are defined as those occurring on one or more occasions in at least 1/100 patients; infrequent adverse events are those occurring in 1/100–1/1000 patients; and rare events are those occurring in fewer than 1/1000 patients.

Event frequencies are calculated as the number of patients reporting an event divided by the total number of patients (N=1334) exposed to Felbatol®.

Dosage Table (adults)

	WEEK 1	WEEK 2	WEEK 3
Dosage reduction of concomitant AEDs	REDUCE original dose by 20–33%*	REDUCE original dose by up to an additional 1/3*	REDUCE as clinically indicated
Felbatol® Dosage	1200 mg/day Initial dose	2400 mg/day Therapeutic dosage range	3600 mg/day Therapeutic dosage range

* See ***Adjunctive*** and ***Conversion to Monotherapy*** sections.

Body as a Whole: *Frequent:* Weight increase, asthenia, malaise, influenza-like symptoms; *Rare:* anaphylactoid reaction, chest pain substernal.
Cardiovascular: *Frequent:* Palpitation, tachycardia; *Rare:* supraventricular tachycardia.
Central Nervous System: *Frequent:* Agitation, psychological disturbance, aggressive reaction; *Infrequent:* hallucination, euphoria, suicide attempt, migraine.
Digestive: *Frequent:* SGOT increased; *Infrequent:* esophagitis, appetite increased; *Rare:* GGT elevated.
Hematologic: *Infrequent:* Lymphadenopathy, leukopenia, leukocytosis, thrombocytopenia, granulocytopenia; *Rare:* antinuclear factor test positive, qualitative platelet disorder, agranulocytosis.
Metabolic/Nutritional: *Infrequent:* Hypokalemia, hyponatremia, LDH increased, alkaline phosphatase increased, hypophosphatemia; *Rare:* creatinine phosphokinase increased.
Musculoskeletal: *Infrequent:* Dystonia.
Dermatological: *Frequent:* Pruritus; *Infrequent:* urticaria, bullous eruption; *Rare:* buccal mucous membrane swelling, Stevens-Johnson Syndrome.
Special Senses: *Rare:* Photosensitivity allergic reaction.

Postmarketing Adverse Event Reports:

Voluntary reports of adverse events in patients taking Felbatol® (usually in conjunction with other drugs) have been received since market introduction and may have no causal relationship with the drug(s). These include the following by body system:

Body as a Whole: neoplasm, sepsis, L.E. syndrome, SIDS, sudden death, edema, hypothermia, rigors, hyperpyrexia.
Cardiovascular: atrial fibrillation, atrial arrhythmia, cardiac arrest, torsade de pointes, cardiac failure, hypotension, hypertension, flushing, thrombophlebitis, ischemic necrosis, gangrene, peripheral ischemia, bradycardia, Henoch-Schönlein purpura (vasculitis).
Central & Peripheral Nervous System: delusion, paralysis, mononeuritis, cerebrovascular disorder, cerebral edema, coma, manic reaction, encephalopathy, paranoid reaction, nystagmus, choreoathetosis, extrapyramidal disorder, confusion, psychosis, status epilepticus, dyskinesia, dysarthria, respiratory depression, apathy, concentration impaired.
Dermatological: abnormal body odor, sweating, lichen planus, livedo reticularis, alopecia, toxic epidermal necrolysis.
Digestive: (Refer to **WARNINGS**) hepatitis, hepatic failure, G.I. hemorrhage, hyperammonemia, pancreatitis, hematemesis, gastritis, rectal hemorrhage, flatulence, gingival bleeding, acquired megacolon, ileus, intestinal obstruction, enteritis, ulcerative stomatitis, glossitis, dysphagia, jaundice, gastric ulcer, gastric dilatation, gastroesophageal reflux.
Fetal Disorders: fetal death, microcephaly, genital malformation, anencephaly, encephalocele.
Hematologic: (Refer to **WARNINGS**) increased and decreased prothrombin time, anemia, hypochromic anemia, aplastic anemia, pancytopenia, hemolytic uremic syndrome, increased mean corpuscular volume (mcv) with and without anemia, coagulation disorder, embolism-limb, disseminated intravascular coagulation, eosinophilia, hemolytic anemia, leukemia, including myelogenous leukemia, and lymphoma, including T-cell and B-cell lymphoproliferative disorders.
Metabolic/Nutritional: hypernatremia, hypoglycemia, SIADH, hypomagnesemia, dehydration, hyperglycemia, hypocalcemia.
Musculoskeletal: arthralgia, muscle weakness, involuntary muscle contraction, rhabdomyolysis.
Respiratory: dyspnea, pneumonia, pneumonitis, hypoxia, epistaxis, pleural effusion, respiratory insufficiency, pulmonary hemorrhage, asthma.
Special Senses: hemianopsia, decreased hearing, conjunctivitis.
Urogenital: menstrual disorder, acute renal failure, hepatorenal syndrome, hematuria, urinary retention, nephrosis, vaginal hemorrhage, abnormal renal function, dysuria, placental disorder.

DRUG ABUSE AND DEPENDENCE

Abuse: Abuse potential was not evaluated in human studies.

Dependence: Rats administered felbamate orally at doses 8.3 times the recommended human dose 6 days each week for 5 consecutive weeks demonstrated no signs of physical dependence as measured by weight loss following drug withdrawal on day 7 of each week.

OVERDOSAGE

Four subjects inadvertently received Felbatol® (felbamate) as adjunctive therapy in dosages ranging from 5400 to 7200 mg/day for durations between 6 and 51 days. One subject who received 5400 mg/day as monotherapy for 1 week reported no adverse experiences. Another subject attempted suicide by ingesting 12,000 mg of Felbatol® in a 12-hour period. The only adverse experiences reported were mild gastric distress and a resting heart rate of 100 bpm. No serious adverse reactions have been reported.

General supportive measures should be employed if overdosage occurs. It is not known if felbamate is dialyzable.

DOSAGE AND ADMINISTRATION

Felbatol® (felbamate) has been studied as monotherapy and adjunctive therapy in adults and as adjunctive therapy in children with seizures associated with Lennox-Gastaut syndrome. As Felbatol® is added to or substituted for existing AEDs, it is strongly recommended to reduce the dosage of those AEDs in the range of 20–33% to minimize side effects (see **Drug Interactions** subsection).

Felbamate should be used with caution in patients with renal dysfunction. Adjunctive therapy with medications which affect felbamate plasma concentrations, especially AEDS, may warrant further reductions in felbamate daily doses in patients with renal dysfunction.

Adults (14 years of age and over)

The majority of patients received 3600 mg/day in clinical trials evaluating its use as both monotherapy and adjunctive therapy.

Monotherapy: (Initial therapy) Felbatol® (felbamate) has not been systematically evaluated as initial monotherapy. Initiate Felbatol® at 1200 mg/day in divided doses three or four times daily. The prescriber is advised to titrate previously untreated patients under close clinical supervision, increasing the dosage in 600-mg increments every 2 weeks to 2400 mg/day based on clinical response and thereafter to 3600 mg/day if clinically indicated.

Conversion to Monotherapy: Initiate Felbatol® at 1200 mg/day in divided doses three or four times daily. Reduce the dosage of concomitant AEDs by one-third at initiation of Felbatol® therapy. At week 2, increase the Felbatol® dosage to 2400 mg/day while reducing the dosage of other AEDs up to an additional one-third of their original dosage. At week 3, increase the Felbatol® dosage up to 3600 mg/day and continue to reduce the dosage of other AEDs as clinically indicated.

Adjunctive Therapy: Felbatol® should be added at 1200 mg/day in divided doses three or four times daily while reducing present AEDs by 20% in order to control plasma concentrations of concurrent phenytoin, valproic acid, phenobarbital, and carbamazepine and its metabolites. Further reductions of the concomitant AEDs dosage may be necessary to minimize side effects due to drug interactions. Increase the dosage of Felbatol® by 1200 mg/day increments at weekly intervals to 3600 mg/day. Most side effects seen during Felbatol® adjunctive therapy resolve as the dosage of concomitant AEDs is decreased.

[See table above]

While the above Felbatol® conversion guidelines may result in a Felbatol® 3600 mg/day dose within 3 weeks, in some patients titration to a 3600 mg/day Felbatol® dose has been achieved in as little as 3 days with appropriate adjustment of other AEDs.

Children with Lennox-Gastaut Syndrome (Ages 2–14 years)

Adjunctive Therapy: Felbatol® should be added at 15 mg/kg/day in divided doses three or four times daily while reducing present AEDs by 20% in order to control plasma levels of concurrent phenytoin, valproic acid, phenobarbital, and carbamazepine and its metabolites. Further reductions of the concomitant AEDs dosage may be necessary to minimize side effects due to drug interactions. Increase the dosage of Felbatol® by 15 mg/kg/day increments at weekly intervals to 45 mg/kg/day. Most side effects seen during Felbatol® adjunctive therapy resolve as the dosage of concomitant AEDs is decreased.

HOW SUPPLIED

Felbatol® (felbamate) Tablets, 400 mg, are yellow, scored, capsule-shaped tablets, debossed "0430" on one side and "WALLACE" on the other; available in Bottles of 100 (NDC 0037-0430-01) and Unit Dose 100's (NDC 0037-0430-11).

Felbatol® (felbamate) Tablets, 600 mg, are peach-colored, scored, capsule-shaped tablets, debossed "0431" on one side and "WALLACE" on the other; available in Bottles of 100 (NDC 0037-0431-01) and Unit Dose 100's (NDC 0037-0431-11). Felbatol® (felbamate) Oral Suspension, 600 mg/5 mL, is peach-colored; available in 8 oz bottles (NDC 0037-0442-67) and 32 oz bottles (NDC 0037-0442-17).

Shake suspension well before using. Store at controlled room temperature 20°–25°C (68°–77°F). Dispense in tight container.

WALLACE LABORATORIES, Division of Carter-Wallace, Inc. Cranbury, NJ 08512

PATIENT INFORMATION/CONSENT

FELBATOL® (felbamate) SHOULD NOT BE USED BY PATIENTS UNTIL THERE HAS BEEN A COMPLETE

Continued on next page

Felbatol—Cont.

DISCUSSION OF THE RISKS AND WRITTEN INFORMED CONSENT HAS BEEN OBTAINED.

IMPORTANT INFORMATION AND WARNING:

Felbatol®, taken by itself or with other prescription and/or non-prescription drugs, can result in severe, potentially fatal blood abnormality ("aplastic anemia") and/or severe, potentially fatal liver damage.

PATIENT CONSENT:

My [My son, daughter, ward, ____________________

______________________________________'s] treatment with Felbatol® has been personally explained to me by Dr. ________________________.

The following points of information, among others, have been specifically discussed and made clear and I have had the opportunity to ask any questions concerning this information:

1. I, ____________________________________ (Patient's Name), understand that Felbatol® is used to treat certain types of seizures and my physician has told me that I have this type(s) of seizures;
INITIALS: __________

2. I understand that Felbatol® is being used since my seizures have not been satisfactorily treated with other antiepileptic drugs;
INITIALS: __________

3. I understand that there is a serious risk that I could develop aplastic anemia and/or liver failure, both of which are potentially fatal, by using Felbatol®;
INITIALS: __________

4. I understand that there are no laboratory tests which will predict if I am at an increased risk for one of the potentially fatal conditions;
INITIALS: __________

5. I understand that I should have the recommended blood work before my treatment with Felbatol® is begun or continued and then every 1–2 weeks while taking Felbatol®. I understand that although this blood work may help detect if I develop one of these conditions, it may do so only after significant, irreversible and potentially fatal damage has already occurred;
INITIALS: __________

6. If I am currently taking another antiepileptic drug, I understand that the manufacturer of Felbatol® recommends that the dosage of these other drugs be decreased by a certain amount when Felbatol® is started; if my physician determines that this should not be done in my case, he/she has explained the reason(s) for this decision;
INITIALS: __________

7. I understand that I must immediately report any unusual symptoms to Dr. ________________________ and be especially aware of any rashes, easy bruising, bleeding, sore throats, fever, and/or dark urine;
INITIALS: __________

I now authorize Dr. ____________________ to begin my treatment with Felbatol®; OR, if my treatment has already begun with Felbatol®, to continue such treatment.

____
Patient, Parent, or Guardian

____
Address

____
Telephone

PHYSICIAN STATEMENT:

I have fully explained to the patient, ____________________

____, the nature and purpose of the treatment with Felbatol® (felbamate) and the potential risks associated with that treatment. I have asked the patient if he/she has any questions regarding this treatment or the risks and have answered those questions to the best of my ability. I also acknowledge that I have read and understand the prescribing information listed above.

____
Physician Date

NOTE TO PHYSICIAN: It is strongly recommended that you retain a signed copy of the informed consent with the patient's medical records.

SUPPLY OF PATIENT INFORMATION/CONSENT FORMS:

A supply of "Patient Information/Consent" forms as printed above is available, free of charge, from your local Wallace representative, or may be obtained by calling 609-655-6147. Permission to use the above Patient Information/Consent by photocopy reproduction is also hereby granted by Carter-Wallace, Inc.

IN-00431-10 Rev. 2/99

Shown in Product Identification Guide, page 339

LUFYLLIN® ℞
(dyphylline)
Elixir

LUFYLLIN® Tablets ℞
(dyphylline tablets, USP, 200 mg)

LUFYLLIN®-400 Tablets ℞
(dyphylline tablets, USP, 400 mg)

DESCRIPTION

LUFYLLIN (dyphylline), a xanthine derivative, is a bronchodilator available for oral administration as tablets containing 200 mg and 400 mg of dyphylline. Other ingredients: magnesium stearate, microcrystalline cellulose.

Chemically, dyphylline is 7-(2,3-dihydroxypropyl)-theophylline, a white, extremely bitter, amorphous powder that is freely soluble in water and soluble in alcohol to the extent of 2 g/100 mL. Dyphylline forms a neutral solution that is stable in gastrointestinal fluids over a wide range of pH.

The molecular formula for dyphylline is $C_{10}H_{14}N_4O_4$ with a molecular weight of 254.25. Its structural formula is:

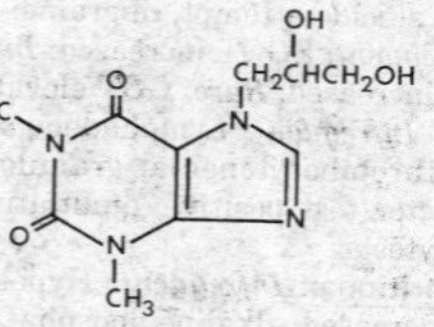

CLINICAL PHARMACOLOGY

Dyphylline is a xanthine derivative with pharmacologic actions similar to theophylline and other members of this class of drugs. Its primary action is that of bronchodilation, but it also exhibits peripheral vasodilatory and other smooth muscle relaxant activity to a lesser degree. The bronchodilatory action of dyphylline, as with other xanthines, is thought to be mediated through competitive inhibition of phosphodiesterase with a resulting increase in cyclic AMP producing relaxation of bronchial smooth muscle.

LUFYLLIN is well tolerated and produces less nausea than aminophylline and other alkaline theophylline compounds when administered orally. Unlike the hydrolyzable salts of theophylline, dyphylline is not converted to free theophylline *in vivo*. It is absorbed rapidly in therapeutically active form and in healthy volunteers reaches a mean peak plasma concentration of 17.1 mcg/mL in approximately 45 minutes following a single oral dose of 1000 mg of LUFYLLIN.

Dyphylline exerts its bronchodilatory effects directly and, unlike theophylline, is excreted unchanged by the kidneys without being metabolized by the liver. Because of this, dyphylline pharmacokinetics and plasma levels are not influenced by various factors that affect liver function and hepatic enzyme activity, such as smoking, age, congestive heart failure, or concomitant use of drugs which affect liver function.

The elimination half-life of dyphylline is approximately two hours (1.8–2.1 hr) and approximately 88% of a single oral dose can be recovered from the urine unchanged. The renal clearance would be correspondingly reduced in patients with impaired renal function. In anuric patients, the half-life may be increased 3 to 4 times normal.

Dyphylline plasma levels are dose-related and generally predictable. The range of plasma levels within which dyphylline can be expected to produce effective bronchodilation has not been determined.

Dyphylline plasma concentrations can be accurately determined using high pressure liquid chromatography (HPLC)* or gas-liquid chromatography (GLC).

INDICATIONS AND USAGE

For relief of acute bronchial asthma and for reversible bronchospasm associated with chronic bronchitis and emphysema.

CONTRAINDICATIONS

Hypersensitivity to dyphylline or related xanthine compounds.

WARNINGS

LUFYLLIN is not indicated in the management of status asthmaticus, which is a serious medical emergency.

Although the relationship between plasma levels of dyphylline and appearance of toxicity is unknown, excessive doses may be expected to be associated with an increased risk of adverse effects.

PRECAUTIONS

General: Use LUFYLLIN with caution in patients with severe cardiac disease, hypertension, hyperthyroidism, acute myocardial injury, or peptic ulcer.

Drug interactions: Synergism between xanthine bronchodilators (e.g., theophylline), ephedrine, and other sympathomimetic bronchodilators has been reported. This should be considered whenever these agents are prescribed concomitantly.

Concurrent administration of dyphylline and probenecid, which competes for tubular secretion, has been shown to increase the plasma half-life of dyphylline (see Clinical Pharmacology).

Carcinogenesis, mutagenesis, impairment of fertility: No long-term animal studies have been performed with LUFYLLIN.

Pregnancy: Teratogenic effects—Pregnancy Category C. Animal reproduction studies have not been conducted with LUFYLLIN. It is also not known if LUFYLLIN can cause fetal harm when administered to a pregnant woman or can affect reproduction capacity. LUFYLLIN should be given to a pregnant woman only if clearly needed.

*See Valia, *et al.*, *J. Chromatogr.* **221**: 170 (1980). Small quantities of pure dyphylline powder may be obtained from Wallace Laboratories, Cranbury, N.J. The internal standard, β-hydroxyethyl-theophylline, may be obtained from companies supplying analytical chemicals.

Nursing mothers: Dyphylline is present in human milk at approximately twice the maternal plasma concentration. Caution should be exercised when LUFYLLIN is administered to a nursing woman.

Pediatric use: Safety and effectiveness in children have not been established.

ADVERSE REACTIONS

Adverse reactions with the use of LUFYLLIN have been infrequent, relatively mild, and rarely required reduction in dosage or withdrawal of therapy.

The following adverse reactions which have been reported with other xanthine bronchodilators, and which have most often been related to excessive drug plasma levels, should be considered as potential adverse effects when dyphylline is administered:

Gastrointestinal: nausea, vomiting, epigastric pain, hematemesis, diarrhea.

Central nervous system: headache, irritability, restlessness, insomnia, hyperexcitability, agitation, muscle twitching, generalized clonic and tonic convulsions.

Cardiovascular: palpitation, tachycardia, extrasystoles, flushing, hypotension, circulatory failure, ventricular arrhythmias.

Respiratory: tachypnea.

Renal: albuminuria, gross and microscopic hematuria, diuresis.

Other: hyperglycemia, inappropriate ADH syndrome.

OVERDOSAGE

There have been no reports, in the literature, of overdosage with LUFYLLIN. However, the following information based on reports of theophylline overdosage are considered typical of the xanthine class of drugs and should be kept in mind.

Signs and symptoms: Restlessness, anorexia, nausea, vomiting, diarrhea, insomnia, irritability, and headache. Marked overdosage with resulting severe toxicity has produced agitation, severe vomiting, dehydration, excessive thirst, tinnitus, cardiac arrhythmias, hyperthermia, diaphoresis, and generalized clonic and tonic convulsions. Cardiovascular collapse has also occurred, with some fatalities. Seizures have occurred in some cases associated with very high theophylline plasma concentrations, without any premonitory symptoms of toxicity.

Treatment: There is no specific antidote for overdosage with drugs of the xanthine class. Symptomatic treatment and general supportive measures should be instituted with careful monitoring and maintenance of vital signs, fluids, and electrolytes. The stomach should be emptied by inducing emesis if the patient is conscious and responsive, or by gastric lavage, taking care to protect against aspiration, especially in stuporous or comatose patients. Maintenance of an adequate airway is essential in case oxygen or assisted respiration is needed. Sympathomimetic agents should be avoided but sedatives such as short-acting barbiturates may be useful.

Dyphylline is dialyzable and, although not recommended as a routine procedure in overdosage cases, hemodialysis may be of some benefit when severe intoxication is present or when the patient has not responded to general supportive and symptomatic treatment.

DOSAGE AND ADMINISTRATION

Dosage should be individually titrated according to the severity of the condition and the response of the patient.

Usual adult dosage: Up to 15 mg/kg every six hours.

Appropriate dosage adjustments should be made in patients with impaired renal function (see Clinical Pharmacology).

HOW SUPPLIED

LUFYLLIN Tablets contain 200 mg dyphylline and are white, rectangular, scored on one side and imprinted WALLACE 521 on the other side. The tablets are available in bottles of 100 (NDC 0037-0521-92), 1000 (NDC 0037-0521-97), and 5000 (NDC 0037-0521-98).

LUFYLLIN-400 Tablets contain 400 mg dyphylline and are white, capsule-shaped, scored on one side and imprinted WALLACE 731 on the other side. The tablets are available in bottles of 100 (NDC 0037-0731-92), 1000 (NDC 0037-0731-97), and 2500 (NDC 0037-0731-99).

Storage: Store at controlled room temperature 20°–25°C (68°–77°F).

Dispense in a tight container.

WALLACE LABORATORIES
Division of
Carter-Wallace, Inc.
Cranbury, New Jersey 08512

IN-0521-07 Rev. 9/98

LUFYLLIN®-GG ℞
(dyphylline and guaifenesin tablets and elixir, USP)
Tablets and Elixir

DESCRIPTION

LUFYLLIN®-GG is a bronchodilator/expectorant combination available for oral administration as *Tablets* and *Elixir*.

Each Tablet contains:

Dyphylline	200 mg
Guaifenesin	200 mg

Other ingredients: corn starch, D&C Yellow No. 10, magnesium aluminum silicate, magnesium stearate, microcrystalline cellulose.

Each 15 mL (one tablespoonful) of Elixir contains:

Dyphylline	100 mg
Guaifenesin	100 mg
Alcohol (by volume)	17%

Other ingredients: citric acid, FD&C Yellow No. 6, flavor (artificial), purified water, saccharin sodium, sodium citrate, sucrose.

Dyphylline is 7-(2,3-dihydroxypropyl)-theophylline, a white, extremely bitter, amorphous powder that is fully soluble in water and soluble in alcohol to the extent of 2g/100 mL. Dyphylline forms a neutral solution that is stable in gastrointestinal fluids over a wide range of pH.

CLINICAL PHARMACOLOGY

Dyphylline is a xanthine derivative with pharmacologic actions similar to theophylline and other members of this class of drugs. Its primary action is that of bronchodilation, but it also exhibits peripheral vasodilatory and other smooth muscle relaxant activity to a lesser degree. The bronchodilatory action of dyphylline, as with other xanthines, is thought to be mediated through competitive inhibition of phosphodiesterase with a resulting increase in cyclic AMP producing relaxation of bronchial smooth muscle.

Dyphylline in LUFYLLIN-GG is well tolerated and produces less nausea than aminophylline and other alkaline theophylline compounds when administered orally. Unlike the hydrolyzable salts of theophylline, dyphylline is not converted to free theophylline *in vivo*. It is absorbed rapidly in therapeutically active form and in healthy volunteers reaches a mean peak plasma concentration of 17.1 mcg/mL in approximately 45 minutes following a single oral dose of 1000 mg of dyphylline.

Dyphylline exerts its bronchodilatory effects directly and, unlike theophylline, is excreted unchanged by the kidneys without being metabolized by the liver. Because of this, dyphylline pharmacokinetics and plasma levels are not influenced by various factors that affect liver function and hepatic enzyme activity, such as smoking, age, or concomitant use of drugs which affect liver function.

The elimination half-life of dyphylline is approximately two hours (1.8–2.1 hr) and approximately 88% of a single oral dose can be recovered from the urine unchanged. The renal clearance would be correspondingly reduced in patients with impaired renal function. In anuric patients, the half-life may be increased 3 to 4 times normal.

Dyphylline plasma levels are dose-related and generally predictable. The therapeutic range of plasma levels within which dyphylline can be expected to produce effective bronchodilation has not been determined.

Dyphylline plasma concentrations can be accurately determined using high pressure liquid chromatography (HPLC)* or gas-liquid chromatography (GLC).

Guaifenesin is an expectorant whose action helps increase the output of thin respiratory tract fluid to facilitate mucociliary clearance and removal of inspissated mucus.

INDICATIONS AND USAGE

For relief of acute bronchial asthma and for reversible bronchospasm associated with chronic bronchitis and emphysema.

CONTRAINDICATIONS

Hypersensitivity to any of the ingredients or related compounds.

WARNINGS

LUFYLLIN-GG is not indicated in the management of status asthmaticus, which is a serious medical emergency.

Although the relationship between plasma levels of dyphylline and appearance of toxicity is unknown, excessive doses may be expected to be associated with an increased risk of adverse effects.

PRECAUTIONS

General: Use LUFYLLIN-GG with caution in patients with severe cardiac disease, hypertension, hyperthyroidism, acute myocardial injury or peptic ulcer.

Drug interactions: Synergism between xanthine bronchodilators (e.g., theophylline), ephedrine and other sympathomimetic bronchodilators has been reported. This should be considered whenever these agents are prescribed concomitantly.

* *See* Valia, *et al*, *J. Chromatogr.* **221**: 170 (1980). Small quantities of pure dyphylline powder may be obtained from Wallace Laboratories, Cranbury, N.J. The internal standard, β-hydroxyethyl-theophylline may be obtained from companies supplying analytical chemicals.

Concurrent administration of dyphylline and probenecid, which competes for tubular secretion, has been shown to increase plasma half-life of dyphylline (see Clinical Pharmacology).

Carcinogenesis, mutagenesis, impairment of fertility: No long-term animal studies have been performed with LUFYLLIN-GG.

Pregnancy: Teratogenic effects — Pregnancy Category C. Animal reproduction studies have not been conducted with LUFYLLIN-GG. It is also not known whether the product can cause fetal harm when administered to a pregnant woman or can affect reproduction capacity. LUFYLLIN-GG should be given to a pregnant woman only if clearly needed.

Nursing mothers: Dyphylline is present in human milk at approximately twice the maternal plasma concentration. Caution should be exercised when LUFYLLIN-GG is administered to a nursing woman.

Pediatric Use: Safety and effectiveness in children below the age of six have not been established. Use caution when administering to children six years of age or older.

ADVERSE REACTIONS

LUFYLLIN-GG may cause nausea, headache, cardiac palpitation and CNS stimulation. Postprandial administration may help avoid gastric discomfort.

The following adverse reactions which have been reported with other xanthine bronchodilators, and which have most often been related to excessive drug plasma levels, should be considered as potential adverse effects when dyphylline is administered:

Gastrointestinal: nausea, vomiting, epigastric pain, hematemesis, diarrhea.

Central nervous system: headache, irritability, restlessness, insomnia, hyperexcitability, agitation, muscle twitching, generalized clonic and tonic convulsions.

Cardiovascular: palpitation, tachycardia, extrasystoles, flushing, hypotension, circulatory failure, ventricular arrhythmias.

Respiratory: tachypnea.

Renal: albuminuria, gross and microscopic hematuria, diuresis.

Other: hyperglycemia, inappropriate ADH syndrome.

OVERDOSAGE

There have been no reports, in the literature, of overdosage with LUFYLLIN-GG. However, the following information based on reports of theophylline overdosage are considered typical of the xanthine class of drugs and should be kept in mind.

Signs & Symptoms: Restlessness, anorexia, nausea, vomiting, diarrhea, insomnia, irritability, and headache. Marked overdosage with resulting severe toxicity has produced agitation, severe vomiting, dehydration, excessive thirst, tinnitus, cardiac arrhythmias, hyperthermia, diaphoresis, and generalized clonic and tonic convulsions. Cardiovascular collapse has also occurred, with some fatalities. Seizures have occurred in some cases associated with very high theophylline plasma concentrations, without any premonitory symptoms of toxicity.

Treatment: There is no specific antidote for overdosage with drugs of the xanthine class. Symptomatic treatment and general supportive measures should be instituted with careful monitoring and maintenance of vital signs, fluids and electrolytes. The stomach should be emptied by inducing emesis if the patient is conscious and responsive, or by gastric lavage, taking care to protect against aspiration, especially in stuporous or comatose patients. Maintenance of an adequate airway is essential in case oxygen or assisted respiration is needed. Sympathomimetic agents should be avoided but sedatives such as short-acting barbiturates may be useful.

Dyphylline is dialyzable and, although not recommended as a routine procedure in overdosage cases, hemodialysis may be of some benefit when severe intoxication is present or when the patient has not responded to general supportive and symptomatic treatment.

DOSAGE AND ADMINISTRATION

Dosage should be individually titrated according to the severity of the condition and the response of the patient.

Usual adult dosage:

One tablet or 30 mL (two tablespoonfuls) elixir, four times daily.

Children above age six:

One-half to one tablet or 15 to 30 mL (one to two tablespoonfuls) elixir, three or four times daily.

Not recommended for use in children below age six: (see Precautions).

HOW SUPPLIED

LUFYLLIN-GG Tablets (dyphylline 200 mg and guaifenesin 200 mg) are round, convex, light yellow, scored on one side and imprinted on the other side with WALLACE 541. The tablets are available in bottles of 100 (NDC 0037-0541-92), 1000 (NDC 0037-0541-97), and 3000 (NDC 0037-0541-96), and in boxes of 100 unit-dose (NDC 0037-0541-85).

LUFYLLIN-GG Elixir (dyphylline 100 mg, guaifenesin 100 mg and alcohol 17% by volume per 15 mL) is a clear, light yellow-orange liquid with a mild wine-like odor and taste. The elixir is available in bottles of one pint (NDC 0037-0545-68) and one gallon (NDC 0037-0545-69).

Storage:

Tablets and Elixir — Store at controlled room temperature 20°–25°C (68°–77°F).

Dispense in a tight container.

Tablets-Protect from moisture.

WALLACE LABORATORIES

Division of

CARTER-WALLACE, INC.

Cranbury, New Jersey 08512

IN-054107 Rev. 9/98

MALTSUPEX® OTC

(malt soup extract)

Powder, Liquid, Tablets

(See PDR For Nonprescription Drugs.)

MILTOWN® ©IV ℞

(meprobamate tablets, USP)

DESCRIPTION

Meprobamate is a white powder with a *characteristic odor* and a bitter taste. It is slightly soluble in water, freely soluble in acetone and alcohol, and sparingly soluble in ether. The structural formula of meprobamate is:

$$NH_2COOCH_2-\overset{\displaystyle CH_3}{\underset{\displaystyle CH_2CH_2CH_3}{\overset{|}{\underset{|}{C}}}}-CH_2OOCNH_2$$

'Miltown'-200 contains 200 mg meprobamate per tablet. Other ingredients: acacia, carnauba wax, corn starch, gelatin, magnesium carbonate, magnesium stearate, methylcellulose shellac, sugar, talc, titanium dioxide, white wax and other ingredients.

'Miltown'-400 contains 400 mg meprobamate per tablet. Other ingredients: corn starch, magnesium stearate, methylcellulose.

ACTIONS

Meprobamate is a carbamate derivative which has been shown in animal studies to have effects at multiple sites in the central nervous system, including the thalamus and limbic system.

INDICATIONS

'Miltown' (meprobamate) is indicated for the management of anxiety disorders or for the short-term relief of the symptoms of anxiety. Anxiety or tension associated with the stress of everyday life usually do not require treatment with an anxiolytic.

The effectiveness of 'Miltown' in long-term use, that is, more than 4 months, has not been assessed by systematic clinical studies. The physician should periodically reassess the usefulness of the drug for the individual patient.

CONTRAINDICATIONS

Acute intermittent porphyria as well as allergic or idiosyncratic reactions to meprobamate or related compounds such as carisoprodol, mebutamate, tybamate or carbromal.

WARNINGS

Drug Dependence

Physical dependence, psychological dependence, and abuse have occurred. When chronic intoxication from prolonged use occurs, it usually involves ingestion of greater than recommended doses and is manifested by ataxia, slurred speech, and vertigo. Therefore, careful supervision of dose and amounts prescribed is advised, as well as avoidance of prolonged administration, especially for alcoholics and other patients with a known propensity for taking excessive quantities of drugs.

Sudden withdrawal of the drug after prolonged and excessive use may precipitate recurrence of pre-existing symptoms, such as anxiety, anorexia, or insomnia, or withdrawal reactions, such as vomiting, ataxia, tremors, muscle twitching, confusional states, hallucinosis, and, rarely, convulsive seizures. Such seizures are more likely to occur in persons with central nervous system damage or pre-existent or latent convulsive disorders. Onset of withdrawal symptoms occurs usually within 12 to 48 hours after discontinuation of meprobamate; symptoms usually cease within the next 12 to 48 hours.

When excessive dosage has continued for weeks or months, dosage should be reduced gradually over a period of one or two weeks rather than abruptly stopped. Alternatively, a long-acting barbiturate may be substituted, then gradually withdrawn.

Potentially Hazardous Tasks

Patients should be warned that this drug may impair the mental and/or physical abilities required for the performance of potentially hazardous tasks such as driving a motor vehicle or operating machinery.

Additive Effects

Since the effects of meprobamate and alcohol or meprobamate and other CNS depressants or psychotropic drugs may be additive, appropriate caution should be exercised with patients who take more than one of these agents simultaneously.

Usage in Pregnancy and Lactation

An increased risk of congenital malformations associated with the use of minor tranquilizers (meprobamate, chlordiazepoxide, and diazepam) during the first trimester of pregnancy has been suggested in several studies. Because use of these drugs is rarely a matter of urgency, their use during this period should almost always be avoided. The possibility that a woman of childbearing potential may be pregnant at the time of institution of therapy should be considered. Patients should be advised that if they become pregnant during therapy or intend to become pregnant they should communicate with their physician about the desirability of discontinuing the drug.

Meprobamate passes the placental barrier. It is present both in umbilical cord blood at or near maternal plasma levels and in breast milk of lactating mothers at concentra-

Continued on next page

Miltown—Cont.

tions two to four times that of maternal plasma. When use of meprobamate is contemplated in breast-feeding patients, the drug's higher concentration in breast milk as compared to maternal plasma levels should be considered.

Usage in Children

'Miltown'-200 and 'Miltown'-400 should not be administered to children under age six, since there is a lack of documented evidence for safety and effectiveness in this age group.

PRECAUTIONS

The lowest effective dose should be administered, particularly to elderly and/or debilitated patients, in order to preclude oversedation.

The possibility of suicide attempts should be considered and the least amount of drug feasible should be dispensed at any one time.

Meprobamate is metabolized in the liver and excreted by the kidney; to avoid its excess accumulation, caution should be exercised in administration to patients with compromised liver or kidney function.

Meprobamate occasionally may precipitate seizures in epileptic patients.

Geriatric Use

Clinical studies of Miltown did not include sufficient numbers of subjects aged 65 and over to determine whether they respond differently from younger subjects. Other reported clinical experience has not identified differences in responses between the elderly and younger patients. In general, dose selection for an elderly patient should be cautious, usually starting at the low end of the dosing range, reflecting the greater frequency of decreased hepatic, renal, or cardiac function, and of concomitant disease or other drug therapy.

ADVERSE REACTIONS

Central Nervous System

Drowsiness, ataxia, dizziness, slurred speech, headache, vertigo, weakness, paresthesias, impairment of visual accommodation, euphoria, overstimulation, paradoxical excitement, fast EEG activity.

Gastrointestinal

Nausea, vomiting, diarrhea.

Cardiovascular

Palpitations, tachycardia, various forms of arrhythmia, transient ECG changes, syncope; also, hypotensive crises (including one fatal case).

Allergic or Idiosyncratic

Allergic or idiosyncratic reactions are usually seen within the period of the first to fourth dose in patients having had no previous contact with the drug. Milder reactions are characterized by an itchy, urticarial, or erythematous maculopapular rash which may be generalized or confined to the groin. Other reactions have included leukopenia, acute nonthrombocytopenic purpura, petechiae, ecchymoses, eosinophilia, peripheral edema, adenopathy, fever, fixed drug eruption with cross reaction to carisoprodol, and cross sensitivity between meprobamate/mebutamate and meprobamate/carbromal.

More severe hypersensitivity reactions, rarely reported, include hyperpyrexia, chills, angioneurotic edema, bronchospasm, oliguria, and anuria. Also, anaphylaxis, erythema multiforme, exfoliative dermatitis, stomatitis, proctitis, Stevens-Johnson syndrome, and bullous dermatitis, including one fatal case of the latter following administration of meprobamate in combination with prednisolone.

In case of allergic or idiosyncratic reactions to meprobamate, discontinue the drug and initiate appropriate symptomatic therapy, which may include epinephrine, antihistamines, and in severe cases corticosteroids. In evaluating possible allergic reactions, also consider allergy to excipients.

Hematologic

(See also **Allergic or Idiosyncratic.**) Agranulocytosis and aplastic anemia have been reported. These cases rarely were fatal. Rare cases of thrombocytopenic purpura have been reported.

Other

Exacerbation of porphyric symptoms.

DOSAGE AND ADMINISTRATION

'Miltown'-200 and 400:

The usual adult daily dosage is 1200 mg to 1600 mg, in three or four divided doses; a daily dosage above 2400 mg is not recommended. The usual daily dosage for children ages six to twelve is 200 mg to 600 mg, in two or three divided doses.

Not recommended for children under age 6 (see **Usage in Children**).

OVERDOSAGE

Suicidal attempts with meprobamate have resulted in drowsiness, lethargy, stupor, ataxia, coma, shock, vasomotor and respiratory collapse. Some suicidal attempts have been fatal.

The following data on meprobamate tablets have been reported in the literature and from other sources. These data are not expected to correlate with each case (considering factors such as individual susceptibility and length of time from ingestion to treatment), but represent the **usual ranges** reported.

Acute simple overdose (meprobamate alone): Death has been reported with ingestion of as little as 12 g meprobamate and survival with as much as 40 g.

Blood Levels:

0.5–2.0 mg% represents the usual blood level range of meprobamate after therapeutic doses. The level may occasionally be as high as 3.0 mg%.

3–10 mg% usually corresponds to findings of mild to moderate symptoms of overdosage, such as stupor or light coma.

10–20 mg% usually corresponds to deeper coma, requiring more intensive treatment. Some fatalities occur.

At levels greater than 20%, more fatalities than survivals can be expected.

Acute combined overdose (meprobamate with alcohol or other CNS depressants or psychotropic drugs): Since effects can be additive, a history of ingestion of a low dose of meprobamate plus any of these compounds (or of a relative low blood or tissue level) cannot be used as a prognostic indicator.

In cases where excessive doses have been taken, sleep ensues rapidly and blood pressure, pulse, and respiratory rates are reduced to basal levels. Any drug remaining in the stomach should be removed and symptomatic therapy given. Should respiration or blood pressure become compromised, respiratory assistance, central nervous system stimulants, and pressor agents should be administered cautiously as indicated. Meprobamate is metabolized in the liver and excreted by the kidney. Diuresis, osmotic (mannitol) diuresis, peritoneal dialysis, and hemodialysis have been used successfully. Careful monitoring of urinary output is necessary and caution should be taken to avoid overhydration. Relapse and death, after initial recovery, have been attributed to incomplete gastric emptying and delayed absorption. Meprobamate can be measured in biological fluids by two methods: colorimetric (Hoffman, A.J. and Ludwig, B.J.: *J Amer Pharm Assn 48:* 740, 1959) and gas chromatographic (Douglas, J.F. et al.: *Anal Chem 39:* 956, 1967).

HOW SUPPLIED

'Miltown'-200: 200 mg white, sugar-coated tablets coded 37-1101 and Wallace; available in bottles of 100 (NDC 0037-1101-01).

'Miltown'-400: 400 mg white, scored tablets coded 37-1001 and Wallace; available in bottles of 100 (NDC 0037-1001-01), and 1000 (NDC 0037-1001-02).

Storage: Store at controlled room temperature 20°–25°C (68°–77°F). Dispense in a tight container.

WALLACE LABORATORIES
Division of CARTER-WALLACE, INC.
Cranbury, New Jersey 08512
IN-070J2-10 Rev. 4/99

ORGANIDIN® NR* (*Newly Reformulated) Tablets, Liquid (guaifenesin) ℞
TUSSI-ORGANIDIN® NR* (*Newly Reformulated) Liquid Ⓒ ℞
TUSSI-ORGANIDIN®-S† NR* (*Newly Reformulated) Liquid (guaifenesin, codeine phosphate) Ⓒ ℞
TUSSI-ORGANIDIN® DM NR* (*Newly Reformulated) Liquid ℞
TUSSI-ORGANIDIN® DM-S† NR* (*Newly Reformulated) Liquid (guaifenesin, dextromethorphan hydrobromide) ℞

Professional Labeling Information and Directions for Use These products labeled for sale on prescription only.

DESCRIPTION

Guaifenesin (glyceryl guaiacolate) has the chemical name 3-(2-methoxyphenoxy)-1,2-propanediol. Its molecular formula is $C_{10}H_{14}O_4$ with a molecular weight of 198.21. It is a white or slightly gray crystalline substance with a slightly bitter aromatic taste. One gram dissolves in 20 mL water at 25°C; it is freely soluble in ethanol. Guaifenesin is readily absorbed from the GI tract and is rapidly metabolized and excreted in the urine. Guaifenesin has a plasma half-life of one hour. The major urinary metabolite is β-(2-methoxyphenoxy) lactic acid.

ORGANIDIN® NR* (*Newly Reformulated) (guaifenesin) is an expectorant available for oral administration as:

Tablets — each containing 200 mg guaifenesin, USP.

Other ingredients: Corn starch, croscarmellose sodium, FD&C Red No. 40, magnesium stearate, microcrystalline cellulose.

Liquid — each teaspoonful (5 mL) containing 100 mg guaifenesin, USP.

Other ingredients: Caramel, citric acid, flavor (raspberry), glycerin, propylene glycol, purified water, saccharin sodium, sodium benzoate, sorbitol solution.

TUSSI-ORGANIDIN® NR* (*Newly Reformulated) and TUSSI-ORGANIDIN® DM NR* (*Newly Reformulated) are antitussive-expectorant combinations available for oral administration as liquids.

TUSSI-ORGANIDIN® NR* (*Newly Reformulated) is a clear red liquid with a raspberry flavor. Each teaspoonful (5 mL) contains guaifenesin, USP 100 mg and codeine phosphate, USP 10 mg.

Other ingredients: Citric acid, FD&C Red No. 40, flavor (artificial), glycerin, propylene glycol, purified water, saccharin sodium, sodium benzoate, sorbitol.

TUSSI-ORGANIDIN® DM NR* (*Newly Reformulated) Liquid is a clear yellow liquid with a raspberry flavor. Each teaspoonful (5 mL) contains guaifenesin, USP 100 mg and dextromethorphan hydrobromide, USP 10 mg.

Other ingredients: Citric acid, D&C Yellow No. 10, FD&C Red No. 40, flavor (artificial), glycerin, propylene glycol, purified water, saccharin sodium, sodium benzoate, sorbitol.

CLINICAL PHARMACOLOGY

ORGANIDIN® NR* (*Newly Reformulated) (guaifenesin) is an expectorant, the action of which promotes or facilitates the removal of secretions from the respiratory tract. By increasing sputum volume and making sputum less viscous, guaifenesin facilitates expectoration of retained secretions.

TUSSI-ORGANIDIN® NR* (*Newly Reformulated) combines the expectorant, guaifenesin, and the cough suppressant, codeine. Codeine is a centrally acting antitussive agent.

TUSSI-ORGANIDIN® DM NR* (*Newly Reformulated) combines the expectorant, guaifenesin, and the cough suppressant, dextromethorphan hydrobromide. Dextromethorphan is a synthetic nonopioid cough suppressant, the dextro isomer of the codeine analogue of levorphanol. Dextromethorphan acts centrally to elevate the threshold for coughing but does not have addictive, analgesic or sedative actions and does not produce respiratory depression with usual doses.

INDICATIONS AND USAGE

ORGANIDIN® NR* (*Newly Reformulated): Helps loosen phlegm (mucus) and thin bronchial secretions to rid the bronchial passageways of bothersome mucus, drain bronchial tubes and make coughs more productive. Helps loosen phlegm and thin bronchial secretions in patients with stable chronic bronchitis.

TUSSI-ORGANIDIN® NR* (*Newly Reformulated) and TUSSI-ORGANIDIN® DM NR* (*Newly Reformulated): Temporarily relieves cough due to minor throat and bronchial irritation as may occur with the common cold or inhaled irritants. Calms the cough control center and relieves coughing.

CONTRAINDICATIONS

Hypersensitivity to any of the ingredients.

The use of dextromethorphan-containing products are contraindicated in patients receiving monoamine oxidase inhibitors (MAOIs).

PRECAUTIONS

Carcinogenesis, Mutagenesis, Impairment of Fertility: Animal studies to assess the long-term carcinogenic and mutagenic potential or the effect on fertility in animals or humans have not been performed.

Pregnancy:

Teratogenic Effects—Pregnancy Category C: Animal reproduction studies have not been conducted. Safe use in pregnancy has not been established relative to possible adverse effects on fetal development. Therefore, these products should not be used in pregnant patients unless, in the judgment of the physician, the potential benefits outweigh possible hazards.

Nonteratogenic Effects: Dependence has been reported in newborns whose mothers took opiates regularly during pregnancy. Withdrawal signs include irritability, excessive crying, tremors, hyperreflexia, fever, vomiting, and diarrhea. Signs usually appear during the first few days of life.

Labor and Delivery: Narcotic analgesics cross the placental barrier. The closer to delivery and the larger the dose used, the greater the possibility of respiratory depression in the newborn. Narcotic analgesics should be avoided during labor if delivery of a premature infant is anticipated. If the mother has received narcotic analgesics during labor, newborn infants should be observed closely for signs of respiratory depression. Resuscitation may be required.

Nursing Mothers: It is not known whether guaifenesin or dextromethorphan is excreted in human milk. Because many drugs are excreted in human milk, caution should be exercised when these products are administered to a nursing woman and a decision should be made whether to discontinue nursing or to discontinue the drug, taking into account the importance of the drug to the mother.

TUSSI-ORGANIDIN® NR* (*Newly Reformulated): Because the hepatic enzyme system, which acts to conjugate codeine to an inactive glucuronide (an important inactivation pathway), is not fully developed in infants less than 6 months of age, the use of codeine is contraindicated in nursing mothers.

Laboratory Test Interactions: Guaifenesin or its metabolites may cause color interference with the VMA (vanillylmandelic acid) test for catechols. It may also falsely elevate the level of urinary 5-HIAA (5-hydroxyindoleacetic acid) in certain serotonin metabolite chemical tests because of color interference.

Information for Patients: TUSSI-ORGANIDIN® NR* (*Newly Reformulated): Patients should be warned about engaging in activities requiring mental alertness, such as driving a car or operating dangerous machinery.

TUSSI-ORGANIDIN® DM NR* (*Newly Reformulated): Patients should be warned not to use this product if they are now taking a prescription monoamine oxidase inhibitor (MAOI) (certain drugs for depression, psychiatric or emotional conditions, or Parkinson's disease), or for 2 weeks after stopping the MAOI drug. If patients are uncertain whether a prescription drug contains an MAOI, they should be instructed to consult a health professional before taking such a product.

Drug Interactions: TUSSI-ORGANIDIN® NR* (*Newly Reformulated): The use of codeine may result in additive CNS depressant effects when coadministered with alcohol, antihistamines, psychotropics or other drugs that produce CNS depression.
TUSSI-ORGANIDIN® DM NR* (*Newly Reformulated): Serious toxicity may result if dextromethorphan is coadministered with monoamine oxidase inhibitors (MAOIs). The use of dextromethorphan hydrobromide may result in additive CNS depressant effects when coadministered with alcohol, antihistamines, psychotropics or other drugs that produce CNS depression.

ADVERSE REACTIONS

Guaifenesin is well tolerated and has a wide margin of safety. Side effects have been generally mild and infrequent. Nausea and vomiting are the side effects that occur most commonly. Dizziness, headache, and rash (including urticaria) have been reported rarely.
Codeine [TUSSI-ORGANIDIN® NR* (*Newly Reformulated)]: Nausea, vomiting, constipation, drowsiness, and miosis have been reported. Higher doses may induce euphoria, light-headedness, dizziness, drowsiness and depression of respiration. Pruritus and skin rashes have been rare.
Dextromethorphan [TUSSI-ORGANIDIN® DM NR* (*Newly Reformulated)]: Rare drowsiness or mild gastrointestinal disturbances are the only side effects associated with dextromethorphan in clinical use. [*see also* Drug Interactions]

DRUG ABUSE AND DEPENDENCE

TUSSI-ORGANIDIN® NR* (*Newly Reformulated) Liquid: Controlled Substance—Schedule V.
Dependence—Codeine may be habit-forming.

OVERDOSAGE

In massive overdosage the stomach should be emptied (emesis and/or gastric lavage) and further absorption prevented. Treatment is symptomatic and supportive.
The acute toxicity of **guaifenesin** is low and overdosage is unlikely to produce serious toxic effects. In laboratory animals no toxicity resulted when guaifenesin was administered by stomach tube in doses up to 5 grams/kg.
Severe intoxication with **codeine** may result in dyspnea, vertigo, double vision, delusions, hallucinations, speech disturbances, excitement, restlessness, delirium, constricted pupils, respiratory depression (slow and shallow breathing), Cheyne-Stokes respiration, circulatory collapse, stupor and coma.
Treatment of overdosage consists primarily of support of vital functions, especially management of codeine-induced respiratory depression. The narcotic antagonist naloxone is a specific antidote for respiratory depression that may result from overdose or unusual sensitivity from narcotics.
Overdosage with **dextromethorphan** may produce excitement and mental confusion. Very high doses may produce respiratory depression. One case of toxic psychosis (hyperactivity, marked visual and auditory hallucinations) after ingestion of a single 300 mg dose of dextromethorphan has been reported.

DOSAGE AND ADMINISTRATION

ORGANIDIN® NR* (*Newly Reformulated) (guaifenesin)
Tablets — Adults and children 12 years of age and older:
One to 2 tablets (200 mg to 400 mg) every four hours, not to exceed 2400 mg (12 tablets) in 24 hours.
Liquid — Adults and children 12 years of age and older:
Two to four teaspoonfuls (200 mg to 400 mg) every four hours, not to exceed 2400 mg (24 teaspoonfuls) in 24 hours.
Children 6 years to under 12 years of age: One to two teaspoonfuls (100 mg to 200 mg) every four hours, not to exceed 1200 mg (12 teaspoonfuls) in 24 hours.
Children 2 years to under 6 years of age: 1/2 to 1 teaspoonful (50 mg to 100 mg) every four hours, not to exceed 600 mg (6 teaspoonfuls) in 24 hours.
Children 6 mo. to under 2 years of age: A common dosage is 1/4 to 1/2 teaspoonful (25 mg to 50 mg) every four hours, not to exceed 300 mg (3 teaspoonfuls) in 24 hours. Individualized dosage should be determined by evaluation of patient.
TUSSI-ORGANIDIN® NR* (*Newly Reformulated) Liquid
Adults and children 12 years of age and older: 2 teaspoonfuls (10 mL) every four hours, not to exceed 12 teaspoonfuls (60 mL) in 24 hours.
Children 6 years to under 12 years of age: 1 teaspoonful (5 mL) every four hours, not to exceed 6 teaspoonfuls (30 mL) in a 24 hour period.
Children 2 to under 6 years of age: Oral dosage is based on 1 mg/kg/day of codeine administered in four equal divided doses.
The average body weight for each age group may also be used to determine codeine dosage as follows:
For children 2 years of age (average body weight 12 kg): The oral dosage is 1.5 mL (3 mg codeine + 30 mg guaifenesin) TUSSI-ORGANIDIN® NR* (*Newly Reformulated) Liquid every 4–6 hr, not to exceed 6 mL (12 mg codeine + 120 mg guaifenesin) in a 24 hr period.
For children 3 years of age (average 14 kg): 1.75 mL (3.5 mg codeine + 35 mg guaifenesin) every 4–6 hours, not to exceed 7 mL (14 mg codeine + 140 mg guaifenesin) in 24 hours.
For children 4 years of age (average 16 kg): 2 mL (4 mg codeine + 40 mg guaifenesin) every 4–6 hours, not to exceed 8 mL (16 mg codeine + 160 mg guaifenesin) in 24 hours.
For children 5 years of age (average 18 kg): 2.25 mL (4.5 mg codeine + 45 mg guaifenesin) every 4–6 hours, not to exceed 9 mL (18 mg codeine + 180 mg guaifenesin) in 24 hours.
Patients should be instructed to obtain and use a dispensing device (such as a dropper calibrated for age or weight) to administer the drug to a child, to use extreme care in measuring dosage, and not to exceed the recommended daily dosage.
CODEINE IS NOT RECOMMENDED FOR USE IN CHILDREN UNDER 2 YEARS OF AGE.
Children under 2 years of age may be more susceptible to the respiratory depressant effects of codeine, including respiratory arrest, coma and death.
TUSSI-ORGANIDIN® DM NR* (*Newly Reformulated) Liquid
Adults and children 12 years of age and older: 2 teaspoonfuls (10 mg) every four hours not to exceed 12 teaspoonfuls (60 mL) in 24 hours.
Children 6 years to under 12 years of age: 1 teaspoonful (5 mL) every four hours not to exceed 6 teaspoonfuls (30 mL) in 24 hours.
Children 2 to under 6 years of age: 1/2 teaspoonful (2.5 mL) every four hours not to exceed 3 teaspoonfuls (15 mL) in 24 hours.
Children 6 mo. to under 2 years of age: A common dosage is 1/8 teaspoonful to 1/4 teaspoonful (0.6 mL to 1.25 mL) every 4 hours or 1/2 teaspoonful (2.5 mL) every 6–8 hours, not to exceed 1.5 teaspoonfuls (7.5 mL) in 24 hours. Individualized dosage should be determined by evaluation of patient.
PATIENTS SHOULD BE ADVISED TO KEEP THESE AND ALL DRUGS OUT OF THE REACH OF CHILDREN AND TO SEEK PROFESSIONAL ASSISTANCE OR CONTACT A POISON CONTROL CENTER IMMEDIATELY IN CASE OF ACCIDENTAL OVERDOSE.

HOW SUPPLIED

ORGANIDIN® NR* (*Newly Reformulated) (guaifenesin)
Tablets — Each round, scored, rose-colored tablet contains 200 mg guaifenesin USP—available in bottles of 100 (NDC 0037-4312-01)
Liquid — 100 mg guaifenesin per teaspoonful (5 mL)—available as a clear amber liquid in bottles of 1 pint (NDC 0037-4214-10)
TUSSI-ORGANIDIN® NR* (*Newly Reformulated) Liquid — Guaifenesin 100 mg and codeine phosphate 10 mg per teaspoonful (5 mL) of clear red liquid in bottles of one pint (NDC 0037-4814-10) and 4 fl oz (NDC 0037-4814-01) labeled TUSSI-ORGANIDIN®-S† NR*
TUSSI-ORGANIDIN® DM NR* (*Newly Reformulated) Liquid — Guaifenesin 100 mg and dextromethorphan hydrobromide 10 mg per teaspoonful (5 mL) of clear yellow liquid in bottles of one pint (NDC 0037-4714-10) and 4 fl oz (NDC 0037-4714-01) labeled TUSSI-ORGANIDIN® DM-S† NR*
†TUSSI-ORGANIDIN®-S NR* and TUSSI-ORGANIDIN® DM-S NR* are TUSSI-ORGANIDIN® NR* and TUSSI-ORGANIDIN® DM NR* Liquids, respectively, either in 4 fl oz unit of use containers with a 10 mL graduated oral syringe and fitment or in 30 mL sample containers.
STORAGE—Store at controlled room temperature 20°–25°C (68°–77°F). Protect tablets from moisture. Keep bottle tightly closed.

WALLACE LABORATORIES
Division of Carter-Wallace, Inc.
Cranbury, NJ 08512
IN-046J2-04 Rev. 1/98

Shown in Product Identification Guide, page 339

RYNA®
(Liquid)
RYNA–C® Ⓒ
(Liquid)

(See PDR For Nonprescription Drugs.)

RYNA-12™ S ℞
Suspension

DESCRIPTION

RYNA-12™ S Suspension is an antihistamine/nasal decongestant combination available for oral administration as a *Suspension*. Each 5 mL (one teaspoonful) of the pink-colored, natural strawberry- artificial currant flavored Suspension contains:

Phenylephrine Tannate	5 mg
Pyrilamine Tannate	30 mg

Other ingredients: benzoic acid, FD&C Red No. 3, flavors (natural and artificial), glycerin, kaolin, magnesium aluminum silicate, methylparaben, pectin, purified water, saccharin sodium, sucrose.

CLINICAL PHARMACOLOGY

RYNA-12™ S Suspension combines the sympathomimetic decongestant effect of phenylephrine with the antihistaminic action of pyrilamine.

INDICATIONS AND USAGE

RYNA-12™ S Suspension is indicated for symptomatic relief of the coryza and nasal congestion associated with the common cold, sinusitis, allergic rhinitis and other upper respiratory tract conditions. Appropriate therapy should be provided for the primary disease.

CONTRAINDICATIONS

RYNA-12™ S Suspension is contraindicated for newborns, nursing mothers and patients sensitive to any of the ingredients or related compounds.

WARNINGS

Use with caution in patients with hypertension, cardiovascular disease, hyperthyroidism, diabetes, narrow angle glaucoma or prostatic hypertrophy. Use with caution or avoid use in patients taking monoamine oxidase (MAO) inhibitors, or within 14 days of stopping such treatment. This product contains an antihistamine which may cause drowsiness and may have additive central nervous system (CNS) effects with alcohol or other CNS depressants (e.g., hypnotics, sedatives, tranquilizers).

PRECAUTIONS

General: Antihistamines are more likely to cause dizziness, sedation and hypotension in elderly patients. Antihistamines may cause excitation, particularly in children, but their combination with sympathomimetics may cause either mild stimulation or mild sedation.
Information for patients: Caution patients against drinking alcoholic beverages or engaging in potentially hazardous activities requiring alertness, such as driving a car or operating machinery while using this product. Patients should be warned not to use this product if they are now taking a prescription monoamine oxidase inhibitor (MAOI) (certain drugs for depression, psychiatric or emotional conditions, or Parkinson's disease), or for 2 weeks after stopping the MAOI drug. If patients are uncertain whether a prescription drug contains an MAOI, they should be instructed to consult a health professional before taking such a product.
Drug interactions: MAO inhibitors may prolong and intensify the anticholinergic effects of antihistamines and the overall effects of sympathomimetic agents.
Carcinogenesis, mutagenesis, impairment of fertility: No long term animal studies have been performed with RYNA-12™ S Suspension.
Pregnancy: Teratogenic effects: Pregnancy Category C. Animal reproduction studies have not been conducted with RYNA-12™ S Suspension. It is also not known whether RYNA-12™ S Suspension can cause fetal harm when administered to a pregnant woman or can affect reproduction capacity. RYNA-12™ S Suspension should be given to a pregnant woman only if clearly needed.
Nursing mothers: RYNA-12™ S Suspension should not be administered to a nursing woman.

ADVERSE REACTIONS

Adverse effects associated with RYNA-12™ S Suspension at recommended doses have been minimal. The most common have been drowsiness, sedation, dryness of mucous membranes, and gastrointestinal effects. Serious side effects with oral antihistamines or sympathomimetics have been rare.

OVERDOSAGE

Signs & symptoms: May vary from CNS depression to stimulation (restlessness to convulsions). Antihistamine overdosage in young children may lead to convulsions and death. Atropine-like signs and symptoms may be prominent.
Treatment: Induce vomiting if it has not occurred spontaneously. Precautions must be taken against aspiration especially in infants, children and comatose patients. If gastric lavage is indicated, isotonic or half-isotonic saline solution is preferred. Stimulants should not be used. If hypotension is a problem, vasopressor agents may be considered.

DOSAGE AND ADMINISTRATION

Administer the recommended dose every 12 hours.
RYNA-12™ S Suspension: *Children over six years of age*—5 to 10 mL (1 to 2 teaspoonfuls); *Children two to six years of age*—2.5 to 5 mL (½ to 1 teaspoonful); *Children under two years of age*—Titrate dose individually.

HOW SUPPLIED

RYNA-12™ S Suspension (phenylephrine tannate 5 mg, and pyrilamine tannate 30 mg, per 5 mL) in 4 fl oz **unit of use** container with a 10 mL graduated oral syringe and fitment (NDC 0037-0655-04).
Storage: Store at controlled room temperature 20°-25°C (68°-77°F).

WALLACE LABORATORIES
Division of
CARTER-WALLACE, INC.
Cranbury, New Jersey 08512
IN-0655-02 Rev. 4/99

Shown in Product Identification Guide, page 339

RYNATAN® ℞
(azatadine maleate, USP and pseudoephedrine sulfate, USP)
Long-Acting Antihistamine/ Decongestant Tablets

DESCRIPTION

RYNATAN® Long-Acting Antihistamine/Decongestant Tablets contain 1 mg azatadine maleate, USP in the tablet coat-

Continued on next page

Rynatan/Rynatan-S—Cont.

ing and 120 mg pseudoephedrine sulfate, USP, equally distributed between the tablet coating and the barrier-coated core. Following ingestion, the two active components in the coating are quickly liberated; release of the decongestant in the core is delayed for several hours.

Azatadine maleate is an antihistamine having the empirical formula, $C_{20}H_{22}N_2 \bullet 2C_4H_4O_4$, the chemical name, 6,11-Dihydro-11-(-methyl-4-piperidylidene)-5*H*-benzo [5,6] cyclohepta [1,2-*b*] pyridine maleate (1:2), and the chemical structure:

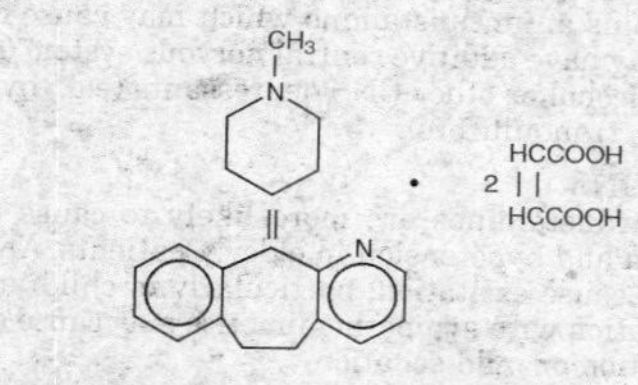

The molecular weight of azatadine maleate is 522.54. Azatadine maleate is a white to off-white powder and is very soluble in water and soluble in alcohol.

Pseudoephedrine sulfate, a sympathomimetic amine, is a salt of pseudoephedrine, one of the naturally occurring alkaloids obtained from various species of the plant *Ephedra*. The empirical formula for pseudoephedrine sulfate is $(C_{10}H_{15}NO)_2 \bullet H_2SO_4$; the chemical name is Benzenemethanol, α-[1-(methylamino)ethyl]-, [S-(R*,R*)]-, sulfate (2:1) (salt), and the chemical structure is:

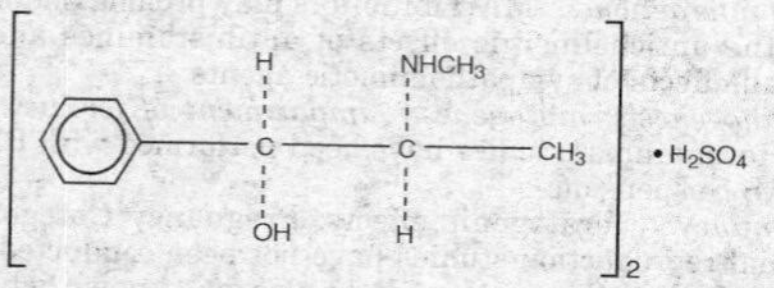

The molecular weight of pseudoephedrine sulfate is 428.56. It is a white to off-white crystal or powder, very soluble in water, freely soluble in alcohol, and sparingly soluble in chloroform.

The inactive ingredients for RYNATAN® Tablets are: acacia, butylparaben, calcium sulfate, carnauba wax, corn starch, D&C Red No. 30 Al Lake, FD&C Yellow No. 6 Al Lake, gelatin, lactose, magnesium stearate, neutral soap, oleic acid, povidone, rosin, sugar, talc, white wax, and zein.

CLINICAL PHARMACOLOGY

Azatadine maleate is an antihistamine, related to cyproheptadine, with antiserotonin, anticholinergic (drying), and sedative effects. Antihistamines appear to compete with histamine for histamine H_1-receptor sites on effector cells. The antihistamines antagonize those pharmacological effects of histamine which are mediated through activation of H_1-receptor sites and thereby reduce the intensity of allergic reactions and tissue injury response involving histamine release. Antihistamines antagonize the vasodilator effect of endogenously released histamine, especially in small vessels, and mitigate the effect of histamine which results in increased capillary permeability and edema formation. As consequences of these actions, antihistamines antagonize the physiological manifestations of histamine release in the nose following antigen-antibody interaction, such as congestion related to vascular engorgement, mucosal edema, and profuse, watery secretion, and irritation and sneezing resulting from histamine action of afferent nerve terminals.

Pseudoephedrine sulfate (d-isoephedrine sulfate) is an orally effective nasal decongestant which appears to exert its sympathomimetic effect indirectly, predominantly through release of adrenergic mediators from postganglionic nerve terminals. In effective recommended oral dosage, pseudoephedrine sulfate produces minimal other sympathomimetic effects, such as pressor activity and CNS stimulation. Use of an orally administered vasoconstrictor for shrinkage of congested nasal mucosa has several advantages: a) it produces a gradual but sustained decongestant effect, causing little, if any "rebound" congestion; b) it facilitates shrinkage of swollen mucosa in upper respiratory areas that are relatively inaccessible to topically applied sprays or drops; c) it relieves nasal obstruction without the additional irritation that may result from local medication.

Pseudoephedrine passes through the blood-brain and placental barriers. While the antihistamines have not been studied systematically for passage through these barriers, the occurrence of pharmacologic effects in the central nervous system and in newborns indicate presence of the drug.

Following administration of the two drugs to normal volunteers in either a single RYNATAN® Tablet or similar doses in two conventional pseudoephedrine sulfate tablets and a conventional tablet of azatadine maleate, the blood levels of pseudoephedrine and the urinary excretion of azatadine showed that the RYNATAN® Tablets are bioequivalent to the conventional dosage forms. The apparent elimination half-life of pseudoephedrine in RYNATAN® Tablets was approximately 6½ hours. The apparent elimination half-life of azatadine maleate (available from the outer layer of the RYNATAN® Tablets or from the conventional azatadine maleate tablet) was approximately 12 hours.

INDICATIONS AND USAGE

RYNATAN® Long-Acting Antihistamine/Decongestant Tablets are indicated for the relief of the symptoms of upper respiratory mucosal congestion in perennial and allergic rhinitis, and for the relief of nasal congestion and eustachian tube congestion. Analgesics, antibiotics, or both may be administered concurrently, when indicated.

CONTRAINDICATIONS

Antihistamines should not be used to treat lower respiratory tract symptoms, including asthma.

This product is contraindicated in patients with narrow-angle glaucoma or urinary retention, and in patients receiving monoamine oxidase (MAO) inhibitor therapy or within 2 weeks of stopping such treatment. (See **Drug Interactions** section.) It is also contraindicated in patients with severe hypertension, severe coronary artery disease, hyperthyroidism, and in those who have shown hypersensitivity or idiosyncrasy to its components, to adrenergic agents, or to other drugs of similar chemical structures. Manifestations of patient idiosyncrasy to adrenergic agents include: insomnia, dizziness, weakness, tremor, or arrhythmias.

WARNINGS

RYNATAN® Tablets should be used with considerable caution in patients with: stenosing peptic ulcer, pyloroduodenal obstruction, urinary bladder obstruction due to symptomatic prostatic hypertrophy, or narrowing of the bladder neck. It should also be administered with caution to patients with: cardiovascular disease, including hypertension or ischemic heart disease; increased intraocular pressure (see **CONTRAINDICATIONS**); diabetes mellitus; or in patients receiving digitalis or oral anticoagulants.

Central nervous system stimulation and convulsions or cardiovascular collapse with accompanying hypotension may be produced by sympathomimetics.

Do not exceed recommended dosage.

Use in Activities Requiring Mental Alertness: Patients should be warned about engaging in activities requiring mental alertness, such as driving a car or operating appliances, machinery, etc.

Use in Patients Approximately 60 Years and Older: Antihistamines are more likely to cause dizziness, sedation, and hypotension in patients over 60 years of age. In these patients, sympathomimetics are also more likely to cause adverse reactions, such as confusion, hallucinations, convulsions, CNS depression and death. For this reason, before considering the use of a repeat-action formulation, the safe use of a short-acting sympathomimetic in that particular patient should be demonstrated.

PRECAUTIONS

General: Because of the atropine-like action of antihistamines, this product should be used with caution in patients with a history of bronchial asthma.

Information for Patients:

1. Products containing antihistamines may cause drowsiness.
2. Patients should not engage in activities requiring mental alertness, such as driving or operating machinery or appliances.
3. Alcohol or other sedative drugs may enhance the drowsiness caused by antihistamines.
4. Patients should not take RYNATAN® Tablets if they are receiving a monoamine oxidase inhibitor or within 2 weeks of stopping such treatment, or if they are receiving oral anticoagulants.
5. This medication should not be given to children less than 12 years of age.

Drug Interactions: MAO inhibitors prolong and intensify the effects of antihistamines. Concomitant use of antihistamines with alcohol, tricyclic antidepressants, barbiturates, or other central nervous system depressants may have an additive effect.

When sympathomimetic drugs are given to patients receiving monoamine oxidase inhibitors, hypertensive reactions, including hypertensive crises, may occur. The antihypertensive effects of methyldopa, mecamylamine, reserpine, and veratrum alkaloids may be reduced by sympathomimetics. Beta-adrenergic blocking agents may also interact with sympathomimetics. Increased ectopic pacemaker activity can occur when pseudoephedrine is used concomitantly with digitalis. Antacids increase the rate of absorption of pseudoephedrine, while kaolin decreases it.

Drug/Laboratory Test Interactions: The *in vitro* addition of pseudoephedrine to sera containing the cardiac isoenzyme MB of serum creatine phosphokinase progressively inhibits the activity of the enzyme. The inhibition becomes complete over 6 hours.

Carcinogenesis, Mutagenesis, and Impairment of Fertility: There is no animal or laboratory study of the mixture of azatadine maleate and pseudoephedrine sulfate to evaluate carcinogenesis or mutagenesis. Reproduction studies of this mixture in rats showed no evidence of impaired fertility.

Pregnancy Category C: Retarded fetal development and the presence of angulated hyoid wings were seen in the offspring of pregnant rabbits administered RYNATAN® Tablets at about 12.5 times and 5 times the recommended human dosage, respectively; increased resorption was noted at about 25 times the human dosage. A decreased survival rate at day 21 was seen in rat pups born of mothers given RYNATAN® Tablets during pregnancy at a dose about 12.5 times the human dosage. There are no adequate and well-controlled studies in pregnant women. RYNATAN® Tablets should be used during pregnancy only if the potential benefits to the mother justify the potential risks to the infant. (See **Nonteratogenic Effects**.)

Nonteratogenic Effects: Antihistamines should not be used in the third trimester of pregnancy because newborns and premature infants may have severe reactions to them, such as convulsions.

Nursing Mothers: It is not known whether these drugs are excreted in human milk. However, certain antihistamines and sympathomimetics are known to be excreted in human milk. Because of the higher risks of antihistamines for infants generally and for newborns and prematures in particular, a decision should be made whether to discontinue nursing or to discontinue the drug, taking into account the importance of the drug to the mother.

There is a report of irritability, excessive crying, and disturbed sleeping patterns in a nursing infant whose mother had taken a product containing an antihistamine and pseudoephedrine.

Pediatric Use: Safety and effectiveness in children below the age of 12 years have not been established.

ADVERSE REACTIONS

The following adverse reactions are associated with antihistamine and sympathomimetic drugs. (Those adverse reactions which occur most frequently with the antihistamines are underlined.)

General: Urticaria, drug rash; anaphylactic shock; photosensitivity; excessive perspiration; chills; dryness of mouth, nose, and throat.

Cardiovascular: Hypertension (see **CONTRAINDICATIONS** and **WARNINGS**), hypotension, arrhythmias and cardiovascular collapse, headache, palpitations, extrasystoles, tachycardia, angina.

Hematologic: Hemolytic anemia, hypoplastic anemia, thrombocytopenia, agranulocytosis.

Central Nervous System: Sedation, sleepiness, dizziness, vertigo, tinnitus, acute labyrinthitis, disturbed coordination, fatigue, mydriasis, confusion, restlessness, excitation, nervousness, tension, tremor, irritability, insomnia, euphoria, paresthesias, blurred vision, hysteria, neuritis, convulsions, fear, anxiety, hallucinations, CNS depression, weakness, pallor.

Gastrointestinal: Epigastric distress, anorexia, nausea, vomiting, diarrhea, constipation, abdominal cramps.

Genitourinary: Urinary frequency, urinary retention, dysuria, early menses.

Respiratory: Thickening of bronchial secretions, tightness of chest and wheezing, nasal stuffiness, respiratory difficulty.

DRUG ABUSE AND DEPENDENCE

There is no information to indicate that abuse or dependency occurs with azatadine maleate.

Pseudoephedrine, like other central nervous system stimulants, has been abused. At high doses, subjects commonly experience an elevation of mood, a sense of increased energy and alertness, and decreased appetite. Some individuals become anxious, irritable, and loquacious. In addition to the marked euphoria, the user experiences a sense of markedly enhanced physical strength and mental capacity. With continued use, tolerance develops, the user increases the dose, and toxic signs and symptoms appear. Depression may follow rapid withdrawal.

OVERDOSAGE

In the event of overdosage, emergency treatment should be started immediately.

Manifestations of overdosage may vary from central nervous system depression (sedation, apnea, diminished mental alertness, cyanosis, coma, cardiovascular collapse) to stimulation (insomnia, hallucinations, tremors, or convulsions) to death. Other signs and symptoms may be euphoria, excitement, tachycardia, palpitations, thirst, perspiration, nausea, dizziness, tinnitus, ataxia, blurred vision, and hypertension or hypotension. Stimulation is particularly likely in children, as are atropine-like signs and symptoms (dry mouth; fixed, dilated pupils; flushing; hyperthermia; and gastrointestinal symptoms).

In large doses sympathomimetics may give rise to giddiness, headache, nausea, vomiting, sweating, thirst, tachycardia, precordial pain, palpitations, difficulty in micturition, muscular weakness and tenseness, anxiety, restlessness, and insomnia. Many patients can present a toxic psychosis with delusions and hallucinations. Some may develop cardiac arrhythmias, circulatory collapse, convulsions, coma, and respiratory failure.

The oral LD_{50} of the mixture of the two drugs in mature rats and mice was greater than 1700 mg/kg and 600 mg/kg, respectively.

Treatment—The patient should be induced to vomit, even if emesis has occurred spontaneously. Pharmacologically induced vomiting by the administration of ipecac syrup is a preferred method. However, vomiting should not be induced in patients with impaired consciousness. The action of ipecac is facilitated by physical activity and by the administration of eight to twelve fluid ounces of water. If emesis does not occur within 15 minutes, the dose of ipecac should be repeated. Precautions against aspiration must be taken, especially in infants and children. Following emesis, any drug remaining in the stomach may be absorbed by activated charcoal administered as a slurry with water. If vomiting is unsuccessful or contraindicated, gastric lavage should be performed. Isotonic and one-half isotonic saline are the lavage solutions of choice. Saline cathartics, such as milk of

magnesia, draw water into the bowel by osmosis and therefore may be valuable for their action in rapid dilution of bowel content. Dialysis is of little value in antihistamine poisoning. After emergency treatment the patient should continue to be medically monitored.
Treatment of the signs and symptoms of overdosage is symptomatic and supportive. Stimulants (analeptic agents) should not be used. Vasopressors may be used to treat hypotension. Short-acting barbiturates, diazepam, or paraldehyde, may be administered to control seizures. Hyperpyrexia, especially in children, may require treatment with tepid water sponge baths or a hypothermic blanket. Apnea is treated with ventilatory support.

DOSAGE AND ADMINISTRATION

RYNATAN® Tablets ARE NOT INTENDED FOR USE IN CHILDREN UNDER 12 YEARS OF AGE. The usual adult dosage is one tablet twice a day.

HOW SUPPLIED

RYNATAN® Tablets contain 1 mg azatadine maleate and 120 mg pseudoephedrine sulfate. RYNATAN® Tablets are coral-colored, sugar-coated tablets branded in black with the product name (RYNATAN) and product identification numbers, 711, bottle of 100 (NDC 0037-0711-10).
Store between 2° and 30°C (36° and 86°F).
MANUFACTURED BY
Key Pharmaceuticals, Inc.
Kenilworth, NJ 07033 USA
DISTRIBUTED BY
WALLACE LABORATORIES
Division of Carter-Wallace, Inc.
Cranbury, NJ 08512
IN-0711-02 Rev. 4/99

Shown in Product Identification Guide, page 339

RYNATAN®-P ℞
Pediatric Suspension

DESCRIPTION

RYNATAN®-P is an antihistamine/nasal decongestant combination available for oral administration as *Pediatric Suspension*. Each 5 mL (one teaspoonful) of the pink-colored natural strawberry- artificial currant flavored Pediatric Suspension contains:

Phenylephrine Tannate	5 mg
Chlorpheniramine Tannate	2 mg
Pyrilamine Tannate	12.5 mg

Other ingredients: benzoic acid, FD&C Red No. 3, flavors (natural and artificial), glycerin, kaolin, magnesium aluminum silicate, methylparaben, pectin, purified water, saccharin sodium, sucrose.

CLINICAL PHARMACOLOGY

RYNATAN®-P Pediatric Suspension combines the sympathomimetic decongestant effect of phenylephrine with the antihistaminic actions of chlorpheniramine and pyrilamine.

INDICATIONS AND USAGE

RYNATAN®-P Pediatric Suspension is indicated for symptomatic relief of the coryza and nasal congestion associated with the common cold, sinusitis, allergic rhinitis and other upper respiratory tract conditions. Appropriate therapy should be provided for the primary disease.

CONTRAINDICATIONS

RYNATAN®-P Pediatric Suspension is contraindicated for newborns, nursing mothers and patients sensitive to any of the ingredients or related compounds.

WARNINGS

Use with caution in patients with hypertension, cardiovascular disease, hyperthyroidism, diabetes, narrow angle glaucoma or prostatic hypertrophy. Use with caution or avoid use in patients taking monoamine oxidase (MAO) inhibitors, or within 14 days of stopping such treatment. This product contains antihistamines which may cause drowsiness and may have additive central nervous system (CNS) effects with alcohol or other CNS depressants (e.g., hypnotics, sedatives, tranquilizers).

PRECAUTIONS

General: Antihistamines are more likely to cause dizziness, sedation and hypotension in elderly patients. Antihistamines may cause excitation, particularly in children, but their combination with sympathomimetics may cause either mild stimulation or mild sedation.
Information for patients: Caution patients against drinking alcoholic beverages or engaging in potentially hazardous activities requiring alertness, such as driving a car or operating machinery while using this product. Patients should be warned not to use this product if they are now taking a prescription monoamine oxidase inhibitor (MAOI) (certain drugs for depression, psychiatric or emotional conditions, or Parkinson's disease), or for 2 weeks after stopping the MAOI drug. If patients are uncertain whether a prescription drug contains an MAOI, they should be instructed to consult a health professional before taking such a product.
Drug interactions: MAO inhibitors may prolong and intensify the anticholinergic effects of antihistamines and the overall effects of sympathomimetic agents.
Carcinogenesis, mutagenesis, impairment of fertility: No long term animal studies have been performed with RYNATAN®-P Pediatric Suspension.
Pregnancy: Teratogenic effects: Pregnancy Category C. Animal reproduction studies have not been conducted with RYNATAN®-P Pediatric Suspension. It is also not known whether RYNATAN®-P Pediatric Suspension can cause fetal harm when administered to a pregnant woman or can affect reproduction capacity. RYNATAN®-P Pediatric Suspension should be given to a pregnant woman only if clearly needed.
Nursing mothers: RYNATAN®-P Pediatric Suspension should not be administered to a nursing woman.

ADVERSE REACTIONS

Adverse effects associated with RYNATAN®-P Pediatric Suspension at recommended doses have been minimal. The most common have been drowsiness, sedation, dryness of mucous membranes, and gastrointestinal effects. Serious side effects with oral antihistamines or sympathomimetics have been rare.

OVERDOSAGE

Signs & symptoms: May vary from CNS depression to stimulation (restlessness to convulsions). Antihistamine overdosage in young children may lead to convulsions and death. Atropine-like signs and symptoms may be prominent.
Treatment: Induce vomiting if it has not occurred spontaneously. Precautions must be taken against aspiration especially in infants, children and comatose patients. If gastric lavage is indicated, isotonic or half-isotonic saline solution is preferred. Stimulants should not be used. If hypotension is a problem, vasopressor agents may be considered.

DOSAGE AND ADMINISTRATION

Administer the recommended dose every 12 hours.
RYNATAN®-P Pediatric Suspension: *Children over six years of age*—5 to 10 mL (1 to 2 teaspoonfuls): *Children two to six years of age*—2.5 to 5 mL (1/2 to 1 teaspoonful); *Children under two years of age*—Titrate dose individually.

HOW SUPPLIED

RYNATAN®-P Pediatric Suspension (phenylephrine tannate 5 mg, chlorpheniramine tannate 2 mg, and pyrilamine tannate 12.5 mg per 5 mL); in pint bottles (NDC 0037-0715-68).
Storage: Store at controlled room temperature 20°–25°C (68°–77°F).
Dispense in a tight container.

Produced under license from
Jame Fine Chemicals, Inc.
Bound Brook, NJ, USA

WALLACE LABORATORIES
Division of
CARTER-WALLACE, INC.
Cranbury, New Jersey 08512
IN-0715-02 Rev. 1/00

Shown in Product Identification Guide, page 339

RYNATUSS® ℞
Tablets
Pediatric Suspension

DESCRIPTION

RYNATUSS® is an antitussive/antihistamine/nasal decongestant/bronchodilator combination available for oral administration as *Tablets* and as *Pediatric Suspension*
Each tablet contains:

Carbetapentane Tannate	60 mg
Chlorpheniramine Tannate	5 mg
Ephedrine Tannate	10 mg
Phenylephrine Tannate	10 mg

Other ingredients: corn starch, dibasic calcium phosphate, FD&C Blue No. 1, FD&C Red No. 40, magnesium stearate, methylcellulose, polygalacturonic acid, povidone, talc.
Each 5 mL (one teaspoonful) of the Pediatric Suspension contains:

Carbetapentane Tannate	30 mg
Chlorpheniramine Tannate	4 mg
Ephedrine Tannate	5 mg
Phenylephrine Tannate	5 mg

Other ingredients: benzoic acid, FD&C Blue No. 1, FD&C Red No. 3, FD&C Red No. 40, FD&C Yellow No. 5 (see Precautions), flavors (natural and artificial), glycerin, Kaolin, magnesium aluminum silicate, methylparaben, pectin, purified water, saccharin sodium, sucrose.

CLINICAL PHARMACOLOGY

RYNATUSS combines the antitussive action of carbetapentane, the sympathomimetic decongestant effect of phenylephrine, the antihistaminic action of chlorpheniramine, and the bronchodilator action of ephedrine.

INDICATIONS AND USAGE

RYNATUSS is indicated for the symptomatic relief of cough associated with respiratory tract conditions such as the common cold, bronchial asthma, acute and chronic bronchitis. Appropriate therapy should be provided for the primary disease.

CONTRAINDICATIONS

RYNATUSS is contraindicated for newborns, nursing mothers, and patients who are sensitive to any of the ingredients or related compounds.

WARNINGS

Use with caution in patients with hypertension, cardiovascular disease, hyperthyroidism, diabetes, narrow angle glaucoma, or prostatic, hypertrophy. Do not use in patients taking monoamine oxidase (MAO) inhibitors, or for 14 days after stopping treatment with an MAOI.
This product contains antihistamines which may cause drowsiness and may have additive central nervous system (CNS) effects with alcohol or other CNS depressants (e.g., hypnotics, sedatives, tranquilizers).

PRECAUTIONS

For RYNATUSS Pediatric Suspension only: This product contains FD&C Yellow No. 5 (tartrazine) which may cause allergic-type reactions (including bronchial asthma) in certain susceptible individuals. Although the overall incidence of FD&C Yellow No. 5 (tartrazine) sensitivity in the general population is low, it is frequently seen in patients who also have aspirin hypersensitivity.
General: Antihistamines are more likely to cause dizziness, sedation, and hypotension in elderly patients. Antihistamines may cause excitation, particularly in children, but their combination with sympathomimetics may cause either mild stimulation or mild sedation.
Information for patients: Caution patients against drinking alcoholic beverages or engaging in potentially hazardous activities requiring alertness, such as driving a car or operating machinery, while using this product. Patients should be warned not to use this product if they are now taking a prescription monoamine oxidase inhibitor (MAOI) (certain drugs for depression, psychiatric or emotional conditions, or Parkinson's disease), or for 2 weeks after stopping the MAOI drug. If patients are uncertain whether a prescription drug contains an MAOI, they should be instructed to consult a health professional before taking such a product.
Drug Interactions: MAO inhibitors may prolong and intensify the anticholinergic effects of antihistamines and the overall effects of sympathomimetic agents.
Carcinogenesis, mutagenesis, impairment of fertility: No long term animal studies have been performed with RYNATUSS.
Pregnancy: Teratogenic effects: Pregnancy Category C. Animal reproduction studies have not been conducted with RYNATUSS. It is also not known whether RYNATUSS can cause fetal harm when administered to a pregnant woman or can affect reproduction capacity. RYNATUSS should be given to a pregnant woman only if clearly needed.
Nursing mothers: RYNATUSS should not be administered to a nursing woman.

ADVERSE REACTIONS

Adverse effects associated with RYNATUSS at recommended doses have been minimal. The most common have been drowsiness, sedation, dryness of mucous membranes, and gastrointestinal effects. Serious side effects with oral antihistamines or sympathomimetics have been rare.

OVERDOSAGE

Signs and symptoms: May vary from CNS depression to stimulation (restlessness to convulsions). Antihistamine overdosage in young children may lead to convulsions and death. Atropine-like signs and symptoms may be prominent.
Treatment: Induce vomiting if it has not occurred spontaneously. Precautions must be taken against aspiration especially in infants, children, and comatose patients. If gastric lavage is indicated, isotonic or half-isotonic saline solution is preferred. Stimulants should not be used. If hypotension is a problem, vasopressor agents may be considered.

DOSAGE AND ADMINISTRATION

Administer the recommended dose every 12 hours.
RYNATUSS Tablets: Adults – 1 to 2 tablets.
RYNATUSS Pediatric Suspension: *Children over six years of age*– 5 to 10 mL (1 to 2 teaspoonfuls); *Children two to six years of age*– 2.5 to 5 mL (1/2 to 1 teaspoonful); *Children under two years of age*– Titrate dose individually.

HOW SUPPLIED

RYNATUSS® Tablets are mauve, capsule-shaped, scored on one side and imprinted WALLACE 717 on the other side, containing in each tablet: carbetapentane tannate 60 mg, chlorpheniramine tannate 5 mg, ephedrine tannate 10 mg, phenylephrine tannate 10 mg, available in bottles of 100 (NDC 0037-0717-92), 500 (NDC 0037-0717-96), and 2000 (NDC 0037-0717-95).
RYNATUSS® Pediatric Suspension is pink with strawberry-currant flavor, containing in each 5 mL (one teaspoonful): carbetapentane tannate 30 mg, chlorpheniramine tannate 4 mg, ephedrine tannate 5 mg, phenylephrine tannate 5 mg, available in bottles of 8 fl oz (NDC 0037-0718-67) and one pint (NDC 0037-0718-68).
Storage: RYNATUSS Tablets and RYNATUSS Pediatric Suspension: Store at controlled room temperature 15°–30°C (59°–86°F).
Dispense in a tight container.
WALLACE LABORATORIES
Division of CARTER-WALLACE, INC.
Cranbury, New Jersey 08512
IN-0717-05 Rev: 1/95

Shown in Product Identification Guide, page 339

Continued on next page

SOMA®
(carisoprodol)
Tablets, USP ℞

DESCRIPTION

'SOMA' (carisoprodol) Tablets, USP is available as 350 mg round, white tablets. Chemically, carisoprodol is N-isopropyl-2-methyl-2-propyl-1,3-propanediol dicarbamate. Carisoprodol is a white, crystalline powder, having a mild, characteristic odor and a bitter taste. It is very slightly soluble in water; freely soluble in alcohol, in chloroform, and in acetone; its solubility is practically independent of pH. Carisoprodol is present as a racemic mixture. The molecular formula is $C_{12}H_{24}N_2O_4$, with a molecular weight of 260.33. The structural formula is:

$$H_2NCOOCH_2C(CH_2CH_2CH_3)(CH_3)CH_2OOCNHCH(CH_3)_2$$

Other ingredients: alginic acid, magnesium stearate, potassium sorbate, starch, tribasic calcium phosphate.

ACTIONS

Carisoprodol produces muscle relaxation in animals by blocking interneuronal activity in the descending reticular formation and spinal cord. The onset of action is rapid and effects last four to six hours.

INDICATIONS

Carisoprodol is indicated as an adjunct to rest, physical therapy, and other measures for the relief of discomfort associated with acute, painful musculoskeletal conditions. The mode of action of this drug has not been clearly identified, but may be related to its sedative properties. Carisoprodol does not directly relax tense skeletal muscles in man.

CONTRAINDICATIONS

Acute intermittent porphyria as well as allergic or idiosyncratic reactions to carisoprodol or related compounds.

WARNINGS

Idiosyncratic Reactions—On very rare occasions, the first dose of carisoprodol has been followed by idiosyncratic symptoms appearing within minutes or hours. Symptoms reported include: extreme weakness, transient quadriplegia, dizziness, ataxia, temporary loss of vision, diplopia, mydriasis, dysarthria, agitation, euphoria, confusion, and disorientation. Symptoms usually subside over the course of the next several hours. Supportive and symptomatic therapy, including hospitalization, may be necessary.

Usage in Pregnancy and Lactation—Safe usage of this drug in pregnancy or lactation has not been established. Therefore, use of this drug in pregnancy, in nursing mothers, or in women of childbearing potential requires that the potential benefits of the drug be weighed against the potential hazards to mother and child. Carisoprodol is present in breast milk of lactating mothers at concentrations two to four times that of maternal plasma. This factor should be taken into account when use of the drug is contemplated in breast-feeding patients.

Usage in Children—Because of limited clinical experience, 'SOMA' is not recommended for use in patients under 12 years of age.

Potentially Hazardous Tasks—Patients should be warned that this drug may impair the mental and/or physical abilities required for the performance of potentially hazardous tasks such as driving a motor vehicle or operating machinery.

Additive Effects—Since the effects of carisoprodol and alcohol or carisoprodol and other CNS depressants or psychotropic drugs may be additive, appropriate caution should be exercised with patients who take more than one of these agents simultaneously.

Drug Dependence—In dogs, no withdrawal symptoms occurred after abrupt cessation of carisoprodol from dosages as high as 1 gm/kg/day. In a study in man, abrupt cessation of 100 mg/kg/day (about five times the recommended daily adult dosage) was followed in some subjects by mild withdrawal symptoms such as abdominal cramps, insomnia, chilliness, headache, and nausea. Delirium and convulsions did not occur. In clinical use, psychological dependence and abuse have been rare, and there have been no reports of significant abstinence signs. Nevertheless, the drug should be used with caution in addiction-prone individuals.

PRECAUTIONS

Carisoprodol is metabolized in the liver and excreted by the kidney; to avoid its excess accumulation, caution should be exercised in administration to patients with compromised liver or kidney function.

ADVERSE REACTIONS

Central Nervous System —Drowsiness and other CNS effects may require dosage reduction. Also observed: dizziness, vertigo, ataxia, tremor, agitation, irritability, headache, depressive reactions, syncope, and insomnia. (See also Idiosyncratic Reactions under "Warnings.")

Allergic or Idiosyncratic —Allergic or idiosyncratic reactions occasionally develop. They are usually seen within the period of the first to fourth dose in patients having had no previous contact with the drug. Skin rash, erythema multiforme, pruritus, eosinophilia, and fixed drug eruption with cross reaction to meprobamate have been reported with carisoprodol. Severe reactions have been manifested by asthmatic episodes, fever, weakness, dizziness, angioneurotic edema, smarting eyes, hypotension, and anaphylactoid shock. (See also Idiosyncratic Reactions under "Warnings.") In case of allergic or idiosyncratic reactions to carisoprodol, discontinue the drug and initiate appropriate symptomatic therapy, which may include epinephrine, antihistamines, and in severe cases corticosteroids. In evaluating possible allergic reactions, also consider allergy to excipients (information on excipients is available to physicians on request).

Cardiovascular —Tachycardia, postural hypotension, and facial flushing.

Gastrointestinal —Nausea, vomiting, hiccup, and epigastric distress.

Hematologic —Leukopenia, in which other drugs or viral infection may have been responsible, and pancytopenia, attributed to phenylbutazone, have been reported. No serious blood dyscrasias have been attributed to carisoprodol.

DOSAGE AND ADMINISTRATION

The usual adult dosage of 'SOMA' (carisoprodol) Tablets, USP is one 350 mg tablet, three times daily and at bedtime. Usage in patients under age 12 is not recommended.

OVERDOSAGE

Overdosage of carisoprodol has produced stupor, coma, shock, respiratory depression, and, very rarely, death. The effects of an overdosage of carisoprodol and alcohol or other CNS depressants or psychotropic agents can be additive even when one of the drugs has been taken in the usual recommended dosage. Any drug remaining in the stomach should be removed and symptomatic therapy given. Should respiration or blood pressure become compromised, respiratory assistance, central nervous system stimulants, and pressor agents should be administered cautiously as indicated. Carisoprodol is metabolized in the liver and excreted by the kidney. Although carisoprodol overdosage experience is limited, the following types of treatment have been used successfully with the related drug meprobamate: diuresis, osmotic (mannitol) diuresis, peritoneal dialysis, and hemodialysis (carisoprodol is dialyzable). Careful monitoring of urinary output is necessary and caution should be taken to avoid overhydration. Observe for possible relapse due to incomplete gastric emptying and delayed absorption. Carisoprodol can be measured in biological fluids by gas chromatography (Douglas, J. F. et al.: *J Pharm Sci 58:* 145, 1969).

HOW SUPPLIED

'SOMA' (carisoprodol) Tablets, USP 350 mg: Round, convex, white tablets, inscribed with 'SOMA' on one side and 37-WALLACE 2001 on the other side, are available in bottles of 100 (NDC 0037-2001-01) and 500 (NDC 0037-2001-03), and unit-dose packages of 100 (NDC 0037-2001-85).

Storage: Store at controlled room temperature 15°–30°C (59°–86°F).

Dispense in a tight container.

WALLACE LABORATORIES
Division of CARTER-WALLACE, INC.
Cranbury, New Jersey 08512
IN-090H2-10 Rev. 9/94

Shown in Product Identification Guide, page 339

SOMA® COMPOUND ℞
(carisoprodol and aspirin tablets, USP)
carisoprodol 200 mg + aspirin 325 mg
TABLETS

DESCRIPTION

SOMA Compound is a combination product containing carisoprodol, a centrally-acting muscle relaxant, plus aspirin, an analgesic with antipyretic and anti-inflammatory properties. It is available as a two-layered, white and orange, round tablet for oral administration. Each tablet contains carisoprodol, USP 200 mg and aspirin 325 mg. Chemically, carisoprodol is N-isopropyl-2-methyl-2-propyl-1,3-propanediol dicarbamate. Its empirical formula is $C_{12}H_{24}N_2O_4$, with a molecular weight of 260.33. The structural formula is:

$$H_2NCOOCH_2C(CH_2CH_2CH_3)(CH_3)CH_2OOCNHCH(CH_3)_2$$

Other ingredients: croscarmellose sodium, FD&C Red #40, FD&C Yellow #6, hydroxypropyl methylcellulose, magnesium stearate, microcrystalline cellulose, povidone, starch, stearic acid.

CLINICAL PHARMACOLOGY

Carisoprodol: Carisoprodol is a centrally-acting muscle relaxant that does not directly relax tense skeletal muscles in man. The mode of action of carisoprodol in relieving acute muscle spasm of local origin has not been clearly identified, but may be related to its sedative properties. In animals, carisoprodol has been shown to produce muscle relaxation by blocking interneuronal activity and depressing transmission of polysynaptic neurons in the spinal cord and in the descending reticular formation of the brain. The onset of action is rapid and lasts four to six hours.

Carisoprodol is metabolized in the liver and is excreted by the kidneys. It is dialyzable by peritoneal and hemodialysis.

Aspirin: Aspirin is a nonnarcotic analgesic with anti-inflammatory and antipyretic activity. Inhibition of prostaglandin biosynthesis appears to account for most of its anti-inflammatory and for at least part of its analgesic and antipyretic properties.

Aspirin is rapidly absorbed and almost totally hydrolyzed to salicylic acid following oral administration. Although aspirin has a half-life of only about 15 minutes, the apparent biologic half-life of salicylic acid in the therapeutic plasma concentration range is between 6 and 12 hours. Salicylic acid is eliminated by renal excretion and by biotransformation to inactive metabolites. Clearance of salicylic acid in the high-dose range is sensitive to urinary pH (see *Drug Interactions*) and is reduced by renal dysfunction.

INDICATIONS AND USAGE

SOMA Compound is indicated as an adjunct to rest, physical therapy, and other measures for the relief of pain, muscle spasm, and limited mobility associated with acute, painful musculoskeletal conditions.

CONTRAINDICATIONS

Acute intermittent porphyria; bleeding disorders; allergic or idiosyncratic reactions to carisoprodol, aspirin or related compounds.

WARNINGS

On very rare occasions, the first dose of carisoprodol has been followed by an idiosyncratic reaction with symptoms appearing within minutes or hours. These may include extreme weakness, transient quadriplegia, dizziness, ataxia, temporary loss of vision, diplopia, mydriasis, dysarthria, agitation, euphoria, confusion, and disorientation. Although symptoms usually subside over the course of the next several hours, discontinue SOMA Compound and initiate appropriate supportive and symptomatic therapy, which may include epinephrine and/or antihistamines. In severe cases, corticosteroids may be necessary. Severe reactions have been manifested by asthmatic episodes, fever, weakness, dizziness, angioneurotic edema, smarting eyes, hypotension, and anaphylactoid shock.

The effects of carisoprodol with agents such as alcohol, other CNS depressants, or psychotropic drugs may be additive. Appropriate caution should be exercised with patients who may take one or more of these agents simultaneously with SOMA Compound.

PRECAUTIONS

General: To avoid excessive accumulation of carisoprodol, aspirin, or their metabolites, use SOMA Compound with caution in patients with compromised liver or kidney function, or in elderly or debilitated patients (see CLINICAL PHARMACOLOGY).

Use with caution in patients with history of gastritis or peptic ulcer, in patients on anticoagulant therapy, and in addiction-prone individuals.

Information for Patients: Caution patients that this drug may impair the mental and/or physical abilities required for the performance of potentially hazardous tasks such as driving a motor vehicle or operating machinery.

Caution patients with a predisposition for gastrointestinal bleeding that concomitant use of aspirin and alcohol may have an additive effect in this regard.

Caution patients that dosage of medications used for gout, arthritis, or diabetes may have to be adjusted when aspirin is administered or discontinued (see *Drug Interactions*).

Drug Interactions: Clinically important interactions may occur when certain drugs are administered concomitantly with aspirin or aspirin-containing drugs.

1. *Oral Anticoagulants*—By interfering with platelet function or decreasing plasma prothrombin concentration, aspirin enhances the potential for bleeding in patients on anticoagulants.
2. *Methotrexate*—aspirin enhances the toxic effects of this drug.
3. *Probenecid and Sulfinpyrazone*—large doses of aspirin reduce the uricosuric effect of both drugs. Renal excretion of salicylate may also be reduced.
4. *Oral Antidiabetic Drugs*—enhancement of hypoglycemia may occur.
5. *Antacids*—to the extent that they raise urinary pH, antacids may substantially decrease plasma salicylate concentrations; conversely, their withdrawal can result in a substantial increase.
6. *Ammonium Chloride*—this and other drugs that acidify a relatively alkaline urine can elevate plasma salicylate concentrations.
7. *Ethyl Alcohol*—enhanced aspirin-induced fecal blood loss has been reported.
8. *Corticosteroids*—salicylate plasma levels may be decreased when adrenal corticosteroids are given, and may be increased substantially when they are discontinued.

Carcinogenesis, Mutagenesis, Impairment of Fertility: No long-term studies have been done with SOMA Compound.

***Pregnancy—Teratogenic Effects:* Pregnancy Category C.** Adequate animal reproduction studies have not been conducted with SOMA Compound. It is also not known whether SOMA Compound can cause fetal harm when administered to a pregnant woman or can affect reproduction capacity. SOMA Compound should be given to a pregnant woman only if clearly needed.

Studies in rodents have shown salicylates to be teratogenic when given in early gestation, and embryocidal when given in later gestation in doses considerably greater than usual therapeutic doses in humans. Studies in women who took aspirin during pregnancy have not demonstrated an increased incidence of congenital abnormalities in the offspring.

Labor and Delivery: Ingestion of aspirin near term or prior to delivery may prolong delivery or lead to bleeding in mother, fetus, or neonate.

Nursing Mothers: Carisoprodol is excreted in human milk in concentrations two-to-four times that in maternal plasma. Aspirin is excreted in human milk in moderate amounts and can produce a bleeding tendency in nursing infants. Because of the potential for serious adverse reactions in nursing infants, a decision should be made whether to discontinue nursing or the drug, taking into account the importance of the drug to the mother.

Pediatric Use: Safety and effectiveness in children below the age of twelve have not been established.

ADVERSE REACTIONS

If severe reactions occur, discontinue SOMA Compound and initiate appropriate symptomatic and supportive therapy. The following side effects which have occurred with the administration of the individual ingredients alone may also occur with the combination.

Carisoprodol: Central Nervous System—Drowsiness is the most frequent complaint and along with other CNS effects may require dosage reduction. Observed less frequently are dizziness, vertigo and ataxia. Tremor, agitation, irritability, headache, depressive reactions, syncope, and insomnia have been infrequent or rare.

Idiosyncratic—Idiosyncratic reactions are very rare. They are usually seen within the period of the first to fourth dose in patients having had no previous contact with the drug (see WARNINGS).

Allergic—Skin rash, erythema multiforme, pruritus, eosinophilia, and fixed drug eruptions with cross-reaction to meprobamate have been reported. If allergic reactions occur, discontinue SOMA Compound and treat symptomatically. In evaluating possible allergic reactions, also consider allergy to excipients (information on excipients is available to physicians on request).

Cardiovascular—Tachycardia, postural hypotension, and facial flushing.

Gastrointestinal—Nausea, vomiting, epigastric distress, and hiccup.

Hematologic—No serious blood dyscrasias have been attributed to carisoprodol alone. Leukopenia and pancytopenia have been reported, very rarely, in situations in which other drugs or viral infections may have been responsible.

Aspirin: The most common adverse reactions associated with the use of aspirin have been gastrointestinal, including nausea, vomiting, gastritis, occult bleeding, constipation, and diarrhea. Gastric erosion, angioedema, asthma, rash, pruritus and urticaria have been reported less commonly. Tinnitus is a sign of high serum salicylate levels (see OVERDOSAGE).

Aspirin Intolerance—Allergic type reactions in aspirin-sensitive individuals may involve the respiratory tract or the skin. Symptoms of the former range from rhinorrhea and shortness of breath to severe asthma, and the latter may consist of urticaria, edema, rash, or angioedema (giant hives). These may occur independently or in combination.

DRUG ABUSE AND DEPENDENCE

Abuse: In clinical use, abuse has been rare.

Dependence: In clinical use, dependence with SOMA Compound has been rare, and there have been no reports of significant abstinence signs. Nevertheless, the following information on the individual ingredients should be kept in mind.

Carisoprodol—In dogs, no withdrawal symptoms occurred after abrupt cessation of carisoprodol from dosages as high as 1 gm/kg/day. In a study in man, abrupt cessation of 100 mg/kg/day (about five times the recommended daily adult dosage) was followed in some subjects by mild withdrawal symptoms such as abdominal cramps, insomnia, chills, headache, and nausea. Delirium and convulsions did not occur (see PRECAUTIONS).

OVERDOSAGE

Signs and Symptoms: Any of the following which have been reported with the individual ingredients may occur and may be modified to a varying degree by the effects of the other ingredients present in SOMA Compound.

Carisoprodol—Stupor, coma, shock, respiratory depression, and, very rarely, death. Overdosage with carisoprodol in combination with alcohol, other CNS depressants, or psychotropic agents can have additive effects, even when one of the agents has been taken in the usually recommended dosage.

Aspirin—Headache, tinnitus, hearing difficulty, dim vision, dizziness, lassitude, hyperpnea, rapid breathing, thirst, nausea, vomiting, sweating and occasionally diarrhea are characteristic of mild to moderate salicylate poisoning. Salicylate poisoning should be considered in children with symptoms of vomiting, hyperpnea, and hyperthermia.

Hyperpnea is an early sign of salicylate poisoning, but dyspnea supervenes at plasma levels above 50 mg/dL. These respiratory changes eventually lead to serious acid-base disturbances. Metabolic acidosis is a constant finding in infants but occurs in older children only with severe poisoning; adults usually exhibit respiratory alkalosis initially and acidosis terminally.

Other symptoms of severe salicylate poisoning include hyperthermia, dehydration, delirium, and mental disturbances. Skin eruptions, GI hemorrhage, or pulmonary edema are less common. Early CNS stimulation is replaced by increasing depression, stupor, and coma. Death is usually due to respiratory failure or cardiovascular collapse.

Treatment: *General:* Provide symptomatic and supportive treatment, as indicated. Any drug remaining in the stomach should be removed using appropriate procedures and caution to protect the airway and prevent aspiration, especially in the stuporous or comatose patient. Incomplete gastric emptying with delayed absorption of carisoprodol has been reported as a cause for relapse. Should respiration or blood pressure become compromised, respiratory assistance, central nervous system stimulants, and pressor agents should be administered cautiously, as indicated.

Carisoprodol: The following have been used successfully in overdosage with the related drug meprobamate: diuretics, osmotic (mannitol) diuresis, peritoneal dialysis, and hemodialysis (see CLINICAL PHARMACOLOGY). Careful monitoring of urinary output is necessary and caution should be taken to avoid overhydration. Carisoprodol can be measured in biological fluid by gas chromatography (Douglas, J. F., et al: *J Pharm Sci 58:* 145, 1969).

Aspirin—Since there are no specific antidotes for salicylate poisoning, the aim of treatment is to enhance elimination of salicylate and prevent or reduce further absorption; to correct any fluid, electrolyte or metabolic imbalance; and to provide general and cardiorespiratory support. If acidosis is present, intravenous sodium bicarbonate must be given, along with adequate hydration, until salicylate levels decrease to within the therapeutic range. To enhance elimination, forced diuresis and alkalinization of the urine may be beneficial. The need for hemoperfusion or hemodialysis is rare and should be used only when other measures have failed.

DOSAGE AND ADMINISTRATION

Usual Adult Dosage: 1 or 2 tablets, four times daily.

Not recommended for use in children under age twelve (see PRECAUTIONS).

HOW SUPPLIED

SOMA Compound Tablets (carisoprodol, USP 200 mg and aspirin 325 mg) are round, convex, two-layered and inscribed on the white layer with SOMA C and on the light orange layer with WALLACE 2103. The tablets are available in bottles of 100 (NDC 0037-2103-01) and 500 (NDC 0037-2103-03) and unit-dose packages of 100 (NDC 0037-2103-85).

Storage: Store at controlled room temperature 15°–30°C (59°–86°F). Protect from moisture.

Dispense in a tight container.

WALLACE LABORATORIES
Division of CARTER-WALLACE, INC.
Cranbury, New Jersey 08512
IN-094E2-12 Rev. 9/93
Patent No. 4534973

Shown in Product Identification Guide, page 339

SOMA® COMPOUND with CODEINE ㊂ ℞

(carisoprodol, aspirin and codeine phosphate tablets, USP)

carisoprodol 200 mg + aspirin 325 mg + codeine phosphate 16 mg—Warning: May be habit-forming TABLETS

DESCRIPTION

'Soma' Compound with Codeine is a combination product containing carisoprodol, a centrally-acting muscle relaxant, plus aspirin, an analgesic with antipyretic and anti-inflammatory properties and codeine phosphate, a centrally-acting narcotic analgesic. It is available as a two-layered, white and yellow, oval-shaped tablet for oral administration. Each tablet contains carisoprodol 200 mg, aspirin 325 mg, and codeine phosphate 16 mg. Chemically, carisoprodol is N-isopropyl-2-methyl-2-propyl-1,3-propanediol dicarbamate. Its empirical formula is $C_{12}H_{24}N_2O_4$, with a molecular weight of 260.33. The structural formula is:

$$\begin{array}{c} CH_2CH_2CH_3 \\ | \\ H_2NCOOCH_2CCH_2OOCNHCH(CH_3)_2 \\ | \\ CH_3 \end{array}$$

Other ingredients: croscarmellose sodium, D&C Yellow #10, hydroxypropyl methylcellulose, magnesium stearate, microcrystalline cellulose, povidone, sodium metabisulfite, starch, stearic acid.

CLINICAL PHARMACOLOGY

Carisoprodol: Carisoprodol is a centrally-acting muscle relaxant that does not directly relax tense skeletal muscles in man. The mode of action of carisoprodol in relieving acute muscle spasm of local origin has not been clearly identified, but may be related to its sedative properties. In animals, carisoprodol has been shown to produce muscle relaxation by blocking interneuronal activity and depressing transmission of polysynaptic neurons in the spinal cord and in the descending reticular formation of the brain. The onset of action is rapid and lasts four to six hours.

Carisoprodol is metabolized in the liver and is excreted by the kidneys. It is dialyzable by peritoneal and hemodialysis.

Aspirin: Aspirin is a non-narcotic analgesic with anti-inflammatory and antipyretic activity. Inhibition of prostaglandin biosynthesis appears to account for most of its anti-inflammatory and for at least part of its analgesic and antipyretic properties.

Aspirin is rapidly absorbed and almost totally hydrolyzed to salicylic acid following oral administration. Although aspirin has a half-life of only about 15 minutes, the apparent biologic half-life of salicylic acid in the therapeutic plasma concentration range is between 6 and 12 hours. Salicylic acid is eliminated by renal excretion and by biotransformation to inactive metabolites. Clearance of salicylic acid in the high-dose range is sensitive to urinary pH (see *Drug Interactions*) and is reduced by renal dysfunction.

Codeine Phosphate: Codeine phosphate is a centrally-acting narcotic-analgesic. Its actions are qualitatively similar to morphine, but its potency is substantially less.

Clinical studies have shown that combining aspirin and codeine produces a significant additive effect in analgesic efficacy.

INDICATIONS AND USAGE

'Soma' Compound with Codeine is indicated as an adjunct to rest, physical therapy, and other measures for the relief of pain, muscle spasm, and limited mobility associated with acute, painful musculoskeletal conditions when the additional action of codeine is desired.

CONTRAINDICATIONS

Acute intermittent porphyria; bleeding disorders; allergic or idiosyncratic reactions to carisoprodol, aspirin, codeine, or related compounds.

WARNINGS

On very rare occasions, the first dose of carisoprodol has been followed by idiosyncratic reactions, with symptoms appearing within minutes or hours. These may include extreme weakness, transient quadriplegia, dizziness, ataxia, temporary loss of vision, diplopia, mydriasis, dysarthria, agitation, euphoria, confusion, and disorientation. Although symptoms usually subside over the course of the next several hours, discontinue 'Soma' Compound with Codeine and initiate appropriate supportive and symptomatic therapy, which may include epinephrine and/or antihistamines. In severe cases, corticosteroids may be necessary. Severe reactions have been manifested by asthmatic episodes, fever, weakness, dizziness, angioneurotic edema, smarting eyes, hypotension, and anaphylactoid shock.

The effects of carisoprodol with agents such as alcohol, other CNS depressants, or psychotropic drugs may be additive. Appropriate caution should be exercised with patients who take one or more of these agents simultaneously with Soma Compound with Codeine.

Contains sodium metabisulfite, a sulfite that may cause allergic-type reactions including anaphylactic symptoms and life-threatening or less severe asthmatic episodes in certain susceptible people. The overall prevalence of sulfite sensitivity in the general population is unknown and probably low. Sulfite sensitivity is seen more frequently in asthmatic than in nonasthmatic people.

PRECAUTIONS

General: To avoid excessive accumulation of carisoprodol, aspirin, or their metabolites, use 'Soma' Compound with Codeine with caution in patients with compromised liver or kidney function, or in elderly or debilitated patients (see CLINICAL PHARMACOLOGY).

Use with caution in patients with history of gastritis or peptic ulcer, in patients on anticoagulant therapy, and in addiction-prone individuals.

Information for Patients: Caution patients that this drug may impair the mental and/or physical abilities required for the performance of potentially hazardous tasks such as driving a motor vehicle or operating machinery.

Caution patients with a predisposition for gastrointestinal bleeding that concomitant use of aspirin and alcohol may have an additive effect in this regard.

Caution patients that dosage of medications used for gout, arthritis, or diabetes may have to be adjusted when aspirin is administered or discontinued (see ***Drug Interactions***).

Drug Interactions: Clinically important interactions may occur when certain drugs are administered concomitantly with aspirin or aspirin-containing drugs.

1. *Oral Anticoagulants* —By interfering with platelet function or decreasing plasma prothrombin concentration, aspirin enhances the potential for bleeding in patients on anticoagulants.
2. *Methotrexate* —aspirin enhances the toxic effects of this drug.
3. *Probenecid and Sulfinpyrazone* —large doses of aspirin reduce the uricosuric effect of both drugs. Renal excretion of salicylate may also be reduced.
4. *Oral Antidiabetic Drugs* —enhancement of hypoglycemia may occur.
5. *Antacids* —to the extent that they raise urinary pH, antacids may substantially decrease plasma salicylate con-

Continued on next page

Soma Compound w/Codeine—Cont.

centrations; conversely, their withdrawal can result in a substantial increase.

6. *Ammonium Chloride* —this and other drugs that acidify a relatively alkaline urine can elevate plasma salicylate concentrations.
7. *Ethyl Alcohol* —enhanced aspirin-induced fecal blood loss has been reported.
8. *Corticosteroids* —salicylate plasma levels may be decreased when adrenal corticosteroids are given, and may be increased substantially when they are discontinued.

Carcinogenesis, Mutagenesis, Impairment of Fertility: No long-term studies have been done with 'Soma' Compound with Codeine.

Pregnancy—Teratogenic Effects: **Pregnancy Category C.** Adequate animal reproduction studies have not been conducted with 'Soma' Compound with Codeine. It is also not known whether 'Soma' Compound with Codeine can cause fetal harm when administered to a pregnant woman or can affect reproduction capacity. 'Soma' Compound with Codeine should be given to a pregnant woman only if clearly needed. Studies in rodents have shown salicylates to be teratogenic when given in early gestation, and embryocidal when given in later gestation in doses considerably greater than usual therapeutic doses in humans. Studies in women who took aspirin during pregnancy have not demonstrated an increased incidence of congenital abnormalities in the offspring.

Labor and Delivery: Ingestion of aspirin near term or prior to delivery may prolong delivery or lead to bleeding in mother, fetus, or neonate.

Nursing Mothers: Carisoprodol is excreted in human milk in concentrations two-to-four times that in maternal plasma. Aspirin is excreted in human milk in moderate amounts and can produce a bleeding tendency in nursing infants. Because of the potential for serious adverse reactions in nursing infants, a decision should be made whether to discontinue nursing or the drug, taking into account the importance of the drug to the mother.

Pediatric Use: Safety and effectiveness in children below the age of twelve have not been established.

ADVERSE REACTIONS

If severe reactions occur, discontinue 'Soma' Compound with Codeine and initiate appropriate symptomatic and supportive therapy.

The following side effects which have occurred with the administration of the individual ingredients alone may also occur with the combination.

Carisoprodol: *Central Nervous System*—Drowsiness is the most frequent complaint and along with other CNS effects may require dosage reduction. Observed less frequently are dizziness, vertigo and ataxia. Tremor, agitation, irritability, headache, depressive reactions, syncope, and insomnia have been infrequent or rare.

Idiosyncratic—Idiosyncratic reactions are very rare. They are usually seen within the period of the first to fourth dose in patients having had no previous contact with the drug (see WARNINGS).

Allergic—Skin rash, erythema multiforme, pruritus, eosinophilia, and fixed drug eruptions with cross-reaction to meprobamate have been reported. If allergic reactions occur, discontinue 'Soma' Compound with Codeine and treat symptomatically. In evaluating possible allergic reactions, also consider allergy to excipients (information on excipients is available to physicians on request).

Cardiovascular—Tachycardia, postural hypotension, and facial flushing.

Gastrointestinal—Nausea, vomiting, epigastric distress and hiccup.

Hematologic—No serious blood dyscrasias have been attributed to carisoprodol alone. Leukopenia and pancytopenia have been reported, very rarely, in situations in which other drugs or viral infections may have been responsible.

Aspirin: The most common adverse reactions associated with the use of aspirin have been gastrointestinal, including nausea, vomiting, gastritis, occult bleeding, constipation and diarrhea. Gastric erosion, angioedema, asthma, rash, pruritus and urticaria have been reported less commonly. Tinnitus is a sign of high serum salicylate levels (see OVERDOSAGE).

Aspirin Intolerance—Allergic type reactions in aspirin-sensitive individuals may involve the respiratory tract or the skin. Symptoms of the former range from rhinorrhea and shortness of breath to severe asthma, and the latter may consist of urticaria, edema, rash, or angioedema (giant hives). These may occur independently or in combination.

Codeine Phosphate: Nausea, vomiting, constipation, miosis, sedation, and dizziness have been reported.

DRUG ABUSE AND DEPENDENCE

Controlled Substance: Schedule C-III (see PRECAUTIONS).

Abuse: In clinical use, abuse has been rare.

Dependence: In clinical use, dependence with 'Soma' Compound with Codeine has been rare and there have been no reports of significant abstinence signs. Nevertheless, the following information on the individual ingredients should be kept in mind.

Carisoprodol—In dogs, no withdrawal symptoms occurred after abrupt cessation of carisoprodol from dosages as high as 1 gm/kg/day. In a study in man, abrupt cessation of 100 mg/kg/day (about five times the recommended daily adult dosage) was followed in some subjects by mild withdrawal symptoms such as abdominal cramps, insomnia, chills, headache, and nausea. Delirium and convulsions did not occur (see PRECAUTIONS).

Codeine Phosphate—Drug dependence of the morphine type may result.

OVERDOSAGE

Signs and Symptoms: Any of the following which have been reported with the individual ingredients may occur and may be modified to a varying degree by the effects of the other ingredients present in 'Soma' Compound with Codeine.

Carisoprodol—Stupor, coma, shock, respiratory depression and, very rarely, death. Overdosage with carisoprodol in combination with alcohol, other CNS depressants, or psychotropic agents can have additive effects, even when one of the agents has been taken in the usually recommended dosage.

Aspirin—Headache, tinnitus, hearing difficulty, dim vision, dizziness, lassitude, hyperpnea, rapid breathing, thirst, nausea, vomiting, sweating and occasionally diarrhea are characteristic of mild to moderate salicylate poisoning. Salicylate poisoning should be considered in children with symptoms of vomiting, hyperpnea, and hyperthermia.

Hyperpnea is an early sign of salicylate poisoning, but dyspnea supervenes at plasma levels above 50 mg/dl. These respiratory changes eventually lead to serious acid-base disturbances. Metabolic acidosis is a constant finding in infants but occurs in older children only with severe poisoning; adults usually exhibit respiratory alkalosis initially and acidosis terminally.

Other symptoms of severe salicylate poisoning include hyperthermia, dehydration, delirium, and mental disturbances. Skin eruptions, GI hemorrhage, or pulmonary edema are less common. Early CNS stimulation is replaced by increasing depression, stupor, and coma. Death is usually due to respiratory failure or cardiovascular collapse.

Codeine Phosphate—pinpoint pupils, CNS depression, coma, respiratory depression, and shock.

Treatment: *General*—Provide symptomatic and supportive treatment, as indicated. Any drug remaining in the stomach should be removed using appropriate procedures and caution to protect the airway and prevent aspiration, especially in the stuporous or comatose patient. Incomplete gastric emptying with delayed absorption of carisoprodol has been reported as a cause for relapse. Should respiration or blood pressure become compromised, respiratory assistance, central nervous system stimulants, and pressor agents should be administered cautiously, as indicated.

Carisoprodol—The following have been used successfully in overdosage with the related drug meprobamate: diuretics, osmotic (mannitol) diuresis, peritoneal dialysis, and hemodialysis (see CLINICAL PHARMACOLOGY). Careful monitoring of urinary output is necessary and caution should be taken to avoid overhydration. Carisoprodol can be measured in biological fluid by gas chromatography (Douglas, J. F., et al: *J Pharm Sci 58:* 145, 1969).

Aspirin—Since there are no specific antidotes for salicylate poisoning, the aim of treatment is to enhance elimination of salicylate and prevent or reduce further absorption; to correct any fluid, electrolyte or metabolic imbalance; and to provide general and cardiorespiratory support. If acidosis is present, intravenous sodium bicarbonate must be given, along with adequate hydration, until salicylate levels decrease to within the therapeutic range. To enhance elimination, forced diuresis and alkalinization of the urine may be beneficial. The need for hemoperfusion or hemodialysis is rare and should be used only when other measures have failed.

Codeine Phosphate—Narcotic antagonists, such as nalorphine and levallorphan, may be indicated.

DOSAGE AND ADMINISTRATION

Usual Adult Dosage: 1 or 2 tablets, four times daily. Not recommended for use in children under age twelve.

HOW SUPPLIED

'Soma' Compound with Codeine Tablets (carisoprodol, USP 200 mg, aspirin 325 mg, and codeine phosphate, USP 16 mg) are oval, convex, two-layered and inscribed on the white layer with SOMA CC and on the yellow layer with WALLACE 2403. The tablets are available in bottles of 100 (NDC 0037-2403-01).

Storage: Store at controlled room temperature 15°–30°C (59°–86°F). Protect from moisture.

Dispense in a tight container.

WALLACE LABORATORIES
Division of CARTER-WALLACE, INC.
Cranbury, New Jersey 08512
IN-095E2–12

Rev. 9/93
Patent No. 4534974

Shown in Product Identification Guide, page 339

TUSSI-12®
Tablets
Suspension

℞

DESCRIPTION

TUSSI-12® is an antitussive/antihistamine/nasal decongestant combination available for oral administration as Tablets and as a Suspension.

Each tablet contains:

Carbetapentane Tannate	60 mg
Chlorpheniramine Tannate	5 mg
Phenylephrine Tannate	10 mg

Other ingredients: corn starch, dibasic calcium phosphate, FD&C Blue No. 1, FD&C Red No. 40, magnesium stearate, methylcellulose, polygalacturonic acid, povidone, talc.

Each 5 mL (one teaspoonful) of the suspension contains:

Carbetapentane Tannate	30 mg
Chlorpheniramine Tannate	4 mg
Phenylephrine Tannate	5 mg

Other ingredients: benzoic acid, FD&C Blue No. 1, FD&C Red No. 3, FD&C Red No. 40, FD&C Yellow No. 5 (see Precautions), flavors (natural and artificial), glycerin, kaolin, magnesium aluminum silicate, methylparaben, pectin, purified water, saccharin sodium, sucrose.

CLINICAL PHARMACOLOGY

TUSSI-12 Tablets and Suspension combine the antitussive action of carbetapentane, the sympathomimetic decongestant effect of phenylephrine, and the antihistaminic action of chlorpheniramine.

INDICATIONS AND USAGE

TUSSI-12 Tablets and Suspension are indicated for the symptomatic relief of cough associated with respiratory tract conditions such as the common cold, bronchial asthma, acute and chronic bronchitis. Appropriate therapy should be provided for the primary disease.

CONTRAINDICATIONS

TUSSI-12 Tablets and Suspension are contraindicated for newborns, nursing mothers, and patients who are sensitive to any of the ingredients or related compounds.

WARNINGS

Use with caution in patients with hypertension, cardiovascular disease, hyperthyroidism, diabetes, narrow angle glaucoma, or prostatic hypertrophy. Do not use in patients taking monoamine oxidase (MAO) inhibitors, or for 14 days after stopping treatment with an MAOI.

These products contain an antihistamine which may cause drowsiness and may have additive central nervous system (CNS) effects with alcohol or other CNS depressants (e.g., hypnotics, sedatives, tranquilizers).

PRECAUTIONS

TUSSI-12 Suspension contains FD&C Yellow No. 5 (tartrazine) which may cause allergic-type reactions (including bronchial asthma) in certain susceptible individuals. Although the overall incidence of FD&C Yellow No. 5 (tartrazine) sensitivity in the general population is low, it is frequently seen in patients who also have aspirin hypersensitivity.

General: Antihistamines are more likely to cause dizziness, sedation, and hypotension in elderly patients. Antihistamines may cause excitation, particularly in children, but their combination with sympathomimetics may cause either mild stimulation or mild sedation.

Information for patients: Caution patients against drinking alcoholic beverages or engaging in potentially hazardous activities requiring alertness, such as driving a car or operating machinery, while using these products. Patients should be warned not to use these products if they are now taking a prescription monoamine oxidase inhibitor (MAOI) (certain drugs for depression, psychiatric or emotional conditions, or Parkinson's disease), or for 2 weeks after stopping the MAOI drug. If patients are uncertain whether a prescription drug contains an MAOI, they should be instructed to consult a health professional before taking such a product.

Drug interactions: MAO inhibitors may prolong and intensify the anticholinergic effects of antihistamines and the overall effects of sympathomimetic agents.

Carcinogenesis, mutagenesis, impairment of fertility: No long term animal studies have been performed with TUSSI-12 Tablets or Suspension.

Pregnancy: Teratogenic effects: Pregnancy Category C. Animal reproduction studies have not been conducted with TUSSI-12 Tablets or Suspension. It is also not known whether TUSSI-12 Tablets or Suspension can cause fetal harm when administered to a pregnant woman or can affect reproduction capacity. TUSSI-12 Tablets or Suspension should be given to a pregnant woman only if clearly needed.

Nursing mothers: TUSSI-12 Tablets or Suspension should not be administered to a nursing woman.

ADVERSE REACTIONS

Adverse effects associated with TUSSI-12 Tablets or Suspension at recommended doses have been minimal. The most common have been drowsiness, sedation, dryness of mucous membranes, and gastrointestinal effects. Serious side effects with oral antihistamines or sympathomimetics have been rare.

OVERDOSAGE

Signs and symptoms: May vary from CNS depression to stimulation (restlessness to convulsions). Antihistamine overdosage in young children may lead to convulsions and death. Atropine-like signs and symptoms may be prominent.

Treatment: Induce vomiting if it has not occurred spontaneously. Precautions must be taken against aspiration especially in infants, children, and comatose patients. If gastric lavage is indicated, isotonic or half-isotonic saline solution is preferred. Stimulants should not be used. If hypotension is a problem, vasopressor agents may be considered.

DOSAGE AND ADMINISTRATION

Administer the recommended dose every 12 hours.
TUSSI-12® Tablets: Adults—1 to 2 tablets.
TUSSI-12 Suspension: *Over six years of age*—5 to 10 mL (1 to 2 teaspoonfuls); *Children two to six years of age*—2.5 to 5 mL (1/2 to 1 teaspoonful); *Children under two years of age*—Titrate dose individually.

HOW SUPPLIED

TUSSI-12® Tablets are mauve, capsule-shaped, scored on one side and imprinted WALLACE 0640 on the other side, containing in each tablet: carbetapentane tannate 60 mg, chlorpheniramine tannate 5 mg, phenylephrine tannate 10 mg, available in bottles of 100 (NDC 0037-0640-10).
TUSSI-12® Suspension is pink with strawberry-currant flavor, containing in each 5 mL (one teaspoonful): carbetapentane tannate 30 mg, chlorpheniramine tannate 4 mg, phenylephrine tannate 5 mg, available in pint bottles (NDC 0037-0642-16).
Storage: Store at controlled room temperature 20°–25°C (68°–77°F).
Dispense in a tight container.
PATENT PENDING

WALLACE LABORATORIES
Division of
CARTER-WALLACE, INC.
Cranbury, New Jersey 08512

IN-0642-04 Rev. 7/99
Shown in Product Identification Guide, page 339 & 340

VASCOR® ℞
brand of bepridil hydrochloride
Tablets

Marketed jointly by McNeil Pharmaceutical and Wallace Laboratories. See McNeil Pharmaceutical for product information.

VōSoL® HC ℞
OTIC SOLUTION
(hydrocortisone and acetic acid otic solution, USP)

DESCRIPTION

VōSoL HC (hydrocortisone and acetic acid otic solution, USP) is a solution containing hydrocortisone (1%) and acetic acid (2%), in a propylene glycol vehicle containing propylene glycol diacetate (3%), benzethonium chloride (0.02%), sodium acetate (0.015%) and citric acid (0.05%). The empirical formulas for acetic acid and hydrocortisone are CH_3COOH and $C_{21}H_{30}O_5$, with a molecular weight of 60.05 and 362.46, respectively. The structural formulas are:

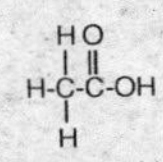

Acetic Acid

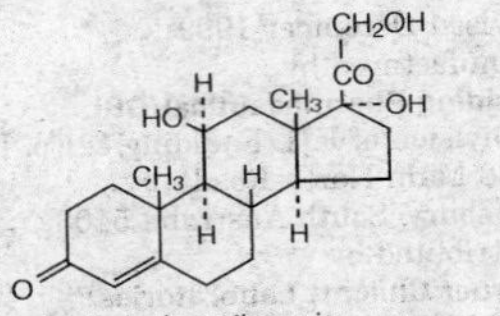

Chemically, hydrocortisone is: Pregn-4-ene-3,20-dione, 11, 17, 21-trihydroxy-, (11β)-.

VōSoL HC is available as a nonaqueous otic solution buffered at pH 3 for use in the external ear canal.

CLINICAL PHARMACOLOGY

Acetic acid is antibacterial and antifungal; hydrocortisone is antiinflammatory, antiallergic and antipruritic; propylene glycol is hydrophilic and provides a low surface tension; benzethonium chloride is a surface active agent that promotes contact of the solution with tissues.

INDICATIONS AND USAGE

For the treatment of superficial infections of the external auditory canal caused by organisms susceptible to the action of the antimicrobial, complicated by inflammation.

CONTRAINDICATIONS

Hypersensitivity to VōSoL HC or any of the ingredients; herpes simplex, vaccinia and varicella. Performated tympanic membrane is considered a contraindication to the use of any medication in the external ear canal.

WARNINGS

Discontinue promptly if sensitization or irritation occurs.

PRECAUTIONS

Transient stinging or burning may be noted occasionally when the solution is first instilled into the acutely inflamed ear.

PEDIATRIC USE

Safety and effectiveness in pediatric patients below the age of 3 years have not been established.

ADVERSE REACTIONS

Stinging or burning may be noted occasionally; local irritation has occurred very rarely.

DOSAGE AND ADMINISTRATION

Carefully remove all cerumen and debris to allow VōSoL HC to contact infected surfaces directly. To promote continuous contact, insert a wick of cotton saturated with VōSoL HC into the ear canal; the wick may also be saturated after insertion. Instruct the patient to keep the wick in for at least 24 hours and to keep it moist by adding 3 to 5 drops of VōSoL HC every 4 to 6 hours. The wick may be removed after 24 hours but the patient should continue to instill 5 drops of VōSoL HC 3 or 4 times daily thereafter, for as long as indicated. In pediatric patients, 3 to 4 drops may be sufficient due to the smaller capacity of the ear canal.

HOW SUPPLIED

VōSoL HC (Hydrocortisone and acetic acid otic solution, USP), containing hyrocortisone (1%) and acetic acid (2%), is available in 10 mL, measured-drop, safety-tip plastic bottles (NDC 0037-3811-12).

STORAGE

Store at room temperature, 20°–25°C (68°–77°F). Keep container tightly closed.

WALLACE LABORATORIES
Division of CARTER-WALLACE, INC.
Cranbury, New Jersey 08512
IN-056H9-05D Rev. 12/97

Warner Chilcott Laboratories

ROCKAWAY 80 CORPORATE CENTER
100 ENTERPRISE DRIVE
SUITE 280
ROCKAWAY, NJ 07866

Direct Inquiries to:
(800) 521-8813
Product/Medical Information:
(800) 521-8813
(973) 442-3236
Medical Emergency Contact:
After hours and weekends
(303) 739-1110

Following is the list of products

CHOLEDYL SA® ℞
[Ko ′-le-dil]
Oxtriphylline Extended-release Tablets, USP
400mg, 600mg

DORYX® ℞
[Dor ′-ix]
Coated Doxycycline Hyclate Pellet filled Capsules
100mg

ERYC® ℞
[Er ′ik]
Erythromycin delayed-release Capsules, USP
250mg

ESTRACE® ℞
[Es′ trāce]
(Estradiol Vaginal Cream, USP, 0.01%)

MANDELAMINE® ℞
[Man-del ′-a-meen]
Methenamine Mandelate Tablets, USP
.5gm, 1gm

OVCON® 35 0.4/35 ℞
[Ov-cŏn]
OVCON® 50
(Norethindrone and Ethinyl Estradiol Tablets, USP)
21- and 28-DAY REGIMENS

PYRIDIUM® ℞
[Per-i ′-deum]
Phenazopyridine Hydrochloride Tablets, USP
100mg, 200mg

PYRIDIUM® PLUS ℞
Phenazopyridine HCl, hyoscyamine HBr, butabarbital Tablets

NATAFORT®
Prenatal Multivitamin Tablet with Iron

NATACHEW™
Chewable Prenatal Multivitamin Tablet with Iron

DORYX ℞
[dor′-ix]
(Coated Doxycycline Hyclate Pellets)

DESCRIPTION

DORYX® Capsules contain specially coated pellets of doxycycline hyclate for oral administration. Also contains lactose, NF; microcrystalline cellulose, NF; povidone, USP. The capsule shell and/or band contains FD and C blue No. 1; FD and C yellow No. 6; D and C yellow No. 10; gelatin, NF; silicon dioxide; sodium lauryl sulfate, NF; titanium dioxide, USP. Doxycycline is a broad-spectrum antibiotic synthetically derived from oxytetracycline and available as doxycycline hyclate. The chemical designation of this light-yellow crystalline powder is alpha-6-desoxy-5-oxytetra-cycline. Doxycycline has a high degree of lipoid solubility and a low affinity for calcium binding. It is highly stable in normal human serum. Doxycycline will not degrade into an epianhydro form.

CLINICAL PHARMACOLOGY

Tetracyclines are readily absorbed and are bound to plasma proteins in varying degree. They are concentrated by the liver in the bile and excreted in the urine and feces at high concentrations and in a biologically active form.
Doxycycline is virtually completely absorbed after oral administration. Following a 200 mg dose, normal adult volunteers averaged peak serum levels of 2.6 mcg/mL of doxycycline at 2 hours decreasing to 1.45 mcg/mL at 24 hours. Excretion of doxycycline by the kidney is about 40%/72 hours in individuals with normal function (creatinine clearance about 75 mL/min). This percentage excretion may fall as low as 1–5%/72 hours in individuals with severe renal insufficiency (creatinine clearance below 10 mL/min). Studies have shown no significant difference in serum half-life of doxycycline (range 18–22 hours) in individuals with normal and severely impaired renal function.
Hemodialysis does not alter serum half-life.
Microbiology: Doxycycline is primarily bacteriostatic and is thought to exert its antimicrobial effect by the inhibition of protein synthesis. Doxycycline is active against a wide range of gram-positive and gram-negative organisms. The drugs in the tetracycline class have closely similar antimicrobial spectra and cross resistance among them is common.
Susceptibility Tests: Diffusion Techniques: The use of antibiotic disc susceptibility test methods which measure zone diameter gives an accurate estimation of susceptibility of organisms to DORYX®. One such standard procedure[1] has been recommended for use with discs for testing antimicrobials. Doxycycline 30 mcg discs should be used for the determination of the susceptibility of organisms to doxycycline.
With this type of procedure, a report of "susceptible" from the laboratory indicates that the infecting organism is likely to respond to therapy. A report of "intermediate susceptibility" suggests that the organism would be susceptible if high dosage is used or if the infection is confined to tissue and fluids (e.g., urine) in which high antibiotic levels are obtained. A report of "resistant" indicates that the infecting organism is not likely to respond to therapy. With the doxycycline disc, a zone of 16 mm or greater indicates susceptibility, zone sizes of 12 mm or less indicate resistance, and zone sizes of 13 to 15 mm indicate intermediate susceptibility.
Standardized procedures require the use of laboratory control organisms. The 30 mcg tetracycline disc should give zone diameters between 19 and 28 mm for *S. aureus* ATCC 25923 and between 18 and 25 mm for *E. coli* ATCC 25922. The 30 mcg doxycycline disc should give zone diameters between 23 and 29 mm for *S. aureus* ATCC 25923, and between 18 and 24 mm for *E. coli* ATCC 25922.
Dilution Techniques: A bacterial isolate may be considered susceptible if the MIC (minimal inhibitory concentration) value for doxycycline is less than 4 mcg/mL.
Organisms are considered resistant if the MIC is greater than 12.5 mcg/mL. MICs greater than 4.0 mcg/mL and less than 12.5 mcg/mL indicate intermediate susceptibility.
As with standard diffusion methods, dilution procedures require the use of laboratory control mechanisms. Standard doxycycline powder should give MIC values in the range of 0.25 mcg/mL and 1.0 mcg/mL for *S. aureus* ATCC 25923. For *E. coli* ATCC 25922 the MIC range should be between 1.0 mcg/mL and 4.0 mcg/mL.

INDICATIONS AND USAGE

Doxycycline is indicated in infections caused by the following microorganisms:

- Rickettsiae (Rocky Mountain spotted fever, typhus fever and the typhus group, Q fever, rickettsialpox and tick fevers).
- *Mycoplasma pneumoniae* (PPLO, Eaton's agent)
- Agents of psittacosis and ornithosis.
- Agents of lymphogranuloma venereum and granuloma inguinale.
- The spirochetal agent of relapsing fever (*Borrelia recurrentis*).

The following gram-negative microorganisms:

- *Haemophilus ducreyi* (chancroid)
- *Yersinia pestis* (formerly *Pasteurella pestis*)
- *Francisella tularensis* (formerly *Pasteurella tularensis*)
- *Bartonella bacilliformis*
- *Bacteroides* species
- *Vibrio cholerae* (formerly *Vibrio comma*)
- *Campylobacter fetus* (formerly *Vibrio fetus*)
- *Brucella* species (in conjunction with streptomycin)

Because many strains of the following groups of microorganisms have been shown to be resistant to tetracyclines, culture and susceptibility testing are recommended.
Doxycycline is indicated for treatment of infections caused by the following gram-negative microorganisms, when bacteriological testing indicates appropriate susceptibility to the drug:

Continued on next page

Doryx—Cont.

Escherichia coli
Enterobacter aerogenes (formerly *Aerobacter aerogenes*)
Shigella species
Mima species and *Herellea* species
Haemophilus influenzae (respiratory infections)
Klebsiella species (respiratory and urinary infections)

Doxycycline is indicated for treatment of infections caused by the following gram-positive microorganisms when bacteriological testing indicates appropriate susceptibility to the drug:

Streptococcus species:

Up to 44 percent of strains of *Streptococcus pyogenes* and 74 percent of *Streptococcus faecalis* have been found to be resistant to tetracycline drugs.

Therefore, tetracyclines should not be used for streptococcal disease unless the organism has been demonstrated to be susceptible.

For upper respiratory infections due to group A beta-hemolytic streptococci, penicillin is the usual drug of choice, including prophylaxis of rheumatic fever.

Diplococcus pneumoniae.

Staphylococcus aureus (respiratory, skin and soft-tissue infections). Tetracyclines are not the drug of choice in the treatment of any type of staphylococcal infection.

When penicillin is contraindicated, doxycycline is an alternative drug in the treatment of infections due to:

Treponema pallidum and *Treponema pertenue* (syphilis and yaws)
Listeria monocytogenes
Clostridium species
Bacillus anthracis
Fusobacterium fusiforme (Vincent's infection)
Actinomyces species

In acute intestinal amebiasis, doxycycline may be a useful adjunct to amebicides.

In severe acne, doxycycline may be useful adjunctive therapy.

Doxycycline is indicated in the treatment of trachoma, although the infectious agent is not always eliminated, as judged by immunofluorescence.

Inclusion conjunctivitis may be treated with oral doxycycline alone, or with a combination of topical agents.

Doxycycline is indicated for the treatment of uncomplicated urethral, endocervical or rectal infections in adults caused by *Chlamydia trachomatis.*[2]

Doxycycline is indicated for the treatment of nongonococcal urethritis caused by *Chlamydia trachomatis* and *Ureaplasma urealyticum* and for the treatment of acute epididymo-orchitis caused by *Chlamydia trachomatis.*[2]

Doxycycline is indicated for the treatment of uncomplicated gonococcal infections in adults (except for anorectal infections in men), the gonococcal arthritis-dermatitis syndrome and acute epididymo-orchitis caused by *N. gonorrhoeae.*[2]

CONTRAINDICATIONS

The drug is contraindicated in persons who have shown hypersensitivity to any of the tetracyclines.

WARNINGS

THE USE OF DRUGS OF THE TETRACYCLINE CLASS DURING TOOTH DEVELOPMENT (LAST HALF OF PREGNANCY, INFANCY AND CHILDHOOD TO THE AGE OF 8 YEARS) MAY CAUSE PERMANENT DISCOLORATION OF THE TEETH (YELLOW-GRAY-BROWN). This adverse reaction is more common during long term use of the drugs but has been observed following repeated short term courses. Enamel hypoplasia has also been reported. TETRACYCLINE DRUGS, THEREFORE, SHOULD NOT BE USED IN THIS AGE GROUP UNLESS OTHER DRUGS ARE NOT LIKELY TO BE EFFECTIVE OR ARE CONTRAINDICATED.

Results of animal studies indicate that tetracyclines cross the placenta, are found in fetal tissues and can have toxic effects on the developing fetus (often related to retardation of skeletal development). Evidence of embryotoxicity has been noted in animals treated early in pregnancy. If any tetracycline is used during pregnancy or if the patient becomes pregnant while taking these drugs, the patient should be apprised of potential hazard to the fetus.

As with other tetracyclines, doxycycline forms a stable calcium complex in any bone-forming tissue. A decrease in the fibula growth rate has been observed in prematures given oral tetracycline in doses of 25 mg/kg every six hours. This reaction was shown to be reversible when the drug was discontinued.

Photosensitivity manifested by an exaggerated sunburn reaction has been observed in some individuals taking tetracyclines. Patients apt to be exposed to direct sunlight or ultraviolet light should be advised that this reaction can occur with tetracycline drugs, and treatment should be discontinued at the first evidence of skin erythema.

The antianabolic action of the tetracyclines may cause an increase in BUN. Studies to date indicate that this does not occur with the use of doxycycline in patients with impaired renal function.

PRECAUTIONS

As with other antibiotic preparations, use of this drug may result in overgrowth of nonsusceptible organisms, including fungi. If superinfection occurs, the antibiotic should be discontinued and appropriate therapy instituted.

All infections due to group A beta-hemolytic streptococci should be treated for at least 10 days.

Laboratory tests: In venereal disease when coexistent syphilis is suspected, dark-field examination should be done before treatment is started and the blood serology repeated monthly for at least 4 months.

In long term therapy, periodic laboratory evaluation of organ systems, including hematopoietic, renal and hepatic studies should be performed.

Drug Interactions: Because tetracyclines have been shown to depress plasma prothrombin activity, patients who are on anticoagulant therapy may require downward adjustment of their anticoagulant dosage.

Since bacteriostatic drugs may interfere with the bactericidal action of penicillin, it is advisable to avoid giving tetracyclines in conjunction with penicillin.

For concomitant therapy with antacids or iron-containing preparations and food see DOSAGE AND ADMINISTRATION section.

Carcinogenesis, mutagenesis, impairment of fertility: Long-term studies are currently being conducted to determine whether tetracyclines have carcinogenic potential. Animal studies conducted in rats and mice have not provided conclusive evidence that tetracyclines may be carcinogenic or that they impair fertility. In two mammalian cell assays (L51784 mouse lymphoma and Chinese hamster lung cells *in vitro*), positive responses for mutagenicity occurred at concentrations of 60 and 10 mcg/mL, respectively. In humans, no association between tetracyclines and these effects have been made.

Pregnancy: Pregnancy Category D (see WARNINGS section).

Nursing mothers: Tetracyclines are present in the milk of lactating women who are taking a drug in this class. Because of the potential for serious adverse reactions in nursing infants from the tetracyclines, a decision should be made whether to discontinue nursing or discontinue the drug, taking into account the importance of the drug to the mother (see WARNINGS section).

Pediatric use: See WARNINGS and DOSAGE AND ADMINISTRATION sections.

ADVERSE REACTIONS

Due to oral doxycycline's virtually complete absorption, side effects to the lower bowel, particularly diarrhea, have been infrequent. The following adverse reactions have been observed in patients receiving tetracyclines:

Gastrointestinal: Anorexia, nausea, vomiting, diarrhea, glossitis, dysphagia, enterocolitis, and inflammatory lesions (with monilial overgrowth) in the anogenital region. These reactions have been caused by both the oral and parenteral administration of tetracyclines. Rare instances of esophagitis and esophageal ulcerations have been reported in patients receiving capsule and tablet forms of drugs in the tetracycline class. Most of these patients took medications immediately before going to bed (see DOSAGE AND ADMINISTRATION section).

Skin: Maculopapular and erythematous rashes. Exfoliative dermatitis has been reported but is uncommon. Photosensitivity is discussed above (see WARNINGS section).

Renal toxicity: Rise in BUN has been reported and is apparently dose-related (see WARNINGS section).

Hypersensitivity reactions: Urticaria, angioneurotic edema, anaphylaxis, anaphylactoid purpura, pericarditis, and exacerbation of systemic lupus erythematosus.

Bulging fontenals in infants and benign intracranial hypertension in adults have been reported in individuals receiving tetracyclines. These conditions disappeared when the drug was discontinued.

Blood: Hemolytic anemia, thrombocytopenia, neutropenia, and eosinophilia have been reported with tetracyclines.

When given over prolonged periods, tetracyclines have been reported to produce brown-black microscopic discoloration of thyroid glands. No abnormalities of thyroid function are known to occur.

DOSAGE AND ADMINISTRATION

THE USUAL DOSAGE AND FREQUENCY OF ADMINISTRATION OF DOXYCYCLINE DIFFERS FROM THAT OF THE OTHER TETRACYCLINES. EXCEEDING THE RECOMMENDED DOSAGE MAY RESULT IN AN INCREASED INCIDENCE OF SIDE EFFECTS.

Adults: The usual dose of oral doxycycline is 200 mg on the first day of treatment (administered 100 mg every 12 hours) followed by a maintenance dose of 100 mg/day. The maintenance dose may be administered as a single dose or as 50 mg every 12 hours. In the management of more severe infections (particularly chronic infections of the urinary tract), 100 mg every 12 hours is recommended.

For pediatric patients above eight years of age: The recommended dosage schedule for pediatric patients weighing 100 pounds or less is 2 mg/lb of body weight divided into two doses on the first day of treatment, followed by 1 mg/lb of body weight given as a single daily dose or divided into two doses on subsequent days. For more severe infections up to 2 mg/lb of body weight may be used. For pediatric patients over 100 pounds, the usual adult dose should be used.

Uncomplicated gonococcal infections in adults (except anorectal infections in men): 100 mg, by mouth, twice-a-day for 7 days.[2] As an alternate single visit dose, administer 300 mg stat followed in one hour by a second 300 mg dose. The dose may be administered with food, including milk or carbonated beverage, as required.

Acute epididymo-orchitis caused by *N. gonorrhoeae:* 100 mg, by mouth, twice-a-day for at least 10 days.[2]

Primary and secondary syphilis: 300 mg a day in divided doses for at least 10 days.[2]

Uncomplicated urethral, endocervical, or rectal infection in adults caused by *Chlamydia trachomatis:* 100 mg by mouth, twice-a-day for at least 7 days.[2]

Nongonococcal urethritis caused by *C. trachomatis* and *U. urealyticum:* 100 mg, by mouth, twice-a-day for at least 7 days.[2]

Acute epididymo-orchitis caused by *C. trachomatis:* 100 mg, by mouth, twice-a-day for at least 10 days.[2]

The therapeutic antibacterial serum activity will usually persist for 24 hours following recommended dosage.

When used in streptococcal infections, therapy should be continued for 10 days.

Administration of adequate amounts of fluid along with capsule and tablet forms of drugs in the tetracycline class is recommended to wash down the drugs and reduce the risk of esophageal irritation and ulceration (see ADVERSE REACTIONS section).

If gastric irritation occurs, it is recommended that doxycycline be given with food or milk. The absorption of doxycycline is not markedly influenced by simultaneous ingestion of food or milk.

Concomitant therapy: Antacids containing aluminum, calcium or magnesium, sodium bicarbonate, and iron-containing preparations should not be given to patients taking oral tetracyclines.

Studies to date have indicated that administration of doxycycline at the usual recommended doses does not lead to excessive accumulation of the antibiotic in patients with renal impairment.

HOW SUPPLIED

DORYX® Capsules have a yellow transparent body with light blue opaque cap; the capsule bearing the inscription "DORYX" in white. Pellets are colored yellow. Each capsule contains specially coated pellets of doxycycline hyclate equivalent to 100 mg of doxycycline, supplied in:

Bottles of 50 capsules .... N 0430-0838-19

STORAGE CONDITIONS

Store at controlled room temperature below 25°C (77°F).

References:

1. NCCLS Approved Standard:
M2-A3, Vol. 4, Performance Standards for Antimicrobial Disk Susceptibility Tests, Third Edition: available from the National Committee for Clinical Laboratory Standards, 771 East Lancaster Avenue, Villanova, Pa. 19085
2. CDC Sexuality Transmitted Diseases Treatment Guidelines 1982

Rx only

Revised December 1999
Manufactured by
Faulding Pharmaceutical/DBL
A Division of F.H. Faulding & Co. Limited
1538 Main North Road
Salisbury, South Australia 5108
Distributed by
Warner Chilcott Laboratories™
WARNER CHILCOTT, INC.
100 Enterprise Drive
Rockaway, NJ 07866 USA

ESTRACE® ℞

[es'trāce]

(ESTRADIOL VAGINAL CREAM, USP, 0.01%)

Rx only

WARNINGS

1. **ESTROGENS HAVE BEEN REPORTED TO INCREASE THE RISK OF ENDOMETRIAL CARCINOMA IN POST-MENOPAUSAL WOMEN.**
   Close clinical surveillance of all women taking estrogens is important. Adequate diagnostic measures, including endometrial sampling when indicated, should be undertaken to rule out malignancy in all cases of undiagnosed persistent or recurring abnormal vaginal bleeding. There is no evidence that "natural" estrogens are more or less hazardous than "synthetic" estrogens at equi-estrogenic doses.
2. **ESTROGENS SHOULD NOT BE USED DURING PREGNANCY.**
   There is no indication for estrogen therapy during pregnancy or during the immediate postpartum period. Estrogens are ineffective for the prevention or treatment of threatened or habitual abortion. Estrogens are not indicated for the prevention of postpartum breast engorgement.
   Estrogen therapy during pregnancy is associated with an increased risk of congenital defects in the reproductive organs of the fetus, and possibly other birth defects. Studies of women who received diethylstilbestrol (DES) during pregnancy have shown that female offspring have an increased risk of vaginal adenosis, squamous cell dysplasia of the uterine cervix, and clear cell vaginal cancer later in life; male off-

spring have an increased risk of urogenital abnormalities and possibly testicular cancer later in life. The 1985 DES Task Force concluded that use of DES during pregnancy is associated with a subsequent increased risk of breast cancer in the mothers, although a causal relationship remains unproven and the observed level of excess risk is similar to that for a number of other breast cancer risk factors.

DESCRIPTION

Each gram of ESTRACE® (ESTRADIOL VAGINAL CREAM, USP, 0.01%) contains 0.1 mg estradiol in a nonliquefying base containing purified water, propylene glycol, stearyl alcohol, white ceresin wax, glyceryl monostearate, hydroxypropyl methylcellulose, 2208 4000 cps, sodium lauryl sulfate, methylparaben, edetate di-sodium and *tertiary*-butylhydroquinone. Estradiol is chemically described as estra-1,3,5(10)-triene-3, 17β-diol. It has an empirical formula of $C_{18}H_{24}O_2$ and molecular weight of 272.37. The structural formula is:

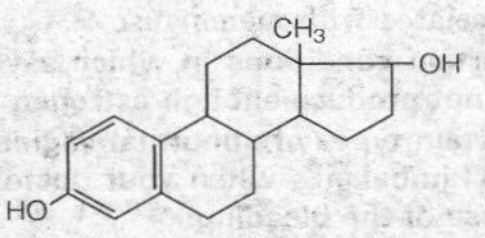

CLINICAL PHARMACOLOGY

Estrogen drug products act by regulating the transcription of a limited number of genes. Estrogens diffuse through cell membranes, distribute themselves throughout the cell, and bind to and activate the nuclear estrogen receptor, a DNA-binding protein which is found in estrogen-responsive tissues. The activated estrogen receptor binds to specific DNA sequences, or hormone-response elements, which enhance the transcription of adjacent genes and in turn lead to the observed effects. Estrogen receptors have been identified in tissues of the reproductive tract, breast, pituitary, hypothalamus, liver, and bone of women.

Estrogens are important in the development and maintenance of the female reproductive system and secondary sex characteristics. By a direct action, they cause growth and development of the uterus, fallopian tubes, and vagina. With other hormones, such as pituitary hormones and progesterone, they cause enlargement of the breasts through promotion of ductal growth, stromal development, and the accretion of fat. Estrogens are intricately involved with other hormones, especially progesterone, in the processes of the ovulatory menstrual cycle and pregnancy, and affect the release of pituitary gonadotropins. They also contribute to the shaping of the skeleton, maintenance of tone and elasticity of urogenital structures, changes in the epiphyses of the long bones that allow for the pubertal growth spurt and its termination, and pigmentation of the nipples and genitals.

Estrogens occur naturally in several forms. The primary source of estrogen in normally cycling adult women is the ovarian follicle, which secretes 70 to 500 micrograms of estradiol daily, depending on the phase of the menstrual cycle. This is converted primarily to estrone, which circulates in roughly equal proportion to estradiol, and to small amounts of estriol. After menopause, most endogenous estrogen is produced by conversion of androstenedione, secreted by the adrenal cortex, to estrone by peripheral tissues. Thus, estrone—especially in its sulfate ester form—is the most abundant circulating estrogen in postmenopausal women.

Although circulating estrogens exist in a dynamic equilibrium of metabolic interconversions, estradiol is the principal intracellular human estrogen and is substantially more potent than estrone or estriol at the receptor.

Estrogens used in therapy are well absorbed through the skin, mucous membranes, and gastrointestinal tract. When applied for a local action, absorption is usually sufficient to cause systemic effects. When conjugated with aryl and alkyl groups for parenteral administration, the rate of absorption of oily preparations is slowed with a prolonged duration of action, such that a single intramuscular injection of estradiol valerate or estradiol cypionate is absorbed over several weeks.

Administered estrogens and their esters are handled within the body essentially the same as the endogenous hormones. Metabolic conversion of estrogens occurs primarily in the liver (first pass effect), but also at local target tissue sites. Complex metabolic processes result in a dynamic equilibrium of circulating conjugated and unconjugated estrogenic forms which are continually interconverted, especially between estrone and estradiol and between esterified and non-esterified forms. Although naturally-occurring estrogens circulate in the blood largely bound to sex hormone-binding globulin and albumin, only unbound estrogens enter target tissue cells. A significant proportion of the circulating estrogen exists as sulfate conjugates, especially estrone sulfate, which serves as a circulating reservoir for the formation of more active estrogenic species. A certain proportion of the estrogen is excreted into the bile and then reabsorbed from the intestine. During this enterohepatic recirculation, estrogens are desulfated and resulfated and undergo degradation through conversion to less active estrogens (estriol and other estrogens), oxidation to nonestrogenic substances (catecholestrogens, which interact with catecholamine metabolism, especially in the central nervous system), and conjugation with glucuronic acids (which are then rapidly excreted in the urine).

When given orally, naturally-occurring estrogens and their esters are extensively metabolized (first pass effect) and circulate primarily as estrone sulfate, with smaller amounts of other conjugated and unconjugated estrogenic species. This results in limited oral potency. By contrast, synthetic estrogens, such as ethinyl estradiol and the nonsteroidal estrogens, are degraded very slowly in the liver and other tissues, which results in their high intrinsic potency. Estrogen drug products administered by non-oral routes are not subject to first-pass metabolism, but also undergo significant hepatic uptake, metabolism, and enterohepatic recycling.

INDICATIONS AND USAGE

ESTRACE (ESTRADIOL VAGINAL CREAM, USP, 0.01%) is indicated in the treatment of vulval and vaginal atrophy.

CONTRAINDICATIONS

Estrogens should not be used in individuals with any of the following conditions:

1. Known or suspected pregnancy (see **BOXED WARNINGS**).
   Estrogens may cause fetal harm when administered to a pregnant woman.
2. Undiagnosed abnormal genital bleeding.
3. Known or suspected cancer of the breast except in appropriately selected patients being treated for metastatic disease.
4. Known or suspected estrogen-dependent neoplasia.
5. Active thrombophlebitis or thromboembolic disorders.

WARNINGS

1. Induction of malignant neoplasms.

Endometrial cancer. The reported endometrial cancer risk among unopposed estrogen users is about 2 to 12 fold greater than in non-users, and appears dependent on duration of treatment and on estrogen dose. Most studies show no significant increased risk associated with use of estrogens for less than one year. The greatest risk appears associated with prolonged use—with increased risks of 15 to 24-fold for five to ten years or more. In three studies, persistence of risk was demonstrated for 8 to over 15 years after cessation of estrogen treatment. In one study a significant decrease in the incidence of endometrial cancer occurred six months after estrogen withdrawal. Concurrent progestin therapy may offset this risk but the overall health impact in postmenopausal women is not known (see **PRECAUTIONS**).

Breast cancer. While the majority of studies have not shown an increased risk of breast cancer in women who have ever used estrogen replacement therapy, some have reported a moderately increased risk (relative risks of 1.3–2.0) in those taking higher doses or those taking lower doses for prolonged periods of time, especially in excess of 10 years. Other studies have not shown this relationship.

While the effects of added progestins on the risk of breast cancer are also unknown, available epidemiological evidence suggests that progestins do not reduce, and may enhance, the moderately increased breast cancer incidence that has been reported with prolonged estrogen replacement therapy (see **PRECAUTIONS**).

Congenital lesions with malignant potential. Estrogen therapy during pregnancy is associated with an increased risk of fetal congenital reproductive tract disorders, and possibly other birth defects. Studies of women who received DES during pregnancy have shown that female offspring have an increased risk of vaginal adenosis, squamous cell dysplasia of the uterine cervix, and clear cell vaginal cancer later in life; male offspring have an increased risk of urogenital abnormalities and possibly testicular cancer later in life. Although some of these changes are benign, others are precursors of malignancy.

2. Gallbladder disease. Two studies have reported a 2- to 4-fold increase in the risk of gallbladder disease requiring surgery in women receiving postmenopausal estrogens.

3. Cardiovascular disease. Large doses of estrogen (5 mg conjugated estrogens per day), comparable to those used to treat cancer of the prostate and breast, have been shown in a large prospective clinical trial in men to increase the risks of nonfatal myocardial infarction, pulmonary embolism, and thrombophlebitis. These risks cannot necessarily be extrapolated from men to women. However, to avoid the theoretical cardiovascular risk to women caused by high estrogen doses, the dose for estrogen replacement therapy should not exceed the lowest effective dose.

4. Elevated blood pressure. Occasional blood pressure increases during estrogen replacement therapy have been attributed to idiosyncratic reactions to estrogens. More often, blood pressure has remained the same or has dropped. One study showed that postmenopausal estrogen users have higher blood pressure than nonusers. Two other studies showed slightly lower blood pressure among estrogen users compared to nonusers. Postmenopausal estrogen use does not increase the risk of stroke. Nonetheless, blood pressure should be monitored at regular intervals with estrogen use.

5. Hypercalcemia. Administration of estrogens may lead to severe hypercalcemia in patients with breast cancer and bone metastases. If this occurs, the drug should be stopped and appropriate measures taken to reduce the serum calcium level.

PRECAUTIONS

A. General

1. Addition of a progestin. Studies of the addition of a progestin for 10 or more days of a cycle of estrogen administration have reported a lowered incidence of endometrial hyperplasia than would be induced by estrogen treatment alone. Morphological and biochemical studies of endometria suggest that 10 to 14 days of progestin are needed to provide maximal maturation of the endometrium and to reduce the likelihood of hyperplastic changes.

There are, however, possible risks which may be associated with the use of progestins in estrogen replacement regimens. These include: (1) adverse effects on lipoprotein metabolism (lowering HDL and raising LDL) which could diminish the purported cardioprotective effect of estrogen therapy (see **PRECAUTIONS** below); (2) impairment of glucose tolerance; and (3) possible enhancement of mitotic activity in breast epithelial tissue, although few epidemiological data are available to address this point (see **WARNINGS**).

The choice of progestin, its dose, and its regimen may be important in minimizing these adverse effects, but these issues will require further study before they are clarified.

2. Cardiovascular risk. *A causal relationship between estrogen replacement therapy and reduction of cardiovascular disease in postmenopausal women has not been proven. Furthermore, the effect of added progestins on this putative benefit is not yet known.*

In recent years many published studies have suggested that there may be a cause-effect relationship between postmenopausal oral estrogen replacement therapy *without added progestins* and a decrease in cardiovascular disease in women. Although most of the observational studies which assessed this statistical association have reported a 20% to 50% reduction in coronary heart disease risk and associated mortality in estrogen takers, the following should be considered when interpreting these reports:

(1) Because only one of these studies was randomized and it was too small to yield statistically significant results, all relevant studies were subject to selection bias. Thus, the apparently reduced risk of coronary artery disease cannot be attributed with certainty to estrogen replacement therapy. It may instead have been caused by life-style and medical characteristics of the women studied with the result that healthier women were selected for estrogen therapy. In general, treated women were of higher socioeconomic and educational status, more slender, more physically active, more likely to have undergone surgical menopause, and less likely to have diabetes than the untreated women. Although some studies attempted to control for these selection factors, it is common for properly designed randomized trials to fail to confirm benefits suggested by less rigorous study designs. Thus, ongoing and future large-scale randomized trials may fail to confirm this apparent benefit.

(2) Current medical practice often includes the use of concomitant progestin therapy in women with intact uteri (see **PRECAUTIONS** and **WARNINGS**). While the effects of added progestins on the risk of ischemic heart disease are not known, all available progestins reverse at least some of the favorable effects of estrogens on HDL and LDL levels.

3. Physical examination. A complete medical and family history should be taken prior to the initiation of any estrogen therapy. The pretreatment and periodic physical examinations should include special reference to blood pressure, breasts, abdomen, and pelvic organs, and should include a Papanicolaou smear. As a general rule, estrogen should not be prescribed for longer than one year without reexamining the patient.

4. Hypercoagulability. Some studies have shown that women taking estrogen replacement therapy have hypercoagulability, primarily related to decreased antithrombin activity. This effect appears dose- and duration-dependent and is less pronounced than that associated with oral contraceptive use. Also, postmenopausal women tend to have increased coagulation parameters at baseline compared to premenopausal women. There is some suggestion that low dose postmenopausal mestranol may increase the risk of thromboembolism, although the majority of studies (of primarily conjugated estrogens users) report no such increase. There is insufficient information on hypercoagulability in women who have had previous thromboembolic disease.

5. Familial hyperlipoproteinemia. Estrogen therapy may be associated with massive elevations of plasma triglycerides leading to pancreatitis and other complications in patients with familial defects of lipoprotein metabolism.

6. Fluid retention. Because estrogens may cause some degree of fluid retention, conditions which might be exacerbated by this factor, such as asthma, epilepsy, migraine, and cardiac or renal dysfunction, require careful observation.

7. Uterine bleeding and mastodynia. Certain patients may develop undesirable manifestations of estrogenic stimulation, such as abnormal uterine bleeding and mastodynia.

8. Impaired liver function. Estrogens may be poorly metabolized in patients with impaired liver function and should be administered with caution.

B. Information for the Patient. See text of Patient Package Insert below.

Advise patients that the number of doses per tube will vary with dosage requirement and patient handling.

C. Laboratory Tests. Estrogen administration should generally be guided by clinical response at the smallest dose, rather than laboratory monitoring, for relief of symptoms for those indications in which symptoms are observable.

D. Drug/Laboratory Test Interactions.

1. Accelerated prothrombin time, partial thromboplastin time, and platelet aggregation time; increased platelet count; increased factors II, VII antigen, VIII antigen,

Continued on next page

Estrace—Cont.

VIII coagulant activity, IX, X, XII, VII-X complex, II-VII-X complex, and beta-thromboglobulin; decreased levels of anti-factor Xa and antithrombin III, decreased antithrombin III activity; increased levels of fibrinogen and fibrinogen activity; increased plasminogen antigen and activity.

2. Increased thyroid-binding globulin (TBG) leading to increased circulating total thyroid hormone, as measured by protein-bound iodine (PBI), T4 levels (by column or by radioimmunoassay) or T3 levels by radioimmunoassay. T3 resin uptake is decreased, reflecting the elevated TBG. Free T4 and free T3 concentrations are unaltered.
3. Other binding proteins may be elevated in serum, i.e., corticosteroid binding globulin (CBG), sex hormone-binding globulin (SHBG), leading to increased circulating corticosteroids and sex steroids, respectively. Free or biologically active hormone concentrations are unchanged. Other plasma proteins may be increased (angiotensinogen/renin substrate, alpha-1-antitrypsin, ceruloplasmin).
4. Increased plasma HDL and HDL-2 subfraction concentrations, reduced LDL cholesterol concentration, increased triglycerides levels.
5. Impaired glucose tolerance.
6. Reduced response to metyrapone test.
7. Reduced serum folate concentration.

E. Carcinogenesis, Mutagenesis, and Impairment of Fertility.
Long term continuous administration of natural and synthetic estrogens in certain animal species increases the frequency of carcinomas of the breast, uterus, cervix, vagina, testis, and liver. See **CONTRAINDICATIONS** and **WARNINGS**.

F. Pregnancy Category X.
Estrogens should not be used during pregnancy. See **CONTRAINDICATIONS** and **BOXED WARNINGS**.

G. Nursing Mothers. As a general principle, the administration of any drug to nursing mothers should be done only when clearly necessary since many drugs are excreted in human milk. In addition, estrogen administration to nursing mothers has been shown to decrease the quantity and quality of the milk.

H. Pediatric Use. Safety and effectiveness in pediatric patients have not been established. Large and repeated doses of estrogen over an extended period of time have been shown to accelerate epiphyseal closure, resulting in short adult stature if treatment is initiated before the completion of physiologic puberty in normally developing children. In patients in whom bone growth is not complete, periodic monitoring of bone maturation and effects on epiphyseal centers is recommended.
Estrogen treatment of prepubertal children also induces premature breast development and vaginal cornification, and may potentially induce vaginal bleeding in girls. In boys, estrogen treatment may modify the normal pubertal process. All other physiological and adverse reactions shown to be associated with estrogen treatment of adults could potentially occur in the pediatric population, including thromboembolic disorders and growth stimulation of certain tumors. Therefore, estrogens should only be administered to pediatric patients when clearly indicated and the lowest effective dose should always be utilized.

ADVERSE REACTIONS

The following additional adverse reactions have been reported with estrogen therapy (see **WARNINGS** regarding induction of neoplasia, adverse effects on the fetus, increased incidence of gallbladder disease, cardiovascular disease, elevated blood pressure, and hypercalcemia).

1. Genitourinary system.
Changes in vaginal bleeding pattern and abnormal withdrawal bleeding or flow; breakthrough bleeding, spotting.
Increase in size of uterine leiomyomata.
Vaginal candidiasis.
Change in amount of cervical secretion.

2. Breasts.
Tenderness, enlargement.

3. Gastrointestinal.
Nausea, vomiting.
Abdominal cramps, bloating.
Cholestatic jaundice.
Increased incidence of gallbladder disease.

4. Skin.
Chloasma or melasma that may persist when drug is discontinued.
Erythema multiforme.
Erythema nodosum.
Hemorrhagic eruption.
Loss of scalp hair.
Hirsutism.

5. Eyes.
Steepening of corneal curvature.
Intolerance to contact lenses.

6. Central Nervous System.
Headache, migraine, dizziness.
Mental depression.
Chorea.

7. Miscellaneous.
Increase or decrease in weight.
Reduced carbohydrate tolerance.
Aggravation of prophyria.
Edema.
Changes in libido.

OVERDOSAGE

Serious ill effects have not been reported following acute ingestion of large doses of estrogen-containing oral contraceptives by young children. Overdosage of estrogen may cause nausea and vomiting, and withdrawal bleeding may occur in females.

DOSAGE AND ADMINISTRATION

For treatment of vulval and vaginal atrophy associated with the menopause, the lowest dose and regimen that will control symptoms should be chosen and medication should be discontinued as promptly as possible.
Attempts to discontinue or taper medication should be made at 3-month to 6-month intervals.
Usual Dosage: The usual dosage range is 2 to 4 g (marked on the applicator) daily for one or two weeks, then gradually reduced to one half initial dosage for a similar period. A maintenance dosage of 1 g, one to three times a week, may be used after restoration of the vaginal mucosa has been achieved.
NOTE: The number of doses per tube will vary with dosage requirements and patient handling.
Patients with intact uteri should be monitored closely for signs of endometrial cancer and appropriate diagnostic measures should be taken to rule out malignancy in the event of persistent or recurring abnormal vaginal bleeding.

HOW SUPPLIED

ESTRACE® (ESTRADIOL VAGINAL CREAM, USP, 0.01%).
NDC 0430-3754-14: Tube containing 1½ oz (42.5 g) with a calibrated plastic applicator for delivery of 1, 2, 3, or 4 g.
NDC 0430-3754-11: Carton containing four 0.42 oz (12 g) refill tubes.
Store at room temperature. Protect from temperatures in excess of 40°C (104°F).
Manufactured by:
Bristol-Myers
Squibb Company
Princeton, NJ 08543
Manufactured for:
Warner Chilcott, Inc
Rockaway, NJ 07866
Revised: April 1998

J4-503E

ESTRACE® (ESTRADIOL VAGINAL CREAM, USP, 0.01%)

INFORMATION FOR THE PATIENT
Rx only
NOTE: The number of doses per tube will vary with dosage requirements and patient handling.

INTRODUCTION
This leaflet describes when and how to use estrogens, and the risks and benefits of estrogen treatment.
Estrogens have important benefits but also some risks. You must decide, with your doctor, whether the risks to you of estrogen use are acceptable because of their benefits. If you use estrogens, check with your doctor to be sure you are using the lowest possible dose that works, and that you don't use them longer than necessary. How long you need to use estrogens will depend on the reason for use.

WARNINGS

1. **ESTROGENS INCREASE THE RISK OF CANCER OF THE UTERUS IN WOMEN WHO HAVE HAD THEIR MENOPAUSE ("CHANGE OF LIFE").**
If you use any estrogen-containing drug, it is important to visit your doctor regularly and report any unusual vaginal bleeding right away. Vaginal bleeding after menopause may be a warning sign of uterine cancer. Your doctor should evaluate any unusual vaginal bleeding to find out the cause.
2. **ESTROGENS SHOULD NOT BE USED DURING PREGNANCY.**
Estrogens do not prevent miscarriage (spontaneous abortion) and are not needed in the days following childbirth. If you take estrogens during pregnancy, your unborn child has a greater than usual chance of having birth defects. The risk of developing these defects is small, but clearly larger than the risk in children whose mothers did not take estrogens during pregnancy. These birth defects may affect the baby's urinary system and sex organs. Daughters born to mothers who took DES (an estrogen drug) have a higher than usual chance of developing cancer of the vagina or cervix when they become teenagers or young adults. Sons may have a higher than usual chance of developing cancer of the testicles when they become teenagers or young adults.

USES OF ESTROGEN
(Not every estrogen drug is approved for every use listed in this section. If you want to known which of these possible uses are approved for the medicine prescribed for you, ask your doctor or pharmacist to show you the professional labeling. You can also look up the specific estrogen product in a book called the "Physicians' Desk Reference", which is available in many book stores and public libraries. Generic drugs carry virtually the same labeling information as their brand name versions.)

- **To reduce moderate or severe menopausal symptoms.**
Estrogens are hormones made by the ovaries of normal women. Between ages 45 and 55, the ovaries normally stop making estrogens. This leads to a drop in body estrogen levels which causes the "change of life" or menopause (the end of monthly menstrual periods). If both ovaries are removed during an operation before natural menopause takes place, the sudden drop in estrogen levels causes "surgical menopause".
When the estrogen levels begin dropping, some women develop very uncomfortable symptoms, such as feelings of warmth in the face, neck, and chest, or sudden intense episodes of heat and sweating ("hot flashes" or "hot flushes"). Using estrogen drugs can help the body adjust to lower estrogen levels and reduce these symptoms. Most women have only mild menopausal symptoms or none at all and do not need to use estrogen drugs for these symptoms. Others may need to take estrogens for a few months while their bodies adjust to lower estrogen levels. The majority of women do not need estrogen replacement for longer than six months for these symptoms.
- **To treat vulval and vaginal atrophy** (itching, burning, dryness in or around the vagina, difficulty or burning on urination) associated with menopause.
- **To treat certain conditions in which a young woman's ovaries do not produce enough estrogen naturally.**
- **To treat certain types of abnormal vaginal bleeding due to hormonal imbalance when your doctor has found no serious cause of the bleeding.**
- **To treat certain cancers in special situations, in men and women.**
- **To prevent thinning of bones.**
Osteoporosis is a thinning of the bones that makes them weaker and allows them to break more easily. The bones of the spine, wrists and hips break most often in osteoporosis. Both men and women start to lose bone mass after about age 40, but women lose bone mass faster after the menopause. Using estrogens after the menopause slows down bone thinning and may prevent bones from breaking. Lifelong adequate calcium intake, either in the diet (such as dairy products) or by calcium supplements (to reach a total daily intake of 1000 milligrams per day before menopause or 1500 milligrams per day after menopause), may help to prevent osteoporosis. Regular weight-bearing exercise (like walking and running for an hour, two or three times a week) may also help to prevent osteoporosis. Before you change your calcium intake or exercise habits, it is important to discuss these lifestyle changes with your doctor to find out if they are safe for you.
Since estrogen use has some risks, only women who are likely to develop osteoporosis should use estrogens for prevention. Women who are likely to develop osteoporosis often have the following characteristics: white or Asian race, slim, cigarette smokers, and a family history of osteoporosis in a mother, sister, or aunt. Women who have relatively early menopause, often because their ovaries were removed during an operation ("surgical menopause"), are more likely to develop osteoporosis than women whose menopause happens at the average age.

WHO SHOULD NOT USE ESTROGENS
Estrogens should not be used:

- **During pregnancy (see Boxed Warnings).**
If you think you may be pregnant, do not use any form of estrogen-containing drug. Using estrogens while you are pregnant may cause your unborn child to have birth defects. Estrogens do not prevent miscarriage.
- **If you have unusual vaginal bleeding which has not been evaluated by your doctor (see Boxed Warnings).**
Unusual vaginal bleeding can be a warning sign of cancer of the uterus, especially if it happens after menopause. Your doctor must find out the cause of the bleeding so that he or she can recommend the proper treatment. Taking estrogens without visiting your doctor can cause you serious harm if your vaginal bleeding is caused by cancer of the uterus.
- **If you have had cancer.**
Since estrogens increase the risk of certain types of cancer, you should not use estrogens if you have ever had cancer of the breast or uterus, unless your doctor recommends that the drug may help in the cancer treatment. (For certain patients with breast or prostate cancer, estrogens may help.)
- **If you have any circulation problems.**
Estrogen drugs should not be used except in unusually special situations in which your doctor judges that you need estrogen therapy so much that the risks are acceptable. Men and women with abnormal blood clotting conditions should avoid estrogen use (see **DANGERS OF ESTROGENS**, below).
- **When they do not work.**
During menopause, some women develop nervous symptoms or depression. Estrogens do not relieve these symptoms. You may have heard that taking estrogens for years after menopause will keep your skin soft and supple and keep you feeling young. There is no evidence for these claims and such long-term estrogen use may have serious risks.
- **After childbirth or when breastfeeding a baby.**
Estrogens should not be used to try to stop the breasts from filling with milk after a baby is born. Such treatment may increase the risk of developing blood clots (see **DANGERS OF ESTROGENS**, below).
If you are breastfeeding, you should avoid using any drugs because many drugs pass through to the baby in

the milk. While nursing a baby, you should take drugs only on the advice of your health care provider.

DANGERS OF ESTROGENS

- **Cancer of the uterus.**
  Your risk of developing cancer of the uterus gets higher the longer you use estrogens and the larger doses you use. One study showed that after women stop taking estrogens, this higher cancer risk quickly returns to the usual level of risk (as if you had never used estrogen therapy). Three other studies showed that the cancer risk stayed high for 8 to more than 15 years after stopping estrogen treatment. Because of this risk, **IT IS IMPORTANT TO TAKE THE LOWEST DOSE THAT WORKS AND TO TAKE IT ONLY AS LONG AS YOU NEED IT.**
  Using progestin therapy together with estrogen therapy may reduce the higher risk of uterine cancer related to estrogen use (but see **OTHER INFORMATION**, below).
  If you have had your uterus removed (total hysterectomy), there is no danger of developing cancer of the uterus.
- **Cancer of the breast.**
  Most studies have not shown a higher risk of breast cancer in women who have ever used estrogens. However, some studies have reported that breast cancer developed more often (up to twice the usual rate) in women who used estrogens for long periods of time (especially more than 10 years), or who used higher doses for shorter time periods.
  Regular breast examinations by a health professional and monthly self-examination are recommended for all women.
- **Gallbladder disease.**
  Women who use estrogens after menopause are more likely to develop gallbladder disease needing surgery than women who do not use estrogens.
- **Abnormal blood clotting.**
  Taking estrogens may cause changes in your blood clotting system. These changes allow the blood to clot more easily, possibly allowing clots to form in your bloodstream. If blood clots do form in your bloodstream, they can cut off the blood supply to vital organs, causing serious problems. These problems may include a stroke (by cutting off blood to the brain), a heart attack (by cutting off blood to the heart), a pulmonary embolus (by cutting off blood to the lungs), or other problems. Any of these conditions may cause death or serious long term disability. However, most studies of low dose estrogen usage by women do not show an increased risk of these complications.

SIDE EFFECTS

In addition to the risks listed above, the following side effects have been reported with estrogen use:
Nausea and vomiting.
Breast tenderness or enlargement.
Enlargement of benign tumors ("fibroids") of the uterus.
Retention of excess fluid. This may make some conditions worsen, such as asthma, epilepsy, migraine, heart disease, or kidney disease.
A spotty darkening of the skin, particularly on the face.

REDUCING RISK OF ESTROGEN USE

If you use estrogens, you can reduce your risks by doing these things:

- **See your doctor regularly.**
  While you are using estrogens, it is important to visit your doctor at least once a year for a check-up. If you develop vaginal bleeding while taking estrogens, you may need further evaluation. If members of your family have had breast cancer or if you have ever had breast lumps or an abnormal mammogram (breast x-ray), you may need to have more frequent breast examinations.
- **Reassess your need for estrogens.**
  You and your doctor should reevaluate whether or not you still need estrogens at least every six months.
- **Be alert for signs of trouble.**
  If any of these warning signals (or any other unusual symptoms) happen while you are using estrogens, call your doctor immediately:

Abnormal bleeding from the vagina (possible uterine cancer)
Pains in the calves or chest, sudden shortness of breath, or coughing blood (possible clot in the legs, heart, or lungs)
Severe headache or vomiting, dizziness, faintness, changes in vision or speech, weakness or numbness of an arm or leg (possible clot in the brain or eye)
Breast lumps (possible breast cancer; ask your doctor or health professional to show you how to examine your breasts monthly)
Yellowing of the skin or eyes (possible liver problem)
Pain, swelling, or tenderness in the abdomen (possible gallbladder problem)

OTHER INFORMATION

1. Estrogens increase the risk of developing a condition (endometrial hyperplasia) that may lead to cancer of the lining of the uterus. Taking progestins, another hormone drug, with estrogens lower the risk of developing this condition. Therefore, if your uterus has not been removed, your doctor may prescribe a progestin for you to take together with the estrogen.
You should know, however, that taking estrogens **with** progestins may have additional risks. These include: (a) unhealthy effects on blood fats (especially the lowering of HDL blood cholesterol, the "good" blood fat which protects against heart disease); (b) unhealthy effects on blood sugar (which might make a diabetic condition worse); and (c) a possible further increase in breast cancer risk which may be associated with long-term estrogen use.
Some research has shown that estrogens taken **without** progestins may protect women against developing heart disease. However, this is not certain. The protection shown may have been caused by the characteristics of the estrogen-treated women, and not by the estrogen treatment itself. In general, treated women were slimmer, more physically active, and were less likely to have diabetes than the untreated women. These characteristics are known to be associated with a reduced risk for heart disease.
You are cautioned to discuss very carefully with your doctor or health care provider all the possible risks and benefits of long-term estrogen and progestin treatment as they affect you personally.
2. Your doctor has prescribed this drug for you and you alone. Do not give the drug to anyone else.
3. If you will be taking calcium supplements as part of the treatment to help prevent osteoporosis, check with your doctor about how much to take.
4. Keep this and all drugs out of the reach of children. In case of overdose, call your doctor, hospital or poison control center immediately.
5. This leaflet provides a summary of the most important information about estrogens. If you want more information, ask your doctor or pharmacist to show you the professional labeling. The professional labeling is also published in a book called the "Physicians' Desk Reference," which is available in book stores and public libraries. Generic drugs carry virtually the same labeling information as their brand name versions.

HOW SUPPLIED

ESTRACE® (ESTRADIOL VAGINAL CREAM, USP, 0.01%).
NDC 0430-3754-14: Tube containing 1½ oz (42.5 g) with a calibrated plastic applicator for delivery of 1, 2, 3, or 4 g.
NDC 0430-3754-11: Carton containing four 0.42 oz (12 g) refill tubes.
NOTE: The number of doses per tube will vary with dosage requirements and patient handling.
Store at room temperature. Protect from temperatures in excess of 40°C (104°F).

Manufactured by:
Bristol-Myers
Squibb Company
Princeton, NJ 08543
Manufactured for:
Warner Chilcott, Inc.
100 Enterprise Drive
Rockaway, NJ 08766
Revised: June 2000 J4690 or 03-6052
3754G010

NATACHEW™ ℞

CHEWABLE PRENATAL MULTIVITAMIN TABLET WITH IRON

Each wildberry-flavored chewable tablet contains:

VITAMINS	
Vitamin A (as beta-carotene)	1000 IU
Vitamin D_3 (cholecalciferol)	400 IU
Vitamin E (dl-alpha tocopheryl acetate)	11 IU
Vitamin C (as sodium ascorbate and ascorbic acid)	120 mg
Folic Acid	1 mg
Thiamine Mononitrate (vitamin B_1)	2 mg
Riboflavin (vitamin B_2)	3 mg
Niacinamide	20 mg
Vitamin B_6 (pyridoxine HCl)	10 mg
Vitamin B_{12} (cyanocobalamin)	12 mcg
MINERAL	
Iron (as ferrous fumarate)	29 mg

INDICATIONS

To provide vitamin and mineral supplementation throughout pregnancy and during the postnatal period, for both the lactating and non-lactating mother. It is also useful for improving nutritional status prior to conception.

DOSAGE

One tablet daily, or as directed by a physician.

WARNING: Accidental overdose of iron-containing products is a leading cause of fatal poisoning in children under 6. Keep this product out of the reach of children. In case of accidental overdose, call a doctor or poison control center immediately.

CAUTION: Folic acid may partially correct the hematological damage due to Vitamin B_{12} deficiency of pernicious anemia, while the associated neurological damage progresses. In rare instances, allergic hypersensitivity has been reported following administration of folic acid.

HOW SUPPLIED

NataChew Tablets are round, tan, speckled and wildberry flavored. They are debossed "WC" with a bisect on one side and "227" on the other side. NataChew Tablets are supplied as follows: N 0430-0227-23, bottles of 90 tablets.
DISPENSE: In a tight, light-resistant container as defined by the USP.
STORAGE: Store at controlled room temperature 15°–30°C (59°–86°F). Protect from moisture and excessive heat. Note that contact with moisture may produce surface discoloration of the tablet.
KEEP THIS AND ALL MEDICATIONS OUT OF THE REACH OF CHILDREN.

Rx only
Issued 9/99
Manufactured by: Amide Pharmaceutical, Inc.
Little Falls, NJ 07424
Manufactured for: Warner Chilcott, Inc.
100 Enterprise Drive Rockaway, NJ 07866 USA
0227C010
US Patent 4,684,534 Patent Pending

OVCON® 35 0.4/35 ℞

[ov-cŏn]

OVCON® 50

(NORETHINDRONE AND ETHINYL ESTRADIOL TABLETS, USP)
21- and 28-DAY REGIMENS
Rx only

Patients should be counseled that this product does not protect against HIV-infection (AIDS) and other sexually transmitted diseases.

DESCRIPTION

21-Day OVCON® 35 provides a regimen for oral contraception derived from 21 tablets composed of norethindrone and ethinyl estradiol. The chemical name for norethindrone is 17-hydroxy-19-nor-17α-pregn-4-en-20-yn-3-one and for ethinyl estradiol the chemical name is 19-nor-17α-pregna-1,3,5 (10)-trien-20-yne-3,17-diol.
28-Day OVCON® 35 and OVCON® 50 (norethindrone and ethinyl estradiol tablets, USP) provide a continuous regimen for oral contraception derived from 21 tablets composed of norethindrone and ethinyl estradiol to be followed by 7 green tablets of inert ingredients. The structural formulas are:

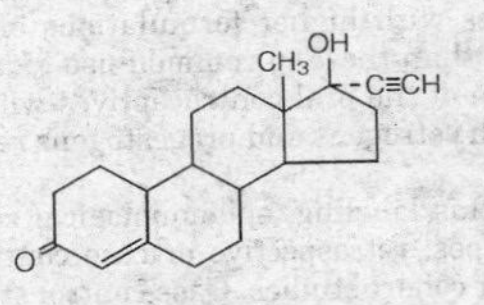

NORETHINDRONE

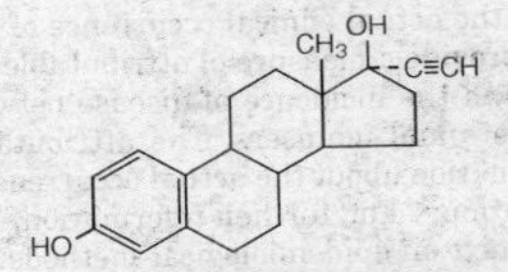

ETHINYL ESTRADIOL

The active OVCON 35 tablets contain 0.4 mg norethindrone and 0.035 mg ethinyl estradiol. The active OVCON 50 tablets contain 1 mg norethindrone and 0.05 mg ethinyl estradiol.
The green tablets contain inert ingredients.
OVCON 35, 21-Day contains the following inactive ingredients: dibasic calcium phosphate, FD&C Yellow No. 6 (aluminum lake), lactose, magnesium stearate, povidone, sodium starch glycolate.
OVCON 35, 28-Day contains the following inactive ingredients: acacia, dibasic calcium phosphate, D&C Yellow No. 10 (aluminum lake), FD&C Blue No. 1 (aluminum lake), FD&C Yellow No. 6 (aluminum lake), lactose, magnesium stearate, povidone, sodium starch glycolate, starch (corn), and talc.
OVCON 50, 28-Day contains the following inactive ingredients: acacia, dibasic calcium phosphate, D&C Yellow No. 10 (aluminum lake), FD&C Blue No. 1 (aluminum lake), FD&C Yellow No. 6 (aluminum lake), lactose, magnesium stearate, povidone, sodium starch glycolate, starch (corn), and talc.

CLINICAL PHARMACOLOGY

Combination oral contraceptives act by suppression of gonadotropins. Although the primary mechanism of this action is inhibition of ovulation, other alterations include changes in the cervical mucus (which increase the difficulty of sperm entry into the uterus) and the endometrium (which reduce the likelihood of implantation).

INDICATIONS AND USAGE

Oral contraceptives are indicated for the prevention of pregnancy in women who elect to use this product as a method of contraception. Oral contraceptive products such as OVCON 50, 28-Day, which contain 50 mcg of estrogen, should not be used unless medically indicated.
Oral contraceptives are highly effective. Table 1 lists the typical accidental pregnancy rates for users of combination oral contraceptives and other methods of contraception. The efficacy of these contraceptive methods, except sterilization, depends upon the reliability with which they are used. Correct and consistent use of methods can result in lower failure rates.
[See table at top of next page]

CONTRAINDICATIONS

Oral contraceptives should not be used in women who currently have the following conditions:

- Thrombophlebitis or thromboembolic disorders
- A past history of deep vein thrombophlebitis or thromboembolic disorders

Continued on next page

Ovcon—Cont.

- Cerebrovascular or coronary artery disease
- Known or suspected carcinoma of the breast
- Carcinoma of the endometrium or other known or suspected estrogen-dependent neoplasia
- Undiagnosed abnormal genital bleeding
- Cholestatic jaundice of pregnancy or jaundice with prior pill use
- Hepatic adenomas or carcinomas
- Known or suspected pregnancy

WARNINGS

Cigarette smoking increases the risk of serious cardiovascular side effects from oral contraceptive use. This risk increases with age and with heavy smoking (15 or more cigarettes per day) and is quite marked in women over 35 years of age. Women who use oral contraceptives should be strongly advised not to smoke.

The use of oral contraceptives is associated with increased risk of several serious conditions including myocardial infarction, thromboembolism, stroke, hepatic neoplasia, and gallbladder disease, although the risk of serious morbidity or mortality is very small in healthy women without underlying risk factors. The risk of morbidity and mortality increases significantly in the presence of other underlying risk factors such as hypertension, hyperlipidemias, obesity and diabetes.

Practitioners prescribing oral contraceptives should be familiar with the following information relating to these risks.

The information contained in this package insert is principally based on studies carried out in patients who used oral contraceptives with higher formulations of estrogens and progestogens than those in common use today. The effect of long-term use of the oral contraceptives with lower formulations of both estrogens and progestogens remains to be determined.

Throughout this labeling, epidemiological studies reported are of two types: retrospective or case control studies and prospective or cohort studies. Case control studies provide a measure of the relative risk of a disease, namely, a *ratio* of the incidence of a disease among oral contraceptive users to that among nonusers. The relative risk does not provide information on the actual clinical occurrence of a disease. Cohort studies provide a measure of attributable risk, which is the *difference* in the incidence of disease between oral contraceptive users and nonusers. The attributable risk does provide information about the actual occurrence of a disease in the population.* For further information, the reader is referred to a text on epidemiological methods.

*Adapted from Stadel BB: Oral contraceptives and cardiovascular disease. *N Engl J Med*, 1981;305:612–618, 672–677; with author's permission.

1. THROMBOEMBOLIC DISORDERS AND OTHER VASCULAR PROBLEMS

The physician should be alert to the earliest manifestations of thromboembolic thrombotic disorders as discussed below. Should any of these occur or be suspected the drug should be discontinued immediately.

a. Myocardial Infarction

An increased risk of myocardial infarction has been attributed to oral contraceptive use. This risk is primarily in smokers or women with other underlying risk factors for coronary artery disease such as hypertension, hypercholesterolemia, morbid obesity, and diabetes. The relative risk of heart attack for current oral contraceptive users has been estimated to be two to six. The risk is very low under the age of 30.

Smoking in combination with oral contraceptive use has been shown to contribute substantially to the incidence of myocardial infarctions in women in their mid-thirties or older, with smoking accounting for the majority of excess cases. Mortality rates associated with circulatory disease have been shown to increase substantially in smokers over the age of 35 and nonsmokers over the age of 40 (Figure 1) among women who use oral contraceptives.

FIGURE 1
CIRCULATORY DISEASE MORTALITY RATES PER 100,000 WOMEN-YEARS BY AGE, SMOKING STATUS AND ORAL CONTRACEPTIVE USE

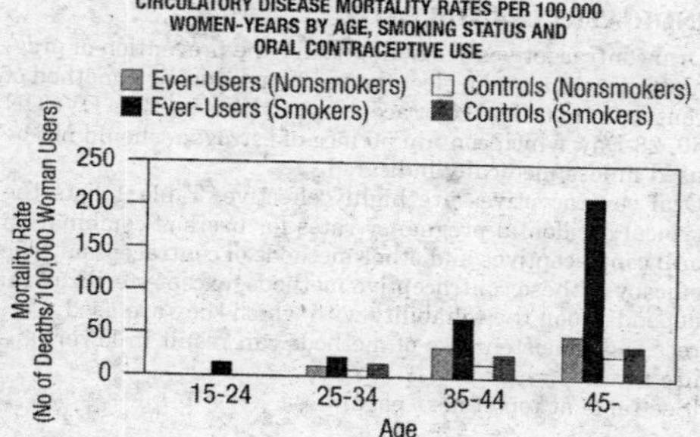

Layde PM, Beral V: Further analyses of mortality in oral contraceptive users: Royal College of General Practitioners' oral contraception study. (Table 5) *Lancet* 1981;1:541–546.

Oral contraceptives may compound the effects of well-known risk factors, such as hypertension, diabetes, hyperlipidemias, age, and obesity. In particular, some progestogens are known to decrease HDL cholesterol and cause glucose intolerance, while estrogens may create a state of hyperinsulinism. Oral contraceptives have been shown to increase blood pressure among users (see section 9 in Warnings). Such increases in risk factors have been associated with an increased risk of heart disease and the risk increases with the number of risk factors present. Oral contraceptives must be used with caution in women with cardiovascular disease risk factors.

b. Thromboembolism

An increased risk of thromboembolic and thrombotic disease associated with the use of oral contraceptives is well established. Case control studies have found the relative risk of users compared to non-users to be 3 for the first episode of superficial venous thrombosis, 4 to 11 for deep vein thrombosis or pulmonary embolism, and 1.5 to 6 for women with predisposing conditions for venous thromboembolic disease. Cohort studies have been shown the relative risk to be somewhat lower, about 3 for new cases and about 4.5 for new cases requiring hospitalization. The risk of thromboembolic disease due to oral contraceptives is not related to length of use and disappears after pill use is stopped.

A two- to four-fold increase in relative risk of postoperative thromboembolic complications has been reported with the use of oral contraceptives. The relative risk of venous thrombosis in women who have predisposing conditions is twice that of women without such medical conditions. If feasible, oral contraceptives should be discontinued at least four weeks prior to and for two weeks after elective surgery of a type associated with an increase in risk of thromboembolism and during and following prolonged immobilization. Since the immediate postpartum period is also associated with an increased risk of thromboembolism, oral contraceptives should be started no earlier than four to six weeks after delivery in women who elect not to breastfeed.

c. Cerebrovascular diseases

Oral contraceptives have been shown to increase both the relative and attributable risk of cerebrovascular events (thrombotic and hemorrhagic strokes); although, in general, the risk is greatest among older (>35 years), hypertensive women who also smoke. Hypertension was found to be a risk factor for both users and nonusers, for both types of strokes, while smoking interacted to increase the risk for hemorrhagic strokes.

In a large study, the relative risk of thrombotic strokes has been shown to range from 3 for normotensive users to 14 for users with severe hypertension. The relative risk of hemorrhagic stroke is reported to be 1.2 for nonsmokers who used oral contraceptives, 2.6 for smokers who did not use oral contraceptives, 7.6 for smokers who used oral contraceptives, 1.8 for normotensive users and 25.7 for users with severe hypertension. The attributable risk is also greater in older women.

d. Dose-related risk of vascular disease from oral contraceptives

A positive association has been observed between the amount of estrogen and progestogen in oral contraceptives and the risk of vascular disease. A decline in serum high density lipoproteins (HDL) has been reported with many progestational agents. A decline in serum high density lipoproteins has been associated with an increased incidence of ischemic heart disease. Because estrogens increase HDL cholesterol, the net effect of an oral contraceptive depends on a balance achieved between doses of estrogen and progestogen and the nature and absolute amount of progestogens used in the contraceptive. The amount of both hormones should be considered in the choice of an oral contraceptive.

Minimizing exposure to estrogen and progestogen is in keeping with good principles of therapeutics. For any particular estrogen/progestogen combination, the dosage regimen prescribed should be one which contains the least amount of estrogen and progestogen that is compatible with a low failure rate and the needs of the individual patient. New acceptors of oral contraceptive agents should be started on preparations containing 0.05 mg or less of estrogen. Products containing 50 mcg estrogen should be used only when medically indicated.

e. Persistence of risk

There are two studies which have shown persistence of risk of vascular disease for ever-users of oral contraceptives. In a study in the United States, the risk of developing myocardial infarction after discontinuing oral contraceptives persists for at least 9 years for women 40–49 years old who had used oral contraceptives for five or more years, but this increased risk was not demonstrated in other age groups. In another study in Great Britain, the risk of developing cerebrovascular disease persisted for at least 6 years after discontinuation of oral contraceptives, although excess risk was very small. However, both studies were performed with oral contraceptive formulations containing 50 micrograms or higher of estrogens.

2. ESTIMATES OF MORTALITY FROM CONTRACEPTIVE USE

One study gathered data from a variety of sources which have estimated the mortality rate associated with different methods of contraception at different ages (Table 2).

[See table at top of next page]

These estimates include the combined risk of death associated with contraceptive methods plus the risk attributable to pregnancy in the event of method failure. Each method of contraception has its specific benefits and risk. The study concluded that with the exception of oral contraceptive users 35 and older who smoke and 40 and older who do not smoke, mortality associated with all methods of birth control is low and below that associated with childbirth.

The observation of a possible increase in risk of mortality with age for oral contraceptive users is based on data gathered in the 1970s–but not reported until 1983. However, current clinical practice involves the use of lower estrogen dose formulations combined with careful restriction of oral contraceptive use to women who do not have the various risk factors listed in this labeling.

Because of these changes in practice and, also, because of some limited new data which suggest that the risk of cardiovascular disease with the use of oral contraceptives may now be less than previously observed (Porter JB, Hunter J, Jick H, et al. Oral contraceptives and nonfatal vascular disease. *Obstet Gynecol* 1985;66:1–4 and Porter JB, Jick H, Walker AM. Mortality among oral contraceptive users. *Obstet Gynecol* 1987;70:29–32), the Fertility and Maternal Health Drugs Advisory Committee was asked to review the topic in 1989. The Committee concluded that although car-

TABLE 1
LOWEST EXPECTED AND TYPICAL FAILURE RATES DURING THE FIRST YEAR OF CONTINUOUS USE OF A METHOD
% of Women Experiencing an Accidental Pregnancy in the First Year of Continuous Use

Method	Lowest Expected*	Typical**
(No contraception)	(85)	(85)
Oral contraceptives		
combined	0.1	3***
progestin only	0.5	3***
Diaphragm with spermicidal cream or jelly	6	18
Spermicides alone (foam, creams, jellies and vaginal suppositories)	3	21
Vaginal sponge		
nulliparous	6	18
multiparous	9	28
IUD	0.8–2.0	3#
Condom without spermicides	2	12
Periodic abstinence (all methods)	1–9	20
Injectable progestogen	0.3–0.4	0.3–0.4
Implants		
6 capsules	0.04	0.04
2 rods	0.03	0.03
Female sterilization	0.2	0.4
Male sterilization	0.1	0.15

Reproduced with permission of the Population Council from J. Trussel, et al: Contraceptive failure in the United States: An update. Studies in Family Planning, 21(1), January-February 1990.

*The authors' best guess of the percentage of women expected to experience an accidental pregnancy among couples who initiate a method (not necessarily for the first time) and who use it consistently and correctly during the first year if they do not stop for any reason other than pregnancy.

**This term represents "typical" couples who initiate use of a method (not necessarily for the first time), who experience an accidental pregnancy during the first year if they do not stop use for any reason other than pregnancy.

***Combined typical rate for both combined and progestin only.

#Combined typical rate for both medicated and nonmedicated IUD.

diovascular disese risk may be increased with oral contraceptive use after age 40 in healthy nonsmoking women (even with the newer low-dose formulations), there are greater potential health risks associated with pregnancy in older women and with the alternative surgical and medical procedures which may be necessary if such women do not have access to effective and acceptable means of contraception.

Therefore, the Committee recommended that the benefits of oral contraceptive use by healthy nonsmoking women over 40 may outweigh the possible risks. Of course, older women, as all women who take oral contraceptives, should take the lowest possible dose formulation that is effective.

3. CARCINOMA OF THE REPRODUCTIVE ORGANS

Numerous epidemiological studies have been performed on the incidence of breast, endometrial, ovarian, and cervical cancer in women using oral contraceptives. The overwhelming evidence in the literature suggests that use of oral contraceptives is not associated with an increase in the risk of developing breast cancer, regardless of the age and parity of first use or with most of the marketed brands and doses. The Cancer and Steroid Hormone (CASH) study also showed no latent effect on the risk of breast cancer for at least a decade following long-term use. A few studies have shown a slightly increased relative risk of developing breast cancer, although the methodology of these studies, which included differences in examination of users and nonusers and differences in age at start of use, has been questioned. Some studies suggest that oral contraceptive use has been associated with an increase in the risk of cervical intraepithelial neoplasia in some populations of women.

However, there continues to be controversy about the extent to which such findings may be due to differences in sexual behavior and other factors.

In spite of many studies of the relationship between oral contraceptive use and breast cancer and cervical cancers, a cause-and-effect relationship has not been established.

4. HEPATIC NEOPLASIA

Benign hepatic adenomas are associated with oral contraceptive use, although their occurrence is rare in the United States. Indirect calculations have estimated the attributable risk to be in the range of 3.3 cases/100,000 for users, a risk that increases after four or more years of use. Rupture of hepatic adenomas may cause death through intra-abdominal hemorrhage.

Studies from Britain have shown an increased risk of developing hepatocellular carcinoma in long-term (>8 years) oral contraceptive users. However, these cancers are extremely rare in the U.S. and the attributable risk (the excess incidence) of liver cancers in oral contraceptive users approaches less than one per million users.

5. OCULAR LESIONS

There have been clinical case reports of retinal thrombosis associated with the use of oral contraceptives. Oral contraceptives should be discontinued if there is unexplained partial or complete loss of vision; onset of proptosis or diplopia; papilledema; or retinal vascular lesions. Appropriate diagnostic and therapeutic measures should be undertaken immediately.

6. ORAL CONTRACEPTIVE USE BEFORE OR DURING EARLY PREGNANCY

Extensive epidemiological studies have revealed no increased risk of birth defects in women who have used oral contraceptives prior to pregnancy. Studies also do not suggest a teratogenic effect, particularly in so far as cardiac anomalies and limb reduction defects are concerned, when taken inadvertently during early pregnancy.

The administration of oral contraceptives to induce withdrawal bleeding should not be used as a test for pregnancy. Oral contraceptives should not be used during pregnancy to treat threatened or habitual abortion.

It is recommended that for any patient who has missed two consecutive periods, pregnancy should be ruled out before continuing oral contraceptive use. If the patient has not adhered to the prescribed schedule, the possibility of pregnancy should be considered at the time of the first missed period. Oral contraceptive use should be discontinued if pregnancy is confirmed.

7. GALLBLADDER DISEASE

Earlier studies have reported an increased lifetime relative risk of gallbladder surgery in users of oral contraceptives and estrogens. More recent studies, however, have shown that the relative risk of developing gallbladder disease among oral contraceptive users may be minimal.

The recent findings of minimal risk may be related to the use of oral contraceptive formulations containing lower hormonal doses of estrogens and progestogens.

8. CARBOHYDRATE AND LIPID METABOLIC EFFECTS

Oral contraceptives have been shown to cause glucose intolerance in a significant percentage of users. Oral contraceptives containing greater than 75 micrograms of estrogens cause hyperinsulinism, while lower doses of estrogen cause less glucose intolerance. Progestogens increase insulin secretion and create insulin resistance, this effect varying with different progestational agents.

However, in the nondiabetic woman, oral contraceptives appear to have no effect on fasting blood glucose. Because of these demonstrated effects, prediabetic and diabetic women should be carefully observed while taking oral contraceptives.

A small proportion of women will have persistent hypertriglyceridemia while on the pill. As discussed earlier (see Warnings 1.a. and 1.d.), changes in serum triglycerides and lipoprotein levels have been reported in oral contraceptive users.

TABLE 2
ANNUAL NUMBER OF BIRTH-RELATED OR METHOD-RELATED DEATHS ASSOCIATED WITH CONTROL OF FERTILITY PER 100,000 NONSTERILE WOMEN, BY FERTILITY CONTROL METHOD ACCORDING TO AGE

Method of control and outcome	AGE 15–19	20–24	25–29	30–34	35–39	40–44
No fertility control methods*	7.0	7.4	9.1	14.8	25.7	28.2
Oral contraceptives nonsmoker**	0.3	0.5	0.9	1.9	13.8	31.6
Oral contraceptives smoker**	2.2	3.4	6.6	13.5	51.1	117.2
IUD**	0.8	0.8	1.0	1.0	1.4	1.4
Condom*	1.1	1.6	0.7	0.2	0.3	0.4
Diaphragm/spermicide*	1.9	1.2	1.2	1.3	2.2	2.8
Periodic abstinence*	2.5	1.6	1.6	1.7	2.9	3.6

*Deaths are birth related
**Deaths are method related

Ory HW: Mortality associated with fertility and fertility control: 1983. *Fam Plann Perspect* 1983; 15:50–56.

9. ELEVATED BLOOD PRESSURE

An increase in blood pressure has been reported in women taking oral contraceptives and this increase is more likely in older oral contraceptive users and with continued use. Data from the Royal College of General Practitioners and subsequent randomized trials have shown that the incidence of hypertension increases with increasing concentrations of progestogens.

Women with a history of hypertension or hypertension-related diseases, or renal disease should be encouraged to use another method of contraception. If women elect to use oral contraceptives, they should be monitored closely and if significant elevation of blood pressure occurs, oral contraceptives should be discontinued. For most women, elevated blood pressure will return to normal after stopping oral contraceptives, and there is no difference in the occurrence of hypertension among ever- and never-users.

10. HEADACHE

The onset or exacerbation of migraine or development of headache with a new pattern which is recurrent, persistent, or severe requires discontinuation of oral contraceptives and evaluation of the cause.

11. BLEEDING IRREGULARITIES

Breakthrough bleeding and spotting are sometimes encountered in patients on oral contraceptives, especially during the first three months of use. Nonhormonal causes should be considered and adequate diagnostic measures taken to rule out malignancy or pregnancy in the event of breakthrough bleeding, as in the case of any abnormal vaginal bleeding. If pathology has been excluded, time or a change to another formulation may solve the problem. In the event of amenorrhea, pregnancy should be ruled out.

Women with a history of oligomenorrhea or secondary amenorrhea or young women without regular cycles prior to taking oral contraceptives may again have irregular bleeding or amenorrhea after discontinuation of oral contraceptives.

PRECAUTIONS

1. SEXUALLY-TRANSMITTED DISEASES

Patients should be counseled that this product does not protect against HIV infection (AIDS) and other sexually transmitted diseases.

2. PHYSICAL EXAMINATION AND FOLLOW-UP

It is good medical practice for all women to have annual history and physical examinations, including women using oral contraceptives. The physical examination, however, may be deferred until after initiation of oral contraceptives if requested by the woman and judged appropriate by the clinician. The physical examination should include special reference to blood pressure, breasts, abdomen and pelvic organs, including cervical cytology, and relevant laboratory tests. In case of undiagnosed, persistent or recurrent abnormal vaginal bleeding, appropriate measures should be conducted to rule out malignancy. Women with a strong family history of breast cancer or who have breast nodules should be monitored with particular care.

3. LIPID DISORDERS

Women who are being treated for hyperlipidemias should be followed closely if they elect to use oral contraceptives. Some progestogens may elevate LDL levels and may render the control of hyperlipidemias more difficult.

4. LIVER FUNCTION

If jaundice develops in any woman receiving such drugs, the medication should be discontinued. Steroid hormones may be poorly metabolized in patients with impaired liver function.

5. FLUID RETENTION

Oral contraceptives may cause some degree of fluid retention. They should be prescribed with caution, and only with carefuly monitoring, in patients with conditions which might be aggravated by fluid retention.

6. EMOTIONAL DISORDERS

Women with a history of depression should be carefully observed and the drug discontinued if depression recurs to a serious degree.

Patients becoming significantly depressed while taking oral contraceptives should stop the medication and use an alternate method of contraception in an attempt to determine whether the symptom is drug related.

7. CONTACT LENSES

Contact lens wearers who develop visual changes or changes in lens tolerance should be assessed by an ophthalmologist.

8. DRUG INTERACTIONS

Reduced efficacy and increased incidence of breakthrough bleeding and menstrual irregularities have been associated with concomitant use of rifampin. A similar association, though less marked, has been suggested with barbiturates, phenylbutazone, phenytoin sodium, and possibly with griseofulvin, ampicillin, and tetracyclines.

9. INTERACTIONS WITH LABORATORY TESTS

Certain endocrine and liver function tests and blood components may be affected by oral contraceptives:

a. Increased prothrombin and factors VII, VIII, IX, and X; decreased antithrombin 3; increased norepinephrine-induced platelet aggregability.

b. Increased thyroid-binding globulin (TBG) leading to increased circulating total thyroid hormone, as measured by protein-bound iodine (PBI), T4 by column or by radioimmunoassay. Free T3 resin uptake is decreased, reflecting the elevated TBG, free T4 concentration is unaltered.

c. Other binding proteins may be elevated in serum.

d. Sex-binding globulins are increased and result in elevated levels of total circulating sex steroids and corticoids; however, free or biologically active levels remain unchanged.

e. Triglycerides may be increased.

f. Glucose tolerance may be decreased.

g. Serum folate levels may be depressed by oral contraceptive therapy. This may be of clinical significance if a woman becomes pregnant shortly after discontinuing oral contraceptives.

10. CARCINOGENESIS

See **WARNINGS** section.

11. PREGNANCY

Pregnancy Category X. See **CONTRAINDICATIONS** and **WARNINGS** sections.

12. NURSING MOTHERS

Small amounts of oral contraceptive steroids have been identified in the milk of nursing mothers and a few adverse effects on the child have been reported, including jaundice and breast enlargement. In addition, oral contraceptives given in the postpartum period may interfere with lactation by decreasing the quantity and quality of breast milk. If possible, the nursing mother should be advised not to use oral contraceptives but to use other forms of contraception until she has completely weaned her child.

13. VOMITING AND/OR DIARRHEA

Although a cause-and-effect relationship has not been clearly established, several cases of oral contraceptive failure have been reported in association with vomiting and/or diarrhea. If significant gastrointestinal disturbance occurs in any woman receiving contraceptive steroids, the use of a back-up method of contraception for the remainder of that cycle is recommended.

14. PEDIATRIC USE

Safety and efficacy of OVCON® 35 and OVCON® 50 have been established in women of reproductive age. Safety and efficacy are expected to be the same in postpubertal adolescents under the age of 16 years and in users ages 16 years and older. Use of this product before menarche is not indicated.

INFORMATION FOR THE PATIENT

See Patient Labeling Printed Below

ADVERSE REACTIONS

An increased risk of the following serious adverse reactions has been associated with the use of oral contraceptives (see Warnings section):

- Thrombophlebitis
- Arterial thromboembolism
- Pulmonary embolism
- Myocardial infarction
- Cerebral hemorrhage
- Cerebral thrombosis
- Hypertension
- Gallbladder disease
- Hepatic adenomas or benign liver tumors

Continued on next page

Ovcon—Cont.

There is evidence of an association between the following conditions and the use of oral contraceptives, although additional confirmatory studies are needed:

- Mesenteric thrombosis
- Retinal thrombosis

The following adverse reactions have been reported in patients receiving oral contraceptives and are believed to be drug related:

- Nausea
- Vomiting
- Gastrointestinal symptoms (such as abdominal cramps and bloating)
- Breakthrough bleeding
- Spotting
- Change in menstrual flow
- Amenorrhea
- Temporary infertility after discontinuation of treatment
- Edema
- Melasma which may persist
- Breast changes: tenderness, enlargement, and secretion
- Change in weight (increase or decrease)
- Change in cervical ectropion and secretion
- Possible diminution in lactation when given immediately postpartum
- Cholestatic jaundice
- Migraine
- Rash (allergic)
- Mental depression
- Reduced tolerance to carbohydrates
- Vaginal candidiasis
- Change in corneal curvature (steepening)
- Intolerance to contact lenses

The following adverse reactions have been reported in users of oral contraceptives, and the association has been neither confirmed nor refuted:

- Premenstrual syndrome
- Cataracts
- Changes in appetite
- Cystitis-like syndrome
- Headache
- Nervousness
- Dizziness
- Hirsutism
- Loss of scalp hair
- Erythema multiforme
- Erythema nodosum
- Hemorrhagic eruption
- Vaginitis
- Porphyria
- Impaired renal function
- Hemolytic uremic syndrome
- Budd/Chiari syndrome
- Acne
- Changes in libido
- Colitis

OVERDOSAGE

Serious ill effects have not been reported following acute ingestion of large doses of oral contraceptives by young children. Overdosage may cause nausea, and withdrawal bleeding may occur in females.

NONCONTRACEPTIVE HEALTH EFFECTS

The following noncontraceptive health benefits related to the use of oral contraceptives are supported by epidemiological studies which largely utilized oral contraceptive formulations containing estrogen doses exceeding 0.035 mg of ethinyl estradiol or 0.05 mg of mestranol.

Effects on menses:

- Increased menstrual cycle regularity
- Decreased blood loss and decreased incidence of iron deficiency anemia
- Decreased incidence of dysmenorrhea

Effects related to inhibition of ovulation:

- Decreased incidence of functional ovarian cysts
- Decreased incidence of ectopic pregnancies

Effects from long-term use:

- Decreased incidence of fibroadenomas and fibrocystic disease of the breast
- Decreased incidence of acute pelvic inflammatory disease
- Decreased incidence of endometrial cancer
- Decreased incidence of ovarian cancer

DOSAGE AND ADMINISTRATION

The following is a summary of the instructions given to the patient in the "HOW TO TAKE THE PILL" section of the DETAILED PATIENT PACKAGE INSERT.

The patient is given instructions in five (5) categories.

1. IMPORTANT POINTS TO REMEMBER: The patient is told (a) that she should take one pill every day at the same time, (b) many women have spotting or light bleeding or gastric distress during the first one to three cycles, (c) missing pills can also cause spotting or light bleeding, (d) she should use a back-up method for contraception if she has vomiting or diarrhea or takes some concomitant medications, and/or if she has trouble remembering the pill, (e) if she has any other questions, she should consult her physician.
2. BEFORE SHE STARTS TAKING HER PILLS: She should decide what time of day she wishes to take the pill, check whether her pill pack has 21 or 28 pills, and note the order in which she should take the pills (diagrammatic drawings of the pill pack are included in the patient insert).
3. WHEN SHE SHOULD START THE FIRST PACK: The Day-One start is listed as the first choice and the Sunday start (the Sunday after her period starts) is given as the second choice. If she uses the Sunday start she should use a back-up method in the first cycle if she has intercourse before she has taken seven pills.
4. WHAT TO DO DURING THE CYCLE: The patient is advised to take one pill at the same time every day until the pack is empty. If she is on a 21-day regimen, she should wait seven days to start the next pack. If she is on the 28-day regimen, she should start the next pack the day after the last inactive tablet and not wait any days between packs.
5. WHAT TO DO IF SHE MISSES A PILL OR PILLS: The patient is given instructions about what she should do if she misses one, two or more than two pills at varying times in her cycle for both the Day-One and the Sunday start. The patient is warned that she may become pregnant if she has unprotected intercourse in the seven days after missing pills. To avoid this, she must use another birth control method such as condom, foam, or sponge in these seven days.

HOW SUPPLIED

OVCON® 35 (norethindrone and ethinyl estradiol tablets, USP) is available in 21- and 28-day regimens. Each package contains 21 round, peach tablets of 0.4 mg norethindrone and 0.035 mg ethinyl estradiol, imprinted with **MJ** on one side and **583** on the other. Each round, green tablet in the 28-day regimen contains inert ingredients and is imprinted with **MJ** on one side and **850** on the other.

OVCON 35, 21-Day
NDC 0430-0583-11 Carton of 6 compacts

OVCON 35, 28-Day
NDC 0430-0582-14 Carton of 6 compacts

OVCON® 50 (norethindrone and ethinyl estradiol tablets, USP) is available in 28-day regimens. Each package contains 21 round, yellow tablets of 1.0 mg norethindrone and 0.05 mg ethinyl estradiol, imprinted with **MJ** on one side and **584** on the other. Each round, green tablet in the 28-day regimen contains inert ingredients and is imprinted with **MJ** on one side and **850** on the other.

OVCON 50, 28-Day
NDC 0430-0585-14 Carton of 6 compacts

Store below 30° C (86° F).

References are available upon request.

PATIENT PACKAGE INSERT BRIEF SUMMARY

This product (like all oral contraceptives) is intended to prevent pregnancy. It does not protect against HIV infection (AIDS) and other sexually transmitted diseases.

Oral contraceptives, also known as "birth control pills" or "the pill," are taken to prevent pregnancy and when taken correctly, have a failure rate of about 1% per year when used without missing any pills. The typical failure rate of large numbers of pill users is less than 3% per year when women who miss pills are included.

Oral contraceptive use is associated with certain serious diseases that can be life-threatening or may cause temporary or permanent disability. The risks associated with taking oral contraceptives increase significantly if you:

- Smoke
- Have high blood pressure, diabetes, high cholesterol
- Have or have had clotting disorders, heart attack, stroke, angina pectoris, cancer of the breast or sex organs, jaundice or malignant or benign liver tumors.

You should not take the pill if you suspect you are pregnant or have unexplained vaginal bleeding.

Cigarette smoking increases the risk of serious cardiovascular side effects from oral contraceptive use. This risk increases with age and with heavy smoking (15 or more cigarettes per day) and is quite marked in women over 35 years of age. Women who use oral contraceptives are strongly advised not to smoke.

Most side effects of the pill are not serious. The most common such effects are nausea, vomiting, bleeding between menstrual period, weight gain, breast tenderness, and difficulty wearing contact lenses. These side effects, especially nausea and vomiting, may subside within the first three months of use.

The serious side effects of the pill occur very infrequently, especially if you are in good health and are young. However, you should know that the following medical conditions have been associated with or made worse by the pill:

1. Blood clots in the legs (thrombophlebitis), lungs (pulmonary embolism), stoppage or rupture of a blood vessel in the brain (stroke), blockage of blood vessels in the heart (heart attack or angina pectoris), or other organs of the body. As mentioned above, smoking increases the risk of heart attacks and strokes and subsequent serious medical consequences.
2. Liver tumors, which may rupture and cause severe bleeding. A possible but not definite association has been found with the pill and liver cancer. However, liver cancers are extremely rare. The chance of developing liver cancer from using the pill is thus even rarer.
3. High blood pressure, although blood pressure usually returns to normal when the pill is stopped.

The symptoms associated with these serious side effects are discussed in the detailed leaflet given to you with your supply of pills. Notify your doctor or health care provider if you notice any unusual physical disturbances while taking the pill. In addition, drugs such as rifampin, as well as some anticonvulsants and some antibiotics may decrease oral contraceptive effectiveness.

Studies to date of women taking the pill have not shown an increase in the incidence of cancer of the breast or cervix. There is, however, insufficient evidence to rule out the possibility that the pill may cause such cancers.

Taking the pill provides some important noncontraceptive effects. These include less painful menstruation, less menstrual blood loss and anemia, fewer pelvic infections, and fewer cancers of the ovary and the lining of the uterus.

Be sure to discuss any medical condition you may have with your health care provider. Your health care provider will take a medical and family history before prescribing oral contraceptives and will examine you. The physical examination may be delayed to another time if you request it and the health care provider believes that it is a good medical practice to postpone it. You should be reexamined at least once a year while taking oral contraceptives. The detailed patient information booklet gives you further information which you should read and discuss with your health care professional.

DOSAGE AND ADMINISTRATION

HOW TO TAKE THE PILL

The instructions given in the DETAILED PATIENT PACKAGE INSERT are also given in the **BRIEF SUMMARY** included inside each compact. In the event the patient may read only the brief summary, these instructions include the directions on starting the first pack on Day-One (first choice) of her period and the Sunday start (Sunday after period starts). The patient is advised that, if she used the Sunday start, she should use a back-up method in the first cycle if she has intercourse before she has taken seven pills. The patient is also instructed as to what she should do if she misses a pill or pills. The patient is warned that she may become pregnant if she misses a pill or pills and that she should use a back-up method of birth control in the event she has intercourse any time during the seven day period following the missed pill or pills.

A diagrammatic drawing of the specific pill pack is included in the **BRIEF SUMMARY**.

PATIENT PACKAGE INSERT

This product (like all oral contraceptives) is intended to prevent pregnancy. It does not protect against HIV infection (AIDS) and other sexually transmitted diseases.

INTRODUCTION

You should not use OVCON 50 (norethindrone and ethinyl estradiol tablets, USP), 28-Day, which contains higher doses of estrogen than other oral contraceptives, unless specifically recommended by your health care provider.

Any woman who considers using oral contraceptives (the birth control pill or the pill) should understand the benefits and risks of using this form of birth control.

Although the oral contraceptives have important advantages over other methods of contraception, they have certain risks that no other method has and some of these risks may continue after you have stopped using the oral contraceptive. This booklet will give you much of the information you will need to make this decision and will also help you determine if you are at risk of developing any of the serious side effects of the pill. It will tell you how to use the pill properly so that it will be as effective as possible. However, this booklet is not a replacement for a careful discussion between you and your health care professional. You should discuss the information provided in this booklet with him or her, both when you first start taking the pill and during your revisits. You should also follow your health care professional's advice with regard to regular check-ups while you are on the pill.

EFFECTIVENESS OF ORAL CONTRACEPTIVES

Oral contraceptives or "birth control pills" or "the pill" are used to prevent pregnancy and are more effective than other nonsurgical methods of birth control. The chance of becoming pregnant is less than 1% (1 pregnancy per 100 women per year of use) when the pills are used correctly and no pills are missed. Typical failure rates are actually 3% per year. The chance of becoming pregnant increases with each missed pill during a menstrual cycle.

In comparison, typical accidental pregnancy rates for other nonsurgical methods of birth control during the first year of use are as follows:

IUD: 3%
Diaphragm with spermicides: 18%
Spermicides alone: 21%
Vaginal sponge: 18% to 28%
Condom alone: 12%
Periodic abstinence: 20%
Injectable progestogen: 0.3% to 0.4%
Implants: 0.03 to 0.04%
No methods: 85%.

WHO SHOULD NOT TAKE ORAL CONTRACEPTIVES

Cigarette smoking increases the risk of serious cardiovascular side effects from oral contraceptive use. This risk increases with age and with heavy smoking (15 or more cigarettes per day) and is quite marked in women over 35 years of age. Women who use oral contraceptives should not smoke.

Some women should not use the pill. For example, you should not take the pill if you are pregnant or think you may be pregnant. You should also not use the pill if you have or have ever had any of the following conditions:

- A history of heart attack or stroke
- Blood clots in the legs (thrombophlebitis), lungs (pulmonary embolism), or eyes
- A history of blood clots in the deep veins of your legs
- Chest pain (angina pectoris)
- Known or suspected breast cancer or cancer of the lining of the uterus
- Unexplained vaginal bleeding (until a diagnosis is reached by your doctor)
- Yellowing of the whites of the eyes or of the skin (jaundice) during pregnancy or during previous use of the pill
- Liver tumor (benign or cancerous)

Tell your health care professional if you have ever had any of these conditions. Your health care professional can recommend a safer method of birth control.

OTHER CONSIDERATIONS BEFORE TAKING ORAL CONTRACEPTIVES

Tell your health care professional if you have:

- Breast nodules, fibrocystic disease of the breast or an abnormal breast x-ray or mammogram
- Diabetes
- Elevated cholesterol or triglycerides
- High blood pressure
- Migraine or other headaches or epilepsy
- Mental depression
- Gallbladder, heart, or kidney disease
- History of scanty or irregular menstrual periods

Women with any of these conditions should be checked often by their health care professional if they choose to use oral contraceptives.

Also, be sure to inform your doctor or health care professional if you smoke or are on any medications.

RISKS OF TAKING ORAL CONTRACEPTIVES

1. Risks of developing blood clots

Blood clots and blockage of blood vessels are the most serious side effects of taking oral contraceptives. In particular, a clot in the legs can cause thrombophlebitis and a clot that travels to the lungs can cause a sudden blocking of the vessel carrying blood to the lungs. Either of these can cause death or disability. Rarely, clots occur in the blood vessels of the eye and may cause blindness, double vision, or impaired vision.

If you take oral contraceptives and need elective surgery, need to stay in bed for a prolonged illness, or have recently delivered a baby, you may be at risk of developing blood clots. You should consult your doctor about stopping oral contraceptives three to four weeks before surgery and not taking oral contraceptives for two weeks after surgery or during bed rest. You should also not take oral contraceptives soon after delivery of a baby. It is advisable to wait for at least four weeks after delivery if you are not breastfeeding. If you are breastfeeding see the section on Breastfeeding in General Precautions.

2. Heart attacks and strokes

Oral contraceptives may increase the tendency to develop strokes (stoppage or rupture of blood vessels in the brain) and angina pectoris and heart attacks (blockage of blood vessels in the heart). Any of these conditions can cause death or disability.

Smoking greatly increases the possibility of suffering heart attacks and strokes. Furthermore, smoking and the use of oral contraceptives greatly increase the chances of developing and dying of heart disease.

3. Gallbladder disease

Oral contraceptive users probably have a greater risk than nonusers of having gallbladder disease, although this risk may be related to pills containing high doses of estrogens.

4. Liver tumors

In rare cases, oral contraceptives can cause benign but dangerous liver tumors. These benign liver tumors can rupture and cause fatal internal bleeding. In addition, a possible, but not definite, association has been found with the pill and liver cancers in two studies, in which a few women who developed these very rare cancers were found to have used oral contraceptives for long periods. However, liver cancers in general are extremely rare and the chance of developing liver cancer from using the pill is thus even rarer.

5. Cancer of the reproductive organs

There is, at present, no confirmed evidence that oral contraceptives increase the risk of cancer of the reproductive organs and breasts in human studies. Several studies have found no overall increase in the risk of developing breast cancer. However, women who use oral contraceptives and have a strong family history of breast cancer, or who have breast nodules or abnormal mammograms, should be closely followed by their doctors.

Some studies have found an increase in the incidence of cancer of the cervix in women who use oral contraceptives. However, this finding may be related to factors other than the use of oral contraceptives.

ESTIMATED RISK OF DEATH FROM A BIRTH CONTROL METHOD OR PREGNANCY

All methods of birth control and pregnancy are associated with a risk of developing certain diseases which may lead to disability or death. An estimate of the number of deaths associated with different methods of birth control and pregnancy has been calculated and is shown in the following table.

[See table above]

ANNUAL NUMBER OF BIRTH-RELATED OR METHOD-RELATED DEATHS ASSOCIATED WITH CONTROL OF FERTILITY PER 100,000 NONSTERILE WOMEN, BY FERTILITY CONTROL METHOD ACCORDING TO AGE

Method of control and outcome	AGE 15–19	20–24	25–29	30–34	35–39	40–44
No fertility control methods*	7.0	7.4	9.1	14.8	25.7	28.2
Oral contraceptives nonsmoker**	0.3	0.5	0.9	1.9	13.8	31.6
Oral contraceptives smoker**	2.2	3.4	6.6	13.5	51.1	117.2
IUD**	0.8	0.8	1.0	1.0	1.4	1.4
Condom*	1.1	1.6	0.7	0.2	0.3	0.4
Diaphragm/spermicide*	1.9	1.2	1.2	1.3	2.2	2.8
Periodic abstinence*	2.5	1.6	1.6	1.7	2.9	3.6

*Deaths are birth related

**Deaths are method related

It can be seen in the table that for women aged 15 to 39, the risk of death was highest with pregnancy (7–26 deaths per 100,000 women, depending on age). Among pill users who do not smoke, the risk of death was always lower than that associated with pregnancy for any age group, although over the age of 40, the risk increases to 32 deaths per 100,000 women, compared to 28 associated with pregnancy at that age. However, for pill users who smoke and are over the age of 35, the estimated number of deaths exceeds those for other methods of birth control. If a women is over the age of 40 and smokes, her estimated risk of death is four times higher (117/100,000 women) than the estimated risk associated with pregnancy (28/100,000 women) in that age group.

The suggestion that women over 40 who don't smoke should not take oral contraceptives is based on information from older high-dose pills and on less selective use of pills than is practiced today.

An Advisory Committee of the FDA discussed this issue in 1989 and recommended that the benefits of oral contraceptive use by healthy, nonsmoking women over 40 years of age may outweigh the possible risks. However, all women, especially older women, are cautioned to use the lowest dose pill that is effective.

In the above table, the risk of death from any birth control method is less than the risk of childbirth, except for oral contraceptive users over the age of 35 who smoke and pill users over the age of 40 even if they do not smoke.

You should discuss this information with your health care professional.

WARNING SIGNALS

If any of these adverse conditions occur while you are taking oral contraceptives, call your doctor immediately:

- Sharp chest pain, coughing of blood, or sudden shortness of breath (indicating a possible clot in the lung)
- Pain in the calf (indicating a possible clot in the leg)
- Crushing chest pain or heaviness in the chest (indicating a possible heart attack)
- Sudden severe headache or vomiting, dizzinesss or fainting, disturbances of vision or speech, weakness, or numbness in an arm or leg (indicating a possible stroke)
- Sudden partial or complete loss of vision (indicating a possible clot in the eye)
- Breast lumps (indicating possible breast cancer or fibrocystic disease of the breast; ask your doctor or health care professional to show you how to examine your breasts)
- Severe pain or tenderness in the stomach area (indicating a possibly ruptured liver tumor)
- Difficulty in sleeping, weakness, lack of energy, fatigue, or change in mood (possibly indicating severe depression)
- Jaundice or a yellowing of the skin or eyeballs, accompanied frequently by fever, fatigue, loss of appetite, dark-colored urine, or light-colored bowel movements (indicating possible liver problems)
- Abnormal vaginal bleeding (See Side Effects of Oral Contraceptives, 1. Vaginal bleeding, below.)

SIDE EFFECTS OF ORAL CONTRACEPTIVES

In addition to the risks and more serious side effects discussed above (See Risks of Taking Oral Contraceptives, Estimated Risk of Death from a Birth Control Method or Pregnancy and Warning Signals section, above.), the following may also occur:

1. Vaginal bleeding

Irregular vaginal bleeding or spotting may occur while you are taking the pills. Irregular bleeding may vary from slight staining between menstrual periods to breakthrough bleeding which is a flow much like a regular period. Irregular bleeding occurs most often during the first few months of oral contraceptive use, but may also occur after you have been taking the pill for some time. Such bleeding may be temporary and usually does not indicate any serious problems. It is important to continue taking your pills on schedule. If the bleeding occurs in more than one cycle or lasts for more than a few days, talk to your doctor or health care professional.

2. Gastrointestinal effects

The most frequent, unpleasant side effects are nausea and vomiting, stomach cramps, bloating, and a change in appetite.

3. Contact lenses

If you wear contact lenses and notice a change in vision or an inability to wear your lenses, contact your doctor or health care professional.

4. Fluid retention

Oral contraceptives may cause edema (fluid retention) with swelling of the fingers or ankles and may raise your blood pressure. If you experience fluid retention, conntact your doctor or health care professional.

5. Melasma

A spotty darkening of the skin is possible, particuarly of the face.

6. Other side effects

Other side effects may include change in appetite, headache, nervousness, depression, dizziness, loss of scalp hair, rash, and vaginal infections.

If any of these side effects bother you, call your doctor or health care professional.

GENERAL PRECAUTIONS

1. Missed periods and use of oral contraceptives before or during early pregnancy

There may be times when you may not menstruate regularly after you have completed taking a cycle of pills. If you have taken your pills regularly and miss one menstrual period, continue taking your pills for the next cycle but be sure to inform your health care professional before doing so. If you have not taken the pills daily as instructed and missed a menstrual period, or if you missed two consecutive menstrual periods, you may be pregnant. Check with your health care professional immediately to determine whether you are pregnant. Do not continue to take oral contraceptives until you are sure you are not pregnant, but continue to use another method of contraception.

There is no conclusive evidence that oral contraceptive use is associated with an increase in birth defects, when taken inadvertently during early pregnancy. Previously, a few studies had reported that oral contraceptives might be associated with birth defects, but these studies have not been confirmed. Nevertheless, oral contraceptives or any other drugs should not be used during pregnancy unless clearly necessary and prescribed by your doctor. You should check with your doctor about risks to your unborn child of any medication taken during pregnancy.

2. While breastfeeding

If you are breastfeeding, consult your doctor before starting oral contraceptives. Some of the drug will be passed on to the child in the milk. A few adverse effects on the child have been reported, including yellowing of the skin (jaundice) and breast enlargement. In addition, oral contraceptives may decrease the amount and quality of your milk. If possible, do not use oral contraceptives while breastfeeding. You should use another method of contraception since breastfeeding provides only partial protection from becoming pregnant and this partial protection decreases significantly as you breastfeed for longer periods of time. You should consider starting oral contraceptives only after you have weaned your child completely.

3. Laboratory tests

If you are scheduled for any laboratory tests, tell your doctor you are taking birth control pills. Certain blood tests may be affected by birth control pills.

4. Drug interactions

Certain drugs may interact with birth control pills to make them less effective in preventing pregnancy or cause an increase in breakthrough bleeding. Such drugs include rifampin, drugs used for epilepsy such as barbiturates (for example, phenobarbital) and phenytoin (Dilantin is one brand of this drug), phenylbutazone (Butazolidin is one brand) and possibly ampicillin and tetracyclines (several brand names). You may need to use an additional method of contraception when you take drugs which can make oral contraceptives less effective.

HOW TO TAKE THE PILL

IMPORTANT POINTS TO REMEMBER

SEXUALLY-TRANSMITTED DISEASES

This product (like all oral contraceptives) is intended to prevent pregnancy. It does not protect against transmission of HIV (AIDS) and other sexually transmitted diseases such as chlamydia, genital herpes, genital warts, gonorrhea, hepatitis B, and syphilis.

Continued on next page

Ovcon—Cont.

***BEFORE* YOU START TAKING YOUR PILLS:**

1. BE SURE TO READ THESE DIRECTIONS:
   Before you start taking your pills.
   Anytime you are not sure what to do.
2. THE RIGHT WAY TO TAKE THE PILL IS TO TAKE ONE PILL EVERY DAY AT THE SAME TIME.
   If you miss pills you could get pregnant. This includes starting the pack late. The more pills you miss, the more likely you are to get pregnant.
3. MANY WOMEN HAVE SPOTTING OR LIGHT BLEEDING, OR MAY FEEL SICK TO THEIR STOMACH DURING THE FIRST 1–3 PACKS OF PILLS.
   If you do feel sick to your stomach, do not stop taking the pill. The problem will usually go away. If it doesn't go away, check with your doctor or clinic.
4. MISSING PILLS CAN ALSO CAUSE SPOTTING OR LIGHT BLEEDING, even when you make up these missed pills.
   On the days you take 2 pills to make up for missed pills, you could also feel a little sick to your stomach.
5. IF YOU HAVE VOMITING OR DIARRHEA, for any reasons, or IF YOU TAKE SOME MEDICINES, including some antibiotics, your pills may not work as well. Use a back-up method (such as condoms, foam, or sponge) until you check with your doctor or clinic.
6. IF YOU HAVE TROUBLE REMEMBERING TO TAKE THE PILL, talk to your doctor or clinic about how to make pill-taking easier or about using another method of birth control.
7. IF YOU HAVE ANY QUESTIONS OR ARE UNSURE ABOUT THE INFORMATION IN THIS LEAFLET, call your doctor or clinic.

***BEFORE* YOU START TAKING YOUR PILLS**

1. DECIDE WHAT TIME OF DAY YOU WANT TO TAKE YOUR PILL.
   It is important to take it at about the same time every day.
2. LOOK AT YOUR PILL PACK TO SEE IF IT HAS 21 OR 28 PILLS:
   The *21-pill pack* has 21 "active" peach pills (with hormones) to take for 3 weeks, followed by one week without pills.
   The *28-pill pack* has 21 "active" peach or yellow pills (with hormones) to take for 3 weeks, followed by 1 week of reminder green pills (without hormones).

0.4/35 OVCON® 35
(Norethindrone and Ethinyl Estradiol Tablets, USP)

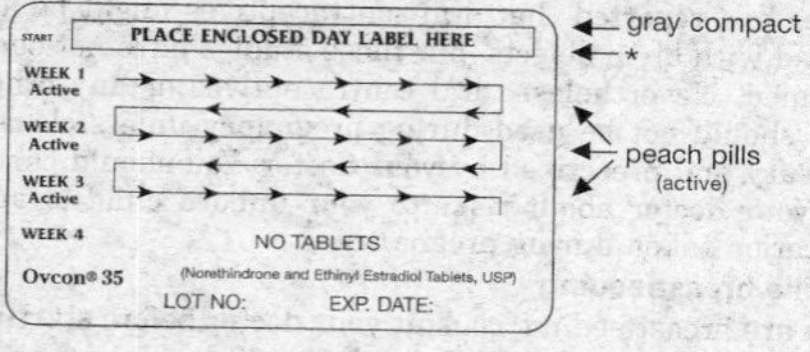

21-pill pack

Each of the 21 **peach** pills contains norethindrone (0.4 mg) and ethinyl estradiol (0.035 mg).

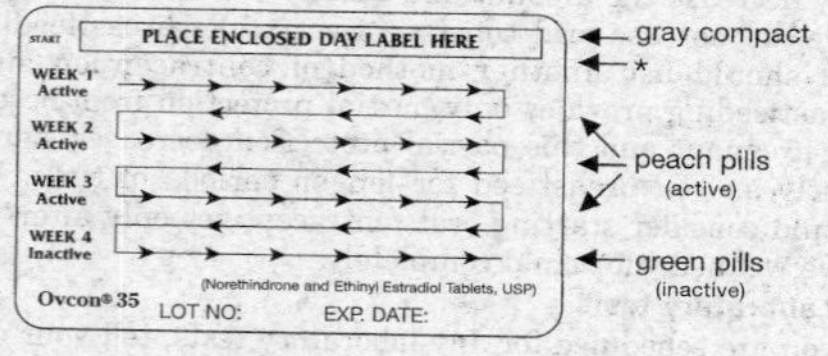

28-pill pack

Each of the 21 **peach** pills contains norethindrone (0.4 mg) and ethinyl estradiol (0.035 mg). Each green pill in the 28-day regimen contains inert ingredients.

OVCON® 50
(Norethindrone and Ethinyl Estradiol Tablets, USP)

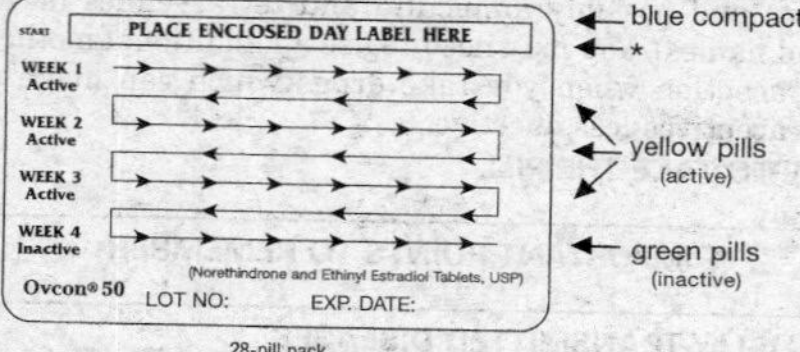

28-pill pack

Each of the 21 **yellow** pills contains norethindrone (1 mg) and ethinyl estradiol (0.05 mg).
Each green pill in the 28–day regimen contains inert ingredients.
*For use of day labels, see **WHEN TO START THE *FIRST* PACK OF PILLS** below.

3. BE SURE YOU HAVE READY AT ALL TIMES:
   ANOTHER KIND OF BIRTH CONTROL (such as condoms, foam, or sponge) to use as a back-up in case you miss pills.
   AN EXTRA, FULL PILL PACK.

WHEN TO START THE *FIRST* PACK OF PILLS

You have a choice of which day to start taking your first pack of pills. Decide with your doctor or clinic which is the best day for you. Once you have decided which day you will begin taking your pills, immediately do the following: remove the Brief Summary from inside the compact and look for the day label sheet attached; peel the label from the sheet which has the start day printed on the left hand side; affix the label to the blister card in the designated location. Take your pill daily in the order indicated by the arrows on the blister card. Pick a time of day which will be easy to remember.

DAY 1 START:

1. Take the first "active" peach or yellow pill of the first pack during the *first 24 hours* of your period.
2. You will not need to use a back-up method of birth control, since you are starting the pill at the beginning of your period.

SUNDAY START:

1. Take the first "active" peach or yellow pill of the first pack on the *Sunday after your period starts*, even if you are still bleeding. If your period begins on Sunday, start the pack that same day.
2. *Use another method of birth control* as a back-up method if you have sex anytime from the Sunday you start your first pack until the next Sunday (7 days). Condoms, foam, or the sponge are good back-up methods of birth control.

WHAT TO DO DURING THE MONTH

1. TAKE ONE PILL AT THE SAME TIME EVERY DAY UNTIL THE PACK IS EMPTY.
   Do not skip pills even if you are spotting or bleeding between monthly periods or feel sick to your stomach (nausea).
   Do not skip pills even if you do not have sex very often.
2. WHEN YOU FINISH A PACK OR SWITCH YOUR BRAND OF PILLS:
   21 pills: Wait 7 days to start the next pack. You will probably have your period during that week. Be sure that no more than 7 days pass between 21-day packs.
   28 pills: Start the next pack on the day after your last "reminder" pill. Do not wait any days between packs.

WHAT TO DO IF YOU MISS PILLS

If you MISS 1 peach or yellow "active" pill:

1. Take it as soon as you remember. Take the next pill at your regular time. This means you may take 2 pills in 1 day.
2. You do not need to use a back-up birth control method if you have sex.

If you MISS 2 peach or yellow "active" pills in a row in WEEK 1 OR WEEK 2 of your pack:

1. Take 2 pills on the day you remember and 2 pills the next day.
2. Then take 1 pill a day until you finish the pack.
3. You MAY BECOME PREGNANT if you have sex in the *7 days* after you miss pills. You MUST use another birth control method (such as condoms, foam, or sponge) as a back-up for those 7 days.

If you MISS 2 peach or yellow "active" pills in a row in THE 3rd WEEK:

1. If you are a Day 1 Starter:
   THROW OUT the rest of the pill pack and start a new pack that same day.
   If you are a Sunday Starter:
   Keep taking 1 pill every day until Sunday.
   On Sunday, THROW OUT the rest of the pack and start a new pack of pills that same day.
2. You may not have your period this month but this is expected. However, if you miss your period 2 months in a row, call your doctor or clinic because you might be pregnant.
3. You MAY BECOME PREGNANT if you have sex in the *7 days* after you miss pills. You MUST use another birth control method (such as condoms, foam, or sponge) as a back-up for those 7 days.

If you MISS 3 OR MORE peach or yellow "active" pills in a row (during the first 3 weeks):

1. If you are a Day 1 Starter:
   THROW OUT the rest of the pill pack and start a new pack that same day.
   If you are a Sunday Starter:
   Keep taking 1 pill every day until Sunday.
   On Sunday, THROW OUT the rest of the pack and start a new pack of pills that same day.
2. You may not have your period this month but this is expected. However, if you miss your period 2 months in a row, call your doctor or clinic because you might be pregnant.
3. You MAY BECOME PREGNANT if you have sex in the *7 days* after you miss pills. You MUST use another birth control method (such as condoms, foam, or sponge) as a back-up for those 7 days.

A REMINDER FOR THOSE ON 28-DAY PACKS:
If you forget any of the 7 green "reminder" pills in Week 4:
THROW AWAY the pills you missed.
Keep taking 1 pill each day until the pack is empty.
You do not need a back-up method.

FINALLY, IF YOU ARE STILL NOT SURE WHAT TO DO ABOUT THE PILLS YOU HAVE MISSED:
Use a BACK-UP METHOD anytime you have sex.
KEEP TAKING ONE "ACTIVE" PILL EACH DAY until you can reach your doctor or clinic.

GENERAL

1. Pregnancy due to pill failure
The incidence of pill failure resulting in pregnancy is approximately 1% (ie, one pregnancy per 100 women per year) if taken every day as directed, but more typical failure rates are about 3%. If failure does occur, the risk to the fetus is minimal.

2. Pregnancy after stopping the pill
There may be some delay in becoming pregnant after you stop using oral contraceptives, especially if you had irregular menstrual cycles before you used oral contraceptives. It may be advisable to postpone conception until you begin menstruating regularly once you have stopped taking the pill and desire pregnancy.
There does not appear to be any increase in birth defects in newborn babies when pregnancy occurs soon after stopping the pill.

Other

a. Overdosage
Serious ill effects have not been reported following ingestion of large doses of oral contraceptives by young children. Overdosage may cause nausea and withdrawal bleeding in females. In case of overdosage, contact your poison control center, health care professional, or nearest emergency room.
KEEP THIS DRUG AND ALL DRUGS OUT OF THE REACH OF CHILDREN.

b. General medical information
Your health care professional will take a medical and family history before prescribing oral contraceptives and will examine you. The physical examination may be delayed to another time if you request it and the health care provider believes that it is a good medical practice to postpone it. You should be reexamined at least once a year. Be sure to inform your health care professional if there is a family history of any of the conditions listed previously in this leaflet. Be sure to keep all appointments with your health care professional, because this is a time to determine if there are early signs of side effects of oral contraceptive use.
Do not use this drug for any condition other than the one for which it was prescribed. This drug has been prescribed specifically for you; do not give it to others who may want birth control pills.

NONCONTRACEPTIVE EFFECTS OF ORAL CONTRACEPTIVES

In addition to preventing pregnancy, use of oral contraceptives may provide certain benefits. They are:

- Menstrual cycles may become more regular
- Blood flow during menstruation may be lighter and less iron may be lost. Therefore, anemia due to iron deficiency is less likely to occur.
- Pain or other symptoms during menstruation may be encountered less frequently
- Ectopic (tubal) pregnancy may occur less frequently
- Noncancerous cysts or lumps in the breast may occur less frequently
- Acute pelvic inflammatory disease may occur less frequently
- Oral contraceptive use may provide some protection against developing two forms of cancer: cancer of the ovaries and cancer of the lining of the uterus.

If you want more information about birth control pills, ask your doctor or pharmacist. They have a more technical leaflet called the Professional Labeling, which you may wish to read.

Manufactured by: Bristol-Myers Squibb Company
Princeton, NJ 08543
Manufactured for: Warner Chilcott, Inc.
100 Enterprise Drive
Rockaway, NJ 07866 USA
0582G050 Revised March 2000

IDENTIFICATION PROBLEM?
Turn to the **Product Identification Guide,** where you'll find more than 1600 products pictured in actual size and full color.

Warner Lambert Consumer Group of Pfizer Inc.

182 TABOR ROAD
MORRIS PLAINS, NJ 07950

DIRECT MEDICAL EMERGENCIES AND INQUIRIES TO:
Consumer Relations Group
800-723-7529
FAX: 973-385-6667

BONINE®
(Meclizine hydrochloride)
Chewable Tablets

ACTION
BONINE (meclizine) is an H_1 histamine receptor blocker of the piperazine side chain group. It exhibits its action by an effect on the Central Nervous System (CNS), possibly by its ability to block muscarinic receptors in the brain.

INDICATIONS
BONINE is effective in the management of nausea, vomiting and dizziness associated with motion sickness.

CONTRAINDICATIONS
Do not take this product, unless directed by a doctor, if you have a breathing problem such as emphysema or chronic bronchitis, or if you have glaucoma or difficulty in urination due to enlargement of the prostate gland.

WARNINGS
May cause drowsiness; alcohol, sedatives and tranquilizers may increase the drowsiness effect. Avoid alcoholic beverages while taking this product. Do not take this product if you are taking sedatives or tranquilizers without first consulting your doctor. Do not drive or operate dangerous machinery while taking this medication.

Usage In Children
Clinical studies establishing safety and effectiveness in children have not been done; therefore, usage is not recommended in children under 12 years of age.

Usage in Pregnancy
As with any drug, if you are pregnant or nursing a baby, seek advice of a health care professional before taking this product.

ADVERSE REACTIONS
Drowsiness, dry mouth, and on rare occasions, blurred vision have been reported.

DOSAGE AND ADMINISTRATION
For motion sickness, take one or two tablets of Bonine once daily, one hour before travel starts, for up to 24 hours of protection against motion sickness. The tablet can be chewed with or without water or swallowed whole with water. Thereafter, the dose may be repeated every 24 hours for the duration of the travel.

HOW SUPPLIED
BONINE (meclizine HCl) is available in convenient packets of 8 and 16 chewable tablets of 25 mg. meclizine HCl.

INACTIVE INGREDIENTS
FD&C Red #40, Lactose, Magnesium Stearate, Purified Siliceous Earth, Raspberry Flavor, Saccharin Sodium, Starch, Talc.

UNISOM® SleepTabs™
[yu 'na-som]
Nighttime Sleep Aid
(doxylamine succinate)

PRODUCT OVERVIEW

KEY FACTS
Unisom is an ethanolamine antihistamine (doxylamine) which characteristically shows a high incidence of sedation. It produces a reduced latency to end of wakefulness and early onset of sleep.

MAJOR USES
Unisom has been shown to be clinically effective as a sleep aid when 1 tablet is given 30 minutes before retiring.

SAFETY INFORMATION
Unisom is contraindicated in pregnancy and nursing mothers. It is also contraindicated in patients with asthma, glaucoma, and enlargement of the prostate. Caution should be used if taken when alcohol is being consumed. Caution is also indicated when taken concurrently with other medications due to the anticholinergic properties of antihistamines.

DESCRIPTION
Pale blue oval scored tablets containing 25 mg. of doxylamine succinate, 2-[α-(2-dimethylaminoethoxy)α-methylbenzyl]pyridine succinate.

INACTIVE INGREDIENTS
Dibasic Calcium Phosphate, FD&C Blue #1 Aluminum Lake, Magnesium Stearate, Microcrystalline Cellulose, Sodium Starch Glycolate.

ADMINISTRATION AND DOSAGE
One tablet 30 minutes before going to bed. Take once daily or as directed by a doctor. Not for children under 12 years of age.

WARNINGS
Do not take this product, unless directed by a doctor, if you have a breathing problem such as emphysema or chronic bronchitis, or if you have glaucoma or difficulty in urination due to enlargement of the prostate gland. Do not take this product if pregnant or nursing a baby.
- If sleeplessness persists continuously for more than two weeks, consult your doctor. Insomnia may be a symptom of a serious underlying medical illness.
- Do not take this product if presently taking any other drug, without consulting your doctor or pharmacist.
- Take this product with caution if alcohol is being consumed.
- For adults only. Do not give to children under 12 years of age.
- Keep this and all medications out of the reach of children. This product contains an antihistamine and will cause drowsiness. It should be used only at bedtime.

SIDE EFFECTS
Occasional anticholinergic effects may be seen.

ATTENTION
Use only if tablet blister seals are unbroken.

HOW SUPPLIED
Boxes of 8, 16, 32 or 48 tablets.

MAXIMUM STRENGTH UNISOM® SLEEPGELS®
Nighttime Sleep Aid

DESCRIPTION
Maximum Strength Unisom SleepGels are liquid-filled, blue soft gelatin capsules.

ACTIVE INGREDIENT
Diphenhydramine Hydrochloride 50 mg.

INACTIVE INGREDIENTS
FD&C Blue No. 1, Gelatin, Glycerin, Pharmaceutical Glaze, Polyethylene Glycol, Propylene Glycol, Purified Water, Sorbitol, Titanium Dioxide.

INDICATIONS
Helps to reduce difficulty falling asleep.

ACTION
Diphenhydramine Hydrochloride is an ethanolamine antihistamine with anticholinergic and sedative effects.

ADMINISTRATION AND DOSAGE
Adults and children 12 years of age and over: Oral dosage is one softgel (50 mg) at bedtime if needed, or as directed by a doctor.

WARNINGS
Do not take this product, unless directed by a doctor, if you have a breathing problem such as emphysema or chronic bronchitis, or if you have glaucoma or difficulty in urination due to enlargement of the prostate gland. Do not take this product if pregnant or nursing a baby.
- Do not give to children under 12 years of age.
- If sleeplessness persists continuously for more than two weeks, consult your doctor. Insomnia may be a symptom of serious underlying medical illness.
- Avoid alcoholic beverages while taking this product. Do not take this product if you are taking sedatives or tranquilizers, without first consulting your doctor.
- **Do Not Use:** with any other product containing diphenhydramine, including one applied topically.
- Keep this and all drugs out of the reach of children.
- In case of accidental overdose, seek professional assistance or contact a poison control center immediately.

DRUG INTERACTION
Monoamine oxidase (MAO) inhibitors prolong and intensify the anticholinergic effects of antihistamines. The CNS depressant effect is heightened by alcohol and other CNS depressant drugs.

SYMPTOMS OF ORAL OVERDOSAGE
Antihistamine overdosage reactions may vary from central nervous system depression to stimulation.
Stimulation is particularly likely in children. Atropine-like signs and symptoms, such as dry mouth, fixed and dilated pupils, flushing, and gastrointestinal symptoms, may also occur.

ATTENTION
Use only if softgel blister seals are unbroken.

HOW SUPPLIED
Boxes of 16 liquid filled softgels in child resistant blisters and boxes of 8 with non-child resistant packaging. Also in a 32 count easy to open child resistant bottle.
Store between 15° and 30°C (59° and 86°F)

Warner-Lambert

Consumer Healthcare
Warner-Lambert Company
201 TABOR ROAD
MORRIS PLAINS, NJ 07950

Direct Inquiries and For Medical Information Contact:
Consumer Affairs
1-(800) 223-0182
(See PDR For Nonprescription Drugs)

ACTIFED® COLD & ALLERGY Tablets OTC
[ăk 'tŭh-fĕd]
Pseudoephedrine HCl (60 mg)
Triprolidine HCl (2.5 mg)
Nasal Decongestant/Antihistamine

ACTIFED® Cold & Sinus Caplets OTC
[ak'tuh-fed]
New Formula
Acetaminophen (500 mg)
Pseudoephedrine Hydrochloride (30 mg)
Chlorpheniramine Maleate (2 mg)

ANUSOL® HC-1 Ointment OTC
[ă'nū-sōl"]
Hydrocortisone Acetate (equivalent to 1% Hydrocortisone)
Hydrocortisone Anti-Itch Ointment

ANUSOL® Hemorrhoidal Ointment OTC
[ă'nū-sōl"]
Pramoxine HCl (1%)
Zinc Oxide (12.5%)
Mineral Oil
Protectant/External Analgesic

ANUSOL® Hemorrhoidal Suppositories OTC
[ă'nū-sōl"]
Topical Starch (51%)
Protectant

BENADRYL® ALLERGY CHEWABLES OTC
[bĕ '-nă-drĭl]
Diphenhydramine HCl (12.5 mg)
Antihistamine

BENADRYL® ALLERGY/COLD Tablets OTC
[bĕ '-nă-drĭl]
Acetaminophen (500 mg)
Diphenhydramine HCl (12.5 mg)
Pseudoephedrine HCl (30 mg)
Pain Reliever-Fever Reducer/
Antihistamine/Nasal Decongestant

BENADRYL®ALLERGY/CONGESTION Tablets OTC
[bĕ '-nă-drĭl]
Diphenhydramine HCl (25 mg)
Pseudoephedrine HCl (60 mg)
Antihistamine/Nasal Decongestant

BENADRYL® ALLERGY/CONGESTION Liquid Medication OTC
[bĕ 'nă-drĭl]
Diphenhydramine HCl (12.5 mg)
Pseudoephedrine HCl (30 mg)
Antihistamine/Nasal Decongestant

BENADRYL® ALLERGY Ultratab™ Tablets and Kapseal® Capsules OTC
[bĕ '-nă-drĭl]
Diphenhydramine HCl (25 mg)
Antihistamine

Continued on next page

BENADRYL® ALLERGY Liquid Medication OTC
[*bĕ 'nă-drĭl*]

Diphenhydramine HCl (12.5 mg)
Antihistamine

BENADRYL® ALLERGY/SINUS Headache Caplets & Gelcaps OTC
[*bĕ 'nă-drĭl*]

Acetaminophen (500 mg)
Diphenhydramine HCl (12.5 mg)
Pseudoephedrine HCl (30 mg)
Pain Reliever/Antihistamine/Nasal Decongestant

BENADRYL® DYE-FREE ALLERGY Liqui-gels® Softgel OTC
[*bĕ 'nă-drĭl*]

Diphenhydramine HCl (25 mg)
Antihistamine

BENADRYL® DYE-FREE ALLERGY Liquid Medication OTC
[*bĕ 'nă-drĭl*]

Diphenhydramine HCl (12.5 mg)
Antihistamine

BENADRYL® Itch Relief Stick Extra Strength OTC
[*bĕ '-nă-drĭl*]

Diphenhydramine HCl (2%)
Zinc Acetate (0.1%)
Topical Analgesic/Skin Protectant

BENADRYL® Itch Stopping Cream OTC
[*bĕ '-nă-drĭl*]

Original Strength
Diphenhydramine HCl (1%)
Zinc Acetate (0.1%)
Topical Analgesic/Skin Protectant
Extra Strength
Diphenhydramine HCl (2%)
Zinc Acetate (0.1%)
Topical Analgesic/Skin Protectant

BENADRYL® Itch Stopping Gel OTC
[*bĕ '-nă-drĭl*]

Original Strength
Diphenhydramine HCl (1%)
Topical Analgesic
Extra Strength
Diphenhydramine HCl (2%)
Topical Analgesic

BENADRYL® Itch Stopping Spray OTC
[*bĕ '-nă-drĭl*]

Original Strength
Diphenhydramine HCl (1%)
Zinc Acetate (0.1%)
Topical Analgesic/Skin Protectant
Extra Strength
Diphenyhydramine HCl (2%)
Zinc Acetate (0.1%)
Topical Analgesic/Skin Protectant

BENYLIN® ADULT Formula OTC
[*bĕ '-nă-lĭn*]

Dextromethorphan HBr (15 mg)
Cough Suppressant

BENYLIN® EXPECTORANT OTC
[*bĕ '-nă-lĭn*]

Dextromethorphan HBr (5 mg)
Guaifenesin (100 mg)
Cough Suppressant/Expectorant

BENYLIN® MULTI SYMPTOM OTC
[*bĕ 'nă-lĭn*]

Dextromethorphan HBr (5 mg)
Guaifenesin (100 mg)
Pseudoephedrine HCl (15 mg)
Cough Suppressant/Expectorant/Nasal Decongestant

BENYLIN® PEDIATRIC OTC
[*bĕ '-nă-lĭn*]

Dextromethorphan HBr (7.5 mg)
Cough Suppressant

CALADRYL® CLEAR Lotion OTC
[*kăl '-ă-drĭl*]

Pramoxine HCl (1%)
Zinc Acetate (0.1%)
Skin Protectant/External Analgesic

CALADRYL® Cream for Kids OTC
[*kăl '-ă-drĭl*]

Calamine (8%)
Pramoxine HCl (1%)
External Analgesic/Skin Protectant

CALADRYL® Lotion OTC
[*kăl '-ă-drĭl*]

Calamine (8%)
Pramoxine HCl (1%)
External Analgesic/Skin Protectant

COOL MINT LISTERINE® OTC
[*lĭs 'tərĕn*]

Eucalyptol (0.092%)
Menthol (0.042%)
Methyl Salicylate (0.060%)
Thymol (0.064%)
Antiseptic

FRESHBURST LISTERINE® OTC
[*lĭs 'tərĕn*]

Eucalyptol (0.092%)
Menthol (0.042%)
Methyl Salicylate (0.060%)
Thymol (0.064%)
Antiseptic

LISTERINE® Antiseptic OTC
[*lĭs 'tərĕn*]

Eucalyptol (0.092%)
Menthol (0.042%)
Methyl Salicylate (0.060%)
Thymol (0.064%)
Antiseptic

TARTAR CONTROL LISTERINE® Antiseptic OTC
[*lĭs'tərĕn*]

Eucalyptol (0.092%)
Menthol (0.042%)
Methyl Salicylate (0.060%)
Thymol (0.064%)
Antiseptic

LISTERMINT® Alcohol-Free Mouthwash OTC
[*lĭs 'tər mĭnt*]

LUBRIDERM® Daily UV Lotion with Sunscreen OTC
[*lū brĭ dĕrm*]

Octyl Methoxycinnamate (7.5%)
Octyl Salicylate (4%)
Oxybenzone (3%)
Moisturizer/Sun Protection

NEOSPORIN® Ointment OTC
[*nē'uh-spō'rŭn*]

Bacitracin Zinc (400 units)
Neomycin (3.5 mg)
Polymyxin B Sulfate (5000 units)
First Aid Antibiotic

NEOSPORIN® + PAIN RELIEF Maximum Strength Cream OTC
[*nē 'uh-spō 'rŭn*]

Neomycin (3.5 mg)
Polymyxin B Sulfate (10,000 units)
Pramoxine HCl (10 mg)
First Aid Antibiotic/Pain Relieving Cream

NEOSPORIN® + PAIN RELIEF Maximum Strength Ointment OTC
[*nē"uh-spŏ'rŭn*]

Bacitracin Zinc (500 units)
Neomycin (3.5 mg)
Polymyxin B Sulfate (10,000 units)
Pramoxine HCl (10 mg)
First Aid Antibiotic/Pain Relieving Ointment

NIX® Creme Rinse OTC
[*nĭks*]

Permethrin (280 mg)
Lice Treatment

NIX® Lice Control Spray For Bedding and Furniture OTC
[*niks*]

Permethrin 0.25%
NOT FOR USE IN HUMANS

POLYSPORIN® Ointment OTC
[*pŏl 'ē-spō 'rŭn*]

Bacitracin Zinc (500 Units in a special White Petrolatum Base)
Polymyxin B Sulfate (10,000 Units)
First Aid Antibiotic

POLYSPORIN® Powder OTC
[*pŏl 'ē-spō 'rŭn*]

Bacitracin Zinc (500 units in a Lactose Base)
Polymyxin B Sulfate (10,000 units)
First Aid Antibiotic

SINUTAB® Non-Drying Liquid Caps OTC
[*sĭn 'ū tăb*]

Guaifenesin (200 mg)
Pseudoephedrine HCl (30 mg)
Expectorant/Nasal Decongestant

SINUTAB® SINUS ALLERGY Medication Maximum Strength Tablets & Caplets OTC
[*sĭn 'ū tăb*]

Acetaminophen (500 mg)
Chlorpheniramine Maleate (2 mg)
Pseudoephedrine HCl (30 mg)
Pain Reliever/Antihistamine/Nasal Decongestant

SINUTAB® SINUS Medication Maximum Strength Without Drowsiness Tablets & Caplets OTC
[*sĭn 'ū tăb*]

Acetaminophen (500 mg)
Pseudoephedrine HCl (30 mg)
Pain Reliever/Nasal Decongestant

SUDAFED® 12 Hour Tablets OTC
[*sū 'duh-fĕd"*]

Pseudoephedrine HCl (120 mg)
Long Acting Nasal Decongestant

SUDAFED® 24 Hour Tablets OTC
[*sū 'duh-fĕd*]

Pseudoephedrine HCl (240 mg)
Long-Acting Nasal Decongestant

SUDAFED® COLD & ALLERGY Tablets OTC
[*sū 'dah-fĕd"*]

Chlorpheniramine Maleate (4 mg)
Pseudoephedrine HCl (60 mg)
Antihistamine/Nasal Decongestant

SUDAFED® COLD & COUGH Liquid Caps OTC
[*sū 'dah-fĕd"*]

Acetaminophen (250 mg)
Dextromethorphan HBr (10 mg)

Guaifenesin (100 mg)
Pseudoephedrine HCl (30 mg)
Pain Reliever-Fever Reducer/Cough Suppressant/Expectorant/Nasal Decongestant

SUDAFED® Cold & Sinus Liquid Caps OTC
[*sū 'dah-fĕd"*]

Acetaminophen (325 mg)
Pseudoephedrine HCl (30 mg)
Pain Reliever-Fever Reducer/
Nasal Decongestant

SUDAFED® Severe Cold Formula Caplets & Tablets OTC
[*sū 'dah-fĕd"*]

Acetaminophen (500 mg)
Dextromethorphan Hydrobromide (15 mg)
Pseudoephedrine HCl (30 mg)
Pain Reliever-Fever Reducer/
Cough Suppressant/Nasal Decongestant

SUDAFED® NASAL DECONGESTANT 30 mg Tablets OTC
[*sū 'dah-fĕd"*]

Pseudoephedrine HCl (30 mg)
Nasal Decongestant

SUDAFED® NON-DRYING SINUS Liquid Caps OTC
[*sū 'dah-fĕd"*]

Guaifenesin (200 mg)
Pseudoephedrine HCl (30 mg)
Expectorant/Nasal Decongestant

SUDAFED® SINUS Maximum Strength Caplets and Tablets OTC
[*sū 'dah-fĕd"*]

Acetaminophen (500 mg)
Pseudoephedrine HCl (30 mg)
Pain Reliever/Nasal Decongestant

CHILDREN'S SUDAFED® COLD & COUGH Liquid OTC
[*sū 'dah-fĕd"*]

Dextromethorphan HBr (5 mg)
Pseudoephedrine HCl (15 mg)
Cough Suppressant/Nasal Decongestant

CHILDREN'S SUDAFED® NASAL DECONGESTANT Chewables OTC
[*sū 'dah-fĕd"*]

Pseudoephedrine HCl (15 mg)
Nasal Decongestant

CHILDREN'S SUDAFED® NASAL DECONGESTANT Liquid OTC
[*sū 'dah-fĕd*]

Pseudoephedrine HCl (15 mg)
Nasal Decongestant

TUCKS® Pre-moistened Hemorrhoidal Vaginal Pads OTC
[*tŭks*]

Witch Hazel (50%)
Astringent

TUCKS® Take Alongs Towelettes OTC
[*tŭks*]

Witch Hazel (50%)
Astringent

ZANTAC® 75 TABLETS OTC
[*zan ' tak*]

Ranitidine Hydrochloride (84 mg)
(equivalent to 75 mg ranitidine)
Acid Reducer

Watson Laboratories, Inc.

**311 BONNIE CIRCLE
CORONA, CA 92880**

Address Inquiries to:
Customer Service Department
Telephone: 800/272-5525
FAX: 909/735-2871

The following list of Watson Laboratories products is provided to facilitate identification. It includes the color(s) and identification codes for all tablets and capsules.

PRODUCT	IDENTIFICATION CODE
GENERIC NAME Description *Color(s), Shape*	(Front/Back*)
ACEBUTOLOL HYDROCHLORIDE Capsules, 200 mg ℞ *Red/Gray*	WATSON 437
ACEBUTOLOL HYDROCHLORIDE Capsules, 400 mg ℞ *Maroon/Green*	WATSON 438
ACETAMINOPHEN AND CODEINE PHOSPHATE Tablets, USP, 300 mg/15 mg (C-III) ℞ *White, round*	WATSON/850 *Scored*
ACETAMINOPHEN AND CODEINE PHOSPHATE Tablets, USP, 300 mg/30 mg (C-III) ℞ *White, round*	WATSON/851 *Scored*
ACETAMINOPHEN AND CODEINE PHOSPHATE Tablets, USP, 300 mg/60 mg (C-III) ℞ *White, round*	WATSON/852 *Scored*
ACYCLOVIR Tablets, USP, 400 mg ℞ *White oval*	WATSON 335
ACYCLOVIR Tablets, USP, 800 mg ℞ *White oval*	WATSON 336
ALPRAZOLAM Tablets, USP, 0.25 mg (C-IV) ℞ *White, Oval*	WATSON 682/0.25 *BiConvex, Scored*
ALPRAZOLAM Tablets, USP, 0.5 mg (C-IV) ℞ *Peach, Oval*	WATSON 683/0.5 *BiConvex, Scored*
ALPRAZOLAM Tablets, USP, 1 mg (C-IV) ℞ *Blue, Oval,*	WATSON 684/1.0 *BiConvex, Scored*
AMILORIDE HCl & HCTZ Tablets, USP, 5mg/50 mg ℞ *Peach, Round*	WATSON 685/5-50 *Scored*
AMOXAPINE Tablets, USP, 25 mg ℞ *White, Round*	WATSON 379/Bisected
AMOXAPINE Tablets, USP, 50 mg ℞ *Salmon, Round*	WATSON 380/Bisected
AMOXAPINE Tablets, USP, 100 mg ℞ *Blue, Round*	WATSON 381/Bisected
AMOXAPINE Tablets, USP, 150 mg ℞ *Peach, Round*	WATSON 382/Bisected
BACLOFEN Tablets, USP, 10 mg ℞ *White, Oval*	WATSON 686/10 *Scored*
BACLOFEN Tablets, USP, 20 mg ℞ *White, Round*	WATSON 687/20 *Scored*
BUTALBITAL, ASPIRIN, CAFFEINE, and CODEINE PHOSPHATE Capsules, USP 50 mg/325 mg/40 mg/30 mg (C-III) ℞ *Blue/Yellow*	WATSON/425
BUTALBITAL/ACETAMINOPHEN/CAFFEINE Tablets, USP 50 mg/500 mg/40 mg ℞ *Blue, Capsule-shaped*	WATSON/613
CAPTOPRIL Tablets, USP, 12.5 mg ℞ *White, Capsule-shaped*	WATSON 688/12.5 *Scored*
CAPTOPRIL Tablets, USP, 25 mg ℞ *White, Round*	WATSON 689/25 *Quadrisect-Scored*
CAPTOPRIL Tablets, USP, 50 mg ℞ *White, Football shaped*	WATSON 690/50 *Scored*
CAPTOPRIL Tablets, USP, 100 mg ℞ *White, Football shaped*	WATSON 691/100 *Scored*
CARISOPRODOL Tablets, 350 mg ℞ *white round*	WATSON/784
CHLORDIAZEPOXIDE HCL Capsules, 5 mg (C-IV) ℞ *green op/yellow op*	WATSON/785
10 mg (C-IV) ℞ *black op/green op*	WATSON/786
25 mg (C-IV) ℞ *green op/white op*	WATSON/787
CHLORZOXAZONE Tablets, USP, 500 mg ℞ *Green, Capsule-shaped*	WATSON 693/500 *Partial-Scored*
CLOMIPHENE CITRATE Tablets, 50 mg ℞ *off white round*	WATSON/781
CLOMIPRAMINE HYDROCHLORIDE Capsules, 25 mg ℞ *Opaque Blue/Opaque Blue*	WATSON 594/25 mg
CLOMIPRAMINE HYDROCHLORIDE Capsules, 50 mg ℞ *Opaque Yellow/Opaque Yellow*	WATSON 595/50 mg
CLOMIPRAMINE HYDROCHLORIDE Capsules, 75 mg ℞ *Opaque Green/Opaque Green*	WATSON 596/75 mg
CLONAZEPAM Tablets, USP, 0.5 mg (C-IV) ℞ *yellow/round*	WATSON 746 *Biconvex, Scored*
CLONAZEPAM Tablets, USP, 1 mg (C-IV) ℞ *aqua/round*	WATSON 747 *Biconvex, Scored*
CLONAZEPAM Tablets, USP, 2 mg (C-IV) ℞ *white/round*	WATSON 748 *Biconvex, Scored*
CLORAZEPATE DIPOTASSIUM Tablets, 3.75 mg (C-IV) ℞ *Light Blue, Triangular*	*Scored* WATSON 835
CLORAZEPATE DIPOTASSIUM Tablets, 7.5 mg (C-IV) ℞ *Light Peach, Triangular*	*Scored* WATSON 836
CLORAZEPATE DIPOTASSIUM Tablets, 15 mg (C-IV) ℞ *Lavender, Triangular*	WATSON 837
CYCLOBENZAPRINE HYDROCHLORIDE ℞ Tablets, USP, 10 mg *White, round*	WATSON/418
DESIPRAMINE HCL Tablets, 25 mg ℞ *yellow round*	WATSON/808
50 mg ℞ *green round*	WATSON/809
100 mg ℞ *peach round*	WATSON/545
DICLOFENAC POTASSIUM Tablets, 50 mg ℞ *Light brown, round*	WATSON/585
DICLOFENAC SODIUM DELAYED RELEASE Tablets, USP, 50 mg ℞ *White round*	WATSON 338
DICLOFENAC SODIUM DELAYED RELEASE Tablets, USP, 75 mg ℞ *White round*	WATSON 339
DICYCLOMINE HCL Capsules, 10 mg ℞ *dk blue/dk blue*	WATSON/794 cap 10 mg body
Tablets 20 mg ℞ *blue round*	WATSON/795
DIETHYLPROPION HCL Tablets, 25 mg ℞ (C-IV) *white round*	WATSON/783
DIETHYLPROPION HCL Extended Release Tablets, 75 mg ℞ (C-IV) *white capsule shaped*	WATSON/782
DILTIAZEM Extended release Capsules, 120 mg *Pink, white*	120/WATSON/662
DILTIAZEM Extended release Capsules, 180 mg *Pink, white*	180/WATSON/663
DILTIAZEM Extended release Capsule, 240 mg *Red, white*	240/WATSON/664
DILTIAZEM HCL Tablets, 30 mg ℞ *blue round*	WATSON/775
60 mg ℞ *white round*	WATSON/776
90 mg ℞ *blue oblong*	WATSON/777
120 mg ℞ *white oblong*	WATSON/778
DOXEPIN HYDROCHLORIDE Capsules, USP, 10 mg ℞ *Scarlet/Pink Opaque*	WATSON 695/10
DOXEPIN HYDROCHLORIDE Capsules, USP, 25 mg ℞ *Blue/Pink Opaque*	WATSON 696/25
DOXEPIN HYDROCHLORIDE Capsules, USP, 50 mg ℞ *Pink/Flesh Opaque*	WATSON 697/50
ESTAZOLAM Tablets, 1 mg (C-IV) ℞ White, diamond shaped	WATSON 744/1 Scored
ESTAZOLAM Tablets, 2 mg (C-IV) ℞ Dark Pink, diamond shaped	WATSON 745/2 Scored

Continued on next page

Product Listing-Watson—Cont.

ESTRADIOL WATSON 528/Scored
Tablets, USP, 0.5 mg ℞
White, Round

ESTRADIOL WATSON 487/Scored
Tablets, USP, 1 mg ℞
Gray, Round

ESTRADIOL WATSON 488/Scored
Tablets, USP, 2 mg ℞
Light Green, Round

ESTROPIPATE WATSON 414/Scored
Tablets, USP, 0.75 mg ℞
(calculated as sodium
estrone sulfate 0.625 mg)
Yellow, Round

ESTROPIPATE WATSON 415/Scored
Tablets, USP, 1.5 mg ℞
(calculated as sodium
estrone sulfate 1.25 mg)
Peach, Round

ESTROPIPATE WATSON 416/Scored
Tablets, USP, 3 mg ℞
(calculated as sodium
estrone sulfate 2.5 mg)
Blue, Round

ETODOLAC WATSON 735/200
Capsules, 200 mg ℞
Gray/Brown opaque

ETODOLAC WATSON 736/300
Capsules, 300 mg ℞
Gray/Red

ETODOLAC WATSON 667/400
Tablets, 400 mg ℞
Yellow Capsule Shaped, Film Coated, Biconvex

ETODOLAC WATSON 728/500
Tablets, 500 mg ℞
Blue, Capsule-Shaped, Film-coated Biconvex

FUROSEMIDE WATSON 300
Tablets, USP, 20 mg ℞
White, Round

FUROSEMIDE WATSON/311
Tablets, USP, 20 mg ℞
White, Oval

FUROSEMIDE WATSON 301/Scored
Tablets, USP, 40 mg ℞
White, Round

FUROSEMIDE WATSON 302/Scored
Tablets, USP, 80 mg ℞
White, Round

GLIPIZIDE WATSON 460/Scored
Tablets, USP, 5 mg ℞
White, Round

GLIPIZIDE WATSON 461/Scored
Tablets, USP, 10 mg ℞
White, Round

GUANABENZ ACETATE WATSON 451
Tablets, USP, 4 mg ℞
Orange, Round

GUANABENZ ACETATE WATSON 452
Tablets, USP, 8 mg ℞
Grey, Round

GUANFACINE HYDROCHLORIDE WATSON 444
Tablets, 1 mg ℞ USP
Pink, Round, Biconvex

GUANFACINE HYDROCHLORIDE WATSON 453
Tablets, 2 mg ℞ USP
Peach, Round, Biconvex

HYDROCODONE BITARTRATE and APAP WATSON
Tablets, USP, 2.5 mg/500 mg CIII ℞ 388/Bisected
White, Oblong

HYDROCODONE BITARTRATE and APAP WATSON
Tablets, USP, 5 mg/ 500 mg CIII ℞ 349/Bisected
White, Capsule-shaped

HYDROCODONE BITARTRATE and APAP WATSON
Tablets, USP, 7.5 mg/500 mg CIII ℞ 385/Bisected
White, Capsule-shaped

HYDROCODONE BITARTRATE and APAP WATSON
Tablets, USP, 7.5 mg/650 mg CIII ℞ 502/Bisected
Pink, Capsule-shaped

HYDROCODONE BITARTRATE and APAP WATSON
Tablets, USP, 7.5 mg/ 750 mg CIII ℞ 387/Bisected
White, Oblong

HYDROCODONE BITARTRATE and APAP WATSON
Tablets, USP, 10 mg/500 mg CIII ℞ 540/Bisected
Blue, Capsule-Shaped

HYDROCODONE BITARTRATE and APAP WATSON
Tablets, USP, 10 mg/650mg CIII ℞ 503/Bisected
Light Green, Capsule-Shaped

HYDROXYCHLOROQUINE
SULFATE WATSON 698/200
Tablets, USP, 200 mg ℞
White/Off-White, Oval

HYDROXYZINE
HYDROCHLORIDE WATSON 699/10
Tablets, USP, 10 mg ℞
Orange, Round, Film-coated

HYDROXYZINE
HYDROCHLORIDE WATSON 700/25
Tablets, USP, 25 mg ℞
Green, Round, Film-coated

HYDROXYZINE WATSON 704/50
HYDROCHLORIDE
Tablets, USP, 50 mg ℞
Yellow, Round, Film-coated

HYDROXYZINE PAMOATE
Capsules, 25 mg ℞ WATSON/800
dk green op/lt green
50 mg ℞ WATSON/801
green op/white op

INDAPAMIDE WATSON 527
Tablets, USP, 1.25 mg ℞
Orange, Film Coated, Round

INDAPAMIDE WATSON 504
Tablets, USP, 2.5 mg ℞
White, Film Coated, Round

KETOROLAC TROMETHAMINE
Tablets, USP, 10 mg ℞
White round WATSON 858

LABETALOL HYDROCHLORIDE WATSON/605
Tablets, 100 mg ℞
Beige, Round, Film-coated, Scored

LABETALOL HYDROCHLORIDE WATSON/606
Tablets, 200 mg ℞
White, Round, Film-coated, Scored

LABETALOL HYDROCHLORIDE WATSON/607
Tablets, 300 mg ℞
Blue, Round, Film-coated, Scored

LORAZEPAM WATSON/240 Scored 0.5
Tablets, USP, 0.5 mg CIV ℞
White, Round

LORAZEPAM WATSON/241 Scored 1
Tablets, USP, 1 mg CIV ℞
White, Round

LORAZEPAM WATSON/242 Scored 2
Tablets, USP, 2 mg CIV ℞
White, Round

LOXAPINE WATSON 369/5 mg
Capsules, USP, 5 mg ℞
White/white

LOXAPINE WATSON 370/10 mg
Capsules, USP, 10 mg ℞
Yellow/white

LOXAPINE WATSON 371/25 mg
Capsules, USP, 25 mg ℞
Green/white

LOXAPINE WATSON 372/50 mg
Capsules, USP, 50 mg ℞
Blue/white

MAPROTILINE HYDROCHLORIDE WATSON/373
Tablets, USP, 25 mg ℞ (Partial Bisect)
Peach, Film Coated, Oval

MAPROTILINE HYDROCHLORIDE WATSON
Tablets, USP, 50 mg ℞ 374/Scored
Peach, Film Coated, Round

MAPROTILINE HYDROCHLORIDE WATSON/375
Tablets, USP, 75 mg ℞ (Partial Bisect)
White, Film Coated, Oval

MECLIZINE HCL
25 mg ℞ WATSON/803
yellow/white oval

MEPERIDINE HYDROCHLORIDE
Tablets, 50 mg USP ℞ CII WATSON/726/50
white, round, biconvex

MEPIRIDINE HYDROCHLORIDE
Tablets, 100 mg USP ℞ CII WATSON/727/100
white, round, biconvex

MEPROBAMATE
Tablets, 200 mg ℞ CIV WATSON/804
white round scored
400 mg ℞ CIV WATSON/805
white round convex

METHOCARBAMOL
Tablets, 500 mg ℞ WATSON/806
white round scored
750 mg ℞ WATSON/807
white capsule shaped

METHYLPREDNISOLONE
Tablets, 4 mg ℞ WATSON/790
white oval quadrisect

METOPROLOL TARTRATE WATSON 462/Scored
Tablets, USP, 50 mg ℞
Pink, Film Coated, Round

METOPROLOL TARTRATE WATSON 463/Scored
Tablets, USP, 100 mg ℞
Light Blue, Film Coated, Round

MEXILETINE HYDROCHLORIDE WATSON 491/150 mg
Capsules, USP, 150 mg ℞
Brown/Light Brown

MEXILETINE HYDROCHLORIDE WATSON 492/200 mg
Capsules, USP, 200 mg ℞
Brown/Brown

MEXILETINE HYDROCHLORIDE WATSON 493/250 mg
Capsules, USP, 250 mg ℞
Brown/Light Green

NAPROXEN
Tablets, 250 mg ℞ WATSON/821
white round
375 mg ℞ WATSON/822
gray capsule shaped
500 mg ℞ WATSON/791
white capsule shaped

NAPROXEN SODIUM
Tablets, 275 mg ℞ WATSON/792
white oval
550 mg ℞ WATSON/793
green oval

OXYBUTYNIN CHLORIDE
Tablets, 5 mg ℞ WATSON/779
pale blue round

OXYCODONE and
ACETAMINOPHEN WATSON 737/5–500 mg
Capsules, USP 5 mg/500 mg CII ℞
Opaque White and Opaque Red

OXYCODONE and ACETAMINOPHEN WATSON/749
Tablets, USP 5 mg/325 mg CII ℞ *Scored*
White, Round, Bisected

OXYCODONE HYDROCHLORIDE
Tablets, 5 mg USP CII ℞ WATSON/774
white, round *Scored on one side*

OXYCODONE and ASPIRIN
Tablets 4.5 mg/0.38 mg/325 mg USP CII ℞ WATSON/820
Yellow, Round, Biconvex *Scored*

PENTAZOCINE &
NALOXONE HCl WATSON 395/50/0.5
Tablets, USP, 50 mg/0.5 CIV ℞ *Scored*
Light Green, Capsule Shaped

PERPHENAZINE/AMITRIPTYLINE
HYDROCHLORIDE WATSON 706/2–10
Tablets, USP, 2 mg/10 mg ℞ *Biconvex*
Blue, Round, Film-coated

PERPHENAZINE/AMITRIPTYLINE
HYDROCHLORIDE WATSON 707/2–25
Tablets, USP, 2 mg/25 mg ℞ *Biconvex*
Light Orange, Round, Film-coated

PERPHENAZINE/AMITRIPTYLINE
HYDROCHLORIDE WATSON 708/4–10
Tablets, USP, 4 mg/10 mg ℞ *Biconvex*
Beige, Round, Film-coated

PERPHENAZINE/AMITRIPTYLINE
HYDROCHLORIDE WATSON 709/4–25
Tablets, USP, 4 mg/25 mg ℞ *Biconvex*
Yellow, Round,Film-coated

PIROXICAM WATSON 712/10 mg
Capsules, USP, 10 mg ℞
Light Blue/White

PIROXICAM WATSON 713/20 mg
Capsules, USP, 20 mg ℞
Light Blue/Light Blue

PREDNISONE
Tablets, 5 mg ℞ WATSON/830
white round
10 mg ℞ WATSON/831
white round
20 mg ℞ WATSON/832
peach round
50 mg ℞ WATSON/797
white round

PROPOXYPHENE HYDROCHLORIDE
& ACETAMINOPHEN WATSON 714/65–650
Tablets USP 65/650 mg CIV
Orange, Oblong

PROPRANOLOL HYDROCHLORIDE WATSON 305/
Tablets, USP, 10 mg ℞ Scored
Orange, Round

PROPRANOLOL HYDROCHLORIDE WATSON 306/
Tablets, USP, 20 mg ℞ Scored
Blue, Round

PROPRANOLOL HYDROCHLORIDE WATSON 307/
Tablets, USP, 40 mg ℞ Scored
Green, Round

PROPRANOLOL HYDROCHLORIDE WATSON 352/
Tablets, USP, 60 mg ℞ Scored
Pink, Round

PROPRANOLOL HYDROCHLORIDE WATSON 308/
Tablets, USP, 80 mg ℞ Scored
Yellow, Round

QUININE SULFATE WATSON 716/325 mg
Capsules, USP, 325 mg ℞
Opaque White/Opaque White

QUININE SULFATE WATSON 715/260 mg
Tablets, USP, 260 mg ℞
White, Round

RANITIDINE
Tablets, 150 mg ℞ WATSON/760
beige round
300 mg ℞ WATSON/761
beige capsule shaped

SELEGILINE HYDROCHLORIDE WATSON/137
Capsules, 5 mg ℞
Aqua Blue/Dark Blue

SELEGILINE HYDROCHLORIDE WATSON/136
Tablets, 5 mg ℞
White, Shield-shaped

SILVER SULFADIAZINE
Cream, 1% ℞
white

SUCRALFATE
Tablets, 1 gm ℞ WATSON/780
lt blue oblong

SULFASALAZINE
Tablets, 500 mg ℞ WATSON/796
mustard round bisect

TRIAMTERENE and
HYDROCHLOROTHIAZIDE WATSON 424/Scored
Tablets, USP, 37.5 mg/25 mg ℞
Light green, Round

TRIAMTERENE and
HYDROCHLOROTHIAZIDE WATSON 348/Scored
Tablets, USP, 75 mg/50 mg ℞
Yellow, Round

TRIHEXYPHENIDYL HYDROCHLORIDE — WATSON/575
Tablets, USP, 2 mg ℞
White, Round, Scored

TRIHEXYPHENIDYL HYDROCHLORIDE — WATSON 576
Tablets, USP, 5 mg ℞
White, Round, Scored

VALPROIC ACID
Syrup, 250 mg/5 mL ℞
Red

VERAPAMIL HYDROCHLORIDE — WATSON 404
Tablets, USP, 40 mg ℞
Light Peach, Film Coated, Round

VERAPAMIL HYDROCHLORIDE — WATSON 343/Scored
Tablets, USP, 80 mg ℞
White, Film Coated, Round

VERAPAMIL HYDROCHLORIDE — WATSON 344/Scored
Tablets, USP, 80 mg ℞
Light peach, Film Coated, Round

VERAPAMIL HYDROCHLORIDE — WATSON 345/Scored
Tablets, USP, 120 mg ℞
White, Film Coated, Round

VERAPAMIL HYDROCHLORIDE — WATSON 346/Scored
Tablets, USP, 120 mg ℞
Peach, Film Coated, Round

YOHIMBINE HYDROCHLORIDE — WATSON 717/5.4 *Biconvex, Scored*
Tablets, 5.4 mg ℞
White, Round

ORAL CONTRACEPTIVE PRODUCTS:
(available in 21 day and 28 day packs)

NORETHINDRONE
NOR-QD® Tablets
(norethindrone 0.35 mg)

NORETHINDRONE AND ETHINYL ESTRADIOL TABLETS USP: ℞
BREVICON®
NORINYL® 1+35
NORINYL® 1+50
TRI-NORINYL®
NECON® 0.5/35 — WATSON/507
(0.5 mg norethindrone and 35 mcg ethinyl estradiol)
NECON® 1/35 — WATSON/508
(1 mg norethindrone and 35 mcg ethinyl estradiol)
NECON® 10/11 — 10 tablets of WATSON/507 and 11 tablets of WATSON/508
(10 tablets—each contains 0.5 mg norethindrone and 35 mcg ethinyl estradiol; 11 tablets—each contains 1 mg norethindrone and 35 mcg ethinyl estradiol.)

NORETHINDRONE AND MESTRANOL TABLETS USP: ℞
NECON® 1/50 — WATSON/510
(1 mg norethindrone and 50 mcg mestranol)

NORGESTREL AND ETHINYL ESTRADIOL TABLETS USP: ℞
OGESTREL
(0.5 mg norgestrel and 0.05 mg ethinyl estradiol)
LOW-OGESTREL — 21 tablets of WATSON/847 and 7 tablets of P1
(0.3 mg norgestrel and 0.03 mg ethinyl estradiol)

ETHYNODIOL DIACETATE AND ETHINYL ESTRADIOL TABLETS USP: ℞
ZOVIA® 1/35E — WATSON 383/Blank
(1 mg ethynodiol diacetate and 35 mcg ethinyl estradiol)
ZOVIA® 1/50E — WATSON 384/Blank
(1 mg ethynodiol diacetate and 50 mcg ethinyl estradiol)

LEVONORGESTREL AND ETHINYL ESTRADIOL TABLETS USP: ℞
LEVORA® 0.15/30–28
(levonoregestrel and ethinyl estradiol tablets, USP)
TRIVORA®-28
(levonorgestrel and ethinyl estradiol tablets, USP)

ALORA® ℞
estradiol transdermal system
Continuous Delivery for Twice Weekly Dosing

PRESCRIBING INFORMATION

1. ESTROGENS HAVE BEEN REPORTED TO INCREASE THE RISK OF ENDOMETRIAL CARCINOMA IN POSTMENOPAUSAL WOMEN.
Close clinical surveillance of all women taking estrogens is important. Adequate diagnostic measures, including endometrial sampling when indicated, should be undertaken to rule out malignancy in all cases of undiagnosed persistent or recurring abnormal vaginal bleeding. There is currently no evidence that "natural" estrogens are more or less hazardous than "synthetic" estrogens at equi-estrogenic doses.

2. ESTROGENS SHOULD NOT BE USED DURING PREGNANCY.
There is no indication for estrogen therapy during pregnancy or during the immediate postpartum period. Estrogens are ineffective for the prevention or treatment of threatened or habitual abortion. Estrogens are not indicated for the prevention of postpartum breast engorgement.
Estrogen therapy during pregnancy is associated with an increased risk of congenital defects in the reproductive organs of the fetus, and possibly other birth defects. Studies of women who received diethylstilbestrol (DES) during pregnancy have shown that female offspring have an increased risk of vaginal adenosis, squamous cell dysplasia of the uterine cervix, and clear cell vaginal cancer later in life; male offspring have an increased risk of urogenital abnormalities and possibly testicular cancer later in life. The 1985 DES Task Force concluded that use of DES during pregnancy is associated with a subsequent increased risk of breast cancer in the mothers, although a causal relationship remains unproven and the observed level of excess risk is similar to that for a number of other breast cancer risk factors.

DESCRIPTION

Alora estradiol transdermal system is designed to deliver 17β-estradiol continuously and consistently over a 3 or 4-day interval upon application to intact skin. Three strengths of **Alora** systems are available, having nominal *in vivo* delivery of 0.05, 0.075, and 0.1 mg estradiol per day through skin of average permeability (inter-individual variation in skin permeability is approximately 20%). **Alora** systems have contact surface areas of 18, 27, and 36 cm^2 and contain 1.5, 2.3, and 3.0 mg of estradiol, USP, respectively. The composition of the systems per unit active surface area is identical. Estradiol, USP (17β-estradiol) is a white, crystalline powder that is chemically described as estra-1,3,5(10)-triene-3,17β-diol, has an empirical formula of $C_{18}H_{24}O_2$ and has molecular weight of 272.37. The structural formula is:

Estradiol

The **Alora** system consists of three layers. Proceeding from the polyethylene backing film as shown in the cross-sectional view below, the adhesive matrix drug reservoir that is in contact with the skin consists of estradiol, USP and sorbitan monooleate dissolved in an acrylic adhesive matrix. The polyester overlapped release liner protects the adhesive matrix during storage and is removed prior to application of the system to the skin.

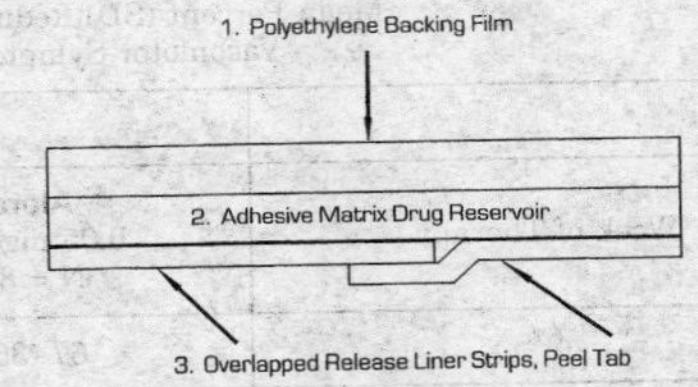

CLINICAL PHARMACOLOGY

Alora provides systemic estrogen replacement therapy by delivering estradiol, the major estrogenic hormone secreted by the human ovary, through the area of intact skin covered by the system. Estrogens are important in the development and maintenance of the female reproductive system and secondary sex characteristics. By a direct action, they cause growth and development of the uterus, Fallopian tubes, and vagina. With other hormones, such as pituitary hormones and progesterone, they cause enlargement of the breasts through promotion of ductal growth, stromal development, and the accretion of fat. They also contribute to the shaping of skeleton, maintenance of tone and elasticity of urogenital structures, changes in the epiphyses of the long bones that allow for the pubertal growth spurt and its termination, and pigmentation of the nipples and genitals.
Circulating estrogen concentration modulates the pituitary secretion of the gonadotrophins luteinizing hormone (LH) and follicle stimulating hormone (FSH) through a negative feedback mechanism and estrogen replacement therapy acts to reduce the elevated levels of these hormones seen in the postmenopausal woman. In a multiple dose study in 22 postmenopausal women, **Alora** 0.1 mg/day reduced circulating concentrations of LH and FSH by 34% and 45%, respectively, by the end of the third dose.
Estrogens occur naturally in several forms. The primary source of estrogen in normally cycling adult women is the ovarian follicle, which secretes 70 to 500 micrograms of estradiol daily, depending on the phase of the menstrual cycle. This is converted primarily to estrone, which circulates in roughly equal proportion to estradiol, and to a small amount of estriol. After menopause, most endogenous estrogen is produced by conversion of androstenedione, secreted by the adrenal cortex, to estrone by peripheral tissues. Thus, estrone (especially in its sulfate ester form) is the most abundant circulating estrogen in postmenopausal women. Although circulating estrogens exist in a dynamic equilibrium of metabolic interconversions, estradiol is the principal intracellular human estrogen and is substantially more potent than estrone or estriol at the receptor level.
Estrogen drug products act by regulating the transcription of a limited number of genes. Estrogens diffuse through cell membranes, distribute themselves throughout the cell, and bind to, and activate the nuclear estrogen receptor, a DNA-binding protein which is found in estrogen-responsive tissues. The activated estrogen receptor binds to specific DNA sequences, or hormone-response elements, which enhance the transcription of adjacent genes and in turn leads to the observed effects. Estrogen receptors have been identified in tissues of the reproductive tract, breast, pituitary, hypothalamus, liver, and in bone of women.
Estrogens used in therapy are well absorbed through the skin, mucous membranes, and gastrointestinal tract. When applied for a local action, absorption is usually sufficient to cause systemic effects. When conjugated with aryl and alkyl groups for parenteral administration, the rate of systemic absorption of injected oily preparations is slowed with a prolonged duration of action, such that a single intramuscular injection of estradiol valerate or estradiol cypionate is absorbed over several weeks.
Administered estrogens and their esters are handled within the body essentially the same as the endogenous hormones. Metabolic conversion of estrogens occurs primarily in the liver (first pass effect), but also at local target tissue sites. Complex metabolic processes result in a dynamic equilibrium of circulating conjugated and unconjugated estrogenic forms which are continually interconverted, especially between estrone and estradiol and between esterified and non-esterified forms. Although naturally-occurring estrogens circulate in the blood largely bound to sex hormone-binding globulin and albumin, only unbound estrogens enter target tissue cells. A significant proportion of the circulating estrogen exists as sulfate conjugates, especially estrone sulfate, which serves as a circulating reservoir for the formation of more active estrogenic species. A certain proportion of the estrogen is excreted into the bile and then reabsorbed from the intestine. During this enterohepatic recirculation, estrogens are desulfated and resulfated and undergo degradation through conversion to less active estrogens (estriol and other estrogens), oxidation to non-estrogenic substances (catecholestrogens, which interact with catecholamine metabolism, especially in the central nervous system), and conjugation with glucuronic acids (which are then rapidly excreted in the urine).
Loss of ovarian estradiol secretion after menopause can result in instability of thermoregulation, causing hot flushes associated with sleep disturbance and excessive sweating, and urogenital atrophy, causing dyspareunia and urinary incontinence. Estradiol replacement therapy alleviates many of these symptoms of estradiol deficiency in the menopausal woman.

Pharmacokinetics

Transdermal administration of **Alora** produces mean serum concentrations of estradiol comparable to those produced by premenopausal women in the early follicular phase of the ovulatory cycle. The pharmacokinetics and metabolism of transdermally administered estradiol using **Alora** have been evaluated in a total of 123 healthy postmenopausal women in three dose-range finding studies and in three definitive studies.

Absorption

Estradiol is transported across intact skin and into the systemic circulation by a passive diffusion process, the rate of diffusion across the stratum corneum being the principal factor. **Alora** presents sufficient concentration of estradiol to the surface of the skin to maintain continuous transport over the 3 to 4 day dosing interval.
Direct measurement of total absorbed dose of estradiol through analysis of residual estradiol content of systems worn over a continuous four day interval during 251 separate occasions in 123 postmenopausal women demonstrated that the average daily dose absorbed from **Alora** was 0.003 ± 0.001 mg estradiol per cm^2 active surface area. The nominal mean *in vivo* daily delivery rates of estradiol calculated from these data are 0.054 mg/day, 0.081 mg/day, and 0.11 mg/day for the 18 cm^2, 27 cm^2, and 36 cm^2 **Alora** systems, respectively.
In one multiple dose study, 22 postmenopausal women were treated with three consecutive **Alora** 0.1 mg/day systems on abdominal sites of application in a twice weekly dosing regimen and 3 consecutive Estraderm®[1] 0.1 estradiol transdermal systems in the same dosing regimen. During the third **Alora** dose, serum concentrations of estradiol increased above steady state baseline within 4 hours, achieved mean maximum concentration of 133 pg/ml within 18–24 hours, and remained relatively constant between 70 and 100 pg/ml until system removal at 96 hours. In contrast, Estraderm 0.1 mg/day produced higher fluctuations in estradiol serum concentrations, achieving and maintaining serum concentrations greater than 70 pg/ml only during the first 36 hours of the dosing period. Thereafter, serum estradiol concentrations declined steadily to a mean level of 22 pg/ml at system removal at 96 hours of the third dosing interval. The mean steady state estradiol serum concentration profiles for **Alora**

Continued on next page

Alora—Cont.

0.1 mg/day and Estraderm 0.1 mg/day are shown in Figure 1.

Figure 1

Mean steady state estradiol serum concentration during the third twice weekly dose of **Alora** 0.1 mg/day compared to Estraderm 0.1 mg/day in 22 postmenopausal women.

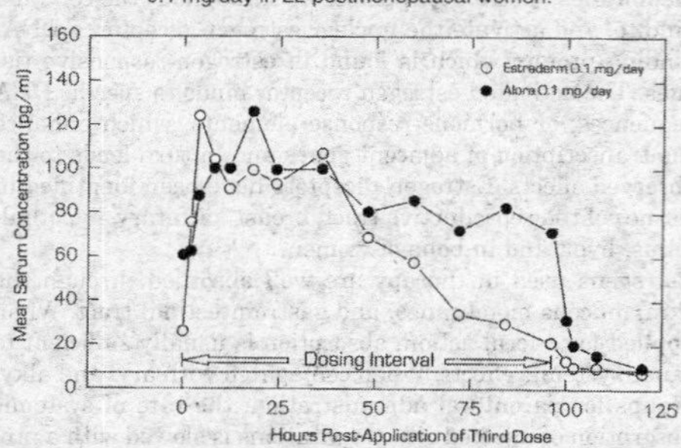

In another study, 20 women also were treated with three consecutive doses of **Alora** 0.05 mg/day, **Alora** 0.075 mg/day and **Alora** 0.1 mg/day on abdominal application sites. Mean steady state estradiol serum concentrations observed over the dosing interval are shown in Figure 2.

Figure 2

Mean steady state estradiol serum concentration during the third twice weekly dose of **Alora** 0.1 mg/day, **Alora** 0.075 mg/day, and **Alora** 0.05 mg/day in 20 postmenopausal women.

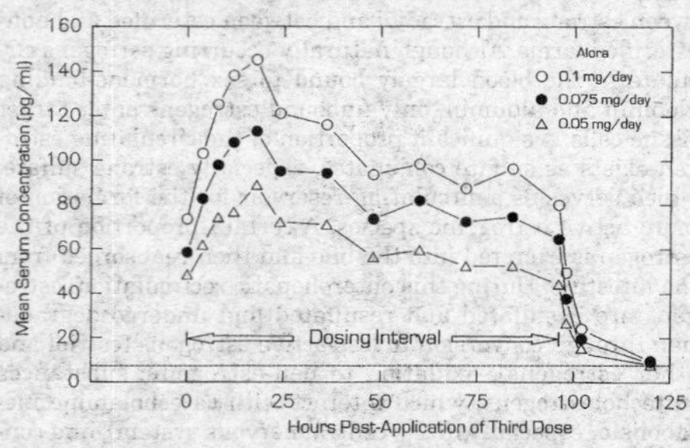

In a single dose randomized crossover study conducted to compare the effect of site of **Alora** application, 31 postmenopausal women wore single **Alora** 0.05 mg/day for four day periods on the lower abdomen, upper quadrant of the buttocks, and outside aspect of the hip. The estradiol serum concentration profiles are shown in Figure 3.

Figure 3

Mean estradiol serum concentration during a single 4 day wearing of **Alora** 0.05 mg/day applied by 31 postmenopausal women to the lower abdomen, upper quadrant of the buttocks or outer aspect of the hip.

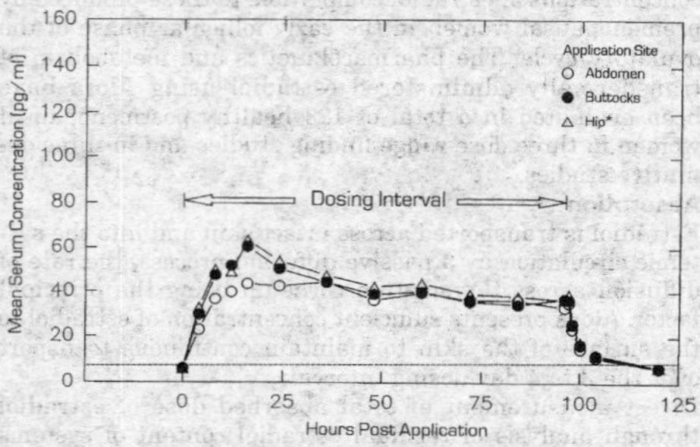

* C_{max} and C_{avg} statistically different from abdomen

Table 1 provides a summary of the estradiol pharmacokinetic parameters studied during biopharmaceutic evaluation of **Alora**.

[See table 1 above]

Distribution

No specific investigation of the tissue distribution of estradiol absorbed from **Alora** in humans has been conducted. However, a significant body of literature exists that indicates that estradiol is widely distributed in the body and is generally found in higher concentrations in the sex hormone target organs. Estradiol in blood is distributed between free estradiol, albumin bound estradiol, and sex hormone binding globulin (SHBG) bound estradiol. Serum concentrations reported here are expressed as total estradiol concentrations.

Metabolism

Since transdermally absorbed estradiol is not subject to first pass liver metabolism, the ratio of serum concentrations of estradiol to either of its major metabolites, estrone or estrone sulfate, is significantly greater than that seen for the oral route of administration. The clinical relevance of the estradiol to estrone ratio is presently unknown.

In controlled clinical trials using **Alora** compared to orally administered conjugated equine estrogens (CEE), the serum concentrations of estradiol and its metabolites were measured after 12 weeks therapy and are given in Table 2. The overall mean (SD) ratio of estradiol to estrone was 1.26 (0.80) for **Alora** and was 0.30 (0.39) for CEE.

[See table 2 above]

Elimination

No specific studies of elimination of estradiol have been performed using **Alora**. However, elimination of estradiol is known to be primarily through liver metabolism and conjugation to more hydrophilic compounds such as sulfates and glucuronides which are then cleared through renal elimination. Because estradiol has a short half-life, transdermal administration of estradiol allows for rapid decline in blood levels after **Alora** is removed. The apparent mean (SD) serum half-life of estradiol determined from biopharmaceutic studies conducted with **Alora** is 1.75 ± 2.87 hours.

Special Populations

Alora has been studied only in postmenopausal women.

CONTROLLED CLINICAL STUDIES

Efficacy and safety of **Alora** have been studied in two double blind/double dummy, randomized, parallel group trials involving a total of 594 postmenopausal women over a 12 week dosing period. In both studies, measures of efficacy included reduction in weekly number of moderate-to-severe vasomotor symptoms when compared to a weekly baseline average determined during a 2-week pre-dosing screening period. Only women having estradiol and FSH serum concentrations in the postmenopausal range and who exhibited a weekly average of at least 60 moderate-to-severe hot flushes during the screening period were enrolled in the studies.

In a positive control study, each patient received unopposed estrogen for a duration of 12 weeks in the form of **Alora** 0.05 mg/day, **Alora** 0.1 mg/day, administered twice weekly; or once daily oral administration of conjugated equine estrogens (CEE) 0.625 mg, or CEE 1.25 mg. In this study, the population was primarily caucasian (88%), had a mean age of 50.4 years (range 29–75 years), and had undergone either natural menopause (46%) or surgical menopause (54%) at an average age of 42.5 years (range 19–62 years). Mean baseline frequency of moderate-to-severe vasomotor symptoms was 95 per week in the overall population studied. Mean percent reduction in frequency of moderate-to-severe hot flushes is shown in Table 3.

[See table 3 above]

In a placebo-controlled study, each patient received either **Alora** 0.05 mg/day, **Alora** 0.1 mg/day, or matching placebo unopposed and dosed twice weekly over a 12 week duration. In this study, the population was also primarily caucasian (88%), had a mean age of 50.9 years (range 31–70 years), and had undergone either natural menopause (44%) or surgical menopause (56%) at an average age of 43.0 years (range 16–58 years). Mean baseline frequency of moderate-to-severe vasomotor symptoms was 89 per week in the overall population studied. Mean percent reduction in frequency of moderate-to-severe hot flushes is shown in Table 4.

[See table 4 above]

Table 1
Mean (SD) Pharmacokinetic Profile of **Alora**
Over an 84 Hour Dosing Interval

Alora (mg/day)	Application Site	N	Dosing	C_{max} (pg/ml)	C_{min} (pg/ml)	C_{avg} (pg/ml)	CL (L/hr)
0.05	Abdomen	20	Multiple	92 (33)	43 (12)	64 (19)	54 (18)
0.075	Abdomen	20	Multiple	120 (60)	53 (23)	86 (40)	53 (12)
0.1	Abdomen	42	Multiple	144 (57)	58 (20)	98 (38)	61 (18)
0.05	Abdomen	31	Single	53 (23)	—	41 (18)	69 (22)
	Buttock	31	Single	67 (45)	—	45 (21)	66 (23)
	Hip*	31	Single	69 (30)	—	48 (17)	62 (18)

* C_{max} and C_{avg} statistically different from abdomen

Table 2
Mean (SD) Serum Concentration of Estradiol and its Metabolites
After 12 Weeks Therapy with **Alora** or CEE

	Concentrations after 12 Weeks Therapy			
	Alora 0.05 mg/day	CEE 0.625 mg/day	**Alora** 0.1 mg/day	CEE 1.25 mg/day
Estradiol (pg/ml)	49 (52)	25 (32)	105 (89)	52 (66)
Estrone (pg/ml)	43 (23)	89 (42)	69 (37)	232 (210)
Estrone Sulfate (pg/ml)	765 (710)	1714 (1112)	1243 (960)	2741 (2655)

Table 3
Mean Percent (SD) Reduction in Frequency of Moderate-to-Severe
Vasomotor Symptoms for **Alora** Compared to CEE

	Mean Percent Reduction (SD)			
Week of Therapy	**Alora** 0.05 mg/day N = 79	CEE 0.625 mg/day N = 78	**Alora** 0.1 mg/day N = 79	CEE 1.25 mg/day N = 78
4 *	72 (26)	78 (30)	83 (28)	86 (20)
8 *	81 (24)	88 (21)	91 (22)	92 (18)
12	87 (20)	91 (18)	92 (20)	96 (11)

Analysis includes all randomized patients who received at least one dose of study drug and who had a post-baseline measurement of efficacy. At weeks 4 and 8, * indicates statistically significant differences ($p<0.05$) between **Alora** 0.05 mg/day and CEE 0.625 mg/day.

Table 4
Mean Percent (SD) Reduction in Frequency of Moderate-to-Severe
Vasomotor Symptoms for **Alora** Compared to Placebo

	Mean Percent Reduction (SD)		
Week of Therapy	**Alora** 0.05 mg/day N = 87	**Alora** 0.1 mg/day N = 91	Placebo N = 90
4 *	67 (36)	81 (32)	50 (41)
8 *	77 (42)	89 (27)	55 (42)
12*	80 (40)	90 (25)	60 (43)

Analysis includes all randomized patients who received at least one dose of study drug and who had a post-baseline measurement of efficacy. At weeks 4, 8, and 12, * indicates statistically significant differences ($p<0.05$) between both strengths of **Alora** and placebo.

In the two clinical trials, vaginal cytology was obtained predosing and at last visit in a total of 103 women treated with **Alora** 0.05 mg/day, in 88 women treated with **Alora** 0.1 mg/day and in 46 women in the placebo group. Superficial cells increased by a mean of 15.4%, 26.6% and 8.1% for the **Alora** 0.05 mg/day, **Alora** 0.1 mg/day, and placebo groups, respectively. Corresponding reductions in basal/parabasal and intermediate cells were also observed.

INDICATIONS AND USAGE

Alora is indicated in:

1. Treatment of moderate-to-severe vasomotor symptoms associated with the menopause. There is no adequate evidence that estrogens are effective for nervous symptoms or depression which might occur during menopause and they should not be used to treat these conditions.
2. Treatment of vulval and vaginal atrophy.
3. Treatment of hypoestrogenism due to hypogonadism, castration or primary ovarian failure.

CONTRAINDICATIONS

Estrogens should not be used in individuals with any of the following conditions:

1. Known or suspected pregnancy (see Boxed Warning): Estrogens may cause fetal harm when administered to a pregnant woman.
2. Undiagnosed abnormal genital bleeding;
3. Known or suspected cancer of the breast;
4. Known or suspected estrogen-dependent neoplasia;
5. Active thrombophlebitis, or thromboembolic disorders.
6. Known hypersensitivity to any of the components of **Alora**.

WARNINGS

1. Induction of malignant neoplasms.
   Endometrial cancer. The reported endometrial cancer risk among unopposed estrogen users is about 2 to 12 fold greater than in nonusers, and appears dependent on duration of treatment and on estrogen dose. Most studies show no significant increased risk associated with use of estrogens for less than one year. The greatest risk appears associated with prolonged use—with increased risks of 15 to 24-fold for five to ten years or more. In three studies, persistence of risk was demonstrated for 8 to over 15 years after cessation of estrogen treatment. In one study a significant decrease in the incidence of endometrial cancer occurred six months after estrogen withdrawal. Concurrent progestin therapy may offset this risk but the overall health impact in postmenopausal women is not known (see PRECAUTIONS).
   Breast cancer. Some studies have suggested a possible increased incidence of breast cancer in those women taking estrogen therapy at higher doses or for prolonged periods of time. While the majority of studies have not shown an increased risk of breast cancer in women who have ever used estrogen replacement therapy, some have reported a moderately increased risk (relative risks of 1.3–2.0) in those taking higher doses or those taking lower doses for prolonged periods of time, especially in excess of 10 years. On the other hand, other studies have not shown this relationship.
   Congenital lesions with malignant potential. Estrogen therapy during pregnancy is associated with an increased risk of fetal congenital reproductive tract disorders, and possibly other birth defects. Studies of women who received DES during pregnancy have shown that female offspring have an increased risk of vaginal adenosis, squamous cell dysplasia of the uterine cervix, and clear cell vaginal cancer later in life; male offspring have an increased risk of urogenital abnormalities and possibly testicular cancer later in life. Although some of these changes are benign, others are precursors of malignancy.
2. Gallbladder disease. Two studies have reported a 2- to 4-fold increase in the risk of gallbladder disease requiring surgery in women receiving oral estrogen replacement therapy, similar to the 2-fold increase previously noted in users of oral contraceptives.
3. Cardiovascular disease: Large doses of estrogen (5 mg conjugated estrogens per day), comparable to those used to treat cancer of the prostate and breast, have been shown in a large prospective clinical trial in men to increase the risk of nonfatal myocardial infarction, pulmonary embolism, and thrombophlebitis. These risks cannot necessarily be extrapolated from men to women. However, to avoid the theoretical cardiovascular risk to women caused by high estrogen doses, the dose for estrogen replacement therapy should not exceed the lowest effective dose.
4. Elevated blood pressure: Occasional blood pressure increases during estrogen replacement therapy have been attributed to idiosyncratic reactions to estrogens. More often, blood pressure has remained the same or has dropped. One study showed that postmenopausal estrogen users have higher blood pressure than nonusers. Two other studies showed slightly lower blood pressure among estrogen users compared to nonusers. Postmenopausal estrogen use does not increase the risk of stroke. Nonetheless, blood pressure should be monitored at regular intervals during estrogen use.
5. Hypercalcemia: Administration of estrogens may lead to severe hypercalcemia in patients with breast cancer and bone metastases. If hypercalcemia occurs, use of the drug should be stopped and appropriate measures should be taken to reduce the serum calcium level.

PRECAUTIONS

A. General

1. Addition of a progestin. Studies of the addition of a progestin for 10 or more days of a cycle of estrogen administration have reported a lowered incidence of endometrial hyperplasia than would be induced by estrogen treatment alone. Morphologic and biochemical studies of endometrium suggest that 10 to 14 days of progestin are needed to provide maximal maturation of the endometrium and to reduce the likelihood of hyperplastic changes.
   There are, however, possible risks which may be associated with the use of progestins in estrogen replacement regimens. These include:
   (1) adverse effects on lipoprotein metabolism (lowering HDL and raising LDL) which could diminish the purported cardioprotective effect of estrogen therapy (see PRECAUTIONS below).
   (2) impairment of glucose tolerance; and
   (3) possible enhancement of mitotic activity in breast epithelial tissue, although few epidemiological data are available to address this point (see PRECAUTIONS below).
   The choice of progestin, its dose, and its regimen may be important in minimizing these adverse effects, but these issues will require further study before they are clarified.
2. Cardiovascular risk. A causal relationship between estrogen replacement therapy and reduction of cardiovascular disease in postmenopausal women has not been proven. Furthermore, the effect of added progestins on this putative benefit is not yet known. In recent years, many published studies have suggested that there may be a cause-effect relationship between postmenopausal oral estrogen replacement therapy without added progestins and a decrease in cardiovascular disease in women. Although most of the observational studies which assess this statistical association have reported a 20% to 50% reduction in coronary heart disease risk and associated mortality in estrogen users, the following should be considered when interpreting these reports:
   (1) Because only one of these studies was randomized and it was too small to yield statistically significant results, all relevant studies were subject to selection bias. Thus, the apparently reduced risk of coronary disease cannot be attributed with certainty to estrogen replacement therapy. It may instead have been caused by life-style and medical characteristics of the women studied with the results that healthier women were selected for estrogen therapy. In general, treated women were of higher socioeconomic and educational status, more slender, more physically active, more likely to have undergone surgical menopause, and less likely to have diabetes than the untreated women. Although some studies attempted to control for these selection factors, it is common for properly designed randomized trials to fail to confirm benefits suggested by less rigorous study designs. Thus, ongoing and future large-scale randomized trials may fail to confirm this apparent benefit.
   (2) Current medical practice often includes the use of concomitant progestin therapy in women with intact uteri. (See PRECAUTIONS and WARNINGS). While the effects of added progestins on the risk of ischemic heart disease are not known, all available progestins reverse at least some of the favorable effects of estrogens on HDL and LDL levels.
   (3) While effects of added progestins on the risk of breast cancer are also unknown, available epidemiological evidence suggests that progestins do not reduce, and may enhance, the moderately increased breast cancer incidence that has been reported with prolonged estrogen replacement therapy (see WARNINGS above).

Because relatively long-term use of estrogens by a woman with a uterus has been shown to increase the risk of endometrial cancer, physicians often recommend that women who are deemed candidates for hormone replacement should take progestins as well as estrogens. When considering prescribing concomitant estrogens and progestins for hormone replacement therapy, physicians and patients are advised to carefully weigh the potential benefits and risks of the added progestin. Large-scale randomized, placebo-controlled, prospective clinical trials are required to clarify these issues.

3. Physical Examination. A complete medical and family history should be taken before initiation of any estrogen therapy. The pre-treatment and periodic physical examinations should include special reference to blood pressure, breasts, abdomen and pelvic organs, as well as a cervical Papanicolaou test. As a general rule, estrogen should be prescribed for no longer than 1 year without another physical examination being performed.
4. Hypercoagulability. Some studies have shown that women taking estrogen replacement therapy have hypercoagulability, primarily related to decreased antithrombin activity. This effect appears dose-and duration-dependent and is less pronounced than that associated with oral contraceptive use. Also postmenopausal women tend to have increased coagulation parameters at baseline compared to premenopausal women. There is some suggestion that low dose postmenopausal mestranol may increase the risk of thromboembolism, although the majority of studies (primarily of oral conjugated estrogen users) report no such increase. There is insufficient information on hypercoagulability in women who have had previous thromboembolic disease.
5. Familial hyperlipoproteinemia. Estrogen therapy may be associated with massive elevations of plasma triglycerides leading to pancreatitis and other complications in patients with familial defects of lipoprotein metabolism.
6. Fluid retention. Because estrogens may cause some degree of fluid retention, careful observation is required when conditions that might be influenced by this factor are present (e.g., asthma, epilepsy, migraine, and cardiac or renal dysfunction).
7. Uterine bleeding and mastodynia. Certain patients may develop undesirable manifestations of estrogenic stimulation, such as abnormal uterine bleeding and mastodynia.
8. Impaired liver function. Estrogens may be poorly metabolized in patients with impaired liver function and should be administered with caution in such patients.

B. Information for the Patient

See Patient Package Insert printed below.

C. Laboratory Tests

Estrogen administration should generally be guided by clinical response at the smallest dose, rather than laboratory monitoring, for relief of symptoms for those indications in which symptoms are observable.

D. Drug/Laboratory Test Interactions

1. Accelerated prothrombin time, partial thromboplastin time, and platelet aggregation time; increased platelet count; increased factors II, VII antigen, VIII antigen, VIII coagulant activity, IX, X, XII, VII-X complex, and beta-thromboglobulin; decreased levels of anti-factor Xa and antithrombin III, decreased antithrombin III activity; increased levels of fibrinogen and fibrinogen activity; increased plasminogen antigen and activity.
2. Increased thyroid-binding globulin (TBG) leading to increased circulating total thyroid hormone, as measured by protein-bound iodine (PBI), T4 levels (by column or by radioimmunoassay) or T3 levels by radioimmunoassay. T3 resin uptake is decreased, reflecting the elevated TBG. Free T4 and free T3 concentrations are unaltered.
3. Other binding proteins may be elevated in serum, i.e., corticosteroid binding globulin (CBG), sex hormone-binding globulin (SHBG), leading to increased circulating corticosteroids and sex steroids, respectively. Free or biologically active hormone concentrations are unchanged. Other plasma proteins may be increased (angiotensinogen/renin substrate, alpha-1-antitrypsin, ceruloplasmin).
4. Increased plasma HDL and HDL-2 subfraction concentrations, reduced LDL cholesterol concentration, increased triglycerides levels.
5. Impaired glucose tolerance.
6. Reduced response to the metapyrone test.
7. Reduced serum folate concentration.

E. Carcinogenesis, Mutagenesis, Impairment of Fertility

Long-term continuous administration of natural and synthetic estrogens in certain animal species increases the frequency of carcinomas of the breast, uterus, cervix, vagina, testis, and liver (see CONTRAINDICATIONS and WARNINGS).

F. Pregnancy Category X

Estrogens should not be used during pregnancy (see CONTRAINDICATIONS and Boxed Warnings).

G. Nursing Mothers

As a general principle, the administration of any drug to nursing mothers should be done only when clearly necessary since many drugs are excreted in human milk. In addition, estrogen administration to nursing mothers has been shown to decrease the quantity and quality of the milk.

H. Geriatric Use

The safety and effectiveness in geriatric patients (over age 65) have not been established.

ADVERSE REACTIONS

Alora has been studied in two well-controlled clinical trials. One study compared twice weekly dosing of **Alora** at 0.05 mg/day and 0.1 mg/day to once daily dosing of 0.625 mg and 1.25 mg of orally administered conjugated equine estrogens (CEE) in the intent-to-treat population of 321 postmenopausal women. In addition, the same **Alora** doses were studied in a placebo-controlled study in an intent-to-treat population of 273 postmenopausal women. Incidence of adverse experiences $> 5\%$ of each treatment group is given below in Table 5.

[See table 5 at top of next page]

Vaginal Bleeding

Overall in these two studies, 232 of the 594 patients enrolled possessed a partially or fully intact uterus. Fifty five (24%) of these women experienced at least one instance of vaginal bleeding during treatment. Of those patients receiving placebo, 12.9% of patients experienced at least one vaginal bleeding episode. The incidence of vaginal bleeding among estrogen treated patients increased with increasing

Continued on next page

Alora—Cont.

dose of all estrogen treatments: 8.7% of those receiving **Alora** 0.05 mg/day, 20.0% of those receiving CEE 0.625 mg/day, 33.3% of those receiving CEE 1.25 mg/day, and 33.3% of those receiving **Alora** 0.1 mg/day.

Skin Irritation

In the total population of 594 postmenopausal women exposed to either placebo and/or **Alora** systems in these studies, a total of 46 (7.7%) patients reported cases of skin reaction at the site of transdermal system application. The majority of these cases were mild and resolved spontaneously. Overall, therapy was discontinued by 13 (2.2%) patients due to system application site reaction, 8 (2.3%) of those receiving both placebo and **Alora** and 5 (2.0%) of those receiving only placebo systems.

The following additional adverse reactions have been reported with estrogen therapy (see WARNINGS regarding induction of neoplasia, adverse effects on the fetus, increased incidence of gallbladder disease, cardiovascular disease, elevated blood pressure, and hypercalcemia).

1. Genitourinary System. Changes in vaginal bleeding pattern and abnormal withdrawal bleeding or flow; breakthrough bleeding, spotting. Increase in size of uterine leiomyomata; vaginal candidiasis; change in amount of cervical secretion.
2. Breasts. Tenderness, enlargement.
3. Gastrointestinal. Nausea, vomiting, abdominal cramps, bloating; cholestatic jaundice; increased incidence of gallbladder disease.
4. Skin. Chloasma or melasma that may persist when the drug is discontinued, erythema multiforme, erythema nodosum, hemorrhagic eruption, loss of scalp hair, hirsutism.
5. Eyes. Steepening of corneal curvature; intolerance to contact lenses.
6. Central Nervous System. Headache, migraine, dizziness, mental depression, chorea.
7. Miscellaneous. Increase or decrease in weight, reduced carbohydrate tolerance, aggravation of porphyria, edema, changes in libido.

OVERDOSAGE

Serious ill effects have not been reported following acute ingestion of large doses of estrogen containing oral contraceptives by young children. Overdosage of estrogen may cause nausea and vomiting, and withdrawal bleeding may occur in females.

DOSAGE AND ADMINISTRATION

Alora should be administered twice weekly, as instructed. The adhesive side of the **Alora** system should be placed on a clean, dry area of skin. The recommended application site is the lower abdomen. In addition, the upper quadrant of the buttocks or outer aspect of the hip may be used. ***Alora should not be applied to the breasts.*** The sites of application should be rotated, with an interval of at least 1 week allowed between applications to a particular site. The area selected should not be oily, damaged, or irritated. The waistline should be avoided, since tight clothing may rub the system off. The system should be applied immediately after opening the pouch and removing the protective liner. The system should be pressed firmly in place with the palm of the hand for about 10 seconds, making sure there is good contact, especially around the edges.

In the event that a system should fall off, the same system may be reapplied. If necessary, a new system may be applied. In either case, the original treatment schedule should be maintained.

Initiation of Therapy

Three **Alora** strengths having nominal estradiol *in vivo* delivery rates of 0.05 mg/day, 0.075 mg/day, and 0.1 mg/day (differentiated by the physical size of **Alora**) are available for treatment of moderate-to-severe vasomotor symptoms, vulval and vaginal atrophy associated with the menopause, hypogonadism, castration, or primary ovarian failure. Treatment is usually initiated with **Alora** 0.05 mg/day applied to the skin twice weekly. The dose should be adjusted as necessary and the lowest dose required to control symptoms should be used. Attempts to discontinue or taper medication should be made at 3-month to 6-month intervals.

In women who are not currently taking oral estrogens or in women switching from topical therapy or another transdermal estradiol therapy, treatment with **Alora** can be initiated at once. In women who are currently taking oral estrogens, treatment with **Alora** should be initiated 1 week after withdrawal of oral therapy or sooner if menopausal symptoms reappear in less than 1 week.

Therapeutic Regimen

Alora may be administered in a continuous regimen in patients who do not possess an intact uterus. In those patients with an intact uterus who are not using concomitant progestin therapy, **Alora** can be administered on a cyclic schedule (e.g. 3 weeks of therapy followed by 1 week without).

HOW SUPPLIED

Alora 0.05 mg/day (estradiol transdermal system). Each 18 cm^2 system contains 1.5 mg of estradiol USP for nominal delivery of 0.05 mg of estradiol per day when dosed in a twice weekly regimen.

NDC 52544-471-08 Patient Calendar Box of 8 Systems
NDC 52544-471-23 Patient Calendar Box of 24 Systems

Table 5
Incidence of Adverse Events > 5%
in a Placebo-Controlled Study of **Alora**
Data are Expressed as % of Treatment Group

Adverse Event	**Alora** 0.05 mg/day N = 88	**Alora** 0.1 mg/day N = 94	Placebo N = 91
Infection	17.0	18.1	16.5
Headache	12.5	21.3	23.1
Sinusitis	6.8	10.6	6.6
Pain	6.8	5.3	5.5
Arthralgia	6.8	1.1	4.4
Abdominal Pain	5.7	3.2	3.3
Vaginal Discharge	4.5	5.3	0.0
Breast Pain	4.5	5.3	0.0
Nausea	4.5	4.3	11.0
Vaginal Bleeding	3.4	20.2	4.4
Back Pain	3.4	7.4	3.3
Vaginitis	3.4	3.2	9.9
Accidental Injury	2.3	6.4	4.4
Flatulence	2.3	5.3	1.1
Fibrocystic Breast	1.1	5.3	1.1
Pelvic Pain	0.0	5.3	2.2

Alora 0.075 mg/day (estradiol transdermal system). Each 27 cm^2 system contains 2.3 mg of estradiol USP for nominal delivery of 0.075 mg of estradiol per day when dosed in a twice weekly regimen.

NDC 52544-472-08 Patient Calendar Box of 8 Systems

Alora 0.1 mg/day (estradiol transdermal system). Each 36 cm^2 system contains 3.0 mg of estradiol USP for nominal delivery of 0.1 mg of estradiol per day when dosed in a twice weekly regimen.

NDC 52544-473-08 Patient Calendar Box of 8 Systems

Store at 15°–30°C (59°–86°F).

Do not store unpouched. Apply immediately upon removal from the protective pouch.

Discard used **Alora** in household trash in a manner that prevents accidental application or ingestion by children, pets, or others.

Distributed by: Watson Pharma, Inc.
a subsidiary of Watson Laboratories, Inc.
Corona, CA 92880
REVISED AUGUST 1999

1. Registered trademark of Ciba-Geigy.

PATIENT PACKAGE INSERT

Getting the Best Results with Alora—This Leaflet Can Help

This leaflet describes the correct way to apply and use the **Alora** patch—the key to getting the best results with **Alora**. It also talks about the risks and side effects of estrogen use. If you want to know more after you read it, ask your doctor, pharmacist, or other health care professional.

The **Alora** estradiol transdermal system is a thin, clear, plastic patch that sticks to the skin. Each patch is sealed in a pouch, which protects it until you're ready to put it on. Don't open a pouch or remove a patch until just before you apply it.

What You Need to Do: Checklist

✔ **Put on a new patch twice a week. Use one of the schedules on the inside flap of the patch box.**

For instance, if you apply your first patch on Sunday, take that patch off on Wednesday and put on a new one. Stick with this schedule as long as you use **Alora**. To help remind you, mark the schedule on the inside flap of the patch box. Put a check next to the first day you apply the patch.

✔ **Place the patch on the lower abdomen (below the panty line) when you first start using Alora.**

As you gain more experience applying **Alora**, you may want to try the hips or buttocks to see which area works best for you.

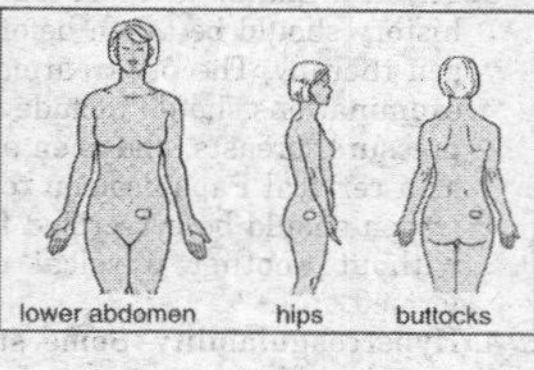

Do not apply **Alora** to your breasts or any other parts of the body.

To help the batch stay in place:

- Try not to disturb the patch while putting on and removing clothes. It may help to place the patch where your underwear will cover it at all times.
- Be careful while changing clothes, washing or drying off, so that you do not catch the patch with your clothes or the towel.
- Try different sites on the lower abdomen, hips, or buttocks area to see what works well with your body and your clothing.
- When you first start using the patch, be conscious of it.
- If the patch starts to lift, simply press it back in place.

When you change your patch, don't put the new one in the same place. For instance, if you had **Alora** on one side of the abdomen, put the new patch on the other side. Wait at least one week before you reuse any spot to help reduce the chance of skin redness or irritation.

✔ **Apply the patch with care. Before you begin, read all the information in these four steps.**

Step 1. Choose a spot for the patch.

Make sure the skin at the spot is:

- Freshly washed, but **dry and cool** (wait a few minutes after taking a hot bath or shower).
- Free of body powder or lotion.
- Free of cuts, rashes, or any other skin problem.

Step 2. Open the pouch that contains the patch.

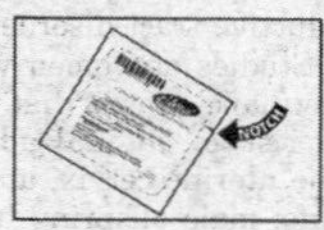
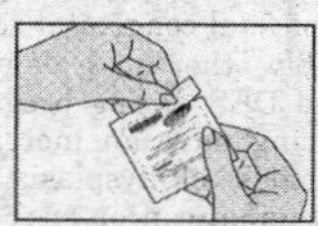

- Locate the notch on the top left or right corner of the pouch.
- Grasp the pouch at the notch and tear off the top edge. Do not cut the pouch with scissors, which might damage the patch inside.
- Pull the patch out.

Step 3. Apply one half of the patch to your skin.

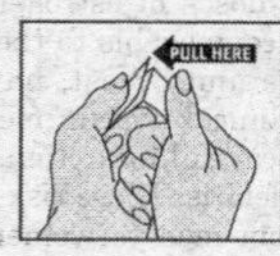

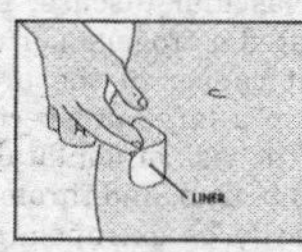

- Remove half of the liner, which covers the sticky surface of the patch. To find the liner, bend the patch in half. Then grab the clear straight edge of the liner and pull that piece off.
- Without touching the sticky surface, press the sticky half of the patch onto your skin. (If you touch the sticky surface, the patch may not stay on as well.)
- Rub the sticky half firmly to ensure full contact with your skin.

Step 4. Apply the second half of the patch to your skin.

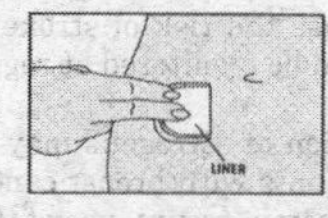

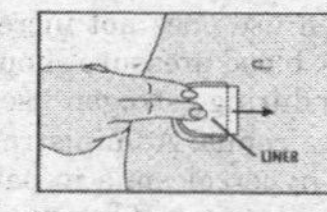

- Bend the patch back over itself. Press down on the liner firmly.

• Push the liner forward a little to loosen the edge.

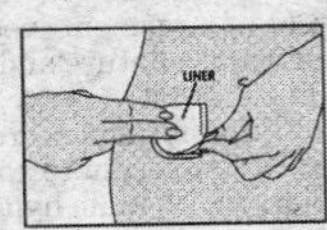

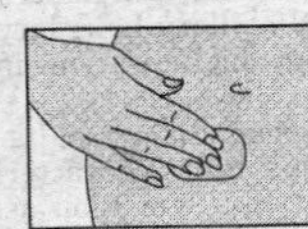

• Grab the loose edge at either corner and peel off the second piece of the liner. Try not to touch the sticky surface of the patch.
• **Press the entire patch firmly onto the skin with your finger tips.** Press for at least 10 seconds to make sure the patch will stay in place. Be sure all of it sticks to your skin, even around the edges.
• **Take off the old patch. Fold it in half (sticky sides together) and throw it away out of the reach of children and pets.**

The skin under the old patch may look pink, but the color should fade away soon. In some cases, the skin may itch or look red; this may last from a couple of hours to a couple of days. Most of the time this is minor, and goes away by itself. But if it bothers you a lot or lasts longer than a few days, call your doctor.

Questions You May Have

Q. Should I take the patch off when I swim or bathe?

A. No. Wear each patch all the time until you put on a new one. Baths, showers, or swimming should not affect the **Alora** patch as long as you don't rub the patch as you wash. Avoid soaking in a hot tub for a long time, though, which can make the patch come off.

Wearing the patch while spending time in the sun should be no problem. Just be sure you put the patch on a spot your clothing or bathing suit covers.

Q. What should I do if the patch comes off?

A. If the patch starts to lift off your skin, apply a little pressure with your fingertips. The patch is designed to restick. Most women find that the **Alora** patch seldom comes off. But if it does, try putting the same patch back on the same spot. If it sticks firmly all over, leave it on. If not, take it off and put a new patch on a new spot. No matter what day this happens, stick to the twice-a-week schedule that you have marked on the patch box for the next patch.

Q. What should I do if I forget to change the patch on the day it's due?

A. Remove the old patch and apply a new one to a new spot as soon as you remember. No matter what day this happens, stick to your twice-a-week schedule for the next patch.

Q. How long should I keep using Alora?

A. The answer will be different for each woman. Talk to your doctor every 6 months about how you are feeling and whether you still need estrogen.

For Best Results, Stick with Your Patch Program

• **Replace your patch twice each week, on the two days you have chosen.** Until it becomes a habit, try:
— Marking your schedule on the inside flap of the patch box;
— Marking the days on your calendar;

SU	M	TU	W	TH	F	SA
Alora			Alora			

— Linking the days you change your patch to other things that always happen on those days (e.g., an exercise class, meetings, etc.)

• **Handle each patch with care.**
— Make sure the skin is clean, dry, and free of lotion and powder.
— Try to avoid touching the sticky surface when applying the patch.
— Be careful while changing clothes, washing or drying off, so that you do not catch the patch with your clothes or the towel.
— When you first start using the patch, be conscious of it.
— If the patch starts to lift, simply press it back in place.

• **Keep working with your doctor, pharmacist, or other health care professional.** Ask questions. If you have concerns, talk them over—don't just stop using the patch on your own. Remember, it may take a little time and some experience to get accustomed to using a patch.
• **Get your refills of the Alora patch before your supply runs out.**

If you would like more information on the **Alora** patch, please call toll free **1-888-ALORA-4-U** (1-888-256-7248).

INFORMATION FOR THE PATIENT

INTRODUCTION

This leaflet describes when and how to use estrogens, and the risks and benefits of estrogen treatment. Your doctor has prescribed the **Alora** estradiol transdermal system for the treatment of your menopausal symptoms. Estradiol is the same hormone that your ovaries produce abundantly before menopause. During menopause, production of estrogen hormones by your body decreases well below the amounts normally produced during your fertile years. In many women this decrease in estrogen production causes uncomfortable symptoms, most noticeably hot flashes and sleep disturbances. Estrogens can be given to reduce or eliminate these symptoms.

Estrogens have important benefits but also some risks. You must decide, with your doctor, whether the benefits of estrogen use outweigh the risks. If you use estrogens, check with your doctor to be sure you are using the lowest possible dose that works and that you don't use them longer than necessary. How long you need to use estrogens will depend on the reason for use.

1. ESTROGENS INCREASE THE RISK OF CANCER OF THE UTERUS IN WOMEN WHO HAVE HAD THEIR MENOPAUSE ("CHANGE OF LIFE")
If you use any estrogen-containing drug, it is important to visit your doctor regularly and report any unusual vaginal bleeding right away. Vaginal bleeding after menopause may be a warning sign of uterine cancer. Your doctor should evaluate any unusual vaginal bleeding to find out the cause.
2. ESTROGENS SHOULD NOT BE USED DURING PREGNANCY
Estrogens do not prevent miscarriage (spontaneous abortion) and are not needed in the days following childbirth. If you take estrogens during pregnancy, your unborn child has a greater than usual chance of having birth defects. The risk of developing these defects is small, but clearly larger than the risk in children whose mothers did not take estrogens during pregnancy. These birth defects may affect the baby's urinary system and sex organs. Daughters born to mothers who took DES (an estrogen drug) have a higher than usual chance of developing cancer of the vagina or cervix when they become teenagers or young adults. Sons may have a higher than usual chance of developing cancer of the testicles when they become teenagers or young adults.

INFORMATION ABOUT ALORA

How Alora Works

The **Alora** estradiol transdermal system that your doctor has prescribed for you releases small amounts of estradiol through the skin and into the blood stream in a continous way. The dose of estradiol you require will depend on your individual response. The dose is adjusted by the size of the **Alora** estradiol transdermal system. **Alora** is available in three sizes.

Benefits of Treatment with Alora

Regular twice weekly use of **Alora** offers relief from moderate-to-severe symptoms of menopause, hot flashes and vaginal dryness. Small quantities of the naturally occurring hormone estradiol are absorbed through the skin from the **Alora** estradiol transdermal system, ensuring a continuous supply of circulating hormone in the body.

When estradiol is administered through the skin, the hormone does not undergo the rapid chemical changes in the liver and stomach that would occur if you were taking it in tablet or capsule form by mouth.

USES OF ESTROGEN

(Not every estrogen drug is approved for every use listed in this section. If you want to know which of these possible uses are approved for the medicine prescribed for you, ask your doctor or pharmacist to show you the professional labeling. You can also look up the specific estrogen product in a book called the "Physician's Desk Reference", which is available in many book stores and public libraries. Generic drugs carry virtually the same labeling information as their brand name versions.)

• **To reduce moderate or severe menopausal symptoms.**
Estrogens are hormones made by the ovaries of women. Between ages 45 and 55, the ovaries normally stop making estrogens. This drop in body estrogen levels causes the "change of life" or menopause (the end of monthly menstrual periods). Sometimes, both ovaries are removed during an operation before natural menopause takes place and the sudden drop in estrogen levels causes "surgical menopause."
When estrogen levels begin dropping, some women develop very uncomfortable symptoms, such as feelings of warmth in the face, neck, and chest, or sudden intense episodes of heat and sweating ("hot flashes" or "hot flushes"). Using estrogen drugs can help the body adjust to lower estrogen levels and reduce these symptoms. Some women have only mild menopausal symptoms, or none at all, and do not need estrogen therapy for these symptoms. Other women may need estrogens for a few months while their bodies adjust to lower estrogen levels. For the treatment of menopausal symptoms, the majority of women need estrogen replacement therapy for no longer than 6 months. Since every woman is different, you and your doctor should periodically reevaluate your need for continued estrogen use.
• **To treat vulval and vaginal atrophy** (itching, burning, dryness in or around the vagina, difficulty or burning on urination) associated with menopause.
• **To treat certain conditions in which a young woman's ovaries do not produce enough estrogen naturally.**
• **To treat certain types of abnormal vaginal bleeding due to hormonal imbalance when your doctor has found no serious cause of the bleeding.**
• **To treat certain cancers in special situations, in men and women.**
• **To prevent thinning of bones.**
Osteoporosis is a thinning of the bones that makes them weaker and allows them to break more easily. The bones of the spine, wrists, and hips break most often in osteporosis. Both men and women start to lose bone mass after about age 40, but women lose bone mass faster after menopause. Using estrogens after menopause slows down bone thinning and may prevent bones from breaking. Lifelong adequate calcium intake, either in the diet (such as dairy products) or by calcium supplements (to reach a total daily intake of 1000 milligrams before menopause or 1500 milligrams after menopause) may help to prevent osteoporosis. Regular weight-bearing exercise (like walking or running for an hour, two or three times a week) may also help to prevent osteoporosis. Before you change your calcium intake or exercise habits, it is important to discuss these lifestyle changes with your doctor to find out if they are safe for you.
Since estrogen use has some risks, only women who are likely to develop osteoporosis should use estrogens to prevent this condition. Women who are likely to develop osteoporosis often have the following characteristics: white or Asian race, slim, cigarette smokers, and a family history of osteoporosis in a mother, sister, or aunt. Women who have relatively early menopause, often because their ovaries were surgically removed, are more likely to develop osteoporosis than women whose menopause happens at the average age (about 45 to 55 years).

WHO SHOULD NOT USE ESTROGENS

Estrogens shoult not be used:

• **During pregnancy (see boxed Warning).**
If you think you may be pregnant, do not use any form of estrogen-containing drug. Using estrogens while you are pregnant may cause your unborn child to have birth defects. Estrogens do not prevent miscarriage.
• **If you have unusual vaginal bleeding which has not been evaluated by your doctor (see boxed Warning).**
Unusual vaginal bleeding can be a warning sign of cancer of the uterus, especially if it happens after menopause. Your doctor must find out the cause of the bleeding so that he or she can recommend the proper treatment. Taking estrogens without visiting your doctor can cause you serious harm if your vaginal bleeding is caused by cancer of the uterus.
• **If you have had cancer.**
Since estrogens increase the risk of certain types of cancer, you should not use estrogens if you have ever had cancer of the breast or uterus, unless your doctor recommends that the drug may help in the cancer treatment. (For certain patients with breast or prostate cancer, estrogens may help.)
• **If you have any circulation problems.**
Estrogen therapy should not be used except in unusually special situations and only after consultation with your doctor and only in recommended doses. Patients with a tendency for abnormal blood clotting should avoid estrogen use (see DANGERS OF ESTROGENS, below).
• **When they do not work.**
During menopause, some women develop nervous symptoms or depression. Estrogens do not relieve these symptoms. You may have heard that taking estrogens for years afer menopause will keep your skin soft and supple and keep you feeling young. There is no evidence for these claims and such long-term estrogen use may have serious risks.
• **After childbirth or when breast-feeding a baby.**
Estrogens should not be used to try to stop the breasts from filling with milk after a baby is born. Such treatment may increase the risk of developing blood clots (see DANGERS OF ESTROGENS, below).
If you are breast-feeding, you should avoid using any drugs because many drugs pass through to the baby in the milk. While nursing a baby, you should take drugs only on the advice of your health care provider.

DANGERS OF ESTROGENS

• **Cancer of the uterus.**
The risk of developing cancer of the uterus gets higher the longer estrogens are used and when larger doses are taken. One study showed that when estrogens are discontinued, this increased risk of cancer seems to fall off quickly. Three other studies showed that the risk for uterine cancer stayed high for 8 to more than 15 years after stopping estrogen treatment. Because of this risk, **IT IS IMPORTANT TO TAKE THE LOWEST DOSE THAT WORKS AND TO TAKE IT ONLY AS LONG AS YOU NEED IT.**
Using progestin therapy together with estrogen therapy may reduce the higher risk of uterine cancer related to estrogen use (see OTHER INFORMATION, below.)
If you have had your uterus removed (total hysterectomy), there is no danger of developing cancer of the uterus.
• **Cancer of the breast.**
Most studies have shown no association between the usual doses used for estrogen replacement therapy and breast cancer. However, some studies have reported that breast cancer developed more often (up to twice the usual rate) in women who used estrogens for long periods of time (especially longer than 10 years), or who used higher doses for shorter periods of time.
Regular breast examinations by a health professional and monthly self-examination are recommended for women receiving estrogen therapy, as they are for all women.
• **Gallbladder disease.**
Women who use esrogens after menopause are more likely to develop gallbladder disease needing surgery than women who do not use estrogens.
• **Abnormal blood clotting.**
Taking estrogens may increase the risk of blood clots. These changes allow the blood to clot more easily, possibly

Continued on next page

Alora—Cont.

allowing clots to form in your bloodstream. If blood clots do form in your bloodstream, they can cut off the blood supply to vital organs, causing serious problems. These clots can cause a stroke (by cutting off blood to the brain), heart attack (by cutting off blood to the heart), a pulmonary embolus (by cutting off blood to the lungs), or other problems. Any of these conditions may be fatal or cause serious long-term disability. However, most studies of low-dose estrogen usage by women do not show an increased risk of these complications.

SIDE EFFECTS

In addition to the risks listed above, the following side effects have been reported with estrogen use:

- Nausea and vomiting.
- Breast tenderness or enlargement.
- Enlargement benign tumors ("fibroids") of the uterus.
- Retention of excess fluid. This may make some conditions worsen, such as asthma, epilepsy, migraine, heart disease, or kidney disease.
- A spotty darkening of the skin, particularly on the face.
- Skin irritation, redness, or rash may occur at the site of application.

REDUCING RISK OF ESTROGEN USE

If you use estrogens, you can reduce your risks by doing these things:

- **See your doctor regularly.**
  While you are using estrogens, it is important to visit your doctor at least once a year for a check-up. If you develop vaginal bleeding while taking estrogens, you may need further evaluation. If members of your family have had breast cancer or if you have ever had breast lumps or an abnormal mammogram (breast x-ray), you may need to have more frequent breast examinations.
- **Reassess your need for estrogens.**
  You and your doctor should reevaluate whether or not you still need estrogens at least every six months.
- **Be alert for signs of trouble.**
  If any of these warning signals (or any other unusual symptoms) happen while you are using estrogens, call your doctor immediately:
  — Abnormal bleeding from the vagina (possible uterine cancer).
  — Pains in the calves or chest, sudden shortness of breath, or coughing blood (possible clots in the legs, heart or lungs).
  — Severe headache or vomiting, dizziness, faintness, changes in vision or speech, weakness or numbness of an arm or leg (possible clot in the brain or eye).
  — Breast lumps (possible breast cancer; ask your doctor or health professional to show you how to examine your breasts monthly).
  — Yellowing of the skin or eyes (possible liver problem).
  — Pain, swelling or tenderness in the abdomen (possible gallbladder problem).

OTHER INFORMATION

1. Estrogens increase the risk of developing a condition (endometrial hyperplasia) that may lead to cancer of the lining of the uterus. If your uterus has not been removed, your doctor may choose to prescribe a progestin, a different hormone drug to be used in association with estrogen treatment. Progestin lowers the risk of developing endometrial hyperplasia, a possible precancerous condition of the uterine lining, which may occur while using estrogen. There may be additional risks associated with the use of progestin together with estrogen treatment. The possible risks include:
   - unfavorable effects on blood fats (especially the lowering of HDL blood cholesterol, the "good" cholesterol which protects against heart disease);
   - unhealthy effects on blood sugar (which might make a diabetic condition worse); and
   - a possible further increase in breast cancer risk which may be associated with long-term estrogen use.

   Some research has suggested that estrogen taken without progestin may protect women against developing heart disease. However, this effect of estrogen is not certain because the estrogen-treated women had characteristics known to protect against heart disease; they were slimmer, more physicaly active, and less likely to have diabetes.

   You are cautioned to discuss very carefully with your doctor or healthcare provider all the possible risks and benefits of long-term estrogen and progestin treatment, as they affect you personally.
2. Your doctor has prescribed this drug for you and you alone. Do not give the drug to anyone else.
3. If you will be taking calcium supplements as part of the treatment to help prevent osteoporosis, check with your doctor about how much to take.
4. Keep this and all drugs out of the reach of children. In case of overdose, remove the system and call your doctor, hospital, or poison control center immediately. Dispose of used **Alora** estradiol transdermal systems in a manner that prevents accidental application or ingestion by children, pets, or others.

This leaflet provides a summary of the most important information about estrogens. If you want more information, ask your doctor or pharmacist to show you the professional labeling.

HOW SUPPLIED

Alora estradiol transdermal system 0.05 mg/day
Patient Calendar Box of 8 Systems (**NDC** 52544-471-08)
Patient Calendar Box of 24 Systems (**NDC** 52544-471-23)
Alora estradiol transdermal system 0.075 mg/day
Patient Calendar Box of 8 Systems (**NDC** 52544-472-08)
Alora estradiol transdermal system 0.1 mg/day
Patient Calendar Box of 8 Systems (**NDC** 52544-473-08)
Store at 15°–30°C (59°–86°F).
Do not store unpouched.
Apply immediately upon removal from the protective pouch.
Distributed by: Watson Pharma, Inc.
a subsidiary of Watson Laboratories, Inc.
Corona, CA 92880
REVISED AUGUST 1999
U.S. Patent Nos. 5,122,383; 5,227,168; 5,212,199; and 5,164,190

ANDRODERM®

Ⓒ℞

[*an-drō-derm*]

Testosterone Transdermal System
Controlled Delivery for Once-Daily Application

DESCRIPTION

Androderm (testosterone transdermal system) provides continuous delivery of testosterone (the primary endogenous androgen) for 24 hours following application to intact, nonscrotal skin (e.g., back, abdomen, thighs, upper arms).

Two strengths of *Androderm* are available which deliver *in vivo* 2.5 mg or 5 mg of testosterone per day across skin of average permeability.

Androderm has a central drug delivery reservoir surrounded by a peripheral adhesive area. The *Androderm* 2.5 mg system has a total contact surface area of 37 cm² with a 7.5 cm² central drug delivery reservoir containing 12.2 mg testosterone USP, dissolved in an alcohol-based gel. The *Androderm* 5 mg system has a total contact surface area of 44 cm² with a 15 cm² central drug delivery reservoir containing 24.3 mg testosterone USP, dissolved in an alcohol-based gel. Testosterone USP is a white, or creamy white crystalline powder or crystals chemically described as 17β- hydroxyandrost-4-en-3-one.

Testosterone
$C_{19}H_{28}O_2$ mw 288.43

The *Androderm* systems have six components as shown in Figure 1. Proceeding from the top toward the surface attached to the skin, the system is composed of (1) metallized polyester/Surlyn®* (ethylene-methacrylic acid copolymer)/ ethylene vinyl acetate backing film with alcohol resistant ink, (2) a drug reservoir of testosterone USP, alcohol USP, glycerin USP, glycerol monooleate, methyl laurate, and purified water USP, gelled with an acrylic acid copolymer, (3) a permeable polyethylene microporous membrane, and (4) a peripheral layer of acrylic adhesive surrounding the central, active drug delivery area of the system. Prior to opening of the system and application to the skin, the central delivery surface of the system is sealed with a peelable laminate disc (5) composed of a five-layer laminate containing polyester/ polyesterurethane adhesive/aluminum foil/polyesterurethane adhesive/polyethylene. The disc is attached to and removed with the release liner (6), a silicone-coated polyester film, which is removed before the system can be used.

*Surlyn is a registered trademark of E.I. DuPont de Nemours & Company

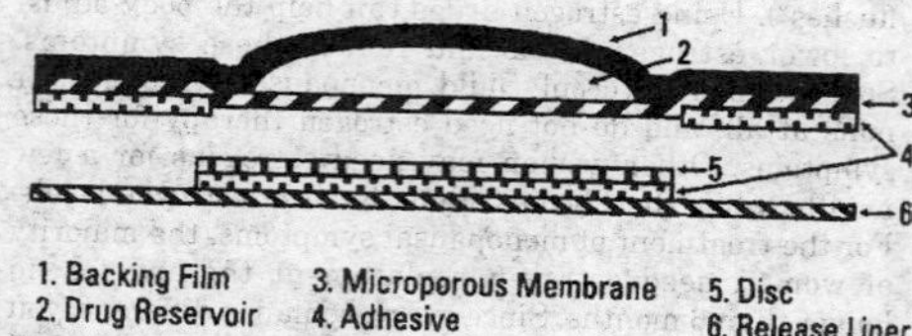

Figure 1: System Schematic

The active ingredient in the system is testosterone. The remaining components of the system are pharmacologically inactive.

CLINICAL PHARMACOLOGY

Androderm (testosterone transdermal system) delivers physiologic amounts of testosterone producing circulating testosterone concentrations that approximate the normal circadian rhythm of healthy young men.

Testosterone

Androderm (testosterone transdermal system) delivers testosterone, the primary androgenic hormone. Testosterone is responsible for the normal growth and development of the male sex organs and for maintenance of secondary sex characteristics. These effects include the growth and maturation of the prostate, seminal vesicles, penis, and scrotum; development of male hair distribution, such as facial, pubic, chest, and axillary hair; laryngeal enlargement; vocal cord thickening; and alterations in body musculature and fat distribution.

Male hypogonadism results from insufficient secretion of testosterone and is characterized by low serum testosterone concentrations. Symptoms associated with male hypogonadism include the following: impotence and decreased sexual desire; fatigue and loss of energy; mood depression; and regression of secondary sexual characteristics.

General Androgen Effects

Androgens promote retention of nitrogen, sodium, potassium, and phosphorus, and decreased urinary excretion of calcium. Androgens have been reported to increase protein anabolism and decrease protein catabolism. Nitrogen balance is improved only when there is sufficient intake of calories and protein.

Androgens are also responsible for the growth spurt of adolescence and for the eventual termination of linear growth that is brought about by the fusion of the epiphyseal growth centers. In children, exogenous androgens accelerate linear growth rates but may cause disproportionate advancement in bone maturation. Use over long periods may result in fusion of the epiphyseal growth centers and termination of the growth process. Androgens have been reported to stimulate the production of red blood cells by enhancing erythropoietin production.

During exogenous administration of androgens, endogenous testosterone release is inhibited through feedback inhibition of pituitary LH secretion. With large doses of exogenous androgens, spermatogenesis may also be suppressed through feedback inhibition of pituitary follicle stimulating hormone (FSH) secretion.

There is a lack of substantial evidence that androgens are effective in accelerating fracture healing or in shortening post-surgical convalescence.

Pharmacokinetics

Absorption

Following Androderm (testosterone transdermal system) application to non-scrotal skin, testosterone is continuously absorbed during the 24-hour dosing period. Daily application of *Androderm* at approximately 10 PM results in a serum testosterone concentration profile that mimics the normal circadian variation observed in healthy young men (Fig. 2 below). Maximum concentrations occur in the early morning hours with minimum concentrations in the evening (Table 1 below).

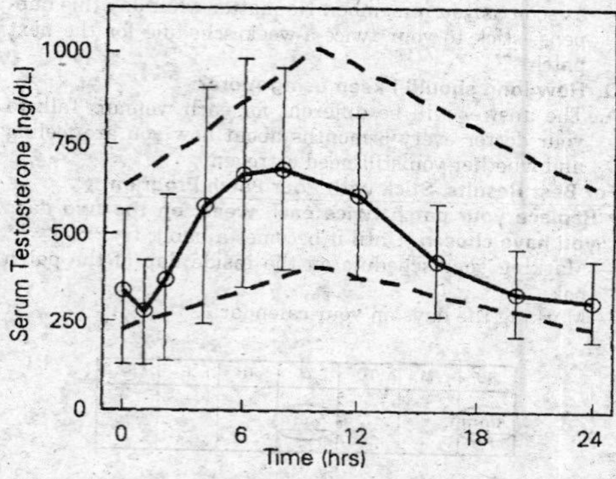

Figure 2: Mean (SD) steady state serum testosterone concentrations during nightly application of *Androderm* 2.5 mg systems in 29 hypogonadal male patients, 27 patients used 2 systems nightly and 2 patients used 3 systems nightly. Area between the dashed lines shows the 95% confidence interval for the circadian variation observed in healthy young men.[1] System application (t=0) at approximately 10 PM.

Table 1: Steady-state serum testosterone pharmacokinetic parameters in hypogonadal men measured during continuous Androderm (testosterone transdermal system) treatment.

Parameter	Units	n	Mean	SD
Cmax	ng/dL	56	753	276
Cavg	ng/dL	56	498	169
Cmin	ng/dL	56	246	120
Tmax	hr	56	7.9	2.2
$T_{1/2}$	min	29	71	32
CL	L/day	49	1304	464

Cmax = maximum serum concentration
Cavg = average serum concentration (AUC/24 hr)
Cmin = minimum serum concentration
Tmax = time of maximum serum concentration
$T_{1/2}$ = elimination half-life
CL = clearance

In a group of 34 hypogonadal men, application of two *Androderm* 2.5 mg systems to the abdomen, back, thighs, or upper arms resulted in average testosterone absorption of 4 to 5 mg over 24 hours. The serum testosterone concentration profiles during application were similar for these sites (Table 2). Applications to the chest and shins resulted in greater inter-individual variability and average 24 hour absorption of 3 to 4 mg.

[See table at top of next page]

In a steady-state study of 12 hypogonadal men, nightly application of 1, 2, or 3 *Androderm* 2.5 mg systems resulted in increases in the mean morning serum testosterone concentrations. These concentrations averaged 424, 584, and 766 ng/dL with the application of 1, 2, and 3 systems, respectively. The mean baseline serum testosterone concentration was 76 ng/dL.

Normal range morning serum testosterone concentrations are reached during the first day of dosing. There is no accumulation of testosterone during continuous treatment.

In a study of 20 hypogonadal patients, two *Androderm* 2.5 mg systems and a single *Androderm* 5 mg system produced equivalent serum testosterone concentration profiles. Average steady state concentrations over 24 hours (Cssavg) were 613±169 and 621±176 ng/dL for the two 2.5 mg and single 5 mg systems, respectively. Cmax values were 925±340 ng/dL for the two 2.5 mg systems and 905±254 ng/dL for the single 5 mg system.

In 16 hypogonadal men, the topical administration of 0.1% triamcinolone cream to the skin under the central drug reservoir prior to application of the *Androderm* system did not significantly alter transdermal absorption of testosterone; however, the rate of complete adherence was lower. In these patients, pretreatment with an ointment formulation significantly reduced testosterone absorption from the system.

Distribution

In serum, testosterone is bound with high affinity to sex hormone binding globulin (SHBG) and with low affinity to albumin. The albumin bound portion easily dissociates and is presumed to be bioactive. The SHBG-bound portion is not considered to be bioactive. The amount of SHBG in serum and the total testosterone concentration determine the distribution of bioactive and non-bioactive androgen.

Bioactive serum testosterone concentrations (BT) measured during Androderm (testosterone transdermal system) treatment paralleled the serum testosterone profile (Figure 2) and remained within the normal reference range.

Metabolism

Inactivation of testosterone occurs primarily in the liver. Testosterone (T) is metabolized to various 17-keto steroids through two different pathways, and the major active metabolites are estradiol (E2) and dihydrotestosterone (DHT). DHT binds with greater affinity to SHBG than does testosterone. In reproductive tissues, DHT is further metabolized to 3-alpha and 3-beta androstanediol.

In many tissues, the activity of testosterone appears to depend on reduction to DHT, which binds to cytosol receptor proteins. The steroid-receptor complex is transported to the nucleus, where it initiates transcription events and cellular changes related to androgen action.

During steady-state pharmacokinetic studies in hypogonadal men treated with *Androderm*, the average DHT:T and E2:T ratios were comparable to those in normal men, approximately 1:10 and 1:200, respectively.

Upon removal of the *Androderm* systems, serum testosterone concentrations decrease with an apparent half-life of approximately 70 minutes. Hypogonadal concentrations are reached within 24 hours following system removal.

Androderm therapy suppresses endogenous testosterone secretion via the pituitary/gonadal axis, resulting in a reduction in baseline serum testosterone concentrations compared to the untreated state.

Excretion

Approximately 90% of a testosterone dose given intramuscularly is excreted in the urine as glucuronide and sulfate conjugates of testosterone and its metabolites; about 6% is excreted in the feces, mostly in unconjugated form.

Special Populations

Geriatric

No age related effects on testosterone pharmacokinetics were observed in clinical trials of *Androderm* in men up to 65 years of age. In a group of 9 elderly testosterone deficient men (65–79 years of age, average baseline testosterone level 184±50 ng/dL), a single application of two *Androderm* 2.5 mg systems to the back resulted in an average testosterone level of 591±121 ng/dL with a Tmax of 14.2±4.2 hours. The total testosterone delivered over the 24-hour application time was 3.8±0.6 mg, approximately 20% less than the average amount delivered in younger patients.

Race

There is insufficient information available from *Androderm* trials to compare testosterone pharmacokinetics in different racial groups.

Renal Insufficiency

There is no experience with use of *Androderm* in patients with renal insufficiency.

Hepatic Insufficiency

There is no experience with use of *Androderm* in patients with hepatic insufficiency.

Drug-Drug Interactions

See "Precautions" below

Clinical Studies

In clinical studies using the *Androderm* 2.5 mg system, 93% of patients were treated with two systems daily, 6% used three systems daily, and 1% used one system daily.

The hormonal effects of Androderm (testosterone transdermal system) as a treatment for male hypogonadism were demonstrated in four open-label trials that included 94 hypogonadal men, ages 15 to 65 years. In these trials, *Androderm* produced average morning serum testosterone concentrations within the normal reference range in 92% of patients. The mean (SD) serum hormone concentrations and percentage of patients who achieved average concentrations within the normal ranges are shown in Table 3 below.

Table 2: Mean serum testosterone concentrations (ng/dL) measured during single-dose applications of two *Androderm* 2.5 mg systems applied at night to different sites in 34 hypogonadal men.

Sample Time (hr)	Abdomen		Back		Thigh		Upper Arm	
	Mean	SD	Mean	SD	Mean	SD	Mean	SD
0	90	82	80	74	85	76	81	69
3	286	201	429	252	271	201	308	226
6	476	236	608	250	489	254	468	245
9	570	234	613	214	592	251	534	204
12	575	244	588	233	594	247	527	199
24	352	164	403	174	367	161	332	124

Table 3: Individual morning serum hormone concentrations (ng/dL) and percent of patients with mean concentrations within the normal range during continuous *Androderm* treatment (n=94).

Normal Range	T (306–1031)	BT (93–420)	DHT (28–85)	E2 (0.9–3.6)
Mean	589	312	47	2.7
SD	209	127	18	1.2
% Normal	92	88	85	77
% High	1	12	2	22
% Low	7	0	13	1

A physiological suppression of the pituitary/gonadal axis occurs during continuous *Androderm* treatment leading to reduced serum LH concentrations. In clinical trials, 10 of 21 (48%) of men with primary (hypergonadotropic) hypogonadism achieved normal range LH concentrations within 6 to 12 months of treatment. LH concentrations may remain elevated in some patients despite serum testosterone concentrations within the normal range.

Twenty-nine patients, previously treated with testosterone, completed 12 months of *Androderm* treatment. Following an 8-week androgen withdrawal period, *Androderm* treatment produced positive effects on fatigue, mood and sexual function. The percent of patients complaining of fatigue decreased from 79% to 10% during treatment ($p<0.001$). The average patient depression score (Beck Depression Inventory) decreased from 6.9 to 3.9 ($p<0.001$). Nocturnal penile tumescence and rigidity monitoring showed an increase in mean duration of erections 0.23 to 0.39 hours per night (p=0.01) and an increase in penile tip rigidity from 18% to 50% ($p<0.001$). The total number of self-reported erections reported increased from 2.3 to 7.8 per week ($p<0.001$).

Comparison with intramuscular testosterone: Sixty-six patients, previously treated with testosterone injections, received *Androderm* or intramuscular testosterone enanthate (200 mg every 2 weeks) treatment for 6 months. The percent of time that serum concentrations measured throughout the dosing interval remained within the normal range were as follows:

	Androderm	IM	*p* value
T	82%	72%	0.05
BT	87%	39%	<0.001
DHT	76%	70%	0.06
E2	81%	35%	<0.001

Sexual function was comparable between groups.

Effect on plasma lipids: In 67 men treated for 6 to 12 months, the average (SE) serum total cholesterol and HDL concentrations were 199 (7.6) ng/dL and 46 (2.3) ng/dL. Compared to baseline values during a hypogonadal state achieved by 8 weeks of androgen withdrawal in 29 patients, the following changes in lipids were observed during 1 year of *Androderm* treatment: Cholesterol decreased 1.2%; HDL decreased 8%; Cholesterol/HDL ratio increased 9%. In these patients, lipids measured during *Androderm* treatment were not significantly different from those measured during prior IM injection treatment.

Effects on the prostate: Prostate size and serum prostate specific antigen (PSA) concentrations during treatment were comparable to values reported for eugonadal men. One case of prostate carcinoma occurred during *Androderm* treatment; two cases were detected during IM treatment.

INDICATIONS AND USAGE

Androderm (testosterone transdermal system) is indicated for testosterone replacement therapy in men for conditions associated with a deficiency or absence of endogenous testosterone.

Primary hypogonadism (congenital or acquired)—Testicular failure due to cryptorchidism, bilateral torsion, orchitis, vanishing testis syndrome, or orchidectomy, Klinefelter's syndrome, chemotherapy, or toxic damage from alcohol or heavy metals. These men usually have low serum testosterone concentrations accompanied by gonadotropins (FSH, LH) above the normal range.

Secondary, i.e., hypogonadotropic hypogonadism (congenital or acquired)—idiopathic gonadotropin or luteinizing hormone-releasing hormone (LHRH) deficiency, or pituitary-hypothalamic injury from tumors, trauma, or radiation. These men have low serum testosterone concentrations without associated elevation in gonadotropins. Appropriate adrenal cortical and thyroid hormone replacement therapy may be necessary in patients with multiple pituitary or hypothalamic abnormalities.

CONTRAINDICATIONS

Androgens are contraindicated in men with carcinoma of the breast or known or suspected carcinoma of the prostate.

Androderm therapy has not been evaluated in women and must not be used in women. Testosterone may cause fetal harm.

Androderm is contraindicated in patients with known hypersensitivity to any of its components.

WARNINGS

Prolonged use of high doses of orally active 17-alpha-alkyl androgens (e.g., methyltestosterone) has been associated with the development of peliosis hepatis, cholestatic jaundice and hepatic neoplasms, including hepatocellular carcinoma (see PRECAUTIONS, Carcinogenesis). Peliosis hepatis can be a life-threatening or fatal complication. Testosterone is not known to produce these adverse effects.

Geriatric patients treated with androgens may be at an increased risk for the development of prostatic hyperplasia.

Geriatric patients and other patients with clinical or demographic characteristics that are recognized to be associated with an increased risk of prostate cancer should be evaluated for the presence of subclinical or clinical prostate cancer prior to initiation of testosterone replacement therapy, because testosterone therapy may promote the growth of existing subclinical foci of prostate cancer.[2]

In men receiving testosterone replacement therapy, surveillance for prostate cancer should be consistent with current practices for eugonadal men (see PRECAUTIONS, Carcinogenesis).

Edema, with or without congestive heart failure, may be a serious complication of androgen treatment in patients with preexisting cardiac, renal, or hepatic disease. In addition to discontinuation of the drug, diuretic therapy may be required.

Gynecomastia frequently develops and occasionally persists in patients being treated for hypogonadism.

PRECAUTIONS

General

The physician should instruct patients to report any of the following side effects of androgens:

- Too frequent or persistent erections of the penis
- Any nausea, vomiting, jaundice, or ankle swelling

Virilization of female sexual partners has been reported with male use of a topical testosterone solution. Topically applied creams leave as much as 90 mg residual testosterone on the skin. The occlusive backing film on Androderm (testosterone transdermal system) prevents the partner from coming in contact with the active material in the system. Transfer of the system to the partner is unlikely.

Changes in body hair distribution, significant increase in acne, or other signs of virilization of the female partner should be brought to the attention of a physician.

Information for Patients

An information brochure is available for patients concerning the use of *Androderm*.

Advise patients of the following:

Androderm should not be applied to the scrotum.

Androderm should not be applied over a bony prominence or on a part of the body that could be subject to prolonged pressure during sleep or sitting. Application to these sites has been associated with burn-like blister reactions.

Androderm does not have to be removed during sexual intercourse, nor while taking a shower or bath.

Androderm systems should be applied nightly.

Laboratory Tests

Hemoglobin and hematocrit should be checked periodically to detect polycythemia in patients who are receiving androgen therapy.

Liver function, prostate specific antigen, total cholesterol and HDL cholesterol should be checked periodically.

Drug Interactions

Anticoagulants: C-17 substituted derivatives of testosterone, such as methandrostenolone, have been reported to decrease the anticoagulant requirements of patients receiving oral anticoagulants. Patients receiving oral anticoagulants require close monitoring especially when androgens are started or stopped.

Oxyphenbutazone: Concurrent administration of oxyphenbutazone and androgens may result in elevated serum levels of oxyphenbutazone.

Insulin: In diabetic patients, the metabolic effects of androgens may decrease blood glucose and, therefore, insulin requirements.

Drug/Laboratory Test Interferences

Androgens may decrease levels of thyroxine-binding globulin, resulting in decreased total T_4 serum levels and increased resin uptake of T_3 and T_4. Free thyroid hormone levels remain unchanged, however, and there is no clinical evidence of thyroid dysfunction.

Carcinogenesis, Mutagenesis, Impairment of Fertility

Animal Data: Testosterone has been tested by subcutaneous injection and implantation in mice and rats. The im-

Continued on next page

Androderm—Cont.

plant induced cervical-uterine tumors in mice, which metastasized in some cases. There is suggestive evidence that injection of testosterone into some strains of female mice increases their susceptibility to hepatoma. Testosterone is also known to increase the number of tumors and decrease the degree of differentiation of chemically induced carcinomas of the liver in rats.

Human Data: There are rare reports of hepatocellular carcinoma in patients receiving long-term therapy with androgens in high doses. Withdrawal of drugs did not lead to regression of the tumors in all cases.

Geriatric patients treated with androgens may be at an increased risk for the development of prostatic hyperplasia. Geriatric patients and other patients with clinical or demographic characteristics that are recognized to be associated with an increased risk of prostate cancer should be evaluated for the presence of subclinical or clinical prostate cancer prior to initiation of testosterone replacement therapy, because testosterone therapy may promote the growth of existing subclinical foci of prostate cancer.[2]

In men receiving testosterone replacement therapy, surveillance for prostate cancer should be consistent with current practices for eugonadal men.

Pregnancy Category X: (See Contraindications).

Teratogenic Effects: *Androderm* must not be used in women.

Nursing Mothers: *Androderm* must not be used in women.

Pediatric Use: *Androderm* has not been evaluated clinically in males under 15 years of age.

ADVERSE REACTIONS

Adverse Events Associated with Androderm (testosterone transdermal system)

In clinical studies of 122 patients treated with *Androderm*, the most common adverse events reported were skin reactions at the site of system application. Transient mild to moderate erythema was observed at the site of application in the majority of patients at some time during treatment. The adverse reactions reported by more than 1% of patients are listed below shown in order of decreasing frequency.

Event	Percent of Patients
pruritus at application site	37%
burn-like blister reaction under system	12%
erythema at application site	7%
vesicles at application site	6%
prostate abnormalities	5%
headache	4%
allergic contact dermatitis to the system	4%
burning at application site	3%
induration at application site	3%
depression	3%
rash	2%
gastrointestinal bleeding	2%

The following reactions occurred in less than 1% of patients: fatigue; body pain; pelvic pain; hypertension; peripheral vascular disease; increased appetite; accelerated growth; anxiety; confusion; decreased libido; paresthesia; thinking abnormalities; vertigo; acne; bullae at application site; mechanical irritation at application site; rash at application site; contamination of application site; prostate carcinoma; dysuria; hematuria; impotence; urinary incontinence; urinary tract infection; testicular abnormalities.

Three types of application site reactions occurred: irritation which included mild to moderate erythema, induration or burning; allergic contact dermatitis; and burn-like blister reactions.

Chronic skin irritation caused 5% of patients to discontinue treatment. Mild skin irritation may be ameliorated by treatment of affected skin with over-the-counter topical hydrocortisone cream applied after system removal.

Applying a small amount of 0.1% triamcinolone acetonide cream (Rx) to the skin under the central drug reservoir of the *Androderm* system has been shown to reduce the incidence and severity of skin irritation. The administration of 0.1% triamcinolone acetonide cream (Rx) does not significantly alter transdermal absorption of testosterone from the system. **Ointment formulations should not be used for pretreatment as they may significantly reduce testosterone absorption.**

Five patients (4%) developed allergic contact dermatitis after 3 to 8 weeks treatment that required discontinuation. These reactions were characterized by pruritus, erythema, induration and in some instances vesicles or bullae, which recurred with each system application. Rechallenge with components of the system showed ethanol sensitization in 4 patients. One patient's reaction was attributed to testosterone. None of these patients had adverse sequelae related to oral alcohol ingestion or to injectable testosterone use. Older patients may be more prone to develop allergic contact dermatitis.

Fourteen patients (12%) had burn-like blister reactions that involved bullae, epidermal necrosis or the development of ulcerated lesions. These reactions typically occurred once, at a single application site; 5 patients experienced a single recurrence. None withdrew from the clinical trials. These reactions occurred at a rate of approximately 1 in 6,500 system applications (1 in 3,250 treatment days). The majority of these lesions were associated with system application over bony prominences or on parts of the body that may have been subject to prolonged pressure during sleep or sitting (e.g., over the deltoid region of the upper arm, the greater trochanter of the femur, or the ischial tuberosity). The more severe lesions healed over several weeks with scarring in some cases. Such lesions should be treated as burns.

Adverse Events Associated with Injection or Oral Treatments

Skin and Appendages: Hirsutism, male pattern of baldness, seborrhea, and acne.

Endocrine and Urogenital: Gynecomastia and excessive frequency and duration of penile erections. Oligospermia may occur at high dosages (see CLINICAL PHARMACOLOGY).

Fluid and Electrolyte Disturbances: Retention of sodium, chloride, water, potassium, calcium, and inorganic phosphates.

Gastrointestinal: Nausea, cholestatic jaundice, alterations in liver function tests. Rare instances of hepatocellular neoplasms and peliosis hepatis have occurred (see WARNINGS).

Hematologic: Suppression of clotting factors II, V, VII and X; bleeding in patients on concomitant anticoagulant therapy and polycythemia.

Nervous System: Increased or decreased libido, headache, anxiety, depression and generalized paresthesia.

Metabolic: Increased serum cholesterol.

Miscellaneous: Rarely, anaphylactoid reactions.

DRUG ABUSE AND DEPENDENCE

Androderm (testosterone transdermal system) is a Schedule III controlled substance under the Anabolic Steroids Control Act.

Oral consumption of the *Androderm* system or the gel contents of the system will not result in clinically significant serum testosterone concentrations in the target organs due to extensive first-pass metabolism.

OVERDOSAGE

There is one report of acute overdosage with testosterone enanthate injection: testosterone levels of up to 11,400 ng/dL were implicated in a cerebrovascular accident.

DOSAGE AND ADMINISTRATION

The usual starting dose is one *Androderm* 5 mg system or two *Androderm* 2.5 mg systems applied nightly for 24 hours, providing a total dose of 5 mg/day.

The adhesive side of the *Androderm* system should be applied to a clean, dry area of the skin on the back, abdomen, upper arms, or thighs. Avoid application over bony prominences or on a part of the body that may be subject to prolonged pressure during sleep or sitting (e.g., the deltoid region of the upper arm, the greater trochanter of the femur, and the ischial tuberosity). DO NOT APPLY TO THE SCROTUM. The sites of application should be rotated, with an interval of 7 days between applications to the same site. The area selected should not be oily, damaged or irritated. (See Table 2.)

The system should be applied immediately after opening the pouch and removing the protective release liner. The system should be pressed firmly in place, making sure there is good contact with the skin, especially around the edges.

To ensure proper dosing, the morning serum testosterone concentration may be measured following system application the previous evening. If the serum concentration is outside the normal range, sampling should be repeated with assurance of proper system adhesion as well as appropriate application time. Confirmed serum concentrations outside the normal range may require increasing the daily dose to 7.5 mg (i.e., one 5 mg and one 2.5 mg systems or three 2.5 mg systems) or decreasing the daily dose to 2.5 mg (i.e., one 2.5 mg system), maintaining nightly application. Because of variability in analytical values among diagnostic laboratories, this laboratory work and any later analyses for assessing the effect of *Androderm* therapy, should be performed at the same laboratory so results can be compared.

Mild skin irritation may be ameliorated by treatment of the affected skin with over-the-counter topical hydrocortisone cream applied after system removal.

Applying a small amount of 0.1% triamcinolone acetonide cream (Rx) to the skin under the central drug reservoir of the *Androderm* system has been shown to reduce the incidence and severity of skin irritation. The administration of 0.1% triamcinolone acetonide cream (Rx) does not significantly alter transdermal absorption of testosterone from the system. **Ointment formulations should not be used for pretreatment as they may significantly reduce testosterone absorption.**

Androderm (testosterone transdermal system) therapy for non-virilized patients may be initiated with one 2.5 mg/day system applied nightly.

HOW SUPPLIED

Androderm (testosterone transdermal system) 2.5 mg/day.

Each system contains 12.2 mg testosterone USP for delivery of 2.5 mg of testosterone per day (see DESCRIPTION).

Cartons of 60 systems NDC 62109-9133-2

Androderm (testosterone transdermal system) 5 mg/day.

Each system contains 24.3 mg testosterone USP for delivery of 5 mg of testosterone per day (see DESCRIPTION).

Cartons of 30 systems NDC 62109-9134-2

Storage and Disposal

Store at room temperature, 15° to 30°C (59° to 86°F). Apply to skin immediately upon removal from the protective pouch. Do not store outside the pouch provided. Damaged systems should not be used. The drug reservoir may be burst by excessive pressure or heat. Discard systems in household trash in a manner that prevents accidental application or ingestion by children, pets or others.

REFERENCES

1. Mazer NA, et al. Mimicking the circadian pattern of testosterone and metabolite levels with an enhanced transdermal delivery system. In Gurney, Junjinger, Peppas, eds. *Pulsatile Drug Delivery: Current Applications and Future Trends.* Stuttgart: Wiss. Verl.-Ges.; 1993, 73–97.

2. Schroeder FH. Androgens and carcinoma of the prostate. In Neischlag E, Behre HM, eds. *Testosterone Action, Deficiency, Substitution.* Berlin/Heidelberg: Springer-Verlag; 1990, 245–260.

Rx only

DATE OF ISSUANCE AUG. 1999

U.S. Patent Nos. 4,849,224, 4,855,294, 4,863,970, 4,983,395, 5,152,997, and 5,164,190.

Distributed by: Watson Pharma, Inc.
a subsidiary of Watson Laboratories, Inc.
Corona, CA 92880

AD:L9

BREVICON® 28-DAY Tablets ℞
(norethindrone and ethinyl estradiol)

NORINYL® 1 + 35 28-DAY Tablets ℞
(norethindrone and ethinyl estradiol)

NORINYL® 1 + 50 28-DAY Tablets ℞
(norethindrone and mestranol)

Patients should be counseled that this product does not protect against HIV infection (AIDS) and other sexually transmitted diseases.

ORAL CONTRACEPTIVE AGENTS

DESCRIPTION

BREVICON 28-DAY Tablets provide a continuous oral contraceptive regimen consisting of 21 blue tablets containing norethindrone 0.5 mg and ethinyl estradiol 0.035 mg and 7 orange tablets containing inert ingredients.

NORINYL 1 + 35 28-DAY Tablets provide a continuous oral contraceptive regimen consisting of 21 yellow-green tablets containing norethindrone 1 mg and ethinyl estradiol 0.035 mg and 7 orange tablets containing inert ingredients.

NORINYL 1 + 50 28-DAY Tablets provide a continuous oral contraceptive regimen consisting of 21 white tablets containing norethindrone 1 mg and mestranol 0.05 mg and 7 orange tablets containing inert ingredients.

Norethindrone is a potent progestational agent with the chemical name 17-Hydroxy-19-Nor-17α-pregn-4-en-20 yn-3-one. Ethinyl estradiol is an estrogen with the chemical name 19-nor-17α-pregna-1,3,5(10)-trien-20-yne-3,17-diol. Mestranol is an estrogen with the chemical name 3-Methoxy-19-nor-17α-pregna-1,3,5(10)-trien-20-yn-17-ol. Their structural formulae follow:

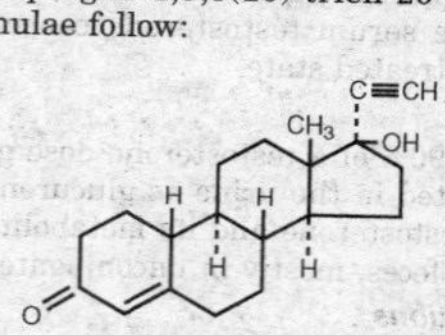

NORETHINDRONE

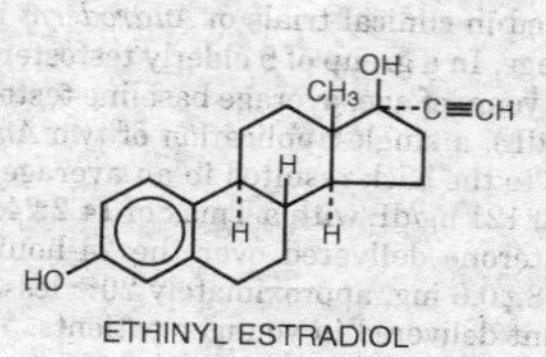

ETHINYL ESTRADIOL

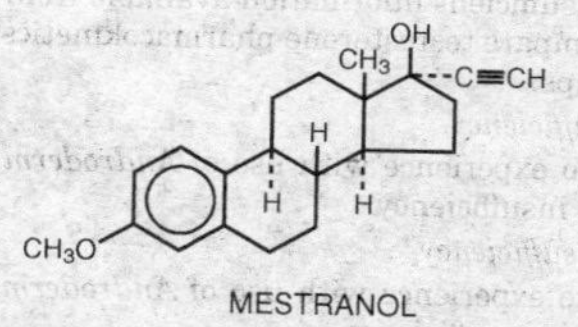

MESTRANOL

The blue BREVICON tablets contain the following inactive ingredients: FD&C Blue No. 1, lactose, magnesium stearate, povidone, and starch.

The yellow-green NORINYL 1 + 35 tablets contain the following inactive ingredients: D&C Green No. 5, D&C Yellow No. 10, lactose, magnesium stearate, povidone, and starch.

The white NORINYL 1 + 50 tablets contain the following inactive ingredients: lactose, magnesium stearate, povidone, and starch.

The inactive orange tablets in the 28-day regimens of BREVICON, NORINYL 1 + 35 and NORINYL 1 + 50 contain the following ingredients: FD&C Yellow No. 6, lactose, magnesium stearate, povidone, and starch.

CLINICAL PHARMACOLOGY

Combination oral contraceptives act by suppression of gonadotrophins. Although the primary mechanism of this action is inhibition of ovulation, other alterations include changes in the cervical mucus (which increase the difficulty of sperm entry into the uterus) and the endometrium (which may reduce the likelihood of implantation).

INDICATIONS AND USAGE

Oral contraceptives are indicated for the prevention of pregnancy in women who elect to use this product as a method of contraception.

Oral contraceptive products such as Norinyl 1 + 50, which contain 50 mcg of estrogen, should not be used unless medically indicated.

Oral contraceptives are highly effective. Table 1 lists the typical accidental pregnancy rates for users of combination oral contraceptives and other methods of contraception.[1] The efficacy of these contraceptive methods, except sterilization, depends upon the reliability with which they are used. Correct and consistent use of methods can result in lower failure rates.

[See table 1 above]

CONTRAINDICATIONS

Oral contraceptives should not be used in women who have the following conditions:

- Thrombophlebitis and thromboembolic disorders
- A past history of deep vein thrombophlebitis or thromboembolic disorders
- Cerebral vascular or coronary artery disease
- Known or suspected carcinoma of the breast
- Carcinoma of the endometrium or other known or suspected estrogen-dependent neoplasia
- Undiagnosed abnormal genital bleeding
- Cholestatic jaundice of pregnancy or jaundice with prior pill use
- Hepatic adenomas, carcinomas or benign liver tumors
- Known or suspected pregnancy

WARNINGS

Cigarette smoking increases the risk of serious cardiovascular side effects from oral contraceptive use. This risk increases with age and with heavy smoking (15 or more cigarettes per day) and is quite marked in women over 35 years of age. Women who use oral contraceptives are strongly advised not to smoke.

The use of oral contraceptives is associated with increased risks of several serious conditions including myocardial infarction, thromboembolism, stroke, hepatic neoplasia, and gallbladder disease, although the risk of serious morbidity or mortality is very small in healthy women without underlying risk factors. The risk of morbidity and mortality increases significantly in the presence of other underlying risk factors such as hypertension, hyperlipidemias, hypercholesterolemia, obesity and diabetes.[2–5]

Practitioners prescribing oral contraceptives should be familiar with the following information relating to these risks.

The information contained in this package insert is principally based on studies carried out in patients who used oral contraceptives with higher formulations of both estrogens than those in common use today. The effect of long-term use of the oral contraceptives with lower formulations of both estrogens and progestogens remains to be determined.

Throughout this labeling, epidemiological studies reported are of two types: retrospective or case control studies and prospective or cohort studies. Case control studies provide a measure of the relative risk of a disease. Relative risk, the *ratio* of the incidence of a disease among oral contraceptive users to that among non-users, cannot be assessed directly from case control studies, but the odds ratio obtained is a measure of relative risk. The relative risk does not provide information on the actual clinical occurrence of a disease. Cohort studies provide not only a measure of relative risk but a measure of attributable risk, which is the *difference* in the incidence of disease between the oral contraceptive users and non-users. The attributable risk does provide information about the actual occurrence of a disease in the population (adapted from ref. 12 and 13 with the author's permission). For further information, the reader is referred to a text on epidemiological methods.

1. THROMBOEMBOLIC DISORDERS AND OTHER VASCULAR PROBLEMS

a. Myocardial Infarction

An increased risk of myocardial infarction has been attributed to oral contraceptive use. This risk is primarily in smokers or women with other underlying risk factors for coronary artery disease such as hypertension, hypercholesterolemia, morbid obesity and diabetes.[2–5, 13] The relative risk of heart attack for current oral contraceptive users has been estimated to be 2 to 6.[2, 14–19] The risk is very low under the age of 30. However, there is the possibility of a risk of cardiovascular disease even in very young women who take oral contraceptives.

Smoking in combination with oral contraceptive use has been shown to contribute substantially to the incidence of myocardial infarctions in women in their mid-thirties or older, with smoking accounting for the majority of excess cases.[20]

Mortality rates associated with circulatory disease have been shown to increase substantially in smokers over the age of 35 and non-smokers over the age of 40 among women who use oral contraceptives (see TALBE II).[16]

Table 1– Percentage of women experiencing an unintended pregnancy during the first year of typical use and the first year of perfect use of contraception and the percentage continuing use at the end of the first year. United States.

Method (1)	% of Women Experiencing an Unintended Pregnancy within the First Year of Use: Typical Use[1] (2)	Perfect Use[2] (3)	% of Women Continuing Use at One Year[3] (4)
Chance[4]	85	85	
Spermicides[5]	26	6	40
Periodic abstinence	25		63
Calendar		9	
Ovulation method		3	
Sympto-thermal[6]		2	
Post-ovulation		1	
Withdrawal	19	4	
Cap[7]			
Parous women	40	26	42
Nulliparous women	20	9	56
Sponge			
Parous women	40	20	42
Nulliparous women	20	9	56
Diaphragm[7]	20	6	56
Condom[8]			
Female (Reality)	21	5	56
Male	14	3	61
Pill	5		71
Progestin only		0.5	
Combined		0.1	
IUD			
Progesterone T	2.0	1.5	81
Copper T 380A	0.8	0.6	78
LNg 20	0.1	0.1	81
Depo-Provera	0.3	0.3	70
Norplant and Norplant-2	0.05	0.05	88
Female sterilization	0.5	0.5	100
Male sterilization	0.15	0.10	100

Emergency Contraceptive Pills: Treatment initiated within 72 hours after unprotected intercourse reduces the risk of pregnancy by at least 75%.[9]

Lactational Amenorrhea Method: LAM is a highly effective, *temporary* method of contraception.[10]

Source: Trussell J. Contraceptive Efficacy Table from Hatcher R.A., Trussell J, Stewart F, Cates W, Stewart GK, Kowal D, Guest F, in Contraceptive Technology: Seventeenth Revised Edition. New York, NY: Irvington Publishers, 1998.

1 Among *typical* couples who initiate use of a method (not necessarily for the first time), the percentage who experience an accidental pregnancy during the first year if they do not stop use for any other reason.

2 Among couples who initiate use of a method (not necessarily for the first time) and who use it *perfectly* (both consistently and correctly), the percentage who experience an accidental pregnancy during the first year if they do not stop use for any other reason.

3 Among couples attempting to avoid pregnancy, the percentage who continue to use a method for one year.

4 The percents becoming pregnant in columns (2) and (3) are based on data from populations where contraception is not used and from women who cease using contraction in order to become pregnant. Among such populations, about 89% become pregnant within one year. This estimate was lowered slightly (to 85%) to represent the percent who would become pregnant within one year among women now relying on reversible methods of contraception if they abandoned contraception altogether.

5 Foams, creams, gels, vaginal suppositories, and vaginal film.

6 Cervical mucus (ovulation) method supplemented by calendar in the pre-ovulatory and basal body temperature in the post-ovulatory phases.

7 With spermicidal cream or jelly.

8 Without spermicides.

9 The treatment schedule is one dose within 72 hours after unprotected intercourse and a second dose 12 hours after the first dose. The Food and Drug Administration has declared the following brands of oral contraceptives to be safe and effective for emergency contraception: Ovral (1 dose is 2 white pills), Aleese (1 dose is 5 pink pills), Nordette or Levlen (1 dose is 2 light-orange pills), Lo/Ovral (1 dose is 4 white pills), Triphasil or Tri-Levlen (1 dose is 4 yellow pills).

10 However, to maintain effective protection against pregnancy, another method of contraception must be used as soon as menstruation resumes, the frequency or duration of breastfeeds is reduced, bottle feeds are introduced, or the baby reaches six months of age.

TABLE II: CIRCULATORY DISEASE MORTALITY RATES PER 100,000 WOMAN YEARS BY AGE, SMOKING STATUS AND ORAL CONTRACEPTIVE USE

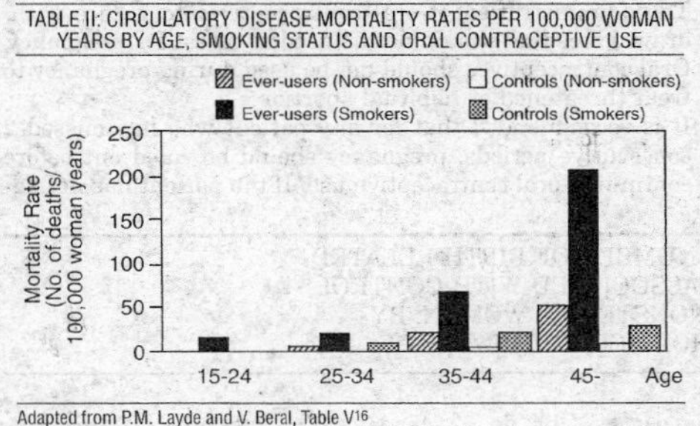

Adapted from P.M. Layde and V. Beral, Table V[16]

Oral contraceptives may compound the effects of well-known risk factors such as hypertension, diabetes, hyperlipidemias, hypercholesterolemia, age and obesity.[3, 13, 21] In particular, some progestogens are known to decrease HDL cholesterol and cause glucose intolerance, while estrogens may create a state of hyperinsulinism.[21–25] Oral contraceptives have been shown to increase blood pressure among users (see **WARNINGS**, section 9). Similar effects on risk factors have been associated with an increased risk of heart disease. Oral contraceptives must be used with caution in women with cardiovascular disease risk factors.

b. Thromboembolism

An increased risk of thromboembolic and thrombotic disease associated with the use of oral contraceptives is well established. Case control studies have found the relative risk of users compared to non-users to be 3 for the first episode of superficial venous thrombosis, 4 to 11 for deep vein thrombosis or pulmonary embolism, and 1.5 to 6 for women with predisposing conditions for venous thromboembolic disease.[12, 13, 26–31] Cohort studies have shown the relative risk to be somewhat lower, and 3 for new cases and about 4.5 for new cases requiring hospitalization.[32] The risk of thromboembolic disease due to oral contraceptives is not related to length of use and disappears after pill use is stopped.[12]

A 2- to 6-fold increase in relative risk of post-operative thromboembolic complications has been reported with the use of oral contraceptives. The relative risk of venous thrombosis in women who have predisposing conditions is twice that of women without such medical conditions.[83] If feasible, oral contraceptives should be discontinued at least 4 weeks prior to and for 2 weeks after elective surgery and during and following prolonged immobilization. Since the immediate post-partum period also is associated with an increased risk of thromboembolism, oral contraceptives should be started no earlier than 4 to 6 weeks after delivery in women who elect not to breast feed.[33]

c. Cerebrovascular diseases

An increase in both the relative and attributable risks of cerebrovascular events (thrombotic and hemorrhagic strokes) has been shown in users of oral contraceptives. In general, the risk is greatest among older (>35 years), hypertensive women who also smoke. Hypertension was found to be a risk factor for both users and non-users for both types of strokes while smoking interacted to increase the risk for hemorrhagic strokes.[34]

In a large study, the relative risk of thrombotic strokes has been shown to range from 3 for normotensive uses to 14 for

Continued on next page

Brevicon/Norinyl—Cont.

users with severe hypertension.[35] The relative risk of hemorrhagic stroke is reported to be 1.2 for non-smokers who used oral contraceptives, 2.6 for smokers who did not use oral contraceptives, 7.6 for smokers who used oral contraceptives, 1.8 for normotensive users, and 25.7 for users with severe hypertension.[35] The attributable risk also is greater in women in their mid-thirties or older and among smokers.[13]

d. Dose-related risk of vascular disease from oral contraceptives

A positive association has been observed between the amount of estrogen and progestogen in oral contraceptives and the risk of vascular disease.[36–38] A decline in serum high density lipoproteins (HDL) has been reported with many progestational agents.[22–24] A decline in serum high density lipoproteins has been associated with an increased incidence of ischemic heart disease.[39] Because estrogens increase HDL cholesterol, the net effect of an oral contraceptive depends on a balance achieved between doses of estrogen and progestogen and the nature and absolute amount of progestogens used in the contraceptives. The amount of both hormones should be considered in the choice of an oral contraceptive.[37]

Minimizing exposure to estrogen and progestogen is in keeping with good principles of therapeutics. For any particular estrogen/progestogen combination, the dosage regimen prescribed should be one which contains the least amount of estrogen and progestogen that is compatible with a low failure rate and the needs of the individual patient. New acceptors of oral contraceptive agents should be started on preparations containing the lowest estrogen content that produces satisfactory results for the individual.

Products containing 50 mcg estrogen should be used only when medically indicated.

e. Persistence of risk of vascular disease

There are three studies which have shown persistence of risk of vascular disease for ever-users of oral contraceptives.[17, 34, 40] In a study in the United States, the risk of developing myocardial infarction after discontinuing oral contraceptives persists for at least 9 years for women 40–49 years who had used oral contraceptives for 5 or more years, but this increased risk was not demonstrated in other age groups.[17] In another study in Great Britain, the risk of developing cerebrovascular disease persisted for at least 6 years after discontinuation of oral contraceptives, although excess risk was very small.[40] There is a significantly increased relative risk of subarachnoid hemorrhage after termination of use of oral contraceptives.[34] However, these studies were performed with oral contraceptive formations containing 50 µg or higher of estrogen.

2. ESTIMATES OF MORTALITY FROM CONTRACEPTIVE USE

One study gathered data from a variety of sources which have estimated the mortality rates associated with different methods of contraception at different ages (see Table III).[41] These estimates include the combined risk of death associated with contraceptive methods plus the risk attributable to pregnancy in the event of method failure. Each method of contraception has its specific benefits and risks. The study concluded that with the exception of oral contraceptive users 35 and older who smoke and 40 and older who do not smoke, mortality associated with all methods of birth control is low and below that associated with childbirth. The observation of a possible increase in risk of mortality with age for oral contraceptive users is based on data gathered in the 1970s—but not reported in the U.S. until 1983.[16, 41] However, current clinical practice involves the use of lower estrogen dose formulations combined with careful restriction of oral contraceptive use to women who do not have the various risk factors listed in this labeling.

Because of these changes in practice and, also, because of some limited new data which suggest that the risk of cardiovascular disease with the use of oral contraceptives may now be less than previously observed,[78, 79] the Fertility and Maternal Health Drugs Advisory Committee was asked to review the topic in 1989. The Committee concluded that although cardiovascular disease risks may be increased with oral contraceptive use after age 40 in healthy non-smoking women (even with the newer low-dose formulations), there are greater potential health risks associated with pregnancy in older women and with the alternative surgical and medical procedures which may be necessary if such women do not have access to effective and acceptable means of contraception.

Therefore, the Committee recommended that the benefits of oral contraceptive use by healthy non-smoking women over 40 may outweigh the possible risks. Of course, older women, as all women who take oral contraceptives, should take the lowest possible dose formulation that is effective.[80]

[See table III below]

3. CARCINOMA OF THE BREAST AND REPRODUCTIVE ORGANS

Numerous epidemiological studies have been performed on the incidence of breast, endometrial, ovarian, and cervical cancer in women using oral contraceptives. The overwhelming evidence in the literature suggests that use of oral contraceptives is not associated with an increase in the risk of developing breast cancer, regardless of the age and parity of first use or with most of the marketed brands and doses.[42–44] The Cancer and Steroid Hormone (CASH) study also showed no latent effect on the risk of breast cancer for at least a decade following long-term use.[43] A few studies have shown a slightly increased relative risk of developing breast cancer,[44–47] although the methodology of these studies, which included differences in examination of users and non-users and differences in age at start of use, has been questioned.[47–49] Some studies have reported an increased relative risk of developing breast cancer, particularly at a younger age. This increased relative risk appears to be related to duration of use.[81, 82]

Some studies suggest that oral contraceptive use has been associated with an increase in the risk of cervical intraepithelial neoplasia in some populations of women.[50–53] However, there continues to be controversy about the extent to which such findings may be due to differences in sexual behavior and other factors.

In spite of many studies of the relationship between oral contraceptive use and breast or cervical cancers, a cause and effect relationship has not been established.

4. HEPATIC NEOPLASIA

Benign hepatic adenomas are associated with oral contraceptive use although the incidence of benign tumors is rare in the United States. Indirect calculations have estimated the attributable risk to be in the range of 3.3 cases per 100,000 for users, a risk that increases after 4 or more years of use.[54] Rupture of rare, benign, hepatic adenomas may cause death through intra-abdominal hemorrhage.[55–56]

Studies in the United States and Britain have shown an increased risk of developing hepatocellular carcinoma in long-term (>8 years) oral contraceptive users.[57–59] However, these cancers are extremely rare in the United States and the attributable risk (the excess incidence) of liver cancers in oral contraceptive users approaches less than 1 per 1,000,000 users.

5. OCULAR LESIONS

There have been clinical case reports of retinal thrombosis associated with the use of oral contraceptives. Oral contraceptives should be discontinued if there is unexplained partial or complete loss of vision; onset of proptosis or diplopia; papilledema; or retinal vascular lesions. Appropriate diagnostic and therapeutic measures should be undertaken immediately.

6. ORAL CONTRACEPTIVE USE BEFORE OR DURING EARLY PREGNANCY

Extensive epidemiological studies have revealed no increased risk of birth defects in women who have used oral contraceptives prior to pregnancy.[60–62] Studies also do not suggest a teratogenic effect, particularly insofar as cardiac anomalies and limb reduction defects are concerned, when taken inadvertently during early pregnancy.[60, 61, 63, 64]

The administration of oral contraceptives to induce withdrawal bleeding should not be used as a test for pregnancy. Oral contraceptives should not be used during pregnancy to treat threatened or habitual abortion.

It is recommended that for any patient who has missed 2 consecutive periods, pregnancy should be ruled out before continuing oral contraceptive use. If the patient has not adhered to the prescribed schedule, the possibility of pregnancy should be considered at the first missed period. Oral contraceptive use should be discontinued if pregnancy is confirmed.

7. GALLBLADDER DISEASE

Earlier studies have reported an increased lifetime relative risk of gallbladder surgery in users of oral contraceptives and estrogens.[65–66] More recent studies, however, have shown that the relative risk of developing gallbladder disease among oral contraceptive users may be minimal.[67] The recent findings of minimal risk may be related to the use of oral contraceptive formulations containing lower hormonal doses of estrogens and progestogens.[68]

8. CARBOHYDRATE AND LIPID METABOLIC EFFECTS

Oral contraceptives have been shown to cause glucose intolerance in a significant percentage of users.[25] Oral contraceptives containing greater than 75 µg of estrogen cause hyperinsulinism, while lower doses of estrogen cause less glucose intolerance.[70] Progestogens increase insulin secretion and create insulin resistance, this effect varying with different progestational agents.[25, 71] However, in the non-diabetic woman, oral contraceptives appear to have no effect on fasting blood glucose.[69] Because of these demonstrated effects, prediabetic and diabetic women should be carefully observed while taking oral contraceptives.

Some women may develop persistent hypertriglyceridemia while on the pill.[72] As discussed earlier (see **WARNINGS**, sections 1a. and 1d.), changes in serum triglycerides and lipoprotein levels have been reported in oral contraceptive users.[23]

9. ELEVATED BLOOD PRESSURE

An increase in blood pressure has been reported in women taking oral contraceptives and this increase is more likely in older oral contraceptive users and with continued use.[73, 84] Data from the Royal College of General Practitioners and subsequent randomized trials have shown that the incidence of hypertension increases with increasing concentrations of progestogens.

Women with a history of hypertension or hypertension-related diseases or renal disease should be encouraged to use another method of contraception. If women elect to use oral contraceptives, they should be monitored closely and if significant elevation of blood pressure occurs oral contraceptives should be discontinued. For most women, elevated blood pressure will return to normal after stopping oral contraceptives and there is no difference in the occurrence of hypertension among ever- and never-users.[73–75]

10. HEADACHE

The onset or exacerbation of migraine or development of headache with a new pattern which is recurrent, persistent or severe requires of discontinuation of oral contraceptives and evaluation of the cause.

11. BLEEDING IRREGULARITIES

Breakthrough bleeding and spotting are sometimes encountered in patients on oral contraceptives, especially during the first 3 months of use. Non-hormonal causes should be considered and adequate diagnostic measures taken to rule out malignancy or pregnancy in the event of breakthrough bleeding, as in the case of any abnormal vaginal bleeding. If pathology has been excluded, time or a change to another formulation may solve the problem. In the event of amenorrhea, pregnancy should be ruled out.

Some women may encounter post-bill amenorrhea or oligomenorrhea, especially when such a condition was pre-existent.

PRECAUTIONS

GENERAL

Patients should be counseled that this product does not protect against HIV infection (AIDS) and other sexually transmitted diseases.

1. PHYSICAL EXAMINATION AND FOLLOW-UP

It is good medical practice for all women to have annual history and physical examinations, including women using oral contraceptives. The physical examination, however, may be deferred until after initiation of oral contraceptives if requested by the woman and judged appropriate by the clinician. The physical examination should include special reference to blood pressure, breasts, abdomen and pelvic organs, including cervical cytology, and relevant laboratory tests. In case of undiagnosed, persistent or recurrent abnormal vaginal bleeding, appropriate measures should be conducted to rule out malignancy. Women with a strong family history of breast cancer or who have breast nodules should be monitored with particular care.

2. LIPID DISORDERS

Women who are being treated for hyperlipidemias should be followed closely if they elect to use oral contraceptives. Some progestogens may elevate LDL levels and may render the control of hyperlipidemias more difficult.

3. LIVER FUNCTION

If jaundice develops in any woman receiving oral contraceptives the medication should be discontinued. Steroid hormones may be poorly metabolized in patients with impaired liver function.

4. FLUID RETENTION

Oral contraceptives may cause some degree of fluid retention. They should be prescribed with caution, and only with careful monitoring, in patients with conditions which might be aggravated by fluid retention.

5. EMOTIONAL DISORDERS

Women with a history of depression should be carefully observed and the drug discontinued if depression recurs to a serious degree.

TABLE III: ESTIMATED ANNUAL NUMBER OF BIRTH-RELATED OR METHOD-RELATED DEATHS ASSOCIATED WITH CONTROL OF FERTILITY PER 100,000 NONSTERILE WOMEN, BY FERTILITY CONTROL METHOD ACCORDING TO AGE

Method of control and outcome	15–19	20–24	25–29	30–34	35–39	40–44
No fertility control methods*	7.0	7.4	9.1	14.8	25.7	2.2
Oral contraceptives non-smoker**	0.3	0.5	0.9	1.9	13.8	31.6
Oral contraceptives smoker**	2.2	3.4	6.6	13.5	51.1	117.2
IUD**	0.8	0.8	1.0	1.0	1.4	1.4
Condom*	1.1	1.6	0.7	0.2	0.3	0.4
Diaphragm/Spermicide*	1.9	1.2	1.2	1.3	2.2	2.8
Periodic abstinence*	2.5	1.6	1.6	1.7	2.9	3.6

*Deaths are birth-related
**Deaths are method-related

Estimates adapted from H.W. Ory, Table 3[41]

6. CONTACT LENSES
Contact lens wearers who develop visual changes or changes in lens tolerance should be assessed by an ophthalmologist.

7. DRUG INTERACTIONS
Reduced efficacy and increased incidence of breakthrough bleeding and menstrual irregularities have been associated with concomitant use of rifampin. A similar association though less marked, has been suggested with barbiturates, phenylbutazone, phenytoin sodium, and possibly with griseofulvin, ampicillin and tetracyclines.[76]

8. INTERACTIONS WITH LABORATORY TESTS
Certain endocrine and liver function tests and blood components may be affected by oral contraceptives:
a. Increased prothrombin and factors, VII, VIII, IX, and X; decreased antithrombin 3; increased norepinephrine-induced platelet aggregability.
b. Increased thyroid binding globulin (TBG) leading to increased circulating total thyroid hormone, as measured by protein-bound iodine (PBI), T4 by column or by radioimmunoassay. Free T3 resin uptake is decreased, reflecting the elevated TBG. Free T4 concentration is unaltered.
c. Other binding proteins may be elevated in serum.
d. Sex steroid binding globulins are increased and result in elevated levels of total circulating sex steroids and corticoids; however, free or biologically active levels remain unchanged.
e. Triglycerides may be increased.
f. Glucose tolerance may be decreased.
g. Serum folate levels may be depressed by oral contraceptive therapy. This may be of clinical significance if a woman becomes pregnant shorty after discontinuing oral contraceptives.

9. CARCINOGENESIS
See **WARNINGS** section.

10. PREGNANCY
Pregnancy Category X. See **CONTRAINDICATIONS** and **WARNINGS** sections.

11. NURSING MOTHERS
Small amounts of oral contraceptive steroids have been identified in the milk of nursing mothers and a few adverse effects on the child have been reported, including jaundice and breast enlargement. In addition, oral contraceptives given in the postpartum period may interfere with lactation by decreasing the quantity and quality of breast milk. If possible, the nursing mother should be advised not to use oral contraceptives but to use other forms of contraception until she has completely weaned her child.

12. PEDIATRIC USE
Safety and efficacy have been established in women of reproductive age. Safety and efficacy are expected to be the same for postpubertal adolescents under the age of 16 and for users 16 years and older. Use of the product before menarche is not indicated.

INFORMATION FOR THE PATIENT

See **PATIENT LABELING** printed below.

ADVERSE REACTIONS

An increased risk of the following serious adverse reactions has been associated with the use of oral contraceptives (see **WARNINGS** section):
- Thrombophlebitis
- Arterial thromboembolism
- Pulmonary embolism
- Myocardial infarction
- Cerebral hemorrhage
- Cerebral thrombosis
- Hypertension
- Gallbladder disease
- Hepatic adenomas, carcinomas or benign liver tumors

There is evidence of an association between the following conditions and the use of oral contraceptives, although additional confirmatory studies are needed:
- Mesenteric thrombosis
- Retinal thrombosis

The following adverse reactions have been reported in patients receiving oral contraceptives and are believed to be drug-related:
- Nausea
- Vomiting
- Gastrointestinal symptoms (such as abdominal cramps and bloating)
- Breakthrough bleeding
- Spotting
- Change in menstrual flow
- Amenorrhea
- Temporary infertility after discontinuation of treatment
- Edema
- Melasma which may persist
- Breast changes: tenderness, enlargement, secretion
- Change in weight (increase or decrease)
- Change in cervical erosion and secretion
- Diminution in lactation when given immediately postpartum
- Cholestatic jaundice
- Migraine
- Rash (allergic)
- Mental depression
- Reduced tolerance to carbohydrates
- Vaginal candidiasis
- Change in corneal curvature (steepening)
- Intolerance to contact lenses

The following adverse reactions have been reported in users of oral contraceptives and the association has been neither confirmed nor refuted:
- Pre-menstrual syndrome
- Cataracts
- Changes in appetite
- Cystitis-like syndrome
- Headache
- Nervousness
- Dizziness
- Hirsutism
- Loss of scalp hair
- Erythema multiforme
- Erythema nodosum
- Hemorrhagic eruption
- Vaginitis
- Porphyria
- Impaired renal function
- Hemolytic uremic syndrome
- Budd-Chiari syndrome
- Acne
- Changes in libido
- Colitis

OVERDOSAGE

Serious ill effects have not been reported following acute ingestion of large doses of oral contraceptives by young children. Overdosage may cause nausea, and withdrawal bleeding may occur in females.

NON-CONTRACEPTIVE HEALTH BENEFITS

The following non-contraceptive health benefits related to the use of oral contraceptives are supported by epidemiological studies which largely utilized oral contraceptive formulations containing estrogen doses exceeding 0.035 mg of ethinyl estradiol or 0.05 mg of menstranol.[6–11]
Effects on menses:
- increased menstrual cycle regularity
- Decreased blood loss and decreased incidence of iron deficiency anemia
- Decreased incidence of dysmenorrhea

Effects related to inhibition of ovulation:
- Decreased incidence of functional ovarian cysts
- Decreased incidence of ectopic pregnancies

Effects from long-term use:
- Decreased incidence of fibroadenomas and fibrocystic disease of the breast
- Decreased incidence of acute pelvic inflammatory disease
- Decreased incidence of endometrial cancer
- Decreased incidence of ovarian cancer

Keep this and all medication out of the reach of children.

DOSAGE AND ADMINISTRATION

To achieve maximum contraceptive effectiveness, oral contraceptives must be taken exactly as directed and at intervals not exceeding 24 hours.
28-Day Schedule: For a DAY 1 START, count the first day of menstrual flow as Day 1 and the first tablet (white or yellow-green or blue) is then taken on Day 1. For a SUNDAY START when menstrual flow begins on or before Sunday, the first tablet (white or yellow-green or blue) is taken on that day. With either a Day 1 START or SUNDAY START, 1 tablet (white or yellow-green or blue) is taken each day at the same time for 21 days. Then the orange tablets are taken for 7 days, whether bleeding has stopped or not. After all 28 tablets have been taken whether bleeding has stopped or not, the same dosage schedule is repeated beginning on the following day.

INSTRUCTIONS TO PATIENTS

- To achieve maximum contraceptive effectiveness, the oral contraceptive pill must be taken exactly as directed and at intervals not exceeding 24 hours.
- Important: Women should be instructed to use an additional method of protection until after the first 7 days of administration *in the initial cycle.*
- Due to the normally increased risk of thromboemoblism occurring postpartum, women should be instructed not to initiate treatment with oral contraceptives earlier than 4–6 weeks after a full-term delivery. If pregnancy is terminated in the first 12 weeks, the patient should be instructed to start oral contraceptives immediately or within 7 days. If pregnancy is terminated after 12 weeks, the patient should be instructed to start oral contraceptives after 2 weeks.[33, 77]
- If spotting or breakthrough bleeding should occur, the patient should continue the medication according to the schedule. Should spotting or breakthrough bleeding persist, the patient should notify her physician.
- If the patient misses 1 pill, she should be instructed to take it as soon as she remembers and then take the next pill at the regular time. The patient should be advised that missing a pill can cause spotting or light bleeding and that she may be a little sick to her stomach on the days she takes the missed pill with her regularly scheduled pill. If the patient has missed more than one pill, see DETAILED PATIENT LABELING: HOW TO TAKE THE PILL, WHAT TO DO IF YOU MISS PILLS.
- Use of oral contraceptives in the event of a missed menstrual period:
  1. If the patient has not adhered to the prescribed dosage regimen, the possibility or pregnancy should be considered after the first missed period and oral contraceptives should be withheld until pregnancy has been ruled out.
  2. If the patient has adhered to the prescribed regimen and misses 2 consecutive periods, pregnancy should be ruled out before continuing the contraceptive regimen.

HOW SUPPLIED

Brevicon® 28-Day tablets (norethindrone and ethinyl estradiol) are available in 28-tablet blister cards with a WALLETTE® tablet dispenser. Six blister cards are repackaged in a carton. Each dispenser contains 21 contains Blue active tablets, round in shape with "Watson" debossed on one-side and 254 on the other side and 7 orange inert tablets. The 7 orange inert tablets are round in shape with "Watson" debossed on one side and "P" on the other side.
Norinyl® 1 + 35, 28-Day tablets (norethindrone and ethinyl estradiol) are available in 28-tablet blister cards with a WALLETTE® tablet dispenser. Six blister cards are repackaged in a carton. Each dispenser contains 21 contains Yellow-Green active tablets, round in shape with "Watson" debossed on one-side and 259 on the other side and 7 orange inert tablets. The 7 orange inert tablets are round in shape with "Watson" debossed on one side and "P" on the other side.
Norinyl® 1 + 50, 28-Day tablets (norethindrone and ethinyl estradiol) are available in 28-tablet blister cards with a WALLETTE® tablet dispenser. Six blister cards are repackaged in a carton. Each dispenser contains 21 contains White active tablets, round in shape with "Watson" debossed on one-side and 265 on the other side and 7 orange inert tablets. The 7 orange inert tablets are round in shape with "Watson" debossed on one side and "P" on the other side.

REFERENCES

1. Trussell J. Contraceptive Efficacy Table from Hatcher R.A., Trussell J, Stewart F, Cates W, Stewart GK, Kowal D, Guest F, in Contraceptive Technology: Seventeenth Revised Edition. New York, NY: Irvington Publishers, 1998. **2.** Mann, J., et al.: *Br Med J* 2(5956):241–245, 1975. **3.** Knopp, R.H.: *J Reprod Med* 31(9):913–921, 1986. **4.** Mann, J.I., et al.: *Br Med J* 2:445–447, 1976. **5.** Ory, H.: *JAMA* 237:2619–2622, 1977. **6.** The Cancer and Steroid Hormone Study of the Centers for Disease Control: *JAMA* 249(2):1596–1599, 1983. **7.** The Cancer and Steroid Hormone Study of the Centers for Disease Control: *JAMA* 257(6):796–800, 1987. **8.** Ory, H.W.: *JAMA* 228(1):68–69, 1974. **9.** Ory, H.W., et al.: *N Engl J Med* 294:419–422, 1976. **10.** Ory, H.W.: *Fam Plann Perspect* 14:182–184, 1982. **11.** Ory, H.W., et al.: *Making Choices*, New York, The Alan Guttmacher Institute, 1983. **12.** Stadel, B.: *N Engl J Med* 305(11):612–618, 1981. **13.** Stadel, B.: *N Engl J Med* 305(12):672–677, 1981. **14.** Adam, S., et al.: *Br J Obstet Gynaecol* 88:838–845, 1981. **15.** Mann, J., et al.: *Br Med J* 2(5965):245–248, 1975. **16.** Royal College of General Practitioners' Oral Contraceptive Study: *Lancet* 1:541–546, 1981. **17.** Slone, D., et al.: *N Engl J Med* 305(8):420–424, 1981. **18.** Vessey, M.P.: *Br J Fam Plann* 6 (Supplement):1–12, 1980. **19.** Russell-Briefel, R., et al.: *Prev Med* 15:352–362, 1986. **20.** Goldbaum, G., et al.: *JAMA* 258(10):1339–1342, 1987. **21.** LaRosa, J.C.: *J Reprod Med* 31 (9):906–912, 1986. **22.** Krauss, R.M., et al.: *Am J Obstet Gynecol* 145:446–452, 1983. **23.** Wahl, P., et al.: *N Engl J Med* 308(15):862–867, 1983. **24.** Wynn, V., et al.: *Am J Obstet Gynecol* 142(6):766–771, 1982. **25.** Wynn V., et al.: *J Reprod Med* 31(9):892–897, 1986. **26.** Inman, W.H., et al.: *Br Med J* 2(5599):193–199, 1968. **27.** Maguire, M.G., et al.: *Am J Epidemiol* 110(2):188–195, 1979. **28.** Petitti, D., et al.: *JAMA* 242(11):1150–1154, 1979. **29.** Vessey, M.P., et al.: *Br Med J* 2(5599):199–205, 1968. **30.** Vessey, M.P., et al.: *Br Med J* 2(5658):651–657, 1969. **31.** Porter, J.B., et al.: *Obstet Gynecol* 59(3):299–302, 1982. **32.** Vessey, M.P., et al.: *J Biosoc Sci* 8:373–427, 1976. **33.** Mishell, D.R., et al.: *Reproductive Endocrinology,* Philadelphia, F.A. Davis Co., 1979. **34.** Petitti, D.B., et al.: *Lancet* 2:234–236, 1978. **35.** Collaborative Group for the Study of Stroke in Young Women: *JAMA* 231(7):718–722, 1975. **36.** Inman, W.H., et al.: *Br Med J* 2:203–209, 1970. **37.** Meade, T.W., et al.: *Br Med J* 280(6224):1157–1161, 1980. **38.** Kay, C.R.: *Am J Obstet Gynecol* 142(6):762–765, 1982. **39.** Gordon, T., et al.: *Am J Med* 62:707–714, 1977. **40.** Royal College of General Practitioners' Oral Contraception Study: *J Coll Gen Pract* 33:75–82, 1983. **41.** Ory, H.W.: *Fam Plann Perspect* 15(2):57–63, 1983. **42.** Paul, C., et al.: *Br Med J* 293:723–725, 1986. **43.** The Cancer and Steroid Hormone Study of the Centers for Disease Control: *N Engl J Med* 315(7):405–411, 1986. **44.** Pike, M.C., et al.: *Lancet* 2:926–929, 1983. **45.** Miller, D.R., et al.: *Obstet Gynecol* 68:863–868, 1986. **46.** Olsson, H., et al.: *Lancet* 2:748–749, 1985. **47.** McPherson, K., et al.: *Br J Cancer* 56:653–660, 1987. **48.** Huggins, G.R., et al.: *Fertil Steril* 47(5):733–761, 1987. **49.** McPherson, K., et al.: *Br Med J* 293:709–710, 1986. **50.** Ory, H., et al.: *Am J Obstet Gynecol* 124(6):573–577, 1976. **51.** Vessey, M.P., et al.: *Lancet* 2:930, 1983. **52.** Brinton, L.A., et al.: *Int J Cancer* 38:339–344, 1986. **53.** WHO Collaborative Study of Neoplasia and Steroid Contraceptives: *Br Med J* 290:961–965, 1985. **54.** Rooks, J.B., et al.: *JAMA* 242(7):644–648, 1979. **55.** Bein, N.N., et al.: *Br J Surg* 64:433–435, 1977. **56.** Klatskin, G.: *Gastroenterology* 73:386–394, 1977. **57.** Henderson, B.E., et al.: *Br J Cancer* 48:437–440, 1983. **58.** Neuberger, J., et al.: *Br Med J* 292:1355–1357, 1986. **59.** Forman D., et al.: *Br Med J* 292:1357–1361, 1986. **60.** Harlap, S., et al.: *Obstet Gynecol* 55(4):447–452, 1980. **61.** Savolainen, E., et al.: *Am J Obstet Gynecol* 140(5):521–524,

Continued on next page

Brevicon/Norinyl—Cont.

1981. **62.** Janerich, D.T., et al.: *Am J Epideminol* 112(1):73–79, 1980. **63.** Ferencz, C., et al.: *Teratology* 21:225–239, 1980. **64.** Rothman, K.J., et al.: *Am J Epidemiol* 109(4): 433–439, 1979. **65.** Boston Collaborative Drug Surveillance Program: *Lancet* 1:1399–1404, 1973. **66.** Royal College of General Practitioners: *Oral contraceptives and health.* New York, Pittman, 1974. **67.** Rome Group for the Epidemiology and Prevention of Cholelithiasis: *Am J Epidemiol* 119(5): 796–805, 1984. **68.** Strom, B.L., et al.: *Clin Pharmacol Ther* 39(3):335–341, 1986. **69.** Perlman, J.A., et al.: *J Chronic Dis* 38(10):857–864, 1985. **70.** Wynn, V., et al.: *Lancet* 1:1045–1049, 1979. **71.** Wynn, V.: *Progesterone and Progestin*, New York, Raven Press, 1983. **72.** Wynn, V., et al.: *Lancet* 2:720–723, 1966. **73.** Fisch, I.R., et al.: *JAMA* 237(23): 2499–2503, 1977. **74.** Laragh, J.H.: *Am J Obstet Gynecol* 126(1):141–147, 1976. **75.** Ramcharan, S., et al.: *Pharmacology of Steroid Contraceptive Drugs,* New York, Raven Press, 1977. **76.** Stockley, I.: *Pharm J* 216:140–143, 1976. **77.** Dickey, R.P.: *Managing Contraceptive Pill Patients,* Oklahoma, Creative Informatics Inc., 1984. **78.** Porter J.B., Hunter J., Jick H., et al.: *Obstet Gynecol* 1985:66:1–4. **79.** Porter J.B., Hershel J., Walker A.M.: *Obstet Gynecol* 1987;70:29–32. **80.** Fertility and Maternal Heatlh Drugs Advisory Committee, F.D.A., October, 1989. **81.** Schlesselman J., Stadel B.V., Murray P., Lai S.: *Breast cancer in relation to early use of oral contraceptives.* JAMA 1988:259: 1828–1833. **82.** Hennekens C.H., Speizer F.E., Lipnick R.J., Rosner B., Bain C., Belanger C., Stampfer M.J., Willett W., Peto R.: *A case-control study of oral contraceptive use and breast cancer.* JNCI 1984:72:39–42. **83.** Royal College of General Practitioners: *Oral contraceptives, venous thrombosis, and varicose veins. J Coll Gen Pract* 28:393–399, 1978. **84.** Royal College of General Practitioners' Oral Contraception Study: *Effect on Hypertension and benign breast disease of progestogen component in combined oral contraceptives. Lancet* 1:624, 1977.

DETAILED PATIENT LABELING

This product (like all oral contraceptives) is intended to prevent pregnancy. It does not protect against HIV infection (AIDS) and other sexually transmitted diseases.

INTRODUCTION

You should not use Norinyl 1 + 50, which contains higher doses of estrogen than other oral contraceptives, unless specifically recommended by your health care provider.

Any woman who considers using oral contraceptives ("birth control pills" or "the pill") should understand the benefits and risks of using this form of birth control. This leaflet will give you much of the information you will need to make this decision and also will help you determine if you are at risk of developing any of the serious side effects of the pill. It will tell you how to use the pill properly so that it will be as effective as possible. However, this leaflet is not a replacement for a careful discussion between you are your health care provider. You should discuss the information provided in this leaflet with him or her, both when you first start taking the pill and during your regular visits. You also should follow the advice of your health care provider with regard to regular checkups while you are on the pill.

EFFECTIVENESS OF ORAL CONTRACEPTIVES

Oral contraceptives are used to prevent pregnancy and are more effective than other non-surgical methods of birth control. When they are taken correctly, without missing any pills, the chance of becoming pregnant is less than 1% (1 pregnancy per 100 women per year of use). Typical failure rates are actually 3% per year. The chance of becoming pregnant increases with each missed pill during a menstrual cycle.

In comparison, typical failure rates for other nonsurgical methods of birth control during the first year are as follows: [See table below]

Table 1– Percentage of women experiencing an unintended pregnancy during the first year of typical use and the first year of perfect use of contraception and the percentage continuing use at the end of the first year. United States.

Method (1)	% of Women Experiencing an Unintended Pregnancy within the First Year of Use: Typical Use[1] (2)	Perfect Use[2] (3)	% of Women Continuing Use at One Year[3] (4)
Chance[4]	85	85	
Spermicides[5]	26	6	40
Periodic abstinence	25		63
Calendar		9	
Ovulation method		3	
Sympto-thermal[6]		2	
Post-ovulation		1	
Withdrawal	19	4	
Cap[7]			
Parous women	40	26	42
Nulliparous women	20	9	56
Sponge			
Parous women	40	20	42
Nulliparous women	20	9	56
Diaphragm[7]	20	6	56
Condom[8]			
Female (Reality)	21	5	56
Male	14	3	61
Pill	5		71
Progestin only		0.5	
Combined		0.1	
IUD			
Progesterone T	2.0	1.5	81
Copper T 380A	0.8	0.6	78
LNg 20	0.1	0.1	81
Depo-Provera	0.3	0.3	70
Norplant and Norplant-2	0.05	0.05	88
Female sterilization	0.5	0.5	100
Male sterilization	0.15	0.10	100

Emergency Contraceptive Pills: Treatment initiated within 72 hours after unprotected intercourse reduces the risk of pregnancy by at least 75%.[9]

Lactational Amenorrhea Method: LAM is a highly effective, *temporary* method of contraception.[10]

Source: Trussell J. Contraceptive Efficacy Table from Hatcher R.A., Trussell J, Stewart F, Cates W, Stewart GK, Kowal D, Guest F, in Contraceptive Technology: Seventeenth Revised Edition. New York, NY: Irvington Publishers, 1998.

1 Among *typical* couples who initiate use of a method (not necessarily for the first time), the percentage who experience an accidental pregnancy during the first year if they do not stop use for any other reason.

2 Among couples who initiate use of a method (not necessarily for the first time) and who use it *perfectly* (both consistently and correctly), the percentage who experience an accidental pregnancy during the first year if they do not stop use for any other reason.

3 Among couples attempting to avoid pregnancy, the percentage who continue to use a method for one year.

4 The percents becoming pregnant in columns (2) and (3) are based on data from populations where contraception is not used and from women who cease using contraction in order to become pregnant. Among such populations, about 89% become pregnant within one year. This estimate was lowered slightly (to 85%) to represent the percent who would become pregnant within one year among women now relying on reversible methods of contraception if they abandoned contraception altogether.

5 Foams, creams, gels, vaginal suppositories, and vaginal film.

6 Cervical mucus (ovulation) method supplemented by calendar in the pre-ovulatory and basal body temperature in the post-ovulatory phases.

7 With spermicidal cream or jelly.

8 Without spermicides.

9 The treatment schedule is one dose within 72 hours after unprotected intercourse and a second dose 12 hours after the first dose. The Food and Drug Administration has declared the following brands of oral contraceptives to be safe and effective for emergency contraception: Ovral (1 dose is 2 white pills), Aleese (1 dose is 5 pink pills). Nordette or Levlen (1 dose is 2 light-orange pills), Lo/Ovral (1 dose is 4 white pills), Triphasil or Tri-Levlen (1 dose is 4 yellow pills).

10 However, to maintain effective protection against pregnancy, another method of contraception must be used as soon as menstruation resumes, the frequency or duration of breastfeeds is reduced, bottle feeds are introduced, or the baby reaches six months of age.

WHO SHOULD NOT TAKE ORAL CONTRACEPTIVES

Cigarette smoking increases the risk of serious cardiovascular side effects from oral contraceptive use. This risk increases with age and with heavy smoking (15 or more cigarettes per day) and is quite marked in women over 35 years of age. Women who use oral contraceptives are strongly advised not to smoke.

Some women should not use the pill. For example, you should not take the pill if you are pregnant or think you may be pregnant. You also should not use the pill if you have any of the following conditions:

- A history of heart attack or stroke
- Blood clots in the legs (thrombophlebitis), brain (stroke), lungs (pulmonary embolism) or eyes
- A history of blood clots in the deep veins of your legs
- Chest pain (angina pectoris)
- Known or suspected breast cancer or cancer of the lining of the uterus, cervix or vagina
- Unexplained vaginal bleeding (until a diagnosis is reached by your doctor)
- Yellowing of the whites of the eyes or of the skin (jaundice) during pregnancy or during previous use of the pill
- Liver tumor (benign or cancerous)
- Known or suspected pregnancy

Tell your health care provider if you have ever had any of these conditions. Your health care provider can recommend a safer method of birth control.

OTHER CONSIDERATIONS BEFORE TAKING ORAL CONTRACEPTIVES

Tell your health care provider if you have or have had:

- Breast nodules, fibrocystic disease of the breast, an abnormal breast x-ray or mammogram
- Diabetes
- Elevated cholesterol or triglycerides
- High blood pressure
- Migraine or other headaches or epilepsy
- Mental depression
- Gallbladder, heart or kidney disease
- History of scanty or irregular menstrual periods

Women with any of these conditions should be checked often by their health care provider if they choose to use oral contraceptives.

Also, be sure to inform your doctor or health care provider if you smoke or are on any medications.

RISKS OF TAKING ORAL CONTRACEPTIVES

1. Risk of developing blood clots

Blood clots and blockage of blood vessels are the most serious side effects of taking oral contraceptives. In particular, a clot in the legs can cause thrombophlebitis and a clot that travels to the lungs can cause a sudden blocking of the vessel carrying blood to the lungs. Rarely, clots occur in the blood vessels of the eye and may cause blindness, double vision, or impaired vision.

If you take oral contraceptives and need elective surgery, need to stay in bed for a prolonged illness or have recently delivered a baby, you may be at risk of developing blood clots. You should consult your doctor about stopping oral contraceptives three to four weeks before surgery and not taking oral contraceptives for two weeks after surgery or during bed rest. You should also not take oral contraceptives soon after delivery of a baby. It is advisable to wait for at least four weeks after delivery if you are not breast feeding. If you are breast feeding, you should wait until you have weaned your child before using the pill (see **GENERAL PRECAUTIONS, While Breast Feeding**).

2. Heart attacks and strokes

Oral contraceptives may increase the tendency to develop strokes (stoppage or rupture of blood vessels in the brain) and angina pectoris and heart attacks (blockage of blood vessels in the heart). Any of these conditions can cause death or temporary or permanent disability.

Smoking greatly increases the possibility of suffering heart attacks and strokes. Furthermore, smoking and the use of oral contraceptives greatly increase the changes of developing and dying of heart disease.

3. Gallbladder disease

Oral contraceptive users may have a greater risk than nonusers of having gallbladder disease, although this risk may be related to pills containing high doses of estrogen.

4. Liver tumors

In rare cases, oral contraceptives can cause benign but dangerous liver tumors. These benign liver tumors can rupture and cause fatal internal bleeding. In addition, a possible but not definite association has been found with the pill and liver cancers in 2 studies in which a few women who develop these very rare cancers were found to have used oral contraceptives for long periods. However, liver cancers are extremely rare. The change of developing liver cancer from using the pill is thus even rarer.

5. Cancer of the breast and reproductive organs

There is, at present, no confirmed evidence that oral contraceptives increase the risk of cancer of the reproductive organs in human studies. Several studies have found no overall increase in the risk of developing breast cancer. However, women who use oral contraceptives and have a strong family history of breast cancer or who have breast nodules or abnormal mammograms should be followed closely by their doctors. Some studies have reported an increase in the risk of developing breast cancer, particularly at a younger age. This increased risk appears to be related to duration of use.

Some studies have found an increase in the incidence of cancer of the cervix in women who use oral contraceptives. However, this finding may be related to factors other than the use of oral contraceptives.

ESTIMATED RISK OF DEATH FROM A BIRTH CONTROL METHOD OR PREGNANCY

All methods of birth control and pregnancy are associated with a risk of developing certain diseases which may lead to disability or death. An estimate of the number of deaths associated with different methods of birth control and pregnancy has been calculated and is shown in the following table:

[See table above]

In the above table, the risk of death from any birth control method is less than the risk of childbirth except for oral contraceptive users over the age of 35 who smoke and pill users over the age of 40 even if they do not smoke. It can be seen from the table that for women aged 15 to 39 the risk of death is highest with pregnancy (7–26 deaths per 100,000 women, depending on age). Among pill users who do not smoke the risk of death is always lower than that associated with pregnancy for any age group, although over the age of 40 the risk increases to 32 deaths per 100,000 women compared to 28 associated with pregnancy at that age. However, for pill users who smoke and are over the age of 35 the estimated number of deaths exceeds those for other methods of birth control. If a woman is over the age of 40 and smokes, her estimated risk of death is 4 times higher (117/100,000 women) than the estimated risk associated with pregnancy (28/100,000 women) in that age group.

The suggestion that women over 40 who don't smoke should not take oral contraceptives is based on information from older high-dose pills and on less selective use of pills than is practiced today. An Advisory Committee of the FDA discussed this issue in 1989 and recommended that the benefits of oral contraceptive use by healthy, non-smoking women over 40 years of age may outweigh the possible risks. However, all women, especially older women, are cautioned to use the lowest dose pill that is effective.

WARNING SIGNALS

If any of these adverse effects occur while you are taking oral contraceptives, call your doctor immediately:

- Sharp chest pain, coughing of blood or sudden shortness of breath (indicating a possible clot in the lung)
- Pain in the calf (indicating a possible clot in the leg)
- Crushing chest pain or heaviness in the chest (indicating a possible heart attack)
- Sudden severe headache or vomiting, dizziness or fainting, disturbances of vision or speech, weakness or numbness in an arm or leg (indicating a possible stroke)
- Sudden partial or complete loss of vision (indicating a possible clot in the eye)
- Breast lumps (indicating possible breast cancer or fibrocystic disease of the breast: ask your doctor or health care provider to show you how to examine your breasts)
- Severe pain or tenderness in the stomach area (indicating a possible ruptured liver tumor)
- Difficulty in sleeping, weakness, lack of energy, fatigue or change in mood (possibly indicating severe depression)
- Jaundice or a yellowing of the skin or eyeballs, accompanied frequently by fever, fatigue, loss of appetite, dark color urine or light colored bowel movements (indicating possible liver problems)

SIDE EFFECTS OF ORAL CONTRACEPTIVES

1. Vaginal bleeding

Irregular vaginal bleeding or spotting may occur while you are taking the pill. Irregular bleeding may vary from slight staining between menstrual periods to breakthrough bleeding which is a flow much like a regular period. Irregular bleeding occurs most often during the first few months of oral contraceptive use but may also occur after you have been taking the pill for some time. Such bleeding may be temporary and usually does not indicate any serious problem. It is important to continue taking your pills on schedule. If the bleeding occurs in more than 1 cycle or lasts for more than a few days, talk to your doctor or health care provider.

2. Contact lenses

If you wear contact lenses and notice a change in vision or an inability to wear your lenses, contact your doctor or health care provider.

3. Fluid retention

Oral contraceptives may cause edema (fluid retention) with swelling of the fingers or ankles and may raise your blood pressure. If you experience fluid retention, contact your doctor or health care provider.

4. Melasma (Mask of Pregnancy)

A spotty darkening of the skin is possible, particularly of the face.

5. Other side effects

Other side effects may include change in appetite, headache, nervousness, depression, dizziness, loss of scalp hair, rash and vaginal infections.

If any of these side effects occur, contact your doctor or health care provider.

TABLE III. ESTIMATED ANNUAL NUMBER OF BIRTH-RELATED OR METHOD-RELATED DEATHS ASSOCIATED WITH CONTROL OF FERTILITY PER 100,000 NONSTERILE WOMEN, BY FERTILITY CONTROL METHOD ACCORDING TO AGE

Method of control and outcome	15–19	20–24	25–29	30–34	35–39	40–44
No fertility control methods*	7.0	7.4	9.1	14.8	25.7	28.2
Oral contraceptives non-smoker**	0.3	0.5	0.9	1.9	13.8	31.6
Oral contraceptives smoker**	2.2	3.4	6.6	13.5	51.1	117.2
IUD**	0.8	0.8	1.0	1.0	1.4	1.4
Condom*	1.1	1.6	0.7	0.2	0.3	0.4
Diaphragm/Spermicide*	1.9	1.2	1.2	1.3	2.2	2.8
Periodic abstinence*	2.5	1.6	1.6	1.7	2.9	3.6

*Deaths are birth-related
**Deaths are method-related

Estimates adapted from W.H. Ory, Table 3[41]

GENERAL PRECAUTIONS

1. Missed periods and use of oral contraceptives before or during early pregnancy

At times you may not menstruate regularly after you have completed taking a cycle of pills. If you have taken your pills regularly and miss 1 menstrual period, continue taking your pills for the next cycle but be sure to inform your health care provider before doing so. If you have not taken the pills daily as instructed and miss 1 menstrual period, or if you miss 2 consecutive menstrual periods, you may be pregnant. Check with your health care provider immediately to determine whether you are pregnant. Do not continue to take oral contraceptives until your are sure you are not pregnant, but continue to use another method of birth control.

There is no conclusive evidence that oral contraceptive use is associated with an increase in birth defects when taken inadvertently during early pregnancy. Previously, a few studies had reported that oral contraceptives might be associated with birth defects but these studies have not been confirmed. Nevertheless, oral contraceptives or any other drugs should not be used during pregnancy unless clearly necessary and prescribed by your doctor. You should check with your doctor about risks to your unborn child from any medication taken during pregnancy.

2. While breast feeding

If you are breast feeding, consult your doctor before starting oral contraceptives. Some of the drug will be passed on to the child in the milk. A few adverse effects on the child have been reported, including yellowing of the skin (jaundice) and breast enlargement. In addition, oral contraceptives may decrease the amount and quality of your milk. If possible, do not use oral contraceptives and use another method of contraception while breast feeding. You should consider starting oral contraceptives only after you have weaned your child completely.

3. Laboratory tests

If you are scheduled for any laboratory tests, tell your doctor you are taking birth control pills. Certain blood tests may be affected by birth control pills.

4. Drug interactions

Certain drugs may interact with birth control pills to make them less effective in preventing pregnancy or cause an increase in breakthrough bleeding. Such drugs include rifampin; drugs used for epilepsy such as barbiturates (for example phenobarbital) and phenytoin (Dilantin is one brand of this drug); phenylbutazone (Butazolidin is one brand of this drug) and possibly certain antibiotics. You may need to use additional contraception when you take drugs which can make oral contraceptives less effective.

5. This product (like all oral contraceptives) is intended to prevent pregnancy. It does not protect against transmission of HIV (AIDS) and other sexually transmitted diseases such as chlamydia, genital herpes, genital warts, gonorrhea, hepatitis B, and syphilis.

HOW TO TAKE THE PILL

IMPORTANT POINTS TO REMEMBER

BEFORE YOU START TAKING YOUR PILLS:

1. BE SURE TO READ THESE DIRECTIONS:
   Before you start taking your pills.
   Anytime you are not sure what to do.
2. THE RIGHT WAY TO TAKE THE PILLS IS TO TAKE ONE PILL EVERY DAY AT THE SAME TIME.
   If you miss pills you could get pregnant. This includes starting the pack late. The more pills you miss, the more likely you are to get pregnant.
3. MANY WOMEN HAVE SPOTTING OR LIGHT BLEEDING, OR MAY FEEL SICK TO THEIR STOMACH DURING THE FIRST 1–3 PACKS OF PILLS.
   If you feel sick to your stomach, do not stop taking the Pill. The problem will usually go away. If it doesn't go away, check with your doctor or clinic.
4. MISSING PILLS CAN ALSO CAUSE SPOTTING OR LIGHT BLEEDING, even when you make up these missed pills.
   On the days you take 2 pills to make up for missed pills, you could also feel a little sick to your stomach.
5. IF YOU HAVE VOMITING OR DIARRHEA, for any reason, or if you take some medicines, including some antibiotics, your pills may not work as well. Use a back-up method (such as condoms, foam, or sponge) until you check with your doctor or clinic.
6. IF YOU HAVE TROUBLE REMEMBERING TO TAKE THE PILL, talk to your doctor or clinic about how to make pill-taking easier or about using another method of birth control.
7. IF YOU HAVE ANY QUESTIONS OR ARE UNSURE ABOUT THE INFORMATION IN THIS LEAFLET, call your doctor or clinic.

BEFORE YOU START TAKING YOUR PILLS

1. DECIDE WHAT TIME OF DAY YOU WANT TO TAKE YOUR PILL.
   It is important to take it at about the same time every day.
2. LOOK AT YOUR PILL PACK TO SEE IF IT HAS 28 PILLS:
   The 28-pill pack has 21 "active" white or yellow-green or blue pills (with hormones) to take for 3 weeks, followed by 1 week of reminder orange pills (without hormones).
3. ALSO FIND:
   1) where on the pack to start taking pills,
   2) in what order to take the pills (follow the arrows).

Brevicon, Norinyl 1 + 35, Norinyl 1 + 50
Active Pill Colors: White or Yellow-Green or Blue
Reminder Pill Color: Orange

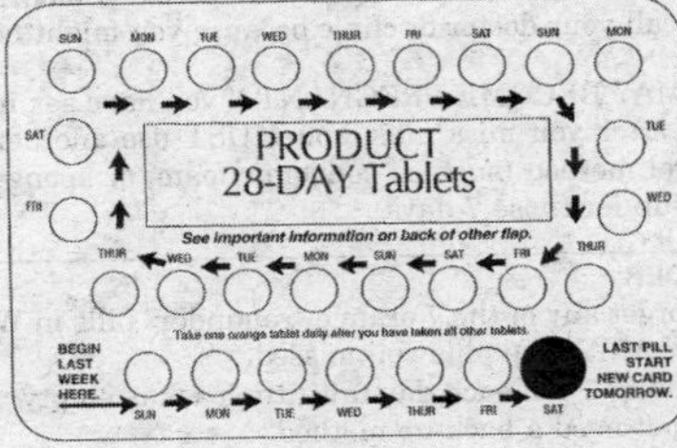

4. BE SURE YOU HAVE READY AT ALL TIMES:
   ANOTHER KIND OF BIRTH CONTROL (such as condoms, foam, or sponge) to use as a back-up in case you miss pills.
   AN EXTRA, FULL PILL PACK.

WHEN TO START THE FIRST PACK OF PILLS

You have a choice of which day to start taking your first pack of pills. Decide with your doctor or clinic which is the best day for you. Pick a time of day which will be easy to remember.

DAY 1 START:

1. Take the first "active" white or yellow-green or blue pill of the first pack during the first 24 hours of your period.
2. You will not need to use a back-up method of birth control, since you are starting the pill at the beginning of your period.

SUNDAY START:

1. Take the first "active" white or yellow-green or blue pill of the first pack on the Sunday after your period starts, even if you are still bleeding. If your period begins on Sunday, start the pack that same day.
2. Use another method of birth control as a back-up method if you have sex anytime from the Sunday you start your first pack until the next Sunday (7 days). Condoms, foam, or the sponge are good back-up methods of birth control.

WHAT TO DO DURING THE MONTH

1. **TAKE ONE PILL AT THE SAME TIME EVERY DAY UNTIL THE PACK IS EMPTY**
   Do not skip pills if you are spotting or bleeding between monthly periods or feel sick to your stomach (nausea).
   Do not skip pills even if you do not have sex very often.

Continued on next page

Brevicon/Norinyl—Cont.

2. **WHEN YOU FINISH A PACK OR SWITCH YOUR BRAND OF PILLS:**
 28 pills: Start the next pack on the day after your last "reminder" pill. Do no wait any days between packs.

WHAT TO DO IF YOU MISS PILLS

If you **MISS 1** white or yellow-green or blue "active" pill:
1. Take it as soon as you remember. Take the next pill at your regular time. This means you may take 2 pills in 1 day.
2. You do not need to use a back-up birth control method if you have sex.

If you **MISS 2** white or yellow-green or blue "active" pills in a row in **WEEK 1 OR WEEK 2** of your pack:
1. Take 2 pills on the day you remember and 2 pills the next day.
2. Then take 1 pill a day until you finish the pack.
3. You MAY BECOME PREGNANT if you have sex in the 7 days after you miss pills. You MUST use another birth control method (such as condoms, foam, or sponge) as a back-up for those 7 days.

If you **MISS 2** white or yellow-green or blue "active" pills in a row in **THE 3rd WEEK**:
1. ***If you are a Day 1 Starter:***
 THROW OUT the rest of the pill pack and start a new pack that same day.
 If you are a Sunday Starter:
 Keep taking 1 pill every day until Sunday.
 On Sunday, THROW OUT the rest of the pack and start a new pack of pills that same day.
2. You may not have your period this month but this is expected. However, if you miss your period 2 months in a row, call your doctor or clinic because you might be pregnant.
3. You MAY BECOME PREGNANT if you have sex in the 7 days after you miss pills. You MUST use another birth control method (such as condoms, foam, or sponge) as a back-up for those 7 days.

If you **MISS 3 OR MORE** white or yellow-green or blue "active" pills in a row (during the first 3 weeks):
1. ***If you are a Day 1 Starter:***
 THROW OUT the rest of the pill pack and start a new pack of pills that same day.

If you are a Sunday Starter:
Keep taking 1 pill every day until Sunday.
On Sunday, THROW OUT the rest of the pack and start a new pack of pills that same day.
2. You may not have your period this month but this is expected. However, if you miss your period 2 months in a row, call your doctor or clinic because you might be pregnant.
3. You MAY BECOME PREGNANT if you have sex in the 7 days after you miss pills. You MUST use another birth control method (such as condoms, foam, or sponge) as a back-up for those 7 days.

REMINDER:
If you forget any of the 7 orange "reminder" pills in Week 4:
THROW AWAY the pills you missed.
Keep taking 1 pill each day until the pack is empty.
You do not need a back-up method.

FINALLY, IF YOU ARE STILL NOT SURE WHAT TO DO ABOUT THE PILLS YOU HAVE MISSED:
Use a BACK-UP METHOD anytime you have sex.
KEEP TAKING ONE "ACTIVE" PILL EACH DAY until you can reach your doctor or clinic.

6. Missed periods, spotting or light bleeding
At times, you may not have a period after you have completed a pack of pills. If you miss 1 period but you have taken the pills exactly as you were supposed to, continue as usual into the next cycle. If you have not taken the pills correctly, and have missed a period, you may be pregnant and you should stop taking the Pill until your doctor or clinic determines whether or not you are pregnant. Until you can talk to your doctor or clinic, use an appropriate back-up birth control method. If you miss 2 consecutive periods, you should stop taking the Pill until it is determined that you are not pregnant.
Even if spotting or light bleeding should occur, continue taking the Pill according to the schedule. Should spotting or light bleeding persist, you should notify your doctor or clinic.

7. Stopping the pill before surgery or prolonged bed rest
If you are scheduled for surgery or you need to stay in bed for a long period of time you should tell your doctor that you are on the Pill. You should stop taking the Pill four weeks before your operation to avoid an increased risk of blood clots. Talk to your doctor about when you may start taking the Pill again.

8. Starting the pill after pregnancy
After you have a baby it is advisable to wait 4–6 weeks before starting to take the Pill. Talk to your doctor about when you may start taking the Pill after pregnancy.

9. Pregnancy due to pill failure
When the Pill is taken correctly, the expected pregnancy rate is approximately 1% (i.e., 1 pregnancy per 100 women per year). If pregnancy occurs while taking the Pill, there is little risk to the fetus. The typical failure rate of large numbers of pill users is less than 3% when women who have missed pills are included. If you become pregnant, you should discuss your pregnancy with your doctor.

10. Pregnancy after stopping the pill
There may be some delay in becoming pregnant after you stop taking the Pill, especially if you had irregular periods before you started using the Pill. Your doctor may recommend that you delay becoming pregnant until you have had one or more regular periods.
There does not appear to be any increase in birth defects in newborn babies when pregnancy occurs soon after stopping the Pill.

11. Overdosage
There are no reports of serious illness or side effects in young children who have swallowed a large number of pills. In adults, overdosage may cause nausea and/or bleeding in females. In case of overdosage, contact your doctor, clinic or pharmacist.

12. Other information
Your doctor or clinic will take a medical and family history and will examine you before prescribing the Pill. The physical examination may be delayed to another time if you request it and the health care provider believes that it is a good medical practice to postpone it. You should be reexamined at least once a year. Be sure to inform your doctor or clinic if there is a family history of any of the conditions listed previously in this leaflet. Be sure to keep all appointments with your doctor or clinic because this is a time to determine if there are early signs of side effects from using the Pill.
Do not use the Pill for any condition other than the one for which it was prescribed. The Pill has been prescribed specifically for you, do not give it to others who may want birth control pills.
If you want more information about birth control pills, ask your doctor or clinic. They have a more technical leaflet called **PHYSICIAN LABELING** which you might want to read.

NON-CONTRACEPTIVE HEALTH BENEFITS

In addition to preventing pregnancy, use of oral contraceptives may provide certain non-contraceptive health benefits:
- Menstrual cycles may become more regular
- Blood flow during menstruation may be lighter and less iron may be lost. Therefore, anemia due to iron deficiency is less likely to occur
- Pain or other symptoms during menstruation may be encountered less frequently
- Ectopic (tubal) pregnancy may occur less frequently
- Non-cancerous cysts or lumps in the breast may occur less frequently
- Acute pelvic inflammatory disease may occur less frequently
- Oral contraceptive use may provide some protection against developing two forms of cancer: cancer of the ovaries and cancer of the lining of the uterus
- If you want more information about birth control pills, ask your doctor or pharmacist. They have a more technical leaflet called the Professional Labeling, which you may wish to read.

Keep this and all medication out of the reach of children.
Store at controlled room temperature 15°C to 25°C (59°F to 77°F).

BRIEF SUMMARY
PATIENT PACKAGE INSERT

This product (like all oral contraceptives) is intended to prevent pregnancy. It does not protect against HIV infection (AIDS) and other sexually transmitted diseases.
Oral contraceptives, also known as "birth control pills" or "the pill," are taken to prevent pregnancy and, when taken correctly, have a failure rate of about 1% per year when used without missing any pills. The typical failure rate of large numbers of pill users is less than 3% per year when women who miss pills are included. For most women, oral contraceptives are also free of serious or unpleasant side effects. However, forgetting to take oral contraceptives considerably increases the chances of pregnancy.
For the majority of women, oral contraceptives can be taken safely, but there are some women who are at high risk of developing certain serious diseases that can be life-threatening or may cause temporary or permanent disability. The risks associated with taking oral contraceptives increase significantly if you:
- Smoke
- Have high blood pressure, diabetes or high cholesterol
- Have or have had clotting disorders, heart attack, stroke, angina pectoris, cancer of the breast or sex organs, jaundice or malignant or benign liver tumors

You should not take the pill if you suspect you are pregnant or have unexplained vaginal bleeding.

Cigarette smoking increases the risk of serious cardiovascular side effects from oral contraceptive use. This risk increases with age and with heavy smoking (15 or more cigarettes per day) and is quite marked in women over 35 years of age. Women who use oral contraceptives are strongly advised not to smoke.

Most side effects of the pill are not serious. The most common such effects are nausea, vomiting, bleeding between menstrual periods, weight gain, breast tenderness and difficulty wearing contact lenses. These side effects, especially nausea and vomiting, may subside within the first 3 months of use.
The serious side effects of the pill occur very infrequently, especially if you are in good health and are young. However, you should know that the following medical conditions have been associated with or made worse by the pill:
1. Blood clots in the legs (thrombophlebitis) or lungs (pulmonary embolism), stoppage or rupture of a blood vessel in the brain (stroke), blockage of blood vessels in the heart (heart attack or angina pectoris), eye or other organs of the body. As mentioned above, smoking increases the risk of heart attacks and strokes and subsequent serious medical consequences.
2. Liver tumors, which may rupture and cause severe bleeding. A possible but not definite association has been found with the pill and liver cancer. However, liver cancers are extremely rare. The chance of developing liver cancer from using the pill is thus even rarer.
3. High blood pressure, although blood pressure usually returns to normal when the pill is stopped.

The symptoms associated with these serious side effects are discussed in the detailed leaflet given to you with your supply of pills. Notify your doctor or health care provider if you notice any unusual physical disturbances while taking the pill. In addition, drugs such as rifampin, as well as some anti-convulsants and some antibiotics, may decrease oral contraceptive effectiveness.
Studies to date of women taking the pill have not shown an increase in the incidence of cancer of the breast or cervix. There is, however, insufficient evidence to rule out the possibility that the pill may cause such cancers. Some studies have reported an increase in the risk of developing breast cancer, particularly at a younger age. This increased risk appears to be related to duration of use.
Taking the pill provides some important non-contraceptive health benefits. These include less painful menstruation, less menstrual blood loss and anemia, fewer pelvic infections and fewer cancers of the ovary and the lining of the uterus.
Be sure to discuss any medical condition you may have with your health care provider. Your health care provider will take a medical and family history before prescribing oral contraceptives and will examine you. The physical examination may be delayed to another time if you request it and the health care provider believes that it is a good medical practice to postpone it. You should be reexamined at least once a year while taking oral contraceptives. The detailed patient information leaflet gives you further information which you should read and discuss with your health care provider.

HOW TO TAKE THE PILL

See full text of HOW TO TAKE THE PILL which is printed in full in the Detailed Patient Labeling.

Rx only
WATSONPHARMA
Manufactured for:
Watson Pharma, Inc.
a subsidiary of
Watson Laboratories, Inc.
Corona, CA 92880
by: ICN Puerto Rico, Inc.
Humacao, PR 00791
Address medical inquiries to:
WATSONPHARMA Medical Information
PO BOX 1900
Corona, CA 92878-1900
800-272-5525

Revised: April 10, 2000

A08829-3

Shown in Product Identification Guide, page 340

LEVORA® 0.15/30-21 Tablets ℞
[lē-vŏra]
(levonorgestrel and ethinyl estradiol tablets, USP)
LEVORA® 0.15/30-28 Tablets
[lē-vŏra]
(levonorgestrel and ethinyl estradiol tablets, USP)
Part Number A08917-1

Patients should be counseled that this product does not protect against HIV infection (AIDS) and other sexually transmitted diseases.

ORAL CONTRACEPTIVE AGENTS

DESCRIPTION

Levora® 0.15/30-21 Tablets provide an oral contraceptive regimen consisting of 21 white tablets containing levonorgestrel 0.15 mg and ethinyl estradiol 0.03 mg.
Levora® 0.15/30-28 Tablets provide an oral contraceptive regimen consisting of 21 white tablets containing levonorgestrel 0.15 mg and ethinyl estradiol 0.03 mg followed by 7 peach tablets containing inert ingredients.
Levonorgestrel is a totally synthetic progestogen with the chemical name (-)-13-Ethyl-17-hydroxy-18,19-dinor-17α-pregn-4-en-20-yn-3-one. Ethinyl estradiol is an estrogen with the chemical name 19-Nor-17α-pregna-1,3,5(10)-trien-20-yne-3,17-diol. Their structural formula follow:

C_2H_5 OH C≡CH H H H H O

LEVONORGESTREL

ETHINYL ESTRADIOL

The white Levora® 0.15/30 tablets contain the following inactive ingredients: croscarmellose sodium, lactose, magnesium stearate, microcrystalline cellulose, and povidone. The inactive peach tablets in the 28-day regimen of Levora® 0.15/30 contain the following inactive ingredients: FD&C Yellow No. 6, lactose, magnesium stearate, and starch (corn).

CLINICAL PHARMACOLOGY

Combination oral contraceptives act by suppression of gonadotrophins. Although the primary mechanism of this action is inhibition of ovulation, other alterations include changes in the cervical mucus (which increase the difficulty of sperm entry into the uterus) and the endometrium (which may reduce the likelihood of implantation).

INDICATIONS AND USAGE

Oral contraceptives are indicated for the prevention of pregnancy in women who elect to use this product as a method of contraception

Oral contraceptives are highly effective. Table I lists the typical accidental pregnancy rates for users of combination oral contraceptives and other methods of contraception.[1] The efficacy of these contraceptive methods, except sterilization, depends upon the reliability with which they are used. Correct and consistent use of methods can result in lower failure rates.

TABLE I: PERCENTAGE OF WOMEN EXPERIENCING A CONTRACEPTIVE FAILURE DURING THE FIRST YEAR OF PERFECT USE AND FIRST YEAR OF TYPICAL USE

	% of Women Experiencing an Accidental Pregnancy within the First Year of Use	
Method	Typical Use[a]	Percent Use[b]
Chance	85	85
Spermicides	21	6
Periodic abstinence	20	1-9
Withdrawal	19	4
Cap		
Parous	36	26
Nulliparous	18	9
Sponge		
Parous	36	20
Nulliparous	18	9
Diaphragm	18	6
Condom		
Female	21	5
Male	12	3
Pill	3	
Progestin only		0.5
Combined		0.1
IUD		
Progesterone	2	1.5
Copper T 380A	0.8	0.6
Injection (Depo-Provera)	0.3	0.3
Implants (Norplant)	0.09	0.09
Female sterilization	0.4	0.4
Male sterilization	0.15	0.10

Adapted with permission.[1]

[a] Among *typical* couples who initiate use of a method (not necessarily for the first time), the percentage who experience an accidental pregnancy during the first year if they do not stop use for any other reason.

[b] Among couples who initiate use of a method (not necessarily for the first time) and who use it *perfectly* (both consistently and correctly), the percentage who experience an accidental pregnancy during the first year if they do not stop use for any other reason.

CONTRAINDICATIONS

Oral contraceptives should not be used in women who have the following conditions:

- Thrombophlebitis or thromboembolic disorders
- A past history of deep vein thrombophlebitis or thromboembolic disorders
- Cerebral vascular or coronary artery disease
- Known or suspected carcinoma of the breast
- Carcinoma of the endometrium or other known or suspected estrogen-dependent neoplasia
- Undiagnosed abnormal genital bleeding
- Cholestatic jaundice of pregnancy or jaundice with prior pill use
- Hepatic adenomas, carcinomas or benign liver tumors
- Known or suspected pregnancy

WARNINGS

Cigarette smoking increases the risk of serious cardiovascular side effects from oral contraceptive use. This risk increases with age and with heavy smoking (15 or more cigarettes per day) and is quite marked in women over 35 years of age. Women who use oral contraceptives should be strongly advised not to smoke.

The use of oral contraceptives is associated with increased risks of several serious conditions including myocardial infraction, thromboembolism, stroke, hepatic neoplasia, and gallbladder disease, although the risk of serious morbidity or mortality is very small in healthy women without underlying risk factors. The risk of morbidity and mortality increases significantly in the presence of other underlying risk factors such as hypertension, hyperlipidemias, hypercholesterolemia, obesity and diabetes.[2-5]

Practitioners prescribing oral contraceptives should be familiar with the following information relating to these risks.

The information contained in this package insert is principally based on studies carried out in patients who used oral contraceptives with higher formulations of both estrogens and progestogens than those in common use today. The effect of long-term use of the oral contraceptives with lower formulations of both estrogens and progestogens remains to be determined.

Throughout this labeling, epidemiological studies reported are of two types: retrospective or case control studies and prospective or cohort studies.[6-11] Case control studies provide a measure of the relative risk of a disease. Relative risk, the *ratio* of the incidence of a disease among oral contraceptive users to that among non-users, cannot be assessed directly from case control studies, but the odds ratio obtained is a measure of relative risk. The relative risk does not provide information on the actual clinical occurrence of a disease. Cohort studies provide not only a measure of the relative risk but of a measure of attributable risk, which is the *difference* in the incidence of disease between oral contraceptive users and non-users. The attributable risk does provide information about the actual occurrence of a disease in the population. (Adapted from ref. 12 and 13 with the author's permission.) For further information, the reader is referred to a text on epidemiological methods.

1. THROMBOEMBOLIC DISORDERS AND OTHER VASCULAR PROBLEMS

a. Myocardial infarction

An increased risk of myocardial infarction has been attributed to oral contractive use. This risk is primarily in smokers or women with other underlying risk factors for coronary artery disease such as hypertension, hypercholesterolemia, morbid obesity and diabetes.[2-5, 13] The relative risk of heart attack for current oral contraceptive users has been estimated to be 2 to 6.[2, 14-19] The risk is very low under the age of 30. However, there is the possibility of a risk of cardiovascular disease even in very young women who take oral contraceptives.

Smoking in combination with oral contraceptive use has been shown to contribute substantially to the incidence of myocardial infractions in women in their mid-thirties or older, with smoking accounting for the majority of excess cases.[20]

Mortality rates associated with circulatory disease have been shown to increase substantially in smokers over the age of 35 and non-smokers over the age of 40 among women who use oral contraceptives (see Table II).[16]

TABLE II: CIRCULATORY DISEASE MORTALITY RATES PER 100, 000 WOMAN YEARS BY AGE, SMOKING STATUS AND ORAL CONTRACEPTIVE USE

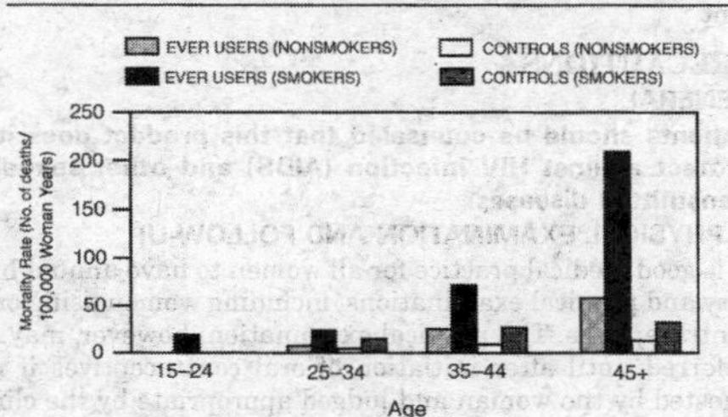

Adapted from P.M. Layde and V. Beral, Table V[16]

Oral contraceptives may compound the effects of well-known risk factors such as hypertension, diabetes, hyperlipidemias, hypercholesterolemia age and obesity.[3, 13, 21] In particular, some progestogens are known to decrease HDL cholesterol and cause glucose intolerance, while estrogens may create a state of hyperinsulinism.[21-25] Oral contraceptives have been shown to increase blood pressure among users (see **WARNINGS**, section 9). Similar effects on risk factors have been associated with an increased risk of heart disease. Oral contraceptives must be used with caution in women with cardiovascular disease risk factors.

b. Thromboembolism

An increased risk of thromboembolic and thrombotic disease associated with the use of oral contraceptives is well established. Case control studies have found the relative risk of users compared to non-users to be 3 for the first episode of superficial venous thrombosis, 4 to 11 for deep vein thrombosis or pulmonary embolism, and 1.5 to 6 for women with predisposing conditions for venous thromboembolic disease.[12, 13, 26-31] Cohort studies have shown the relative risk to be somewhat lower, about 3 for new cases and about 4.5 for new cases requiring hospitalization.[32] The risk of thromboembolic disease due to oral contraceptives is not related to length of use and disappears after pill use is stopped.[12]

A 2- to 6-fold increase in relative risk of post-operative thromboembolic complications has been reported with the use of oral contraceptives. The relative risk of venous thrombosis in women who have predisposing conditions is twice that of women without such medical conditions.[83] If feasible, oral contraceptives should be discontinued at least 4 weeks prior to and for 2 weeks after elective surgery and during and following prolonged immobilization. Since the immediate postpartum period also is associated with an increased risk of thromboembolism, oral contraceptives should be started no earlier than 4 to 6 weeks after delivery in women who elect not to breast feed.[33]

c. Cerebrovascular diseases

An increase in both the relative and attributable risks of cerebrovascular events (thrombotic and hemorrhagic strokes) has been shown in users of oral contraceptives. In general, the risk is greatest among older (>35 years), hypertensive women who also smoke. Hypertension was found to be a risk factor for both users and non-users for both types of strokes while smoking interacted to increase the risk for hemorrhagic strokes.[34]

In a large study, the relative risk of thrombotic strokes has been shown to range from 3 for normotensive users to 14 for users with severe hypertension.[35] The relative risk of hemorrhagic stroke is reported to be 1.2 for non-smokers who used oral contraceptives, 2.6 for smokers who did not use oral contraceptives, 7.6 for smokers who used oral contraceptives, 1.8 for normotensive users and 25.7 for users with severe hypertension.[35] The attributable risk also is greater in women in their mid-thirties or older and among smokers.[13]

d. Dose-related risk of vascular disease with oral contraceptives

A positive association has been observed between the amount of estrogen and progestogen in oral contraceptives and the risk of vascular disease.[36-38] A decline in serum high-density lipoproteins (HDL) has been reported with many progestational agents.[22-24] A decline in serum high-density lipoproteins has been associated with an increased incidence of ischemic heart disease.[39] Because estrogens increase HDL cholesterol, the net effect of an oral contraceptive depends on a balance achieved between doses of estrogen and progestogen and the nature and absolute amount of progestogens used in the contraceptives. The amount of both hormones should be considered in the choice of an oral contraceptive.[37]

Minimizing exposure to estrogen and progestogen is in keeping with good principles of therapeutics. For any particular estrogen/progestogen combination, the dosage regimen prescribed should be one which contains the least amount of estrogen and progestogen that is compatible with a low failure rate and the needs of the individual patient. New acceptors of oral contraceptive agents should be started on preparations containing the lowest estrogen content that produces satisfactory results for the individual.

e. Persistence of risk of vascular disease

There are three studies which have shown persistence of risk of vascular disease for ever-users of oral contraceptives.[17, 34, 40] In a study in the United States, the risk of developing myocardial infarction after discontinuing oral contraceptives persists for at least 9 years for women 40-49 years who had used oral contraceptives for 5 or more years, but this increased risk was not demonstrated in other age groups.[17] In another study in Great Britain, the risk of developing cerebrovascular disease persisted for at least 6 years after discontinuation of oral contraceptives, although excess risk was very small.[40] There is a significantly increased relative risk of subarachnoid hemorrhage after termination of use of oral contraceptives.[34] However, these studies were performed with oral contraceptive formulations containing 50 mcg or higher of estrogen.

2. ESTIMATES OF MORTALITY FROM CONTRACEPTIVE USE

One study gathered data from a variety of sources which have estimated the mortality rates associated with different methods of contraception at different ages (see Table III).[41] These estimates include the combined risk of death associated with contraceptive methods plus the risk attributable to pregnancy in the event of method failure. Each method of contraception has its specific benefits and risks. The study concluded that with the exception of oral contraceptive users 35 and older who smoke and 40 and older who do not smoke, mortality associated with all methods of birth control is low and below that associated with childbirth. The observation of a possible increase in risk of mortality with age for oral contraceptive users is based on data gathered in the 1970's–but not reported in the U.S. until 1983.[16, 41] However, current clinical practice involves the use of lower estrogen dose formulations combined with careful restriction of oral contraceptive use to women who do not have the various risk factors listed in this labeling.

Because of these changes in practice and, also, because of some limited new data which suggest that the risk of cardiovascular disease with the use of oral contraceptives may now be less than previously observed,[78, 79] the Fertility and Maternal Health Drugs Advisory Committee was asked to review the topic in 1989. The Committee concluded that al-

Continued on next page

Levora—Cont.

though cardiovascular disease risks may be increased with oral contraceptive use after age 40 in healthy non-smoking women (even with the newer low-dose formulations), there are greater potential health risks associated with pregnancy in older women and with the alternative surgical and medical procedures which may be necessary if such women do not have access to effective and acceptable means of contraception.

Therefore, the Committee recommended that the benefits of oral contraceptive use by healthy non-smoking women over 40 may outweigh the possible risks. Of course, older women, as all women who take oral contraceptives, should take the lowest possible dose formulation that is effective.[80]

[See table below]

3. CARCINOMA OF THE BREAST AND REPRODUCTIVE ORGANS

Numerous epidemiological studies have been performed on the incidence of breast, endometrial, ovarian and cervical cancer in women using oral contraceptives. The overwhelming evidence in the literature suggests that use of oral contraceptives is not associated with an increase in the risk of developing breast cancer, regardless of the age and parity of first use or with most of the marketed brands and doses.[42-44]

The Cancer and Steroid Hormone (CASH) study also showed no latent effect on the risk of breast cancer for at least a decade following long-term use.[43] A few studies have shown a slightly increased relative risk of developing breast cancer,[44-47] although the methodology of these studies, which included differences in examination of users and nonusers and differences in age at start of use, has been questioned.[47-49] Some studies have reported an increased relative risk of developing breast cancer, particularly at a younger age. This increased relative risk appears to be related to duration of use.[81-82]

Some studies suggest that oral contraceptive use has been associated with an increase in the risk of cervical intraepithelial neoplasia in some populations of women.[50-53] However, there continues to be controversy about the extent to which such findings may be due to differences in sexual behavior and other factors.

In spite of many studies of the relationship between oral contraceptive use and breast or cervical cancers, a cause and effect relationship has not been established.

4. HEPATIC NEOPLASIA

Benign hepatic adenomas are associated with oral contraceptive use although the incidence of benign tumors is rare in the United States. Indirect calculations have estimated the attributable risk to be in the range of 3.3 cases per 100,000 for users, a risk that increases after 4 or more years of use.[54] Rupture of rare, benign, hepatic adenomas may cause death through intra-abdominal hemorrhage.[55-56]

Studies in the United States and Britain have shown an increased risk of developing hepatocellular carcinoma in long-term (>8 years) oral contraceptive users.[57-59] However, these cancers are extremely rare in the United States and the attributable risk (the excess incidence) of liver cancers in oral contraceptive users approaches less than 1 per 1,000,000 users.

5. OCULAR LESIONS

There have been clinical case reports of retinal thrombosis associated with the use of oral contraceptives. Oral contraceptives should be discontinued if there is unexplained partial or complete loss of vision; onset of proptosis or diplopia; papilledema; or retinal vascular lesions. Appropriate diagnostic and therapeutic measures should be undertaken immediately.

6. ORAL CONTRACEPTIVE USE BEFORE OR DURING EARLY PREGNANCY

Extensive epidemiological studies have revealed no increased risk of birth defects in women who have used oral contraceptives prior to pregnancy.[60-62] Studies also do not suggest a teratogenic effect, particularly insofar as cardiac anomalies and limb reduction defects are concerned, when taken inadvertently during early pregnancy.[60,61,63,64]

The administration of oral contraceptives to induce withdrawal bleeding should not be used as a test for pregnancy. Oral contraceptives should not be used during pregnancy to treat threatened or habitual abortion.

It is recommended that for any patient who has missed 2 consecutive periods, pregnancy should be ruled out before continuing oral contraceptives use. If the patient has not adhered to the prescribed schedule, the possibility of pregnancy should be considered at the first missed period. Oral contraceptive use should be discontinued if pregnancy is confirmed.

7. GALLBLADDER DISEASE

Earlier studies have reported an increased lifetime relative risk of gallbladder surgery in users of oral contraceptives and estrogens.[65-66] More recent studies, however, have shown that the relative risk of developing gallbladder disease among oral contraceptive users may be minimal.[67] The recent findings of minimal risk may be related to the use of oral contraceptive formulations containing lower hormonal doses of estrogens and progestogens.[68]

8. CARBOHYDRATE AND LIPID METABOLIC EFFECTS

Oral contraceptives have been shown to cause glucose intolerance in a significant percentage of users.[25] Oral contraceptives containing greater than 75 mcg of estrogen cause hyperinsulinism, while lower doses of estrogen cause less glucose intolerance.[70] Progestogens increase insulin secretion and create insulin resistance, this effect varying with different progestational agents.[25, 71] However, in the nondiabetic woman, oral contraceptives appear to have no effect on fasting blood glucose.[69] Because of these demonstrated effects, prediabetic and diabetic women should be carefully observed while taking oral contraceptives.

Some women may develop persistent hypertriglyceridemia while on the pill.[72] As discussed earlier (see **WARNINGS**, sections 1a. and 1d.), changes in serum triglycerides and lipoprotein levels have been reported in oral contraceptive users.[23]

9. ELEVATED BLOOD PRESSURE

An increase in blood pressure have been reported in women taking oral contraceptives and this increase is more likely in older oral contraceptive users and with continued use.[73, 84] Data from the Royal College of General Practitioners and subsequent randomized trials have shown that the incidence of hypertension increases with increasing concentrations of progestogens.

Women with a history of hypertension or hypertension-related diseases or renal disease should be encouraged to use another method of contraception. If women elect to use oral contraceptives, they should be monitored closely and if significant elevation of blood pressure occurs, oral contraceptives should be discontinued. For most women, elevated blood pressure will return to normal after stopping oral contraceptives and there is no difference in the occurrence of hypertension among ever-and never-users.[73-75]

10. HEADACHE

The onset or exacerbation of migraine or development of headache with a new pattern which is recurrent, persistent or severe requires discontinuation of oral contraceptives and evaluation of the cause.

11. BLEEDING IRREGULARITIES

Breakthrough bleeding and spotting are sometimes encountered in patients on oral contraceptives, especially during the first 3 months of use. Non-hormonal causes should be considered and adequate diagnostic measures taken to rule out malignancy or pregnancy in the event of breakthrough bleeding, as in the case of any abnormal vaginal bleeding. If pathology has been excluded, time or a change to another formulation may solve the problem. In the event of amenorrhea, pregnancy should be ruled out.

Some woman may encounter post-pill amenorrhea or oligomenorrhea, especially when such a condition was pre-existent.

PRECAUTIONS

GENERAL

Patients should be counseled that this product does not protect against HIV infection (AIDS) and other sexually transmitted diseases.

1. PHYSICAL EXAMINATION AND FOLLOW-UP

It is good medical practice for all women to have annual history and physical examinations, including women using oral contraceptives. The physical examination, however, may be deferred until after initiation of oral contraceptives if requested by the woman and judged appropriate by the clinician. The physical examination should include special reference to blood pressure, breasts, abdomen and pelvic organs, including cervical cytology, and relevant laboratory tests. In case of undiagnosed, persistent or recurrent abnormal vaginal bleeding, appropriate measures should be conducted to rule out malignancy. Women with a strong family history of breast cancer or who have breast nodules should be monitored with particular care.

2. LIPID DISORDERS

Women who are being treated for hyperlipidemias should be followed closely if they elect to use oral contraceptives. Some progestogens may elevate LDL levels and may render the control of hyperlipidemias more difficult.

3. LIVER FUNCTION

If jaundice develops in any woman receiving oral contraceptives the medication should be discontinued. Steroid hormones may be poorly metabolized in patients with impaired liver function.

4. FLUID RETENTION

Oral contraceptives may cause some degree of fluid retention. They should be prescribed with caution, and only with careful monitoring, in patients with conditions which might be aggravated by fluid retention.

5. EMOTIONAL DISORDERS

Women with a history of depression should be carefully observed and the drug discontinued if depression recurs to a serious degree.

6. CONTACT LENSES

Contact lens wearers who develop visual changes or changes in lens tolerance should be assessed by an ophthalmologist.

7. DRUG INTERACTIONS

Reduced efficacy and increased incidence of breakthrough bleeding and menstrual irregularities have been associated with concomitant use of rifampin. A similar association, though less marked, has been suggested with barbiturates, phenylbutazone, phenytoin sodium, and possibly with griseofulvin, ampicillin and tetracyclines.[76]

8. INTERACTIONS WITH LABORATORY TESTS

Certain endocrine and liver function tests and blood components may be affected by oral contraceptives:

a. Increased prothrombin and factors VII, VIII, IX and X; decreased antithrombin 3; increased norepinephrine-induced platelet aggregability.

b. Increased thyroid binding globulin (TBG) leading to increased circulating total thyroid hormone, as measured by protein-bound iodine (PBI), T4 by column or by radioimmunoassay. Free T3 resin uptake is decreased, reflecting the elevated TBG. Free T4 concentration is unaltered.

c. Other binding proteins may be elevated in the serum.

d. Sex steroid binding globulins are increased and result in elevated levels of total circulating sex steroids and corticoids; however, free or biologically active levels remain unchanged.

e. Triglycerides may be increased.

f. Glucose tolerance may be decreased.

g Serum folate levels may be depressed by oral contraceptive therapy. This may be of clinical significance if a woman becomes pregnant shortly after discontinuing oral contraceptives.

9. CARCINOGENESIS

See **WARNINGS** section.

10. PREGNANCY

Pregnancy Category X. See **CONTRAINDICATIONS** and **WARNINGS** sections.

11. NURSING MOTHERS

Small amounts of oral contraceptive steroids have been identified in the milk of nursing mothers and a few adverse effects on the child have been reported, including jaundice and breast enlargement. In addition, oral contraceptives given in the postpartum period may interfere with lactation by decreasing the quantity and quality of breast milk. If possible, the nursing mother should be advised not to use oral contraceptives but to use other forms of contraception until she has completely weaned her child.

INFORMATION FOR THE PATIENT

See **PATIENT LABELING** printed below.

ADVERSE REACTIONS

An increased risk of the following serious adverse reactions has been associated with the use of oral contraceptives (see **WARNINGS** section):

- Thrombophlebitis
- Arterial thromboembolism
- Pulmonary embolism
- Myocardial infarction
- Cerebral hemorrhage
- Cerebral thrombosis
- Hypertension
- Gallbladder disease
- Hepatic adenomas, carcinomas or benign liver tumors

There is evidence of an association between the following conditions and the use of oral contraceptives, although additional confirmatory studies are needed:

- Mesenteric thrombosis
- Retinal thrombosis

The following adverse reactions have been reported in patients receiving oral contraceptives and are believed to be drug-related:

- Nausea
- Vomiting
- Gastrointestinal symptoms (such as abdominal cramps and bloating)
- Breakthrough bleeding
- Spotting
- Change in menstrual flow
- Amenorrhea
- Temporary infertility after discontinuation of treatment
- Edema

TABLE III: ESTIMATED ANNUAL NUMBER OF BIRTH-RELATED OR METHOD-RELATED DEATHS ASSOCIATED WITH CONTROL OF FERTILITY PER 100,000 NONSTERILE WOMEN, BY FERTILITY CONTROL METHOD ACCORDING TO AGE

Method of control and outcome	15–19	20–24	25–29	30–34	35–39	40–44
No fertility control methods*	7.0	7.4	9.1	14.8	25.7	28.2
Oral contraceptives non-smoker**	0.3	0.5	0.9	1.9	13.8	31.6
Oral contraceptives smoker**	2.2	3.4	6.6	13.5	51.1	117.2
IUD**	0.8	0.8	1.0	1.0	1.4	1.4
Condom*	1.1	1.6	0.7	0.2	0.3	0.4
Diaphragm/Spermicide*	1.9	1.2	1.2	1.3	2.2	2.8
Periodic abstinence*	2.5	1.6	1.6	1.7	2.9	3.6

*Deaths are birth-related

**Deaths are method-related

Estimates adapted from H.W. Ory, Table 3[41]

- Melasma which may persist
- Breast changes: tenderness, enlargement, secretion
- Change in weight (increase or decrease)
- Change in cervical erosion and secretion
- Diminution in lactation when given immediately postpartum
- Cholestatic jaundice
- Migraine
- Rash (allergic)
- Mental depression
- Reduced tolerance to carbohydrates
- Vaginal candidiasis
- Change in corneal curvature (steepening)
- Intolerance to contact lenses

The following adverse reactions have been reported in users of oral contraceptives and the association has been neither confirmed nor refuted:

- Pre-menstrual syndrome
- Cataracts
- Changes in appetite
- Cystitis-like syndrome
- Headache
- Nervousness
- Dizziness
- Hirsutism
- Loss of scalp hair
- Erythema multiforme
- Erythema nodosum
- Hemorrhagic eruption
- Vaginitis
- Porphyria
- Impaired renal function
- Hemolytic uremic syndrome
- Budd-Chiari syndrome
- Acne
- Changes in libido
- Colitis

OVERDOSAGE

Serious ill effects have not been reported following acute ingestion of large doses of oral contraceptives by young children. Overdosage may cause nausea, and withdrawal bleeding may occur in females.

NON-CONTRACEPTIVE HEALTH BENEFITS

The following non-contraceptive health benefits related to the use of oral contraceptives are supported by epidemiological studies which largely utilized oral contraceptive formulations containing estrogen doses exceeding 0.035 mg of ethinyl estradiol or 0.05 mg of mestranol.[6-11]

Effects on menses:

- Increased menstrual cycle regularity
- Decreased blood loss and decreased incidence of iron deficiency anemia
- Decreased incidence of dysmenorrhea

Effects related to inhibition of ovulation:

- Decreased incidence of functional ovarian cysts
- Decreased incidence of ectopic pregnancies

Effects from long-term use:

- Decreased incidence of fibroadenomas and fibrocystic disease of the breast
- Decreased incidence of acute pelvic inflammatory disease
- Decreased incidence of endometrial cancer
- Decreased incidence of ovarian cancer

DOSAGE AND ADMINISTRATION

To achieve maximum contraceptive effectiveness, oral contraceptives must be taken exactly as directed and at intervals not exceeding 24 hours.

21-Day Schedule: For a DAY 1 START, count the first day of menstrual flow as Day 1 and the first tablet (white) is then taken on Day 1. For a SUNDAY START when menstrual flow begins on or before Sunday, the first tablet (white) is taken on that day. With either a DAY 1 START or SUNDAY START, 1 tablet is taken each day at the same time for 21 days. No tablets are taken for 7 days, then, whether bleeding has stopped or not, a new course is started of 1 tablet a day for 21 days. This institutes a 3 weeks on, 1 week off dosage regimen.

28-Day Schedule: For a DAY 1 START, count the first day of menstrual flow as Day 1 and the first tablet (white) is then taken on Day 1. For a SUNDAY START when menstrual flow begins on or before Sunday, the first tablet (white) is taken on that day. With either a DAY 1 START or SUNDAY START, 1 tablet (white) is taken each day at the same time for 21 days. Then the peach tablets are taken for 7 days, whether bleeding has stopped or not. After all 28 tablets have been taken, whether bleeding has stopped or not, the same dosage schedule is repeated beginning on the following day.

INSTRUCTIONS TO PATIENTS

- To achieve maximum contraceptive effectiveness, the oral contraceptive pill must be taken exactly as directed and at intervals not exceeding 24 hours.
- Important: Women should be instructed to use an additional method of protection until after the first 7 days of administration *in the initial cycle.*
- Due to the normally increased risk of thromboembolism occurring postpartum, women should be instructed not to initiate treatment with oral contraceptives earlier than 4 weeks after a full-term delivery. If pregnancy is terminated in the first 12 weeks, the patient should be instructed to start oral contraceptives immediately or within 7 days. If pregnancy is terminated after 12 weeks, the patient should be instructed to start oral contraceptives after 2 weeks.[33, 77]
- If spotting or breakthrough bleeding should occur, the patient should continue the medication according to the schedule. Should spotting or breakthrough bleeding persist, the patient should notify her physician.
- If the patient misses 1 pill, she should be instructed to take it as soon as she remembers and then take the next pill at the regular time. The patient should be advised that missing a pill can cause spotting or light bleeding and that she may be a little sick to her stomach on the days she takes the missed pill with her regularly scheduled pill. If the patient has missed more than one pill, see DETAILED PATIENT LABELING: HOW TO TAKE THE PILL, WHAT TO DO IF YOU MISS PILLS.
- Use of oral contraceptives in the event of a missed menstrual period:
  1. If the patient has not adhered to the prescribed dosage regimen, the possibility of pregnancy should be considered after the first missed period and oral contraceptives should be withheld until pregnancy has been ruled out.
  2. If the patient has adhered to the prescribed regimen and misses 2 consecutive periods, pregnancy should be ruled out before continuing the contraceptive regimen.

HOW SUPPLIED

Levora® 0.15/30-21 Tablets (levonorgestrel and ethinyl estradiol tablets, USP): Each white tablet is unscored, round in shape, with "15/30" debossed on one side and "WATSON" on the other side, and contains 0.15 mg levonorgestrel and 0.03 mg ethinyl estradiol. Levora® 0.15/30-21 is packaged in cartons of six tablet dispensers. Each dispenser contains 21 white (active) tablets.

Levora® 0.15/30-28 Tablets (levonorgestrel and ethinyl estradiol tablets, USP): Each white tablet is unscored, round in shape, with "15/30" debosssed on one side and "WATSON" on the other side, and contains 0.15 mg levonorgestrel and 0.03 mg ethinyl estradiol. Levora® 0.15/30-28 is packaged in cartons of six tablet dispensers. Each tablet dispenser contains 21 white (active) tablets and 7 peach (inert) tablets. Inert tablets are unscored, round in shape with "WATSON" debossed on one side and PI on the other side.

Rx only

Store at controlled room temperature 15°-25°C (59°-77°F).

REFERENCES

1. Hatcher, R.A., Trussell, J., Stewart, F., et al.: *Contraceptive Technology: Sixteenth Revised Edition*, New York, NY, 1994. **2.** Mann, J., et al.: *Br Med J* 2(5956)241-245, 1975. **3.** Knopp, R.H.: *J Reprod Med* 31(9):913-921, 1986. **4.** Mann, J.I., et al.: *Br Med J* 2:445-447, 1976. **5.** Ory, H.: *JAMA* 237: 2619-2622, 1977. **6.** The Cancer and Steroid Hormone Study of the Centers for Disease Control: *JAMA* 249(2): 1596-1599, 1983. **7.** The Cancer and Steroid Hormone Study of the Centers for Disease Control: *JAMA* 257(6):796-800, 1987. **8.** Ory, H.W.: *JAMA* 228(1):68-69, 1974. **9.** Ory, H.W., et al.: *N Eng J Med* 294:419-422, 1976. **10.** Ory, H.W.: *Fam Plann Perspect* 14:182-184, 1982. **11.** Ory, H.W., et al.: *Making Choices*, New York, The Alan Guttmacher Institute, 1983. **12.** Stadel, B.: *N Eng J Med* 305(11):612-618, 1981. **13.** Stadel, B.: *N Eng J Med* 305(12):672-677, 1981. **14.** Adam, S., et al.: *Br J Obstet Gynaecol* 88:838-845, 1981. **15.** Mann, J., et al.: *Br Med J* 2(5965):245-248, 1975. **16.** Royal College of General Practitioners' Oral Contraceptive Study: *Lancet* 1:541-546, 1981. **17.** Slone, D., et al.: *N Eng J Med* 305(8):420-424, 1981. **18.** Vessey, M.P.: *Br J Fam Plann* 6(supplement):1-12, 1980. **19.** Russell-Briefel, R., et al.: *Prev Med* 15:352-362, 1986. **20.** Goldbaum, G., et al.: *JAMA* 258(10):1339-1342, 1987. **21.** LaRosa, J.C.: *J Reprod Med* 31(9):906-912, 1986. **22.** Krauss, R.M., et al.: *Am J Obstet Gynecol* 145:446-452, 1983. **23.** Wahl, P., et al.: *N Eng J Med* 308(15):862-867, 1983. **24.** Wynn, V., et al.: *Am J Obstet Gynecol* 142(6):766-771, 1982. **25.** Wynn, V., et al.: *J Reprod Med* 31(9):892-897, 1986. **26.** Inman, W.H., et al.: *Br Med J* 2(5599):193-199, 1968. **27.** Maguire, M.G., et al.: *Am J Epidemiol* 110 (2):188-195, 1979. **28.** Petitti, D., et al.: *JAMA* 242(11):1150-1154, 1979. **29.** Vessey, M.P., et al.: *Br Med J* 2(5599):199-205, 1968. **30.** Vessey, M.P., et al.: *Br Med J* 2(5658):651-657, 1969. **31.** Porter, J.B., et al.: *Obstet Gynecol* 59(3):299-302, 1982. **32.** Vessey, M.P., et al.: *J Biosoc Sci* 8:373-427, 1976. **33.** Mishell, D.R., et al.: *Reproductive Endocrinology*, Philadelphia, F.A. Davis Co., 1979. **34.** Pettiti, D.B., et al.: *Lancet* 2:234-236, 1978. **35.** Collaborative Group for the Study of Stroke in Young Women: *JAMA* 231(7):718-722, 1975. **36.** Inman, W.H., et al.: *Br Med J* 2:203-209, 1970. **37.** Meade, T.W., et al.: *Br Med J* 280(6224):1157-1161, 1980. **38.** Kay, C.R., *Am J Obstet Gynecol* 142(6):762-765, 1982. **39.** Gordon, T., et al.: *Am J Med* 62:707-714, 1977. **40.** Royal College of General Practitioners' Oral Contraception Study: *J Coll Gen Pract* 33:75-82, 1983. **41.** Ory, H.W.: *Fam Plann Perspect* 15(2):57-63, 1983. **42.** Paul, C., et al.: *Br Med J* 293:723-725, 1986. **43.** The Cancer and Steroid Hormone Study of the Centers for Disease Control: *N Eng J Med* 315(7):405-411, 1986. **44.** Pike, M.C., et al.: *Lancet* 2:926-929, 1983. **45.** Miller, D.R., et al.: *Obstet Gynecol* 68:863-868, 1986. **46.** Olsson, H., et al.: *Lancet* 2:748-749, 1985. **47.** McPherson, K., et al.: *Br J Cancer* 56:653-660, 1987. **48.** Huggins, G.R., et al.: *Fetil Steril* 47(5):733-761, 1987. **49.** McPherson, K., et al.: *Br Med J* 293:709-710, 1986. **50.** Ory, H., et al.: *Am J Obstet Gynecol* 124(6):573-577, 1976. **51.** Vessey, M.P., et al.: *Lancet* 2:930, 1983. **52.** Brinton, L.A., et al.: *Int J Cancer* 38: 339-344, 1986. **53.** WHO Collaborative Study of Neoplasia and Steroid Contraceptives: *Br Med J* 290:961-965, 1985. **54.** Rooks, J.B., et al.: *JAMA* 242(7):644-648, 1979.**55.** Bein, N.N., et al.: *Br J Surg* 64: 433-435, 1977. **56.** Klatskin, G.: *Gastroenterology* 73:386-394, 1977. **57.** Henderson, B.E., et al.: *Br J Cancer* 48:437-440, 1983. **58.** Neuberger, J., et al.: *Br Med J* 292:1355-1357, 1986. **59.** Forman, D., et al.: *Br Med J* 292:1357-1361, 1986. **60.** Harlap, S., et al.: *Obstet Gynecol* 55(4):447-452, 1980. **61.** Savolainen, E., et al.: *Am J Obstet Gynecol* 140(5):521-524, 1981. **62.** Janerich, D.T., et al.: *Am J Epidemiol* 112(1):73-79, 1980. **63.** Ferencz, C., et al.: *Teratology* 21:225-259, 1980. **64.** Rothman, K.J., et al.: *Am J Epidemiol*, 109(4):433-439, 1979. **65.** Boston Collaborative Drug Surveillance Program: *Lancet* 1:1399-1404, 1973. **66.** Royal College of General Practioners: *Oral contraceptives and health*. New York, Pittman, 1974. **67.** Rome Group for the Epidemiology and Prevention of Cholelithiasis: *Am J Epidemiol* 119(5):796-805, 1984. **68.** Strom, B.L., et al.: *Clin Pharmacol Ther* 39(3):335-341, 1986. **69.** Perlman, J.A., et al.: *J Chronic Dis* 38(10):857-864, 1985. **70.** Wynn, V., et al.: *Lancet* 1:1045-1049, 1979. **71.** Wynn, V.: *Progesterone and Progestin*, New York, Raven Press, 1983. **72.** Wynn, V., et al.: *Lancet* 2:720-723, 1966. **73.** Fisch, I.R., et al.: *JAMA* 237(23):2499-2503, 1977. **74.** Laragh, J.H.: *Am J Obstet Gynecol* 126(1):141-147, 1976. **75.** Ramcharan, S., et al.: *Pharmacology of Steroid Contraceptive Drugs*, New York, Raven Press, 1977. **76.** Stockley, I:, *Pharm J* 216: 140-143, 1976. **77.** Dickey, R.P.: *Managing Contraceptive Pill Patients*, Oklahoma, Creative Informatics Inc., 1984. **78.** Porter, J.B., Hunter, J., Jick, H., et al.: *Obstet Gynecol* 1985;66:1-4. **79.** Porter, J.B., Hershel, J., Walker, A.M.: *Obstet Gynecol* 1987;70:29-32. **80.** Fertility and Maternal Health Drugs Advisory Committee, F.D.A., October, 1989. **81.** Schlesselman, J., Stadel, B.V., Murray, P., Lai, S.: *Breast cancer in relation to early use of oral contraceptives. JAMA* 1988;259:1828-1833. **82.** Hennekens, C.H., Speizer, F.E., Lipnick, R.J., Rosner, B., Bain, C., Belanger, C., Stampfer, M.J., Willett, W., Peto, R.: *A case—control study of oral contraceptive use and breast cancer.* JNCI 1984;72:39-42. **83.** Royal College of General Practitioners: *Oral contraceptives, venous thrombosis, and varicose veins. J Coll Gen Pract* 28:393-399, 1978. **84.** Royal College of General Practitioners' Oral Contraception Study: *Effect on hypertension and benign breast disease of progestogen component in combined oral contraceptives, Lancet* 1:624, 1977.

Manufactured for
WATSON PHARMA, INC.
a subsidiary of
Watson Laboratories, Inc.
Corona, CA 91720
By Patheon Inc.
Mississauga, ON L5N 7K9 CANADA

Address medical inquiries to:
WATSON PHARMA, INC.
Medical Information
PO Box 1900
Corona, CA 91718

WATSON PHARMA

A08917-1 Printed in USA

Shown in Product Identification Guide, page 340

LOW-OGESTREL®-28 ℞

[lō-ōgĕstrĕl]

(norgestrel and ethinyl estradiol tablets USP, 0.3 mg/0.03 mg)

Rx only

Patients should be counseled that this product does not protect against HIV infection (AIDS) and other sexually transmitted diseases.

ORAL CONTRACEPTIVE AGENTS

DESCRIPTION

Low-Ogestrel®-28 Tablets (norgestrel and ethinyl estradiol tablets USP, 0.3 mg/0.03 mg) provide an oral contraceptive regimen consisting of 21 white tablets followed by 7 peach tablets.

Each white tablet, for oral administration contains 0.3 mg of norgestrel and 0.03 mg ethinyl estradiol and the following inactive ingredients: croscarmellose sodium, lactose, magnesium stearate, microcrystalline cellulose, and povidone.

Each inactive peach tablet, for oral administration, in the 28 day regimen contains the following inactive ingredients: lactose monohydrate, microcrystalline cellulose, anhydrous lactose, FD&C Yellow No. 6 Lake, and magnesium stearate.

Norgestrel is a totally synthetic progestogen, insoluble in water, freely soluble in chloroform, sparingly soluble in alcohol with the chemical name (±)-13-Ethyl-17-hydroxy-18, 19-dinor-17α-preg-4-en-20-yn-3-one. Ethinyl estradiol is an estrogen, insoluble in water, soluble in alcohol, in chloroform, in ether, in vegetable oils, and in solutions of fixed alkali hydroxides with the chemical name 19-nor-17α-pregna-1,3,5(10)-trien-20-yne-3,17-diol. Their structural formulae follow:

[See chemical structures at top of next column]

Therapeutic class: Oral contraceptive.

Continued on next page

Low-Ogestrel—Cont.

NORGESTREL
$C_{21}H_{28}O_2$
MW 312.45

ETHINYL ESTRADIOL
$C_{20}H_{24}O_2$
MW 296.41

CLINICAL PHARMACOLOGY

Combination oral contraceptives act by suppression of gonadotrophins. Although the primary mechanism of this action is inhibition of ovulation, other alterations include changes in the cervical mucus (which increase the difficulty of sperm entry into the uterus) and the endometrium (which may reduce the likelihood of implantation).

INDICATIONS AND USAGE

Low-Ogestrel® (norgestrel and ethinyl estradiol tablets, USP, 0.3 mg/0.03 mg) are indicated for the prevention of pregnancy in women who elect to use this product as a method of contraception.

Oral contraceptives are highly effective. Table I lists the typical accidental pregnancy rates for users of combination oral contraceptives and other methods of contraception.[1] The efficacy of these contraceptive methods, except sterilization, depends upon the reliability with which they are used. Correct and consistent use of methods can result in lower failure rates.

[See table below]

CONTRAINDICATIONS

Oral contraceptives should not be used in women who have the following conditions:

- Thrombophlebitis or thromboembolic disorders
- A past history of deep vein thrombophlebitis or thromboembolic disorders
- Cerebral vascular or coronary artery disease
- Known or suspected carcinoma of the breast
- Carcinoma of the endometrium or other known or suspected estrogen-dependent neoplasia
- Undiagnosed abnormal genital bleeding
- Cholestatic jaundice of pregnancy or jaundice with prior pill use
- Hepatic adenomas, carcinomas or benign liver tumors
- Known or suspected pregnancy

WARNINGS

Cigarette smoking increases the risk of serious cardiovascular side effects from oral contraceptive use. This risk increases with age and with heavy smoking (15 or more cigarettes per day) and is quite marked in women over 35 years of age. Women who use oral contraceptives are strongly advised not to smoke.

The use of oral contraceptives is associated with increased risks of several serious conditions including myocardial infarction, thromboembolism, stroke, hepatic neoplasia, and gallbladder disease, although the risk of serious morbidity or mortality is very small in healthy women without underlying risk factors. The risk of morbidity and mortality increases significantly in the presence of other underlying risk factors such as hypertension, hyperlipidemias, hypercholesterolemia, obesity and diabetes.[2–5]

Practitioners prescribing oral contraceptives should be familiar with the following information relating to these risks.

The information contained in this package insert is principally based on studies carried out in patients who used oral contraceptives with higher formulations of both estrogens and progestogens than those in common use today. The effect of long-term use of the oral contraceptives with lower formulations of both estrogens and progestogens remains to be determined.

Throughout this labeling, epidemiological studies reported are of two types: retrospective or case control studies and prospective or cohort studies. Case control studies provide a measure of the relative risk of a disease. Relative risk, the *ratio* of the incidence of a disease among oral contraceptive users to that among non-users, cannot be assessed directly from case control studies, but the odds ratio obtained is a measure of relative risk. The relative risk does not provide information on the actual clinical occurrence of a disease. Cohort studies provide not only a measure of relative risk but a measure of attributable risk, which is the *difference* in the incidence of disease between the oral contraceptive users and non-users. The attributable risk does provide information about the actual occurrence of a disease in the population. (Adapted from ref. 12 and 13 with the author's permission.) For further information, the reader is referred to a text on epidemiological methods.

1. THROMBOEMBOLIC DISORDERS AND OTHER VASCULAR PROBLEMS

a. Myocardial Infarction

An increased risk of myocardial infarction has been attributed to oral contraceptive use. This risk is primarily in smokers or women with other underlying risk factors for coronary artery disease such as hypertension, hypercholesterolemia, morbid obesity and diabetes.[2–5, 13] The relative risk of heart attack for current oral contraceptive users has been estimated to be 2 to 6.[2, 14–19] The risk is very low under the age of 30. However, there is the possibility of a risk of cardiovascular disease even in very young women who take oral contraceptives. Smoking in combination with oral contraceptive use has been shown to contribute substantially to the incidence of myocardial infarctions in women in their mid-thirties or older, with smoking accounting for the majority of excess cases.[20]

Mortality rates associated with circulatory disease have been shown to increase substantially in smokers over the age of 35 and non-smokers over the age of 40 among women who use oral contraceptives (see Table II).[16]

TABLE II: CIRCULATORY DISEASE MORTALITY RATES PER 100,000 WOMAN YEARS BY AGE, SMOKING STATUS AND ORAL CONTRACEPTIVE USE

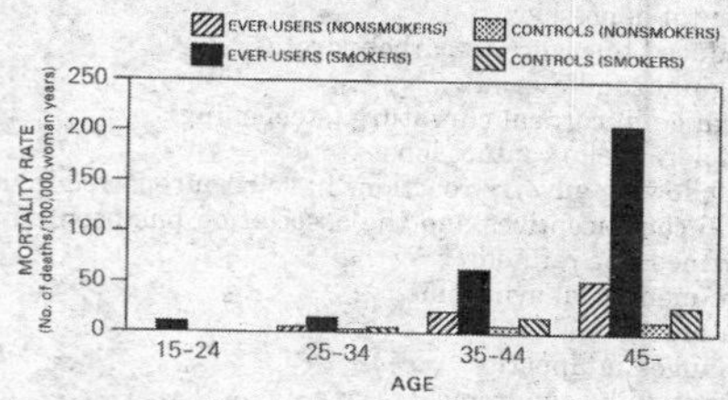

Adapted from P.M. Layde and V. Beral, Table V[16]

Oral contraceptives may compound the effects of well-known risk factors such as hypertension, diabetes, hyperlipidemias, hypercholesterolemia, age and obesity.[3, 13, 21] In particular, some progestogens are known to decrease HDL cholesterol and cause glucose intolerance, while estrogens may create a state of hyperinsulinism.[21–25] Oral contraceptives have been shown to increase blood pressure among users (see ***WARNINGS***, section 9). Similar effects on risk factors have been associated with an increased risk of heart disease. Oral contraceptives must be used with caution in women with cardiovascular disease risk factors.

b. Thromboembolism

An increased risk of thromboembolic and thrombotic disease associated with the use of oral contraceptives is well established. Case control studies have found the relative risk of users compared to non-users to be 3 for the first episode of superficial venous thrombosis, 4 to 11 for deep vein thrombosis or pulmonary embolism, and 1.5 to 6 for women with predisposing conditions for venous thromboembolic disease.[12, 13, 26–31] Cohort studies have shown the relative risk to be somewhat lower, about 3 for new cases and about 4.5 for new cases requiring hospitalization.[32] The risk of thromboembolic disease due to oral contraceptives is not related to length of use and disappears after pill use is stopped.[12]

A 2- to 6-fold increase in relative risk of post-operative thromboembolic complications has been reported with the use of oral contraceptives. The relative risk of venous thrombosis in women who have predisposing conditions is twice that of women without such medical conditions.[83] If feasible, oral contraceptives should be discontinued at least 4 weeks prior to and for 2 weeks after elective surgery and during and following prolonged immobilization. Since the immediate postpartum period also is associated with an increased risk of thromboembolism, oral contraceptives should be started no earlier than 4 to 6 weeks after delivery in women who elect not to breast feed.[33]

c. Cerebrovascular diseases

An increase in both the relative and attributable risks of cerebrovascular events (thrombotic and hemorrhagic strokes) has been shown in users of oral contraceptives. In general, the risk is greatest among older (>35 years), hypertensive women who also smoke. Hypertension was found to be a risk factor for both users and non-users for both types of strokes while smoking interacted to increase the risk for hemorrhagic strokes.[34]

In a large study, the relative risk of thrombotic strokes has been shown to range from 3 for normotensive users to 14 for users with severe hypertension.[35] The relative risk of hemorrhagic stroke is reported to be 1.2 for non-smokers who used oral contraceptives, 2.6 for smokers who did not use oral contraceptives, 7.6 for smokers who used oral contraceptives, 1.8 for normotensive users and 25.7 for users with severe hypertension.[35] The attributable risk also is greater in women in their mid-thirties or older and among smokers.[13]

d. Dose-related risk of vascular disease from oral contraceptives

A positive association has been observed between the amount of estrogen and progestogen in oral contraceptives and the risk of vascular disease.[36–38] A decline in serum high density lipoproteins (HDL) has been reported with many progestational agents.[22–24] A decline in serum high density lipoproteins has been associated with an increased incidence of ischemic heart disease.[39] Because estrogens increase HDL cholesterol, the net effect of an oral contraceptive depends on a balance achieved between doses of estrogen and progestogen and the nature and absolute amount of progestogens used in the contraceptives. The amount of both hormones should be considered in the choice of an oral contraceptive.[37]

Minimizing exposure to estrogen and progestogen is in keeping with good principles of therapeutics. For any particular estrogen/progestogen combination, the dosage regimen prescribed should be one which contains the least amount of estrogen and progestogen that is compatible with a low failure rate and the needs of the individual patient. New acceptors of oral contraceptive agents should be started on preparations containing the lowest estrogen content that produces satisfactory results for the individual.

TABLE I: PERCENTAGE OF WOMEN EXPERIENCING A CONTRACEPTIVE FAILURE DURING THE FIRST YEAR OF PERFECT USE AND FIRST YEAR OF TYPICAL USE

Method	Percentage of women experiencing an accidental pregnancy within the first year of use	
	Typical use[a]	Perfect use[b]
Chance	85	85
Spermicides	21	6
Periodic abstinence	20	1-9
Withdrawal	19	4
Cap		
Parous	36	26
Nulliparous	18	9
Sponge		
Parous	36	20
Nulliparous	18	9
Diaphragm	18	6
Condom		
Female	21	5
Male	12	3
Pill	3	
Progestin only		0.5
Combined		0.1
IUD		
Progesterone	2	1.5
Copper T 380A	0.8	0.6
Injection (Depo-Provera)	0.3	0.3
Implants (Norplant)	0.09	0.09
Female sterilization	0.4	0.4
Male sterilization	0.15	0.10

Adapted with permission[1].

a Among *typical* couples who initiate use of a method (not necessarily for the first time), the percentage who experience an accidental pregnancy during the first year if they do not stop use for any other reason.

b Among couples who initiate use of a method (not necessarily for the first time) and who use it *perfectly* (both consistently and correctly), the percentage who experience an accidental pregnancy during the first year if they do not stop use for any other reason.

e. Persistence of risk of vascular disease

There are three studies which have shown persistence of risk of vascular disease for ever-users of oral contraceptives.[17, 34, 40] In a study in the United States, the risk of developing myocardial infarction after discontinuing oral contraceptives persists for at least 9 years for women 40–49 years who had used oral contraceptives for 5 or more years, but this increased risk was not demonstrated in other age groups.[17] In another study in Great Britain, the risk of developing cerebrovascular disease persisted for at least 6 years after discontinuation of oral contraceptives, although excess risk was very small.[40] There is a significantly increased relative risk of subarachnoid hemorrhage after termination of use of oral contraceptives.[34] However, these studies were performed with oral contraceptive formulations containing 50 µg or higher of estrogen.

2. ESTIMATES OF MORTALITY FROM CONTRACEPTIVE USE

One study gathered data from a variety of sources which have estimated the mortality rates associated with different methods of contraception at different ages (see Table III).[41] These estimates include the combined risk of death associated with contraceptive methods plus the risk attributable to pregnancy in the event of method failure. Each method of contraception has its specific benefits and risks. The study concluded that with the exception of oral contraceptive users 35 and older who smoke and 40 and older who do not smoke, mortality associated with all methods of birth control is low and below that associated with childbirth. The observation of a possible increase in risk of mortality with age for oral contraceptive users is based on data gathered in the 1970s—but not reported in the U.S. until 1983.[16, 41] However, current clinical practice involves the use of lower estrogen dose formulations combined with careful restriction of oral contraceptive use to women who do not have the various risk factors listed in this labeling.

Because of these changes in practice and, also, because of some limited new data which suggest that the risk of cardiovascular disease with the use of oral contraceptives may now be less than previously observed.[78, 79] the fertility and Maternal Health Drugs Advisory Committee was asked to review the topic in 1989. The Committee concluded that although cardiovascular disease risks may be increased with oral contraceptive use after age 40 in healthy non-smoking women (even with the newer low-dose formulations), there are greater potential health risks associated with pregnancy in older women and with the alternative surgical and medical procedures which may be necessary if such women do not have access to effective and acceptable means of contraception.

Therefore, the Committee recommended that the benefits of oral contraceptive use by healthy non-smoking women over 40 may outweigh the possible risks. Of course, older women, as all women who take oral contraceptives, should take the lowest possible dose formulation that is effective.[80]

[See table above]

TABLE III: ESTIMATED ANNUAL NUMBER OF BIRTH-RELATED OR METHOD-RELATED DEATHS ASSOCIATED WITH CONTROL OF FERTILITY PER 100,000 NONSTERILE WOMEN, BY FERTILITY CONTROL METHOD ACCORDING TO AGE

Method of control and outcome	15-19	20-24	25-29	30-34	35-39	40-44
No fertility control methods*	7.0	7.4	9.1	14.8	25.7	28.2
Oral contraceptives non-smoker**	0.3	0.5	0.9	1.9	13.8	31.6
Oral contraceptives smoker**	2.2	3.4	6.6	13.5	51.1	117.2
IUD**	0.8	0.8	1.0	1.0	1.4	1.4
Condom*	1.1	1.6	0.7	0.2	0.3	0.4
Diaphragm/Spermicide*	1.9	1.2	1.2	1.3	2.2	2.8
Periodic abstinence*	2.5	1.6	1.6	1.7	2.9	3.6

*Deaths are birth-related
**Deaths are method-related

Estimates adapted from H.W. Ory, Table 3[41]

3. CARCINOMA OF THE BREAST AND REPRODUCTIVE ORGANS

Numerous epidemiological studies have been performed on the incidence of breast, endometrial, ovarian and cervical cancer in women using oral contraceptives. The overwhelming evidence in the literature suggests that the use of oral contraceptives is not associated with an increase in the risk of developing breast cancer, regardless of the age and parity of first use or with most of the marketed brands and doses.[42–44] The Cancer and Steroid Hormone (CASH) study also showed no latent effect on the risk of breast cancer for at least a decade following long-term use.[43] A few studies have shown a slightly increased relative risk of developing breast cancer,[44–47] although the methodology of these studies, which included differences in examination of users and non-users and differences in age at start of use, has been questioned.[47–49] Some studies have reported an increased relative risk of developing breast cancer, particularly at a younger age. This increased relative risk appears to be related to duration of use.[81, 82]

Some studies suggest that oral contraceptive use has been associated with an increase in the risk of cervical intraepithelial neoplasia in some populations of women.[50–53] However, there continued to be controversy about the extent to which such findings may be due to differences in sexual behavior and other factors.

In spite of many studies of the relationship between oral contraceptive use and breast or cervical cancers, a cause and effect relationship has not been established.

4. HEPATIC NEOPLASIA

Benign hepatic adenomas are associated with oral contraceptive use although the incidence of benign tumors is rare in the United States. Indirect calculations have estimated the attributable risk to be in the range of 3.3 cases per 100,000 for users, a risk that increases after 4 or more years of use.[54] Rupture of rare, benign, hepatic adenomas may cause death through intra-abdominal hemorrhage.[55–56]

Studies in the United States and Britain have shown an increased risk of developing hepatocellular carcinoma in long-term (>8 years) oral contraceptive users.[57–59] However, these cancers are extremely rare in the United States and the attributable risk (the excess incidence) of liver cancers in oral contraceptive users approaches less than 1 per 1,000,000 users.

5. OCULAR LESIONS

There have been clinical case reports of retinal thrombosis associated with the use of oral contraceptives. Oral contraceptives should be discontinued if there is unexplained partial or complete loss of vision; onset of proptosis or diplopia; papilledema; or retinal vascular lesions. Appropriate diagnostic and therapeutic measures should be undertaken immediately.

6. ORAL CONTRACEPTIVE USE BEFORE OR DURING EARLY PREGNANCY

Extensive epidemiological studies have revealed no increased risk of birth defects in women who have used oral contraceptives prior to pregnancy.[60–62] Studies also do not suggest a teratogenic effect, particularly insofar as cardiac anomalies and limb reduction defects are concerned, when taken inadvertently during early pregnancy.[60, 61, 63, 64] The administration of oral contraceptives to induce withdrawal bleeding should not be used as a test for pregnancy. Oral contraceptives should not be used during pregnancy to treat threatened or habitual abortion.

It is recommended that for any patient who has missed 2 consecutive periods, pregnancy should be ruled out before continuing oral contraceptive use. If the patient has not adhered to the prescribed schedule, the possibility of pregnancy should be considered at the first missed period. Oral contraceptive use should be discontinued if pregnancy is confirmed.

7. GALLBLADDER DISEASE

Earlier studies have reported an increased lifetime relative risk of gallbladder surgery in users of oral contraceptives and estrogens.[65–66] More recent studies, however, have shown that the relative risk of developing gallbladder disease among oral contraceptive users may be minimal.[67] The recent findings of minimal risk may be related to the use of oral contraceptive formulations containing lower hormonal doses of estrogens and progestogens.[68]

8. CARBOHYDRATE AND LIPID METABOLIC EFFECTS

Oral contraceptives have been shown to cause glucose intolerance in a significant percentage of users.[25] Oral contraceptives containing greater than 75 µg of estrogen cause hyperinsulinism, while lower doses of estrogen cause less glucose intolerance.[70] Progestogens increase insulin secretion and create insulin resistance, this effect varying with different progestational agents.[25, 71] However, in the non-diabetic woman, oral contraceptives appear to have no effect on fasting blood glucose.[69] Because of these demonstrated effects, pre-diabetic and diabetic women should be carefully observed while taking oral contraceptives.

Some women may develop persistent hypertriglyceridemia while on the pill.[72] As discussed earlier (see ***WARNINGS***, sections 1a. and 1d.), changes in serum triglycerides and lipoprotein levels have been reported in oral contraceptive users.[23]

9. ELEVATED BLOOD PRESSURE

An increase in blood pressure has been reported in women taking oral contraceptives and this increase is more likely in older oral contraceptive users and with continued use.[73, 84] Data from the Royal College of General Practitioners and subsequent randomized trials have shown that the incidence of hypertension increases with increasing concentrations of progestogens.

Women with a history of hypertension or hypertension-related diseases or renal disease should be encouraged to use another method of contraception. If women elect to use oral contraceptives, they should be monitored closely and if significant elevation of blood pressure occurs oral contraceptives should be discontinued. For most women, elevated blood pressure will return to normal after stopping oral contraceptives and there is no difference in the occurrence of hypertension among ever- and never-users.[73–75]

10. HEADACHE

The onset or exacerbation of migraine or development of headache with a new pattern which is recurrent, persistent or severe requires discontinuation of oral contraceptives and evaluation of the cause.

11. BLEEDING IRREGULARITIES

Breakthrough bleeding and spotting are sometimes encountered in patients on oral contraceptives, especially during the first 3 months of use. Non-hormonal causes should be considered and adequate diagnostic measures taken to rule out malignancy or pregnancy in the event of breakthrough bleeding, as in the case of any abnormal vaginal bleeding. If pathology, has been excluded, time or a change to another formulation may solve the problem. In the event of amenorrhea, pregnancy should be ruled out.

Some women may encounter post-pill amenorrhea or oligomenorrhea, especially when such a condition was pre-existent.

PRECAUTIONS

GENERAL

Patients should be counseled that this product does not protect against HIV infection (AIDS) and other sexually transmitted diseases.

1. PHYSICAL EXAMINATION AND FOLLOW-UP

It is good medical practice for all women to have annual history and physical examinations, including women using oral contraceptives. The physical examination, however, may be deferred until after initiation of oral contraceptives if requested by the woman and judged appropriate by the clinician. The physical examination should include special reference to blood pressure, breasts, abdomen and pelvic organs, including cervical cytology, and relevant laboratory tests. In case of undiagnosed, persistent or recurrent abnormal vaginal bleeding, appropriate measures should be conducted to rule out malignancy. Women with a strong family history of breast cancer or who have breast nodules should be monitored with particular care.

2. LIPID DISORDERS

Women who are being treated for hyperlipidemias should be followed closely if they elect to use oral contraceptives. Some progestogens may elevate LDL levels and may render the control of hyperlipidemias more difficult.

3. LIVER FUNCTION

If jaundice develops in any woman receiving oral contraceptives the medication should be discontinued. Steroid hormones may be poorly metabolized in patients with impaired liver function.

4. FLUID RETENTION

Oral contraceptives may cause some degree of fluid retention. They should be prescribed with caution, and only with careful monitoring, in patients with conditions which might be aggravated by fluid retention.

5. EMOTIONAL DISORDERS

Women with a history of depression should be carefully observed and the drug discontinued if depression recurs to a serious degree.

6. CONTACT LENSES

Contact lens wearers who develop visual changes or changes in lens tolerance should be assessed by an ophthalmologist.

7. DRUG INTERACTIONS

Reduced efficacy and increased incidence of breakthrough bleeding and menstrual irregularities have been associated with concomitant use of rifampin. A similar association though less marked, has been suggested with barbiturates, phenylbutazone, phenytoin sodium, and possibly with griseofulvin, ampicillin and tetracyclines.[76]

8. INTERACTIONS WITH LABORATORY TESTS

Certain endocrine and liver function tests and blood components may be affected by oral contraceptives:

- **a.** Increased prothrombin and factors VII, VIII, IX, and X: decreased antithrombin 3; increased norepinephrine-induced platelet aggregability.
- **b.** Increased thyroid binding globulin (TBG) leading to increased circulating total thyroid hormone, as measured by protein-bound iodine (PBI), T4 by column or by radioimmunoassay. Free T3 resin uptake is decreased, reflecting the elevated TBG. Free T4 concentration is unaltered.
- **c.** Other binding proteins may be elevated in serum.
- **d.** Sex steroid binding globulins are increased and result in elevated levels of total circulating sex steroids and corticoids; however, free or biologically active levels remain unchanged.
- **e.** Triglycerides may be increased.
- **f.** Glucose tolerance may be decreased.
- **g.** Serum folate levels may be depressed by oral contraceptive therapy. This may be of clinical significance if a woman becomes pregnant shortly after discontinuing oral contraceptives.

Continued on next page

Low-Ogestrel—Cont.

9. CARCINOGENESIS
See ***WARNINGS*** section.
10. PREGNANCY
Pregnancy Category X. See *CONTRAINDICATIONS* and ***WARNINGS*** sections.
11. NURSING MOTHERS
Small amounts of oral contraceptive steroids have been identified in the milk of nursing mothers and a few adverse effects on the child have been reported, including jaundice and breast enlargement. In addition, oral contraceptives given in the postpartum period may interfere with lactation by decreasing the quantity and quality of breast milk. If possible, the nursing mother should be advised not to use oral contraceptives but to use other forms of contraception until she has completely weaned her child.

INFORMATION FOR THE PATIENT
See ***PATIENT LABELING*** printed below.

ADVERSE REACTIONS

An increased risk of the following serious adverse reactions has been associated with the use of oral contraceptives (see ***WARNINGS*** section):
- Thrombophlebitis
- Arterial thromboembolism
- Pulmonary embolism
- Myocardial infarction
- Cerebral hemorrhage
- Cerebral thrombosis
- Hypertension
- Gallbladder disease
- Hepatic adenomas, carcinomas or benign liver tumors

There is evidence of an association between the following conditions and the use of oral contraceptives, although additional confirmatory studies are needed:
- Mesenteric thrombosis
- Retinal thrombosis

The following adverse reactions have been reported in patients receiving oral contraceptives and are believed to be drug-related:
- Nausea
- Vomiting
- Gastrointestinal symptoms (such as abdominal cramps and bloating)
- Breakthrough bleeding
- Spotting
- Change in menstrual flow
- Amenorrhea
- Temporary infertility after discontinuation of treatment
- Edema
- Melasma which may persist
- Breast changes: tenderness, enlargement, secretion
- Change in weight (increase or decrease)
- Change in cervical erosion and secretion
- Diminution in lactation when given immediately postpartum
- Cholestatic jaundice
- Migraine
- Rash (allergic)
- Mental depression
- Reduced tolerance to carbohydrates
- Vaginal candidiasis
- Change in corneal curvature (steepening)
- Intolerance to contact lenses

The following adverse reactions have been reported in users of oral contraceptives and the association has been neither confirmed nor refuted:
- Pre-menstrual syndrome
- Cataracts
- Changes in appetite
- Cystitis-like syndrome
- Headache
- Nervousness
- Dizziness
- Hirsutism
- Loss of scalp hair
- Erythema multiforme
- Erythema nodosum
- Hemorrhagic eruption
- Vaginitis
- Porphyria
- Impaired renal function
- Hemolytic uremic syndrome
- Budd-Chiari syndrome
- Acne
- Changes in libido
- Colitis

OVERDOSAGE

Serious ill effects have not been reported following acute ingestion of large doses of oral contraceptives by young children. Overdosage may cause nausea, and withdrawal bleeding may occur in females.

NON-CONTRACEPTIVE HEALTH BENEFITS
The following non-contraceptive health benefits related to the use of oral contraceptives are supported by epidemiological studies which largely utilized oral contraceptive formulations containing estrogen doses exceeding 0.035 mg of ethinyl estradiol or 0.05 mg of mestranol.[6–11]
Effect on menses:
- Increased menstrual cycle regularity
- Decreased blood loss and decreased incidence of iron deficiency anemia
- Decreased incidence of dysmenorrhea

Effects related to inhibition of ovulation:
- Decreased incidence of functional ovarian cysts
- Decreased incidence of ectopic pregnancies

Effects from long-term use:
- Decreased incidence of fibroadenomas and fibrocystic disease of the breast
- Decreased incidence of acute pelvic inflammatory disease
- Decreased incidence of endometrial cancer
- Decreased incidence of ovarian cancer

DOSAGE AND ADMINISTRATION

To achieve maximum contraceptive effectiveness, oral contraceptives must be taken exactly as directed and at intervals not exceeding 24 hours.

28-Day Schedule: For a DAY 1 START, count the first day of menstrual flow as Day 1 and the first tablet (white) is then taken on Day 1. For a SUNDAY START when menstrual flow begins on or before Sunday, the first tablet (white) is taken on that day. With either a DAY 1 START or SUNDAY START, 1 tablet (white) is taken each day at the same time for 21 days. Then the peach tablets are taken for 7 days, whether bleeding has stopped or not. After all 28 tablets have been taken, whether bleeding has stopped or not, the same dosage schedule is repeated beginning on the following day.

INSTRUCTIONS TO PATIENTS
- To achieve maximum contraceptive effectiveness, the oral contraceptive pill must be taken exactly as directed and at intervals not exceeding 24 hours.
- Important: Women should be instructed to use an additional method of protection until after the first 7 days of administration *in the initial* cycle.
- Due to the normally increased risk of thromboembolism occurring postpartum, women should be instructed not to initiate treatment with oral contraceptives earlier than 4–6 weeks after a full-term delivery. If pregnancy is terminated in the first 12 weeks, the patient should be instructed to start oral contraceptives immediately or within 7 days. If pregnancy is terminated after 12 weeks, the patient should be instructed to start oral contraceptives after 2 weeks.[33, 77]
- If spotting or breakthrough bleeding should occur, the patient should continue the medication according to the schedule. Should spotting or breakthrough bleeding persist, the patients should notify her physician.
- If the patient misses 1 pill, she should be instructed to take it as soon as she remembers and then take the next pill at the regular time. The patient should be advised that missing a pill can cause spotting or light bleeding and that she may be a little sick to her stomach on the days she takes the missed pill with her regularly scheduled pill. If the patient has *missed more than one pill, see* ***DETAILED PATIENT LABELING:*** *HOW TO TAKE THE PILL, WHAT TO DO IF YOU MISS PILLS.*
- Use of oral contraceptives in the event of a missed menstrual period:
  1. If the patient has not adhered to the prescribed dosage regimen, the possibility of pregnancy should be considered after the first missed period and oral contraceptives should be withheld until pregnancy has been ruled out.
  2. If the patient has adhered to the prescribed regimen and misses 2 consecutive periods, pregnancy should be ruled out before continuing the contraceptive regimen.

HOW SUPPLIED

Low-Ogestrel®-28 Tablets (norgestrel and ethinyl estradiol tablets USP, 0.3 mg/0.03 mg): Each white tablet is unscored, round in shape, with "847" debossed on one side and "WATSON" on the other side, and contains 0.3 mg norgestrel and 0.03 mg ethinyl estradiol. Low-Ogestrel®-28 is packaged in cartons of six tablet dispensers. Each tablet dispenser contains 21 white (active) tablets and 7 peach (inert) tablets. Inert tablets are unscored, round in shape with "WATSON" debossed on one side and "P1" on the other side.

Rx only

Store at controlled room temperature 15°C to 25°C (59°F to 77°F).

Keep this and all medications out of the reach of children.

REFERENCES

1. Hatcher, R.A. Trussel, J. Stewart, F., et al.: *Contraceptive Technology: Sixteenth Revised Edition*, New York, NY, 1994. **2.** Mann, J., et al.: *Br Med J* 2(5956): 241–245, 1975. **3.** Knopp, R.H.: *J Reprod Med* 31(9): 913–921, 1986. **4.** Mann, J.I., et al.: *Br Med J* 2: 445–447, 1976. **5.** Ory, H.: *JAMA* 237: 2619–2622, 1977. **6.** The Cancer and Steroid Hormone Study of the Centers for Disease Control: *JAMA* 249(2): 1596–1599, 1983. **7.** The Cancer and Steroid Hormone Study of the Centers for Disease Control: *JAMA* 257(6): 796–800, 1987. **8.** Ory, H.W.: *JAMA* 228(1):68–69, 1974. **9.** Ory, H.W.: et al.: *N Engl J Med* 294: 419–422, 1976. **10.** Ory, H.W.: *Fam Plann Perspect* 14: 182–184, 1982. **11.** Ory, H.W., et al.: *Making Choices*, New York, The Alan Guttmacher Institute, 1983. **12.** Stadel, B.: *N Engl J Med* 305(11): 612–618, 1981. **13.** Stadel, B.: *N Engl J Med* 305(12): 672–677, 1981. **14.** Adam, S., et al: *Br J Obstet Gynaecol* 88: 838–845, 1981. **15.** Mann, J., et al.: *Br Med J* 2(5965): 245–248, 1975. **16.** Royal College of General Practitioners' Oral Contraceptive Study: *Lancet* 1: 541–546, 1981. **17.** Slone, D., et al.: *N Engl J Med* 305(8): 420–424, 1981. **18.** Vessey, M.P.: *Br J Fam Plann* 6 (Supplement): 1–12, 1980. **19.** Russell-Briefel, R., et al.: *Prev Med* 15: 352–362, 1986. **20.** Goldbaum, G., et al.: *JAMA* 258(10): 1339–1342, 1987. **21.** LaRosa, J.C.: *J Reprod Med* 31 (9): 906–912, 1986. **22.** Krauss, R.M., et al.: *Am J Obstet Gynecol* 145: 446–452, 1983. **23.** Wahl, P., et al.: *N Engl J Med* 308(15): 862–867. 1983. **24.** Wynn, V., et al.: *Am J Obstet Gynecol* 142(6): 766–771, 1982. **25.** Wynn V., et al.: *J Reprod Med* 31(9): 892–897, 1986. **26.** Inman, W.H., et al.: *Br Med J* 2(5599): 193–199, 1968. **27.** Maguire, M.G., et al.: *Am J Epidemiol* 110(2): 188–195, 1979. **28.** Petitti, D., et al.: *JAMA* 242(11): 1150–1154, 1979. **29.** Vessey, M.P., et al.: *Br Med J* 2(5599): 199–205, 1968. **30.** Vessey, M.P.; et al.: *Br Med J* 2(5658): 651–657, 1969. **31.** Porter, J.B., et al.: *Obstet Gynecol* 59(3): 299–302, 1982. **32.** Vessey, M.P., et al.: *J Biosoc Sci* 8: 373–427, 1976. **33.** Mishell, D.R., et al.: *Reproductive Endocrinology*, Philadelphia, F.A. Davis Co., 1979. **34.** Petitti, D.B., et al.: *Lancet* 2:234–236, 1978. **35.** Collaborative Group for the Study of Stroke in Young Women: *JAMA* 231(7): 718–722, 1975. **36.** Inman, W.H., et al.: *Br Med J* 2: 203–209, 1970. **37.** Meade, T.W., et al.: *Br Med J* 280(6224): 1157–1161, 1980. **38.** Kay, C.R.: *Am J Obstet Gynecol* 142(6): 762–765, 1982. **39.** Gordon, T., et al.: *Am J Med* 62: 707–714, 1977. **40.** Royal College of General Practitioners' Oral Contraception Study: *J Coll Gen Pract* 33: 75–82, 1983. **41.** Ory, H.W.: *Fam Plann Perspect* 15(2): 57–63, 1983. **42.** Paul, C., et al.: *Br Med J* 293: 723–725, 1986. **43.** The Cancer and Steroid Hormone Study of the Centers for Disease Control: *N Engl J Med* 315(7): 405–411, 1986. **44.** Pike, M.C., et al.: *Lancet* 2: 926–929, 1983. **45.** Miller, D.R., et al.: *Obstet Gynecol* 68: 863–868, 1986. **46.** Olsson, H., et al.: *Lancet* 2: 748–749, 1985. **47.** McPherson, K., et al.: *Br J Cancer* 56: 653–660, 1987. **48.** Huggins, G.R., et al.: *Fertil Steril* 47(5): 733–761, 1987. **49.** McPherson, K., et al.: *Br Med J* 293: 709–710, 1986. **50.** Ory, H., et al.: *Am J Obstet Gynecol* 124(6): 573–577, 1976. **51.** Vessey, M.P., et al.: *Lancet* 2: 930, 1983. **52.** Brinton, L.A., et al.: *Int J Cancer* 38:339–344, 1986. **53.** WHO Collaborative Study of Neoplasia and Steroid Contraceptives: *Br Med J* 290: 961–965, 1985. **54.** Rooks, J.B., et al.: *JAMA* 242(7): 644–648, 1979. **55.** Bein, N.N., et al.: *Br J Surg* 64: 433–435, 1977. **56.** Klatskin, G.: *Gastroenterology* 73: 386–394, 1977. **57.** Henderson, B.E., et al.: *Br J Cancer* 48: 437–440, 1983. **58.** Neuberger, J., et al.: *Br Med J* 292: 1355–1357, 1986. **59.** Forman, D., et al.: *Br Med J* 292: 1357–1361, 1986. **60.** Harlap, S., et al.: *Obstet Gynecol* 55(4): 447–452, 1980. **61.** Savolainen, E., et al.: *Am J Obstet Gynecol* 140(5): 521–524, 1981. **62.** Janerich, D.T., et al.: *Am J Epidemiol* 112(1): 73–79, 1980. **63.** Ferencz, C., et al.: *Teratology* 21: 225–239, 1980. **64.** Rothman, K.J., et al.: *Am J Epidemiol* 109(4): 433–439, 1979. **65.** Boston Collaborative Drug Surveillance Program: *Lancet* 1: 1399–1404, 1973. **66.** Royal College of General Practitioners: *Oral contraceptives and health*, New York, Pittman, 1974. **67.** Rome Group for the Epidemiology and Prevention of Cholelithiasis: *Am J Epidemiol* 119(5): 796–805, 1984. **68.** Strom, B.L., et al: *Clin Pharmacol Ther* 39(3): 335–341, 1986. **69.** Perlman, J.A., et al.: *J Chronic Dis* 38(10): 857–864, 1985. **70.** Wynn, V., et al.: *Lancet* 1: 1045–1049, 1979. **71.** Wynn, V.: *Progesterone and Progestin*, New York, Raven Press, 1983. **72.** Wynn, V., et al.: *Lancet* 2: 720–723, 1966. **73.** Fisch, I.R., et al.: *JAMA* 237(23): 2499–2503, 1977. **74.** Laragh, J.H.: *Am J Obstet Gynecol* 126(1): 141–147, 1976. **75.** Ramcharan, S., et al.: *Pharmacology of Steroid Contraceptive Drugs*, New York, Raven Press, 1977. **76.** Stockley, I.: *Pharm J* 216: 140–143, 1976. **77.** Dickey, R.P.: *Managing Contraceptive Pill Patients*, Oklahoma, Creative Informatics Inc., 1984. **78.** Porter J.B., Hunter J., Jick H., et al.: *Obstet Gynecol* 1985;66: 1–4. **79.** Porter J.B., Hershel J., Walker A.M.: *Obstet Gynecol* 1987;70: 29–32. **80.** Fertility and Maternal Health Drugs Advisory Committee, F.D.A., October, 1989. **81.** Schlessman J., Stadel B.V., Murray P., Lai S.: *Breast cancer in relation to early use of oral contraceptives.* JAMA 1988;259: 1828–1833. **82.** Hennekens C.H., Speizer F.E., Lipnick R.J., Rosner B., Bain C., Belanger C., Stampfer M.J., Willett W., Peto R.: *A case-control study of oral contraceptive use and breast cancer.* JNCI 1984;72: 39–42. **83.** Royal College of General Practitioners: *Oral contraceptives, venous thrombosis, and varicose veins. J Coll Gen Pract* 28: 393–399, 1978. **84.** Royal College of General Practitioners' Oral Contraception Study: *Effect on Hypertension and benign breast disease of progestogen component in combined oral contraceptives. Lancet* 1: 624, 1977.

DETAILED PATIENT LABELING

This product (like all oral contraceptives) is intended to prevent pregnancy. It does not protect against HIV infection (AIDS) and other sexually transmitted diseases.

INTRODUCTION

Any woman who considers using oral contraceptives ("birth control pills" or "the pill") should understand the benefits and risks of using this form of birth control. This leaflet will give you much of the information you will need to make this decision and also will help you determine if you are at risk of developing any of the serious side effects of the pill. It will tell you how to use the pill properly so that it will be as effective as possible. However, this leaflet is not a replacement for a careful discussion between you and your health care provider. You should discuss the information provided in this leaflet with him or her, both when you first start taking the pill and during your regular visits. You also should follow the advice of your health care provider with regard to regular checkups while you are on the pill.

EFFECTIVENESS OF ORAL CONTRACEPTIVES

Oral contraceptives are used to prevent pregnancy and are more effective than other non-surgical methods of birth con-

trol. When they are taken correctly, without missing any pills, the chance of becoming pregnant is less than 1% (1 pregnancy per 100 women per year of use). Typical failure rates are actually 3% per year. The chance of becoming pregnant increases with each missed pill during a menstrual cycle.
In comparison, typical failure rates for other nonsurgical methods of birth control during the first year are as follows: [See first table in next column]

WHO SHOULD NOT TAKE ORAL CONTRACEPTIVES

Cigarette smoking increases the risk of serious cardiovascular side effects from oral contraceptive use. This risk increases with age and with heavy smoking (15 or more cigarettes per day) and is quite marked in women over 35 years of age. Women who use oral contraceptives are strongly advised not to smoke.

Some women should not use the pill. For example, you should not take the pill if you are pregnant or think you may be pregnant. You also should not use the pill if you have any of the following conditions:
- A history of heart attack or stroke
- Blood clots in the legs (thrombophlebitis), brain (stroke), lungs (pulmonary embolism) or eyes
- A history of blood clots in the deep veins of your legs
- Chest pain (angina pectoris)
- Known or suspected breast cancer or cancer of the lining of the uterus, cervix or vagina
- Unexplained vaginal bleeding (until a diagnosis is reached by your doctor)
- Yellowing of the whites of the eyes or of the skin (jaundice) during pregnancy or during previous use of the pill
- Liver tumor (benign or cancerous)
- Known or suspected pregnancy

Tell your health care provider if you have ever had any of these conditions. Your health care provider can recommend a safer method of birth control.

OTHER CONSIDERATIONS BEFORE TAKING ORAL CONTRACEPTIVES

Tell your health care provider if you have or have had:
- Breast nodules, fibrocystic disease of the breast, an abnormal breast x-ray or mammogram
- Diabetes
- Elevated cholesterol or triglycerides
- High blood pressure
- Migraine or other headaches or epilepsy
- Mental depression
- Gallbladder, heart or kidney disease
- History of scanty or irregular menstrual periods

Women with any of these conditions should be checked often by their health care provider if they choose to use oral contraceptives. Also, be sure to inform your doctor or health care provider if you smoke or are on any medications.

RISKS OF TAKING ORAL CONTRACEPTIVES

1. Risk of developing blood clots
Blood clots and blockage of blood vessels are the most serious side effects of taking oral contraceptives. In particular, a clot in the legs can cause thrombophlebitis and a clot that travels to the lungs can cause a sudden blocking of the vessel carrying blood to the lungs. Rarely, clots occur in the blood vessels of the eye and may cause blindness, double vision, or impaired vision.
If you take oral contraceptives and need elective surgery, need to stay in bed for a prolonged illness or have recently delivered a baby, you may be at risk of developing blood clots. You should consult your doctor about stopping oral contraceptives three to four weeks before surgery and not taking oral contraceptives for two weeks after surgery or during bed rest. You should also no take oral contraceptives soon after delivery of a baby. It is advisable to wait for at least four weeks after delivery if you are not breast feeding. If you are breast feeding, you should wait until you have weaned your child before using the pill (see *GENERAL PRECAUTIONS—While breast feeding*).

2. Heart attacks and strokes
Oral contraceptives may increase the tendency to develop strokes (stoppage or rupture of blood vessels in the brain) and angina pectoris and heart attacks (blockage of blood vessels in the heart). Any of these conditions can cause death or temporary or permanent disability.
Smoking greatly increases the possibility of suffering heart attacks and strokes. Furthermore, smoking and the use of oral contraceptives greatly increase the chances of developing and dying of heart disease.

3. Gallbladder disease
Oral contraceptive users may have a greater risk than nonusers of having gallbladder disease, although this risk may be related to pills containing high doses of estrogen.

4. Liver tumors
In rare cases, oral contraceptives can cause benign but dangerous liver tumors. These benign liver tumors can rupture and cause fatal internal bleeding. In addition, a possible but not definite association has been found with the pill and liver cancers in 2 studies in which a few women who developed these very rare cancers were found to have used oral contraceptives for long periods. However, liver cancers are extremely rare. The chance of developing liver cancer from using the pill is thus even rarer.

5. Cancer of the breast and reproductive organs
There is, at present, no confirmed evidence that oral contraceptives increase the risk of cancer of the reproductive organs in human studies. Several studies have found no overall increase in the risk of developing breast cancer. However, women who use oral contraceptives and have a strong family history of breast cancer or who have breast nodules or abnormal mammograms should be followed closely by their doctors. Some studies have reported an increase in the risk of developing breast cancer, particularly at a younger age. This increased risk appears to be related to duration of use.
Some studies have found an increase in the incidence of cancer of the cervix in women who use oral contraceptives. However, this finding may be related to factors other than the use of oral contraceptives.

ESTIMATED RISK OF DEATH FROM A BIRTH CONTROL METHOD OR PREGNANCY

All methods of birth control and pregnancy are associated with a risk of developing certain diseases which may lead to disability or death. An estimate of the number of deaths associated with different methods of birth control and pregnancy has been calculated and is shown in the following table:
[See second table above]
In the above table, the risk of death from any birth control method is less than the risk of childbirth except for oral contraceptive users over the age or 35 who smoke and pill users over the age of 40 even if they do not smoke. It can be seen from the table that for women aged 15 to 39 the risk of death is highest with pregnancy (7–26 deaths per 100,000 women, depending on age). Among pill users who do not smoke the risk of death is always lower than that associated with pregnancy for any age group, although over the age of 40 the risk increases to 32 deaths per 100,000 women compared to 28 associated with pregnancy at that age. However, for pill users who smoke and are over the age of 35 the estimated number of deaths exceeds those for other methods of birth control. If a woman is over the age of 40 and smokes, her estimated risk of death is 4 times higher (117/100,00 women) than the estimated risk associated with pregnancy (28/100,000 women) in that age group.
The suggestion that women over 40 who don't smoke should not take oral contraceptives is based on information from older high-dose pills and on less selective use of pills than is practiced today. An Advisory Committee of the FDA discussed this issue in 1989 and recommended that the benefits of oral contraceptive use by healthy, non-smoking women over 40 years of age may outweigh the possible risks. However, all women, especially older women, are cautioned to use the lowest dose pill that is effective.

Comparison of reversible contraceptive methods: Percentage of women experiencing a contraceptive failure (pregnancy) during the first year of use.

Method	Percentage of women experiencing a pregnancy within the first year of use: Average use	Correct use
No contraception	85	85
Spermicides	21	6
Periodic abstinence	20	1-9[a]
Withdrawal	19	4
Cap		
Given birth	36	26
Never given birth	18	9
Sponge		
Given birth	36	20
Never given birth	18	9
Diaphragm	18	6
Condom		
Female	21	5
Male	12	3
Pill		3
Progestin only		0.5
Combined		0.1
IUD		
Progesterone	2	1.5
Copper T 380A	0.8	0.6
Injectables	0.3	0.3
Implant	0.09	0.09

Adapted with permission—Hatcher, R.A. Trussell, J. Stewart, F., et al.: *Contraceptive Technology: Sixteenth Revised Edition*, New York, NY, 1994.

[a]Depending on method (calendar, ovulation, symptom-thermal)

ESTIMATED ANNUAL NUMBER OF BIRTH-RELATED OR METHOD-RELATED DEATHS ASSOCIATED WITH CONTROL OF FERTILITY PER 100,000 NONSTERILE WOMEN, BY FERTILITY CONTROL METHOD ACCORDING TO AGE

Method of control and outcome	15-19	20-24	25-29	30-34	35-39	40-44
No fertility control methods*	7.0	7.4	9.1	14.8	25.7	28.2
Oral contraceptives non-smoker**	0.3	0.5	0.9	1.9	13.8	31.6
Oral contraceptives smoker**	2.2	3.4	6.6	13.5	51.1	117.2
IUD**	0.8	0.8	1.0	1.0	1.4	1.4
Condom*	1.1	1.6	0.7	0.2	0.3	0.4
Diaphragm/Spermicide*	1.9	1.2	1.2	1.3	2.2	2.8
Periodic abstinence*	2.5	1.6	1.6	1.7	2.9	3.6

*Deaths are birth-related
**Deaths are method-related

WARNING SIGNALS

If any of these adverse effects occur while you are taking oral contraceptives, call your doctor immediately.
- Sharp chest pain, coughing of blood or sudden shortness of breath (indicating a possible clot in the lung)
- Pain in the calf (indicating a possible clot in the leg)
- Crushing chest pain or heaviness in the chest (Indicating a possible heart attack)
- Sudden severe headache or vomiting, dizziness or fainting, disturbances of vision or speech, weakness or numbness in an arm or leg (indicating a possible stroke)
- Sudden partial or complete loss of vision (indicating a possible clot in the eye)
- Breast lumps (indicating possible breast cancer or fibrocystic disease of the breast: ask your doctor or health care provider to show you how to examine your breasts)
- Severe pain or tenderness in the stomach area (indicating a possible ruptured liver tumor)
- Difficulty in sleeping, weakness, lack of energy, fatigue or change in mood (possibly indicating severe depression)
- Jaundice or a yellowing of the skin or eyeballs, accompanied frequently by fever, fatigue, loss of appetite, dark colored urine or light colored bowel movements (indicating possible liver problems)
-

SIDE EFFECTS OF ORAL CONTRACEPTIVES

1. Vaginal bleeding
Irregular vaginal bleeding or spotting may occur while you are taking the pill. Irregular bleeding may vary from slight staining between menstrual periods to breakthrough bleeding which is a flow much like a regular period. Irregular bleeding occurs most often during the first few months of oral contraceptive use but may also occur after you have been taking the pill for some time. Such bleeding may be temporary and usually does not indicate any serious problem. It is important to continue taking your pills on schedule. If the bleeding occurs in more than 1 cycle or lasts for more than a few days, talk to your doctor or health care provider.

2. Contact lenses
If you wear contact lenses and notice a change in vision or an inability to wear your lenses, contact your doctor or health care provider.

3. Fluid retention
Oral contraceptives may cause edema (fluid retention) with swelling of the fingers or ankles and may raise your blood

Continued on next page

Low-Ogestrel—Cont.

pressure. If you experience fluid retention, contact your doctor or health care provider.

4. Melasma (Mask of Pregnancy)
A spotty darkening of the skin is possible, particularly of the face.

5. Other side effects
Other side effects may include change in appetite, headache, nervousness, depression, dizziness, loss of scalp hair, rash and vaginal infections.
If any of these side effects occur, contact your doctor or health care provider.

GENERAL PRECAUTIONS

1. Missed periods and use of oral contraceptives before or during early pregnancy
At times you may not menstruate regularly after you have completed taking a cycle of pills. If you have taken your pills regularly and miss 1 menstural period, continue taking your pills for the next cycle but be sure to inform your health care provider before doing so. If you have not taken the pills daily as instructed and miss 1 menstrual period, or if you miss 2 consecutive menstrual periods, you may be pregnant. Check with your health care provider immediately to determine whether you are pregnant. Do not continue to take oral contraceptives until you are sure you are not pregnant, but continue to use another method of birth control.
There is no conclusive evidence that oral contraceptive use is associated with an increase in birth defects when taken inadvertently during early pregnancy. Previously, a few studies had reported that oral contraceptives might be associated with birth defects but these studies have not been confirmed. Nevertheless, oral contraceptives or any other drugs should not be used during pregnancy unless clearly necessary and prescribed by your doctor. You should check with your doctor about risks to your unborn child from any medication taken during pregnancy.

2. While breast feeding
If you are breast feeding, consult your doctor before starting oral contraceptives. Some of the drug will be passed on to the child in the milk. A few adverse effects on the child have been reported, including yellowing of the skin (jaundice) and breast enlargement. In addition, oral contraceptives may decrease the amount and quality of your milk. If possible, do not use oral contraceptives and use another method of contraception while breast feeding. You should consider starting oral contraceptives only after you have weaned your child completely.

3. Laboratory tests
If you are scheduled for any laboratory tests, tell your doctor you are taking birth control pills. Certain blood tests may be affected by birth control pills.

4. Drug Interactions
Certain drugs may interact with birth control pills to make them less effective in preventing pregnancy or cause an increase in breakthrough bleeding. Such drugs include rifampin; drugs used for epilepsy such as barbiturates (for example phenobarbital) and phenytoin (Dilantin is one brand of this drug); phenylbutazone (Butazolidin is one brand of this drug) and possible certain antibiotics. You may need to use additional contraception when you take drugs which can make oral contraceptives less effective.

5. This product (like all oral contraceptives) is intended to prevent pregnancy. It does not protect against transmission of HIV (AIDS) and other sexually transmitted diseases such as chlamydia, genital herpes, genital warts, gonorrhea, hepatitis B, and syphilis.

HOW TO TAKE THE PILL

IMPORTANT POINTS TO REMEMBER

BEFORE YOU START TAKING YOUR PILLS:

1. BE SURE TO READ THESE DIRECTIONS:
   Before you start taking your pills.
   Anytime you are not sure what to do.
2. THE RIGHT WAY TO TAKE THE PILL IS TO TAKE ONE PILL EVERY DAY AT THE SAME TIME.
   If you miss pills you could get pregnant. This includes starting the pack late.
   The more pills you miss, the more likely you are to get pregnant.
3. MANY WOMEN HAVE SPOTTING OR LIGHT BLEEDING, OR MAY FEEL SICK TO THEIR STOMACH DURING THE FIRST 1–3 PACKS OF PILLS.
   If you feel sick to your stomach, do not stop taking the Pill. The problem will usually go away. If it doesn't go away, check with your doctor or clinic.
4. MISSING PILLS CAN ALSO CAUSE SPOTTING OR LIGHT BLEEDING, even when you make up these missed pills.
   On the days you take 2 pills to make up for missed pills, you could also feel a little sick to your stomach.
5. IF YOU HAVE VOMITING OR DIARRHEA, for any reason, or IF YOU TAKE SOME MEDICINES, including some antibiotics, your pills may not work as well.
   Use a back-up method (such as condoms, foam, or sponge) until you check with your doctor or clinic.
6. IF YOU HAVE TROUBLE REMEMBERING TO TAKE THE PILL, talk to your doctor or clinic about how to make pill-taking easier or about using another method of birth control.
7. IF YOU HAVE ANY QUESTIONS OR ARE UNSURE ABOUT THE INFORMATION IN THIS LEAFLET, call your doctor or clinic.

BEFORE YOU START TAKING YOU PILLS

1. DECIDE WHAT TIME OF DAY YOU WANT TO TAKE YOUR PILL.
   It is important to take it at about the same time every day.
2. LOOK AT YOUR PILL PACK:
   The pill pack has 21 "active" white (with hormones) pills to take for 3 weeks, followed by 1 weeks of reminder peach pills (without hormones).
3. ALSO FIND:
   1) where on the pack to start taking pills, and
   2) in what order to take the pills (follow the arrows).

Active Pill Color: White
Reminder Pill Color: Peach

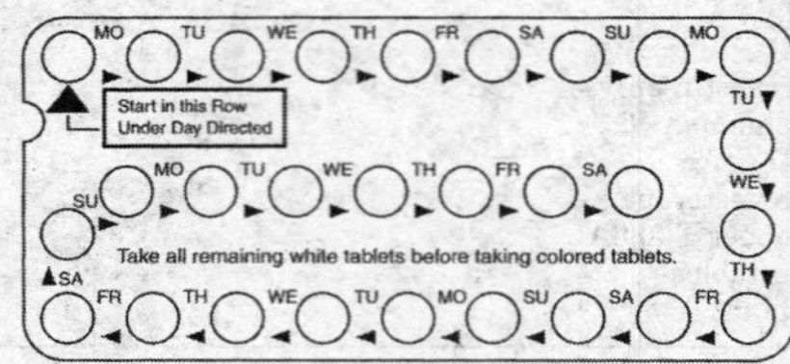

4. BE SURE TO HAVE READY AT ALL TIMES:
   ANOTHER KIND OF BIRTH CONTROL (such as condoms, foam, or sponge) to use as a back-up in case you miss pills.
   AN EXTRA, FULL PILL PACK.

WHEN TO START THE FIRST PACK OF PILLS

You have a choice of which day to start taking your first pack of pills. Decide with your doctor or clinic which is the best day for you. Pick a time of day which will be easy to remember.

DAY 1 START:

1. Take the first "active" white pill of the first pack during the first 24 hours of your period.
2. You will not need to use a back-up method of birth control, since you are starting the pill at the beginning of your period.

SUNDAY START:

1. Take the first "active" white pill of the first pack on the Sunday after your period starts, even if you are still bleeding. If your period begins on Sunday, start the pack that same day.
2. Use another method of birth control as a back-up method if you have sex anytime from the Sunday you start your first pack until the next Sunday (7 days). Condoms, foam, or the sponge are good back-up methods of birth control.

WHAT TO DO DURING THE MONTH

1. **TAKE ONE PILL AT THE SAME TIME EVERY DAY UNTIL THE PACK IS EMPTY.**
   Do not skip pills even if you are spotting or bleeding between monthly periods or feel sick to your stomach (nausea).
   Do not skip pills even if you do not have sex very often.
2. **WHEN YOU FINISH A PACK OR SWITCH YOUR BRAND OF PILLS:**
   Start the next pack on the day after your last "reminder" pill. Do not wait any days between packs.

WHAT TO DO IF YOU MISS PILLS

If you **MISS 1** white "active" pill:

1. Take it as soon as you remember. Take the next pill at your regular time. This means you may take 2 pills in 1 day.
2. You do not need to use a back-up birth control method if you have sex.

If you **MISS 2** white "active" pills in a row in **WEEK 1 OR WEEK 2** of your pack:

1. Take 2 pills on the day you remember and 2 pills the next day.
2. Then take 1 pill a day until you finish the pack.
3. You MAY BECOME PREGNANT if you have sex in the 7 days after you miss pills. You MUST use another birth control method (such as condoms, foam, or sponge) as a back-up for those 7 days.

If you **MISS 2** white "active" pills in row in **THE 3rd WEEK:**

1. ***If you are a Day 1 Starter:***
   THROW OUT the rest of the pill pack and start a new pack that same day.
   If you are a Sunday Starter:
   Keep taking 1 pill every day until Sunday.
   On Sunday, THROW OUT the rest of the pack and start a new pack of pills that same day.
2. You may not have your period this month but this is expected. However, if you miss your period 2 months in a row, call your doctor or clinical because you might be pregnant.
3. You MAY BECOME PREGNANT if you have sex in the 7 days after you miss pills. You MUST use another birth control methods (such as condoms, foam, or sponge) as a back-up for those 7 days.

If you **MISS 3 OR MORE** white "active" pills in a row (during the first 3 weeks):

1. ***If you are a Day 1 Starter:***
   THROW OUT the rest of the pill pack and start a new pack of pills that same day.
   If you are a Sunday Starter:
   Keep taking 1 pill every day until Sunday.
   On Sunday, THROW OUT the rest of the pack and start a new pack of pills that same day.
2. You may not have your period this month but this is expected. However, if you miss your period 2 months in a row, call your doctor or clinic because you might be pregnant.
3. You MAY BECOME PREGNANT if you have sex in the 7 days after you miss pills. You MUST use another birth control method (such as condoms, foam, or sponge) as a back-up for those 7 days.

REMINDER:
If you forget any of the 7 peach "reminder" pills in Week 4:
THROW AWAY the pills you missed.
Keep taking 1 pill each day until the pack is empty.
You do not need a back-up method.

FINALLY, IF YOU ARE STILL NOT SURE WHAT TO DO ABOUT THE PILLS YOU HAVE MISSED:
Use a BACK-UP METHOD anytime you have sex.
KEEP TAKING ONE "ACTIVE" PILL EACH DAY until you can reach your doctor or clinic.

6. Missed periods, spotting or light bleeding
At times, you may not have a period after you have completed a pack of pills. If you miss 1 period but you have taken the pills exactly as you were supposed to, continue as usual into the next cycle. If you have not taken the pills correctly, and have missed a period, you may be pregnant and you should stop taking the Pill until your doctor or clinic determines whether or not you are pregnant. Until you can talk to your doctor or clinic, use an appropriate back-up birth control method. If you miss 2 consecutive periods, you should stop taking the Pill until it is determined that you are not pregnant.
Even if spotting or light bleeding should occur, continue taking the Pill according to the schedule. Should spotting or light bleeding persist, you should notify your doctor or clinic.

7. Stopping the pill before surgery or prolonged bed rest
If you are scheduled for surgery or you need to stay in bed for a long period of time you should tell your doctor that you are on the Pill. You should stop taking the Pill four weeks before your operation to avoid an increased risk of blood clots. Talk to your doctor about when you may start taking the Pill again.

8. Starting the pill after pregnancy
After you have a baby it is advisable to wait 4–6 weeks before starting to take the Pill. Talk to your doctor about when you may start taking the Pill after pregnancy.

9. Pregnancy due to pill failure
When the pill is taken correctly, the expected pregnancy rate is approximately 1% (ie, 1 pregnancy per 100 women per year). If pregnancy occurs while taking the Pill, there is little risk to the fetus. The typical failure rate of large numbers of pill users is less than 3% when women who have missed pills are included. If you become pregnant, you should discuss your pregnancy with your doctor.

10. Pregnancy after stopping the pill
There may be some delay in becoming pregnant after you stop taking the Pill, especially if you had irregular periods before you started using the Pill. Your doctor may recommend that you delay becoming pregnant until you have had one or more regular periods.
There does not appear to be any increase in birth defects in newborn babies when pregnancy occurs soon after stopping the Pill.

11. Overdosage
There are no reports of serious illness or side effects in young children who have swallowed a large number of pills. In adults, overdosage may cause nausea and/or bleeding in females. In case of overdosage, contact your doctor, clinic or pharmacist.

12. Other information
Your doctor or clinic will take a medical and family history and will examine you before prescribing the Pill. The physical examination may be delayed to another time if you request it and the health care provider believes that it is a good medical practice to postpone it. You should be reexamined at least once a year. Be sure to inform your doctor or clinic if there is a family history of any of the conditions listed previously in this leaflet. Be sure to keep all appointments with your doctor or clinic because this is a time to determine if there are early signs of side effects from using the Pill.
Do not use the Pill for any condition other than the one for which it was prescribed. The Pill has been prescribed specifically for you, do not give it to others who may want birth control pills.
If you want more information about birth control pills, ask your doctor or clinic. They have a more technical leaflet called ***PHYSICIAN LABELING*** which you might want to read.

NON-CONTRACEPTIVE HEALTH BENEFITS

In addition to preventing pregnancy, use of oral contraceptives may provide certain non-contraceptive health benefits:

- Menstrual cycles may become more regular
- Blood flow during menstruation may be lighter and less iron may be lost. Therefore, anemia due to iron deficiency is less likely to occur

- Pain or other symptoms during menstruation may be encountered less frequently
- Ectopic (tubal) pregnancy may occur less frequently
- Non-cancerous cysts or lumps in the breast may occur less frequently
- Acute pelvic inflammatory disease may occur less frequently
- Oral contraceptive use may provide some protection against developing two forms of cancer: cancer of the ovaries and cancer of the lining of the uterus
- If you want more information about birth control pills, ask your doctor or pharmacist. They have a more technical leaflet called the Professional Labeling, which you may wish to read.

Store at controlled room temperature 15°C to 25°C (59°F to 77°F).
Keep this and all medications out of the reach of children.

BRIEF SUMMARY
PATIENT PACKAGE INSERT

This product (like all oral contraceptives) is intended to prevent pregnancy. It does not protect against HIV infection (AIDS) and other sexually transmitted diseases.

Oral contraceptives, also known as "birth control pills" or "the pill" are taken to prevent pregnancy and, when taken correctly, have a failure rate of about 1% per year when used without missing any pills. The typical failure rate of large numbers of pill users is less than 3% per year when women who miss pills are included. For most women, oral contraceptives are also free of serious or unpleasant side effects. However, forgetting to take oral contraceptives considerably increases the chances of pregnancy.

For the majority of women, oral contraceptives can be taken safely, but there are some women who are at high risk of developing certain serious diseases that can be life-threatening or may cause temporary or permanent disability. The risks associated with taking oral contraceptives increase significantly if you:

- Smoke
- Have high blood pressure, diabetes or high cholesterol
- Have or have had clotting disorders, heart attack, stroke, angina pectoris, cancer of the breast or sex organs, jaundice or malignant or benign liver tumors

You should not take the pill if you suspect you are pregnant or have unexplained vaginal bleeding.

Cigarette smoking increases the risk of serious cardiovascular side effects from oral contraceptive use. This risk increases with age and with heavy smoking (15 or more cigarettes per day) and is quite marked in women over 35 years of age. Women who use oral contraceptives are strongly advised not to smoke.

Most side effects of the pill are not serious. The most common such effects are nausea, vomiting, bleeding between menstrual periods, weight gain, breast tenderness and difficulty wearing contact lenses. These side effects, especially nausea and vomiting, may subside with the first 3 months of use.

The serious side effects of the pill occur very infrequently, especially if you are in good health and are young. However, you should know that the following medical conditions have been associated with or made worse by the pill:

1. Blood clots in the legs (thrombophlebitis) or lungs (pulmonary embolism), stoppage or rupture of a blood vessel in the brain (stroke), blockage of blood vessels in the heart (heart attack or angina pectoris), eye or other organs of the body. As mentioned above, smoking increases the risk of heart attacks and strokes and subsequent serious medical consequences.
2. Liver tumors, which may rupture and cause severe bleeding. A possible but not definite association has been found with the pill and liver cancer. However, liver cancers are extremely rare. The chance of developing liver cancer from using the pill is thus even rarer.
3. High blood pressure, although blood pressure usually returns to normal when the pill is stopped.

The symptoms associated with these serious side effects are discussed in the detailed leaflet given to you with your supply of pills. Notify your doctor or health care provider if you notice any unusual physical disturbances while taking the pill. In addition, drugs such as rifampin, as well as some anti-convulsants and some antibiotics, may decrease oral contraceptive effectiveness.

Studies to date of women taking the pill have not shown an increase in the incidence of cancer of the breast or cervix. There is, however, insufficient evidence to rule out the possibility that the pill may cause such cancers. Some studies have reported an increase in the risk of developing breast cancer, particularly at a younger age. This increased risk appears to be related to duration of use.

Taking the pill provides some important non-contraceptive health benefits. These include less painful menstruation, less menstrual blood loss and anemia, fewer pelvic infections and fewer cancers of the ovary and the lining of the uterus.

Be sure to discuss any medical condition you may have with your health care provider. Your health care provider will take a medical and family history before prescribing oral contraceptives and will examine you. The physical examination may be delayed to another time if you request it and the health care provider believes that it is a good medical practice to postpone it. You should be reexamined at least once a year while taking oral contraceptives. The detailed patient information leaflet give you further information which you should read and discuss with your health care provider.

HOW TO TAKE THE PILL

See full text of HOW TO TAKE THE PILL which is printed in full in the ***DETAILED PATIENT LABELING***.

Keep this and all medications out of the reach of children.
Rx only

Revised: March 25, 1999
Address medical inquiries to:
WATSON PHARMA, INC.
Medical Information
PO Box 1900
Corona, CA 92878-1900
Mfg. by: Searle & Co., San Juan PR 00936
for: WATSON PHARMA, INC.
a subsidiary of Watson Laboratories, Inc.
Corona, CA 92880

Shown in Product Identification Guide, page 340

LOXITANE® ℞
LOXAPINE SUCCINATE
Capsules

LOXITANE® C ℞
LOXAPINE HYDROCHLORIDE
Oral Concentrate
For Oral Use

LOXITANE® IM ℞
LOXAPINE HYDROCHLORIDE
For Intramuscular Use Only

DESCRIPTION

LOXITANE loxapine, a dibenzoxazepine compound, represents a subclass of tricyclic antipsychotic agents, chemically distinct from the thioxanthenes, butyrophenones, and phenothiazines. Chemically, it is 2-Chloro-11-(4-methyl-1-piperazinyl)-dibenz[*b,f*] [1,4]oxazepine. It is present in capsules as the succinate salt, and in the concentrate and parenteral primarily as the hydrochloride salt.

LOXAPINE BASE

CAPSULES — Each capsule contains loxapine succinate equivalent to 5, 10, 25, or 50 mg of loxapine base and the following inactive ingredients: Blue 1, Gelatin, Lactose, Magnesium Stearate, Titanium Dioxide, and Yellow 10. Additionally, the 5 mg capsule contains Red 33, the 10 mg capsule contains Red 28 and Red 33, and the 25 mg capsule contains FD&C Yellow No. 6.

ORAL CONCENTRATE — Each mL contains loxapine hydrochloride equivalent to 25 mg of loxapine base and propylene glycol as an inactive ingredient.

Hydrochloric acid and, if necessary, sodium hydroxide are used to adjust pH to approximately 5.8 during manufacture.

INTRAMUSCULAR — (Sterile) - Not for Intravenous Use - Each mL contains loxapine hydrochloride equivalent to 50 mg of loxapine base. Inactive Ingredients: Polysorbate 80 NF 5% w/v, Propylene Glycol 70% v/v, and Water for Injection qs ad 100% v.

Hydrochloric acid and, if necessary, sodium hydroxide are used to adjust pH to approximately 5.5 during manufacture.

CLINICAL PHARMACOLOGY

Pharmacodynamics

Pharmacologically, loxapine is a tranquilizer for which the exact mode of action has not been established. However, changes in the level of excitability of subcortical inhibitory areas have been observed in several animal species in association with such manifestations of tranquilization as calming effects and suppression of aggressive behavior.

In normal human volunteers, signs of sedation were seen within 20 to 30 minutes after administration, were most pronounced within 1 1/2 to three hours, and lasted through 12 hours. Similar timing of primary pharmacologic effects was seen in animals.

Absorption, Distribution, Metabolism, and Excretion

After administration of LOXITANE as an oral solution, systemic bioavailability of the parent drug was only about one third that after an equivalent intramuscular dose (25 mg base) in male volunteers. C_{max} for the parent drug was similar for the IM and oral administrations, whereas T_{max} was significantly longer for the IM administration than the oral administration (approximately 5 vs 1 hour). The lower systemic availability of the parent drug after oral administration as compared to the IM administration may be due to first pass metabolism of the oral form.

This is supported by the finding that two metabolites found in serum (8-hydroxyloxapine and 8-hydroxydesmethylloxapine) were formed to a lesser extent after IM administration of loxapine as compared to oral administration.

The apparent half-life of loxapine after oral and IM administration is approximately four hours (range, 1 to 14 hours) and 12 hours (range, 8 to 23 hours), respectively. The extended half-life for the IM administration as compared to the oral administration may be explained by prolonged absorption of loxapine from the muscle during the concurrent elimination process.

Loxapine is extensively metabolized, and urinary recovery over 48 hours resulted in recoveries of approximately 30% and 40% of an IM and orally administered loxapine dose as five metabolites.

INDICATIONS AND USAGE

LOXITANE is indicated for the management of the manifestations of psychotic disorders. The antipsychotic efficacy of LOXITANE was established in clinical studies which enrolled newly hospitalized and chronically hospitalized acutely ill schizophrenic patients as subjects.

CONTRAINDICATIONS

LOXITANE is contraindicated in comatose or severe drug-induced depressed states (alcohol, barbiturates, narcotics, etc.).

LOXITANE is contraindicated in individuals with known hypersensitivity to dibenzoxazepines.

WARNINGS

Tardive Dyskinesia

Tardive dyskinesia, a syndrome consisting of potentially irreversible, involuntary, dyskinetic movements may develop in patients treated with neuroleptic (antipsychotic) drugs. Although the prevalence of the syndrome appears to be highest among the elderly, especially elderly women, it is impossible to rely upon prevalence estimates to predict, at the inception of neuroleptic treatment, which patients are likely to develop the syndrome. Whether neuroleptic drug products differ in their potential to cause tardive dyskinesia is unknown.

Both the risk of developing the syndrome and the likelihood that it will become irreversible are believed to increase as the duration of treatment and the total cumulative dose of neuroleptic drugs administered to the patient increase. However, the syndrome can develop, although much less commonly, after relatively brief treatment periods at low doses.

There is no known treatment for established cases of tardive dyskinesia, although the syndrome may remit, partially or completely, if neuroleptic treatment is withdrawn. Neuroleptic treatment itself, however, may suppress (or partially suppress) the signs and symptoms of the syndrome and thereby may possibly mask the underlying disease process. The effect that symptomatic suppression has upon the long-term course of the syndrome is unknown.

Given these considerations, neuroleptics should be prescribed in a manner that is most likely to minimize the occurrence of tardive dyskinesia. Chronic neuroleptic treatment should generally be reserved for patients who suffer from a chronic illness that, (1) is known to respond to neuroleptic drugs, and (2) for whom alternative, equally effective, but potentially less harmful treatments are *not* available or appropriate. In patients who do require chronic treatment, the smallest dose and the shortest duration of treatment producing a satisfactory clinical response should be sought. The need for continued treatment should be reassessed periodically.

If signs and symptoms of tardive dyskinesia appear in a patient on neuroleptics, drug discontinuation should be considered. However, some patients may require treatment despite the presence of the syndrome. (See **ADVERSE REACTIONS** and **Information for Patients** sections.)

Neuroleptic Malignant Syndrome (NMS)

A potentially fatal symptom complex sometimes referred to as Neuroleptic Malignant Syndrome (NMS) has been reported in association with antipsychotic drugs. Clinical manifestations of NMS are hyperpyrexia, muscle rigidity, altered mental status, and evidence of autonomic instability (irregular pulse or blood pressure, tachycardia, diaphoresis, and cardiac dysrhythmias).

The diagnostic evaluation of patients with this syndrome is complicated. In arriving at a diagnosis, it is important to identify cases where the clinical presentation includes both serious medical illness (e.g., pneumonia, systemic infection, etc.) and untreated or inadequately treated extrapyramidal signs and symptoms (EPS). Other important considerations in the differential diagnosis include central anticholinergic toxicity, heat stroke, drug fever, and primary central nervous system (CNS) pathology.

The management of NMS should include: (1) immediate discontinuation of antipsychotic drugs and other drugs not essential to concurrent therapy, (2) intensive symptomatic treatment and medical monitoring, and (3) treatment of any concomitant serious medical problems for which specific treatments are available. There is no general agreement about specific pharmacological treatment regimens for uncomplicated NMS.

If a patient requires antipsychotic drug treatment after recovery from NMS, the potential reintroduction of drug therapy should be carefully considered. The patient should be carefully monitored, since recurrences of NMS have been reported.

LOXITANE, like other tranquilizers, may impair mental and/or physical abilities, especially during the first few days of therapy. Therefore, ambulatory patients should be warned about activities requiring alertness (e.g., operating vehicles or machinery) and about concomitant use of alcohol and other CNS depressants.

Continued on next page

Loxitane—Cont.

LOXITANE has not been evaluated for the management of behavioral complications in patients with mental retardation, and therefore, it cannot be recommended.

PRECAUTIONS

General

LOXITANE should be used with extreme caution in patients with a history of convulsive disorders since it lowers the convulsive threshold. Seizures have been reported in patients receiving LOXITANE at antipsychotic dose levels, and may occur in epileptic patients even with maintenance of routine anticonvulsant drug therapy.

LOXITANE has an antiemetic effect in animals. Since this effect may also occur in man, LOXITANE may mask signs of overdosage of toxic drugs and may obscure conditions such as intestinal obstruction and brain tumor.

LOXITANE should be used with caution in patients with cardiovascular disease. Increased pulse rates have been reported in the majority of patients receiving antipsychotic doses; transient hypotension has been reported. In the presence of severe hypotension requiring vasopressor therapy, the preferred drugs may be norepinephrine or angiotensin. Usual doses of epinephrine may be ineffective because of inhibition of its vasopressor effect by LOXITANE.

The possibility of ocular toxicity from loxapine cannot be excluded at this time. Therefore, careful observation should be made for pigmentary retinopathy and lenticular pigmentation since these have been observed in some patients receiving certain other antipsychotic drugs for prolonged periods.

Because of possible anticholinergic action, the drug should be used cautiously in patients with glaucoma or a tendency to urinary retention, particularly with concomitant administration of anticholinergic-type antiparkinson medication.

Experience to date indicates the possibility of a slightly higher incidence of extrapyramidal effects following intramuscular administration than normally anticipated with oral formulations. The increase may be attributable to higher plasma levels following intramuscular injection.

Neuroleptic drugs elevate prolactin levels; the elevation persists during chronic administration. Tissue culture experiments indicate that approximately one third of human breast cancers are prolactin dependent *in vitro*, a factor of potential importance if the prescription of these drugs is contemplated in a patient with a previously detected breast cancer. Although disturbances such as galactorrhea, amenorrhea, gynecomastia, and impotence have been reported, the clinical significance of elevated serum prolactin levels is unknown for most patients. An increase in mammary neoplasms has been found in rodents after chronic administration of neuroleptic drugs. Neither clinical studies nor epidemiologic studies conducted to date, however, have shown an association between chronic administration of these drugs and mammary tumorigenesis; the available evidence is considered too limited to be conclusive at this time.

Information for Patients

Given the likelihood that some patients exposed chronically to neuroleptics will develop tardive dyskinesia, it is advised that all patients in whom chronic use is contemplated be given, if possible, full information about this risk. The decision to inform patients and/or their guardians must obviously take into account the clinical circumstances and the competency of the patient to understand the information provided.

Drug Interactions

There have been rare reports of significant respiratory depression, stupor and/or hypotension with the concomitant use of loxapine and lorazepam.

The risk of using loxapine in combination with CNS-active drugs has not been systematically evaluated. Therefore, caution is advised if the concomitant administration of loxapine and CNS-active drugs is required.

Usage in Pregnancy

Safe use of LOXITANE during pregnancy or lactation has not been established; therefore, its use in pregnancy, in nursing mothers, or in women of childbearing potential requires that the benefits of treatment be weighed against the possible risks to mother and child. No embryotoxicity or teratogenicity was observed in studies in rats, rabbits or dogs although, with the exception of one rabbit study, the highest dosage was only two times the maximum recommended human dose and in some studies it was below this dose. Perinatal studies have shown renal papillary abnormalities in offspring of rats treated from midpregnancy with doses of 0.6 and 1.8 mg/kg, doses which approximate the usual human dose but which are considerably below the maximum recommended human dose.

Nursing Mothers

The extent of the excretion of LOXITANE or its metabolites in human milk is not known. However, LOXITANE and its metabolites have been shown to be transported into the milk of lactating dogs. LOXITANE administration to nursing women should be avoided if clinically possible.

Pediatric Use

Safety and effectiveness of LOXITANE in pediatric patients have not been established.

ADVERSE REACTIONS

CNS Effects: Manifestations of adverse effects on the central nervous system, other than extrapyramidal effects, have been seen infrequently. Drowsiness, usually mild, may occur at the beginning of therapy or when dosage is increased. It usually subsides with continued LOXITANE® therapy. The incidence of sedation has been less than that of certain aliphatic phenothiazines and slightly more than the piperazine phenothiazines. Dizziness, faintness, staggering gait, shuffling gait, muscle twitching, weakness, insomnia, agitation, tension, seizures, akinesia, slurred speech, numbness, and confusional states have been reported. Neuroleptic malignant syndrome (NMS) has been reported (see **WARNINGS**).

Extrapyramidal Reactions - Neuromuscular (extrapyramidal) reactions during the administration of LOXITANE have been reported frequently, often during the first few days of treatment. In most patients, these reactions involved parkinsonian-like symptoms such as tremor, rigidity, excessive salivation, and masked facies. Akathisia (motor restlessness) also has been reported relatively frequently. These symptoms are usually not severe and can be controlled by reduction of LOXITANE dosage or by administration of antiparkinson drugs in usual dosage. Dystonic and dyskinetic reactions have occurred less frequently, but may be more severe. Dystonias include spasms of muscles of the neck and face, tongue protrusion, and oculogyric movement. Dyskinetic reactions have been described in the form of choreoathetoid movements. These reactions sometimes require reduction or temporary withdrawal of loxapine dosage in addition to appropriate counteractive drugs.

Persistent Tardive Dyskinesia - As with all antipsychotic agents, tardive dyskinesia may appear in some patients on long-term therapy or may appear after drug therapy has been discontinued. The risk appears to be greater in elderly patients on high-dose therapy, especially females. The symptoms are persistent and in some patients appear to be irreversible. The syndrome is characterized by rhythmical involuntary movement of the tongue, face, mouth, or jaw (e.g., protrusion of tongue, puffing of cheeks, puckering of mouth, chewing movements). Sometimes these may be accompanied by involuntary movements of extremities.

There is no known effective treatment for tardive dyskinesia; antiparkinson agents usually do not alleviate the symptoms of this syndrome. It is suggested that all antipsychotic agents be discontinued if these symptoms appear. Should it be necessary to reinstitute treatment, or increase the dosage of the agent, or switch to a different antipsychotic agent, the syndrome may be masked. It has been suggested that fine vermicular movements of the tongue may be an early sign of the syndrome, and if the medication is stopped at that time the syndrome may not develop.

Cardiovascular Effects: Tachycardia, hypotension, hypertension, orthostatic hypotension, light-headedness, and syncope have been reported.

A few cases of ECG changes similar to those seen with phenothiazines have been reported. It is not known whether these were related to LOXITANE administration.

Hematologic: Rarely, agranulocytosis, thrombocytopenia, leukopenia.

Skin: Dermatitis, edema (puffiness of face), pruritus, rash, alopecia, and seborrhea have been reported with loxapine.

Anticholinergic Effects: Dry mouth, nasal congestion, constipation, blurred vision, urinary retention, and paralytic ileus have occurred.

Gastrointestinal: Nausea and vomiting have been reported in some patients. Hepatocellular injury (i.e., SGOT/SGPT elevation) has been reported in association with loxapine administration and rarely, jaundice and/or hepatitis questionably related to LOXITANE treatment.

Other Adverse Reactions: Weight gain, weight loss, dyspnea, ptosis, hyperpyrexia, flushed facies, headache, paresthesia, and polydipsia have been reported in some patients. Rarely, galactorrhea, amenorrhea, gynecomastia, and menstrual irregularity of uncertain etiology have been reported.

OVERDOSAGE

Signs and symptoms of overdosage will depend on the amount ingested and individual patient tolerance. As would be expected from the pharmacologic actions of the drug, the clinical findings may range from mild depression of the CNS and cardiovascular systems to profound hypotension, respiratory depression, and unconsciousness. The possibility of occurrence of extrapyramidal symptoms and/or convulsive seizures should be kept in mind. Renal failure following loxapine overdosage has also been reported.

The treatment of overdosage is essentially symptomatic and supportive. Early gastric lavage and extended dialysis might be expected to be beneficial. Centrally-acting emetics may have little effect because of the antiemetic action of loxapine. In addition, emesis should be avoided because of the possibility of aspiration of vomitus. Avoid analeptics, such as pentylenetetrazol, which may cause convulsions. Severe hypotension might be expected to respond to the administration of levarterenol or phenylephrine. EPINEPHRINE SHOULD NOT BE USED SINCE ITS USE IN A PATIENT WITH PARTIAL ADRENERGIC BLOCKADE MAY FURTHER LOWER THE BLOOD PRESSURE. Severe extrapyramidal reactions should be treated with anticholinergic antiparkinson agents or diphenhydramine hydrochloride, and anticonvulsant therapy should be initiated as indicated. Additional measures include oxygen and intravenous fluids.

DOSAGE AND ADMINISTRATION

LOXITANE is administered, usually in divided doses, two to four times a day. Daily dosage (in terms of base equivalents) should be adjusted to the individual patient's needs as assessed by the severity of symptoms and previous history of response to antipsychotic drugs.

Oral Administration

Initial dosage of 10 mg twice daily is recommended, although in severely disturbed patients initial dosage up to a total of 50 mg daily may be desirable. Dosage should then be increased fairly rapidly over the first seven to ten days until there is effective control of psychotic symptoms. The usual therapeutic and maintenance range is 60 to 100 mg daily. However, as with other antipsychotic drugs, some patients respond to lower dosage and others require higher dosage for optimal benefit. Daily dosage higher than 250 mg is not recommended.

LOXITANE C Oral Concentrate should be mixed with orange or grapefruit juice shortly before administration. Use only the enclosed calibrated (10 mg, 15 mg, 25 mg, 50 mg) dropper for dosage.

Maintenance Therapy

For maintenance therapy, dosage should be reduced to the lowest level compatible with symptom control; many patients have been maintained satisfactorily at dosages in the range of 20 to 60 mg daily.

Intramuscular Administration

LOXITANE IM is utilized for prompt symptomatic control in the acutely agitated patient and in patients whose symptoms render oral medication temporarily impractical. During clinical trial there were only rare reports of significant local tissue reaction.

LOXITANE IM is administered by intramuscular (not intravenous) injection in doses of 12.5 mg (1/4 mL) to 50 mg (1 mL) at intervals of four to six hours or longer, both dose and interval depending on patient response. Many patients have responded satisfactorily to twice-daily dosage. As described above for oral administration, attention is directed to the necessity for dosage adjustment on an individual basis over the early days of loxapine administration.

Once the desired symptomatic control is achieved and the patient is able to take medication orally, loxapine should be administered in capsule or oral concentrate form. Usually this should occur within five days.

HOW SUPPLIED

LOXITANE®, loxapine succinate, Capsules are available in the following base equivalent strengths:

5 mg - Hard shell, opaque, dark-green capsules printed with "Ⓦ" over "WATSON" on one half and "LOXITANE" over "5 mg" on the other, are supplied as follows: NDC 52544-811-01 - Bottle of 100s

10 mg - Hard shell, opaque, with yellow body and a dark-green cap, printed with "Ⓦ" over "WATSON" on one half and "LOXITANE" over "10 mg" on the other, are supplied as follows:
NDC 52544-812-01 - Bottle of 100s
NDC 52544-812-10 - Bottle of 1000s

25 mg - Hard shell, opaque, with a light-green body and a dark-green cap, printed with "Ⓦ" over "WATSON" on one half and "LOXITANE" over "25 mg" on the other, are supplied as follows:
NDC 52544-813-01 - Bottle of 100s
NDC 52544-813-10 - Bottle of 1000s

50 mg - Hard shell, opaque, with a blue body and a dark-green cap, printed with "Ⓦ" over "WATSON" on one half and "LOXITANE" over "50 mg" on the other, are supplied as follows:
NDC 52544-814-01 - Bottle of 100s
NDC 52544-814-10 - Bottle of 1000s

Store at controlled room temperature 15°–30°C (59°–86°F).

LOXITANE® C, loxapine hydrochloride, Oral Concentrate is supplied as follows:

NDC 52544-815-34 - 4 fl oz (120 mL) with calibrated dropper.

Each mL contains loxapine HCl equivalent to 25 mg of loxapine base.

Store at controlled room temperature 20°–25°C (68°–77°F).

DO NOT FREEZE.

mfd for: WATSON PHARMA, INC.
a subsidiary of Watson Laboratories, Inc.
Corona, CA 92880
by: LEDERLE PHARMACEUTICAL DIVISION
of American Cyanamid Company
Pearl River, NY 10965

LOXITANE® IM, loxapine hydrochloride, for intramuscular use only is supplied as follows:

NDC 52544-816-79 - 10 mL multi-dose vial

Each mL contains loxapine HCl equivalent to 50 mg of loxapine base.

Keep package closed to protect from light. Intensification of the straw color to a light amber will not alter potency or therapeutic efficacy; if noticeably discolored, ampul or vial should not be used.

Store at controlled room temperature 15°–30°C (59°–86°F).

DO NOT FREEZE.

Rx only

mfd for: WATSON PHARMA, INC.
a subsidiary of Watson Laboratories, Inc.
Corona, CA 92880
by: LEDERLE PARENTERALS, INC.
Carolina, Puerto Rico 00987
CI 5062-1 Issued July 16, 1998

Shown in Product Identification Guide, page 340

MICROZIDE™ Capsules ℞

(Hydrochlorothiazide 12.5 mg)

Rx only

DESCRIPTION

Microzide™ (hydrochlorothiazide 12.5 mg) is the 3,4-dihydro derivative of chlorothiazide. Its chemical name is

6-chloro-3,4-dihydro-2*H*-1,2,4-benzothiadiazine-7-sulfonamide 1,1-dioxide. Its empirical formula is $C_7H_8ClN_3O_4S_2$; its molecular weight is 297.72; and its structural formula is:

It is a white, or practically white, crystalline powder which is slightly soluble in water, but freely soluble in sodium hydroxide solution.

MICROZIDE is supplied as 12.5 mg capsules for oral use. Each capsule contains the following inactive ingredients: colloidal silicon dioxide, corn starch, D&C Red #28, D&C Yellow #10, FD&C Blue #1, gelatin, lactose monohydrate, magnesium stearate, titanium dioxide and other ingredients.

CLINICAL PHARMACOLOGY

Hydrochlorothiazide blocks the reabsorption of sodium and chloride ions, and it thereby increases the quantity of sodium traversing the distal tubule and the volume of water excreted. A portion of the additional sodium presented to the distal tubule is exchanged there for potassium and hydrogen ions. With continued use of hydrochlorothiazide and depletion of sodium, compensatory mechanisms tend to increase this exchange and may produce excessive loss of potassium, hydrogen and chloride ions. Hydrochlorothiazide also decreases the excretion of calcium and uric acid, may increase the excretion of iodide and may reduce glomerular filtration rate. Metabolic toxicities associated with excessive electrolyte changes caused by hydrochlorothiazide have been shown to be dose-related.

Pharmacokinetics and Metabolism: Hydrochlorothiazide is well absorbed (65% to 75%) following oral administration. Absorption of hydrochlorothiazide is reduced in patients with congestive heart failure.

Peak plasma concentrations are observed within 1 to 5 hours of dosing, and range from 70 to 490 ng/mL following oral doses of 12.5 to 100 mg. Plasma concentrations are linearly related to the administered dose. Concentrations of hydrochlorothiazide are 1.6 to 1.8 times higher in whole blood than in plasma. Binding to serum proteins has been reported to be approximately 40% to 68%. The plasma elimination half-life has been reported to be 6 to 15 hours. Hydrochlorothiazide is eliminated primarily by renal pathways. Following oral doses of 12.5 to 100 mg, 55% to 77% of the administered dose appears in urine and greater than 95% of the absorbed dose is excreted in urine as unchanged drug. In patients with renal disease, plasma concentrations of hydrochlorothiazide are increased and the elimination half-life is prolonged.

When MICROZIDE is administered with food, its bioavailability is reduced by 10%, the maximum plasma concentration is reduced by 20%, and the time to maximum concentration increases from 1.6 to 2.9 hours.

Pharmacodynamics: Acute antihypertensive effects of thiazides are thought to result from a reduction in blood volume and cardiac output, secondary to a natriuretic effect, although a direct vasodilatory mechanism has also been proposed. With chronic administration, plasma volume returns toward normal, but peripheral vascular resistance is decreased. The exact mechanism of the antihypertensive effect of hydrochlorothiazide is not known.

Thiazides do not affect normal blood pressure. Onset of action occurs within 2 hours of dosing, peak effect is observed at about 4 hours, and activity persists for up to 24 hours.

Clinical Studies: In an 87 patient 4-week double-blind, placebo controlled, parallel group trial, patients who received MICROZIDE had reductions in seated systolic and diastolic blood pressure that were significantly greater than those seen in patients who received placebo. In published placebo-controlled trials comparing 12.5 mg of hydrochlorothiazide to 25 mg, the 12.5 mg dose preserved most of the placebo-corrected blood pressure reduction seen with 25 mg.

INDICATIONS AND USAGE

MICROZIDE is indicated in the management of hypertension either as the sole therapeutic agent, or in combination with other antihypertensives. Unlike potassium sparing combination diuretic products, MICROZIDE may be used in those patients in whom the development of hyperkalemia cannot be risked, including patients taking ACE inhibitors.

Usage in Pregnancy: The routine use of diuretics in an otherwise healthy woman is inappropriate and exposes mother and fetus to unnecessary hazard. Diuretics do not prevent development of toxemia of pregnancy, and there is no satisfactory evidence that they are useful in the treatment of developed toxemia.

Edema during pregnancy may arise from pathological causes or from the physiologic and mechanical consequences of pregnancy. Diuretics are indicated in pregnancy when edema is due to pathologic causes, just as they are in the absence of pregnancy. Dependent edema in pregnancy resulting from restriction of venous return by the expanded uterus is properly treated through elevation of the lower extremities and use of support hose; use of diuretics to lower intravascular volume in this case is illogical and unnecessary. There is hypervolemia during normal pregnancy which is harmful to neither the fetus nor the mother (in the absence of cardiovascular disease), but which is associated with edema, including generalized edema in the majority of pregnant women. If this edema produces discomfort, increased recumbency will often provide relief. In rare instances this edema may cause extreme discomfort which is not relieved by rest. In these cases a short course of diuretics may provide relief and may be appropriate.

CONTRAINDICATIONS

Hydrochlorothiazide is contraindicated in patients with anuria. Hypersensitivity to this product or other sulfonamide derived drugs is also contraindicated.

WARNINGS

Diabetes and Hypoglycemia: Latent diabetes mellitus may become manifest and diabetic patients given thiazides may require adjustment of their insulin dose.

Renal Disease: Cumulative effects of the thiazides may develop in patients with impaired renal function. In such patients, thiazides may precipitate azotemia.

PRECAUTIONS

Electrolyte and Fluid Balance Status: In published studies, clinically significant hypokalemia has been consistently less common in patients who received 12.5 mg of hydrochlorothiazide than in patients who received higher doses. Nevertheless, periodic determination of serum electrolytes should be performed in patients who may be at risk for the development of hypokalemia. Patients should be observed for signs of fluid or electrolyte disturbances, i.e. hyponatremia, hypochloremic alkalosis, and hypokalemia and hypomagnesemia.

Warning signs or symptoms of fluid and electrolyte imbalance include dryness of mouth, thirst, weakness, lethargy, drowsiness, restlessness, muscle pains or cramps, muscular fatigue, hypotension, oliguria tachycardia, and gastrointestinal disturbances such as nausea and vomiting.

Hypokalemia may develop, especially with brisk diuresis when severe cirrhosis is present, during concomitant use of corticosteroid or adrenocorticotropic hormone (ACTH) or after prolonged therapy. Interference with adequate oral electrolyte intake will also contribute to hypokalemia. Hypokalemia and hypomagnesemia can provoke ventricular arrhythmias or sensitize or exaggerate the response of the heart to the toxic effects of digitalis. Hypokalemia may be avoided or treated by potassium supplementation or increased intake of potassium rich foods.

Dilutional hyponatremia is life-threatening and may occur in edematous patients in hot weather; appropriate therapy is water restriction rather than salt administration, except in rare instances when the hyponatremia is life-threatening. In actual salt depletion, appropriate replacement is the therapy of choice.

Hyperuricemia: Hyperuricemia or acute gout may be precipitated in certain patients receiving thiazide diuretics.

Impaired Hepatic Function: Thiazides should be used with caution in patients with impaired hepatic function. They can precipitate hepatic coma in patients with severe liver disease.

Parathyroid Disease: Calcium excretion is decreased by thiazides, and pathologic changes in the parathyroid glands, with hypercalcemia and hypophosphatemia, have been observed in a few patients on prolonged thiazide therapy.

Drug Interactions: When given concurrently the following drugs may interact with thiazide diuretics:

Alcohol, barbiturates, or narcotics—potentiation of orthostatic hypotension may occur.

Antidiabetic drugs—(oral agents and insulin) dosage adjustment of the antidiabetic drug may be required.

Other antihypertensive drugs—additive effect or potentiation.

Cholestyramine and colestipol resins—Cholestyramine and colestipol resins bind the hydrochlorothiazide and reduce its absorption from the gastrointestinal tract by up to 85 and 43 percent, respectively.

Corticosteroid, ACTH—intensified electrolyte depletion, particularly hypokalemia.

Pressor amines (e.g., norepinephrine)—possible decreased response to pressor amines but not sufficient to preclude their use.

Skeletal muscle relaxants, nondepolarizing (e.g., tubocurarine)—possible increased responsiveness to the muscle relaxant

Lithium—generally should not be given with diuretics. Diuretic agents reduce the renal clearance of lithium and greatly increase the risk of lithium toxicity. Refer to the package insert for lithium preparations before use of such preparations with MICROZIDE.

Non-steroidal anti-inflammatory drugs—In some patients, the administration of a non-steroidal anti-inflammatory agent can reduce the diuretic, natriuretic, and antihypertensive effects of loop, potassium-sparing and thiazide diuretics. When MICROZIDE and non-steroidal anti-inflammatory agents are used concomitantly, the patients should be observed closely to determine if the desired effect of the diuretic is obtained.

Drug/Laboratory Test Interactions: Thiazides should be discontinued before carrying out tests for parathyroid function (see PRECAUTIONS, *General*).

Carcinogenesis, Mutagenesis, Impairment of Fertility: Two-year feeding studies in mice and rats conducted under the auspices of the National Toxicology Program (NTP) uncovered no evidence of a carcinogenic potential of hydrochlorothiazide in female mice (at doses of up to approximately 600 mg/kg/day) or in male and female rats (at doses of approximately 100 mg/kg/day). The NTP, however, found equivocal evidence for hepatocarcinogenicity in male mice. Hydrochlorothiazide was not genotoxic *in vitro* in the Ames mutagenicity assay of *Salmonella typhimurium* strains TA 98, TA 100, TA 1535, TA 1537, and TA 1538 and in the Chinese Hamster Ovary (CHO) test for chromosomal aberrations, or *in vivo* in assays using mouse germinal cell chromosomes, Chinese hamster bone marrow chromosomes, and the *Drosophila* sex-linked recessive lethal trait gene. Positive test results were obtained only in the *in vitro* CHO Sister Chromatid Exchange (clastogenicity) and in the Mouse Lymphoma Cell (mutagenicity) assays, using concentrations of hydrochlorothiazide from 43 to 1300 µg/mL, and in the *Aspergillus nidulans* non-disjunction assay at an unspecified concentration.

Hydrochlorothiazide had no adverse effects on the fertility of mice and rats of either sex in studies wherein these species were exposed, via their diet, to doses of up to 100 and 4 mg/kg, respectively, prior to conception and throughout gestation.

Pregnancy:

Teratogenic Effects —Pregnancy Category B: Studies in which hydrochlorothiazide was orally administered to pregnant mice and rats during their respective periods of major organogenesis at doses up to 3000 and 1000 mg hydrochlorothiazide/kg, respectively, provided no evidence of harm to the fetus.

There are, however, no adequate and well-controlled studies in pregnant women. Because animal reproduction studies are not always predictive of human response, this drug should be used during pregnancy only if clearly needed.

Nonteratogenic Effects: Thiazides cross the placental barrier and appear in cord blood. There is a risk of fetal or neonatal jaundice, thrombocytopenia, and possibly other adverse reactions that have occurred in adults.

Nursing Mothers: Thiazides are excreted in breast milk. Because of the potential for serious adverse reactions in nursing infants, a decision should be made whether to discontinue nursing or to discontinue hydrochlorothiazide, taking into account the importance of the drug to the mother.

Pediatric Use: Safety and effectiveness in pediatric patients have not been established.

Elderly Use: A greater blood pressure reduction and an increase in side effects may be observed in the elderly (i.e. >65 years) with hydrochlorothiazide. Starting treatment with the lowest available dose of hydrochlorothiazide (12.5 mg) is therefore recommended. If further titration is required, 12.5 mg increments should be utilized.

ADVERSE REACTIONS

The adverse reactions associated with hydrochlorothiazide have been shown to be dose related. In controlled clinical trials, the adverse events reported with doses of 12.5 mg hydrochlorothiazide once daily were comparable to placebo. The following adverse reactions have been reported for doses of hydrochlorothiazide 25 mg and greater and, within each category, are listed in the order of decreasing severity.

Body as a whole: Weakness.

Cardiovascular: Hypotension including orthostatic hypotension (may be aggravated by alcohol, barbiturates, narcotics or antihypertensive drugs).

Digestive: Pancreatitis, jaundice (intrahepatic cholestatic jaundice), diarrhea, vomiting, sialadenitis, cramping, constipation, gastric irritation, nausea, anorexia.

Hematologic: Aplastic anemia, agranulocytosis, leukopenia, hemolytic anemia, thrombocytopenia.

Hypersensitivity: Anaphylactic reactions, necrotizing angiitis (vasculitis and cutaneous vasculitis), respiratory distress including pneumonitis and pulmonary edema, photosensitivity, fever, urticaria, rash, purpura.

Metabolic: Electrolyte imbalance (see **PRECAUTIONS**), hyperglycemia, glycosuria, hyperuricemia.

Musculoskeletal: Muscle spasm.

Nervous System/Psychiatric: Vertigo, paresthesia, dizziness, headache, restlessness.

Renal: Renal failure, renal dysfunction, interstitial nephritis (See **WARNINGS**).

Skin: Erythema multiforme including Stevens-Johnson syndrome, exfoliative dermatitis including toxic epidermal necrolysis, alopecia.

Special Senses: Transient blurred vision, xanthopsia.

Urogenital: Impotence.

Whenever adverse reactions are moderate or severe, thiazide dosage should be reduced or therapy withdrawn.

OVERDOSAGE

The most common signs and symptoms observed are those caused by electrolyte depletion (hypokalemia, hypochloremia, hyponatremia) and dehydration resulting from excessive diuresis. If digitalis has also been administered, hypokalemia may accentuate cardiac arrhythmias.

In the event of overdosage, symptomatic and supportive measures should be employed. Emesis should be induced or gastric lavage performed. Correct dehydration, electrolyte imbalance, hepatic coma and hypotension by established procedures. If required, give oxygen or artificial respiration

Continued on next page

Microzide—Cont.

for respiratory impairment. The degree to which hydrochlorothiazide is removed by hemodialysis has not been established.

The oral LD_{50} of hydrochlorothiazide is greater than 10 g/kg in the mouse and rat.

DOSAGE AND ADMINISTRATION

For Control of Hypertension: The adult initial dose of MICROZIDE is one capsule given once daily whether given alone or in combination with other antihypertensives. Total daily doses greater than 50 mg are not recommended.

HOW SUPPLIED

MICROZIDE capsules are #4 Teal Opaque/Teal Opaque two piece hard gelatin capsules imprinted with MICROZIDE and 12.5 mg in black ink. They are supplied in bottles of 100 with child resistant closures (NDC 52544-622-01).

Storage: Keep container tightly closed. Protect from light, moisture, freezing, −20°C (−4°F) and store at room temperature, 15–30°C (59–86°F).

Watson Pharma, Inc.
A subsidiary of
Watson Laboratories, Inc.
Corona, CA 92880
13304-3
R3 10/99

Shown in Product Identification Guide, page 340

NECON® ℞

[nē-con]
(norethindrone and ethinyl estradiol tablets, USP)

12621-2
Necon 1/35-21
Necon 1/35-28
(norethindrone and ethinyl estradiol tablets, USP)
Necon 10/11-21
Necon 10/11-28
(norethindrone and ethinyl estradiol tablets, USP)
Necon 0.5/35-21
Necon 0.5/35-28
(norethindrone and ethinyl estradiol tablets, USP)
Necon 1/50-21
Necon 1/50-28
(norethindrone and mestranol tablets, USP)

Patients should be counseled that this product does not protect against HIV infection (AIDS) and other sexually transmitted diseases.

DESCRIPTION

Necon 1/35-21 and *Necon 1/35-28 (Norethindrone and Ethinyl Estradiol Tablets, USP).* Each dark yellow tablet contains 1 mg of norethindrone and 35 mcg of ethinyl estradiol, and the inactive ingredients include microcrystalline cellulose, lactose (anhydrous), magnesium stearate, polacrilin potassium and povidone. In addition, the coloring agent is D&C Yellow No. 10. Each white tablet in the Necon 1/35-28 package is a placebo containing no active ingredients and the inactive ingredients include microcrystalline cellulose, lactose (anhydrous), and magnesium stearate.

Necon 0.5/35-21 and *Necon 0.5/35-28 (Norethindrone and Ethinyl Estradiol Tablets, USP).* Each light yellow tablet contains 0.5 mg of norethindrone and 35 mcg of ethinyl estradiol, and the inactive ingredients include microcrystalline cellulose, lactose (anhydrous), magnesium stearate, polacrilin potassium and povidone. In addition, the coloring agent is D&C Yellow No. 10. Each white tablet in the Necon 0.5/35-28 package is a placebo containing no active ingredients and the inactive ingredients include microcrystalline cellulose, lactose (anhydrous), and magnesium stearate.

Necon 10/11-21 and *Necon 10/11-28 (Norethindrone and Ethinyl Estradiol Tablets, USP).* Each light yellow tablet (10) contains 0.5 mg of norethindrone and 35 mcg of ethinyl estradiol. Each dark yellow tablet (11) contains 1 mg of norethindrone and 35 mcg of ethinyl estradiol. The inactive ingredients include microcrystalline cellulose, lactose (anhydrous), magnesium stearate, polacrilin potassium and povidone. In addition, the coloring agent is D&C Yellow No. 10. Each white tablet in the Necon 10/11-28 package is a placebo containing no active ingredients and the inactive ingredients include microcrystalline cellulose, lactose (anhydrous), and magnesium stearate.

Necon 1/50-21 and *Necon 1/50-28 (Norethindrone and Mestranol Tablets, USP).* Each light blue tablet contains 1 mg of norethindrone and 50 mcg of mestranol, and the inactive ingredients include microcrystalline cellulose, lactose (anhydrous), magnesium stearate, polacrilin potassium and povidone. In addition, the coloring agent is FD&C Blue No. 1 Aluminum Lake. Each white tablet in the Necon 1/50-28 package is a placebo containing no active ingredients and the inactive ingredients include microcrystalline cellulose, lactose (anhydrous), and magnesium stearate.

The chemical name for norethindrone is 17-hydroxy-19-*nor*-17α-pregn-4-en-20-yn-3-one. The chemical name of ethinyl estradiol is 19-nor-17α-pregna-1, 3, 5(10)-trien-20-yne-3, 17-diol. The chemical name for mestranol is 3-methoxy-19-nor-17α-pregna-1, 3, 5(10)-trien-20-yn-17-ol. The structural formulas are as follows:

NORETHINDRONE
M.W. = 298.43

ETHINYL ESTRADIOL
M.W. = 296.41

MESTRANOL
M.W. = 310.44

CLINICAL PHARMACOLOGY

Combination oral contraceptives act primarily by suppression of gonadotropins. Although the primary mechanism of this action is inhibition of ovulation, other alterations in the genital tract, including changes in the cervical mucus (which increase the difficulty of sperm entry into the uterus) and the endometrium (which may reduce the likelihood of implantation).

INDICATIONS AND USAGE

Necon 1/35, Necon 0.5/35, Necon 10/11 and Necon 1/50 are indicated for the prevention of pregnancy in women who elect to use oral contraceptives as a method of contraception.

Oral contraceptives are highly effective. Table I lists the typical accidental pregnancy rates for users of combination oral contraceptives and other methods of contraception. The efficacy of these contraceptive methods, except sterilization, depends upon the reliability with which they are used. Correct and consistent use of methods can result in lower failure rates.

[See table at left]

CONTRAINDICATIONS

Oral contraceptives should not be used in women who have the following conditions:

- Thrombophlebitis or thromboembolic disorders
- A past history of deep vein thrombophlebitis or thromboembolic disorders
- Cerebral vascular disease, myocardial infarction or coronary artery disease, or a past history of these conditions
- Known or suspected carcinoma of the breast, or a history of this condition
- Known or suspected carcinoma of the female reproductive organs or suspected estrogen-dependent neoplasia, or a history of these conditions
- Undiagnosed abnormal genital bleeding
- History of cholestatic jaundice of pregnancy or jaundice with prior oral contraceptive use
- Past or present, benign or malignant liver tumors
- Known or suspected pregnancy

WARNINGS

Cigarette smoking increases the risk of serious adverse effects on the heart and blood vessels from oral contraceptive use. This risk increases with age and with heavy smoking (15 or more cigarettes per day) and is quite marked in women over 35 years of age. Women who use oral contraceptives are strongly advised not to smoke.

The use of oral contraceptives is associated with increased risk of several serious conditions including venous and arterial thromboembolism, thrombotic and hemorrhagic stroke, myocardial infarction, liver tumors or other liver lesions, and gallbladder disease. The risk of morbidity and mortality increases significantly in the presence of other risk factors such as hypertension, hyperlipidemia, obesity, and diabetes mellitus.

Practitioners prescribing oral contraceptives should be familiar with the following information relating to these and other risks. The information contained herein is principally based on studies carried out in patients who use oral contraceptives with formulations containing higher amounts of estrogens and progestogens than those in common use today. The effect of long-term use of the oral contraceptives with lesser amounts of both estrogens and progestogens remains to be determined.

Throughout this labeling, epidemiological studies reported are of two types: retrospective case-control studies and pro-

Method (1)	% of Women Experiencing an Unintended Pregnancy within the First Year of Use: Typical Use[1] – (2)	Perfect Use[2] – (3)	% of Women Continuing Use at One Year[3] – (4)
Chance[4] –	85	85	
Spermicides[5] –	26	6	40
Periodic abstinence	25		63
Calendar		9	
Ovulation Method		3	
Sympto-Thermal[6] –		2	
Post-Ovulation		1	
Withdrawal	19	4	
Cap[7] –			
Parous Women	40	26	42
Nulliparous Women	20	9	56
Sponge			
Parous Women	40	20	42
Nulliparous Women	20	9	56
Diaphragm[7] –	20	6	56
Condom[8] –			
Female (Reality)	21	5	56
Male	14	3	61
Pill	5		71
Progestin Only		0.5	
Combined		0.1	
IUD			
Progesterone T	2.0	1.5	81
Copper T380A	0.8	0.6	78
LNg 20	0.1	0.1	81
Depo-Provera	0.3	0.3	70
Norplant and Norplant-2	0.05	0.05	88
Female Sterilization	0.5	0.5	100
Male Sterilization	0.15	0.10	100

Adapted from Hatcher et al., 1998 Ref. #1.

1 Among *typical* couples who initiate use of a method (not necessarily for the first time), the percentage who experience an accidental pregnancy during the first year if they do not stop use for any other reason.
2 Among couples who initiate use of a method (not necessarily for the first time) and who use it *perfectly* (both consistently and correctly), the percentage who experience an accidental pregnancy during the first year if they do not stop use for any other reason.
3 Among couples attempting to avoid pregnancy, the percentage who continue to use a method for one year.
4 The percents becoming pregnant in columns (2) and (3) are based on data from populations where contraception is not used and from women who cease using contraception in order to become pregnant. Among such populations, about 89% become pregnant within one year. This estimate was lowered slightly (to 85%) to represent the percent who would become pregnant within one year among women now relying on reversible methods of contraception if they abandoned contraception altogether.
5 Foams, creams, gels, vaginal suppositories, and vaginal film.
6 Cervical mucus (ovulation) method supplemented by calendar in the pre-ovulatory and basal body temperature in the post-ovulatory phases.
7 With spermicidal cream or jelly.
8 Without spermicides.

spective cohort studies. Case-control studies provide an estimate of the relative risk of a disease, which is defined as the *ratio* of the incidence of a disease among oral contraceptive users to that among nonusers. The relative risk (or odds ratio) does not provide information about the actual clinical occurrence of a disease. Cohort studies provide a measure of both the relative risk and the attributable risk. The latter is the *difference* in the incidence of disease between oral contraceptive users and nonusers. The attributable risk does provide information about the actual occurrence or incidence of a disease in the subject population. For further information, the reader is referred to a text on epidemiological methods.

1. Thromboembolic disorders and other vascular problems

a. Myocardial infarction

An increased risk of myocardial infarction has been associated with oral contraceptive use.[2–21] This increased risk is primarily in smokers or in women with other underlying risk factors for coronary artery disease such as hypertension, obesity, diabetes, and hypercholesterolemia. The relative risk for myocardial infarction in current oral contraceptive users has been estimated to be 2 to 6. The risk is very low under the age of 30. However, there is the possibility of a risk of cardiovascular disease even in very young women who take oral contraceptives.

Smoking in combination with oral contraceptive use has been reported to contribute substantially to the risk of myocardial infarction in women in the mid-thirties or older, with smoking accounting for the majority of excess cases.[22] Mortality rates associated with circulatory disease have been shown to increase substantially in smokers, especially in those 35 years of age and older among women who use oral contraceptives.(Table II.)

TABLE II. CIRCULATORY DISEASE MORTALITY RATES PER 100,000 WOMEN—YEARS BY AGE, SMOKING STATUS, AND ORAL CONTRACEPTIVE USE.[14]

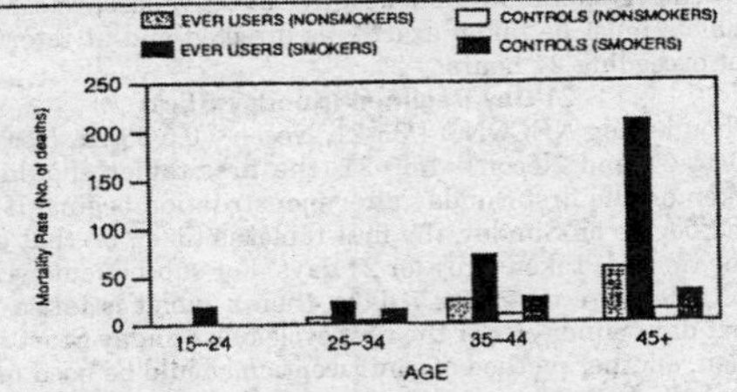

Adapted from P.M. Layde and V. Beral, Ref. # 12.

Oral contraceptives may compound the effects of well-known cardiovascular risk factors such as hypertension, diabetes, hyperlipidemias, hypercholesterolemia, age, cigarette smoking, and obesity. In particular, some progestogens decrease HDL cholesterol[23–31] and cause glucose intolerance, while estrogens may create a state of hyperinsulinism.[32] Oral contraceptives have been shown to increase blood pressure among some users (see **WARNING** No. 9). Similar effects on risk factors have been associated with an increased risk of heart disease.

b. Thromboembolism

An increased risk of thromboembolic and thrombotic disease associated with the use of oral contraceptives is well established.[17, 33–51] Case-control studies have estimated the relative risk to be 3 for the first episode of superficial venous thrombosis, 4 to 11 for deep vein thrombosis or pulmonary embolism, and 1.5 to 6 for women with predisposing conditions for venous thromboembolic disease.[34–37, 45, 46] Cohort studies have shown the relative risk to be somewhat lower, about 3 for new cases (subjects with no past history of venous thrombosis or varicose veins) and about 4.5 for new cases requiring hospitalization.[42, 47, 48] The risk of venous thromboembolic disease associated with oral contraceptives is not related to duration of use.

A two- to seven-fold increase in relative risk of postoperative thromboembolic complications has been reported with the use of oral contraceptives.[38, 39] The relative risk of venous thrombosis in women who have predisposing conditions is about twice that of women without such medical conditions.[43] If feasible, oral contraceptives should be discontinued at least 4 weeks prior to and for 2 weeks after elective surgery of a type associated with an increased risk of thromboembolism, and also during and following prolonged immobilization. Since the immediate postpartum period is also associated with an increased risk of thromboembolism, oral contraceptives should be started no earlier than 4 to 6 weeks after delivery in women who elect not to breast feed.

c. Cerebrovascular disease

Both the relative and attributable risks of cerebrovascular events (thrombotic and hemorrhagic strokes) have been reported to be increased with oral contraceptive use,[14, 17, 18, 34, 42, 46, 52–59] although, in general, the risk was greatest among older (over 35 years) hypertensive women who also smoked. Hypertension was reported to be a risk factor for both users and nonusers for both types of strokes, while smoking increased the risk factor for both users and nonusers for both types of strokes, while smoking increased the risk for hemorrhagic strokes.

In one large study,[52] the relative risk for thrombotic stroke was reported as 9.5 times greater in users than in nonusers. It ranged from 3 for normotensive users to 14 for users with severe hypertension.[54] The relative risk for hemorrhagic stroke was reported to be 1.2 for nonsmokers who used oral

TABLE III. ANNUAL NUMBER OF BIRTH-RELATED OR METHOD-RELATED DEATHS ASSOCIATED WITH CONTROL OF FERTILITY PER 100,000 NONSTERILE WOMEN, BY FERTILITY CONTROL METHOD ACCORDING TO AGE.[67]

Method of control	Age 15–19	20–24	25–29	30–34	35–39	40–44
No fertility control methods*	7.0	7.4	9.1	14.8	25.7	28.2
Oral contraceptives						
nonsmoker**	0.3	0.5	0.9	1.9	13.8	31.6
smoker**	2.2	3.4	6.6	13.5	51.1	117.2
IUD**	0.8	0.8	1.0	1.0	1.4	1.4
Condom*	1.1	1.6	0.7	0.2	0.3	0.4
Diaphragm/spermicide*	1.9	1.2	1.2	1.3	2.2	2.8
Periodic abstinence*	2.5	1.6	1.6	1.7	2.9	3.6

* Deaths are birth-related
** Deaths are method-related
Adapted from H.W. Ory, ref. #35.

contraceptives, 1.9 to 2.6 for smokers who did not use oral contraceptives, 6.1 to 7.6 for smokers who used oral contraceptives, 1.8 for normotensive users, and 25.7 for users with severe hypertension. The risk is also greater in older women and among smokers.

d. Dose-related risk of vascular disease with oral contraceptives

A positive association has been reported between the amount of estrogen and progestogen in oral contraceptives and the risk of vascular disease.[41, 43, 53, 59–64] A decline in serum high density lipoproteins (HDL) has been reported with many progestogens.[23–31] A decline in serum high density lipoproteins has been associated with an increased incidence of ischemic heart disease.[65] Because estrogens increase HDL-cholesterol, the net effect of an oral contraceptive depends on the balance achieved between doses of estrogen and progestogen and the nature and absolute amount of progestogens used in the contraceptives. The amount of both steroids should be considered in the choice of an oral contraceptive.

Minimizing exposure to estrogen and progestogen is in keeping with good principles of therapeutics. For any particular estrogen-progestogen combination, the dosage regimen prescribed should be one that contains the least amount of estrogen and progestogen that is compatible with a low failure rate and the needs of the individual patient. New acceptors of oral contraceptives should be started on preparations containing the lowest estrogen content that produces satisfactory results in the individual.

e. Persistence of risk of vascular disease

There are three studies that have shown persistence of risk of vascular disease for users of oral contraceptives. In a study in the United States, the risk of developing myocardial infarction after discontinuing oral contraceptives persisted for at least 9 years for women 40–49 years old who had used oral contraceptives for 5 or more years, but this increased risk was not demonstrated in other age groups.[16] Another American study reported former use of oral contraceptives was significantly associated with increased risk of subarachnoid hemorrhage.[57] In another study, in Great Britain, the risk of developing non-rheumatic heart disease plus hypertension, subanoid hemorrhage, cerebral thrombosis, and transient ischemic attacks persisted for at least 6 years after discontinuation of oral contraceptives, although the excess risk was small.[14, 18, 66] It should be noted that these studies were performed with oral contraceptive formulations containing 50 mcg or more of estrogens.

2. Estimates of mortality from contraceptive use

One study[67] gathered data from a variety of sources that have estimated the mortality rates associated with different methods of contraception at different ages. (Table 2). These estimates include the combined risk of death associated with contraceptive methods plus the risk attributable to pregnancy in the event of method failure. Each method of contraception has its specific benefits and risks. The study concluded that, with the exception of oral contraceptive users 35 and older who smoke and 40 and older who do not smoke, mortality associated with all methods of birth control is low and below that associated with childbirth. The observation of a possible increase in risk of mortality with age of oral contraceptive users is based on data gathered in the 1970's, but not reported until 1983.[67] However, current clinical practice involves the use of lower estrogen dose formulations combined with careful restriction of oral contraceptive use to women who do not have various risk factors listed in this labeling.

Because of these changes in practice and, also, because of some limited new data that suggest that the risk of cardiovascular disease with the use of oral contraceptives may now be less than previously observed,[48, 152] the Fertility and Maternal Health Drugs Advisory Committee was asked to review the topic in 1989. The Committee concluded that, although cardiovascular disease risks may be increased with oral contraceptive use after age 40 in healthy, nonsmoking women (even with the newer low-dose formulations), there are greater potential health risks associated with pregnancy in older women and with the alternative surgical and medical procedures that may be necessary if such women do not have access to effective and acceptable means of contraception.

Therefore, the Committee recommended that the benefits of oral contraceptive use by healthy nonsmoking women over 40 may outweigh the possible risks. Of course, older women, as all women who take oral contraceptives, should take the lowest possible dose formulation that is effective.

[See table above]

3. Carcinoma of the breast and reproductive organs

Numerous epidemiological studies have been performed on the incidence of breast, endometrial, ovarian, and cervical cancer in women using oral contraceptives. While there are conflicting reports, most studies suggest that the use of oral contraceptives is not associated with an overall increase in the risk of developing breast cancer. A meta-analysis of 54 studies reports that women who are currently using combined oral contraceptives or have used them in the past 10 years are at slightly increased risk of having breast cancer diagnosed although the additional cancers tend to be localized to the breast. There is no evidence of an increased risk of having breast cancer diagnosed 10 or more years after cessation of use.

Some studies suggested that oral contraceptive use was associated with an increase in the risk of cervical intraepithelial neoplasia, dysplasia, erosion, carcinoma, or microglandular dysplasia in some populations of women.[17, 50, 103–115] However, there continues to be controversy about the extent to which such findings may be due to differences in sexual behavior and other factors.

4. Hepatic neoplasia

Benign hepatic adenomas are associated with oral contraceptive use, although the incidence of benign tumors is rare in the United States. Indirect calculations have estimated the attributable risk to be in the range of 3.3 cases per 100,000 for users, a risk that increases after four or more years of use, especially with oral contraceptives of higher dose (49). Rupture of benign, hepatic adenomas may cause death through intraabdominal hemorrhage (50, 51).

Studies have shown an increased risk of developing hepatocellular carcinoma in oral contraceptive users. However, these cancers are rare in the United States, and the attributable risk (the excess incidence) of liver cancers in oral contraceptive users approaches less than one per million users.

5. OCULAR LESIONS

There have been clinical case reports of retinal thrombosis associated with the use of oral contraceptives. Oral contraceptives should be discontinued if there is unexplained partial or complete loss of vision; onset of proptosis or diplopia; papilledema; or retinal vascular lesions. Appropriate diagnostic and therapeutic measures should be undertaken immediately.

6. ORAL CONTRACEPTIVE USE BEFORE OR DURING EARLY PREGNANCY

Extensive epidemiological studies have revealed no increased risk of birth defects in women who have used oral contraceptives prior to pregnancy (56,57). The majority of recent studies also do not indicate a teratogenic effect, particularly in so far as cardiac anomalies and limb reduction defects are concerned, (55, 56, 58, 59), when taken inadvertently during early pregnancy.

The administration of oral contraceptives to induce withdrawal bleeding should not be used as a test for pregnancy. Oral contraceptives should not be used during pregnancy to treat threatened or habitual abortion.

It is recommended that for any patient who has missed two consecutive periods, pregnancy should be ruled out before continuing oral contraceptive use. If the patient has not adhered to the prescribed schedule, the possibility of pregnancy should be considered at the time of the first missed period. Oral contraceptive use should be discontinued if pregnancy is ruled out.

7. GALLBLADDER DISEASE

Earlier studies have reported an increased lifetime relative risk of gallbladder surgery in users of oral contraceptives and estrogens (60,61). More recent studies, however, have shown that the relative risk of developing gallbladder disease among oral contraceptive users may be minimal (62–64). The recent findings of minimal risk may be related to the use of oral contraceptive formulations containing lower hormonal doses of estrogens and progestogens.

8. CARBOHYDRATE AND LIPID METABOLIC EFFECTS

Oral contraceptives have been shown to cause a decrease in glucose tolerance in a significant percentage of users (17). This effect has been shown to be directly related to estrogen dose (65). Progestogens increase insulin secretion and create insulin resistance, this effect varying with different progestational agents (17,66). However, in the non-diabetic woman, oral contraceptives appear to have no effect on fast-

Continued on next page

Necon—Cont.

ing blood glucose (67). Because of these demonstrated effects, prediabetic and diabetic women in particular should be carefully monitored while taking oral contraceptives.
A small proportion of women will have persistent hypertriglyceridemia while on the pill. As discussed earlier (see **WARNINGS** 1a and 1d), changes in serum triglycerides and lipoprotein levels have been reported in oral contraceptive users.
9. ELEVATED BLOOD PRESSURE
An increase in blood pressure has been reported in women taking oral contraceptives (68) and this increase is more likely in older oral contraceptive users (69) and with extended duration of use (61). Data from the Royal College of General Practitioners (12) and subsequent randomized trials have shown that the incidence of hypertension increases with increasing progestational activity.
Women with a history of hypertension or hypertension-related diseases, or renal disease (70) should be encouraged to use another method of contraception. If women elect to use oral contraceptives, they should be monitored closely and if significant elevation of blood pressure occurs, oral contraceptives should be discontinued. For most women, elevated blood pressure will return to normal after stopping oral contraceptives, and there is no difference in the occurrence of hypertension between former and never users (68–71).
10. HEADACHE
The onset or exacerbation of migraine or development of headache with a new pattern which is recurrent, persistent, or severe requires discontinuation of oral contraceptives and evaluation of the cause.
11. BLEEDING IRREGULARITIES
Breakthrough bleeding and spotting are sometimes encountered in patients on oral contraceptives, especially during the first three months of use. Non-hormonal causes should be considered and adequate diagnostic measures taken to rule out malignancy or pregnancy in the event of breakthrough bleeding, as in the case of any abnormal vaginal bleeding. If pathology has been excluded, time or a change to another formulation may solve the problem. In the event of amenorrhea, pregnancy should be ruled out. Some women may encounter post-pill amenorrhea or oligomenorrhea, especially when such a condition was preexistent.
12. ECTOPIC PREGNANCY
Ectopic as well as intrauterine pregnancy may occur in contraceptive failures. However, in progestogen-only oral contraceptive failures, the ratio of ectopic to intrauterine pregnancies is higher than in women who are not receiving oral contraceptives, since the drugs are more effective in preventing intrauterine than ectopic pregnancies.

PRECAUTIONS

1. PHYSICAL EXAMINATION AND FOLLOW-UP
It is good medical practice for all women to have annual history and physical examinations, including women using oral contraceptives. The physical examination, however, may be deferred until after initiation of oral contraceptives if requested by the woman and judged appropriate by the clinician. The physical examination should include special reference to blood pressure, breasts, abdomen, and pelvic organs, including cervical cytology, and relevant laboratory tests. In case of undiagnosed, persistent, or recurrent abnormal vaginal bleeding, appropriate measures should be conducted to rule out malignancy. Women with a strong family history of breast cancer or who have breast nodules should be monitored with particular care.
2. LIPID DISORDERS
Women who are being treated for hyperlipidemias should be followed closely if they elect to use oral contraceptives. Some progestogens may elevate LDL levels and may render the control of hyperlipidemias more difficult.
3. LIVER FUNCTION
If jaundice develops in any woman receiving such drugs, the medication should be discontinued. Steroid hormones may be poorly metabolized in patients with impaired liver function.
4. FLUID RETENTION
Oral contraceptives may cause some degree of fluid retention. They should be prescribed with caution, and only with careful monitoring, in patients with conditions which might be aggravated by fluid retention.
5. EMOTIONAL DISORDERS
Women with a history of depression should be carefully observed and the drug discontinued if depression recurs to a serious degree.
6. CONTACT LENSES
Contact lens wearers who develop visual changes or changes in lens tolerance should be assessed by an ophthalmologist.
7. DRUG INTERACTIONS
Reduced efficacy and increased incidence of breakthrough bleeding and menstrual irregularities have been associated with concomitant use of rifampin. A similar association, though less marked, has been suggested with barbiturates, phenylbutazone, phenytoin sodium, carbamazepine, and possibly with griseofulvin, ampicillin, and tetracyclines (72).
8. INTERACTIONS WITH LABORATORY TESTS
Certain endocrine and liver function tests and blood components may be affected by oral contraceptives:

a. Increased prothrombin and factors VII, VIII, IX and X; decreased antithrombin 3; increased norepinephrine-induced platelet aggregability.
b. Increased thyroid binding globulin (TBG) leading to increased circulating total thyroid hormone, as measured by protein-bound iodine (PBI), T_4 by column or by radioimmunoassay. Free T_3 resin uptake is decreased, reflecting the elevated TBG; free T_4 concentration is unaltered.
c. Other binding proteins may be elevated in the serum.
d. Sex-binding globulins are increased and result in elevated levels of total circulating sex steroids and corticoids; however, free or biologically active levels remain unchanged.
e. Triglycerides may be increased.
f. Glucose tolerance may be decreased.
g. Serum folate levels may be depressed by oral contraceptive therapy. This may be of clinical significance if a woman becomes pregnant shortly after discontinuing oral contraceptives.

9. CARCINOGENESIS
See **WARNINGS** section.
10. PREGNANCY
Pregnancy Category X. See **CONTRAINDICATIONS** and **WARNINGS** sections.
11. NURSING MOTHERS
Small amounts of oral contraceptive steroids have been identified in the milk of nursing mothers and a few adverse effects on the child have been reported, including jaundice and breast enlargement. In addition, combination oral contraceptives given in the postpartum period may interfere with lactation by decreasing the quantity and quality of breast milk. If possible, the nursing mother should be advised not to use combination oral contraceptives but to use other forms of contraception until she has completely weaned her child.
12. SEXUALLY TRANSMITTED DISEASES
Patients should be counseled that this product does not protect against HIV infection (AIDS) and other sexually transmitted diseases.
13. PEDIATRIC USE
Safety and efficacy of NECON Tablets has been established in women of reproductive age. Safety and efficacy are expected to be the same for postpubertal adolescents under the age of 16 and for users 16 years and older. Use of this product before menarche is not indicated.

INFORMATION FOR THE PATIENT

See Patient Labeling Printed Below.

ADVERSE REACTIONS

An increased risk of the following serious adverse reactions has been associated with the use of oral contraceptives (see **WARNINGS** section).

- Thrombophlebitis and venous thrombosis with or without embolism
- Arterial thromboembolism
- Pulmonary embolism
- Myocardial infarction
- Cerebral hemorrhage
- Cerebral thrombosis
- Hypertension
- Gallbladder disease
- Hepatic adenomas or benign liver tumors

The following adverse reactions have been reported in patients receiving oral contraceptives and are believed to be drug-related:

- Nausea
- Vomiting
- Gastrointestinal symptoms (such as abdominal cramps and bloating)
- Breakthrough bleeding
- Spotting
- Changes in menstrual flow
- Amenorrhea
- Temporary infertility after discontinuation of treatment
- Edema
- Melasma which may persist
- Breast changes: tenderness, enlargement, secretion
- Change in weight (increase or decrease)
- Change in cervical erosion or secretion
- Diminution in lactation when given immediately postpartum
- Cholestatic jaundice
- Migraine
- Rash (allergic)
- Mental depression
- Reduced tolerance to carbohydrates
- Vaginal candidiasis
- Change in corneal curvature (steepening)
- Intolerance to contact lenses

The following adverse reactions have been reported in users of oral contraceptives and the association has been neither confirmed nor refuted:

- Pre-menstrual syndrome
- Cataracts
- Changes in appetite
- Cystitis-like syndrome
- Headache
- Nervousness
- Dizziness
- Hirsutism
- Loss of scalp hair
- Erythema multiforme
- Erythema nodosum
- Hemorrhagic eruption
- Vaginitis
- Porphyria
- Impaired renal function
- Hemolytic uremic syndrome
- Acne
- Changes in libido
- Colitis
- Budd-Chiari syndrome

OVERDOSAGE

Serious ill effects have not been reported following acute ingestion of large doses of oral contraceptives by young children. Overdosage may cause nausea, and withdrawal bleeding may occur in females.

NON-CONTRACEPTIVE HEALTH BENEFITS

The following non-contraceptive health benefits related to the use of combination oral contraceptives are supported by epidemiological studies which largely utilized oral contraceptive formulations containing estrogen doses exceeding 0.035 mg of ethinyl estradiol or 0.05 mg of mestranol (73–78).
Effects on menses:
- increased menstrual cycle regularity
- decreased blood loss and decreased risk of iron-deficiency anemia
- decreased frequency of dysmenorrhea

Effects related to inhibition of ovulation:
- decreased incidence of functional ovarian cysts
- decreased incidence of ectopic pregnancies

Other effects:
- decreased incidence of fibroadenomas and fibrocystic disease of the breast
- decreased incidence of acute pelvic inflammatory disease
- decreased incidence of endometrial cancer
- decreased incidence of ovarian cancer

DOSAGE AND ADMINISTRATION

To achieve maximum contraceptive effectiveness, Necon®™ Tablets must be taken exactly as directed and at intervals not exceeding 24 hours.

21-Day Regimen (Sunday Start)

When taking NECON® 1/35-21, Necon® 0.5/35-21, Necon® 10/11-21 and Necon® 1/50-21, the first tablet should be taken on the first Sunday after menstruation begins. If period begins on Sunday, the first tablet is taken on that day. One tablet is taken daily for 21 days. For subsequent cycles, no tablets are taken for 7 days, then a tablet is taken the next day (Sunday). For the first cycle of a Sunday Start regimen, another method of contraception should be used until after the first 7 consecutive days of administration.
If the patient misses one (1) active tablet in Weeks 1, 2, or 3, the tablet should be taken as soon as she remembers. If the patient misses two (2) active tablets in Week 1 or Week 2, the patient should take two (2) tablets the day she remembers and two (2) tablets the next day; and then continue taking one (1) tablet a day until she finishes the dispenser. The patient should be instructed to use a back-up method of birth control if she has sex in the seven (7) days after missing pills. If the patient misses two (2) active tablets in the third week or misses three (3) or more active tablets in a row, the patient should continue taking one tablet every day until Sunday. On Sunday, the patient should throw out the rest of the dispenser and start a new dispenser that same day. The patient should be instructed to use a back-up method of birth control if she has sex in the seven (7) days after missing pills.
Complete instructions to facilitate a patient counseling on proper pill usage may be found in the Detailed Patient Labeling ("How to Take the Pill" section).

21-Day Regimen (Day 1 Start)

The dosage of Necon® 1/35-21, Necon® 0.5/35-21, Necon® 10/11-21 and Necon® 1/50-21, for the initial cycle of therapy is one tablet adminstered daily from the 1st day through the 21st day of the menstrual cycle, counting the first day of menstrual flow "Day 1". For subsequent cycles, no tablets are taken for 7 days, then a new course is started of one tablet a day for 21 days. The dosage regimen then continues with 7 days of no medication, followed by 21 days of medication, instituting a three-weeks-on, one-week-off dosage regimen.
If the patient misses one (1) active tablet in Weeks 1, 2, or 3, the tablet should be taken as soon as she remembers. If the patient misses two (2) active tablets in Week 1 or Week 2, the patient should take two (2) tablets the day she remembers and two (2) tablets the next day; and then continue taking one (1) tablet a day until she finishes the dispenser. The patient should be instructed to use a back-up method of birth control if she has sex in the seven (7) days after missing pills. If the patient misses two (2) active tablets in the 3rd week or misses three (3) or more active tablets in a row, the patient should throw out the rest of the dispenser and start a new dispenser that same day. The patient should be instructed to use a back-up method of birth control if she has sex in the seven (7) days after missing pills.
Complete instructions to facilitate patient counseling on proper pill usage may be found in the Detailed Patient Labeling ("How to Take the Pill" section).

28-Day Regimen (Sunday Start)

When taking Necon® 1/35-28, Necon® 0.5/35-28, Necon® 10/11-28 and Necon® 1/50-28, the first tablet should be taken on the first Sunday after menstruation begins. If period begins on Sunday, the first tablet should be taken that day. Take one active tablet daily for 21 days followed by one white placebo tablet daily for 7 days. After 28 tablets have been taken, a new course is started the next day (Sunday).

For the first cycle of a Sunday Start regimen, another method of contraception should be used until after the first 7 consecutive days of administration.
If the patient misses one (1) active tablet in Weeks 1, 2, or 3, the tablet should be taken as soon as she remembers. If the patient misses two (2) active tablets in Week 1 or Week 2, the patient should take two (2) tablets the day she remembers and two (2) tablets the next day; and then continue taking one (1) tablet a day until she finishes the dispenser. The patient should be instructed to use a back-up method of birth control if she has sex in the seven (7) days after missing pills. If the patient misses two (2) active tablets in the third week or misses three (3) or more active tablets in a row, the patient should continue taking one tablet every day until Sunday. On Sunday, the patient should throw out the rest of the dispenser and start a new dispenser that same day. The patient should be instructed to use a back-up method of birth control if she has sex in the seven (7) days after missing pills.
Complete instructions to facilitate patient counseling on proper pill usage may be found in the Detailed Patient Labeling ("How to Take the Pill" section).

28-Day Regimen (Day 1 Start)

The dosage of Necon® 1/35 -28, Necon® 0.5/35-28, Necon® 10/11-28 and Necon® 1/50-28, for the initial cycle of therapy is one active tablet administered daily from the 1st through the 21st day of the menstrual cycle, counting the first day of menstrual flow as "Day 1" followed by one white tablet daily for 7 days. Tablets are taken without interruption for 28 days. After 28 tablets have been taken, a new course is started the next day.
If the patient misses one (1) active tablet in Weeks 1, 2, or 3, the tablet should be taken as soon as she remembers. If the patient misses two (2) active tablets in Week 1 or Week 2, the patient should take two (2) tablets the day she remembers and two (2) tablets the next day; and then continue taking one (1) tablet a day until she finishes the dispenser. The patient should be instructed to use a back-up method of birth control if she has sex in the seven (7) days after missing pills. If the patient misses two (2) active tablets in the third week or misses three (3) or more active tablets in a row, the patient should throw out the rest of the dispenser and start a new dispenser that same day. The patient should be instructed to use a back-up method of birth control if she has sex in the seven (7) days after missing pills.
Complete instructions to facilitate patient counseling on proper pill usage may be found in the Detailed Patient Labeling ("How to Take the Pill" section).
The use of Necon® 1/35, Necon® 0.5/35, Necon® 10/11 and Necon® 1/50 for contraception may be initiated 4 weeks postpartum in women who elect not to breast feed. When the tablets are administered during the postpartum period, the increased risk of thromboembolic disease associated with the postpartum period must be considered. (See **CONTRAINDICATIONS** and **WARNINGS** concerning thromboembolic disease. See also **PRECAUTIONS** for "Nursing Mothers".) The possibility of ovulation and conception prior to initiation of medication should be considered.
(See Discussion of Dose-Related Risk of Vascular Disease from Oral Contraceptives.)

ADDITIONAL INSTRUCTIONS FOR ALL DOSING REGIMENS

Breakthrough bleeding, spotting, and amenorrhea are frequent reasons for patients discontinuing oral contraceptives. In breakthrough bleeding, as in all cases of irregular bleeding from the vagina, nonfunctional causes should be borne in mind. In undiagnosed persistent or recurrent abnormal bleeding from the vagina, adequate diagnostic measures are indicated to rule out pregnancy or malignancy. If pathology has been excluded, time or a change to another formulation may solve the problem. Changing to an oral contraceptive with a higher estrogen content, while potentially useful in minimizing menstrual irregularity, should be done only if necessary since this may increase the risk of thromboembolic disease.
Use of oral contraceptives in the event of a missed menstrual period:

1. If the patient has not adhered to the prescribed schedule, the possibility of pregnancy should be considered at the time of the first missed period and oral contraceptive use should be discontinued until pregnancy is ruled out.
2. If the patient has adhered to the prescribed regimen and misses two consecutive periods, pregnancy should be ruled out before continuing oral contraceptive use.

HOW SUPPLIED

Necon® 1/35: (Norethindrone and Ethinyl Estradiol Tablets, USP)
Each dark yellow Necon® 1/35 tablets is round in shape, unscored, with a debossed **WATSON** on one side and 508 on the other side, and contains 1 mg of norethindrone and 0.035 mg of ethinyl estradiol.
Necon® 1/35-21 (NDC 52544-508-21) is packaged in cartons of six tablet dispensers of 21 tablets each.
Necon® 1/35-28 (NDC 52544-552-28) is packaged in cartons of six tablet dispensers. Each dispenser contains 21 dark yellow tablets and 7 white placebo tablets. (Placebo tablets have a debossed **WATSON** on one side and P on the other side.)
Necon® 0.5/35: (Norethindrone and Ethinyl Estradiol Tablets, USP)
Each light yellow Necon® 0.5/35 tablet is round in shape, unscored, with a debossed **WATSON** on one side and 507 on the other side, and contains 0.5 mg of norethindrone and 0.035 mg of ethinyl estradiol.
Necon® 0.5/35-21 (NDC 52554-507-21) is packaged in cartons of six tablet dispensers of 21 tablets each.
Necon® 0.5/35-28 (NDC 52544-550-28) is packaged in cartons of six tablet dispensers. Each dispenser contains 21 light yellow tablets and 7 white placebo tablets (Placebo tablets have a debossed **WATSON** on one side and P on the other side.)
Necon® 10/11: (Norethindrone and Ethinyl Estradiol Tablets, USP)
Each light yellow Necon® 10/11 tablet is round in shape, with a debossed **WATSON** on one side and 507 on the other side, and contains 0.5 mg of norethindrone and 0.035 mg of ethinyl estradiol. Each dark yellow Necon® 10/11 tablet is round in shape, with a debossed **WATSON** on one side and 508 on the other side, and contains 1 mg of norethindrone and 0.035 mg of ethinyl estradiol.
Necon® 10/11-21 (NDC 5244-553-21) is packaged in cartons of six tablet dispensers. Each dispenser contains 10 light yellow tablets and 11 dark yellow tablets.
Necon® 10/11-28 (NDC 52544-554-28) is packaged in cartons of six tablet dispensers. Each dispenser contains 10 light yellow tablets and 11 dark yellow tablets, and 7 white placebo tablets. (Placebo tablets have a debossed **WATSON** on one side and P on the other side.)
Necon® 1/50: (Norethindrone and Mestranol Tablets, USP)
Each light blue Necon® 1/50 tablet is round in shape, unscored, with a debossed **WATSON** on one side and 510 on the other side, and contains 1 mg of norethindrone and 0.050 mg of mestranol. Necon® 1/50-21 (NDC 52544-510-21) is packaged in cartons of six tablet dispensers of 21 tablets each.
Necon® 1/50-28 (NDC 52544-56-28) is packaged in cartons of six tablet dispensers. Each dispenser contains 21 light blue tablets and 7 white placebo tablets. (Placebo tablets have a debossed **WATSON** on one side and P on the other side.)
Store at controlled room temperature 15°C to 30°C (59°F to 86°F).
Rx only

REFERENCES

1. Source: Trussell J. Contraceptive Efficacy Table from Hatcher RA, Trussell J, Stewart F, Cates W, Stewart GK, Kowal D, Guest F, in Contraceptive Technology: Seventeenth Revised Edition. New York, NY: Irvington Publishers, 1998. **2.** Stadel BV, Oral contraceptives and cardiovascular disease. (Pt. 1). *N Engl J Med* 1981; 305:612–618. **3.** Stadel BV, Oral contraceptives and cardiovascular disease. (Pt. 2). *N Engl J Med* 1981; 305:672–677. **4.** Adam SA, Thorogood M. Oral contraception and myocardial infarction revisited: the effects of new preparations and prescribing patterns. *Br J Obstet Gynaecol* 1981; 88:838–845. **5.** Mann JI, Inman WH, Oral contraceptives and death from myocardial infarction. *Br Med J* 1975; 2(5965):245–248. **6.** Mann JI, Vessey MP, Thorogood M, Doll R. Myocardial infarction in young women with special reference to oral contraceptive practice. *Br Med J* 1975; 2(5956):241–245. **7.** Royal College of General Practitioners' Oral Contraception Study: Further analyses of mortality in oral contraceptive users. *Lancet* 1981; 1:541–546. **8.** Stone D, Shapiro S, Kaufman DW, Rosenberg L, Miettinen OS, Stolley PD. Risk of myocardial infarction in relation to current and discontinued use of oral contraceptives. *N Engl J Med* 1981: 305:420–424. **9.** Vessey MP. Female hormones and vascular disease-an epidemiological overview. *Br J Fam Plann* 1980; 6(Supplement): 1–12. **10.** Russell-Briefel RG, Ezzati TM, Fulwood R, Perlman JA, Murphy RS. Cardiovascular risk status and oral contraceptive use, United States 1976–1980. *Prevent Med* 1986; 15: 352–362. **11.** Goldbaum GM, Kendrick JS, Hogelin GC, Gentry EM. The relative impact of smoking and oral contraceptive use on women in the United States. *JAMA* 1987; 258:1339–1342. **12.** Layde PM, Beral V. Further analyses of mortality in oral contraceptive users; Royal College of General Practitioners' Oral Contraception Study. (Table 5) *Lancet* 1981; 1:541–546. **13.** Knopp RH. Arteriosclerosis risk: the roles of oral contraceptives and postmenopausal estrogens. *J Reprod Med* 1986; 31(9) (Supplement) :913–921. **14.** Krauss RM, Roy S, Mishell DR, Casagrande J, Pike MC. Effects of two low-dose oral contraceptives on serum lipids and lipoproteins: Differential changes in high-density lipoproteins subclasses. *Am J Obstet* 1983; 145;446–452. **15.** Wahl P, Walden C, Knopp R, Hoover J, Wallace R, Heiss G, Rifkind B. Effect of estrogen/progestin potency on lipid/lipoprotein cholesterol. *N Engl J Med* 1983; 308:862–867. **16.** Wynn V, Niththyananthan R. The effect of progestin in combined oral contraceptives on serum lipids with special reference to high density lipoproteins. *Am J Obstet Gynecol* 1982; 142: 766–771. **17.** Wynn V, Godsland I. Effects of oral contraceptives on carbohydrate metabolism. *J Reprod Med* 1986; 31 (9) (Supplement) :892–897. **18.** LaRosa JC. Atherosclerotic risk factors in cardiovascular disease. *J Reprod Med* 1986; 31 (9) (Supplement): 906–912. **19.** Inman WH, Vessey MP. Investigation of death from pulmonary, coronary, and cerebral thrombosis and embolism in women of child-bearing age. *Br Med J* 1968; 2(5599): 193–199. **20.** Maguire MG, Tonascia J, Sartwell PE, Stolley PD, Tockman MS. Increased risk of thrombosis due to oral contraceptives: a further report. *Am J Epidemiol* 1979; 110(2): 188–195. **21.** Petitti DB, Wingerd J, Pellegrin F, Ramacharan S. Risk of vascular disease in women: smoking, oral contraceptives, noncontraceptive estrogens, and other factors. *JAMA* 1979; 242: 1150–1154. **22.** Vessey MP, Doll R. Investigation of relation between use of oral contraceptives and thromboembolic disease. *Br Med J* 1968;2(5599) :199–205. **23.** Vessey MP, Doll R. Investigation of relation between use of oral contraceptives and thromboembolic disease. A further report. *Br Med J* 1969; 2(5658): 651–657. **24.** Porter JB, Hunter JR, Danielson DA, Jick H, Stergachis A. Oral contraceptives and non-fatal vascular disease-recent experience. *Obstet Gyneco* 1982; 59 (3):299–302. **25.** Vessey M, Doll R, Peto R, Johnson B, Wiggins P. A long-term follow-up study of women using different methods of contraception: an interim report. *J Bio-social Sci* 1976; 8: 375–427. **26.** Royal College of General Practitioners: Oral Contraceptives, venous thrombosis, and varicose veins. *J Royal Coll Gen Pract* 1978;28: 393–399. **27.** Collaborative Group for the Study of Stroke in Young Women: Oral contraception and increased risk of cerebral ischemia or thrombosis. *N Engl J Med* 1973; 288:871–878. **28.** Petitti DB, Wingerd J. Use of oral contraceptives, cigarette smoking, and risk of subarachnoid hemorrhage. *Lancet* 1978; 2: 234–236. **29.** Inman WH. Oral contraceptives and fatal subarachnoid hemorrhage. *Br Med J* 1979; 2 (6203): 1468–1470. **30.** Collaborative Group for the Study of Stroke in Young Women: Oral Contraceptives and stroke in young women: associated risk factors. *JAMA* 1975; 231: 718–722. **31.** Inman WH, Vessey MP, Westerholm B, Engelund A. Thromboembolic disease and the steroidal content of oral contraceptives. A report to the Committee on Safety of Drugs. *Br Med J* 1970; 2: 203–209. **32.** Meade TW, Greenberg G, Thompson SG. Progestogens and cardiovascular reactions associated with oral contraceptives and a comparison of the safety of 50- and 35-mcg oestrogen preparations. *Br Med J* 1980; 280 (6224): 1157–1161. **33.** Kay CR. Progestogens and arterial disease-evidence from the Royal College of General Practitioners' Study. *Am J Obstet Gynecol* 1982; 142: 762–675. **34.** Royal College of General Practitioners: Incidence of arterial disease among oral contraceptive users. *J Royal Coll Gen Pract* 1983; 33: 75–82. **35.** Ory HW. Mortality associated with fertility and fertility control: 1983. *Family Planning Perspectives* 1983; 15: 50–56. **36.** The Cancer and Steroid Hormone Study of the Centers for Disease Control and the National Institute of Child Health and Human Development: Oral contraceptive use and the risk of breast cancer. *N Engl J Med* 1986; 315: 405–411. **37.** Pike MC, Henderson BE, Krailo MD, Duke A, Roy S. Breast cancer in young women and use of oral contraceptives: possible modifying effect of formulation and age at use. *Lancet* 1983; 2: 926–929. **38.** Paul C, Skegg DG, Spears GFS, Kaldor JM. Oral contraceptives and breast cancer: A national study. *Br Med J* 1986; 293: 723–725. **39.** Miller DR, Rosenberg L, Kaufman W, Schottenfeld D, Stolley PD, Shapiro S. Breast cancer risk in relation to early oral contraceptive use. *Obstet Gynecol* 1986; 68: 863–868. **40.** Olson H, Olson KL, Moller TR, Ranstam J, Holm P. Oral contraceptive use and breast cancer in young women in Sweden (letter). *Lancet* 1985; 2: 748–749. **41.** McPherson K, Vessey M, Neil A, Doll R, Jones L, Roberts M. Early contraceptive use and breast cancer: Results of another case-control study. *Br J Cancer* 1987; 56: 653–660. **42.** Huggins GR, Zucker PF. Oral contraceptives and neoplasia: 1987 update. *Fertil Steril* 1987; 47: 733–761. **43.** McPherson K, Drife JO. The pill and breast cancer: why the uncertainty? *Br Med J* 1986; 293: 709–710. **44.** Shapiro S. Oral contraceptives-time to take stock. *N Engl J Med* 1987; 315: 450–451. **45.** Ory H, Naib Z, Conger SB, Hatcher RA, Tyler CW. Contraceptive choice and prevalence of cervical dysplasia and carcinoma in situ. *Am J Obstet Gynecol* 1976; 124: 573–577. **46.** Vessey MP, Lawless M, McPherson K, Yeates D. Neoplasia of the cervix uteri and contraception: a possible adverse effect of the pill. *Lancet* 1983; 2: 930. **47.** Brinton LA, Huggins GR, Lehman HF, Malli K, Savitz DA, Trapido E, Rosenthal J, Hoover R. Long term use of oral contraceptives and risk of invasive cervical cancer. *Int J Cancer* 1986; 38: 399–344. **48.** WHO Collaborative Study of Neoplasia and Steroid Contraceptives: Invasive cervical cancer and combined oral contraceptives. *Br Med J* 1985; 290: 961–965. **49.** Rooks JB, Ory HW, Ishak KG, Strauss LT, Greenspan JR, Hill AP, Tyler CW. Epidemiology of hepatocellular adenoma; the role of oral contraceptive use. *JAMA* 1979; 242: 644–648. **50.** Bein NN, Goldsmith HS. Recurrent massive hemorrhage from benign hepatic tumors secondary to oral contraceptives. *Br J Surg* 1977; 64: 433–435. **51.** Klatskin G. Hepatic tumors: possible relationship to use of oral contraceptives. *Gastroenterology* 1977; 73: 386–394. **52.** Henderson BE, Preston-Martin S, Edmondson HA, Peters RL, Pike MC. Hepatocellular carcinoma and oral contraceptives. *Br J Cancer* 1983; 48: 437–440. **53.** Neuberger J, Forman D, Doll R, Williams R. Oral contraceptives and hepatocellular carcinoma. *Br Med J* 1986; 292: 1355–1357. **54.** Forman D, Vincent TJ, Doll R. Cancer of the liver and oral contraceptives. *Br Med J* 1986; 292: 1357–1361. **55.** Harlap S, Eldor J. Births following oral contraceptive failures. *Obstet Gynecol* 1980; 55: 447–452. **56.** Savolainen E, Saksela E, Saxen L. Teratogenic hazards of oral contraceptives analyzed in a national malformation register. *Am J Obstet Gynecol* 1981; 140: 521–524. **57.** Janerich DT, Piper JM, Glebatis DM. Oral contraceptives and birth defects. *Am J Epidemiol* 1980; 112: 73–79. **58.** Ferencz C, Matanoski GM, Wilson PD, Rubin JD, Neill CA, Gutberlet R. Maternal hormone therapy and congenital heart disease. *Teratology* 1980; 21: 225–239. **59.** Rothman KJ, Fyler DC, Goldblatt A, Kreidberg MB. Exogenous hormones and other drug exposures of children with congenital heart disease. *Am J Epidemiol* 1979; 109: 433–

Continued on next page

Necon—Cont.

439. **60.** Boston Collaborative Drug Surveillance Program: Oral contraceptives and venous thromboembolic disease, surgically confirmed gallbladder disease, and breast tumors. *Lancet* 1973; 1:1399–1404. **61.** Royal College of General Practitioners: Oral contraceptives and health. *New York, Pittman* 1974. **62.** Layde PM, Vessey MP, Yeates D. Risk of gallbladder disease: a cohort study of young women attending family planning clinics. *J Epidemiol Community Health* 1982; 36: 274–278. **63.** Rome Group for Epidemiology and Prevention of Cholelithiasis (GREPCO): Prevalence of gallstone disease in an Italian adult female population. *Am J Epidemiol* 1984; 119: 796–805. **64.** Storm BL, Tamragouri RT, Morse ML, Lazar EL, West SL, Stolley PD, Jones JK. Oral contraceptives and other risk factors for gallbladder disease. *Clin Pharmacol Ther* 1986; 39: 335–341. **65.** Wynn V, Adams PW, Godsland IF, Melrose J, Niththyananthan R, Oakley NW, Seedj A. Comparison of effects of different combined oral contraceptive formulations on carbohydrate and lipid metabolism. *Lancet* 1979; 1: 1045–1049. **66.** Wynn V. Effetct of progesterone and progestins on carbohydrate metabolism. In: Progesterone and Progestin. Bardin CW, Milgrom E, Mauvis-Jarvis P, eds. *New York, Raven Press* 1983; pp.395–410. **67.** Perlman JA, Roussell-Briefel RG, Ezzati TM, Lieberknecht G. Oral glucose tolerance and the potency of oral contraceptive progestogens. *J Chronic Dis* 1985; 38: 857–864. **68.** Royal College of General Practitioners' Oral Contraception Study: Effect on hypertension and benign breast disease of progestogen component in combined oral contraceptives. *Lancet* 1977; 1: 624. **69.** Fisch IR, Frank J. Oral contraceptives and blood pressure. *JAMA* 1977; 237: 2499–2503. **70.** Laragh AJ. Oral contraceptive induced hypertension – nine years later. *Am J Obstet Gynecol* 1976; 126: 141–147. **71.** Ramcharan S, Peritz E, Pellegrin FA, Williams WT. Incidence of hypertension in the Walnut Creek Contraceptive Drug Study cohort: In: Pharmacology of steroid-contraceptive drugs. Garattini S, Berendes HW. eds. *New York, Raven Press* 1977; pp. 277–288. (Monographs of the Mario Negri Institute for Pharmacological Research Milan.) **72.** Stockley I. Interactions with oral contraceptives. *J Pharm* 1976; 216: 140–143. **73.** The Cancer and Steroid Hormone Study of the Centers for Disease Control and the National Institute of Child Health and Human Development: Oral contraceptive use and the risk of ovarian cancer. *JAMA* 1983; 249: 1596–1599. **74.** The Cancer and Steroid Hormone Study of the Centers for Disease Control and the National Institute of Child Health and Human Development: Combination oral contraceptive use and the risk of endometrial cancer. *JAMA* 1987; 257: 796–800. **75.** Ory HW. Functional ovarian cysts and oral contraceptives: negative association confirmed surgically. *JAMA* 1974; 228: 68–69. **76.** Ory HW, Cole P, MacMahon B, Hoover R. Oral contraceptives and reduced risk of benign breast disease. *N Engl J Med* 1976; 294: 419–422. **77.** Ory HW. The noncontraceptive health benefits from oral contraceptive use. *Fam Plann Perspect* 1982; 14: 182–184. **78.** Ory HW, Forrest JD, Lincoln R. Making choices: Evaluating the health risks and benefits of birth control methods. *New York, The Alan Guttmacher Institute* 1983: p. 1. **79.** Schlesselman J, Stadel BV, Murray P, Lai S. Breast cancer in relation to early use of oral contraceptives. *JAMA* 1988; 259: 1828–1833. **80.** Hennekens CH, Speizer FE, Lipnick RJ, Rosner B, Bain C, Belanger C, Stampfer MJ, Willett W, Peto R. A case-control study of oral contraceptive use and breast cancer. *JNCI* 1984; 72: 39–42. **81.** La Vecchia C, Decarli A, Fasoli M, Franceschi S, Gentile A, Negri E, Parazzini F, Tognoni G. Oral contraceptives and cancers of the breast and of the female genital tract. Interim results from a case-control study. *Br J Cancer* 1986; 54: 311–317. **82.** Meirik O, Lund E, Adami H, Bergstrom R, Christoffersen T, Bergsjo P. Oral contraceptive use and breast cancer in young women. A Joint National Case-control study in Sweden and Norway. *Lancet* 1986; II: 650–654. **83.** Kay CR, Hannaford PC. Breast cancer and the pill—A further report from the Royal College of General Practitioners' oral contraception study. *Br J Cancer* 1988; 58: 675–680. **84.** Stadel BV, Lai S, Schlesselman JJ, Murray P. Oral contraceptives and premenopausal breast cancer in nulliparous women. *Contraception* 1988; 38: 287–299. **85.** Miller DR, Rosenberg L, Kaufman DW, Stolley P, Warshauer ME, Shapiro S. Breast cancer before age 45 and oral contraceptive use: New Findings. *Am J Epidemiol* 1989; 129: 269–280. **86.** The UK National Case-Control Study Group. Oral contraceptive use and breast cancer risk in young women. *Lancet* 1989; 1: 973–982. **87.** Schlesselman JJ. Cancer of the breast and reproductive tract in relation to use of oral contraceptives. *Contraception* 1989; 40: 1–38. **88.** Vessey MP, McPherson K, Villard-Mackintosh L, Yeates D. Oral contraceptives and breast cancer latest findings in a large cohort study. *Br J Cancer* 1989; 59: 613–617. **89.** Jick SS, Walker AM, Stergachis A, Jick H. Oral contraceptives and breast cancer. *Br J Cancer* 1989; 59: 618–621.

BRIEF SUMMARY PATIENT PACKAGE INSERT

Oral contraceptives, also known as "birth control pills" or "the pill," are taken to prevent pregnancy and when taken correctly, have a failure rate of less than 1% per year when used without missing any pills. The typical failure rate of large numbers of pill users is less than 3% per year when women who miss pills are included. For most women oral contraceptives are also free of serious or unpleasant side effects. However, forgetting to take pills considerably increases the chances of pregnancy.

For the majority of women, oral contraceptives can be taken safely. But there are some women who are at high risk of developing certain serious diseases that can be fatal or may cause temporary or permanent disability. The risks associated with taking oral contraceptives increase significantly if you:

- smoke
- have high blood pressure, diabetes, high cholesterol
- have or have had clotting disorders, heart attack, stroke, angina pectoris, cancer of the breast or sex organs, jaundice or malignant or benign liver tumors.

Although cardiovascular disease risks may be increased with oral contraceptive use after age 40 in healthy, non-smoking women (even with the newer low-dose formulations), there are also greater potential health risks associated with pregnancy in older women.

You should not take the pill if you suspect you are pregnant or have unexplained vaginal bleeding.

Cigarette smoking increases the risk of serious cardiovascular side effects from oral contraceptive use. This risk increases with age and with heavy smoking (15 or more cigarettes per day) and is quite marked in women over 35 years of age. Women who use oral contraceptives are strongly advised not to smoke.

Most side effects of the pill are not serious. The most common such effects are nausea, vomiting, bleeding between menstrual periods, weight gain, breast tenderness, and difficulty wearing contact lenses. These side effects, especially nausea and vomiting, may subside within the first three months of use.

The serious side effects of the pill occur very infrequently, especially if you are in good health and are young. However, you should know that the following medical conditions have been associated with or made worse by the pill:

1. Blood clots in the legs (thrombophlebitis), lungs (pulmonary embolism), stoppage or rupture of blood vessel in the brain (stroke), blockage of blood vessels in the heart (heart attack or angina pectoris), or other organs of the body. As mentioned above, smoking increases the risk of heart attacks and strokes and subsequent serious medical consequences.
2. Liver tumors, which may rupture and cause severe bleeding. A possible, but not definite association has also been found with the pill and liver cancer. However, liver cancers are extremely rare. The chance of developing liver cancer from using the pill is thus even rarer.
3. High blood pressure, although blood pressure usually returns to normal when the pill is stopped.

The symptoms associated with these serious side effects are discussed in the detailed leaflet given to you with your supply of pills. Notify your doctor or health care provider if you notice any unusual physical disturbances while taking the pill. In addition, drugs such as rifampin, as well as some anti-convulsants and some antibiotics may decrease oral contraceptive effectiveness. There is conflict among studies regarding breast cancer and oral contraceptive use. Some studies have reported an increase in the risk of developing breast cancer, particularly at a younger age. This increased risk appears to be related to duration of use. The majority of studies have found no overall increase in the risk of developing breast cancer. Some studies have found an increase in the incidence of cancer of the cervix in women who use oral contraceptives. However, this finding may be related to factors other than the use of oral contraceptives. There is insufficient evidence to rule out the possibility pills may cause such cancers.

Taking the combination pill provides some important non-contraceptive benefits. These include less painful menstruation, less menstrual blood loss and anemia, fewer pelvic infections, and fewer cancers of the ovary and the lining of the uterus.

Be sure to discuss any medical condition you may have with your health care provider. Your health care provider will take a medical and family history before prescribing oral contraceptives and will examine you. The physical examination may be delayed to another time if you request it and the health care provider believes that it is a good medical practice to postpone it. You should be reexamined at least once a year while taking oral contraceptives. Your pharmacist should have given you the detailed patient information labeling which gives you further information which you should read and discuss with your health care provider.

This product (like all oral contraceptives) is intended to prevent pregnancy. It does not protect against transmission of HIV (AIDS) and other sexually transmitted diseases such as chlamydia, genital herpes, genital warts, gonorrhea, hepatitis B, and syphilis.

DETAILED PATIENT LABELING

PLEASE NOTE: This labeling is revised from time to time as important new medical information becomes available. Therefore, please review this labeling carefully.

The following oral contraceptive products contain a combination of estrogen and progestogen, the two kinds of female hormones.

Necon® 1/35-21 and Necon® 1/35-28

Each dark yellow tablet contains 1 mg norethindrone and 0.035 mg ethinyl estraidol. Each white tablet in Necon® 1/35-28 contains inert ingredients.

Necon® 0.5/35-21 and Necon® 0.5/35-28

Each light yellow tablet contains 0.5 mg norethindrone and 0.035 mg ethinyl estradiol. Each white tablet in Necon® 0.5/35-28 contains inert ingredients.

Necon® 10/11-21 and Necon® 10/11-28

Each light yellow tablet contains 0.5 mg norethindrone and 0.035 mg ethinyl estradiol. Each dark yellow tablet contains 1 mg norethindrone and 0.035 mg ethinyl estradiol. Each white tablet in Necon® 10/11-28 contains inert ingredients.

Necon® 1/50-21 and Necon® 1/50-28

Each light blue tablet contains 1 mg norethindrone and 0.05 mg mestranol. Each white tablet in Necon® 1/50-28 contains inert ingredients.

INTRODUCTION

Any woman who considers using oral contraceptives (the birth control pill or the pill) should understand the benefits and risks of using this form of birth control. This patient labeling will give you much of the information you will need to make this decision and will also help you determine if you are at risk of developing any of the serious side effects of the pill. It will tell you how to use the pill properly so that it will be as effective as possible. However, this labeling is not a replacement for a careful discussion between you and your health care provider. You should discuss the information provided in this labeling with him or her, both when you first start taking the pill and during your revisits. You should also follow your health care provider's advice with regard to regular check-ups while you are on the pill.

EFFECTIVENESS OF ORAL CONTRACEPTIVES

Oral contraceptives or "birth control pills" or "the pill" are used to prevent pregnancy and are more effective than other non-surgical methods of birth control. When they are taken correctly, the chance of becoming pregnant is less than 1% (1 pregnancy per 100 women per year of use) when used perfectly, without missing any pills. Typical failure rates are actually 3% per year. The chance of becoming pregnant increases with each missed pill during a menstrual cycle.

In comparison, typical failure rates for other non-surgical methods of birth control during the first year of use are as follows:

Implant: < 1%
Injection: <1%
IUD: 1 to 2%
Diaphragm with spermicides: 18%
Spermicides alone: 21%
Vaginal sponge: 18 to 36%
Cervical Cap: 18 to 36%
Condom alone (male): 12%
Condom alone (female): 21%
Periodic abstinence: 20%
No methods: 85%

WHO SHOULD NOT TAKE ORAL CONTRACEPTIVES

Cigarette smoking increases the risk of serious cardiovascular side effects from oral contraceptive use. This risk increases with age and with heavy smoking (15 or more cigarettes per day) and is quite marked in women over 35 years of age. Women who use oral contraceptives are strongly advised not to smoke.

Some women should not use the pill. For example, you should not take the pill if you are pregnant or think you may be pregnant. You should also not use the pill if you have any of the following conditions

- A history of heart attack or stroke
- Blood clots in the legs (thrombophlebitis), lungs (pulmonary embolism), or eyes
- A history of blood clots in the deep veins of your legs
- Chest pain (angina pectoris)
- Known or suspected breast cancer or cancer of the lining of the uterus, cervix, or vagina
- Unexplained vaginal bleeding (until a diagnosis is reached by your doctor)
- Yellowing of the whites of the eyes or of the skin (jaundice) during pregnancy or during previous use of the pill
- Liver tumor (benign or cancerous)
- Known or suspected pregnancy

Tell your health care provider if you have ever had any of these conditions. Your health care provider can recommend a safe method of birth control.

OTHER CONSIDERATIONS BEFORE TAKING ORAL CONTRACEPTIVES

Tell your health care provider if you have or have had:

- Breast nodules, fibrocystic disease of the breast, an abnormal breast x-ray or mammogram
- Diabetes
- Elevated cholesterol or triglycerides
- High blood pressure
- Migraine or other headaches or epilepsy
- Mental depression
- Gallbladder, heart or kidney disease
- History of scanty or irregular menstrual periods

Women with any of these conditions should be checked often by their health care provider if they choose to use oral contraceptives.

Also be sure to inform your doctor or health care provider if you smoke or are on any medications.

FINALLY, IF YOU ARE STILL NOT SURE WHAT TO DO ABOUT THE PILLS YOU HAVE MISSED:

Use a BACK-UP METHOD anytime you have sex. KEEP TAKING ONE "ACTIVE" PILL EACH DAY until you can reach your doctor or clinic.

PREGNANCY DUE TO PILL FAILURE

The incidence of pill failure resulting in pregnancy is approximately one percent (i.e., one pregnancy per 100 women per year) if taken every day as directed, but more typical failure rates are about 3%. If failure does occur, the risk to the fetus is minimal.

PREGNANCY AFTER STOPPING THE PILL

There may be some delay in becoming pregnant after you stop using oral contraceptives, especially if you had irregular menstrual cycles before you used oral contraceptives. It may be advisable to postpone conception until you begin menstruating regularly once you have stopped taking the pill and desire pregnancy.

There does not appear to be any increase in birth defects in newborn babies when pregnancy occurs soon after stopping the pill.

OVERDOSAGE

Serious ill effects have not been reported following ingestion of large doses of oral contraceptives by young children. Overdosage may cause nausea and withdrawal bleeding in females. In case of overdosage, contact your health care provider or pharmacist.

OTHER INFORMATION

Your health care provider will take a medical and family history before prescribing oral contraceptives and will examine you. The physical examination may be delayed to another time if you request it and the health care provider believes that it is a good medical practice to postpone it. You should be reexamined at least once a year. Be sure to inform your health care provider if there is a family history of any of the conditions listed previously in this leaflet. Be sure to keep all appointments with your health care provider, because this is a time to determine if there are early signs of side effects of oral contraceptive use.

Do not use the drug for any condition other than the one for which it was prescribed. This drug has been prescribed specifically for you; do not give it to others who may want birth control pills.

HEALTH BENEFITS FROM ORAL CONTRACEPTIVES

In addition to preventing pregnancy, use of combination oral contraceptives may provide certain benefits. They are:

- menstrual cycles may become more regular
- blood flow during menstruation may be lighter and less iron may be lost. Therefore, anemia due to iron deficiency is less likely to occur.
- pain or other symptoms during menstruation may be encountered less frequently
- ectopic (tubal) pregnancy may occur less frequently
- noncancerous cysts or lumps in the breast may occur less frequently
- acute pelvic inflammatory disease may occur less frequently
- oral contraceptive use may provide some protection against developing two forms of cancer: cancer of the ovaries and cancer of the lining of the uterus.

If you want more information about birth control pills, ask your doctor or pharmacist. They have a more technical leaflet called the Professional Labeling, which you may wish to read. The Professional Labeling is also published in a book entitled Physicians' Desk Reference, available in many book stores and public libraries.

Manufactured by
Watson Laboratories, Inc.
a subsidiary of Watson Pharmaceuticals, Inc.
Corona, CA 92880

Revised: September 30, 1999

Necon® 1/35-21
Necon® 1/35-28
Necon® 0.5/35-21
Necon® 0.5/35-28
Necon® 10/11-21
Necon® 10/11-28
(norethindrone and ethinyl estradiol tablets USP)
Necon® 1/50-21
Necon® 1/50-28
(norethindrone and mestranol tablets USP)

12621-2

GENERAL PRECAUTIONS

1. Missed periods and use of oral contraceptives before or during early pregnancy

There may be times when you may not menstruate regularly after you have completed taking a cycle of pills. If you have taken your pills regularly and miss one menstrual period, continue taking your pills for the next cycle but be sure to inform your health care provider before doing so. If you have not taken the pills daily as instructed and missed a menstrual period, you may be pregnant. If you missed two consecutive menstrual periods and it is 45 days or more from the start of your last menstrual period, you may be pregnant. Check with your health care provider immediately to determine whether you are pregnant. Do not continue to take oral contraceptives until you are sure you are not pregnant, but continue to use another method of contraception.

There is no conclusive evidence that oral contraceptive use is associated with an increase in birth defects, when taken inadvertently during early pregnancy. Previously, a few studies had reported that oral contraceptives might be associated with birth defects, but these findings have not been seen in more recent studies. Nevertheless, oral contraceptives or any other drugs should not be used during pregnancy unless clearly necessary and prescribed by your doctor. You should check with your doctor about risks to your unborn child of any medication taken during pregnancy.

2. While breast feeding

If you are breast feeding, consult your doctor before starting oral contraceptives. Some of the drug will be passed on to the child in the milk. A few adverse effects on the child have been reported, including yellowing of the skin (jaundice) and breast enlargement. In addition, oral contraceptives may decrease the amount and quality of your milk. If possible, do not use oral contraceptives while breast feeding. You should use another method of contraception since breast feeding provides only partial protection from becoming pregnant and this partial protection decreases significantly as you breast feed for longer periods of time. You should consider starting oral contraceptives only after you have weaned your child completely.

3. Laboratory tests

If you are scheduled for any laboratory tests, tell your doctor you are taking birth control pills. Certain blood tests may be affected by birth control pills.

4. Drug interactions

Certain drugs may interact with birth control pills to make them less effective in preventing pregnancy or cause an increase in breakthrough bleeding. Such drugs include rifampin, drugs used for epilepsy such a barbiturates (for example, phenobarbital), anticonvulsants such as carbamazepine (Tegretol is one brand of this drug), phenytoin (Dilantin is one brand of this drug), phenylbutazone (Butazolidin is one brand), and possibly certain antibiotics. You may need to use additional contraception when you take drugs which can make oral contraceptives less effective.

5. Sexually transmitted diseases

This product (like all oral contraceptives) is intended to prevent pregnancy. It does not protect against transmission of HIV (AIDS) and other sexually transmitted diseases such as chlamydia, genital herpes, genital warts, gonorrhea, hepatitis B, and syphilis.

HOW TO TAKE THE PILL

IMPORTANT POINTS TO REMEMBER

BEFORE YOU START TAKING THE PILLS:

1. BE SURE TO READ THESE DIRECTIONS:
   Before you start taking your pills.
   Anytime you are not sure what to do.
2. THE RIGHT WAY TO TAKE THE PILL IS TO TAKE ONE PILL EVERY DAY AT THE SAME TIME.
   If you miss pills you could get pregnant. This includes starting the dispenser late. The more pills you miss, the more likely you are to get pregnant.
3. MANY WOMEN HAVE SPOTTING OR LIGHT BLEEDING, OR MAY FEEL SICK TO THEIR STOMACH DURING THE FIRST 1–3 DISPENSERS OF PILLS. If you feel sick to your stomach, do not stop taking the pill. The problem will usually go away. If it doesn't go away, check with your doctor or clinic.
4. MISSING PILLS CAN ALSO CAUSE SPOTTING OR LIGHT BLEEDING, even when you make up these missed pills.
   On the days you take 2 pills to make up for missed pills you could also feel a little sick to your stomach.
5. IF YOU HAVE VOMITING OR DIARRHEA, for any reason, or IF YOU TAKE SOME MEDICATION, including some antibiotics, your pills may not work as well. Use a back-up method (such as condoms, foam, or sponge) until you check with your doctor or clinic.
6. IF YOU HAVE TROUBLE REMEMBERING TO TAKE THE PILL, talk to your doctor or clinic about how to make pill-taking easier or about using another method of birth control.
7. IF YOU HAVE ANY QUESTIONS OR ARE UNSURE ABOUT THE INFORMATION IN THIS LEAFLET, call your doctor or clinic.

BEFORE YOU START TAKING YOUR PILLS

1. DECIDE WHAT TIME OF DAY YOU WANT TO TAKE YOUR PILL. It is important to take it at about the same time every day.
2. LOOK AT YOUR PILL DISPENSER TO SEE IF IT HAS 21 OR 28 PILLS.
   The 21-pill dispenser has 21 "active" pills (with hormones) to take for 3 weeks. This is followed by 1 week without pills.
   The 28-pill dispenser has 21 "active" pills (with hormones) to take for 3 weeks. This is followed by 1 week of reminder white pills (without hormones).
   Necon® 10/11: There are 10 light yellow "active" pills and 11 dark yellow "active" pills
   Necon® 1/35: There are 21 dark yellow "active" pills.
   Necon® 0.5/35: There are 21 light yellow "active" pills.
   Necon® 1/50: There are 21 light blue "active" pills.
3. ALSO FIND:
   1) where on the dispenser to start taking pills,
   2) in what order to take the pills
   CHECK ADDITIONAL INSTRUCTIONS FOR USING THIS DISPENSER IN THE BRIEF SUMMARY PATIENT PACKAGE INSERT.
4. BE SURE YOU HAVE READY AT ALL TIMES ANOTHER KIND OF BIRTH CONTROL (such as condoms, foam or sponge) to use as a back-up in case you miss pills. AN EXTRA, FULL PILL DISPENSER.

WHEN TO START THE FIRST DISPENSER OF PILLS:

You have a choice of which day to start taking your first dispenser of pills. Decide with your doctor or clinic which is the best day for you. Pick a time of day which will be easy to remember.

SUNDAY START:

Necon® 10/11: Take the first "active" light yellow pill of the first dispenser on the Sunday after your period starts, even if you are still bleeding. If your period begins on Sunday, start the dispenser the same day.

Necon® 1/35: Take the first "active" dark yellow pill of the first dispenser on the Sunday after your period starts, even if you are still bleeding. If your period begins on Sunday, start the dispenser the same day.

Necon® 0.5/35: Take the first "active" light yellow pill of the first dispenser on the Sunday after your period starts, even if you are still bleeding. If your period begins on Sunday, start the dispenser the same day.

Necon® 1/50: Take the first "active" light blue pill of the first dispenser on the Sunday after your period starts, even if you are still bleeding. If your period begins on Sunday, start the dispenser the same day.

Use another method of birth control as back-up method if you have sex anytime from the Sunday you start your first dispenser until the next Sunday (7 days). Condoms, foam, or the sponge are good back-up methods of birth control.

DAY 1 START:

Necon® 10/11: Take the first "active" light yellow pill of the first dispenser during the first 24 hours of your period.

Necon® 1/35: Take the first "active" dark yellow pill of the first dispenser during the first 24 hours of your period.

Necon® 0.5/35: Take the first "active" light yellow pill of the first dispenser during the first 24 hours of your period.

Necon® 1/50: Take the first "active" light blue pill of the first dispenser during the first 24 hours of your period.

You will not need to use a back-up method of birth control, since you are starting the pill at the beginning of your period.

WHAT TO DO DURING THE MONTH:

1. **TAKE ONE PILL AT THE SAME TIME EVERY DAY UNTIL THE DISPENSER IS EMPTY.**
   Do not skip pills even if you are spotting or bleeding between monthly periods or feel sick to your stomach (nausea).
   Do not skip pills even if you do not have sex very often.
2. **WHEN YOU FINISH A DISPENSER OR SWITCH YOUR BRAND OF PILLS:**
   21 pills: Wait 7 days to start the next dispenser. You will probably have your period during that week. Be sure that no more than 7 days pass betwen 21-day dispensers.
   28 pills: Start the next dispenser on the day after your last "reminder" pill. Do not wait any days between dispensers.

WHAT TO DO IF YOU MISS PILLS:

Necon® 10/11:

If you MISS 1 light yellow or dark yellow "active" pill:

1. Take it as soon as you remember. Take the next pill at your regular time. This means you may take 2 pills in 1 day.
2. You do not need to use a back-up birth control method if you have sex.

If you MISS 2 light yellow or dark yellow "active" pills in a row in WEEK 1 or WEEK 2 of your dispenser:

1. Take 2 pills on the day you remember and 2 pills the next day.
2. Then take 1 pill a day until you finish the dispenser.
3. You MAY BECOME PREGNANT if you have sex in the 7 days after you miss pills. You MUST use another birth control method (such as condoms, foam, or sponge) as a back-up method for those 7 days.

If you MISS 2 dark yellow "active" pills in a row in THE 3RD WEEK:

1. **If you are a Sunday Starter:**
   Keep taking 1 pill every day until Sunday. On Sunday, THROW OUT the rest of the dispenser and start a new dispenser of pills that same day.
   If you are a Day 1 Starter:
   THROW OUT the rest of the pill dispenser and start a new dispenser that same day.
2. You may not have your period this month but this is expected. However, if you miss your period 2 months in a row, call your doctor or clinic because you might be pregnant.

Continued on next page

Necon—Cont.

3. You MAY BECOME PREGNANT if you have sex in the 7 days after you miss pills. You MUST use another birth control method (such as condoms, foam, or sponge) as a back-up method for those 7 days.

If you MISS 3 OR MORE light yellow or dark yellow "active" pills in a row (during the first 3 weeks):

1. **If you are a Sunday Starter:**
   Keep taking 1 pill every day until Sunday. On Sunday, THROW OUT the rest of the dispenser and start a new dispenser of pills that same day.
   If you are a Day 1 Starter:
   THROW OUT the rest of the pill dispenser and start a new dispenser of pills that same day.
2. You may not have your period this month but this is expected. However, if you miss your period 2 months in a row, call your doctor or clinic because you might be pregnant.
3. You MAY BECOME PREGNANT if you have sex in the 7 days after you miss pills. You MUST use another birth control method (such as condoms, foam, or sponge) as a back-up method for those 7 days.

Necon® 1/35:

If you MISS 1 dark yellow "active" pill:

1. Take it as soon as you remember. Take the next pill at your regular time. This means you may take 2 pills in 1 day.
2. You do not need to use a back-up birth control method if you have sex.

If you MISS 2 dark yellow "active" pills in a row in WEEK 1 or WEEK 2 of your dispenser:

1. Take 2 pills on the day you remember and 2 pills the next day.
2. Then take 1 pill a day until you finish the dispenser.
3. You MAY BECOME PREGNANT if you have sex in the 7 days after you miss pills. You MUST use another birth control method (such as condoms, foam, or sponge) as a back-up method for those 7 days.

If you MISS 2 dark yellow "active" pills in a row in THE 3RD WEEK:

1. **If you are a Sunday Starter:**
   Keep taking 1 pill every day until Sunday. On Sunday, THROW OUT the rest of the dispenser and start a new dispenser of pills that same day.
   If you are a Day 1 Starter:
   THROW OUT the rest of the pill dispenser and start a new dispenser that same day.
2. You may not have your period this month but this is expected. However, if you miss your period 2 months in a row, call your doctor or clinic because you might be pregnant.
3. You MAY BECOME PREGNANT if you have sex in the 7 days after you miss pills. You MUST use another birth control method (such as condoms, foam, or sponge) as a back-up method for those 7 days.

If you MISS 3 OR MORE dark yellow "active" pills in a row (during the first 3 weeks):

1. **If you are a Sunday Starter:**
   Keep taking 1 pill every day until Sunday. On Sunday, THROW OUT the rest of the dispenser and start a new dispenser of pills that same day.
   If you are a Day 1 Starter:
   THROW OUT the rest of the pill dispenser and start a new dispenser of pills that same day.
2. You may not have your period this month but this is expected. However, if you miss your period 2 months in a row, call your doctor or clinic because you might be pregnant.
3. You MAY BECOME PREGNANT if you have sex in the 7 days after you miss pills. You MUST use another birth control method (such as condoms, foam, or sponge) as a back-up method for those 7 days.

Necon® 0.5/35:

If you MISS 1 light yellow "active" pill:

1. Take it as soon as you remember. Take the next pill at your regular time. This means you may take 2 pills in 1 day.
2. You do not need to use a back-up birth control method if you have sex.

If you MISS light yellow "active" pills in a row in WEEK 1 or WEEK 2 of your dispenser:

1. Take 2 pills on the day you remember and 2 pills the next day.
2. Then take 1 pill a day until you finish the dispenser.
3. You MAY BECOME PREGNANT if you have sex in the 7 days after you miss pills. You MUST use another birth control method (such as condoms, foam, or sponge) as a back-up method for those 7 days.

If you MISS 2 light yellow "active" pills in a row in THE 3RD WEEK:

1. **If you are a Sunday Starter:**
   Keep taking 1 pill every day until Sunday. On Sunday, THROW OUT the rest of the dispenser and start a new dispenser of pills that same day.
   If you are a Day 1 Starter:
   THROW OUT the rest of the pill dispenser and start a new dispenser that same day.
2. You may not have your period this month but this is expected. However, if you miss your period 2 months in a row, call your doctor or clinic because you might be pregnant.

ANNUAL NUMBER OF BIRTH-RELATED OR METHOD-RELATED DEATHS ASSOCIATED WITH CONTROL OF FERTILITY PER 100,000 NONSTERILE WOMEN, BY FERTILITY CONTROL METHOD ACCORDING TO AGE.

Method of control and outcome	15-19	20-24	25-29	30-34	35-39	40-44
No fertility control methods*	7.0	7.4	9.1	14.8	25.7	28.2
Oral contraceptives non-smoker**	0.3	0.5	0.9	1.9	13.8	31.6
Oral contraceptives smoker**	2.2	3.4	6.6	13.5	51.1	117.2
IUD**	0.8	0.8	1.0	1.0	1.4	1.4
Condom*	1.1	1.6	0.7	0.2	0.3	0.4
Diaphragm/spermicide*	1.9	1.2	1.2	1.3	2.2	2.8
Periodic abstinence*	2.5	1.6	1.6	1.7	2.9	3.6

* Deaths are birth-related
**Deaths are method-related
Adapted from H.W. Ory, ref. #35

3. You MAY BECOME PREGNANT if you have sex in the 7 days after you miss pills. You MUST use another birth control method (such as condoms, foam, or sponge) as a back-up method for those 7 days.

If you MISS 3 OR MORE light yellow "active" pills in a row (during the first 3 weeks):

1. **If you are a Sunday Starter:**
   Keep taking 1 pill every day until Sunday. On Sunday, THROW OUT the rest of the dispenser and start a new dispenser of pills that same day.
   If you are a Day 1 Starter:
   THROW OUT the rest of the pill dispenser and start a new dispenser of pills that same day.
2. You may not have your period this month but this is expected. However, if you miss your period 2 months in a row, call your doctor or clinic because you might be pregnant.
3. You MAY BECOME PREGNANT if you have sex in the 7 days after you miss pills. You MUST use another birth control method (such as condoms, foam, or sponge) as a back-up method for those 7 days.

Necon® 1/50:

If you MISS 1 light blue "active" pill:

1. Take it as soon as you remember. Take the next pill at your regular time. This means you may take 2 pills in 1 day.
2. You do not need to use a back-up birth control method if you have sex.

If you MISS 2 light blue "active" pills in a row in WEEK 1 or WEEK 2 of your dispenser:

1. Take 2 pills on the day you remember and 2 pills the next day.
2. Then take 1 pill a day until you finish the dispenser.
3. You MAY BECOME PREGNANT if you have sex in the 7 days after you miss pills. You MUST use another birth control method (such as condoms, foam, or sponge) as a back-up method for those 7 days.

If you MISS 2 light blue "active" pills in a row in THE 3RD WEEK:

1. **If you are a Sunday Starter:**
   Keep taking 1 pill every day until Sunday. On Sunday, THROW OUT the rest of the dispenser and start a new dispenser of pills that same day.
   If you are a Day 1 Starter:
   THROW OUT the rest of the pill dispenser and start a new dispenser that same day.
2. You may not have your period this month but this is expected. However, if you miss your period 2 months in a row, call your doctor or clinic because you might be pregnant.
3. You MAY BECOME PREGNANT if you have sex in the 7 days after you miss pills. You MUST use another birth control method (such as condoms, foam, or sponge) as a back-up method for those 7 days.

If you MISS 3 OR MORE light blue "active" pills in a row (during the first 3 weeks):

1. **If you are a Sunday Starter:**
   Keep taking 1 pill every day until Sunday. On Sunday, THROW OUT the rest of the dispenser and start a new dispenser of pills that same day.
   If you are a Day 1 Starter:
   THROW OUT the rest of the pill dispenser and start a new dispenser of pills that same day.
2. You may not have your period this month but this is expected. However, if you miss your period 2 months in a row, call your doctor or clinic because you might be pregnant.
3. You MAY BECOME PREGNANT if you have sex in the 7 days after you miss pills. You MUST use another birth control method (such as condoms, foam, or sponge) as a back-up method for those 7 days.

A REMINDER FOR THOSE ON 28-DAY DISPENSERS

If you forget any of the 7 white "reminder" pills in Week 4:
THROW AWAY the pills you missed.
Keep taking 1 pill each day until the dispenser is empty.
You do not need a back-up method.

RISKS OF TAKING ORAL CONTRACEPTIVES

1. Risk of developing blood clots

Blood clots and blockage of blood vessels are one of the most serious side effects of taking oral contraceptives and can cause death or serious disability. In particular, a clot in the leg can cause thrombophlebitis and a clot that travels to the lungs can cause a sudden blocking of the vessel carrying blood to the lungs. Rarely, clots occur in the blood vessels of the eye and may cause blindness, double vision, or impaired vision.

If you take oral contraceptives and need elective surgery, need to stay in bed for a prolonged illness or have recently delivered a baby, you may be at risk of developing blood clots. You should consult your doctor about stopping oral contraceptives three to four weeks before surgery and not taking oral contraceptives for two weeks after surgery or during bed rest. You should also not take oral contraceptives soon after delivery of a baby. It is advisable to wait for at least four weeks after delivery if you are breast feeding or four weeks after a second trimester abortion. If you are breast feeding, you should wait until you have weaned your child before using the pill. (See also the section on Breast Feeding in General Precautions.)

The risk of circulatory disease in oral contraceptive users may be higher in users of high-dose pills and may be greater with longer duration of oral contraceptive use. In addition, some of these increased risks may continue for a number of years after stopping oral contraceptives. The risk of abnormal blood clotting increases with age in both users and nonusers of oral contraceptives, but the increased risk from the oral contraceptive appears to be present at all ages. For women aged 20 to 44, it is estimated that about 1 in 2,000 using oral contraceptives will be hospitalized each year because of abnormal clotting. Among nonusers in the same age group, about 1 in 20,000 would be hospitalized each year. For oral contraceptive users in general, it has been estimated that in women between the ages of 15 and 34 the risk of death due to a circulatory disorder is about 1 in 12,000 per year, whereas for nonusers the rate is about 1 in 50,000 per year. In the age group 35 to 44, the risk is estimated to be about 1 in 2,500 per year for oral contraceptive users and about 1 in 10,000 per year for nonusers.

2. Heart attacks and strokes

Oral contraceptives may increase the tendency to develop strokes (stoppage or rupture of blood vessels in the brain) and angina pectoris and heart attacks (blockage of blood vessels in the heart). Any of these conditions can cause death or serious disability.

Smoking greatly increases the possibility of suffering heart attacks and strokes. Furthermore, smoking and the use of oral contraceptives greatly increases the chances of developing and dying of heart disease.

3. Gallbladder disease

Oral contraceptive users probably have a greater risk than nonusers of having gallbladder disease, although this risk may be related to pills containing high doses of estrogens.

4. Liver tumors

In rare cases, oral contraceptives can cause benign but dangerous liver tumors. These benign liver tumors can rupture and cause fatal internal bleeding. In addition, a possible but not definite association has been found with the pill and liver cancers in two studies, in which a few women who developed these very rare cancers were found to have used oral contraceptives for long periods. However, liver cancers are rare.

5. Cancer of the reproductive organs and breasts

There is conflict among studies regarding breast cancer and oral contraceptive use. Some studies have reported an increase in the risk of developing breast cancer, particularly at a younger age. This increased risk appears to be related to duration of use. The majority of studies have found no overall increase in the risk of developing breast cancer. Some studies have found an increase in the incidence of cancer of the cervix in women who use oral contraceptives. However, this finding may be related to factors other than the use of oral contraceptives. There is insufficient evidence to rule out the possibility that pills may cause such cancers.

ESTIMATED RISK OF DEATH FROM A BIRTH CONTROL METHOD OR PREGNANCY

All methods of birth control and pregnancy are associated with a risk of developing certain diseases that may lead to disability or death. An estimate of the number of deaths associated with different methods of birth control and pregnancy has been calculated and is shown in the following table:
[See table above]

In the above table, the risk of death from any birth control method is less than the risk of childbirth, except for oral contraceptive users over the age of 35 who smoke and pill users over the age of 40 even if they do not smoke. It can be seen in the table that for women aged 15 to 39, the risk of death was highest with pregnancy (7–26 deaths per 100,000 women, depending on age). Among pill users who do not smoke, the risk of death was always lower than that associated with pregnancy for any age group, although over the age of 40, the risk increases to 32 deaths per 100,000 women, compared to 28 associated with pregnancy at that age. However, for pill users who smoke and are over the age of 35, the estimated number of deaths exceeds those for other methods of birth control. If a woman is over the age of 40 and smokes, her estimated risk of death is four times higher (117/100,000 women) than the estimated risk associated with pregnancy (28/100,000) in that age group.

The suggestion that women over 40 who do not smoke should not take oral contraceptives is based on information from older, higher dose pills. An Advisory Committee of the FDA discussed this issue in 1989 and recommended that the benefits of low-dose oral contraceptive use by healthy, non-smoking women over 40 years of age may outweigh the possible risks.

WARNING SIGNALS

If any of these adverse effects occur while you are taking oral contraceptives, call your doctor immediately:

- Sharp chest pain, coughing of blood, or sudden shortness of breath (indicating a possible clot in the lung)
- Pain in the calf (indicating a possible clot in the leg)
- Crushing chest pain or heaviness in the chest (indicating a possible heart attack)
- Sudden severe headache or vomiting, dizziness or fainting, disturbances of vision or speech, weakness, or numbness in an arm or leg (indicating a possible stroke)
- Sudden partial or complete loss of vision (indicating a possible clot in the eye)
- Breast lumps (indicating possible breast cancer or fibrocystic disease of the breast; ask your doctor or health care provider to show you how to examine your breasts)
- Severe pain or tenderness in the stomach area (indicating a possible ruptured liver tumor)
- Difficulty in sleeping, weakness, lack of energy, fatigue, or change in mood (possibly indicating severe depression)
- Jaundice or a yellowing of the skin or eyeballs, accompanied frequently by fever, fatigue, loss of appetite, dark-colored urine, or light-colored bowel movements (indicating possible liver problems)

SIDE EFFECTS OF ORAL CONTRACEPTIVES

1. Vaginal bleeding

Irregular vaginal bleeding or spotting may occur while you are taking the pills. Irregular bleeding may vary from slight staining between menstrual periods to breakthrough bleeding which is a flow much like a regular period. Irregular bleeding occurs most often during the first few months of oral contraceptive use, but may also occur after you have been taking the pill for some time. Such bleeding may be temporary and usually does not indicate any serious problems. It is important to continue taking your pills on schedule. If the bleeding occurs in more than one cycle or lasts for more than a few days, talk to your doctor or health care provider.

2. Contact lenses

If you wear contact lenses and notice a change in vision or an inability to wear you lenses, contact your doctor or health care provider.

3. Fluid retention

Oral contraceptives may cause edema (fluid retention) with swelling of the fingers or ankles and may raise your blood pressure. If you experience fluid retention, contact your doctor or health care provider.

4. Melasma

A spotty darkening of the skin is possible, particularly of the face, which may persist.

5. Other side effects

Other side effects may include nausea and vomiting, change in appetite, headache, nervousness, depression, dizziness, loss of scalp hair, rash, and vaginal infections. If any of these side effects bother you, call your doctor or health care provider.

Shown in Product Identification Guide, page 340

NOR-QD® Tablets ℞
(norethindrone 0.35 mg)
Part Number: 13536

PHYSICIAN LABELING

Patients should be counseled that this product does not protect against HIV infection (AIDS) and other sexually transmitted diseases.

DESCRIPTION

Each yellow NOR-QD® tablet provides a continuous oral contraceptive regimen of 0.35 mg norethindrone daily, and the inactive ingredients include D&C Yellow No. 10, FD&C Yellow No. 6, lactose, magnesium stearate, povidone, and starch.

The chemical name for norethindrone is 17-Hydroxy-19-Nor-17α-pregn-4-en-20-yn-3-one. The structural formula follows:

[See chemical structure at top of next column]

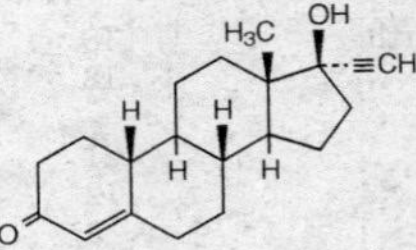

norethindrone

Therapeutic class = oral contraceptive.

CLINICAL PHARMACOLOGY

1. Mode of Action. NOR-QD® progestin-only oral contraceptives prevent conception by suppressing ovulation in approximately half of users, thickening the cervical mucus to inhibit sperm penetration, lowering the midcycle LH and FSH peaks, slowing the movement of the ovum through the fallopian tubes, and altering the endometrium.

2. Pharmacokinetics. Serum progestin levels peak about two hours after oral administration, followed by rapid distribution and elimination. By 24 hours after drug ingestion, serum levels are near baseline, making efficacy dependent upon rigid adherence to the dosing schedule. There are large variations in serum levels among individual users. Progestin-only administration results in lower steady-state serum progestin levels and a shorter elimination half-life than concomitant administration with estrogens.

INDICATIONS AND USAGE

1. Indications. Progestin-only oral contraceptives are indicated for the prevention of pregnancy.

2. Efficacy. If used perfectly, the first-year failure rate for progestin-only oral contraceptives is 0.5%. However, the typical failure rate is estimated to be closer to 5%, due to late or omitted pills. The following table lists the pregnancy rates for users of all major methods of contraception.

Table 1.
Comparison of reversible contraceptive methods:
Percent of women experiencing a contraceptive failure (pregnancy) during the first year of use.

Method	Percent of women experiencing a pregnancy within the first year of use Average Use	Perfect Use
No contraception	85	85
Spermicides	21	6
Periodic abstinence	20	1–9[1]
Withdrawal	19	4
Cervical caps		
Given birth	36	26
Never given birth	18	9
Diaphragms	18	6
Condoms		
Female	21	5
Male	12	3
Pills	3	
Progestin-only		0.5
Combined		0.1
IUDs		
Progesterone	2	1.5
Copper T 380A	0.8	0.6
Injectables	0.3	0.3
Implant	0.09	0.09

Adapted with permission.[2]

1. Depending on method (calendar, ovulation, symptom-thermal, post-ovulation)
2. Hatcher RA, Trussel J, Stewart F, Stewart GK, Kowal D, Guest F, Cates W, Pollcar M. Contraceptive Technology 1994-1996, New York, NY: Irvington Publishers, 1994.

CONTRAINDICATIONS

Progestin-only oral contraceptives should not be used by women who currently have the following conditions:

- Known or suspected pregnancy
- Known or suspected carcinoma of the breast
- Undiagnosed abnormal genital bleeding
- Hypersensitivity to any component of this product
- Benign or malignant liver tumors
- Acute liver disease

WARNINGS

Cigarette smoking greatly increases the possibility of suffering heart attacks and strokes. Women who use oral contraceptives are strongly advised not to smoke.

Nor-QD does not contain estrogen and, therefore, this insert does not discuss the serious health risks that have been associated with the estrogen component of combined oral contraceptives. The health care provider is referred to the prescribing information of combined oral contraceptives for a discussion of those risks, including, but not limited to, an increased risk of serious cardiovascular disease in women who smoke, carcinoma of the breast and reproductive organs, hepatic neoplasia, and changes in carbohydrates and lipid metabolism. The relationship between progestin-only oral contraceptives and these risks have not been established and there are no studies definitely linking progestin-only pill (POP) use to an increased risk of heart attack or stroke.

The physician should remain alert to the earliest manifestation of symptoms of any serious disease and discontinue oral contraceptive therapy when appropriate.

1. Ectopic pregnancy. The incidence of ectopic pregnancies for progestin-only oral contraceptive users is 5 per 1000 woman-years. Up to 10% of pregnancies reported in clinical studies of progestin-only oral contraceptive users are extra-uterine. Although symptoms of ectopic pregnancy should be watched for, a history of ectopic pregnancy need not be considered a contraindication to use of this contraceptive method. Health providers should be alert to the possibility of an ectopic pregnancy in women who become pregnant or complain of lower abdominal pain while on progestin-only oral contraceptives.

2. Delayed follicular atresia/Ovarian cysts. If follicular development occurs, atresia of the follicle is sometimes delayed, and the follicle may continue to grow beyond the size it would attain in a normal cycle. Generally these enlarged follicles disappear spontaneously. Often they are asymptomatic; in some cases they are associated with mild abdominal pain. Rarely they may twist or rupture, requiring surgical intervention.

3. Irregular genital bleeding. Irregular menstrual patterns are common among women using progestin-only oral contraceptives. If genital bleeding is suggestive of infection, malignancy or other abnormal conditions, such nonpharmacologic causes should be ruled out. If prolonged amenorrhea occurs, the possibility of pregnancy should be evaluated.

4. Carcinoma of the breast and reproductive organs. Some epidemiologic studies of oral contraceptive users have reported an increased relative risk of developing breast cancer, particularly at a younger age and apparently related to duration of use. These studies have predominantly involved combined oral contraceptives and there is insufficient data to determine whether the use of POPs similarly increases the risk. Women with breast cancer should not use oral contraceptives because the role of female hormones in breast cancer has not been fully determined.

Some studies suggest that oral contraceptive use has been associated with an increase in the risk of cervical intraepithelial neoplasia in some populations of women. However, there continues to be controversy about the extent to which such findings may be due to differences in sexual behavior and other factors. There is insufficient data to determine whether the use of POPs increases the risk of developing cervical intraepithelial neoplasia.

5. Hepatic neoplasia. Benign hepatic adenomas are associated with combined oral contraceptive use, although the incidence of benign tumors is rare in the United States. Rupture of benign, hepatic adenomas may cause death through intraabdominal hemorrhage.

Studies from Britain and the U.S. have shown an increased risk of developing hepatocellular carcinoma in combined oral contraceptive users. However, these cancers are rare. There is insufficient data to determine whether POPs increase the risk of developing hepatic neoplasia.

PRECAUTIONS

1. General. Patients should be counseled that this product does not protect against HIV infection (AIDS) and other sexually transmitted diseases.

2. Physical examination and followup. It is considered good medical practice for sexually active women using oral contraceptives to have annual history and physical examinations. The physical examination may be deferred until after initiation of oral contraceptives if requested by the woman and judged appropriate by the clinician.

3. Carbohydrates and lipid metabolism. Some users may experience slight deterioration in glucose tolerance, with increases in plasma insulin but women with diabetes mellitus who use progestin-only oral contraceptives do not generally experience changes in their insulin requirements. Nonetheless, prediabetic and diabetic women in particular should be carefully monitored while taking POPs.

Lipid metabolism is occasionally affected in that HDL, HDL_2, and apolipoprotein A-I and A-II may be decreased; hepatic lipase may be increased. There is no effect on total cholesterol, HDL_3, LDL, or VLDL.

4. Drug interactions. The effectiveness of progestin-only pills is reduced by hepatic enzyme-inducing drugs such as the anticonvulsants phenytoin, carbamazepine, and barbiturates, and the antituberculosis drug rifampin. No significant interaction has been found with broad-spectrum antibiotics.

5. Interactions with laboratory tests. The following endocrine tests may be affected by progestin-only oral contraceptive use:

- Sex hormone-binding globulin (SHBG) concentrations may be decreased.
- Thyroxine concentrations may be decreased, due to a decrease in thyroid binding globulin (TBG).

6. Carcinogenesis. See **WARNINGS** section.

7. Pregnancy. Many studies have found no effects on fetal development associated with long-term use of contraceptive doses of oral progestins. The few studies of infant growth and development that have been conducted have not demonstrated significant adverse effects. It is nonetheless prudent to rule out suspected pregnancy before initiating any hormonal contraceptive use.

8. Nursing mothers. No adverse effects have been found on breastfeeding performance or on the health, growth or development of the infant. Small amounts of progestin pass into the breast milk, resulting in steroid levels in infant plasma of 1–6% of the levels of maternal plasma.

9. Fertility following discontinuation: The limited available data indicate a rapid return of normal ovulation and

Continued on next page

Nor-QD—Cont.

fertility following discontinuation of progestin-only oral contraceptives.

10. Headache. The onset or exacerbation of migraine or the development of severe headache with focal neurological symptoms which is recurrent or persistent requires discontinuation of progestin-only contraceptives and evaluation of the cause.

11. Pediatric use. Safety and efficacy of Nor-QD have been established in women of reproductive age. Safety and efficacy are expected to be the same for postpubertal adolescents under the age of 16 and for users 16 years and older. Use of this product before menarche is not indicated.

INFORMATION FOR THE PATIENT

1. See **PATIENT LABELING** for detailed information.
2. **Counseling issues.** The following points should be discussed with prospective users before prescribing progestin-only oral contraceptives.

- The necessity of taking pills at the same time every day, including throughout all bleeding episodes.
- The need to use a backup method such as condoms and spermicides for the next 48 hours whenever a progestin-only contraceptive is taken 3 or more hours late.
- The potential side effects of progestin-only oral contraceptives, particularly menstrual irregularities.
- The need to inform the clinician of prolonged episodes of bleeding, amenorrhea or severe abdominal pain.
- The importance of using a barrier method in addition to progestin-only oral contraceptives if a woman is at risk of contracting or transmitting STDs/HIV.

ADVERSE REACTIONS

- Menstrual irregularity is the most frequently reported side effect.
- Frequent and irregular bleeding are common, while long duration of bleeding episodes and amenorrhea are less likely.
- Headache, breast tenderness, nausea, and dizziness are increased among progestin-only oral contraceptive users in some studies.
- Androgenic side effects such as acne, hirsutism, and weight gain occur rarely.

OVERDOSAGE

There have been no reports of serious ill effects from overdosage, including ingestion by children.

DOSAGE AND ADMINISTRATION

To achieve maximum contraceptive effectiveness, NOR-QD® must be taken exactly as directed. One tablet is taken every day, at the same time. Administration is continuous, with no interruption between pill packs. See **PATIENT LABELING** for detailed instructions.

HOW SUPPLIED

NOR-QD® (norethindrone) tablets are available in 28-tablet dispensers.

Rx only

STORAGE

Store at controlled room temperature 15°–25°C (59°–77°F).

REFERENCE

McCann M, and Potter L. Progestin-Only Oral Contraceptives: A Comprehensive Review. Contraception, 50:60 (Suppl. 1), December 1994.

DETAILED INFORMATION FOR THE PATIENT

This product (like all oral contraceptives) is used to prevent pregnancy. It does not protect against HIV infection (AIDS) and other sexually transmitted diseases.

INTRODUCTION

This leaflet is about birth control pills that contain one hormone, a progestin. Please read this leaflet before you begin to take your pills. It is meant to be used along with talking with your doctor or clinic.

Progestin-only pills are often called "POPs" or "the minipill." POPs have less progestin than the combined birth control pill (or "the pill") which contains both an estrogen and a progestin.

HOW EFFECTIVE ARE POPS?

About 1 in 200 POPs users will get pregnant in the first year if they all take POPs perfectly (that is, on time, every day). About 1 in 20 "typical" POPs users (including women who are late taking pills or miss pills) gets pregnant in the first year of use. The following table will help you compare the efficacy of different methods.

Table 1.

Comparison of reversible contraceptive methods: Percent of women who become pregnant during the first year of use.

Method	Percent of women experiencing a pregnancy within the first year of use: Average Use	Perfect Use
No contraception	85	85
Spermicides	21	6
Periodic abstinence	20	1–9[1]
Withdrawal	19	4
Cervical caps		
Given birth	36	26
Never given birth	18	9
Diaphragms	18	6
Condoms		
Female	21	5
Male	12	3
Pills	3	
POPs		0.5
Combined pills		0.1
IUDs		
Progesterone	2	1.5
Copper T 380A	0.8	0.6
Injectables	0.3	0.3
Implant	0.09	0.09

Adapted with permission.[2]

1. Depending on method (calendar, ovulation, symptom-thermal, post-ovulation)
2. Hatcher RA, Trussel J, Stewart F, Stewart GK, Kowal D, Guest F, Cates W, Pollcar M. Contraceptive Technology 1994-1996. New York, NY: Irvington Publishers, 1994.

HOW DO POPS WORK?

- They make the cervical mucus at the entrance to the womb (the uterus) too thick for the sperm to get through to the egg.
- They prevent ovulation (release of the egg from the ovary) in about half the time.
- They also affect other hormones, the fallopian tubes and the lining of the uterus.

YOU SHOULD NOT TAKE POPS

- If there is any chance you may be pregnant.
- If you have breast cancer.
- If you have bleeding between your periods which has not been diagnosed.
- If you are taking certain drugs for epilepsy (seizures) or for TB. (See **USING POPS WITH OTHER MEDICINES** below.)
- If you are hypersensitive or allergic to any component of this product.
- If you have liver tumors, either benign or cancerous.
- If you have acute liver disease.

RISKS OF TAKING POPS

WARNING: If you have sudden or severe pain in your lower abdomen or stomach area, you may have an ectopic pregnancy or an ovarian cyst. If this happens, you should contact your doctor or clinic immediately.

1. Ectopic pregnancy. An ectopic pregnancy is a pregnancy outside the womb. Because POPs protect against pregnancy, the chance of having a pregnancy outside the womb is very low. If you do get pregnant while taking POPs, you have a slightly higher chance that the pregnancy will be ectopic than do users of some other birth control methods.

2. Ovarian cysts. These cysts are small sacs of fluid in the ovary. They are more common among POP users than among users of most other birth control methods. They usually disappear without treatment and rarely cause problems.

3. Cancer of the reproductive organs and breasts. Some studies in women who use combined oral contraceptives that contain both estrogen and a progestin have reported an increase in the risk of developing breast cancer, particularly at a younger age and apparently related to duration of use. There is insufficient data to determine whether the use of POPs similarly increases this risk.

Some studies have found an increase in the incidence of cancer of the cervix in women who use oral contraceptives. However, this finding may be related to factors other than the use of oral contraceptives and there is insufficient data to determine whether the use of POPs increases the risk of developing cancer of the cervix.

4. Liver tumors. In rare cases, combined oral contraceptives can cause benign but dangerous liver tumors. These benign liver tumors can rupture and cause fatal internal bleeding. In addition, a possible but not definite association has been found with combined oral contraceptives and liver cancers in studies in which a few women who developed these very rare cancers were found to have used combined oral contraceptives for long periods of time. There is insufficient data to determine whether POPs increase the risk of liver tumors.

SEXUALLY-TRANSMITTED DISEASES (STDS)

WARNING: POPs do not protect against getting or giving someone HIV (AIDS) or any other STD, such as chlamydia, gonorrhea, genital warts or herpes.

SIDE EFFECTS

1. Irregular bleeding. The most common side effect of POPs is a change in menstrual bleeding. Your periods may be either early or late, and you may have some spotting between periods. Taking pills late or missing pills can also result in some spotting or bleeding.

2. Other side effects. Less common side effects include headaches, tender breasts, nausea and dizziness. Weight gain, acne and extra hair on your face and body have been reported, but are rare.

If you are concerned about any of these side effects, check with your doctor or clinic.

USING POPS WITH OTHER MEDICINES

Before taking a POP, inform your health care provider of any other medication, including over-the-counter medicine, that you may be taking.

If you are taking medicines for seizures (epilepsy) or tuberculosis (TB), tell your doctor or clinic. These medicines can make POPs less effective:

Medicines for seizures:
- Phenytoin (Dilantin®)
- Carbamazepine (Tegretol®)
- Phenobarbital

Medicine for TB:
- Rifampin (Rifampicin)

Before you begin taking any new medicines be sure your doctor or clinic knows you are taking birth control pills that contain a progestin.

HOW TO TAKE POPS

IMPORTANT POINTS TO REMEMBER

- POPs must be taken at the same time every day, so choose a time and then take the pill at that same time every day. Every time you take a pill late, and especially if you miss a pill, you are more likely to get pregnant.
- Start the next pack the day after the last pack is finished. There is no break between packs. Always have your next pack of pills ready.
- You may have some menstrual spotting between periods. Do not stop taking your pills if this happens.
- If you vomit soon after taking a pill, use a backup method (such as condom and/or spermicide) for 48 hours.
- If you want to stop taking POPs, you can do so at any time, but, if you remain sexually active and don't wish to become pregnant, be certain to use another birth control method.
- If you are not sure about how to take POPs, ask your doctor or clinic.

STARTING POPS

- It's best to take your first POP on the first day of your menstrual period.
- If you decide to take your first POP on another day, use a backup method (such as condom and/or spermicide) every time you have sex during the next 48 hours.
- If you have had a miscarriage or an abortion, you can start POPs the next day.

IF YOU ARE LATE OR MISS TAKING YOUR POPS

- If you are more than 3 hours late or you miss one or more POPs:
  1. TAKE a missed pill as soon as you remember that you missed it,
  2. THEN go back to taking POPs at your regular time,
  3. BUT be sure to use a backup method (such as condom and/or spermicide) every time you have sex for the next 48 hours.
- If you are not sure what to do about the pills you have missed, keep taking POPs and use a backup method until you can talk to your doctor or clinic.

IF YOU ARE BREASTFEEDING

- If you are fully breastfeeding (not giving your baby any food or formula), you may start your pills 6 weeks after delivery.
- If you are partially breastfeeding (giving your baby some food or formula), you should start taking pills by 3 weeks after delivery.

IF YOU ARE SWITCHING PILLS

- If you are switching from the combined pills to POPs, take the first POP the day after you finish the last active combined pill. Do not take any of the 7 inactive pills from the combined pill pack. You should know that many women have irregular periods after switching to POPs, but this is normal and to be expected.
- If you are switching from POPs to the combined pills, take the first active combined pill on the first day of your period, even if your POPs pack is not finished.
- If you switch to another brand of POPs, start the new brand anytime.
- If you are breastfeeding, you can switch to another method of birth control at any time, except do not switch to the combined pills until you stop breastfeeding or at least until 6 months after delivery.

PREGNANCY WHILE ON THE PILL

If you become pregnant, or think you might be, stop taking POPs and contact your physician. Even though research has shown that POPs do not cause harm to the unborn baby, it is always best not to take any drugs or medicines that you don't need when you are pregnant.

You should get a pregnancy test:
- If your period is late and you took one or more pills late or missed taking them and had sex without a backup method.
- Anytime you miss 2 periods in a row.

WILL POPS AFFECT YOUR ABILITY TO GET PREGNANT LATER?

If you want to become pregnant, simply stop taking POPs. POPs will not delay your ability to get pregnant.

BREASTFEEDING

If you are breastfeeding, POPs will not affect the quality or amount of your breastmilk or the health of your nursing baby.

OVERDOSE

No serious problems have been reported when many pills were taken by accident, even by a small child, so there is usually no reason to treat an overdose.

OTHER QUESTIONS OR CONCERNS

Cigarette smoking greatly increases the possibility of suffering heart attacks and strokes. Women who use oral contraceptives are strongly advised not to smoke.

Diabetic women taking POPs do not generally require changes in the amount of insulin they are taking. However, your physician may monitor you more closely under these conditions.

If you have any questions or concerns, check with your doctor or clinic. You can also ask for the more detailed "professional package labeling" written for doctors and other health care providers.

HOW TO STORE YOUR POPs

Store your POPs at room temperature 15°–25°C (59°–77°F).

Be certain to read new revisions of this leaflet. You may check the date of the most recent revision by phoning the manufacturer toll-free at 1-800-272-5525 or by writing to the address below:

Revised: July 1, 1998

Address medical inquiries to:
Medical Information Department
Watson Laboratories, Inc.
311 Bonnie Circle
Corona, CA 92880
Manufactured for:
WATSON PHARMA
A Division of Watson Laboratories, Inc.
Corona, CA 92880
by Syntex Inc.
Humacao, PR 00791

Shown in Product Identification Guide, page 340

NORCO® TABLETS Ⓒ℞

DESCRIPTION

NORCO® (Hydrocodone bitartrate and acetaminophen) is supplied in tablet form for oral administration.

Hydrocodone bitartrate is an opioid analgesic and antitussive and occurs as fine, white crystals or as a crystalline powder. It is affected by light. The chemical name is 4,5α-epoxy-3-methoxy-17-methylmorphinan-6-one tartrate (1:1) hydrate (2:5). It has the following structural formula:

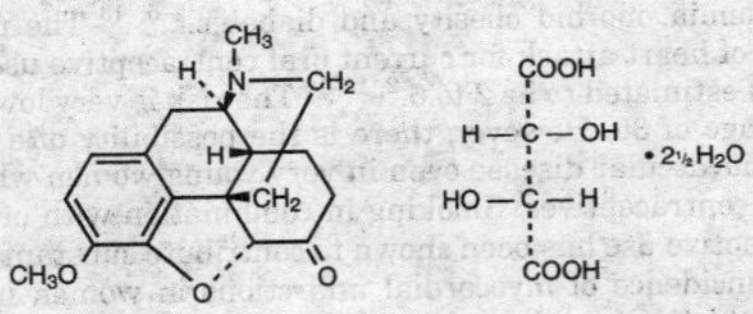

$C_{18}H_{21}NO_3 \cdot C_4H_6O_6 \cdot 2^1/_2H_2O$ MW=494.50

Acetaminophen, 4-hydroxyacetanilide, a slightly bitter, white, odorless, crystalline powder, is a non-opiate, non-salicylate analgesic and antipyretic. It has the following structural formula:

CH_3CONH–⟨benzene ring⟩–OH

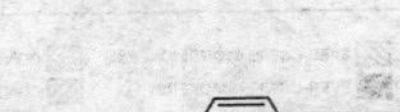

$C_8H_9NO_2$ MW=151.17

Each NORCO® 10/325 tablet contains:

Hydrocodone Bitartrate	10 mg
Acetaminophen	325 mg

In addition, each tablet contains the following inactive ingredients: croscarmellose sodium, crospovidone, D&C yellow #10 aluminum lake, magnesium stearate, microcrystalline cellulose, starch, povidone and stearic acid.

CLINICAL PHARMACOLOGY

Hydrocodone is a semisynthetic narcotic analgesic and antitussive with multiple actions qualitatively similar to those of codeine. Most of these involve the central nervous system and smooth muscle. The precise mechanism of action of hydrocodone and other opiates is not known, although it is believed to relate to the existence of opiate receptors in the central nervous system. In addition to analgesia, narcotics may produce drowsiness, changes in mood and mental clouding.

The analgesic action of acetaminophen involves peripheral influences, but the specific mechanism is as yet undetermined. Antipyretic activity is mediated through hypothalamic heat regulating centers. Acetaminophen inhibits prostaglandin synthetase. Therapeutic doses of acetaminophen have negligible effects on the cardiovascular or respiratory systems; however, toxic doses may cause circulatory failure and rapid, shallow breathing.

Pharmacokinetics: The behavior of the individual components is described below.

Hydrocodone: Following a 10 mg oral dose of hydrocodone administered to five adult male subjects, the mean peak concentration was 23.6 ± 5.2 ng/mL. Maximum serum levels were achieved at 1.3 ± 0.3 hours and the half-life was determined to be 3.8 ± 0.3 hours. Hydrocodone exhibits a complex pattern of metabolism including O-demethylation, N-demethylation and 6-keto reduction to the corresponding 6-α- and 6-β-hydroxymetabolites.

See **OVERDOSAGE** for toxicity information.

Acetaminophen: Acetaminophen is rapidly absorbed from the gastrointestinal tract and is distributed throughout most body tissues. The plasma half-life is 1.25 to 3 hours, but may be increased by liver damage and following overdosage. Elimination of acetaminophen is principally by liver metabolism (conjugation) and subsequent renal excretion of metabolites. Approximately 85% of an oral dose appears in the urine within 24 hours of administration, most as the glucuronide conjugate, with small amounts of other conjugates and unchanged drug.

See **OVERDOSAGE** for toxicity information.

INDICATIONS AND USAGE

NORCO® Tablets are indicated for the relief of moderate to moderately severe pain.

CONTRAINDICATIONS

NORCO® Tablets should not be administered to patients who have previously exhibited hypersensitivity to hydrocodone or acetaminophen.

WARNINGS

Respiratory Depression: At high doses or in sensitive patients, hydrocodone may produce dose-related respiratory depression by acting directly on the brain stem respiratory center. Hydrocodone also affects the center that controls respiratory rhythm, and may produce irregular and periodic breathing.

Head Injury and Increased Intracranial Pressure: The respiratory depressant effects of narcotics and their capacity to elevate cerebrospinal fluid pressure may be markedly exaggerated in the presence of head injury, other intracranial lesions or a pre-existing increase in intracranial pressure. Furthermore, narcotics produce adverse reactions which may obscure the clinical course of patients with head injuries.

Acute Abdominal Conditions: The administration of narcotics may obscure the diagnosis or clinical course of patients with acute abdominal conditions.

PRECAUTIONS

General: Special Risk Patients: As with any narcotic analgesic agent, NORCO® Tablets should be used with caution in elderly or debilitated patients, and those with severe impairment of hepatic or renal function, hypothyroidism, Addison's disease, prostatic hypertrophy or urethral stricture. The usual precautions should be observed and the possibility of respiratory depression should be kept in mind.

Cough reflex: Hydrocodone suppresses the cough reflex; as with all narcotics, caution should be exercised when NORCO® Tablets are used postoperatively and in patients with pulmonary disease.

Information for Patients: NORCO® Tablets, like all narcotics, may impair mental and/or physical abilities required for the performance of potentially hazardous tasks such as driving a car or operating machinery; patients should be cautioned accordingly.

Alcohol and other CNS depressants may produce an additive CNS depression, when taken with this combination product, and should be avoided.

Hydrocodone may be habit-forming. Patients should take the drug only for as long as it is prescribed, in the amounts prescribed, and no more frequently than prescribed.

Laboratory Tests: In patients with severe hepatic or renal disease, effects of therapy should be monitored with serial liver and/or renal function tests.

Drug Interactions: Patients receiving narcotics, antihistamines, antipsychotics, antianxiety agents, or other CNS depressants (including alcohol) concomitantly with NORCO® Tablets may exhibit an additive CNS depression. When combined therapy is contemplated, the dose of one or both agents should be reduced.

The use of MAO inhibitors or tricyclic antidepressants with hydrocodone preparations may increase the effect of either the antidepressant or hydrocodone.

Drug/Laboratory Test Interactions: Acetaminophen may produce false-positive test results for urinary 5-hydroxyindoleacetic acid.

Carcinogenesis, Mutagenesis, Impairment of Fertility: No adequate studies have been conducted in animals to determine whether hydrocodone or acetaminophen have a potential for carcinogenesis, mutagenesis, or impairment of fertility.

Pregnancy:

Teratogenic Effects: Pregnancy Category C: There are no adequate and well-controlled studies in pregnant women. NORCO® Tablets should be used during pregnancy only if the potential benefit justifies the potential risk to the fetus.

Nonteratogenic Effects: Babies born to mothers who have been taking opioids regularly prior to delivery will be physically dependent. The withdrawal signs include irritability and excessive crying, tremors, hyperactive reflexes, increased respiratory rate, increased stools, sneezing, yawning, vomiting and fever. The intensity of the syndrome does not always correlate with the duration of maternal opioid use or dose. There is no consensus on the best method of managing withdrawal.

Labor and Delivery: As with all narcotics, administration of NORCO® Tablets to the mother shortly before delivery may result in some degree of respiratory depression in the newborn, especially if higher doses are used.

Nursing Mothers: Acetaminophen is excreted in breast milk in small amounts, but the significance of its effects on nursing infants is not known. It is not known whether hydrocodone is excreted in human milk. Because many drugs are excreted in human milk and because of the potential for serious adverse reactions in nursing infants from NORCO® Tablets, a decision should be made whether to discontinue nursing or to discontinue the drug, taking into account the importance of the drug to the mother.

Pediatric Use: Safety and effectiveness in pediatric patients have not been established.

ADVERSE REACTIONS

The most frequently reported adverse reactions are lightheadedness, dizziness, sedation, nausea and vomiting. These effects seem to be more prominent in ambulatory than in nonambulatory patients, and some of these adverse reactions may be alleviated if the patient lies down.

Other adverse reactions include:

Central Nervous System: Drowsiness, mental clouding, lethargy, impairment of mental and physical performance, anxiety, fear, dysphoria, psychic dependence, mood changes.

Gastrointestinal System: Prolonged administration of NORCO® Tablets may produce constipation.

Genitourinary System: Ureteral spasm, spasm of vesical sphincters and urinary retention have been reported with opiates.

Respiratory Depression: Hydrocodone bitartrate may produce dose-related respiratory depression by acting directly on brain stem respiratory centers (see **OVERDOSAGE**).

Dermatological: Skin rash, pruritus.

The following adverse drug events may be borne in mind as potential effects of acetaminophen: allergic reactions, rash, thrombocytopenia, agranulocytosis.

Potential effects of high dosage are listed in the **OVERDOSAGE** section.

DRUG ABUSE AND DEPENDENCE

Controlled Substance: NORCO® Tablets are classified as a Schedule III controlled substance.

Abuse and Dependence: Psychic dependence, physical dependence, and tolerance may develop upon repeated administration of narcotics; therefore, NORCO® Tablets should be prescribed and administered with caution. However, psychic dependence is unlikely to develop when NORCO® Tablets are used for a short time for the treatment of pain.

Physical dependence, the condition in which continued administration of the drug is required to prevent the appearance of a withdrawal syndrome, assumes clinically significant proportions only after several weeks, of continued narcotic use, although some mild degree of physical dependence may develop after a few days of narcotic therapy. Tolerance, in which increasingly large doses are required in order to produce the same degree of analgesia, is manifested initially by a shortened duration of analgesic effect, and subsequently by decreases in the intensity of analgesia. The rate of development of tolerance varies among patients.

OVERDOSAGE

Following an acute overdosage, toxicity may result from hydrocodone or acetaminophen.

Signs and Symptoms

Hydrocodone: Serious overdose with hydrocodone is characterized by respiratory depression (a decrease in respiratory rate and/or tidal volume, Cheyne-Stokes respiration, cyanosis), extreme somnolence progressing to stupor or coma, skeletal muscle flaccidity, cold and clammy skin, and sometimes bradycardia and hypotension. In severe overdosage, apnea, circulatory collapse, cardiac arrest and death may occur.

Acetaminophen: In acetaminophen overdosage: dose-dependent, potentially fatal hepatic necrosis is the most serious adverse effect. Renal tubular necrosis, hypoglycemic coma and thrombocytopenia may also occur.

Early symptoms following a potentially hepatotoxic overdose may include: nausea, vomiting, diaphoresis and general malaise. Clinical and laboratory evidence of hepatic toxicity may not be apparent until 48 to 72 hours post-ingestion.

In adults, hepatic toxicity has rarely been reported with acute overdoses of less than 10 grams, or fatalities with less than 15 grams.

Treatment: A single or multiple overdose with hydrocodone and acetaminophen is a potentially lethal polydrug overdose, and consultation with a regional poison control center is recommended.

Continued on next page

Norco—Cont.

Immediate treatment includes support of cardiorespiratory function and measures to reduce drug absorption. Vomiting should be induced mechanically, or with syrup of ipecac, if the patient is alert (adequate pharyngeal and laryngeal reflexes). Oral activated charcoal (1 g/kg) should follow gastric emptying. The first dose should be accompanied by an appropriate cathartic. If repeated doses are used, the cathartic might be included with alternate doses as required. Hypotension is usually hypovolemic and should respond to fluids. Vasopressors and other supportive measures should be employed as indicated. A cuffed endo-tracheal tube should be inserted before gastric lavage of the unconscious patient and, when necessary, to provide assisted respiration.

Meticulous attention should be given to maintaining adequate pulmonary ventilation. In severe cases of intoxication, peritoneal dialysis, or preferably hemodialysis may be considered. If hypoprothrombinemia occurs due to acetaminophen overdose, vitamin K should be administered intravenously.

Naloxone, a narcotic antagonist, can reverse respiratory depression and coma associated with opioid overdose. Naloxone hydrochloride 0.4 mg to 2 mg is given parenterally. Since the duration of action of hydrocodone may exceed that of the naloxone, the patient should be kept under continuous surveillance and repeated doses of the antagonist should be administered as needed to maintain adequate respiration. A narcotic antagonist should not be administered in the absence of clinically significant respiratory or cardiovascular depression.

If the dose of acetaminophen may have exceeded 140 mg/kg, acetylcysteine should be administered as early as possible. Serum acetaminophen levels should be obtained, since levels four or more hours following ingestion help predict acetaminophen toxicity. Do not await acetaminophen assay results before initiating treatment. Hepatic enzymes should be obtained initially, and repeated at 24-hour intervals.

Methemoglobinemia over 30% should be treated with methylene blue by slow intravenous administration.

The toxic dose for adults for acetaminophen is 10 g.

DOSAGE AND ADMINISTRATION

Dosage should be adjusted according to the severity of the pain and the response of the patient. However, it should be kept in mind that tolerance to hydrocodone can develop with continued use and that the incidence of untoward effects is dose related.

The usual adult dosage is one tablet every four to six hours as needed for pain. The total daily dosage should not exceed 6 tablets.

HOW SUPPLIED

NORCO® 10/325 is supplied as a yellow, capsule-shaped tablet containing 10 mg hydrocodone bitartrate and 325 mg acetaminophen, bisected on one side and debossed with "NORCO 539" on the other side.

Bottles of 100 NDC 52544-539-01

Bottles of 500 NDC 52544-539-05

Store at controlled room temperature, 15° to 30°C (59°F to 86°F)

Dispense in a tight, light-resistant container with a child-resistant closure.

Rx only

WATSON PHARMA, INC.
a subsidiary of
Watson Laboratories, Inc.
Corona, CA 92880

Revised March 14, 2000
13095-3

Shown in Product Identification Guide, page 340

OGESTREL® 0.5/50–28 ℞

[ō'gĕstrĕl]

(norgestrel and ethinyl estradiol tablets USP, 0.5 mg/0.05 mg)

Rx only

Patients should be counseled that this product does not protect against HIV infection (AIDS) and other sexually transmitted diseases.

ORAL CONTRACEPTIVE AGENTS

DESCRIPTION

Ogestrel® 0.5/50–28 Tablets (norgestrel and ethinyl estradiol tablets USP, 0.5 mg/0.05 mg) provide an oral contraceptive regimen consisting of 21 white tablets followed by 7 peach inert tablets.

Each white tablet, for oral administration contains 0.5 mg of norgestrel and 0.05 mg ethinyl estradiol and the following inactive ingredients: croscarmellose sodium, lactose, magnesium stearate, microcrystalline cellulose, and povidone.

Each inactive peach tablet, for oral administration, in the 28 day regimen contains the following inactive ingredients: lactose monohydrate, microcrystalline cellulose, anhydrous lactose, FD&C Yellow No. 6 Lake, and magnesium stearate.

Norgestrel is a totally synthetic progestogen, insoluble in water, freely soluble in chloroform, sparingly soluble in alcohol with the chemical name (±)-13-Ethyl-17-hydroxy-18, 19-dinor-17α-pregn-4-en-20-yn-3-one. Ethinyl estradiol is an estrogen, insoluble in water, soluble in alcohol, in chloroform, in ether, in vegetable oils, and in solutions of fixed alkali hydroxides with the chemical name 19-nor-17α-pregna-1,3,5(10)-trien-20-yne-3, 17-diol. Their structure formulae follow:

NORGESTREL
$C_{21}H_{28}O_2$
MW 312.45

ETHINYL ESTRADIOL
$C_{20}H_{24}O_2$
MW 296.41

Therapeutic class: Oral contraceptive.

CLINICAL PHARMACOLOGY

Combination oral contraceptives act by suppression of gonadotrophins. Although the primary mechanism of this action is inhibition of ovulation, other alterations include changes in the cervical mucus (which increase the difficulty of sperm entry into the uterus) and the endometrium (which may reduce the likelihood of implantation).

INDICATIONS AND USAGE

Ogestrel® (norgestrel and ethinyl estradiol tablets USP, 0.5 mg/0.05 mg) are indicated for the prevention of pregnancy in women who elect to use this product as a method of contraception.

Oral contraceptives are highly effective. Table I lists the typical accidental pregnancy rates for users of combination oral contraceptives and other methods of contraception.[1] The efficacy of these contraceptive methods, except sterilization, depends upon the reliability with which they are used. Correct and consistent use of methods can result in lower failure rates.

TABLE I: PERCENTAGE OF WOMEN EXPERIENCING A CONTRACEPTIVE FAILURE DURING THE FIRST YEAR OF PERFECT USE AND FIRST YEAR OF TYPICAL USE

Method	Percentage of women experiencing an accidental pregnancy within the first year of use	
	Typical use[a]	Perfect use[b]
Chance	85	85
Spermicides	21	6
Periodic abstinence	20	1–9
Withdrawal	19	4
Cap		
Parous	36	26
Nulliparous	18	9
Sponge		
Parous	36	20
Nulliparous	18	9
Diaphragm	18	6
Condom		
Female	21	5
Male	12	3
Pill	3	
Progestin only		0.5
Combined		0.1
IUD		
Progesterone	2	1.5
Copper T 380A	0.8	0.6
Injection (Depo-Provera)	0.3	0.3
Implants (Norplant)	0.09	0.09
Female sterilization	0.4	0.4
Male sterilization	0.15	0.10

Adapted with permission[1].

[a] Among *typical* couples who initiate use of a method (not necessarily for the first time), the percentage who experience an accidental pregnancy during the first year if they do not stop use for any other reason.

[b] Among couples who initiate use of a method (not necessarily for the first time) and who use it *perfectly* (both consistently and correctly), the percentage who experience an accidental pregnancy during the first year if they do not stop use for any other reason.

CONTRAINDICATIONS

Oral contraceptives should not be used in women who have the following conditions:

- Thrombophlebitis or thromboembolic disorders
- A past history of deep vein thrombophlebitis or thromboembolic disorders
- Cerebral vascular or coronary artery disease
- Known or suspected carcinoma of the breast
- Carcinoma of the endometrium or other known or suspected estrogen-dependent neoplasia
- Undiagnosed abnormal genital bleeding
- Cholestatic jaundice of pregnancy or jaundice with prior pill use
- Hepatic adenomas, carcinomas or benign liver tumors
- Known or suspected pregnancy

WARNINGS

Cigarette smoking increases the risk of serious cardiovascular side effects from oral contraceptive use. This risk increases with age and with heavy smoking (15 or more cigarettes per day) and is quite marked in women over 35 years of age. Women who use oral contraceptives should be strongly advised not to smoke.

The use of oral contraceptives is associated with increased risks of several serious conditions including myocardial infarction, thromboembolism, stroke, hepatic neoplasia, and gallbladder disease, although the risk of serious morbidity or mortality is very small in healthy women without underlying risk factors. The risk of morbidity and mortality increases significantly in the presence of other underlying risk factors such as hypertension, hyperlipidemias, hypercholesterolemia, obesity, and diabetes.[2–5]

Practitioners prescribing oral contraceptives should be familiar with the following information relating to these risks.

The information contained in this package insert is principally based on studies carried out in patients who used oral contraceptives with higher formulations of both estrogens and progestogens than those in common use today. The effect of long-term use of the oral contraceptives with lower formulations of both estrogens and progestogens remains to be determined.

Throughout this labeling, epidemiological studies reported are of two types: retrospective or case control studies and prospective or cohort studies. Case control studies provide a measure of the relative risk of a disease. Relative risk, the *ratio* of the incidence of a disease among oral contraceptive users to that among non-users, cannot be assessed directly from case control studies, but the odds ratio obtained is a measure of relative risk. The relative risk does not provide information on the actual clinical occurrence of a disease. Cohort studies provide not only a measure of relative risk but a measure of attributable risk, which is the *difference* in the incidence of disease between the oral contraceptive users and non-users. The attributable risk does provide information about the actual occurrence of a disease in the population. (Adapted from ref. 12 and 13 with the author's permission.) For further information, the reader is referred to a text on epidemiological methods.

1. THROMBOEMBOLIC DISORDERS AND OTHER VASCULAR PROBLEMS

a. Myocardial Infarction

An increased risk of myocardial infarction has been attributed to oral contraceptive use. This risk is primarily in smokers or women with other underlying risk factors for coronary artery disease such as hypertension, hypercholesterolemia, morbid obesity and diabetes.[2–5, 13] The relative risk of heart attack for current oral contraceptive users has been estimated to be 2 to 6.[2, 14–19] The risk is very low under the age of 30. However, there is the possibility of a risk of cardiovascular disease even in very young women who take oral contraceptives. Smoking in combination with oral contraceptive use has been shown to contribute substantially to the incidence of myocardial infarctions in women in their mid-thirties or older, with smoking accounting for the majority of excess cases.[20]

Mortality rates associated with circulatory disease have been shown to increase substantially in smokers over the age of 35 and non-smokers over the age of 40 among women who use oral contraceptives (see Table II).[16]

TABLE II: CIRCULATORY DISEASE MORTALITY RATES PER 100,000 WOMAN YEARS BY AGE, SMOKING STATUS AND ORAL CONTRACEPTIVE USE

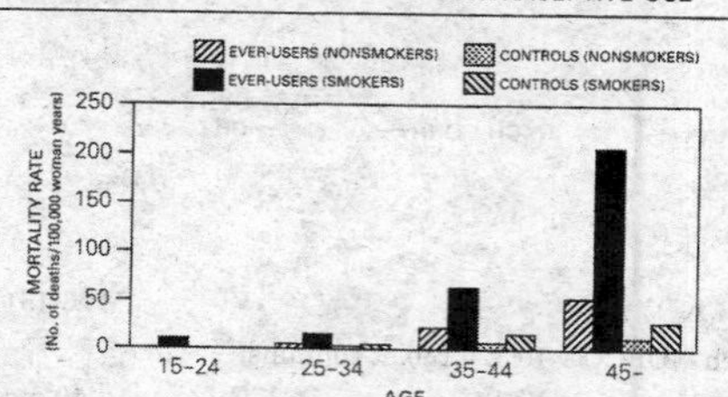

Adapted from P.M. Layde and V. Beral, Table V[16]

Oral contraceptives may compound the effects of well-known risk factors such as hypertension, diabetes, hyperlipidemias, hypercholesterolemia, age, and obesity.[3, 13, 21] In particular, some progestogens are known to decrease HDL cholesterol and cause glucose intolerance, while estrogens may create a state of hyperinsulinism.[21–25] Oral contraceptives have been shown to increase blood pressure among users (see ***WARNINGS***, section 9). Similar effects on risk factors have been associated with an increased risk of heart disease. Oral contraceptives must be used with caution in women with cardiovascular disease risk factors.

b. Thromboembolism
An increased risk of thromboembolic and thrombotic disease associated with the use of oral contraceptives is well established. Case control studies have found the relative risk of users compared to non-users to be 3 for the first episode of superficial venous thrombosis, 4 to 11 for deep vein thrombosis or pulmonary embolism, and 1.5 to 6 for women with predisposing conditions for venous thromboembolic disease.[12, 13, 26–31] Cohort studies have shown the relative risk to be somewhat lower, about 3 for new cases and about 4.5 for new cases requiring hospitalization.[32] The risk of thromboembolic disease due to oral contraceptives is not related to length of use and disappears after pill use is stopped.[12]
A 2- to 6-fold increase in relative risk of post-operative thromboembolic complications has been reported with the use of oral contraceptives. The relative risk of venous thrombosis in women who have predisposing conditions is twice that of women without such medical conditions.[83] If feasible, oral contraceptives should be discontinued at least 4 weeks prior to and for 2 weeks after elective surgery and during and following prolonged immobilization. Since the immediate postpartum period also is associated with an increased risk of thromboembolism, oral contraceptives should be started no earlier than 4 to 6 weeks after delivery in women who elect not to breast feed.[33]

c. Cerebrovascular diseases
An increase in both the relative and attributable risks of cerebrovascular events (thrombotic and hemorrhagic strokes) has been shown in users of oral contraceptives. In general, the risk is greatest among older (>35 years), hypertensive women who also smoke. Hypertension was found to be a risk factor for both users and non-users for both types of strokes while smoking interacted to increase the risk for hemorrhagic strokes.[34]
In a large study, the relative risk of thrombotic strokes has been shown to range from 3 for normotensive users to 14 for users with severe hypertension.[35] The relative risk of hemorrhagic stroke is reported to be 1.2 for non-smokers who used oral contraceptives, 2.6 for smokers who did not use oral contraceptives, 7.6 for smokers who used oral contraceptives, 1.8 for normotensive users and 25.7 for users with severe hypertension.[35] The attributable risk also is greater in women in their mid-thirties or older and among smokers.[13]

d. Dose-related risk of vascular disease from oral contraceptives
A positive association has been observed between the amount of estrogen and progestogen in oral contraceptives and the risk of vascular disease.[36–38] A decline in serum high density lipoproteins (HDL) has been reported with many progestational agents.[22–24] A decline in serum high density lipoproteins has been associated with an increased incidence of ischemic heart disease.[39] Because estrogens increase HDL cholesterol, the net effect of an oral contraceptive depends on a balance achieved between doses of estrogen and progestogen and the nature and absolute amount of progestogens used in the contraceptives. The amount of both hormones should be considered in the choice of an oral contraceptive.[37]
Minimizing exposure to estrogen and progestogen is in keeping with good principles of therapeutics. For any particular estrogen/progestogen combination, the dosage regimen prescribed should be one which contains the least amount of estrogen and progestogen that is compatible with a low failure rate and the needs of the individual patient. New acceptors of oral contraceptive agents should be started on preparations containing the lowest estrogen content that produces satisfactory results for the individual.

e. Persistence of risk of vascular disease
There are three studies which have shown persistence of risk of vascular disease for ever-users of oral contraceptives.[17, 34, 40] In a study in the United States, the risk of developing myocardial infarction after discontinuing oral contraceptives persists for at least 9 years for women 40–49 years who has used oral contraceptives for 5 or more years, but this increased risk was not demonstrated in other age groups.[17] In another study in Great Britain, the risk of developing cerebrovascular disease persisted for at least 6 years after discontinuation of oral contraceptives, although excess risk was very small.[40] There is a significantly increased relative risk of subarachnoid hemorrhage after termination of use of oral contraceptives.[34] However, these studies were performed with oral contraceptives formulations containing 50 µg or higher of estrogen.

2. ESTIMATES OF MORTALITY FROM CONTRACEPTIVE USE
One study gathered data from a variety of sources which have estimated the mortality rates associated with different methods of contraception at different ages (see Table III).[41] These estimates include the combined risk of death associated with contraceptive methods plus the risk attributable to pregnancy in the event of method failure. Each method of contraception has its specific benefits and risks. The study concluded that with the exception of oral contraceptive users 35 and older who smoke and 40 and older who do not smoke, mortality associated with all methods of birth control is low and below that associated with childbirth. The observation of a possible increase in risk of mortality with age for oral contraceptive users is based on data gathered in the 1970s—but not reported in the U.S. until 1983.[16, 41] However, current clinical practice involves the use of lower estrogen dose formulations combined with careful restriction of oral contraceptive use to women who do not have the various risk factors listed in this labeling.

TABLE III: ESTIMATED ANNUAL NUMBER OF BIRTH-RELATED OR METHOD-RELATED DEATHS ASSOCIATED WITH CONTROL OF FERTILITY PER 100,000 NONSTERILE WOMEN, BY FERTILITY CONTROL METHOD ACCORDING TO AGE

Method of control and outcome	15–19	20–24	25–29	30–34	35–39	40–44
No fertility control methods*	7.0	7.4	9.1	14.8	25.7	28.2
Oral contraceptives non-smoker**	0.3	0.5	0.9	1.9	13.8	31.6
Oral contraceptives smoker**	2.2	3.4	6.6	13.5	51.1	117.2
IUD**	0.8	0.8	1.0	1.0	1.4	1.4
Condom*	1.1	1.6	0.7	0.2	0.3	0.4
Diaphragm/Spermicide*	1.9	1.2	1.2	1.3	2.2	2.8
Periodic abstinence*	2.5	1.6	1.6	1.7	2.9	3.6

*Deaths are birth-related
**Deaths are method-related

Estimates adapted from H.W. Ory, Table 3[41]

Because of these changes in practice and, also, because of some limited new data which suggest that the risk of cardiovascular disease with the use of oral contraceptives may now be less than previously observed,[78, 79] the Fertility and Maternal Health Drugs Advisory Committee was asked to review the topic in 1989. The Committee concluded that although cardiovascular disease risks may be increased with oral contraceptive use after age 40 in healthy non-smoking women (even with the newer low-dose formulations), there are greater potential health risks associated with pregnancy in older women and with the alternative surgical and medical procedures which may be necessary if such women do not have access to effective and acceptable means of contraception.
Therefore, the Committee recommended that the benefits of oral contraceptive use by healthy non-smoking women over 40 may outweigh the possible risks. Of course, older women, as all women who take oral contraceptives, should take the lowest possible dose formulation that is effective.[80]
[See table above]

3. CARCINOMA OF THE BREAST AND REPRODUCTIVE ORGANS
Numerous epidemiological studies have been performed on the incidence of breast, endometrial, ovarian, and cervical cancer in women using oral contraceptives. The overwhelming evidence in the literature suggests that use of oral contraceptives is not associated with an increase in the risk of developing breast cancer, regardless of the age and parity of first use or with most of the marketed brands and doses.[42–44] The Cancer and Steroid Hormone (CASH) study also showed no latent effect on the risk of breast cancer for at least a decade following long-term use.[43] A few studies have shown a slightly increased relative risk of developing breast cancer,[44–47] although the methodology of these studies, which included differences in examination of users and non-users and differences in age at start of use, has been questioned.[47–49] Some studies have reported an increased relative risk of developing breast cancer, particularly at a younger age. This increased relative risk appears to be related to duration of use.[81, 82]
Some studies suggest that oral contraceptive use has been associated with an increase in the risk of cervical intraepithelial neoplasia in some populations of women.[50–53] However, there continues to be controversy about the extent to which such findings may be due to differences in sexual behavior and other factors.
In spite of many studies of the relationship between oral contraceptive use and breast or cervical cancers, a cause and effect relationship has not been established.

4. HEPATIC NEOPLASIA
Benign hepatic adenomas are associated with oral contraceptive use although the incidence of benign tumors is rare in the United States. Indirect calculations have estimated the attributable risk to be in the range of 3.3 cases per 100,000 for users, a risk that increases after 4 or more years of use.[54] Rupture of rare, benign, hepatic adenomas may cause death through intra-abdominal hemorrhage.[55–56]
Studies in the United States and Britain have shown an increased risk of developing hepatocellular carcinoma in long-term (>8 years) oral contraceptive users.[57–59] However, these cancers are extremely rare in the United States and the attributable risk (the excess incidence) of liver cancers in oral contraceptive users approaches less than 1 per 1,000,000 users.

5. OCULAR LESIONS
There have been clinical case reports of retinal thrombosis associated with the use of oral contraceptives. Oral contraceptives should be discontinued if there is unexplained partial or complete loss of vision; onset of proptosis or diplopia; papilledema; or retinal vascular lesions. Appropriate diagnostic and therapeutic measures should be undertaken immediately.

6. ORAL CONTRACEPTIVE USE BEFORE OR DURING EARLY PREGNANCY
Extensive epidemiological studies have revealed no increased risk of birth defects in women who have used oral contraceptives prior to pregnancy.[60–62] Studies also do not suggest a teratogenic effect, particularly insofar as cardiac anomalies and limb reduction defects are concerned, when taken inadvertently during early pregnancy.[60, 61, 63, 64] The administration of oral contraceptives to induce withdrawal bleeding should not be used as a test for pregnancy. Oral contraceptives should not be used during pregnancy to treat threatened or habitual abortion.
It is recommended that for any patient who has missed 2 consecutive periods, pregnancy should be ruled out before continuing oral contraceptive use. If the patient has not adhered to the prescribed schedule, the possibility of pregnancy should be considered at the first missed period. Oral contraceptive use should be discontinued if pregnancy is confirmed.

7. GALLBLADDER DISEASE
Earlier studies have reported an increased lifetime relative risk of gallbladder surgery in users of oral contraceptives and estrogens.[65–66] More recent studies, however, have shown that the relative risk of developing gallbladder disease among oral contraceptive users may be minimal.[67] The recent findings of minimal risk may be related to the use of oral contraceptive formulations containing lower hormonal doses of estrogens and progestogens.[68]

8. CARBOHYDRATE AND LIPID METABOLIC EFFECTS
Oral contraceptives have been shown to cause glucose intolerance in a significant percentage of users.[25] Oral contraceptives containing greater than 75 µg of estrogen cause hyperinsulinism, while lower doses of estrogen cause less glucose intolerance.[70] Progestogens increase insulin secretion and create insulin resistance, this effect varying with different progestational agents.[25, 71] However, in the non-diabetic woman, oral contraceptives appear to have no effect on fasting blood glucose.[69] Because of these demonstrated effects, pre-diabetic and diabetic women should be carefully observed while taking oral contraceptives.
Some women may develop persistent hypertriglyceridemia while on the pill.[72] As discussed earlier (see ***WARNINGS***, sections 1a. and 1d.), changes in serum triglycerides and lipoprotein levels have been reported in oral contraceptive users.[23]

9. ELEVATED BLOOD PRESSURE
An increase in blood pressure has been reported in women taking oral contraceptives and this increase is more likely in older oral contraceptive users and with continued use.[73, 84] Data from the Royal College of General Practitioners and subsequent randomized trials have shown that the incidence of hypertension increases with increasing concentrations of progestogens.
Women with a history of hypertension or hypertension-related diseases or renal disease should be encouraged to use another method of contraception. If women elect to use oral contraceptives, they should be monitored closely and if significant elevation of blood pressure occurs oral contraceptives should be discontinued. For most women, elevated blood pressure will return to normal after stopping oral contraceptives and there is no difference in the occurrence of hypertension among ever- and never-users.[73–75]

10. HEADACHE
The onset or exacerbation of migraine or development of headache with a new pattern which is recurrent, persistent or severe requires discontinuation of oral contraceptives and evaluation of the cause.

11. BLEEDING IRREGULARITIES
Breakthrough bleeding and spotting are sometimes encountered in patients on oral contraceptives, especially during the first 3 months of use. Non-hormonal causes should be considered and adequate diagnostic measures taken to rule out malignancy or pregnancy in the event of breakthrough bleeding, as in the case of any abnormal vaginal bleeding. If pathology has been excluded, time or a change to another formulation may solve the problem. In the event of amenorrhea, pregnancy should be ruled out.
Some women may encounter post-pill amenorrhea or oligomenorrhea, especially when such a condition was pre-existent.

PRECAUTIONS

GENERAL
Patients should be counseled that this product does not protect against HIV infection (AIDS) and other sexually transmitted diseases.

Continued on next page

Ogestrel—Cont.

1. PHYSICAL EXAMINATION AND FOLLOW-UP
It is good medical practice for all women to have annual history and physical examinations, including women using oral contraceptives. The physical examination, however, may be deferred until after initiation of oral contraceptives if requested by the woman and judged appropriate by the clinician. The physical examination should include special reference to blood pressure, breasts, abdomen and pelvic organs, including cervical cytology, and relevant laboratory tests. In case of undiagnosed, persistent or recurrent abnormal vaginal bleeding, appropriate measures should be conducted to rule out malignancy. Women with a strong family history of breast cancer or who have breast nodules should be monitored with particular care.

2. LIPID DISORDERS
Women who are being treated for hyperlipidemias should be followed closely if they elect to use oral contraceptives. Some progestogens may elevate LDL levels and may render the control of hyperlipidemias more difficult.

3. LIVER FUNCTION
If jaundice develops in any woman receiving oral contraceptives the medication should be discontinued. Steroid hormones may be poorly metabolized in patients with impaired liver function.

4. FLUID RETENTION
Oral contraceptives may cause some degree of fluid retention. They should be prescribed with caution, and only with careful monitoring, in patients with conditions which might be aggravated by fluid retention.

5. EMOTIONAL DISORDERS
Women with a history of depression should be carefully observed and the drug discontinued if depression recurs to a serious degree.

6. CONTACT LENSES
Contact lens wearers who develop visual changes or changes in lens tolerance should be assessed by an ophthalmologist.

7. DRUG INTERACTIONS
Reduced efficacy and increased incidence of breakthrough bleeding and menstrual irregularities have been associated with concomitant use of rifampin. A similar association though less marked, has been suggested with barbiturates, phenylbutazone, phenytoin sodium, and possibly with griseofulvin, ampicillin, and tetracyclines.[76]

8. INTERACTIONS WITH LABORATORY TESTS
Certain endocrine and liver function tests and blood components may be affected by oral contraceptives:

a. Increased prothrombin and factors VII, VIII, IX, and X; decreased antithrombin 3; increased norepinephrine-induced platelet aggregability.
b. Increased thyroid binding globulin (TBG) leading to increased circulating total thyroid hormone, as measured by protein-bound iodine (PBI), T4 by column or by radioimmunoassay. Free T3 resin uptake is decreased, reflecting the elevated TBG. Free T4 concentration is unaltered.
c. Other binding proteins may be elevated in serum.
d. Sex steroid binding globulins are increased and result in elevated levels of total circulating sex steroids and corticoids; however, free or biologically active levels remain unchanged.
e. Triglycerides may be increased.
f. Glucose tolerance may be decreased.
g. Serum folate levels may be depressed by oral contraceptive therapy. This may be of clinical significance if a woman becomes pregnant shortly after discontinuing oral contraceptives.

9. CARCINOGENESIS
See ***WARNINGS*** section.

10. PREGNANCY
Pregnancy Category X. See ***CONTRAINDICATIONS*** and ***WARNINGS*** sections.

11. NURSING MOTHERS
Small amounts of oral contraceptive steroids have been identified in the milk of nursing mothers and a few adverse effects on the child have been reported, including jaundice and breast enlargement. In addition, oral contraceptives given in the postpartum period may interfere with lactation by decreasing the quantity and quality of breast milk. If possible, the nursing mother should be advised not to use oral contraceptives but to use other forms of contraception until she has completely weaned her child.

INFORMATION FOR THE PATIENT
See ***PATIENT LABELING*** printed below.

ADVERSE REACTIONS

An increased risk of the following serious adverse reactions has been associated with the use of oral contraceptives (see ***WARNINGS*** section):
- Thrombophlebitis
- Arterial thromboembolism
- Pulmonary embolism
- Myocardial infarction
- Cerebral hemorrhage
- Cerebral thrombosis
- Hypertension
- Gallbladder disease
- Hepatic adenomas, carcinomas or benign liver tumors

There is evidence of an association between the following conditions and the use of oral contraceptives, although additional confirmatory studies are needed:
- Mesenteric thrombosis
- Retinal thrombosis

The following adverse reactions have been reported in patients receiving oral contraceptives and are believed to be drug-related:
- Nausea
- Vomiting
- Gastrointestinal symptoms (such as abdominal cramps and bloating)
- Breakthrough bleeding
- Spotting
- Change in menstrual flow
- Amenorrhea
- Temporary infertility after discontinuation of treatment
- Edema
- Melasma which may persist
- Breast changes: tenderness, enlargement, secretion
- Change in weight (increase or decrease)
- Change in cervical erosion and secretion
- Diminution in lactation when given immediately postpartum
- Cholestatic jaundice
- Migraine
- Rash (allergic)
- Mental depression
- Reduced tolerance to carbohydrates
- Vaginal candidiasis
- Change in corneal curvature (steepening)
- Intolerance to contact lenses

The following adverse reactions have been reported in users of oral contraceptives and the association has been neither confirmed nor refuted:
- Pre-menstrual syndrome
- Cataracts
- Changes in appetite
- Cystitis-like syndrome
- Headache
- Nervousness
- Dizziness
- Hirsutism
- Loss of scalp hair
- Erythema multiforme
- Erythema nodosum
- Hemorrhagic eruption
- Vaginitis
- Porphyria
- Impaired renal function
- Hemolytic uremic syndrome
- Budd-Chiari syndrome
- Acne
- Changes in libido
- Colitis

OVERDOSAGE

Serious ill effects have not been reported following acute ingestion of large doses of oral contraceptives by young children. Overdosage may cause nausea, and withdrawal bleeding may occur in females.

NON-CONTRACEPTIVE HEALTH BENEFITS
The following non-contraceptive health benefits related to the use of oral contraceptives are supported by epidemiological studies which largely utilized oral contraceptive formulations containing estrogen doses exceeding 0.035 mg of ethinyl estradiol or 0.5 mg of mestranol.[6–11]
Effects on menses:
- Increased menstrual cycle regularity
- Decreased blood loss and decreased incidence of iron deficiency anemia
- Decreased incidence of dysmenorrhea

Effects related to inhibition of ovulation:
- Decreased incidence of functional ovarian cysts
- Decreased incidence of ectopic pregnancies

Effects from long-term use:
- Decreased incidence of fibroadenomas and fibrocystic disease of the breast
- Decreased incidence of acute pelvic inflammatory disease
- Decreased incidence of endometrial cancer
- Decreased incidence of ovarian cancer

DOSAGE AND ADMINISTRATION

To achieve maximum contraceptive effectiveness, oral contraceptives must be taken exactly as directed and at intervals not exceeding 24 hours.

28-Day Schedule: For a DAY 1 START, count the first day of menstrual flow as Day 1 and the first tablet (white) is then taken on Day 1. For a SUNDAY START when menstrual flow begins on or before Sunday, the first tablet (white) is taken on that day. With either a DAY 1 START or SUNDAY START, 1 tablet (white) is taken each day at the same time for 21 days. Then the peach tablets are taken for 7 days, whether bleeding has stopped or not. After all 28 tablets have been taken, whether bleeding has stopped or not, the same dosage schedule is repeated beginning on the following day.

INSTRUCTIONS TO PATIENTS
- To achieve maximum contraceptive effectiveness, the oral contraceptive pill must be taken exactly as directed and at intervals not exceeding 24 hours.
- Important: Women should be instructed to use an additional method of protection until after the first 7 days of administration *in the initial cycle.*
- Due to the normally increased risk of thromboembolism occurring postpartum, women should be instructed not to initiate treatment with oral contraceptives earlier than 4–6 weeks after a full-term delivery. If pregnancy is terminated in the first 12 weeks, the patient should be instructed to start oral contraceptives immediately or within 7 days. If pregnancy is terminated after 12 weeks, the patient should be instructed to start oral contraceptives after 2 weeks.[33, 77]
- If spotting or breakthrough bleeding should occur, the patient should continue the medication according to the schedule. Should spotting or breakthrough bleeding persist, the patient should notify her physician.
- If the patient misses 1 pill, she should be instructed to take it as soon as she remembers and then take the next pill at the regular time. The patient should be advised that missing a pill can cause spotting or light bleeding and that she may be a little sick to her stomach on the days she takes the missed pill with her regularly scheduled pill. If the patient has missed more than one pill, see ***DETAILED PATIENT LABELING: HOW TO TAKE THE PILL, WHAT TO DO IF YOU MISS PILLS.***
- Use of oral contraceptives in the event of a missed menstrual period:
  1. If the patient has not adhered to the prescribed dosage regimen, the possibility of pregnancy should be considered after the first missed period and oral contraceptives should be withheld until pregnancy has been ruled out.
  2. If the patient has adhered to the prescribed regimen and misses 2 consecutive periods, pregnancy should be ruled out before continuing the contraceptive regimen.

HOW SUPPLIED

Ogestrel® 0.5/50-28 Tablets (norgestrel and ethinyl estradiol tablets USP, 0.5 mg/0.05 mg): Each white tablet is unscored, round in shape, with "5/50" debossed on one side and "SCS" on the other side, and contains 0.5 mg norgestrel and 0.05 mg ethinyl estradiol. Ogestrel® 0.5/50-28 is packaged in cartons of three tablet dispensers. Each tablet dispenser contains 21 white (active) tablets and 7 peach (inert) tablets. Inert tablets are unscored, round in shape with "SCS" debossed on one side and "P" on the other side.

Rx only

Store between 15°C to 25°C (59°F to 77°F).

Keep this and all medications out of the reach of children.

REFERENCES

1. Hatcher, R.A. Trussell, J. Stewart, F., et al.: *Contraceptive Technology: Sixteenth Revised Edition*, New York, NY, 1994. **2.** Mann, J., et al.: *Br Med J* 2(5956): 241–245, 1975. **3.** Knopp, R.H.: *J Reprod Med* 31(9): 913–921, 1986. **4.** Mann, J.I., et al.: *Br Med J* 2: 445–447, 1976 **5.** Ory, H.: *JAMA* 237: 2619–2622, 1977. **6.** The Cancer and Steroid Hormone Study of the Centers for Disease Control: *JAMA* 249(2): 1596–1599, 1983. **7.** The Cancer and Steroid Hormone Study of the Centers for Disease Control: *JAMA* 257(6): 796–800, 1987. **8.** Ory, H.W.: *JAMA* 228(1): 68–69, 1974. **9.** Ory, H.W., et al.: *N Engl J Med* 294: 419–422, 1976. **10.** Ory, H.W.: *Fam Plann Perspect* 14: 182–184, 1982 **11.** Ory, H.W., et al.: *Making Choices*, New York, The Alan Guttmacher Institute, 1983. **12.** Stadel, B.: *N Engl J Med* 305(11): 612–618, 1981. **13.** Stadel, B.: *N Engl J Med* 305(12): 672–677, 1981. **14.** Adam, S., et al.: *Br J Obstet Gynaecol* 88: 838–845, 1981. **15.** Mann, J., et al.: *Br Med J* 2(5965): 245–248, 1975. **16.** Royal College of General Practitioners' Oral Contraceptive Study: *Lancet* 1: 541–546, 1981. **17.** Slone, D., et al.: *N Engl J Med* 305(8): 420–424, 1981. **18.** Vessey, M.P.: *Br J Fam Plann* 6 (Supplement): 1–12, 1980. **19.** Russell-Briefel, R., et al.: *Prev Med* 15: 352–362, 1986. **20.** Goldbaum, G., et al.: *JAMA* 258(10): 1339–1342, 1987. **21.** LaRosa, J.C.: *J Reprod Med* 31 (9): 906–912, 1986. **22.** Krauss, R.M., et al.: *Am J Obstet Gynecol* 145: 446–452, 1983. **23.** Wahl, P., et al.: *N Engl J Med* 308(15): 862–867. 1983. **24.** Wynn, V., et al.: *Am J Obstet Gynecol* 142(6): 766–771, 1982. **25.** Wynn V., et al.: *J Reprod Med* 31(9): 892–897, 1986. **26.** Inman, W.H., et al.: *Br Med J* 2(5599): 193–199, 1968. **27.** Maguire, M.G., et al.: *Am J Epidemiol* 110(2): 188–195, 1979. **28.** Petitti, D., et al.: *JAMA* 242(11): 1150–1154, 1979. **29.** Vessey, M.P., et al.: *Br Med J* 2(5599): 199–205, 1968. **30.** Vessey, M.P., et al.: *Br Med J* 2(5658): 651–657, 1969. **31.** Porter, J.B., et al.: *Obstet Gynecol* 59(3): 299–302, 1982. **32.** Vessey, M.P., et al.: *J Biosoc Sci* 8: 373–427, 1976. **33.** Mishell, D.R., et al.: *Reproductive Endocrinology*, Philadelphia, F.A. Davis Co., 1979. **34.** Petitti, D.B., et al.: *Lancet* 2: 234–236, 1978. **35.** Collaborative Group for the Study of Stroke in Young Women: *JAMA* 231(7): 718–722, 1975. **36.** Inman, W.H., et al.: *Br Med J* 2: 203–209, 1970. **37.** Meade, T.W., et al.: *Br Med J* 280(6224): 1157–1161, 1980. **38.** Kay, C.R.: *Am J Obstet Gynecol* 142(6): 762–765, 1982. **39.** Gordon, T., et al.: *Am J Med* 62: 707–714, 1977. **40.** Royal College of General Practitioners' Oral Contraception Study: *J Coll Gen Pract* 33: 75–82, 1983. **41.** Ory, H.W.: *Fam Plann Perspect* 15(2): 57–63, 1983. **42.** Paul, C., et al.: *Br Med J* 293: 723–725, 1986. **43.** The Cancer and Steroid Hormone Study of the Centers for Disease Control: *N Engl J Med* 315(7): 405–411, 1986. **44.** Pike, M.C., et al.: *Lancet* 2: 926–929, 1983. **45.** Miller, D.R., et al.: *Obstet Gynecol* 68: 863–868, 1986. **46.** Olsson, H., et al.: *Lancet* 2: 748–749, 1985. **47.** McPherson, K., et al.: *Br J Cancer* 56: 653–660, 1987. **48.** Huggins, G.R., et al.: *Fertil Steril* 47(5): 733–761, 1987. **49.** McPherson, K., et al.: *Br Med J* 293: 709–710, 1986. **50.** Ory, H., et al.: *Am J Obstet Gynecol* 124(6): 573–577, 1976. **51.** Vessey, M.P., et al.: *Lancet* 2: 930, 1983. **52.** Brinton, L.A., et al.: *Int J Cancer* 38: 339–344, 1986. **53.** WHO Collaborative Study of Neoplasia and Steroid Contraceptives: *Br Med J* 290: 961–965, 1985.

ESTIMATED ANNUAL NUMBER OF BIRTH-RELATED OR METHOD-RELATED DEATHS ASSOCIATED WITH CONTROL OF FERTILITY PER 100,000 NON-STERILE WOMEN, BY FERTILITY CONTROL METHOD ACCORDING TO AGE

Method of control and outcome	15–19	20–24	25–29	30–34	35–39	40–44
No fertility control methods*	7.0	7.4	9.1	14.8	25.7	28.2
Oral contraceptives non-smoker**	0.3	0.5	0.9	1.9	13.8	31.6
Oral contraceptives smoker**	2.2	3.4	6.6	13.5	51.1	117.2
IUD**	0.8	0.8	1.0	1.0	1.4	1.4
Condom*	1.1	1.6	0.7	0.2	0.3	0.4
Diaphragm/Spermicide*	1.9	1.2	1.2	1.3	2.2	2.8
Periodic abstinence*	2.5	1.6	1.6	1.7	2.9	3.6

*Deaths are birth-related
**Deaths are method-related

54. Rooks, J.B., et al.: *JAMA* 242(7): 644–648, 1979. **55.** Bein, N.N., et al.: *Br J Surg* 64: 433–435, 1977. **56.** Klatskin, G.: *Gastroenterology* 73: 386–394, 1977. **57.** Henderson, B.E., et al.: *Br J Cancer* 48: 437–440, 1983. **58.** Neuberger, J., et al.: *Br Med J* 292: 1355–1357, 1986. **59.** Forman, D., et al.: *Br Med J* 292: 1357–1361, 1986. **60.** Harlap, S., et al.: *Obstet Gynecol* 55(4): 447–452, 1980. **61.** Savolainen, E., et al.: *Am J Obstet Gynecol* 140(5): 521–524, 1981. **62.** Janerich, D.T., et al.: *Am J Epidemiol* 112(1): 73–79, 1980. **63.** Ferencz, C., et al.: *Teratology* 21: 225–239, 1980. **64.** Rothman, K.J., et al.: *Am J Epidemiol* 109(4): 433–439, 1979. **65.** Boston Collaborative Drug Surveillance Program: *Lancet* 1: 1399–1404, 1973. **66.** Royal College of General Practitioners: *Oral contraceptives and health*. New York, Pittman, 1974. **67.** Rome Group for the Epidemiology and Prevention of Cholelithiasis: *Am J Epidemiol* 119(5): 796–805, 1984. **68.** Strom, B.L., et al.: *Clin Pharmacol Ther* 39(3): 335–341, 1986. **69.** Perlman, J.A., et al.: *J Chronic Dis* 38(10): 857–864, 1985. **70.** Wynn, V., et al.: *Lancet* 1: 1045–1049, 1979. **71.** Wynn, V.: *Progesterone and Progestin*, New York, Raven Press, 1983. **72.** Wynn, V., et al.: *Lancet* 2: 720–723, 1966. **73.** Fisch, I.R., et al: *JAMA* 237(23): 2499–2503, 1977. **74.** Laragh, J.H.: *Am J Obstet Gynecol* 126(1): 141–147, 1976. **75.** Ramcharan, S., et al.: *Pharmacology of Steroid Contraceptive Drugs*, New York, Raven Press, 1977. **76.** Stockley, I.: *Pharm J* 216: 140–143, 1976. **77.** Dickey, R.P.: *Managing Contraceptive Pill Patients*, Oklahoma, Creative Informatics Inc., 1984. **78.** Porter J.B., Hunter J., Jick H., et al.: *Obstet Gynecol* 1985;66: 1–4. **79.** Porter J.B., Hershel J., Walker A.M.: *Obstet Gynecol* 1987;70: 29–32. **80.** Fertility and Maternal Health Drugs Advisory Committee, F.D.A., October, 1989. **81.** Schlesselman J., Stadel B.V., Murray P., Lai S.: *Breast cancer in relation to early use of oral contraceptives.* JAMA 1988;259: 1828–1833. **82.** Henekens C.H., Speizer F.E., Lipnick R.J., Rosner B., Bain C., Belanger C., Stampfer M.J., Willett W., Peto R.: *A case-control study of oral contraceptive use and breast cancer.* JNCI 1984; 72: 39–42. **83.** Royal College of General Practitioners: *Oral contraceptives, venous thrombosis, and varicose veins. J Coll Gen Pract* 28: 393–399, 1978. **84.** Royal College of General Practitioners' Oral Contraception Study: *Effect on Hypertension and benign breast disease of progestogen component in combined oral contraceptives. Lancet* 1: 624, 1977.

DETAILED PATIENT LABELING

This product (like all oral contraceptives) is intended to prevent pregnancy. It does not protect against HIV infection (AIDS) and other sexually transmitted diseases.

INTRODUCTION

Any woman who considers using oral contraceptives ("birth control pills" or "the pill") should understand the benefits and risks of using this form of birth control. This leaflet will give you much of the information you will need to make this decision and also will help you determine if you are at risk of developing any of the serious side effects of the pill. It will tell you how to use the pill properly so that it will be as effective as possible. However, this leaflet is not a replacement for a careful discussion between you and your health care provider. You should discuss the information provided in this leaflet with him or her, both when you first start taking the pill and during your regular visits. You also should follow the advice of your health care provider with regard to regular checkups while you are on the pill.

EFFECTIVENESS OF ORAL CONTRACEPTIVES

Oral contraceptives are used to prevent pregnancy and are more effective than other non-surgical methods of birth control. When they are taken correctly, without missing any pills, the chance of becoming pregnant is less than 1% (1 pregnancy per 100 women per year of use). Typical failure rates are actually 3% per year. The chance of becoming pregnant increases with each missed pill during a menstrual cycle.

In comparison, typical failure rates for other nonsurgical methods of birth control during the first year are as follows:

Comparison of reversible contraceptive methods: Percentage of women experiencing a contraceptive failure (pregnancy) during the first year of use.

Method	Percentage of women experiencing an accidental pregnancy within the first year of use	
	Average use	Correct use
No contraception	85	85
Spermicides	21	6
Periodic abstinence	20	1–9[a]
Withdrawal	19	4
Cap		
Given birth	36	26
Never given birth	18	9
Sponge		
Given birth	36	20
Never given birth	18	9
Diaphragm	18	6
Condom		
Female	21	5
Male	12	3
Pill		
Progestin only		0.5
Combined		0.1
IUD		
Progesterone	2	1.5
Copper T 380A	0.8	0.6
Injectables	0.3	0.3
Implant	0.09	0.09

Adapted with permission—Hatcher, R.A. Trussell, J. Stewart, F., et al.: *Contraceptive Technology: Sixteenth Revised Edition*, New York, NY, 1994.

[a]Depending on method (calendar, ovulation, symptom-thermal)

WHO SHOULD NOT TAKE ORAL CONTRACEPTIVES

Cigarette smoking increases the risk of serious cardiovascular side effects from oral contraceptive use. This risk increases with age and with heavy smoking (15 or more cigarettes per day) and is quite marked in women over 35 years of age. Women who use oral contraceptives are strongly advised not to smoke.

Some women should not use the pill. For example, you should not take the pill if you are pregnant or think you may be pregnant. You also should not use the pill if you have any of the following conditions:

- A history of heart attack or stroke
- Blood clots in the legs (thrombophlebitis), brain (stroke), lungs (pulmonary embolism) or eyes
- A history of blood clots in the deep veins of your legs
- Chest pain (angina pectoris)
- Known or suspected breast cancer or cancer of the lining of the uterus, cervix or vagina
- Unexplained vaginal bleeding (until a diagnosis is reached by your doctor)
- Yellowing of the whites of the eyes or of the skin (jaundice) during pregnancy or during previous use of the pill
- Liver tumor (benign or cancerous)
- Known or suspected pregnancy

Tell your health care provider if you have ever had any of these conditions. Your health care provider can recommend a safer method of birth control.

OTHER CONSIDERATIONS BEFORE TAKING ORAL CONTRACEPTIVES

Tell your health care provider if you have or have had:

- Breast nodules, fibrocystic disease of the breast, an abnormal breast x-ray or mammogram
- Diabetes
- Elevated cholesterol or triglycerides
- High blood pressure
- Migraine or other headaches or epilepsy
- Mental depression
- Gallbladder, heart or kidney disease
- History of scanty or irregular menstrual periods

Women with any of these conditions should be checked often by their health care provider if they choose to use oral contraceptives. Also, be sure to inform your doctor or health care provider if you smoke or are on any medications.

RISKS OF TAKING ORAL CONTRACEPTIVES

1. Risk of developing blood clots

Blood clots and blockage of blood vessels are the most serious side effects of taking oral contraceptives. In particular, a clot in the legs can cause thrombophlebitis and a clot that travels to the lungs can cause sudden blocking of the vessel carrying blood to the lungs. Rarely, clots occur in the blood vessels of the eye and may cause blindness, double vision, or impaired vision.

If you take oral contraceptives and need elective surgery, need to stay in bed for a prolonged illness or have recently delivered a baby, you may be at risk of developing blood clots. You should consult your doctor about stopping oral contraceptives three to four weeks before surgery and not taking oral contraceptives for two weeks after surgery or during bed rest. You should also not take oral contraceptives soon after the delivery of a baby. It is advisable to wait for at least four weeks after delivery if you are not breast feeding. If you are breast feeding, you should wait until you have weaned your child before using the pill (see ***GENERAL PRECAUTIONS—While breast feeding***).

2. Heart attacks and strokes

Oral contraceptives may increase the tendency to develop strokes (stoppage or rupture of blood vessels in the brain) and angina pectoris and heart attacks (blockage of blood vessels in the heart). Any of these conditions can cause death or temporary or permanent disability.

Smoking greatly increases the possibility of suffering heart attacks and strokes. Furthermore, smoking and the use of oral contraceptives greatly increase the chances of developing and dying of heart disease.

3. Gallbladder disease

Oral contraceptive users may have a greater risk than nonusers of having gallbladder disease, although this risk may be related to pills containing high doses of estrogen.

4. Liver tumors

In rare cases, oral contraceptives can cause benign but dangerous liver tumors. These benign liver tumors can rupture and cause fatal internal bleeding. In addition, a possible but not definite association has been found with the pill and liver cancers in 2 studies in which a few women who developed these very rare cancers were found to have used oral contraceptives for long periods. However, liver cancers are extremely rare. The chance of developing liver cancer from using the pill is thus even rarer.

5. Cancer of the breast and reproductive organs

There is, at present, no confirmed evidence that oral contraceptives increase the risk of cancer of the reproductive organs in human studies. Several studies have found no overall increase in the risk of developing breast cancer. However, women who use oral contraceptives and have a strong family history of breast cancer or who have breast nodules or abnormal mammograms should be followed closely by their doctors. Some studies have reported an increase in the risk of developing breast cancer, particularly at a younger age. This increased risk appears to be related to duration of use.

Some studies have found an increase in the incidence of cancer of the cervix in women who use oral contraceptives. However, this finding may be related to factors other than the use of oral contraceptives.

ESTIMATED RISK OF DEATH FROM A BIRTH CONTROL METHOD OR PREGNANCY

All methods of birth control and pregnancy are associated with a risk of developing certain diseases which may lead to disability or death. An estimate of the number of deaths associated with different methods of birth control and pregnancy has been calculated and is shown in the following table:

[See table above]

In the above table, the risk of death from any birth control method is less than the risk of childbirth except for oral contraceptive users over the age of 35 who smoke and pill users over the age of 40 even if they do not smoke. It can be seen from the table that for women aged 15 to 39 the risk of death is highest with pregnancy (7–26 deaths per 100,000 women, depending on age). Among pill users who do not smoke the risk of death is always lower than that associated with pregnancy for any age group, although over the age of 40 the risk increases to 32 deaths per 100,000 women compared to 28 associated with pregnancy at that age. However, for pill users who smoke and are over the age of 35 the estimated number of deaths exceeds those for other methods of birth control. If a woman is over the age of 40 and smokes, her estimated risk of death is 4 times higher (117/100,000 women) than the estimated risk associated with pregnancy (28/100,000) in that age group.

The suggestion that women over 40 who don't smoke should not take oral contraceptives is based on information from older high-dose pills and on less selective use of pills than is practiced today. An Advisory Committee of the FDA discussed this issue in 1989 and recommended that the benefits of oral contraceptive use by healthy, non-smoking women over 40 years of age may outweigh the possible risks. However, all women, especially older women, are cautioned to use the lowest dose pill that is effective.

Continued on next page

Ogestrel—Cont.

WARNING SIGNALS

If any of these adverse effects occur while you are taking oral contraceptives, call your doctor immediately:

- Sharp chest pain, coughing of blood or sudden shortness of breath (indicating a possible clot in the lung)
- Pain in the calf (indicating a possible clot in the leg)
- Crushing chest pain or heaviness in the chest (indicating a possible heart attack)
- Sudden severe headache or vomiting, dizziness or fainting, disturbances of vision or speech, weakness or numbness in an arm or leg (indicating a possible stroke)
- Sudden partial or complete loss of vision (indicating a possible clot in the eye)
- Breast lumps (indicating possible breast cancer or fibrocystic disease of the breast: ask your doctor or health care provider to show you how to examine your breasts)
- Severe pain or tenderness in the stomach area (indicating a possible ruptured liver tumor)
- Difficulty in sleeping, weakness, lack of energy, fatigue or change in mood (possibly indicating severe depression)
- Jaundice or a yellowing of the skin or eyeballs, accompanied frequently by fever, fatigue, loss of appetite, dark colored urine or light colored bowel movements (indicating possible liver problems)

SIDE EFFECTS OF ORAL CONTRACEPTIVES

1. Vaginal bleeding

Irregular vaginal bleeding or spotting may occur while you are taking the pill. Irregular bleeding may vary from slight staining between menstrual periods to breakthrough bleeding which is a flow much like a regular period. Irregular bleeding occurs most often during the first few months of oral contraceptive use but may also occur after you have been taking the pill for some time. Such bleeding may be temporary and usually does not indicate any serious problem. It is important to continue taking your pills on schedule. If the bleeding occurs in more than 1 cycle or lasts for more than a few days, talk to your doctor or health care provider.

2. Contact lenses

If you wear contact lenses and notice a change in vision or an inability to wear your lenses, contact your doctor or health care provider.

3. Fluid retention

Oral contraceptives may cause edema (fluid retention) with swelling of the fingers or ankles and may raise your blood pressure. If you experience fluid retention, contact your doctor or health care provider.

4. Melasma (Mask of Pregnancy)

A spotty darkening of the skin is possible, particularly of the face.

5. Other side effects

Other side effects may include change in appetite, headache, nervousness, depression, dizziness, loss of scalp hair, rash and vaginal infections.

If any of these side effects occur, contact your doctor or health care provider.

GENERAL PRECAUTIONS

1. Missed periods and use of oral contraceptives before or during early pregnancy

At times you may not menstruate regularly after you have completed taking a cycle of pills. If you have taken your pills regularly and miss 1 menstrual period, continue taking your pills for the next cycle but be sure to inform your health care provider before doing so. If you have not taken the pills daily as instructed and miss 1 menstrual period, or if you miss 2 consecutive menstrual periods, you may be pregnant. Check with your health care provider immediately to determine whether you are pregnant. Do not continue to take oral contraceptives until you are sure you are not pregnant, but continue to use another method of birth control.

There is no conclusive evidence that oral contraceptive use is associated with an increase in birth defects when taken inadvertently during early pregnancy. Previously, a few studies had reported that oral contraceptives might be associated with birth defects but these studies have not been confirmed. Nevertheless, oral contraceptives or any other drugs should not be used during pregnancy unless clearly necessary and prescribed by your doctor. You should check with your doctor about risks to your unborn child from any medication taken during pregnancy.

2. While breast feeding

If you are breast feeding, consult your doctor before starting oral contraceptives. Some of the drug will be passed on to the child in the milk. A few adverse effects on the child have been reported, including yellowing of the skin (jaundice) and breast enlargement. In addition, oral contraceptives may decrease the amount and quality of your milk. If possible, do not use oral contraceptives and use another method of contraception while breast feeding. You should consider starting oral contraceptives only after you have weaned your child completely.

3. Laboratory tests

If you are scheduled for any laboratory tests, tell your doctor you are taking birth control pills. Certain blood tests may be affected by birth control pills.

4. Drug interactions

Certain drugs may interact with birth control pills to make them less effective in preventing pregnancy or cause an increase in breakthrough bleeding. Such drugs include rifampin; drugs used for epilepsy such as barbiturates (for example phenobarbital) and phenytoin (Dilantin is one brand of this drug); phenylbutazone (Butazolidin is one brand of this drug) and possibly certain antibiotics. You may need to use additional contraception when you take drugs which can make oral contraceptives less effective.

5. This product (like all oral contraceptives) is intended to prevent pregnancy. It does not protect against transmission of HIV (AIDS) and other sexually transmitted diseases such as chlamydia, genital herpes, genital warts, gonorrhea, hepatitis B, and syphilis.

HOW TO TAKE THE PILL

IMPORTANT POINTS TO REMEMBER

BEFORE YOU START TAKING YOUR PILLS:

1. BE SURE TO READ THESE DIRECTIONS:
   Before you start taking your pills.
   Anytime you are not sure what to do.
2. THE RIGHT WAY TO TAKE THE PILL IS TO TAKE ONE PILL EVERY DAY AT THE SAME TIME.
   If you miss pills you could get pregnant. This includes starting the pack late.
   The more pills you miss, the more likely you are to get pregnant.
3. MANY WOMEN HAVE SPOTTING OR LIGHT BLEEDING, OR MAY FEEL SICK TO THEIR STOMACH DURING THE FIRST 1–3 PACKS OF PILLS.
   If you feel sick to your stomach, do not stop taking the Pill. The problem will usually go away. If it doesn't go away, check with your doctor or clinic.
4. MISSING PILLS CAN ALSO CAUSE SPOTTING OR LIGHT BLEEDING, even when you make up these missed pills.
   On the days you take 2 pills to make up for missed pills, you could also feel a little sick to your stomach.
5. IF YOU HAVE VOMITING OR DIARRHEA, for any reason, or IF YOU TAKE SOME MEDICINES, including some antibiotics, your pills may not work as well.
   Use a back-up method (such as condoms, foam, or sponge) until you check with your doctor or clinic.
6. IF YOU HAVE TROUBLE REMEMBERING TO TAKE THE PILL, talk to your doctor of clinic about how to make pill-taking easier or about using another method of birth control.
7. IF YOU HAVE ANY QUESTIONS OR ARE UNSURE ABOUT THE INFORMATION IN THIS LEAFLET, call your doctor or clinic.

BEFORE YOU START TAKING YOUR PILLS

1. DECIDE WHAT TIME OF DAY YOU WANT TO TAKE YOUR PILL.

It is important to take it at about the same time every day.

2. LOOK AT YOUR PILL PACK:

The pill pack has 21 "active" white (with hormones) pills to take for 3 weeks, followed by 1 week of reminder peach pills (without hormones).

3. ALSO FIND:
   1) where on the pack to start taking pills, and
   2) in what order to take the pills (follow the arrows).

Active Pill Color: White
Reminder Pill Color: Peach

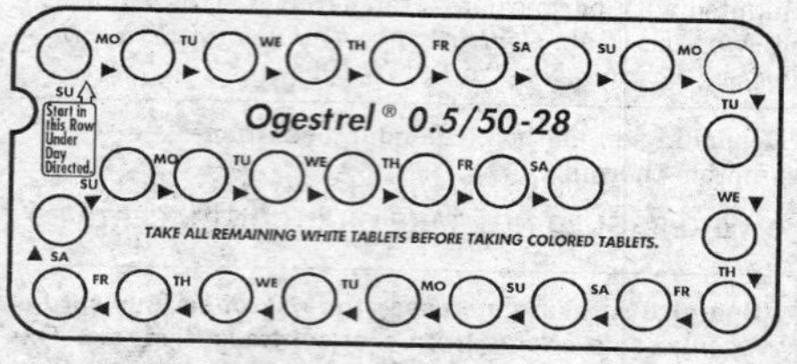

Ogestrel® 0.5/50-28
Start in this Row Under Day Directed
TAKE ALL REMAINING WHITE TABLETS BEFORE TAKING COLORED TABLETS.

4. BE SURE YOU HAVE READY AT ALL TIMES ANOTHER KIND OF BIRTH CONTROL (such as condoms, foam, or sponge) to use as a back-up in case you miss pills.
   AN EXTRA, FULL PILL PACK

WHEN TO START THE FIRST PACK OF PILLS

You have a choice of which day to start taking your first pack of pills. Decide with your doctor or clinic which is the best day for you. Pick a time of day which will be easy to remember.

DAY 1 START:

1. Take the first "active" white pill of the first pack during the first 24 hours of your period.
2. You will not need to use a back-up method of birth control, since you are starting the pill at the beginning of your period.

SUNDAY START:

1. Take the first "active" white pill of the first pack on the Sunday after your period starts, even if you are still bleeding. If your period begins on Sunday, start the pack that same day.
2. Use another method of birth control as a back-up method if you have sex anytime from the Sunday you start your first pack until the next Sunday (7 days). Condoms, foam, or the sponge are good back-up methods of birth control.

WHAT TO DO DURING THE MONTH

1. **TAKE ONE PILL AT THE SAME TIME EVERY DAY UNTIL THE PACK IS EMPTY.**
   Do not skip pills even if you are spotting or bleeding between monthly periods or feel sick to your stomach (nausea).
   Do not skip pills even if you do not have sex very often.
2. **WHEN YOU FINISH A PACK OR SWITCH YOUR BRAND OF PILLS:**
   Start the next pack on the day after your last "reminder" pill. Do not wait any days between packs.

WHAT TO DO IF YOU MISS PILLS

If you **MISS 1** white "active" pill:

1. Take it as soon as you remember. Take the next pill at your regular time. This means you may take 2 pills in 1 day.
2. You do not need to use a back-up birth control method if you have sex.

If you **MISS 2** white "active" pills in a row in **WEEK 1 OR WEEK 2** of your pack:

1. Take 2 pills on the day you remember and 2 pills the next day.
2. Then take 1 pill a day until you finish the pack.
3. You MAY BECOME PREGNANT if you have sex in the 7 days after you miss pills. You MUST use another birth control method (such as condoms, foam, or sponge) as a back-up for those 7 days.

If you **MISS 2** white "active" pills in a row in **THE 3rd WEEK:**

1. ***If you are a Day 1 Starter:***
   THROW OUT the rest of the pill pack and start a new pack that same day.
   If you are a Sunday Starter:
   Keep taking 1 pill every day until Sunday.
   On Sunday, THROW OUT the rest of the pack and start a new pack of pills that same day.
2. You may not have your period this month but this is expected.
   However, if you miss your period 2 months in a row, call your doctor or clinic because you might be pregnant.
3. You MAY BECOME PREGNANT if you have sex in the 7 days after you miss pills. You MUST use another birth control method (such as condoms, foams, or sponge) as a back-up for those 7 days.

If you **MISS 3 OR MORE** white "active" pills in a row (during the first 3 weeks):

1. ***If you are a Day 1 Starter:***
   THROW OUT the rest of the pill pack and start a new pack of pills that same day.
   If you are a Sunday Starter:
   Keep taking 1 pill every day until Sunday.
   On Sunday, THROW OUT the rest of the pack and start a new pack of pills that same day.
2. You may not have your period this month but this is expected.
   However, if you miss your period 2 months in a row, call your doctor or clinic because you might be pregnant.
3. You MAY BECOME PREGNANT if you have sex in the 7 days after you miss pills. You MUST use another birth control method (such as condoms, foam, or sponge) as a back-up for those 7 days.

REMINDER:

If you forget any of the 7 peach "reminder" pills in Week 4
THROW AWAY the pills you missed.
Keep taking 1 pill each day until the pack is empty.
You do not need a back-up method.

FINALLY, IF YOU ARE STILL NOT SURE WHAT TO DO ABOUT THE PILLS YOU HAVE MISSED:

Use a BACK-UP METHOD anytime you have sex.
KEEP TAKING ONE "ACTIVE" PILL EACH DAY until you can reach your doctor or clinic.

6. Missed periods, spotting or light bleeding

At times, you may not have a period after you have completed a pack of pills. If you miss 1 period but you have taken the pills exactly as you were supposed to, continue as usual into the next cycle. If you have not taken the pills correctly, and have missed a period, you may be pregnant and you should stop taking the Pill until your doctor or clinic determines whether or not you are pregnant. Until you can talk to your doctor or clinic, use an appropriate back-up birth control method. If you miss 2 consecutive periods, you should stop taking the Pill until it is determined that you are not pregnant.

Even if spotting or light bleeding should occur, continue taking the Pill according to the schedule. Should spotting or light bleeding persist, you should notify your doctor or clinic.

7. Stopping the pill before surgery or prolonged bed rest

If you are scheduled for surgery or you need to stay in bed for a long period of time you should tell your doctor that you are on the Pill. You should stop taking the Pill four weeks before your operation to avoid an increased risk of blood clots. Talk to your doctor about when you may start taking the Pill again.

8. Starting the pill after pregnancy

After you have a baby it is advisable to wait 4–6 weeks before starting to take the Pill. Talk to your doctor about when you may start taking the Pill after pregnancy.

9. Pregnancy due to pill failure

When the Pill is taken correctly, the expected pregnancy rate is approximately 1% (i.e., 1 pregnancy per 100 women per year). If pregnancy occurs while taking the Pill, there is little risk to the fetus. The typical failure rate of large numbers of pill users is less than 3% when women who have missed pills are included. If you become pregnant, you should discuss your pregnancy with your doctor.

10. Pregnancy after stopping the pill

There may be some delay in becoming pregnant after you stop taking the Pill, especially if you had irregular periods

before you started using the Pill. Your doctor may recommend that you delay becoming pregnant until you have had one or more regular periods.
There does not appear to be any increase in birth defects in newborn babies when pregnancy occurs soon after stopping the Pill.

11. Overdosage
There are no reports of serious illness or side effects in young children who have swallowed a large number of pills. In adults, overdosage may cause nausea and/or bleeding in females. In case of overdosage, contact your doctor, clinic or pharmacist.

12. Other Information
Your doctor or clinic will take a medical and family history and will examine you before prescribing the Pill. The physical examination may be delayed to another time if you request it and the health care provider believes that it is a good medical practice to postpone it. You should be reexamined at least once a year. Be sure to inform your doctor or clinic if there is a family history of any of the conditions listed previously in this leaflet. Be sure to keep all appointments with your doctor or clinic because this is a time to determine if there are early signs of side effects from using the Pill.
Do not use the Pill for any condition other than the one for which it was prescribed. The Pill has been prescribed specifically for you, do not give it to others who may want birth control pills.
If you want more information about birth control pills, ask your doctor or clinic. They have a more technical leaflet called ***PHYSICIAN LABELING*** which you might want to read.

NON-CONTRACEPTIVE HEALTH BENEFITS

In addition to preventing pregnancy, use of oral contraceptives may provide certain non-contraceptive health benefits:
- Menstrual cycles may become more regular
- Blood flow during menstruation may be lighter and less iron may be lost. Therefore, anemia due to iron deficiency is less likely to occur
- Pain or other symptoms during menstruation may be encountered less frequently
- Ectopic (tubal) pregnancy may occur less frequently
- Non-cancerous cysts or lumps in the breast may occur less frequently
- Acute pelvic inflammatory disease may occur less frequently
- Oral contraceptive use may provide some protection against developing two forms of cancer: cancer of the ovaries and cancer of the lining of the uterus
- If you want more information about birth control pills, ask your doctor or pharmacist. They have a more technical leaflet called the Professional Labeling, which you may wish to read.

Store between 15°C to 25°C (59°F to 77°F).
Keep this and all medication out of the reach of children.

BRIEF SUMMARY
PATIENT PACKAGE INSERT

This product (like all oral contraceptives) is intended to prevent pregnancy. It does not protect against HIV infection (AIDS) and other sexually transmitted diseases.
Oral contraceptives, also known as "birth control pills" or "the pill," are taken to prevent pregnancy and, when taken correctly, have a failure rate of about 1% per year when used without missing any pills. The typical failure rate of large numbers of pill users is less than 3% per year when women who miss pills are included. For most women, oral contraceptives are also free of serious or unpleasant side effects. However, forgetting to take oral contraceptives considerably increases the chances of pregnancy.
For the majority of women, oral contraceptives can be taken safely, but there are some women who are at high risk of developing certain serious diseases that can be life-threatening or may cause temporary or permanent disability. The risks associated with taking oral contraceptives increase significantly if you:
- Smoke
- Have high blood pressure, diabetes or high cholesterol
- Have or have had clotting disorders, heart attack, stroke, angina pectoris, cancer of the breast or sex organs, jaundice or malignant or benign liver tumors

You should not take the pill if you suspect you are pregnant or have unexplained vaginal bleeding.

Cigarette smoking increases the risk of serious cardiovascular side effects from oral contraceptive use. This risk increases with age and with heavy smoking (15 or more cigarettes per day) and is quite marked in women over 35 years of age. Women who use oral contraceptives are strongly advised not to smoke.

Most side effects of the pill are not serious. The most common such effects are nausea, vomiting, bleeding between menstrual periods, weight gain, breast tenderness and difficulty wearing contact lenses. These side effects, especially nausea and vomiting, may subside within the first 3 months of use.
The serious side effects of the pill occur very infrequently, especially if you are in good health and are young. However, you should know that the following medical conditions have been associated with or made worse by the pill:
1. Blood clots in the legs (thrombophlebitis) or lungs (pulmonary embolism), stoppage or rupture of a blood vessel in the brain (stroke), blockage of blood vessels in the heart (heart attack or angina pectoris), eye or other organs of the body. As mentioned above, smoking increases the risk of heart attacks and strokes and subsequent serious medical consequences.
2. Liver tumors, which may rupture and cause severe bleeding. A possible but not definite association has been found with the pill and liver cancer. However, liver cancers are extremely rare. The chance of developing liver cancer from using the pill is thus even rarer.
3. High blood pressure, although blood pressure usually returns to normal when the pill is stopped.

The symptoms associated with these serious side effects are discussed in the detailed leaflet given to you with your supply of pills. Notify your doctor or health care provider if you notice any unusual physical disturbances while taking the pill. In addition, drugs such as rifampin, as well as some anti-convulsants and some antibiotics, may decrease oral contraceptive effectiveness.
Studies to date of women taking the pill have not shown an increase in the incidence of cancer of the breast or cervix. There is, however, insufficient evidence to rule out the possibility that the pill may cause such cancers. Some studies have reported an increase in the risk of developing breast cancer, particularly at a younger age. This increased risk appears to be related to duration of use.
Taking the pill provides some important non-contraceptive health benefits. These include less painful menstruation, less menstrual blood loss and anemia, fewer pelvic infections and fewer cancers of the ovary and the lining of the uterus.
Be sure to discuss any medical condition you may have with your health care provider. Your health care provider will take a medical and family history before prescribing oral contraceptives and will examine you. The physical examination may be delayed to another time if you request it and the health care provider believes that it is a good medical practice to postpone it. You should be reexamined at least once a year while taking oral contraceptives. The detailed patient information leaflet gives you further information which you should read and discuss with your health care provider.

HOW TO TAKE THE PILL

See full text of *HOW TO TAKE THE PILL* which is printed in full in the ***DETAILED PATIENT LABELING.***
Keep this and all medication out of the reach of children.
Rx only

Revised: Jan. 06, 2000

Address medical inquiries to:
WATSON PHARMA, INC.
Medical Information
PO Box 1900
Corona, CA 92878-1900

Mfg. by: Searle & Co.
San Juan, PR 00936
for: WATSON PHARMA, INC.
a subsidiary of Watson Laboratories, Inc.
Corona, CA 92880

TRI-NORINYL®-28 ℞

(norethindrone and ethinyl estradiol)
Rx only

Patients should be counseled that this product does not protect against HIV infection (AIDS) and other sexually transmitted diseases.

ORAL CONTRACEPTIVE AGENTS

DESCRIPTION

Tri-Norinyl-28 provides a continuous oral contraceptive regimen of 7 blue tablets, 9 yellow-green tablets, 5 more blue tablets, and then 7 orange tablets. Each blue tablet contains norethindrone 0.5 mg and ethinyl estradiol 0.035 mg, each yellow-green tablet contains norethindrone 1 mg and ethinyl estradiol 0.035 mg, and each orange tablet contains inert ingredients.
Norethindrone is a potent progestational agent with the chemical name 17-Hydroxy-19-nor-17α-pregn-4-en-20-yn-3-one. Ethinyl estradiol is an estrogen with the chemical name 19-Nor-17α-pregna-1,3,5(10)-trien-20-yne-3,17-diol. Their structural formulae follow:

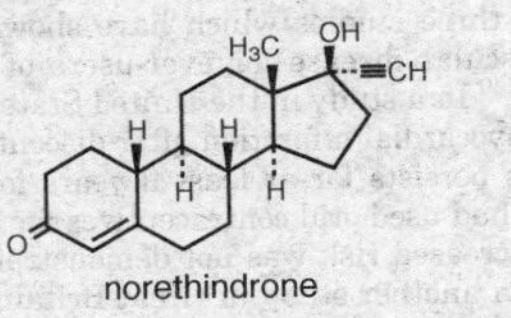

norethindrone

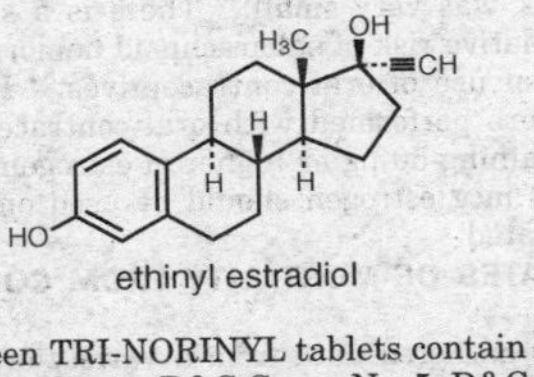

ethinyl estradiol

The yellow-green TRI-NORINYL tablets contain the following inactive ingredients: D&C Green No. 5, D&C Yellow No. 10, lactose, magnesium stearate, povidone, and starch.
The blue TRI-NORINYL tablets contain the following inactive ingredients: FD&C Blue No. 1, lactose, magnesium stearate, povidone, and starch.
The inactive orange tablets in the 28-day regimen contain the following inactive ingredients: FD&C Yellow No. 6, lactose, magnesium stearate, povidone, and starch.

CLINICAL PHARMACOLOGY

Combination oral contraceptives act by suppression of gonadotrophins. Although the primary mechanism of this action is inhibition of ovulation, other alterations include changes in the cervical mucus (which increase the difficulty of sperm entry into the uterus) and the endometrium (which may reduce the likelihood of implantation).

INDICATIONS AND USAGE

Oral contraceptives are indicated for the prevention of pregnancy in women who elect to use this product as a method of contraception.
Oral contraceptive products such as Norinyl, which contain 50 mcg of estrogen, should not be used unless medically indicated.
Oral contraceptives are highly effective. Table 1 lists the typical accidental pregnancy rates for users of combination oral contraceptives and other methods of contraception.[1] The efficacy of these contraceptive methods, except sterilization, depends upon the reliability with which they are used. Correct and consistent use of methods can result in lower failure rates.
[See table at top of next page]

CONTRAINDICATIONS

Oral contraceptives should not be used in women who have the following conditions:
- Thrombophlebitis or thromboembolic disorders
- A past history of deep vein thrombophlebitis or thromboembolic disorders
- Cerebral vascular or coronary artery disease
- Known or suspected carcinoma of the breast
- Carcinoma of the endometrium or other known or suspected estrogen-dependent neoplasia
- Undiagnosed abnormal genital bleeding
- Cholestatic jaundice of pregnancy or jaundice with prior pill use
- Hepatic adenomas, carcinomas or benign liver tumors
- Known or suspected pregnancy

WARNINGS

Cigarette smoking increases the risk of serious cardiovascular side effects from oral contraceptive use. This risk increases with age and with heavy smoking (15 or more cigarettes per day) and is quite marked in women over 35 years of age. Women who use oral contraceptives should be strongly advised not to smoke.

The use of oral contraceptives is associated with increased risks of several serious conditions including myocardial infarction, thromboembolism, stroke, hepatic neoplasia, and gallbladder disease, although the risk of serious morbidity or mortality is very small in healthy women without underlying risk factors. The risk of morbidity and mortality increases significantly in the presence of other underlying risk factors such as hypertension, hyperlipidemias, hypercholesterolemia, obesity and diabetes.[2–5]
Practitioners prescribing oral contraceptives should be familiar with the following information relating to these risks.
The information contained in this package insert is principally based on studies carried out in patients who used oral contraceptives with higher formulations of both estrogens and progestogens than those in common use today.[6–11] The effect of long-term use of the oral contraceptives with lower formulations of both estrogens and progestogens remains to be determined.
Throughout this labeling, epidemiological studies reported are of two types: retrospective or case control studies and prospective or cohort studies. Case control studies provide a measure of the relative risk of a disease. Relative risk, the *ratio* of the incidence of a disease among oral contraceptive users to that among non-users, cannot be assessed directly from case control studies, but the odds ratio obtained is a measure of relative risk. The relative risk does not provide information on the actual clinical occurrence of a disease. Cohort studies provide not only a measure of the relative risk but a measure of attributable risk, which is the *difference* in the incidence of disease between oral contraceptive users and non-users. The attributable risk does provide information about the actual occurrence of a disease in the population (adapted from ref. 12 and 13 with the author's permission). For further information, the reader is referred to a text on epidemiological methods.

1. THROMBOEMBOLIC DISORDERS AND OTHER VASCULAR PROBLEMS

a. Myocardial Infarction
An increased risk of myocardial infarction has been attributed to oral contraceptive use. This risk is primarily in smokers or women with other underlying risk factors for coronary artery disease such as hypertension, hypercholesterolemia, morbid obesity and diabetes.[2–5, 13] The relative risk of heart attack for current oral contraceptive users has been estimated to be 2 to 6.[2, 14–19] The risk is very low under the age of 30. However, there is the possibility of a risk of cardiovascular disease even in very young women who take oral contraceptives.

Continued on next page

Tri-Norinyl—Cont.

Smoking in combination with oral contraceptive use has been shown to contribute substantially to the incidence of myocardial infarctions in women in their mid-thirties or older, with smoking accounting for the majority of excess cases.[20]

Mortality rates associated with circulatory disease have been shown to increase substantially in smokers over the age of 35 and non-smokers over the age of 40 among women who use oral contraceptives (see Table II).[16]

TABLE II: CIRCULATORY DISEASE MORTALITY RATES PER 100,000 WOMAN YEARS BY AGE, SMOKING STATUS AND ORAL CONTRACEPTIVE USE

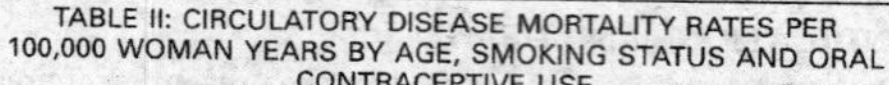

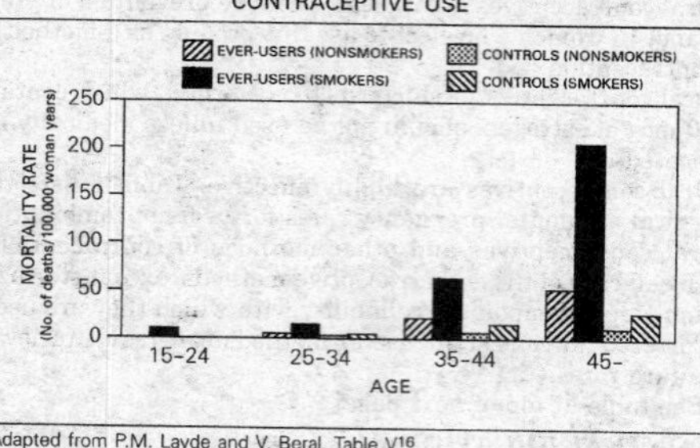

Adapted from P.M. Layde and V. Beral, Table V[16]

Oral contraceptives may compound the effects of well-known risk factors such as hypertension, diabetes, hyperlipidemias, hypercholesterolemia, age and obesity.[3, 13, 21] In particular, some progestogens are known to decrease HDL cholesterol and cause glucose intolerance, while estrogens may create a state of hyperinsulinism.[21–25] Oral contraceptives have been shown to increase blood pressure among users (see ***WARNINGS,*** section 9). Similar effects on risk factors have been associated with an increased risk of heart disease. Oral contraceptives must be used with caution in women with cardiovascular disease risk factors.

b. Thromboembolism

An increased risk of thromboembolic and thrombotic disease associated with the use of oral contraceptives is well established. Case control studies have found the relative risk of users compared to nonusers to be 3 for the first episode of superficial venous thrombosis, 4 to 11 for deep vein thrombosis or pulmonary embolism, and 1.5 to 6 for women with predisposing conditions for venous thromboembolic disease.[12, 13, 26–31] Cohort studies have shown the relative risk to be somewhat lower, about 3 for new cases and about 4.5 for new cases requiring hospitalization.[32] The risk of thromboembolic disease due to oral contraceptives is not related to length of use and disappears after pill use is stopped.[12]

A 2- to 6-fold increase in relative risk of post-operative thromboembolic complications has been reported with the use of oral contraceptives. The relative risk of venous thrombosis in women who have predisposing conditions is twice that of women without such medical conditions.[83] If feasible, oral contraceptives should be discontinued at least 4 weeks prior to and for 2 weeks after elective surgery and during and following prolonged immobilization. Since the immediate postpartum period also is associated with an increased risk of thromboembolism, oral contraceptives should be started no earlier than 4 to 6 weeks after delivery in women who elect not to breast feed.[33]

c. Cerebrovascular diseases

An increase in both the relative and attributable risks of cerebrovascular events (thrombotic and hemorrhagic strokes) has been shown in users of oral contraceptives. In general, the risk is greatest among older (>35 years), hypertensive women who also smoke. Hypertension was found to be a risk factor for both users and non-users for both types of strokes while smoking interacted to increase the risk for hemorrhagic strokes.[34]

In a large study, the relative risk of thrombotic strokes has been shown to range from 3 for normotensive users to 14 for users with severe hypertension.[35] The relative risk of hemorrhagic stroke is reported to be 1.2 for non-smokers who used oral contraceptives, 2.6 for smokers who did not use oral contraceptives, 7.6 for smokers who used oral contraceptives, 1.8 for normotensive users and 25.7 for users with severe hypertension.[35] The attributable risk also is greater in women in their mid-thirties or older and among smokers.[13]

d. Dose-related risk of vascular disease from oral contraceptives

A positive association has been observed between the amount of estrogen and progestogen in oral contraceptives and the risk of vascular disease.[36–38] A decline in serum high density lipoproteins (HDL) has been reported with many progestational agents.[22–24] A decline in serum high density lipoproteins has been associated with an increased incidence of ischemic heart disease.[39] Because estrogens increase HDL cholesterol, the net effect of an oral contraceptive depends on a balance achieved between doses of estrogen and progestogen and the nature and absolute amount of progestogens used in the contraceptives. The amount of both hormones should be considered in the choice of an oral contraceptive.[37]

Minimizing exposure to estrogen and progestogen is in keeping with good principles of therapeutics. For any particular estrogen/progestogen combination, the dosage regimen prescribed should be one which contains the least amount of estrogen and progestogen that is compatible with a low failure rate and the needs of the individual patient. New acceptors of oral contraceptive agents should be started on preparations containing the lowest estrogen content that produces satisfactory results for the individual. Products containing 50 mcg estrogen should be used only when medically indicated.

e. Persistence of risk of vascular disease

There are three studies which have shown persistence of risk of vascular disease for ever-users of oral contraceptives.[17, 34, 40] In a study in the United States, the risk of developing myocardial infarction after discontinuing oral contraceptives persists for at least 9 years for women 40–49 years who had used oral contraceptives for 5 or more years, but this increased risk was not demonstrated in other age groups.[17] In another study in Great Britain, the risk of developing cerebrovascular disease persisted for at least 6 years after discontinuation of oral contraceptives, although excess risk was very small.[40] There is a significantly increased relative risk of subarachnoid hemorrhage after termination of use of oral contraceptives.[34] However, these studies were performed with oral contraceptive formulations containing 50 μg or higher of estrogen. Products containing 50 mcg estrogen should be used only when medically indicated.

2. ESTIMATES OF MORTALITY FROM CONTRACEPTIVE USE

One study gathered data from a variety of sources which have estimated the mortality rates associated with different methods of contraception at different ages (see Table III).[41] These estimates include the combined risk of death associated with contraceptive methods plus the risk attributable to pregnancy in the event of method failure. Each method of contraception has its specific benefits and risks. The study concluded that with the exception of oral contraceptive users 35 and older who smoke and 40 and older who do not smoke, mortality associated with all methods of birth control is low and below that associated with childbirth. The observation of a possible increase in risk of mortality with age for oral contraceptive users is based on data gathered in the 1970s—but not reported in the U.S. until 1983.[16, 41] However, current clinical practice involves the use of lower estrogen dose formulations combined with careful restriction of oral contraceptive use to women who do not have the various risk factors listed in this labeling.

Because of these changes in practice and, also because of some limited new data which suggest that the risk of cardiovascular disease with the use of oral contraceptives may now be less than previously observed,[78, 79] the Fertility and Maternal Health Drugs Advisory Committee was asked to review the topic in 1989. The Committee concluded that although cardiovascular disease risks may be increased with oral contraceptive use after age 40 in healthy nonsmoking women (even with the newer low-dose formulations), there are greater potential health risks associated with pregnancy in older women and with the alternative surgical and medical procedures which may be necessary if such women do not have access to effective and acceptable means of contraception.

Therefore, the Committee recommended that the benefits of oral contraceptive use by healthy non-smoking women over 40 may outweigh the possible risks. Of course, older women, as all women who take oral contraceptives, should take the lowest possible dose formulation that is effective.[80]

Table 1- Percentage of women experiencing an unintended pregnancy during the first year of typical use and the first year of perfect use of contraception and the percentage continuing use at the end of the first year. United States.

Method (1)	% of Women Experiencing an Unintended Pregnancy within the First Year of Use: Typical use[1] (2)	Perfect use[2] (3)	% of Women Continuing Use at One Year[3] (4)
Chance[4]	85	85	
Spermicides[5]	26	6	40
Periodic abstinence	25		63
Calendar		9	
Ovulation method		3	
Sympto-thermal[6]		2	
Post-ovulation		1	
Withdrawal	19	4	
Cap[7]			
Parous women	40	26	42
Nulliparous women	20	9	56
Sponge			
Parous women	40	20	42
Nulliparous women	20	9	56
Diaphragm[7]	20	6	56
Condom[8]			
Female (Reality)	21	5	56
Male	14	3	61
Pill	5		71
Progestin only		0.5	
Combined		0.1	
IUD			
Progesterone T	2.0	1.5	81
Copper T 380A	0.8	0.6	78
LNg 20	0.1	0.1	81
Depo-Provera	0.3	0.3	70
Norplant and Norplant-2	0.05	0.05	88
Female sterilization	0.5	0.5	100
Male sterilization	0.15	0.10	100

Emergency Contraceptive Pills: Treatment initiated within 72 hours after unprotected intercourse reduces the risk of pregnancy by at least 75%.[9]

Lactational Amenorrhea Method: LAM is a highly effective, *temporary* method of contraception.[10]

Source: Trussell J. Contraceptive Efficacy Table from Hatcher R.A., Trussell J. Stewart F, Cates W. Stewart GK, Kowal D, Guest F, in Contraceptive Technology: Seventeenth Revised Edition. New York, NY: Irvington Publishers, 1998.

1 Among *typical* couples who initiate use of a method (not necessarily for the first time), the percentage who experience an accidental pregnancy during the first year if they do not stop use for any other reason.

2 Among couples who initiate use of a method (not necessarily for the first time) and who use it *perfectly* (both consistently and correctly), the percentage who experience an accidental pregnancy during the first year if they do not stop use for any other reason.

3 Among couples attempting to avoid pregnancy, the percentage who continue to use a method for one year.

4 The percentage becoming pregnant in columns (2) and (3) are based on data from populations where contraception is not used and from women who cease using contraception in order to become pregnant. Among such populations, about 89% become pregnant within one year. This estimate was lowered slightly (to 85%) to represent the percent who would become pregnant within one year among women now relying on reversible methods of contraception if they abandoned contraception altogether.

5 Foams, creams, gels, vaginal suppositories, and vaginal film.

6 Cervical mucus (ovulation) method supplemented by calendar in the pre-ovulatory and basal body temperature in the post-ovulatory phases.

7 With spermicidal cream or jelly.

8 Without spermicides.

9 The treatment schedule is one dose within 72 hours after unprotected intercourse and a second dose 12 hours after the first dose. The Food and Drug Administration has declared the following brands of oral contraceptives to be safe and effective for emergency contraception: Ovral (1 dose is 2 white pills). Aleese (1 dose is 5 pink pills), Nordette or Levlen (1 dose is 2 light-orange pills), Lo/Ovral (1 dose is 4 white pills), Triphasil or Tri-Levlen (1 dose is 4 yellow pills).

10 However, to maintain effective protection against pregnancy, another method of contraception must be used as soon as menstruation resumes, the frequency or duration of breastfeeds is reduced, bottle feeds are introduced, or the baby reaches six months of age.

TABLE III: ESTIMATED ANNUAL NUMBER OF BIRTH-RELATED OR METHOD-RELATED DEATHS ASSOCIATED WITH CONTROL OF FERTILITY PER 100,000 NONSTERILE WOMEN, BY FERTILITY CONTROL METHOD ACCORDING TO AGE

Method of control and outcome	15–19	20–24	25–29	30–34	35–39	40–44
No fertility control methods*	7.0	7.4	9.1	14.8	25.7	28.2
Oral contraceptives non-smoker**	0.3	0.5	0.9	1.9	13.8	31.6
Oral contraceptives smoker**	2.2	3.4	6.6	13.5	51.1	117.2
IUD**	0.8	0.8	1.0	1.0	1.4	1.4
Condom*	1.1	1.6	0.7	0.2	0.3	0.4
Diaphragm/Spermicide*	1.9	1.2	1.2	1.3	2.2	2.8
Periodic abstinence*	2.5	1.6	1.6	1.7	2.9	3.6

*Deaths are birth-related
**Deaths are method-related

Estimates adapted from H.W. Ory, Table 3[41]

[See table at right]

3. CARCINOMA OF THE BREAST AND REPRODUCTIVE ORGANS

Numerous epidemiological studies have been performed on the incidence of breast, endometrial, ovarian and cervical cancer in women using oral contraceptives. The overwhelming evidence in the literature suggests that use of oral contraceptives is not associated with an increase in the risk of developing breast cancer, regardless of the age and parity of first use or with most of the marketed brands and doses.[42–44] The Cancer and Steroid Hormone (CASH) study also showed no latent effect on the risk of breast cancer for at least a decade following long-term use.[43] A few studies have shown a slightly increased relative risk of developing breast cancer,[44–47] although the methodology of these studies, which included differences in examination of users and non-users and differences in age at start of use, has been questioned.[47–49] Some studies have reported an increased relative risk of developing breast cancer, particularly at a younger age. This increased relative risk appears to be related to duration of use.[81, 82]

Some studies suggest that oral contraceptive use has been associated with an increase in the risk of cervical intraepithelial neoplasia in some populations of women.[50–53] However, there continues to be controversy about the extent to which such findings may be due to differences in sexual behavior and other factors.

In spite of many studies of the relationship between oral contraceptive use and breast or cervical cancers, a cause and effect relationship has not been established.

4. HEPATIC NEOPLASIA

Benign hepatic adenomas are associated with oral contraceptive use although the incidence of benign tumors is rare in the United States. Indirect calculations have estimated the attributable risk to be in the range of 3.3 cases per 100,000 for users, a risk that increases after 4 or more years of use.[54] Rupture of rare, benign, hepatic adenomas may cause death through intra-abdominal hemorrhage.[55–56]

Studies in the United States and Britain have shown an increased risk of developing hepatocellular carcinoma in long-term (>8 years) oral contraceptive users.[57–59] However, these cancers are extremely rare in the United States and the attributable risk (the excess incidence) of liver cancers in oral contraceptive users approaches less than 1 per 1,000,000 users.

5. OCULAR LESIONS

There have been clinical case reports of retinal thrombosis associated with the use of oral contraceptives. Oral contraceptives should be discontinued if there is unexplained partial or complete loss of vision; onset of proptosis or diplopia; papilledema; or retinal vascular lesions. Appropriate diagnostic and therapeutic measures should be undertaken immediately.

6. ORAL CONTRACEPTIVE USE BEFORE OR DURING EARLY PREGNANCY

Extensive epidemiological studies have revealed no increased risk of birth defects in women who have used oral contraceptives prior to pregnancy.[60–62] Studies also do not suggest a teratogenic effect, particulary insofar as cardiac anomalies and limb reduction defects are concerned, when taken inadvertently during early pregnancy.[60,61,63,64]

The administration of oral contraceptives to induce withdrawal bleeding should not be used as a test for pregnancy. Oral contraceptives should not be used during pregnancy to treat threatened or habitual abortion.

It is recommended that for any patient who has missed 2 consecutive periods, pregnancy should be ruled out before continuing oral contraceptive use. If the patient has not adhered to the prescribed schedule, the possibility of pregnancy should be considered at the first missed period. Oral contraceptive use should be discontinued if pregnancy is confirmed.

7. GALLBLADDER DISEASE

Earlier studies have reported an increased lifetime relative risk of gallbladder surgery in users of oral contraceptives and estrogens.[65–66] More recent studies, however, have shown that the relative risk of developing gallbladder disease among oral contraceptive users may be minimal.[67] The recent findings of minimal risk may be related to the use of oral contraceptive formulations containing lower hormonal doses of estrogens and progestogens.[68]

8. CARBOHYDRATE AND LIPID METABOLIC EFFECTS

Oral contraceptives have been shown to cause glucose intolerance in a significant percentage of users.[25] Oral contraceptives containing greater than 75 µg of estrogen cause hyperinsulinism, while lower doses of estrogen cause less glucose intolerance.[70] Progestogens increase insulin secretion and create insulin resistance, this effect varying with different progestational agents.[25, 71] However, in the non-diabetic woman, oral contraceptives appear to have no effect on fasting blood glucose.[69] Because of these demonstrated effects, prediabetic and diabetic women should be carefully observed while taking oral contraceptives.

Some women may develop persistent hypertriglyceridemia while on the pill.[72] As discussed earlier (see ***WARNINGS,*** sections 1a. and 1d.), changes in serum triglycerides and lipoprotein levels have been reported in oral contraceptive users.[23]

9. ELEVATED BLOOD PRESSURE

An increase in blood pressure has been reported in women taking oral contraceptives and this increase is more likely in older oral contraceptive users and with continued use.[73, 84] Data from the Royal College of General Practitioners and subsequent randomized trials have shown that the incidence of hypertension increases with increasing concentrations of progestogens.

Women with a history of hypertension or hypertension-related diseases or renal disease should be encouraged to use another method of contraception. If women elect to use oral contraceptives, they should be monitored closely and if significant elevation of blood pressure occurs oral contraceptives should be discontinued. For most women, elevated blood pressure will return to normal after stopping oral contraceptives and there is no difference in the occurrence of hypertension among ever- and never-users.[73–75]

10. HEADACHE

The onset or exacerbation of migraine or development of headache with a new pattern which is recurrent, persistent or severe requires discontinuation of oral contraceptives and evaluation of the cause.

11. BLEEDING IRREGULARITIES

Breakthrough bleeding and spotting are sometimes encountered in patients on oral contraceptives, especially during the first 3 months of use. Non-hormonal causes should be considered and adequate diagnostic measures taken to rule out malignancy or pregnancy in the event of breakthrough bleeding, as in the case of any abnormal vaginal bleeding. If pathology has been excluded, time or a change to another formulation may solve the problem. In the event of amenorrhea, pregnancy should be ruled out.

Some women may encounter post-pill amenorrhea or oligomenorrhea, especially when such a condition was pre-existent.

PRECAUTIONS

GENERAL

Patients should be counseled that this product does not protect against HIV infection (AIDS) and other sexually transmitted diseases.

1. PHYSICAL EXAMINATION AND FOLLOW-UP

It is good medical practice for all women to have annual history and physical examinations, including women using oral contraceptives. The physical examination, however, may be deferred until after initiation of oral contraceptives if requested by the woman and judged appropriate by the clinician. The physical examination should include special reference to blood pressure, breasts, abdomen and pelvic organs, including cervical cytology, and relevant laboratory tests. In case of undiagnosed, persistent or recurrent abnormal vaginal bleeding, appropriate measures should be conducted to rule out malignancy. Women with a strong family history of breast cancer or who have breast nodules should be monitored with particular care.

2. LIPID DISORDERS

Women who are being treated for hyperlipidemias should be followed closely if they elect to use oral contraceptives. Some progestogens may elevate LDL levels and may render the control of hyperlipidemias more difficult.

3. LIVER FUNCTION

If jaundice develops in any woman receiving oral contraceptives the medication should be discontinued. Steroid hormones may be poorly metabolized in patients with impaired liver function.

4. FLUID RETENTION

Oral contraceptives may cause some degree of fluid retention. They should be prescribed with caution, and only with careful monitoring, in patients with conditions which might be aggravated by fluid retention.

5. EMOTIONAL DISORDERS

Women with a history of depression should be carefully observed and the drug discontinued if depression recurs to a serious degree.

6. CONTACT LENSES

Contact lens wearers who develop visual changes or changes in lens tolerance should be assessed by an ophthalmologist.

7. DRUG INTERACTIONS

Reduced efficacy and increased incidence of breakthrough bleeding and menstrual irregularities have been associated with concomitant use of rifampin. A similar association though less marked, has been suggested with barbiturates, phenylbutazone, phenytoin sodium, and possibly with griseofulvin, ampicillin and tetracyclines.[76]

8. INTERACTIONS WITH LABORATORY TESTS

Certain endocrine and liver function tests and blood components may be affected by oral contraceptives:

a. Increased prothrombin and factors VII, VIII, IX, and X; decreased antithrombin 3; increased norepinephrine-induced platelet aggregability.
b. Increased thyroid binding globulin (TBG) leading to increased circulating total thyroid hormone, as measured by protein-bound iodine (PBI), T4 by column or by radioimmunoassay. Free T3 resin uptake is decreased, reflecting the elevated TBG. Free T4 concentration is unaltered.
c. Other binding proteins may be elevated in serum.
d. Sex steroid binding globulins are increased and result in elevated levels of total circulating sex steroids and corticoids; however, free or biologically active levels remain unchanged.
e. Triglycerides may be increased.
f. Glucose tolerance may be decreased.
g. Serum folate levels may be depressed by oral contraceptive therapy. This may be of clinical significance if a woman becomes pregnant shortly after discontinuing oral contraceptives.

9. CARCINOGENESIS

See ***WARNINGS*** section.

10. PREGNANCY

Pregnancy Category X. See ***CONTRAINDICATIONS*** and ***WARNINGS*** sections.

11. NURSING MOTHERS

Small amounts of oral contraceptive steroids have been identified in the milk of nursing mothers and a few adverse effects on the child have been reported, including jaundice and breast enlargement. In addition, oral contraceptives given in the postpartum period may interfere with lactation by decreasing the quantity and quality of breast milk. If possible, the nursing mother should be advised not to use oral contraceptives but to use other forms of contraception until she has completely weaned her child.

12. PEDIATRIC USE

Safety and efficacy of Tri-Norinyl have been established in women of reproductive age. Safety and efficacy are expected to be the same for postpubertal adolescents under the age of 16 and for users 16 years and older. Use of the product before menarche is not indicated.

INFORMATION FOR THE PATIENT

See ***PATIENT LABELING*** printed below.

ADVERSE REACTIONS

An increased risk of the following serious adverse reactions has been associated with the use of oral contraceptives (see ***WARNINGS*** section):

- Thrombophlebitis
- Arterial thromboembolism
- Pulmonary embolism
- Myocardial infarction
- Cerebral hemorrhage
- Cerebral thrombosis
- Hypertension
- Gallbladder disease
- Hepatic adenomas, carcinomas or benign liver tumors

There is evidence of an association between the following conditions and the use of oral contraceptives, although additional confirmatory studies are needed:

- Mesenteric thrombosis
- Retinal thrombosis

The following adverse reactions have been reported in patients receiving oral contraceptives and are believed to be drug-related:

- Nausea
- Vomiting
- Gastrointestinal symptoms (such as abdominal cramps and bloating)
- Breakthrough bleeding
- Spotting
- Change in menstrual flow
- Amenorrhea
- Temporary infertility after discontinuation of treatment
- Edema
- Melasma which may persist
- Breast changes: tenderness, enlargement, secretion

Continued on next page

Tri-Norinyl—Cont.

- Change in weight (increase or decrease)
- Change in cervical erosion and secretion
- Diminution in lactation when given immediately postpartum
- Cholestatic jaundice
- Migraine
- Rash (allergic)
- Mental depression
- Reduced tolerance to carbohydrates
- Vaginal candidiasis
- Change in corneal curvature (steepening)
- Intolerance to contact lenses

The following adverse reactions have been reported in users of oral contraceptives and the association has been neither confirmed nor refuted:

- Pre-menstrual syndrome
- Cataracts
- Changes in appetite
- Cystitis-like syndrome
- Headache
- Nervousness
- Dizziness
- Hirsutism
- Loss of scalp hair
- Erythema multiforme
- Erythema nodosum
- Hemorrhagic eruption
- Vaginitis
- Porphyria
- Impaired renal function
- Hemolytic uremic syndrome
- Budd-Chiari syndrome
- Acne
- Changes in libido
- Colitis

OVERDOSAGE

Serious ill effects have not been reported following acute ingestion of large doses of oral contraceptives by young children. Overdosage may cause nausea, and withdrawal bleeding may occur in females.

NON-CONTRACEPTIVE HEALTH BENEFITS

The following non-contraceptive health benefits related to the use of oral contraceptives are supported by epidemiological studies which largely utilized oral contraceptive formulations containing estrogen doses exceeding 0.035 mg of ethinyl estradiol or 0.05 mg of mestranol.[6–11]

Effects on menses:

- Increased menstrual cycle regularity
- Decreased blood loss and decreased incidence of iron deficiency anemia
- Decreased incidence of dysmenorrhea

Effects related to inhibition of ovulation:

- Decreased incidence of functional ovarian cysts
- Decreased incidence of ectopic pregnancies

Effects from long-term use:

- Decreased incidence of fibroadenomas and fibrocystic disease of the breast
- Decreased incidence of acute pelvic inflammatory disease
- Decreased incidence of endometrial cancer
- Decreased incidence of ovarian cancer

Keep this and all medication out of the reach of children.

DOSAGE AND ADMINISTRATION

To achieve maximum contraceptive effectiveness, oral contraceptives must be taken exactly as directed and at intervals not exceeding 24 hours.

28-Day Schedule: For a DAY 1 START, count the first day of menstrual flow as Day 1 and the first blue tablet is then taken on Day 1. For a SUNDAY START when menstrual flow begins on or before Sunday, the first blue tablet is taken on that day. With either a DAY 1 START or SUNDAY START, 1 blue tablet is taken for 7 days, then 1 yellow-green tablet for 9 days, then 1 blue tablet for 5 days, then 1 orange tablet (inert) for 7 days, whether bleeding has stopped or not. With either a DAY 1 START or SUNDAY START 1 tablet is taken each day at the same time for 28 days. After all 28 tablets are taken, whether bleeding has stopped or not, the same dosage schedule is repeated beginning on the following day.

INSTRUCTIONS TO PATIENTS

- To achieve maximum contraceptive effectiveness, the oral contraceptive pill must be taken exactly as directed and at intervals not exceeding 24 hours.
- Important: Women should be instructed to use an additional method of protection until after the first 7 days of administration *in the initial cycle.*
- Due to the normally increased risk of thromboembolism occurring postpartum, women should be instructed not to initiate treatment with oral contraceptives earlier than 4 weeks after a full-term delivery. If pregnancy is terminated in the first 12 weeks, the patient should be instructed to start oral contraceptives immediately or within 7 days. If pregnancy is terminated after 12 weeks, the patient should be instructed to start oral contraceptives after 2 weeks.[33, 77]
- If spotting or breakthrough bleeding should occur, the patient should continue the medication according to the schedule. Should spotting or breakthrough bleeding persist, the patient should notify her physician.
- If the patient misses 1 pill, she should be instructed to take it as soon as she remembers and then take the next pill at the regular time. The patient should be advised that missing a pill can cause spotting or light bleeding and that she may be a little sick to her stomach on the days she takes the missed pill with her regularly scheduled pill. If the patient has missed more than one pill, see ***DETAILED PATIENT LABELING: HOW TO TAKE THE PILL, WHAT TO DO IF YOU MISS PILLS.***
- Use of oral contraceptives in the event of a missed menstrual period:
  1. If the patient has not adhered to the prescribed dosage regimen, the possibility of pregnancy should be considered after the first missed period and oral contraceptives should be withheld until pregnancy has been ruled out.
  2. If the patient has adhered to the prescribed regimen and misses 2 consecutive periods, pregnancy should be ruled out before continuing the contraceptive regimen.

HOW SUPPLIED

Tri-Norinyl®-28 tablets (norethindrone and ethinyl estradiol) are available in 28-tablet blister cards with a WALLETTE® tablet dispenser. Six blister cards are repackaged in a carton.

Tri-Norinyl®-28 (norethindrone and ethinyl estradiol) are available in 28-tablet blister cards with a WALLETTE® tablet dispenser. Six blister cards are repackaged in a carton. Each dispenser contains 7 blue active tablets; 9 yellow-green active tablets; 5 more blue active tablets; round in shape with "Watson" debossed on one side and "274" on the other side and 7 orange inert tablets with "Watson" on one side and "P" on the otherside.

Store at controlled room temperature 15°C to 25°C (59°F to 77°F).

REFERENCES

1. Hatcher, R.A. Trussell, J. Stewart, F., et al.: *Contraceptive Technology: Sixteenth Revised Edition*, New York, NY, 1998. **2.** Mann, J., et al.: *Br Med J* 2(5956): 241–245, 1975. **3.** Knopp, R.H.: *J Reprod Med* 31(9): 913–921, 1986. **4.** Mann, J.I., et al.: *Br Med J* 2: 445–447, 1976. **5.** Ory, H.: *JAMA* 237: 2619–2622, 1977. **6.** The Cancer and Steroid Hormone Study of the Centers for Disease Control: *JAMA* 249(2): 1596–1599, 1983. **7.** The Cancer and Steroid Hormone Study of the Centers for Disease Control: *JAMA* 257(6): 796–800, 1987. **8.** Ory, H.W.: *JAMA* 228(1): 68–69, 1974. **9.** Ory, H.W., et al.: *N Engl J Med* 294: 419–422, 1976. **10.** Ory, H.W.: *Fam Plann Perspect* 14: 182–184, 1982. **11.** Ory, H.W., et al.: *Making Choices*, New York, The Alan Guttmacher Institute, 1983. **12.** Stadel, B.: *N Engl J Med* 305(11): 612–618, 1981. **13.** Stadel, B.: *N Engl J Med* 305(12): 672–677, 1981. **14.** Adam, S., et al.: *Br J Obstet Gynaecol* 88: 838–845, 1981. **15.** Mann, J., et al.: *Br Med J* 2(5965): 245–248, 1975. **16.** Royal College of General Practitioners' Oral Contraceptive Study: *Lancet* 1: 541–546, 1981. **17.** Slone, D., et al.: *N Engl J Med* 305(8): 420–424, 1981. **18.** Vessey, M.P.: *Br J Fam Plann* 6 (supplement): 1–12, 1980. **19.** Russell-Briefel, R., et al.: *Prev Med* 15: 352–362, 1986. **20.** Goldbaum, G., et al.: *JAMA* 258(10): 1339–1342, 1987. **21.** LaRosa, J.C.: *J Reprod Med* 31 (9): 906–912, 1986. **22.** Krauss, R.M., et al.: *Am J Obstet Gynecol* 145: 446–452, 1983. **23.** Wahl, P., et al.: *N Engl J Med* 308(15): 862–867, 1983. **24.** Wynn, V., et al.: *Am J Obstet Gynecol* 142(6): 766–771, 1982. **25.** Wynn, V., et al.: *J Reprod Med* 31(9): 892–897, 1986. **26.** Inman, W.H., et al.: *Br Med J* 2(5599): 193–199, 1968. **27.** Maguire, M.G., et al.: *Am J Epidemiol* 110(2): 188–195, 1979. **28.** Petitti, D., et al.: *JAMA* 242(11): 1150–1154, 1979. **29.** Vessey, M.P., et al.: *Br Med J* 2(5599): 199–205, 1968. **30.** Vessey, M.P., et al.: *Br Med J* 2(5658): 651–657, 1969. **31.** Porter, J.B., et al.: *Obstet Gynecol* 59(3): 299–302, 1982. **32.** Vessey, M.P., et al.: *J Biosoc Sci* 8: 373–427, 1976. **33.** Mishell, D.R., et al.: *Reproductive Endocrinology*, Philadelphia, F.A. Davis Co., 1979. **34.** Petitti, D.B., et al.: *Lancet* 2: 234–236, 1978. **35.** Collaborative Group for the Study of Stroke in Young Women: *JAMA* 231(7): 718–722, 1975. **36.** Inman, W.H., et al.: *Br Med J* 2: 203–209, 1970. **37.** Meade, T.W., et al.: *Br Med J* 280(6224): 1157–1161, 1980. **38.** Kay, C.R.: *Am J Obstet Gynecol* 142(6): 762–765, 1982. **39.** Gordon, T., et al.: *Am J Med* 62: 707–714, 1977. **40.** Royal College of General Practitioners' Oral Contraception Study: *J Coll Gen Pract* 33: 75–82, 1983. **41.** Ory, H.W.: *Fam Plann Perspect* 15(2) :57–63, 1983. **42.** Paul, C., et al.: *Br Med J* 293: 723–725, 1986. **43.** The Cancer and Steroid Hormone Study of the Centers for Disease Control: *N Engl J Med* 315(7): 405–411, 1986. **44.** Pike, M.C., et al.: *Lancet* 2: 926–929, 1983. **45.** Miller, D.R., et al.: *Obstet Gynecol* 68 :863–868, 1986. **46.** Olsson, H., et al.: *Lancet* 2: 748–749, 1985. **47.** McPherson, K., et al.: *Br J Cancer* 56: 653–660, 1987. **48.** Huggins, G.R., et al.: *Fertil Steril* 47(5): 733–761, 1987. **49.** McPherson, K., et al.: *Br Med J* 293: 709–710, 1986. **50.** Ory, H., et al.: *Am J Obstet Gynecol* 124(6): 573–577, 1976. **51.** Vessey, M.P., et al.: *Lancet* 2: 930, 1983. **52.** Brinton, L.A., et al.: *Int J Cancer* 38: 339–344, 1986. **53.** WHO Collaborative Study of Neoplasia and Steroid Contraceptives: *Br Med J* 290: 961–965, 1985. **54.** Rooks, J.B., et al.: *JAMA* 242(7): 644–648, 1979. **55.** Bein, N.N., et al.: *Br J Surg* 64: 433–435, 1977. **56.** Klatskin, G.: *Gastroenterology* 73: 386–394, 1977. **57.** Henderson, B.E., et al.: *Br J Cancer* 48: 437–440, 1983. **58.** Neuberger, J., et al.: *Br Med J* 292: 1355–1357, 1986. **59.** Forman, D., et al.: *Br Med J* 292: 1357–1361, 1986. **60.** Harlap, S., et al.: *Obstet Gynecol* 55(4): 447–452, 1980. **61.** Savolainen, E., et al.: *Am J Obstet Gynecol* 140(5): 521–524, 1981. **62.** Janerich, D.T., et al.: *Am J Epidemiol* 112(1): 73–79, 1980. **63.** Ferencz, C., et al.: *Teratology* 21: 225–239, 1980. **64.** Rothman, K.J., et al.: *Am J Epidemiol* 109(4): 433–439, 1979. **65.** Boston Collaborative Drug Surveillance Program: *Lancet* 1: 1399–1404, 1973. **66.** Royal College of General Practitioners: *Oral contraceptives and health.* New York, Pittman, 1974. **67.** Rome Group for the Epidemiology and Prevention of Cholelithiasis: *Am J Epidemiol* 119(5): 796–805, 1984. **68.** Strom, B.L., et al.: *Clin Pharmacol Ther* 39(3): 335–341, 1986. **69.** Perlman, J.A., et al.: *J Chronic Dis* 38(10): 857–864, 1985. **70.** Wynn, V., et al.: *Lancet* 1: 1045–1049, 1979. **71.** Wynn, V.: *Progesterone and Progestin*, New York, Raven Press, 1983. **72.** Wynn, V., et al.: *Lancet* 2: 720–723, 1966. **73.** Fisch, I.R., et al.: *JAMA* 237(23): 2499–2503, 1977.**74.** Laragh, J.H.: *Am J Obstet Gynecol* 126(1): 141–147, 1976. **75.** Ramcharan, S., et al.: *Pharmacology of Steroid Contraceptive Drugs*, New York, Raven Press, 1977. **76.** Stockley, I.: *Pharm J* 216: 140–143, 1976. **77.** Dickey, R.P.: *Managing Contraceptive Pill Patients*, Oklahoma, Creative Informatics Inc., 1984. **78.** Porter J.B., Hunter J., Jick H., et al.: *Obstet Gynecol* 1985;66: 1–4. **79.** Porter J.B., Hershel J., Walker A.M.: *Obstet Gynecol* 1987;70: 29–32. **80.** Fertility and Maternal Health Drugs Advisory Committee, F.D.A., October, 1989. **81.** Schlesselman J., Stadel B.V., Murray P., Lai S.: *Breast cancer in relation to early use of oral contraceptives.* JAMA 1988;259: 1828–1833. **82.** Hennekens C.H., Speizer F.E., Lipnick R.J., Rosner B., Bain C., Belanger C., Stampfer M.J., Willett W., Peto R.: *A case-control study of oral contraceptive use and breast cancer. JNCI* 1984; 72: 39–42. **83.** Royal College of General Practitioners: *Oral contraceptives, venous thrombosis, and varicose veins. J Coll Gen Pract* 28: 393–399, 1978. **84.** Royal College of General Practitioners' Oral Contraception Study: *Effect on Hypertension and benign breast disease of progestogen component in combined oral contraceptives. Lancet* 1: 624, 1977.

DETAILED PATIENT LABELING

This product (like all oral contraceptives) is intended to prevent pregnancy. It does not protect against HIV infection (AIDS) and other sexually transmitted diseases.

INTRODUCTION

Any woman who considers using oral contraceptives ("birth control pills" or "the pill") should understand the benefits and risks of using this form of birth control. This leaflet will give you much of the information you will need to make this decision and also will help you determine if you are at risk of developing any of the serious side effects of the pill. It will tell you how to use the pill properly so that it will be as effective as possible. However, this leaflet is not a replacement for a careful discussion between you and your health care provider. You should discuss the information provided in this leaflet with him or her, both when you first start taking the pill and during your regular visits. You also should follow the advice of your health care provider with regard to regular checkups while you are on the pill.

EFFECTIVENESS OF ORAL CONTRACEPTIVES

Oral contraceptives are used to prevent pregnancy and are more effective than other non-surgical methods of birth control. When they are taken correctly, without missing any pills, the chance of becoming pregnant is less than 1% (1 pregnancy per 100 women per year of use). Typical failure rates are actually 3% per year. The chance of becoming pregnant increases with each missed pill during a menstrual cycle.

In comparison, typical failure rates for other nonsurgical methods of birth control during the first year are as follows:

[See table 1 at top of next page]

WHO SHOULD NOT TAKE ORAL CONTRACEPTIVES

Cigarette smoking increases the risk of serious cardiovascular side effects from oral contraceptive use. This risk increases with age and with heavy smoking (15 or more cigarettes per day) and is quite marked in women over 35 years of age. Women who use oral contraceptives are strongly advised not to smoke.

Some women should not use the pill. For example, you should not take the pill if you are pregnant or think you may be pregnant. You also should not use the pill if you have any of the following conditions:

- A history of heart attack or stroke
- Blood clots in the legs (thrombophlebitis), brain (stroke), lungs (pulmonary embolism) or eyes
- A history of blood clots in the deep veins of your legs
- Chest pain (angina pectoris)
- Known or suspected breast cancer or cancer of the lining of the uterus, cervix or vagina
- Unexplained vaginal bleeding (until a diagnosis is reached by your doctor)
- Yellowing of the whites of the eyes or of the skin (jaundice) during pregnancy or during previous use of the pill
- Liver tumor (benign or cancerous)
- Known or suspected pregnancy

Tell your health care provider if you have ever had any of these conditions. Your health care provider can recommend a safer method of birth control.

OTHER CONSIDERATIONS BEFORE TAKING ORAL CONTRACEPTIVES

Tell your health care provider if you have or have had:

- Breast nodules, fibrocystic disease of the breast, an abnormal breast x-ray or mammogram
- Diabetes
- Elevated cholesterol or triglycerides
- High blood pressure
- Migraine or other headaches or epilepsy
- Mental depression
- Gallbladder, heart or kidney disease
- History of scanty or irregular menstrual periods

Table 1- Percentage of women experiencing an unintended pregnancy during the first year of typical use and the first year of perfect use of contraception and the percentage continuing use at the end of the first year. United States.

Method (1)	% of Women Experiencing an Unintended Pregnancy within the First Year of Use: Typical use[1] (2)	% of Women Experiencing an Unintended Pregnancy within the First Year of Use: Perfect use[2] (3)	% of Women Continuing Use at One Year[3] (4)
Chance[4]	85	85	
Spermicides[5]	26	6	40
Periodic abstinence	25		63
Calendar		9	
Ovulation method		3	
Sympto-thermal[6]		2	
Post-ovulation		1	
Withdrawal	19	4	
Cap[7]			
Parous women	40	26	42
Nulliparous women	20	9	56
Sponge			
Parous women	40	20	42
Nulliparous women	20	9	56
Diaphragm[7]	20	6	56
Condom[8]			
Female (Reality)	21	5	56
Male	14	3	61
Pill	5		71
Progestin only		0.5	
Combined		0.1	
IUD			
Progesterone T	2.0	1.5	81
Copper T 380A	0.8	0.6	78
LNg 20	0.1	0.1	81
Depo-Provera	0.3	0.3	70
Norplant and Norplant-2	0.05	0.05	88
Female sterilization	0.5	0.5	100
Male sterilization	0.15	0.10	100

Emergency Contraceptive Pills: Treatment initiated within 72 hours after unprotected intercourse reduces the risk of pregnancy by at least 75%.[9]

Lactational Amenorrhea Method: LAM is a highly effective, *temporary* method of contraception.[10]

Source: Trussell J. Contraceptive Efficacy Table from Hatcher R.A., Trussell J. Stewart F, Cates W. Stewart GK, Kowal D, Guest F, in Contraceptive Technology: Seventeenth Revised Edition. New York, NY: Irvington Publishers, 1998.

1 Among *typical* couples who initiate use of a method (not necessarily for the first time), the percentage who experience an accidental pregnancy during the first year if they do not stop use for any other reason.

2 Among couples who initiate use of a method (not necessarily for the first time) and who use it *perfectly* (both consistently and correctly), the percentage who experience an accidental pregnancy during the first year if they do not stop use for any other reason.

3 Among couples attempting to avoid pregnancy, the percentage who continue to use a method for one year.

4 The percentage becoming pregnant in columns (2) and (3) are based on data from populations where contraception is not used and from women who cease using contraception in order to become pregnant. Among such populations, about 89% become pregnant within one year. This estimate was lowered slightly (to 85%) to represent the percent who would become pregnant within one year among women now relying on reversible methods of contraception if they abandoned contraception altogether.

5 Foams, creams, gels, vaginal suppositories, and vaginal film.

6 Cervical mucus (ovulation) method supplemented by calendar in the pre-ovulatory and basal body temperature in the post-ovulatory phases.

7 With spermicidal cream or jelly.

8 Without spermicides.

9 The treatment schedule is one dose within 72 hours after unprotected intercourse and a second dose 12 hours after the first dose. The Food and Drug Administration has declared the following brands of oral contraceptives to be safe and effective for emergency contraception: Ovral (1 dose is 2 white pills). Aleese (1 dose is 5 pink pills), Nordette or Levlen (1 dose is 2 light-orange pills), Lo/Ovral (1 dose is 4 white pills), Triphasil or Tri-Levlen (1 dose is 4 yellow pills).

10 However, to maintain effective protection against pregnancy, another method of contraception must be used as soon as menstruation resumes, the frequency or duration of breastfeeds is reduced, bottle feeds are introduced, or the baby reaches six months of age.

ESTIMATED ANNUAL NUMBER OF BIRTH-RELATED OR METHOD-RELATED DEATHS ASSOCIATED WITH CONTROL OF FERTILITY PER 100,000 NONSTERILE WOMEN, BY FERTILITY CONTROL METHOD ACCORDING TO AGE

Method of control and outcome	15–19	20–24	25–29	30–34	35–39	40–44
No fertility control methods*	7.0	7.4	9.1	14.8	25.7	28.2
Oral contraceptives non-smoker**	0.3	0.5	0.9	1.9	13.8	31.6
Oral contraceptives smoker**	2.2	3.4	6.6	13.5	51.1	117.2
IUD**	0.8	0.8	1.0	1.0	1.4	1.4
Condom*	1.1	1.6	0.7	0.2	0.3	0.4
Diaphragm/Spermicide*	1.9	1.2	1.2	1.3	2.2	2.8
Periodic abstinence*	2.5	1.6	1.6	1.7	2.9	3.6

*Deaths are birth-related
**Deaths are method-related

Estimates adapted from H.W. Ory, Table 3[41].

Women with any of these conditions should be checked often by their health care provider if they choose to use oral contraceptives.

Also, be sure to inform your doctor or health care provider if you smoke or are on any medications.

RISKS OF TAKING ORAL CONTRACEPTIVES

1. Risk of developing blood clots

Blood clots and blockage of blood vessels are the most serious side effects of taking oral contraceptives. In particular, a clot in the legs can cause thrombophlebitis and a clot that travels to the lungs can cause a sudden blocking of the vessel carrying blood to the lungs. Rarely, clots occur in the blood vessels of the eye and may cause blindness, double vision, or impaired vision.

If you take oral contraceptives and need elective surgery, need to stay in bed for a prolonged illness or have recently delivered a baby, you may be at risk of developing blood clots. You should consult your doctor about stopping oral contraceptives three to four weeks before surgery and not taking oral contraceptives for two weeks after surgery or during bed rest. You should also not take oral contraceptives soon after delivery of a baby. It is advisable to wait for at least four weeks after delivery if you are not breast feeding. If you are breast feeding, you should wait until you have weaned your child before using the pill (see *GENERAL PRECAUTIONS—While breast feeding*).

2. Heart attacks and strokes

Oral contraceptives may increase the tendency to develop strokes (stoppage or rupture of blood vessels in the brain) and angina pectoris and heart attacks (blockage of blood vessels in the heart). Any of these conditions can cause death or temporary or permanent disability.

Smoking greatly increases the possibility of suffering heart attacks and strokes. Furthermore, smoking and the use of oral contraceptives greatly increase the chances of developing and dying of heart disease.

3. Gallbladder disease

Oral contraceptive users may have a greater risk than nonusers of having gallbladder disease, although this risk may be related to pills containing high doses of estrogen.

4. Liver tumors

In rare cases, oral contraceptives can cause benign but dangerous liver tumors. These benign liver tumors can rupture and cause fatal internal bleeding. In addition, a possible but not definite association has been found with the pill and liver cancers in 2 studies in which a few women who developed these very rare cancers were found to have used oral contraceptives for long periods. However, liver cancers are extremely rare. The chance of developing liver cancer from using the pill is thus even rarer.

5. Cancer of the breast and reproductive organs

There is, at present, no confirmed evidence that oral contraceptives increase the risk of cancer of the reproductive organs in human studies. Several studies have found no overall increase in the risk of developing breast cancer. However, women who use oral contraceptives and have a strong family history of breast cancer or who have breast nodules or abnormal mammograms should be followed closely by their doctors. Some studies have reported an increase in the risk of developing breast cancer, particularly at a younger age. This increased risk appears to be related to duration of use.

Some studies have found an increase in the incidence of cancer of the cervix in women who use oral contraceptives. However, this finding may be related to factors other than the use of oral contraceptives.

ESTIMATED RISK OF DEATH FROM A BIRTH CONTROL METHOD OR PREGNANCY

All methods of birth control and pregnancy are associated with a risk of developing certain diseases which may lead to disability or death. An estimate of the number of deaths associated with different methods of birth control and pregnancy has been calculated and is shown in the following table:

[See table below]

In the above table, the risk of death from any birth control method is less than the risk of childbirth except for oral contraceptive users over the age of 35 who smoke and pill users over the age of 40 even if they do not smoke. It can be seen from the table that for women aged 15 to 39 the risk of death is highest with pregnancy (7–26 deaths per 100,000 women, depending on age). Among pill users who do not smoke the risk of death is always lower than that associated with pregnancy for any age group, although over the age of 40 the risk increases to 32 deaths per 100,000 women compared to 28 associated with pregnancy at that age. However, for pill users who smoke and are over the age of 35 the estimated number of deaths exceeds those for other methods of birth control. If a woman is over the age of 40 and smokes, her estimated risk of death is 4 times higher (117/100,000 women) than the estimated risk associated with pregnancy (28/100,000 women) in that age group.

The suggestion that women over 40 who don't smoke should not take oral contraceptives is based on information from older high-dose pills and on less selective use of pills than is practiced today. An Advisory Committee of the FDA discussed this issue in 1989 and recommended that the benefits of oral contraceptive use by healthy, non-smoking women over 40 years of age may outweigh the possible risks. However, all women, especially older women, are cautioned to use the lowest dose pill that is effective.

WARNING SIGNALS

If any of these adverse effects occur while you are taking oral contraceptives, call your doctor immediately:

- Sharp chest pain, coughing of blood or sudden shortness of breath (indicating a possible clot in the lung)
- Pain in the calf (indicating a possible clot in the leg)
- Crushing chest pain or heaviness in the chest (indicating a possible heart attack)
- Sudden severe headache or vomiting, dizziness or fainting, disturbances of vision or speech, weakness or numbness in an arm or leg (indicating a possible stroke)
- Sudden partial or complete loss of vision (indicating a possible clot in the eye)
- Breast lumps (indicating possible breast cancer of fibrocystic disease of the breast: ask your doctor or health care provider to show you how to examine your breasts)
- Severe pain or tenderness in the stomach area (indicating a possible ruptured liver tumor)
- Difficulty in sleeping, weakness, lack of energy, fatigue or change in mood (possibly indicating severe depression)
- Jaundice or a yellowing of the skin or eyeballs, accompanied frequently by fever, fatigue, loss of appetite, dark colored urine or ligh colored bowel movements (indicating possible liver problems)

SIDE EFFECTS OF ORAL CONTRACEPTIVES

1. Vaginal bleeding

Irregular vaginal bleeding or spotting may occur while you are taking the pill. Irregular bleeding may vary from slight

Continued on next page

Tri-Norinyl—Cont.

staining between menstrual periods to breakthrough bleeding which is a flow much like a regular period. Irregular bleeding occurs most often during the first few months of oral contraceptive use but may also occur after you have been taking the pill for some time. Such bleeding may be temporary and usually does not indicate any serious problem. It is important to continue taking your pills on schedule. If the bleeding occurs in more than 1 cycle or lasts for more than a few days, talk to your doctor or health care provider.

2. Contact lenses

If you wear contact lenses and notice a change in vision or an inability to wear your lenses, contact your doctor or health care provider.

3. Fluid retention

Oral contraceptives may cause edema (fluid retention) with swelling of the fingers or ankles and may raise your blood pressure. If you experience fluid retention, contact your doctor or health care provider.

4. Melasma (Mask of Pregnancy)

A spotty darkening of the skin is possible, particularly of the face.

5. Other side effects

Other side effects may include change in appetite, headache, nervousness, depression, dizziness, loss of scalp hair, rash and vaginal infections

If any of these side effects occurs, contact your doctor or health care provider.

GENERAL PRECAUTIONS

1. Missed periods and use of oral contraceptives before or during early pregnancy

At times you may not menstruate regularly after you have completed taking a cycle of pills. If you have taken your pills regularly and miss 1 menstrual period, continue taking your pills for the next cycle but be sure to inform your health care provider before doing so. If you have not taken the pills daily as instructed and miss 1 menstrual period, or if you miss 2 consecutive menstrual periods, you may be pregnant. Check with your health care provider immediately to determine whether you are pregnant. Do not continue to take oral contraceptives until you are sure you are not pregnant, but continue to use another method of birth control.

There is no conclusive evidence that oral contraceptive use is associated with an increase in birth defects when taken inadvertently during early pregnancy. Previously, a few studies had reported that oral contraceptives might be associated with birth defects but these studies have not been confirmed. Nevertheless, oral contraceptives or any other drugs should not be used during pregnancy unless clearly necessary and prescribed by your doctor. You should check with your doctor about risks to your unborn child from any medication taken during pregnancy.

2. While breast feeding

If you are breast feeding, consult your doctor before starting oral contraceptives. Some of the drug will be passed on to the child in the milk. A few adverse effects on the child have been reported, including yellowing of the skin (jaundice) and breast enlargement. In addition, oral contraceptives may decrease the amount and quality of your milk. If possible, do not use oral contraceptives and use another method of contraception while breast feeding. You should consider starting oral contraceptives only after you have weaned your child completely.

3. Laboratory tests

If you are scheduled for any laboratory tests, tell your doctor you are taking birth control pills. Certain blood tests may be affected by birth control pills.

4. Drug interactions

Certain drugs may interact with birth control pills to make them less effective in preventing pregnancy or cause an increase in breakthrough bleeding. Such drugs include rifampin; drugs used for epilepsy such as barbiturates (for example phenobarbital) and phenytoin (Dilantin is one brand of this drug); phenylbutazone (Butazolidin is one brand of this drug) and possibly certain antibiotics. You may need to use additional contraception when you take drugs which can make oral contraceptives less effective.

5. This product (like all oral contraceptives) is intended to prevent pregnancy. It does not protect against transmission of HIV (AIDS) and other sexually transmitted diseases such as chlamydia, genital herpes, genital warts, gonorrhea, hepatitis B, and syphilis.

HOW TO TAKE THE PILL

IMPORTANT POINTS TO REMEMBER

BEFORE YOU START TAKING YOUR PILLS:

1. BE SURE TO READ THESE DIRECTIONS:
   Before you start taking your pills.
   Anytime you are not sure what to do.
2. THE RIGHT WAY TO TAKE THE PILL IS TO TAKE ONE PILL EVERY DAY AT THE SAME TIME.
   If you miss pills you could get pregnant. This includes starting the pack late.
   The more pills you miss, the more likely you are to get pregnant.
3. MANY WOMEN HAVE SPOTTING OR LIGHT BLEEDING, OR MAY FEEL SICK TO THEIR STOMACH DURING THE FIRST 1–3 PACKS OF PILLS.
   If you feel sick to your stomach, do not stop taking the Pill. The problem will usually go away. If it doesn't go away, check with your doctor or clinic.
4. MISSING PILLS CAN ALSO CAUSE SPOTTING OR LIGHT BLEEDING, even when you make up these missed pills.
   On the days you take 2 pills to make up for missed pills, you could also feel a little sick to your stomach.
5. IF YOU HAVE VOMITING OR DIARRHEA, for any reason, or IF YOU TAKE SOME MEDICINES, including some antibiotics, your pills may not work as well.
   Use a back-up method (such as condoms, foam, or sponge) until you check with your doctor or clinic.
6. IF YOU HAVE TROUBLE REMEMBERING TO TAKE THE PILL, talk to your doctor or clinic about how to make pill-taking easier or about using another method of birth control.
7. IF YOU HAVE ANY QUESTIONS OR ARE UNSURE ABOUT THE INFORMATION IN THIS LEAFLET, call your doctor or clinic.

BEFORE YOU START TAKING YOUR PILLS

1. DECIDE WHAT TIME OF DAY YOU WANT TO TAKE YOUR PILL.
   It is important to take it at about the same time every day.
2. LOOK AT YOUR PILL PACK TO SEE IF IT HAS 28 PILLS:
   The 28-pill pack has 21 "active" blue and yellow-green pills (with hormones) to take for 3 weeks, followed by 1 week of reminder orange pills (without hormones).
3. ALSO FIND:
   1) where on the pack to start taking pills,
   2) in what order to take the pills (follow the arrows) and
   3) the week numbers as shown in the pictures below.

Active pill colors: blue and yellow-green
Reminder pill color: orange

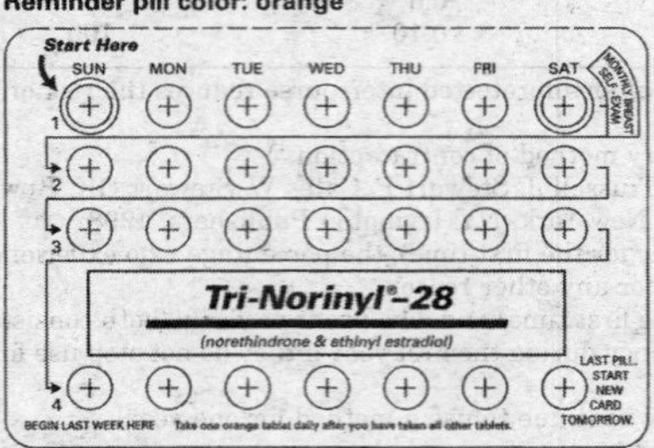

4. BE SURE YOU HAVE READY AT ALL TIMES:
   ANOTHER KIND OF BIRTH CONTROL (such as condoms, foam, or sponge) to use as a back-up in case you miss pills.
   AN EXTRA, FULL PILL PACK.

WHEN TO START THE FIRST PACK OF PILLS

You have a choice of which day to start taking your first pack of pills. Decide with your doctor or clinic which is the best day for you. Pick a time of day which will be easy to remember.

DAY 1 START:

1. Take the first "active" blue pill of the first pack during the first 24 hours of your period.
2. You will not need to use a back-up method of birth control, since you are starting the pill at the beginning of your period.

SUNDAY START:

1. Take the first "active" blue pill of the first pack on the Sunday after your period starts, even if you are still bleeding. If your period begins on Sunday, start the pack that same day.
2. Use another method of birth control as a back-up method if you have sex anytime from the Sunday you start your first pack until the next Sunday (7 days). Condoms, foam, or the sponge are good back-up methods of birth control.

WHAT TO DO DURING THE MONTH

1. **TAKE ONE PILL AT THE SAME TIME EVERY DAY UNTIL THE PACK IS EMPTY.**
   Do not skip pills even if you are spotting or bleeding between monthly periods or feel sick to your stomach (nausea).
   Do not skip pills even if you do not have sex very often.
2. **WHEN YOU FINISH A PACK OR SWITCH YOUR BRAND OF PILLS:**
   28 pills: Start the next pack on the day after your last "reminder" pill. Do not wait any days between packs.

WHAT TO DO IF YOU MISS PILLS

If you **MISS 1** blue or yellow-green "active" pill:

1. Take it as soon as you remember. Take the next pill at your regular time. This means you may take 2 pills in 1 day.
2. You do not need to use a back-up birth control method if you have sex.

If you **MISS 2** blue or yellow-green "active" pills in a row in **WEEK 1 OR WEEK 2** of your pack:

1. Take 2 pills on the day you remember and 2 pills the next day.
2. Then take 1 pill a day until you finish the pack.
3. You MAY BECOME PREGNANT if you have sex in the 7 days after you miss pills. You MUST use another birth control method (such as condoms, foam, or sponge) as a back-up for those 7 days.

If you **MISS 2** blue or yellow-green "active" pills in a row in **THE 3rd WEEK:**

1. ***If you are a Day 1 Starter:***
   THROW OUT the rest of the pill pack and start a new pack that same day.

If you are a Sunday Starter:
Keep taking 1 pill every day until Sunday.
On Sunday, THROW OUT the rest of the pack and start a new pack of pills that same day.

2. You may not have your period this month but this is expected. However, if you miss your period 2 months in a row, call your doctor or clinic because you might be pregnant.
3. You MAY BECOME PREGNANT if you have sex in the 7 days after you miss pills. You MUST use another birth control method (such as condoms, foam, or sponge) as a back-up for those 7 days.

If you **MISS 3 OR MORE** blue or yellow-green "active" pills in a row (during the first 3 weeks):

1. ***If you are a Day 1 Starter:***
   THROW OUT the rest of the pill pack and start a new pack that same day.

If you are a Sunday Starter:
Keep taking 1 pill every day until Sunday.
On Sunday, THROW OUT the rest of the pack and start a new pack of pills that same day.

2. You may not have your period this month but this is expected. However, if you miss your period 2 months in a row, call your doctor or clinic because you might be pregnant.
3. You MAY BECOME PREGNANT if you have sex in the 7 days after you miss pills. You MUST use another birth control method (such as condoms, foam, or sponge) as a back-up for those 7 days.

A REMINDER:

If you forget any of the 7 orange "reminder" pills in Week 4:
THROW AWAY the pills you missed.
Keep taking 1 pill each day until the pack is empty.
You do not need a back-up method.

FINALLY, IF YOU ARE STILL NOT SURE WHAT TO DO ABOUT THE PILLS YOU HAVE MISSED:

Use a BACK-UP METHOD anytime you have sex.
KEEP TAKING ONE "ACTIVE" PILL EACH DAY until you can reach your doctor or clinic.

6. Missed periods, spotting or light bleeding

At times, you may not have a period after you have completed a pack of pills. If you miss 1 period but you have taken the pills exactly as you were supposed to, continue as usual into the next cycle. If you have not taken the pills correctly, and have missed a period, you may be pregnant and you should stop taking the Pill until your doctor or clinic determines whether or not you are pregnant. Until you can talk to your doctor or clinic, use an appropriate back-up birth control method. If you miss 2 consecutive periods, you should stop taking the Pill until it is determined that you are not pregnant.

Even if spotting or light bleeding should occur, continue taking the Pill according to the schedule. Should spotting or light bleeding persist, you should notify your doctor or clinic.

7. Stopping the pill before surgery or prolonged bed rest

If you are scheduled for surgery or you need to stay in bed for a long period of time you should tell your doctor that you are on the Pill. You should stop taking the Pill four weeks before your operation to avoid an increased risk of blood clots. Talk to your doctor about when you may start taking the Pill again.

8. Starting the pill after pregnancy

After you have a baby it is advisable to wait 4–6 weeks before starting to take the Pill. Talk to your doctor about when you may start taking the Pill after pregnancy.

9. Pregnancy due to pill failure

When the Pill is taken correctly, the expected pregnancy rate is approximately 1% (ie, 1 pregnancy per 100 women per year). If pregnancy occurs while taking the Pill, there is little risk to the fetus. The typical failure rate of large numbers of pill users is less than 3% when women who have missed pills are included. If you become pregnant, you should discuss your pregnancy with your doctor.

10. Pregnancy after stopping the pill

There may be some delay in becoming pregnant after you stop taking the Pill, especially if you had irregular periods before you started using the pill. Your doctor may recommend that you delay becoming pregnant until you have had one or more regular periods.

There does not appear to be any increase in birth defects in newborn babies when pregnancy occurs soon after stopping the Pill.

11. Overdosage

There are no reports of serious illness or side effects in young children who have swallowed a large number of pills. In adults, overdosage may cause nausea and/or bleeding in females. In case of overdosage, contact your doctor, clinic or pharmacist.

12. Other information

Your doctor or clinic will take a medical and family history and will examine you before prescribing the Pill. The physical examination may be delayed to another time if you request it and the health care provider believes that it is a good medical practice to postpone it. You should be reexamined at least once a year. Be sure to inform your doctor or clinic if there is a family history of any of the conditions listed previously in this leaflet. Be sure to keep all appointments with your doctor or clinic because this is a time to determine if there are early signs of side effects from using the Pill.

Do not use the Pill for any condition other than the one for which it was prescribed. The Pill has been prescribed specifically for you, do not give it to others who may want birth control pills.

If you want more information about birth control pills, ask your doctor or clinic. They have a more technical leaflet called ***PHYSICIAN LABELING*** which you might want to read.

NON-CONTRACEPTIVE HEALTH BENEFITS

In addition to preventing pregnancy, use of oral contraceptives may provide certain non-contraceptive health benefits:

- Menstrual cycles may become more regular
- Blood flow during menstruation may be lighter and less iron may be lost. Therefore, anemia due to iron deficiency is less likely to occur
- Pain or other symptoms during menstruation may be encountered less frequently
- Ectopic (tubal) pregnancy may occur less frequently
- Non-cancerous cysts or lumps in the breast may occur less frequently
- Acute pelvic inflammatory disease may occur less frequently
- Oral contraceptive use may provide some protection against developing two forms of cancer: cancer of the ovaries and cancer of the lining of the uterus

Keep this and all medication out of the reach of children.

Store at controlled room temperature 15°C to 25°C (59°F to 77°F).

BRIEF SUMMARY
PATIENT PACKAGE INSERT

This product (like all oral contraceptives) is intended to prevent pregnancy. It does not protect against HIV infection (AIDS) and other sexually transmitted diseases.

Oral contraceptives, also known as "birth control pills" or "the pill", are taken to prevent pregnancy and, when taken correctly, have a failure rate of about 1% per year when used without missing any pills. The typical failure rate of large numbers of pill users is less than 3% per year when women who miss pills are included. For most women, oral contraceptives are also free of serious or unpleasant side effects. However, forgetting to take oral contraceptives considerably increases the chances of pregnancy.

For the majority of women, oral contraceptives can be taken safely, but there are some women who are at high risk of developing certain serious diseases that can be life-threatening or may cause temporary or permanent disability. The risks associated with taking oral contraceptives increase significantly if you:

- Smoke
- Have high blood pressure, diabetes or high cholesterol
- Have or have had clotting disorders, heart attack, stroke, angina pectoris, cancer of the breast or sex organs, jaundice or malignant or benign liver tumors

You should not take the pill if you suspect you are pregnant or have unexplained vaginal bleeding.

Cigarette smoking increases the risk of serious cardiovascular side effects from oral contraceptive use. This risk increases with age and with heavy smoking (15 or more cigarettes per day) and is quite marked in women over 35 years of age. Women who use oral contraceptives are strongly advised not to smoke.

Most side effects of the pill are not serious. The most common such effects are nausea, vomiting, bleeding between menstrual periods, weight gain, breast tenderness and difficulty wearing contact lenses. These side effects, especially nausea and vomiting, may subside within the first 3 months of use.

The serious side effects of the pill occur very infrequently, especially if you are in good health and are young. However, you should know that the following medical conditions have been associated with or made worse by the pill:

1. Blood clots in the legs (thrombophlebitis) or lungs (pulmonary embolism), stoppage or rupture of a blood vessels in the brain (stroke), blockage of blood vessels in the heart (heart attack or angina pectoris), eye or other organs of the body. As mentioned above, smoking increases the risk of heart attacks and strokes and subsequent serious medical consequences.
2. Liver tumors, which may rupture and cause severe bleeding. A possible but not definite association has been found with the pill and liver cancer. However, liver cancers are extremely rare. The chance of developing liver cancer from using the pill is thus even rarer.
3. High blood pressure, although blood pressure usually returns to normal when the pill is stopped. The symptoms associated with these serious side effects are discussed in the detailed leaflet given to you with your supply of pills. Notify your doctor or health care provider if you notice any unusual physical disturbances while taking the pill. In addition, drugs such as rifampin, as well as some anti-convulsants and some antibiotics, may decrease oral contraceptive effectiveness.

Studies to date of women taking the pill have not shown an increase in the incidence of cancer of the breast or cervix. There is, however, insufficient evidence to rule out the possibility that the pill may cause such cancers. Some studies have reported an increase in the risk of developing breast cancer, particularly at a younger age. This increased risk appears to be related to duration of use.

Taking the pill provides some important non-contraceptive health benefits. These include less painful menstruation, less menstrual blood loss and anemia, fewer pelvic infections and fewer cancers of the ovary and the lining of the uterus.

Be sure to discuss any medical condition you may have with your health care provider. Your health care provider will take a medical and family history before prescribing oral contraceptives and will examine you. The physical examination may be delayed to another time if you request it and the health care provider believes that it is a good medical practice to postpone it. You should be reexamined at least once a year while taking oral contraceptives. The detailed patient information leaflet gives you further information which you should read and discuss with your health care provider.

HOW TO TAKE THE PILL

See full text of *HOW TO TAKE THE PILL* which is printed in full in the ***DETAILED PATIENT LABELING.***

Revised: April 6, 2000

Manufactured for:
Watson Pharma, Inc.
a subsidiary of
Watson Laboratories, Inc.
Corona, CA 92880
by ICN Puerto Rico, Inc.
Humacao, PR 00791
Address medical inquiries to:
WATSONPHARMA
Medical Information
PO Box 1900
Corona, CA 92878-1900
800-272-5525

A08826-3

TRIVORA® –21 Tablets –28 Tablets ℞

(levonorgestrel and ethinyl estradiol tablets, USP)–triphasic regimen

Part Number: A08916

Patients should be counseled that this product does not protect against HIV infection (AIDS) and other sexually transmitted diseases.

ORAL CONTRACEPTIVE AGENTS

DESCRIPTION

Trivora-21 Tablets provide an oral contraceptive regimen of 6 blue tablets followed by 5 white tablets and 10 pink tablets. Each blue tablet contains levonorgestrel 0.05 mg and ethinyl estradiol 0.03 mg, each white tablet contains levonogestrel 0.075 mg and ethinyl estradiol 0.04 mg and each pink tablet contains levonorgestrel 0.125 mg and ethinyl estradiol 0.03 mg.

Trivora-28 tablets provide a continuous oral contraceptive regimen of 6 blue tablets, 5 white tablets, 10 pink tablets and then 7 peach tablets. Each blue tablet contains levonorgestrel 0.05 mg and ethinyl estradiol 0.03 mg, each white tablet contains levonorgestrel 0.075 mg and ethinyl estradiol 0.04 mg, each pink tablet contains levonorgestrel 0.125 mg and ethinyl estradiol 0.03 mg and each peach tablet contains inert ingredients.

Levonorgestrel is a totally synthetic progestogen with the chemical name (–)-13-Ethyl-17-hydroxy-18, 19-dinor-17α-pregn-4-en-20-yn-3-one. Ethinyl estradiol is an estrogen with the chemical name 19-Nor-17α-pregna-1,3,5(10)-trien-20-yne-3,17-diol. Their structural formulae follow:

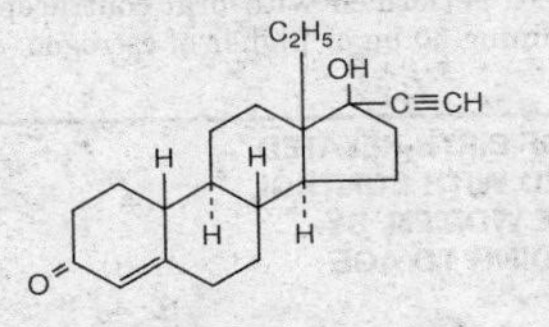

LEVONORGESTREL
$C_{21}H_{28}O_2$
M.W. = 312.45

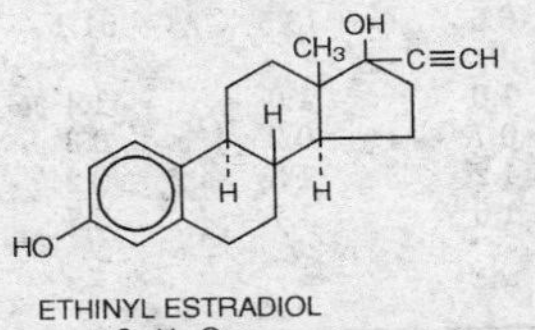

ETHINYL ESTRADIOL
$C_{20}H_{24}O_2$
M.W. = 296.41

The inactive ingredients present in all the tablets are lactose monohydrate, magnesium stearate, povidone, starch (corn) plus the following dyes:

Blue tablet: FD&C Blue #1
Pink tablet: FD&C Red #40
Peach tablet: FD&C Yellow #6

CLINICAL PHARMACOLOGY

Combination oral contraceptives act by suppression of gonadotrophins. Although the primary mechanism of this action is inhibition of ovulation, other alterations include changes in the cervical mucus (which increase the difficulty of sperm entry into the uterus) and the endometrium (which may reduce the likelihood of implantation).

INDICATIONS AND USAGE

Oral contraceptives are indicated for the prevention of pregnancy in women who elect to use this product as a method of contraception.

Oral contraceptives are highly effective. Table I lists the typical accidental pregnancy rates for users of combination oral contraceptives and other methods of oral contraception.[1] The efficacy of these contraceptive methods, except sterilization, depends upon the reliability with which they are used. Correct and consistent use of methods can result in lower failure rates.

[See table I at top of next page]

CONTRAINDICATIONS

Oral contraceptives should not be used in women who have the following conditions:

- Thrombophlebitis or thromboembolic disorders
- A past history of deep vein thrombophlebitis or thromboembolic disorders
- Cerebral vascular or coronary artery disease
- Known or suspected carcinoma of the breast
- Carcinoma of the endometrium or other known or suspected estrogen-dependent neoplasia
- Undiagnosed abnormal genital bleeding
- Cholestatic jaundice of pregnancy or jaundice with prior pill use
- Hepatic adenomas, carcinomas or benign liver tumors
- Known or suspected pregnancy

WARNINGS

Cigarette smoking increases the risk of serious cardiovascular side effects from oral contraceptive use. This risk increases with age and with heavy smoking (15 or more cigarettes per day) and is quite marked in women over 35 years of age. Women who use oral contraceptives should be strongly advised not to smoke.

The use of oral contraceptives is associated with increased risks of several serious conditions, including myocardial infarction, thromboembolism, stroke, hepatic neoplasia, and gallbladder disease, although the risk of serious morbidity or mortality is very small in healthy women without underlying risk factors. The risk of morbidity and mortality increases significantly in the presence of other underlying risk factors such as hypertension, hyperlipidemias, hypercholesterolemia, obesity and diabetes.[2–5]

Practitioners prescribing oral contraceptives should be familiar with the following information relating to these risks.

The information contained in this package insert is principally based on studies carried out in patients who used oral contraceptives with higher formulations of both estrogens and progestogens than those in common use today. The effect of long-term use of the oral contraceptives with lower formulations of both estrogens and progestogens remains to be determined.

Throughout this labeling, epidemiological studies reported are of two types: retrospective or case control studies and prospective or cohort studies. Case control studies provide a measure of the relative risk of a disease. Relative risk, the *ratio* of the incidence of a disease among oral contraceptive users to that among non-users, cannot be assessed directly from case control studies, but the odds ratio obtained is a measure of relative risk. The relative risk does not provide information on the actual clinical occurrence of a disease. Cohort studies provide not only a measure of the relative risk but a measure of attributable risk, which is the *difference* in the incidence of disease between oral contraceptive users and non-users. The attributable risk does not provide information about the actual occurrence of a disease in the population. (Adapted from ref. 12 and 13 with the author's permission.) For further information, the reader is referred to a text on epidemiological methods.

1. THROMBOEMBOLIC DISORDERS AND OTHER VASCULAR PROBLEMS

a. Myocardial Infarction

An increased risk of myocardial infarction has been attributed to oral contraceptive use. This risk is primarily in smokers or women with other underlying risk factors for coronary artery disease such as hypertension, hypercholesterolemia, morbid obesity and diabetes.[2–5, 13] The relative risk of heart attack for current oral contraceptive users has been estimated to be 2 to 6.[2, 14–19] The risk is very low under the age of 30. However, there is the possibility of a risk of cardiovascular disease even in very young women who take oral contraceptives.

Smoking in combination with oral contraceptive use has been shown to contribute substantially to the incidence of

Continued on next page

Trivora—Cont.

myocardial infarctions in women in their mid-thirties or older, with smoking accounting for the majority of excess cases.[20]

Mortality rates associated with circulatory disease have been shown to increase substantially in smokers over the age of 35 and non-smokers over the age of 40 among women who use oral contraceptives (see Table II).[16]

TABLE II: CIRCULATORY DISEASE MORTALITY RATES PER 100,000 WOMAN YEARS BY AGE, SMOKING STATUS AND ORAL CONTRACEPTIVE USE

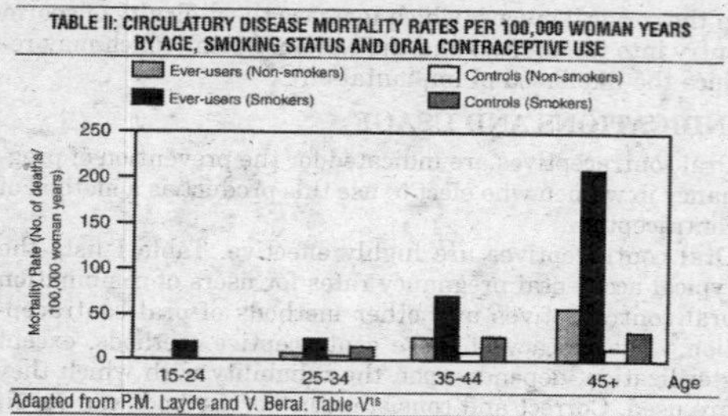

Adapted from P.M. Layde and V. Beral. Table V[18]

Oral contraceptives may compound the effects of well-known risk factors such as hypertension, diabetes, hyperlipidemias, hypercholesterolemia, age and obesity.[3, 13, 21] In particular, some progestogens are known to decrease HDL cholesterol and cause glucose intolerance, while estrogens may create a state of hyperinsulinism.[21–25] Oral contraceptives have been shown to increase blood pressure among users (see **WARNINGS,** section 9). Similar effects on risk factors have been associated with an increased risk of heart disease. Oral contraceptives must be used with caution in women with cardiovascular disease risk factors.

b. Thromboembolism

An increased risk of thromboembolic and thrombotic disease associated with the use of oral contraceptives is well established. Case control studies have found the relative risk of users compared to nonusers to be 3 for the first episode of superficial venous thrombosis, 4 to 11 for deep vein thrombosis or pulmonary embolism, and 1.5 to 6 for women with predisposing conditions for venous thromboembolic disease.[12, 13, 26–31] Cohort studies have shown the relative risk to be somewhat lower, about 3 for new cases and about 4.5 for new cases requiring hospitalization.[32] The risk of thromboembolic disease due to oral contraceptives is not related to length of use and disappears after pill use is stopped.[12]

A 2- to 6-fold increase in relative risk of post-operative thromboembolic complications has been reported with the use of oral contraceptives. The relative risk of venous thrombosis in women who have predisposing conditions is twice that of women without such medical conditions.[83] If feasible, oral contraceptives should be discontinued at least 4 weeks prior to and for 2 weeks after elective surgery and during and following prolonged immobilization. Since the immediate postpartum period also is associated with an increased risk of thromboembolism, oral contraceptives should be started no earlier than 4 to 6 weeks after delivery in women who elect not to breast feed.[33]

c. Cerebrovascular diseases

An increase in both the relative and attributable risks of cerebrovascular events (thrombotic and hemorrhagic strokes) has been shown in users of oral contraceptives. In general, the risk is greatest among older (>35 years), hypertensive women who also smoke. Hypertension was found to be a risk factor for both users and non-users for both types of strokes while smoking interacted to increase the risk for hemorrhagic strokes.[34]

In a large study, the relative risk of thrombotic strokes has been shown to range from 3 for normotensive users to 14 for users with severe hypertension.[35] The relative risk of hemorrhagic stroke is reported to be 1.2 for non-smokers who used oral contraceptives, 2.6 for smokers who did not use oral contraceptives, 7.6 for smokers who used oral contraceptives, 1.8 for normotensive users and 25.7 for users with severe hypertension.[35] The attributable risk also is greater in women in their mid-thirties or older and among smokers.[13]

TABLE I: PERCENTAGE OF WOMEN EXPERIENCING A CONTRACEPTIVE FAILURE DURING THE FIRST YEAR OF PERFECT USE AND FIRST YEAR OF TYPICAL USE

Method	% of Women Experiencing an Accidental Pregnancy within the First Year of Use	
	Typical Use[a]	Perfect Use[b]
Chance	85	85
Spermicides	21	6
Periodic abstinence	20	1-9
Withdrawal	19	4
Cap		
Parous	36	26
Nulliparous	18	9
Sponge		
Parous	36	20
Nulliparous	18	9
Diaphragm	18	6
Condom		
Female	21	5
Male	12	3
Pill	3	
Progestin only		0.5
Combined		0.1
IUD		
Progesterone	2	1.5
Copper T 380A	0.8	0.6
Injection (Depo-Provera)	0.3	0.3
Implants (Norplant)	0.09	0.09
Female Sterilization	0.4	0.4
Male Sterilization	0.15	0.10

Adapted with permission[1].

[a]Among *typical* couples who initiate use of a method (not necessarily for the first time), the percentage who experience an accidental pregnancy during the first year if they do not stop use for any other reason.

[b]Among couples who initiate use of a method (not necessarily for the first time) and who use it *perfectly* (both consistently and correctly), the percentage who experience an accidental pregnancy during the first year if they do not stop use for any other reason.

d. Dose-related risk of vascular disease from oral contraceptives

A positive association has been observed between the amount of estrogen and progestogen in oral contraceptives and the risk of vascular disease.[36–38] A decline in serum high-density lipoproteins (HDL) has been reported with many progestational agents.[22–24] A decline in serum high-density lipoproteins has been associated with an increased incidence of ischemic heart disease.[39] Because estrogens increase HDL cholesterol, the net effect of an oral contraceptive depends on a balance achieved between doses of estrogen and progestogen and the nature and absolute amount of progestogens used in the contraceptives. The amount of both hormones should be considered in the choice of an oral contraceptive.[37]

Minimizing exposure to estrogen and progestogen is in keeping with good principles of therapeutics. For any particular estrogen/progestogen combination, the dosage regimen prescribed should be one which contains the least amount of estrogen and progestogen that is compatible with a low failure rate and the needs of the individual patient. New acceptors of oral contraceptive agents should be started on preparations containing the lowest estrogen content that produces satisfactory results for the individual.

e. Persistence of risk of vascular disease

There are three studies which have shown persistence of risk of vascular disease for ever-users of oral contraceptives.[17, 34, 40] In a study in the United States, the risk of developing myocardial infarction after discontinuing oral contraceptives persists for at least 9 years for women 40–49 years who had used oral contraceptives for 5 or more years, but this increased risk was not demonstrated in other age groups.[17] In another study in Great Britain, the risk of developing cerebrovascular disease persisted for at least 6 years after discontinuation of oral contraceptives, although excess risk was very small.[40] There is a significantly increased relative risk of subarachnoid hemorrhage after termination of use of oral contraceptives.[34] However, these studies were performed with oral contraceptive formulations containing 50 µg or higher of estrogen.

2. ESTIMATES OF MORTALITY FROM CONTRACEPTIVE USE

One study gathered data from a variety of sources which have estimated the mortality rates associated with different methods of contraception at different ages (see Table III).[41] These estimates include the combined risk of death associated with contraceptive methods plus the risk attributable to pregnancy in the event of method failure. Each method of contraception has its specific benefits and risks. The study concluded that with the exception of oral contraceptive users 35 and older who smoke and 40 and older who do not smoke, mortality associated with all methods of birth control is low and below that associated with childbirth. The observation of a possible increase in risk of mortality with age for oral contraceptive users is based on data gathered in the 1970s – but not reported in the U.S. until 1983.[16, 41] However, current clinical practice involves the use of lower estrogen dose formulations combined with careful restriction of oral contraceptive use to women who do not have the various risk factors listed in this labeling.

Because of these changes in practice and, also, because of some limited new data which suggest that the risk of cardiovascular disease with the use of oral contraceptives may now be less than previously observed,[78, 79] the Fertility and Maternal Health Drugs Advisory Committee was asked to review the topic in 1989. The Committee concluded that although cardiovascular disease risks may be increased with oral contraceptive use after age 40 in healthy non-smoking women (even with the newer low-dose formulations), there are greater potential health risks associated with pregnancy in older women and with the alternative surgical and medical procedures which may be necessary if such women do not have access to effective and acceptable means of contraception.

Therefore, the Committee recommended that the benefits of oral contraceptive use by healthy non-smoking women over 40 may outweigh the possible risks. Of course, older women, as all women who take oral contraceptives, should take the lowest possible dose formulation that is effective.[80]

[See table III below]

3. CARCINOMA OF THE REPRODUCTIVE ORGANS AND BREASTS

Numerous epidemiological studies have been performed on the incidence of breast, endometrial, ovarian and cervical cancer in women using oral contraceptives. The overwhelming evidence in the literature suggests that use of oral contraceptives is not associated with an increase in the risk of developing breast cancer, regardless of the age and parity of first use or with most of the marketed brands and doses.[42–44] The Cancer and Steroid Hormone (CASH) study also showed no latent effect on the risk of breast cancer for at least a decade following long-term use.[43] A few studies have shown increased relative risk of developing breast cancer,[44–47] although the methodology of these studies, which included differences in examination of users and non-users and differences in age at start of use, has been questioned.[47–49] Some studies have reported an increased relative risk of developing breast cancer, particularly at a younger age. This increased relative risk appears to be related to duration of use.[81, 82]

Some studies suggest that oral contraceptive use has been associated with an increase in the risk of cervical intraepithelial neoplasia in some populations of women.[50–53] How-

TABLE III: ESTIMATED ANNUAL NUMBER OF BIRTH-RELATED OR METHOD-RELATED DEATHS ASSOCIATED WITH CONTROL OF FERTILITY PER 100,000 NONSTERILE WOMEN, BY FERTILITY CONTROL METHOD ACCORDING TO AGE

Method of control and outcome	15-19	20-24	25-29	30-34	35-39	40-44
No fertility control methods*	7.0	7.4	9.1	14.8	25.7	28.2
Oral contraceptives non-smoker**	0.3	0.5	0.9	1.9	13.8	31.6
Oral contraceptives smoker**	2.2	3.4	6.6	13.5	51.1	117.2
IUD**	0.8	0.8	1.0	1.0	1.4	1.4
Condom*	1.1	1.6	0.7	0.2	0.3	0.4
Diaphragm/Spermicide*	1.9	1.2	1.2	1.3	2.2	2.8
Periodic abstinence*	2.5	1.6	1.6	1.7	2.7	3.6

*Deaths are birth-related

**Deaths are method-related

Estimates adapted from H.W. Ory, Table 3[41]

ever, there continues to be controversy about the extent to which such findings may be due to differences in sexual behavior and other factors.

In spite of many studies of the relationship between oral contraceptive use and breast or cervical cancer, a cause and effect relationship has not been established.

4. HEPATIC NEOPLASIA

Benign hepatic adenomas are associated with oral contraceptive use although the incidence of benign tumors is rare in the United States. Indirect calculations have estimated the attributable risk to be in the range of 3.3 cases per 100,000 for users, a risk that increases after 4 or more years of use.[54] Rupture of rare, benign, hepatic adenomas may cause death through intra-abdominal hemorrhage.[55–56]

Studies in the United States and Britain have shown an increased risk of developing hepatocellular carcinoma in the long-term (>8 years) oral contraceptive users.[57–59] However, these cancers are extremely rare in the United States and the attributable risk (the excess incidence) of liver cancers in oral contraceptive users approaches less than 1 per 1,000,000 users.

5. OCULAR LESIONS

There have been clinical case reports of retinal thrombosis associated with the use of oral contraceptives. Oral contraceptives should be discontinued if there is unexplained partial or complete loss of vision; onset of proptosis or diplopia; papilledema; or retinal vascular lesions. Appropriate diagnostic and therapeutic measures should be undertaken immediately.

6. ORAL CONTRACEPTIVE USE BEFORE OR DURING EARLY PREGNANCY

Extensive epidemiological studies have revealed no increased risk of birth defects in women who have used oral contraceptives prior to pregnancy.[60–62] Studies also do not suggest a teratogenic effect, particularly insofar as cardiac anomalies and limb reduction defects are concerned, when taken inadvertently during early pregnancy.[60, 61, 63, 64]

The administration of oral contraceptives to induce withdrawal bleeding should not be used as a test for pregnancy. Oral contraceptives should not be used during pregnancy to treat threatened or habitual abortion.

It is recommended that for any patient who has missed 2 consecutive periods, pregnancy should be ruled out before continuing oral contraceptive use. If the patient has not adhered to the prescribed schedule, the possibility of pregnancy should be considered at the first missed period. Oral contraceptive use should be discontinued if pregnancy is confirmed.

7. GALLBLADDER DISEASE

Earlier studies have reported an increased lifetime relative risk of gallbladder surgery in users of oral contraceptives and estrogens.[65–66] More recent studies, however, have shown that the relative risk of developing gallbladder disease among oral contraceptive users may be minimal.[67] The recent findings of minimal risk may be related to the use of oral contraceptive formulations containing lower hormonal doses of estrogens and progestogens.[68]

8. CARBOHYDRATE AND LIPID METABOLIC EFFECTS

Oral contraceptives have been shown to cause glucose intolerance in a significant percentage of users.[25] Oral contraceptives containing greater than 75 µg of estrogen cause hyperinsulinism, while lower doses of estrogen cause less glucose intolerance.[70] Progestogens increase insulin secretion and create insulin resistance, this effect varying with different progestational agents.[25, 71] However, in the non-diabetic woman, oral contraceptives appear to have no effect on fasting blood glucose.[69] Because of these demonstrated effects, prediabetic and diabetic women should be carefully observed while taking oral contraceptives.

Some women may develop persistent hypertriglyceridemia while on the pill.[72] As discussed earlier (see **WARNINGS**, sections 1a. and 1d.), changes in serum triglycerides and lipoprotein levels have been reported in oral contraceptive users.[23]

9. ELEVATED BLOOD PRESSURE

An increase in blood pressure has been reported in women taking oral contraceptives and this increase is more likely in older oral contraceptive users and with continued use.[73,84] Data from the Royal College of General Practitioners and subsequent randomized trials have shown that the incidence of hypertension increases with increasing concentrations of progestogens.

Women with a history of hypertension or hypertension-related diseases or renal disease should be encouraged to use another method of contraception. If women elect to use oral contraceptives, they should be monitored closely and if significant elevation of blood pressure occurs, oral contraceptives should be discontinued. For most women, elevated blood pressure will return to normal after stopping oral contraceptives and there is no difference in the occurrence of hypertension among ever- and never-users.[73–75]

10. HEADACHE

The onset or exacerbation of migraine or development of headache with a new pattern which is recurrent, persistent or severe requires discontinuation of oral contraceptives and evaluation of the cause.

11. BLEEDING IRREGULARITIES

Breakthrough bleeding and spotting are sometimes encountered in patients on oral contraceptives, especially during the first 3 months of use. Non-hormonal causes should be considered and adequate diagnostic measures taken to rule out malignancy or pregnancy in the event of breakthrough bleeding, as in the case of any abnormal vaginal bleeding. If pathology has been excluded, time or a change to another formulation may solve the problem. In the event of amenorrhea, pregnancy should be ruled out.

Some women may encounter post-pill amenorrhea or oligomenorrhea, especially when such a condition was pre-existent.

PRECAUTIONS

GENERAL

Patients should be counseled that this product does not protect against HIV infection (AIDS) and other sexually transmitted diseases.

1. PHYSICAL EXAMINATION AND FOLLOW-UP

It is good medical practice for all women to have annual history and physical examinations, including women using oral contraceptives. The physical examination, however, may be deferred until after initiation of oral contraceptives if requested by the woman and judged appropriate by the clinician. The physical examination should include special reference to blood pressure, breasts, abdomen and pelvic organs, including cervical cytology, and relevant laboratory tests. In case of undiagnosed, persistent or recurrent abnormal vaginal bleeding, appropriate measures should be conducted to rule out malignancy. Women with a strong family history of breast cancer or who have breast nodules should be monitored with particular care.

2. LIPID DISORDERS

Women who are being treated for hyperlipidemias should be followed closely if they elect to use oral contraceptives. Some progestogens may elevate LDL levels and may render the control of hyperlipidemias more difficult.

3. LIVER FUNCTION

If jaundice develops in any woman receiving oral contraceptives the medication should be discontinued. Steroid hormones may be poorly metabolized in patients with impaired liver function.

4. FLUID RETENTION

Oral contraceptives may cause some degree of fluid retention. They should be prescribed with caution, and only with careful monitoring, in patients with conditions which might be aggravated by fluid retention.

5. EMOTIONAL DISORDERS

Women with a history of depression should be carefully observed and the drug discontinued if depression recurs to a serious degree.

6. CONTACT LENSES

Contact lens wearers who develop visual changes or changes in lens tolerance should be assessed by an ophthalmologist.

7. DRUG INTERACTIONS

Reduced efficacy and increased incidence of breakthrough bleeding and menstrual irregularities have been associated with concomitant use of rifampin. A similar association though less marked, has been suggested with barbiturates, phenylbutazone, phenytoin sodium, and possibly with griseofulvin, ampicillin and tetracyclines.[76]

8. INTERACTIONS WITH LABORATORY TESTS

Certain endocrine and liver function tests and blood components may be affected by oral contraceptives:

- **a.** Increased prothrombin and factors VII, VIII, IX, and X; decreased antithrombin 3; increased norepinephrine-induced platelet aggregability.
- **b.** Increased thyroid binding globulin (TBG) leading to increased circulating total thyroid hormone, as measured by protein-bound iodine (PBI), T4 by column or by radioimmunoassay. Free T3 resin uptake is decreased, reflecting the elevated TBG. Free T4 concentration is unaltered.
- **c.** Other binding proteins may be elevated in serum.
- **d.** Sex steroid binding globulins are increased and result in elevated levels of total circulating sex steroids and corticoids; however, free or biologically active levels remain unchanged.
- **e.** Triglycerides may be increased.
- **f.** Glucose tolerance may be decreased.
- **g.** Serum folate levels may be depressed by oral contraceptive therapy. This may be of clinical significance if a woman becomes pregnant shortly after discontinuing oral contraceptives.

9. CARCINOGENESIS

See **WARNINGS** section.

10. PREGNANCY

Pregnancy Category X. See **CONTRAINDICATIONS** and **WARNINGS** sections.

11. NURSING MOTHERS

Small amounts of oral contraceptive steroids have been identified in the milk of nursing mothers and a few adverse effects on the child have been reported, including jaundice and breast enlargement. In addition, oral contraceptives given in the postpartum period may interfere with lactation by decreasing the quantity and quality of breast milk. If possible, the nursing mother should be advised not to use oral contraceptives while breast feeding. She should use another method of contraception since breast feeding provides only partial protection from becoming pregnant and this partial protection decreases significantly as she breast feeds for longer periods of time. The nursing mother should consider starting oral contraceptives only after she has weaned her child completely.

INFORMATION FOR THE PATIENT

See **PATIENT LABELING** printed below.

ADVERSE REACTIONS

An increased risk of the following serious adverse reactions has been associated with the use of oral contraceptives (see **WARNINGS** section):

- Thrombophlebitis
- Arterial thromboembolism
- Pulmonary embolism
- Myocardial infarction
- Cerebral hemorrhage
- Cerebral thrombosis
- Hypertension
- Gallbladder disease
- Hepatic adenomas, carcinomas or benign liver tumors

There is evidence of an association between the following conditions and the use of oral contraceptives, although additional confirmatory studies are needed:

- Mesenteric thrombosis
- Retinal thrombosis

The following adverse reactions have been reported in patients receiving oral contraceptives and are believed to be drug-related:

- Nausea
- Vomiting
- Gastrointestinal symptoms (such as abdominal cramps and bloating)
- Breakthrough bleeding
- Spotting
- Changes in menstrual flow
- Amenorrhea
- Temporary infertility after discontinuation of treatment
- Edema
- Melasma which may persist
- Breast changes; tenderness, enlargement, secretion
- Change in weight (increase or decrease)
- Change in cervical erosion and secretion
- Diminution in lactation when given immediately postpartum
- Cholestatic jaundice
- Migraine
- Rash (allergic)
- Mental depression
- Reduced tolerance to carbohydrates
- Vaginal candidiasis
- Change in corneal curvature (steepening)
- Intolerance to contact lenses

The following adverse reactions have been reported in users of oral contraceptives and the association has been neither confirmed nor refuted:

- Pre-menstrual syndrome
- Cataracts
- Changes in appetite
- Cystitis-like syndrome
- Headache
- Nervousness
- Dizziness
- Hirsutism
- Loss of scalp hair
- Erythema multiforme
- Erythema nodosum
- Hemorrhagic eruption
- Vaginitis
- Porphyria
- Impaired renal function
- Hemolytic uremic syndrome
- Budd-Chiari syndrome
- Acne
- Changes in libido
- Colitis

OVERDOSAGE

Serious ill effects have not been reported following acute ingestion of large doses of oral contraceptives by young children. Overdosage may cause nausea, and withdrawal bleeding may occur in females.

HEALTH BENEFITS FROM ORAL CONTRACEPTIVES

The following health benefits related to the use of oral contraceptives are supported by epidemiological studies which largely utilized oral contraceptive formulations containing estrogen doses exceeding 0.035 mg of ethinyl estradiol or 0.05 mg of mestranol.[6–11]

Effects on menses:

- Increased menstrual cycle regularity
- Decreased blood loss and decreased incidence of iron deficiency anemia
- Decreased incidence of dysmenorrhea

Effects related to inhibition of ovulation:

- Decreased incidence of functional ovarian cysts
- Decreased incidence of ectopic pregnancies

Effects from long-term use:

- Decreased incidence of fibroadenomas and fibrocystic disease of the breast
- Decreased incidence of acute pelvic inflammatory disease
- Decreased incidence of endometrial cancer
- Decreased incidence of ovarian cancer.

DOSAGE AND ADMINISTRATION

To achieve maximum contraceptive effectiveness, oral contraceptives must be taken exactly as directed and at intervals exceeding 24 hours.

Continued on next page

Trivora—Cont.

21-Day Schedule: For a DAY 1 START, count the first day of menstrual flow as Day 1 and first blue tablet is then taken on Day 1. For a SUNDAY START, when menstrual flow begins on or before Sunday, the first blue tablet is taken on that day. With either a DAY 1 START or SUNDAY START, 1 blue tablet is taken for 6 days, then 1 white tablet for 5 days, then 1 pink tablet for 10 days. With either a DAY 1 START or SUNDAY START, 1 tablet is taken each day at the same time for 21 days. No tablets are taken for 7 days, then, whether bleeding has stopped or not, a new course is started of 1 tablet a day for 21 days. This institutes 3 weeks on, 1 week off dosage regimen.

28-Day Schedule: For a DAY 1 START, count the first day of menstrual flow as Day 1 and the first blue tablet is then taken on Day 1. For a SUNDAY START when menstrual flow begins on or before Sunday, the first blue tablet is taken on that day. With either a DAY 1 START or SUNDAY START, 1 blue tablet is taken for 6 days, then 1 white tablet for 5 days, then 1 pink tablet for 10 days, then 1 peach (inert) tablet for 7 days. With either a DAY 1 START or SUNDAY START, 1 tablet is taken each day at the same time for 28 days. After all 28 tablets are taken, whether bleeding has stopped or not, the same dosage schedule is repeated beginning on the following day.

INSTRUCTIONS TO PATIENTS

- To achieve maximum contraceptive effectiveness, the oral contraceptive pill must be taken exactly as directed and at intervals not exceeding 24 hours.
- Important: Women should be instructed to use an additional method of protection until after the first 7 days of administration *in the initial cycle.*
- Due to the normally increased risk of thromboembolism occurring postpartum, women should be instructed not to initiate treatment with oral contraceptives earlier than 4 weeks after a full-term delivery. If pregnancy is terminated in the first 12 weeks, the patient should be instructed to start oral contraceptives immediately or within 7 days. If pregnancy is terminated after 12 weeks, the patient should be instructed to start oral contraceptives after 2 weeks.[33, 77]
- If spotting or breakthrough bleeding should occur, the patient should continue the medication according to the schedule. Should spotting or breakthrough bleeding persist, the patient should notify her physician.
- If the patient misses 1 pill, she should be instructed to take it as soon as she remembers and then take the next pill at the regular time. The patient should be advised that missing a pill can cause spotting or light bleeding and that she may be a little sick to her stomach on the days she takes the missed pill with her regularly scheduled pill. If the patient has missed more than one pill, see DETAILED PATIENT LABELING: HOW TO TAKE THE PILL, WHAT TO DO IF YOU MISS PILLS.
- Use of oral contraceptives in the event of a missed menstrual period:

1. If the patient has not adhered to the prescribed dosage regimen, the possibility of pregnancy should be considered after the first missed period and oral contraceptives should be withheld until pregnancy has been ruled out.
2. If the patient has adhered to the prescribed regimen and misses 2 consecutive periods, pregnancy should be ruled out before continuing the contraceptive regimen.

HOW SUPPLIED

Trivora®-21 Tablets are available in 21-tablet blister cards. Six blister cards are packaged in a carton. All the tablets are unscored, round in shape. The blue tablets are debossed with "WATSON" on one side and "50/30" on the other side. The white tablets are debossed with "WATSON" on one side and "75/40" on the other side. The pink tablets are debossed with "WATSON" on one side and "125/30" on the other side. Trivora®-28 Tablets are available in 28-tablet blister cards. Six blister cards are packaged in a carton. Trivora®-28 Tablets contain the same 21 active tablets as Trivora®-21 Tablets with 7 additional inert tablets. The peach inert tablets are unscored, round in shape with "WATSON" on one side and "P1" on the other side.

Rx only

Store at controlled room temperature 15°–30°C (59°–86°F).

REFERENCES

1. Hatcher, R.A. Trussell, J., Stewart, F., et al.: *Contraceptive Technology: Sixteenth Revised Edition,* New York, NY 1994.
2. Mann, J., et al.: *Br Med J* 2(5956):241–245, 1975.
3. Knopp, R.H.: *J Reprod Med* 31(9):913–921, 1986.
4. Mann, J.I., et al.: *Br Med J* 2:445–447, 1976.
5. Ory, H.: *JAMA* 237:2619–2622, 1977.
6. The Cancer and Steroid Hormone Study of the Centers for Disease Control: *JAMA* 249(2):1596–1599, 1983.
7. The Cancer and Steroid Hormone Study of the Centers for Disease Control: *JAMA* 257(6):796–800. 1987.
8. Ory, H.W.: *JAMA* 228(1):68–69, 1974.
9. Ory, H.W., et al.: *N Engl J Med* 294:419–422, 1976.
10. Ory, H.W.: *Fam Plann Perspect* 14:182–184, 1982.
11. Ory, H.W. et al.: *Making Choices,* New York, The Alan Guttmacher Institute, 1983.
12. Stadel, B.: *N Engl J Med* 305(11):612–618, 1981.
13. Stadel, B.: *N Engl J Med* 305(12):672–677, 1981.
14. Adam, S., et al.: *Br J Obstet Gynaecol* 88:838–845, 1981.
15. Mann, J., et al.: *Br Med J* 2(5965):245–248, 1975.
16. Royal College of General Practitioners' Oral Contraceptive Study: *Lancet* 1:541–546, 1981.
17. Slone, D., et al.: *N Engl J Med* 305(8):420–424, 1981.
18. Vessey, M.P.: *Br J Fam Plann* 6 (supplement):1–12, 1980.
19. Russell-Briefel, R., et al.: *Prev Med* 15:352–362, 1986.
20. Goldbaum, G., et al.: *JAMA* 258(10):1339–1342, 1987.
21. LaRosa, J.C.: *J Reprod Med* 31 (9):906–912, 1986.
22. Krauss, R.M., et al.: *Am J Obstet Gynecol* 145:446–452, 1983.
23. Wahl, P., et al.: *N Engl J Med* 308(15)862–867, 1983.
24. Wynn, V., et al.: *Am J Obstet Gynecol* 142(6):766–771, 1982.
25. Wynn, V., et al.: *J Reprod Med* 31(9):892–897, 1986.
26. Inman, W.H., et al.: *Br Med J* 2(5599):193–199, 1968.
27. Maguire, M.G., et al.: *Am J Epidemiol* 110(2):188–195, 1979.
28. Petitti, D., et al.: *JAMA* 242(11):1150–1154, 1979.
29. Vessey, M.P., et al.: *Br Med J* 2(5599):199–205, 1968.
30. Vessey, M.P., et al.: *Br Med J* 2(5658):651–657, 1969.
31. Porter, J.B., et al.: *Obstet Gynecol* 59(3):299–302, 1982.
32. Vessey, M.P., et al.: *J Biosoc Sci* 8:373–427, 1976.
33. Mishell, D.R., et al.: *Reproductive Endocrinology,* Philadelphia, F.A. Davis Co., 1979.
34. Petitti, D.B., et al.: *Lancet* 2:234–236, 1978.
35. Collaborative Group for the Study of Stroke in Young Women: *JAMA* 231(7):718–722, 1975.
36. Inman, W.H., et al.: *Br Med J* 2:203–209, 1970.
37. Meade, T.W., et al.: *Br Med J* 280(6224):1157–1161, 1980.
38. Kay, C.R.: *Am J Obstet Gynecol* 142(6):762–765, 1982.
39. Gordon, T., et al.: *Am J Med* 62:707–714, 1977.
40. Royal College of General Practitioners' Oral Contraception Study: *J Coll Gen Pract* 33:75–82, 1983.
41. Ory, H.W.: *Fam Plann Perspect* 15(2):57–63, 1983.
42. Paul, C., et al.: *Br Med J* 293:723–725, 1986.
43. The Cancer and Steroid Hormone Study of the Centers for Disease Control: *N Engl J Med* 315(7):405–411, 1986.
44. Pike, M.C., et al.: *Lancet* 2:926–929, 1983.
45. Miller, D.R., et al.: *Obstet Gynecol* 68:863–868, 1986.
46. Olsson, H., et al.: *Lancet* 2:748–749, 1985.
47. McPherson, K., et al.: *Br J Cancer* 56:653–660, 1987.
48. Huggins, G.R., et al.: *Fertil Steril* 47(5):733–761, 1987.
49. McPherson, K., et al.: *Br Med J* 293:709–710, 1986.
50. Ory, H., et al.: *Am J Obstet Gynecol* 124(6):573–577, 1976.
51. Vessey, M.P., et al.: *Lancet* 2:930, 1983.
52. Brinton, L.A., et al.: *Int J Cancer* 38:339–344, 1986.
53. WHO Collaborative Study of Neoplasia and Steroid Contraceptives: *Br Med J* 290:961–965, 1985.
54. Rooks, J.B., et al.: *JAMA* 242(7):644–648, 1979.
55. Bein, N.N., et al.: *Br J Surg* 64:433–435, 1977.
56. Klatskin, G., *Gastroenterology* 73:386–394, 1977.
57. Henderson, B.E., et al.: *Br J Cancer* 48:437–440, 1983.
58. Neuberger, J., et al.: *Br Med J* 292:1355–1357, 1986.
59. Forman, D., et al.: *Br Med J* 292:1357–1361, 1986.
60. Harlap, S., et al.: *Obstet Gynecol* 55(4):447–452, 1980.
61. Savolainen, E., et al.: *Am J Obstet Gynecol* 140(5):521–524, 1981.
62. Janerich, D.T., et al.: *Am J Epidemiol* 112(1):73–79, 1980.
63. Ferencz, C., et al., *Teratology* 21:225–239, 1980.
64. Rothman, K.J., et al.: *Am J Epidemiol* 109(4):433–439, 1979.
65. Boston Collaborative Drug Surveillance Program: *Lancet* 1:1399–1404, 1973.
66. Royal College of General Practitioners: *Oral contraceptives and health,* New York, Pittman, 1974.
67. Rome Group for the Epidemiology and Prevention of Cholelithiasis: *Am J Epidemiol* 119(5):796–805, 1984.
68. Strom, B.L., et al.: *Clin Pharmacol Ther* 39(3):335–341, 1986.
69. Perlman, J.A., et al.: *J Chronic Dis* 38(10):857–864, 1985.
70. Wynn, V., et al.: *Lancet* 1:1045–1049, 1979.
71. Wynn, V.: *Progesterone and Progestin,* New York, Raven Press, 1983.
72. Wynn, V., et al.: *Lancet* 2:720–723, 1966.
73. Fisch, I.R., et al.: *JAMA* 237(23):2499–2503, 1977.
74. Laragh, J.H.: *Am J Obstet Gynecol* 126(1):141–147, 1976.
75. Ramcharan, S., et al.: *Pharmacology of Steroid Contraceptive Drugs,* New York, Raven Press, 1977.
76. Stockley, I.: *Pharm J* 216:140–143, 1976.
77. Dickey, R.P.: *Managing Contraceptive Pill Patients,* Oklahoma, Creative Informatics Inc., 1984.
78. Porter, J.B., Hunter, J., Jick, H., et al.: *Obstet Gynecol* 1985:66:1–4.
79. Porter, J.B., Hershel, J., Walker, A.M.: *Obstet Gynecol* 1987:70:29–32.
80. Fertility and Maternal Health Drugs Advisory Committee, F.D.A., October, 1989.
81. Schlesselman, J., Stadel, B.V., Murray, P., Lai, S.: *Breast cancer in relation to early use of oral contraceptives.* JAMA 1988:259:1828–1833.
82. Hennekens, C.H., Speizer, F.E., Lipnick, R.J., Rosner, B., Bain, C., Belanger, C., Stampfer, M.J., Willett, W., Peto, R.: *A case-control study of oral contraceptive use and breast cancer.* JNCI 1984; 72:39–42.
83. Royal College of General Practitioners: *Oral contraceptives, venous thrombosis, and varicose veins. J Coll Gen Pract* 28:393–399, 1978.
84. Royal College of General Practitioners' Oral Contraception Study: *Effect on hypertension and benign breast disease of progestogen component in combined oral contraceptives. Lancet* 1:624, 1977.

Manufactured for Watson Pharma, INC. a subsidiary of Watson Laboratories, Inc.
Corona, CA 92880 (USA)
By Syntex (FP) Inc.
Humacao, PR 00791
Revised: Feb. 26, 1998
Trivora®-21 Tablets
Trivora®-28 Tablets
(levonorgestrel and ethinyl estradiol tablets, USP)–triphasic regimen

Shown in Product Identification Guide, page 340

ZOVIA ℞

[zō vĭa]

(ethynodiol diacetate and ethinyl estradiol tablets, USP)
Rx only

Zovia 1/35E-21
Zovia 1/35E-28
Zovia 1/50E-21
Zovia 1/50E-28

(Ethynodiol Diacetate and Ethinyl Estradiol Tablets, USP)

Patients should be counseled that this product does not protect against HIV infection (AIDS) and other sexually transmitted diseases.

DESCRIPTION

Zovia 1/35E-21 and Zovia 1/35E-28. Each light pink tablet contains 1 mg of ethynodiol diacetate and 35 mcg of ethinyl estradiol, and the inactive ingredients include microcrystalline cellulose, lactose (anhydrous), magnesium stearate, polacrilin potassium and povidone. In addition, the coloring agents are D&C Yellow No. 10 and D&C Red No. 30. Each white tablet in the Zovia 1/35E-28 package is a placebo containing no active ingredients and the inactive ingredients include microcrystalline cellulose, lactose (anhydrous) and magnesium stearate.

Zovia 1/50E-21 and Zovia 1/50E-28. Each pink tablet contains 1 mg of ethynodiol diacetate and 50 mcg of ethinyl estradiol, and the inactive ingredients iinclude microcrystalline cellulose, lactose (anhydrous), magnesium stearate, polacrilin piotassium and povidone. In addition, the coloring agents are D&C Yellow No. 10 and D&C Red No. 30. Each white tablet in the Zovia 1/50E-28 package is a placebo containing no active ingredients, and the inactive ingredients include microcrystalline cellulose, lactose (anhydrous) and magnesium stearate.

The chemical name for ethynodiol diacetate is 19-nor-17α-pregn-4-en-20-yne-3β, 17-diol diacetate, and for ethinyl estradiol it is 19-nor-17α-pregn-1, 3, 5 (10)-trien-20-yne-3, 17-diol. The structural formulas are as follows:

Therapeutic class: Oral contraceptive

ethynodiol diacetate
M.W. = 384.51

ethinyl estradiol
M.W. = 296.41

CLINICAL PHARMACOLOGY

Combination oral contraceptives act primarily by suppression of gonadotropins. Although the primary mechanism of this action is inhibition of ovulation, other alterations in the genital tract, including changes in the cervical mucus (which increase the difficulty of sperm entry into the uterus) and the endometrium (which may reduce the likelihood of implantation) may also contribute to contraceptive effectiveness.

INDICATIONS AND USAGE

Zovia 1/35E and Zovia 1/50E are indicated for the prevention of pregnancy in women who elect to use oral contraceptives as a method of contraception.

Oral contraceptives are highly effective. Table 1 lists the typical accidental pregnancy rates for users of combination oral contraceptives and other methods of contraception. The efficacy of these contraceptive methods, except sterilization and progestogen implants and injections, depends upon the reliability with which they are used. Correct and consistent use of methods can result in lower failure rates.

Table 1. Lowest expected and typical failure rates during the first year of continuous use of a method. Percent of women experiencing an accidental pregnancy in the first year of continuous use.[1, 1a]

Method	Lowest Expected*	Typical**
No contraception	85	85
Oral contraceptives		
Combined	0.1	N/A***
Progestogen only	0.5	N/A***
Diaphragm with spermicidal cream or jelly	6	18
Spermicides alone (foam, creams, jellies and vaginal suppositories	3	21
Vaginal sponge		
Nulliparous	6	18
Parous	9	28
IUD (medicated)		
Progesterone	2	N/A***
Copper T 380A	0.8	N/A***
Condom without spermicides	2	12
Periodic abstinence (all methods)	1-9	20
Progestogen injections	0.3	0.3
Progestogen implants	0.2	0.2
Female sterilization	0.2	0.4
Male sterilization	0.1	0.15

Adapted from Trussel et al[1]

* The authors' best guess of the percentage of women expected to experience an accidental pregnancy among couples who initiate a method (not necessarily for the first time) and who use it consistently and correctly during the first year if they do not stop for any other reason.

** This term represents "typical" couples who initiate use of a method (not necessarily for the first time), who experience an accidental pregnancy during the first year if they do not stop for any other reason.

*** N/A—Data not available

CONTRAINDICATIONS

Oral contraceptives should not be used in women who have the following conditions:

- Thrombophlebitis or thromboembolic disorders
- A past history of deep vein thrombophlebitis or thromboembolic disorders
- Cerebral vascular disease, myocardial infarction, or coronary artery disease, or a past history of these conditions
- Known or suspected carcinoma of the breast, or a history of this condition
- Known or suspected carcinoma of the female reproductive organs or suspected estrogen-dependent neoplasia, or a history of these conditions
- Undiagnosed abnormal genital bleeding
- History of cholestatic jaundice of pregnancy or jaundice with prior oral contraceptive use
- Past or present, benign or malignant liver tumors
- Known or suspected pregnancy

WARNINGS

Cigarette smoking increases the risk of serious cardiovascular side effects from oral contraceptive use. This risk increases with age and with heavy smoking (15 or more cigarettes per day) and is quite marked in women over 35 years of age. Women who use oral contraceptives should be strongly advised not to smoke.

The use of oral contraceptives is associated with increased risk of several serious conditions including venous and arterial thromboembolism, thrombotic and hemorrhagic stroke, myocardial infarction, liver tumors or other liver lesions, and gallbladder disease. The risk of morbidity and mortality increases signficantly in the presence of other risk factors such as hypertension, hyperlipidemia, obesity, and diabetes mellitus.

Practitioners prescribing oral contraceptives should be familiar with the following information relating to these and other risks.

The information contained herein is principally based on studies carried out in patients who use oral contraceptives with formulations containing higher amounts of estrogens and progestogens than those in common use today. The effect of long-term use of the oral contraceptives with lesser amounts of both estrogens and progestogens remains to be determined.

Throughout this labeling, epidemiological studies reported are of two types: retrospective case-control studies and prospective cohort studies. Case-control studies provide an estimate of the relative risk of a disease, which is defined as the *ratio* of the incidence of a disease among oral contraceptive users to that among nonusers. The relative risk (or odds ratio) does not provide information about the actual clinical occurrence of a disease. Cohort studies provide a measure of both the relative risk and the attributable risk. the latter is the *difference* in the incidence of disease between oral contraceptive users and nonusers. The attributable risk does provide information about the actual occurrence or incidence of a disease in the subject population. For further information, the reader is referred to a text on epidemiological methods.

1. Thromboembolic disorders and other vascular problems.

a. Myocardial infarction. An increased risk of myocardial infarction has been associated with oral contraceptive use.[2–21] This increased risk is primarily in smokers or in women with other underlying risk factors for coronary artery disease such as hypertension, obesity, diabetes, and hypercholesterolemia. The relative risk for myocardial infarction in current oral contraceptive users has been estimated to be 2 to 6. The risk is very low under the age of 30. However, there is the possibility of a risk of cardiovascular disease even in very young women who take oral contraceptives.

Smoking in combination with oral contraceptive use has been reported to contribute substantially to the risk of myocardial infarction in women in their mid-thirties or older, with smoking accounting for the majority of excess cases.[22] Mortality rates associated with circulatory disease have been shown to increase substantially in smokers, especially in those 35 years of age and older among women who use oral contraceptives (see Figure 1, Table 2).

Figure 1. Circulatory disease mortality rates per 100,000 women—years by age, smoking status, and oral contraceptive use.[14]

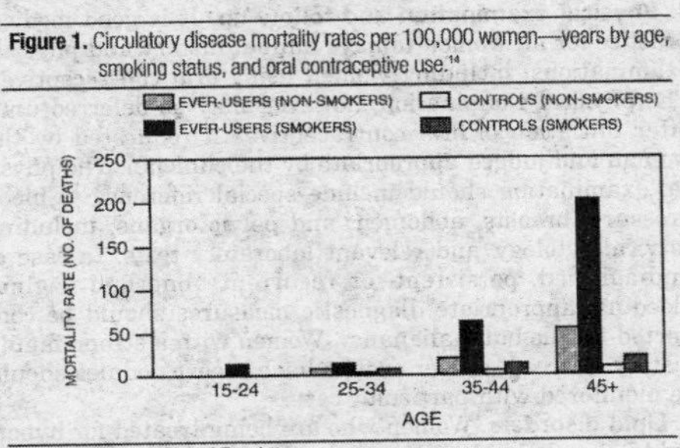

Adapted from Layde and Beral.[14]

Oral contraceptives may compound the effects of well-known cardiovascular risk factors such as hypertension, diabetes, hyperlipidemias, hypercholesterolemia, age, cigarette smoking, and obesity. In particular, some progestogens decrease HDL cholesterol[23–31] and cause glucose intolerance, while estrogens may create a state of hyperinsulinism.[32] Oral contraceptives have been shown to increase blood pressure among some users (see **WARNING** No. 9). Similar effects on risk factors have been associated with an increased risk of heart disease.

b. Thromboembolism. An increased risk of thromboembolic and thrombolic disease associated with the use of oral contraceptives is well established.[17, 33–51] Case-control studies have estimated the relative risk to be 3 for the first episode of superficial venous thrombosis, 4 to 11 for deep vein thrombosis or pulmonary embolism, and 1.5 to 6 for women with predisposing conditions for venous thromboembolic disease.[34–37, 45, 46] Cohort studies have shown the relative risk to be somewhat lower, about 3 for new cases (subjects with no past history of venous thrombosis or varicose veins) and about 4.5 for new cases requiring hospitalization.[42, 47, 48] The risk of venous thromboemblic disease associated with oral contraceptives is not related to duration of use.

A two- to seven-fold increase in relative risk of postoperative thromboembolic complications has been reported with the use of oral contraceptives.[38, 39] The relative risk of venous thrombosis in women who have predisposing conditions is about twice that of women without such medical conditions.[43] If feasible, oral contraceptives should be discontinued at least 4 weeks prior to and for 2 weeks after elective surgery of a type associated with an increased risk of thromboembolism, and also during and following prolonged immobilization. Since the immediate postpartum period is also associated with an increased risk of thromboembolism, oral contraceptives should be started no earlier than 4 to 6 weeks after delivery in women who elect not to breast feed.

c. Cerebrovascular diseases. Both the relative and attributable risks of cerebrovascular events (thrombotic and hemorrhagic strokes) have been reported to be increased with oral contraceptive use,[14, 17, 18, 34, 42, 46, 52–59] although, in general, the risk was greatest among older (over 35 years) hypertensive women who also smoked. Hypertension was reported to be a risk factor for both users and nonusers, for both types of strokes, while smoking increased the risk for hemorrhagic strokes.

In one large study,[52] the relative risk for thrombotic stroke was reported as 9.5 times greater in users than in nonusers. It ranged from 3 for normotensive users to 14 for users with severe hypertension.[54] The relative risk for hemorrhagic stroke was reported to be 1.2 for nonsmokers who used oral contraceptives, 1.9 to 2.6 for smokers who did not use oral contraceptives, 6.1 to 7.6 for smokers who used oral contraceptives, 1.8 for normotensive users, and 25.7 for users with severe hypertension. The risk is also greater in older women and among smokers.

d. Dose-related risk of vascular disease with oral contraceptives. A positive association has been reported between the amount of estrogen and progestogen in oral contraceptives and the risk of vascular disease.[41, 43, 53, 59–64] A decline in serum high density lipoproteins (HDL) has been reported with many progestogens.[23–31] A decline in serum high density lipoproteins has been associated with an increased incidence of ischemic heart disease.[65] Because estrogens increase HDL-cholesterol, the net effect of an oral contraceptive depends on the balance achieved between doses of estrogen and progestogen and the nature and absolute amount of progestogens used in the contraceptives. The amount of both steroids should be considered in the choice of an oral contraceptive.

Minimizing exposure to estrogen and progestogen is in keeping with good principles of therapeutics. For any particular estrogen-progestogen combination, the dosage regimen prescribed should be one that contains the least amount of estrogen and progestogen that is compatible with a low failure rate and the needs of the individual patient. New acceptors of oral contraceptives should be started on preparations containing the lowest estrogen content that produces satisfactory results in the individual.

e. Persistance of risk of vascular disease. There are three studies that have shown persistence of risk of vascular disease for users of oral contraceptives. In a study in the United States, the risk of developing myocardial infarction after discontinuing oral contraceptives persisted for at least 9 years for women 40–49 years old who had used oral contraceptives for 5 or more years, but this increased risk was not demonstrated in other age groups.[16] Another American study reported former use of oral contraceptives was significantly associated with increased risk of subaracnoid hemorrhage.[57] In another study, in Great Britain, the risk of developing nonrheumatic heart disease plus hypertension, subarachnoid hemorrhage, cerebral thrombosis, and transient ischemic attacks persisted for at least 6 years after discontinuation of oral contraceptives, although the excess risk was small.[14, 18, 66] It should be noted that these studies were performed with oral contraceptive formulations containing 50 mcg or more of estrogens.

2. Estimates of mortality from contraceptive use. One study[67] gathered data from a variety of sources that have estimated the mortality rates associated with different methods of contraception at different ages. (Table 2). These estimates include the combined risk of death associated with contraceptive methods plus the risk attributable to pregnancy in the event of method failure. Each method of contraception has its specific benefits and risks. The study concluded that, with the exception of oral contraceptive users 35 and older who smoke and 40 or older who do not smoke, mortality associated with all methods of birth control is low and below that associated with childbirth. The observation of a possible increase in risk of mortality with age of oral contraceptive users is based on data gathered in the 1970's, but not reported until 1983.[67] However, current clinical practice involves the use of lower estrogen dose formulations combined with careful restriction of oral contraceptive use to women who do not have the various risk factors listed in this labeling.

Because of these changes in practice and, also, because of some limited new data that suggest that the risk of cardiovascular disease with the use of oral contraceptives may now be less than previously observed,[48, 152] the Fertility and Maternal Health Drugs Advisory Committee was asked to review the topic in 1989. The Committee concluded that, although cardiovascular disease risks may be increased with oral contraceptive use after age 40 in healthy nonsmoking women (even with the newer low-dose formulations), there are greater potential health risks associated with pregnancy in older women and with the alternative surgical and medical procedures that may be necessary if such women do not have access to effective and acceptable means of contraception.

Therefore, the Committee recommended that the benefits of oral contraceptive use by healthy nonsmoking women over 40 may outweigh the possible risks. Of course, older women, as all women who take oral contraceptives, should take the lowest possible dose formulation that is effective.

[See table at top of next page]

3. Carcinoma of the breast and reproductive organs. Numerous epidemiological studies have been performed on the incidence of breast, endometrial, ovarian, and cervical cancer in women using oral contraceptives. While there are conflicting reports, most studies suggest that the use of oral contraceptives is not associated with an overall increase in the risk of developing breast cancer.[17, 40, 68–78] Some studies have reported an increased relative risk of developing breast cancer, particularly at a young age.[79–102, 151] This increased relative risk appears to be related to duration of use.

Some studies suggested that oral contraceptive use was associated with an increase in the risk of cervical intraepithelial neoplasia, dysplasia, erosion, carcinoma, or microglandular dysplasia in some populations of women.[17, 50, 103–115] However, there continues to be controversy about the extent to which such findings may be due to differences in sexual behavior and other factors.

In spite of many studies of the relationship between oral contraceptive use and breast and cervical cancers, a cause and effect relationship has not been established.

Continued on next page

Zovia—Cont.

4. Hepatic neoplasia. Benign hepatic adenomas and other hepatic lesions have been associated with oral contraceptive use,[116–121] although the incidence of such benign tumors is rare in the United States. Indirect calculations have estimated the attributable risk to be in the range of 3.3 cases per 100,000 for users, a risk that increases after 4 or more years of use.[120] Rupture of benign, hepatic adenomas or other lesions may cause death through intraabdominal hemorrhage. Therefore, such lesions should be considered in women presenting with abdominal pain and tenderness, abdominal mass, or shock. About one quarter of the cases presented because of abdominal masses, up to one half had signs and symptoms of acute intraperitoneal hemorrhage.[121] Diagnosis may prove difficult.

Studies from the U.S.,[122, 150] Great Britain,[123, 124] and Italy[125] have shown an increased risk of hepatocellular carcinoma in long-term (>8 years; relative risk of 7–20) oral contraceptive users. However, these cancers are rare in the United States, and the attributable risk (the excess incidence) of liver cancers in oral contraceptive users approaches less than 1 per 1,000,000 users.

5. Ocular lesions. There have been reports of retinal thrombosis and other ocular lesions associated with the use of oral contraceptives. Oral contraceptives should be discontinued if there is unexplained, gradual or sudden, partial or complete loss of vision; onset of proptosis or diplopia; papilledema; or any evidence of retinal vascular lesions. Appropriate diagnostic and therapeutic measures should be undertaken immediately.

6. Oral contraceptive use before or during pregnancy. Extensive epidemiological studies have revealed no increased risk of birth defects in women who have used oral contraceptives prior to pregnancy.[126, 129] The majority of recent studies also do not suggest a teratogenic effect, particularly insofar as cardiac anomalies and limb reduction defects are concerned,[126, 129] when the pill is taken inadvertently during early pregnancy.

The administration of oral contraceptives to induce withdrawal bleeding should not be used as a test for pregnancy. Oral contraceptives should not be used during pregnancy to treat threatened or habitual abortion. It is recommended that for any patient who has missed two consecutive periods, pregnancy should be ruled out before continuing oral contraceptive use. If the patient has not adhered to the prescribed schedule, the possibility of pregnancy should be considered at the time of the first missed period and further use of oral contraceptives should be withheld until pregnancy has been ruled out. Oral contraceptive use should be discontinued if pregnancy is confirmed.

7. Gallbladder disease. Earlier studies reported an increased lifetime relative risk of gallbladder surgery in users of oral contraceptives and estrogens.[40, 42, 53, 70] More recent studies, however, have shown that the relative risk of developing gallbladder disease among oral contraceptive users may be minimal.[130–132] The recent findings of minimal risk may be related to the use of oral contraceptive formulations containing lower doses of estrogens and progestogens.

8. Carbohydrate and lipid metabolic effects. Oral contraceptives have been shown to cause a decrease in glucose tolerance in a signficant percentage of users.[32] This effect has been shown to be directly related to estrogen dose.[133] Progestogens increase insulin secretion and create insulin resistance, the effect varying with different progestational agents.[32, 134] However, in the nondiabetic woman, oral contraceptives appear to have no effect on fasting blood glucose. Because of these demonstrated effects, prediabetic and diabetic women should be carefully observed while taking oral contraceptives.

Some women may have persistent hypertriglyceridemia while on the pill. As discussed earlier (see **WARNINGS** 1a and 1d), changes in serum triglycerides and lipoprotein levels have been reported in oral contraceptive users.[23–31, 135, 136]

9. Elevated blood pressure. An increase in blood pressure has been reported in women taking oral contraceptives[50, 53, 137–139] and this increase is more likely in older oral contraceptive users[137] and with extended duration of use.[53] Data from the Royal College of General Practitioners[138] and subsequent randomized trials have shown that the incidence of hypertension increases with increasing concentration of progestogens.

Women with a history of hypertension or hypertension-related disease, or renal disease[139] should be encouraged to use another method of contraception. If such women elect to use oral contraceptives, they should be monitored closely and if significant elevation of blood pressure occurs, oral contraceptives should be discontinued. For most women, elevated blood pressure will return to normal after stopping oral contraceptives,[137] and there is no difference in the occurrence of hypertension among ever- and never-users.[140]

10. Headache. The onset or exacerbation of migraine or the development of headache of a new pattern that is recurrent, persistent, or severe requires discontinuation of oral contraceptives and evaluation of the cause.

11. Bleeding irregularities. Breakthrough bleeding and spotting are sometimes encountered in patients on oral contraceptives, especially during the first three months of use. Nonhormonal causes should be considered and adequate diagnostic measures taken to rule out malignancy or pregnancy in the event of breakthrough bleeding, as in the case of any abnormal vaginal bleeding. If a pathologic basis has been excluded, time alone or a change to another formulation may solve the problem. In the event of amenorrhea, pregnancy should be ruled out.

TABLE 2. Annual number of birth-related or method-related deaths associated with control of fertility per 100,000 nonsterile women, by fertility control method according to age.[67]

Method of control	15–19	20–24	25–29	30–34	35–39	40–44
No fertility control methods*	7.0	7.4	9.1	14.8	25.7	28.2
Oral contraceptives						
nonsmoker**	0.3	0.5	0.9	1.9	13.8	31.6
smoker**	2.2	3.4	6.6	13.5	51.1	117.2
IUD**	0.8	0.8	1.0	1.0	1.4	1.4
Condom*	1.1	1.6	0.7	0.2	0.3	0.4
Diaphragm/Spermicide*	1.9	1.2	1.2	1.3	2.2	2.8
Periodic abstinence*	2.5	1.6	1.6	1.7	2.9	3.6

Adapted from Ory.[67]

* Deaths are birth-related
** Deaths are method-related

PRECAUTIONS

1. Physical examination and follow-up. It is good medical practice for all women to have annual history and physical examinations, including women using oral contraceptives. The physical examination, however, may be deferred until after initiation of oral contraceptives if requested by the woman and judged appropriate by the clinician. The physical examination should include special reference to blood pressure, breasts, abdomen, and pelvic organs, including cervical cytology, and relevant laboratory tests. In case of undiagnosed, persistent, or recurrent abnormal vaginal bleeding, appropriate diagnostic measures should be conducted to rule out malignancy. Women with a strong family history of breast cancer or who have breast nodules should be monitored with particular care.

2. Lipid disorders. Women who are being treated for hyperlipidemias should be folowed closely if they elect to use oral contraceptives. Some progestogens may elevate LDL levels and may render the control of hyperlipidemias more difficult.

3. Liver function. If jaundice develops in any woman receiving oral contraceptives, they should be discontinued. Steroids may be poorly metabolized in patients with impaired liver function and should be administered with caution in such patients. Cholestatic jaundice has been reported after combined treatment with oral contraceptives and troleandomycin. Hepatotoxicity following a combination of oral contraceptives and and cyclosporine has also been reported.

4. Fluid retention. Oral contraceptives may cause some degree of fluid retention. They should be prescribed with caution, and only with careful monitoring, in patients with conditions that might be aggravated by fluid retention, such as convulsive disorders, migraine syndrome, asthma, or cardiac, hepatic, or renal dysfunction.

5. Emotional disorders. Women with a history of depression should be carefully observed and the drug discontinued if depression recurs to a serious degree.

6. Contact lenses. Contact lens wearers who develop visual changes or changes in lens tolerance should be assessed by an ophthalmologist.

7. Drug Interactions. Reduced efficacy and increased incidence of breakthrough bleeding and menstrual irregularities have been associated with concomitant use of rifampin. A similar association, though less marked, has been suggested for barbiturates, phenylbutazone, phenytoin sodium, and possibly with griseofulvin, ampicillin, and tetracyclines.

8. Laboratory test interactions. Certain endocrine and liver function tests and blood components may be affected by oral contraceptives:

a. Increased prothrombin and factors VII, VIII, IX and X; decreased antithrombin III; increased platelet aggregability.
b. Increased thyroid binding globulin (TBG), leading to increased circulating total thyroid hormone as measured by protein-bound iodine (PBI), T_4 by column or by radioimmunoassay. Free T_3 resin uptake is decreased, reflecting the elevated TBG; free T_4 concentration is unaltered.
c. Other binding proteins may be elevated in the serum.
d. Sex-steroid binding globulins are increased and result in elevated levels of total circulating sex steroids and corticoids; however, free or biologically active levels remain unchanged.
e. Triglycerides and phospholipids may be increased.
f. Glucose tolerance may be decreased.
g. Serum folate levels may be depressed. This may be of clinical signficance if a woman becomes pregnant shortly after discontinuing oral contraceptives.
h. Increased sulfobromophthalein and other abnormalities in liver function tests may occur.
i. Plasma levels of trace minerals may be altered.
j. Response to the metyrapone test may be reduced.

9. Carcinogenesis. See **WARNINGS.**

10. Pregnancy. Pregnancy Category X. See **CONTRAINDICATIONS** and **WARNINGS.**

11. Nursing mother. Small amounts of oral contraceptive steroids have been identified in the milk of nursing mothers[141–143] and a few adverse effects on the child have been reported, including jaundice and breast enlargement. In addition, oral contraceptives give in the postpartum period may interfere with lactation by decreasing the quantity and quality of breast milk. If possible, the nursing mother should be advised not to use oral contraceptives, but to use other forms of contraception until she has completely weaned her child.

12. Venereal diseases. Oral contraceptives are of no value in the prevention or treatment of venereal disease. The prevalence of cervical *Chlamydia trachomatis* and *Neisseria gonorrhoeae* in oral contraceptive users is increased severalfold.[144, 145] It should not be assumed that oral contraceptives afford protection against pelvic inflammatory disease from chlamydia.[144] Patients should be counseled that this product does not protect against HIV infection (AIDS) and other sexually transmitted diseases.

13. General.

a. The pathologist should be advised of oral contraceptive therapy when relevant specimens are submitted.
b. Treatment with oral contraceptives may mask the onset of the climacteric. (See **WARNINGS** regarding risks in this age group.)

INFORMATION FOR THE PATIENT

See patient labeling printed below.

ADVERSE REACTIONS

An increased risk of the following serious adverse reactions has been associated with the use of oral contraceptives (see **WARNINGS**):

- Thrombophlebitis and thrombosis
- Arterial thromboembolism
- Pulmonary embolism
- Myocardial infarction and coronary thrombosis
- Cerebral hemorrhage
- Cerebral thrombosis
- Hypertension
- Gallbladder disease
- Benign and malignant liver tumors, and other hepatic lesions

There is evidence of an association between the following conditions and the use of oral contraceptives, although additional confirmatory studies are needed:

- Mesenteric thrombosis
- Neuro-ocular lesions (e.g., retinal thrombosis and optic neuritis)

The following adverse reactions have been reported in patients receiving oral contraceptives and are believed to be drug-related:

- Nausea
- Vomiting
- Gastrointestinal symptoms (such as abdominal cramps and bloating)
- Breakthrough bleeding
- Spotting
- Change in menstrual flow
- Amenorrhea during or after use
- Temporary infertility after discontinuation of use
- Edema
- Chloasma or melasma, which may persist
- Breast changes: tenderness, enlargement, secretion
- Change in weight (increase or decrease)
- Change in cervical erosion or secretion
- Diminution in lactation when given immediately postpartum
- Cholestatic jaundice
- Migraine
- Rash (allergic)
- Mental depression
- Reduced tolerance to carbohydrates
- Vaginal candidiasis
- Change in corneal curvature (steepening)
- Intolerance to contact lenses

The following adverse reactions or conditions have been reported in users of oral contraceptives and the association has been neither confirmed nor refuted:

- Premenstrual syndrome
- Cataracts
- Changes in appetite
- Cystitis-like syndrome
- Headache
- Nervousness
- Dizziness
- Hirsutism
- Loss of scalp hair
- Erythema multiforme
- Erythema nodosum
- Hemorrhagic eruption
- Vaginitis
- Porphyria
- Impaired renal function
- Hemolytic uremic syndrome
- Acne
- Changes in libido
- Colitis
- Budd-Chiari syndrome
- Endocervical hyperplasia or ectropion

OVERDOSAGE

Serious ill effects have not been reported following acute ingestion of large doses of oral contraceptives by young children.[180, 181] Overdosage may cause nausea, and withdrawal bleeding may occur in females.

NON-CONTRACEPTIVE HEALTH BENEFITS

The following non-contraceptive health benefits related to the use of oral contraceptives are supported by epidemiological studies that largely utilized oral contraceptive formulations containing estrogen doses exceeding 35 mcg of ethinyl estradiol or 50 mcg of mestranol.[148, 149]

Effects on menses:
- Increased menstrual cycle regularity
- Decreased blood loss and decreased risk of iron-deficiency anemia
- Decreased frequency of dysmenorrhea

Effects related to inhibition of ovulation:
- Decreased risk of functional ovarian cysts
- Decreasd risk of ectopic pregnancies

Effects from long-term use:
- Decreased risk of fibroadenomas and fibrocystic disease of the breast
- Decreased risk of acute pelvic inflammatory disease
- Decreased risk of endometrial cancer
- Decreased risk of ovarian cancer
- Decreased risk of uterine fibroids

DOSAGE AND ADMINISTRATION

To achieve maximum contraceptive effectiveness, oral contraceptives must be taken exactly as directed and at intervals of 24 hours.

IMPORTANT: If the Sunday start schedule is selected, the patient should be instructed to use an additional method of protection until after the first week of administration *in the initial cycle.*

The possibility of ovulation and conception prior to initiation of use should be considered.

Zovia 1/35E-21 and Zovia 1/35E-28
Zovia 1/50E-21 and Zovia 1/50E-28

Dosage Schedules

The Zovia 1/35E-21 and Zovia 1/50E-21 tablet dispensers contain 21 tablets arranged in three numbered rows of 7 tablets each.

The Zovia 1/35E-28 and Zovia 1/50E-28 tablet dispensers contain 21 colored active tablets arranged in three numbered rows of 7 tablets each, followed by a fourth row of 7 white placebo tablets.

Days of the week are printed above the tablets, starting with Sunday on the left.

Two dosage schedules are described, one of which may be more convenient or suitable than the other for an individual patient.

Schedule #1: Sunday start. The patient begins taking Zovia 1/35E-21, Zovia 1/35E-28, Zovia 1/50E-21, or Zovia 1/50E-28 from the first row of her package, one tablet daily, starting on the first Sunday after the onset of menstruation. If the patient's period begins on a Sunday she takes her first tablet that very same day. The 21st tablet or the 28th tablet, depending on whether the patient is taking the 21- or 28-tablet course, will be taken on a Saturday.

Subsequent cycles:

21-tablet course—The patient begins a new 21-tablet course on the eighth day. Sunday, after taking her last tablet. All subsequent cycles will also begin on Sunday, one tablet being taken each day for 3 weeks followed by a week of no pill-taking.

28-tablet course—The patient begins a new 28-tablet course on the next day, Sunday, and all subsequent cycles will also begin on Sunday, one tablet being taken each and every day. With a Sunday-start schedule, a woman whose period begins on the day of or 1 to 4 days before taking the first tablet should expect a diminution of flow and fewer menstrual days. The initial cycle will likely be shortened by from 1 to 5 days. Thereafter, cycles should be about 28 days in length.

Schedule #2: Day 1 start. The patient begins taking Zovia 1/35E-21 or Zovia 1/50E-21 from the first row of her package, one tablet daily, starting with the pill day which corresponds to day 1 of her menstrual cycle; the first day of menstruation is counted as day 1. After the last (Saturday) tablet in row #3 has been taken, if any remain in the first row, the patient completes her 21-tablet schedule starting with Sunday in row #1.

Subsequent cycles: The patient begins a new 21-tablet course on the eighth day after taking her last tablet, again starting the same day of the week on which she began her first course. All subsequent cycles will also begin on that same day, one tablet being taken each day for 3 weeks followed by a week of no pill-taking.

Special notes

Spotting, breakthrough bleeding, or nausea. If spotting (bleeding insufficient to require a pad), breakthrough bleeding (heavier bleeding similar to a menstrual flow), or nausea occurs the patient should continue taking her tablets as directed. The incidence of spotting, breakthrough bleeding or nausea is minimal, most frequently occurring in the first cycle. Ordinarily spotting or breakthrough bleeding will stop within a week. Usually the patient will begin to cycle regularly within two to three courses of tablet-taking. In the event of spotting or breakthrough bleeding organic causes should be borne in mind. (see **WARNING** No. 11)

Missed menstrual periods. Withdrawal flow will normally occur 2 or 3 days after the last active tablet is taken. Failure of withdrawal bleeding ordinarily does not mean that the patient is pregnant, providing the dosage schedule has been correctly followed. (See **WARNING** No. 6)

If the patient has *not* adhered to the prescribed dosage regimen, the possibility of pregnancy should be considered after the first missed period, and oral contraceptives should be withheld until pregnancy has been ruled out.

If the patient has adhered to the prescribed regimen and misses two consecutive periods, pregnancy should be ruled out before continuing the contraceptive regimen.

The first intermenstrual interval after discontinuing the tablets is usually prolonged; consequently, a patient for whom a 28-day cycle is usual might not begin to menstruate for 35 days or longer. Ovulation in such prolonged cycles will occur correspondingly later in the cycle. Posttreatment cycles after the first one, however, are usually typical for the individual woman prior to taking tablets. (See **WARNING** No. 11)

Missed tablets. If a woman misses taking one active tablet, the missed tablet should be taken as soon as it is remembered. In addition, the next tablet should be taken at the usual time. If two consecutive active tablets are missed in week 1 or week 2 of the dispenser, the dosage should be doubled for the next 2 days. The regular schedule should then be resumed, but an additional method of protection must be used as backup for the next 7 days if she has sex during that time or she may become pregnant.

If two consecutive active tablets are missed in week 3 of the dispenser or three consecutive active tablets are misssed during any of the first 3 weeks of the dispenser, direct the patient to do one of the following: Day 1 Starters should discard the rest of the dispenser and begin a new dispenser that same day; Sunday Starters should continue to take 1 tablet daily until Sunday, discard the rest of the dispenser and begin a new dispenser that same day. The patient may not have a period this month; however, if she has missed two consecutive periods, pregnancy should be ruled out. An additional method of protection must be used as a backup for the next 7 days after the tablets are missed if she has sex during that time or she may become pregnant.

While there is little likelihood of ovulation if only one active tablet is missed, the possibility of spotting or breakthrough bleeding is increased and should be expected if two or more successive active tablets are missed. However, the possibility of ovulation increases with each successive day that scheduled active tablets are missed.

If one or more placebo tablets of Zovia 1/35E-28 or Zovia 1/50E-28 are missed, the Zovia 1/35E-28 or Zovia 1/50E-28 schedule should be resumed on the following Sunday (the eighth day after the last colored tablet was taken). Omission of placebo tablets in the 28-tablet courses does not increase the possibility of conception provided that this schedule is followed.

HOW SUPPLIED

Zovia 1/35E: Each light pink Zovia 1/35E tablet is round in shape, unscored, debossed with WATSON 383 and contains 1 mg of ethynodiol diacetate and 35 mcg of ethinyl estradiol.

Zovia 1/35E-21 (NDC 52544-532-21) is packaged in cartons of six tablet dispensers of 21 tablets each.

Zovia 1/35E-28 (NDC 52544-383-28) is packaged in cartons of six tablet dispensers. Each dispenser contains 21 light pink tablet and 7 white placebo tablets. (Placebo tablets have a debossed WATSON on one side and P on the other side.)

Zovia 1/50E: Each pink Zovia 1/50E tablet is round in shape, unscored, debossed with WATSON 384 and contains 1 mg of ethynodiol diacetate and 50 mcg of ethinyl estradiol.

Zovia 1/50E-21 (NDC 52544-533-21) is packaged in cartons of six tablet dispensers of 21 tablets each.

Zovia 1/50E-28 (NDC 52544-384-28) is packaged in cartons of six tablet dispensers. Each dispenser contains 21 pink tablets and 7 white placebo tablets. (Placebo tablets have a debosssed WATSON on one side and P on the other side).

Store at controlled room temperature 15°C to 30°C (59°F to 86°F).

REFERENCES

1. Trussel J, et al. *Stud Fam Plann.* 1987;18(Sept-Oct); and 1990;21(Jan-Feb):51. **1a.** *Physicians' Desk Reference* 47th ed. Orudell, NJ: Medical Economics Co Inc; 1993;2598–2601. **2.** Mann JI, et al. *Br Med J.* 1975;2(May 3):241. **3.** Mann JI, et al. *Br Med J.* 1975;3(Sept13):631. **4.** Mann JI, et al. *Br Med J.* 1975;2(May 3):245. **5.** Mann JI, et al. Br Med J. 1976;2(Aug 21):445. **6.** Arthes FG, et al. *Chest.* 1976;70(Nov):574. **7.** Jain AK, *Am J Obstet Gynecol.* 1976;301(Oct 1):126 and *Stud Fam Plann.* 1977;8(March): 50. **8.** Ory HW. *JAMA.* 1977;237(June 13);2619. **9.** Jick H, et al. *JAMA.* 1978;239(April 3):1403, 1407. **10.** Jick H, et al. *JAMA.* 1978;240(Dec 1):2548. **11.** Shapiro S, et al. *Lancet.* 1979;1(April 7):743. **12.** Rosenberg L, et al. *Am J Epidemiol.* 1980;111(Jan):59. **13.** Krueger DE, et al. *Am J Epidemiol.* 1980;111(June):655. **14.** Layde P, et al. *Lancet.* 1981;1(March 7):541. **15.** Adam SA, et al. *Br J Obstet Gynaecol.* 1981;88(Aug):838. **16.** Slone D, et al. *N Engl J Med* 1981;305(Aug 20):420. **17.** Ramcharan S, et al. *The Walnut Creek Contraceptive Drug Study. Vol 3.* US Govt Ptg Off. 1981; and *J Reprod Med.* 1980;25(Dec):346. **18.** Layde PM, et al. *J R Coll Gen Pract.* 1983;33(Feb):75. **19.** Rosenberg L, et al. *JAMA.* 1985;253(May 24/31):2965. **20.** Mant D, et al. *J Epidemiol Community Health.* 1987;41(Sept):215. **21.** Croft P, et al. *Br Med J.* 1989;298(Jan 21):165. **22.** Goldbaum GM, et al. *JAMA.* 1987;258(Sept 11):1339. **23.** Bradley DD, et al. *N Engl J Med.* 1978;299(July 6):17. **24.** Tikkanen MJ. *J Reprod Med.* 1986;31(Sept suppl):898. **25.** Lipson A, et al. *Contraception.* 1986;34(Aug):121. **26.** Burkman RT, et al. *Obstet Gynecol.* 1988; 71(Jan):33. **27.** Knopp RH, *J Reprod Med.* 1986;31(Sept suppl):913. **28.** Krauss RM, et al. *Am J Obstet Gynecol.* 1983;145(Feb 15):446. **29.** Wahl P, et al. *N Engl J Med.* 1983;308(April 14):862. **30.** Wynn V, et al. *Am J Obstet Gynecol.* 1982;142(March 15):766. **31.** LaRosa JC. *J Reprod Med.* 1986;31(Sept suppl):906. **32.** Wynn V, et al. *J Reprod Med.* 1986;31(Sept suppl):892. **33.** Royal College of General Practitioners. *JR Coll Gen Pract.* 1967;13(May):267. **34.** Inman WHW, et al. *Br Med J.* 1968;(April 27):193. **35.** Vessey MP, et al. *Br Med J.* 1968;2(April 27):199. **36.** Vessey MP, et al. *Br Med J.* 1969;2(June14):651. **37.** Sartwell PE, et al. *Am J Epidemiol.* 1969;90(Nov):365. **38.** Vessey MP, et al. *Br Med J.* 1970;3(July 18):123. **39.** Greene GR, et al. *Am J Public Health.* 1972;62(May):680. **40.** Boston Collaborative Drug Surveillance Programme. *Lancet.* 1973;1(June 23):1399. **41.** Stolley PD, et al, *Am J Epidemiol.* 1975;102(Sept):197. **42.** Vessey MP, et al. *J Biosoc Sci.* 1976;8(Oct):373. **43.** Kay CR, *Jr Coll Gen Pract.* 1978;28(July):393. **44.** Petitti DB, et al. *Am J Epidemiol.* 1978;108(Dec):480. **45.** Maguire MG, et al. *Am J Epidemiol.* 1979;110(Aug):188. **46.** Petitti DB, et al. *JAMA.* 1979;242(Sept 14):1150. **47.** Porter JB, et al. *Obstet Gynecol.* 1982;59(March):299. **48.** Porter JB, et al. *Obstet Gynecol.* 1985;66(July):1. **49.** Vessey MP, et al. *Br Med J.* 1986;292(Feb 22):526. **50.** Hoover R, et al. *Am J Public Health.* 1978;68(April):335. **51.** Vessey MP, *Br J Fam Plann.* 1980;6(Oct suppl):1. **52.** Collaborative Group for the Study of Stroke in Young Women. *N Engl J Med.* 1973;288(April 26):871. **53.** Royal College of General Practitioners. *Oral Contraceptives and Health.* New York, NY: Pitman Publ Corp; May 1974. **54.** Collaborative Group for the Study of Stroke in Young Women. *JAMA.* 1975;231(Feb 17):718. **55.** Beral V. *Lancet.* 1976;2(Nov 13):1047. **56.** Vessey MP, et al. *Lancet.* 1977;2(Oct 8):731; and 1981;1(March 7):549. **57.** Petitti DB, et al. *Lancet.* 1978;2(July 29):234. **58.** Inman WHW. *Br Med J.* 1979;2(Dec 8):1468. **59.** Vessy MP, et al. *Br Med J.* 1984;289(Sept 1):530. **60.** Inman WHW, et al. *Br Med J.* 1970;2(April 25):203. **61.** Meade TW, et al. *Br Med J.* 1980;280(May 10):1157. **62.** Bottiger LE, et al. *Lancet.* 1980;1(May 24):1097. **63.** Kay CR, *Am J Obstet Gynecol.* 1982;142(March 15):762. **64.** Vessey MP, et al. *Br Med J.* 1986;292(Feb 22):526. **65.** Gordon T, et al. *Am J Med.* 1977;62(May):707. **66.** Beral V, et al. *Lancet.* 1977;2 (Oct 8): 727. **67.** Ory H. *Fam Plann Perspect.* 1983;15(March-April): 57. **68.** Arthes FG, et al. *Cancer.* 1971;28(Dec):1391. **69.** Vessey MP, et al. *Br Med J.* 1972;3(Sept 23):719. **70.** Boston Collaborative Drug Surveilance Program. *N Engl J Med.* 1974;290(Jan3):15. **71.** Vessey MP, et al. *Lancet.* 1975;1(April 26):941. **72.** Casagrande J, et al. *J Natl Cancer Inst.* 1976;56(April):839. **73.** Kelsey, JL, et al. *Am J Epidemiol.* 1978;107(March):236. **74.** Kay CR, *Br Med J.* 1981;282(June 27):2089. **75.** Vessey MP, et al. *Br Med J.* 1981;282(June 27):2093. **76.** The Cancer and Steroid Hormone Study of the Center for Disease Control and the National Institute of Child Health and Human Development. Oral contraceptive use and the risk of breast cancer. *N Engl J Med.* 1986;315(Aug 14):405. **77.** Paul C, et al. *Br Med J.* 1986; 293(Sept 20):723. **78.** Miller DR, et al. *Obstet Gynecol.* 1986;68(Dec):863. **79.** Pike MC, et al. *Lancet.* 1983;2(Oct 22):926. **80.** McPherson K, et al. *Br J Cancer.* 1987;56(Nov): 653. **81.** Hoover R, et al. *N Engl J Med.* 1976;295(Aug 19): 401. **82.** Lees AW, et al. *Int J Cancer.* 1978;22(Dec):700. **83.** Brinton LA, et al. *J Natl Cancer Inst.* 1979;62(Jan):37. **84.** Black MM, *Pathol Res Pract.* 1980;166:491; and *Cancer.* 1980;46(Dec):2747; and *Cancer.* 1983;51 June):2147. **85.** Clavel F, et al. *Bull Cancer* (Paris). 1981;68(Dec):449. **86.** Brinton LA, et al. *Int J Epidemiol.* 1982;11(Dec):316. **87.** Harris NV, et al. *Am J Epidemiol.* 1982;116(Oct):643. **88.** Jick H, et al. *Am J Epidemiol.* 1980;112(Nov):577. **89.** McPherson K, et al. *Lancet.* 1983;2(Dec 17):1414. **90.** Hoover R, et al. *J Natl Cancer Inst.* 1981;67(Oct):815. **91.** Jick H, et al. *Am J Epidemiol.* 1980;112(Nov):586. **92.** Meirik O, et al. *Lancet.* 1986;2(Sept 20):650. **93.** Fasal E, et al. *J Natl Cancer Inst.* 1975;55(Oct):767. **94.** Paffenbarger RS, et al. *Cancer.* 1977;39(April suppl):1887. **95.** Stadel BV, et al. *Contraception.* 1988;38(Sept): 287. **96.** Miller DR, et al. *Am J Epidemiol.* 1989;129(Feb):269. **97.** Kay CR, et al. *Br J Cancer.* 1988;58(Nov):675. **98.** Miller DR, et al. *Obstet Gynecol.* 1986;68(Dec):863. **99.** Olsson H, et al. *Lancet.* 1985;1(March 30):748. **100.** Chilvers C, et al. *Lancet.* 1989;1(May 6):973. **101.** Huggins GR, et al. *Fertil Steril.* 1987;47(May):733. **102.** Pike MC, et al. *Br J Cancer.* 1981;43(Jan):72. **103.** Ory H, et al. *Am J Obstet Gynecol.* 1976;124(March 15):573. **104.** Stern E, et al. *Science.* 1977;196(June 24):1460. **105.** Pertiz E, et al. *Am J Epidemiol.* 1977;106(Dec):462. **106.** Ory HW, et al. In: Garattini S, Berendes H, eds. *Pharmacology of Ste-*

Continued on next page

Zovia—Cont.

roid Contraceptive Drugs. New York, NY: Raven Press; 1977;211-224. **107.** Meisels A, et al. *Cancer*. 1977;40(Dec): 3076. **108.** Goldacre MJ, et al. *Br Med J*. 1978;1(March 25): 748. **109.** Swan SH, et al. *Am J Obstet Gynecol*. 1981;139(Jan 1):52. **110.** Vessey MP, et al. *Lancet*. 1983;2(Oct 22):930. **111.** Dallenbach-Hellweg G. *Pathol Res Pract*. 1984:179:38. **112.** Thomas DB, et al. *Br Med J*. 1985;290(March 30):961. **113.** Brinton LA, et al. *Int J Cancer*. 1986;38 (Sept):339. **114.** Ebeling K, et al. *Int J Cancer*. 1987;39(April):427. **115.** Beral V, et al. *Lancet*. 1988;2(Dec 10):1331. **116.** Baum JK, et al. *Lancet*. 1973;2(Oct 27):926. **117.** Edmondson HA, et al. *N Engl J Med*. 1976;294(Feb 26): 470. **118.** Bein NN, et al. *Br J Surg*. 1977;64(June):433. **119.** Klatskin G. *Gastroenterology*. 1977;73 (Aug):386. **120.** Rooks JB, et al. *JAMA*. 1979;242(Aug 17):644. **121.** Sturtevant FM. In: Moghissi K, ed. *Controversies in Contraception*.. Baltimore, MD: Williams & Wilkins; 1979:93-150. **122.** Henderson BE, et al. *Br J Cancer*. 1983;48(July):437. **123.** Neuberger J, et al. *Br Med J*. 1986;292(May 24):1355. **124.** Forman D, et al. *Br Med J*. 1986;292(May 24):1357. **125.** La Vecchia C, et al. *Br J Cancer*. 1989;59(March):460. **126.** Savolainen E, et al. *Am J Obstet Gynecol*. 1981;140(July 1): 521. **127.** Ferencz C, et al. *Teratology*. 1980;21(April):225. **128.** Rothman KJ, et al. *Am J Epidemiol*. 1979;109(April): 433. **129.** Harlap S, et al. *Obstet Gynecol*. 1980;55(April): 447. **130.** Layde PM, et al. *J Epidemiol Community Health*. 1982;36(Dec):274. **131.** Rome Group for the Epidemiology and Prevention of Cholelithiasis (GREPCO). *Am J Epidemiol*. 1984;119(May):796. **132.** Strom BL, et al. *Clin Pharmacol Ther*. 1986;39(March):335. **133.** Wynn V. In: Bardin CE, et al. eds. *Progesterone and Progestins*. New York, NY: Raven Press;1983:395-410. **134.** Perlman JA, et al. *J Chron Dis*. 1985;38(Oct)857. **135.** Powell MG, et al. *Obstet Gynecol*. 1984;63(June):764. **136.** Wynn V, et al. *Lancet*. 1966;2(Oct 1):720. **137.** Firsch IR, et al. *JAMA*. 1977;237(June 6):2499. **138.** Kay CR. *Lancet*. 1977;1(March 19):624. **139.** Laragh JH, *Am J Obstet Gynecol*. 1976;126(Sept 1):141. **140.** Ramcharan S. In: Garattini S, Berendes HW, eds. *Pharmacology of Steroid Contraceptive Drugs*. New York, NY: Raven Press; 1977:277-288. **141.** Laumas KR, et al. *Am J Obstet Gynecol*. 1967;98(June 1):411. **142.** Saxena BN, et al. *Contraception*. 1977;16(Dec):605. **143.** Nilsson S. et al. *Contraception*. 1978;17(Feb):131. **144.** Washington AE, et al. *JAMA*. 1985;253(April 19):2246. **145.** Louv WC, et al. *Am J Obstet Gynecol*. 1989;160(Feb):396. **146.** Francis WG, et al. *Can Med Assoc J*. 1965;92(Jan 23):191. **147.** Verhulst HL, et al. *J Clin Pharmacol*. 1967;7(Jan-Feb):9. **148.** Ory HW, *Fam Plann Perspect*. 1982;14(July-Aug):182.**149.** Ory HW, et al. *Making Choices Evaluating the Health Risks and Benefits of Birth Control Methods*. New York, NY: The Alan Guttmacher Institute; 1983. **150.** Palmer JR, et al. *Am J Epidemiol*. 1989;130(Nov):878. **151.** Romieu I, et al. *J Natl Cancer Inst*. 1989;81(Sept):1313. **152.** Porter JB, et al. *Obstet Gynecol*. 1987;70(July):29.

Manufactured by
Watson Laboratories, Inc.,
Corona, CA 92880 12178-3

Revised, October 14, 1999

Zovia 1/35E-21
Zovia 1/35E-28
Zovia 1/50E-21
Zovia 1/50E-28
(Ethynodiol Diacetate and Ethinyl Estradiol Tablets, USP)
Shown in Product Identification Guide, page 340

WE Pharmaceuticals, Inc.

P.O. BOX 1142
RAMONA, CA, 92065

Direct Inquiries to:
(760) 788-9155
For Medical Emergencies Contact:
(760) 788-9155

AH-CHEW® Chewable Tablets ℞

Each tablet contains chlorpheniramine maleate 2mg. phenylephrine HCl 10mg. methscopolamine nitrate 1.25mg.

DOSAGE

12 yrs. & Older 1 or 2 Tabs (Q.I.D.), 6–12 yrs. 1 Tab (Q.I.D.).

HOW SUPPLIED

Bottles of 100, NDC# 59196-003-01

AH-CHEW®D Chewable Tablets ℞

Each tablet contains phenylephrine HCl 10mg.

DOSAGE

12 yrs. & Older 1 or 2 Tabs (Q.I.D.), 6–12 yrs. 1 Tab (Q.I.D.)

HOW SUPPLIED

Bottles of 100, NDC# 59196-007-01

D-FEDA™ II Tablets ℞

Each tablet contains pseudoephedrine HCl 60 mg, guaifenesin 600 mg.

DOSAGE

12 yrs. & Older 1 or 2 Tabs (B.I.D.), 6–12 yrs. 1 Tab (B.I.D.), 2–6 Yrs. $^1/_2$ Tab (B.I.D.).

HOW SUPPLIED

Bottles of 100, NDC #59196-005-01

E-Z SPACER® ℞

Portable Drug Delivery System for use with metered dose inhalers.

HOW SUPPLIED

One Unit plus Instructions for Single Patient Use.
NDC #59196-009-01

E-Z SPACER® and MASK ℞

DESCRIPTION

Portable Drug Delivery System for use with metered dose inhalers. Mask contains no latex.

HOW SUPPLIED

One Unit plus Instructions for Single Patient Use
NDC # 59196-029-01

E-Z SPACER® MASK (SMALL) ℞

For use with E-Z Spacer Drug Delivery System (contains no Latex)

HOW SUPPLIED

One mask plus instructions for Single Patient Use.
NDC #59196-020-01

OMNIHIST® L.A. Tablets ℞

Each tablet contains chlorpheniramine maleate 8 mg, phenylephrine HCl 20 mg, methscopolamine nitrate 2.5 mg.

DOSAGE

12 yrs. & Older 1 Tab (B.I.D.), 6–12 yrs. $^1/_2$ Tab (B.I.D.)

HOW SUPPLIED

Bottles of 100, NDC #59196-002-01

PREDNISOLONE SYRUP, USP ℞

DESCRIPTION

Contains Prednisolone 15 mg per 5 mL.

HOW SUPPLIED

Prednisolone Syrup, USP, is a cherry flavored red liquid containing 15 mg of Prednisolone in each 5 mL (teaspoonful) and is supplied in 240 mL bottles (NDC 59196-0010-24) and 480 mL bottles (NDC 59196-0010-48).

SINUVENT® Tablets ℞

Each tablet contains phenylpropanolamine HCl 75mg, guaifenesin 600mg.

DOSAGE

12 yrs. & Older 1 Tab (B.I.D.), 6–12 yrs. $^1/_2$ Tab (B.I.D.)

HOW SUPPLIED

Bottles of 100, NDC# 59196-001-01

ULTRABROM® Capsules ℞

Each capsule contains brompheniramine maleate 12mg. pseudoephedrine HCl 120mg.

DOSAGE

12 yrs. and Older 1 Cap (B.I.D.)

HOW SUPPLIED

Bottles of 100, NDC# 59196-006-01

ULTRABROM® PD Capsules ℞

Each capsule contains brompheniramine maleate 6mg, pseudoephedrine HCl 60mg.

DOSAGE

12 yrs. & Older 1 or 2 Caps B.I.D., 6–12 yrs. 1 Cap B.I.D.

HOW SUPPLIED

Bottles of 100, NDC# 59196-004-01

WellSpring Pharmaceutical Corporation

172 COUNTY ROUTE 537E
COLTS NECK, NJ 07722

Direct Inquiries to:
(732) 460-9788

DIBENZYLINE® ℞

brand of
phenoxybenzamine hydrochloride
Capsules
Rx only

DESCRIPTION

Each *Dibenzyline* capsule, with red cap and rod body, is imprinted SKF and E33 and contains phenoxybenzamine hydrochloride, 10 mg Inactive ingredients consist of benzyl alcohol, cetylpyridinium chloride, D&C Red No. 33, FD&C Red No. 3, FD&C Yellow No. 6, gelatin, lactose, sodium lauryl sulfate and trace amounts of other inactive ingredients. *Dibenzyline* is N-(2 Chloroethyl)-N-(1-methyl-2-phenoxyethyl)benzylamine hydrochloride:

CH_3
—CH_2NCHCH_2O— • HCl
CH_2CH_2Cl

Phenoxybenzamine hydrochloride is a colorless, crystalline powder with a molecular weight of 340.3 which melts between 136° and 141°C. It is soluble in water, alcohol and chloroform; insoluble in ether.

CLINICAL PHARMACOLOGY

Dibenzyline (phenoxybenzamine hydrochloride) is a long-acting, adrenergic, *alpha*-receptor blocking agent which can produce and maintain "chemical sympathectomy" by oral administration. It increases blood flow to the skin, mucosa and abdominal viscera, and lowers both supine and erect blood pressures. It has no effect on the parasympathetic system.

Twenty to 30 percent of orally administered phenoxybenzamine appears to be absorbed in the active form.[1]

The half-life of orally administered phenoxybenzamine hydrochloride is not known; however, the half-life of intravenously administered drug is approximately 24 hours. Demonstrable effects with intravenous administration persist for at least 3 to 4 days, and the effects of daily administration are cumulative for nearly a week.[1]

INDICATION AND USAGE

Pheochromocytoma, to control episodes of hypertension and sweating. If tachycardia is excessive, it may be necessary to use a beta-blocking agent concomitantly.

CONTRAINDICATIONS

Conditions where a fall in blood pressure may be undesirable.

WARNING

Dibenzyline-induced *alpha*-adrenergic blockade leaves *beta*-adrenergic receptors unopposed. Compounds that stimulate both types of receptors may therefore produce an exaggerated hypotensive response and tachycardia.

PRECAUTIONS

General—Administer with caution in patients with marked cerebral or coronary arteriosclerosis or renal damage. Adrenergic blocking effect may aggravate symptoms of respiratory infections.

Drug Interactions[2]—Dibenzyline (phenoxybenzamine hydrochloride) may interact with compounds that stimulate both *alpha*- and *beta*-adrenergic receptors (i.e., epinephrine) to produce an exaggerated hypotensive response and tachycardia (See WARNING.)

Dibenzyline blocks hyperthermia production by levarterenol, and blocks hypothermia production by reserpine.

Carcinogenesis, Mutagenesis, Impairment of Fertility—Phenoxybenzamine hydrochloride has shown *in vitro* mutagenic activity in the Ames test and in the mouse lymphoma assay; it has not shown mutagenic activity in the micronucleus test in mice. In rats and mice repeated intraperitoneal administration of phenoxybenzamine hydrochloride resulted in peritoneal sarcomas. Chronic oral dosing in rats has produced malignant tumors in the gastrointestinal tract. The majority of these tumors were found in the nonglandular stomach of the rats.

In chronic oral studies in rats, ulcerative and/or erosive gastritis of the glandular stomach occurred which was probably drug related.

Pregnancy-Teratogenic Effects—Pregnancy Category C. Adequate reproductive studies have not been performed with Dibenzyline (phenoxybenzamine hydrochloride). It is also not known whether *Dibenzyline* can cause fetal harm when administered to a pregnant woman. *Dibenzyline* should be given to a pregnant woman only if clearly needed.

Nursing Mothers—It is not known whether this drug is excreted in human milk. Because many drugs are excreted in human milk, and because of the potential for serious adverse reactions from phenoxybenzamine hydrochloride, a decision should be made whether to discontinue nursing or to discontinue the drug, taking into account the importance of the drug to the mother.

Pediatric Use—Safety and effectiveness in pediatric patients have not been established.

ADVERSE REACTIONS

The following adverse reactions have been observed, but there are insufficient data to support an estimate of their frequency.

Autonomic Nervous System*: Postural hypotension, tachycardia, inhibition of ejaculation, nasal congestion, miosis.

Miscellaneous: Gastrointestinal irritation, drowsiness, fatigue.

OVERDOSAGE

SYMPTOMS—These are largely the result of block of the sympathetic nervous system and of the circulating epinephrine. They may include postural hypotension resulting in dizziness or fainting; tachycardia, particularly postural; vomiting, lethargy; shock.

*These so-called "side effects" are actually evidence of adrenergic blockade and vary according to the degree of blockade.

TREATMENT—When symptoms and signs of overdosage exist, discontinue the drug. Treatment of circulatory failure, if present, is a prime consideration in cases of mild overdosage, recumbent position with legs elevated usually restores cerebral circulation. In the more severe cases, the usual measures to combat shock should be instituted. Usual pressor agents are *not* effective. Epinephrine is contraindicated because it stimulates both *alpha* and *beta* receptors; since *alpha* receptors are blocked, the net effect of epinephrine administration is vasodilation and a further drop in blood pressure (epinephrine reversal).

The patient may have to be kept flat for 24 hours or more in the case of overdose, as the effect of the drug is prolonged. Leg bandages and an abdominal binder may shorten the period of disability.

I.V. infusion of levarterenol bitartrate* may be used to combat severe hypotensive reactions, because it stimulates *alpha* receptors primarily. Although Dibenzyline (phenoxybenzamine hydrochloride) is an *alpha*-adrenergic blocking agent, a sufficient dose of levarterenol bitartrate will overcome this effect.

The oral LD_{50} for phenoxybenzamine hydrochloride is approximately 2000 mg/kg in rats and approximately 500 mg/kg in guinea pigs.

DOSAGE AND ADMINISTRATION

The dosage should be adjusted to fit the needs of each patient. Small initial doses should be *slowly* increased until the desired effect is obtained or the side effects from blockade become troublesome. *After each increase, the patient should be observed on that level before instituting another increase.* The dosage should be carried to a point where symptomatic relief and/or objective improvement are obtained, but not so high that the side effects from blockade become troublesome.

Initially, 10 mg of Dibenzyline (phenoxybenzamine hydrochloride) twice a day. Dosage should be increased every other day, usually to 20 to 40 mg 2 or 3 times a day, until an optimal dosage is obtained, as judged by blood pressure control.

STORAGE

Store between 15° and 30°C (59° and 86°F).

HOW SUPPLIED

Dibenzyline (phenoxybenzamine hydrochloride) capsules, 10 mg, in bottles of 100 (*NDC* 65197-001-01).

REFERENCES

1. Weiner, N.: Drugs That Inhibit Adrenergic Nerves and Block Adrenergic Receptors, in Goodman, L., and Gilman, A., *The Pharmacological Basis of Therapeutics*, ed. 6, New York, Macmillan Publishing Co., 1980, p. 179; p. 182.
2. Martin, E.W.: *Drug Interactions Index* 1978/1979, Philadelphia, J.B. Lippincott Co., 1978, pp. 209–210.

*Available as Levophed® Bitartrate (brand of norepinephrine bitartrate) from Sanofi Winthrop Pharmaceuticals.

DATE OF ISSUANCE DEC. 1999

Manufactured for
WellSpring Pharmaceutical Corporation
Colts Neck, NJ 07722 USA
by **SmithKline Beecham Pharmaceuticals**
Cidra, Puerto Rico
DI:L1
/31031

DYRENIUM® ℞
brand of
triamterene
Capsules
50 mg and 100 mg
potassium-sparing diuretic
Rx only

DESCRIPTION

Dyrenium (triamterene) is a potassium-sparing diuretic.

Structural Formula

Triamterene

Triamterene is 2, 4, 7-triamino-6-phenyl-pteridine. Its molecular weight is 253.27. At 50°C, triamterene is slightly soluble in water. It is soluble in dilute ammonia, dilute aqueous sodium hydroxide and dimethylformamide. It is sparingly soluble in methanol.

Each capsule for oral use, with opaque red cap and body, contains triamterene, 50 or 100 mg, and is imprinted with the product name DYRENIUM, strength (50 or 100) and SKF. Inactive ingredients consist of benzyl alcohol, cetylpyridmium chloride, D&C Red No. 33, FD&C Yellow No. 6, gelatin, lactose, magnesium stearate, povidone, sodium lauryl sulfate, titanium dioxide and trace amounts of other inactive ingredients.

CLINICAL PHARMACOLOGY

Triamterene has a unique mode of action; it inhibits the reabsorption of sodium ions in exchange for potassium and hydrogen ions at that segment of the distal tubule under the control of adrenal mineralocorticoids (especially aldosterone). This activity is not directly related to aldosterone secretion or antagonism; it is a result of a direct effect on the renal tubule.

The fraction of filtered sodium reaching this distal tubular exchange site is relatively small, and the amount which is exchanged depends on the level of mineralocorticoid activity. Thus, the degree of natriuresis and diresis produced by inhibition of the exchange mechanism is necessarily limited. Increasing the amount of available sodium and the level of mineralocorticoid activity by the use of more proximally acting diuretics will increase the degree of diuresis and potassium conservation.

Triamterene occasionally causes increases in serum potassium which can result in hyperkalemia. It does not produce alkalosis because it does not cause excessive excretion of titratable acid and ammonium.

Triamterene has been shown to cross the placental barrier and appear in the cord blood of animals.

Pharmacokinetics

Onset of action is 2 to 4 hours after ingestion. In normal volunteers the mean peak serum levels were 30 ng/mL at 3 hours. The average percent of drug recovered in the urine (0 to 48 hours) was 21%. Triamterene is primarily metabolized to the sulfate conjugate of hydroxytriamterene. Both the plasma and urine levels of this metabolite greatly exceed triamterene levels. Triamterene is rapidly absorbed, with somewhat less than 50% of the oral dose reaching the urine. Most patients will respond to Dyrenium (triamterene) during the first day of treatment. Maximum therapeutic effect, however, may not be seen for several days. Duration of diuresis depends on several factors, especially renal function, but it generally tapers off 7 to 9 hours after administration.

INDICATIONS AND USAGE

Dyrenium (triamterene) is indicated in the treatment of edema associated with congestive heart failure, cirrhosis of the liver and the nephrotic syndrome; also in steroid-induced edema, idiopathic edema and edema due to secondary hyperaldosteronism.

Dyrenium may be used alone or with other diuretics either for its added diuretic effect or its potassium-sparing potential. It also promotes increased diuresis when patients prove resistant or only partially responsive to thiazides or other diuretics because of secondary hyperaldosteronism.

Usage in Pregnancy. The routine use of diuretics in an otherwise healthy woman is inappropriate and exposes mother and fetus to unnecessary hazard. Diuretics do not prevent development of toxemia of pregnancy, and there is no satisfactory evidence that they are useful in the treatment of developed toxemia.

Edema during pregnancy may arise from pathological causes or from the physiologic and mechanical consequences of pregnancy. Diuretics are indicated in pregnancy when edema is due to pathologic causes, just as they are in the absence of pregnancy (however, see PRECAUTIONS below). Dependent edema in pregnancy, resulting from restriction of venous return by the expanded uterus, is properly treated through elevation of the lower extremities and use of support hose; use of diuretics to lower intravascular volume in this case is illogical and unnecessary. There is hypervolemia during normal pregnancy which is harmful to neither the fetus nor the mother (in the absence of cardiovascular disease), but which is associated with edema, including generalized edema, in the majority of pregnant women. If this edema produces discomfort, increased recumbency will often provide relief. In rare instances, this edema may cause extreme discomfort which is not relieved by rest. In these cases, a short course of diuretics may provide relief and may be appropriate.

CONTRAINDICATIONS

Anuria. Severe or progressive kidney disease or dysfunction with the possible exception of nephrosis.

Severe hepatic disease. Hypersensitivity to the drug.

Dyrenium (triamterene) should not be used in patients with pre-existing elevated serum potassium, as is sometimes seen in patients with impaired renal function or azotemia, or in patients who develop hyperkalemia while on the drug. Patients should not be placed on dietary potassium supplements, potassium salts or potassium-containing salt substitutes in conjunction with *Dyrenium*.

Dyrenium should not be given to patients receiving other potassium-sparing agents such as spironolactone, amiloride hydrochloride or other formulations containing triamterene. Two deaths have been reported in patients receiving concomitant spironolactone and *Dyrenium* or Dyazide®. Although dosage recommendations were exceeded in one case and in the other serum electrolytes were not properly monitored, these two drugs should not be given concomitantly.

WARNINGS

Abnormal elevation of serum potassium levels (greater than or equal to 5.5 mEq/liter) can occur with all potassium-sparing agents, including *Dyrenium*. Hyperkalemia is more likely to occur in patients with renal impairment and diabetes (even without evidence of renal impairment), and in the elderly or severely ill. Since uncorrected hyperkalemia may be fatal, serum potassium levels must be monitored at frequent intervals especially in patients receiving *Dyrenium*, when dosages are changed or with any illness that may influence renal function.

There have been isolated reports of hypersensitivity reactions; therefore, patients should be observed regularly for the possible occurrence of blood dyscrasias, liver damage or other idiosyncratic reactions.

Periodic BUN and serum potassium determinations should be made to check kidney function, especially in patients with suspected or confirmed renal insufficiency. It is particularly important to make serum potassium determinations in elderly or diabetic patients receiving the drug; these patients should be observed carefully for possible serum potassium increases.

If hyperkalemia is present or suspected, an electrocardiogram should be obtained. If the ECG shows no widening of the QRS or arrhythmia in the presence of hyperkalemia, it is usually sufficient to discontinue Dyrenium (triamterene) and any potassium supplementation and substitute a thiazide alone. Sodium polystyrene sulfonate (Kayexalate®, Winthrop) may be administered to enhance the excretion of excess potassium. **The presence of a widened QRS complex or arrhythmia in association with hyperkalemia requires prompt additional therapy.** For tachyarrhythmia, infuse 44 mEq of sodium bicarbonate or 10 mL of 10% calcium gluconate or calcium chloride over several minutes. For asystole, bradycardia or A-V block transvenous pacing is also recommended.

The effect of calcium and sodium bicarbonate is transient and repeated administration may be required. When indicated by the clinical situation, excess K^+ may be removed by dialysis or oral or rectal administration of Kayexalate®. Infusion of glucose and insulin has also been used to treat hyperkalemia.

PRECAUTIONS

General

Dyrenium (triamterene) tends to conserve potassium rather than to promote the excretion as do many diuretics and, occasionally, can cause increases in serum potassium which, in some instances, can result in hyperkalemia. In rare instances, hyperkalemia has been associated with cardiac irregularities.

Electrolyte imbalance often encountered in such diseases as congestive heart failure, renal disease or cirrhosis may be aggravated or caused independently by any effective diuretic agent including *Dyrenium*. The use of full doses of a diuretic when salt intake is restricted can result in a low-salt syndrome.

Triamterene can cause mild nitrogen retention which is reversible upon withdrawal of the drug and is seldom observed with intermittent (every-other-day) therapy.

Triamterene may cause a decreasing alkali reserve with the possibility of metabolic acidosis.

By the very nature of their illness, cirrhotics with splenomegaly sometimes have marked variations in their blood pictures. Since triamterene is a weak folic acid antagonist, it may contribute to the appearance of megaloblastosis in cases where folic acid stores have been depleted. Therefore, periodic blood studies in these patients are recommended. They should also be observed for exacerbations of underlying liver disease.

Triamterene has elevated uric acid, especially in persons predisposed to gouty arthritis.

Triamterene has been reported in renal stones in association with other calculus components. *Dyrenium* should be used with caution in patients with histories of renal stones.

Information for Patients

To help avoid stomach upset, it is recommended that the drug be taken after meals.

If a single daily dose is prescribed, it may be preferable to take it in the morning to minimize the effect of increased frequency of urination on nighttime sleep.

If a dose is missed, the patient should not take more than the prescribed dose at the next dosing interval.

Laboratory Tests

Hyperkalemia will rarely occur in patients with adequate urinary output, but it is a possibility if large doses are used for considerable periods of time. If hyperkalemia is ob-

Continued on next page

Dyrenium—Cont.

served, Dyrenium (triamterene) should be withdrawn. The normal adult range of serum potassium is 3.5 to 5.0 mEq per liter with 4.5 mEq often being used for a reference point. Potassium levels persistently above 6 mEq per liter require careful observation and treatment. Normal potassium levels tend to be higher in neonates (7.7 mEq per liter) than in adults.

Serum potassium levels do not necessarily indicate true body potassium concentration. A rise in plasma pH may cause a decrease in plasma potassium concentration and an increase in the intracellular potassium concentration. Because *Dyrenium* conserves potassium, it has been theorized that in patients who have received intensive therapy or been given the drug for prolonged periods, a rebound kaliuresis could occur upon abrupt withdrawal. In such patients withdrawal of *Dyrenium* should be gradual.

Drug Interactions

Caution should be used when lithium and diuretics are used concomitantly because diuretic-induced sodium loss may reduce the renal clearance of lithium and increase serum lithium levels with risk of lithium toxicity. Patients receiving such combined therapy should have serum lithium levels monitored closely and the lithium dosage adjusted if necessary.

A possible interaction resulting in acute renal failure has been reported in a few subjects when indomethacin, a nonsteroidal anti-inflammatory agent, was given with triamterene. Caution is advised in administering nonsteroidal anti-inflammatory agents with triamterene.

The effects of the following drugs may be potentiated when given together with triamterene: antihypertensive medication, other diuretics, preanesthetic and anesthetic agents, skeletal muscle relaxants (nondepolarizing).

Potassium-sparing agents should be used with caution in conjunction with angiotensin-converting enzyme (ACH) inhibitors due to an increased risk of hyperkalemia.

The following agents, given together with triamterene, may promote serum potassium accumulation and possibly result in hyperkalemia because of the potassium-sparing nature of triamterene, especially in patients with renal insufficiency: blood from blood bank (may contain up to 30 mEq of potassium per liter of plasma or up to 65 mEq per liter of whole blood when stored for more than 10 days); low-salt milk (may contain up to 60 mEq of potassium per liter); potassium-containing medications (such as parenteral penicillin G potassium); salt substitutes (most contain substantial amounts of potassium).

Dyrenium (triamterene) may raise blood glucose levels; for adult onset diabetes, dosage adjustments of hypoglycemic agents may be necessary during and after therapy; concurrent use with chlorpropamide may increase the risk of severe hyponatremia.

Drug/Laboratory Test Interactions

Triamterene and quinidine have similar fluorescence spectra; thus, triamterene will interfere with the fluorescent measurement of quinidine.

Carcinogenesis, Mutagenesis, Impairment of Fertility

Carcinogenesis: In studies conducted under the auspices of the National Toxicology Program, groups of rats were fed diets containing 0, 150, 300 or 600 ppm triamterene, and groups of mice were fed diets containing 0, 100, 200 or 400 ppm triamterene. Male and female rats exposed to the highest tested concentration received triamterene at about 25 and 30 mg/kg/day, respectively. Male and female mice exposed to the highest tested concentration received triamterene at about 45 and 60 mg/kg/day, respectively.

There was an increased incidence of hepatocellular neoplasia (primarily adenomas) in male and female mice at the highest dosage level. These doses represent 7.5X and 10X the Maximum Recommended Human Dose (MRHD) of 300 mg/kg/day (or 6 mg/kg/day based on a 50 kg patient) for male and female mice, respectively, when based on body weight and 0.7X and 0.9X the MRHD when based on body-surface area.

Although hepatocellular neoplasia (exclusively adenomas) in the rat study was limited to triamterene-exposed males, incidence was not dose-dependent and there was no statistically significant difference from control incidence at any dose level.

Mutagenesis: Triamterene was not mutagenic in bacteria (*Salmonella typhimurium* strains TA98, TA100, TA1535 or TA1537) with or without metabolic activation. It did not induce chromosomal aberrations in Chinese hamster ovary (CHO) cells *in vitro* with or without metabolic activation, but it did induce sister chromatid exchanges in CHO cells *in vitro* with and without metabolic activation.

Impairment of Fertility: Studies of the effects of triamterene on animal reproductive function have not been conducted.

Pregnancy: Category C

Teratogenic Effects: Reproduction studies have been performed in rats at doses as high as 20 times the Maximum Recommended Human Dose (MRHD) on the basis of body weight, and 6 times the MRHD on the basis of body surface area without evidence of harm to the fetus due to triamterene. Because animal reproduction studies are not always predictive of human response, this drug should be used during pregnancy only if clearly needed.

Nonteratogenic Effects: Triamterene has been shown to cross the placental barrier and appear in the cord blood. The use of triamterene in pregnant women requires that the anticipated benefits be weighed against possible hazards to the fetus. These possible hazards include adverse reactions which have occurred in the adult.

Nursing Mothers: Triamterene has not been studied in nursing mothers. Triamterene appears in animal milk and is likely present in human milk. If use of the drug product is deemed essential, the patient should stop nursing.

Pediatric Use: Safety and effectiveness in pediatric patients have not been established.

ADVERSE REACTIONS

Adverse effects are listed in decreasing order of frequency, however, the most serious adverse effects are listed first regardless of frequency. All adverse effects occur rarely (that is, 1 in 1000, or less).

Hypersensitivity: anaphylaxis, rash, photosensitivity.

Metabolic: hyperkalemia, hypokalemia.

Renal: azotemia, elevated BUN and creatinine, renal stones, acute interstitial nephritis (rare), acute renal failure (one case of irreversible renal failure has been reported).

Gastrointestinal: jaundice and/or liver enzyme abnormalities, nausea and vomiting, diarrhea.

Hematologic: thrombocytopenia, megaloblastic anemia.

Central Nervous System: weakness, fatigue, dizziness, headache, dry mouth.

OVERDOSAGE

In the event of overdosage it can be theorized that electrolyte imbalance would be the major concern, with particular attention to possible hyperkalemia. Other symptoms that might be seen would be nausea and vomiting, other GI disturbances and weakness. It is conceivable that some hypotension could occur. As with an overdosage of any drug, immediate evacuation of the stomach should be induced through emesis and gastric lavage. Careful evaluation of the electrolyte pattern and fluid balance should be made. There is no specific antidote.

Reversible acute renal failure following ingestion of 50 tablets of a product containing a combination of 50 mg triamterane and 25 mg hydrochlorothiazide has been reported.

The oral LD_{50} in mice is 380 mg/kg. The amount of drug in a single dose ordinarily associated with symptoms of overdose or likely to be life-threatening is not known.

Although triamterene is 67% protein-bound, there may be some benefit to dialysis in cases of overdosage.

DOSAGE AND ADMINISTRATION

Adult Dosage

Dosage should be titrated to the needs of the individual patient. When used alone, the usual starting dose is 100 mg twice daily after meals. When combined with another diuretic or antihypertensive agent, the total daily dosage of each agent should usually be lowered initially and then adjusted to the patient's needs. The total daily dosage should not exceed 300 mg. Please refer to PRECAUTIONS—General.

When Dyrenium (triamterene) is added to other diuretic therapy or when patients are switched to *Dyrenium* from other diuretics, all potassium supplementation should be discontinued.

HOW SUPPLIED

Capsules: 50 mg in bottles of 100 and 100 mg in bottles of 100.

Store between 15° and 30°C (59° and 86°F). Protect from light.

50 mg 100's: NDC 65197-002-01
100 mg 100's: NDC 65197-003-01
DATE OF ISSUANCE DEC. 1999

Manufactured for
WellSpring Pharmaceutical Corporation
Colts Neck, NJ 07722 USA
by **SmithKline Beecham Pharmaceuticals**
Cidra, Puerto Rico
DY:L1
731026

Westlake Laboratories, Inc.

24700 CENTER RIDGE ROAD
CLEVELAND, OH 44145

Direct Inquiries to:
Customer Service
(888) WSTLAKE (978–5253)
Fax (440) 835–2177
Internet: www.westlake-labs.com

BEVITAMEL OTC

[*bē-vĭt 'ə-mĕl*]
Melatonin-B-Vitamin Supplement

DESCRIPTION

Each tablet contains:

	Amount	% U.S.RDA*
Melatonin	3 mg	***
Vitamin B12	1000 µg	16667
Folic Acid	400 µg	100

* U.S. Recommended Daily Amount (RDA) established by the U.S. Food and Drug Administration (FDA).
*** The U.S.RDA has not been established by the U.S. FDA.

INDICATIONS

Bevitamel can be used to enhance the natural sleep process. Vitamin B12 and Folic Acid can be used to assist the metabolism of blood homocysteine.

CONTRAINDICATIONS

Product NOT intended for the treatment of Pernicious anemia

WARNINGS

Keep out of reach of children and store in a cool dry place. Tamper-resistant package, do not use if outer seal is missing or broken.

PRECAUTIONS

The dose size and timing may need to be adjusted by the physician to provide maximum effect for individual patients.

Individuals taking other medications, or with autoimmune, seizure or endocrine disorders and pregnant or lactating women, should consult a physician prior to use.

ADVERSE REACTIONS

None known.

DOSAGE AND ADMINISTRATION

One tablet sub-lingual approximately 30 minutes before bedtime as directed by a physician. Fractional tablets may be taken when indicated.

OVERDOSAGE

None known.

HOW SUPPLIED

BEVITAMEL is supplied as a pink bisected sub-lingual tablet (60 per bottle).

Westwood-Squibb Pharmaceuticals, Inc.

100 FOREST AVENUE
BUFFALO, NY 14213

For Medical Information Contact:
Generally:
Consumer Affairs Department:
1-800-494-7258
Adverse Drug Experiences
and Product Defects Reporting call during business hours only:
1-800-494-7258

DOVONEX® ℞

[*dōvă-nex*]
(calcipotriene cream)
Cream, 0.005%
FOR TOPICAL DERMATOLOGIC USE ONLY.
Not for Ophthalmic, Oral or Intravaginal Use.

DESCRIPTION

Dovonex (calcipotriene cream) Cream contains calcipotriene monohydrate, a synthetic vitamin D_3 derivative, for topical dermatological use.

Chemically, calcipotriene monohydrate is (5Z,7E,22E,24S)-24-cyclopropyl-9, 10-secochola-5,7,10(19), 22-tetraene-1α,3β,24-triol monohydrate, with empirical formula $C_{27}H_{40}O_3 \cdot H_2O$, a molecular weight of 430.6, and the following structural formula:

Calcipotriene monohydrate is a white or off-white crystalline substance. Dovonex Cream contains calcipotriene monohydrate equivalent to 50 µg/g anhydrous calcipotriene in a cream base of cetearyl alcohol, ceteth-20, diazolidinyl urea, dichlorobenzyl alcohol, dibasic sodium phosphate, edetate disodium, glycerin, mineral oil, petrolatum, and water.

CLINICAL PHARMACOLOGY

In humans, the natural supply of vitamin D depends mainly on exposure to the ultraviolet rays of the sun for conversion of 7-dehydrocholesterol to vitamin D_3 (cholecalciferol) in the skin. Calcipotriene is a synthetic analog of vitamin D_3.

Clinical studies with radiolabelled calcipotriene ointment indicate that approximately 6% (±3%, SD) of the applied dose of calcipotriene is absorbed systemically when the ointment is applied topically to psoriasis plaques, or 5% (±2.6%, SD) when applied to normal skin, and much of the absorbed active is converted to inactive metabolites within 24 hours of application. Systemic absorption of the cream has not been studied.

Vitamin D and its metabolites are transported in the blood, bound to specific plasma proteins. The active form of the vitamin, 1,25-dihydroxy vitamin D_3 (calcitriol) is known to be recycled via the liver and excreted in the bile. Calcipotriene metabolism following systemic uptake is rapid, and occurs via a similar pathway to the natural hormone.

CLINICAL STUDIES

Adequate and well-controlled trials of patients treated with Dovonex Cream have demonstrated improvement usually beginning after 2 weeks of therapy. This improvement continued with approximately 50% of patients showing at least marked improvement in the signs and symptoms of psoriasis after 8 weeks of therapy, but only approximately 4% showed complete clearing.

INDICATIONS AND USAGE

Dovonex (calcipotriene cream) Cream, 0.005%, is indicated for the treatment of plaque psoriasis. The safety and effectiveness of topical calcipotriene in dermatoses other than psoriasis have not been established.

CONTRAINDICATIONS

Dovonex Cream is contraindicated in those patients with a history of hypersensitivity to any of the components of the preparation. It should not be used by patients with demonstrated hypercalcemia or evidence of vitamin D toxicity. Dovonex Cream should not be used on the face.

PRECAUTIONS

General: Use of Dovonex Cream may cause transient irritation of both lesions and surrounding uninvolved skin. If irritation develops, Dovonex Cream should be discontinued. Reversible elevation of serum calcium has occurred with use of topical calcipotriene. If elevation in serum calcium outside the normal range should occur, discontinue treatment until normal calcium levels are restored.

Information for Patients: Patients using Dovonex Cream should receive the following information and instructions:

1. This medication is to be used only as directed by the physician. It is for external use only. Avoid contact with the face or eyes. As with any topical medication, patients should wash their hands after application.
2. This medication should not be used for any disorder other than that for which it was prescribed.
3. Patients should report to their physician any signs of adverse reactions.

Carcinogenesis, Mutagenesis, Impairment of Fertility: Animal studies have not been conducted to evaluate the carcinogenic potential of calcipotriene. Studies in rats at doses up to 54 μg/kg/day (318 μg/m²/day) of calcipotriene indicated no impairment of fertility or general reproductive performance.

Calcipotriene did not elicit any mutagenic effects in the Ames mutagenicity assay, the mouse lymphoma TK locus assay, the human lymphocyte chromosome aberration test, or the mouse micronucleus test.

Pregnancy: Teratogenic Effects: Pregnancy Category C. Studies of teratogenicity were done by the oral route where bioavailability is expected to be approximately 40–60% of the administered dose. Increased rabbit maternal and fetal toxicity was noted at 12 μg/kg/day (132 μg/m²/day). Rabbits administered 36 μg/kg/day (396 μg/m²/day) resulted in fetuses with a significant increase in the incidence of pubic bones, forelimb phalanges, and incomplete bone ossification. In a rat study, oral doses of 54 μg/kg/day (318 μg/m²/day) resulted in a significantly higher incidence of skeletal abnormalities consisting primarily of enlarged fontanelles and extra ribs. The enlarged fontanelles are most likely due to calcipotriene's effect upon calcium metabolism. The maternal and fetal calculated no-effect exposures in the rat (43.2 μg/m²/day) and rabbit (17.6 μg/m²/day) studies are approximately equal to the expected human systemic exposure level (18.5 μg/m²/day) from dermal applicatioin. There are no adequate and well-controlled studies in pregnant women. Therefore, Dovonex Cream should be used during pregnancy only if the potential benefit justifies the potential risk to the fetus.

Nursing Mothers: There is evidence that maternal 1,25-dihydroxy vitamin D_3 (calcitriol) may enter the fetal circulation, but it is not known whether it is excreted in human milk. The systemic disposition of calcipotriene is expected to be similar to that of the naturally occurring vitamin. Because many drugs are excreted in human milk, caution should be exercised when Dovonex Cream is administered to a nursing woman.

Pediatric Use: Safety and effectiveness of Dovonex Cream in pediatric patients have not been established. Because of a higher ratio of skin surface area to body mass, pediatric patients are at greater risk than adults of systemic adverse effects when they are treated with topical medication.

Geriatric Use: Of the total number of patients in clinical studies of calcipotriene cream, approximately 15% were 65 or older, while approximately 3% were 75 and over. There were no significant differences in adverse events for subjects over 65 years compared to those under 65 years of age. However, the greater sensitivity of older individuals cannot be ruled out.

ADVERSE REACTIONS

In controlled clinical trials, the most frequent adverse experiences reported for Dovonex Cream were cases of skin irritation which occurred in approximately 10–15% of patients. Rash, pruritus, dermatitis, and worsening of psoriasis were reported in 1 to 10% of patients.

OVERDOSAGE

Topically applied calcipotriene can be absorbed in sufficient amounts to produce systemic effects. Elevated serum calcium has been observed with excessive use of topical calcipotriene. If elevation in serum calcium should occur, discontinue treatment until normal calcium levels are restored (See **PRECAUTIONS**).

DOSAGE AND ADMINISTRATION

Apply a thin layer of Dovonex Cream to the affected skin twice daily and rub in gently and completely. The safety and efficacy of Dovonex Cream have been demonstrated in patients treated for eight weeks.

HOW SUPPLIED

Dovonex® (calcipotriene cream) Cream 0.005% is available in: 60 gram aluminum tubes (NDC 0072-0260-06) and 100 gram aluminum tubes (NDC 0072-0260-10).

STORAGE

Store at controlled room temperature 15°–25°C (59°–77°F). Do not freeze.

Manufactured by
Leo Laboratories Ltd.,
Dublin, Ireland

A Bristol-Myers Squibb Company J4-687
Princeton, NJ, 08543 USA E6-B001A-04-00
US Patent No. 4,866,048
Revised May 2000

DONOVEX® ℞

[*dō vă-nex*]

(calcipotriene ointment), 0.005%

For topical dermatologic use only. Not for ophthalmic, oral or intravaginal use.

DESCRIPTION

Donovex (calcipotriene ointment) contains the compound calcipotriene, a synthetic vitamin D_3 derivative for topical dermatological use.

Chemically, calcipotriene is (5Z, 7E, 22E, 24S)-24-cyclopropyl-9,10-secochola-5,7,10(19),22-tetraene-1α, 3β, 24-triol-, with the empirical formula $C_{27}H_{40}O_3$, a molecular weight of 412.6, and the following structural formula:

Calcipotriene is a white or off-white crystalline substance. Donovex contains calcipotriene 50 μg/g in an ointment base of dibasic sodium phosphate, edetate disodium, mineral oil, petrolatum, propylene glycol, tocopherol, steareth-2 and water.

CLINICAL PHARMACOLOGY

In humans, the natural supply of vitamin D depends mainly on exposure to the ultraviolet rays of the sun for conversion of 7-dehydrocholesterol to vitamin D_3 (cholecalciferol) in the skin. Calcipotriene is a synthetic analog of vitamin D_3.

Clinical studies with radiolabelled ointment indicate that approximately 6% (±3%, SD) of the applied dose of calcipotriene is absorbed systemically when the ointment is applied topically to psoriasis plaques, or 5% (±2.6%, SD) when applied to normal skin, and much of the absorbed active is converted to inactive metabolites within 24 hours of application.

Vitamin D and its metabolites are transported in the blood, bound to specific plasma proteins. The active form of the vitamin, 1,25-dihydroxy vitamin D_3 (calcitriol), is known to be recycled via the liver and excreted in the bile. Calcipotriene metabolism following systemic uptake is rapid, and occurs via a similar pathway to the natural hormone. The primary metabolites are much less potent than the parent compound.

There is evidence that maternal 1,25-dihydroxy vitamin D_3 (calcitriol) may enter the fetal circulation, but it is not known whether it is excreted in human milk. The systemic disposition of calcipotriene is expected to be similar to that of the naturally occurring vitamin.

CLINICAL STUDIES: Adequate and well-controlled trials of patients treated with Donovex have demonstrated improvement usually beginning after two weeks of therapy. This improvement continued in patients using Donovex once daily and twice daily. After 8 weeks of once daily Donovex, 56.7% of patients showed at least marked improvements (6.4% showed complete clearing). After 8 weeks of twice daily Donovex, 70.0% of patients showed at least marked improvement (11.3% showed complete clearing).

Subtracting percentages of patients using placebo (vehicle only) from percentages of patients using Donovex who had at least marked improvements after 8 weeks yields 39.9% for once daily and 49.6% for twice daily. This adjustment for placebo effect indicates that what might appear to be differences between once and twice daily use may reflect differences in the studies independent from the frequency of dosing. Although there was a numerical difference in comparison across studies, twice daily dosing has not been shown to be superior in efficacy to once daily dosing.

Over 400 patients have been treated in open label clinical studies of Donovex for periods of up to one year. In half of these studies, patients who previously had not responded well to Donovex were excluded. The adverse events in these extended studies included skin irritation in approximately 25% of patients and worsening of psoriasis in approximately 10% of patients. In one of these open label studies, half of the patients no longer required Donovex by 16 weeks of treatment, because of satisfactory therapeutic results.

INDICATIONS AND USAGE

Donovex (calcipotriene ointment), 0.005%, is indicated for the treatment of moderate plaque psoriasis in adults. The safety and effectiveness of topical calcipotriene in dermatoses other than psoriasis have not been established.

CONTRAINDICATIONS

Donovex is contraindicated in those patients with a history of hypersensitivity to any of the components of the preparation. It should not be used by patients with demonstrated hypercalcemia or evidence of vitamin D toxicity. Donovex should not be used on the face.

PRECAUTIONS

General

Use of Donovex may cause irritation of lesions and surrounding uninvolved skin. If irritation develops, Donovex should be discontinued.

Transient, rapidly reversible elevation of serum calcium has occurred with use of Donovex. If elevation in serum calcium outside the normal range should occur, discontinue treatment until normal calcium levels are restored.

Information for patients: Patients using Donovex should receive the following information and instructions:

1. This medication is to be used only as directed by the physician. It is for external use only. Avoid contact with the face or eyes. As with any topical medication, patients should wash hands after application.
2. This medication should not be used for any disorder other than that for which it was prescribed.
3. Patients should report to their physician any signs of local adverse reactions.

Carcinogenesis, Mutagenesis, Impairment of Fertility: Long-term animal studies have not been conducted to evaluate the carcinogenic potential of calcipotriene. Studies in rats at doses up to 54 μg/kg/day (318 μg/m²/day) of calcipotriene indicated no impairment of fertility or general reproductive performance.

Calcipotriene did not elicit any mutagenic effects in the Ames mutagenicity assay, the mouse lymphoma TK locus assay, the human lymphocyte chromosome aberration test or the mouse micronucleus test.

Pregnancy; Teratogenic Effects; Pregnancy Category C. Studies of teratogenicity were done by the oral route where bioavailability is expected to be approximately 40–60% of the administered dose. In rabbits, increased maternal and fetal toxicity were noted at a dosage of 12 μg/kg/day (132 μg/m²/day); a dosage of 36 μg/kg/day (396 μg/m²/day) resulted in a significant increase in the incidence of incomplete ossification of the pubic bones and forelimb phalanges of fetuses. In a rat study, a dosage of 54 μg/kg/day (318 μg/m²/day) resulted in a significantly increased incidence of skeletal abnormalities (enlarged fontanelles and extra ribs). The enlarged fontanelles are most likely due to calcipotriene's effect upon calcium metabolism. The estimated maternal and fetal no-effect exposure levels in the rat (43.2 μg/m²/day) and rabbit (17.6 μg/m²/day) studies are approximately equal to the expected human systemic exposure level (18.5 μg/m²/day) from dermal application. There are no adequate and well-controlled studies in pregnant women. Therefore, Donovex Ointment should be used during pregnancy only if the potential benefit justifies the potential risk to the fetus.

Nursing mothers: It is not known whether calcipotriene is excreted in human milk. Because many drugs are excreted in human milk, caution should be exercised when Donovex is administered to a nursing woman.

Pediatric Use: Safety and effectiveness of Donovex in children have not been established. Because of a higher ratio of skin surface area to body mass, children are at greater risk than adults of systemic adverse effects when they are treated with topical medication.

Geriatric Use: Of the total number of patients in clinical studies of calcipotriene ointment, approximately 12 % were 65 or older, while approximately 4% were 75 and over. The results of an analysis of severity of skin-related adverse events showed a statistically significant difference for subjects over 65 years (more severe) compared to those under 65 years (less severe).

ADVERSE REACTIONS

In controlled clinical trials, the most frequent adverse reactions reported for Donovex were burning, itching, and skin irritation, which occurred in approximately 10–15% of patients. Erythema, dry skin, peeling, rash, dermatitis, worsening of psoriasis including development of facial/scalp pso-

Continued on next page

Dovonex—Cont.

riasis were reported in 1 to 10% of patients. Other experiences reported in less than 1% of patients included skin atrophy, hyperpigmentation, hypercalcemia, and folliculitis. Once daily dosing has not been shown to be superior in safety to twice daily dosing.

OVERDOSAGE

Topically applied Donovex can be absorbed in sufficient amounts to produce systemic effects. Elevated serum calcium has been observed with excessive use of Donovex.

DOSAGE AND ADMINISTRATION

Apply a thin layer of Donovex to the affected skin once or twice daily, and rub in gently and completely.

HOW SUPPLIED

Donovex (calcipotriene ointment) Ointment, 0.005% is available in 30 g, 60 g, and 100 g aluminum tubes. Store at controlled room temperature 15°–25° C (59°–77° F). Do not freeze.

Rx only.

Manufactured by Leo Laboratories Ltd.,
Dublin, Ireland 5/97
©1997 Distributed by
Westwood-Squibb Pharmaceuticals Inc.
Princeton, NJ USA 08543
A Bristol-Myers Squibb Company
Revised August 1999
E6-B001B-08-99
03-6013-3C

DOVONEX® ℞ only

(calcipotriene solution)
Scalp Solution, 0.005%

FOR TOPICAL DERMATOLOGIC USE ONLY. Not for ophthalmic, oral or intravaginal use.

DESCRIPTION

Dovonex (calcipotriene solution) Scalp Solution 0.005%, is a colorless topical solution containing 0.005% calcipotriene in a vehicle of isopropanol (51% v/v) propylene glycol, hydroxypropyl cellulose, sodium citrate, menthol and water.

The chemical name of calcipotriene is (5Z, 7E, 22E, 24S)-24-cyclopropyl-9, 10-secochola-5,7,10(19), 22-tetraene-1α, 3β, 24-triol, with the empirical formula $C_{27}H_{40}O_3$, a molecular weight of 412.6, and the following structural formula:

OH H H HO OH

CLINICAL PHARMACOLOGY

In humans, the natural supply of vitamin D depends mainly on exposure to the ultraviolet rays of the sun for conversion of 7-dehydrocholesterol to vitamin D_3 (cholecalciferol) in the skin. Calcipotriene is a synthetic analog of vitamin D_3.

Although the precise mechanism of calcipotriene's antipsoriatic action is not fully understood, *in vitro* evidence suggests that calcipotriene is roughly equipotent to the natural vitamin in its effects on proliferation and differentiation of a variety of cell types. Calcipotriene has also been shown, in animal studies, to be 100–200 times less potent in its effects on calcium utilization than the natural hormone.

Clinical studies with radiolabelled calcipotriene solution indicate that less than 1% of the applied dose of calcipotriene is absorbed through the scalp when the solution (2.0 mL) is applied topically to normal skin or psoriasis plaques (160 cm^2) for 12 hours, and that much of the absorbed calcipotriene is converted to inactive metabolites within 24 hours of application.

Vitamin D and its metabolites are transported in the blood, bound to specific plasma proteins. The active form of the vitamin, 1,25-dihydroxy vitamin D_3 (calcitriol), is known to be recycled via the liver and excreted in the bile. Calcipotriene metabolism following systemic uptake is rapid, and occurs via a similar pathway to the natural hormone. The primary metabolites are much less potent than the parent compound.

There is evidence that maternal 1,25-dihydroxy vitamin D_3 (calcitriol) may enter the fetal circulation, but it is not known whether it is excreted in human milk. The systemic disposition of calcipotriene is expected to be similar to that of the naturally occurring vitamin.

CLINICAL STUDIES

Adequate and well-controlled trials of patients treated with Dovonex Scalp Solution, 0.005%, have demonstrated improvement usually beginning after 2 weeks of therapy. This improvement continued with approximately 31% of patients appearing either cleared (14%) or almost cleared (17%) after 8 weeks of therapy.

INDICATIONS AND USAGE

Dovonex (calcipotriene solution) Scalp Solution, 0.005%, is indicated for the topical treatment of chronic, moderately severe psoriasis of the scalp. The safety and effectiveness of topical calcipotriene in dermatoses other than psoriasis have not been established.

CONTRAINDICATIONS

Dovonex Scalp Solution, 0.005%, is contraindicated in those patients with acute psoriatic eruptions or a history of hypersensitivity to any of the components of the preparation. It should not be used by patients with demonstrated hypercalcemia or evidence of vitamin D toxicity.

WARNINGS

Avoid contact with the eyes or mucous membranes. Discontinue use if a sensitivity reaction occurs or if excessive irritation develops on uninvolved skin areas.

Drug product is flammable. Keep away from open flame.

PRECAUTIONS

General: Use of Dovonex Scalp Solution, 0.005%, may cause transient irritation of both lesions and surrounding uninvolved skin. If irritation develops, Dovonex Scalp Solution, 0.005% should be discontinued.

For external use only. Keep out of the reach of children. Always wash hands thoroughly after use.

Reversible elevation of serum calcium has occurred with use of topical calcipotriene. If elevation in serum calcium outside the normal range should occur, discontinue treatment until normal calcium levels are restored.

Information for Patients: Patients using Dovonex Scalp Solution, 0.005% should receive the following information and instructions:

1. This medication is to be used only as directed by the physician. It is for external use only. Avoid contact with the face or eyes. As with any topical medication, patients should wash their hands after application.
2. This medication should not be used for any disorder other than that for which it was prescribed.
3. Patients should report to their physician any signs of adverse reactions.

Carcinogenesis, Mutagenesis, Impairment of Fertility: Animal studies have not been conducted to evaluate the carcinogenic potential of calcipotriene. Studies in rats at doses up to 54 µg/kg/day (318 µg/m^2/day) of calcipotriene indicated no impairment of fertility or general reproductive performance.

Calcipotriene did not elicit any mutagenic effects in the Ames mutagenicity assay, the mouse lymphoma TK locus assay, the human lymphocyte chromosome aberration test or the mouse micronucleus test.

Pregnancy; Teratogenic Effects; Pregnancy Category C: Studies of teratogenicity were done by the oral route where bioavailability is expected to be approximately 40–60% of the administered dose. Increased rabbit maternal and fetal toxicity was noted at 12 µg/kg/day (132 µg/m^2/day). Rabbits administered 36 µg/kg/day (396 µg/m^2/day) resulted in fetuses with a significant increase in the incidences of pubic bones, forelimb phalanges, and incomplete bone ossification. In a rat study, oral doses of 54 µg/kg/day (318 µg/m^2/day) resulted in a significantly higher incidence of skeletal abnormalities consisting primarily of enlarged fontanelles and extra ribs. The enlarged fontanelles are most likely due to calcipotriene's effect upon calcium metabolism. The maternal and fetal calculated no-effect exposures in the rat (43.2 µg/m^2/day) and rabbit (17.6 µg/m^2/day) studies are greater than the expected human systemic exposure level (0.13 µg/m^2/day) from dermal application. There are no adequate and well-controlled studies in pregnant women. Therefore, Dovonex Scalp Solution, 0.005%, should be used during pregnancy only if the potential benefit justifies the potential risk to the fetus.

Nursing Mothers: There is evidence that maternal 1,25-dihydroxy vitamin D_3 (calcitriol) may enter the fetal circulation, but it is not known whether it is excreted in human milk. The systemic disposition of calcipotriene is expected to be similar to that of the naturally occurring vitamin. Because many drugs are excreted in human milk, caution should be exercised when Dovonex Scalp solution, 0.005%, is administered to a nursing woman.

Pediatric Use: Safety and effectiveness of Dovonex Scalp Solution, 0.005%, in pediatric patients have not been specifically established. Because of a higher ratio of skin surface area to body mass, pediactic patients are at greater risk than adults of systemic adverse effects when they are treated with topical medication.

Geriatric Use

Of the total number of patients in clinical studies of calcipotriene solution, approximately 16% were 65 or older, while approximately 4% were 75 and over. The results of an analysis of severity of skin-related adverse events showed no differences for subjects over 65 years compared to those under 65 years, but greater sensitivity of some older individuals cannot be ruled out.

ADVERSE REACTIONS

In controlled clinical trials, the most frequent adverse reactions reported to be related to Dovonex Scalp Solution, 0.005%, use were transient burning, stinging and tingling, which occurred in approximately 23% of patients. Rash was reported in about 11% of patients. Dry skin, irritation and worsening of psoriasis was reported in 1–5% of patients. Skin atrophy, hyperpigmentation, hypercalcemia, and folliculitis were not observed in these studies, but cannot be excluded.

OVERDOSAGE

Topically applied calcipotriene can be absorbed in sufficient amounts to produce systemic effects. Elevated serum calcium has been observed with excessive use of topical calcipotriene. If elevation in serum calcium should occur, discontinue treatment until normal calcium levels are restored. (See **PRECAUTIONS.**)

DOSAGE AND ADMINISTRATION

Comb the hair to remove scaly debris and after suitably parting, apply Dovonex Scalp Solution, 0.005% twice daily, only to the lesions, and rub in gently and completely, taking care to prevent the solution spreading onto the forehead. The safety and efficacy of Dovonex Scalp Solution, 0.005%, have been demonstrated in patients treated for eight weeks. **Keep Dovonex Scalp Solution, 0.005%, well away from the eyes.** Avoid application of the solution to uninvolved scalp margins. **Always wash hands thoroughly after use.**

HOW SUPPLIED

Dovonex® (calcipotriene solution) Scalp Solution, 0.005%, is available in 60 mL plastic bottles (NDC 0072-1160-06).

STORAGE

Store at controlled room temperature 15°C–25°C (59°F–77°F). Avoid sunlight. Do not freeze.

Rx only.

Manufactured by Leo Pharmaceutical Products, Ltd., Ballerup, Denmark
©1995 Distributed by Westwood-Squibb Pharmaceuticals Inc., Princeton, NJ 08543, U.S.A.
A Bristol-Myers Squibb Company
E6-B001C-04-00 Revised May 2000
J4-686

LAC-HYDRIN® 12%* ℞

(ammonium lactate cream) Cream
For Dermatologic use only. Not for ophthalmic, oral or intravaginal use.

Rx only

DESCRIPTION

*Lac-Hydrin is a formulation of 12% lactic acid neutralized with ammonium hydroxide, as ammonium lactate, with a pH of 4.4-5.4.Lac-Hydrin Cream also contains water, light mineral oil, glyceryl stearate, polyoxyl 100 stearate, propylene glycol, polyoxyl 40 stearate, glycerin, cetyl alcohol, magnesium aluminum silicate, laureth-4, methyl and propyl parabens, and methylcellulose. Lactic acid is a racemic mixture of 2-hydroxypropanoic acid and has the following structural formula:

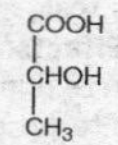

CLINICAL PHARMACOLOGY

Lactic acid is an alpha-hydroxy acid. It is a normal constituent of tissues and blood. The alpha-hydroxy acids (and their salts) are felt to act as humectants when applied to the skin. This property may influence hydration of the stratum corneum. In addition, lactic acid, when applied to the skin, may act to decrease corneocyte cohesion. The mechanism(s) by which this is accomplished is not yet known.

An *in vitro* study of percutaneous absorption of Lac-Hydrin Cream using human cadaver skin indicates that approximately 6.1% of the material was absorbed after 68 hours.

INDICATIONS AND USAGE

Lac-Hydrin Cream is indicated for the treatment of ichthyosis vulgaris and xerosis.

CONTRAINDICATIONS

None known.

WARNING

Use of this product should be discontinued if hypersensitivity to any of the ingredients is noted. Sun exposure (natural or artificial sunlight) to areas of the skin treated with Lac-Hydrin Cream should be minimized or avoided (see Precautions section).

PRECAUTIONS

General: For external use only. Stinging or burning may occur when applied to skin with fissures, erosions, or that is otherwise abraded (for example, after shaving the legs). Caution is advised when used on the face because of the potential for irritation. The potential for post-inflammatory hypo- or hyperpigmentation has not been studied.

Information for patients: Patients using Lac-Hydrin Cream should receive the following information and instructions:

1. This medication is to be used as directed by the physician, and should not be used for any disorder other than for which it was prescribed. Caution is advised when used on the face because of the potential for irritation. It is for external use only. Avoid contact with eyes, lips, or mucous membranes.
2. Patients should minimize or avoid use of this product on areas of the skin that may be exposed to natural or artificial sunlight, including the face. If sun exposure is unavoidable, clothing should be worn to protect the skin.

3. This medication may cause stinging or burning when applied to skin with fissures, erosions, or abrasions (for example, after shaving the legs).
4. If the skin condition worsens with treatment, the medication should be promptly discontinued.

Carcinogenesis, Mutagenesis, Impairment of Fertility: Carcinogenesis: A long-term photocarcinogenicity study in hairless albino mice suggested that topically applied 12% ammonium lactate cream enhanced the rate of ultraviolet light-induced skin tumor formation. Although the biologic significance of these results to humans is not clear, patients should minimize or avoid use of this product on areas of the skin that may be exposed to natural or artificial sunlight, including the face. Long-term dermal carcinogenicity studies in animals have not been conducted to evaluate the carcinogenic potential of ammonium lactate.

Pregnancy: Teratogenic effects: Pregnancy Category C. Animal reproduction studies have not been conducted with Lac-Hydrin Cream. It is also not known whether Lac-Hydrin Cream can cause fetal harm when administered to a pregnant woman or can affect reproduction capacity. Lac-Hydrin Cream should be given to a pregnant woman only if clearly needed.

Nursing Mothers: Although lactic acid is a normal constituent of blood and tissues, it is not known to what extent this drug affects normal lactic acid levels in human milk. Because many drugs are excreted in human milk, caution should be exercised when Lac-Hydrin Cream is administered to a nursing woman.

Pediatric Use: The safety and effectiveness of Lac-Hydrin Cream have not been established in pediatric patients less than 12 years old. Potential systemic toxicity from percutaneous absorption has not been studied. Because of the increased surface area to body weight ratio in pediatric patients, the systemic burden of lactic acid may be increased.

ADVERSE REACTIONS

In controlled clinical trials of patients with ichthyosis vulgaris, the most frequent adverse reactions in patients treated with Lac-Hydrin Cream were rash (including erythema and irritation) and burning/stinging. Each was reported in approximately 10-15% of patients. In addition, itching was reported in approximately 5% of patients.

In controlled clinical trials of patients with xerosis, the most frequent adverse reactions in patients treated with Lac-Hydrin Cream were transient burning, in about 3% of patients, stinging, dry skin and rash, each reported in approximately 2% of patients.

DOSAGE AND ADMINISTRATION

Apply to the affected areas and rub in thoroughly. Use twice daily or as directed by a physician.

HOW SUPPLIED

Lac-Hydrin Cream is available in cartons of 280 g (2-140 g plastic tubes). Store at controlled room temperature, 15-30°C (59-86°F).

Princeton, NJ, USA 08543 03-2954-0
A Bristol-Myers Squibb Company Revised August 1999
E7-B001A-08-99

LAC–HYDRIN® 12%* ℞

(ammonium lactate)
Lotion
For topical use only. Not for ophthalmic use.

RX only.

DESCRIPTION

*Lac-Hydrin, specially formulates 12% lactic acid, neutralized with ammonium hydroxide, as ammonium lactate to provide a lotion pH of 4.5–5.5. Lac-Hydrin also contains light mineral oil, glyceryl stearate, PEG-100 stearate, propylene glycol, polyoxyl 40 stearate, glycerin, magnesium aluminum silicate, laureth-4, cetyl alcohol, methyl and propylparabens, methylcellulose, fragrance, and water. Lactic acid is a racemic mixture of 2-hydroxypropanoic acid and has the following structural formula:

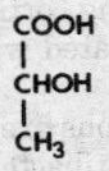

CLINICAL PHARMACOLOGY

It is generally accepted that the water content of the stratum corneum is a controlling factor in maintaining skin flexibility. When the stratum corneum contains more than 10% water it remains soft and pliable; however, when the water content drops below 10% the stratum corneum becomes less flexible and rough, and may exhibit scaling and cracking and the underlying skin may become irritated.

Symptomatic relief of dry skin is provided by skin protectants containing hygroscopic substances (humectants) which increase skin moisture. Lactic acid, an α-hydroxy acid, is reported to be one of the most effective naturally occurring humectants in the skin. The α-hydroxy acids (and their salts), in addition to having beneficial effects on dry skin, have also been shown to reduce excessive epidermal keratinization in patients with hyperkeratotic conditions (e.g., ichthyosis).

Pharmacokinetics: The mechanism of action of topically applied neutralized lactic acid is not yet known.

INDICATIONS AND USAGE

Lac-Hydrin is indicated for the treatment of dry, scaly skin (xerosis) and ichthyosis vulgaris and for temporary relief of itching associated with these conditions.

CONTRAINDICATIONS

Known hypersensitivity to any of the label ingredients.

PRECAUTIONS

General: For external use only. Avoid contact with eyes, lips or mucous membranes. Stinging or burning may occur when applied to skin with fissures, erosions or that is otherwise abraded (for example, after shaving the legs). Caution is advised when used on the face because of the potential for irritation. The potential for post-inflammatory hypo- or hyperpigmentation has not been studied.

Information for Patients: Patients using Lac-Hydrin (ammonium lactate) Lotion should receive the following information and instructions:

1. This medication is to be used as directed by the physician, and should not be used for any disorder other than for which it was prescribed. Caution is advised when used on the face because of the potential for irritation. It is for external use only. Avoid contact with eyes, lips, or mucous membranes.
2. Patients should minimize or avoid use of this product on areas of the skin that may be exposed to natural or artificial sunlight, including the face. If sun exposure is unavoidable, clothing should be worn to protect the skin.
3. This medication may cause transient stinging or burning when applied to skin with fissures, erosions, or abrasions (for example, after shaving the legs).
4. If the skin condition worsens with treatment, the medication should be promptly discontinued.

Carcinogenesis, Mutagenesis, Impairment of Fertility: A long-term photocarcinogenicity study in hairless albino mice suggested that topically applied 12% ammonium lactate cream enhanced the rate of ultraviolet light-induced skin tumor formation. Although the biological significance of these results to humans is not clear, patients should minimize or avoid use of this product on areas of the skin that may be exposed to natural or artificial sunlight, including the face. Long-term dermal carcinogenicity studies in animals have not been conducted to evaluate the carcinogenic potential of ammonium lactate.

Pregnancy (Category C): Animal reproduction studies have not been conducted with Lac-Hydrin. It is also not known whether Lac-Hydrin can cause fetal harm when administered to a pregnant woman or can affect reproduction capacity. Lac-Hydrin should be given to a pregnant woman only if clearly needed.

Nursing Mothers: Although lactic acid is a normal constituent of blood and tissues, it is not known to what extent this drug affects normal lactic acid levels in human milk. Because many drugs are excreted in human milk, caution should be exercised when Lac-Hydrin is administered to a nursing woman.

Pediatric Use: Safety and effectiveness of Lac-Hydrin have been demonstrated in infants and children. No unusual toxic effects were reported.

ADVERSE REACTIONS

The most frequent adverse experiences in patients with xerosis are transient stinging (1 in 30 patients), burning (1 in 30 patients), erythema (1 in 50 patients) and peeling (1 in 60 patients). Other adverse reactions which occur less frequently are irritation, eczema, petechiae, dryness and hyperpigmentation.

Due to the more severe initial skin conditions associated with ichthyosis, there was a higher incidence of transient stinging, burning and erythema (each occurring in 1 in 10 patients).

OVERDOSAGE

The oral administration of Lac-Hydrin to rats and mice showed this drug to be practically non-toxic (LD_{50}>15 mL/kg).

DOSAGE AND ADMINISTRATION

Shake well. Apply to the affected areas and rub in thoroughly. Use twice daily or as directed by a physician.

HOW SUPPLIED

225g (NDC 0072-5712-08; NSN 6505-01-216-6274) plastic bottle and 400g (NDC 0072-5712-14) plastic bottle.
Store at controlled room temperature (15°–30°C; 59°–86°F).

REFERENCES

1. Blank IH: Further observation on factors which influence the water content of the stratum corneum. *J Invest Dermatol* 21:259–271, 1953.
2. Blank IH: Factors which influence the water content of the stratum corneum. *J Invest Dermatol* 18:433–440, 1952.
3. Middleton JD: Sodium lactate as a moisturizer. *Cosmetics and Toiletries* 93:85–86, 1978.
4. VanScott EJ and Yu RJ: Modulations of keratinization with α-hydroxy acids and related compounds. In *Recent Advances in Dermatopharmacology*, P. Frost, E.E. Gomez and N. Zaias (eds) Spectrum Publications, Inc. NY, 211–217, 1977.

Princeton, NJ USA 08543 Revised August 1999
A Bristol-Myers Squibb Company E7-B001B-08-99
03-2963-0

ULTRAVATE® ℞

(halobetasol propionate cream)
Cream, 0.05%
For Dermatological Use Only. Not for Ophthalmic Use.

Rx only.

DESCRIPTION

ULTRAVATE (halobetasol propionate cream) Cream contains halobetasol propionate, a synthetic corticosteroid for topical dermatological use. The corticosteroids constitute a class of primarily synthetic steroids used topically as an anti-inflammatory and antipruritic agent.

Chemically halobetasol propionate is 21-chloro-6α, 9-difluoro-11β, 17-dihydroxy-16β-methylpregna-1, 4-diene-3-20-dione, 17 propionate, $C_{25}H_{31}ClF_2O_5$. It has the following structural formula:

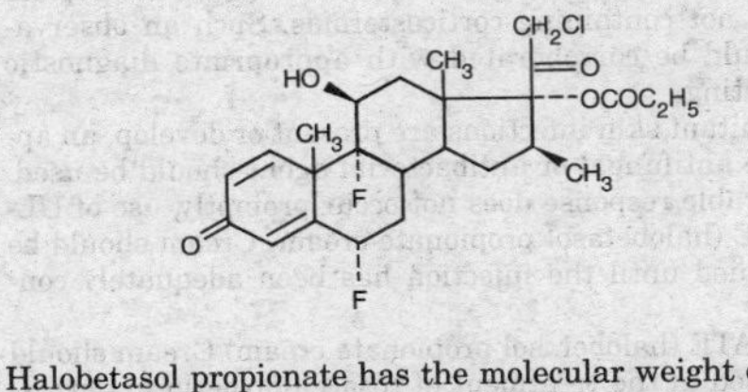

Halobetasol propionate has the molecular weight of 485. It is a white crystalline powder insoluble in water.

Each gram of ULTRAVATE Cream contains 0.5 mg/g of halobetasol propionate in a cream base of cetyl alcohol, glycerin, isopropyl isostearate, isopropyl palmitate, steareth-21, diazolidinyl urea, methylchloroisothiazolinone, methylisothiazolinone and water.

CLINICAL PHARMACOLOGY

Like other topical corticosteroids, halobetasol propionate has anti-inflammatory, antipruritic and vasoconstrictive actions. The mechanism of the anti-inflammatory activity of the topical corticosteroids, in general, is unclear. However, corticosteroids are thought to act by the induction of phospholipase A_2 inhibitory proteins, collectively called lipocortins. It is postulated that these proteins control the biosynthesis of potent mediators of inflammation such as prostaglandins and leukotrienes by inhibiting the release of their common precursor arachidonic acid. Arachidonic acid is released from membrane phospholipids by phospholipase A_2.

Pharmacokinetics—The extent of percutaneous absorption of topical corticosteroids is determined by many factors including the vehicle and the integrity of the epidermal barrier. Occlusive dressings with hydrocortisone for up to 24 hours have not been demonstrated to increase penetration; however, occlusion of hydrocortisone for 96 hours markedly enhances penetration. Topical corticosteroids can be absorbed from normal intact skin. Inflammation and/or other disease processes in the skin may increase percutaneous absorption.

Human and animal studies indicate that less than 6% of the applied dose of halobetasol propionate enters the circulation with 96 hours following topical administration of the cream. Studies performed with ULTRAVATE (halobetasol propionate cream) Cream indicate that it is in the super-high range of potency as compared with other topical corticosteroids.

INDICATIONS AND USAGE

ULTRAVATE (halobetasol propionate cream) Cream 0.05% is a super-high potency corticosteroid indicated for the relief of the inflammatory and pruritic manifestations of corticosteroid-responsive dermatoses. Treatment beyond two consecutive weeks is not recommended, and the total dosage should not exceed 50 g/week because of the potential for the drug to suppress the hypothalamic-pituitary-adrenal (HPA) axis.

CONTRAINDICATIONS

ULTRAVATE (halobetasol propionate cream) Cream is contraindicated in those patients with a history of hypersensitivity to any of the components of the preparation.

PRECAUTIONS

General: Systemic absorption of topical corticosteroids can produce reversible hypothalamic-pituitary-adrenal (HPA) axis suppression with the potential for glucocorticosteroid insufficiency after withdrawal of treatment. Manifestations of Cushing's syndrome, hyperglycemia, and glucosuria can also be produced in some patients by systemic absorption of topical corticosteroids while on treatment.

Patients applying a topical steroid to a large surface area or to areas under occlusion should be evaluated periodically for evidence of HPA axis suppression. This may be done by using the ACTH stimulation, A.M. plasma cortisol, and urinary free-cortisol tests. Patients receiving super potent corticosteroids should not be treated for more than 2 weeks at a time and only small areas should be treated at any one time due to increased risk of HPA suppression.

ULTRAVATE (halobetasol propionate cream) Cream produced HPA axis suppression when used in divided doses at 7

Continued on next page

Ultravate Cream—Cont.

grams per day for one week in patients with psoriasis. These effects were reversible upon discontinuation of treatment.

If HPA axis suppression is noted, an attempt should be made to withdraw the drug, to reduce the frequency of application, or to substitute a less potent corticosteroid. Recovery of HPA axis function is generally prompt upon discontinuation of topical corticosteroids. Infrequently, signs and symptoms of glucocorticosteroids insufficiency may occur requiring supplemental systemic corticosteroids. For information on systemic supplementation, see prescribing information for those products.

Pediatric patients may be more susceptible to systemic toxicity from equivalent doses due to their larger skin surface to body mass ratios (See PRECAUTIONS: Pediatric Use).

If irritation develops, ULTRAVATE (halobetasol propionate cream) Cream should be discontinued and appropriate therapy instituted. Allergic contact dermatitis with corticosteroids is usually diagnosed by observing failure to heal rather than noting a clinical exacerbation as with most topical products not containing corticosteroids. Such an observation should be corroborated with appropriate diagnostic patch testing.

If concomitant skin infections are present or develop, an appropriate antifungal or antibacterial agent should be used. If a favorable response does not occur promptly, use of ULTRAVATE (halobetasol propionate cream) Cream should be discontinued until the infection has been adequately controlled.

ULTRAVATE (halobetasol propionate cream) Cream should not be used in the treatment of rosacea or perioral dermatitis, and it should not be used on the face, groin, or in the axillae.

Information for Patients: Patients using topical corticosteroids should receive the following information and instructions:

1. The medication is to be used as directed by the physician. It is for external use only. Avoid contact with the eyes.
2. The medication should not be used for any disorder other than that for which it was prescribed.
3. The treated skin area should not be bandaged, otherwise covered or wrapped, so as to be occlusive unless directed by the physician.
4. Patients should report to the their physician any signs of local adverse reactions.
5. Parents of pediatric patients should be advised not to use tight-fitting diapers or plastic pants on a child being treated in the diaper area, as these garments may constitute occlusive dressing.

Laboratory Tests: The following tests may be helpful in evaluating patients for HPA axis suppression: ACTH-stimulation test; A.M. plasma cortisol test; Urinary free-cortisol test.

Carcinogenesis, mutagenesis, and Impairment of fertility: Long-term animal studies have not been performed to evaluate the carcinogenic potential of halobetasol propionate.

Positive mutagenicity effects were observed in two genotoxicity assays. Halobetasol propionate was positive in a Chinese hamster micronucleus test, and in a mouse lymphoma gene mutation assay *in vitro*.

Studies in the rat following oral administration at dose levels up to 50 µg/kg/day indicated no impairment of fertility or general reproductive performance.

In other genotoxicity testing, halobetasol propionate was not found to be genotoxic in the Ames/Salmonella assay, in the sister chromatid exchange test in somatic cells of the Chinese hamster, in chromosome aberration studies of germinal and somatic cells of rodents, and in a mammalian spot test to determine point mutations.

Pregnancy: *Teratogenic effects: Pregnancy Category C:* Corticosteroids have been shown to be teratogenic in laboratory animals when administered systemically at relatively low dosage levels. Some corticosteroids have been shown to be teratogenic after dermal application in laboratory animals. Halobetasol propionate has been shown to be teratogenic in SPF rats and chinchilla-type rabbits when given systemically during gestation at doses of 0.04 to 0.1 mg/kg in rats and 0.01 mg/kg in rabbits. These doses are approximately 13.33 and 3 times, respectively, the human topical dose of ULTRAVATE (halobetasol propionate cream) Cream. Halobetasol propionate was embryotoxic in rabbits but not in rats.

Cleft palate was observed in both rats and rabbits. Omphalocele was seen in rats, but not in rabbits.

There are no adequate and well-controlled studies of the teratogenic potential of halobetasol propionate in pregnant women. ULTRAVATE (halobetasol propionate cream) Cream should be used during pregnancy only if the potential benefit justifies the potential risk to the fetus.

Nursing Mothers: Systemically administered corticosteroids appear in human milk and could suppress growth, interfere with endogenous corticosteroid production, or cause other untoward effects. It is not known whether topical administration of corticosteroids could result in sufficient systemic absorption to produce detectable quantities in human milk. Because many drugs are excreted in human milk, caution should be exercised when ULTRAVATE (halobetasol propionate cream) Cream is administered to a nursing woman.

Pediatric Use: Safety and effectiveness of ULTRAVATE (halobetasol propionate cream) Cream in pediatric patients have not been established and use in pediatric patients under 12 is not recommended. Because of a higher ratio of skin surface area to body mass, pediatric patients are at a greater risk than adults of HPA axis suppression and Cushing's syndrome when they are treated with topical corticosteroids. They are therefore also at greater risk of adrenal insufficiency during or after withdrawal of treatment. Adverse effects including striae have been reported with inappropriate use of topical corticosteroids in infants and children.

HPA axis suppression, Cushing's syndrome, linear growth retardation, delayed weight gain and intracranial hypertension have been reported in children receiving topical corticosteroids. Manifestations of adrenal suppression in children include low plasma cortisol levels and an absence of response to ACTH stimulation. Manifestations of intracranial hypertension include bulging fontanelles, headaches, and bilateral papilledema.

ADVERSE REACTIONS

In controlled clinical trials, the most frequent adverse events reported for ULTRAVATE (halobetasol propionate cream) Cream included stinging, burning or itching in 4.4% of the patients. Less frequently reported adverse reactions were dry skin, erythema, skin atrophy, leukoderma, vesicles and rash.

The following additional local adverse reactions are reported infrequently with topical corticosteroids, and they may occur more frequently with high potency corticosteroids, such as ULTRAVATE (halobetasol propionate cream) Cream. These reactions are listed in an approximate decreasing order of occurrence: folliculitis, hypertrichosis, acneiform eruptions, hypopigmentation, perioral dermatitis, allergic contact dermatitis, secondary infection, striae and miliaria.

OVERDOSAGE

Topically applied ULTRAVATE (halobetasol propionate cream) Cream can be absorbed in sufficient amounts to produce systemic effects (see PRECAUTIONS).

DOSAGE AND ADMINISTRATION

Apply a thin layer of ULTRAVATE (halobetasol propionate cream) Cream to the affected skin once or twice daily, as directed by your physician, and rub in gently and completely.

ULTRAVATE (halobetasol propionate cream) Cream is a high potency topical corticosteroids; therefore, treatment should be limited to two weeks, and amounts greater than 50 g/wk should not be used. As with other corticosteroids, therapy should be discontinued when control is achieved. If no improvement is seen within 2 weeks, reassessment of diagnosis may be necessary.

ULTRAVATE (halobetasol propionate cream) Cream should not be used with occlusive dressings.

HOW SUPPLIED

ULTRAVATE CREAM, 0.05% is supplied in the following tube sizes:

15 g (NDC 0072-1400-15)

50 g (NDC 0072-1400-50)

Store between 15° and 30°C (59° and 86°F).

WESTWOOD SQUIBB™

A Bristol-Myers Squibb Company
Buffalo, New York U.S.A. 14213 03-5994-1

ULTRAVATE® ℞

(halobetasol propionate ointment)
Ointment, 0.05%
For Dermatological Use Only. Not for Ophthalmic Use.

Rx only.

DESCRIPTION

ULTRAVATE (halobetasol propionate ointment) Ointment contains halobetasol propionate, a synthetic corticosteroid for topical dermatological use. The corticosteroids constitute a class of primarily synthetic steroids used topically as an anti-inflammatory and antipruritic agent.

Chemically halobetasol propionate is 21-chloro-6α, 9-difluro-11β, 17-dihydroxy-16β-methylpregna-1, 4-diene-3-20-dione, 17-propionate, $C_{25}H_{31}ClF_2O_5$. It has the following structural formula:

CH$_2$Cl, HO, CH$_3$, =O, ---OCOC$_2$H$_5$, CH$_3$, CH$_3$, F, O, F

Halobetasol propionate has the molecular weight of 485. It is a white crystalline powder insoluble in water.

Each gram of ULTRAVATE Ointment contains 0.5 mg/g of halobetasol propionate in a base of aluminum stearate, beeswax, pentaerythritol cocoate, petrolatum, propylene glycol, sorbitan sesquioleate, and stearyl citrate.

CLINICAL PHARMACOLOGY

Like other topical corticosteroids, halobetasol propionate has anti-inflammatory, antipruritic and vasoconstrictive actions. The mechanism of the anti-inflammatory activity of the topical corticosteroids, in general, is unclear. However, corticosteroids are thought to act by the induction of phospholipase A_2 inhibitory proteins, collectively called lipocortins. It is postulated that these proteins control the biosynthesis of potent mediators of inflammation such as prostaglandins and leukotrienes by inhibiting the release of their common precursor arachidonic acid. Arachidonic acid is released from membrane phospholipids by phospholipase A_2.

Pharmacokinetics

The extent of percutaneous absorption of topical corticosteroids is determined by many factors including the vehicle and the integrity of the epidermal barrier. Occlusive dressings with hydrocortisone for up to 24 hours have not been demonstrated to increase penetration; however, occlusion of hydrocortisone for 96 hours markedly enhances penetration. Topical corticosteroids can be absorbed from normal intact skin. Inflammation and/or other disease processes in the skin may increase percutaneous absorption.

Human and animal studies indicate that less than 6% of the applied dose of halobetasol propionate enters the circulation within 96 hours following topical administration of the ointment.

Studies performed with ULTRAVATE (halobetasol propionate ointment) Ointment indicate that it is in the super-high range of potency as compared with other topical corticosteroids.

INDICATIONS AND USAGE

ULTRAVATE (halobetasol propionate ointment) Ointment 0.05% is a super-high potency corticosteroid indicated for the relief of the inflammatory and pruritic manifestations of corticosteroid-responsive dermatoses. Treatment beyond two consecutive weeks is not recommended, and the total dosage should not exceed 50 g/week because of the potential for the drug to suppress the hypothalamic-pituitary-adrenal (HPA) axis.

CONTRAINDICATIONS

ULTRAVATE (halobetasol propionate ointment) Ointment is contraindicated in those patients with a history of hypersensitivity to any of the components of the preparation.

PRECAUTIONS

General: Systemic absorption of topical corticosteroids can produce reversible hypothalamic-pituitary-adrenal (HPA) axis suppression with the potential for glucocorticosteroid insufficiency after withdrawal of treatment. Manifestations of Cushing's syndrome, hyperglycemia, and glucosuria can also be produced in some patients by systemic absorption of topical corticosteroids while on treatment.

Patients applying a topical steroid to a large surface area or to areas under occlusion should be evaluated periodically for evidence of HPA axis suppression. This may be done by using the ACTH stimulation, A.M. plasma cortisol, and urinary free-cortisol tests. Patients receiving super potent corticosteroids should not be treated for more than 2 weeks at a time and only small areas should be treated at any one time due to the increased risk of HPA suppression.

ULTRAVATE (halobetasol propionate ointment) Ointment produced HPA axis suppression when used in divided doses at 7 grams per day for one week in patients with psoriasis. These effects were reversible upon discontinuation of treatment.

If HPA axis suppression is noted, an attempt should be made to withdraw the drug, to reduce the frequency of application, or to substitute a less potent corticosteroid. Recovery of HPA axis function is generally prompt upon discontinuation of topical corticosteroids. Infrequently, signs and symptoms of glucocorticosteroid insufficiency may occur requiring supplemental systemic corticosteroids. For information on systemic supplementation, see prescribing information for those products.

Pediatric patients may be more susceptible to systemic toxicity from equivalent doses due to their larger skin surface to body mass ratios (See PRECAUTIONS: Pediatric Use).

If irritation develops, ULTRAVATE (halobetasol propionate ointment) Ointment should be discontinued and appropriate therapy instituted. Allergic contact dermatitis with corticosteroids is usually diagnosed by observing failure to heal rather than noting a clinical exacerbation as with most topical products not containing corticosteroids. Such an observation should be corroborated with appropriate diagnostic patch testing.

If concomitant skin infections are present or develop, an appropriate antifungal or antibacterial agent should be used. If a favorable response does not occur promptly, use of ULTRAVATE (halobetasol propionate ointment) Ointment should be discontinued until the infection has been adequately controlled.

ULTRAVATE (halobetasol propionate ointment) Ointment should not be used in the treatment of rosacea or perioral dermatitis, and it should not be used on the face, groin, or in the axillae.

Information for Patients

Patients using topical corticosteroids should receive the following information and instructions:

1. The medication is to be used as directed by the physician. It is for external use only. Avoid contact with the eyes.
2. The medication should not be used for any disorder other than that for which it was prescribed.
3. The treated skin area should not be bandaged, otherwise covered or wrapped, so as to be occlusive unless directed by the physician.

4. Patients should report to their physician any signs of local adverse reactions.
5. Parents of pediatric patients should be advised not to use tight-fitting diapers or plastic pants on a child being treated in the diaper area, as these garments may constitute occlusive dressing.

Laboratory Tests

The following tests may be helpful in evaluating patients for HPA axis suppression: ACTH-stimulation test; A.M. plasma cortisol test; Urinary free-cortisol test.

Carcinogenesis, mutagenesis, and Impairment of fertility

Long-term animal studies have not been performed to evaluate the carcinogenic potential of halobetasol propionate.

Positive mutagenicity effects were observed in two genotoxicity assays. Halobetasol propionate was positive in a Chinese hamster micronucleus test, and in a mouse lymphoma gene mutation assay *in vitro*.

Studies in the rat following oral administration at dose levels up to 50 µg/kg/day indicated no impairment of fertility or general reproductive performance.

In other genotoxicity testing, halobetasol propionate was not found to be genotoxic in the Ames/Salmonella assay, in the sister chromatid exchange test in somatic cells of the Chinese hamster, in chromosome aberration studies of germinal and somatic cells of rodents, and in a mammalian spot test to determine point mutations.

Pregnancy

Teratogenic effects: Pregnancy Category C: Corticosteroids have been shown to be teratogenic in laboratory animals when administered systemically at relatively low dosage levels. Some corticosteroids have been shown to be teratogenic after dermal application in laboratory animals.

Halobetasol propionate has been shown to be teratogenic in SPF rats and chinchilla-type rabbits when given systematically during gestation at doses of 0.04 to 0.1 mg/kg in rats and 0.01 mg/kg in rabbits. These doses are approximately 13, 33 and 3 times, respectively, the human topical dose of ULTRAVATE (halobetasol propionate ointment) Ointment. Halobetasol propionate was embryotoxic in rabbits but not in rats.

Cleft palate was observed in both rats and rabbits. Omphalocele was seen in rats, but not in rabbits.

There are no adequate and well-controlled studies of the teratogenic potential of halobetasol propionate in pregnant women. ULTRAVATE (halobetasol propionate ointment) Ointment should be used during pregnancy only if the potential benefit justifies the potential risk to the fetus.

Nursing Mothers

Systematically administered corticosteroids appear in human milk and could suppress growth, interfere with endogenous corticosteroid production, or cause other untoward effects. It is not known whether topical administration of corticosteroids could result in sufficient systemic absorption to produce detectable quantities in human milk. Because many drugs are excreted in human milk, caution should be exercised when ULTRAVATE (halobetasol propionate ointment) Ointment is administered to a nursing woman.

Pediatric Use

Safety and effectiveness of ULTRAVATE (halobetasol propionate ointment) Ointment in pediatric patients have not been established and use in pediatric patients under 12 is not recommended. Because of a higher ratio of skin surface area to body mass, pediatric patients are at a greater risk than adults of HPA axis suppression and Cushing's syndrome when they are treated with topical corticosteroids. They are therefore also at greater risk of adrenal insufficiency during or after withdrawal of treatment. Adverse effects including striae have been reported with inappropriate use of topical corticosteroids in infants and children.

HPA axis suppression, Cushing's syndrome, linear growth retardation, delayed weight gain and intracranial hypertension have been reported in children receiving topical corticosteroids. Manifestations of adrenal suppression in children include low plasma cortisol levels and an absence of response to ACTH stimulation. Manifestations of intracranial hypertension include bulging fontanelles, headaches, and bilateral papilledema.

ADVERSE REACTIONS

In controlled clinical trials, the most frequent adverse events reported for ULTRAVATE (halobetasol propionate ointment) Ointment included stinging or burning in 1.6% of the patients. Less frequently reported adverse reactions were pustulation, erythema, skin atrophy, leukoderma, acne, itching, secondary infection, telangiectasia, urticaria, dry skin, miliaria, paresthesia, and rash.

The following additional local adverse reactions are reported infrequently with topical corticosteroids, and they may occur more frequently with high potency corticosteroids, such as ULTRAVATE (halobetasol propionate ointment) Ointment. These reactions are listed in an approximate decreasing order of occurrence: folliculitis, hypertrichosis, acneiform eruptions, hypopigmentation, perioral dermatitis, allergic contact dermatitis, secondary infection, striae and miliaria.

OVERDOSAGE

Topically applied ULTRAVATE (halobetasol propionate ointment) Ointment can be absorbed in sufficient amounts to produce systemic effects (see **PRECAUTIONS**).

DOSAGE AND ADMINISTRATION

Apply a thin layer of ULTRAVATE (halobetasol propionate ointment) Ointment to the affected skin once or twice daily, as directed by your physician, and rub in gently and completely.

ULTRAVATE (halobetasol propionate ointment) Ointment is a high potency topical corticosteroid; therefore, treatment should be limited to two weeks, and amounts greater than 50 g/wk should not be used. As with other corticosteroids, therapy should be discontinued when control is achieved. If no improvement is seen within 2 weeks, reassessment of diagnosis may be necessary.

ULTRAVATE (halobetasol propionate ointment) Ointment should not be used with occlusive dressings.

HOW SUPPLIED

ULTRAVATE OINTMENT, 0.05% is supplied in the following tube sizes:

15 g (NDC 0072-1450-15)
50 g (NDC 0072-1450-50)

Store between 15° and 30°C (59° and 86°F).

WESTWOOD SQUIBB™

A Bristol-Myers Squibb Company
Buffalo, New York U.S.A. 14213 03-5995-2

Women First HealthCare, Inc.

12220 EL CAMINO REAL
SUITE 400
SAN DIEGO, CA 92130

Direct Inquiries to:
Ph: (888) 796-3631
Fax: (858) 509-0853

ESCLIM™ ℞

[ĕs-clīm]

estradiol transdermal system
Continuous delivery for twice-weekly application

Prescribing Information

1. **ESTROGENS HAVE BEEN REPORTED TO INCREASE THE RISK OF ENDOMETRIAL CARCINOMA IN POSTMENOPAUSAL WOMEN.**

   Close clinical surveillance of all women taking estrogens is important. Adequate diagnostic measures, including endometrial sampling when indicated, should be undertaken to rule out malignancy in all cases of undiagnosed persistent or recurring abnormal vaginal bleeding. There is no evidence that "natural" estrogens are more or less hazardous than "synthetic" estrogens at equiestrogenic doses.

2. **ESTROGENS SHOULD NOT BE USED DURING PREGNANCY.**

   There is no indication for estrogen therapy during pregnancy or during the immediate postpartum period. Estrogens are ineffective for the prevention or treatment of threatened or habitual abortion. Estrogens are not indicated for the prevention of postpartum breast engorgement.

   Estrogen therapy during pregnancy is associated with an increased risk of congenital defects in the reproductive organs of the fetus and possibly other birth defects. Studies of women who received diethylstilbestrol (DES) during pregnancy have shown that female offspring have an increased risk of vaginal adenosis, squamous cell dysplasia of the uterine cervix, and clear cell vaginal cancer later in life; male offspring have an increased risk of urogenital abnormalities and possibly testicular cancer later in life. The 1985 DES Task Force concluded that use of DES during pregnancy is associated with a subsequent increased risk of breast cancer in the mothers, although a causal relationship remains unproven, and the observed level of excess risk is similar to that for a number of other breast cancer risk factors.

DESCRIPTION

The Esclim™ estradiol transdermal system contains estradiol in a polymeric adhesive. The system is designed to release 17β-estradiol continuously upon application to intact skin.

Five systems are available to provide nominal *in vivo* delivery of 0.025, 0.0375, 0.05, 0.075, or 0.1 mg of estradiol per day via skin of average permeability. Each corresponding system having an active surface area of 11, 16.5, 22, 33, or 44 cm^2 contains 5, 7.5, 10, 15, or 20 mg of estradiol USP, respectively.

The composition of the systems per unit area is identical.

Estradiol USP (17β-estradiol) is a white, crystalline powder, chemically described as estra-1, 3, 5 (10)-triene-3, 17β-diol.

The structural formula is:

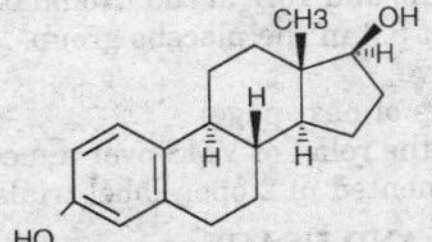

The molecular formula of estradiol is $C_{18}H_{24}O_2$. The molecular weight is 272.39.

Esclim transdermal systems are composed of a soft, flexible, rectangular foam backing material with rounded corners, covered on 1 side with a self-adhesive polymer matrix which contains estradiol and pharmacologically inactive components. The adhesive surface is covered by a transparent protective release liner as shown in the diagram below.

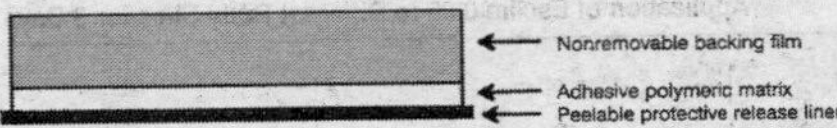

The active component of the system is estradiol. The remaining components of the system (EVA copolymers, ethylcellulose, octyldodecanol, dipropylene glycol, polyester protective release liner) are pharmacologically inactive.

CLINICAL PHARMACOLOGY

Estrogens are largely responsible for the development and maintenance of the female reproductive system and secondary sexual characteristics. Although circulating estrogens exist in a dynamic equilibrium of metabolic interconversions, estradiol is the principal intracellular human estrogen and is substantially more potent than its metabolites, estrone and estriol, at the receptor level. The primary source of estrogen in normally cycling adult women is the ovarian follicle, which secretes 70 to 500 µg of estradiol daily, depending on the phase of the menstrual cycle. After menopause, most endogenous estrogen is produced by conversion of androstenedione, secreted by the adrenal cortex, to estrone by peripheral tissues. Thus, estrone and the sulfate conjugated form, estrone sulfate, are the most abundant circulating estrogens in postmenopausal women.

Circulating estrogens modulate the pituitary secretion of the gonadotropins, luteinizing hormone (LH) and follicle stimulating hormone (FSH) through a negative feedback mechanism, and estrogen replacement therapy acts to reduce the elevated levels of these hormones seen in postmenopausal women.

Pharmacokinetics

The pharmacokinetics of transdermally administered estradiol using Esclim have been evaluated in a total of 138 healthy postmenopausal women in 9 clinical pharmacology and biopharmaceutic studies.

Absorption

Transdermal administration of estradiol produces therapeutic serum concentrations of estradiol with lower circulating concentrations of estrone and estrone conjugates and requires smaller total doses than does oral therapy.

The *in vivo* estradiol daily delivery rate from Esclim was estimated using the baseline adjusted average serum concentrations determined from pharmacokinetic studies and an estradiol clearance value of 1600 L/day. The estimated mean *in vivo* transdermal delivery rates of estradiol are 0.020 mg/day, 0.051 mg/day, and 0.101 mg/day for the 11 cm^2, 22 cm^2, and 44 cm^2 Esclim systems, respectively.

The bioavailability of estradiol from Esclim was compared with Vivelle™ in a 4-day single application randomized crossover study of Esclim 0.05 (22 cm^2), Esclim 0.1 (44 cm^2) and Vivelle 0.05 in 23 postmenopausal women. The mean maximum serum estradiol concentrations of 62 pg/mL and 124 pg/mL were obtained at a mean T_{max} of 27 hours following application of Esclim 0.05 and Esclim 0.1, respectively. In this study, serum estradiol concentration profiles (Figure 1) and pharmacokinetic parameters (C_{max} and AUC) obtained with the Esclim 0.1 system were twice as high as those produced by the Esclim 0.05 system.

Figure 1: Mean Uncorrected Serum Estradiol Concentrations After Application of Esclim 0.05, Esclim 0.1 and Vivelle 0.05 for 4 Days

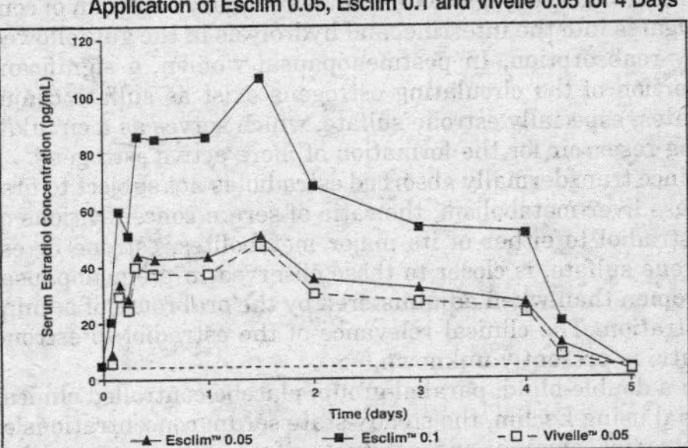

In a 3-week multiple application study in 18 postmenopausal women, Esclim 0.05 (22 cm^2) applied to the buttocks increased serum estradiol concentrations within 4 hours and maintained an average serum estradiol concentration of approximately 51 pg/mL above baseline. Trough values of approximately 27 to 35 pg/mL above the baseline were observed at the end of each application interval (3 or 4 days). Nearly identical serum estradiol concentration profiles were seen during each successive week, indicating little or no accumulation of estradiol in the body.

In a 3-day, single-application, crossover study in 12 postmenopausal women, estradiol serum concentrations were compared following application of the Esclim 0.05 system to sites on the buttocks (site used in clinical trials), the femoral triangle, and the upper arm. The profiles of serum estradiol concentrations from these different application sites are

Continued on next page

Esclim—Cont.

shown in Figure 2, and the pharmacokinetic results derived from each site are presented in Table 1.

Figure 2: Mean Uncorrected Serum Estradiol Concentrations After Application of Esclim 0.05 to Different Body Sites for 3 Days

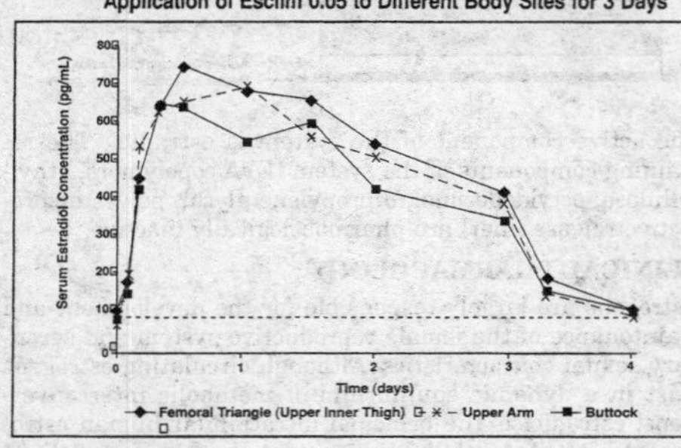

[See table 1 above]
Linear pharmacokinetics have been demonstrated for the Esclim transdermal system. Serum estradiol concentrations following a 4-day application of the Esclim 0.025, 0.05, and 0.1 systems are shown in Figure 3, while the mean values for pharmacokinetic parameters from these applications are summarized in Table 2. Results for the Esclim 0.025 system are from 1 study, while results for Esclim 0.05 and 0.1 systems are from a separate study. C_{max} occurred at approximately 30 hours.

Figure 3: Mean Uncorrected Serum Estradiol Concentrations After Application of Esclim 0.025, Esclim 0.05, and Esclim 0.1 for 4 Days

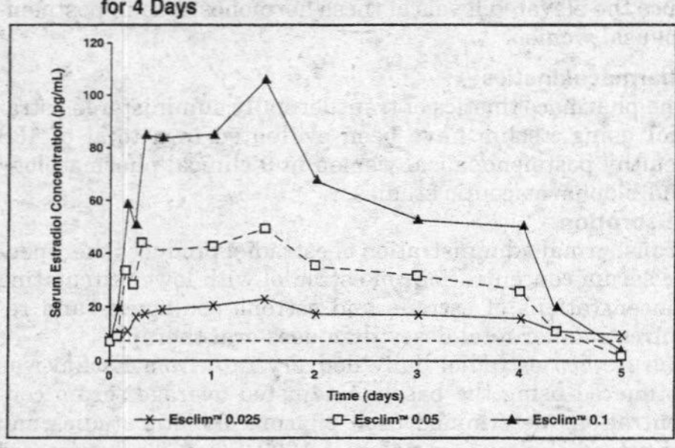

[See table 2 above]

Distribution

The distribution of exogenous estrogens is similar to that of endogenous estrogens. Estrogens are widely distributed in the body and are generally found in higher concentrations in the sex hormone target organs. Estradiol and other naturally occurring estrogens are bound mainly to sex hormone binding globulin (SHBG), and to lesser degree to albumin.

Metabolism

Exogenous estrogens are metabolized in the same manner as endogenous estrogens. Circulating estrogens exist in a dynamic equilibrium of metabolic interconversions. These transformations take place mainly in the liver. Estradiol is converted reversibly to estrone, and both can be converted to estriol, which is the major urinary metabolite. Estrogens also undergo enterohepatic recirculation via sulfate and glucuronide conjugation in the liver, biliary secretion of conjugates into the intestine, and hydrolysis in the gut followed by reabsorption. In postmenopausal women, a significant portion of the circulating estrogens exist as sulfate conjugates, especially estrone sulfate, which serves as a circulating reservoir for the formation of more active estrogens.
Since transdermally absorbed estradiol is not subject to first pass liver metabolism, the ratio of serum concentrations of estradiol to either of its major metabolites, estrone or estrone sulfate, is closer to those observed in premenopausal women than when administered by the oral route of administration. The clinical relevance of the estradiol to estrone ratio is presently unknown.
In a double-blind, parallel-group, placebo-controlled clinical trial using Esclim, the steady-state serum concentrations of estradiol, etsrone, and estrone sulfate were measured between 24 and 72 hours after application of patch at week 13 and are presented in Table 3.
[See table 3 above]

Excretion

Estradiol, estrone, and estriol are excreted in the urine along with glucuronide and sulfate conjugates. Serum concentrations of estradiol and estrone returned to baseline values within 12 to 24 hours after removal of Esclim.

Special Populations

No specific studies have been conducted using Esclim in any special populations.

Drug Interactions

No specific drug interaction studies have been conducted using Esclim.

Clinical Trials

In a 12-week, double-blind study evaluating the efficacy and safety of Esclim 0.025, 0.05, and 0.1 versus placebo in symptomatic women (average of 8 or more moderate to severe hot flushes per day), reduction in the frequency of these vasomotor symptoms was demonstrated within 4 weeks. Results from this trial are presented in Table 4 and Figure 4.
After 4 weeks of treatment, the mean reduction in the moderate to severe vasomotor symptoms (MSVS) was up to 8.6 MSVS per day in the Esclim 0.025 group, 9.2 and 10.2 in the Esclim 0.05, and Esclim 0.1 groups respectively, compared with 5.3 in the placebo group. After 12 weeks of treatment, this increased to 9.9 in the Esclim 0.025 group, 10.4 in the Esclim 0.05 group, and 10.7 in the Esclim 0.1 group and remained stable at 5.2 in the placebo group.
[See table 4 above]
[See figure at top of next page]
Maintenance of the relief of VMS over a median period of 2 years was documented in 2 open-label trials.

Table 1: Mean Uncorrected Estradiol Pharmacokinetic Parameters After Application of Esclim 0.05 Patches to Different Body Sites

Parameter	Femoral Triangle	Upper Arm	Buttock
C_{max} (pg/mL)	80.1 ± 34.9	80.2 ± 44.1	72.6 ± 36.2
C_{min72} (pg/mL)	41.6 ± 18.3	38.7 ± 15.2	34.5 ± 18.8
C_{av72} (pg/mL)	49.0 ± 24.6	47.4 ± 24.3	42.8 ± 20.7
C_{av96} (pg/mL)	42.8 ± 20.5	40.8 ± 19.7	37.3 ± 17.1
$AUC_{(0-72)}$ (pg•hr/mL)	4106 ± 1826	3825 ± 1897	3477 ± 1530
$AUC_{(0-96)}$ (pg•hr/mL)	4578 ± 1938	4306 ± 1925	3885 ± 1622

Table 2: Mean ± SD Uncorrected Estradiol Pharmacokinetic Parameters for Esclim Transdermal Systems Applied to the Buttocks (N = 23)

Surface Area (cm²)	Estradiol Dose (mg/day)	C_{max} (pg/mL)	C_{min}[a] (pg/mL)	C_{avg} (pg/mL)
11	0.025	24.5 ± 11[b]	15.5 ± 6.1[b]	17.8 ± 6.6[b]
22	0.05	61.6 ± 33	26.3 ± 14	38.6 ± 21
44	0.1	124 ± 66	51.4 ± 29	74.0 ± 43

[a]C_{min}=Serum estradiol concentration at 96 hours following application.[b]N = 17.

Table 3: Mean ± SD Steady State Serum Concentration of Estradiol and Its Metabolites at Week 13 Following the Application of Esclim

Patch	Steady State Serum Concentration		
	Estradiol (pg/mL)	Estrone (pg/mL)	Estrone Sulfate (ng/dL)
Placebo	19.6 ± 14.0 31[a]	20.7 ± 11.7 31	42.9 ± 24.0 30
0.025 mg/day	48.2 ± 27.4 22	38.7 ± 21.5 22	152.6 ± 129.7 22
0.05 mg/day	102.8 ± 63.6 24	49.0 ± 28.0 24	236.1 ± 147.1 22
0.1 mg/day	165.3 ± 116.1 28	64.9 ± 31.7 28	373.6 ± 272.0 28

[a]number of subjects

Table 4: Changes From Baseline in Frequency of MSVS

Week	Placebo (N = 54)	Esclim 0.025 mg/day (N = 48)	Esclim 0.05 mg/day (N = 47)	Esclim 0.1 mg/day (N = 47)
Week 0 (Baseline) Mean ± SD	11.4 ± 3.7	11.6 ± 5.4	10.9 ± 4.2	11.2 ± 2.8
Week 4 Mean Reduction ± SD (% Reduction)	-5.3 ± 4.1 (-48.9%)	-8.6 ± 5.7* (-72.6%)	-9.2 ± 4.5* (-84.4%)	-10.2 ± 2.9* (-92.0%)
Week 8 Mean Reduction ± SD (% Reduction)	-5.5 ± 4.7 (-51.5%)	-9.4 ± 5.7* (-79.8%)	-10.3 ± 4.3* (-94.0%)	-10.6 ± 2.8* (-95.4%)
Week 12 Mean Reduction ± SD (% Reduction)	-5.2 ± 5.1 (-50.3%)	-9.9 ± 5.8* (-83.4%)	-10.4 ± 4.2* (-95.3%)	-10.7 ± 2.8* (-95.6%)

*Statistically different from placebo in mean reduction (Dunnett's test)

INDICATIONS AND USAGE

Esclim (estradiol transdermal system) is indicated in the following:

1. Treatment of moderate to severe vasomotor symptoms associated with menopause. There is no adequate evidence that estrogens are effective for nervous symptoms of depression that might occur during menopause, and they should not be used to treat these conditions.
2. Treatment of vulval and vaginal atrophy.
3. Treatment of hypoestrogenism due to hypogonadism, castration, or primary ovarian failure.

CONTRAINDICATIONS

Patients with known hypersensitivity to any of the components of the therapeutic system should not use Esclim. Estrogens should not be used in individuals with any of the following conditions:

1. Known or suspected pregnancy (see Boxed Warning). Estrogen may cause fetal harm when administered to a pregnant woman.

Figure 4: Reduction of MSVS During Double-Blind, Placebo-Controlled Study

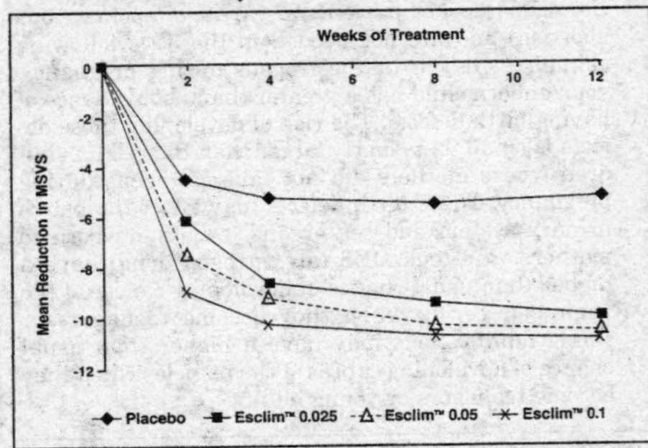

2. Undiagnosed abnormal genital bleeding.
3. Known or suspected cancer of the breast except in appropriately selected patients being treated for metastatic disease.
4. Known or suspected estrogen-dependent neoplasia.
5. Active thrombophlebitis or thromboembolic disorders.

WARNINGS

1. *Induction of Malignant Neoplasms.* Some studies have suggested a possible increased incidence of breast cancer in those women taking estrogen therapy at higher doses or for prolonged periods of time. The majority of studies, however, have not shown an association with the usual doses used for estrogen replacement therapy. Women on this therapy should have regular breast examinations and should be instructed in breast self-examination. The reported endometrial cancer risk among unopposed estrogen users is about 2- to 12-fold greater than in nonusers and appears dependent on duration of treatment and on estrogen dose. Most studies show no significant increased risk associated with the use of estrogens for less than 1 year. The greatest risk appears associated with prolonged use with increased risks of 15- to 24-fold for 5 to 10 years or more. In 3 studies, persistence of risk was demonstrated for 8 to over 15 years after cessation of estrogen treatment. In 1 study, a significant decrease in the incidence of endometrial cancer occurred 6 months after estrogen withdrawal. Concurrent progestin therapy may offset this risk, but the overall health impact in postmenopausal women is not known (see PRECAUTIONS). Estrogen therapy during pregnancy is associated with an increased risk of fetal congenital reproductive tract disorders. In female offspring, there is an increased risk of vaginal adenosis, squamous cell dysplasia of the cervix, and clear cell vaginal cancer later in life; in males, urogenital and possibly testicular abnormalities. Although some of these changes are benign, it is not known whether they are precursors of malignancy.
2. *Gallbladder Disease.* Two studies have reported a 2- to 4-fold increase in the risk of surgically confirmed gallbladder disease in postmenopausal women receiving oral estrogen replacement therapy, similar to the 2-fold increase previously noted in users of oral contraceptives.
3. *Cardiovascular Disease.* Large doses of estrogen (5 mg conjugated estrogens per day), comparable to those used to treat cancer of the prostate and breast, have been shown in a large prospective clinical trial in men to increase the risks of nonfatal myocardial infarction, pulmonary embolism, and thrombophlebitis.
These risks cannot necessarily be extrapolated from men to women. However, to avoid the theoretical cardiovascular risk to women caused by high estrogen doses, the dose for estrogen replacement therapy should not exceed the lowest effective dose.
4. *Elevated Blood Pressure.* Occasional blood pressure increases during estrogen replacement therapy have been attributed to idiosyncratic reactions to estrogens. More often, blood pressure has remained the same or has dropped. Postmenopausal estrogen use does not increase the risk of stroke. Nonetheless, blood pressure should be monitored at regular intervals with estrogen use, especially if high doses are used. Ethinyl estradiol and conjugated estrogens have been shown to increase renin substrate. In contrast to these oral estrogens, transdermally-administered estradiol does not affect renin substrate.
5. *Hypercalcemia.* Administration of estrogen may lead to severe hypercalcemia in patients with breast cancer and bone metastases. If this occurs, the drug should be stopped and appropriate measures taken to reduce the serum calcium level.

PRECAUTIONS

General

1. *Addition of a Progestin.* Studies of the addition of a progestin for 10 or more days of a cycle of estrogen administration have reported a lowered incidence of endometrial hyperplasia than would be induced by estrogen treatment alone. Morphological and biochemical studies of endometria suggest that 10 to 14 days of progestin are needed to provide maximal maturation of the endometrium and to reduce the likelihood of hyperplastic changes.
There are, however, possible risks that may be associated with the use of progestins in estrogen replacement regimens. These include:

Table 5: Incidence of Adverse Events >5% in a Placebo-Controlled Study of Esclim Data Are Expressed as % of Treatment Group

Adverse Event	Placebo (N = 54)	Esclim 0.025 mg/day (N = 48)	Esclim 0.05 mg/day (N = 47)	Esclim 0.1 mg/day (N = 47)
Breast Pain	3.7	25.0	44.7	46.8
Headache	22.2	18.8	8.5	6.4
Infection	7.4	10.4	10.6	8.5
Injury Accident	3.7	10.4	4.3	2.1
Anxiety	0	8.3	2.1	0
Emotional Lability	1.9	8.3	2.1	6.4
Arthralgia	1.9	6.3	2.1	4.3
Flu Syndrome	7.4	6.3	6.4	8.5
Joint Disorder	0	6.3	0	0
Pruritus	1.9	6.3	12.8	0
Rhinitis	1.9	6.3	4.3	4.3
Abdominal Pain	9.3	4.2	10.6	2.1
General Edema	1.9	4.2	6.4	6.4
Monilia Vagina	5.6	4.2	8.5	4.3
Nausea	1.9	4.2	10.6	8.5
Peripheral Edema	0	4.2	2.1	6.4
Sinusitis	7.4	4.2	2.1	4.3
Asthenia	1.9	2.1	10.6	6.4
Back Pain	3.7	2.1	2.1	6.4
Diarrhea	1.9	2.1	8.5	0
Dysmenorrhea	0	2.1	2.1	6.4
Enlarged Abdomen	0	2.1	2.1	6.4
Enlarged Breast	0	2.1	2.1	8.5
Rash	5.6	2.1	4.3	2.1
Anemia	0	0	6.4	4.3
Gastroenteritis	1.9	0	0	6.4
Hyperlipemia	5.6	0	0	2.1
Leukorrhea	0	0	12.8	0
Paresthesia	1.9	0	6.4	0

(1) adverse effects on lipoprotein metabolism (lowering HDL and raising LDL), which could diminish the purported cardioprotective effect of estrogen therapy (see PRECAUTIONS, below);
(2) impairment of glucose tolerance; and
(3) possible enhancement of mitotic activity in breast epithelial tissue, although few epidemiological data are available to address this point (see PRECAUTIONS, below).
The choice of progestin, its dose, and its regimen may be important in minimizing these adverse effects, but these issues will require further study before they are clarified.

2. *Cardiovascular Risk.* A causal relationship between estrogen replacement therapy and reduction of cardiovascular disease in postmenopausal women has not been proven. Furthermore, the effect of added progestins on this putative benefit is not yet known.
In recent years, many published studies have suggested that there may be a cause-effect relationship between postmenopausal oral estrogen replacement therapy *without added progestins* and a decrease in cardiovascular disease in women. Although most of the observational studies which assessed this statistical association have reported a 20% to 50% reduction in coronary heart disease risk and associated mortality in estrogen takers, the following should be considered when interpreting these reports:
(1) Because only 1 of these studies was randomized, and it was too small to yield statistically significant results, all relevant studies were subject to selection bias. Thus, the apparently reduced risk of coronary artery disease cannot be attributed with certainty to estrogen replacement therapy. It may instead have been caused by lifestyle and medical characteristics of the women studied with the result that healthier women were selected for estrogen therapy. In general, treated women were of higher socio-economic and educational status, more slender, more physically active, more likely to have undergone surgical menopause, and less likely to have diabetes than the untreated women. Although some studies attempted to control for these selection factors, it is common for properly-designed randomized trials to fail to confirm benefits suggested by less rigorous study designs. Thus ongoing and future large-scale randomized trials may fail to confirm this apparent benefit.
(2) Current medical practice often includes the use of concomitant progestin therapy in women with intact uteri (see PRECAUTIONS and WARNINGS). While the effects of added progestins on the risk of ischemic heart disease are not known, all available progestins reverse at least some of the favorable effects of estrogens on HDL and LDL levels.
(3) While the effects of added progestins on the risk of breast cancer are also unknown, available epidemiologic evidence suggests that progestins do not reduce, and may enhance, the moderately increased breast cancer incidence that has been reported with prolonged estrogen replacement therapy (see WARNINGS, above).
Because relatively long-term use of estrogens by a woman with a uterus has been shown to induce endometrial cancer, physicians often recommend that women who are deemed candidates for hormone replacement should take progestins as well as estrogens. When considering prescribing concomitant estrogens and progestins for hormone replacement therapy, physicians and patients are advised to carefully weigh the potential benefits and risks of the added progestin. Large-scale randomized, placebo-controlled, prospective clinical trials are required to clarify these issues.

3. *Physical Examination.* A complete medical and family history should be taken prior to the initiation of any estrogen therapy. The pre-treatment and periodic physical examinations should include special reference to blood pressure, breasts, abdomen, and pelvic organs and should include a Papanicolaou smear. As a general rule, estrogen should not be prescribed for longer than 1 year without re-examining the patient.
4. *Hypercoagulability.* Some studies have shown that women taking estrogen replacement therapy have hypercoagulability, primarily related to decreased antithrombin activity. This effect appears dose and duration dependent and is less pronounced than that associated with oral contraceptive use. Also, postmenopausal women tend to have increased coagulation parameters at baseline compared to premenopausal women. There is some suggestion that low-dose postmenopausal mestranol may increase the risk of thromboembolism, although the majority of studies (primarily of users of conjugated estrogens) report no such increase. There is insufficient information on hypercoagulability in women who have had previous thromboembolic disease.
5. *Familial Hyperlipoproteinemia.* Estrogen therapy may be associated with massive elevations of plasma triglycerides leading to pancreatitis and other complications in patients with familial defects of lipoprotein metabolism.
6. *Fluid Retention.* Because estrogens may cause some degree of fluid retention, conditions that might be exacerbated by this factor, such as asthma, epilepsy, migraine, and cardiac or renal dysfunction, require careful observation.
7. *Uterine Bleeding and Mastodynia.* Certain patients may develop undesirable manifestations of estrogenic stimulation, such as abnormal uterine bleeding and mastodynia.
8. *Impaired Liver Function.* Estrogens may be poorly metabolized in patients with impaired liver function and should be administered with caution.

Information for the Patient

See text of Patient Package Insert, which appears after the HOW SUPPLIED section.

Laboratory Tests

Estrogen administration should generally be guided by clinical response at the smallest dose, rather than laboratory monitoring, for relief of symptoms for those indications in which symptoms are observable.

Drug/Laboratory Test Interactions

Some of these drug/laboratory test interactions have been observed only with estrogen-progestin combinations (oral contraceptives):

1. Accelerated prothrombin time, partial thromboplastin time, and platelet aggregation time; increased platelet count; increased factors II, VII antigen, VIII antigen, VIII coagulant activity, IX, X, XII, VII-X complex, II-VII-X complex; and beta-thromboglobulin; decreased levels of anti-factor Xa and antithrombin III; decreased antithrombin III activity; increased levels of fibrinogen and fibrinogen activity; increased plasminogen antigen and activity.

Continued on next page

Esclim—Cont.

2. Increased thyroid-binding globulin (TBG) leading to increased circulating total thyroid hormone, as measured by protein-bound iodine (PBI), T_4 levels (by column or by radioimmunoassay) or T_3 levels by radioimmunoassay. T_3 resin uptake is decreased, reflecting the elevated TBG. Free T_4 and free T_3 concentrations are unaltered.
3. Other binding proteins may be elevated in serum, i.e. corticosteroid binding globulin (CBG), sex hormone-binding globulin (SHBG), leading to increased circulating corticosteroids and sex steroids respectively. Free or biologically active hormone concentrations are unchanged. Other plasma proteins may be increased (angiotensinogen/renin substrate, alpha-1-antitrypsin, ceruloplasmin).
4. Increased plasma HDL and HDL-2 subfraction concentrations, reduced LDL cholesterol concentration, increased triglyceride levels.
5. Impaired glucose tolerance.
6. Reduced response to metyrapone test.
7. Reduced serum folate concentration.

Carcinogenesis, Mutagenesis, Impairment of Fertility
Long-term, continuous administration of natural and synthetic estrogens in certain animal species increases the frequency of carcinomas of the breast, uterus, cervix, vagina, testis, and liver (see CONTRAINDICATIONS and WARNINGS).

Pregnancy Category X
Estrogens should not be used during pregnancy (see CONTRAINDICATIONS and Boxed Warning).

Nursing Mothers
As a general principle, the administration of any drug to nursing mothers should be done only when clearly necessary since many drugs are excreted in human milk. In addition, estrogen administration to nursing mothers has been shown to decrease the quantity and quality of the milk.

ADVERSE REACTIONS

See WARNINGS and Boxed Warning regarding the potential adverse effects on the fetus, the induction of malignant neoplasms, gallbladder disease, cardiovascular disease, elevated blood pressure, and hypercalcemia.
Skin irritation: In controlled clinical studies with Esclim, the most commonly reported adverse events were topical reactions of erythema and/or pruritus at the application site. In general these reactions caused patients little or no discomfort, and led to premature discontinuation of treatment in 0.9% (3/317) of patients in these trials. The rate of application site reactions, based on 8,135 applications of the 0.025, 0.05, and 0.1 Esclim systems in these trials was 6.1 per 100 applications (4.9, 5.4, 10.7 for the 3 Esclim doses respectively) compared to 6.2 in the placebo treated patients (2,014 applications).
In a placebo-controlled trial of Esclim 0.025, 0.05, and 0.1 conducted in 196 patients in the US, the adverse events reported by at least 5% of patients in 1 or more of the treatment groups are shown in Table 5.
[See table 5 at top of previous page]
Urogenital Adverse Events (See Precautions: Addition of a progestin): In the US placebo-controlled study, 72 patients were included who had intact uteri. As expected, after 12–13 weeks of continuous unopposed therapy, findings of endometrial hyperplasia (diagnosed either by endometrial biopsy and/or ultrasonography) were increased with increasing doses of estradiol (placebo: 0/18 patients; Esclim 0.025: 1/14 (7.1%); Esclim 0.05: 12/22 (54.5%); Esclim 0.1: 10/18 (55.6%). In the 86 patients who had not previously undergone a total hysterectomy, vaginal bleeding was also increased with increasing doses of estradiol [placebo: 2/21 patients (9.5%); Esclim 0.025: 6/19 (31.6%); Esclim 0.05: 14/25 (56.0%); Esclim 0.1: 12/21 (57.1%)].
In 2 long-term studies involving a total of 488 patients treated for a mean duration of 618 days and up to 3.5 years, the nature and incidence of adverse events did not change with prolonged duration of treatment.
The following additional adverse reactions have been reported with estrogen therapy:

1. *Genitourinary System.* Changes in vaginal bleeding pattern and abnormal withdrawal bleeding or flow; breakthrough bleeding, spotting; increase in size of uterine leiomyomata; vaginal candidiasis; change in amount of cervical secretion.
2. *Breasts.* Tenderness, enlargement.
3. *Gastrointestinal.* Nausea, vomiting; abdominal cramps, bloating; cholestatic jaundice; gallbladder disease.
4. *Skin.* Chloasma or melasma that may persist when drug is discontinued; erythema multiforme; erythema nodosum; hemorrhagic eruption; loss of scalp hair; hirsutism.
5. *Eyes.* Steepening of corneal curvature: intolerance to contact lenses.
6. *Central Nervous System.* Headache, migraine, dizziness; mental depression; chorea.
7. *Miscellaneous.* Increase or decrease in weight; reduced carbohydrate tolerance; aggravation of porphyria; edema; changes in libido.

OVERDOSAGE

Serious ill effects have not been reported following acute ingestion of large doses of estrogen containing oral contraceptives by young children. Overdosage of estrogen may cause nausea and vomiting, and withdrawal bleeding may occur in females.

DOSAGE AND ADMINISTRATION

The adhesive side of Esclim system should be placed on a clean, dry area of the skin on buttocks, femoral triangle (upper inner thigh), or upper arm, but *Esclim should not be applied to the breasts or other parts of the body.* The Esclim transdermal system should be replaced every 3 to 4 days (twice a week). The sites of application must be rotated, with an interval of at least 1 week allowed between applications to a particular site. The area selected should not be oily, damaged, or irritated. The waistline should be avoided, since tight clothing may rub the system off. The system should be applied immediately after opening the pouch and removing the protective liner. The system should be pressed firmly in place with the palm of the hand for about 10 seconds, making sure there is good contact, especially around the edges. In the unlikely event that a system should fall off, the same system may be reapplied. If necessary, a new system may be applied. In either case, the original treatment schedule should be continued.

Initiation of Therapy
For the treatment of moderate to severe vasomotor symptoms, and vulval and vaginal atrophy associated with menopause, and of hypoestrogenism due to hypogonadism, castration, or primary ovarian failure, treatment is generally initiated with the Esclim 0.025 transdermal system applied to the skin twice weekly, but the initial selection of the dose should be based on the evaluation of the severity of the patient's symptomatology and responsiveness to estrogen treatment. Depending upon the clinical response to treatment, the dosage can then be titrated up or down to individual needs. In order to use the lowest dosage necessary for the control of symptoms, decisions to increase dosage should not be made until after the first 2 or 3 weeks of therapy. Attempts to discontinue or taper medication should be made at 3-month to 6-month intervals.
In women not currently taking oral estrogens or in women switching from another estradiol transdermal therapy, treatment with the Esclim estradiol transdermal system may be initiated at once.
In women who are currently taking oral estrogens, treatment with the Esclim estradiol transdermal system should be initiated 1 week after withdrawal of oral hormone replacement therapy, or sooner if menopausal symptoms reappear in less than 1 week.

Therapeutic Regimen
Esclim may be given continuously in patients who do not have an intact uterus. In those patients with an intact uterus, Esclim may be given on a cyclic schedule (e.g., 3 weeks on drug followed by 1 week off drug).

HOW SUPPLIED

Esclim™ estradiol transdermal system 0.025 mg/day
(Each 11 cm^2 system contains 5 mg of estradiol USP)
Patient Pack of 8 systems .... NDC 64248-310-01
Esclim™ estradiol transdermal system 0.0375 mg/day
(Each 16.5 cm^2 system contains 7.5 mg of estradiol USP)
Patient Pack of 8 systems .... NDC 64248-320-01
Esclim™ estradiol transdermal system 0.05 mg/day
(Each 22 cm^2 system contains 10 mg of estradiol USP)
Patient Pack of 8 systems .... NDC 64248-330-01
Esclim™ estradiol transdermal system 0.075 mg/day
(Each 33 cm^2 system contains 15 mg of estradiol USP)
Patient Pack of 8 systems .... NDC 64248-340-01
Esclim™ estradiol transdermal system 0.1 mg/day
(Each 44 cm^2 system contains 20 mg of estradiol USP)
Patient Pack of 8 systems .... NDC 64248-350-01
Store at 25°C (77°F); excursion permitted to 15–30°C (59–86°F). [See USP Controlled Room Temperature.] Do not store unpouched. Apply immediately upon removal from the protective pouch.
Rx only.

ESCLIM™

estradiol transdermal system
Information for the Patient

INTRODUCTION

The Esclim™ system that your doctor has prescribed for you releases small amounts of estradiol through the skin in a continuous way. Estradiol is the same hormone that your ovaries produce abundantly before menopause. The dose of estradiol you require will depend on your individual response. The dose is adjusted by the size of the Esclim system used; the systems are available in 5 sizes.
This leaflet describes when and how to use estrogens, and the risks and benefits of estrogen treatment.
Estrogens have important benefits but also some risks. You must decide, with your doctor, whether the risks to you of estrogen use are acceptable because of their benefits. If you use estrogens, check with your doctor to be sure you are using the lowest possible dose that works, and that you don't use them longer than necessary. How long you need to use estrogens will depend on the reason for use.

1. ESTROGENS INCREASE THE RISK OF CANCER OF THE UTERUS IN WOMEN WHO HAVE HAD THEIR MENOPAUSE ("CHANGE OF LIFE").
If you use any estrogen-containing drug, it is important to visit your doctor regularly and report any unusual vaginal bleeding right away. Vaginal bleeding after menopause may be a warning sign of uterine cancer. Your doctor should evaluate any unusual vaginal bleeding to find out the cause.

2. ESTROGENS SHOULD NOT BE USED DURING PREGNANCY.
Estrogens do not prevent miscarriage (spontaneous abortion) and are not needed in the days following childbirth. It you take estrogens during pregnancy, your unborn child has a greater than usual chance of having birth defects. The risk of developing these defects is small, but clearly larger than the risk in children whose mothers did not take estrogens during pregnancy. These birth defects may affect the baby's urinary system and sex organs. Daughters born to mothers who took DES (an estrogen drug) have a higher than usual chance of developing cancer of the vagina or cervix when they become teenagers or young adults. Sons may have a higher than usual chance of developing cancer of the testicles when they become teenagers or young adults.

INFORMATION ABOUT ESCLIM

How the Esclim™ System Works
The Esclim system contains 17β-estradiol. When applied to the skin as directed below, the Esclim system releases 17β-estradiol continuously through the skin into the bloodstream.

How and Where to Apply the Esclim System
Each Esclim system is individually sealed in a protective pouch. Tear open this pouch at the indentation (do not use scissors) and remove the system. The system is made up of a self-adhesive matrix, which contains the estradiol. The adhesive surface is covered by a transparent protective release liner. The adhesive side will be placed against your skin. This liner must be removed before applying the system.

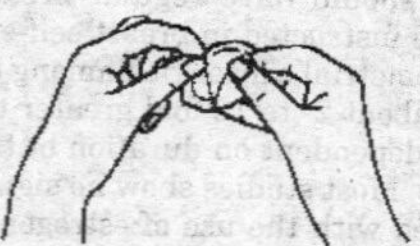

Remove the protective liner and discard it. Try to avoid touching the adhesive. Apply the adhesive side of the Esclim system to a clean, dry area of the skin on your upper arm, buttocks, or upper inner thigh. ***Do not apply Esclim to your breasts or other parts of your body.*** The sites of application must be rotated, with an interval of at least 1 week allowed between applications to a particular site. The area selected should not be oily, damaged, or irritated. The waistline should be avoided, since tight clothing may rub and remove the system. The system should be applied immediately after opening the pouch and removing the protective foil liner. The system should be pressed firmly in place with the palm of the hand for about 10 seconds, making sure there is good contact, especially around the edges.

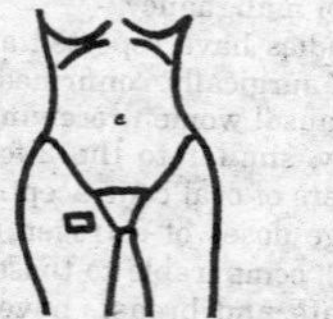

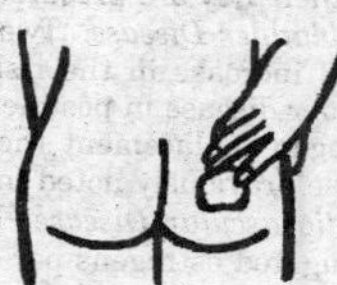

The Esclim system should be worn continuously until it is time to replace it with a new system. You may wish to experiment with different locations when applying the system, to find ones that are most comfortable for you and where clothing will not rub on the system.

When to Apply the Esclim System
The Esclim system should be changed every 3 to 4 days, 2 times per week, on the same 2 days of the week.
When changing the system, remove the used Esclim system. After removal, fold the patch in half so that the adhesive sides are together and discard. Any adhesive that might remain on your skin can be easily rubbed off. Then place the new Esclim system on a different skin site. (The same skin site should not be used again for at least 1 week after removal of the system.)
Contact with water when you are bathing, swimming, or showering will not affect the system. In the event that a system should fall off, the same system may be reapplied. If necessary, a new system may be applied. In either case, the original treatment schedule should be continued.

USES OF ESTROGEN

(Not every estrogen drug is approved for every use listed in this section. If you want to know which of these possible uses are approved for the medicine prescribed for you, ask your doctor or pharmacist to show you the professional labeling. You can also look up the specific estrogen product in a book called the "Physicians' Desk Reference," which is available in many book stores and public libraries. Generic drugs carry virtually the same labeling information as their brand name versions.)

— **To reduce moderate or severe menopausal symptoms.**
Estrogens are hormones made by the ovaries of normal women. Between ages 45 and 55, the ovaries normally stop making estrogens. This leads to a drop in body estrogen levels which causes the "change of life" or menopause (the end of monthly menstrual periods). If both ovaries are removed during an operation before natural

menopause takes place, the sudden drop in estrogen levels causes "surgical menopause."

When the estrogen levels begin dropping, some women develop very uncomfortable symptoms, such as feelings of warmth in the face, neck, and chest, or sudden intense episodes of heat and sweating ("hot flashes" or "hot flushes"). Using estrogen drugs can help the body adjust to lower estrogen levels and reduce these symptoms. Most women have only mild menopausal symptoms or none at all and do not need to use estrogen drugs for these symptoms. Others may need to take estrogens for a few months while their bodies adjust to lower estrogen levels. The majority of women do not need estrogen replacement for longer than 6 months for these symptoms.

— **To treat vulval and vaginal atrophy** (itching, burning, dryness in or around the vagina, difficulty or burning on urination) associated with menopause.

— **To treat certain conditions in which a young woman's ovaries do not produce enough estrogen naturally.**

— **To treat certain types of abnormal vaginal bleeding due to hormonal imbalance when your doctor has found no serious cause of the bleeding.**

— **To treat certain cancers in special situations, in men and women.**

— **To prevent thinning of bones.**

WHO SHOULD NOT USE ESTROGENS

Estrogens should not be used:

— **During pregnancy (see Boxed Warning).**
If you think you may be pregnant, do not use any form of estrogen-containing drug. Using estrogens while you are pregnant may cause your unborn child to have birth defects. Estrogens do not prevent miscarriage.

— **If you have unusual vaginal bleeding which has not been evaluated by your doctor (see Boxed Warning).**
Unusual vaginal bleeding can be a warning sign of cancer of the uterus, especially if it happens after menopause. Your doctor must find the cause of the bleeding so that he or she can recommend the proper treatment. Taking estrogens without visiting your doctor can cause you serious harm if your vaginal bleeding is caused by cancer of the uterus.

— **If you have had cancer.**
Since estrogens increase the risk of certain types of cancer, you should not use estrogens if you have ever had cancer of the breast or uterus, unless your doctor recommends that the drug may help in the cancer treatment. (For certain patients with breast or prostate cancer, estrogens may help.)

— **If you have any circulation problems.**
Estrogen drugs should not be used except in unusually special situations in which your doctor judges that you need estrogen therapy so much that the risks are acceptable. Men and women with abnormal blood clotting conditions should avoid estrogen use (see Dangers of Estrogens, below).

— **When they do not work.**
During menopause, some women develop nervous symptoms or depression. Estrogens do not relieve these symptoms. You may have heard that taking estrogens for years after menopause will keep your skin soft and supple and keep you feeling young. There is no evidence for these claims and such long-term estrogen use may have serious risks.

— **After childbirth or when breastfeeding a baby.**
Estrogens should not be used to try to stop the breasts from filling with milk after a baby is born. Such treatment may increase the risk of developing blood clots (see Dangers of Estrogens, below).
If you are breastfeeding, you should avoid using any drugs because many drugs pass through to the baby in the milk. While nursing a baby, you should take drugs only on the advice of your health care provider.

DANGERS OF ESTROGENS

— **Cancer of the uterus.**
Your risk of developing cancer of the uterus gets higher the longer you use estrogens and the larger doses you use. One study showed that after women stop taking estrogens, this higher cancer risk quickly returns to the usual level of risk (as if you had never used estrogen therapy). Three other studies showed that the cancer risk stayed high for 8 to more than 15 years after stopping estrogen treatment. Because of the risk, **IT IS IMPORTANT TO TAKE THE LOWEST DOSE THAT WORKS AND TO TAKE IT ONLY AS LONG AS YOU NEED IT.**
Using progestin therapy together with estrogen therapy may reduce the higher risk of uterine cancer related to estrogen use (but see Other Information, below).
If you have had your uterus removed (total hysterectomy), there is no danger of developing cancer of the uterus.

— **Cancer of the breast.**
Most studies have not shown a higher risk of breast cancer in women who have ever used estrogens. However, some studies have reported that breast cancer developed more often (up to twice the usual rate) in women who used estrogens for long periods of time (especially more than 10 years), or who used higher doses for shorter time periods.
Regular breast examinations by a health professional and monthly self-examination are recommended for all women.

— **Gallbladder disease.**
Women who use estrogens after menopause are more likely to develop gallbladder disease needing surgery than women who do not use estrogens.

— **Abnormal blood clotting.**
Taking estrogens may cause changes in your blood clotting system. These changes allow the blood to clot more easily, possibly allowing clots to form in your bloodstream. If blood clots do form in your bloodstream, they can cut off the blood supply to vital organs, causing serious problems. These problems may include a stroke (by cutting off blood to the brain), a heart attack (by cutting off blood to the heart), a pulmonary embolus (by cutting off blood to the lungs), or other problems. Any of these conditions may cause death or serious long-term disability. However, most studies of low dose estrogen usage by women do not show an increased risk of these complications.

SIDE EFFECTS

In addition to the risks listed above, the following side effects have been reported with estrogen use:

— Headaches.
— Nausea and vomiting.
— Breast tenderness or enlargement.
— Enlargement of benign tumors ("fibroids") of the uterus.
— Retention of excess fluid. This may make some conditions worsen, such as asthma, epilepsy, migraine, heart disease, or kidney disease.
— A spotty darkening of the skin, particularly on the face.
— Skin irritation, redness, or rash may occur at the application site.

REDUCING RISK OF ESTROGEN USE

If you use estrogens, you can reduce your risks by doing these things:

— **See your doctor regularly.**
While you are using estrogens, it is important to visit your doctor at least once a year for a check-up. If you develop vaginal bleeding while taking estrogens, you may need further evaluation. If members of your family have had breast cancer or if you have ever had breast lumps or an abnormal mammogram (breast X-ray), you may need to have more frequent breast examinations.

— **Reassess your need for estrogens.**
You and your doctor should reevaluate whether or not you still need estrogens at least every 6 months.

— **Be alert for signs of trouble.**
If any of these warning signals (or any other unusual symptoms) happen while you are using estrogens, call your doctor immediately:
Abnormal bleeding from the vagina (possible uterine cancer).
Pains in the calves or chest, sudden shortness of breath, or coughing blood (possible clot in the legs, heart, or lungs).
Severe headache or vomiting, dizziness, faintness, changes in vision or speech, weakness or numbness of an arm or leg (possible clot in the brain or eye).
Breast lumps (possible breast cancer; ask your doctor or health professional to show you how to examine your breasts monthly).
Yellowing of the skin or eyes (possible liver problem).
Pain, swelling, or tenderness in the abdomen (possible gallbladder problem).
Skin irritation.

OTHER INFORMATION

1. Estrogens increase the risk of developing a condition (endometrial hyperplasia) that may lead to cancer of the lining of the uterus. Taking progestins, another hormone drug, with estrogens lowers the risk of developing this condition. Therefore, if your uterus has not been removed, your doctor may prescribe a progestin for you to take together with your estrogen.
You should know, however, that taking estrogens *with* progestins may have additional risks. These include:
— Unhealthy effects on blood fats (especially a lowering of HDL blood cholesterol, the "good" blood fat which protects against heart disease).
— Unhealthy effects on blood sugar (which might make a diabetic condition worse).
— A possible further increase in breast cancer risk which may be associated with long-term estrogen use.

Some research has shown that estrogens taken *without* progestins may protect women against developing heart disease. However, this is not certain. The protection shown may have been caused by the characteristics of the estrogen-treated women, and not by the estrogen treatment itself. In general, treated women were slimmer, more physically active, and were less likely to have diabetes than the untreated women. These characteristics are known to protect against heart disease.

You are cautioned to discuss very carefully with your doctor or health care provider all the possible risks and benefits of long-term estrogen and progestin treatment as they affect you personally.

2. Your doctor has prescribed this drug for you and you alone. Do not give the drug to anyone else.
3. Keep this and all drugs out of the reach of children. In case of overdose, call your doctor, hospital, or poison control center immediately.
4. This leaflet provides a summary of the most important information about estrogens. If you want more information, ask your doctor or pharmacist to show you the professional labeling. The professional labeling is also published in a book called the "Physicians' Desk Reference," which is available in book stores and public libraries. Generic drugs carry virtually the same labeling information as their brand name versions.

Store at 25°C (77°F); excursions permitted to 15°–30°C (59°–86°F). Do not store unpouched. Apply immediately upon removal from the protective pouch.

Rx only.

Distributed by:
WOMEN FIRST HEALTHCARE, INC.
San Diego, CA 92130
Manufactured by:
Laboratoires Fournier S.A.
21000 Dijon, France
Made in France
July 1999
©WFHC 1999 PN0303

ORTHO-EST® ℞
(estropipate tablets, USP)

WARNINGS:

1. ESTROGENS HAVE BEEN REPORTED TO INCREASE THE RISK OF ENDOMETRIAL CARCINOMA IN POSTMENOPAUSAL WOMEN.

Close clinical surveillance of all women taking estrogens is important. Adequate diagnostic measures, including endometrial sampling when indicated, should be undertaken to rule out malignancy in all cases of undiagnosed persistent or recurring abnormal vaginal bleeding. There is no evidence that "natural" estrogens are more or less hazardous than "synthetic" estrogens at equi-estrogenic doses.

2. ESTROGENS SHOULD NOT BE USED DURING PREGNANCY.

There is no indication for estrogen therapy during pregnancy or during the immediate postpartum period. Estrogens are ineffective for the prevention or treatment of threatened, or habitual abortion. Estrogens are not indicated for the prevention of postpartum breast engorgement.

Estrogen therapy during pregnancy is associated with an increased risk of congenital defects in the reproductive organs of the fetus, and possibly other birth defects. Studies of women who received diethylstilbestrol (DES) during pregnancy have shown that female offspring have an increased risk of vaginal adenosis, squamous cell dysplasia of the uterine cervix, and clear cell vaginal cancer later in life; male offspring have an increased risk of urogenital abnormalities and possibly testicular cancer later in life. The 1985 DES Task Force concluded that use of DES during pregnancy is associated with a subsequent increased risk of breast cancer in the mothers, although a causal relationship remains unproven and the observed level of excess risk is similar to that for a number of other breast cancer risk factors.

DESCRIPTION ORTHO-EST (estropipate tablets USP), (formerly piperazine estrone sulfate), is a natural estrogenic substance prepared from purified crystalline estrone, solubilized as the sulfate and stabilized with piperazine. It is appreciably soluble in water and has almost no odor or taste—properties which are ideally suited for oral administration. The amount of piperazine in ORTHO-EST is not sufficient to exert a pharmacological action. Its addition ensures solubility, stability and uniform potency of the estrone sulfate. Chemically, estropipate, molecular weight: 436.56, is represented by estra-1,3,5(10)-trien-17-one, 3-(sulfooxy)-, compound with piperazine (1:1). The structural formula may be represented as follows:

ORTHO-EST is available as tablets for oral administration containing either 0.75 mg (ORTHO-EST .625) or 1.5 mg (ORTHO-EST 1.25) estropipate. (Calculated as sodium estrone sulfate .625 mg and 1.25 mg respectively).

Inactive Ingredients:
Each tablet contains: Lactose, magnesium stearate and pregelatinized starch. ORTHO-EST 1.25 also contains: D&C Red No. 7 Calcium Lake, FD&C Blue No. 2 Aluminium Lake.

CLINICAL PHARMACOLOGY

Estrogen drug products act by regulating the transcription of a limited number of genes. Estrogens diffuse through cell membranes, distribute themselves throughout the cell, and bind to and activate the nuclear estrogen receptor, a DNA-binding protein which is found in estrogen-responsive tissues. The activated estrogen receptor binds to specific DNA sequences, or hormone-response elements, which enhance the transcription of adjacent genes and in turn lead to the observed effects. Estrogen receptors have been identified in tissues of the reproductive tract, breast, pituitary, hypothalamus, liver, and bone of women.

Continued on next page

Ortho-Est—Cont.

Estrogens are important in the development and maintenance of the female reproductive system and secondary sex characteristics. By a direct action, they cause growth and development of the uterus, Fallopian tubes, and vagina. With other hormones, such as pituitary hormones and progesterone, they cause enlargement of the breasts through promotion of ductal growth, stromal development, and the accretion of fat. Estrogens are intricately involved with other hormones, especially progesterone, in the processes of the ovulatory menstrual cycle and pregnancy, and affect the release of pituitary gonadotropins. They also contribute to the shaping of the skeleton, maintenance of tone and elasticity of urogenital structures, changes in the epiphyses of the long bones that allow for the pubertal growth spurt and its termination, and pigmentation of the nipples and genitals.

Estrogens occur naturally in several forms. The primary source of estrogen in normally cycling adult women is the ovarian follicle, which secretes 70 to 500 micrograms of estradiol daily, depending on the phase of the menstrual cycle. This is converted primarily to estrone, which circulates in roughly equal proportion to estradiol, and to small amounts of estriol. After menopause, most endogenous estrogen is produced by conversion of androstenedione, secreted by the adrenal cortex, to estrone by peripheral tissues. Thus, estrone-especially in its sulfate ester form—is the most abundant circulating estrogen in postmenopausal women. Although circulating estrogens exist in a dynamic equilibrium of metabolic interconversions, estradiol is the principal intracellular human estrogen and is substantially more potent than estrone or estriol at the receptor.

Estrogens used in therapy are well absorbed through the skin, mucous membranes, and gastrointestinal tract. When applied for a local action, absorption is usually sufficient to cause systemic effects. When conjugated with aryl and alkyl groups for parenteral administration, the rate of absorption of oily preparations is slowed with a prolonged duration of action, such that a single intramuscular injection of estradiol valerate or estradiol cypionate is absorbed over several weeks.

Administered estrogens and their esters are handled within the body essentially the same as the endogenous hormones. Metabolic conversion of estrogens occurs primarily in the liver (first pass effect), but also at local target tissue sites. Complex metabolic processes result in a dynamic equilibrium of circulating conjugated and unconjugated estrogenic forms which are continually interconverted, especially between estrone and estradiol and between esterified and unesterified forms. Although naturally-occurring estrogens circulate in the blood largely bound to sex hormone-binding globulin and albumin, only unbound estrogens enter target tissue cells. A significant proportion of the circulating estrogen exists as sulfate conjugates, especially estrone sulfate, which serves as a circulating reservoir for the formation of more active estrogenic species. A certain proportion of the estrogen is excreted into the bile and then reabsorbed from the intestine. During this enterohepatic recirculation, estrogens are desulfated and resulfated and undergo degradation through conversion to less active estrogens (estriol and other estrogens), oxidation to nonestrogenic substances (catecholestrogens, which interact with catecholamine metabolism, especially in the central nervous system), and conjugation with glucuronic acids (which are then rapidly excreted in the urine).

When given orally, naturally-occurring estrogens and their esters are extensively metabolized (first pass effect) and circulate primarily as estrone sulfate, with smaller amounts of other conjugated and unconjugated estrogenic species. This results in limited oral potency. By contrast, synthetic estrogens, such as ethinyl estradiol and the nonsteroidal estrogens, are degraded very slowly in the liver and other tissues, which results in their high intrinsic potency. Estrogen drug products administered by non-oral routes are not subject to first-pass metabolism, but also undergo significant hepatic uptake, metabolism, and enterohepatic recycling.

INDICATIONS AND USAGE

Estrogen drug products are indicated in the:

1. Treatment of moderate to severe vasomotor symptoms associated with the menopause. There is no adequate evidence that estrogens are effective for nervous symptoms or depression which might occur during menopause and they should not be used to treat these conditions.
2. Treatment of vulval and vaginal atrophy.
3. Treatment of hypoestrogenism due to hypogonadism, castration or primary ovarian failure.
4. Prevention of osteoporosis.

Since estrogen administration is associated with risk, selection of patients should ideally be based on prospective identification of risk factors for developing osteoporosis. Unfortunately, there is no certain way to identify those women who will develop osteoporotic fractures. Most prospective studies of efficacy for this indication have been carried out in white menopausal women, without stratification by other risk factors, and tend to show a universally salutary effect on bone. Thus, patient selection must be individualized based on the balance of risks and benefits. A more favorable risk/benefit ratio exists in a hysterectomized woman because she has no risk of endometrial cancer (see BOXED WARNINGS).

Estrogen replacement therapy reduces bone resorption and retards or halts postmenopausal bone loss. Case-control studies have shown an approximately 60 percent reduction in hip and wrist fractures in women whose estrogen replacement was begun within a few years of menopause. Studies also suggest that estrogen reduces the rate of vertebral fractures. Even when started as late as 6 years after menopause, estrogen prevents further loss of bone mass for as long as the treatment is continued. The results of a double-blind, placebo-controlled two-year study have shown that treatment with one tablet of estropipate .75 daily for 25 days (of a 31-day cycle per month) prevents vertebral bone mass loss in postmenopausal women. When estrogen therapy is discontinued, bone mass declines at a rate comparable to the immediate postmenopausal period. There is no evidence that estrogen replacement therapy restores bone mass to premenopausal levels.

At skeletal maturity there are sex and race differences in both the total amount of bone present and its density, in favor of men and blacks. Thus, women are at higher risk than men because they start with less bone mass and, for several years following natural or induced menopause, the rate of bone mass decline is accelerated. White and Asian women are at higher risk than black women.

Early menopause is one of the strongest predictors for the development of osteoporosis. In addition, other factors affecting the skeleton which are associated with osteoporosis include genetic factors (small build, family history), endocrine factors (nulliparity, thyrotoxicosis, hyperparathyroidism, Cushing's syndrome, hyperprolactinemia, Type I diabetes), lifestyle (cigarette smoking, alcohol abuse, sedentary exercise habits) and nutrition (below average body weight, dietary calcium intake).

The mainstays of prevention and management of osteoporosis are estrogen, an adequate lifetime calcium intake, and exercise. Postmenopausal women absorb dietary calcium less efficiently than premenopausal women and require an average of 1500 mg/day of elemental calcium to remain in neutral calcium balance. By comparison, premenopausal women require about 1000 mg/day and the average calcium intake in the USA is 400-600 mg/day. Therefore, when not contraindicated, calcium supplementation may be helpful.

Weight-bearing exercise and nutrition may be important adjuncts to the prevention and management of osteoporosis. Immobilization and prolonged bed rest produce rapid bone loss, while weight-bearing exercise has been shown both to reduce bone loss and to increase bone mass. The optimal type and amount of physical activity that would prevent osteoporosis have not been established, however in two studies an hour of walking and running exercises twice or three times weekly significantly increased lumbar spine bone mass.

CONTRAINDICATIONS

Estrogens should not be used in individuals with any of the following conditions:

1. Known or suspected pregnancy (see BOXED WARNINGS). Estrogens may cause fetal harm when administered to a pregnant woman.
2. Undiagnosed abnormal genital bleeding.
3. Known or suspected cancer of the breast except in appropriately selected patients being treated for metastatic disease.
4. Known or suspected estrogen-dependent neoplasia.
5. Active thrombophlebitis or thromboembolic disorders.

WARNINGS

1. ***Induction of malignant neoplasms.***

Endometrial cancer. The reported endometrial cancer risk among unopposed estrogen users is about 2- to 12-fold greater than in nonusers, and appears dependent on duration of treatment and on estrogen dose. Most studies show no significant increased risk associated with use of estrogens for less than one year. The greatest risk appears associated with prolonged use—with increased risks of 15-to 24-fold for five to ten years or more. In three studies, persistence of risk was demonstrated for 8 to over 15 years after cessation of estrogen treatment. In one study a significant decrease in the incidence of endometrial cancer occurred six months after estrogen withdrawal. Concurrent progestin therapy may offset this risk but the overall health impact in postmenopausal women is not known (see PRECAUTIONS).

Breast cancer. While the majority of studies have not shown an increased risk of breast cancer in women who have ever used estrogen replacement therapy, some have reported a moderately increased risk (relative risks of 1.3- 2.0) in those taking higher doses or those taking lower doses for prolonged periods of time, especially in excess of 10 years. Other studies have not shown this relationship.

Congenital lesions with malignant potential. Estrogen therapy during pregnancy is associated with an increased risk of fetal congenital reproductive tract disorders, and possibly other birth defects. Studies of women who received DES during pregnancy have shown that female offspring have an increased risk of vaginal adenosis, squamous cell dysplasia of the uterine cervix, and clear cell vaginal cancer later in life; male offspring have an increased risk of urogenital abnormalities and possibly testicular cancer later in life. Although some of these changes are benign, others are precursors of malignancy.

2. ***Gallbladder disease.*** Two studies have reported a 2- to 4-fold increase in the risk of gallbladder disease requiring surgery in women receiving postmenopausal estrogens.

3. ***Cardiovascular disease.*** Large doses of estrogen (5 mg conjugated estrogens per day), comparable to those used to treat cancer of the prostate and breast, have been shown in a large prospective clinical trial in men to increase the risks of nonfatal myocardial infarction, pulmonary embolism, and thrombophlebitis. These risks cannot necessarily be extrapolated from men to women. However, to avoid the theoretical cardiovascular risk to women caused by high estrogen doses, the dose for estrogen replacement therapy should not exceed the lowest effective dose.

4. ***Elevated blood pressure.*** Occasional blood pressure increases during estrogen replacement therapy have been attributed to idiosyncratic reactions to estrogens. More often, blood pressure has remained the same or has dropped. One study showed that postmenopausal estrogen users have higher blood pressure than nonusers. Two other studies showed slightly lower blood pressure among estrogen users compared to nonusers. Postmenopausal estrogen use does not increase the risk of stroke. Nonetheless, blood pressure should be monitored at regular intervals with estrogen use.

5. ***Hypercalcemia.*** Administration of estrogens may lead to severe hypercalcemia in patients wtih breast cancer and bone metastases. If this occurs, the drug should be stopped and appropriate measures taken to reduce the serum calcium level.

PRECAUTIONS

A. *General*

1. **Addition of a progestin.** Studies of the addition of a progestin for seven or more days of a cycle of estrogen administration have reported a lowered incidence of endometrial hyperplasia which would otherwise be induced by estrogen treatment. Morphological and biochemical studies of endometrium suggest that 10 to 14 days of progestin are needed to provide maximal maturation of the endometrium and to eliminate any hyperplastic changes. There are possible additional risks which may be associated with the inclusion of progestins in estrogen replacement regimens. These include: (1) adverse effects on lipoprotein metabloism (lowering HDL and raising LDL) which may diminish the possible cardioprotective effect of estrogen therapy (see PRECAUTIONS, D.4., below); (2) impairment of glucose tolerance; and (3) possible enhancement of mitotic activity in breast epithelial tissue (although few epidemiological data are available to address this point). The choice of progestin, its dose, and its regimen may be important in minimizing these adverse effects, but these issues remain to be clarified.

2. **Physical examination.** A complete medical and family history should be taken prior to the initiation of any estrogen therapy. The pretreatment and periodic physical examinations should include special reference to blood pressure, breasts, abdomen, and pelvic organs, and should include a Papanicolaou smear. As a general rule, estrogen should not be prescribed for longer than one year without reexamining the patient.

3. **Hypercoagulability.** Some studies have shown that women taking estrogen replacement therapy have hypercoagulability, primarily related to decreased antithrombin activity. This effect appears dose- and duration-dependent and is less pronounced than that associated with oral contraceptive use. Also, postmenopausal women tend to have increased coagulation parameters at baseline compared to premenopausal women. There is some suggestion that low dose postmenopausal mestranol may increase the risk of thromboembolism, although the majority of studies (of primarily conjugated estrogens users) report no such increase. There is insufficient information on hypercoagulability in women who have had previous thromboembolic disease.

4. **Familial hyperlipoproteinemia.** Estrogen therapy may be associated with massive elevations of plasma triglycerides leading to pancreatitis and other complications in patients with familial defects of lipoprotein metabolism.

5. **Fluid retention.** Because estrogens may cause some degree of fluid retention, conditions which might be exacerbated by this factor, such as asthma, epilepsy, migraine, and cardiac or renal dysfunction, require careful observation.

6. **Uterine bleeding and mastodynia.** Certain patients may develop undesirable manifestations of estrogenic stimulation, such as abnormal uterine bleeding and mastodynia.

7. **Impaired liver function.** Estrogen may be poorly metabolized in patients with impaired liver function and should be administered with caution.

B. *Information for the Patient.* See text of Patient Package Insert below.

C. *Laboratory Tests.* Estrogen administration should generally be guided by clinical response at the smallest dose, rather than laboratory monitoring, for relief of symptoms for those indications in which symptoms are observable.

D. *Drug/Laboratory Test Interactions.*

Accelerated prothrombin time, partial thromboplastin time, and platelet aggregation time; increased platelet count; increased factors II, VII antigen, VIII antigen, VIII coagulant activity, IX, X, XII, VII—X complex, II—VII—X complex, and beta-thromboglobulin; decreased levels of anti-factor Xa and antithrombin III, decreased antithrombin III activity; increased levels of fibrinogen and fibrinogen activity; increased plasminogen antigen and activity.

Increased thyroid-binding globulin (TBG) leading to increased circulating total thyroid hormone, as measured by protein-bound iodine (PBI), T4 levels (by column or by radioimmunoassay) or T3 levels by radioimmunoassay. T3 resin uptake is decreased, reflecting the elevated TBG. Free T4 and free T3 concentrations are unaltered.

Other binding proteins may be elevated in serum, i.e., corticosteroid binding globulin (CBG), sex hormone-binding globulin (SHBG), leading to increased circulating corticosteroids and sex steroids respectively. Free or biologically active hormone concentrations are unchanged. Other plasma proteins may be increased (angiotensinogen/renin substrate, alpha-I-antitrypsin, ceruloplasmin).
Increased plasma HDL and HDL-2 subfraction concentrations, reduced LDL cholesterol concentration, increased triglycerides levels.
Impaired glucose tolerance.
Reduced response to metyrapone test.
Reduced serum folate concentration.
E. *Carcinogenesis, Mutagenesis, and Impairment of Fertility.* Long-term continuous administration of natural and synthetic estrogens in certain animal species increases the frequency of carcinomas of the breast, uterus, cervix, vagina, testis, and liver. See "CONTRAINDICATIONS" and "WARNINGS" sections.
F. *Pregnancy Category X.* Estrogens should not be used during pregnancy. See "CONTRAINDICATIONS" and BOXED WARNING.
G. *Nursing Mothers.* As a general principle, the administration of any drug to nursing mothers should be done only when clearly necessary since many drugs are excreted in human milk. In addition, estrogen administration to nursing mothers has been shown to decrease the quantity and quality of the milk.

ADVERSE REACTIONS

The following additional adverse reactions have been reported with estrogen therapy (see WARNINGS regarding induction of neoplasia, adverse effects on the fetus, increased incidence of gallbladder disease, cardiovascular disease, elevated blood pressure, and hypercalcemia).

1. *Genitourinary system.*
   Changes in vaginal bleeding pattern and abnormal withdrawal bleeding or flow; breakthrough bleeding, spotting.
   Increase in size of uterine leiomyomata.
   Vaginal candidiasis.
   Change in amount of cervical secretion.
2. *Breast.*
   Tenderness, enlargement.
3. *Gastrointestinal.*
   Nausea, vomiting.
   Abdominal cramps, bloating.
   Cholestatic jaundice.
   Increased incidence of gallbladder disease.
4. *Skin.*
   Chloasma or melasma that may persist when drug is discontinued.
   Erythema multiforme.
   Erythema nodosum.
   Hemorrhagic eruption.
   Loss of scalp hair.
   Hirsutism.
5. *Eyes.*
   Steepening of corneal curvature.
   Intolerance to contact lenses.
6. *Central Nervous System.*
   Headache, migraine, dizziness.
   Mental depression.
   Chorea.
7. *Miscellaneous.*
   Increase or decrease in weight.
   Reduced carbohydrate tolerance.
   Aggravation of porphyria.
   Edema.
   Changes in libido.

OVERDOSAGE

Serious ill effects have not been reported following acute ingestion of large doses of estrogen-containing oral contraceptives by young children. Overdosage of estrogen may cause nausea and vomiting, and withdrawal bleeding may occur in females.

DOSAGE AND ADMINISTRATION

1. For treatment of moderate to severe vasomotor symptoms, vulval and vaginal atrophy associated with the menopause, the lowest dose and regimen that will control symptoms should be chosen and medication should be discontinued as promptly as possible.
Attempts to discontinue or taper medication should be made at 3-month to 6-month intervals.
Usual dosage ranges:
Vasomotor symptoms—0.75 mg to 6 mg estropipate per day. The lowest dose that will control symptoms should be chosen. If the patient has not menstruated within the last two months or more, cyclic administration is started arbitrarily. If the patient is menstruating, cyclic administration is started on day 5 of bleeding.
Vulval and vaginal atrophy—0.75 mg to 6 mg estropipate daily, depending upon the tissue response of the individual patient. The lowest dose that will control symptoms should be chosen. Administer cyclically.
2. For treatment of female hypoestrogenism due to hypogonadism, castration, or primary ovarian failure.
Usual dosage ranges:
Female hypogonadism—A daily dose of 1.5 mg to 9 mg estropipate may be given for the first three weeks of a theoretical cycle, followed by a rest period of eight to ten days. The lowest dose that will control symptoms should be chosen. If bleeding does not occur by the end of this period, the same dosage schedule is repeated. The number of courses of estrogen therapy necessary to produce bleeding may vary depending on the responsiveness of the endometrium. If satisfactory withdrawal bleeding does not occur, an oral progestogen may be given in addition to estrogen during the third week of the cycle.
Female castration or primary ovarian failure—A daily dose of 1.5 mg to 9 mg estropipate may be given for the first three weeks of a theoretical cycle, followed by a rest period of eight to ten days. Adjust dosage upward or downward according to the severity of symptoms and response of the patient. For maintenance, adjust dosage to lowest level that will provide effective control.
Treated patients with an intact uterus should be monitored closely for signs of endometrial cancer and appropriate diagnostic measures should be taken to rule out malignancy in the event of persistent or recurring abnormal vaginal bleeding.
3. For prevention of osteoporosis. A daily dose of one ORTHO-EST .625 (0.75 mg estropipate) tablet for 25 days of a 31-day cycle per month.

HOW SUPPLIED

ORTHO-EST (estropipate tablets, USP) is supplied as ORTHO-EST .625 (0.75 mg estropipate; calculated as sodium estrone sulfate 0.625 mg), white, diamond-shaped tablets, scored on one side and imprinted with WFHC 101 on the other, NDC 64248-101-01; and ORTHO-EST 1.25 (1.5 mg estropipate; calculated as sodium estrone sulfate 1.25 mg), lavender, diamond-shaped tablets, scored on one side and imprinted with WFHC 102 on the other, NDC 64248-102-01. Both tablet sizes are available in bottles of 100.
Tablets are standardized to provide uniform estrone activity and are scored to provide dosage flexibility.
Dispense in tight, light-resistant containers as defined in the USP.
Store below 30°C (86°F).

PATIENT INFORMATION

WHAT YOU SHOULD KNOW ABOUT ESTROGENS

ORTHO-EST
(estropipate tablets, USP)

INTRODUCTION

This leaflet describes when and how to use estrogens, and the risks and benefits of estrogen treatment.
Estrogens have important benefits but also some risks. You must decide, with your doctor, whether the risks to you of estrogen use are acceptable because of their benefits. If you use estrogens, check with your doctor to be sure you are using the lowest possible dose that works, and that you do not use them longer than necessary. How long you need to use estrogens will depend on the reason for use.

WARNINGS
ESTROGENS INCREASE THE RISK OF CANCER OF THE UTERUS IN WOMEN WHO HAVE HAD THEIR MENOPAUSE ("CHANGE OF LIFE").
If you use any estrogen-containing drug, it is important to visit your doctor regularly and report any unusual vaginal bleeding right away. Vaginal bleeding after menopause may be a warning sign of uterine cancer. Your doctor should evaluate any unusual vaginal bleeding to find out the cause.
ESTROGENS SHOULD NOT BE USED DURING PREGNANCY.
Estrogens do not prevent miscarriage (spontaneous abortion) and are not needed in the days following childbirth. If you take estrogens during pregnancy, your unborn child has a greater than usual chance of having birth defects. The risk of developing these defects is small, but clearly larger than the risk in children whose mothers did not take estrogens during pregnancy. These birth defects may affect the baby's urinary system and sex organs. Daughters born to mothers who took DES (an estrogen drug) have a higher than usual chance of developing cancer of the vagina or cervix when they become teenagers or young adults. Sons may have a higher than usual chance of developing cancer of the testicles when they become teenagers or young adults.

USES OF ESTROGEN

(Not every estrogen drug is approved for every use listed in this section. If you want to know which of these possible uses are approved for the medicine prescribed for you, ask your doctor or pharmacist to show you the professional labeling. You can also look up the specific estrogen product in a book called the "Physicians' Desk Reference", which is available in many book stores and public libraries. Generic drugs carry virtually the same labeling information as their brand name versions.)

- **To reduce moderate or severe menopausal symptoms.** Estrogens are hormones made by the ovaries of normal women. Between ages 45 and 55, the ovaries normally stop making estrogens. This leads to a drop in body estrogen levels which causes the "change of life" or menopause (the end of monthly menstrual periods). If both ovaries are removed during an operation before natural menopause takes place, the sudden drop in estrogen levels causes "surgical menopause".

When the estrogen levels begin dropping, some women develop very uncomfortable symptoms, such as feelings of warmth in the face, neck, and chest, or sudden intense episodes of heat and sweating ("hot flashes" or "hot flushes"). Using estrogen drugs can help the body adjust to lower estrogen levels and reduce these symptoms. Most women have only mild menopausal symptoms or none at all and do not need to use estrogen drugs for these symptoms. Others may need to take estrogens for a few months while their bodies adjust to lower estrogen levels. The majority of women do not need estrogen replacement for longer than six months for these symptoms.

- **To treat vulval and vaginal atrophy** (itching, burning, dryness in or around the vagina, difficulty or burning on urination) associated with menopause.
- **To treat certain conditions in which a young women's ovaries do not produce enough estrogen naturally.**
- **To treat certain types of abnormal vaginal bleeding due to hormonal imbalance when your doctor has found no serious cause of the bleeding.**
- **To treat certain cancers in special situations, in men and women.**
- **To prevent thinning of bones.**

Osteoporosis is a thinning of the bones that makes them weaker and allows them to break more easily. The bones of the spine, wrists and hips break more often in osteoporosis. Both men and women start to lose bone mass after about age 40, but women lose bone mass faster after the menopause. Using estrogens after the menopause slows down bone thinning and may prevent bones from breaking. Lifelong adequate calcium intake, either in the diet (such as dairy products) or by calcium supplements (to reach a total daily intake of 1000 milligrams per day before menopause or 1500 milligrams per day after menopause), may help to prevent osteoporosis. Regular weight-bearing exercise (like walking and running for an hour, two or three times a week) may also help to prevent osteoporosis. Before you change your calcium intake or exercise habits, it is important to discuss these lifestyle changes with your doctor to find out if they are safe for you.
Since estrogen use has some risks, only women who are likely to develop osteoporosis should use estrogens for prevention. Women who are likely to develop osteoporosis often have the following characteristics: white or Asian race, slim, cigarette smokers, and a family history of osteoporosis in a mother, sister, or aunt. Women who have relatively early menopause, often because their ovaries were removed during an operation ("surgical menopause"), are more likely to develop osteoporosis than women whose menopause happens at the average age.

WHO SHOULD NOT USE ESTROGENS

Estrogens should not be used:

- **During pregnancy (see BOXED WARNING).**

If you think you may be pregnant, do not use any form of estrogen-containing drug. Using estrogens while you are pregnant may cause your unborn child to have birth defects. Estrogens do not prevent miscarriage.

- **If you have unusual vaginal bleeding which has not been evaluated by your doctor (see BOXED WARNING).**
- Unusual vaginal bleeding can be a warning sign of cancer of the uterus, especially if it happens after menopause. Your doctor must find out the cause of the bleeding so that he or she can recommend the proper treatment. Taking estrogens without visiting your doctor can cause you serious harm if your vaginal bleeding is caused by cancer of the uterus.
- **If you have had cancer.**

Since estrogens increase the risk of certain types of cancer, you should not use estrogens if you have ever had cancer of the breast or uterus, unless your doctor recommends that the drug may help in the cancer treatment. (For certain patients with breast or prostate cancer, estrogens may help.)

- **If you have any circulation problems.**

Estrogen drugs should not be used except in unusually special situations in which your doctor judges that you need estrogen therapy so much that the risks are acceptable. Men and women with abnormal blood clotting conditions should avoid estrogen use (see DANGERS OF ESTROGENS, below).

- **When they do not work.**

During menopause, some women develop nervous symptoms or depression. Estrogens do not relieve these symptoms. You may have heard that taking estrogens for years after menopause will keep your skin soft and supple and keep you feeling young. There is no evidence for these claims and such long-term estrogen use may have serious risks.

- **After childbirth or when breastfeeding a baby.**

Estrogens should not be used to try to stop the breasts from filling with milk after a baby is born. Such treatment may increase the risk of developing blood clots (see DANGERS OF ESTROGENS, below).
If you are breastfeeding, you should avoid using any drugs because many drugs pass through to the baby in the milk. While nursing a baby, you should take drugs only on the advice of your health care provider.

DANGERS OF ESTROGENS

- **Cancer of the uterus.**

Your risk of developing cancer of the uterus gets higher the longer you use estrogens and the larger doses you use. One study showed that after women stop taking estrogens, this higher cancer risk quickly returns to the usual level of risk (as if you had never used estogen therapy). Three other studies showed that the cancer risk stayed high for 8 to more than 15 years after stopping estrogen treatment. Be-

Continued on next page

Ortho-Est—Cont.

cause of this risk, IT IS IMPORTANT TO TAKE THE LOWEST DOSE THAT WORKS AND TO TAKE IT ONLY AS LONG AS YOU NEED IT.

Using progestin therapy together with estrogen therapy may reduce the higher risk of uterine cancer related to estrogen use (but see OTHER INFORMATION, below).

If you have had your uterus removed (total hysterectomy), there is no danger of developing cancer of the uterus.

• **Cancer of the breast.**

Most studies have not shown a higher risk of breast cancer in women who have ever used estrogens. However, some studies have reported that breast cancer developed more often (up to twice the usual rate) in women who used estrogens for long periods of time (especially more than 10 years), or who used higher doses for shorter time periods. Regular breast examinations by a health professional and monthly self-examination are recommended for all women.

• **Gallbladder disease.**

Women who use estrogens after menopause are more likely to develop gallbladder disease needing surgery than women who do not use estrogens.

• **Abnormal blood clotting.**

Taking estrogens may cause changes in your blood clotting system. These changes allow the blood to clot more easily, possibly allowing clots to form in your bloodstream. If blood clots do form in your bloodstream, they can cut off the blood supply to vital organs, causing serious problems. These problems may include a stroke (by cutting off blood to the brain), a heart attack (by cutting off blood to the heart), a pulmonary embolus (by cutting off blood to the lungs), or other problems. Any of these conditions may cause death or serious long-term disability. However, most studies of low dose estrogen usage by women do not show an increased risk of these complications.

SIDE EFFECTS

In addition to the risks listed above, the following side effects have been reported with estrogen use:

Nausea and vomiting

Breast tenderness or enlargement.

Enlargement of benign tumors ("fibroids") of the uterus.

Retention of excess fluid. This may make some conditions worsen, such as asthma, epilepsy, migraine, heart disease, or kidney disease.

A spotty darkening of the skin, particularly on the face.

REDUCING RISK OF ESTROGEN USE

If you use estrogens, you can reduce your risks by doing these things:

- **See your doctor regularly.** While you are using estrogens, it is important to visit your doctor at least once a year for a check up. If you develop vaginal bleeding while taking estrogens, you may need further evaluation. If members of your family have had breast cancer or if you have ever had breast lumps or an abnormal mammogram (breast X ray), you may need to have more frequent breast examinations.
- **Reassess your need for estrogens.** You and your doctor should reevaluate whether or not you still need estrogens at least every six months.
- **Be alert for signs of trouble.** If any of these warning signals (or any other unusual symptoms) happen while you are using estrogens, call your doctor immediately:

Abnormal bleeding from the vagina (possible uterine cancer).

Pains in the calves or chest, sudden shortness of breath, or coughing blood (possible clot in the legs, heart, or lungs).

Severe headache or vomiting, dizziness, faintness, changes in vision or speech, weakness or numbness of an arm or leg (possible clot in the brain or eye).

Breast lumps (possible breast cancer, ask your doctor or health professional to show you how to examine your breasts monthly).

Yellowing of the skin or eyes (possible liver problem).

Pain, swelling, or tenderness in the abdomen (possible gallbladder problem).

OTHER INFORMATION

Some doctors may choose to prescribe a progestin, a different hormonal drug, for you to take together with your estrogen treatment. Progestins lower your risk of developing endometrial hyperplasia (a possible pre-cancerous condition of the uterus) while using estrogens. Taking estrogens and progestins together may also protect you from the higher risk of uterine cancer, but this has not been clearly established. Combined use of progestin and estrogen treatment may have additional risks, however. The possible risks include unhealthy effects on blood fats (especially a lowering of HDL cholesterol, the "good" blood fat which protects against heart disease risk), unhealthy effects on blood sugar (which might worsen a diabetic condition), and a possible further increase in the breast cancer risk which may be associated with long-term estrogen use. The type of progestin drug used and its dosage schedule may be important in minimizing these effects.

Your doctor has prescribed this drug for you and you alone. Do not give the drug to anyone else.

If you will be taking calcium supplements as part of the treatment to help prevent osteoporosis, check with your doctor about how much to take.

Keep this and all drugs out of the reach of children. In case of overdose, call your doctor, hospital or poison control center immediately.

This leaflet provides a summary of the most important information about estrogens. If you want more information, ask your doctor or pharmacist to show you the professional labeling. The professional labeling is also published in a book called the "Physicians' Desk Reference," which is available in book stores and public libraries. Generic drugs carry virtually the same labeling information as their brand name versions.

HOW SUPPLIED

ORTHO-EST .625 (estropipate tablets USP, 0.75 mg) is a white, diamond-shaped tablet.

ORTHO-EST 1.25 (estropipate tablets USP, 1.5 mg) is a lavender, diamond-shaped tablet.

Distributed by:
Women First HealthCare, Inc.
San Diego, CA 92130
Manufactured by:
OMJ Pharmaceuticals, Inc.
Manati, Puerto Rico 00674
© OMJ 1998
634-20-181-1

Shown in Product Identification Guide, page 341

Wyeth-Ayerst Pharmaceuticals

Division of American Home Products Corporation
P.O. BOX 8299
PHILADELPHIA, PA 19101

Direct General Inquiries to:
(610) 688-4400

For Medical Information Contact:
Medical Affairs
Day: (800) 934-5556
8:30 AM to 4:30 PM (Eastern Standard Time),
Weekdays only

In Emergencies:
Day: (800) 934-5556
Night: (610) 688-4400
(Emergencies only;
non-emergencies should wait until the next day)

For prescribing information for products of Elkins-Sinn Incorporated, see page 1193 of the 2001 PDR; ESI Lederle Inc. see page 1218; Lederle Laboratories, see page 1653; and page 2707 for products of A.H. Robins Company. Information for these products can also be obtained by writing to Professional Service, Wyeth-Ayerst Pharmaceuticals, P.O. Box 8299, Philadelphia, PA 19101, or by contacting your local Wyeth-Ayerst representative.

Product Identification Codes

The following is a numerical list of National Drug Code (NDC) numbers with their corresponding product names for all oral solid dosage forms listed under Wyeth-Ayerst Pharmaceuticals.

Numerical Listing

PRODUCTS MANUFACTURED BY WYETH LABORATORIES

Product Ident. Code	Product
1	Equanil® (meprobamate) Tablet 400 mg. Ⓒ IV
2	Equanil® (meprobamate) Tablet 200 mg. Ⓒ IV
19	Phenergan® (promethazine HCl) Tablet 12.5 mg.
27	Phenergan® (promethazine HCl) Tablet 25 mg.
56	Ovral® (each tablet contains 0.5 mg. norgestrel with 0.05 mg. ethinyl estradiol) Tablet, white
62	Ovrette® (norgestrel) Tablet
64	Ativan® (lorazepam) Tablet 1 mg. Ⓒ IV
65	Ativan® (lorazepam) Tablet 2 mg. Ⓒ IV
73	Wytensin® (guanabenz acetate) Tablet 4 mg.
74	Wytensin® (guanabenz acetate) Tablet 8 mg.
78	Lo/Ovral® (each tablet contains 0.3 mg. norgestrel with 0.03 mg. ethinyl estradiol) Tablet, white
81	Ativan® (lorazepam) Tablet 0.5 mg. Ⓒ IV
85	Wygesic® (each tablet contains 65 mg. propoxyphene HCl, U.S.P., and 650 mg. acetaminophen, U.S.P.) Tablet Ⓒ IV
91	Equagesic® (meprobamate with aspirin) Tablet
227	Phenergan® (promethazine HCl) Tablet 50 mg.
261	Mepergan® Fortis (meperidine HCl and promethazine HCl) Capsule Ⓒ II
445	Ovral®-28 pink inert tablet
486	Lo/Ovral®-28 pink inert tablet
650	Alesse™-28 green inert tablet
690	Oruvail® (ketoprofen extended-release capsules) 200 mg.
701	Effexor® (venlafaxine HCl) Tablet 25 mg.
703	Effexor® (venlafaxine HCl) Tablet 50 mg.
704	Effexor® (venlafaxine HCl) Tablet 75 mg.
705	Effexor® (venlafaxine HCl) Tablet 100 mg.
771	Ismo® (isosorbide dinitrate) Tablet 20 mg.
781	Effexor® (venlafaxine HCl) Tablet 37.5 mg.
821	Oruvail® (ketoprofen extended-release capsules) 100 mg.
822	Oruvail® (ketoprofen extended-release capsules) 150 mg.
833	Effexor® XR (venlafaxine HCl) Extended-Release Capsules, 75 mg.
836	Effexor® XR (venlafaxine HCl) Extended-Release Capsules, 150 mg.
837	Effexor® XR (venlafaxine HCl) Extended-Release Capsules, 37.5 mg.
925	Sonata® (zaleplon) Capsule 5 mg
926	Sonata® (zaleplon) Capsule 10 mg
912	Alesse™ (each tablet contains 0.10 mg levonorgestrel and 0.02 mg ethinyl estradiol), pink
2511	Ovral®-28 Pilpak® (21 white tablets each containing 0.5 mg. norgestrel with 0.05 mg. ethinyl estradiol and 7 pink inert tablets)
2514	Lo/Ovral®-28 Pilpak® (21 white tablets each containing 0.3 mg. norgestrel with 0.03 mg. ethinyl estradiol and 7 pink inert tablets)
2535	Triphasil®-21 Tablets (levonorgestrel and ethinyl estradiol tablets—triphasic regimen)
2536	Triphasil®-28 Tablets (levonorgestrel and ethinyl estradiol tablets—triphasic regimen)
4126	Isordil® Sublingual Tablet 5 mg
4130	Trecator®-SC (ethionamide) Tablet 250 mg
4132	Surmontil® (trimipramine maleate) Capsule 25 mg
4133	Surmontil® (trimipramine maleate) Capsule 50 mg
4139	Isordil® (isosorbide dinitrate) Sublingual Tablet 2.5 mg
4152	Isordil® (isosorbide dinitrate) 5 Titradose Tablet 5 mg
4153	Isordil® (isosorbide dinitrate) 10 Titradose Tablet 10 mg
4154	Isordil® (isosorbide dinitrate) 20 Titradose Tablet 20 mg
4158	Surmontil® (trimipramine) Capsule 100 mg
4159	Isordil® (isosorbide dinitrate) 30 Titradose Tablet 30 mg
4161	Isordil® (isosorbide dinitrate) Sublingual Tablet 10 mg
4177	Sectral® (acebutolol HCl) Capsule 200 mg
4179	Sectral® (acebutolol HCl) Capsule 400 mg
4181	Orudis® (ketoprofen capsule) 50 mg
4186	Orudis® (ketoprofen capsule) 25 mg
4187	Orudis® (ketoprofen capsule) 75 mg
4188	Cordarone® (amiodarone) Tablet 200 mg
4191	Synalgos®-DC (each capsule contains 16 mg. dihydrocodeine bitartrate, 356.4 mg. aspirin, and 30 mg. caffeine) Capsule
4192	Isordil® (isosorbide dinitrate) 40 Titradose Tablet 40 mg

PRODUCTS MANUFACTURED BY AYERST LABORATORIES INC.

Product Ident. Code	Product
243	Atromid-S® (clofibrate) Capsule 500 mg.
421	Inderal® (propranolol HCl) Tablet 10 mg.
422	Inderal® (propranolol HCl) Tablet 20 mg.
424	Inderal® (propranolol HCl) Tablet 40 mg.
426	Inderal® (propranolol HCl) Tablet 60 mg.
428	Inderal® (propranolol HCl) Tablet 80 mg.
443	Grisactin® 250 (griseofulvin, microsize) Capsule 250 mg.
444	Grisactin® 500 (griseofulvin, microsize) Tablet 500 mg.
455	Inderide® LA (each capsule contains 80 mg. Inderal® LA [propranolol HCl] and 50 mg. hydrochlorothiazide) Capsule
457	Inderide® LA (each capsule contains 120 mg. Inderal® LA [propranolol HCl] and 50 mg. hydrochlorothiazide) Capsule
459	Inderide® LA (each capsule contains 160 mg. Inderal® LA [propranolol HCl] and 50 mg. hydrochlorothiazide) Capsule
470	Inderal® LA (propranolol HCl) Capsule 60 mg.
471	Inderal® LA (propranolol HCl) Capsule 80 mg.
473	Inderal® LA (propranolol HCl) Capsule 120 mg.
479	Inderal® LA (propranolol HCl) Capsule 160 mg.
484	Inderide® (each tablet contains 40 mg. Inderal® [propranolol HCl] and 25 mg. hydrochlorothiazide) Tablet
488	Inderide® (each tablet contains 80 mg. Inderal® [propranolol HCl] and 25 mg. hydrochlorothiazide) Tablet
702	Diucardin® (hydroflumethiazide) Tablet 50 mg.
738	Lodine® (etodolac capsule) 200 mg.
739	Lodine® (etodolac capsule) 300 mg.
761	Lodine® (etodolac tablet) 400 mg.
787	Lodine® (etodolac tablet) 500 mg.
809	Antabuse® (disulfiram) Tablet 250 mg.
829	Lodine® XL (etodolac extended-release tablet) 400 mg.
831	Lodine® XL (etodolac extended-release tablet) 600 mg.
839	Lodine® XL (etodolac extended-release tablet) 500 mg.
864	Premarin® (conjugated estrogens tablets, USP) Tablet 0.9 mg.
865	Premarin® (conjugated estrogens tablets, USP) Tablet 2.5 mg.
866	Premarin® (conjugated estrogens tablets, USP) Tablet 1.25 mg.

867 Premarin® (conjugated estrogens tablets, USP) Tablet 0.625 mg.

868 Premarin® (conjugated estrogens tablets, USP) Tablet 0.3 mg.

875 Prempro™ (conjugated estrogens/medroxyprogesterone acetate 0.625 mg./2.5 mg. [continuous regimen] Tablets)

975 Prempro™ (conjugated estrogens/medroxyprogesterone acetate 0.625 mg./5 mg. [continuous regimen] Tablets)

2573 Premphase® (conjugated estrogens/medroxyprogesterone acetate 0.625 mg./5 mg. [cyclic regimen] Tablets)

ALESSE™-21 Tablets ℞

[ă 'lĕs]

levonorgestrel and ethinyl estradiol tablets

Patients should be counseled that this product does not protect against HIV infection (AIDS) and other sexually transmitted diseases.

DESCRIPTION

21 pink active tablets each containing 0.10 mg of levonorgestrel, d(-)-13β-ethyl-17α-ethinyl-17β-hydroxygon-4-en-3-one, a totally synthetic progestogen, and 0.02 mg of ethinyl estradiol, 17α-ethinyl-1,3,5(10)-estratriene-3, 17β-diol. The inactive ingredients present are cellulose, hydroxypropyl methylcellulose, iron oxide, lactose, magnesium stearate, polacrilin potassium, polyethylene glycol, titanium dioxide, and wax E.

Levonorgestrel

Ethinyl Estradiol

CLINICAL PHARMACOLOGY

Combination oral contraceptives act by suppression of gonadotropins. Although the primary mechanism of this action is inhibition of ovulation, other alterations include changes in the cervical mucus (which increase the difficulty of sperm entry into the uterus) and the endometrium (which reduce the likelihood of implantation).

PHARMACOKINETICS

Absorption

No specific investigation of the absolute bioavailability of Alesse in humans has been conducted. However, literature indicates that levonorgestrel is rapidly and completely absorbed after oral administration (bioavailability about 100%) and is not subject to first-pass metabolism. Ethinyl estradiol is rapidly and almost completely absorbed from the gastrointestinal tract but, due to first-pass metabolism in gut mucosa and liver, the bioavailability of ethinyl estradiol is between 38% and 48%.

After a single dose of Alesse to 22 women under fasting conditions, maximum serum concentrations of levonorgestrel are 2.8 ± 0.9 ng/mL (mean ± SD) at 1.6 ± 0.9 hours. At steady state, attained from day 19 onwards, maximum levonorgestrel concentrations of 6.0 ± 2.7 ng/mL are reached at 1.5 ± 0.5 hours after the daily dose. The minimum serum levels of levonorgestrel at steady state are 1.9 ± 1.0 ng/mL. Observed levonorgestrel concentrations increased from day 1 (single dose) to days 6 and 21 (multiple doses) by 34% and 96%, respectively (Figure 1). Unbound levonorgestrel concentrations increased from day 1 to days 6 and 21 by 25% and 83%, respectively. The kinetics of total levonorgestrel are non-linear due to an increase in binding of levonorgestrel to sex hormone binding globulin (SHBG), which is attributed to increased SHBG levels that are induced by the daily administration of ethinyl estradiol.

Following a single dose, maximum serum concentrations of ethinyl estradiol of 62 ± 21 pg/mL are reached at 1.5 ± 0.5 hours. At steady state, attained from at least day 6 onwards, maximum concentrations of ethinyl estradiol were 77 ± 30 pg/mL and were reached at 1.3 ± 0.7 hours after the daily dose. The minimum serum levels of ethinyl estradiol at steady state are 10.5 ± 5.1 pg/mL. Ethinyl estradiol concentrations did not increase from days 1 to 6, but did increase by 19% from days 1 to 21 (Figure 1).

[See figure 1 above]

Table I provides a summary of levonorgestrel and ethinyl estradiol pharmacokinetic parameters.

[See table 1 above]

Distribution

Levonorgestrel in serum is primarily bound to SHBG. Ethinyl estradiol is about 97% bound to plasma albumin. Ethinyl estradiol does not bind to SHBG, but induces SHBG synthesis.

FIGURE 1

Mean (SE) levonorgestrel and ethinyl estradiol serum concentrations in 22 subjects receiving Alesse (100 µg levonorgestrel and 20 µg ethinyl estradiol)

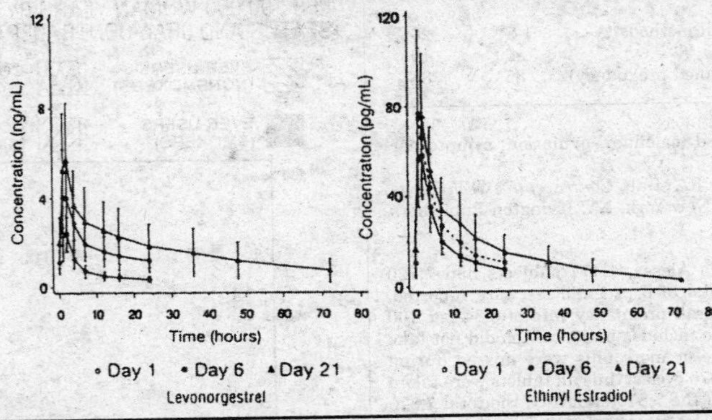

TABLE 1: MEAN (SD) PHARMACOKINETIC PARAMETERS OF ALESSE OVER A 21-DAY DOSING PERIOD

Day	C_{max} ng/mL	T_{max} h	AUC ng·h/mL	CL/F mL/h/kg	Vλz/F L/kg	SHBG nmol/L
			Levonorgestrel			
1	2.75 (0.88)	1.6 (0.9)	35.2 (12.8)	53.7 (20.8)	2.66 (1.09)	57 (18)
6	4.52 (1.79)	1.5 (0.7)	46.0 (18.8)	40.8 (14.5)	2.05 (0.86)	81 (25)
21	6.00 (2.65)	1.5 (0.5)	68.3 (32.5)	28.4 (10.3)	1.43 (0.62)	93 (40)
			Unbound Levonorgestrel			
	pg/mL	h	pg·h/mL	L/h/kg	L/kg	fu %
1	51.2 (12.9)	1.6 (0.9)	654 (201)	2.79 (0.97)	135.9 (41.8)	1.92 (0.30)
6	77.9 (22.0)	1.5 (0.7)	794 (240)	2.24 (0.59)	112.4 (40.5)	1.80 (0.24)
21	103.6 (36.9)	1.5 (0.5)	1177 (452)	1.57 (0.49)	78.6 (29.7)	1.78 (0.19)
			Ethinyl Estradiol			
	pg/mL	h	pg·h/mL	mL/h/kg	L/kg	
1	62.0 (20.5)	1.5 (0.5)	653 (227)	567 (204)	14.3 (3.7)	
6	76.7 (29.9)	1.3 (0.7)	604 (231)	610 (196)	15.5 (4.0)	
21	82.3 (33.2)	1.4 (0.6)	776 (308)	486 (179)	12.4 (4.1)	

Metabolism

Levonorgestrel: The most important metabolic pathway occurs in the reduction of the Δ4-3-oxo group and hydroxylation at positions 2α, 1β, and 16β, followed by conjugation. Most of the metabolites that circulate in the blood are sulfates of 3α,5β-tetrahydro-levonorgestrel, while excretion occurs predominantly in the form of glucuronides. Some of the parent levonorgestrel also circulates as 17β-sulfate. Metabolic clearance rates may differ among individuals by several-fold, and this may account in part for the wide variation observed in levonorgestrel concentrations among users.

Ethinyl estradiol: Cytochrom P450 enzymes (CYP3A4) in the liver are responsible for the 2-hydroxylation that is the major oxidative reaction. The 2-hydroxy metabolite is further transformed by methylation and glucuronidation prior to urinary and fecal excretion. Levels of Cytochrome P450 (CYP3A) vary widely among individuals and can explain the variation in rates of ethinyl estradiol 2-hydroxylation. Ethinyl estradiol is excreted in the urine and feces as glucuronide and sulfate conjugates, and undergoes enterohepatic circulation.

Excretion

The elimination half-life for levonorgestrel is approximately 36 ± 13 hours at steady state. Levonorgestrel and its metabolites are primarily excreted in the urine (40% to 68%) and about 16% to 48% are excreted in feces. The elimination half-life of ethinyl estradiol is 18 ± 4.7 hours at steady state.

SPECIAL POPULATIONS

Race

Based on the pharmacokinetic study with Alesse, there are no apparent differences in pharmacokinetic parameters among women of different races.

Hepatic Insufficiency

No formal studies have evaluated the effect of hepatic disease on the disposition of Alesse. However, steroid hormones may be poorly metabolized in patients with impaired liver function.

Renal Insufficiency

No formal studies have evaluated the effect of renal disease on the disposition of Alesse.

Drug-Drug Interactions

Interactions between ethinyl estradiol and other drugs have been reported in the literature.

- *Interactions with Absorption:* Diarrhea may increase gastrointestinal motility and reduce hormone absorption. Similarly, any drug which reduces gut transit time may reduce hormone concentrations in the blood.
- *Interactions with Metabolism:*
  Gastrointestinal wall: Sulfation of ethinyl estradiol has been shown to occur in the gastrointestinal (GI) wall. Therefore, drugs which act as competitive inhibitors for sulfation in the GI wall may increase ethinyl estradiol bioavailability (e.g., ascorbic acid).
  Hepatic metabolism: Interactions can occur with drugs that induce microsomal enzymes which can decrease ethinyl estradiol concentrations (e.g., rifampin, barbiturates, phenylbutazone, phenytoin, griseofulvin).
- *Interference with Enterohepatic Circulation:* Some clinical reports suggest that enterohepatic circulation of estrogens may decrease when certain antibiotic agents are given, which may reduce ethinyl estradiol concentrations (e.g., ampicillin, tetracycline).
- *Interference in the Metabolism of Other Drugs:* Ethinyl estradiol may interfere with the metabolism of other drugs by inhibiting hepatic microsomal enzymes or by inducing hepatic drug conjugation, particularly glucuronidation. Accordingly, plasma and tissue concentrations may either be increased or decreased, respectively (e.g., cyclosporin, theophylline).

INDICATIONS AND USAGE

Oral contraceptives are indicated for the prevention of pregnancy in women who elect to use this product as a method of contraception.

Oral contraceptives are highly effective. Table II lists the typical accidental pregnancy rates for users of combination oral contraceptives and other methods of contraception. The efficacy of these contraceptive methods, except sterilization, the IUD, and Norplant® System, depends upon the reliability with which they are used. Correct and consistent use of methods can result in lower failure rates.

TABLE II: PERCENTAGE OF WOMEN EXPERIENCING AN UNINTENDED PREGNANCY DURING THE FIRST YEAR OF USE OF A CONTRACEPTIVE METHOD

Method	Perfect Use	Typical Use
Norplant® System (6 capsules)	0.1	0.1
Male sterilization	0.1	0.15
Female sterilization	0.4	0.4
Depo-Provera® (injectable progestogen)	0.3	0.3
Oral contraceptives		
Combined	0.1	NA
Progestin only	0.5	NA
IUD		
Progesterone	1.5	2.0
Copper T 380A	0.6	0.8
Condom (male) without spermicide	3	12
(female) without spermicide	5	21
Cervical cap		
Nulliparous women	9	18
Parous women	26	36
Diaphragm with spermicidal cream or jelly	6	18
Spermicides alone (foam, creams, jellies, and vaginal suppositories)	6	21

Continued on next page

Alesse-21—Cont.

Periodic abstinence (all methods)	1-9*	20
Withdrawal	4	19
No contraception (planned pregnancy)	85	85

NA - not available
*Depending on method (calendar, ovulation, symptothermal, post-ovulation)
Adapted from Hatcher RA et al., *Contraceptive Technology*, 16th Revised Edition. New York, NY: Irvington Publishers, 1994.

In a clinical trial with Alesse, 1,477 subjects had 7,720 cycles of use and a total of 5 pregnancies were reported. This represents an overall pregnancy rate of 0.84 per 100 woman-years. This rate includes patients who did not take the drug correctly. One or more pills were missed during 1,479 (18.8%) of the 7,870 cycles; thus all tablets were taken during 6,391 (81.2%) of the 7,870 cycles. Of the total 7,870 cycles, a total of 150 cycles were excluded from the calculation of the Pearl index due to the use of backup contraception and/or missing 3 or more consecutive pills.

CONTRAINDICATIONS

Oral contraceptives should not be used in women with any of the following conditions:
Thrombophlebitis or thromboembolic disorders
A past history of deep-vein thrombophlebitis or thromboembolic disorders
Cerebrovascular or coronary artery disease
Known or suspected carcinoma of the breast
Carcinoma of the endometrium or other known or suspected estrogen-dependent neoplasia
Undiagnosed abnormal genital bleeding
Cholestatic jaundice of pregnancy or jaundice with prior pill use
Hepatic adenomas or carcinomas
Known or suspected pregnancy

WARNINGS

Cigarette smoking increases the risk of serious cardiovascular side effects from oral-contraceptive use. This risk increases with age and with heavy smoking (15 or more cigarettes per day) and is quite marked in women over 35 years of age. Women who use oral contraceptives should be strongly advised not to smoke.

The use of oral contraceptives is associated with increased risks of several serious conditions including myocardial infarction, thromboembolism, stroke, hepatic neoplasia, gallbladder disease, and hypertension, although the risk of serious morbidity or mortality is very small in healthy women without underlying risk factors. The risk of morbidity and mortality increases significantly in the presence of other underlying risk factors such as hypertension, hyperlipidemias, obesity and diabetes.
Practitioners prescribing oral contraceptives should be familiar with the following information relating to these risks.
The information contained in this package insert is principally based on studies carried out in patients who used oral contraceptives with higher formulations of estrogens and progestogens than those in common use today. The effect of long-term use of the oral contraceptives with lower doses of both estrogens and progestogens remains to be determined.
Throughout this labeling, epidemiological studies reported are of two types: retrospective or case control studies and prospective or cohort studies. Case control studies provide a measure of the relative risk of disease, namely, a ratio of the incidence of a disease among oral-contraceptive users to that among nonusers. The relative risk does not provide information on the actual clinical occurrence of a disease. Cohort studies provide a measure of attributable risk, which is the difference in the incidence of disease between oral-contraceptive users and nonusers. The attributable risk does provide information about the actual occurrence of a disease in the population. For further information, the reader is referred to a text on epidemiological methods.

1. THROMBOEMBOLIC DISORDERS AND OTHER VASCULAR PROBLEMS

a. *Myocardial Infarction*
An increased risk of myocardial infarction has been attributed to oral-contraceptive use. This risk is primarily in smokers or women with other underlying risk factors for coronary-artery disease such as hypertension, hypercholesterolemia, morbid obesity, and diabetes. The relative risk of heart attack for current oral-contraceptive users has been estimated to be two to six. The risk is very low under the age of 30.
Smoking in combination with oral-contraceptive use has been shown to contribute substantially to the incidence of myocardial infarction in women in their mid-thirties or older with smoking accounting for the majority of excess cases. Mortality rates associated with circulatory disease have been shown to increase substantially in smokers over the age of 35 and nonsmokers over the age of 40 (Table III) among women who use oral contraceptives.
[See figure at top of next column]

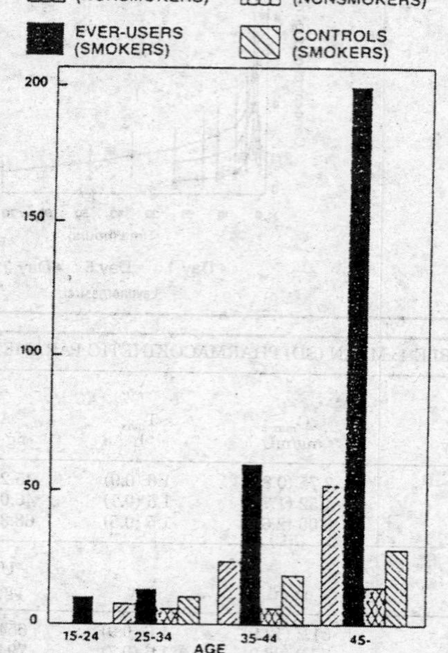

TABLE III (Adapted from P.M. Layde and V. Beral, Lancet, I: 541-546, 1981.)

Oral contraceptives may compound the effects of well-known risk factors, such as hypertension, diabetes, hyperlipidemias, age and obesity. In particular, some progestogens are known to decrease HDL cholesterol and cause glucose intolerance, while estrogens may create a state of hyperinsulinism. Oral contraceptives have been shown to increase blood pressure among users (see section 9 in **"Warnings"**). Similar effects on risk factors have been associated with an increased risk of heart disease. Oral contraceptives must be used with caution in women with cardiovascular disease risk factors.

b. *Thromboembolism*
An increased risk of thromboembolic and thrombotic disease associated with the use of oral contraceptives is well established. Case control studies have found the relative risk of users compared to non-users to be 3 for the first episode of superficial venous thrombosis, 4 to 11 for deep-vein thrombosis or pulmonary embolism, and 1.5 to 6 for women with predisposing conditions for venous thromboembolic disease. Cohort studies have shown the relative risk to be somewhat lower, about 3 for new cases and about 4.5 for new cases requiring hospitalization. The risk of thromboembolic disease due to oral contraceptives is not related to length of use and disappears after pill use is stopped.
A two- to four-fold increase in relative risk of postoperative thromboembolic complications has been reported with the use of oral contraceptives. The relative risk of venous thrombosis in women who have predisposing conditions is twice that of women without such medical conditions. If feasible, oral contraceptives should be discontinued at least four weeks prior to and for two weeks after elective surgery of a type associated with an increase in risk of thromboembolism and during and following prolonged immobilization. Since the immediate postpartum period is also associated with an increased risk of thromboembolism, oral contraceptives should be started no earlier than four to six weeks after delivery in women who elect not to breast-feed, or a midtrimester pregnancy termination.

c. *Cerebrovascular diseases*
Oral contraceptives have been shown to increase both the relative and attributable risks of cerebrovascular events (thrombotic and hemorrhagic strokes), although, in general, the risk is greatest among older (>35 years), hypertensive women who also smoke. Hypertension was found to be a risk factor for both users and nonusers, for both types of strokes, while smoking interacted to increase the risk for hemorrhagic strokes.
In a large study, the relative risk of thrombotic strokes has been shown to range from 3 for normotensive users to 14 for users with severe hypertension. The relative risk of hemorrhagic stroke is reported to be 1.2 for nonsmokers who used oral contraceptives, 2.6 for smokers who did not use oral contraceptives, 7.6 for smokers who used oral contraceptives, 1.8 for normotensive users and 25.7 for users with severe hypertension. The attributable risk is also greater in older women.

d. *Dose-related risk of vascular disease from oral contraceptives*
A positive association has been observed between the amount of estrogen and progestogen in oral contraceptives and the risk of vascular disease. A decline in serum high-density lipoproteins (HDL) has been reported with many progestational agents. A decline in serum high-density lipoproteins has been associated with an increased incidence of ischemic heart disease. Because estrogens increase HDL cholesterol, the net effect of an oral contraceptive depends on a balance achieved between doses of estrogen and progestogen and the nature and absolute amount of progestogen used in the contraceptive. The amount of both hormones should be considered in the choice of an oral contraceptive.
Minimizing exposure to estrogen and progestogen is in keeping with good principles of therapeutics. For any particular estrogen/progestogen combination, the dosage regimen prescribed should be one which contains the least amount of estrogen and progestogen that is compatible with a low failure rate and the needs of the individual patient. New acceptors of oral-contraceptive agents should be started on preparations containing less than 50 mcg of estrogen.

e. *Persistence of risk of vascular disease*
There are two studies which have shown persistence of risk of vascular disease for ever-users of oral contraceptives. In a study in the United States, the risk of developing myocardial infarction after discontinuing oral contraceptives persists for at least 9 years for women 40–49 years who had used oral contraceptives for five or more years, but this increased risk was not demonstrated in other age groups. In another study in Great Britain, the risk of developing cerebrovascular disease persisted for at least 6 years after discontinuation of oral contraceptives, although excess risk was very small. However, both studies were performed with oral contraceptive formulations containing 50 micrograms or higher of estrogens.

2. ESTIMATES OF MORTALITY FROM CONTRACEPTIVE USE

One study gathered data from a variety of sources which have estimated the mortality rate associated with different methods of contraception at different ages (Table IV). These estimates include the combined risk of death associated with contraceptive methods plus the risk attributable to pregnancy in the event of method failure. Each method of contraception has its specific benefits and risks. The study concluded that with the exception of oral-contraceptive users 35 and older who smoke and 40 and older who do not smoke, mortality associated with all methods of birth control is less than that associated with childbirth. The observation of a possible increase in risk of mortality with age for oral-contraceptive users is based on data gathered in the 1970's—but not reported until 1983. However, current clinical practice involves the use of lower estrogen dose formulations combined with careful restriction of oral-contraceptive use to women who do not have the various risk factors listed in this labeling.
Because of these changes in practice and, also, because of some limited new data which suggest that the risk of cardiovascular disease with the use of oral contraceptives may now be less than previously observed, the Fertility and Maternal Health Drugs Advisory Committee was asked to review the topic in 1989. The Committee concluded that although cardiovascular disease risks may be increased with oral-contraceptive use after age 40 in healthy nonsmoking women (even with the newer low-dose formulations), there are greater potential health risks associated with pregnancy in older women and with the alternative surgical and medical procedures which may be necessary if such women do not have assess to effective and acceptable means of contraception.
Therefore, the Committee recommended that the benefits of oral-contraceptive use by healthy nonsmoking women over 40 may outweigh the possible risks. Of course, older women, as all women who take oral contraceptives, should take the lowest possible dose formulation that is effective.

TABLE IV: ANNUAL NUMBER OF BIRTH-RELATED OR METHOD-RELATED DEATHS ASSOCIATED WITH CONTROL OF FERTILITY PER 100,000 NONSTERILE WOMEN, BY FERTILITY-CONTROL METHOD AND ACCORDING TO AGE

Method of control and outcome	15-19	20-24	25-29	30-34	35-39	40-44
No fertility-control methods*	7.0	7.4	9.1	14.8	25.7	28.2
Oral contraceptives nonsmoker**	0.3	0.5	0.9	1.9	13.8	31.6
Oral contraceptives smoker**	2.2	3.4	6.6	13.5	51.1	117.2
IUD**	0.8	0.8	1.0	1.0	1.4	1.4
Condom*	1.1	1.6	0.7	0.2	0.3	0.4
Diaphragm/ spermicide*	1.9	1.2	1.2	1.3	2.2	2.8
Periodic abstinence*	2.5	1.6	1.6	1.7	2.9	3.6

* Deaths are birth related
** Deaths are method related
Adapted from H.W. Ory, Family Planning Perspectives, *15*: 57-63, 1983.

3. CARCINOMA OF THE REPRODUCTIVE ORGANS

Numerous epidemiological studies have been performed on the incidence of breast, endometrial, ovarian and cervical cancer in women using oral contraceptives. The overwhelming evidence in the literature suggests that use of oral contraceptives is not associated with an increase in the risk of developing breast cancer, regardless of the age and parity of first use or with most of the marketed brands and doses. The Cancer and Steroid Hormone (CASH) study also showed no latent effect on the risk of breast cancer for at least a decade following long-term use. A few studies have shown a slightly increased relative risk of developing breast cancer, although the methodology of these studies, which included differences in examination of users and nonusers and differences in age at start of use, has been questioned. Some studies suggest that oral-contraceptive use has been associated with an increase in the risk of cervical intraepithelial neoplasia in some populations of women. However, there continues to be controversy about the extent to which such findings may be due to differences in sexual behavior and other factors.

In spite of many studies of the relationship between oral-contraceptive use and breast and cervical cancers, a cause-and-effect relationship has not been established.

4. HEPATIC NEOPLASIA

Benign hepatic adenomas are associated with oral-contraceptive use, although the incidence of these benign tumors is rare in the United States. Indirect calculations have estimated the attributable risk to be in the range of 3.3 cases/100,000 for users, a risk that increases after four or more years of use. Rupture of rare, benign, hepatic adenomas may cause death through intra-abdominal hemorrhage.

Studies from Britain have shown an increased risk of developing hepatocellular carcinoma in long-term (>8 years) oral-contraceptive users. However, these cancers are extremely rare in the U.S. and the attributable risk (the excess incidence) of liver cancers in oral-contraceptive users approaches less than one per million users.

5. OCULAR LESIONS

There have been clinical case reports of retinal thrombosis associated with the use of oral contraceptives. Oral contraceptives should be discontinued if there is unexplained partial or complete loss of vision; onset of proptosis or diplopia; papilledema; or retinal vascular lesions. Appropriate diagnostic and therapeutic measures should be undertaken immediately.

6. ORAL-CONTRACEPTIVE USE BEFORE OR DURING EARLY PREGNANCY

Extensive epidemiological studies have revealed no increased risk of birth defects in women who have used oral contraceptives prior to pregnancy. Studies also do not suggest a teratogenic effect, particularly in so far as cardiac anomalies and limb-reduction defects are concerned, when taken inadvertently during early pregnancy.

The administration of oral contraceptives to induce withdrawal bleeding should not be used as a test for pregnancy. Oral contraceptives should not be used during pregnancy to treat threatened or habitual abortion.

It is recommended that for any patient who has missed two consecutive periods, pregnancy should be ruled out before continuing oral-contraceptive use. If the patient has not adhered to the prescribed schedule, the possibility of pregnancy should be considered at the time of the first missed period. Oral-contraceptive use should be discontinued if pregnancy is confirmed.

7. GALLBLADDER DISEASE

Earlier studies have reported an increased lifetime relative risk of gallbladder surgery in users of oral contraceptives and estrogens. More recent studies, however, have shown that the relative risk of developing gallbladder disease among oral-contraceptive users may be minimal. The recent findings of minimal risk may be related to the use of oral-contraceptive formulations containing lower hormonal doses of estrogens and progestogens.

8. CARBOHYDRATE AND LIPID METABOLIC EFFECTS

Oral contraceptives have been shown to cause glucose intolerance in a significant percentage of users. Oral contraceptives containing greater than 75 micrograms of estrogens cause hyperinsulinism, while lower doses of estrogen cause less glucose intolerance. Progestogens increase insulin secretion and create insulin resistance, this effect varying with different progestational agents. However, in the nondiabetic woman, oral contraceptives appear to have no effect on fasting blood glucose. Because of these demonstrated effects, prediabetic and diabetic women should be carefully observed while taking oral contraceptives.

A small proportion of women will have persistent hypertriglyceridemia while on the pill. As discussed earlier (see "**Warnings**" 1a. and 1d.), changes in serum triglycerides and lipoprotein levels have been reported in oral-contraceptive users.

9. ELEVATED BLOOD PRESSURE

An increase in blood pressure has been reported in women taking oral contraceptives and this increase is more likely in older oral-contraceptive users and with continued use. Data from the Royal College of General Practitioners and subsequent randomized trials have shown that the incidence of hypertension increases with increasing quantities of progestogens.

Women with a history of hypertension or hypertension-related diseases, or renal disease should be encouraged to use another method of contraception. If women with hypertension elect to use oral contraceptives, they should be monitored closely and if significant elevation of blood pressure occurs, oral contraceptives should be discontinued. For most women, elevated blood pressure will return to normal after stopping oral contraceptives, and there is no difference in the occurrence of hypertension among ever- and never-users.

10. HEADACHE

The onset or exacerbation of migraine or development of headache with a new pattern that is recurrent, persistent or severe requires discontinuation of oral contraceptives and evaluation of the cause.

11. BLEEDING IRREGULARITIES

Breakthrough bleeding and spotting are sometimes encountered in patients on oral contraceptives, especially during the first three months of use. The type and dose of progestogen may be important. Nonhormonal causes should be considered and adequate diagnostic measures taken to rule out malignancy or pregnancy in the event of breakthrough bleeding, as in the case of any abnormal vaginal bleeding. If pathology has been excluded, time or a change to another formulation may solve the problem. In the event of amenorrhea, pregnancy should be ruled out.

Some women may encounter post-pill amenorrhea or oligomenorrhea, especially when such a condition was preexistent.

PRECAUTIONS

Patients should be counseled that this product does not protect against HIV infection (AIDS) and other sexually transmitted diseases.

1. PHYSICAL EXAMINATION AND FOLLOW-UP

A periodic history and physical examination is appropriate for all women, including women using oral contraceptives. The physical examination, however, may be deferred until after initiation of oral contraceptives if requested by the woman and judged appropriate by the clinician. The physical examination should include special reference to blood pressure, breasts, abdomen and pelvic organs, including cervical cytology, and relevant laboratory tests. In case of undiagnosed, persistent or recurrent abnormal vaginal bleeding, appropriate diagnostic measures should be conducted to rule out malignancy. Women with a strong family history of breast cancer or who have breast nodules should be monitored with particular care.

2. LIPID DISORDERS

Women who are being treated for hyperlipidemias should be followed closely if they elect to use oral contraceptives. Some progestogens may elevate LDL levels and may render the control of hyperlipidemias more difficult. (See "**Warnings**," 1d.)

3. LIVER FUNCTION

If jaundice develops in any woman receiving such drugs, the medication should be discontinued. Steroid hormones may be poorly metabolized in patients with impaired liver function.

4. FLUID RETENTION

Oral contraceptives may cause some degree of fluid retention. They should be prescribed with caution, and only with careful monitoring, in patients with conditions which might be aggravated by fluid retention.

5. EMOTIONAL DISORDERS

Patients becoming significantly depressed while taking oral contraceptives should stop the medication and use an alternative method of contraception in an attempt to determine whether the symptom is drug related. Women with a history of depression should be carefully observed and the drug discontinued if depression recurs to a serious degree.

6. CONTACT LENSES

Contact-lens wearers who develop visual changes or changes in lens tolerance should be assessed by an ophthalmologist.

7. DRUG INTERACTIONS

Reduced efficacy and increased incidence of breakthrough bleeding and menstrual irregularities have been associated with concomitant use of rifampin. A similar association, though less marked, has been suggested with barbiturates, phenylbutazone, phenytoin, and possibly with griseofulvin, ampicillin, and tetracyclines.

8. INTERACTIONS WITH LABORATORY TESTS

Certain endocrine- and liver-function tests and blood components may be affected by oral contraceptives:

a. Increased prothrombin and factors VII, VIII, IX, and X; decreased antithrombin 3; increased norepinephrine-induced platelet aggregability.

b. Increased thyroid-binding globulin (TBG) leading to increased circulating total thyroid hormone, as measured by protein-bound iodine (PBI), T4 by column or by radioimmunoassay. Free T3 resin uptake is decreased, reflecting the elevated TBG; free T4 concentration is unaltered.

c. Other binding proteins may be elevated in serum.

d. Sex-hormone binding globulins are increased and result in elevated levels of total circulating sex steroids; however, free or biologically active levels remain unchanged.

e. Triglycerides may be increased.

f. Glucose tolerance may be decreased.

g. Serum folate levels may be depressed by oral-contraceptive therapy. This may be of clinical significance if a woman becomes pregnant shortly after discontinuing oral contraceptives.

9. CARCINOGENESIS

See "**Warnings**" section.

10. PREGNANCY

Pregnancy Category X. See "**Contraindications**" and "**Warnings**" sections.

11. NURSING MOTHERS

Small amounts of oral-contraceptive steroids have been identified in the milk of nursing mothers, and a few adverse effects on the child have been reported, including jaundice and breast enlargement. In addition, oral contraceptives given in the postpartum period may interfere with lactation by decreasing the quantity and quality of breast milk. If possible, the nursing mother should be advised not to use oral contraceptives but to use other forms of contraception until she has completely weaned her child.

INFORMATION FOR THE PATIENT

See Patient Labeling Printed Below.

ADVERSE REACTIONS

An increased risk of the following serious adverse reactions has been associated with the use of oral contraceptives (see "**Warnings**" section):

Thrombophlebitis
Arterial thromboembolism
Pulmonary embolism
Myocardial infarction
Cerebral hemorrhage
Cerebral thrombosis
Hypertension
Gallbladder disease
Hepatic adenomas or benign liver tumors

There is evidence of an association between the following conditions and the use of oral contraceptives, although additional confirmatory studies are needed:

Mesenteric thrombosis
Retinal thrombosis

The following adverse reactions have been reported in patients receiving oral contraceptives and are believed to be drug related:

Nausea
Vomiting
Gastrointestinal symptoms (such as abdominal cramps and bloating)
Breakthrough bleeding
Spotting
Change in menstrual flow
Amenorrhea
Temporary infertility after discontinuation of treatment
Edema
Melasma which may persist
Breast changes: tenderness, enlargement, secretion
Change in weight (increase or decrease)
Change in cervical erosion and secretion
Diminution in lactation when given immediately postpartum
Cholestatic jaundice
Migraine
Rash (allergic)
Mental depression
Reduced tolerance to carbohydrates
Vaginal candidiasis
Change in corneal curvature (steepening)
Intolerance to contact lenses

The following adverse reactions have been reported in users of oral contraceptives and the association has been neither confirmed nor refuted:

Premenstrual syndrome
Cataracts
Optic neuritis
Changes in appetite
Cystitis-like syndrome
Headache
Nervousness
Dizziness
Hirsutism
Loss of scalp hair
Erythema multiforme
Erythema nodosum
Hemorrhagic eruption
Vaginitis
Porphyria
Impaired renal function
Hemolytic uremic syndrome
Budd-Chiari syndrome
Acne
Changes in libido
Colitis

OVERDOSAGE

Serious ill effects have not been reported following acute ingestion of large doses of oral contraceptives by young children. Overdosage may cause nausea, and withdrawal bleeding may occur in females.

Noncontraceptive Health Benefits

The following noncontraceptive health benefits related to the use of oral contraceptives are supported by epidemiological studies which largely utilized oral-contraceptive formulations containing doses exceeding 0.035 mg of ethinyl estradiol or 0.05 mg of mestranol.

Effects on menses:
Increased menstrual cycle regularity
Decreased blood loss and decreased incidence of iron-deficiency anemia
Decreased incidence of dysmenorrhea

Effects related to inhibition of ovulation:
Decreased incidence of functional ovarian cysts
Decreased incidence of ectopic pregnancies

Effects from long-term use:
Decreased incidence of fibroadenomas and fibrocystic disease of the breast
Decreased incidence of acute pelvic inflammatory disease
Decreased incidence of endometrial cancer
Decreased incidence of ovarian cancer

DOSAGE AND ADMINISTRATION

To achieve maximum contraceptive effectiveness, Alesse™ must be taken exactly as directed and at intervals not exceeding 24 hours. The dispenser should be kept in the wallet supplied to avoid possible fading of the pills. If the pills fade, patients should continue to take them as directed.

Continued on next page

Alesse-21—Cont.

The dosage of Alesse-21 is one pink tablet daily for 21 consecutive days, followed by 7 days when no tablets are taken. It is recommended that Alesse-21 tablets be taken at the same time each day.

Sunday start:

During the first cycle of medication, the patient is instructed to begin taking Alesse-21 on the first Sunday after the onset of menstruation. If menstruation begins on a Sunday, the first tablet (pink) is taken that day. One pink tablet should be taken daily for 21 consecutive days, followed by seven days when no tablet is taken. Withdrawal bleeding should usually occur within three days following discontinuation of pink tablets. During the first cycle, contraceptive reliance should not be placed on Alesse-21 until a pink tablet has been taken daily for 7 consecutive days. The possibility of ovulation and conception prior to initiation of medication should be considered.

The patient begins her next and all subsequent 21-day courses of tablets on the same day of the week (Sunday) on which she began her first course, following the same schedule: 21 days on pink tablets—7 days when no tablets are taken. If in any cycle the patient starts tablets later than the proper day, she should protect herself against pregnancy by using another method of birth control until she has taken a pink tablet daily for 7 consecutive days.

Day 1 start:

During the first cycle of medication, the patient is instructed to begin taking Alesse-21 during the first 24 hours of her period (day one of her menstrual cycle). One pink tablet should be taken daily for 21 consecutive days. Withdrawal bleeding should usually occur within three days following discontinuation of pink tablets. If medication is begun on day one of the menstrual cycle, no back-up contraception is necessary. If Alesse-21 tablets are started later than day one of the first menstrual cycle or postpartum, contraceptive reliance should not be placed on Alesse-21 tablets until after the first 7 consecutive days of administration. The possibility of ovulation and conception prior to initiation of medication should be considered.

When the patient is switching from a 21-day regimen of tablets, she should wait 7 days after her last tablet before she starts Alesse. She will probably experience withdrawal bleeding during that week. She should be sure that no more than 7 days pass after her previous 21-day regimen. When the patient is switching from a 28-day regimen of tablets, she should start her first pack of Alesse on the day after her last tablet. She should not wait any days between packs.

If spotting or breakthrough bleeding occur, the patient is instructed to continue on the same regimen. This type of bleeding is usually transient and without significance; however, if the bleeding is persistent or prolonged, the patient is advised to consult her physician. While there is little likelihood of ovulation occurring if only one or two pink tablets are missed, the possibility of ovulation increases with each successive day that scheduled pink tablets are missed. Although the occurrence of pregnancy is unlikely if Alesse is taken according to directions, if withdrawal bleeding does not occur, the possibility of pregnancy must be considered. If the patient has not adhered to the prescribed schedule (missed one or more tablets or started taking them on a day later than she should have), the probability of pregnancy should be considered at the time of the first missed period and appropriate diagnostic measures taken before the medication is resumed. If the patient has adhered to the prescribed regimen and misses two consecutive periods, pregnancy should be ruled out before continuing the contraceptive regimen.

The risk of pregnancy increases with each active (pink) tablet missed. For additional patient instructions regarding missed tablets, see the "WHAT TO DO IF YOU MISS PILLS" section in the **DETAILED PATIENT LABELING** below.

In the nonlactating mother, Alesse may be initiated postpartum, for contraception. When the tablets are administered in the postpartum period, the increased risk of thromboembolic disease associated with the postpartum period must be considered (See "**Contraindications**", "**Warnings**", and "**Precautions**" concerning thromboembolic disease).

HOW SUPPLIED

Alesse™-21 tablets (0.10 mg levonorgestrel and 0.02 mg ethinyl estradiol) are available in packages of 3 MINI-PACK™ dispensers of 21 tablets each, NDC 0008-0912-02, as follows:

21 active tablets. NDC 0008-0912, pink, round tablet marked "**W**" and "912".

Store at controlled room temperature 20°-25° C (68°-77° F). References available upon request.

Brief Summary Patient Package Insert

This product (like all oral contraceptives) is intended to prevent pregnancy. It does not protect against HIV infection (AIDS) and other sexually transmitted diseases.

Oral contraceptives, also known as "birth-control pills" or "the pill", are taken to prevent pregnancy, and when taken correctly, have a failure rate of less than 1.0% per year when used without missing any pills. The typical failure rate of large numbers of pill users is less than 3.0% per year when women who miss pills are included. For most women oral contraceptives are also free of serious or unpleasant side effects. However, forgetting to take pills considerably increases the chances of pregnancy.

For the majority of women, oral contraceptives can be taken safely. But there are some women who are at high risk of developing certain serious diseases that can be life-threatening or may cause temporary or permanent disability or death. The risks associated with taking oral contraceptives increase significantly if you:

- smoke.
- have high blood pressure, diabetes, high cholesterol.
- have or have had clotting disorders, heart attack, stroke, angina pectoris, cancer of the breast or sex organs, jaundice, or malignant or benign liver tumors.

You should not take the pill if you suspect you are pregnant or have unexplained vaginal bleeding.

Cigarette smoking increases the risk of serious adverse effects on the heart and blood vessels from oral-contraceptive use. This risk increases with age and with heavy smoking (15 or more cigarettes per day) and is quite marked in women over 35 years of age. Women who use oral contraceptives should not smoke.

Most side effects of the pill are not serious. The most common such effects are nausea, vomiting, bleeding between menstrual periods, weight gain, breast tenderness, and difficulty wearing contact lenses. These side effects, especially nausea and vomiting, may subside within the first three months of use.

The serious side effects of the pill occur very infrequently, especially if you are in good health and do not smoke. However, you should know that the following medical conditions have been associated with or made worse by the pill:

1. Blood clots in the legs (thrombophlebitis), lungs (pulmonary embolism), stoppage or rupture of a blood vessel in the brain (stroke), blockage of blood vessels in the heart (heart attack and angina pectoris) or other organs of the body. As mentioned above, smoking increases the risk of heart attacks and strokes and subsequent serious medical consequences.

2. Liver tumors, which may rupture and cause severe bleeding. A possible but not definite association has been found with the pill and liver cancer. However, liver cancers are extremely rare. The chance of developing liver cancer from using the pill is thus even rarer.

3. High blood pressure, although blood pressure usually returns to normal when the pill is stopped.

The symptoms associated with these serious side effects are discussed in the detailed leaflet given to you with your supply of pills. Notify your doctor or health-care provider if you notice any unusual physical disturbances while taking the pill. In addition, drugs such as rifampin, as well as some anticonvulsants and some antibiotics, may decrease oral-contraceptive effectiveness.

Studies to date of women taking the pill have not shown an increase in the incidence of cancer of the breast or cervix. There is, however, insufficient evidence to rule out the possibility that pills may cause such cancers.

Taking the pill provides some important noncontraceptive benefits. These include less painful menstruation, less menstrual blood loss and anemia, fewer pelvic infections, and fewer cancers of the ovary and the lining of the uterus.

Be sure to discuss any medical condition you may have with your health-care provider. Your health-care provider will take a medical and family history before prescribing oral contraceptives and will examine you. The physical examination may be delayed to another time if you request it and the health-care provider believes that it is appropriate to postpone it. You should be reexamined at least once a year while taking oral contraceptives. The detailed patient information leaflet gives you further information which you should read and discuss with your health-care provider.

This product (like all oral contraceptives) is intended to prevent pregnancy. It does not protect against transmission of HIV (AIDS) and other sexually transmitted diseases such as chlamydia, genital herpes, genital warts, gonorrhea, hepatitis B, and syphilis.

DETAILED PATIENT LABELING

This product (like all oral contraceptives) is intended to prevent pregnancy. It does not protect against HIV infection (AIDS) and other sexually transmitted diseases.

INTRODUCTION

Any woman who considers using oral contraceptives (the birth-control pill or the pill) should understand the benefits and risks of using this form of birth control. This leaflet will give you much of the information you will need to make this decision and will also help you determine if you are at risk of developing any of the serious side effects of the pill. It will tell you how to use the pill properly so that it will be as effective as possible.

However, this leaflet is not a replacement for a careful discussion between you and your health-care provider. You should discuss the information provided in this leaflet with him or her, both when you first start taking the pill and during your revisits. You should also follow your health-care provider's advice with regard to regular check-ups while you are on the pill.

EFFECTIVENESS OF ORAL CONTRACEPTIVES

Oral contraceptives or "birth-control pills" or "the pill" are used to prevent pregnancy and are more effective than other nonsurgical methods of birth control. When they are taken correctly, the chance of becoming pregnant is less than 1.0% per year when used perfectly, without missing any pills. Typical failure rates are less than 3.0% per year. The chance of becoming pregnant increases with each missed pill during the menstrual cycle.

In comparison, typical failure rates for other methods of birth control during the first year of use are as follows:

IUD: 3%
Depo-Provera® (injectable progestogen): 0.3%
Norplant® System (implants): 0.1%
Diaphragm with spermicides: 18%
Spermicides alone: 21%
Male condom alone: 12%
Female condom alone: 21%
Cervical cap
  Nulliparous women: 18%
  Parous women: 36%
Periodic abstinence: 20%
No methods: 85%

WHO SHOULD NOT TAKE ORAL CONTRACEPTIVES

Cigarette smoking increases the risk of serious adverse effects on the heart and blood vessels from oral-contraceptive use. This risk increases with age and with heavy smoking (15 or more cigarettes per day) and is quite marked in women over 35 years of age. Women who use oral contraceptives should not smoke.

Some women should not use the pill. For example, you should not take the pill if you are pregnant or think you may be pregnant. You should also not use the pill if you have had any of the following conditions:

- Heart attack or stroke.
- Blood clots in the legs (thrombophlebitis), lungs (pulmonary embolism), or eyes.
- Blood clots in the deep veins of your legs.
- Known or suspected breast cancer or cancer of the lining of the uterus, cervix or vagina.
- Liver tumor (benign or cancerous).

Or, if you have any of the following:

- Chest pain (angina pectoris).
- Unexplained vaginal bleeding (until a diagnosis is reached by your doctor).
- Yellowing of the whites of the eyes or of the skin (jaundice) during pregnancy or during previous use of the pill
- Known or suspected pregnancy.

Tell your health-care provider if you have ever had any of these conditions. Your health-care provider can recommend another method of birth control.

OTHER CONSIDERATIONS BEFORE TAKING ORAL CONTRACEPTIVES

Tell your health-care provider if you or any family member has ever had:

- Breast nodules, fibrocystic disease of the breast, an abnormal breast X ray or mammogram.
- Diabetes.
- Elevated cholesterol or triglycerides.
- High blood pressure.
- Migraine or other headaches or epilepsy.
- Mental depression.
- Gallbladder, heart or kidney disease.
- History of scanty or irregular menstrual periods.

Women with any of these conditions should be checked often by their health-care provider if they choose to use oral contraceptives. Also, be sure to inform your doctor or health-care provider if you smoke or are on any medications.

RISKS OF TAKING ORAL CONTRACEPTIVES

1. *Risk of developing blood clots*

Blood clots and blockage of blood vessels are the most serious side effects of taking oral contraceptives and can be fatal. In particular, a clot in the legs can cause thrombophlebitis and a clot that travels to the lungs can cause a sudden blocking of the vessel carrying blood to the lungs. Rarely, clots occur in the blood vessels of the eye and may cause blindness, double vision, or impaired vision.

If you take oral contraceptives and need elective surgery, need to stay in bed for a prolonged illness, or have recently delivered a baby, you may be at risk of developing blood clots. You should consult your doctor about stopping oral contraceptives three to four weeks before surgery and not taking oral contraceptives for two weeks after surgery or during bed rest. You should also not take oral contraceptives soon after delivery of a baby or a midtrimester pregnancy termination. It is advisable to wait for at least four weeks after delivery if you are not breast-feeding. If you are breast-feeding, you should wait until you have weaned your child before using the pill (See also the section on breast-feeding in "GENERAL PRECAUTIONS.")

2. *Heart attacks and strokes*

Oral contraceptives may increase the tendency to develop strokes (stoppage or rupture of blood vessels in the brain) and angina pectoris and heart attacks (blockage of blood vessels in the heart). Any of these conditions can cause death or serious disability.

Smoking greatly increases the possibility of suffering heart attacks and strokes. Furthermore, smoking and the use of oral contraceptives greatly increase the chances of developing and dying of heart disease.

3. *Gallbladder disease*

Oral-contraceptive users probably have a greater risk than nonusers of having gallbladder disease, although this risk may be related to pills containing high doses of estrogens.

4. *Liver tumors*

In rare cases, oral contraceptives can cause benign but dangerous liver tumors. These benign liver tumors can rupture and cause fatal internal bleeding. In addition, a possible but not definite association has been found with the pill and liver cancers in two studies in which a few women who developed these very rare cancers were found to have used oral contraceptives for long periods. However, liver cancers are extremely rare. The chance of developing liver cancer from using the pill is thus even rarer.

5. *Cancer of the reproductive organs*

There is, at present, no confirmed evidence that oral contraceptives increase the risk of cancer of the reproductive organs in human studies. Several studies have found no overall increase in the risk of developing breast cancer. However, women who use oral contraceptives and have a strong family history of breast cancer or who have breast nodules or abnormal mammograms should be closely followed by their doctors.

Some studies have found an increase in the incidence of cancer of the cervix in women who use oral contraceptives. However, this finding may be related to factors other than the use of oral contraceptives.

ESTIMATED RISK OF DEATH FROM A BIRTH CONTROL METHOD OR PREGNANCY

All methods of birth control and pregnancy are associated with a risk of developing certain diseases which may lead to disability or death. An estimate of the number of deaths associated with different methods of birth control and pregnancy has been calculated and is shown in the following table.

ANNUAL NUMBER OF BIRTH-RELATED OR METHOD-RELATED DEATHS ASSOCIATED WITH CONTROL OF FERTILITY PER 100,000 NONSTERILE WOMEN, BY FERTILITY-CONTROL METHOD AND ACCORDING TO AGE

Method of control and outcome	15-19	20-24	25-29	30-34	35-39	40-44
No fertility-control methods*	7.0	7.4	9.1	14.8	25.7	28.2
Oral contraceptives nonsmoker**	0.3	0.5	0.9	1.9	13.8	31.6
Oral contraceptives smoker**	2.2	3.4	6.6	13.5	51.1	117.2
IUD**	0.8	0.8	1.0	1.0	1.4	1.4
Condom*	1.1	1.6	0.7	0.2	0.3	0.4
Diaphragm/ spermicide*	1.9	1.2	1.2	1.3	2.2	2.8
Periodic abstinence*	2.5	1.6	1.6	1.7	2.9	3.6

* Deaths are birth related
**Deaths are method related

In the above table, the risk of death from any birth-control method is less than the risk of childbirth, except for oral-contraceptive users over the age of 35 who smoke and pill users over the age of 40 even if they do not smoke. It can be seen in the table that for women aged 15 to 39, the risk of death was highest with pregnancy (7 to 26 deaths per 100,000 women, depending on age). Among pill users who do not smoke, the risk of death was always lower than that associated with pregnancy for any age group, except for those women over the age of 40, when the risk increases to 32 deaths per 100,000 women, compared to 28 associated with pregnancy at that age. However, for pill users who smoke and are over the age of 35, the estimated number of deaths exceeds those for other methods of birth control. If a woman is over the age of 40 and smokes, her estimated risk of death is four times higher (117/100,000 women) than the estimated risk associated with pregnancy (28/100,000 women) in that age group.

The suggestion that women over 40 who don't smoke should not take oral contraceptives is based on information from older high-dose pills and on less-selective use of pills than is practiced today. An Advisory Committee of the FDA discussed this issue in 1989 and recommended that the benefits of oral-contraceptive use by healthy, nonsmoking women over 40 years of age may outweigh the possible risks. However, all women, especially older women, are cautioned to use the lowest-dose pill that is effective.

WARNING SIGNALS

If any of these adverse effects occur while you are taking oral contraceptives, call your doctor immediately:

- Sharp chest pain, coughing of blood, or sudden shortness of breath (indicating a possible clot in the lung).
- Pain in the calf (indicating a possible clot in the leg).
- Crushing chest pain or heaviness in the chest (indicating a possible heart attack).
- Sudden severe headache or vomiting, dizziness or fainting, disturbances of vision or speech, weakness, or numbness in an arm or leg (indicating a possible stroke).
- Sudden partial or complete loss of vision (indicating a possible clot in the eye).
- Breast lumps (indicating possible breast cancer or fibrocystic disease of the breast; ask your doctor or health-care provider to show you how to examine your breasts).
- Severe pain or tenderness in the stomach area (indicating a possibly ruptured liver tumor).
- Difficulty in sleeping, weakness, lack of energy, fatigue, or change in mood (possibly indicating severe depression).
- Jaundice or a yellowing of the skin or eyeballs, accompanied frequently by fever, fatigue, loss of appetite, dark-colored urine, or light-colored bowel movements (indicating possible liver problems).

SIDE EFFECTS OF ORAL CONTRACEPTIVES

1. *Vaginal bleeding*

Irregular vaginal bleeding or spotting may occur while you are taking the pills. Irregular bleeding may vary from slight staining between menstrual periods to breakthrough bleeding which is a flow much like a regular period. Irregular bleeding occurs most often during the first few months of oral-contraceptive use, but may also occur after you have been taking the pill for some time. Such bleeding may be temporary and usually does not indicate any serious problems. It is important to continue taking your pills on schedule. If the bleeding occurs in more than one cycle or lasts for more than a few days, talk to your doctor or health-care provider.

2. *Contact lenses*

If you wear contact lenses and notice a change in vision or an inability to wear your lenses, contact your doctor or health-care provider.

3. *Fluid retention*

Oral contraceptives may cause edema (fluid retention) with swelling of the fingers or ankles and may raise your blood pressure. If you experience fluid retention, contact your doctor or health-care provider.

4. *Melasma*

A spotty darkening of the skin is possible, particularly of the face.

5. *Other side effects*

Other side effects may include change in appetite, headache, nervousness, depression, dizziness, loss of scalp hair, rash, and vaginal infections.

If any of these side effects bother you, call your doctor or health-care provider.

GENERAL PRECAUTIONS

1. *Missed periods and use of oral contraceptives before or during early pregnancy.*

There may be times when you may not menstruate regularly after you have completed taking a cycle of pills. If you have taken your pills regularly and miss one menstrual period, continue taking your pills for the next cycle but be sure to inform your health-care provider before doing so. If you have not taken the pills daily as instructed and missed a menstrual period, or if you missed two consecutive menstrual periods, you may be pregnant. Check with your health-care provider immediately to determine whether you are pregnant. Do not continue to take oral contraceptives until you are sure you are not pregnant, but continue to use another method of contraception.

There is no conclusive evidence that oral-contraceptive use is associated with an increase in birth defects, when taken inadvertently during early pregnancy. Previously, a few studies had reported that oral contraceptives might be associated with birth defects, but these studies have not been confirmed. Nevertheless, oral contraceptives or any other drugs should not be used during pregnancy unless clearly necessary and prescribed by your doctor. You should check with your doctor about risks to your unborn child of any medication taken during pregnancy.

2. *While breast-feeding*

If you are breast-feeding, consult your doctor before starting oral contraceptives. Some of the drug will be passed on to the child in the milk. A few adverse effects on the child have been reported, including yellowing of the skin (jaundice) and breast enlargement. In addition, oral contraceptives may decrease the amount and quality of your milk. If possible, do not use oral contraceptives while breast-feeding. You should use another method of contraception since breast-feeding provides only partial protection from becoming pregnant and this partial protection decreases significantly as you breast-feed for longer periods of time. You should consider starting oral contraceptives only after you have weaned your child completely.

3. *Laboratory tests*

If you are scheduled for any laboratory tests, tell your doctor you are taking birth-control pills. Certain blood tests may be affected by birth-control pills.

4. *Drug interactions*

Certain drugs may interact with birth-control pills to make them less effective in preventing pregnancy or cause an increase in breakthrough bleeding. Such drugs include rifampin, drugs used for epilepsy such as barbiturates (for example, phenobarbital) and phenytoin (Dilantin is one brand of this drug), phenylbutazone (Butazolidin is one brand) and possibly certain antibiotics. You may need to use an additional method of contraception during any cycle in which you take drugs that can make oral contraceptives less effective.

This product (like all oral contraceptives) is intended to prevent pregnancy. It does not protect against transmission of HIV (AIDS) and other sexually transmitted diseases such as chlamydia, genital herpes, genital warts, gonorrhea, hepatitis B, and syphilis.

HOW TO TAKE THE PILL

This product (like all oral contraceptives) is intended to prevent pregnancy. It does not protect against transmission of HIV (AIDS) and other sexually transmitted diseases such as chlamydia, genital herpes, genital warts, gonorrhea, hepatitis B, and syphilis.

IMPORTANT POINTS TO REMEMBER

BEFORE YOU START TAKING YOUR PILLS:

1. BE SURE TO READ THESE DIRECTIONS:
Before you start taking your pills.
And
Anytime you are not sure what to do.

2. THE RIGHT WAY TO TAKE THE PILL IS TO TAKE ONE PILL EVERY DAY AT THE SAME TIME.
If you miss pills you could get pregnant. This includes starting the pack late. The more pills you miss, the more likely you are to get pregnant.

3. MANY WOMEN HAVE SPOTTING OR LIGHT BLEEDING, OR MAY FEEL SICK TO THEIR STOMACH DURING THE FIRST 1–3 PACKS OF PILLS.
If you feel sick to your stomach, do not stop taking the pill. The problem will usually go away. If it doesn't go away, check with your doctor or clinic.

4. MISSING PILLS CAN ALSO CAUSE SPOTTING OR LIGHT BLEEDING, even when you make up these missed pills. On the days you take 2 pills to make up for missed pills, you could also feel a little sick to your stomach.

5. IF YOU HAVE VOMITING OR DIARRHEA, for any reason, or IF YOU TAKE SOME MEDICINES, including some antibiotics, your pills may not work as well.
Use a back-up method (such as condoms or foam) until you check with your doctor or clinic.

6. IF YOU HAVE TROUBLE REMEMBERING TO TAKE THE PILL, talk to your doctor or clinic about how to make pill-taking easier or about using another method of birth control.

7. IF YOU HAVE ANY QUESTIONS OR ARE UNSURE ABOUT THE INFORMATION IN THIS LEAFLET, call your doctor or clinic.

***BEFORE* YOU START TAKING YOUR PILLS**

1. DECIDE WHAT TIME OF DAY YOU WANT TO TAKE YOUR PILL. It is important to take it at about the same time every day.

2. LOOK AT YOUR PILL PACK TO SEE IF IT HAS 21 OR 28 PILLS.
The *21-pill pack* has 21 "active" pink pills (with hormones) to take for 3 weeks, followed by 1 week without pills.
The *28-pill pack* has 21 "active" pink pills (with hormones) to take for 3 weeks, followed by 1 week of reminder light-green pills (without hormones).

3. ALSO FIND:
1) where on the pack to start taking pills, and
2) in what order to take the pills (follow the arrow).

4. BE SURE YOU HAVE READY AT ALL TIMES:
ANOTHER KIND OF BIRTH CONTROL (such as condoms or foam) to use as a back-up in case you miss pills.

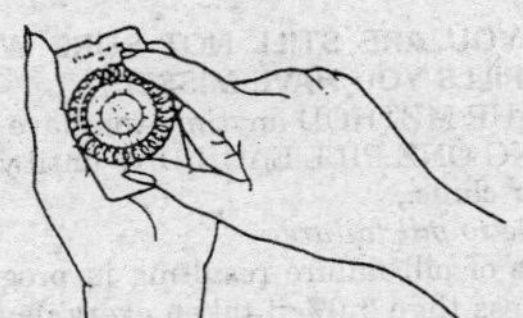

AN EXTRA, FULL PILL PACK.

WHEN TO START THE *FIRST* PACK OF PILLS:

You have a choice of which day to start taking your first pack of pills.

Decide with your doctor or clinic which is the best day for you. Pick a time of day which will be easy to remember.

DAY 1 START:

1. Take the first "active" pink pill of the first pack during the *first 24 hours of your period.*
2. You will not need to use a back-up method of birth control, since you are starting the pill at the beginning of your period.

SUNDAY START:

1. Take the first "active" pink pill of the first pack on the *Sunday after your period starts,* even if you are still bleeding. If your period begins on Sunday, start the pack that same day.
2. *Use another method of birth control* as a back-up method if you have sex anytime from the Sunday you start your first pack until the next Sunday (7 days). Condoms or foam are good back-up methods of birth control.

WHAT TO DO DURING THE MONTH

1. TAKE ONE PILL AT THE SAME TIME EVERY DAY UNTIL THE PACK IS EMPTY.

Do not skip pills even if you are spotting or bleeding between monthly periods or feel sick to your stomach (nausea).

Do not skip pills even if you do not have sex very often.

2. WHEN YOU FINISH A PACK OR SWITCH YOUR BRAND OF PILLS:

21 pills: Wait 7 days to start the next pack. You will probably have your period during that week. Be sure that no more than 7 days pass between 21-day packs.

28 pills: Start the next pack on the day after your last "reminder" pill. Do not wait any days between packs.

WHAT TO DO IF YOU MISS PILLS

If you **MISS 1** pink "active" pill:

1. Take it as soon as you remember. Take the next pill at your regular time. This means you take 2 pills in 1 day.
2. You do not need to use a back-up birth-control method if you have sex.

If you **MISS 2** pink "active" pills in a row in **WEEK 1 OR WEEK 2** of your pack:

Continued on next page

Alesse-21—Cont.

1. Take 2 pills on the day you remember and 2 pills the next day.
2. Then take 1 pill a day until you finish the pack.
3. You MAY BECOME PREGNANT if you have sex in the 7 *days* after you miss pills. You MUST use another birth-control method (such as condoms or foam) as a back-up for those 7 days.

If you **MISS 2** pink "active" pills in a row in **THE 3rd WEEK:**
1. ***If you are a Day 1 Starter:***
THROW OUT the rest of the pill pack and start a new pack that same day.
If you are a Sunday Starter:
Keep taking 1 pill every day until Sunday.
On Sunday, THROW OUT the rest of the pack and start a new pack of pills that same day.
2. You may not have your period this month but this is expected.
However, if you miss your period 2 months in a row, call your doctor or clinic because you might be pregnant.
3. You MAY BECOME PREGNANT if you have sex in the 7 *days* after you miss pills. You MUST use another birth-control method (such as condoms or foam) as a back-up for those 7 days.

If you **MISS 3 OR MORE** pink "active" pills in a row (during the first 3 weeks):
1. ***If you are a Day 1 Starter:***
THROW OUT the rest of the pill pack and start a new pack that same day.
If you are a Sunday Starter:
Keep taking 1 pill every day until Sunday.
On Sunday, THROW OUT the rest of the pack and start a new pack of pills that same day.
2. You may not have your period this month but this is expected.
However, if you miss your period 2 months in a row, call your doctor or clinic because you might be pregnant.
3. You MAY BECOME PREGNANT if you have sex in the 7 *days* after you miss pills. You MUST use another birth-control method (such as condoms or foam) as a back-up for those 7 days.

A REMINDER FOR THOSE ON 28-DAY PACKS:
If you forget any of the 7 light-green "reminder" pills in Week 4:
THROW AWAY the pills you missed.
Keep taking 1 pill each day until the pack is empty.
You do not need a back-up method if you start your next pack on time.

FINALLY, IF YOU ARE STILL NOT SURE WHAT TO DO ABOUT THE PILLS YOU HAVE MISSED:
Use a BACK-UP METHOD anytime you have sex.
KEEP TAKING ONE PILL EACH DAY until you can reach your doctor or clinic.

Pregnancy due to pill failure
The incidence of pill failure resulting in pregnancy is approximately less than 1.0% if taken every day as directed, but more typical failure rates are less than 3.0%. If failure does occur, the risk to the fetus is minimal.

RISKS TO THE FETUS
If you do become pregnant while using oral contraceptives, the risk to the fetus is small, on the order of no more than one per thousand. You should, however, discuss the risks to the developing child with your doctor.

Pregnancy after stopping the pill
There may be some delay in becoming pregnant after you stop using oral contraceptives, especially if you had irregular menstrual cycles before you used oral contraceptives. It may be advisable to postpone conception until you begin menstruating regularly once you have stopped taking the pill and desire pregnancy.
There does not appear to be any increase in birth defects in newborn babies when pregnancy occurs soon after stopping the pill.

Overdosage
Serious ill effects have not been reported following ingestion of large doses of oral contraceptives by young children. Overdosage may cause nausea and withdrawal bleeding in females. In case of overdosage, contact your health-care provider or pharmacist.

Other information
Your health-care provider will take a medical and family history before prescribing oral contraceptives and will examine you. The physical examination may be delayed to another time if you request it and the health-care provider believes that it is appropriate to postpone it. You should be reexamined at least once a year. Be sure to inform your health-care provider if there is a family history of any of the conditions listed previously in this leaflet. Be sure to keep all appointments with your health-care provider, because this is a time to determine if there are early signs of side effects of oral-contraceptive use.
Do not use the drug for any condition other than the one for which it was prescribed. This drug has been prescribed specifically for you; do not give it to others who may want birth-control pills.

HEALTH BENEFITS FROM ORAL CONTRACEPTIVES
In addition to preventing pregnancy, use of oral contraceptives may provide certain benefits. They are:
- Menstrual cycles may become more regular.
- Blood flow during menstruation may be lighter, and less iron may be lost. Therefore, anemia due to iron deficiency is less likely to occur.
- Pain or other symptoms during menstruation may be encountered less frequently.
- Ovarian cysts may occur less frequently.
- Ectopic (tubal) pregnancy may occur less frequently.
- Noncancerous cysts or lumps in the breast may occur less frequently.
- Acute pelvic inflammatory disease may occur less frequently.
- Oral-contraceptive use may provide some protection against developing two forms of cancer: cancer of the ovaries and cancer of the lining of the uterus.

If you want more information about birth-control pills, ask your doctor or pharmacist. They have a more technical leaflet called the Professional Labeling which you may wish to read.
Manufactured by:
Wyeth Laboratories
A Wyeth-Ayerst Company
Philadelphia, PA 19101
CI 4843-2 Revised April 24, 1997
Shown in Product Identification Guide, page 341

ALESSE™-28 ℞
[*ă 'lĕs*]
levonorgestrel and ethinyl estradiol tablets

Patients should be counseled that this product does not protect against HIV infection (AIDS) and other sexually transmitted diseases.

DESCRIPTION
21 pink active tablets each containing 0.10 mg of levonorgestrel, d(-)-13β-ethyl-17α-ethinyl-17β-hydroxygon-4-en-3-one, a totally synthetic progestogen, and 0.02 mg of ethinyl estradiol, 17α-ethinyl-1,3,5(10)-estratriene-3, 17β-diol. The inactive ingredients present are cellulose, hydroxypropyl methylcellulose, iron oxide, lactose, magnesium stearate, polacrilin potassium, polyethylene glycol, titanium dioxide, and wax E.
7 light-green inert tablets, each containing cellulose, FD&C blue no. 1, hydroxypropyl methylcellulose, iron oxide, lactose, magnesium stearate, polacrilin potassium, polyethylene glycol, titanium dioxide, and wax E.

Levonorgestrel

Ethinyl Estradiol

CLINICAL PHARMACOLOGY
See ALESSE™-21.

INDICATIONS AND USAGE
See ALESSE-21.

CONTRAINDICATIONS
See ALESSE-21.

WARNINGS
See ALESSE-21.

PRECAUTIONS
See ALESSE-21.
Drug Interactions: See ALESSE-21.
Carcinogenesis: See ALESSE-21.
Pregnancy: See ALESSE-21.
Nursing Mothers: See ALESSE-21.
Information for the Patient: See Alesse-21.

ADVERSE REACTIONS
See Alesse-21.

OVERDOSAGE
See Alesse-21.

NONCONTRACEPTIVE HEALTH BENEFITS
See Alesse-21.

DOSAGE AND ADMINISTRATION
To achieve maximum contraceptive effectiveness, Alesse™ must be taken exactly as directed and at intervals not exceeding 24 hours. The dispenser should be kept in the wallet supplied to avoid possible fading of the pills. If the pills fade, patients should continue to take them as directed.
The dosage of Alesse-28 is one pink tablet daily for 21 consecutive days, followed by one light-green inert tablet daily for 7 consecutive days, according to the prescribed schedule. It is recommended that Alesse-28 tablets be taken at the same time each day.

Sunday start:
During the first cycle of medication, the patient is instructed to begin taking Alesse-28 on the first Sunday after the onset of menstruation. If menstruation begins on a Sunday, the first tablet (pink) is taken that day. One pink tablet should be taken daily for 21 consecutive days, followed by one light-green inert tablet daily for seven consecutive days. Withdrawal bleeding should usually occur within three days following discontinuation of pink tablets. During the first cycle, contraceptive reliance should not be placed on Alesse-28 until a pink tablet has been taken daily for 7 consecutive days. The possibility of ovulation and conception prior to initiation of medication should be considered.
The patient begins her next and all subsequent 28-day courses of tablets on the same day of the week (Sunday) on which she began her first course, following the same schedule: 21 days on pink tablets—7 days on light-green inert tablets. If in any cycle the patient starts tablets later than the proper day, she should protect herself against pregnancy by using another method of birth control until she has taken a pink tablet daily for 7 consecutive days.

Day 1 start:
During the first cycle of medication, the patient is instructed to begin taking Alesse-28 during the first 24 hours of her period (day one of her menstrual cycle). One pink tablet should be taken daily for 21 consecutive days, followed by one light-green inert tablet daily for seven consecutive days. Withdrawal bleeding should usually occur within three days following discontinuation of pink tablets. If medication is begun on day one of the menstrual cycle, no back-up contraception is necessary. If Alesse-28 tablets are started later than day one of the first menstrual cycle or postpartum, contraceptive reliance should not be placed on Alesse-28 tablets until after the first 7 consecutive days of administration. The possibility of ovulation and conception prior to initiation of medication should be considered.
When the patient is switching from a 21-day regimen of tablets, she should wait 7 days after her last tablet before she starts Alesse. She will probably experience withdrawal bleeding during that week. She should be sure that no more than 7 days pass after her previous 21-day regimen. When the patient is switching from a 28-day regimen of tablets, she should start her first pack of Alesse on the day after her last tablet. She should not wait any days between packs.
If spotting or breakthrough bleeding occur, the patient is instructed to continue on the same regimen. This type of bleeding is usually transient and without significance; however, if the bleeding is persistent or prolonged, the patient is advised to consult her physician. While there is little likelihood of ovulation occurring if only one or two pink tablets are missed, the possibility of ovulation increases with each successive day that scheduled pink tablets are missed. Although the occurrence of pregnancy is unlikely if Alesse is taken according to directions, if withdrawal bleeding does not occur, the possibility of pregnancy must be considered. If the patient has not adhered to the prescribed schedule (missed one or more tablets or started taking them on a day later than she should have), the probability of pregnancy should be considered at the time of the first missed period and appropriate diagnostic measures taken before the medication is resumed. If the patient has adhered to the prescribed regimen and misses two consecutive periods, pregnancy should be ruled out before continuing the contraceptive regimen.
The risk of pregnancy increases with each active (pink) tablet missed. For additional patient instructions regarding missed tablets, see the "WHAT TO DO IF YOU MISS PILLS" section in the **DETAILED PATIENT LABELING** below.
In the nonlactating mother, Alesse may be initiated postpartum, for contraception. When the tablets are administered in the postpartum period, the increased risk of thromboembolic disease associated with the postpartum period must be considered (See "**Contraindications**", "**Warnings**", and "**Precautions**" concerning thromboembolic disease).

HOW SUPPLIED
Alesse™-28 tablets (0.10 mg levonorgestrel and 0.02 mg ethinyl estradiol) are available in packages of 3 MINI-PACK™ dispensers of 28 tablets each, NDC 0008-2576-02, as follows:
21 active tablets, NDC 0008-0912, pink, round tablet marked "W" and "912".
7 inert tablets, NDC 0008-0650, light-green, round tablet marked "W" and "650".
Store at controlled room temperature 20°–25° C (68°–77° F).
References available upon request.

BRIEF SUMMARY PATIENT PACKAGE INSERT
See Alesse-21.

DETAILED PATIENT LABELING
See Alesse-21.
Manufactured by:
Wyeth Laboratories
A Wyeth-Ayerst Company
Philadelphia, PA 19101
CI 4844-2 Revised April 24, 1997
Shown in Product Identification Guide, page 341

AMPHOJEL® OTC
[*am 'fo-jel*]
(aluminum hydroxide gel)
ORAL SUSPENSION

COMPOSITION
Suspension—Peppermint flavored—Each teaspoonful (5 ml) contains 320 mg of aluminum hydroxide [$Al(OH)_3$] as a gel,

and not more than 0.10 mEq of sodium. The inactive ingredients present are calcium benzoate, glycerin, hydroxypropyl methylcellulose, menthol, peppermint oil, potassium butylparaben, potassium propylparaben, saccharin, simethicone, sorbitol solution, and water.

INDICATIONS

For the symptomatic relief of hyperacidity associated with the diagnosis of peptic ulcer, gastritis, peptic esophagitis, gastric hyperacidity, and hiatal hernia.

DOSAGE

Suspension—two teaspoonfuls followed by a sip of water if desired, five or six times daily, between meals and on retiring. Two teaspoonfuls have the capacity to neutralize 20 mEq of acid.

WARNINGS

Patients are advised not to take more than 12 teaspoonfuls (60 ml) in a 24-hour period or use this maximum dosage for more than two weeks except under the advice and supervision of a physician. Prolonged use of aluminum-containing antacids in patients with renal failure may result in or worsen dialysis osteomalacia. Elevated tissue aluminum levels contribute to the development of dialysis encephalopathy and osteomalacia syndromes. Also, a number of cases of dialysis encephalopathy have been associated with elevated aluminum levels in the dialysate water. Small amounts of aluminum are absorbed from the gastrointestinal tract and reneal excretion of aluminum is impaired in renal failure. Prolonged use of aluminum-containing antacids in such patients may contribute to increased plasma levels of aluminum. Aluminum is not well removed by dialysis because it is bound to albumin and transferrin, which do not cross dialysis membranes. As a result, aluminum is deposited in bone, and dialysis osteomalacia may develop when large amounts of aluminum are ingested orally by patients with impaired renal function. Pregnant women and nursing mothers are advised to seek the advice of a health professional before using this product.

PRECAUTION

May cause constipation.

DRUG INTERACTION PRECAUTIONS

Antacids may interact with certain prescription drugs.
This product must not be taken if the patient is presently taking a prescription antibiotic drug containing any form of tetracycline.
If patients are presently taking a prescription drug, they are advised to check with their physicians before taking this product.
Keep tightly closed and store at room temperature, Approx. 77°F (25°C). Suspension should be shaken well before use. Avoid freezing. Keep this and all drugs out of the reach of children.

HOW SUPPLIED

Suspension—Peppermint flavored—bottles of 12 fluidounces.
Manufactured by:
Wyeth Laboratories
A Wyeth-Ayerst Company
Philadelphia, PA 19101

ANTABUSE® ℞

[ăn 'tăh-būse]
(disulfiram)
IN ALCOHOLISM
Rx only

> **WARNING**
> Antabuse should *never* be administered to a patient when he is in a state of alcohol intoxication, or without his full knowledge.
> The physician should instruct relatives accordingly.

DESCRIPTION

CHEMICAL NAME: bis(diethylthiocarbamoyl) disulfide
STRUCTURAL FORMULA:

$$(C_2H_5)_2N-\underset{\underset{S}{\|}}{C}-S-S-\underset{\underset{S}{\|}}{C}-N(C_2H_5)_2$$

Antabuse occurs as a white to off-white, odorless, and almost tasteless powder, soluble in water to the extent of about 20 mg in 100 mL, and in alcohol to the extent of about 3.8 g in 100 mL.
Antabuse contains these inactive ingredients: magnesium aluminum silicate; magnesium stearate, NF; povidone, USP; starch, NF.

ACTION

Antabuse produces a sensitivity to alcohol which results in a highly unpleasant reaction when the patient under treatment ingests even small amounts of alcohol.
Antabuse blocks the oxidation of alcohol at the acetaldehyde stage. During alcohol metabolism following Antabuse intake, the concentration of acetaldehyde occurring in the blood may be 5- to 10-times higher than that found during metabolism of the same amount of alcohol alone.
Accumulation of acetaldehyde in the blood produces a complex of highly unpleasant symptoms referred to hereinafter as the Antabase-alcohol reaction. This reaction, which is proportional to the dosage of both Antabuse and alcohol, will persist as long as alcohol is being metabolized. Antabuse does not appear to influence the rate of alcohol elimination from the body.
Antabuse is absorbed slowly from the gastrointestinal tract and eliminated slowly from the body. One (or even two) weeks after a patient has taken his last dose of Antabuse, ingestion of alcohol may produce unpleasant symptoms.
Prolonged administration of Antabuse does not produce tolerance; the longer a patient remains on therapy, the more exquisitely sensitive he becomes to alcohol.

INDICATION

Antabuse is an aid in the management of selected chronic alcoholic patients who *want* to remain in a state of enforced sobriety so that supportive and psychotherapeutic treatment may be applied to best advantage.
Antabuse is not a cure for alcoholism. When used alone, without proper motivation and supportive therapy, it is unlikely that it will have any substantive effect on the drinking pattern of the chronic alcoholic.

CONTRAINDICATIONS

Patients who are receiving or have recently received metronidazole, paraldehyde, alcohol, or alcohol-containing preparations, e.g., cough syrups, tonics and the like, should not be given Antabuse.
Antabuse is contraindicated in the presence of severe myocardial disease or coronary occlusion, psychoses, and hypersensitivity to disulfiram or to other thiuram derivatives used in pesticides and rubber vulcanization.

WARNINGS

> Antabuse should *never* be administered to a patient when he is in a state of alcohol intoxication, or without his full knowledge.
> The physician should instruct relatives accordingly.

The patient must be fully informed of the Antabuse-alcohol reaction. He must be strongly cautioned against surreptitious drinking while taking the drug, and he must be fully aware of possible consequences. He should be warned to avoid alcohol in disguised form, i.e., in sauces, vinegars, cough mixtures, and even aftershave lotions and back rubs. He should also be warned that reactions may occur with alcohol up to 14 days after ingesting Antabuse.

The Antabuse-Alcohol Reaction

Antabuse plus alcohol, even small amounts, produces flushing, throbbing in head and neck, throbbing headache, respiratory difficulty, nausea, copious vomiting, sweating, thirst, chest pain, palpitation, dyspnea, hyperventilation, tachycardia, hypotension, syncope, marked uneasiness, weakness, vertigo, blurred vision, and confusion. In severe reactions there may be respiratory depression, cardiovascular collapse, arrhythmias, myocardial infarction, acute congestive heart failure, unconsciousness, convulsions, and death.
The intensity of the reaction varies with each individual but is generally proportional to the amounts of Antabuse and alcohol ingested. Mild reactions may occur in the sensitive individual when the blood alcohol concentration is increased to as little as 5 to 10 mg per 100 mL. Symptoms are fully developed at 50 mg per 100 mL, and unconsciousness usually results when the blood alcohol level reaches 125 to 150 mg.
The duration of the reaction varies from 30 to 60 minutes, to several hours in the more severe cases, or as long as there is alcohol in the blood.

Drug Interactions

Disulfiram appears to decrease the rate at which certain drugs are metabolized and therefore may increase the blood levels and the possibility of clinical toxicity of drugs given concomitantly.
DISULFIRAM SHOULD BE USED WITH CAUTION IN THOSE PATIENTS RECEIVING PHENYTOIN AND ITS CONGENERS, SINCE THE CONCOMITANT ADMINISTRATION OF THESE TWO DRUGS CAN LEAD TO PHENYTOIN INTOXICATION. PRIOR TO ADMINISTERING DISULFIRAM TO A PATIENT ON PHENYTOIN THERAPY, A BASELINE PHENYTOIN SERUM LEVEL SHOULD BE OBTAINED. SUBSEQUENT TO INITIATION OF DISULFIRAM THERAPY, SERUM LEVELS OF PHENYTOIN SHOULD BE DETERMINED ON DIFFERENT DAYS FOR EVIDENCE OF AN INCREASE OR FOR A CONTINUING RISE IN LEVELS. INCREASED PHENYTOIN LEVELS SHOULD BE TREATED WITH APPROPRIATE DOSAGE ADJUSTMENT.
It may be necessary to adjust the dosage of oral anticoagulants upon beginning or stopping disulfiram, since disulfiram may prolong prothrombin time.
Patients taking isoniazid when disulfiram is given should be observed for the appearance of unsteady gait or marked changes in mental status; the disulfiram should be discontinued if such signs appear.
In rats, simultaneous ingestion of disulfiram and nitrite in the diet for 78 weeks has been reported to cause tumors, and it has been suggested that disulfiram may react with nitrites in the rat stomach to form a nitrosamine, which is tumorigenic. Disulfiram alone in the rats' diet did not lead to such tumors. The relevance of this finding to humans is not known at this time.

Concomitant Conditions

Because of the possibility of an accidental Antabuse-alcohol reaction, Antabuse should be used with extreme caution in patients with any of the following conditions: diabetes mellitus, hypothyroidism, epilepsy, cerebral damage, chronic and acute nephritis, hepatic cirrhosis or insufficiency.

Usage in Pregnancy

The safe use of this drug in pregnancy has not been established. Therefore, Antabuse should be used during pregnancy only when, in the judgment of the physician, the probable benefits outweigh the possible risks.

PRECAUTIONS

Patients with a history of rubber contact dermatitis should be evaluated for hypersensitivity to thiuram derivatives before receiving Antabuse (see "**CONTRAINDICATIONS**").
It is suggested that every patient under treatment carry an *Identification Card*, stating that he is receiving Antabuse and describing the symptoms most likely to occur as a result of the Antabuse-alcohol reaction. In addition, this card should indicate the physician or institution to be contacted in an emergency. (Cards may be obtained from Wyeth-Ayerst Laboratories upon request.)
Alcoholism may accompany or be followed by dependence on narcotics or sedatives. Barbiturates and Antabuse have been administered concurrently without untoward effects; the possibility of initiating a new abuse should be considered.
Hepatic toxicity including hepatic failure resulting in transplantation or death have been reported. Severe and sometimes fatal hepatitis associated with disulfiram therapy may develop even after many months of therapy. Hepatic toxicity has occurred in patients with or without prior history of abnormal liver function. Patients should be advised to immediately notify their physician of any early symptoms of hepatitis, such as fatigue, weakness, malaise, anorexia, nausea, vomiting, jaundice, or dark urine.
Baseline and follow-up liver function tests (10 to 14 days) are suggested to detect any hepatic dysfunction that may result with Antabuse® therapy. In addition, a complete blood count and serum chemistries, including liver function tests, should be monitored.
Patients taking Antabuse Tablets should not be exposed to ethylene dibromide or its vapors. This precaution is based on preliminary results of animal research currently in progress that suggest a toxic interaction between inhaled ethylene dibromide and ingested disulfiram resulting in a higher incidence of tumors and mortality in rats. A correlation between this finding and humans, however, has not been demonstrated.

ADVERSE REACTIONS

(See "**CONTRAINDICATIONS**," "**WARNINGS**," and "**PRECAUTIONS**.")
OPTIC NEURITIS, PERIPHERAL NEURITIS, POLYNEURITIS, AND PERIPHERAL NEUROPATHY MAY OCCUR FOLLOWING ADMINISTRATION OF ANTABUSE.
Multiple cases of hepatitis, including both cholestatic and fulminant hepatitis, as well as hepatic failure resulting in transplantation or death, have been reported with administration of Antabuse.
Occasional skin eruptions are, as a rule, readily controlled by concomitant administration of an antihistaminic drug.
In a small number of patients, a transient mild drowsiness, fatigability, impotence, headache, acneform eruptions, allergic dermatitis, or a metallic or garlic-like aftertaste may be experienced during the first two weeks of therapy. These complaints usually disappear spontaneously with the continuation of therapy, or with reduced dosage.
Psychotic reactions have been noted, attributable in most cases to high dosage, combined toxicity (with metronidazole or isoniazid), or to the unmasking of underlying psychoses in patients stressed by the withdrawal of alcohol.

DOSAGE AND ADMINISTRATION

Antabuse should never be administered until the patient has abstained from alcohol for at least 12 hours.

Initial Dosage Schedule

In the first phase of treatment, a *maximum* of 500 mg daily is given in a single dose for one to two weeks. Although usually taken in the morning, Antabuse may be taken on retiring by patients who experience a sedative effect. Alternatively, to minimize, or eliminate, the sedative effect, dosage may be adjusted downward.

Maintenance Regimen

The average maintenance dose is 250 mg daily (range, 125 to 500 mg); it should not exceed 500 mg daily.

Note: Occasionally patients, while seemingly on adequate maintenance doses of Antabuse, report that they are able to drink alcoholic beverages with impunity and without any symptomatology. All appearances to the contrary, such patients must be presumed to be disposing of their tablets in some manner without actually taking them. Until such patients have been observed reliably taking their daily Antabuse Tablets (preferably crushed and well mixed with liquid), it cannot be concluded that Antabuse is ineffective.

Duration of Therapy

The daily, uninterrupted administration of Antabuse must be continued until the patient is fully recovered socially and a basis for permanent self-control is established. Depending on the individual patient, maintenance therapy may be required for months, or even years.

Continued on next page

Antabuse—Cont.

Trial with Alcohol

During early experience with Antabuse, it was thought advisable for each patient to have at least one supervised alcohol-drug reaction. More recently, the test reaction has been largely abandoned. Furthermore, such a test reaction should never be administered to a patient over 50 years of age. A clear, detailed, and convincing description of the reaction is felt to be sufficient in most cases.

However, where a test reaction is deemed necessary, the suggested procedure is as follows:

After the first one to two weeks' therapy with 500 mg daily, a drink of 15 mL ($^1/_2$ oz) of 100 proof whiskey, or equivalent, is taken slowly. This test dose of alcoholic beverage may be repeated once only, so that the total dose does not exceed 30 mL (1 oz) of whiskey. Once a reaction develops, no more alcohol should be consumed. Such tests should be carried out only when the patient is hospitalized, or comparable supervision and facilities, including oxygen, are available.

Management Of Antabuse-Alcohol Reaction

In severe reactions, whether caused by an excessive test dose or by the patient's unsupervised ingestion of alcohol, supportive measures to restore blood pressure and treat shock should be instituted. Other recommendations include: oxygen, carbogen (95% oxygen and 5% carbon dioxide), vitamin C intravenously in massive doses (1 g), and ephedrine sulfate. Antihistamines have also been used intravenously. Potassium levels should be monitored, particularly in patients on digitalis, since hypokalemia has been reported.

HOW SUPPLIED

Antabuse® (disulfiram) Tablets are available in the following dosage strength:

250 mg, NDC 0046-0809-81, white-to-off-white, octagonal-shaped, scored, compressed tablet, embossed with a stylized "A" on one side and imprinted with "ANTABUSE" and "250" on the scored reverse side, in bottles of 100 tablets.

Store at room temperature, approximately 25°C.

Dispense in a tight, light-resistant container as defined in the USP

Manufactured by:
Ayerst Laboratories Inc.
A Wyeth-Ayerst Company
Philadelphia, PA 19101
CI 5190-2 Revised May 22, 2000

Shown in Product Identification Guide, page 341

ANTIVENIN ℞
(Micrurus fulvius)
[an "te ven 'in]
(equine origin)
North American Coral Snake Antivenin

COMPOSITION

Each combination package contains one vial of lyophilized Antivenin (Micrurus fulvius) with 0.25% phenol and 0.005% thimerosal (mercury derivative) as preservatives (before lyophilization); one vial of diluent containing 10 mL of Bacteriostatic Water for Injection, U.S.P., with phenylmercuric nitrate (0.001%) as preservative.

HOW SUPPLIED

Combination packages as described (not returnable).

Manufactured by Wyeth Laboratories, A Wyeth-Ayerst Company, Marietta, PA 17547.

CI 3280-1 Issued January 13, 1983

For prescribing information write to Professional Service, Wyeth-Ayerst Pharmaceuticals, P.O. Box 8299, Philadelphia, PA 19101, or contact your local Wyeth-Ayerst representative.

A.P.L.® ℞
(chorionic gonadotropin for injection, USP)
For Intramuscular Injection Only

Rx only

DESCRIPTION

Human chorionic gonadotropin (HCG), a polypeptide hormone produced by the human placenta, is composed of an alpha and a beta subunit. The alpha subunit is essentially identical to the alpha subunits of the human pituitary gonadotropins, luteinizing hormone (LH) and follicle-stimulating hormone (FSH), as well as to the alpha subunit of human thyroid stimulating hormone (TSH). The beta subunits of these hormones differ in amino acid sequence.

A.P.L. (chorionic gonadotropin, USP) is a gonad-stimulating principle obtained from the urine of pregnant women. It is a sterile, amorphous powder prepared by cryodesiccation, and is freely soluble in water.

When reconstituted with the accompanying 10 mL of sterile diluent water, each SECULE® vial contains:

5,000 USP units of chorionic gonadotropin, 2.0% benzyl alcohol, 0.9% lactose, and not more than 0.2% phenol;

10,000 USP units of chorionic gonadotropin, 2.0% benzyl alcohol, 1.8% lactose, and not more than 0.2% phenol;

20,000 USP units of chorionic gonadotropin, 2.0% benzyl alcohol, 3.6% lactose, and not more than 0.2% phenol.

The pH is adjusted with sodium hydroxide or hydrochloric acid.

After reconstitution, store refrigerated and use within 30 days.

THIS PRODUCT IS FOR INTRAMUSCULAR INJECTION ONLY.

HOW SUPPLIED

A.P.L.® (chorionic gonadotropin for injection, USP)

NDC 0046-0970-10 — Each package provides:
(1) One vial containing 5,000 USP units chorionic gonadotropin in dry form, and
(2) One 10 mL ampul sterile diluent.

NDC 0046-0971-10 — Each package provides:
(1) One vial containing 10,000 USP units chorionic gonadotropin in dry form, and
(2) One 10 mL ampul sterile diluent.

NDC 0046-0972-10 — Each package provides:
(1) One vial containing 20,000 USP units chorionic gonadotropin in dry form, and
(2) One 10 mL ampul sterile diluent.

The product is assayed in accord with USP method; USP potency units are defined in terms of the USP Chorionic Gonadotropin Reference Standard.

When reconstituted with 10 mL of accompanying sterile diluent, the resulting solutions also contain 2.0% benzyl alcohol, not more than 0.2% phenol, and the following concentrations of lactose: No. 970, 0.9%; No. 971, 1.8%; No. 972, 3.6%. The pH is adjusted with sodium hydroxide or hydrochloric acid.

Directions for Reconstitution

Withdraw sterile air from lyophilized vial. Remove 10 mL from diluent ampule and add to lyophilized vial; agitate gently until powder is completely dissolved.

MAY BE STORED FOR 30 DAYS IN A REFRIGERATOR AFTER RECONSTITUTION.

Manufactured by:
Ayerst Laboratories Inc.
A Wyeth-Ayerst Company
Philadelphia, PA 19101
CI 4379-4 Revised April 24, 1998

For prescribing information write to Professional Service, Wyeth-Ayerst Pharmaceuticals, P.O. Box 8299, Philadelphia, PA 19101, or contact your local Wyeth-Ayerst representative.

ATIVAN® Ⓒ ℞
[ăt ĭ-văn]
(lorazepam)
Injection

DESCRIPTION

Lorazepam, a benzodiazepine with antianxiety, sedative, and anticonvulsant effects, is intended for intramuscular or intravenous routes of administration. It has the chemical formula: 7-chloro-5(2-chlorophenyl)-1,3-dihydro-3-hydroxy-*2H*-1,4-benzodiazepin-2-one. The molecular weight is 321.16, and the C.A.S. No. is [846-49-1].

Lorazepam is a nearly white powder almost insoluble in water. Each mL of sterile injection contains either 2.0 or 4.0 mg of lorazepam, 0.18 mL polyethylene glycol 400 in propylene glycol with 2.0% benzyl alcohol as preservative.

CLINICAL PHARMACOLOGY

Lorazepam interacts with the γ-aminobutyric acid (GABA)-benzodiazepine receptor complex, which is widespread in the brain of humans as well as other species. This interaction is presumed to be responsible for lorazepam's mechanism of action. Lorazepam exhibits relatively high and specific affinity for its recognition site but does not displace GABA. Attachment to the specific binding site enhances the affinity of GABA for its receptor site on the same receptor complex. The pharmacodynamic consequences of benzodiazepine agonist actions include antianxiety effects, sedation, and reduction of seizure activity. The intensity of action is directly related to the degree of benzodiazepine receptor occupancy.

Effects in Pre-Operative Patients

Intravenous or intramuscular administration of the recommended dose of 2 mg to 4 mg of Ativan Injection to adult patients is followed by dose-related effects of sedation (sleepiness or drowsiness), relief of preoperative anxiety, and lack of recall of events related to the day of surgery in the majority of patients. The clinical sedation (sleepiness or drowsiness) thus noted is such that the majority of patients are able to respond to simple instructions whether they give the appearance of being awake or asleep. The lack of recall is relative rather than absolute, as determined under conditions of careful patient questioning and testing, using props designed to enhance recall. The majority of patients under these reinforced conditions had difficulty recalling perioperative events or recognizing props from before surgery. The lack of recall and recognition was optimum within 2 hours following intramuscular administration and 15 to 20 minutes after intravenous injection.

The intended effects of the recommended adult dose of Ativan Injection usually last 6 to 8 hours. In rare instances, and where patients received greater than the recommended dose, excessive sleepiness and prolonged lack of recall were noted. As with other benzodiazepines, unsteadiness, enhanced sensitivity to CNS-depressant effects of ethyl alcohol and other drugs were noted in isolated and rare cases for greater than 24 hours.

Physiologic Effects in Healthy Adults

Studies in healthy adult volunteers reveal that intravenous lorazepam in doses up to 3.5 mg/70 kg does not alter sensitivity to the respiratory stimulating effect of carbon dioxide and does not enhance the respiratory-depressant effects of doses of meperidine up to 100 mg/70 kg (also determined by carbon dioxide challenge) as long as patients remain sufficiently awake to undergo testing. Upper airway obstruction has been observed in rare instances where the patient received greater than the recommended dose and was excessively sleepy and difficult to arouse (see **WARNINGS** and **ADVERSE REACTIONS.**)

Clinically employed doses of Ativan Injection do not greatly affect the circulatory system in the supine position or employing a 70-degree tilt test. Doses of 8 mg to 10 mg of intravenous lorazepam (2 to $2^1/_2$ times the maximum recommended dosage) will produce loss of lid reflexes within 15 minutes.

Studies in 6 healthy young adults who received lorazepam injection and no other drugs revealed that visual tracking (the ability to keep a moving line centered) was impaired for a mean of 8 hours following administration of 4 mg of intramuscular lorazepam and 4 hours following administration of 2 mg intramuscularly with considerable subject variation. Similar findings were noted with pentobarbital, 150 and 75 mg. Although this study showed that both lorazepam and pentobarbital interfered with eye-hand coordination, the data are insufficient to predict when it would be safe to operate a motor vehicle or engage in a hazardous occupation or sport.

Pharmacokinetics and Metabolism

Absorption

Intravenous

A 4-mg dose provides an initial concentration of 70 ng/mL.

Intramuscular

Following intramuscular administration, lorazepam is completely and rapidly absorbed reaching peak concentrations within 3 hours. A 4-mg dose provides a C_{max} of approximately 48 ng/mL. Following administration of 1.5 to 5.0 mg of lorazepam IM, the amount of lorazepam delivered to the circulation is proportional to the dose administered.

Distribution/Metabolism/Elimination

At clinically relevant concentrations, lorazepam is 91±2% bound to plasma proteins; its volume of distribution is approximately 1.3 L/kg. Unbound lorazepam penetrates the blood/brain barrier freely by passive diffusion, a fact confirmed by CSF sampling. Following parenteral administration, the terminal half-life and total clearance averaged 14.5±5 hours and 1.1±0.4 mL/min/kg, respectively.

Lorazepam is extensively conjugated to the 3-O-phenolic glucuronide in the liver and is known to undergo enterohepatic recirculation. Lorazepam glucuronide is an inactive metabolite and is eliminated mainly by the kidneys.

Following a single 2-mg oral dose of ^{14}C-lorazepam to 8 healthy subjects, 88±4% of the administered dose was recovered in urine and 7±2% was recovered in feces. The percent of administered dose recovered in urine as lorazepam glucuronide was 74±4%. Only 0.3% of the dose was recovered as unchanged lorazepam, and the remainder of the radioactivity represented minor metabolites.

Special Populations

Effect of Age

Pediatrics

NEONATES (BIRTH TO 1 MONTH)

Following a single 0.05 mg/kg (n=4) or 0.1 mg/kg (n=6) intravenous dose of lorazepam, *mean total clearance normalized to body weight was reduced by 80% compared to normal adults*, terminal half-life was prolonged 3-fold, and volume of distribution was decreased by 40% in neonates with asphyxia neonatorum compared to normal adults. All neonates were of ≥ 37 weeks of gestational age.

INFANTS (1 MONTH UP TO 2 YEARS)

There is no information on the pharmacokinetic profile of lorazepam in infants in the age range of 1 month to 2 years.

CHILDREN (2 YEARS TO 12 YEARS)

Total (bound and unbound) lorazepam had a 50% higher mean volume of distribution (normalized to body-weight) and a 30% longer mean half-life in children with acute lymphocytic leukemia in complete remission (2 to 12 years, n=37) compared to normal adults (n=10). *Unbound* lorazepam clearance normalized to body-weight was comparable in children and adults.

ADOLESCENTS (12 YEARS TO 18 YEARS)

Total (bound and unbound) lorazepam had a 50% higher mean volume of distribution (normalized to body-weight) and a mean half-life that has two fold greater in adolescents with acute lymphocytic leukemia in complete remission (12 to 18 years, n=13) compared to normal adults (n=10). *Unbound* lorazepam clearance normalized to body-weight was comparable in adolescents and adults.

Elderly

Following single intravenous doses of 1.5 to 3 mg of Ativan Injection, mean total body clearance of lorazepam decreased by 20% in 15 elderly subjects of 60 to 84 years of age compared to that in 15 younger subjects of 19 to 38 years of age. Consequently, no dosage adjustment appears to be necessary in elderly subjects based solely on their age.

Effect of Gender

Gender has no effect on the pharmacokinetics of lorazepam.

Effect of Race

Young Americans (n=15) and Japanese subjects (n=7) had very comparable mean total clearance value of 1.0 mL/min/

kg. However, elderly Japanese subjects had a 20% lower mean total clearance than elderly Americans, 0.59 mL/min/kg vs. 0.77 mL/min/kg, respectively.

Patients with Renal Insufficiency

Because the kidney is the primary route of elimination of lorazepam glucuronide, renal impairment would be expected to compromise its clearance. This should have no direct effect on the glucuronidation (and inactivation) of lorazepam. There is a possibility that the enterohepatic circulation of lorazepam glucuronide leads to a reduced efficiency of the net clearance of lorazepam in this population. Six normal subjects, six patients with renal impairment (Cl_{cr} of 22±9 mL/min), and four patients on chronic maintenance hemodialysis were given single 1.5 to 3.0 mg intravenous doses of lorazepam. Mean volume of distribution and terminal half-life values of lorazepam were 40% and 25% higher, respectively, in renally impaired patients than in normal subjects. Both parameters were 75% higher in patients undergoing hemodialysis than in normal subjects. Overall, though, in this group of subjects the mean total clearance of lorazepam did not change. About 8% of the administered intravenous dose was removed as intact lorazepam during the 6-hour dialysis session.

The kinetics of lorazepam glucuronide were markedly affected by renal dysfunction. The mean terminal half-life was prolonged by 55% and 125% in renally impaired patients and patients under hemodialysis, respectively, as compared to normal subjects. The mean metabolic clearance decreased by 75% and 90% in renally impaired patients and patients under hemodialysis, respectively, as compared with normal subjects. About 40% of the administered lorazepam intravenous dose was removed as glucuronide conjugate during the 6-hour dialysis session.

Hepatic Disease

Because cytochrome oxidation is not involved with the metabolism of lorazepam, liver disease would not be expected to have an effect on metabolic clearance. This prediction is supported by the observation that following a single 2 mg intravenous dose of lorazepam, cirrhotic male patients (n=13) and normal male subjects (n=11) exhibited no substantive difference in their ability to clear lorazepam.

Effect of Smoking

Administration of a single 2 mg intravenous dose of lorazepam showed that there was no difference in any of the pharmacokinetic parameters of lorazepam between cigarette smokers (n=10, mean=31 cigarettes per day) and nonsmoking subjects (n=10) who were matched for age, weight and gender.

Clinical Studies

The effectiveness of Ativan Injection in status epilepticus was established in two multi-center controlled trials in 177 patients. With rare exceptions, patients were between 18 and 65 years of age. More than half the patients in each study had tonic-clonic status epilepticus; patients with simple partial and complex partial status epilepticus comprised the rest of the population studied, along with a smaller number of patients who had the absence status.

One study (n=58) was a double-blind active-control trial comparing Ativan Injection and diazepam. Patients were randomized to receive Ativan 2 mg IV (with an additional 2 mg IV if needed) or diazepam 5 mg IV (with an additional 5 mg IV if needed). The primary outcome measure was a comparison of the proportion of responders in each treatment group, where a responder was defined as a patient whose seizures stopped within 10 minutes after treatment and who continued seizure-free for at least an additional 30 minutes. Twenty-four of the 30 (80%) patients were deemed responders to Ativan and 16/28 (57%) patients were deemed responders to diazepam (p=0.04). Of the 24 Ativan responders, 23 received both 2 mg infusions.

Non-responders to Ativan 4 mg were given an additional 2 to 4 mg Ativan; non-responders to diazepam 10 mg were given an additional 5 to 10 mg diazepam. After this additional dose administration, 28/30 (93%) of patients randomized to Ativan and 24/28 (86%) of patients randomized to diazepam were deemed responders, a difference that was not statistically significant.

Although this study provides support for the efficacy of Ativan as the treatment for status epilepticus, it cannot speak reliably or meaningfully to the comparative performance of either diazepam (Valium) or lorazepam (Ativan Injection) under the conditions of actual use.

A second study (n=119) was a double-blind dose-comparison trial with 3 doses of Ativan Injection: 1 mg, 2 mg, and 4 mg. Patients were randomized to receive one of the three doses of Ativan. The primary outcome and definition of responder were as in the first study. Twenty-five of 41 patients (61%) responded to 1 mg Ativan; 21/37 patients (57%) responded to 2 mg Ativan; and 31/41 (76%) responded to 4 mg Ativan. The p-value for a statistical test of the difference between the Ativan 4 mg dose group and the Ativan 1-mg dose group was 0.08 (two-sided). Data from all randomized patients were used in this test.

Although analyses failed to detect an effect of age, sex, or race on the effectiveness of Ativan in status epilepticus, the numbers of patients evaluated were too few to allow a definitive conclusion about the role these factors may play.

INDICATIONS AND USAGE

Status Epilepticus

Ativan Injection is indicated for the treatment of status epilepticus.

Preanesthetic

Ativan Injection is indicated in adult patients for preanesthetic medication, producing sedation (sleepiness or drowsiness), relief of anxiety, and a decreased ability to recall events related to the day of surgery. It is most useful in those patients who are anxious about their surgical procedure and who would prefer to have diminished recall of the events of the day of surgery (see **PRECAUTIONS, Information for Patients**).

CONTRAINDICATIONS

Ativan Injection is contraindicated in patients with a known sensitivity to benzodiazepines or its vehicle (polyethylene glycol, propylene glycol and benzyl alcohol), in patients with acute narrow-angle glaucoma, or in patients with sleep apnea syndrome. It is also contraindicated in patients with severe respiratory insufficiency, except in those patients requiring relief of anxiety and/or diminished recall of events while being mechanically ventilated. The use of Ativan Injection intra-arterially is contraindicated because, as with other injectable benzodiazepines, inadvertent intra-arterial injection may produce arteriospasm resulting in gangrene which may require amputation (see **WARNINGS**).

WARNINGS

Use in Status Epilepticus

Management of Status Epilepticus

Status epilepticus is a potentially life-threatening condition associated with a high risk of permanent neurological impairment, if inadequately treated. The treatment of status, however, requires far more than the administration of an anticonvulsant agent. It involves observation and management of all parameters critical to maintaining vital function and the capacity to provide support of those functions as required. Ventilatory support must be readily available. The use of benzodiazepines, like Ativan Injection, is ordinarily only one step of a complex and sustained intervention which may require additional interventions (e.g., concomitant intravenous administration of phenytoin). Because status epilepticus may result from a correctable acute cause such as hypoglycemia, hyponatremia, or other metabolic or toxic derangement, such an abnormality must be immediately sought and corrected. Furthermore, patients who are susceptible to further seizure episodes should receive adequate maintenance antiepileptic therapy.

Any health care professional who intends to treat a patient with status epilepticus should be familiar with this package insert and the pertinent medical literature concerning current concepts for the treatment of status epilepticus. A comprehensive review of the considerations critical to the informed and prudent management of status epilepticus cannot be provided in drug product labeling. The archival medical literature contains many informative references on the management of status epilepticus, among them the report of the working group on status epilepticus of the Epilepsy Foundation of America "Treatment of Convulsive Status Epilepticus" (JAMA 1993; 270:854–859). As noted in the report just cited, it may be useful to consult with a neurologist if a patient fails to respond (e.g., fails to regain consciousness).

For the treatment of status epilepticus, the usual recommended dose of Ativan Injection is 4 mg given slowly (2 mg/min) for patients 18 years and older. If seizures cease, no additional Ativan Injection is required. If seizures continue or recur after a 10- to 15- minute observation period, an additional 4 mg intravenous dose may be slowly administered. *Experience with further doses of Ativan is very limited.* The usual precautions in treating status epilepticus should be employed. An intravenous infusion should be started, vital signs should be monitored, an unobstructed airway should be maintained, and artificial ventilation equipment should be available.

Respiratory Depression

The most important risk associated with the use of Ativan Injection in status epilepticus is respiratory depression. Accordingly, airway patency must be assured and respiration monitored closely. Ventilatory support should be given as required.

Excessive Sedation

Because of its prolonge duration of action, the prescriber should be alert to the possibility, especially when multiple doses have been given, that the sedative effects of lorazepam may add to the impairment of consciousness seen in the post-ictal state.

Preanesthetic Use

AIRWAY OBSTRUCTION MAY OCCUR IN HEAVILY SEDATED PATIENTS. INTRAVENOUS LORAZEPAM AT ANY DOSE, WHEN GIVEN EITHER ALONE OR IN COMBINATION WITH OTHER DRUGS ADMINISTERED DURING ANESTHESIA, MAY PRODUCE HEAVY SEDATION; THEREFORE, EQUIPMENT NECESSARY TO MAINTAIN A PATENT AIRWAY AND TO SUPPORT RESPIRATION/VENTILATION SHOULD BE AVAILABLE.

As is true of similar CNS-acting drugs, the decision as to when patients who have received injectable lorazepam, particularly on an outpatient basis, may again operate machinery, drive a motor vehicle, or engage in hazardous or other activities requiring attention and coordination must be individualized. It is recommended that no patient engage in such activities for a period of 24 to 48 hours or until the effects of the drug, such as drowsiness, have subsided, whichever is longer. Impairment of performance may persist for greater intervals because of extremes of age, concomitant use of other drugs, stress of surgery, or the general condition of the patient.

Clinical trials have shown that patients over the age of 50 years may have a more profound and prolonged sedation with intravenous lorazepam (see also **DOSAGE AND ADMINISTRATION, Preanesthetic**).

As with all central-nervous-system-depressant drugs, care should be exercised in patients given injectable lorazepam as premature ambulation may result in injury from falling. There is no added beneficial effect from the addition of scopolamine to injectable lorazepam, and their combined effect may result in an increased incidence of sedation, hallucination and irrational behavior.

General (All Uses)

PRIOR TO INTRAVENOUS USE, ATIVAN INJECTION MUST BE DILUTED WITH AN EQUAL AMOUNT OF COMPATIBLE DILUENT (see **DOSAGE AND ADMINISTRATION**). INTRAVENOUS INJECTION SHOULD BE MADE SLOWLY AND WITH REPEATED ASPIRATION. CARE SHOULD BE TAKEN TO DETERMINE THAT ANY INJECTION WILL NOT BE INTRA-ARTERIAL AND THAT PERIVASCULAR EXTRAVASATION WILL NOT TAKE PLACE. IN THE EVENT THAT A PATIENT COMPLAINS OF PAIN DURING INTENDED INTRAVENOUS INJECTION OF ATIVAN INJECTION, THE INJECTION SHOULD BE STOPPED IMMEDIATELY TO DETERMINE IF INTRA-ARTERIAL INJECTION OR PERIVASCULAR EXTRAVASATION HAS TAKEN PLACE.

Since the liver is the most likely site of conjugation of lorazepam and since excretion of conjugated lorazepam (glucuronide) is a renal function, this drug is not recommended for use in patients with hepatic and/or renal *failure*. Ativan should be used with caution in patients with mild-to-moderate hepatic or renal disease (see **DOSAGE AND ADMINISTRATION**).

Pregnancy

ATIVAN MAY CAUSE FETAL DAMAGE WHEN ADMINISTERED TO PREGNANT WOMEN. Ordinarily, Ativan Injection should not be used during pregnancy except in serious or life-threatening conditions where safer drugs cannot be used or are ineffective. Status epilepticus may represent such a serioius life-threatening condition.

An increased risk of congenital malformations associated with the use of minor tranquilizers (chlordiazepoxide, diazepam and meprobamate) during the first trimester of pregnancy has been suggested in several studies. In humans, blood levels obtained from umbilical cord blood indicate placental transfer of lorazepam and lorazepam glucuronide.

Reproductive studies in animals were performed in mice, rats, and two strains of rabbits. Occasional anomalies (reduction of tarsals, tibia, metatarsals, malrotated limbs, gastroschisis, malformed skull, and microphthalmia) were seen in drug-treated rabbits without relationship to dosage. Although all of these anomalies were not present in the concurrent control group, they have been reported to occur randomly in historical controls. At doses of 40 mg/kg orally or 4 mg/kg intravenously and higher, there was evidence of fetal resorption and increased fetal loss in rabbits which was not seen at lower doses.

The possibility that a woman of childbearing potential may be pregnant at the time of therapy should be considered. There are insufficient data regarding obstetrical safety of parenteral lorazepam, including use in cesarean section. Such use, therefore, is not recommended.

Endoscopic Procedures

There are insufficient data to support the use of Ativan Injection for outpatient endoscopic procedures. Inpatient endoscopic procedures require adequate recovery room observation time.

When Ativan Injection is used for peroral endoscopic procedures, adequate topical or regional anesthesia is recommended to minimize reflex activity associated with such procedures.

PRECAUTIONS

General

The additive central-nervous-system effects of other drugs, such as phenothiazines, narcotic analgesics, barbiturates, antidepressants, scopolamine, and monoamine-oxidase inhibitors, should be borne in mind when these other drugs are used concomitantly with or during the period of recovery from Ativan Injection (see **CLINICAL PHARMACOLOGY** and **WARNINGS**).

Extreme caution must be used when administering Ativan Injection to elderly patients, very ill patients, or to patients with limited pulmonary reserve because of the possibility that hypoventilation and/or hypoxic cardiac arrest may occur. Resuscitative equipment for ventilatory support should be readily available (see **WARNINGS** and **DOSAGE AND ADMINISTRATION**).

When lorazepam injection is used IV as the premedicant prior to regional or local anesthesia, the possibility of excessive sleepiness or drowsiness may interfere with patient cooperation in determining levels of anesthesia. This is most likely to occur when greater than 0.05 mg/kg is given and when narcotic analgesics are used concomitantly with the recommended dose (see **ADVERSE REACTIONS**).

As with all benzodiazepines, paradoxical reactions may occur in rare instances and in an unpredictable fashion (see **ADVERSE REACTIONS**). In these instances, further use of the drug in these patients should be considered with caution.

There have been reports of possible propylene glycol toxicity (e.g., lactic acidosis, hyperosmolality, hypotension) and pos-

Continued on next page

Ativan Injection—Cont.

sible polyethylene glycol toxicity (e.g., acute tubular necrosis) during administration of Ativan Injection at higher than recommended doses. Symptoms may be more likely to develop in patients with renal impairment.

Information for Patients

Patients should be informed of the pharmacological effects of the drug, including sedation, relief of anxiety, and lack of recall, the duration of these effects (about 8 hours), and be apprised of the risks as well as the benefits of therapy.

Patients who receive Ativan Injection as a premedicant should be cautioned that driving a motor vehicle, operating machinery, or engaging in hazardous or other activities requiring attention and coordination, should be delayed for 24 to 48 hours following the injection or until the effects of the drug, such as drowsiness, have subsided, whichever is longer. Sedatives, tranquilizers and narcotic analgesics may produce a more prolonged and profound effect when administered along with injectable Ativan. This effect may take the form of excessive sleepiness or drowsiness and, on rare occasions, interfere with recall and recognition of events of the day of surgery and the day after.

Patients should be advised that getting out of bed unassisted may result in falling and injury if undertaken within 8 hours of receiving lorazepam injection. Since tolerance for CNS depressants will be diminished in the presence of Ativan Injection, these substances should either be avoided or taken in reduced dosage. Alcoholic beverages should not be consumed for at least 24 to 48 hours after receiving lorazepam injectable due to the additive effects on central-nervous-system depression seen with benzodiazepines in general. Elderly patients should be told that Ativan Injection may make them very sleepy for a period longer than 6 to 8 hours following surgery.

Laboratory Tests

In clinical trials, no laboratory test abnormalities were identified with either single or multiple doses of Ativan Injection. These tests included: CBC, urinalysis, SGOT, SGPT, bilirubin, alkaline phosphatase, LDH, cholesterol, uric acid, BUN, glucose, calcium, phosphorus, and total proteins.

Drug Interactions

Ativan Injection, like other injectable benzodiazepines, produces additive depression of the central nervous system when administered with other CNS depressants such as ethyl alcohol, phenothiazines, barbiturates, MAO inhibitors, and other antidepressants.

When scopolamine is used concomitantly with injectable lorazepam, an increased incidence of sedation, hallucinations and irrational behavior has been observed.

There have been rare reports of significant respiratory depression, stupor and/or hypotension with the concomitant use of loxapine and lorazepam.

Marked sedation, excessive salivation, ataxia, and, rarely, death have been reported with the concomitant use of clozapine and lorazepam.

Apnea, coma, bradycardia, arrhythmia, heart arrest, and death have been reported with the concomitant use of haloperidol and lorazepam.

The risk of using lorazepam in combination with scopolamine, loxapine, clozapine, haloperidol, or other CNS-depressant drugs has not been systematically evaluated. Therefore, caution is advised if the concomitant administration of lorazepam and these drugs is required.

Concurrent administration of any of the following drugs with lorazepam had no effect on the pharmacokinetics of lorazepam; metoprolol, cimetidine, ranitidine, disulfiram, propranolol, metronidazole, and propoxyphene. No change in Ativan dosage is necessary when concomitantly given with any of these drugs.

Lorazepam-Valproate Interaction

Concurrent administration of lorazepam (2 mg intravenously) with valproate (250 mg twice daily orally for 3 days) to 6 healthy male subjects resulted in decreased total clearance of lorazepam by 40% and decreased formation rate of lorazepam glucuronide by 55%, as compared with lorazepam administered alone. Accordingly, lorazepam plasma concentrations were about two-fold higher for at least 12 hours post-dose administration during valproate treatment. Lorazepam dosage should be reduced to 50% of the normal adult dose when this drug combination is prescribed in patients (see also **DOSAGE AND ADMINISTRATION**).

Lorazepam-Oral Contraceptive Steroids Interaction

Coadministration of lorazepam (2 mg intravenously) with oral contraceptive steroids (norethindrone acetate, 1 mg, and ethinyl estradiol, 50 µg, for at least 6 months) to healthy females (n=7) was associated with a 55% decrease in half-life, a 50% increase in the volume of distribution, thereby resulting in an almost 3.7-fold increase in total clearance of lorazepam as compared with control healthy females (n=8). It may be necessary to increase the dose of Ativan in female patients who are concomitantly taking oral contraceptives (see also **DOSAGE AND ADMINISTRATION**).

Lorazepam-Probenecid Interaction

Concurrent administration of lorazepam (2 mg intravenously) with probenecid (500 mg orally every 6 hours) to 9 healthy volunteers resulted in a prolongation of lorazepam half-life by 130% and a decrease in its total clearance by 45%. No change in volume of distribution was noted during probenecid co-treatment. Ativan dosage needs to be reduced by 50% when coadministered with probenecid (see also **DOSAGE AND ADMINISTRATION**).

Drug/Laboratory Test Interactions

No laboratory test abnormalities were identified when lorazepam was given alone or concomitantly with another drug, such as narcotic analgesics, inhalation anesthetics, scopolamine, atropine, and a variety of tranquilizing agents.

Carcinogenesis, Mutagenesis, Impairment of Fertility

No evidence of carcinogenic potential emerged in rats and mice during an 18-month study with oral lorazepam. No studies regarding mutagenesis have been performed. The results of a pre-implantation study in rats, in which the oral lorazepam dose was 20 mg/kg dose, showed no impairment of fertility.

Pregnancy

Teratogenic Effects—Pregnancy Category D (See **WARNINGS**.)

Labor and Delivery

There are insufficient data to support the use of Ativan Injection during labor and delivery, including cesarean section; therefore, its use in this clinical circumstance is not recommended.

Nursing Mothers

Lorazepam has been detected in human breast milk, Therefore, lorazepam should not be administered to nursing mothers because, like other benzodiazepines, the possibility exists that lorazepam may sedate or otherwise adversely affect the infant.

Pediatric Use

Status Epilepticus

The safety of Ativan in pediatric patients with status epilepticus has not been systematically evaluated.

Open-label studies described in the medical literature included 273 pediatric/adolescent patients; the age range was from a few hours old to 18 years of age. Paradoxical excitation was observed in 10% to 30% of the pediatric patients under 8 years of age and was characterized by tremors, agitation, euphoria, logorrhea, and brief episodes of visual hallucinations. Parodoxical excitation in pediatric patients also has been reported with other benzodiazepines when used for status epilepticus, as an anesthesia, or for pre-chemotherapy treatment.

Pediatric patients (as well as adults) with atypical petit mal status epilepticus have developed brief tonic-clonic seizures shortly after Ativan was given. This "paradoxical" effect was also reported for diazepam and clonazepam. Nevertheless, the development of seizures after treatment with benzodiazepines is probably rare, based on the incidence in the uncontrolled treatment series reported (i.e., seizures were not observed for 112 pediatric patients and 18 adults or during approximately 400 doses.).

Preanesthetic

There are insufficient data to support the efficacy of injectable lorazepam as a preanesthetic agent in patients less than 18 years of age.

General

Seizure activity and myoclonus have been reported to occur following administration of Ativan Injection, especially in very low birth weight neonates.

Pediatric patients may exhibit a sensitivity to benzyl alcohol, polyethelene glycol and propylene glycol, components of Ativan Injection (see also **CONTRAINDICATIONS**). The "gasping syndrome," characterized by central nervous system depression, metabolic acidosis, gasping respirations, and high levels of benzyl alcohol and its metabolites found in the blood and urine, has been associated with benzyl alcohol dosages >99 mg/kg/day in neonates and low-birth-weight neonates. Additional symptoms may include gradual neurological deterioration, seizures, intracranial hemorrhage, hematologic abnormalities, skin breakdown, hepatic and renal failure, hypotension, bradycardia, and cardiovascular collapse. Central nervous system toxicity, including seizures and intraventricular hemorrhage, as well as unresponsiveness, tachypnea, tachycardia, and diaphoresis have been associated with propylene glycol toxicity. Although normal therapeutic doses of Ativan Injection contain very small amounts of these compounds, premature and low-birth-weight infants as well as pediatric patients receiving high dosages may be more susceptible to their effects.

Geriatric Use

Status Epilepticus

Age over 65 years may be associated with a greater incidence of central nervous system depression and more respiratory depression.

ADVERSE REACTIONS

Status Epilepticus

The most important adverse clinical event caused by the use of Ativan Injection is repiratory depression (see **WARNINGS**).

The adverse clinical events most commonly observed with the use of Ativan Injection in clinical trials evaluating its use in status epilepticus were hypotension, somnolence, and respiratory failure.

Incidence in Controlled Clinical Trials

All adverse events were recorded during the trials by the clinical investigators using terminology of their own choosing. Similar types of events were grouped into standardized categories using modified COSTART dictionary terminology. These categories are used in the table and listings below with the frequencies representing the proportion of individuals exposed to Ativan Injection or to comparative therapy.

The prescriber should be aware that these figures cannot be used to predict the frequency of adverse events in the course of usual medical practice where patient characteristics and other factors may differ from those prevailing during clinical studies. Similarly, the cited frequencies cannot be directly compared with figures obtained from other clinical investigators involving different treatment, uses, or investigators. An inspection of these frequencies, however, does provide the prescribing physician with one basis to estimate the relative contribution of drug and nondrug factors to the adverse event incidences in the population studied.

Commonly Observed Adverse Events in a Controlled Dose-Comparison Clinical Trial

Table 1 lists the treatment-emergent adverse events that occurred in the patients treated with Ativan Injection in a dose-comparison trial of Ativan 1 mg, 2 mg, and 4 mg.

TABLE 1. NUMBER (%) OF STUDY EVENTS IN A DOSE COMPARISON CLINICAL TRIAL

Body System Event	Ativen Injection (n=130)[a]
Any Study Event (1 or more)[b]	16 (12.3%)
Body as a whole	
Infection	1 (<1%)
Cardiovascular system	
Hypotension	2 (1.5%)
Digestive system	
Liver function tests abnormal	1 (<1%)
Nausea	1 (<1%)
Vomiting	1 (<1%)
Metabolic and Nutritional	
Acidosis	1 (<1%)
Nervous system	
Brain edema	1 (<1%)
Coma	1 (<1%)
Convulsion	1 (<1%)
Somnolence	2 (1.5%)
Thinking abnormal	1 (<1%)
Respiratory system	
Hyperventilation	1 (<1%)
Hypoventilation	1 (<1%)
Respiratory failure	2 (1.5%)
Terms not classifiable	
Injection site reaction	1 (<1%)
Urogenital system	
Cystitis	1 (<1%)

a: One hundred and thirty (130) patients received Ativan Injection.

b: Totals are not necessarily the sum of the individual study events because a patient may report two or more different study events in the same body system.

Commonly Observed Adverse Events in Active-Controlled Clinical Trials

In two studies, patients who completed the course of treatment for status epilepticus were permitted to be reenrolled and to receive treatment for a second status episode, given that there was a sufficient interval between the two episodes. Safety was determined from all treatment episodes for all intent-to-treat patients, i.e., from all "patient-episodes." Table 2 lists the treatment emergent adverse events that occurred in at least 1% of the patient-episodes in which Ativan Injection or diazepam was given. The table represents the pooling of results from the two controlled trials.

[See table at bottom of next page]

These trials were not designed or intended to demonstrate the comparative safety of the two treatments.

The overall adverse experience profile for Ativan was similar between women and men. There are insufficient data to support a statement regarding the distribution of adverse events by race. Generally, age greater than 65 years may be associated with a greater incidence of central-nervous-system depression and more respiratory depression.

Other Events Observed During the Pre-marketing Evaluation of Ativan Injection for the Treatment of Status Epilepticus

Ativan Injection, active comparators, and Ativan Injection in combination with a comparator were administered to 488 individuals during controlled and open-label clinical trials. Because of reenrollments, these 488 patients participated in a total of 521 patient-episodes. Ativan Injection alone was given in 69% of these patient-episodes (n=360). The safety information below is based on data available from 326 of these patient-episodes in which Ativan Injection was given alone.

All adverse events that were seen once are listed, except those already included in previous listings (Table 1 and Table 2).

Study events were classified by body system in descending frequency by using the following definitions: frequent adverse events were those that occurred in at least 1/100 individuals; infrequent study events were those that occurred in 1/100 to 1/1000 individuals.

Frequent and Infrequent Study Events

BODY AS A WHOLE-	Infrequent: asthenia, chills, headache, infection.
DIGESTIVE SYSTEM-	Infrequent: abnormal liver function test, increased salivation, nausea, vomiting.
METABOLIC AND NUTRITIONAL-	Infrequent: acidosis, alkaline phosphatase increased.
NERVOUS SYSTEM-	Infrequent: agitation, ataxia, brain edema, coma, confusion, convulsion, hallucinations, myoclonus, stupor, thinking abnormal, tremor.
RESPIRATORY SYSTEM-	Frequent: apnea; Infrequent: hyperventilation, hypoventilation, respiratory disorder.
TERMS NOT CLASSIFIABLE-	Infrequent: injection site reaction.
UROGENITAL SYSTEM-	Infrequent: cystitis.

Preanesthetic

Central Nervous System

The most frequent adverse drug event reported with injectable lorazepam is a central-nervous-system-depression. The incidence varied from one study to another, depending on the dosage, route of administration, use of other central-nervous-system depressants, and the investigator's opinion concerning the degree and duration of desired sedation. Excessive sleepiness and drowsiness were the most common consequence of CNS depression. This interfered with patient cooperation in approximately 6% (25/446) of patients undergoing regional anesthesia, causing difficulty in assessing levels of anesthesia. Patients over 50 years of age had a higher incidence of excessive sleepiness or drowsiness when compared with those under 50 (21/106 versus 24/245) when lorazepam was given intravenously (see **DOSAGE AND ADMINISTRATION**). On rare occasion (3/1580) the patient was unable to give personal identification in the operating room on arrival, and one patient fell when attempting premature ambulation in the postoperative period.

Symptoms such as restlessness, confusion, depression, crying, sobbing, and delirium occurred in about 1.3% (20/1580). One patient injured himself by picking at his incision during the immediate postoperative period.

Hallucinations were present in about 1% (14/1580) of patients and were visual and self-limiting.

An occasional patient complained of dizziness, diplopia and/or blurred vision. Depressed hearing was infrequently reported during the peak-effect period.

An occasional patient had a prolonged recovery room stay, either because of excessive sleepiness or because of some form of inappropriate behavior. The latter was seen most commonly when scopolamine was given concomitantly as a premedicant.

Limited information derived from patients who were discharged the day after receiving injectable lorazepam showed one patient complained of some unsteadiness of gait and a reduced ability to perform complex mental functions. Enhanced sensitivity to alcoholic beverages has been reported more than 24 hours after receiving injectable lorazepam, similar to experience with other benzodiazepines.

Local Effects

Intramuscular injection of lorazepam has resulted in pain at the injection site, a sensation of burning, or observed redness in the same area in a very variable incidence from one study to another. The overall incidence of pain and burning was about 17% (146/859) in the immediate postinjection period and about 1.4% (12/859) at the 24-hour observation time. Reactions at the injection site (redness) occurred in approximately 2% (17/859) in the immediate postinjection period and were present 24 hours later in about 0.8% (7/859).

Intravenous administration of lorazepam resulted in painful responses in 13/771 patients or approximately 1.6% in the immediate postinjection period, and 24 hours later 4/771 patients or about 0.5% still complained of pain. Redness did not occur immediately following intravenous injection but was noted in 19/771 patients at the 24-hour observation period. This incidence is similar to that observed with an intravenous infusion before lorazepam is given. Intra-arterial injection may produce arteriospasm resulting in gangrene which may require amputation (see **CONTRAINDICATIONS**).

Cardiovascular System

Hypertension (0.1%) and hypotension (0.1%) have occasionally been observed after patients have received injectable lorazepam.

Respiratory System

Five patients (5/446) who underwent regional anesthesia were observed to have airway obstruction. This was believed due to excessive sleepiness at the time of the procedure and resulted in temporary hypoventilation. In this instance, appropriate airway management may become necessary (see also **CLINICAL PHARMACOLOGY, WARNINGS** and **PRECAUTIONS**).

Other Adverse Experiences

Skin rash, nausea and vomiting have occasionally been noted in patients who have received injectable lorazepam combined with other drugs during anesthesia and surgery.

Paradoxical Reactions

As with all benzodiazepines, parodoxical reactions such as stimulation, mania, irritability, restlessness, agitation, aggression, psychosis, hostility, rage, or hallucinations may occur in rare instances and in an unpredictable fashion. In these instances, further use of the drug in these patients should be considered with caution (see **PRECAUTIONS, General**).

Postmarketing Reports

Voluntary reports of other adverse events temporally associated with the use of Ativan Injection that have been received since market introduction and that may have no causal relationship with the use of Ativan Injection include the following: acute brain syndrome, aggravation of pheochromocytoma, amnesia, apnea/respiratory arrest, arrhythmia, bradycardia, brain edema, coagulation disorder, coma, convulsion, gastrointestinal hemorrhage, heart arrest/failure, heart block, liver damage, lung edema, lung hemorrhage, nervousness, neuroleptic malignant syndrome, paralysis, pericardial effusion, pneumothorax, pulmonary hypertension, tachycardia, thrombocytopenia, urinary incontinence, ventricular arrhythmia.

Fatalities also have been reported, usually in patients on concomitant medications (e.g., respiratory depressants) and/or with other medical conditions (e.g., obstructive sleep apnea).

DRUG ABUSE AND DEPENDENCE

Controlled Substance Class

Lorazepam is a controlled substance in Schedule IV.

Abuse and Physical and Psychological Dependence

As with other benzodiazepines, Ativan Injection has a potential for abuse and may lead to dependence. Physicians should be aware that repeated doses over a prolonged period of time may result in physical and psychological dependence and withdrawal symptoms, following abrupt discontinuance, similar in character to those noted with barbiturates and alcohol.

OVERDOSAGE

Symptoms

Overdosage of benzodiazepines is usually manifested by varying degrees of central-nervous-system depression, ranging from drowsiness to coma. In mild cases symptoms include drowsiness, mental confusion and lethargy. In more serious examples, symptoms may include ataxia, hypotonia, hypotension, hypnosis, stages one (1) to three (3) coma, and, very rarely, death.

Treatment

Treatment of overdosage is mainly supportive until the drug is eliminated from the body. Vital signs and fluid balance should be carefully monitored in conjunction with close observation of the patient. An adequate airway should be maintained and assisted respiration used as needed. With normally functioning kidneys, forced diuresis with intravenous fluids and electrolytes may accelerate elimination of benzodiazepines from the body. In addition, osmotic diuretics, such as mannitol, may be effective as adjunctive measures. In more critical situations, renal dialysis and exchange blood transfusions may be indicated. Lorazepam does not appear to be removed in significant quantities by dialysis, although lorazepam glucuronide may be highly dialyzable. The value of dialysis has not been adequately determined for lorazepam.

The benzodiazepine antagonist flumazenil may be used in hospitalized patients as an adjunct to, not as a substitute for, proper management of benzodiazepine overdose. **The prescriber should be aware of a risk of seizure in association with flumazenil treatment, particularly in long-term benzodiazepine users and in cyclic antidepressant overdose.** The complete flumazenil package insert including **CONTRAINDICATIONS, WARNINGS** and **PRECAUTIONS** should be consulted prior to use.

DOSAGE AND ADMINISTRATION

Ativan must never be used without individualization of dosage particularly when used with other medications capable of producing central-nervous-system depression.

EQUIPMENT NECESSARY TO MAINTAIN A PATENT AIRWAY SHOULD BE IMMEDIATELY AVAILABLE PRIOR TO INTRAVENOUS ADMINISTRATION OF LORAZEPAM (see **WARNINGS**).

Status Epilepticus

General Advice

Status epilepticus is a potentially life-threatening condition associated with a high risk of permanent neurological impairment, if inadequately treated. The treatment of status, however, requires far more than the administration of an anticonvulsant agent. It involves observation and management of all parameters critical to maintaining vital function and the capacity to provide support of those functions as required. Ventilatory support must be readily available. The use of benzodiazepines, like Ativan Injection, is ordinarily only an initial step of a complex and sustained intervention which may require additional interventions, (e.g., concomitant intravenous administration of phenytoin). Because status epilepticus may result from a correctable acute cause such as hypoglycemia, hyponatremia, or other metabolic or toxic derangement, such an abnormality must be immediately sought and corrected. Furthermore, patients who are susceptible to further seizure episodes should receive adequate maintenance antiepileptic therapy.

Any health care professional who intends to treat a patient with status epilepticus should be familiar with this package insert and the pertinent medical literature concerning current concepts for the treatment of status epilepticus. A comprehensive review of the considerations critical to the informed and prudent management of status epilepticus cannot be provided in drug product labeling. The archival medical literature contains many informative references on the management of status epilepticus, among them the report of the working group on status epilepticus of the Epilepsy Foundation of America "Treatment of Convulsive Status Epilepticus" (JAMA 1993; 270:854–859). As noted in the report just cited, it may be useful to consult with a neurologist if a patient fails to respond (e.g., fails to regain consciousness).

Intravenous Injection

For the treatment of status epilepticus, the usual recommended dose of Ativan Injection is 4 mg given slowly (2 mg/min) for patients 18 years and older. If seizures cease, no additional Ativan Injection is required. If seizures continue or recur after a 10- to 15-minute observation period, an additional 4 mg intravenous dose may be slowly administered. *Experience with further doses of Ativan is very limited.* The usual precautions in treating status epilepticus should be employed. An intravenous infusion should be started, vital signs should be monitored, an unobstructed airway should be maintained, and artificial ventilation equipment should be available.

Intramuscular Injection

IM Ativan is not preferred in the treatment of status epilepticus because therapeutic lorazepam levels may not be reached as quickly as with IV administration. However,

TABLE 2. NUMBER (%) OF STUDY EVENTS IN ACTIVE CONTROLLED CLINICAL TRIALS

Body System Event	Ativan Injection (n=85)[a]	Diazepam (n=80)[a]
Any Study Event (1 or more)[b]	14 (16.5%)	11 (13.8%)
Body as a whole		
Headache	1 (1.2%)	1 (1.3%)
Cardiovascular system		
Hypotension	2 (2.4%)	0
Hemic and lymphatic system		
Hypochromic anemia	0	1 (1.3%)
Leukocytosis	0	1 (1.3%)
Thrombocythemia	0	1 (1.3%)
Nervous system		
Coma	1 (1.2%)	1 (1.3%)
Somnolence	3 (3.5%)	3 (3.8%)
Stupor	1 (1.2%)	0
Respiratory system		
Hypoventilation	1 (1.2%)	2 (2.5%)
Apnea	1 (1.2%)	1 (1.3%)
Respiratory failure	2 (2.4%)	1 (1.3%)
Respiratory disorder	1 (1.2%)	0

a: The number indicates the number of "patient-episodes." Patient-episodes were used rather than "patients" because a total of 7 patients were reenrolled for the treatment of a second episode of status: 5 patients received Ativan Injection on two occasions that were far enough apart to establish the diagnosis of status epilepticus for each episode, and, using the same time criterion, 2 patients received diazepam on two occasions.

b: Totals are not necessarily the sum of the individual study events because a patient may report two or more different study events in the same body system.

Continued on next page

Ativan Injection—Cont.

when an intravenous port is not available, the IM route may prove useful (see **CLINICAL PHARMACOLOGY, Pharmacokinetics and Metabolism**).

Pediatric

The safety of Ativan in pediatric patients has not been established.

Preanesthetic

Intramuscular Injection

For the designated indications as a premedicant, the usual recommended dose of lorazepam for intramuscular injection is 0.05 mg/kg up to a maximum of 4 mg. As with all premedicant drugs, the dose should be individualized (see also **CLINICAL PHARMACOLOGY, WARNINGS, PRECAUTIONS**, and **ADVERSE REACTIONS**). Doses of other central-nervous-system-depressant drugs ordinarily should be reduced (see **PRECAUTIONS**). *For optimum effect, measured as lack of recall, intramuscular lorazepam should be administered at least 2 hours before the anticipated operative procedure.* Narcotic analgesics should be administered at their usual preoperative time.

There are insufficient data to support efficacy or make dosage recommendations for intramuscular lorazepam in patients less than 18 years of age; therefore, such use is not recommended.

Intravenous Injection

For the primary purpose of sedation and relief of anxiety, the usual recommended initial dose of lorazepam for intravenous injection is 2 mg total, or 0.02 mg/lb (0.044 mg/kg), whichever is smaller. This dose will suffice for sedating most adult patients and ordinarily should not be exceeded in patients over 50 years of age. In those patients in whom a greater likelihood of lack of recall for perioperative events would be beneficial, larger doses as high as 0.05 mg/kg up to a total of 4 mg may be administered (see **CLINICAL PHARMACOLOGY, WARNINGS, PRECAUTIONS**, and **ADVERSE REACTIONS**). Doses of other injectable central-nervous-system-depressant drugs ordinarily should be reduced (see **PRECAUTIONS**). *For optimum effect, measured as lack of recall, intravenous lorazepam should be administered 15 to 20 minutes before the anticipated operative procedure.*

There are insufficient data to support efficacy or make dosage recommendations for intravenous lorazepam in patients less than 18 years of age; therefore, such use is not recommended.

Dose Administration in Special Populations

Elderly Patients and Patients with Hepatic Disease

No dosage adjustments are needed in elderly patients and in patients with hepatic disease.

Patients with Renal Disease

For acute dose administration, adjustment is not needed for patients with renal disease. However, in patients with renal disease, caution should be exercised if frequent doses are given over relatively short periods of time (see also **CLINICAL PHARMACOLOGY**).

Dose Adjustment Due to Drug Interactions

The dose of Ativan should be reduced by 50% when coadministered with probenecid or valproate (see **PRECAUTIONS, Drug Interactions**).

It may be necessary to increase the dose of Ativan in female patients who are concomitantly taking oral contraceptives.

Administration

The **TUBEX® BLUNT POINTE**™ Sterile Cartridge Unit is suitable for substances to be administered intravenously. It is intended for use with injection sets specifically manufactured as "needle-less" injection systems. As of the date of this circular, **TUBEX BLUNT POINTE** is compatible with LifeShield® Prepierced Reseal injection site, InterLink® Injection Site, SafeLine® Injection Site, User-Gard® Intermittent Injection Cap, and SafSite® reflux valve.

The **TUBEX** Sterile Cartridge-Needle Unit is suitable for substances to be administered intravenously or intramuscularly.

When given intramuscularly, Ativan Injection, undiluted, should be injected deep in the muscle mass.

Injectable Ativan can be used with atropine sulfate, narcotic analgesics, other parenterally used analgesics, commonly used anesthetics, and muscle relaxants.

Immediately prior to intravenous use, Ativan Injection must be diluted with an equal volume of compatible solution. Contents should be mixed thoroughly by gently inverting the container repeatedly until a homogenous solution results. Do not shake vigorously, as this will result in air entrapment. When properly diluted, the drug may be injected directly into a vein or into the tubing of an existing intravenous infusion (see above for tubing products compatible with the **BLUNT POINTE** Sterile Cartridge Unit). The rate of injection should not exceed 2.0 mg per minute.

Parenteral drug products should be inspected visually for particulate matter and discoloration prior to administration, whenever solution and container permit. Do not use if solution is discolored or contains a precipitate.

Ativan Injection is compatible for dilution purposes with the following solutions: Sterile Water for Injection, USP; Sodium Chloride Injection, USP; 5% Dextrose Injection, USP.

HOW SUPPLIED

Ativan® (lorazepam) Injection is available in **TUBEX® BLUNT POINTE**™ Sterile Cartridge Units and Sterile Cartridge-Needle Units (22 gauge × 1¼ inch needle), in boxes of 10 **TUBEX®** as follows:

1 mg per 0.5 mL, NDC 0008-0581-50, 0.5 mL fill in 1 mL size **BLUNT POINTE**™

1 mg per 0.5 mL, NDC 0008-0581-07, 0.5 mL fill in 1 mL size

2 mg per mL, NDC 0008-0581-52, 1 mL fill in 2 mL size **BLUNT POINTE**™

2 mg per mL, NDC 0008-0581-02, 1 mL fill in 2 mL size

4 mg per mL, NDC 0008-0570-50, 1 mL fill in 2 mL size **BLUNT POINTE**™

4 mg per mL, NDC 0008-0570-02, 1 mL fill in 2 mL size and in boxes of 50 **TUBEX®** as follows:

For IM or IV injection.

2 mg per mL, NDC 0008-0581-55, 1 mL fill in 2 mL size

Protect from light.

Store in a refrigerator.

Use carton to protect contents from light.

ALSO AVAILABLE

TUBEX® BLUNT POINTE™ Sterile Cartridge Units and Sterile Cartridge-Needle Units (22 gauge × 1¼ inch needle), packaged in boxes of 10 **TUBEX®** in TAMP-R-TEL® tamper-resistant packages as follows:

1 mg per 0.5 mL, NDC 0008-0581-51, 0.5 mL fill in 1 mL size **BLUNT POINTE**™

1 mg per 0.5 mL, NDC 0008-0581-05, 0.5 mL fill in 1 mL size

2 mg per mL, NDC 0008-0581-53, 1 mL fill in 2 mL size **BLUNT POINTE**™

2 mg per mL, NDC 0008-0581-06, 1 mL fill in 2 mL size

4 mg per mL, NDC 0008-0570-51, 1 mL fill in 2 mL size **BLUNT POINTE**™

4 mg per mL, NDC 0008-0570-05, 1 mL fill in 2 mL size

Single-dose and multiple-dose vials are available as follows:

2 mg per mL, NDC 0008-0581-15, 1 mL vial and NDC 0008-0581-13, 10 mL vial

4 mg per mL, NDC 0008-0570-15, 1 mL vial and NDC 0008-0570-13, 10 mL vial

TUBEX is a registered trademark of Wyeth-Ayerst Laboratories. **BLUNT POINTE** is a trademark of Wyeth-Ayerst Laboratories.

InterLink is a registered trademark of Baxter International, Inc.

LifeShield is a registered trademark of Abbott Laboratories.

SafeLine is a registered trademark of McGaw, Inc.

SafSite is a registered trademark of B. Braun Medical, Inc.

User-Gard is a registered trademark of Arrow International, Inc.

Manufactured by:
Wyeth Laboratories
A Wyeth-Ayerst Company
Philadelphia, PA 19101
CI 5072-2 Revised March 26, 1999

ATIVAN® Ⓒ ℞
[ăt 'ĭ-văn]
(lorazepam)
Tablets

DESCRIPTION

Ativan (lorazepam), an antianxiety agent, has the chemical formula, 7-chloro-5-(*o*-chlorophenyl)-1,3-dihydro-3-hydroxy-2*H*-1,4-benzodiazepin-2-one.

It is a nearly white powder almost insoluble in water. Each Ativan (lorazepam) tablet, to be taken orally, contains 0.5 mg, 1 mg, or 2 mg of lorazepam. The inactive ingredients present are lactose and other ingredients.

CLINICAL PHARMACOLOGY

Studies in healthy volunteers show that in single high doses Ativan (lorazepam) has a tranquilizing action on the central nervous system with no appreciable effect on the respiratory or cardiovascular systems.

Ativan (lorazepam) is readily absorbed with an absolute bioavailability of 90 percent. Peak concentrations in plasma occur approximately 2 hours following administration. The peak plasma level of lorazepam from a 2 mg dose is approximately 20 ng/mL.

The mean half-life of unconjugated lorazepam in human plasma is about 12 hours and for its major metabolite, lorazepam glucuronide, about 18 hours. At clinically relevant concentrations, lorazepam is approximately 85% bound to plasma proteins. Ativan (lorazepam) is rapidly conjugated at its 3-hydroxy group into lorazepam glucuronide which is then excreted in the urine. Lorazepam glucuronide has no demonstrable CNS activity in animals.

The plasma levels of lorazepam are proportional to the dose given. There is no evidence of accumulation of lorazepam on administration up to six months.

Studies comparing young and elderly subjects have shown that the pharmacokinetics of lorazepam remain unaltered with advancing age.

INDICATIONS AND USAGE

Ativan (lorazepam) is indicated for the management of anxiety disorders or for the short-term relief of the symptoms of anxiety or anxiety associated with depressive symptoms. Anxiety or tension associated with the stress of everyday life usually does not require treatment with an anxiolytic.

The effectiveness of Ativan (lorazepam) in long-term use, that is, more than 4 months, has not been assessed by systematic clinical studies. The physician should periodically reassess the usefulness of the drug for the individual patient.

CONTRAINDICATIONS

Ativan (lorazepam) is contraindicated in patients with known sensitivity to the benzodiazepines or with acute narrow-angle glaucoma.

WARNINGS

Ativan (lorazepam) is not recommended for use in patients with a primary depressive disorder or psychosis. As with all patients on CNS-acting drugs, patients receiving lorazepam should be warned not to operate dangerous machinery or motor vehicles and that their tolerance for alcohol and other CNS depressants will be diminished.

Physical and Psychological Dependence

Withdrawal symptoms, similar in character to those noted with barbiturates and alcohol (convulsions, tremor, abdominal and muscle cramps, vomiting, and sweating), have occurred following abrupt discontinuance of lorazepam. The more severe withdrawal symptoms have usually been limited to those patients who received excessive doses over an extended period of time. Generally milder withdrawal symptoms (e.g., dysphoria and insomnia) have been reported following abrupt discontinuance of benzodiazepines taken continuously at therapeutic levels for several months. Consequently, after extended therapy, abrupt discontinuation should generally be avoided and a gradual dosage-tapering schedule followed. Addiction-prone individuals (such as drug addicts or alcoholics) should be under careful surveillance when receiving lorazepam or other psychotropic agents because of the predisposition of such patients to habituation and dependence.

PRECAUTIONS

In patients with depression accompanying anxiety, a possibility for suicide should be borne in mind.

For elderly or debilitated patients, the initial daily dosage should not exceed 2 mg in order to avoid oversedation.

The usual precautions for treating patients with impaired renal or hepatic function should be observed.

In patients where gastrointestinal or cardiovascular disorders coexist with anxiety, it should be noted that lorazepam has not been shown to be of significant benefit in treating the gastrointestinal or cardiovascular component.

Esophageal dilation occurred in rats treated with lorazepam for more than one year at 6 mg/kg/day. The no-effect dose was 1.25 mg/kg/day (approximately 6 times the maximum human therapeutic dose of 10 mg per day). The effect was reversible only when the treatment was withdrawn within two months of first observation of the phenomenon. The clinical significance of this is unknown. However, use of lorazepam for prolonged periods and in geriatric patients requires caution, and there should be frequent monitoring for symptoms of upper G.I. disease.

Safety and effectiveness of Ativan (lorazepam) in children of less than 12 years have not been established.

Information for Patients

To assure the safe and effective use of Ativan (lorazepam), patients should be informed that, since benzodiazepines may produce psychological and physical dependence, it is advisable that they consult with their physician before either increasing the dose or abruptly discontinuing this drug.

Essential Laboratory Tests

Some patients on Ativan (lorazepam) have developed leukopenia, and some have had elevations of LDH. As with other benzodiazepines, periodic blood counts and liver-function tests are recommended for patients on long-term therapy.

Clinically Significant Drug Interactions

The benzodiazepines, including Ativan (lorazepam), produce CNS-depressant effects when administered with such medications as barbiturates or alcohol.

Carcinogenesis and Mutagenesis

No evidence of carcinogenic potential emerged in rats during an 18-month study with Ativan (lorazepam). No studies regarding mutagenesis have been performed.

Pregnancy

Reproductive studies in animals were performed in mice, rats, and two strains of rabbits. Occasional anomalies (reduction of tarsals, tibia, metatarsals, malrotated limbs, gastroschisis, malformed skull, and microphthalmia) were seen in drug-treated rabbits without relationship to dosage. Although all of these anomalies were not present in the concurrent control group, they have been reported to occur randomly in historical controls. At doses of 40 mg/kg and higher, there was evidence of fetal resorption and increased fetal loss in rabbits which was not seen at lower doses.

The clinical significance of the above findings is not known. However, an increased risk of congenital malformations associated with the use of minor tranquilizers (chlordiazepoxide, diazepam, and meprobamate) during the first trimester of pregnancy has been suggested in several studies. Because the use of these drugs is rarely a matter of urgency, the use of lorazepam during this period should almost always be avoided. The possibility that a woman of childbearing potential may be pregnant at the time of institution of therapy should be considered. Patients should be advised that if they become pregnant, they should communicate with their physician about the desirability of discontinuing the drug.

In humans, blood levels obtained from umbilical cord blood indicate placental transfer of lorazepam and lorazepam glucuronide.

Nursing Mothers

It is not known whether oral lorazepam is excreted in human milk like the other benzodiazepine tranquilizers. As a general rule, nursing should not be undertaken while a patient is on a drug, since many drugs are excreted in human milk.

ADVERSE REACTIONS

Adverse reactions, if they occur, are usually observed at the beginning of therapy and generally disappear on continued medication or upon decreasing the dose. In a sample of about 3,500 anxious patients, the most frequent adverse reaction to Ativan (lorazepam) is sedation (15.9%), followed by dizziness (6.9%), weakness (4.2%), and unsteadiness (3.4%). Less frequent adverse reactions are disorientation, depression, nausea, change in appetite, headache, sleep disturbance, agitation, dermatological symptoms, eye-function disturbance, together with various gastrointestinal symptoms and autonomic manifestations. The incidence of sedation and unsteadiness increased with age.

Small decreases in blood pressure have been noted but are not clinally significant, probably being related to the relief of anxiety produced by Ativan (lorazepam).

Transient amnesia or memory impairment has been reported in association with the use of benzodiazepines.

OVERDOSAGE

In the management of overdosage with any drug, it should be borne in mind that multiple agents may have been taken.

Symptoms

Overdosage of benzodiazepines is usually manifested by varing degrees of central nervous system depression ranging from drowsiness to coma. In mild cases, symptoms include drowsiness, mental confusion and lethary. In more serious cases, and especially when other drugs or alcohol were ingested, symptoms may include ataxia, hypotonia, hypotension, hypnotic state, stage one (1) to three (3) coma, and very rarely, death.

Management

Induced vomiting and/or gastric lavage should be undertaken, followed by general supportive care, monitoring of vital signs, and close observation of the patient. Hypotension, though unlikely, usually may be controlled with norepinephrine bitartrate injection. The value of dialysis has not been adequately determined for lorazepam.

The benzodiazepine antagonist flumazenil may be used in hospitalized patients as an adjunct to, not as a substitute for, proper management of benzodiazepine overdose. **The prescriber should be aware of a risk of seizure in association with flumazenil treatment, particularly in long-term benzodiazepine users and in cyclic antidepressant overdose.** The complete flumazenil package insert including "**CONTRAINDICATIONS**," "**WARNINGS**," and "**PRECAUTIONS**" should be consulted prior to use.

DOSAGE AND ADMINISTRATION

Ativan (lorazepam) is administered orally. For optimal results, dose, frequency of administration, and duration of therapy should be individualized according to patient response. To facilitate this, 0.5 mg, 1 mg, and 2 mg tablets are available.

The usual range is 2 to 6 mg/day given in divided doses, the largest dose being taken before bedtime, but the daily dosage may vary from 1 to 10 mg/day.

For anxiety, most patients require an initial dose of 2 to 3 mg/day given b.i.d. or t.i.d.

For insomnia due to anxiety or transient situational stress, a single daily dose of 2 to 4 mg may be given, usually at bedtime.

For elderly or debilitated patients, an initial dosage of 1 to 2 mg/day in divided doses is recommended, to be adjusted as needed and tolerated.

The dosage of Ativan (lorazepam) should be increased gradually when needed to help avoid adverse effects. When higher dosage is indicated, the evening dose should be increased before the daytime doses.

HOW SUPPLIED

Ativan® (lorazepam) Tablets are available in the following dosage strengths:

0.5 mg, NDC 0008-0081, white, five-sided tablet with a raised "A" on one side and "WYETH" and "81" on reverse side, in bottles of 100 and 500 tablets.

1 mg, NDC 0008-0064, white, five-sided tablet with a raised "A" on one side and "WYETH" and "64" on scored reverse side, in bottles of 100, 500, and 1000 tablets.

2 mg, NDC 0008-0065, white, five-sided tablet with a raised "A" on one side and "WYETH" and "65" on scored reverse side, in bottles of 100, 500, and 1000 tablets.

BOTTLES:

Keep tightly closed.

Store at controlled room temperature.

Dispense in tight container.

The appearance of ATIVAN tablets is a registered trademark of Wyeth-Ayerst Laboratories.

Manufactured by:
Wyeth Laboratories
A Wyeth-Ayerst Company
Philadelphia, PA 19101

CI 5181-1 Issued February 17, 1999

Shown in Product Identification Guide, page 341

ATROMID-S® ℞

[ă 'trō-mid s]

Capsules

(clofibrate capsules)

Antilipidemic agent for reduction of elevated serum lipids

Rx only

DESCRIPTION

Atromid-S Capsules (clofibrate capsules) is ethyl 2-(p-chlorophenoxy)-2-methyl-propionate, an antilipidemic agent.

structural formula

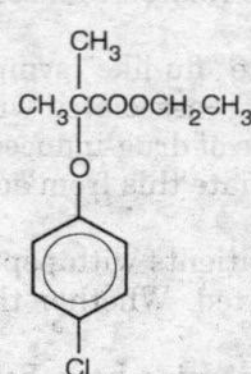

Its molecular formula is $C_{12}H_{15}O_3Cl$, molecular weight 242.7, and boiling point 148–150°C at 25 mm Hg. It is a stable, colorless to pale-yellow liquid with a faint odor and characteristic taste, soluble in common solvents but not in water. Each Atromid-S Capsule contains 500 mg clofibrate for oral administration.

Atromid-S Capsules contain the following inactive ingredients: D&C Red No. 28, D&C Red No. 30, D&C Yellow No. 10, FD&C Blue No. 1, FD&C Red No. 28, FD&C Red No. 40, FD&C Yellow No. 6, gelatin.

CLINICAL PHARMACOLOGY

Atromid-S is an antilipidemic agent. It acts to lower elevated serum lipids by reducing the very low-density lipoprotein fraction (S_f 20–400) rich in triglycerides. Serum cholesterol may be decreased, particularly in those patients whose cholesterol elevation is due to the presence of IDL as a result of Type III hyperlipoproteinemia.

The mechanism of action has not been established definitively. Clofibrate may inhibit the hepatic release of lipoproteins (particularly VLDL), potentiate the action of lipoprotein lipase, and increase the fecal excretion of neutral sterols.

Between 95% and 99% of an oral dose of clofibrate is excreted in the urine as free and conjugated clofibric acid; thus, the absorption of clofibrate is virtually complete. The half-life of clofibric acid in normal volunteers averages 18 to 22 hours (range 14 to 35 hours) but can vary by up to 7 hours in the same subject at different times. Clofibric acid is highly protein-bound (95% to 97%). In subjects undergoing continuous clofibrate treatment, 1 g q12h, plasma concentrations of clofibric acid range from 120 to 125 mcg/mL to an approximate peak of 200 mcg/mL.

Several investigators have observed in their studies that clofibrate may produce a decrease in cholesterol linoleate but an increase in palmitoleate and oleate, the latter being considered atherogenic in experimental animals. The significance of this finding is unknown at this time.

Reduction of triglycerides in some patients treated with clofibrate or certain of its chemically and clinically similar analogs may be associated with an increase in LDL cholesterol. Increase in LDL cholesterol has been observed in patients whose cholesterol is initially normal.

Animal studies suggest that clofibrate interrupts cholesterol biosynthesis prior to mevalonate formation.

INDICATIONS AND USAGE

The initial treatment of choice for hyperlipidemia is dietary therapy specific for the type of hyperlipidemia.[1]

Excess body weight and alcoholic intake may be important factors in hypertriglyceridemia and should be addressed prior to any drug therapy. Physical exercise can be an important ancillary measure. Estrogen therapy, some beta-blockers, and thiazide diuretics may also be associated with increases in plasma triglycerides. Discontinuation of such products may obviate the need for specific antilipidemic therapy. Contributory diseases such as hypothyroidism or diabetes mellitus should be looked for and adequately treated. The use of drugs should be considered only when reasonable attempts have been made to obtain satisfactory results with nondrug methods. If the decision ultimately is to use drugs, the patient should be instructed that this does not reduce the importance of adhering to diet.

Because Atromid-S is associated with certain serious adverse findings reported in two large clinical trials (see "**WARNINGS**"), agents other than clofibrate may be more suitable for a particular patient.

Atromid-S is indicated for Primary Dysbetalipoproteinemia (Type III hyperlipidemia) that does not respond adequately to diet.

Atromid-S may be considered for the treatment of adult patients with very high serum-triglyceride levels (Type IV and V hyperlipidemia) who present a risk of abdominal pain and pancreatitis and who do not respond adequately to a determined dietary effort to control them. Patients who present such risk typically have serum triglycerides over 2000 mg/dl and have elevations of VLDL-cholesterol as well as fasting chylomicrons (Type V hyperlipidemia). Subjects who consistently have total serum or plasma triglycerides below 1000 mg/dl are unlikely to present a risk of pancreatitis. Atromid-S therapy may be considered for those subjects with triglyceride elevations between 1000 and 2000 mg/dl who have a history of pancreatitis or of recurrent abdominal pain typical of pancreatitis. It is recognized that some Type IV patients with triglycerides under 1000 mg/dl may, through dietary or alcoholic indiscretion, convert to a Type V pattern with massive triglyceride elevations accompanying fasting chylomicronemia, but the influence of Atromid-S therapy on the risk of pancreatitis in such situations has not been adequately studied.

Atromid-S is not useful for the hypertriglyceridemia of Type I hyperlipidemia, where elevations of chylomicrons and plasma triglycerides are accompanied by normal levels of very low-density lipoprotein (VLDL). Inspection of plasma refrigerated for 12 to 14 hours is helpful in distinguishing Types I, IV, and V hyperlipoproteinemia.[2]

Atromid-S has not been shown to be effective for prevention of coronary heart disease.

The biochemical response to Atromid-S is variable, and it is not always possible to predict from the lipoprotein type or other factors which patients will obtain favorable results. LDL cholesterol, as well as triglycerides, should be rechecked during the first several months of therapy in order to detect rises in LDL cholesterol that often accompany fibric-acid-type drug-induced reductions in elevated triglycerides. It is essential that lipid levels be reassessed periodically and that the drug be discontinued in any patient in whom lipids do not show significant improvement.

CONTRAINDICATIONS

Clofibrate is contraindicated in pregnant women. While teratogenic studies have not demonstrated any effect attributable to clofibrate, it is known that serum of the rabbit fetus accumulates a higher concentration of clofibrate than that found in maternal serum, and it is possible that the fetus may not have developed the enzyme system required for the excretion of clofibrate.

It is contraindicated in patients with clinically significant hepatic or renal dysfunction. Rhabdomyolysis and severe hyperkalemia have been reported in association with preexisting renal insufficiency.

It is contraindicated in patients with primary biliary cirrhosis, since it may raise the already elevated cholesterol in these cases.

It is contraindicated in patients with a known hypersensitivity to clofibrate.

It is contraindicated in nursing women (see "**PRECAUTIONS**").

WARNINGS

In a large study involving 5,000 patients in a clofibrate-treated group and 5,000 in a placebo-treated group followed for an average of five years on drug or placebo and one year beyond (the WHO study), there was a statistically significant 44% higher age-adjusted total mortality in the clofibrate-treated group than in a comparable placebo group. The excess deaths were due to noncardiovascular causes; half of this difference was due to malignancy; other causes of death included postcholecystectomy complications and pancreatitis.[3] In another prospective study involving 1,000 clofibrate- and 3,000 placebo-treated patients followed for an average of six years on drug or placebo (the Coronary Drug Project study), the noncardiovascular mortality rate, including that of malignancy, was not significantly different in the clofibrate- and placebo-treated groups.[4] This should not be interpreted to mean that clofibrate is not associated with an increased risk of noncardiovascular death, because the patients in the Coronary Drug Project were much older than those in the WHO study and they all had had a previous myocardial infarction, so that the deaths in the Coronary Drug Project were overwhelmingly due to cardiovascular causes, and it would have been very difficult to discern a clofibrate-associated risk of death due to noncardiovascular causes if it existed. Both studies demonstrated that clofibrate users have twice the risk of developing cholelithiasis and cholecystitis requiring surgery as do nonusers.

A potential benefit of clofibrate was, however, reported in the WHO study which involved patients with hypercholesterolemia and no history of myocardial infarction or angina pectoris. In this study, there was a statistically significant 25% decrease in subsequent nonfatal myocardial infarctions in the clofibrate-treated group when compared with the placebo group. There was no difference in incidence of fatal myocardial infarction in the two groups. In the Coronary Drug Project study, which involved patients with or without hypercholesterolemia and/or hypertriglyceridemia and with a history of previous myocardial infarction, there was no significant difference in incidence of either nonfatal or fatal myocardial infarction between the clofibrate- and placebo-treated groups.[3]

As a result of these and other studies, the following can be stated:

1. Clofibrate, in general, causes a relatively modest reduction of serum cholesterol and a somewhat greater reduction of serum triglycerides. In Type III hyperlipidemia, however, substantial reductions of both cholesterol and triglycerides can occur with clofibrate use.
2. No study to date has shown a convincing reduction in incidence of *fatal* myocardial infarction.
3. A significantly increased incidence of cholelithiasis has been demonstrated consistently in clofibrate-treated groups, and an increase in morbidity from this complication and mortality from cholecystectomy must be anticipated during clofibrate treatment.

Continued on next page

Atromid-S—Cont.

4. Several types of other undesirable events have been associated in a statistically significant way with clofibrate administration in the WHO and the Coronary Drug Project studies. There was an increase in incidence of noncardiovascular deaths reported in the WHO study. There was an increase in cardiac arrhythmias, intermittent claudication, and definite or suspected thromboembolic events, and angina reported in the Coronary Drug Project, which was not, however, reported in the WHO study.

5. Administration of clofibrate to mice and rats in long-term studies at 1 to 2 times the maximum recommended human dose (based on surface area, mg/m^2), resulted in a higher incidence of benign and malignant liver tumors than in controls.

There was an increase in benign Leydig cell tumors in male rats treated at 400 mg/kg/day or 2 times the maximum recommended human dose in one study.

A comparative carcinogenicity study was also done in rats comparing three drugs in this class: fenofibrate (10 and 60 mg/kg; 0.3 and 1.6 times the human dose), clofibrate (400 mg/kg; 1.6 times the human dose), and gemfibrozil (250 mg/kg; 1.7 times the human dose). Pancreatic acinar adenomas were increased in males and females on fenofibrate; hepatocellular carcinoma and pancreatic acinar adenomas were increased in males and hepatic neoplastic nodules in females treated with clofibrate; hepatic neoplastic nodules were increased in males and females treated with gemfibrozil while testicular interstitial cell tumors were increased in males on all three drugs.

6. Administration of clofibrate to male monkeys at dosages of 1 to 2 times the maximum recommended human dose resulted in increases in mortality of 2- to 5-fold. As in the case of men in the WHO study, no single cause of death was identified.

BECAUSE OF THE TUMORIGENICITY OF CLOFIBRATE IN RODENTS AND THE POSSIBLE INCREASED RISK OF MALIGNANCY ASSOCIATED WITH CLOFIBRATE IN THE HUMAN, AS WELL AS THE INCREASED RISK OF CHOLELITHIASIS, AND BECAUSE THERE IS NOT, TO DATE, SUBSTANTIAL EVIDENCE OF A BENEFICIAL EFFECT ON CARDIOVASCULAR MORTALITY FROM CLOFIBRATE, THIS DRUG SHOULD BE UTILIZED ONLY FOR THOSE PATIENTS DESCRIBED IN THE "**INDICATIONS AND USAGE**" SECTION, AND SHOULD BE DISCONTINUED IF SIGNIFICANT LIPID RESPONSE IS NOT OBTAINED.

Concomitant Anticoagulants

CAUTION SHOULD BE EXERCISED WHEN ANTICOAGULANTS ARE GIVEN IN CONJUNCTION WITH ATROMID-S®. THE DOSAGE OF THE ANTICOAGULANT SHOULD BE REDUCED USUALLY BY ONE-HALF (DEPENDING ON THE INDIVIDUAL CASE) TO MAINTAIN THE PROTHROMBIN TIME AT THE DESIRED LEVEL TO PREVENT BLEEDING COMPLICATIONS. FREQUENT PROTHROMBIN DETERMINATIONS ARE ADVISABLE UNTIL IT HAS BEEN DEFINITELY DETERMINED THAT THE PROTHROMBIN LEVEL HAS BEEN STABILIZED.

Skeletal Muscle

Myalgia, myositis, myopathy, and rhabdomyolysis with or without elevation of CPK have been associated with Atromid-S therapy. Consideration should be given to withholding or discontinuing drug therapy in any patient with a risk factor predisposing to the development of renal failure secondary to rhabdomyolysis, including: severe acute infection; hypotension; major surgery; trauma; severe metabolic, endocrine, or electrolyte disorders; and uncontrolled seizures.

Atromid-S therapy should be discontinued if markedly elevated CPK levels occur or myositis is diagnosed.

Avoidance of Pregnancy

Strict birth-control procedures must be exercised by women of child-bearing potential. In patients who plan to become pregnant, clofibrate should be withdrawn several months before conception. Because of the possibility of pregnancy occurring despite birth-control precautions in patients taking clofibrate, the possible benefits of the drug to the patient must be weighed against possible hazards to the fetus. (See **"Pregnancy"** section.)

PRECAUTIONS

General

Before instituting therapy with clofibrate, attempts should be made to control serum lipids with appropriate dietary regimens, weight loss in obese patients, control of diabetes mellitus, etc.

Because of the long-term administration of a drug of this nature, adequate baseline studies should be performed to determine that the patient has significantly elevated serum lipid levels. Frequent determinations of serum lipids should be obtained during the first few months of Atromid-S administration, and periodic determinations made thereafter. The drug should be withdrawn after three months if response is inadequate. However, in the case of xanthoma tuberosum, the drug should be employed for longer periods (even up to one year) provided that there is a reduction in the size and/or number of the xanthomata.

Since cholelithiasis is a possible side effect of clofibrate therapy, appropriate diagnostic procedures should be performed if signs and symptoms related to disease of the biliary system should occur.

Clofibrate may produce "flu-like" symptoms (muscular aching, soreness, cramping) associated with increased creatine kinase levels indicative of drug-induced myopathy. The physician should differentiate this from actual viral and/or bacterial disease.

Use with caution in patients with peptic ulcer, since reactivation has been reported. Whether this is drug related is unknown.

Various cardiac arrhythmias have been reported with the use of clofibrate.

Laboratory Tests

Subsequent serum lipid determinations should be done to detect a paradoxical rise in serum cholesterol or triglyceride levels. Clofibrate will not alter the seasonal variations of serum cholesterol: peak elevations in midwinter and late summer and decreases in fall and spring. If the drug is discontinued, the patient should be continued on an appropriate hypolipidemic diet, and serum lipids should be monitored until stabilized, as a rise in these values to or above the original baseline may occur.

During clofibrate therapy, frequent serum-transaminase determinations and other liver-function tests should be performed, since the drug may produce abnormalities in these parameters. These effects are usually reversible when the drug is discontinued. Hepatic biopsies are usually within normal limits. If the hepatic-function tests steadily rise or show excessive abnormalities, the drug should be withdrawn. Therefore, use with caution in those patients with a past history of jaundice or hepatic disease.

Complete blood counts should be done periodically since anemia, and more frequently, leukopenia have been reported in patients who have been taking clofibrate.

Drug Interactions

Caution should be exercised when anticoagulants are given in conjunction with Atromid-S. Usually, the dosage of the anticoagulant should be reduced by one-half (depending on the individual case) to maintain the prothrombin time at the desired level to prevent bleeding complications. Frequent prothrombin determinations are advisable until it has been determined definitely that the prothrombin level has been stabilized.

Atromid-S may displace acidic drugs such as phenytoin or tolbutamide from their binding sites. Caution should be exercised when treating patients with either of these drugs or other highly protein-bound drugs and Atromid-S. The hypoglycemic effect of tolbutamide has been reported to increase when Atromid-S is given concurrently.

Fulminant rhabdomyolysis has been seen as early as three weeks after initiation of combined therapy with another fibrate and lovastatin but may be seen after several months. For these reasons, it is felt that, in most subjects who have had an unsatisfactory lipid response to either drug alone, the possible benefits of combined therapy with lovastatin and a fibrate do not outweigh the risks of severe myopathy, rhabdomyolysis, and acute renal failure. While it is not known whether this interaction occurs with fibrates other than gemfibrozil, myopathy and rhabdomyolysis have occasionally been associated with the use of fibrates alone, including clofibrate. Therefore, the combined use of lovastatin with fibrates should generally be avoided.

Carcinogenesis, Mutagenesis, Impairment of Fertility

See "**WARNINGS**" section for information on carcinogenesis and mutagenesis.

Arrest of spermatogenesis has been seen in both dogs and monkeys at doses approximately 2 times the maximum recommended human dose (based on surface area).

Electron microscopy studies have demonstrated peroxisomal proliferation following clofibrate administration to the rat. Changes in peroxisome morphology and numbers have been observed in humans after treatment with several members of the fibrate class, including clofibrate, when liver biopsies were compared before and after treatment in the same individual.

Pregnancy

Teratogenic effects

Pregnancy Category C. Animal reproduction studies have not been conducted with Atromid-S. It is also not known whether Atromid-S can cause fetal harm when administered to a pregnant woman or can affect reproductive capacity. However, animal reproduction studies with clofibrate plus androsterone showed increases in neonatal deaths and pup mortality during lactation.

Nursing Mothers

Atromid-S is contraindicated in lactating women, since an active metabolite (CPIB) has been measured in breast milk.

Pediatric Use

Safety and efficacy in pediatric patients have not been established.

ADVERSE REACTIONS

The most common is nausea. Less frequently encountered gastrointestinal reactions are vomiting, loose stools, dyspepsia, flatulence, and abdominal distress. Reactions reported less often than gastrointestinal ones are headache, dizziness, and fatigue; muscle cramping, aching, and weakness; skin rash, urticaria, and pruritus; dry brittle hair, and alopecia.

The following reported adverse reactions are listed alphabetically by systems:

Cardiovascular

Increased or decreased angina.
Cardiac arrhythmias.
Both swelling and phlebitis at site of xanthomas.

Dermatologic

Allergic reactions including urticaria.
Skin rash.
Pruritus.
Dry skin and dry, brittle hair.
Alopecia.
Toxic epidermal necrolysis.
Erythema multiforme.
Stevens-Johnson syndrome.

Gastrointestinal

Gallstones.
Nausea.
Vomiting.
Diarrhea.
Gastrointestinal upset (bloating, flatulence, abdominal distress).
Hepatomegaly (not associated with hepatotoxicity).
Stomatitis and gastritis.

Genitourinary

Findings consistent with renal dysfunction as evidenced by dysuria, hematuria, proteinuria, decreased urine output. One patient's renal biopsy suggested "allergic reaction."
Impotence and decreased libido.

Hematologic

Leukopenia.
Potentiation of anticoagulant effect.
Anemia.
Eosinophilia.
Agranulocytosis.

Musculoskeletal

Myalgia (muscle cramping, aching, weakness).
"Flu-like" symptoms.
Myositis.
Myopathy.
Rhabdomyolysis in the setting of preexisting renal insufficiency.
Arthralgia.

Neurologic

Fatigue, weakness, drowsiness.
Dizziness.
Headache.

Miscellaneous

Weight gain.
Polyphagia.

Laboratory Findings

Abnormal liver-function tests as evidenced by increased transaminase (SGOT and SGPT), BSP retention, and increased thymol turbidity.
Proteinuria.
Increased creatine phosphokinase.
Hyperkalemia in association with renal insufficiency and continuous ambulatory peritoneal dialysis treatment.

Reported adverse reactions whose direct relationship with the drug has not been established: peptic ulcer, gastrointestinal hemorrhage, rheumatoid arthritis, tremors, increased perspiration, systemic lupus erythematosus, blurred vision, gynecomastia, thrombocytopenic purpura.

OVERDOSAGE

While there has been no reported case of overdosage, should it occur, symptomatic supportive measures should be taken.

DOSAGE AND ADMINISTRATION

Initial: The recommended dosage for adults is 2 g daily in divided doses. Some patients may respond to a lower dosage.

Maintenance: Same as for initial dosage.

HOW SUPPLIED

Atromid-S Capsules (clofibrate capsules)—Each orange, oblong, soft-gelatin capsule contains 500 mg clofibrate, in bottles of 100 (NDC 0046-0243-81).

The appearance of these orange, oblong, soft-gelatin capsules is a trademark of Wyeth-Ayerst Laboratories.

Store at room temperature, approximately 25° C (77° F).

Dispense in a well-closed, light-resistant container as defined in the USP.

Avoid freezing and excessive heat.

REFERENCES

1. Coronary Risk Handbook (1973). American Heart Association.
2. Nikkila, EA: Familial lipoprotein lipase deficiency and related disorders of chylomicron metabolism. In Stanbury JB et al (eds): The Metabolic Basis of Inherited Disease, 5th ed., McGraw-Hill, 1983, Chap. 30. p.622–642.
3. Report from the Committee of Principal Investigators: A cooperative trial in the primary prevention of ischaemic heart disease using clofibrate. Br Heart J *40* :1069, 1978.
4. The Coronary Drug Project Research Group: Clofibrate and niacin in coronary heart disease. JAMA *231* :360, 1975.

Manufactured for
Ayerst Laboratories Inc.
A Wyeth-Ayerst Company
Philadelphia, PA 19101
CI 3770-7 Revised June 19, 1996

Shown in Product Identification Guide, page 341

PEDIATRIC USE
Safety and efficacy in patients under the age of 18 have not been established.
USE IN THE ELDERLY
No significant difference has been observed in the antihypertensive effect of Cardene I.V. in elderly patients (≥65 years) compared with other adult patients in clinical studies.

ADVERSE EXPERIENCES

Two hundred forty-four patients participated in two multicenter, double-blind, placebo controlled trials of Cardene I.V. Adverse experiences were generally not serious and most were expected consequences of vasodilation. Adverse experiences occasionally required dosage adjustment. Therapy was discontinued in approximately 12% of patients, mainly due to hypotension, headache, and tachycardia.
[See table at top of previous page]
RARE EVENTS
The following rare events have been reported in clinical trials or in the literature in association with the use of intravenously administered nicardipine.
Body as a Whole: fever, neck pain
Cardiovascular: angina pectoris, atrioventricular block, ST segment depression, inverted T wave, deep-vein thrombophlebitis
Digestive: dyspepsia
Hemic and Lymphatic: thrombocytopenia
Metabolic and Nutritional: hypophosphatemia, peripheral edema
Nervous: confusion, hypertonia
Respiratory: respiratory disorder
Special Senses: conjunctivitis, ear disorder, tinnitus
Urogenital: urinary frequency
Sinus node dysfunction and myocardial infarction, which may be due to disease progression, have been seen in patients on chronic therapy with orally administered nicardipine.

OVERDOSAGE

Several overdosages with orally administered nicardipine have been reported. One adult patient allegedly ingested 600 mg of nicardipine [standard (immediate release) capsules], and another patient, 2160 mg of the sustained release formulation of nicardipine. Symptoms included marked hypotension, bradycardia, palpitations, flushing, drowsiness, confusion and slurred speech. All symptoms resolved without sequelae. An overdosage occurred in a one year old child who ingested half of the powder in a 30 mg nicardipine standard capsule. The child remained asymptomatic. Based on results obtained in laboratory animals, lethal overdose may cause systemic hypotension, bradycardia (following initial tachycardia) and progressive atrioventricular conduction block. Reversible hepatic function abnormalities and sporadic focal hepatic necrosis were noted in some animal species receiving very large doses of nicardipine.
For treatment of overdosage, standard measures including monitoring of cardiac and respiratory functions should be implemented. The patient should be positioned so as to avoid cerebral anoxia. Frequent blood pressure determinations are essential. Vasopressors are clinically indicated for patients exhibiting profound hypotension. Intravenous calcium gluconate may help reverse the effects of calcium entry blockade.

DOSAGE AND ADMINISTRATION

Cardene I.V. (nicardipine hydrochloride) is intended for intravenous use. DOSAGE MUST BE INDIVIDUALIZED depending upon the severity of hypertension and the response of the patient during dosing.
Blood pressure should be monitored both during and after the infusion; too rapid or excessive reduction in either systolic or diastolic blood pressure during parenteral treatment should be avoided.
PREPARATION
WARNING: AMPULS MUST BE DILUTED BEFORE INFUSION
Dilution: Cardene I.V. is administered by slow continuous infusion at a CONCENTRATION OF 0.1 MG/ML. Each ampul (25 mg) should be diluted with 240 mL of compatible intravenous fluid (see below), resulting in 250 mL of solution at a concentration of 0.1 mg/mL.
Cardene I.V. has been found to be compatible and stable in glass or polyvinyl chloride containers for 24 hours at controlled room temperature with:
Dextrose (5%) Injection, USP
Dextrose (5%) and Sodium Chloride (0.45%) Injection, USP
Dextrose (5%) and Sodium Chloride (0.9%) Injection, USP
Dextrose (5%) with 40 mEq Potassium, USP
Sodium Chloride (0.45%) Injection, USP
Sodium Chloride (0.9%) Injection, USP
Cardene I.V. is NOT compatible with Sodium Bicarbonate (5%) Injection, USP, or Lactated Ringer's Injection, USP.
THE DILUTED SOLUTION IS STABLE FOR 24 HOURS AT ROOM TEMPERATURE.
Inspection: As with all parenteral drugs, Cardene I.V. should be inspected visually for particulate matter and discoloration prior to administration, whenever solution and container permit. Cardene I.V. is normally light yellow in color.

DOSAGE
As a Substitute for Oral Nicardipine Therapy
The intravenous infusion rate required to produce an average plasma concentration equivalent to a given oral dose at steady state is shown in the following table:

Oral Cardene Dose	Equivalent I.V. Infusion Rate
20 mg q8h	0.5 mg/hr
30 mg q8h	1.2 mg/hr
40 mg q8h	2.2 mg/hr

For Initiation of Therapy in a Drug Free Patient
The time course of blood pressure decrease is dependent on the initial rate of infusion and the frequency of dosage adjustment.
Cardene I.V. is administered by slow continuous infusion at a CONCENTRATION OF 0.1 MG/ML. With constant infusion, blood pressure begins to fall within minutes. It reaches about 50% of its ultimate decrease in about 45 minutes and does not reach final steady state for about 50 hours.
When treating acute hypertensive episodes in patients with chronic hypertension, discontinuation of infusion is followed by a 50% offset of action in 30±7 minutes but plasma levels of drug and gradually decreasing antihypertensive effects exist for about 50 hours.
Titration: For gradual reduction in blood pressure, initiate therapy at 50 mL/hr (5.0 mg/hr). If desired blood pressure reduction is not achieved at this dose, the infusion rate may be increased by 25 mL/hr (2.5 mg/hr) every 15 minutes up to a maximum of 150 mL/hr (15.0 mg/hr), until desired blood pressure reduction is achieved. For more rapid blood pressure reduction, initiate therapy at 50 mL/hr (5.0 mg/hr). If desired blood pressure reduction is not achieved at this dose, the infusion rate may be increased by 25 mL/hr (2.5 mg/hr) every 5 minutes up to a maximum of 150 mL/hr (15.0 mg/hr), until desired blood pressure reduction is achieved. Following achievement of the blood pressure goal, the infusion rate should be decreased to 30 mL/hr (3 mg/hr).
Maintenance: The rate of infusion should be adjusted as needed to maintain desired response.
CONDITIONS REQUIRING INFUSION ADJUSTMENT
Hypotension or Tachycardia: If there is concern of impending hypotension or tachycardia, the infusion should be discontinued. When blood pressure has stabilized, infusion of Cardene I.V. may be restarted at low doses such as 30–50 mL/hr (3.0–5.0 mg/hr) and adjusted to maintain desired blood pressure.
Infusion Site Changes: Cardene I.V. should be continued as long as blood pressure control is needed. The infusion site should be changed every 12 hours if administered via peripheral vein.
Impaired Cardiac, Hepatic, or Renal Function: Caution is advised when titrating Cardene I.V. in patients with congestive heart failure or impaired hepatic or renal function (see "Precautions").
TRANSFER TO ORAL ANTIHYPERTENSIVE AGENTS
If treatment includes transfer to an oral antihypertensive agent other than Cardene capsules, therapy should generally be initiated upon discontinuation of Cardene I.V. If Cardene capsules are to be used, the first dose of a TID regimen should be administered 1 hour prior to discontinuation of the infusion.

HOW SUPPLIED

Cardene I.V. (nicardipine hydrochloride) is available in packages of 10 ampuls of 10 mL as follows:
25 mg (2.5 mg/mL), NDC 0008-0812-02.
Store at controlled room temperature, 20°–25° C (68°–77° F).
Freezing does not adversely affect the product, but exposure to elevated temperatures should be avoided.
Protect from light. Store ampuls in carton until used.
Caution: Federal law prohibits dispensing without prescription.
U.S. Patent Nos. 3,985,758; 4,880,823; and 5,164,405
Cardene® is a registered trademark of Syntex (U.S.A.) Inc.
Manufactured under license
from Syntex (U.S.A.) Inc. by
Wyeth Laboratories
A Wyeth-Ayerst Company
Philadelphia, PA 19101
CI 4806-1 Issued November 27, 1996

CEROSE®–DM OTC
[se-rōs ' DM]

(See PDR For Nonprescription Drugs and Dietary Supplements.)

CHOLERA VACCINE ℞
USP

DESCRIPTION

Cholera Vaccine, USP is a sterile suspension of equal parts of Ogawa and Inaba serotypes of killed *Vibrio cholerae (V. comma)* in buffered sodium chloride injection. The Inaba and Ogawa strains of *V. cholerae* are grown on trypticase soy agar medium, removed from the medium with buffered sodium chloride injection and killed by the addition of 0.5 percent phenol. Phenol in a concentration of 0.5 percent is also used as the preservative in the finished vaccine. The vaccine contains 8 units of each serotype antigen (Ogawa and Inaba) per milliliter.
Cholera vaccine may be injected intracutaneously (intradermally), subcutaneously or intramuscularly.

CLINICAL PHARMACOLOGY

Cholera vaccine is used for active immunization against cholera. Field studies carried out in endemic cholera areas have shown cholera vaccines to be approximately 50% effective in reducing incidence of disease and for only 3 to 6 months. Use of cholera vaccine does not prevent transmission of infection.

INDICATION AND USAGE

Active immunization against cholera is indicated only for individuals traveling to or residing in countries where cholera is endemic or epidemic.

CONTRAINDICATIONS

Use of cholera vaccine should be postponed in the presence of any acute illness.
A history of severe systemic reaction or allergic response following a prior dose of cholera vaccine is a contraindication to further use.

WARNINGS

DO NOT INJECT INTRAVENOUSLY.
Cholera vaccine should not be administered intramuscularly to persons with thrombocytopenia or any coagulation disorder that would contraindicate intramuscular injection.

PRECAUTIONS

GENERAL
A separate, sterilized syringe and needle should be used for each patient to prevent transmission of hepatitis B virus and other infectious agents from one person to another.
Before delivering the dose intramuscularly or subcutaneously, aspirate to help avoid inadvertent injection into a blood vessel.
Before the injection of any biological, the physician should take all precautions known for prevention of allergic or other side reactions. This should include: a review of the patient's history regarding possible sensitivity; and a knowledge of the recent literature pertaining to the use of the biological concerned.
Epinephrine (1:1000) should be available for immediate use when this product is injected.
DRUG INTERACTIONS
Some data suggest that administration of cholera and yellow fever vaccines within three weeks of each other may result in decreased levels of antibody response to both vaccines as compared with administration at longer intervals. However, there is no evidence that protection to either disease is diminished following simultaneous administration.[1]
It is currently recommended that, when feasible, cholera and yellow fever vaccines should be administered at a minimal interval of three weeks, unless time constraints preclude this. If the vaccines cannot be administered at least three weeks apart, they should be given simultaneously.[2]
PREGNANCY
Pregnancy Category C
Animal reproduction studies have not been conducted with cholera vaccine. It is also not known whether cholera vaccine can cause fetal harm when administered to a pregnant woman or can affect reproductive capacity. However, as with other inactivated bacterial vaccines, its use is not contraindicated during pregnancy unless the intended recipient has manifested significant systemic or allergic reaction following administration of prior doses. Use of cholera vaccine during pregnancy should be individualized to reflect actual need.[1,3]

ADVERSE REACTIONS

Local reactions manifested by erythema, induration, pain, and tenderness at the site of injection occur in most recipients, and such local reactions may persist for a few days. Recipients frequently develop malaise, headache, and mild-to-moderate temperature elevations which may persist for 1 to 2 days.[1,4]

DOSAGE AND ADMINISTRATION

Shake vial vigorously before withdrawing each dose.
Parenteral drug products should be inspected visually for presence of particulate matter and discoloration prior to use.
The primary immunizing course consists of two doses administered one week to one month or more apart. The table below summarizes the recommended doses for both primary and booster immunizations by age, volume (mL), and route of administration.[3,5] The intracutaneous (intradermal) route is satisfactory for persons 5 years of age and older, but higher levels of antibody may be achieved in children less than 5 years old by the subcutaneous or intramuscular routes.

Dose number	Route & Age			
	Intra-dermal	Subcutaneous or Intramuscular		
	5 years and over	6 mos-4 years	5–10 years	Over 10 years
1 & 2 Boosters	0.2 mL 0.2 mL	0.2 mL 0.2 mL	0.3 mL 0.3 mL	0.5 mL 0.5 mL

In areas where cholera is epidemic or endemic, booster doses should be given every six months.

Continued on next page

Cholera Vaccine—Cont.

The primary immunizing series need never be repeated for booster doses to be effective.
Before injection, the rubber diaphragm of the vial and the skin over the site to be injected should be cleansed and prepared with a suitable germicide.

HOW SUPPLIED

Cholera Vaccine, USP, is supplied as 1.5 and 20 mL vials.

STORAGE

Keep between 2° and 8°C (35° and 46°F).
Keep from freezing.

REFERENCES

1. Recommendation of the Immunization Practices Advisory Committee (ACIP). General recommendations on immunization. MMWR 32(1):1, 1983.
2. Recommendations of the Immunization Practices Advisory Committee (ACIP). Yellow fever vaccine. MMWR 32(52):679, 1984.
3. Recommendation of the Public Health Service Advisory Committee on Immunization Practices—Cholera Vaccine. MMWR 27(20):173, 1978.
4. GANGAROSA, E. and FAICH, G.: Cholera: The risk to American travelers. Ann. Int. Med. 74:412, 1971.
5. Report of the Committee on Infectious Diseases, American Academy of Pediatrics, 1982 (Red Book).

Manufactured by:
Wyeth Laboratories
A Wyeth-Ayerst Company
Marietta, PA 17547
U S Gov't License No. 3
CI 4228-1 Issued April 25, 1994

CORDARONE® ℞

[kŏr 'dă-rōn]
(amiodarone HCl)
Tablets

DESCRIPTION

Cordarone is a member of a new class of antiarrhythmic drugs with predominantly Class III (Vaughan Williams' classification) effects, available for oral administration as pink, scored tablets containing 200 mg of amiodarone hydrochloride. The inactive ingredients present are colloidal silicon dioxide, lactose, magnesium stearate, povidone, starch, and FD&C Red 40. Cordarone is a benzofuran derivative: 2-butyl -3-benzofuranyl 4-[2-(diethylamino)-ethoxy]-3,5-diiodophenyl ketone hydrochloride. It is not chemically related to any other available antiarrhythmic drug.
The structural formula is as follows:

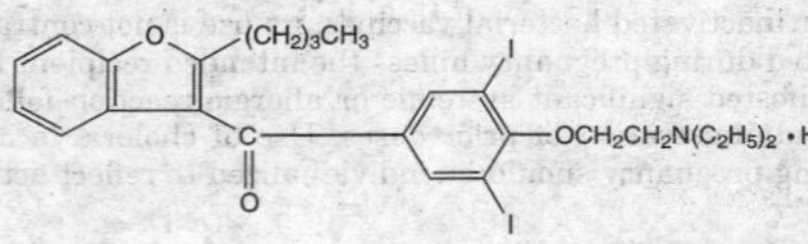

$C_{25}H_{29}I_2NO_3 \cdot HCl$ Molecular Weight: 681.8

Amiodarone HCl is a white to cream-colored crystalline powder. It is slightly soluble in water, soluble in alcohol, and freely soluble in chloroform. It contains 37.3% iodine by weight.

CLINICAL PHARMACOLOGY

Electrophysiology/Mechanisms of Action

In animals, Cordarone is effective in the prevention or suppression of experimentally-induced arrhythmias. The antiarrhythmic effect of Cordarone may be due to at least two major properties: 1) a prolongation of the myocardial cell-action potential duration and refractory period and 2) noncompetitive α- and β-adrenergic inhibition.
Cordarone prolongs the duration of the action potential of all cardiac fibers while causing minimal reduction of dV/dt (maximal upstroke velocity of the action potential). The refractory period is prolonged in all cardiac tissues. Cordarone increases the cardiac refractory period without influencing resting membrane potential, except in automatic cells where the slope of the prepotential is reduced, generally reducing automaticity. These electrophysiologic effects are reflected in a decreased sinus rate of 15 to 20%, increased PR and QT intervals of about 10%, the development of U-waves, and changes in T-wave contour. These changes should not require discontinuation of Cordarone as they are evidence of its pharmacological action, although Cordarone can cause marked sinus bradycardia or sinus arrest and heart block. On rare occasions, QT prolongation has been associated with worsening of arrhythmia (see "**WARNINGS**").

Hemodynamics

In animal studies and after intravenous dosing in man, Cordarone relaxes vascular smooth muscle, reduces peripheral vascular resistance (afterload), and slightly increases cardiac index. After oral dosing, however, Cordarone produces no significant change in left ventricular ejection fraction (LVEF), even in patients with depressed LVEF. After acute intravenous dosing in man, Cordarone may have a mild negative inotropic effect.

Pharmacokinetics

Following oral administration in man, Cordarone is slowly and variably absorbed. The bioavailability of Cordarone is approximately 50%, but has varied between 35 and 65% in various studies. Maximum plasma concentrations are attained 3 to 7 hours after a single dose. Despite this, the onset of action may occur in 2 to 3 days, but more commonly takes 1 to 3 weeks, even with loading doses. Plasma concentrations with chronic dosing at 100 to 600 mg/day are approximately dose proportional, with a mean 0.5 mg/L increase for each 100 mg/day. These means, however, include considerable individual variability. Food increases the rate and extent of absorption of Cordarone. The effects of food upon the bioavailability of Cordarone have been studied in 30 healthy subjects who received a single 600-mg dose immediately after consuming a high fat meal and following an overnight fast. The area under the plasma concentration-time curve (AUC) and the peak plasma concentration (C_{max}) of amiodarone increased by 2.3 (range 1.7 to 3.6) and 3.8 (range 2.7 to 4.4) times, respectively, in the presence of food. Food also increased the rate of absorption of amiodarone, decreasing the time to peak plasma concentration (T_{max}) by 37%. The mean AUC and mean C_{max} of desethylamiodarone increased by 55% (range 58 to 101%) and 32% (range 4 to 84%), respectively, but there was no change in the T_{max} in the presence of food.
Cordarone has a very large but variable volume of distribution, averaging about 60 L/kg, because of extensive accumulation in various sites, especially adipose tissue and highly perfused organs, such as the liver, lung, and spleen. One major metabolite of Cordarone, desethylamiodarone (DEA), has been identified in man; it accumulates to an even greater extent in almost all tissues. No data are available on the activity of DEA in humans, but in animals, it has significant electrophysiologic and antiarrhythmic effects generally similar to amiodarone itself. DEA's precise role and contribution to the antiarrhythmic activity of oral amiodarone are not certain. The development of maximal ventricular class III effects after oral Cordarone administration in humans correlates more closely with DEA accumulation over time than with amiodarone accumulation.
Amiodarone is eliminated primarily by hepatic metabolism and biliary excretion and there is negligible excretion of amiodarone or DEA in urine. Neither amiodarone nor DEA is dialyzable.
In clinical studies of 2 to 7 days, clearance of amiodarone after intravenous administration in patients with VT and VF ranged between 220 and 440 ml/hr/kg. Age, sex, renal disease, and hepatic disease (cirrhosis) do not have marked effects on the disposition of amiodarone or DEA. Renal impairment does not influence the pharmacokinetics of amiodarone. After a single dose of intravenous amiodarone in cirrhotic patients, significantly lower C_{max} and average concentration values are seen for DEA, but mean amiodarone levels are unchanged. Normal subjects over 65 years of age show lower clearances (about 100 ml/hr/kg) than younger subjects (about 150 ml/hr/kg) and an increase in $t_{1/2}$ from about 20 to 47 days. In patients with severe left ventricular dysfunction, the pharmacokinetics of amiodarone are not significantly altered but the terminal disposition $t_{1/2}$ of DEA is prolonged. Although no dosage adjustment for patients with renal, hepatic, or cardiac abnormalities has been defined during chronic treatment with Cordarone, close clinical monitoring is prudent for elderly patients and those with severe left ventricular dysfunction.
Following single dose administration in 12 healthy subjects, Codarone exhibited multi-compartmental pharmcokinetics with mean apparent plasma terminal elimination half-life of 58 days (range 15 to 142 days) for amiodarone and 36 days (range 14 to 75 days) for the active metabolite (DEA). In patients, following discontinuation of chronic oral therapy, Cordarone has been shown to have a biphasic elimination with an initial one-half reduction of plasma levels after 2.5 to 10 days. A much slower terminal plasma-elimination phase shows a half-life of the parent compound ranging from 26 to 107 days, with a mean of approximately 53 days and most patients in the 40- to 55-day range. In the absence of a loading-dose period, steady-state plasma concentrations, at constant oral dosing, would therefore be reached between 130 and 535 days, with an average of 265 days. For the metabolite, the mean plasma-elimination half-life was approximately 61 days. These data probably reflect an initial elimination of the drug from well-perfused tissue (the 2.5- to 10-day half-life phase), followed by a terminal phase representing extremely slow elimination from poorly perfused tissue compartments such as fat.
The considerable intersubject variation in both phases of elimination, as well as uncertainty as to what compartment is critical to drug effect, requires attention to individual responses once arrhythmia control is achieved with loading doses because the correct maintenance dose is determined, in part, by the elimination rates. Daily maintenance doses of Cordarone should be based on individual patient requirements (see "**DOSAGE AND ADMINISTRATION**").
Cordarone and its metabolite have a limited transplacental transfer of approximately 10 to 50%. The parent drug and its metabolite have been detected in breast milk.
Cordarone is highly protein-bound (approximately 96%).
Although electrophysiologic effects, such as prolongation of QTc, can be seen within hours after a parenteral dose of Cordarone, effects on abnormal rhythms are not seen before 2 to 3 days and usually require 1 to 3 weeks, even when a loading dose is used. There may be a continued increase in effect for longer periods still. There is evidence that the time to effect is shorter when a loading-dose regimen is used.
Consistent with the slow rate of elimination, antiarrhythmic effects persist for weeks or months after Cordarone is discontinued, but the time of recurrence is variable and unpredictable. In general, when the drug is resumed after recurrence of the arrhythmia, control is established relatively rapidly compared to the initial response, presumably because tissue stores were not wholly depleted at the time of recurrence.

Pharmacodynamics

There is no well-established relationship of plasma concentration to effectiveness, but it does appear that concentrations much below 1 mg/L are often ineffective and that levels above 2.5 mg/L are generally not needed. Within individuals dose reductions and ensuing decreased plasma concentrations can result in loss of arrhythmia control. Plasma-concentration measurements can be used to identify patients whose levels are unusually low, and who might benefit from a dose increase, or unusually high, and who might have dosage reduction in the hope of minimizing side effects. Some observations have suggested a plasma concentration, dose, or dose/duration relationship for side effects such as pulmonary fibrosis, liver-enzyme elevations, corneal deposits and facial pigmentation, peripheral neuropathy, gastrointestinal and central nervous system effects.

Monitoring Effectiveness

Predicting the effectiveness of any antiarrhythmic agent in long-term prevention of recurrent ventricular tachycardia and ventricular fibrillation is difficult and controversial, with highly qualified investigators recommending use of ambulatory monitoring, programmed electrical stimulation with various stimulation regimens, or a combination of these, to assess response. There is no present consensus on many aspects of how best to assess effectiveness, but there is a reasonable consensus on some aspects:

1. If a patient with a history of cardiac arrest does not manifest a hemodynamically unstable arrhythmia during electrocardiographic monitoring prior to treatment, assessment of the effectiveness of Cordarone requires some provocative approach, either exercise or programmed electrical stimulation (PES).
2. Whether provocation is also needed in patients who do manifest their life-threatening arrhythmia spontaneously is not settled, but there are reasons to consider PES or other provocation in such patients. In the fraction of patients whose PES-inducible arrhythmia can be made noninducible by Cordarone (a fraction that has varied widely in various series from less than 10% to almost 40%, perhaps due to different stimulation criteria), the prognosis has been almost uniformly excellent, with very low recurrence (ventricular tachycardia or sudden death) rates. More controversial is the meaning of continued inducibility. There has been an impression that continued inducibility in Cordarone patients may not foretell a poor prognosis but, in fact, many observers have found greater recurrence rates in patients who remain inducible than in those who do not. A number of criteria have been proposed, however, for identifying patients who remain inducible but who seem likely nonetheless to do well on Cordarone. These criteria include increased difficulty of induction (more stimuli or more rapid stimuli), which has been reported to predict a lower rate of recurrence, and ability to tolerate the induced ventricular tachycardia without severe symptoms, a finding that has been reported to correlate with better survival but not with lower recurrence rates. While these criteria require confirmation and further study in general, *easier* inducibility or *poorer* tolerance of the induced arrhythmia should suggest consideration of a need to revise treatment.

Several predictors of success not based on PES have also been suggested, including complete elimination of all nonsustained ventricular tachycardia on ambulatory monitoring and very low premature ventricular-beat rates (less than 1 VPB/1,000 normal beats).
While these issues remain unsettled for Cordarone, as for other agents, the prescriber of Cordarone should have access to (direct or through referral), and familiarity with, the full range of evaluatory procedures used in the care of patients with life-threatening arrhythmias.
It is difficult to describe the effectiveness rates of Cordarone, as these depend on the specific arrhythmia treated, the success criteria used, the underlying cardiac disease of the patient, the number of drugs tried before resorting to Cordarone, the duration of follow-up, the dose of Cordarone, the use of additional antiarrhythmic agents, and many other factors. As Cordarone has been studied principally in patients with refractory life-threatening ventricular arrhythmias, in whom drug therapy must be selected on the basis of response and cannot be assigned arbitrarily, randomized comparisons with other agents or placebo have not been possible. Reports of series of treated patients with a history of cardiac arrest and mean follow-up of one year or more have given mortality (due to arrhythmia) rates that were highly variable, ranging from less than 5% to over 30%, with most series in the range of 10 to 15%. Overall arrhythmia-recurrence rates (fatal and nonfatal) also were highly variable (and, as noted above, depended on response to PES and other measures), and depend on whether patients who do not seem to respond initially are included. In most cases, considering only patients who

seemed to respond well enough to be placed on long-term treatment, recurrence rates have ranged from 20 to 40% in series with a mean follow-up of a year or more.

INDICATIONS AND USAGE

Because of its life-threatening side effects and the substantial management difficulties associated with its use (see "**WARNINGS**" below), Cordarone is indicated only for the treatment of the following documented, life-threatening recurrent ventricular arrhythmias when these have not responded to documented adequate doses of other available antiarrhythmics or when alternative agents could not be tolerated.

1. Recurrent ventricular fibrillation.
2. Recurrent hemodynamically unstable ventricular tachycardia.

As is the case for other antiarrhythmic agents, there is no evidence from controlled trials that the use of Cordarone favorably affects survival.

Cordarone should be used only by physicians familiar with and with access to (directly or through referral) the use of all available modalities for treating recurrent life-threatening ventricular arrhythmias, and who have access to appropriate monitoring facilities, including in-hospital and ambulatory continuous electrocardiographic monitoring and electrophysiologic techniques. Because of the life-threatening nature of the arrhythmias treated, potential interactions with prior therapy, and potential exacerbation of the arrhythmia, initiation of therapy with Cordarone should be carried out in the hospital.

CONTRAINDICATIONS

Cordarone is contraindicated in severe sinus-node dysfunction, causing marked sinus bradycardia; second- and third-degree atrioventricular block; and when episodes of bradycardia have caused syncope (except when used in conjunction with a pacemaker).

Cordarone is contraindicated in patients with a known hypersensitivity to the drug.

WARNINGS

Cordarone is intended for use only in patients with the indicated life-threatening arrhythmias because its use is accompanied by substantial toxicity.

Cordarone has several potentially fatal toxicities, the most important of which is pulmonary toxicity (hypersensitivity pneumonitis or interstitial/alveolar pneumonitis) that has resulted in clinically manifest disease at rates as high as 10 to 17% in some series of patients with ventricular arrhythmias given doses around 400 mg/day, and as abnormal diffusion capacity without symptoms in a much higher percentage of patients. Pulmonary toxicity has been fatal about 10% of the time. Liver injury is common with Cordarone, but is usually mild and evidenced only by abnormal liver enzymes. Overt liver disease can occur, however, and has been fatal in a few cases. Like other antiarrhythmics, Cordarone can exacerbate the arrhythmia, e.g., by making the arrhythmia less well tolerated or more difficult to reverse. This has occurred in 2 to 5% of patients in various series, and significant heart block or sinus bradycardia has been seen in 2 to 5%. All of these events should be manageable in the proper clinical setting in most cases. Although the frequency of such proarrhythmic events does not appear greater with Cordarone than with many other agents used in this population, the effects are prolonged when they occur. Even in patients at high risk of arrhythmic death, in whom the toxicity of Cordarone is an acceptable risk, Cordarone poses major management problems that could be life-threatening in a population at risk of sudden death, so that every effort should be made to utilize alternative agents first.

The difficulty of using Cordarone effectively and safely itself poses a significant risk to patients. Patients with the indicated arrhythmias must be hospitalized while the loading dose of Cordarone is given, and a response generally requires at least one week, usually two or more. Because absorption and elimination are variable, maintenance-dose selection is difficult, and it is not unusual to require dosage decrease or discontinuation of treatment. In a retrospective survey of 192 patients with ventricular tachyarrhythmias, 84 required dose reduction and 18 required at least temporary discontinuation because of adverse effects, and several series have reported 15 to 20% overall frequencies of discontinuation due to adverse reactions. The time at which a previously controlled life-threatening arrhythmia will recur after discontinuation or dose adjustment is unpredictable, ranging from weeks to months. The patient is obviously at great risk during this time and may need prolonged hospitalization. Attempts to substitute other antiarrhythmic agents when Cordarone must be stopped will be made difficult by the gradually, but unpredictably, changing amiodarone body burden. A similar problem exists when Cordarone is not effective; it still poses the risk of an interaction with whatever subsequent treatment is tried.

Mortality

In the National Heart, Lung and Blood Institute's Cardiac Arrhythmia Suppression Trial (CAST), a long-term, multi-centered, randomized, double-blind study in patients with asymptomatic non-life-threatening ventricular arrhythmias who had had myocardial infarctions more than six days but less than two years previously, an excessive mortality or non-fatal cardiac arrest rate was seen in patients treated with encainide or flecainide (56/730) compared with that seen in patients assigned to matched placebo-treated groups (22/725). The average duration of treatment with encainide or flecainide in this study was ten months.

Cordarone therapy was evaluated in two multi-centered, randomized, double-blind, placebo-controlled trials involving 1202 (Canadian Amiodarone Myocardial Infarction Arrhythmia Trial; CAMIAT) and 1486 (European Myocardial Infarction Amiodarone Trial; EMIAT) post-MI patients followed for up to 2 years. Patients in CAMIAT qualified with ventricular arrhythmias, and those randomized to amiodarone received weight- and response-adjusted doses of 200 to 400 mg/day. Patients in EMIAT qualified with ejection fraction <40%, and those randomized to amiodarone received fixed doses of 200 mg/day. Both studies had weeks-long loading dose schedules. Intent-to-treat all-cause mortality results were as follows:

[See table above]

	Placebo		Amiodarone		Relative Risk	
	N	Deaths	N	Deaths		95% CI
EMIAT	743	102	743	103	0.99	0.76–1.31
CAMIAT	596	68	606	57	0.88	0.58–1.16

These data are consistent with the results of a pooled analysis of smaller, controlled studies involving patients with structural heart disease (including myocardial infarction).

Pulmonary Toxicity

Cordarone may cause a clinical syndrome of cough and progressive dyspnea accompanied by functional, radiographic, gallium-scan, and pathological data consistent with pulmonary toxicity, the frequency of which varies from 2 to 7% in most published reports, but is as high as 10 to 17% in some reports. Therefore, when Cordarone therapy is initiated, a baseline chest X ray and pulmonary-function tests, including diffusion capacity, should be performed. The patient should return for a history, physical exam, and chest X ray every 3 to 6 months.

Preexisting pulmonary disease does not appear to increase the risk of developing pulmonary toxicity; however, these patients have a poorer prognosis if pulmonary toxicity does develop.

Pulmonary toxicity secondary to Cordarone seems to result from either indirect or direct toxicity as represented by hypersensitivity pneumonitis or interstitial/alveolar pneumonitis, respectively.

Hypersensitivity pneumonitis usually appears earlier in the course of therapy, and rechallenging these patients with Cordarone results in a more rapid recurrence of greater severity. Bronchoalveolar lavage is the procedure of choice to confirm this diagnosis, which can be made when a T suppressor/cytotoxic (CD8-positive) lymphocytosis is noted. Steroid therapy should be instituted and Cordarone therapy discontinued in these patients.

Interstitial/alveolar pneumonitis may result from the release of oxygen radicals and/or phospholipidosis and is characterized by findings of diffuse alveolar damage, interstitial pneumonitis or fibrosis in lung biopsy specimens. Phospholipidosis (foamy cells, foamy macrophages), due to inhibition of phospholipase, will be present in most cases of Cordarone-induced pulmonary toxicity; however, these changes also are present in approximately 50% of all patients on Cordarone therapy. These cells should be used as markers of therapy, but not as evidence of toxicity. A diagnosis of Cordarone-induced interstitial/alveolar pneumonitis should lead, at a minimum, to dose reduction or, preferably, to withdrawal of the Cordarone to establish reversibility, especially if other acceptable antiarrhythmic therapies are available. Where these measures have been instituted, a reduction in symptoms of amiodarone-induced pulmonary toxicity was usually noted within the first week, and a clinical improvement was greatest in the first two to three weeks. Chest X ray changes usually resolve within two to four months. According to some experts, steroids may prove beneficial. Prednisone in doses of 40 to 60 mg/day or equivalent doses of other steroids have been given and tapered over the course of several weeks depending upon the condition of the patient. In some cases rechallenge with Cordarone at a lower dose has not resulted in return of toxicity. Recent reports suggest that the use of lower loading and maintenance doses of Cordarone are associated with a decreased incidence of Cordarone-induced pulmonary toxicity.

In a patient receiving Cordarone, any new respiratory symptoms should suggest the possibility of pulmonary toxicity, and the history, physical exam, chest X ray, and pulmonary-function tests (with diffusion capacity) should be repeated and evaluated. A 15% decrease in diffusion capacity has a high sensitivity but only a moderate specificity for pulmonary toxicity; as the decrease in diffusion capacity approaches 30%, the sensitivity decreases but the specificity increases. A gallium-scan also may be performed as part of the diagnostic workup.

Fatalities, secondary to pulmonary toxicity, have occurred in approximately 10% of cases. However, in patients with life-threatening arrhythmias, discontinuation of Cordarone therapy due to suspected drug-induced pulmonary toxicity should be undertaken with caution, as the most common cause of death in these patients is sudden cardiac death. Therefore, every effort should be made to rule out other causes of respiratory impairment (i.e., congestive heart failure with Swan-Ganz catheterization if necessary, respiratory infection, pulmonary embolism, malignancy, etc.) before discontinuing Cordarone in these patients. In addition, bronchoalveolar lavage, transbronchial lung biopsy and/or open lung biopsy may be necessary to confirm the diagnosis, especially in those cases where no acceptable alternative therapy is available.

If a diagnosis of Cordarone-induced hypersensitivity pneumonitis is made, Cordarone should be discontinued, and treatment with steroids should be instituted. If a diagnosis of Cordarone-induced interstitial/alveolar pneumonitis is made, steroid therapy should be instituted and, preferably, Cordarone discontinued or, at a minimum, reduced in dosage. Some cases of Cordarone-induced interstitial/alveolar pneumonitis may resolve following a reduction in Cordarone dosage in conjunction with the administration of steroids. In some patients, rechallenge at a lower dose has not resulted in return of interstitial/alveolar pneumonitis; however, in some patients (perhaps because of severe alveolar damage) the pulmonary lesions have not been reversible.

Worsened Arrhythmia

Cordarone, like other antiarrhythmics, can cause serious exacerbation of the presenting arrhythmia, a risk that may be enhanced by the presence of concomitant antiarrhythmics. Exacerbation has been reported in about 2 to 5% in most series, and has included new ventricular fibrillation, incessant ventricular tachycardia, increased resistance to cardioversion, and polymorphic ventricular tachycardia associated with QT prolongation (Torsade de Pointes). In addition, Cordarone has caused symptomatic bradycardia or sinus arrest with suppression of escape foci in 2 to 4% of patients.

Liver Injury

Elevations of hepatic enzyme levels are seen frequently in patients exposed to Cordarone and in most cases are asymptomatic. If the increase exceeds three times normal, or doubles in a patient with an elevated baseline, discontinuation of Cordarone or dosage reduction should be considered. In a few cases in which biopsy has been done, the histology has resembled that of alcoholic hepatitis or cirrhosis. Hepatic failure has been a rare cause of death in patients treated with Cordarone.

Loss of Vision

Cases of optic neuropathy and/or optic neuritis, usually resulting in visual impairment, have been reported in patients treated with amiodarone. In some cases, visual impairment has progressed to permanent blindness. Optic neuropathy and/or neuritis may occur at any time following initiation of therapy. A causal relationship to the drug has not been clearly established. If symptoms of visual impairment appear, such as changes in visual acuity and decreases in peripheral vision, prompt ophthalmic examination is recommended. Appearance of optic neuropathy and/or neuritis calls for re-evaluation of Cordarone therapy. The risks and complications of antiarrhythmic therapy with Cordarone must be weighed against its benefits in patients whose lives are threatened by cardiac arrhythmias. Regular ophthalmic examination, including fundoscopy and slit-lamp examination, is recommended during administration of Cordarone. (See "**ADVERSE REACTIONS.**")

Neonatal Hypo- or Hyperthyroidism

Cordarone can cause fetal harm when administered to a pregnant woman. Although Cordarone use during pregnancy is uncommon, there have been a small number of published reports of congenital goiter/hypothyroidism and hyperthyroidism. If Cordarone is used during pregnancy, or if the patient becomes pregnant while taking Cordarone, the patient should be apprised of the potential hazard to the fetus.

In general, Cordarone® should be used during pregnancy only if the potential benefit to the mother justifies the unknown risk to the fetus.

In pregnant rats and rabbits, amiodarone HCl in doses of 25 mg/kg/day (approximately 0.4 and 0.9 times, respectively, the maximum recommended human maintenance dose*) had no adverse effects on the fetus. In the rabbit, 75 mg/kg/day (approximately 2.7 times the maximum recommended human maintenance dose*) caused abortions in greater than 90% of the animals. In the rat, doses of 50 mg/kg/day or more were associated with slight displacement of the testes and an increased incidence of incomplete ossification of some skull and digital bones; at 100 mg/kg/day or more, fetal body weights were reduced; at 200 mg/kg/day, there was an increased incidence of fetal resportion. (These doses in the rat are approximately 0.8, 1.6 and 3.2 times the maximum recommended human maintenance dose.*) Adverse effects on fetal growth and survival also were noted in one of two strains of mice at a dose of 5 mg/kg/day (approximately 0.04 times the maximum recommended human maintenance dose*).

*600 mg in a 50 kg patient (doses compared on a body surface area basis)

PRECAUTIONS

Impairment of Vision

Optic Neuropathy and/or Neuritis

Cases of optic neuropathy and optic neuritis have been reported (see "**WARNINGS**").

Continued on next page

Cordarone Tablets—Cont.

Corneal Microdeposits
Corneal microdeposits appear in the majority of adults treated with Cordarone. They are usually discernible only by slit-lamp examination, but give rise to symptoms such as visual halos or blurred vision in as many as 10% of patients. Corneal microdeposits are reversible upon reduction of dose or termination of treatment. Asymptomatic microdeposits alone are not a reason to reduce dose or discontinue treatment (see "**ADVERSE REACTIONS**").

Neurologic
Chronic administration of oral amiodarone in rare instances may lead to the development of peripheral neuropathy that may resolve when amiodarone is discontinued, but this resolution has been slow and incomplete.

Photosensitivity
Cordarone has induced photosensitization in about 10% of patients; some protection may be afforded by the use of sun-barrier creams or protective clothing. During long-term treatment, a blue-gray discoloration of the exposed skin may occur. The risk may be increased in patients of fair complexion or those with excessive sun exposure, and may be related to cumulative dose and duration of therapy.

Thyroid Abnormalities
Cordarone inhibits peripheral conversion of thyroxine (T_4) to triiodothyronine (T_3) and may cause increased thyroxine levels, decreased T_3 levels, and increased levels of inactive reverse T_3 (rT_3) in clinically euthyroid patients. It is also a potential source of large amounts of inorganic iodine. Because of its release of inorganic iodine, or perhaps for other reasons, Cordarone can cause either hypothyroidism or hyperthyroidism. Thyroid function should be monitored prior to treatment and periodically thereafter, particularly in elderly patients, and in any patient with a history of thyroid nodules, goiter, or other thyroid dysfunction. Because of the slow elimination of Cordarone and its metabolites, high plasma iodide levels, altered thyroid function, and abnormal thyroid-function tests may persist for several weeks or even months following Cordarone withdrawal.

Hypothyroidism has been reported in 2 to 4% of patients in most series, but in 8 to 10% in some series. This condition may be identified by relevant clinical symptoms and particularly by elevated serum TSH levels. In some clinically hypothyroid amiodarone-treated patients, free thyroxine index values may be normal. Hypothyroidism is best managed by Cordarone dose reduction and/or thyroid hormone supplement. However, therapy must be individualized, and it may be necessary to discontinue Cordarone in some patients.

Hyperthyroidism occurs in about 2% of patients receiving Cordarone, but the incidence may be higher among patients with prior inadequate dietary iodine intake. Cordarone-induced hyperthyroidism usually poses a greater hazard to the patient than hypothyroidism because of the possibility of arrhythmia breakthrough or aggravation. In fact, IF ANY NEW SIGNS OF ARRHYTHMIA APPEAR, THE POSSIBILITY OF HYPERTHYROIDISM SHOULD BE CONSIDERED. Hyperthyroidism is best identified by relevant clinical symptoms and signs, accompanied usually by abnormally elevated levels of serum T_3 RIA, and further elevations of serum T_4, and a subnormal serum TSH level (using a sufficiently sensitive TSH assay). The finding of a flat TSH response to TRH is confirmatory of hyperthyroidism and may be sought in equivocal cases. Since arrhythmia breakthroughs may accompany Cordarone-induced hyperthyrodism, aggressive medical treatment is indicated, including, if possible, dose reduction or withdrawal of Cordarone. The institution of antithyroid drugs, β-adrenergic blockers and/or temporary corticosteroid therapy may be necessary. The action of antithyroid drugs may be especially delayed in amiodarone-induced thyrotoxicosis because of substantial quantities of preformed thyroid hormones stored in the gland. Radioactive iodine therapy is contraindicated because of the low radioiodine uptake associated with amiodarone-induced hyperthyroidism. Experience with thyroid surgery in this setting is extremely limited, and this form of therapy runs the theoretical risk of inducing thyroid storm. Cordarone-induced hyperthyroidism may be followed by a transient period of hypothyroidism.

Surgery
Volatile Anesthetic Agents: Close perioperative monitoring is recommended in patients undergoing general anesthesia who are on amiodarone therapy as they may be more sensitive to the myocardial depressant and conduction effects of halogenated inhalational anesthetics.

Hypotension Postbypass: Rare occurrences of hypotension upon discontinuation of cardiopulmonary bypass during open-heart surgery in patients receiving Cordarone have been reported. The relationship of this event to Cordarone therapy is unknown.

Adult Respiratory Distress Syndrome (ARDS): Postoperatively, occurrences of ARDS have been reported in patients receiving Cordarone therapy who have undergone either cardiac or noncardiac surgery. Although patients usually respond well to vigorous respiratory therapy, in rare instances the outcome has been fatal. Until further studies have been performed, it is recommended that FiO_2 and the determinants of oxygen delivery to the tissues (e.g., SaO_2, PaO_2) be closely monitored in patients on Cordarone.

Laboratory Tests
Elevations in liver enzymes (SGOT and SGPT) can occur. Liver enzymes in patients on relatively high maintenance doses should be monitored on a regular basis. Persistent significant elevations in the liver enzymes or hepatomegaly should alert the physician to consider reducing the maintenance dose of Cordarone or discontinuing therapy.
Cordarone alters the results of thyroid-function tests, causing an increase in serum T_4 and serum reverse T_3, and a decline in serum T_3 levels. Despite these biochemical changes, most patients remain clinically euthyroid.

Drug Interactions
Although only a small number of drug-drug interactions with Cordarone have been explored formally, most of these have shown such an interaction. The potential for other interactions should be anticipated, particularly for drugs with potentially serious toxicity, such as other antiarrhythmics. If such drugs are needed, their dose should be reassessed and, where appropriate, plasma concentration measured.
In view of the long and variable half-life of Cordarone, potential for drug interactions exists not only with concomitant medication but also with drugs administered after discontinuation of Cordarone.

Cyclosporine
Concomitant use of amiodarone and cyclosporine has been reported to produce persistently elevated plasma concentrations of cyclosporine resulting in elevated creatinine, despite reduction in dose of cyclosporine.

Digitalis
Administration of Cordarone to patients receiving digoxin therapy regularly results in an increase in the serum digoxin concentration that may reach toxic levels with resultant clinical toxicity. **On initiation of Cordarone, the need for digitalis therapy should be reviewed and the dose reduced by approximately 50% or discontinued.** If digitalis treatment is continued, serum levels should be closely monitored and patients observed for clinical evidence of toxicity. These precautions probably should apply to digitoxin administration as well.

Anticoagulants
Potentiation of warfarin-type anticoagulant response is almost always seen in patients receiving Cordarone and can result in serious or fatal bleeding. **The dose of the anticoagulant should be reduced by one-third to one-half, and prothrombin times should be monitored closely.**

Antiarrhythmic Agents
Other antiarrhythmic drugs, such as quinidine, procainamide, disopyramide, and phenytoin, have been used concurrently with Cordarone.
There have been case reports of increased steady-state levels of quinidine, procainamide, and phenytoin during concomitant therapy with Cordarone. In general, any added antiarrhythmic drug should be initiated at a lower than usual dose with careful monitoring.
In general, combination of Cordarone with other antiarrhythmic therapy should be reserved for patients with life-threatening ventricular arrhythmias who are incompletely responsive to a single agent or incompletely responsive to Cordarone. During transfer to Cordarone the dose levels of previously administered agents should be reduced by 30 to 50% several days after the addition of Cordarone, when arrhythmia suppression should be beginning. The continued need for the other antiarrhythmic agent should be reviewed after the effects of Cordarone have been established, and discontinuation ordinarily should be attempted. If the treatment is continued, these patients should be particularly carefully monitored for adverse effects, especially conduction disturbances and exacerbation of tachyarrhythmias, as Cordarone is continued. In Cordarone-treated patients who require additional antiarrhythmic therapy, the initial dose of such agents should be approximately half of the usual recommended dose.
Cordarone should be used with caution in patients receiving β-blocking agents or calcium antagonists because of the possible potentiation of bradycardia, sinus arrest, and AV block; if necessary, Cordarone can continue to be used after insertion of a pacemaker in patients with severe bradycardia or sinus arrest.

Volatile Anesthetic Agents (See "**PRECAUTIONS, Surgery**, *Volatile Anesthetic Agents.*")
[See table below]

SUMMARY OF DRUG INTERACTIONS WITH CORDARONE

Concomitant Drug	Interaction: Onset (days)	Interaction: Magnitude	Recommended Dose Reduction of Concomitant Drug
Warfarin	3 to 4	Increases prothrombin time by 100%	↓ 1/3 to 1/2
Digoxin	1	Increases serum concentration by 70%	↓ 1/2
Quinidine	2	Increases serum concentration by 33%	↓ 1/3 to 1/2 (or discontinue)
Procainamide	<7	Increases plasma concentration by 55%; NAPA* concentration by 33%	↓ 1/3 (or discontinue)

*NAPA = n-acetyl procainamide.

Electrolyte Disturbances
Since antiarrhythmic drugs may be ineffective or may be arrhythmogenic in patients with hypokalemia, any potassium or magnesium deficiency should be corrected before instituting Cordarone therapy.

Carcinogenesis, Mutagenesis, Impairment of Fertility
Amiodarone HCl was associated with a statistically significant, dose-related increase in the incidence of thyroid tumors (follicular adenoma and/or carcinoma) in rats. The incidence of thyroid tumors was greater than control even at the lowest dose level tested, i.e., 5 mg/kg/day (approximately 0.08 times the maximum recommended human maintenance dose*).
Mutagenicity studies (Ames, micronucleus, and lysogenic tests) with Cordarone were negative.
In a study in which amiodarone HCl was administered to male and female rats, beginning 9 weeks prior to mating, reduced fertility was observed at a dose level of 90 mg/kg/day (approximately 1.4 times the maximum recommended human maintenance dose*).

*600 mg in a 50 kg patient (dose compared on a body surface area basis)

Pregnancy: Pregnancy Category D
See "**WARNINGS, Neonatal Hypo- or Hyperthyroidism.**"

Labor and Delivery
It is not known whether the use of Cordarone during labor or delivery has any immediate or delayed adverse effects. Preclinical studies in rodents have not shown any effect of Cordarone on the duration of gestation or on parturition.

Nursing Mothers
Cordarone is excreted in human milk, suggesting that breast-feeding could expose the nursing infant to a significant dose of the drug. Nursing offspring of lactating rats administered Cordarone have been shown to be less viable and have reduced body-weight gains. Therefore, when Cordarone therapy is indicated, the mother should be advised to discontinue nursing.

Pediatric Use
The safety and effectiveness of Cordarone in pediatric patients have not been established.

Geriatric Use
Clinical studies of Cordarone Tablets did not include sufficient numbers of subjects aged 65 and over to determine whether they respond differently from younger subjects. Other reported clinical experience has not identified differences in responses between the elderly and younger patients. In general, dose selection for an elderly patient should be cautious, usually starting at the low end of the dosing range, reflecting the greater frequency of decreased hepatic, renal, or cardiac function, and of concomitant disease or other drug therapy.

ADVERSE REACTIONS

Adverse reactions have been very common in virtually all series of patients treated with Cordarone for ventricular arrhythmias with relatively large doses of drug (400 mg/day and above), occurring in about three-fourths of all patients and causing discontinuation in 7 to 18%. The most serious reactions are pulmonary toxicity, exacerbation of arrhythmia, and rare serious liver injury (see "**WARNINGS**"), but other adverse effects constitute important problems. They are often reversible with dose reduction or cessation of Cordarone treatment. Most of the adverse effects appear to become more frequent with continued treatment beyond six months, although rates appear to remain relatively constant beyond one year. The time and dose relationships of adverse effects are under continued study.
Neurologic problems are extremely common, occurring in 20 to 40% of patients and including malaise and fatigue, tremor and involuntary movements, poor coordination and gait, and peripheral neuropathy; they are rarely a reason to stop therapy and may respond to dose reductions or discontinuation (see "**PRECAUTIONS**").
Gastrointestinal complaints, most commonly nausea, vomiting, constipation, and anorexia, occur in about 25% of patients but rarely require discontinuation of drug. These commonly occur during high-dose administration (i.e., loading dose) and usually respond to dose reduction or divided doses.
Ophthalmic abnormalities including optic neuropathy and/or optic neuritis, in some cases progressing to permanent blindness, papilledema, corneal degeneration, photosensitivity, eye discomfort, scotoma, lens opacities, and macular degeneration have been reported. (See "**WARNINGS.**")
Asymptomatic corneal microdeposits are present in virtually all adult patients who have been on drug for more than 6 months. Some patients develop eye symptoms of halos, photophobia, and dry eyes. Vision is rarely affected and drug discontinuation is rarely needed.
Dermatological adverse reactions occur in about 15% of patients, with photosensitivity being most common (about 10%). Sunscreen and protection from sun exposure may be helpful, and drug discontinuation is not usually necessary. Prolonged exposure to Cordarone occasionally results in a blue-gray pigmentation. This is slowly and occasionally incompletely reversible on discontinuation of drug but is of cosmetic importance only.

	Loading Dose (Daily)	Adjustment and Maintenance Dose (Daily)	
Ventricular Arrhythmias	1 to 3 weeks	~1 month	usual maintenance
	800 to 1,600 mg	600 to 800 mg	400 mg

Cardiovascular adverse reactions, other than exacerbation of the arrhythmias, include the uncommon occurrence of congestive heart failure (3%) and bradycardia. Bradycardia usually responds to dosage reduction but may require a pacemaker for control. CHF rarely requires drug discontinuation. Cardiac conduction abnormalities occur infrequently and are reversible on discontinuation of drug.

Hepatitis, cholestatic hepatitis, cirrhosis, epididymitis, vasculitis, pseudotumor cerebri, thrombocytopenia, angioedema, bronchiolitis obliterans organizing pneumonia (possibly fatal), pleuritis, pancreatitis, toxic epidermal necrolysis, pancytopenia, and neutropenia also have been reported in patients receiving Cordarone.

The following side-effect rates are based on a retrospective study of 241 patients treated for 2 to 1,515 days (mean 441.3 days).

The following side effects were reported in 10 to 33% of patients:

Gastrointestinal: Nausea and vomiting.

The following side effects were each reported in 4 to 9% of patients:

Dermatologic: Solar dermatitis/photosensitivity.

Neurologic: Malaise and fatigue, tremor/abnormal involuntary movements, lack of coordination, abnormal gait/ataxia, dizziness, paresthesias.

Gastrointestinal: Constipation, anorexia.

Ophthalmologic: Visual disturbances.

Hepatic: Abnormal liver-function tests.

Respiratory: Pulmonary inflammation or fibrosis.

The following side effects were each reported in 1 to 3% of patients:

Thyroid: Hypothyroidism, hyperthyroidism.

Neurologic: Decreased libido, insomnia, headache, sleep disturbances.

Cardiovascular: Congestive heart failure, cardiac arrhythmias, SA node dysfunction.

Gastrointestinal: Abdominal pain.

Hepatic: Nonspecific hepatic disorders.

Other: Flushing, abnormal taste and smell, edema, abnormal salivation, coagulation abnormalities.

The following side effects were each reported in less than 1% of patients:

Blue skin discoloration, rash, spontaneous ecchymosis, alopecia, hypotension, and cardiac conduction abnormalities.

In surveys of almost 5,000 patients treated in open U.S. studies and in published reports of treatment with Cordarone, the adverse reactions most frequently requiring discontinuation of Cordarone included pulmonary infiltrates or fibrosis, paroxysmal ventricular tachycardia, congestive heart failure, and elevation of liver enzymes. Other symptoms causing discontinuations less often included visual disturbances, solar dermatitis, blue skin discoloration, hyperthyroidism and hypothyroidism.

OVERDOSAGE

There have been a few reported cases of Cordarone overdose in which 3 to 8 grams were taken. There were no deaths or permanent sequelae. The acute oral LD_{50} of amiodarone HCl in mice and rats is greater than 3,000 mg/kg.

In addition to general supportive measures, the patient's cardiac rhythm and blood pressure should be monitored, and if bradycardia ensues, a β-adrenergic agonist or a pacemaker may be used. Hypotension with inadequate tissue perfusion should be treated with positive inotropic and/or vasopressor agents. Neither Cordarone nor its metabolite is dialyzable.

DOSAGE AND ADMINISTRATION

BECAUSE OF THE UNIQUE PHARMACOKINETIC PROPERTIES, DIFFICULT DOSING SCHEDULE, AND SEVERITY OF THE SIDE EFFECTS IF PATIENTS ARE IMPROPERLY MONITORED, CORDARONE SHOULD BE ADMINISTERED ONLY BY PHYSICIANS WHO ARE EXPERIENCED IN THE TREATMENT OF LIFE-THREATENING ARRHYTHMIAS WHO ARE THOROUGHLY FAMILIAR WITH THE RISKS AND BENEFITS OF CORDARONE THERAPY, AND WHO HAVE ACCESS TO LABORATORY FACILITIES CAPABLE OF ADEQUATELY MONITORING THE EFFECTIVENESS AND SIDE EFFECTS OF TREATMENT.

In order to insure that an antiarrhythmic effect will be observed without waiting several months, loading doses are required. A uniform, optimal dosage schedule for administration of Cordarone has not been determined. Because of the food effect on absorption, Cordarone should be administered consistently with regard to meals (see "**CLINICAL PHARMACOLOGY**"). Individual patient titration is suggested according to the following guidelines.

For life-threatening ventricular arrhythmias, such as ventricular fibrillation or hemodynamically unstable ventricular tachycardia: Close monitoring of the patients is indicated during the loading phase, particularly until risk of recurrent ventricular tachycardia or fibrillation has abated. Because of the serious nature of the arrhythmia and the lack of predictable time course of effect, loading should be performed in a hospital setting. Loading doses of 800 to 1,600 mg/day are required for 1 to 3 weeks (occasionally longer) until initial therapeutic response occurs. (Administration of Cordarone in divided doses with meals is suggested for total daily doses of 1,000 mg or higher, or when gastrointestinal intolerance occurs.) If side effects become excessive, the dose should be reduced. Elimination of recurrence of ventricular fibrillation and tachycardia usually occurs within 1 to 3 weeks, along with reduction in complex and total ventricular ectopic beats.

Upon starting Cordarone therapy, an attempt should be made to gradually discontinue prior antiarrhythmic drugs (see section on "**Drug Interactions**"). When adequate arrhythmia control is achieved, or if side effects become prominent, Cordarone dose should be reduced to 600 to 800 mg/day for one month and then to the maintenance dose, usually 400 mg/day (see "**CLINICAL PHARMACOLOGY—Monitoring Effectiveness**"). Some patients may require larger maintenance doses, up to 600 mg/day, and some can be controlled on lower doses. Cordarone may be administered as a single daily dose, or in patients with severe gastrointestinal intolerance, as a b.i.d. dose. In each patient, the chronic maintenance dose should be determined according to antiarrhythmic effect as assessed by symptoms, Holter recordings, and/or programmed electrical stimulation and by patient tolerance. Plasma concentrations may be helpful in evaluating nonresponsiveness or unexpectedly severe toxicity (see "**CLINICAL PHARMACOLOGY**").

The lowest effective dose should be used to prevent the occurrence of side effects. In all instances, the physician must be guided by the severity of the individual patient's arrhythmia and response to therapy.

When dosage adjustments are necessary, the patient should be closely monitored for an extended period of time because of the long and variable half-life of Cordarone and the difficulty in predicting the time required to attain a new steady-state level of drug. Dosage suggestions are summarized below:

[See table above]

HOW SUPPLIED

Cordarone® (amiodarone HCl) Tablets are available in bottles of 60 tablets and in Redipak® cartons containing 100 tablets (10 blister strips of 10) as follows:

200 mg, NDC 0008-4188, round, convex-faced, pink tablets with a raised "C" and marked "200" on one side, with reverse side scored and marked "Wyeth" and "4188."

Keep tightly closed.

Store at room temperature, approximately 25°C (77°F).

Protect from light.

Dispense in a light-resistant, tight container.

Use carton to protect contents from light.

Rx only.

Manufactured for
Wyeth Laboratories
A Wyeth-Ayerst Company
Philadelphia, PA 19101
by Sanofi Winthrop Industrie
1, rue de la Vierge
33440 Ambares, France
CI 6036-1 Issued August 26, 1999

Shown in Product Identification Guide, page 341

CORDARONE® INTRAVENOUS ℞

(amiodarone hydrochloride)
Rx only

DESCRIPTION

Cordarone Intravenous (Cordarone I.V.) contains amiodarone HCl ($C_{25}H_{29}I_2NO_3 \cdot HCl$), a class III antiarrhythmic drug. Amiodarone HCl is (2-butyl-3-benzofuranyl)[4-[2-(diethylamino)ethoxy]-3,5-diiodophenyl]methanone hydrochloride. Amiodarone HCl has the following structural formula:

Amiodarone HCl is a white to slightly yellow crystalline powder, and is very slightly soluble in water. It has a molecular weight of 681.78 and contains 37.3% iodine by weight. Cordarone I.V. is a sterile clear, pale-yellow solution visually free from particulates. Each milliliter of the Cordarone I.V. formulation contains 50 mg of amiodarone HCl, 20.2 mg of benzyl alcohol, 100 mg of polysorbate 80, and water for injection.

CLINICAL PHARMACOLOGY

Mechanisms of Action

Amiodarone is generally considered a class III antiarrhythmic drug, but it possesses electrophysiologic characteristics of all four Vaughan Williams classes. Like class I drugs, amiodarone blocks sodium channels at rapid pacing frequencies, and like class II drugs, it exerts a noncompetitive antisympathetic action. One of its main effects, with prolonged administration, is to lengthen the cardiac action potential, a class III effect. The negative chronotropic effect of amiodarone in nodal tissues is similar to the effect of class IV drugs. In addition to blocking sodium channels, amiodarone blocks myocardial potassium channels, which contributes to slowing of conduction and prolongation of refractoriness. The antisympathetic action and the block of calcium and potassium channels are responsible for the negative dromotropic effects on the sinus node and for the slowing of conduction and prolongation of refractoriness in the atrioventricular (AV) node. Its vasodilatory action can decrease cardiac workload and consequently myocardial oxygen consumption.

Cordarone I.V. administration prolongs intranodal conduction (Atrial-His, AH) and refractoriness of the atrioventricular node (ERP AVN), but has little or no effect on sinus cycle length (SCL), refractoriness of the right atrium and right ventricle (ERP RA and ERP RV), repolarization (QTc), intraventricular conduction (QRS), and infranodal conduction (His-ventricular, HV). A comparison of the electrophysiologic effects of Cordarone I.V. and oral Cordarone is shown in the table below.

EFFECTS OF INTRAVENOUS AND ORAL CORDARONE ON ELECTROPHYSIOLOGIC PARAMETERS

Formulation	SCL	QRS	QTc	AH	HV	ERP RA	ERP RV	ERP AVN
I.V.	↔	↔	↔	↑	↔	↔	↔	↑
Oral	↑	↔	↑	↑	↔	↑	↑	↑

↔No change

At higher doses (>10 mg/kg) of Cordarone I.V., prolongation of the ERP RV and modest prolongation of the QRS have been seen. These differences between oral and intravenous administration suggest that the initial acute effects of Cordarone I.V. may be predominantly focused on the AV node, causing an intranodal conduction delay and increased nodal refractoriness due to slow channel blockade (class IV activity) and noncompetitive adrenergic antagonism (class II activity).

Pharmacokinetics and Metabolism

Amiodarone exhibits complex disposition characteristics after intravenous administration. Peak serum concentrations after single 5 mg/kg 15-minute intravenous infusions in healthy subjects range between 5 and 41 mg/L. Peak concentrations after 10-minute infusions of 150 mg Cordarone I.V. in patients with ventricular fibrillation (VF) or hemodynamically unstable ventricular tachycardia (VT) range between 7 and 26 mg/L. Due to rapid distribution, serum concentrations decline to 10% of peak values within 30 to 45 minutes after the end of the infusion. In clinical trials, after 48 hours of continued infusions (125, 500, or 1000 mg/day) plus supplemental (150 mg) infusions (for recurrent arrhythmias), amiodarone mean serum concentrations between 0.7 to 1.4 mg/L were observed (n=260).

N-desethylamiodarone (DEA) is the major active metabolite of amiodarone in humans. DEA serum concentrations above 0.05 mg/L are not usually seen until after several days of continuous infusion but with prolonged therapy reach approximately the same concentration as amiodarone. The enzymes responsible for the N-deethylation are believed to be the cytochrome P-450 3A (CYP3A) subfamily, principally CYP3A4. This isozyme is present in both the liver and intestines. The highly variable systemic availability of oral amiodarone may be attributed potentially to large interindividual variability in CYP3A4 activity.

Amiodarone is eliminated primarily by hepatic metabolism and biliary excretion and there is negligible excretion of amiodarone or DEA in urine. Neither amiodarone nor DEA is dialyzable. Amiodarone and DEA cross the placenta and both appear in breast milk.

No data are available on the activity of DEA in humans, but in animals, it has significant electrophysiologic and antiarrhythmic effects generally similar to amiodarone itself. DEA's precise role and contribution to the antiarrhythmic activity of oral amiodarone are not certain. The development of maximal ventricular class III effects after oral Cordarone administration in humans correlates more closely with DEA accumulation over time than with amiodarone accumulation. On the other hand (see CLINICAL TRIALS), after Cordarone I.V. administration, there is evidence of activity well before significant concentrations of DEA are attained.

The following table summarizes the mean ranges of pharmacokinetic parameters of amiodarone reported in single dose i.v. (5 mg/kg over 15 min) studies of healthy subjects.

PHARMACOKINETIC PROFILE AFTER I.V. AMIODARONE ADMINISTRATION

Drug	Clearance (mL/h/kg)	V_c (L/kg)	V_{ss} (L/kg)	$t_{1/2}$ (days)
Amiodarone	90–158	0.2	40–84	20–47
Desethylamiodarone	197–290	—	68–168	≥AMI $t_{1/2}$

Notes: V_c and V_{ss} denote the central and steady-state volumes of distribution from i.v. studies.
"—" denotes not available.

Continued on next page

Cordarone Intravenous—Cont.

Desethylamiodarone clearance and volume involve an unknown biotransformation factor.
The systemic availability of ***oral*** amiodarone in healthy subjects ranges between 33% and 65%.
From *in vitro* studies, the protein binding of amiodarone is >96%.
In clinical studies of 2 to 7 days, clearance of amiodarone after intravenous administration in patients with VT and VF ranged between 220 and 440 mL/h/kg. Age, sex, renal disease, and hepatic disease (cirrhosis) do not have marked effects on the disposition of amiodarone or DEA. Renal impairment does not influence the pharmacokinetics of amiodarone. After a single dose of Cordarone I.V. in cirrhotic patients, significantly lower C_{max} and average concentration values are seen for DEA, but mean amiodarone levels are unchanged. Normal subjects over 65 years of age show lower clearances (about 100 mL/hr/kg) than younger subjects (about 150 mL/hr/kg) and an increase in $t_{1/2}$ from about 20 to 47 days. In patients with severe left ventricular dysfunction, the pharmacokinetics of amiodarone are not significantly altered but the terminal disposition $t_{1/2}$ of DEA is prolonged. Although no dosage adjustment for patients with renal, hepatic, or cardiac abnormalities has been defined during chronic treatment with ***oral*** Cordarone, close clinical monitoring is prudent for elderly patients and those with severe left ventricular dysfunction.
There is no established relationship between drug concentration and therapeutic response for short-term intravenous use. Steady-state amiodarone concentrations of 1 to 2.5 mg/L have been associated with antiarrhythmic effects and acceptable toxicity following chronic ***oral*** Cordarone therapy.

Pharmacodynamics

Cordarone I.V. has been reported to produce negative inotropic and vasodilatory effects in animals and humans. In clinical studies of patients with refractory VF or hemodynamically unstable VT, treatment-emergent, drug-related hypotension occurred in 288 of 1836 patients (16%) treated with Cordarone I.V. No correlations were seen between the baseline ejection fraction and the occurrence of clinically significant hypotension during infusion of Cordarone I.V.

Clinical Trials

Apart from studies in patients with VT or VF, described below, there are two other studies of amiodarone showing an antiarrhythmic effect before significant levels of DEA could have accumulated. A placebo-controlled study of i.v. amiodarone (300 mg over 2 hours followed by 1200 mg/day) in post-coronary artery bypass graft patients with supraventricular and 2- to 3-consecutive-beat ventricular arrhythmias showed a reduction in arrhythmias from 12 hours on. A baseline-controlled study using a similar i.v. regimen in patients with recurrent, refractory VT/VF also showed rapid onset of antiarrhythmic activity; amiodarone therapy reduced episodes of VT by 85% compared to baseline.
The acute effectiveness of Cordarone I.V. in suppressing recurrent VF or hemodynamically unstable VT is supported by two randomized, parallel, dose-response studies of approximately 300 patients each. In these studies, patients with at least two episodes of VF or hemodynamically unstable VT in the preceding 24 hours were randomly assigned to receive doses of approximately 125 or 1000 mg over the first 24 hours, an 8-fold difference. In one study, a middle dose of approximately 500 mg was evaluated. The dose regimen consisted of an initial rapid loading infusion, followed by a slower 6-hour loading infusion, and then an 18-hour maintenance infusion. The maintenance infusion was continued up to hour 48. Additional 10-minute infusions of 150 mg Cordarone I.V. were given for "breakthrough" VT/VF more frequently to the 125-mg dose group, thereby considerably reducing the planned 8-fold differences in total dose to 1.8- and 2.6- fold, respectively, in the two studies.
The prospectively defined primary efficacy end point was the rate of VT/VF episodes per hour. For both studies, the median rate was 0.02 episodes per hour in patients receiving the high dose and 0.07 episodes per hour in patients receiving the low dose, or approximately 0.5 versus 1.7 episodes per day (p=0.07, 2-sided, in both studies). In one study, the time to first episode of VT/VF was significantly prolonged (approximately 10 hours in patients receiving the low dose and 14 hours in patients receiving the high dose). In both studies, significantly fewer supplemental infusions were given to patients in the high-dose group. Mortality was not affected in these studies; at the end of double-blind therapy or after 48 hours, all patients were given open access to whatever treatment (including Cordarone I.V.) was deemed necessary.

INDICATIONS AND USAGE

Cordarone I.V. is indicated for initiation of treatment and prophylaxis of frequently recurring ventricular fibrillation and hemodynamically unstable ventricular tachycardia in patients refractory to other therapy. Cordarone I.V. also can be used to treat patients with VT/VF for whom oral Cordarone is indicated, but who are unable to take oral medication. During or after treatment with Cordarone I.V., patients may be transferred to oral Cordarone theray (see **DOSAGE AND ADMINISTRATION**).
Cordarone I.V. should be used for acute treatment until the patient's ventricular arrhythmias are stabilized. Most patients will require this therapy for 48 to 96 hours, but Cordarone I.V. may be safely administered for longer periods if necessary.

CONTRAINDICATIONS

Cordarone I.V. is contraindicated in patients with known hypersensitivity to any of the components of Cordarone I.V., or in patients with cardiogenic shock, marked sinus bradycardia, and second- or third-degree AV block unless a functioning pacemaker is available.

WARNINGS

Hypotension

Hypotension is the most common adverse effect seen with Cordarone I.V. In clinical trials, treatment-emergent, drug-related hypotension was reported as an adverse effect in 288 (16%) of 1836 patients treated with Cordarone I.V. Clinically significant hypotension during infusions was seen most often in the first several hours of treatment and was not dose related, but appeared to be related to the rate of infusion. Hypotension necessitating alterations in Cordarone I.V. therapy was reported in 3% of patients, with permanent discontinuation required in less than 2% of patients. Hypotension should be treated initially by slowing the infusion; additional standard therapy may be needed, including the following: vasopressor drugs, positive inotropic agents, and volume expansion. ***The initial rate of infusion should be monitored closely and should not exceed that prescribed in* DOSAGE AND ADMINISTRATION.**

Bradycardia and AV Block

Drug-related bradycardia occurred in 90 (4.9%) of 1836 patients in clinical trials while they were receiving Cordarone I.V. for life-threatening VT/VF; it was not dose-related. Bradycardia should be treated by slowing the infusion rate or discontinuing Cordarone I.V. In some patients, inserting a pacemaker is required. Despite such measures, bradycardia was progressive and terminal in 1 patient during the controlled trials. Patients with a known predisposition to bradycardia or AV block should be treated with Cordarone I.V. in a setting where a temporary pacemaker is available.

Long-Term Use

See labeling for oral Cordarone. There has been limited experience in patients receiving Cordarone I.V. for longer than 3 weeks.

Neonatal Hypo- or Hyperthyroidism

Although ***oral*** Cordarone use during pregnancy is uncommon, there have been a small number of published reports of congenital goiter/hypothyroidism and hyperthyroidism. If Cordarone I.V. is administered during pregnancy, the patient should be apprised of the potential hazard to the fetus. In pregnant rats and rabbits, ***oral*** amiodarone HCl in doses of 25 mg/kg/day (approximately 0.4 and 0.9 times, respectively, the maximum recommended human maintenance dose*) had no adverse effects on the fetus. In the rabbit, 75 mg/kg/day (approximately 2.7 times the maximum recommended human maintenance dose*) caused abortions in greater than 90% of the animals. In the rat, doses of 50 mg/kg/day or more were associated with slight displacement of the testes and an increased incidence of incomplete ossification of some skull and digital bones; at 100 mg/kg/day or more, fetal body weights were reduced; at 200 mg/kg/day, there was an increased incidence of fetal resorption. (These doses in the rat are approximately 0.8, 1.6 and 3.2 times the maximum recommended human maintenance dose.*) Adverse effects on fetal growth and survival also were noted in one of two strains of mice at a dose of 5 mg/kg/day (approximately 0.04 times the maximum recommended human maintenance dose*)
*600 mg in a 50 kg patient (doses compared on a body surface area basis)

PRECAUTIONS

Cordarone I.V. should be administered only by physicians who are experienced in the treatment of life-threatening arrhythmias, who are thoroughly familiar with the risks and benefits of Cordarone therapy, and who have access to facilities adequate for monitoring the effectiveness and side effects of treatment.

Liver Enzyme Elevations

Elevations of blood hepatic enzyme values—alanine aminotransferase (ALT), aspartate aminotransferase (AST), and gamma-glutamyl transferase (GGT)—are seen commonly in patients with immediately life-threatening VT/VF. Interpreting elevated AST activity can be difficult because the values may be elevated in patients who have had recent myocardial infarction, congestive heart failure, or multiple electrical defibrillations. Approximately 54% of patients receiving Cordarone I.V. in clinical studies had baseline liver enzyme elevations, and 13% had clinically significant elevations. In 81% of patients with both baseline and on-therapy data available, the liver enzyme elevations either improved during therapy or remained at baseline levels. Baseline abnormalities in hepatic enzymes are not a contraindication to treatment.
Two (2) cases of fatal hepatocellular necrosis after treatment with Cordarone I.V. have been reported. The patients, one 28 years of age and the other 60 years of age, were treated for atrial arrhythmias with an initial infusion of 1500 mg over 5 hours, a rate much higher than recommended. Both patients developed hepatic and renal failure within 24 hours after the start of Cordarone I.V. treatment and died on day 14 and day 4, respectively. Because these episodes of hepatic necrosis may have been due to the rapid rate of infusion with possible rate-related hypotension, ***the initial rate of infusion should be monitored closely and should not exceed that prescribed in* DOSAGE AND ADMINISTRATION.**
In patients with life-threatening arrhythmias, the potential risk of hepatic injury should be weighed against the potential benefit of Cordarone I.V. therapy, but patients receiving Cordarone I.V. should be monitored carefully for evidence of progressive hepatic injury. Consideration should be given to reducing the rate of administration or withdrawing Cordarone I.V. in such cases.

Proarrhythmia

Like all antiarrhythmic agents, Cordarone I.V. may cause a worsening of existing arrhythmias or precipitate a new arrhythmia. Proarrhythmia, primarily torsades de pointes, has been associated with prolongation by Cordarone I.V. of the QTc interval to 500 ms or greater. Although QTc prolongation occurred frequently in patients receiving Cordarone I.V., torsades de pointes or new-onset VF occurred infrequently (less than 2%). Patients should be monitored for QTc prolongation during infusion with Cordarone I.V.

Pulmonary Disorders

ARDS

Two percent (2%) of patients were reported to have adult respiratory distress syndrome (ARDS) during clinical studies. ARDS is a disorder characterized by bilateral, diffuse pulmonary infiltrates with pulmonary edema and varying degrees of respiratory insufficiency. The clinical and radiographic picture can arise after a variety of lung injuries, such as those resulting from trauma, shock, prolonged cardiopulmonary resuscitation, and aspiration pneumonia, conditions present in many of the patients enrolled in the clinical studies. It is not possible to determine what role, if any, Cordarone I.V. played in causing or exacerbating the pulmonary disorder in those patients.
Postoperatively, occurrences of ARDS have been reported in patients receiving ***oral*** Cordarone therapy who have undergone either cardiac or noncardiac surgery. Although patients usually respond well to vigorous respiratory therapy, in rare instances the outcome has been fatal. Until further studies have been performed, it is recommended that FiO_2 and the determinants of oxygen delivery to the tissues (e.g., SaO_2, PaO_2) be closely monitored in patients on Cordarone.

Pulmonary fibrosis

Only 1 of more than 1000 patients treated with Cordarone I.V. in clinical studies developed pulmonary fibrosis. In that patient, the condition was diagnosed 3 months after treatment with Cordarone I.V., during which time she received ***oral*** Cordarone. Pulmonary toxicity is a well-recognized complication of long-term Cordarone use (see labeling for oral Cordarone).

Surgery

Close perioperative monitoring is recommended in patients undergoing general anesthesia who are on amiodarone therapy as they may be more sensitive to the myocardial depressant and conduction defects of halogenated inhalational anesthetics.

Drug Interactions

Amiodarone can inhibit metabolism mediated by cytochrome P-450 enzymes, probably accounting for the significant effects of oral Cordarone (and presumably Cordarone I.V.) on the pharmacokinetics of various therapeutic agents including digoxin, quinidine, procainamide, warfarin (CYP2C9), dextromethorphan (CYP2D6), and cyclosporine (CYP3A4). Hemodynamic and electrophysiologic interactions have also been observed after concomitant administration with propranolol, diltiazem, and verapamil. Conversely, agents producing a significant effect on amiodarone pharmacokinetics include phenytoin, cimetidine, and cholestyramine. Because of the long half-life of amiodarone, drug interactions may persist long after discontinuation of drug administration. Few data are available on drug interactions with Cordarone I.V. Except as noted, the following tables summarize the important interactions between ***oral*** Cordarone and other therapeutic agents.

SUMMARY OF DRUG INTERACTIONS WITH CORDARONE

Drugs Whose Effects May Be Increased by Cordarone

Concomitant Drug	Interaction
Warfarin	Increases prothrombin time.
Digoxin	Increases serum concentration.
Quinidine	Increases serum concentration.
Procainamide	Increases serum concentration, NAPA concentration.
Disopyramide	Increases QT prolongation which could cause arrhythmia.
Fentanyl	May cause hypotension, bradycardia, decreased cardiac output.
Flecainide	Reduces the dose of flecainide needed to maintain therapeutic plasma concentrations.
Lidocaine	**Oral**: Sinus bradycardia was observed in a patient receiving oral Cordarone who was given lidocaine for local anesthesia. **I.V.**: Seizure associated with increased lidocaine concentrations was observed in one patient.
Cyclosporine	Produces persistently elevated plasma concentrations of cyclosporine resulting in elevated creatinine, despite reduction in dose of cyclosporine.

SUMMARY OF DRUG INTERACTIONS WITH CORDARONE

Drugs that May Interfere with the Actions of Cordarone

Concomitant Drug	Interaction
Cholestyramine	Increases enterohepatic elimination of amiodarone and may reduce serum levels and $t_{1/2}$.
Cimetidine	Increases serum amiodarone levels.
Phenytoin	Decreases serum amiodarone levels.

Potential drug class interactions with Cordarone

Beta Blockers: Since Cordarone has weak beta blocking activity, use with beta blocking agents could increase risk of hypotension and bradycardia.

Calcium Channel Blockers: Cordarone inhibits atrioventricular conduction and decreases myocardial contractility, increasing the risk of AV block with verapamil or diltiazem or of hypotension with any calcium channel blocker.

Volatile Anesthetic Agents: (see **PRECAUTIONS—Surgery**).

In addition to the interactions noted above, chronic (>2 weeks) ***oral*** Cordarone administration impairs metabolism of phenytoin, dextromethorphan, and methotrexate.

Electrolyte Disturbances

Patients with hypokalemia or hypomagnesemia should have the condition corrected whenever possible before being treated with Cordarone I.V., as these disorders can exaggerate the degree of QTc prolongation and increase the potential for torsades de pointes. Special attention should be given to electrolyte and acid-base balance in patients experiencing severe or prolonged diarrhea or in patients receiving concomitant diuretics.

Carcinogenesis, Mutagenesis, Impairment of Fertility

No carcinogenicity studies were conducted with Cordarone I.V. However, ***oral*** Cordarone caused a statistically significant, dose-related increase in the incidence of thyroid tumors (follicular adenoma and/or carcinoma) in rats. The incidence of thyroid tumors in rats was greater than the incidence in controls even at the lowest dose level tested i.e., 5 mg/kg/day (approximately 0.08 times the maximum recommended human maintenance dose*).

Mutagenicity studies conducted with amiodarone HCl (Ames, micronucleus, and lysogenic induction tests) were negative.

No fertility studies were conducted with Cordarone I.V. However, in a study in which ***oral*** amiodarone HCl was administered to male and female rats, beginning 9 weeks prior to mating, reduced fertility was observed at a dose level of 90 mg/kg/day (approximately 1.4 times the maximum recommended human maintenance dose*).

*600 mg in a 50 kg patient (dose compared on a body surface area basis)

Pregnancy

Category D. See **WARNINGS** and **Neonatal Hypo- or Hyperthyroidism.**

In addition to causing infrequent congenital goiter/hypothyroidism and hyperthyroidism, amiodarone has caused a variety of adverse effects in animals.

In a reproductive study in which amiodarone was given intravenously to rabbits at dosages of 5, 10, or 25 mg/kg per day (about 0.1, 0.3, and 0.7 times the maximum recommended human dose [MRHD] on a body surface area basis), maternal deaths occurred in all groups, including controls. Embryotoxicity (as manifested by fewer full-term fetuses and increased resorptions with concomitantly lower litter weights) occurred at dosages of 10 mg/kg and above. No evidence of embryotoxicity was observed at 5 mg/kg and no teratogenicity was observed at any dosages.

In a teratology study in which amiodarone was administered by continuous i.v. infusion to rats at dosages of 25, 50, or 100 mg/kg per day (about 0.4, 0.7, and 1.4 times the MRHD when compared on a body surface area basis), maternal toxicity (as evidenced by reduced weight gain and food consumption) and embryotoxicity (as evidenced by increased resorptions, decreased live litter size, reduced body weights, and retarded sternum and metacarpal ossification) were observed in the 100 mg/kg group.

Cordarone I.V. should be used during pregnancy only if the potential benefit to the mother justifies the risk to the fetus.

Nursing Mothers

Amiodarone is excreted in human milk, suggesting that breast-feeding could expose the nursing infant to a significant dose of the drug. Nursing offspring of lactating rats administered amiodarone have demonstrated reduced viability and reduced body weight gains. The risk of exposing the infant to amiodarone should be weighed against the potential benefit of arrhythmia suppression in the mother. The mother should be advised to discontinue nursing.

Labor and Delivery

It is not known whether the use of Cordarone during labor or delivery has any immediate or delayed adverse effects. Preclinical studies in rodents have not shown any effect on the duration of gestation or on parturition.

Pediatric Usage

The safety and efficacy of Cordarone in the pediatric population have not been established; therefore, its use in pediatric patients is not recommended.

SUMMARY TABULATION OF TREATMENT-EMERGENT DRUG-RELATED STUDY EVENTS IN PATIENTS RECEIVING CORDARONE I.V. IN CONTROLLED AND OPEN-LABEL STUDIES (≥2% INCIDENCE)

Study Event	Controlled Studies (n=814)	Open-Label Studies (n=1022)	Total (n=1836)
Body as a Whole			
Fever	24 (2.9%)	13 (1.2%)	37 (2.0%)
Cardiovascular System			
Bradycardia	49 (6.0%)	41 (4.0%)	90 (4.9%)
Congestive heart failure	18 (2.2%)	21 (2.0%)	39 (2.1%)
Heart arrest	29 (3.5%)	26 (2.5%)	55 (2.9%)
Hypotension	165 (20.2%)	123 (12.0%)	288 (15.6%)
Ventricular tachycardia	15 (1.8%)	30 (2.9%)	45 (2.4%)
Digestive System			
Liver function tests abnormal	35 (4.2%)	29 (2.8%)	64 (3.4%)
Nausea	29 (3.5%)	43 (4.2%)	72 (3.9%)

AMIODARONE HCl SOLUTION STABILITY

Solution	Concentration (mg/mL)	Container	Comments
5% Dextrose in Water (D_5W)	1.0–6.0	PVC	Physically compatible, with amiodarone loss <10% at 2 hours.
5% Dextrose in Water (D_5W)	1.0–6.0	Polyolefin, Glass	Physically compatible, with no amiodarone loss at 24 hours.

Y-SITE INJECTION INCOMPATIBILITY

Drug	Vehicle	Amiodarone Concentration	Comments
Aminophylline	D_5W	4 mg/mL	Precipitate
Cefamandole Nafate	D_5W	4 mg/mL	Precipitate
Cefazolin Sodium	D_5W	4 mg/mL	Precipitate
Mezlocillin Sodium	D_5W	4 mg/mL	Precipitate
Heparin Sodium	D_5W	—	Precipitate
Sodium Bicarbonate	D_5W	3 mg/mL	Precipitate

ADVERSE REACTIONS

In a total of 1836 patients in controlled and uncontrolled clinical trials, 14% of patients received Cordarone I.V. for at least 1 week, 5% received it for at least 2 weeks, 2% received it for at least 3 weeks, and 1% received it for more than 3 weeks, without an increased incidence of severe adverse reactions. The mean duration of therapy in these studies was 5.6 days; median exposure was 3.7 days.

The most important treatment-emergent adverse effects were hypotension, asystole/cardiac arrest/electromechanical dissociation (EMD), cardiogenic shock, congestive heart failure, bradycardia, liver function test abnormalities, VT, and AV block. Overall, treatment was discontinued for about 9% of the patients because of adverse effects. The most common adverse effects leading to discontinuation of Cordarone I.V. therapy were hypotension (1.6%), asystole/cardiac arrest/EMD (1.2%), VT (1.1%), and cardiogenic shock (1%).

The following table lists the most common (incidence ≥2%) treatment-emergent adverse events during Cordarone I.V. therapy considered at least possibly drug-related. These data were collected from the Wyeth-Ayerst clinical trials involving 1836 patients with life-threatening VT/VF. Data from all assigned treatment groups are pooled because none of the adverse events appeared to be dose-related.

[See first table above]

Other treatment-emergent possibly drug-related adverse events reported in less than 2% of patients receiving Cordarone I.V. in Wyeth-Ayerst controlled and uncontrolled studies included the following: abnormal kidney function, atrial fibrillation, diarrhea, increased ALT, increased AST, lung edema, nodal arrhythmia, prolonged QT interval, respiratory disorder, shock, sinus bradycardia, Stevens-Johnson syndrome, thrombocytopenia, VF, and vomiting.

In postmarketing surveillance, toxic epidermal necrolysis, pancytopenia, neutropenia, angioedema, and anaphylactic shock also has been reported with amiodarone therapy.

OVERDOSAGE

The most likely effects of an inadvertent overdose of Cordarone I.V. are hypotension, cardiogenic shock, bradycardia, AV block, and hepatotoxicity. Hypotension and cardiogenic shock should be treated by slowing the infusion rate or with standard therapy: vasopressor drugs, positive inotropic agents, and volume expansion. Bradycardia and AV block may require temporary pacing. Hepatic enzyme concentrations should be monitored closely. Amiodarone is not dialyzable. The acute ***oral*** LD_{50} of amiodarone HCl in mice and rats is greater than 3,000 mg/kg.

DOSAGE AND ADMINISTRATION

Amiodarone shows considerable interindividual variation in response. Thus, although a starting dose adequate to suppress life-threatening arrhythmias is needed, close monitoring with adjustment of dose as needed is essential. The recommended starting dose of Cordarone I.V. is about 1000 mg over the first 24 hours of therapy, delivered by the following infusion regimen:

CORDARONE I.V. DOSE RECOMMENDATIONS — FIRST 24 HOURS —

Loading infusions	
***First* Rapid:**	**150 mg over the FIRST 10 minutes (15 mg/min).** Add 3 mL of Cordarone I.V. (150 mg) to 100 mL D_5W (concentration = 1.5 mg/mL). Infuse 100 mL over 10 minutes.
***Followed by* Slow:**	**360 mg over the NEXT 6 hours (1 mg/min).** Add 18 mL of Cordarone I.V. (900 mg) to 500 mL D_5W (concentration = 1.8 mg/mL).
Maintenance infusion	**540 mg over the REMAINING 18 hours (0.5 mg/min).** Decrease the rate of the slow loading infusion to 0.5 mg/min.

After the first 24 hours, the maintenance infusion rate of 0.5 mg/min (720 mg/24 hours) should be continued utilizing a concentration of 1 to 6 mg/mL (Cordarone I.V. concentrations greater than 2 mg/mL should be administered via a central venous catheter). In the event of breakthrough episodes of VF or hemodynamically unstable VT, 150-mg supplemental infusions of Cordarone I.V. mixed in 100 mL of D_5W may be administered. Such infusions should be administered over 10 minutes to minimize the potential for hypotension. The rate of the maintenance infusion may be increased to achieve effective arrhythmia suppression.

The first 24-hour dose may be individualized for each patient; however, in controlled clinical trials, mean daily doses above 2100 mg were associated with an increased risk of hypotension. The initial infusion rate should not exceed 30 mg/min.

Based on the experience from clinical studies of Cordarone I.V., a maintenance infusion of up to 0.5 mg/min can be cautiously continued for 2 to 3 weeks regardless of the patient's age, renal function, or left ventricular function. There has been limited experience in patients receiving Cordarone I.V. for longer than 3 weeks.

The surface properties of solutions containing injectable amiodarone are altered such that the drop size may be reduced. This reduction may lead to underdosage of the patient by up to 30% if drop counter infusion sets are used. Cordarone I.V. must be delivered by a volumetric infusion pump.

Cordarone I.V. should, whenever possible, be administered through a central venous catheter dedicated to that purpose. An in-line filter should be used during administration. Cordarone I.V. concentrations greater than 3 mg/mL in D_5W have been associated with a high incidence of peripheral vein phlebitis; however, concentrations of 2.5 mg/mL or less appear to be less irritating. Therefore, for infusions longer than 1 hour, Cordarone I.V. concentrations should not exceed 2 mg/mL unless a central venous catheter is used.

Continued on next page

Cordarone Intravenous—Cont.

Cordarone I.V. infusions exceeding 2 hours must be administered in glass or polyolefin bottles containing D_5W. Use of **evacuated glass containers** for admixing Cordarone I.V. is not recommended as incompatibility with a buffer in the container may cause precipitation.
It is well known that amiodarone adsorbs to polyvinyl chloride (PVC) tubing and the clinical trial dose administration schedule was designed to account for this adsorption. All of the clinical trials were conducted using PVC tubing and its use is therefore recommended. The concentrations and rates of infusion provided in **DOSAGE AND ADMINISTRATION** reflect doses identified in these studies. It is important that the recommended infusion regimen be followed closely.
Cordarone I.V. does not need to be protected from light during administration.
[See second table at top of previous page]

Admixture Incompatibility
Cordarone I.V. in D_5W is incompatible with the drugs shown below.
[See third table at top of previous page]

Intravenous to Oral Transition
Patients whose arrhythmias have been suppressed by Cordarone I.V. may be switched to oral Cordarone. The optimal dose for changing from intravenous to oral administration of Cordarone will depend on the dose of Cordarone I.V. already administered, as well as the bioavailability of oral Cordarone. When changing to oral Cordarone therapy, clinical monitoring is recommended, particularly for elderly patients.
The following table provides suggested doses of oral Cordarone to be initiated after varying durations of Cordarone I.V. administration. These recommendations are made on the basis of a comparable total body amount of amiodarone delivered by the intravenous and oral routes, based on 50% bioavailability of oral amiodarone.

RECOMMENDATIONS FOR ORAL DOSAGE AFTER I.V. INFUSION

Duration of Cordarone I.V. Infusion#	Initial Daily Dose of Oral Cordarone
<1 week	800–1600 mg
1—3 weeks	600–800 mg
>3 weeks*	400 mg

Assuming a 720 mg/day infusion (0.5 mg/min).
* Cordarone I.V is not intended for maintenance treatment.

HOW SUPPLIED
Cordarone® I.V. (amiodarone HCl) is available in packages of 10 ampuls (2 cartons each containing 5 ampuls), 3 mL each, as follows:
50 mg per mL, NDC 0008-0814-01.
Store at room temperature, 15° to 25°C (59° to 77°F).
Protect from light and excessive heat.
Use carton to protect contents from light until used.
Manufactured by:
Wyeth Laboratories
A Wyeth-Ayerst Company
Philadelphia, PA 19101
by arrangement with Sanofi S.A.
CI 5032-3 Revised May 7, 1999

DIUCARDIN® ℞
[*dī "ū-căr 'dĭn*]
(hydroflumethiazide tablets, USP)

DESCRIPTION
Diucardin (hydroflumethiazide) is an oral thiazide (benzothiadiazide) diuretic-antihypertensive agent.
Diucardin is available as 50 mg tablets for oral administration.
Chemical name: 3,4-Dihydro-6-(trifluoromethyl)-2H-1,2,4-benzothiadiazine-7-sulfonamide 1,1-dioxide.
Structural formula:

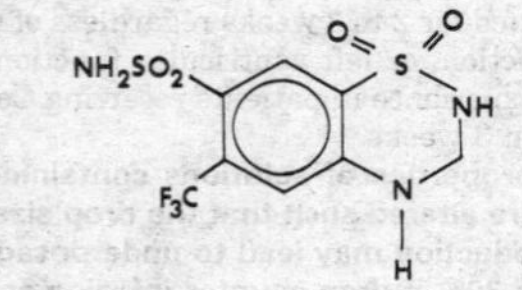

Hydroflumethiazide is an odorless white to cream-colored, finely divided, crystalline powder. It has a melting point between 270° and 275° C. Hydroflumethiazide is freely soluble in acetone, soluble in alcohol, and very slightly soluble in water.
The inactive ingredients contained in Diucardin tablets are: lactose, magnesium stearate, microcrystalline cellulose, povidone, and starch.

CLINICAL PHARMACOLOGY
Hydroflumethiazide is incompletely but fairly rapidly absorbed from the gastrointestinal tract. It appears to have a biphasic biological half-life with an estimated alpha-phase of about 2 hours and an estimated beta-phase of about 17 hours; it has a metabolite with a longer half-life, which is extensively bound to the red blood cells. Hydroflumethiazide is excreted in the urine; its metabolite has also been detected in the urine.
The mechanism of action results in an interference with the renal tubular mechanism of electrolyte reabsorption. At maximal therapeutic dosage, all thiazides are approximately equal in their diuretic potency. The mechanism whereby thiazides function in the control of hypertension is unknown.

INDICATIONS AND USAGE
Diucardin is indicated as adjunctive therapy in edema associated with congestive heart failure, hepatic cirrhosis, and corticosteroid and estrogen therapy.
Diucardin has also been found useful in edema due to various forms of renal dysfunction such as: nephrotic syndrome; acute glomerulonephritis; and chronic renal failure.
Diucardin is indicated in the management of hypertension either as the sole therapeutic agent or to enhance the effect of other antihypertensive drugs in the more severe forms of hypertension.
USAGE IN PREGNANCY
The routine use of diuretics in an otherwise healthy woman is inappropriate and exposes mother and fetus to unnecessary hazard. Diuretics do not prevent development of toxemia of pregnancy, and there is no satisfactory evidence that they are useful in the treatment of developed toxemia.
Edema during pregnancy may arise from pathological causes or from the physiologic and mechanical consequences of pregnancy. Thiazides are indicated in pregnancy when edema is due to pathologic causes just as they are in the absence of pregnancy (however, see "**PRECAUTIONS**—PREGNANCY" below).
Dependent edema in pregnancy, resulting from restriction of venous return by the expanded uterus, is properly treated through elevation of the lower extremities and use of support hose. Use of diuretics to lower intravascular volume in this case is illogical and unnecessary. There is hypervolemia during normal pregnancy which is harmful to neither the fetus nor the mother (in absence of cardiovascular disease), but which is associated with edema, including generalized edema, in the majority of pregnant women. If this edema produces discomfort, increased recumbency will often provide relief. In rare instances, this edema may cause extreme discomfort which is not relieved by rest. In these cases, a short course of diuretics may provide relief and may be appropriate.

CONTRAINDICATIONS
Anuria.
Hypersensitivity to this or other sulfonamide-derived drugs.

WARNINGS
Diucardin should be used with caution in severe renal disease. In patients with renal disease, thiazides may precipitate azotemia. Cumulative effects of the drug may develop in patients with impaired renal function.
Thiazides should be used with caution in patients with impaired hepatic function or progressive liver disease, since minor alterations of fluid and electrolyte balance may precipitate hepatic coma.
Thiazides may add to or potentiate the action of other antihypertensive drugs. Potentiation occurs with ganglionic or peripheral adrenergic blocking drugs.
Sensitivity reactions may occur in patients with a history of allergy or bronchial asthma.
The possibility of exacerbation or activation of systemic lupus erythematosus has been reported.

PRECAUTIONS
GENERAL
All patients receiving thiazide therapy should be observed for clinical signs of fluid or electrolyte imbalance; namely, hyponatremia, hypochloremic alkalosis, and hypokalemia. Serum and urine electrolyte determinations are particularly important when the patient is vomiting excessively or receiving parenteral fluids. Medication such as digitalis may also influence serum electrolytes. Warning signs, irrespective of cause, are: dryness of mouth, thirst, weakness, lethargy, drowsiness, restlessness, muscle pains or cramps, muscular fatigue, hypotension, oliguria, tachycardia, and gastrointestinal disturbances such as nausea and vomiting.
Hypokalemia may develop with thiazides as with any other potent diuretic, especially with brisk diuresis, when severe cirrhosis is present, or during concomitant use of corticosteroids or ACTH.
Interference with adequate oral electrolyte intake will also contribute to hypokalemia. Digitalis therapy may exaggerate metabolic effects of hypokalemia, especially with reference to myocardial activity.
Any chloride deficit is generally mild and usually does not require specific treatment except under extraordinary circumstances (as in liver disease or renal disease). Dilutional hyponatremia may occur in edematous patients in hot weather; appropriate therapy is water restriction, rather than administration of salt, except in rare instances when the hyponatremia is life-threatening. In actual salt depletion, appropriate replacement is the therapy of choice.
Hyperuricemia may occur or frank gout may be precipitated in certain patients receiving thiazide therapy.
Insulin requirements in diabetic patients may be increased, decreased, or unchanged. Latent diabetes mellitus may become manifested during thiazide administration.
The antihypertensive effects of the drug may be enhanced in the post-sympathectomy patient.
If progressive renal impairment becomes evident, as indicated by a rising creatinine or blood urea nitrogen, a careful reappraisal of therapy is necessary with consideration given to withholding or discontinuing diuretic therapy.
Thiazides may decrease serum PBI levels without signs of thyroid disturbance.
Lithium generally should not be given with diuretics because they reduce its renal clearance and increase the risk of lithium toxicity. Read circulars for lithium preparations before use of such concomitant therapy with Diucardin.
Thiazides have been shown to increase the urinary excretion of magnesium; this may result in hypomagnesemia.
Calcium excretion is decreased by thiazides. Pathological changes in the parathyroid gland with hypercalcemia and hypophosphatemia have been observed in a few patients on prolonged thiazide therapy. The common complications of hyperparathyroidism, such as renal lithiasis, bone resorption, and peptic ulceration, have not been seen.
LABORATORY TESTS
Periodic determination of serum electrolytes to detect possible electrolyte imbalance should be performed at appropriate intervals.
DRUG INTERACTIONS
Anticoagulants, oral
(Effects may be decreased when used concurrently with thiazide diuretics; dosage adjustments may be necessary.)
Antigout medications
(Thiazide diuretics may raise the level of blood uric acid; dosage adjustment of antigout medications may be necessary to control hyperuricemia and gout.)
Antihypertensive medications, other, especially diazoxide, or preanesthetic and anesthetic agents used in surgery or skeletal-muscle relaxants, nondepolarizing, used in surgery
(Effects may be potentiated when used concurrently with thiazide diuretics; dosage adjustments may be necessary.)
Amphotericin B or Corticosteroids or Corticotropin (ACTH)
(Concurrent use with thiazide diuretics may intensify electrolyte imbalance, particularly hypokalemia.)
Cardiac glycosides
(Concurrent use with thiazide diuretics may enhance the possibility of digitalis toxicity associated with hypokalemia.)
Colestipol
(May inhibit gastrointestinal absorption of the thiazide diuretics; administration 1 hour before or 4 hours after colestipol is recommended.)
Hypoglycemics
(Thiazide diuretics may raise blood glucose levels; for adult-onset diabetics, dosage adjustment of hypoglycemic medications may be necessary during and after thiazide diuretic therapy; insulin requirements may be increased, decreased, or unchanged.)
Lithium salts
(Concurrent use with thiazide diuretics is not recommended, as they may provoke lithium toxicity because of reduced renal clearance.)
Methenamine
(Effectiveness may be decreased when used concurrently with thiazide diuretics because of alkalinization of the urine.)
Nonsteroidal anti-inflammatory agents
(In some patients, the steroidal anti-inflammatory agent can reduce the diuretic, natriuretic, and antihypertensive effects of loop, potassium sparing, and thiazide diuretics. Therefore, when hydroflumethiazide and nonsteroidal anti-inflammatory agents are used concomitantly, the patient should be observed closely to determine if the desired effect of the diuretic is obtained.)
Norepinephrine
(Thiazides may decrease arterial responsiveness to norepinephrine. This diminution is not sufficient to preclude effectiveness of the pressor agent for therapeutic use.)
Tubocurarine
(Thiazide drugs may increase the responsiveness to tubocurarine.)
DIAGNOSTIC INTERFERENCE—With expected physiologic effects:
Blood and urine glucose levels (usually only in patients with a predisposition for glucose intolerance) and
Serum bilirubin levels (by displacement from albumin binding) and
Serum calcium levels (thiazide diuretics should be discontinued before parathyroid-function tests are carried out) and
Serum uric acid levels (may be increased)
Serum magnesium, potassium, and sodium levels (may be decreased; serum magnesium levels may increase in uremic patients)
Serum protein-bound iodine (PBI) levels (may be decreased)
Thiazides should be discontinued before carrying out tests for parathyroid function (see "**PRECAUTIONS**—GENERAL, Calcium excretion").
CARCINOGENESIS, MUTAGENESIS, IMPAIRMENT OF FERTILITY
No studies have been performed to evaluate carcinogenic or mutagenic potential of Diucardin or the potential of Diucardin to impair fertility.
PREGNANCY
Teratogenic Effects—Pregnancy Category C
Animal reproduction studies have not been conducted with Diucardin. It is also not known whether Diucardin can

cause fetal harm when administered to a pregnant woman or can affect reproduction capacity. Diucardin should be given to a pregnant woman only if clearly needed.

Nonteratogenic Effects

Fetal or neonatal jaundice, thrombocytopenia, and possibly other adverse reactions which have occurred in the adult.

NURSING MOTHERS

Thiazides appear in breast milk. If use of the drug is deemed essential, the patient may consider stopping nursing.

PEDIATRIC USE

Safety and effectiveness in children have not been established.

ADVERSE REACTIONS

The following adverse reactions have been observed, but there is not enough systematic collection of data to support an estimate of their frequency.

GASTROINTESTINAL SYSTEMS

Anorexia, gastric irritation, nausea, vomiting, cramping, diarrhea, constipation, jaundice (intrahepatic cholestatic jaundice), pancreatitis, sialadenitis.

CENTRAL NERVOUS SYSTEM

Dizziness, vertigo, paresthesias, headache, xanthopsia.

HEMATOLOGIC

Leukopenia, agranulocytosis, thrombocytopenia, aplastic anemia, hemolytic anemia.

CARDIOVASCULAR

Orthostatic hypotension (may be aggravated by alcohol, barbiturates, or narcotics).

DERMATOLOGIC—HYPERSENSITIVITY

Purpura, photosensitivity, rash, urticaria, necrotizing angiitis (vasculitis, cutaneous vasculitis), fever, respiratory distress including pneumonitis, anaphylactic reactions.

OTHER

Hyperglycemia, glycosuria, hyperuricemia, muscle spasm, weakness, restlessness, transient blurred vision.

Whenever adverse reactions are moderate or severe, thiazide dosage should be reduced or therapy withdrawn.

OVERDOSAGE

SIGNS AND SYMPTOMS

Diuresis, lethargy progressing to coma, with minimal cardiorespiratory depression and with or without significant serum electrolyte changes or dehydration; GI irritation; hypermotility; transient elevation in BUN level.

TREATMENT

Empty stomach by gastric lavage, taking care to avoid aspiration. Monitor serum electrolyte levels and renal function, and institute supportive measures, as required to maintain hydration, electrolyte balance, respiration, and cardiovascular and renal function. Treat GI effects symptomatically.

DOSAGE AND ADMINISTRATION

The average adult diuretic dose is 25 to 200 mg per day. The average adult antihypertensive dose is 50 to 100 mg per day. Therapy should be individualized according to patient response. This therapy should be titrated to gain maximal response as well as the minimal dose possible to maintain that therapeutic response.

HOW SUPPLIED

Diucardin®—Each scored, white oval compressed tablet, inscribed "DIUCARDIN 50," contains 50 mg hydroflumethiazide, in bottles of 100 (NDC 0046-0702-81).

Store at room temperature (approximately 25° C)

Dispense in a well-closed container as defined in the USP

Caution: Federal law prohibits dispensing without prescription.

Manufactured by:
Ayerst Laboratories Inc.
A Wyeth-Ayerst Company
Philadelphia, PA 19101
CI 4104-4 Revised July 27, 1995

Shown in Product Identification Guide, page 341

EFFEXOR® ℞

[*ĕf-fĕks 'ŏr*]
(venlafaxine hydrochloride)
Tablets

DESCRIPTION

Effexor (venlafaxine hydrochloride) is a structurally novel antidepressant for oral administration. It is chemically unrelated to tricyclic, tetracyclic, or other available antidepressant agents. It is designated (R/S)-1-[2-(dimethylamino)-1-(4-methoxyphenyl)ethyl] cyclohexanol hydrochloride or (±)-1-[α-[(dimethylamino)methyl]-p-methoxybenzyl] cyclohexanol hydrochloride and has the empirical formula of $C_{17}H_{27}NO_2$ HCl. Its molecular weight is 313.87. The structural formula is shown below.

venlafaxine hydrochloride

Venlafaxine hydrochloride is a white to off-white crystalline solid with a solubility of 572 mg/mL in water (adjusted to ionic strength of 0.2 M with sodium chloride). Its octanol: water (0.2 M sodium chloride) partition coefficient is 0.43.

Compressed tablets contain venlafaxine hydrochloride equivalent to 25 mg, 37.5 mg, 50 mg, 75 mg, or 100 mg venlafaxine. Inactive ingredients consist of cellulose, iron oxides, lactose, magnesium stearate, and sodium starch glycolate.

CLINICAL PHARMACOLOGY

Pharmacodynamics

The mechanism of the antidepressant action of venlafaxine in humans is believed to be associated with its potentiation of neurotransmitter activity in the CNS. Preclinical studies have shown that venlafaxine and its active metabolite, O-desmethylvenlafaxine (ODV), are potent inhibitors of neuronal serotonin and norepinephrine reuptake and weak inhibitors of dopamine reuptake. Venlafaxine and ODV have no significant affinity for muscarinic, histaminergic, or α-1 adrenergic receptors *in vitro*. Pharmacologic activity at these receptors is hypothesized to be associated with the various anticholinergic, sedative, and cardiovascular effects seen with other psychotropic drugs. Venlafaxine and ODV do not possess monoamine oxidase (MAO) inhibitory activity.

Pharmacokinetics

Venlafaxine is well absorbed and extensively metabolized in the liver. O-desmethylvenlafaxine (ODV) is the only major active metabolite. On the basis of mass balance studies, at least 92% of a single dose of venlafaxine is absorbed. Approximately 87% of a venlafaxine dose is recovered in the urine within 48 hours as either unchanged venlafaxine (5%), unconjugated ODV (29%), conjugated ODV (26%), or other minor inactive metabolites (27%). Renal elimination of venlafaxine and its metabolites is the primary route of excretion. The relative bioavailability of venlafaxine from a tablet was 100% when compared to an oral solution. Food has no significant effect on the absorption of venlafaxine or on the formation of ODV.

The degree of binding of venlafaxine to human plasma is 27%±2% at concentrations ranging from 2.5 to 2215 ng/mL. The degree of ODV binding to human plasma is 30%±12% at concentrations ranging from 100 to 500 ng/mL. Protein-binding-induced drug interactions with venlafaxine are not expected.

Steady-state concentrations of both venlafaxine and ODV in plasma were attained within 3 days of multiple-dose therapy. Venlafaxine and ODV exhibited linear kinetics over the dose range of 75 to 450 mg total dose per day (administered on a q8h schedule). Plasma clearance, elimination half-life and steady-state volume of distribution were unaltered for both venlafaxine and ODV after multiple-dosing. Mean±SD steady-state plasma clearance of venlafaxine and ODV is 1.3±0.6 and 0.4±0.2 L/h/kg, respectively; elimination half-life is 5±2 and 11±2 hours, respectively; and steady-state volume of distribution is 7.5±3.7 L/kg and 5.7±1.8 L/kg, respectively. When equal daily doses of venlafaxine were administered as either b.i.d. or t.i.d. regimens, the drug exposure (AUC) and fluctuation in plasma levels of venlafaxine and ODV were comparable following both regimens.

Age and Gender

A pharmacokinetic analysis of 404 venlafaxine-treated patients from two studies involving both b.i.d. and t.i.d. regimens showed that dose-normalized trough plasma levels of either venlafaxine or ODV were unaltered due to age or gender differences. Dosage adjustment based upon the age or gender of a patient is generally not necessary (see "**DOSAGE AND ADMINISTRATION**").

Liver Disease

In 9 patients with hepatic cirrhosis, the pharmacokinetic disposition of both venlafaxine and ODV was significantly altered after oral administration of venlafaxine. Venlafaxine elimination half-life was prolonged by about 30%, and clearance decreased by about 50% in cirrhotic patients compared to normal subjects. ODV elimination half-life was prolonged by about 60% and clearance decreased by about 30% in cirrhotic patients compared to normal subjects. A large degree of intersubject variability was noted. Three patients with more severe cirrhosis had a more substantial decrease in venlafaxine clearance (about 90%) compared to normal subjects.

Dosage adjustment is necessary in these patients (see "**DOSAGE AND ADMINISTRATION**").

Renal Disease

In a renal impairment study, venlafaxine elimination half-life after oral administration was prolonged by about 50% and clearance was reduced by about 24% in renally impaired patients (GFR =10-70 mL/min), compared to normal subjects. In dialysis patients, venlafaxine elimination half-life was prolonged by about 180% and clearance was reduced by about 57% compared to normal subjects. Similarly, ODV elimination half-life was prolonged by about 40% although clearance was unchanged in patients with renal impairment (GFR =10-70 mL/min) compared to normal subjects. In dialysis patients, ODV elimination half-life was prolonged by about 142% and clearance was reduced by about 56%, compared to normal subjects. A large degree of intersubject variability was noted.

Dosage adjustment is necessary in these patients (see "**DOSAGE AND ADMINISTRATION**").

CLINICAL TRIALS

The efficacy of Effexor (venlafaxine hydrochloride) as a treatment for depression was established in 5 placebo-controlled, short-term trials. Four of these were 6-week trials in outpatients meeting DSM-III or DSM-III-R criteria for major depression: two involving dose titration with Effexor in a range of 75 to 225 mg/day (t.i.d. schedule), the third involving fixed Effexor doses of 75, 225, and 375 mg/day (t.i.d. schedule), and the fourth involving doses of 25, 75, and 200 mg/day (b.i.d. schedule). The fifth was a 4-week study of inpatients meeting DSM-III-R criteria for major depression with melancholia whose Effexor doses were titrated in a range of 150 to 375 mg/day (t.i.d schedule). In these 5 studies, Effexor was shown to be significantly superior to placebo on at least 2 of the following 3 measures: Hamilton Depression Rating Scale (total score), Hamilton depressed mood item, and Clinical Global Impression—Severity of Illness rating. Doses from 75 to 225 mg/day were superior to placebo in outpatient studies and a mean dose of about 350 mg/day was effective in inpatients. Data from the 2 fixed-dose outpatient studies were suggestive of a dose-response relationship in the range of 75 to 225 mg/day. There was no suggestion of increased response with doses greater than 225 mg/day.

While there were no efficacy studies focusing specifically on an elderly population, elderly patients were included among the patients studied. Overall, approximately $^2/_3$ of all patients in these trials were women. Exploratory analyses for age and gender effects on outcome did not suggest any differential responsiveness on the basis of age or sex.

INDICATIONS AND USAGE

Effexor (venlafaxine hydrochloride) is indicated for the treatment of depression.

The efficacy of Effexor in the treatment of depression was established in 6-week controlled trials of outpatients whose diagnoses corresponded most closely to the DSM-III or DSM-III-R category of major depressive disorder and in a 4-week controlled trial of inpatients meeting diagnostic criteria for major depressive disorder with melancholia (see "**CLINICAL PHARMACOLOGY**").

A major depressive episode implies a prominent and relatively persistent depressed or dysphoric mood that usually interferes with daily functioning (nearly every day for at least 2 weeks); it should include at least 4 of the following 8 symptoms: change in appetite, change in sleep, psychomotor agitation or retardation, loss of interest in usual activities or decrease in sexual drive, increased fatigue, feelings of guilt or worthlessness, slowed thinking or impaired concentration, and a suicide attempt or suicidal ideation.

The effectiveness of Effexor in long-term use, that is, for more than 4 to 6 weeks, has not been systematically evaluated in controlled trials. Therefore, the physician who elects to use Effexor for extended periods should periodically re-evaluate the long-term usefulness of the drug for the individual patient.

CONTRAINDICATIONS

Effexor (venlafaxine hydrochloride) is contraindicated in patients known to be hypersensitive to it.

Concomitant use in patients taking monoamine oxidase inhibitors (MAOIs) is contraindicated (see "**WARNINGS**").

WARNINGS

Potential for Interaction with Monoamine Oxidase Inhibitors

Adverse reactions, some of which were serious, have been reported in patients who have recently been discontinued from a monoamine oxidase inhibitor (MAOI) and started on Effexor, or who have recently had Effexor therapy discontinued prior to initiation of an MAOI. These reactions have included tremor, myoclonus, diaphoresis, nausea, vomiting, flushing, dizziness, hyperthermia with features resembling neuroleptic malignant syndrome, seizures, and death. In patients receiving antidepressants with pharmacological properties similar to venlafaxine in combination with a monoamine oxidase inhibitor, there have also been reports of serious, sometimes fatal, reactions. For a selective serotonin reuptake inhibitor, these reactions have included hyperthermia, rigidity, myoclonus, autonomic instability with possible rapid fluctuations of vital signs, and mental status changes that include extreme agitation progressing to delirium and coma. Some cases presented with features resembling neuroleptic malignant syndrome. Severe hyperthermia and seizures, sometimes fatal, have been reported in association with the combined use of tricyclic antidepressants and MAOIs. These reactions have also been reported in patients who have recently discontinued these drugs and have been started on an MAOI. Therefore, it is recommended that Effexor not be used in combination with an MAOI, or within at least 14 days of discontinuing treatment with an MAOI. Based on the half-life of Effexor, at least 7 days should be allowed after stopping Effexor before starting an MAOI.

Sustained Hypertension

Venlafaxine treatment is associated with sustained increases in blood pressure. (1) In a premarketing study comparing three fixed doses of venlafaxine (75, 225, and 375 mg/day) and placebo, a mean increase in supine diastolic blood pressure (SDBP) of 7.2 mm Hg was seen in the 375 mg/day group at week 6 compared to essentially no changes in the 75 and 225 mg/day groups and a mean decrease in SDBP of 2.2 mm Hg in the placebo group. (2) An analysis for patients meeting criteria for sustained hypertension (defined as treatment-emergent SDBP ≥ 90 mm Hg *and* ≥ 10 mm Hg

Continued on next page

Effexor—Cont.

above baseline for 3 consecutive visits) revealed a dose-dependent increase in the incidence of sustained hypertension for venlafaxine:

Probability of Sustained Elevation in SDBP (Pool of Premarketing Venlafaxine Studies)	
Treatment Group	Incidence of Sustained Elevation in SDBP
Venlafaxine	
<100 mg/day	3%
101–200 mg/day	5%
201–300 mg/day	7%
>300 mg/day	13%
Placebo	2%

An analysis of the patients with sustained hypertension and the 19 venlafaxine patients who were discontinued from treatment because of hypertension (<1% of total venlafaxine-treated group) revealed that most of the blood pressure increases were in a modest range (10–15 mm Hg, SDBP). Nevertheless, sustained increases of this magnitude could have adverse consequences. Therefore, it is recommended that patients receiving venlafaxine have regular monitoring of blood pressure. For patients who experience a sustained increase in blood pressure while receiving venlafaxine, either dose reduction or discontinuation should be considered.

PRECAUTIONS

General

Anxiety and Insomnia

Treatment-emergent anxiety, nervousness, and insomnia were more commonly reported for venlafaxine-treated patients compared to placebo-treated patients in a pooled analysis of short-term, double-blind, placebo-controlled depression studies:

Symptom	Venlafaxine n = 1033	Placebo n = 609
Anxiety	6%	3%
Nervousness	13%	6%
Insomnia	18%	10%

Anxiety, nervousness, and insomnia led to drug discontinuation in 2%, 2%, and 3%, respectively, of the patients treated with venlafaxine in the phase 2–3 depression studies.

Changes in Appetite and Weight

Treatment-emergent anorexia was more commonly reported for venlafaxine-treated (11%) than placebo-treated patients (2%) in the pool of short-term, double-blind, placebo-controlled depression studies. A dose-dependent weight loss was often noted in patients treated with venlafaxine for several weeks. Significant weight loss, especially in underweight depressed patients, may be an undesirable result of venlafaxine treatment. A loss of 5% or more of body weight occurred in 6% of patients treated with venlafaxine compared with 1% of patients treated with placebo and 3% of patients treated with another antidepressant. However, discontinuation for weight loss associated with venlafaxine was uncommon (0.1% of venlafaxine-treated patients in the phase 2–3 depression trials).

Activation of Mania/Hypomania

During phase 2–3 trials, hypomania or mania occurred in 0.5% of patients treated with venlafaxine. Activation of mania/hypomania has also been reported in a small proportion of patients with major affective disorder who were treated with other marketed antidepressants. As with all antidepressants, Effexor (venlafaxine hydrochloride) should be used cautiously in patients with a history of mania.

Hyponatremia

Hyponatremia and/or the syndrome of inappropriate antidiuretic hormone secretion (SIADH) may occur with venlafaxine. This should be taken into consideration in patients who are, for example, volume-depleted, elderly, or taking diuretics.

Mydriasis.

Mydriasis has been reported in association with venlafaxine; therefore patients with raised intraocular pressure or at risk of acute narrow angle glaucoma should be monitored.

Seizures

During premarketing testing, seizures were reported in 0.26% (8/3082) of venlafaxine-treated patients. Most seizures (5 of 8) occurred in patients receiving doses of 150 mg/day or less. Effexor should be used cautiously in patients with a history of seizures. It should be discontinued in any patient who develops seizures.

Skin and Mucous Membrane Bleeding

The risk of skin and mucous membrane bleeding may be increased in patients taking venlafaxine. As with other serotonin-reuptake inhibitors, venlafaxine should be used cautiously in patients predisposed to bleeding at these sites.

Suicide

The possibility of a suicide attempt is inherent in depression and may persist until significant remission occurs. Close supervision of high-risk patients should accompany initial drug therapy. Prescriptions for Effexor should be written for the smallest quantity of tablets consistent with good patient management in order to reduce the risk of overdose.

Use in Patients with Concomitant Illness

Clinical experience with Effexor in patients with concomitant systemic illness is limited. Caution is advised in administering Effexor to patients with diseases or conditions that could affect hemodynamic responses or metabolism.

Effexor has not been evaluated or used to any appreciable extent in patients with a recent history of myocardial infarction or unstable heart disease. Patients with these diagnoses were sytematically excluded from many clinical studies during the product's premarketing testing. Evaluation of the electrocardiograms for 769 patients who received Effexor in 4- to 6-week double-blind placebo-controlled trials, however, showed that the incidence of trial-emergent conduction abnormalities did not differ from that with placebo. The mean heart rate in Effexor-treated patients was increased relative to baseline by about 4 beats per minute.

The electrocardiograms for 357 patients who received Effexor XR (the extended-release form of venlafaxine) and 285 patients who received placebo in 8- to 12-week double-blind, placebo-controlled trials were analyzed. The mean change from baseline in corrected QT interval (QTc) for Effexor XR-treated patients was increased relative to that for placebo-treated patients (increase of 4.7 msec for Effexor XR and decrease of 1.9 msec for placebo). In these same trials, the mean change from baseline in heart rate for Effexor XR-treated patients was significantly higher than that for placebo (a mean increase of 4 beats per minute for Effexor XR and 1 beat per minute for placebo). The clinical significance of these changes is unknown.

In patients with renal impairment (GFR=10-70 mL/min) or cirrhosis of the liver, the clearances of venlafaxine and its active metabolite were decreased, thus prolonging the elimination half-lives of these substances. A lower dose may be necessary (see **"DOSAGE AND ADMINISTRATION"**). Effexor (venlafaxine hydrochloride), like all antidepressants, should be used with caution in such patients.

Information for Patients

Physicians are advised to discuss the following issues with patients for whom they prescribe Effexor:

Interference with Cognitive and Motor Performance

Clinical studies were performed to examine the effects of venlafaxine on behavioral performance of healthy individuals. The results revealed no clinically significant impairment of psychomotor, cognitive, or complex behavior performance. However, since any psychoactive drug may impair judgment, thinking, or motor skills, patients should be cautioned about operating hazardous machinery, including automobiles, until they are reasonably certain that Effexor therapy does not adversely affect their ability to engage in such activities.

Pregnancy

Patients should be advised to notify their physician if they become pregnant or intend to become pregnant during therapy.

Nursing

Patients should be advised to notify their physician if they are breast-feeding an infant.

Concomitant Medication

Patients should be advised to inform their physicians if they are taking, or plan to take, any prescription or over-the-counter drugs, since there is a potential for interactions.

Alcohol

Although Effexor has not been shown to increase the impairment of mental and motor skills caused by alcohol, patients should be advised to avoid alcohol while taking Effexor.

Allergic Reactions

Patients should be advised to notify their physician if they develop a rash, hives, or a related allergic phenomenon.

Laboratory Tests

There are no specific laboratory tests recommended.

Drug Interactions

As with all drugs, the potential for interaction by a variety of mechanisms is a possibility.

Alcohol

A single dose of ethanol (0.5 g/kg) had no effect on the pharmacokinetics of venlafaxine or ODV when venlafaxine was administered at 150 mg/day in 15 healthy male subjects. Additionally, administration of venlafaxine in a stable regimen did not exaggerate the psychomotor and psychometric effects induced by ethanol in these same subjects when they were not receiving venlafaxine.

Cimetidine

Concomitant administration of cimetidine and venlafaxine in a steady-state for both drugs resulted in inhibition of first-pass metabolism of venlafaxine in 18 healthy subjects. The oral clearance of venlafaxine was reduced by about 43%, and the exposure (AUC) and maximum concentration (C_{max}) of the drug were increased by about 60%. However, co-administration of cimetidine had no apparent effect on the pharmacokinetics of ODV, which is present in much greater quantity in the circulation than is venlafaxine. The overall pharmacological activity of venlafaxine plus ODV is expected to increase only slightly, and no dosage adjustment should be necessary for most normal adults. However, for patients with pre-existing hypertension, and for elderly patients or patients with hepatic dysfunction, the interaction associated with the concomitant use of venlafaxine and cimetidine is not known and potentially could be more pronounced. Therefore, caution is advised with such patients.

Diazepam

Under steady-state conditions for venlafaxine administered at 150 mg/day, a single 10 mg dose of diazepam did not appear to affect the pharmacokinetics of either venlafaxine or ODV in 18 healthy male subjects. Venlafaxine also did not have any effect on the pharmacokinetics of diazepam or its active metabolite, desmethyldiazepam, or affect the psychomotor and psychometric effects induced by diazepam.

Haloperidol

Venlafaxine administered under steady-state conditions at 150 mg/day in 24 healthy subjects decreased total oral-dose clearance (Cl/F) of a single 2 mg dose of haloperidol by 42%, which resulted in a 70% increase in haloperidol AUC. In addition, the haloperidol C_{max} increased 88% when coadministered with venlafaxine, but the haloperidol elimination half-life ($t_{1/2}$) was unchanged. The mechanism explaining this finding is unknown.

Lithium

The steady-state pharmacokinetics of venlafaxine administered at 150 mg/day were not affected when a single 600 mg oral dose of lithium was administered to 12 healthy male subjects. O-desmethylvenlafaxine (ODV) also was unaffected. Venlafaxine had no effect on the pharmacokinetics of lithium.

Drugs Highly Bound to Plasma Protein

Venlafaxine is not highly bound to plasma proteins; therefore, administration of Effexor to a patient taking another drug that is highly protein bound should not cause increased free concentrations of the other drug.

Drugs that Inhibit Cytochrome P450 Isoenzymes

CYP2D6 Inhibitors: *In vitro* and *in vivo* studies indicate that venlafaxine is metabolized to its active metabolite, ODV, by CYP2D6, the isoenzyme that is responsible for the genetic polymorphism seen in the metabolism of many antidepressants. Therefore, the potential exists for a drug interaction between drugs that inhibit CYP2D6-mediated metabolism and venlafaxine. However, although imipramine partially inhibited the CYP2D6-mediated metabolism of venlafaxine, resulting in higher plasma concentrations of venlafaxine and lower plasma concentrations of ODV, the total concentration of active compounds (venlafaxine plus ODV) was not affected. Additionally, in a clinical study involving CYP2D6-poor and -extensive metabolizers, the total concentration of active compounds (venlafaxine plus ODV), was similar in the two metabolizer groups. Therefore, no dosage adjustment is required when venlafaxine is coadministered with a CYP2D6 inhibitor.

CYP3A4 Inhibitors: *In vitro* studies indicate that venlafaxine is likely metabolized to a minor, less active metabolite, N-desmethylvenlafaxine, by CYP3A4. Because CYP3A4 is typically a minor pathway relative to CYP2D6 in the metabolism of venlafaxine, the potential for a clinically significant drug interaction between drugs that inhibit CYP3A4-mediated metabolism and venlafaxine is small.

The concomitant use of venlafaxine with a drug treatment(s) that potently inhibits both CYP2D6 and CYP3A4, the primary metabolizing enzymes for venlafaxine, has not been studied. Therefore, caution is advised should a patient's therapy include venlafaxine and any agent(s) that produce potent simultaneous inhibition of these two enzyme systems.

Drugs Metabolized by Cytochrome P450 Isoenzymes

CYP2D6: *In vitro* studies indicate that venlafaxine is a relatively weak inhibitor of CYP2D6. These findings have been confirmed in a clinical drug interaction study comparing the effect of venlafaxine to that of fluoxetine on the CYP2D6-mediated metabolism of dextromethorphan to dextrorphan.

Imipramine—Venlafaxine did not affect the pharmacokinetics of imipramine and 2-OH-imipramine. However, desipramine AUC, C_{max}, and C_{min} increased by about 35% in the presence of venlafaxine. The 2-OH-desipramine AUC's increased by at least 2.5 fold (with venlafaxine 37.5 mg q12h) and by 4.5 fold (with venlafaxine 75 mg q12h). Imipramine did not affect the pharmacokinetics of venlafaxine and ODV. The clinical significance of elevated 2-OH-desipramine levels is unknown.

Risperidone—Venlafaxine administered under steady-state conditions at 150 mg/day slightly inhibited the CYP2D6-mediated metabolism of risperidone (administered as a single 1 mg oral dose) to its active metabolite, 9-hydroxyrisperidone, resulting in an approximate 32% increase in risperidone AUC. However, venlafaxine coadministration did not significantly alter the pharmacokinetic profile of the total active moiety (risperidone plus 9-hydroxyrisperidone).

CYP3A4: Venlafaxine did not inhibit CYP3A4 *in vitro.* This finding was confirmed *in vivo* by clinical drug interaction studies in which venlafaxine did not inhibit the metabolism of several CYP3A4 substrates, including alprazolam, diazepam, and terfenadine.

Indinavir—In a study of 9 health volunteers, venlafaxine administered under steady-state conditions at 150 mg/day resulted in a 28% decrease in the AUC of a single 800 mg oral dose of indinavir and a 36% decrease in indinavir C_{max}. Indinavir did not affect the pharmacokinetics of venlafaxine and ODV. The clinical significance of this finding is unknown.

CYP1A2: Venlafaxine did not inhibit CYP1A2 *in vitro.* This finding was confirmed *in vivo* by a clinical drug interaction study in which venlafaxine did not inhibit the metabolism of caffeine, a CYP1A2 substrate.

CYP2C9: Venlafaxine did not inhibit CYP2C9 *in vitro.* The clinical significance of this finding is unknown.

CYP2C19: Venlafaxine did not inhibit the metabolism of diazepam which is partially metabolized by CYP2C19 (see "*Diazepam*" above).

Monoamine Oxidase Inhibitors

See **"CONTRAINDICATIONS"** and **"WARNINGS."**

CNS-Active Drugs

The risk of using venlafaxine in combination with other CNS-active drugs has not been systematically evaluated (except in the case of those CNS-active drugs noted above). Consequently, caution is advised if the concomitant administration of venlafaxine and such drugs is required.

Electroconvulsive Therapy

There are no clinical data establishing the benefit of electroconvulsive therapy combined with Effexor treatment.

Postmarketing Spontaneous Drug Interaction Reports

See **"ADVERSE REACTIONS, Postmarketing Reports."**

Carcinogenesis, Mutagenesis, Impairment of Fertility

Carcinogenesis

Venlafaxine was given by oral gavage to mice for 18 months at doses up to 120 mg/kg per day, which was 16 times, on a mg/kg basis, and 1.7 times on a mg/m^2 basis, the maximum recommended human dose. Venlafaxine was also given to rats by oral gavage for 24 months at doses up to 120 mg/kg per day. In rats receiving the 120 mg/kg dose, plasma levels of venlafaxine were 1 times (male rats) and 6 times (female rats) the plasma levels of patients receiving the maximum recommended human dose. Plasma levels of the O-desmethyl metabolite were lower in rats than in patients receiving the maximum recommended dose. Tumors were not increased by venlafaxine treatment in mice or rats.

Mutagenicity

Venlafaxine and the major human metabolite, O-desmethylvenlafaxine (ODV), were not mutagenic in the Ames reverse mutation assay in Salmonella bacteria or the CHO/HGPRT mammalian cell forward gene mutation assay. Venlafaxine was also not mutagenic in the *in vitro* BALB/c-3T3 mouse cell transformation assay, the sister chromatid exchange assay in cultured CHO cells, or the *in vivo* chromosomal aberration assay in rat bone marrow. ODV was not mutagenic in the *in vitro* CHO cell chromosomal aberration assay. There was a clastogenic response in the *in vivo* chromosomal aberration assay in rat bone marrow in male rats receiving 200 times, on a mg/kg basis, or 50 times, on a mg/m^2 basis, the maximum human daily dose. The no effect dose was 67 times (mg/kg) or 17 times (mg/m^2) the human dose.

Impairment of Fertility

Reproduction and fertility studies in rats showed no effects on male or female fertility at oral doses of up to 8 times the maximum recommended human daily dose on a mg/kg basis, or up to 2 times on a mg/m^2 basis.

Pregnancy

Teratogenic Effects—Pregnancy Category C

Venlafaxine did not cause malformations in offspring of rats or rabbits given doses up to 11 times (rat) or 12 times (rabbit) the maximum recommended human daily dose on a mg/kg basis, or 2.5 times (rat) and 4 times (rabbit) the human daily dose on a mg/m^2 basis. However, in rats, there was a decrease in pup weight, an increase in stillborn pups, and an increase in pup deaths during the first 5 days of lactation, when dosing began during pregnancy and continued until weaning. The cause of these deaths is not known. These effects occurred at 10 times (mg/kg) or 2.5 times (mg/m^2) the maximum human daily dose. The no effect dose for rat pup mortality was 1.4 times the human dose on a mg/kg basis or 0.25 times the human dose on a mg/m^2 basis. There are no adequate and well-controlled studies in pregnant women. Because animal reproduction studies are not always predictive of human response, this drug should be used during pregnancy only if clearly needed.

Labor and Delivery

The effect of Effexor® (venlafaxine hydrochloride) on labor and delivery in humans is unknown.

Nursing Mothers

Venlafaxine and ODV have been reported to be excreted in human milk. Because of the potential for serious adverse reactions in nursing infants from Effexor, a decision should be made whether to discontinue nursing or to discontinue the drug, taking into account the importance of the drug to the mother.

Usage in Children

Safety and effectiveness in individuals below 18 years of age have not been established.

Geriatric Use

Of the 2,897 patients in phase 2–3 depression studies with Effexor, 12% (357) were 65 years of age or over. No overall differences in effectiveness or safety were observed between these patients and younger patients, and other reported clinical experience generally has not identified differences in response between the elderly and younger patients. However, greater sensitivity of some older individuals cannot be ruled out. As with other antidepressants, several cases of hyponatremia and syndrome of inappropriate antidiuretic hormone secretion (SIADH) have been reported, usually in the elderly.

The pharmacokinetics of venlafaxine and ODV are not substantially altered in the elderly (see **"CLINICAL PHARMACOLOGY"**). No dose adjustment is recommended for the elderly on the basis of age alone, although other clinical circumstances, some of which may be more common in the elderly, such as renal or hepatic impairment, may warrant a dose reduction (see **"DOSAGE AND ADMINISTRATION"**).

TABLE 1
Treatment-Emergent Adverse Experience Incidence in 4- to 8-Week Placebo-Controlled Clinical Trials[1]

Body System	Preferred Term	Effexor (n=1033)	Placebo (n=609)
Body as a Whole	Headache	25%	24%
	Asthenia	12%	6%
	Infection	6%	5%
	Chills	3%	—
	Chest pain	2%	1%
	Trauma	2%	1%
Cardiovascular	Vasodilatation	4%	3%
	Increased blood pressure/hypertension	2%	—
	Tachycardia	2%	—
	Postural hypotension	1%	—
Dermatological	Sweating	12%	3%
	Rash	3%	2%
	Pruritus	1%	—
Gastrointestinal	Nausea	37%	11%
	Constipation	15%	7%
	Anorexia	11%	2%
	Diarrhea	8%	7%
	Vomiting	6%	2%
	Dyspepsia	5%	4%
	Flatulence	3%	2%
Metabolic	Weight loss	1%	—
Nervous System	Somnolence	23%	9%
	Dry mouth	22%	11%
	Dizziness	19%	7%
	Insomnia	18%	10%
	Nervousness	13%	6%
	Anxiety	6%	3%
	Tremor	5%	1%
	Abnormal dreams	4%	3%
	Hypertonia	3%	2%
	Paresthesia	3%	2%
	Libido decreased	2%	—
	Agitation	2%	—
	Confusion	2%	1%
	Thinking abnormal	2%	1%
	Depersonalization	1%	—
	Depression	1%	—
	Urinary retention	1%	—
	Twitching	1%	—
Respiration	Yawn	3%	—
Special Senses	Blurred vision	6%	2%
	Taste perversion	2%	—
	Tinnitus	2%	—
	Mydriasis	2%	—
Urogenital System	Abnormal ejaculation/orgasm	12%[2]	—[2]
	Impotence	6%[2]	—[2]
	Urinary frequency	3%	2%
	Urination impaired	2%	—
	Orgasm disturbance	2%[3]	—[3]
	Menstrual disorder	1%[3]	—[3]

[1] Events reported by at least 1% of patients treated with Effexor (venlafaxine hydrochloride) are included, and are rounded to the nearest %. Events for which the Effexor incidence was equal to or less than placebo are not listed in the table, but included the following: abdominal pain, pain, back pain, flu syndrome, fever, palpitation, increased appetite, myalgia, arthralgia, amnesia, hypesthesia, rhinitis, pharyngitis, sinusitis, cough increased, urinary tract infection, and dysmenorrhea[3]

—Incidence less than 1%.

[2] Incidence based on number of male patients.

[3] Incidence based on number of female patients.

ADVERSE REACTIONS

Associated with Discontinuation of Treatment

Nineteen percent (537/2897) of venlafaxine patients in phase 2–3 depression studies discontinued treatment due to an adverse event. The more common events (≥1%) associated with discontinuation and considered to be drug-related (i.e., those events associated with dropout at a rate approximately twice or greater for venlafaxine compared to placebo) included:

	Venlafaxine	Placebo
CNS		
Somnolence	3%	1%
Insomnia	3%	1%
Dizziness	3%	—
Nervousness	2%	—
Dry mouth	2%	—
Anxiety	2%	1%
Gastrointestinal		
Nausea	6%	1%
Urogenital		
Abnormal ejaculation*	3%	—
Other		
Headache	3%	1%
Asthenia	2%	—
Sweating	2%	—

* Percentages based on the number of males.

— Less than 1%

Incidence in Controlled Trials

Commonly Observed Adverse Events in Controlled Clinical Trials

The most commonly observed adverse events associated with the use of Effexor® (incidence of 5% or greater) and not seen at an equivalent incidence among placebo-treated patients (i.e., incidence for Effexor at least twice that for placebo), derived from the 1% incidence table below, were asthenia, sweating, nausea, constipation, anorexia, vomiting, somnolence, dry mouth, dizziness, nervousness, anxiety, tremor, and blurred vision as well as abnormal ejaculation/orgasm and impotence in men.

Adverse Events Occurring at an Incidence of 1% or More Among Effexor-Treated Patients

The table that follows enumerates adverse events that occurred at an incidence of 1% or more, and were more frequent than in the placebo group, among Effexor-treated patients who participated in short-term (4- to 8-week) placebo-controlled trials in which patients were administered doses in a range of 75 to 375 mg/day. This table shows the percentage of patients in each group who had at least one episode of an event at some time during their treatment. Reported adverse events were classified using a standard COSTART-based Dictionary terminology.

The prescriber should be aware that these figures cannot be used to predict the incidence of side effects in the course of usual medical practice where patient characteristics and other factors differ from those which prevailed in the clinical trials. Similarly, the cited frequencies cannot be compared with figures obtained from other clinical investigations involving different treatments, uses and investigators. The cited figures, however, do provide the prescribing physician with some basis for estimating the relative contribution of drug and nondrug factors to the side effect incidence rate in the population studied.

[See table above]

Dose Dependency of Adverse Events

A comparison of adverse event rates in a fixed-dose study comparing Effexor (venlafaxine hydrochloride) 75, 225, and

Continued on next page

Effexor—Cont.

375 mg/day with placebo revealed a dose dependency for some of the more common adverse events associated with Effexor use, as shown in the table that follows. The rule for including events was to enumerate those that occurred at an incidence of 5% or more for at least one of the venlafaxine groups and for which the incidence was at least twice the placebo incidence for at least one Effexor group. Tests for potential dose relationships for these events (Cochran-Armitage Test, with a criterion of exact 2-sided p-value ≤0.05) suggested a dose-dependency for several adverse events in this list, including chills, hypertension, anorexia, nausea, agitation, dizziness, somnolence, tremor, yawning, sweating, and abnormal ejaculation.

[See table below]

Adaptation to Certain Adverse Events

Over a 6-week period, there was evidence of adaptation to some adverse events with continued therapy (e.g., dizziness and nausea), but less to other effects (e.g., abnormal ejaculation and dry mouth).

Vital Sign Changes

Effexor (venlafaxine hydrochloride) treatment (averaged over all dose groups) in clinical trials was associated with a mean increase in pulse rate of approximately 3 beats per minute, compared to no change for placebo. It was associated with mean increases in diastolic blood pressure ranging from 0.7 to 2.5 mm Hg averaged over all dose groups, compared to mean decreases ranging from 0.9 to 3.8 mm Hg for placebo. However, there is a dose dependency for blood pressure increase (see **"WARNINGS"**).

Laboratory Changes

Of the serum chemistry and hematology parameters monitored during clinical trials with Effexor, a statistically significant difference with placebo was seen only for serum cholesterol. In pre-marketing trials, treatment with Effexor tablets was associated with a mean final on-therapy increase in total cholesterol of 3 mg/dL. Patients treated with Effexor tablets for at least 3 months in placebo-controlled 12-month extension trials had a mean final on-therapy increase in total cholesterol of 9.1 mg/dL. This increase was duration dependent over the 12-month study period and tended to be greater with higher doses. An increase in serum cholesterol from baseline by ≥ 50 mg/dL and to values > 260 mg/dL at any time after baseline, has been recorded in 8.1% of patients.

ECG Changes

In an analysis of ECGs obtained in 769 patients treated with Effexor and 450 patients treated with placebo in controlled clinical trials, the only statistically significant difference observed was for heart rate, i.e., a mean increase from baseline of 4 beats per minute for Effexor (see **"PRECAUTIONS"**, **General**, *Use in Patients with Concomitant Illness*").

Other Events Observed During the Premarketing Evaluation of Venlafaxine

During its premarketing assessment, multiple doses of Effexor were administered to 2897 patients in phase 2 and 3 studies. In addition, in premarketing assessment of Effexor XR (the extended release form of venlafaxine), multiple doses were administered to 705 patients in phase 3 depression studies and Effexor was administered to 96 patients. During its premarketing assessment for Generalized Anxiety Disorder, multiple doses of Effexor XR was administered to 476 patients in phase 3 studies. The conditions and duration of exposure to venlafaxine in both development programs varied greatly, and included (in overlapping categories) open and double-blind studies, uncontrolled and controlled studies, inpatient (Effexor only) and outpatient studies, fixed-dose and titration studies. Untoward events associated with this exposure were recorded by clinical investigators using terminology of thier own choosing. Consequently, it is not possible to provide a meaningful estimate of the proportion of individuals experiencing adverse events without first grouping similar types of untoward events into a smaller number of standardized event categories.

In the tabulations that follow, reported adverse events were classified using a standard COSTART-based Dictionary terminology. The frequencies presented, therefore, represent the proportion of the 4174 patients exposed to multiple doses of either formulation of venlafaxine who experienced an event of the type cited on at least one occasion while receiving venlafaxine. All reported events are included except those already listed in Table 1 and those events for which a drug cause was remote. If the COSTART term for an event was so general as to be uninformative, it was replaced with a more informative term. It is important to emphasize that, although the events reported occurred during treatment with venlafaxine, they were not necessarily caused by it.

Events are further categorized by body system and listed in order of decreasing frequency using the following definitions: **frequent** adverse events are defined as those occurring on one or more occasions in at least 1/100 patients; **infrequent** adverse events are those occurring in 1/100 to 1/1000 patients; **rare** events are those occurring in fewer than 1/1000 patients.

Body as a whole—**Frequent:** chest pain substernal, neck pain; **Infrequent:** face edema, intentional injury, malaise, moniliasis, neck rigidity, pelvic pain, photosensitivity reaction, suicide attempt; **Rare:** appendicitis, carcinoma, cellulitis, withdrawal syndrome.

Cardiovascular system—**Frequent:** migraine; **Infrequent:** angina pectoris, arrhythmia, extrasystoles, hypotension, peripheral vascular disorder (mainly cold feet and/or cold hands), syncope, thrombophlebitis; **Rare:** arteritis, first-degree atrioventricular block, bigeminy, bradycardia, bundle branch block, cerebrial ischemia, coronary artery disease, congestive heart failure, heart arrest, mitral valve disorder, mucocutaneous hemorrhage, myocardial infarct, pallor.

Digestive system—**Frequent:** eructation; **Infrequent:** bruxism, colitis, dysphagia, tongue edema, esophagitis, gastritis, gastroenteritis, gastrointestinal ulcer, gingivitis, glossitis, rectal hemorrhage, hemorrhoids, melena, stomatitis, mouth ulceration; **Rare:** cheilitis, cholecystitis, cholelithiasis, hematemesis, gastrointestinal hemorrhage, gum hemorrhage, hepatitis, ileitis, jaundice, intestinal obstruction, oral moniliasis, proctitis, increased salivation, soft stools, tongue discoloration

Endocrine system—**Rare:** goiter, hyperthyroidism, hypothyroidism, thyroid nodule, thyroiditis.

Hemic and lymphatic system—**Frequent:** ecchymosis; **Infrequent:** anemia, leukocytosis, leukopenia, lymphadenopathy, thrombocythemia, thrombocytopenia; **Rare:** basophilia, cyanosis, eosinophilia, lymphocytosis.

Metabolic and nutritional—**Frequent:** edema, weight gain; **Infrequent:** alkaline phosphatase increased, glycosuria, hypercholesteremia, hyperglycemia, hyperuricemia, hypoglycemia, hypokalemia, SGOT increased, thirst; **Rare:** alcohol intolerance, bilirubinemia, BUN increased, creatinine increased, diabetes mellitus, dehydration, gout, hemochromatosis, hypercalcinuria, hyperkalemia, hyperlipemia, hyperphosphatemia, hyponatremia, hypophosphatemia, hypoproteinemia, SGPT increased, uremia.

Musculoskeletal system—**Infrequent:** arthritis, arthrosis, bone pain, bone spurs, bursitis, leg cramps, myasthenia, tenosynovitis; **Rare:** pathological fracture, myopathy, osteoporosis, osteosclerosis, rheumatoid arthritis, tendon rupture.

Nervous system—**Frequent:** emotional lability, trismus, vertigo; **Infrequent:** apathy, ataxia, circumoral paresthesia, CNS stimulation, euphoria, hallucinations, hostility, hyperesthesia, hyperkinesia, hypotonia, incoordination, libido increased, manic reaction, myoclonus, neuralgia, neuropathy, paranoid reaction, psychosis, psychotic seizure, abnormal speech, stupor; **Rare:** akathisia, akinesia, alcohol abuse, aphasia, bradykinesia, buccoglossal syndrome, cerebrovascular accident, loss of consciousness, delusions, dementia, dystonia, facial paralysis, abnormal gait, Guillain-Barre Syndrome, hypokinesia, neuritis, nystagmus, psychotic depression, reflexes decreased, reflexes increased, suicidal ideation, torticollis.

Respiratory system—**Frequent:** bronchitis, dyspnea; **Infrequent:** asthma, chest congestion, epistaxis, hyperventilation, laryngismus, laryngitis, pneumonia, voice alteration; **Rare:** atelectasis, hemoptysis, hypoventilation, hypoxia, pleurisy, pulmonary embolus, sleep apnea.

Skin and appendages—**Infrequent:** acne, alopecia, brittle nails, contact dermatitis, dry skin, eczema, skin hypertrophy, maculopapular rash, psoriasis, urticaria; **Rare:** erythemia nodosum, exfoliative dermatitis, lichenoid dermatitis, hair discoloration, skin discoloration, furunculosis, hirsutism, leukoderma, pustular rash, vesiculobullous rash, seborrhea, skin atrophy, skin striae.

Special senses—**Frequent:** abnormality of accommodation, abnormal vision; **Infrequent:** cataract, conjunctivitis, corneal lesion, diplopia, dry eyes, exophthalmos, eye pain, hyperacusis, otitis media, parosmia, photophobia, taste loss, visual field defect; **Rare:** blepharitis, chromatopsia, conjunctival edema, deafness, glaucoma, retinal hemorrhage, subconjunctival hemorrhage, keratitis, labyrinthitis, miosis, papilledema, decreased pupillary reflex, otitis externa, scleritis, uveitis.

Urogenital system—**Frequent:** metrorrhagia,* prostatitis,* vaginitis*; **Infrequent:** albuminuria, amenorrhea*, cystitis, dysuria, hematuria, female lactation,* leukorrhea,* menorrhagia,* nocturia, bladder pain, breast pain, polyuria, pyuria, urinary incontinence, urinary urgency, vaginal hemorrhage*; **Rare:** abortion,* anuria, breast engorgement, breast enlargement, fibrocystic breast, calcium crystalluria, cervicitis,* ovarian cyst,* prolonged erection,* gynecomastia (male),* hypomenorrhea,* kidney calculus, kidney pain, kidney function abnormal, mastitis, menopause,* pyelonephritis, oliguria, salpingitis,* urolithiasis, uterine hemorrhage,* uterine spasm.*

* Based on the number of men and women as appropriate.

Postmarketing Reports

Voluntary reports of other adverse events temporally associated with the use of Effexor that have been received since market introduction and that may have no causal relationship with the use of Effexor include the following: agranulocytosis, anaphylaxis, aplastic anemia, catatonia, congenital anomalies, CPK increased, deep vein thrombophlebitis, dehydration, delirium, EKG abnormalities (such as atrial fibrillation, supraventricular tachycardia, ventricular extrasystole, ventricular tachycardia), epidermal necrosis/Stevens-Johnson Syndrome, erythema multiforme, extrapyramidal symptoms (including tardive dyskinesia), fatigue, hemorrhage (including eye and gastrointestinal bleeding), hepatic events (including GGT elevation; abnormalities of unspecified liver function tests; liver damage, necrosis, or failure; and fatty liver), involuntary movement, LDH increased, neuroleptic malignant syndrome-like events (including a case of a 10-year-old who may have been taking methylphenidate, was treated and recovered), pancreatitis, panic, prolactin increased, renal failure, serotonin syndrome, shock-like electrical sensations (in some cases, subsequent to the discontinuation of Effexor or tapering of dose), and syndrome of inappropriate antidiuretic hormone secretion (usually in the elderly).

There have been reports of elevated clozapine levels that were temporally associated with adverse events, including

TABLE 2
Treatment-Emergent Adverse Experience Incidence in a Dose Comparison Trial

Body System/ Preferred Term	Placebo (n=92)	Effexor (mg/day) 75 (n=89)	225 (n=89)	375 (n=88)
Body as a Whole				
Abdominal pain	3.3%	3.4%	2.2%	8.0%
Asthenia	3.3%	16.9%	14.6%	14.8%
Chills	1.1%	2.2%	5.6%	6.8%
Infection	2.2%	2.2%	5.6%	2.3%
Cardiovascular System				
Hypertension	1.1%	1.1%	2.2%	4.5%
Vasodilatation	0.0%	4.5%	5.6%	2.3%
Digestive System				
Anorexia	2.2%	14.6%	13.5%	17.0%
Dyspepsia	2.2%	6.7%	6.7%	4.5%
Nausea	14.1%	32.6%	38.2%	58.0%
Vomiting	1.1%	7.9%	3.4%	6.8%
Nervous System				
Agitation	0.0%	1.1%	2.2%	4.5%
Anxiety	4.3%	11.2%	4.5%	2.3%
Dizziness	4.3%	19.1%	22.5%	23.9%
Insomnia	9.8%	22.5%	20.2%	13.6%
Libido decreased	1.1%	2.2%	1.1%	5.7%
Nervousness	4.3%	21.3%	13.5%	12.5%
Somnolence	4.3%	16.9%	18.0%	26.1%
Tremor	0.0%	1.1%	2.2%	10.2%
Respiratory System				
Yawn	0.0%	4.5%	5.6%	8.0%
Skin and Appendages				
Sweating	5.4%	6.7%	12.4%	19.3%
Special Senses				
Abnormality of accommodation	0.0%	9.1%	7.9%	5.6%
Urogenital System				
Abnormal ejaculation/orgasm	0.0%	4.5%	2.2%	12.5%
Impotence	0.0%	5.8%	2.1%	3.6%
(Number of men)	(n=63)	(n=52)	(n=48)	(n=56)

seizures, following the addition of venlafaxine. There have been reports of increases in prothrombin time, partial thromboplastin time, or INR when venlafaxine was given to patients receiving warfarin therapy.

DRUG ABUSE AND DEPENDENCE

Controlled Substance Class

Effexor (venlafaxine hydrochloride) is not a controlled substance.

Physical and Psychological Dependence

In vitro studies revealed that venlafaxine has virtually no affinity for opiate, benzodiazepine, phencyclidine (PCP), or N-methyl-D-aspartic acid (NMDA) receptors.

Venlafaxine was not found to have any significant CNS stimulant activity in rodents. In primate drug discrimination studies, venlafaxine showed no significant stimulant or depressant abuse liability.

Discontinuation effects have been reported in patients receiving venlafaxine (see "**DOSAGE AND ADMINISTRATION**").

While Effexor has not been systematically studied in clinical trials for its potential for abuse, there was no indication of drug-seeking behavior in the clinical trials. However, it is not possible to predict on the basis of premarketing experience the extent to which a CNS active drug will be misused, diverted, and/or abused once marketed. Consequently, physicians should carefully evaluate patients for history of drug abuse and follow such patients closely, observing them for signs of misuse or abuse of Effexor (e.g., development of tolerance, incrementation of dose, drug-seeking behavior).

OVERDOSAGE

Human Experience

There were 14 reports of acute overdose with Effexor (venlafaxine hydrochloride), either alone or in combination with other drugs and/or alcohol, among the patients included in the premarketing evaluation. The majority of the reports involved ingestions in which the total dose of Effexor taken was estimated to be no more than several-fold higher than the usual therapeutic dose. The 3 patients who took the highest doses were estimated to have ingested approximately 6.75 g, 2.75 g, and 2.5 g. The resultant peak plasma levels of venlafaxine for the latter 2 patients were 6.24 and 2.35 µg/mL, respectively, and the peak plasma levels of O-desmethylvenlafaxine were 3.37 and 1.30 µg/mL, respectively. Plasma venlafaxine levels were not obtained for the patient who ingested 6.75 g of venlafaxine. All 14 patients recovered without sequelae. Most patients reported no symptoms. Among the remaining patients, somnolence was the most commonly reported symptom. The patient who ingested 2.75 g of venlafaxine was observed to have 2 generalized convulsions and a prolongation of QTc to 500 msec, compared with 405 msec at baseline. Mild sinus tachycardia was reported in 2 of the other patients.

In postmarketing experience, overdose with venlafaxine has occurred predominantly in combination with alcohol and/or other drugs. Electrocardiogram changes (e.g., prolongation of QT interval, bundle branch block, QRS prolongation), sinus and ventricular tachycardia, bradycardia, hypotension, altered level of consciousness (ranging from somnolence to coma), seizures, vertigo, and death have been reported.

Management of Overdosage

Treatment should consist of those general measures employed in the management of overdosage with any antidepressant.

Ensure an adequate airway, oxygenation, and ventilation. Monitor cardiac rhythm and vital signs. General supportive and symptomatic measures are also recommended. Induction of emesis is not recommended. Gastric lavage with a large-bore orogastric tube with appropriate airway protection, if needed, may be indicated if performed soon after ingestion or in symptomatic patients. Activated charcoal should be administered. Due to the large volume of distribution of venlafaxine hydrochloride, forced diuresis, dialysis, hemoperfusion and exchange transfusion are unlikely to be of benefit. No specific antidotes for Effexor are known.

In managing overdosage, consider the possibility of multiple drug involvement. The physician should consider contacting a poison control center on the treatment of any overdose. Telephone numbers of certified poison control centers are listed in the *Physicians' Desk Reference* (PDR).

DOSAGE AND ADMINISTRATION

Initial Treatment

The recommended starting dose for Effexor is 75 mg/day, administered in two or three divided doses, taken with food. Depending on tolerability and the need for further clinical effect, the dose may be increased to 150 mg/day. If needed, the dose should be further increased up to 225 mg/day. When increasing the dose, increments of up to 75 mg/day should be made at intervals of no less than 4 days. In outpatient settings there was no evidence of usefulness of doses greater than 225 mg/day for moderately depressed patients, but more severely depressed inpatients responded to a mean dose of 350 mg/day. Certain patients, including more severely depressed patients, may therefore respond more to higher doses, up to a maximum of 375 mg/day, generally in three divided doses.

Dosage for Patients with Hepatic Impairment

Given the decrease in clearance and increase in elimination half-life for both venlafaxine and ODV that is observed in patients with hepatic cirrhosis compared to normal subjects (see "**CLINICAL PHARMACOLOGY**"), it is recommended that the total daily dose be reduced by 50% in patients with moderate hepatic impairment. Since there was much individual variability in clearance between patients with cirrhosis, it may be necessary to reduce the dose even more than 50%, and individualization of dosing may be desirable in some patients.

Dosage for Patients with Renal Impairment

Given the decrease in clearance for venlafaxine and the increase in elimination half-life for both venlafaxine and ODV that is observed in patients with renal impairment (GFR = 10-70 mL/min) compared to normals (see "**CLINICAL PHARMACOLOGY**"), it is recommended that the total daily dose be reduced by 25% in patients with mild to moderate renal impairment. It is recommended that the total daily dose be reduced by 50% and the dose be withheld until the dialysis treatment is completed (4 hrs) in patients undergoing hemodialysis. Since there was much individual variability in clearance between patients with renal impairment, individualization of dosing may be desirable in some patients.

Dosage for Elderly Patients

No dose adjustment is recommended for elderly patients on the basis of age. As with any antidepressant, however, caution should be exercised in treating the elderly. When individualizing the dosage, extra care should be taken when increasing the dose.

Maintenance/Continuation/Extended Treatment

There is no body of evidence available to answer the question of how long a patient should continue to be treated with Effexor. It is generally agreed that acute episodes of major depression require several months or longer of sustained pharmacologic therapy. Whether the dose of antidepressant needed to induce remission is identical to the dose needed to maintain and/or sustain euthymia is unknown.

Discontinuing Effexor (venlafaxine hydrochloride)

When discontinuing Effexor after more than 1 week of therapy, it is generally recommended that the dose be tapered to minimize the risk of discontinuation symptoms. Patients who have received Effexor for 6 weeks or more should have their dose tapered gradually over at least a 2-week period. Discontinuation symptoms have been systematically evaluated in patients taking venlafaxine, to include prospective analyses of clinical trials in Generalized Anxiety Disorder and retrospective surveys of trials in depression. Abrupt discontinuation or dose reduction of venlafaxine at various doses has been found to be associated with the appearance of new symptoms, the frequency of which increased with increased dose level and with longer duration of treatment. Reported symptoms include agitation, anorexia, anxiety, confusion, coordination impaired, diarrhea, dizziness, dry mouth, dysphoric mood, fasciculation, fatigue, headaches, hypomania, insomnia, nausea, nervousness, nightmares, sensory disturbances (including shock-like electrical sensations), somnolence, sweating, tremor, vertigo, and vomiting. It is therefore recommended that the dosage of Effexor be tapered gradually and the patient monitored. The period required for tapering may depend on the dose, duration of therapy and the individual patient. Discontinuation effects are well known to occur with antidepressants.

SWITCHING PATIENTS TO OR FROM A MONOAMINE OXIDASE INHIBITOR

At least 14 days should elapse between discontinuation of an MAOI and initiation of therapy with Effexor. In addition, at least 7 days should be allowed after stopping Effexor before starting an MAOI (see "**CONTRAINDICATIONS**" and "**WARNINGS**").

HOW SUPPLIED

Effexor® (venlafaxine hydrochloride) Tablets are available as follows:

25 mg, peach, shield-shaped tablet with "25" and a "**W**" on one side and "701" on scored reverse side.

NDC 0008-0701-01, bottle of 100 tablets.

NDC 0008-0701-02, carton of 10 Redipak® blister strips of 10 tablets each.

37.5 mg, peach, shield-shaped tablet with "37.5" and a "**W**" on one side and "781" on scored reverse side.

NDC 0008-0781-01, bottle of 100 tablets.

NDC 0008-0781-02, carton of 10 Redipak® blister strips of 10 tablets each.

50 mg, peach, shield-shaped tablet with "50" and a "**W**" on one side and "703" on scored reverse side.

NDC 0008-0703-01, bottle of 100 tablets.

NDC 0008-0703-02, carton of 10 Redipak® blister strips of 10 tablets each.

75 mg, peach, shield-shaped tablet with "75" and a "**W**" on one side and "704" on scored reverse side.

NDC 0008-0704-01, bottle of 100 tablets.

NDC 0008-0704-02, carton of 10 Redipak® blister strips of 10 tablets each.

100 mg, peach, shield-shaped tablet with "100" and a "**W**" on one side and "705" on scored reverse side.

NDC 0008-0705-01, bottle of 100 tablets.

NDC 0008-0705-02, carton of 10 Redipak® blister strips of 10 tablets each.

The appearance of these tablets is a trademark of Wyeth-Ayerst Laboratories.

Store at controlled room temperature, 20°C to 25°C (68°F to 77°F), in a dry place.

Dispense in a well-closed container as defined in the USP.

Manufactured by:
Wyeth Laboratories
A Wyeth-Ayerst Company
Philadelphia, PA 19101
CI 6027-3 Revised April 14, 2000

Shown in Product Identification Guide, page 341

EFFEXOR® XR ℞

[ĕf-fĕks'ŏr XR]
(venlafaxine hydrochloride)
Extended-Release Capsules

DESCRIPTION

Effexor XR is an extended-release capsule for oral administration that contains venlafaxine hydrochloride, a structurally novel antidepressant. Venlafaxine hydrochloride is chemically unrelated to tricyclic, tetracyclic, or other available antidepressants and to other agents used to treat Generalized Anxiety Disorder. It is designated (R/S)-1-[2-(dimethylamino)-1-(4-methoxyphenyl)ethyl] cyclohexanol hydrochloride or (±)-1-[α-[(dimethylamino)methyl]-p-methoxybenzyl] cyclohexanol hydrochloride and has the empirical formula of $C_{17}H_{27}NO_2$ hydrochloride. Its molecular weight is 313.87. The structural formula is shown below.

venlafaxine hydrochloride

Venlafaxine hydrochloride is a white to off-white crystalline solid with a solubility of 572 mg/mL in water (adjusted to ionic strength of 0.2 M with sodium chloride). Its octanol: water (0.2 M sodium chloride) partition coefficient is 0.43.

Effexor XR is formulated as an extended-release capsule for once-a-day oral administration. Drug release is controlled by diffusion through the coating membrane on the spheroids and is not pH dependent. Capsules contain venlafaxine hydrochloride equivalent to 37.5 mg, 75 mg, or 150 mg venlafaxine. Inactive ingredients consist of cellulose, ethylcellulose, gelatin, hydroxypropyl methylcellulose, iron oxide, and titanium dioxide. The 37.5 mg capsule also contains D&C Red #28, D&C Yellow #10, and FD&C Blue #1.

CLINICAL PHARMACOLOGY

Pharmacodynamics

The mechanism of the antidepressant action of venlafaxine in humans is believed to be associated with its potentiation of neurotransmitter activity in the CNS. Preclinical studies have shown that venlafaxine and its active metabolite, O-desmethylvenlafaxine (ODV), are potent inhibitors of neuronal serotonin and norepinephrine reuptake and weak inhibitors of dopamine reuptake. Venlafaxine and ODV have no significant affinity for muscarinic cholinergic, H_1-histaminergic, or α_1-adrenergic receptors *in vitro*. Pharmacologic activity at these receptors is hypothesized to be associated with the various anticholinergic, sedative, and cardiovascular effects seen with other psychotropic drugs. Venlafaxine and ODV do not possess monoamine oxidase (MAO) inhibitory activity.

Pharmacokinetics

Steady-state concentrations of venlafaxine and ODV in plasma are attained within 3 days of oral multiple dose therapy. Venlafaxine and ODV exhibited linear kinetics over the dose range of 75 to 450 mg/day. Mean±SD steady-state plasma clearance of venlafaxine and ODV is 1.3±0.6 and 0.4±0.2 L/h/kg, respectively; apparent elimination half-life is 5±2 and 11±2 hours, respectively; and apparent (steady-state) volume of distribution is 7.5±3.7 and 5.7±1.8 L/kg, respectively. Venlafaxine and ODV are minimally bound at therapeutic concentrations to plasma proteins (27 and 30%, respectively).

Absorption

Venlafaxine is well absorbed and extensively metabolized in the liver. O-desmethylvenlafaxine (ODV) is the only major active metabolite. On the basis of mass balance studies, at least 92% of a single oral dose of venlafaxine is absorbed. The absolute bioavailability of venlafaxine is about 45%.

Administration of Effexor XR (150 mg q24 hours) generally resulted in lower C_{max} (150 ng/mL for venlafaxine and 260 ng/mL for ODV) and later T_{max} (5.5 hours for venlafaxine and 9 hours for ODV) than for immediate release venlafaxine tablets ($C_{max's}$ for immediate release 75 mg q12 hours were 225 ng/mL for venlafaxine and 290 ng/mL for ODV; $T_{max's}$ were 2 hours for venlafaxine and 3 hours for ODV). When equal daily doses of venlafaxine were administered as either an immediate release tablet or the extended-release capsule, the exposure to both venlafaxine and ODV was similar for the two treatments, and the fluctuation in plasma concentrations was slightly lower with the Effexor XR capsule. Effexor XR, therefore, provides a slower rate of absorption, but the same extent of absorption compared with the immediate release tablet.

Food did not affect the bioavailability of venlafaxine or its active metabolite, ODV. Time of administration (AM vs PM) did not affect the pharmacokinetics of venlafaxine and ODV from the 75 mg Effexor XR capsule.

Metabolism and Excretion

Following absorption, venlafaxine undergoes extensive presystemic metabolism in the liver, primarily to ODV, but also to N-desmethylvenlafaxine, N,O-didesmethylvenlafaxine, and other minor metabolites. *In vitro* studies indicate that the formation of ODV is catalyzed by CYP2D6; this has been confirmed in a clinical study showing that patients with low CYP2D6 levels ("poor metabolizers") had increased

Continued on next page

Effexor-XR—Cont.

levels of venlafaxine and reduced levels of ODV compared to people with normal CYP2D6 ("extensive metabolizers"). The differences between the CYP2D6 poor and extensive metabolizers, however, are not expected to be clinically important because the sum of venlafaxine and ODV is similar in the two groups and venlafaxine and ODV are pharmacologically approximately equiactive and equipotent.

Approximately 87% of a venlafaxine dose is recovered in the urine within 48 hours as unchanged venlafaxine (5%), unconjugated ODV (29%), conjugated ODV (26%), or other minor inactive metabolites (27%). Renal elimination of venlafaxine and its metabolites is thus the primary route of excretion.

Special Populations

Age and Gender: A population pharmacokinetic analysis of 404 venlafaxine-treated patients from two studies involving both b.i.d. and t.i.d. regimens showed that dose-normalized trough plasma levels of either venlafaxine or ODV were unaltered by age or gender differences. Dosage adjustment based on the age or gender of a patient is generally not necessary (see "**DOSAGE AND ADMINISTRATION**").

Extensive/Poor Metabolizers: Plasma concentrations of venlafaxine were higher in CYP2D6 poor metabolizers than extensive metabolizers. Because the total exposure (AUC) of venlafaxine and ODV was similar in poor and extensive metabolizer groups, however, there is no need for different venlafaxine dosing regimens for these two groups.

Liver Disease: In 9 patients with hepatic cirrhosis, the pharmacokinetic disposition of both venlafaxine and ODV was significantly altered after oral administration of venlafaxine. Venlafaxine elimination half-life was prolonged by about 30%, and clearance decreased by about 50% in cirrhotic patients compared to normal subjects. ODV elimination half-life was prolonged by about 60%, and clearance decreased by about 30% in cirrhotic patients compared to normal subjects. A large degree of intersubject variability was noted. Three patients with more severe cirrhosis had a more substantial decrease in venlafaxine clearance (about 90%) compared to normal subjects. Dosage adjustment is necessary in these patients (see "**DOSAGE AND ADMINISTRATION**").

Renal Disease: In a renal impairment study, venlafaxine elimination half-life after oral administration was prolonged by about 50% and clearance was reduced by about 24% in renally impaired patients (GFR=10–70 mL/min), compared to normal subjects. In dialysis patients, venlafaxine elimination half-life was prolonged by about 180% and clearance was reduced by about 57% compared to normal subjects. Similarly, ODV elimination half-life was prolonged by about 40% although clearance was unchanged in patients with renal impairment (GFR=10–70 mL/min) compared to normal subjects. In dialysis patients, ODV elimination half-life was prolonged by about 142% and clearance was reduced by about 56% compared to normal subjects. A large degree of intersubject variability was noted. Dosage adjustment is necessary in these patients (see "**DOSAGE AND ADMINISTRATION**").

Clinical Trials

Depression

The efficacy of Effexor XR (venlafaxine hydrochloride) extended-release capsules as a treatment for depression was established in two placebo-controlled, short-term, flexible-dose studies in adult outpatients meeting DSM-III-R or DSM-IV criteria for major depression.

A 12-week study utilizing Effexor XR doses in a range 75–150 mg/day (mean dose for completers was 136 mg/day) and an 8-week study utilizing Effexor XR doses in a range 75–225 mg/day (mean dose for completers was 177 mg/day) both demonstrated superiority of Effexor XR over placebo on the HAM-D total score, HAM-D Depressed Mood Item, the MADRS total score, the Clinical Global Impressions (CGI) Severity of Illness item, and the CGI Global Improvement item. In both studies, Effexor XR was also significantly better than placebo for certain factors of the HAM-D, including the anxiety/somatization factor, the cognitive disturbance factor, and the retardation factor, as well as for the psychic anxiety score.

A 4-week study of inpatients meeting DSM-III-R criteria for major depression with melancholia utilizing Effexor (the immediate release form of venlafaxine) in a range of 150 to 375 mg/day (t.i.d. schedule) demonstrated superiority of Effexor over placebo. The mean dose in completers was 350 mg/day.

Examination of gender subsets of the population studied did not reveal any differential responsiveness on the basis of gender.

Generalized Anxiety Disorder

The efficacy of Effexor XR capsules as a treatment for Generalized Anxiety Disorder (GAD) was established in two 8-week, placebo-controlled, fixed-dose studies in outpatients meeting DSM-IV criteria for GAD.

One study evaluating Effexor XR doses of 75, 150, and 225 mg/day, and placebo showed that the 225 mg/day dose was more effective than placebo on the Hamilton Rating Scale for Anxiety (HAM-A) total score, both the HAM-A anxiety and tension items, and the Clinical Global Impressions (CGI) scale. While there was also evidence for superiority over placebo for the 75 and 150 mg/day doses, these doses were not as consistently effective as the highest dose.

A second study evaluating Effexor XR doses of 75 and 150 mg/day and placebo showed that both doses were more effective than placebo on some of these same outcomes, however, the 75 mg/day dose was more consistently effective than the 150 mg/day dose. A dose-response relationship for effectiveness in GAD was not clearly established in the 75-225 mg/day dose range utilized in these two studies.

Examination of gender subsets of the population studied did not reveal any differential responsiveness on the basis of gender.

INDICATIONS AND USAGE

Depression

Effexor XR (venlafaxine hydrochloride) extended-release capsules is indicated for the treatment of depression.

The efficacy of Effexor XR in the treatment of depression was established in 8- and 12-week controlled trials of outpatients whose diagnoses corresponded most closely to the DSM-III-R or DSM-IV category of major depressive disorder (see "**Clinical Trials**").

A major depressive episode (DSM-IV) implies a prominent and relatively persistent (nearly every day for at least 2 weeks) depressed mood or the loss of interest or pleasure in nearly all activities, representing a change from previous functioning, and includes the presence of at least five of the following nine symptoms during the same two-week period: depressed mood, markedly diminished interest or pleasure in usual activities, significant change in weight and/or appetite, insomnia or hypersomnia, psychomotor agitation or retardation, increased fatigue, feelings of guilt or worthlessness, slowed thinking or impaired concentration, a suicide attempt or suicidal ideation.

The efficacy of Effexor (the immediate release form of venlafaxine) in the treatment of depression in inpatients meeting diagnostic criteria for major depressive disorder with melancholia was established in a 4-week controlled trial (see "**Clinical Trials**"). The safety and efficacy of Effexor XR in hospitalized depressed patients have not been adequately studied.

The effectiveness of Effexor XR in long-term use, that is, for more than 12 weeks, has not been systematically evaluated in controlled trials. The physician who elects to use Effexor XR for extended periods should periodically re-evaluate the long-term usefulness of the drug for the individual patient (see "**DOSAGE AND ADMINISTRATION**").

Generalized Anxiety Disorder

Effexor XR is indicated for the treatment of Generalized Anxiety Disorder (GAD) as defined in DSM-IV. Anxiety or tension associated with the stress of everyday life usually does not require treatment with an anxiolytic.

The efficacy of Effexor XR in the treatment of GAD was established in 8-week placebo-controlled trials in outpatients diagnosed with GAD according to DSM-IV criteria (See "**Clinical Trials**").

Generalized Anxiety Disorder (DSM-IV) is characterized by excessive anxiety and worry (apprehensive expectation) that is persistent for at least 6 months and which the person finds difficult to control. It must be associated with at least 3 of the following 6 symptoms: restlessness or feeling keyed up or on edge, being easily fatigued, difficulty concentrating or mind going blank, irritability, muscle tension, sleep disturbance.

The effectiveness of Effexor XR in the long-term treatment of GAD, that is, for more than 8 weeks, has not been systematically evaluated in controlled trials. The physician who elects to use Effexor XR for extended periods should periodically re-evaluate the long-term usefulness of the drug for the individual patient (See "**DOSAGE AND ADMINISTRATION**").

CONTRAINDICATIONS

Effexor XR (venlafaxine hydrochloride) extended-release capsules is contraindicated in patients known to be hypersensitive to venlafaxine hydrochloride.

Concomitant use in patients taking monoamine oxidase inhibitors (MAOIs) is contraindicated (see "**WARNINGS**").

WARNINGS

Potential for Interaction with Monoamine Oxidase Inhibitors

Adverse reactions, some of which were serious, have been reported in patients who have recently been discontinued from a monoamine oxidase inhibitor (MAOI) and started on venlafaxine, or who have recently had venlafaxine therapy discontinued prior to initiation of an MAOI. These reactions have included tremor, myoclonus, diaphoresis, nausea, vomiting, flushing, dizziness, hyperthermia with features resembling neuroleptic malignant syndrome, seizures, and death. In patients receiving antidepressants with pharmacological properties similar to venlafaxine in combination with an MAOI, there have also been reports of serious, sometimes fatal, reactions. For a selective serotonin reuptake inhibitor, these reactions have included hyperthermia, rigidity, myoclonus, autonomic instability with possible rapid fluctuations of vital signs, and mental status changes that include extreme agitation progressing to delirium and coma. Some cases presented with features resembling neuroleptic malignant syndrome. Severe hyperthermia and seizures, sometimes fatal, have been reported in association with the combined use of tricyclic antidepressants and MAOIs. These reactions have also been reported in patients who have recently discontinued these drugs and have been started on an MAOI. The effects of combined use of venlafaxine and MAOIs have not been evaluated in humans or animals. Therefore, because venlafaxine is an inhibitor of both norepinephrine and serotonin reuptake, it is recommended that Effexor XR (venlafaxine hydrochloride) extended-release capsules not be used in combination with an MAOI, or within at least 14 days of discontinuing treatment with an MAOI. Based on the half-life of venlafaxine, at least 7 days should be allowed after stopping venlafaxine before starting an MAOI.

Sustained Hypertension

Venlafaxine is associated with sustained increases in blood pressure in some patients. Among patients treated with 75–375 mg per day of Effexor XR in premarketing studies, 3% (19/705) experienced sustained hypertension [defined as treatment-emergent supine diastolic blood pressure (SDBP) ≥90 mm Hg and ≥10 mm Hg above baseline for 3 consecutive on-therapy visits]. Among patients treated with 75–225 mg per day of Effexor XR in premarketing GAD studies, 0.4% (2/476) experienced sustained hypertension. Experience with the immediate-release venlafaxine showed that sustained hypertension was dose-related, increasing from 3–7% at 100–300 mg per day to 13% at doses above 300 mg per day. An insufficient number of patients received mean doses of Effexor XR over 300 mg/day to fully evaluate the incidence of sustained increases in blood pressure at these higher doses.

In placebo-controlled premarketing depression studies with Effexor XR 75–225 mg/day, a final on-drug mean increase in supine diastolic blood pressure (SDBP) of 1.2 mm Hg was observed for Effexor XR-treated patients compared with a mean decrease of 0.2 mm Hg for placebo-treated patients. In placebo-controlled premarketing GAD studies with Effexor XR 75–225 mg/day, a final on-drug mean increase in SDBP of 1.1 mm Hg was observed for Effexor XR-treated patients compared with a mean decrease of 0.9 mm Hg for placebo-treated patients.

In premarketing depression and GAD studies, 0.7% (5/705) and 0.4% (2/476) of the Effexor XR-treated patients, respectively, discontinued treatment because of elevated blood pressure. Among these patients, most of the blood pressure increases were in a modest range (12–16 mm Hg, SDBP in depression studies; 22 mm Hg for the two patients discontinuing for hypertension in GAD studies).

Sustained increases of SDBP could have adverse consequences. Therefore, it is recommended that patients receiving Effexor XR have regular monitoring of blood pressure. For patients who experience a sustained increase in blood pressure while receiving venlafaxine, either dose reduction or discontinuation should be considered.

PRECAUTIONS

General

Insomnia and Nervousness

Treatment-emergent insomnia and nervousness were more commonly reported for patients treated with Effexor XR (venlafaxine hydrochloride) extended-release capsules than with placebo in pooled analyses of short-term depression and GAD studies, as shown in Table 1.

[See table below]

Insomnia and nervousness each led to drug discontinuation in 0.9% of the patients treated with Effexor XR in Phase 3 depression studies.

In Phase 3 GAD trials, insomnia and nervousness led to drug discontinuation in 5% and 3%, respectively, of the patients treated with Effexor XR.

Changes in Appetite and Weight

Treatment-emergent anorexia was more commonly reported for Effexor XR-treated (8%) than placebo-treated patients (4%) in the pool of short-term depression studies. Significant weight loss, especially in underweight depressed patients, may be an undesirable result of Effexor XR treatment. A loss of 5% or more of body weight occurred in 7% of Effexor XR-treated and 2% of placebo-treated patients in placebo-controlled depression trials. Discontinuation rates for anorexia and weight loss associated with Effexor XR were low (1.0% and 0.1%, respectively, of Effexor XR-treated patients in Phase 3 depression studies).

In the pool of short-term GAD studies, treatment-emergent anorexia was reported in 13% and 2% of patients receiving Effexor XR and placebo, respectively. A loss of 7% or more of body weight occurred in 3% of the Effexor XR-treated and 0% of the placebo-treated patients in these trials. Discontinuation rates for anorexia and weight loss were low (1.7% and 0.2% respectively, of Effexor XR-treated patients).

TABLE 1
Incidence of Insomnia and Nervousness in Placebo-Controlled Depression and GAD Trials

	Depression		GAD	
Symptom	Effexor XR n = 357	Placebo n = 285	Effexor XR n = 476	Placebo n = 201
Insomnia	17%	11%	22%	11%
Nervousness	10%	5%	12%	5%

Activation of Mania/Hypomania
During premarketing depression studies, mania or hypomania occurred in 0.3% of Effexor XR-treated patients and 0.0% placebo patients. In premarketing GAD studies, 0.0% of Effexor XR-treated patients and 0.5% of placebo-treated patients experienced mania or hypomania. In all premarketing depression trials with Effexor, mania or hypomania occurred in 0.5% of venlafaxine-treated patients compared with 0% of placebo patients. Mania/hypomania has also been reported in a small proportion of patients with mood disorders who were treated with other marketed antidepressants. As with all antidepressants, Effexor XR should be used cautiously in patients with a history of mania.
Hyponatremia
Hyponatremia and/or the syndrome of inappropriate antidiuretic hormone secretion (SIADH) may occur with venlafaxine. This should be taken into consideration in patients who are, for example, volume-depleted, elderly, or taking diuretics.
Mydriasis
Mydriasis has been reported in association with venlafaxine; therefore patients with raised intra-ocular pressure or at risk of acute narrow angle glaucoma should be monitored.
Seizures
During premarketing experience, no seizures occurred among 705 Effexor XR-treated patients in the depression studies or among 476 Effexor XR-treated patients in GAD studies. In all premarketing depression trials with Effexor, seizures were reported at various doses in 0.3% (8/3082) of venlafaxine-treated patients. Effexor XR, like many antidepressants, should be used cautiously in patients with a history of seizures and should be discontinued in any patient who develops seizures.
Skin and Mucous Membrane Bleeding
The risk of skin and mucous membrane bleeding may be increased in patients taking venlafaxine. As with other serotonin-reuptake inhibitors, venlafaxine should be used cautiously in patients predisposed to bleeding at these sites.
Suicide
The possibility of a suicide attempt is inherent in depression and may persist until significant remission occurs. Close supervision of high-risk patients should accompany initial drug therapy. Prescriptions for Effexor XR should be written for the smallest quantity of capsules consistent with good patient management in order to reduce the risk of overdose.
The same precautions observed when treating patients with depression should be observed when treating patients with GAD.
Use in Patients With Concomitant Illness
Premarketing experience with venlafaxine in patients with concomitant systemic illness is limited. Caution is advised in administering Effexor XR to patients with diseases or conditions that could affect hemodynamic responses or metabolism.
Venlafaxine has not been evaluated or used to any appreciable extent in patients with a recent history of myocardial infarction or unstable heart disease. Patients with these diagnoses were systematically excluded from many clinical studies during venlafaxine's premarketing testing. The electrocardiograms for 357 patients who received Effexor XR and 285 patients who received placebo in 8- to 12-week double-blind, placebo-controlled trials in depression and the electrocardiograms for 311 patients who received Effexor XR and 153 patients who received placebo in 8-week double-blind, placebo-controlled trials in GAD were analyzed. The mean change from baseline in corrected QT interval (QT_c) for Effexor XR-treated patients in depression studies was increased relative to that for placebo-treated patients (increase of 4.7 msec for Effexor XR and decrease of 1.9 msec for placebo). The clinical significance of these changes is unknown. The mean change from baseline in corrected QT interval (QT_c) for Effexor XR-treated patients in the GAD studies did not differ significantly from that with placebo.
In these same trials, the mean change from baseline in heart rate for Effexor XR-treated patients in the depression studies was significantly higher than that for placebo (a mean increase of 4 beats per minute for Effexor XR and 1 beat per minute for placebo). The mean change from baseline in heart rate for Effexor XR-treated patients in the GAD studies was significantly higher than that for placebo (a mean increase of 3 beats per minute for Effexor XR and no change for placebo). The clinical significance of these changes is unknown.
Evaluation of the electrocardiograms for 769 patients who received immediate release Effexor in 4- to 6-week double-blind, placebo-controlled trials showed that the incidence of trial-emergent conduction abnormalities did not differ from that with placebo. In patients with renal impairment (GFR=10–70 mL/min) or cirrhosis of the liver, the clearances of venlafaxine and its active metabolites were decreased, thus prolonging the elimination half-lives of these substances. A lower dose may be necessary (see "**DOSAGE AND ADMINISTRATION**"). Effexor XR, like all antidepressants, should be used with caution in such patients.

Information for Patients
Physicians are advised to discuss the following issues with patients for whom they prescribe Effexor XR (venlafaxine hydrochloride) extended-release capsules:
Interference with Cognitive and Motor Performance
Clinical studies were performed to examine the effects of venlafaxine on behavioral performance of healthy individuals. The results revealed no clinically significant impairment of psychomotor, cognitive, or complex behavior performance. However, since any psychoactive drug may impair judgment, thinking, or motor skills, patients should be cautioned about operating hazardous machinery, including automobiles, until they are reasonably certain that venlafaxine therapy does not adversely affect their ability to engage in such activities.
Concomitant Medication
Patients should be advised to inform their physicians if they are taking, or plan to take, any prescription or over-the-counter drugs, since there is a potential for interactions.
Alcohol
Although venlafaxine has not been shown to increase the impairment of mental and motor skills caused by alcohol, patients should be advised to avoid alcohol while taking venlafaxine.
Allergic Reactions
Patients should be advised to notify their physician if they develop a rash, hives, or a related allergic phenomenon.
Pregnancy
Patients should be advised to notify their physician if they become pregnant or intend to become pregnant during therapy.
Nursing
Patients should be advised to notify their physician if they are breast-feeding an infant.

Laboratory Tests
There are no specific laboratory tests recommended.

Drug Interactions
As with all drugs, the potential for interaction by a variety of mechanisms is a possibility.
Alcohol
A single dose of ethanol (0.5 g/kg) had no effect on the pharmacokinetics of venlafaxine or O-desmethylvenlafaxine (ODV) when venlafaxine was administered at 150 mg/day in 15 healthy male subjects. Additionally, administration of venlafaxine in a stable regimen did not exaggerate the psychomotor and psychometric effects induced by ethanol in these same subjects when they were not receiving venlafaxine.
Cimetidine
Concomitant administration of cimetidine and venlafaxine in a steady-state study for both drugs resulted in inhibition of first-pass metabolism of venlafaxine in 18 healthy subjects. The oral clearance of venlafaxine was reduced by about 43%, and the exposure (AUC) and maximum concentration (C_{max}) of the drug were increased by about 60%. However, co-administration of cimetidine had no apparent effect on the pharmacokinetics of ODV, which is present in much greater quantity in the circulation than venlafaxine. The overall pharmacological activity of venlafaxine plus ODV is expected to increase only slightly, and no dosage adjustment should be necessary for most normal adults. However, for patients with pre-existing hypertension, and for elderly patients or patients with hepatic dysfunction, the interaction associated with the concomitant use of venlafaxine and cimetidine is not known and potentially could be more pronounced. Therefore, caution is advised with such patients.
Diazepam
Under steady-state conditions for venlafaxine administered at 150 mg/day, a single 10 mg dose of diazepam did not appear to affect the pharmacokinetics of either venlafaxine or ODV in 18 healthy male subjects. Venlafaxine also did not have any effect on the pharmacokinetics of diazepam or its active metabolite, desmethyldiazepam, or affect the psychomotor and psychometric effects induced by diazepam.
Haloperidol
Venlafaxine administered under steady-state conditions at 150 mg/day in 24 healthy subjects decreased total oral-dose clearance (Cl/F) of a single 2 mg dose of haloperidol by 42%, which resulted in a 70% increase in haloperidol AUC. In addition, the haloperidol C_{max} increased 88% when coadministered with venlafaxine, but the haloperidol elimination half-life ($t_{1/2}$) was unchanged. The mechanism explaining this finding is unknown.
Lithium
The steady-state pharmacokinetics of venlafaxine administered at 150 mg/day were not affected when a single 600 mg oral dose of lithium was administered to 12 healthy male subjects. ODV also was unaffected. Venlafaxine had no effect on the pharmacokinetics of lithium.
Drugs Highly Bound to Plasma Proteins
Venlafaxine is not highly bound to plasma proteins; therefore, administration of Effexor XR to a patient taking another drug that is highly protein bound should not cause increased free concentrations of the other drug.
Drugs that Inhibit Cytochrome P450 Isoenzymes
CYP2D6 Inhibitors: *In vitro* and *in vivo* studies indicate that venlafaxine is metabolized to its active metabolite, ODV, by CYP2D6, the isoenzyme that is responsible for the genetic polymorphism seen in the metabolism of many antidepressants. Therefore, the potential exists for a drug interaction between drugs that inhibit CYP2D6-mediated metabolism of venlafaxine, reducing the metabolism of venlafaxine to ODV, resulting in increased plasma concentrations of venlafaxine and decreased concentrations of the active metabolite. CYP2D6 inhibitors such as quinidine would be expected to do this, but the effect would be similar to what is seen in patients who are genetically CYP2D6 poor metabolizers (See "*Metabolism and Excretion*" under "**CLINICAL PHARMACOLOGY**"). Therefore, no dosage adjustment is required when venlafaxine is coadministered with a CYP2D6 inhibitor.
The concomitant use of venlafaxine with a drug treatment(s) that potently inhibits both CYP2D6 and CYP3A4, the primary metabolizing enzymes for venlafaxine, has not been studied. Therefore, caution is advised should a patient's therapy include venlafaxine and any agent(s) that produce simultaneous inhibition of these two enzyme systems.
Drugs Metabolized by Cytochrome P450 Isoenzymes
CYP2D6: *In vitro* studies indicate that venlafaxine is a relatively weak inhibitor of CYP2D6. These findings have been confirmed in a clinical drug interaction study comparing the effect of venlafaxine with that of fluoxetine on the CYP2D6-mediated metabolism of dextromethorphan to dextrorphan.
Imipramine—Venlafaxine did not affect the pharmacokinetics of imipramine and 2-OH-imipramine. However, desipramine AUC, C_{max}, and C_{min} increased by about 35% in the presence of venlafaxine. The 2-OH-desipramine AUC's increased by at least 2.5 fold (with venlafaxine 37.5 mg q12h) and by 4.5 fold (with venlafaxine 75 mg q12h). Imipramine did not affect the pharmacokinetics of venlafaxine and ODV. The clinical significance of elevated 2-OH-desipramine levels is unknown.
Risperidone—Venlafaxine administered under steady-state conditions at 150 mg/day slightly inhibited the CYP2D6-mediated metabolism of risperidone (administered as a single 1 mg oral dose) to its active metabolite, 9-hydroxyrisperidone, resulting in an approximate 32% increase in risperidone AUC. However, venlafaxine coadministration did not significantly alter the pharmacokinetic profile of the total active moiety (risperidone plus 9-hydroxyrisperidone).
CYP3A4: Venlafaxine did not inhibit CYP3A4 *in vitro*. This finding was confirmed *in vivo* by clinical drug interaction studies in which venlafaxine did not inhibit the metabolism of several CYP3A4 substrates, including alprazolam, diazepam, and terfenadine.
Indinavir—In a study of 9 healthy volunteers, venlafaxine administered under steady-state conditions at 150 mg/day resulted in a 28% decrease in the AUC of a single 800 mg oral dose of indinavir and a 36% decrease in indinavir C_{max}. Indinavir did not affect the pharmacokinetics of venlafaxine and ODV. The clinical significance of this finding is unknown.
CYP1A2: Venlafaxine did not inhibit CYP1A2 *in vitro*. This finding was confirmed *in vivo* by a clinical drug interaction study in which venlafaxine did not inhibit the metabolism of caffeine, a CYP1A2 substrate.
CYP2C9: Venlafaxine did not inhibit CYP2C9 *in vitro*. The clinical significance of this finding is unknown.
CYP2C19: Venlafaxine did not inhibit the metabolism of diazepam, which is partially metabolized by CYP2C19 (see "*Diazepam*" above).
Monoamine Oxidase Inhibitors
See "**CONTRAINDICATIONS**" and "**WARNINGS**."
CNS-Active Drugs
The risk of using venlafaxine in combination with other CNS-active drugs has not been systematically evaluated (except in the case of those CNS-active drugs noted above). Consequently, caution is advised if the concomitant administration of venlafaxine and such drugs is required.
Electroconvulsive Therapy
There are no clinical data establishing the benefit of electroconvulsive therapy combined with Effexor XR (venlafaxine hydrochloride) extended-release capsules treatment.
Postmarketing Spontaneous Drug Interaction Reports
See **"ADVERSE REACTIONS," "Postmarketing Reports."**

Carcinogenesis, Mutagenesis, Impairment of Fertility
Carcinogenesis
Venlafaxine was given by oral gavage to mice for 18 months at doses up to 120 mg/kg per day, which was 1.7 times the maximum recommended human dose on a mg/m^2 basis. Venlafaxine was also given to rats by oral gavage for 24 months at doses up to 120 mg/kg per day. In rats receiving the 120 mg/kg dose, plasma concentrations of venlafaxine at necropsy were 1 times (male rats) and 6 times (female rats) the plasma concentrations of patients receiving the maximum recommended human dose. Plasma levels of the O-desmethyl metabolite were lower in rats than in patients receiving the maximum recommended dose. Tumors were not increased by venlafaxine treatment in mice or rats.
Mutagenesis
Venlafaxine and the major human metabolite, O-desmethylvenlafaxine (ODV), were not mutagenic in the Ames reverse mutation assay in Salmonella bacteria or the Chinese hamster ovary/HGPRT mammalian cell forward gene mutation assay. Venlafaxine was also not mutagenic or clastogenic in the *in vitro* BALB/c-3T3 mouse cell transformation assay, the sister chromatid exchange assay in cultured Chinese hamster ovary cells, or in the *in vivo* chromosomal aberration assay in rat bone marrow. ODV was not clastogenic in the *in vitro* Chinese hamster ovary cell chromosomal aberration assay, but elicited a clastogenic response in the *in vivo* chromosomal aberration assay in rat bone marrow.
Impairment of Fertility
Reproduction and fertility studies in rats showed no effects on male or female fertility at oral doses of up to 2 times the maximum recommended human dose on a mg/m^2 basis.

Continued on next page

Effexor-XR—Cont.

Pregnancy

Teratogenic Effects—Pregnancy Category C

Venlafaxine did not cause malformations in offspring of rats or rabbits given doses up to 2.5 times (rat) or 4 times (rabbit) the maximum recommended human daily dose on a mg/m^2 basis. However, in rats, there was a decrease in pup weight, an increase in stillborn pups, and an increase in pup deaths during the first 5 days of lactation, when dosing began during pregnancy and continued until weaning. The cause of these deaths is not known. These effects occurred at 2.5 times (mg/m^2) the maximum human daily dose. The no effect dose for rat pup mortality was 0.25 times the human dose on a mg/m^2 basis. There are no adequate and well-controlled studies in pregnant women. Because animal reproduction studies are not always predictive of human response, this drug should be used during pregnancy only if clearly needed.

Labor and Delivery

The effect of venlafaxine on labor and delivery in humans is unknown.

Nursing Mothers

Venlafaxine and ODV have been reported to be excreted in human milk. Because of the potential for serious adverse reactions in nursing infants from Effexor XR, a decision should be made whether to discontinue nursing or to discontinue the drug, taking into account the importance of the drug to the mother.

Pediatric Use

Safety and effectiveness in pediatric patients have not been established.

Geriatric Use

Approximately 4% (14/357) and 3% (14/476) of Effexor XR-treated patients in placebo-controlled premarketing depression and GAD trials, respectively, were 65 years of age or over. Of 2,897 Effexor-treated patients in premarketing phase depression studies, 12% (357) were 65 years of age or over. No overall differences in effectiveness or safety were observed between geriatric patients and younger patients, and other reported clinical experience generally has not identified differences in response between elderly and younger patients. However, greater sensitivity of some older individuals cannot be ruled out. As with other antidepressants, several cases of hyponatremia and syndrome of inappropriate antidiuretic hormone secretion (SIADH) have been reported, usually in the elderly.

The pharmacokinetics of venlafaxine and ODV are not substantially altered in the elderly (see **"CLINICAL PHARMACOLOGY"**). No dose adjustment is recommended for the elderly on the basis of age alone, although other clinical circumstances, some of which may be more common in the elderly, such as renal or hepatic impairment, may warrant a dose reduction (see **"DOSAGE AND ADMINISTRATION"**).

ADVERSE REACTIONS

The information included in the Adverse Findings Observed in Short-Term, Placebo-Controlled Studies with Effexor® XR subsection is based on data from a pool of three 8- and 12-week controlled clinical trials in depression (includes two U.S. trials and one European trial) and from a pool of two 8-week controlled clinical trials in GAD with Effexor XR. Information on additional adverse events associated with Effexor XR in the entire development program for the formulation and with Effexor (the immediate release formulation of venlafaxine) is included in the "**Other Adverse Events Observed During the Premarketing Evaluation of Effexor and Effexor XR**" subsection (See also **"WARNINGS"** and **"PRECAUTIONS"**).

Adverse Findings Observed in Short-Term, Placebo-Controlled Studies with Effexor XR

Adverse Events Associated with Discontinuation of Treatment

Approximately 11% of the 357 patients who received Effexor XR (venlafaxine hydrochloride) extended-release capsules in placebo-controlled clinical trials for depression discontinued treatment due to an adverse experience, compared with 6% of the 285 placebo-treated patients in those studies. Approximately 23% of the 476 patients who received Effexor XR capsules in placebo-controlled clinical trials for GAD discontinued treatment due to an adverse experience, compared with 10% of the 201 placebo-treated patients in those studies. The most common events leading to discontinuation and considered to be drug-related (i.e., leading to discontinuation in at least 1% of the Effexor XR-treated patients at a rate at least twice that of placebo for either indication) are shown in Table 2.

[See table below]

Adverse Events Occurring at an Incidence of 2% or More Among Effexor XR-Treated Patients

Tables 3 and 4 enumerate the incidence, rounded to the nearest percent, of treatment-emergent adverse events that occurred during acute therapy of depression (up to 12 weeks) and of GAD (up to 8 weeks), respectively, in 2% or more of patients treated with Effexor XR (dose range of 75 to 225 mg/day) where the incidence in patients treated with Effexor XR was greater than the incidence for the respective placebo-treated patients. The table shows the percentage of patients in each group who had at least one episode of an event at some time during their treatment. Reported adverse events were classified using a standard COSTART-based Dictionary terminology.

The prescriber should be aware that these figures cannot be used to predict the incidence of side effects in the course of usual medical practice where patient characteristics and other factors differ from those which prevailed in the clinical trials. Similarly, the cited frequencies cannot be compared with figures obtained from other clinical investigations involving different treatments, uses and investigators. The cited figures, however, do provide the prescribing physician with some basis for estimating the relative contribution of drug and nondrug factors to the side effect incidence rate in the population studied.

Commonly Observed Adverse Events from Tables 3 and 4:

Depression

Note in particular the following adverse events that occurred in at least 5% of Effexor XR patients and at a rate at least twice that of the placebo group for all placebo-controlled trials for the depression indication (Table 3): Abnormal ejaculation, gastrointestinal complaints (nausea, dry mouth, and anorexia), CNS complaints (dizziness, somnolence, and abnormal dreams), and sweating. In the two U.S. placebo-controlled trials, the following additional events occurred in at least 5% of Effexor XR-treated patients (n=192) and at a rate at least twice that of the placebo group: Abnormalities of sexual function (impotence in men, anorgasmia in women, and libido decreased), gastrointestinal complaints (constipation and flatulence), CNS complaints (insomnia, nervousness, and tremor), problems of special senses (abnormal vision), cardiovascular effects (hypertension and vasodilatation), and yawning.

Generalized Anxiety Disorder

Note in particular the following adverse events that occurred in at least 5% of Effexor XR patients and at a rate at least twice that of the placebo group for all placebo-controlled trials for the GAD indication (Table 4): Abnormalities of sexual function (abnormal ejaculation and impotence in men, and libido decreased), gastrointestinal complaints (nausea, dry mouth, anorexia, constipation, and vomiting), CNS complaints (insomnia and nervousness), problems of special senses (abnormal vision), cardiovascular complaints (vasodilatation), yawning, and sweating.

TABLE 3
Treatment-Emergent Adverse Event Incidence in Short-Term Placebo-Controlled Effexor XR Clinical Trials in Depressed Patients[1,2]

Body System / Preferred Term	% Reporting Event Effexor XR (n=357)	Placebo (n=285)
Body as a Whole		
Asthenia	8%	7%
Cardiovascular System		
Vasodilatation[3]	4%	2%
Hypertension	4%	1%
Digestive System		
Nausea	31%	12%
Constipation	8%	5%
Anorexia	8%	4%
Vomiting	4%	2%
Flatulence	4%	3%
Metabolic/Nutritional		
Weight Loss	3%	0%
Nervous System		
Dizziness	20%	9%
Somnolence	17%	8%
Insomnia	17%	11%
Dry Mouth	12%	6%
Nervousness	10%	5%
Abnormal Dreams[4]	7%	2%
Tremor	5%	2%
Depression	3%	<1%
Paresthesia	3%	1%
Libido Decreased	3%	<1%
Agitation	3%	1%
Respiratory System		
Pharyngitis	7%	6%
Yawn	3%	0%
Skin		
Sweating	14%	3%
Special Senses		
Abnormal Vision[5]	4%	<1%
Urogenital System		
Abnormal Ejaculation (male)[6,7]	16%	<1%
Impotence[7]	4%	<1%
Anorgasmia (female)[8,9]	3%	<1%

[1] Incidence, rounded to the nearest %, for events reported by at least 2% of patients treated with Effexor XR, except the following events which had an incidence equal to or less than placebo: abdominal pain, accidental injury, anxiety, back pain, bronchitis, diarrhea, dysmenorrhea, dyspepsia, flu syndrome, headache, infection, pain, palpitation, rhinitis, and sinusitis.

[2] <1% indicates an incidence greater than zero but less than 1%.

[3] Mostly "hot flashes."

[4] Mostly "vivid dreams," "nightmares," and "increased dreaming."

[5] Mostly "blurred vision" and "difficulty focusing eyes."

[6] Mostly "delayed ejaculation."

[7] Incidence is based on the number of male patients.

[8] Mostly "delayed orgasm" or "anorgasmia."

[9] Incidence is based on the number of female patients.

[See table at bottom of next page]

Vital Sign Changes

Effexor XR (venlafaxine hydrochloride) extended-release capsules treatment for up to 12 weeks in premarketing placebo-controlled depression trials was associated with a mean final on-therapy increase in pulse rate of approximately 2 beats per minute, compared with 1 beat per minute for placebo. Effexor XR treatment for up to 8 weeks in premarketing placebo-controlled GAD trials was associated with a mean final on-therapy increase in pulse rate of approximately 2 beats per minute, compared with less than 1 beat per minute for placebo. (See the "**Sustained Hypertension**" section of "**WARNINGS**" for effects on blood pressure.)

Laboratory Changes

Effexor XR (venlafaxine hydrochloride) extended-release capsules treatment for up to 12 weeks in premarketing placebo-controlled depression trials and for up to 8 weeks in premarketing placebo-controlled GAD trials was associated with mean final on-therapy increases in serum cholesterol concentration of approximately 1.5 mg/dL and 2.5 mg/dL, respectively.

Patients treated with Effexor tablets (the immediate-release form of venlafaxine) for at least 3 months in placebo-controlled 12-month extension trials had a mean final on-therapy increase in total cholesterol of 9.1 mg/dL. This increase was duration dependent over the 12-month study period and tended to be greater with higher doses. An in-

Table 2
Common Adverse Events Leading to Discontinuation of Treatment in Placebo-Controlled Trials[1]

Adverse Event	Percentage of Patients Discontinuing Due to Adverse Event: Depression Indication[2] Effexor XR n=357	Depression Indication Placebo n=285	GAD Indication Effexor XR n=476	GAD Indication Placebo n=201
Body as a Whole				
Headache	—	—	4%	<1%
Asthenia	—	—	3%	<1%
Cardiovascular System				
Vasodilatation	—	—	1%	0%
Digestive System				
Nausea	4%	<1%	10%	<1%
Anorexia	1%	<1%	2%	<1%
Dry Mouth	1%	0%	2%	<1%
Nervous System				
Dizziness	2%	1%	4%	1%
Insomnia	1%	<1%	5%	2%
Nervousness	—	—	3%	<1%
Somnolence	2%	<1%	4%	<1%
Thinking abnormal	—	—	1%	0%
Tremor	—	—	1%	0%
Special Senses				
Abnormal Vision	—	—	1%	0%

[1] Two of the depression studies were flexible dose and one was fixed dose. The two GAD studies were fixed dose.

[2] In U.S. placebo-controlled trials for depression, the following were also common events leading to discontinuation and were considered to be drug-related for Effexor XR-treated patients (% Effexor XR [n = 192], % Placebo [n = 202]: hypertension (1%, <1%); diarrhea (1%, 0%); paresthesia (1%, 0%); tremor (1%, 0%); abnormal vision, mostly blurred vision (1%, 0%); and abnormal, mostly delayed, ejaculation (1%, 0%).

crease in serum cholesterol from baseline by ≥50 mg/dL and to values >260 mg/dL, at any time after baseline, has been recorded in 8.1% of patients.

ECG Changes

(See the "*Use in Patients with Concomitant Illnesses*" section of "**PRECAUTIONS**").

Other Adverse Events Observed During the Premarketing Evaluation of Effexor and Effexor XR

During its premarketing assessment, multiple doses of Effexor XR were administered to 705 patients in phase 3 depression studies and Effexor was administered to 96 patients. During its premarketing assessment, multiple doses of Effexor XR were administered to 476 patients in phase 3 GAD studies. In addition, in premarketing assessment of Effexor, multiple doses were administered to 2897 patients in phase 2–3 depression studies. The conditions and duration of exposure to venlafaxine in both development programs varied greatly, and included (in overlapping categories) open and double-blind studies, uncontrolled and controlled studies, inpatient (Effexor only) and outpatient studies, fixed-dose, and titration studies. Untoward events associated with this exposure were recorded by clinical investigators using terminology of their own choosing. Consequently, it is not possible to provide a meaningful estimate of the proportion of individuals experiencing adverse events without first grouping similar types of untoward events into a smaller number of standardized event categories.

In the tabulations that follow, reported adverse events were classified using a standard COSTART-based Dictionary terminology. The frequencies presented, therefore, represent the proportion of the 4174 patients exposed to multiple doses of either formulation of venlafaxine who experienced an event of the type cited on at least one occasion while receiving venlafaxine. All reported events are included except those already listed in Tables 3 and 4 and those events for which a drug cause was remote. If the COSTART term for an event was so general as to be uninformative, it was replaced with a more informative term. It is important to emphasize that, although the events reported occurred during treatment with venlafaxine, they were not necessarily caused by it.

Events are further categorized by body system and listed in order of decreasing frequency using the following definitions: **frequent** adverse events are those occurring on one or more occasions in at least 1/100 patients; **infrequent** adverse events are those occurring in 1/100 to 1/1000 patients; **rare** events are those occurring in fewer than 1/1000 patients.

Body as a whole - **Frequent:** chest pain substernal; **Infrequent:** face edema, intentional injury, malaise, moniliasis, neck rigidity, pelvic pain, photosensitivity reaction, suicide attempt; **Rare:** appendicitis, carcinoma, cellulitis, withdrawal syndrome.

Cardiovascular system - **Frequent:** migraine, postural hypotension; **Infrequent:** angina pectoris, arrhythmia, extrasystoles, hypotension, peripheral vascular disorder (mainly cold feet and/or cold hands), syncope, thrombophlebitis; **Rare:** arteritis, first-degree atrioventricular block, bigeminy, bradycardia, bundle branch block, cerebral ischemia, coronary artery disease, congestive heart failure, heart arrest, mitral valve disorder, mucocutaneous hemorrhage, myocardial infarct, pallor.

TABLE 4
Treatment-Emergent Adverse Event Incidence in Short-Term Placebo-Controlled Effexor XR Clinical Trials in GAD Patients[1,2]

Body System Preferred Term	% Reporting Event Effexor XR (n=476)	 Placebo (n=201)
Body as a Whole		
Asthenia	16%	9%
Infection[3]	10%	9%
Abdominal Pain	6%	5%
Fever	3%	<1%
Neck Pain	3%	2%
Chills	3%	<1%
Cardiovascular System		
Vasodilatation[4]	6%	2%
Tachycardia	3%	2%
Digestive System		
Nausea	43%	11%
Anorexia	13%	2%
Diarrhea	12%	10%
Constipation	12%	5%
Vomiting	6%	2%
Flatulence	3%	1%
Musculoskeletal System		
Myalgia	4%	3%
Nervous System		
Dry Mouth	23%	5%
Insomnia	22%	11%
Dizziness	20%	11%
Somnolence	20%	11%
Nervousness	12%	5%
Libido Decreased	6%	2%
Abnormal Dreams[5]	4%	2%
Tremor	4%	<1%
Paresthesia	3%	<1%
Thinking Abnormal[6]	2%	1%
Trismus	2%	0%
Twitching	2%	<1%
Respiratory System		
Rhinitis	8%	6%
Yawn	6%	<1%
Cough Increased	3%	2%
Skin		
Sweating	11%	<1%
Special Senses		
Abnormal Vision[7]	8%	0%
Urogenital System		
Abnormal Ejaculation (male)[8,9]	17%	0%
Impotence[9]	6%	1%
Dysmenorrhea[10]	6%	5%
Orgasmic Dysfunction (female)[10,11]	4%	0%
Urinary Frequency	3%	2%

[1] Incidence, rounded to the nearest %, for events reported by at least 2% of patients treated with Effexor XR, except the following events which had an incidence equal to or less than placebo: accidental injury, agitation, back pain, depression, dyspepsia, flu syndrome, headache, hypertonia, pain, palpitation, pharyngitis, sinusitis, and tinnitus.
[2] <1% indicates an incidence greater than zero but less than 1%.
[3] Mostly upper respiratory infections.
[4] Mostly "hot flashes."
[5] Mostly "vivid dreams," "nightmares," and "increased dreaming."
[6] Mostly "difficulty concentrating."
[7] Mostly "blurred vision" and "difficulty focusing eyes."
[8] Mostly "delayed ejaculation," includes "anorgasmia."
[9] Incidence is based on the number of male patients.
[10] Incidence is based on the number of female patients.
[11] Mostly "delayed orgasm" and includes "abnormal orgasm" and "anorgasmia."

Digestive system - **Frequent:** eructation, increased appetite; **Infrequent:** bruxism, colitis, dysphagia, tongue edema, esophagitis, gastritis, gastroenteritis, gastrointestinal ulcer, gingivitis, glossitis, rectal hemorrhage, hemorrhoids, melena, stomatitis, mouth ulceration; **Rare:** cheilitis, cholecystitis, cholelithiasis, hematemesis, gastrointestinal hemorrhage, gum hemorrhage, hepatitis, ileitis, jaundice, intestinal obstruction, oral moniliasis, proctitis, increased salivation, soft stools, tongue discoloration.

Endocrine system - **Rare:** goiter, hyperthyroidism, hypothyroidism, thyroid nodule, thyroiditis.

Hemic and lymphatic system - **Frequent:** ecchymosis; **Infrequent:** anemia, leukocytosis, leukopenia, lymphadenopathy, thrombocythemia, thrombocytopenia; **Rare:** basophilia, cyanosis, eosinophilia, lymphocytosis.

Metabolic and nutritional - **Frequent:** edema, weight gain; **Infrequent:** alkaline phosphatase increased, glycosuria, hypercholesteremia, hyperglycemia, hyperuricemia, hypoglycemia, hypokalemia, SGOT increased, thirst; **Rare:** alcohol intolerance, bilirubinemia, BUN increased, creatinine increased, diabetes mellitus, dehydration, gout, hemochromatosis, hypercalcinuria, hyperkalemia, hyperlipemia, hyperphosphatemia, hyponatremia, hypophosphatemia, hypoproteinemia, SGPT increased, uremia.

Musculoskeletal system - **Frequent:** arthralgia; **Infrequent:** arthritis, arthrosis, bone pain, bone spurs, bursitis, leg cramps, myasthenia, tenosynovitis; **Rare:** pathological fracture, myopathy, osteoporosis, osteosclerosis, rheumatoid arthritis, tendon rupture.

Nervous system - **Frequent:** amnesia, confusion, depersonalization, emotional lability, hypesthesia, vertigo; **Infrequent:** apathy, ataxia, circumoral paresthesia, CNS stimulation, euphoria, hallucinations, hostility, hyperesthesia, hyperkinesia, hypotonia, incoordination, libido increased, manic reaction, myoclonus, neuralgia, neuropathy, paranoid reaction, psychosis, seizure, abnormal speech, stupor; **Rare:** akathisia, akinesia, alcohol abuse, aphasia, bradykinesia, buccoglossal syndrome, cerebrovascular accident, loss of consciousness, delusions, dementia, dystonia, facial paralysis, abnormal gait, Guillain-Barré Syndrome, hypokinesia, neuritis, nystagmus, psychotic depression, reflexes decreased, reflexes increased, suicidal ideation, torticollis.

Respiratory system - **Frequent:** dyspnea; **Infrequent:** asthma, chest congestion, epistaxis, hyperventilation, laryngismus, laryngitis, pneumonia, voice alteration; **Rare:** atelectasis, hemoptysis, hypoventilation, hypoxia, pleurisy, pulmonary embolus, sleep apnea.

Skin and appendages- **Frequent:** rash, pruritus; **Infrequent:** acne, alopecia, brittle nails, contact dermatitis, dry skin, eczema, skin hypertrophy, maculopapular rash, psoriasis, urticaria; **Rare:** erythema nodosum, exfoliative dermatitis, lichenoid dermatitis, hair discoloration, skin discoloration, furunculosis, hirsutism, leukoderma, pustular rash, vesiculobullous rash, seborrhea, skin atrophy, skin striae.

Special senses- **Frequent:** abnormality of accommodation, mydriasis, taste perversion; **Infrequent:** cataract, conjunctivitis, corneal lesion, diplopia, dry eyes, exophthalmos, eye pain, hyperacusis, otitis media, parosmia, photophobia, taste loss, visual field defect; **Rare:** blepharitis, chromatopsia, conjunctival edema, deafness, glaucoma, retinal hemorrhage, subconjunctival hemorrhage, keratitis, labyrinthitis, miosis, papilledema, decreased pupillary reflex, otitis externa, scleritis, uveitis.

Urogenital system- **Frequent:** metrorrhagia,* prostatitis,* urination impaired, vaginitis*; **Infrequent:** albuminuria, amenorrhea,* cystitis, dysuria, hematuria, female lactation,* leukorrhea,* menorrhagia,* nocturia, bladder pain, breast pain, polyuria, pyuria, urinary incontinence, urinary retention, urinary urgency, vaginal hemorrhage*; **Rare:** abortion,* anuria, breast engorgement, breast enlargement, fibrocystic breast, calcium crystalluria, cervicitis,* ovarian cyst,* prolonged erection,* gynecomastia (male),* hypomenorrhea,* kidney calculus, kidney pain, kidney function abnormal, mastitis, menopause,* pyelonephritis, oliguria, salpingitis,* urolithiasis, uterine hemorrhage,* uterine spasm.*

*Based on the number of men and women as appropriate.

Postmarketing Reports

Voluntary reports of other adverse events temporally associated with the use of Effexor (the immediate release form of venlafaxine) that have been received since market introduction and that may have no causal relationship with the use of Effexor include the following; agranulocytosis, anaphylaxis, aplastic anemia, catatonia, congenital anomalies, CPK increased, deep vein thrombophlebitis, delirium, EKG abnormalities (such as atrial fibrillation, supraventricular tachycardia, ventricular extrasystoles, ventricular tachycardia), epidermal necrosis/Stevens-Johnson Syndrome, erythema multiforme, extrapyramidal symptoms (including tardive dyskinesia), hemorrhage (including eye and gastrointestinal bleeding), hepatic events (including GGT elevation; abnormalities of unspecified liver function tests; liver damage, necrosis, or failure; and fatty liver), involuntary movements, LDH increased, neuroleptic malignant syndrome-like events (including a case of a 10-year-old who may have been taking methylphenidate, was treated and recovered), pancreatitis, panic, prolactin increased, renal failure, serotonin syndrome, shock-like electrical sensations (in some cases, subsequent to the discontinuation of Effexor or tapering of dose), and syndrome of inappropriate antidiuretic hormone secretion (usually in the elderly).

Continued on next page

Effexor-XR—Cont.

There have been reports of elevated clozapine levels that were temporally associated with adverse events, including seizures, following the addition of venlafaxine. There have been reports of increases in prothrombin time, partial thromboplastin time, or INR when venlafaxine was given to patients receiving warfarin therapy.

DRUG ABUSE AND DEPENDENCE

Controlled Substance Class

Effexor XR (venlafaxine hydrochloride) extended-release capsules is not a controlled substance.

Physical and Psychological Dependence

In vitro studies revealed that venlafaxine has virtually no affinity for opiate, benzodiazepine, phencyclidine (PCP), or N-methyl-D-aspartic acid (NMDA) receptors.

Venlafaxine was not found to have any significant CNS stimulant activity in rodents. In primate drug discrimination studies, venlafaxine showed no significant stimulant or depressant abuse liability.

Discontinuation effects have been reported in patients receiving venlafaxine (see "**DOSAGE AND ADMINISTRATION**").

While venlafaxine has not been systematically studied in clinical trials for its potential for abuse, there was no indication of drug-seeking behavior in the clinical trials. However, it is not possible to predict on the basis of premarketing experience the extent to which a CNS active drug will be misused, diverted, and/or abused once marketed. Consequently, physicians should carefully evaluate patients for history of drug abuse and follow such patients closely, observing them for signs of misuse or abuse of venlafaxine (e.g., development of tolerance, incrementation of dose, drug-seeking behavior).

OVERDOSAGE

Human Experience

Among the patients included in the premarketing evaluation of Effexor XR, there were 2 reports of acute overdosage with Effexor XR in depression trials, either alone or in combination with other drugs. One patient took a combination of 6 g of Effexor XR and 2.5 mg of lorazepam. This patient was hospitalized, treated symptomatically, and recovered without any untoward effects. The other patient took 2.85 g of Effexor XR. This patient reported paresthesia of all four limbs but recovered without sequelae.

There were 2 reports of acute overdose with Effexor XR in GAD trials. One patient took a combination of 0.75 g of Effexor XR and 200 mg of paroxetine and 50 mg of zolpidem. This patient was described as being alert, able to communicate, and a little sleepy. This patient was hospitalized, treated with activated charcoal, and recovered without any untoward effects. The other patient took 1.2 g of Effexor XR. This patient recovered and no other specific problems were found. The patient had moderate dizziness, nausea, numb hands and feet, and hot-cold spells 5 days after the overdose. These symptoms resolved over the next week.

Among the patients included in the premarketing evaluation with Effexor, there were 14 reports of acute overdose with venlafaxine, either alone or in combination with other drugs and/or alcohol. The majority of the reports involved ingestion in which the total dose of venlafaxine taken was estimated to be no more than several-fold higher than the usual therapeutic dose. The 3 patients who took the highest doses were estimated to have ingested approximately 6.75 g, 2.75 g, and 2.5 g. The resultant peak plasma levels of venlafaxine for the latter 2 patients were 6.24 and 2.35 µg/mL, respectively, and the peak plasma levels of O-desmethylvenlafaxine were 3.37 and 1.30 µg/mL, respectively. Plasma venlafaxine levels were not obtained for the patient who ingested 6.75 g of venlafaxine. All 14 patients recovered without sequelae. Most patients reported no symptoms. Among the remaining patients, somnolence was the most commonly reported symptom. The patient who ingested 2.75 g of venlafaxine was observed to have 2 generalized convulsions and a prolongation of QTc to 500 msec, compared with 405 msec at baseline. Mild sinus tachycardia was reported in 2 of the other patients.

In postmarketing experience, overdose with venlafaxine has occurred predominantly in combination with alcohol and/or other drugs. Electrocardiogram changes (e.g., prolongation of QT interval, bundle branch block, QRS prolongation), sinus and ventricular tachycardia, bradycardia, hypotension, altered level of consciousness (ranging from somnolence to coma), seizures, vertigo, and death have been reported.

Management of Overdosage

Treatment should consist of those general measures employed in the management of overdosage with any antidepressant.

Ensure an adequate airway, oxygenation, and ventilation. Monitor cardiac rhythm and vital signs. General supportive and symptomatic measures are also recommended. Induction of emesis is not recommended. Gastric lavage with a large bore orogastric tube with appropriate airway protection, if needed, may be indicated if performed soon after ingestion or in symptomatic patients.

Activated charcoal should be administered. Due to the large volume of distribution of venlafaxine, forced diuresis, dialysis, hemoperfusion and exchange transfusion are unlikely to be of benefit. No specific antidotes for venlafaxine are known.

In managing overdosage, consider the possibility of multiple drug involvement. The physician should consider contacting a poison control center for additional information on the treatment of any overdose. Telephone numbers for certified poison control centers are listed in the *Physicians' Desk Reference* (PDR).

DOSAGE AND ADMINISTRATION

Effexor XR should be administered in a single dose with food either in the morning or in the evening at approximately the same time each day. Each capsule should be swallowed whole with fluid and not divided, crushed, chewed, or placed in water.

Initial Treatment

Depression

For most patients, the recommended starting dose for Effexor XR is 75 mg/day, administered in a single dose. In the clinical trials establishing the efficacy of Effexor XR in moderately depressed outpatients, the initial dose of venlafaxine was 75 mg/day. For some patients, it may be desirable to start at 37.5 mg/day for 4 to 7 days, to allow new patients to adjust to the medication before increasing to 75 mg/day. While the relationship between dose and antidepressant response for Effexor XR has not been adequately explored, patients not responding to the initial 75 mg/day dose may benefit from dose increases to a maximum of approximately 225 mg/day. Dose increases should be in increments of up to 75 mg/day, as needed, and should be made at intervals of not less than 4 days, since steady state plasma levels of venlafaxine and its major metabolites are achieved in most patients by day 4. In the clinical trials establishing efficacy, upward titration was permitted at intervals of 2 weeks or more; the average doses were about 140–180 mg/day (see "**Clinical Trials**" under "**CLINICAL PHARMACOLOGY**").

It should be noted that, while the maximum recommended dose for moderately depressed outpatients is also 225 mg/day for Effexor (the immediate release form of venlafaxine), more severely depressed inpatients in one study of the development program for that product responded to a mean dose of 350 mg/day (range of 150 to 375 mg/day). Whether or not higher doses of Effexor XR are needed for more severely depressed patients is unknown; however, the experience with Effexor XR doses higher than 225 mg/day is very limited.

Generalized Anxiety Disorder

For most patients, the recommended starting dose for Effexor XR is 75 mg/day, administered in a single dose. In clinical trials establishing the efficacy of Effexor XR in outpatients with Generalized Anxiety Disorder (GAD), the initial dose of venlafaxine was 75 mg/day. For some patients, it may be desirable to start at 37.5 mg/day for 4 to 7 days, to allow new patients to adjust to the medication before increasing to 75 mg/day. Although a dose-response relationship for effectiveness in GAD was not clearly established in fixed-dose studies, certain patients not responding to the initial 75 mg/day dose may benefit from dose increases to a maximum of approximately 225 mg/day. Dose increases should be in increments of up to 75 mg/day, as needed, and should be made at intervals of not less than 4 days.

Switching Patients from Effexor Tablets

Depressed patients who are currently being treated at a therapeutic dose with Effexor may be switched to Effexor XR at the nearest equivalent dose (mg/day), e.g., 37.5 mg venlafaxine two-times-a-day to 75 mg Effexor XR once daily. However, individual dosage adjustments may be necessary.

Patients with Hepatic Impairment

Given the decrease in clearance and increase in elimination half-life for both venlafaxine and ODV that is observed in patients with hepatic cirrhosis compared with normal subjects (see "**CLINICAL PHARMACOLOGY**"), it is recommended that the starting dose be reduced by 50% in patients with moderate hepatic impairment. Because there was much individual variability in clearance between patients with cirrhosis, individualization of dosage may be desirable in some patients.

Patients with Renal Impairment

Given the decrease in clearance for venlafaxine and the increase in elimination half-life for both venlafaxine and ODV that is observed in patients with renal impairment (GFR = 10–70 mL/min) compared with normal subjects (see "**CLINICAL PHARMACOLOGY**"), it is recommended that the total daily dose be reduced by 25%–50%. In patients undergoing hemodialysis, it is recommended that the total daily dose be reduced by 50% and that the dose be withheld until the dialysis treatment is completed (4 hrs). Because there was much individual variability in clearance between patients with renal impairment, individualization of dosage may be desirable in some patients.

Elderly Patients

No dose adjustment is recommended for elderly patients solely on the basis of age. As with any drug for the treatment of depression or generalized anxiety disorder, however, caution should be exercised in treating the elderly. When individualizing the dosage, extra care should be taken when increasing the dose.

Maintenance/Extended Treatment

There is no body of evidence available from controlled trials to indicate how long patients with depression or generalized anxiety disorder should be treated with Effexor XR.

It is generally agreed, however, that pharmacological treatment for acute episodes of depression should continue for up to six months or longer. Whether the dose of antidepressant needed to induce remission is identical to the dose needed to maintain euthymia is unknown

In patients with Generalized Anxiety Disorder, there are no efficacy data beyond eight weeks of treatment with Effexor XR. The need for continuing medication in patients with GAD who improve with Effexor XR treatment should be periodically reassessed.

Discontinuing Effexor XR

When discontinuing Effexor XR after more than 1 week of therapy, it is generally recommended that the dose be tapered to minimize the risk of discontinuation symptoms. Patients who have received Effexor XR for 6 weeks or more should have their dose tapered over at least a 2-week period. In clinical trials with Effexor XR, tapering was achieved by reducing the daily dose by 75 mg at 1 week intervals. Individualization of tapering may be necessary. Discontinuation symptoms have been systematically evaluated in patients taking venlafaxine, to include prospective analyses of clinical trials in Generalized Anxiety Disorder and retrospective surveys of trials in depression. Abrupt discontinuation or dose reduction of venlafaxine at various doses has been found to be associated with the appearance of new symptoms, the frequency of which increased with increased dose level and with longer duration of treatment. Reported symptoms include agitation, anorexia, anxiety, confusion, coordination impaired, diarrhea, dizziness, dry mouth, dysphoric mood, fasciculation, fatigue, headaches, hypomania, insomnia, nausea, nervousness, nightmares, sensory disturbances (including shock-like electrical sensations), somnolence, sweating, tremor, vertigo, and vomiting. It is therefore recommended that the dosage of Effexor XR be tapered gradually and the patient monitored. The period required for tapering may depend on the dose, duration of therapy and the individual patient. Discontinuation effects are well known to occur with antidepressants.

Switching Patients To or From a Monoamine Oxidase Inhibitor

At least 14 days should elapse between discontinuation of an MAOI and initiation of therapy with Effexor XR. In addition, at least 7 days should be allowed after stopping Effexor XR before starting an MAOI (see "**CONTRAINDICATIONS**" and "**WARNINGS**").

HOW SUPPLIED

Effexor® XR (venlafaxine hydrochloride) extended-release capsules are available as follows:

37.5 mg, grey cap/peach body with "**W**" and "Effexor XR" on the cap and "37.5" on the body.

NDC 0008-0837-01, bottle of 100 capsules.

NDC 0008-0837-03, carton of 10 Redipak® blister strips of 10 capsules each.

Store at controlled room temperature, 20°C to 25°C (68°F to 77°F).

Bottles: Protect from light. Dispense in light-resistant container.

Blisters: Protect from light. Use blister carton to protect contents from light.

75 mg, peach cap and body with "**W**" and "Effexor XR" on the cap and "75" on the body.

NDC 0008-0833-01, bottle of 100 capsules.

NDC 0008-0833-03, carton of 10 Redipak® blister strips of 10 capsules each.

Store at controlled room temperature, 20°C to 25°C (68°F to 77°F).

150 mg, dark orange cap and body with "**W**" and "Effexor XR" on the cap and "150" on the body.

NDC 0008-0836-01, bottle of 100 capsules.

NDC 0008-0836-03, carton of 10 Redipak® blister strips of 10 capsules each.

Store at controlled room temperature, 20°C to 25°C (68°F to 77°F).

The appearance of these capsules is a trademark of Wyeth-Ayerst Laboratories.

Manufactured by:
Wyeth Laboratories
A Wyeth-Ayerst Company
Philadelphia, PA 19101

CI 5044-5 Revised April 14, 2000

Shown in Product Identification Guide, page 341

ENBREL® ℞

[ĕn' brĕl]

etanercept

DESCRIPTION

ENBREL (etanercept) is a dimeric fusion protein consisting of the extracellular ligand-binding portion of the human 75 kilodalton (p75) tumor necrosis factor receptor (TNFR) linked to the Fc portion of human IgG1. The Fc component of etanercept contains the C_H2 domain, the C_H3 domain and hinge region, but not the C_H1 domain of IgG1. Etanercept is produced by recombinant DNA technology in a Chinese hamster ovary (CHO) mammalian cell expression system. It consists of 935 amino acids and has an apparent molecular weight of approximately 150 kilodaltons.

ENBREL is supplied as a sterile, white, preservative-free, lyophilized powder for parenteral administration after reconstitution with 1 mL of the supplied Sterile Bacteriostatic Water for Injection, USP (containing 0.9% benzyl alcohol). Following reconstitution, the solution of ENBREL is clear and colorless, with a pH of 7.4 ± 0.3. Each single-use vial of ENBREL contains 25 mg etanercept, 40 mg mannitol, 10 mg sucrose, and 1.2 mg tromethamine.

CLINICAL PHARMACOLOGY

General

Etanercept binds specifically to tumor necrosis factor (TNF) and blocks its interaction with cell surface TNF receptors. TNF is a naturally occurring cytokine that is involved in normal inflammatory and immune responses. It plays an important role in the inflammatory processes of rheumatoid arthritis (RA), polyarticular-course juvenile rheumatoid arthritis (JRA) and the resulting joint pathology.[1,2] Elevated levels of TNF are found in the synovial fluid of RA patients.[3] Two distinct receptors for TNF (TNFRs), a 55 kilodalton protein (p55) and a 75 kilodalton protein (p75), exist naturally as monomeric molecules on cell surfaces and in soluble forms.[4] Biological activity of TNF is dependent upon binding to either cell surface TNFR.

Etanercept is a dimeric soluble form of the p75 TNF receptor that can bind to two TNF molecules. It inhibits the activity of TNF in vitro and has been shown to affect several animal models of inflammation, including murine collagen-induced arthritis.[5,6] Etanercept inhibits binding of both TNFα and TNFβ (lymphotoxin alpha [LTα]) to cell surface TNFRs, rendering TNF biologically inactive.[6] Cells expressing transmembrane TNF that bind ENBREL are not lysed in vitro in the presence or absence of complement.[6]

Etanercept can also modulate biological responses that are induced or regulated by TNF, including expression of adhesion molecules responsible for leukocyte migration (i.e., E-selectin and to a lesser extent intercellular adhesion molecule-1 [ICAM-1]), serum levels of cytokines (e.g., IL-6), and serum levels of matrix metalloproteinase-3 (MMP-3 or stromelysin).[6]

Pharmacokinetics

After administration of 25 mg of ENBREL by a single subcutaneous (SC) injection to three patients with RA, a median half-life of 115 hours (range 98 to 300 hours) was observed with a clearance of 89 mL/hr (52 mL/hr/m^2). A maximum serum concentration (Cmax) of 1.2 mcg/mL (range 0.6 to 1.5 mcg/mL) and time to Cmax of 72 hours (range 48 to 96 hours) was observed in these patients. After continued dosing of RA patients (N = 25) with ENBREL for 6 months with 25 mg twice weekly, the median observed level was 3.0 mcg/mL (range 1.7 to 5.6 mcg/mL). Based on the available data, individual patients may undergo a two- to five-fold increase in serum levels with repeated dosing. Serum concentrations in patients with RA have not been measured for periods of dosing that exceed 6 months.

Pharmacokinetic parameters were not different between men and women and did not vary with age in adult patients. No formal pharmacokinetic studies have been conducted to examine the effects of renal or hepatic impairment or interactions with methotrexate.

Pediatric patients with JRA (ages 4 to 17 years) were administered 0.4 mg/kg of ENBREL for up to 18 weeks. The average serum concentration after repeated dosing was 2.1 mcg/mL, with a range of 0.7 to 4.3 mcg/mL. Preliminary data suggest that the clearance of ENBREL is reduced slightly in children ages 4 to 8 years. Children <4 years of age have not been studied.

CLINICAL STUDIES

Adult Rheumatoid Arthritis

The safety and efficacy of ENBREL were assessed in two randomized, double-blind, controlled studies. Study I evaluated 234 patients with active RA who were ≥ 18 years old, had failed therapy with at least one but no more than four disease-modifying antirheumatic drugs (DMARDs; e.g., hydroxychloroquine, oral or injectable gold, methotrexate [MTX], azathioprine, D-penicillamine, sulfasalazine), and had ≥ 12 tender joints, ≥ 10 swollen joints, and either ESR ≥ 28 mm/hour, CRP > 2.0 mg/dL, or morning stiffness for ≥ 45 minutes. Doses of 10 mg or 25 mg ENBREL or placebo were administered SC twice a week for 6 consecutive months. Results from patients receiving 25 mg are presented below.

Study II evaluated 89 patients with similar inclusion criteria to Study I except that subjects in Study II had additionally received MTX for at least 6 months with a stable dose (12.5 to 25 mg/wk) for at least 4 weeks and they had at least 6 tender or painful joints. Subjects in Study II received a dose of 25 mg ENBREL or placebo SC twice a week for 6 months in addition to their stable MTX dose.

Study III compared the efficacy of ENBREL to MTX in patients with active RA. This study evaluated 632 patients who were ≥ 18 years old with early (≤ 3 years disease duration) active RA; had never received treatment with MTX; and had ≥ 12 tender joints, ≥ 10 swollen joints, and either ESR ≥ 28 mm/hr, CRP > 2.0 mg/dL, or morning stiffness for ≥ 45 minutes. Doses of 10 mg or 25 mg ENBREL were administered SC twice a week for 12 consecutive months. Results from patients receiving 25 mg are presented below. MTX tablets (escalated from 7.5 mg/week to a maximum of 20 mg/week over the first 8 weeks of the trial) or placebo tablets were given once a week on the same day as the injection of placebo or ENBREL doses, respectively.

The results of all 3 trials were expressed in percentage of patients with improvement in RA using American College of Rheumatology (ACR) response criteria.[7]

Clinical Response

The percent of ENBREL-treated patients receiving ACR 20, 50, and 70 responses was consistent across all 3 trials. The results of the three trials are summarized in Table 1.

[See table 1 above]

Table 1
ACR Responses in Placebo- and Active-Controlled Trials
(Percent of Patients)

	Placebo Controlled				Active Controlled	
	Study I		Study II		Study III	
Response	Placebo N = 80	ENBREL[a] N = 78	MTX/Placebo N = 30	MTX/ENBREL[a] N = 59	MTX N = 217	ENBREL[a] N = 207
ACR 20						
Month 3	23%	62%[b]	33%	66%[b]	56%	62%
Month 6	11%	59%[b]	27%	71%[b]	58%	65%
Month 12	NA	NA	NA	NA	65%	72%
ACR 50						
Month 3	8%	41%[b]	0%	42%[b]	24%	29%
Month 6	5%	40%[b]	3%	39%[b]	32%	40%
Month 12	NA	NA	NA	NA	43%	49%
ACR 70						
Month 3	4%	15%[b]	0	15%[b]	7%	13%[c]
Month 6	1%	15%[b]	0	15%[b]	14%	21%[c]
Month 12	NA	NA	NA	NA	22%	25%

a. 25 mg ENBREL SC twice weekly.
b. $p < 0.01$, ENBREL vs. placebo.
c. $p < 0.05$, ENBREL vs. MTX.

The time course for ACR 20 response rates for patients receiving placebo or 25 mg ENBREL in Studies I and II is summarized in Figure 1. The time course of responses to ENBREL in Study III were similar.

Figure 1
Time Course of ACR 20 Responses

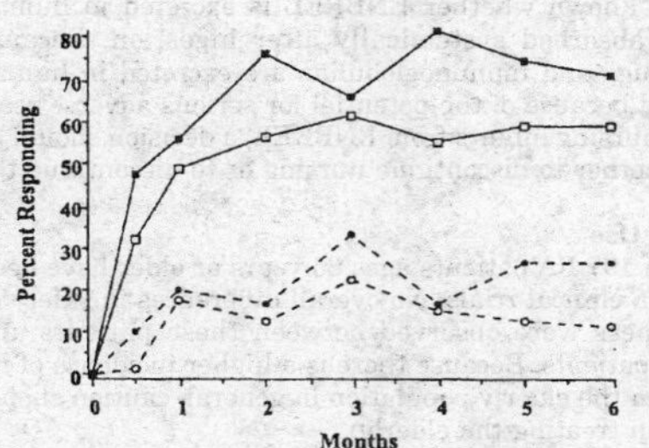

Among patients receiving ENBREL, the clinical responses generally appeared within 1 to 2 weeks after initiation of therapy and nearly always occurred by 3 months. A dose response was seen in Studies I and III; 25 mg ENBREL was more effective than 10 mg (10 mg was not evaluated in Study II). ENBREL was significantly better than placebo in all components of the ACR criteria as well as other measures of RA disease activity not included in the ACR response criteria, such as morning stiffness.

In Study III, approximately 10% of patients treated with ENBREL achieved a major clinical response, defined as maintenance of an ACR 70 response over a 6-month period.

The results of the components of the ACR response criteria for Study I are shown in Table 2. Findings were similar in Studies II and III for patients treated with ENBREL.

[See table 2 above]

Table 2
Components of ACR Response in Study I

	Placebo N = 80		ENBREL[a] N = 78	
Parameter (median)	Baseline	3 Months	Baseline	3 Months*
Number of tender joints[b]	34.0	29.5	31.2	10.0[f]
Number of swollen joints[c]	24.0	22.0	23.5	12.6[f]
Physician global assessment[d]	7.0	6.5	7.0	3.0[f]
Patient global assessment[d]	7.0	7.0	7.0	3.0[f]
Pain[d]	6.9	6.6	6.9	2.4[f]
Diability index[e]	1.7	1.8	1.6	1.0[f]
ESR (mm/hr)	31.0	32.0	28.0	15.5[f]
CRP (mg/dL)	2.8	3.9	3.5	0.9[f]

* Results at 6 months showed similar improvement.
a. 25 mg ENBREL SC twice weekly.
b. Scale 0-71.
c. Scale 0-68.
d. Visual analog scale; 0 = best, 10 = worst.
e. Health assessment questionnaire; 0 = best, 3 = worst; includes eight categories: dressing and grooming, arising, eating, walking, hygiene, reach, grip, and activities.
f. $p < 0.01$, ENBREL vs. placebo, based on mean percent change from baseline.

After discontinuation of ENBREL, symptoms of arthritis generally returned within a month. Reintroduction of treatment with ENBREL after discontinuations of up to 18 months resulted in the same magnitudes of response as patients who received ENBREL without interruption of therapy based on results of open-label studies. Continued durable responses have been seen for up to 36 months in open-label extension treatment trials when patients received ENBREL without interruption.

A Health Assessment Questionnaire (HAQ),[8] which included disability, vitality, mental health, general health status, and arthritis-associated health status subdomains, was administered every 3 months during Studies I and III. All subdomains of the HAQ were improved in patients treated with ENBREL.

In Study III, health outcome measures were assessed by the SF-36 questioinnaire. The eight subscales of the SF-36 were combined into two summary scales, the physical component summary (PCS) and the mental component sumary (MCS).[9] At 12 months, patients treated with 25 mg ENBREL showed significantly more improvement in the PCS compared to the 10 mg ENBREL group, but not in the MCS.

Radiographic Response

In Study III, structural joint damage was assessed radiographically and expressed as change in total Sharp score (TSS) and its components, the erosion score and joint space narrowing (JSN) score. Radiographs of hands/wrists and forefeet were read at baseline, 6 months, and 12 months. The results are shown in Table 3. A significant difference for change in erosion score was observed at 6 months and maintained at 12 months.

[See table 3 at top of next page]

Polyarticular-Course Juvenile Rheumatoid Arthritis (JRA)

The safety and efficacy of ENBREL were assessed in a two-part study of 69 children with polyarticular-course JRA who had a variety of JRA onset types. Patients ages 4 to 17 years with moderately to severely active polyarticular-course JRA refractory to or intolerant of methotrexate were enrolled; patients remained on a stable dose of a single nonsteroidal anti-inflammatory drug and/or prednisone (≤ 0.2 mg/kg/day or 10 mg maximum). In part 1, all patients received 0.4 mg/kg (maximum 25 mg per dose) ENBREL SC twice weekly. In part 2, patients with a clinical response at day 90 were randomized to remain on ENBREL or receive placebo for four months and assessed for disease flare. Responses were measured using the JRA Definition of Improvement (DOI),[10] defined as ≥ 30% improvement in at least three of six and ≥ 30% worsening in no more than one of six JRA core set criteria, including active joint count, limitation of motion, physician and patient/parent global assessments, functional assessment, and ESR. Disease flare was defined as a ≥ 30% worsening in three of six JRA core set criteria and ≥ 30% improvement in not more than one of six JRA core set criteria and a minimum of two active joints.

In part 1 of the study, 51 of 69 (74%) patients demonstrated a clinical response and entered part 2.[11] In part 2, 6 of 25 (24%) patients remaining on ENBREL experienced a disease flare compared to 20 of 26 (77%) patients receiving placebo (p=0.007). From the start of part 2, the median time to flare was ≥ 116 days for patients who received ENBREL and 28 days for patients who received placebo. Each component of the JRA core set criteria worsened in the arm that

Continued on next page

Enbrel—Cont.

received placebo and remained stable or improved in the arm that continued on ENBREL. The data suggested the possibility of a higher flare rate among those patients with a higher baseline ESR. Of patients who demonstrated a clinical response at 90 days and entered part 2 of the study, some of the patients remaining on ENBREL continued to improve from month 3 through month 7, while those who received placebo did not improve.

The majority of JRA patients who developed a disease flare in part 2 and reintroduced ENBREL treatment up to 4 months after discontinuation re-responded to ENBREL therapy, in open-label studies. Most of the responding patients who continued ENBREL therapy without interruption have maintained responses for up to 18 months.

Studies have not been done in patients with polyarticular-course JRA to assess the effects of continued ENBREL therapy in patients who do not respond within 3 months of initiating ENBREL therapy, or to assess the combination of ENBREL with methotrexate.

Immunogenicity

Patients were tested at multiple timepoints for antibodies to ENBREL. Antibodies to ENBREL, all non-neutralizing, were detected at least once in sera of 16% of adult rheumatoid arthritis patients. No apparent correlation of antibody development to clinical response or adverse events was observed. Results from JRA patients were similar to those seen in adult RA patients treated with ENBREL. The long-term immunogenicity of ENBREL is unknown.

The data reflect the percentage of patients whose test results were considered positive for antibodies to ENBREL in an ELISA assay, and are highly dependent on the sensitivity and specificity of the assay. Additionally, the observed incidence of antibody positivity in an assay may be influenced by several factors including sample handling, concomitant medications, and underlying disease. For these reasons, comparison of the incidence of antibodies to ENBREL with the incidence of antibodies to other products may be misleading.

INDICATIONS AND USAGE

ENBREL is indicated for reducing signs and symptoms and delaying structural damage in patients with moderately to severely active rheumatoid arthritis. ENBREL can be used in combination with methotrexate in patients who do not respond adequately to methotrexate alone.

ENBREL is indicated for reducing signs and symptoms of moderately to severely active polyarticular-course juvenile rheumatoid arthritis in patients who have had an inadequate response to one or more DMARDs.

CONTRAINDICATIONS

ENBREL should not be administered to patients with sepsis or with known hypersensitivity to ENBREL or any of its components.

WARNINGS

IN POST-MARKETING REPORTS, SERIOUS INFECTIONS AND SEPSIS, INCLUDING FATALITIES, HAVE BEEN REPORTED WITH THE USE OF ENBREL. MANY OF THESE SERIOUS EVENTS HAVE OCCURRED IN PATIENTS WITH UNDERLYING DISEASES THAT IN ADDITION TO THEIR RHEUMATOID ARTHRITIS COULD PREDISPOSE THEM TO INFECTIONS. PATIENTS WHO DEVELOP A NEW INFECTION WHILE UNDERGOING TREATMENT WITH ENBREL SHOULD BE MONITORED CLOSELY. ADMINISTRATION OF ENBREL SHOULD BE DISCONTINUED IF A PATIENT DEVELOPS A SERIOUS INFECTION OR SEPSIS. TREATMENT WITH ENBREL SHOULD NOT BE INITIATED IN PATIENTS WITH ACTIVE INFECTIONS, INCLUDING CHRONIC OR LOCALIZED INFECTIONS. PHYSICIANS SHOULD EXERCISE CAUTION WHEN CONSIDERING THE USE OF ENBREL IN PATIENTS WITH A HISTORY OF RECURRING INFECTIONS, OR WITH UNDERLYING CONDITIONS WHICH MAY PREDISPOSE PATIENTS TO INFECTIONS, SUCH AS ADVANCED OR POORLY CONTROLLED DIABETES (see **PRECAUTIONS, ADVERSE REACTIONS, Infections**).

PRECAUTIONS

General

Allergic reactions associated with administration of ENBREL during clinical trials have been reported in < 2% of patients. If an anaphylactic reaction or other serious allergic reaction occurs, administration of ENBREL should be discontinued immediately and appropriate therapy initiated.

Information to Patients

If a patient or caregiver is to self-administer ENBREL, he/she should be instructed in injection techniques and how to measure the correct dose to help ensure the proper administration of ENBREL (see **How to Use ENBREL, Instructions for Preparing and Giving an Injection.**) The first injection should be performed under the supervision of a qualified health care professional. The patient's or caregiver's ability to self-inject subcutaneously should be assessed. A puncture-resistant container for disposal of needles and syringes should be used. Patients and caregivers should be instructed in the technique as well as proper syringe and needle disposal, and be cautioned against reuse of these items.

Immunosuppression

The possibility exists for anti-TNF therapies, including ENBREL, to affect host defenses against infections and malignancies since TNF mediates inflammation and modulates cellular immune responses. In a study of 49 patients with RA treated with ENBREL, there was no evidence of depression of delayed-type hypersensitivity, depression of immunoglobulin levels, or change in enumeration of effector cell populations. The impact of treatment with ENBREL on the development and course of malignancies, as well as active and/or chronic infections is not fully understood (see **WARNINGS, ADVERSE REACTIONS, Infections** and **Malignancies**). The safety and efficacy of ENBREL in patients with immunosuppression or chronic infections have not been evaluated.

Table 3
Mean Radiographic Change Over 6 and 12 Months in Study III

		MTX	25 mg Enbrel	MTX - ENBREL (95% Confidence Interval*)	P value
12 Months	Total Sharp score	1.59	1.00	0.59 (−0.12, 1.30)	0.110
	Erosion score	1.03	0.47	0.56 (0.11, 1.00)	0.002
	JSN score	0.56	0.52	0.04 (−0.39, 0.46)	0.529
6 Months	Total Sharp score	1.06	0.57	0.49 (0.06, 0.91)	0.001
	Erosion score	0.68	0.30	0.38 (0.09, 0.66)	0.001
	JSN score	0.38	0.27	0.11 (−0.14, 0.35)	0.585

* 95% confidence intervals for the differences in change scores between MTX and ENBREL

Immunizations

No data are available on the effects of vaccination in patients receiving ENBREL. Live vaccines should not be given concurrently with ENBREL. No data are available on the secondary transmission of infection by live vaccines in patients receiving ENBREL (see **PRECAUTIONS, Immunosuppression**).

It is recommended that JRA patients, if possible, be brought up to date with all immunizations in agreement with current immunization guidelines prior to initiating ENBREL therapy. Two JRA patients developed varicella infection and signs and symptoms of aseptic meningitis, which resolved without sequelae. Patients with a significant exposure to varicella virus should temporarily discontinue ENBREL therapy and be considered for prophylactic treatment with Varicella Zoster Immune Globulin.

Autoantibody Formation

Treatment with ENBREL may result in the formation of autoimmune antibodies (see **ADVERSE REACTIONS, Autoantibodies**).

Drug Interactions

Specific drug interactions studies have not been conducted with ENBREL.

Carcinogenesis, Mutagenesis, and Impairment of Fertility

Long-term animal studies have not been conducted to evaluate the carcinogenic potential of ENBREL or its effect on fertility. Mutagenesis studies were conducted in vitro and in vivo, and no evidence of mutagenic activity was observed.

Pregnancy (Category B)

Developmental toxicity studies have been performed in rats and rabbits at doses ranging from 60- to 100-fold higher than the human dose and have revealed no evidence of harm to the fetus due to ENBREL. There are, however, no studies in pregnant women. Because animal reproduction studies are not always predictive of human response, this drug should be used during pregnancy only if clearly needed.

Nursing Mothers

It is not known whether ENBREL is excreted in human milk or absorbed systemically after ingestion. Because many drugs and immunoglobulins are excreted in human milk, and because of the potential for serious adverse reactions in nursing infants from ENBREL, a decision should be made whether to discontinue nursing or to discontinue the drug.

Geriatric Use

A total of 197 RA patients ages 65 years or older have been studied in clinical trials. No overall differences in safety or effectiveness were observed between these patients and younger patients. Because there is a higher incidence of infections in the elderly population in general, caution should be used in treating the elderly.

Pediatric Use

ENBREL is indicated for treatment of polyarticular-course juvenile rheumatoid arthritis in patients who have had an inadequate response to one or more DMARDs. For issues relevant to pediatric patients, in addition to other sections of the label, see also **PRECAUTIONS, Immunizations**, and **ADVERSE REACTIONS, Adverse Reactions in Pediatric Patients.** ENBREL has not been studied in children < 4 years of age.

ADVERSE REACTIONS

ENBREL has been studied in 1197 patients with RA, followed for up to 36 months. The proportion of patients who discontinued treatment due to adverse events was approximately 4% in both ENBREL and placebo-treated patients.

Injection Site Reactions

In controlled trials, 37% of patients treated with ENBREL developed injection site reactions. All injection site reactions were described as mild to moderate (erythema and/or itching, pain, or swelling) and generally did not necessitate drug discontinuation. Injection site reactions generally occurred in the first month and subsequently decreased in frequency. The mean duration of injection site reactions was 3 to 5 days. Seven percent of patients experienced redness at a previous injection site when subsequent injections were given.

Infections

In controlled trials, there were no differences in rates of infection among patients treated with ENBREL and those treated with placebo or MTX. The most common type of infection was upper respiratory infection, which occurred in 16% of placebo-treated patients and 29% of patients treated with ENBREL. When the longer observation of patients on ENBREL was accounted for, the event rate was similar in both groups.

In placebo-controlled trials in DMARD-refractory RA, no increase in the incidence of serious infections was observed (approximately 1% in both placebo and ENBREL-treated groups). The rates of infections for the ENBREL arm in Study III were similar. In all clinical trials in RA, 50 of 1197 subjects exposed to ENBREL for up to 36 months experienced serious infections, including pyelonephritis, bronchitis, septic arthritis, abdominal abscess, cellulitis, osteomyelitis, wound infection, pneumonia, foot abscess, leg ulcer, diarrhea, sinusitis, and sepsis. Serious infections, including sepsis and death, have also been reported during post-marketing use of ENBREL. Some have occurred within a few weeks after initiating treatment with ENBREL. Many of the patients had underlying conditions (e.g., diabetes, congestive heart failure, history of active or chronic infections) in addition to their rheumatoid arthritis. (See **WARNINGS**). Data from a sepsis clinical trial not specifically in patients with RA suggest that ENBREL treatment may increase mortality in patients with established sepsis.[12]

Malignancies

Seventeen malignancies of various types were observed in 1197 RA patients treated in clinical trials with ENBREL for up to 36 months. The observed rates and incidences were similar to those expected for the population studied.

Autoantibodies

Patients had serum samples tested for autoantibodies at multiple timepoints. In Studies I and II, the percentage of the patients evaluated for antinuclear antibodies (ANA), the percentage of patients who developed new positive ANA (≥ 1:40) was higher in patients treated with ENBREL (11%) than in placebo-treated patients (5%). The percentage of patients who developed new positive anti–double-stranded DNA antibodies was also higher by radioimmunoassay (15% of patients treated with ENBREL compared to 4% of placebo-treated patients) and by crithidia lucilae assay (3% of patients treated with ENBREL compared to none of placebo-treated patients). The proportion of patients treated with ENBREL who developed anticardiolipin antibodies was similarly increased compared to placebo-treated patients. In Study III, no pattern of increased autoantibody development was seen in ENBREL patients compared to MTX patients.

No patients in placebo- and active-controlled trials developed clinical signs suggestive of a lupus-like syndrome. The impact of long-term treatment with ENBREL on the development of autoimmune diseases is unknown.

Other Adverse Reactions

Table 4 summarizes events reported in at least 3% of all patients with higher incidence in patients treated with ENBREL compared to controls in placebo-controlled RA trials (including the combination methotrexate trial) and relevant events from Study III.

[See table 4 at bottom of next page]

Among patients with rheumatoid arthritis treated in placebo-controlled trials, serious adverse events occurred at a frequency of 4% in 349 patients treated with ENBREL compared to 5% of 152 placebo-treated patients. In Study III, serious adverse events occurred at a frequency of 6% in 415 patients treated with ENBREL compared to 8% of 217 MTX-treated patients. Among patients with RA in placebo-controlled, active-controlled, and open-label trials of ENBREL, malignancies (see **ADVERSE REACTIONS, Malignancies**) and infections (see **ADVERSE REACTIONS, Infections**) were the most common serious adverse events observed. Other infrequent serious adverse events observed included heart failure, myocardial infarction, myocardial ischemia, cerebral ischemia, hypertension, hypotension, cholecystitis, pancreatitis, gastrointestinal hemorrhage, bursitis, depression, dyspnea, deep vein thrombosis, pulmonary embolism, membranous glomerulonephropathy, polymyositis, and thrombophlebitis.

Adverse Reactions in Pediatric Patients

In general, the adverse events in pediatric patients were similar in frequency and type as those seen in adult patients. Differences from adults and other special considerations are discussed in the following paragraphs.

Severe adverse reactions reported in 69 JRA patients ages 4 to 17 years included varicella (see also **PRECAUTIONS – Immunizations**), gastroenteritis, depression/personality disorder, cutaneous ulcer, esophagitis/gastritis, group A streptococcal septic shock, type I diabetes mellitus, and soft tissue and post-operative wound infection.

Forty-three of 69 (62%) children with JRA experienced an infection while receiving ENBREL during 3 months of study (part 1 open-label), and the frequency and severity of infections was similar in 58 patients completing 12 months of open-label extension therapy. The types of infections reported in JRA patients were generally mild and consistent with those commonly seen in outpatient pediatric populations.

The following adverse events were reported more commonly in 69 JRA patients receiving 3 months of ENBREL compared to the 349 adult RA patients in placebo-controlled trials. These included headache (19% of patients, 1.7 events per patient year), nausea (9%, 1.0 events per patient year), abdominal pain (19%, 0.74 events per patient year), and vomiting (13%, 0.74 events per patient year).

OVERDOSAGE

The maximum tolerated dose of ENBREL has not been established in humans. Toxicology studies have been performed in monkeys at doses up to 30 times the human dose with no evidence of dose-limiting toxicities. No dose-limiting toxicities have been observed during clinical trials of ENBREL. Single IV doses up to 60 mg/m^2 have been administered to healthy volunteers in an endotoxemia study without evidence of dose-limiting toxicities. The highest dose level evaluated in RA patients has been a single IV loading dose of 32 mg/m^2 followed by SC doses of 16 mg/m^2 (~25 mg) administered twice weekly. In one RA trial, one patient mistakenly self-administered 62 mg ENBREL SC twice weekly for 3 weeks without experiencing adverse effects.

DOSAGE AND ADMINISTRATION

The recommended dose of ENBREL for adult patients with rheumatoid arthritis is 25 mg given twice weekly as a subcutaneous injection 72–96 hours apart (see **Clinical Studies**). Methotrexate, glucocorticoids, salicylates, nonsteroidal anti-inflammatory drugs (NSAIDs), or analgesics may be continued during treatment with ENBREL. Higher doses of ENBREL have not been studied.

The recommended dose of ENBREL for pediatric patients ages 4 to 17 years with active polyarticular-course JRA is 0.4 mg/kg (up to a maximum 25 mg per dose) given twice weekly as a subcutaneous injection 72–96 hours apart. Glucocorticoids, nonsteroidal anti-inflammatory drugs (NSAIDs), or analgesics may be continued during treatment with ENBREL. Concurrent use with methotrexate and higher doses of ENBREL have not been studied in pediatric patients.

Preparation of ENBREL

ENBREL is intended for use under the guidance and supervision of a physician. Patients may self-inject only if their physician determines that it is appropriate and with medical follow-up, as necessary, after proper training in how to measure the correct dose and in injection technique.

Note: The needle cover of the diluent syringe contains dry natural rubber (latex), which should not be handled by persons sensitive to this substance.

ENBREL should be reconstituted aseptically with 1 mL of the supplied Sterile Bacteriostatic Water for Injection, USP (0.9% benzyl alcohol) giving a solution of 1.0 mL containing 25 mg of ENBREL. During reconstitution of ENBREL, the diluent should be injected very slowly into the vial. Some foaming will occur. This is normal. To avoid excessive foaming, **do not shake or vigorously agitate**. The contents should be swirled gently during dissolution. Generally, dissolution of ENBREL takes less than 10 minutes. The reconstituted solution should be clear and colorless and used within 6 hours (see **Storage and Stability**).

Visually inspect the solution for particulate matter and discoloration prior to administration. The solution should not be used if discolored or cloudy, or if particulate matter remains. Withdraw the solution into the syringe, removing only the dose to be given from the vial. Some foam or bubbles may remain in the vial.

No other medications should be added to solutions containing ENBREL, and do not reconstitute ENBREL with other diluents. Do not filter reconstituted solution during preparation or administration.

Rotate sites for self-injection (thigh, abdomen, or upper arm). New injections should be given at least one inch from an old site and never into areas where the skin is tender, bruised, red, or hard. (See **How to Use ENBREL, Instructions for Preparing and Giving an Injection** instruction sheet.)

Storage and Stability

Do not use a dose tray beyond the date stamped on the carton dose tray label, vial label, or diluent syringe label. The dose tray containing ENBREL (sterile powder) must be refrigerated at 2–8°C (36–46°F). DO NOT FREEZE.

Administer reconstituted solutions as soon as possible after reconstitution. If not administered immediately after reconstitution, ENBREL may be stored in the vial at 2–8°C (36–46°F) for up to 6 hours. **ANY ENBREL NOT USED WITHIN 6 HOURS OF RECONSTITUTION SHOULD BE DISCARDED, PRODUCT STABILITY AND STERILITY CANNOT BE ASSURED.**

HOW SUPPLIED

ENBREL is supplied in a carton containing four dose trays (NDC 58406-425-34). Each dose tray contains one 25 mg single-use vial of etanercept, one syringe (1 mL Sterile Bacteriostatic Water for Injection, USP, containing 0.9% benzyl alcohol), one plunger, and two alcohol swabs.

Rx only

REFERENCES

1. Feldman M, Brennan FM, Maini RN. The role of cytokines in rheumatoid arthritis. Ann Rev Immunol 1996;14:397.
2. Grom A, Murray KF, Luyrink L et al. Patterns of expression of tumor necrosis factor α, tumor necrosis factor β, and their receptors in synovia of patients with juvenile rheumatoid arthritis and juvenile spondyloarthropathy. Arthritis Rheum 1996;39;1703.
3. Saxne T, Palladino Jr MA, Heinegard D, et al. Detection of tumor necrosis factor alpha but not tumor necrosis factor beta in rheumatoid arthritis synovial fluid and serum. Arthritis Rheum 1998;31:1041.
4. Smith CA, Farrah T, Goodwin RG. The TNF receptor superfamily of cellular and viral proteins: activation, costimulation, and death. Cell 1994;75:959.
5. Wooley PH, Dutcher J, Widmer MB, et al. Influence of a recombinant human soluble tumor necrosis factor receptor FC fusion protein on type II collagen-induced arthritis in mice. J Immunol 1993;151:6602.
6. Data on file, Immunex Corporation.
7. Felson DT, Anderson JJ, Boers M, et al. American College of Rheumatology preliminary definition of improvement in rheumatoid arthritis. Arthritis Rheum 1995;6:727.
8. Ramey DR, Fries JF, Singh G. The Health Assessment Questionnaire 1995 – Status and Review. In: Spilker B, ed. "Quality of Life and Pharmacoeconomics in Clinical Trials." 2nd ed. Philadelphia, PA. Lippincott-Raven;1996.
9. Ware JE, Gandek, B. Overview of the SF-36 Health Survey and the International Quality of Life Assessment (IQOLA) Project. J Clin Epidemiol 1998; 51(11):903–12.
10. Giannini EH, Ruperto N, Ravelli A, et al. Preliminary definition of improvement in juvenile arthritis. Arthr Rheum 1997;40(7):1202.
11. Lovell DJ, Giannini EH, Reiff A, et al. Etanercept in children with polyarticular juvenile rheumatoid arthritis. N Engl J Med 2000; 342(11):763–9.
12. Fisher CJ Jr, Agosti JM, Opal SM, et al. Treatment of septic shock with the tumor necrosis factor receptor:Fc fusion protein. The Soluble TNF Receptor Sepsis Study Group. N Engl J Med 1996;334(26):1697.

0311-04
Issue Date 06/2000
Manufactured by:
Immunex Corporation
Seattle, Washington 98101
U.S. License Number 1132
Marketed by Immunex Corporation and Wyeth-Ayerst Pharmaceuticals
Immunex U.S. Patent Numbers:
5,605,690; 5,712,155; 5,395,760; 5,945,397

Table 4
Percent of RA Patients Reporting Adverse Events in Controlled Clinical Trials*

Event	Placebo Controlled		Active Controlled (Study III)	
	Percent of patients		Percent of patients	
	Placebo† (n = 152)	ENBREL (n = 349)	MTX (n = 217)	ENBREL (n = 415)
Injection site reaction	10	37	7	34
Infection	32	35	72	64
Non-upper respiratory infection**	32	38	60	51
Upper respiratory infection**	16	29	39	31
Headache	13	17	27	24
Nausea	10	9	29	15
Rhinitis	8	12	14	16
Dizziness	5	7	11	8
Pharyngitis	5	7	9	6
Cough	3	6	6	5
Asthenia	3	5	12	11
Abdominal Pain	3	5	10	10
Rash	3	5	23	14
Peripheral edema	3	2	4	8
Respiratory disorder	1	5	NA	NA
Dyspepsia	1	4	10	11
Sinusitis	2	3	3	5
Vomiting	-	3	8	5
Mouth ulcer	1	2	14	6
Alopecia	1	1	12	6
Pneumonitis ("MTX lung")	-	-	2	0

* Includes data from the 6-month study in which patients received concurrent MTX therapy.
† The duration of exposure for patients receiving placebo was less than the ENBREL-treated patients.
** Includes data from two of the three placebo controlled trials.

EQUAGESIC® Ⓒ ℞

[ek "wa-je 'zik]
(meprobamate with aspirin)

DESCRIPTION

Each tablet of Equagesic contains 200 mg meprobamate and 325 mg aspirin. The inactive ingredients present are cellulose, D&C Yellow 10, FD&C Red 3, FD&C Yellow 6, hydrogenated vegetable oil, magnesium stearate, polacrilin potassium, and starch.

HOW SUPPLIED

Equagesic® (meprobamate with aspirin) Tablets, 200 mg meprobamate and 325 mg aspirin, are available as follows: NDC 0008-0091, pink and yellow, double-layer, round, scored tablet marked "WYETH" and "91", in bottles of 100 tablets.

Store at room temperature, approx. 25°C (77°F).
Keep tightly closed.
Protect from light.
Dispense in light-resistant, tight container.

The appearance of EQUAGESIC tablets is a registered trademark of Wyeth-Ayerst Laboratories.

Manufactured by:
Wyeth Laboratories Inc.
A Wyeth-Ayerst Company
Philadelphia, PA 19101
CI 3343-6 Revised November 18, 1994

For full prescribing information write to Professional Service, Wyeth-Ayerst Pharmaceuticals, P.O. Box 8299, Philadelphia, PA 19101, or contact your local Wyeth-Ayerst representative.

EQUANIL® Ⓒ ℞

[ek 'wah-nil]
(meprobamate)
Tablets

DESCRIPTION

Meprobamate is a white powder with a characteristic odor and a bitter taste. It is slightly soluble in water, freely soluble in acetone and alcohol, and sparingly soluble in ether. Equanil tablets contain 200 mg or 400 mg meprobamate. The inactive ingredients present are lactose, methylcellulose, polacrilin potassium, and stearic acid.

HOW SUPPLIED

Equanil® (meprobamate) Tablets are available in the following dosage strengths:

200 mg, NDC 0008-0002, white, five-sided tablet marked "WYETH" and "2", in bottles of 100 tablets.

400 mg, NDC 0008-0001, white, round, scored tablet marked "WYETH" and "1", in bottles of 100 and 500 tablets.

Keep tightly closed.
Dispense in tight container.
Store at room temperature, approximately 25°C (77°F).

Manufactured by:
Wyeth Laboratories Inc.
A Wyeth-Ayerst Company
Philadelphia, PA 19101
CI 3313-6 Revised January 18, 1994

For prescribing information write to Professional Service, Wyeth-Ayerst Pharmaceuticals, P.O. Box 8299, Philadelphia, PA 19101, or contact your local Wyeth-Ayerst representative.

FACTREL® ℞

[făc-trĕl ']
(gonadorelin hydrochloride)
Synthetic Luteinizing Hormone Releasing Hormone (LH-RH)
DIAGNOSTIC USE ONLY

HOW SUPPLIED

LYOPHILIZED POWDER

in single-dose Secule® vials containing 100 mcg (NDC 0046-0507-05) and 500 mcg (NDC 0046-0509-05) gonadorelin as

Continued on next page

Factrel—Cont.

the hydrochloride with 100 mg lactose, USP. Each Secule® vial is accompanied by one ampul containing 2 mL sterile diluent of 2% benzyl alcohol in sterile water.
Secule® —Registered trademark to designate a vial containing an injectable preparation in dry form.
CI 4992-1 Issued July 25, 1997
For full prescribing information turn to the Diagnostic Product Information section of this edition of the PDR.

FLUOTHANE® ℞

[flū 'o-thān]
(halothane, USP)
Inhalation

Caution: Federal law prohibits dispensing without prescription.

DESCRIPTION

Fluothane (halothane, USP) is supplied as a liquid and is vaporized for use as an inhalation anesthetic. It is 2-bromo-2-chloro-1, 1, 1-trifluoro-ethane and has the following structural formula:

```
     Br  F
     |   |
  H—C—C—F
     |   |
     Cl  F
```

$C_2HBrClF_3$

The molecular weight is 197.38. The drug substance halothane molecule has an asymmetric carbon atom; the commercial product is a racemic mixture. Resolution of the mixture has not been reported.*

*Klaus Florey, editor, Analytical Profiles of Drug Substances, Vol. 1, page 127, (1972).

Halothane is miscible with alcohol, chloroform, ether, and other fat solvents.
The specific gravity is 1.872–1.877 at 20°C, and the boiling point (range) is 49°C–51°C at 760 mm Hg. The vapor pressure is 243 mm Hg at 20°C. The blood/gas coefficient is 2.5 at 37°C, and the olive oil/water coefficient is 220 at 37°C. Vapor concentrations within anesthetic range are nonirritating and have a pleasant odor.
Fluothane is nonflammable, and its vapors mixed with oxygen in proportions from 0.5 to 50% (v/v) are not explosive. Fluothane does not decompose in contact with warm soda lime. When moisture is present, the vapor attacks aluminum, brass, and lead, but not copper. Rubber, some plastics, and similar materials are soluble in Fluothane; such materials will deteriorate rapidly in contact with Fluothane vapor or liquid. Stability of Fluothane is maintained by the addition of 0.01% thymol (w/w), up to 0.00025% ammonia (w/w).

CLINICAL PHARMACOLOGY

Fluothane is an inhalation anesthetic. Induction and recovery are rapid, and depth of anesthesia can be rapidly altered. Fluothane progressively depresses respiration. There may be tachypnea with reduced tidal volume and alveolar ventilation. Fluothane is not an irritant to the respiratory tract, and no increase in salivary or bronchial secretions ordinarily occurs. Pharyngeal and laryngeal reflexes are rapidly obtunded. It causes bronchodilation. Hypoxia, acidosis, or apnea may develop during deep anesthesia.
Fluothane reduces the blood pressure and frequently decreases the pulse rate. The greater the concentration of the drug, the more evident these changes become. Atropine may reverse the bradycardia. Fluothane does not cause the release of catecholamines from adrenergic stores. Fluothane also causes dilation of the vessels of the skin and skeletal muscles.
Cardiac arrhythmias may occur during Fluothane anesthesia. These include nodal rhythm, AV dissociation, ventricular extrasystoles, and asystole. Fluothane sensitizes the myocardial conduction system to the action of epinephrine and norepinephrine, and the combination may cause serious cardiac arrhythmias. Fluothane increases cerebrospinal-fluid pressure. Fluothane produces moderate muscular relaxation. Muscle relaxants are used as adjuncts in order to maintain lighter levels of anesthesia. Fluothane augments the action of nondepolarizing relaxants and ganglionic-blocking agents. Fluothane is a potent uterine relaxant.
The mechanism(s) whereby Fluothane and other substances induce general anesthesia is unknown. Fluothane is a very potent anesthetic in humans, with a minimum alveolar concentration (MAC) determined to be 0.64%. The MAC has been found to decrease with age (see MAC table in "Dosage and Administration").

INDICATIONS AND USAGE

Fluothane (halothane, USP) is indicated for the induction and maintenance of general anesthesia.

CONTRAINDICATIONS

Fluothane is not recommended for obstetrical anesthesia except when uterine relaxation is required.

WARNINGS

When previous exposure to Fluothane was followed by unexplained hepatic dysfunction and/or jaundice, consideration should be given to the use of other agents.

PRECAUTIONS

GENERAL
Fluothane should be used in vaporizers that permit a reasonable approximation of output, and preferably of the calibrated type. The vaporizer should be placed out of circuit in closed-circuit rebreathing systems; otherwise, overdosage is difficult to avoid. The patient should be closely observed for signs of overdosage, i.e., depression of blood pressure, pulse rate, and ventilation, particularly during assisted or controlled ventilation.
Fluothane increases cerebrospinal-fluid pressure. Therefore, in patients with markedly raised intracranial pressure, if Fluothane is indicated, administration should be preceded by measures ordinarily used to reduce cerebrospinal-fluid pressure. Ventilation should be carefully assessed, and it may be necessary to assist or control ventilation to ensure adequate oxygenation and carbon dioxide removal.
In susceptible individuals, halothane anesthesia may trigger a skeletal-muscle hypermetabolic state leading to a high oxygen demand and the clinical syndrome known as malignant hyperthermia. The syndrome includes nonspecific features such as muscle rigidity, tachycardia, tachypnea, cyanosis, arrhythmias, and unstable blood pressure. (It should also be noted that many of these nonspecific signs may appear with light anesthesia, acute hypoxia, etc.) An increase in overall metabolism may be reflected in an elevated temperature (which may rise rapidly, early or late in the case, but usually is not the first sign of augmented metabolism) and an increased usage of the CO_2 absorption system (hot canister). PaO_2 and pH may decrease, and hyperkalemia and a base deficit may appear. Treatment includes discontinuance of triggering agents (e.g., halothane), administration of intravenous dantrolene, and application of supportive therapy. Such therapy includes vigorous efforts to restore body temperature to normal, respiratory and circulatory support as indicated, and management of electrolyte-fluid-acid-base derangements. Renal failure may appear later, and urine flow should be sustained if possible. It should be noted that the syndrome of malignant hyperthermia secondary to halothane appears to be rare.
INFORMATION FOR PATIENTS
When appropriate, as in some cases where discharge is anticipated soon after general anesthesia, patients should be cautioned not to drive automobiles, operate hazardous machinery, or engage in hazardous sports for 24 hours or more (depending on the total dose of Fluothane, condition of the patient, and consideration given to other drugs administered after anesthesia).
DRUG INTERACTIONS
Epinephrine or norepinephrine should be employed cautiously, if at all, during Fluothane (halothane, USP) anesthesia, since their simultaneous use may induce ventricular tachycardia or fibrillation.
Nondepolarizing relaxants and ganglionic-blocking agents should be administered cautiously, since their actions are augmented by Fluothane (halothane, USP).
Clinical experience and animal experiments suggest that pancuronium should be given with caution to patients receiving chronic tricyclic antidepressant therapy who are anesthetized with halothane, because severe ventricular arrhythmias may result from such usage.
CARCINOGENESIS, MUTAGENESIS, IMPAIRMENT OF FERTILITY
An 18-month inhalational carcinogenicity study of halothane at 0.05% in the mouse revealed no evidence of anesthetic-related carcinogenicity. This concentration is equivalent to 24 hours of 1% halothane.
Mutagenesis testing of halothane revealed both positive and negative results. In the rat, one-year exposure to trace concentrations of halothane (1 and 10 ppm) and nitrous oxide produced chromosomal damage to spermatogonia cells and bone marrow cells. Negative mutagenesis tests included: Ames bacterial assay, Chinese hamster lung fibroblast assay, sister chromatid exchange in Chinese hamster ovary cells, and human leukocyte culture assay.
Reproduction studies of halothane (10 ppm) and nitrous oxide in the rat caused decreased fertility. This trace concentration corresponds to 1/1000 the human maintenance dose.
PREGNANCY
Teratogenic Effects: Pregnancy Category C. Some studies have shown Fluothane to be teratogenic, embryotoxic, and fetotoxic in the mouse, rat, hamster, and rabbit at subanesthetic and/or anesthetic concentrations. There are no adequate and well-controlled studies in pregnant women. Fluothane should be used during pregnancy only if the potential benefit justifies the potential risk to the fetus.
LABOR AND DELIVERY
The uterine relaxation obtained with Fluothane, unless carefully controlled, may fail to respond to ergot derivatives and oxytocic posterior pituitary extract.
NURSING MOTHERS
It is not known whether this drug is excreted in human milk. Because many drugs are excreted in human milk, caution should be exercised when Fluothane is administered to a nursing woman.
PEDIATRIC USE
Extensive clinical experience reveals that maintenance concentrations of halothane are generally higher in infants and children, and that maintenance requirements decrease with age. See MAC table, based upon age, in "Dosage and Administration."

ADVERSE REACTIONS

The following adverse reactions have been reported: mild, moderate, and severe hepatic dysfunction (including hepatic necrosis); cardiac arrest; hypotension; respiratory arrest; cardiac arrhythmias; hyperpyrexia; shivering; nausea; and emesis.

OVERDOSAGE

In the event of overdosage, or what may appear to be overdosage, drug administration should be stopped, and assisted or controlled ventilation with pure oxygen initiated.

DOSAGE AND ADMINISTRATION

Fluothane may be administered by the nonrebreathing technique, partial rebreathing, or closed technique. The induction dose varies from patient to patient but is usually within the range of 0.5% to 3%. The maintenance dose varies from 0.5% to 1.5%.
Fluothane may be administered with either oxygen or a mixture of oxygen and nitrous oxide.
Fluothane should not be kept indefinitely in vaporizer bottles not specifically designed for its use. Thymol does not volatilize along with Fluothane and, therefore, accumulates in the vaporizer and may, in time, impart a yellow color to the remaining liquid or to wicks in vaporizers. The development of such discoloration may be used as an indicator that the vaporizer should be drained and cleaned, and the discolored Fluothane (halothane, USP) discarded. Accumulation of thymol may be removed by washing with diethyl ether. After cleaning a wick or vaporizer, make certain all the diethyl ether has been removed before reusing the equipment to avoid introducing ether into the system.
Because of the more rapid uptake of Fluothane and the increased blood concentration required for anesthesia in younger patients, the minimum alveolar concentration (MAC)[1] values will decrease with age as follows:

Age	MAC %
Infants	1.08
3 yrs.	0.91
10 yrs.	0.87
15 yrs.	0.92
24 yrs.	0.84
42 yrs.	0.76
81 yrs.	0.64

HOW SUPPLIED

Fluothane® (halothane, USP) is available in unit packages of 125 mL (NDC 0046-3125-81) and 250 mL (NDC 0046-3125-82) of halothane, USP, stabilized with 0.01% thymol (w/w) and up to 0.00025% ammonia (w/w).
HANDLING AND STORAGE
Store at room temperature (approximately 25°C) in a tight, closed container.
Protect from light.
Use carton to protect contents from light.

PHYSICIAN REFERENCE

1. Gregory, GA et al: *Anesthesiology* 1969; *30*(*5*):488–491.

Manufactured for:
Ayerst Laboratories Inc.
A Wyeth-Ayerst Company
Philadelphia, PA 19101
By ICI Chemicals and Polymers Ltd.
Runcorn, Cheshire, U.K.
CI 3816-6 Revised June 23, 1994

GRISACTIN® ℞

[griz-ăc 'tĭn]
(griseofulvin) microsize

Caution: Federal law prohibits dispensing without prescription.

DESCRIPTION

Griseofulvin is an oral fungistatic antibiotic for the treatment of superficial mycoses. It is derived from a species of *Penicillium.*
Grisactin is produced by a special process that fractures griseofulvin particles into minute crystals of irregular shape offering a greater and more effective surface area for increased gastrointestinal absorption.
Grisactin Capsules and Tablets contain the following inactive ingredients:
— 250 mg capsules: black iron oxide, D&C Yellow No. 10, FD&C Blue No. 2, FD&C Red No. 40, FD&C Yellow No. 6, gelatin, lactose, magnesium stearate, titanium dioxide, water.
— 500 mg tablets: calcium carboxymethylcellulose, D&C Red No. 36, gelatin, magnesium stearate, starch.

HOW SUPPLIED

Grisactin (griseofulvin) microsize—
Grisactin 250, each capsule contains 250 mg, in bottles of 100 (NDC 0046-0443-81) and 500 (NDC 0046-0443-85).
Grisactin 500, each tablet (scored) contains 500 mg, in bottles of 60 (NDC 0046-0444-60).
Store at room temperature (approximately 25°C)
Dispense in a well-closed container as defined in the USP
Manufactured by:
Ayerst Laboratories Inc.
A Wyeth-Ayerst Company
Philadelphia, PA 19101
CI 4103-3 Revised February 11, 1994

For prescribing information write to Professional Service, Wyeth-Ayerst Pharmaceuticals, P.O. Box 8299, Philadelphia, PA 19101, or contact your local Wyeth-Ayerst representative.
Shown in Product Identification Guide, page 341

HEPARIN ℞

[hep 'ăh-rĭn]

Lock Flush Solution, USP

Caution: Federal law prohibits dispensing without prescription.

Heparin Lock Flush Solution is intended for maintenance of patency of intravenous injection devices only and is not to be used for anticoagulant therapy.

DESCRIPTION

TUBEX® Heparin Lock Flush Solution, USP is a sterile solution. Each mL contains either 10 or 100 USP units heparin sodium derived from porcine intestinal mucosa (standardized for use as an anticoagulant) in normal saline solution, and not more than 10 mg benzyl alcohol as a preservative. The pH range is 5.0 to 7.5.

The potency is determined by biological assay using a USP reference standard based upon units of heparin activity per milligram.

Heparin is a heterogenous group of straight-chain anionic mucopolysaccharides, called glycosaminoglycans, having anticoagulant properties. Although others may be present, the main sugars occurring in heparin are: (1) α-L-iduronic acid 2-sulfate, (2) 2-deoxy-2-sulfamino-α-D-glucose 6-sulfate, (3) β-D-glucuronic acid, (4) 2-acetamido-2-deoxy-α-D-glucose, and (5) α-L-iduronic acid. These sugars are present in decreasing amounts, usually in the order (2) > (1) > (4) > (3) > (5), and are joined by glycosidic linkages forming polymers of varying sizes. Heparin is strongly acidic because of its content of covalently linked sulfate and carboxylic acid groups. In heparin sodium, the acidic protons of the sulfate units are partially replaced by sodium ions.

STRUCTURE OF HEPARIN SODIUM (representative subunits):

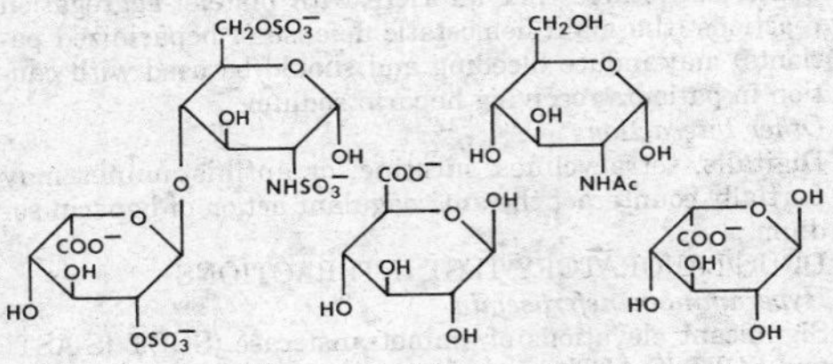

CLINICAL PHARMACOLOGY

Heparin inhibits reactions that lead to the clotting of blood and the formation of fibrin clots both *in vitro* and *in vivo.* Heparin acts at multiple sites in the normal coagulation systems. Small amounts of heparin in combination with antithrombin III (heparin cofactor) can inhibit thrombosis by inactivating activated Factor X and inhibiting the conversion of prothrombin to thrombin. Once active thrombosis has developed, larger amounts of heparin can inhibit further coagulation by inactivating thrombin and preventing the conversion of fibrinogen to fibrin. Heparin also prevents the formation of a stable fibrin clot by inhibiting the activation of the fibrin stabilizing factor.

Bleeding time is usually unaffected by heparin. Clotting time is prolonged by full therapeutic doses of heparin; in most cases, it is not measurably affected by low doses of heparin.

Loglinear plots of heparin plasma concentrations with time, for a wide range of dose levels, are linear which suggests the absence of zero order processes. Liver and the reticuloendothelial system are the sites of biotransformation. The biphasic elimination curve, a rapidly declining alpha phase ($t_{1/2}$ = 10 min.), and after the age of 40 a slower beta phase, indicates uptake in organs. The absence of a relationship between anticoagulant half-life and concentration half-life may reflect factors such as protein binding of heparin.

Heparin does not have fibrinolytic activity; therefore, it will not lyse existing clots.

INDICATIONS AND USAGE

Heparin Lock Flush Solution, USP is intended to maintain patency of an indwelling venipuncture device designed for intermittent injection or infusion therapy or blood sampling. Heparin Lock Flush Solution, USP may be used following initial placement of the device in the vein, after each injection of a medication or after withdrawal of blood for laboratory tests. (See "**Dosage and Administration,** MAINTENANCE OF PATENCY OF INTRAVENOUS DEVICES," for direction for use.)

Heparin Lock Flush Solution, USP is not to be used for anticoagulant therapy.

CONTRAINDICATIONS

Heparin sodium should not be used in patients with the following conditions:

severe thrombocytopenia; an uncontrollable active bleeding state (see **"Warnings"**), except when this is due to disseminated intravascular coagulation.

WARNINGS

This product contains benzyl alcohol as a preservative. Benzyl alcohol has been reported to be associated with a fatal "Gasping Syndrome" in premature neonates.

Neonatologists do not advise the use of 100 units/mL concentration because of the risk of bleeding, especially in low birth weight neonates.

Heparin is not intended for intramuscular use.

HYPERSENSITIVITY

Patients with documented hypersensitivity to heparin should be given the drug only in clearly life-threatening situations. (See "**Adverse Reactions**, HYPERSENSITIVITY.")

HEMORRHAGE

Hemorrhage can occur at virtually any site in patients receiving heparin. An unexplained fall in hematocrit, fall in blood pressure or any other unexplained symptom should lead to serious consideration of a hemorrhagic event.

Heparin sodium should be used with extreme caution in infants and in patients with disease states in which there is increased danger of hemorrhage. Some of the conditions in which increased danger of hemorrhage exists are:

Cardiovascular—subacute bacterial endocarditis, severe hypertension.

Surgical—during and immediately following (a) spinal tap or spinal anesthesia or (b) major surgery, especially involving the brain, spinal cord, or eye.

Hematologic—conditions associated with increased bleeding tendencies, such as hemophilia, thrombocytopenia and some vascular purpuras.

Gastrointestinal—ulcerative lesions and continuous tube drainage of the stomach or small intestine.

Other—menstruation, liver disease with impaired hemostasis.

THROMBOCYTOPENIA

Thrombocytopenia has been reported to occur in patients receiving heparin with a reported incidence of 0 to 30%. Mild thrombocytopenia (count greater than 100,000/mm^3) may remain stable or reverse even if heparin is continued. However, thrombocytopenia of any degree should be monitored closely. If the count falls below 100,000/mm^3 or if recurrent thrombosis develops (see **Precautions**, GENERAL, *White-clot Syndrome*"), the heparin product should be discontinued. If continued heparin therapy is essential, administration of heparin from a different organ source can be reinstituted with caution.

PRECAUTIONS

GENERAL

In infants, the cumulative amounts of heparin and benzyl alcohol received from the frequent administration of Heparin Lock Flush Solution, USP during a 24–hour period should be considered.

Precautions must be exercised when drugs which are incompatible with heparin are administered through an indwelling intravenous catheter containing Heparin Lock Flush Solution, USP. (See "**Dosage and Administration**, MAINTENANCE OF PATENCY OF INTRAVENOUS DEVICES.")

White-clot Syndrome

It has been reported that patients on heparin may develop new thrombus formation in association with thrombocytopenia, resulting from irreversible aggregation of platelets induced by heparin, the so-called "white-clot syndrome." The process may lead to severe thromboembolic complications like skin necrosis, gangrene of the extremities that may lead to amputation, myocardial infarction, pulmonary embolism, stroke, and possibly death. Therefore, heparin administration should be promptly discontinued if a patient develops new thrombosis in association with thrombocytopenia.

Increased Risk in Older Women

A higher incidence of bleeding has been reported in women over 60 years of age.

LABORATORY TESTS

Periodic platelet counts, hematocrits and tests for occult blood in stool are recommended during the entire course of heparin use (see **"Dosage and Administration"**).

DRUG INTERACTIONS

Platelet Inhibitors

Drugs such as acetylsalicylic acid, dextran, phenylbutazone, ibuprofen, indomethacin, dipyridamole, hydroxychloroquine, and others that interfere with platelet-aggregation reactions (the main hemostatic defense of heparinized patients) may induce bleeding and should be used with caution in patients receiving heparin sodium.

Other Interactions

Digitalis, tetracyclines, nicotine, or antihistamines may partially counteract the anticoagulant action of heparin sodium.

CARCINOGENESIS, MUTAGENESIS, IMPAIRMENT OF FERTILITY

No long-term studies in animals have been performed to evaluate carcinogenic potential of heparin sodium. Also, no reproduction studies in animals have been performed concerning mutagenesis or impairment of fertility.

PREGNANCY

Teratogenic Effects —Pregnancy Category C

Animal reproduction studies have not been conducted with heparin sodium. It is also not known whether heparin sodium can cause fetal harm when administered to a pregnant woman or can affect reproduction capacity. Heparin sodium should be given to a pregnant woman only if clearly needed.

Nonteratogenic Effects

Heparin does not cross the placental barrier.

NURSING MOTHERS

Heparin is not excreted in human milk.

PEDIATRIC USE

Heparin Lock Flush Solution, USP is not recommended for use in the neonate (see **"Warnings"**).

ADVERSE REACTIONS

HEMORRHAGE

Hemorrhage is the chief complication that may result from heparin use (see **"Warnings,** HEMORRHAGE"). An overly prolonged clotting time or minor bleeding during therapy can usually be controlled by withdrawing the drug (see **"Overdosage"**).

LOCAL IRRITATION

Local irritation and erythema have been reported with the use of Heparin Lock Flush Solution, USP.

HYPERSENSITIVITY

Generalized hypersensitivity reactions have been reported, with chills, fever, and urticaria as the most usual manifestations, and asthma, rhinitis, lacrimation, headache, nausea and vomiting, and anaphylactoid reactions, including shock, occurring more rarely. Itching and burning, especially on the plantar side of the feet, may occur.

Thrombocytopenia has been reported to occur in patients receiving heparin with a reported incidence of 0 to 30%. While often mild and of no obvious clinical significance, such thrombocytopenia can be accompanied by severe thromboembolic complications, such as skin necrosis, gangrene of the extremities that may lead to amputation, myocardial infarction, pulmonary embolism, stroke, and possibly death. (See **"Warnings"** and **"Precautions."**)

Certain episodes of painful, ischemic and cyanosed limbs have been attributed, in the past, to allergic vasospastic reactions. Whether these are, in fact, identical to the thrombocytopenia-associated complications remains to be determined.

OVERDOSAGE

SYMPTOMS

Bleeding is the chief sign of heparin overdosage. Nosebleeds, blood in urine, or tarry stools may be noted as the first sign of bleeding. Easy bruising or petechial formations may precede frank bleeding.

TREATMENT—Neutralization of Heparin Effect

When clinical circumstances (bleeding) require reversal of heparinization, protamine sulfate (1% solution) by slow infusion will neutralize heparin sodium. No more than 50 mg should be administered, very slowly, in any 10-minute period. Each mg of protamine sulfate neutralizes approximately 100 USP heparin units. The amount of protamine required decreases over time as heparin is metabolized. Although the metabolism of heparin is complex, it may, for the purpose of choosing a protamine dose, be assumed to have a half-life of about $^1/_2$ hour after intravenous injection.

Administration of protamine sulfate can cause severe hypotensive and anaphylactoid reactions. Because fatal reactions, often resembling anaphylaxis, have been reported, the drug should be given only when resuscitation techniques and treatment of anaphylactoid shock are readily available.

For additional information consult the labeling of Protamine Sulfate Injection, USP products.

DOSAGE AND ADMINISTRATION

Parenteral drug products should be inspected visually for particulate matter and discoloration prior to administration, whenever solution and container permit. Slight discoloration does not alter potency.

Heparin Lock Flush Solution, USP is **not recommended for use in the neonate** (see **"Warnings"**).

MAINTENANCE OF PATENCY OF INTRAVENOUS DEVICES

To prevent clot formation in a heparin lock set or central venous catheter following its proper insertion, Heparin Lock Flush Solution, USP is injected via the injection hub in a quantity sufficient to fill the entire device. This solution should be replaced each time the device is used. Aspirate before administering any solution via the device in order to confirm patency and location of needle or catheter tip. If the drug to be administered is incompatible with heparin, the entire device should be flushed with normal saline before and after the medication is administered; following the second saline flush, Heparin Lock Flush Solution, USP may be reinstilled into the device. The device manufacturer's instructions should be consulted for specifics concerning its use. Usually this dilute heparin solution will maintain anticoagulation within the device for up to 4 hours.

Note: Since repeated injections of small doses of heparin can alter tests for activated partial thromboplastin time (APTT), a baseline value for APTT should be obtained prior to insertion of an intravenous device.

WITHDRAWAL OF BLOOD SAMPLES

Heparin Lock Flush Solution, USP may also be used after each withdrawal of blood for laboratory tests. When heparin would interfere with or alter the results of blood tests, the heparin solution should be cleared from the device by aspirating and discarding it before withdrawing the blood sample.

The **TUBEX® BLUNT POINTE**™ Sterile Cartridge Unit is suitable for substances to be administered intravenously. It is intended for use with injection sets specifically manu-

Continued on next page

Heparin Lock Flush—Cont.

factured as "needle-less" injection systems. As of the date of this circular, **TUBEX BLUNT POINTE** is compatible with LifeShield® Prepierced Reseal injection site, Interlink® Injection Site, and SafeLine® Injection Site, User-Gard® Intermittent Injection Cap, and Safesite® reflux valve.

HOW SUPPLIED

Heparin Lock Flush Solution, USP is available in **TUBEX® BLUNT POINTE**™ Sterile Cartridge Units and in **TUBEX®** Sterile Cartridge-Needle Units.

Each 1 mL size **TUBEX®** contains one of the following concentrations of heparin sodium, in packages of 50 **TUBEX®**:
10 USP Units per mL:
NDC 0008-0523-50, **BLUNT POINTE**™.
NDC 0008-0523-01, (25 gauge × 5/8 inch needle).
100 USP Units per mL:
NDC 0008-0487-50, **BLUNT POINTE**™.
NDC 0008-0487-01, (25 gauge × 5/8 inch needle).
Each 2.5 mL size **TUBEX®** contains one of the following concentrations of heparin sodium in packages of 50 **TUBEX®**:
25 USP Units per **TUBEX®** (10 USP Units per mL):
NDC 0008-0523-51, **BLUNT POINTE**™.
NDC 0008-0523-02, (25 gauge × 5/8 inch needle).
250 USP Units per **TUBEX®** (100 USP Units per mL):
NDC 0008-0487-51, **BLUNT POINTE**™.
NDC 0008-0487-03, (25 gauge × 5/8 inch needle).
Do not use if solution is discolored or contains a precipitate
Store at controlled room temperature, 20° to 25°C (68° to 77°F) [see USP].
Do not freeze
Single use only. Discard any unused solution after initial use.
TUBEX is a registered trademark of Wyeth-Ayerst Laboratories.
BLUNT POINTE is a trademark of Wyeth-Ayerst Laboratories.
InterLink is a registered trademark of Baxter International, Inc.
LifeShield is a registered trademark of Abbott Laboratories.
SafeLine is a registered trademark of McGaw, Inc.
SafSite is a registered trademark of B. Braun Medical, Inc.
User-Gard is a registered trademark of Arrow International, Inc.
Manufactured by:
Wyeth Laboratories
A Wyeth-Ayerst Company
Philadelphia, PA 19101
CI 4202-2 Revised May 9, 1997

HEPARIN ℞
[*hĕp 'ăh-rĭn*]
Sodium Injection, USP

Caution: Federal law prohibits dispensing without prescription.

DESCRIPTION

TUBEX® Heparin Sodium Injection, USP, is a sterile solution. Each mL contains 1,000, 2,500, 5,000, 7,500, 10,000, 15,000, or 20,000 USP units heparin sodium, derived from porcine intestinal mucosa (standardized for use as an anticoagulant), in water for injection, and not more than 10 mg benzyl alcohol as a preservative.
The potency is determined by biological assay, using a USP reference standard based upon units of heparin activity per milligram.
The pH range is 5.0 to 7.5.
Heparin is a heterogenous group of straight-chain anionic mucopolysaccharides, called glycosaminoglycans, having anticoagulant properties. Although others may be present, the main sugars occurring in heparin are: (1) α-L-iduronic acid 2-sulfate, (2) 2-deoxy-2-sulfamino-α-D-glucose 6-sulfate, (3) β-D-glucuronic acid, (4) 2-acetamido-2-deoxy-α-D-glucose, and (5) α-L-iduronic acid. These sugars are present in decreasing amounts, usually in the order (2) > (1) > (4) > (3) > (5), and are joined by glycosidic linkages, forming polymers of varying sizes. Heparin is strongly acidic because of its content of covalently linked sulfate and carboxylic acid groups. In heparin sodium, the acidic protons of the sulfate units are partially replaced by sodium ions.
STRUCTURE OF HEPARIN SODIUM (representative subunits):

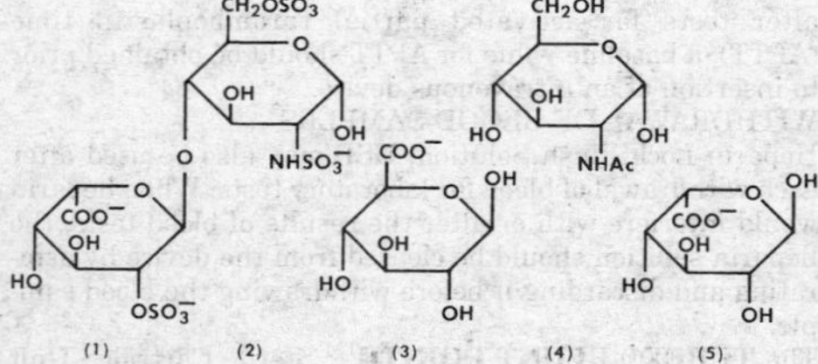

CLINICAL PHARMACOLOGY

Heparin inhibits reactions that lead to the clotting of blood and the formation of fibrin clots both *in vitro* and *in vivo.* Heparin acts at multiple sites in the normal coagulation system. Small amounts of heparin in combination with antithrombin III (heparin cofactor) can inhibit thrombosis by inactivating activated Factor X and inhibiting the conversion of prothrombin to thrombin. Once active thrombosis has developed, larger amounts of heparin can inhibit further coagulation by inactivating thrombin and preventing the conversion of fibrinogen to fibrin. Heparin also prevents the formation of a stable fibrin clot by inhibiting the activation of the fibrin-stabilizing factor.
Bleeding time is usually unaffected by heparin. Clotting time is prolonged by full therapeutic doses of heparin; in most cases, it is not measurably affected by low doses of heparin.
Peak plasma levels of heparin are achieved 2 to 4 hours following subcutaneous administration, although there are considerable individual variations. Loglinear plots of heparin plasma concentrations with time, for a wide range of dose levels, are linear which suggests the absence of zero order processes. Liver and the reticulo-endothelial system are the sites of biotransformation. The biphasic elimination curve, a rapidly declining alpha phase ($t_{1/2}$ = 10 min.), and after the age of 40 a slower beta phase, indicates uptake in organs. The absence of a relationship between anticoagulant half-life and concentration half-life may reflect factors such as protein binding of heparin.
Heparin does not have fibrinolytic activity; therefore, it will not lyse existing clots.

INDICATIONS AND USAGE

Heparin sodium injection is indicated for anticoagulant therapy in prophylaxis and treatment of venous thrombosis and its extension, in low-dose regimen for prevention of postoperative deep venous thrombosis and pulmonary embolism in patients undergoing major abdominothoracic surgery who are at risk of developing thromboembolic disease (see "**Dosage and Administration**"); for prophylaxis and treatment of pulmonary embolism, in atrial fibrillation with embolization, for diagnosis and treatment of acute and chronic consumptive coagulopathies (disseminated intravascular coagulation), for prevention of clotting in arterial and cardiac surgery, and for prophylaxis and treatment of peripheral arterial embolism.
Heparin may also be employed as an anticoagulant in blood transfusions, extracorporeal circulation, dialysis procedures, and in blood samples for laboratory purposes.

CONTRAINDICATIONS

Heparin sodium should not be used in patients:
with severe thrombocytopenia;
in whom suitable blood-coagulation tests—e.g., the whole-blood clotting time, partial thromboplastin time, etc.—cannot be performed at appropriate intervals (this contraindication refers to full-dose heparin; there is usually no need to monitor coagulation parameters in patients receiving low-dose heparin);
with an uncontrollable active bleeding state (see "**Warnings**"), except when this is due to disseminated intravascular coagulation.

WARNINGS

Heparin is not intended for intramuscular use.
HYPERSENSITIVITY
Patients with documented hypersensitivity to heparin should be given the drug only in clearly life-threatening situations.
HEMORRHAGE
Hemorrhage can occur at virtually any site in patients receiving heparin. An unexplained fall in hematocrit, fall in blood pressure or any other unexplained symptom should lead to serious consideration of a hemorrhagic event.
Heparin sodium should be used with extreme caution in disease states in which there is increased danger of hemorrhage. Some of the conditions in which increased danger of hemorrhage exists are:
Cardiovascular —subacute bacterial endocarditis, severe hypertension.
Surgical —during and immediately following (a) spinal tap or spinal anesthesia or (b) major surgery, especially involving the brain, spinal cord or eye.
Hematologic —conditions associated with increased bleeding tendencies, such as hemophilia, thrombocytopenia and some vascular purpuras.
Gastrointestinal —ulcerative lesions and continuous tube drainage of the stomach or small intestine.
Other —Menstruation, liver disease with impaired hemostasis.
COAGULATION TESTING
When heparin sodium is administered in therapeutic amounts, its dosage should be regulated by frequent blood-coagulation tests. If the coagulation test is unduly prolonged or if hemorrhage occurs, heparin sodium should be discontinued promptly (see "**Overdosage**").
THROMBOCYTOPENIA
Thrombocytopenia has been reported to occur in patients receiving heparin with a reported incidence of 0 to 30%. Mild thrombocytopenia (count greater than 100,000/mm^3) may remain stable or reverse even if heparin is continued. However, thrombocytopenia of any degree should be monitored closely. If the count falls below 100,000/mm^3 or if recurrent thrombosis develops (see "**PRECAUTIONS**, GENERAL *White-clot Syndrome,*"), the heparin product should be discontinued. If continued heparin therapy is essential, administration of heparin from a different organ source can be reinstituted with caution.
MISCELLANEOUS
This product contains benzyl alcohol as preservative. Benzyl alcohol has been reported to be associated with a fatal "Gasping Syndrome" in premature neonates.

PRECAUTIONS

GENERAL
White-clot Syndrome
It has been reported that patients on heparin may develop new thrombus formation in association with thrombocytopenia, resulting from irreversible aggregation of platelets induced by heparin, the so-called "white-clot syndrome." The process may lead to severe thromboembolic complications like skin necrosis, gangrene of the extremities that may lead to amputation, myocardial infarction, pulmonary embolism, stroke, and possibly death. Therefore, heparin administration should be promptly discontinued if a patient develops new thrombosis in association with thrombocytopenia.
Heparin Resistance
Increased resistance to heparin is frequently encountered in fever, thrombosis, thrombophlebitis, infections with thrombosing tendencies, myocardial infarction, cancer, and in postsurgical patients.
Increased Risk in Older Women
A higher incidence of bleeding has been reported in women over 60 years of age.
LABORATORY TESTS
Periodic platelet counts, hematocrits and tests for occult blood in stool are recommended during the entire course of heparin therapy, regardless of the route of administration (see "**Dosage and Administration**").
DRUG INTERACTIONS
Oral Anticoagulants
Heparin sodium may prolong the one-stage prothrombin time. Therefore, when heparin sodium is given with dicumarol or warfarin sodium, a period of at least 5 hours after the last intravenous dose or 24 hours after the last subcutaneous dose should elapse before blood is drawn if a valid prothrombin time is to be obtained.
Platelet Inhibitors
Drugs such as acetylsalicylic acid, dextran, phenylbutazone, ibuprofen, indomethacin, dipyridamole, hydroxychloroquine, and others that interfere with platelet-aggregation reactions (the main hemostatic defense of heparinized patients) may induce bleeding and should be used with caution in patients receiving heparin sodium.
Other Interactions
Digitalis, tetracyclines, nicotine, or antihistamines may partially counteract the anticoagulant action of heparin sodium.
DRUG/LABORATORY TEST INTERACTIONS
Hyperaminotransferasemia
Significant elevations of aminotransferase (SGOT [S-AST] and SGPT [S-ALT]) levels have occurred in a high percentage of patients (and healthy subjects) who have received heparin. Since aminotransferase determinations are important in the differential diagnosis of myocardial infarction, liver disease and pulmonary emboli, increases that might be caused by drugs (like heparin) should be interpreted with caution.
CARCINOGENESIS, MUTAGENESIS, IMPAIRMENT OF FERTILITY
No long-term studies in animals have been performed to evaluate carcinogenic potential of heparin. Also, no reproduction studies in animals have been performed concerning mutagenesis or impairment of fertility.
PREGNANCY
Teratogenic Effects—Pregnancy Category C
Animal reproduction studies have not been conducted with heparin sodium. It is also not known whether heparin sodium can cause fetal harm when administered to a pregnant woman or can affect reproduction capacity. Heparin sodium should be given to a pregnant woman only if clearly needed.
Nonteratogenic Effects
Heparin does not cross the placental barrier.
NURSING MOTHERS
Heparin is not excreted in human milk.
PEDIATRIC USE
See "**Dosage and Administration.**"

ADVERSE REACTIONS

HEMORRHAGE
Hemorrhage is the chief complication that may result from heparin therapy (see "**Warnings**").
An overly prolonged clotting time or minor bleeding during therapy can usually be controlled by withdrawing the drug (see "**Overdosage**"). It should be appreciated that gastrointestinal- or urinary-tract bleeding during anticoagulant therapy may indicate the presence of an underlying occult lesion. Bleeding can occur at any site but certain specific hemorrhagic complications may be difficult to detect:

a. Adrenal hemorrhage, with resultant acute adrenal insufficiency, has occurred during anticoagulant therapy. Therefore, such treatment should be discontinued in patients who develop signs and symptoms of acute adrenal hemorrhage and insufficiency. Initiation of corrective therapy should not depend on laboratory confirmation of the diagnosis, since any delay in an acute situation may result in the patient's death.
b. Ovarian (corpus luteum) hemorrhage developed in a number of women of reproductive age receiving short- or long-term anticoagulant therapy. This complication, if unrecognized, may be fatal.

c. Retroperitoneal hemorrhage.

LOCAL IRRITATION

Local irritation, erythema, mild pain, hematoma, or ulceration may follow deep, subcutaneous (intrafat) injection of heparin sodium. These complications are much more common after intramuscular use, and such use is not recommended.

HYPERSENSITIVITY

Generalized hypersensitivity reactions have been reported, with chills, fever, and urticaria as the most usual manifestations, and asthma, rhinitis, lacrimation, headache, nausea and vomiting, and anaphylactoid reactions, including shock, occurring more rarely. Itching and burning, especially on the plantar side of the feet, may occur.

Thrombocytopenia has been reported to occur in patients receiving heparin with a reported incidence of 0 to 30%. While often mild and of no obvious clinical significance, such thrombocytopenia can be accompanied by severe thromboembolic complications such as skin necrosis, gangrene of the extremities that may lead to amputation, myocardial infarction, pulmonary embolism, stroke, and possibly death. (See "**Warnings**," and "**Precautions**.")

Certain episodes of painful, ischemic and cyanosed limbs have been attributed, in the past, to allergic vasospastic reactions. Whether these are, in fact, identical to the thrombocytopenia-associated complications remains to be determined.

MISCELLANEOUS

Osteoporosis following long-term administration of high doses of heparin, cutaneous necrosis after systemic administration, suppression of aldosterone synthesis, delayed transient alopecia, priapism, and rebound hyperlipemia on discontinuation of heparin sodium have also been reported.

Significant elevations of aminotransferase (SGOT [S-AST] and SGPT [S-ALT]) levels have occurred in a high percentage of patients (and healthy subjects) who have received heparin.

OVERDOSAGE

SYMPTOMS

Bleeding is the chief sign of heparin overdosage. Nosebleeds, blood in urine, or tarry stools may be noted as the first sign of bleeding. Easy bruising or petechial formations may precede frank bleeding.

TREATMENT—Neutralization of Heparin Effect

When clinical circumstances (bleeding) require reversal of heparinization, protamine sulfate (1% solution) by slow infusion will neutralize heparin sodium. No more than 50 mg should be administered, very slowly, in any 10-minute period. Each mg of protamine sulfate neutralizes approximately 100 USP heparin units. The amount of protamine required decreases over time as heparin is metabolized. Although the metabolism of heparin is complex, it may, for the purpose of choosing a protamine dose, be assumed to have a half-life of about 1/2 hour after intravenous injection.

Administration of protamine sulfate can cause severe hypotensive and anaphylactoid reactions. Because fatal reactions, often resembling anaphylaxis, have been reported, the drug should be given only when resuscitation techniques and treatment of anaphylactoid shock are readily available.

For additional information consult the labeling of Protamine Sulfate Injection, USP, products.

DOSAGE AND ADMINISTRATION

Parenteral drug products should be inspected visually for particulate matter and discoloration prior to administration, whenever solution and container permit. Slight discoloration does not alter potency.

When heparin is added to an infusion solution for continuous intravenous administration, the container should be inverted at least six times to insure adequate mixing and prevent pooling of the heparin in the solution.

Heparin sodium is not effective by oral administration and should be given by intermittent intravenous injection, intravenous infusion, or deep subcutaneous (intrafat, i.e., above the iliac crest or abdominal fat layer) injection. *The intramuscular route of administration should be avoided because of the frequent occurrence of hematoma at the injection site.*

The **TUBEX® BLUNT POINTE™** Sterile Cartridge Unit is suitable for substances to be administered intravenously. It is intended for use with injection sets specifically manufactured as "needle-less" injection systems. As of the date of this circular, **TUBEX BLUNT POINTE** is compatible with LifeShield® Prepierced Reseal injection site, InterLink® Injection Site, and SafeLine® Injection Site, User-Gard® Intermittent Injection Cap, and SafSite® reflux valve.

The dosage of heparin sodium should be adjusted according to the patient's coagulation-test results. When heparin is given by continuous intravenous infusion, the coagulation time should be determined approximately every 4 hours in the early stages of treatment. When the drug is administered intermittently by intravenous injection, coagulation tests should be performed before each injection during the early stages of treatment and at appropriate intervals thereafter. Dosage is considered adequate when the activated partial thromboplastin time (APTT) is 1.5 to 2 times normal or when the whole-blood clotting time is elevated approximately 2.5 to 3 times the control value. After deep subcutaneous (intrafat) injections, tests for adequacy of dosage are best performed on samples drawn 4 to 6 hours after the injections.

Method of Administration	Frequency	Recommended Dose [based on 150 lb (68 kg) patient]
Deep, Subcutaneous (Intrafat Injection)	Initial Dose	5,000 units by IV injection followed by 10,000–20,000 units of a concentrated solution, subcutaneously
A different site should be used for each injection to prevent the development of massive hematoma.	Every 8 hours	8,000–10,000 units of a concentrated solution
	(or) Every 12 hours	15,000–20,000 units of a concentrated solution
Intermittent Intravenous Injection	Initial Dose	10,000 units, either undiluted or in 50–100 mL isotonic sodium chloride injection
	Every 4 to 6 hours	5,000–10,000 units, either undiluted or in 50–100 mL isotonic sodium chloride injection
Intravenous Infusion	Initial Dose	5,000 units by IV injection
	Continuous	20,000–40,000 units in 1,000 mL of isotonic sodium chloride solution for infusion/day

Periodic platelet counts, hematocrits and tests for occult blood in stool are recommended during the entire course of heparin therapy, regardless of the route of administration.

CONVERTING TO ORAL ANTICOAGULANT

When an oral anticoagulant of the coumarin or similar type is to be begun in patients already receiving heparin sodium, baseline and subsequent tests of prothrombin activity must be determined at a time when heparin activity is too low to affect the prothrombin time. This is about 5 hours after the last IV bolus and 24 hours after the last subcutaneous dose. If continuous IV heparin infusion is used, prothrombin time can usually be measured at any time.

In converting from heparin to an oral anticoagulant, the dose of the oral anticoagulant should be the usual initial amount, and thereafter prothrombin time should be determined at the usual intervals. To ensure continuous anticoagulation, it is advisable to continue full heparin therapy for several days after the prothrombin time has reached the therapeutic range. Heparin therapy may then be discontinued without tapering.

THERAPEUTIC ANTICOAGULANT EFFECT WITH FULL-DOSE HEPARIN

Although dosage must be adjusted for the individual patient according to the results of suitable laboratory tests, the following dosage schedules may be used as guidelines:

[See table above]

PEDIATRIC USE

Follow recommendations of appropriate pediatric reference texts. In general, the following dosage schedule may be used as a guideline.

Initial Dose: 50 units/kg (IV, drip).

Maintenance Dose: 100 units/kg (IV, drip) every four hours, or 20,000 units/M^2/24 hours continuously.

SURGERY OF THE HEART AND BLOOD VESSELS

Patients undergoing total body perfusion for open-heart surgery should receive an initial dose of not less than 150 units of heparin sodium per kilogram of body weight. Frequently, a dose of 300 units of heparin sodium per kilogram of body weight is used for procedures estimated to last less than 60 minutes or 400 units per kilogram for those estimated to last longer than 60 minutes.

LOW-DOSE PROPHYLAXIS OF POSTOPERATIVE THROMBOEMBOLISM

A number of well-controlled clinical trials have demonstrated that low-dose heparin prophylaxis, given just prior to and after surgery, will reduce the incidence of postoperative deep-vein thrombosis in the legs, as measured by the I-125 fibrinogen technique and venography, and of clinical pulmonary embolism. The most widely used dosage has been 5,000 units 2 hours before surgery and 5,000 units every 8 to 12 hours thereafter for 7 days or until the patient is fully ambulatory, whichever is longer. The heparin is given by deep subcutaneous injection in the arm or abdomen with a fine needle (25 to 26 gauge) to minimize tissue trauma. A concentrated solution of heparin sodium is recommended. Such prophylaxis should be reserved for patients over 40 undergoing major surgery. Patients with bleeding disorders, those having neurosurgery, spinal anesthesia, eye surgery, or potentially sanguineous operations should be excluded, as well as patients receiving oral anticoagulants or platelet-active drugs (see "**Warnings**"). The value of such prophylaxis in hip surgery has not been established. The possibility of increased bleeding during surgery or postoperatively should be borne in mind. If such bleeding occurs, discontinuance of heparin and neutralization with protamine sulfate is advisable. If clinical evidence of thromboembolism develops despite low-dose prophylaxis, full therapeutic doses of anticoagulants should be given unless contraindicated. All patients should be screened prior to heparinization to rule out bleeding disorders, and monitoring should be performed with appropriate coagulation tests just prior to surgery. Coagulation-test values should be normal or only slightly elevated. There is usually no need for daily monitoring of the effect of low-dose heparin in patients with normal coagulation parameters.

EXTRACORPOREAL DIALYSIS USE

Follow equipment manufacturer's operating directions carefully.

BLOOD TRANSFUSION

Addition of 400 to 600 USP units per 100 mL of whole blood. Usually, 7,500 USP units of heparin sodium are added to 100 mL of Sterile Sodium Chloride Injection (or 75,000 USP units per 1,000 mL of Sterile Sodium Chloride Injection) and mixed, and from this sterile solution, 6 to 8 mL is added per 100 mL of whole blood.

LABORATORY SAMPLES

Addition of 70 to 150 units of heparin sodium per 10 to 20 mL sample of whole blood is usually employed to prevent coagulation of the sample. Leukocyte counts should be performed on heparinized blood within two hours after addition of the heparin. Heparinized blood should not be used for isoagglutinin, complement, erythrocyte fragility tests, or platelet counts.

HOW SUPPLIED

Heparin Sodium Injection, USP, is available in **TUBEX®** Sterile Cartridge-Needle Units.

Each 1 mL size **TUBEX** contains one of the following concentrations of heparin sodium:

1,000 USP Units per mL
NDC 0008–0275–01, (22 gauge × 1 1/4 inch needle), in packages of 10 **TUBEX**.

2,500 USP Units per mL
NDC 0008–0482–01, (25 gauge × 5/8 inch needle), in packages of 10 **TUBEX**.

5,000 USP Units per 0.5 mL (10,000 USP Units per mL)
NDC 0008–0277–02, (25 gauge ×5/8 inch needle), in packages of 10 **TUBEX**.
NDC 0008–0277–03, (25 gauge × 5/8 inch needle), in packages of 50 **TUBEX**.

5,000 USP Units per mL
NDC 0008–0278–02, (25 gauge × 5/8 inch needle), in packages of 10 **TUBEX**.

7,500 USP Units per mL
NDC 0008–0293–01, (25 gauge × 5/8 inch needle), in packages of 10 **TUBEX**.

10,000 USP Units per mL
NDC 0008–0277–01, (25 gauge × 5/8 inch needle), in packages of 10 **TUBEX**.

20,000 USP Units per mL
NDC 0008–0276–01, (25 gauge × 5/8 inch needle), in packages of 10 **TUBEX**.

Heparin Sodium Injection, USP, 1,000 USP Units per mL, is also available in packages of 10 **TUBEX® BLUNT POINTE™** Sterile Cartridge Units, NDC 0008–0275–50.

Store at controlled room temperature, 20°–25°C (68°–77°F) [see USP].

Do not freeze.

Do not use if solution is discolored or contains a precipitate.

Manufactured by:
Wyeth Laboratories
A Wyeth-Ayerst Company
Philadelphia, PA 19101
CI 3465-8 Revised April 30, 1997

INDERAL® ℞

[ĭn 'der-al]

(propranolol hydrochloride)

Rx only

DESCRIPTION

Inderal (propranolol hydrochloride) is a synthetic beta-adrenergic receptor blocking agent chemically described as 1-(Isopropylamino)-3-(1-naphthyloxy)-2-propanol hydrochloride. Its structural formula is

OH
$OCH_2CHCH_2NHCH(CH_3)_2$
· HCl

Continued on next page

Inderal—Cont.

Propranolol hydrochloride is a stable, white, crystalline solid which is readily soluble in water and ethanol. Its molecular weight is 295.81.

Inderal is available as 10 mg, 20 mg, 40 mg, 60 mg, and 80 mg tablets for oral administration and as a 1 mg/mL sterile injectable solution for intravenous administration.

The inactive ingredients contained in Inderal Tablets are: lactose, magnesium stearate, microcrystalline cellulose, and stearic acid. In addition, Inderal 10 mg and 80 mg Tablets contain FD&C Yellow No. 6 and D&C Yellow No. 10; Inderal 20 mg Tablets contain FD&C Blue No. 1; Inderal 40 mg Tablets contain FD&C Blue No. 1, FD&C Yellow No. 6, and D&C Yellow No. 10; Inderal 60 mg Tablets contain D&C Red No. 30.

CLINICAL PHARMACOLOGY

Inderal is a nonselective beta-adrenergic receptor blocking agent possessing no other autonomic nervous system activity. It specifically competes with beta-adrenergic receptor stimulating agents for available receptor sites. When access to beta-receptor sites is blocked by Inderal, the chronotropic, inotropic, and vasodilator responses to beta-adrenergic stimulation are decreased proportionately.

Propranolol is almost completely absorbed from the gastrointestinal tract, but a portion is immediately bound by the liver. Peak effect occurs in one to one- and one-half hours. The biologic half-life is approximately four hours.

There is no simple correlation between dose or plasma level and therapeutic effect, and the dose-sensitivity range as observed in clinical practice is wide. The principal reason for this is that sympathetic tone varies widely between individuals. Since there is no reliable test to estimate sympathetic tone or to determine whether total beta blockade has been achieved, proper dosage requires titration.

The mechanism of the antihypertensive effect of Inderal has not been established. Among the factors that may be involved in contributing to the antihypertensive action are (1) decreased cardiac output, (2) inhibition of renin release by the kidneys, and (3) diminution of tonic sympathetic nerve outflow from vasomotor centers in the brain. Although total peripheral resistance may increase initially, it readjusts to or below the pretreatment level with chronic use. Effects on plasma volume appear to be minor and somewhat variable.

Inderal has been shown to cause a small increase in serum potassium concentration when used in the treatment of hypertensive patients.

In angina pectoris, propranolol generally reduces the oxygen requirement of the heart at any given level of effort by blocking the catecholamine-induced increases in the heart rate, systolic blood pressure, and the velocity and extent of myocardial contraction. Propranolol may increase oxygen requirements by increasing left ventricular fiber length, end diastolic pressure, and systolic ejection period. The net physiologic effect of beta-adrenergic blockade is usually advantageous and is manifested during exercise by delayed onset of pain and increased work capacity. Propranolol exerts its antiarrhythmic effects in concentrations associated with beta-adrenergic blockade, and this appears to be its principal antiarrhythmic mechanism of action. In dosages greater than required for beta blockade, Inderal also exerts a quinidine-like or anesthetic-like membrane action, which affects the cardiac action potential. The significance of the membrane action in the treatment of arrhythmias is uncertain.

The mechanism of the antimigraine effect of propranolol has not been established. Beta-adrenergic receptors have been demonstrated in the pial vessels of the brain.

The specific mechanism of Inderal's antitremor effects has not been established, but beta-2 (noncardiac) receptors may be involved. A central effect is also possible. Clinical studies have demonstrated that Inderal is of benefit in exaggerated physiological and essential (familial) tremor.

Beta-receptor blockade can be useful in conditions in which, because of pathologic or functional changes, sympathetic activity is detrimental to the patient. But there are also situations in which sympathetic stimulation is vital. For example, in patients with severely damaged hearts, adequate ventricular function is maintained by virtue of sympathetic drive, which should be preserved. In the presence of AV block greater than first degree, beta blockade may prevent the necessary facilitating effect of sympathetic activity on conduction. Beta blockade results in bronchial constriction by interfering with adrenergic bronchodilator activity, which should be preserved in patients subject to bronchospasm.

Propranolol is not significantly dialyzable.

The Beta-Blocker Heart Attack Trial (BHAT) was a National Heart, Lung and Blood Institute-sponsored multicenter, randomized, double-blind, placebo-controlled trial conducted in 31 U.S. centers (plus one in Canada) in 3,837 persons without history of severe congestive heart failure or presence of recent heart failure; certain conduction defects; angina since infarction, who had survived the acute phase of myocardial infarction. Propranolol was administered at either 60 or 80 mg t.i.d. based on blood levels achieved during an initial trial of 40 mg t.i.d. Therapy with Inderal, begun 5 to 21 days following infarction, was shown to reduce overall mortality up to 39 months, the longest period of follow-up. This was primarily attributable to a reduction in cardiovascular mortality. The protective effect of Inderal was consistent regardless of age, sex, or site of infarction. Compared with placebo, total mortality was reduced 39% at 12 months and 26% over an average follow-up period of 25 months. The Norwegian Multicenter Trial in which propranolol was administered at 40 mg q.i.d. gave overall results which support the findings in the BHAT.

Although the clinical trials used either t.i.d. or q.i.d. dosing, clinical, pharmacologic, and pharmacokinetic data provide a reasonable basis for concluding that b.i.d. dosing with propranolol should be adequate in the treatment of postinfarction patients.

Clinical

In the BHAT, patients on Inderal were prescribed either 180 mg/day (82% of patients) or 240 mg/day (18% of patients). Patients were instructed to take the medication 3 times a day at mealtimes. This dosing schedule would result in an overnight dosing interval of 12 to 14 hours which is similar to the dosing interval for a b.i.d regimen. In addition, blood samples were drawn at various times and analyzed for propranolol. When the patients were grouped into tertiles based on the blood levels observed and the mortality in the upper and lower tertiles was compared, there was no evidence that blood levels affected mortality.

Pharmacologic

Studies in normal volunteers have shown that a 90 mg b.i.d. regimen maintains beta blockade at, or above, the minimum for 60 mg t.i.d. dosing for 24 hours even though differences occurred at two time intervals. At 10 to 12 hours after the first dose of the day, t.i.d. dosing gave more beta blockade than b.i.d. dosing; at 20 to 24 hours the trend of the relationship was reversed. These relationships were similar in direction to those observed for plasma propranolol levels. (See **"Pharmacokinetic."**)

Pharmacokinetic

A bioavailability study in normal volunteers showed that the blood levels produced by 180 mg/day given b.i.d. are below those provided by the same daily dosage given t.i.d. at 10 to 12 hours after the first dose of the day, but above those of a t.i.d. regimen at 20 to 24 hours. However, the blood levels produced by b.i.d. dosing were always equivalent to or above the minimum for t.i.d. dosing throughout the 24 hours. In addition, the mean AUC on the fourth day for the b.i.d. regimen was about 17% greater than for the t.i.d. regimen (1,194 *vs.* 1,024 ng/mL·hr).

INDICATIONS AND USAGE

Hypertension

Inderal is indicated in the management of hypertension. It may be used alone or used in combination with other antihypertensive agents, particularly a thiazide diuretic. Inderal is not indicated in the management of hypertensive emergencies.

Angina Pectoris Due to Coronary Atherosclerosis

Inderal is indicated for the long-term management of patients with angina pectoris.

Cardiac Arrhythmias

1) Supraventricular arrhythmias
   a) Paroxysmal atrial tachycardias, particularly those arrhythmias induced by catecholamines or digitalis or associated with the Wolff-Parkinson-White syndrome. (See W-P-W under **"WARNINGS."**)
   b) Persistent sinus tachycardia which is noncompensatory and impairs the well-being of the patient.
   c) Tachycardias and arrhythmias due to thyrotoxicosis when causing distress or increased hazard and when immediate effect is necessary as adjunctive, short-term (2 to 4 weeks) therapy. May be used with, but not in place of, specific therapy. (See **"Thyrotoxicosis"** under **"WARNINGS."**)
   d) Persistent atrial extrasystoles which impair the well-being of the patient and do not respond to conventional measures.
   e) Atrial flutter and fibrillation when ventricular rate cannot be controlled by digitalis alone, or when digitalis is contraindicated.
2) Ventricular tachycardias.
   Ventricular arrhythmias do not respond to propranolol as predictably as do the supraventricular arrhythmias.
   a) Ventricular tachycardias
   With the exception of those induced by catecholamines or digitalis, Inderal is not the drug of first choice. In critical situations when cardioversion techniques or other drugs are not indicated or are not effective, Inderal may be considered. If, after consideration of the risks involved, Inderal is used, it should be given intravenously in low dosage and very slowly. (See **"DOSAGE AND ADMINISTRATION."**) *Care in the administration of* Inderal *with constant electrocardiographic monitoring is essential as the failing heart requires some sympathetic drive for maintenance of myocardial tone.*
   b) Persistent premature ventricular extrasystoles which do not respond to conventional measures and impair the well-being of the patient.
3) Tachyarrhythmias of digitalis intoxication
   If digitalis-induced tachyarrhythmias persist following discontinuance of digitalis and correction of electrolyte abnormalities, they are usually reversible with *oral* Inderal. Severe bradycardia may occur. (See **"Overdosage."**)
   Intravenous propranolol hydrochloride is reserved for life-threatening arrhythmias. Temporary maintenance with oral therapy may be indicated. (See **"DOSAGE AND ADMINISTRATION."**)
4) Resistant tachyarrhythmias due to excessive catecholamine action during anesthesia
   Tachyarrhythmias due to excessive catecholamine action during anesthesia may sometimes arise because of release of endogenous catecholamines or administration of catecholamines. When usual measures fail in such arrhythmias, Inderal may be given intravenously to abolish them. All general inhalation anesthetics produce some degree of myocardial depression. Therefore, when Inderal is used to treat arrhythmias during anesthesia, it should be used with extreme caution and constant ECG and central venous pressure monitoring. (See **"WARNINGS."**)

Myocardial Infarction

Inderal is indicated to reduce cardiovascular mortality in patients who have survived the acute phase of myocardial infarction and are clinically stable.

Migraine

Inderal is indicated for the prophylaxis of common migraine headache. The efficacy of propranolol in the treatment of a migraine attack that has started has not been established, and propranolol is not indicated for such use.

Essential Tremor

Inderal is indicated in the management of familial or hereditary essential tremor. Familial or essential tremor consists of involuntary, rhythmic, oscillatory movements, usually limited to the upper limbs. It is absent at rest but occurs when the limb is held in a fixed posture or position against gravity and during active movement. Inderal causes a reduction in the tremor amplitude but not in the tremor frequency. Inderal is not indicated for the treatment of tremor associated with Parkinsonism.

Hypertrophic Subaortic Stenosis

Inderal is useful in the management of hypertrophic subaortic stenosis, especially for treatment of exertional or other stress-induced angina, palpitations, and syncope. Inderal also improves exercise performance. The effectiveness of propranolol hydrochloride in this disease appears to be due to a reduction of the elevated outflow pressure gradient, which is exacerbated by beta-receptor stimulation. Clinical improvement may be temporary.

Pheochromocytoma

After primary treatment with an alpha-adrenergic blocking agent has been instituted, Inderal may be useful as *adjunctive* therapy if the control of tachycardia becomes necessary before or during surgery. It is hazardous to use Inderal unless alpha-adrenergic blocking drugs are already in use, since this would predispose to serious blood pressure elevation. Blocking only the peripheral dilator (beta) action of epinephrine leaves its constrictor (alpha) action unopposed. In the event of hemorrhage or shock, there is a disadvantage in having both beta and alpha blockade since the combination prevents the increase in heart rate and peripheral vasoconstriction needed to maintain blood pressure.

With inoperable or metastatic pheochromocytoma, Inderal may be useful as an adjunct to the management of symptoms due to excessive beta-receptor stimulation.

CONTRAINDICATIONS

Inderal is contraindicated in 1) cardiogenic shock, 2) sinus bradycardia and greater than first degree block, 3) bronchial asthma, 4) congestive heart failure (see **"WARNINGS"**) unless the failure is secondary to a tachyarrhythmia treatable with Inderal.

WARNINGS

Cardiac Failure

Sympathetic stimulation may be a vital component supporting circulatory function in patients with congestive heart failure, and its inhibition by beta blockade may precipitate more severe failure. Although beta blockers should be avoided in overt congestive heart failure, if necessary, they can be used with close follow-up in patients with a history of failure who are well compensated and are receiving digitalis and diuretics. Beta-adrenergic blocking agents do not abolish the inotropic action of digitalis on heart muscle.

In Patients Without a History of Heart Failure, continued use of beta blockers can, in some cases, lead to cardiac failure. Therefore, at the first sign or symptom of heart failure, the patient should be digitalized and/or treated with diuretics, and the response observed closely, or Inderal should be discontinued (gradually, if possible).

In Patients with Angina Pectoris, there have been reports of exacerbation of angina and, in some cases, myocardial infarction, following *abrupt* discontinuance of Inderal therapy. Therefore, when discontinuance of Inderal is planned, the dosage should be gradually reduced over at least a few weeks and the patient should be cautioned against interruption or cessation of therapy without the physician's advice. If Inderal therapy is interrupted and exacerbation of angina occurs, it usually is advisable to reinstitute Inderal therapy and take other measures appropriate for the management of unstable angina pectoris. Since coronary artery disease may be unrecognized, it may be prudent to follow the above advice in patients considered at risk of having occult atherosclerotic heart disease who are given propranolol for other indications.

NONALLERGIC BRONCHOSPASM (E.G., CHRONIC BRONCHITIS, EMPHYSEMA)

PATIENTS WITH BRONCHOSPASTIC DISEASES SHOULD IN GENERAL NOT RECEIVE BETA BLOCK-

ERS. Inderal should be administered with caution since it may block bronchodilation produced by endogenous and exogenous catecholamine stimulation of beta receptors.

Major Surgery

The necessity or desirability of withdrawal of beta-blocking therapy prior to major surgery is controversial. It should be noted, however, that the impaired ability of the heart to respond to reflex adrenergic stimuli may augment the risks of general anesthesia and surgical procedures.

Inderal, like other beta blockers, is a competitive inhibitor of beta-receptor agonists and its effects can be reversed by administration of such agents, e.g., dobutamine or isoproterenol. However, such patients may be subject to protracted severe hypotension. Difficulty in starting and maintaining the heartbeat has also been reported with beta blockers.

Diabetes and Hypoglycemia

Beta-adrenergic blockade may prevent the appearance of certain premonitory signs and symptoms (pulse rate and pressure changes) of acute hypoglycemia in labile insulin-dependent diabetes. In these patients, it may be more difficult to adjust the dosage of insulin. Hypoglycemic attacks may be accompanied by a precipitous elevation of blood pressure in patients on propranolol.

Propranolol therapy, particularly in infants and children, diabetic or not, has been associated with hypoglycemia especially during fasting as in preparation for surgery. Hypoglycemia also has been found after this type of drug therapy and prolonged physical exertion and has occurred in renal insufficiency, both during dialysis and sporadically, in subjects on propranolol.

Thyrotoxicosis

Beta blockade may mask certain clinical signs of hyperthyroidism. Therefore, abrupt withdrawal of propranolol may be followed by an exacerbation of symptoms of hyperthyroidism, including thyroid storm. Propranolol may change thyroid-function tests, increasing T_4 and reverse T_3 and decreasing T_3.

In Patients With Wolff-Parkinson-White Syndrome, several cases have been reported in which, after propranolol, the tachycardia was replaced by a severe bradycardia requiring a demand pacemaker. In one case this resulted after an initial dose of 5 mg propranolol.

PRECAUTIONS

General

Propranolol should be used with caution in patients with impaired hepatic or renal function. Inderal is not indicated for the treatment of hypertensive emergencies.

Beta-adrenoreceptor blockade can cause reduction of intraocular pressure. Patients should be told that Inderal may interfere with the glaucoma screening test. Withdrawal may lead to a return of increased intraocular pressure.

Risk of anaphylactic reaction. While taking beta blockers, patients with a history of severe anaphylactic reaction to a variety of allergens may be more reactive to repeated challenge, either accidental, diagnostic, or therapeutic. Such patients may be unresponsive to the usual doses of epinephrine used to treat allergic reaction.

Clinical Laboratory Tests

Elevated blood urea levels in patients with severe heart disease, elevated serum transaminase, alkaline phosphatase, lactate dehydrogenase.

Drug Interactions

Patients receiving catecholamine-depleting drugs such as reserpine should be closely observed if Inderal is administered. The added catecholamine-blocking action may produce an excessive reduction of resting sympathetic nervous activity, which may result in hypotension, marked bradycardia, vertigo, syncopal attacks, or orthostatic hypotension.

Caution should be exercised when patients receiving a beta blocker are administered a calcium-channel blocking drug, especially intravenous verapamil, for both agents may depress myocardial contractility or atrioventricular conduction. On rare occasions, the concomitant intravenous use of a beta blocker and verapamil has resulted in serious adverse reactions, especially in patients with severe cardiomyopathy, congestive heart failure or recent myocardial infarction.

Blunting of the antihypertensive effect of beta-adrenoceptor blocking agents by nonsteroidal anti-inflammatory drugs has been reported.

Hypotension and cardiac arrest have been reported with the concomitant use of propranolol and haloperidol.

Aluminum hydroxide gel greatly reduces intestinal absorption of propranolol.

Ethanol slows the rate of absorption of propranolol.

Phenytoin, phenobarbitone, and *rifampin* accelerate propranolol clearance.

Chlorpromazine, when used concomitantly with propranolol, results in increased plasma levels of both drugs.

Antipyrine and *lidocaine* have reduced clearance when used concomitantly with propranolol.

Thyroxine may result in a lower than expected T_3 concentration when used concomitantly with propranolol.

Cimetidine decreases the hepatic metabolism of propranolol, delaying elimination and increasing blood levels.

Theophylline clearance is reduced when used concomitantly with propranolol.

Carcinogenesis, Mutagenesis, Impairment of Fertility

In dietary administration studies in which mice and rats were treated with propranolol for up to 18 months at doses of up to 150 mg/kg/day, there was no evidence of drug-related tumorigenesis. In a study in which both male and female rats were exposed to propranolol in their diets at concentrations of up to 0.05%, from 60 days prior to mating and throughout pregnancy and lactation for two generations, there were no effects on fertility. Based on differing results from Ames Tests performed by different laboratories, there is equivocal evidence for a genotoxic effect of propranolol in bacteria (*S. typhimurium* strain TA 1538).

Pregnancy: Pregnancy Category C

In a series of reproductive and developmental toxicology studies, propranolol was given to rats by gavage or in the diet throughout pregnancy and lactation. At doses of 150 mg/kg/day (> 10 times the maximum recommended human daily dose of propranolol on a body weight basis), but not at doses of 80 mg/kg/day, treatment was associated with embryotoxicity (reduced litter size and increased resorption sites) as well as neonatal toxicity (deaths). Propranolol also was administered (in the feed) to rabbits (throughout pregnancy and lactation) at doses as high as 150 mg/kg/day (> 15 times the maximum recommended daily human dose). No evidence of embryo or neonatal toxicity was noted.

There are no adequate and well-controlled studies in pregnant women. Intrauterine growth retardation has been reported in neonates whose mothers received propranolol during pregnancy. Neonates whose mothers are receiving propranolol at parturition have exhibited bradycardia, hypoglycemia and respiratory depression. Adequate facilities for monitoring these infants at birth should be available. Inderal should be used during pregnancy only if the potential benefit justifies the potential risk to the fetus.

Nursing Mothers

Inderal is excreted in human milk. Caution should be exercised when Inderal is administered to a nursing woman.

Pediatric Use

High serum propranolol levels have been noted in patients with Down's syndrome (trisomy 21), suggesting that the bioavailability of propranolol may be increased in patients with this condition.

Evaluation of the effects of propranolol in pediatric patients, relative to the drug's efficacy and safety, has not been as systematically performed as in adults. Information is available in the medical literature to allow fair estimates, and specific dosing information has been reasonably studied.

Cardiovascular diseases that are common to adults and children are generally as responsive to propranolol intervention in children as they are in adults.

Adverse reactions are also similar: for example, bronchospasm and congestive heart failure related to propranolol therapy have been reported in pediatric patients and occur through the same mechanisms as previously described in adults.

The normal echocardiogram evolves through a series of changes as the heart matures during growth and development in pediatric patients. Should echocardiography be used to monitor propranolol therapy in pediatric patients, the age-related changes in the echocardiogram need to be borne in mind.

Geriatric Use

Clinical studies of propranolol did not include sufficient numbers of subjects aged 65 and over to determine whether they respond differently from younger subjects. Other reported clinical experience has not identified differences in responses between the elderly and younger patients. In general, dose selection for an elderly patient should be cautious, usually starting at the low end of the dosing range, reflecting the greater frequency of the decreased hepatic, renal or cardiac function, and of concomitant disease or other drug therapy.

ADVERSE REACTIONS

Most adverse effects have been mild and transient and have rarely required the withdrawal of therapy.

Cardiovascular: Bradycardia; congestive heart failure; intensification of AV block; hypotension; paresthesia of hands; thrombocytopenic purpura; arterial insufficiency, usually of the Raynaud type.

Central Nervous System: Light-headedness; mental depression manifested by insomnia, lassitude, weakness, fatigue; reversible mental depression progressing to catatonia; visual disturbances; hallucinations, vivid dreams, an acute reversible syndrome characterized by disorientation for time and place, short-term memory loss, emotional lability, slightly clouded sensorium, and decreased performance on neuropsychometrics. Total daily doses above 160 mg (when administered as divided doses of greater than 80 mg each) may be associated with an increased incidence of fatigue, lethargy, and vivid dreams.

Gastrointestinal: Nausea, vomiting, epigastric distress, abdominal cramping, diarrhea, constipation, mesenteric arterial thrombosis, ischemic colitis.

Allergic: Pharyngitis and agranulocytosis, erythematous rash, fever combined with aching and sore throat, laryngospasm, and respiratory distress.

Respiratory: Bronchospasm.

Hematologic: Agranulocytosis, nonthrombocytopenic purpura, thrombocytopenic purpura.

Autoimmune: In extremely rare instances, systemic lupus erythematosus has been reported.

Miscellaneous: Alopecia, LE-like reactions, psoriasiform rashes, dry eyes, male impotence, and Peyronie's disease have been reported rarely. Oculomucocutaneous reactions involving the skin, serous membranes and conjunctivae reported for a beta blocker (practolol) have not been associated with propranolol.

DOSAGE AND ADMINISTRATION

The dosage range for Inderal is different for each indication.

Oral

Hypertension—*Dosage must be individualized.*

The usual initial dosage is 40 mg Inderal twice daily, whether used alone or added to a diuretic. Dosage may be increased gradually until adequate blood pressure control is achieved. The usual maintenance dosage is 120 mg to 240 mg per day. In some instances a dosage of 640 mg a day may be required. The time needed for full antihypertensive response to a given dosage is variable and may range from a few days to several weeks.

While twice-daily dosing is effective and can maintain a reduction in blood pressure throughout the day, some patients, especially when lower doses are used, may experience a modest rise in blood pressure toward the end of the 12-hour dosing interval. This can be evaluated by measuring blood pressure near the end of the dosing interval to determine whether satisfactory control is being maintained throughout the day. If control is not adequate, a larger dose, or 3-times-daily therapy may achieve better control.

Angina Pectoris—*Dosage must be individualized.*

Total daily doses of 80 mg to 320 mg, when administered orally, twice a day, three times a day, or four times a day, have been shown to increase exercise tolerance and to reduce ischemic changes in the ECG. If treatment is to be discontinued, reduce dosage gradually over a period of several weeks. (See "**WARNINGS**.")

Arrhythmias—10 mg to 30 mg three or four times daily, before meals and at bedtime.

Myocardial Infarction—The recommended daily dosage is 180 mg to 240 mg per day in divided doses. Although a t.i.d. regimen was used in the Beta-Blocker Heart Attack Trial and a q.i.d. regimen in the Norwegian Multicenter Trial, there is a reasonable basis for the use of either a t.i.d. or b.i.d. regimen (see "**CLINICAL PHARMACOLOGY**"). The effectiveness and safety of daily dosages greater than 240 mg for prevention of cardiac mortality have not been established. However, higher dosages may be needed to effectively treat coexisting diseases such as angina or hypertension (see above).

Migraine—*Dosage must be individualized.*

The initial oral dose is 80 mg Inderal daily in divided doses. The usual effective dose range is 160 mg to 240 mg per day. The dosage may be increased gradually to achieve optimum migraine prophylaxis. If a satisfactory response is not obtained within four to six weeks after reaching the maximum dose, Inderal therapy should be discontinued. It may be advisable to withdraw the drug gradually over a period of several weeks.

Essential Tremor—*Dosage must be individualized.*

The initial dosage is 40 mg Inderal twice daily. Optimum reduction of essential tremor is usually achieved with a dose of 120 mg per day. Occasionally, it may be necessary to administer 240 mg to 320 mg per day.

Hypertrophic Subaortic Stenosis—20 mg to 40 mg three or four times daily, before meals and at bedtime.

Pheochromocytoma—*Preoperatively*—60 mg daily in divided doses for three days prior to surgery, concomitantly with an alpha-adrenergic blocking agent.

—*Management of inoperable tumor* —30 mg daily in divided doses.

Use in Pediatric Patients: Intravenous administration of Inderal is not recommended in pediatric patients. Oral dosage for treating hypertension requires individual titration, beginning with a 1.0 mg per kg (body weight) per day dosage regimen (i.e., 0.5 mg per kg b.i.d.).

The usual pediatric dosage range is 2 mg to 4 mg per kg per day in two equally divided doses (i.e., 1.0 mg per kg b.i.d. to 2.0 mg per kg b.i.d.). Pediatric dosage calculated by weight (recommended) generally produces propranolol plasma levels in a therapeutic range similar to that in adults. On the other hand, pediatric doses calculated on the basis of body surface area (*not* recommended) usually result in plasma levels above the mean adult therapeutic range. Doses above 16 mg per kg per day should not be used in pediatric patients. If treatment with Inderal is to be discontinued, a gradually decreasing dose titration over a 7- to 14-day period is necessary.

Intravenous

Parenteral drug products should be inspected visually for particulate matter and discoloration prior to administration, whenever solution and container permit.

Intravenous administration is reserved for life-threatening arrhythmias or those occurring under anesthesia. The usual dose is from 1 mg to 3 mg administered under careful monitoring, e.g., electrocardiographic, central venous pressure. The rate of administration should not exceed 1 mg (1 mL) per minute to diminish the possibility of lowering blood pressure and causing cardiac standstill. Sufficient time should be allowed for the drug to reach the site of action even when a slow circulation is present. If necessary, a second dose may be given after two minutes. Thereafter, additional drug should not be given in less than four hours. Additional Inderal should not be given when the desired alteration in rate and/or rhythm is achieved.

Transference to oral therapy should be made as soon as possible.

Continued on next page

Inderal—Cont.

The intravenous administration of Inderal has not been evaluated adequately in the management of hypertensive emergencies.

Overdosage

Inderal is not significantly dialyzable. In the event of overdosage or exaggerated response, the following measures should be employed:

General—If ingestion is or may have been recent, evacuate gastric contents, taking care to prevent pulmonary aspiration.

Bradycardia—ADMINISTER ATROPINE (0.25 mg to 1.0 mg); IF THERE IS NO RESPONSE TO VAGAL BLOCKADE, ADMINISTER ISOPROTERENOL CAUTIOUSLY.

Cardiac Failure—DIGITALIZATION AND DIURETICS.

Hypotension — VASOPRESSORS, *e.g.*, LEVARTERENOL OR EPINEPHRINE (THERE IS EVIDENCE THAT EPINEPHRINE IS THE DRUG OF CHOICE).

Bronchospasm — ADMINISTER ISOPROTERENOL AND AMINOPHYLLINE.

HOW SUPPLIED

Inderal®
(propranolol hydrochloride)

Tablets

INDERAL 10—Each hexagonal-shaped, orange, scored tablet, embossed with an "I" and imprinted with "INDERAL 10", contains 10 mg propranolol hydrochloride, in bottles of 100 (NDC 0046-0421-81); 1,000 (NDC 0046-0421-91); and 5,000 (NDC 0046-0421-95). Also in Unit Dose packages of 100 (NDC 0046-0421-99).

Store at room temperature (approximately 25° C).

Dispense in a well-closed container as defined in the USP.

INDERAL 20—Each hexagonal-shaped, blue, scored tablet, embossed with an "I" and imprinted with "INDERAL 20", contains 20 mg propranolol hydrochloride, in bottles of 100 (NDC 0046-0422-81); 1,000 (NDC 0046-0422-91); and 5,000 (NDC 0046-0422-95).

Store at room temperature (approximately 25° C).

Dispense in a well-closed, light-resistant container as defined in the USP.

Protect from light.

Use carton to protect contents from light.

INDERAL 40—Each hexagonal-shaped, green, scored tablet, embossed with an "I" and imprinted with "INDERAL 40", contains 40 mg propranolol hydrochloride, in bottles of 100 (NDC 0046-0424-81); 1,000 (NDC 0046-0424-91); and 5,000 (NDC 0046-0424-95).

Store at room temperature (approximately 25° C).

Dispense in a well-closed, light-resistant container as defined in the USP.

Protect from light.

Use carton to protect contents from light.

INDERAL 60—Each hexagonal-shaped, pink, scored tablet, embossed with an "I" and imprinted with "INDERAL 60", contains 60 mg propranolol hydrochloride, in bottles of 100 (NDC 0046-0426-81).

Store at room temperature (approximately 25° C).

Dispense in a well-closed container as defined in the USP.

INDERAL 80—Each hexagonal-shaped, yellow, scored tablet, embossed with an "I" and imprinted with "INDERAL 80", contains 80 mg propranolol hydrochloride, in bottles of 100 (NDC 0046-0428-81); 1,000 (NDC 0046-0428-91); and 5,000 (NDC 0046-0428-95).

Store at room temperature (approximately 25° C).

Dispense in a well-closed container as defined in the USP.

The appearance of these tablets is a registered trademark of Wyeth-Ayerst Laboratories.

Injectable

—Each mL contains 1 mg of propranolol hydrochloride in Water for Injection. The pH is adjusted with citric acid. Supplied as: 1 mL ampuls in boxes of 10 (NDC 0046-3265-10).

Store at room temperature (approximately 25°C).

Protect from freezing or excessive heat.

Manufactured by:
Ayerst Laboratories Inc.
A Wyeth-Ayerst Company
Philadelphia, PA 19101
CI 3791-9 Revised April 13, 1999

Shown in Product Identification Guide, page 341

INDERAL® LA ℞

[ĭn 'der-al]
(propranolol hydrochloride)
Long-Acting Capsules

Rx only

DESCRIPTION

Inderal (propranolol hydrochloride) is a synthetic beta-adrenergic receptor-blocking agent chemically described as 1-(Isopropylamino)-3-(1-naphthyloxy)-2-propanol hydrochloride. Its structural formula is

[See chemical structure at top of next column]

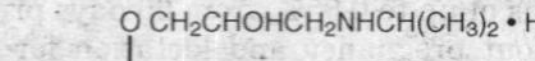

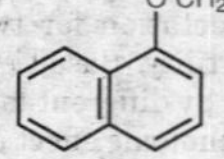

Propranolol hydrochloride is a stable, white, crystalline solid which is readily soluble in water and ethanol. Its molecular weight is 295.81.

Inderal LA is formulated to provide a sustained release of propranolol hydrochloride. Inderal LA is available as 60 mg, 80 mg, 120 mg, and 160 mg capsules.

Inderal LA capsules contain the following inactive ingredients: cellulose, ethylcellulose, gelatin capsules, hydroxypropyl methylcellulose, and titanium dioxide. In addition, Inderal LA 60 mg, 80 mg, and 120 mg capsules contain D&C Red No. 28 and FD&C Blue No. 1; Inderal LA 160 mg capsules contain FD&C Blue No. 1.

These capsules comply with USP Drug Release Test 1.

CLINICAL PHARMACOLOGY

Inderal is a nonselective, beta-adrenergic receptor-blocking agent possessing no other autonomic nervous system activity. It specifically competes with beta-adrenergic receptor-stimulating agents for available receptor sites. When access to beta-receptor sites is blocked by Inderal, the chronotropic, inotropic, and vasodilator responses to beta-adrenergic stimulation are decreased proportionately.

Inderal LA Capsules (60, 80, 120, and 160 mg) release propranolol HCl at a controlled and predictable rate. Peak blood levels following dosing with Inderal LA occur at about 6 hours, and the apparent plasma half-life is about 10 hours. When measured at steady state over a 24-hour period the areas under the propranolol plasma concentration-time curve (AUCs) for the capsules are approximately 60% to 65% of the AUCs for a comparable divided daily dose of Inderal Tablets. The lower AUCs for the capsules are due to greater hepatic metabolism of propranolol, resulting from the slower rate of absorption of propranolol. Over a twenty-four (24) hour period, blood levels are fairly constant for about twelve (12) hours, then decline exponentially.

Inderal LA should not be considered a simple mg-for-mg substitute for conventional propranolol and the blood levels achieved do not match (are lower than) those of two to four times daily dosing with the same dose. When changing to Inderal LA from conventional propranolol, a possible need for retitration upwards should be considered, especially to maintain effectiveness at the end of the dosing interval. In most clinical settings, however, such as hypertension or angina where there is little correlation between plasma levels and clinical effect, Inderal LA has been therapeutically equivalent to the same mg dose of conventional Inderal as assessed by 24-hour effects on blood pressure and on 24-hour exercise responses of heart rate, systolic pressure, and rate pressure product. Inderal LA can provide effective beta blockade for a 24-hour period.

The mechanism of the antihypertensive effect of Inderal has not been established. Among the factors that may be involved in contributing to the antihypertensive action are: (1) decreased cardiac output, (2) inhibition of renin release by the kidneys, and (3) diminution of tonic sympathetic nerve outflow from vasomotor centers in the brain. Although total peripheral resistance may increase initially, it readjusts to or below the pretreatment level with chronic use. Effects on plasma volume appear to be minor and somewhat variable. Inderal has been shown to cause a small increase in serum potassium concentration when used in the treatment of hypertensive patients.

In angina pectoris, propranolol generally reduces the oxygen requirement of the heart at any given level of effort by blocking the catecholamine-induced increases in the heart rate, systolic blood pressure, and the velocity and extent of myocardial contraction. Propranolol may increase oxygen requirements by increasing left ventricular fiber length, end diastolic pressure, and systolic ejection period. The net physiologic effect of beta-adrenergic blockade is usually advantageous and is manifested during exercise by delayed onset of pain and increased work capacity.

In dosages greater than required for beta blockade, Inderal also exerts a quinidine-like or anesthetic-like membrane action which affects the cardiac action potential. The significance of the membrane action in the treatment of arrhythmias is uncertain.

The mechanism of the antimigraine effect of propranolol has not been established. Beta-adrenergic receptors have been demonstrated in the pial vessels of the brain.

Beta-receptor blockade can be useful in conditions in which, because of pathologic or functional changes, sympathetic activity is detrimental to the patient. But there are also situations in which sympathetic stimulation is vital. For example, in patients with severely damaged hearts, adequate ventricular function is maintained by virtue of sympathetic drive, which should be preserved. In the presence of AV block, greater than first degree, beta blockade may prevent the necessary facilitating effect of sympathetic activity on conduction. Beta blockade results in bronchial constriction by interfering with adrenergic bronchodilator activity, which should be preserved in patients subject to bronchospasm.

Propranolol is not significantly dialyzable.

INDICATIONS AND USAGE

Hypertension

Inderal LA is indicated in the management of hypertension; it may be used alone or used in combination with other antihypertensive agents, particularly a thiazide diuretic. Inderal LA is not indicated in the management of hypertensive emergencies.

Angina Pectoris Due to Coronary Atherosclerosis

Inderal LA is indicated for the long-term management of patients with angina pectoris.

Migraine

Inderal LA is indicated for the prophylaxis of common migraine headache. The efficacy of propranolol in the treatment of a migraine attack that has started has not been established, and propranolol is not indicated for such use.

Hypertrophic Subaortic Stenosis

Inderal LA is useful in the management of hypertrophic subaortic stenosis, especially for treatment of exertional or other stress-induced angina, palpitations, and syncope. Inderal LA also improves exercise performance. The effectiveness of propranolol hydrochloride in this disease appears to be due to a reduction of the elevated outflow pressure gradient which is exacerbated by beta-receptor stimulation. Clinical improvement may be temporary.

CONTRAINDICATIONS

Inderal is contraindicated in 1) cardiogenic shock; 2) sinus bradycardia and greater than first-degree block; 3) bronchial asthma; 4) congestive heart failure (see **"WARNINGS"**), unless the failure is secondary to a tachyarrhythmia treatable with Inderal.

WARNINGS

Cardiac Failure: Sympathetic stimulation may be a vital component supporting circulatory function in patients with congestive heart failure, and its inhibition by beta blockade may precipitate more severe failure. Although beta blockers should be avoided in overt congestive heart failure, if necessary, they can be used with close follow-up in patients with a history of failure who are well compensated and are receiving digitalis and diuretics. Beta-adrenergic blocking agents do not abolish the inotropic action of digitalis on heart muscle.

In Patients without a History of Heart Failure, continued use of beta blockers can, in some cases, lead to cardiac failure. Therefore, at the first sign or symptom of heart failure, the patient should be digitalized and/or treated with diuretics, and the response observed closely, or Inderal should be discontinued (gradually, if possible).

In Patients with Angina Pectoris, there have been reports of exacerbation of angina and, in some cases, myocardial infarction, following *abrupt* discontinuance of Inderal therapy. Therefore, when discontinuance of Inderal is planned, the dosage should be gradually reduced over at least a few weeks, and the patient should be cautioned against interruption or cessation of therapy without the physician's advice. If Inderal therapy is interrupted and exacerbation of angina occurs, it usually is advisable to reinstitute Inderal therapy and take other measures appropriate for the management of unstable angina pectoris. Since coronary artery disease may be unrecognized, it may be prudent to follow the above advice in patients considered at risk of having occult atherosclerotic heart disease who are given propranolol for other indications.

Nonallergic Bronchospasm (e.g., Chronic Bronchitis, Emphysema)—PATIENTS WITH BRONCHOSPASTIC DISEASES SHOULD IN GENERAL NOT RECEIVE BETA BLOCKERS. Inderal should be administered with caution since it may block bronchodilation produced by endogenous and exogenous catecholamine stimulation of beta receptors.

Major Surgery: The necessity or desirability of withdrawal of beta-blocking therapy prior to major surgery is controversial. It should be noted, however, that the impaired ability of the heart to respond to reflex adrenergic stimuli may augment the risks of general anesthesia and surgical procedures.

Inderal, like other beta blockers, is a competitive inhibitor of beta-receptor agonists and its effects can be reversed by administration of such agents, e.g., dobutamine or isoproterenol. However, such patients may be subject to protracted severe hypotension. Difficulty in starting and maintaining the heartbeat has also been reported with beta blockers.

Diabetes and Hypoglycemia: Beta-adrenergic blockade may prevent the appearance of certain premonitory signs and symptoms (pulse rate and pressure changes) of acute hypoglycemia in labile insulin-dependent diabetes. In these patients, it may be more difficult to adjust the dosage of insulin. Hypoglycemic attacks may be accompanied by a precipitous elevation of blood pressure in patients on propranolol.

Propranolol therapy, particularly in infants and children, diabetic or not, has been associated with hypoglycemia especially during fasting as in preparation for surgery. Hypoglycemia also has been found after this type of drug therapy and prolonged physical exertion and has occurred in renal insufficiency, both during dialysis and sporadically, in patients on propranolol.

Thyrotoxicosis: Beta blockade may mask certain clinical signs of hyperthyroidism. Therefore, abrupt withdrawal of propranolol may be followed by an exacerbation of symptoms of hyperthyroidism, including thyroid storm. Propranolol may change thyroid-function tests, increasing T_4 and reverse T_3, and decreasing T_3.

In Patients with Wolff-Parkinson-White Syndrome, several cases have been reported in which, after propranolol, the tachycardia was replaced by a severe bradycardia requiring a demand pacemaker. In one case this resulted after an initial dose of 5 mg propranolol.

PRECAUTIONS

General

Propranolol should be used with caution in patients with impaired hepatic or renal function. Inderal is not indicated for the treatment of hypertensive emergencies.

Beta-adrenoreceptor blockade can cause reduction of intraocular pressure. Patients should be told that Inderal may interfere with the glaucoma screening test. Withdrawal may lead to a return of increased intraocular pressure.

Risk of anaphylactic reaction. While taking beta blockers, patients with a history of severe anaphylactic reaction to a variety of allergens may be more reactive to repeated challenge, either accidental, diagnostic, or therapeutic. Such patients may be unresponsive to the usual doses of epinephrine used to treat allergic reaction.

Clinical Laboratory Tests

Elevated blood urea levels in patients with severe heart disease, elevated serum transaminase, alkaline phosphatase, lactate dehydrogenase.

Drug Interactions

Patients receiving catecholamine-depleting drugs such as reserpine should be closely observed if Inderal is administered. The added catecholamine-blocking action may produce an excessive reduction of resting sympathetic nervous activity which may result in hypotension, marked bradycardia, vertigo, syncopal attacks, or orthostatic hypotension.

Caution should be exercised when patients receiving a beta blocker are administered a calcium-channel-blocking drug, especially intravenous verapamil, for both agents may depress myocardial contractility or atrioventricular conduction. On rare occasions, the concomitant intravenous use of a beta blocker and verapamil has resulted in serious adverse reactions, especially in patients with severe cardiomyopathy, congestive heart failure or recent myocardial infarction.

Blunting of the antihypertensive effect of beta-adrenoceptor blocking agents by nonsteroidal anti-inflammatory drugs has been reported.

Hypotension and cardiac arrest have been reported with the concomitant use of propranolol and haloperidol.

Aluminum hydroxide gel greatly reduces intestinal absorption of propranolol.

Ethanol slows the rate of absorption of propranolol.

Phenytoin, phenobarbitone, and *rifampin* accelerate propranolol clearance.

Chlorpromazine, when used concomitantly with propranolol, results in increased plasma levels of both drugs.

Antipyrine and *lidocaine* have reduced clearance when used concomitantly with propranolol.

Thyroxine may result in a lower than expected T_3 concentration when used concomitantly with propranolol.

Cimetidine decreases the hepatic metabolism of propranolol, delaying elimination and increasing blood levels.

Theophylline clearance is reduced when used concomitantly with propranolol.

Carcinogenesis, Mutagenesis, Impairment of Fertility

In dietary administration studies in which mice and rats were treated with propranolol for up to 18 months at doses of up to 150 mg/kg/day, there was no evidence of drug-related tumorigenesis. In a study in which both male and female rats were exposed to propranolol in their diets at concentrations of up to 0.05%, from 60 days prior to mating and throughout pregnancy and lactation for two generations, there were no effects on fertility. Based on differing results from Ames Tests performed by different laboratories, there is equivocal evidence for a genotoxic effect of propranolol in bacteria (*S. typhimurium* strain TA 1538).

Pregnancy: Pregnancy Category C

In a series of reproductive and developmental toxicology studies, propranolol was given to rats by gavage or in the diet throughout pregnancy and lactation. At doses of 150 mg/kg/day (> 10 times the maximum recommended human daily dose of propranolol on a body weight basis), but not at doses of 80 mg/kg/day, treatment was associated with embryotoxicity (reduced litter size and increased resorption sites) as well as neonatal toxicity (deaths). Propranolol also was administered (in the feed) to rabbits (throughout pregnancy and lactation) at doses as high as 150 mg/kg/day (> 15 times the maximum recommended daily human dose). No evidence of embryo or neonatal toxicity was noted.

There are no adequate and well-controlled studies in pregnant women. Intrauterine growth retardation has been reported in neonates whose mothers received propranolol during pregnancy. Neonates whose mothers are receiving propranolol at parturition have exhibited bradycardia, hypoglycemia and respiratory depression. Adequate facilities for monitoring these infants at birth should be available. Inderal should be used during pregnancy only if the potential benefit justifies the potential risk to the fetus.

Nursing Mothers

Inderal is excreted in human milk. Caution should be exercised when Inderal is administered to a nursing woman.

Pediatric Use

Safety and effectiveness in pediatric patients have not been established.

Geriatric Use

Clinical studies of propranolol did not include sufficient numbers of subjects aged 65 and over to determine whether they respond differently from younger subjects. Other reported clinical experience has not identified differences in responses between the elderly and younger patients. In general, dose selection for an elderly patient should be cautious, usually starting at the low end of the dosing range, reflecting the greater frequency of the decreased hepatic, renal or cardiac function, and of concomitant disease or other drug therapy.

ADVERSE REACTIONS

Most adverse effects have been mild and transient and have rarely required the withdrawal of therapy.

Cardiovascular: Bradycardia; congestive heart failure; intensification of AV block; hypotension; paresthesia of hands; thrombocytopenic purpura; arterial insufficiency, usually of the Raynaud type.

Central Nervous System: Light-headedness, mental depression manifested by insomnia, lassitude, weakness, fatigue; reversible mental depression progressing to catatonia; visual disturbances; hallucinations; vivid dreams; an acute reversible syndrome characterized by disorientation for time and place, short-term memory loss, emotional lability, slightly clouded sensorium, and decreased performance on neuropsychometrics. For immediate formulations, fatigue, lethargy, and vivid dreams appear dose related.

Gastrointestinal: Nausea, vomiting, epigastric distress, abdominal cramping, diarrhea, constipation, mesenteric arterial thrombosis, ischemic colitis.

Allergic: Pharyngitis and agranulocytosis; erythematous rash, fever combined with aching and sore throat; laryngospasm, and respiratory distress.

Respiratory: Bronchospasm.

Hematologic: Agranulocytosis, nonthrombocytopenic purpura, thrombocytopenic purpura.

Autoimmune: In extremely rare instances, systemic lupus erythematosus has been reported.

Miscellaneous: Alopecia, LE-like reactions, psoriasiform rashes, dry eyes, male impotence, and Peyronie's disease have been reported rarely. Oculomucocutaneous reactions involving the skin, serous membranes and conjunctivae reported for a beta blocker (practolol) have not been associated with propranolol.

DOSAGE AND ADMINISTRATION

Inderal LA provides propranolol hydrochloride in a sustained-release capsule for administration once daily. If patients are switched from Inderal Tablets to Inderal LA Capsules, care should be taken to assure that the desired therapeutic effect is maintained. Inderal LA should not be considered a simple mg-for-mg substitute for Inderal. Inderal LA has different kinetics and produces lower blood levels. Retitration may be necessary, especially to maintain effectiveness at the end of the 24-hour dosing interval.

Hypertension

Dosage must be individualized. The usual initial dosage is 80 mg Inderal LA once daily, whether used alone or added to a diuretic. The dosage may be increased to 120 mg once daily or higher until adequate blood pressure control is achieved. The usual maintenance dosage is 120 to 160 mg once daily. In some instances a dosage of 640 mg may be required. The time needed for full hypertensive response to a given dosage is variable and may range from a few days to several weeks.

Angina Pectoris

Dosage must be individualized. Starting with 80 mg Inderal LA once daily, dosage should be gradually increased at three- to seven-day intervals until optimal response is obtained. Although individual patients may respond at any dosage level, the average optimal dosage appears to be 160 mg once daily. In angina pectoris, the value and safety of dosage exceeding 320 mg per day have not been established. If treatment is to be discontinued, reduce dosage gradually over a period of a few weeks (see **"WARNINGS"**).

Migraine

Dosage must be individualized. The initial oral dose is 80 mg Inderal LA once daily. The usual effective dose range is 160 to 240 mg once daily. The dosage may be increased gradually to achieve optimal migraine prophylaxis. If a satisfactory response is not obtained within four to six weeks after reaching the maximal dose, Inderal LA therapy should be discontinued. It may be advisable to withdraw the drug gradually over a period of several weeks.

Hypertrophic Subaortic Stenosis

80 to 160 mg Inderal LA once daily.

Pediatric Dosage

At this time the data on the use of the drug in this age group are too limited to permit adequate directions for use.

OVERDOSAGE

Inderal is not significantly dialyzable. In the event of overdosage or exaggerated response, the following measures should be employed:

General

If ingestion is, or may have been, recent, evacuate gastric contents, taking care to prevent pulmonary aspiration.

Bradycardia

ADMINISTER ATROPINE (0.25 to 1.0 mg); IF THERE IS NO RESPONSE TO VAGAL BLOCKADE, ADMINISTER ISOPROTERENOL CAUTIOUSLY.

Cardiac Failure

DIGITALIZATION AND DIURETICS.

Hypotension

VASOPRESSORS, e.g., LEVARTERENOL OR EPINEPHRINE (THERE IS EVIDENCE THAT EPINEPHRINE IS THE DRUG OF CHOICE).

Bronchospasm

ADMINISTER ISOPROTERENOL AND AMINOPHYLLINE.

HOW SUPPLIED

Inderal® LA Capsules (propranolol hydrochloride)

Each white/light-blue capsule, identified by 3 narrow bands, 1 wide band, and "INDERAL LA 60," contains 60 mg of propranolol hydrochloride in bottles of 100 (NDC 0046-0470-81) and in bottles of 1,000 (NDC 0046-0470-91).

Each light-blue capsule, identified by 3 narrow bands, 1 wide band, and "INDERAL LA 80," contains 80 mg of propranolol hydrochloride in bottles of 100 (NDC 0046-0471-81) and in bottles of 1,000 (NDC 0046-0471-91).

Each light-blue/dark-blue capsule, identified by 3 narrow bands, 1 wide band, and "INDERAL LA 120," contains 120 mg of propranolol hydrochloride in bottles of 100 (NDC 0046-0473-81) and in bottles of 1,000 (NDC 0046-0473-91).

Each dark-blue capsule, identified by 3 narrow bands, 1 wide band, and "INDERAL LA 160," contains 160 mg of propranolol hydrochloride in bottles of 100 (NDC 0046-0479-81) and in bottles of 1,000 (NDC 0046-0479-91).

The appearance of these capsules is a registered trademark of Wyeth-Ayerst Laboratories.

Store at room temperature (approximately 25° C).

Protect from light, moisture, freezing, and excessive heat.

Dispense in a tight, light-resistant container as defined in the USP.

Use carton to protect contents from light.

Manufactured by:
Ayerst Laboratories Inc.
A Wyeth-Ayerst Company
Philadelphia, PA 19101
CI 4628-3 Revised March 17, 1999

Shown in Product Identification Guide, page 341

INDERIDE® ℞

[*in 'de-rīde*]
(propranolol hydrochloride [INDERAL®] and hydrochlorothiazide)

Caution: Federal law prohibits dispensing without prescription.

DESCRIPTION

Inderide Tablets for oral administration combine two antihypertensive agents: Inderal (propranolol hydrochloride), a beta-adrenergic blocking agent, and hydrochlorothiazide, a thiazide diuretic-antihypertensive. Inderide 40/25 Tablets contain 40 mg propranolol hydrochloride and 25 mg hydrochlorothiazide; Inderide 80/25 Tablets contain 80 mg propranolol hydrochloride and 25 mg hydrochlorothiazide.

Inderal (propranolol hydrochloride) is a synthetic beta-adrenergic receptor-blocking agent chemically described as 1-(Isopropylamino)-3-(1-naphthyloxy)-2-propanol hydrochloride. Its structural formula is:

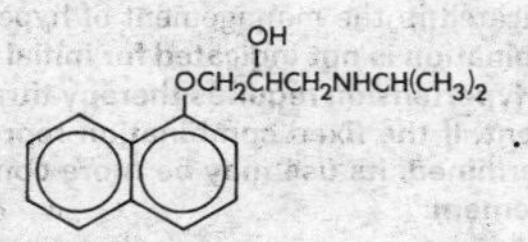

Propranolol hydrochloride is a stable, white, crystalline solid which is readily soluble in water and ethanol. Its molecular weight is 295.81.

Hydrochlorothiazide is a white, or practically white, practically odorless, crystalline powder. It is slightly soluble in water; freely soluble in sodum hydroxide solution; sparingly soluble in methanol; insoluble in ether, chloroform, benzene, and dilute mineral acids. Its chemical name is: 6-Chloro-3,4-dihydro-2H-1,2,4-benzothiadiazine-7-sulfonamide1,1-dioxide. Its structural formula is:

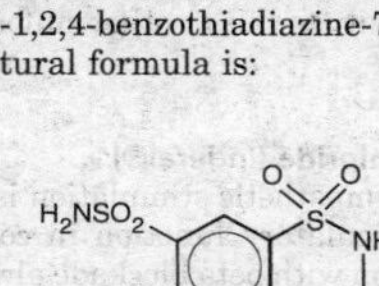

The inactive ingredients contained in Inderide Tablets are lactose, magnesium stearate, microcrystalline cellulose, stearic acid, and yellow ferric oxide.

CLINICAL PHARMACOLOGY

Propranolol hydrochloride (Inderal®)

Propranolol hydrochloride is a nonselective beta-adrenergic receptor blocking agent possessing no other autonomic nervous system activity. It specifically competes with beta-adrenergic receptor stimulating agents for available receptor sites. When access to beta-receptor sites is blocked by propranolol, the chronotropic, inotropic, and vasodilator responses to beta-adrenergic stimulation are decreased proportionately.

Propranolol is almost completely absorbed from the gastrointestinal tract, but a portion is immediately metabolized by the liver on its first pass through the portal circulation.

Peak effect occurs in one to one-and-one-half hours. The biologic half-life is approximately four hours. Propranolol is not significantly dialyzable. There is no simple correlation between dose or plasma level and therapeutic effect, and the dose-sensitivity range, as observed in clinical practice, is

Continued on next page

Inderide—Cont.

wide. The principal reason for this is that sympathetic tone varies widely between individuals. Since there is no reliable test to estimate sympathetic tone or to determine whether total beta blockade has been achieved, proper dosage requires titration.

The mechanism of the antihypertensive effects of propranolol has not been established. Among the factors that may be involved in contributing to the antihypertensive action are (1) decreased cardiac output, (2) inhibition of renin release by the kidneys, and (3) diminution of tonic sympathetic nerve outflow from vasomotor centers in the brain. Although total peripheral resistance may increase initially, it readjusts to, or below, the pretreatment level with chronic use. Effects on plasma volume appear to be minor and somewhat variable. Propranolol has been shown to cause a small increase in serum potassium concentration when used in the treatment of hypertensive patients. Propranolol hydrochloride decreases heart rate, cardiac output, and blood pressure.

Beta-receptor blockade can be useful in conditions in which, because of pathologic or functional changes, sympathetic activity is detrimental to the patient. But there are also situations in which sympathetic stimulation is vital. For example, in patients with severely damaged hearts, adequate ventricular function is maintained by virtue of sympathetic drive, which should be preserved. In the presence of AV block greater than first degree, beta blockade may prevent the necessary facilitating effect of sympathetic activity on conduction. Beta blockade results in bronchial constriction by interfering with adrenergic bronchodilator activity, which should be preserved in patients subject to bronchospasm.

The proper objective of beta-blockade therapy is to decrease adverse sympathetic stimulation, but not to the degree that may impair necessary sympathetic support.

Hydrochlorothiazide

Hydrochlorothiazide is a benzothiadiazine (thiazide) diuretic closely related to chlorothiazide. The mechanism of the antihypertensive effect of the thiazides is unknown. Thiazides do not affect normal blood pressure.

Thiazides affect the renal tubular mechanism of electrolyte reabsorption. At maximal therapeutic dosage, all thiazides are approximately equal in their diuretic potency.

Thiazides increase excretion of sodium and chloride in approximately equivalent amounts. Natriuresis causes a secondary loss of potassium and bicarbonate. Onset of diuretic action of hydrochlorothiazide occurs in two hours, and the peak effect in about four hours. Its action persists for approximately six to 12 hours. Thiazides are eliminated rapidly by the kidney.

INDICATIONS AND USAGE

Inderide is indicated in the management of hypertension. **This fixed combination is not indicated for initial therapy of hypertension. Hypertension requires therapy titrated to the individual patient. If the fixed combination represents the dosage so determined, its use may be more convenient in patient management.**

CONTRAINDICATIONS

Propranolol hydrochloride (Inderal®)

Propranolol is contraindicated in: 1) cardiogenic shock; 2) sinus bradycardia and greater than first-degree block; 3) bronchial asthma; 4) congestive heart failure (see **WARNINGS**) unless the failure is secondary to a tachyarrhythmia treatable with propranolol.

Hydrochlorothiazide

Hydrochlorothiazide is contraindicated in patients with anuria or hypersensitivity to this or other sulfonamide-derived drugs.

WARNINGS

Propranolol hydrochloride (Inderal®)

Cardiac Failure: Sympathetic stimulation is a vital component supporting circulatory function in congestive heart failure, and inhibition with beta blockade always carries the potential hazard of further depressing myocardial contractility and precipitating cardiac failure. Propranolol acts selectively without abolishing the inotropic action of digitalis on the heart muscle (i.e., that of supporting the strength of myocardial contractions). In patients already receiving digitalis, the positive inotropic action of digitalis may be reduced by propranolol's negative inotropic effect. The effects of propranolol and digitalis are additive in depressing AV conduction.

Patients Without a History of Heart Failure: Continued depression of the myocardium over a period of time can, in some cases, lead to cardiac failure. In rare instances, this has been observed during propranolol therapy. Therefore, at the first sign or symptom of impending cardiac failure, patients should be fully digitalized and/or given additional diuretic, and the response observed closely: a) if cardiac failure continues, despite adequate digitalization and diuretic therapy, propranolol therapy should be withdrawn (gradually, if possible); b) if tachyarrhythmia is being controlled, patients should be maintained on combined therapy and the patient closely followed until threat of cardiac failure is over.

Angina Pectoris: There have been reports of exacerbation of angina and, in some cases, myocardial infarction following *abrupt* discontinuation of propranolol therapy. Therefore, when discontinuance of propranolol is planned, the dosage should be gradually reduced and the patient should be carefully monitored. In addition, when propranolol is prescribed for angina pectoris, the patient should be cautioned against interruption or cessation of therapy without the physician's advice. If propranolol therapy is interrupted and exacerbation of angina occurs, it usually is advisable to reinstitute propranolol therapy and take other measures appropriate for the management of unstable angina pectoris. Since coronary artery disease may be unrecognized, it may be prudent to follow the above advice in patients considered at risk of having occult atherosclerotic heart disease, who are given propranolol for other indications.

Nonallergic Bronchospasm (e.g., chronic bronchitis, emphysema): PATIENTS WITH BRONCHOSPASTIC DISEASES SHOULD, IN GENERAL, NOT RECEIVE BETA BLOCKERS. Propranolol should be administered with caution since it may block bronchodilation produced by endogenous and exogenous catecholamine stimulation of beta receptors.

Major Surgery: The necessity or desirability of withdrawal of beta-blocking therapy prior to major surgery is controversial. It should be noted, however, that the impaired ability of the heart to respond to reflex adrenergic stimuli may augment the risks of general anesthesia and surgical procedures.

Propranolol, like other beta blockers, is a competitive inhibitor of beta-receptor agonists, and its effects can be reversed by administration of such agents, e.g., dobutamine or isoproterenol. However, such patients may be subject to protracted severe hypotension. Difficulty in starting and maintaining the heartbeat has also been reported with beta blockers.

Diabetes and Hypoglycemia: Beta-adrenergic blockade may prevent the appearance of certain premonitory signs and symptoms (pulse rate and pressure changes) of acute hypoglycemia in labile insulin-dependent diabetes. In these patients, it may be more difficult to adjust the dosage of insulin. Hypoglycemic attack may be accompanied by a precipitous elevation of blood pressure.

Propranolol therapy, particularly in infants and children, diabetic or not, has been associated with hypoglycemia especially during fasting as in preparation for surgery. Hypoglycemia also has been found after this type of drug therapy and prolonged physical exertion and has occurred in renal insufficiency, both during dialysis and sporadically, in subjects on propranolol.

Thyrotoxicosis: Beta blockade may mask certain clinical signs of hyperthyroidism. Therefore, abrupt withdrawal of propranolol may be followed by an exacerbation of symptoms of hyperthyroidism, including thyroid storm. Propranolol may change thyroid-function tests, increasing T_4 and reverse T_3, and decreasing T_3.

Wolff-Parkinson-White Syndrome: Several cases have been reported in which, after propranolol, the tachycardia was replaced by a severe bradycardia requiring a demand pacemaker. In one case this resulted after an initial dose of 5 mg propranolol.

Hydrochlorothiazide

Thiazides should be used with caution in severe renal disease. In patients with renal disease, thiazides may precipitate azotemia. In patients with impaired renal function, cumulative effects of the drug may develop.

Thiazides should also be used with caution in patients with impaired hepatic function or progressive liver disease, since minor alterations of fluid and electrolyte balance may precipitate hepatic coma.

Thiazides may add to or potentiate the action of other antihypertensive drugs. Potentiation occurs with ganglionic or peripheral adrenergic-blocking drugs.

Sensitivity reactions may occur in patients with a history of allergy or bronchial asthma. The possibility of exacerbation or activation of systemic lupus erythematosus has been reported.

PRECAUTIONS

General

Propranolol hydrochloride (Inderal®)

Propranolol should be used with caution in patients with impaired hepatic or renal function. Inderide is not indicated for the treatment of hypertensive emergencies.

Risk of anaphylactic reaction: While taking beta blockers, patients with a history of severe anaphylactic reaction to a variety of allergens may be more reactive to repeated challenge, either accidental, diagnostic, or therapeutic. Such patients may be unresponsive to the usual doses of epinephrine used to treat allergic reaction.

Hydrochlorothiazide

All patients receiving thiazide therapy should be observed for clinical signs of fluid or electrolyte imbalance, namely hyponatremia, hypochloremic alkalosis, and hypokalemia. Serum and urine electrolyte determinations are particularly important when the patient is vomiting excessively or receiving parenteral fluids. Medication such as digitalis may also influence serum electrolytes. Warning signs, irrespective of cause, are: dryness of mouth, thirst, weakness, lethargy, drowsiness, restlessness, muscle pains or cramps, muscular fatigue, hypotension, oliguria, tachycardia, and gastrointestinal disturbances such as nausea and vomiting.

Hypokalemia may develop, especially with brisk diuresis or when severe cirrhosis is present.

Interference with adequate oral electrolyte intake will also contribute to hypokalemia. Hypokalemia can sensitize or exaggerate the response of the heart to the toxic effects of digitalis (e.g., increased ventricular irritability).

Hypokalemia may be avoided or treated by use of potassium supplements or foods with a high potassium content.

Any chloride deficit is generally mild, and usually does not require specific treatment except under extraordinary circumstances (as in liver or renal disease). Dilutional hyponatremia may occur in edematous patients in hot weather; appropriate therapy is water restriction rather than administration of salt, except in rare instances when the hyponatremia is life-threatening. In actual salt depletion, appropriate replacement is the therapy of choice.

Hyperuricemia may occur or frank gout may be precipitated in certain patients receiving thiazide therapy.

Diabetes mellitus which has been latent may become manifest during thiazide administration.

The antihypertensive effects of the drug may be enhanced in the postsympathectomy patient.

If progressive renal impairment becomes evident, consider withholding or discontinuing diuretic therapy.

Calcium excretion is decreased by thiazides. Pathologic changes in the parathyroid gland with hypercalcemia and hypophosphatemia have been observed in a few patients on prolonged thiazide therapy. The common complications of hyperparathyroidism, such as renal lithiasis, bone resorption, and peptic ulceration, have not been seen.

Information for Patients

Beta-adrenoreceptor blockade can cause reduction of intraocular pressure. Patients should be told that Inderide may interfere with the glaucoma screening test. Withdrawal may lead to a return of increased intraocular pressure.

Laboratory Tests

Propranolol hydrochloride (Inderal®)

Elevated blood urea levels in patients with severe heart disease, elevated serum transaminase, alkaline phosphatase, lactate dehydrogenase.

Hydrochlorothiazide

Periodic determination of serum electrolytes to detect possible electrolyte imbalance should be performed at appropriate intervals.

Drug/Drug Interactions

Propranolol hydrochloride (Inderal®)

Patients receiving catecholamine-depleting drugs such as reserpine should be closely observed if Inderide is administered. The added catecholamine-blocking action may produce an excessive reduction of resting sympathetic nervous activity, which may result in hypotension, marked bradycardia, vertigo, syncopal attacks, or orthostatic hypotension.

Caution should be exercised when patients receiving a beta blocker are administered a calcium-channel blocking drug, especially intravenous verapamil, for both agents may depress myocardial contractility or atrioventricular conduction. On rare occasions, the concomitant intravenous use of a beta blocker and verapamil has resulted in serious adverse reactions, especially in patients with severe cardiomyopathy, congestive heart failure, or recent myocardial infarction.

Blunting of the antihypertensive effect of beta-adrenoceptor blocking agents by nonsteroidal anti-inflammatory drugs has been reported.

Hypotension and cardiac arrest have been reported with the concomitant use of propranolol and haloperidol.

Aluminum hydroxide gel greatly reduces intestinal absorption of propranolol.

Ethanol slows the rate of absorption of propranolol.

Phenytoin, phenobarbitone, and rifampin accelerate propranolol clearance.

Chlorpromazine, when used concomitantly with propranolol, results in increased plasma levels of both drugs.

Antipyrine and *lidocaine* have reduced clearance when used concomitantly with propranolol.

Thyroxine may result in a lower than expected T_3 concentration when used concomitantly with propranolol.

Cimetidine decreases the hepatic metabolism of propranolol, delaying elimination and increasing blood levels.

Theophylline clearance is reduced when used concomitantly with propranolol.

Hydrochlorothiazide

Thiazide drugs may increase the responsiveness to tubocurarine.

Thiazides may decrease arterial responsiveness to norepinephrine. This diminution is not sufficient to preclude effectiveness of the pressor agent for therapeutic use.

Insulin requirements in diabetic patients may be increased, decreased, or unchanged.

Hypokalemia may develop during concomitant use of corticosteroids or ACTH.

Drug/Laboratory Test Interactions

Hydrochlorothiazide

Thiazides may decrease serum PBI levels without signs of thyroid disturbance.

Thiazides should be discontinued before carrying out tests for parathyroid function (see **"PRECAUTIONS—General"**).

Carcinogenesis, Mutagenesis, Impairment of Fertility

Combinations of propranolol and hydrochlorothiazide have not been evaluated for carcinogenic or mutagenic potential or for potential to adversely affect fertility.

Propranolol hydrochloride (Inderal®)

In dietary administration studies in which mice and rats were treated with propranolol for up to 18 months at doses of up to 150 mg/kg/day, there was no evidence of drug-related tumorigenesis. In a study in which both male and female rats were exposed to propranolol in their diets at concentrations of up to 0.05%, from 60 days prior to mating and throughout pregnancy and lactation for two generations, there were no effects on fertility. Based on differing results from Ames Tests performed by different laboratories, there is equivocal evidence for a genotoxic effect of propranolol in bacteria (*S. typhimurium* strain TA 1538).

Hydrochlorothiazide

Two-year feeding studies in mice and rats conducted under the auspices of the National Toxicology Program (NTP) uncovered no evidence of a carcinogenic potential of hydrochlorothiazide in female mice (at doses of up to approximately 600 mg/kg/day) or in male and female rats (at doses of up to approximately 100 mg/kg/day). The NTP, however, found equivocal evidence for hepatocarcinogenicity in male mice.

Hydrochlorothiazide was not genotoxic *in vitro* in the Ames bacterial mutagen assay (*S. typhimurium* strains TA 98, TA 100, TA 1535, TA 1537 and TA 1538) or in the Chinese Hamster Ovary (CHO) test for chromosomal aberrations. Nor was it genotoxic *in vivo* in assays using mouse germinal cell chromosomes, Chinese hamster bone marrow chromosomes, and the *Drosophila* sex-linked recessive lethal trait gene. Positive test results were obtained in the *in vitro* CHO Sister Chromatid Exchange (clastogenicity), Mouse Lymphoma Cell (mutagenicity) and *Aspergillus nidulans* non-disjunction assays.

Hydrochlorothiazide had no adverse effects on the fertility of mice and rats of either sex in studies wherein these species were exposed, via their diet, to doses of up to 100 mg/kg and 4 mg/kg, respectively, prior to mating and throughout gestation.

Pregnancy: Pregnancy Category C

Combinations of propranolol and hydrochlorothiazide have not been evaluated for effects on pregnancy in animals. Nor are there adequate and well-controlled studies of propranolol, hydrochlorothiazide, or Inderide in pregnant women. Inderide should be used during pregnancy only if the potential benefit justifies the potential risk to the fetus.

Propranolol hydrochloride (Inderal®)

In a series of reproduction and developmental toxicology studies, propranolol was given to rats by gavage or in the diet throughout pregnancy and lactation. At doses of 150 mg/kg/day (>30 times the dose of propranolol contained in the maximum recommended human daily dose of Inderide), but not at doses of 80 mg/kg/day, treatment was associated with embryotoxicity (reduced liter size and increased resorption sites) as well as neonatal toxicity (deaths). Propranolol also was administered (in the feed) to rabbits (throughout pregnancy and lactation) at doses as high as 150 mg/kg/day (>45 times the dose of propranolol contained in the maximum recommended daily human dose of Inderide). No evidence of embryo or neonatal toxicity was noted.

Intrauterine growth retardation has been reported in human neonates whose mothers received propranolol during pregnancy. Neonates whose mothers received propranolol at parturition have exhibited bradycardia, hypoglycemia and respiratory depression. Adequate facilities for monitoring these infants at birth should be available.

Hydrochlorothiazide

Studies in which hydrochlorothiazide was orally administered to pregnant mice and rats at doses of up to 3000 and 1000 mg/kg/day, respectively, provided no evidence of harm to the fetus.

Thiazides cross the placental barrier and appear in cord blood. The use of thiazides in pregnant women requires that the anticipated benefit be weighed against possible hazards to the fetus. These hazards include fetal or neonatal jaundice, thrombocytopenia, and possibly other adverse reactions that have occurred in the adult.

Nursing Mothers

Propranolol hydrochloride (Inderal®)

Propranolol is excreted in human milk. Caution should be exercised when Inderide is administered to a nursing woman.

Hydrochlorothiazide

Thiazides appear in breast milk. If the use of drug is deemed essential, the patient should stop nursing.

Pediatric Use

Safety and effectiveness in pediatric patients have not been established.

ADVERSE REACTIONS

The following adverse reactions have been observed, but there is not enough systematic collection of data to support an estimate of their frequency. Within each category, adverse reactions are listed in decreasing order of severity. Although many side effects are mild and transient, some require discontinuation of therapy.

Propranolol hydrochloride (Inderal®)

Cardiovascular: Congestive heart failure; hypotension; intensification of AV block; bradycardia; thrombocytopenic purpura; arterial insufficiency, usually of the Raynaud type; paresthesia of hands.

Central Nervous System: Reversible mental depression progressing to catatonia; mental depression manifested by insomnia, lassitude, weakness, fatigue; an acute reversible syndrome characterized by disorientation for time and place, short-term memory loss, emotional lability, slightly clouded sensorium, decreased performance on neuropsychometrics; hallucinations; visual disturbances; vivid dreams; light-headedness. Total daily doses above 160 mg (when administered as divided doses of greater than 80 mg each) may be associated with an increased incidence of fatigue, lethargy, and vivid dreams.

Gastrointestinal: Mesenteric arterial thrombosis; ischemic colitis; nausea, vomiting, epigastric distress, abdominal cramping, diarrhea, constipation.

Allergic: Laryngospasm and respiratory distress; pharyngitis and agranulocytosis; fever combined with aching and sore throat; erythematous rash.

Respiratory: Bronchospasm.

Hematologic: Agranulocytosis; nonthrombocytopenic purpura; thrombocytopenic purpura.

Autoimmune: In extremely rare instances, systemic lupus erythematosus has been reported.

Miscellaneous: Male impotence. Alopecia, LE-like reactions, psoriasiform rashes, dry eyes, and Peyronie's disease have been reported rarely. Oculomucocutaneous reactions involving the skin, serous membranes, and conjunctivae reported for a beta blocker (practolol) have not been associated with propranolol.

Hydrochlorothiazide

Cardiovascular: Orthostatic hypotension (may be aggravated by alcohol, barbiturates or narcotics).

Central Nervous System: Dizziness, vertigo, headache, xanthopsia, paresthesias.

Gastrointestinal: Pancreatitis; jaundice (intrahepatic cholestatic jaundice); sialadenitis; anorexia, nausea, vomiting, gastric irritation, cramping, diarrhea, constipation.

Hypersensitivity: Anaphylactic reactions; necrotizing angiitis (vasculitis, cutaneous vasculitis); respiratory distress including pneumonitis; fever; urticaria, rash, purpura, photosensitivity.

Hematologic: Aplastic anemia, agranulocytosis, leukopenia, thrombocytopenia.

Miscellaneous: Hyperglycemia, glycosuria; hyperuricemia; muscle spasm; weakness; restlessness; transient blurred vision.

Whenever adverse reactions are moderate or severe, thiazide dosage should be reduced or therapy withdrawn.

OVERDOSAGE

The propranolol hydrochloride component may cause bradycardia, cardiac failure, hypotension, or bronchospasm. Propranolol is not significantly dialyzable.

The hydrochlorothiazide component can be expected to cause diuresis. Lethargy of varying degree may appear and may progress to coma within a few hours, with minimal depression of respiration and cardiovascular function, and in the absence of significant serum electrolyte changes or dehydration. The mechanism of central nervous system depression with thiazide overdosage is unknown. Gastrointestinal irritation and hypermotility can occur, temporary elevation of BUN has been reported, and serum electrolyte changes could occur, especially in patients with impairment of renal function.

The oral LD_{50} dosages in rats and mice for propranolol, hydrochlorothiazide, and combined propranolol/hydrochlorothiazide (40/25, 80/25) are 364 to 533 mg/kg, greater than 2,750 to 5,000 mg/kg, and 538 to 845 mg/kg, respectively.

Treatment

The following measures should be employed:

General—If ingestion is, or may have been, recent, evacuate gastric contents, taking care to prevent pulmonary aspiration.

Bradycardia—Administer atropine (0.25 to 1.0 mg). If there is no response to vagal blockade, administer isoproterenol cautiously.

Cardiac Failure—Digitalization and diuretics.

Hypotension—Vasopressors, e.g., levarterenol or epinephrine.

Bronchospasm—Administer isoproterenol and aminophylline.

Stupor or Coma—Administer supportive therapy as clinically warranted.

Gastrointestinal Effects—Though usually of short duration, these may require symptomatic treatment.

Abnormalities in BUN and/or Serum Electrolytes—Monitor serum electrolyte levels and renal function; institute supportive measures as required individually to maintain hydration, electrolyte balance, respiration, and cardiovascular-renal function.

DOSAGE AND ADMINISTRATION

The dosage must be determined by individual titration.

Hydrochlorothiazide can be given at doses of 12.5 to 50 mg per day when used alone. The initial dose of propranolol is 80 mg daily, and it may be increased gradually until optimal blood pressure control is achieved. The usual effective dose when used alone is 160 to 480 mg per day.

One Inderide Tablet twice daily can be used to administer up to 160 mg of propranolol and 50 mg of hydrochlorothiazide. For doses of propranolol greater than 160 mg the combination products are not appropriate, because their use would lead to an excessive dose of the thiazide component.

When necessary, another antihypertensive agent may be added gradually beginning with 50 percent of the usual recommended starting dose to avoid an excessive fall in blood pressure.

HOW SUPPLIED

Inderide 40/25

Each hexagonal-shaped, off-white, scored tablet, embossed with an "I" and imprinted with "INDERIDE 40/25," contains 40 mg propranolol hydrochloride (Inderal®) and 25 mg hydrochlorothiazide, in bottles of 100 (NDC 0046-0484-81) and 1,000 (NDC 0046-0484-91).

Inderide 80/25

Each hexagonal-shaped, off-white, scored tablet, embossed with an "I" and imprinted with "INDERIDE 80/25," contains 80 mg propranolol hydrochloride (Inderal®) and 25 mg hydrochlorothiazide, in bottles of 100 (NDC 0046-0488-81).

Store at room temperature (approximately 25° C).

Protect from moisture, freezing, and excessive heat.

Dispense in a well-closed container as defined in the USP.

The appearance of these tablets is a registered trademark of Wyeth-Ayerst Laboratories.

Manufactured by:
Ayerst Laboratories Inc.
A Wyeth-Ayerst Company
Philadelphia, PA 19101

CI 4982-1 Issued June 19, 1997

Shown in Product Identification Guide, page 341

INDERIDE® LA ℞

[*in 'de-rīde*]

(propranolol hydrochloride and hydrochlorothiazide)

Long-Acting Capsules

No. 455—Each Inderide® LA 80/50 Capsule contains:

Propranolol hydrochloride (Inderal® LA)	80 mg
Hydrochlorothiazide	50 mg

No. 457—Each Inderide® LA 120/50 Capsule contains:

Propranolol hydrochloride (Inderal® LA)	120 mg
Hydrochlorothiazide	50 mg

No. 459—Each Inderide® LA 160/50 Capsule contains:

Propranolol hydrochloride (Inderal® LA)	160 mg
Hydrochlorothiazide	50 mg

Caution: Federal law prohibits dispensing without prescription.

DESCRIPTION

Inderide LA is indicated in the once-daily management of hypertension.

Inderide LA combines two antihypertensive agents: Inderal (propranolol hydrochloride), a beta-adrenergic receptor-blocking agent, and hydrochlorothiazide, a thiazide diuretic-antihypertensive. Inderide LA is formulated to provide a sustained release of propranolol hydrochloride. Hydrochlorothiazide in Inderide LA exists in a conventional (not sustained-release) formulation.

Inderal (propranolol hydrochloride) is a synthetic beta-adrenergic receptor-blocking agent chemically described as 1-(Isopropylamino)-3-(1-naphthyloxy)-2-propanol hydrochloride. Its structural formula is:

$OCH_2CH(OH)CH_2NHCH(CH_3)_2 \cdot HCl$

Propranolol hydrochloride is a stable, white, crystalline solid which is readily soluble in water and ethanol. Its molecular weight is 295.81.

Hydrochlorothiazide is a white, or practically white, practically odorless, crystalline powder. It is slightly soluble in water; freely soluble in sodium hydroxide solution; sparingly soluble in methanol; insoluble in ether, chloroform, benzene, and dilute mineral acids. Its chemical name is 6-Chloro-3,4-dihydro-2H-1,2,4-benzothiadiazine-7-sulfonamide 1,1-dioxide. Its structural formula is:

H_2NO_2S … NH … Cl … N

Inderide LA contains the following inactive ingredients: calcium carbonate, ethylcellulose, gelatin capsules, hydroxypropyl methylcellulose, lactose, magnesium stearate, microcrystalline cellulose, sodium lauryl sulfate, sodium starch glycolate, titanium dioxide, and D&C Yellow No. 10. In addition, Inderide LA 80/50 mg and 120/50 mg Capsules contain D&C Red No. 33; Inderide LA 120/50 mg and 160/50 mg Capsules contain FD&C Blue No. 1 and FD&C Red No. 40.

CLINICAL PHARMACOLOGY

Propranolol Hydrochloride (Inderal®)

Inderal is a nonselective, beta-adrenergic receptor-blocking agent possessing no other autonomic nervous system activity. It specifically competes with beta-adrenergic receptor-stimulating agents for available receptor sites. When access

Continued on next page

Inderide LA—Cont.

to beta-receptor sites is blocked by Inderal, the chronotropic, inotropic, and vasodilator responses to beta-adrenergic stimulation are decreased proportionately.
Inderide LA Capsules (80/50, 120/50, and 160/50 mg) release propranolol hydrochloride at a controlled and predictable rate. Peak propranolol blood levels following dosing with Inderide LA occur at about 6 hours, and the apparent plasma half-life is about 10 hours. Over a 24-hour period, propranolol blood levels are fairly constant for about 12 hours, then decline exponentially. When measured at steady state over a 24-hour period, the areas under the propranolol plasma concentration-time curve (AUCs) for the capsules are approximately 60% to 65% of the AUCs for a comparable divided daily dose of Inderal Tablets. The lower AUCs for the capsules are due to greater hepatic metabolism of propranolol resulting from the slower rate of absorption of propranolol.
Inderide LA should not be considered a simple mg-for-mg substitute for conventional Inderide Tablets, and the propranolol blood levels achieved do not match (are lower than) those of twice-daily dosing of Inderide Tablets with the same dose. When changing to Inderide LA from conventional Inderide Tablets, a possible need for retitration upwards should be considered.
The mechanism of the antihypertensive effect of propranolol has not been established. Among the factors that may be involved in contributing to the antihypertensive action are: (1) decreased cardiac output, (2) inhibition of renin release by the kidneys, and (3) diminution of tonic sympathetic nerve outflow from vasomotor centers in the brain.
Propranolol hydrochloride decreases heart rate, cardiac output, and blood pressure. Although total peripheral vascular resistance may increase initially, it readjusts to or below the pretreatment level with chronic usage. Effects on plasma volume appear to be minor and somewhat variable. Inderal has been shown to cause a small increase in serum potassium concentration when used in the treatment of hypertensive patients.
Beta-receptor blockade is useful in conditions in which, because of pathologic or functional changes, sympathetic activity is excessive or inappropriate, and detrimental to the patient. But there are also situations in which sympathetic stimulation is vital. For example, in patients with severely damaged hearts, adequate ventricular function is maintained by virtue of sympathetic drive, which should be preserved. In the presence of AV block, beta blockade may prevent the necessary facilitating effect of sympathetic activity on conduction. Beta blockade results in bronchial constriction by interfering with adrenergic bronchodilator activity, which should be preserved in patients subject to bronchospasm.
The proper objective of beta-blockade therapy is to decrease adverse sympathetic stimulation, but not to the degree that may impair necessary sympathetic support.
Hydrochlorothiazide
Hydrochlorothiazide is a benzothiadiazine (thiazide) diuretic closely related to chlorothiazide. The mechanism of the antihypertensive effect of the thiazides is unknown. Thiazides usually do not affect normal blood pressure.
Thiazides affect the renal tubular mechanism of electrolyte reabsorption. At maximal therapeutic dosage, all thiazides are approximately equal in their diuretic efficacy.
Thiazides increase excretion of sodium and chloride in approximately equivalent amounts. Natriuresis causes a secondary loss of potassium and bicarbonate.
Onset of diuretic action of thiazides occurs in 2 hours, and the peak effect in about 4 hours. Its action persists for approximately 6 to 12 hours. Thiazides are eliminated rapidly by the kidney. The hydrochlorothiazide in Inderide LA is a conventional (not sustained-release) formulation.

INDICATIONS AND USAGE

Inderide LA is indicated in the management of hypertension.
This fixed-combination drug is not indicated for initial therapy of hypertension. Hypertension requires therapy titrated to the individual patient. If the fixed combination represents the dosage so determined, its use may be more convenient in patient management. The treatment of hypertension is not static, but must be reevaluated as conditions in each patient warrant.

CONTRAINDICATIONS

Propranolol Hydrochloride (Inderal®)
Propranolol is contraindicated in: 1) cardiogenic shock; 2) sinus bradycardia and greater than first-degree block; 3) bronchial asthma; 4) congestive heart failure (see **WARNINGS**), unless the failure is secondary to a tachyarrhythmia treatable with propranolol.
Hydrochlorothiazide
Hydrochlorothiazide is contraindicated in patients with anuria or hypersensitivity to this or other sulfonamide-derived drugs.

WARNINGS

Propranolol Hydrochloride (Inderal®)
Cardiac Failure: Sympathetic stimulation may be a vital component supporting circulatory function in patients with congestive heart failure, and its inhibition by beta blockade may precipitate more severe failure. Although beta blockers should be avoided in overt congestive heart failure, if necessary, they can be used with close follow-up in patients with a history of failure who are well compensated and are receiving digitalis and diuretics. Beta-adrenergic blocking agents do not abolish the inotropic action of digitalis on heart muscle.
In Patients Without a History of Heart Failure, continued use of beta blockers can, in some cases, lead to cardiac failure. Therefore, at the first sign or symptom of heart failure, the patient should be digitalized and/or treated with diuretics, and the response observed closely, or propranolol should be discontinued (gradually, if possible).

In Patients with Angina Pectoris, there have been reports of exacerbation of angina and, in some cases, myocardial infarction, following *abrupt* discontinuance of propranolol therapy. Therefore, when discontinuance of propranolol is planned, the dosage should be gradually reduced and the patient carefully monitored. In addition, when propranolol is prescribed for angina pectoris, the patient should be cautioned against interruption or cessation of therapy without the physician's advice. If propranolol therapy is interrupted and exacerbation of angina occurs, it usually is advisable to reinstitute propranolol therapy and take other measures appropriate for the management of unstable angina pectoris. Since coronary artery disease may be unrecognized, it may be prudent to follow the above advice in patients considered at risk of having occult atherosclerotic heart disease who are given propranolol for other indications.

Thyrotoxicosis: Beta blockade may mask certain clinical signs of hyperthyroidism. Therefore, abrupt withdrawal of propranolol may be followed by an exacerbation of symptoms of hyperthyroidism, including thyroid storm. Propranolol does not distort thyroid function tests.
In Patients With Wolff-Parkinson-White Syndrome, several cases have been reported in which, after propranolol, the tachycardia was replaced by a severe bradycardia requiring a demand pacemaker. In one case this resulted after an initial dose of 5 mg propranolol.
Major Surgery: The necessity or desirability of withdrawal of beta-blocking therapy prior to major surgery is controversial. It should be noted, however, that the impaired ability of the heart to respond to reflex adrenergic stimuli may augment the risks of general anesthesia and surgical procedures.
Nonallergic Bronchospasm *(e.g., chronic bronchitis, emphysema):* PATIENTS WITH BRONCHOSPASTIC DISEASES SHOULD, IN GENERAL, NOT RECEIVE BETA BLOCKERS. Inderal should be administered with caution since it may block bronchodilation produced by endogenous and exogenous catecholamine stimulation of beta receptors.
Diabetes and Hypoglycemia: Beta-adrenergic blockade may prevent the appearance of certain premonitory signs and symptoms (pulse rate and pressure changes) of acute hypoglycemia in labile insulin-dependent diabetes. In these patients, it may be more difficult to adjust the dosage of insulin. Hypoglycemic attacks may be accompanied by a precipitous elevation of blood pressure.
Propranolol therapy, particularly in infants and children, diabetic or not, has been associated with hypoglycemia especially during fasting as in preparation for surgery. Hypoglycemia also has been found after this type of drug therapy and prolonged physical exertion and has occurred in renal insufficiency, both during dialysis and sporadically, in subjects on propranolol.
Hydrochlorothiazide
Thiazides should be used with caution in severe renal disease. In patients with renal disease, thiazides may precipitate azotemia. In patients with impaired renal function, cumulative effects of the drug may develop.
Thiazides should also be used with caution in patients with impaired hepatic function or progressive liver disease, since minor alterations of fluid and electrolyte balance may precipitate hepatic coma.
Thiazides may add to or potentiate the action of other antihypertensive drugs. Potentiation occurs with ganglionic or peripheral adrenergic-blocking drugs.
Sensitivity reactions may occur in patients with a history of allergy or bronchial asthma. The possibility of exacerbation or activation of systemic lupus erythematosus has been reported.

PRECAUTIONS

General
Propranolol Hydrochloride (Inderal®)
Propranolol should be used with caution in patients with impaired hepatic or renal function. Propranolol is not indicated for the treatment of hypertensive emergencies.
Beta-adrenoreceptor blockade can cause reduction of intraocular pressure. Patients should be told that propranolol may interfere with the glaucoma screening test. Withdrawal may lead to a return of increased intraocular pressure.
Risk of anaphylactic reaction: While taking beta blockers, patients with a history of severe anaphylactic reaction to a variety of allergens may be more reactive to repeated challenge, either accidental, diagnostic, or therapeutic. Such patients may be unresponsive to the usual doses of epinephrine used to treat allergic reaction.
Hydrochlorothiazide
All patients receiving thiazide therapy should be observed for clinical signs of fluid or electrolyte imbalance, namely: Hyponatremia, hypochloremic alkalosis, and hypokalemia. Serum and urine electrolyte determinations are particularly important when the patient is vomiting excessively or receiving parenteral fluids. Medication such as digitalis may also influence serum electrolytes. Warning signs irrespective of cause are: Dryness of mouth, thirst, weakness, lethargy, drowsiness, restlessness, muscle pains or cramps, muscular fatigue, hypotension, oliguria, tachycardia, and gastrointestinal disturbances such as nausea and vomiting.
Hypokalemia may develop, especially with brisk diuresis, when severe cirrhosis is present or during concomitant use of corticosteroids or ACTH.
Interference with adequate oral electrolyte intake will also contribute to hypokalemia. Hypokalemia can sensitize or exaggerate the response of the heart to the toxic effect of digitalis (e.g., increased ventricular irritability).
Hypokalemia may be avoided or treated by use of potassium supplements, such as foods with a high potassium content.
Any chloride deficit is generally mild and usually does not require specific treatment, except under extraordinary circumstances (as in liver or renal disease). Dilutional hyponatremia may occur in edematous patients in hot weather; appropriate therapy is water restriction, rather than administration of salt, except in rare instances when the hyponatremia is life-threatening. In actual salt depletion, appropriate replacement is the therapy of choice.
Hyperuricemia may occur or frank gout may be precipitated in certain patients receiving thiazide therapy.
Insulin requirements in diabetic patients may be increased, decreased, or unchanged. Diabetes mellitus which has been latent may become manifest during thiazide administration.
If progressive renal impairment becomes evident, consider withholding or discontinuing diuretic therapy.
Thiazides may decrease serum PBI levels without signs of thyroid disturbance.
Calcium excretion is decreased by thiazides. Pathologic changes in the parathyroid gland with hypercalcemia and hypophosphatemia have been observed in a few patients on prolonged thiazide therapy. The common complications of hyperparathyroidism, such as renal lithiasis, bone resorption, and peptic ulceration have not been seen. Thiazides should be discontinued before carrying out tests for parathyroid function.
Clinical Laboratory Tests
Propranolol Hydrochloride (Inderal®)
Elevated blood urea levels in patients with severe heart disease, elevated serum transaminase, alkaline phosphatase, lactate dehydrogenase.
Hydrochlorothiazide
Periodic determination of serum electrolytes to detect possible electrolyte imbalance should be performed at appropriate intervals.
Drug Interactions
Propranolol Hydrochloride (Inderal®)
Patients receiving catecholamine-depleting drugs, such as reserpine, should be closely observed if propranolol is administered. The added catecholamine-blocking action may produce an excessive reduction of resting sympathetic nervous activity, which may result in hypotension, marked bradycardia, vertigo, syncopal attacks, or orthostatic hypotension.
Blunting of the antihypertensive effect of beta-adrenoceptor blocking agents by nonsteroidal anti-inflammatory drugs has been reported.
Hypotension and cardiac arrest have been reported with the concomitant use of propranolol and haloperidol.
Hydrochlorothiazide
Thiazide drugs may increase the responsiveness to tubocurarine.
The antihypertensive effects of thiazides may be enhanced in the postsympathectomy patient. Thiazides may decrease arterial responsiveness to norepinephrine. This diminution is not sufficient to preclude effectiveness of the pressor agent for therapeutic use.
Carcinogenesis, Mutagenesis, Impairment of Fertility
Combinations of propranolol and hydrochlorothiazide have not been evaluated for carcinogenic or mutagenic potential or for potential to adversely affect fertility.
Propranolol Hydrochloride (Inderal®)
In dietary administration studies in which mice and rats were treated with propranolol for up to 18 months at doses of up to 150 mg/kg/day, there was no evidence of drug-related tumorigenesis. In a study in which both male and female rats were exposed to propranolol in their diets at concentrations of up to 0.05%, from 60 days prior to mating and throughout pregnancy and lactation for two generations, there were no effects on fertility. Based on differing results from Ames Tests performed by different laboratories, there is equivocal evidence for a genotoxic effect of propranolol in bacteria (*S. typhimurium* strain TA 1538).
Hydrochlorothiazide
Two-year feeding studies in mice and rats conducted under the auspices of the National Toxicology Program (NTP) uncovered no evidence of a carcinogenic potential of hydrochlorothiazide in female mice (at doses of up to approximately 600 mg/kg/day) or in male and female rats (at doses of up to approximately 100 mg/kg/day). The NTP, however, found equivocal evidence for hepatocarcinogenicity in male mice.
Hydrochlorothiazide was not genotoxic *in vitro* in the Ames bacterial mutagen assay (*S. typhimurium* strains TA 98, TA 100, TA 1535, TA 1537 and TA 1538) or in the Chinese Hamster Ovary (CHO) test for chromosomal aberrations. Nor was it genotoxic *in vivo* in assays using mouse germinal cell

chromosomes, Chinese hamster bone marrow chromosomes, and the *Drosophila* sex-linked recessive lethal trait gene. Positive test results were obtained in the *in vitro* CHO Sister Chromatid Exchange (clastogenicity). Mouse Lymphoma Cell (mutagenicity) and *Aspergillus nidulans* non-disjunction assays.

Hydrochlorothiazide had no adverse effects on the fertility of mice and rats of either sex in studies wherein these species were exposed, via their diets, to doses of up to 100 mg/kg and 4 mg/kg, respectively, prior to mating and throughout gestation.

Pregnancy: Pregnancy Category C

Combinations of propranolol and hydrochlorothiazide have not been evaluated for effects on pregnancy in animals. Nor are there adequate and well-controlled studies of propranolol, hydrochlorothiazide, or Inderide in pregnant women. Inderide should be used during pregnancy only if the potential benefit justifies the potential risk to the fetus.

Propranolol Hydrochloride (Inderal®)

In a series of reproductive and developmental toxicology studies, propranolol was given to rats by gavage or in the diet throughout pregnancy and lactation. At doses of 150 mg/kg/day (>30 times the dose of propranolol contained in the maximum recommended human daily dose of Inderide), but not at doses of 80 mg/kg/day, treatment was associated with embryotoxicity (reduced litter size and increased resorption sites) as well as neonatal toxicity (deaths). Propranolol also was administered (in the feed) to rabbits (throughout pregnancy and lactation) at doses as high as 150 mg/kg/day (>45 times the dose of propranolol contained in the maximum recommended daily human dose of Inderide). No evidence of embryo or neonatal toxicity was noted. Intrauterine growth retardation has been reported in human neonates whose mothers received propranolol during pregnancy. Neonates whose mothers received propranolol at parturition have exhibited bradycardia, hypoglycemia and respiratory depression. Adequate facilities for monitoring these infants at birth should be available.

Hydrochlorothiazide

Studies in which hydrochlorothiazide was orally administered to pregnant mice and rats at doses of up to 3000 and 1000 mg/kg/day, respectively, provided no evidence of harm to the fetus.

Thiazides cross the placental barrier and appear in cord blood. The use of thiazides in pregnant women requires that the anticipated benefit be weighed against possible hazards to the fetus. These hazards include fetal or neonatal jaundice, thrombocytopenia, and possibly other adverse reactions that have occurred in the adult.

Nursing Mothers

Propranolol and thiazides are excreted in human milk. Caution should be exercised when Inderide LA is administered to a nursing woman.

Pediatric Use

Safety and effectiveness in pediatric patients have not been established.

ADVERSE REACTIONS

Propranolol Hydrochloride (Inderal®)

Most adverse effects have been mild and transient and have rarely required the withdrawal of therapy.

Cardiovascular: Bradycardia; congestive heart failure; intensification of AV block; hypotension; paresthesia of hands; thrombocytopenic purpura; arterial insufficiency, usually of the Raynaud type.

Central Nervous System: Light-headedness; mental depression manifested by insomnia, lassitude, weakness, fatigue; reversible mental depression progressing to catatonia; visual disturbances; hallucinations; an acute reversible syndrome characterized by disorientation for time and place, short-term memory loss, emotional lability, slightly clouded sensorium, and decreased performance on neuropsychometrics.

Gastrointestinal: Nausea, vomiting, epigastric distress, abdominal cramping, diarrhea, constipation, mesenteric arterial thrombosis, ischemic colitis.

Allergic: Pharyngitis and agranulocytosis; erythematous rash; fever combined with aching and sore throat; laryngospasm and respiratory distress.

Respiratory: Bronchospasm.

Hematologic: Agranulocytosis; nonthrombocytopenic purpura, thrombocytopenic purpura.

Autoimmune: In extremely rare instances, systemic lupus erythematosus has been reported.

Miscellaneous: Alopecia, LE-like reactions; psoriasiform rashes; dry eyes; male impotence; and Peyronie's disease have been reported rarely. Oculomucocutaneous reactions involving the skin, serous membranes, and conjunctivae reported for a beta blocker (practolol) have not been associated with propranolol.

Hydrochlorothiazide

Gastrointestinal: Anorexia, gastric irritation, nausea, vomiting, cramping; diarrhea; constipation; jaundice (intrahepatic cholestatic jaundice); pancreatitis; sialadenitis.

Central Nervous System: Dizziness, vertigo; paresthesias; headache; xanthopsia.

Hematologic: Leukopenia; agranulocytosis; thrombocytopenia; aplastic anemia.

Cardiovascular: Orthostatic hypotension (may be aggravated by alcohol, barbiturates, or narcotics).

Hypersensitivity: Purpura; photosensitivity; rash; urticaria; necrotizing angiitis (vasculitis, cutaneous vasculitis); fever; respiratory distress, including pneumonitis; anaphylactic reactions.

Other: Hyperglycemia; glycosuria; hyperuricemia; muscle spasm; weakness; restlessness; transient blurred vision.

Whenever adverse reactions are moderate or severe, thiazide dosage should be reduced or therapy withdrawn.

OVERDOSAGE OR EXAGGERATED RESPONSE

The propranolol hydrochloride (Inderal) component may cause bradycardia, cardiac failure, hypotension, or bronchospasm.

The hydrochlorothiazide component can be expected to cause diuresis. Lethargy of varying degree may appear and may progress to coma within a few hours, with minimal depression of respiration and cardiovascular function, and in the absence of significant serum electrolyte changes or dehydration. The mechanism of central nervous system depression with thiazide overdosage is unknown. Gastrointestinal irritation and hypermotility can occur; temporary elevation of BUN has been reported and serum electrolyte changes could occur, especially in patients with impairment of renal function.

Treatment

The following measures should be employed:

General: If ingestion is, or may have been, recent, evacuate gastric contents, taking care to prevent pulmonary aspiration.

Bradycardia: Administer atropine (0.25 to 1.0 mg). If there is no response to vagal blockade, administer isoproterenol cautiously.

Cardiac Failure: Digitalization and diuretics.

Hypotension: Vasopressors, e.g., levarterenol or epinephrine.

Bronchospasm: Administer isoproterenol and aminophylline.

Stupor or Coma: Administer supportive therapy as clinically warranted.

Gastrointestinal Effects: Though usually of short duration, these may require symptomatic treatment.

Abnormalities in BUN and/or Serum Electrolytes: Monitor serum electrolyte levels and renal function; institute supportive measures, as required individually, to maintain hydration, electrolyte balance, respiration, and cardiovascular function.

DOSAGE AND ADMINISTRATION

The dosage must be determined by individual titration.

Hydrochlorothiazide can be given at doses of 12.5 to 50 mg per day when used alone. The initial dose of propranolol is 80 mg daily, and it may be increased gradually until optimal blood pressure control is achieved. The usual effective dose, when used alone, is 160 to 480 mg per day.

One Inderide LA Capsule once a day can be used to administer up to 160 mg of propranolol and 50 mg of hydrochlorothiazide. For doses of propranolol greater than 160 mg, the combination products are not appropriate because their use would lead to an excessive dose of the thiazide component.

Inderide LA provides propranolol hydrochloride in a sustained-release form and hydrochlorothiazide in conventional formulation, for once-daily administration. If patients are switched from Inderide Tablets (or Inderal plus hydrochlorothiazide) to Inderide LA, care should be taken to ensure that the desired therapeutic effect is maintained. Inderide LA should not be considered a mg-for-mg substitute for Inderide or Inderal plus hydrochlorothiazide. Inderide LA has different kinetics and produces lower blood levels. Retitration may be necessary, especially to maintain effectiveness at the end of the 24-hour dosing interval.

When necessary, another antihypertensive agent may be added gradually, beginning with 50% of the usual recommended starting dose, to avoid an excessive fall in blood pressure.

HOW SUPPLIED

Each beige capsule, identified by one wide band and 3 narrow bands, all in gold, and "Inderide LA 80/50", contains 80 mg of propranolol hydrochloride (Inderal® LA) and 50 mg of hydrochlorothiazide, in bottles of 100 (NDC 0046- 0455-81).

Each beige/brown capsule, identified by one wide band and 3 narrow bands, all in gold, and "Inderide LA 120/50", contains 120 mg of propranolol hydrochloride (Inderal® LA) and 50 mg of hydrochlorothiazide, in bottles of 100 (NDC 0046-0457-81).

Each brown capsule, identified by one wide band and 3 narrow bands, all in gold, and "Inderide LA 160/50", contains 160 mg of propranolol hydrochloride (Inderal® LA) and 50 mg of hydrochlorothiazide, in bottles of 100 (NDC 0046-0459-81).

Store at room temperature (approximately 25° C).

Protect from light, moisture, freezing, and excessive heat. Dispense in a tight, light-resistant container as defined in the USP.

The appearance of these capsules is a registered trademark of Wyeth-Ayerst Laboratories.

Manufactured by:
Ayerst Laboratories
A Wyeth-Ayerst Company
Philadelphia, PA 19101
CI 3764-8 Issued June 23, 1997

Shown in Product Identification Guide, page 341

INFLUENZA VIRUS VACCINE, TRIVALENT, TYPES A AND B ℞

(Purified Subvirion)

FluShield®

[flū' sheeld]

2000-2001 formula

DO NOT INJECT INTRAVENOUSLY

Rx only

DESCRIPTION

FluShield® (Influenza Virus Vaccine, Trivalent, Types A and B [Purified Subvirion]) is a sterile injectable for administration intramuscularly.

FluShield® is prepared from the allantoic fluids of chick embryos inoculated with a specific type of influenza virus. During processing, not more than 5 µg of gentamicin sulfate per mL is added. The harvested virus is concentrated, purified, then inactivated with formaldehyde.

The viral antigens contained in FluShield®, Trivalent (Purified Subvirion), are concentrated and refined by a column-chromatographic procedure. At the same time, addition of tri(n)butylphosphate and Polysorbate 80, USP, to the column-eluting fluids effects inactivation and disruption of a significant proportion of the virus to smaller subunit particles. The recovered subvirion (split-virus) suspension is freed of substantial portions of the disrupting agents by dialysis and of other undesirable materials by selective filtration through membranes of controlled pore size.

The viral antigen content has been standardized by immunodiffusion tests, according to current U.S. Public Health Service (PHS) requirements. Each dose (0.5 mL) contains the proportions and not less than the microgram amounts of hemagglutinin antigens (µg HA) representative of the specific components recommended for the 2000-2001 season: 15 µg HA of A/New Caledonia/20/99 (H1N1)-like, 15 µg HA of A/Panama/2007/99 (H3N2) (A/Moscow/10/99 [H3N2]-like), and 15 µg HA of B/Yamanashi/166/98 (B/Beijing/184/93-like).

The vaccine contains 1:10,000 thimerosal (mercury derivative; 25 µg mercury per 0.5 mL dose) as a preservative. Gentamicin sulfate is used during manufacturing, but is not detectable in the final product by assay procedures. The product appears as a slightly opalescent solution.

CLINICAL PHARMACOLOGY

The administration of inactivated influenza virus vaccine each year before the influenza season is the single most important influenza-control measure.[1]

The injection of antigens prepared from inactivated influenza virus stimulates the production of specific antibodies. Any protection afforded is only against those strains of virus from which the vaccine is prepared or closely related strains. With the passing of time, there may be major antigenic changes in the prevalent strains, or there may be continuous and progressive antigenic variation within a given virus subtype over time (antigenic drift), so that infection or immunization with one strain may not induce immunity to distantly related strains. Influenza A and B are the two types of influenza viruses that cause epidemic human disease. Influenza A viruses are further classified into subtypes on the basis of two surface antigens: hemagglutinin (H) and neuraminidase (N). A person's immunity to the surface antigens, especially hemagglutinin, reduces the likelihood of infection and the severity of disease if infection occurs. Influenza virus vaccine prevents illness in approximately 70% to 90% of healthy persons younger than 65 years when the antigenic match between vaccine and circulating viruses is close.[1] The PHS regularly reviews the antigenic characteristics of circulating strains in order to select those to be included in the contemporary vaccine.

Based upon the epidemiological data available through the early months of 2000 the Federal Government determined, after consultation with advisory groups, that the influenza virus vaccines to be distributed in 2000-2001 will be trivalent, including 15 µg HA each of strains that are antigenically similar to A/Moscow/10/99, A/New Caledonia/20/99, and B/Beijing/184/93.

INDICATIONS AND USAGE

FluShield® is indicated for active immunization against the specific influenza virus strains contained in the 2000-2001 formulation. FluShield® is recommended for 1) individuals 6 months of age or older at high-risk for developing complications from influenza virus infections which may result in hospitalization or death and for their medical care providers or household contacts and 2) anyone who wishes to reduce his or her chances of acquiring influenza. FluShield® should only be administered if it is prescribed by a healthcare professional whose license includes the prescribing of biologicals.

Elderly persons and persons with certain chronic diseases may develop lower postvaccination antibody titers than healthy young adults and thus may remain susceptible to influenza-related upper respiratory tract infections. However, even if such persons develop influenza illness despite vaccination, the vaccine has been shown to be effective in helping to prevent lower respiratory tract involvement or other secondary complications, thereby reducing the risk of hospitalization and death.[1]

Guidelines for the use of influenza virus vaccine among different groups are given below.

Target Groups for Vaccination

Groups at increased risk for influenza-related complications:

1. Persons 50 years of age or older (see **PRECAUTIONS—Geriatric Use**).

Continued on next page

FluShield—Cont.

2. Residents of nursing homes and other chronic-care facilities housing patients of any age with chronic medical conditions.
3. Adults and children with chronic disorders of the pulmonary or cardiovascular systems, including asthma.
4. Adults and children who have required regular medical follow-up or hospitalization during the preceding year because of chronic metabolic diseases (including diabetes mellitus), renal dysfunction, hemoglobinopathies, or immunosuppression (including immunosuppression caused by medications or by human immunodeficiency virus).
5. Children and teenagers (aged 6 months to 18 years) who are receiving long-term aspirin therapy and, therefore, might be at risk of developing Reye's syndrome after influenza infection.
6. Women who will be in the second or third trimester of pregnancy during the influenza season.[1]

Pregnant Women

Although animal reproductive studies have not been conducted, the prescribing healthcare professional should be aware of the recommendations of the Advisory Committee on Immunization Practices (ACIP), which are incorporated below. Influenza-associated excess mortality among pregnant women has not been documented, except during the pandemics of 1918–19 and 1957–58. However, because death-certificate data often do not indicate whether a woman was pregnant at the time of death, studies conducted during interpandemic periods may underestimate the impact of influenza in this population. Case reports and limited studies suggest that pregnancy may increase the risk for serious medical complications of influenza as a result of increases in heart rate, stroke volume and oxygen consumption, decreases in lung capacity, and changes in immunologic function. A study of the impact of influenza during 17 interpandemic influenza seasons demonstrated that the relative risk for hospitalization for selected cardiorespiratory conditions among pregnant women increased from 1.4 during weeks 14 to 20 of gestation to 4.7 during weeks 37 to 42 compared with rates among women who were 1 to 6 months postpartum. Women in their third trimester of pregnancy were hospitalized at a rate comparable to that of nonpregnant women who have high-risk medical conditions for whom influenza virus vaccine has traditionally been recommended. Using data from this study, it was estimated that an average of 1 to 2 hospitalizations among pregnant women could be prevented for every 1,000 pregnant women immunized.[1]

On the basis of these and other data that suggest that influenza infection may cause increased morbidity in women during the second and third trimesters of pregnancy, the ACIP recommends that women who will be beyond the first trimester of pregnancy (≥14 weeks' gestation) during the influenza season be vaccinated. Pregnant women who have medical conditions that increase their risk for complications from influenza should be vaccinated before the influenza season, regardless of the stage of pregnancy. A study of influenza immunization of more than 2,000 pregnant women have demonstrated no adverse fetal effects associated with influenza virus vaccine; however, more data are needed (see "**PRECAUTIONS—Pregnancy**").[1]

Persons who can transmit influenza to persons at high risk:

Persons who are clinically or subclinically infected can transmit influenza virus to persons at high risk whom they care for or with whom they live. Some persons at high risk, e.g., the elderly, transplant recipients, and persons with acquired immunodeficiency syndrome (AIDS), can have a low antibody response to influenza virus vaccine. Efforts to help protect these members of high-risk groups against influenza might be improved by reducing the likelihood of influenza exposure from their caregivers. Therefore, the following groups should be vaccinated:

1. Physicians, nurses, and other personnel in both hospital and outpatient settings.
2. Employees of nursing homes and chronic-care facilities who have contact with patients or residents.
3. Employees of assisted living and other residences for persons in high-risk groups.
4. Providers of home care to high-risk persons (e.g., visiting nurses, volunteer workers).
5. Household members (including children) of persons in high-risk groups.[1]

Vaccination of Other Groups

General population:

Physicians should administer influenza virus vaccine to any person who wishes to reduce the likelihood of becoming ill with influenza caused by the strains incorporated into this year's vaccine. Persons who provide essential community services should be considered for vaccination to minimize disruption of essential activities during influenza outbreaks. Students or other persons in institutional settings (e.g., those who reside in dormitories) should be encouraged to receive vaccine to minimize the disruption of routine activities during epidemics.[1]

Persons infected with human immunodeficiency virus (HIV):

Limited information exists regarding the frequency and severity of influenza illness among HIV-infected persons, but reports suggest that symptoms might be prolonged and the risk of complications increased for some HIV-infected persons. Influenza virus vaccine has produced substantial antibody titers against influenza in vaccinated HIV-infected persons who have minimal AIDS-related symptoms and high CD4+ T-lymphocyte cell counts. In patients who have advanced HIV disease and low CD4+ T-lymphocyte cell counts, however, influenza virus vaccine may not induce protective antibody titers; a second dose of vaccine does not improve the immune response for these persons.

Studies have examined the effect on influenza vaccination on replication of HIV type 1 (HIV-1). Although some studies have demonstrated a transient (i.e., 2- to 4-week) increase in replication of HIV-1 in the plasma or peripheral blood mononuclear cells of HIV-infected persons after vaccine administration, other studies using similar laboratory techniques have not indicated any substantial increase in replication. Deterioration of CD4+ T-lymphocyte cell counts and progression of clinical HIV disease have not been demonstrated among HIV-infected persons who receive vaccine.

Because influenza can result in serious illness and complications and because influenza vaccination may result in protective antibody titers, vaccination will benefit many HIV-infected patients.[1]

Travelers:

The risk of exposure to influenza during foreign travel varies, depending on season and destination. Influenza can occur throughout the year in the tropics; the season of greatest influenza activity in the Southern Hemisphere is April through September. Because of the short incubation period for influenza, exposure to the virus during travel can result in clinical illness that begins during travel, an inconvenience or potential danger, especially for persons at increased risk for complications. Persons preparing to travel to the tropics at any time of year, or travel with large organized tourist groups containing persons from areas of the world where influenza viruses are circulating, or travel to the Southern Hemisphere from April through September should review their vaccination histories. If they were not vaccinated the previous fall or winter, they should consider influenza vaccination prior to travel. Persons in the high-risk categories especially should be encouraged to receive the most current vaccine. Persons at high risk who received the previous season's vaccine prior to travel should be revaccinated in the fall or winter with the current vaccine.[1]

Immunization programs:

If this product is to be used in an immunization program sponsored by an organization WHERE A TRADITIONAL PHYSICIAN/PATIENT RELATIONSHIP DOES NOT EXIST, each participant (or legal guardian) should be made aware of the possible risks and adverse events that have been associated with the use of influenza virus vaccines, including the possible risk of a form of paralysis sometimes known as Guillain-Barré syndrome. Information about possible side effects and adverse events is presented below, and informed consent, preferably written, should be obtained from the intended recipient (or legal guardian) before vaccine administration. FluShield® is a prescription product and shall only be administered upon prescription by a healthcare professional who is licensed to prescribe biologicals. The prescribing healthcare professional should be familiar with the text of this insert, including the **CONTRAINDICATIONS**, **WARNINGS**, **PRECAUTIONS**, and **ADVERSE REACTIONS** sections.

Simultaneous Administration of Pneumococcal or Pediatric Vaccines

The target groups for influenza and pneumococcal polysaccharide vaccination overlap considerably. For persons at high risk who have not previously been vaccinated with pneumococcal polysaccharide vaccine, healthcare professionals should strongly consider administering pneumococcal and influenza virus vaccine concurrently. These vaccines can be administered at the same time at different sites without increasing side effects.[1] However, influenza virus vaccine is given annually, whereas pneumococcal polysaccharide vaccine is not.[2]

Children at high risk for influenza-related complications can receive influenza virus vaccine at the same time as they receive other routine vaccinations, with administration at different sites recommended.

As with any vaccine, FluShield® may not protect 100% of individuals receiving the vaccine.

CONTRAINDICATIONS

FLUSHIELD® SHOULD NOT BE ADMINISTERED TO INDIVIDUALS WITH A HISTORY OF HYPERSENSITIVITY (ALLERGY) TO CHICKEN EGG OR TO ANY COMPONENT(S) OF INFLUENZA VIRUS VACCINE, INCLUDING THIMEROSAL, WITHOUT FIRST CONSULTING A PHYSICIAN (see **ADVERSE REACTIONS**). Before being vaccinated, persons known to be hypersensitive to egg protein or other components should be given a skin test or other allergy-evaluating test, using the influenza virus vaccine as the antigen. Persons with adverse reactions to such testing should not be vaccinated. Chemoprophylaxis may be indicated for prevention of influenza A in such persons. However, persons with a history of anaphylactic hypersensitivity to vaccine components but who are also at highest risk for complications of influenza infections may benefit from vaccine after appropriate allergy evaluation and desensitization.[1]

Persons with a past history of Guillain-Barré syndrome (GBS) should not be given influenza virus vaccine (see **ADVERSE REACTIONS**).

Persons with acute febrile illnesses usually should not be vaccinated until their symptoms have abated. However, minor illnesses with or without fever should not contraindicate the use of influenza virus vaccine, particularly in children with a mild upper respiratory tract infection or allergic rhinitis.[1,3]

WARNINGS

Patients with impaired immune responsiveness, whether due to the use of immunosuppressive therapy (including irradiation, large amounts of corticosteroids, antimetabolites, alkylating agents, and cytotoxic agents), a genetic defect, HIV infection, leukemia, lymphoma, generalized malignancy, or other causes, may have a reduced antibody response to active immunization procedures. Short-term (less than 2 weeks) oral corticosteroid therapy or administration via topical (skin or eyes) or inhalational routes, or intra-articular, bursal, or tendon injections is thought not to be immunosuppressive.[4] Inactivated vaccines are not a risk to immunocompromised individuals, although their efficacy may be substantially reduced. Because patients with immunodeficiencies may not have an adequate response to immunizing agents, they may remain susceptible despite having received an appropriate vaccine. If feasible, specific serum antibody titers or other immunologic responses may be determined after immunization to assess immunity.[3] Chemoprophylaxis may be indicated for high-risk persons who are expected to have a poor antibody response to influenza virus vaccine.[1]

Healthcare professionals should prescribe and/or administer this product with caution to patients with a possible history of latex sensitivity since this packaging contains dry natural rubber.

PRECAUTIONS

General

Care should be taken by the healthcare professional for the effective use of this product.

1. Prior to the administration of any dose of FluShield®, the patient, parent, or guardian should be asked about the personal history, family history, and recent health status of the vaccine recipient. The healthcare professional should ascertain previous immunization history, current health status, and occurrence of any symptoms and/or signs of an adverse event after previous immunization in order to determine the existance of any contraindication to immunization with FluShield® and to allow an assessment of benefits and risks.
2. Influenza virus is remarkably capricious antigenically, and significant changes may occur from time to time. *It is known definitely that influenza virus vaccine, as now constituted, is not effective against all possible strains of influenza virus. Any protection afforded is only against those strains of virus from which the vaccine is prepared or against closely related strains.*
3. Influenza virus vaccine often contains one or more antigens used in previous years. However, immunity declines during the year following immunization. Therefore, revaccination on a yearly basis is necessary to provide optimal protection for the current season. REMAINING 1999-2000 VACCINE SHOULD NOT BE USED.
4. Before the injection of any biological, the healthcare professional should take all precautions known for the prevention of allergic or any other side reactions. This should include: a review of the patient's history regarding sensitivity; the ready availability of epinephrine injection (1:1000) and other appropriate agents used for control of immediate or delayed allergic reactions; and a knowledge of recent literature pertaining to use of the biological concerned, including the nature of side effects and adverse reactions that may follow its use.
5. A separate sterile syringe and needle or sterile disposable unit should be used for each patient to prevent transmission of hepatitis or other infectious agents from one person to another. Reusable glass syringes and needles should be heat-sterilized. Needles should be disposed of properly and should not be recapped.
6. Special care should be taken to prevent injection into or near a blood vessel or nerve.
7. Vaccine sterility and stability cannot be assured if unit doses are withdrawn from the multidose vial and allowed to remain in syringes for longer than a few minutes prior to injection into patients.
8. Guidance should be provided to the patient, parent, or guardian on measures to be taken should suspected adverse events occur, such as antipyretic measures for elevated temperatures and the need to report any suspected adverse occurrence to the healthcare professional.
9. Healthcare professionals should administer FluShield® with caution to patients with a possible history of latex sensitivity, since this packaging contains dry natural rubber.

Drug Interactions

There have been conflicting reports[5–15] on the effects of influenza virus vaccine on the elimination of some drugs metabolized by the hepatic cytochrome P-450 system. Hypoprothrombinemia in patients receiving warfarin and elevated theophylline serum concentrations have occurred. Most studies have failed to show any adverse effects of influenza virus vaccine in patients receiving these drugs. Nevertheless, monitoring for possible enhanced drug effect or toxicity is indicated for those persons taking theophylline preparations or warfarin sodium.

Individuals receiving therapy with immunosuppressive agents (large amounts of corticosteroids, antimetabolites, alkylating agents, cytotoxic agents) may not respond optimally to active immunization procedures (see **WARNINGS**).

As with other intramuscular injections, this product should be given with caution to a person on anticoagulant therapy.

Carcinogenesis, Mutagenesis, Impairment of Fertility
FluShield® has not been evaluated for its carcinogenic or mutagenic potential or for impairment of fertility.

Pregnancy
Pregnancy Category C:
Animal reproduction studies have not been conducted with influenza virus vaccine. It is also not known whether influenza virus vaccine can cause fetal harm when administered to a pregnant woman or can affect reproductive capacity. Influenza virus vaccine should be given to a pregnant woman only if clearly needed. The benefits of preventing influenza-related complications versus the theoretical risk of fetal harm should be considered, and discussed with the patient before administering influenza virus vaccine to a pregnant woman. The ACIP states that, if used during pregnancy, administration of influenza virus vaccine after 14 weeks of gestation may be preferable to avoid coincidental association of the vaccine with early pregnancy loss[1] (see **INDICATIONS AND USAGE**, **Target Groups for Vaccination**).

Nursing mothers:
Influenza virus vaccine does not affect the safety of breastfeeding for mothers or infants. Breastfeeding does not adversely affect immune response and is not a contraindication for vaccination.[1]

Geriatric Use
The effectiveness of influenza virus vaccine in preventing or attenuating illness varies, depending primarily on the age and immunocompetence of the vaccine recipient and the degree of similarity between the virus strains included in the vaccine and those that circulate during the influenza season. Studies have indicated that the effectiveness of influenza virus vaccine in preventing hospitalization for pneumonia and influenza among elderly persons living in settings other than nursing homes or similar chronic-care facilities ranges from 30% to 70% when a good match exists between vaccine and circulating viruses.[1]
Among elderly persons residing in nursing homes, influenza virus vaccine is most effective in preventing severe illness, secondary complications, and death. Studies of this population have indicated that the vaccine can be 50% to 60% effective in preventing hospitalization and pneumonia and 80% effective in preventing death, even though efficacy in preventing influenza may often be in the range of 30% to 40% among the frail elderly. Achieving a high rate of vaccination among nursing home residents can reduce the spread of infection in a facility, thus preventing disease through herd immunity. Vaccination of healthcare workers in nursing homes also has been effective in reducing the impact of influenza among residents.[1]

Pediatric Use
The safety and effectiveness of influenza virus vaccine in pediatric patients under 6 months of age have not been established. However, the ACIP recommends influenza vaccination in certain circumstances for persons 6 months of age or older (see **INDICATIONS AND USAGE**, **Target Groups for Vaccination** and **DOSAGE AND ADMINISTRATION**).[1]

ADVERSE REACTIONS

BECAUSE INFLUENZA VIRUS VACCINE CONTAINS ONLY NONINFECTIOUS VIRUSES, IT CANNOT CAUSE INFLUENZA. Occasional cases of respiratory disease following vaccination represent coincidental illnesses unrelated to influenza vaccination.[1]
The most frequent side effect of vaccination is soreness at the vaccination site for up to 2 days. These local reactions generally are mild and rarely interfere with the ability to conduct usual daily activities.[1] With vaccines in general, it is not uncommon for patients to note at or around the injection site the following minor reactions: swelling or edema; pain or tenderness; redness, erythema, inflammation, or skin discoloration; induration or mass; or hypersensitivity reaction.
In addition, the following types of systemic reactions have occurred:
Fever, malaise, myalgia, and other systemic symptoms can occur following vaccination and most often affect persons who have had no exposure to the influenza virus antigens in the vaccine (e.g., young children). These reactions begin 6 to 12 hours after vaccination and can persist for 1 or 2 days.[1]
One report of delayed anaphylaxis or delayed onset of severe asthma or hypersensitivity reaction in a known asthmatic after administration of FluShield® has been received. The reaction began approximately 6 hours following receipt of influenza virus vaccine and resulted in death within the next hour. Other systemic events that have been reported include: arthralgia, asthenia, chills, dizziness, headache, lymphadenopathy, pruritus, rash, vomiting, diarrhea, and pharyngitis. Recent placebo-controlled trials suggest that in elderly persons and healthy young adults, split-virus influenza vaccine is not associated with higher rates of systemic symptoms (e.g., fever, malaise, myalgia, and headache) when compared with placebo injections.[1] Other events that have been reported include angiopathy and vasculitis.[16–18]
Immediate, presumably allergic, reactions such as hives, angioedema, allergic asthma, or systemic anaphylaxis occur rarely after influenza vaccination. These reactions probably result from hypersensitivity to some vaccine component—the majority of reactions are most likely related to residual egg protein. Although current influenza virus vaccines contain only a small quantity of egg protein, this protein can induce immediate hypersensitivity reactions among persons who have severe egg allergy. Persons who have developed hives, have had swelling of the lips or tongue, or experienced acute respiratory distress or collapse after eating eggs should consult a physician for appropriate evaluation to help determine if vaccine should be administered. Persons who have documented immunoglobulin E (IgE)-mediated hypersensitivity to eggs, including those who have had occupational asthma or other allergic responses due to exposure to egg protein, might also be at increased risk for reactions from influenza virus vaccine and similar consultation should be considered. The protocol for influenza vaccination developed by Murphy and Strunk may be considered for patients who have egg allergies and medical conditions that place them at increased risk for influenza-associated complications.[19] Hypersensitivity reactions to any vaccine component can occur. Although exposure to vaccines containing thimerosal can lead to induction of hypersensitivity, most patients do not develop reactions to thimerosal when administered as a component of vaccines even when patch or intradermal tests for thimerosal indicate hypersensitivity. When reported, hypersensitivity to thimerosal has usually consisted of local, delayed-type hypersensitivity reactions.[1] One study has reported a decrease in pulmonary function in some asthmatics who received influenza vaccine.[20] However, another study suggested that influenza vaccination was not associated with clinically significant asthma exacerbation or worsening of asthma symptoms in vaccines with acute exacerbation or with stable asthma.[21]
There have been rare reports of Guillain-Barré syndrome (GBS) following receipt of influenza virus vaccine. GBS is an uncommon illness characterized by ascending paralysis which is usually self-limited and reversible. Though most persons with GBS recover without residual weakness, approximately 5% of cases are fatal. Before 1976, no association of GBS with influenza virus vaccine use was recognized.
Information from the Centers for Disease Control and Prevention ACIP Recommendations regarding GBS is incorporated below. Although the 1976 swine influenza virus vaccine was associated with an increased frequency of GBS, evidence for a causal relationship of GBS with subsequent vaccines prepared from other virus strains is less clear. However, obtaining strong evidence for a possible small increase in risk is difficult for a rare condition such as GBS, which has an annual background incidence of only 1 to 2 cases per 100,000 adults. During three of four influenza seasons studied from 1977 through 1991, the point estimates of the overall relative risk for GBS after influenza vaccination were slightly elevated but were not statistically significant in any of these studies. However, in a recent study of the 1992-1993 and 1993-1994 seasons, the overall relative risk for GBS was 1.7 (95% confidence interval=1.0 to 2.8, p=0.04) during the 6 weeks following vaccination, representing an excess of slightly more than one additional case of GBS per million persons vaccinated; the combined number of GBS cases peaked 2 weeks after vaccination.[22] The increase in the relative risk and the increased number of cases in the second week after vaccination may be the result of vaccination but also could be due to other factors (e.g., confounding or diagnostic bias) rather than a true vaccine-related risk.[1]
Even if GBS were a true side effect of vaccination in the years after 1976, the estimated risk for GBS of slightly more than one additional case per million persons vaccinated is substantially less than that for severe influenza, which could be prevented by vaccination in all age groups, especially for persons aged ≥65 years and those who have medical indications for influenza vaccination.[1] During different epidemics occurring from 1972 through 1981, estimated rates of influenza-associated hospitalization have ranged from approximately 200 to 300 hospitalizations per million population for previously healthy persons aged 5 to 44 years and from 2,000 to >10,000 hospitalizations per million population for persons aged ≥65 years. During epidemics from 1972-73 through 1994-95, estimated rates of influenza-associated death have ranged from approximately 300 to >1,500 per million persons aged ≥65 years, which account for more than 90% of all influenza-associated deaths.
The average case-fatality ratio of GBS is 6% and increases with age. However, no evidence indicates that the case-fatality ratio for GBS differs among vaccinated and non-vaccinated persons.
Whereas the incidence of GBS in the general population is very low, persons with a history of GBS have a substantially greater likelihood of subsequently developing GBS than persons without such a history. Thus, the likelihood of coincidentally developing GBS after influenza vaccination is expected to be greater among persons with a history of GBS than among persons with no history of this syndrome. Whether influenza vaccination might be causally associated with this risk for recurrence is not known.[1] Avoiding subsequent influenza vaccination of persons known to have developed GBS within 6 weeks of a previous influenza vaccination seems prudent. Candidates for influenza virus vaccine should be made aware of the possible risks, including GBS, and the benefits of administration.
Other neurologic disorders not defined as GBS, including encephalopathies, facial paralysis, unspecified neuritis, encephalitis, peripheral nerve disease, brachial neuritis, optic neuritis, demyelinating disease, labyrinthitis and meningitis have been temporally associated with influenza vaccination.[23] Rarely, transverse myelitis has been reported.[24]

ADVERSE EVENT REPORTING
The manufacturer and lot number of the vaccine administered should be recorded in the vaccine recipient's permanent medical record, along with the date of administration of the vaccine and the name, address, and title of the person administering the vaccine. Any adverse events following immunizations should be reported by the healthcare professional to the U.S. Department of Health and Human Services (DHHS).
The U.S. DHHS has established the Vaccine Adverse Event Reporting System (VAERS) to accept all reports of suspected adverse events after administration of any vaccine. The toll-free number for VAERS forms and information is 800-822-7967.

DOSAGE AND ADMINISTRATION

FOR INTRAMUSCULAR USE ONLY

AGE GROUP	DOSAGE SCHEDULE
9 years and older	0.5 mL (one dose)
3 to 8 years	0.5 mL (1 or 2 doses)*
6 to 35 months	0.25 mL (1 or 2 doses)*

*Two doses are recommended for children under 9 years who are receiving influenza virus vaccine for the first time. With the 2-dose regimen, allow 4 weeks or more between doses. Both doses are recommended for maximum protection.

For those under 13 years, only split-virus (subvirion) vaccine is recommended. Immunogenicity and reactogenicity of split- and whole-virus vaccines are similar in adults when used according to the recommended dosage.[1]
Although influenza virus vaccine often contains one or more antigens used in previous years, immunity declines during the year following vaccination. Therefore, a history of vaccination in any previous year with a vaccine containing one or more antigens included in the current vaccine does NOT preclude the need for revaccination for the 2000-2001 influenza season to help provide optimal protection. REMAINING 1999-2000 VACCINE SHOULD NOT BE USED.
Influenza virus vaccine may be offered to high-risk persons presenting for routine care or hospitalization beginning in September, but not until new vaccine is available (see **INDICATIONS AND USAGE**, **Vaccination of Other Groups**, *Travelers* for travel-related exceptions). Opportunities to vaccinate persons at high risk for complications of influenza should not be missed. In the United States, influenza activity generally peaks between late December and early March, and high levels of influenza activity infrequently occur in the contiguous 48 states before December. Although the optimal time for vaccination for high-risk persons usually is the period from October through mid-November, vaccine should continue to be offered to both children and adults up to and even after influenza virus activity is documented in a community.[1] In facilities such as nursing homes it is particularly important to avoid administering vaccine too far in advance of the influenza season because antibody levels may begin to decline within a few months of vaccination.[1]
Children less than 9 years of age who have not been vaccinated previously should receive two doses with at least 1 month between doses to maximize the chance of a satisfactory antibody response to all three vaccine antigens. The second dose should be given before December, if possible.
Parenteral drug products should be inspected visually for particulate matter and discoloration prior to administration. The product should not be used if particulate matter or discoloration is found. The product appears as a slightly opalescent solution.
DO NOT INJECT INTRAVENOUSLY. Injections of FluShield® are recommended to be given intramuscularly. The recommended site is the deltoid muscle for adults and older children.[1] The preferred site for infants and young children is the anterolateral aspect of the thigh musculature. Because of lack of adequate evaluation of other routes in high-risk persons, the preferred route of vaccination is intramuscular whenever possible. Before injection, the skin over the site to be injected should be cleansed with a suitable germicide. After insertion of the needle, aspirate and wait to see if any blood appears in the syringe, which will help avoid inadvertent injection into a blood vessel. If blood appears, withdraw the needle and prepare for a new injection at another site.

HOW SUPPLIED

Influenza Virus Vaccine, Trivalent, Types A and B, (Purified Subvirion), FluShield®, is available in vials of 5 mL as follows:
NDC 0008-0985-01
ALSO AVAILABLE
TUBEX® Sterile Cartridge-Needle Units, 0.5 mL fill in 1 mL size (25 gauge × 5/8 inch needle), in packages of 10 TUBEX as follows:
NDC 0008-0985-02

Storage
Store between 2°C to 8°C (36°F to 46°F). Potency is destroyed by freezing; do not use FluShield® that has been frozen.

REFERENCES

1. Prevention and control of influenza: Recommendations of the Advisory Committee on Immunization Practices (ACIP). MMWR-April 14, 2000;*48 (RR-5)*.
2. Prevention of Pneumococcal Disease: Recommendations of the Advisory Committee on Immunization Practices (ACIP). MMWR-April 4, 1997; *46 (No. RR-8)*.
3. American Academy of Pediatrics: Report of the Committee on Infectious Diseases. 24th ed. Elk Grove Village, IL, American Academy of Pediatrics, 1997.

Continued on next page

FluShield—Cont.

4. Recommendations of the Advisory Committee on Immunization Practices (ACIP): Use of vaccines and immune globulins in persons with altered immunocompetence. MMWR-April 9, 1993; *42 (No. RR-4)*.
5. KRAMER, P., and McCLAIN, C.: Depression of aminopyrine metabolism by influenza vaccination. NEJM 1981; *305*: 1262.
6. RENTON, K. et al: Decreased elimination of theophylline after influenza vaccination. Can Med Assoc J 1980; *123*: 288.
7. GOLDSTEIN, R.S. et al: Decreased elimination of theophylline after influenza vaccination. Can Med Assoc J 1982; *126*: 470.
8. BRITTON, L. and RUBEN, F.L.: Serum and theophylline levels after influenza vaccination. Can Med Assoc J 1982; *126*: 1375.
9. FISCHER, R.G. et al: Influence of trivalent influenza vaccine on serum theophylline levels. Can Med Assoc J 1982; *126*: 1312–13.
10. SAN JOAQUIN, V.H., REYES, S., AND MARKS, M.I.: Influenza vaccination in asthmatic children on maintenance theophylline therapy. Clin Pediatrics 1982; *21*: 724–6.
11. STULTS, B. AND HASISAKI, P.: Influenza vaccination and theophylline pharmacokinetics in patients with chronic obstructive lung disease. West J Med 1983; *139*: 651–4.
12. PATRIARCA, P.A. et al: Influenza vaccination and warfarin or theophylline toxicity in nursing-home residents. NEJM 1983; *308*: 1601.
13. MEREDITH, C.G. et al: Effects of influenza virus vaccine on hepatic drug metabolism. Clin Pharm Ther 1985; *37*: 396–401.
14. LIPSKY, B.A. et al: Influenza vaccination and warfarin anticoagulation. Ann Int Med 1984; *100*: 835–7.
15. KRAMER, P. et al: Effect of influenza vaccine on warfarin anticoagulation. Clin Pharmacol Ther 1984; *35*: 416.
16. HULL, T.P. and BATES, J.H.: Optic neuritis after influenza vaccination. Am J Ophthalmol 1997; *124(5)*:703–704.
17. KAWASAKI, A. et al: Bilateral anterior ischemic optic neuropathy following influenza vaccination. J Neuro-Ophthalmol 1988; *18(1)*:56–59.
18. KELSALL, J.T.: Microscopic polyangitis following influenza vaccination. J Rheumatol 1997; *24*:7.
19. MURPHY, K.R. and STRUNK, R.L.: Safe administration of influenza vaccine in asthmatic children hypersensitive to egg proteins. J Pediatr 1985; *106*: 931–3.
20. NICHOLSON, K. et al: Randomised placebo-controlled crossover trial on effect of inactivated influenza vaccine on pulmonary function in asthma. Lancet 1998; *351*:326–331.
21. PARK, C.L. and FRANK, A.: Does influenza vaccination exacerbate asthma? Drug Safety 1998; *19*(2):83–88.
22. LASKY, T et al: The Guillian Barré syndrome and the 1992-1993 and 1993-1994 influenza vaccines. NEJM 1998, *339(25)*:1797–1802.
23. RETAILLIAU, H. et al: Illness after influenza vaccination reported through a nationwide surveillance system, 1976–1977. Am J Epidemiol 1980; *111*: 170.
24. BAKSHI, R. AND MAZZIOTTA, J.C.: Acute transverse myelitis after influenza vaccination: Magnetic resonance imaging findings. J Neuroimaging 1996; *6*: 248–250.

Manufactured by:
Wyeth Laboratories
A Wyeth-Ayerst Company
Marietta, PA 17547
U.S. Gov't. License No. 3
CI 6146-1 Issued July 13, 2000

ISMO® ℞

[*īs 'mō*]
(isosorbide mononitrate)
20 mg tablets

DESCRIPTION

Isosorbide mononitrate is 1,4:3,6-dianhydro-D-glucitol,5-nitrate, an organic nitrate whose structural formula is:

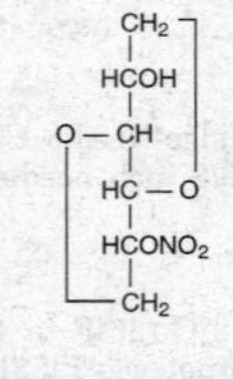

and whose molecular weight is 191.14. The organic nitrates are vasodilators, active on both arteries and veins.

Each Ismo® tablet contains 20 mg of isosorbide mononitrate. The inactive ingredients in each tablet are D&C Yellow 10 Aluminum Lake, FD&C Yellow 6 Aluminum Lake, hydroxypropyl methylcellulose, lactose, magnesium stearate, microcrystalline cellulose, polyethylene glycol, polysorbate 20, povidone, silicon dioxide, sodium starch glycolate, titanium dioxide and hydroxypropyl cellulose.

CLINICAL PHARMACOLOGY

Isosorbide mononitrate is the major active metabolite of isosorbide dinitrate (ISDN), and most of the clinical activity of the dinitrate is attributable to the mononitrate.

The principal pharmacological action of isosorbide mononitrate, due to its nitric oxide metabolite, is direct relaxation of vascular smooth muscle. The result is dilatation of peripheral arteries and veins, especially the latter. Dilation of the veins promotes peripheral pooling of blood and decreases venous return to the heart, thereby reducing left ventricular end-diastolic pressure and pulmonary capillary wedge pressure (preload). Arteriolar relaxation reduces systemic vascular resistance, systolic arterial pressure, and mean arterial pressure (afterload). Dilatation of the coronary arteries also occurs. The relative importance of preload reduction, afterload reduction, and coronary dilatation remains undefined.

Pharmacodynamics

Dosing regimens for most chronically used drugs are designed to provide plasma concentrations that are continuously greater than a minimally effective concentration. This strategy is inappropriate for organic nitrates. Several well-controlled clinical trials have used exercise testing to assess the antianginal efficacy of continuously delivered nitrates. In the large majority of these trials, active agents were indistinguishable from placebo after 24 hours (or less) of continuous therapy. Attempts to overcome tolerance by dose escalation, even to doses far in excess of those used acutely, have consistently failed. Only after nitrates have been absent from the body for several hours has their antianginal efficacy been restored.

The drug-free interval sufficient to avoid tolerance to isosorbide mononitrate has not been completely defined. In the only regimen of twice-daily isosorbide mononitrate that has been shown to avoid development of tolerance, the two doses of Ismo tablets are given 7 hours apart, so there is a gap of 17 hours between the second dose of each day and the first dose of the next day. Taking account of the relatively long half-life of isosorbide mononitrate this result is consistent with those obtained for other organic nitrates.

The same twice-daily regimen of Ismo tablets successfully avoided significant rebound/withdrawal effects. The incidence and magnitude of such phenomena have appeared, in studies of other nitrates, to be highly dependent upon the schedule of nitrate administration.

Pharmacokinetics

In humans, isosorbide mononitrate is not subject to first pass metabolism in the liver. The absolute bioavailability of isosorbide mononitrate from Ismo tablets is nearly 100%. Maximum serum concentrations of isosorbide mononitrate are achieved 30 to 60 minutes after ingestion of Ismo.

The volume of distribution of isosorbide mononitrate is approximately 0.6 L/kg, and less than 4% is bound to plasma proteins. It is cleared from the serum by denitration to isosorbide; glucuronidation to the mononitrate glucuronide; and denitration/hydration to sorbitol. None of these metabolites is vasoactive. Less than 1% of administered isosorbide mononitrate is eliminated in the urine.

The overall elimination half-life of isosorbide mononitrate is about 5 hours; the rate of clearance is the same in healthy young adults, in patients with various degrees of renal, hepatic, or cardiac dysfunction, and in the elderly. In a single-dose study, the pharmacokinetics of isosorbide mononitrate were dose-proportional up to at least 60 mg.

Clinical Trials

Controlled trials of single doses of Ismo tablets have demonstrated that antianginal activity is present about 1 hour after dosing, with peak effect seen from 1 to 4 hours after dosing.

In placebo-controlled trials lasting 2 to 3 weeks, Ismo tablets were administered twice daily, in asymmetric regimens (with interdosing intervals of 7 and 17 hours) designed to avoid tolerance. One trial tested doses of 10 mg and 20 mg; one trial tested doses of 20 mg, 40 mg, and 60 mg; and three trials tested only doses of 20 mg. In each trial, the subjects were persons with known chronic stable angina, and the primary measure of efficacy was exercise tolerance on a standardized treadmill test. After initial dosing and for at least 3 weeks, exercise tolerance in patients treated with Ismo 20 mg tablets was significantly greater than that seen in patients treated with placebo, although there was some attenuation of effect with time. Treatment with Ismo tablets was superior to placebo for at least 12 hours after the first dose (i.e., 5 hours after the second dose) of each day. Significant tolerance and rebound phenomena were not observed.

The 10-mg dose was not unequivocally superior to placebo, while the effect of the 40-mg dose was similar to that of the 20-mg dose. The 60-mg dose appeared to be less effective, and it was associated with a rebound phenomenon (early-morning worsening).

INDICATIONS AND USAGE

Ismo tablets are indicated for the prevention of angina pectoris due to coronary artery disease. The onset of action of oral isosorbide mononitrate is not sufficiently rapid for this product to be useful in aborting an acute anginal episode.

CONTRAINDICATIONS

Allergic reactions to organic nitrates are extremely rare, but they do occur. Isosorbide mononitrate is contraindicated in patients who are allergic to it.

WARNINGS

Amplification of the vasodilatory effects of Ismo by sildenafil can result in severe hypotension. The time course and dose dependence of this interaction have not been studied. Appropriate supportive care has not been studied, but it seems reasonable to treat this as a nitrate overdose, with elevation of the extremities and with central volume expansion.

The benefits of isosorbide mononitrate in patients with acute myocardial infarction or congestive heart failure have not been established. Because the effects of isosorbide mononitrate are difficult to terminate rapidly, this drug is not recommended in these settings.

If isosorbide mononitrate is used in these conditions, careful clinical or hemodynamic monitoring must be used to avoid the hazards of hypotension and tachycardia.

PRECAUTIONS

General

Severe hypotension, particularly with upright posture, may occur with even small doses of isosorbide mononitrate. This drug should therefore be used with caution in patients who may be volume depleted or who, for whatever reason, are already hypotensive. Hypotension induced by isosorbide mononitrate may be accompanied by paradoxical bradycardia and increased angina pectoris.

Nitrate therapy may aggravate the angina caused by hypertrophic cardiomyopathy.

In industrial workers who have had long-term exposure to unknown (presumably high) doses of organic nitrates, tolerance clearly occurs. Chest pain, acute myocardial infarction, and even sudden death have occurred during temporary withdrawal of nitrates from these workers, demonstrating the existence of true physical dependence. The importance of these observations to the routine, clinical use of oral isosorbide mononitrate is not known.

Information for Patients

Patients should be told that the antianginal efficacy of Ismo tablets can be maintained by carefully following the prescribed schedule of dosing (two doses taken 7 hours apart). For most patients, this can be accomplished by taking the first dose on awakening and the second dose 7 hours later.

As with other nitrates, daily headaches sometimes accompany treatment with isosorbide mononitrate. In patients who get these headaches, the headaches are a marker of the activity of the drug. Patients should resist the temptation to avoid headaches by altering the schedule of their treatment with isosorbide mononitrate, since loss of headache may be associated with simultaneous loss of antianginal efficacy. Aspirin and/or acetaminophen, on the other hand, often successfully relieve isosorbide mononitrate-induced headaches with no deleterious effect on isosorbide mononitrate's antianginal efficacy.

Treatment with isosorbide mononitrate may be associated with light-headedness on standing, especially just after rising from a recumbent or seated position. This effect may be more frequent in patients who have also consumed alcohol.

Drug Interactions

The vasodilating effects of isosorbide mononitrate may be additive with those of other vasodilators. Alcohol, in particular, has been found to exhibit additive effects of this variety.

Marked symptomatic orthostatic hypotension has been reported when calcium channel blockers and organic nitrates were used in combination. Dose adjustments of either class of agents may be necessary.

Carcinogenesis, Mutagenesis, and Impairment of Fertility

No carcinogenic effects were observed in mice exposed to oral isosorbide mononitrate for 104 weeks at doses of up to 900 mg/kg/day (102 × the human exposure comparing body surface area). Rats treated with 900 mg/kg/day for 26 weeks (225 × the human exposure comparing body surface area) and 500 mg/kg/day for the remaining 95 to 111 weeks (males and females, respectively) showed no evidence of tumors.

No mutagenic activity was seen in a variety of *in vitro* and *in vivo* assays.

No adverse effects on fertility were observed when isosorbide mononitrate was administered to male and female rats at doses up to 500 mg/kg/day (125 × the human exposure comparing body surface area).

Pregnancy Category C

Isosorbide mononitrate has been shown to be associated with stillbirths and neonatal death in rats receiving 500 mg/kg/day of isosorbide mononitrate (125 × the human exposure comparing body surface area). At 250 mg/kg/day, no adverse effects on reproduction and development were reported.

In rats and rabbits receiving isosorbide mononitrate at up to 250 mg/kg/day, no developmental abnormalities, fetal abnormalities, or other effects upon reproductive performance were detected; these doses are larger than the maximum recommended human dose by factors between 70 (body-surface-area basis in rabbits) and 310 (body-weight basis, either species). In rats receiving 500 mg/kg/day, there were small but statistically significant increases in the rates of prolonged gestation, prolonged parturition, stillbirth, and neonatal death; and there were small but statistically significant decreases in birth weight, live litter size, and pup survival.

There are no adequate and well-controlled studies in pregnant women. Isosorbide mononitrate should be used during pregnancy only if the potential benefit justifies the potential risk to the fetus.

Nursing Mothers

It is not known whether isosorbide mononitrate is excreted in human milk. Because many drugs are excreted in human milk, caution should be exercised when isosorbide mononitrate is administered to a nursing woman.

Pediatric Use
Safety and effectiveness of isosorbide mononitrate in pediatric patients have not been established.
Geriatric Use
Clinical studies of Ismo® did not include sufficient numbers of subjects aged 65 and over to determine whether they respond differently from younger subjects. Other reported clinical experience has not identified differences in responses between the elderly and younger patients. In general, dose selection for an elderly patient should be cautious, usually starting at the low end of the dosing range, although age, renal, hepatic or cardiac dysfunction do not appear to have a clinically significant effect on the clearance of Ismo®.

ADVERSE REACTIONS

The table below shows the frequencies of the adverse reactions observed in more than 1% of the subjects (a) in 6 placebo-controlled domestic studies in which patients in the active-treatment arm received 20 mg of isosorbide mononitrate twice daily, and (b) in all studies in which patients received isosorbide mononitrate in a variety of regimens. In parentheses, the same table shows the frequencies with which these adverse reactions led to discontinuation of treatment. Overall, 11% of the patients who received isosorbide mononitrate in the six controlled U.S. studies discontinued treatment because of adverse reactions. Most of these discontinued because of headache. "Dizziness" and nausea were also frequently associated with withdrawal from these studies.

Frequency of Adverse Reactions (Discontinuations)*

	6 Controlled Studies		92 Clinical Studies
Dose	Placebo	20 mg	(varied)
Patients	204	219	3344
Headache	9% (0%)	38% (9%)	19% (4.3%)
Dizziness	1% (0%)	5% (1%)	3% (0.2%)
Nausea, Vomiting	<1% (0%)	4% (3%)	2% (0.2%)

* Some individuals discontinued for multiple reasons.

Other adverse reactions, each reported by fewer than 1% of exposed patients, and in many cases of uncertain relation to drug treatment, were:
Cardiovascular: angina pectoris, arrhythmias, atrial fibrillation, hypotension, palpitations, postural hypotension, premature ventricular contractions, supraventricular tachycardia, syncope.
Dermatologic: pruritus, rash.
Gastrointestinal: abdominal pain, diarrhea, dyspepsia, tenesmus, tooth disorder, vomiting.
Genitourinary: dysuria, impotence, urinary frequency.
Miscellaneous: asthenia, blurred vision, cold sweat, diplopia, edema, malaise, neck stiffness, rigors.
Musculoskeletal: arthralgia.
Neurological: agitation, anxiety, confusion, dyscoordination, hypoesthesia, hypokinesia, increased appetite, insomnia, nervousness, nightmares.
Respiratory: bronchitis, pneumonia, upper-respiratory tract infection.
Extremely rarely, ordinary doses of organic nitrates have caused methemoglobinemia in normal-seeming patients; for further discussion of its diagnosis and treatment see under **OVERDOSAGE.**

OVERDOSAGE

Hemodynamic Effects
The ill effects of isosorbide mononitrate overdose are generally the results of isosorbide mononitrate's capacity to induce vasodilatation, venous pooling, reduced cardiac output, and hypotension. These hemodynamic changes may have protean manifestations, including increased intracranial pressure, with any or all of persistent throbbing headache, confusion, and moderate fever; vertigo; palpitations; visual disturbances; nausea and vomiting (possibly with colic and even bloody diarrhea); syncope (especially in the upright posture); air hunger and dyspnea, later followed by reduced ventilatory effort; diaphoresis, with the skin either flushed or cold and clammy; heart block and bradycardia; paralysis; coma; seizures and death.
Laboratory determinations of serum levels of isosorbide mononitrate and its metabolites are not widely available, and such determinations have, in any event, no established role in the management of isosorbide mononitrate overdose.
There are no data suggesting what dose of isosorbide mononitrate is likely to be life-threatening in humans. In rats and mice, there is significant lethality at doses of 2000 mg/kg and 3000 mg/kg, respectively.
No data are available to suggest physiological maneuvers (e.g., maneuvers to change the pH of the urine) that might accelerate elimination of isosorbide mononitrate. In particular, dialysis is known to be ineffective in removing isosorbide mononitrate from the body.
No specific antagonist to the vasodilator effects of isosorbide mononitrate is known, and no intervention has been subject to controlled study as a therapy of isosorbide mononitrate overdose. Because the hypotension associated with isosorbide mononitrate overdose is the result of venodilatation and arterial hypovolemia, prudent therapy in this situation should be directed toward an increase in central fluid volume. Passive elevation of the patient's legs may be sufficient, but intravenous infusion of normal saline or similar fluid may also be necessary.
The use of epinephrine or other arterial vasoconstrictors in this setting is likely to do more harm than good.
In patients with renal disease or congestive heart failure, therapy resulting in central volume expansion is not without hazard. Treatment of isosorbide mononitrate overdose in these patients may be subtle and difficult, and invasive monitoring may be required.
Methemoglobinemia
Methemoglobinemia has been reported in patients receiving other organic nitrates, and it probably could also occur as a side effect of isosorbide mononitrate. Certainly nitrate ions liberated during metabolism of isosorbide mononitrate can oxidize hemoglobin into methemoglobin. Even in patients totally without cytochrome b_5 reductase activity, however, and even assuming that the nitrate moiety of isosorbide mononitrate is quantitatively applied to oxidation of hemoglobin, about 2 mg/kg of isosorbide mononitrate should be required before any of these patients manifests clinically significant ($\geq$ 10%) methemoglobinemia. In patients with normal reductase function, significant production of methemoglobin should require even larger doses of isosorbide mononitrate. In one study in which 36 patients received 2 to 4 weeks of continuous nitroglycerin therapy at 3.1 to 4.4 mg/hr (equivalent, in total administered dose of nitrate ions, to 7.8 to 11.1 mg of isosorbide mononitrate per hour), the average methemoglobin level measured was 0.2%; this was comparable to that observed in parallel patients who received placebo.
Notwithstanding these observations, there are case reports of significant methemoglobinemia in association with moderate overdoses of organic nitrates. None of the affected patients had been thought to be unusually susceptible.
Methemoglobin levels are available from most clinical laboratories. The diagnosis should be suspected in patients who exhibit signs of impaired oxygen delivery despite adequate cardiac output and adequate arterial pO_2. Classically, methemoglobinemic blood is described as chocolate brown, without color change on exposure to air.
When methemoglobinemia is diagnosed, the treatment of choice is methylene blue, 1 to 2 mg/kg intravenously.

DOSAGE AND ADMINISTRATION

The recommended regimen of Ismo tablets is 20 mg (one tablet) twice daily, with the two doses given 7 hours apart. For most patients, this can be accomplished by taking the first dose on awakening and the second dose 7 hours later. Dosage adjustments are not necessary for elderly patients or patients with altered renal or hepatic function.
As noted above (**CLINICAL PHARMACOLOGY**), multiple studies of organic nitrates have shown that maintenance of continuous 24-hour plasma levels results in refractory tolerance. The dosing regimen for Ismo tablets provides a daily nitrate-free interval to avoid the development of this tolerance.
As also noted under **CLINICAL PHARMACOLOGY,** well-controlled studies have shown that tolerance to Ismo tablets is avoided when using the twice-daily regimen in which the two doses are given 7 hours apart. This regimen has been shown to have antianginal efficacy beginning 1 hour after the first dose and lasting at least 5 hours after the second dose. The duration (if any) of antianginal activity beyond 12 hours has not been studied; large controlled studies with other nitrates suggest that no dosing regimen should be expected to provide more than about 12 hours of continuous antianginal efficacy per day.
In clinical trials, Ismo tablets have been administered in a variety of regimens. Single doses less than 20 mg have not been adequately studied, while single doses greater than 20 mg have demonstrated no greater efficacy than doses of 20 mg.

HOW SUPPLIED

Ismo® (isosorbide mononitrate) tablets, 20 mg, are available in bottles of 100 (NDC 0008-0771-01) and in unit dose packages of 10 blister strips of 10 tablets (NDC 0008-0771-02). Each orange, round, film-coated tablet is engraved "ISMO 20" on one side and scored on the reverse side.
Store at controlled room temperature between 20°C and 25°C (68°F and 77°F).
Dispense in tight container.
Manufactured by:
Wyeth Laboratories
A Wyeth-Ayerst Company
Philadelphia, PA 19101
Distributed jointly with:
Boehringer Mannheim Pharmaceuticals Corp.
Rockville, MD 20850
CI 4130-8 Revised March 16, 2000
Shown in Product Identification Guide, page 341

ISORDIL® ℞
[*ī'sŏr-dĭl*]
(isosorbide dinitrate)
Sublingual Tablets

DESCRIPTION

Isosorbide dinitrate (ISDN) is 1,4:3,6-dianhydro-D-glucitol 2,5-dinitrate, an organic nitrate whose structural formula is
[See chemical structure at top of next column]

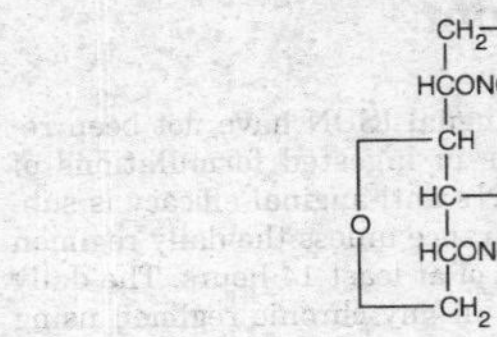

and whose molecular weight is 236.14. The organic nitrates are vasodilators, active on both arteries and veins.
Isosorbide dinitrate is a white, crystalline, odorless compound which is stable in air and in solution, has a melting point of 70°C and has an optical rotation of +134° (c=1.0, alcohol, 20°C). Isosorbide dinitrate is freely soluble in organic solvents such as acetone, alcohol, and ether, but is only sparingly soluble in water.
Each Isordil® Sublingual tablet contains 2.5, 5, or 10 mg of isosorbide dinitrate. The inactive ingredients in each tablet are cellulose, lactose, magnesium stearate, and starch. The 2.5 mg dosage strength also contains D&C Yellow 10 and FD&C Yellow 6, and the 5 mg dosage strength also contains FD&C Red 40.

CLINICAL PHARMACOLOGY

The principal pharmacological action of isosorbide dinitrate is relaxation of vascular smooth muscle and consequent dilatation of peripheral arteries and veins, especially the latter. Dilatation of the veins promotes peripheral pooling of blood and decreases venous return to the heart, thereby reducing left ventricular end-diastolic pressure and pulmonary capillary wedge pressure (preload). Arteriolar relaxation reduces systemic vascular resistance, systolic arterial pressure, and mean arterial pressure (afterload). Dilatation of the coronary arteries also occurs. The relative importance of preload reduction, afterload reduction, and coronary dilatation remains undefined.
Dosing regimens for most chronically used drugs are designed to provide plasma concentrations that are continuously greater than a minimally effective concentration. This strategy is inappropriate for organic nitrates. Several well-controlled clinical trials have used exercise testing to assess the anti-anginal efficacy of continuously-delivered nitrates. In the large majority of these trials, active agents were no more effective than placebo after 24 hours (or less) of continuous therapy. Attempts to overcome nitrate tolerance by dose escalation, even to doses far in excess of those used acutely, have consistently failed. Only after nitrates have been absent from the body for several hours has their anti-anginal efficacy been restored.
Pharmacokinetics
Bioavailability of ISDN after single sublingual doses is 40 to 50%. Multiple-dose studies of sublingual ISDN pharmacokinetics have not been reported; multiple-dose studies of ingested ISDN have observed progressive increases in bioavailability during chronic therapy. Serum levels of ISDN reach their maxima 10 to 15 minutes after sublingual dosing.
Once absorbed, the volume of distribution of isosorbide dinitrate is 2 to 4 L/kg, and this volume is cleared at the rate of 2 to 4 L/min, so ISDN's half-life in serum is about an hour. Since the clearance exceeds hepatic blood flow, considerable extrahepatic metabolism must also occur. Clearance is affected primarily by denitration to the 2-mononitrate (15 to 25%) and the 5-mononitrate (75 to 85%).
Both metabolites have biological activity, especially the 5-mononitrate. With an overall half-life of about 5 hours, the 5-mononitrate is cleared from the serum by denitration to isosorbide, glucuronidation to the 5-mononitrate glucuronide, and denitration/hydration to sorbitol. The 2-mononitrate has been less well studied, but it appears to participate in the same metabolic pathways, with a half-life of about 2 hours.
The daily dose-free interval sufficient to avoid tolerance to organic nitrates has not been well defined. Studies of nitroglycerin (an organic nitrate with a very short half-life) have shown that daily dose-free intervals of 10 to 12 hours are usually sufficient to minimize tolerance. Daily dose-free intervals that have succeeded in avoiding tolerance during trials of moderate doses (*e.g.,* 30 mg) of immediate-release ISDN have generally been somewhat longer (at least 14 hours), but this is consistent with the longer half-lives of ISDN and its active metabolites.
Few well-controlled clinical trials of organic nitrates have been designed to detect rebound or withdrawal effects. In one such trial, however, subjects receiving nitroglycerin had *less* exercise tolerance at the end of the daily dose-free interval than the parallel group receiving placebo. The incidence, magnitude, and clinical significance of similar phenomena in patients receiving ISDN have not been studied.
Clinical Trials
In a controlled trial in which 0.4 mg of sublingual nitroglycerin took 1.9 minutes to begin to produce an anti-anginal effect, 5 mg of sublingual ISDN took 3.4 minutes to begin to produce a similar effect. In the same trial, the anti-anginal effect of the sublingual nitroglycerin was evident for about an hour, while that of the sublingual ISDN lasted about 2 hours.
In other controlled trials, the anti-anginal efficacy of sublingual ISDN has persisted for periods ranging from 30 minutes up to 4 hours.

Continued on next page

Isordil Tablets—Cont.

Multiple-dose trials of sublingual ISDN have not been reported. Multiple-dose trials of ingested formulations of ISDN have shown that ISDN's anti-anginal efficacy is substantially attenuated by tolerance unless the daily regimen includes a dose-free interval of at least 14 hours. The daily dose-free interval necessary in any chronic regimen using sublingual ISDN is not known.
From large, well-controlled studies of other nitrates, it is reasonable to believe that the maximal achievable daily duration of anti-anginal effect from isosorbide dinitrate is about 12 hours. No dosing regimen for isosorbide dinitrate has, however, ever actually been shown to achieve this duration of effect. In the absence of data from multiple-dose trials, and considering the capacity of organic nitrates to induce tolerance, it is not reasonable to assume that multiple sublingual ISDN tablets taken during the course of a day will all have similar effects.

INDICATIONS AND USAGE

Isordil Sublingual tablets are indicated for the prevention and treatment of angina pectoris due to coronary artery disease. However, because the onset of action of sublingual ISDN is significantly slower than that of sublingual nitroglycerin, sublingual ISDN is not the drug of first choice for abortion of an acute anginal episode.

CONTRAINDICATIONS

Allergic reactions to organic nitrates are extremely rare, but they do occur. Isordil is contraindicated in patients who are allergic to isosorbide dinitrate or any of its other ingredients.

WARNINGS

Amplification of the vasodilatory effects of Isordil by sildenafil can result in severe hypotension. The time course and dose dependence of this interaction have not been studied. Appropriate supportive care has not been studied, but it seems reasonable to treat this as a nitrate overdose, with elevation of the extremities and with central volume expansion.
The benefits of sublingual isosorbide dinitrate in patients with acute myocardial infarction or congestive heart failure have not been established. If one elects to use isosorbide dinitrate in these conditions, careful clinical or hemodynamic monitoring must be used to avoid the hazards of hypotension and tachycardia.

PRECAUTIONS

General
Severe hypotension, particularly with upright posture, may occur with even small doses of isosorbide dinitrate. This drug should therefore be used with caution in patients who may be volume depleted or who, for whatever reason, are already hypotensive. Hypotension induced by isosorbide dinitrate may be accompanied by paradoxical bradycardia and increased angina pectoris.
Nitrate therapy may aggravate the angina caused by hypertrophic cardiomyopathy.
As tolerance to isosorbide dinitrate develops, the effect of sublingual nitroglycerin on exercise tolerance, although still observable, is somewhat blunted.
Some clinical trials in angina patients have provided nitroglycerin for about 12 continuous hours of every 24-hour day. During the daily dose-free interval in some of these trials, anginal attacks have been more easily provoked than before treatment, and patients have demonstrated hemodynamic rebound and *decreased* exercise tolerance. The importance of these observations to the routine, clinical use of sublingual isosorbide dinitrate is not known.
In industrial workers who have had long-term exposure to unknown (presumably high) doses of organic nitrates, tolerance clearly occurs. Chest pain, acute myocardial infarction, and even sudden death have occurred during temporary withdrawal of nitrates from these workers, demonstrating the existence of true physical dependence.

Information for Patients
Patients should be told that the anti-anginal efficacy of isosorbide dinitrate is strongly related to its dosing regimen, so the prescribed schedule of dosing should be followed carefully. In particular, daily headaches sometimes accompany treatment with isosorbide dinitrate. In patients who get these headaches, the headaches are a marker of the activity of the drug. Patients should resist the temptation to avoid headaches by altering the schedule of their treatment with isosorbide dinitrate, since loss of headache may be associated with simultaneous loss of anti-anginal efficacy. Aspirin and/or acetaminophen, on the other hand, often successfully relieve isosorbide dinitrate-induced headaches with no deleterious effect on isosorbide dinitrate's anti-anginal efficacy.
Treatment with isosorbide dinitrate may be associated with lightheadedness on standing, especially just after rising from a recumbent or seated position. This effect may be more frequent in patients who have also consumed alcohol.

Drug Interactions
The vasodilating effects of isosorbide dinitrate may be additive with those of other vasodilators. Alcohol, in particular, has been found to exhibit additive effects of this variety.

Carcinogenesis, Mutagenesis, Impairment of Fertility
No long-term studies in animals have been performed to evaluate the carcinogenic potential of isosorbide dinitrate. In a modified two-litter reproduction study, there was no remarkable gross pathology and no altered fertility or gestation among rats fed isosorbide dinitrate at 25 or 100 mg/kg/day.

Pregnancy Category C
At oral doses 35 and 150 times the maximum recommended human daily dose, isosorbide dinitrate has been shown to cause a dose-related increase in embryotoxicity (increase in mummified pups) in rabbits. There are no adequate, well-controlled studies in pregnant women. Isosorbide dinitrate should be used during pregnancy only if the potential benefit justifies the potential risk to the fetus.

Nursing Mothers
It is not known whether isosorbide dinitrate is excreted in human milk. Because many drugs are excreted in human milk, caution should be exercised when isosorbide dinitrate is administered to a nursing woman.

Pediatric Use
Safety and effectiveness in pediatric patients have not been established.

ADVERSE REACTIONS

Adverse reactions to isosorbide dinitrate are generally dose-related, and almost all of these reactions are the result of isosorbide dinitrate's activity as a vasodilator. Headache, which may be severe, is the most commonly reported side effect. Headache may be recurrent with each daily dose, especially at higher doses. Transient episodes of lightheadedness, occasionally related to blood pressure changes, may also occur. Hypotension occurs infrequently, but in some patients it may be severe enough to warrant discontinuation of therapy. Syncope, crescendo angina, and rebound hypertension have been reported but are uncommon.
Extremely rarely, ordinary doses of organic nitrates have caused methemoglobinemia in normal-seeming patients. Methemoglobinemia is so infrequent at these doses that further discussion of its diagnosis and treatment is deferred (see **OVERDOSAGE**).
Data are not available to allow estimation of the frequency of adverse reactions during treatment with Isordil® Sublingual tablets.

OVERDOSAGE

Hemodynamic Effects
The ill effects of isosorbide dinitrate overdose are generally the results of isosorbide dinitrate's capacity to induce vasodilatation, venous pooling, reduced cardiac output, and hypotension. These hemodynamic changes may have protean manifestations, including increased intracranial pressure, with any or all of persistent throbbing headache, confusion, and moderate fever; vertigo; palpitations; visual disturbances; nausea and vomiting (possibly with colic and even bloody diarrhea); syncope (especially in the upright posture); air hunger and dyspnea, later followed by reduced ventilatory effort; diaphoresis, with the skin either flushed or cold and clammy; heart block and bradycardia; paralysis; coma; seizures; and death.
Laboratory determinations of serum levels of isosorbide dinitrate and its metabolites are not widely available, and such determinations have, in any event, no established role in the management of isosorbide dinitrate overdose.
There are no data suggesting what dose of isosorbide dinitrate is likely to be life-threatening in humans. In rats, the median acute lethal dose (LD_{50}) was found to be 1100 mg/kg.
No data are available to suggest physiological maneuvers (*e.g.*, maneuvers to change the pH of the urine) that might accelerate elimination of isosorbide dinitrate and its active metabolites. Similarly, it is not known which, if any, of these substances can usefully be removed from the body by hemodialysis.
No specific antagonist to the vasodilator effects of isosorbide dinitrate is known, and no intervention has been subject to controlled studies as a therapy for isosorbide dinitrate overdose. Because the hypotension associated with isosorbide dinitrate overdose is the result of venodilatation and arterial hypovolemia, prudent therapy in this situation should be directed toward increase in central fluid volume. Passive elevation of the patient's legs may be sufficient, but intravenous infusion of normal saline or similar fluid may also be necessary.
The use of epinephrine or other arterial vasoconstrictors in this setting is likely to do more harm than good.
In patients with renal disease or congestive heart failure, therapy resulting in central volume expansion is not without hazard. Treatment of isosorbide dinitrate overdose in these patients may be subtle and difficult, and invasive monitoring may be required.

Methemoglobinemia
Nitrate ions liberated during metabolism of isosorbide dinitrate can oxidize hemoglobin into methemoglobin. Even in patients totally without cytochrome b_5 reductase activity, however, and even assuming that the nitrate moieties of isosorbide dinitrate are quantitatively applied to oxidation of hemoglobin, about 1 mg/kg of isosorbide dinitrate should be required before any of these patients manifests clinically significant ($\geq$10%) methemoglobinemia. In patients with normal reductase function, significant production of methemoglobin should require even larger doses of isosorbide dinitrate. In one study in which 36 patients received 2 to 4 weeks of continuous nitroglycerin therapy at 3.1 to 4.4 mg/hr (equivalent, in total administered dose of nitrate ions, to 4.8 to 6.9 mg of bioavailable isosorbide dinitrate per hour), the average methemoglobin level measured was 0.2%; this was comparable to that observed in parallel patients who received placebo.
Notwithstanding these observations, there are case reports of significant methemoglobinemia in association with moderate overdoses of organic nitrates. None of the affected patients had been thought to be unusually susceptible.
Methemoglobin levels are available from most clinical laboratories. The diagnosis should be suspected in patients who exhibit signs of impaired oxygen delivery despite adequate cardiac output and adequate arterial pO_2. Classically, methemoglobinemic blood is described as chocolate brown, without color change on exposure to air.
When methemoglobinemia is diagnosed, the treatment of choice is methylene blue, 1 to 2 mg/kg intravenously.

DOSAGE AND ADMINISTRATION

As noted under **CLINICAL PHARMACOLOGY**, multiple-dose studies with ISDN and other nitrates have shown that maintenance of continuous 24-hour plasma levels results in refractory tolerance. Every dosing regimen for ISDN must provide a daily dose-free interval to minimize the development of this tolerance. In the case of sublingual tablets, it is probably true that one of the daily dose-free intervals must be somewhat longer than 14 hours.
As also noted under **CLINICAL PHARMACOLOGY**, the efficacy of daily doses after the first dose has never been demonstrated.
Large controlled studies with other nitrates suggest that no dosing regimen with Isordil Sublingual tablets should be expected to provide more than about 12 hours of continuous anti-anginal efficacy per day.
A patient anticipating activity likely to cause angina should take one Isordil Sublingual tablet (2.5 to 5 mg) about 15 minutes before the activity is expected to begin. Isordil Sublingual tablets may be used to abort an acute anginal episode, but its use is recommended only in patients who fail to respond to sublingual nitroglycerin.

HOW SUPPLIED

Isordil® (isosorbide dinitrate) Sublingual Tablets are available as follows:
2.5 mg, round, yellow tablets imprinted "2.5" on one side and "W" on reverse side:
NDC 0008-4139-01, bottles of 100.
NDC 0008-4139-03, bottles of 500.
NDC 0008-4139-05, Redipak® cartons of 100 (10 blister strips of 10).
5 mg, round, pink tablets imprinted "5" on one side and "W" on reverse side:
NDC 0008-4126-01, bottles of 100.
NDC 0008-4126-03, bottles of 500.
NDC 0008-4126-07, Redipak cartons of 100 (10 blister strips of 10).
Store at room temperature, approximately 25°C (77°F)
Protect from light
Keep bottles tightly closed
Dispense in a light-resistant, tight container
Use carton to protect blisters from light
10 mg, round, white tablets imprinted "10" on one side and "Wyeth" on reverse side:
NDC 0008-4161-01, bottles of 100.
Store at room temperature, approximately 25°C (77°F)
Keep tightly closed
Dispense in a tight container
ALSO AVAILABLE
Oral Titradose® Tablets in the following dosage strengths:
5 mg, NDC 0008-4152, in bottles of 100, 500 or 1,000 and in Redipak cartons of 100 (10 blister strips of 10).
10 mg, NDC 0008-4153, in bottles of 100, 500 or 1,000 and in Redipak cartons of 100 (10 blister strips of 10).
20 mg, NDC 0008-4154, in bottles of 100 or 500 and in Redipak cartons of 100 (10 blister strips of 10).
30 mg, NDC 0008-4159, in bottles of 100 or 500 and in Redipak cartons of 100 (10 blister strips of 10).
40 mg, NDC 0008-4192, in bottles of 100 and in Redipak cartons of 100 (10 blister strips of 10).
Manufactured by:
Wyeth Laboratories
A Wyeth-Ayerst Company
Philadelphia, PA 19101
CI 4370-2 Revised February 9, 1999
Shown in Product Identification Guide, page 341

ISORDIL® TITRADOSE® ℞

[ī 'sŏr-dĭl]
(isosorbide dinitrate)
Tablets

DESCRIPTION

Isosorbide dinitrate (ISDN) is 1,4:3,6-dianhydro-D-glucitol 2,5-dinitrate, an organic nitrate whose structural formula is

and whose molecular weight is 236.14. The organic nitrates are vasodilators, active on both arteries and veins.

Isosorbide dinitrate is a white, crystalline, odorless compound which is stable in air and in solution, has a melting point of 70°C and has an optical rotation of +134° (c=1.0, alcohol, 20°C). Isosorbide dinitrate is freely soluble in organic solvents such as acetone, alcohol, and ether, but is only sparingly soluble in water.

Each Isordil® Titradose® tablet contains 5, 10, 20, 30, or 40 mg of isosorbide dinitrate. The inactive ingredients in each tablet are lactose, cellulose, and magnesium stearate. The 5 mg, 20 mg, 30 mg, and 40 mg dosage strengths also contain the following: 5 mg—FD&C Red 40; 20 mg and 40 mg—D&C Yellow 10, FD&C Blue 1, and FD&C Yellow 6; 30 mg—FD&C Blue 1.

CLINICAL PHARMACOLOGY

The principal pharmacological action of isosorbide dinitrate is relaxation of vascular smooth muscle and consequent dilatation of peripheral arteries and veins, especially the latter. Dilatation of the veins promotes peripheral pooling of blood and decreases venous return to the heart, thereby reducing left ventricular end-diastolic pressure and pulmonary capillary wedge pressure (preload). Arteriolar relaxation reduces systemic vascular resistance, systolic arterial pressure, and mean arterial pressure (afterload). Dilatation of the coronary arteries also occurs. The relative importance of preload reduction, afterload reduction, and coronary dilatation remains undefined.

Dosing regimens for most chronically used drugs are designed to provide plasma concentrations that are continuously greater than a minimally effective concentration. This strategy is inappropriate for organic nitrates. Several well-controlled clinical trials have used exercise testing to assess the anti-anginal efficacy of continuously-delivered nitrates. In the large majority of these trials, active agents were no more effective than placebo after 24 hours (or less) of continuous therapy. Attempts to overcome nitrate tolerance by dose escalation, even to doses far in excess of those used acutely, have consistently failed. Only after nitrates have been absent from the body for several hours has their anti-anginal efficacy been restored.

Pharmacokinetics

Absorption of isosorbide dinitrate after oral dosing is nearly complete, but bioavailability is highly variable (10% to 90%), with extensive first-pass metabolism in the liver. Serum levels reach their maxima about an hour after ingestion. The average bioavailability of ISDN is about 25%; most studies have observed progressive increases in bioavailability during chronic therapy.

Once absorbed, the volume of distribution of isosorbide dinitrate is 2 to 4 L/kg, and this volume is cleared at the rate of 2 to 4 L/min, so ISDN's half-life in serum is about an hour. Since the clearance exceeds hepatic blood flow, considerable extrahepatic metabolism must also occur. Clearance is affected primarily by denitration to the 2-mononitrate (15 to 25%) and the 5-mononitrate (75 to 85%).

Both metabolites have biological activity, especially the 5-mononitrate. With an overall half-life of about 5 hours, the 5-mononitrate is cleared from the serum by denitration to isosorbide, glucuronidation to the 5-mononitrate glucuronide, and denitration/hydration to sorbitol. The 2-mononitrate has been less well studied, but it appears to participate in the same metabolic pathways, with a half-life of about 2 hours.

The daily dose-free interval sufficient to avoid tolerance to organic nitrates has not been well defined. Studies of nitroglycerin (an organic nitrate with a very short half-life) have shown that daily dose-free intervals of 10 to 12 hours are usually sufficient to minimize tolerance. Daily dose-free intervals that have succeeded in avoiding tolerance during trials of moderate doses (*e.g.*, 30 mg) of immediate-release ISDN have generally been somewhat longer (at least 14 hours), but this is consistent with the longer half-lives of ISDN and its active metabolites.

Few well-controlled clinical trials of organic nitrates have been designed to detect rebound or withdrawal effects. In one such trial, however, subjects receiving nitroglycerin had *less* exercise tolerance at the end of the daily dose-free interval than the parallel group receiving placebo. The incidence, magnitude, and clinical significance of similar phenomena in patients receiving ISDN have not been studied.

Clinical Trials

In clinical trials, immediate-release oral isosorbide dinitrate has been administered in a variety of regimens, with total daily doses ranging from 30 mg to 480 mg. Controlled trials of single oral doses of isosorbide dinitrate have demonstrated effective reductions in exercise-related angina for up to 8 hours. Anti-anginal activity is present about 1 hour after dosing.

Most controlled trials of multiple-dose oral ISDN taken every 12 hours (or more frequently) for several weeks have shown statistically significant anti-anginal efficacy for only 2 hours after dosing. Once-daily regimens, and regimens with one daily dose-free interval of at least 14 hours (*e.g.*, a regimen providing doses at 0800, 1400, and 1800 hours), have shown efficacy after the first dose of each day that was similar to that shown in the single-dose studies cited above. The effects of the second and later doses have been smaller and shorter-lasting than the effect of the first.

From large, well-controlled studies of other nitrates, it is reasonable to believe that the maximum achievable daily duration of anti-anginal effect from isosorbide dinitrate is about 12 hours. No dosing regimen for isosorbide dinitrate has, however, ever actually been shown to achieve this duration of effect. One study of 8 patients, who were administered a pretitrated dose (average 27.5 mg) of immediate-release ISDN at 0800, 1300, and 1800 hours for 2 weeks, revealed that significant anti-anginal effectiveness was discontinuous and totaled about 6 hours in a 24 hour period.

INDICATIONS AND USAGE

Isordil Titradose tablets are indicated for the prevention of angina pectoris due to coronary artery disease. The onset of action of immediate-release oral isosorbide dinitrate is not sufficiently rapid for this product to be useful in aborting an acute anginal episode.

CONTRAINDICATIONS

Allergic reactions to organic nitrates are extremely rare, but they do occur. Isordil Titradose is contraindicated in patients who are allergic to isosorbide dinitrate or any of its other ingredients.

WARNINGS

Amplification of the vasodilatory effects of Isordil by sildenafil can result in severe hypotension. The time course and dose dependence of this interaction have not been studied. Appropriate supportive care has not been studied, but it seems reasonable to treat this as a nitrate overdose, with elevation of the extremities and with central volume expansion.

The benefits of immediate-release oral isosorbide dinitrate in patients with acute myocardial infarction or congestive heart failure have not been established. If one elects to use isosorbide dinitrate in these conditions, careful clinical or hemodynamic monitoring must be used to avoid the hazards of hypotension and tachycardia. Because the effects of oral isosorbide dinitrate are so difficult to terminate rapidly, this formulation is not recommended in these settings.

PRECAUTIONS

General

Severe hypotension, particularly with upright posture, may occur with even small doses of isosorbide dinitrate. This drug should therefore be used with caution in patients who may be volume depleted or who, for whatever reason, are already hypotensive. Hypotension induced by isosorbide dinitrate may be accompanied by paradoxical bradycardia and increased angina pectoris.

Nitrate therapy may aggravate the angina caused by hypertrophic cardiomyopathy.

As tolerance to isosorbide dinitrate develops, the effect of sublingual nitroglycerin on exercise tolerance, although still observable, is somewhat blunted.

Some clinical trials in angina patients have provided nitroglycerin for about 12 continuous hours of every 24-hour day. During the daily dose-free interval in some of these trials, anginal attacks have been more easily provoked than before treatment, and patients have demonstrated hemodynamic rebound and *decreased* exercise tolerance. The importance of these observations to the routine, clinical use of immediate-release oral isosorbide dinitrate is not known.

In industrial workers who have had long-term exposure to unknown (presumably high) doses of organic nitrates, tolerance clearly occurs. Chest pain, acute myocardial infarction, and even sudden death have occurred during temporary withdrawal of nitrates from these workers, demonstrating the existence of true physical dependence.

Information for Patients

Patients should be told that the anti-anginal efficacy of isosorbide dinitrate is strongly related to its dosing regimen, so the prescribed schedule of dosing should be followed carefully. In particular, daily headaches sometimes accompany treatment with isosorbide dinitrate. In patients who get these headaches, the headaches are a marker of the activity of the drug. Patients should resist the temptation to avoid headaches by altering the schedule of their treatment with isosorbide dinitrate, since loss of headache may be associated with simultaneous loss of anti-anginal efficacy. Aspirin and/or acetaminophen, on the other hand, often successfully relieve isosorbide dinitrate-induced headaches with no deleterious effect on isosorbide dinitrate's anti-anginal efficacy. Treatment with isosorbide dinitrate may be associated with lightheadedness on standing, especially just after rising from a recumbent or seated position. This effect may be more frequent in patients who have also consumed alcohol.

Drug Interactions

The vasodilating effects of isosorbide dinitrate may be additive with those of other vasodilators. Alcohol, in particular, has been found to exhibit additive effects of this variety.

Carcinogenesis, Mutagenesis, Impairment of Fertility

No long-term studies in animals have been performed to evaluate the carcinogenic potential of isosorbide dinitrate. In a modified two-litter reproduction study, there was no remarkable gross pathology and no altered fertility or gestation among rats fed isosorbide dinitrate at 25 or 100 mg/kg/day.

Pregnancy Category C

At oral doses 35 and 150 times the maximum recommended human daily dose, isosorbide dinitrate has been shown to cause a dose-related increase in embryotoxicity (increase in mummified pups) in rabbits. There are no adequate, well-controlled studies in pregnant women. Isosorbide dinitrate should be used during pregnancy only if the potential benefit justifies the potential risk to the fetus.

Nursing Mothers

It is not known whether isosorbide dinitrate is excreted in human milk. Because many drugs are excreted in human milk, caution should be exercised when isosorbide dinitate is administered to a nursing woman.

Pediatric Use

Safety and effectiveness in pediatric patients have not been established.

ADVERSE REACTIONS

Adverse reactions to isosorbide dinitrate are generally dose-related, and almost all of these reactions are the result of isosorbide dinitrate's activity as a vasodilator. Headache, which may be severe, is the most commonly reported side effect. Headache may be recurrent with each daily dose, especially at higher doses. Transient episodes of lightheadedness, occasionally related to blood pressure changes, may also occur. Hypotension occurs infrequently, but in some patients it may be severe enough to warrant discontinuation of therapy. Syncope, crescendo angina, and rebound hypertension have been reported but are uncommon.

Extremely rarely, ordinary doses of organic nitrates have caused methemoglobinemia in normal-seeming patient. Methemoglobinemia is so infrequent at these doses that further discussion of its diagnosis and treatment is deferred (see "**OVERDOSAGE**").

Data are not available to allow estimation of the frequency of adverse reactions during treatment with Isordil® Titradose® tablets.

OVERDOSAGE

Hemodynamic Effects

The ill effects of isosorbide dinitrate overdose are generally the results of isosorbide dinitrate's capacity to induce vasodilatation, venous pooling, reduced cardiac output, and hypotension. These hemodynamic changes may have protean manifestations, including increased intracranial pressure, with any or all of persistent throbbing headache, confusion, and moderate fever; vertigo; palpitations; visual disturbances; nausea and vomiting (possibly with colic and even bloody diarrhea); syncope (especially in the upright posture); air hunger and dyspnea, later followed by reduced ventilatory effort; diaphoresis, with the skin either flushed or cold and clammy; heart block and bradycardia; paralysis; coma; seizures; and death.

Laboratory determinations of serum levels of isosorbide dinitrate and its metabolites are not widely available, and such determinations have, in any event, no established role in the management of isosorbide dinitrate overdose.

There are no data suggesting what dose of isosorbide dinitrate is likely to be life-threatening in humans. In rats, the median acute lethal dose (LD_{50}) was found to be 1100 mg/kg.

No data are available to suggest physiological maneuvers (*e.g.*, maneuvers to change the pH of the urine) that might accelerate elimination of isosorbide dinitrate and its active metabolites. Similarly, it is not known which, if any, of these substances can usefully be removed from the body by hemodialysis.

No specific antagonist to the vasodilator effects of isosorbide dinitrate is known, and no intervention has been subject to controlled studies as a therapy for isosorbide dinitrate overdose. Because the hypotension associated with isosorbide dinitrate overdose is the result of venodilatation and arterial hypovolemia, prudent therapy in this situation should be directed toward increase in central fluid volume. Passive elevation of the patient's legs may be sufficient, but intravenous infusion of normal saline or similar fluid may also be necessary.

The use of epinephrine or other arterial vasoconstrictors in this setting is likely to do more harm than good.

In patients with renal disease or congestive heart failure, therapy resulting in central volume expansion is not without hazard. Treatment of isosorbide dinitrate overdose in these patients may be subtle and difficult, and invasive monitoring may be required.

Methemoglobinemia

Nitrate ions liberated during metabolism of isosorbide dinitrate can oxidize hemoglobin into methemoglobin. Even in patients totally without cytochrome b_5 reductase activity, however, and even assuming that the nitrate moieties of isosorbide dinitrate are quantitatively applied to oxidation of hemoglobin, about 1 mg/kg of isosorbide dinitrate should be required before any of these patients manifests clinically significant (≥10%) methemoglobinemia. In patients with normal reductase function, significant production of methemoglobin should require even larger doses of isosorbide dinitrate. In one study in which 36 patients received 2 to 4 weeks of continuous nitroglycerin therapy at 3.1 to 4.4 mg/hr (equivalent, in total administered dose of nitrate ions, to 4.8 to 6.9 mg of bioavailable isosorbide dinitrate per hour), the average methemoglobin level measured was 0.2%; this was comparable to that observed in parallel patients who received placebo.

Notwithstanding these observations, there are case reports of significant methemoglobinemia in association with moderate overdoses of organic nitrates. None of the affected patients had been thought to be unusually susceptible.

Methemoglobin levels are available from most clinical laboratories. The diagnosis should be suspected in patients who exhibit signs of impaired oxygen delivery despite adequate cardiac output and adequate arterial pO_2. Classically, methemoglobinemic blood is described as chocolate brown, without color change on exposure to air.

When methemoglobinemia is diagnosed, the treatment of choice is methylene blue, 1 to 2 mg/kg intravenously.

Continued on next page

Isordil Titradose—Cont.

DOSAGE AND ADMINISTRATION

As noted under "**CLINICAL PHARMACOLOGY**," multiple-dose studies with ISDN and other nitrates have shown that maintenance of continuous 24-hour plasma levels results in refractory tolerance. Every dosing regimen for Isordil Titradose tablets must provide a daily dose-free interval to minimize the development of this tolerance. With immediate-release ISDN, it appears that one daily dose-free interval must be at least 14 hours long.

As also noted under "**CLINICAL PHARMACOLOGY**," the effects of the second and later doses have been smaller and shorter-lasting than the effects of the first.

Large controlled studies with other nitrates suggest that no dosing regimen with Isordil Titradose tablets should be expected to provide more than about 12 hours of continuous anti-anginal efficacy per day.

As with all titratable drugs, it is important to administer the minimum dose which produces the desired clinical effect. The ususal starting dose of Isordil Titradose is 5 mg to 20 mg, two or three times daily. For maintenance therapy, 10 mg to 40 mg, two or three times daily is recommended. Some patients may require higher doses. A daily dose-free interval of at least 14 hours is advisable to minimize tolerance. The optimal interval will vary with the individual patient, dose and regimen.

HOW SUPPLIED

Isordil® (isosorbide dinitrate) Oral Titradose® Tablets are available as follows:

5 mg, round, pink tablets imprinted "WYETH 4152" on one side and deeply scored on reverse side:
NDC 0008-4152-01, bottles of 100.
NDC 0008-4152-02, bottles of 500.
NDC 0008-4152-03, bottles of 1,000.
NDC 0008-4152-05, Redipak® cartons of 100 (10 blister strips of 10).

Store at room temperature, approximately 25°C (77°F)
Protect from light
Keep bottles tightly closed
Dispense in a light-resistant, tight container
Use carton to protect blisters from light

10 mg, round, white tablets imprinted "WYETH 4153" on one side and deeply scored on reverse side:
NDC 0008-4153-01, bottles of 100.
NDC 0008-4152-02, bottles of 500.
NDC 0008-4153-03, bottles of 1,000.
NDC 0008-4153-05, Redipak cartons of 100 (10 blister strips of 10).

Store at room temperature, approximately 25°C (77°F)
Keep bottles tightly closed
Dispense in a tight container

20 mg, round, green tablets imprinted "WYETH 4154" on one side and deeply scored on reverse side:
NDC 0008-4154-01, bottles of 100.
NDC 0008-4154-02, bottles of 500.
NDC 0008-4154-05, Redipak cartons of 100 (10 blister strips of 10).

30 mg, round, blue tablets imprinted "WYETH 4159" on one side and deeply scored on reverse side:
NDC 0008-4159-01, bottles of 100.
NDC 0008-4159-02, bottles of 500.
NDC 0008-4159-04, Redipak cartons of 100 (10 blister strips of 10).

40 mg, round, light green tablets imprinted "WYETH 4192" on one side and deeply scored on reverse side:
NDC 0008-4192-01, bottles of 100.
NDC 0008-4192-04, Redipak cartons of 100 (10 blister strips of 10).

Store at room temperature, approximately 25°C (77°F)
Protect from light
Keep bottles tightly closed
Dispense in a light-resistant, tight container
Use carton to protect blisters from light

US Pat No. Re. 29077

The appearances of these tablets are trademarks of Wyeth-Ayerst Laboratories.

ALSO AVAILABLE

Sublingual Tablets, 2.5 mg, NDC 0008-4139, in bottles of 100 or 500 and in Redipak cartons of 100 (10 blister strips of 10).

Sublingual Tablets, 5 mg, NDC 0008-4126, in bottles of 100 or 500 and in Redipak cartons of 100 (10 blister strips of 10).

Sublingual Tablets, 10 mg, NDC 0008-4161, in bottles of 100.

Manufactured by:
Wyeth Laboratories
A Wyeth-Ayerst Company
Philadelphia, PA 19101

CI 5182-1 Issued February 17, 1999

Shown in Product Identification Guide, page 341

LODINE® ℞

[lō 'deen]

(etodolac capsules and tablets)

DESCRIPTION

Lodine® (etodolac capsules and tablets) is a pyranocarboxylic acid chemically designated as (±) 1,8-diethyl-1,3,4,9-tetrahydropyrano-[3,4-b]indole-1-acetic acid. The structural formula for etodolac is shown below:

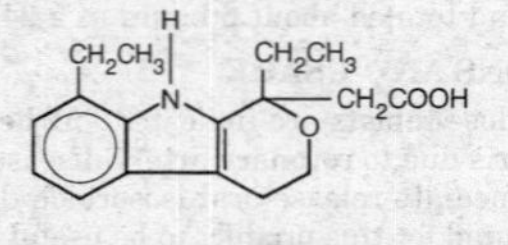

The empirical formula for etodolac is $C_{17}H_{21}NO_3$. The molecular weight of the base is 287.37. It has a pKa of 4.65 and an n-octanol:water partition coefficient of 11.4 at pH 7.4. Etodolac is a white crystalline compound, insoluble in water but soluble in alcohols, chloroform, dimethyl sulfoxide, and aqueous polyethylene glycol.

Inactive ingredients are:

— *in capsules:* cellulose, gelatin, iron oxides, lactose, magnesium stearate, povidone, sodium lauryl sulfate, sodium starch glycolate, and titanium dioxide.

— *in tablets:* cellulose, hydroxypropyl methylcellulose, lactose, magnesium stearate, polyethylene glycol, polysorbate 80, povidone, sodium starch glycolate, and titanium dioxide. The 400 mg tablets contain D&C Yellow #10, FD&C Blue #2, and FD&C Yellow #6 as color additives. The 500 mg tablets contain FD&C Blue #2 only.

Lodine is available in 200 and 300 mg capsules, and 400 and 500 mg tablets, for oral administration.

CLINICAL PHARMACOLOGY

PHARMACOLOGY

Etodolac is a nonsteroidal anti-inflammatory drug (NSAID) that exhibits anti-inflammatory, analgesic, and antipyretic activities in animal models. The mechanism of action of etodolac, like that of other NSAIDs, is not known but is believed to be associated with the inhibition of prostaglandin biosynthesis.

Lodine is a racemic mixture of [-]R- and [+]S-etodolac. As with other NSAIDs, it has been demonstrated in animals that the [+]S-form is biologically active. Both enantiomers are stable and there is no [-]R to [+]S conversion *in vivo*.

PHARMACODYNAMICS

Analgesia was demonstrable ½ hour following single doses of 200 to 400 mg Lodine, with the peak effect occurring in 1 to 2 hours. The analgesic effect generally lasted for 4 to 6 hours (see **Clinical Trials**).

PHARMACOKINETICS

The pharmacokinetics of etodolac have been evaluated in 267 normal subjects, 44 elderly patients (>65 years old), 19 patients with renal failure (creatinine clearance 37 to 88 mL/min), 9 patients on hemodialysis, and 10 patients with compensated hepatic cirrhosis.

Etodolac, when administered orally, exhibits kinetics that are well described by a two-compartment model with first-order absorption.

Lodine has no apparent pharmacokinetic interaction when administered with phenytoin, glyburide, furosemide or hydrochlorothiazide.

ABSORPTION

Etodolac is well absorbed and had a relative bioavailability of 100% when 200 mg capsules were compared with a solution of etodolac. Based on mass balance studies, the systemic availability of etodolac from either the tablet or capsule formulation, is at least 80%. Etodolac does not undergo significant first-pass metabolism following oral administration. Mean (± 1 SD) peak plasma concentrations range from approximately 14 ± 4 to 37 ± 9 μg/mL after 200 to 600 mg single doses and are reached in 80 ± 30 minutes (see Table 1 for summary of pharmacokinetic parameters). The dose-proportionality based on AUC (the area under the plasma concentration-time curve) is linear following doses up to 600 mg every 12 hours. Peak concentrations are dose proportional for both total and free etodolac following doses up to 400 mg every 12 hours, but following a 600 mg dose, the peak is about 20% higher than predicted on the basis of lower doses.

Table 1. Etodolac Steady-State Pharmacokinetic Parameters

(N=267)

Kinetic Parameters	Mean ± SD
Extent of oral absorption (bioavailability) [F]	≥80%
Oral-dose clearance [CL/F]	47 ± 16 mL/h/kg
Steady-state volume [V_{ss}/F]	362 ± 129 mL/kg
Distribution half-life [$t_{1/2}, \alpha$]	0.71 ± 0.50 h
Terminal half-life [$t_{1/2}, \beta$]	7.3 ± 4.0 h

Antacid Effects

The extent of absorption of etodolac is not affected when Lodine is administered with an antacid. Coadministration with an antacid decreases the peak concentration reached by about 15 to 20%, with no measurable effect on time-to-peak.

Food Effects

The extent of absorption of etodolac is not affected when Lodine is administered after a meal. Food intake, however, reduces the peak concentration reached by approximately one half and increases the time-to-peak concentration by 1.4 to 3.8 hours.

Distribution

Etodolac has an apparent steady-state volume of distribution about 0.362 L/kg. Within the therapeutic dose range, etodolac is more than 99% bound to plasma proteins. The free fraction is less than 1% and is independent of etodolac total concentration over the dose range studied.

Metabolism

Etodolac is extensively metabolized in the liver, with renal elimination of etodolac and its metabolites being the primary route of excretion. The intersubject variability of etodolac plasma levels, achieved after recommended doses, is substantial.

Protein Binding

Data from *in vitro* studies, using peak serum concentrations at reported therapeutic doses in humans, show that the etodolac free fraction is not significantly altered by acetaminophen, ibuprofen, indomethacin, naproxen, piroxicam, chlorpropamide, glipizide, glyburide, phenytoin, and probenecid.

Elimination

The mean plasma clearance of etodolac, following oral dosing is 47 (± 16) mL/h/kg, and terminal disposition half-life is 7.3 (± 4.0) hours. Approximately 72% of the administered dose is recovered in the urine as the following, indicated as % of the administered dose:

— etodolac, unchanged	1%
— etodolac glucuronide	13%
— hydroxylated metabolites (6-, 7-, and 8-OH)	5%
— hydroxylated metabolite glucuronides	20%
— unidentified metabolites	33%

Fecal excretion accounted for 16% of the dose.

SPECIAL POPULATIONS

Elderly Patients

In clinical studies, etodolac clearance was reduced by about 15% in older patients (>65 years of age). In these studies, age was shown not to have any effect on etodolac half-life or protein binding, and there was no change in expected drug accumulation. No dosage adjustment is generally necessary in the elderly on the basis of pharmacokinetics. The elderly may need dosage adjustment, however, on the basis of body size (see **Precautions**—GERIATRIC POPULATION), as they may be more sensitive to antiprostaglandin effects than younger patients (see **Precautions**—GERIATRIC POPULATION).

Renal Impairment

Studies in patients with mild-to-moderate renal impairment (creatinine clearance 37 to 88 mL/min) showed no significant differences in the disposition of total and free etodolac. In patients undergoing hemodialysis, there was a 50% greater apparent clearance of total etodolac, due to a 50% greater unbound fraction. Free etodolac clearance was not altered, indicating the importance of protein binding in etodolac's disposition. Nevertheless, etodolac is not dialyzable.

Hepatic Impairment

In patients with compensated hepatic cirrhosis, the disposition of total and free etodolac is not altered. Although no dosage adjustment is generally required in this patient population, etodolac clearance is dependent on hepatic function and could be reduced in patients with severe hepatic failure.

CLINICAL TRIALS

ANALGESIA

Controlled clinical trials in analgesia were single-dose, randomized, double-blind, parallel studies in three pain models, including dental extractions. The analgesic effective dose for Lodine established in these acute pain models was 200 to 400 mg. The onset of analgesia occurred approximately 30 minutes after oral administration. Lodine 200 mg provided efficacy comparable to that obtained with aspirin (650 mg). Lodine 400 mg provided efficacy comparable to that obtained with acetaminophen with codeine (600 mg + 60 mg). The peak analgesic effect was between 1 to 2 hours. Duration of relief averaged 4 to 5 hours for 200 mg of Lodine and 5 to 6 hours for 400 mg of Lodine as measured by when approximately half of the patients required remedication.

OSTEOARTHRITIS

The use of Lodine in managing the signs and symptoms of osteoarthritis of the hip or knee was assessed in double-blind, randomized, controlled clinical trials in 341 patients. In patients with osteoarthritis of the knee, Lodine, in doses of 600 to 1000 mg/day, was better than placebo in two studies. The clinical trials in osteoarthritis used b.i.d. dosage regimens.

RHEUMATOID ARTHRITIS

In a 3-month study with 426 patients, Lodine 300 mg b.i.d. was effective in management of rheumatoid arthritis and comparable in efficacy to piroxicam 20 mg/day. In a long-term study with 1,446 patients in which 60% of patients completed 6 months of therapy and 20% completed 3 years of therapy, Lodine in a dose of 500 mg b.i.d. provided efficacy comparable to that obtained with ibuprofen 600 mg q.i.d. In clinical trials of rheumatoid arthritis patients, Lodine has been used in combination with gold, d-penicillamine, chloroquine, corticosteroids, and methotrexate.

INDICATIONS AND USAGE

Lodine is indicated for acute and long-term use in the management of signs and symptoms of osteoarthritis and rheumatoid arthritis. Lodine is also indicated for the management of pain.

CONTRAINDICATIONS

Lodine is contraindicated in patients with known hypersensitivity to etodolac. Lodine should not be given to patients who have experienced asthma, urticaria, or other allergic-type reactions after taking aspirin or other NSAIDs. Severe, rarely fatal, anaphylactic-like reactions to Lodine have been reported in such patients (see **Warnings**—ANAPHYLACTOID REACTIONS).

WARNINGS

RISK OF GASTROINTESTINAL (GI) ULCERATION, BLEEDING, AND PERFORATION WITH NONSTEROIDAL, ANTI-INFLAMMATORY DRUG (NSAID) THERAPY

Serious GI toxicity, such as bleeding, ulceration, and perforation, can occur at any time, with or without warning symptoms, in patients treated chronically with NSAIDs. Although minor upper GI problems, such as dyspepsia, are common, usually developing early in therapy, physicians should remain alert for ulceration and bleeding in patients treated chronically with NSAIDs, even in the absence of previous GI-tract symptoms. In patients observed in clinical trials of such agents for several months' to 2 years' duration, symptomatic upper GI ulcers, gross bleeding, or perforation appears to occur in approximately 1% of patients treated for 3 to 6 months and in about 2% to 4% of patients treated for 1 year. Physicians should inform patients about the signs and/or symptoms of serious GI toxicity and what steps to take if they occur.

Studies to date have not identified any subset of patients not at risk of developing peptic ulceration and bleeding. Except for a prior history of serious GI events and other risk factors known to be associated with peptic ulcer disease, such as alcoholism, smoking, etc., no risk factors (e.g., age, sex) have been associated with increased risk. Elderly or debilitated patients seem to tolerate ulceration or bleeding less well than other individuals, and most spontaneous reports of fatal GI events are in this population. Studies to date are inconclusive concerning the relative risk of various NSAIDs in causing such reactions. High doses of any NSAID probably carry a greater risk of these reactions, although controlled clinical trials showing this do not exist in most cases. In considering the use of relatively large doses (within the recommended dosage range), sufficient benefit should be anticipated to offset the potential increased risk of GI toxicity.

ANAPHYLACTOID REACTIONS

Anaphylactoid reactions may occur in patients without prior exposure to etodolac. Lodine should not be given to patients with the aspirin triad. The triad typically occurs in asthmatic patients who experience rhinitis with or without nasal polyps, or who exhibit severe, potentially fatal bronchospasm after taking aspirin or other nonsteroidal anti-inflammatory drugs. Fatal reactions have been reported in such patients (see **Contraindications** and **Precautions**—*Pre-existing Asthma*). Emergency help should be sought in cases where an anaphylactoid reaction occurs.

ADVANCED RENAL DISEASE

In cases with advanced kidney disease, as with other NSAIDs, treatment with Lodine should only be initiated with close monitoring of the patient's kidney function (see **Precautions**—*Renal Effects*).

PREGNANCY

In late pregnancy, as with other NSAIDs, Lodine should be avoided because it may cause premature closure of the ductus arteriosus (see **Precautions**—*Teratogenic Effects—Pregnancy Category C*).

PRECAUTIONS

GENERAL PRECAUTIONS

Renal Effects

As with other NSAIDs, long-term administration of etodolac to rats has resulted in renal papillary necrosis and other renal medullary changes. Renal pelvic transitional epithelial hyperplasia, a spontaneous change occurring with variable frequency, was observed with increased frequency in treated male rats in a 2-year chronic study.

A second form of renal toxicity encountered with Lodine, as with other NSAIDs, is seen in patients with conditions in which renal prostaglandins have a supportive role in the maintenance of renal perfusion. In these patients, administration of a nonsteroidal anti-inflammatory drug may cause a dose-dependent reduction in prostaglandin formation and, secondarily, in renal blood flow, which may precipitate overt renal decompensation. Patients at greatest risk of this reaction are those with impaired renal function, heart failure, or liver dysfunction; those taking diuretics; and the elderly. Discontinuation of nonsteroidal anti-inflammatory drug therapy is usually followed by recovery to the pretreatment state.

Etodolac metabolites are eliminated primarily by the kidneys. The extent to which the inactive glucuronide metabolites may accumulate in patients with renal failure has not been studied. As with other drugs whose metabolites are excreted by the kidney, the possibility that adverse reactions (not listed in **Adverse Reactions**) may be attributable to these metabolites should be considered.

Hepatic Effects

Borderline elevations of one or more liver tests may occur in up to 15% of patients taking NSAIDs, including Lodine. These abnormalities may disappear, remain essentially unchanged, or progress with continued therapy. Meaningful elevations of ALT or AST (approximately three or more times the upper limit of normal) have been reported in approximately 1% of patients in clinical trials with Lodine. A patient with symptoms and/or signs suggesting liver dysfunction, or in whom an abnormal liver test has occurred, should be evaluated for evidence of the development of a more severe hepatic reaction while on therapy with Lodine. Rare cases of liver necrosis and hepatic failure, some of them with fatal outcomes have been reported. If clinical signs and symptoms consistent with liver disease develop, or if systemic manifestations occur (e.g. eosinophilia, rash, etc.), Lodine should be discontinued.

Hematological Effects

Anemia is sometimes seen in patients receiving NSAIDs including Lodine. This may be due to fluid retention, GI blood loss, or an incompletely described effect upon erythropoiesis. Patients on long-term treatment with NSAIDs, including Lodine, should have their hemoglobin or hematocrit checked if they exhibit any signs or symptoms of anemia.

All drugs which inhibit the biosynthesis of prostaglandins may interfere to some extent with platelet function and vascular responses to bleeding.

Fluid Retention and Edema

Fluid retention and edema have been observed in some patients taking NSAIDs, including Lodine. Therefore, Lodine should be used with caution in patients with fluid retention, hypertension, or heart failure.

Pre-existing Asthma

About 10% of patients with asthma may have aspirin-sensitive asthma. The use of aspirin in patients with aspirin-sensitive asthmas has been associated with severe bronchospasm which can be fatal. Since cross reactivity, including bronchospasm, between aspirin and other nonsteroidal anti-inflammatory drugs has been reported in such aspirin-sensitive patients, etodolac should not be administered to patients with this form of aspirin sensitivity and should be used with caution in all patients with pre-existing asthma.

INFORMATION FOR PATIENTS

Lodine, like other drugs of its class, can cause discomfort and, rarely, more serious side effects, such as gastrointestinal bleeding, which may result in hospitalization and even fatal outcomes.

Physicians may wish to discuss with their patients the potential risks (see **Warnings**, **Precautions**, **Adverse Reactions**) and likely benefits of nonsteroidal anti-inflammatory drug treatment.

Patients on Lodine should report to their physicians signs or symptoms of gastrointestinal ulceration or bleeding, blurred vision or other eye symptoms, skin rash, weight gain, or edema.

Because serious gastrointestinal tract ulcerations and bleeding can occur without warning symptoms, physicians should follow chronically treated patients for the signs and symptoms of ulcerations and bleeding and should inform them of the importance of this follow-up (see **Warnings**—RISK OF GI ULCERATION, BLEEDING AND PERFORATION WITH NONSTEROIDAL ANTI-INFLAMMATORY THERAPY).

Patients should also be instructed to seek medical emergency help in case of an occurrence of anaphylactoid reactions (see **Warnings**).

LABORATORY TESTS

Patients on long-term treatment with Lodine, as with other NSAIDs, should have their hemoglobin or hematocrit checked periodically for signs or symptoms of anemia. Appropriate measures should be taken in case such signs of anemia occur.

If clinical signs and symptoms consistent with liver disease develop or if systematic manifestations occur (e.g., eosinophilia, rash, etc.) and if abnormal liver tests are detected, persist or worsen, Lodine should be discontinued.

DRUG INTERACTIONS

Antacids

The concomitant administration of antacids has no apparent effect on the extent of absorption of Lodine. However, antacids can decrease the peak concentration reached by 15% to 20% but have no detectable effect on the time-to-peak.

Aspirin

When Lodine is administered with aspirin, its protein binding is reduced, although the clearance of free etodolac is not altered. The clinical significance of this interaction is not known; however, as with other NSAIDs, concomitant administration of Lodine and aspirin is not generally recommended because of the potential of increased adverse effects.

Warfarin

Short-term pharmacokinetic studies have demonstrated that concomitant administration of warfarin and Lodine results in reduced protein binding of warfarin, but there was no change in the clearance of free warfarin. There was no significant difference in the pharmacodynamic effect of warfarin administered alone and warfarin administered with Lodine as measured by prothrombin time. Thus, concomitant therapy with warfarin and Lodine should not require dosage adjustment of either drug. However, there have been a few spontaneous reports of prolonged prothrombin times in Lodine-treated patients receiving concomitant warfarin therapy. Caution should be exercised because interactions have been seen with other NSAIDs.

Cyclosporin, Digoxin, Lithium, Methotrexate

Lodine, like other NSAIDs, through effects on renal prostaglandins, may cause changes in the elimination of these drugs leading to elevated serum levels of digoxin, lithium, and methotrexate and increased toxicity. Nephrotoxicity associated with cyclosporine may also be enhanced. Patients receiving these drugs who are given Lodine, or any other NSAID, and particularly those patients with altered renal function, should be observed for the development of the specific toxicities of these drugs.

Phenylbutazone

Phenylbutazone causes increase (by about 80%) in the free fraction of etodolac. Although *in vivo* studies have not been done to see if etodolac clearance is changed by coadministration of phenylbutazone, it is not recommended that they be coadministered.

DRUG/LABORATORY TEST INTERACTIONS

The urine of patients who take Lodine can give a false-positive reaction for urinary bilirubin (urobilin) due to the presence of phenolic metabolites of etodolac. Diagnostic dip-stick methodology, used to detect ketone bodies in urine, has resulted in false-positive findings in some patients treated with Lodine. Generally, this phenomenon has not been associated with other clinically significant events. No dose relationship has been observed.

Lodine treatment is associated with a small decrease in serum uric acid levels. In clinical trials, mean decreases of 1 to 2 mg/dL were observed in arthritic patients receiving etodolac (600 mg to 1000 mg/day) after 4 weeks of therapy. These levels then remained stable for up to 1 year of therapy.

CARCINOGENESIS, MUTAGENESIS, AND IMPAIRMENT OF FERTILITY

No carcinogenic effect of etodolac was observed in mice or rats receiving oral doses of 15 mg/kg/day (45 to 89 mg/m^2, respectively) or less for periods of 2 years or 18 months, respectively. Etodolac was not mutagenic in *in vitro* tests performed with *S. typhimurium* and mouse lymphoma cells as well as in an *in vivo* mouse micronucleus test. However, data from the *in vitro* human peripheral lymphocyte test showed an increase in the number of gaps (3.0 to 5.3% unstained regions in the chromatid without dislocation) among the Lodine-treated cultures (50 to 200 µg/mL) compared to negative controls (2.0%); no other difference was noted between the controls and drug-treated groups. Etodolac showed no impairment of fertility in male and female rats up to oral doses of 16 mg/kg (94 mg/m^2). However, reduced implantation of fertilized eggs occurred in the 8 mg/kg group.

PREGNANCY

Teratogenic Effects—Pregnancy Category C

In teratology studies, isolated occurrences of alterations in limb development were found and included polydactyly, oligodactyly, syndactyly, and unossified phalanges in rats and oligodactyly and synostosis of metatarsals in rabbits. These were observed at dose levels (2 to 14 mg/kg/day) close to human clinical doses. However, the frequency and the dosage group distribution of these findings in initial or repeated studies did not establish a clear drug or dose-response relationship.

There are no adequate or well-controlled studies in pregnant women. Lodine should be used during pregnancy only if the potential benefits justify the potential risk to the fetus. Because of the known effects of NSAIDs on parturition and on the human fetal cardiovascular system with respect to closure of the ductus arteriosus, use during late pregnancy should be avoided.

LABOR AND DELIVERY

In rat studies with etodolac, as with other drugs known to inhibit prostaglandin synthesis, an increased incidence of dystocia, delayed parturition, and decreased pup survival occurred. The effects of Lodine on labor and delivery in pregnant women are unknown.

NURSING MOTHERS

It is not known whether etodolac is excreted in human milk. Because many drugs are excreted in human milk and because of the potential for serious adverse reactions in nursing infants from etodolac, a decision should be made whether to discontinue nursing or to discontinue the drug taking into account the importance of the drug to the mother.

PEDIATRIC USE

Safety and effectiveness in pediatric patients have not been established.

GERIATRIC POPULATION

As with any NSAID, however, caution should be exercised in treating the elderly, and when individualizing their dosage, extra care should be taken when increasing the dose because the elderly seem to tolerate NSAID side effects less well than younger patients. In patients 65 years and older, no substantial differences in the side effect profile of Lodine were seen compared with the general population (see **Clinical Pharmacology**—PHARMACOKINETICS.)

ADVERSE REACTIONS

Adverse-reaction information for Lodine was derived from 2,629 arthritic patients treated with Lodine in double-blind and open-label clinical trials of 4 to 320 weeks in duration and worldwide postmarketing surveillance studies. In clinical trials, most adverse reactions were mild and transient. The discontinuation rate in controlled clinical trials, because of adverse events, was up to 10% for patients treated with Lodine.

New patient complaints (with an incidence greater than or equal to 1%) are listed below by body system. The incidences were determined from clinical trials involving 465 patients with osteoarthritis treated with 300 to 500 mg of Lodine b.i.d. (i.e., 600 to 1000 mg/day).

INCIDENCE GREATER THAN OR EQUAL TO 1%—PROBABLY CAUSALLY RELATED

Body as a whole—Chills and fever.

Continued on next page

Lodine—Cont.

Digestive system—Dyspepsia (10%), abdominal pain*, diarrhea*, flatulence*, nausea*, constipation, gastritis, melena, vomiting.
Nervous system—Asthenia/malaise*, dizziness*, depression, nervousness.
Skin and appendages—Pruritus, rash.
Special senses—Blurred vision, tinnitus.
Urogenital system—Dysuria, urinary frequency.
*Drug-related patient complaints occurring in 3 to 9% of patients treated with Lodine.
Drug-related patient-complaints occurring in fewer than 3%, but more than 1%, are unmarked.
INCIDENCE LESS THAN 1%—PROBABLY CAUSALLY RELATED
(Adverse reactions reported only in worldwide postmarketing experience, not seen in clinical trials, are considered rarer and are italicized)
Body as a whole—*Allergic reaction, anaphylactoid reaction.*
Cardiovascular system—Hypertension, congestive heart failure, flushing, palpitations, syncope, *vasculitis (including necrotizing and allergic).*
Digestive system—Thirst, dry mouth, ulcerative stomatitis, anorexia, eructation, elevated liver enzymes, *cholestatic hepatitis,* hepatitis, *cholestatic jaundice, duodenitis, jaundice, hepatic failure, liver necrosis,* peptic ulcer with or without bleeding and/or perforation, *intestinal ulceration, pancreatitis.*
Hemic and lymphatic system—Ecchymosis, anemia, thrombocytopenia, bleeding time increased, *agranulocytosis, hemolytic anemia, leukopenia, neutropenia, pancytopenia.*
Metabolic and nutritional—Edema, serum creatinine increase, *hyperglycemia in previously controlled diabetic patients.*
Nervous system—Insomnia, somnolence.
Respiratory system—Asthma.
Skin and appendages—Angioedema, sweating, urticaria, vesiculobullous rash, *cutaneous vasculitis with purpura, Stevens-Johnson Syndrome,* hyperpigmentation, *erythema multiforme.*
Special senses—Photophobia, transient visual disturbances.
Urogenital system—*Elevated BUN, renal failure, renal insufficiency, renal papillary necrosis.*
INCIDENCE LESS THAN 1%—CAUSAL RELATIONSHIP UNKNOWN (Medical events occurring under circumstances where causal relationship to Lodine is uncertain. These reactions are listed as alerting information for physicians)
Body as a whole—Infection, headache.
Cardiovascular system—Arrhythmias, myocardial infarction, cerebrovascular accident.
Digestive system—Esophagitis with or without stricture or cardiospasm, colitis.
Metabolic and nutritional—Change in weight.
Nervous system—Paresthesia, confusion.
Respiratory system—Bronchitis, dyspnea, pharyngitis, rhinitis, sinusitis.
Skin and appendages—Alopecia, maculopapular rash, photosensitivity, skin peeling.
Special senses—Conjunctivitis, deafness, taste perversion.
Urogenital system—Cystitis, hematuria, leukorrhea, renal calculus, interstitial nephritis, uterine bleeding irregularities.

OVERDOSAGE

Symptoms following acute NSAID overdose are usually limited to lethargy, drowsiness, nausea, vomiting, and epigastric pain, which are generally reversible with supportive care. Gastrointestinal bleeding can occur and coma has occurred following massive ibuprofen or mefenamic-acid overdose. Hypertension, acute renal failure, and respiratory depression may occur but are rare. Anaphylactoid reactions have been reported with therapeutic ingestion of NSAIDs, and may occur following overdose.
Patients should be managed by symptomatic and supportive care following an NSAID overdose. There are no specific antidotes. Gut decontamination may be indicated in patients seen within 4 hours of ingestion with symptoms or following a large overdose (5 to 10 times the usual dose). This should be accomplished via emesis and/or activated charcoal (60 to 100 g in adults, 1 to 2 g/kg in children) with an osmotic cathartic. Forced diuresis, alkalinization of the urine, hemodialysis, or hemoperfusion would probably not be useful due to etodolac's high protein binding.

DOSAGE AND ADMINISTRATION

As with other NSAIDs, the lowest dose and longest dosing interval should be sought for each patient. Therefore, after observing the response to initial therapy with Lodine, the dose and frequency should be adjusted to suit an individual patient's needs.
Dosage adjustment of Lodine is generally not required in patients with mild to moderate renal impairment. Etodolac should be used with caution in such patients, because, as with other NSAIDs, it may further decrease renal function in some patients with impaired renal function. (see **Precautions**—GENERAL PRECAUTIONS, *Renal Effects).*
ANALGESIA
The recommended total daily dose of Lodine for acute pain is up to 1000 mg, given as 200–400 mg every 6 to 8 hours. In some patients, if the potential benefits outweigh the risks; the dose may be increased to 1200 mg/day in order to achieve a therapeutic benefit that might not have been achieved with 1000 mg/day. Doses of etodolac greater than 1000 mg/day have not been adequately evaluated in well-controlled clinical trials.
OSTEOARTHRITIS AND RHEUMATOID ARTHRITIS
The recommended starting dose of Lodine for the management of the signs and symptoms of osteoarthritis or rheumatoid arthritis is: 300 mg b.i.d., t.i.d., or 400 mg b.i.d., or 500 mg b.i.d. During long-term administration, the dose of Lodine may be adjusted up or down depending on the clinical response of the patient. A lower dose of 600 mg/day may suffice for long-term administration. In patients who tolerate 1000 mg/day, the dose may be increased to 1200 mg/day when a higher level of therapeutic activity is required. When treating patients with higher doses, the physician should observe sufficient increased clinical benefit to justify the higher dose. Physicians should be aware that doses above 1000 mg/day have not been adequately evaluated in well-controlled clinical trials.
In chronic conditions, a therapeutic response to therapy with Lodine is sometimes seen within one week of therapy, but most often is observed by two weeks. After a satisfactory response has been achieved, the patient's dose should be reviewed and adjusted as required.

HOW SUPPLIED

Lodine (etodolac capsules and tablets) is available as:
Lodine® (etodolac capsules) Capsules
200 mg capsules (light gray with one wide red band with LODINE 200/white with two narrow red bands)
— in bottles of 100, NDC 0046-0738-81
— in unit-dose packages of 100, NDC 0046-0738-99
300 mg capsules (light gray with one red band with LODINE 300/light gray with two narrow red bands)
— in bottles of 100, NDC 0046-0739-81
— in unit-dose packages of 100, NDC 0046-0739-99
Store at controlled room temperature 20°–25°C (68°–77°F), protected from moisture.
Lodine® (etodolac tablets) Tablets
400 mg tablets (yellow-orange, oval, film-coated tablet, debossed LODINE 400 on one side)
— in bottles of 100, NDC 0046-0761-81
— in unit-dose packages of 100, NDC 0046-0761-99
Store at controlled room temperature 20°–25°C (68°–77°F). Store tablets in original container until ready to use. Dispense in light-resistant container.
500 mg tablets (blue, oval, film-coated tablet, branded LODINE 500 on one side)
— in bottles of 100, NDC 0046-0787-81
— in unit-dose packages of 100, NDC 0046-0787-99
Store at controlled room temperature 20°–25°C (68°–77°F). Store tablets in original container until ready to use. Dispense in light-resistant container.
The appearance of these capsules is a registered trademark of Wyeth-Ayerst Laboratories and the appearance of these tablets is a trademark of Wyeth-Ayerst Laboratories.
Caution: Federal law prohibits dispensing without prescription.
Manufactured by:
Ayerst Laboratories
A Wyeth-Ayerst Company
Philadelphia, PA 19101
CI 4861-1 Issued June 14, 1996
Shown in Product Identification Guide, page 341

LODINE® XL ℞
[lō 'deen XL]
(etodolac extended-release tablets)
400 mg, 500 mg, 600 mg

DESCRIPTION

Lodine XL contains etodolac, which is a member of the pyranocarboxylic acid group of nonsteroidal anti-inflammatory drugs (NSAIDs). Each tablet contains etodolac for oral administration. Etodolac is a racemic mixture of [+]S and [−]R-enantiomers. It is a white crystalline compound, insoluble in water, but soluble in alcohols, chloroform, dimethyl sulfoxide, and aqueous polyethylene glycol.
The chemical name is (±) 1,8-diethyl-1,3,4,9-tetrahydropyrano-[3,4-b]indole-1-acetic acid. The molecular weight is 287.37. Its molecular formula is $C_{17}H_{21}NO_3$ and it has the following structural formula:

The inactive ingredients in Lodine XL include: dibasic sodium phosphate, ethylcellulose, hydroxypropyl methylcellulose, lactose, magnesium stearate, polyethylene glycol, and titanium dioxide. In addition, the 400 mg tablets also contain FD&C Red #40, and FD&C Yellow #6 as color additives and polysorbate 80. The 500 mg tablets also contain D&C Yellow #10, FD&C Blue #2, and iron oxide as color additives and polysorbate 80. The 600 mg tablets also contain hydroxypropyl cellulose and iron oxide.

CLINICAL PHARMACOLOGY

PHARMACODYNAMICS
Lodine XL is a nonsteroidal anti-inflammatory drug (NSAID) that exhibits anti-inflammatory, analgesic, and antipyretic activities in animal models. The mechanism of action of Lodine XL, like that of other NSAIDs, is not completely understood, but may be related to prostaglandin synthetase inhibition.
PHARMACOKINETICS
Absorption
Lodine XL and Lodine both contain etodolac, but differ in their release characteristics. The systemic availability of etodolac from Lodine XL is generally greater than 80%. Etodolac does not undergo significant first-pass metabolism following oral administration. After oral administration of Lodine XL in doses up to 800 mg once daily, peak concentrations occur approximately 6 hours after dosing and are dose proportional for both total and free etodolac. Peak concentrations following 1200 mg Lodine XL once daily were about 20% lower than that predicted by lower doses.
Table 1 shows the comparison of etodolac pharmacokinetic parameters after the administration of Lodine and Lodine XL.
Table 2 shows the etodolac pharmacokinetic parameters in various populations. The data from patients with renal and hepatic impairment were obtained following administration of (immediate-release) Lodine.
[See table 1 & 2 at bottom of next page]
Food / Antacid Effects
Food has no significant effect on the extent of Lodine XL absorption, however, food significantly increased C_{max} (54%) following a 600 mg dose.
The extent of absorption of etodolac is not affected when etodolac is administered with antacid. Coadministration, with an antacid, decreases the peak concentration reached by about 15 to 20% with no measurable effect on time-to-peak.
Distribution
The mean apparent volume of distribution (Vd/F) of etodolac following administration of Lodine XL is 566 mL/kg. Etodolac is more than 99% bound to plasma proteins, primarily to albumin, and is independent of etodolac concentration over the dose range studied. It is not known whether etodolac is excreted in human milk. However, based on its physical-chemical properties, excretion into breast milk is expected.
Metabolism
Etodolac metabolites do not contribute significantly to the pharmacological activity of Lodine XL.
Following administration of immediate-release etodolac, several metabolites have been identified in human plasma and urine. Other metabolites remain to be identified. The metabolites include 6-, 7-, and 8-hydroxylated etodolac and etodolac glucuronide. After a single dose of ^{14}C-etodolac, hydroxylated metabolites accounted for less than 10% of total drug in serum. On chronic dosing, hydroxylated-etodolac metabolites do not accumulate in the plasma of patients with normal renal function. The extent of accumulation of hydroxylated-etodolac metabolites in patients with renal dysfunction has not been studied. The role, if any, of a specific cytochrome P450 system in the metabolism of etodolac is unknown. The hydroxylated-etodolac metabolites undergo further glucuronidation followed by renal excretion and partial elimination in the feces.
Excretion
The mean oral clearance of etodolac following oral Lodine XL dosing is 47 (±17) mL/h/kg. The terminal half-life ($t_{1/2}$) of etodolac after Lodine XL administration is 8.4 hours compared to 6.4 hours for Lodine. Approximately 1% of a Lodine dose is excreted unchanged in the urine, with 72% of the dose excreted into the urine as parent drug plus metabolites:

—etodolac, unchanged	1%
—etodolac glucuronide	13%
—hydroxylated metabolites (6-, 7-, and 8-OH)	5%
—hydroxylated metabolite glucuronides	20%
—unidentified metabolites	33%

Fecal excretion accounted for 16% of the dose.

SPECIAL POPULATIONS

Geriatric
In clinical studies, etodolac clearance was reduced by about 15% in older patients (>65 years of age). In these studies, age was not shown to have any effect on half-life or protein binding, and demonstrated no change in expected drug accumulation. No dosage adjustment is generally necessary in the elderly on the basis of pharmacokinetics. The elderly may need dosage adjustment, however, as they may be more sensitive to antiprostaglandin effects than younger patients (see **Precautions**—GERIATRIC POPULATION).
Pediatric
Lodine XL has not been investigated in pediatric patients.
Race
Pharmacokinetic differences due to race have not been identified. Clinical studies included patients of many races, all of whom responded in a similar fashion.
Hepatic Insufficiency
The pharmacokinetics of etodolac following administration of Lodine XL have not been investigated in subjects with hepatic insufficiency. Following administration of Lodine,

the plasma protein binding and disposition of total and free etodolac were unchanged in the presence of compensated hepatic cirrhosis. Although no dosage adjustment is generally required in patients with chronic hepatic diseases, etodolac clearance is dependent on liver function and could be reduced in patients with severe hepatic failure.

Renal Insufficiency

The pharmacokinetics of etodolac following administration of Lodine XL have not been investigated in subjects with renal insufficiency. Etodolac renal clearance following administration of Lodine was unchanged in the presence of mild-to-moderate renal failure (creatinine clearance, 37 to 88 mL/min). Although renal elimination is a significant pathway of excretion for etodolac metabolites, no dosing adjustment in patients with mild to moderate renal dysfunction is generally necessary. Etodolac plasma protein binding decreases in patients with severe renal deficiency. Etodolac should be used with caution in such patients because, as with other NSAIDs, it may further decrease renal function in some patients. Etodolac is not significantly removed from the blood in patients undergoing hemodialysis.

CLINICAL TRIALS

ARTHRITIS

The use of Lodine XL in managing the signs and symptoms of osteoarthritis of the knee and rheumatoid arthritis was assessed in double-blind, randomized, parallel, controlled clinical trials in 1552 patients. In these trials, Lodine XL in doses of 400 mg to 1200 mg, given once daily, provided efficacy comparable to etodolac given 300 mg b.i.d. to 400 mg t.i.d.

INDICATIONS AND USAGE

Lodine XL is indicated:

For the management of the signs and symptoms of osteoarthritis.

For the management of the signs and symptoms of rheumatoid arthritis.

CONTRAINDICATIONS

Lodine XL is contraindicated in patients with known hypersensitivity to etodolac. Lodine XL should not be given to patients who have experienced asthma, urticaria, or other allergic-type reactions after taking aspirin or other NSAIDs. Severe, rarely fatal, anaphylactic-like reactions to NSAIDs have been reported in such patients (see **Warnings**—ANAPHYLACTOID REACTIONS, and **Precautions**—*Pre-existing Asthma*).

WARNINGS

Gastrointestinal (GI) Effects—Risk of GI Ulceration, Bleeding, and Perforation:

Serious gastrointestinal toxicity, such as inflammation, bleeding, ulceration, and perforation of the stomach, small intestine or large intestine, can occur at any time, with or without warning symptoms, in patients treated with nonsteroidal anti-inflammatory drugs (NSAIDs). Minor upper gastrointestinal problems, such as dyspepsia, are common and may also occur at any time during NSAID therapy. Therefore, physicians and patients should remain alert for ulceration and bleeding, even in the absence of previous GI-tract symptoms. Patients should be informed about the signs and/or symptoms of serious GI toxicity and the steps to take if they occur. The utility of periodic laboratory monitoring has not been demonstrated, nor has it been adequately assessed. Only one in five patients who develop a serious upper GI adverse event on NSAID therapy is symptomatic. It has been demonstrated that upper GI ulcers, gross bleeding, or perforation, caused by NSAIDs, appear to occur in approximately 1% of patients treated for 3–6 months and in about 2%–4% of patients treated for 1 year. These trends continue thus, increasing the likelihood of developing a serious GI event at some time during the course of therapy. However, even short-term therapy is not without risk.

NSAIDs should be prescribed with extreme caution in those with a prior history of ulcer disease or gastrointestinal bleeding. Most spontaneous reports of fatal GI events are in elderly or debilitated patients and therefore special care should be taken in treating this population. **To minimize the potential risk for an adverse GI event, the lowest effective dose should be used for the shortest possible duration.** For high risk patients, alternate therapies that do not involve NSAIDs should be considered.

Studies have shown that patients with a *prior history of peptic ulcer disease and/or gastrointestinal bleeding* and who use NSAIDs, have a greater than 10-fold risk for developing a GI bleed than patients with neither of these risk factors. In addition to a past history of ulcer disease, pharmacoepidemiological studies have identified several other co-therapies or co-morbid conditions that may increase the risk for GI bleeding such as: treatment with oral corticosteroids, treatment with anticoagulants, longer duration of NSAID therapy, smoking, alcoholism, older age, and poor general health status.

ANAPHYLACTOID REACTIONS

As with other NSAIDs, anaphylactoid reaction may occur in patients without known prior exposure to Lodine XL. Lodine XL should not be given to patients with the aspirin triad. This symptom complex typically occurs in asthmatic patients who experience rhinitis with or without nasal polyps, or who exhibit severe, potentially fatal bronchospasm after taking aspirin or other NSAIDs. (see **Contraindications** and **Precautions**—*Pre-existing Asthma*). Emergency help should be sought in cases where an anaphylactoid reaction occurs.

ADVANCED RENAL DISEASE

In cases with advanced kidney disease, treatment with Lodine XL is not recommended. If NSAID therapy, however, must be initiated, close monitoring of the patient's kidney function is advisable (see **Precautions**—*Renal Effects*).

PREGNANCY

In late pregnancy, as with other NSAIDs, Lodine XL should be avoided because it may cause premature closure of the ductus arteriosus (see **Precautions**—*Nonteratogenic Effects*).

PRECAUTIONS

GENERAL

Lodine XL cannot be expected to substitute for corticosteroids or to treat corticosteroid insufficiency. Abrupt discontinuation of corticosteroids may lead to disease exacerbation. Patients on prolonged corticosteroid therapy should have their therapy tapered slowly if a decision is made to discontinue corticosteroids.

The pharmacological activity of Lodine XL in reducing fever and inflammation may diminish the utility of the diagnostic signs in detecting complications of presumed noninfectious, painful conditions.

Hepatic Effects

Borderline elevations of one or more liver tests may occur in up to 15% of patients taking NSAIDs, including Lodine XL. These laboratory abnormalities may progress, may remain unchanged, or may be transient with continued therapy. Notable elevations of ALT or AST (approximately three or more times the upper limit of normal) have been reported in approximately 1% of patients in clinical trials with NSAIDs. In addition, rare cases of severe hepatic reactions, including jaundice and fatal fulminant hepatitis, liver necrosis and hepatic failure, some of them with fatal outcomes, have been reported.

A patient with symptoms and/or signs suggesting liver dysfunction, or in whom an abnormal liver test has occurred, should be evaluated for evidence of the development of a more severe hepatic reaction while on therapy with Lodine XL. If clinical signs and symptoms consistent with liver disease develop, or if systemic manifestations occur (e.g., eosinophilia, rash, etc.), Lodine XL should be discontinued.

Renal Effects

Caution should be used when initiating treatment with Lodine XL in patients with considerable dehydration. It is advisable to rehydrate patients first and then start therapy with Lodine XL.

Caution is also recommended in patients with pre-existing kidney disease (see **Warnings**—ADVANCED RENAL DISEASE).

As with other NSAIDs, long-term administration of Lodine XL has resulted in renal papillary necrosis and other renal medullary changes. Renal toxicity has also been seen in patients in which renal prostaglandins have a compensatory role in the maintenance of renal perfusion. In these patients, administration of a nonsteroidal anti-inflammatory drug may cause a dose-dependent reduction in prostaglandin formation and, secondarily, in renal blood flow, which may precipitate overt renal decompensation. Patients at greatest risk of this reaction are those with impaired renal function, heart failure, liver dysfunction, those taking diuretics and ACE inhibitors, and the elderly. Discontinuation of nonsteroidal anti-inflammatory drug therapy is usually followed by recovery to the pretreatment state.

Lodine XL metabolites are eliminated primarily by the kidneys. The extent to which the metabolites may accumulate in patients with renal failure has not been studied. As with other NSAIDs, metabolites of which are excreted by the kidney, patients with significantly impaired renal function should be more closely monitored.

Hematological Effects

Anemia is sometimes seen in patients receiving NSAIDs, including Lodine XL. This may be due to fluid retention, GI blood loss, or an incompletely described effect upon erythropoiesis. Patients on long-term treatment with NSAIDs, including Lodine XL, should have their hemoglobin or hematocrit checked if they develop signs or symptoms of anemia. All drugs which inhibit the biosynthesis of prostaglandins may interfere to some extent with platelet function and vascular responses to bleeding.

NSAIDs inhibit platelet aggregation and have been shown to prolong bleeding time in some patients. Unlike aspirin, their effect on platelet function is quantitatively less, of shorter duration, and reversible. Patients receiving Lodine XL who may be adversely affected by alterations in platelet function, such as those with coagulation disorders or patients receiving anticoagulants, should be carefully monitored.

Fluid Retention and Edema

Fluid retention and edema have been observed in some patients taking NSAIDs. Therefore, as with other NSAIDS, Lodine XL should be used with caution in patients with fluid retention, hypertension, or heart failure.

Pre-existing Asthma

Patients with asthma may have aspirin-sensitive asthma. The use of aspirin in patients with aspirin-sensitive asthma has been associated with severe bronchospasm, which can be fatal. Since cross reactivity, including bronchospasm, between aspirin and other nonsteroidal anti-inflammatory drugs has been reported in such aspirin-sensitive patients, Lodine XL should not be administered to patients with this form of aspirin-sensitivity and should be used with caution in all patients with pre-existing asthma.

INFORMATION FOR PATIENTS

Lodine XL, like other drugs of its class, can cause discomfort and, rarely, more serious side effects, such as gastrointestinal bleeding, which may result in hospitalization and even fatal outcomes. Although serious GI tract ulcerations and bleeding can occur without warning symptoms, patients should be alert for the signs and symptoms of ulcerations and bleeding, and should ask for medical advice when observing any indicative sign or symptoms. Patients should be apprised of the importance of this follow-up (see **Warnings, Risk of Gastrointestinal Ulceration, Bleeding and Perforation**).

Table 1

Pharmacokinetic Parameters	Mean (CV)% Lodine	Lodine XL
Extent of Oral Absorption (Bioavailability) [F]	≥ 80%	≥ 80%
Time to Peak Concentration (T_{max}), h	1.4 (61%)	6.7 (47%)
Oral Clearance (CL/F), mL/h/kg	49.1 (33%)	46.8 (37%)
Apparent Volume of Distribution (Vd/F), mL/kg	393 (29%)	566 (26%)
Terminal Half-life ($t_{1/2}$), h	6.4 (22%)	8.4 (30%)

† % Coefficient of variation

Table 2 Mean (CV%)† Pharmacokinetic Parameters of Etodolac in Normal Healthy Adults and Various Special Populations

PK Parameters	Lodine XL: Normal Healthy Adults (18–44)* (n=116)	Lodine XL: Healthy Males (18–43) (n=102)	Lodine XL: Healthy Females (25–44) (n=14)	Lodine XL: Elderly (>65 yr) (66–88) (n=24)	Lodine: Hemodialysis‡ (24–65) (n=9) Dialysis On	Lodine: Hemodialysis‡ (24–65) (n=9) Dialysis Off	Lodine: Renal Impairment‡ (46–73) (n=10)	Lodine: Hepatic Impairment‡ (34–60) (n=9)
T_{max}, h	6.7 (47%)†	6.8 (45%)	4.5 (56%)	6.2 (51%)	1.7 (88%)	0.9 (67%)	2.1 (46%)	1.1 (15%)
Oral Clearance, mL/h/kg (CL/F)	46.8 (37%)	46.8 (37%)	47.2 (38%)	51.6 (40%)	NA	NA	58.3 (19%)	42.0 (43%)
Apparent Volume of Distribution, mL/kg (Vd/F)	566 (26%)	580 (26%)	459 (28%)	552 (34%)	NA	NA	NA	NA
Terminal Half-life, h	8.4 (30%)	8.4 (29%)	7.6 (45%)	7.8 (26%)	5.1 (22%)	7.5 (34%)	NA	5.7 (24%)

† % Coefficient of variation
* Age range (years)
‡ Pharmacokinetic parameters obtained following administration of Lodine
NA = not available

Continued on next page

Lodine XL—Cont.

Patients should report to their physicians signs or symptoms of gastrointestinal ulceration or bleeding, skin rash, weight gain, or edema.
Patients should be informed of the warning signs and symptoms of hepatotoxicity (e.g., nausea, fatigue, lethargy, pruritus, jaundice, right upper quadrant tenderness, and "flu-like" symptoms). If these occur, patients should be instructed to stop therapy and seek immediate medical therapy.
Patients should also be instructed to seek emergency help in case of an anaphylactoid reaction (see **Warnings**).
In late pregnancy, as with other NSAIDs, Lodine XL should be avoided because it may cause premature closure of the ductus arteriosus.
LABORATORY TESTS
Patients on long-term treatment with NSAIDs should have their CBC and blood chemistry profile checked periodically. If clinical signs and symptoms consistent with liver or renal disease develop, systemic manifestations occur (e.g., eosinophilia, rash, etc.), or if abnormal liver tests persist or worsen, Lodine XL should be discontinued.
DRUG INTERACTIONS
Aspirin
When etodolac is administered with aspirin, its protein binding is reduced, although the clearance of free etodolac is not altered. The clinical significance of this interaction is not known; however, as with other NSAIDs, concomitant administration of etodolac and aspirin is not generally recommended because of the potential of increased adverse effects.
Warfarin
The effects of warfarin and NSAIDs on GI bleeding are synergistic, such that users of both drugs together have a risk of serious GI bleeding higher than that of users of either drug alone. Short-term pharmacokinetic studies have demonstrated that concomitant administration of warfarin and etodolac results in reduced protein binding of warfarin, but there was no change in the clearance of free warfarin. There was no significant difference in the pharmacodynamic effect of warfarin administered alone and warfarin administered with etodolac as measured by prothrombin time. Thus, concomitant therapy with warfarin and Lodine XL should not require dosage adjustment of either drug. However, there have been a few spontaneous reports of prolonged prothrombin times in etodolac-treated patients receiving concomitant warfarin therapy. Caution should be exercised because interactions have been seen with other NSAIDs.
Methotrexate
Etodolac has no apparent pharmacokinetic interaction with methotrexate. However, NSAIDs have been reported to competitively inhibit methotrexate accumulation in rabbit kidney slices. This may indicate that they could enhance the toxicity of methotrexate. Caution should be used when NSAIDs are administered concomitantly with methotrexate.
ACE-inhibitors
Reports suggest that NSAIDs may diminish the antihypertensive effect of ACE-inhibitors. This interaction should be given consideration in patients taking NSAIDs concomitantly with ACE-inhibitors.
Diuretics
Etodolac has no apparent pharmacokinetic interaction when administered with furosemide or hydrochlorothiazide. Nevertheless, clinical studies, as well as postmarketing observations, have shown that Lodine XL can reduce the natriuretic effect of furosemide and thiazides in some patients. This response has been attributed to inhibition of renal prostaglandin synthesis. During concomitant therapy with NSAIDs, the patient should be observed closely for signs of renal failure (see **Precautions**—*Renal Effects*), as well as to assure diuretic efficacy.
Lithium
NSAIDs have produced an elevation of plasma lithium levels and a reduction in renal lithium clearance. With NSAIDs, the mean minimum lithium concentration increased 15% and the renal clearance was decreased by approximately 20%. These effects have been attributed to inhibition of renal prostaglandin synthesis by the NSAID. Thus, when NSAIDs and lithium are administered concurrently, subjects should be observed carefully for signs of lithium toxicity.
Cyclosporine, Digoxin
Lodine XL, like other NSAIDs, through effects on renal prostaglandins, may cause changes in the elimination of these drugs, leading to elevated serum levels of cyclosporine and digoxin and increased toxicity. Nephrotoxicity associated with cyclosporine may also be enhanced. Patients receiving these drugs who are given Lodine XL, or any other NSAID, and particularly those patients with altered renal function, should be observed for the development of the specific toxicities of these drugs.
Phenylbutazone
Phenylbutazone causes an increase (by about 80%) in the free fraction of etodolac. Although *in vivo* studies have not been done to see if etodolac clearance is changed by coadministration of phenylbutazone, it is not recommended that they be coadministered.
Glyburide
Etodolac has no apparent pharmacokinetic interaction when administered with glyburide.
Phenytoin
Etodolac has no apparent pharmacokinetic interaction when administered with phenytoin.
DRUG/LABORATORY TEST INTERACTIONS
The urine of patients who take etodolac can give a false-positive reaction for urinary bilirubin (urobilin) due to the presence of phenolic metabolites of etodolac. Diagnostic dipstick methodology, used to detect ketone bodies in urine, has resulted in false-positive findings in some patients treated with etodolac. Generally, this phenomenon has not been associated with other clinically significant events. No dose relationship has been observed.
Etodolac treatment is associated with a small decrease in serum uric acid levels. In clinical trials, mean decreases of 1 to 2 mg/dL were observed in arthritic patients receiving etodolac (600 mg to 1000 mg/day) after 4 weeks of therapy. These levels then remained stable for up to 1 year of therapy.
CARCINOGENESIS, MUTAGENESIS, AND IMPAIRMENT OF FERTILITY
No carcinogenic effect of etodolac was observed in mice or rats receiving oral doses of 15 mg/kg/day (45 to 89 mg/m^2, respectively) or less for periods of 18 months or 2 years, respectively. Etodolac was not mutagenic in *in vitro* tests performed with *S. typhimurium* and mouse lymphoma cells as well as in an *in vivo* mouse micronucleus test. However, data from the *in vitro* human peripheral lymphocyte test showed an increase in the number of gaps (3% to 5% unstained regions in the chromatid without dislocation) among the etodolac-treated cultures (50 to 200 µg/mL) compared to negative controls (2%); no other difference was noted between the controls and drug-treated groups. Etodolac showed no impairment of fertility in male and female rats up to oral doses of 16 mg/kg (94 mg/m^2). However, reduced implantation of fertilized eggs occurred in the 8 mg/kg group.
PREGNANCY
Teratogenic Effects—Pregnancy Category C
In teratology studies, isolated occurrences of alterations in limb development were found and included polydactyly, oligodactyly, syndactyly, and unossified phalanges in rats and oligodactyly and synostosis of metatarsals in rabbits. These were observed at dose levels (2 to 14 mg/kg/day) close to human clinical doses. However, the frequency and the dosage group distribution of these findings in initial or repeated studies did not establish a clear drug or dose-response relationship. Animal reproduction studies are not always predictive of human response.
There are no adequate or well-controlled studies in pregnant women. Lodine XL should be used during pregnancy only if the potential benefit justifies the potential risk to the fetus.
Nonteratogenic Effects
Because of the known effects of nonsteroidal anti-inflammatory drugs on the fetal cardiovascular system (closure of the ductus arteriosus), use during pregnancy (particularly late pregnancy) should be avoided.
LABOR AND DELIVERY
In rat studies with NSAIDs, as with other drugs known to inhibit prostaglandin synthesis, an increased incidence of dystocia, delayed parturition, and decreased pup survival occurred. The effects of Lodine XL on labor and delivery in pregnant women are unknown.
NURSING MOTHERS
It is not known whether this drug is excreted in human milk. Because many drugs are excreted in human milk and because of the potential for serious adverse reactions in nursing infants from Lodine XL, a decision should be made whether to discontinue nursing or to discontinue the drug, taking into account the importance of the drug to the mother.
PEDIATRIC USE
Safety and effectiveness in pediatric patients have not been established.
GERIATRIC USE
As with any NSAID, caution should be exercised in treating the elderly (65 years and older). In patients 65 years and older, no substantial differences in the side effect profile of Lodine XL were seen compared with the general population (see **Clinical Pharmacology**—PHARMACOKINETICS).

ADVERSE REACTIONS

A total of 1552 patients were exposed to Lodine XL in controlled clinical studies of at least 4 weeks in length and using daily doses in the range of 400 to 1200 mg. In the tabulations below, adverse event rates are generally categorized based on the incidence of events in the first 30 days of treatment with Lodine XL. As with other NSAIDs, the cumulative adverse event rates may increase significantly over time with extended therapy.
In patients taking NSAIDs, including Lodine XL, the most frequently reported adverse experiences occurring in approximately 1–10% of patients are:
gastrointestinal experiences including:
abdominal pain
constipation
diarrhea
dyspepsia
flatulence
GI ulcers (gastric/duodenal)*
gross bleeding/perforation*
nausea
vomiting
other events including:
abnormal renal function*
anemia*
asthenia
dizziness
edema*
elevated liver enzymes*
headaches
hypertension
increased bleeding time*
infection
pharyngitis
pruritus
rashes
rhinitis
tinnitus*

*Adverse events that were observed in < 1% of patients in the first 30 days of treatment with Lodine XL in clinical trials.
ADDITIONAL NSAID ADVERSE EXPERIENCES REPORTED OCCASIONALLY WITH NSAIDs OR LODINE XL INCLUDE:
Body as a whole—
allergic reaction, anaphylactoid reaction, chills, fever, sepsis
Cardiovascular system—
congestive heart failure, flushing, palpitations, tachycardia, syncope, vasculitis (including necrotizing and allergic).
Digestive system—
anorexia, cholestatic hepatitis, cholestatic jaundice, dry mouth, duodenitis, eructation, esophagitis, gastritis, gastric/peptic ulcers, glossitis, hepatic failure, hepatitis, hematemesis, intestinal ulceration, jaundice, liver necrosis, melena, pancreatitis, rectal bleeding, stomatitis
Hemic and lymphatic system—
agranulocytosis, ecchymosis, eosinophilia, hemolytic anemia, leukopenia, neutropenia, pancytopenia, purpura, thrombocytopenia
Metabolic and nutritional—
hyperglycemia in previously controlled diabetic patients
Nervous system—
anxiety, confusion, depression, dream abnormalities, insomnia, nervousness, paresthesia, somnolence, tremors, vertigo
Respiratory system—
asthma, dyspnea
Skin and appendages—
angioedema, cutaneous vasculitis with purpura, erythema multiforme, hyperpigmentation, sweating, urticaria, vesiculobullous rash
Special senses—
blurred vision, photophobia, transient visual disturbances
Urogenital system—
dysuria, elevated BUN, oliguria/polyuria, proteinuria, renal failure, renal insufficiency, renal papillary necrosis, serum creatinine increase, urinary frequency
OTHER NSAID ADVERSE REACTIONS, WHICH OCCUR RARELY ARE:
Body as a whole—
anaphylactic reactions, appetite changes, death
Cardiovascular system—
arrhythmia, cerebrovascular accident, hypotension, myocardial infarction
Digestive system—
colitis, esophagitis with or without stricture or cardiospasm, thirst, ulcerative stomatitis
Hemic and lymphatic system—
aplastic anemia, lymphadenopathy
Metabolic and nutritional—
change in weight
Nervous system—
coma, convulsions, hallucinations, meningitis
Respiratory—
bronchitis, pneumonia, respiratory depression, sinusitis
Skin and appendages—
alopecia, exfoliative dermatitis, maculopapular rash, photosensitivity, skin peeling, Stevens-Johnson syndrome, toxic epidermal necrosis
Special senses—
conjunctivitis, deafness, hearing impairment, taste perversion
Urogenital system—
cystitis, hematuria, interstitial nephritis, leukorrhea, renal calculus, uterine bleeding irregularities

OVERDOSAGE

Symptoms following acute NSAID overdose are usually limited to lethargy, drowsiness, nausea, vomiting, and epigastric pain, which are generally reversible with supportive care. Gastrointestinal bleeding can occur. Hypertension, acute renal failure, respiratory depression and coma may occur, but are rare. Anaphylactoid reactions have been reported with therapeutic ingestion of NSAIDs, and may occur following an overdose.
Patients should be managed by symptomatic and supportive care following an NSAID overdose. There are no specific antidotes. Emesis and/or activated charcoal (60 to 100 g in adults, 1 to 2 g/kg in children) and/or osmotic cathartic may be indicated in patients seen within 4 hours of ingestion with symptoms or following a large overdose (5 to 10 times

the usual dose). Forced diuresis, alkalinization of the urine, hemodialysis, or hemoperfusion may not be useful due to high protein binding.

DOSAGE AND ADMINISTRATION

As with other NSAIDs, the lowest dose and longest dosing interval should be sought for each patient. Therefore, after observing the response to initial therapy with Lodine XL, the dose and frequency should be adjusted to suit an individual patient's needs.

For the management of the signs and symptoms of osteoarthritis or rheumatoid arthritis, the recommended starting dose of Lodine XL is 400 to 1000 mg, given once daily. As with other NSAIDs, the lowest effective dose should be sought for each patient. During long-term administration, the dose of Lodine XL may be adjusted up or down, depending on the patient's clinical response, up to a maximum dose of 1200 mg/day. Doses above 1200 mg/day have not been studied, and thus a dose-efficacy relationship at doses beyond 1200 mg/day has not been established. In chronic conditions, a therapeutic response to therapy with Lodine XL is sometimes seen within one week of therapy, but most often is observed by two weeks.

HOW SUPPLIED

Lodine® XL (etodolac extended-release tablets) is available as:

400 mg tablets (orange-red, capsular-oval shaped, biconvex film-coated tablet, branded LODINE XL 400 on one side)
—in bottles of 100, NDC 0046-0829-81
—in unit-dose packages of 100, NDC 0046-0829-99

500 mg tablets (grey-green, capsular-oval shaped, biconvex film-coated tablet, branded Lodine XL 500 on one side)
—in bottles of 100, NDC 0046-0839-81
—in unit-dose packages of 100, NDC 0046-0839-99

600 mg tablets (light grey, capsular-oval shaped, biconvex film-coated tablet, branded LODINE XL 600 on one side)
—in bottles of 100, NDC 0046-0831-81
—in unit-dose packages of 100, NDC 0046-0831-99

Store at 25°C (77°F), excursions permitted to 15–30°C (59–86°F). [See USP Controlled Room Temperature.]
Protect from excessive heat and humidity.

Caution: Federal law prohibits dispensing without prescription.

Manufactured by:
Ayerst Laboratories Inc.
A Wyeth-Ayerst Company
Philadelphia, PA 19101

CI 4848-2 Revised January 21, 1998

Shown in Product Identification Guide, page 341

LO/OVRAL® ℞

[*lōh-ōh 'vral*]
Tablets
(norgestrel and ethinyl estradiol tablets)

Patients should be counseled that this product does not protect against HIV infection (AIDS) and other sexually transmitted diseases.

DESCRIPTION

Each LO/OVRAL tablet contains 0.3 mg of norgestrel (*dl* - 13-beta-ethyl -17- alpha-ethinyl -17- beta - hydroxygon - 4- en -3-one), a totally synthetic progestogen, and 0.03 mg of ethinyl estradiol (19-nor-17α-pregna-1,3,5 (10)-trien-20-yne-3,17-diol). The inactive ingredients present are cellulose, lactose, magnesium stearate, and polacrilin potassium.

CLINICAL PHARMACOLOGY

Combination oral contraceptives act by suppression of gonadotropins. Although the primary mechanism of this action is inhibition of ovulation, other alterations include changes in the cervical mucus (which increase the difficulty of sperm entry into the uterus) and the endometrium (which reduce the likelihood of implantation).

INDICATIONS AND USAGE

Oral contraceptives are indicated for the prevention of pregnancy in women who elect to use this product as a method of contraception.

Oral contraceptives are highly effective. Table I lists the typical accidental pregnancy rates for users of combination oral contraceptives and other methods of contraception. The efficacy of these contraceptive methods, except sterilization and the IUD, depends upon the reliability with which they are used. Correct and consistent use of methods can result in lower failure rates.

TABLE I: LOWEST EXPECTED AND TYPICAL FAILURE RATES DURING THE FIRST YEAR OF CONTINUOUS USE OF A METHOD

% of Women Experiencing an Accidental Pregnancy in the First Year of Continuous Use		
Method	Lowest Expected*	Typical**
(No Contraception)	(85)	(85)
Oral contraceptives		3
combined	0.1	N/A***
progestin only	0.5	N/A***
Diaphragm with spermicidal cream or jelly	6	18
Spermicides alone (foams and vaginal suppositories)	3	21
Vaginal Sponge		
nulliparous	6	18
multiparous	9	28
DEPO-PROVERA® (injectable progestogen)	0.3	0.3
NORPLANT® SYSTEM (implants)	0.2#	0.2#
IUD		3
progesterone	2	N/A***
copper T 380A	0.8	N/A***
Condom without spermicides	2	12
Periodic abstinence (all methods)	1–9	20
Female sterilization	0.2	0.4
Male sterilization	0.1	0.15

Adapted from J. Trussell et al., Table 1, Studies in Family Planning, *21(1): Jan.–Feb. 1990.*

* The authors' best guess of the percentage of women expected to experience an accidental pregnancy among couples who initiate a method (not necessarily for the first time) and who use it consistently and correctly during the first year if they do not stop for any other reason.

** This term represents "typical" couples who initiate use of a method (not necessarily for the first time), who experience an accidental pregnancy during the first year if they do not stop use for any other reason.

*** N/A—Data not available.

\# This data is based on NORPLANT® SYSTEM clinical trials.

CONTRAINDICATIONS

Oral contraceptives should not be used in women with any of the following conditions:

Thrombophlebitis or thromboembolic disorders.
A past history of deep-vein thrombophlebitis or thromboembolic disorders.
Cerebral-vascular or coronary-artery disease.
Known or suspected carcinoma of the breast.
Carcinoma of the endometrium or other known or suspected estrogen-dependent neoplasia.
Undiagnosed abnormal genital bleeding.
Cholestatic jaundice of pregnancy or jaundice with prior pill use.
Hepatic adenomas or carcinomas.
Known or suspected pregnancy.

WARNINGS

Cigarette smoking increases the risk of serious cardiovascular side effects from oral-contraceptive use. This risk increases with age and with heavy smoking (15 or more cigarettes per day) and is quite marked in women over 35 years of age. Women who use oral contraceptives should be strongly advised not to smoke.

The use of oral contraceptives is associated with increased risks of several serious conditions including myocardial infarction, thromboembolism, stroke, hepatic neoplasia, gallbladder disease, and hypertension, although the risk of serious morbidity or mortality is very small in healthy women without underlying factors. The risk of morbidity and mortality increases significantly in the presence of other underlying risk factors such as hypertension, hyperlipidemias, obesity, and diabetes.

Practitioners prescribing oral contraceptives should be familiar with the following information relating to these risks.

The information contained in this package insert is based principally on studies carried out in patients who used oral contraceptives with higher formulations of estrogens and progestogens than those in common use today. The effect of long-term use of the oral contraceptives with lower formulations of both estrogens and progestogens remains to be determined.

Throughout this labeling, epidemiological studies reported are of two types: retrospective or case control studies and prospective or cohort studies. Case control studies provide a measure of the relative risk of disease, namely, a ratio of the incidence of a disease among oral-contraceptive users to that among nonusers. The relative risk does not provide information on the actual clinical occurrence of a disease. Cohort studies provide a measure of attributable risk, which is the difference in the incidence of disease between oral-contraceptive users and nonusers. The attributable risk does provide information about the actual occurrence of a disease in the population. For further information, the reader is referred to a text on epidemiological methods.

1. THROMBOEMBOLIC DISORDERS AND OTHER VASCULAR PROBLEMS

a. *Myocardial infarction*

An increased risk of myocardial infarction has been attributed to oral-contraceptive use. This risk is primarily in smokers or women with other underlying risk factors for coronary-artery disease such as hypertension, hypercholesterolemia, morbid obesity, and diabetes. The relative risk of heart attack for current oral-contraceptive users has been estimated to be two to six. The risk is very low under the age of 30.

Smoking in combination with oral-contraceptive use has been shown to contribute substantially to the incidence of myocardial infarctions in women in their mid-thirties or older with smoking accounting for the majority of excess cases. Mortality rates associated with circulatory disease have been shown to increase substantially in smokers over the age of 35 and nonsmokers over the age of 40 (Table II) among women who use oral contraceptives.

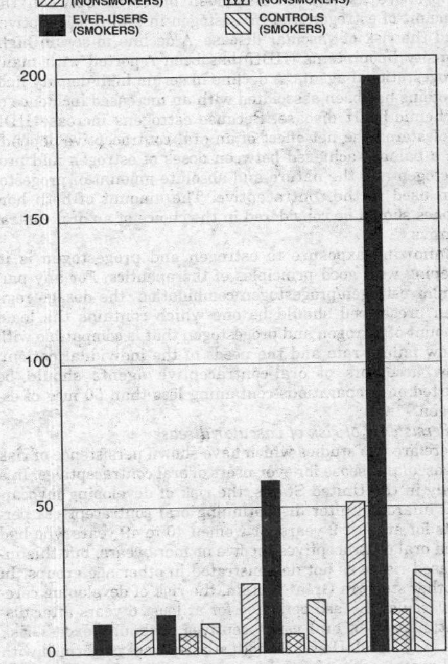

TABLE II. (Adapted from P.M. Layde and V. Beral, Lancet, *1*:541–546, 1981.)

Oral contraceptives may compound the effects of well-known risk factors, such as hypertension, diabetes, hyperlipidemias, age, and obesity. In particular, some progestogens are known to decrease HDL cholesterol and cause glucose intolerance, while estrogens may create a state of hyperinsulinism. Oral contraceptives have been shown to increase blood pressure among users (see section 9 in "Warnings"). Similar effects on risk factors have been associated with an increased risk of heart disease. Oral contraceptives must be used with caution in women with cardiovascular disease risk factors.

b. *Thromboembolism*

An increased risk of thromboembolic and thrombotic disease associated with the use of oral contraceptives is well established. Case control studies have found the relative risk of users compared to nonusers to be 3 for the first episode of superficial venous thrombosis, 4 to 11 for deep-vein thrombosis or pulmonary embolism, and 1.5 to 6 for women with predisposing conditions for venous thromboembolic disease. Cohort studies have shown the relative risk to be somewhat lower, about 3 for new cases and about 4.5 for new cases requiring hospitalization. The risk of thromboembolic disease due to oral contraceptives is not related to length of use and disappears after pill use is stopped.

A two- to four-fold increase in relative risk of postoperative thromboembolic complications has been reported with the use of oral contraceptives. The relative risk of venous thrombosis in women who have predisposing conditions is twice that of women without such medical conditions. If feasible, oral contraceptives should be discontinued at least four weeks prior to and for two weeks after elective surgery of a type associated with an increase in risk of thromboembolism and during and following prolonged immobilization. Since the immediate postpartum period is also associated with an increased risk of thromboembolism, oral contraceptives should be started no earlier than four to six weeks after delivery in women who elect not to breast-feed, or a midtrimester pregnancy termination.

c. *Cerebrovascular diseases*

Oral contraceptives have been shown to increase both the relative and attributable risks of cerebrovascular events (thrombotic and hemorrhagic strokes), although, in general, the risk is greatest among older (>35 years), hypertensive women who also smoke. Hypertension was found to be a risk factor for both users and nonusers, for both types of strokes, while smoking interacted to increase the risk for hemorrhagic strokes.

Continued on next page

Lo/Ovral—Cont.

In a large study, the relative risk of thrombotic strokes has been shown to range from 3 for normotensive users to 14 for users with severe hypertension. The relative risk of hemorrhagic stroke is reported to be 1.2 for nonsmokers who used oral contraceptives, 2.6 for smokers who did not use oral contraceptives, 7.6 for smokers who used oral contraceptives, 1.8 for normotensive users, and 25.7 for users with severe hypertension. The attributable risk is also greater in older women.

d. *Dose-related risk of vascular disease from oral contraceptives*

A positive association has been observed between the amount of estrogen and progestogen in oral contraceptives and the risk of vascular disease. A decline in serum high-density lipoproteins (HDL) has been reported with many progestational agents. A decline in serum high-density lipoproteins has been associated with an increased incidence of ischemic heart disease. Because estrogens increase HDL cholesterol, the net effect of an oral contraceptive depends on a balance achieved between doses of estrogen and progestogen and the nature and absolute amount of progestogen used in the contraceptive. The amount of both hormones should be considered in the choice of an oral contraceptive.

Minimizing exposure to estrogen and progestogen is in keeping with good principles of therapeutics. For any particular estrogen/progestogen combination, the dosage regimen prescribed should be one which contains the least amount of estrogen and progestogen that is compatible with a low failure rate and the needs of the individual patient. New acceptors of oral-contraceptive agents should be started on preparations containing less than 50 mcg of estrogen.

e. *Persistence of risk of vascular disease*

There are two studies which have shown persistence of risk of vascular disease for ever-users of oral contraceptives. In a study in the United States, the risk of developing myocardial infarction after discontinuing oral contraceptives persists for at least 9 years for women 40 to 49 years who had used oral contraceptives for five or more years, but this increased risk was not demonstrated in other age groups. In another study in Great Britain, the risk of developing cerebrovascular disease persisted for at least 6 years after discontinuation of oral contraceptives, although excess risk was very small. However, both studies were performed with oral-contraceptive formulations containing 50 micrograms or higher of estrogens.

2. ESTIMATES OF MORTALITY FROM CONTRACEPTIVE USE

One study gathered data from a variety of sources which have estimated the mortality rate associated with different methods of contraception at different ages (Table III). These estimates include the combined risk of death associated with contraceptive methods plus the risk attributable to pregnancy in the event of method failure. Each method of contraception has its specific benefits and risks. The study concluded that with the exception of oral-contraceptive users 35 and older who smoke and 40 and older who do not smoke, mortality associated with all methods of birth control is less than that associated with childbirth. The observation of a possible increase in risk of mortality with age for oral-contraceptive users is based on data gathered in the 1970's—but not reported until 1983. However, current clinical practice involves the use of lower estrogen dose formulations combined with careful restriction of oral-contraceptive use to women who do not have the various risk factors listed in this labeling.

Because of these changes in practice and, also, because of some limited new data which suggest that the risk of cardiovascular disease with the use of oral contraceptives may now be less than previously observed, the Fertility and Maternal Health Drugs Advisory Committee was asked to review the topic in 1989. The Committee concluded that although cardiovascular-disease risks may be increased with oral-contraceptive use after age 40 in healthy nonsmoking women (even with the newer low-dose formulations), there are greater potential health risks associated with pregnancy in older women and with the alternative surgical and medical procedures which may be necessary if such women do not have access to effective and acceptable means of contraception.

Therefore, the Committee recommended that the benefits of oral-contraceptive use by healthy nonsmoking women over 40 may outweigh the possible risks. Of course, older women, as all women who take oral contraceptives, should take the lowest possible dose formulation that is effective.

[See table below]

3. CARCINOMA OF THE REPRODUCTIVE ORGANS

Numerous epidemiological studies have been performed on the incidence of breast, endometrial, ovarian, and cervical cancer in women using oral contraceptives. The overwhelming evidence in the literature suggests that use of oral contraceptives is not associated with an increase in the risk of developing breast cancer, regardless of the age and parity of first use or with most of the marketed brands and doses. The Cancer and Steroid Hormone (CASH) study also showed no latent effect on the risk of breast cancer for at least a decade following long-term use. A few studies have shown a slightly increased relative risk of developing breast cancer, although the methodology of these studies, which included differences in examination of users and nonusers and differences in age at start of use, has been questioned.

Some studies suggest that oral-contraceptive use has been associated with an increase in the risk of cervical intraepithelial neoplasia in some populations of women. However, there continues to be controversy about the extent to which such findings may be due to differences in sexual behavior and other factors.

In spite of many studies of the relationship between oral-contraceptive use and breast and cervical cancers, a cause-and-effect relationship has not been established.

4. HEPATIC NEOPLASIA

Benign hepatic adenomas are associated with oral-contraceptive use, although the incidence of benign tumors is rare in the United States. Indirect calculations have estimated the attributable risk to be in the range of 3.3 cases/100,000 for users, a risk that increases after four or more years of use. Rupture of rare, benign, hepatic adenomas may cause death through intra-abdominal hemorrhage.

Studies from Britain have shown an increased risk of developing hepatocellular carcinoma in long-term (>8 years) oral-contraceptive users. However, these cancers are extremely rare in the U.S., and the attributable risk (the excess incidence) of liver cancers in oral-contraceptive users approaches less than one per million users.

5. OCULAR LESIONS

There have been clincial case reports of retinal thrombosis associated with the use of oral contraceptives. Oral contraceptives should be discontinued if there is unexplained partial or complete loss of vision; onset of proptosis or diplopia; papilledema; or retinal vascular lesions. Appropriate diagnostic and therapeutic measures should be undertaken immediately.

6. ORAL-CONTRACEPTIVE USE BEFORE OR DURING EARLY PREGNANCY

Extensive epidemiological studies have revealed no increased risk of birth defects in women who have used oral contraceptives prior to pregnancy. Studies also do not suggest a teratogenic effect, particularly insofar as cardiac anomalies and limb-reduction defects are concerned, when taken inadvertently during early pregnancy.

The administration of oral contraceptives to induce withdrawal bleeding should not be used as a test for pregnancy. Oral contraceptives should not be used during pregnancy to treat threatened or habitual abortion.

It is recommended that for any patient who has missed two consecutive periods, pregnancy should be ruled out before continuing oral-contraceptive use. If the patient has not adhered to the prescribed schedule, the possibility of pregnancy should be considered at the time of the first missed period. Oral-contraceptive use should be discontinued if pregnancy is confirmed.

7. GALLBLADDER DISEASE

Earlier studies have reported an increased lifetime relative risk of gallbladder surgery in users of oral contraceptives and estrogens. More recent studies, however, have shown that the relative risk of developing gallbladder disease among oral-contraceptive users may be minimal. The recent findings of minimal risk may be related to the use of oral-contraceptive formulations containing lower hormonal doses of estrogens and progestogens.

8. CARBOHYDRATE AND LIPID METABOLIC EFFECTS

Oral contraceptives have been shown to cause glucose intolerance in a significant percentage of users. Oral contraceptives containing greater than 75 micrograms of estrogens cause hyperinsulinism, while lower doses of estrogen cause less glucose intolerance. Progestogens increase insulin secretion and create insulin resistance, this effect varying with different progestational agents. However, in the nondiabetic woman, oral contraceptives appear to have no effect on fasting blood glucose. Because of these demonstrated effects, prediabetic and diabetic women should be carefully observed while taking oral contraceptives.

A small proportion of women will have persistent hypertriglyceridemia while on the pill. As discussed earlier (see "Warnings," 1a. and 1d.), changes in serum triglycerides and lipoprotein levels have been reported in oral-contraceptive users.

9. ELEVATED BLOOD PRESSURE

An increase in blood pressure has been reported in women taking oral contraceptives, and this increase is more likely in older oral-contraceptive users and with continued use. Data from the Royal College of General Practitioners and subsequent randomized trials have shown that the incidence of hypertension increases with increasing quantities of progestogens.

Women with a history of hypertension or hypertension-related diseases, or renal disease, should be encouraged to use another method of contraception. If women with hypertension elect to use oral contraceptives, they should be monitored closely, and if significant elevation of blood pressure occurs, oral contraceptives should be discontinued. For most women, elevated blood pressure will return to normal after stopping oral contraceptives, and there is no difference in the occurrence of hypertension among ever- and never-users.

10. HEADACHE

The onset or exacerbation of migraine or development of headache with a new pattern that is recurrent, persistent, or severe requires discontinuation of oral contraceptives and evaluation of the cause.

11. BLEEDING IRREGULARITIES

Breakthrough bleeding and spotting are sometimes encountered in patients on oral contraceptives, especially during the first three months of use. The type and dose of progestogen may be important. Nonhormonal causes should be considered and adequate diagnostic measures taken to rule out malignancy or pregnancy in the event of breakthrough bleeding, as in the case of any abnormal vaginal bleeding. If pathology has been excluded, time or a change to another formulation may solve the problem. In the event of amenorrhea, pregnancy should be ruled out.

Some women may encounter post-pill amenorrhea or oligomenorrhea, especially when such a condition was preexistent.

PRECAUTIONS

Patients should be counseled that this product does not protect against HIV infection (AIDS) and other sexually transmitted diseases.

1. PHYSICAL EXAMINATION AND FOLLOW-UP

A periodic history and physical examination is appropriate for all women, including women using oral contraceptives. The physical examination, however, may be deferred until after initiation of oral contraceptives if requested by the woman and judged appropriate by the clinician. The physical examination should include special reference to blood pressure, breasts, abdomen and pelvic organs, including cervical cytology, and relevant laboratory tests. In case of undiagnosed, persistent, or recurrent abnormal vaginal bleeding, appropriate measures should be conducted to rule out malignancy. Women with a strong family history of breast cancer or who have breast nodules should be monitored with particular care.

2. LIPID DISORDERS

Women who are being treated for hyperlipidemias should be followed closely if they elect to use oral contraceptives. Some progestogens may elevate LDL levels and may render the control of hyperlipidemias more difficult. (See "Warnings," 1d.).

3. LIVER FUNCTION

If jaundice develops in any woman receiving such drugs, the medication should be discontinued. Steroid hormones may be poorly metabolized in patients with impaired liver function.

4. FLUID RETENTION

Oral contraceptives may cause some degree of fluid retention. They should be prescribed with caution, and only with careful monitoring, in patients with conditions which might be aggravated by fluid retention.

5. EMOTIONAL DISORDERS

Patients becoming significantly depressed while taking oral contraceptives should stop the medication and use an alternate method of contraception in an attempt to determine whether the symptom is drug related. Women with a history of depression should be carefully observed and the drug discontinued if depression recurs to a serious degree.

6. CONTACT LENSES

Contact-lens wearers who develop visual changes or changes in lens tolerance should be assessed by an ophthalmologist.

TABLE III—ANNUAL NUMBER OF BIRTH-RELATED OR METHOD-RELATED DEATHS ASSOCIATED WITH CONTROL OF FERTILITY PER 100,000 NONSTERILE WOMEN, BY FERTILITY-CONTROL METHOD AND ACCORDING TO AGE

Method of control and outcome	15–19	20–24	25–29	30–34	35–39	40–44
No fertility-control methods*	7.0	7.4	9.1	14.8	25.7	28.2
Oral contraceptives non-smoker**	0.3	0.5	0.9	1.9	13.8	31.6
Oral contraceptives smoker**	2.2	3.4	6.6	13.5	51.1	117.2
IUD**	0.8	0.8	1.0	1.0	1.4	1.4
Condom*	1.1	1.6	0.7	0.2	0.3	0.4
Diaphragm/spermicide*	1.9	1.2	1.2	1.3	2.2	2.8
Periodic abstinence*	2.5	1.6	1.6	1.7	2.9	3.6

* Deaths are birth related
** Deaths are method related
Adapted from H.W. Ory, Family Planning Perspectives, *15*:57–63, 1983.

7. DRUG INTERACTIONS
Reduced efficacy and increased incidence of breakthrough bleeding and menstrual irregularities have been associated with concomitant use of rifampin. A similar association, though less marked, has been suggested with barbiturates, phenylbutazone, phenytoin sodium, and possibly with griseofulvin, ampicillin, and tetracyclines.
8. INTERACTIONS WITH LABORATORY TESTS
Certain endocrine- and liver-function tests and blood components may be affected by oral contraceptives:
a. Increased prothrombin and factors VII, VIII, IX, and X; decreased antithrombin 3; increased norepinephrine-induced platelet aggregability.
b. Increased thyroid-binding globulin (TBG) leading to increased circulating total thyroid hormone, as measured by protein-bound iodine (PBI), T4 by column or by radioimmunoassay. Free T3 resin uptake is decreased, reflecting the elevated TBG; free T4 concentration is unaltered.
c. Other binding proteins may be elevated in serum.
d. Sex-binding globulins are increased and result in elevated levels of total circulating sex steroids and corticoids; however, free or biologically active levels remain unchanged.
e. Triglycerides may be increased.
f. Glucose tolerance may be decreased.
g. Serum folate levels may be depressed by oral-contraceptive therapy. This may be of clinical significance if a woman becomes pregnant shortly after discontinuing oral contraceptives.
9. CARCINOGENESIS
See "Warnings" section.
10. PREGNANCY
Pregnancy Category X. See "Contraindications" and "Warnings" sections.
11. NURSING MOTHERS
Small amounts of oral-contraceptive steroids have been identified in the milk of nursing mothers, and a few adverse effects on the child have been reported, including jaundice and breast enlargement. In addition, oral contraceptives given in the postpartum period may interfere with lactation by decreasing the quantity and quality of breast milk. If possible, the nursing mother should be advised not to use oral contraceptives but to use other forms of contraception until she has completely weaned her child.

INFORMATION FOR THE PATIENT
See Patient Labeling Printed Below.

ADVERSE REACTIONS

An increased risk of the following serious adverse reactions has been associated with the use of oral contraceptives (see "Warnings" section):
Thrombophlebitis.
Arterial thromboembolism.
Pulmonary embolism.
Myocardial infarction.
Cerebral hemorrhage.
Cerebral thrombosis.
Hypertension.
Gallbladder disease.
Hepatic adenomas or benign liver tumors.
There is evidence of an association between the following conditions and the use of oral contraceptives, although additional confirmatory studies are needed:
Mesenteric thrombosis.
Retinal thrombosis.
The following adverse reactions have been reported in patients receiving oral contraceptives and are believed to be drug related:
Nausea.
Vomiting.
Gastrointestinal symptoms (such as abdominal cramps and bloating).
Breakthrough bleeding.
Spotting.
Change in menstrual flow.
Amenorrhea.
Temporary infertility after discontinuation of treatment.
Edema.
Melasma which may persist.
Breast changes: tenderness, enlargement, secretion.
Change in weight (increase or decrease).
Change in cervical erosion and secretion.
Diminution in lactation when given immediately postpartum.
Cholestatic jaundice.
Migraine.
Rash (allergic).
Mental depression.
Reduced tolerance to carbohydrates.
Vaginal candidiasis.
Change in corneal curvature (steepening).
Intolerance to contact lenses.
The following adverse reactions have been reported in users of oral contraceptives, and the association has been neither confirmed nor refuted:
Congenital anomalies.
Premenstrual syndrome.
Cataracts.
Optic neuritis.
Changes in appetite.
Cystitis-like syndrome.
Headache.
Nervousness.
Dizziness.
Hirsutism.
Loss of scalp hair.
Erythema multiforme.
Erythema nodosum.
Hemorrhagic eruption.
Vaginitis.
Porphyria.
Impaired renal function.
Hemolytic uremic syndrome.
Budd-Chiari syndrome.
Acne.
Changes in libido.
Colitis.
Sickle-cell disease.
Cerebral-vascular disease with mitral valve prolapse.
Lupus-like syndromes.

OVERDOSAGE

Serious ill effects have not been reported following acute ingestion of large doses of oral contraceptives by young children. Overdosage may cause nausea, and withdrawal bleeding may occur in females.

NONCONTRACEPTIVE HEALTH BENEFITS

The following noncontraceptive health benefits related to the use of oral contraceptives are supported by epidemiological studies which largely utilized oral-contraceptive formulations containing doses exceeding 0.035 mg of ethinyl estradiol or 0.05 mg of mestranol.
Effects on menses:
Increased menstrual cycle regularity.
Decreased blood loss and decreased incidence of iron-deficiency anemia.
Decreased incidence of dysmenorrhea.
Effects related to inhibition of ovulation:
Decreased incidence of functional ovarian cysts.
Decreased incidence of ectopic pregnancies.
Effects from long-term use:
Decreased incidence of fibroadenomas and fibrocystic disease of the breast.
Decreased incidence of acute pelvic inflammatory disease.
Decreased incidence of endometrial cancer.
Decreased incidence of ovarian cancer.

DOSAGE AND ADMINISTRATION

To achieve maximum contraceptive effectiveness, LO/OVRAL must be taken exactly as directed and at intervals not exceeding 24 hours.
The dosage of LO/OVRAL is one tablet daily for 21 consecutive days per menstrual cycle according to prescribed schedule. Tablets are then discontinued for 7 days (three weeks on, one week off).
It is recommended that LO/OVRAL tablets be taken at the same time each day, preferably after the evening meal or at bedtime.
During the first cycle of medication, the patient is instructed to take one LO/OVRAL tablet daily for twenty-one consecutive days, beginning on the first day (Day 1 Start) of her menstrual cycle or on the Sunday after her period begins (Sunday Start). (The first day of menstruation is day one.) The tablets are then discontinued for one week (7 days). Withdrawal bleeding should usually occur within 3 days following discontinuation of LO/OVRAL. (For Day 1 Start: If LO/OVRAL is first taken later than the first day of the first menstrual cycle of medication or postpartum, contraceptive reliance should not be placed on LO/OVRAL until after the first seven consecutive days of administration. For Sunday Start: Contraceptive reliance should not be placed on LO/OVRAL until after the first seven consecutive days of administration. The possibility of ovulation and conception prior to initiation of medication should be considered.)
The patient begins her next and all subsequent 21-day courses of LO/OVRAL tablets on the same day of the week that she began her first course, following the same schedule: 21 days on—7 days off. She begins taking her tablets on the 8th day after discontinuance, regardless of whether or not a menstrual period has occurred or is still in progress. Any time a new cycle of LO/OVRAL is started later than the 8th day, the patient should be protected by another means of contraception until she has taken a tablet daily for seven consecutive days.
If spotting or breakthrough bleeding occurs, the patient is instructed to continue on the same regimen. This type of bleeding is usually transient and without significance; however, if the bleeding is persistent or prolonged, the patient is advised to consult her physician. Although the occurrence of pregnancy is highly unlikely if LO/OVRAL is taken according to directions, if withdrawal bleeding does not occur, the possibility of pregnancy must be considered. If the patient has not adhered to the prescribed schedule (missed one or more tablets or started taking them on a day later than she should have), the probability of pregnancy should be considered at the time of the first missed period and appropriate diagnostic measures taken before the medication is resumed. If the patient has adhered to the prescribed regimen and misses two consecutive periods, pregnancy should be ruled out before continuing the contraceptive regimen.
For additional patient instructions regarding missed pills, see the "WHAT TO DO IF YOU MISS PILLS" section in the **DETAILED PATIENT LABELING** below.
Any time the patient misses two or more tablets, she should also use another method of contraception until she has taken a tablet daily for seven consecutive days. If breakthrough bleeding occurs following missed tablets, it will usually be transient and of no consequence. While there is little likelihood of ovulation occurring if only one or two tablets are missed, the possibility of ovulation increases with each successive day that scheduled tablets are missed.
In the nonlactating mother, LO/OVRAL may be initiated postpartum, for contraception. When the tablets are administered in the postpartum period, the increased risk of thromboembolic disease associated with the postpartum period must be considered (see "Contraindications," "Warnings, " and "Precautions" concerning thromboembolic disease). It is to be noted that early resumption of ovulation may occur if Parlodel® (bromocriptine mesylate) has been used for the prevention of lactation.

HOW SUPPLIED

LO/OVRAL® Tablets (0.3 mg norgestrel and 0.03 mg ethinyl estradiol) are available in packages of 6 PILPAK® dispensers with 21 tablets each as follows:
NDC 0008-0078, white, round tablet marked "WYETH" and "78".
Store at room temperature, approx. 25°C (77°F).
References available upon request.
Brief Summary Patient Package Insert
This product (like all oral contraceptives) is intended to prevent pregnancy. It does not protect against HIV infection (AIDS) and other sexually transmitted diseases.
Oral contraceptives, also known as "birth-control pills" or "the pill," are taken to prevent pregnancy, and when taken correctly, have a failure rate of less than 1.0% per year when used without missing any pills. The typical failure rate of large numbers of pill users is less than 3.0% per year when women who miss pills are included. For most women oral contraceptives are also free of serious or unpleasant side effects. However, forgetting to take pills considerably increases the chances of pregnancy.
For the majority of women, oral contraceptives can be taken safely. But there are some women who are at high risk of developing certain serious diseases that can be life-threatening or may cause temporary or permanent disability or death. The risks associated with taking oral contraceptives increase significantly if you:
- smoke
- have high blood pressure, diabetes, high cholesterol
- have or have had clotting disorders, heart attack, stroke, angina pectoris, cancer of the breast or sex organs, jaundice, or malignant or benign liver tumors.

You should not take the pill if you suspect you are pregnant or have unexplained vaginal bleeding.

Cigarette smoking increases the risk of serious adverse effects on the heart and blood vessels from oral-contraceptive use. This risk increases with age and with heavy smoking (15 or more cigarettes per day) and is quite marked in women over 35 years of age. Women who use oral contraceptives should not smoke.

Most side effects of the pill are not serious. The most common such effects are nausea, vomiting, bleeding between menstrual periods, weight gain, breast tenderness, and difficulty wearing contact lenses. These side effects, especially nausea and vomiting, may subside within the first three months of use.
The serious side effects of the pill occur very infrequently, especially if you are in good health and do not smoke. However, you should know that the following medical conditions have been associated with or made worse by the pill:
1. Blood clots in the legs (thrombophlebitis), lungs (pulmonary embolism), stoppage or rupture of a blood vessel in the brain (stroke), blockage of blood vessels in the heart (heart attack and angina pectoris) or other organs of the body. As mentioned above, smoking increases the risk of heart attacks and strokes and subsequent serious medical consequences.
2. Liver tumors, which may rupture and cause severe bleeding. A possible but not definite association has been found with the pill and liver cancer. However, liver cancers are extremely rare. The chance of developing liver cancer from using the pill is thus even rarer.
3. High blood pressure, although blood pressure usually returns to normal when the pill is stopped.

The symptoms associated with these serious side effects are discussed in the detailed leaflet given to you with your supply of pills. Notify your doctor or health-care provider if you notice any unusual physical disturbances while taking the pill. In addition, drugs such as rifampin, as well as some anticonvulsants and some antibiotics, may decrease oral contraceptive effectiveness.
Studies to date of women taking the pill have not shown an increase in the incidence of cancer of the breast or cervix. There is, however, insufficient evidence to rule out the possibility that pills may cause such cancers.
Taking the pill provides some important noncontraceptive benefits. These include less painful menstruation, less menstrual blood loss and anemia, fewer pelvic infections, and fewer cancers of the ovary and the lining of the uterus.
Be sure to discuss any medical condition you may have with your health-care provider. Your health-care provider will take a medical and family history before prescribing oral contraceptives and will examine you. The physical examination may be delayed to another time if you request it and the health-care provider believes that it is appropriate to postpone it. You should be reexamined at least once a year while

Continued on next page

Lo/Ovral—Cont.

taking oral contraceptives. The detailed patient information leaflet gives you further information which you should read and discuss with your health-care provider.

DETAILED PATIENT LABELING

This product (like all oral contraceptives) is intended to prevent pregnancy. It does not protect against HIV infection (AIDS) and other sexually transmitted diseases.

INTRODUCTION

Any woman who considers using oral contraceptives (the birth- control pill or the pill) should understand the benefits and risks of using this form of birth control. This leaflet will give you much of the information you will need to make this decision and will also help you determine if you are at risk of developing any of the serious side effects of the pill. It will tell you how to use the pill properly so that it will be as effective as possible. However, this leaflet is not a replacement for a careful discussion between you and your health-care provider. You should discuss the information provided in this leaflet with him or her, both when you first start taking the pill and during your revisits. You should also follow your health-care provider's advice with regard to regular check-ups while you are on the pill.

EFFECTIVENESS OF ORAL CONTRACEPTIVES

Oral contraceptives or "birth-control pills" or "the pill" are used to prevent pregnancy and are more effective than other nonsurgical methods of birth control. When they are taken correctly, the chance of becoming pregnant is less than 1.0% when used perfectly, without missing any pills. Typical failure rates are less than 3.0% per year. The chance of becoming pregnant increases with each missed pill during the menstrual cycle.

In comparison, typical failure rates for other nonsurgical methods of birth control during the first year of use are as follows:

IUD: 3%
DEPO-PROVERA® (injectable progestogen): 0.3%
NORPLANT® SYSTEM (implants): 0.2%
Diaphragm with spermicides: 18%
Spermicides alone: 21%
Male condom alone: 12%
Periodic abstinence: 20%
No methods: 85%

WHO SHOULD NOT TAKE ORAL CONTRACEPTIVES

Cigarette smoking increases the risk of serious adverse effects on the heart and blood vessels from oral-contraceptive use. This risk increases with age and with heavy smoking (15 or more cigarettes per day) and is quite marked in women over 35 years of age. Women who use oral contraceptives should not smoke.

Some women should not use the pill. For example, you should not take the pill if you are pregnant or think you may be pregnant. You should also not use the pill if you have had any of the following conditions:

- Heart attack or stroke.
- Blood clots in the legs (thrombophlebitis), lungs (pulmonary embolism), or eyes.
- Blood clots in the deep veins of your legs.
- Known or suspected breast cancer or cancer of the lining of the uterus, cervix, or vagina.
- Liver tumor (benign or cancerous).

Or, if you have any of the following:

- Chest pain (angina pectoris).
- Unexplained vaginal bleeding (until a diagnosis is reached by your doctor).
- Yellowing of the whites of the eyes or of the skin (jaundice) during pregnancy or during previous use of the pill.
- Known or suspected pregnancy.

Tell your health-care provider if you have ever had any of these conditions. Your health-care provider can recommend another method of birth control.

OTHER CONSIDERATIONS BEFORE TAKING ORAL CONTRACEPTIVES

Tell your health-care provider if you or any family member has ever had:

- Breast nodules, fibrocystic disease of the breast, an abnormal breast X ray or mammogram.
- Diabetes.
- Elevated cholesterol or triglycerides.
- High blood pressure.
- Migraine or other headaches or epilepsy.
- Mental depression.
- Gallbladder, heart, or kidney disease.
- History of scanty or irregular menstrual periods.

Women with any of these conditions should be checked often by their health-care provider if they choose to use oral contraceptives. Also, be sure to inform your doctor or health-care provider if you smoke or are on any medications.

RISKS OF TAKING ORAL CONTRACEPTIVES

1. Risk of developing blood clots

Blood clots and blockage of blood vessels are the most serious side effects of taking oral contraceptives and can be fatal. In particular, a clot in the legs can cause thrombophlebitis and a clot that travels to the lungs can cause a sudden blocking of the vessel carrying blood to the lungs. Rarely, clots occur in the blood vessels of the eye and may cause blindness, double vision, or impaired vision.

If you take oral contraceptives and need elective surgery, need to stay in bed for a prolonged illness, or have recently delivered a baby, you may be at risk of developing blood clots. You should consult your doctor about stopping oral contraceptives three to four weeks before surgery and not taking oral contraceptives for two weeks after surgery or during bed rest. You should also not take oral contraceptives soon after delivery of a baby or a midtrimester pregnancy termination. It is advisable to wait for at least four weeks after delivery if you are not breast-feeding. If you are breast-feeding, you should wait until you have weaned your child before using the pill. (See also the section on breast-feeding in "General Precautions".)

2. Heart attacks and strokes

Oral contraceptives may increase the tendency to develop strokes (stoppage or rupture of blood vessels in the brain) and angina pectoris and heart attacks (blockage of blood vessels in the heart). Any of these conditions can cause death or serious disability.

Smoking greatly increases the possibility of suffering heart attacks and strokes. Furthermore, smoking and the use of oral contraceptives greatly increase the chances of developing and dying of heart disease.

3. Gallbladder disease

Oral-contraceptive users probably have a greater risk than nonusers of having gallbladder disease, although this risk may be related to pills containing high doses of estrogens.

4. Liver tumors

In rare cases, oral contraceptives can cause benign but dangerous liver tumors. These benign liver tumors can rupture and cause fatal internal bleeding. In addition, a possible but not definite association has been found with the pill and liver cancers in two studies in which a few women who developed these very rare cancers were found to have used oral contraceptives for long periods. However, liver cancers are extremely rare. The chance of developing liver cancer from using the pill is thus even rarer.

5. Cancer of the reproductive organs

There is, at present, no confirmed evidence that oral contraceptives increase the risk of cancer of the reproductive organs in human studies. Several studies have found no overall increase in the risk of developing breast cancer. However, women who use oral contraceptives and have a strong family history of breast cancer or who have breast nodules or abnormal mammograms should be closely followed by their doctors.

Some studies have found an increase in the incidence of cancer of the cervix in women who use oral contraceptives. However, this finding may be related to factors other than the use of oral contraceptives.

ESTIMATED RISK OF DEATH FROM A BIRTH-CONTROL METHOD OR PREGNANCY

All methods of birth control and pregnancy are associated with a risk of developing certain diseases which may lead to disability or death. An estimate of the number of deaths associated with different methods of birth control and pregnancy has been calculated and is shown in the following table.

[See table below]

In the above table, the risk of death from any birth-control method is less than the risk of childbirth, except for oral-contraceptive users over the age of 35 who smoke and pill users over the age of 40 even if they do not smoke. It can be seen in the table that for women aged 15 to 39, the risk of death was highest with pregnancy (7 to 26 deaths per 100,000 women, depending on age). Among pill users who do not smoke, the risk of death was always lower than that associated with pregnancy for any age group, except for those women over the age of 40, when the risk increases to 32 deaths per 100,000 women, compared to 28 associated with pregnancy at that age. However, for pill users who smoke and are over the age of 35, the estimated number of deaths exceeds those for other methods of birth control. If a woman is over the age of 40 and smokes, her estimated risk of death is four times higher (117/100,000 women) than the estimated risk associated with pregnancy (28/100,000 women) in that age group.

The suggestion that women over 40 who don't smoke should not take oral contraceptives is based on information from older high-dose pills and on less-selective use of pills than is practiced today. An Advisory Committee of the FDA discussed this issue in 1989 and recommended that the benefits of oral-contraceptive use by healthy, nonsmoking women over 40 years of age may outweigh the possible risks. However, all women, especially older women, are cautioned to use the lowest-dose pill that is effective.

WARNING SIGNALS

If any of these adverse effects occur while you are taking oral contraceptives, call your doctor immediately:

- Sharp chest pain, coughing of blood, or sudden shortness of breath (indicating a possible clot in the lung).
- Pain in the calf (indicating a possible clot in the leg).
- Crushing chest pain or heaviness in the chest (indicating a possible heart attack).
- Sudden severe headache or vomiting, dizziness or fainting, disturbances of vision or speech, weakness, or numbness in an arm or leg (indicating a possible stroke).
- Sudden partial or complete loss of vision (indicating a possible clot in the eye).
- Breast lumps (indicating possible breast cancer or fibrocystic disease of the breast; ask your doctor or health-care provider to show you how to examine your breasts).
- Severe pain or tenderness in the stomach area (indicating a possibly ruptured liver tumor).
- Difficulty in sleeping, weakness, lack of energy, fatigue, or change in mood (possibly indicating severe depression).
- Jaundice or a yellowing of the skin or eyeballs, accompanied frequently by fever, fatigue, loss of appetite, dark-colored urine, or light-colored bowel movements (indicating possible liver problems).

SIDE EFFECTS OF ORAL CONTRACEPTIVES

1. Vaginal bleeding

Irregular vaginal bleeding or spotting may occur while you are taking the pills. Irregular bleeding may vary from slight staining between menstrual periods to breakthrough bleeding which is a flow much like a regular period. Irregular bleeding occurs most often during the first few months of oral-contraceptive use, but may also occur after you have been taking the pill for some time. Such bleeding may be temporary and usually does not indicate any serious problems. It is important to continue taking your pills on schedule. If the bleeding occurs in more than one cycle or lasts for more than a few days, talk to your doctor or health-care provider.

2. Contact lenses

If you wear contact lenses and notice a change in vision or an inability to wear your lenses, contact your doctor or health-care provider.

3. Fluid retention

Oral contraceptives may cause edema (fluid retention) with swelling of the fingers or ankles and may raise your blood pressure. If you experience fluid retention, contact your doctor or health-care provider.

4. Melasma

A spotty darkening of the skin is possible, particularly of the face.

5. Other side effects

Other side effects may include change in appetite, headache, nervousness, depression, dizziness, loss of scalp hair, rash, and vaginal infections.

If any of these side effects bother you, call your doctor or health-care provider.

GENERAL PRECAUTIONS

1. Missed periods and use of oral contraceptives before or during early pregnancy

There may be times when you may not menstruate regularly after you have completed taking a cycle of pills. If you have taken your pills regularly and miss one menstrual period, continue taking your pills for the next cycle but be sure to inform your health-care provider before doing so. If you have not taken the pills daily as instructed and missed a menstrual period, or if you missed two consecutive menstrual periods, you may be pregnant. Check with your health-care provider immediately to determine whether you are pregnant. Do not continue to take oral contraceptives until you are sure you are not pregnant, but continue to use another method of contraception.

ANNUAL NUMBER OF BIRTH-RELATED OR METHOD-RELATED DEATHS ASSOCIATED WITH CONTROL OF FERTILITY PER 100,000 NONSTERILE WOMEN, BY FERTILITY-CONTROL METHOD AND ACCORDING TO AGE

Method of control and outcome	15–19	20–24	25–29	30–34	35–39	40–44
No fertility-control methods*	7.0	7.4	9.1	14.8	25.7	28.2
Oral contraceptives nonsmoker**	0.3	0.5	0.9	1.9	13.8	31.6
Oral contraceptives smoker**	2.2	3.4	6.6	13.5	51.1	117.2
IUD**	0.8	0.8	1.0	1.0	1.4	1.4
Condom*	1.1	1.6	0.7	0.2	0.3	0.4
Diaphragm/spermicide*	1.9	1.2	1.2	1.3	2.2	2.8
Periodic abstinence*	2.5	1.6	1.6	1.7	2.9	3.6

* Deaths are birth related
** Deaths are method related

There is no conclusive evidence that oral-contraceptive use is associated with an increase in birth defects when taken inadvertently during early pregnancy. Previously, a few studies had reported that oral contraceptives might be associated with birth defects, but these studies have not been confirmed. Nevertheless, oral contraceptives or any other drugs should not be used during pregnancy unless clearly necessary and prescribed by your doctor. You should check with your doctor about risks to your unborn child of any medication taken during pregnancy.

2. While breast-feeding

If you are breast-feeding, consult your doctor before starting oral contraceptives. Some of the drug will be passed on to the child in the milk. A few adverse effects on the child have been reported, including yellowing of the skin (jaundice) and breast enlargement. In addition, oral contraceptives may decrease the amount and quality of your milk. If possible, do not use oral contraceptives while breast-feeding. You should use another method of contraception since breast-feeding provides only partial protection from becoming pregnant, and this partial protection decreases significantly as you breast-feed for longer periods of time. You should consider starting oral contraceptives only after you have weaned your child completely.

3. Laboratory tests

If you are scheduled for any laboratory tests, tell your doctor you are taking birth-control pills. Certain blood tests may be affected by birth-control pills.

4. Drug interactions

Certain drugs may interact with birth-control pills to make them less effective in preventing pregnancy or cause an increase in breakthrough bleeding. Such drugs include rifampin, drugs used for epilepsy such as barbiturates (for example, phenobarbital) and phenytoin (Dilantin is one brand of this drug), phenylbutazone (Butazolidin is one brand), and possibly certain antibiotics. You may need to use an additional method of contraception during any cycle in which you take drugs that can make oral contraceptives less effective.

HOW TO TAKE THE PILL

This product (like all oral contraceptives) is intended to prevent pregnancy. It does not protect against transmission of HIV (AIDS) and other sexually transmitted diseases such as chlamydia, genital herpes, genital warts, gonorrhea, hepatitis B, and syphilis.

IMPORTANT POINTS TO REMEMBER

BEFORE YOU START TAKING YOUR PILLS:

1. BE SURE TO READ THESE DIRECTIONS:
Before you start taking your pills.
Anytime you are not sure what to do.

2. THE RIGHT WAY TO TAKE THE PILL IS TO TAKE ONE PILL EVERY DAY AT THE SAME TIME.
If you miss pills you could get pregnant. This includes starting the pack late. The more pills you miss, the more likely you are to get pregnant.

3. MANY WOMEN HAVE SPOTTING OR LIGHT BLEEDING, OR MAY FEEL SICK TO THEIR STOMACH DURING THE FIRST 1-3 PACKS OF PILLS.
If you feel sick to your stomach, do not stop taking the pill. The problem will usually go away. If it doesn't go away, check with your doctor or clinic.

4. MISSING PILLS CAN ALSO CAUSE SPOTTING OR LIGHT BLEEDING, even when you make up these missed pills.
On the days you take 2 pills to make up for missed pills, you could also feel a little sick to your stomach.

5. IF YOU HAVE VOMITING OR DIARRHEA, for any reason, or IF YOU TAKE SOME MEDICINES, including some antibiotics, your pills may not work as well. Use a back-up method (such as condoms or foam) until you check with your doctor or clinic.

6. IF YOU HAVE TROUBLE REMEMBERING TO TAKE THE PILL, talk to your doctor or clinic about how to make pill-taking easier or about using another method of birth control.

7. IF YOU HAVE ANY QUESTIONS OR ARE UNSURE ABOUT THE INFORMATION IN THIS LEAFLET, call your doctor or clinic.

NORDETTE®- 21, OVRAL®, LO/OVRAL®, NORDETTE®-28, OVRAL®-28, AND LO/OVRAL®-28

***BEFORE* YOU START TAKING YOUR PILLS**

1. DECIDE WHAT TIME OF DAY YOU WANT TO TAKE YOUR PILL.
It is important to take it at about the same time every day.

2. LOOK AT YOUR PILL PACK TO SEE IF IT HAS 21 OR 28 PILLS:
The *21-pill pack* has 21 "active" white or light-orange pills (with hormones) to take for 3 weeks, followed by 1 week without pills.
The *28-pill pack* has 21 "active" white or light-orange pills (with hormones) to take for 3 weeks, followed by 1 week of reminder pink pills (without hormones).

3. ALSO FIND:
1) where on the pack to start taking pills, and
2) in what order to take the pills (follow the arrows).
[See figure at top of next column]

4. BE SURE YOU HAVE READY AT ALL TIMES:
ANOTHER KIND OF BIRTH CONTROL (such as condoms or foam) to use as a back-up in case you miss pills.
AN EXTRA, FULL PILL PACK.

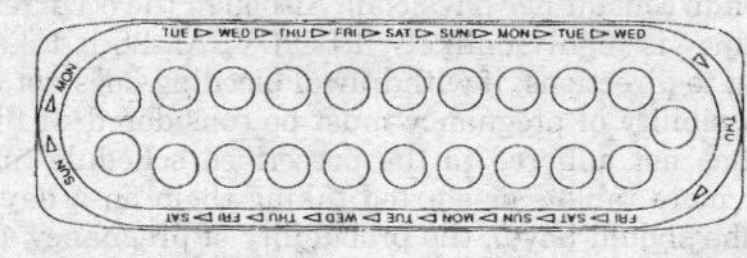

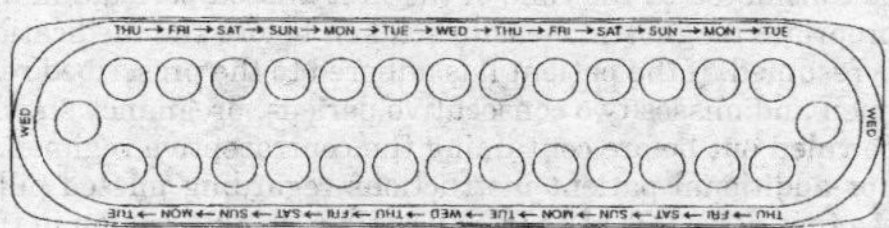

WHEN TO START THE *FIRST* PACK OF PILLS

For the 21-day pill pack you have two choices of which day to start taking your first pack of pills. (See **DAY 1 START** or **SUNDAY START** directions below.) Decide with your doctor or clinic which is the best day for you. The 28-day pill pack accommodates a **SUNDAY START** only. For either pill pack pick a time of day which will be easy to remember.

DAY 1 START:

These instructions are for the 21-day pill pack only. The 28-day pill pack does not accommodate a **DAY 1 START** dosage regimen.

1. Take the first "active" white or light-orange pill of the first pack during the *first 24 hours of your period.*
2. You will not need to use a back-up method of birth control, since you are starting the pill at the beginning of your period.

SUNDAY START:

These instructions are for either the 21-day or the 28-day pill pack.

1. Take the first "active" white or light-orange pill of the first pack on the *Sunday after your period starts,* even if you are still bleeding. If your period begins on Sunday, start the pack that same day.
2. *Use another method of birth control* as a back-up method if you have sex anytime from the Sunday you start your first pack until the next Sunday (7 days). Condoms or foam are good back-up methods of birth control.

WHAT TO DO DURING THE MONTH

1. TAKE ONE PILL AT THE SAME TIME EVERY DAY UNTIL THE PACK IS EMPTY.

Do not skip pills even if you are spotting or bleeding between monthly periods or feel sick to your stomach (nausea).
Do not skip pills even if you do not have sex very often.

2. WHEN YOU FINISH A PACK OR SWITCH YOUR BRAND OF PILLS:

21 pills: Wait 7 days to start the next pack. You will probably have your period during that week. Be sure that no more than 7 days pass between 21-day packs.
28 pills: Start the next pack on the day after your last "reminder" pill. Do not wait any days between packs.

WHAT TO DO IF YOU MISS PILLS

If you **MISS** 1 white or light-orange "active" pill:
1. Take it as soon as you remember. Take the next pill at your regular time. This means you take 2 pills in 1 day.
2. You do not need to use a back-up birth control method if you have sex.

If you **MISS 2** white or light-orange "active" pills in a row in **WEEK 1 or WEEK 2** of your pack:
1. Take 2 pills on the day you remember and 2 pills the next day.
2. Then take 1 pill a day until you finish the pack.
3. You MAY BECOME PREGNANT if you have sex in the 7 *days* after you miss pills. You MUST use another birth control method (such as condoms or foam) as a back-up for those 7 days.

If you **MISS 2** white or light-orange "active" pills in a row in **THE 3rd WEEK:**
The ***Day 1 Starter*** instructions are for the 21-day pill pack only. The 28-day pill pack does not accommodate a **DAY 1 START** dosage regimen. The ***Sunday Starter*** instructions are for either the 21-day or 28-day pill pack.

1. ***If you are a Day 1 Starter:***
THROW OUT the rest of the pill pack and start a new pack that same day.
If you are a Sunday Starter:
Keep taking 1 pill every day until Sunday.
On Sunday, THROW OUT the rest of the pack and start a new pack of pills that same day.
2. You may not have your period this month but this is expected. However, if you miss your period 2 months in a row, call your doctor or clinic because you might be pregnant.
3. You MAY BECOME PREGNANT if you have sex in the 7 *days* after you miss pills. You MUST use another birth control method (such as condoms or foam) as a back-up for those 7 days.

If you **MISS 3 OR MORE** white or light-orange "active" pills in a row (during the first 3 weeks):
The ***Day 1 Starter*** instructions are for the 21-day pill pack only. The 28-day pill pack does not accommodate a **DAY 1 START** dosage regimen. The ***Sunday Starter*** instructions are for either the 21-day or 28-day pill pack.

1. ***If you are a Day 1 Starter:***
THROW OUT the rest of the pill pack and start a new pack that same day.
If you are a Sunday Starter:
Keep taking 1 pill every day until Sunday.
On Sunday, THROW OUT the rest of the pack and start a new pack of pills that same day.
2. You may not have your period this month but this is expected. However, if you miss your period 2 months in a row, call your doctor or clinic because you might be pregnant.
3. You MAY BECOME PREGNANT if you have sex in the 7 *days* after you miss pills. You MUST use another birth control method (such as condoms or foam) as a back-up for those 7 days.

A REMINDER FOR THOSE ON 28-DAY PACKS:

If you forget any of the 7 pink "reminder" pills in Week 4:
THROW AWAY the pills you missed.
Keep taking 1 pill each day until the pack is empty.
You do not need a back-up method if you start your next pack on time.

FINALLY, IF YOU ARE STILL NOT SURE WHAT TO DO ABOUT THE PILLS YOU HAVE MISSED:

Use a BACK-UP METHOD anytime you have sex.
KEEP TAKING ONE PILL EACH DAY until you can reach your doctor or clinic.

OVRETTE®

Ovrette is administered on a continuous daily dosage schedule, one tablet each day, every day of the year. Take the first tablet on the first day of your menstrual period. Tablets should be taken at the same time every day, without interruption, whether bleeding occurs or not. If bleeding is prolonged (more than 8 days) or unusually heavy, you should contact your doctor.

Forgotten pills

The risk of pregnancy increases with each tablet missed. Therefore, it is very important that you take one tablet daily as directed. If you miss one tablet, take it as soon as you remember and also take your next tablet at the regular time. If you miss two tablets, take one of the missed tablets as soon as you remember, as well as your regular tablet for that day at the proper time. Furthermore, you should use another method of birth control in addition to taking Ovrette until you have taken fourteen days (2 weeks) of medication.

If more than two tablets have been missed, Ovrette should be discontinued immediately and another method of birth control used until the start of your next menstrual period. Then you may resume taking Ovrette.

Pregnancy due to pill failure

The incidence of pill failure resulting in pregnancy is approximately less than 1.0% if taken every day as directed, but more typical failure rates are less than 3.0%. If failure does occur, the risk to the fetus is minimal.

RISKS TO THE FETUS

If you do become pregnant while using oral contraceptives, the risk to the fetus is small, on the order of no more than one per thousand. You should, however, discuss the risks to the developing child with your doctor.

Pregnancy after stopping the pill

There may be some delay in becoming pregnant after you stop using oral contraceptives, especially if you had irregular menstrual cycles before you used oral contraceptives. It may be advisable to postpone conception until you begin menstruating regularly once you have stopped taking the pill and desire pregnancy.

There does not appear to be any increase in birth defects in newborn babies when pregnancy occurs soon after stopping the pill.

Overdosage

Serious ill effects have not been reported following ingestion of large doses of oral contraceptives by young children. Overdosage may cause nausea and withdrawal bleeding in females. In case of overdosage, contact your health-care provider or pharmacist.

Other information

Your health-care provider will take a medical and family history before prescribing oral contraceptives and will examine you. The physical examination may be delayed to another time if you request it and the health-care provider believes that it is appropriate to postpone it. You should be reexamined at least once a year. Be sure to inform your health-care provider if there is a family history of any of the conditions listed previously in this leaflet. Be sure to keep all appointments with your health-care provider, because this is a time to determine if there are early signs of side effects of oral-contraceptive use.

Do not use the drug for any condition other than the one for which it was prescribed. This drug has been prescribed specifically for you; do not give it to others who may want birth-control pills.

HEALTH BENEFITS FROM ORAL CONTRACEPTIVES

In addition to preventing pregnancy, use of oral contraceptives may provide certain benefits. They are:

- Menstrual cycles may become more regular
- Blood flow during menstruation may be lighter, and less iron may be lost. Therefore, anemia due to iron deficiency is less likely to occur.

Continued on next page

Lo/Ovral—Cont.

- Pain or other symptoms during menstruation may be encountered less frequently
- Ovarian cysts may occur less frequently
- Ectopic (tubal) pregnancy may occur less frequently
- Noncancerous cysts or lumps in the breast may occur less frequently
- Acute pelvic inflammatory disease may occur less frequently
- Oral-contraceptive use may provide some protection against developing two forms of cancer: cancer of the ovaries and cancer of the lining of the uterus.

If you want more information about birth-control pills, ask your doctor or pharmacist. They have a more technical leaflet called the Professional Labeling which you may wish to read.

Manufactured by:
Wyeth Laboratories
A Wyeth-Ayerst Company
Philadelphia, PA 19101
CI 4257-3 Revised August 14, 1996

Shown in Product Identification Guide, page 341

LO/OVRAL®-28 ℞

[*lōh-ōh 'vrăl-28*]
Tablets
(norgestrel and ethinyl estradiol tablets)

Patients should be counseled that this product does not protect against HIV infection (AIDS) and other sexually transmitted diseases.

DESCRIPTION

21 white LO/OVRAL tablets, each containing 0.3 mg of norgestrel (*dl* -13-beta-ethyl-17-alpha-ethinyl-17-beta-hydroxygon-4-en-3-one), a totally synthetic progestogen, and 0.03 mg of ethinyl estradiol (19-nor-17α-pregna-1,3,5(10)-trien-20-yne-3,17-diol), and 7 pink inert tablets. The inactive ingredients present are cellulose, D&C Red 30, lactose, magnesium stearate, and polacrilin potassium.

CLINICAL PHARMACOLOGY

See LO/OVRAL®.

INDICATIONS AND USAGE

See LO/OVRAL.

CONTRAINDICATIONS

See LO/OVRAL.

WARNINGS

See LO/OVRAL.

PRECAUTIONS

See LO/OVRAL.
Drug Interactions: See LO/OVRAL.
Carcinogenesis: See LO/OVRAL.
Pregnancy: See LO/OVRAL.
Nursing Mothers: See LO/OVRAL.
Information for the Patient: See LO/OVRAL.

ADVERSE REACTIONS

See LO/OVRAL.

OVERDOSAGE

See LO/OVRAL.

NONCONTRACEPTIVE HEALTH BENEFITS

See LO/OVRAL.

DOSAGE AND ADMINISTRATION

To achieve maximum contraceptive effectiveness, LO/OVRAL-28 must be taken exactly as directed and at intervals not exceeding 24 hours.
The dosage of LO/OVRAL-28 is one white tablet daily for 21 consecutive days, followed by one pink inert tablet daily for 7 consecutive days, according to prescribed schedule. It is recommended that tablets be taken at the same time each day, preferably after the evening meal or at bedtime.
During the first cycle of medication, the patient is instructed to begin taking LO/OVRAL-28 on the first Sunday after the onset of menstruation. If menstruation begins on a Sunday, the first tablet (white) is taken that day. One white tablet should be taken daily for 21 consecutive days followed by one pink inert tablet daily for 7 consecutive days. Withdrawal bleeding should usually occur within three days following discontinuation of white tablets. During the first cycle, contraceptive reliance should not be placed on LO/OVRAL-28 until a white tablet has been taken daily for 7 consecutive days. The possibility of ovulation and conception prior to initiation of medication should be considered.
The patient begins her next and all subsequent 28-day courses of tablets on the same day of the week (Sunday) on which she began her first course, following the same schedule: 21 days on white tablets—7 days on pink inert tablets. If in any cycle the patient starts tablets later than the proper day, she should protect herself by using another method of birth control until she has taken a white tablet daily for 7 consecutive days.
If spotting or breakthrough bleeding occurs, the patient is instructed to continue on the same regimen. This type of bleeding is usually transient and without significance; however, if the bleeding is persistent or prolonged, the patient is advised to consult her physician. Although the occurrence of pregnancy is highly unlikely if LO/OVRAL-28 is taken according to directions, if withdrawal bleeding does not occur, the possibility of pregnancy must be considered. If the patient has not adhered to the prescribed schedule (missed one or more tablets or started taking them on a day later than she should have), the probability of pregnancy should be considered at the time of the first missed period and appropriate diagnostic measures taken before the medication is resumed. If the patient has adhered to the prescribed regimen and misses two consecutive periods, pregnancy should be ruled out before continuing the contraceptive regimen.
For additional patient instructions regarding missed pills, see the "WHAT TO DO IF YOU MISS PILLS" section in the **DETAILED PATIENT LABELING** for LO/OVRAL.
Any time the patient misses two or more white tablets, she should also use another method of contraception until she has taken a white tablet daily for seven consecutive days. If the patient misses one or more pink tablets, she is still protected against pregnancy **provided** she begins taking white tablets again on the proper day.
If breakthrough bleeding occurs following missed white tablets, it will usually be transient and of no consequence. While there is little likelihood of ovulation occurring if only one or two white tablets are missed, the possibility of ovulation increases with each successive day that scheduled white tablets are missed.
In the nonlactating mother, LO/OVRAL-28 may be initiated postpartum, for contraception. When the tablets are administered in the postpartum period, the increased risk of thromboembolic disease associated with the postpartum period must be considered (see "Contraindications," "Warnings," and "Precautions" concerning thromboembolic disease). It is to be noted that early resumption of ovulation may occur if Parlodel® (bromocriptine mesylate) has been used for the prevention of lactation.

HOW SUPPLIED

LO/OVRAL®-28 Tablets (0.3 mg norgestrel and 0.03 mg ethinyl estradiol) are available in packages of 6 PILPAK® dispensers, each containing 28 tablets as follows:
21 active tablets, NDC 0008-0078, white, round tablet marked "WYETH" and "78".
7 inert tablets, NDC 0008-0486, pink, round tablet marked "WYETH" and "486".
ALSO AVAILABLE:
LO/OVRAL®-28 Tablets (0.3 mg norgestrel and 0.03 mg ethinyl estradiol) are available in packages of 12 PILPAK® dispensers for clinic use only, each containing 28 tablets as follows:
21 active tablets, NDC 0008-0078, white, round tablet marked "WYETH" and "78".
7 inert tablets, NDC 0008-0486, pink, round tablet marked "WYETH" and "486".
Store at room temperature, approx. 25°C (77°F).

References available upon request.

Brief Summary Patient Package Insert: See LO/OVRAL.
DETAILED PATIENT LABELING: See LO/OVRAL.

HOW TO TAKE THE PILL

For Lo/Ovral-28 PILPAK® Dispenser, See LO/OVRAL.
For Lo/Ovral-28 Clinic Pilpak®, See below.
HOW TO TAKE THE PILL
This product (like all oral contraceptives) is intended to prevent pregnancy. It does not protect against transmission of HIV (AIDS) and other sexually transmitted diseases such as chlamydia, genital herpes, genital warts, gonorrhea, hepatitis B, and syphilis.

IMPORTANT POINTS TO REMEMBER

BEFORE YOU START TAKING YOUR PILLS:
1. BE SURE TO READ THESE DIRECTIONS:
Before you start taking your pills.
Anytime you are not sure what to do.
2. THE RIGHT WAY TO TAKE THE PILL IS TO TAKE ONE PILL EVERY DAY AT THE SAME TIME.
If you miss pills you could get pregnant. This includes starting the pack late. The more pills you miss, the more likely you are to get pregnant.
3. MANY WOMEN HAVE SPOTTING OR LIGHT BLEEDING, OR MAY FEEL SICK TO THEIR STOMACH DURING THE FIRST 1–3 PACKS OF PILLS.
If you feel sick to your stomach, do not stop taking the pill. The problem will usually go away. If it doesn't go away, check with your doctor or clinic.
4. MISSING PILLS CAN ALSO CAUSE SPOTTING OR LIGHT BLEEDING, even when you make up these missed pills.
On the days you take 2 pills to make up for missed pills, you could also feel a little sick to your stomach.
5. IF YOU HAVE VOMITING OR DIARRHEA, for any reason, or IF YOU TAKE SOME MEDICINES, including some antibiotics, your pills may not work as well. Use a back-up method (such as condoms or foam) until you check with your doctor or clinic.
6. IF YOU HAVE TROUBLE REMEMBERING TO TAKE THE PILL, talk to your doctor or clinic about how to make pill-taking easier or about using another method of birth control.
7. IF YOU HAVE ANY QUESTIONS OR ARE UNSURE ABOUT THE INFORMATION IN THIS LEAFLET, call your doctor or clinic.

NORDETTE®-21, OVRAL®, LO/OVRAL®, NORDETTE®-28, OVRAL®-28, AND LO/OVRAL®-28

***BEFORE* YOU START TAKING YOUR PILLS**

1. DECIDE WHAT TIME OF DAY YOU WANT TO TAKE YOUR PILL.
It is important to take it at about the same time every day.
2. LOOK AT YOUR PILL PACK TO SEE IF IT HAS 21 OR 28 PILLS:
The *21-pill pack* has 21 "active" white or light-orange pills (with hormones) to take for 3 weeks, followed by 1 week without pills.
The *28-pill pack* has 21 "active" white or light-orange pills (with hormones) to take for 3 weeks, followed by 1 week of reminder pink pills (without hormones).
3. ALSO FIND:
1) where on the pack to start taking pills,
2) in what order to take the pills (follow the arrows), and
3) the week numbers as shown in the picture below.

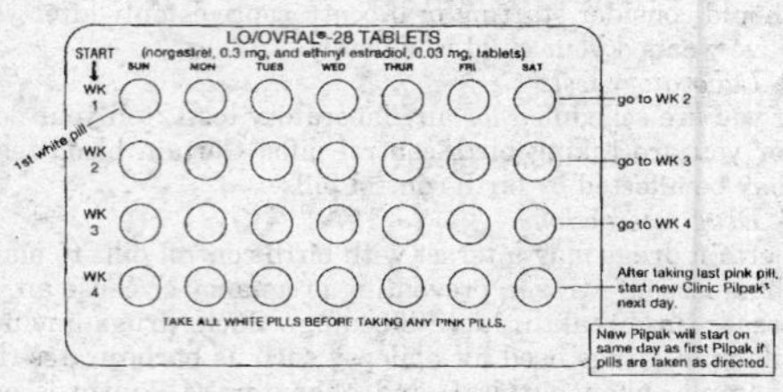

4. BE SURE YOU HAVE READY AT ALL TIMES:
ANOTHER KIND OF BIRTH CONTROL (such as condoms or foam) to use as a back-up in case you miss pills.
AN EXTRA, FULL PILL PACK.

WHEN TO START THE *FIRST* PACK OF PILLS:

For the 21-day pill pack you have two choices of which day to start taking your first pack of pills. (See **DAY 1 START** or **SUNDAY START** directions below.) Decide with your doctor or clinic which is the best day for you. The 28-day pill pack accommodates a **SUNDAY START** only. For either pill pack pick a time of day which will be easy to remember.
DAY 1 START:
These instructions are for the 21-day pill pack only. The 28-day pill pack does not accommodate a **DAY 1 START** dosage regimen.
1. Take the first "active" white or light-orange pill of the first pack during the *first 24 hours of your period.*
2. You will not need to use a back-up method of birth control, since you are starting the pill at the beginning of your period.
SUNDAY START:
These instructions are for either the 21-day or the 28-day pill pack.
1. Take the first "active" white or light-orange pill of the first pack on the *Sunday after your period starts,* even if you are still bleeding. If your period begins on Sunday, start the pack that same day.
2. *Use another method of birth control* as a back-up method if you have sex anytime from the Sunday you start your first pack until the next Sunday (7 days). Condoms or foam are good back-up methods of birth control.

WHAT TO DO DURING THE MONTH:

1. TAKE ONE PILL AT THE SAME TIME EVERY DAY UNTIL THE PACK IS EMPTY.
Do not skip pills even if you are spotting or bleeding between monthly periods or feel sick to your stomach (nausea).
Do not skip pills even if you do not have sex very often.
2. WHEN YOU FINISH A PACK OR SWITCH YOUR BRAND OF PILLS:
21 pills: Wait 7 days to start the next pack. You will probably have your period during that week. Be sure that no more than 7 days pass between 21-day packs.
28 pills: Start the next pack on the day after your last "reminder" pill. Do not wait any days between packs.

WHAT TO DO IF YOU MISS PILLS

If you **MISS 1** white or light-orange "active" pill:
1. Take it as soon as you remember. Take the next pill at your regular time. This means you take 2 pills in 1 day.
2. You do not need to use a back-up birth control method if you have sex.
If you **MISS 2** white or light-orange "active" pills in a row in **WEEK 1 OR WEEK 2** of your pack:
1. Take 2 pills on the day you remember and 2 pills the next day.
2. Then take 1 pill a day until you finish the pack.
3. You MAY BECOME PREGNANT if you have sex in the 7 *days* after you miss pills. You MUST use another birth control method (such as condoms or foam) as a back-up for those 7 days.
If you **MISS 2** white or light-orange "active" pills in a row in **THE 3rd WEEK:**

The ***Day 1 Starter*** instructions are for the 21-day pill pack only. The 28-day pill pack does not accommodate a **DAY 1 START** dosage regimen. The ***Sunday Starter*** instructions are for either the 21-day or 28-day pill pack.

1. ***If you are a Day 1 Starter:***
THROW OUT the rest of the pill pack and start a new pack that same day.
If you are a Sunday Starter:
Keep taking 1 pill every day until Sunday.
On Sunday, THROW OUT the rest of the pack and start a new pack of pills that same day.
2. You may not have your period this month but this is expected.
However, if you miss your period 2 months in a row, call your doctor or clinic because you might be pregnant.
3. You MAY BECOME PREGNANT if you have sex in the 7 *days* after you miss pills. You MUST use another birth control method (such as condoms or foam) as a back-up for those 7 days.

If you **MISS 3 OR MORE** white or light-orange "active" pills in a row (during the first 3 weeks):
The ***Day 1 Starter*** instructions are for the 21-day pill pack only. The 28-day pill pack does not accommodate a **DAY 1 START** dosage regimen. The ***Sunday Starter*** instructions are for either the 21-day or 28-day pill pack.

1. ***If you are a Day 1 Starter:***
THROW OUT the rest of the pill pack and start a new pack that same day.
If you are a Sunday Starter:
Keep taking 1 pill every day until Sunday.
On Sunday, THROW OUT the rest of the pack and start a new pack of pills that same day.
2. You may not have your period this month but this is expected.
However, if you miss your period 2 months in a row, call your doctor or clinic because you might be pregnant.
3. You MAY BECOME PREGNANT if you have sex in the 7 *days* after you miss pills. You MUST use another birth control method (such as condoms or foam) as a back-up for those 7 days.

A REMINDER FOR THOSE ON 28-DAY PACKS:
If your forget any of the 7 pink "reminder" pills in Week 4:
THROW AWAY the pills you missed.
Keep taking 1 pill each day until the pack is empty.
You do not need a back-up method if you start your next pack on time.

FINALLY, IF YOU ARE STILL NOT SURE WHAT TO DO ABOUT THE PILLS YOU HAVE MISSED:
Use a BACK-UP METHOD anytime you have sex.
KEEP TAKING ONE PILL EACH DAY until you can reach your doctor or clinic.

OVRETTE®
Ovrette is administered on a continuous daily dosage schedule, one tablet each day, every day of the year. Take the first tablet on the first day of your menstrual period. Tablets should be taken at the same time every day without interruption, whether bleeding occurs or not. If bleeding is prolonged (more than 8 days) or unusually heavy, you should contact your doctor.

Forgotten pills
The risk of pregnancy increases with each tablet missed. Therefore, it is very important that you take one tablet daily as directed. If you miss one tablet, take it as soon as you remember and also take your next tablet at the regular time. If you miss two tablets, take one of the missed tablets as soon as you remember, as well as your regular tablet for that day at the proper time. Furthermore, you should use another method of birth control in addition to taking Ovrette until you have taken fourteen days (2 weeks) of medication.
If more than two tablets have been missed, Ovrette should be discontinued immediately and another method of birth control used until the start of your next menstrual period. Then you may resume taking Ovrette.

Pregnancy due to pill failure
The incidence of pill failure resulting in pregnancy is approximately less than 1.0% if taken every day as directed, but more typical failure rates are less than 3.0%. If failure does occur, the risk to the fetus is minimal.

RISKS TO THE FETUS
If you do become pregnant while using oral contraceptives, the risk to the fetus is small, on the order of no more than one per thousand. You should, however, discuss the risks to the developing child with your doctor.

Pregnancy after stopping the pill
There may be some delay in becoming pregnant after you stop using oral contraceptives, especially if you had irregular menstrual cycles before you used oral contraceptives. It may be advisable to postpone conception until you begin menstruating regularly once you have stopped taking the pill and desire pregnancy.
There does not appear to be any increase in birth defects in newborn babies when pregnancy occurs soon after stopping the pill.

Overdosage
Serious ill effects have not been reported following ingestion of large doses of oral contraceptives by young children. Overdosage may cause nausea and withdrawal bleeding in females. In case of overdosage, contact your health-care provider or pharmacist.

Other information
Your health-care provider will take a medical and family history before prescribing oral contraceptives and will examine you. The physical examination may be delayed to another time if you request it and the health-care provider believes that it is appropriate to postpone it. You should be reexamined at least once a year. Be sure to inform your health-care provider if there is a family history of any of the conditions listed previously in this leaflet. Be sure to keep all appointments with your health-care provider, because this is a time to determine if there are early signs of side effects of oral-contraceptive use.
Do not use the drug for any condition other than the one for which it was prescribed. This drug has been prescribed specifically for you; do not give it to others who may want birth-control pills.

HEALTH BENEFITS FROM ORAL CONTRACEPTIVES:
See LO/OVRAL.

Manufactured by:
Wyeth Laboratories
A Wyeth-Ayerst Company
Philadelphia, PA 19101

Shown in Product Identification Guide, page 341

CI 4259-3 Revised August 14, 1996

MEPERGAN®

Ⓒ ℞

[*mep 'er-gan*]
(meperidine HCl and promethazine HCl) Injection

DESCRIPTION
This product is available in concentration providing 25 mg each of meperidine hydrochloride and promethazine hydrochloride per mL with 0.1 mg edetate disodium, 0.04 mg calcium chloride, and not more than 0.75 mg sodium formaldehyde sulfoxylate, 0.25 mg sodium metabisulfite, and 5 mg phenol with sodium acetate buffer.

ACTIONS
Meperidine hydrochloride is a narcotic analgesic with multiple actions qualitatively similar to those of morphine. Phenergan®, promethazine HCl, is a phenothiazine derivative that has several different pharmacologic properties including antihistaminic, sedative, and antiemetic actions.

INDICATIONS
As a preanesthetic medication when analgesia and sedation are indicated. As an adjunct to local and general anesthesia.

CONTRAINDICATIONS
Hypersensitivity to meperidine or promethazine.
Under no circumstances should Mepergan be given by intra-arterial injection, due to the likelihood of severe arteriospasm and the possibility of resultant gangrene (see "**Warnings**").
Mepergan should not be given by the subcutaneous route; evidence of chemical irritation has been noted, and necrotic lesions have resulted on rare occasions following subcutaneous injection. The preferred parenteral route of administration is by deep intramuscular injection.
Meperidine is contraindicated in patients who are receiving monoamine oxidase inhibitors (MAOI) or those who have received such agents within 14 days. Therapeutic doses of meperidine have inconsistently precipitated unpredictable, severe, and occasionally fatal reactions in patients who have received such agents within 14 days. The mechanism of these reactions is unclear. Some have been characterized by coma, severe respiratory depression, cyanosis, and hypotension and have resembled the syndrome of acute narcotic overdose. In other reactions the predominant manifestations have been hyperexcitability, convulsions, tachycardia, hyperpyrexia, and hypertension. Although it is not known that other narcotics are free of the risk of such reactions, virtually all of the reported reactions have occurred with meperidine. If a narcotic is needed in such patients, a sensitivity test should be performed in which repeated, small, incremental doses of morphine are administered over the course of several hours while the patient's condition and vital signs are under careful observation.
(Intravenous hydrocortisone or prednisolone have been used to treat severe reactions, with the addition of intravenous chlorpromazine in those cases exhibiting hypertension and hyperpyrexia. The usefulness and safety of narcotic antagonists in the treatment of these reactions is unknown.)

WARNINGS
Mepergan Injection contains sodium metabisulfite, a sulfite that may cause allergic-type reactions, including anaphylactic symptoms and life-threatening or less severe asthmatic episodes, in certain susceptible people. The overall prevalence of sulfite sensitivity in the general population is unknown and probably low. Sulfite sensitivity is seen more frequently in asthmatic than in nonasthmatic people.

Tolerance and Addiction Liability
Warning—may be habit-forming

DRUG DEPENDENCE
Meperidine can produce drug dependence of the morphine type and therefore has the potential for being abused. Psychic dependence, physical dependence, and tolerance may develop upon repeated administration of meperidine, and it should be prescribed and administered with the same degree of caution appropriate to the use of morphine. Like other narcotics, meperidine is subject to the provisions of the Federal narcotic laws.

INTERACTION WITH OTHER CENTRAL NERVOUS SYSTEM DEPRESSANTS
Meperidine should be used with great caution and in reduced dosage in patients who are concurrently receiving other narcotic analgesics, general anesthetics, phenothiazines, other tranquilizers, sedative-hypnotics, tricyclic antidepressants, and other CNS depressants (including alcohol). Respiratory depression, hypotension, and profound sedation or coma may result.
The sedative action of promethazine hydrochloride is additive to the sedative effects of central nervous system depressants; therefore, agents such as alcohol, barbiturates, and narcotic analgesics should either be eliminated or given in reduced dosage in the presence of promethazine hydrochloride. When given concomitantly with promethazine hydrochloride, the dose of barbiturates should be reduced by at least one-half and the dose of analgesic depressants, such as morphine or meperidine, should be reduced by one-quarter to one-half.

HEAD INJURY AND INCREASED INTRACRANIAL PRESSURE
The respiratory-depressant effects of meperidine and its capacity to elevate cerebrospinal-fluid pressure may be markedly exaggerated in the presence of head injury, other intracranial lesions, or a preexisting increase in intracranial pressure. Furthermore, narcotics produce adverse reactions which may obscure the clinical course of patients with head injuries. In such patients, meperidine must be used with extreme caution and only if its use is deemed essential.

INADVERTENT INTRA-ARTERIAL INJECTION
Due to the close proximity of arteries and veins in the areas most commonly used for intravenous injection, extreme care should be exercised to avoid perivascular extravasation or inadvertent intra-arterial injection of Mepergan. Reports compatible with inadvertent intra-arterial injection suggest that pain, severe chemical irritation, severe spasm of distal vessels, and resultant gangrene requiring amputation is likely under such circumstances. Intravenous injection was intended in all the cases reported, but perivascular extravasation or arterial placement of the needle is now suspect. There is no proven successful management of this condition after it occurs, although sympathetic block and heparinization are commonly employed during the acute management because of the results of animal experiments with other known arteriolar irritants. Aspiration of dark blood does not preclude intra-arterial needle placement, because blood is discolored upon contact with promethazine. Use of syringes with rigid plungers or of small bore needles might obscure typical arterial backflow if this is relied upon alone.

INTRAVENOUS USE
If necessary, meperidine may be given intravenously, but the injection should be given very slowly, preferably in the form of a diluted solution. Rapid intravenous injection of narcotic analgesics, including meperidine, increases the incidence of adverse reactions; severe respiratory depression, apnea, hypotension, peripheral circulatory collapse, and cardiac arrest have occurred. Meperidine should not be administered intravenously unless a narcotic antagonist and the facilities for assisted or controlled respiration are immediately available. When meperidine is given parenterally, especially intravenously, the patient should be lying down.
When used intravenously, Mepergan should be given at a rate not to exceed 1 mL (25 mg of each component) per minute. When administering any irritant drug intravenously, it is usually preferable to inject it through the tubing of an intravenous infusion set that is known to be functioning satisfactorily. In the event that a patient complains of pain during intended intravenous injection of Mepergan, the injection should immediately be stopped to provide for evaluation of possible arterial placement or perivascular extravasation.

ASTHMA AND OTHER RESPIRATORY CONDITIONS
Meperidine should be used with extreme caution in patients having an acute asthmatic attack, patients with chronic obstructive pulmonary disease or cor pulmonale, patients having a substantially decreased respiratory reserve, and patients with preexisting respiratory depression, hypoxia, or hypercapnia. In such patients, even usual therapeutic doses of narcotics may decrease respiratory drive while simultaneously increasing airway resistance to the point of apnea.

HYPOTENSIVE EFFECT
The administration of meperidine may result in severe hypotension in an individual whose ability to maintain his blood pressure has already been compromised by a depleted blood volume or concurrent administration of drugs such as the phenothiazines or certain anesthetics.

USAGE IN AMBULATORY PATIENTS
Meperidine may impair the mental and/or physical abilities required for the performance of potentially hazardous tasks, such as driving a car or operating machinery. The patient should be cautioned accordingly.
Meperidine, like other narcotics, may produce orthostatic hypotension in ambulatory patients.

USAGE IN PREGNANCY AND LACTATION
Meperidine should not be used in pregnant women prior to the labor period, unless in the judgment of the physician the potential benefits outweigh the possible hazards, because

Continued on next page

Mepergan—Cont.

safe use in pregnancy prior to labor has not been established relative to possible adverse effects on fetal development.
When used as an obstetrical analgesic, meperidine crosses the placental barrier and can produce respiratory depression in the newborn; resuscitation may be required (see "**Overdosage**").
Meperidine appears in the milk of nursing mothers receiving the drug.

PRECAUTIONS

SUPRAVENTRICULAR TACHYCARDIAS
Meperidine should be used with caution in patients with atrial flutter and other supraventricular tachycardias because of a possible vagolytic action which may produce a significant increase in the ventricular response rate.
CONVULSIONS
Meperidine may aggravate preexisting convulsions in patients with convulsive disorders. If dosage is escalated substantially above recommended levels because of tolerance development, convulsions may occur in individuals without a history of convulsive disorders.
ACUTE ABDOMINAL CONDITIONS
The administration of meperidine or other narcotics may obscure the diagnosis or clinical course in patients with acute abdominal conditions.
SPECIAL-RISK PATIENTS
Meperidine should be given with caution, and the initial dose should be reduced in certain patients, such as the elderly or debilitated, and those with severe impairment of hepatic or renal function, hypothyroidism, Addison's disease, and prostatic hypertrophy or urethral stricture.
Antiemetics may mask the symptoms of an unrecognized disease and thereby interfere with diagnosis.
Patients in pain who have received inadequate or no analgesia have been noted to develop "athetoid-like" movements of the upper extremities following the parenteral administration of promethazine. These symptoms usually disappear upon adequate control of the pain.
Ambulatory patients should be cautioned against driving automobiles or operating dangerous machinery until it is known that they do not become drowsy or dizzy from promethazine hydrochloride therapy.

ADVERSE REACTIONS

The major hazards of meperidine, as with other narcotic analgesics, are respiratory depression and, to a lesser degree, circulatory depression; respiratory arrest, shock, and cardiac arrest have occurred.
The most frequently observed adverse reactions include light-headedness, dizziness, sedation, nausea, vomiting, and sweating. These effects seem to be more prominent in ambulatory patients and in those who are not experiencing severe pain. In such individuals, lower doses are advisable. Some adverse reactions in ambulatory patients may be alleviated if the patient lies down.
Other adverse reactions include:
CENTRAL NERVOUS SYSTEM
Euphoria, dysphoria, weakness, headache, agitation, tremor, uncoordinated muscle movements, transient hallucinations and disorientation, visual disturbances and, rarely, extrapyramidal reactions.
GASTROINTESTINAL
Dry mouth, constipation, biliary-tract spasm.
CARDIOVASCULAR
Flushing of the face, tachycardia, bradycardia, palpitation, faintness, syncope.
Cardiovascular effects from promethazine have been rare. Minor increases in blood pressure and occasional mild hypotension have been reported. Venous thrombosis at the injection site has been reported. Intra-arterial injection of Mepergan may result in gangrene of the affected extremity (see "**Warnings**").
GENITOURINARY
Urinary retention.
ALLERGIC
Pruritus, urticaria, other skin rashes, wheal and flare over the vein with IV injection.
Photosensitivity, although extremely rare, has been reported. Occurrence of photosensitivity may be a contraindication to further treatment with promethazine or related drugs.
OTHER
Pain at injection site; local tissue irritation, induration, and possible tissue necrosis, particularly when injection is repeated at same site; antidiuretic effect.
Patients may occasionally complain of autonomic reactions, such as dryness of the mouth, blurring of vision and, rarely, dizziness following the use of promethazine.
Very rare cases have been reported where patients receiving promethazine have developed leukopenia. In one instance agranulocytosis has been reported. In nearly every instance reported, other toxic agents known to have caused these conditions have been associated with the administration of promethazine.

DOSAGE AND ADMINISTRATION

Parenteral drug products should be inspected visually for particulate matter and discoloration prior to administration, whenever solution and container permit.
WARNING—BARBITURATES ARE NOT CHEMICALLY COMPATIBLE IN SOLUTION WITH MEPERGAN (MEPERIDINE HYDROCHLORIDE AND PROMETHAZINE HYDROCHLORIDE) AND SHOULD NOT BE MIXED IN THE SAME SYRINGE.
Mepergan is usually administered intramuscularly. However, in certain specific situations, the intravenous route may be employed. INADVERTENT INTRA-ARTERIAL INJECTION CAN RESULT IN GANGRENE OF THE AFFECTED EXTREMITY (see "**Warnings**"). SUBCUTANEOUS ADMINISTRATION IS CONTRAINDICATED, AS IT MAY RESULT IN TISSUE NECROSIS (see "**Contraindications**"). INJECTION INTO OR NEAR PERIPHERAL NERVES MAY RESULT IN PERMANENT NEUROLOGICAL DEFICIT.
When used intravenously, the rate should not be greater than 1 mL of Mepergan (25 mg of each component) per minute; it is preferable to inject through the tubing of an intravenous infusion set that is known to be functioning satisfactorily.
The TUBEX® BLUNT POINTE™ Sterile Cartridge Unit is suitable for substances to be administered intravenously only. It is intended for use with injection sets specifically manufactured as "needle-less" injection systems. TUBEX® BLUNT POINTE™ is compatible with Abbott's LifeShield® prepierced reseal injection site, Baxter's InterLink® Injection Site, and B. Braun Medical's SafSite® Reflux Valve, Consult manufacturer's recommendations regarding "Directions for Use" of the "needle-less" system. It is also intended for admixture with, and convenient administration of various medicaments when using Drug Vial Adapters for "needle-less" injection systems.
The TUBEX® Sterile Cartridge-Needle Unit is suitable for substances to be administered intravenously or intramuscularly.
The TUBEX® Sterile Cartridge-Needle Unit is designed for single-dose use. VIALS should be used when required doses are fractions of a milliliter, as indicated below.
ADULT DOSE: 1 to 2 mL (25 to 50 mg of each component) per single injection, which can be repeated every 3 to 4 hours.
CHILDREN 12 YEARS OF AGE AND UNDER: 0.5 mg of each component per pound of body weight. The dosage may be repeated every 3 to 4 hours as necessary.
For preanesthetic medication the usual adult dose is 2 mL (50 mg of each component) intramuscularly with or without appropriate atropine-like drug. Atropine sulfate, 0.3 to 0.4 mg, or scopolamine hydrobromide, 0.25 to 0.4 mg, in sterile solution may be mixed in the same syringe with Mepergan. Repeat doses of 50 mg or less of both promethazine and meperidine may be administered by either route at 3- to 4-hour intervals, as necessary. As an adjunct to local or general anesthesia, the usual dose is 2 mL (50 mg each of meperidine and promethazine).

OVERDOSAGE

SYMPTOMS
Serious overdose with meperidine is characterized by respiratory depression (a decrease in respiratory rate and/or tidal volume, Cheyne-Stokes respiration, cyanosis), extreme somnolence progressing to stupor or coma, skeletal muscle flaccidity, cold and clammy skin, and sometimes bradycardia and hypotension. In severe overdosage, particularly by the intravenous route, apnea, circulatory collapse, cardiac arrest, and death may occur.
TREATMENT
Primary attention should be given to the reestablishment of adequate respiratory exchange through provision of a patent airway and institution of assisted or controlled ventilation. The narcotic antagonist, naloxone hydrochloride, is a specific antidote against respiratory depression which may result from overdosage or unusual sensitivity to narcotics, including meperidine. The usual initial adult dose of naloxone is 0.4 to 2.0 mg, administered intravenously. If the desired degree of counteraction and improvement in respiratory functions is not obtained, this dosage can be repeated at two- to three-minute intervals while resuscitation efforts continue. If 10 mg of naloxone have been administered without an improvement in the clinical situation, the diagnosis of Mepergan overdose should be questioned.
An antagonist should not be administered in absence of clinically significant respiratory or cardiovascular depression. Oxygen, intravenous fluids, vasopressors, and other supportive measures should be employed as indicated.
NOTE: In an individual physically dependent on narcotics, the administration of the usual dose of a narcotic antagonist will precipitate an acute withdrawal syndrome. The severity of this syndrome will depend on the degree of physical dependence and the dose of antagonist administered. The use of narcotic antagonists in such individuals should be avoided if possible. If a narcotic antagonist must be used to treat serious respiratory depression in the physically dependent patient, the antagonist should be administered with extreme care and only one-tenth to one-fifth the usual initial dose administered.
Attempted suicides with promethazine have resulted in deep sedation, coma, rarely convulsions and cardiorespiratory symptoms compatible with the depth of sedation present. Extrapyramidal reactions may be treated with anticholinergic antiparkinson agents, diphenhydramine, or barbiturates.
If severe hypotension occurs, levarterenol or phenylephrine may be indicated. Epinephrine is probably best avoided, since it has been suggested that promethazine overdosage could produce a partial alpha-adrenergic blockade.
A paradoxical reaction, characterized by hyperexcitability and nightmares, has been reported in children receiving large single doses of promethazine.

HOW SUPPLIED

Mepergan® (meperidine HCl and promethazine HCl) Injection is available in TUBEX® BLUNT POINTE™ Sterile Cartridge Units and Sterile Cartridge-Needle Units, in boxes of 10 TUBEX in TAMP-R-TEL® tamper-resistant packages as follows:
NDC 0008-0235-50, 2 mL size Blunt Pointe™
NDC 0008-0235-01, 2 mL size (22 gauge x 1-1/4 inch needle).
Mepergan (meperidine HCl and promethazine HCl) Injection is also available in vials as follows:
NDC 0008-0234, 10 mL vial.
Do not use if solution is discolored or contains a precipitate.
Protect from light
Use carton to protect contents from light
Store at room temperature, approximately 25° C (77° F)
Manufactured by:
Wyeth Laboratories
A Wyeth-Ayerst Company
Philadelphia, PA 19101
CI 4213-3 Revised March 22, 1995

MYLOTARG™ ℞

[*mī 'lō-tărg*]
(gemtuzumab ozogamicin for Injection)
FOR INTRAVENOUS USE ONLY

> **WARNINGS**
> Mylotarg should be administered under the supervision of a physician who is experienced in the use of cancer chemotherapeutic agents.
> Severe myelosuppression occurs when Mylotarg is used at recommended doses.

DESCRIPTION

Mylotarg™ (gemtuzumab ozogamicin for Injection) is a chemotherapy agent composed of a recombinant humanized IgG_4, kappa antibody conjugated with a cytotoxic antitumor antibiotic, calicheamicin, isolated from fermentation of a bacterium, *Micromonospora echinospora* ssp. *calichensis*. The antibody portion of Mylotarg binds specifically to the CD33 antigen, a sialic acid-dependent adhesion protein found on the surface of leukemic blasts and immature normal cells of myelomonocytic lineage, but not on normal hematopoietic stem cells.
The anti-CD33 hP67.6 antibody is produced by mammalian cell suspension culture using a myeloma NSO cell line and is purified under conditions which remove or inactivate viruses. Three separate and independent steps in the hP67.6 antibody purification process achieve retrovirus inactivation and removal. These include low pH treatment, DEAE-Sepharose chromatography, and viral filtration. Mylotarg contains amino acid sequences of which approximately 98.3% are of human origin. The constant region and framework regions contain human sequences while the complementarity-determining regions are derived from a murine antibody (p67.6) that binds CD33. This antibody is linked to N-acetyl-gamma calicheamicin via a bifunctional linker. Gemtuzumab ozogamicin has approximately 50% of the antibody loaded with 4–6 moles calicheamicin per mole of antibody. The remaining 50% of the antibody is not linked to the calicheamicin derivative. Gemtuzumab ozogamicin has a molecular weight of 151 to 153 kDa.

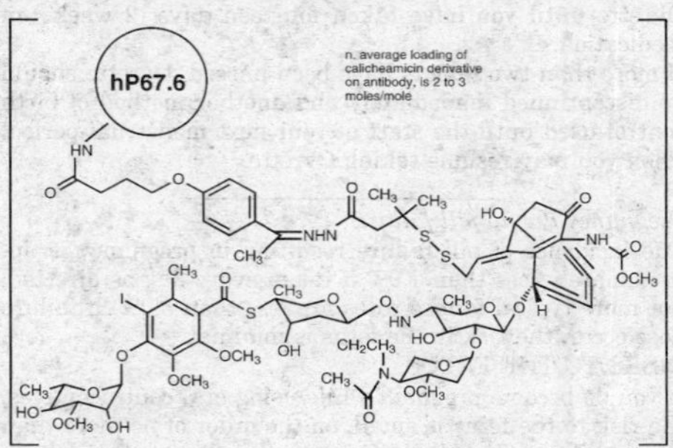

Mylotarg is a sterile, white, preservative-free lyophilized powder containing 5 mg of drug conjugate (protein equivalent) in a 20-mL amber vial. The drug product is light sensitive and must be protected from direct and indirect sunlight and unshielded fluorescent light during the preparation and administration of the infusion. The inactive ingredients are: dextran 40; sucrose; sodium chloride; monobasic and dibasic sodium phosphate.

CLINICAL PHARMACOLOGY

General
Gemtuzumab ozogamicin binds to the CD33 antigen. This antigen is expressed on the surface of leukemic blasts in more than 80% of patients with acute myeloid leukemia (AML). CD33 is also expressed on normal and leukemic myeloid colony-forming cells, including leukemic clonogenic precursors, but it is not expressed on pluripotent hematopoietic stem cells or on nonhematopoietic cells.

Mechanism of Action: Mylotarg is directed against the CD33 antigen expressed by hematopoietic cells. Binding of the anti-CD33 antibody portion of Mylotarg with the CD33 antigen results in the formation of a complex that is internalized. Upon internalization, the calicheamicin derivative is released inside the lysosomes of the myeloid cell. The released calicheamicin derivative binds to DNA in the minor groove resulting in DNA double strand breaks and cell death.

Gemtuzumab ozogamicin is cytotoxic to the CD33 positive HL-60 human leukemia cell line. Gemtuzumab ozogamicin produces significant inhibition of colony formation in cultures of adult leukemic bone marrow cells. The cytotoxic effect on normal myeloid precursors leads to substantial myelosuppression, but this is reversible because pluripotent hematopoietic stem cells are spared. In preclinical animal studies, gemtuzumab ozogamicin demonstrates antitumor effects in the HL-60 human promyelocytic leukemia xenograft tumor in athymic mice.

Human Pharmacokinetics

After administration of the first recommended 9 mg/m^2 dose of gemtuzumab ozogamicin, given as a 2 hour infusion, the elimination half lives of total and unconjugated calicheamicin were about 45 and 100 hours, respectively. After the second 9 mg/m^2 dose, the half life of total calicheamicin was increased to about 60 hours and the area under the concentration-time curve (AUC) was about twice that in the first dose period. The pharmacokinetics of unconjugated calicheamicin did not appear to change from period one to two. Metabolic studies indicate hydrolytic release of the calicheamicin derivative from gemtuzumab ozogamicin. Many metabolites of this derivative were found after *in vitro* incubation of gemtuzumab ozogamicin in human liver microsomes and cytosol, and in HL-60 promyelocytic leukemia cells. Metabolic studies characterizing the possible isozymes involved in the metabolic pathway of Mylotarg have not been performed.

CLINICAL STUDIES

The efficacy and safety of Mylotarg as a single agent have been evaluated in 142 patients in three single arm open-label studies in patients with CD33 positive AML in first relapse. The studies included 65, 40, and 37 patients. In studies 1 and 2 patients were ≥ 18 years of age with a first remission duration of at least 6 months. In study 3, only patients ≥ 60 were enrolled and their first remission had to have lasted for at least 3 months. Patients with secondary leukemia or white blood cell (WBC) counts ≥ 30,000/µL were excluded. Some patients were leukoreduced with hydroxyurea or leukophoresis to lower WBC counts below 30,000/µL in order to minimize the risk of tumor lysis syndrome. The treatment course included two 9 mg/m^2 doses separated by 14 days and a 28-day follow-up after the last dose. Although smaller doses had elicited responses in earlier studies, the 9 mg/m^2 was chosen because it would be expected to saturate all CD33 sites regardless of leukemic burden. A total of 80 patients were 60 years of age and older. The primary endpoint of the three clinical studies was the rate of complete remission (CR), which was defined as

a) leukemic blasts absent from the peripheral blood;

b) ≤ 5% blasts in the bone marrow, as measured by morphology studies;

c) hemoglobin (Hgb) ≥ 9 g/dL, platelets ≥ 100,000/µL, absolute neutrophil count (ANC) ≥ 1500/µL; and

d) red cell and platelet-transfusion independence (no red cell transfusions for 2 weeks; no platelet transfusions for 1 week).

In addition to CR, a second response category, CRp, was defined as patients satisfying the definition of CR, including platelet transfusion independence, with the exception of platelet recovery ≥100,000/µL. This category was added because Mylotarg appears to delay platelet recovery in some patients. Most of these patients (18/19) achieved platelet counts of at least 25,000/µL and about two-thirds (13/19) achieved platelet counts of at least 50,000/µL, before any additional therapy was administered. It is not yet clear whether CR and CRp responses are clinically equivalent; but survival in the two groups appeared similar.

All patients were pre-medicated with acetaminophen 650–1000 mg and diphenhydramine 50 mg to decrease acute transfusion-related symptoms. Growth factors and cytokines were not permitted. Use of prophylactic antibiotics was not specified.

Response Rate

The overall response (OR) rate for the three pooled monotherapy studies was 30% (42/142) consisting of 16% (23/142) of patients with CR and 13% (19/142) of patients with CRp. The median time to remission was 60 days for both CR and CRp. Remission rates in the individual studies are shown in Table 1.

[See table 1 above]

Two of the most important determinants of response following relapse are age and duration of first remission. Remission rates by prognostic category are outlined in Table 2; the impact of age and duration of first remission in these patients was minimal:

[See table 2 above]

Among patients < 60 years of age the overall response rate was 34%; among patients ≥ 60 years of age the overall response rate was 26%. The overall response rates were similar for females and males: 31% of females and 29% of males achieved remission.

TABLE 1: PERCENTAGE OF PATIENTS BY REMISSION CATEGORY

	Study 1	Study 2	Study 3[a]	All Studies
Type of Remission	n = 65	n = 40	n = 37	n = 142
CR (95% CI)	17 (9, 28)	20 (9, 36)	11 (3, 25)	16 (11, 23)
CRp (95% CI)	15 (8, 26)	13 (4, 27)	11 (3, 25)	13 (8, 20)
OR (CR + CRp) (95% CI)	32 (21, 45)	33 (19, 49)	22 (10, 38)	30 (22, 38)

a: Patients 60 years of age or greater

TABLE 2: PERCENTAGE OF PATIENTS BY REMISSION CATEGORY AND PROGNOSTIC GROUP

	Age < 60 years	Age ≥ 60 years	First Remission ≥ 1 yr	First Remission < 1 yr
Type of Remission	n = 62	n = 80	n = 62	n = 80
CR (95% CI)	18 (9, 30)	15 (8, 25)	21 (12, 33)	13 (6, 22)
CRp (95% CI)	16 (8, 28)	11 (5, 20)	11 (5, 22)	15 (8, 25)
OR (CR + CRp) (95% CI)	34 (22, 47)	26 (17, 37)	32 (21, 45)	28 (18, 39)

TABLE 3: SUMMARY OF RELAPSE-FREE SURVIVAL[a] FOR PATIENTS WITH CR AND CRp

Remission Group	n	No. Relapsed	Median months	Min-Max months[b]
CR	23	14	7.2	0.5–24.8
CRp	19	9	4.4	0.33[b]–21.5
OR[c]	42	23	6.8	0.33[b]–24.8

a: Number of months after achieving CR or CRp.
b: Data are limited by data cut-off date; first event occurred in 0.83 months for CRp and in 0.5 months for OR.
c: Six OR patients (1 CR and 5 CRp) had a relapse-free survival of > 12 months.

The majority of patients (94%) in the Phase 2 clinical trials were white, only 6% were non-white. All 42 of the responding patients were white.

Relapse-Free Survival

Relapse-free survival was calculated from the date of initial therapy (Table 3).

[See table 3 above]

Overall Survival

Median duration of overall survival for the 142 patients was 5.9 months and 55/142 patients were alive as of the data cutoff date.

Post-Remission Therapy

Fifteen (15/42, 36%) OR patients (8 CRs and 7 CRps) received hematopoietic stem cell transplantation. The survival of these 15 patients ranged from 3.5 to 26.9 months as of the data cut-off date. Nine OR patients (4 CR and 5 CRp) had an overall survival of > 12 months as of the data cut-off date.

Repeat Courses

Five patients have received a second treatment course of Mylotarg in clinical trials. These patients were initially treated with Mylotarg, achieved remission, then subsequently relapsed. One of these patients (≥ 60 years of age) achieved a second CR after receiving the second course of Mylotarg. Prolonged severe myelosuppression was observed in four patients receiving a third dose.

Overview of Clinical Data

Available single arm trial data do not provide valid comparisons with various cytotoxic regimens that have been used in relapsed acute myeloid leukemia. Response rates are in the range of rates reported with such regimens only if the CRp responses are included.

Nevertheless, treatment with Mylotarg can provide responses, including some of reasonable duration. The data support its use in patients for whom aggressive cytotoxic regimens would be considered unsuitable, such as many patients 60 years of age or older.

INDICATIONS AND USAGE

Mylotarg is indicated for the treatment of patients with CD33 positive acute myeloid leukemia in first relapse who are 60 years of age or older and who are not considered candidates for cytotoxic chemotherapy. The safety and efficacy of Mylotarg in patients with poor performance status and organ dysfunction has not been established.

The effectiveness of Mylotarg is based on OR rates (see **CLINICAL STUDIES** section). There are no controlled trials demonstrating a clinical benefit, such as improvement in disease-related symptoms or increased survival, compared to any other treatment.

CONTRAINDICATIONS

Mylotarg is contraindicated in patients with a known hypersensitivity to gemtuzumab ozogamicin or any of its components: anti-CD33 antibody (hP67.6), calicheamicin derivatives, or inactive ingredients.

WARNINGS

Mylotarg is intended for administration under the supervision of a physician who is experienced in the use of cancer chemotherapeutic agents.

Myelosuppression: Severe myelosuppression will occur in all patients given the recommended dose of this agent. Careful hematologic monitoring is required. Systemic infections should be treated.

Use in Patients with Hepatic Impairment: Mylotarg has not been studied in patients with bilirubin > 2 mg/dL. Caution should be exercised when administering Mylotarg in patients with hepatic impairment (see **ADVERSE REACTIONS** section).

Allergic Reactions: Mylotarg can produce a post-infusion symptom complex of fever and chills, and less commonly hypotension and dyspnea that may occur during the first 24 hours after administration. Grade 3 or 4 non-hematologic infusion-related adverse events included chills, fever, hypotension, hypertension, hyperglycemia, hypoxia, and dyspnea. Most patients received the following prophylactic medications before administration: diphenhydramine 50 mg po and acetaminophen 650–1000 mg po; thereafter, two additional doses of acetaminophen 650–1000 mg po, one every 4 hours as needed. Vital signs should be monitored during infusion for the four hours following infusion.

Anaphylaxis was not reported in the three phase II clinical studies (see **CLINICAL STUDIES** section). However, Mylotarg contains a humanized anti-CD33 antibody. As with any product, the possibility of anaphylaxis cannot be excluded.

Pregnancy: Mylotarg may cause fetal harm when administered to a pregnant woman. Daily treatment of pregnant rats with gemtuzumab ozogamicin during organogenesis caused dose-related decreases in fetal weight in association with dose-related decreases in fetal skeletal ossification beginning at 0.025 mg/kg/day. Doses of 0.060 mg/kg/day (approximately 0.04 times the recommended human single dose on a mg/m^2 basis) produced increased embryo-fetal mortality (increased numbers of resorptions and decreased numbers of live fetuses per litter). Gross external, visceral, and skeletal alterations at the 0.060 mg/kg/day dose level included digital malformations (ectrodactyly, brachydactyly) in one or both hind feet, absence of the aortic arch, wavy ribs, anomalies of the long bones in the forelimb(s) (short/thick humerus, misshapen radius and ulna, and short/thick ulna), misshapen scapula, absence of vertebral centrum, and fused sternebrae. This dose was also associated with maternal toxicity (decreased weight gain, decreased food consumption). There are no adequate and well-controlled studies in pregnant women. If Mylotarg is used in pregnancy, or if the patient becomes pregnant while taking it, the patient should be apprised of the potential hazard to the fetus. Women of childbearing potential should be advised to avoid becoming pregnant while receiving treatment with Mylotarg.

Continued on next page

Mylotarg—Cont.

PRECAUTIONS

DO NOT ADMINISTER AS AN INTRAVENOUS PUSH OR BOLUS

General

Treatment by Experienced Physicians: Treatment should be initiated by and remain under the supervision of a physician who is experienced in the use of cancer chemotherapeutic agents.

Tumor Lysis Syndrome: Tumor lysis syndrome may be a consequence of leukemia treatment. Physicians should consider leukoreduction with hydroxyurea or leukophoresis to reduce the peripheral white blood count to <30,000/µL prior to administration of Mylotarg (see **CLINICAL STUDIES** section). Appropriate measures, (e.g. hydration and allopurinol), must be taken to prevent hyperuricemia.

Laboratory Monitoring: Electrolytes, tests of hepatic function, complete blood counts (CBCs) and platelet counts should be monitored during Mylotarg therapy.

Drug Interactions: There have been no formal drug-interaction studies performed with Mylotarg.

Laboratory Test Interactions: Mylotarg is not known to interfere with any routine diagnostic tests.

Carcinogenesis, Mutagenesis, Impairment of Fertility: No long-term studies in animals have been performed to evaluate the carcinogenic potential of Mylotarg. Gemtuzumab ozogamicin was clastogenic in the mouse *in vivo* micronucleus test. This positive result is consistent with the known ability of calicheamicin to cause double-stranded breaks in DNA. Formal fertility studies were not conducted in animals. When given weekly for 6 doses to rats, gemtuzumab ozogamicin caused atrophy of the seminiferous tubules, oligospermia, desquamate cells in the epididymis, and hyperplasia of the interstitial cells at the dose of 1.2 mg/kg/week (approximately 0.9 times the human dose on a mg/m^2 basis). These findings did not resolve following a 5-week recovery period.

Pregnancy Category D: See **WARNINGS** section.

Nursing Mothers: It is not known if Mylotarg is excreted in human milk. Because many drugs, including immunoglobulins, are excreted in human milk, and because of the potential for serious adverse reactions in nursing infants from Mylotarg, a decision should be made whether to discontinue nursing or to discontinue the drug, taking into account the importance of the drug to the mother.

Pediatric Use: The safety and effectiveness of Mylotarg in pediatric patients have not been studied.

Use in Patients with Renal Impairment: Patients with renal impairment were not studied.

ADVERSE REACTIONS

Mylotarg has been administered to 142 patients with relapsed AML at 9 mg/m^2. Mylotarg was generally given as two intravenous infusions separated by 14 days.

Acute Infusion-Related Events (Table 4)

TABLE 4: PERCENTAGE OF PATIENTS REPORTED TO HAVE ACUTE INFUSION-RELATED ADVERSE EVENTS

Adverse Event	(%) Any Severity	(%) Grade 3 or 4
Chills	62	11
Fever	61	7
Nausea	38	<1
Vomiting	32	<1
Headache	12	<1
Hypotension	11	4
Hypertension	6	3
Hypoxia	6	2
Dyspnea	4	1
Hyperglycemia	2	2

These symptoms generally occurred after the end of the 2-hour intravenous infusion and resolved after 2 to 4 hours with a supportive therapy of acetaminophen, diphenhydramine, and IV fluids (see **WARNINGS** section). Fewer infusion-related events were observed after the second dose.

Antibody Formation: Antibodies to gemtuzumab ozogamicin were not detected in a total of 142 patients in the Phase 2 clinical studies. Two patients in a Phase 1 study developed antibody titers against the calicheamicin/calicheamicin-linker portion of gemtuzumab ozogamicin after three doses. One patient experienced transient fever, hypotension and dyspnea; the other patient had no clinical symptoms. No patient developed antibody responses to the hP67.6 antibody portion of Mylotarg™.

Myelosuppression: Severe myelosuppression is the major toxicity associated with Mylotarg. During the treatment phase, 137/140 (98%) patients experienced Grade 3 or Grade 4 neutropenia. Responding patients recovered ANCs to 500/µL by a median of 40.5 days after the first dose of Mylotarg.

Anemia, Thrombocytopenia: During the treatment phase, 139/141 (99%) patients experienced Grade 3 or Grade 4 thrombocytopenia. Responding patients recovered platelet counts to 25,000/µL by a median of 39 days after the first dose of Mylotarg. 66/141 (47%) patients experienced Grade 3 or Grade 4 anemia.

Infection: During the treatment phase, 40/142 (28%) patients experienced Grade 3 or Grade 4 infections, including opportunistic infections. The most frequent Grade 3 or Grade 4 infection-related treatment-emergent adverse events (TEAEs) were sepsis (16%) and pneumonia (7%). Herpes simplex infection was reported in 22% of the patients.

Bleeding: During the treatment phase, 21/142 (15%) patients experienced Grade 3 or Grade 4 bleeding. The most frequent severe TEAE was epistaxis (3%). There were also reports of cerebral hemorrhage (2%), disseminated intravascular coagulation (2%), intracranial hemorrhage (2%), and hematuria (1%).

Transfusions: During the treatment phase, more transfusions were required in the NR and CRp patients compared with the CRs (Table 5):

[See table 5 above]

TABLE 5: NUMBER OF TRANSFUSIONS BY RESPONSE GROUP

Transfusions	All Patients	CR	CRp	NR
	n = 142	n = 23	n = 19	n = 100
Platelet transfusions				
Mean (SD)	14 (23)	5.4 (6)	14.8 (12)	15.8 (27)
(95% CI)	(10.2, 17.8)	(3, 7.8)	(9.3, 20.4)	(10.6, 21.1)
RBC transfusions				
Mean	8.2 (26)	2.6 (2)	6.2 (5)	9.9 (31)
(95% CI)	(3.9, 12.6)	(1.7, 3.5)	(4, 8.4)	(3.7, 16)

Mucositis: A total of 50/142 (35%) patients were reported to have a TEAE consistent with oral mucositis or stomatitis. During the treatment phase, 5/142 (4%) patients experienced Grade 3 or 4 stomatitis/mucositis after the first dose. The mucositis events for the remaining 45/142 (32%) patients were categorized as Grade 1 or 2.

Hepatotoxicity: Abnormalities of liver function were transient and generally reversible. In clinical studies, 33/141 (23%) patients experienced Grade 3 or Grade 4 hyperbilirubinemia. Nine percent (12/141) of patients experienced Grade 3 or Grade 4 abnormalities in levels of ALT, and 24/141 (17%) patients experienced Grade 3 or Grade 4 abnormalities in levels of AST. Thirteen patients had concurrent elevations of transaminases (grade 3 to 4) and bilirubin. One patient died with liver failure in the setting of tumor lysis syndrome and multisystem organ failure 22 days after treatment. Another patient died after an episode of persistent jaundice and hepatosplenomegaly 156 days after treatment. Among 27 patients who received hematopoietic stem cell transplantation following Mylotarg, four (3 NRs and 1 CR) died of hepatic veno-occlusive disease (VOD) 22 to 392 days following transplantation.

Skin: No patients experienced alopecia. A nonspecific rash was reported in 22%.

Retreatment Events: Five (5) patients have received more than one course of Mylotarg, 4 of these patients at 9 mg/m^2. The adverse event profile for retreated patients was similar to that following their initial treatment. One of the repeat dose patients was in a Phase 1 study and received a first course of 3 doses at 1 mg/m^2 and 2 doses of a second course at 6 mg/m^2. This patient was discontinued from further dose administration as a result of an immune response to the calicheamicin/calicheamicin-linker portion of gemtuzumab ozogamicin. The 4 other retreated patients did not experience an immune response.

Dose Relationship for Adverse Events: Dose-relationship data were generated from a small dose-escalation study. The most common clinical adverse event observed in this study was an infusion-related symptom complex of fever and chills. In general, the severity of fever, but not chills, increased as the dose level increased. Only one dose level of Mylotarg was studied in the Phase 2 clinical trials in relapsed AML.

Treatment-Emergent Adverse Events (TEAE): TEAEs (Grades 1–4) that occurred in ≥ 10% of the patients regardless of causality are listed in Table 6.

TABLE 6. NUMBER (%) OF PATIENTS REPORTING TREATMENT-EMERGENT ADVERSE EVENTS[a]-ALL GRADES (INCIDENCE ≥ 10%[b])

Adverse Event	Efficacy and Safety Studies All Patients (n = 142)	Age ≥ 60 (n = 80)
Body as a whole		
Abdomen enlarged	13 (9)	9 (11)
Abdominal pain	52 (37)	23 (29)
Asthenia	63 (44)	36 (45)
Back pain	22 (15)	14 (18)
Chills	104 (73)	53 (66)
Fever	121 (85)	64 (80)
Headache	50 (35)	21 (26)
Neutropenic fever	30 (21)	16 (20)
Pain	30 (21)	20 (25)
Sepsis	36 (25)	19 (24)
Cardiovascular system		
Hemorrhage	14 (10)	6 (8)
Hypertension	29 (20)	16 (20)
Hypotension	28 (20)	13 (16)
Tachycardia	15 (11)	8 (10)
Digestive system		
Anorexia	41 (29)	25 (31)
Constipation	36 (25)	22 (28)
Diarrhea	54 (38)	30 (38)
Dyspepsia	16 (11)	9 (11)
Nausea	100 (70)	51 (64)
Stomatitis	45 (32)	20 (25)
Vomiting	89 (63)	44 (55)
Hemic and lymphatic system		
Ecchymosis	18 (13)	12 (15)
Metabolic		
Hypokalemia	44 (31)	24 (30)
Hypomagnesemia	14 (10)	3 (4)
Lactic dehydrogenase increased	19 (13)	14 (18)
Musculoskeletal system		
Arthralgia	12 (8)	8 (10)
Nervous system		
Depression	13 (9)	8 (10)
Dizziness	22 (15)	9 (11)
Insomnia	22 (15)	14 (18)
Respiratory system		
Cough increased	28 (20)	15 (19)
Dyspnea	46 (32)	29 (36)
Epistaxis	44 (31)	23 (29)
Pharyngitis	20 (14)	11 (14)
Pneumonia	14 (10)	8 (10)
Pulmonary physical finding[c]	16 (11)	10 (13)
Rhinitis	14 (10)	8 (10)
Skin and appendages		
Herpes simplex	31 (22)	12 (15)
Rash	31 (22)	18 (23)
Local reaction	35 (25)	20 (25)
Peripheral edema	23 (16)	17 (21)
Petechiae	28 (20)	17 (21)
Urogenital system[d]		
Hematuria	14 (10)	8 (10)
Vaginal hemorrhage	7 (12)	2 (7)

a: Does not include changes in laboratory values reported as adverse events for events included in the NCI common toxicity scale.

b: ≥ 10% limit specifies the minimum percentage threshold from at least 1 column for an event to be displayed in the table.

c: Includes rales, rhonchi, and changes in breath sounds.

d: Percentages for sex-specific adverse events are based on the number of patients of the relevant sex.

TEAE with a Grade 3 or 4 severity are listed in Table 7.

TABLE 7. PERCENT (%) OF PATIENTS REPORTED TO HAVE SEVERE OR NCI GRADE 3 OR 4 TREATMENT-EMERGENT ADVERSE EVENTS[a] (INCIDENCE ≥ 5%)[b]

Body System Adverse Event	Efficacy and Safety Studies All Patients (n = 142)	Age ≥ 60 (n = 80)
Any adverse event	129 (91)	70 (88)
Body as a whole		
Asthenia	10 (7)	8 (10)
Chills	18 (13)	12 (15)
Fever	21 (15)	11 (14)
Neutropenic fever	10 (7)	4 (5)
Sepsis	23 (16)	12 (16)
Cardiovascular system		
Hypertension	13 (9)	9 (11)
Hypotension	11 (8)	6 (8)
Digestive system		
Nausea	13 (9)	6 (8)
Metabolic		
Hypokalemia	4 (3)	4 (5)
Lactic dehydrogenase increased	6 (4)	6 (8)

Respiratory system		
Dyspnea	13 (9)	10 (13)
Pneumonia	10 (7)	5 (6)

a: Does not include changes in laboratory values reported as adverse events for events included in the NCI common toxicity scale.
b: ≥ 5% limit specifies the minimum percentage threshold from at least 1 column for an event to be displayed in the table.

Clinically important laboratory abnormalities with a Grade 3 or 4 severity are listed in Table 8.

TABLE 8. NUMBER (%[a]) OF PATIENTS WITH LABORATORY TEST RESULTS OF GRADE 3 OR 4 SEVERITY[b]

	Efficacy and Safety Studies Grades 3–4	
Test	All Patients (n = 142)	Age ≥ 60 (n = 80)
Hematologic		
Hemoglobin	66/141 (47)	36/80 (45)
WBC	136/141 (96)	75/80 (94)
Total neutrophils, absolute	137/140 (98)	78/79 (99)
Lymphocytes	130/140 (93)	70/79 (89)
Platelet count	139/141 (99)	79/80 (99)
Prothrombin time	2/47 (4)	1/23 (4)
Partial thromboplastin time	1/79 (1)	1/42 (2)
Non-hematologic		
Glucose	17/140 (12)	9/79 (11)
Creatinine	2/141 (1)	0/80
Total bilirubin	33/141 (23)	18/80 (23)
AST	24/141 (17)	12/80 (15)
ALT	12/141 (9)	7/80 (9)
Alkaline phosphatase	5/141 (4)	1/80 (1)
Calcium	17/141 (12)	5/80 (6)

a: Percentage is based on the number of patients receiving a particular laboratory test during the study as is indicated for each test.
b: Severity as defined by NCI common toxicity scale version 1.

There were considered to be no clinically important differences in TEAEs between patients < 60 years of age and those patients ≥ 60. Laboratory parameters associated with hepatic dysfunction (e.g., elevated levels of bilirubin, AST, and ALT) were more consistently observed in patients ≥ 60 years old than in those < 60 years old.
There were considered to be no clinically important differences in TEAEs between female and male patients.

OVERDOSAGE

No cases of overdose with Mylotarg were reported in clinical experience. Single doses higher than 9 mg/m^2 in adults were not tested. When a single dose of Mylotarg was administered to animals, mortality was observed in rats at the dose of 2 mg/kg (approximately 1.3-times the recommended human dose on a mg/m^2 basis), and in male monkeys at the dose of 4.5 mg/kg (approximately 6-times the recommended human dose on a mg/m^2 basis).
Signs and Symptoms: Signs of overdose with Mylotarg are unknown.
Recommended Treatment: General supportive measures should be followed in case of overdose. Blood pressure and blood counts should be carefully monitored. Gemtuzumab ozogamicin is not dialyzable.

DOSAGE AND ADMINISTRATION

The recommended dose of Mylotarg is 9 mg/m^2, administered as a 2-hour intravenous infusion. Patients should receive the following prophylactic medications one hour before Mylotarg administration: diphenhydramine 50 mg po and acetaminophen 650–1000 mg po; thereafter, two additional doses of acetaminophen 605–1000 mg po, one every 4 hours as needed. Vital signs should be monitored during infusion and for four hours following infusion. The recommended treatment course with Mylotarg is a total of 2 doses with 14 days between the doses. Full recovery from hematologic toxicities is not a requirement for administration of the second dose. Mylotarg may be administered in an outpatient setting.
Hepatic Insufficiency: Patients with hepatic impairment were not included in the clinical studies. See **WARNINGS** section.
Renal Insufficiency: Patients with renal impairment were not included in the clinical studies.
Instructions for Reconstitution
The drug product is light sensitive and must be protected from direct and indirect sunlight and unshielded fluorescent light during the preparation and administration of the infusion. **All preparation should take place in a biologic safety hood with the fluorescent light off.** Prior to reconstitution, allow drug vials to come to room temperature. Reconstitute the contents of each vial with 5 mL Sterile Water for Injection, USP, using sterile syringes. Gently swirl each vial. Each vial should be inspected for complete solution and for particulate. The final concentration of drug in the vial is 1 mg/mL. While in the vial, the reconstituted drug may be stored refrigerated (2–8° C) and protected from light for up to 8 hours.
Instructions for Dilution
Withdraw the desired volume from each vial and inject into a 100 mL IV bag of 0.9% Sodium Chloride Injection. Place the 100-mL IV bag into an UV protectant bag. The resulting drug solution in the IV bag should be used immediately.
Administration
DO NOT ADMINISTER AS AN INTRAVENOUS PUSH OR BOLUS
Once the reconstituted Mylotarg is diluted into the IV bag containing normal saline, the resulting solution should be infused over a 2-hour period. A separate IV line equipped with a low protein-binding 1.2-micron terminal filter must be used for administration of the drug. Mylotarg may be given peripherally or through a central line. Premedication, consisting of acetaminophen and diphenhydramine, should be given before each infusion to reduce the incidence of a post-infusion symptom complex (see **ADVERSE REACTIONS, Acute Infusion-Related Events**).
Stability and Storage: Mylotarg should be stored refrigerated (2–8° C, 36–46° F and protected from light).
Instructions for Use, Handling and for Disposal: Mylotarg should be inspected visually for particular matter and discoloration, following reconstitution and prior to administration. Protect from light and use an UV protective bag over the IV bag during infusion. Procedures for handling and disposal of anticancer drugs should be considered. Several guidelines on this subject have been published.[1,2,3]

HOW SUPPLIED

Mylotarg™ (gemtuzumab ozogamicin for Injection) is supplied as a single-vial package with an amber glass vial containing 5 mg of Mylotarg lyophilized powder. Single-unit 5 mg package: each 20 mL vial contains 5 mg of Mylotarg. NDC 0008-4510-01.

REFERENCES

1. Recommendation for the Safe Handling of Parenteral Antineoplastic Drugs. NIH Publication No. 83-2621. For Sale by the Superintendent of Documents, US Government Printing Office, Washington, DC 20402.
2. AMA Council Report. Guidelines for Handling Parenteral Antineoplastics. JAMA 1985; 253 (11): 1590–1592.
3. National Study Commission on Cytotoxic Exposure—Recommendations for Handling Cytotoxic Agents. Available from Louis P. Jeffrey, ScD, Chairman, National Study Commission on Cytotoxic Exposure, Massachusetts College of Pharmacy and Allied Health Sciences, 179 Longwood Avenue, Boston, Massachusetts 02115.

Manufactured by:
Wyeth Laboratories
Division of Wyeth-Ayerst Pharmaceuticals Inc.
Philadelphia, PA 19101
CI 6125-3 Revised June 2000

NORPLANT® SYSTEM ℞

[*nŏr ′ plănt*]
(levonorgestrel implants)

Patients should be counseled that this product does not protect against HIV infection (AIDS) and other sexually transmitted diseases.
Prescribing Information

DESCRIPTION

The NORPLANT SYSTEM kit contains levonorgestrel implants, a set of six flexible closed capsules made of silicone rubber tubing (Silastic®, dimethylsiloxane/methylvinylsiloxane copolymer), each containing 36 mg of the progestin levonorgestrel contained in an insertion kit to facilitate implantation. The capsules are sealed with Silastic (polydimethylsiloxane) adhesive and sterilized. Each capsule is 2.4 mm in diameter and 34 mm in length. The capsules are inserted in a superficial plane beneath the skin of the upper arm.
Information contained herewith regarding safety and efficacy was derived from studies which used two slightly different Silastic tubing formulations. The formulation being used in the NORPLANT SYSTEM has slightly higher release rates of levonorgestrel and at least comparable efficacy.
Evidence indicates that the dose of levonorgestrel provided by the NORPLANT SYSTEM is initially about 85 mcg/day followed by a decline to about 50 mcg/day by 9 months and to about 35 mcg/day by 18 months with a further decline thereafter to about 30 mcg/day. The NORPLANT SYSTEM is a progestin-only product and does not contain estrogen.
Levonorgestrel, (d(-)-13-beta-ethyl-17-alpha-ethinyl-17-beta-hydroxygon-4-en-3-one), the active ingredient in the NORPLANT SYSTEM, has a molecular weight of 312.45 and the following structural formula:

Levonorgestrel

CLINICAL PHARMACOLOGY

Levonorgestrel is a totally synthetic and biologically active progestin which exhibits no significant estrogenic activity and is highly progestational. The absolute configuration conforms to that of D-natural steroids. Levonorgestrel is not subjected to a "first-pass" effect and is virtually 100% bioavailable. Plasma concentrations average approximately 0.30 ng/mL over 5 years but are highly variable as a function of individual metabolism and body weight.
Diffusion of levonorgestrel through the wall of each capsule provides a continuous low dose of the progestin. Resulting blood levels are substantially below those generally observed among users of combination oral contraceptives containing the progestins norgestrel or levonorgestrel. Because of the range of variability in blood levels and variation in individual response, blood levels alone are not predictive of the risk of pregnancy in an individual woman.
At least two mechanisms are active in preventing pregnancy: ovulation inhibition and thickening of the cervical mucus. Other mechanisms may add to these contraceptive effects.
Levonorgestrel concentrations among women show considerable variation depending on individual clearance rates, body weight, and possibly other factors. Levonorgestrel concentrations reach a maximum, or near maximum, within 24 hours after placement with mean values of 1600 ± 1100 pg/mL. They decline rapidly over the first month partially due to a circulating protein, SHBG, that binds levonorgestrel and which is depressed by the presence of levonorgestrel. At 3 months, mean levels decline to values of around 400 pg/mL while concentrations normalized to a 60 kg body weight were 327 ± 119 (SD) pg/mL at 12 months with further decline by 1.4 pg/mL/month to reach 258 ± 95 (SD) pg/mL at 60 months. Concentrations decreased with increasing body weight by a mean of 3.3 pg/mL/kg. After capsule removal, mean concentrations drop to below 100 pg/mL by 96 hours and to below assay sensitivity (50 pg/mL) by 5 to 14 days. Fertility rates return to levels comparable to those seen in the general population of women using no method of contraception. Circulating concentrations can be used to forecast the risk of pregnancy only in a general statistical sense. Mean concentrations associated with pregnancy have been 210 ± 60 (SD) pg/mL. However, in clinical studies, 20 percent of women had one or more values below 200 pg/mL but an average annual gross pregnancy rate of less than 1.0 per 100 women through 5 years.
Although lipoprotein levels were altered in several clinical studies with the NORPLANT SYSTEM, the long-term clinical effects of these changes have not been determined. A decrease in total cholesterol levels has been reported in all lipoprotein studies and reached statistical significance in several. Both increases and decreases in high-density lipoprotein (HDL) levels have been reported in clinical trials. No statistically significant increases have been reported in the ratio of total cholesterol to HDL-cholesterol. Low-density lipoprotein (LDL) levels decreased during NORPLANT SYSTEM use. Triglyceride levels also decreased from pretreatment values.

INDICATIONS AND USAGE

The NORPLANT SYSTEM is indicated for the prevention of pregnancy and is a long-term (up to 5 years) reversible contraceptive system. The capsules should be removed by the end of the 5th year. New capsules may be inserted at that time if continuing contraceptive protection is desired.
In multicenter trials with the NORPLANT SYSTEM, involving 2470 women, the relationship between body weight and efficacy was investigated. Tabulated below is the preg-

Continued on next page

TABLE 1
Annual and Five-Year Cumulative Pregnancy Rates
Per 100 Users by Weight Class

Weight class	year 1	year 2	year 3	year 4	year 5	Cumulative
<50 kg (<110 lbs)	0.2	0	0	0	0	0.2
50–59 kg (110–130 lbs)	0.2	0.5	0.4	2.0	0.4	3.4
60–69 kg (131–153 lbs)	0.4	0.5	1.6	1.7	0.8	5.0
≥70 kg (≥154 lbs)	0	1.1	5.1	2.5	0	8.5
All	0.2	0.5	1.2	1.6	0.4	3.9

Norplant—Cont.

nancy experience as a function of body weight. Because NORPLANT SYSTEM is a long-term method of contraception, this is reported over five years of use.

[See table at bottom of previous page]

Typically, pregnancy rates with contraceptive methods are reported for only the first year of use as shown below. The efficacy of these contraceptive methods, except the IUD and sterilization, depends in part on the reliability of use. The efficacy of the NORPLANT SYSTEM does not depend on patient compliance. However, no contraceptive method is 100% effective.

TABLE 2
Lowest Expected and Typical Failure Rates (%)
During the First Year of Use of a Contraceptive Method

Method	Lowest Expected	Typical
NORPLANT SYSTEM (6 capsules)	0.09	0.09
Male Sterilization	0.1	0.15
Female Sterilization	0.4	0.4
DEPO-PROVERA® (injectable progestogen)	0.3	0.3
Oral contraceptives		3
Combined	0.1	NA
Progestin only	0.5	NA
IUD		
Progesterone	1.5	2.0
Copper T 380A	0.6	0.8
Condom (male) without spermicide	3	12
(female) without spermicide	5	21
Cervical Cap		
Nulliparous women	9	18
Parous women	26	36
Diaphragm with spermicidal cream or jelly	6	18
Spermicides alone (foam, creams, jellies, and vaginal suppositories)	6	21
Periodic abstinence (all methods)	1–9*	20
Withdrawal	4	19
No contraception (planned pregnancy)	85	85

NA—not available

* Depending on method (calendar, ovulation, symptothermal, post-ovulation) Adapted from Hatcher, RA et al. *Contraceptive Technology*, 16th Revised Edition. New York, NY: Irvington Publishers, 1994.

NORPLANT SYSTEM gross annual discontinuation and continuation rates are summarized in Table 3.

[See table below]

CONTRAINDICATIONS

1. Active thrombophlebitis or thromboembolic disorders. There is insufficient information regarding women who have had previous thromboembolic disease.
2. Undiagnosed abnormal genital bleeding.
3. Known or suspected pregnancy.
4. Acute liver disease; benign or malignant liver tumors.
5. Known or suspected carcinoma of the breast.
6. History of idiopathic intracranial hypertension.
7. Hypersensitivity to levonorgestrel or any of the other components of the NORPLANT SYSTEM.

WARNINGS

A. **Warnings Based on Experience with the NORPLANT SYSTEM**

1. *Insertion and Removal Complications*

A surgical incision is required to insert NORPLANT SYSTEM capsules. Complications related to insertion such as pain, edema, and bruising may occur. There also have been reports of infection (including cellulitis and abscess formation), blistering, ulcerations, sloughing, excessive scarring, phlebitis, and hyperpigmentation at the insertion site. There have been reports of arm pain, numbness, and tingling following the insertion and removal procedures. There also have been reports of nerve injury, most commonly associated with deep placement and removal. Expulsion of capsules has been reported more frequently when placement of the capsules was shallow or too close to the incision or when infection was present. There have been reports of capsule displacement (i.e., movement), most of which involved minor changes in the positioning of the capsules. However, infrequent reports (< 1%) of significant displacement (a few to several inches) have been received. Some of these reports have been associated with pain and difficult removal. Removal is also a surgical procedure and may take longer, be more difficult, and/or cause more pain than insertion and may be associated with difficulty locating capsules. These complications may lead to the need for additional incisions and/or office visits. See also **"PRECAUTIONS"** and **"ADVERSE REACTIONS."**

2. *Bleeding Irregularities*

Most women can expect some variation in menstrual bleeding patterns. Irregular menstrual bleeding, intermenstrual spotting, prolonged episodes of bleeding and spotting, and amenorrhea occur in some women. Irregular bleeding patterns associated with the NORPLANT SYSTEM could mask symptoms of cervical or endometrial cancer. Overall, these irregularities diminish with continuing use. Since some NORPLANT SYSTEM users experience periods of amenorrhea, missed menstrual periods cannot serve as the only means of identifying early pregnancy. Pregnancy tests should be performed whenever a pregnancy is suspected. Six (6) weeks or more of amenorrhea after a pattern of regular menses may signal pregnancy. If pregnancy occurs, the capsules must be removed.

Although bleeding irregularities have occurred in clinical trials, proportionately more women had increases rather than decreases in hemoglobin concentrations, a difference that was highly statistically significant. This finding generally indicates that reduced menstrual blood loss is associated with the use of the NORPLANT SYSTEM. In rare instances, patients experienced heavy bleeding that resulted in hemoglobin values consistent with anemia.

3. *Ovarian Cysts (Delayed Follicular Atresia)*

If follicular development occurs with the NORPLANT SYSTEM, atresia of the follicle is sometimes delayed, and the follicle may continue to grow beyond the size it would attain in a normal cycle. These enlarged follicles cannot be distinguished clinically from ovarian cysts. In the majority of women, enlarged follicles will spontaneously disappear and should not require surgery. Rarely, they may twist or rupture, sometimes causing abdominal pain, and surgical intervention may be required.

4. *Ectopic Pregnancies*

Ectopic pregnancies have occurred among NORPLANT SYSTEM users, although clinical studies have shown no increase in the rate of ectopic pregnancies per year among NORPLANT SYSTEM users as compared with users of no method or of IUDs. The incidence among NORPLANT SYSTEM users was 1.3 per 1000 woman-years, a rate significantly below the rate that has been estimated for noncontraceptive users in the United States (2.7 to 3.0 per 1000 woman-years). The risk of ectopic pregnancy may increase with the duration of NORPLANT SYSTEM use and possibly with increased weight of the user. Physicians should be alert to the possibility of an ectopic pregnancy among women using the NORPLANT SYSTEM who become pregnant or complain of lower-abdominal pain. Any patient who presents with lower-abdominal pain must be evaluated to rule out ectopic pregnancy.

5. *Foreign-body Carcinogenesis*

Rarely, cancers have occurred at the site of foreign-body intrusions or old scars. None has been reported in NORPLANT SYSTEM clinical trials. In rodents, which are highly susceptible to such cancers, the incidence decreases with decreasing size of the foreign body. Because of the resistance of human beings to these cancers and because of the small size of the capsules, the risk to users of the NORPLANT SYSTEM is judged to be minimal.

6. *Thromboembolic Disorders and Other Vascular Problems*

An increased risk of thromboembolic and thrombotic disease (pulmonary embolism, superficial venous thrombosis, and deep-vein thrombosis) has been found to be associated with the use of combination oral contraceptives. The relative risk has been estimated to be 4- to 11-fold higher for users than for nonusers. There have also been post-marketing reports of these events coincident with NORPLANT SYSTEM use. The reports of thrombophlebitis and superficial phlebitis have more commonly occurred in the arm of insertion. Some of these cases have been associated with trauma to that arm.

Cerebrovascular Disorders: Combination oral contraceptives have been shown to increase both the relative and attributable risks of cerebrovascular events (thrombotic and hemorrhagic strokes), although, in general, the risk is greatest among older (>35 years) hypertensive women who also smoke. Hypertension was found to be a risk factor for both users and nonusers for both types of strokes, while smoking interacted to increase the risk for hemorrhagic strokes. There have been post-marketing reports of stroke coincident with NORPLANT SYSTEM use.

Myocardial Infarction: An increased risk of myocardial infarction has been attributed to combination oral-contraceptive use. This is thought to be primarily thrombotic in origin and is related to the estrogen component of combination oral contraceptives. This increased risk occurs primarily in smokers or in women with other underlying risk factors for coronary-artery disease, such as family history of coronary-artery disease, hypertension, hypercholesterolemia, morbid obesity, and diabetes. The current relative risk of heart attack for combination oral-contraceptive users has been estimated as 2 to 6 times the risk for nonusers. The absolute risk is very low for women under 30 years of age.

Studies indicate a significant trend toward higher rates of myocardial infarctions and strokes with increasing doses of progestin in combination oral contraceptives. However, a recent study showed no increased risk of myocardial infarction associated with the past use of levonorgestrel-containing combination oral contraceptives. There have been post-marketing reports of myocardial infarction coincident with NORPLANT SYSTEM use.

Patients who develop active thrombophlebitis or thromboembolic disease should have the NORPLANT SYSTEM capsules removed. Removal should also be considered in women who will be subjected to prolonged immobilization due to surgery or other illnesses.

7. *Use Before or During Early Pregnancy*

Extensive epidemiological studies have revealed no increased risk of birth defects in women who have used oral contraceptives prior to pregnancy. Studies also do not suggest a teratogenic effect, particularly insofar as cardiac anomalies and limb-reduction defects are concerned, when taken inadvertently during early pregnancy. There is no evidence suggesting that the risk associated with NORPLANT SYSTEM use is different.

There have been rare reports of congenital anomalies in offspring of women who were using the NORPLANT SYSTEM inadvertently during early pregnancy. A cause and effect relationship is not believed to exist.

8. *Idiopathic Intracranial Hypertension*

Idiopathic intracranial hypertension (pseudotumor cerebri, benign intracranial hypertension) is a disorder of unknown etiology which is seen most commonly in obese females of reproductive age. There have been reports of idiopathic intracranial hypertension in NORPLANT SYSTEM users. A cardinal sign of idiopathic intracranial hypertension is papilledema; early symptoms may include headache (associated with a change in frequency, pattern, severity, or persistence; of particular importance are those headaches that are unremitting in nature) and visual disturbances. Patients with these symptoms, particularly obese patients or those with recent weight gain, should be screened for papilledema and, if present, the patient should be referred to a neurologist for further diagnosis and care. NORPLANT SYSTEM should be removed from patients experiencing this disorder.

B. **Warnings Based on Experience with Combination (Progestin plus Estrogen) Oral Contraceptives**

1. *Cigarette Smoking*

Cigarette smoking increases the risk of serious cardiovascular side effects from the use of combination oral contraceptives. This risk increases with age and with heavy smoking (15 or more cigarettes per day) and is quite marked in women over 35 years old. While this is believed to be an estrogen-related effect, it is not known whether a similar risk exists with progestin-only methods such as the NORPLANT SYSTEM; however, women who use the NORPLANT SYSTEM should be advised not to smoke.

2. *Elevated Blood Pressure*

Increased blood pressure has been reported in users of combination oral contraceptives. The prevalence of elevated blood pressure increases with long exposure. Although there were no statistically significant trends among NORPLANT SYSTEM users in clinical trials, physicians should be aware of the possibility of elevated blood pressure with the NORPLANT SYSTEM.

3. *Carcinoma*

Numerous epidemiological studies have been performed to determine the incidence of breast, endometrial, ovarian, and cervical cancer in women using combination oral contraceptives. Recent evidence in the literature suggests that use of combination oral contraceptives is not associated with an increased risk of developing breast cancer in the overall population of users. The Cancer and Steroid Hormone (CASH) study also showed no latent effect on the risk of breast cancer for at least a decade following long-term use. However, some of these same recent studies have shown an increased relative risk of breast cancer in certain subgroups of combination oral-contraceptive users, although no consistent pattern of findings has been identified. This information should be considered when prescribing the NORPLANT SYSTEM.

Some studies suggest that combination oral-contraceptive use has been associated with an increase in the risk of cervical intraepithelial neoplasia in some populations of women. However, there continues to be controversy about the extent to which such findings may be due to differences in sexual behavior and other factors. In spite of many studies of the relationship between combination oral-contraceptive use and breast and cervical cancers, a cause-and-effect relationship has not been established.

Evidence indicates that combination oral contraceptives may decrease the risk of ovarian and endometrial cancer.

TABLE 3
Annual and Five-Year Cumulative Rates
per 100 Users

	year 1	year 2	year 3	year 4	year 5	Cumulative
Pregnancy	0.2	0.5	1.2	1.6	0.4	3.9
Bleeding Irregularities	9.1	7.9	4.9	3.3	2.9	25.1
Medical (excl. bleeding irreg.)	6.0	5.6	4.1	4.0	5.1	22.4
Personal	4.6	7.7	11.7	10.7	11.7	38.7
Continuation	81.0	77.4	79.2	76.7	77.6	29.5

Irregular bleeding patterns associated with the NORPLANT SYSTEM could mask symptoms of cervical or endometrial cancer.

4. *Hepatic Tumors*
Hepatic adenomas have been found to be associated with the use of combination oral contraceptives with an estimated incidence of about 3 occurrences per 100,000 users per year, a risk that increases after 4 or more years of use. Although benign, hepatic adenomas may rupture and cause death through intra-abdominal hemorrhage. The contribution of the progestin component of oral contraceptives to the development of hepatic adenomas is not known.

5. *Ocular Lesions*
There have been clinical case reports of retinal thrombosis associated with the use of oral contraceptives. Although it is believed that this adverse reaction is related to the estrogen component of oral contraceptives, the NORPLANT SYSTEM capsules should be removed if there is unexplained partial or complete loss of vision; onset of proptosis or diplopia; papilledema; or retinal vascular lesions. Appropriate diagnostic and therapeutic measures should be undertaken immediately.

6. *Gallbladder Disease*
Earlier studies have reported an increased lifetime relative risk of gallbladder surgery in users of oral contraceptives and estrogens. More recent studies, however, have shown that the relative risk of developing gallbladder disease among oral-contraceptive users may be minimal. The recent findings of minimal risk may be related to the use of oral-contraceptive formulations containing lower hormonal doses of estrogens and progestins. The association of this risk with use of the NORPLANT SYSTEM progestin-only method is not known.

PRECAUTIONS

General

Patients should be counseled that this product does not protect against HIV infection (AIDS) and other sexually transmitted diseases.

1. *Physical Examination and Follow-Up*
A complete medical history and physical examination should be taken prior to the implantation or reimplantation of NORPLANT SYSTEM capsules and at least annually during its use. These physical examinations should include special reference to the implant site, blood pressure, breasts, abdomen and pelvic organs, including cervical cytology and relevant laboratory tests. In case of undiagnosed, persistent or recurrent abnormal vaginal bleeding, appropriate diagnostic measures should be conducted to rule out malignancy. Women with a strong family history of breast cancer or who have breast nodules should be monitored with particular care.

2. *Insertion and Removal*
To be sure that the woman is not pregnant at the time of capsule placement and to assure contraceptive effectiveness during the first cycle of use, it is advisable that insertion be done during the first 7 days of the menstrual cycle or immediately following an abortion. However, NORPLANT SYSTEM capsules may be inserted at any time during the cycle provided pregnancy has been excluded and a nonhormonal contraceptive method is used for at least 7 days following insertion. Insertion is not recommended before 6 weeks postpartum in breast-feeding women.

Insertion and removal instructions must be followed closely. It is strongly advised that all health-care professionals who insert and remove NORPLANT SYSTEM capsules be instructed in the procedures before they attempt them. Proper insertion just under the skin will facilitate removal.

If infection develops after insertion, suitable treatment should be instituted. If infection persists, capsules should be removed.

In the case of capsule expulsion, the expelled capsule must be replaced using a new sterile capsule, as contraceptive efficacy may be inadequate with fewer than 6 capsules. If infection is present, it should be treated and cured before capsule replacement.

Removal should be done upon patient request, for medical indications, or at the end of 5 years of use, by personnel instructed in the removal technique. If the capsules were placed deeply, they may be harder to remove. The use of general anesthesia during removal should generally be avoided.

Before initiating the removal procedure, all NORPLANT SYSTEM capsules should be located via palpation. If all 6 capsules cannot be located by palpation, they may be localized by ultrasound (7 MHz), X ray, or compression mammography. If all capsules cannot be removed at the first attempt, removal should be attempted later when the site has healed.

Upon removal, NORPLANT SYSTEM capsules should be disposed of in accordance with the Center for Disease Control and Prevention guidelines for the handling of biohazardous waste.

See also **"WARNINGS," "ADVERSE REACTIONS"** and **"INSTRUCTIONS FOR INSERTION AND REMOVAL—Removal Procedure."**

3. *Carbohydrate and Lipid Metabolism*
An altered glucose tolerance characterized by decreased insulin sensitivity following glucose loading has been found in some users of combination and progestin-only oral contraceptives. The effects of the NORPLANT SYSTEM on carbohydrate metabolism appear to be minimal. In a study in which pretreatment serum-glucose levels were compared with levels after 1 and 2 years of NORPLANT SYSTEM use, no statistically significant differences in mean serum-glucose levels were evident 2 hours after glucose loading. The clinical significance of these findings is unknown, but diabetic patients should be carefully observed while using the NORPLANT SYSTEM.

Women who are being treated for hyperlipidemias should be followed closely if they elect to use the NORPLANT SYSTEM. Some progestins may elevate LDL levels and may render the control of hyperlipidemias more difficult. (See **"WARNINGS,"** A.6.)

4. *Liver Function*
If jaundice develops in any women while using the NORPLANT SYSTEM, consideration should be given to removing the capsules. Steroid hormones may be poorly metabolized in patients with impaired liver function.

5. *Fluid Retention*
Steroid contraceptives may cause some degree of fluid retention. They should be prescribed with caution, and only with careful monitoring, in patients with conditions which might be aggravated by fluid retention.

6. *Emotional Disorders*
Consideration should be given to removing NORPLANT SYSTEM capsules in women who become significantly depressed since the symptom may be drug-related. Women with a history of depression should be carefully observed and removal considered if depression recurs to a serious degree.

7. *Contact Lenses*
Contact-lens wearers who develop visual changes or changes in lens tolerance should be assessed by an ophthalmologist.

8. *Autoimmune Disease*
Autoimmune diseases such as scleroderma, systemic lupus erythematosus and rheumatoid arthritis occur in the general population and more frequently among women of childbearing age. There have been rare reports of various autoimmune diseases, including the above, in NORPLANT SYSTEM users; however, the rate of reporting is significantly less than the expected incidence for these diseases. Studies have raised the possibility of developing antibodies against silicone-containing devices; however, the specificity and clinical relevance of these antibodies are unknown. While it is believed that the occurrence of autoimmune disease among NORPLANT SYSTEM users is coincidental, health-care providers should be alert to the earliest manifestations.

Drug Interactions

Reduced efficacy (pregnancy) has been reported for NORPLANT SYSTEM users taking phenytoin and carbamazepine. These drugs may increase the metabolism of levonorgestrel through induction of microsomal liver enzymes. NORPLANT SYSTEM users should be warned of the possibility of decreased efficacy with the use of drugs exhibiting enzyme-inducing activity such as those noted above and rifampin. For women receiving long-term therapy with hepatic enzyme inducers, another method of contraception should be considered.

Drug/Laboratory Test Interactions

Certain endocrine tests may be affected by NORPLANT SYSTEM use:

1. Sex-hormone-binding globulin concentrations are decreased.
2. Thyroxine concentrations may be slightly decreased and triiodothyronine uptake increased.

Carcinogenesis

See **"WARNINGS"** section.

Pregnancy

Pregnancy Category X. See **"WARNINGS"** section.

Nursing Mothers

Steroids are not considered the contraceptives of first choice for breast-feeding women. Levonorgestrel has been identified in the breast milk. The health of breast-fed infants whose mothers began using the NORPLANT SYSTEM during the 5th to 7th week postpartum was evaluated; no significant effects were observed on the growth or development of infants who were followed to 12 months of age. No data are available on use in breast-feeding mothers earlier than this after parturition.

Pediatric Use

Safety and efficacy of the NORPLANT SYSTEM have been established in women of reproductive age. Safety and efficacy are expected to be similar for postpubertal adolescents under 16 and users 16 and older. Use of this product before menarche is not indicated.

Information for the Patient

See Patient Labeling.

Two copies of the Patient Labeling are included to help describe the characteristics of the NORPLANT SYSTEM to the patient. One copy should be provided to the patient. Patients should also be advised that the Prescribing Information is available to them at their request. It is recommended that propective users be fully informed about the risks and benefits associated with use of the NORPLANT SYSTEM, with other forms of contraception, and with no contraception at all. It is also recommended that prospective users be fully informed about the insertion and removal procedures. Health-care providers may wish to obtain informed consent from all patients in light of the techniques involved with insertion and removal.

ADVERSE REACTIONS

The following adverse reactions have been associated with the NORPLANT SYSTEM during the first year of use. They include:

Many bleeding days or prolonged bleeding	27.6%
Spotting	17.1%
Amenorrhea	9.4%
Irregular (onsets of) bleeding	7.6%
Frequent bleeding onsets	7.0%
Scanty bleeding	5.2%
Pain or itching near implant site (usually transient)	3.7%
Infection at implant site	0.7%

In addition, removal difficulties affecting subjects (including multiple incisions, capsule fragments remaining, pain, multiple visits, deep placement, lengthy removal procedure, or other) have been reported with a frequency of 6.2%, which is based on 849 removals occurring through 5 years of use. See **"WARNINGS"** and **"PRECAUTIONS."**

Clinical studies comparing NORPLANT® SYSTEM users with other contraceptive method users suggest that the following adverse reactions occurring during the first year are probably associated with NORPLANT SYSTEM use. These adverse reactions have also been reported post-marketing:

Headache
Nervousness/Anxiety
Nausea/Vomiting
Dizziness
Adnexal enlargement
Dermatitis/Rash
Acne
Change of appetite
Mastalgia
Weight gain
Hirsutism, hypertrichosis, and scalp-hair loss

In addition, the following adverse reactions have been reported with a frequency of 5% or greater during the first year and are possibly related to NORPLANT SYSTEM use:

Breast discharge
Cervicitis
Musculoskeletal pain
Abdominal discomfort
Leukorrhea
Vaginitis

The following adverse reactions have been reported post-marketing with an incidence of less than 1% and are possibly related to NORPLANT SYSTEM use:

Emotional lability
Idiopathic intracranial hypertension (IIH, pseudotumor cerebri, benign intracranial hypertension)
Induration
Bruising
Abscess, cellulitis
Dysmenorrhea
Migraine
Arm pain
Numbness
Tingling
Depression
Excessive scarring
Hyperpigmentation
Nerve injury

The following adverse reactions have been reported post-marketing with an incidence of less than 1%. These events occurred under circumstances where a causal relationship to the NORPLANT SYSTEM is unknown. These reactions are listed as information for physicians:

Congenital anomalies
Pulmonary embolism
Superficial venous thrombosis
Deep-vein thrombosis
Myocardial infarction
Blistering, ulcerations, and sloughing
Thrombotic thrombocytopenic purpura (TTP)
Stroke
Pruritus
Urticaria
Asthenia (fatigue/weakness)
Phlebitis

OVERDOSAGE

Overdosage can result if more than six capsules of the NORPLANT SYSTEM are in situ. All implanted NORPLANT SYSTEM capsules should be removed before inserting a new set of NORPLANT SYSTEM capsules. Overdosage may cause fluid retention with its associated effects and uterine bleeding irregularities.

DOSAGE AND ADMINISTRATION

The NORPLANT SYSTEM consists of six Silastic® capsules, each containing 36 mg of the progestin, levonorgestrel. The total administered (implanted) dose is 216 mg. Implantation of all six capsules should be performed during the first 7 days of the onset of menses by a health-care professional instructed in the NORPLANT SYSTEM insertion technique. Insertion is subdermal in the midportion of the upper arm about 8 to 10 cm above the elbow crease. Distribution should be in a fanlike pattern, about 15 degrees apart, for a total of 75 degrees. Proper insertion will facilitate later removal. (See section on Insertion/Removal.)

HOW SUPPLIED

The NORPLANT SYSTEM Kit includes the following items:
1 NORPLANT SYSTEM (levonorgestrel implants), a set of six implants (capsules)
1 NORPLANT SYSTEM trocar
1 Scalpel
1 Forceps
1 Syringe
2 Syringe needles
1 Package of skin closures

Continued on next page

Norplant—Cont.

3 Packages of gauze sponges
1 Stretch bandage
1 Surgical drape (fenestrated)
2 Surgical drapes

Store at room temperature away from excess heat and moisture.

Note: The indented statement below is required by the Federal government's Clean Air Act for all products containing or manufactured with chlorofluorocarbons (CFC's).

> **WARNING:** Manufactured with dichlorodifluoromethane, a substance which harms public health and environment by destroying ozone in the upper atmosphere.

A notice similar to the above WARNING has been placed in the patient information leaflet of this product under Environmental Protection Agency (EPA) regulations. The patient's warning states that the patient should consult his or her physician if there are questions about alternatives.
Dichlorodifluoromethane is a chemical used in the sterilization process of the NORPLANT SYSTEM and is not contained in the product itself.

NDC 0008-2564-01

References available upon request.

INSTRUCTIONS FOR INSERTION AND REMOVAL

The NORPLANT SYSTEM consists of six levonorgestrel-releasing capsules that are inserted subdermally in the medial aspect of the upper arm.
The NORPLANT SYSTEM provides up to 5 years of effective contraceptive protection.
The basis for successful use and subsequent removal of NORPLANT SYSTEM capsules is a correct and carefully performed subdermal insertion of the six capsules. It is recommended that health-care professionals performing insertions or removals of NORPLANT SYSTEM capsules avail themselves of instruction and supervision in the proper technique prior to attempting these procedures. During insertion, special attention should be given to the following:
— asepsis.
— correct subdermal placement of the capsules.
— careful technique to minimize tissue trauma.
This will help to avoid infections and excessive scarring at the insertion area and will help keep the capsules from being inserted deeply in the tissue. If the capsules are placed deeply, they will be more difficult to remove than correctly placed subdermal capsules.

Insertion Procedure

Insertion should be performed within seven days from the onset of menses. However, NORPLANT SYSTEM capsules may be inserted at any time during the cycle provided pregnancy has been excluded and a nonhormonal contraceptive method is used for at least 7 days following insertion. It is recommended that a complete history and physical examination, including a gynecologic examination, be performed before the insertion of NORPLANT SYSTEM capsules. Determine if the subject has any allergies to the antiseptic or anesthetic to be used or contraindications to progestin-only contraception. If none are found, the capsules are inserted using the procedure outlined below.
One NORPLANT SYSTEM set consists of six capsules in a sterile pouch. The insertion is performed under aseptic conditions using a trocar to place the capsules under the skin.

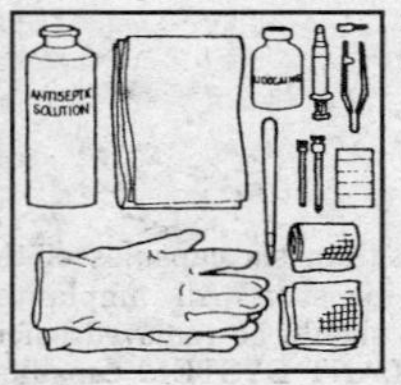

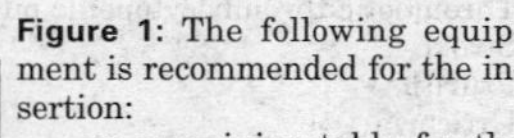

Figure 1: The following equipment is recommended for the insertion:
—an examining table for the patient to lie on.
—sterile surgical drapes, sterile gloves (free of talc), antiseptic solution.
—local anesthetic, needles, and syringe.
—#11 scalpel, #10 trocar, forceps
—skin closure, sterile gauze, and compresses.

The plastic cover and tray are NOT STERILE.

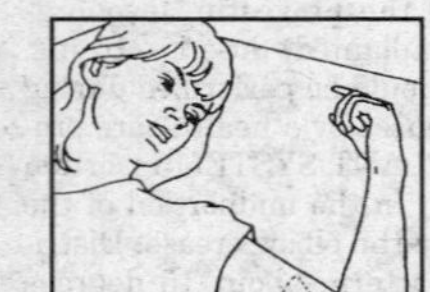

Figure 2: Have the patient lie on her back on the examination table with her left arm (if the patient is left-handed, the right arm) flexed at the elbow and externally rotated so that her hand is lying by her head. The capsules will be inserted subdermally through a small 2-mm incision and positioned in a fanlike manner with the fan opening towards the shoulder.

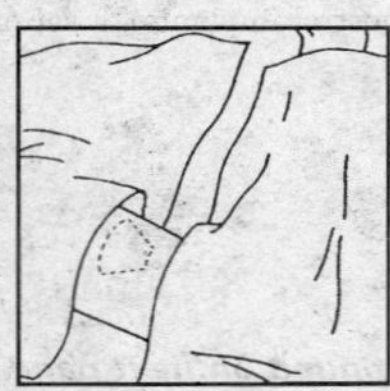

Figure 3: Prep the patient's upper arm with antiseptic solution; cover the arm above and below the insertion area with a sterile cloth. The optimal insertion area is in the inside of the upper arm about 8 to 10 cm above the elbow crease.

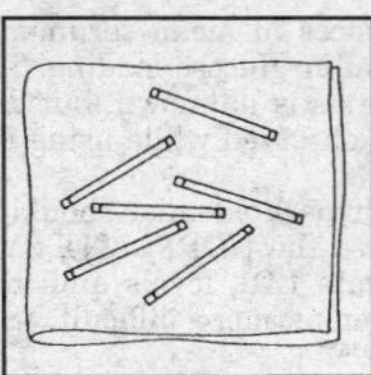

Figure 4: Open the sterile NORPLANT SYSTEM package carefully by pulling apart the sheets of the pouch, allowing the capsules to fall onto a sterile drape. Count the six capsules.

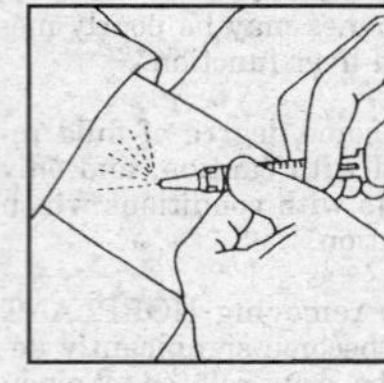

Figure 5: After determining the absence of known allergies to the anesthetic agent or related drugs, fill a 5-mL syringe with the local anesthetic. Since blood loss is minimal with this procedure, use of epinephrine-containing anesthetics is not considered necessary. Anesthetize the insertion area by first inserting the needle under the skin and injecting a small amount of anesthetic. Then anesthetize six areas about 4 to 4.5 cm long, to mimic the fanlike position of the implanted capsules.

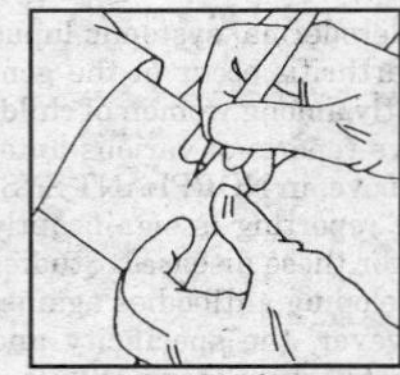

Figure 6: Use the scalpel to make a small incision (about 2 mm) just through the dermis of the skin. Alternatively, the trocar may be inserted directly through the skin without making an incision with the scapel. The bevel of the trocar should always face up during the insertion.

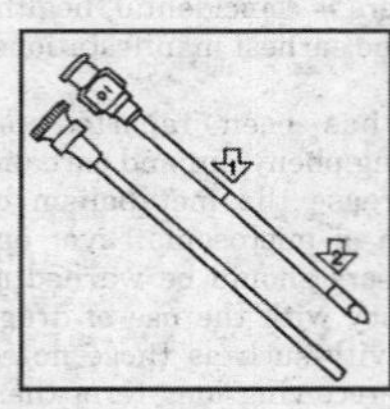

Figure 7: The trocar has two marks on it. The first mark is closer to the hub and indicates how far the trocar should be introduced under the skin before the loading of each capsule. The second mark is close to the tip and indicates how much of the trocar should remain under the skin following the insertion of each implant.

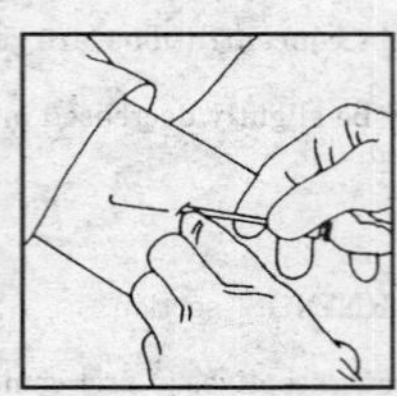

Figure 8: Insert the tip of the trocar through the incision beneath the skin at a shallow angle. Once the trocar is inserted, it should be oriented with the the bevel up toward the skin to keep the capsules in a superficial plane. It is important to keep the trocar subdermal by tenting the skin with the trocar, as failure to do so may result in deep placement of the capsules and could make removal more difficult.

Advance the trocar gently under the skin to the first mark near the hub of the trocar. The tip of the trocar is now at a distance of about 4 to 4.5 cm from the incision.
Do not force the trocar, and if resistance is felt, try another direction.

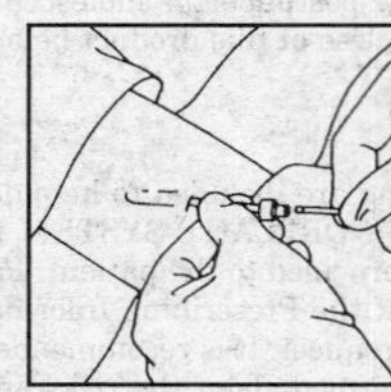

Figure 9: When the trocar has been inserted the appropriate distance, remove the obturator and load the first capsule into the trocar using the thumb and forefinger.

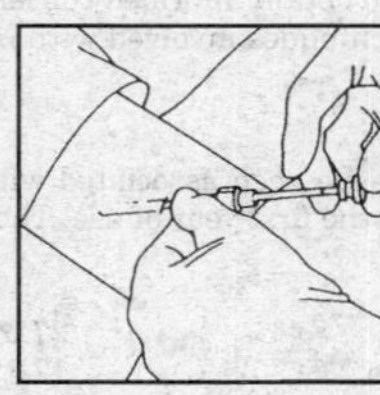

Figure 10: Gently advance the capsule with the obturator towards the tip of the trocar until you feel resistance. Never force the obturator.

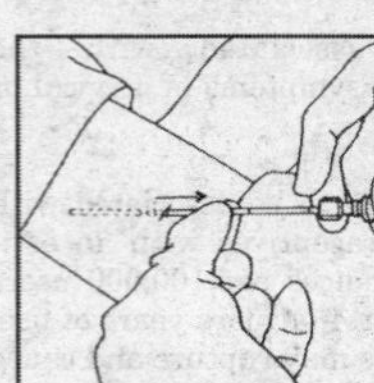

Figure 11: Hold the obturator steady, and bring the trocar back until it touches the handle of the obturator.

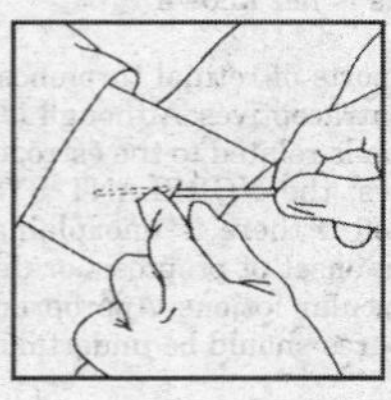

Figure 12: The capsule should have been released under the skin when the mark close to the tip of the trocar is visible in the incision. Release of the capsule can be checked by palpation. It is important to keep the obturator steady and not to push the capsule into the tissue.

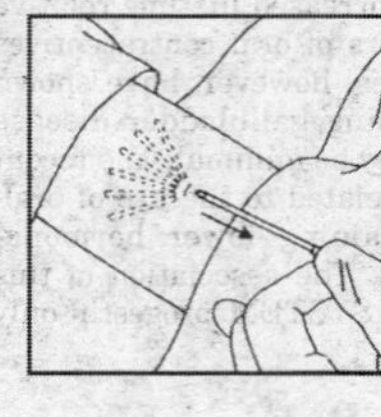

Figure 13: Do not remove the trocar from the incision until all capsules have been inserted. The trocar is withdrawn only to the mark close to its tip. Each succeeding capsule is always inserted next to the previous one, to form a fanlike shape. Fix the position of the previous capsule with the forefinger and and middle finger of the free hand, and advance the trocar along the tips of the fingers. This will ensure a suitable distance of about 15 degrees between capsules and keep the trocar from puncturing any of the previously inserted capsules.

Leave a distance of about 5 mm between the incision and the tips of the capsules. This will help avoid spontaneous expulsions. The correct position of the capsules can be ensured by feeling them with the fingers after the insertion has been completed.

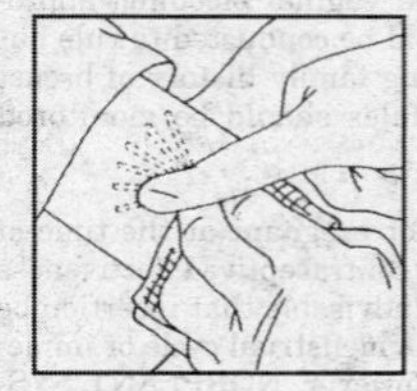

Figure 14: After placement of the sixth capsule, a sterile gauze may be used to apply pressure briefly to the insertion site to ensure hemostasis. Palpate the distal ends of the capsules to make sure that all six have been properly placed.

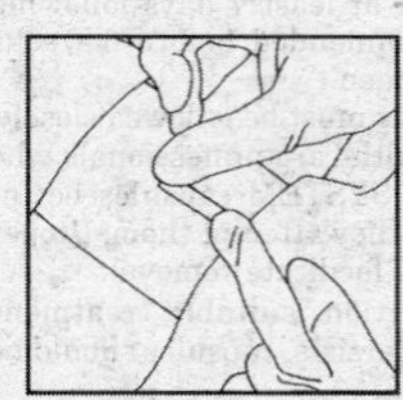

Figure 15: Press the edges of the incision together, and close the incision with a skin closure. Suturing the incision should not be necessary.

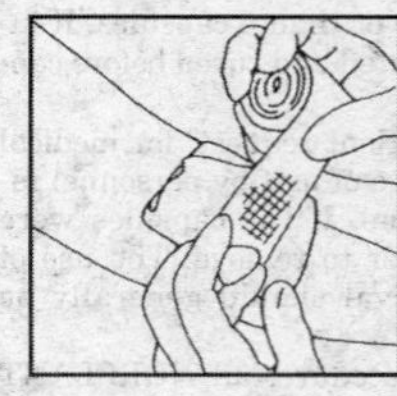

Figure 16: Cover the insertion area with a dry compress, and wrap gauze around the arm to ensure hemostasis.
Observe the patient for a few minutes for signs of syncope or bleeding from the incision before she is discharged.
Advise the patient to keep the insertion area dry and avoid heavy lifting for 2 to 3 days. The gauze may be removed after 1 day, and the butterfly bandage as soon as the incision has healed, i.e., normally in 3 days.

Removal Procedure

Described below is a removal procedure which was developed and used during the clinical trials for the NORPLANT SYSTEM. As with many surgical procedures, variations of the technique have appeared and some have been published. No one particular procedure routinely appears to have any advantage over another.
It is recommended that removals be prescheduled so that preparations for carrying out the procedure can be facilitated.
Removal of the capsules should be performed very gently and will usually take more time and may be more difficult and/or more painful than insertion. Capsules are sometimes nicked, cut, or broken during removal, or may be difficult to

locate. The incidence of overall removal difficulties, including those that did not result in patient complaints (e.g., damage to the capsules) was 13.2%. Less than half of these removal difficulties have caused inconvenience to the patient. If the removal of some of the capsules proves difficult, have the patient return for another visit. The remaining capsule(s) will be easier to remove after the area is healed. It may be appropriate to seek consultation or provide referral for patients in whom initial attempts at capsule removal prove difficult. If contraception is still desired, a barrier method should be advised until all capsules are removed. The position of the patient and the asepsis are the same as for insertion.

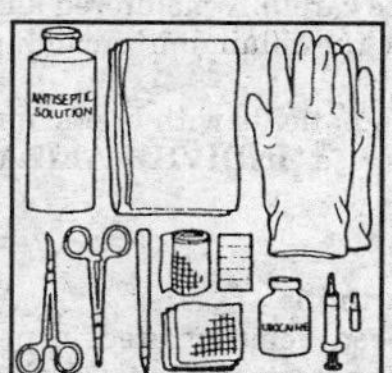

Figure 17: The following equipment is needed for the removal:
- —an examining table for the patient to lie on.
- —sterile surgical drapes, sterile gloves (free of talc), antiseptic solution.
- —local anesthetic, needles, and syringe.
- —#11 scalpel, forceps (straight and curved mosquito).
- —skin closure, sterile gauze, and compresses.

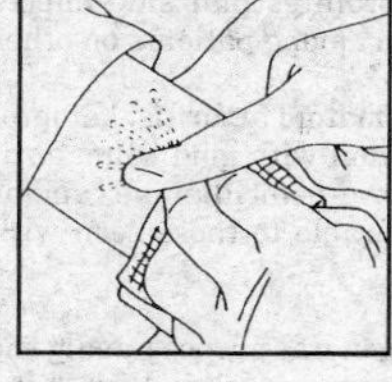

Figure 18: Palpate the capsules to make sure that all six capsules have been located, marking their position with a sterile marker. If all six capsules cannot be located by palpation, they may be localized by ultrasound (7 MHz), X ray, or compression mammography.

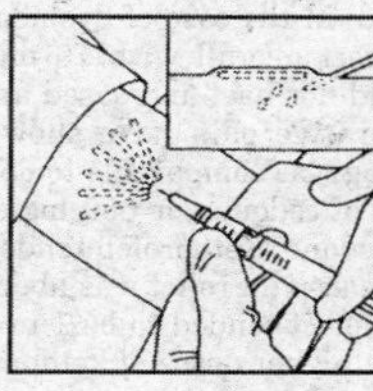

Figure 19: Once all six capsules are located, apply a small amount of local anesthetic *under* the capsule ends nearest the original incision site. This will serve to raise the ends of the capsules. Anesthetic injected over the capsules will obscure them and make removal more difficult. Additional small amounts of the anesthetic can be used for the removal of each of the capsules, if required.

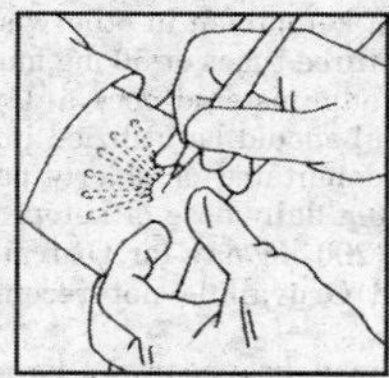

Figure 20: Make a 4-mm incision with the scalpel close to the ends of the capsules. Do not make a large incision.

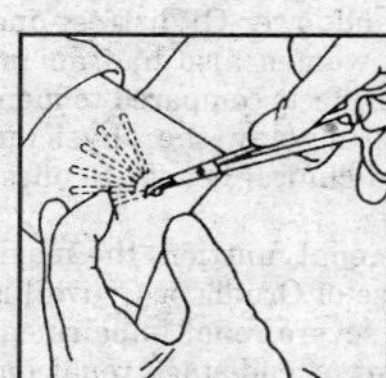

Figure 21: Push each capsule gently towards the incision with the fingers. When the tip is visible or near to the incision, grasp it with a mosquito forceps.

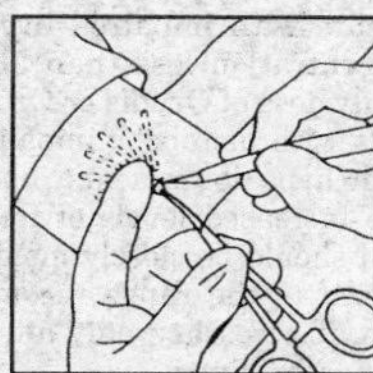

Figure 22: Use the scalpel, forceps, or gauze to very gently open the tissue sheath that has formed around the capsule.

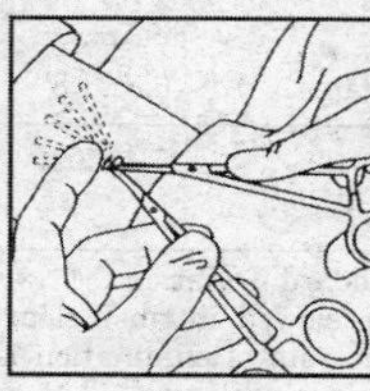

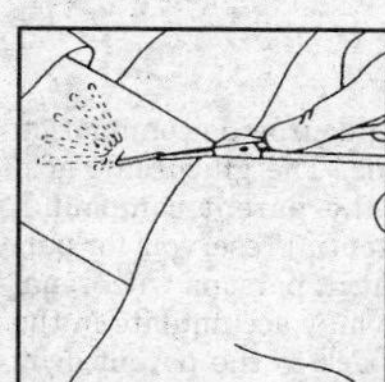

Figures 23 and 24: Remove the capsule from the incision with the second forceps.

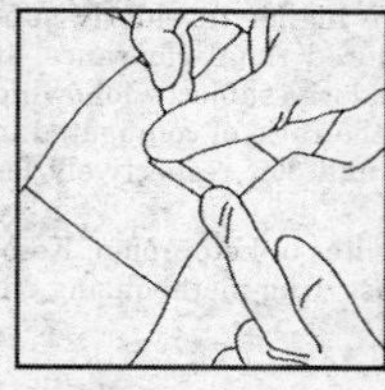

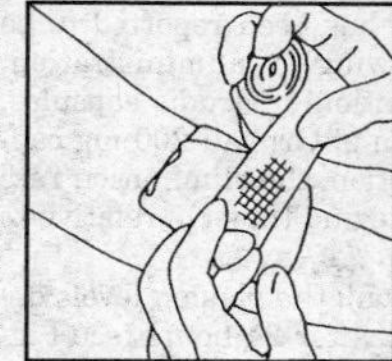

Figures 25 and 26: After the procedure is completed, the incision is closed and bandaged as with insertion. The upper arm should be kept dry for a few days.

Following removal, fertility rates return to levels comparable to those seen in the general population of women using no method of contraception, and a pregnancy may occur at any time. If the patient wishes to continue using the method, a new set of NORPLANT SYSTEM capsules can be inserted through the same incision in the same or opposite direction.

HINTS

Insertion

- — Counseling of the patient on the benefits and side effects of the method prior to insertion will greatly increase patient satisfaction.
- — Correct subdermal placement of the capsules will facilitate removal.
- — Before insertion, apply the anesthetic just beneath the skin so as to raise the dermis above the underlying tissue.
- — Never force the trocar.
- — To ensure subdermal placement, the trocar with bevel up should be supported by the index finger and should visibly raise the skin at all times during insertion.
- — To avoid damaging the previous implanted capsule, stabilize the capsule with your forefinger and middle finger and advance the trocar alongside the finger tips at an angle of 15 degrees.
- — After insertion, make a drawing for the patient's file showing the location of the 6 capsules and describe any variations in placement. This will greatly aid removal.

REMOVAL

- — Alternate removal techniques have been developed.
- — The removal of the implants will usually take more time and may be more difficult and/or more painful than the insertion. Capsules are sometimes nicked, cut, or broken during removal, or may be difficult to locate.
- — Before initiating removal, all capsules should be located by palpation. If all six capsules cannot be located by palpation, they may be localized via ultrasound (7 MHz), X ray, or compression mammography.
- — Before removal, apply the anesthetic *under* the capsule ends nearest the original incision site.
- — If the removal of some of the capsules proves difficult, interrupt the procedure and have the patient return for another visit. The remaining capsule(s) will be easier to remove after the area is healed.
- — It may be appropriate to seek consultation or provide referral for patients in whom initial attempts at capsule removal prove difficult.

Distributed by
Wyeth Laboratories
A Wyeth-Ayerst Company
Philadelphia, PA 19101
CI 4064-8 Revised December 11, 1998

Shown in Product Identification Guide, page 341

ORUDIS® ℞
[ō ′roo ′dĭs]
(ketoprofen)
Capsules

ORUVAIL® ℞
[or ′ü vāl]
(ketoprofen)
Extended-Release
Capsules

DESCRIPTION

Ketoprofen is a nonsteroidal anti-inflammatory drug. The chemical name for ketoprofen is 2–(3-benzoylphenyl)-propionic acid with the following structural formula:

Its empirical formula is $C_{16}H_{14}O_3$, with a molecular weight of 254.29. It has a pKa of 5.94 in methanol:water (3:1) and an n-octanol:water partition coefficient of 0.97 (buffer pH 7.4).

Ketoprofen is a white or off-white, odorless, nonhygroscopic, fine to granular powder, melting at about 95° C. It is freely soluble in ethanol, chloroform, acetone, ether and soluble in benzene and strong alkali, but practically insoluble in water at 20° C.

Orudis capsules contain 25 mg, 50 mg, or 75 mg of ketoprofen for oral administration. The inactive ingredients present are D&C Yellow 10, FD&C Blue 1, FD&C Yellow 6, gelatin, lactose, magnesium stearate, and titanium dioxide. The 25 mg dosage strength also contains D&C Red 28 and FD&C Red 40.

Each Oruvail 100 mg, 150 mg, or 200 mg capsule contains ketoprofen in the form of hundreds of coated pellets. The dissolution of the pellets is pH dependent with optimum dissolution occurring at pH 6.5–7.5. There is no dissolution at pH 1.

In addition to the active ingredient, each 100 mg, 150 mg, or 200 mg capsule of Oruvail contains the following inactive ingredients: D&C Red 22, D&C Red 28, FD&C Blue 1, ethyl cellulose, gelatin, shellac, silicon dioxide, sodium lauryl sulfate, starch, sucrose, talc, titanium dioxide, and other proprietary ingredients. The 100 and 150 mg capsules also contain D&C Yellow 10 and FD&C Green 3.

CLINICAL PHARMACOLOGY

Ketoprofen is a nonsteroidal anti-inflammatory drug with analgesic and antipyretic properties.

The anti-inflammatory, analgesic, and antipyretic properties of ketoprofen have been demonstrated in classical animal and *in vitro* test systems. In anti-inflammatory models ketoprofen has been shown to have inhibitory effects on prostaglandin and leukotriene synthesis, to have antibradykinin activity, as well as to have lysosomal membrane-stabilizing action. However, its mode of action, like that of other nonsteroidal anti-inflammatory drugs, is not fully understood.

PHARMACODYNAMICS

Ketoprofen is a racemate with only the S enantiomer possessing pharmacological activity. The enantiomers have similar concentration time curves and do not appear to interact with one another.

An analgesic effect-concentration relationship for ketoprofen was established in an oral surgery pain study with Orudis. The effect-site rate constant (k_{e0}) was estimated to be 0.9 $hour^{-1}$ (95% confidence limits: 0 to 2.1), and the concentration (Ce_{50}) of ketoprofen that produced one-half the maximum PID (pain intensity difference) was 0.3 µg/mL (95% confidence limits: 0.1 to 0.5). Thirty-three (33) to 68% of patients had an onset of action (as measured by reporting some pain relief) within 30 minutes following a single oral dose in postoperative pain and dysmenorrhea studies. Pain relief (as measured by remedication) persisted for up to 6 hours in 26 to 72% of patients in these studies.

PHARMACOKINETICS

General

Orudis and Oruvail capsules both contain ketoprofen. They differ only in their release characteristics. Orudis capsules release drug in the stomach whereas the pellets in Oruvail capsules are designed to resist dissolution in the low pH of gastric fluid but release drug at a controlled rate in the higher pH environment of the small intestine (see **"DESCRIPTION"**).

Irrespective of the pattern of release, the systemic availability (F_s) when either oral formulation is compared with IV administration is approximately 90% in humans. For 75 to 200 mg single doses, the area under the curve has been shown to be dose proportional. The figure depicts the plasma time curves associated with both products.

Ketoprofen is >99% bound to plasma proteins, mainly to albumin.

Separate sections follow which delineate differences between Orudis and Oruvail capsules.

Absorption

Orudis capsules—Ketoprofen is rapidly and well-absorbed, with peak plasma levels occurring within 0.5 to 2 hours.

Oruvail capsules—Ketoprofen is also well-absorbed from this dosage form, although an observable increase in

Continued on next page

Orudis/Oruvail—Cont.

plasma levels does not occur until approximately 2 to 3 hours after taking the formulation. Peak plasma levels are usually reached 6 to 7 hours after dosing. (See Figure and Table, below).

When ketoprofen is administered with food, its total bioavailability (AUC) is not altered; however, the rate of absorption from either dosage form is slowed.

Orudis capsules—Food intake reduces C_{max} by approximately one-half and increases the mean time to peak concentration (t_{max}) from 1.2 hours for fasting subjects (range, 0.5 to 3 hours) to 2.0 hours for fed subjects (range, 0.75 to 3 hours). The fluctuation of plasma peaks may also be influenced by circadian changes in the absorption process.

Concomitant administration of magnesium hydroxide and aluminum hydroxide does not interfere with absorption of ketoprofen from Orudis capsules.

Oruvail capsules—Administration of Oruvail with a high-fat meal causes a delay of about 2 hours in reaching the C_{max}; neither the total bioavailability (AUC) nor the C_{max} is affected. Circardian changes in the absorption process have not been studied.

The administration of antacids or other drugs which may raise stomach pH would not be expected to change the rate or extent of absorption of ketoprofen from Oruvail capsules.

Multiple Dosing

Steady-state concentrations of ketoprofen are attained within 24 hours after commencing treatment with Orudis or Oruvail capsules. In studies with healthy male volunteers, trough levels at 24 hours following administration of Oruvail 200 mg capsules were 0.4 mg/L compared with 0.07 mg/L at 24 hours following administration of Orudis 50 mg capsules QID (12 hours) or 0.13 mg/L following administration of Orudis 75 mg capsules TID for 12 hours. Thus, relative to the peak plasma concentration, the accumulation of ketoprofen after multiple doses of Oruvail or Orudis capsules is minimal.

The figure below shows a reduction in peak height and area after the second 50 mg dose. This is probably due to a combination of food effects, circadian effects, and plasma sampling times. It is unclear to what extent each factor contributes to the loss of peak height and area.

The shaded area represents ±1 standard deviation (S.D.) around the mean for Orudis or Oruvail.

KETOPROFEN PLASMA CONCENTRATIONS IN SUBJECTS RECEIVING 200 MG OF ORUVAIL ONCE A DAY (QD), OR ORUDIS 50 MG EVERY 4 HOURS FOR 16 HOURS

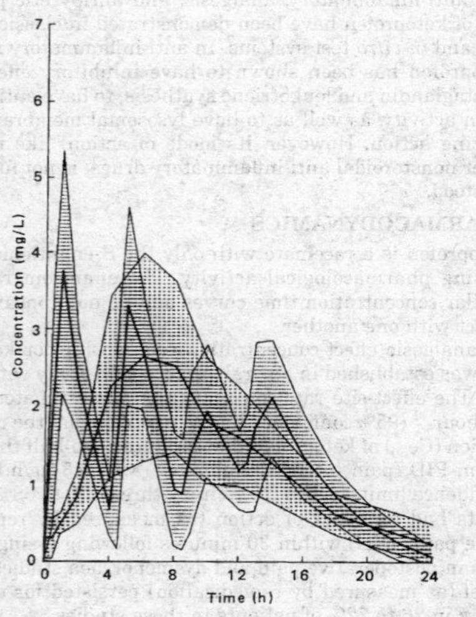

COMPARISON OF PHARMACOKINETIC PARAMETERS# FOR ORUDIS AND ORUVAIL

Kinetic Parameters	Orudis (4×50 mg)	Oruvail (1×200 mg)
Extent of oral absorption (bioavailability) F_s (%)	90	90
Peak plasma levels C_{max} (mg/L)		
Fasted	3.9±1.3	3.1±1.2
Fed	2.4±1.0	3.4±1.3
Time to peak concentration t_{max} (h)		
Fasted	1.2±0.6	6.8±2.1
Fed	2.0±0.8	9.2±2.6
Area under plasma concentration-time curve AUC_{0-24h}(mg·h/L)		
Fasted	32.1±7.2	30.1±7.9
Fed	36.6±8.1	31.3±8.1
Oral-dose clearance CL/F (L/h)	6.9±0.8	6.8±1.8
Half-life $t_{1/2}$ (h) [See footnote 1]	2.1±1.2	5.4±2.2

Values expressed are mean ± standard deviation

[1] In the case of Oruvail, absorption is slowed, intrinsic clearance is unchanged, but because the rate of elimination is dependent on absorption, the half-life is prolonged.

Metabolism

The metabolic fate of ketoprofen is glucuronide conjugation to form an unstable acyl-glucuronide. The glucuronic acid moiety can be converted back to the parent compound. Thus, the metabolite serves as a potential reservoir for parent drug, and this may be important in persons with renal insufficiency, whereby the conjugate may accumulate in the serum and undergo deconjugation back to the parent drug (see "**Special Populations**: *Renally impaired*").The conjugates are reported to appear only in trace amounts in plasma in healthy adults, but are higher in elderly subjects—presumably because of reduced renal clearance. It has been demonstrated that in elderly subjects following multiple doses (50 mg every 6 h), the ratio of conjugated to parent ketoprofen AUC was 30% and 3%, respectively for the S & R enantiomers.

There are no known active metabolites of ketoprofen. Ketoprofen has been shown not to induce drug-metabolizing enzymes.

Elimination

The plasma clearance of ketoprofen is approximately 0.08 L/kg/h with a V_d of 0.1 L/kg after IV administration. The elimination half-life of ketoprofen has been reported to be 2.05±0.58 h (Mean ± S.D.) following IV administration, from 2 to 4 h following administration of Orudis capsules, and 5.4±2.2 h after administration of Oruvail 200 mg capsules. In cases of slow drug absorption, the elimination rate is dependent on the absorption rate and thus $t_{1/2}$ relative to an IV dose appears prolonged.

After a single 200 mg dose of Oruvail, the plasma levels decline slowly, and average 0.4 mg/L after 24 hours (see Figure above).

In a 24-hour period, approximately 80% of an administered dose of ketoprofen is excreted in the urine, primarily as the glucuronide metabolite.

Enterohepatic recirculation of the drug has been postulated, although biliary levels have never been measured to confirm this.

Special Populations

Elderly: Clearance and unbound fraction

The plasma and renal clearance of ketoprofen is reduced in the elderly (mean age, 73 years) compared to a younger normal population (mean age, 27 years). Hence, ketoprofen peak concentration and AUC increase with increasing age. In addition, there is a corresponding increase in unbound fraction with increasing age. Data from one trial suggest that the increase is greater in women than in men. It has not been determined whether age-related changes in absorption among the elderly contribute to the changes in bioavailability of ketoprofen.

Orudis capsules—In a study conducted with young and elderly men and women, results for subjects older than 75 years of age showed that free drug AUC increased by 40% and C_{max} increased by 60% as compared with estimates of the same parameters in young subjects (those younger than 35 years of age; see "**INDIVIDUALIZATION OF DOSAGE**").

Also in the elderly, the ratio of intrinsic clearance/availability decreased by 35% and plasma half-life was prolonged by 26%. This reduction is thought to be due to a decrease in hepatic extraction associated with aging.

Oruvail capsules—The effects of age and gender on ketoprofen disposition were investigated in 2 small studies in which elderly male and female subjects received Oruvail 200 mg capsules. The results were compared with those from another study conducted in healthy young men.

Compared to the younger subject group, the elimination half-life in the elderly was prolonged by 54% and total drug C_{max} and AUC were 40% and 70% higher, respectively. Plasma concentrations in the elderly after single doses and at steady state were essentially the same. Thus, no drug accumulation occurs.

In comparison to younger subjects taking the immediate-release formulation (Orudis), there was a decrease of 16% and 25% in total drug C_{max} and AUC, respectively, among the elderly. Free drug data are not available for Oruvail.

Renally impaired

Studies of the effects of renal-function impairment have been small. They indicate a decrease in clearance in patients with impaired renal function. In 23 patients with renal impairment, free ketoprofen peak concentration was not significantly elevated, but free ketoprofen clearance was reduced from 15 L/kg/h for normal subjects to 7 L/kg/h in patients with mildly impaired renal function, and to 4 L/kg/h in patients with moderately to severely impaired renal function. The elimination $t_{1/2}$ was prolonged from 1.6 hours in normal subjects to approximately 3 hours in patients with mild renal impairment, and to approximately 5 to 9 hours in patients with moderately to severely impaired renal function.

No studies have been conducted in patients with renal impairment taking Oruvail capsules (see "**INDIVIDUALIZATION OF DOSAGE**").

Hepatically impaired

For patients with alcoholic cirrhosis, no significant changes in the kinetic disposition of Orudis capsules were observed relative to age-matched normal subjects: the plasma clearance of drug was 0.07 L/kg/h in 26 hepatically impaired patients. The elimination half-life was comparable to that observed for normal subjects. However, the unbound (biologically active) fraction was approximately doubled, probably due to hypoalbuminemia and high variability which was observed in the pharmacokinetics for cirrhotic patients. Therefore, these patients should be carefully monitored and daily doses of ketoprofen kept at the minimum providing the desired therapeutic effect.

No studies have been conducted in patients with heptic impairment taking Oruvail capsules (see "**INDIVIDUALIZATION OF DOSAGE**").

CLINICAL TRIALS

Rheumatoid Arthritis and Osteoarthritis

The efficacy of ketoprofen has been demonstrated in patients with rheumatoid arthritis and osteoarthritis. Using standard assessments of therapeutic response, there were no detectable differences in effectiveness or in the incidence of adverse events in crossover comparison of Orudis and Oruvail. In other trials, ketoprofen demonstrated effectiveness comparable to aspirin, ibuprofen, naproxen, piroxicam, diclofenac and indomethacin. In some of these studies there were more dropouts due to gastrointestinal side effects among patients on ketoprofen than among patients on other NSAIDs.

In studies with patients with rheumatoid arthritis, ketoprofen was administered in combination with gold salts, antimalarials, low-dose methotrexate, d-penicillamine, and/or corticosteroids with results comparable to those seen with control nonsteroidal drugs.

Management of Pain

The effectiveness of Orudis as a general-purpose analgesic has been studied in standard pain models which have shown the effectiveness of doses of 25 to 150 mg. Doses of 25 mg were superior to placebo. Doses larger than 25 mg generally could not be shown to be significantly more effective, but there was a tendency toward faster onset and greater duration of action with 50 mg, and, in the case of dysmenorrhea, a significantly greater effect overall with 75 mg. Doses greater than 50 to 75 mg did not have increased analgesic effect. Studies in postoperative pain have shown that Orudis in doses of 25 to 100 mg was comparable to 650 mg of acetaminophen with 60 mg of codeine, or 650 mg of acetaminophen with 10 mg of oxycodone. Ketoprofen tended to be somewhat slower in onset; peak pain relief was about the same and the duration of the effect tended to be 1 to 2 hours longer, particularly with the higher doses of ketoprofen.

The use of Oruvail in patients with acute pain is not recommended, since, in comparison to Orudis, Oruvail would be expected to have a delayed analgesic response due to its extended-release characteristics.

INDIVIDUALIZATION OF DOSAGE

The recommended starting dose of ketoprofen in otherwise healthy patients is Orudis, 75 mg three times or 50 mg four times a day, or Oruvail, 200 mg administered once a day. Smaller doses of Orudis or Oruvail should be utilized initially in small individuals or in debilitated or elderly patients. The recommended maximum daily dose of ketoprofen is 300 mg/day for Orudis or 200 mg/day for Oruvail. Concomitant use of Orudis and Oruvail is not recommended.

If minor side effects appear, they may disappear at a lower dose which may still have an adequate therapeutic effect. If well tolerated but not optimally effective, the dosage may be increased. Individual patients may show a better response to 300 mg of Orudis daily as compared to 200 mg, although in well-controlled clinical trials patients on 300 mg did not show greater mean effectiveness. They did, however, show an increased frequency of upper- and lower-GI distress and headaches. It is of interest that women also had an increased frequency of these adverse effects compared to men. When treating patients with 300 mg/day, the physician should observe sufficient increased clinical benefit to offset potential increased risk.

In patients with mildly impaired renal function, the maximum recommended total daily dose of Orudis or Oruvail is 150 mg. In patients with a more severe renal impairment (GFR less than 25 mL/min/1.73 m^2 or end-stage renal impairment), the maximum total daily dose of Orudis or Oruvail should not exceed 100 mg.

In elderly patients, renal function may be reduced with apparently normal serum creatinine and/or BUN levels. Therefore, it is recommended that the initial dosage of Orudis or Oruvail should be reduced for patients over 75 years of age.

It is recommended that for patients with impaired liver function and serum albumin concentration less than 3.5 g/dL, the maximum initial total daily dose of Orudis or Oruvail should be 100 mg. All patients with metabolic impairment, particularly those with both hypoalbuminemia and reduced renal function, may have increased levels of free (biologically active) ketoprofen and should be closely monitored. The dosage may be increased to the range recommended for the general population, if necessary, only after good individual tolerance has been ascertained.

Because hypoalbuminemia and reduced renal function both increase the fraction of free drug (biologically active form), patients who have both conditions may be at greater risk of adverse effects. Therefore, it is recommended that such patients also be started on lower doses of Orudis or Oruvail and closely monitored.

As with other nonsteroidal anti-inflammatory drugs, the predominant adverse effects of ketoprofen are gastrointestinal. To attempt to minimize these effects, physicians may wish to prescribe that Orudis or Oruvail be taken with antacids, food, or milk. Although food delays the absorption of both formulations (see "**CLINICAL PHARMACOLOGY**"), in most of the clinical trials ketoprofen was taken with food or milk.

Physicians may want to make specific recommendations to patients about when they should take Orudis or Oruvail in relation to food and/or what patients should do if they experience minor GI symptoms associated with either formulation.

INDICATIONS AND USAGE

Orudis or Oruvail are indicated for the management of the signs and symptoms of rheumatoid arthritis and osteoarthritis. Oruvail is not recommended for treatment of acute pain because of its extended-release characteristics (see "**PHARMACOKINETICS**").

Orudis is indicated for the management of pain. Orudis is also indicated for treatment of primary dysmenorrhea.

CONTRAINDICATIONS

Ketoprofen is contraindicated in patients who have shown hypersensitivity to it. Ketoprofen should not be given to patients in whom aspirin or other nonsteroidal anti-inflammatory drugs induce asthma, urticaria, or other allergic-type reactions, because severe, rarely fatal, anaphylactic reactions to ketoprofen have been reported in such patients.

WARNINGS

Risk of GI Ulceration, Bleeding and Perforation with NSAID Therapy

Serious gastrointestinal toxicity, such as bleeding, ulceration, and perforation, can occur at any time with or without warning symptoms, in patients treated chronically with NSAID therapy. Although minor upper-gastrointestinal problems, such as dyspepsia, are common, usually developing early in therapy, physicians should remain alert for ulceration and bleeding in patients treated chronically with NSAIDs even in the absence of previous GI-tract symptoms. In patients observed in clinical trials of several months to two years' duration, symptomatic upper-GI ulcers, gross bleeding, or perforation appear to occur in approximately 1% of patients treated for 3 to 6 months, and in about 2–4% of patients treated for one year. Physicians should inform patients about the signs and/or symptoms of serious GI toxicity and what steps to take if they occur.

Studies to date have not identified any subset of patients not at risk of developing peptic ulceration and bleeding. Except for a prior history of serious GI events and other risk factors known to be associated with peptic ulcer disease, such as alcoholism, smoking, etc., no other risk factors (e.g., age, sex) have been associated with increased risk. Elderly or debilitated patients seem to tolerate ulceration or bleeding less well than other individuals, and most spontaneous reports of fatal GI events are in this population. Studies to date are inconclusive concerning the relative risk of various NSAIDs in causing such reactions. High doses of any NSAID probably carry a greater risk of these reactions, although controlled clinical trials showing this do not exist in most cases. In considering the use of relatively large doses (within the recommended dosage range), sufficient benefit should be anticipated to offset the potential increased risk of GI toxicity.

GENERAL PRECAUTIONS

Ketoprofen and other nonsteroidal anti-inflammatory drugs cause nephritis in mice and rats associated with chronic administration. Rare cases of interstitial nephritis or nephrotic syndrome have been reported in humans with ketoprofen since it has been marketed.

A second form of renal toxicity has been seen in patients with conditions leading to a reduction in renal blood flow or blood volume, where renal prostaglandins have a supportive role in the maintenance of renal blood flow. In these patients, administration of a nonsteroidal anti-inflammatory drug results in a dose-dependent decrease in prostaglandin synthesis and, secondarily, in renal blood flow which may precipitate overt renal failure. Patients at greatest risk of this reaction are those with impaired renal function, heart failure, liver dysfunction, those taking diuretics, and the elderly. Discontinuation of nonsteroidal anti-inflammatory drug therapy is typically followed by recovery to the pretreatment state.

Since ketoprofen is primarily eliminated by the kidneys and its pharmacokinetics are altered by renal failure (see "**CLINICAL PHARMACOLOGY**"), patients with significantly impaired renal function should be closely monitored, and a reduction of dosage should be anticipated to avoid accumulation of ketoprofen and/or its metabolites (see "**INDIVIDUALIZATION OF DOSAGE**").

As with other nonsteroidal anti-inflammatory drugs, borderline elevations of one or more liver function tests may occur in up to 15% of patients. These abnormalities may progress, may remain essentially unchanged, or may disappear with continued therapy. The ALT (SGPT) test is probably the most sensitive indicator of liver dysfunction. Meaningful (3 times the upper limit of normal) elevations of ALT or AST (SGOT) occurred in controlled clinical trials in less than 1% of patients. A patient with symptoms and/or signs suggesting liver dysfunction, or in whom an abnormal liver test has occurred, should be evaluated for evidence of the development of a more severe hepatic reaction while on therapy with ketoprofen. Serious hepatic reactions, including jaundice, have been reported from post-marketing experience with ketoprofen as well as with other nonsteroidal anti-inflammatory drugs.

In patients with chronic liver disease with reduced serum albumin levels, ketoprofen's pharmacokinetics are altered (see "**CLINICAL PHARMACOLOGY**"). Such patients should be closely monitored, and a reduction of dosage should be anticipated to avoid high blood levels of ketoprofen and/or its metabolites (see "**INDIVIDUALIZATION OF DOSAGE**").

If steroid dosage is reduced or eliminated during therapy, it should be reduced slowly and the patients observed closely for any evidence of adverse effects, including adrenal insufficiency and exacerbation of symptoms of arthritis.

Anemia is commonly observed in rheumatoid arthritis and is sometimes aggravated by nonsteroidal anti-inflammatory drugs, which may produce fluid retention or significant gastrointestinal blood loss in some patients. Patients on long-term treatment with NSAIDs, including Orudis or Oruvail, should have their hemoglobin or hematocrit checked if they develop signs or symptoms of anemia.

Peripheral edema has been observed in approximately 2% of patients taking ketoprofen. Therefore, as with other nonsteroidal anti-inflammatory drugs, ketoprofen should be used with caution in patients with fluid retention, hypertension, or heart failure.

Information for Patients

Orudis or Oruvail contain ketoprofen. Like other drugs of its class, ketoprofen is not free of side effects. The side effects of these drugs can cause discomfort and, rarely, there are more serious side effects, such as gastrointestinal bleeding, which may result in hospitalization and even fatal outcomes.

NSAIDs are often essential agents in the management of arthritis and have a major role in the treatment of pain, but they also may be commonly employed for conditions which are less serious. Physicians may wish to discuss with their patients the potential risks (see "**WARNINGS,**" "**GENERAL PRECAUTIONS,**" and "**ADVERSE REACTIONS**" sections) and likely benefits of NSAID treatment, particularly when the drugs are used for less serious conditions where treatment without NSAIDs may represent an acceptable alternative to both the patient and physician.

Because aspirin causes an increase in the level of unbound ketoprofen, patients should be advised not to take aspirin while taking ketoprofen (see "**Drug Interactions**"). It is possible that minor adverse symptoms of gastric intolerance may be prevented by administering Orudis with antacids, food, or milk. Oruvail has not been studied with antacids. Because food and milk do affect the rate but not the extent of absorption (see "**CLINICAL PHARMACOLOGY**"), physicians may want to make specific recommendations to patients about when they should take ketoprofen in relation to food and/or what patients should do if they experience minor GI symptoms associated with ketoprofen therapy.

Laboratory Tests

Because serious GI-tract ulceration and bleeding can occur without warning symptoms, physicians should follow chronically treated patients for the signs and symptoms of ulceration and bleeding and should inform them of the importance of this follow-up (see "**WARNINGS—Risk of GI Ulceration, Bleeding and Perforation with NSAID Therapy**").

Drug Interactions

The following drug interactions were studied with ketoprofen doses of 200 mg/day. The possibility of increased interaction should be kept in mind when Orudis doses greater than 50 mg as a single dose or 200 mg of ketoprofen per day are used concomitantly with highly bound drugs.

1. *Antacids*

Concomitant administration of magnesium hydroxide and aluminum hydroxide does not interfere with the rate or extent of the absorption of ketoprofen administered as Orudis.

2. *Aspirin*

Ketoprofen does not alter aspirin absorption; however, in a study of 12 normal subjects, concurrent administration of aspirin decreased ketoprofen protein binding and increased ketoprofen plasma clearance from 0.07 L/kg/h without aspirin to 0.11 L/kg/h with aspirin. The clinical significance of these changes has not been adequately studied. Therefore, concurrent use of aspirin and ketoprofen is not recommended.

3. *Diuretic*

Hydrochlorothiazide, given concomitantly with ketoprofen, produces a reduction in urinary potassium and chloride excretion compared to hydrochlorothiazide alone. Patients taking diuretics are at greater risk of developing renal failure secondary to a decrease in renal blood flow caused by prostaglandin inhibition (see "**GENERAL PRECAUTIONS**").

4. *Digoxin*

In a study in 12 patients with congestive heart failure where ketoprofen and digoxin were concomitantly administered, ketoprofen did not alter the serum levels of digoxin.

5. *Warfarin*

In a short-term controlled study in 14 normal volunteers, ketoprofen did not significantly interfere with the effect of warfarin on prothrombin time. Bleeding from a number of sites may be a complication of warfarin treatment and GI bleeding a complication of ketoprofen treatment. Because prostaglandins play an important role in hemostasis and ketoprofen has an effect on platelet function as well (see "DRUG/LABORATORY TEST INTERACTIONS: EFFECT ON BLOOD COAGULATION"), concurrent therapy with ketoprofen and warfarin requires close monitoring of patients on both drugs.

6. *Probenecid*

Probenecid increases both free and bound ketoprofen by reducing the plasma clearance of ketoprofen to about one-third, as well as decreasing its protein binding. Therefore, the combination of ketoprofen and probenecid is not recommended.

7. *Methotrexate*

Ketoprofen, like other NSAIDs, may cause changes in the elimination of methotrexate leading to elevated serum levels of the drug and increased toxicity.

8. *Lithium*

Nonsteroidal anti-inflammatory agents have been reported to increase steady-state plasma lithium levels. It is recommended that plasma lithium levels be monitored when ketoprofen is co-administered with lithium.

Drug/Laboratory Test Interactions: Effect on Blood Coagulation

Ketoprofen decreases platelet adhesion and aggregation. Therefore, it can prolong bleeding time by approximately 3 to 4 minutes from baseline values. There is no significant change in platelet count, prothrombin time, partial thromboplastin time, or thrombin time.

Carcinogenesis, Mutagenesis, Impairment of Fertility

Chronic oral toxicity studies in mice (up to 32 mg/kg/day; 96 mg/m^2/day) did not indicate a carcinogenic potential for ketoprofen. The maximum recommended human therapeutic dose is 300 mg/day for a 60 kg patient with a body surface area of 1.6 m^2, which is 5 mg/kg/day or 185 mg/m^2/day. Thus the mice were treated at 0.5 times the maximum human daily dose based on surface area.

A 2-year carcinogenicity study in rats, using doses up to 6.0 mg/kg/day (36 mg/m^2/day), showed no evidence of tumorigenic potential. All groups were treated for 104 weeks except the females receiving 6.0 mg/kg/day (36 mg/m^2/day) where the drug treatment was terminated in week 81 because of low survival; the remaining rats were sacrificed after week 87. Their survival in the groups treated for 104 weeks was within 6% of the control group. An earlier 2-year study with doses up to 12.5 mg/kg/day (75 mg/m^2/day) also showed no evidence of tumorigenicity, but the survival rate was low and the study was therefore judged inconclusive.

Ketoprofen did not show mutagenic potential in the Ames Test. Ketoprofen administered to male rats (up to 9 mg/kg/day; or 54 mg/m^2/day) had no significant effect on reproductive performance or fertility. In female rats administered 6 or 9 mg/kg/day (36 or 54 mg/m^2/day), a decrease in the number of implantation sites has been noted. The dosages of 36 mg/m^2/day in rats represent 0.2 times the maximum recommended human dose of 185 mg/m^2/day (see above).

Abnormal spermatogenesis or inhibition of spermatogenesis developed in rats and dogs at high doses, and a decrease in the weight of the testes occurred in dogs and baboons at high doses.

Teratogenic Effects: Pregnancy Category B

In teratology studies ketoprofen administered to mice at doses up to 12 mg/kg/day (36 mg/m^2/day) and rats at doses up to 9 mg/kg/day (54 mg/m^2/day), the approximate equivalent of 0.2 times the maximum recommended therapeutic dose of 185 mg/m^2/day, showed no teratogenic or embryotoxic effects. In separate studies in rabbits, maternally toxic doses were associated with embryotoxicity but not teratogenicity.

There are no adequate and well-controlled studies in pregnant women. Because animal teratology studies are not always predictive of the human response, ketoprofen should be used during pregnancy only if the potential benefit justifies the risk.

Labor and Delivery

The effects of ketoprofen on labor and delivery in pregnant women are unknown. Studies in rats have shown ketoprofen at doses of 6 mg/kg (36 mg/m^2/day, approximately equal to 0.2 times the maximum recommended human dose) prolongs pregnancy when given before the onset of labor. Because of the known effects of prostaglandin-inhibiting drugs on the fetal cardiovascular system (closure of ductus arteriosus), use of ketoprofen during late pregnancy should be avoided.

Nursing Mothers

Data on secretion in human milk after ingestion of ketoprofen do not exist. In rats, ketoprofen at doses of 9 mg/kg (54 mg/m^2/day; approximately 0.3 times the maximum human therapeutic dose) did not affect perinatal development. Upon administration to lactating dogs, the milk concentration of ketoprofen was found to be 4 to 5% of the plasma drug level. As with other drugs that are excreted in milk, ketoprofen is not recommended for use in nursing mothers.

Pediatric Use

Ketoprofen is not recommended for use in pediatric patients, because its safety and effectiveness have not been studied in the pediatric population.

ADVERSE REACTIONS

The incidence of common adverse reactions (above 1%) was obtained from a population of 835 Orudis-treated patients

Continued on next page

Orudis/Oruvail—Cont.

in double-blind trials lasting from 4 to 54 weeks and in 622 Oruvail-treated (200 mg/day) patients in trials lasting from 4 to 16 weeks.
Minor gastrointestinal side effects predominated; upper gastrointestinal symptoms were more common than lower gastrointestinal symptoms. In crossover trials in 321 patients with rheumatoid arthritis or osteoarthritis, there was no difference in either upper or lower gastrointestinal symptoms between patients treated with 200 mg of Oruvail once a day or 75 mg of Orudis TID (225 mg/day). Peptic ulcer or GI bleeding occurred in controlled clinical trials in less than 1% of 1,076 patients; however, in open label continuation studies in 1,292 patients the rate was greater than 2%.
The incidence of peptic ulceration in patients on NSAIDs is dependent on many risk factors including age, sex, smoking, alcohol use, diet, stress, concomitant drugs such as aspirin and corticosteroids, as well as the dose and duration of treatment with NSAIDs (see "**WARNINGS**").
Gastrointestinal reactions were followed in frequency by central nervous system side effects, such as headache, dizziness, or drowsiness. The incidence of some adverse reactions appears to be dose-related (see "**DOSAGE AND ADMINISTRATION**"). Rare adverse reactions (incidence less than 1%) were collected from one or more of the following sources: foreign reports to manufacturers and regulatory agencies, publications, and U.S. clinical trials, and/or U.S. postmarketing spontaneous reports.
Reactions are listed below under body system, then by incidence or number of cases in decreasing incidence.

Incidence Greater than 1% (Probable Causal Relationship)
Digestive: Dyspepsia (11%), nausea*, abdominal pain*, diarrhea*, constipation*, flatulence*, anorexia, vomiting, stomatitis.
Nervous System: Headache*, dizziness, CNS inhibition (i.e., pooled reports of somnolence, malaise, depression, etc.) or excitation (i.e., insomnia, nervousness, dreams, etc.)*.
Special Senses: Tinnitus, visual disturbance.
Skin and Appendages: Rash.
Urogenital: Impairment of renal function (edema, increased BUN)*, signs or symptoms of urinary-tract irritation.
*Adverse events occurring in 3 to 9% of patients.

Incidence Less than 1% (Probable Causal Relationship)
Body as a Whole: Chills, facial edema, infection, pain, allergic reaction, anaphylaxis.
Cardiovascular: Hypertension, palpitation, tachycardia, congestive heart failure, peripheral vascular disease, vasodilation.
Digestive: Appetite increased, dry mouth, eructation, gastritis, rectal hemorrhage, melena, fecal occult blood, salivation, peptic ulcer, gastrointestinal perforation, hematemesis, intestinal ulceration, hepatic dysfunction, hepatitis, cholestatic hepatitis, jaundice.
Hemic: Hypocoagulability, agranulocytosis, anemia, hemolysis, purpura, thrombocytopenia.
Metabolic and Nutritional: Thirst, weight gain, weight loss, hyponatremia.
Musculoskeletal: Myalgia.
Nervous System: Amnesia, confusion, impotence, migraine, paresthesia, vertigo.
Respiratory: Dyspnea, hemoptysis, epistaxis, pharyngitis, rhinitis, bronchospasm, laryngeal edema.
Skin and Appendages: Alopecia, eczema, pruritus, purpuric rash, sweating, urticaria, bullous rash, exfoliative dermatitis, photosensitivity, skin discoloration, onycholysis, toxic epidermal necrolysis, erythema multiforme, Stevens-Johnson syndrome.
Special Senses: Conjunctivitis, conjunctivitis sicca, eye pain, hearing impairment, retinal hemorrhage and pigmentation change, taste perversion.
Urogenital: Menometrorrhagia, hematuria, renal failure, interstitial nephritis, nephrotic syndrome.

Incidence Less than 1% (Causal Relationship Unknown)
The following rare adverse reactions, whose causal relationship to ketoprofen is uncertain, are being listed to serve as alerting information to the physician.
Body as a Whole: Septicemia, shock.
Cardiovascular: Arrhythmias, myocardial infarction.
Digestive: Buccal necrosis, ulcerative colitis, microvesicular steatosis, pancreatitis.
Endocrine: Diabetes mellitus (aggravated).
Nervous System: Dysphoria, hallucination, libido disturbance, nightmares, personality disorder, aseptic meningitis.
Urogenital: Acute tubulopathy, gynecomastia.

OVERDOSAGE

Signs and symptoms following acute NSAID overdose are usually limited to lethargy, drowsiness, nausea, vomiting, and epigastric pain, which are generally reversible with supportive care. Respiratory depression, coma, or convulsions have occurred following large ketoprofen overdoses. Gastrointestinal bleeding, hypotension, hypertension, or acute renal failure may occur, but are rare.
Patients should be managed by symptomatic and supportive care following an NSAID overdose. There are no specific antidotes. Gut decontamination may be indicated in patients with symptoms seen within 4 hours (longer for sustained-release products) or following a large overdose (5 to 10 times the usual dose). This should be accomplished via emesis and/or activated charcoal (60 to 100 g in adults, 1 to 2 g/kg in children) with a saline cathartic or sorbitol added to the first dose. Forced diuresis, alkalinization of the urine, hemodialysis or hemoperfusion would probably not be useful due to ketoprofen's high protein binding.
Case reports include twenty-six overdoses: 6 were in children, 16 in adolescents, and 4 in adults. Five of these patients had minor symptoms (vomiting in 4, drowsiness in 1 child). A 12-year-old girl had tonic-clonic convulsions 1–2 hours after ingesting an unknown quantity of ketoprofen and 1 or 2 tablets of acetaminophen with hydrocodone. Her ketoprofen level was 1128 mg/L (56 times the upper therapeutic level of 20 mg/L) 3–4 hours post ingestion. Full recovery ensued 18 hours after ingestion following management with intubation, diazepam, and activated charcoal. A 45-year-old woman ingested twelve 200 mg Oruvail and 375 mL vodka, was treated with emesis and supportive measures 2 hours after ingestion, and recovered completely with her only complaint being mild epigastric pain.

DOSAGE AND ADMINISTRATION

Rheumatoid Arthritis and Osteoarthritis
The recommended starting dose of ketoprofen in otherwise healthy patients is for Orudis 75 mg three times or 50 mg four times a day, or for Oruvail 200 mg administered once a day. Smaller doses of Orudis or Oruvail should be utilized initially in small individuals, in debilitated or elderly patients. The recommended maximum daily dose of ketoprofen is 300 mg/day for Orudis or 200 mg/day for Oruvail (see "**INDIVIDUALIZATION OF DOSAGE**").
Dosages higher than 300 mg/day of Orudis or 200 mg/day of Oruvail are not recommended because they have not been studied. Concomitant use of Orudis and Oruvail is not recommended. Relatively smaller people may need smaller doses (See "**INDIVIDUALIZATION OF DOSAGE**").

Management of Pain and Dysmenorrhea
The usual dose of Orudis recommended for mild-to-moderate pain and dysmenorrhea is 25 to 50 mg every 6 to 8 hours as necessary. A smaller dose should be utilized initially in small individuals, in debilitated or elderly patients, or in patients with renal or liver disease (see "**GENERAL PRECAUTIONS**"). A larger dose may be tried if the patient's response to a previous dose was less than satisfactory, but doses above 75 mg have not been shown to give added analgesia. Daily doses above 300 mg are not recommended because they have not been adequately studied. Because of its typical nonsteroidal anti-inflammatory drug-side-effect profile, including as its principal adverse effect GI side effects (see "**WARNINGS**" and "**ADVERSE REACTIONS**"), higher doses of Orudis should be used with caution and patients receiving them observed carefully (see "**INDIVIDUALIZATION OF DOSAGE**").
Oruvail is not recommended for use in treating acute pain because of its extended-release characteristics.

HOW SUPPLIED

Orudis® (ketoprofen) Capsules are available as follows:
25 mg, NDC 0008-4186, dark-green and red capsule marked "WYETH 4186" on one side and "ORUDIS 25" on the reverse side, in bottles of 100 capsules.
50 mg, NDC 0008-4181, dark-green and light-green capsule marked "WYETH 4181" on one side and "ORUDIS 50" on the reverse side, in bottles of 100 capsules.
75 mg, NDC 0008-4187, dark-green and white capsule marked "WYETH 4187" on one side and "ORUDIS 75" on the reverse side, in bottles of 100 and 500 capsules, and in Redipak® cartons of 100, each containing 10 blister strips of 10 capsules.
Oruvail® (ketoprofen) Extended-Release Capsules are available as follows:
100 mg, NDC 0008-0821, opaque pink and dark-green capsule marked with two radial bands and "ORUVAIL 100" in bottles of 100 capsules.
150 mg, NDC 0008-0822, opaque pink and light-green capsule marked with two radial bands and "ORUVAIL 150" in bottles of 100 capsules.
200 mg, NDC 0008-0690, opaque pink and off-white capsule marked with two radial bands and "ORUVAIL 200" in bottles of 100 capsules and in Redipak® cartons each containing 10 blister strips of 10 capsules.
Keep tightly closed.
Store at room temperature, approximately 25° C (77° F).
Dispense in a tight container.
Oruvail capsules should be protected from direct light and excessive heat and humidity.
The appearance of these capsules is a registered trademark of Wyeth-Ayerst Laboratories.
Caution: Federal law prohibits dispensing without prescription.
By arrangement with Rhone-Poulenc Rorer France.
Orudis Capsules manufactured and distributed by Wyeth Laboratories.
Oruvail Capsules distributed by Wyeth Laboratories.
Wyeth Laboratories
A Wyeth-Ayerst Company
Philadelphia, PA 19101
CI 4808-2 Revised November 26, 1997
Shown in Product Identification Guide, page 341 & 342

OVRAL® ℞
[ōh 'vrăl]
TABLETS
(norgestrel and ethinyl estradiol tablets)

Patients should be counseled that this product does not protect against HIV infection (AIDS) and other sexually transmitted diseases.

DESCRIPTION

Each Ovral tablet contains 0.5 mg of norgestrel (*dl* -13-beta-ethyl-17-alpha-ethinyl -17- beta-hydroxygon -4- en -3- one), a totally synthetic progestogen, and 0.05 mg of ethinyl estradiol (19-nor-17α-pregna-1,3,5 (10)-trien-20-yne-3,17-diol). The inactive ingredients present are cellulose, lactose, magnesium stearate, and polacrilin potassium.

CLINICAL PHARMACOLOGY

See LO/OVRAL®.

INDICATIONS AND USAGE

Oral contraceptives are indicated for the prevention of pregnancy in women who elect to use this product as a method of contraception.
Oral contraceptive products such as Ovral or Ovral®-28, which contain 50 mcg of estrogen, should not be used unless medically indicated.
Oral contraceptives are highly effective. Table I lists the typical accidental pregnancy rates for users of combination oral contraceptives and other methods of contraception. The efficacy of these contraceptive methods, except sterilization and the IUD, depends upon the reliability with which they are used. Correct and consistent use of methods can result in lower failure rates.

TABLE I: LOWEST EXPECTED AND TYPICAL FAILURE RATES DURING THE FIRST YEAR OF CONTINUOUS USE OF A METHOD

% of Women Experiencing an Accidental Pregnancy in the First Year of Continuous Use

Method	Lowest Expected*	Typical**
(No Contraception)	(85)	(85)
Oral contraceptives		3
combined	0.1	N/A***
progestin only	0.5	N/A***
Diaphragm with spermicidal cream or jelly	6	18
Spermicides alone (foams and vaginal suppositories)	3	21
Vaginal Sponge		
nulliparous	6	18
multiparous	9	28
DEPO-PROVERA® (injectable progestogen)	0.3	0.3
NORPLANT® SYSTEM (implants)	0.2#	0.2#
IUD		3
progesterone	2	N/A***
copper T 380A	0.8	N/A***
Condom without spermicides	2	12
Periodic abstinence (all methods)	1–9	20
Female sterilization	0.2	0.4
Male sterilization	0.1	0.15

Adapted from J. Trussell et al., Table 1, Studies in Family Planning, *21(1)*: Jan.–Feb. 1990.

* The authors' best guess of the percentage of women expected to experience an accidental pregnancy among couples who initiate a method (not necessarily for the first time) and who use it consistently and correctly during the first year if they do not stop use for any other reason.
** This term represents "typical" couples who initiate use of a method (not necessarily for the first time), who experience an accidental pregnancy during the first year if they do not stop use for any other reason.
*** N/A—Data not available
\# This data is based on NORPLANT® SYSTEM clinical trials.

CONTRAINDICATIONS

See LO/OVRAL.

WARNINGS

See LO/OVRAL.
1. THROMBOEMBOLIC DISORDERS AND OTHER VASCULAR PROBLEMS.
a. *Myocardial infarction:* See LO/OVRAL.
b. *Thromboembolism:* See LO/OVRAL.
c. *Cerebrovascular diseases:* See LO/OVRAL.
d. *Dose-related risk of vascular disease from oral contraceptives*
A positive association has been observed between the amount of estrogen and progestogen in oral contraceptives and the risk of vascular disease. A decline in serum high-density lipoproteins (HDL) has been reported with many progestational agents. A decline in serum high-density lipoproteins has been associated with an increased incidence of ischemic heart disease. Because estrogens increase HDL cholesterol, the net effect of an oral contraceptive depends on a balance achieved between doses of estrogen and progestogen and the nature and absolute amount of progestogen used in the contraceptive. The amount of both hormones should be considered in the choice of an oral contraceptive.
Minimizing exposure to estrogen and progestogen is in keeping with good principles of therapeutics. For any particular estrogen/progestogen combination, the dosage regimen prescribed should be one which contains the least

amount of estrogen and progestogen that is compatible with a low failure rate and the needs of the individual patient. New acceptors of oral-contraceptive agents should be started on preparations containing less than 50 mcg of estrogen. Products containing 50 mcg of estrogen should be used only when medically indicated.

e. *Persistence of risk of vascular disease:* See LO/OVRAL.

2. ESTIMATES OF MORTALITY FROM ORAL CONTRACEPTIVE USE: See LO/OVRAL.
3. CARCINOMA OF THE REPRODUCTIVE ORGANS: See LO/OVRAL.
4. HEPATIC NEOPLASIA: See LO/OVRAL.
5. OCULAR LESIONS: See LO/OVRAL.
6. ORAL-CONTRACEPTIVE USE BEFORE OR DURING EARLY PREGNANCY: See LO/OVRAL.
7. GALLBLADDER DISEASE: See LO/OVRAL.
8. CARBOHYDRATE AND LIPID METABOLIC EFFECTS: See LO/OVRAL.
9. ELEVATED BLOOD PRESSURE: See LO/OVRAL.
10. HEADACHE: See LO/OVRAL.
11. BLEEDING IRREGULARITIES: See LO/OVRAL.

PRECAUTIONS

See LO/OVRAL.

Drug Interactions: See LO/OVRAL.
Carcinogenesis: See LO/OVRAL.
Pregnancy: See LO/OVRAL.
Nursing Mothers: See LO/OVRAL.
Information For The Patient: See LO/OVRAL.

ADVERSE REACTIONS

See LO/OVRAL.

OVERDOSAGE

See LO/OVRAL.

NONCONTRACEPTIVE HEALTH BENEFITS

See LO/OVRAL.

DOSAGE AND ADMINISTRATION

To achieve maximum contraceptive effectiveness, Ovral must be taken exactly as directed and at intervals not exceeding 24 hours.

The dosage of Ovral is one tablet daily for 21 consecutive days per menstrual cycle according to prescribed schedule. Tablets are then discontinued for 7 days (three weeks on, one week off).

It is recommended that Ovral tablets be taken at the same time each day, preferably after the evening meal or at bedtime.

During the first cycle of medication, the patient is instructed to take one Ovral tablet daily for twenty-one consecutive days, beginning on the first day (Day 1 Start) of her menstrual cycle or on the Sunday after her period begins (Sunday Start). (The first day of menstruation is day one.) The tablets are then discontinued for one week (7 days). Withdrawal bleeding should usually occur within 3 days following discontinuation of Ovral. (For Day 1 Start: If Ovral is first taken later than the first day of the first menstrual cycle of medication or postpartum, contraceptive reliance should not be placed on Ovral until after the first seven consecutive days of administration. For Sunday Start: Contraceptive reliance should not be placed on Ovral until after the first seven consecutive days of administration. The possibility of ovulation and conception prior to initiation of medication should be considered.) The patient begins her next and all subsequent 21-day courses of Ovral tablets on the same day of the week that she began her first course, following the same schedule: 21 days on—7 days off. She begins taking her tablets on the 8th day after discontinuance, regardless of whether or not a menstrual period has occurred or is still in progress. Any time a new cycle of Ovral is started later than the 8th day, the patient should be protected by another means of contraception until she has taken a tablet daily for seven consecutive days.

If spotting or breakthrough bleeding occurs, the patient is instructed to continue on the same regimen. This type of bleeding is usually transient and without significance; however, if the bleeding is persistent or prolonged, the patient is advised to consult her physician. Although the occurrence of pregnancy is highly unlikely if Ovral is taken according to directions, if withdrawal bleeding does not occur, the possibility of pregnancy must be considered. If the patient has not adhered to the prescribed schedule (missed one or more tablets or started taking them on a day later than she should have), the probability of pregnancy should be considered at the time of the first missed period and appropriate diagnostic measures taken before the medication is resumed. If the patient has adhered to the prescribed regimen and misses two consecutive periods, pregnancy should be ruled out before continuing the contraceptive regimen.

For additional patient instructions regarding missed pills, see the "WHAT TO DO IF YOU MISS PILLS" section in the **DETAILED PATIENT LABELING** for LO/OVRAL.

Any time the patient misses two or more tablets, she should also use another method of contraception until she has taken a tablet daily for seven consecutive days. If breakthrough bleeding occurs following missed tablets, it will usually be transient and of no consequence. While there is little likelihood of ovulation occurring if only one or two tablets are missed, the possibility of ovulation increases with each successive day that scheduled tablets are missed.

In the nonlactating mother, Ovral may be initiated postpartum, for contraception. When the tablets are administered in the postpartum period, the increased risk of thromboembolic disease associated with the postpartum period must be considered (see "Contraindications," "Warnings," and "Precautions" concerning thromboembolic disease). It is to be noted that early resumption of ovulation may occur if Parlodel® (bromocriptine mesylate) has been used for the prevention of lactation.

HOW SUPPLIED

Ovral® Tablets (0.5 mg norgestrel and 0.05 mg ethinyl estradiol) are available in packages of 6 PILPAK® dispensers with 21 tablets each as follows:

NDC 0008-0056-01, white, round tablet marked "WYETH" and "56".

Store at room temperature, approx. 25° C (77° F).

References available upon request.

Brief Summary Patient Package Insert: See LO/OVRAL.

DETAILED PATIENT LABELING

This product (like all oral contraceptives) is intended to prevent pregnancy. It does not protect against HIV infection (AIDS) and other sexually transmitted diseases.

INTRODUCTION

You should not use Ovral or Ovral-28, which contain higher doses of estrogen than other oral contraceptives, unless specifically recommended by your health-care provider. Any woman who considers using oral contraceptives (the birth-control pill or the pill) should understand the benefits and risks of using this form of birth control. This leaflet will give you much of the information you will need to make this decision and will also help you determine if you are at risk of developing any of the serious side effects of the pill. It will tell you how to use the pill properly so that it will be as effective as possible. However, this leaflet is not a replacement for a careful discussion between you and your health-care provider. You should discuss the information provided in this leaflet with him or her, both when you first start taking the pill and during your revisits. You should also follow your health-care provider's advice with regard to regular check-ups while you are on the pill.

EFFECTIVENESS OF ORAL CONTRACEPTIVES: See LO/OVRAL.

WHO SHOULD NOT TAKE ORAL CONTRACEPTIVES: See LO/OVRAL.

OTHER CONSIDERATIONS BEFORE TAKING ORAL CONTRACEPTIVES: See LO/OVRAL.

RISKS OF TAKING ORAL CONTRACEPTIVES: See LO/OVRAL.

ESTIMATED RISK OF DEATH FROM A BIRTH-CONTROL METHOD OR PREGNANCY: See LO/OVRAL.

WARNING SIGNALS: See LO/OVRAL.

SIDE EFFECTS OF ORAL CONTRACEPTIVES: See LO/OVRAL.

GENERAL PRECAUTIONS: See LO/OVRAL.

HOW TO TAKE THE PILL: See LO/OVRAL.

RISKS TO THE FETUS: See LO/OVRAL.

HEALTH BENEFITS FROM ORAL CONTRACEPTIVES: See LO/OVRAL.

Manufactured by:
Wyeth Laboratories
A Wyeth-Ayerst Company
Philadelphia, PA 19101
CI 4255-4 Revised February 19, 1997

Shown in Product Identification Guide, page 342

OVRAL®-28 ℞

[*ōh 'vral-28*]
Tablets
(norgestrel and ethinyl estradiol tablets)

Patients should be counseled that this product does not protect against HIV infection (AIDS) and other sexually transmitted diseases.

DESCRIPTION

21 white Ovral tablets, each containing 0.5 mg of norgestrel (*dl* -13-beta-ethyl-17-alpha-ethinyl-17-beta-hydroxygon-4-en-3-one), a totally synthetic progestogen, and 0.05 mg of ethinyl estradiol (19-nor-17α-pregna-1,3,5 (10)-trien-20-yne-3,17-diol), and 7 pink inert tablets. The inactive ingredients present are cellulose, D&C Red 30, lactose, magnesium stearate, and polacrilin potassium.

CLINICAL PHARMACOLOGY

See LO/OVRAL®.

INDICATIONS AND USAGE

See OVRAL®.

CONTRAINDICATIONS

See LO/OVRAL.

WARNINGS

See OVRAL.

PRECAUTIONS

See LO/OVRAL.

Drug Interactions: See LO/OVRAL.
Carcinogenesis: See LO/OVRAL.
Pregnancy: See LO/OVRAL.
Nursing Mothers: See LO/OVRAL.
Information for the Patient: See LO/OVRAL.

ADVERSE REACTIONS

See LO/OVRAL.

OVERDOSAGE

See LO/OVRAL.

NONCONTRACEPTIVE HEALTH BENEFITS

See LO/OVRAL

DOSAGE AND ADMINISTRATION

To achieve maximum contraceptive effectiveness, Ovral-28 must be taken exactly as directed and at intervals not exceeding 24 hours.

The dosage of Ovral-28 is one white tablet daily for 21 consecutive days, followed by one pink inert tablet daily for 7 consecutive days, according to prescribed schedule.

It is recommended that Ovral-28 tablets be taken at the same time each day, preferably after the evening meal or at bedtime.

During the first cycle of medication, the patient is instructed to begin taking Ovral-28 on the first Sunday after the onset of menstruation. If menstruation begins on a Sunday, the first tablet (white) is taken that day. One white tablet should be taken daily for 21 consecutive days followed by one pink inert tablet daily for 7 consecutive days. Withdrawal bleeding should usually occur within three days following discontinuation of white tablets. During the first cycle, contraceptive reliance should not be placed on Ovral-28 until a white tablet has been taken daily for 7 consecutive days. The possibility of ovulation and conception prior to initiation of medication should be considered.

The patient begins her next and all subsequent 28-day courses of tablets on the same day of the week (Sunday) on which she began her first course, following the same schedule: 21 days on white tablets—7 days on pink inert tablets. If in any cycle the patient starts tablets later than the proper day, she should protect herself by using another method of birth control until she has taken a white tablet daily for 7 consecutive days.

If spotting or breakthrough bleeding occurs, the patient is instructed to continue on the same regimen. This type of bleeding is usually transient and without significance; however, if the bleeding is persistent or prolonged, the patient is advised to consult her physician. Although the occurrence of pregnancy is highly unlikely if Ovral-28 is taken according to directions, if withdrawal bleeding does not occur, the possibility of pregnancy must be considered. If the patient has not adhered to the prescribed schedule (missed one or more tablets or started taking them on a day later than she should have), the probability of pregnancy should be considered at the time of the first missed period and appropriate diagnostic measures taken before the medication is resumed. If the patient has adhered to the prescribed regimen and misses two consecutive periods, pregnancy should be ruled out before continuing the contraceptive regimen.

For additional patient instructions regarding missed pills, see the "WHAT TO DO IF YOU MISS PILLS" section in the **DETAILED PATIENT LABELING** for LO/OVRAL.

Any time the patient misses two or more white tablets, she should also use another method of contraception until she has taken a white tablet daily for seven consecutive days. If the patient misses one or more pink tablets, she is still protected against pregnancy **provided** she begins taking white tablets again on the proper day.

If breakthrough bleeding occurs following missed white tablets, it will usually be transient and of no consequence. While there is little likelihood of ovulation occurring if only one or two white tablets are missed, the possibility of ovulation increases with each successive day that scheduled white tablets are missed.

In the nonlactating mother, Ovral-28 may be initiated postpartum, for contraception. When the tablets are administered in the postpartum period, the increased risk of thromboembolic disease associated with the postpartum period must be considered (see "Contraindications", "Warnings", and "Precautions" concerning thromboembolic disease). It is to be noted that early resumption of ovulation may occur if Parlodel® (bromocriptine mesylate) has been used for the prevention of lactation.

HOW SUPPLIED

Ovral®-28 Tablets (0.5 mg norgestrel and 0.05 mg ethinyl estradiol) are available in packages of 6 PILPAK® dispensers, each containing 28 tablets as follows:

21 active tablets, NDC 0008-0056, white, round tablet marked "WYETH" and "56".

7 inert tablets, NDC 0008-0445, pink, round tablet marked "WYETH" and "445".

Store at room temperature, approx. 25°C (77°F).

References available upon request.

Brief Summary Patient Package Insert: See LO/OVRAL.
DETAILED PATIENT LABELING: See OVRAL.

Manufactured by:
Wyeth Laboratories
A Wyeth-Ayerst Company
Philadelphia, PA 19101.
CI 4258-4 March 14, 1997

Shown in Product Identification Guide, page 342

OVRETTE® ℞

[*oh-vret '*]
Tablets
(norgestrel tablets)

Patients should be counseled that this product does not protect against HIV infection (AIDS) and other sexually transmitted diseases.

Each OVRETTE tablet contains 0.075 mg of norgestrel (*dl* -13-beta-ethyl-17-alpha-ethinyl-17-beta-hydroxygon-4-en-3-

Continued on next page

Ovrette—Cont.

one). The inactive ingredients present are cellulose, FD&C Yellow 5, lactose, magnesium stearate, and polacrilin potassium.

DESCRIPTION

Each OVRETTE tablet contains 0.075 mg of a single active steroid ingredient, norgestrel, a totally synthetic progestogen. The available data suggest that the d (-)enantiomeric form of norgestrel is the biologically active portion. This form amounts to 0.0375 mg per OVRETTE tablet.

CLINICAL PHARMACOLOGY

The primary mechanism through which OVRETTE prevents conception is not known, but progestogen-only contraceptives are known to alter the cervical mucus, exert a progestational effect on the endometrium, interfering with implantation, and, in some patients, suppress ovulation.

INDICATIONS AND USAGE

See LO/OVRAL®.

CONTRAINDICATIONS

See LO/OVRAL.

WARNINGS

See LO/OVRAL.

PRECAUTIONS

See LO/OVRAL.

INFORMATION FOR THE PATIENT

See LO/OVRAL.

DRUG INTERACTIONS

See LO/OVRAL.

CARCINOGENESIS

See LO/OVRAL.

PREGNANCY

See LO/OVRAL.

NURSING MOTHERS

See LO/OVRAL.

ADVERSE REACTIONS

See LO/OVRAL.

OVERDOSAGE

See LO/OVRAL.

DOSAGE AND ADMINISTRATION

To achieve maximum contraceptive effectiveness, OVRETTE must be taken exactly as directed and at intervals not exceeding 24 hours.

OVRETTE is administered on a continuous daily dosage regimen starting on the first day of menstruation, i.e., one tablet each day, every day of the year.

Tablets should be taken at the same time each day and continued daily, without interruption, whether bleeding occurs or not. The patient should be advised that, if prolonged bleeding occurs, she should consult her physician. In the nonlactating mother, OVRETTE may be initiated postpartum, for contraception. When the tablets are administered in the postpartum period, the increased risk of thromboembolic disease associated with the postpartum period must be considered (see "Contraindications," "Warnings," and "Precautions" concerning thromboembolic disease). It is to be noted that early resumption of ovulation may occur if Parlodel® (bromocriptine mesylate) has been used for the prevention of lactation.

The risk of pregnancy increases with each tablet missed. If the patient misses one tablet, she should be instructed to take it as soon as she remembers and to also take her next tablet at the regular time. If she misses two tablets, she should take one of the missed tablets as soon as she remembers, as well as taking her regular tablet for that day at the proper time. Furthermore, she should use a method of nonhormonal contraception in addition to taking OVRETTE until fourteen tablets have been taken. If more than 2 tablets have been missed, OVRETTE should be discontinued immediately and a method of nonhormonal contraception should be used until menses has appeared or pregnancy has been excluded. If menses does not appear within 45 days from the last period, a method of nonhormonal contraception should be substituted until the start of the next menstrual period or an appropriate diagnostic procedure is performed to rule out pregnancy.

HOW SUPPLIED

OVRETTE® Tablets (0.075 mg norgestrel) are available in packages of 6 PILPAK® dispensers with 28 tablets each as follows: NDC 0008-0062-01, yellow, round tablet marked "WYETH" and "62".

Store at room temperature, approx. 25°C (77°F).

References available upon request.

Brief Summary Patient Package Insert: See LO/OVRAL

DETAILED PATIENT LABELING: See LO/OVRAL.

HOW TO TAKE THE PILL

This product (like all oral contraceptives) is intended to prevent pregnancy. It does not protect against transmission of HIV (AIDS) and other sexually transmitted diseases such as chlamydia, genital herpes, genital warts, gonorrhea, hepatitis B, and syphillis.

1. *General Instructions*

You must take your pill every day according to the instructions. Oral contraceptives are most effective if taken no more than 24 hours apart. Take your pill at the same time every day so that you are less likely to forget to take it. You will then maintain an effective dose of the oral contraceptive in your body.

If your doctor has scheduled you for surgery, or you need prolonged bed rest, he or she may suggest that you stop taking the pill four weeks before surgery to avoid an increased risk of blood clots. It is also advisable not to start oral contraceptives sooner than four weeks after delivery of a baby or a midtrimester pregnancy termination.

Ovrette is administered on a continuous daily dosage schedule, one tablet each day, every day of the year. Take the first tablet on the first day of your menstrual period. Tablets should be taken at the same time every day, without interruption, whether bleeding occurs or not. If bleeding is prolonged (more than 8 days) or unusually heavy, you should contact your doctor.

SPOTTING OR BREAKTHROUGH BLEEDING

Spotting is slight staining between menstrual periods which may not even require a pad. Breakthrough bleeding is a flow much like a regular period, requiring sanitary protection. Spotting is more common than breakthrough bleeding, and both occur more often in the first few cycles than in later cycles. These types of bleeding are usually temporary and without significance. It is important to continue taking your pills on schedule. If the bleeding persists for more than a few days, consult your doctor.

2. *If you forget to take your pill*

The risk of pregnancy increases with each tablet missed. Therefore, it is very important that you take one tablet daily as directed. If you miss one tablet, take it as soon as you remember and also take your next tablet at the regular time. If you miss two tablets, take one of the missed tablets as soon as you remember, as well as your regular tablet for that day at the proper time. Furthermore, you should use another method of birth control in addition to taking Ovrette until you have taken fourteen days (2 weeks) of medication.

If more than two tablets have been missed, Ovrette should be discontinued immediately and another method of birth control used until the start of your next menstrual period. Then you may resume taking Ovrette.

At times there may be no menstrual period after a cycle of pills. Therefore, if you miss one menstrual period but have taken the pills **exactly as you were supposed to,** continue as usual into the next cycle. If you have not taken the pills correctly and miss a menstrual period, or if it is 45 days or more from the start of your last menstrual period, you may be pregnant and should stop taking oral contraceptives until your doctor determines whether or not you are pregnant. Until you can get to your doctor, use another form of nonhormonal contraception. If two consecutive menstrual periods are missed, you should stop taking pills until it is determined by a physician whether you are pregnant.

3. *Pregnancy due to pill failure*

The incidence of pill failure resulting in pregnancy is approximately less than 1.0% if taken every day as directed, but more typical failure rates are less than 3.0%. If failure does occur, the risk to the fetus is minimal.

4. *Risks to the fetus*

If you do become pregnant while using oral contraceptives, the risk to the fetus is small, on the order of no more than one per thousand. You should, however, discuss the risks to the developing child with your doctor.

5. *Pregnancy after stopping the pill*

There may be some delay in becoming pregnant after you stop using oral contraceptives, especially if you had irregular menstrual cycles before you used oral contraceptives. It may be advisable to postpone conception until you begin menstruating regularly once you have stopped taking the pill and desire pregnancy.

There does not appear to be any increase in birth defects in newborn babies when pregnancy occurs soon after stopping the pill.

6. *Overdosage*

Serious ill effects have not been reported following ingestion of large doses of oral contraceptives by young children. Overdosage may cause nausea and withdrawal bleeding in females. In case of overdosage, contact your health-care provider or pharmacist.

7. *Other information*

Your health-care provider will take a medical and family history before prescribing oral contraceptives and will examine you. The physical examination may be delayed to another time if you request it and the health-care provider believes that it is appropriate to postpone it. You should be reexamined at least once a year. Be sure to inform your health-care provider if there is a family history of any of the conditions listed previously in this leaflet. Be sure to keep all appointments with your health-care provider, because this is a time to determine if there are early signs of side effects of oral-contraceptive use.

Do not use the drug for any condition other than the one for which it was prescribed. This drug has been prescribed specifically for you; do not give it to others who may want birth control pills.

HEALTH BENEFITS FROM ORAL CONTRACEPTIVES

In addition to preventing pregnancy, use of oral contraceptives may provide certain benefits.

They are:

- Menstrual cycles may become more regular.
- Blood flow during menstruation may be lighter, and less iron may be lost. Therefore, anemia due to iron deficiency is less likely to occur.
- Pain or other symptoms during menstruation may be encountered less frequently.
- Ovarian cysts may occur less frequently.
- Ectopic (tubal) pregnancy may occur less frequently.
- Noncancerous cysts or lumps in the breast may occur less frequently.
- Acute pelvic inflammatory disease may occur less frequently.
- Oral-contraceptive use may provide some protection against developing two forms of cancer: cancer of the ovaries and cancer of the lining of the uterus.

If you want more information about birth-control pills, ask your doctor or pharmacist. They have a more technical leaflet called the Professional Labeling which you may wish to read.

Manufactured by:
Wyeth Laboratories
A Wyeth-Ayerst Company
Philadelphia, PA 19101
CI 4271-2 Revised August 14, 1996

PHENERGAN® ℞

[fĕn 'ĕr-găn]
(promethazine HCl Injection, USP)
INJECTION

DESCRIPTION

Phenergan (promethazine HCl) Injection, is a sterile, pyrogen-free solution for deep intramuscular or intravenous administration. Promethazine HCl (10*H*-phenothiazine-10-ethanamine, *N,N*,α-trimethyl-, monohydrochloride, (±)-) is a racemic compound and has the following structural formula:

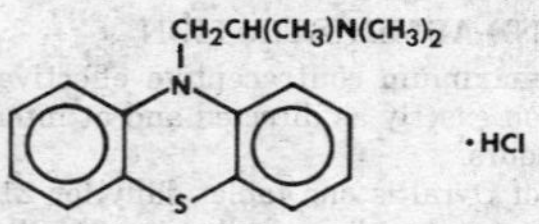

$C_{17}H_{21}ClN_2S$ MW=320.89

Each mL of ampul contains either 25 mg or 50 mg promethazine HCl with 0.1 mg edetate disodium, 0.04 mg calcium chloride, 0.25 mg sodium metabisulfite, and 5 mg phenol in Water for Injection. The pH range is 4.0 to 5.5, buffered with acetic acid-sodium acetate, and it is sealed under nitrogen. Each mL of the **TUBEX®** and **TUBEX® BLUNT POINTE™** Sterile Cartridge Units contains either 25 mg or 50 mg promethazine HCl with 0.1 mg edetate disodium, 0.04 mg calcium chloride, not more than 5 mg monothioglycerol; and 5 mg phenol in Water for Injection. The pH range is 4.0 to 5.5, buffered with sodium acetate-acetic acid, and it is sealed under nitrogen.

Phenergan (promethazine HCl) Injection is a clear, colorless solution. The product is light sensitive. It should be inspected before use and discarded if either color or particulate is observed.

CLINICAL PHARMACOLOGY

Promethazine HCl is a phenothiazine derivative which possesses antihistaminic, sedative, antimotion-sickness, antiemetic, and anticholinergic effects. Promethazine is a competitive H_1 receptor antagonist, but does not block the release of histamine. Structural differences from the neuroleptic phenothiazines results in its relative lack (1/10) of dopamine antagonist properties. In therapeutic doses, promethazine HCl produces no significant effects on the cardiovascular system. Clinical effects are generally apparent within 5 minutes of an intravenous injection and within 20 minutes of an intramuscular injection. Duration of action is four to six hours, although effects may persist up to 12 hours. Promethazine HCl is metabolized in the liver, with the sulfoxides of promethazine and N-desmethylpromethazine being the predominant metabolites appearing in the urine. Following intravenous administration in healthy volunteers, the plasma half-life for promethazine has been reported to range from 9 to 16 hours. The mean plasma half-life for promethazine after intramuscular administration in healthy volunteers has been reported to be 9.8±3.4 hours.

INDICATIONS AND USAGE

Phenergan Injection is indicated for the following conditions:

1. Amelioration of allergic reactions to blood or plasma.
2. In anaphylaxis as an adjunct to epinephrine and other standard measures after the acute symptoms have been controlled.
3. For other uncomplicated allergic conditions of the immediate type when oral therapy is impossible or contraindicated.
4. For sedation and relief of apprehension and to produce light sleep from which the patient can be easily aroused.
5. Active treatment of motion sickness.
6. Prevention and control of nausea and vomiting associated with certain types of anesthesia and surgery.
7. As an adjunct to analgesics for the control of postoperative pain.
8. Preoperative, postoperative, and obstetric (during labor) sedation.
9. Intravenously in special surgical situations, such as repeated bronchoscopy, ophthalmic surgery, and poor-risk pa-

tients, with reduced amounts of meperidine or other narcotic analgesic as an adjunct to anesthesia and analgesia.

CONTRAINDICATIONS

Phenergan Injection is contraindicated in comatose states and in patients who have demonstrated an idiosyncrasy or hypersensitivity to promethazine or other phenothiazines.

Under no circumstances should Phenergan Injection be given by intra-arterial injection due to the likelihood of severe arteriospasm and the possibility of resultant gangrene (see **"WARNINGS—Inadvertent Intra-arterial Injection"**).

Phenergan Injection should not be given by the subcutaneous route; evidence of chemical irritation has been noted, and necrotic lesions have resulted on rare occasions following subcutaneous injection. The preferred parenteral route of administration is by deep intramuscular injection.

WARNINGS

Sulfite Sensitivity

Phenergan Injection (ampuls only) contains sodium metabisulfite, a sulfite that may cause allergic-type reactions, including anaphylactic symptoms and life-threatening or less severe asthma episodes, in certain susceptible people. The overall prevalence of sulfite sensitivity in the general population is unknown and probably low. Sulfite sensitivity is seen more frequently in asthmatic than in nonasthmatic people.

CNS Depression

Phenergan Injection may impair the mental and physical abilities required for the performance of potentially hazardous tasks, such as driving a vehicle or operating machinery. The impairment may be amplified by concomitant use of other central-nervous-system depressants such as alcohol, sedative-hypnotics (including barbiturates), general anesthetics, narcotics, narcotic analgesics, tranquilizers, etc. (see **"PRECAUTIONS—Information for Patients"**).

Lower Seizure Threshold

Phenergan Injection may lower seizure threshold and should be used with caution in persons with seizure disorders or in persons who are using concomitant medications, such as narcotics or local anesthetics, which may also affect seizure threshold.

Bone-Marrow Depression

Phenergan Injection should be used with caution in patients with bone-marrow depression. Leukopenia and agranulocytosis have been reported, usually when Phenergan has been used in association with other known marrow-toxic agents.

Use in Pediatric Patients

PHENERGAN INJECTION IS NOT RECOMMENDED FOR USE IN PEDIATRIC PATIENTS LESS THAN TWO YEARS OF AGE.

CAUTION SHOULD BE EXERCISED WHEN ADMINISTERING PHENERGAN INJECTION TO PEDIATRIC PATIENTS 2 YEARS OF AGE AND OLDER. ANTIEMETICS ARE NOT RECOMMENDED FOR TREATMENT OF UNCOMPLICATED VOMITING IN PEDIATRIC PATIENTS, AND THEIR USE SHOULD BE LIMITED TO PROLONGED VOMITING OF KNOWN ETIOLOGY. THE EXTRAPYRAMIDAL SYMPTOMS WHICH CAN OCCUR SECONDARY TO PHENERGAN INJECTION ADMINISTRATION MAY BE CONFUSED WITH THE CNS SIGNS OF UNDIAGNOSED PRIMARY DISEASE, e.g., ENCEPHALOPATHY OR REYE'S SYNDROME. THE USE OF PHENERGAN INJECTION SHOULD BE AVOIDED IN PEDIATRIC PATIENTS WHOSE SIGNS AND SYMPTOMS MAY SUGGEST REYE'S SYNDROME OR OTHER HEPATIC DISEASES.

Excessively large dosages of antihistamines, including Phenergan Injection, in pediatric patients may cause hallucinations, convulsions, and sudden death. In pediatric patients who are acutely ill associated with dehydration, there is an increased susceptibility to dystonias with the use of Phenergan Injection.

Inadvertent Intra-arterial Injection

Due to the close proximity of arteries and veins in the areas most commonly used for intravenous injection, extreme care should be exercised to avoid perivascular extravasation or inadvertent intra-arterial injection. Reports compatible with inadvertent intra-arterial injection of Phenergan Injection, usually in conjunction with other drugs intended for intravenous use, suggest that pain, severe chemical irritation, severe spasm of distal vessels, and resultant gangrene requiring amputation are likely under such circumstances. Intravenous injection was intended in all the cases reported but perivascular extravasation or arterial placement of the needle is now suspect. There is no proven successful management of this condition after it occurs, although sympathetic block and heparinization are commonly employed during the acute management because of the results of animal experiments with other known arteriolar irritants. Aspiration of dark blood does not preclude intra-arterial needle placement, because blood is discolored upon contact with Phenergan Injection. Use of syringes with rigid plungers or of small bore needles might obscure typical arterial backflow if this is relied upon alone.

When used intravenously, Phenergan Injection should be given in a concentration no greater than 25 mg per mL and at a rate not to exceed 25 mg per minute. When administering any irritant drug intravenously, it is usually preferable to inject it through the tubing of an intraveous infusion set that is known to be functioning satisfactorily. In the event that a patient complains of pain during intended intravenous injection of Phenergan Injection, the injection should be stopped immediately to provide for evaluation of possible arterial placement or perivascular extravasation.

Visual Inspection

This product is light sensitive and should be inspected before use and discarded if either color or particulate is observed.

Other Considerations

Sedative drugs or CNS depressants should be avoided in patients with a history of sleep apnea.

Administration of promethazine has been associated with reported cholestatic jaundice.

PRECAUTIONS

General

Drugs having anticholingeric properties should be used with caution in patients with narrow-angle glaucoma, prostatic hypertrophy, stenosing peptic ulcer, pyloroduodenal obstruction, and bladder-neck obstruction.

Phenergan Injection should be used cautiously in persons with cardiovascular disease or impairment of liver function.

Information for Patients

Phenergan Injection may cause marked drowsiness or impair the mental or physical abilities required for the performance of potentially hazardous tasks, such as driving a vehicle or operating machinery. The use of alcohol, sedative-hypnotics (including barbiturates), general anesthetics, narcotics, narcotic analgesics, tranquilizers, etc, with Phenergan Injection may enhance impairment. Pediatric patients should be supervised to avoid potential harm in bike riding or in other hazardous activities.

Patients should be advised to report any involuntary muscle movements.

Persistent or worsening pain or burning at the injection site should be reported immediately.

Avoid prolonged exposure to the sun.

Drug Interactions

CNS Depressants—Phenergan Injection may increase, prolong, or intensify the sedative action of central-nervous-system depressants, such as alcohol, sedative-hypnotics (including barbiturates), general anesthetics, narcotics, narcotic analgesics, tranquilizers, etc. When given concomitanty with Phenergan Injection, the dose of barbiturates should be reduced by at least one-half, and the dose of narcotics should be reduced by one-quarter to one-half. Dosage must be individualized. Excessive amounts of Phenergan Injection relative to a narcotic may lead to restlessness and motor hyperactivity in the patient with pain; these symptoms usually disappear with adequate control of the pain.

Epinephrine—Although reversal of the vasopressor effect of epinephrine has not been reported with Phenergan Injection, it is recommended that epinephrine NOT be used in the case of Phenergan Injection overdose.

Anticholinergics—Concomitant use of other agents with anticholinergic properties should be undertaken with caution.

Monoamine Oxidase Inhibitors (MAOI)—Drug interactions, including an increased incidence of extrapyramidal effects, have been reported when some MAOI and phenothiazines are used conomitantly. Although such a reaction has not been reported with Phenergan Injection, the possibility should be considered.

Laboratory Test Interactions

The following laboratory tests may be affected in patients who are receiving therapy with Phenergan Injection:

Pregnancy Tests—Diagnostic pregnancy tests based on immunological reactions between HCG and anti-HCG may result in false-negative or false-positive interpretations.

Glucose Tolerance Test—An increase in glucose tolerance has been reported in patients receiving promethazine HCl.

Carcinogenesis, Mutagenesis and Impairment of Fertility

Long term animal studies have not been performed to assess the carcinogenic potential of Phenergan Injection, nor are there other animal or human data concerning carcinogenicity, mutagenicity, or impairment of fertility. Phenergan Injection was nonmutagenic in the Ames *Salmonella* test system.

Pregnancy

Teratogenic Effects—Pregnancy Category C

Teratogenic effects have not been demonstrated in rat-feeding studies at doses of 6.25 and 12.5 mg/kg (approximately 2.1 and 4.2 times the maximum recommended human daily dose) of Phenergan Injection. Daily doses of 25 mg/kg intraperitoneally have been found to produce fetal mortality in rats.

There are no adequate and well-controlled studies of Phenergan Injection in pregnant women. Because animal reproduction studies are not always predictive of human response, Phenergan Injection should be used during pregnancy only if the potential benefit justifies the potential risk to the fetus.

Adequate studies to determine the action of the drug on parturition, lactation and development of the animal neonate have not been conducted.

Nonteratogenic Effects

Phenergan Injection received within two weeks of delivery may inhibit platelet aggregation in the newborn.

Labor and Delivery

Phenergan Injection may be used alone or as an adjunct to narcotic analgesics during labor (see **"DOSAGE AND ADMINISTRATION"**). Limited data suggest that use of Phenergan Injection during labor and delivery does not have an appreciable effect on the duration of labor or delivery and does not increase the risk of need for intervention in the newborn. The effect on later growth and development of the newborn is unknown. (See also *"Nonteratogenic Effects."*)

Nursing Mothers

It is not known whether Phenergan Injection is excreted in human milk. Because many drugs are excreted in human milk, caution should be exercised when Phenergan Injection is administered to a nursing woman.

Pediatric Use

Safety and effectiveness in pediatric patients under 2 years of age have not been established.

Phenergan Injection should be used with caution in pediatric patients 2 years of age and older (see **"WARNINGS—Use in Pediatric Patients"**).

Use in Geriatric Patients (approximately 60 years or older)

Since therapeutic requirements for sedative drugs tend to be less in geriatric patients, the dosage should be reduced for these patients.

ADVERSE REACTIONS

CNS Effects

Drowsiness is the most prominent CNS effect of the drug. Extrapyramidal reactions may occur with high doses; this is almost always responsive to a reduction in dosage. Other reported reactions include dizziness, lassitude, tinnitus, incoordination, fatigue, blurred vision, euphoria, diplopia, nervousness, insomnia, tremors, convulsive seizures, oculogyric crises, excitation, catatonic-like states, hysteria, and hallucinations.

Cardiovascular Effects

Tachycardia, bradycardia, faintness, dizziness, and increases and decreases in blood pressure have been reported following the use of Phenergan Injection. Venous thrombosis at the injection site has been reported. INTRA-ARTERIAL INJECTION MAY RESULT IN GANGRENE OF THE AFFECTED EXTREMITY (see **"WARNINGS—Inadvertent Intra-arterial Injection"**).

Gastrointestinal Effects

Nausea and vomiting have been reported, usually in association with surgical procedures and combination drug therapy.

Allergic Reactions

These include urticaria, dermatitis, asthma, and photosensitivity. Angioneurotic edema has been reported.

Other Reported Reactions

Leukopenia and agranulocytosis, usually when Phenergan has been used in association with other known marrow-toxic agents, have been reported. Thrombocytopenic purpura and jaundice of the obstructive type have been associated with the use of Phenergan. The jaundice is usually reversible on discontinuation of the drug. Subcutaneous injection has resulted in tissue necrosis. Nasal stuffiness may occur. Dry mouth has been reported.

Paradoxical Reactions (Overdosage)

Hyperexcitability and abnormal movements, which have been reported in pediatric patients following a single administration of Phenergan Injection, may be manifestations of relative overdosage, in which case, consideration should be given to the discontinuation of Phenergan Injection and to the use of other drugs. Respiratory depression, nightmares, delirium, and agitated behavior have also been reported in some of these patients.

OVERDOSAGE

Signs and symptoms of overdosage range from mild depression of the central nervous system and cardiovascular system to profound hypotension, respiratory depression, and unconsciousness.

Stimulation may be evident, especially in pediatric patients and geriatric patients. Convulsions may rarely occur. A paradoxical reaction has been reported in pediatric patients receiving single doses of 75 mg to 125 mg orally, characterized by hyperexcitability and nightmares.

Atropine-like and symptoms—dry mouth, fixed, dilated pupils, flushing, etc., as well as gastrointestinal symptoms, may occur.

Treatment

Treatment of overdosage is essentially symptomatic and supportive. Only in cases of extreme overdosage or individual sensitivity do vital signs, including respiration, pulse, blood pressure, temperature, and EKG, need to be monitored. Attention should be given to the reestablishment of adequate respiratory exchange through provision of a patent airway and institution of assisted or controlled ventilation. Diazepam may be used to control convulsions. Acidosis and electrolyte losses should be corrected. Note that any depressant effects of Phenergan Injection are not reversed by naloxone.

Avoid analeptics, which may cause convulsions. The treatment of choice for resulting hypotension is administration of intravenous fluids, accompanied by repositioning if indicated. In the event that vasopressors are considered for the management of severe hypotension which does not respond to intravenous fluids and repositioning, the administration of levarterenol or phenylephrine should be considered. EPINEPHRINE SHOULD NOT BE USED, since its use in a patient with partial adrenergic blockade may further lower the blood pressure. Extrapyramidal reactions may be treated with anticholinergic antiparkinson agents, diphenhydramine, or barbiturates. Oxygen may also be administered. Limited experience with dialysis indicates that it is not helpful.

DOSAGE AND ADMINISTRATION

Parenteral drug products should be inspected visually for particulate matter and discoloration prior to administration, whenever solution and container permit.

Continued on next page

Phenergan—Cont.

Do not use Phenergan Injection if solution has developed color or contains precipitate.
To avoid the possibility of physical and/or chemical incompatibility, consult specialized literature before diluting with any injectable solution or combining with any other medication. Do not use if there is a precipitate or any sign of incompatibility.

Important Notes on Administration
The preferred parenteral route of administration for Phenergan Injection is by deep intramuscular injection. The proper intravenous administration of this product is well-tolerated, but use of this route is not without some hazard. Not for subcutaneous administration.

INADVERTENT INTRA-ARTERIAL INJECTION CAN RESULT IN GANGRENE OF THE AFFECTED EXTREMITY (see "WARNINGS—Inadvertent Intra-arterial Injection"). SUBCUTANEOUS INJECTION IS CONTRAINDICATED, AS IT MAY RESULT IN TISSUE NECROSIS (see "CONTRAINDICATIONS").
Injection into or near a nerve may result in permanent tissue damage.
When used intravenously, Phenergan Injection should be given in concentration no greater than 25 mg/mL as at rate not to exceed 25 mg per minute; it is preferable to inject through the tubing of an intravenous infusion set that is known to be functioning satisfactorily.
The **TUBEX® BLUNT POINTE™** Sterile Cartridge Unit is suitable for substances to be administered intravenously. It is intended for use with injection sets specifically manufactured as "needle-less" injection systems. As of the date of this circular, the **TUBEX BLUNT POINTE** is compatible with LifeShield® Prepierced Reseal injection site, Inter-Link® Injection Site, Safe Line® Injection Site, User-Gard® Intermittent Injection Cap, and SafSite® reflux valve.
The TUBEX® Sterile Cartridge Needle Unit is suitable for substances to be administered intravenously or intramuscularly.

Allergic Conditions
The average adult dose is 25 mg. This dose may be repeated within two hours if necessary, but continued therapy, if indicated, should be via the oral route as soon as existing circumstances permit. After initiation of treatment, dosage should be adjusted to the smallest amount adequate to relieve symptoms. The average adult dose for amelioration of allergic reactions to blood or plasma is 25 mg.

Sedation
In hospitalized adult patients, nighttime sedation may be achieved by a dose of 25 to 50 mg of Phenergan Injection.

Nausea and Vomiting
For control of nausea and vomiting, the usual adult dose is 12.5 to 25 mg, not to be repeated more frequently than every four hours. When used for control of postoperative nausea and vomiting, the medication may be administered either intramuscularly or intravenously and dosage of analgesics and barbiturates reduced accordingly.

Preoperative and Postoperative Use
As an adjunct to preoperative or postoperative medication, 25 to 50 mg Phenergan Injection in adults may be combined with appropriately reduced doses of analgesics and atropine-like drugs as desired. Dosage of concomitant analgesic or hypnotic medication should be reduced accordingly.

Obstetrics
Phenergan Injection in doses of 50 mg will provide sedation and relieve apprehension in the early stages of labor. When labor is definitely established, 25 to 75 mg (average dose, 50 mg) Phenergan Injection may be given intramuscularly or intravenously with an appropriately reduced dose of any desired narcotic. If necessary. Phenergan Injection with a reduced dose of analgesic may be repeated once or twice at four-hour intervals in the course of a normal labor. A maximum total dose of 100 mg of Phenergan Injection may be administered during a 24-hour period to patients in labor.

Pediatric Patients
Phenergan Injection is not recommended for use in pediatric patients less than two year of age.
In pediatric patients 2 years of age and older, the dosage should not exceed half that of the suggested adult dose. As an adjunct to premedication, the suggested dose is 0.5 mg per lb. of body weight in combination with an appropriately reduced dose of narcotic or barbiturate and the appropriate dose of an atropine-like drug. Antiemetics should not be used in vomiting of unknown etiology in pediatric patients (see **"WARNINGS—Use in Pediatric Patients)**.

HOW SUPPLIED
Phenergan® (promethazine HCl) Injection is available in 1 mL ampuls, in packages of 25 ampuls, as follows:
25 mg per mL, NDC 0008-0630-01
50 mg per mL, NDC 0008-0746-01
Store at controlled room temperature 15°–30°C (59°–86°F). Protect from light. Keep covered in carton until time of use. Do not use if solution has developed color or contains a precipitate.
Also Available:
Phenergan Injection is also available in the following dosage strengths in **TUBEX® BLUNT POINTE™** Sterile Cartridge Units and Sterile Cartridge-Needle Units, packaged in boxes of 10 **TUBEX®** as follows:
25 mg per mL, NDC 0008-0416-50, 1 mL size **BLUNT POINTE™.**
25 mg per mL, NDC 0008-0416-01, 1 mL size (22 gauge × 1-1/4 inch needle).
50 mg per mL, NDC 0008-0417-01, 1 mL size (22 gauge × 1-1/4 inch needle).
TUBEX is a registered trademark of Wyeth-Ayerst Laboratories. **BLUNT POINTE** is a trademark of Wyeth-Ayerst Laboratories.
InterLink is a registered trademark of Baxter International, Inc.
LifeShield is a registered trademark of Abbott Laboratories.
SafeLine is a registered trademark of McGaw, Inc.
SafSite is a registered trademark of B. Braun Medical, Inc.
User-Gard is a registered trademark of Arrow International, Inc.
Manufactured by:
Wyeth Laboratories Inc.
A Wyeth-Ayerst Company
Philadelphia PA 19101
CI 3727-7 Revised January 10, 2000

PHENERGAN® ℞
[fĕn 'ĕr-găn]
(promethazine hydrochloride)
Syrup Plain and

PHENERGAN® ℞
(promethazine hydrochloride)
Syrup Fortis

DESCRIPTION
Each teaspoon (5 mL) of Phenergan Syrup Plain contains 6.25 mg promethazine hydrochloride in a flavored syrup base with a pH between 4.7 and 5.2. Alcohol 7%. The inactive ingredients present are artificial and natural flavors, citric acid, D&C Red 33, D&C Yellow 10, FD&C Blue 1, FD&C Yellow 6, glycerin, saccharin sodium, sodium benzoate, sodium citrate, sodium propionate, water, and other ingredients.
Each teaspoon (5 mL) of Phenergan Syrup Fortis contains 25 mg promethazine hydrochloride in a flavored syrup base with a pH between 5.0 and 5.5. Alcohol 1.5%. The inactive ingredients present are artificial and natural flavors, citric acid, saccharin sodium, sodium benzoate, sodium propionate, water, and other ingredients.
Promethazine hydrochloride is a racemic compound; the empirical formula is $C_{17}H_{20}N_2S{\cdot}HCl$ and its molecular weight is 320.88.
Promethazine hydrochloride, a phenothiazine derivative, is designated chemically as 10*H*-Phenothiazine-10-ethanamine, *N,N*,α-trimethyl-, monohydrochloride, (±)- with the following structural formula:

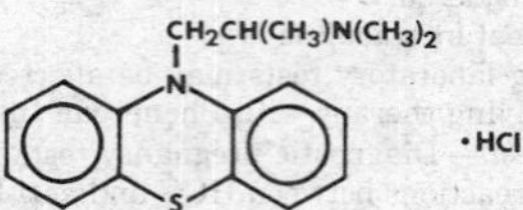

Promethazine hydrochloride occurs as a white to faint yellow, practically odorless, crystalline powder which slowly oxidizes and turns blue on prolonged exposure to air. It is soluble in water and freely soluble in alcohol.

CLINICAL PHARMACOLOGY
Promethazine is a phenothiazine derivative which differs structurally from the antipsychotic phenothiazines by the presence of a branched side chain and no ring substitution. It is thought that this configuration is responsible for its relative lack (1/10 that of chlorpromazine) of dopaminergic (CNS) action.
Promethazine is an H_1 receptor blocking agent. In addition to its antihistaminic action, it provides clinically useful sedative and antiemetic effects. In therapeutic dosage, promethazine produces no significant effects on the cardiovascular system.
Promethazine is well absorbed from the gastrointestinal tract. Clinical effects are apparent within 20 minutes after oral administration and generally last four to six hours, although they may persist as long as 12 hours. Promethazine is metabolized by the liver to a variety of compounds; the sulfoxides of promethazine and N-demethylpromethazine are the predominant metabolites appearing in the urine.

INDICATIONS AND USAGE
Phenergan is useful for:
Perennial and seasonal allergic rhinitis.
Vasomotor rhinitis.
Allergic conjunctivitis due to inhalant allergens and foods.
Mild, uncomplicated allergic skin manifestations of urticaria and angioedema.
Amelioration of allergic reactions to blood or plasma.
Dermographism.
Anaphylactic reactions, as adjunctive therapy to epinephrine and other standard measures, after the acute manifestations have been controlled.
Preoperative, postoperative, or obstetric sedation.
Prevention and control of nausea and vomiting associated with certain types of anesthesia and surgery.
Therapy adjunctive to meperidine or other analgesics for control of postoperative pain.
Sedation in both children and adults, as well as relief of apprehension and production of light sleep from which the patient can be easily aroused.
Active and prophylactic treatment of motion sickness.
Antiemetic therapy in postoperative patients.

CONTRAINDICATIONS
Promethazine is contraindicated in individuals known to be hypersensitive or to have had an idiosyncratic reaction to promethazine or to other phenothiazines.
Antihistamines are contraindicated for use in the treatment of lower respiratory tract symptoms including asthma.

WARNINGS
Promethazine may cause marked drowsiness. Ambulatory patients should be cautioned against such activities as driving or operating dangerous machinery until it is known that they do not become drowsy or dizzy from promethazine therapy.
The sedative action of promethazine hydrochloride is additive to the sedative effects of central nervous system depressants; therefore, agents such as alcohol, narcotic analgesics, sedatives, hypnotics, and tranquilizers should either be eliminated or given in reduced dosage in the presence of promethazine hydrochloride. When given concomitantly with promethazine hydrochloride, the dose of barbiturates should be reduced by at least one-half, and the dose of analgesic depressants, such as morphine or meperidine, should be reduced by one-quarter to one-half.
Promethazine may lower seizure threshold. This should be taken into consideration when administering to persons with known seizure disorders or when giving in combination with narcotics or local anesthetics which may also affect seizure threshold.
Sedative drugs or CNS depressants should be avoided in patients with a history of sleep apnea.
Antihistamines should be used with caution in patients with narrow-angle glaucoma, stenosing peptic ulcer, pyloroduodenal obstruction, and urinary bladder obstruction due to symptomatic prostatic hypertrophy and narrowing of the bladder neck.
Administration of promethazine has been associated with reported cholestatic jaundice.

PRECAUTIONS
GENERAL
Promethazine should be used cautiously in persons with cardiovascular disease or with impairment of liver function.
INFORMATION FOR PATIENTS
Phenergan may cause marked drowsiness or impair the mental and/or physical abilities required for the performance of potentially hazardous tasks, such as driving a vehicle or operating machinery. Ambulatory patients should be told to avoid engaging in such activities until it is known that they do not become drowsy or dizzy from Phenergan therapy. Children should be supervised to avoid potential harm in bike riding or in other hazardous activities.
The concomitant use of alcohol or other central nervous system depressants, including narcotic analgesics, sedatives, hypnotics, and tranquilizers, may have an additive effect and should be avoided or their dosage reduced.
Patients should be advised to report any involuntary muscle movements or unusual sensitivity to sunlight.
DRUG INTERACTIONS
The sedative action of promethazine is additive to the sedative effects of other central nervous system depressants, including alcohol, narcotic analgesics, sedatives, hypnotics, tricyclic antidepressants, and tranquilizers; therefore, these agents should be avoided or administered in reduced dosage to patients receiving promethazine.
DRUG/LABORATORY TEST INTERACTIONS
The following laboratory tests may be affected in patients who are receiving therapy with promethazine hydrochloride:
Pregnancy Tests
Diagnostic pregnancy tests based on immunological reactions between HCG and anti-HCG may result in false-negative or false-positive interpretations.
Glucose Tolerance Test
An increase in blood glucose has been reported in patients receiving promethazine.
CARCINOGENESIS, MUTAGENESIS, IMPAIRMENT OF FERTILITY
Long-term animal studies have not been performed to assess the carcinogenic potential of promethazine, nor are there other animal or human data concerning carcinogenicity, mutagenicity, or impairment of fertility with this drug. Promethazine was nonmutagenic in the *Salmonella* test system of Ames.
PREGNANCY
Teratogenic Effects —Pregnancy Category C
Teratogenic effects have not been demonstrated in rat-feeding studies at doses of 6.25 and 12.5 mg/kg of promethazine. These doses are from approximately 2.1 to 4.2 times the maximum recommended total daily dose of promethazine for a 50-kg subject, depending upon the indication for which the drug is prescribed. Specific studies to test the action of the drug on parturition, lactation, and development of the animal neonate were not done, but a general preliminary study in rats indicated no effect on these parameters. Although antihistamines, including promethazine, have been

found to produce fetal mortality in rodents, the pharmacological effects of histamine in the rodent do not parallel those in man. There are no adequate and well-controlled studies of promethazine in pregnant women. Phenergan should be used during pregnancy only if the potential benefit justifies the potential risk to the fetus.

Nonteratogenic Effects

Promethazine taken within two weeks of delivery may inhibit platelet aggregation in the newborn.

LABOR AND DELIVERY

Phenergan, in appropriate dosage form, may be used alone or as an adjunct to narcotic analgesics during labor and delivery. (See "**Indications and Usage**" and "**Dosage and Administration**.")

See also "*Nonteratogenic Effects*."

NURSING MOTHERS

It is not known whether promethazine is excreted in human milk. Caution should be exercised when promethazine is administered to a nursing woman.

PEDIATRIC USE

This product should not be used in children under 2 years of age because safety for such use has not been established.

ADVERSE REACTIONS

Nervous System —Sedation, sleepiness, occasional blurred vision, dryness of mouth, dizziness; rarely confusion, disorientation, and extrapyramidal symptoms such as oculogyric crisis, torticollis, and tongue protrusion (usually in association with parenteral injection or excessive dosage).

Cardiovascular —Increased or decreased blood pressure.

Dermatologic —Rash, rarely photosensitivity.

Hematologic —Rarely leukopenia, thrombocytopenia; agranulocytosis (1 case).

Gastrointestinal —Nausea and vomiting.

OVERDOSAGE

Signs and symptoms of overdosage with promethazine range from mild depression of the central nervous system and cardiovascular system to profound hypotension, respiratory depression, and unconsciousness.

Stimulation may be evident, especially in children and geriatric patients. Convulsions may rarely occur. A paradoxical reaction has been reported in children receiving single doses of 75 mg to 125 mg orally, characterized by hyperexcitability and nightmares.

Atropinelike signs and symptoms—dry mouth, fixed, dilated pupils, flushing, as well as gastrointestinal symptoms, may occur.

TREATMENT

Treatment of overdosage is essentially symptomatic and supportive. Only in cases of extreme overdosage or individual sensitivity do vital signs, including respiration, pulse, blood pressure, temperature, and EKG need to be monitored. Activated charcoal orally or by lavage may be given, or sodium or magnesium sulfate orally as a cathartic. Attention should be given to the reestablishment of adequate respiratory exchange through provision of a patent airway and institution of assisted or controlled ventilation. Diazepam may be used to control convulsions. Acidosis and electrolyte losses should be corrected. Note that any depressant effects of promethazine are not reversed by naloxone. Avoid analeptics which may cause convulsions.

Severe hypotension usually responds to the administration of norepinephrine or phenylephrine. EPINEPHRINE SHOULD NOT BE USED, since its use in patients with partial adrenergic blockade may further lower the blood pressure.

Limited experience with dialysis indicates that it is not helpful.

DOSAGE AND ADMINISTRATION

ALLERGY

The average oral dose is 25 mg taken before retiring; however, 12.5 mg may be taken before meals and on retiring, if necessary. Children tolerate this product well. Single 25-mg doses at bedtime or 6.25 to 12.5 mg taken three times daily will usually suffice. After initiation of treatment in children or adults, dosage should be adjusted to the smallest amount adequate to relieve symptoms.

Phenergan Rectal Suppositories may be used if the oral route is not feasible, but oral therapy should be resumed as soon as possible if continued therapy is indicated.

The administration of promethazine hydrochloride in 25-mg doses will control minor transfusion reactions of an allergic nature.

MOTION SICKNESS

The average adult dose is 25 mg taken twice daily. The initial dose should be taken one-half to one hour before anticipated travel and be repeated 8 to 12 hours later, if necessary. On succeeding days of travel, it is recommended that 25 mg be given on arising and again before the evening meal. For children, Phenergan Tablets, Syrup, or Rectal Suppositories, 12.5 to 25 mg, twice daily, may be administered.

NAUSEA AND VOMITING

The average effective dose of Phenergan for the active therapy of nausea and vomiting in children or adults is 25 mg. When oral medication cannot be tolerated, the dose should be given parenterally (cf. Phenergan Injection) or by rectal suppository. 12.5- to 25-mg doses may be repeated, as necessary, at 4- to 6-hour intervals.

For nausea and vomiting in children, the usual dose is 0.5 mg per pound of body weight, and the dose should be adjusted to the age and weight of the patient and the severity of the condition being treated.

For prophylaxis of nausea and vomiting, as during surgery and the postoperative period, the average dose is 25 mg repeated at 4- to 6-hour intervals, as necessary.

SEDATION

This product relieves apprehension and induces a quiet sleep from which the patient can be easily aroused. Administration of 12.5 to 25 mg Phenergan by the oral route or by rectal suppository at bedtime will provide sedation in children. Adults usually require 25 to 50 mg for nighttime, presurgical, or obstetrical sedation.

PRE- AND POSTOPERATIVE USE

Phenergan in 12.5- to 25-mg doses for children and 50-mg doses for adults the night before surgery relieves apprehension and produces a quiet sleep.

For preoperative medication children require doses of 0.5 mg per pound of body weight in combination with an equal dose of meperidine and the appropriate dose of an atropine-like drug.

Usual adult dosage is 50 mg Phenergan with an equal amount of meperidine and the required amount of a belladonna alkaloid.

Postoperative sedation and adjunctive use with analgesics may be obtained by the administration of 12.5 to 25 mg in children and 25- to 50-mg doses in adults.

Phenergan Syrup Plain and Phenergan Syrup Fortis are not recommended for children under 2 years of age.

HOW SUPPLIED

Phenergan® (Promethazine Hydrochloride) Syrup Plain is a clear, green solution supplied as follows:

NDC 0008-0549-02, case of 24 bottles of 4 fl. oz. (118 mL).

NDC 0008-0549-03, bottle of 1 pint (473 mL).

Phenergan® (Promethazine Hydrochloride) Syrup Fortis is a clear, light straw-colored solution supplied as follows:

NDC 0008-0231-01, bottle of 1 pint (473 mL).

Keep bottles tightly closed.

Store at Room Temperature, between 15° C and 25° C (59° F and 77° F).

Protect from light.

Dispense in light-resistant, glass, tight containers.

Manufactured by:

Wyeth Laboratories

A Wyeth-Ayerst Company

Philadelphia, PA 19101

CI 4871-1 Issued July 8, 1996

PHENERGAN® ℞

[fĕn ′ĕr-găn]

(promethazine HCl)

TABLETS •

SUPPOSITORIES

DESCRIPTION

Each tablet of Phenergan contains 12.5 mg, 25 mg, or 50 mg promethazine hydrochloride. The inactive ingredients present are lactose, magnesium stearate, and methylcellulose. Each dosage strength also contains the following:

12.5 mg—FD&C Yellow 6 and saccharin sodium;

25 mg—saccharin sodium;

50 mg—FD&C Red 40.

Each rectal suppository of Phenergan contains 12.5 mg, 25 mg, or 50 mg promethazine hydrochloride with ascorbyl palmitate, silicon dioxide, white wax, and cocoa butter.

Promethazine hydrochloride is a racemic compound; the empirical formula is $C_{17}H_{20}N_2S{\cdot}HCl$ and its molecular weight is 320.88.

Promethazine hydrochloride, a phenothiazine derivative, is designated chemically as 10*H*-Phenothiazine-10-ethanamine, *N,N,*α-trimethyl-, monohydrochloride, (±)- with the following structural formula:

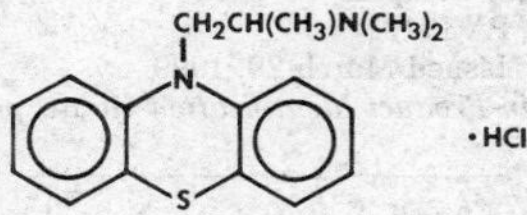

Promethazine hydrochloride occurs as a white to faint yellow, practically odorless, crystalline powder which slowly oxidizes and turns blue on prolonged exposure to air. It is soluble in water and freely soluble in alcohol.

CLINICAL PHARMACOLOGY

Promethazine is a phenothiazine derivative which differs structurally from the antipsychotic phenothiazines by the presence of a branched side chain and no ring substitution. It is thought that this configuration is responsible for its relative lack ($^1/_{10}$ that of chlorpromazine) of dopaminergic (CNS) action.

Promethazine is an H_1 receptor blocking agent. In addition to its antihistaminic action, it provides clinically useful sedative and antiemetic effects. In therapeutic dosage, promethazine produces no significant effects on the cardiovascular system.

Promethazine is well absorbed from the gastrointestinal tract. Clinical effects are apparent within 20 minutes after oral administration and generally last four to six hours, although they may persist as long as 12 hours. Promethazine is metabolized by the liver to a variety of compounds; the sulfoxides of promethazine and N-demethylpromethazine are the predominant metabolites appearing in the urine.

INDICATIONS AND USAGE

Phenergan, either orally or by suppository, is useful for:

Perennial and seasonal allergic rhinitis.

Vasomotor rhinitis.

Allergic conjunctivitis due to inhalant allergens and foods.

Mild, uncomplicated allergic skin manifestations of urticaria and angioedema.

Amelioration of allergic reactions to blood or plasma.

Dermographism.

Anaphylactic reactions, as adjunctive therapy to epinephrine and other standard measures, after the acute manifestations have been controlled.

Preoperative, postoperative, or obstetric sedation.

Prevention and control of nausea and vomiting associated with certain types of anesthesia and surgery.

Therapy adjunctive to meperidine or other analgesics for control of postoperative pain.

Sedation in both children and adults, as well as relief of apprehension and production of light sleep from which the patient can be easily aroused.

Active and prophylactic treatment of motion sickness.

Antiemetic therapy in postoperative patients.

CONTRAINDICATIONS

Promethazine is contraindicated in individuals known to be hypersensitive or to have had an idiosyncratic reaction to promethazine or to other phenothiazines.

Antihistamines are contraindicated for use in the treatment of lower respiratory tract symptoms including asthma.

WARNINGS

Promethazine may cause marked drowsiness. Ambulatory patients should be cautioned against such activities as driving or operating dangerous machinery until it is known that they do not become drowsy or dizzy from promethazine therapy.

The sedative action of promethazine hydrochloride is additive to the sedative effects of central nervous system depressants; therefore, agents such as alcohol, narcotic analgesics, sedatives, hypnotics, and tranquilizers should either be eliminated or given in reduced dosage in the presence of promethazine hydrochloride. When given concomitantly with promethazine hydrochloride, the dose of barbiturates should be reduced by at least one-half, and the dose of analgesic depressants, such as morphine or meperidine, should be reduced by one-quarter to one-half.

Promethazine may lower seizure threshold. This should be taken into consideration when administering to persons with known seizure disorders or when giving in combination with narcotics and local anesthetics which may also affect seizure threshold.

Sedative drugs or CNS depressants should be avoided in patients with a history of sleep apnea.

Antihistamines should be used with caution in patients with narrow-angle glaucoma, stenosing peptic ulcer, pyloroduodenal obstruction, and urinary bladder obstruction due to symptomatic prostatic hypertrophy and narrowing of the bladder neck.

Administration of promethazine has been associated with reported cholestatic jaundice.

PRECAUTIONS

General

Promethazine should be used cautiously in persons with cardiovascular disease or with impairment of liver function.

Information for Patients

Phenergan may cause marked drowsiness or impair the mental and/or physical abilities required for the performance of potentially hazardous tasks, such as driving a vehicle or operating machinery. Ambulatory patients should be told to avoid engaging in such activities until it is known that they do not become drowsy or dizzy from Phenergan therapy. Children should be supervised to avoid potential harm in bike riding or in other hazardous activities.

The concomitant use of alcohol or other central nervous system depressants, including narcotic analgesics, sedatives, hypnotics, and tranquilizers, may have an additive effect and should be avoided or their dosage reduced.

Patients should be advised to report any involuntary muscle movements or unusual sensitivity to sunlight.

Drug Interactions

The sedative action of promethazine is additive to the sedative effects of other central nervous system depressants, including alcohol, narcotic analgesics, sedatives, hypnotics, tricyclic antidepressants, and tranquilizers; therefore, these agents should be avoided or administered in reduced dosage to patients receiving promethazine.

Drug/Laboratory Test Interactions

The following laboratory tests may be affected in patients who are receiving therapy with promethazine hydrochloride:

Pregnancy Tests

Diagnostic pregnancy tests based on immunological reactions between HCG and anti-HCG may result in false-negative or false-positive interpretations.

Glucose Tolerance Test

An increase in blood glucose has been reported in patients receiving promethazine.

Carcinogenesis, Mutagenesis, Impairment of Fertility

Long-term animal studies have not been performed to assess the carcinogenic potential of promethazine, nor are there other animal or human data concerning carcinogenic-

Continued on next page

Phenergan Tabs/Supposits—Cont.

ity, mutagenicity, or impairment of fertility with this drug. Promethazine was nonmutagenic in the *Salmonella* test system of Ames.

Pregnancy

Teratogenic Effects —Pregnancy Category C

Teratogenic effects have not been demonstrated in rat-feeding studies at doses of 6.25 and 12.5 mg/kg of promethazine. These doses are from approximately 2.1 to 4.2 times the maximum recommended total daily dose of promethazine for a 50-kg subject, depending upon the indication for which the drug is prescribed. Specific studies to test the action of the drug on parturition, lactation, and development of the animal neonate were not done, but a general preliminary study in rats indicated no effect on these parameters. Although antihistamines, including promethazine, have been found to produce fetal mortality in rodents, the pharmacological effects of histamine in the rodent do not parallel those in man. There are no adequate and well-controlled studies of promethazine in pregnant women. Phenergan® should be used during pregnancy only if the potential benefit justifies the potential risk to the fetus.

Nonteratogenic Effects

Promethazine taken within two weeks of delivery may inhibit platelet aggregation in the newborn.

Labor and Delivery

Phenergan, in appropriate dosage form, may be used alone or as an adjunct to narcotic analgesics during labor and delivery. (See "**INDICATIONS AND USAGE**" and "**DOSAGE AND ADMINISTRATION**.")

See also *"Nonteratogenic Effects."*

Nursing Mothers

It is not known whether promethazine is excreted in human milk. Caution should be exercised when promethazine is administered to a nursing woman.

Pediatric Use

This product should not be used in children under 2 years of age because safety for such use has not been established.

ADVERSE REACTIONS

Nervous System —Sedation, sleepiness, occasional blurred vision, dryness of mouth, dizziness; rarely confusion, disorientation, and extrapyramidal symptoms such as oculogyric crisis, torticollis, and tongue protrusion (usually in association with parenteral injection or excessive dosage).

Cardiovascular —Increased or decreased blood pressure.

Dermatologic —Rash, rarely photosensitivity.

Hematologic —Rarely leukopenia, thrombocytopenia; agranulocytosis (1 case).

Gastrointestinal —Nausea and vomiting.

OVERDOSAGE

Signs and symptoms of overdosage with promethazine range from mild depression of the central nervous system and cardiovascular system to profound hypotension, respiratory depression, and unconsciousness.

Stimulation may be evident, especially in children and geriatric patients. Convulsions may rarely occur. A paradoxical reaction has been reported in children receiving single doses of 75 mg to 125 mg orally, characterized by hyperexcitability and nightmares.

Atropine-like signs and symptoms—dry mouth, fixed, dilated pupils, flushing, as well as gastrointestinal symptoms, may occur.

TREATMENT

Treatment of overdosage is essentially symptomatic and supportive. Only in cases of extreme overdosage or individual sensitivity do vital signs, including respiration, pulse, blood pressure, temperature, and EKG, need to be monitored. Activated charcoal orally or by lavage may be given, or sodium or magnesium sulfate orally as a cathartic. Attention should be given to the reestablishment of adequate respiratory exchange through provision of a patent airway and institution of assisted or controlled ventilation. Diazepam may be used to control convulsions. Acidosis and electrolyte losses should be corrected. Note that any depressant effects of promethazine are not reversed by naloxone. Avoid analeptics which may cause convulsions.

Severe hypotension usually responds to the administration of norepinephrine or phenylephrine. EPINEPHRINE SHOULD NOT BE USED, since its use in patients with partial adrenergic blockade may further lower the blood pressure.

Limited experience with dialysis indicates that it is not helpful.

DOSAGE AND ADMINISTRATION

Allergy

The average oral dose is 25 mg taken before retiring; however, 12.5 mg may be taken before meals and on retiring, if necessary. Children tolerate this product well. Single 25-mg doses at bedtime or 6.25 to 12.5 mg taken three times daily will usually suffice. After initiation of treatment in children or adults, dosage should be adjusted to the smallest amount adequate to relieve symptoms. The administration of promethazine hydrochloride in 25-mg doses will control minor transfusion reactions of an allergic nature.

Motion Sickness

The average adult dose is 25 mg taken twice daily. The initial dose should be taken one-half to one hour before anticipated travel and be repeated 8 to 12 hours later, if necessary. On succeeding days of travel, it is recommended that 25 mg be given on arising and again before the evening meal. For children, Phenergan Tablets, Syrup, or Rectal Suppositories, 12.5 to 25 mg, twice daily, may be administered.

Nausea and Vomiting

The average effective dose of Phenergan for the active therapy of nausea and vomiting in children or adults is 25 mg. When oral medication cannot be tolerated, the dose should be given parenterally (cf. Phenergan Injection) or by rectal suppository. 12.5- to 25-mg doses may be repeated, as necessary, at 4- to 6-hour intervals.

For nausea and vomiting in children, the usual dose is 0.5 mg per pound of body weight, and the dose should be adjusted to the age and weight of the patient and the severity of the condition being treated.

For prophylaxis of nausea and vomiting, as during surgery and the postoperative period, the average dose is 25 mg repeated at 4- to 6-hour intervals, as necessary.

Sedation

This product relieves apprehension and induces a quiet sleep from which the patient can be easily aroused. Administration of 12.5 to 25 mg Phenergan by the oral route or by rectal suppository at bedtime will provide sedation in children. Adults usually require 25 to 50 mg for nighttime, presurgical, or obstetrical sedation.

Pre- and Postoperative Use

Phenergan in 12.5- to 25-mg doses for children and 50-mg doses for adults the night before surgery relieves apprehension and produces a quiet sleep.

For preoperative medication children require doses of 0.5 mg per pound of body weight in combination with an equal dose of meperidine and the appropriate dose of an atropine-like drug.

Usual adult dosage is 50 mg Phenergan with an equal amount of meperidine and the required amount of a belladonna alkaloid.

Postoperative sedation and adjunctive use with analgesics may be obtained by the administration of 12.5 to 25 mg in children and 25- to 50-mg doses in adults.

Phenergan Tablets and Phenergan Rectal Suppositories are not recommended for children under 2 years of age.

HOW SUPPLIED

Phenergan® (promethazine HCl) Tablets are available as follows:

12.5 mg, orange tablet with "WYETH" on one side and "19" on the scored reverse side.

NDC 0008-0019-01, bottle of 100 tablets.

25 mg, white tablet with "WYETH" and "27" on one side and scored on the reverse side.

NDC 0008-0027-02, bottle of 100 tablets.

NDC 0008-0027-07, Redipak® carton of 100 tablets (10 blister strips of 10).

50 mg, pink tablet with "WYETH" on one side and "227" on the other side.

NDC 0008-0227-01, bottle of 100 tablets.

Keep tightly closed.

Store at room temperature, between 15°C and 25°C (59°F and 77°F).

Protect from light.

Dispense in light-resistant, tight container.

Use carton to protect contents from light.

Phenergan® (promethazine HCl) Rectal Suppositories are available in boxes of 12 as follows:

12.5 mg, ivory, torpedo-shaped suppository wrapped in copper-colored foil, NDC 0008-0498-01.

25 mg, ivory, torpedo-shaped suppository wrapped in light-green foil, NDC 0008-0212-01.

50 mg, ivory, torpedo-shaped suppository wrapped in blue foil, NDC 0008-0229-01.

Store refrigerated between 2°–8°C (36°–46°F).

Dispense in well-closed container.

Manufactured by:
Wyeth Laboratories
A Wyeth-Ayerst Company
Philadelphia, PA 19101

CI 5184-1 Issued March 29, 1999

Shown in Product Identification Guide, page 342

PHENERGAN® Ⓒ ℞

[fĕn 'ĕr-găn]

with codeine

(Promethazine Hydrochloride and Codeine Phosphate) Syrup

DESCRIPTION

Each teaspoon (5 mL) of Phenergan with codeine contains 10 mg codeine phosphate (Warning—may be habit-forming) and 6.25 mg promethazine hydrochloride in a flavored syrup base with a pH between 4.8 to 5.4. Alcohol 7%. The inactive ingredients present are artificial and natural flavors, citric acid, D&C Red 33, FD&C Blue 1, FD&C Yellow 6, glycerine, saccharin sodium, sodium benzoate, sodium citrate, sodium propionate, water, and other ingredients.

Codeine is one of the naturally occurring phenanthrene alkaloids of opium derived from the opium poppy; it is classified pharmacologically as a narcotic analgesic. Codeine phosphate may be chemically named as (5α,6α)-7,8-didehydro-4, 5-epoxy-3-methoxy-17-methylmorphinan-6-ol phosphate (1:1) (salt) hemihydrate with the following structural formula:

[See chemical structure at top of next column]

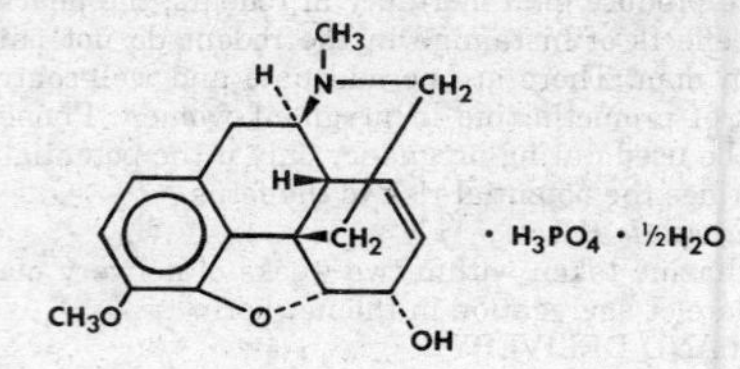

$\cdot H_3PO_4 \cdot \frac{1}{2}H_2O$

The phosphate salt of codeine occurs as white, needle-shaped crystals or white crystalline powder. Codeine phosphate is freely soluble in water and slightly soluble in alcohol, with a molecular weight of 406.37. The empirical formula is $C_{18}H_{21}NO_3 \cdot H_3PO_4 \cdot {}^1/_2H_2O$, and the stereochemistry is 5α, 6α isomer as indicated in the structure.

Promethazine hydrochloride is a racemic compound; the empirical formula is $C_{17}H_{20}N_2S \cdot HCl$ and its molecular weight is 320.88.

Promethazine hydrochloride, a phenothiazine derivative, is designated chemically as 10*H*-Phenothiazine-10-ethanamine, *N,N*,α-trimethyl-, monohydrochloride, (±)-. with the following structural formula:

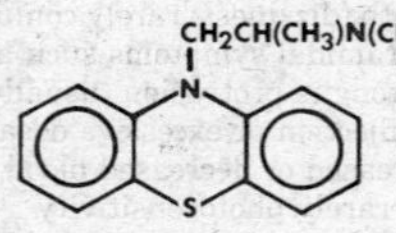

$CH_2CH(CH_3)N(CH_3)_2$ $\cdot HCl$

Promethazine hydrochloride occurs as a white to faint yellow, practically odorless, crystalline powder which slowly oxidizes and turns blue on prolonged exposure to air. It is soluble in water and freely soluble in alcohol.

CLINICAL PHARMACOLOGY

Codeine

Narcotic analgesics, including codeine, exert their primary effects on the central nervous system and gastrointestinal tract. The analgesic effects of codeine are due to its central action; however, the precise sites of action have not been determined, and the mechanisms involved appear to be quite complex. Codeine resembles morphine both structurally and pharmacologically, but its actions at the doses of codeine used therapeutically are milder, with less sedation, respiratory depression, and gastrointestinal, urinary, and pupillary effects. Codeine produces an increase in biliary tract pressure, but less than morphine or meperidine. Codeine is less constipating than morphine.

Codeine has good antitussive activity, although less than that of morphine at equal doses. It is used in preference to morphine, because side effects are infrequent at the usual antitussive dose of codeine.

Codeine in oral therapeutic dosage does not usually exert major effects on the cardiovascular system.

Narcotic analgesics may cause nausea and vomiting by stimulating the chemoreceptor trigger zone (CTZ); however, they also depress the vomiting center, so that subsequent doses are unlikely to produce vomiting. Nausea is minimal after usual oral doses of codeine.

Narcotic analgesics cause histamine release, which appears to be responsible for wheals or urticaria sometimes seen at the site of injection on parenteral administration. Histamine release may also produce dilation of cutaneous blood vessels, with resultant flushing of the face and neck, pruritus, and sweating.

Codeine and its salts are well absorbed following both oral and parenteral administration. Codeine is about 2/3 as effective orally as parenterally. Codeine is metabolized primarily in the liver by enzymes of the endoplasmic reticulum, where it undergoes O-demethylation, N-demethylation, and partial conjugation with glucuronic acid. The drug is excreted primarily in the urine, largely as inactive metabolites and small amounts of free and conjugated morphine. Negligible amounts of codeine and its metabolites are found in the feces.

Following oral or subcutaneous administration of codeine, the onset of analgesia occurs within 15 to 30 minutes and lasts for four to six hours.

The cough-depressing action, in animal studies, was observed to occur 15 minutes after oral administration of codeine, peak action at 45 to 60 minutes after ingestion. The duration of action, which is dose-dependent, usually did not exceed 3 hours.

Promethazine

Promethazine is a phenothiazine derivative which differs structurally from the antipsychotic phenothiazines by the presence of a branched side chain and no ring substitution. It is thought that this configuration is responsible for its lack (1/10 that of chlorpromazine) of dopaminergic (CNS) action.

Promethazine is an H_1 receptor blocking agent. In addition to its antihistaminic action, it provides clinically useful sedative and antiemetic effects. In therapeutic dosages, promethazine produces no significant effects on the cardiovascular system.

Promethazine is well absorbed from the gastrointestinal tract. Clinical effects are apparent within 20 minutes after oral administration and generally last four to six hours, although they may persist as long as 12 hours. Promethazine is metabolized by the liver to a variety of compounds; the sulfoxides of promethazine and N-demethylpromethazine are the predominant metabolites appearing in the urine.

INDICATIONS AND USAGE

Phenergan with codeine is indicated for the temporary relief of coughs and upper respiratory symptoms associated with allergy or the common cold.

CONTRAINDICATIONS

Codeine is contraindicated in patients with a known hypersensitivity to the drug.

Promethazine is contraindicated in individuals known to be hypersensitive or to have had an idiosyncratic reaction to promethazine or to other phenothiazines.

Antihistamines and codeine are both contraindicated for use in the treatment of lower respiratory tract symptoms, including asthma.

WARNINGS

Codeine

Dosage of codeine SHOULD NOT BE INCREASED if cough fails to respond; an unresponsive cough should be reevaluated in 5 days or sooner for possible underlying pathology, such as foreign body or lower respiratory tract disease.

Codeine may cause or aggravate constipation.

Respiratory depression leading to arrest, coma, and death has occurred with the use of codeine antitussives in young children, particularly in the under-one-year infants whose ability to deactivate the drug is not fully developed.

Administration of codeine may be accompanied by histamine release and should be used with caution in atopic children.

Head Injury and Increased Intracranial Pressure

The respiratory-depressant effects of narcotic analgesics and their capacity to elevate cerebrospinal fluid pressure may be markedly exaggerated in the presence of head injury, intracranial lesions, or a preexisting increase in intracranial pressure. Narcotics may produce adverse reactions which may obscure the clinical course of patients with head injuries.

Asthma and Other Respiratory Conditions

Narcotic analgesics or cough suppressants, including codeine, should not be used in asthmatic patients (see "Contraindications"). Nor should they be used in acute febrile illness associated with productive cough or in chronic respiratory disease where interference with ability to clear the tracheobronchial tree of secretions would have a deleterious effect on the patient's respiratory function.

Hypotensive Effect

Codeine may produce orthostatic hypotension in ambulatory patients.

Promethazine

Promethazine may cause marked drowsiness. Ambulatory patients should be cautioned against such activities as driving or operating dangerous machinery until it is known that they do not become drowsy or dizzy from promethazine therapy.

The sedative action of promethazine hydrochloride is additive to the sedative effects of central nervous system depressants; therefore, agents such as alcohol, narcotic analgesics, sedatives, hypnotics, and tranquilizers should either be eliminated or given in reduced dosage in the presence of promethazine hydrochloride. When given concomitantly with promethazine hydrochloride, the dose of barbiturates should be reduced by at least one-half, and the dose of analgesic depressants, such as morphine or meperidine, should be reduced by one-quarter to one-half.

Promethazine may lower seizure threshold. This should be taken into consideration when administering to persons with known seizure disorders or when giving in combination with narcotics or local anesthetics which may also affect seizure threshold.

Sedative drugs or CNS depressants should be avoided in patients with a history of sleep apnea.

Antihistamines should be used with caution in patients with narrow-angle glaucoma, stenosing peptic ulcer, pyloroduodenal obstruction, and urinary bladder obstruction due to symptomatic prostatic hypertrophy and narrowing of the bladder neck.

Administration of promethazine has been associated with reported cholestatic jaundice.

PRECAUTIONS

Animal reproduction studies have not been conducted with the drug combination—promethazine and codeine. It is not known whether this drug combination can cause fetal harm when administered to a pregnant woman or can affect reproduction capacity. Phenergan with codeine should be given to a pregnant woman only if clearly needed.

General

Narcotic analgesics, including codeine, should be administered with caution and the initial dose reduced in patients with acute abdominal conditions, convulsive disorders, significant hepatic or renal impairment, fever, hypothyroidism, Addison's disease, ulcerative colitis, prostatic hypertrophy, in patients with recent gastrointestinal or urinary tract surgery, and in the very young or elderly or debilitated patients.

Promethazine should be used cautiously in persons with cardiovascular disease or with impairment of liver function.

Information for Patients

Phenergan with codeine may cause marked drowsiness or may impair the mental and/or physical abilities required for the performance of potentially hazardous tasks, such as driving a vehicle or operating machinery. Ambulatory patients should be told to avoid engaging in such activities until it is known that they do not become drowsy or dizzy from

PHENERGAN WITH CODEINE

Adults	1 teaspoon (5 mL) every 4 to 6 hours, not to exceed 30.0 mL in 24 hours.
Children 6 years to under 12 years	1/2 to 1 teaspoon (2.5 to 5 mL) every 4 to 6 hours, not to exceed 30.0 mL in 24 hours.
Children under 6 years (weight: 18 kg or 40 lbs)	1/4 to 1/2 teaspoon (1.25 to 2.5 mL) every 4 to 6 hours, not to exceed 9.0 mL in 24 hours.
Children under 6 years (weight: 16 kg or 35 lbs)	1/4 to 1/2 teaspoon (1.25 to 2.5 mL) every 4 to 6 hours, not to exceed 8.0 mL in 24 hours.
Children under 6 years (weight: 14 kg or 30 lbs)	1/4 to 1/2 teaspoon (1.25 to 2.5 mL) every 4 to 6 hours, not to exceed 7.0 mL in 24 hours.
Children under 6 years (weight: 12 kg or 25 lbs)	1/4 to 1/2 teaspoon (1.25 to 2.5 mL) every 4 to 6 hours, not to exceed 6.0 mL in 24 hours.

Phenergan with codeine is not recommended for children under 2 years of age.

Phenergan with codeine therapy. Children should be supervised to avoid potential harm in bike riding or in other hazardous activities.

The concomitant use of alcohol or other central nervous system depressants, including narcotic analgesics, sedatives, hypnotics, and tranquilizers, may have an additive effect and should be avoided or their dosage reduced.

Patients should be advised to report any involuntary muscle movements or unusual sensitivity to sunlight.

Codeine, like other narcotic analgesics, may produce orthostatic hypotension in some ambulatory patients. Patients should be cautioned accordingly.

Drug Interactions

Codeine

In patients receiving MAO inhibitors, an initial small test dose is advisable to allow observation of any excessive narcotic effects or MAOI interaction.

Promethazine

The sedative action of promethazine is additive to the effects of other central nervous system depressants, including alcohol, narcotic analgesics, sedatives, hypnotics, tricyclic antidepressants, and tranquilizers; therefore, these agents should be avoided or administered in reduced dosage to patients receiving promethazine.

Drug/Laboratory Test Interactions

Because narcotic analgesics may increase biliary tract pressure, with resultant increases in plasma amylase or lipase levels, determination of these enzyme levels may be unreliable for 24 hours after a narcotic analgesic has been given.

The following laboratory tests may be affected in patients who are receiving therapy with promethazine hydrochloride:

Pregnancy Tests

Diagnostic pregnancy tests based on immunological reactions between HCG and anti-HCG may result in false-negative or false-positive interpretations.

Glucose Tolerance Test

An increase in blood glucose has been reported in patients receiving promethazine.

Carcinogenesis, Mutagenesis, Impairment of Fertility

Long-term animal studies have not been performed to assess the carcinogenic potential of codeine or of promethazine, nor are there other animal or human data concerning carcinogenicity, mutagenicity, or impairment of fertility with these agents. Codeine has been reported to show no evidence of carcinogenicity or mutagenicity in a variety of test systems, including the micronucleus and sperm abnormality assays and the *Salmonella* assay. Promethazine was nonmutagenic in the *Salmonella* test system of Ames.

Pregnancy

Teratogenic Effects —Pregnancy Category C

Codeine

A study in rats and rabbits reported no teratogenic effect of codeine administered during the period of organogenesis in doses ranging from 5 to 120 mg/kg. In the rat, doses at the 120-mg/kg level, in the toxic range for the adult animal, were associated with an increase in embryo resorption at the time of implantation. In another study a single 100-mg/kg dose of codeine administered to pregnant mice reportedly resulted in delayed ossification in the offspring.

There are no studies in humans, and the significance of these findings to humans, if any, is not known.

Promethazine

Teratogenic effects have not been demonstrated in rat-feeding studies at doses of 6.25 and 12.5 mg/kg of promethazine. These doses are 8.3 and 16.7 times the maximum recommended total daily dose of promethazine for a 50-kg subject. Specific studies to test the action of the drug on parturition, lactation, and development of the animal neonate were not done, but a general preliminary study in rats indicated no effect on these parameters. Although antihistamines, including promethazine, have been found to produce fetal mortality in rodents, the pharmacological effects of histamine in the rodent do not parallel those in man. There are no adequate and well-controlled studies of promethazine in pregnant women.

Phenergan® with codeine should be used during pregnancy only if the potential benefit justifies the potential risk to the fetus.

Nonteratogenic Effects

Dependence has been reported in newborns whose mothers took opiates regularly during pregnancy. Withdrawal signs include irritability, excessive crying, tremors, hyperreflexia, fever, vomiting, and diarrhea. Signs usually appear during the first few days of life.

Promethazine taken within two weeks of delivery may inhibit platelet aggregation in the newborn.

Labor and Delivery

Narcotic analgesics cross the placental barrier. The closer to delivery and the larger the dose used, the greater the possibility of respiratory depression in the newborn. Narcotic analgesics should be avoided during labor if delivery of a premature infant is anticipated. If the mother has received narcotic analgesics during labor, newborn infants should be observed closely for signs of respiratory depression. Resuscitation may be required (see "**OVERDOSAGE**"). The effect of codeine, if any, on the later growth, development, and functional maturation of the child is unknown.

See also "*Nonteratogenic Effects.*"

Nursing Mothers

Some studies, but not others, have reported detectable amounts of codeine in breast milk. The levels are probably not clinically significant after usual therapeutic dosage. The possibility of clinically important amounts being excreted in breast milk in individuals abusing codeine should be considered.

It is not known whether promethazine is excreted in human milk.

Caution should be exercised when Phenergan with codeine is administered to a nursing woman.

Pediatric Use

This product should not be used in children under 2 years of age because safety for such use has not been established.

ADVERSE REACTIONS

Codeine

Nervous System —CNS depression, particularly respiratory depression, and to a lesser extent circulatory depression; light-headedness, dizziness, sedation, euphoria, dysphoria, headache, transient hallucination, disorientation, visual disturbances, and convulsions.

Cardiovascular —Tachycardia, bradycardia, palpitation, faintness, syncope, orthostatic hypotension (common to narcotic analgesics).

Gastrointestinal —Nausea, vomiting, constipation, and biliary tract spasm. Patients with chronic ulcerative colitis may experience increased colonic motility; in patients with acute ulcerative colitis, toxic dilation has been reported.

Genitourinary —Oliguria, urinary retention; antidiuretic effect has been reported (common to narcotic analgesics).

Allergic —Infrequent pruritus, giant urticaria, angioneurotic edema, and laryngeal edema.

Other —Flushing of the face, sweating and pruritus (due to opiate-induced histamine release); weakness.

Promethazine

Nervous System —Sedation, sleepiness, occasional blurred vision, dryness of mouth, dizziness; rarely confusion, disorientation, and extrapyramidal symptoms such as oculogyric crisis, torticollis, and tongue protrusion (usually in association with parenteral injection or excessive dosage).

Cardiovascular —Increased or decreased blood pressure.

Dermatologic —Rash, rarely photosensitivity.

Hematologic —Rarely leukopenia, thrombocytopenia; agranulocytosis (1 case).

Gastrointestinal —Nausea and vomiting.

DRUG ABUSE AND DEPENDENCE

Controlled Substance

Phenergan with codeine is a Schedule V Controlled Substance.

Abuse

Codeine is known to be subject to abuse; however, the abuse potential of oral codeine appears to be quite low. Even parenteral codeine does not appear to offer the psychic effects sought by addicts to the same degree as heroin or morphine. However, codeine must be administered only under close supervision to patients with a history of drug abuse or dependence.

Dependence

Psychological dependence, physical dependence, and tolerance are known to occur with codeine.

OVERDOSAGE

Codeine

Serious overdose with codeine is characterized by respiratory depression (a decrease in respiratory rate and/or tidal volume, Cheyne-Stokes respiration, cyanosis), extreme somnolence progressing to stupor or coma, skeletal muscle flaccidity, cold and clammy skin, and sometimes bradycardia and hypotension. The triad of coma, pinpoint pupils, and respiratory depression is strongly suggestive of opiate poisoning. In severe overdosage, particularly by the intravenous route, apnea, circulatory collapse, cardiac arrest, and death may occur. Promethazine is additive to the depressant effects of codeine.

It is difficult to determine what constitutes a standard toxic or lethal dose. However, the lethal oral dose of codeine in an adult is reported to be in the range of 0.5 to 1.0 gram. In-

Continued on next page

Phenergan w/Codeine—Cont.

fants and children are believed to be relatively more sensitive to opiates on a body-weight basis. Elderly patients are also comparatively intolerant to opiates.

Promethazine

Signs and symptoms of overdosage with promethazine range from mild depression of the central nervous system and cardiovascular system to profound hypotension, respiratory depression, and unconsciousness.

Stimulation may be evident, especially in children and geriatric patients. Convulsions may rarely occur. A paradoxical reaction has been reported in children receiving single doses of 75 mg to 125 mg orally, characterized by hyperexcitability and nightmares.

Atropine-like signs and symptoms—dry mouth, fixed, dilated pupils, flushing, as well as gastrointestinal symptoms, may occur.

Treatment

The treatment of overdosage with Phenergan with codeine is essentially symptomatic and supportive. Only in cases of extreme overdosage or individual sensitivity do vital signs including respiration, pulse, blood pressure, temperature, and EKG need to be monitored. Activated charcoal orally or by lavage may be given, or sodium or magnesium sulfate orally as a cathartic. Attention should be given to the reestablishment of adequate respiratory exchange through provision of a patent airway and institution of assisted or controlled ventilation. The narcotic antagonist, naloxone hydrochloride, may be administered when significant respiratory depression occurs with Phenergan with codeine; any depressant effects of promethazine are not reversed with naloxone. Diazepam may be used to control convulsions. Avoid analeptics, which may cause convulsions. Acidosis and electrolyte losses should be corrected. A rise in temperature or pulmonary complications may signal the need for institution of antibiotic therapy.

Severe hypotension usually responds to the administration of norepinephrine or phenylephrine. EPINEPHRINE SHOULD NOT BE USED, since its use in a patient with partial adrenergic blockade may further lower the blood pressure.

Limited experience with dialysis indicates that it is not helpful.

DOSAGE AND ADMINISTRATION

The average effective dose is given in the following table:
[See table at top of previous page]

HOW SUPPLIED

Phenergan® with codeine is a clear, purple solution supplied as follows:
NDC 0008-0550-02, case of 24 bottles of 4 fl. oz. (118 mL).
NDC 0008-0550-03, bottle of 1 pint (473 mL).

Keep tightly closed—Store at room temperature, between 15° C and 25° C (59° F and 77° F).
Protect from light.
Dispense in light-resistant, glass, tight container.

Manufactured by:
Wyeth Laboratories
A Wyeth-Ayerst Company
Philadelphia, PA 19101
CI 4868-2 Revised July 22, 1998

PHENERGAN® ℞

[fĕn 'ĕr-găn]
with dextromethorphan
(Promethazine Hydrochloride and Dextromethorphan Hydrobromide)
Syrup

DESCRIPTION

Each teaspoon (5 mL) of Phenergan with dextromethorphan contains 6.25 mg promethazine hydrochloride and 15 mg dextromethorphan hydrobromide in a flavored syrup base with a pH between 4.7 and 5.2. Alcohol 7%. The inactive ingredients present are artificial and natural flavors, citric acid, D&C Yellow 10, FD&C Yellow 6, glycerin, saccharin sodium, sodium benzoate, sodium citrate, sodium propionate, water, and other ingredients.

Promethazine hydrochloride is a racemic compound; the empirical formula is $C_{17}H_{20}N_2S{\cdot}HCl$ and its molecular weight is 320.88.

Promethazine hydrochloride, a phenothiazine derivative, is designated chemically as 10*H*-Phenothiazine-10-ethanamine, *N,N*,α-trimethyl-, monohydrochloride, (±)-, with the following structural formula:

$CH_2CH(CH_3)N(CH_3)_2$ · HCl

Promethazine hydrochloride occurs as a white to faint yellow, practically odorless, crystalline powder which slowly oxidizes and turns blue on prolonged exposure to air. It is soluble in water and freely soluble in alcohol.

Dextromethorphan hydrobromide is a salt of the methyl ether of the dextrorotatory isomer of levorphanol, a narcotic analgesic. It is chemically named as 3-methoxy-17-methyl-9α, 13α, 14α-morphinan hydrobromide monohydrate with the following structural formula:

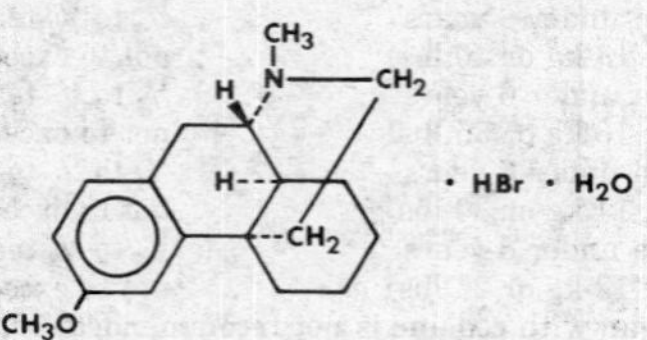

Dextromethorphan hydrobromide monohydrate occurs as white crystals, is sparingly soluble in water, and is freely soluble in alcohol. The empirical formula is $C_{18}H_{25}NO{\cdot}HBr{\cdot}H_2O$, and the molecular weight of the monohydrate is 370.33. Dextromethorphan HBr monohydrate is dextrorotatory with a specific rotation of +27.6 degrees in water (20 degrees C, sodium D-line).

CLINICAL PHARMACOLOGY

PROMETHAZINE

Promethazine is a phenothiazine derivative which differs structurally from the antipsychotic phenothiazines by the presence of a branched side chain and no ring substitution. It is thought that this configuration is responsible for its relative lack (1/10 that of chlorpromazine) of dopaminergic (CNS) action.

Promethazine is an H_1 receptor blocking agent. In addition to its antihistaminic action, it provides clinically useful sedative and antiemetic effects. In therapeutic dosages, promethazine produces no significant effects on the cardiovascular system.

Promethazine is well absorbed from the gastrointestinal tract. Clinical effects are apparent within 20 minutes after oral administration and generally last four to six hours, although they may persist as long as 12 hours. Promethazine is metabolized by the liver to a variety of compounds; the sulfoxides of promethazine and N-demethylpromethazine are the predominant metabolites appearing in the urine.

DEXTROMETHORPHAN

Dextromethorphan is an antitussive agent and, unlike the isomeric levorphanol, it has no analgesic or addictive properties.

The drug acts centrally and elevates the threshold for coughing. It is about equal to codeine in depressing the cough reflex. In therapeutic dosage dextromethorphan does not inhibit ciliary activity.

Dextromethorphan is rapidly absorbed from the gastrointestinal tract and exerts its effect in 15 to 30 minutes. The duration of action after oral administration is approximately three to six hours. Dextromethorphan is metabolized primarily by liver enzymes undergoing O-demethylation, N-demethylation, and partial conjugation with glucuronic acid and sulfate. In humans, (+)-3-hydroxy-N-methylmorphinan, (+)-3-hydroxymorphinan, and traces of unmetabolized drug were found in urine after oral administration.

INDICATIONS AND USAGE

Phenergan with dextromethorphan is indicated for the temporary relief of coughs and upper respiratory symptoms associated with allergy or the common cold.

CONTRAINDICATIONS

Promethazine is contraindicated in individuals known to be hypersensitive or to have had an idiosyncratic reaction to promethazine or to other phenothiazines.

Antihistamines are contraindicated for use in the treatment of lower respiratory tract symptoms, including asthma.

Dextromethorphan should not be used in patients receiving a monoamine oxidase inhibitor (MAOI) (see "PRECAUTIONS—DRUG INTERACTIONS").

WARNINGS

PROMETHAZINE

Promethazine may cause marked drowsiness. Ambulatory patients should be cautioned against such activities as driving or operating dangerous machinery until it is known that they do not become drowsy or dizzy from promethazine therapy.

The sedative action of promethazine hydrochloride is additive to the sedative effects of central nervous system depressants; therefore, agents such as alcohol, narcotic analgesics, sedatives, hypnotics, and tranquilizers should either be eliminated or given in reduced dosage in the presence of promethazine hydrochloride. When given concomitantly with promethazine hydrochloride, the dose of barbiturates should be reduced by at least one-half, and the dose of analgesic depressants, such as morphine or meperidine, should be reduced by one-quarter to one-half.

Promethazine may lower seizure threshold. This should be taken into consideration when administering to persons with known seizure disorders or when giving in combination with narcotics or local anesthetics which may also affect seizure threshold.

Sedative drugs or CNS depressants should be avoided in patients with a history of sleep apnea.

Antihistamines should be used with caution in patients with narrow-angle glaucoma, stenosing peptic ulcer, pyloroduodenal obstruction, and urinary bladder obstruction due to symptomatic prostatic hypertrophy and narrowing of the bladder neck.

Administration of promethazine has been associated with reported cholestatic jaundice.

DEXTROMETHORPHAN

Administration of dextromethorphan may be accompanied by histamine release and should be used with caution in atopic children.

PRECAUTIONS

Animal reproduction studies have not been conducted with the drug combination—promethazine and dextromethorphan. It is not known whether this drug combination can cause fetal harm when administered to a pregnant woman or can affect reproduction capacity. Phenergan with dextromethorphan should be given to a pregnant woman only if clearly needed.

GENERAL

Promethazine should be used cautiously in persons with cardiovascular disease or with impairment of liver function. Dextromethorphan should be used with caution in sedated patients, in the debilitated, and in patients confined to the supine position.

INFORMATION FOR PATIENTS

Phenergan with dextromethorphan may cause marked drowsiness or impair the mental and/or physical abilities required for the performance of potentially hazardous tasks, such as driving a vehicle or operating machinery. Ambulatory patients should be told to avoid engaging in such activities until it is known that they do not become drowsy or dizzy from Phenergan with dextromethorphan therapy. Children should be supervised to avoid potential harm in bike riding or in other hazardous activities.

The concomitant use of alcohol or other central nervous system depressants, including narcotic analgesics, sedatives, hypnotics, and tranquilizers, may have an additive effect and should be avoided or their dosage reduced.

Patients should be advised to report any involuntary muscle movements or unusual sensitivity to sunlight.

DRUG INTERACTIONS

Hyperpyrexia, hypotension, and death have been reported coincident with the coadministration of monoamine oxidase (MAO) inhibitors and products containing dextromethorphan. Thus, concomitant administration of Phenergan with dextromethorphan and MAO inhibitors should be avoided (see "**Contraindications**").

The sedative action of promethazine is additive to the sedative effects of other central nervous system depressants, including alcohol, narcotic analgesics, sedatives, hypnotics, tricyclic antidepressants, and tranquilizers; therefore, these agents should be avoided or administered in reduced dosage to patients receiving promethazine.

DRUG/LABORATORY TEST INTERACTIONS

The following laboratory tests may be affected in patients who are receiving therapy with promethazine hydrochloride:

Pregnancy Tests

Diagnostic pregnancy tests based on immunological reactions between HCG and anti-HCG may result in false-negative or false-positive interpretations.

Glucose Tolerance Test

An increase in blood glucose has been reported in patients receiving promethazine.

CARCINOGENESIS, MUTAGENESIS, IMPAIRMENT OF FERTILITY

Long-term animal studies have not been performed to assess the carcinogenic potential of promethazine or of dextromethorphan. There are no animal or human data concerning the carcinogenicity, mutagenicity, or impairment of fertility with these drugs. Promethazine was nonmutagenic in the *Salmonella* test system of Ames.

PREGNANCY

Teratogenic Effects —Pregnancy Category C

Teratogenic effects have not been demonstrated in rat-feeding studies at doses of 6.25 and 12.5 mg/kg of promethazine. These doses are 8.3 and 16.7 times the maximum recommended total daily dose for a 50-kg subject. Specific studies to test the action of the drug on parturition, lactation, and development of the animal neonate were not done, but a general preliminary study in rats indicated no effect on these parameters. Although antihistamines, including promethazine, have been found to produce fetal mortality in rodents, the pharmacological effects of histamine in the rodent do not parallel those in man. There are no adequate and well-controlled studies of promethazine in pregnant women.

Phenergan with dextromethorphan should be used during pregnancy only if the potential benefit justifies the potential risk to the fetus.

Nonteratogenic Effects

Promethazine taken within two weeks of delivery may inhibit platelet aggregation in the newborn.

LABOR AND DELIVERY

See "*Nonteratogenic Effects.*"

NURSING MOTHERS

It is not known whether promethazine or dextromethorphan is excreted in human milk. Caution should be exercised when Phenergan with dextromethorphan is administered to a nursing woman.

PEDIATRIC USE

This product should not be used in children under 2 years of age because safety for that use has not been established.

ADVERSE REACTIONS

PROMETHAZINE

Nervous System —Sedation, sleepiness, occasional blurred vision, dryness of mouth, dizziness; rarely confusion, disori-

entation, and extrapyramidal symptoms such as oculogyric crisis, torticollis, and tongue protrusion (usually in association with parenteral injection or excessive dosage).
Cardiovascular —Increased or decreased blood pressure.
Dermatologic —Rash, rarely photosensitivity.
Hematologic —Rarely leukopenia, thrombocytopenia; agranulocytosis (1 case).
Gastrointestinal —Nausea and vomiting.
DEXTROMETHORPHAN
Dextromethorphan hydrobromide occasionally causes slight drowsiness, dizziness, and gastrointestinal disturbances.

DRUG ABUSE AND DEPENDENCE

According to the WHO Expert Committee on Drug Dependence, dextromethorphan could produce very slight psychic dependence but no physical dependence.

OVERDOSAGE

PROMETHAZINE
Signs and symptoms of overdosage with promethazine range from mild depression of the central nervous system and cardiovascular system to profound hypotension, respiratory depression, and unconsciousness.
Stimulation may be evident, especially in children and geriatric patients. Convulsions may rarely occur. A paradoxical reaction has been reported in children receiving single doses of 75 mg to 125 mg orally, characterized by hyperexcitability and nightmares.
Atropine-like signs and symptoms—dry mouth, fixed, dilated pupils, flushing, as well as gastrointestinal symptoms, may occur.
DEXTROMETHORPHAN
Dextromethorphan may produce central excitement and mental confusion. Very high doses may produce respiratory depression. One case of toxic psychosis (hyperactivity, marked visual and auditory hallucinations) after ingestion of a single dose of 20 tablets (300 mg) of dextromethorphan has been reported.
TREATMENT
Treatment of overdosage with Phenergan with dextromethorphan is essentially symptomatic and supportive. Only in cases of extreme overdosage or individual sensitivity do vital signs including respiration, pulse, blood pressure, temperature, and EKG need to be monitored. Activated charcoal orally or by lavage may be given, or sodium or magnesium sulfate orally as a cathartic. Attention should be given to the reestablishment of adequate respiratory exchange through provision of a patent airway and institution of assisted or controlled ventilation. Diazepam may be used to control convulsions. Acidosis and electrolyte losses should be corrected. The antidotal efficacy of narcotic antagonists to dextromethorphan has not been established; note that any of the depressant effects of promethazine are not reversed by naloxone. Avoid analeptics, which may cause convulsions.
Severe hypotension usually responds to the administration of norepinephrine or phenylephrine. EPINEPHRINE SHOULD NOT BE USED, since its use in a patient with partial adrenergic blockade may further lower the blood pressure.
Limited experience with dialysis indicates that it is not helpful.

DOSAGE AND ADMINISTRATION

The average effective dose for adults is one teaspoon (5 mL) every 4 to 6 hours, not to exceed 30.0 mL in 24 hours. For children 6 years to under 12 years of age, the dose is one-half to one teaspoon (2.5 to 5.0 mL) every 4 to 6 hours, not to exceed 20.0 mL in 24 hours. For children 2 years to under 6 years of age, the dose is one-quarter to one-half teaspoon (1.25 to 2.5 mL) every 4 to 6 hours, not to exceed 10.0 mL in 24 hours.
Phenergan with dextromethorphan is not recommended for children under 2 years of age.

HOW SUPPLIED

Phenergan® with dextromethorphan (Promethazine Hydrochloride and Dextromethorphan Hydrobromide) Syrup is a clear, yellow solution supplied as follows:
NDC 0008-0548-02, case of 24 bottles of 4 fl. oz. (118 mL).
NDC 0008-0548-03, bottle of 1 pint (473 mL).
Keep bottles tightly closed and store at room temperature between 15° and 25°C (59° and 77°F).
Protect from light.
Dispense in light-resistant, glass, tight containers.
Manufactured by:
Wyeth Laboratories
A Wyeth-Ayerst Company
Philadelphia, PA 19101
CI 4872-1 Issued September 6, 1996

PHENERGAN® VC ℞

[fĕn ′ĕr-găn]
(Promethazine Hydrochloride and Phenylephrine Hydrochloride) Syrup

DESCRIPTION

Each teaspoon (5 mL) of Phenergan VC contains 6.25 mg promethazine hydrochloride and 5 mg phenylephrine hydrochloride in a flavored syrup base with a pH between 4.7 and 5.2. Alcohol 7%. The inactive ingredients present are artificial and natural flavors, citric acid, FD&C Yellow 6, glycerin, saccharin sodium, sodium benzoate, sodium citrate, sodium propionate, water, and other ingredients.
Promethazine hydrochloride is a racemic compound; the empirical formula is $C_{17}H_{20}N_2S{\cdot}HCl$ and its molecular weight is 320.88.
Promethazine hydrochloride, a phenothiazine derivative, is designated chemically as 10*H*-Phenothiazine-10-ethanamine. *N,N*,α-trimethyl-, monohydrochloride, (±)- with the following structural formula:

[Structural formula: phenothiazine ring with N–CH₂CH(CH₃)N(CH₃)₂ · HCl]

Promethazine hydrochloride occurs as white to faint yellow, practically odorless, crystalline powder which slowly oxidizes and turns blue on prolonged exposure to air. It is soluble in water and freely soluble in alcohol.
Phenylephrine hydrochloride is a sympathomimetic amine salt. It may be chemically named as 3-hydroxy-α-[(methylamino)methyl]-benzenemethanol hydrochloride and has the following chemical formula:

[Structural formula: 3-hydroxyphenyl–C(OH)(H)–CH₂NHCH₃ · HCl]

Phenylephrine hydrochloride occurs as white or nearly white crystals, having a bitter taste. It is freely soluble in water and alcohol, with a molecular weight of 203.67. The empirical formula is $C_9H_{13}NO_2{\cdot}HCl$, and the stereochemistry is R-isomer as indicated in the structure; Specific Rotation—between −42° and −47.5°. Phenylephrine hydrochloride is subject to oxidation and must be protected from light and air.

CLINICAL PHARMACOLOGY

PROMETHAZINE
Promethazine is a phenothiazine derivative which differs structurally from the antipsychotic phenothiazines by the presence of a branched side chain and no ring substitution. It is thought that this configuration is responsible for its relative lack (1/10 that of chlorpromazine) of dopaminergic (CNS) action.
Promethazine is an H_1 receptor blocking agent. In addition to its antihistaminic action, it provides clinically useful sedative and antiemetic effects. In therapeutic dosages, promethazine produces no significant effects on the cardiovascular system.
Promethazine is well absorbed from the gastrointestinal tract. Clinical effects are apparent within 20 minutes after oral administration and generally last four to six hours, although they may persist as long as 12 hours. Promethazine is metabolized by the liver to a variety of compounds; the sulfoxides of promethazine and N-demethylpromethazine are the predominant metabolites appearing in the urine.
PHENYLEPHRINE
Phenylephrine is a potent postsynaptic α-receptor agonist with little effect on β receptors of the heart. Phenylephrine has no effect on β-adrenergic receptors of the bronchi or peripheral blood vessels. A direct action at receptors accounts for the greater part of its effects, only a small part being due to its ability to release norepinephrine.
Therapeutic doses of phenylephrine mainly cause vasoconstriction. Phenylephrine increases resistance and, to a lesser extent, decreases capacitance of blood vessels. Total peripheral resistance is increased, resulting in increased systolic and diastolic blood pressure. Pulmonary arterial pressure is usually increased, and renal blood flow is usually decreased. Local vasoconstriction and hemostasis occur following topical application or infiltration of phenylephrine into tissues.
The main effect of phenylephrine on the heart is bradycardia; it produces a positive inotropic effect on the myocardium in doses greater than those usually used therapeutically. Rarely, the drug may increase the irritability of the heart, causing arrhythmias. Cardiac output is decreased slightly. Phenylephrine increases the work of the heart by increasing peripheral arterial resistance.
Phenylephrine has a mild central stimulant effect.
Following oral administration or topical application of phenylephrine to the mucosa, constriction of blood vessels in the nasal mucosa relieves nasal congestion associated with allergy or head colds. Following oral administration, nasal decongestion may occur within 15 or 20 minutes and may persist for up to 4 hours.
Phenylephrine is irregularly absorbed from and readily metabolized in the gastrointestinal tract. Phenylephrine is metabolized in the liver and intestine by monoamine oxidase. The metabolites and their route and rate of excretion have not been identified. The pharmacologic action of phenylephrine is terminated at least partially by uptake of the drug into tissues.

INDICATIONS AND USAGE

Phenergan VC is indicated for the temporary relief of upper respiratory symptoms, including nasal congestion, associated with allergy or the common cold.

CONTRAINDICATIONS

Promethazine is contraindicated in individuals known to be hypersensitive or to have had an idiosyncratic reaction to promethazine or to other phenothiazines.
Antihistamines are contraindicated for use in the treatment of lower respiratory tract symptoms or asthma.
Phenylephrine is contraindicated in patients with hypertension or with peripheral vascular insufficiency (ischemia may result with risk of gangrene or thrombosis of compromised vascular beds). Phenylephrine should not be used in patients known to be hypersensitive to the drug or in those receiving a monoamine oxidase inhibitor (MAOI).

WARNINGS

PROMETHAZINE
Promethazine may cause marked drowsiness. Ambulatory patients should be cautioned against such activities as driving or operating dangerous machinery until it is known that they do not become drowsy or dizzy from promethazine therapy.
The sedative action of promethazine hydrochloride is additive to the sedative effects of central nervous system depressants; therefore, agents such as alcohol, narcotic analgesics, sedatives, hypnotics, and tranquilizers should either be eliminated or given in reduced dosage in the presence of promethazine hydrochloride. When given concomitantly with promethazine hydrochloride, the dose of barbiturates should be reduced by at least one-half, and the dose of analgesic depressants, such as morphine or meperidine, should be reduced by one-quarter to one-half.
Promethazine may lower seizure threshold. This should be taken into consideration when administering to persons with known seizure disorders or when giving in combination with narcotics or local anesthetics which may also affect seizure threshold.
Sedative drugs or CNS depressants should be avoided in patients with a history of sleep apnea.
Antihistamines should be used with caution in patients with narrow-angle glaucoma, stenosing peptic ulcer, pyloroduodenal obstruction, and urinary bladder obstruction due to symptomatic prostatic hypertrophy and narrowing of the bladder neck.
Administration of promethazine has been associated with reported cholestatic jaundice.
PHENYLEPHRINE
Because phenylephrine is an adrenergic agent, it should be given with caution to patients with thyroid diseases, diabetes mellitus, and heart diseases or those receiving tricyclic antidepressants.
Men with symptomatic, benign prostatic hypertrophy can experience urinary retention when given oral nasal decongestants.
Phenylephrine can cause a decrease in cardiac output, and extreme caution should be used when administering the drug, parenterally or orally, to patients with arteriosclerosis, to elderly individuals, and/or to patients with initially poor cerebral or coronary circulation.
Phenylephrine should be used with caution in patients taking diet preparations, such as amphetamines or phenylpropanolamine, because synergistic adrenergic effects could result in serious hypertensive response and possible stroke.

PRECAUTIONS

Animal reproduction studies have not been conducted with the drug combination—promethazine and phenylephrine. It

PHENERGAN VC

PHENYLEPHRINE

Drug	Effect
Phenylephrine with prior administration of monoamine oxidase inhibitors (MAOI).	Cardiac pressor response potentiated. May cause acute hypertensive crisis.
Phenylephrine with tricyclic antidepressants.	Pressor response increased.
Phenylephrine with ergot alkaloids.	Excessive rise in blood pressure.
Phenylephrine with bronchodilator sympathomimetic agents and with epinephrine or other sympathomimetics.	Tachycardia or other arrhythmias may occur.
Phenylephrine with prior administration of propranolol or other β-adrenergic blockers.	Cardiostimulating effects blocked.
Phenylephrine with atropine sulfate.	Reflex bradycardia blocked; pressor response enhanced.
Phenylephrine with prior administration of phentolamine or other α-adrenergic blockers.	Pressor response decreased.
Phenylephrine with diet preparations, such as amphetamines or phenylpropanolamine.	Synergistic adrenergic response.

Continued on next page

Phenergan VC—Cont.

is not known whether this drug combination can cause fetal harm when administered to a pregnant woman or can affect reproduction capacity. Phenergan VC should be given to a pregnant woman only if clearly needed.

GENERAL

Promethazine should be used cautiously in persons with cardiovascular disease or impairment of liver function.

Phenylephrine should be used with caution in patients with cardiovascular disease, particularly hypertension.

INFORMATION FOR PATIENTS

Phenergan VC may cause marked drowsiness or impair the mental and/or physical abilities required for the performance of potentially hazardous tasks, such as driving a vehicle or operating machinery. Ambulatory patients should be told to avoid engaging in such activities until it is known that they do not become drowsy or dizzy from Phenergan VC therapy. Children should be supervised to avoid potential harm in bike riding or other hazardous activities.

The concomitant use of alcohol or other central nervous system depressants, including narcotic analgesics, sedatives, hypnotics, and tranquilizers, may have an additive effect and should be avoided or their dosage reduced.

Patients should be advised to report any involuntary muscle movements or unusual sensitivity to sunlight.

DRUG INTERACTIONS

PROMETHAZINE

The sedative action of promethazine is additive to the sedative effects of other central nervous system depressants, including alcohol, narcotic analgesics, sedatives, hypnotics, tricyclic antidepressants, and tranquilizers; therefore, these agents should be avoided or administered in reduced dosage to patients receiving promethazine.

[See table at top of previous page]

DRUG/LABORATORY TEST INTERACTIONS

The following laboratory tests may be affected in patients who are receiving therapy with promethazine hydrochloride:

Pregnancy Tests

Diagnostic pregnancy tests based on immunological reactions between HCG and anti-HCG may result in false-negative or false-positive interpretations.

Glucose Tolerance Test

An increase in blood glucose has been reported in patients receiving promethazine.

CARCINOGENESIS, MUTAGENESIS, IMPAIRMENT OF FERTILITY

PROMETHAZINE

Long-term animal studies have not been performed to assess the carcinogenic potential of promethazine, nor are there other animal or human data concerning carcinogenicity, mutagenicity, or impairment of fertility with this drug. Promethazine was nonmutagenic in the *Salmonella* test system of Ames.

PHENYLEPHRINE

A study which followed the development of cancer in 143,574 patients over a four-year period indicated that in 11,981 patients who received phenylephrine (systemic or topical), there was no statistically significant association between the drug and cancer at any or all sites.

Long-term animal studies have not been performed to assess the carcinogenic potential of phenylephrine, nor are there other animal or human data concerning mutagenicity.

A study of the effects of adrenergic drugs on ovum transport in rabbits indicated that treatment with phenylephrine did not alter incidence of pregnancy; the number of implantations was significantly reduced when high doses of the drug were used.

PREGNANCY

Teratogenic Effects —Pregnancy Category C

PROMETHAZINE

Teratogenic effects have not been demonstrated in rat-feeding studies at doses of 6.25 and 12.5 mg/kg of promethazine. These doses are 8.3 and 16.7 times the maximum recommended total daily dose of promethazine for a 50-kg subject. Specific studies to test the action of the drug on parturition, lactation, and development of the animal neonate were not done, but a general preliminary study in rats indicated no effect on these parameters. Although antihistamines, including promethazine, have been found to produce fetal mortality in rodents, the pharmacological effects of histamine in the rodent do not parallel those in man. There are no adequate and well-controlled studies of promethazine in pregnant women.

PHENYLEPHRINE

A study in rabbits indicated that continued moderate overexposure to phenylephrine (3 mg/day) during the second half of pregnancy (22nd day of gestation to delivery) may contribute to perinatal wastage, prematurity, premature labor, and possibly fetal anomalies; when phenylephrine (3 mg/day) was given to rabbits during the first half of pregnancy (3rd day after mating for seven days), a significant number gave birth to litters of low birth weight. Another study showed that phenylephrine was associated with anomalies of aortic arch and with ventricular septal defect in the chick embryo.

Phenergan VC should be used during pregnancy only if the potential benefit justifies the potential risk to the fetus.

Nonteratogenic Effects

Promethazine taken within two weeks of delivery may inhibit platelet aggregation in the newborn.

LABOR AND DELIVERY

Administration of phenylephrine to patients in late pregnancy or labor may cause fetal anoxia or bradycardia by increasing contractility of the uterus and decreasing uterine blood flow.

See also "*Nonteratogenic Effects*."

NURSING MOTHERS

It is not known whether promethazine or phenylephrine is excreted in human milk.

Caution should be exercised when Phenergan VC is administered to a nursing woman.

PEDIATRIC USE

This product should not be used in children under 2 years of age because safety for such use has not been established.

ADVERSE REACTIONS

PROMETHAZINE

Nervous System —Sedation, sleepiness, occasional blurred vision, dryness of mouth, dizziness; rarely confusion, disorientation, and extrapyramidal symptoms such as oculogyric crisis, torticollis, and tongue protrusion (usually in association with parenteral injection or excessive dosage).

Cardiovascular —Increased or decreased blood pressure.

Dermatologic —Rash, rarely photosensitivity.

Hematologic —Rarely leukopenia, thrombocytopenia; agranulocytosis (1 case).

Gastrointestinal —Nausea and vomiting.

PHENYLEPHRINE

Nervous System —Restlessness, anxiety, nervousness, and dizziness.

Cardiovascular —Hypertension (see "**Warnings**").

Other —Precordial pain, respiratory distress, tremor, and weakness.

OVERDOSAGE

PROMETHAZINE

Signs and symptoms of overdosage with promethazine range from mild depression of the central nervous system and cardiovascular system to profound hypotension, respiratory depression, and unconsciousness.

Stimulation may be evident, especially in children and geriatric patients. Convulsions may rarely occur. A paradoxical reaction has been reported in children receiving single doses of 75 mg to 125 mg orally, characterized by hyperexcitability and nightmares.

Atropine-like signs and symptoms—dry mouth, fixed, dilated pupils, flushing, as well as gastrointestinal symptoms, may occur.

PHENYLEPHRINE

Signs and symptoms of overdosage with phenylephrine include hypertension, headache, convulsions, cerebral hemorrhage, and vomiting. Ventricular premature beats and short paroxysms of ventricular tachycardia may also occur. Headache may be a symptom of hypertension. Bradycardia may also be seen early in phenylephrine overdosage through stimulation of baroreceptors.

TREATMENT

Treatment of overdosage with Phenergan VC is essentially symptomatic and supportive. Only in cases of extreme overdosage or individual sensitivity do vital signs including respiration, pulse, blood pressure, temperature, and EKG need to be monitored. Activated charcoal orally or by lavage may be given, or sodium or magnesium sulfate orally as a cathartic. Attention should be given to the reestablishment of adequate respiratory exchange through provision of a patent airway and institution of assisted or controlled ventilation. Diazepam may be used to control convulsions. Acidosis and electrolyte losses should be corrected. Note that any depressant effects of promethazine are not reversed by naloxone. Avoid analeptics which may cause convulsions.

Severe hypotension usually responds to the administration of norepinephrine or phenylephrine. EPINEPHRINE SHOULD NOT BE USED, since its use in patients with partial adrenergic blockade may further lower the blood pressure.

Limited experience with dialysis indicates that it is not helpful.

DOSAGE AND ADMINISTRATION

The recommended adult dose is one teaspoon (5 mL) every 4 to 6 hours, not to exceed 30.0 mL in 24 hours. For children 6 years to under 12 years of age, the dose is one-half to one teaspoon (2.5 to 5.0 mL) repeated at 4- to 6-hour intervals, not to exceed 30.0 mL in 24 hours. For children 2 years to under 6 years of age, the dose is one-quarter to one-half teaspoon (1.25 to 2.5 mL) every 4 to 6 hours.

Phenergan VC is not recommended for children under 2 years of age.

HOW SUPPLIED

Phenergan® VC (Promethazine Hydrochloride and Phenylephrine Hydrochloride) Syrup, is a clear, orange-yellow solution supplied as follows:

NDC 0008-0551-02, case of 24 bottles of 4 fl. oz. (118 mL).

NDC 0008-0551-03, bottle of 1 pint (473 mL).

Keep bottles tightly closed and store at room temperature between 15° and 25°C (59° and 77°F).

Protect from light.

Dispense in light-resistant, glass, tight containers.

Manufactured by:
Wyeth Laboratories
A Wyeth-Ayerst Company
Philadelphia, PA 19101
CI 4869-1 Issued July 8, 1996

PHENERGAN® VC ℂ ℞

[fĕn 'ĕr-gan]

with codeine
(Promethazine Hydrochloride, Phenylephrine Hydrochloride, and Codeine Phosphate) Syrup

DESCRIPTION

Each teaspoon (5 mL) of Phenergan VC with codeine contains 10 mg codeine phosphate (Warning—may be habit-forming), 6.25 mg promethazine hydrochloride, and 5 mg phenylephrine hydrochloride in a flavored syrup base with a pH between 4.8 to 5.4. Alcohol 7%. The inactive ingredients present are artificial and natural flavors, citric acid, D&C Red 33, FD&C Yellow 6, glycerin, saccharin sodium, sodium benzoate, sodium citrate, sodium propionate, water, and other ingredients.

Codeine is one of the naturally occurring phenanthrene alkaloids of opium derived from the opium poppy; it is classified pharmacologically as a narcotic analgesic. Codeine phosphate may be chemically named as (5α,6α)–7,8–didehydro –4,5– epoxy –3– methoxy –17– methylmorphinan –6– ol phosphate (1:1) (salt) hemihydrate with the following structural formula:

$\cdot\ H_3PO_4 \cdot \frac{1}{2}H_2O$

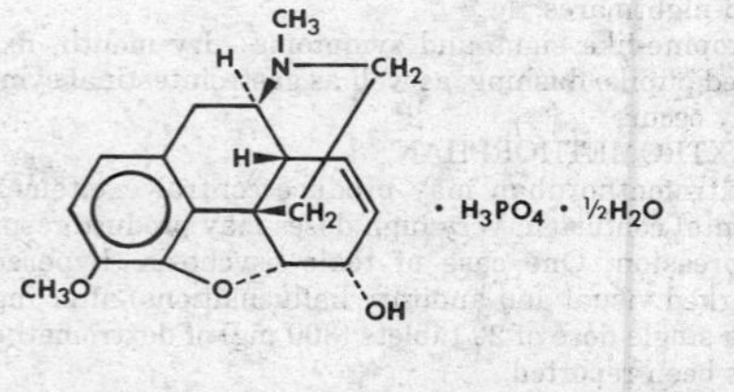

The phosphate salt of codeine occurs as white, needle-shaped crystals or white crystalline powder. Codeine phosphate is freely soluble in water and slightly soluble in alcohol, with a molecular weight of 406.37. The empirical formula is $C_{18}H_{21}NO_3 \cdot H_3PO_4 \cdot {}^1/_2H_2O$, and the stereochemistry is 5α, 6α isomer as indicated in the structure.

Promethazine hydrochloride is a racemic compound; the empirical formula is $C_{17}H_{20}N_2S \cdot HCl$ and its molecular weight is 320.88.

Promethazine hydrochloride, a phenothiazine derivative, is designated chemically as 10*H*-Phenothiazine-10-ethanamine, *N,N*,α-trimethyl-, monohydrochloride, (±)- with the following structural formula:

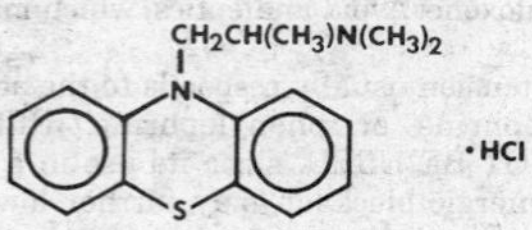

$CH_2CH(CH_3)N(CH_3)_2 \quad \cdot HCl$

Promethazine hydrochloride occurs as a white to faint yellow, practically odorless, crystalline powder which slowly oxidizes and turns blue on prolonged exposure to air. It is soluble in water and freely soluble in alcohol.

Phenylephrine hydrochloride is a sympathomimetic amine salt. It may be chemically named as 3-hydroxy-α-[(methylamino)methyl]-benzenemethanol hydrochloride and has the following chemical formula:

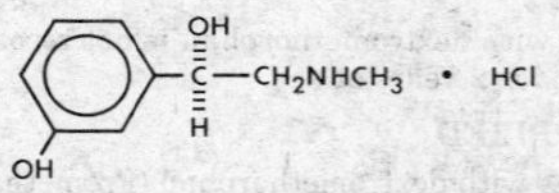

$-CH_2NHCH_3 \cdot HCl$

Phenylephrine hydrochloride occurs as white or nearly white crystals, having a bitter taste. It is freely soluble in water and alcohol, with a molecular weight of 203.67. The empirical formula is $C_9H_{13}NO_2 \cdot HCl$, and the stereochemistry is R-isomer as indicated in the structure; Specific Rotation—between −42° and −47.5°. Phenylephrine hydrochloride is subject to oxidation and must be protected from light and air.

CLINICAL PHARMACOLOGY

Codeine

Narcotic analgesics, including codeine, exert their primary effects on the central nervous system and gastrointestinal tract. The analgesic effects of codeine are due to its central action; however, the precise sites of action have not been determined, and the mechanisms involved appear to be quite complex. Codeine resembles morphine both structurally and pharmacologically, but its actions at the doses of codeine used therapeutically are milder, with less sedation, respiratory depression, and gastrointestinal, urinary, and pupillary effects. Codeine produces an increase in biliary tract pressure, but less than morphine or meperidine. Codeine is less constipating than morphine.

Codeine has good antitussive activity, although less than that of morphine at equal doses. It is used in preference to morphine, because side effects are infrequent at the usual antitussive dose of codeine.

Codeine in oral therapeutic dosage does not usually exert major effects on the cardiovascular system.
Narcotic analgesics may cause nausea and vomiting by stimulating the chemoreceptor trigger zone (CTZ); however, they also depress the vomiting center, so that subsequent doses are unlikely to produce vomiting. Nausea is minimal after usual oral doses of codeine.
Narcotic analgesics cause histamine release, which appears to be responsible for wheals or urticaria sometimes seen at the site of injection on parenteral administration. Histamine release may also produce dilation of cutaneous blood vessels, with resultant flushing of the face and neck, pruritus, and sweating.
Codeine and its salts are well absorbed following both oral and parenteral administration. Codeine is about $^2/_3$ as effective orally as parenterally. Codeine is metabolized primarily in the liver by enzymes of the endoplasmic reticulum, where it undergoes O-demethylation, N-demethylation, and partial conjugation with glucuronic acid. The drug is excreted primarily in the urine, largely as inactive metabolites and small amounts of free and conjugated morphine. Negligible amounts of codeine and its metabolites are found in the feces.
Following oral or subcutaneous administration of codeine, the onset of analgesia occurs within 15 to 30 minutes and lasts for four to six hours.
The cough-depressing action, in animal studies, was observed to occur 15 minutes after oral administration of codeine, peak action at 45 to 60 minutes after ingestion. The duration of action, which is dose-dependent, usually did not exceed 3 hours.

Promethazine

Promethazine is a phenothiazine derivative which differs structurally from the antipsychotic phenothiazines by the presence of a branched side chain and no ring substitution. It is thought that this configuration is responsible for its relative lack ($^1/_{10}$ that of chlorpromazine) of dopaminergic (CNS) action.
Promethazine is an H_1 receptor blocking agent. In addition to its antihistaminic action, it provides clinically useful sedative and antiemetic effects. In therapeutic dosages, promethazine produces no significant effects on the cardiovascular system.
Promethazine is well absorbed from the gastrointestinal tract. Clinical effects are apparent within 20 minutes after oral administration and generally last four to six hours, although they may persist as long as 12 hours. Promethazine is metabolized by the liver to a variety of compounds; the sulfoxides of promethazine and N-demethylpromethazine are the predominant metabolites appearing in the urine.

Phenylephrine

Phenylephrine is a potent postsynaptic α-receptor agonist with little effect on β receptors of the heart. Phenylephrine has no effect on β-adrenergic receptors of the bronchi or peripheral blood vessels. A direct action at receptors accounts for the greater part of its effects, only a small part being due to its ability to release norepinephrine.
Therapeutic doses of phenylephrine mainly cause vasoconstriction. Phenylephrine increases resistance and, to a lesser extent, decreases capacitance of blood vessels. Total peripheral resistance is increased, resulting in increased systolic and diastolic blood pressure. Pulmonary arterial pressure is usually increased, and renal blood flow is usually decreased. Local vasoconstriction and hemostasis occur following topical application or infiltration of phenylephrine into tissues.
The main effect of phenylephrine on the heart is bradycardia; it produces a positive inotropic effect on the myocardium in doses greater than those usually used therapeutically. Rarely, the drug may increase the irritability of the heart, causing arrhythmias. Cardiac output is decreased slightly. Phenylephrine increases the work of the heart by increasing peripheral arterial resistance.
Phenylephrine has a mild central stimulant effect.
Following oral administration or topical application of phenylephrine to the mucosa, constriction of blood vessels in the nasal mucosa relieves nasal congestion associated with allergy or head colds. Following oral administration, nasal decongestion may occur within 15 or 20 minutes and may persist for up to 4 hours.
Phenylephrine is irregularly absorbed from and readily metabolized in the gastrointestinal tract. Phenylephrine is metabolized in the liver and intestine by monoamine oxidase. The metabolites and their route and rate of excretion have not been identified. The pharmacologic action of phenylephrine is terminated at least partially by uptake of the drug into tissues.

INDICATIONS AND USAGE

Phenergan VC with codeine is indicated for the temporary relief of coughs and upper respiratory symptoms, including nasal congestion, associated with allergy or the common cold.

CONTRAINDICATIONS

Codeine is contraindicated in patients with a known hypersensitivity to the drug.
Promethazine is contraindicated in individuals known to be hypersensitive or to have had an idiosyncratic reaction to promethazine or to other phenothiazines.
Phenylephrine is contraindicated in patients with hypertension or with peripheral vascular insufficiency (ischemia may result with risk of gangrene or thrombosis of compromised

PHENERGAN VC WITH CODEINE
Phenylephrine

Drug	Effect
Phenylephrine with prior administration of monoamine oxidase inhibitors (MAOI).	Cardiac pressor response potentiated. May cause acute hypertensive crisis.
Phenylephrine with tricyclic antidepressants.	Pressor response increased.
Phenylephrine with ergot alkaloids.	Excessive rise in blood pressure.
Phenylephrine with bronchodilator sympathomimetic agents and with epinephrine or other sympathomimetics.	Tachycardia or other arrhythmias may occur.
Phenylephrine with prior administration of propranolol or other β-adrenergic blockers.	Cardiostimulating effects blocked.
Phenylephrine with atropine sulfate.	Reflex bradycardia blocked; pressor response enhanced.
Phenylephrine with prior administration of phentolamine or other α-adrenergic blockers.	Pressor response decreased.
Phenylephrine with diet preparations, such as amphetamines or phenylpropanolamine.	Synergistic adrenergic response.

vascular beds). Phenylephrine should not be used in patients known to be hypersensitive to the drug or in those receiving a monoamine oxidase inhibitor (MAOI).
Antihistamines and codeine are both contraindicated for use in the treatment of lower respiratory tract symptoms, including asthma.

WARNINGS

Codeine

Dosage of codeine SHOULD NOT BE INCREASED if cough fails to respond; an unresponsive cough should be reevaluated in 5 days or sooner for possible underlying pathology, such as foreign body or lower respiratory tract disease.
Codeine may cause or aggravate constipation.
Respiratory depression leading to arrest, coma, and death has occurred with the use of codeine antitussives in young children, particularly in the under-one-year infants whose ability to deactivate the drug is not fully developed.
Administration of codeine may be accompanied by histamine release and should be used with caution in atopic children.

Head Injury and Increased Intracranial Pressure

The respiratory-depressant effects of narcotic analgesics and their capacity to elevate cerebrospinal fluid pressure may be markedly exaggerated in the presence of head injury, intracranial lesions, or a preexisting increase in intracranial pressure. Narcotics may produce adverse reactions which may obscure the clinical course of patients with head injuries.

Asthma and Other Respiratory Conditions

Narcotic analgesics or cough suppressants, including codeine, should not be used in asthmatic patients (see "**CONTRAINDICATIONS**"). Nor should they be used in acute febrile illness associated with productive cough or in chronic respiratory disease where interference with ability to clear the tracheobronchial tree of secretions would have a deleterious effect on the patient's respiratory function.

Hypotensive Effect

Codeine may produce orthostatic hypotension in ambulatory patients.

Promethazine

Promethazine may cause marked drowsiness. Ambulatory patients should be cautioned against such activities as driving or operating dangerous machinery until it is known that they do not become drowsy or dizzy from promethazine therapy.
The sedative action of promethazine hydrochloride is additive to the sedative effects of central nervous system depressants; therefore, agents such as alcohol, narcotic analgesics, sedatives, hypnotics, and tranquilizers should either be eliminated or given in reduced dosage in the presence of promethazine hydrochloride. When given concomitantly with promethazine hydrochloride, the dose of barbiturates should be reduced by at least one-half, and the dose of analgesic depressants, such as morphine or meperidine, should be reduced by one-quarter to one-half.
Promethazine may lower seizure threshold. This should be taken into consideration when administering to persons with known seizure disorders or when giving in combination with narcotics or local anesthetics which may also affect seizure threshold.
Sedative drugs or CNS depressants should be avoided in patients with a history of sleep apnea. Antihistamines should be used with caution in patients with narrow-angle glaucoma, stenosing peptic ulcer, pyloroduodenal obstruction, and urinary bladder obstruction due to symptomatic prostatic hypertrophy and narrowing of the bladder neck.
Administration of promethazine has been associated with reported cholestatic jaundice.

Phenylephrine

Because phenylephrine is an adrenergic agent, it should be given with caution to patients with thyroid diseases, diabetes mellitus, and heart diseases or those receiving tricyclic antidepressants.
Men with symptomatic, benign prostatic hypertrophy can experience urinary retention when given oral nasal decongestants.
Phenylephrine can cause a decrease in cardiac output, and extreme caution should be used when administering the drug, parenterally or orally, to patients with arteriosclerosis, to elderly individuals, and/or to patients with initially poor cerebral or coronary circulation.
Phenylephrine should be used with caution in patients taking diet preparations, such as amphetamines or phenylpropanolamine, because synergistic adrenergic effects could result in serious hypertensive response and possible stroke.

PRECAUTIONS

Animal reproduction studies have not been conducted with the drug combination—promethazine, phenylephrine, and codeine. It is not known whether this drug combination can cause fetal harm when administered to a pregnant woman or can affect reproduction capacity. Phenergan VC with codeine should be given to a pregnant woman only if clearly needed.

General

Narcotic analgesics, including codeine, should be administered with caution and the initial dose reduced in patients with acute abdominal conditions, convulsive disorders, significant hepatic or renal impairment, fever, hypothyroidism, Addison's disease, ulcerative colitis, prostatic hypertrophy, in patients with recent gastrointestinal or urinary tract surgery, and in the very young or elderly or debilitated patients.
Promethazine should be used cautiously in persons with cardiovascular disease or with impairment of liver function.
Phenylephrine should be used with caution in patients with cardiovascular disease, particularly hypertension.

Information for Patients

Phenergan VC with codeine may cause marked drowsiness or impair the mental and/or physical abilities required for the performance of potentially hazardous tasks, such as driving a vehicle or operating machinery. Ambulatory patients should be told to avoid engaging in such activities until it is known that they do not become drowsy or dizzy from Phenergan VC with codeine therapy. Children should be supervised to avoid potential harm in bike riding or in other hazardous activities.
The concomitant use of alcohol or other central nervous system depressants, including narcotic analgesics, sedatives, hypnotics, and tranquilizers, may have an additive effect and should be avoided or their dosage reduced.
Patients should be advised to report any involuntary muscle movements or unusual sensitivity to sunlight.
Codeine, like other narcotic analgesics, may produce orthostatic hypotension in some ambulatory patients. Patients should be cautioned accordingly.

Drug Interactions

Codeine

In patients receiving MAO inhibitors, an initial small test dose is advisable to allow observation of any excessive narcotic effects or MAOI interaction.

Promethazine

The sedative action of promethazine is additive to the effects of other central nervous system depressants, including alcohol, narcotic analgesics, sedatives, hypnotics, tricyclic antidepressants, and tranquilizers; therefore, these agents should be avoided or administered in reduced dosage to patients receiving promethazine.
[See table above]

Drug/Laboratory Test Interactions

Because narcotic analgesics may increase biliary tract pressure, with resultant increases in plasma amylase or lipase levels, determination of these enzyme levels may be unreliable for 24 hours after a narcotic analgesic has been given.
The following laboratory tests may be affected in patients who are receiving therapy with promethazine hydrochloride:

Pregnancy Tests

Diagnostic pregnancy tests based on immunological reactions between HCG and anti-HCG may result in false-negative or false-positive interpretations.

Glucose Tolerance Test

An increase in blood glucose has been reported in patients receiving promethazine.

Carcinogenesis, Mutagenesis, Impairment of Fertility

Codeine and Promethazine

Long-term animal studies have not been performed to assess the carcinogenic potential of codeine or of promethazine, nor are there other animal or human data concerning carcinogenicity, mutagenicity, or impairment of fertility with these agents. Codeine has been reported to show no evidence of carcinogenicity or mutagenicity in a variety of test systems, including the micronucleus and sperm abnormality assays and the *Salmonella* assay. Promethazine was nonmutagenic in the *Salmonella* test system of Ames.

Phenylephrine

A study which followed the development of cancer in 143,574 patients over a four-year period indicated that in

Continued on next page

Phenergan VC w/Codeine—Cont.

11,981 patients who received phenylephrine (systemic or topical), there was no statistically significant association between the drug and cancer at any or all sites.
Long-term animal studies have not been performed to assess the carcinogenic potential of phenylephrine, nor are there other animal or human data concerning mutagenicity.
A study of the effects of adrenergic drugs on ovum transport in rabbits indicated that treatment with phenylephrine did not alter incidence of pregnancy; the number of implantations was significantly reduced when high doses of the drug were used.

Pregnancy

Teratogenic Effects —Pregnancy Category C

Codeine

A study in rats and rabbits reported no teratogenic effect of codeine administered during the period of organogenesis in doses ranging from 5 to 120 mg/kg. In the rat, doses at the 120-mg/kg level, in the toxic range for the adult animal, were associated with an increase in embryo resorption at the time of implantation. In another study a single 100-mg/kg dose of codeine administered to pregnant mice reportedly resulted in delayed ossification in the offspring.
There are no studies in humans, and the significance of these findings to humans, if any, is not known.

Promethazine

Teratogenic effects have not been demonstrated in rat-feeding studies at doses of 6.25 and 12.5 mg/kg of promethazine. These doses are 8.3 and 16.7 times the maximum recommended total daily dose for a 50-kg subject. Specific studies to test the action of the drug on parturition, lactation, and development of the animal neonate were not done, but a general preliminary study in rats indicated no effect on these parameters. Although antihistamines, including promethazine, have been found to produce fetal mortality in rodents, the pharmacological effects of histamine in the rodent do not parallel those in man. There are no adequate and well-controlled studies of promethazine in pregnant women.

Phenylephrine

A study in rabbits indicated that continued moderate overexposure to phenylephrine (3 mg/day) during the second half of pregnancy (22nd day of gestation to delivery) may contribute to perinatal wastage, prematurity, premature labor, and possibly fetal anomalies; when phenylephrine (3 mg/day) was given to rabbits during the first half of pregnancy (3rd day after mating for seven days), a significant number gave birth to litters of low birth weight. Another study showed that phenylephrine was associated with anomalies of aortic arch and with ventricular septal defect in the chick embryo.
Phenergan® VC with codeine should be used during pregnancy only if the potential benefit justifies the potential risk to the fetus.

Nonteratogenic Effects

Dependence has been reported in newborns whose mothers took opiates regularly during pregnancy. Withdrawal signs include irritability, excessive crying, tremors, hyperreflexia, fever, vomiting, and diarrhea. Signs usually appear during the first few days of life.
Promethazine taken within two weeks of delivery may inhibit platelet aggregation in the newborn.

Labor And Delivery

Narcotic analgesics cross the placental barrier. The closer to delivery and the larger the dose used, the greater the possibility of respiratory depression in the newborn. Narcotic analgesics should be avoided during labor if delivery of a premature infant is anticipated. If the mother has received narcotic analgesics during labor, newborn infants should be observed closely for signs of respiratory depression. Resuscitation may be required (see "**OVERDOSAGE**"). The effect of codeine, if any, on the later growth, development, and functional maturation of the child is unknown.
Administration of phenylephrine to patients in late pregnancy or labor may cause fetal anoxia or bradycardia by increasing contractility of the uterus and decreasing uterine blood flow.
See also "*Nonteratogenic Effects*."

Nursing Mothers

Some studies, but not others, have reported detectable amounts of codeine in breast milk. The levels are probably not clinically significant after usual therapeutic dosage. The possibility of clinically important amounts being excreted in breast milk in individuals abusing codeine should be considered.
It is not known whether either phenylephrine or promethazine is excreted in human milk.
Caution should be exercised when Phenergan VC with codeine is administered to a nursing woman.

Pediatric Use

This product should not be used in children under 2 years of age because safety for such use has not been established.

ADVERSE REACTIONS

Codeine

Nervous System —CNS depression, particularly respiratory depression, and to a lesser extent circulatory depression; light-headedness, dizziness, sedation, euphoria, dysphoria, headache, transient hallucination, disorientation, visual disturbances, and convulsions.
Cardiovascular —Tachycardia, bradycardia, palpitation, faintness, syncope, orthostatic hypotension (common to narcotic analgesics).
Gastrointestinal —Nausea, vomiting, constipation, and biliary tract spasm. Patients with chronic ulcerative colitis may experience increased colonic motility; in patients with acute ulcerative colitis, toxic dilation has been reported.
Genitourinary —Oliguria, urinary retention; antidiuretic effect has been reported (common to narcotic analgesics).
Allergic —Infrequent pruritus, giant urticaria, angioneurotic edema, and laryngeal edema.
Other —Flushing of the face, sweating and pruritus (due to opiate-induced histamine release); weakness.

Promethazine

Nervous System —Sedation, sleepiness, occasional blurred vision, dryness of mouth, dizziness; rarely confusion, disorientation, and extrapyramidal symptoms such as oculogyric crisis, torticollis, and tongue protrusion (usually in association with parenteral injection or excessive dosage).
Cardiovascular —Increased or decreased blood pressure.
Dermatologic —Rash, rarely photosensitivity.
Hematologic —Rarely leukopenia, thrombocytopenia; agranulocytosis (1 case).
Gastrointestinal —Nausea and vomiting.

Phenylephrine

Nervous System —Restlessness, anxiety, nervousness, and dizziness.
Cardiovascular —Hypertension (see "**WARNINGS**").
Other —Precordial pain, respiratory distress, tremor, and weakness.

DRUG ABUSE AND DEPENDENCE

Controlled Substance

Phenergan VC with codeine is a Schedule V Controlled Substance.

Abuse

Codeine is known to be subject to abuse; however, the abuse potential of oral codeine appears to be quite low. Even parenteral codeine does not appear to offer the psychic effects sought by addicts to the same degree as heroin or morphine. However, codeine must be administered only under close supervision to patients with a history of drug abuse or dependence.

Dependence

Psychological dependence, physical dependence, and tolerance are known to occur with codeine.

OVERDOSAGE

Codeine

Serious overdose with codeine is characterized by respiratory depression (a decrease in respiratory rate and/or tidal volume, Cheyne-Stokes respiration, cyanosis), extreme somnolence progressing to stupor or coma, skeletal muscle flaccidity, cold and clammy skin, and sometimes bradycardia and hypotension. The triad of coma, pinpoint pupils, and respiratory depression is strongly suggestive of opiate poisoning. In severe overdosage, particularly by the intravenous route, apnea, circulatory collapse, cardiac arrest, and death may occur. Promethazine is additive to the depressant effects of codeine.
It is difficult to determine what constitutes a standard toxic or lethal dose. However, the lethal oral dose of codeine in an adult is reported to be in the range of 0.5 to 1.0 gram. Infants and children are believed to be relatively more sensitive to opiates on a body-weight basis. Elderly patients are also comparatively intolerant to opiates.

Promethazine

Signs and symptoms of overdosage with promethazine range from mild depression of the central nervous system and cardiovascular system to profound hypotension, respiratory depression, and unconsciousness.
Stimulation may be evident, especially in children and geriatric patients. Convulsions may rarely occur. A paradoxical reaction has been reported in children receiving single doses of 75 mg to 125 mg orally, characterized by hyperexcitability and nightmares.
Atropine-like signs and symptoms—dry mouth, fixed, dilated pupils, flushing, as well as gastrointestinal symptoms, may occur.

Phenylephrine

Signs and symptoms of overdosage with phenylephrine include hypertension, headache, convulsions, cerebral hemorrhage, and vomiting. Ventricular premature beats and short paroxysms of ventricular tachycardia may also occur. Headache may be a symptom of hypertension. Bradycardia may also be seen early in phenylephrine overdosage through stimulation of baroreceptors.

Treatment

Treatment of overdosage with Phenergan VC with codeine is essentially symptomatic and supportive. Only in cases of extreme overdosage or individual sensitivity do vital signs including respiration, pulse, blood pressure, temperature, and EKG need to be monitored. Activated charcoal orally or by lavage may be given, or sodium or magnesium sulfate orally as a cathartic. Attention should be given to the reestablishment of adequate respiratory exchange through provision of a patent airway and institution of assisted or controlled ventilation. The narcotic antagonist, naloxone hydrochloride, may be administered when significant respiratory depression occurs with Phenergan VC with codeine; any depressant effects of promethazine are not reversed by naloxone. Diazepam may be used to control convulsions. Avoid analeptics, which may cause convulsions. Acidosis and electrolyte losses should be corrected. A rise in temperature or pulmonary complications may signal the need for institution of antibiotic therapy.
Severe hypotension usually responds to the administration of norepinephrine or phenylephrine. EPINEPHRINE SHOULD NOT BE USED, since its use in a patient with partial adrenergic blockade may further lower the blood pressure.
Limited experience with dialysis indicates that it is not helpful.

DOSAGE AND ADMINISTRATION

The average effective dose is given in the following table:
[See table below]

PHENERGAN VC WITH CODEINE

Adults	1 teaspoon (5 mL) every 4 to 6 hours, not to exceed 30.0 mL in 24 hours.
Children 6 years to under 12 years	1/2 to 1 teaspoon (2.5 to 5 mL) every 4 to 6 hours, not to exceed 30.0 mL in 24 hours.
Children under 6 years (weight: 18 kg or 40 lbs)	1/4 to 1/2 teaspoon (1.25 to 2.5 mL) every 4 to 6 hours, not to exceed 9.0 mL in 24 hours.
Children under 6 years (weight: 16 kg or 35 lbs)	1/4 to 1/2 teaspoon (1.25 to 2.5 mL) every 4 to 6 hours, not to exceed 8.0 mL in 24 hours.
Children under 6 years (weight: 14 kg or 30 lbs)	1/4 to 1/2 teaspoon (1.25 to 2.5 mL) every 4 to 6 hours, not to exceed 7.0 mL in 24 hours.
Children under 6 years (weight: 12 kg or 25 lbs)	1/4 to 1/2 teaspoon (1.25 to 2.5 mL) every 4 to 6 hours, not to exceed 6.0 mL in 24 hours.

Phenergan VC with codeine is not recommended for children under 2 years of age.

HOW SUPPLIED

Phenergan® VC with codeine is a clear, reddish-orange solution supplied as follows:
NDC 0008-0552-02, case of 24 bottles of 4 fl. oz. (118 mL).
NDC 0008-0552-03, bottle of 1 pint (473 mL).

Keep tightly closed—Stored at room temperature, between 15° C and 25° C (59° F and 77° F).

Protect from light.

Dispense in light-resistant, glass, tight container.

Manufactured by:
Wyeth Laboratories
A Wyeth-Ayerst Company
Philadelphia, PA 19101
CI 4870-2 Revised July 22, 1998

PREMARIN® INTRAVENOUS ℞

[prĕm 'a-rĭn]

(conjugated estrogens, USP)

for Injection

Specially prepared for Intravenous & Intramuscular use

Rx only

1. ESTROGENS HAVE BEEN REPORTED TO INCREASE THE RISK OF ENDOMETRIAL CARCINOMA.

Three independent, case-controlled studies have reported an increased risk of endometrial cancer in postmenopausal women exposed to exogenous estrogens for more than one year.[1–3] This risk was independent of the other known risk factors for endometrial cancer. These studies are further supported by the finding that incidence rates of endometrial cancer have increased sharply since 1969 in eight different areas of the United States with population-based cancer-reporting systems, an increase which may be related to the rapidly expanding use of estrogens during the last decade.[4]
The three case-controlled studies reported that the risk of endometrial cancer in estrogen users was about 4.5 to 13.9 times greater than in nonusers. The risk appears to depend on both duration of treatment[1] and on estrogen dose.[3] In view of these findings, when estrogens are used for the treatment of menopausal symptoms, the lowest dose that will control symptoms should be utilized and medication should be discontinued as soon as possible. When prolonged treatment is medically indicated, the patient should be reassessed, on at least a semiannual basis, to determine the need for continued therapy. Although the evidence must be considered preliminary, one study suggests that cyclic administration of low doses of estrogen may carry less risk than continuous administration.[3] It therefore appears prudent to utilize such a regimen.
Close clinical surveillance of all women taking estrogens is important. In all cases of undiagnosed persistent or recurring abnormal vaginal bleeding, adequate diagnos-

tic measures should be undertaken to rule out malignancy.
There is no evidence at present that "natural" estrogens are more or less hazardous than "synthetic" estrogens at equiestrogenic doses.
2. ESTROGENS SHOULD NOT BE USED DURING PREGNANCY.
The use of female sex hormones, both estrogens and progestogens, during early pregnancy may seriously damage the offspring. It has been shown that females exposed *in utero* to diethylstilbestrol, a nonsteroidal estrogen, have an increased risk of developing, in later life, a form of vaginal or cervical cancer that is ordinarily extremely rare.[5,6] This risk has been estimated as not greater than 4 per 1,000 exposures.[7] Furthermore, a high percentage of such exposed women (from 30% to 90%) have been found to have vaginal adenosis,[8–12] epithelial changes of the vagina and cervix. Although these changes are histologically benign, it is not known whether they are precursors of malignancy. Although similar data are not available with the use of other estrogens, it cannot be presumed they would not induce similar changes.
Several reports suggest an association between intrauterine exposure to female sex hormones and congenital anomalies, including congenital heart defects and limb-reduction defects.[13–16] One case-controlled study[16] estimated a 4.7-fold increased risk of limb-reduction defects in infants exposed *in utero* to sex hormones (oral contraceptives, hormone withdrawal tests for pregnancy, or attempted treatment for threatened abortion). Some of these exposures were very short and involved only a few days of treatment. The data suggest that the risk of limb-reduction defects in exposed fetuses is somewhat less than 1 per 1,000.
In the past, female sex hormones have been used during pregnancy in an attempt to treat threatened or habitual abortion. There is considerable evidence that estrogens are ineffective for these indications, and there is no evidence from well-controlled studies that progestogens are effective for these uses.
If Premarin Intravenous (conjugated estrogens, USP) for injection is used during pregnancy, or if the patient becomes pregnant while taking this drug, she should be apprised of the potential risks to the fetus, and the advisability of pregnancy continuation.

DESCRIPTION

Each Secule® vial contains 25 mg of conjugated estrogens, USP, in a sterile lyophilized cake which also contains lactose 200 mg, sodium citrate 12.2 mg, and simethicone 0.2 mg. The pH is adjusted with sodium hydroxide or hydrochloric acid. A sterile diluent (5 mL) containing 2% benzyl alcohol in sterile water is provided for reconstitution. The reconstituted solution is suitable for intravenous or intramuscular injection.
Premarin (conjugated estrogens, USP) is a mixture of estrogens, obtained exclusively from natural sources, occurring as the sodium salts of water-soluble estrogen sulfates blended to represent the average composition of material derived from pregnant mares' urine. It contains estrone, equilin, and 17 α-dihydroequilin, together with smaller amounts of 17 α-estradiol, equilenin, and 17 α-dihydroequilenin as salts of their sulfate esters.

CLINICAL PHARMACOLOGY

Estrogens are important in the development and maintenance of the female reproductive system and secondary sex characteristics. They promote growth and development of the vagina, uterus, and fallopian tubes, and enlargement of the breasts. Indirectly, they contribute to the shaping of the skeleton, maintenance of tone and elasticity of urogenital structures, changes in the epiphyses of the long bones that allow for the pubertal growth spurt and its termination, growth of axillary and pubic hair, and pigmentation of the nipples and genitals. Decline of estrogenic activity at the end of the menstrual cycle can bring on menstruation, although the cessation of progesterone secretion is the most important factor in the mature ovulatory cycle. However, in the preovulatory or nonovulatory cycle, estrogen is the primary determinant in the onset of menstruation. Estrogens also affect the release of pituitary gonadotropins.
The pharmacologic effects of conjugated estrogens are similar to those of endogenous estrogens. They are soluble in water and may be administered by intravenous or intramuscular injection.
In responsive tissues (female genital organs, breasts, hypothalamus, pituitary) estrogens enter the cell and are transported into the nucleus. As a result of estrogen action, specific RNA and protein synthesis occurs.
Metabolism and inactivation occur primarily in the liver. Some estrogens are excreted into the bile; however, they are reabsorbed from the intestine and returned to the liver through the portal venous system. Water-soluble estrogen conjugates are strongly acidic and, therefore, ionized in body fluids, which favor excretion through the kidneys since tubular reabsorption is minimal.

INDICATION

Premarin Intravenous (conjugated estrogens, USP) for injection is indicated in the treatment of abnormal uterine bleeding due to hormonal imbalance in the absence of organic pathology.

CONTRAINDICATIONS

Estrogens should not be used in women with any of the following conditions:
1. Known or suspected cancer of the breast, except in appropriately selected patients being treated for metastatic disease.
2. Known or suspected estrogen-dependent neoplasia.
3. Known or suspected pregnancy (see Boxed Warning).
4. Undiagnosed abnormal genital bleeding.
5. Active thrombophlebitis or thromboembolic disorders.
6. A past history of thrombophlebitis, thrombosis, or thromboembolic disorders associated with previous estrogen use (except when used in treatment of breast malignancy).

WARNINGS

1. *Induction of malignant neoplasms.* Long-term, continuous administration of natural and synthetic estrogens in certain animal species increases the frequency of carcinomas of the breast, cervix, vagina, and liver. There are now reports that estrogens increase the risk of carcinoma of the endometrium in humans (see Boxed Warning).
At the present time there is no satisfactory evidence that estrogens given to postmenopausal women increase the risk of cancer of the breast,[17] although a recent long-term follow-up of a single physician's practice has raised this possibility.[18] Because of the animal data, there is a need for caution in prescribing estrogens for women with a strong family history of breast cancer, or who have breast nodules, fibrocystic disease, or abnormal mammograms.
2. *Gallbladder disease.* A recent study has reported a 2- to 3-fold increase in the risk of surgically confirmed gallbladder disease in women receiving postmenopausal estrogens,[17] similar to the 2-fold increase previously noted in users of oral contraceptives.[19,24a]
3. *Effects similar to those caused by estrogen-progestogen oral contraceptives.* There are several serious adverse effects of oral contraceptives, some of which have not, up to now, been documented as consequences of postmenopausal estrogen therapy. This may reflect the comparatively low doses of estrogen used in postmenopausal women. It would be expected that the larger doses of estrogen used to treat prostatic or breast cancer are more likely to result in these adverse effects, and, in fact, it has been shown that there is an increased risk of thrombosis in men receiving estrogens for prostatic cancer.[20–23]
a. *Thromboembolic disease.* It is now well established that users of oral contraceptives have an increased risk of various thromboembolic and thrombotic vascular diseases, such as thrombophlebitis, pulmonary embolism, stroke, and myocardial infarction.[24–31] Cases of retinal thrombosis, mesenteric thrombosis, and optic neuritis have been reported in oral-contraceptive users. There is evidence that the risk of several of these adverse reactions is related to the dose of the drug.[32,33] An increased risk of postsurgery thromboembolic complications has also been reported in users of oral contraceptives.[34,35] If feasible, estrogen should be discontinued at least 4 weeks before surgery of the type associated with an increased risk of thromboembolism, or during periods of prolonged immobilization.
In some studies, women on estrogen replacement therapy, given alone or in combination with a progestin, have been reported to have an increased risk of thrombophlebitis, and/or thromboembolic disease. The physician should be aware of the possibility of thrombotic disorders (thrombophlebitis, retinal thrombosis, cerebral embolism, and pulmonary embolism) during estrogen replacement therapy and be alert to their earliest manifestations. Should any of these occur or be suspected, estrogen replacement therapy should be discontinued immediately. Patients who have risk factors for thrombotic disorders should be kept under careful observation. Subgroups of women who have underlying risk factors, or who are receiving relatively large doses of estrogens, may have increased risk. Therefore, estrogens should not be used in persons with active thrombophlebitis or thromboembolic disorders, and they should not be used (except in treatment of malignancy) in persons with a history of such disorders in association with estrogen use. They should be used with caution in patients with cerebral vascular or coronary artery disease and only for those in whom estrogens are clearly needed.
Large doses of estrogen (5 mg conjugated estrogens per day), comparable to those used to treat cancer of the prostate and breast, have been shown in a large prospective clinical trial in men[36] to increase the risk of nonfatal myocardial infarction, pulmonary embolism, and thrombophlebitis. When estrogen doses of this size are used, any of the thromboembolic and thrombotic adverse effects associated with oral contraceptives or estrogen replacement therapy should be considered a clear risk.
b. *Hepatic adenoma.* Benign hepatic adenomas appear to be associated with the use of oral contraceptives.[37–39] Although benign, and rare, these may rupture and may cause death through intra-abdominal hemorrhage. Such lesions have not yet been reported in association with other estrogen or progestogen preparations but should be considered in estrogen users having abdominal pain and tenderness, abdominal mass, or hypovolemic shock. Hepatocellular carcinoma has also been reported in women taking estrogen-containing oral contraceptives.[38] The relationship of this malignancy to these drugs is not known at this time.
c. *Elevated blood pressure.* Women using oral contraceptives sometimes experience increased blood pressure which, in most cases, returns to normal on discontinuing the drug. There is now a report that this may occur with use of estrogens in the menopause[40] and blood pressure should be monitored with estrogen use, especially if high doses are used.
d. *Glucose tolerance.* A worsening of glucose tolerance has been observed in a significant percentage of patients on estrogen-containing oral contraceptives. For this reason, diabetic patients should be carefully observed while receiving estrogen.
4. *Hypercalcemia.* Administration of estrogens may lead to severe hypercalcemia in patients with breast cancer and bone metastases. If this occurs, the drug should be stopped and appropriate measures taken to reduce the serum calcium level.

PRECAUTIONS

A. General Precautions

1. A complete medical and family history should be taken prior to the initiation of any estrogen therapy. The pretreatment and periodic physical examinations should include special reference to blood pressure, breasts, abdomen, and pelvic organs, and should include a Papanicolaou smear. As a general rule, estrogen should not be prescribed for longer than one year without another physical examination being performed.
2. Fluid retention—Because estrogens may cause some degree of fluid retention, conditions which might be influenced by this factor such as asthma, epilepsy, migraine, and cardiac or renal dysfunction, require careful observation.
3. Certain patients may develop undesirable manifestations of excessive estrogenic stimulation, such as abnormal or excessive uterine bleeding, mastodynia, etc.
4. Oral contraceptives appear to be associated with an increased incidence of mental depression.[24a] Although it is not clear whether this is due to the estrogenic or progestogenic component of the contraceptive, patients with a history of depression should be carefully observed.
5. Preexisting uterine leiomyomata may increase in size during estrogen use.
6. The pathologist should be advised of estrogen therapy when relevant specimens are submitted.
7. Patients with a past history of jaundice during pregnancy have an increased risk of recurrence of jaundice while receiving estrogen-containing oral-contraceptive therapy. If jaundice develops in any patient receiving estrogen, the medication should be discontinued while the cause is investigated.
8. Estrogens may be poorly metabolized in patients with impaired liver function and they should be administered with caution in such patients.
9. Because estrogens influence the metabolism of calcium and phosphorus, they should be used with caution in patients with metabolic bone diseases that are associated with hypercalcemia or in patients with renal insufficiency.
10. Because of the effects of estrogens on epiphyseal closure, they should be used judiciously in young patients in whom bone growth is not yet complete.
11. Certain endocrine and liver function tests may be affected by estrogen-containing oral contraceptives. The following similar changes may be expected with larger doses of estrogen:
a. Increased sulfobromophthalein retention.
b. Increased prothrombin and factors VII, VIII, IX, and X; decreased antithrombin 3; increased norepinephrine-induced platelet aggregability.
c. Increased thyroid binding globulin (TBG) leading to increased circulating total thyroid hormone, as measured by PBI, T4 by column, or T4 by radioimmunoassay. Free T3 resin uptake is decreased, reflecting the elevated TBG; free T4 concentration is unaltered.
d. Impaired glucose tolerance.
e. Decreased pregnanediol excretion.
f. Reduced response to metyrapone test.
g. Reduced serum folate concentration.
h. Increased serum triglyceride and phospholipid concentration.
12. Familial hyperlipoproteinemia. Estrogen therapy may be associated with massive elevations of plasma triglycerides leading to pancreatitis and other complications in patients with familial defects of lipoprotein metabolism.

B. Information for the Patient

See text which appears after the "PHYSICIAN REFERENCES."

C. Pregnancy Category X

See **"CONTRAINDICATIONS"** and Boxed Warning.

D. Nursing Mothers

As a general principle, the administration of any drug to nursing mothers should be done only when clearly necessary, since many drugs are excreted in human milk.

ADVERSE REACTIONS

(See **"WARNINGS"** regarding induction of neoplasia, adverse effects on the fetus, increased incidence of gallbladder disease, and adverse effects similar to those of oral contraceptives, including thromboembolism.) The following additional adverse reactions have been reported with estrogenic therapy, including oral contraceptives:
1. *Genitourinary system:* Breakthrough bleeding, spotting, change in menstrual flow; dysmenorrhea; premenstrual-like syndrome; amenorrhea during and after treatment; increase in size of uterine fibromyomata; vaginal candidiasis; change in cervical erosion and in degree of cervical secretion; cystitis-like syndrome.
2. *Breasts:* Tenderness, enlargement, secretion.
3. *Gastrointestinal:* Nausea, vomiting; abdominal cramps, bloating; cholestatic jaundice; pancreatitis.
4. *Skin:* Chloasma or melasma which may persist when drug is discontinued; erythema multiforme; erythema nodosum; hemorrhagic eruption; loss of scalp hair; hirsutism.

Continued on next page

Premarin Intravenous—Cont.

5. *Cardiovascular:* Venous thromboembolism; pulmonary embolism.
6. *Eyes:* Steepening of corneal curvature; intolerance to contact lenses.
7. *CNS:* Headache, migraine, dizziness; mental depression; chorea.
8. *Miscellaneous:* Increase or decrease in weight; reduced carbohydrate tolerance; aggravation of porphyria; edema; changes in libido.

ACUTE OVERDOSAGE

Numerous reports of ingestion of large doses of estrogen-containing oral contraceptives by young children indicate that acute serious ill effects do not occur. Overdosage of estrogens may cause nausea, and withdrawal bleeding may occur in females.

DOSAGE AND ADMINISTRATION

Abnormal uterine bleeding due to hormonal imbalance: One 25 mg injection, intravenously or intramuscularly. Intravenous use is preferred since more rapid response can be expected from this mode of administration.
Repeat in 6 to 12 hours if necessary. The use of Premarin® Intravenous (conjugated estrogens, USP) for injection does not preclude the advisability of other appropriate measures. The usual precautionary measures governing intravenous administration should be adhered to. Injection should be made SLOWLY to obviate the occurrence of flushes.
Infusion of Premarin Intravenous (conjugated estrogens, USP) for injection with other agents is not generally recommended. In emergencies, however, when an infusion has already been started it may be expedient to make the injection into the tubing just distal to the infusion needle. If so used, compatibility of solutions must be considered.
Compatibility of solutions: Premarin Intravenous is compatible with normal saline, dextrose, and invert sugar solutions. IT IS NOT COMPATIBLE WITH PROTEIN HYDROLYSATE, ASCORBIC ACID, OR ANY SOLUTION WITH AN ACID pH.
Treated patients with an intact uterus should be monitored closely for signs of endometrial cancer, and appropriate diagnostic measures should be taken to rule out malignancy in the event of persistent or recurring abnormal vaginal bleeding.

Directions For Storage and Reconstitution

Storage before reconstitution: Store package in refrigerator, 2°–8°C (36°–46°F).
To reconstitute: First withdraw air from Secule® vial so as to facilitate introduction of sterile diluent. Then, flow the sterile diluent slowly against side of Secule® vial and agitate gently. DO NOT SHAKE VIOLENTLY.
Storage after reconstitution: It is common practice to utilize the reconstituted solution within a few hours. If it is necessary to keep the reconstituted solution for more than a few hours, store the reconstituted solution under refrigeration (2°–8°C). Under these conditions, the solution is stable for 60 days, and is suitable for use unless darkening or precipitation occurs.

HOW SUPPLIED

NDC 0046-0749-05—Each package provides: (1) One Secule® vial containing 25 mg of conjugated estrogens, USP, for injection (also lactose 200 mg, sodium citrate 12.2 mg, and simethicone 0.2 mg). The pH is adjusted with sodium hydroxide or hydrochloric acid. (2) One 5 mL ampul sterile diluent with 2% benzyl alcohol in sterile water.
Premarin Intravenous (conjugated estrogens, USP) for injection is prepared by cryodesiccation.
SECULE®—Registered trademark to designate a vial containing an injectable preparation in dry form.

PHYSICIAN REFERENCES

1. Ziel, H. K. *et al.*: N. Engl. J. Med. *293* :1167–1170, 1975.
2. Smith, D. C. *et al.*: N. Engl. J. Med. *293* :1164–1167, 1975.
3. Mack, T. M. *et al.*: N. Engl. J. Med. *294* :1262–1267, 1976.
4. Weiss, N. S. *et al.*: N. Engl. J. Med. *294* :1259–1262, 1976.
5. Herbst, A. L. *et al.*: N. Engl. J. Med. *284* :878–881, 1971.
6. Greenwald, P. *et al.*: N. Engl. J. Med. *285* :390–392, 1971.
7. Lanier, A. *et al.*: Mayo Clin. Proc. *48* :793–799, 1973.
8. Herbst, A. *et al.*: Obstet. Gynecol. *40* :287–298, 1972.
9. Herbst, A. *et al.*: Am. J. Obstet. Gynecol. *118* :607–615, 1974.
10. Herbst, A. *et al.*: N. Engl. J. Med. *292* :334–339, 1975.
11. Stafl, A. *et al.*: Obstet. Gynecol. *43* :118–128, 1974.
12. Sherman, A. I. *et al.*: Obstet. Gynecol. *44* :531–545, 1974.
13. Gal, I. *et al.*: Nature *216* :83, 1967.
14. Levy, E. P. *et al.*: Lancet *1* :611, 1973.
15. Nora, J. *et al.*: Lancet *1* :941–942, 1973.
16. Janerich, D. T. *et al.*: N. Engl. J. Med. *291* :697–700, 1974.
17. Boston Collaborative Drug Surveillance Program: N. Engl. J. Med. *290* :15–19, 1974.
18. Hoover, R. *et al.*: N. Engl. J. Med. *295* :401–405, 1976.
19. Boston Collaborative Drug Surveillance Program: Lancet *1* :1399–1404, 1973.
20. Daniel, D. G. *et al.*: Lancet *2* :287–289, 1967.
21. The Veterans Administration Cooperative Urological Research Group: J. Urol. *98* :516–522, 1967.
22. Bailar, J. C.: Lancet *2* :560, 1967.
23. Blackard, C. *et al.*: Cancer *26* :249–256, 1970.
24. Royal College of General Practitioners: J. R. Coll. Gen. Pract. *13* :267–279, 1967.
24a. Royal College of General Practitioners: Oral Contraceptives and Health, New York, Pitman Corp., 1974.
25. Inman, W. H. W. *et al.*: Br. Med. J. *2* :193–199, 1968.
26. Vessey, M. P. *et al.*: Br. Med. J. *2* :651–657, 1969.
27. Sartwell, P. E. *et al.*: Am. J. Epidemiol. *90* :365–380, 1969.
28. Collaborative Group for the Study of Stroke in Young Women: N. Engl. J. Med. *288* :871–878, 1973.
29. Collaborative Group for the Study of Stroke in Young Women: J.A.M.A. *231* :718–722, 1975.
30. Mann, J. I. *et al.*: Br. Med. J. *2* :245–248, 1975.
31. Mann, J. I. *et al.*: Br. Med. J. *2* :241–245, 1975.
32. Inman, W. H. W. *et al.*: Br. Med. J. *2* :203–209, 1970.
33. Stolley, P. D. *et al.*: Am. J. Epidemiol. *102* :197–208, 1975.
34. Vessey, M. P. *et al.*: Br. Med. J. *3* :123–126, 1970.
35. Greene, G. R., *et al.*: Am. J. Public Health *62* :680–685, 1972.
36. Coronary Drug Project Research Group: J.A.M.A. *214* : 1303–1313, 1970.
37. Baum, J. *et al.*: Lancet *2* :926–928, 1973.
38. Mays, E. T. *et al.*: J.A.M.A. *235* :730–732, 1976.
39. Edmondson, H. A. *et al.*: N. Engl. J. Med. *294* :470–472, 1976.
40. Pfeffer, R. I. *et al.*: Am. J. Epidemiol. *103* :445–456, 1976.

INFORMATION FOR THE PATIENT

What You Should Know About Estrogens

Estrogens are female hormones produced by the ovaries. The ovaries make several different kinds of estrogens. In addition, scientists have been able to make a variety of synthetic estrogens. As far as we know, all these estrogens have similar properties and, therefore, much the same usefulness, side effects, and risks. This leaflet is intended to help you understand what estrogens are used for, the risks involved in their use, and how to use them as safely as possible.
This leaflet includes the most important information about estrogens, but not all the information. If you want to know more, you should ask your doctor for more information, or you can ask your doctor or pharmacist to let you read the package insert prepared for the doctor.

Uses of Estrogen

THERE IS NO PROPER USE OF ESTROGENS IN A PREGNANT WOMAN. Estrogens are prescribed by doctors for a number of purposes, including:
1. To provide estrogen during a period of adjustment when a woman's ovaries stop producing a majority of her estrogens, in order to prevent certain uncomfortable symptoms of estrogen deficiency. (With the menopause, which generally occurs between the ages of 45 and 55, women produce a much smaller amount of estrogens.)
2. To prevent symptoms of estrogen deficiency when a woman's ovaries have been removed surgically before the natural menopause.
3. To prevent pregnancy. (Estrogens are given along with a progestogen, another female hormone; these combinations are called oral contraceptives, or birth-control pills. Patient labeling is available to women taking oral contraceptives and they will not be discussed in this leaflet.)
4. To treat certain cancers in women and men.

Estrogens in the Menopause

In the natural course of their lives, all women eventually experience a decrease in estrogen production. This usually occurs between ages 45 and 55, but may occur earlier or later. Sometimes the ovaries may need to be removed before natural menopause by an operation, producing a "surgical menopause."
When the amount of estrogen in the blood begins to decrease, many women may develop typical symptoms: feelings of warmth in the face, neck, and chest, or sudden intense episodes of heat and sweating throughout the body (called "hot flashes" or "hot flushes"). These symptoms are sometimes very uncomfortable. Some women may also develop changes in the vagina (called "atrophic vaginitis") that cause discomfort, especially during and after intercourse.
Estrogens can be prescribed to treat these symptoms of the menopause. It is estimated that considerably more than half of all women undergoing the menopause have only mild symptoms or no symptoms at all and, therefore, do not need estrogens. Other women may need estrogens for a few months, while their bodies adjust to lower estrogen levels. Sometimes the need will be for periods longer than six months. In an attempt to avoid overstimulation of the uterus (womb), estrogens are usually given cyclically during each month of use, such as three weeks of pills followed by one week without pills.
Sometimes women experience nervous symptoms or depression during menopause. There is no evidence that estrogens are effective for such symptoms without associated vasomotor symptoms. In the absence of vasomotor symptoms, estrogens should not be used to treat nervous symptoms, although other treatment may be needed.
You may have heard that taking estrogens for long periods (years) after the menopause will keep your skin soft and supple and keep you feeling young. There is no evidence that this is so, however, and such long-term treatment carries important risks.

The Dangers of Estrogens

1. *Endometrial cancer.* There are reports that if estrogens are used in the postmenopausal period for more than a year, there is an increased risk of *endometrial cancer* (cancer of the lining of the uterus). Women taking estrogens have roughly 5- to 10-times as great a chance of getting this cancer as women who take no estrogens. To put this another way, while a postmenopausal woman not taking estrogens has 1 chance in 1,000 each year of getting endometrial cancer, a woman taking estrogens has 5 to 10 chances in 1,000 each year. For this reason *it is important to take estrogens only when they are really needed.*
The risk of this cancer is greater the longer estrogens are used and when larger doses are taken. Therefore, you should not take more estrogen than your doctor prescribes. *It is important to take the lowest dose of estrogen that will control symptoms and to take it only as long as it is needed.* If estrogens are needed for longer periods of time, your doctor will want to reevaluate your need for estrogens at least every six months.
Women using estrogens should report any vaginal bleeding to their doctors; such bleeding may be of no importance, but it can be an early warning of endometrial cancer. If you have undiagnosed vaginal bleeding, you should not use estrogens until a diagnosis is made and you are certain there is no endometrial cancer.
Note: If you have had your uterus removed (total hysterectomy), there is no danger of developing endometrial cancer.
2. *Other possible cancers.* Estrogens can cause development of other tumors in animals, such as tumors of the breast, cervix, vagina, or liver, when given for a long time. At present there is no good evidence that women using estrogens in the menopause have an increased risk of such tumors, but there is no way yet to be sure they do not; and one study raises the possibility that use of estrogens in the menopause may increase the risk of breast cancer many years later. This is a further reason to use estrogens only when clearly needed. While you are taking estrogens, it is important that you go to your doctor at least once a year for a physical examination. Also, if members of your family have had breast cancers, or if you have breast nodules, or abnormal mammograms (breast X rays), your doctor may wish to carry out more frequent examinations of your breasts.
3. *Gallbladder disease.* Women who use estrogens after menopause are more likely to develop gallbladder disease needing surgery than women who do not use estrogens. Birth-control pills have a similar effect.
4. *Abnormal blood clotting.* Taking estrogens may increase the risk of blood clotting in various parts of the body. This can result in a stroke (if the clot is in the brain), a heart attack (a clot in a blood vessel of the heart), or a pulmonary embolus (a clot which forms in the legs or pelvis, then breaks off and travels to the lungs). Any of these can be fatal.
It is recommended that if you have had clotting in the legs or lungs, or a heart attack or stroke, while you were using estrogens or birth-control pills, you should not use estrogens (unless they are being used to treat cancer of the breast or prostate). If you have had a stroke or heart attack, or if you have angina pectoris, estrogens should be used with great caution and only if clearly needed (for example, if you have severe symptoms of the menopause).
5. *Inflammation of the pancreas (Pancreatitis).* Women with high triglyceride levels may have an increased risk of developing inflammation of the pancreas.

Special Warning About Pregnancy

You should not receive estrogen if you are pregnant. If this should occur, there is a greater than usual chance that the developing child will be born with a birth defect, although the possibility remains fairly small. A female child may have an increased risk of developing cancer of the vagina or cervix later in life (in the teens or twenties). Every possible effort should be made to avoid exposure to estrogens during pregnancy. If exposure occurs, see your doctor.

Other Effects of Estrogens

In addition to the serious known risks of estrogens described above, estrogens have the following side effects and potential risks:
1. *Nausea and vomiting.* The most common side effect of estrogen therapy is nausea. Vomiting is less common.
2. *Effects on breasts.* Estrogens may cause breast tenderness or enlargement and may cause the breasts to secrete a liquid. These effects are not dangerous.
3. *Effects on the uterus.* Estrogens may cause benign fibroid tumors of the uterus to get larger.
4. *Effects on liver.* Women taking oral contraceptives develop, on rare occasions, a tumor of the liver which can rupture and bleed into the abdomen and may cause death. So far, these tumors have not been reported in women using estrogens in the menopause, but you should report any swelling or unusual pain or tenderness in the abdomen to your doctor immediately.
Women with a past history of jaundice (yellowing of the skin and white parts of the eyes) may get jaundice again during estrogen use. If this occurs, stop taking estrogens and see your doctor.
5. *Other effects.* Estrogens may cause excess fluid to be retained in the body. This may make some conditions worse, such as asthma, epilepsy, migraine, heart disease, or kidney disease.

Summary

Estrogens have important uses, but they have serious risks as well. You must decide, with your doctor, whether the

risks are acceptable to you in view of the benefits of treatment. Except where your doctor has prescribed estrogens for use in special cases of cancer of the breast or prostate, you should not use estrogens if you have cancer of the breast or uterus, are pregnant, have undiagnosed abnormal vaginal bleeding, clotting in the legs or lungs, or have had a stroke, heart attack or angina, or clotting in the legs or lungs in the past while you were taking estrogens.
You can use estrogens as safely as possible by understanding that your doctor will require regular physical examinations while you are taking them, will try to discontinue the drug as soon as possible, and use the smallest dose possible. Be alert for signs of trouble including:
1. Abnormal bleeding from the vagina.
2. Pains in the calves or chest, or sudden shortness of breath, or coughing blood.
3. Severe headache, dizziness, faintness, or changes in vision.
4. Breast lumps (you should ask your doctor how to examine your own breasts).
5. Jaundice (yellowing of the skin).
6. Mental depression.

Your doctor has prescribed this drug for you and you alone. Do not give the drug to anyone else.

HOW SUPPLIED

Premarin® (conjugated estrogens tablets, USP) tablets for oral administration.
Premarin® Vaginal Cream—Premarin® in a nonliquefying base, designed for vaginal use.
Premarin® Intravenous—Premarin® specially prepared for intravenous and intramuscular use.
Manufactured by:
Ayerst Laboratories Inc.
A Wyeth-Ayerst Company
Philadelphia, PA 19101
CI 3902-6 Revised April 29, 1998

PREMARIN® ℞

[*prĕm 'a-rĭn*]
(conjugated estrogens tablets, USP)

Rx only

1. **ESTROGENS HAVE BEEN REPORTED TO INCREASE THE RISK OF ENDOMETRIAL CARCINOMA IN POST-MENOPAUSAL WOMEN.**
Close clinical surveillance of all women taking estrogens is important. Adequate diagnostic measures, including endometrial sampling when indicated, should be undertaken to rule out malignancy in all cases of undiagnosed persistent or recurring abnormal vaginal bleeding. There is no evidence that "natural" estrogens are more or less hazardous than "synthetic" estrogens at equiestrogenic doses.
2. **ESTROGENS SHOULD NOT BE USED DURING PREGNANCY.**
There is no indication for estrogen therapy during pregnancy or during the immediate postpartum period. Estrogens are ineffective for the prevention or treatment of threatened or habitual abortion. Estrogens are not indicated for the prevention of postpartum breast engorgement.
Estrogen therapy during pregnancy is associated with an increased risk of congenital defects in the reproductive organs of the fetus, and possibly other birth defects. Studies of women who received diethylstilbestrol (DES) during pregnancy have shown that female offspring have an increased risk of vaginal adenosis, squamous cell dysplasia of the uterine cervix, and clear cell vaginal cancer later in life; male offspring have an increased risk of urogenital abnormalities and possibly testicular cancer later in life. The 1985 DES Task Force concluded that use of DES during pregnancy is associated with a subsequent increased risk of breast cancer in the mothers, although a causal relationship remains unproven and the observed level of excess risk is similar to that for a number of other breast cancer risk factors.

DESCRIPTION

Premarin (conjugated estrogens tablets, USP) for oral administration contains a mixture of estrogens obtained exclusively from natural sources, occurring as the sodium salts of water-soluble estrogen sulfates blended to represent the average composition of material derived from pregnant mares' urine. It is a mixture of sodium estrone sulfate and sodium equilin sulfate. It contains as concomitant components, as sodium sulfate conjugates, 17 α-dihydroequilin, 17 α-estradiol, and 17 β-dihydroequilin. Tablets for oral administration are available in 0.3 mg, 0.625 mg, 0.9 mg, 1.25 mg, and 2.5 mg strengths of conjugated estrogens.
Premarin Tablets contain the following inactive ingredients: calcium phosphate tribasic, calcium sulfate, carnauba wax, cellulose, glyceryl monooleate, lactose, magnesium stearate, methylcellulose, pharmaceutical glaze, polyethylene glycol, stearic acid, sucrose, titanium dioxide.
— 0.3 mg tablets also contain: D&C Yellow No. 10, FD&C Blue No. 1, FD&C Blue No. 2, FD&C Yellow No. 6; these tablets comply with USP Drug Release Test 1.
— 0.625 mg tablets also contain: FD&C Blue No. 2, D&C Red No. 27, FD&C Red No. 40; these tablets comply with USP Drug Release Test 1.
— 0.9 mg tablets also contain: D&C Red No. 6, D&C Red No. 7; these tablets comply with USP Drug Release Test 2.
— 1.25 mg tablets also contain: black iron oxide, D&C Yellow No. 10, FD&C Yellow No. 6, talc; these tablets comply with USP Drug Release Test 3.
— 2.5 mg tablets also contain: FD&C Blue No. 2, D&C Red No. 7, talc; these tablets comply with USP Drug Release Test 3.

TABLE 1. PHARMACOKINETIC PARAMETERS FOR PREMARIN

Pharmacokinetic Profile of Unconjugated Estrogens Following a Dose of 2 x 0.625 mg

Drug	C_{max} (pg/mL)	t_{max} (h)	$t_{1/2}$ (h)	AUC (pg•h/mL)
estrone	139	8.8	28.0	5016
baseline-adjusted estrone	120	8.8	17.4	2956
equilin	66	7.9	13.6	1210

Pharmacokinetic Profile of Conjugated Estrogens Following a Dose of 2 x 0.625 mg

Drug	C_{max} (ng/mL)	t_{max} (h)	$t_{1/2}$ (h)	AUC (ng•h/mL)
total estrone	7.3	7.3	15.0	134
baseline-adjusted total estrone	7.1	7.3	13.6	122
total equilin	5.0	6.2	10.1	65

CLINICAL PHARMACOLOGY

Estrogen drug products act by regulating the transcription of a limited number of genes.
Estrogens diffuse through cell membranes, distribute themselves throughout the cell, and bind to and activate the nuclear estrogen receptor, a DNA-binding protein which is found in estrogen-responsive tissues. The activated estrogen receptor binds to specific DNA sequences, or hormone-response elements, which enhance the transcription of adjacent genes and in turn lead to the observed effects. Estrogen receptors have been identified in tissues of the reproductive tract, breast, pituitary, hypothalamus, liver, and bone of women.
Estrogens are important in the development and maintenance of the female reproductive system and secondary sex characteristics. By a direct action, they cause growth and development of the uterus, fallopian tubes, and vagina. With other hormones, such as pituitary hormones and progesterone, they cause enlargement of the breasts through promotion of ductal growth, stromal development, and the accretion of fat. Estrogens are intricately involved with other hormones, especially progesterone, in the processes of the ovulatory menstrual cycle and pregnancy, and affect the release of pituitary gonadotropins. They also contribute to the shaping of the skeleton, maintenance of tone and elasticity of urogenital structures, changes in the epiphyses of the long bones that allow for the pubertal growth spurt and its termination, and pigmentation of the nipples and genitals.
Estrogens occur naturally in several forms. The primary source of estrogen in normally cycling adult women is the ovarian follicle, which secretes 70 to 500 micrograms of estradiol daily, depending on the phase of the menstrual cycle. This is converted primarily to estrone, which circulates in roughly equal proportion to estradiol, and to small amounts of estriol. After menopause, most endogenous estrogen is produced by conversion of androstenedione, secreted by the adrenal cortex, to estrone by peripheral tissues. Thus, estrone—especially in its sulfate ester form—is the most abundant circulating estrogen in postmenopausal women. Although circulating estrogens exist in a dynamic equilibrium of metabolic interconversions, estradiol is the principal intracellular human estrogen and is substantially more potent than estrone or estriol at the receptor.

Information Regarding Lipid Effects

The results of a clinical trial conducted in a 97% Caucasian population at low risk for cardiovascular disease show that Premarin significantly increases HDL-C and the HDL_2-C subfraction and significantly decreases LDL-C.
The following table summarizes mean percent changes from baseline lipid parameter values after 1 year of treatment with Premarin.

MEAN PERCENT CHANGE FROM BASELINE LIPID PROFILE VALUES AFTER ONE YEAR OF TREATMENT

Lipid Parameter	Premarin 0.625 mg Dose
Total Cholesterol	0.2
HDL-C	14.1*
HDL_2-C	70.8*
LDL-C	-7.7*
Triglycerides	39.4*

* Significantly ($p \leq 0.05$) different from baseline value.

PHARMACOKINETICS

Absorption

Conjugated estrogens used in therapy are soluble in water and are well absorbed from the gastrointestinal tract after release from the drug formulation. Maximum plasma concentrations of the various conjugated and unconjugated estrogens are attained within 4 to 10 hours after oral administration.
Estrogens used in therapy are also well absorbed through the skin and mucous membranes. When applied for a local action, absorption is usually sufficient to cause systemic effects. When conjugated with aryl and alkyl groups for parenteral administration, the rate of absorption of oily preparations is slowed with a prolonged duration of action, such that a single intramuscular injection of estradiol valerate or estradiol cypionate is absorbed over several weeks.

Distribution

Although naturally-occurring estrogens circulate in the blood largely bound to sex hormone-binding globulin (SHBG) and albumin, only unbound estrogens enter target tissue cells. (Conjugated estrogens bind mainly to albumin; unconjugated estrogens bind to both albumin and SHBG). The apparent terminal-phase disposition half-life ($t_{1/2}$) of the various estrogens is prolonged by the slow absorption from Premarin and ranges from 10 to 24 hours.

Metabolism

Administered estrogens and their esters are handled within the body essentially the same as the endogenous hormones. Metabolic conversion of estrogens occurs primarily in the liver (first-pass effect), but also at local target tissue sites. Complex metabolic processes result in a dynamic equilibrium of circulating conjugated and unconjugated estrogenic forms which are continually interconverted, especially between estrone and estradiol and between esterified and non-esterified forms. A significant proportion of the circulating estrogen exists as sulfate conjugates, especially estrone sulfate, which serves as a circulating reservoir for the formation of more active estrogenic species. A certain proportion of the estrogen is excreted into the bile, then reabsorbed from the intestine and returned to the liver through the portal venous system. During this enterohepatic recirculation, estrogens are desulfated and resulfated and undergo degradation through conversion to less active estrogens (estriol and other estrogens), oxidation to nonestrogenic substances (catecholestrogens, which interact with catecholamine metabolism, especially in the central nervous system), and conjugation with glucuronic acids (which are then rapidly excreted in the urine).
When given orally, naturally-occurring estrogens and their esters are extensively metabolized (first-pass effect) and circulate primarily as estrone sulfate, with smaller amounts of other conjugated and unconjugated estrogenic species. This results in limited oral potency. By contrast, synthetic estrogens, such as ethinyl estradiol and the nonsteroidal estrogens, are degraded very slowly in the liver and other tissues, which results in their high intrinsic potency. Estrogen drug products administered by non-oral routes are not subject to first-pass metabolism, but also undergo significant hepatic uptake, metabolism, and enterohepatic recycling.

Excretion

Water-soluble estrogen conjugates are strongly acidic and are ionized in body fluids, which favor excretion through the kidneys since tubular reabsorption is minimal.
[See table above]

INDICATIONS AND USAGE

Estrogen drug products are indicated in the:
1. Treatment of moderate to severe vasomotor symptoms associated with the menopause. There is no adequate evidence that estrogens are effective for nervous symptoms or depression which might occur during menopause and they should not be used to treat these conditions.
2. Treatment of vulvar and vaginal atrophy.
3. Treatment of hypoestrogenism due to hypogonadism, castration or primary ovarian failure.
4. Treatment of breast cancer (for palliation only) in appropriately selected women and men with metastatic disease.
5. Treatment of advanced androgen-dependent carcinoma of the prostate (for palliation only).
6. Prevention of osteoporosis. Since estrogen administration is associated with risk, selection of patients ideally should be based on prospective identification of risk factors for developing osteoporosis. Unfortunately, there is no certain way to identify those women who will develop osteoporotic fractures. Most prospective studies of efficacy for this indication have been carried out in white menopausal women, without stratification by other risk factors, and tend to show a universally salutary effect on bone. Thus, patient selection

Continued on next page

Premarin Tablets—Cont.

must be individualized based on the balance of risks and benefits. A more favorable risk/benefit ratio exists in a hysterectomized woman because she has no risk of endometrial cancer (see Boxed Warning).

Estrogen replacement therapy reduces bone resorption and retards or halts postmenopausal bone loss. Case-control studies have shown an approximately 60 percent reduction in hip and wrist fractures in women whose estrogen replacement was begun within a few years of menopause. Studies also suggest that estrogen reduces the rate of vertebral fractures. Even when started as late as 6 years after menopause, estrogen prevents further loss of bone mass for as long as the treatment is continued. When estrogen therapy is discontinued, bone mass declines at a rate comparable to the immediate postmenopausal period. There is no evidence that estrogen replacement therapy restores bone mass to premenopausal levels.

At skeletal maturity there are sex and race differences in both the total amount of bone present and its density, in favor of men and blacks. Thus, women are at higher risk than men because they start with less bone mass and, for several years following natural or induced menopause, the rate of bone mass decline is accelerated. White and Asian women are at higher risk than black women.

Early menopause is one of the strongest predictors for the development of osteoporosis. In addition, other factors affecting the skeleton which are associated with osteoporosis include genetic factors (small build, family history), endocrine factors (nulliparity, thyrotoxicosis, hyperparathyroidism, Cushing's syndrome, hyperprolactinemia, Type I diabetes), lifestyle (cigarette smoking, alcohol abuse, sedentary exercise habits), and nutrition (below average body weight, dietary calcium intake).

The mainstays of prevention and management of osteoporosis are estrogen, an adequate lifetime calcium intake, and exercise. Postmenopausal women absorb dietary calcium less efficiently than premenopausal women and require an average of 1500 mg/day of elemental calcium to remain in neutral calcium balance. By comparison, premenopausal women require about 1,000 mg/day and the average calcium intake in the USA is 400–600 mg/day. Therefore, when not contraindicated, calcium supplementation may be helpful.

Weight-bearing exercise and nutrition may be important adjuncts to the prevention and management of osteoporosis. Immobilization and prolonged bed rest produce rapid bone loss, while weight-bearing exercise has been shown both to reduce bone loss and to increase bone mass. The optimal type and amount of physical activity that would prevent osteoporosis have not been established, however in two studies an hour of walking and running exercises twice or three times weekly significantly increased lumbar spine bone mass.

CONTRAINDICATIONS

Estrogens should not be used in individuals with any of the following conditions:

1. Known or suspected pregnancy (see Boxed Warning). Estrogen may cause fetal harm when administered to a pregnant woman.
2. Undiagnosed abnormal genital bleeding.
3. Known or suspected cancer of the breast except in appropriately selected patients being treated for metastatic disease.
4. Known or suspected estrogen-dependent neoplasia.
5. Active thrombophlebitis or thromboembolic disorders. There is insufficient information regarding women who have had previous thromboembolic disease.
6. Premarin Tablets should not be used in patients hypersensitive to their ingredients.

WARNINGS

1. *Induction of malignant neoplasms.*

Breast cancer. While the majority of studies have not shown an increased risk of breast cancer in women who have ever used estrogen replacement therapy, there are conflicting data whether there is an increased risk in women using estrogens for prolonged periods of time, especially in excess of 10 years.

In the three year clinical Postmenopausal Estrogen Progestin Intervention (PEPI) trial of 875 women to assess differences among placebo, unopposed Premarin, and three different combination hormone therapy regimens, one (1) new case of breast cancer was detected in the placebo group (n=174), one in the Premarin alone group (n=175), none in the continuous Premarin plus continuous medroxyprogesterone acetate group (n=174), and two (2) in the continuous Premarin plus cyclic medroxyprogesterone acetate group (n=174).

Women on this therapy should have regular breast examinations and should be instructed in breast self-examination, and women over the age of 40 should have regular mammograms.

Endometrial cancer. The reported endometrial cancer risk among unopposed estrogen users is about 2- to 12-fold greater than in non-users, and appears dependent on duration of treatment and on estrogen dose. Most studies show no significant increased risk associated with use of estrogens for less than one year. The greatest risk appears associated with prolonged use, with increased risks of 15- to 24-fold for five to ten years or more. In three studies, persistence of risk was demonstrated for 8 to over 15 years after cessation of estrogen treatment. In one study a significant decrease in the incidence of endometrial cancer occurred six months after estrogen withdrawal. Concurrent progestin therapy may offset this risk but the overall health impact in postmenopausal women is not known (see **PRECAUTIONS**).

Congenital lesions with malignant potential. Estrogen therapy during pregnancy is associated with an increased risk of fetal congenital reproductive tract disorders, and possibly other birth defects. Studies of women who received DES during pregnancy have shown that female offspring have an increased risk of vaginal adenosis, squamous cell dysplasia of the uterine cervix, and clear cell vaginal cancer later in life; male offspring have an increased risk of urogenital abnormalities and possibly testicular cancer later in life. Although some of these changes are benign, others are precursors of malignancy.

2. *Gallbladder disease.* Two studies have reported a 2- to 4-fold increase in the risk of gallbladder disease requiring surgery in women receiving postmenopausal estrogens.

3. *Thromboembolic disorders and other vascular problems.* In some studies, women on estrogen replacement therapy, given alone or in combination with a progestin, have been reported to have an increased risk of thrombophlebitis, and/or thromboembolic disease. Large doses of estrogen (5 mg conjugated estrogens per day), comparable to those used to treat cancer of the prostate and breast, have been shown in a large prospective clinical trial in men to increase the risk of nonfatal myocardial infarction, pulmonary embolism, and thrombophlebitis. The physician should be aware of the possibility of thrombotic disorders (thrombophlebitis, retinal thrombosis, cerebral embolism, and pulmonary embolism) during estrogen replacement therapy and be alert to their earliest manifestations. Should any of these occur or be suspected, estrogen replacement therapy should be discontinued immediately. Patients who have risk factors for thrombotic disorders should be kept under careful observation.

4. *Elevated blood pressure.* Occasional blood pressure increases during estrogen replacement therapy have been attributed to idiosyncratic reactions to estrogens. More often, blood pressure has remained the same or has dropped. One study showed that postmenopausal estrogen users have higher blood pressure than nonusers. Two other studies showed slightly lower blood pressure among estrogen users compared to nonusers. Blood pressure should be monitored at regular intervals with estrogen use.

5. *Hypercalcemia.* Administration of estrogens may lead to severe hypercalcemia in patients with breast cancer and bone metastases. If this occurs, the drug should be stopped and appropriate measures taken to reduce the serum calcium level.

PRECAUTIONS

A. **General**

1. *Addition of a progestin.* Studies of the addition of a progestin for 10 or more days of a cycle of estrogen administration have reported a lowered incidence of endometrial hyperplasia than would be induced by estrogen treatment alone. Morphological and biochemical studies of endometria suggest that 10 to 14 days of progestin are needed to provide maximal maturation of the endometrium and to reduce the likelihood of any hyperplastic changes.

There are, however, possible risks which may be associated with the use of progestins in estrogen replacement regimens. The potential risks include adverse effects on lipoprotein metabolism, impairment of glucose tolerance, and possible enhancement of mitotic activity in breast epithelial tissue, although few epidemiological data are available to address this point (see **PRECAUTIONS** below).

The choice of progestin, its dose, and its regimen may be important in minimizing these adverse effects, but these issues will require further study before they are clarified.

2. *Cardiovascular risk.* A causal relationship between estrogen replacement therapy and reduction of cardiovascular disease in postmenopausal women has not been proven. Futhermore, the effect of added progestins on this putative benefit is not yet known.

In recent years many published studies have suggested that there may be a cause-effect relationship between postmenopausal oral estrogen replacement therapy *without added progestins* and a decrease in cardiovascular disease in women. Although most of the observational studies which assessed this statistical association have reported a 20% to 50% reduction in coronary heart disease risk and associated mortality in estrogen takers, the following should be considered when interpreting these reports:

(1) Because only one of these studies was randomized and it was too small to yield statistically significant results, all relevant studies were subject to selection bias. Thus, the apparently reduced risk of coronary artery disease cannot be attributed with certainty to estrogen replacement therapy. It may instead have been caused by life-style and medical characteristics of the women studied with the result that healthier women were selected for estrogen therapy. In general, treated women were of higher socioeconomic and educational status, more slender, more physically active, more likely to have undergone surgical menopause, and less likely to have diabetes than the untreated women. Although some studies attempted to control for these selection factors, it is common for properly designed randomized trials to fail to confirm benefits suggested by less rigorous study designs. Thus, ongoing and future large-scale randomized trials may fail to confirm this apparent benefit.

(2) Current medical practice often includes the use of concomitant progestin therapy in women with intact uteri (see **PRECAUTIONS** and **WARNINGS**). While the effects of added progestins on the risk of ischemic heart disease are not known, all available progestins reverse at least some of the favorable effects of estrogens on HDL and LDL cholesterol levels.

(3) While the effects of added progestins on the risk of breast cancer are also unknown, available epidemiological evidence suggests that progestins do not reduce, and may enhance, the moderately increased breast cancer incidence that has been reported with prolonged estrogen replacement therapy (see **WARNINGS**).

Because relatively long-term use of estrogens by a woman with a uterus has been shown to increase the risk of endometrial cancer, physicians often recommend that these women should take progestins as well as estrogens. When considering prescribing concomitant estrogens and progestins for hormone replacement therapy, physicians and patients are advised to carefully weigh the potential benefits and risks of the added progestin. Large-scale randomized, placebo-controlled, clinical trials and future epidemiological studies are required to clarify these issues.

3. *Physical examination.* A complete medical and family history should be taken prior to the initiation of any estrogen therapy. The pretreatment and periodic physical examinations should include special reference to blood pressure, breasts, abdomen, and pelvic organs, and should include a Papanicolaou smear. As a general rule, estrogen should not be prescribed for longer than one year without reexamining the patient.

4. *Hypercoagulability.* Some studies have shown that women taking estrogen replacement therapy have hypercoagulability, primarily related to decreased antithrombin activity. This effect appears dose- and duration-dependent and is less pronounced than that associated with oral contraceptive use. Also, postmenopausal women tend to have increased coagulation parameters at baseline compared to premenopausal women. There is some suggestion that low dose postmenopausal mestranol may increase the risk of thromboembolism. There is insufficient information on hypercoagulability in women who have had previous thromboembolic disease.

5. *Familial hyperlipoproteinemia.* Estrogen therapy may be associated with massive elevations of plasma triglycerides leading to pancreatitis and other complications in patients with familial defects of lipoprotein metabolism.

6. *Fluid retention.* Because estrogens may cause some degree of fluid retention, conditions which might be exacerbated by this factor, such as asthma, epilepsy, migraine, and cardiac or renal dysfunction, require careful observation.

7. *Exacerbation of endometriosis.* Endometriosis may be exacerbated with administration of estrogen therapy.

8. *Uterine bleeding and mastodynia.* Certain patients may develop undesirable manifestations of estrogenic stimulation, such as abnormal uterine bleeding and mastodynia.

9. *Impaired liver function.* Estrogens may be poorly metabolized in patients with impaired liver function and should be administered with caution.

10. *Uterine fibroids.* Pre-existing uterine leiomyomata may increase in size during estrogen use.

11. *Hypocalcemia.* Estrogens should be used with caution in individuals with metabolic bone disease associated with severe hypocalcemia.

B. **Information for the Patient.** See text of Patient Package Insert which appears after the **HOW SUPPLIED** section.

C. **Laboratory Tests.**

Estrogen administration should generally be guided by clinical response at the smallest dose, rather than laboratory monitoring, for relief of symptoms for those indications in which symptoms are observable. For prevention of osteoporosis, however, see **DOSAGE AND ADMINISTRATION** section.

D. **Drug/Laboratory Test Interactions.**

1. Accelerated prothrombin time, partial thromboplastin time, and platelet aggregation time; increased platelet count; increased factors II, VII antigen, VIII antigen, VIII coagulant activity, IX, X, XII, VII-X complex, II-VII-X complex, and beta-thromboglobulin; decreased levels of anti-factor Xa and antithrombin III, decreased antithrombin III activity; increased levels of fibrinogen and fibrinogen activity; increased plasminogen antigen and activity.
2. Increased thyroid-binding globulin (TBG) leading to increased circulating total thyroid hormone, as measured by protein-bound iodine (PBI), T4 levels (by column or by radioimmunoassay) or T3 levels by radioimmunoassay. T3 resin uptake is decreased, reflecting the elevated TBG. Free T4 and free T3 concentrations are unaltered.
3. Other binding proteins may be elevated in serum, i.e., corticosteroid binding globulin (CBG), sex hormone-binding globulin (SHBG), leading to increased circulating corticosteroids and sex steroids respectively. Free or biologically active hormone concentrations are unchanged. Other plasma proteins may be increased (angiotensinogen/renin substrate, alpha-1-antitrypsin, ceruloplasmin).
4. Increased plasma HDL and HDL-2 subfraction concentrations, reduced LDL cholesterol concentration, increased triglyceride levels.
5. Impaired glucose tolerance.
6. Reduced response to metyrapone test.
7. Reduced serum folate concentration.

E. **Carcinogenesis, Mutagenesis, and Impairment of Fertility.** Long-term continuous administration of natural and synthetic estrogens in certain animal species increases the frequency of carcinomas of the breast, uterus, cervix, vagina, testis, and liver. See **CONTRAINDICATIONS** and **WARNINGS**.

F. **Pregnancy Category X.** Estrogens should not be used during pregnancy. See **CONTRAINDICATIONS** and Boxed Warning.

G. **Nursing Mothers.**

As a general principle, the administration of any drug to nursing mothers should be done only when clearly necessary since many drugs are excreted in human milk. In addition, estrogen administration to nursing mothers has been shown to decrease the quantity and quality of the milk.

H. **Pediatric Use.** See **DOSAGE AND ADMINISTRATION.**

ADVERSE REACTIONS

The following additional adverse reactions have been reported with estrogen therapy (see **WARNINGS** regarding induction of malignant neoplasms, gallbladder disease, thromboembolic disorders and other vascular problems, elevated blood pressure, and hypercalcemia; see **PRECAUTIONS** regarding cardiovascular risk).

1. *Genito-urinary system.*
   Changes in vaginal bleeding pattern and abnormal withdrawal bleeding or flow; breakthrough bleeding, spotting.
   Increase in size of uterine leiomyomata.
   Vaginal candidiasis.
   Change in amount of cervical secretion.
2. *Breasts.*
   Tenderness, enlargement.
3. *Gastrointestinal.*
   Nausea, vomiting.
   Abdominal cramps, bloating.
   Cholestatic jaundice.
   Increased incidence of gallbladder disease.
   Pancreatitis.
4. *Skin.*
   Chloasma or melasma that may persist when drug is discontinued.
   Erythema multiforme.
   Erythema nodosum.
   Hemorrhagic eruption.
   Loss of scalp hair.
   Hirsutism.
5. *Cardiovascular.*
   Venous thromboembolism.
   Pulmonary embolism.
6. *Eyes.*
   Steepening of corneal curvature.
   Intolerance to contact lenses.
7. *Central Nervous System.*
   Headache.
   Migraine.
   Dizziness.
   Mental depression.
   Chorea.
8. *Miscellaneous.*
   Increase or decrease in weight.
   Reduced carbohydrate tolerance.
   Aggravation of porphyria.
   Edema.
   Changes in libido.
   Anaphylactoid/anaphylactic reactions.

OVERDOSAGE

Serious ill effects have not been reported following acute ingestion of large doses of estrogen-containing oral contraceptives by young children. Overdosage of estrogen may cause nausea and vomiting, and withdrawal bleeding may occur in females.

DOSAGE AND ADMINISTRATION

1. For treatment of moderate to severe vasomotor symptoms, and/or vulvar and vaginal atrophy associated with the menopause, the lowest dose and regimen that will control symptoms should be chosen and medication should be discontinued as promptly as possible.

Vasomotor symptoms—0.625 mg daily.

Vulvar and vaginal atrophy—0.3 mg to 1.25 mg or more daily, depending upon the tissue response of the individual patient.

Premarin® therapy may be given continuously with no interruption in therapy, or in cyclical regimens (regimens such as 25 days on drug followed by five days off drug) as is medically appropriate on an individualized basis.

Attempts to discontinue or taper medication should be made at 3-month to 6-month intervals.

2. For treatment of female hypoestrogenism due to hypogonadism, castration, or primary ovarian failure:

Female hypogonadism—0.3 mg to 0.625 mg daily, administered cyclically (e.g., three weeks on and one week off). Doses are adjusted depending on the severity of symptoms and responsiveness of the endometrium.

In clinical studies of delayed puberty due to female hypogonadism, breast development was induced by doses as low as 0.15 mg. The dosage may be gradually titrated upward at 6 to 12 month intervals as needed to achieve appropriate bone age advancement and eventual epiphyseal closure. Clinical studies suggest that doses of 0.15 mg, 0.3 mg, and 0.6 mg are associated with mean ratios of bone age advancement to chronological age progression $\Delta BA/\Delta CA$) of 1.1, 1.5, and 2.1, respectively. (Premarin in the dose strength of 0.15 mg is not available commercially). Available data suggest that chronic dosing with 0.625 mg is sufficient to induce artificial cyclic menses with sequential progestin treatment and to maintain bone mineral density after skeletal maturity is achieved.

Female castration or primary ovarian failure—1.25 mg daily, cyclically. Adjust dosage, upward or downward, according to severity of symptoms and response of the patient. For maintenance, adjust dosage to lowest level that will provide effective control.

3. For treatment of breast cancer, for palliation only, in appropriately selected women and men with metastatic disease:

Suggested dosage is 10 mg three times daily for a period of at least three months.

4. For treatment of advanced androgen-dependent carcinoma of the prostate, for palliation only:

1.25 mg to 2.5 mg three times daily. The effectiveness of therapy can be judged by phosphatase determinations as well as by symptomatic improvement of the patient.

5. For prevention of osteoporosis:

0.625 mg daily. Premarin therapy may be given continuously with no interruption in therapy, or in cyclical regimens (regimens such as 25 days on drug followed by five days off drug) as is medically appropriate on an individualized basis.

HOW SUPPLIED

Premarin® (conjugated estrogens tablets, USP)

— Each oval purple tablet contains 2.5 mg, in bottles of 100 (NDC 0046-0865-81) and 1,000 (NDC 0046-0865-91).

— Each oval yellow tablet contains 1.25 mg, in bottles of 100 (NDC 0046-0866-81); 1,000 (NDC 0046-0866-91); 5,000 (NDC 0046-0866-95); and Unit-Dose packages of 100 (NDC 0046-0866-99).

— Each oval white tablet contains 0.9 mg, in bottles of 100 (NDC 0046-0864-81).

— Each oval maroon tablet contains 0.625 mg, in bottles of 100 (NDC 0046-0867-81); 1,000 (NDC 0046-0867-91); 5,000 (NDC 0046-0867-95); and Unit-Dose packages of 100 (NDC 0046-0867-99).

— Each oval green tablet contains 0.3 mg, in bottles of 100 (NDC 0046-0868-81) and 1,000 (NDC 0046-0868-91).

The appearance of these tablets is a trademark of Wyeth-Ayerst Laboratories.

Store at room temperature (approximately 25° C).

Dispense in a well-closed container as defined in the USP.

INFORMATION FOR THE PATIENT

INTRODUCTION

This leaflet describes when and how to use estrogens and the risks of estrogen treatment.

Estrogens have important benefits but also some risks. You must decide, with your doctor, whether the risks to you of estrogen use are acceptable because of their benefits. If you decide to start taking estrogens, check with your doctor to make sure you are using the lowest possible effective dose, and that you use them for only as long as necessary. How long you need to use estrogens will depend upon the reason for use.

1. ESTROGENS INCREASE THE RISK OF CANCER OF THE UTERUS IN WOMEN WHO HAVE HAD THEIR MENOPAUSE ("CHANGE OF LIFE").

If you use any estrogen-containing drug, it is important to visit your doctor regularly and report any unusual vaginal bleeding right away. Vaginal bleeding after menopause may be a warning sign of uterine cancer. Your doctor should evaluate any unusual vaginal bleeding to find out the cause.

2. ESTROGENS SHOULD NOT BE USED DURING PREGNANCY.

Estrogens do not prevent miscarriage (spontaneous abortion) and are not needed in the days following childbirth. If you take estrogens during pregnancy, your unborn child has a greater than usual chance of having birth defects. The risk of developing these defects is small, but clearly larger than the risk in children whose mothers did not take estrogens during pregnancy. These birth defects may affect the baby's urinary system and sex organs. Daughters born to mothers who took DES (an estrogen drug) have a higher than usual change of developing cancer of the vagina or cervix when they become teenagers or young adults. Sons may have a higher than usual chance of developing cancer of the testicles when they become teenagers or young adults.

USES OF ESTROGEN

(Not every estrogen drug is approved for every use listed in this section. If you want to know which of these possible uses are approved for the medicine prescribed for you, ask your doctor or pharmacist to show you the professional labeling. You can also look up the specific estrogen product in a book called *The Physicians' Desk Reference*, which is available in many book stores and public libraries. Generic drugs carry virtually the same labeling information as their brand name versions.)

To reduce moderate to severe menopausal symptoms.

Estrogens are hormones made by the ovaries of normal women. Between ages 45 and 55, the ovaries normally stop making estrogens. This leads to a drop in body estrogen levels which causes the "change of life" or menopause (the end of monthly menstrual periods). If both ovaries are removed during an operation before natural menopause takes place, the sudden drop in estrogen levels causes "surgical menopause."

When the estrogen levels begin dropping, some women develop very uncomfortable symptoms, such as feeling of warmth in the face, neck, and chest, or sudden intense episodes of heat and sweating ("hot flashes" or "hot flushes"). Using estrogen drugs can help the body adjust to lower estrogen levels and reduce these symptoms. In some women the symptoms are mild; in others they can be severe. These symptoms may last only a few months or longer. Taking Premarin can alleviate these symptoms. If you are not taking estrogen for other reasons, such as the prevention of osteoporosis, you should take Premarin only as long as you need it for relief from your menopausal symptoms.

To treat vulvar and vaginal atrophy (itching, burning, dryness in or around the vagina, difficulty or burning on urination) associated with menopause.

To treat certain conditions in which a young woman's ovaries do not produce enough estrogen naturally.

To treat certain types of abnormal uterine bleeding due to hormonal imbalance when your doctor has found no serious cause of the bleeding.

To treat certain cancers in special situations, in men and women.

To prevent thinning of bones.

Osteoporosis is a thinning of the bones that makes them weaker and allows them to break more easily. The bones of the spine, wrists and hips break most often in osteoporosis. Both men and women start to lose bone mass after about age 40, but women lose bone mass faster after the menopause. Using estrogens after the menopause slows down bone thinning and may prevent bones from breaking. Lifelong adequate calcium intake, either in the diet (such as dairy products) or by calcium supplements (to reach a total daily intake of 1000 milligrams per day before menopause or 1500 milligrams per day after menopause), may help to prevent osteoporosis. Regular weight-bearing exercise (like walking and running for an hour, two or three times a week) may also help to prevent osteoporosis. Before you change your calcium intake or exercise habits, it is important to discuss these lifestyle changes with your doctor to find out if they are safe for you. Since estrogen use has some risks, only women who are likely to develop osteoporosis should use estrogens for prevention. Women who are likely to develop osteoporosis often have the following characteristics: white or Asian race, slim, cigarette smokers, and a family history of osteoporosis in a mother, sister, or aunt. Women who have relatively early menopause, often because their ovaries were removed during an operation ("surgical menopause"), are more likely to develop osteoporosis than women whose menopause happens at the average age.

WHO SHOULD NOT USE ESTROGENS

Estrogens should not be used:

During pregnancy (see Boxed Warning).

If you think you may be pregnant, do not use any form of estrogen-containing drug. Using estrogens while you are pregnant may cause your unborn child to have birth defects. Estrogens do not prevent miscarriage.

If you have unusual vaginal bleeding which has not been evaluated by your doctor (see Boxed Warning).

Unusual vaginal bleeding can be a warning sign of cancer of the uterus, especially if it happens after menopause. Your doctor must find out the cause of the bleeding so that he or she can recommend the proper treatment. Taking estrogens without visiting your doctor can cause you serious harm if your vaginal bleeding is caused by cancer of the uterus.

If you have had cancer.

Since estrogens increase the risk of certain types of cancer, you should not use estrogens if you have ever had cancer of the breast or uterus, unless your doctor recommends that the drug may help in the cancer treatment. (For certain patients with breast or prostate cancer, estrogens may help.)

If you have any circulation problems.

Estrogen drugs should not be used except in unusually special situations in which your doctor judges that you need estrogen therapy so much that the risks are acceptable. Men and women with abnormal blood clotting conditions should avoid estrogen use (see **RISKS OF ESTROGENS**, below).

When they do not work.

During menopause, some women develop nervous symptoms or depression. Estrogens do not relieve these symptoms. You may have heard that taking estrogens for years after menopause will keep your skin soft and supple and keep you feeling young. There is no evidence for these claims and such long-term estrogen use may have serious risks.

After childbirth or when breastfeeding a baby.

Estrogens should not be used to try to stop the breasts from filling with milk after a baby is born. Such treatment may increase the risk of developing blood clots (see **RISKS OF ESTROGENS**, below).

If you are breastfeeding, you should avoid using any drugs because many drugs pass through to the baby in the milk. While nursing a baby, you should take drugs only on the advice of your health-care provider.

RISKS OF ESTROGENS

Cancer of the uterus.

Your risk of developing cancer of the uterus gets higher the longer you use estrogens and the larger doses you use. One study showed that after women stop taking estrogens, this higher cancer risk quickly returns to the usual level of risk (as if you had never used estrogen therapy). Three other

Continued on next page

Premarin Tablets—Cont.

studies showed that the cancer risk stayed high for 8 to more than 15 years after stopping estrogen treatment. Because of this risk, **IT IS IMPORTANT TO TAKE THE LOWEST DOSE THAT WORKS AND TO TAKE IT ONLY AS LONG AS YOU NEED IT.**
Using progestin therapy together with estrogen therapy may reduce the higher risk of uterine cancer related to estrogen use (but see **OTHER INFORMATION**, below).
If you have had your uterus removed (total hysterectomy), there is no risk of developing cancer of the uterus.

Cancer of the breast.
Most studies have ***not*** shown a higher risk of breast cancer in women who have ever used estrogens at some time in their lifetimes. However, some studies suggest there may be a higher risk of breast cancer in women who use estrogens for long periods of time, especially more than 10 years.
All women should do monthly self-exams of their breasts and have regular breast exams by a health professional. Women ages 40 and above should have periodic mammograms to check for early signs of breast cancer.
Ask your health professional how to do a breast self-exam.
Gallbladder disease.
Women who use estrogens after menopause are more likely to develop gallbladder disease needing surgery than women who do not use estrogens.
Inflammation of the pancreas (Pancreatitis).
Women with high triglyceride levels may have an increased risk of developing inflammation of the pancreas.
Abnormal blood clotting.
Taking estrogens may cause changes in your blood clotting system. These changes allow the blood to clot more easily, possibly allowing clots to form in your bloodstream. If blood clots do form in your bloodstream, they can cut off the blood supply to vital organs, causing serious problems. These problems may include a stroke (by cutting off blood to the brain), a heart attack (by cutting off blood to the heart), a pulmonary embolus (by cutting off blood to the lungs), or other problems. Any of these conditions may cause death or serious long term disability.
Endometriosis.
Administration of estrogens may worsen endometriosis. If you have had endometriosis, speak with your health professional.

SIDE EFFECTS
In addition to the risks listed above, the following side effects have been reported with estrogen use:
Nausea and vomiting.
Breast tenderness or enlargement.
Enlargement of benign tumors ("fibroids") of the uterus.
Retention of excess fluid. This may make some conditions worsen, such as asthma, epilepsy, migraine, heart disease, or kidney disease.
A spotty darkening of the skin, particularly on the face.

REDUCING RISK OF ESTROGEN USE
If you use estrogens, you can reduce your risks by doing these things:
See your doctor regularly.
While you are using estrogens, it is important to visit your doctor at least once a year for a checkup. If you develop vaginal bleeding while taking estrogens, you may need further evaluation. If members of your family have had breast cancer or if you have ever had breast lumps or an abnormal mammogram (breast x-ray), you may need to have more frequent breast examinations.
Reassess your need for estrogens.
You and your doctor should reevaluate whether or not you still need estrogens at least every six months.
Be alert for signs of trouble.
If any of these warning signals (or any other unusual symptoms) happen while you are using estrogens, call your doctor immediately:

- Abnormal bleeding from the vagina (possible uterine cancer)
- Pains in the calves or chest, sudden shortness of breath, or coughing blood (possible clot in the legs, heart, or lungs)
- Severe headache or vomiting, dizziness, faintness, changes in vision or speech, weakness or numbness of an arm or leg (possible clot in the brain or eye)
- Breast lumps (possible breast cancer; ask your doctor or health professional to show you how to examine your breasts monthly)
- Yellowing of the skin or eyes (possible liver problem)
- Pain, swelling, or tenderness in the abdomen (possible gallbladder problem)

OTHER INFORMATION
1. Estrogens increase the risk of developing a condition (endometrial hyperplasia) that may lead to cancer of the lining of the uterus. Taking progestins, another hormonal drug, with estrogens lowers the risk of developing this condition. Therefore, if your uterus has not been removed, your doctor may prescribe a progestin for you to take together with the estrogen.
You should know, however, that taking estrogens *with* progestins may have additional risks. These may include unhealthy effects on blood fats (especially the lowering of HDL blood cholesterol, the "good" blood fat which protects against heart disease). However, while it has been reported that some estrogen and progestin combinations have an unfavorable effect on blood fats, studies of Premarin given with medroxyprogesterone acetate (MPA) (0.625 mg Premarin with either 2.5 mg MPA continuously or 5 mg of MPA cyclically) have shown decreases in LDL ("bad" cholesterol) and increases in HDL ("good" cholesterol). Other risks include unhealthy effects on blood sugars, which might make a diabetic condition worse, and a possible further increase in breast cancer risk which may be associated with long-term estrogen use.
Some research has shown that estrogens taken *without* progestins may protect women against developing heart disease. However, this is not certain. The protection shown may have been caused by the characteristics of the estrogen-treated women, and not by the estrogen treatment itself. In general, treated women were slimmer, more physically active, and were less likely to have diabetes than the untreated women. These characteristics are known to protect against heart disease.
You are cautioned to discuss very carefully with your doctor or health-care provider all the possible risks and benefits of long-term estrogen and progestin treatment as they affect you personally.
2. Your doctor has prescribed this drug for you and you alone. Do not give the drug to anyone else.
3. If you will be taking calcium supplements as part of the treatment to help prevent osteoporosis, check with your doctor about the amounts recommended.
4. Keep this and all drugs out of the reach of children. In case of overdose, call your doctor, hospital or poison control center immediately.
5. This leaflet provides a summary of the most important information about estrogens. If you want more information, ask your doctor or pharmacist to show you the professional labeling. The professional labeling is also published in a book called *The Physicians' Desk Reference*, which is available in bookstores and public libraries. Generic drugs carry virtually the same labeling information as their brand name versions.

HOW SUPPLIED
Premarin® (conjugated estrogens tablets, USP)—tablets for oral administration.
Each oval purple tablet contains 2.5 mg.
Each oval yellow tablet contains 1.25 mg.
Each oval white tablet contains 0.9 mg.
Each oval maroon tablet contains 0.625 mg.
Each oval green tablet contains 0.3 mg.
The appearance of these tablets is a trademark of Wyeth-Ayerst Laboratories.
Manufactured by:
Ayerst Laboratories Inc.
A Wyeth-Ayerst Company
Philadelphia, PA 19101
CI 6045-3 Revised April 17, 2000
Shown in Product Identification Guide, page 342

PREMARIN® ℞
[prĕm 'a-rin]
(conjugated estrogens)
VAGINAL CREAM
in a nonliquefying base
Rx only

1. ESTROGENS HAVE BEEN REPORTED TO INCREASE THE RISK OF ENDOMETRIAL CARCINOMA.
Three independent, case-controlled studies have reported an increased risk of endometrial cancer in postmenopausal women exposed to exogenous estrogens for more than one year.[1–3] This risk was independent of the other known risk factors for endometrial cancer. These studies are further supported by the finding that incidence rates of endometrial cancer have increased sharply since 1969 in eight different areas of the United States with population-based cancer-reporting systems, an increase which may be related to the rapidly expanding use of estrogens during the last decade.[4]
The three case-controlled studies reported that the risk of endometrial cancer in estrogen users was about 4.5 to 13.9 times greater than in nonusers. The risk appears to depend on both duration of treatment[1] and on estrogen dose.[3] In view of these findings, when estrogens are used for the treatment of menopausal symptoms, the lowest dose that will control symptoms should be utilized and medication should be discontinued as soon as possible. When prolonged treatment is medically indicated, the patient should be reassessed, on at least a semiannual basis, to determine the need for continued therapy. Although the evidence must be considered preliminary, one study suggests that cyclic administration of low doses of estrogen may carry less risk than continuous administration.[3] It therefore appears prudent to utilize such a regimen.
Close clinical surveillance of all women taking estrogens is important. In all cases of undiagnosed persistent or recurring abnormal vaginal bleeding, adequate diagnostic measures should be undertaken to rule out malignancy.
There is no evidence at present that "natural" estrogens are more or less hazardous than "synthetic" estrogens at equiestrogenic doses.
2. ESTROGENS SHOULD NOT BE USED DURING PREGNANCY.
The use of female sex hormones, both estrogens and progestogens, during early pregnancy may seriously damage the offspring. It has been shown that females exposed *in utero* to diethylstilbestrol, a nonsteroidal estrogen, have an increased risk of developing, in later life, a form of vaginal or cervical cancer that is ordinarily extremely rare.[5,6] This risk has been estimated as not greater than 4 per 1,000 exposures.[7] Furthermore, a high percentage of such exposed women (from 30% to 90%) have been found to have vaginal adenosis,[8–12] epithelial changes of the vagina and cervix. Although these changes are histologically benign, it is not known whether they are precursors of malignancy. Although similar data are not available with the use of other estrogens, it cannot be presumed they would not induce similar changes.
Several reports suggest an association between intrauterine exposure to female sex hormones and congenital anomalies, including congenital heart defects and limb reduction defects.[13–16] One case-controlled study[16] estimated a 4.7-fold increased risk of limb reduction defects in infants exposed *in utero* to sex hormones (oral contraceptives, hormone withdrawal tests for pregnancy, or attempted treatment for threatened abortion). Some of these exposures were very short and involved only a few days of treatment. The data suggest that the risk of limb-reduction defects in exposed fetuses is somewhat less than 1 per 1,000.
In the past, female sex hormones have been used during pregnancy in an attempt to treat threatened or habitual abortion. There is considerable evidence that estrogens are ineffective for these indications, and there is no evidence from well-controlled studies that progestogens are effective for these uses.
If Premarin (conjugated estrogens) Vaginal Cream is used during pregnancy, or if the patient becomes pregnant while taking this drug, she should be apprised of the potential risks to the fetus, and the advisability of pregnancy continuation.

DESCRIPTION
Each gram of Premarin® (conjugated estrogens) Vaginal Cream contains 0.625 mg conjugated estrogens, USP in a nonliquefying base containing cetyl esters wax, cetyl alcohol, white wax, glyceryl monostearate, propylene glycol monostearate, methyl stearate, benzyl alcohol, sodium lauryl sulfate, glycerin, and mineral oil. Premarin Vaginal Cream is applied intravaginally.
Premarin (conjugated estrogens) is a mixture of estrogens obtained exclusively from natural sources, occurring as the sodium salts of water-soluble estrogen sulfates blended to represent the average composition of material derived from pregnant mares' urine. It contains estrone, equilin, and 17 α-dihydroequilin, together with smaller amounts of 17 α-estradiol, equilenin, and 17 α-dihydroequilenin as salts of their sulfate esters.

CLINICAL PHARMACOLOGY
Estrogens are important in the development and maintenance of the female reproductive system and secondary sex characteristics. They promote growth and development of the vagina, uterus, and fallopian tubes, and enlargement of the breasts. Indirectly, they contribute to the shaping of the skeleton, maintenance of tone and elasticity of urogenital structures, changes in the epiphyses of the long bones that allow for the pubertal growth spurt and its termination, growth of axillary and pubic hair, and pigmentation of the nipples and genitals. Decline of estrogenic activity at the end of the menstrual cycle can bring on menstruation, although the cessation of progesterone secretion is the most important factor in the mature ovulatory cycle. However, in the preovulatory or nonovulatory cycle, estrogen is the primary determinant in the onset of menstruation. Estrogens also affect the release of pituitary gonadotropins.
The pharmacologic effects of conjugated estrogens are similar to those of endogenous estrogens. They are soluble in water and may be absorbed from mucosal surfaces after local administration.
In responsive tissues (female genital organs, breasts, hypothalamus, pituitary) estrogens enter the cell and are transported into the nucleus. As a result of estrogen action, specific RNA and protein synthesis occurs.
Metabolism and inactivation occur primarily in the liver. Some estrogens are excreted into the bile; however, they are reabsorbed from the intestine and returned to the liver through the portal venous system. Water-soluble estrogen conjugates are strongly acidic and, therefore, ionized in body fluids, which favor excretion through the kidneys since tubular reabsorption is minimal.

INDICATIONS AND USAGE
Premarin (conjugated estrogens) Vaginal Cream is indicated in the treatment of atrophic vaginitis and kraurosis vulvae.
Premarin Vaginal Cream HAS NOT BEEN SHOWN TO BE EFFECTIVE FOR ANY PURPOSE DURING PREGNANCY AND ITS USE MAY CAUSE SEVERE HARM TO THE FETUS (SEE BOXED WARNING).

CONTRAINDICATIONS
Estrogens should not be used in women with any of the following conditions:
1. Known or suspected cancer of the breast except in appropriately selected patients being treated for metastatic disease.

2. Known or suspected estrogen-dependent neoplasia.
3. Known or suspected pregnancy (see Boxed Warning).
4. Undiagnosed abnormal genital bleeding.
5. Active thrombophlebitis or thromboembolic disorders.
6. A past history of thrombophlebitis, thrombosis, or thromboembolic disorders associated with previous estrogen use (except when used in treatment of breast malignancy).

Premarin Vaginal Cream should not be used in patients hypersensitive to its ingredients.

WARNINGS

1. *Induction of malignant neoplasms.* Long-term, continuous administration of natural and synthetic estrogens in certain animal species increases the frequency of carcinomas of the breast, cervix, vagina, and liver. There are now reports that estrogens increase the risk of carcinoma of the endometrium in humans (see Boxed Warning).

At the present time there is no satisfactory evidence that estrogens given to postmenopausal women increase the risk of cancer of the breast,[17] although a recent long-term follow-up of a single physician's practice has raised this possibility.[18] Because of the animal data, there is a need for caution in prescribing estrogens for women with a strong family history of breast cancer or who have breast nodules, fibrocystic disease, or abnormal mammograms.

2. *Gallbladder disease.* A recent study has reported a 2- to 3-fold increase in the risk of surgically confirmed gallbladder disease in women receiving postmenopausal estrogens,[17] similar to the 2-fold increase previously noted in users of oral contraceptives.[19,24a]

3. *Effects similar to those caused by estrogen-progestogen oral contraceptives.* There are several serious adverse effects of oral contraceptives, some of which have not, up to now, been documented as consequences of postmenopausal estrogen therapy. This may reflect the comparatively low doses of estrogen used in postmenopausal women. It would be expected that the larger doses of estrogen used to treat prostatic or breast cancer are more likely to result in these adverse effects, and, in fact, it has been shown that there is an increased risk of thrombosis in men receiving estrogens for prostatic cancer.[20–23]

a. *Thromboembolic disease.* It is now well established that users of oral contraceptives have an increased risk of various thromboembolic and thrombotic vascular diseases, such as thrombophlebitis, pulmonary embolism, stroke, and myocardial infarction.[24–31] Cases of retinal thrombosis, mesenteric thrombosis, and optic neuritis have been reported in oral-contraceptive users. There is evidence that the risk of several of these adverse reactions is related to the dose of the drug.[32,33] An increased risk of postsurgery thromboembolic complications has also been reported in users of oral contraceptives.[34,35] If feasible, estrogen should be discontinued at least 4 weeks before surgery of the type associated with an increased risk of thromboembolism, or during periods of prolonged immobilization.

In some studies, women on estrogen replacement therapy, given alone or in combination with a progestin, have been reported to have an increased risk of thrombophlebitis, and/or thromboembolic disease. The physician should be aware of the possibility of thrombotic disorders (thrombophlebitis, retinal thrombosis, cerebral embolism, and pulmonary embolism) during estrogen replacement therapy and be alert to their earliest manifestations. Should any of these occur or be suspected, estrogen replacement therapy should be discontinued immediately. Patients who have risk factors for thrombotic disorders should be kept under careful observation. Subgroups of women who have underlying risk factors, or who are receiving relatively large doses of estrogens, may have increased risk. Therefore, estrogens should not be used in persons with active thrombophlebitis or thromboembolic disorders, and they should not be used (except in treatment of malignancy) in persons with a history of such disorders in association with estrogen use. They should be used with caution in patients with cerebral vascular or coronary artery disease and only for those in whom estrogens are clearly needed.

Large doses of estrogen (5 mg conjugated estrogens per day), comparable to those used to treat cancer of the prostate and breast, have been shown in a large prospective clinical trial in men[36] to increase the risk of nonfatal myocardial infarction, pulmonary embolism, and thrombophlebitis. When estrogen doses of this size are used, any of the thromboembolic and thrombotic adverse effects associated with oral contraceptives or estrogen replacement therapy should be considered a clear risk.

b. *Hepatic adenoma.* Benign hepatic adenomas appear to be associated with the use of oral contraceptives.[37–39] Although benign, and rare, these may rupture and may cause death through intra-abdominal hemorrhage. Such lesions have not yet been reported in association with other estrogen or progestogen preparations but should be considered in estrogen users having abdominal pain and tenderness, abdominal mass, or hypovolemic shock. Hepatocellular carcinoma has also been reported in women taking estrogen-containing oral contraceptives.[38] The relationship of this malignancy to these drugs is not known at this time.

c. *Elevated blood pressure.* Women using oral contraceptives sometimes experience increased blood pressure which, in most cases, returns to normal on discontinuing the drug. There is now a report that this may occur with use of estrogens in the menopause[40] and blood pressure should be monitored with estrogen use, especially if high doses are used.

d. *Glucose tolerance.* A worsening of glucose tolerance has been observed in a significant percentage of patients on estrogen-containing oral contraceptives. For this reason, diabetic patients should be carefully observed while receiving estrogen.

4. *Hypercalcemia.* Administration of estrogens may lead to severe hypercalcemia in patients with breast cancer and bone metastases. If this occurs, the drug should be stopped and appropriate measures taken to reduce the serum calcium level.

PRECAUTIONS

A. **General Precautions.**

1. A complete medical and family history should be taken prior to the initiation of any estrogen therapy. The pretreatment and periodic physical examinations should include special reference to blood pressure, breasts, abdomen, and pelvic organs, and should include a Papanicolaou smear. As a general rule, estrogens should not be prescribed for longer than one year without another physical examination being performed.
2. Fluid retention—Because estrogens may cause some degree of fluid retention, conditions which might be influenced by this factor, such as asthma, epilepsy, migraine, and cardiac or renal dysfunction, require careful observation.
3. Familial hyperlipoproteinemia—Estrogen therapy may be associated with massive elevations of plasma triglycerides leading to pancreatitis and other complications in patients with familial defects of lipoprotein metabolism.
4. Certain patients may develop undesirable manifestations of excessive estrogenic stimulation, such as abnormal or excessive uterine bleeding, mastodynia, etc.
5. Prolonged administration of unopposed estrogen therapy has been reported to increase the risk of endometrial hyperplasia in some patients.
6. Oral contraceptives appear to be associated with an increased incidence of mental depression.[24a] Although it is not clear whether this is due to the estrogenic or progestogenic component of the contraceptive, patients with a history of depression should be carefully observed.
7. Preexisting uterine leiomyomata may increase in size during estrogen use.
8. The pathologist should be advised of estrogen therapy when relevant specimens are submitted.
9. Patients with a past history of jaundice during pregnancy have an increased risk of recurrence of jaundice while receiving estrogen-containing oral-contraceptive therapy. If jaundice develops in any patient receiving estrogen, the medication should be discontinued while the cause is investigated.
10. Estrogens may be poorly metabolized in patients with impaired liver function and should be administered with caution in such patients.
11. Because estrogens influence the metabolism of calcium and phosphorus, they should be used with caution in patients with metabolic bone diseases that are associated with hypercalcemia or in patients with renal insufficiency.
12. Because of the effects of estrogens on epiphyseal closure, they should be used judiciously in young patients in whom bone growth is not yet complete.
13. Barrier contraceptives - Premarin Vaginal Cream exposure has been reported to weaken latex condoms. The potential for Premarin Vaginal Cream to weaken and contribute to the failure of condoms, diaphragms, or cervical caps made of latex or rubber should be considered.

Concomitant Progestin Use:

The lowest effective dose appropriate for the specific indication should be utilized. Studies of the addition of a progestin for 7 or more days of a cycle of estrogen administration have reported a lowered incidence of endometrial hyperplasia. Morphological and biochemical studies of the endometrium suggest that 10 to 13 days of progestin are needed to provide maximal maturation of the endometrium and to eliminate any hyperplastic changes. Whether this will provide protection from endometrial carcinoma has not been clearly established. There are possible additional risks which may be associated with the inclusion of progestin in estrogen replacement regimens. If concomitant progestin therapy is used, potential risks may include adverse effects on carbohydrate and lipid metabolism. The choice of progestin and dosage may be important in minimizing these adverse effects.

B. **Information For Patients**

(See text which appears after the **PHYSICIAN REFERENCES**.)

C. **Drug/Laboratory Test Interactions**

Certain endocrine and liver function tests may be affected by estrogen-containing oral contraceptives. The following similar changes may be expected with larger doses of estrogen:

a. Increased sulfobromophthalein retention.
b. Increased prothrombin and factors VII, VIII, IX, and X; decreased antithrombin 3; increased norepinephrine-induced platelet aggregability.
c. Increased thyroid binding globulin (TBG) leading to increased circulating total thyroid hormone, as measured by PBI, T_4 by column, or T_4 by radioimmunoassay. Free T_3 resin uptake is decreased, reflecting the elevated TBG; free T_4 concentration is unaltered.
d. Impaired glucose tolerance.
e. Decreased pregnanediol excretion.
f. Reduced response to metyrapone test.
g. Reduced serum folate concentration.
h. Increased serum triglyceride and phospholipid concentration.

D. **Carcinogenesis, Mutagenesis, Impairment Of Fertility**

(See **WARNINGS** section for information on carcinogenesis.)

E. **Pregnancy Category X**

(See **CONTRAINDICATIONS** and Boxed Warning.)

F. **Nursing Mothers**

It is not known whether this drug is excreted in human milk. Because many drugs are excreted in human milk and because of the potential for serious adverse reactions in nursing infants from estrogens, a decision should be made whether to discontinue nursing or to discontinue the drug, taking into account the importance of the drug to the mother.

G. **Pediatric Use**

Safety and effectiveness in pediatric patients have not been established.

ADVERSE REACTIONS

(See **WARNINGS** regarding induction of neoplasia, adverse effects on the fetus, increased incidence of gallbladder disease, and adverse effects similar to those of oral contraceptives, including thromboembolism.) The following additional adverse reactions have been reported with estrogenic therapy, including oral contraceptives:

1. *Genitourinary system:* Breakthrough bleeding, spotting, change in menstrual flow; dysmenorrhea; premenstrual-like syndrome; amenorrhea during and after treatment; increase in size of uterine fibromyomata; vaginal candidiasis; change in cervical erosion and in degree of cervical secretion; cystitis-like syndrome.
2. *Breasts:* Tenderness, enlargement, secretion.
3. *Gastrointestinal:* Nausea, vomiting, abdominal cramps, bloating; cholestatic jaundice, pancreatitis.
4. *Skin:* Chloasma or melasma which may persist when drug is discontinued; erythema multiforme; erythema nodosum; hemorrhagic eruption; loss of scalp hair; hirsutism.
5. *Cardiovascular:* Venous thromboembolism, pulmonary embolism.
6. *Eyes:* Steepening of corneal curvature; intolerance to contact lenses.
7. *CNS:* Headache, migraine, dizziness; mental depression; chorea.
8. *Miscellaneous:* Increase or decrease in weight; reduced carbohydrate tolerance; aggravation of porphyria; edema; changes in libido.

OVERDOSAGE

Numerous reports of ingestion of large doses of estrogen-containing oral contraceptives by young children indicate that acute serious ill effects do not occur. Overdosage of estrogens may cause nausea, and withdrawal bleeding may occur in females.

DOSAGE AND ADMINISTRATION

Given cyclically for short-term use only:

For treatment of atrophic vaginitis, or kraurosis vulvae.

The lowest dose that will control symptoms should be chosen and medication should be discontinued as promptly as possible.

Administration should be cyclic (e.g., three weeks on and one week off).

Attempts to discontinue or taper medication should be made at three- to six-month intervals.

Usual Dosage Range:

$^1/_2$ to 2 g daily, intravaginally, depending on the severity of the condition.

Treated patients with an intact uterus should be monitored closely for signs of endometrial cancer, and appropriate diagnostic measures should be taken to rule out malignancy in the event of persistent or recurring abnormal vaginal bleeding.

Instructions for Use of Gentle Measure™ Applicator:

1. Remove cap from tube.
2. Screw nozzle end of applicator onto tube.
3. *Gently* squeeze tube from the *bottom* to force sufficient cream into the barrel to provide the prescribed dose. Use the marked stopping points on the applicator as a guideline to measure the correct dose.
4. Unscrew applicator from tube.
5. Lie on back with knees drawn up. To deliver medication, gently insert applicator deeply into vagina and press plunger downward to its original position.

TO CLEANSE: Pull plunger to remove it from barrel. Wash with mild soap and warm water.

DO NOT BOIL OR USE HOT WATER.

HOW SUPPLIED

Premarin® (conjugated estrogens) Vaginal Cream—Each gram contains 0.625 mg conjugated estrogens, USP.

Combination package: Each contains Net Wt. 1$^1/_2$ oz (42.5 g) tube with one plastic applicator calibrated in $^1/_2$ g increments to a maximum of 2 g (NDC 0046-0872-93).

Also Available—Refill package: Each contains Net Wt. 1$^1/_2$ oz (42.5 g) tube (NDC 0046-0872-01).

Store at room temperature (approximately 25° C).

PHYSICIAN REFERENCES

1. Ziel, H. K. et al: N. Engl. J. Med. *293* :1167–1170, 1975.
2. Smith, D. C. et al: N. Engl. J. Med. *293* :1164–1167, 1975.
3. Mack, T. M. et al: N. Engl. J. Med *294* :1262–1267, 1976.

Continued on next page

Premarin Vaginal Cream—Cont.

4. Weiss, N. S. et al: N. Engl. J. Med. *294* :1259–1262, 1976.
5. Herbst, A. L. et al: N. Engl. J. Med. *284* :878–881, 1971.
6. Greenwald, P. et al: N. Engl. J. Med. *285* :390–392, 1971.
7. Lanier, A. et al: Mayo Clin. Proc. *48* :793–799, 1973.
8. Herbst, A. et al: Obstet. Gynecol. *40* :287–298, 1972.
9. Herbst, A. et al: Am. J. Obstet. Gynecol. *118* :607–615, 1974.
10. Herbst, A. et al: N. Engl. J. Med. *292* :334–339, 1975.
11. Stafl, A. et al: Obstet. Gynecol. *43* :118–128, 1974.
12. Sherman, A. I. et al: Obstet. Gynecol. *44* :531–545, 1974.
13. Gal, I. et al: Nature *216* :83, 1967.
14. Levy, E. P. et al: Lancet *1* :611, 1973.
15. Nora, J. et al: Lancet *1* :941–942, 1973.
16. Janerich, D. T. et al: N. Engl. J. Med. *291* :697–700, 1974.
17. Boston Collaborative Drug Surveillance Program: N. Engl. J. Med. *290* :15–19, 1974.
18. Hoover, R. et al: N. Engl. J. Med. *295* :401–405, 1976.
19. Boston Collaborative Drug Surveillance Program: Lancet *1* :1399–1404, 1973.
20. Daniel, D. G. et al: Lancet *2* :287–289, 1967.
21. The Veterans Administration Cooperative Urological Research Group: J. Urol. *98* :516–522, 1967.
22. Bailar, J. C.: Lancet *2* :560, 1967.
23. Blackard, C. et al: Cancer *26* :249–256, 1970.
24. Royal College of General Practitioners: J. R. Coll. Gen. Pract. *13* :267–279, 1967.
24a. Royal College of General Practitioners: Oral Contraceptives and Health, New York, Pitman Corp., 1974.
25. Inman, W. H. W. et al: Br. Med. J. *2* :193–199, 1968.
26. Vessey, M. P. et al: Br. Med. J. *2* :651–657, 1969.
27. Sartwell, P. E. et al: Am. J. Epidemiol. *90* :365–380, 1969.
28. Collaborative Group for the Study of Stroke in Young Women: N. Engl. J. Med. *288* :871–878, 1973.
29. Collaborative Group for the Study of Stroke in Young Women: J.A.M.A. *231* :718–722, 1975.
30. Mann, J. I. et al: Br. Med. J. *2* :245–248, 1975.
31. Mann, J. I. et al: Br. Med. J. *2* :241–245, 1975.
32. Inman, W. H. W. et al: Br. Med. J. *2* :203–209, 1970.
33. Stolley, P. D. et al: Am. J. Epidemiol. *102* :197–208, 1975.
34. Vessey, M. P. et al: Br. Med. J. *3* :123–126, 1970.
35. Greene, G. R. et al: Am. J. Public Health *62* :680–685, 1972.
36. Coronary Drug Project Research Group: J.A.M.A. *214* : 1303–1313, 1970.
37. Baum, J. et al: Lancet *2* :926–928, 1973.
38. Mays, E. T. et al: J.A.M.A. *235* :730–732, 1976.
39. Edmondson, H. A. et al: N. Engl. J. Med. *294* :470–472, 1976.
40. Pfeffer, R. I. et al: Am. J. Epidemiol. *103* :445–456, 1976.

INFORMATION FOR THE PATIENT
WHAT YOU SHOULD KNOW ABOUT ESTROGENS

Estrogens are female hormones produced by the ovaries. The ovaries make several different kinds of estrogens. In addition, scientists have been able to make a variety of synthetic estrogens. As far as we know, all these estrogens have similar properties and, therefore, much the same usefulness, side effects, and risks. This leaflet is intended to help you understand what estrogens are used for, the risks involved in their use, and how to use them as safely as possible.

This leaflet includes the most important information about estrogens, but not all the information. If you want to know more, you should ask your doctor for more information or you can ask your doctor or pharmacist to let you read the package insert prepared for the doctor.

USES OF ESTROGEN

THERE IS NO PROPER USE OF ESTROGENS IN A PREGNANT WOMAN.

Estrogens are prescribed by doctors for a number of purposes, including:

1. To provide estrogen during a period of adjustment when a woman's ovaries stop producing a majority of her estrogens, in order to prevent certain uncomfortable symptoms of estrogen deficiency. (With the menopause, which generally occurs between the ages of 45 and 55, women produce a much smaller amount of estrogens.)
2. To prevent symptoms of estrogen deficiency when a woman's ovaries have been removed surgically before the natural menopause.
3. To prevent pregnancy. (Estrogens are given along with a progestogen, another female hormone; these combinations are called oral contraceptives, or birth-control pills. Patient labeling is available to women taking oral contraceptives and they will not be discussed in this leaflet.)
4. To treat certain cancers in women and men.

ESTROGENS IN THE MENOPAUSE

In the natural course of their lives, all women eventually experience a decrease in estrogen production. This usually occurs between ages 45 and 55, but may occur earlier or later. Sometimes the ovaries may need to be removed before natural menopause by an operation, producing a "surgical menopause."

When the amount of estrogen in the blood begins to decrease, many women may develop typical symptoms: feelings of warmth in the face, neck, and chest, or sudden intense episodes of heat and sweating throughout the body (called "hot flashes" or "hot flushes"). These symptoms are sometimes very uncomfortable. Some women may also develop changes in the vagina (called "atrophic vaginitis") that cause discomfort, especially during and after intercourse.

Estrogens can be prescribed to treat these symptoms of the menopause. It is estimated that considerably more than half of all women undergoing the menopause have only mild symptoms or no symptoms at all and, therefore, do not need estrogens. Other women may need estrogens for a few months, while their bodies adjust to lower estrogen levels. Sometimes the need will be for periods longer than six months. In an attempt to avoid overstimulation of the uterus (womb), estrogens are usually given cyclically during each month of use, such as three weeks of pills followed by one week without pills.

Sometimes women experience nervous symptoms or depression during menopause. There is no evidence that estrogens are effective for such symptoms without associated vasomotor symptoms. In the absence of vasomotor symptoms, estrogens should not be used to treat nervous symptoms, although other treatment may be needed.

You may have heard that taking estrogens for long periods (years) after the menopause will keep your skin soft and supple and keep you feeling young. There is no evidence that this is so, however, and such long-term treatment carries important risks.

THE DANGERS OF ESTROGENS

1. *Endometrial cancer.* There are reports that if estrogens are used in the postmenopausal period for more than a year, there is an increased risk of *endometrial cancer* (cancer of the lining of the uterus). Women taking estrogens have roughly 5- to 10-times as great a chance of getting this cancer as women who take no estrogens. To put this another way, while a postmenopausal woman not taking estrogens has 1 chance in 1,000 each year of getting endometrial cancer, a woman taking estrogens has 5 to 10 chances in 1,000 each year. For this reason *it is important to take estrogens only when they are really needed.*

The risk of this cancer is greater the longer estrogens are used and when larger doses are taken. Therefore, you should not take more estrogen than your doctor prescribes. *It is important to take the lowest dose of estrogen that will control symptoms and to take it only as long as it is needed.* If estrogens are needed for longer periods of time, your doctor will want to reevaluate your need for estrogens at least every six months.

Women using estrogens should report any vaginal bleeding to their doctors; such bleeding may be of no importance, but it can be an early warning of endometrial cancer. If you have undiagnosed vaginal bleeding, you should not use estrogens until a diagnosis is made and you are certain there is no endometrial cancer.

Note: If you have had your uterus removed (total hysterectomy), there is no danger of developing endometrial cancer.

2. *Other possible cancers.* Estrogens can cause development of other tumors in animals, such as tumors of the breast, cervix, vagina, or liver, when given for a long time. At present there is no good evidence that women using estrogens in the menopause have an increased risk of such tumors, but there is no way yet to be sure they do not; and one study raises the possibility that use of estrogens in the menopause may increase the risk of breast cancer many years later. This is a further reason to use estrogens only when clearly needed. While you are taking estrogens, it is important that you go to your doctor at least once a year for a physical examination. Also, if members of your family have had breast cancers or if you have breast nodules, or abnormal mammograms (breast X rays), your doctor may wish to carry out more frequent examinations of your breasts.

3. *Gallbladder disease.* Women who use estrogens after menopause are more likely to develop gallbladder disease needing surgery than women who do not use estrogens. Birth-control pills have a similar effect.

4. *Abnormal blood clotting.* Taking estrogens may increase the risk of blood clotting in various parts of the body. This can result in a stroke (if the clot is in the brain), a heart attack (a clot in a blood vessel of the heart), or a pulmonary embolus (a clot which forms in the legs or pelvis, then breaks off and travels to the lungs). Any of these can be fatal.

It is recommended that if you have had clotting in the legs or lungs, or a heart attack or stroke while you were using estrogens or birth-control pills, you should not use estrogens (unless they are being used to treat cancer of the breast or prostate). If you have had a stroke or heart attack, or if you have angina pectoris, estrogens should be used with great caution and only if clearly needed (for example, if you have severe symptoms of the menopause).

5. *Inflammation of the pancreas (Pancreatitis).* Women with high triglyceride levels may have increased risk of developing inflammation of the pancreas.

SPECIAL WARNING ABOUT PREGNANCY

You should not receive estrogen if you are pregnant. If this should occur, there is a greater than usual chance that the developing child will be born with a birth defect, although the possibility remains fairly small. A female child may have an increased risk of developing cancer of the vagina or cervix later in life (in the teens or twenties). Every possible effort should be made to avoid exposure to estrogens during pregnancy. If exposure occurs, see your doctor.

OTHER EFFECTS OF ESTROGENS

In addition to the serious known risks of estrogens described above, estrogens have the following side effects and potential risks:

1. *Nausea and vomiting.* The most common side effect of estrogen therapy is nausea. Vomiting is less common.
2. *Effects on breasts.* Estrogens may cause breast tenderness or enlargement and may cause the breasts to secrete a liquid. These effects are not dangerous.
3. *Effects on the uterus.* Estrogens may cause benign fibroid tumors of the uterus to get larger.
4. *Effects on liver.* Women taking oral contraceptives develop, on rare occasions, a tumor of the liver which can rupture and bleed into the abdomen and may cause death. So far, these tumors have not been reported in women using estrogens in the menopause, but you should report any swelling or unusual pain or tenderness in the abdomen to your doctor immediately.

Women with a past history of jaundice (yellowing of the skin and white parts of the eyes) may get jaundice again during estrogen use. If this occurs, stop taking estrogens and see your doctor.

5. *Other effects.* Estrogens may cause excess fluid to be retained in the body. This may make some conditions worse, such as asthma, epilepsy, migraine, heart disease, or kidney disease.

SUMMARY

Estrogens have important uses, but they have serious risks as well. You must decide, with your doctor, whether the risks are acceptable to you in view of the benefits of treatment. Except where your doctor has prescribed estrogens for use in special cases of cancer of the breast or prostate, you should not use estrogens if you have cancer of the breast or uterus, are pregnant, have undiagnosed abnormal vaginal bleeding, clotting in the legs or lungs, or have had a stroke, heart attack or angina, or clotting in the legs or lungs in the past while you were taking estrogens.

You can use estrogens as safely as possible by understanding that your doctor will require regular physical examinations while you are taking them, will try to discontinue the drug as soon as possible, and will use the smallest dose possible. Be alert for signs of trouble including:

1. Abnormal bleeding from the vagina.
2. Pains in the calves or chest, sudden shortness of breath, or coughing blood.
3. Severe headache, dizziness, faintness, or changes in vision.
4. Breast lumps (you should ask your doctor how to examine your own breasts).
5. Jaundice (yellowing of the skin).
6. Mental depression.

Your doctor has prescribed this drug for you and you alone. Do not give the drug to anyone else.

Premarin Vaginal Cream exposure has been reported to weaken latex condoms. The potential for Premarin Vaginal Cream to weaken and contribute to the failure of condoms, diaphragms, or cervical caps made of latex or rubber should be considered.

HOW SUPPLIED

Premarin® (conjugated estrogens) Vaginal Cream—Each gram contains 0.625 mg conjugated estrogens, USP.

Combination package: Each contains Net Wt. $1^1/_2$ oz (42.5 g) tube with one plastic applicator calibrated in $^1/_2$ g increments to a maximum of 2 g (NDC 0046-0872-93).

Also Available—Refill package: Each contains Net Wt. $1^1/_2$ oz (42.5 g) tube (NDC 0046-0872-01).

Store at room temperature (approximately 25° C).

INSTRUCTIONS FOR USE OF PREMARIN®
(conjugated estrogens)
Vaginal Cream Gentle Measure™ Applicator:

The Gentle Measure Applicator has been specifically designed for comfortable, easy use.

1. Remove cap from tube.
2. Screw nozzle end of applicator onto tube.
3. *Gently* squeeze tube from the *bottom* to force sufficient cream into the barrel to provide the prescribed dose. Use the marked stopping points on the applicator as a guideline to measure the correct dose.
4. Unscrew applicator from tube.
5. Lie on back with knees drawn up. To deliver medication, gently insert applicator deeply into vagina and press plunger downward to its original position.

TO CLEANSE: Pull plunger to remove it from barrel. Wash with mild soap and warm water.

DO NOT BOIL OR USE HOT WATER.

Manufactured by:
Ayerst Laboratories Inc.
A Wyeth-Ayerst Company
Philadelphia, PA 19101
CI 4856-3 Revised May 5, 1998

Shown in Product Identification Guide, page 342

PREMPRO™ ℞
(conjugated estrogens/medroxyprogesterone acetate tablets)

PREMPHASE®
(conjugated estrogens/medroxyprogesterone acetate tablets)

Caution: Federal law prohibits dispensing without prescription.

Table 1. PHARMACOKINETIC PARAMETERS FOR UNCONJUGATED AND CONJUGATED ESTROGENS (CE), AND MEDROXYPROGESTERONE ACETATE

DRUG	2 × 0.625 mg CE/2.5 mg MPA Combination Tablets (n=54)				2 × 0.625 mg CE/5 mg MPA Combination Tablets (n=51)			
PK Parameter Geometric Mean (SD)	C_{max} (pg/mL)	t_{max} (h)	$t_{1/2}$ (h)	AUC (pg•h/mL)	C_{max} (pg/mL)	t_{max} (h)	(h)	AUC (pg•h/mL)
Unconjugated Estrogens								
Estrone	175 (41)	7.6 (1.8)	31.6 (7.4)	5358 (1840)	124 (53)	10 (3.5)	62.2 (85.2)	6303 (2542)
BA*-Estrone	159 (41)	7.6 (1.8)	16.9 (5.8)	3313 (1310)	104 (51)	10 (3.5)	26.0 (25.9)	3136 (1598)
Equilin	71 (22)	5.8 (2.0)	9.9 (3.5)	951 (413)	52 (23)	8.9 (3.0)	15.5 (8.2)	1179 (540)
PK Parameter Geometric Mean (SD)	C_{max} (ng/mL)	t_{max} (h)	$t_{1/2}$ (h)	AUC (ng•h/mL)	C_{max} (ng/mL)	t_{max} (h)	$t_{1/2}$ (h)	AUC (ng•h/mL)
Conjugated Estrogens								
Total Estrone	6.6 (2.5)	6.1 (1.7)	20.7 (7.0)	116 (68)	6.3 (3.0)	9.1 (2.6)	23.6 (8.4)	151 (63)
BA*-Total Estrone	6.4 (2.5)	6.1 (1.7)	15.4 (5.2)	100 (57)	6.2 (3.0)	9.1 (2.6)	20.6 (7.3)	139 (56)
Total Equilin	5.1 (2.3)	4.6 (1.6)	11.4 (2.9)	50 (35)	4.2 (2.2)	7.0 (2.5)	17.2 (22.6)	72 (36)
Medroxyprogesterone Acetate	C_{max} (ng/mL)	t_{max} (h)	$t_{1/2}$ (h)	Cl/F (L/h/kg)	C_{max} (ng/mL)	t_{max} (h)	$t_{1/2}$ (h)	Cl/F (L/h/kg)
MPA	1.5 (0.6)	2.8 (1.5)	37.6 (11.2)	2.3 (0.7)	48 (1.5)	2.4 (1.2)	46.3 (18.0)	1.6 (0.5)

BA* = Baseline Adjusted
C_{max} = peak plasma concentration
t_{max} = time peak concentration occurs
$t_{1/2}$ = terminal-phase disposition half-life ($0.693/\lambda_z$)
AUC = total area under the curve
Cl/F = apparent oral clearance

DESCRIPTION

PREMPRO therapy consists of a single tablet containing 0.625 mg of the conjugated estrogens found in Premarin® tablets and 2.5 mg or 5 mg of medroxyprogesterone acetate (MPA) for oral administration.

PREMPHASE therapy consists of two separate tablets, a maroon Premarin tablet containing 0.625 mg of conjugated estrogens which is taken orally on days 1 through 14 and a light-blue tablet containing 0.625 mg of the conjugated estrogens found in Premarin tablets and 5 mg of medroxyprogesterone acetate (MPA) which is taken orally on days 15 through 28.

The conjugated estrogens found in Premarin tablets are a mixture of sodium estrone sulfate and sodium equilin sulfate. They contain as concomitant components, as sodium sulfate conjugates, 17α-dihydroequilin, 17α-estradiol and 17β-dihydroequilin.

Medroxyprogesterone acetate is a derivative of progesterone. It is a white to off-white, odorless, crystalline powder, stable in air, melting between 200° C and 210° C. It is freely soluble in chloroform, soluble in acetone and in dioxane, sparingly soluble in alcohol and in methanol, slightly soluble in ether, and insoluble in water. The chemical name for MPA is pregn-4-ene-3,20-dione, 17-(acetyloxy)-6-methyl-, (6α)-. Its molecular formula is $C_{24}H_{34}O_4$, with a molecular weight of 386.53. Its structural formula is:

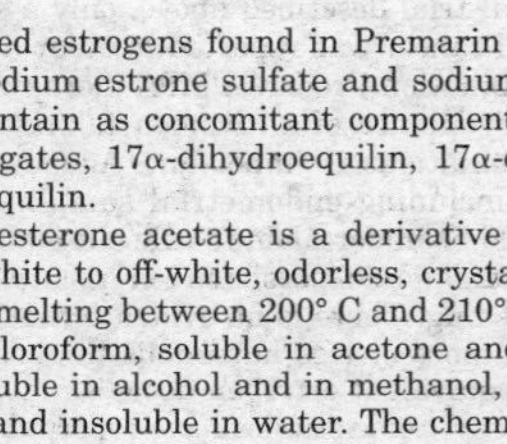

<u>PREMPRO 2.5 mg</u>

Each peach tablet for oral administration contains 0.625 mg conjugated estrogens, 2.5 mg of medroxyprogesterone acetate and the following inactive ingredients: calcium phosphate tribasic, calcium sulfate, carnauba wax, cellulose, glyceryl monooleate, lactose, magnesium stearate, methylcellulose, pharmaceutical glaze, polyethylene glycol, sucrose, povidone, titanium dioxide, and red ferric oxide.

<u>PREMPRO 5.0 mg</u>

Each light-blue tablet for oral administration contains 0.625 mg conjugated estrogens, 5 mg of medroxyprogesterone acetate and the following inactive ingredients: calcium phosphate tribasic, calcium sulfate, carnauba wax, cellulose, glyceryl monooleate, lactose, magnesium stearate, methylcellulose, pharmaceutical glaze, polyethylene glycol, sucrose, povidone, titanium dioxide, FD&C Blue No. 2.

<u>PREMPHASE</u>

Each maroon Premarin tablet for oral administration contains 0.625 mg of conjugated estrogens and the following inactive ingredients: calcium phosphate tribasic, calcium sulfate, carnauba wax, cellulose, glyceryl monooleate, lactose, magnesium stearate, methylcellulose, pharmaceutical glaze, polyethylene glycol, stearic acid, sucrose, titanium dioxide, FD&C Blue No.2, D&C Red No. 27, FD&C Red No. 40. These tablets comply with USP Drug Release Test 1.

Each light-blue tablet for oral administration contains 0.625 mg of conjugated estrogens and 5 mg of medroxyprogesterone acetate and the following inactive ingredients: calcium phosphate tribasic, calcium sulfate, carnauba wax, cellulose, glyceryl monooleate, lactose, magnesium stearate, methylcellulose, pharmaceutical glaze, polyethylene glycol, sucrose, povidone, titanium dioxide, FD&C Blue No.2.

CLINICAL PHARMACOLOGY

Estrogens are largely responsible for the development and maintenance of the female reproductive system and secondary sexual characteristics. By a direct action, they cause growth and development of the uterus, fallopian tubes, and vagina. With other hormones, such as pituitary hormones and progesterone, they cause enlargement of the breasts through promotion of ductal growth, stromal development, and the accretion of fat. Estrogens are intricately involved with other hormones, especially progesterone, in the processes of the ovulatory menstrual cycle and pregnancy and affect the release of pituitary gonadotropins. They also contribute to the shaping of the skeleton, maintenance of tone and elasticity of urogenital structures, changes in the epiphyses of the long bones that allow for the pubertal growth spurt and its termination, and pigmentation of the nipples and genitals.

Although circulating estrogens exist in a dynamic equilibrium of metabolic interconversions, estradiol is the principal intracellular human estrogen and is substantially more potent than its metabolites, estrone and estriol at the receptor level. The primary source of estrogen in normally cycling adult women is the ovarian follicle, which secretes 70 to 500 µg of estradiol daily, depending on the phase of the menstrual cycle. After menopause, most endogenous estrogen is produced by interconversion of androstenedione, secreted by the adrenal cortex, to estrone by peripheral tissues. Thus, estrone and the sulfate conjugated form, estrone sulfate, are the most abundant circulating estrogens in postmenopausal women.

Circulating estrogens modulate the pituitary secretion of gonadotropins, luteinizing hormone (LH) and follicle stimulating hormone (FSH) through a negative feedback mechanism. Estrogen replacement therapy acts to reduce the elevated levels of these hormones seen in postmenopausal women.

The pharmacologic effects of the administered conjugated estrogens are similar to those of endogenous estrogens. In responsive tissue (female genital organs, breasts, hypothalamus, pituitary) estrogens enter the cell and are transported into the nucleus. As a result of the estrogen action, specific RNA and protein synthesis occurs.

The use of unopposed estrogen therapy has been associated with an increased risk of endometrial hyperplasia, a possible precursor of endometrial adenocarcinoma. The results of clinical studies indicate that the addition of a progestin to an estrogen replacement regimen for more than 10 days per cycle reduces the incidence of endometrial hyperplasia and the attendant risk of adenocarcinoma in women with intact uteri. The addition of a progestin to an estrogen replacement regimen has not been shown to interfere with the efficacy of estrogen replacement therapy for its approved indications.

Androgenic and anabolic effects of medroxyprogesterone acetate (MPA) have been noted, but the drug is apparently devoid of significant estrogenic activity. Parenterally administered MPA inhibits gonadotropin production, which in turn prevents follicular maturation and ovulation, although available data indicate that this does not occur when the usually recommended oral dosage is given as single daily doses. MPA may achieve its beneficial effect on the endometrium in part by decreasing nuclear estradiol receptors and suppression of epithelial DNA synthesis in endometrial tissue.

PHARMACOKINETICS

Absorption

Conjugated estrogens are soluble in water and are well absorbed from the gastrointestinal tract after release from the drug formulation. However, PREMPRO and PREMPHASE contain a formulation of MPA that is immediately released and a modified-release formulation of conjugated estrogens that slowly releases estrogens over several hours. Maximum plasma concentrations of the various conjugated and unconjugated estrogens are attained within 4 to 10 hours after dose administration. MPA is well absorbed from the gastrointestinal tract, and maximum MPA plasma concentrations are attained within 2 to 4 hours after dose administration. Table 1 summarizes the mean pharmacokinetic parameters for unconjugated and conjugated estrogens, and medroxyprogesterone acetate following administration of 0.625 mg/2.5 mg and 0.625 mg/5mg tablets to healthy postmenopausal women.

Food-Effect: Single dose studies in healthy, postmenopausal women were conducted to investigate any potential drug interaction when PREMPRO or PREMPHASE is administered with a high fat breakfast. Administration with food decreased the C_{max} of total estrone by 18 to 34% and increased total equilin C_{max} by 38% compared to the fasting state, with no other effect on the rate or extent of absorption of other conjugated or unconjugated estrogens. Administration with food approximately doubles MPA C_{max} and increases MPA AUC by approximately 20 to 30%.

Dose Proportionality: The C_{max} and AUC values for MPA observed in two separate pharmacokinetic studies conducted with PREMPRO or PREMPHASE 2 × 0.625 mg/2.5 mg and 2 × 0.625 mg/5mg tablets exhibited nonlinear dose proportionality; doubling the MPA dose from 2 × 2.5 to 2 × 5.0 mg increased the mean C_{max} and AUC by 3.2 and 2.8 folds, respectively. The apparent clearance (Cl/F) of MPA obtained with 2 × 0.625 mg/5 mg tablets was lower than that observed with 2 × 0.625 mg/2.5 mg tablets.

[See table above]

Distribution

The conjugated estrogens bind mainly to albumin, but the unconjugated estrogens bind to both albumin and sex-hormone-binding globulin (SHBG). MPA is approximately 90% bound to plasma proteins but does not bind to SHBG.

Metabolism

Metabolism and inactivation of estrogens occur primarily in the liver. Some estrogens are excreted into the bile; however, they are reabsorbed from the intestine and returned to the liver through the portal venous system. Metabolism and elimination of MPA occurs primarily in the liver via hydroxylation, with subsequent conjugation and elimination in the urine.

Excretion

Water-soluble estrogen conjugates are strongly acidic and are ionized in body fluids, which favor excretion through the kidneys since tubular reabsorption is minimal. The apparent terminal-phase disposition half-life ($t_{1/2}$) of the various estrogens is prolonged by the slow absorption from PREMPRO and PREMPHASE and ranges from 10 to 24 hours. Most metabolites of MPA are excreted as glucuronide conjugates with only minor amounts excreted as sulfates. MPA has a $t_{1/2}$ ranging from 38 to 46 hours.

Drug-Interactions

Coadministration of conjugated estrogens with MPA does not affect the pharmacokinetic profile of MPA. Similarly, MPA does not affect the pharmacokinetic profile of the conjugated or unconjugated estrogens.

CLINICAL STUDIES

In a 1-year clinical trial of 1376 women randomized to PREMPRO 0.625 mg/2.5 mg (Regimen A, n=340), PREMPRO 0.625 mg/5 mg (Regimen B, n=338), PREMPHASE 0.625 mg/5 mg (Regimen C, n=351), or Premarin 0.625 mg alone (n=347), results of evaluable biopsies at 12 months

Continued on next page

Prempro—Cont.

(n=279 for Regimen A, 274 for Regimen B, 277 for Regimen C, and 283 for Premarin alone) showed a reduced risk of endometrial hyperplasia in the two PREMPRO treatment groups (less than 1%) and in the PREMPHASE treatment group (less than 1%; 1% when focal hyperplasia was included) compared to the Premarin group (8%; 20% when focal hyperplasia was included). See Table 2.

[See table 2 at right]

In this clinical trial the incidence of amenorrhea increased over time in both PREMPRO groups. Seventeen percent of the patients randomized to Regimen A experienced amenorrhea during the entire 13 cycles of the study, and 15 percent of the patients on Regimen B experienced amenorrhea during the entire 13 cycles of the study. The following two figures describe cumulative amenorrhea which is defined as amenorrhea continuing from a given cycle to the end of the study.

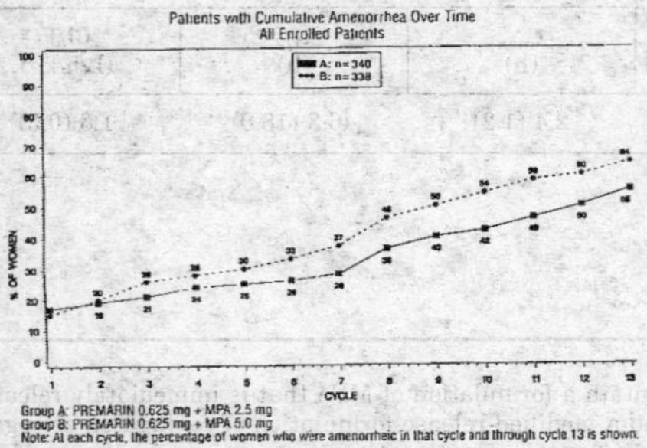

Group A: PREMARIN 0.625 mg + MPA 2.5 mg
Group B: PREMARIN 0.625 mg + MPA 5.0 mg
Note: At each cycle, the percentage of women who were amenorrheic in that cycle and through cycle 13 is shown.

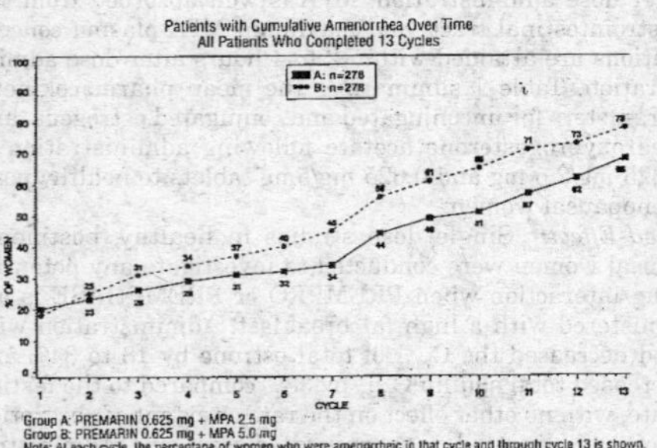

Group A: PREMARIN 0.625 mg + MPA 2.5 mg
Group B: PREMARIN 0.625 mg + MPA 5.0 mg
Note: At each cycle, the percentage of women who were amenorrheic in that cycle and through cycle 13 is shown.

Information Regarding Lipid Effects

The results of a clinical trial conducted in a 97% Caucasian population at low risk for cardiovascular disease, showed that the increases in HDL-C and HDL_2-C subfraction were significantly less for PREMPRO and PREMPHASE than Premarin alone, but decreases in LDL-C were comparable with Premarin alone. Compared with Premarin, total Cholesterol concentrations were significantly lower after 1 year of treatment than at baseline among patients receiving PREMPRO or PREMPHASE.

The following table summarizes mean percent changes from baseline lipid parameter values after 1 year of treatment with the combined regimens.

[See table 3 above]

For information regarding cardiovascular effects in the general population as well as in women with documented coronary heart disease, see **PRECAUTIONS, General**—*Cardiovascular Risk*.

Table 2. INCIDENCE OF ENDOMETRIAL HYPERPLASIA AFTER ONE YEAR OF TREATMENT

	– – – – Groups – – – –			
Patient	PREMPRO 0.625 mg/2.5 mg	PREMPRO 0.625 mg/5 mg	PREMPHASE 0.625 mg/5 mg	Premarin 0.625 mg
Total number of patients	340	338	351	347
Number of patients with evaluable biopsies	279	274	277	283
No. (%) of patients with biopsies				
• all focal and non-focal hyperplasia	2 (<1)*	0 (0)*	3 (1)*	57 (20)
• excluding focal cystic hyperplasia	2 (<1)*	0 (0)*	1 (<1)*	25 (8)

*Significant ($p < 0.001$) in comparison with Premarin (0.625 mg) alone.

Table 3. MEAN PERCENT CHANGE FROM BASELINE LIPID PROFILE VALUES AFTER ONE YEAR OF TREATMENT

	– – – – – – Treatment Groups – – – – – –			
	PREMPRO 0.625 mg/2.5 mg n=90	PREMPRO 0.625 mg/5 mg n=84	PREMPHASE 0.625 mg/5 mg n=95	Premarin 0.625 mg n=86
Lipid Parameter				
Total Cholesterol	-4.7†	-4.2†	-3.5†	0.2
HDL-C	3.5†	3.7†	4.4†	14.1
HDL_2-C	34.7†	40.1†	30.3†	70.8
LDL-C	-10.3	-8.8	-8.7	-7.7
Triglycerides	24.1†	19.1†	27.5†	39.4

†Significantly ($p \leq 0.05$) different from Premarin alone.

INDICATIONS AND USAGE

PREMPRO or PREMPHASE therapy is indicated in women with an intact uterus for the:

1. Treatment of moderate to severe vasomotor symptoms associated with the menopause. There is no adequate evidence that estrogens are effective for nervous symptoms or depression which might occur during menopause and they should not be used to treat these conditions.
2. Treatment of vulvar and vaginal atrophy.
3. Prevention of osteoporosis.

Since estrogen administration is associated with risks as well as benefits, selection of patients ideally should be based on prospective identification of risk factors for developing osteoporosis. Unfortunately, there is no certain way to identify those women who will develop osteoporotic fractures. Most prospective studies of efficacy for this indication have been carried out in white menopausal women, without stratification by other risk factors, and tend to show a universally salutary effect on bone. Thus, patient selection must be individualized based on the balance of risks and benefits.

Estrogen replacement therapy reduces bone resorption and retards or halts postmenopausal bone loss. Case-control studies have shown an approximately 60% reduction in hip and wrist fractures in women whose estrogen replacement was begun within a few years of menopause. Studies also suggest that estrogen reduces the rate of vertebral fractures. Even when started as late as 6 years after menopause, estrogen may prevent further loss of bone mass for as long as the treatment is continued. When estrogen therapy is discontinued, bone mass declines at a rate comparable to that in the immediate postmenopausal period. There is no evidence that estrogen replacement therapy restores bone mass to premenopausal levels.

At skeletal maturity there are sex and race differences in both the total amount of bone present and its density, in favor of men and blacks. Thus, women are at higher risk than men because they start with less bone mass and, for several years following natural or induced menopause, the rate of bone mass decline is accelerated. White and Asian women are at higher risk than black women.

Early menopause is one of the strongest predictors for the development of osteoporosis. In addition, other factors affecting the skeleton which are associated with osteoporosis include genetic factors (small build, family history), endocrine factors (nulliparity, thyrotoxicosis, hyperparathyroidism, Cushing's syndrome, hyperprolactinemia, type I diabetes), lifestyle (cigarette smoking, alcohol abuse, sedentary exercise habits) and nutrition (below average body weight, dietary calcium intake).

The mainstays of prevention and management of osteoporosis are estrogen, an adequate lifetime calcium intake, and exercise. Postmenopausal women absorb dietary calcium less efficiently than premenopausal women and require an average of 1500 mg/day of elemental calcium to remain in neutral calcium balance. By comparison, premenopausal women require about 1000 mg/day and the average calcium intake in the USA is 400–600 mg/day. Therefore, when not contraindicated, calcium supplementation may be helpful.

Weight-bearing exercise and nutrition may be important adjuncts to the prevention and management of osteoporosis. Immobilization and prolonged bed rest produce rapid bone loss, while weight-bearing exercise has been shown both to reduce bone loss and to increase bone mass. The optimal type and amount of physical activity that would prevent osteoporosis have not been established; however, in two studies an hour of walking and running exercises twice or three times weekly significantly increased lumbar spine bone mass.

CONTRAINDICATIONS

Estrogens/progestins combined should not be used in women under any of the following conditions or circumstances:

1. Known or suspected pregnancy, including use for missed abortion or as a diagnostic test for pregnancy. Estrogen or progestin may cause fetal harm when administered to a pregnant woman.
2. Known or suspected cancer of the breast.
3. Known or suspected estrogen-dependent neoplasia.
4. Undiagnosed abnormal genital bleeding.
5. Active or past history of thrombophlebitis, thromboembolic disorders, or stroke.
6. Liver dysfunction or disease.

PREMPRO or PREMPHASE therapy should not be used in patients hypersensitive to the ingredients contained in the tablets.

WARNINGS

ALL WARNINGS BELOW PERTAIN TO THE USE OF THIS COMBINATION PRODUCT.

Based on experience with estrogens and/or progestins:

1. *Induction of malignant neoplasms*

Endometrial cancer. The reported endometrial cancer risk among users of unopposed estrogen was about 2- to 12-fold greater than in nonusers and appears dependent on duration of treatment and on estrogen dose. There is no significant increased risk associated with the use of estrogens for less than one year. The greatest risk appears associated with prolonged use, with increased risks of 15- to 24-fold for five years or more. In three studies, persistence of risk was demonstrated for 8 to over 15 years after cessation of estrogen treatment. In one study, a significant decrease in the incidence of endometrial cancer occurred six months after estrogen withdrawal.

A large clinical trial has demonstrated that when MPA is administered with Premarin, there is a markedly reduced incidence of endometrial hyperplasia, a possible precursor of endometrial cancer. Endometrial hyperplasia has been reported in a large clinical trial to occur at a rate of approximately 1% or less with PREMPRO AND PREMPHASE. Studies have also demonstrated a reduced risk of endometrial cancer when a progestin is administered with estrogen replacement therapy. In the large clinical trial described above, only a single case of endometrial cancer was reported to occur among women taking combination Premarin/MPA therapy.

Clinical surveillance of all women taking estrogen/progestin combinations is important. Adequate diagnostic measures, including endometrial sampling when indicated, should be undertaken to rule out malignancy in all cases of undiagnosed persistent or recurring abnormal vaginal bleeding. There is no evidence that "natural" estrogens are more or less hazardous than "synthetic" estrogens at equivalent estrogen doses.

Breast cancer. Some studies have reported a moderately increased risk of breast cancer (relative risk of 1.3 to 2.0) in those women on estrogen replacement therapy taking higher doses, or in those taking lower doses for prolonged periods of time, especially in excess of 10 years. The majority of studies, however, have not shown an association in women who have ever used estrogen replacement therapy.

The effect of added progestins on the risk of breast cancer is unknown, although a moderately increased risk in those taking combination estrogen/progestin therapy has been reported. Other studies have not shown this relationship. In a one year clinical trial of PREMPRO, PREMPHASE and Premarin alone, 5 new cases of breast cancer were detected among 1377 women who received the combination treatments, while no new cases were detected among 347 women who received Premarin alone. The overall incidence of breast cancer in this clinical trial does not exceed that expected in the general population. In the three year clinical Postmenopausal Estrogen Progestin Intervention (PEPI) trial of 875 women to assess differences among placebo, unopposed Premarin, and three different combination hormone therapy regimens, one (1) new case of breast cancer was detected in the placebo group (n=174), one in the Premarin alone group (n=175), none in the continuous Premarin plus continuous medroxyprogesterone acetate group (n=174), and two (2) in the continuous Premarin plus cyclic medroxyprogesterone acetate group (n=174).

Women on hormone replacement therapy should have regular breast examinations and should be instructed in breast self-examination, and women over the age of 50 should have regular mammograms.

2. *Thromboembolic Disorders and Other Vascular Problems.* In some studies, women on estrogen replacement therapy, given alone or in combination with a progestin, have been reported to have an increased risk of thrombophlebitis, and/or thromboembolic disease. The physician should be aware of the possibility of thrombotic disorders (thrombophlebitis, retinal thrombosis, cerebral embolism, and pulmonary embolism) during hormone replacement therapy and be alert to their earliest manifestations. Should any of these occur or be suspected, hormone replacement therapy should be discontinued immediately. Women who have risk factors for thrombotic disorders should be kept under careful observation.
3. *Effects during pregnancy.* Use in pregnancy is not recommended.

4. *Gallbladder disease.* Two studies have reported a 2- to 4-fold increase in the risk of surgically confirmed gallbladder disease in women receiving postmenopausal estrogens. In a large clinical trial, 5 of 1376 subjects taking Premarin alone or Premarin/Cycrin® at doses comparable to PREMPRO or PREMPHASE developed cholecystitis with cholelithiasis that required cholecystectomy.
5. *Elevated blood pressure.* Occasional blood pressure increases during estrogen replacement therapy have been attributed to idiosyncratic reactions to estrogens. More often, blood pressure has remained the same or has dropped. One study showed that postmenopausal estrogen users have higher blood pressure than nonusers. In a large clinical trial, transient elevations from baseline of 40 mm Hg or more systolic and 20 mm Hg or more diastolic were reported in less than 2% and 4% of postmenopausal subjects, respectively. Two other studies showed slightly lower blood pressure among estrogen users compared to nonusers. Postmenopausal estrogen use does not increase the risk of stroke. Nonetheless, blood pressure should be monitored at regular intervals with estrogen use.
6. *Hypercalcemia.* Administration of estrogens may lead to severe hypercalcemia in patients with breast cancer and bone metastases. If this occurs, the drugs should be stopped and appropriate measures taken to reduce the serum calcium level.
7. *Visual abnormalities.* Discontinue medication pending examination if there is sudden partial or complete loss of vision, or a sudden onset of proptosis, diplopia, or migraine. If examination reveals papilledema or retinal vascular lesions, medication should be withdrawn.

PRECAUTIONS

General

Based on experience with estrogens and/or progestins:
1. *Cardiovascular Risk.* A causal relationship between estrogen replacement therapy and reduction of cardiovascular disease in postmenopausal women has not been proven. Furthermore, the effect of added progestins on this putative benefit is not yet known.
Current medical practice often includes the use of concomitant progestin therapy in women with intact uteri. While the effects of added progestins on the risk of ischemic heart disease are not known, medroxyprogesterone acetate at the doses in PREMPRO or PREMPHASE attenuates much of the favorable effect of conjugated estrogens on HDL levels, although it maintains the favorable effect of conjugated estrogens on LDL levels (see **CLINICAL STUDIES**).
Studies in the General Population:
In recent years many published studies have suggested that there may be a cause-effect relationship between postmenopausal oral estrogen replacement therapy *without added progestins* and a decrease in cardiovascular disease in women. Although most of the observational studies which assessed this statistical association have reported a 20% to 50% reduction in coronary heart disease risk and associated mortality in estrogen takers, the following should be considered when interpreting these reports.
Because only one of these studies was randomized and it was too small to yield statistically significant results, all relevant studies were subject to selection bias. Thus, the apparently reduced risk of coronary heart disease cannot be attributed with certainty to estrogen replacement therapy. It may instead have been caused by life-style and medical characteristics of the women studied with the result that healthier women were selected for estrogen therapy. In general, treated women were of higher socioeconomic and educational status, more slender, more physically active, more likely to have undergone surgical menopause, and less likely to have diabetes than the untreated women. Although some studies attempted to control for these selection factors, it is common for properly designed randomized trials to fail to confirm benefits suggested by less rigorous study designs. Ongoing large-scale trials are intended to further explore this relationship.
The safety data regarding PREMPRO and PREMPHASE were obtained primarily from clinical trials and epidemiologic studies of postmenopausal Caucasian women, who were at generally low risk for cardiovascular disease and higher than average risk for osteoporosis. The safety profile of PREMPRO and PREMPHASE derived from these study populations cannot necessarily be extrapolated to other populations of diverse racial and/or demographic composition.
Stuides in Women with Documented Coronary Heart Disease:
In the Heart and Estrogen/progestin Replacement Study (HERS), 2763 postmenopausal women with documented coronary heart disease (CHD) who were taking their usual cardiac medications were randomized to Prempro 0.625 mg/2.5 mg or placebo. Documented CHD was defined as the presence of one or more of the following: previous myocardial infarction, previous percutaneous mechanical revascularization, previous coronary artery bypass graft surgery, or angiographic evidence of greater than 50% occlusion of one or more major coronary arteries. During an average follow-up of 4.1 years, treatment with Prempro did not reduce the overall rate of recurrent coronary heart disease events, defined as CHD death or nonfatal myocardial infarctions, in this predominantly elderly population (average age 66.7 years) with established coronary disease. There were more CHD events in the hormone group than in the placebo group in year 1 and fewer events in years 3 through 5.
When considering prescribing an estrogen/progestin regimen, such as PREMPRO or PREMPHASE, physicians are advised to weigh the potential benefits and risks of therapy as applicable to each individual patient.
2. *Use in hysterectomized women.* Existing data do not support the use of the combination of estrogen and progestin in postmenopausal women without a uterus. There are possible risks which may be associated with the inclusion of progestin in estrogen replacement regimens. The potential risks include some deterioration in glucose tolerance, as reported in a large clinical trial of PREMPRO and PREMPHASE, and less favorable effects on lipid metabolism as compared to the lipid effects of Premarin alone (see **CLINICAL STUDIES**).
3. *Physical examination.* A complete medical and family history should be taken prior to the initiation of any estrogen/progestin therapy. The pretreatment and periodic physical examinations should include special reference to blood pressure, breasts, abdomen, and pelvic organs, and should include a Papanicolaou smear. As a general rule, estrogen should not be prescribed for longer than one year without another physical examination being performed.
4. *Fluid retention.* Because estrogens/progestins may cause some degree of fluid retention, conditions which might be influenced by this factor, such as asthma, epilepsy, migraine, and cardiac or renal dysfunction, require careful observation.
5. *Uterine bleeding.* Certain patients may develop abnormal uterine bleeding. In cases of undiagnosed abnormal uterine bleeding, adequate diagnostic measures are indicated. (See **WARNINGS**.)
6. The pathologist should be advised of estrogen/progestin therapy when relevant specimens are submitted.
Based on experience with estrogens:
1. *Familial hyperlipoproteinemia.* Estrogen therapy may be associated with massive elevations of plasma triglycerides leading to pancreatitis and other complications in patients with familial defects of lipoprotein metabolism.
2. *Hypercoagulability.* Some epidemiological studies have shown that women taking estrogen replacement therapy have hypercoagulability primarily related to decreased antithrombin activity. This effect appears dose- and duration-dependent and is less pronounced than that associated with oral contraceptive use. Also, postmenopausal women tend to have changes in levels of coagulation parameters at baseline compared to premenopausal women. There is some suggestion that low-dose mestranol may increase the risk of thromboembolism in postmenopausal women. There is insufficient information on hypercoagulability in women who have had previous thromboembolic disease. In a clinical trial of 1724 patients, in which 204 PREMPRO™-treated patients and 107 PREMPHASE®-treated patients had metabolic studies performed, factors VII and X concentrations and plasminogen activity increased at the end of 1 year, and antithrombin III activity decreased in women receiving PREMPRO 0.625 mg/2.5 mg MPA or PREMPHASE 0.625 mg/5 mg MPA at the end of the year. At the end of the year, antithrombin III activity increased slightly in women receiving PREMPRO 0.625 mg/5.0 mg MPA.
3. *Mastodynia.* Certain patients may develop undesirable manifestations of estrogenic stimulation such as mastodynia. In a large clinical trial of PREMPRO, PREMPHASE, and Premarin®, approximately one third of the subjects receiving PREMPRO and approximately one third of the subjects receiving PREMPHASE reported breast pain during treatment versus 12% for Premarin alone.
Based on experience with progestins:
1. *Lipoprotein metabolism.* See **CLINICAL STUDIES.**
2. *Impaired glucose tolerance.* See *Use in hysterectomized women,* above.
3. *Depression.* Patients who have a history of depression should be observed and the drugs discontinued if the depression recurs to a serious degree.

Information for the Patient

See text of Patient Package Insert which appears after the **HOW SUPPLIED** section.

Drug/Laboratory Test Interactions

1. Accelerated prothrombin time, partial thromboplastin time, and platelet aggregation time; increased platelet count; increased factors II, VII antigen, VIII coagulant activity, IX, X, XII, VII-X complex, II-VII-X complex, and beta-thromboglobulin; decreased levels of anti-factor Xa and antithrombin III, decreased antithrombin III activity; increased levels of fibrinogen and fibrinogen activity; increased plasminogen antigen and activity.
2. Increased thyroid-binding globulin (TBG) leading to increased circulating total thyroid hormone, as measured by protein-bound iodine (PBI), T_4 levels (by column or by radioimmunoassay) or T_3 levels by radioimmunoassay, T_3 resin uptake is decreased, reflecting the elevated TBG. Free T_4 and free T_3 concentrations are unaltered.
3. Other binding proteins may be elevated in serum, i.e., corticosteroid binding globulin (CBG), sex hormone-binding globulin (SHBG), leading to increased circulating corticosteroids and sex steroids respectively. Free or biologically active hormone concentrations are unchanged. Other plasma proteins may be increased (angiotensinogen/renin substrate, alpha-1-antitrypsin, ceruloplasmin).
4. Increased plasma HDL and HDL-2 subfraction concentrations, reduced LDL cholesterol concentration, increased triglyceride levels.
5. Impaired glucose tolerance. For this reason, diabetic patients should be carefully observed while receiving estrogen/progestin therapy.
6. Reduced response to metyrapone test.
7. Reduced serum folate concentration.
8. Aminoglutethimide administered concomitantly with MPA may significantly depress the bioavailability of MPA.

Carcinogenesis, Mutagenesis, and Impairment of Fertility.

Long term continuous administration of natural and synthetic estrogens in certain animal species increases the frequency of carcinomas of the breasts, uterus, cervix, vagina, testis, and liver. (See **CONTRAINDICATIONS** and **WARNINGS**.)
In a two-year oral study of MPA in which female rats were exposed to dosages of up to 5000 µg/kg/day in their diets (50 times higher—based on AUC values—than the level observed experimentally in women taking 10 mg of MPA), a dose-related increase in pancreatic islet cell tumors (adenomas and carcinomas) occurred. Pancreatic tumor incidence was increased at 1000 and 5000 µg/kg/day, but not at 200 µg/kg/day.
A decreased incidence of spontaneous mammary gland tumors was observed in all three MPA-treated groups, compared to controls, in the two-year rat study. The mechanism for the decreased incidence of mammary gland tumors observed in the MPA-treated rats may be linked to the significant decrease in serum prolactin concentration observed in rats.
Beagle dogs treated with MPA developed mammary nodules, some of which were malignant. Although nodules occasionally appeared in control animals, they were intermittent in nature, whereas the nodules in the drug-treated animals were larger, more numerous, persistent, and there were some breast malignancies with metastases. It is known that progestogens stimulate synthesis and release of growth hormone in dogs. The growth hormone, along with the progestogen, stimulates mammary growth and tumors. In contrast, growth hormone in humans is not increased, nor does growth hormone have any significant mammotrophic role. Therefore, the MPA-induced increase of mammary tumors in dogs probably has no significance to humans. No pancreatic tumors occurred in dogs.

Pregnancy Category X

Estrogens/progestins should not be used during pregnancy. See **CONTRAINDICATIONS**.

Nursing Mothers

As a general principle, the administration of any drug to nursing mothers should be done only when clearly necessary since many drugs are excreted in human milk. Estrogen administration to nursing mothers has been shown to decrease the quantity and quality of the milk. Detectable amounts of progestin have been identified in the milk of mothers receiving the drug. The effect of this on the nursing infant has not been determined.

ADVERSE REACTIONS

(See **WARNINGS** regarding induction of neoplasia, adverse effects on the fetus, increased incidence of gallbladder disease, elevated blood pressure, thromboembolic disorders, visual abnormalities, and hypercalcemia and **PRECAUTIONS** for cardiovascular disease.)
In a one year clinical trial that included 678 women treated with PREMPRO, 351 women treated with PREMPHASE, and 347 women treated with Premarin, the following adverse events occurred at a rate ≥ 5% (see Table 4):
[See table at top of next page]
The following adverse reactions also have been reported with estrogen and/or progestin therapy:
Genitourinary system. Changes in vaginal bleeding pattern and abnormal withdrawal bleeding or flow, breakthrough bleeding, spotting, change in amount of cervical secretion, premenstrual-like syndrome, cystitis-like syndrome, increase in size of uterine leiomyomata, vaginal candidiasis, amenorrhea, changes in cervical erosion.
Breasts. Tenderness, enlargement, galactorrhea.
Gastrointestinal. Nausea, cholestatic jaundice, changes in appetite, vomiting, abdominal cramps, bloating, increased incidence of gallbladder disease, pancreatitis.
Skin. Chloasma or melasma that may persist when drug is discontinued, erythema multiforme, erythema nodosum, hemorrhagic eruption, loss of scalp hair, hirsutism, itching, urticaria, pruritus, generalized rash, rash (allergic) with and without pruritus, acne.
Cardiovascular. In susceptible individuals, change in blood pressure, thrombophlebitis, pulmonary embolism, cerebral thrombosis and embolism.
CNS. Headache, dizziness, mental depression, nervousness, migraine, chorea, insomnia, somnolence.
Eyes. Neuro-ocular lesions, e.g., retinal thrombosis and optic neuritis. Steepening of corneal curvature, intolerance of contact lenses.
Miscellaneous. Increase or decrease in weight, edema, changes in libido, fatigue, backache, reduced carbohydrate tolerance, aggravation of porphyria, pyrexia, anaphylactoid reactions, anaphylaxis.

ACUTE OVERDOSAGE

Serious ill effects have not been reported following acute ingestion of large doses of estrogen/progestin-containing oral contraceptives by young children. Overdosage may cause nausea and vomiting, and withdrawal bleeding may occur in females.

DOSAGE AND ADMINISTRATION

PREMPRO therapy consists of a single tablet to be taken once daily.

Continued on next page

Prempro—Cont.

1. For treatment of moderate-to-severe vasomotor symptoms and vulval and vaginal atrophy associated with menopause, patients should be started at the lowest effective dose—PREMPRO 0.625 mg/2.5 mg daily. Patients should be reevaluated at 3-month to 6-month intervals to determine if treatment for symptoms is still necessary. Adequate diagnostic measures, including endometrial sampling when indicated, should be undertaken to rule out malignancy in cases of undiagnosed persistent or recurring abnormal vaginal bleeding. In patients where bleeding or spotting remains a problem, after appropriate evaluation, consideration should be given to increasing the MPA dose to PREMPRO 0.625 mg/5 mg daily. This dose can be periodically reassessed by the health care provider.
2. For prevention of osteoporosis—PREMPRO 0.625 mg/2.5 mg daily. Patients should be monitored closely for signs of endometrial cancer, and appropriate diagnostic measures should be taken to rule out malignancy in the event of persistent or recurring abnormal vaginal bleeding. In patients where bleeding or spotting remains a problem, after appropriate evaluation, consideration should be given to increasing the MPA dose to PREMPRO 0.625 mg/5 mg daily. This dose can be periodically reassessed by the health care provider.

PREMPHASE therapy consists of two separate tablets; one maroon 0.625 mg Premarin tablet taken daily on days 1 through 14 and one light-blue tablet, containing 0.625 mg conjugated estrogens and 5 mg of medroxyprogesterone acetate, taken on days 15 through 28.

1. For treatment of moderate to severe vasomotor symptoms and vulvar and vaginal atrophy associated with menopause. Patients should be reevaluated at 3-month to 6-month intervals to determine if treatment for symptoms is still necessary. Adequate diagnostic measures, including endometrial sampling when indicated, should be undertaken to rule out malignancy in cases of undiagnosed persistent or recurring abnormal vaginal bleeding.
2. For prevention of osteoporosis. Treated patients with an intact uterus should be monitored closely for signs of endometrial cancer, and appropriate diagnostic measures should be taken to rule out malignancy in the event of persistent or recurring abnormal vaginal bleeding.

HOW SUPPLIED

PREMPRO™ therapy consists of a single tablet to be taken once daily.

PREMPRO 0.625 mg/2.5 mg

Each carton includes 3 EZ DIAL™ dispensers containing 28 tablets. One EZ DIAL™ dispenser contains 28 oval, peach tablets containing 0.625 mg of the conjugated estrogens found in Premarin® tablets and 2.5 mg of medroxyprogesterone acetate for oral administration.

PREMPRO 0.625 mg/5 mg

Each carton includes 3 EZ DIAL™ dispensers containing 28 tablets. One EZ DIAL™ dispenser contains 28 oval, light-blue tablets containing 0.625 mg of the conjugated estrogens found in Premarin® tablets and 5 mg of medroxyprogesterone acetate for oral administration.

PREMPHASE® therapy consists of two separate tablets; one maroon Premarin® tablet taken daily on days 1 through 14 and one light-blue tablet taken on days 15 through 28.

Each carton includes 3 EZ DIAL™ dispensers containing 28 tablets. One EZ DIAL™ dispenser contains 14 oval, maroon Premarin tablets containing 0.625 mg of conjugated estrogens and 14 oval, light-blue tablets that contain 0.625 mg of the conjugated estrogens found in Premarin tablets and 5 mg of medroxyprogesterone acetate (MPA) for oral administration.

The appearance of PREMPRO™ tablets is a trademark of Wyeth-Ayerst Laboratories.

The appearance of Premarin® tablets is a trademark of Wyeth-Ayerst Laboratories. The appearance of the conjugated estrogens/medroxyprogesterone acetate combination tablets is a registered trademark.

Store at controlled room temperature 20°C–25°C (68°F–77°F).

INFORMATION FOR THE PATIENT

Your physician has prescribed PREMPRO or PREMPHASE, a combination of two hormones, an estrogen and a progestin. This leaflet describes the major benefits and risks of your treatment, as well as how and when treatment should be taken.

PREMPRO and PREMPHASE replace the hormones in your body which naturally decrease at menopause. The hormone combination you will be taking has been shown to provide the benefits of estrogen replacement therapy while lowering the frequency of a possible precancerous condition of the uterine lining. This therapy is not intended for women who have had a hysterectomy (surgical removal of the uterus).

Estrogens have several important uses but also some risks. You must decide, with your doctor, whether the risks of estrogens are acceptable when weighed against their benefits. The length of treatment with estrogens can vary from woman to woman. Check with your doctor to make sure you are using the lowest possible effective dose.

With PREMPRO or PREMPHASE therapy several menstrual-like bleeding patterns may occur. These may range from absence of bleeding to irregular bleeding. If bleeding occurs, it is frequently light spotting or moderate menstrual-like bleeding, but it may be heavy. If you experience vaginal bleeding while taking PREMPRO or PREMPHASE, you should discuss your bleeding pattern with your doctor and set up an appropriate schedule for follow-up care.

Table 4. ALL TREATMENT EMERGENT STUDY EVENTS REGARDLESS OF DRUG RELATIONSHIP REPORTED AT A FREQUENCY ≥ 5%

	Regimen A PREMPRO 0.625 mg/2.5 mg continuous (n=340)	Regimen B PREMPRO 0.625 mg/5.0 mg continuous (n=338)	Regimen C PREMPHASE 0.625 mg/5.0 mg cyclic sequential (n=351)	Regimen E PREMARIN 0.625 mg (n=347)
Body as a whole				
abdominal pain	16%	21%	23%	17%
accidental injury	5%	4%	5%	5%
asthenia	6%	8%	10%	8%
back pain	14%	13%	16%	14%
flu syndrome	10%	13%	12%	14%
headache	36%	28%	37%	38%
infection	16%	16%	18%	14%
pain	11%	13%	12%	13%
pelvic pain	4%	5%	5%	5%
Digestive system				
diarrhea	6%	6%	5%	10%
dyspepsia	6%	6%	5%	5%
flatulence	8%	9%	8%	5%
nausea	11%	9%	11%	11%
Metabolic and Nutritional				
peripheral edema	4%	4%	3%	5%
Musculoskeletal system				
arthralgia	9%	7%	9%	7%
leg cramps	3%	4%	5%	4%
Nervous system				
depression	6%	11%	11%	10%
dizziness	5%	3%	4%	6%
hypertonia	4%	3%	3%	7%
Respiratory system				
pharyngitis	11%	11%	13%	12%
rhinitis	8%	6%	8%	7%
sinusitis	8%	7%	7%	5%
Skin and appendages				
pruritus	10%	8%	5%	4%
rash	4%	6%	4%	3%
Urogenital system				
breast pain	33%	38%	32%	12%
cervix disorder	4%	4%	5%	5%
dysmenorrhea	8%	5%	13%	5%
leukorrhea	6%	5%	9%	8%
vaginal hemorrhage	2%	1%	3%	6%
vaginitis	7%	7%	5%	3%

USES OF ESTROGEN

To reduce moderate to severe menopausal symptoms. Estrogens are hormones produced by the ovaries of normal women. When a woman is between the ages of 45 and 55, the ovaries normally stop making estrogens. This leads to a drop in body estrogen levels that causes the "change of life" or menopause (the end of monthly menstrual periods). A sudden drop in estrogen levels also occurs if both ovaries are removed during an operation before natural menopause takes place. This is referred to as "surgical menopause."

When the estrogen levels begin dropping, some women develop very uncomfortable symptoms, such as feelings of warmth in the face, neck, and chest, or sudden intense episodes of heat and sweating ("hot flashes" or "hot flushes"). Using estrogen drugs can help the body adjust to lower estrogen levels and reduce these symptoms. In some women the symptoms are mild; in others they can be severe. These symptoms may last only a few months or longer. Taking PREMPRO or PREMPHASE can alleviate these symptoms. If you are not taking hormones for other reasons, such as the prevention of osteoporosis, you should take PREMPRO or PREMPHASE only as long as you need it for relief from your menopausal symptoms.

To prevent thinning of bones. Osteoporosis is a thinning of the bones that makes them weaker and allows them to break more easily. The bones of the spine, wrists, and hips break most often in osteoporosis. Both men and women start to lose bone mass after about age 40, but women lose bone mass faster after the menopause. Using estrogens after the menopause slows down bone thinning and may prevent bones from breaking. Lifelong adequate calcium intake, either from diet (such as dairy products) or from calcium supplements (to reach a total daily intake of 1000 milligrams per day before menopause or 1500 milligrams per day after menopause), may help to prevent osteoporosis. Regular weight-bearing exercise (like walking and running for an hour, two or three times a week) may also help to prevent osteoporosis. Before you change your calcium intake or exercise habits, it is important to discuss these lifestyle changes with your doctor to find out if they are safe for you.

Since estrogen use has some risks, only women who are likely to develop osteoporosis should use estrogens for prevention. Women who are likely to develop osteoporosis often have the following characteristics:

- White or Asian race
- Small, slim body frame
- Cigarette-smoking habit
- Family history of osteoporosis (in a mother, sister, or aunt)
- Early menopause either natural or because of surgical removal of ovaries ("surgical menopause")

To treat vulvar and vaginal atrophy (itching, burning, dryness in or around the vagina, difficulty or burning on urination) associated with menopause.

WHO SHOULD NOT USE ESTROGENS

During pregnancy. If you think you may be pregnant, do not use any form of estrogen-containing drug. Using estrogens while you are pregnant may cause your unborn child to have birth defects. Estrogens do not prevent miscarriage.

If you have unusual vaginal bleeding which has not been evaluated by your doctor. Unusual vaginal bleeding can be a warning sign of cancer of the uterus, especially if it happens after menopause. Your doctor must find out the cause of the bleeding so that he or she can recommend the proper treatment. Taking estrogens without visiting your doctor can cause you serious harm if your vaginal bleeding is caused by cancer of the uterus.

If you have had cancer. Since estrogens increase the risk of certain types of cancer, you should not use estrogens if you have ever had cancer of the breast or uterus.

If you have any circulation problems. Estrogen drugs should not be used except in unusually special situations in which your doctor decides that you need estrogen therapy so much that the risks are acceptable. Women with abnormal blood clotting conditions should avoid estrogen use (see **RISKS OF ESTROGENS AND/OR PROGESTINS**).

When they do not work. During menopause, some women develop nervous symptoms or depression. Estrogens do not relieve these symptoms. You may have heard that taking estrogens for years after menopause will keep your skin soft and supple and keep you feeling young. There is no evidence for these claims and such long-term estrogen use may have serious risks.

After childbirth or when breastfeeding a baby. Estrogen should not be used to try to stop the breast from filling with milk after a baby is born. Such treatment may increase the risk of developing blood clots (see **RISKS OF ESTROGENS AND/OR PROGESTINS**).

If you are breastfeeding, you should avoid using any drugs because many drugs pass through to the baby in the milk. While nursing a baby, you should take drugs only on the advice of your health-care provider.

RISKS OF ESTROGENS AND/OR PROGESTINS

Cancer of the uterus. If you use any drug which contains estrogen, it is important to visit your doctor regularly and

report any unusual vaginal bleeding right away. Vaginal bleeding after menopause may be a warning sign of uterine cancer. Your doctor should evaluate any unusual vaginal bleeding to find out the cause.
The risk of cancer of the uterus increases when estrogens are used alone, the longer they are used, and when larger doses are taken. There is a higher risk of cancer of the uterus if you are overweight, diabetic, or have high blood pressure. The hormone combination you will be taking contains estrogen and progestin. This combination has been shown to provide the benefits of estrogen replacement therapy for the **USES OF ESTROGEN** listed above, while reducing the risk of a precancerous condition of the uterine lining (see **OTHER INFORMATION,** below).
However, additional risks may be associated with the inclusion of a progestin in estrogen treatment. The possible risks include less favorable effects on blood fats as compared to Premarin alone, unfavorable effects on blood sugars, and a possible increase in breast cancer risk (see *Cancer of the breast*, below). Usually, the smaller the dose and the shorter the duration of treatment, the more these effects are minimized. Check with your doctor to make sure you are using the lowest effective dose and only for as long as you need it.
If you have had your uterus removed, there is no risk of developing cancer of the uterus and no benefit to be gained by using a combination estrogen/progestin product.
Cancer of the breast. Most studies have not shown a higher risk of breast cancer in women who have ever used estrogens. However, some studies have reported that breast cancer developed more often (up to twice the usual rate) in women who used estrogens for long periods of time (especially more than 10 years), or who used high doses for shorter time periods. The effects of added progestin on the risk of breast cancer are unknown. Some studies have reported a somewhat increased risk, even higher than the possible risk associated with estrogens alone. Others have not. Regular breast examinations by a health professional and monthly self-examination are recommended for all women. Regular mammograms are recommended for all women over 50 years of age.
Gallbladder disease. Women who use estrogens after menopause are more likely to develop gallbladder disease needing surgery than women who do not use estrogens.
Inflammation of the Pancreas. Women with high triglyceride levels may have an increased risk of developing inflammation of the pancreas.
Abnormal blood clotting. Taking estrogens may cause changes in your blood clotting system. These changes allow the blood to clot more easily, possibly allowing clots to form in your bloodstream. If blood clots do form in your bloodstream, they can cut off the blood supply to vital organs, causing serious problems. These problems may include a stroke (by cutting off blood to the brain), a heart attack (by cutting off blood to the heart), a pulmonary embolus (by cutting off blood to the lungs), or other problems. Any of these conditions may cause death or serious long-term disability.
Heart Disease. A recent 4-year study suggests that women with a history of coronary heart disease may have an increased risk of serious cardiac events during the first year of treatment with estrogen/progestin therapy. Therefore, if you have had a heart attack, or you have been told you have blocked coronary arteries (arteries to your heart) or have any heart problem, you should consult your physician regarding the potential benefits and risks of estrogen/progestin therapy.
Excess calcium in the blood. Taking estrogens may lead to severe hypercalcemia in women with breast and/or bone cancer.
During pregnancy. There is an increased risk of birth defects in children whose mothers take this drug during the first four months of pregnancy. Several reports suggest an association between mothers who take these drugs in the first trimester of pregnancy and genital abnormalities in male and female babies. The risk to the male baby is the possibility of being born with a condition in which the opening of the penis is on the underside rather than the tip of the penis (hypospadias). Hypospadias occurs in about 5 to 8 per 1,000 male births and is about doubled with exposure to these drugs. There is not enough information to quantify the risk to exposed female fetuses. However, enlargement of the clitoris and fusion of the labia may occur, although rarely.
Therefore, since drugs of this type may induce mild masculinization of the external genitalia of the female fetus, as well as hypospadias in the male fetus, it is wise to avoid using the drug during the first trimester of pregnancy. These drugs have been used as a test for pregnancy, but such use is no longer considered safe because of possible damage to a developing baby. Also, more rapid methods for testing for pregnancy are now available. If you take PREMPRO or PREMPHASE and later find you were pregnant when you took it, be sure to discuss this with your doctor as soon as possible.

SIDE EFFECTS WITH ESTROGENS AND/OR PROGESTINS

In addition to the risks listed above, the following side effects have been reported with estrogen and/or progestin use:
- Nausea, vomiting, pain, cramps, swelling, or tenderness in the abdomen.
- Yellowing of the skin and/or whites of the eyes.
- Breast tenderness or enlargement.
- Enlargement of benign tumors ("fibroids") of the uterus.
- Irregular bleeding or spotting.
- Change in amount of cervical secretion.
- Vaginal yeast infections.
- Retention of excess fluid. This may make some conditions worsen, such as asthma, epilepsy, migraine, heart disease, or kidney disease.
- A spotty darkening of the skin, particularly on the face; reddening of the skin; skin rashes.
- Worsening of porphyria.
- Headache, migraines, dizziness, faintness, or changes in vision (including intolerance to contact lenses).
- Mental depression.
- Involuntary muscle spasms.
- Hair loss or abnormal hairiness.
- Increase or decrease in weight.
- Changes in sex drive.
- Possible changes in blood sugar.

REDUCING THE RISKS OF ESTROGEN/PROGESTIN

If you decide to take an estrogen/progestin combination, you can reduce your risks by carefully monitoring your treatment.
See your doctor regularly. While you are taking PREMPRO or PREMPHASE, it is important to visit your doctor at least once a year for a checkup. If you develop vaginal bleeding while taking estrogens, you may need further evaluation. If members of your family have had breast cancer or if you have ever had breast lumps or an abnormal mammogram (breast X ray), you may need to have more frequent breast examinations.
Reassess your need for treatment. You and your doctor should reevaluate whether or not you still need estrogens at least every six months.
Be alert for signs of trouble. If any of these warning signals (or any other unusual symptoms) happen while you are using estrogen/progestin, call your doctor immediately:
- Abnormal bleeding from the vagina (possible uterine abnormality).
- Pains in the calves or chest, a sudden shortness of breath or coughing blood (indicating possible clots in the legs, heart, or lungs).
- Severe headache or vomiting, dizziness, faintness, or changes in vision or speech, weakness or numbness of an arm or leg (indicating possible clots in the brain or eye).
- Breast lumps (possible breast cancer; ask your doctor or health professional to show you how to examine your breasts monthly).
- Yellowing of the skin and/or whites of the eyes (possible liver problems).
- Pain, swelling, or tenderness in the abdomen (possible gallbladder problem).

OTHER INFORMATION

1. Estrogens increase the risk of developing a condition (endometrial hyperplasia) that may lead to cancer of the lining of the uterus. Taking progestins, another hormonal drug, with estrogens lowers the risk of developing this condition. Therefore, since your uterus has not been removed, your doctor has prescribed PREMPRO or PREMPHASE, which includes both a progestin and estrogens.
You should know, however, that taking estrogens *with* progestins may have unhealthy effects on blood sugar, which might make a diabetic condition worse. Additional risks include a possible further increase in breast cancer risk which may be associated with long-term estrogen use. Some research has shown that estrogens taken *without* progestins may protect women against developing heart disease. However, this is not certain. The protection shown may have been caused by the characteristics of the estrogen-treated women and not by the estrogen treatment itself. In general, treated women were slimmer, more physically active, and were less likely to have diabetes than the untreated women. These characteristics are known to protect against heart disease.
You are cautioned to discuss very carefully with your doctor or health-care provider all the possible risks and benefits of long-term estrogen and progestin treatment as they affect you personally.
2. Your doctor has prescribed this drug for you and you alone. Do not give the drug to anyone else.
3. If you will be taking calcium supplements as part of the treatment to help prevent osteoporosis, check with your doctor about the amounts recommended.
4. Keep this and all drugs out of the reach of children. In case of overdose, call your doctor, hospital, or poison control center immediately.
5. This leaflet provides the most important information about PREMPRO and PREMPHASE. If you want to read more, ask your doctor or pharmacist to let you read the professional labeling. The professional labeling is also published in a book called *The Physicians' Desk Reference*, which is available in bookstores and public libraries.

HOW SUPPLIED

PREMPRO™ is a combination of the conjugated estrogens found in Premarin® tablets and medroxyprogesterone acetate (MPA). Depending on the dosage strength, PREMPRO therapy consists of either a single peach tablet or a single light-blue tablet to be taken once daily.
PREMPRO 0.625 mg/2.5 mg
Each carton includes 3 EZ DIAL™ dispensers containing 28 tablets. One EZ DIAL™ dispenser contains 28 oval, peach tablets containing 0.625 mg of the conjugated estrogens found in Premarin® tablets and 2.5 mg of medroxyprogesterone acetate for oral administration.
PREMPRO 0.625 mg/5 mg
Each carton includes 3 EZ DIAL™ dispensers containing 28 tablets. One EZ DIAL™ dispenser contains 28 oval, light-blue tablets containing 0.625 mg of the conjugated estrogens found in Premarin® tablets and 5 mg of medroxyprogesterone acetate for oral administration.
The appearance of PREMPRO™ tablets is a trademark of Wyeth-Ayerst Laboratories.
PREMPHASE® is a combination of two separate tablets; one maroon Premarin® tablet taken daily on days 1 through 14 and one light-blue tablet taken on days 15 through 28. Each carton includes 3 EZ DIAL™ dispensers containing 28 tablets. One EZ DIAL™ dispenser contains 14 oval, maroon Premarin tablets containing 0.625 mg of conjugated estrogens and 14 oval, light-blue tablets that contain 0.625 mg of the conjugated estrogens found in Premarin tablets and 5 mg of medroxyprogesterone acetate (MPA) for oral administration.
The appearance of Premarin® tablets is a trademark of Wyeth-Ayerst Laboratories. The appearance of the conjugated estrogens/medroxyprogesterone acetate combination tablets is a registered trademark.
Keep out of reach of children.
Store at controlled room temperature 20° C–25° C (68° F–77° F).
U.S. Patent Nos. 5,547,948; 5,210,081; Re. 36,247
Manufactured by:
Ayerst Laboratories Inc.
A Wyeth-Ayerst Company
Philadelphia, PA 19101
CI 6096-1 Issued January 6, 2000

Shown in Product Identification Guide, page 342

PROTONIX® ℞
[*prō 'tŏn-ĭks*]
(pantoprazole sodium)
Delayed-Release Tablets

DESCRIPTION

The active ingredient in PROTONIX® (pantoprazole sodium) Delayed-Release Tablets is a substituted benzimidazole, sodium 5-(difluoromethoxy)-2-[[(3,4-dimethoxy-2-pyridinyl)methyl] sulfinyl]-1*H*-benzimidazole sesquihydrate, a compound that inhibits gastric acid secretion. Its empirical formula is $C_{16}H_{14}F_2N_3NaO_4S \times 1.5\ H_2O$, with a molecular weight of 432.4. The structural formula is:

Pantoprazole sodium sesquihydrate is a white to off-white crystalline powder and is racemic. Pantoprazole has weakly basic and acidic properties. Pantoprazole sodium sesquihydrate is freely soluble in water, very slightly soluble in phosphate buffer at pH 7.4, and practically insoluble in n-hexane.
The stability of the compound in aqueous solution is pH-dependent. The rate of degradation increases with decreasing pH. At ambient temperature, the degradation half-life is approximately 2.8 hours at pH 5.0 and approximately 220 hours at pH 7.8.
PROTONIX is supplied as a delayed-release tablet for oral administration. Each delayed-release tablet contains 45.1 mg of pantoprazole sodium sesquihydrate (equivalent to 40 mg pantoprazole) with the following inactive ingredients: anhydrous sodium carbonate NF, mannitol USP, crospovidone NF, povidone USP, calcium stearate NF, hydroxypropyl methylcellulose USP, titanium dioxide USP, yellow iron oxide NF, propylene glycol USP, methacrylic acid copolymer NF, polysorbate 80 NF, sodium lauryl sulfate NF, and triethyl citrate NF.

CLINICAL PHARMACOLOGY

Pharmacokinetics

Protonix is prepared as an enteric-coated tablet so that absorption of pantoprazole begins only after the tablet leaves the stomach. Peak serum concentration (C_{max}) and area under the serum concentration time curve (AUC) increase in a manner proportional to oral and intravenous doses from 10 mg to 80 mg. Pantoprazole does not accumulate and its pharmacokinetics are unaltered with multiple daily dosing. Following oral or intravenous administration, the serum concentration of pantoprazole declines biexponentially with a terminal elimination half-life of approximately one hour.
In extensive metabolizers (see Metabolism section) with normal liver function receiving an oral dose of the enteric-coated 40 mg pantoprazole tablet, the peak concentration (C_{max}) is 2.4 (µg/mL, the time to reach the peak concentration (t_{max}) is 2.4 h and the total area under the plasma concentration versus time curve (AUC) is 4.8 (µg•hr/mL). When pantoprazole is given with food, its t_{max} is highly variable and may increase significantly. Following intravenous administration of pantoprazole to extensive metabolizers, its total clearance is 7.6–14.0 L/h and its apparent volume of distribution is 11.0–23.6L.

Continued on next page

Protonix—Cont.

Effect of Single Doses of Oral Pantoprazole on Intragastric pH

Time	Median pH: Placebo	20 mg	40 mg	80 mg
8 a.m. - 8 a.m. (24 hours)	1.3	2.9*	3.8*#	3.9*#
8 a.m. - 10 p.m. (Daytime)	1.6	3.2*	4.4*#	4.8*#
10 p.m. - 8 a.m. (Nighttime)	1.2	2.1*	3.0*	2.6*

* Significantly different from placebo
\# Signifcantly different from 20 mg

Erosive Esophagitis Healing Rates (per protocol)

Week	PROTONIX 10 mg QD (n = 153)	PROTONIX 20 mg QD (n = 158)	PROTONIX 40 mg QD (n = 162)	Placebo (n = 68)
4	45.6%+	58.4%+#	75.0%+*	14.3%
8	66.0%+	83.5%+#	92.6%+*	39.7%

+ ($p < 0.001$) PROTONIX versus placebo.
* ($p <0.05$) versus 10 mg, or 20 mg PROTONIX
\# ($p <0.05$) versus 10 mg PROTONIX

Absorption

The absorption of pantoprazole is rapid, with a C_{max} of 2.5 µg/mL that occurs approximately 2.5 hours after single or multiple oral 40-mg doses. Pantoprazole is well absorbed; it undergoes little first-pass metabolism resulting in an absolute bioavailability of approximately 77%. Pantoprazole absorption is not affected by concomitant administration of antacids. Administration of pantoprazole with food may delay its absorption up to 2 hours or longer; however, the C_{max} and the extent of pantoprazole absorption (AUC) are not altered. Thus, pantoprazole may be taken without regard to timing of meals.

Distribution

The apparent volume of distribution of pantoprazole is approximately 11.0–23.6L, distributing mainly in extracellular fluid. The serum protein binding of pantoprazole is about 98%, primarily to albumin.

Metabolism

Pantoprazole is extensively metabolized in the liver through the cytochrome P450 (CYP) system. Pantoprazole metabolism is independent of the route of administration (intravenous or oral). The main metabolic pathway is demethylation, by CYP2C19, with subsequent sulfation; other metabolic pathways include oxidation by CYP3A4. There is no evidence that any of the pantoprazole metabolites have significant pharmacologic activity. CYP2C19 displays a known genetic polymorphism due to its deficiency in some subpopulations (e.g. 3% of Caucasians and African-Americans and 17–23% of Asians). Although these sub-populations of slow pantoprazole metabolizers have elimination half-life values of 3.5 to 10.0 hours, they still have minimal accumulation (≤ 23%) with once daily dosing.

Elimination

After a single oral or intravenous dose of ^{14}C-labeled pantoprazole to healthy, normal metabolizer volunteers, approximately 71% of the dose was excreted in the urine with 18% excreted in the feces through biliary excretion. There was no renal excretion of unchanged pantoprazole.

Special Populations

Geriatric

Only slight to moderate increases in pantoprazole AUC (43%) and C_{max} (26%) were found in elderly volunteers (64 to 76 years of age) after repeated oral administration, compared with younger subjects. No dosage adjustment is recommended based on age.

Pediatric

The pharmacokinetics of pantoprazole have not been investigated in patients <18 years of age.

Gender

There is a modest increase in pantoprazole AUC and C_{max} in women compared to men. However, weight-normalized clearance values are similar in women and men. No dosage adjustment is needed based on gender (Also see Use in Women).

Renal Impairment

In patients with severe renal impairment, pharmacokinetic parameters for pantoprazole were similar to those of healthy subjects. No dosage adjustment is necessary in patients with renal impairment or in patients undergoing hemodialysis.

Hepatic Impairment

In patients with mild to moderate hepatic impairment, maximum pantoprazole concentrations increased only slightly (1.5-fold) relative to healthy subjects. Although serum half-life values increased to 7–9 hours and AUC values increased by 5- to 7-fold in hepatic-impaired patients, these increases were no greater than those observed in slow CYP2C19 metabolizers, where no dosage frequency adjustment is warranted. These pharmacokinetic changes in hepatic-impaired patients result in minimal drug accumulation following once daily multiple-dose administration. No dosage adjustment is needed in patients with mild or moderate hepatic impairment. The pharmacokinetics of pantoprazole have not yet been well characterized in patients with severe hepatic impairment. Therefore, the potential for modest drug accumulation (≤ 21%) when dosed once daily needs to be weighed against the potential for reduced acid control when dosed every other day in these patients.

Drug-Drug Interactions

Pantoprazole is metabolized mainly by CYP2C19 and to minor extents by CYPs 3A4, 2D6 and 2C9. In *in vivo* drug-drug interaction studies with CYP2C19 substrates (diazepam [also a CYP3A4 substrate] and phenytoin [also a CYP3A4 inducer]), nifedipine (a CYP3A4 substrate), metoprolol (a CYP2D6 substrate), diclofenac (a CYP2C9 substrate) and theophylline (a CYP1A2 substrate) in healthy subjects, the pharmacokinetics of pantoprazole were not significantly altered. It is, therefore, expected that other drugs metabolized by CYPs 2C19, 3A4, 2D6, 2C9 and 1A2 would not significantly affect the pharmacokinetics of pantoprazole. *In vivo* studies also suggest that pantoprazole does not significantly affect the kinetics of other drugs (cisapride, theophylline, diazepam [and its active metabolite, desmethyldiazepam], phenytoin, warfarin, metoprolol, nifedipine, carbamazepine and oral contraceptives) metabolized by CYPs 2C19, 3A4, 2C9, 2D6 and 1A2. Therefore, it is expected that pantoprazole would not significantly affect the pharmacokinetics of other drugs metabolized by these isozymes. Dosage adjustment of such drugs is not necessary when they are coadministered with pantoprazole. In other *in vivo* studies, digoxin, ethanol, glyburide, antipyrine, and caffeine had no clinically relevant interactions with pantoprazole.

Pharmacodynamics

Mechanism of Action

Pantoprazole is a proton pump inhibitor (PPI) that suppresses the final step in gastric acid production by forming a covalent bond to two sites of the (H^+,K^+)-ATPase enzyme system at the secretory surface of the gastric parietal cell. This effect is dose-related and leads to inhibition of both basal and stimulated gastric acid secretion irrespective of the stimulus. The binding to the (H^+,K^+)-ATPase results in a duration of antisecretory effect that persists longer than 24 hours.

Antisecretory Activity

Under maximal acid stimulatory conditions using pentagastrin, a dose-dependent decrease in gastric acid output occurs after a single dose of oral (20–80 mg) or a single dose of intravenous (20–120 mg) pantoprazole in healthy volunteers. Pantoprazole given once daily results in increasing inhibition of gastric acid secretion. Following the initial oral dose of 40 mg pantoprazole, a 51% mean inhibition was achieved by 2.5 hours. With once a day dosing for 7 days the mean inhibition was increased to 85%. Pantoprazole suppressed acid secretion in excess of 95% in half of the subjects. Acid secretion had returned to normal within a week after the last dose of pantoprazole; there was no evidence of rebound hypersecretion.

In a series of dose-response studies pantoprazole, at oral doses ranging from 20 to 120 mg, caused dose-related increases in median basal gastric pH and in the percent of time gastric pH was > 3 and > 4. Treatment with 40 mg of pantoprazole produced optimal increases in gastric pH which were significantly greater than the 20-mg dose. Doses higher than 40 mg (60, 80, 120 mg) did not result in further significant increases in median gastric pH. The effects of pantoprazole on median pH from one double-blind crossover study are shown below.

[See first table above]

A double-blind crossover study compared pantoprazole 40 mg with omeprazole 20 mg once daily for 7 days. For both one day and one week treatment periods, pantoprazole administered in the morning produced significantly greater increases in median pH during 24 hours than did omeprazole.

Serum Gastrin Effects

Fasting serum gastrin levels were assessed in two double-blind studies of the acute healing of erosive esophagitis (EE) in which 682 patients with gastroesophageal reflux disease (GERD) received 10, 20, or 40 mg of pantoprazole for up to 8 weeks. At 4 weeks of treatment there was an increase in mean gastrin levels of 7%, 35%, and 72% over pretreatment values in the 10, 20 and 40 mg treatment groups, respectively. A similar increase in serum gastrin levels was noted at the 8 week visit with mean increases of 3%, 26%, and 84% for the three pantoprazole dose groups.

In long term studies involving over 800 patients, a 2- to 3-fold mean increase from the pretreatment fasting serum gastrin level was observed in the initial months of treatment with pantoprazole at doses of 40 mg per day during GERD maintenance studies and 40 mg or higher per day in patients with refractory GERD. Fasting serum gastrin levels generally remained at approximately 2 to 3 times baseline for up to 4 years of periodic follow-up in clinical trials. Following healing of gastric or duodenal ulcers with pantoprazole treatment, elevated gastrin levels return to normal by at least 3 months.

Enterochromaffin-Like (ECL) Cell Effects

In 39 patients treated with oral pantoprazole 40 mg to 240 mg daily (majority receiving 40 mg to 80 mg) for up to 5 years, there was a moderate increase in ECL-cell density starting after the first year of use which appeared to plateau after 4 years.

In a nonclinical study in Sprague-Dawley rats, lifetime exposure (24 months) to pantoprazole at doses of 0.5 to 200 mg/kg/day resulted in dose-related increases in gastric ECL-cell proliferation and gastric neuroendocrine (NE)-cell tumors. Gastric NE-cell tumors in rats may result from chronic elevation of serum gastrin levels. The high density of ECL cells in the rat stomach makes this species highly susceptible to the proliferative effects of elevated gastrin levels produced by proton pump inhibitors.

However, there were no observed elevations in serum gastrin following the administration of pantoprazole at a dose of 0.5 mg/kg/day. In a separate study, a gastric NE-cell tumor without concomitant ECL-cell proliferative changes was observed in 1 female rat following 12 months of dosing with pantoprazole at 5 mg/kg/day and a 9 month off-dose recovery. (See **PRECAUTIONS**, Carcinogenesis, Mutagenesis, Impairment of Fertility).

Other Effects

No clinically relevant effects of pantoprazole on cardiovascular, respiratory, ophthalmic, or central nervous system function have been detected. In a clinical pharmacology study, pantoprazole 40 mg given once daily for 2 weeks had no effect on the levels of the following hormones: cortisol, testosterone, triiodothyronine (T3), thyroxine (T4), thyroid-stimulating hormone, thyronine-binding protein, parathyroid hormone, insulin, glucagon, renin, aldosterone, follicle-stimulating hormone, luteinizing hormone, prolactin and growth hormone.

Clinical Studies

PROTONIX Delayed-Release Tablets were used in all clinical trials.

Erosive Esophagitis (EE) Associated with Gastroesophageal Reflux Disease (GERD)

A US multicenter double-blind, placebo-controlled study of PROTONIX 10 mg, 20 mg or 40 mg once daily was conducted in 603 patients with reflux symptoms and endoscopically diagnosed EE of grade 2 or above (Hetzel-Dent scale). In this study, approximately 25% of enrolled patients had severe EE of grade 3 and 10% had grade 4. The percentages of patients healed (per protocol, n=541) in this study were as follows:

[See second table above]

In this study, all PROTONIX treatment groups had significantly greater healing rates than the placebo group. This was true regardless of *H. pylori* status for the 20-mg and 40-mg PROTONIX treatment groups. The 40-mg dose of PROTONIX resulted in healing rates significantly greater than those found with either the 20- or 10-mg dose.

A significantly greater proportion of patients taking PROTONIX 40 mg experienced complete relief of daytime and nighttime heartburn and the absence of regurgitation starting from the first day of treatment compared with placebo. Patients taking PROTONIX consumed significantly fewer antacid tablets per day than those taking placebo.

PROTONIX 20 mg and 40 mg once daily was also compared with nizatidine 150 mg twice daily in a US multicenter, double-blind study of 243 patients with reflux symptoms and endoscopically diagnosed EE of grade 2 or above. The percentages of patients healed (per protocol, n=212) were as follows:

[See first table at top of next page]

Once daily treatment with PROTONIX 20 or 40 mg resulted in significantly superior rates of healing at both 4 and 8 weeks compared with twice daily treatment with 150 mg of nizatidine. For the 40 mg treatment group, significantly greater healing rates compared to nizatidine were achieved regardless of the *H. pylori* status.

A significantly greater proportion of the patients in the PROTONIX treatment groups experienced complete relief of nighttime heartburn and regurgitation starting on the first day and of daytime heartburn on the second day compared with those taking nizatidine 150 mg twice daily. Patients taking PROTONIX consumed significantly fewer antacid tablets per day than those taking nizatidine.

INDICATIONS AND USAGE

Short-Term Treatment of Erosive Esophagitis Associated With Gastroesophageal Reflux Disease (GERD)

PROTONIX Delayed-Release Tablets are indicated for the short-term treatment (up to 8 weeks) in the healing and symptomatic relief of erosive esophagitis. For those patients who have not healed after 8 weeks of treatment, an additional 8 week course of PROTONIX may be considered.

The safety and efficacy of PROTONIX for maintenance therapy (e.g., beyond 16 weeks) have not been established. (see **PRECAUTIONS**).

CONTRAINDICATIONS

PROTONIX Delayed-Release Tablets are contraindicated in patients with known hypersensitivity to any component of the formulation.

PRECAUTIONS

General

Symptomatic response to therapy with pantoprazole does not preclude the presence of gastric malignancy.

In rodents, pantoprazole is carcinogenic and caused rare types of gastrointestinal tumors. The relevance of these animal findings to humans is unknown. The safety and efficacy of PROTONIX for maintenance therapy (e.g., beyond 16 weeks) have not been established. PROTONIX is not indicated for maintenance therapy (see **INDICATIONS AND USAGE**).

No dosage adjustment is necessary in patients with mild or moderate hepatic impairment. The pharmacokinetics of pantoprazole has not been well characterized in patients with severe hepatic impairment. Therefore, the potential for modest drug accumulation (≤21%) when dosed once daily needs to be weighed against the potential for reduced acid control when dosed every other day in these patients.

Information for Patients

Patients should be cautioned that PROTONIX Delayed-Release Tablets should not be split, crushed or chewed. The tablets should be swallowed whole, with or without food in the stomach. Concomitant administration of antacids does not affect the absorption of pantoprazole.

Drug Interactions

Pantoprazole is metabolized through the cytochrome P450 system, primarily the CYP2C19 and CYP3A4 isozymes, and subsequently undergoes Phase II conjugation. Based on studies evaluating possible interactions of pantoprazole with other drugs metabolized by the cytochrome P450 system, no dosage adjustment is needed with concomitant use of the following drugs: theophylline, cisapride, antipyrine, caffeine, carbamazepine, diazepam, diclofenac, digoxin, ethanol, glyburide, an oral contraceptive (levonorgestrel/ethinyl estradiol), metoprolol, nifedipine, phenytoin, or warfarin. Clinically relevant interactions of pantoprazole with other drugs with the same metabolic pathways are not expected. Therefore, when co-administered with pantoprazole, adjustment of the dosage of pantoprazole or of such drugs may not be necessary. There was also no interaction with concomitantly administered antacids.

Because of profound and long lasting inhibition of gastric acid secretion, it is theoretically possible that pantoprazole may interfere with absorption of drugs where gastric pH is an important determinant of their bioavailability (e.g., ketoconazole, ampicillin esters, and iron salts).

Carcinogenesis, Mutagenesis, Impairment of Fertility

In a 24-month carcinogenicity study, Sprague-Dawley rats were treated orally with doses of 0.5 to 200 mg/kg/day, about 0.1 to 40 times the exposure on a body surface area basis, of a 50-kg person dosed at 40 mg/day. In the gastric fundus, treatment at 0.5 to 200 mg/kg/day produced enterochromaffin-like (ECL) cell hyperplasia and benign and malignant neuroendocrine cell tumors in a dose-related manner. In the forestomach, treatment at 50 and 200 mg/kg/day (about 10 and 40 times the recommended human dose on a body surface area basis) produced benign squamous cell papillomas and malignant squamous cell carcinomas. Rare gastrointestinal tumors associated with pantoprazole treatment included an adenocarcinoma of the duodenum at 50 mg/kg/day, and benign polyps and adenocarcinomas of the gastric fundus at 200 mg/kg/day. In the liver, treatment at 0.5 to 200 mg/kg/day produced dose-related increases in the incidences of hepatocellular adenomas and carcinomas. In the thyroid gland, treatment at 200 mg/kg/day produced increased incidences of follicular cell adenomas and carcinomas for both male and female rats.

Sporadic occurrences of hepatocellular adenomas and a hepatocellular carcinoma were observed in Sprague-Dawley rats exposed to pantoprazole in 6-month and 12-month toxicity studies.

In a 24-month carcinogenicity study, Fischer 344 rats were treated orally with doses of 5 to 50 mg/kg/day, approximately 1 to 10 times the recommended human dose based on body surface area. In the gastric fundus, treatment at 5 to 50 mg/kg/day produced enterochromaffin-like (ECL) cell hyperplasia and benign and malignant neuroendocrine cell tumors. Dose selection for this study may not have been adequate to comprehensively evaluate the carcinogenic potential of pantoprazole.

In a 24-month carcinogenicity study, B6C3F1 mice were treated orally with doses of 5 to 150 mg/kg/day, 0.5 to 15 times the recommended human dose based on body surface area. In the liver, treatment at 150 mg/kg/day produced increased incidences of combined hepatocellular adenomas and carcinomas in female mice. Treatment at 5 to 150 mg/kg/day also produced gastric fundic ECl cell hyperplasia.

Pantoprazole was positive in the *in vitro* human lymphocyte chromosomal aberration assays, in one of two mouse micronucleus tests for clastogenic effects, and in the *in vitro* Chinese hamster ovarian cell/HGPRT forward mutation assay for mutagenic effects. Equivocal results were observed in the *in vivo* rat liver DNA covalent binding assay. Pantoprazole was negative in the *in vitro* Ames mutation assay, the *in vitro* unscheduled DNA synthesis (UDS) assay with rat hepatocytes, the *in vitro* AS52/GPT mammalian cell-forward gene mutation assay, the *in vitro* thymidine kinase mutation test with mouse lymphoma L5178Y cells, and the *in vivo* rat bone marrow cell chromosomal aberration assay.

Erosive Esophagitis Healing Rates (per protocol)

Week	PROTONIX 20 mg QD (n = 72)	PROTONIX 40 mg QD (n = 70)	Nizatidine 150 mg BID (n = 70)
4	61.4%[+]	64.0%[+]	22.2%
8	79.2%[+]	82.9%[+]	41.4%

[+] ($p < 0.001$) PROTONIX versus nizatidine.

Most Frequent Adverse Events Reported as Drug Related in Short-term Domestic Trials

	% Incidence			
	Study 300-US		Study 301-US	
Study Event	PROTONIX (n = 521)	Placebo (n = 82)	PROTONIX (n = 161)	Nizatidine (n = 82)
Headache	6	6	9	13
Diarrhea	4	1	6	6
Flatulence	2	2	4	0
Abdominal pain	1	2	4	4
Rash	<1	0	2	0
Eructation	1	1	0	0
Insomnia	<1	2	1	1
Hyperglycemia	1	0	<1	0

Note: Only adverse events with an incidence greater than or equal to the comparators are shown.

Adverse Events in GERD Patients in Short-term International Trials

	% Incidence			
Study Event	Pantoprazole Total (N=2805)	Ranitidine 300 mg (N=594)	Omeprazole 20 mg (N=474)	Famotidine 40 mg (N=239)
Headache	2	3	2	1
Diarrhea	2	2	2	<1
Abdominal Pain	1	1	<1	<1

Pantoprazole at oral doses up to 500 mg/kg/day in male rats (98 times the recommended human dose based on body surface area) and 450 mg/kg/day in female rats (88 times the recommended human dose based on body surface area) was found to have no effect on fertility and reproductive performance.

Pregnancy

Teratogenic Effects

Pregnancy Category B.

Teratology studies have been performed in rats at oral doses up to 450 mg/kg/day (88 times the recommended human dose based on body surface area) and rabbits at oral doses up to 40 mg/kg/day (16 times the recommended human dose based on body surface area) and have revealed no evidence of impaired fertility or harm to the fetus due to pantoprazole. There are, however, no adequate and well-controlled studies in pregnant women. Because animal reproduction studies are not always predictive of human response, this drug should be used during pregnancy only if clearly needed.

Nursing Mothers

Pantoprazole and its metabolites are excreted in the milk of rats. It is not known whether pantoprazole is excreted in human milk. Many drugs which are excreted in human milk have a potential for serious adverse reactions in nursing infants. Based on the potential for tumorigenicity shown for pantoprazole in rodent carcinogenicity studies, a decision should be made whether to discontinue nursing or to discontinue the drug, taking into account the benefit of the drug to the mother.

Pediatric Use

Safety and effectiveness in pediatric patients have not been established.

Use in Women

Erosive esophagitis healing rates in the 221 women treated with pantoprazole in US clinical trials were similar to those found in men. The incidence rates of adverse events were also similar between men and women.

Use in Elderly

Erosive esophagitis healing rates in the 107 elderly patients (≥ 65 years old) treated with pantoprazole in US clinical trials were similar to those found in patients under the age of 65. The incidence rates of adverse events and laboratory abnormalities in patients aged 65 years and older were similar to those associated with patients younger than 65 years of age. The healing rates of the 25 patients at least 75 years old were 80% for those treated with 10 mg of pantoprazole and 100% for those patients treated with either 20 or 40 mg. In addition, the safety profile in patients 65 years and older was similar to that of patients younger than 65 years of age.

ADVERSE REACTIONS

Worldwide, more than 11,100 patients have been treated with pantoprazole in clinical trials involving various dosages and duration of treatment. In general, pantoprazole has been well tolerated in both short-term and long-term trials.

In two US controlled clinical trials involving PROTONIX 10-, 20-, or 40-mg doses for up to 8 weeks, there were no dose-related effects on the incidence of adverse events. The following adverse events considered by investigators to be possibly, probably or definitely related to drug occurred in 1% or more in the individual studies of GERD patients on therapy with PROTONIX.

[See second table above]

In addition, in these short-term domestic trials, the following treatment-emergent events, regardless of causality, occurred at a rate of (≥ 1% in PROTONIX-treated patients: asthenia, back pain, chest pain, neck pain, flu syndrome, infection, pain, migraine, constipation, dyspepsia, gastroenteritis, gastrointestinal disorder, nausea, rectal disorder, vomiting, hyperlipemia, liver function tests abnormal, SGPT increased, arthralgia, anxiety, dizziness, hypertonia, bronchitis, cough increased, dyspnea, pharyngitis, rhinitis, sinusitis, upper respiratory tract infection, urinary frequency, and urinary tract infection.

In international short-term double-blind or open-label, clinical trials involving 20- to 80 mg per day, the following adverse events were reported to occur in 1% or more of 2805 GERD patients receiving pantoprazole for up to 8 weeks.

[See third table above]

Additional adverse experiences occurring in <1% of GERD patients based on pooled results from either short-term domestic or international trials are shown below within each body system. In most instances the relationship to pantoprazole was unclear.

BODY AS A WHOLE: abscess, allergic reaction, chills, cyst, face edema, fever, generalized edema, heat stroke, hernia, laboratory test abnormal, malaise, moniliasis, neoplasm, non-specified drug reaction.

CARDIOVASCULAR SYSTEM: angina pectoris, arrhythmia, cardiovascular disorder, chest pain substernal, congestive heart failure, electrocardiogram abnormal, hemorrhage, hypertension, hypotension, myocardial ischemia, palpitation, retinal vascular disorder, syncope, tachycardia, thrombophlebitis, thrombosis, vasodilatation.

DIGESTIVE SYSTEM: anorexia, aphthous stomatitis, cardiospasm, colitis, dry mouth, duodenitis, dysphagia, enteritis, esophageal hemorrhage, esophagitis, gastrointestinal carcinoma, gastrointestinal hemorrhage, gastrointestinal moniliasis, gingivitis, glossitis, halitosis, hematemesis, increased appetite, melena, mouth ulceration, oral moniliasis, periodontal abscess, periodontitis, rectal hemorrhage, stomach ulcer, stomatitis, stools abnormal, tongue discoloration, ulcerative colitis.

ENDOCRINE SYSTEM: diabetes mellitus, glycosuria, goiter.

HEPATO-BILIARY SYSTEM: biliary pain, bilirubinemia, cholecystitis, cholelithiasis, cholestatic jaundice, hepatitis, alkaline phosphatase increased, gamma glutamyl transpeptidase increased, SGOT increased.

HEMIC AND LYMPHATIC SYSTEM: anemia, ecchymosis, eosinophilia, hypochromic anemia, iron deficiency anemia, leukocytosis, leukopenia, thrombocytopenia.

METABOLIC AND NUTRITIONAL: dehydration, edema, gout, peripheral edema, thirst, weight gain, weight loss.

MUSCULOSKELETAL SYSTEM: arthritis, arthrosis, bone disorder, bone pain, bursitis, joint disorder, leg cramps, neck rigidity, myalgia, tenosynovitis.

Continued on next page

Protonix—Cont.

NERVOUS SYSTEM: abnormal dreams, confusion, convulsion, depression, dry mouth, dysarthria, emotional lability, hallucinations, hyperkinesia, hypesthesia, libido decreased, nervousness, neuralgia, neuritis, paresthesia, reflexes decreased, sleep disorder, somnolence, thinking abnormal, tremor, vertigo.
RESPIRATORY SYSTEM: asthma, epistaxis, hiccup, laryngitis, lung disorder, pneumonia, voice alteration.
SKIN AND APPENDAGES: acne, alopecia, contact dermatitis, dry skin, eczema, fungal dermatitis, hemorrhage, herpes simplex, herpes zoster, lichenoid dermatitis, maculopapular rash, pain, pruritus, skin disorder, skin ulcer, sweating, urticaria.
SPECIAL SENSES: abnormal vision, amblyopia, cataract specified, deafness, diplopia, ear pain, extraocular palsy, glaucoma, otitis externa, taste perversion, tinnitus.
UROGENITAL SYSTEM: albuminuria, balanitis, breast pain, cystitis, dysmenorrhea, dysuria, epididymitis, hematuria, impotence, kidney calculus, kidney pain, nocturia, prostatic disorder, pyelonephritis, scrotal edema, urethral pain, urethritis, urinary tract disorder, urination impaired, vaginitis.

Postmarketing Reports

There have been spontaneous reports of adverse events with the post-marketing use of pantoprazole. These reports include anaphylaxis; angioedema (Quincke's edema); anterior ischemic optic neuropathy; severe dermatologic reactions, including erythema multiforme, Stevens-Johnson syndrome, and toxic epidermal necrolysis (TEN, some fatal); and pancreatitis.
In addition, also observed have been jaundice, confusion, hypokinesia, speech disorder, increased salivation, vertigo, nausea, and tinnitus.

Laboratory Values

In two US controlled trials, 0.4% of the patients on 40 mg pantoprazole experienced SGPT elevations of greater than three times the upper limit of normal at the final treatment visit. Except in those patients where there was a clear alternative explanation for a laboratory value change, such as intercurrent illness, the elevations tended to be mild and sporadic. The following changes in laboratory parameters were reported as adverse events: creatinine increased, hypercholesterolemia, and hyperuricemia.

OVERDOSAGE

Some reports of overdosage with pantoprazole have been received. A spontaneous report of a suicide involving an overdosage of pantoprazole (560 mg) has been received; however, the death was more reasonably attributed to the unknown doses of chloroquine and zopiclone which were also taken since two other reported cases of pantoprazole overdosage involved similar amounts of pantoprazole (400 and 600 mg) with no adverse effects observed. One patient in a flexible dosing study of refractory peptic ulcer disease received a dose of 320 mg per day for 3 months; treatment was well tolerated. Doses of up to 240 mg per day, given intravenously for seven days, have been administered to healthy subjects and have been well tolerated.
Pantoprazole is not removed by hemodialysis.
Single oral doses of pantoprazole at 709 mg/kg, 798 mg/kg and 887 mg/kg were lethal to mice, rats and dogs, respectively. The symptoms of acute toxicity were hypoactivity, ataxia, hunched sitting, limb-splay, lateral position, segregation, absence of ear reflex, and tremor.

DOSAGE AND ADMINISTRATION

Treatment of Erosive Esophagitis

The recommended adult oral dose is 40 mg given once daily for up to 8 weeks. For those patients who have not healed after 8 weeks of treatment, an additional 8-week course of PROTONIX may be considered. (See **INDICATIONS AND USAGE**)
No dosage adjustment is necessary in patients with mild, moderate or severe renal insufficiency or in elderly patients. No dosage adjustment is necessary in patients undergoing hemodialysis. No dosage adjustment is needed in patients with mild or moderate hepatic impairment. The pharmacokinetics of pantoprazole have not yet been well characterized in patients with severe hepatic impairment. Therefore, the potential for modest drug accumulation (≤ 21%) when dosed once daily needs to be weighed against the potential for reduced acid control when dosed every other day in these patients.
PROTONIX Delayed-Release Tablets should be swallowed whole, with or without food in the stomach. Concomitant administration of antacids does not affect the absorption of PROTONIX.
Patients should be cautioned that PROTONIX Delayed-Release Tablets should not be split, chewed or crushed.

HOW SUPPLIED

PROTONIX is supplied as 40 mg yellow oval biconvex delayed-release tablets imprinted with PROTONIX (brown ink) on one side.
They are available as follows:
NDC 0008-0841-81 bottles of 90

Storage

Store PROTONIX Delayed-Release Tablets at 20°–25°C (68°–77°F); excursion permitted to 15°–30°C (59°–86°F). [See USP Controlled Room Temperature].
Rx only
US Patent No. 4,758,579

Manufactured for Wyeth Laboratories
A Wyeth-Ayerst Company
Philadelphia, PA 19101
under license from
Byk Gulden Pharmaceuticals
D78467 Konstanz, Germany
CI 6004-1 Issued March 1, 2000

PROTOPAM® CHLORIDE ℞
(pralidoxime chloride)
Lyophilized Powder for Injection

Caution: Federal law prohibits dispensing without prescription.

DESCRIPTION

Chemical name: 2-formyl-1-methylpyridinium chloride oxime. Available in the United States as Protopam Chloride, pralidoxime chloride is frequently referred to as 2-PAM Chloride.
Structural formula:

$$\left[\text{pyridinium ring: } N^{+}\text{-}CH_3,\ 2\text{-}CH{=}NOH \right] Cl^{-}$$

Pralidoxime chloride occurs as an odorless, white, nonhygroscopic, crystalline powder which is soluble in water to the extent of 1 g in less than 1 mL. Stable in air, it melts between 215° and 225°C, with decomposition.
The specific activity of the drug resides in the 2-formyl-1-methylpyridinium ion and is independent of the particular salt employed. The chloride is preferred because of physiologic compatibility, excellent water solubility at all temperatures, and high potency per gram, due to its low (173) molecular weight.
Pralidoxime chloride is a cholinesterase reactivator.
Protopam Chloride for intravenous injection or infusion is prepared by cryodesiccation. Each vial contains 1 g of sterile pralidoxime chloride, and NaOH to adjust pH, to be reconstituted with 20 mL of Sterile Water for Injection, USP. The pH of the reconstituted solution is 3.5 to 4.5. Intramuscular or subcutaneous injection may be used when intravenous injection is not feasible.

CLINICAL PHARMACOLOGY

The principal action of pralidoxime is to reactivate cholinesterase (mainly outside of the central nervous system) which has been inactivated by phosphorylation due to an organophosphate pesticide or related compound. The destruction of accumulated acetylcholine can then proceed, and neuromuscular junctions will again function normally. Pralidoxime also slows the process of "aging" of phosphorylated cholinesterase to a nonreactivatable form, and detoxifies certain organophosphates by direct chemical reaction. The drug has its most critical effect in relieving paralysis of the muscles of respiration. Because pralidoxime is less effective in relieving depression of the respiratory center, atropine is always required concomitantly to block the effect of accumulated acetylcholine at this site. Pralidoxime relieves muscarinic signs and symptoms, salivation, bronchospasm, etc., but this action is relatively unimportant since atropine is adequate for this purpose.
Pralidoxime is distributed throughout the extracellular water; it is not bound to plasma protein. The drug is rapidly excreted in the urine partly unchanged, and partly as a metabolite produced by the liver. Consequently, pralidoxime is relatively short acting, and repeated doses may be needed, especially where there is any evidence of continuing absorption of the poison.
The minimum therapeutic concentration of pralidoxime in plasma is 4 μg/mL; this level is reached in about 16 minutes after a single injection of 600 mg Protopam Chloride. The apparent half-life of Protopam Chloride is 74 to 77 minutes.
It has been reported[1] that the supplemental use of oxime cholinesterase reactivators (such as pralidoxime) reduces the incidence and severity of developmental defects in chick embryos exposed to such known teratogens as parathion, bidrin, carbachol, and neostigmine. This protective effect of the oximes was shown to be dose related.

INDICATIONS AND USAGE

Protopam is indicated as an antidote: (1) in the treatment of poisoning due to those pesticides and chemicals of the organophosphate class which have anticholinesterase activity and (2) in the control of overdosage by anticholinesterase drugs used in the treatment of myasthenia gravis.
The principal indications for the use of pralidoxime are muscle weakness and respiratory depression. In severe poisoning, respiratory depression may be due to muscle weakness.

CONTRAINDICATIONS

There are no known absolute contraindications for the use of Protopam. Relative contraindications include known hypersensitivity to the drug and other situations in which the risk of its use clearly outweighs possible benefit (see **"Precautions"**).

WARNINGS

Protopam is not effective in the treatment of poisoning due to phosphorus, inorganic phosphates, or organophosphates not having anticholinesterase activity
Protopam is **not** indicated as an antidote for intoxication by pesticides of the carbamate class since it may increase the toxicity of carbaryl.

PRECAUTIONS

GENERAL

Pralidoxime has been very well tolerated in most cases, but it must be remembered that the desperate condition of the organophosphate-poisoned patient will generally mask such minor signs and symptoms as have been noted in normal subjects.
Intravenous administration of Protopam should be carried out slowly and, preferably, by infusion, since certain side effects, such as tachycardia, laryngospasm, and muscle rigidity, have been attributed in a few cases to a too-rapid rate of injection. (See **"Dosage and Administration"**.)
Protopam should be used with great caution in treating organophosphate overdosage in cases of myasthenia gravis since it may precipitate a myasthenic crisis.
Because pralidoxime is excreted in the urine, a decrease in renal function will result in increased blood levels of the drug. Thus, the dosage of pralidoxime should be reduced in the presence of renal insufficiency.

LABORATORY TESTS

Treatment of organophosphate poisoning should be instituted without waiting for the results of laboratory tests. Red blood cell, plasma cholinesterase, and urinary paranitrophenol measurements (in the case of parathion exposure) may be helpful in confirming the diagnosis and following the course of the illness. A reduction in red blood cell cholinesterase concentration to below 50% of normal has been seen only with organophosphate ester poisoning.

DRUG INTERACTIONS

When atropine and pralidoxime are used together, the signs of atropinization (flushing, mydriasis, tachycardia, dryness of the mouth and nose) may occur earlier than might be expected when atropine is used alone. This is especially true if the total dose of atropine has been large and the administration of pralidoxime has been delayed.[2-4]
The following precautions should be kept in mind in the treatment of anticholinesterase poisoning, although they do not bear directly on the use of pralidoxime: since barbiturates are potentiated by the anticholinesterases, they should be used cautiously in the treatment of convulsions; morphine, theophylline, aminophylline, succinylcholine, reserpine, and phenothiazine-type tranquilizers should be avoided in patients with organophosphate poisoning.

CARCINOGENESIS, MUTAGENESIS, IMPAIRMENT OF FERTILITY

Since pralidoxime chloride is indicated for short-term emergency use only, no investigations of its potential for carcinogenesis, mutagenesis, or impairment of fertility have been conducted by the manufacturer, or reported in the literature.

PREGNANCY

Teratogenic Effects —Pregnancy Category C:
Animal reproduction studies have not been conducted with pralidoxime. It is also not known whether pralidoxime can cause fetal harm when administered to a pregnant woman or can affect reproduction capacity. Pralidoxime should be given to a pregnant woman only if clearly needed.

NURSING MOTHERS

It is not known whether this drug is excreted in human milk. Because many drugs are excreted in human milk, caution should be exercised when pralidoxime is administered to a nursing woman.

PEDIATRIC USE

Safety and effectiveness in pediatric patients have not been estabished.

ADVERSE REACTIONS

Forty to 60 minutes after intramuscular injection, mild to moderate pain may be experienced at the site of injection. Pralidoxime may cause blurred vision, diplopia and impaired accommodation, dizziness, headache, drowsiness, nausea, tachycardia, increased systolic and diastolic blood pressure, hyperventilation, and muscular weakness when given parenterally to normal volunteers who have not been exposed to anticholinesterase poisons. In patients, it is very difficult to differentiate the toxic effects produced by atropine or the organophosphate compounds from those of the drug.
Elevations in SGOT and/or SGPT enzyme levels were observed in 1 of 6 normal volunteers given 1200 mg of pralidoxime chloride intramuscularly, and in 4 of 6 volunteers given 1800 mg intramuscularly. Levels returned to normal in about 2 weeks. Transient elevations in creatine phosphokinase were observed in all normal volunteers given the drug. A single intramuscular injection of 330 mg in 1 mL in rabbits caused myonecrosis, inflammation, and hemorrhage.
When atropine and pralidoxime are used together, the signs of atropinization may occur earlier than might be expected when atropine is used alone. This is especially true if the total dose of atropine has been large and the administration of pralidoxime has been delayed.[2-4] Excitement and manic behavior immediately following recovery of consciousness have been reported in several cases. However, similar behavior has occurred in cases of organophosphate poisoning that were not treated with pralidoxime.[3,5,6]

DRUG ABUSE AND DEPENDENCE

Pralidoxime chloride is not subject to abuse and possesses no known potential for dependence.

OVERDOSAGE

MANIFESTATIONS OF OVERDOSAGE

Observed in normal subjects only: dizziness, blurred vision, diplopia, headache, impaired accommodation, nausea, slight tachycardia. In therapy it has been difficult to differentiate side effects due to the drug from those due to the effects of the poison.

TREATMENT OF OVERDOSAGE

Artificial respiration and other supportive therapy should be administered as needed.

ACUTE TOXICITY

IV—man TDLo: 14 mg/kg (toxic effects: CNS)
IV—rat LD50: 96 mg/kg
IM—rat LD50: 150 mg/kg
ORAL—mouse LD50: 4100 mg/kg
IP—mouse LD50: 155 mg/kg
IV—mouse LD50: 90 mg/kg
IM—mouse LD50: 180 mg/kg
IV—rabbit LD50: 95 mg/kg
IM—guinea pig LD50: 168 mg/kg

DOSAGE AND ADMINISTRATION

ORGANOPHOSPHATE POISONING

"Pralidoxime is most effective if administered immediately after poisoning. Generally, little is accomplished if the drug is given more than 36 hours after termination of exposure. When the poison has been ingested, however, exposure may continue for some time due to slow absorption from the lower bowel, and fatal relapses have been reported after initial improvement. Continued administration for several days may be useful in such patients. Close supervision of the patient is indicated for at least 48 to 72 hours. If dermal exposure has occurred, clothing should be removed and the hair and skin washed thoroughly with sodium bicarbonate or alcohol as soon as possible. Diazepam may be given cautiously if convulsions are not controlled by atropine."[7]

Severe poisoning (coma, cyanosis, respiratory depression) requires intensive management. This includes the removal of secretions, airway management, the correction of acidosis, and hypoxemia.

Atropine should be given as soon as possible after hypoxemia is improved. Atropine should not be given in the presence of significant hypoxia due to the risk of atropine-induced ventricular fibrillation. In adults, atropine may be given intravenously in doses of 2 to 4 mg. This should be repeated at 5- to 10-minute intervals until full atropinization (secretions are inhibited) or signs of atropine toxicity appear (delirium, hyperthermia, muscle twitching).

Some degree of atropinization should be maintained for at least 48 hours, and until any depressed blood cholinesterase activity is reversed.

Morphine, theophylline, aminophylline, and succinylcholine are contraindicated. Tranquilizers of the reserpine or phenothiazine type are to be avoided.

After the effects of atropine become apparent, Protopam may be administered.

PROTOPAM CHLORIDE INJECTION

Parenteral drug products should be inspected visually for particulate matter and discoloration prior to administration, whenever solution and container permit.

Discard unused solution after a dose has been withdrawn.

In adults, inject an initial dose of 1 to 2 g of Protopam, preferably as an infusion in 100 mL of saline, over a 15- to 30-minute period. If this is not practical or if pulmonary edema is present, the dose should be given slowly by intravenous injection as a 5 percent solution in water over not less than five minutes. After about an hour, a second dose of 1 to 2 g will be indicated if muscle weakness has not been relieved. Additional doses may be given cautiously if muscle weakness persists.

Too-rapid administration may result in temporary worsening of cholinergic manifestations. Injection rate should not exceed 200 mg/minute. If intravenous administration is not feasible, intramuscular or subcutaneous injection should be used.

In severe cases, especially after ingestion of the poison, it may be desirable to monitor the effect of therapy electrocardiographically because of the possibility of heart block due to the anticholinesterase. Where the poison has been ingested, it is particularly important to take into account the likelihood of continuing absorption from the lower bowel since this constitutes new exposure. In such cases, additional doses of Protopam (pralidoxime) may be needed every three to eight hours. In effect, the patient should be "titrated" with Protopam as long as signs of poisoning recur. As in all cases of organophosphate poisoning, care should be taken to keep the patient under observation for at least 24 hours.

If convulsions interfere with respiration, they may be controlled by the slow intravenous injection of diazepam, up to 20 mg in adults.

ANTICHOLINESTERASE OVERDOSAGE

As an antagonist to such anticholinesterases as neostigmine, pyridostigmine, and ambenonium, which are used in the treatment of myasthenia gravis, Protopam may be given in a dosage of 1 to 2 g intravenously followed by increments of 250 mg every five minutes.

HOW SUPPLIED

NDC 0046-0374-06—*Hospital Package:* This contains six 20 mL vials of 1 g each of sterile Protopam Chloride (pralidoxime chloride) white to off-white porous cake*, without diluent or syringe. Solution may be prepared by adding 20 mL of Sterile Water for Injection, USP. These are single-dose vials for intravenous injection or for intravenous infusion after further dilution with physiologic saline. Intramuscular or subcutaneous injection may be used when intravenous injection is not feasible.

*When necessary, sodium hydroxide is added during processing to adjust the pH.

Store at room temperature (approximately 25°C).

ANIMAL PHARMACOLOGY AND TOXICOLOGY

The following table lists chemical and trade or generic names of pesticides, chemicals, and drugs against which Protopam (usually administered in conjunction with atropine) has been found to have antidotal activity on the basis of animal experiments. All compounds listed are organophosphates having anticholinesterase activity. A great many additional substances are in industrial use but have been omitted because of lack of special information.

AAT—see PARATHION

AFLIX®—see FORMOTHION

ALKRON®—See PARATHION

AMERICAN CYANAMID 3422—see PARATHION

AMITON—diethyl-S-(2-diethylaminoethyl)phosphorothiolate

ANTHIO®—see FORMOTHION

APHAMITE—see PARATHION

ARMIN—ethyl-4-nitrophenylethylphosphonate

AZINPHOS-METHYL—dimethyl-S-[(4-oxo-1,2,3,-benzotriazin-3 (4H)-yl)methyl] phosphorodithioate

MORPHOTHION—dimethyl-S-2-keto-2-(N-morpholyl)ethylphosphorodithioate

NEGUVON®—see TRICHLOROFON

NIRAN®—see PARATHION

NITROSTIGMINE—see PARATHION

O,O-DIETHYL-O-p-NITROPHENYL PHOSPHOROTHIOATE—see PARATHION

O,O-DIETHYL-O-p-NITROPHENYLTHIO PHOSPHATE—see PARATHION

OR 1191—see PHOSPHAMIDON

OS 1836—see VINYLPHOS

OXYDEMETONMETHYL—dimethyl-S-2-(ethylsulfinyl) ethyl phosphorothiolate

PARAOXON—diethyl (4-nitrophenyl) phosphate

PARATHION—diethyl (4-nitrophenyl) phosphorothionate

PENPHOS—see PARATHION

PHENCAPTON—diethyl-S-(2,5-dichlorophenylmercaptomethyl) phosphorodithioate

PHOSDRIN®—see MEVINPHOS

PHOS-KIL—see PARATHION

PHOSPHAMIDON—1-chloro-1-diethylcarbamoyl-1-propen-2-yl-dimethylphosphate

PHOSPHOLINE IODIDE®—see echothiophate iodide

PHOSPHOROTHIOIC ACID, O,O-DIETHYL-O-p-NITROPHENYL ESTER—see PARATHION

PLANTHION—see PARATHION

QUELETOX—see FENTHION

RHODIATOX®—see PARATHION

RUELENE®—4-tert-butyl-2-chlorophenylmethyl-N-methylphosphoroamidate

SARIN—isopropyl-methylphosphonofluoridate

SHELL OS 1836—see VINYLPHOS

SHELL 2046—see MEVINPHOS

SNP—see PARATHION

SOMAN—pinacolyl-methylphosphonofluoridate

SYSTOX®—diethyl-(2-ethylmercaptoethyl) phosphorothionate

TEP—see TEPP

TEPP—tetraethylpyro phosphate

THIOPHOS®—see PARATHION

TIGUVON—see FENTHION

TRICHLOROFON—dimethyl-1-hydroxy-2,2,2-trichloroethylphosphonate

VAPONA®—see DICHLORVOS

VAPOPHOS—see PARATHION

VINYLPHOS—diethyl-2-chloro-vinylphosphate

PROTOPAM appears to be ineffective, or marginally effective, against poisoning by:
CIODRIN® (alpha-methylbenzyl-3[dimethoxyphosphinyloxy]-ciscrotonate)
DIMEFOX (tetramethylphosphorodiamidic fluoride)
DIMETHOATE (dimethyl-S-[N-methylcarbamoylmethyl]phosphorodithioate)
METHYL DIAZINON (dimethyl-[2-isopropyl-4-methylpyrimidyl]-phosphorothionate)
METHYL PHENCAPTON (dimethyl-S-[2,5-dichlorophenylmercaptomethyl]phosphorodithioate)
PHORATE (diethyl-S-ethylmercaptomethylphosphorodithioate)
SCHRADAN (octamethylpyrophosphoramide)
WEPSYN® (5-amino-1-[bis-(dimethylamino) phosphinyl]-3-phenyl-1,2,4-triazole).

The use of Protopam should, nevertheless, be considered in any life-threatening situation resulting from poisoning by these compounds, since the limited and arbitrary conditions of pharmacologic screening do not always accurately reflect the usefulness of Protopam in the clinical situation.

CLINICAL STUDIES

The use of Protopam (pralidoxime) has been reported in the treatment of human cases of poisoning by the following substances:
Azodrin
Diazinon
Dichlorvos (DDVP) with chlordane
Disulfoton
EPN
Isoflurophate
Malathion
Metasystox I® and Fenthion
Methyldemeton
Methylparathion
Mevinphos
Parathion
Parathion and Mevinphos
Phosphamidon
Sarin
Systox®
TEPP

Of these cases, over 100 were due to parathion, about a dozen each to malathion, diazinon, and mevinphos, and a few to each of the other compounds.

REFERENCES

1. LANDAUER, W.: Cholinomimetic teratogens. V. The effect of oximes and related cholinesterase reactivators, *Teratology 15* :33 (Feb) 1977.
2. MOLLER, K.O., JENSEN-HOLM, J., and LAUSEN, H.H.: *Ugeskr. Laeg. 123* :501, 1961.
3. NAMBA, T., NOLTE, C.T., JACKREL, J. and GROB, D.: Poisoning due to organophosphate insecticides. Acute and chronic manifestations, *Amer. J. Med. 50* :475 (Apr), 1971.
4. ARENA, J.M.: Poisoning, Toxicology Symptoms, Treatments, ed. 4, Springfield, IL, Charles C. Thomas, 1979, p. 133.
5. BRACHFELD, J., and ZAVON, M.R.: Organic phosphate (Phosdrin®) intoxication. Report of a case and the results of treatment with 2-PAM, *Arch. Environ. Health 11* :859, 1965.
6. HAYES, W.J., Jr.: Toxicology of Pesticides, Baltimore, The Williams & Wilkins Company, 1975, p. 416.
7. AMA Department of Drugs: AMA Drug Evaluations, ed. 4, Chicago, American Medical Association, 1980, p. 1455.

Manufactured by:
Ayerst Laboratories Inc.
A Wyeth-Ayerst Company
Philadelphia, PA 19101
CI 3799-6 Revised June 25, 1996

RAPAMUNE® ORAL SOLUTION ℞
[răp 'ă-mūn]
sirolimus

WARNING:
Increased susceptibility to infection and the possible development of lymphoma may result from immunosuppression. Only physicians experienced in immunosup-

Continued on next page

Rapamune—Cont.

pressive therapy and management of renal transplant patients should use Rapamune®. Patients receiving the drug should be managed in facilities equipped and staffed with adequate laboratory and supportive medical resources. The physician responsible for maintenance therapy should have complete information requisite for the follow-up of the patient.

DESCRIPTION

Rapamune® (sirolimus) is an immunosuppressive agent. Sirolimus is a macrocyclic lactone produced by *Streptomyces hygroscopicus*. The chemical name of sirolimus (also known as rapamycin) is (3*S*,6*R*,7*E*,9*R*,10*R*,12*R*,14*S*,15*E*,17*E*,19*E*,21*S*,23*S*,26*R*,27*R*,34a*S*) - 9,10,12,13,14,21,22,23,24,25,26,27,32,33,34,34a- hexadecahydro -9,27-dihydroxy-3-[(1*R*)-2-[(1*S*,3*R*,4*R*)-4-hydroxy-3-methoxycyclohexyl]-1-methylethyl]-10,21-dimethoxy-6,8,12,14,20,26 - hexamethyl-23,27-epoxy-3*H*-pyrido[2,1-*c*][1,4] oxaazacyclohentriacontine-1,5,11,28,29 (4*H*,6*H*,31*H*)-pentone. Its molecular formula is $C_{51}H_{79}NO_{13}$ and its molecular weight is 914.2. The structural formula of sirolimus is shown below.

Sirolimus is a white to off-white powder and is insoluble in water but freely soluble in benzyl alcohol, chloroform, acetone, and acetonitrile.

Each mL of Rapamune® Oral Solution contains 1 mg sirolimus; inactive ingredients are Phosal 50 PG® (phosphatidylcholine, propylene glycol, monodiglycerides, ethanol, soy fatty acids, and ascorbyl palmitate) and Polysorbate 80, NF. Rapamune Oral Solution contains 1.5%–2.5% ethanol.

CLINICAL PHARMACOLOGY

Mechanism of Action

Sirolimus inhibits T lymphocyte activation and proliferation that occurs in response to antigenic and cytokine (Interleukin [IL]-2, IL-4, and IL-15) stimulation by a mechanism that is distinct from that of other immunosuppressants. Sirolimus also inhibits antibody production. In cells, sirolimus binds to the immunophilin, FK Binding Protein-12 (FKBP-12), to generate an immunosuppressive complex. The sirolimus: FKBP-12 complex has no effect on calcineurin activity. This complex binds to and inhibits the activation of the mammalian Target Of Rapamycin (mTOR), a key regulatory kinase. This inhibition suppresses cytokine-driven T-cell proliferation, inhibiting the progression from the G_1 to the S phase of the cell cycle.

Studies in experimental models show that sirolimus prolongs allograft (kidney, heart, skin, islet, small bowel, pancreatico-duodenal, and bone marrow) survival in mice, rats, pigs, and/or primates. Sirolimus reverses acute rejection of heart and kidney allografts in rats and prolonged the graft survival in presensitized rats. In some studies, the immunosuppressive effect of sirolimus lasted up to 6 months after discontinuation of therapy. This tolerization effect is alloantigen specific.

In rodent models of autoimmune disease, sirolimus suppresses immune-mediated events associated with systemic lupus erythematosus, collagen-induced arthritis, autoimmune type I diabetes, autoimmune myocarditis, experimental allergic encephalomyelitis, graft-versus-host disease, and autoimmune uveoretinitis.

Pharmacokinetics

Sirolimus pharmacokinetic activity has been determined following oral administration in healthy subjects, pediatric dialysis patients, hepatically-impaired patients and renal transplant patients.

Absorption

Following oral administration, sirolimus is rapidly absorbed, with a mean-time-to-peak concentration of approximately 1 hour after a single dose in healthy subjects and approximately 2 hours after multiple oral doses in renal transplant recipients. The systemic availability of sirolimus was estimated to be approximately 14%. Sirolimus concentrations in stable renal transplant patients are dose proportional between 3 and 12 mg/m^2.

Food effects: In 22 healthy volunteers, a high fat breakfast (1.88 kcal, 54.7% fat) altered the bioavailability characteristics of sirolimus. Compared to fasting, a 34% decrease in the peak blood sirolimus concentration (C_{max}), a 3.5-fold increase in the time-to-peak concentration (t_{max}), and a 35% increase in total exposure (AUC) was observed. To minimize variability, Rapamune should be taken consistently with or without food (see **DOSAGE AND ADMINISTRATION**).

SIROLIMUS PHARMACOKINETIC PARAMETERS (MEAN ±SD) IN RENAL TRANSPLANT PATIENTS (MULTIPLE DOSE)[a, b]

n	Dose	$C_{max,ss}$[c] (ng/mL)	$t_{max,ss}$ (h)	$AUC_{\tau,ss}$[c] (ng•h/mL)	CL/F/WT[d] (mL/h/kg)
19	2 mg	12.2 ± 6.2	3.01 ± 2.40	158 ± 70	182 ± 72
23	5 mg	37.4 ± 21	1.84 ± 1.30	396 ± 193	221 ± 143

a: Sirolimus administered four hours after cyclosporine oral solution (MODIFIED) (e.g., Neoral® Oral Solution) and/or cyclosporine capsules (MODIFIED) (e.g., Neoral® Soft Gelatin Capsules).
b: As measured by the Liquid Chromatographic/Tandem Mass Spectrometric Method (LC/MS/MS)
c: These parameters were dose normalized prior to the statistical comparison.
d: CL/F/WT = oral dose clearance.

SIROLIMUS PHARMACOKINETIC PARAMETERS (MEAN ±SD) IN 18 HEALTHY SUBJECTS AND 18 PATIENTS WITH HEPATIC IMPAIRMENT (15 MG SINGLE DOSE)

Population	$C_{max,ss}$[a] (ng/mL)	t_{max} (h)	$AUC_{0-\infty}$ (ng•h/mL)	CL/F/WT (mL/h/kg)
Healthy subjects	78.2 ± 18.3	0.82 ± 0.17	970 ± 272	215 ± 76
Hepatic impairment	77.9 ± 23.1	0.84 ± 0.17	1567 ± 616	144 ± 62

a: As measured by (LC/MS/MS)

SIROLIMUS PHARMACOKINETIC PARAMETERS (MEAN ± SD) IN PEDIATRIC PATIENTS WITH STABLE CHRONIC RENAL FAILURE MAINTAINED ON HEMODIALYSIS OR PERITONEAL DIALYSIS (1, 3, 9, 15 MG/M^2 SINGLE DOSE)

Age Group (y)	n	t_{max} (h)	$t_{1/2}$ (h)	CL/F/WT (mL/h/kg)
5–11	9	1.1 ± 0.5	71 ± 40	580 ± 450
12–18	11	0.79 ± 0.17	55 ± 18	450 ± 232

Distribution

The mean (± SD) blood-to-plasma ratio of sirolimus was 36 (± 17.9) in stable renal allograft recipients, indicating that sirolimus is extensively partitioned into formed blood elements. The mean volume of distribution (V_{SS}/F) of sirolimus is 12 ± 7.52 L/kg. Sirolimus is extensively bound (approximately 92%) to human plasma proteins. In man, the binding of sirolimus was shown mainly to be associated with serum albumin (97%), α_1-acid glycoprotein, and lipoproteins.

Metabolism

Sirolimus is a substrate for both cytochrome P450 IIIA4 (CYP3A4) and P-glycoprotein. Sirolimus is extensively metabolized by O-demethylation and/or hydroxylation. Seven (7) major metabolites, including hydroxy, demethyl, and hydroxydemethyl, are identifiable in whole blood. Some of these metabolites are also detectable in plasma, fecal, and urine samples. Glucuronide and sulfate conjugates are not present in any of the biologic matrices. Sirolimus is the major component in human whole blood and contributes to greater than 90% of the immunosuppressive activity.

Excretion

After a single dose of [^{14}C]sirolimus in healthy volunteers, the majority (91%) of radioactivity was recovered from the feces, and only a minor amount (2.2%) was excreted in urine.

Pharmacokinetics in renal transplant patients

Pharmacokinetic parameters for sirolimus oral solution given daily in combination with cyclosporine and corticosteroids in renal transplant patients are summarized below based on data collected at months 1, 3, and 6 after transplantation. There were no significant differences in any of these parameters with respect to treatment group or month.
[See first table above]
Whole blood sirolimus trough concentrations, as measured by immunoassay, (mean ± SD) for the 2 mg/day and 5 mg/day dose groups were 8.59 ± 4.01 (n = 226) and 17.3 ± 7.4 (n = 219), respectively. Whole blood trough sirolimus concentrations, as measured by LC/MS/MS, were significantly correlated (r^2 = 0.96) with $AUC_{\tau,ss}$. Upon repeated twice daily administration without an initial loading dose in a multiple-dose study, the average trough concentration of sirolimus increases approximately 2 to 3-fold over the initial 6 days of therapy at which time steady state is reached. A loading dose of 3 times the maintenance dose will provide near steady state concentrations within 1 day in most patients. The mean ± SD terminal elimination half life ($t_{1/2}$) of sirolimus after multiple dosing in stable renal transplant patients was estimated to be about 62 ± 16 hours.

Special Populations

Hepatic impairment: Sirolimus (15 mg) was administered as a single oral dose to 18 subjects with normal hepatic function and to 18 patients with Child-Pugh classification A or B hepatic impairment, in which hepatic impairment was primary and not related to an underlying systemic disease. Shown below are the mean ± SD pharmacokinetic parameters following the administration of sirolimus oral solution.
[See second table above]
Compared with the values in the normal hepatic group, the hepatic impairment group had higher mean values for sirolimus AUC (61%) and $t_{1/2}$ (43%) and had lower mean values for sirolimus CL/F/WT (33%). The mean $t_{1/2}$ increased from 79 ± 12 hours in subjects with normal hepatic function to 113 ± 41 hours in patients with impaired hepatic function. The rate of absorption of sirolimus was not altered by hepatic disease, as evidenced by C_{max} and t_{max} values. However, hepatic diseases with varying etiologies may show different effects and the pharmacokinetics of sirolimus in patients with severe hepatic dysfunction is unknown. Dosage adjustment is recommended for patients with mild to moderate hepatic impairment (see **DOSAGE AND ADMINISTRATION**).

Renal impairment: The effect of renal impairment on the pharmacokinetics of sirolimus is not known. However, there is minimal (2.2%) renal excretion of the drug or its metabolites.

Pediatric: Limited pharmacokinetic data are available in pediatric patients. The table below summarizes pharmacokinetic data obtained in pediatric dialysis patients with chronically impaired renal function.
[See third table above]

Geriatric: Clinical studies of Rapamune did not include a sufficient number of patients > 65 years of age to determine whether they will respond differently than younger patients. Sirolimus trough concentration data in 35 renal transplant patients > 65 years of age were similar to those in the adult population (n=822) from 18 to 65 years of age.

Gender: Sirolimus oral dose clearance in males was 12% lower than that in females; male subjects had a significantly longer $t_{1/2}$ than did female subjects (72.3 hours versus 61.3 hours). These pharmacokinetic differences do not require dose adjustment based on gender.

Race: In large phase III trials using Rapamune and cyclosporine oral solution (MODIFIED) (e.g., Neoral® Oral Solution) and/or cyclosporine capsules (MODIFIED) (e.g., Neoral® Soft Gelatin Capsules), there were no significant differences in mean trough sirolimus concentrations over time between black (n = 139) and non-black (n = 724) patients during the first 6 months after transplantation at sirolimus doses of 2 mg/day and 5 mg/day.

CLINICAL STUDIES

The safety and efficacy of Rapamune for the prevention of organ rejection following renal transplantation were assessed in two randomized, double-blind, multicenter, controlled trials. These studies compared two dose levels of Rapamune oral solution (2 mg and 5 mg, once daily) with azathioprine (Study 1) or placebo (Study 2) when administered in combination with cyclosporine and corticosteroids. Study 1 was conducted in the United States at 38 sites. Seven hundred nineteen (719) patients were enrolled in this trial and randomized following transplantation; 284 were randomized to receive Rapamune 2 mg/day, 274 were randomized to receive Rapamune 5 mg/day, and 161 to receive azathioprine 2–3 mg/kg/day. Study 2 was conducted in Australia, Canada, Europe, and the United States, at a total of 34 sites. Five hundred seventy-six (576) patients were enrolled in this trial and randomized before transplantation; 227 were randomized to receive Rapamune 2 mg/day, 219 were randomized to receive Rapamune 5 mg/day, and 130 to receive placebo. In both studies, the use of antilymphocyte antibody induction therapy was prohibited. In both studies, the primary efficacy endpoint was the rate of efficacy failure in the first 6 months after transplantation. Efficacy failure was defined as the first occurrence of an acute rejection episode (confirmed by biopsy), graft loss, or death.

The tables below summarize the results of the primary efficacy analyses from these trials. Rapamune, at doses of 2 mg/day and 5 mg/day, significantly reduced the incidence of efficacy failure (statistically significant at the <0.025 level; nominal significance level adjusted for multiple [2] dose comparisons) at 6 months following transplantation compared to both azathioprine and placebo.
[See first & second table at top of next page]
Patient and graft survival at 1 year were co-primary endpoints. The table below shows graft and patient survival at

1 year in Study 1 and Study 2. The graft and patient survival rates at 1 year were similar in the Rapamune- and comparator-treated patients.

[See third table above]

The reduction in the incidence of first biopsy-confirmed acute rejection episodes in Rapamune-treated patients compared to the control groups included a reduction in all grades of rejection.

[See fourth table above]

In Study 1, which was prospectively stratified by race within center, efficacy failure was similar for Rapamune 2 mg/day and lower for Rapamune 5 mg/day compared to azathioprine in black patients. In Study 2, which was not prospectively stratified by race, efficacy failure was similar for both Rapamune doses compared to placebo in black patients. The decision to use the higher dose of Rapamune in black patients must be weighed against the increased risk of dose dependent adverse events that were observed with the Rapamune 5 mg dose (see **ADVERSE REACTIONS**).

[See fifth table above]

Mean glomerular filtration (GFR) at one year post transplant were calculated using the Nankivell equation for all subjects in Studies 1 and 2 who had serum creatinine measured at 12 months. In Studies 1 and 2 mean GFR, at 12 months, were lower in patients treated with cyclosporine and Rapamune compared to those treated with cyclosporine and the respective azathioprine or placebo control.

Within each treatment group in Studies 1 and 2, mean GFR at one year post transplant was lower in patients who experienced at least 1 episode of biopsy-proven acute rejection, compared to those who did not.

Renal function should be monitored and appropriate adjustment of the immunosuppression regimen should be considered in patients with elevated serum creatinine levels (see **PRECAUTIONS**).

INDICATIONS AND USAGE

Repamune is indicated for the prophylaxis of organ rejection in patients receiving renal transplants. It is recommended that Rapamune be used in a regimen with cyclosporine and corticosteroids.

CONTRAINDICATIONS

Rapamune is contraindicated in patients with a hypersensitivity to sirolimus or its derivatives or any component of the drug product.

WARNINGS

Increased susceptibility to infection and the possible development of lymphoma and other malignancies, particularly of the skin, may result from immunosuppression (see **ADVERSE REACTIONS**). Oversuppression of the immune system can also increase susceptibility to infection including opportunistic infections, fatal infections, and sepsis. Only physicians experienced in immunosuppressive therapy and management of organ transplant patients should use Rapamune. Patients receiving the drug should be managed in facilities equipped and staffed with adequate laboratory and supportive medical resources. The physician responsible for maintenance therapy should have complete information requisite for the follow-up of the patient.

As usual for patients with increased risk for skin cancer, exposure to sunlight and UV light should be limited by wearing protective clothing and using sunscreen with a high protection factor.

Increased serum cholesterol and triglycerides that may require treatment occurred more frequently in patients treated with Rapamune compared to azathioprine or placebo controls. (see **PRECAUTIONS**).

In phase III studies, mean serum creatinine was increased and mean glomerular filtration rate was decreased in patients treated with Rapamune and cyclosporine compared to those treated with cyclosporine and placebo or azathioprine controls (see **CLINICAL STUDIES**). Renal function should be monitored during the administration of maintenance immunosuppression regimens including Rapamune in combination with cyclosporine, and appropriate adjustment of the immunosuppression regimen should be considered in patients with elevated serum creatinine levels. Caution should be exercised when using agents which are known to impair renal function (see **PRECAUTIONS**).

In clinical trials, Rapamune has been administered concurrently with corticosteroids and with the following formulations of cyclosporine:

Sandimmune® Injection (cyclosporine injection)

Sandimmune® Oral Solution (cyclosporine oral solution)

Neoral® Soft Gelatin Capsules (cyclosporine capsules [MODIFIED])

Neoral® Oral Solution (cyclosporine oral solution [MODIFIED])

The efficacy and safety of the use of Rapamune in combination with other immunosuppressive agents has not been determined.

PRECAUTIONS

General

Rapamune is intended for oral administration only.

Lymphocele, a known surgical complication of renal transplantation, occurred significantly more often in a dose-related fashion in Rapamune-treated patients. Appropriate post-operative measures should be considered to minimize this complication.

Lipids

The use of Rapamune in renal transplant patients was associated with increased serum cholesterol and triglycerides that may require treatment.

INCIDENCE (%) OF THE PRIMARY ENDPOINT AT 6 MONTHS: STUDY 1[a]

	Rapamune® 2 mg/day (n = 284)	Rapamune® 5 mg/day (n = 274)	Azathioprine 2–3 mg/kg/day (n = 161)
Efficacy failure at 6 months	18.7	16.8	32.3
Components of efficacy failure			
Biopsy-proven acute rejection	16.5	11.3	29.2
Graft loss	1.1	2.9	2.5
Death	0.7	1.8	0
Lost to follow-up	0.4	0.7	0.6

a: Patients received cyclosporine and corticosteroids.

INCIDENCE (%) OF THE PRIMARY ENDPOINT AT 6 MONTHS: STUDY 2[a]

	Rapamune® 2 mg/day (n = 227)	Rapamune® 5 mg/day (n = 219)	Placebo (n = 130)
Efficacy failure at 6 months	30.0	25.6	47.7
Components of efficacy failure			
Biopsy-proven acute rejection	24.7	19.2	41.5
Graft loss	3.1	3.7	3.9
Death	2.2	2.7	2.3
Lost to follow-up	0	0	0

a: Patients received cyclosporine and corticosteroids.

1 YEAR GRAFT AND PATIENT SURVIVAL (%)[a]

		Rapamune® 2 mg/day	Rapamune® 5 mg/day	Azathioprine 2–3 mg/kg/day	Placebo
Study 1		(n = 284)	(n = 274)	(n = 161)	
	Graft survival	94.7	92.7	93.8	
	Patient survival	97.2	96.0	98.1	
Study 2		(n = 227)	(n = 219)		(n = 130)
	Graft survival	89.9	90.9		87.7
	Patient survival	96.5	95.0		94.6

a: Patients received cyclosporine and corticosteroids.

PERCENTAGE OF EFFICACY FAILURE BY RACE AT 6 MONTHS

	Rapamune® 2 mg/day	Rapamune® 5 mg/day	Azathioprine 2–3 mg/kg/day	Placebo
Study 1				
Black (n=166)	34.9 (n=63)	18.0 (n=61)	33.3 (n=42)	
Nonblack (n=553)	14.0 (n=221)	16.4 (n=213)	31.9 (n=119)	
Study 2				
Black (n=66)	30.8 (n=26)	33.7 (n=27)		38.5 (n=13)
Nonblack (n=510)	29.9 (n=201)	24.5 (n=192)		48.7 (n=117)

OVERALL CALCULATED GLOMERULAR FILTRATION RATES (CC/MIN) BY NANKIVELL EQUATION AT 12 MONTHS POST TRANSPLANT

	Rapamune® 2 mg/day	Rapamune® 5 mg/day	Azathioprine 2–3 mg/kg/day	Placebo
Study 1	(n=233)	(n=226)	(n=127)	
Mean (SE)	57.4 (1.28)	55.1 (1.28)	65.9 (1.69)	
Study 2	(n=190)	(n=175)		(n=101)
Mean (SE)	54.9 (1.26)	52.9 (1.46)		61.7 (1.81)

In phase III clinical trials, in *de novo* renal transplant recipients who began the study with normal, fasting, total serum cholesterol (fasting serum cholesterol < 200 mg/dL), there was an increased incidence of patients who developed hypercholesterolemia (fasting serum cholesterol > 240 mg/dL) in patients receiving both Rapamune 2 mg and Rapamune 5 mg compared to azathioprine and placebo controls.

In phase III clinical trials, in *de novo* renal transplant recipients who began the study with normal, fasting, total serum triglycerides (fasting serum triglycerides < 200 mg/dL), there was an increased incidence of patients who developed hypertriglyceridemia (fasting serum triglycerides > 500 mg/dL) in patients receiving Rapamune 2 mg and Rapamune 5 mg compared to azathioprine and placebo controls.

Treatment of new-onset hypercholesterolemia, with lipid-lowering agents, was required in 42–52% of patients enrolled in the Rapamune arms of the study compared to 16% of patients in the placebo arm and 22% of patients in the azathioprine arm.

Renal transplant patients have a higher prevalence of clinically significant hyperlipidemia. Accordingly, the risk/benefit should be carefully considered in patients with established hyperlipidemia before initiating an immunosuppressive regimen including Rapamune.

Any patient who is administered Rapamune should be monitored for hyperlipidemia using laboratory tests and if hyperlipidemia is detected, subsequent interventions such as diet, exercise, and lipid-lowering agents, as outlined by the National Cholesterol Education Program guidelines, should be initiated.

In the limited number of patients studied, the concomitant administration of Rapamune and HMG-CoA reductase inhibitors and/or fibrates appeared to be well tolerated. Nevertheless, all patients administered Rapamune with cyclosporine, in conjunction with an HMG-CoA reductase inhibitor, should be monitored for the development of rhabdomyolysis.

Renal Function

Patients treated with cyclosporine and Rapamune were noted to have higher serum creatinine levels and lower glomerular filtration rates compared to patients treated with cyclosporine and placebo or azathioprine controls. Renal function should be monitored during the administration of maintenance immunosupression regimens including Rapamune in combination with cyclosporine, and appropriate adjustment of the immunosupression regimen should be considered in patients with elevated serum creatinine levels. Caution should be exercised when using agents (e.g. aminoglycosides, and amphotericin B) which are known to have a deleterious effect on renal function.

Antimicrobial Prophylaxis

Cases of *Pneumocystis carinii* pneumonia have been reported in patients not receiving antimicrobial prophylaxis. Therefore, antimicrobial prophylaxis for *Pneumocystis carinii* pneumonia should be administered for 1 year following transplantation.

Cytomegalovirus (CMV) prophylaxis is recommended for 3 months after transplantation, particularly for patients at increased risk for CMV disease.

Information for Patients

Patients should be given complete dosage instructions (see **PATIENT INSTRUCTIONS**). Women of childbearing potential should be informed of the potential risks during pregnancy and that they should use effective contraception prior to initiation of Rapamune therapy, during Rapamune therapy and for 12 weeks after Rapamune therapy has been stopped (see **PRECAUTIONS: Pregnancy**).

Continued on next page

Rapamune—Cont.

Patients should be told that exposure to sunlight and UV light should be limited by wearing protective clothing and using a sunscreen with a high protection factor because of the increased risk for skin cancer (see **WARNINGS**).

Laboratory Tests

It is prudent to monitor blood sirolimus levels in patients likely to have altered drug metabolism, in patients ≥ 13 years who weigh less than 40 kg, in patients with hepatic impairment, and during concurrent administration of potent CYP3A4 inducers and inhibitors (see **PRECAUTIONS: Drug Interactions**).

Drug Interactions

Sirolimus is known to be a substrate for both cytochrome CYP3A4 and P-glycoprotein. The pharmacokinetic interaction between sirolimus and concomitantly administered drugs is discussed below. Drug interaction studies have not been conducted with drugs other than those described below.

Cyclosporine capsules MODIFIED: In a single dose drug-drug interaction study, 24 healthy volunteers were administered 10 mg sirolimus either simultaneously or 4 hours after a 300 mg dose of Neoral® Soft Gelatin Capsules (cyclosporine capsules [MODIFIED]). For simultaneous administration, mean C_{max} and AUC of sirolimus were increased by 116% and 230% respectively relative to administration of sirolimus alone. However, when given 4 hours after Neoral® Soft Gelatin Capsules (cyclosporine capsules [MODIFIED]) administration, sirolimus C_{max} and AUC were increased by 37% and 80% respectively compared to administration of sirolimus alone.

Mean cyclosporine C_{max} and AUC were not significantly affected when sirolimus was given simultaneously or when administered 4 hours after Neoral® Soft Gelatin Capsules (cyclosporine capsules [MODIFIED]). However, after multiple-dose administration of sirolimus given 4 hours after Neoral® in renal post-transplant patients over 6 months, cyclosporine oral-dose clearance was reduced, and lower doses of Neoral® Soft Gelatin Capsules (cyclosporine capsules [MODIFIED]) were needed to maintain target cyclosporine concentration.

Because of the effect of cyclosporine capsules (MODIFIED) it is recommended that sirolimus should be taken 4 hours after administration of cyclosporine oral solution (MODIFIED) and/or cyclosporine capsules (MODIFIED), (see DOSAGE AND ADMINISTRATION).

Cyclosporine oral solution: In a multiple-dose study in 150 psoriasis patients, sirolimus 0.5, 1.5, and 3 mg/m^2/day was administered simultaneously with Sandimmune® Oral Solution (cyclosporine oral solution) 1.25 mg/kg/day. The increase in average sirolimus trough concentrations ranged between 67%–86% relative to when sirolimus was administered without cyclosporine. The intersubject variability (%CV) for sirolimus trough concentrations ranged from 39.7% to 68.7%. There was no significant effect of multiple-dose sirolimus on cyclosporine trough concentrations following Sandimmune® Oral Solution (cyclosporine oral solution) administration. However, the %CV was higher (range 85.9%–165%) than those from previous studies.

Sandimmune® Oral Solution (cyclosporine oral solution) is not bioequivalent to Neoral® Oral Solution (cyclosporine oral solution [MODIFIED]) and should not be used interchangeably. Although there is no published data comparing Sandimmune® Oral Solution (cyclosporine oral solution) to SangCya® Oral Solution (cyclosporine oral solution [MODIFIED]), they should not be used interchangeably. Likewise, Sandimmune Soft Gelatin Capsules (cyclosporine capsules) are not bioequivalent to Neoral® Soft Gelatin Capsules (cyclosporine capsules [MODIFIED] and should not be used interchangeably.

Diltiazem: The simultaneous oral administration of 10 mg of sirolimus oral solution and 120 mg of diltiazem to 18 healthy volunteers significantly affected the bioavailability of sirolimus. Sirolimus C_{max}, t_{max}, and AUC were increased 1.4-, 1.3-, and 1.6-fold, respectively. Sirolimus did not affect the pharmacokinetics of either diltiazem or its metabolites desacetyldiltiazem and desmethyldiltiazem. If diltiazem is administered, sirolimus should be monitored and a dose adjustment may be necessary.

Ketoconazole: Multiple-dose ketoconazole administration significantly affected the rate and extent of absorption and sirolimus exposure, as reflected by increases in sirolimus C_{max}, t_{max}, and AUC of 4.3-fold, 38%, and 10.9-fold, respectively. However, the terminal $t_{1/2}$ of sirolimus was not changed. Single-dose sirolimus did not affect steady-state 12-hour plasma ketoconazole concentrations. It is recommended that sirolimus should not be coadministered with ketoconazole.

Rifampin: Pretreatment of 14 healthy volunteers with multiple doses of rifampin, 600 mg daily for 14 days, followed by a single 20 mg-dose of sirolimus, greatly increased sirolimus oral-dose clearance by 5.5-fold (range = 2.8 to 10), which represents mean decreases in AUC and C_{max} of about 82% and 71%, respectively. In patients where rifampin is indicated, alternative therapeutic agents with less enzyme induction potential should be considered.

Drugs which may be coadministered without dose adjustment

Clinically significant pharmacokinetic drug-drug interactions were not observed in studies of drugs listed below. A synopsis of the type of study performed for each drug is provided. Sirolimus and these drugs may be coadministered without dose adjustments.

Acyclovir: Acyclovir, 200 mg, was administered once daily for 3 days followed by a single 10-mg dose of sirolimus oral solution on day 3 in 20 adult healthy volunteers.

Digoxin: Digoxin, 0.25 mg, was administered daily for 8 days and a single 10-mg dose of sirolimus oral solution was given on day 8 to 24 healthy volunteers.

Glyburide: A single 5-mg dose of glyburide and a single 10-mg dose of sirolimus oral solution were administered to 24 healthy volunteers. Sirolimus did not affect the hypoglycemic action of glyburide.

Nifedipine: A single 60-mg dose of nifedipine and a single 10-mg dose of sirolimus oral solution were administered to 24 healthy volunteers.

Norgestrel/ethinyl estradiol (Lo/Ovral®): Sirolimus oral solution, 2 mg, was given daily for 7 days to 21 healthy female volunteers on norgestrel/ethinyl estradiol.

Prednisolone: Pharmacokinetic information was obtained from 42 stable renal transplant patients receiving daily doses of prednisone (5–20 mg/day) and either single or multiple doses of sirolimus oral solution (0.5–5 mg/m^2 q 12h).

Sulfamethoxazole/trimethoprim (Bactrim®): A single oral dose of sulfamethoxazole (400 mg)/trimethoprim, (80 mg) was given to 15 renal transplant patients receiving daily oral doses of sirolimus (8 to 25 mg/m^2).

Other drug interactions

Sirolimus is extensively metabolized by the CYP3A4 isoenzyme in the gut wall and liver. Therefore, absorption and the subsequent elimination of systematically absorbed sirolimus may be influenced by drugs that affect this isoenzyme. Inhibitors of CYP3A4 may decrease the metabolism of sirolimus and increase sirolimus levels, while inducers of CYP3A4 may increase the metabolism of sirolimus and decrease sirolimus levels.

Drugs that may increase sirolimus blood concentrations include:

- Calcium channel blockers: nicardipine, verapamil.
- Antifungal agents: clotrimazole, fluconazole, itraconazole.
- Macrolide antibiotics: clarithromycin, erythromycin, troleandomycin.
- Gastrointestinal prokinetic agents: cisapride, metoclopramide.
- Other drugs: bromocriptine, cimetidine, danazol, HIV-protease inhibitors (e.g., ritonavir, indinavir)

Drugs that may decrease sirolimus levels include:

- Anticonvulsants: carbamazepine, phenobarbital, phenytoin.
- Antibiotics: rifabutin, rifapentine.

This list is not all inclusive.

Care should be exercised when drugs that are metabolized by CYP3A4 are administered concomitantly with Rapamune. Grapefruit juice reduces CYP3A4-mediated metabolism of Rapamune and must not be used for dilution (see **DOSAGE AND ADMINISTRATION**).

Vaccination

Immunosuppressants may affect response to vaccination. Therefore, during treatment with Rapamune, vaccination may be less effective. The use of live vaccines should be avoided; live vaccines may include, but are not limited to measles, mumps, rubella, oral polio, BCG, yellow fever, varicella, and TY21a typhoid.

Drug-Laboratory Test Interactions

There are no studies on the interactions of sirolimus in commonly employed clinical laboratory tests.

Carcinogenesis, Mutagenesis, and Impairment of Fertility

Sirolimus was not genotoxic in the *in vitro* bacterial reverse mutation assay, the Chinese hamster ovary cell chromosomal aberration assay, the mouse lymphoma cell forward mutation assay, or the *in vivo* mouse micronucleus assay.

Carcinogenicity studies were conducted in female mice and male and female rats. Carcinogenicity studies have not been completed in male mice. In the 86-week female mouse study at dosages of 0, 12.5, 25 and 50/6 (dosage lowered from 50 to 6 mg/kg/day at week 31 due to infection secondary to immunosuppression) there was a statistically significant increase in malignant lymphoma at all dosages (approximately 6 to 135 times the clinical doses adjusted for body surface area) compared to controls. In the 104-week rat study at dosages of 0, 0.05, 0.1, and 0.2 mg/kg/day, there was a statistically significant increased incidence of testicular adenoma in the 0.2 mg/kg/day group (approximately 0.4 to 1 times the clinical doses adjusted for body surface area).

There was no effect on fertility in female rats following the administration of sirolimus at dosages up to 0.5 mg/kg (approximately 1 to 3 times the clinical doses adjusted for body surface area). In male rats, there was no significant difference in fertility rate compared to controls at a dosage of 2 mg/kg (approximately 4 to 11 times the clinical doses adjusted for body surface area). Reductions in testicular weights and/or histological lesions (e.g., tubular atrophy and tubular giant cells) were observed in rats following dosages of 0.65 mg/kg (approximately 1 to 3 times the clinical doses adjusted for body surface area) and above and in a monkey study at 0.1 mg/kg (approximately 0.4 to 1 times the clinical doses adjusted for body surface area) and above. Sperm counts were reduced in male rats following the administration of sirolimus for 13 weeks at a dosage of 6 mg/kg (approximately 12 to 32 times the clinical doses adjusted for body surface area), but showed improvement by 3 months after dosing was stopped.

Pregnancy

Pregnancy Category C: Sirolimus was embryo/feto toxic in rats at dosages of 0.1 mg/kg and above (approximately 0.2 to 0.5 the clinical doses adjusted for body surface area). Embryo/feto toxicity was manifested as mortality and reduced fetal weights (with associated delays in skeletal ossification). However, no teratogenesis was evident. In combination with cyclosporine, rats had increased embryo/feto mortality compared to Rapamune alone. There were no effects on rabbit development at the maternally toxic dosage of 0.05 mg/kg (approximately 0.3 to 0.8 times the clinical doses adjusted for body surface area). There are no adequate and well controlled studies in pregnant women. Effective contraception must be initiated before Rapamune therapy, during Rapamune therapy, and for 12 weeks after Rapamune therapy has been stopped. Rapamune should be used during pregnancy only if the potential benefit outweighs the potential risk to the embryo/fetus.

Use during lactation

Sirolimus is excreted in trace amounts in milk of lactating rats. It is not known whether sirolimus is excreted in human milk. The pharmacokinetic and safety profiles of sirolimus in infants are not known. Because many drugs are excreted in human milk and because of the potential for adverse reactions in nursing infants from sirolimus, a decision should be made whether to discontinue nursing or to discontinue the drug, taking into account the importance of the drug to the mother.

Pediatric use

The safety and efficacy of Rapamune in pediatric patients below the age of 13 years have not been established.

Geriatric use

Clinical studies of Rapamune did not include sufficient numbers of patients aged 65 and over to determine whether safety and efficacy differ in this population from younger patients. Data pertaining to sirolimus trough concentrations suggest that dose adjustments based upon age in geriatric renal patients are not necessary.

ADVERSE REACTIONS

The incidence of adverse reactions was determined in two randomized, double-blind, multicenter controlled trials in which 499 renal transplant patients received Rapamune® 2 mg/day, 477 received Rapamune 5 mg/day, 160 received azathioprine, and 124 received placebo. All patients were treated with cyclosporine and corticosteroids. Data (≥ 12 months post-transplant) presented in the table below show the adverse reactions that occurred in any treatment group with an incidence of ≥ 20%.

Specific adverse reactions associated with the administration of Rapamune occurred at a significantly higher frequency than with the respective control group. For both Rapamune 2 mg/day and 5 mg/day these include hypercholesterolemia, hyperlipemia, hypertension, and rash; for Rapamune 2 mg/day: acne; and for Rapamune 5 mg/day: anemia, arthralgia, diarrhea, hypokalemia, and thrombocytopenia. The elevations of triglycerides and cholesterol and decreases in platelets and hemoglobin occurred in a dose related manner in patients receiving Rapamune.

Patients maintained on Rapamune 5 mg/day, when compared to patients on Rapamune 2 mg/day, demonstrated an increased incidence of the following adverse events: anemia, leukopenia, thrombocytopenia, hypokalemia, hyperlipemia, fever, and diarrhea.

[See first table at bottom of next page]

At 12 months, there were no significant differences in incidence rates for clinically important opportunistic or common transplant-related infections across treatment groups, with the exception of mucosal infections with *Herpes simplex*, which occurred at a significantly greater rate in patients treated with Rapamune 5 mg/day than in both of the comparator groups.

The table below summarizes the incidence of malignancies in the two controlled trials for the prevention of acute rejection. At 12 months following transplantation there was a very low incidence of malignancies and there were no significant differences among treatment groups.

[See second table at bottom of next page]

Among the adverse events that were reported at a rate of ≥ 3% and < 20%, the following were more prominent in patients maintained on Rapamune 5 mg/day, when compared to patients on Rapamune 2 mg/day; epistaxis, lymphocele, insomnia, thrombotic thrombocytopenic purpura (hemolytic-uremic syndrome), skin ulcer, increased LDH, hypotension, facial edema.

The following adverse events were reported with ≥ 3% and < 20% incidence in patients in any Rapamune treatment group in the two controlled clinical trials for the prevention of acute rejection: BODY AS A WHOLE: abdomen enlarged, abscess, ascites, cellulitis, chills, face edema, flu syndrome, generalized edema, hernia, *Herpes* zoster, infection, lymphocele, malaise, pelvic pain, peritonitis, sepsis; CARDIOVASCULAR SYSTEM: atrial fibrillation, congestive heart failure, hemorrhage, hypervolemia, hypotension, palpitation, peripheral vascular disorder, postural hypotension, syncope, tachycardia, thrombophlebitis, thrombosis, vasodilatation; DIGESTIVE SYSTEM: anorexia, dysphagia, eructation, esophagitis, flatulence, gastritis, gastroenteritis, gingivitis, gum hyperplasia, ileus, liver function tests abnormal, mouth ulceration, oral moniliasis, stomatitis; ENDOCRINE SYSTEM: Cushing's syndrome, diabetes mellitus, glycosuria; HEMIC AND LYMPHATIC SYSTEM: ecchymosis, leukocytosis, lymphadenopathy, polycythemia, thrombotic thrombocytopenic purpura (hemolytic-uremic syndrome); METABOLIC AND NUTRITIONAL: acidosis, alkaline phosphatase increased. BUN increased, creatine phosphokinase increased, dehydration, healing abnormal, hypercalcemia, hyperglycemia, hyperphosphatemia, hypocalcemia, hypoglycemia, hypomagnesemia, hyponatremia, lactic dehydrogenase increased, SGOT increased, SGPT increased, weight loss; MUSCULOSKELETAL SYSTEM: arthrosis, bone necrosis, leg cramps, myalgia, osteoporosis, tetany; NERVOUS SYSTEM: anxiety, confusion, depression, dizziness, emotional lability, hypertonia, hypesthesia, hypotonia, insomnia, neuropathy, paresthesia, somnolence; RESPIRATORY SYSTEM: asthma, atelectasis, bronchitis, cough increased, epistaxis, hypoxia, lung edema, pleural effusion, pneumonia, rhinitis, sinusitis; SKIN AND APPENDAGES: fungal dermatitis, hirsutism, pruritus, skin hypertrophy, skin ulcer, sweating; SPECIAL SENSES: abnormal vision, cataract, conjunctivitis, deafness, ear pain, otitis media, tinnitus; UROGENITAL SYSTEM: albuminuria, bladder pain, dysuria, hematuria, hydronephrosis, impotence, kidney pain, kidney tubular necrosis, nocturia, oliguria, pyelonephritis, pyuria, scrotal edema, testis disorder, toxic nephropathy, urinary frequency, urinary incontinence, urinary retention.

Less frequently occurring adverse events included: Mycobacterial infections, Epstein-Barr virus infections, and pancreatitis.

Other clinical experience: Cases of pneumonitis with no identified infectious etiology, sometimes with an interstitial pattern, have occurred in patients receiving immunosuppressive regimens including Rapamune. In some cases, pneumonitis has resolved upon discontinuation of Rapamune; however, a causal relationship is uncertain.

OVERDOSAGE

There is minimal experience with overdose. During clinical trials, there were two accidental Rapamune ingestions, of 120 mg and 150 mg. One patient, receiving 150 mg, experienced an episode of transient atrial fibrillation. The other patient experienced no adverse effects. General supportive measures should be followed in all cases of overdose. Based on the poor aqueous solubility and high erythrocyte binding of Rapamune, it is anticipated that Rapamune is not dialyzable to any significant extent.

In mice and rats, the acute oral LD_{50} was greater than 800 mg/kg.

DOSAGE AND ADMINISTRATION

It is recommended that Rapamune be used in a regimen with cyclosporine and corticosteroids. Rapamune is to be administered orally once daily. The initial dose of Rapamune should be administered as soon as possible after transplantation. For de novo transplant recipients, a loading dose of Rapamune of 3 times the maintenance dose should be given. A daily maintenance dose of 2 mg is recommended for use in renal transplant patients, with a loading dose of 6 mg. Although a daily maintenance dose of 5 mg, with a loading dose of 15 mg, was used in clinical trials and was shown to be safe and effective, no efficacy advantage over the 2 mg dose could be established for renal transplant patients. Patients receiving 2 mg of Rapamune per day demonstrated an overall better safety profile than did patients receiving 5 mg of Rapamune per day.

ADVERSE EVENTS OCCURRING AT A FREQUENCY OF ≥ 20% IN ANY TREATMENT GROUP IN PREVENTION OF ACUTE RENAL REJECTION TRIALS (%)[a] AT ≥ 12 MONTHS POST-TRANSPLANTATION FOR STUDIES 1 AND 2

Body System	Rapamune® —2 mg/day—		Rapamune® —5 mg/day—		Azathioprine 2–3 mg/kg/day	Placebo
Adverse Event	Study 1 (n = 281)	Study 2 (n = 218)	Study 1 (n = 269)	Study 2 (n = 208)	Study 1 (n = 160)	Study 2 (n = 124)
Body As A Whole						
Abdominal pain	28	29	30	36	29	30
Asthenia	38	22	40	28	37	28
Back pain	16	23	26	22	23	20
Chest pain	16	18	19	24	16	19
Fever	27	23	33	34	33	35
Headache	23	34	27	34	21	31
Pain	24	33	29	29	30	25
Cardiovascular System						
Hypertension	43	45	39	49	29	48
Digestive System						
Constipation	28	36	34	38	37	31
Diarrhea	32	25	42	35	28	27
Dyspepsia	17	23	23	25	24	34
Nausea	31	25	36	31	39	29
Vomiting	21	19	25	25	31	21
Hemic And Lymphatic System						
Anemia	27	23	37	33	29	21
Leukopenia	9	9	15	13	20	8
Thrombocytopenia	13	14	20	30	9	9
Metabolic And Nutritional						
Creatinine increased	35	39	37	40	28	38
Edema	24	20	16	18	23	15
Hypercholesteremia (See **WARNINGS** and **PRECAUTIONS**)	38	43	42	46	33	23
Hyperkalemia	15	17	12	14	24	27
Hyperlipemia (See **WARNINGS** and **PRECAUTIONS**)	38	45	44	57	28	23
Hypokalemia	17	11	21	17	11	9
Hypophosphatemia	20	15	23	19	20	19
Peripheral edema	60	54	64	58	58	48
Weight gain	21	11	15	8	19	15
Musculoskeletal System						
Arthralgia	25	25	27	31	21	18
Nervous System						
Insomnia	14	13	22	14	18	8
Tremor	31	21	30	22	28	19
Respiratory System						
Dyspnea	22	24	28	30	23	30
Pharyngitis	17	16	16	21	17	22
Upper respiratory infection	20	26	24	23	13	23
Skin And Appendages						
Acne	31	22	20	22	17	19
Rash	12	10	13	20	6	6
Urogenital System						
Urinary tract infection	20	26	23	33	31	26

a: Patients received cyclosporine and corticosteroids.

INCIDENCE (%) OF MALIGNANCIES IN PREVENTION OF ACUTE RENAL REJECTION TRIALS: AT 12 MONTHS POST-TRANSPLANT[a]

Malignancy	Rapamune® 2 mg/day (n = 511)	Rapamune® 5 mg/day (n = 493)	Azathioprine 2–3 mg/kg/day (n = 161)	Placebo (n = 130)
Lymphoma/lymphoproliferative disease	0.4	1.4	0.6	0
Non-melanoma skin carcinoma	0.4	1.4	1.2	3.1
Other malignancy	0.6	0.6	0	0

a: Patients received cyclosporine and corticosteroids.

To minimize the variability of exposure to Rapamune, this drug should be taken consistently with or without food. Grapefruit juice reduces CYP3A4-mediated metabolism of Rapamune and must not be administered with Rapamune or used for dilution.

It is recommended that sirolimus must be taken 4 hours after administration of cyclosporine oral solution (MODIFIED) and/or cyclosporine capsules (MODIFIED).

Dosage Adjustments

The initial dosage in patients ≥ 13 years who weigh less than 40 kg should be adjusted, based on body surface area, to 1 mg/m^2/day. The loading dose should be 3 mg/m^2.

It is recommended that the maintenance dose of Rapamune be reduced by approximately one third in patients with hepatic impairment. It is not necessary to modify the Rapamune loading dose. Dosage need not be adjusted because of impaired renal function.

Blood Concentration Monitoring

Routine therapeutic drug level monitoring is not required in most patients. Blood sirolimus levels should be monitored in pediatric patients; in patients with hepatic impairment; during concurrent administration of strong CYP3A4 inducers and inhibitors; and/or if cyclosporine dosing is markedly reduced or discontinued. In controlled clinical trials with concomitant cyclosporine, mean sirolimus whole blood trough levels, as measured by immunoassay, were 9 ng/mL (range 4.5–14 ng/mL [10th to 90th percentile]) for the 2 mg/day treatment group, and 17 ng/mL (range 10–28 ng/mL [10th to 90th percentile]) for the 5 mg/day dose.

Results from other assays may differ from those with an immunoassay. On average, chromatographic methods (HPLC UV or LC/MS/MS) yield results that are approximately 20% lower than the immunoassay whole blood concentration determinations. Adjustments to the targeted range should be made according to the assay utilized to determine sirolimus trough concentrations. Therefore, comparison between concentrations in the published literature and an individual patient concentration using current assays must be made with detailed knowledge of the assay methods employed. A discussion of the different assay methods is contained in *Clinical Therapeutics*, Volume 22, Supplement B, April 2000.

Instructions for Dilution and Administration

Bottles

The amber oral dose syringe should be used to withdraw the prescribed amount of Rapamune® Oral Solution from the bottle. Empty the correct amount of Rapamune from the syringe into only a glass or plastic container holding at least two (2) ounces (1/4 cup, 60 mL) of water or orange juice. No other liquids, including grapefruit juice, should be used for dilution. Stir vigorously and drink at once. Refill the container with an additional volume (minimum of four [4] ounces (1/2 cup, 120 mL)) of water or orange juice, stir vigorously, and drink at once.

Pouches

When using the pouch, squeeze the entire contents of the pouch into only a glass or plastic container holding at least two (2) ounces (1/4 cup, 60 mL) of water or orange juice. No other liquids, including grapefruit juice, should be used for dilution. Stir vigorously and drink at once. Refill the container with an additional volume (minimum of four [4] ounces (1/2 cup, 120 mL)) of water or orange juice, stir vigorously, and drink at once.

Handling and Disposal

Since Rapamune is not absorbed through the skin, there are no special precautions. However, if direct contact with the skin or mucous membranes occurs, wash thoroughly with soap and water; rinse eyes with plain water.

HOW SUPPLIED

Rapamune® Oral Solution is supplied at a concentration of 1 mg/ml in:

1. Cartons:
   NDC# 0008-1030-06, containing a 2 oz (60ml fill) amber glass bottle
   NDC# 0008-1030-15, containing a 5 oz (150ml fill) amber glass bottle

In addition to the bottles, each carton is supplied with an oral syringe adapter for fitting into the neck of the bottle, sufficient disposable amber oral syringes and caps for daily dosing, and a carrying case.

2. Cartons:
   NDC# 0008-1030-03, containing 30 unit-of-use laminated aluminum pouches of 1ml
   NDC# 0008-1030-07, containing 30 unit-of-use laminated aluminum pouches of 2ml
   NDC# 0008-1030-08, containing 30 unit-of-use laminated aluminum pouches of 5ml

Storage

Rapamune® Oral Solution bottles and pouches should be stored protected from light and refrigerated at 2° C to 8° C (36° F to 46° F). Once the bottle is opened, the contents should be used within one month. If necessary, the patient may store both the pouches and the bottles at room temperatures up to 25° C (77° F) for a short period of time (e.g., several days, but not longer than 30 days).

An amber syringe and cap are provided for dosing and the product may be kept in the syringe for a maximum of 24 hours at room temperatures up to 25° C (77° F) or refrigerated at 2° C to 8° C (36° F to 46° F). The syringe should be discarded after one use. After dilution, the preparation should be used immediately.

Continued on next page

Rapamune—Cont.

Rapamune Oral Solution provided in bottles may develop a slight haze when refrigerated. If such a haze occurs allow the product to stand at room temperature and shake gently until the haze disappears. The presence of this haze does not affect the quality of the product.

℞ only

US Pat. Nos.: 5,100,899; 5,212,155; 5,308,847; 5,403,833; 5,536,729.

PATIENT INSTRUCTIONS FOR RAPAMUNE® ADMINISTRATION

Bottles

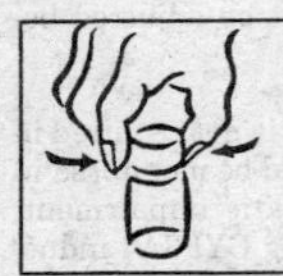

1. Open the solution bottle. Remove the safety cap by squeezing the tabs on the cap and twisting counterclockwise.

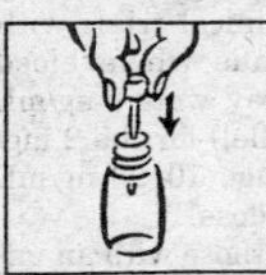

2. Upon first use, insert the adapter assembly (plastic tube with stopper) tightly into the bottle until it is even with the top of the bottle. Do not remove the adapter assembly from the bottle once inserted.

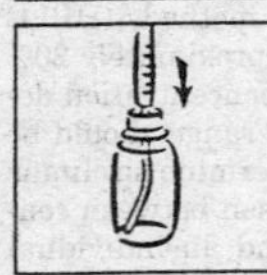

3. For each use, tightly insert one of the amber syringes with the plunger fully depressed into the opening in the adapter.

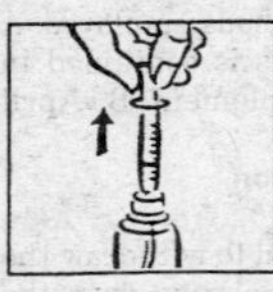

4. Withdraw the prescribed amount of Rapamune® oral solution by gently pulling out the plunger of the syringe until the bottom of the black line of the plunger is even with the appropriate mark on the syringe. Always keep the bottle in an upright position. If bubbles form in the syringe, empty the syringe into the bottle and repeat the procedure.

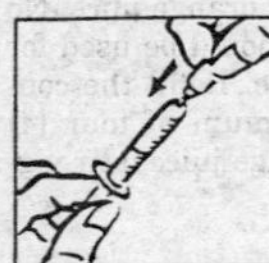

5. You may have been instructed to carry your medication with you. If it is necessary to carry the filled syringe, place a cap securely on the syringe—the cap should snap into place.

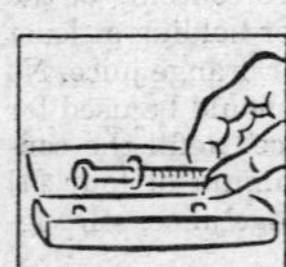

6. Then place the capped syringe in the enclosed carrying case. Once in the syringe, the medication may be kept at room temperature or refrigerated and should be used within 24 hours. Extreme temperature (below 36° F and above 86° F) should be avoided. Remember to keep this medication out of the reach of children.

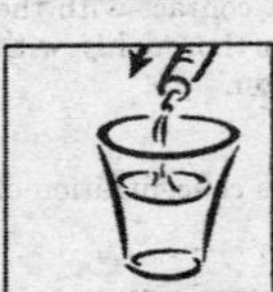

7. Empty the syringe into a glass or plastic cup containing at least 2 ounces (1/4 cup; 60 mL) of water or orange juice, stir vigorously for one (1) minute and drink immediately. Refill the container with at least 4 ounces (1/2 cup; 120 mL) of water or orange juice, stir vigorously again and drink the rinse solution. Apple juice, grapefruit juice, or other liquids are NOT to be used. Only glass or plastic cups should be used to dilute Rapamune® oral solution. The syringe and cap should be used once and then discarded.

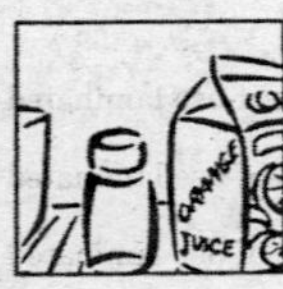

8. Always store the bottles of medication in the refrigerator. When refrigerated, a slight haze may develop in the solution. The presence of a haze does not affect the quality of the product. If this happens, bring the Rapamune® oral solution to room temperature and shake until the haze disappears. If it is necessary to wipe clean the mouth of the bottle before returning the product to the refrigerator, wipe with a dry cloth to avoid introducing water, or any other liquid, into the bottle.

PATIENTS INSTRUCTIONS FOR RAPAMUNE® ADMINISTRATION

Pouches

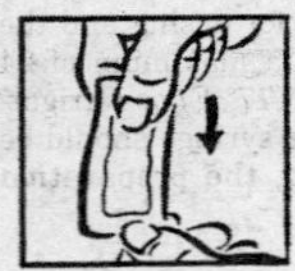

1. Before opening the pouch, squeeze the pouch from the neck area to push the contents into the lower part of the pouch.

2. Carefully open the pouch by folding the marked area and then cutting with a scissors along the marked line near the top of the pouch.

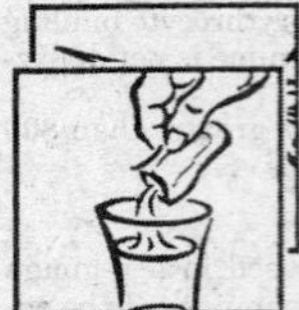

3. Squeeze the entire contents of the pouch into a glass or plastic cup containing at least 2 ounces (1/4 cup; 60 mL) of water or orange juice, stir vigorously for one (1) minute and drink immediately. Refill the container with at least 4 ounces (1/2 cup, 120 mL) of water or orange juice, stir vigorously again and drink the rinse solution. Apple juice, grapefruit juice or other liquids are NOT to be used. Only glass or plastic cups should be used to dilute RAPAMUNE® oral solution.

4. Unused pouches should be stored in the refrigerator.

Manufactured by:
Wyeth Laboratories
Division of Wyeth-Ayerst Pharmaceuticals Inc.
Philadelphia PA 19101
CI 6019-3 Revised May 17, 2000

SECTRAL® ℞

[*sĕk 'trăl*]
(acebutolol hydrochloride)
Capsules

DESCRIPTION

Sectral (acebutolol HCl) is a selective, hydrophilic beta-adrenoreceptor blocking agent with mild intrinsic sympathomimetic activity for use in treating patients with hypertension and ventricular arrhythmias. It is marketed in capsule form for oral administration. Sectral capsules are provided in two dosage strengths which contain 200 or 400 mg of acebutolol as the hydrochloride salt. The inactive ingredients present are D&C Red 22, FD&C Blue 1, FD&C Yellow 6, gelatin, povidone, starch, stearic acid, and titanium dioxide. The 200 mg dosage strength also contains D&C Red 28 and the 400 mg dosage strength also contains FD&C Red 40.

Acebutolol HCl has the following structural formula:

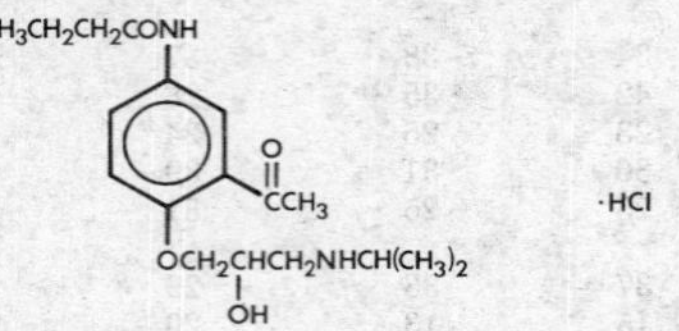

$C_{18}H_{28}N_2O_4 \cdot HCl$ M.W. 372.9

Acebutolol HCl is a white or slightly off-white powder freely soluble in water, and less soluble in alcohol. Chemically it is defined as the hydrochloride salt ±N-[3-Acetyl-4-[2-hydroxy-3-[(1-methylethyl)amino]propoxy]phenyl]butanamide, or (±)-3'-Acetyl-4'-[2-hydroxy -3- (isopropylamino) propoxy] butyranilide.

CLINICAL PHARMACOLOGY

Sectral is a cardioselective, β -adrenoreceptor blocking agent, which possesses mild intrinsic sympathomimetic activity (ISA) in its therapeutically effective dose range.

Pharmacodynamics

β_1-cardioselectivity has been demonstrated in experimental animal studies. In anesthetized dogs and cats, Sectral is more potent in antagonizing isoproterenol-induced tachycardia (β_1) than in antagonizing isoproterenol-induced vasodilatation (β_2). In guinea pigs and cats, it is more potent in antagonizing this tachycardia than in antagonizing isoproterenol-induced bronchodilatation (β_2). ISA of Sectral has been demonstrated in catecholamine-depleted rats by tachycardia induced by intravenous administration of this agent. A membrane-stabilizing effect has been detected in animals, but only with high concentrations of Sectral.

Clinical studies have demonstrated β_1-blocking activity at the recommended doses by: a) reduction in the resting heart rate and decrease in exercise-induced tachycardia; b) reduction in cardiac output at rest and after exercise; c) reduction of systolic and diastolic blood pressures at rest and postexercise; d) inhibition of isoproterenol-induced tachycardia.

The β_1-selectivity of Sectral has also been demonstrated on the basis of the following vascular and bronchial effects:

Vascular Effects: Sectral has less antagonistic effects on peripheral vascular β_2-receptors at rest and after epinephrine stimulation than nonselective β-antagonists.

Bronchial Effects: In single-dose studies in asthmatics examining effects of various beta-blockers on pulmonary function, low doses of acebutolol produce less evidence of bronchoconstriction and less reduction of beta$_2$ agonist, bronchodilating effects, than nonselective agents like propranolol but more than atenolol.

ISA has been observed with Sectral in man, as shown by a slightly smaller (about 3 beats per minute) decrease in resting heart rate when compared to equivalent β-blocking doses of propranolol, metoprolol or atenolol. Chronic therapy with Sectral induced no significant alteration in the blood lipid profile.

Sectral has been shown to delay AV conduction time and to increase the refractoriness of the AV node without significantly affecting sinus node recovery time, atrial refractory period, or the HV conduction time. The membrane-stabilizing effect of Sectral is not manifest at the doses used clinically.

Significant reductions in resting and exercise heart rates and systolic blood pressures have been observed 1.5 hours after Sectral administration with maximal effects occurring between 3 and 8 hours postdosing in normal volunteers. Sectral has demonstrated a significant effect on exercise-induced tachycardia 24 to 30 hours after drug administration.

There are significant correlations between plasma levels of acebutolol and both the reduction in resting heart rate and the percent of β-blockade of exercise-induced tachycardia.

The antihypertensive effect of Sectral has been shown in double-blind controlled studies to be superior to placebo and similar to propranolol and hydrochlorothiazide. In addition, patients responding to Sectral administered twice daily had a similar response whether the dosage regimen was changed to once daily administration or continued on a b.i.d. regimen. Most patients responded to 400 to 800 mg per day in divided doses.

The antiarrhythmic effect of Sectral was compared with placebo, propranolol, and quinidine. Compared with placebo, Sectral significantly reduced mean total ventricular ectopic beats (VEB), paired VEB, multiform VEB, R-on-T beats, and ventricular tachycardia (VT). Both Sectral and propranolol significantly reduced mean total and paired VEB and VT. Sectral and quinidine significantly reduced resting total and complex VEB; the antiarrhythmic efficacy of Sectral was also observed during exercise.

Pharmacokinetics and Metabolism

Sectral is well absorbed from the GI tract. It is subject to extensive first-pass hepatic biotransformation, with an absolute bioavailability of approximately 40% for the parent compound. The major metabolite, an N-acetyl derivative (diacetolol), is pharmacologically active. This metabolite is equipotent to Sectral and in cats is more cardioselective than Sectral; therefore, this first-pass phenomenon does not attenuate the therapeutic effect of Sectral. Food intake does not have a significant effect on the area under the plasma concentration-time curve (AUC) of Sectral although the rate of absorption and peak concentration decreased slightly.

The plasma elimination half-life of Sectral is approximately 3 to 4 hours, while that of its metabolite, diacetolol, is 8 to 13 hours. The time to reach peak concentration for Sectral is 2.5 hours and for diacetolol, after oral administration of Sectral, 3.5 hours.

Within the single oral dose range of 200 to 400 mg, the kinetics are dose proportional. However, this linearity is not seen at higher doses, probably due to saturation of hepatic biotransformation sites. In addition, after multiple dosing the lack of linearity is also seen by AUC increases of approximately 100% as compared to single oral dosing. Elimination via renal excretion is approximately 30% to 40% and by nonrenal mechanisms 50% to 60%, which includes excretion into the bile and direct passage through the intestinal wall.

Sectral has a low binding affinity for plasma proteins (about 26%). Sectral and its metabolite, diacetolol, are relatively hydrophilic and, therefore, only minimal quantities have been detected in the cerebrospinal fluid (CSF).

Drug interaction studies with tolbutamide and warfarin indicated no influence on the therapeutic effects of these compounds. Digoxin and hydrochlorothiazide plasma levels were not affected by concomitant Sectral administration. The kinetics of Sectral were not significantly altered by concomitant administration of hydrochlorothiazide, hydralazine, sulfinpyrazone, or oral contraceptives.

In patients with renal impairment, there is no effect on the elimination half-life of Sectral, but there is decreased elimination of the metabolite, diacetolol, resulting in a two- to three-fold increase in its half-life. For this reason, the drug should be administered with caution in patients with renal insufficiency (see **PRECAUTIONS**). Sectral and its major metabolite are dialyzable.

Sectral crosses the placental barrier and is secreted in breast milk.

In geriatric patients, the bioavailability of Sectral and its metabolite is increased, approximately two-fold, probably due to decreases in the first-pass metabolism and renal function in the elderly.

INDICATIONS AND USAGE

Hypertension

Sectral is indicated for the management of hypertension in adults. It may be used alone or in combination with other antihypertensive agents, especially thiazide-type diuretics.

Ventricular Arrhythmias

Sectral is indicated in the management of ventricular premature beats; it reduces the total number of premature beats, as well as the number of paired and multiform ventricular ectopic beats, and R-on-T beats.

CONTRAINDICATIONS

Sectral is contraindicated in: 1) persistently severe bradycardia; 2) second- and third-degree heart block; 3) overt cardiac failure; and 4) cardiogenic shock. (See **WARNINGS**.)

WARNINGS

Cardiac Failure
Sympathetic stimulation may be essential for support of the circulation in individuals with diminished myocardial contractility, and its inhibition by β-adrenergic receptor blockade may precipitate more severe failure. Although β-blockers should be avoided in overt cardiac failure, Sectral can be used with caution in patients with a history of heart failure who are controlled with digitalis and/or diuretics. Both digitalis and Sectral impair AV conduction. If cardiac failure persists, therapy with Sectral should be withdrawn.

In Patients Without A History of Cardiac Failure
In patients with aortic or mitral valve disease or compromised left ventricular function, continued depression of the myocardium with β-blocking agents over a period of time may lead to cardiac failure. At the first signs of failure, patients should be digitalized and/or be given a diuretic and the response observed closely. If cardiac failure continues despite adequate digitalization and/or diuretic, Sectral therapy should be withdrawn.

Exacerbation of Ischemic Heart Disease Following Abrupt Withdrawal
Following abrupt cessation of therapy with certain β-blocking agents in patients with coronary artery disease, exacerbation of angina pectoris and, in some cases, myocardial infarction and death have been reported. Therefore, such patients should be cautioned against interruption of therapy without a physician's advice. Even in the absence of overt ischemic heart disease, when discontinuation of Sectral is planned, the patient should be carefully observed, and should be advised to limit physical activity to a minimum while Sectral is gradually withdrawn over a period of about two weeks. (If therapy with an alternative β-blocker is desired, the patient may be transferred directly to comparable doses of another agent without interruption of β-blocking therapy.) If an exacerbation of angina pectoris occurs, antianginal therapy should be restarted immediately in full doses and the patient hospitalized until his condition stabilizes.

Peripheral Vascular Disease
Treatment with β-antagonists reduces cardiac output and can precipitate or aggravate the symptoms of arterial insufficiency in patients with peripheral or mesenteric vascular disease. Caution should be exercised with such patients, and they should be observed closely for evidence of progression of arterial obstruction.

Bronchospastic Diseases
PATIENTS WITH BRONCHOSPASTIC DISEASE SHOULD, IN GENERAL, NOT RECEIVE A β-BLOCKER. Because of its relative β_1-selectivity, however, low doses of Sectral may be used with caution in patients with bronchospastic disease who do not respond to, or who cannot tolerate, alternative treatment. Since β_1-selectivity is not absolute and is dose-dependent, the lowest possible dose of Sectral should be used initially, preferably in divided doses to avoid the higher plasma levels associated with the longer dose-interval. A bronchodilator, such as a theophylline or a β_2-stimulant, should be made available in advance with instructions concerning its use.

Anesthesia and Major Surgery
The necessity, or desirability, of withdrawal of a β-blocking therapy prior to major surgery is controversial. β-adrenergic receptor blockade impairs the ability of the heart to respond to β-adrenergically mediated reflex stimuli. While this might be of benefit in preventing arrhythmic response, the risk of excessive myocardial depression during general anesthesia may be enhanced and difficulty in restarting and maintaining the heart beat has been reported with beta-blockers. If treatment is continued, particular care should be taken when using anesthetic agents which depress the myocardium, such as ether, cyclopropane and trichlorethylene, and it is prudent to use the lowest possible dose of Sectral. Sectral, like other β-blockers, is a competitive inhibitor of β-receptor agonists, and its effect on the heart can be reversed by cautious administration of such agents (e.g., dobutamine or isoproterenol—see **OVERDOSE**).
Manifestations of excessive vagal tone (e.g., profound bradycardia, hypotension) may be corrected with atropine 1 to 3 mg IV in divided doses.

Diabetes and Hypoglycemia
β-blockers may potentiate insulin-induced hypoglycemia and mask some of its manifestations such as tachycardia; however, dizziness and sweating are usually not significantly affected. Diabetic patients should be warned of the possibility of masked hypoglycemia.

Thyrotoxicosis
β-adrenergic blockade may mask certain clinical signs (tachycardia) of hyperthyroidism. Abrupt withdrawal of β-blockade may precipitate a thyroid storm; therefore, patients suspected of developing thyrotoxicosis from whom Sectral therapy is to be withdrawn should be monitored closely.

PRECAUTIONS

Risk of Anaphylactic Reaction
While taking beta-blockers, patients with a history of severe anaphylactic reaction to a variety of allergens may be more reactive to repeated challenge, either accidental, diagnostic, or therapeutic. Such patients may be unresponsive to the usual doses of epinephrine used to treat allergic reaction.

Impaired Renal or Hepatic Function
Studies on the effect of acebutolol in patients with renal insufficiency have not been performed in the U.S. Foreign published experience shows that acebutolol has been used successfully in chronic renal insufficiency. Acebutolol is excreted through the GI tract, but the active metabolite, diacetolol, is eliminated predominantly by the kidney. There is a linear relationship between renal clearance of diacetolol and creatinine clearance. Therefore, the daily dose of acebutolol should be reduced by 50% when the creatinine clearance is less than 50 mL/min and by 75% when it is less than 25 mL/min. Sectral should be used cautiously in patients with impaired hepatic function.
Sectral has been used successfully and without problems in elderly patients in the U.S. clinical trials without specific adjustment of dosage. However, elderly patients may require lower maintenance doses because the bioavailability of both Sectral and its metabolite are approximately doubled in this age group.

TOTAL VOLUNTEERED AND ELICITED (U.S. STUDIES)

Body System/ Adverse Reaction	SECTRAL (N=1002) %	Propranolol (N=424) %	Hydrochlorothiazide (N=178) %	Placebo (N=314) %
Cardiovascular				
Chest Pain	2	4	4	1
Edema	2	2	4	1
Central Nervous System				
Depression	2	1	3	1
Dizziness	6	7	12	2
Fatigue	11	17	10	4
Headache	6	9	13	4
Insomnia	3	6	5	1
Abnormal dreams	2	3	0	1
Dermatologic				
Rash	2	2	4	1
Gastrointestinal				
Constipation	4	2	7	0
Diarrhea	4	5	5	1
Dyspepsia	4	6	3	1
Flatulence	3	4	7	1
Nausea	4	6	3	0
Genitourinary				
Micturition (frequency)	3	1	9	<1
Musculoskeletal				
Arthralgia	2	1	3	2
Myalgia	2	1	4	0
Respiratory				
Cough	1	1	2	0
Dyspnea	4	6	4	2
Rhinitis	2	1	4	<1
Special Senses				
Abnormal Vision	2	2	3	0

Information for Patients
Patients, especially those with evidence of coronary artery disease, should be warned against interruption or discontinuation of Sectral therapy without a physician's supervision. Although cardiac failure rarely occurs in properly selected patients, those being treated with β-adrenergic blocking agents should be advised to consult a physician if they develop signs or symptoms suggestive of impending CHF, or unexplained respiratory symptoms.
Patients should also be warned of possible severe hypertensive reactions from concomitant use of α-adrenergic stimulants, such as the nasal decongestants commonly used in OTC cold preparations and nasal drops.

Clinical Laboratory Findings
Sectral®, like other β-blockers, has been associated with the development of antinuclear antibodies (ANA). In prospective clinical trials, patients receiving Sectral had a dose-dependent increase in the development of positive ANA titers, and the overall incidence was higher than that observed with propranolol. Symptoms (generally persistent arthralgias and myalgias) related to this laboratory abnormality were infrequent (less than 1% with both drugs). Symptoms and ANA titers were reversible upon discontinuation of treatment.

Drug Interactions
Catecholamine-depleting drugs, such as reserpine, may have an additive effect when given with β-blocking agents. Patients treated with Sectral plus catecholamine depletors should, therefore, be observed closely for evidence of marked bradycardia or hypotension which may present as vertigo, syncope/presyncope, or orthostatic changes in blood pressure without compensatory tachycardia. Exaggerated hypertensive responses have been reported from the combined use of β-adrenergic antagonists and α-adrenergic stimulants, including those contained in proprietary cold remedies and vasoconstrictive nasal drops. Patients receiving β-blockers should be warned of this potential hazard.
Blunting of the antihypertensive effect of beta-adrenoceptor blocking agents by nonsteroidal anti-inflammatory drugs has been reported.
No significant interactions with digoxin, hydrochlorothiazide, hydralazine, sulfinpyrazone, oral contraceptives, tolbutamide, or warfarin have been observed.

Carcinogenesis, Mutagenesis, Impairment of Fertility
Chronic oral toxicity studies in rats and mice, employing dose levels as high as 300 mg/kg/day, which is equivalent to 15 times the maximum recommended (60 kg) human dose, did not indicate a carcinogenic potential for Sectral. Diacetolol, the major metabolite of Sectral in man, was without carcinogenic potential in rats when tested at doses as high as 1800 mg/kg/day. Sectral and diacetolol were also shown to be devoid of mutagenic potential in the Ames Test. Sectral, administered orally to two generations of male and female rats at doses of up to 240 mg/kg/day (equivalent to 12 times the maximum recommended therapeutic dose in a 60-kg human) and diacetolol, administered to two generations of male and female rats at doses of up to 1000 mg/kg/day, had no significant impact on reproductive performance or fertility.

Pregnancy
Teratogenic Effects
Pregnancy Category B: Reproduction studies have been performed with Sectral in rats (up to 630 mg/kg/day) and rabbits (up to 135 mg/kg/day). These doses are equivalent to approximately 31.5 and 6.8 times the maximum recommended therapeutic dose in a 60-kg human, respectively. The compound was not teratogenic in either species. In the rabbit, however, doses of 135 mg/kg/day caused slight fetal growth retardation; this effect was considered to be a result of maternal toxicity, as evidenced by reduced food intake, a lowered rate of body weight gain, and mortality. Studies have also been performed in these species with diacetolol (at doses of up to 450 mg/kg/day in rabbits and up to 1800 mg/kg/day in rats.) Other than a significant elevation in postimplantation loss with 450 mg/kg/day diacetolol, a level at which food consumption and body weight gain were reduced in rabbit dams and a nonstatistically significant increase in incidence of bilateral cataract in rat fetuses from dams treated with 1800 mg/kg/day diacetolol, there was no evidence of harm to the fetus. There are no adequate and well-controlled trials in pregnant women. Because animal teratology studies are not always predictive of the human response, Sectral should be used during pregnancy only if the potential benefit justifies the risk to the fetus.
Nonteratogenic Effects
Studies in humans have shown that both acebutolol and diacetolol cross the placenta. Neonates of mothers who have received acebutolol during pregnancy have reduced birth weight, decreased blood pressure, and decreased heart rate. In the newborn the elimination half-life of acebutolol was 6 to 14 hours, while the half-life of diacetolol was 24 to 30 hours for the first 24 hours after birth, followed by a half-life of 12 to 16 hours. Adequate facilities for monitoring these infants at birth should be available.

Labor and Delivery
The effect of Sectral on labor and delivery in pregnant women is unknown. Studies in animals have not shown any effect of Sectral on the usual course of labor and delivery.

Nursing Mothers
Acebutolol and diacetolol also appear in breast milk with a milk:plasma ratio of 7.1 and 12.2, respectively. Use in nursing mothers is not recommended.

Pediatric Use
Safety and effectiveness in pediatric patients have not been established.

Geriatric Use
Clinical studies of Sectral and other reported clinical experience is inadequate to determine whether there are differences in safety or effectiveness between patients above or below age 65.
Elderly subjects evidence greater bioavailability of acebutolol (see **CLINICAL PHARMACOLOGY—Pharmacokinetics and Metabolism**), presumably because of age-related reduction in first-pass metabolism and renal function. Therefore, it may be appropriate to start elderly patients at the low end of the dosing range (see **DOSAGE AND ADMINISTRATION—Use In Older Patients**).

ADVERSE REACTIONS

Sectral is well tolerated in properly selected patients. Most adverse reactions have been mild, not required discontinuation of therapy, and tended to decrease as duration of treatment increases.

Continued on next page

Sectral—Cont.

The following table shows the frequency of treatment-related side effects derived from controlled clinical trials in patients with hypertension, angina pectoris, and arrhythmia. These patients received Sectral, propranolol, or hydrochlorothiazide as monotherapy, or placebo.

[See table at top of previous page]

The following selected (potentially important) side effects were seen in up to 2% of Sectral patients:

Cardiovascular: hypotension, bradycardia, heart failure.
Central Nervous System: anxiety, hyper/hypoesthesia, impotence.
Dermatological: pruritus.
Gastrointestinal: vomiting, abdominal pain.
Genitourinary: dysuria, nocturia.
Liver and Biliary System: A small number of cases of liver abnormalities (increased SGOT, SGPT, LDH) have been reported in association with acebutolol therapy. In some cases increased bilirubin or alkaline phosphatase, fever, malaise, dark urine, anorexia, nausea, headache, and/or other symptoms have been reported. In some of the reported cases, the symptoms and signs were confirmed by rechallenge with acebutolol. The abnormalities were reversible upon cessation of acebutolol therapy.
Musculoskeletal: back pain, joint pain.
Respiratory: pharyngitis, wheezing.
Special Senses: conjunctivitis, dry eye, eye pain.
Autoimmune: In extremely rare instances, systemic lupus erythematosus has been reported.

The incidence of drug-related adverse effects (volunteered and solicited) according to Sectral dose is shown below. (Data from 266 hypertensive patients treated for 3 months on a constant dose.)

Body System	400 mg/day (N=132)	800 mg/day (N=63)	1200 mg/day (N=71)
Cardiovascular	5%	2%	1%
Gastrointestinal	3%	3%	7%
Musculoskeletal	2%	3%	4%
Central Nervous System	9%	13%	17%
Respiratory	1%	5%	6%
Skin	1%	2%	1%
Special Senses	2%	2%	6%
Genitourinary	2%	3%	1%

Potential Adverse Effects

In addition, certain adverse effects not listed above have been reported with other β-blocking agents and should also be considered as potential adverse effects of Sectral.

Central Nervous System: Reversible mental depression progressing to catatonia (an acute syndrome characterized by disorientation for time and place), short-term memory loss, emotional lability, slightly clouded sensorium, and decreased performance (neuropsychometrics).
Cardiovascular: Intensification of AV block (see **CONTRAINDICATIONS**).
Allergic: Erythematous rash, fever combined with aching and sore throat, laryngospasm, and respiratory distress.
Hematologic: Agranulocytosis, nonthrombocytopenic, and thrombocytopenic purpura.
Gastrointestinal: Mesenteric arterial thrombosis and ischemic colitis.
Miscellaneous: Reversible alopecia and Peyronie's disease.

The oculomucocutaneous syndrome associated with the β-blocker practolol has not been reported with Sectral during investigational use and extensive foreign clinical experience.

OVERDOSAGE

No specific information on emergency treatment of overdosage is available for Sectral. However, overdosage with other β-blocking agents has been accompanied by extreme bradycardia, advanced atrioventricular block, intraventricular conduction defects, hypotension, severe congestive heart failure, seizures, and in susceptible patients, bronchospasm and hypoglycemia. Although specific information on the emergency treatment of Sectral overdose is not available, on the basis of the pharmacological actions and the observations in treating overdoses with other β-blockers, the following general measures should be considered:

1. Empty stomach by emesis or lavage.
2. Bradycardia: IV atropine (1 to 3 mg in divided doses). If antivagal response is inadequate, administer isoproterenol cautiously since larger than usual doses of isoproterenol may be required.
3. Persistent hypotension in spite of correction of bradycardia: Administer vasopressor (e.g., epinephrine, levarterenol, dopamine, or dobutamine) with frequent monitoring of blood pressure and pulse rate.
4. Bronchospasm: A theophylline derivative, such as aminophylline and/or parenteral β_2-stimulant, such as terbutaline.
5. Cardiac failure: Digitalize the patient and/or administer a diuretic. It has been reported that glucagon is useful in this situation.

Sectral is dialyzable.

DOSAGE AND ADMINISTRATION

Hypertension

The initial dosage of Sectral in uncomplicated mild-to-moderate hypertension is 400 mg. This can be given as a single daily dose, but in occasional patients twice daily dosing may be required for adequate 24-hour blood-pressure control. An optimal response is usually achieved with dosages of 400 to 800 mg per day, although some patients have been maintained on as little as 200 mg per day. Patients with more severe hypertension or who have demonstrated inadequate control may respond to a total of 1200 mg daily (administered b.i.d.), or to the addition of a second antihypertensive agent. Beta-1 selectivity diminishes as dosage is increased.

Ventricular Arrhythmia

The usual initial dose of Sectral is 400 mg daily given as 200 mg b.i.d. Dosage should be increased gradually until an optimal clinical response is obtained, generally at 600 to 1200 mg per day. If treatment is to be discontinued, the dosage should be reduced gradually over a period of about two weeks.

Use in Older Patients

Older patients have an approximately 2-fold increase in bioavailability and may require lower maintenance doses. Doses above 800 mg/day should be avoided in the elderly.

HOW SUPPLIED

Sectral® (acebutolol HCl) is available in the following dosage strengths:

200 mg, opaque purple and orange capsule marked "WYETH 4177" and "Sectral 200"
NDC 0008-4177-01, in bottles of 100 capsules.
NDC 0008-4177-04, in Redipak® cartons of 100 capsules (10 blister strips of 10).

Keep tightly closed
Store at room temperature, approximately 25° C (77°F)
Protect from light
Dispense in a light-resistant, tight container
Use carton to protect contents from light

400 mg, opaque brown and orange capsule marked "WYETH 4179" and "Sectral 400"
NDC 0008-4179-01, in bottles of 100 capsules.

Keep tightly closed
Store at room temperature, approximately 25°C (77°F)
Dispense in a tight container

The appearance of these capsules is a trademark of Wyeth-Ayerst Laboratories.

by arrangement with Rhone-Poulenc Rorer France
Manufactured by:
Wyeth Laboratories
A Wyeth-Ayerst Company
Philadelphia, PA 19101
CI 5185-1 Issued February 12, 1999

Shown in Product Identification Guide, page 342

SONATA® Ⓒ ℞

[sō 'nă-tă]
(zaleplon)
Capsules

DESCRIPTION

Zaleplon is a nonbenzodiazepine hypnotic from the pyrazolopyrimidine class. The chemical name of zaleplon is N-[3-(3-cyanopyrazolo[1,5-a]pyrimidin-7-yl)phenyl]-N-ethylacetamide. Its empirical formula is $C_{17}H_{15}N_5O$, and its molecular weight is 305.34. The structural formula is shown below.

NC, N, N, N, H_3C, N, CH_2CH_3, O

ZALEPLON

Zaleplon is a white to off-white powder that is practically insoluble in water and sparingly soluble in alcohol or propylene glycol. Its partition coefficient in octanol/water is constant (log PC = 1.23) over the pH range of 1 to 7.

Sonata® capsules contain zaleplon as the active ingredient. Inactive ingredients consist of microcrystalline cellulose, pregelatinized starch, silicon dioxide, sodium lauryl sulfate, magnesium stearate, lactose, gelatin, titanium dioxide, D&C yellow #10, FD&C blue #1, FD&C green #3, and FD&C yellow #5.

CLINICAL PHARMACOLOGY

Pharmacodynamics and Mechanism of Action

While Sonata (zaleplon) is a hypnotic agent with a chemical structure unrelated to benzodiazepines, barbiturates, or other drugs with known hypnotic properties, it interacts with the GABA-BZ receptor complex. Subunit modulation of the GABA-BZ receptor chloride channel macromolecular complex is hypothesized to be responsible for some of the pharmacological properties of benzodiazepines, which include sedative, anxiolytic, muscle relaxant, and anticonvulsive effects in animal models.

Other nonclinical studies have also shown that zaleplon binds selectively to the brain omega-1 receptor situated on the alpha subunit of the $GABA_A$ receptor complex and potentiates t-butyl-bicyclophosphorothionate (TBPS) binding. Studies of binding of zaleplon to purified $GABA_A$ receptors ($\alpha_1\beta_1\gamma_2$ [omega-1] and $\alpha_2\beta_1\gamma_2$ [omega-2]) have shown that zaleplon has a low affinity for these receptors, with preferential binding to the omega-1 receptor.

Pharmacokinetics

The pharmacokinetics of zaleplon have been investigated in more than 500 healthy subjects (young and elderly), nursing mothers, and patients with hepatic disease or renal disease. In healthy subjects, the pharmacokinetic profile has been examined after single doses of up to 60 mg and once-daily administration at 15 and 30 mg for 10 days. Zaleplon was rapidly absorbed with a time to peak concentration (t_{max}) of approximately 1 hour and a terminal-phase elimination half-life ($t_{1/2}$) of approximately 1 hour. Zaleplon does not accumulate with once-daily administration and its pharmacokinetics are dose proportional in the therapeutic range.

Absorption

Zaleplon is rapidly and almost completely absorbed following oral administration. Peak plasma concentrations are attained within approximately 1 hour after oral administration. Although zaleplon is well absorbed, its absolute bioavailability is approximately 30% because it undergoes significant presystemic metabolism.

Distribution

Zaleplon is a lipophilic compound with a volume of distribution of approximately 1.4 L/kg following intravenous (iv) administration, indicating substantial distribution into extravascular tissues. The in vitro plasma protein binding is approximately 60%±15% and is independent of zaleplon concentration over the range of 10 to 1000 ng/mL. This suggests that zaleplon disposition should not be sensitive to alterations in protein binding. The blood to plasma ratio for zaleplon is approximately 1, indicating that zaleplon is uniformly distributed throughout the blood with no extensive distribution into red blood cells.

Metabolism

After oral administration, zaleplon is extensively metabolized, with less than 1% of the dose excreted unchanged in urine. Zaleplon is primarily metabolized by aldehyde oxidase to form 5-oxo-zaleplon. Zaleplon is metabolized to a lesser extent by CYP3A4 to form desethylzaleplon, which is quickly converted, presumably by aldehyde oxidase, to 5-oxo-desethylzaleplon. These oxidative metabolites are then converted to glucuronides and eliminated in urine. All of zaleplon's metabolites are pharmacologically inactive.

Elimination

After either oral or iv administration, zaleplon is rapidly eliminated with mean $t_{1/2}$ of approximately 1 hour. The oral-dose plasma clearance of zaleplon is about 3 L/h/kg and the iv zaleplon plasma clearance is approximately 1 L/h/kg. Assuming normal hepatic blood flow and negligible renal clearance of zaleplon, the estimated hepatic extraction ratio of zaleplon is approximately 0.7, indicating that zaleplon is subject to high first-pass metabolism.

After administration of a radiolabeled dose of zaleplon, 70% of the administered dose is recovered in urine within 48 hours (71% recovered within 6 days), almost all as zaleplon metabolites and their glucuronides. An additional 17% is recovered in feces within 6 days, most as 5-oxo-zaleplon.

Effect of Food

In healthy adults a high-fat/heavy meal prolonged the absorption of zaleplon compared to the fasted state, delaying t_{max} by approximately 2 hours and reducing C_{max} by approximately 35%. Zaleplon AUC and elimination half-life were not significantly affected. These results suggest that the effects of Sonata on sleep onset may be reduced if it is taken with or immediately after a high-fat/heavy meal.

Special Populations

Age: The pharmacokinetics of Sonata have been investigated in three studies with elderly men and women ranging in age from 65 to 85 years. The pharmacokinetics of Sonata in elderly subjects, including those over 75 years of age, are not significantly different from that in young healthy subjects.

Gender: There is no significant difference in the pharmacokinetics of Sonata in men and women.

Race: The pharmacokinetics of zaleplon have been studied in Japanese subjects as representative of Asian populations. For this group, C_{max} and AUC were increased 37% and 64%, respectively. This finding can likely be attributed to differences in body weight, or alternatively, may represent differences in enzyme activities resulting from differences in diet, environment, or other factors. The effects of race on pharmacokinetic characteristics in other ethnic groups have not been well characterized.

Hepatic Impairment: Zaleplon is metabolized primarily by the liver and undergoes significant presystemic metabolism. Consequently, the oral clearance of zaleplon was reduced by 70% and 87% in compensated and decompensated cirrhotic patients, respectively, leading to marked increases in mean C_{max} and AUC (up to 4-fold and 7-fold in compensated and decompensated patients, respectively), in comparison with healthy subjects. The dose of Sonata should therefore be reduced in patients with mild to moderate hepatic impairment (see **DOSAGE AND ADMINISTRATION**). Sonata is not recommended for use in patients with severe hepatic impairment.

Renal Impairment: Because renal excretion of unchanged zaleplon accounts for less than 1% of the administered dose, the pharmacokinetics of zaleplon are not altered in patients with renal insufficiency. No dose adjustment is necessary in patients with mild to moderate renal impairment. Sonata has not been adequately studied in patients with severe renal impairment.

Drug-Drug Interactions

Because zaleplon is primarily metabolized by aldehyde oxidase, and to a lesser extent by CYP3A4, inhibitors of these enzymes might be expected to decrease zaleplon's clearance and inducers of these enzymes might be expected to increase its clearance. Zaleplon has been shown to have minimal effects on the kinetics of warfarin (both R- and S-forms), imipramine, ethanol, ibuprofen, diphenhydramine, thioridazine, and digoxin. However, the effects of zaleplon on inhibition of enzymes involved in the metabolism of other drugs has not been studied. (See **Drug Interactions** under **PRECAUTIONS**).

Clinical Trials

Controlled Trials Supporting Effectiveness

Sonata (typically administered in doses of 5, 10, or 20 mg) has been studied in patients with chronic insomnia (n = 3298) in 11 placebo and active controlled trials. Three of the trials were in elderly patients (n = 1019). It has also been studied in transient insomnia (n=264). Because of its very short half-life, studies focused on decreasing sleep latency, with less attention to duration of sleep and number of awakenings, for which consistent differences from placebo were not demonstrated. Studies were also carried out to examine the time course of effects on memory and psychomotor function, and to examine withdrawal phenomena.

Transient Insomnia

Normal adults experiencing transient insomnia during the first night in a sleep laboratory were evaluated in a double-blind, parallel-group trial comparing the effects of two doses of Sonata (5 and 10 mg) with placebo. Sonata 10 mg, but not 5 mg, was superior to placebo in decreasing latency to persistent sleep (LPS), a polysomnographic measure of time to onset of sleep.

Chronic Insomnia

Non-Elderly Patients:

Adult outpatients with chronic insomnia were evaluated in three double-blind, parallel-group outpatient studies, one of 2 weeks duration and two of 4 weeks duration, that compared the effects of Sonata at doses of 5 (in two studies), 10, and 20 mg with placebo on a subjective measure of time to sleep onset (TSO). Sonata 10 and 20 mg were consistently superior to placebo for TSO, generally for the full duration of all three studies. Although both doses were effective, the effect was greater and more consistent for the 20-mg dose. The 5-mg dose was less consistently effective than were the 10- and 20-mg doses. Sleep latency with Sonata 10 and 20 mg was on the order of 10–20 minutes (15%–30%) less than with placebo in these studies.

Adult outpatients with chronic insomnia were evaluated in five double-blind, parallel-group sleep laboratory studies that varied in duration from a single night up to 28 days. Overall, these studies demonstrated a superiority of Sonata 10 and 20 mg over placebo in reducing latency to persistent sleep (LPS) on the first 2 nights of treatment. A reduction in LPS relative to baseline was observed for all treatment groups, including placebo, at later time points, and, thus, a significant difference from placebo was not seen beyond 2 nights.

Elderly Patients:

Elderly outpatients with chronic insomnia were evaluated in two 2-week, double-blind, parallel-group outpatient studies that compared the effects of Sonata 5 and 10 mg with placebo on a subjective measure of time to sleep onset (TSO). Sonata at both doses was superior to placebo on TSO, generally for the full duration of both studies, with an effect size generally similar to that seen in younger persons. The 10-mg dose tended to have a greater effect in reducing TSO.

Elderly outpatients with chronic insomnia were also evaluated in a 2-night sleep laboratory study involving doses of 5 and 10 mg. Both 5- and 10-mg doses of Sonata were superior to placebo in reducing latency to persistent sleep (LPS).

Generally in these studies, there was a slight increase in sleep duration, compared to baseline, for all treatment groups, including placebo, and thus, a significant difference from placebo on sleep duration was not demonstrated.

Studies Pertinent to Safety Concerns for Sedative/Hypnotic Drugs

Memory Impairment

Studies involving the exposure of normal subject to single fixed doses of Sonata (10 or 20 mg) with structured assessments of short-term memory at fixed times after dosing (eg, 1, 2, 3, 4, 5, 8, and 10 hours) generally revealed the expected impairment of short-term memory at 1 hour, the time of peak exposure to zaleplon, for both doses, with a tendency for the effect to be greater after 20 mg. Consistent with the rapid clearance of zaleplon, memory impairment was no longer present as early as 2 hours post dosing in one study, and in none of the studies after 3–4 hours. Nevertheless, spontaneous reporting of adverse events in larger premarketing clinical trials revealed a difference between Sonata and placebo in the risk of next-day amnesia (3% vs 1%), and an apparent dose-dependency for this event (see **ADVERSE REACTIONS**).

Sedative/Psychomotor Effects

Studies involving the exposure of normal subjects to single fixed doses of Sonata (10 or 20 mg) with structured assessments of sedation and psychomotor function (e.g., reaction time and subjective ratings of alertness) at fixed times after dosing (eg, 1, 2, 3, 4, 5, 8, and 10 hours) generally revealed the expected sedation and impairment of psychomotor function at 1 hour, the time of peak exposure to zaleplon, for both doses. Consistent with the rapid clearance of zaleplon, impairment of psychomotor function was no longer present as early as 2 hours post dosing in one study, and in none of the studies after 3–4 hours. Spontaneous reporting of adverse events in larger premarketing clinical trials did not suggest a difference between Sonata and placebo in the risk of next-day somnolence (see **ADVERSE REACTIONS**).

Withdrawal Emergent Anxiety and Insomnia

During nightly use for an extended period, pharmacodynamic tolerance or adaptation to some effects of hypnotics may develop. If the drug has a short elimination half-life, it is possible that a relative deficiency of the drug or its active metabolites (i.e., in relationship to the receptor site) may occur at some point in the interval between each night's use. This sequence of events is believed to be responsible for two clinical findings reported to occur after several weeks of nightly use of other rapidly eliminated hypnotics: increased wakefulness during the last quarter of the night and the appearance of increased signs of daytime anxiety.

Zaleplon has a short half-life and no active metabolites. There is insufficient evidence to assess whether or not Sonata use is associated with increased wakefulness during the latter part of the night. No increase in the signs of daytime anxiety were observed in clinical trials with Sonata. In two sleep laboratory studies involving 14 and 28 days of nightly Sonata dosing (5 and 10 mg in one study and 10 and 20 mg in the second) and structured assessments of daytime anxiety, no increases in daytime anxiety were detected. Similarly, in a pooled analysis (all the parallel group, placebo controlled studies) of spontaneously reported daytime anxiety, no difference was observed between Sonata and placebo.

Rebound insomnia, defined as a dose-dependent temporary worsening in sleep parameters (latency, total sleep time, and number of awakenings) following discontinuation of treatment, is observed with short- and intermediate-acting hypnotics. Rebound insomnia following discontinuation of Sonata relative to baseline was examined at both nights 1 and 2 following discontinuation in two sleep laboratory studies (14 and 28 nights) and five outpatient studies utilizing patient diaries (14 and 28 nights). Overall, the data suggest that rebound insomnia may be dose dependent. At 20 mg, there appeared to be both objective (PSG) and subjective (diary) evidence of rebound insomnia on the first night after discontinuation of treatment with Sonata. At 5 and 10 mg, there was no objective and minimal subjective evidence of rebound insomnia on the first night after discontinuation of treatment with Sonata. At all doses, the rebound effect appeared to resolve by the second night following withdrawal.

Other Withdrawal-Emergent Phenomena

The potential for other withdrawal phenomena was also assessed for in 14 to 28 day studies, including both the sleep laboratory studies and the outpatient studies, and in open-label studies of 6- and 12-month durations. The Benzodiazepine Withdrawal Symptom Questionnaire was used in several of these studies, both at baseline and then during days 1 and 2 following discontinuation. Withdrawal was operationally defined as the emergence of 3 or more new symptoms after discontinuation. Sonata was not distinguishable from placebo at doses of 5, 10, or 20 mg on this measure, nor was Sonata distinguishable from placebo on spontaneously reported withdrawal emergent adverse events. There were no instances of withdrawal delirium, withdrawal associated hallucinations, or any other manifestations of severe sedative/hypnotic withdrawal.

INDICATIONS AND USAGE

Sonata is indicated for the short-term treatment of insomnia. Sonata has been shown to decrease the time to sleep onset for up to 28 days in controlled clinical studies (see **Clinical Trials** under **CLINICAL PHARMACOLOGY**). It has not been shown to increase total sleep time or decrease the number of awakenings.

Hypnotics should generally be limited to 7 to 10 days of use, and reevaluation of the patient is recommended if they are to be taken for more than 2 to 3 weeks. Sonata should not be prescribed in quantities exceeding a 1-month supply (see **WARNINGS**).

CONTRAINDICATIONS

None known.

WARNINGS

Because sleep disturbances may be the presenting manifestation of a physical and/or psychiatric disorder, symptomatic treatment of insomnia should be initiated only after a careful evaluation of the patient. The failure of insomnia to remit after 7 to 10 days of treatment may indicate the presence of a primary psychiatric and/or medical illness that should be evaluated. Worsening of insomnia or the emergence of new thinking or behavior abnormalities may be the consequence of an unrecognized psychiatric or physical disorder. Such findings have emerged during the course of treatment with sedative/hypnotic drugs, including Sonata. Because some of the important adverse effects of Sonata appear to be dose-related, it is important to use the lowest possible effective dose, especially in the elderly (see **DOSAGE AND ADMINISTRATION**).

A variety of abnormal thinking and behavior changes have been reported to occur in association with the use of sedative/hypnotics. Some of these changes may be characterized by decreased inhibition (e.g., aggressiveness and extroversion that seem out of character), similar to effects produced by alcohol and other CNS depressants. Other reported behavioral changes have included bizarre behavior, agitation, hallucinations, and depersonalization. Amnesia and other neuropsychiatric symptoms may occur unpredictably. In primarily depressed patients, worsening of depression, including suicidal thinking, has been reported in association with the use of sedative/hypnotics.

It can rarely be determined with certainty whether a particular instance of the abnormal behaviors listed above are drug induced, spontaneous in origin, or a result of an underlying psychiatric or physical disorder. Nonetheless, the emergence of any new behavioral sign or symptom of concern requires careful and immediate evaluation.

Following rapid dose decrease or abrupt discontinuation of the use of sedative/hypnotics, there have been reports of signs and symptoms similar to those associated with withdrawal from other CNS-depressant drugs (see **DRUG ABUSE AND DEPENDENCE**).

Sonata, like other hypnotics, has CNS-depressant effects. Because of the rapid onset of action, Sonata should only be ingested immediately prior to going to bed or after the patient has gone to bed and has experienced difficulty falling asleep. Patients receiving Sonata should be cautioned against engaging in hazardous occupations requiring complete mental alertness or motor coordination (e.g., operating machinery or driving a motor vehicle) after ingesting the drug, including potential impairment of the performance of such activities that may occur the day following ingestion of Sonata. Sonata, as well as other hypnotics, may produce additive CNS depressant effects when coadministered with other psychotropic medications, anticonvulsants, antihistamines, ethanol, and other drugs that themselves produce CNS depression. Sonata should not be taken with alcohol. Dosage adjustment may be necessary when Sonata is administered with other CNS depressant agents because of the potentially additive effects.

PRECAUTIONS

General

Timing of Drug Administration

Sonata should be taken immediately before bedtime or after the patient has gone to bed and has experienced difficulty falling asleep. As with all sedative/hypnotics, taking Sonata while still up and about may result in short-term memory impairment, hallucinations, impaired coordinations, dizziness, and lightheadedness.

Use in the elderly and/or debilitated patients:

Impaired motor and/or cognitive performance after repeated exposure or unusual sensitivity to sedative/hypnotic drugs is a concern in the treatment of elderly and/or debilitated patients. A dose of 5 mg is recommended for elderly patients to decrease the possibility of side effects (see **DOSAGE AND ADMINISTRATION**). Elderly and/or debilitated patients should be monitored closely.

Use in patients with concomitant illness:

Clinical experience with Sonata in patients with concomitant systemic illness is limited. Sonata should be used with caution in patients with diseases or conditions that could affect metabolism or hemodynamic responses.

Although preliminary studies did not reveal respiratory depressant effects at hypnotic doses of Sonata in normal subjects, caution should be observed if Sonata is prescribed to patients with compromised respiratory function, because sedative/hypnotics have the capacity to depress respiratory drive. Controlled trials of acute administration of Sonata 10 mg in patients with chronic obstructive pulmonary disease or moderate obstructive sleep apnea showed no evidence of alterations in blood gases or apnea/hypopnea index, respectively. However, patients with compromised respiration due to preexisting illness should be monitored carefully.

The dose of Sonata should be reduced to 5 mg in patients with mild to moderate hepatic impairment (see **DOSAGE AND ADMINISTRATION**). It is not recommended for use in patients with severe hepatic impairment.

No dose adjustment is necessary in patients with mild to moderate renal impairment. Sonata has not been adequately studied in patients with severe renal impairment.

Use in patients with depression:

As with other sedative/hypnotic drugs, Sonata should be administered with caution to patients exhibiting signs or symptoms of depression. Suicidal tendencies may be present in such patients and protective measures may be required. Intentional overdosage is more common in this group of patients (see **OVERDOSAGE**); therefore, the least amount of drug that is feasible should be prescribed for the patient at any one time.

Information for patients

Patient information is printed at the end of this insert. To assure safe and effective use of Sonata, the information and instructions provided in the patient information section should be discussed with patients.

Laboratory Tests

There are no specific laboratory tests recommended.

Drug Interactions

As with all drugs, the potential exists for interaction with other drugs by a variety of mechanisms.

Continued on next page

Sonata—Cont.

CNS-active Drugs

Ethanol: Sonata 10 mg potentiated the CNS-impairing effects of ethanol 0.75 g/kg on balance testing and reaction time for 1 hour after ethanol administration and on the digit symbol substitution test (DSST), symbol copying test, and the variability component of the divided attention test for 2.5 hours after ethanol administration. The potentiation resulted from a CNS pharmacodynamic interaction; zaleplon did not affect the pharmacokinetics of ethanol.

Imipramine: Coadministration of single doses of Sonata 20 mg and imipramine 75 mg produced additive effects on decreased alertness and impaired psychomotor performance for 2 to 4 hours after administration. The interaction was pharmacodynamic with no alteration of the pharmacokinetics of either drug.

Paroxetine: Coadministration of a single dose of Sonata 20 mg and paroxetine 20 mg daily for 7 days did not produce any interaction on psychomotor performance. Additionally, paroxetine did not alter the pharmacokinetics of Sonata, reflecting the absence of a role of CYP2D6 in zaleplon's metabolism.

Thioridazine: Coadministration of single doses of Sonata 20 mg and thioridazine 50 mg produced additive effects of decreased alertness and impaired psychomotor performance for 2 to 4 hours after administration. The interaction was pharmacodynamic with no alteration of the pharmacokinetics of either drug.

Drugs that Induce CYP3A4

Rifampin: CYP3A4 is ordinarily a minor metabolizing enzyme of zaleplon. Multiple-dose administration of the potent CYP3A4 inducer rifampin (600 mg every 24 hours, q24h, for 14 days), however, reduced zaleplon C_{max} and AUC by approximately 80%. The coadministration of a potent CYP3A4 enzyme inducer, although not posing a safety concern, thus could lead to ineffectiveness of zaleplon. An alternative non-CYP3A4 substrate hypnotic agent may be considered in patients taking CYP3A4 inducers such as rifampin, phenytoin, carbamazepine and phenobarbital.

Drugs that Inhibit CYP3A4

CYP3A4 is a minor metabolic pathway for the elimination of zaleplon because the sum of desethylzaleplon (formed via CYP3A4 in vitro) and its metabolites, 5-oxo-desethylzaleplon and 5-oxo-desethylzaleplon glucuronide, account for only 9% of the urinary recovery of a zaleplon dose. The coadministration of a potent, selective CYP3A4 inhibitor is therefore not expected to produce a clinically important pharmacokinetic interaction with zaleplon; however, there are no clinical studies specifically addressing this question.

Drugs that Inhibit Aldehyde Oxidase

The aldehyde oxidase enzyme system is less well studied than the cytochrome P450 enzyme system.

Diphenhydramine: Diphenhydramine is reported to be a weak inhibitor of aldehyde oxidase in rat liver, but its inhibitory effects in human liver are not known. There is no pharmacokinetic interaction between zaleplon and diphenhydramine following the administration of a single dose (10 mg and 50 mg, respectively) of each drug. However, because both of these compounds have CNS effects, an additive pharmacodynamic effect is possible.

Drugs that Inhibit Both Aldehyde Oxidase and CYP3A4

Cimetidine: Cimetidine inhibits both aldehyde oxidase (in vitro) and CYP3A4 (in vitro and in vivo), the primary and secondary enzymes, respectively, responsible for zaleplon metabolism. Concomitant administration of Sonata (10 mg) and cimetidine (800 mg) produced an 85% increase in the mean C_{max} and AUC of zaleplon. An initial dose of 5 mg should be given to patients who are concomitantly being treated with cimetidine (see **DOSAGE AND ADMINISTRATION**).

Drugs Highly Bound to Plasma Protein

Zaleplon is not highly bound to plasma proteins (fraction bound 60%±15%); therefore, the disposition of zaleplon is not expected to be sensitive to alterations in protein binding. In addition, administration of Sonata to a patient taking another drug that is highly protein bound should not cause transient increase in free concentrations of the other drug.

Drugs with a Narrow Therapeutic Index

Digoxin: Sonata (10 mg) did not affect the pharmacokinetic or pharmacodynamic profile of digoxin (0.375 mg q24h for 8 days).

Warfarin: Multiple oral doses of Sonata (20 mg q24h for 13 days) did not affect the pharmacokinetics of warfarin (R+)- or (S-)-enantiomers or the pharmacodynamics (prothrombin time) following a single 25 mg oral dose of warfarin.

Drugs that Alter Renal Excretion

Ibuprofen: Ibuprofen is known to affect renal function and, consequently, alter the renal excretion of other drugs. There was no apparent pharmacokinetic interaction between zaleplon and ibuprofen following single dose administration (10 mg and 600 mg, respectively) of each drug. This was expected because zaleplon is primarily metabolized and renal excretion of unchanged zaleplon accounts for less than 1% of the administered dose.

Carcinogenesis, Mutagenesis, and Impairment of Fertility

Carcinogenesis

Lifetime carcinogenicity studies of zaleplon were conducted in mice and rats. Mice received doses of 25, 50, 100, and 200 mg/kg/day in the diet for two years. These doses are equivalent to 6–49 times the maximum recommended human dose (MRHD) of 20 mg on a mg/m^2 basis. There was a significant increase in the incidence of hepatocellular adenomas in female mice in the high dose group. Rats received doses of 1, 10, and 20 mg/kg/day in the diet for two years. These doses are equivalent to 0.5–10 times the maximum recommended human dose (MRHD) of 20 mg on a mg/m^2 basis. Zaleplon was not carcinogenic in rats.

Mutagenesis

Zaleplon was clastogenic, both in the presence and absence of metabolic activation, causing structural and numerical aberrations (polyploidy and endoreduplication), when tested for chromosomal aberrations in the *in vitro* Chinese hamster ovary cell assay. In the *in vitro* human lymphocyte assay, zaleplon caused numerical but not structural aberrations, only in the presence of metabolic activation at the highest concentrations tested. In other *in vitro* assays, zaleplon was not mutagenic in the Ames bacterial gene mutation assay or the Chinese hamster ovary HGPRT gene mutation assay. Zaleplon was not clastogenic in two *in vivo* assays, the mouse bone marrow micronucleus assay and the rat bone marrow chromosomal aberration assay, and did not cause DNA damage in the rat hepatocyte unscheduled DNA synthesis assay.

Impairment of Fertility

In a fertility and reproductive performance study in rats, mortality and decreased fertility were associated with administration of an oral dose of zaleplon of 100 mg/kg/day to males and females prior to and during mating. This dose is equivalent to 49 times the maximum recommended human dose (MRHD) of 20 mg on a mg/m^2 basis. Follow-up studies indicated that impaired fertility was due to an effect on the female.

Pregnancy: Pregnancy Category C

In embryofetal development studies in rats and rabbits, oral administration of up to 100 and 50 mg/kg/day, respectively, to pregnant animals throughout organogenesis produced no evidence of teratogenicity. These doses are equivalent to 49 (rat) and 48 (rabbit) times the maximum recommended human dose (MRHD) of 20 mg on a mg/m^2 basis. In rats, pre- and postnatal growth was reduced in the offspring of dams receiving 100 mg/kg/day. This dose was also maternally toxic, as evidenced by clinical signs and decreased maternal body weight gain during gestation. The no-effect dose for rat offspring growth reduction was 10 mg/kg (a dose equivalent to 5 times the MRHD of 20 mg on a mg/m^2 basis). No adverse effects on embryofetal development were observed in rabbits at the doses examined.

In a pre- and postnatal development study in rats, increased stillbirth and postnatal mortality, and decreased growth and physical development, were observed in the offspring of females treated with doses of 7 mg/kg/day or greater during the latter part of gestation and throughout lactation. There was no evidence of maternal toxicity at this dose. The no-effect dose for offspring development was 1 mg/kg/day (a dose equivalent to 0.5 times the MRHD of 20 mg on a mg/m^2 basis). When the adverse effects on offspring viability and growth were examined in a cross-fostering study, they appeared to result from both *in utero* and lactational exposure to the drug.

There are no studies of zaleplon in pregnant women; therefore, Sonata is not recommended for use in women during pregnancy.

Labor and Delivery

Sonata has no established use in labor and delivery.

Nursing Mothers

A study in lactating mothers indicated that the clearance and half-life of zaleplon is similar to that in young normal subjects. A small amount of zaleplon is excreted in breast milk, with the highest excreted amount occurring during a feeding at approximately 1 hour after Sonata administration. Since the small amount of the drug from breast milk may result in potentially important concentrations in infants, and because the effects of zaleplon on a nursing infant are not known, it is recommended that nursing mothers not take Sonata.

Pediatric Use

The safety and effectiveness of Sonata in pediatric patients have not been established.

Geriatric Use

A total of 628 patients in double-blind, placebo-controlled, parallel-group clinical trials who received Sonata were at least 65 years of age; of these, 311 received 5 mg and 317 received 10 mg. In both sleep laboratory and outpatient studies, elderly patients with insomnia responded to a 5-mg dose with a reduced sleep latency, and thus 5 mg is the recommended dose in this population. During short-term treatment (14 night studies) of elderly patients with Sonata, no adverse event with a frequency of at least 1% occurred at a significantly higher rate with either 5 mg or 10 mg Sonata than with placebo.

ADVERSE REACTIONS

The premarketing development program for Sonata included zaleplon exposures in patients and/or normal subjects from 2 different groups of studies: approximately 900 normal subjects in clinical pharmacology/pharmacokinetic studies; and approximately 2,800 exposures from patients in placebo-controlled clinical effectiveness studies, corresponding to approximately 450 patient exposure years. The conditions and duration of treatment with Sonata varied greatly and included (in overlapping categories) open-label and double-blind phases of studies, inpatients and outpatients, and short-term or longer-term exposure. Adverse reactions were assessed by collecting adverse events, results of physical examinations, vital signs, weights, laboratory analyses, and ECGs.

Adverse events during exposure were obtained primarily by general inquiry and recorded by clinical investigators using terminology of their own choosing. Consequently, it is not possible to provide a meaningful estimate of the proportion of individuals experiencing adverse events without first grouping similar types of events into a smaller number of standardized event categories. In the tables and tabulations that follow, COSTART terminology has been used to classify reported adverse events.

The stated frequencies of adverse events represent the proportion of individuals who experienced, at least once, a treatment-emergent adverse event of the type listed. An event was considered treatment emergent if it occurred for the first time or worsened while receiving therapy following baseline evaluation.

Adverse Findings Observed in Short-Term, Placebo-Controlled Trials

Adverse Events Associated with Discontinuation of Treatment

In premarketing placebo-controlled, parallel-group phase 2–3 clinical trials, 3.1% of 744 patients who received placebo and 3.5% of 2,069 patients who received Sonata discontinued treatment because of an adverse clinical event. This difference was not statistically significant. No event that resulted in discontinuation occurred at a rate of ≥1%.

Adverse Events Occurring at an Incidence of 1% or more Among Sonata 20 mg-Treated Patients

Table 1 enumerates, for a pool of three placebo-controlled 28-night studies of Sonata at doses of 5 or 10 mg and 20 mg, the incidence of treatment emergent adverse events. The table includes only those events that occurred in 1% or more of patients treated with Sonata 20 mg where the incidence in patients treated with Sonata 20 mg was greater than the incidence in placebo-treated patients.

The prescriber should be aware that these figures cannot be used to predict the incidence of adverse events in the course of usual medical practice where patient characteristics and other factors differ from those which prevailed in the clinical trials. Similarly, the cited frequencies cannot be compared with figures obtained from other clinical investigations involving different treatments, uses, and investigators. The cited figures, however, do provide the prescribing physician with some basis for estimating the relative contribution of drug and non-drug factors to the adverse event incidence rate in the population studied.

Table 1
Incidence (%) of Treatment-Emergent Adverse Events in Long-Term (28 Nights) Placebo-Controlled Clinical Trials of Sonata[1]

Body System Preferred Term	Placebo (n=277)	Sonata 5 or 10 mg (n=513)	Sonata 20 mg (n=273)
Body as a whole			
Abdominal pain	4	5	6
Asthenia	5	5	8
Fever	1	2	2
Headache	31	28	38
Malaise	<1	<1	2
Photosensitivity reaction	<1	<1	1
Digestive system			
Anorexia	<1	<1	2
Colitis	0	0	1
Dyspepsia	5	4	7
Nausea	7	7	8
Metabolic and Nutritional			
Peripheral edema	<1	<1	1
Musculoskeletal system			
Myalgia	4	7	5
Nervous system			
Amnesia	1	2	4
Anxiety	2	<1	3
Depersonalization	<1	<1	2
Dizziness	7	7	8
Hallucinations	<1	<1	1
Hypesthesia	0	<1	2
Paresthesia	1	3	3
Somnolence	3	5	5
Tremor	1	2	2
Vertigo	<1	<1	1
Respiratory system			
Epistaxis	0	<1	1
Special senses			
Abnormal vision	<1	<1	2
Ear pain	0	<1	1
Eye pain	3	4	4
Hyperacusis	<1	2	2
Parosmia	1	<1	2
Urogenital system			
Dysmenorrhea	2	2	4

1: Events for which the incidence for Sonata 20 mg-treated patients was at least 1% and greater than the incidence among placebo-treated patients. Incidence greater than 1% has been rounded to the nearest whole number.

Other Events Observed During the Premarketing Evaluation of Sonata

Following is a list of COSTART terms that reflect treatment-emergent adverse events as defined in the introduction to the **ADVERSE REACTIONS** section reported by patients treated with Sonata at doses in a range of 5 to 20 mg/day during premarketing phase 2 and 3 clinical trials throughout the United States, Canada, and Europe including approximately 2800 patients. All reported events are included except those already listed in Table 1 or elsewhere in labeling, and those events for which a drug cause was remote, and those event terms which were so general as to be uninformative. It is important to emphasize that, although the events reported occurred during treatment with Sonata, they were not necessarily caused by it.

Events are further categorized by body system and listed in order of decreasing frequency according to the following definitions: **frequent** adverse events are those occurring on one or more occasions in at least 1/100 patients; **infrequent** adverse events are those occurring in less than 1/100 patients but at least 1/1,000 patients; **rare** events are those occurring in fewer than 1/1,000 patients.

Body as a whole—**Frequent**: back pain, chest pain; **Infrequent**: chest pain substernal, chills, face edema, generalized edema, hangover effect, neck rigidity.

Cardiovascular system—**Frequent**: migraine; **Infrequent**: angina pectoris, bundle branch block, hypertension, hypotension, palpitation, syncope, tachycardia, vasodilatation, ventricular extrasystoles; **Rare**: bigeminy, cerebral ischemia, cyanosis, pericardial effusion, postural hypotension, pulmonary embolus, sinus bradycardia, thrombophlebitis, ventricular tachycardia.

Digestive system—**Frequent**: constipation, dry mouth; **Infrequent**: eructation, esophagitis, flatulence, gastritis gastroenteritis, gingivitis, glossitis, increased appetite, melena, mouth ulceration, rectal hemorrhage, stomatitis; **Rare**: aphthous stomatitis, biliary pain, bruxism, cardiospasm, cheilitis, cholelithiasis, duodenal ulcer, dysphagia, enteritis, gum hemorrhage, increased salivation, intestinal obstruction, liver function tests abnormal, peptic ulcer, tongue discoloration, tongue edema, ulcerative stomatitis.

Endocrine system—**Rare**: diabetes mellitus, goiter, hypothyroidism.

Hemic and lymphatic system—**Infrequent**: anemia, ecchymosis, lymphadenopathy; **Rare**: eosinophilia, leukocytosis, lymphocytosis, purpura.

Metabolic and nutritional—**Infrequent**: edema, gout, hypercholesteremia, thirst, weight gain; **Rare**: bilirubinemia, hyperglycemia, hyperuricemia, hypoglycemia, hypoglycemic reaction, ketosis, SGOT increased, SGPT increased, weight loss.

Musculoskeletal system—**Frequent**: arthritis; **Infrequent**: arthrosis, bursitis, joint disorder (mainly swelling, stiffness, and pain), myasthenia, tenosynovitis; **Rare**: myositis, osteoporosis.

Nervous system—**Frequent**: depression, hypertonia, nervousness, thinking abnormal (mainly difficulty concentrating); **Infrequent**: abnormal gait, agitation, apathy, ataxia, circumoral paresthesia, confusion, emotional lability, euphoria, hyperesthesia, hyperkinesia, hypotonia, incoordination, insomnia, libido decreased, neuralgia, nystagmus; **Rare**: CNS stimulation, delusions, dysarthria, dystonia, facial paralysis, hostility, hypokinesia, myoclonus, neuropathy, psychomotor retardation, ptosis, reflexes decreased, reflexes increased, sleep talking, sleep walking, slurred speech, stupor, trismus.

Respiratory system—**Frequent**: bronchitis; **Infrequent**: asthma, dyspnea, laryngitis, pneumonia, snoring, voice alteration; **Rare**: apnea, hiccup, hyperventilation, pleural effusion, sputum increased.

Skin and appendages—**Frequent**: pruritus, rash; **Infrequent**: acne, alopecia, contact dermatitis, dry skin, eczema, maculopapular rash, skin hypertrophy, sweating, urticaria, vesiculobullous rash; **Rare**: melanosis, psoriasis, pustular rash, skin discoloration.

Special senses—**Frequent**: conjunctivitis; **Infrequent**: diplopia, dry eyes, photophobia, tinnitus, watery eyes; **Rare**: abnormailty of accommodation, blepharitis, cataract specified, corneal erosion, deafness, eye hemorrhage, glaucoma, labyrinthitis, retinal detachment, taste loss, visual field defect.

Urogenital system—**Infrequent**: bladder pain, breast pain, cystitis, decreased urine stream, dysuria, hematuria, impotence, kidney calculus, kidney pain, menorrhagia, metrorrhagia, urinary frequency, urinary incontinence, urinary urgency, vaginitis; **Rare**: albuminuria, delayed menstrual period, leukorrhea, menopause, urethritis, urinary retention, vaginal hemorrhage.

DRUG ABUSE AND DEPENDENCE

Controlled Substance Class

Sonata is classified as a Schedule IV controlled substance by federal regulation.

Abuse, Dependence, and Tolerance

Abuse

Two studies assessed the abuse liability of Sonata at doses of 25, 50, and 75 mg in subjects with known histories of sedative drug abuse. The results of these studies indicate that Sonata has an abuse potential similar to benzodiazepine and benzodiazepine-like hypnotics.

Dependence

The potential for developing physical dependence on Sonata and a subsequent withdrawal syndrome was assessed in controlled studies of 14- and 28-day durations and in open-label studies of 6- and 12-month duration by examining for the emergence of rebound insomnia following drug discontinuation. Some patients (mostly those treated with 20 mg) experienced a mild rebound insomnia on the first night following withdrawal that appeared to be resolved by the second night. The use of the Benzodiazepine Withdrawal Symptom Questionnaire and examination for any other withdrawal emergent events did not detect any other evidence for a withdrawal syndrome following abrupt discontinuation of Sonata therapy in pre-marketing studies.

However, available data cannot provide a reliable estimate of the incidence of dependence during treatment at recommended doses of Sonata. Other sedative/hypnotics have been associated with various signs and symptoms following abrupt discontinuation, ranging from mild dysphoria and insomnia to a withdrawal syndrome that may include abdominal and muscle cramps, vomiting, sweating, tremors, and convulsions. Seizures have been observed in two patients, one of which had a prior seizure, in clinical trials with Sonata. Seizures and death have been seen following the withdrawal of zaleplon from animals at doses many times higher than those proposed for human use. Because individuals with a history of addiction to, or abuse of, drugs or alcohol are at risk of habituation and dependence, they should be under careful surveillance when receiving Sonata or any other hypnotic.

Tolerance

Possible tolerance to the hypnotic effects of Sonata 10 and 20 mg was assessed by evaluating time to sleep onset for Sonata compared with placebo in two placebo-controlled 28-day studies. No development of tolerance to Sonata was observed for time to sleep onset over 4 weeks.

OVERDOSAGE

There is limited pre-marketing clinical experience with the effects of an overdosage of Sonata. Two cases of overdose were reported. One was the accidental ingestion by a 2 1/2 year old boy of 20–40 mg of zaleplon. The second was a 20 year old man who took 100 mg zaleplon plus 2.25 mg of triazolam. Both were treated and recovered uneventfully.

Signs and Symptoms

Signs and symptoms of overdose effects of CNS depressants can be expected to present as exaggerations of the pharmacological effects noted in preclinical testing. Overdose is usually manifested by degrees of central nervous system depression ranging from drowsiness to coma. In mild cases, symptoms include drowsiness, mental confusion, and lethargy; in more serious cases, symptoms may include ataxia, hypotonia, hypotension, respiratory depression, rarely coma, and very rarely death.

Recommended Treatment

General symptomatic and supportive measures should be used along with immediate gastric lavage where appropriate. Intravenous fluids should be administered as needed. Animal studies suggest that flumazenil is an antagonist to zaleplon. However, there is no pre-marketing clinical experience with the use of flumazenil as an antidote to a Sonata overdose. As in all cases of drug overdose, respiration, pulse, blood pressure, and other appropriate signs should be monitored and general supportive measures employed. Hypotension and CNS depression should be monitored and treated by appropriate medical intervention.

Poison Control Center

As with the management of all overdosage, the possibility of multiple drug ingestion should be considered. The physician may wish to consider contacting a poison control center for up-to-date information on the management of hypnotic drug product overdosage.

DOSAGE AND ADMINISTRATION

The dose of Sonata should be individualized. The recommended dose of Sonata for most nonelderly adults is 10 mg. For certain low weight individuals, 5 mg may be a sufficient dose. Although the risk of certain adverse events associated with the use of Sonata appears to be dose dependent, the 20 mg dose has been shown to be adequately tolerated and may be considered for the occasional patient who does not benefit from a trial of a lower dose. Doses above 20 mg have not been adequately evaluated and are not recommended.

Sonata should be taken immediately before bedtime or after the patient has gone to bed and has experienced difficulty falling asleep (see **PRECAUTIONS**). Taking Sonata with or immediately after a heavy, high-fat meal results in slower absorption and would be expected to reduce the effect of Sonata on sleep latency (see **Pharmacokinetics** under **CLINICAL PHARMACOLOGY**).

Special Population

Elderly patients and debilitated patients appear to be more sensitive to the effects of hypnotics, and respond to 5 mg of Sonata. The recommended dose for these patients is therefore 5 mg. Doses over 10 mg are not recommended.

Hepatic insufficiency: Patients with mild to moderate hepatic impairment should be treated with Sonata 5 mg because clearance is reduced in this population. Sonata is not recommended for use in patients with severe hepatic impairment.

Renal insufficiency: No dose adjustment is necessary in patients with mild to moderate renal impairment. Sonata has not been adequately studied in patients with severe renal impairment.

An initial dose of 5 mg should be given to patients concomitantly taking cimetidine becasue zaleplon clearance is reduced in this population (see **Drug Interactions** under **PRECAUTIONS**).

HOW SUPPLIED

Sonata capsules are available in bottles of 100 capsules in the following dosage strengths:

5 mg, NDC 0008-0925, opaque green cap and opaque pale green body with "5 mg" on the cap and "SONATA" on the body.

10 mg, NDC 0008-0926, opaque green cap and opaque light green body with "10 mg" on the cap and "SONATA" on the body.

The appearance of these capsules is a trademark of Wyeth Laboratories.

STORAGE CONDITIONS

Store at controlled room temperature, 20°–25°C (68°–77°F).

Dispense in a light-resistant container as defined in the USP.

INFORMATION FOR PATIENTS TAKING SONATA

Your doctor has prescribed Sonata to help you sleep. The following information is intended to guide you in the safe use of this medicine. It is not meant to take the place of your doctor's instructions. If you have any questions about Sonata capsules, be sure to ask your doctor or pharmacist.

Sonata is used to treat difficulty in falling asleep. Sonata works very quickly and has its effect during the first part of the night, since it is rapidly eliminated by the body. You should take Sonata immediately before going to bed or after you have gone to bed and are having difficulty falling asleep. If your principal sleep difficulty is awakening prematurely after falling asleep, there is no evidence that Sonata will be helpful to you. For Sonata to help you fall asleep you should not take it with or immediately after a high-fat/heavy meal.

Sonata belongs to a group of medicines known as the "hypnotics", or simply, sleep medicines. There are many different sleep medicines available to help people sleep better. Sleep problems are usually temporary, requiring treatment for only a short time, usually 1 or 2 days up to 1 or 2 weeks. Some people have chronic sleep problems that may require more prolonged use of sleep medicine. However, you should not use these medicines for long periods without talking with your doctor about the risks and benefits of prolonged use.

Side Effects

All medicines have side effects. The most common side effects of sleep medicines are:

- Drowsiness
- Dizziness
- Lightheadedness
- Difficulty with coordination

These side effects with Sonata occur most often within an hour after taking it, so it is especially important to take it only when you are about to go to bed or are already in bed.

Sleep medicines can make you sleepy during the day. How drowsy you feel depends upon how your body reacts to the medicine, which sleep medicine you are taking, and how large a dose your doctor has prescribed. Daytime drowsiness is best avoided by taking the lowest dose possible that will still help you sleep at night. Your doctor will work with you to find the dose of Sonata that is best for you. Sonata generally does not cause next-day sleepiness but a few people have reported this.

To manage these side effects while you are taking this medicine:

— When you first start taking Sonata or any other sleep medicine, until you know whether the medicine will still have some carryover effect in you the next day, use extreme care while doing anything that requires complete alertness, such as driving a car, operating machinery, or piloting an aircraft.

— NEVER drink alcohol while you are being treated with Sonata or any sleep medicine. Alcohol can increase the side effects of Sonata or any other sleep medicine.

— Do not take any other medicines without asking your doctor first. This includes medicines you can buy without a prescription. Some medicines can cause drowsiness and are best avoided while taking Sonata.

— Always take the exact dose of Sonata prescribed by your doctor. Never change your dose without talking to your doctor first.

Special Concerns

There are some special problems that may occur while taking sleep medicines.

Memory Problems:

Sleep medicines may cause a special type of memory loss or "amnesia." When this occurs, a person may not remember what has happened for several hours after taking the medicine. This is usually not a problem since most people fall asleep after taking the medicine. Memory loss can be a problem, however, when sleep medicines are taken while traveling, such as during an airplane flight and the person wakes up before the effect of the medicine is gone. This has been called "traveler's amnesia." Memory problems are not common while taking Sonata. In most instances memory problems can be avoided if you take Sonata only when you are able to get 4 or more hours of sleep before you need to be active again. Be sure to talk to your doctor if you think you are having memory problems.

Tolerance:

When sleep medicines are used every night for more than a few weeks, they may lose their effectiveness to help you sleep. This is known as "tolerance." Development of tolerance to Sonata has not been observed in outpatient clinical studies of up to 4-weeks duration, however, it is unknown if the benefits of Sonata on falling asleep more quickly persist beyond 4 weeks. Sleep medicines should, in most cases, be used only for short periods of time, such as 1 or 2 days and

Continued on next page

Sonata—Cont.

generally no longer than 1 or 2 weeks. If your sleep problems continue, consult your doctor, who will determine whether other measures are needed to overcome your sleep problems.

Dependence:

Sleep medicines can cause dependence, especially when these medicines are used regularly for longer than a few weeks or at high doses. Some people develop a need to continue taking their medicines. This is known as dependence or "addiction."

When people develop dependence, they may have difficulty stopping the sleep medicine. If the medicine is suddenly stopped, the body is not able to function normally and unpleasant symptoms (see ***Withdrawal***) may occur. They may find they have to keep taking the medicine either at the prescribed dose or at increasing doses just to avoid withdrawal symptoms.

All people taking sleep medicines have some risk of becoming dependent on the medicine. However, people who have been dependent on alcohol or other drugs in the past may have a higher change of becoming addicted to sleep medicines. This possibility must be considered before using these medicines for more than a few weeks. If you have been addicted to alcohol or drugs in the past, it is important to tell you doctor before starting Sonata or any sleep medicine.

Withdrawal:

Withdrawal symptoms may occur when sleep medicines are stopped suddenly after being used daily for a long time. In some cases, these symptoms can occur even if the medicine has been used for only a week or two. In mild cases, withdrawal symptome may include unpleasant feelings. In more severe cases, abdominal and muscle cramps, vomiting, sweating, shakiness, and rarely, seizures may occur. These more severe withdrawal symptoms are very uncommon. Although withdrawal symptoms have not been observed in the relatively limited controlled trials experience with Sonata, there is, nevertheless, the risk of such events in association with the use of any sleep medicines.

Another problem that may occur when sleep medicines are stopped in known as "rebound insomnia." This means that a person may have more trouble sleeping the first few nights after the medicine is stopped than before starting the medicine. If you should experience rebound insomnia, do not get discouraged. This problem usually goes away on its own after 1 or 2 nights.

If you have been taking Sonata or any other sleep medicine for more than 1 or 2 weeks, do not stop taking it on your own. Always follow your doctor's directions.

Changes In Behavior and Thinking:

Some people using sleep medicines have experienced unusual change in their thinking and/or behavior. These effects are not common. However, they have included:

— more outgoing or aggressive behavior than normal
— loss of personal identity
— confusion
— strange behavior
— agitation
— hallucinations
— worsening of depression
— suicidal thoughts

How often these effects occur depends on several factors, such as a person's general health, the use of other medicines, and which sleep medicine is being used. Clinical experience with Sonata suggests that it is uncommonly associated with these behavior changes.

It is also important to realize that it is rarely clear whether these behavior changes are caused by the medicine, an illness, or occur on their own. In fact, sleep problems that do not improve may be due to illnesses that were present before the medicine was used. If you or your family notice any changes in your behavior, or if you have any unusual or disturbing thoughts, call your doctor immediately.

Pregnancy and Breastfeeding:

Sleep medicines may cause sedation or other potential effects in the unborn baby when used during the last weeks of pregnancy. Therefore, Sonata is not recommended for use during pregnancy. Be sure to tell your doctor if you are pregnant, if you are planning to become pregnant, or if you become pregnant while taking Sonata.

In addition, a very small amount of Sonata may be present in breast milk after use of the medication. The effects of very small amounts of Sonata on an infant are not known; therefore, as with all other hypnotics, it is recommended that you not take Sonata if you are breastfeeding a baby.

Safe Use of Sleeping Medicines:

To ensure the safe and effective use of Sonata or any other sleep medicine, you should observe the following cautions:

1. Sonata is a prescription medicine and should be used ONLY as directed by your doctor. Follow your doctor's instructions about how to take, when to take, and how long to take Sonata.
2. Never use Sonata or any other sleep medicine for longer than directed by your doctor.
3. If you notice any unusual and/or disturbing thoughts or behavior during treatment with Sonata or any other sleep medicine, contact your doctor.
4. Tell your doctor about any medicines you may be taking, including medicines you may buy without a prescription. You should also tell your doctor if you drink alcohol. DO NOT use alcohol while taking Sonata or any other sleep medicine.
5. Do not take Sonata unless you are able to get 4 or more hours of sleep before you must be active again.
6. Do not increase the prescribed dose of Sonata or any other sleep medicine unless instructed by your doctor.
7. When you first start taking Sonata or any other sleep medicine, until you know whether the medicine will still have some carryover effect in you the next day, use extreme care while doing anything that requires complete alertness, such as driving a car, operating machinery, or piloting an aircraft.
8. Be aware that you may have more sleeping problems the first night or two after stopping any sleep medicine.
9. Be sure to tell your doctor if you are pregnant, if you are planning to become pregnant, if you become pregnant, or are breastfeeding a baby while taking Sonata.
10. As with all prescription medicines, never share Sonata or any other sleep medicine with anyone else. Always store Sonata or any other sleep medicine in the original container and out of reach of children.
11. Be sure to tell your physician if you suffer from depression.
12. Sonata works very quickly. You should only take Sonata immediately before going to bed or after you have gone to bed and are having difficulty falling asleep.
13. For Sonata to work best, you should not take Sonata with or immediately after a high-fat/heavy meal.
14. Some people should start with the lowest dose (5 mg) of Sonata; these include the elderly (i.e., ages 65 and over) and people with liver disease.

Manufactured by:
Wyeth Laboratories
A Wyeth-Ayerst Company
Philadelphia, PA 19101
CI 6001-1 Issued August 13, 1999

Shown in Product Identification Guide, page 342

SURMONTIL® ℞

[*sĭr 'mŏn "tĭll*]
(trimipramine maleate)

DESCRIPTION

Surmontil (trimipramine maleate) is 5-(3-dimethylamino-2-methylpropyl)-10,11-dihydro-5H-dibenz (b,f) azepine acid maleate (racemic form).

$\cdot C_4H_4O_4$

$CH_2—{}^{\bullet}CH(CH_3)—CH_2—N(CH_3)_2$

MOLECULAR FORMULA: $C_{20}H_{26}N_2 \cdot C_4H_4O_4$

MOLECULAR WEIGHT: 410.5

Surmontil capsules contain trimipramine maleate equivalent to 25 mg, 50 mg, or 100 mg of trimipramine as the base. The inactive ingredients present are FD&C Blue 1, gelatin, lactose, magnesium stearate, and titanium dioxide. The 25 mg dosage strength also contains D&C Yellow 10 and FD&C Yellow 6; the 50 mg dosage strength also contains D&C Red 28, FD&C Red 40, and FD&C Yellow 6.

Trimipramine maleate is prepared as a racemic mixture which can be resolved into levorotatory and dextrorotatory isomers. The asymmetric center responsible for optical isomerism is marked in the formula by an asterisk. Trimipramine maleate is an almost odorless, white or slightly cream-colored, crystalline substance, melting at 140–144°C. It is very slightly soluble in ether and water, is slightly soluble in ethyl alcohol and acetone, and freely soluble in chloroform and methanol at 20°C.

CLINICAL PHARMACOLOGY

Surmontil is an antidepressant with an anxiety-reducing sedative component to its action. The mode of action of Surmontil on the central nervous system is not known. However, unlike amphetamine-type compounds it does not act primarily by stimulation of the central nervous system. It does not act by inhibition of the monoamine oxidase system.

INDICATIONS AND USAGE

Surmontil is indicated for the relief of symptoms of depression. Endogenous depression is more likely to be alleviated than other depressive states. In studies with neurotic outpatients, the drug appeared to be equivalent to amitriptyline in the less-depressed patients but somewhat less effective than amitriptyline in the more severely depressed patients. In hospitalized depressed patients, trimipramine and imipramine were equally effective in relieving depression.

CONTRAINDICATIONS

Surmontil is contraindicated in cases of known hypersensitivity to the drug. The possibility of cross-sensitivity to other dibenzazepine compounds should be kept in mind. Surmontil should not be given in conjunction with drugs of the monoamine oxidase inhibitor class (e.g., tranylcypromine, isocarboxazid or phenelzine sulfate). The concomitant use of monoamine oxidase inhibitors (MAOI) and tricyclic compounds similar to Surmontil has caused severe hyperpyretic reactions, convulsive crises, and death in some patients. At least two weeks should elapse after cessation of therapy with MAOI before instituting therapy with Surmontil. Initial dosage should be low and increased gradually with caution and careful observation of the patient. The drug is contraindicated during the acute recovery period after a myocardial infarction.

WARNINGS

General Consideration for Use

Extreme caution should be used when this drug is given to patients with any evidence of cardiovascular disease because of the possibility of conduction defects, arrhythmias, myocardial infarction, strokes, and tachycardia.

Caution is advised in patients with increased intraocular pressure, history of urinary retention, or history of narrow-angle glaucoma because of the drug's anticholinergic properties; hyperthyroid patients or those on thyroid medication because of the possibility of cardiovascular toxicity; patients with a history of seizure disorder, because this drug has been shown to lower the seizure threshold; patients receiving guanethidine or similar agents, since Surmontil may block the pharmacologic effects of these drugs.

Since the drug may impair the mental and/or physical abilities required for the performance of potentially hazardous tasks, such as operating an automobile or machinery, the patient should be cautioned accordingly.

PRECAUTIONS

General

The possibility of suicide is inherent in any severely depressed patient and persists until a significant remission occurs. When a patient with a serious suicidal potential is not hospitalized, the prescription should be for the smallest amount feasible.

In schizophrenic patients activation of the psychosis may occur and require reduction of dosage or the addition of a major tranquilizer to the therapeutic regime.

Manic or hypomanic episodes may occur in some patients, in particular those with cyclic-type disorders. In some cases therapy with Surmontil must be discontinued until the episode is relieved, after which therapy may be reinstituted at lower dosages if still required.

Concurrent administration of Surmontil and electroshock therapy may increase the hazards of therapy. Such treatment should be limited to those patients for whom it is essential. When possible, discontinue the drug for several days prior to elective surgery.

Surmontil should be used with caution in patients with impaired liver function.

Chronic animal studies showed occasional occurrence of hepatic congestion, fatty infiltration, or increased serum liver enzymes at the highest dose of 60 mg/kg/day.

Both elevation and lowering of blood sugar have been reported with tricyclic antidepressants.

Drug Interactions

Cimetidine

There is evidence that cimetidine inhibits the elimination of tricyclic antidepressants. Downward adjustment of Surmontil dosage may be required if cimetidine therapy is initiated; upward adjustment if cimetidine therapy is discontinued.

Alcohol

Patients should be warned that the concomitant use of alcoholic beverages may be associated with exaggerated effects.

Catecholamines/Anticholinergics

It has been reported that tricyclic antidepressants can potentiate the effects of catecholamines. Similarly, atropine-like effects may be more pronounced in patients receiving anticholinergic therapy. Therefore, particular care should be exercised when it is necessary to administer tricyclic antidepressants with sympathomimetic amines, local decongestants, local anesthetics containing epinephrine, atropine or drugs with an anticholinergic effect. In resistant cases of depression in adults, a dose of 2.5 mg/kg/day may have to be exceeded. If a higher dose is needed, ECG monitoring should be maintained during the initiation of therapy and at appropriate intervals during stabilization of dose.

Drugs Metabolized by P450 2D6

The biochemical activity of the drug metabolizing isozyme cytochrome P450 2D6 (debrisoquin hydroxylase) is reduced in a subset of the caucasian population (about 7–10% of caucasians are so called "poor metabolizers"); reliable estimates of the prevalence of reduced P450 2D6 isozyme activity among Asian, African, and other populations are not yet available. Poor metabolizers have higher than expected plasma concentrations of tricyclic antidepressants (TCAs) when given usual doses. Depending on the fraction of drug metabolized by P450 2D6, the increase in plasma concentration may be small, or quite large (8 fold increase in plasma AUC of the TCA).

In addition, certain drugs inhibit the activity of this isozyme and make normal metabolizers resemble poor metabolizers. An individual who is stable on a given dose of TCA may become abruptly toxic when given one of these inhibiting drugs as concomitant therapy. The drugs that inhibit cytochrome P450 2D6 include some that are not metabolized by the enzyme (quinidine; cimetidine) and many that are substrates for P450 2D6 (many other antidepressants, phenothiazines, and the Type 1C antiarrhythmics propafenone and flecainide). While all the selective serotonin reuptake inhibitors (SSRIs), e.g., fluoxetine, sertraline, and paroxetine, inhibit P450 2D6, they may vary in the extent of inhibition. The extent to which SSRI TCA interactions may pose clinical problems will depend on the degree of inhibition and the pharmacokinetics of the SSRI involved. Nevertheless, caution is indicated in the co-administration of TCAs with

any of the SSRIs and also in switching from one class to the other. Of particular importance, sufficient time must elapse before initiating TCA treatment in a patient being withdrawn from fluoxetine, given the long half-life of the parent and active metabolite (at least 5 weeks may be necessary).
Concomitant use of tricyclic antidepressants with drugs that can inhibit cytochrome P450 2D6 may require lower doses than usually prescribed for either the tricyclic antidepressant or the other drug.
Furthermore, whenever one of these other drugs is withdrawn from co-therapy, an increased dose of tricyclic antidepressant may be required. It is desirable to monitor TCA plasma levels whenever a TCA is going to be co-administered with another drug known to be an inhibitor of P450 2D6.

Carcinogenesis, Mutagenesis, Impairment of Fertility
Semen studies in man (four schizophrenics and nine normal volunteers) revealed no significant changes in sperm morphology. It is recognized that drugs having a parasympathetic effect, including tricyclic antidepressants, may alter the ejaculatory response.
Chronic animal studies showed occasional evidence of degeneration of seminiferous tubules at the highest dose of 60 mg/kg/day.

Pregnancy
Teratogenic Effects—Pregnancy Category C
Surmontil has shown evidence of embryo-toxicity and/or increased incidence of major anomalies in rats or rabbits at doses 20 times the human dose. There are no adequate and well-controlled studies in pregnant women. Surmontil® should be used during pregnancy only if the potential benefit justifies the potential risk to the fetus.

Pediatric Use
This drug is not recommended for use in children, since safety and effectiveness in the pediatric age group have not been established.

ADVERSE REACTIONS

Note: The pharmacological similarities among the tricyclic antidepressants require that each of the reactions be considered when Surmontil is administered. Some of the adverse reactions included in this listing have not in fact been reported with Surmontil.

Cardiovascular
Hypotension, hypertension, tachycardia, palpitation, myocardial infarction, arrhythmias, heart block, stroke.

Psychiatric
Confusional states (especially the elderly) with hallucinations, disorientation, delusions; anxiety, restlessness, agitation; insomnia and nightmares; hypomania; exacerbation of psychosis.

Neurological
Numbness, tingling, paresthesias of extremities; incoordination, ataxia, tremors; peripheral neuropathy; extrapyramidal symptoms; seizures, alterations in EEG patterns; tinnitus; syndrome of inappropriate ADH (antidiuretic hormone) secretion.

Anticholinergic
Dry mouth and, rarely, associated sublingual adenitis; blurred vision, disturbances of accommodation, mydriasis, constipation, paralytic ileus; urinary retention, delayed micturition, dilation of the urinary tract.

Allergic
Skin rash, petechiae, urticaria, itching, photosensitization, edema of face and tongue.

Hematologic
Bone-marrow depression including agranulocytosis, eosinophilia; purpura; thrombocytopenia. Leukocyte and differential counts should be performed in any patient who develops fever and sore throat during therapy; the drug should be discontinued if there is evidence of pathological neutrophil depression.

Gastrointestinal
Nausea and vomiting, anorexia, epigastric distress, diarrhea, peculiar taste, stomatitis, abdominal cramps, black tongue.

Endocrine
Gynecomastia in the male; breast enlargement and galactorrhea in the female; increased or decreased libido, impotence; testicular swelling; elevation or depression of blood-sugar levels.

Other
Jaundice (simulating obstructive); altered liver function; weight gain or loss; perspiration; flushing; urinary frequency; drowsiness, dizziness, weakness, and fatigue; headache; parotid swelling; alopecia.

Withdrawal Symptoms
Though not indicative of addiction, abrupt cessation of treatment after prolonged therapy may produce nausea, headache, and malaise.

DOSAGE AND ADMINISTRATION

Dosage should be initiated at a low level and increased gradually, noting carefully the clinical response and any evidence of intolerance.
Lower dosages are recommended for elderly patients and adolescents. Lower dosages are also recommended for outpatients as compared to hospitalized patients who will be under close supervision. It is not possible to prescribe a single dosage schedule of Surmontil that will be therapeutically effective in all patients. The physical psychodynamic factors contributing to depressive symptomatology are very complex; spontaneous remissions or exacerbations of depressive symptoms may occur with or without drug therapy. Consequently, the recommended dosage regimens are furnished as a guide which may be modified by factors such as the age of the patient, chronicity and severity of the disease, medical condition of the patient, and degree of psychotherapeutic support.
Most antidepressant drugs have a lag period of ten days to four weeks before a therapeutic response is noted. Increasing the dose will not shorten this period but rather increase the incidence of adverse reactions.

USUAL ADULT DOSE
Outpatients and Office Patients—Initially, 75 mg/day in divided doses, increased to 150 mg/day. Dosages over 200 mg/day are not recommended. Maintenance therapy is in the range of 50 to 150 mg/day. For convenient therapy and to facilitate patient compliance, the total dosage requirement may be given at bedtime.
Hospitalized Patients—Initially, 100 mg/day in divided doses. This may be increased gradually in a few days to 200 mg/day, depending upon individual response and tolerance. If improvement does not occur in 2 to 3 weeks, the dose may be increased to the maximum recommended dose of 250 to 300 mg/day.
Adolescent and Geriatric Patients—Initially, a dose of 50 mg/day is recommended, with gradual increments up to 100 mg/day, depending upon patient response and tolerance.
Maintenance—Following remission, maintenance medication may be required for a longer period of time, at the lowest dose that will maintain remission. Maintenance therapy is preferably administered as a single dose at bedtime. To minimize relapse, maintenance therapy should be continued for about three months.

OVERDOSAGE

Deaths may occur from overdosage with this class of drugs. Multiple drug ingestion (including alcohol) is common in deliberate tricyclic antidepressant overdose. As the management is complex and changing, it is recommended that the physician contact a poison control center for current information on treatment. Signs and symptoms of toxicity develop rapidly after tricyclic antidepressant overdose, therefore, hospital monitoring is required as soon as possible.

Manifestations
Critical manifestations of overdose include: cardiac dysrhythmias, severe hypotension, convulsions, and CNS depression, including coma. Changes in the electrocardiogram, particularly in QRS axis or width, are clinically significant indicators of tricyclic antidepressant toxicity.
Other signs of overdose may include: confusion, disturbed concentration, transient visual hallucinations, dilated pupils, agitation, hyperactive reflexes, stupor, drowsiness, muscle rigidity, vomiting, hypothermia, hyperpyrexia, or any of the symptoms listed under **Adverse Reactions**.

Management
General
Obtain an ECG and immediately initiate cardiac monitoring. Protect the patient's airway, establish an intravenous line and initiate gastric decontamination. A minimum of six hours of observation with cardiac monitoring and observation for signs of CNS or respiratory depression, hypotension, cardiac dysrhythmias and/or conduction blocks, and seizures is necessary. If signs of toxicity occur at any time during this period, extended monitoring is required. There are case reports of patients succumbing to fatal dysrhythmias late after overdose; these patients had clinical evidence of significant poisoning prior to death and most received inadequate gastrointestinal decontamination. Plasma drug levels may not reflect the severity of the poisoning. Therefore, monitoring of plasma drug levels alone should not guide management of the patient.
Gastrointestinal Decontamination
All patients suspected of tricyclic antidepressant overdose should receive gastrointestinal decontamination. This should include large volume gastric lavage followed by activated charcoal. If consciousness is impaired, the airway should be secured prior to lavage. Emesis is contraindicated.
Cardiovascular
A maximal limb-lead QRS duration of $\geq$0.10 seconds has been associated with an increased incidence of seizures. A QRS duration of $\geq$0.16 seconds has been associated with an increased incidence of ventricular dysrhythmias. Intravenous sodium bicarbonate should be used to maintain the serum pH in the range of 7.45 to 7.55. If the pH response is inadequate, hyperventilation may also be used. Concomitant use of hyperventilation and sodium bicarbonate should be done with extreme caution, with frequent pH monitoring. A pH >7.60 or a pCO_2 <20 mm Hg is undesirable. Dysrhythmias unresponsive to sodium bicarbonate therapy/hyperventilation may respond to lidocaine, bretylium or phenytoin. Type 1A and 1C antiarrhythmics are generally contraindicated (e.g., quinidine, disopyramide, and procainamide).
In rare instances, hemoperfusion may be beneficial in acute refractory cardiovascular instability in patients with acute toxicity. However, hemodialysis, peritoneal dialysis, exchange transfusions, and forced diuresis generally have been reported as ineffective in tricyclic antidepressant poisoning.
CNS
In patients with CNS depression, early intubation is advised because of the potential for abrupt deterioration. Seizures should be controlled with benzodiazepines, or if these are ineffective, other anticonvulsants (e.g., phenobarbital, phenytoin). Physostigmine is not recommended except to treat life-threatening symptoms that have been unresponsive to other therapies, and then only in consultation with a poison control center.
Psychiatric Follow-up
Since overdosage is often deliberate, patients may attempt suicide by other means during the recovery phase. Psychiatric referral may be appropriate.
Pediatric Management
The principles of management of child and adult overdosages are similar. It is strongly recommended that the physician contact the local poison control center for specific pediatric treatment.
**Poisindex® Toxicologic Management*. Topic: Antidepressants, Tricyclic Micromedex Inc. Vol.85.

HOW SUPPLIED

Surmontil® (trimipramine maleate) Capsules are available in the following dosage strengths:
25 mg, NDC 0008-4132, opaque blue and yellow capsule marked "WYETH" and "4132", in bottles of 100 capsules.
50 mg, NDC 0008-4133, opaque blue and orange capsule marked "WYETH" and "4133", in bottles of 100 capsules.
100 mg, NDC 0008-4158, opaque blue and white capsule marked "WYETH" and "4158", in bottles of 100 capsules.
Store at room temperature, approximately 25°C (77°F).
Keep bottles tightly closed.
Dispense in tight container.
Protect capsules packaged in blister strips from moisture.
The appearance of these capsules is a trademark of Wyeth-Ayerst Laboratories.

by arrangement with Rhone-Poulenc Rorer France
Manufactured by:
Wyeth Laboratories
A Wyeth-Ayerst Company
Philadelphia, PA 19101
CI 5187-1 Issued February 17, 1999
Shown in Product Identification Guide, page 342

SYNALGOS®-DC Ⓒ℞

[*sĭn 'al "gōs*]
Capsules

DESCRIPTION

Each Synalgos-DC capsule contains 16 mg drocode (dihydrocodeine) bitartrate (Warning—may be habit-forming), 356.4 mg aspirin, and 30 mg caffeine.
The inactive ingredients present are alginic acid, cellulose, D&C Red 28, FD&C Blue 1, gelatin, iron oxides, stearic acid, and titanium dioxide.

HOW SUPPLIED

Synalgos®-DC Capsules are supplied in bottles of 100 and 500 capsules as follows:
NDC 0008-4191, blue and gray capsule marked "WYETH" and "4191".
Store at room temperature (approximately 25°C).
Keep tightly closed.
Dispense in tight container.
Manufactured by:
Wyeth Laboratories
A Wyeth-Ayerst Company
Philadelphia, PA 19101
CI 3484-3 Revised February 11, 1994
For prescribing information write to Professional Service, Wyeth-Ayerst Pharmaceuticals, P.O. Box 8299, Philadelphia, PA 19101, or contact your local Wyeth-Ayerst representative.

SYNVISC® ℞

[*sĭn' vĭsk*]
(Hylan G-F 20)

Caution: Federal law restricts this device to sale by or on the order of a physician (or properly licensed practitioner).

DESCRIPTION

Synvisc (hylan G-F 20) is an elastoviscous fluid containing hylan polymers produced from chicken combs. Hylans are derivatives of hyaluronan (sodium hyaluronate), a natural complex sugar of the glycosamino-glycan family. Hyaluronan is a long-chain polymer containing repeating disaccharide units of Na-glucuronate-N-acetylglucosamine.

INDICATIONS

Synvisc is indicated for the treatment of pain in osteoarthritis (OA) of the knee in patients who have failed to respond adequately to conservative nonpharmacologic therapy and simple analgesics, e.g., acetaminophen.

CONTRAINDICATIONS

- Do not administer to patients with known hypersensitivity (allergy) to hyaluronan (sodium hyaluronate) preparations.
- Do not inject Synvisc in the knees of patients having knee joint infections or skin diseases or infections in the area of the injection site.

WARNINGS

- Do not concomitantly use disinfectants containing quaternary ammonium salts for skin preparation because hyaluronan can precipitate in their presence.

Continued on next page

Synvisc—Cont.

- Do not inject Synvisc extra-articularly or into the synovial tissues and capsule. One such systemic adverse event occurred following extra-articular injections of Synvisc in clinical use outside the U.S.
- Intravascular injections of Synvisc may cause systemic adverse events.

PRECAUTIONS

General

- The effectiveness of a single treatment cycle of less than three injections of Synvisc has not been established.
- The safety and effectiveness of Synvisc in locations other than the knee and for conditions other than osteoarthritis have not been established.
- Do not inject anesthetics or other medications into the knee joint during Synvisc therapy. Such medications may dilute Synvisc and affect its safety and effectiveness.
- Use caution when injecting Synvisc into patients who are allergic to avian proteins, feathers, and egg products.
- The safety and effectiveness of Synvisc in severely inflamed knee joints have not been established.
- Strict aseptic administration technique must be followed.
- STERILE CONTENTS. The syringe is intended for single use. The contents of the syringe must be used immediately after its packaging is opened. Discard any unused Synvisc.
- Do not use Synvisc if package is opened or damaged. Store in original packaging (protected from light) at room temperature below 86°F (30°C). DO NOT FREEZE.
- Remove synovial fluid or effusion, if present, before injecting Synvisc.
- Synvisc should be used with caution when there is evidence of lymphatic or venous stasis in that leg.

Information for Patients

- Provide patients with a copy of the Patient Labeling prior to use.
- Transient pain and/or swelling of the injected joint may occur after intra-articular injection of Synvisc.
- As with any invasive joint procedure, it is recommended that the patient avoid any strenuous activities or prolonged weight-bearing activities such as jogging or tennis following the intra-articular injection.
- The safety and effectiveness of repeat treatment cycles of Synvisc have not been established.
- The packaging of this product contains dry natural rubber latex.

Use in Specific Populations

- **Pregnancy:** The safety and effectiveness of Synvisc have not been established in pregnant women.
- **Nursing mothers:** It is not known if Synvisc is excreted in human milk. The safety and effectiveness of Synvisc have not been established in lactating women.
- The safety and effectiveness of Synvisc have not been established in children.

ADVERSE EVENTS

A total of 511 patients (559 knees) received 1771 injections in seven clinical trials of Synvisc. There were 39 reports in 37 patients (2.2% of injections, 7.2% of patients) of knee pain and/or swelling after these injections. Ten patients (10 knees) were treated with arthrocentesis and removal of joint effusion. Two additional patients (two knees) received treatment with intra-articular steroids. Two patients (two knees) received NSAIDs. One of these patients also received arthrocentesis. One patient was treated with arthroscopy. The remaining patients with adverse events localized to the knee received no treatment or only analgesics.

Systemic adverse events each occurred in 10 (2.0%) of the Synvisc-treated patients. There was one case each of rash (thorax and back) and itching of the skin following Synvisc injections in these studies. These symptoms did not recur when these patients received additional Synvisc injections. The remaining generalized adverse events reported were calf cramps, hemorrhoid problems, ankle edema, muscle pain, tonsillitis with nausea, tachyarrhythmia, phlebitis with varicosities and low back sprain.

In three concurrently controlled clinical trials with a total of 112 patients who received Synvisc and 110 patients who received either saline or arthrocentesis, there were no statistically significant differences in the numbers or types of adverse events between the group of patients that received Synvisc and the group that received control treatments.

In clinical use in Canada (since 1992) and Sweden (since 1995), the most common adverse events reported have been pain, swelling, and/or effusion in the injected knees. Other adverse events reported were one case each of: generalized urticaria; recurring small hives; pain on one side of the body with nausea, anxiety and listlessness; facial flush with swelling of lips; nausea with dizziness; and shivering with headache, nausea, respiratory difficulties; and prickling in body which did not recur after subsequent Synvisc injections. No cases of anaphylaxis or anaphylactoid reactions have been reported. No deaths have been associated with the use of Synvisc. Intra-articular infections did not occur in any of the clinical trials, but have occurred in clinical use following Synvisc injections.

CLINICAL STUDIES

The safety and effectiveness of Synvisc was studied in patients ≥40 years old in the three concurrently controlled clinical trials referred to in the "Adverse Events" section. The three studies investigated a total of 136 women and 81

TABLE 1
DEMOGRAPHIC DATA[1]

	DEMOGRAPHIC VARIABLE			
	Age	Gender [N[2] (%)]		Duration of Osteoarthritis (years)
		M	F	
German Multicenter[3]				
Synvisc®	62.3	21 (45%)	26 (55%)	5.4
Saline	64.7	13 (25%)	39 (75%)	5.6
P (Synvisc/Saline)	0.3	0.04		0.9
German Single Center				
Synvisc	59.8	10 (71%)	4 (29%)	2.4
Saline	59.5	8 (53%)	7 (47%)	2.5
P (Synvisc/Saline)	0.9	0.3		1.0
U.S. Multicenter[4]				
Synvisc	62.9	17 (39%)	27 (61%)	8.9
Arthrocentesis	67.1	12 (29%)	30 (71%)	7.9
P (Synvisc/Arthrocentesis)	0.06	0.3		0.5

Footnotes:
1 Patients ≥40 years old and received the complete treatment course
2 N = number of patients
3 In addition, 1 male and 3 females were treated with Synvisc in one knee and saline in the other
4 In addition, 4 females were treated with Synvisc in one knee and arthrocentesis in the other

TABLE 2
CONCURRENT OSTEOARTHRITIS THERAPIES[1]

CONCURRENT MEDICATIONS[2]	TREATED KNEES			
	TOTAL	Synvisc	Control	p Synvisc/ Control
German Multicenter	N[3]=109	N=52	N=57	
Medications [N (%)][4]	27 (25%)	5 (10%)	22 (39%)	0.001
NSAIDS	17 (16%)	4 (8%)	13 (23%)	0.03
Acetaminophen	7 (6%)	1 (2%)	6 (11%)	0.07
Other medications[5]	3 (3%)	3 (5%)	0 (0%)	0.09
German Single Center[6]	N=29	N=14	N=15	
Any concurrent medication [N (%)]	NA[7]	NA	NA	NA
U.S. Multicenter[8]	N=103	N=51	N=52	
Acetaminophen [N (%)]	100 (97%)	50 (98%)	50 (96%)	0.6

Footnotes:
1 Patients ≥40 years old and received the complete treatment course
2 Individual patients may be represented by more than one therapy
3 N=number of knees
4 Number and percentage of subjects
5 Medications not approved in the U.S.
6 No concurrent therapies were recorded
7 Data not collected
8 Only acetaminophen was allowed

men. The demographics of trial participants were comparable across treatment groups with regard to age, gender, and duration of osteoarthritis, except that there were a significantly greater (p=0.04) number of men in the Synvisc group and women in the control group in one study (see Table 1).
[See table 1 above]

One study was a multicenter study, conducted at four sites, in Germany. This was a randomized, double-blind prospective clinical trial with two treatment groups. The study compared the safety and effectiveness of three weekly intra-articular injections of Synvisc and of physiological saline in 103 subjects (109 knees) with osteoarthritis of the knee.

A significantly greater number of saline-treated patients took concurrent osteoarthritis medications than did patients treated with Synvisc (See Table 2). While both the Synvisc and the saline-treated groups improved significantly as compared to baseline in all effectiveness measures, the Synvisc group showed a significantly greater improvement in all outcome measures than did the saline-treated patients over a twelve-week period (See Table 3).
[See table 2 above]

A second study conducted at a single-center in Germany was a concurrently controlled, randomized, double-blind prospective clinical trial with two treatment groups. This study compared the safety and effectiveness over a 12-week period of three weekly intra-articular injections of Synvisc and of physiological saline in 29 subjects (29 knees) with osteoarthritis of the knee. The results of the study were similar to those in the German multicenter study, except that the significance levels in most comparisons were smaller (See Tables 3A and 3B).

A third study was a prospective, concurrently controlled, randomized, double-blinded multicenter study conducted in 90 subjects (103 knees) at five U.S. sites. The study compared the safety and effectiveness of three weekly intra-articular injections of Synvisc and of three weekly arthrocenteses in subjects with osteoarthritis of the knee over a four-week period after the first injection or arthrocentesis. Both the Synvisc- and the arthrocentesis-treated groups improved significantly as compared to baseline in all effectiveness measures. However, there were no significant differences between the Synvisc-treated and arthrocentesis-treated patients at any time during the four-week evaluation period (See Tables 3A and 3B).
[See tables 3A & 3B at top of next page]

Covariate analyses with the covariates of center, presence or absence of previous treatments, baseline levels of outcome measures, age, gender, body mass, effusion, baseline X-ray score, duration of osteoarthritis, treatment of contralateral knee, and presence or absence of concurrent therapies, did not reveal any factors that significantly affected the results of any of the three studies.

The German studies and the U.S. study differed in several respects, including inclusion of patients with effusions, length of no treatment period prior to Synvisc injection, nature of control treatment, final evaluation time, mean duration of disease, mean weight, prior treatments for OA, and pain and X-ray inclusion criteria. Thus, German and the U.S. studies, which gave different results, investigated different patient populations and compared Synvisc with different control treatments.

Although success criteria for safety were not specified in any of the three studies, adverse events were enumerated in each study. These events are included in the "Adverse Events" section.

DETAILED DEVICE DESCRIPTION

Synvisc contains hylan A (average molecular weight 6,000,000) and hylan B hydrated gel in a buffered physiological sodium chloride solution, pH 7.2. Synvisc has an

TABLE 3A
EFFECTIVENESS OF WEIGHT-BEARING PAIN[1]
EVALUATED BY PATIENTS

	Baseline	Improvement (Change from Baseline)					
Week	0	1	2	3	4	8	12
German Multicenter							
Synvisc-treated							
Mean[2]	69.7	12.0	26.5	37.9	NA[5]	45.9	46.5
P[3]		0.0001	0.0001	0.0001		0.0001	0.0001
Saline-treated							
Mean	75.1	9.0	17.0	23.0	NA	16.8	16.4
P[3]		0.0001	0.0001	0.0001		0.0001	0.0002
P[4]	0.1	0.3	0.01	0.0008	NA	<0.0001	<0.0001
German Single Center							
Synvisc-treated							
Mean	65.2	10.6	31.8	43.9	NA	51.7	53.5
P[3]		0.02	0.0001	0.0001		0.0001	0.0001
Saline-treated							
Mean	69.8	5.4	19.3	25.4	NA	24.4	26.8
P[3]		0.01	0.0001	0.0001		0.0001	0.0001
P[4]	0.4	0.2	0.03	0.01	NA	0.0001	0.0001
U.S. Multicenter							
Synvisc-treated							
Mean	67.3	12.9	18.9	NA	21.3	NA	NA
P[3]		0.0002	0.0001		0.0001		
Saline-treated							
Mean	69.4	9.4	21.2	NA	19.1	NA	NA
P[3]		0.01	0.0001		0.0002		
P[4]	0.6	0.5	0.7	NA	0.7	NA	NA

Footnotes:
[1] Patients ≥40 years old and received the complete treatment course
[2] Mean of assessments on VAS of 0 to 100 mm
[3] Significance from baseline
[4] Significance between Synvisc and control
[5] NA =no measurement taken

TABLE 3B
EFFECTIVENESS OF NIGHT PAIN[1]
EVALUATED BY PATIENTS

	Baseline	Improvement (Change from Baseline)					
Week	0	1	2	3	4	8	12
German Multicenter							
Synvisc-treated							
Mean[2]	41.6	9.2	20.0	26.4	NA[5]	28.3	29.8
P[3]		0.0001	0.0001	0.0001		0.0001	0.0001
Saline-treated							
Mean	45.7	9.5	15.2	21.2	NA	18.4	17.3
P[3]		0.0001	0.0001	0.0001		0.0001	0.0001
P[4]	0.5	0.9	0.2	0.3	NA	0.05	0.02
German Single Center							
Synvisc-treated							
Mean	31.8	8.4	17.7	24.8	NA	28.9	29.5
P[3]		0.04	0.005	0.004		0.005	0.005
Saline-treated							
Mean	33.3	4.5	13.1	16.1	NA	16.1	17.9
P[3]		0.1	0.001	0.0007		0.0001	0.0001
P[4]	0.9	0.4	0.4	0.3	NA	0.1	0.2
U.S. Multicenter							
Synvisc-treated							
Mean	61.0	19.0	17.9	NA	22.8	NA	NA
P[3]		0.0001	0.0001		0.0001		
Saline-treated							
Mean	76.0	23.3	36.3	NA	29.8	NA	NA
P[3]		0.0001	0.0001		0.0001		
P[4]	0.002	0.5	0.004	NA	0.3	NA	NA

Footnotes:
[1] Patients ≥40 years old and received the complete treatment course
[2] Mean of assessments on VAS of 0 to 100 mm
[3] Significance from baseline
[4] Significance between Synvisc and control
[5] NA =no measurement taken

elasticity (storage modulus G′) at 2.5 Hz of 111 ± 13 Pascals (Pa) and a viscosity (loss modulus G″) of 25 ± 2 Pa (elasticity and viscosity of knee synovial fluid of 18–27 year old humans measured with a comparable method at 2.5 Hz: G′ = 117 ± 13 Pa; G″ = 45 ± 8 Pa.)

Each syringe of Synvisc contains:

Hylan polymers (hylan A + hylan B)	16 mg
Sodium chloride	17 mg
Disodium hydrogen phosphate	0.32 mg
Sodium dihydrogen phosphate monohydrate	0.08 mg
Water for injection	q.s. to 2.0 mL

HOW SUPPLIED

Synvisc® is supplied in a 2.25 mL glass syringe containing 2 mL Synvisc.

Product Number: 0008-9149-02 3 disposable syringes

The contents of the syringe are sterile and nonpyrogenic.

DIRECTIONS FOR USE

Synvisc is administered by intra-articular injection once a week (one week apart) for a total of three injections.

Precaution: Do not use Synvisc if the package has been opened or damaged. Store in original packaging (protected from light) at room temperature below 86°F (30°C). DO NOT FREEZE.

Precaution: Strict aseptic administration technique must be followed.

Precaution: Do not concomitantly use disinfectants containing quaternary ammonium salts for skin preparation because hyaluronan can precipitate in their presence.

Precaution: Remove synovial fluid or effusion, if present, before injecting Synvisc.

Do not use the same syringe for removing synovial fluid and for injecting Synvisc, but the same needle should be used.

Take particular care to remove the tip cap of the syringe and needle aseptically.

Inject Synvisc into the knee joint through an 18 to 22 gauge needle.

Do not inject anesthetics or any other medications intra-articularly into the knee while administering Synvisc therapy. This may dilute Synvisc and affect its safety and effectiveness.

Precaution: The syringe containing Synvisc is intended for single use. The contents of the syringe must be used immediately after the syringe has been removed from its packaging. Inject the full 2 mL in one knee only. If treatment is bilateral, a separate syringe must be used for each knee. Discard any unused Synvisc.

DISTRIBUTED BY:
Wyeth Laboratories Inc.
A Wyeth-Ayerst Company
Philadelphia, Pennsylvania 19101
Telephone: 1-800-99-WYETH
Fax: (610) 964-5999

DEVELOPED BY:
Biomatrix, Inc.
65 Railroad Avenue
Ridgefield, New Jersey 07657
Telephone: (201) 945-9550
Fax: (201) 945-0363

MANUFACTURED BY:
Biomatrix Medical Canada Inc.
275, avenue Labrosse
Pointe-Claire, Québec
Canada H9R 1A3

Covered by U.S. patents #4,636,524, #4,713,448, #5,099,013, #5,143,724.

Synvisc is a registered trademark of Biomatrix, Inc.

REFERENCE

Scale D, Wobig M, and Wolpert W: Viscosupplementation of osteoarthritic knees with hylan: a treatment schedule study. Curr Ther Res; 55:220-232, 1994.

CI 5014-3 Revised August 31, 1998

TRECATOR®-SC ℞

[trěk " ă ' tōre]
(ethionamide tablets, USP)
Sugar-Coated Tablets

DESCRIPTION

Trecator-SC (ethionamide tablets, USP) is used in the treatment of tuberculosis. The chemical name for ethionamide is 2-ethylthioisonicotinamide with the following structural formula:

N, C_2H_5, $S{=}C{-}NH_2$

Ethionamide is a yellow crystalline, nonhygroscopic compound with a faint to moderate sulfide odor and a melting point of 162°C. It is practically insoluble in water and ether, but soluble in methanol and ethanol. It has a partition coefficient (octanol/water) Log P value of 0.3699. Trecator-SC tablets contain 250 mg of ethionamide. The inactive ingredients present are lactose, methylcellulose, magnesium stearate, polacrilin potassium, pharmaceutical glaze, talc, gelatin, acacia, sucrose, calcium carbonate, confectioners sugar, FD&C Yellow #6, povidone, sodium benzoate, titanium dioxide, white wax, and carnauba wax.

CLINICAL PHARMACOLOGY

Ethionamide is essentially completely absorbed following oral administration and is not subjected to any appreciable first pass metabolism.[1] Following a single 250 mg oral dose of ethionamide in healthy volunteers, peak plasma concentrations of about 2 µg/mL were attained at 2 hours in most cases. Normal serum concentrations of 1 to 5 µg/mL are usually seen 2 hours following doses of 250 mg to 500 mg.[2] These concentrations approximate the therapeutic range for this drug when the therapeutic range is defined by those serum concentrations associated with a high probability of success and a low probability of dose-related toxicity. The drug is approximately 30 percent bound to plasma proteins. Trecator-SC is rapidly and widely distributed into body tissues and fluids, with concentrations in plasma and various organs being approximately equal. Significant concentrations also are present in cerebrospinal fluid.

Ethionamide is extensively metabolized to active and inactive metabolites with less than 1% excreted as the free form in urine. Metabolism is presumed to occur in the liver and thus far 6 metabolites have been isolated: 2-ethylisonicotinamide, carbamoyl-dihydropyridine, thiocarbamoyl-dihy-

Continued on next page

Trecator-SC—Cont.

dropyridine, S-oxocarbamoyl dihydropyridine, 2-ethylthio-iso-nicotinamide, and ethionamide sulphoxide. The sulphoxide metabolite has been demonstrated to have antimicrobial activity against *Mycobacterium tuberculosis*. Trecator-SC has a plasma elimination half-life of approximately 2 hours after oral dosing.

Mechanism of Action

Ethionamide may be bacteriostatic or bactericidal in action, depending on the concentration of the drug attained at the site of infection and the susceptibility of the infecting organism. The exact mechanism of action of ethionamide has not been full elucidated, but the drug appears to inhibit peptide synthesis in susceptible organisms.

Microbiology

In Vitro Activity

Ethionamide exhibits bacteriostatic activity against extracellular and intracellular *Mycobacterium tuberculosis* organisms. The development of ethionamide resistant *M. tuberculosis* isolates can be obtained by repeated subculturing in liquid or on solid media containing increasing concentrations of ethionamide. Multi-drug resistant strains of *M. tuberculosis* may have acquired resistance to both isoniazid and ethionamide. However, the majority of *M. tuberculosis* isolates that are resistant to one are usually susceptible to the other. There is no evidence of cross-resistance between ethionamide and para-aminosalicylic acid (PAS), streptomycin, or cycloserine. However, limited data suggest that cross-resistance may exist between ethionamide and thiosemicarbazones (i.e., thiacetazone) as well as isoniazid.

In Vivo Activity

Ethionamide administered orally initially decreased the number of culturable *Mycobacterium tuberculosis* organisms from the lungs of H37Rv infected mice. Drug resistance developed with continued ethionamide monotherapy, but did not occur when mice received ethionamide in combination with streptomycin or isoniazid.

SUSCEPTIBILITY TESTING

Ethionamide susceptibility testing should only be performed by qualified or reference laboratories.

Two standardized *in vitro* susceptibility methods are available for testing ethionamide against *M. tuberculosis* organisms. The modified proportion method (CDC or NCCLS M24-P) utilizes Middlebrook and Cohn 7H10 agar medium impregnated with ethionamide at a final concentration of 5.0 µg/mL. After 2 to 3 weeks of incubation, MIC_{99} values are calculated by comparing the quantity of organisms growing in the medium containing drug to the control cultures. Mycobacterial growth in the presence of drug, of at least 1% of the growth in the control culture, indicates resistance.

The radiometric broth method employs the BACTEC 460 machine to compare the growth index from untreated control cultures to cultures grown in the presence of 5.0 µg/mL of ethionamide. Strict adherence to the manufacturer's instructions for sample processing and data interpretation is required for this assay.

Susceptibility test results obtained by these two different methods cannot be compared unless equivalent drug concentrations are evaluated.

The clinical relevance of *in vitro* susceptibility test results for mycobacterial species other than *M. tuberculosis* using either the radiometric or the proportion method has not been determined.

INDICATIONS AND USAGE

Trecator-SC (ethionamide) is primarily indicated for the treatment of active tuberculosis in patients with *M. tuberculosis* resistant to isoniazid or rifampin, or when there is intolerance on the part of the patient to other drugs. Its use alone in the treatment of tuberculosis results in the rapid development of resistance. It is essential, therefore, to give a suitable companion drug or drugs, the choice being based on the results of susceptibility tests. If the susceptibility tests indicate that the patient's organism is resistant to one of the first-line antituberculosis drugs (i.e., isoniazid or rifampin) yet susceptible to ethionamide, ethionamide should be accompanied by at least one drug to which the *M. tuberculosis* isolate is known to be susceptible.[6] If the tuberculosis is resistant to both isoniazid and rifampin, yet susceptible to ethionamide, ethionamide should be accompanied by at least two other drugs to which the *M. tuberculosis* isolate is known to be susceptible.[6]

Patient nonadherence to prescribed treatment can result in treatment failure and in the development of drug-resistant tuberculosis, which can be life-threatening and lead to other serious health risks. It is, therefore, essential that patients adhere to the drug regimen for the full duration of treatment. Directly observed therapy is recommended for all patients receiving treatment for tuberculosis. Patients in whom drug-resistant *M. tuberculosis* organisms are isolated should be managed in consultation with an expert in the treatment of drug-resistant tuberculosis.

CONTRAINDICATIONS

Ethionamide is contraindicated in patients with severe hepatic impairment and in patients who are hypersensitive to the drug.

WARNINGS

The use of Trecator-SC (ethionamide) alone in the treatment of tuberculosis results in rapid development of resistance. It is essential, therefore, to give a suitable companion drug or drugs, the choice being based on the results of susceptibility testing. However, therapy may be initiated prior to receiving the results of susceptibility tests as deemed appropriate by the physician. Ethionamide should be administered with at least one, sometimes two, other drugs to which the organism is known to be susceptible (see **INDICATIONS AND USAGE**). Drugs which have been used as companion agents are rifampin, ethambutol, pyrazinamide, cycloserine, kanamycin, streptomycin, and isoniazid. The usual warnings, precautions, and dosage regimens for these companion drugs should be observed.

Patient compliance is essential to the success of the antituberculosis therapy and to prevent the emergence of drug-resistant organisms. Therefore, patients should adhere to the drug regimen for the full duration of treatment. It is recommended that directly observed therapy be practiced when patients are receiving antituberculous medication. Additional consultation from experts in the treatment of drug-resistant tuberculosis is recommended when patients develop drug-resistant organisms.

PRECAUTIONS

General

Ethionamide may potentiate the adverse effects of the other anti-tuberculous drugs administered concomitantly (see **Drug Interactions**). Ophthalmologic examinations (including ophthalmoscopy) should be performed before and periodically during therapy with Trecator-SC.

Information For Patients

Patients should be advised to consult their physician should blurred vision or any loss of vision, with or without eye pain, occur during treatment.

Excessive ethanol ingestion should be avoided because a psychotic reaction has been reported.[3]

Laboratory Tests

Determination of serum transaminases (SGOT, SGPT) should be made prior to initiation of therapy and should be monitored monthly. If serum transaminases become elevated during therapy, ethionamide and the companion antituberculosis drug or drugs may be discontinued temporarily until the laboratory abnormalities have resolved. Ethionamide and the companion antituberculosis medication(s) then should be reintroduced sequentially to determine which drug (or drugs) is (are) responsible for the hepatotoxicity.

Blood glucose determinations should be made prior to and periodically throughout therapy with Trecator®-SC. Diabetic patients should be particularly alert for episodes of hypoglycemia.

Periodic monitoring of thyroid function tests is recommended as hypothyroidism, with or without goiter, has been reported with ethionamide therapy.

Drug Interactions

Trecator-SC has been found to temporarily raise serum concentrations of isoniazid. Trecator-SC may potentiate the adverse effects of other antituberculous drugs administered concomitantly. In particular, convulsions have been reported when ethionamide is administered with cycloserine and special care should be taken when the treatment regimen includes both of these drugs. Excessive ethanol ingestion should be avoided because a psychotic reaction has been reported.

Carcinogenesis, Mutagenesis, Impairment of Fertility

Teratogenic Effects: Pregnancy Category C

Animal studies conducted with Trecator (ethionamide) indicate that the drug has teratogenic potential in rabbits and rats. The doses used in these studies on a mg/kg basis were considerably in excess of those recommended in humans. There are no adequate and well-controlled studies in pregnant women. Because of these animal studies, however, it must be recommended that Trecator-SC (ethionamide) be withheld from women who are pregnant, or who are likely to become pregnant while under therapy, unless the prescribing physician considers it to be an essential part of the treatment.

Labor and Delivery

The effect of Trecator-SC on labor and delivery in pregnant women is unknown.

Nursing Mothers

Because no information is available on the excretion of ethionamide in human milk, Trecator-SC should be administered to nursing mothers only if the benefits outweigh the risks. Newborns who are breast-fed by mothers who are taking Trecator-SC should be monitored for adverse effects.

Pediatric Use

Due to the fact that pulmonary tuberculosis resistant to primary therapy is rarely found in neonates, infants, and children, investigations have been limited in these age groups. At present, the drug should not be used in pediatric patients under 12 years of age except when the organisms are definitely resistant to primary therapy and systemic dissemination of the disease, or other life-threatening complications of tuberculosis, is judged to be imminent.

ADVERSE REACTIONS

Gastrointestinal: The most common side effects of ethionamide are gastrointestinal disturbances including nausea, vomiting, diarrhea, abdominal pain, excessive salivation, metallic taste, stomatitis, anorexia and weight loss. Adverse gastrointestinal effects appear to be dose related, with approximately 50% of patients unable to tolerate 1 gm as a single dose. Gastrointestinal effects may be minimized by decreasing dosage, by changing the time of drug administration, or by the concurrent administration of an antiemetic agent.

Nervous System: Psychotic disturbances (including mental depression), drowsiness, dizziness, restlessness, headache, and postural hypotension have been reported with ethionamide. Rare reports of peripheral neuritis, optic neuritis, diplopia, blurred vision, and a pellagra-like syndrome also have been reported. Concurrent administration of pyridoxine has been recommended to prevent or relieve neurotoxic effects.

Hepatic: Transient increases in serum bilirubin, SGOT, SGPT; Hepatitis (with or without jaundice).

Other: Hypersensitivity reactions including rash, photosensitivity, thrombocytopenia and purpura have been reported rarely. Hypoglycemia, gynecomastia, impotence, and acne also have occurred. The management of patients with diabetes mellitus may become more difficult in those receiving ethionamide.

OVERDOSE

No specific information is available on the treatment of overdosage with Trecator-SC. If it should occur, standard procedures to evacuate gastric contents and to support vital functions should be employed.

DOSAGE AND ADMINISTRATION

In the treatment of tuberculosis, a major cause of the emergence of drug-resistant organisms, and thus treatment failure, is patient nonadherence to prescribed treatment. Treatment failure and drug-resistant organisms can be life-threatening and may result in other serious health risks. It is, therefore, important that patients adhere to the drug regimen for the full duration of treatment. Directly observed therapy is recommended when patients are receiving treatment for tuberculosis. Consultation with an expert in the treatment of drug-resistant tuberculosis is advised for patients in whom drug-resistant tuberculosis is suspected or likely. Ethionamide should be administered with at least one, sometimes two, other drugs to which the organism is known to be susceptible (see **INDICATIONS AND USAGE**).

Trecator-SC (ethionamide) is administered orally. The usual adult dose is 15 to 20 mg/kg/day, administered once daily or, if patient exhibits poor gastrointestinal tolerance, in divided doses with a maximum daily dosage of 1 gram. Thus far, there is insufficient evidence to indicate the lowest effective dosage levels. Therefore, in order to minimize the risk of resistance developing to the drug or to the companion drug, the principle of giving the highest tolerated dose (based on gastrointestinal intolerance) has been followed. In the adult this would seem to be between 0.5 and 1.0 gm daily, with an average of 0.75 gm daily.

The optimum dosage for pediatric patients has not been established. However, pediatric dosages of 10 to 20 mg/kg p.o. daily in 2 or 3 divided doses given after meals or 15 mg/kg/24 hrs as a single daily dose have been recommended.[4,5]

As with adults, ethionamide may be administered to pediatric patients once daily. It should be noted that in patients with concomitant tuberculosis and HIV infection, malabsorption syndrome may be present. Drug malabsorption should be suspected in patients who adhere to therapy, but who fail to respond appropriately. In such cases, consideration should be given to therapeutic drug monitoring (see **CLINICAL PHARMACOLOGY**).

The best times of administration are those which the individual patient finds most suitable in order to avoid or minimize gastrointestinal intolerance, which is usually at mealtimes. Every effort should be made to encourage patients to persevere with treatment when gastrointestinal side effects appear, since they may diminish in severity as treatment proceeds.

Initiation of therapy at a dose of 250 mg daily, with gradual titration to optimal doses as tolerated by the patient, also may be beneficial. A regimen of 250 mg daily for 1 or 2 days, followed by 250 mg twice daily for 1 or 2 days with a subsequent increase to 1 gm in 3 or 4 divided doses has been reported.[2]

Concomitant administration of pyridoxine is recommended. Duration of treatment should be based on individual clinical response. In general, continue therapy until bacteriological conversion has become permanent and maximal clinical improvement has occurred.

HOW SUPPLIED

Trecator®-SC (ethionamide tablets, USP) are supplied in bottles of 100 tablets as follows:

250 mg, NDC 0008-4130, reddish orange, sugar-coated tablet marked WYETH and 4130.

Store at room temperature, approximately 25°C (77°F). Dispense in a tight container.

REFERENCES

1) Jenner, P.J.: Plasma Levels of Ethionamide and Prothionamide in a Volunteer Following Intravenous and Oral Dosages, Lepr Rev 58:31–37, 1987.

2) Peloquin, C.A.: Pharmacology of the Antimycobacterial Drugs, Med Clin North Am 77(6):1253–1262, 1993.

3) Lansdown, F.S., Beran, M., Litwak, T.: Psychotoxic Reaction During Ethionamide Therapy, Am Rev Resp Dis 95(6):1053–1055, 1967.

4) Feigin, R.D., and Cherry, J.D.: Textbook of Pediatric Infectious Diseases, 2nd Edition. Philadelphia, W.B. Saunders Co., 1987, pp. 1371–1372.

5) Nelson, W.E., Behrman, R.E., Vaughan, V.C. (eds): Nelson Textbook of Pediatrics, 13th edition. Philadelphia, W.B. Saunders Co., 1987, p.636

6) Treatment of Tuberculosis and Tuberculosis Infection in Adults and Children, Am J Respiratory and Critical Care Medicine, 149:1359–1374. 1994.

Manufactured by:
Wyeth Laboratories
A Wyeth-Ayerst Company
Philadelphia, PA 19101
CI 5188-2 Revised May 9, 2000

TRIPHASIL®–21 ℞
[*trī-fă 'sĭl*]
Tablets
(levonorgestrel and ethinyl estradiol tablets—triphasic regimen)

Patients should be counseled that this product does not protect against HIV infection (AIDS) and other sexually transmitted diseases.

DESCRIPTION

Each Triphasil cycle of 21 tablets consists of three different drug phases as follows: Phase 1 comprised of 6 brown tablets, each containing 0.050 mg of levonorgestrel (d(-)-13 beta-ethyl -17- alpha-ethinyl -17- beta-hydroxygon -4- en -3-one), a totally synthetic progestogen, and 0.030 mg of ethinyl estradiol (19-nor-17α-pregna-1,3,5(10)-trien -20- yne-3,17-diol); phase 2 comprised of 5 white tablets, each containing 0.075 mg levonorgestrel and 0.040 mg ethinyl estradiol; and phase 3 comprised of 10 light-yellow tablets, each containing 0.125 mg levonorgestrel and 0.030 mg ethinyl estradiol. The inactive ingredients present are cellulose, iron oxides, lactose, magnesium stearate, polacrilin potassium, polyethylene glycol, titanium dioxide, and hydroxypropyl methylcellulose.

Levonorgestrel

Ethinyl Estradiol

CLINICAL PHARMACOLOGY

Combination oral contraceptives act by suppression of gonadotropins. Although the primary mechanism of this action is inhibition of ovulation, other alterations include changes in the cervical mucus (which increase the difficulty of sperm entry into the uterus) and the endometrium (which reduce the likelihood of implantation).

INDICATIONS AND USAGE

Oral contraceptives are indicated for the prevention of pregnancy in women who elect to use this product as a method of contraception.
Oral contraceptives are highly effective. Table I lists the typical accidental pregnancy rates for users of combination oral contraceptives and other methods of contraception. The efficacy of these contraceptive methods, except sterilization and the IUD, depends upon the reliability with which they are used. Correct and consistent use of methods can result in lower failure rates.

TABLE I: PERCENTAGE OF WOMEN EXPERIENCING AN UNINTENDED PREGNANCY DURING THE FIRST YEAR OF USE OF A CONTRACEPTIVE METHOD

Method	Perfect Use	Typical Use
Levonorgestrel implants	0.05	0.05
Male sterilization	0.1	0.15
Female sterilization	0.5	0.5
Depo-Provera® (injectable progestogen)	0.3	0.3
Oral contraceptives		5
Combined	0.1	NA
Progestin only	0.5	NA
IUD		
Progesterone	1.5	2.0
Copper T 380A	0.6	0.8
Condom (male) without spermicide	3	14
(Female) without spermicide	5	21
Cervical cap		
Nulliparous women	9	20
Parous women	26	40
Vaginal sponge		
Nulliparous women	9	20
Parous women	20	40
Diaphragm with spermicidal cream or jelly	6	20
Spermicides alone (foam, creams, jellies, and vaginal suppositories)	6	26
Periodic abstinence (all methods)	1-9*	25
Withdrawal	4	19
No contraception (planned pregnancy)	85	85

NA—not available
*Depending on method (calendar, ovulation, symptothermal, post-ovulation)
Adapted from Hatcher RA et al. *Contraceptive Technology: 17th Revised Edition.* NY, NY: Ardent Media, Inc., 1998.

CONTRAINDICATIONS

Oral contraceptives should not be used in women with any of the following conditions:
Thrombophlebitis or thromboembolic disorders.
A past history of deep-vein thrombophlebitis or thromboembolic disorders.
Cerebral-vascular or coronary-artery disease.
Known or suspected carcinoma of the breast.
Carcinoma of the endometrium or other known or suspected estrogen-dependent neoplasia.
Undiagnosed abnormal genital bleeding.
Cholestatic jaundice of pregnancy or jaundice with prior pill use.
Hepatic adenomas or carcinomas.
Known or suspected pregnancy.

WARNINGS

Cigarette smoking increases the risk of serious cardiovascular side effects from oral-contraceptive use. This risk increases with age and with heavy smoking (15 or more cigarettes per day) and is quite marked in women over 35 years of age. Women who use oral contraceptives should be strongly advised not to smoke.

The use of oral contraceptives is associated with increased risks of several serious conditions including myocardial infarction, thromboembolism, stroke, hepatic neoplasia, gallbladder disease, and hypertension, although the risk of serious morbidity or mortality is very small in healthy women without underlying factors. The risk of morbidity and mortality increases significantly in the presence of other underlying risk factors such as hypertension, hyperlipidemias, obesity, and diabetes.
Practitioners prescribing oral contraceptives should be familiar with the following information relating to these risks.
The information contained in this package insert is based principally on studies carried out in patients who used oral contraceptives with higher formulations of estrogens and progestogens than those in common use today. The effect of long-term use of the oral contraceptives with lower formulations of both estrogens and progestogens remains to be determined.
Throughout this labeling, epidemiological studies reported are of two types: retrospective or case control studies and prospective or cohort studies. Case control studies provide a measure of the relative risk of disease, namely, a ratio of the incidence of a disease among oral-contraceptive users to that among nonusers. The relative risk does not provide information on the actual clinical occurrence of a disease. Cohort studies provide a measure of attributable risk, which is the difference in the incidence of disease between oral-contraceptive users and nonusers. The attributable risk does provide information about the actual occurrence of a disease in the population. For further information, the reader is referred to a text on epidemiological methods.
1. THROMBOEMBOLIC DISORDERS AND OTHER VASCULAR PROBLEMS
a. *Myocardial infarction*
An increased risk of myocardial infarction has been attributed to oral-contraceptive use. This risk is primarily in smokers or women with other underlying risk factors for coronary-artery disease such as hypertension, hypercholesterolemia, morbid obesity, and diabetes. The relative risk of heart attack for current oral-contraceptive users has been estimated to be two to six. The risk is very low under the age of 30.
Smoking in combination with oral-contraceptive use has been shown to contribute substantially to the incidence of myocardial infarctions in women in their mid-thirties or older with smoking accounting for the majority of excess cases. Mortality rates associated with circulatory disease have been shown to increase substantially in smokers over the age of 35 and nonsmokers over the age of 40 (Table II) among women who use oral contraceptives.

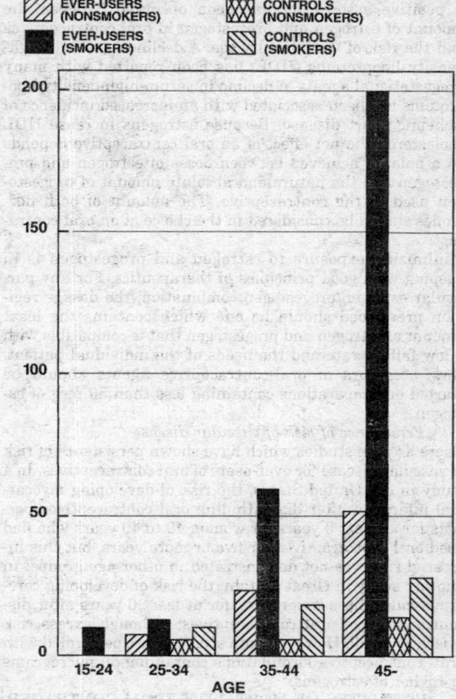

TABLE II. (Adapted from P.M. Layde and V. Beral, Lancet, *1*:541–546, 1981.)

Oral contraceptives may compound the effects of well-known risk factors, such as hypertension, diabetes, hyperlipidemias, age, and obesity. In particular, some progestogens are known to decrease HDL cholesterol and cause glucose intolerance, while estrogens may create a state of hyperinsulinism. Oral contraceptives have been shown to increase blood pressure among users (see section 9 in "Warnings"). Similar effects on risk factors have been associated with an increased risk of heart disease. Oral contraceptives must be used with caution in women with cardiovascular disease risk factors.
b. *Thromboembolism*
An increased risk of thromboembolic and thrombotic disease associated with the use of oral contraceptives is well established. Case control studies have found the relative risk of users compared to nonusers to be 3 for the first episode of superficial venous thrombosis, 4 to 11 for deep-vein thrombosis or pulmonary embolism, and 1.5 to 6 for women with predisposing conditions for venous thromboembolic disease. Cohort studies have shown the relative risk to be somewhat lower, about 3 for new cases and about 4.5 for new cases requiring hospitalization. The risk of thromboembolic disease due to oral contraceptives is not related to length of use and disappears after pill use is stopped.
A two- to four-fold increase in relative risk of postoperative thromboembolic complications has been reported with the use of oral contraceptives. The relative risk of venous thrombosis in women who have predisposing conditions is twice that of women without such medical conditions. If feasible, oral contraceptives should be discontinued at least four weeks prior to and for two weeks after elective surgery of a type associated with an increase in risk of thromboembolism and during and following prolonged immobilization. Since the immediate postpartum period is also associated with an increased risk of thromboembolism, oral contraceptives should be started no earlier than four to six weeks after delivery in women who elect not to breast-feed, or a midtrimester pregnancy termination.
c. *Cerebrovascular diseases*
Oral contraceptives have been shown to increase both the relative and attributable risks of cerebrovascular events (thrombotic and hemorrhagic strokes), although, in general, the risk is greatest among older (>35 years), hypertensive women who also smoke. Hypertension was found to be a risk factor for both users and nonusers, for both types of strokes, while smoking interacted to increase the risk for hemorrhagic strokes.
In a large study, the relative risk of thrombotic strokes has been shown to range from 3 for normotensive users to 14 for users with severe hypertension. The relative risk of hemor-

Continued on next page

Triphasil-21—Cont.

rhagic stroke is reported to be 1.2 for nonsmokers who used oral contraceptives, 2.6 for smokers who did not use oral contraceptives, 7.6 for smokers who used oral contraceptives, 1.8 for normotensive users, and 25.7 for users with severe hypertension. The attributable risk is also greater in older women.

d. *Dose-related risk of vascular disease from oral contraceptives*

A positive association has been observed between the amount of estrogen and progestogen in oral contraceptives and the risk of vascular disease. A decline in serum high-density lipoproteins (HDL) has been reported with many progestational agents. A decline in serum high-density lipoproteins has been associated with an increased incidence of ischemic heart disease. Because estrogens increase HDL cholesterol, the net effect of an oral contraceptive depends on a balance achieved between doses of estrogen and progestogen and the nature and absolute amount of progestogen used in the contraceptive. The amount of both hormones should be considered in the choice of an oral contraceptive.

Minimizing exposure to estrogen and progestogen is in keeping with good principles of therapeutics. For any particular estrogen/progestogen combination, the dosage regimen prescribed should be one which contains the least amount of estrogen and progestogen that is compatible with a low failure rate and the needs of the individual patient. New acceptors of oral-contraceptive agents should be started on preparations containing less than 50 mcg of estrogen.

e. *Persistence of risk of vascular disease*

There are two studies which have shown persistence of risk of vascular disease for ever-users of oral contraceptives. In a study in the United States, the risk of developing myocardial infarction after discontinuing oral contraceptives persists for at least 9 years for women 40 to 49 years who had used oral contraceptives for five or more years, but this increased risk was not demonstrated in other age groups. In another study in Great Britain, the risk of developing cerebrovascular disease persisted for at least 6 years after discontinuation of oral contraceptives, although excess risk was very small. However, both studies were performed with oral- contraceptive formulations containing 50 micrograms or higher of estrogens.

2. ESTIMATES OF MORTALITY FROM CONTRACEPTIVE USE

One study gathered data from a variety of sources which have estimated the mortality rate associated with different methods of contraception at different ages (Table III). These estimates include the combined risk of death associated with contraceptive methods plus the risk attributable to pregnancy in the event of method failure. Each method of contraception has its specific benefits and risks. The study concluded that with the exception of oral-contraceptive users 35 and older who smoke and 40 and older who do not smoke, mortality associated with all methods of birth control is less than that associated with childbirth. The observation of a possible increase in risk of mortality with age for oral-contraceptive users is based on data gathered in the 1970's—but not reported until 1983. However, current clinical practice involves the use of lower estrogen dose formulations combined with careful restriction of oral-contraceptive use to women who do not have the various risk factors listed in this labeling.

Because of these changes in practice and, also, because of some limited new data which suggest that the risk of cardiovascular disease with the use of oral contraceptives may now be less than previously observed, the Fertility and Maternal Health Drugs Advisory Committee was asked to review the topic in 1989. The Committee concluded that although cardiovascular-disease risks may be increased with oral-contraceptive use after age 40 in healthy nonsmoking women (even with the newer low-dose formulations), there are greater potential health risks associated with pregnancy in older women and with the alternative surgical and medical procedures which may be necessary if such women do not have access to effective and acceptable means of contraception.

Therefore, the Committee recommended that the benefits of oral-contraceptive use by healthy nonsmoking women over 40 may outweigh the possible risks. Of course, older women, as all women who take oral contraceptives, should take the lowest possible dose formulation that is effective.

[See table above]

3. CARCINOMA OF THE REPRODUCTIVE ORGANS

Numerous epidemiological studies have been performed on the incidence of breast, endometrial, ovarian, and cervical cancer in women using oral contraceptives. The overwhelming evidence in the literature suggests that the use of oral contraceptives is not associated with an increase in the risk of developing breast cancer, regardless of the age and parity of first use or with most of the marketed brands and doses. The Cancer and Steroid Hormone (CASH) study also showed no latent effect on the risk of breast cancer for at least a decade following long-term use. A few studies have shown a slightly increased relative risk of developing breast cancer, although the methodology of these studies, which included differences in examination of users and nonusers and differences in age at start of use, has been questioned. Some studies suggest that oral-contraceptive use has been associated with an increase in the risk of cervical intraepithelial neoplasia in some populations of women. However, there continues to be controversy about the extent to which such findings may be due to differences in sexual behavior and other factors.

In spite of many studies of the relationship between oral-contraceptive use and breast and cervical cancers, a cause-and-effect relationship has not been established.

TABLE III

ANNUAL NUMBER OF BIRTH-RELATED OR METHOD-RELATED DEATHS ASSOCIATED WITH CONTROL OF FERTILITY PER 100,000 NONSTERILE WOMEN, BY FERTILITY-CONTROL METHOD ACCORDING TO AGE

Method of control and outcome	15–19	20–24	25–29	30–34	35–39	40–44
No fertility-control methods*	7.0	7.4	9.1	14.8	25.7	28.2
Oral contraceptives nonsmoker**	0.3	0.5	0.9	1.9	13.8	31.6
Oral contraceptives smoker**	2.2	3.4	6.6	13.5	51.1	117.2
IUD**	0.8	0.8	1.0	1.0	1.4	1.4
Condom*	1.1	1.6	0.7	0.2	0.3	0.4
Diaphragm/ spermicide*	1.9	1.2	1.2	1.3	2.2	2.8
Periodic abstinence*	2.5	1.6	1.6	1.7	2.9	3.6

* Deaths are birth related

** Deaths are method related

Adapted from H.W. Ory, Family Planning Perspectives, *15*:57–63, 1983.

4. HEPATIC NEOPLASIA

Benign hepatic adenomas are associated with oral-contraceptive use, although the incidence of benign tumors is rare in the United States. Indirect calculations have estimated the attributable risk to be in the range of 3.3 cases/100,000 for users, a risk that increases after four or more years of use. Rupture of rare, benign, hepatic adenomas may cause death through intra-abdominal hemorrhage.

Studies from Britain have shown an increased risk of developing hepatocellular carcinoma in long-term (>8 years) oral-contraceptive users. However, these cancers are extremely rare in the U.S., and the attributable risk (the excess incidence) of liver cancers in oral-contraceptive users approaches less than one per million users.

5. OCULAR LESIONS

There have been clinical case reports of retinal thrombosis associated with the use of oral contraceptives. Oral contraceptives should be discontinued if there is unexplained partial or complete loss of vision; onset of proptosis or diplopia; papilledema; or retinal vascular lesions. Appropriate diagnostic and therapeutic measures should be undertaken immediately.

6. ORAL-CONTRACEPTIVE USE BEFORE OR DURING EARLY PREGNANCY

Extensive epidemiological studies have revealed no increased risk of birth defects in women who have used oral contraceptives prior to pregnancy. Studies also do not suggest a teratogenic effect, particularly insofar as cardiac anomalies and limb-reduction defects are concerned, when taken inadvertently during early pregnancy.

The administration of oral contraceptives to induce withdrawal bleeding should not be used as a test for pregnancy. Oral contraceptives should not be used during pregnancy to treat threatened or habitual abortion.

It is recommended that for any patient who has missed two consecutive periods, pregnancy should be ruled out before continuing oral-contraceptive use. If the patient has not adhered to the prescribed schedule, the possibility of pregnancy should be considered at the time of the first missed period. Oral-contraceptive use should be discontinued if pregnancy is confirmed.

7. GALLBLADDER DISEASE

Earlier studies have reported an increased lifetime relative risk of gallbladder surgery in users of oral contraceptives and estrogens. More recent studies, however, have shown that the relative risk of developing gallbladder disease among oral-contraceptive users may be minimal. The recent findings of minimal risk may be related to the use of oral-contraceptive formulations containing lower hormonal doses of estrogens and progestogens.

8. CARBOHYDRATE AND LIPID METABOLIC EFFECTS

Oral contraceptives have been shown to cause glucose intolerance in a significant percentage of users. Oral contraceptives containing greater than 75 micrograms of estrogens cause hyperinsulinism, while lower doses of estrogen cause less glucose intolerance. Progestogens increase insulin secretion and create insulin resistance, this effect varying with different progestational agents. However, in the nondiabetic woman, oral contraceptives appear to have no effect on fasting blood glucose. Because of these demonstrated effects, prediabetic and diabetic women should be carefully observed while taking oral contraceptives.

A small proportion of women will have persistent hypertriglyceridemia while on the pill. As discussed earlier (see "WARNINGS" 1a. and 1d.), changes in serum triglycerides and lipoprotein levels have been reported in oral-contraceptive users.

9. ELEVATED BLOOD PRESSURE

An increase in blood pressure has been reported in women taking oral contraceptives, and this increase is more likely in older oral-contraceptive users and with continued use. Data from the Royal College of General Practitioners and subsequent randomized trials have shown that the incidence of hypertension increases with increasing quantities of progestogens.

Women with a history of hypertension or hypertension-related diseases, or renal disease, should be encouraged to use another method of contraception. If women with hypertension elect to use oral contraceptives, they should be monitored closely, and if significant elevation of blood pressure occurs, oral contraceptives should be discontinued. For most women, elevated blood pressure will return to normal after stopping oral contraceptives, and there is no difference in the occurrence of hypertension between ever- and never- users.

10. HEADACHE

The onset or exacerbation of migraine or development of headache with a new pattern that is recurrent, persistent, or severe requires discontinuation of oral contraceptives and evaluation of the cause.

11. BLEEDING IRREGULARITIES

Breakthrough bleeding and spotting are sometimes encountered in patients on oral contraceptives, especially during the first three months of use. The type and dose of progestogen may be important. Nonhormonal causes should be considered and adequate diagnostic measures taken to rule out malignancy or pregnancy in the event of breakthrough bleeding, as in the case of any abnormal vaginal bleeding. If pathology has been excluded, time or a change to another formulation may solve the problem. In the event of amenorrhea, pregnancy should be ruled out.

Some women may encounter post-pill amenorrhea or oligomenorrhea, especially when such a condition was preexistent.

PRECAUTIONS

Patients should be counseled that this product does not protect against HIV infection (AIDS) and other sexually transmitted diseases.

1. PHYSICAL EXAMINATION AND FOLLOW-UP

A periodic history and physical examination is appropriate for all women, including women using oral contraceptives. The physical examination, however, may be deferred until after initiation of oral contraceptives if requested by the woman and judged appropriate by the clinician. The physical examination should include special reference to blood pressure, breasts, abdomen and pelvic organs, including cervical cytology, and relevant laboratory tests. In case of undiagnosed, persistent, or recurrent abnormal vaginal bleeding, appropriate measures should be conducted to rule out malignancy. Women with a strong family history of breast cancer or who have breast nodules should be monitored with particular care.

2. LIPID DISORDERS

Women who are being treated for hyperlipidemias should be followed closely if they elect to use oral contraceptives. Some progestogens may elevate LDL levels and may render the control of hyperlipidemias more difficult. (See "Warnings," 1d.)

3. LIVER FUNCTION

If jaundice develops in any woman receiving such drugs, the medication should be discontinued. Steroid hormones may be poorly metabolized in patients with impaired liver function.

4. FLUID RETENTION

Oral contraceptives may cause some degree of fluid retention. They should be prescribed with caution, and only with careful monitoring, in patients with conditions which might be aggravated by fluid retention.

5. EMOTIONAL DISORDERS

Patients becoming significantly depressed while taking oral contraceptives should stop the medication and use an alternate method of contraception in an attempt to determine whether the symptom is drug related.

Women with a history of depression should be carefully observed and the drug discontinued if depression recurs to a serious degree.

6. CONTACT LENSES

Contact-lens wearers who develop visual changes or changes in lens tolerance should be assessed by an ophthalmologist.

7. DRUG INTERACTIONS
Reduced efficacy and increased incidence of breakthrough bleeding and menstrual irregularities have been associated with concomitant use of rifampin. A similar association, though less marked, has been suggested with barbiturates, phenylbutazone, phenytoin sodium, and possibly with griseofulvin, ampicillin, and tetracyclines.
8. INTERACTIONS WITH LABORATORY TESTS
Certain endocrine- and liver-function tests and blood components may be affected by oral contraceptives:
a. Increased prothrombin and factors VII, VIII, IX, and X; decreased antithrombin 3; increased norepinephrine-induced platelet aggregability.
b. Increased thyroid-binding globulin (TBG) leading to increased circulating total thyroid hormone, as measured by protein-bound iodine (PBI), T4 by column or by radioimmunoassay. Free T3 resin uptake is decreased, reflecting the elevated TBG; free T4 concentration is unaltered.
c. Other binding proteins may be elevated in serum.
d. Sex-binding globulins are increased and result in elevated levels of total circulating sex steroids and corticoids; however, free or biologically active levels remain unchanged.
e. Triglycerides may be increased.
f. Glucose tolerance may be decreased.
g. Serum folate levels may be depressed by oral-contraceptive therapy. This may be of clinical significance if a woman becomes pregnant shortly after discontinuing oral contraceptives.
9. CARCINOGENESIS
See "Warnings" section.
10. PREGNANCY
Pregnancy Category X. See "Contraindications" and "Warnings" sections.
11. NURSING MOTHERS
Small amounts of oral-contraceptive steroids have been identified in the milk of nursing mothers, and a few adverse effects on the child have been reported, including jaundice and breast enlargement. In addition, oral contraceptives given in the postpartum period may interfere with lactation by decreasing the quantity and quality of breast milk. If possible, the nursing mother should be advised not to use oral contraceptives but to use other forms of contraception until she has completely weaned her child.
12. PEDIATRIC USE
Safety and efficacy of Triphasil® have been established in women of reproductive age. Safety and efficacy are expected to be the same for postpubertal adolescents under the age of 16 and users 16 and older. Use of this product before menarche is not indicated.

INFORMATION FOR THE PATIENT
See Patient Labeling Printed Below.

ADVERSE REACTIONS

An increased risk of the following serious adverse reactions has been associated with the use of oral contraceptives (see "Warnings" section):
Thrombophlebitis.
Arterial thromboembolism.
Pulmonary embolism.
Myocardial infarction.
Cerebral hemorrhage.
Cerebral thrombosis.
Hypertension.
Gallbladder disease.
Hepatic adenomas or benign liver tumors.
There is evidence of an association between the following conditions and the use of oral contraceptives, although additional confirmatory studies are needed:
Mesenteric thrombosis.
Retinal thrombosis.
The following adverse reactions have been reported in patients receiving oral contraceptives and are believed to be drug-related:
Nausea
Vomiting
Gastrointestinal symptoms (such as abdominal cramps and bloating).
Breakthrough bleeding.
Spotting.
Change in menstrual flow.
Amenorrhea.
Temporary infertility after discontinuation of treatment.
Edema.
Melasma which may persist.
Breast changes: tenderness, enlargement, secretion.
Change in weight (increase or decrease).
Change in cervical erosion and cervical secretion.
Diminution in lactation when given immediately postpartum.
Cholestatic jaundice.
Migraine.
Rash (allergic).
Mental depression.
Reduced tolerance to carbohydrates.
Vaginal candidiasis.
Change in corneal curvature (steepening).
Intolerance to contact lenses.
The following adverse reactions have been reported in users of oral contraceptives, and the association has been neither confirmed nor refuted:
Congenital anomalies.
Premenstrual syndrome.
Cataracts.
Optic neuritis.
Changes in appetite.
Cystitis-like syndrome.
Headache.
Nervousness.
Dizziness.
Hirsutism.
Loss of scalp hair.
Erythema multiforme.
Erythema nodosum.
Hemorrhagic eruption.
Vaginitis.
Porphyria.
Impaired renal function.
Hemolytic uremic syndrome.
Budd-Chiari syndrome.
Acne.
Changes in libido.
Colitis.
Sickle-cell disease.
Cerebral-vascular disease with mitral valve prolapse.
Lupus-like syndromes.

OVERDOSAGE

Serious ill effects have not been reported following acute ingestion of large doses of oral contraceptives by young children. Overdosage may cause nausea, and withdrawal bleeding may occur in females.

NONCONTRACEPTIVE HEALTH BENEFITS

The following noncontraceptive health benefits related to the use of oral contraceptives are supported by epidemiological studies which largely utilized oral-contraceptive formulations containing doses exceeding 0.035 mg of ethinyl estradiol or 0.05 mg of mestranol.
Effects on menses:
Increased menstrual cycle regularity.
Decreased blood loss and decreased incidence of iron-deficiency anemia.
Decreased incidence of dysmenorrhea.
Effects related to inhibition of ovulation:
Decreased incidence of functional ovarian cysts.
Decreased incidence of ectopic pregnancies.
Effects from long-term use:
Decreased incidence of fibroadenomas and fibrocystic disease of the breast.
Decreased incidence of acute pelvic inflammatory disease.
Decreased incidence of endometrial cancer.
Decreased incidence of ovarian cancer.

DOSAGE AND ADMINISTRATION

To achieve maximum contraceptive effectiveness, Triphasil-21 Tablets (levonorgestrel and ethinyl estradiol tablets—triphasic regimen) must be taken exactly as directed and at intervals not exceeding 24 hours.
Triphasil-21 Tablets are a three-phase preparation. The dosage of Triphasil-21 Tablets is one tablet daily for 21 consecutive days per menstrual cycle in the following order: 6 brown tablets (phase 1), followed by 5 white tablets (phase 2), and then followed by the last 10 light-yellow tablets (phase 3), according to the prescribed schedule. Tablets are then discontinued for 7 days (three weeks on, one week off).
It is recommended that Triphasil-21 Tablets be taken at the same time each day, preferably after the evening meal or at bedtime. During the first cycle of medication, the patient should be instructed to take one Triphasil-21 Tablet daily in the order of 6 brown, 5 white and, finally, 10 light-yellow tablets for twenty-one (21) consecutive days, beginning on day one (1) of her menstrual cycle. (The first day of menstruation is day one.) The tablets are then discontinued for one week (7 days). Withdrawal bleeding usually occurs within 3 days following discontinuation of Triphasil-21 Tablets. (If Triphasil-21 Tablets are first taken later than the first day of the first menstrual cycle of medication or postpartum, contraceptive reliance should not be placed on Triphasil-21 Tablets until after the first 7 consecutive days of administration. The possibility of ovulation and conception prior to initiation of medication should be considered.)
When switching from another oral contraceptive, Triphasil-21 Tablets should be started on the first day of bleeding following the last active tablet taken of the previous oral contraceptive.
The patient begins her next and all subsequent 21-day courses of Triphasil-21 Tablets on the same day of the week that she began her first course, following the same schedule: 21 days on—7 days off. She begins taking her brown tablets on the 8th day after discontinuance regardless of whether or not a menstrual period has occurred or is still in progress. Any time the next cycle of Triphasil-21 Tablets is started later than the 8th day, the patient should be protected by another means of contraception until she has taken a tablet daily for seven consecutive days.
If spotting or breakthrough bleeding occurs, the patient is instructed to continue on the same regimen. This type of bleeding is usually transient and without significance; however, if the bleeding is persistent or prolonged, the patient is advised to consult her physician. Although the occurrence of pregnancy is highly unlikely if Triphasil-21 Tablets are taken according to directions, if withdrawal bleeding does not occur, the possibility of pregnancy must be considered. If the patient has not adhered to the prescribed schedule (missed one or more tablets or started taking them on a day later than she should have), the probability of pregnancy should be considered at the time of the first missed period and appropriate diagnostic measures taken before the medication is resumed. If the patient has adhered to the prescribed regimen and misses two consecutive periods, pregnancy should be ruled out before continuing the contraceptive regimen.
The risk of pregnancy increases with each tablet missed. For additional patient instructions regarding missed pills, see the "WHAT TO DO IF YOU MISS PILLS" section in the DETAILED PATIENT LABELING below. If breakthrough bleeding occurs following missed tablets, it will usually be transient and of no consequence.
In the nonlactating mother, Triphasil-21 may be initiated postpartum, for contraception. When the tablets are administered in the postpartum period, the increased risk of thromboembolic disease associated with the postpartum period must be considered (See "Contraindications", "Warnings", and "Precautions" concerning thromboembolic disease). It is to be noted that early resumption of ovulation may occur if Parlodel® (bromocriptine mesylate) has been used for the prevention of lactation.

HOW SUPPLIED

Triphasil®-21 Tablets (levonorgestrel and ethinyl estradiol tablets—triphasic regimen) NDC 0008-2535, are available in packages of 3 dial dispensers. Each cycle contains 21 round, coated tablets as follows:
NDC 0008-0641, six brown tablets marked "W" and "641", each containing 0.050 mg levonorgestrel and 0.030 mg ethinyl estradiol;
NDC 0008-0642, five white to off-white tablets marked "W" and "642", each containing 0.075 mg levonorgestrel and 0.040 mg ethinyl estradiol; and
NDC 0008-0643, ten light-yellow tablets marked "W" and "643", each containing 0.125 mg levonorgestrel and 0.030 mg ethinyl estradiol.
References available upon request.

Brief Summary Patient Package Insert

This product (like all oral contraceptives) is intended to prevent pregnancy. It does not protect against HIV infection (AIDS) and other sexually transmitted diseases.
Oral contraceptives, also known as "birth-control pills" or "the pill," are taken to prevent pregnancy, and when taken correctly, have a failure rate of less than 1.0% per year when used without missing any pills. The typical failure rate of large numbers of pill users is less than 3.0% per year when women who miss pills are included. For most women oral contraceptives are also free of serious or unpleasant side effects. However, forgetting to take pills considerably increases the chances of pregnancy.
For the majority of women, oral contraceptives can be taken safely. But there are some women who are at high risk of developing certain serious diseases that can be life-threatening or may cause temporary or permanent disability or death. The risks associated with taking oral contraceptives increase significantly if you:
- smoke.
- have high blood pressure, diabetes, high cholesterol.
- have or have had clotting disorders, heart attack, stroke, angina pectoris, cancer of the breast or sex organs, jaundice or malignant or benign liver tumors.

You should not take the pill if you suspect you are pregnant or have unexplained vaginal bleeding.

Cigarette smoking increases the risk of serious adverse effects on the heart and blood vessels from oral-contraceptive use. This risk increases with age and with heavy smoking (15 or more cigarettes per day) and is quite marked in women over 35 years of age. Women who use oral contraceptives should not smoke.

Most side effects of the pill are not serious. The most common such effects are nausea, vomiting, bleeding between menstrual periods, weight gain, breast tenderness, and difficulty wearing contact lenses. These side effects, especially nausea and vomiting, may subside within the first three months of use.
The serious side effects of the pill occur very infrequently, especially if you are in good health and do not smoke. However, you should know that the following medical conditions have been associated with or made worse by the pill:
1. Blood clots in the legs (thrombophlebitis), lungs (pulmonary embolism), stoppage or rupture of a blood vessel in the brain (stroke), blockage of blood vessels in the heart (heart attack and angina pectoris) or other organs of the body. As mentioned above, smoking increases the risk of heart attacks and strokes and subsequent serious medical consequences.
2. Liver tumors, which may rupture and cause severe bleeding. A possible but not definite association has been found with the pill and liver cancer. However, liver cancers are extremely rare. The chance of developing liver cancer from using the pill is thus even rarer.
3. High blood pressure, although blood pressure usually returns to normal when the pill is stopped.

The symptoms associated with these serious side effects are discussed in the detailed leaflet given to you with your supply of pills. Notify your doctor or health-care provider if you notice any unusual physical disturbances while taking the pill. In addition, drugs such as rifampin, as well as some anti-convulsants and some antibiotics, may decrease oral-contraceptive effectiveness.

Continued on next page

Triphasil-21—Cont.

Studies to date of women taking the pill have not shown an increase in the incidence of cancer of the breast or cervix. There is, however, insufficient evidence to rule out the possibility that pills may cause such cancers.
Taking the pill provides some important noncontraceptive benefits. These include less painful menstruation, less menstrual blood loss and anemia, fewer pelvic infections, and fewer cancers of the ovary and the lining of the uterus.
Be sure to discuss any medical condition you may have with your health care provider. Your health-care provider will take a medical and family history before prescribing oral contraceptives and will examine you. The physical examination may be delayed to another time if you request it and the health-care provider believes that it is appropriate to postpone it. You should be reexamined at least once a year while taking oral contraceptives. The detailed patient information leaflet gives you further information which you should read and discuss with your health-care provider.

DETAILED PATIENT LABELING

This product (like all oral contraceptives) is intended to prevent pregnancy. It does not protect against HIV infection (AIDS) and other sexually transmitted diseases.

INTRODUCTION

Any woman who considers using oral contraceptives (the birth control pill or the pill) should understand the benefits and risks of using this form of birth control. This leaflet will give you much of the information you will need to make this decision and will also help you determine if you are at risk of developing any of the serious side effects of the pill. It will tell you how to use the pill properly so that it will be as effective as possible. However, this leaflet is not a replacement for a careful discussion between you and your health-care provider. You should discuss the information provided in this leaflet with him or her, both when you first start taking the pill and during your revisits. You should also follow your health-care provider's advice with regard to regular check-ups while you are on the pill.

EFFECTIVENESS OF ORAL CONTRACEPTIVES

Oral contraceptives or "birth-control pills" or "the pill" are used to prevent pregnancy and are more effective than other nonsurgical methods of birth control. When they are taken correctly, the chance of becoming pregnant is less than 1.0% when used perfectly, without missing any pills. Typical failure rates are actually 3.0% per year. The chance of becoming pregnant increases with each missed pill during the menstrual cycle.
In comparison, typical failure rates for other nonsurgical methods of birth control during the first year of use are as follows:

TABLE: PERCENTAGE OF WOMEN EXPERIENCING AN UNINTENDED PREGNANCY DURING THE FIRST YEAR OF USE OF A CONTRACEPTIVE METHOD

Method	Perfect Use	Typical Use
Levonorgestrel implants	0.05	0.05
Male sterilization	0.1	0.15
Female sterilization	0.5	0.5
Depo-Provera® (injectable progestogen)	0.3	0.3
Oral contraceptives		5
Combined	0.1	NA
Progestin only	0.5	NA
IUD		
Progesterone	1.5	2.0
Copper T 380A	0.6	0.8
Condom (male) without spermicide	3	14
(Female) without spermicide	5	21
Cervical cap		
Never given birth	9	20
Given birth	20	40
Vaginal Sponge		
Never given birth	9	20
Given birth	20	40
Diaphragm with spermicidal cream or jelly	6	20
Spermicides alone (foam, creams, jellies, and vaginal suppositories)	6	26
Periodic abstinence (all methods)	1-9*	25
Withdrawal	4	19
No contraception (planned pregnancy)	85	85

NA—not available
*Depending on method (calendar, ovulation, symptothermal, post-ovulation)
Adapted from Hatcher RA et al. *Contraceptive Technology: 17th Revised Edition.* NY, NY: Ardent Media, Inc., 1998

ANNUAL NUMBER OF BIRTH-RELATED OR METHOD-RELATED DEATHS ASSOCIATED WITH CONTROL OF FERTILITY PER 100,000 NONSTERILE WOMEN, BY FERTILITY-CONTROL METHOD ACCORDING TO AGE

Method of control and outcome	15–19	20–24	25–29	30–34	35–39	40–44
No fertility-control methods*	7.0	7.4	9.1	14.8	25.7	28.2
Oral contraceptives nonsmoker**	0.3	0.5	0.9	1.9	13.8	31.6
Oral contraceptives smoker**	2.2	3.4	6.6	13.5	51.1	117.2
IUD**	0.8	0.8	1.0	1.0	1.4	1.4
Condom*	1.1	1.6	0.7	0.2	0.3	0.4
Diaphragm/ spermicide*	1.9	1.2	1.2	1.3	2.2	2.8
Periodic abstinence*	2.5	1.6	1.6	1.7	2.9	3.6

* Deaths are birth related
** Deaths are method related

WHO SHOULD NOT TAKE ORAL CONTRACEPTIVES

Cigarette smoking increases the risk of serious adverse effects on the heart and blood vessels from oral-contraceptive use. This risk increases with age and with heavy smoking (15 or more cigarettes per day) and is quite marked in women over 35 years of age. Women who use oral contraceptives should not smoke.

Some women should not use the pill. For example, you should not take the pill if you are pregnant or think you may be pregnant. You should also not use the pill if you have had any of the following conditions:
- Heart attack or stroke.
- Blood clots in the legs (thrombophlebitis), lungs (pulmonary embolism), or eyes.
- Blood clots in the deep veins of your legs.
- Known or suspected breast cancer or cancer of the lining of the uterus, cervix, or vagina.
- Liver tumor (benign or cancerous).

Or, if you have any of the following:
- Chest pain (angina pectoris).
- Unexplained vaginal bleeding (until a diagnosis is reached by your doctor).
- Yellowing of the whites of the eyes or of the skin (jaundice) during pregnancy or during previous use of the pill.
- Known or suspected pregnancy.

Tell your health-care provider if you have ever had any of these conditions. Your health-care provider can recommend another method of birth control.

OTHER CONSIDERATIONS BEFORE TAKING ORAL CONTRACEPTIVES

Tell your health-care provider if you or any family member has ever had:
- Breast nodules, fibrocystic disease of the breast, an abnormal breast X-ray or mammogram.
- Diabetes.
- Elevated cholesterol or triglycerides.
- High blood pressure.
- Migraine or other headaches or epilepsy.
- Mental depression.
- Gallbladder, heart or kidney disease.
- History of scanty or irregular menstrual periods.

Women with any of these conditions should be checked often by their health-care provider if they choose to use oral contraceptives. Also, be sure to inform your doctor or health-care provider if you smoke or are on any medications.

RISKS OF TAKING ORAL CONTRACEPTIVES

1. *Risk of developing blood clots*

Blood clots and blockage of blood vessels are the most serious side effects of taking oral contraceptives and can be fatal. In particular, a clot in the legs can cause thrombophlebitis and a clot that travels to the lungs can cause a sudden blocking of the vessel carrying blood to the lungs. Rarely, clots occur in the blood vessels of the eye and may cause blindness, double vision, or impaired vision.
If you take oral contraceptives and need elective surgery, need to stay in bed for a prolonged illness, or have recently delivered a baby, you may be at risk of developing blood clots. You should consult your doctor about stopping oral contraceptives three to four weeks before surgery and not taking oral contraceptives for two weeks after surgery or during bed rest. You should also not take oral contraceptives soon after delivery of a baby or a midtrimester pregnancy termination. It is advisable to wait for at least four weeks after delivery if you are not breast-feeding. If you are breast-feeding, you should wait until you have weaned your child before using the pill. (See also the section on breast-feeding in "General Precautions".)

2. *Heart attacks and strokes*

Oral contraceptives may increase the tendency to develop strokes (stoppage or rupture of blood vessels in the brain) and angina pectoris and heart attacks (blockage of blood vessels in the heart). Any of these conditions can cause death or serious disability.
Smoking greatly increases the possibility of suffering heart attacks and strokes. Furthermore, smoking and the use of oral contraceptives greatly increase the chances of developing and dying of heart disease.

3. *Gallbladder disease*

Oral-contraceptive users probably have a greater risk than nonusers of having gallbladder disease, although this risk may be related to pills containing high doses of estrogens.

4. *Liver tumors*

In rare cases, oral contraceptives can cause benign but dangerous liver tumors. These benign liver tumors can rupture and cause fatal internal bleeding. In addition, a possible but not definite association has been found with the pill and liver cancers in two studies in which a few women who developed these very rare cancers were found to have used oral contraceptives for long periods. However, liver cancers are extremely rare. The chance of developing liver cancer from using the pill is thus even rarer.

5. *Cancer of the reproductive organs*

There is, at present, no confirmed evidence that oral contraceptives increase the risk of cancer of the reproductive organs in human studies. Several studies have found no overall increase in the risk of developing breast cancer. However, women who use oral contraceptives and have a strong family history of breast cancer or who have breast nodules or abnormal mammograms should be closely followed by their doctors.
Some studies have found an increase in the incidence of cancer of the cervix in women who use oral contraceptives. However, this finding may be related to factors other than the use of oral contraceptives.

ESTIMATED RISK OF DEATH FROM A BIRTH-CONTROL METHOD OR PREGNANCY

All methods of birth control and pregnancy are associated with a risk of developing certain diseases which may lead to disability or death. An estimate of the number of deaths associated with different methods of birth control and pregnancy has been calculated and is shown in the following table.
[See table above]
In the above table, the risk of death from any birth-control method is less than the risk of childbirth, except for oral-contraceptive users over the age of 35 who smoke and pill users over the age of 40 even if they do not smoke. It can be seen in the table that for women aged 15 to 39, the risk of death was highest with pregnancy (7 to 26 deaths per 100,000 women, depending on age). Among pill users who do not smoke, the risk of death was always lower than that associated with pregnancy for any age group, except for those women over the age of 40, when the risk increases to 32 deaths per 100,000 women, compared to 28 associated with pregnancy at that age. However, for pill users who smoke and are over the age of 35, the estimated number of deaths exceeds those for other methods of birth control. If a woman is over the age of 40 and smokes, her estimated risk of death is four times higher (117/100,000 women) than the estimated risk associated with pregnancy (28/100,000 women) in that age group.
The suggestion that women over 40 who don't smoke should not take oral contraceptives is based on information from older high-dose pills and on less-selective use of pills than is practiced today. An Advisory Committee of the FDA discussed this issue in 1989 and recommended that the benefits of oral-contraceptive use by healthy, nonsmoking women over 40 years of age may outweigh the possible risks. However, all women, especially older women, are cautioned to use the lowest-dose pill that is effective.

WARNING SIGNALS

If any of these adverse effects occur while you are taking oral contraceptives, call your doctor immediately:

- Sharp chest pain, coughing of blood, or sudden shortness of breath (indicating a possible clot in the lung).
- Pain in the calf (indicating a possible clot in the leg).
- Crushing chest pain or heaviness in the chest (indicating a possible heart attack).
- Sudden severe headache or vomiting, dizziness or fainting, disturbances of vision or speech, weakness, or numbness in an arm or leg (indicating a possible stroke).
- Sudden partial or complete loss of vision (indicating a possible clot in the eye).
- Breast lumps (indicating possible breast cancer or fibrocystic disease of the breast; ask your doctor or health care provider to show you how to examine your breasts).
- Severe pain or tenderness in the stomach area (indicating a possibly ruptured liver tumor).
- Difficulty in sleeping, weakness, lack of energy, fatigue, or change in mood (possibly indicating severe depression).
- Jaundice or a yellowing of the skin or eyeballs, accompanied frequently by fever, fatigue, loss of appetite, dark colored urine, or light-colored bowel movements (indicating possible liver problems).

SIDE EFFECTS OF ORAL CONTRACEPTIVES

1. *Vaginal bleeding*

Irregular vaginal bleeding or spotting may occur while you are taking the pills. Irregular bleeding may vary from slight staining between menstrual periods to breakthrough bleeding which is a flow much like a regular period. Irregular bleeding occurs most often during the first few months of oral-contraceptive use, but may also occur after you have been taking the pill for some time. Such bleeding may be temporary and usually does not indicate any serious problems. It is important to continue taking your pills on schedule. If the bleeding occurs in more than one cycle or lasts for more than a few days, talk to your doctor or health-care provider.

2. *Contact lenses*

If you wear contact lenses and notice a change in vision or an inability to wear your lenses, contact your doctor or health-care provider.

3. *Fluid retention*

Oral contraceptives may cause edema (fluid retention) with swelling of the fingers or ankles and may raise your blood pressure. If you experience fluid retention, contact your doctor or health-care provider.

4. *Melasma*

A spotty darkening of the skin is possible, particularly of the face.

5. *Other side effects*

Other side effects may include change in appetite, headache, nervousness, depression, dizziness, loss of scalp hair, rash, and vaginal infections.

If any of these side effects bother you, call your doctor or health-care provider.

GENERAL PRECAUTIONS

1. *Missed periods and use of oral contraceptives before or during early pregnancy*

There may be times when you may not menstruate regularly after you have completed taking a cycle of pills. If you have taken your pills regularly and miss one menstrual period, continue taking your pills for the next cycle but be sure to inform your health-care provider before doing so. If you have not taken the pills daily as instructed and missed a menstrual period, or if you missed two consecutive menstrual periods, you may be pregnant. Check with your health-care provider immediately to determine whether you are pregnant. Do not continue to take oral contraceptives until you are sure you are not pregnant, but continue to use another method of contraception.

There is no conclusive evidence that oral-contraceptive use is associated with an increase in birth defects when taken inadvertently during early pregnancy. Previously, a few studies had reported that oral contraceptives might be associated with birth defects, but these studies have not been confirmed. Nevertheless, oral contraceptives or any other drugs should not be used during pregnancy unless clearly necessary and prescribed by your doctor. You should check with your doctor about risks to your unborn child of any medication taken during pregnancy.

2. *While breast-feeding*

If you are breast-feeding, consult your doctor before starting oral contraceptives. Some of the drug will be passed on to the child in the milk. A few adverse effects on the child have been reported, including yellowing of the skin (jaundice) and breast enlargement. In addition, oral contraceptives may decrease the amount and quality of your milk. If possible, do not use oral contraceptives while breast-feeding. You should use another method of contraception since breast-feeding provides only partial protection from becoming pregnant, and this partial protection decreases significantly as you breast-feed for longer periods of time. You should consider starting oral contraceptives only after you have weaned your child completely.

3. *Laboratory tests*

If you are scheduled for any laboratory tests, tell your doctor you are taking birth-control pills. Certain blood tests may be affected by birth-control pills.

4. *Drug interactions*

Certain drugs may interact with birth-control pills to make them less effective in preventing pregnancy or cause an increase in breakthrough bleeding. Such drugs include rifampin, drugs used for epilepsy such as barbiturates (for example, phenobarbital) and phenytoin (Dilantin is one brand of this drug), phenylbutazone (Butazolidin is one brand), and possibly certain antibiotics. You may need to use an additional method of contraception during any cycle in which you take drugs that can make oral contraceptives less effective.

HOW TO TAKE THE PILL

This product (like all oral contraceptives) is intended to prevent pregnancy. It does not protect against transmission of HIV (AIDS) and other sexually transmitted diseases such as chlamydia, genital herpes, genital warts, gonorrhea, hepatitis B, and syphilis.

IMPORTANT POINTS TO REMEMBER

BEFORE YOU START TAKING YOUR PILLS:

1. BE SURE TO READ THESE DIRECTIONS:

Before you start taking your pills.

Anytime you are not sure what to do.

2. THE RIGHT WAY TO TAKE THE PILL IS TO TAKE ONE PILL EVERY DAY AT THE SAME TIME.

If you miss pills you could get pregnant. This includes starting the pack late. The more pills you miss, the more likely you are to get pregnant.

3. MANY WOMEN HAVE SPOTTING OR LIGHT BLEEDING, OR MAY FEEL SICK TO THEIR STOMACH DURING THE FIRST 1–3 PACKS OF PILLS.

If you feel sick to your stomach, do not stop taking the pill. The problem will usually go away. If it doesn't go away, check with your doctor or clinic.

4. MISSING PILLS CAN ALSO CAUSE SPOTTING OR LIGHT BLEEDING, even when you make up these missed pills.

On the days you take 2 pills to make up for missed pills, you could also feel a little sick to your stomach.

5. IF YOU HAVE VOMITING OR DIARRHEA, for any reason, or IF YOU TAKE SOME MEDICINES, including some antibiotics, your pills may not work as well.

Use a back-up method (such as condoms, foam, or sponge) until you check with your doctor or clinic.

6. IF YOU HAVE TROUBLE REMEMBERING TO TAKE THE PILL, talk to your doctor or clinic about how to make pill-taking easier or about using another method of birth control.

7. IF YOU HAVE ANY QUESTIONS OR ARE UNSURE ABOUT THE INFORMATION IN THIS LEAFLET, call your doctor or clinic.

***BEFORE* YOU START TAKING YOUR PILLS**

1. DECIDE WHAT TIME OF DAY YOU WANT TO TAKE YOUR PILL. It is important to take it at about the same time every day.

2. LOOK AT YOUR PILL PACK TO SEE IF IT HAS 21 OR 28 PILLS:

The *21-pill pack* has 21 "active" brown, white or light-yellow pills (with hormones) to take for 3 weeks, followed by 1 week without pills.

The *28-pill pack* has 21 "active" brown, white or light-yellow pills (with hormones) to take for 3 weeks, followed by 1 week of reminder light-green pills (without hormones).

3. ALSO FIND:

1) where on the pack to start taking pills, and

2) in what order to take the pills (follow the arrow).

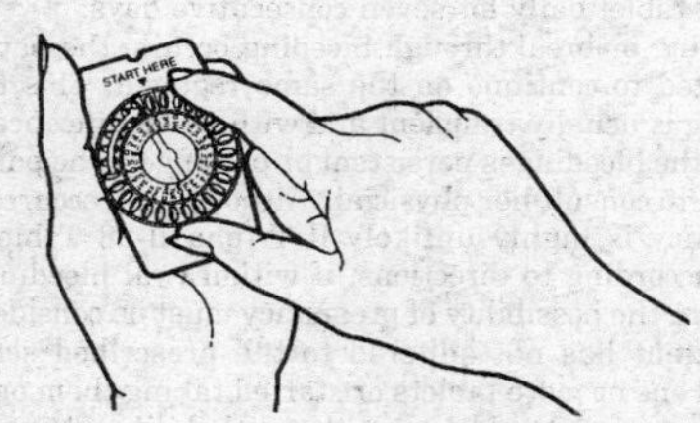

4. BE SURE YOU HAVE READY AT ALL TIMES:

ANOTHER KIND OF BIRTH CONTROL (such as condoms, foam or sponge) to use as a back-up in case you miss pills.

AN EXTRA, FULL PILL PACK.

WHEN TO START THE *FIRST* PACK OF PILLS:

You have a choice of which day to start taking your first pack of pills. Decide with your doctor or clinic which is the best day for you. Pick a time of day which will be easy to remember.

DAY 1 START:

1. Take the first "active" brown pill of the first pack during the *first 24 hours of your period.*

2. You will not need to use a back-up method of birth control, since you are starting the pill at the beginning of your period.

SUNDAY START:

1. Take the first "active" brown pill of the first pack on the *Sunday after your period starts,* even if you are still bleeding. If your period begins on Sunday, start the pack that same day.

2. *Use another method of birth control* as a back-up method if you have sex anytime from the Sunday you start your first pack until the next Sunday (7 days). Condoms, foam, or the sponge are good back-up methods of birth control.

WHAT TO DO DURING THE MONTH:

1. **TAKE ONE PILL AT THE SAME TIME EVERY DAY UNTIL THE PACK IS EMPTY.**

Do not skip pills even if you are spotting or bleeding between monthly periods or feel sick to your stomach (nausea).

Do not skip pills even if you do not have sex very often.

2. **WHEN YOU FINISH A PACK OR SWITCH YOUR BRAND OF PILLS:**

21 pills: Wait 7 days to start the next pack. You will probably have your period during that week. Be sure that no more than 7 days pass between 21-day packs.

28 pills: Start the next pack on the day after your last "reminder" pill. Do not wait any days between packs.

WHAT TO DO IF YOU MISS PILLS

If you **MISS 1** brown, white or light-yellow "active" pill:

1. Take it as soon as you remember. Take the next pill at your regular time. This means you take 2 pills in 1 day.

2. You do not need to use a back-up birth-control method if you have sex.

If you **MISS 2** brown, white or light-yellow "active" pills in a row in **WEEK 1 OR WEEK 2** of your pack:

1. Take 2 pills on the day you remember and 2 pills the next day.

2. Then take 1 pill a day until you finish the pack.

3. You MAY BECOME PREGNANT if you have sex in the 7 *days* after you miss pills. You MUST use another birth-control method (such as condoms, foam, or sponge) as a back-up for those 7 days.

If you **MISS 2** brown, white or light-yellow "active" pills in a row in **THE 3rd WEEK:**

1. ***If you are a Day 1 Starter:***

THROW OUT the rest of the pill pack and start a new pack that same day.

If you are a Sunday Starter:

Keep taking 1 pill every day until Sunday.

On Sunday, THROW OUT the rest of the pack and start a new pack of pills that same day.

2. You may not have your period this month but this is expected. However, if you miss your period 2 months in a row, call your doctor or clinic because you might be pregnant.

3. You MAY BECOME PREGNANT if you have sex in the 7 *days* after you miss pills. You MUST use another birth-control method (such as condoms, foam, or sponge) as a back-up for those 7 days.

If you **MISS 3 OR MORE** brown, white or light-yellow "active" pills in a row (during the first 3 weeks):

1. ***If you are a Day 1 Starter:***

THROW OUT the rest of the pill pack and start a new pack that same day.

If you are a Sunday Starter:

Keep taking 1 pill every day until Sunday.

On Sunday, THROW OUT the rest of the pack and start a new pack of pills that same day.

2. You may not have your period this month but this is expected. However, if you miss your period 2 months in a row, call your doctor or clinic because you might be pregnant.

3. You MAY BECOME PREGNANT if you have sex in the 7 *days* after you miss pills. You MUST use another birth control method (such as condoms, foam, or sponge) as a back-up for those 7 days.

A REMINDER FOR THOSE ON 28-DAY PACKS:

If you forget any of the 7 light-green "reminder" pills in Week 4:

THROW AWAY the pills you missed.

Keep taking 1 pill each day until the pack is empty.

You do not need a back-up method if you start your next pack on time.

FINALLY, IF YOU ARE STILL NOT SURE WHAT TO DO ABOUT THE PILLS YOU HAVE MISSED:

Use a BACK-UP METHOD anytime you have sex.

KEEP TAKING ONE PILL EACH DAY until you can reach your doctor or clinic.

Pregnancy due to pill failure

The incidence of pill failure resulting in pregnancy is approximately less than 1.0% if taken every day as directed, but more typical failure rates are less than 3.0%. If failure does occur, the risk to the fetus is minimal.

RISKS TO THE FETUS

If you do become pregnant while using oral contraceptives, the risk to the fetus is small, on the order of no more than one per thousand. You should, however, discuss the risks to the developing child with your doctor.

Pregnancy after stopping the pill

There may be some delay in becoming pregnant after you stop using oral contraceptives, especially if you had irregular menstrual cycles before you used oral contraceptives. It may be advisable to postpone conception until you begin menstruating regularly once you have stopped taking the pill and desire pregnancy.

There does not appear to be any increase in birth defects in newborn babies when pregnancy occurs soon after stopping the pill.

Overdosage

Serious ill effects have not been reported following ingestion of large doses of oral contraceptives by young children. Overdosage may cause nausea and withdrawal bleeding in females. In case of overdosage, contact your health-care provider or pharmacist.

Other information

Your health-care provider will take a medical and family history before prescribing oral contraceptives and will examine you. The physical examination may be delayed to another time if you request it and the health-care provider believes that it is appropriate to postpone it. You should be reexamined at least once a year. Be sure to inform your health-care provider if there is a family history of any of the conditions listed previously in this leaflet. Be sure to keep all appointments with your health-care provider, because this is a time to determine if there are early signs of side effects of oral-contraceptive use.

Continued on next page

Triphasil-21—Cont.

Do not use the drug for any condition other than the one for which it was prescribed. This drug has been prescribed specifically for you; do not give it to others who may want birth-control pills.

HEALTH BENEFITS FROM ORAL CONTRACEPTIVES

In addition to preventing pregnancy, use of oral contraceptives may provide certain benefits. They are:

- Menstrual cycles may become more regular.
- Blood flow during menstruation may be lighter and less iron may be lost. Therefore, anemia due to iron deficiency is less likely to occur.
- Pain or other symptoms during menstruation may be encountered less frequently.
- Ovarian cysts may occur less frequently.
- Ectopic (tubal) pregnancy may occur less frequently.
- Noncancerous cysts or lumps in the breast may occur less frequently.
- Acute pelvic inflammatory disease may occur less frequently.
- Oral-contraceptive use may provide some protection against developing two forms of cancer: cancer of the ovaries and cancer of the lining of the uterus.

If you want more information about birth-control pills, ask your doctor or pharmacist. They have a more technical leaflet called the Professional Labeling which you may wish to read.

Manufactured by:
Wyeth Laboratories
A Wyeth-Ayerst Company
Philadelphia, PA 19101

CI 4242-3 Revised October 21, 1999

Shown in Product Identification Guide, page 342

TRIPHASIL®-28 ℞

[tri-fā 'sil]

Tablets

(levonorgestrel and ethinyl estradiol tablets—triphasic regimen)

Patients should be counseled that this product does not protect against HIV infection (AIDS) and other sexually transmitted diseases.

DESCRIPTION

Each Triphasil cycle of 28 tablets consists of three different drug phases as follows: Phase 1 comprised of 6 brown tablets, each containing 0.050 mg of levonorgestrel (d(-)-13 beta-ethyl -17- alpha-ethinyl- 17 -beta-hydroxygon-4-en-3-one), a totally synthetic progestogen, and 0.030 mg of ethinyl estradiol (19- nor- 17α-pregna -1,3,5(10)- trien -20- yne-3,17 -diol); phase 2 comprised of 5 white tablets, each containing 0.075 mg levonorgestrel and 0.040 mg ethinyl estradiol; and phase 3 comprised of 10 light-yellow tablets, each containing 0.125 mg levonorgestrel and 0.030 mg ethinyl estradiol; then followed by 7 light-green inert tablets. The inactive ingredients present are cellulose, FD&C Blue 1, iron oxides, lactose, magnesium stearate, polacrilin potassium, polyethylene glycol, titanium dioxide, and hydroxypropyl methylcellulose.

Levonorgestrel

Ethinyl Estradiol

CLINICAL PHARMACOLOGY

See Triphasil®-21.

INDICATIONS AND USAGE

See Triphasil-21.

CONTRAINDICATIONS

See Triphasil-21.

WARNINGS

See Triphasil-21.

PRECAUTIONS

See Triphasil-21.

DRUG INTERACTIONS

See Triphasil-21.

CARCINOGENESIS

See Triphasil-21.

PREGNANCY

See Triphasil-21.

NURSING MOTHERS

See Triphasil-21.

INFORMATION FOR THE PATIENT

See Triphasil-21.

ADVERSE REACTIONS

See Triphasil-21.

OVERDOSAGE

See Triphasil-21.

NONCONTRACEPTIVE HEALTH BENEFITS

See Triphasil-21.

DOSAGE AND ADMINISTRATION

To achieve maximum contraceptive effectiveness, Triphasil-28 Tablets (levonorgestrel and ethinyl estradiol tablets—triphasic regimen) must be taken exactly as directed and at intervals not exceeding 24 hours.

Triphasil-28 Tablets are a three-phase preparation plus 7 inert tablets. The dosage of Triphasil-28 Tablets is **one tablet daily** for 28 consecutive days per menstrual cycle in the following order: 6 brown tablets (phase 1), followed by 5 white tablets (phase 2), followed by 10 light-yellow tablets (phase 3), plus 7 light-green inert tablets, according to the prescribed schedule.

It is recommended that Triphasil-28 Tablets be taken at the same time each day, preferably after the evening meal or at bedtime. During the first cycle of medication, the patient should be instructed to take one Triphasil-28 Tablet daily in the order of 6 brown, 5 white, 10 light-yellow tablets, and then 7 light-green inert tablets for twenty-eight (28) consecutive days, beginning on day one (1) of her menstrual cycle. (The first day of menstruation is day one.) Withdrawal bleeding usually occurs within 3 days following the last light-yellow tablet. (If Triphasil-28 Tablets are first taken later than the first day of the first menstrual cycle of medication or postpartum, contraceptive reliance should not be placed on Triphasil-28 Tablets until after the first 7 consecutive days of administration. The possibility of ovulation and conception prior to initiation of medication should be considered.)

When switching from another oral contraceptive, Triphasil-28 Tablets should be started on the first day of bleeding following the last active tablet taken of the previous oral contraceptive.

The patient begins her next and all subsequent 28-day courses of Triphasil-28 Tablets on the same day of the week that she began her first course, following the same schedule. She begins taking her brown tablets on the next day after ingestion of the last light-green tablet, regardless of whether or not a menstrual period has occurred or is still in progress. Any time a subsequent cycle of Triphasil-28 Tablets is started later than the next day, the patient should be protected by another means of contraception until she has taken a tablet daily for seven consecutive days.

If spotting or breakthrough bleeding occurs, the patient is instructed to continue on the same regimen. This type of bleeding is usually transient and without significance; however, if the bleeding is persistent or prolonged, the patient is advised to consult her physician. Although the occurrence of pregnancy is highly unlikely if Triphasil-28 Tablets are taken according to directions, if withdrawal bleeding does not occur, the possibility of pregnancy must be considered. If the patient has not adhered to the prescribed schedule (missed one or more tablets or started taking them on a day later than she should have), the probability of pregnancy should be considered at the time of the first missed period and appropriate diagnostic measures taken before the medication is resumed. If the patient has adhered to the prescribed regimen and misses two consecutive periods, pregnancy should be ruled out before continuing the contraceptive regimen.

The risk of pregnancy increases with each active (brown, white, or light-yellow) tablet missed. For additional patient instructions regarding missed pills, see the "WHAT TO DO IF YOU MISS PILLS" section in the DETAILED PATIENT LABELING below. If breakthrough bleeding occurs following missed active tablets, it will usually be transient and of no consequence. If the patient misses one or more light-green tablets, she is still protected against pregnancy **provided** she begins taking brown tablets again on the proper day.

In the nonlactating mother, Triphasil-28 may be initiated postpartum, for contraception. When the tablets are administered in the postpartum period, the increased risk of thromboembolic disease associated with the postpartum period must be considered (See "Contraindications", "Warnings", and "Precautions" concerning thromboembolic disease). It is to be noted that early resumption of ovulation may occur if Parlodel® (bromocriptine mesylate) has been used for the prevention of lactation.

HOW SUPPLIED

Triphasil®-28 Tablets (levonorgestrel and ethinyl estradiol tablets—triphasic regimen), NDC 0008-2536, are available in packages of 3 dial dispensers. Each cycle contains 28 round, coated tablets as follows:

NDC 0008-0641, six brown tablets marked "W" and"641", each containing 0.050 mg levonorgestrel and 0.030 mg ethinyl estradiol;

NDC 0008-0642, five white to off-white tablets marked "W" and "642", each containing 0.075 mg levonorgestrel and 0.040 mg ethinyl estradiol;

NDC 0008-0643, ten light-yellow tablets marked "W" and"643", each containing 0.125 mg levonorgestrel and 0.030 mg ethinyl estradiol; and

NDC 0008-0650, seven light-green inert tablets marked "W" and "650".

ALSO AVAILABLE:

Triphasil®-28 Tablets (levonorgestrel and ethinyl estradiol tablets—triphasic regimen), NDC 0008-2536, are available in packages of 50 Pilpak® dispensers for clinic use only. Each cycle contains 28 round, coated tablets as follows:

NDC 0008-0641, six brown tablets marked "W" and"641", each containing 0.050 mg levonorgestrel and 0.030 mg ethinyl estradiol;

NDC 0008-0642, five white to off-white tablets marked "W" and "642", each containing 0.075 mg levonorgestrel and 0.040 mg ethinyl estradiol;

NDC 0008-0643, ten light-yellow tablets marked "W" and"643", each containing 0.125 mg levonorgestrel and 0.030 mg ethinyl estradiol; and

NDC 0008-0650, seven light-green inert tablets marked " W" and "650".

REFERENCES

Available upon request.

Brief Summary Patient Package Insert: See Triphasil-21.

DETAILED PATIENT LABELING: See Triphasil-21.

HOW TO TAKE THE PILL

For Triphasil-28 Dial Dispenser: See Triphasil-21.

For Triphasil-28 Clinic Pilpak®, See below.

HOW TO TAKE THE PILL

This product (like all oral contraceptives) is intended to prevent pregnancy. It does not protect against transmission of HIV (AIDS) and other sexually transmitted diseases such as chlamydia, genital herpes, genital warts, gonorrhea, hepatitis B, and syphilis.

IMPORTANT POINTS TO REMEMBER

BEFORE YOU START TAKING YOUR PILLS:

1. BE SURE TO READ THESE DIRECTIONS:
Before you start taking your pills.
Anytime you are not sure what to do.
2. THE RIGHT WAY TO TAKE THE PILL IS TO TAKE ONE PILL EVERY DAY AT THE SAME TIME.
If you miss pills you could get pregnant. This includes starting the pack late. The more pills you miss, the more likely you are to get pregnant.
3. MANY WOMEN HAVE SPOTTING OR LIGHT BLEEDING, OR MAY FEEL SICK TO THEIR STOMACH DURING THE FIRST 1–3 PACKS OF PILLS.
If you feel sick to your stomach, do not stop taking the pill. The problem will usually go away. If it doesn't go away, check with your doctor or clinic.
4. MISSING PILLS CAN ALSO CAUSE SPOTTING OR LIGHT BLEEDING, even when you make up these missed pills.
On the days you take 2 pills to make up for missed pills, you could also feel a little sick to your stomach.
5. IF YOU HAVE VOMITING OR DIARRHEA, for any reason, or IF YOU TAKE SOME MEDICINES, including some antibiotics, your pills may not work as well.
Use a back-up method (such as condoms, foam, or sponge) until you check with your doctor or clinic.
6. IF YOU HAVE TROUBLE REMEMBERING TO TAKE THE PILL, talk to your doctor or clinic about how to make pill-taking easier or about using another method of birth control.
7. IF YOU HAVE ANY QUESTIONS OR ARE UNSURE ABOUT THE INFORMATION IN THIS LEAFLET, call your doctor or clinic.

***BEFORE* YOU START TAKING YOUR PILLS**

1. DECIDE WHAT TIME OF DAY YOU WANT TO TAKE YOUR PILL.
It is important to take it about the same time every day.
2. LOOK AT YOUR PILL PACK TO SEE IF IT HAS 21 OR 28 PILLS:
The *21-pill pack* has 21 "active" brown, white or light-yellow pills (with hormones) to take for 3 weeks, followed by 1 week without pills.
The *28-pill pack* has 21 "active" brown, white or light-yellow pills (with hormones) to take for 3 weeks, followed by 1 week of reminder light-green pills (without hormones).
3. ALSO FIND:
1) where on the pack to start taking pills.
2) in what order to take the pills (follow the arrows), and
3) the week numbers as shown in the picture below.

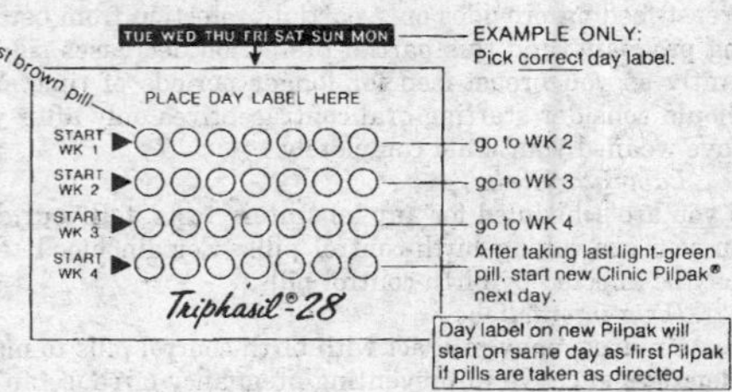

4. BE SURE YOU HAVE READY AT ALL TIMES:
ANOTHER KIND OF BIRTH CONTROL (such as condoms, foam or sponge) to use as a back-up in case you miss pills.
AN EXTRA, FULL PILL PACK.

WHEN TO START THE *FIRST* PACK OF PILLS
You have a choice of which day to start taking your first pack of pills. Decide with your doctor or clinic which is the best day for you. Pick a time of day which will be easy to remember.

DAY 1 START:
1. Take the first "active" brown pill of the first pack during the *first 24 hours of your period.*
2. You will not need to use a back-up method of birth control, since you are starting the pill at the beginning of your period.

SUNDAY START:
1. Take the first "active" brown pill of the first pack on the *Sunday after your period starts,* even if you are still bleeding. If your period begins on Sunday, start the pack that same day.
2. *Use another method of birth control* as a back-up method if you have sex anytime from the Sunday you start your first pack until the next Sunday (7 days). Condoms, foam, or the sponge are good back-up methods of birth control.

WHAT TO DO DURING THE MONTH
1. **TAKE ONE PILL AT THE SAME TIME EVERY DAY UNTIL THE PACK IS EMPTY.**
Do not skip pills even if you are spotting or bleeding between monthly periods or feel sick to your stomach (nausea).
Do not skip pills even if you do not have sex very often.
2. **WHEN YOU FINISH A PACK OR SWITCH YOUR BRAND OF PILLS:**
21 pills: Wait 7 days to start the next pack. You will probably have your period during that week. Be sure that no more than 7 days pass between 21-day packs.
28 pills: Start the next pack on the day after your last "reminder" pill. Do not wait any days between packs.

WHAT TO DO IF YOU MISS PILLS
If you **MISS 1** brown, white or light-yellow "active" pill:
1. Take it as soon as you remember. Take the next pill at your regular time. This means you take 2 pills in 1 day.
2. You do not need to use a back-up birth-control method if you have sex.
If you **MISS 2** brown, white or light-yellow "active" pills in a row in **WEEK 1 OR WEEK 2** of your pack:
1. Take 2 pills on the day you remember and 2 pills the next day.
2. Then take 1 pill a day until you finish the pack.
3. You MAY BECOME PREGNANT if you have sex in the 7 *days* after you miss pills. You MUST use another birth-control method (such as condoms, foam, or sponge) as a back-up for those 7 days.
If you **MISS 2** brown, white or light-yellow "active" pills in a row in **THE 3rd WEEK:**
1. ***If you are a Day 1 Starter.***
THROW OUT the rest of the pill pack and start a new pack that same day.
If you are a Sunday Starter:
Keep taking 1 pill every day until Sunday.
On Sunday, THROW OUT the rest of the pack and start a new pack of pills that same day.
2. You may not have your period this month but this is expected.
However, if you miss your period 2 months in a row, call your doctor or clinic because you might be pregnant.
3. You MAY BECOME PREGNANT if you have sex in the 7 *days* after you miss pills. You MUST use another birth-control method (such as condoms, foam, or sponge) as a back-up for those 7 days.
If you **MISS 3 OR MORE** brown, white or light-yellow "active" pills in a row (during the first 3 weeks):
1. ***If you are a Day 1 Starter:***
THROW OUT the rest of the pill pack and start a new pack that same day.
If you are a Sunday Starter:
Keep taking 1 pill every day until Sunday.
On Sunday, THROW OUT the rest of the pack and start a new pack of pills that same day.
2. You may not have your period this month but this is expected.
However, if you miss your period 2 months in a row, call your doctor or clinic because you might be pregnant.
3. You MAY BECOME PREGNANT if you have sex in the 7 *days* after you miss pills. You MUST use another birth-control method (such as condoms, foam, or sponge) as a back-up for those 7 days.

A REMINDER FOR THOSE ON 28-DAY PACKS
If you forget any of the 7 light-green "reminder" pills in Week 4:
THROW AWAY the pills you missed.
Keep taking 1 pill each day until the pack is empty.
You do not need a back-up method if you start your next pack on time.

FINALLY, IF YOU ARE STILL NOT SURE WHAT TO DO ABOUT THE PILLS YOU HAVE MISSED
Use a BACK-UP METHOD anytime you have sex.
KEEP TAKING ONE PILL EACH DAY until you can reach your doctor or clinic.

Pregnancy due to pill failure
The incidence of pill failure resulting in pregnancy is approximately less than 1.0% if taken every day as directed, but more typical failure rates are less than 3.0%. If failure does occur, the risk to the fetus is minimal.

RISKS TO THE FETUS
If you do become pregnant while using oral contraceptives, the risk to the fetus is small, on the order of no more than one per thousand. You should, however, discuss the risks to the developing child with your doctor.

Pregnancy after stopping the pill
There may be some delay in becoming pregnant after you stop using oral contraceptives, especially if you had irregular menstrual cycles before you used oral contraceptives. It may be advisable to postpone conception until you begin menstruating regularly once you have stopped taking the pill and desire pregnancy.
There does not appear to be any increase in birth defects in newborn babies when pregnancy occurs soon after stopping the pill.

Overdosage
Serious ill effects have not been reported following ingestion of large doses of oral contraceptives by young children. Overdosage may cause nausea and withdrawal bleeding in females. In case of overdosage, contact your health-care provider or pharmacist.

Other information
Your health-care provider will take a medical and family history before prescribing oral contraceptives and will examine you. The physical examination may be delayed to another time if you request it and the health-care provider believes that it is appropriate to postpone it. You should be reexamined at least once a year. Be sure to inform your health-care provider if there is a family history of any of the conditions listed previously in this leaflet. Be sure to keep all appointments with your health-care provider, because this is a time to determine if there are early signs of side effects of oral-contraceptive use.
Do not use the drug for any condition other than the one for which it was prescribed. This drug has been prescribed specifically for you; do not give it to others who may want birth-control pills.

HEALTH BENEFITS FROM ORAL CONTRACEPTIVES: See Triphasil-21.

Manufactured by:
Wyeth Laboratories
A Wyeth-Ayerst Company
Philadelphia, PA 19101
CI 4243-3 Revised October 12, 1999

Shown in Product Identification Guide, page 342

TUBEX® Closed Injection System
[*tū* ′beks]

The TUBEX® closed injection system delivers injectable medication in accurately machine-measured doses with each sterile, prefilled cartridge-needle unit permanently identified up to the moment of injection. Precisely calibrated single-use cartridge-needle units eliminate cross contamination and minimize dosage errors. Super-sharp, siliconized needles minimize penetration pressure. Medication is easily delivered via the TUBEX Injector.
TUBEX sterile cartridge-needle units are ready for instant use, fit easily into the physician's bag, and are readily stored and inventoried in the office.
TAMP-R-TEL® (tamper-resistant package) — a clear, sturdy plastic package for all TUBEX narcotics and barbiturates — adds a new dimension to the handling and record keeping of these controlled drugs. In TAMP-R-TEL, each TUBEX sterile cartridge-needle unit is locked into an individual slot within the package by its own end-lock tab, which is easily broken to release the unit for use. Once the end-lock tab is broken, it is almost impossible to replace it. TAMP-R-TEL thus enhances package integrity, discourages pilferage and facilitates "at a glance" drug count.
The following products are currently available in TUBEX closed injection system. *For prescribing information on products listed, write to Professional Service, Wyeth-Ayerst Pharmaceuticals, P.O. Box 8299, Philadelphia, PA 19101, or contact your local Wyeth-Ayerst representative.*

Product and Needle Size / Units Per Pkg	NDC 0008-
NARCOTICS in TAMP-R-TEL® (tamper-resistant package)	
CODEINE PHOSPHATE, USP (CII) •	
30 mg (1/2 gr.) (25 G × 5/8″) 10—1 mL	0728-01
60 mg (1 gr.) (25 G × 5/8″) 10—1 mL	0729-01
HYDROMORPHONE HYDROCHLORIDE, USP (CII) •	
1 mg (22 G × 1 1/4″) 10—1 mL fill in 2 mL	0387-03
2 mg (1/30 gr.) (22 G × 1 1/4″) 10—1 mL fill in 2 mL	0295-01
4 mg (1/15 gr.) (22 G × 1 1/4″) 10—1 mL fill in 2 mL	0296-01
MEPERGAN® (Meperidine HCl and Promethazine HCl) 25 mg each/mL (CII) • (22 G × 1 1/4″) 10—2 mL	0235-01
10—2 mL TUBEX® BLUNT POINTE™ Sterile Cartridge Units in TAMP-R-TEL®	0235-50
MEPERIDINE HYDROCHLORIDE, USP (CII) •	
25 mg (22 G × 1 1/4″) 10—1 mL fill in 2 mL	0601-02
25 mg 10 TUBEX® BLUNT POINTE™ Sterile Cartridge Units—1 mL fill in 2 mL	0601-50
50 mg (22 G × 1 1/4″) 10—1 mL fill in 2 mL	0602-02
50 mg 10 TUBEX® BLUNT POINTE™ Sterile Cartridge Units—1 mL fill in 2 mL in TAMP-R-TEL®	0602-50
75 mg (22 G × 1 1/4″) 10—1 mL fill in 2 mL	0605-02
75 mg 10 TUBEX® BLUNT POINTE™ Sterile Cartridge Units—1 mL fill in 2 mL in TAMP-R-TEL®	0605-50
100 mg (22 G × 1 1/4″) 10—1 mL fill in 2 mL in TAMP-R-TEL®	0613-02
100 mg 10 TUBEX® BLUNT POINTE™ Sterile Cartridge Units—1 mL fill in 2 mL in TAMP-R-TEL®	0613-50
MORPHINE SULFATE, USP (CII) •	
2 mg (1/30 gr.) (25 G × 5/8″) 10—1 mL	0649-01
2 mg (1/30 gr.) 10 TUBEX® BLUNT POINTE™ Sterile Cartridge Units—2 mL in TAMP-R-TEL®	0649-50
4 mg (1/15 gr.) (25 G × 5/8″) 10—1 mL in TAMP-R-TEL®	0653-01
4 mg (1/15 gr.) 10 TUBEX® BLUNT POINTE™ Sterile Cartridge Units—1 mL in TAMP-R-TEL®	0653-50
8 mg × (1/8 gr.) (25 G × 5/8″) 10—1 mL in TAMP-R-TEL®	0655-03
8 mg (1/8 gr.) 10 TUBEX® BLUNT POINTE™ Sterile Cartridge Units—1 mL fill in 2 mL in TAMP-R-TEL®	0655-50
10 mg (1/6 gr.) (22 G × 1 1/4″) 10—1 mL fill in 1 mL	0656-01
10 mg (1/6 gr.) 10 TUBEX® BLUNT POINTE™ Sterile Cartridge Units—1 mL fill in 2 mL in TAMP-R-TEL®	0656-50
15 mg (1/4 gr.) (22 G × 1 1/4″) 10—1 mL in TAMP-R-TEL®	0657-01
BARBITURATES in TAMP-R-TEL®	
PENTOBARBITAL SODIUM, USP (CII) •	
100 mg (1 1/2 gr.) (22 G × 1 1/4″) 10—2 mL in TAMP-R-TEL®	0303-02
PHENOBARBITAL SODIUM, USP (CIV)	
30 mg (1/2 gr.) (22 G × 1 1/4″) 10—1 mL	0499-01
60 mg (1 gr.) (22 G × 1 1/4″) 10—1 mL in TAMP-R-TEL®	0747-01
130 mg (2 gr.) (22 G × 1 1/4″) 10—1 mL in TAMP-R-TEL®	0304-01

• Narcotic order blank required.

ANTIBIOTICS
BICILLIN® C-R (Penicillin G Benzathine and Penicillin G Procaine Suspension) 300,000 U each/mL
(Marketed and distributed by Monarch Pharmaceuticals)

Product	NDC 0008-
600,000 U (21 G x 1″) (Pediatric use) 10—1 mL	0026-37
1,200,000 U (21 G x 1″) (Pediatric use) 10—2 mL	0026-36
1,200,000 U (21 G x 1 1/4″) 10—2 mL	0026-35
2,400,000 U (18 G × 2″) 10—4 mL (disposable syringe)	0026-22

Continued on next page

Tubex System—Cont.

BICILLIN C-R 900/300
(900,000 units Penicillin G Benzathine and 300,000 units Penicillin G Procaine in suspension)
(Marketed and distributed by Monarch Pharmaceuticals)
1,200,000 U (21 G x 1¼")
10—2 mL 0079-35

1,200,000 U (21 G x 1") (Pediatric use)
10—2 mL 0079-36

BICILLIN LONG-ACTING (Sterile Penicillin G Benzathine Suspension)
(Marketed and distributed by Monarch Pharmaceuticals)
600,000 U (21 G × 1")
10—1 mL 0021-37

1,200,000 U (21 G × 1¼")
10—2 mL 0021-35

2,400,000 U (18 G × 2")
10—4 mL 0021-12
(disposable syringe)

WYCILLIN® (Sterile Penicillin G Procaine Suspension)
(Marketed and distributed by Monarch Pharmaceuticals)
1,200,000 U (20 G × 1¼")
10—2 mL 0018-35

BIOLOGICALS

FluShield®
INFLUENZA VIRUS VACCINE
Trivalent, Types A and B
(chromatograph- and filtered-purified subvirion antigen)
2000-2001 Formula
(25 G × ⅝")
10—0.5 mL 0985-02

CARDIOVASCULAR AGENTS

DIGOXIN, USP
0.25 mg (22 G × 1¼")
10—1 mL 0480-02

EPINEPHRINE, USP (1:1000)
(25 G × ⅝")
10—1 mL 0263-01

HEPARIN SODIUM, USP
1,000 USP units (22 G × 1¼")
10—1 mL 0275-01

1,000 USP units
10 TUBEX® BLUNT POINTE™ Sterile Cartridge Units—1 mL
in TAMP-R-TEL® 0275-50

2,500 USP units (25 G × ⅝")
10—1 mL 0482-01

5,000 USP units (25 G × ⅝")
10—0.5 mL 0277-02

5,000 USP units (25 G × ⅝")
50—0.5 mL 0277-03

5,000 USP units (25 G × ⅝")
10—1.0 mL 0278-02

7,500 USP units (25 G × ⅝")
10—1 mL 0293-01

10,000 USP units (25 G × ⅝")
10—1 mL 0277-01

20,000 USP units (25 G × ⅝")
10—1 mL 0276-01

SPECIAL AGENTS

ATIVAN® (Lorazepam) Ⓒ
2 mg/mL (22 G × 1¼")
10—1 mL fill in 2 mL 0581-02

2 mg/mL (22 G × 1¼")
10—1 mL fill in 2 mL
in TAMP-R-TEL® 0581-06

2 mg/mL
10 TUBEX® BLUNT POINTE™ Sterile Cartridge Units—1 mL fill
in 2 mL 0581-52

2 mg/mL
10 TUBEX® BLUNT POINTE™ Sterile Cartridge Units—1 mL fill
in 2 mL in TAMP-R-TEL® 0581-53

4 mg/mL (22 G × 1¼")
10—1 mL fill in 2 mL 0570-02

4 mg/mL (22 G × 1¼")
10—1 mL fill in 2 mL
in TAMP-R-TEL® 0570-05

4 mg/mL
10 TUBEX® BLUNT POINTE™ Sterile Cartridge Units—1 mL fill
in 2 mL 0570-50

4 mg/mL
10 TUBEX® BLUNT POINTE™ Sterile Cartridge Units—1 mL fill in 2 mL
in TAMP-R-TEL® 0570-51

DIMENHYDRINATE, USP
50 mg (22 G × 1¼")
10—1 mL 0485-01

DIPHENHYDRAMINE HYDROCHLORIDE, USP
50 mg (22 G × 1¼")
10—1 mL 0384-01

HEPARIN LOCK FLUSH Solution, USP
10 USP units per mL (25 G × ⅝")
50—1 mL 0523-01

100 USP units per mL (25 G × ⅝")
50—1 mL 0487-01

10 USP units per mL—25 USP units per TUBEX
(25 G × ⅝")
50—2.5 mL 0523-02

100 USP units per mL—250 USP units per TUBEX
(25 G × ⅝")
50—2.5 mL 0487-03

10 USP units per mL
50 TUBEX® BLUNT POINTE™ Sterile Cartridge Units—1 mL 0523-50

100 USP units per mL
50 TUBEX® BLUNT POINTE™ Sterile Cartridge Units—1 mL 0487-50

10 USP units per mL—25 USP units per TUBEX
50 TUBEX® BLUNT POINTE™ Sterile Cartridge Units—2.5 mL 0523-51

100 USP units per mL—250 USP units per TUBEX
50 TUBEX® BLUNT POINTE™ Sterile Cartridge Units—2.5 mL 0487-51

PHENERGAN® (Promethazine HCl)
25 mg (22 G × 1¼")
10—1 mL 0416-01

50 mg (22 G × 1¼")
10—1 mL 0417-01

SODIUM CHLORIDE, USP (Bacteriostatic)
(25 G × ⅝")
50—1 mL 0333-08

50 TUBEX® BLUNT POINTE™ Sterile Cartridge Units—1 mL 0333-51

(22 G × 1¼")
50—2.5 mL 0333-05

(25 G × ⅝")
50—2.5 mL 0333-02

50 TUBEX® BLUNT POINTE™ Sterile Cartridge Units—2.5 mL 0333-50

Shown in Product Identification Guide, page 342

PLEASE NOTE: THE WYETH-AYERST METAL TUBEX HYPODERMIC SYRINGE AND TUBEX FAST-TRAK SYRINGE HAVE BEEN DISCONTINUED AND REPLACED BY THE TUBEX INJECTOR. EXCHANGE OF THESE DISCONTINUED SYRINGES IS AVAILABLE, FREE OF CHARGE, FROM YOUR WYETH-AYERST AND/OR ELKINS-SINN SALES REPRESENTATIVE, OR FROM WYETH-AYERST DIRECTLY. FOR LOADING AND UNLOADING INFORMATION OF THESE DISCONTINUED SYRINGES, CONTACT THE MEDICAL AFFAIRS DEPARTMENT, AT WYETH-AYERST LABORATORIES, P.O. BOX 8299, PHILADELPHIA, PA 19101.

TUBEX® Injector
NOTE: The TUBEX® Injector is reusable: do not discard.
TUBEX® Sterile Cartridge-Needle Unit

DIRECTIONS FOR USE:

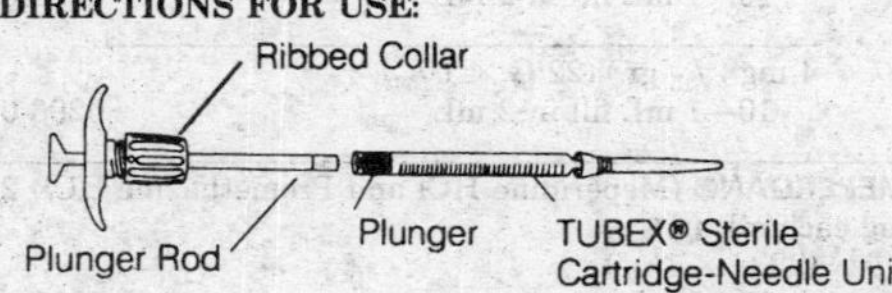

TUBEX® BLUNT POINTE™ Sterile Cartridge Unit

DIRECTIONS FOR USE:

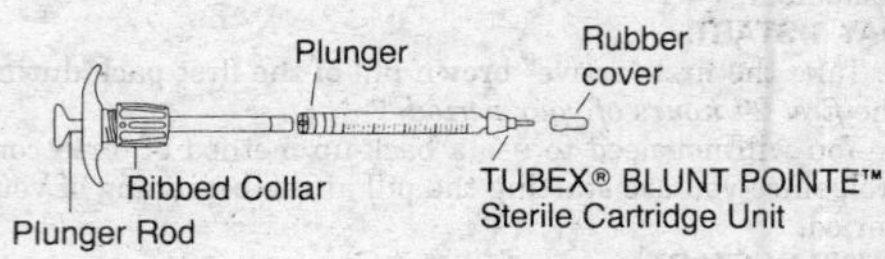

TUBEX® BLUNT POINTE™ Sterile Cartridge Unit is intended for use with injection sets specifically manufactured as "needle-less" injection systems. TUBEX® BLUNT POINTE™ Sterile Cartridge Unit is compatible with Abbott's LifeShield® prepierced reseal injection site, Baxter's Interlink® Injection Site and B. Braun Medical's SafSite® Reflux Valve. Consult manufacturer's recommendations regarding "Directions for Use" of the "needle-less" injection system.

To load a TUBEX® Sterile Cartridge-Needle Unit into the TUBEX® Injector

1. Turn the ribbed collar to the "OPEN" position until it stops.

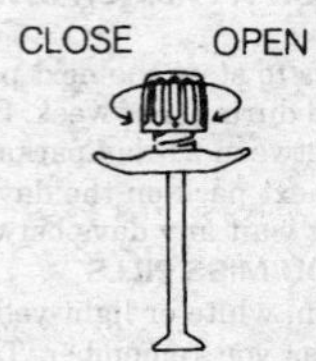

2. Hold the Injector with the open end up and fully insert the TUBEX® Sterile Cartridge Unit.
Firmly tighten the ribbed collar in the direction of the "CLOSE" arrow.

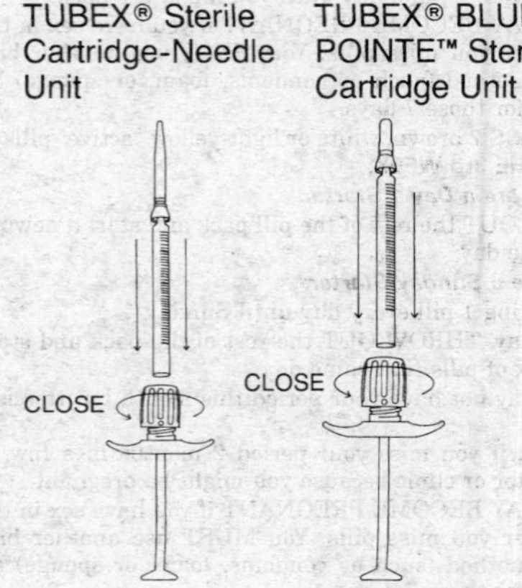

3. Thread the plunger rod into the plunger of the TUBEX® Sterile Cartridge Unit until slight resistance is felt.

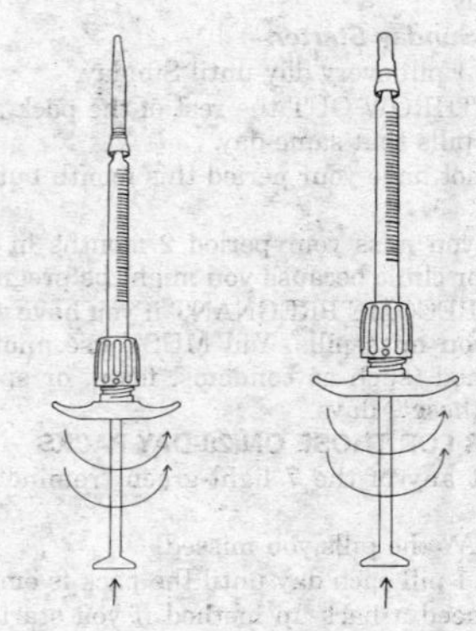

The Injector is now ready for use in the usual manner.

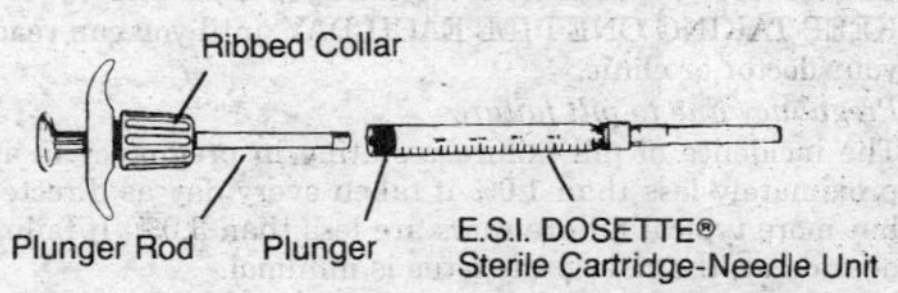

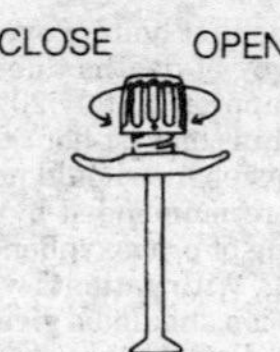

To load an E.S.I. DOSETTE® Sterile Cartridge-Needle Unit into the TUBEX® Injector

1. Turn the ribbed collar to the "OPEN" position until it stops.

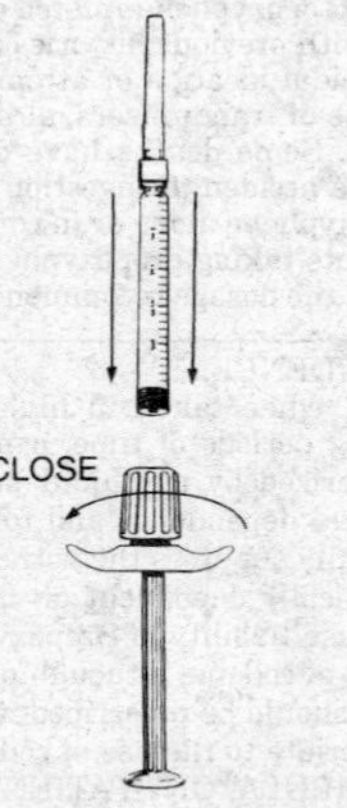

2. Hold the Injector with the open end up and fully insert the DOSETTE® Sterile Cartridge-Needle Unit. Firmly tighten the ribbed collar in the direction of the "CLOSE" arrow.

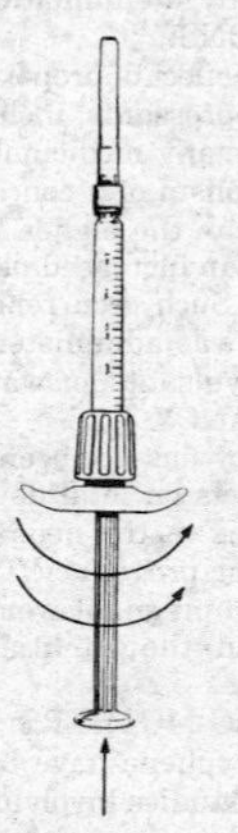

3. Thread the plunger rod into the plunger of the E.S.I. DOSETTE® Sterile Cartridge-Needle Unit until slight resistance is felt.

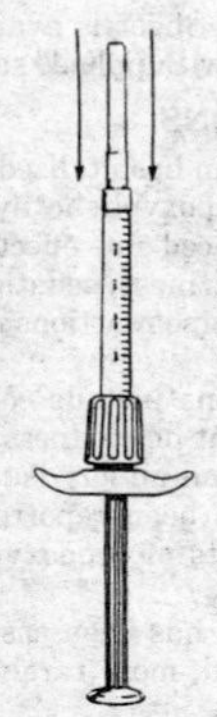

4. Engage the needle-cap assembly by pulling the cap down over the silver cartridge hub. The needle is fully engaged when the silver hub is completely covered.

The Injector is now ready for use in the usual manner.

To administer TUBEX®/DOSETTE® Sterile Cartridge-Needle Units

Method of administration is the same as with conventional syringe. Remove needle cover by grasping it securely; twist and pull. Introduce needle into patient, aspirate by pulling back slightly on the plunger, and inject.

To administer TUBEX® BLUNT POINTE™ Sterile Cartridge Units

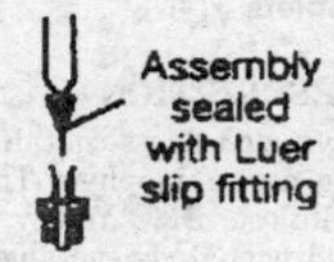

"Needle-less" IV set administration is similar to administration with conventional syringes. Remove rubber cover by grasping it securely; twist and pull. For B. Braun Medical's SafSite® Reflux Valves, aseptically swab the luer slip fitting of the BLUNT POINTE™ sterile cartridge tip assembly with a sterile, individually wrapped, saturated 70% Isopropyl Alcohol swab. This action will remove the lubricant coating from the tip to facilitate a tight seal. Introduce TUBEX® BLUNT POINTE™ Sterile Cartridge Unit into the "needle-less" IV set as per manufacturer's "Directions for Use."

To remove the empty TUBEX®/DOSETTE® Cartridge Unit and dispose into a vertical disposal container

1. Do not recap the needle/point. Disengage the plunger rod.

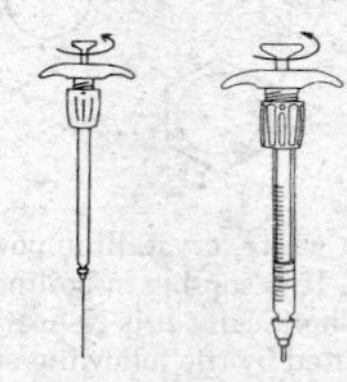

2. Hold the Injector, needle/point pointing down, over a verticle disposal container and loosen the ribbed collar. TUBEX®/DOSETTE® Cartridge Unit will drop into the container.

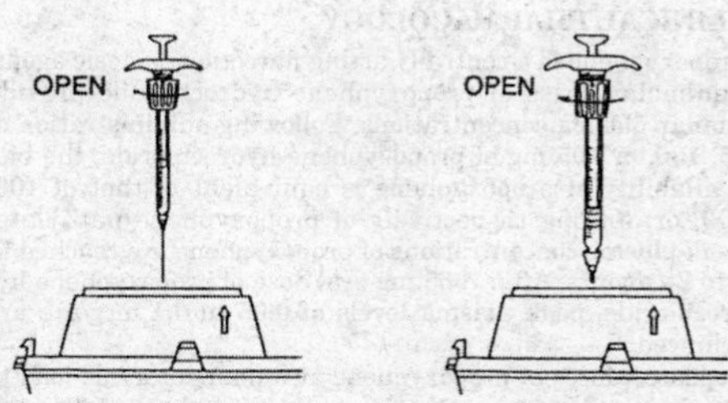

3. Discard the cover.

To remove the empty TUBEX®/DOSETTE® Cartridge Unit and dispose into a horizontal (mailbox) disposal container

1. Do not recap the needle/point. Disengage the plunger rod.
2. Open the horizontal (mailbox) disposal container. Insert TUBEX®/DOSETTE® Cartridge Unit, needle/point pointing down, halfway into container. Close the container lid on cartridge. Loosen ribbed collar; TUBEX®/DOSETTE® Cartridge Unit will drop into the container.

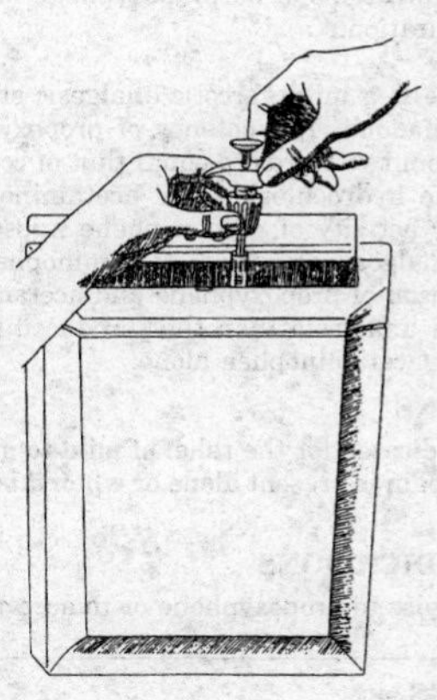

3. Discard the cover.

The TUBEX® Injector is reusable and should not be discarded.

Used TUBEX®/DOSETTE® Cartridge Units should not be employed for successive injections or as multiple-dose containers. They are intended to be used only once and discarded. **NOTE:** Any graduated markings on TUBEX®/DOSETTE® Sterile Cartridge Units are to be used only as a guide in mixing, withdrawing, or administering measured doses.

Wyeth-Ayerst does not recommend and will not accept responsibility for the use of any cartridge-needle units or needle-less system other than TUBEX® or E.S.I. DOSETTE® Cartridge Units in the TUBEX® Injector.

The ESI DOSETTE® cartridge holder has been discontinued. For instructions on its use, contact Medical Affairs, Wyeth-Ayerst Pharmaceuticals, P.O. Box 8299, Phila., PA 19101.

Manufactured by:
Wyeth Laboratories
A Wyeth-Ayerst Company
Philadelphia, Pa 19101

TYPHOID VACCINE USP ℞

DESCRIPTION

Typhoid Vaccine, USP is a saline suspension containing not more than 1000 million Salmonella typhosa (Ty-2 strain) organisms per mL. After growing on veal infusion agar (containing 0.5 percent sodium chloride, 2 percent peptone, and 5 percent agar), the bacteria are washed off the medium, suspended in buffered sodium chloride injection, and killed by a combination of phenol and heat. Phenol (0.5 percent) is added to the final vaccine as preservative. Typhoid Vaccine, USP is tested for safety, potency, and purity and standardized according to F.D.A. Additional Standards for Bacterial Vaccines, 21 C.F.R. 620.10-620.15.

INDICATIONS

Typhoid Vaccine, USP is indicated for active immunization against typhoid fever. Based on data obtained from field studies, it has been estimated that typhoid vaccine is 70% or more effective in preventing typhoid fever, depending in part on the degree of exposure.

Routine immunization against typhoid is no longer recommended for persons residing in the United States. Selective immunization is indicated in the following situations:

1. Intimate exposure to a known typhoid carrier, as would occur with continued household contact.
2. Foreign travel to areas where typhoid fever is endemic.

Although at one time typhoid immunization was suggested for persons attending summer camps or for residents of areas where flooding has occurred, there are no data to support continuation of such practices.[1,2]

CONTRAINDICATIONS

Administration should be postponed in the presence of acute respiratory or other active infection.

A severe systemic or allergic reaction following a prior dose is a contraindication to further use.[3]

PRECAUTIONS

A sterile syringe and needle should be used for each patient to prevent transmission of hepatitis B virus and other infectious agents from one person to another.

Specific information concerning use of typhoid vaccine during pregnancy is not available. However, as with other inactivated bacterial vaccines, its use is not contraindicated during pregnancy unless the intended recipient has manifested significant systemic or allergic reactions following administration of prior doses. Use of typhoid vaccine during pregnancy should be individualized to reflect actual need.

Before the injection of any biological, the physician should take all precautions known for prevention of allergic or any other side reactions. This should include: A review of the patient's history regarding possible sensitivity; the ready availability of epinephrine 1:1000 and other appropriate agents used for control of immediate allergic reactions; and a knowledge of the recent literature pertaining to use of the biological concerned.

REACTIONS

Most recipients of typhoid vaccine experience some degree of local and systemic response, usually beginning within 24 hours of administration and persisting for one or two days. Local reactions are usually manifested by erythema, induration, and tenderness and should be expected in all those injected intracutaneously.

Systemic manifestations may include malaise, headache, myalgia, and elevated temperature.

DOSAGE

PRIMARY IMMUNIZATION

1. Adults and children over 10 years of age:

Two doses of 0.5 mL each, administered subcutaneously, at an interval of four or more weeks.

2. Children less than 10 years of age:

Two doses of 0.25 mL, each administered subcutaneously, at an interval of four or more weeks.

In instances where there is insufficient time for two doses administered at the specified intervals, three doses of the appropriate volume may be given at weekly intervals.

BOOSTER DOSES

1. Adults and children over 10 years of age:

0.5 mL, administered subcutaneously, or 0.1 mL, injected intracutaneously (intradermally).

2. Children 6 months to 10 years of age:

Continued on next page

Typhoid Vaccine—Cont.

0.25 mL, administered subcutaneously, or 0.1 mL, intracutaneously (intradermally)
Under conditions of continued or repeated exposure, a booster dose should be given at least every three years. In instances where an interval of more than three years has elapsed since primary immunization or the last booster dose, a single booster dose is considered sufficient; it is not necessary to repeat the primary immunizing series.

ADMINISTRATION

Shake vial vigorously before withdrawing each dose.
Before injection, the rubber diaphragm of the vial and the skin over the site to be injected should be cleansed and prepared with a suitable germicide.
After insertion of the needle, aspirate to help avoid inadvertent injection into a blood vessel.

HOW SUPPLIED

Typhoid Vaccine, USP is supplied in vials of 5 mL and 10 mL, each containing 8 units per mL.

REFERENCES

1. Recommendations of the Public Health Service Advisory Committee on Immunization Practices—Typhoid Vaccine. Morbidity and Mortality Weekly Report 27 (No. 27): 231, 1978.
2. Report of the Committee on Infectious Diseases, American Academy of Pediatrics, 1982 (Red Book).
3. Recommendations of the Public Health Service Advisory Committee on Immunization Practices—General Recommendations on Immunization. Morbidity and Mortality Weekly Report 29 (No.7): 76, 1980.

Manufactured by:
Wyeth Laboratories
A Wyeth-Ayerst Company
Marietta, PA 17547.
U.S. Gov't License No. 3
CI 4229-1 Issued February 9, 1994

WYDASE® ℞

[*wi-dās*]
(hyaluronidase)

DESCRIPTION

Wydase, a protein enzyme, is a preparation of highly purified bovine testicular hyaluronidase. The exact chemical structure of this enzyme is unknown. Wydase is available in two dosage forms:
Wydase Lyophilized
Hyaluronidase, dehydrated in the frozen state under high vacuum, with lactose and thimerosal (mercury derivative), is supplied as a sterile, white, odorless, amorphous solid and is to be reconstituted with Sodium Chloride Injection, USP, before use, usually in the proportion of one mL per 150 USP units of hyaluronidase (Wydase Lyophilized).
Each vial of 1,500 USP units contains 1.0 mg thimerosal (mercury derivative), added as a preservative, and 13.3 mg lactose. Each vial of 150 USP units contains 0.075 mg thimerosal (mercury derivative), added as a preservative, and 2.66 mg lactose.
Wydase Stabilized Solution
A hyaluronidase injection solution ready for use, colorless and odorless, containing 150 USP units of hyaluronidase per mL with 8.5 mg sodium chloride, 1 mg edetate disodium, 0.4 mg calcium chloride, monobasic sodium phosphate buffer, and not more than 0.1 mg thimerosal (mercury derivative).
The USP and the NF hyaluronidase units are the equivalent to the turbidity-reducing (TR) unit and to the International Unit.

HOW SUPPLIED

Wydase® Lyophilized is supplied as follows:
150 USP (TR) units of hyaluronidase
NDC 0008-0121-01, 1 mL vial, as single vials.
Not Recommended for IV Use.
Store at controlled room temperature in a dry place. Store sterile reconstituted solution below 30°C (86°F). Use within 24 hours.
Following reconstitution, store vial in upright position.
1,500 USP (TR) units of hyaluronidase
NDC 0008-0149-01, 10 mL vial, as single vials.
Not Recommended for IV Use.
Store at controlled room temperature in a dry place. Store sterile reconstituted solution below 30°C (86°F). Use within 14 days.
Following reconstitution, store vial in upright position.
Wydase® Stabilized Solution is supplied as follows:
150 USP (TR) units of hyaluronidase per mL
NDC 0008-0170-01, 1 mL vial, as single vials.
NDC 0008-0170-02, 10 mL vial, as single vials.
Not Recommended for IV Use.
Store in a refrigerator.
Do not use if solution is discolored or contains a precipitate.
Manufactured by:
Wyeth Laboratories
A Wyeth-Ayerst Company
Philadelphia, PA 19101
CI 4224-1 Issued February 8, 1994

For prescribing information write to Professional Service, Wyeth-Ayerst Pharmaceuticals, P.O. Box 8299, Philadelphia, PA 19101, or contact your local Wyeth-Ayerst representative.

WYGESIC® Ⓒ ℞

[*wi-je 'zik*]
(propoxyphene HCl and acetaminophen)
Tablets

DESCRIPTION

Wygesic tablets contain 65 mg propoxyphene HCl and 650 mg acetaminophen. The inactive ingredients present are cellulose, D&C Yellow 10, FD&C Blue 1, FD&C Yellow 6, hydrogenated vegetable oil, hydroxypropyl methylcellulose, methylcellulose, polacrilin potassium, polyethylene glycol, and titanium dioxide.
Propoxyphene hydrochloride is an odorless white crystalline powder with a bitter taste. It is freely soluble in water. Chemically, it is [S-(R*,S*)]-α-[2-(dimethylamino)-1-methylethyl]-α-phenylbenzeneethanol, propanoate (ester), hydrochloride, which can be represented by the following structural formula:

$$(CH_3)_2NCH_2-\overset{CH_3}{\underset{H}{C}}-\overset{OCC_2H_5}{\underset{C_6H_5}{C}}-CH_2-C_6H_5 \cdot HCl$$

Acetaminophen is a white, crystalline powder, possessing a slightly bitter taste. It is soluble in boiling water and freely soluble in alcohol. Chemically, it is N-Acetyl-p-aminophenol, which can be presented by the following structural formula:

$$HO-C_6H_4-NHCOCH_3$$

CLINICAL PHARMACOLOGY

Propoxyphene is a centrally acting narcotic analgesic agent. Equimolar doses of propoxyphene hydrochloride provide similar plasma concentrations. Following administration of 65, 130, or 195 mg of propoxyphene hydrochloride, the bioavailability of propoxyphene is equivalent to that of 100, 200, or 300 mg respectively of propoxyphene napsylate. Peak plasma concentrations of propoxyphene are reached in 2 to 2½ hours. After a 65 mg oral dose of propoxyphene hydrochloride, peak plasma levels of 0.05 to 0.1 mcg/mL are achieved.
Repeated doses of propoxyphene at 6-hour intervals lead to increasing plasma concentrations, with a plateau after the ninth dose at 48 hours.
Propoxyphene is metabolized in the liver to yield norpropoxyphene. Propoxyphene has a half-life of 6 to 12 hours, whereas that of norpropoxyphene is 30 to 36 hours.
Norpropoxyphene has substantially less central nervous system depressant effect than propoxyphene, but a greater local anesthetic effect, which is similar to that of amitriptyline and antiarrhythmic agents, such as lidocaine and quinidine.
In animal studies in which propoxyphene and norpropoxyphene were continuously infused in large amounts, intracardiac conduction time (P-R and QRS intervals) was prolonged. Any intracardiac conduction delay attributable to high concentrations of norpropoxyphene may be of relatively long duration.
ACTIONS
Propoxyphene is a mild narcotic analgesic structurally related to methadone. The potency of propoxyphene hydrochloride is from two-thirds to equal that of codeine.
Propoxyphene hydrochloride and acetaminophen provide the analgesic activity of propoxyphene napsylate and the antipyretic-analgesic activity of acetaminophen.
The combination of propoxyphene and acetaminophen produces greater analgesia than that produced by either propoxyphene or acetaminophen alone.

INDICATIONS

Wygesic is indicated for the relief of mild-to-moderate pain, either when pain is present alone or when it is accompanied by fever.

CONTRAINDICATIONS

Hypersensitivity to propoxyphene or to acetaminophen.

WARNINGS

Do not prescribe propoxyphene for patients who are suicidal or addiction-prone.
Prescribe propoxyphene with caution for patients taking tranquilizers or antidepressant drugs and patients who use alcohol in excess.
Tell your patients not to exceed the recommended dose and to limit their intake of alcohol.
Propoxyphene products in excessive doses, either alone or in combination with other CNS depressants, including alcohol, are a major cause of drug-related deaths. Fatalities within the first hour of overdosage are not uncommon. In a survey of deaths due to overdosage conducted in 1975, in approximately 20% of the fatal cases, death occurred within the first hour (5% occurred within 15 minutes). Propoxyphene should not be taken in doses higher than those recommended by the physician. The judicious prescribing of propoxyphene is essential to the safe use of this drug. With patients who are depressed or suicidal, consideration should be given to the use of nonnarcotic analgesics. Patients should be cautioned about the concomitant use of propoxyphene products and alcohol because of potentially serious CNS-additive effects of these agents. Because of its added depressant effects, propoxyphene should be prescribed with caution for those patients whose medical condition requires the concomitant administration of sedatives, tranquilizers, muscle relaxants, antidepressants, or other CNS-depressant drugs. Patients should be advised of the additive depressant effects of these combinations.
Many of the propoxyphene-related deaths have occurred in patients with previous histories of emotional disturbances or suicidal ideation or attempts as well as histories of misuse of tranquilizers, alcohol, and other CNS-active drugs. Some deaths have occurred as a consequence of the accidental ingestion of excessive quantities of propoxyphene alone or in combination with other drugs. Patients taking propoxyphene should be warned not to exceed the dosage recommended by the physician.

DRUG DEPENDENCE:
Propoxyphene, when taken in higher-than-recommended doses over long periods of time, can produce drug dependence characterized by psychic dependence and, less frequently, physical dependence and tolerance. Propoxyphene will only partially suppress the withdrawal syndrome in individuals physically dependent on morphine or other narcotics. The abuse liability of propoxyphene is qualitatively similar to that of codeine although quantitatively less, and propoxyphene should be prescribed with the same degree of caution appropriate to the use of codeine.
USAGE IN AMBULATORY PATIENTS:
Propoxyphene may impair the mental and/or physical abilities required for the performance of potentially hazardous tasks, such as driving a car or operating machinery. The patient should be cautioned accordingly.

PRECAUTIONS

GENERAL:
Propoxyphene should be administered with caution to patients with hepatic or renal impairment since higher serum concentrations or delayed elimination may occur.
DRUG INTERACTIONS:
The CNS-depressant effect of propoxyphene is additive with that of other CNS depressants, including alcohol.
As is the case with many medicinal agents, propoxyphene may slow the metabolism of a concomitantly administered drug. Should this occur, the higher serum concentrations of that drug may result in increased pharmacologic or adverse effects of that drug. Such occurrences have been reported when propoxyphene was administered to patients on antidepressants, anticonvulsants, or warfarin-like drugs.
USAGE IN PREGNANCY:
Safe use in pregnancy has not been established relative to possible adverse effects on fetal development. Instances of withdrawal symptoms in the neonate have been reported following usage during pregnancy. Therefore, propoxyphene should not be used in pregnant women unless, in the judgment of the physician, the potential benefits outweigh the possible hazards.
USAGE IN NURSING MOTHERS:
Low levels of propoxyphene have been detected in human milk. In postpartum studies involving nursing mothers who were given propoxyphene, no adverse effects were noted in infants receiving mother's milk.
USAGE IN CHILDREN:
Propoxyphene is not recommended for use in children, because documented clinical experience has been insufficient to establish safety and a suitable dosage regimen in the pediatric age group.
A Patient Information Sheet is available for this product. See text following "How Supplied" section below.

ADVERSE REACTIONS

In a survey conducted in hospitalized patients, less than 1% of patients taking propoxyphene hydrochloride at recommended doses experienced side effects. The most frequently reported have been dizziness, sedation, nausea, and vomiting. Some of these adverse reactions may be alleviated if the patient lies down.
Other adverse reactions include constipation, abdominal pain, skin rashes, light-headedness, headache, weakness, euphoria, dysphoria, and minor visual disturbances.
Liver dysfunction has been reported in association with both active components of propoxyphene and acetaminophen tablets.
Propoxyphene therapy has been associated with abnormal liver-function tests and, more rarely, with instances of reversible jaundice.
Hepatic necrosis may result from acute overdoses of acetaminophen (see "Management of Overdosage"). In chronic ethanol abusers, this has been reported rarely with short-term use of acetaminophen doses of 2.5 to 10 g/day. Fatalities have occurred.

MANAGEMENT OF OVERDOSAGE

In all cases of suspected overdosage, call your regional Poison Control Center to obtain the most up-to-date information about the treatment of overdosage. This recommendation is made because, in general, information regarding the treatment of overdosage may change more rapidly than do package inserts.

Initial consideration should be given to the management of the CNS effects of propoxyphene overdosage. Resuscitative measures should be initiated promptly.

SYMPTOMS OF PROPOXYPHENE OVERDOSAGE:

The manifestations of acute overdosage with propoxyphene are those of narcotic overdosage. The patient is usually somnolent, but may be stuporous or comatose and convulsing. Respiratory depression is characteristic. The ventilatory rate and/or tidal volume is decreased, which results in cyanosis and hypoxia. Pupils, initially pinpoint, may become dilated as hypoxia increases. Cheyne-Stokes respiration and apnea may occur. Blood pressure and heart rate are usually normal initially, but blood pressure falls and cardiac performance deteriorates, which ultimately results in pulmonary edema and circulatory collapse unless the respiratory depression is corrected and adequate ventilation is restored promptly. Cardiac arrhythmias and conduction delay may be present. A combined respiratory-metabolic acidosis occurs, owing to retained CO_2 (hypercapnea) and to lactic acid formed during anaerobic glycolysis. Acidosis may be severe if large amounts of salicylates have also been ingested. Death may occur.

TREATMENT OF PROPOXYPHENE OVERDOSAGE:

Attention should be directed first to establishing a patent airway and to restoring ventilation. Mechanically assisted ventilation, with or without oxygen, may be required, and positive-pressure respiration may be desirable if pulmonary edema is present.

The narcotic antagonist naloxone hydrochloride will markedly reduce the degree of respiratory depression, and 0.4 to 2 mg should be administered promptly, preferably intravenously. If the desired degree of counteraction with improvement in respiratory function is not obtained, naloxone should be repeated at 2- to 3-minute intervals. The duration of action of the antagonist may be brief. If no response is observed after 10 mg of naloxone have been administered, the diagnosis of propoxyphene toxicity should be questioned. Naloxone hydrochloride may also be administered by continuous intravenous infusion.

TREATMENT OF PROPOXYPHENE OVERDOSAGE IN CHILDREN:

The usual initial dose of naloxone in children is 0.01 mg/kg body weight given intravenously. If this dose does not result in the desired degree of clinical improvement, a subsequent increased dose of 0.1 mg/kg body weight may be administered. If an IV route of administration is not available, naloxone may be administered IM or subcutaneously in divided doses. If necessary, naloxone can be diluted with sterile water for injection.

Blood gases, pH, and electrolytes should be monitored in order that acidosis and any electrolyte disturbance present may be corrected promptly. Acidosis, hypoxia, and generalized CNS depression predispose to the development of cardiac arrhythmias. Ventricular fibrillation or cardiac arrest may occur and necessitate the full complement of cardiopulmonary resuscitation (CPR) measures. Respiratory acidosis rapidly subsides as ventilation is restored and hypercapnea eliminated, but lactic acidosis may require intravenous bicarbonate for prompt correction.

Electrocardiographic monitoring is essential. Prompt correction of hypoxia, acidosis, and electrolyte disturbance (when present) will help prevent these cardiac complications and will increase the effectiveness of agents administered to restore normal cardiac function.

In addition to the use of a narcotic antagonist, the patient may require careful titration with an anticonvulsant to control convulsions. Analeptic drugs (for example, caffeine or amphetamine) should not be used because of their tendency to precipitate convulsions.

General supportive measures, in addition to oxygen, include, when necessary, intravenous fluids, vasopressor-inotropic compounds, and, when infection is likely, anti-infective agents. Gastric lavage may be useful, and activated charcoal can adsorb a significant amount of ingested propoxyphene. Dialysis is of little value in poisoning due to propoxyphene. Efforts should be made to determine whether other agents, such as alcohol, barbiturates, tranquilizers, or other CNS depressants, were also ingested, since these increase CNS depression as well as cause specific toxic effects.

SYMPTOMS OF ACETAMINOPHEN OVERDOSAGE:

Shortly after oral ingestion of an overdosage of acetaminophen and for the next 24 hours, anorexia, nausea, vomiting, and abdominal pain have been noted. The patient may then present no symptoms, but evidence of liver dysfunction may be apparent during the next 24 to 48 hours, with elevated serum transaminase and lactic dehydrogenase levels, an increase in serum bilirubin concentrations, and a prolonged prothrombin time. Death from hepatic failure may result 3 to 7 days after overdosage.

Acute renal failure may accompany the hepatic dysfunction and has been noted in patients who do not exhibit signs of fulminant hepatic failure. Typically, renal impairment is more apparent 6 to 9 days after ingestion of the overdose.

TREATMENT OF ACETAMINOPHEN OVERDOSAGE: Acetaminophen in massive overdosage may cause hepatic toxicity in some patients. In all cases of suspected overdose, you may wish to call your regional poison center for assistance in diagnosis and for directions in the use of N-acetylcysteine as an antidote.

In adults, hepatic toxicity has rarely been reported with acute overdoses of less than 10 g and fatalities with less than 15 g. Importantly, young children seem to be more resistant than adults to the hepatotoxic effect of an acetaminophen overdose. Despite this, the measures outlined below should be initiated in any adult or child suspected of having ingested an acetaminophen overdose. Clinical and laboratory evidence of hepatic toxicity may not be apparent until 48 to 72 hours postingestion. Early symptoms following a potentially hepatotoxic overdose may include: nausea, vomiting, diaphoresis, and general malaise.

The stomach should be emptied promptly by lavage or by induction of emesis with syrup of ipecac. Patients' estimates of the quantity of a drug ingested are notoriously unreliable. Therefore, if an acetaminophen overdose is suspected, a serum acetaminophen assay should be obtained as early as possible, but no sooner than four hours following ingestion. Liver-function studies should be obtained initially and repeated at 24-hour intervals.

The antidote, N-acetylcysteine, should be administered as early as possible, preferably within 16 hours of the overdose ingestion for optimal results, but in any case, within 24 hours. Following recovery, there are no residual, structural or functional hepatic abnormalities.

ANIMAL TOXICOLOGY:

The acute lethal doses of the hydrochloride and napsylate salts of propoxyphene were determined in 4 species. The results shown in Figure 1 indicate that on a molar basis, the napsylate salt is less toxic than the hydrochloride. This may be due to the relative insolubility and retarded absorption of propoxyphene napsylate.

FIGURE 1
ACUTE ORAL TOXICITY OF PROPOXYPHENE
LD_{50} (mg/kg)±SE
LD_{50} (mMole/kg)

Species	Propoxyphene Hydrochloride	Propoxyphene Napsylate
Mouse	282 ± 39	915 ± 163
	0.75	1.62
Rat	230 ± 44	647 ± 95
	0.61	1.14
Rabbit	ca. 82	>183
	0.22	>0.32
Dog	ca. 100	>183
	0.27	>0.32

Some indication of the relative insolubility and retarded absorption of propoxyphene napsylate was obtained by measuring plasma propoxyphene levels in 2 groups of 4 dogs following oral administration of equimolar doses of the 2 salts. Although none of the animals in this experiment died, 3 of the 4 dogs given propoxyphene hydrochloride exhibited convulsive seizures during the time interval corresponding to the peak plasma levels. The 4 animals receiving the napsylate salt were ataxic but not acutely ill.

DOSAGE AND ADMINISTRATION

The product is given orally. The usual dose is 65 mg propoxyphene HCl and 650 mg acetaminophen every 4 hours as needed for pain. The maximum recommended dose of propoxyphene HCl is 390 mg per day.

Consideration should be given to a reduced total daily dosage in patients with hepatic or renal impairment.

HOW SUPPLIED

Wygesic® (propoxyphene HCl and acetaminophen) Tablets, 65 mg propoxyphene and 650 mg acetaminophen, are available as follows:

NDC 0008-0085, green, capsule-shaped, scored, film-coated tablet marked "WYETH" and "85", in bottles of 100 and 500 tablets, and in REDIPAK® cartons of 100 tablets (10 blister strips of 10).

Keep tightly closed.

Protect from light.

Store at controlled room temperature, 20°–25°C (68°–77°F).

Dispense in tight, light-resistant container as defined in the USP.

PATIENT INFORMATION

Summary

Products containing propoxyphene are used to relieve pain. LIMIT YOUR INTAKE OF ALCOHOL WHILE TAKING THIS DRUG. Make sure your doctor knows if you are taking tranquilizers, sleep aids, antidepressants, antihistamines, or any other drugs that make you sleepy. Combining propoxyphene with alcohol or these drugs in excessive doses is dangerous.

Use care while driving a car or using machines until you see how the drug affects you, because propoxyphene can make you sleepy. Do not take more of the drug than your doctor prescribed. Dependence has occurred when patients have taken propoxyphene for a long period of time at doses greater than recommended.

The rest of this leaflet gives you more information about propoxyphene. Please read it and keep it for further use.

Uses for Propoxyphene

Products containing propoxyphene are used for the relief of mild to moderate pain. Products which contain propoxyphene plus acetaminophen are prescribed for the relief of pain or pain associated with fever.

Before taking Propoxyphene

Make sure your doctor knows if you have ever had an allergic reaction to propoxyphene or acetaminophen.

The effect of propoxyphene in children under 12 has not been studied. Therefore, use of the drug in this age group is not recommended.

How to take Propoxyphene

Follow your doctor's directions exactly. Do not increase the amount you take without your doctor's approval. If you miss a dose of the drug, do not take twice as much the next time.

Pregnancy

Do not take propoxyphene during pregnancy unless your doctor knows you are pregnant and specifically recommends its use. Cases of temporary dependence in the newborn have occurred when the mother has taken propoxyphene consistently in the weeks before delivery. As a general principle, no drug should be taken during pregnancy unless it is clearly necessary.

General Caution

Heavy use of alcohol with propoxyphene is hazardous and may lead to overdosage symptoms (see "Overdosage" below); THEREFORE, LIMIT YOUR INTAKE OF ALCOHOL WHILE TAKING PROPOXYPHENE.

Combinations of excessive doses of propoxyphene, alcohol, and tranquilizers are dangerous. Make sure your doctor knows if you are taking tranquilizers, sleep aids, antidepressant drugs, antihistamines, or any other drugs that make you sleepy. The use of these drugs with propoxyphene increases their sedative effects and may lead to overdosage symptoms, including death (see "Overdosage" below).

Propoxyphene may cause drowsiness or impair your mental and/or physical abilities; therefore, use caution when driving a vehicle or operating dangerous machinery. DO NOT perform any hazardous task until you have seen your response to this drug.

Propoxyphene may increase the concentration in the body of medications such as anticoagulants ("blood thinners"), antidepressants, or drugs used for epilepsy. The result may be excessive or adverse effects of these medications. Make sure your doctor knows if you are taking any of these medications.

Dependence

You can become dependent on propoxyphene if you take it in higher than recommended doses over a long period of time. Dependence is a feeling of need for the drug and a feeling that you cannot perform normally without it.

Overdosage

An overdosage of propoxyphene, alone or in combination with other drugs, including alcohol, may cause weakness, difficulty in breathing, confusion, anxiety, and more severe drowsiness and dizziness. Extreme overdosage may lead to unconsciousness and death.

If the propoxyphene product contains acetaminophen, the overdosage symptoms include nausea, vomiting, lack of appetite, and abdominal pain. Liver damage may occur.

In any suspected overdosage situation, contact your doctor or nearest hospital emergency room. GET EMERGENCY HELP IMMEDIATELY. KEEP THIS AND ALL DRUGS OUT OF THE REACH OF CHILDREN.

Possible Side Effects

When propoxyphene is taken as directed, side effects are infrequent. Among those reported are drowsiness, dizziness, nausea, and vomiting. If these effects occur, it may help if you lie down and rest.

Less frequently reported side effects are constipation, abdominal pain, skin rashes, light-headedness, headache, weakness, minor visual disturbances, and feelings of elation or discomfort.

If side effects occur and concern you, contact your doctor.

Other Information

The safe and effective use of propoxyphene depends on your taking it exactly as directed. This drug has been prescribed specifically for you and your present condition. Do not give this drug to others who may have similar symptoms. Do not use it for any other reason.

If you would like more information about propoxyphene, ask your doctor or pharmacist. They have a more technical leaflet (professional labeling) you may read.

Manufactured by:
Wyeth Laboratories
A Wyeth-Ayerst Company
Philadelphia, PA 19101
CI 3965-4 Revised March 10, 1994

Shown in Product Identification Guide, page 342

WYTENSIN® ℞

[*wi-ten 'sin*]
(guanabenz acetate)

DESCRIPTION

Wytensin (guanabenz acetate), an antihypertensive agent for oral administration, is an aminoguanidine derivative, 2,6-dichlorobenzylideneaminoguanidine acetate, and its structural formula is:

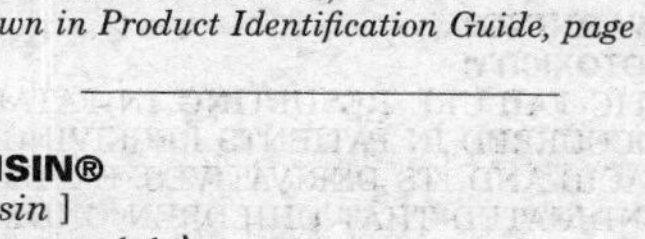

Cl
NH
CH=NNHCNH2 · CH3COOH
Cl

Continued on next page

Wytensin—Cont.

It is an odorless, white to off-white, crystalline substance, sparingly soluble in water and soluble in alcohol, with a molecular weight of 291.14. Each tablet of Wytensin is equivalent to 4 mg or 8 mg of free guanabenz base. The inactive ingredients present are cellulose, iron oxide, lactose, and magnesium stearate. The 8 mg dosage strength also contains FD&C Blue 2.
Wytensin is available as 4 mg or 8 mg tablets for oral administration.

HOW SUPPLIED

Wytensin® (guanabenz acetate) Tablets are available in the following dosage strengths:
4 mg, orange, five-sided tablet with a raised "W"and a "4" under the "W" on one side and "WYETH 73" on reverse side, in bottles of 100 tablets (NDC 0008-0073-01) and 500 tablets (NDC 0008-0073-04) and in Redipak® cartons of 100 tablets (10 blister strips of 10–NDC 0008-0073-05).
8 mg, gray, five-sided tablet with a raised "W" and an "8" under the "W" on one side and "WYETH 74" on scored reverse side, in bottles of 100 tablets (NDC 0008-0074-01).
The appearance of these tablets is a trademark of Wyeth-Ayerst Laboratories.
Keep tightly closed.
Store at room temperature, approximately 25°C (77°F).
Protect from light.
Dispense in light-resistant, tight container.
Manufactured by:
Wyeth Laboratories
A Wyeth-Ayerst Company
Philadelphia, PA 19101
CI 3850-6 Revised February 21, 1997
For prescribing information write to Professional Service, Wyeth-Ayerst Pharmaceuticals, P.O. Box 8299, Philadelphia, PA 19101, or contact your local Wyeth-Ayerst representative.

Zeneca Pharmaceuticals

See AstraZeneca Pharmaceuticals LP

Abbott Laboratories Inc.

Pharmaceutical Products Division
NORTH CHICAGO, IL 60064, U.S.A.

Pharmaceutical Products Division—
Direct Inquiries to:
Customer Service:
(800) 255-5162
Technical Services:
(800) 441-4987
For Medical Information Contact:
Generally:
(800) 633-9110
Adverse Drug Experiences:
(800) 633-9110
Sales and Ordering:
(800) 255-5162
Hospital Products Division—
Direct Inquiries to:
Customer Service:
(800) 222-6883
For Medical Information Contact:
(800) 615-0187
Sales and Ordering
(800) 222-6883

DEPAKOTE® ER ℞
[*dĕp' ă-kōte*]
DIVALPROEX SODIUM EXTENDED-RELEASE TABLETS
℞ only

BOX WARNING:
HEPATOTOXICITY:
HEPATIC FAILURE RESULTING IN FATALITIES HAS OCCURRED IN PATIENTS RECEIVING VALPROIC ACID AND ITS DERIVATIVES. EXPERIENCE HAS INDICATED THAT CHILDREN UNDER THE AGE OF TWO YEARS ARE AT A CONSIDERABLY INCREASED RISK OF DEVELOPING FATAL HEPATOTOXICITY, ESPECIALLY THOSE ON MULTIPLE ANTICONVULSANTS, THOSE WITH CONGENITAL METABOLIC DISORDERS, THOSE WITH SEVERE SEIZURE DISORDERS ACCOMPANIED BY MENTAL RETARDATION, AND THOSE WITH ORGANIC BRAIN DISEASE. WHEN DEPAKOTE IS USED IN THIS PATIENT GROUP, IT SHOULD BE USED WITH EXTREME CAUTION AND AS A SOLE AGENT. THE BENEFITS OF THERAPY SHOULD BE WEIGHED AGAINST THE RISKS. ABOVE THIS AGE GROUP, EXPERIENCE IN EPILEPSY HAS INDICATED THAT THE INCIDENCE OF FATAL HEPATOTOXICITY DECREASES CONSIDERABLY IN PROGRESSIVELY OLDER PATIENT GROUPS.
THESE INCIDENTS USUALLY HAVE OCCURRED DURING THE FIRST SIX MONTHS OF TREATMENT. SERIOUS OR FATAL HEPATOTOXICITY MAY BE PRECEDED BY NON-SPECIFIC SYMPTOMS SUCH AS MALAISE, WEAKNESS, LETHARGY, FACIAL EDEMA, ANOREXIA, AND VOMITING. IN PATIENTS WITH EPILEPSY, A LOSS OF SEIZURE CONTROL MAY ALSO OCCUR. PATIENTS SHOULD BE MONITORED CLOSELY FOR APPEARANCE OF THESE SYMPTOMS. LIVER FUNCTION TESTS SHOULD BE PERFORMED PRIOR TO THERAPY AND AT FREQUENT INTERVALS THEREAFTER, ESPECIALLY DURING THE FIRST SIX MONTHS.
TERATOGENICITY:
VALPROATE CAN PRODUCE TERATOGENIC EFFECTS SUCH AS NEURAL TUBE DEFECTS (E.G., SPINA BIFIDA). ACCORDINGLY, THE USE OF DEPAKOTE TABLETS IN WOMEN OF CHILDBEARING POTENTIAL REQUIRES THAT THE BENEFITS OF ITS USE BE WEIGHED AGAINST THE RISK OF INJURY TO THE FETUS. THIS IS ESPECIALLY IMPORTANT WHEN THE TREATMENT OF A SPONTANEOUSLY REVERSIBLE CONDITION NOT ORDINARILY ASSOCIATED WITH PERMANENT INJURY OR RISK OF DEATH (E.G. MIGRAINE) IS CONTEMPLATED. SEE WARNINGS, INFORMATION FOR PATIENTS.
AN INFORMATION SHEET DESCRIBING THE TERATOGENIC POTENTIAL OF VALPROATE IS AVAILABLE FOR PATIENTS.
PANCREATITIS:
CASES OF LIFE-THREATENING PANCREATITIS HAVE BEEN REPORTED IN BOTH CHILDREN AND ADULTS RECEIVING VALPROATE. SOME OF THE CASES HAVE BEEN DESCRIBED AS HEMORRHAGIC WITH A RAPID PROGRESSION FROM INITIAL SYMPTOMS TO DEATH. CASES HAVE BEEN REPORTED SHORTLY AFTER INITIAL USE AS WELL AS AFTER SEVERAL YEARS OF USE. PATIENTS AND GUARDIANS SHOULD BE WARNED THAT ABDOMINAL PAIN, NAUSEA, VOMITING, AND/OR ANOREXIA CAN BE SYMPTOMS OF PANCREATITIS THAT REQUIRE PROMPT MEDICAL EVALUATION. IF PANCREATITIS IS DIAGNOSED, VALPROATE SHOULD ORDINARILY BE DISCONTINUED. ALTERNATIVE TREATMENT FOR THE UNDERLYING MEDICAL CONDITION SHOULD BE INITIATED AS CLINICALLY INDICATED. (See **WARNINGS** and **PRECAUTIONS**.)

DESCRIPTION

Divalproex sodium is a stable co-ordination compound comprised of sodium valproate and valproic acid in a 1:1 molar relationship and formed during the partial neutralization of valproic acid with 0.5 equivalent of sodium hydroxide. Chemically it is designated as sodium hydrogen bis(2-propylpentanoate). Divalproex sodium has the following structure:

```
 ( CH3CH2CH2–CH–CH2CH2CH3 )
 (             |           )
 (        HO–C=O   Na⊕     )
 (        O=C–O⊖           )
 (             |           )
 ( CH3CH2CH2–CH–CH2CH2CH3 ) n
```

Divalproex sodium occurs as a white powder with a characteristic odor.
DEPAKOTE ER tablets are for oral administration. DEPAKOTE ER tablets contain divalproex sodium in a once-a-day extended-release formulation equivalent to 500 mg of valproic acid.
Inactive Ingredients
DEPAKOTE ER 500 mg Tablets: FD&C Blue No. 1, hydroxypropyl methylcellulose, iron oxide, lactose, microcrystalline cellulose, polydextrose, polyethylene glycol, potassium sorbate, propylene glycol, silicon dioxide, titanium dioxide, and triacetin.

CLINICAL PHARMACOLOGY

Pharmacodynamics
Divalproex sodium dissociates to the valproate ion in the gastrointestinal tract. The mechanisms by which valproate exerts its therapeutic effects have not been established. It has been suggested that its activity in epilepsy is related to increased brain concentrations of gamma-aminobutyric acid (GABA).
Pharmacokinetics
Absorption/Bioavailability
The absolute bioavailability of DEPAKOTE ER TABLETS administered as a single dose after a meal was approximately 90% relative to intravenous infusion.
In two multiple dose studies, when administered either fasting or immediately before smaller meals, the ER tablet produced an average bioavailability of 81–89% relative to DEPAKOTE DELAYED-RELEASE TABLETS given BID. Maximum valproate plasma concentrations (C_{max}) in these studies were achieved on average 7–14 h after DEPAKOTE ER dose intake. In one of these studies, the average C_{max} and minimum plasma concentrations (C_{min}) at steady state of DEPAKOTE ER given fasting and with smaller meals were 74% and 82%, respectively, relative to DEPAKOTE DELAYED-RELEASE TABLETS given BID with smaller meals. In the other study, the average C_{max} and minimum plasma concentrations (C_{min}) at steady state of DEPAKOTE ER were 81% and 85%, respectively, relative to DEPAKOTE DELAYED-RELEASE TABLETS given fasting.
After multiple dosing, DEPAKOTE ER given once daily has been shown to produce percent fluctuation (defined as $100\times[C_{max}-C_{min}]$/[average concentration]) that is 10–20% lower than that of regular DEPAKOTE DELAYED-RELEASE TABLETS given BID. DEPAKOTE ER TABLETS are not bioequivalent to DEPAKOTE DELAYED-RELEASE TABLETS.
Distribution
Protein Binding:
The plasma protein binding of valproate is concentration dependent and the free fraction increases from approximately 10% at 40 μ/mL to 18.5% at 130 μ/mL. Protein binding of valproate is reduced in the elderly, in patients with chronic hepatic diseases, in patients with renal impairment, and in the presence of other drugs (e.g., aspirin). Conversely, valproate may displace certain protein-bound drugs (e.g., phenytoin, carbamazepine, warfarin, and tolbutamide) (see **PRECAUTIONS**, **Drug Interactions** for more detailed information on the pharmacokinetic interactions of valproate with other drugs).
CNS Distribution:
Valproate concentrations in cerebrospinal fluid (CSF) approximate unbound concentrations in plasma (about 10% of total concentration).
Metabolism
Valproate is metabolized almost entirely by the liver. In adult patients on monotherapy, 30–50% of an administered dose appears in urine as a glucuronide conjugate. Mitochondrial β-oxidation is the other major metabolic pathway, typically accounting for over 40% of the dose. Usually, less than 15–20% of the dose is eliminated by other oxidative mechanisms. Less than 3% of an administered dose is excreted unchanged in urine.
The relationship between dose and total valproate concentration is nonlinear; concentration does not increase proportionally with the dose, but rather, increases to a lesser extent due to saturable plasma protein binding. The kinetics of unbound drug are linear.
Elimination
Mean plasma clearance and volume of distribution for total valproate are 0.56 L/hr/1.73 m^2 and 11 L/1.73 m^2, respectively. Mean plasma clearance and volume of distribution for free valproate are 4.6 L/hr/1.73 m^2 and 92 L/1.73 m^2. Mean terminal half-life for valproate monotherapy ranged from 9 to 16 hours following oral dosing regimens of 250 to 1000 mg.
The estimates cited apply primarily to patients who are not taking drugs that affect hepatic metabolizing enzyme systems. For example, patients taking enzyme-inducing antiepileptic drugs (carbamazepine, phenytoin, and phenobarbital) will clear valproate more rapidly.
Special Populations
Elderly—The capacity of elderly patients (age range: 68 to 89 years) to eliminate valproate has been shown to be reduced compared to younger adults (age range: 22 to 26 years). Intrinsic clearance is reduced by 39%; the free fraction is increased by 44%. Accordingly, the initial dosage should be reduced in the elderly (see **DOSAGE AND ADMINISTRATION**).
Effect of Gender:
There are no differences in the body surface area adjusted unbound clearance between males and females (4.8 ± 0.17 and 4.7 ± 0.07 L/hr per 1.73 m^2, respectively).
Effect of Race:
The effects of race on the kinetics of valproate have not been studied.
Effect of Disease:
Liver Disease—(see **BOXED WARNING**, **CONTRAINDICATIONS**, and **WARNINGS**). Liver disease impairs the capacity to eliminate valproate. In one study, the clearance of free valproate was decreased by 50% in 7 patients with cirrhosis and by 16% in 4 patients with acute hepatitis, compared with 6 healthy subjects. In that study, the half-life of valproate was increased from 12 to 18 hours. Liver disease is also associated with decreased albumin concentrations and larger unbound fractions (2 to 2.6 fold increase) of valproate. Accordingly, monitoring of total concentrations may be misleading since free concentrations may be substantially elevated in patients with hepatic disease whereas total concentrations may appear to be normal.
Renal Disease—A slight reduction (27%) in the unbound clearance of valproate has been reported in patients with renal failure (creatinine clearance < 10 mL/minute); however, hemodialysis typically reduces valproate concentrations by about 20%. Therefore, no dosage adjustment appears to be necessary in patients with renal failure. Protein binding in these patients is substantially reduced; thus, monitoring total concentrations may be misleading.
Plasma Levels and Clinical Effect
The relationship between plasma concentration and clinical response is not well documented. One contributing factor is the nonlinear, concentration dependent protein binding of valproate which affects the clearance of the drug. Thus, monitoring of total serum valproate cannot provide a reliable index of the bioactive valproate species.
For example, because the plasma protein binding of valproate is concentration dependent, the free fraction increases from approximately 10% at 40 μg/mL to 18.5% at 130 μg/mL. Higher than expected free fractions occur in the elderly, in hyperlipidemic patients, and in patients with hepatic and renal diseases.

Clinical Trials

The results of a multicenter, randomized, double-blind, placebo-controlled, parallel-group clinical trial demonstrated the effectiveness of DEPAKOTE ER in the prophylactic treatment of migraine headache. This trial recruited patients with a history of migraine headaches with or without aura occurring on average twice or more a month for the preceding three months. Patients with cluster or chronic daily headaches were excluded. Women of childbearing potential were allowed in the trial if they were deemed to be practicing an effective method of contraception.

Patients who experienced ≥2 migraine headaches in the 4-week baseline period were randomized in a 1:1 ratio to DEPAKOTE ER or placebo and treated for 12 weeks. Patients initiated treatment on 500 mg once daily for one week, and were then increased to 1000 mg once daily with an option to permanently decrease the dose back to 500 mg once daily during the second week of treatment if intolerance occurred. Ninety-eight of 114 DEPAKOTE ER-treated patients (86%) and 100 of 110 placebo-treated patients (91%) treated at least two weeks maintained the 1000 mg once daily dose for the duration of their treatment periods. Treatment outcome was assessed on the basis of reduction in 4-week migraine headache rate in the treatment period compared to the baseline period.

Patients (50 male, 187 female) ranging in age from 16 to 69 were treated with DEPAKOTE ER (N=122) or placebo (N=115). Four patients were below the age of 18 and 3 were above the age of 65. Two hundred and two patients (101 in each treatment group) completed the treatment period. The mean reduction in 4-week migraine headache rate was 1.2 from a baseline mean of 4.4 in the DEPAKOTE ER group, versus 0.6 from a baseline mean of 4.2 in the placebo group. The treatment difference was statistically significant (see Figure 1).

Figure 1
Mean Reduction In 4-Week Migraine Headache Rates

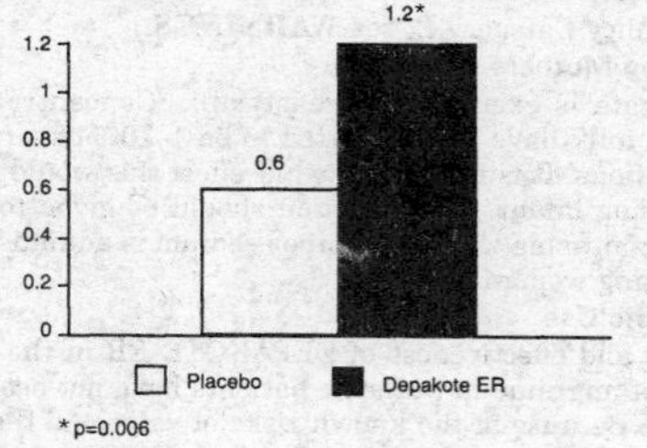

INDICATIONS AND USAGE

DEPAKOTE ER is indicated for prophylaxis of migraine headaches in adults. There is no evidence that DEPAKOTE ER is useful in the acute treatment of migraine headaches. DEPAKOTE ER has not been evaluated for the treatment of mania or epilepsy. Because valproic acid may be a hazard to the fetus, DEPAKOTE ER should be considered for women of childbearing potential only after this risk has been thoroughly discussed with the patient and weighed against the potential benefits of treatment (see **WARNINGS—Usage In Pregnancy**, **PRECAUTIONS—Information for Patients**).

SEE **WARNINGS** FOR STATEMENT REGARDING FATAL HEPATIC DYSFUNCTION.

CONTRAINDICATIONS

DIVALPROEX SODIUM SHOULD NOT BE ADMINISTERED TO PATIENTS WITH HEPATIC DISEASE OR SIGNIFICANT HEPATIC DYSFUNCTION.

Divalproex sodium is contraindicated in patients with known hypersensitivity to the drug.

WARNINGS

Hepatotoxicity

Hepatic failure resulting in fatalities has occurred in patients receiving valproic acid. These incidents usually have occurred during the first six months of treatment. Serious or fatal hepatotoxicity may be preceded by non-specific symptoms such as malaise, weakness, lethargy, facial edema, anorexia, and vomiting. Patients should be monitored closely for appearance of these symptoms. Liver function tests should be performed prior to therapy and at frequent intervals thereafter, especially during the first six months. However, physicians should not rely totally on serum biochemistry since these tests may not be abnormal in all instances, but should also consider the results of careful interim medical history and physical examination. Caution should be observed when administering DEPAKOTE products to patients with a prior history of hepatic disease. Patients on multiple anticonvulsants, children, those with congenital metabolic disorders, those with severe seizure disorders accompanied by mental retardation, and those with organic brain disease may be at particular risk. Experience has indicated that children under the age of two years are at a considerably increased risk of developing fatal hepatotoxicity, especially those with the aforementioned conditions. Above this age group, experience in epilepsy has indicated that the incidence of fatal hepatotoxicity decreases considerably in progressively older patient groups. The use of DEPAKOTE ER in children is not recommended (see PRECAUTIONS—Pediatric Use).

The drug should be discontinued immediately in the presence of significant hepatic dysfunction, suspected or apparent. In some cases, hepatic dysfunction has progressed in spite of discontinuation of drug.

Pancreatitis

Cases of life-threatening pancreatitis have been reported in both children and adults receiving valproate. Some of the cases have been described as hemorrhagic with rapid progression from initial symptoms to death. Some cases have occurred shortly after initial use as well as after several years of use. The rate based upon the reported cases exceeds that expected in the general population and there have been cases in which pancreatitis recurred after rechallenge with valproate. In clinical trials, there were 2 cases of pancreatitis without alternative etiology in 2416 patients, representing 1044 patient-years experience. Patients and guardians should be warned that abdominal pain, nausea, vomiting, and/or anorexia can be symptoms of pancreatitis that require prompt medical evaluation. If pancreatitis is diagnosed, valproate should ordinarily be discontinued. Alternative treatment for the underlying medical condition should be initiated as clinically indicated (see **BOXED WARNING**).

Somnolence in the Elderly

In a double-blind, multicenter trial of valproate in elderly patients with dementia (mean age = 83 years), doses were increased by 125 mg/day to a target dose of 20 mg/kg/day. A significantly higher proportion of valproate patients had somnolence compared to placebo, and although not statistically significant, there was a higher proportion of patients with dehydration. Discontinuations for somnolence were also significantly higher than with placebo. In some patients with somnolence (approximately one-half), there was associated reduced nutritional intake and weight loss. There was a trend for the patients who experienced these events to have a lower baseline albumin concentration, lower valproate clearance, and a higher BUN. In elderly patients, dosage should be increased more slowly and with regular monitoring for fluid and nutritional intake, dehydration, somnolence, and other adverse events. Dose reductions or discontinuation of valproate should be considered in patients with decreased food or fluid intake and in patients with excessive somnolence (see **DOSAGE AND ADMINISTRATION**).

Thrombocytopenia

The frequency of adverse effects (particularly elevated liver enzymes and thrombocytopenia [see **PRECAUTIONS**]) may be dose-related. In a clinical trial of DEPAKOTE (divalproex sodium) as monotherapy in patients with epilepsy, 34/126 patients (27%) receiving approximately 50 mg/kg/day on average, had at least one value of platelets $\leq 75 \times 10^9$/L. Approximately half of these patients had treatment discontinued, with return of platelet counts to normal. In the remaining patients, platelet counts normalized with continued treatment. In this study, the probability of thrombocytopenia appeared to increase significantly at total valproate concentrations of ≥ 110 µg/mL (females) or ≥ 135 µg/mL (males). The therapeutic benefit which may accompany the higher doses should therefore be weighed against the possibility of a greater incidence of adverse effects.

Usage In Pregnancy

ACCORDING TO PUBLISHED AND UNPUBLISHED REPORTS, VALPROIC ACID MAY PRODUCE TERATOGENIC EFFECTS IN THE OFFSPRING OF HUMAN FEMALES RECEIVING THE DRUG DURING PREGNANCY.

THE DATA DESCRIBED BELOW WERE GAINED ALMOST EXCLUSIVELY FROM WOMEN WHO RECEIVED VALPROATE TO TREAT EPILEPSY. THERE ARE MULTIPLE REPORTS IN THE CLINICAL LITERATURE WHICH INDICATE THAT THE USE OF ANTIEPILEPTIC DRUGS DURING PREGNANCY RESULTS IN AN INCREASED INCIDENCE OF BIRTH DEFECTS IN THE OFFSPRING. ALTHOUGH DATA ARE MORE EXTENSIVE WITH RESPECT TO TRIMETHADIONE, PARAMETHADIONE, PHENYTOIN, AND PHENOBARBITAL, REPORTS INDICATE A POSSIBLE SIMILAR ASSOCIATION WITH THE USE OF OTHER ANTIEPILEPTIC DRUGS.

THE INCIDENCE OF NEURAL TUBE DEFECTS IN THE FETUS MAY BE INCREASED IN MOTHERS RECEIVING VALPROATE DURING THE FIRST TRIMESTER OF PREGNANCY. THE CENTERS FOR DISEASE CONTROL (CDC) HAS ESTIMATED THE RISK OF VALPROIC ACID EXPOSED WOMEN HAVING CHILDREN WITH SPINA BIFIDA TO BE APPROXIMATELY 1 TO 2%.

OTHER CONGENITAL ANOMALIES (EG, CRANIOFACIAL DEFECTS, CARDIOVASCULAR MALFORMATIONS AND ANOMALIES INVOLVING VARIOUS BODY SYSTEMS), COMPATIBLE AND INCOMPATIBLE WITH LIFE, HAVE BEEN REPORTED. SUFFICIENT DATA TO DETERMINE THE INCIDENCE OF THESE CONGENITAL ANOMALIES IS NOT AVAILABLE.

THE HIGHER INCIDENCE OF CONGENITAL ANOMALIES IN ANTIEPILEPTIC DRUG-TREATED WOMEN WITH SEIZURE DISORDERS CANNOT BE REGARDED AS A CAUSE AND EFFECT RELATIONSHIP. THERE ARE INTRINSIC METHODOLOGIC PROBLEMS IN OBTAINING ADEQUATE DATA ON DRUG TERATOGENICITY IN HUMANS; GENETIC FACTORS OR THE EPILEPTIC CONDITION ITSELF, MAY BE MORE IMPORTANT THAN DRUG THERAPY IN CONTRIBUTING TO CONGENITAL ANOMALIES.

PATIENTS TAKING VALPROATE MAY DEVELOP CLOTTING ABNORMALITIES. A PATIENT WHO HAD LOW FIBRINOGEN WHEN TAKING MULTIPLE ANTICONVULSANTS INCLUDING VALPROATE GAVE BIRTH TO AN INFANT WITH AFIBRINOGENEMIA WHO SUBSEQUENTLY DIED OF HEMORRHAGE. IF VALPROATE IS USED IN PREGNANCY, THE CLOTTING PARAMETERS SHOULD BE MONITORED CAREFULLY.

HEPATIC FAILURE, RESULTING IN THE DEATH OF A NEWBORN AND OF AN INFANT, HAVE BEEN REPORTED FOLLOWING THE USE OF VALPROATE DURING PREGNANCY.

Animal studies have demonstrated valproate-induced teratogenicity. Increased frequencies of malformations, as well as intrauterine growth retardation and death, have been observed in mice, rats, rabbits, and monkeys following prenatal exposure to valproate. Malformations of the skeletal system are the most common structural abnormalities produced in experimental animals, but neural tube closure defects have been seen in mice exposed to maternal plasma valproate concentrations exceeding approximately 230 µg/mL during susceptible periods of embryonic development. Administration of an oral dose of 200 mg/kg/day or greater (approximately 2 times or greater the maximum human daily dose of 1000 mg/day on a mg/m^2 basis) to pregnant rats during organogenesis produced malformations (skeletal, cardiac, and urogenital) and growth retardation in the offspring. These doses resulted in peak maternal plasma valproate levels of approximately 340 µg/mL or greater. Behavioral deficits have been reported in the offspring of rats given a dose of 200 mg/kg/day throughout most of pregnancy. An oral dose of 350 mg/kg/day (approximately 7 times the maximum human daily dose on a mg/m^2 basis) produced skeletal and visceral malformations in rabbits exposed during organogenesis. Skeletal malformations, growth retardation, and death were observed in rhesus monkeys following administration of an oral dose of 200 mg/kg/day (approximately 4 times the maximum human daily dose on a mg/m^2 basis) during organogenesis. This dose resulted in peak maternal plasma valproate levels of approximately 280 µg/mL.

The prescribing physician will wish to weigh the benefits of therapy against the risks in treating or counseling women of childbearing potential. If this drug is used during pregnancy, or if the patient becomes pregnant while taking this drug, the patient should be apprised of the potential hazard to the fetus.

Tests to detect neural tube and other defects using current accepted procedures should be considered a part of routine prenatal care in childbearing women receiving valproate.

PRECAUTIONS

Hepatic Dysfunction

See **BOXED WARNING**, **CONTRAINDICATIONS** and **WARNINGS**.

Pancreatitis

See **BOXED WARNING** and **WARNINGS**.

General

Because of reports of thrombocytopenia (see **WARNINGS**), inhibition of the secondary phase of platelet aggregation, and abnormal coagulation parameters, (e.g., low fibrinogen), platelet counts and coagulation tests are recommended before initiating therapy and at periodic intervals. It is recommended that patients receiving DEPAKOTE be monitored for platelet count and coagulation parameters prior to planned surgery. In a clinical trial of DEPAKOTE as monotherapy in patients with epilepsy, 34/126 patients (27%) receiving approximately 50 mg/kg/day on average, had at least one value of platelets $\leq 75 \times 10^9$/L. Approximately half of these patients had treatment discontinued, with return of platelet counts to normal. In the remaining patients, platelet counts normalized with continued treatment. In this study, the probability of thrombocytopenia appeared to increase significantly at total valproate concentrations of ≥ 110 µg/mL (females) or ≥ 135 µg/mL (males). Evidence of hemorrhage, bruising, or a disorder of hemostasis/coagulation is an indication for reduction of the dosage or withdrawal of therapy.

Hyperammonemia with or without lethargy or coma has been reported and may be present in the absence of abnormal liver function tests. Asymptomatic elevations of ammonia are more common and when present require more frequent monitoring. If clinically significant symptoms occur, DEPAKOTE therapy should be modified or discontinued.

Since DEPAKOTE may interact with concurrently administered drugs which are capable of enzyme induction, periodic plasma concentration determinations of valproate and concomitant drugs are recommended during the early course of therapy where clinically appropriate (see **PRECAUTIONS—Drug Interactions**).

Valproate is partially eliminated in the urine as a keto-metabolite which may lead to a false interpretation of the urine ketone test.

There have been reports of altered thyroid function tests associated with valproate. The clinical significance of these is unknown.

There are *in vitro* studies that suggest valproate stimulates the replication of the HIV and CMV viruses under certain experimental conditions. The clinical consequence, if any, is not known. Additionally, the relevance of these *in vitro* findings is uncertain for patients receiving maximally suppressive antiretroviral therapy. Nevertheless, these data should be borne in mind when interpreting the results from regular monitoring of the viral load in HIV infected patients receiving valproate or when following CMV infected patients clinically.

Continued on next page

Depakote ER—Cont.

Information for Patients
Patients and guardians should be warned that abdominal pain, nausea, vomiting, and/or anorexia can be symptoms of pancreatitis and, therefore, require further medical evaluation promptly.
Since DEPAKOTE products may produce CNS depression, especially when combined with another CNS depressant (eg, alcohol), patients should be advised not to engage in hazardous activities, such as driving an automobile or operating dangerous machinery, until it is known that they do not become drowsy from the drug.
Since DEPAKOTE has been associated with certain types of birth defects, female patients of child-bearing age considering the use of DEPAKOTE ER for the prevention of migraine should be advised to read the **Patient Information Leaflet**, which appears as the last section of the labeling.
Drug Interactions
Effects of Co-Administered Drugs on Valproate Clearance
Drugs that affect the level of expression of hepatic enzymes, particularly those that elevate levels of glucuronosyltransferases, may increase the clearance of valproate. For example, phenytoin, carbamazepine, and phenobarbital (or primidone) can double the clearance of valproate. Thus, patients on monotherapy will generally have longer half-lives and higher concentrations than patients receiving polytherapy with antiepilepsy drugs.
In contrast, drugs that are inhibitors of cytochrome P450 isozymes, e.g., antidepressants, may be expected to have little effect on valproate clearance because cytochrome P450 microsomal mediated oxidation is a relatively minor secondary metabolic pathway compared to glucuronidation and beta-oxidation.
Because of these changes in valproate clearance, monitoring of valproate and concomitant drug concentrations should be increased whenever enzyme inducing drugs are introduced or withdrawn.
The following list provides information about the potential for an influence of several commonly prescribed medications on valproate pharmacokinetics. The list is not exhaustive nor could it be, since new interactions are continuously being reported.
Drugs for which a potentially important interaction has been observed:
Aspirin—A study involving the co-administration of aspirin at antipyretic doses (11 to 16 mg/kg) with valproate to pediatric patients (n=6) revealed a decrease in protein binding and an inhibition of metabolism of valproate. Valproate free fraction was increased 4-fold in the presence of aspirin compared to valproate alone. The β-oxidation pathway consisting of 2-E-valproic acid, 3-OH-valproic acid, and 3-keto valproic acid was decreased from 25% of total metabolites excreted on valproate alone to 8.3% in the presence of aspirin. DEPAKOTE ER is not indicated for use in children (see **PRECAUTIONS—Pediatric Use**). Whether or not the interaction observed in this study applies to adults is unknown, but caution should be observed if valproate and aspirin are to be co-administered.
Felbamate—A study involving the co-administration of 1200 mg/day of felbamate with valproate to patients with epilepsy (n=10) revealed an increase in mean valproate peak concentration by 35% (from 86 to 115 µg/mL) compared to valproate alone. Increasing the felbamate dose to 2400 mg/day increased the mean valproate peak concentration to 133 µg/mL (another 16% increase). A decrease in valproate dosage may be necessary when felbamate therapy is initiated.
Rifampin—A study involving the administration of a single dose of valproate (7 mg/kg) 36 hours after 5 nights of daily dosing with rifampin (600 mg) revealed a 40% increase in the oral clearance of valproate. Valproate dosage adjustment may be necessary when it is co-administered with rifampin.
Drugs for which either no interaction or a likely clinically unimportant interaction has been observed:
Antacids—A study involving the co-administration of valproate 500 mg with commonly administered antacids (Maalox, Trisogel, and Titralac - 160 mEq doses) did not reveal any effect on the extent of absorption of valproate.
Chlorpromazine—A study involving the administration of 100 to 300 mg/day of chlorpromazine to schizophrenic patients already receiving valproate (200 mg BID) revealed a 15% increase in trough plasma levels of valproate.
Haloperidol—A study involving the administration of 6 to 10 mg/day of haloperidol to schizophrenic patients already receiving valproate (200 mg BID) revealed no significant changes in valproate trough plasma levels.
Cimetidine and Ranitidine—Cimetidine and ranitidine do not affect the clearance of valproate.
Effects of Valproate on Other Drugs
Valproate has been found to be a weak inhibitor of some P450 isozymes, epoxide hydrase, and glucuronyltransferases.
The following list provides information about the potential for an influence of valproate co-administration on the pharmacokinetics or pharmacodynamics of several commonly prescribed medications. The list is not exhaustive, since new interactions are continuously being reported.
Drugs for which a potentially important valproate interaction has been observed:
Amitriptyline/Nortriptyline—Administration of a single oral 50 mg dose of amitriptyline to 15 normal volunteers (10 males and 5 females) who received valproate (500 mg BID) resulted in a 21% decrease in plasma clearance of amitriptyline and a 34% decrease in the net clearance of nortriptyline. Rare postmarketing reports of concurrent use of valproate and amitriptyline resulting in an increased amitriptyline level have been received. Concurrent use of valproate and amitriptyline has rarely been associated with toxicity. Monitoring of amitriptyline levels should be considered for patients taking valproate concomitantly with amitriptyline. Consideration should be given to lowering the dose of amitriptyline/ nortriptyline in the presence of valproate.
Carbamazepine/carbamazepine-10,11-Epoxide—Serum levels of carbamazepine (CBZ) decreased 17% while that of carbamazepine-10,11-epoxide (CBZ-E) increased by 45% upon co-administration of valproate and CBZ to epileptic patients.
Clonazepam—The concomitant use of valproic acid and clonazepam may induce absence status in patients with a history of absence type seizures.
Diazepam—Valproate displaces diazepam from its plasma albumin binding sites and inhibits its metabolism. Co-administration of valproate (1500 mg daily) increased the free fraction of diazepam (10 mg) by 90% in healthy volunteers (n=6). Plasma clearance and volume of distribution for free diazepam were reduced by 25% and 20%, respectively, in the presence of valproate. The elimination half-life of diazepam remained unchanged upon addition of valproate.
Ethosuximide—Valproate inhibits the metabolism of ethosuximide. Administration of a single ethosuximide dose of 500 mg with valproate (800 to 1600 mg/day) to healthy volunteers (n=6) was accompanied by a 25% increase in elimination half-life of ethosuximide and a 15% decrease in its total clearance as compared to ethosuximide alone. Patients receiving valproate and ethosuximide, especially along with other anticonvulsants, should be monitored for alterations in serum concentrations of both drugs.
Lamotrigine—In a steady-state study involving 10 healthy volunteers, the elimination half-life of lamotrigine increased from 26 to 70 hours with valproate co-administration (a 165% increase). The dose of lamotrigine should be reduced when co-administered with valproate.
Phenobarbital—Valproate was found to inhibit the metabolism of phenobarbital. Co-administration of valproate (250 mg BID for 14 days) with phenobarbital to normal subjects (n=6) resulted in a 50% increase in half-life and a 30% decrease in plasma clearance of phenobarbital (60 mg single-dose). The fraction of phenobarbital dose excreted unchanged increased by 50% in presence of valproate.
There is evidence for severe CNS depression, with or without significant elevations of barbiturate or valproate serum concentrations. All patients receiving concomitant barbiturate therapy should be closely monitored for neurological toxicity. Serum barbiturate concentrations should be obtained, if possible, and the barbiturate dosage decreased, if appropriate.
Primidone, which is metabolized to a barbiturate, may be involved in a similar interaction with valproate.
Phenytoin—Valproate displaces phenytoin from its plasma albumin binding sites and inhibits its hepatic metabolism. Co-administration of valproate (400 mg TID) with phenytoin (250 mg) in normal volunteers (n=7) was associated with a 60% increase in the free fraction of phenytoin. Total plasma clearance and apparent volume of distribution of phenytoin increased 30% in the presence of valproate. Both the clearance and apparent volume of distribution of free phenytoin were reduced by 25%.
In patients with epilepsy, there have been reports of breakthrough seizures occurring with the combination of valproate and phenytoin. The dosage of phenytoin should be adjusted as required by the clinical situation.
Tolbutamide—From *in vitro* experiments, the unbound fraction of tolbutamide was increased from 20% to 50% when added to plasma samples taken from patients treated with valproate. The clinical relevance of this displacement is unknown.
Warfarin—In an *in vitro* study, valproate increased the unbound fraction of warfarin by up to 32.6%. The therapeutic relevance of this is unknown; however, coagulation tests should be monitored if DEPAKOTE therapy is instituted in patients taking anticoagulants.
Zidovudine—In six patients who were seropositive for HIV, the clearance of zidovudine (100 mg q8h) was decreased by 38% after administration of valproate (250 or 500 mg q8h); the half-life of zidovudine was unaffected.
Drugs for which either no interaction or a likely clinically unimportant interaction has been observed:
Acetaminophen—Valproate had no effect on any of the pharmacokinetic parameters of acetaminophen when it was concurrently administered to three epileptic patients.
Clozapine—In psychotic patients (n=11), no interaction was observed when valproate was co-administered with clozapine.
Lithium—Co-administration of valproate (500 mg BID) and lithium carbonate (300 mg TID) to normal male volunteers (n=16) had no effect on the steady-state kinetics of lithium.
Lorazepam—Concomitant administration of valproate (500 mg BID) and lorazepam (1 mg BID) in normal male volunteers (n=9) was accompanied by a 17% decrease in the plasma clearance of lorazepam.
Oral Contraceptive Steroids—Administration of a single-dose of ethinyloestradiol (50 µg)/levonorgestrel (250 µg) to 6 women on valproate (200 mg BID) therapy for 2 months did not reveal any pharmacokinetic interaction.

Carcinogenesis, Mutagenesis, Impairment of Fertility
Carcinogenesis
Valproic acid was administered orally to Sprague Dawley rats and ICR (HA/ICR) mice at doses of 80 and 170 mg/kg/day (approximately 0.5 to 2 times of the maximum human daily dose of 1000 mg/day on a mg/m^2 basis) for two years. A variety of neoplasms were observed in both species. The chief findings were a statistically significant increase in the incidence of subcutaneous fibrosarcomas in high dose male rats receiving valproic acid and a statistically significant dose-related trend for benign pulmonary adenomas in male mice receiving valproic acid. The significance of these findings for humans is unknown.
Mutagenesis
Valproate was not mutagenic in an *in vitro* bacterial assay (Ames test), did not produce dominant lethal effects in mice, and did not increase chromosome aberration frequency in an *in vivo* cytogenetic study in rats. Increased frequencies of sister chromatid exchange (SCE) have been reported in a study of epileptic children taking valproate, but this association was not observed in another study conducted in adults. There is some evidence that increased SCE frequencies may be associated with epilepsy. The biological significance of an increase in SCE frequency is not known.
Fertility
Chronic toxicity studies in juvenile and adult rats and dogs demonstrated reduced spermatogenesis and testicular atrophy at oral doses of 400 mg/kg/day or greater in rats (approximately 4 times greater the maximum human daily dose of 1000 mg/day on a mg/m^2 basis) and 150 mg/kg/day or greater in dogs (approximately 5 times or greater the maximum human daily dose on a mg/m^2 basis). Segment I fertility studies in rats have shown oral doses up to 350 mg/kg/day (approximately 3.5 times the maximum human daily dose on a mg/m^2 basis) for 60 days to have no effect on fertility. THE EFFECT OF VALPROATE ON TESTICULAR DEVELOPMENT AND ON SPERM PRODUCTION AND FERTILITY IN HUMANS IS UNKNOWN.
Pregnancy
Pregnancy Category D: see **WARNINGS**.
Nursing Mothers
Valproate is excreted in breast milk. Concentrations in breast milk have been reported to be 1–10% of serum concentrations. It is not known what effect this would have on a nursing infant. Consideration should be given to discontinuing nursing when divalproex sodium is administered to a nursing woman.
Pediatric Use
Safety and effectiveness of DEPAKOTE ER in the prophylaxis of migraine in pediatric patients have not been established. Because of the known risks of valproate therapy in pediatric patients when used for other conditions, the use of DEPAKOTE ER in this population is not recommended.
Experience has indicated that pediatric patients under the age of two years are at a considerably increased risk of developing fatal hepatotoxicity, especially those with the aforementioned conditions (see **BOXED WARNING**). Above the age of 2 years, experience in epilepsy has indicated that the incidence of fatal hepatotoxicity decreases considerably in progressively older patient groups.
The basic toxicology and pathologic manifestations of valproate sodium in neonatal (4-day old) and juvenile (14-day old) rats are similar to those seen in young adult rats. However, additional findings, including renal alterations in juvenile rats and renal alterations and retinal dysplasia in neonatal rats, have been reported. These findings occurred at 240 mg/kg/day, a dosage approximately 2 times the human maximum recommended daily dose of 1000 mg/day on a mg/m^2 basis. They were not seen at 90 mg/kg (approximately equivalent to the maximum human daily dose on a mg/m^2 basis).
Geriatric Use
Safety and effectiveness of DEPAKOTE ER in the prophylaxis of migraine patients over 65 have not been established.
No patients above the age of 65 years were enrolled in double-blind prospective clinical trials of mania associated with bipolar illness using DEPAKOTE DELAYED-RELEASE TABLETS. In a case review study of 583 patients using various valproate products, 72 patients (12%) were greater than 65 years of age. A higher percentage of patients above 65 years of age reported accidental injury, infection, pain, somnolence, and tremor. Discontinuation of valproate was occasionally associated with the latter two events. It is not clear whether these events indicate additional risk or whether they result from preexisting medical illness and concomitant medication use among these patients.
A study of elderly patients with dementia revealed drug related somnolence and discontinuation for somnolence (see **WARNINGS—Somnolence in the Elderly**). The starting dose should be reduced in these patients, and dosage reductions or discontinuation should be considered in patients with excessive somnolence (see **DOSAGE AND ADMINISTRATION**).

ADVERSE REACTIONS
Migraine
Based on the results of one multicenter, randomized, double-blind, placebo-controlled clinical trial, DEPAKOTE ER was well tolerated in the prophylactic treatment of migraine headache. Of the 122 patients exposed to DEPAKOTE ER in the placebo-controlled study, 8% discontinued for adverse events, compared to 9% for the 115 placebo patients.

Based on two placebo-controlled clinical trials and their long term extension, DEPAKOTE DELAYED-RELEASE tablets were generally well tolerated with most adverse events rated as mild to moderate in severity. Of the 202 patients exposed to DEPAKOTE DELAYED-RELEASE tablets in the placebo-controlled trials, 17% discontinued for intolerance. This is compared to a rate of 5% for the 81 placebo patients. Including the long term extension study, the adverse events reported as the primary reason for discontinuation by ≥ 1% of 248 DEPAKOTE DELAYED RELEASE-treated patients were alopecia (6%), nausea and/or vomiting (5%), weight gain (2%), tremor (2%), somnolence (1%), elevated SGOT and/or SGPT (1%), and depression (1%).

Table 1 includes those adverse events reported for patients in the placebo-controlled trial where the incidence rate in the DEPAKOTE ER-treated group was greater than 5% and was greater than that for placebo patients.

Table 1
Adverse Events Reported by >5% of DEPAKOTE ER-Treated Patients During the Migraine Placebo-Controlled Trial with a Greater Incidence than Patients Taking Placebo[1]

Body System Event	Depakote ER (N=122)	Placebo (N=115)
Gastrointestinal System		
Nausea	15%	9%
Dyspepsia	7%	4%
Diarrhea	7%	3%
Vomiting	7%	2%
Abdominal Pain	7%	5%
Nervous System		
Somnolence	7%	2%
Other		
Infection	15%	14%

[1] The following adverse events occurred in greater than 5% of DEPAKOTE ER-treated patients and at a greater incidence for placebo than for DEPAKOTE ER: asthenia and flu syndrome.

The following additional adverse events were reported by greater than 1% but not more than 5% of DEPAKOTE ER-treated patients and with a greater incidence than placebo in the placebo-controlled clinical trial for migraine prophylaxis:

Body as a Whole: Accidental injury, viral infection.
Digestive System: Increased appetite, tooth disorder.
Metabolic and Nutritional Disorders: Edema, weight gain.
Nervous System: Abnormal gait, dizziness, hypertonia, insomnia, nervousness, tremor, vertigo.
Respiratory System: Pharyngitis, rhinitis.
Skin and Appendages: Rash.
Special Senses: Tinnitus.

Table 2 includes those adverse events reported for patients in the placebo-controlled trials where the incidence rate in the DEPAKOTE DELAYED-RELEASE-treated group was greater than 5% and was greater than that for placebo patients.

Table 2
Adverse Events Reported by >5% of DEPAKOTE DELAYED-RELEASE-Treated Patients During Migraine Placebo-Controlled Trials with a Greater Incidence than Patients Taking Placebo[1]

Body System Event	Depakote Delayed Release (N=202)	Placebo (N=81)
Gastrointestinal System		
Nausea	31%	10%
Dyspepsia	13%	9%
Diarrhea	12%	7%
Vomiting	11%	1%
Abdominal Pain	9%	4%
Increased Appetite	6%	4%
Nervous System		
Asthenia	20%	9%
Somnolence	17%	5%
Dizziness	12%	6%
Tremor	9%	0%
Other		
Weight Gain	8%	2%
Back Pain	8%	6%
Alopecia	7%	1%

[1] The following adverse events occurred in greater than 5% of DEPAKOTE DELAYED-RELEASE-treated patients and at a greater incidence for placebo than for DEPAKOTE DELAYED-RELEASE: flu syndrome and pharyngitis.

The following additional adverse events not referred to above were reported by greater than 1% but not more than 5% of DEPAKOTE DELAYED-RELEASE-treated patients and with a greater incidence than placebo in the placebo-controlled clinical trials:

Body as a Whole: Chest pain.
Cardiovascular System: Vasodilatation.
Digestive System: Constipation, dry mouth, flatulence, stomatitis.
Hemic and Lymphatic System: Ecchymosis.
Metabolic and Nutritional Disorders: Peripheral edema.
Musculoskeletal System: Leg cramps.
Nervous System: Abnormal dreams, confusion, paresthesia, speech disorder, thinking abnormalities.
Respiratory System: Dyspnea, sinusitis.
Skin and Appendages: Pruritus.
Urogenital System: Metrorrhagia.

Other Patient Populations

The following adverse events not listed previously were reported by greater than 1% of DEPAKOTE DELAYED-RELEASE-treated patients and with a greater incidence than placebo in placebo-controlled trials of epilepsy or manic episodes associated with bipolar disorder:

Body as a Whole: Chills, chills and fever, drug level increased, fever, headache, malaise, neck rigidity.
Cardiovascular System: Arrhythmia, hypertension, hypotension, palpitation, postural hypotension.
Digestive System: Anorexia, dysphagia, eructation, fecal incontinence, gastroenteritis, glossitis, gum hemorrhage, hematemesis, mouth ulceration, periodontal abscess.
Hemic and Lymphatic System: Anemia, bleeding time increased, leukopenia, petechia.
Metabolic and Nutritional Disorders: Hypoproteinemia, SGOT increased, SGPT increased, weight loss.
Musculoskeletal System: Arthralgia, arthrosis, twitching.
Nervous System: Agitation, amnesia, ataxia, catatonic reaction, depression, diplopia, dysarthria, emotional lability, hallucinations, hypokinesia, incoordination, nystagmus, psychosis, reflexes increased, sleep disorder, tardive dyskinesia.
Respiratory System: Bronchitis, hiccup, pneumonia.
Skin and Appendages: Discoid lupus erythematosis, dry skin, erythema nodosum, furunculosis, maculopapular rash, seborrhea, sweating, vesiculobullous rash.
Special Senses: Amblyopia, conjunctivitis, deafness, dry eyes, eye disorder, eye pain, photophobia, taste perversion.
Urogenital System: Cystitis, dysmenorrhea, menstrual disorder, urinary incontinence, vaginitis.

Adverse events that have been reported with all dosage forms of valproate from epilepsy trials, spontaneous reports, and other sources are listed below by body system.

Gastrointestinal: The most commonly reported side effects at the initiation of therapy are nausea, vomiting, and indigestion. These effects are usually transient and rarely require discontinuation of therapy. Diarrhea, abdominal cramps, and constipation have been reported. Both anorexia with some weight loss and increased appetite with weight gain have also been reported.

CNS Effects: Sedative effects have occurred in patients receiving valproate alone but occur most often in patients receiving concomitant therapy with antiepileptic medication. Sedation usually abates upon reduction of other antiepileptic medication. Tremor (may be dose-related), hallucinations, ataxia, headache, nystagmus, diplopia, asterixis, "spots before eyes", dysarthria, dizziness, confusion, hypesthesia, vertigo, incoordination, and parkinsonism. Rare cases of coma have occurred in patients receiving valproate alone or in conjunction with phenobarbital. In rare instances encephalopathy with fever has developed shortly after the introduction of valproate monotherapy without evidence of hepatic dysfunction or inappropriate plasma levels; all patients recovered after the drug was withdrawn.

Several reports have noted reversible cerebral atrophy and dementia in association with valproate therapy.

Dermatologic: Transient hair loss, skin rash, photosensitivity, generalized pruritus, erythema multiforme, and Stevens-Johnson syndrome. Rare cases of toxic epidermal necrolysis have been reported including a fatal case in a 6 month old infant taking valproate and several other concomitant medications. An additional case of toxic epidermal necrosis resulting in death was reported in a 35 year old patient with AIDS taking several concomitant medications and with a history of multiple cutaneous drug reactions.

Psychiatric: Emotional upset, depression, psychosis, aggression, hyperactivity, hostility, and behavioral deterioration.

Musculoskeletal: Weakness.

Hematologic: Thrombocytopenia and inhibition of the secondary phase of platelet aggregation may be reflected in altered bleeding time, petechiae, bruising, hematoma formation, epistaxis, and frank hemorrhage (see **PRECAUTIONS—General and Drug Interactions**). Relative lymphocytosis, macrocytosis, hypofibrinogenemia, leukopenia, eosinophilia, anemia including macrocytic with or without folate deficiency, bone marrow suppression, pancytopenia, aplastic anemia, and acute intermittent porphyria.

Hepatic: Minor elevations of transaminases (eg, SGOT and SGPT) and LDH are frequent and appear to be dose-related. Occasionally, laboratory test results include increases in serum bilirubin and abnormal changes in other liver function tests. These results may reflect potentially serious hepatotoxicity (see **WARNINGS**).

Endocrine: Irregular menses, secondary amenorrhea, breast enlargement, galactorrhea, and parotid gland swelling. Abnormal thyroid function tests (see **PRECAUTIONS**).

There have been rare spontaneous reports of polycystic ovary disease. A cause and effect relationship has not been established.

Pancreatic: Acute pancreatitis including fatalities (see **WARNINGS**).

Metabolic: Hyperammonemia (see **PRECAUTIONS**), hyponatremia, and inappropriate ADH secretion.

There have been rare reports of Fanconi's syndrome occurring chiefly in children.

Decreased carnitine concentrations have been reported although the clinical relevance is undetermined.

Hyperglycinemia has occurred and was associated with a fatal outcome in a patient with preexistent nonketotic hyperglycinemia.

Genitourinary: Enuresis and urinary tract infection.

Special Senses: Hearing loss, either reversible or irreversible, has been reported; however, a cause and effect relationship has not been established. Ear pain has also been reported.

Other: Anaphylaxis, edema of the extremities, lupus erythematosus, bone pain, cough increased, pneumonia, otitis media, bradycardia, cutaneous vasculitis, and fever.

OVERDOSAGE

Overdosage with valproate may result in somnolence, heart block, and deep coma. Fatalities have been reported; however patients have recovered from valproate levels as high as 2120 μg/mL.

In overdose situations, the fraction of drug not bound to protein is high and hemodialysis or tandem hemodialysis plus hemoperfusion may result in significant removal of drug. The benefit of gastric lavage or emesis will vary with the time since ingestion. General supportive measures should be applied with particular attention to the maintenance of adequate urinary output.

Naloxone has been reported to reverse the CNS depressant effects of valproate overdosage.

DOSAGE AND ADMINISTRATION

DEPAKOTE ER is an extended-release product intended for once-a-day oral administration. DEPAKOTE ER tablets should be swallowed whole and should not be crushed or chewed.

The recommended starting dose is 500 mg once daily for 1 week, thereafter increasing to 1000 mg once daily. Although doses other than 1000 mg once daily of DEPAKOTE ER have not been evaluated in patients with migraine, the effective dose range of DEPAKOTE DELAYED-RELEASE TABLETS in these patients is 500–1000 mg/day. As with other valproate products, doses of DEPAKOTE ER should be individualized and dose adjustment may be necessary. DEPAKOTE ER TABLETS are not bioequivalent to DEPAKOTE DELAYED-RELEASE TABLETS (see **CLINICAL PHARMACOLOGY**, Pharmacokinetics). If a patient requires smaller dose adjustments than that available with DEPAKOTE ER, DEPAKOTE DELAYED-RELEASE TABLETS should be used instead.

General Dosing Advice

Dosing in Elderly Patients—Due to a decrease in unbound clearance of valproate and possibly a greater sensitivity to somnolence in the elderly, the starting dose should be reduced in these patients. Starting doses in the elderly lower than 500 mg can only be achieved by the use of DEPAKOTE DELAYED-RELEASE TABLETS. Dosage should be increased more slowly and with regular monitoring for fluid and nutritional intake, dehydration, somnolence, and other adverse events. Dose reductions or discontinuation of valproate should be considered in patients with decreased food or fluid intake and in patients with excessive somnolence. The ultimate therapeutic dose should be achieved on the basis of both tolerability and clinical response (see **WARNINGS**).

Dose-Related Adverse Events—The frequency of adverse effects (particularly elevated liver enzymes and thrombocytopenia) may be dose-related. The probability of thrombocytopenia appears to increase significantly at total valproate concentrations of ≥ 110 μg/mL (females) or ≥ 135 μg/mL (males) (see **PRECAUTIONS**). The benefit of improved therapeutic effect with higher doses should be weighed against the possibility of a greater incidence of adverse reactions.

G.I. Irritation—Patients who experience G.I. irritation may benefit from administration of the drug with food or by initiating therapy with a lower dose of DEPAKOTE DELAYED-RELEASE TABLETS.

Compliance—Patients should be informed to take DEPAKOTE ER every day as prescribed. If a dose is missed it should be taken as soon as possible, unless it is almost time for the next dose. If a dose is skipped, the patient should not double the next dose.

HOW SUPPLIED

DEPAKOTE ER is available as gray tablets with the corporate logo ᗩ, and the Abbo-Code HC. Each DEPAKOTE ER tablet contains divalproex sodium equivalent to 500 mg of valproic acid in the following packaging sizes:

Bottles of 100 .... (**NDC** 0074-7126-13).
Bottles of 500 .... (**NDC** 0074-7126-53).
ABBO-PAC unit dose packages of 100 . (**NDC** 0074-7126-11).

Recommended storage: Store tablets at 25°C (77°F); excursions permitted to 15-30°C (59-86°F) [see USP Controlled Room Temperature].

Revised: August, 2000

Manufactured by:
ABBOTT LABORATORIES
NORTH CHICAGO, IL 60064, U.S.A.

Patient Information Leaflet

Important Information for Women Who Could Become Pregnant About the Use of Depakote® ER (divalproex sodium) Tablets for Migraine

Continued on next page

Depakote ER—Cont.

Please read this leaflet carefully before you take Depakote® ER (divalproex sodium) tablets. This leaflet provides a summary of important information about taking Depakote ER for migraine to women who could become pregnant. Depakote ER may also be prescribed for uses other than those discussed in this leaflet. If you have any questions or concerns, or want more information about Depakote ER, contact your doctor or pharmacist.

Information For Women Who Could Become Pregnant

Depakote ER is used to prevent or reduce the number of migraines you experience. Depakote ER can be obtained only by prescription from your doctor. The decision to use Depakote ER for the prevention of migraine is one that you and your doctor should make together, taking into account your individual needs and medical condition.

Before using Depakote ER, women who can become pregnant should consider the fact that Depakote has been associated with birth defects, in particular, with spina bifida and other defects related to failure of the spinal canal to close normally. Although the incidence is unknown in migraine patients treated with Depakote, approximately 1 to 2% of children born to women with epilepsy taking Depakote in the first 12 weeks of pregnancy had these defects (based on data from the Centers for Disease Control, a U.S. agency based in Atlanta). The incidence in the general population is 0.1 to 0.2%.

Information For Women Who Are Planning To Get Pregnant

- Women taking Depakote ER for the prevention of migraine who are planning to get pregnant should discuss with their doctor temporarily stopping Depakote ER, before and during their pregnancy.

Information For Women Who Become Pregnant While Taking Depakote ER

- If you become pregnant while taking Depakote ER for the prevention of migraine, you should contact your doctor immediately.

Other Important Information About Depakote ER Tablets

- Depakote ER tablets should be taken exactly as it is prescribed by your doctor to get the most benefits from Depakote ER and reduce the risk of side effects.
- If you have taken more than the prescribed dose of Depakote ER, contact your hospital emergency room or local poison center immediately.
- This medication was prescribed for your particular condition. Do not use it for another condition or give the drug to others.

Facts About Birth Defects

It is important to know that birth defects may occur even in children of individuals not taking any medications or without any additional risk factors.

Facts About Migraine

About 23 million Americans suffer from migraine headaches. About 75% of migraine sufferers are women. A migraine is described as a throbbing headache that gets worse with activity. Migraine may also include nausea and/or vomiting as well as sensitivity to light and sound. Migraine usually happens about once a month, but some people may have them as often as once or twice a week. Often, the symptoms from a migraine can cause people to miss work or school.

If you have frequent migraines, or if acute treatment is not working for you, your doctor may prescribe a preventative therapy. Preventative (prophylactic) treatment is used to prevent attacks and reduce the frequency and severity of headache events.

This summary provides important information about the use of Depakote ER for migraine to women who could become pregnant. If you would like more information about the other potential risks and benefits of Depakote ER, ask your doctor or pharmacist to let you read the professional labeling and then discuss it with them. If you have any questions or concerns about taking Depakote ER, you should discuss them with your doctor.

Revised: August, 2000

Manufactured by:
ABBOTT LABORATORIES
NORTH CHICAGO, IL 60064, U.S.A.

IDENTIFICATION PROBLEM?
Turn to the **Product Identification Guide,**
where you'll find more than
1600 products pictured in actual
size and full color.

ALZA Pharmaceuticals,

A division of ALZA Corporation
1900 CHARLESTON ROAD
MOUNTAIN VIEW, CA 94043

Direct Inquiries to:
Customer Service
(800) 227-9953
FAX: (888) 261-8045

For Medical Information or Medical Emergencies Contact:
Medical Communications
(800) 634-8977 or (800) 506-4959
FAX: (650) 962-2488

CONCERTA™ Ⓒ℞

[cŏn certă]
(methylphenidate HCl)
Extended-release Tablets

DESCRIPTION

CONCERTA™ is a central nervous system (CNS) stimulant. CONCERTA™ is available in two tablet strengths. Each extended-release tablet for once-a-day oral administration contains 18 or 36 mg of methylphenidate HCl USP and is designed to have a 12-hour duration of effect. Chemically, methylphenidate HCl is d,l (racemic) methyl α-phenyl-2-piperidineacetate hydrochloride. Its empirical formula is $C_{14}H_{19}NO_2$•HCl. Its structural formula is:

[Structural formula: O, OCH3, H, N, •HCl]

Methylphenidate HCl USP is a white, odorless crystalline powder. Its solutions are acid to litmus. It is freely soluble in water and in methanol, soluble in alcohol, and slightly soluble in chloroform and in acetone. Its molecular weight is 269.77.

CONCERTA™ also contains the following inert ingredients: butylated hydroxytoluene, carnauba wax, cellulose acetate, hydroxypropyl methylcellulose, lactose, phosphoric acid, poloxamer, polyethylene glycol, polyethylene oxides, povidone, propylene glycol, sodium chloride, stearic acid, succinic acid, synthetic iron oxides, titanium dioxide, and triacetin.

System Components and Performance

CONCERTA™ uses osmotic pressure to deliver methylphenidate HCl at a controlled rate. The system, which resembles a conventional tablet in appearance, comprises an osmotically active trilayer core surrounded by a semipermeable membrane with an immediate-release drug overcoat. The trilayer core is composed of two drug layers containing the drug and excipients, and a push layer containing osmotically active components. There is a precision-laser drilled orifice on the drug-layer end of the tablet. In an aqueous environment, such as the gastrointestinal tract, the drug overcoat dissolves within one hour, providing an initial dose of methylphenidate. Water permeates through the membrane into the tablet core. As the osmotically active polymer excipients expand, methylphenidate is released through the orifice. The membrane controls the rate at which water enters the tablet core, which in turn controls drug delivery. The biologically inert components of the tablet remain intact during gastrointestinal transit and are eliminated in the stool as a tablet shell along with insoluble core components.

CLINICAL PHARMACOLOGY

Pharmacodynamics

Methylphenidate HCl is a central nervous system (CNS) stimulant. The mode of therapeutic action in Attention Deficit Hyperactivity Disorder (ADHD) is not known. Methylphenidate is thought to block the reuptake of norepinephrine and dopamine into the presynaptic neuron and increase the release of these monoamines into the extraneuronal space. Methylphenidate is a racemic mixture comprised of the d- and l-isomers. The d-isomer is more pharmacologically active than the l-isomer.

Pharmacokinetics

Absorption

Methylphenidate is readily absorbed. Following oral administration of CONCERTA™ to adults, plasma methylphenidate concentrations increase rapidly reaching an initial maximum at about 1 to 2 hours, then increase gradually over the next several hours. Peak plasma concentrations are achieved at about 6 to 8 hours after which a gradual decrease in plasma levels of methylphenidate begins. CONCERTA™ qd minimizes the fluctuations between peak and trough concentrations associated with immediate-release methylphenidate tid (see Figure 1). The relative bioavailability of CONCERTA™ qd and methylphenidate tid in adults is comparable.

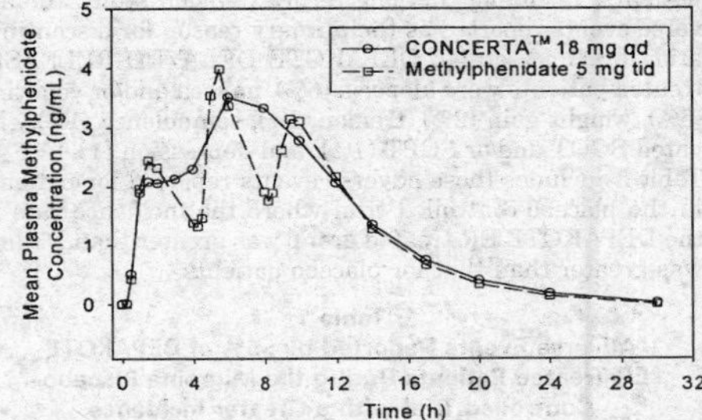

Figure 1. Mean methylphenidate plasma concentrations in 36 adults, following a single dose of CONCERTA™ 18 mg qd and immediate-release methylphenidate 5 mg tid administered every 4 hours.

The mean pharmacokinetic parameters in 36 adults following the administration of CONCERTA™ 18 mg qd and methylphenidate 5 mg tid are summarized in Table 1.
[See table below]

No differences in the pharmacokinetics of CONCERTA™ were noted following single and repeated qd dosing indicating no significant drug accumulation. The AUC and $t_{1/2}$ following repeated qd dosing are similar to those following the first dose of CONCERTA™ 18 mg.

Dose Proportionality

Following administration of CONCERTA™ in single doses of 18, 36, and 54 mg/day to adults, C_{max} and $AUC_{(0\text{-}inf)}$ of d-methylphenidate were proportional to dose, whereas l-methylphenidate C_{max} and $AUC_{(0\text{-}inf)}$ increased disproportionately with respect to dose. Following administration of CONCERTA™, plasma concentrations of the l-isomer were approximately 1/40th the plasma concentrations of the d-isomer.

Distribution

Plasma methylphenidate concentrations in adults decline biexponentially following oral administration. The half-life of methylphenidate in adults following oral administration of CONCERTA™ was approximately 3.5 h.

Metabolism and Excretion

In humans, methylphenidate is metabolized primarily by de-esterification to α-phenyl-piperidine acetic acid (PPA) which has little or no pharmacologic activity. In adults the metabolism of CONCERTA™ qd as evaluated by metabolism to PPA is similar to that of methylphenidate tid. The metabolism of single and repeated qd doses of CONCERTA™ is similar.

After oral dosing of radiolabeled methylphenidate in humans, about 90% of the radioactivity was recovered in urine. The main urinary metabolite was PPA, accounting for approximately 80% of the dose.

Food Effects

In patients, there were no differences in either the pharmacokinetics or the pharmacodynamic performance of CONCERTA™ when administered after a high fat breakfast. There is no evidence of dose dumping in the presence or absence of food.

Special Populations

Gender

In healthy adults, the mean dose-adjusted $AUC_{(0\text{-}inf)}$ values for CONCERTA™ were 36.7 ng•h/mL in men and 37.1 ng•h/mL in women, with no differences noted between the two groups.

Race

In adults receiving CONCERTA™, dose-adjusted $AUC_{(0\text{-}inf)}$ was consistent across ethnic groups; however, the sample size may have been insufficient to detect ethnic variations in pharmacokinetics.

Age

The pharmacokinetics of CONCERTA™ has not been studied in children less than 6 years of age.

Renal Insufficiency

There is no experience with the use of CONCERTA™ in patients with renal insufficiency. After oral administration of radiolabeled methylphenidate in humans, methylphenidate was extensively metabolized and approximately 80% of the radioactivity was excreted in the urine in the form of PPA. Since renal clearance is not an important route of methylphenidate clearance, renal insufficiency is expected to have little effect on the pharmacokinetics of CONCERTA™.

Hepatic Insufficiency

There is no experience with the use of CONCERTA™ in patients with hepatic insufficiency.

Table 1
Mean ± SD Pharmacokinetic Parameters

Parameters	CONCERTA™ (18 mg qd) (n=36)	Methylphenidate (5 mg tid) (n=35)
C_{max} (ng/mL)	3.7 ± 1.0	4.2 ± 1.0
T_{max} (h)	6.8 ± 1.8	6.5 ± 1.8
AUC_{inf} (ng•h/mL)	41.8 ± 13.9	38.0 ± 11.0
$t_{1/2}$ (h)	3.5 ± 0.4	3.0 ± 0.5

Clinical Studies

CONCERTA™ was demonstrated to be effective in the treatment of Attention Deficit Hyperactivity Disorder (ADHD) in three double-blind, active- and placebo-controlled studies in 416 children 6 to 12 years old. The controlled studies compared CONCERTA™ given qd (18, 36, or 54 mg), methylphenidate given tid over 12 hours (15, 30, or 45 mg total daily dose), and placebo in two single-center, 3-week crossover studies (Studies 1 and 2) and in a multicenter, 4-week, parallel-group comparison (Study 3). The primary comparison of interest in all three trials was CONCERTA™ versus placebo.

The Diagnostic and Statistical Manual, 4th edition, of the American Psychiatric Association (DSM-IV) provides criteria for three subtypes of ADHD (Combined Type, Predominantly Inattentive Type, or Predominantly Hyperactive-Impulsive Type). These criteria were used for diagnosis in all three studies.

Symptoms of ADHD were evaluated by community school teachers using the Inattention/Overactivity with Aggression (IOWA) Conners scale. Statistically significant reduction in the Inattention/Overactivity subscale versus placebo was shown consistently across all three controlled studies for CONCERTA™ qd. The scores for CONCERTA™ and placebo for the three studies are presented in Figure 2.

FIGURE 2
Mean (SEM) Community School Teacher IOWA Conners Inattention/Overactivity Scores

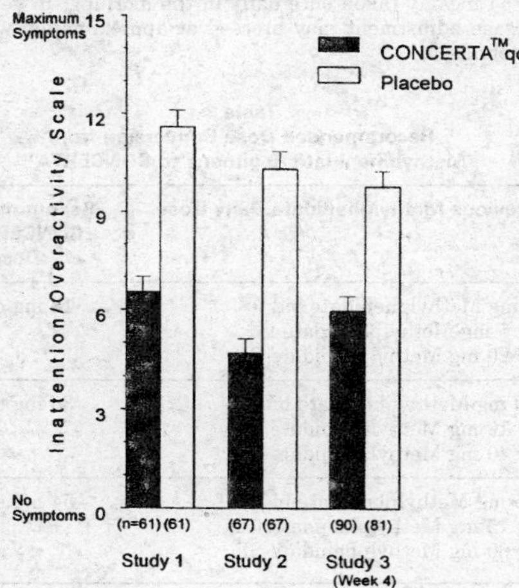

Figure 2: Mean Community School Teacher IOWA Conners Inattention/Overactivity Scores with CONCERTA™ qd (18, 36, or 54 mg) and placebo. Studies 1 and 2 involved a 3-way crossover of 1 week per treatment arm. Study 3 involved 4 weeks of parallel group treatments with a Last Observation Carried Forward analysis at week 4. Error bars represent the mean plus standard error of the mean.

INDICATION AND USAGE

Attention Deficit Hyperactivity Disorder (ADHD)

CONCERTA™ is indicated for the treatment of Attention Deficit Hyperactivity Disorder (ADHD).

The efficacy of CONCERTA™ in the treatment of ADHD was established in three controlled trials of children aged 6 to 12 who met DSM-IV criteria for ADHD (see CLINICAL PHARMACOLOGY).

A diagnosis of Attention Deficit Hyperactivity Disorder (ADHD; DSM-IV) implies the presence of hyperactive-impulsive or inattentive symptoms that caused impairment and were present before age 7 years. The symptoms must cause clinically significant impairment, e.g., in social, academic, or occupational functioning, and be present in two or more settings, e.g., school (or work) and at home. The symptoms must not be better accounted for by another mental disorder. For the Inattentive Type, at least six of the following symptoms must have persisted for at least 6 months: lack of attention to details/careless mistakes; lack of sustained attention; poor listener; failure to follow through on tasks; poor organization; avoids tasks requiring sustained mental effort; loses things; easily distracted; forgetful. For the Hyperactive-Impulsive Type, at least six of the following symptoms must have persisted for at least 6 months: fidgeting/squirming; leaving seat; inappropriate running/climbing; difficulty with quiet activities; "on the go;" excessive talking; blurting answers; can't wait turn; intrusive. The Combined Types requires both inattentive and hyperactive-impulsive criteria to be met.

Special Diagnostic Considerations

Specific etiology of this syndrome is unknown, and there is no single diagnostic test. Adequate diagnosis requires the use not only of medical but of special psychological, educational, and social resources. Learning may or may not be impaired. The diagnosis must be based upon a complete history and evaluation of the child and not solely on the presence of the required number of DSM-IV characteristics.

Need for Comprehensive Treatment Program

CONCERTA™ is indicated as an integral part of a total treatment program for ADHD that may include other measures (psychological, educational, social) for patients with this syndrome. Drug treatment may not be indicated for all children with this syndrome. Stimulants are not intended for use in the child who exhibits symptoms secondary to environmental factors and/or other primary psychiatric disorders, including psychosis. Appropriate educational placement is essential and psychosocial intervention is often helpful. When remedial measures alone are insufficient, the decision to prescribe stimulant medication will depend upon the physician's assessment of the chronicity and severity of the child's symptoms.

Long-Term Use

The effectiveness of CONCERTA™ for long-term use, i.e., for more than 4 weeks, has not been systematically evaluated in controlled trials. Therefore, the physician who elects to use CONCERTA™ for extended periods should periodically re-evaluate the long-term usefulness of the drug for the individual patient (see DOSAGE AND ADMINISTRATION).

CONTRAINDICATIONS

Agitation

CONCERTA™ is contraindicated in patients with marked anxiety, tension, and agitation, since the drug may aggravate these symptoms.

Hypersensitivity to Methylphenidate

CONCERTA™ is contraindicated in patients known to be hypersensitive to methylphenidate or other components of the product.

Glaucoma

CONCERTA™ is contraindicated in patients with glaucoma.

Tics

CONCERTA™ is contraindicated in patients with motor tics or with a family history or diagnosis of Tourette's syndrome (see ADVERSE REACTIONS).

Monoamine Oxidase Inhibitors

CONCERTA™ is contraindicated during treatment with monoamine oxidase inhibitors, and also within a minimum of 14 days following discontinuation of a monoamine oxidase inhibitor (hypertensive crises may result).

WARNINGS

Depression

CONCERTA™ should not be used to treat severe depression.

Fatigue

CONCERTA™ should not be used for the prevention or treatment of normal fatigue states.

Long-Term Suppression of Growth

Sufficient data on the safety of long-term use of methylphenidate in children are not yet available. Although a causal relationship has not been established, suppression of growth (i.e., weight gain, and/or height) has been reported with the long-term use of stimulants in children. Therefore, patients requiring long-term therapy should be carefully monitored. Patients who are not growing or gaining weight as expected should have their treatment interrupted.

Psychosis

Clinical experience suggests that in psychotic patients, administration of methylphenidate may exacerbate symptoms of behavior disturbance and thought disorder.

Seizures

There is some clinical evidence that methylphenidate may lower the convulsive threshold in patients with prior history of seizures, in patients with prior EEG abnormalities in absence of seizures, and, very rarely, in absence of history of seizures and no prior EEG evidence of seizures. In the presence of seizures, the drug should be discontinued.

Potential for Gastrointestinal Obstruction

Because the CONCERTA™ tablet is nondeformable and does not appreciably change in shape in the GI tract, CONCERTA™ should ordinarily not be administered to patients with preexisting severe gastrointestinal narrowing (pathologic or iatrogenic, for example: small bowel inflammatory disease, "short gut" syndrome due to adhesions or decreased transit time, past history of peritonitis, cystic fibrosis, chronic intestinal pseudoobstruction, or Meckel's diverticulum). There have been rare reports of obstructive symptoms in patients with known strictures in association with the ingestion of other drugs in nondeformable controlled-release formulations. Due to the controlled-release design of the tablet, CONCERTA™ should only be used in patients who are able to swallow the tablet whole (see PRECAUTIONS: Information for Patients).

Hypertension and other Cardiovascular Conditions

Use cautiously in patients with hypertension. Blood pressure should be monitored at appropriate intervals in patients taking CONCERTA™, especially patients with hypertension. In the laboratory classroom clinical trials (Studies 1 and 2), both CONCERTA™ and methylphenidate tid increased resting pulse by an average of 2–6 bpm and produced average increases of systolic and diastolic blood pressure of roughly 1–4 mm Hg during the day, relative to placebo. Therefore, caution is indicated in treating patients whose underlying medical conditions might be compromised by increases in blood pressure or heart rate, e.g., those with preexisting hypertension, heart failure, recent myocardial infarction, or hyperthyroidism.

Visual disturbance

Symptoms of visual disturbances have been encountered in rare cases. Difficulties with accommodation and blurring of vision have been reported.

Use in Children Under Six Years of Age

CONCERTA™ should not be used in children under six years, since safety and efficacy in this age group have not been established.

DRUG DEPENDENCE

CONCERTA™ should be given cautiously to patients with a history of drug dependence or alcoholism. Chronic abusive use can lead to marked tolerance and psychological dependence with varying degrees of abnormal behavior. Frank psychotic episodes can occur, especially with parenteral abuse. Careful supervision is required during withdrawal from abusive use since severe depression may occur. Withdrawal following chronic therapeutic use may unmask symptoms of the underlying disorder that may require follow-up.

PRECAUTIONS

Hematologic Monitoring

Periodic CBC, differential, and platelet counts are advised during prolonged therapy.

Information for Patients

Patients should be informed that CONCERTA™ should be swallowed whole with the aid of liquids. Tablets should not be chewed, divided, or crushed. The medication is contained within a nonabsorbable shell designed to release the drug at a controlled rate. The tablet shell, along with insoluble core components, is eliminated from the body; patients should not be concerned if they occasionally notice in their stool something that looks like a tablet.

Patient information is printed at the end of this insert. To assure safe and effective use of CONCERTA™, the information and instructions provided in the patient information section should be discussed with patients.

Drug Interactions

Because of possible effects on blood pressure, CONCERTA™ should be used cautiously with pressor agents.

Human pharmacologic studies have shown that methylphenidate may inhibit the metabolism of coumarin anticoagulants, anticonvulsants (eg, phenobarbital, phenytoin, primidone), and some antidepressants (tricyclics and selective serotonin reuptake inhibitors). Downward dose adjustment of these drugs may be required when given concomitantly with methylphenidate. It may be necessary to adjust the dosage and monitor plasma drug concentrations (or, in the case of coumarin, coagulation times), when initiating or discontinuing concomitant methylphenidate.

Serious adverse events have been reported in concomitant use with clonidine, although no causality for the combination has been established. The safety of using methylphenidate in combination with clonidine or other centrally acting alpha-2 agonists has not been systematically evaluated.

Carcinogenesis, Mutagenesis, and Impairment of Fertility

In a lifetime carcinogenicity study carried out in B6C3F1 mice, methylphenidate caused an increase in hepatocellular adenomas and, in males only, an increase in hepatoblastomas at a daily dose of approximately 60 mg/kg/day. This dose is approximately 30 times and 4 times the maximum recommended human dose of CONCERTA™ on a mg/kg and mg/m^2 basis, respectively. Hepatoblastoma is a relatively rare rodent malignant tumor type. There was no increase in total malignant hepatic tumors. The mouse strain used is sensitive to the development of hepatic tumors, and the significance of these results to humans is unknown.

Methylphenidate did not cause any increases in tumors in a lifetime carcinogenicity study carried out in F344 rats; the highest dose used was approximately 45 mg/kg/day, which is approximately 22 times and 5 times the maximum recommended human dose of CONCERTA™ on a mg/kg and mg/m^2 basis, respectively.

In a 24-week carcinogenicity study in the transgenic mouse strain p53+/−, which is sensitive to genotoxic carcinogens, there was no evidence of carcinogenicity. Male and female mice were fed diets containing the same concentration of methylphenidate as in the lifetime carcinogenicity study; the high-dose groups were exposed to 60 to 74 mg/kg/day of methylphenidate.

Methylphenidate was not mutagenic in the in vitro Ames reverse mutation assay or the in vitro mouse lymphoma cell forward mutation assay. Sister chromatid exchanges and chromosome aberrations were increased, indicative of a weak clastogenic response, in an in vitro assay in cultured Chinese Hamster Ovary cells. Methylphenidate was negative in vivo in males and females in the mouse bone marrow micronucleus assay.

Methylphenidate did not impair fertility in male or female mice that were fed diets containing the drug in an 18-week Continuous Breeding study. The study was conducted at doses up to 160 mg/kg/day, approximately 80-fold and 8-fold the highest recommended human dose of CONCERTA™ on a mg/kg and mg/m^2 basis, respectively.

Pregnancy: Teratogenic Effects

Pregnancy Category C: Methylphenidate has been shown to have teratogenic effects in rabbits when given in doses of 200 mg/kg/day, which is approximately 100 times and 40 times the maximum recommended human dose on a mg/kg and mg/m^2 basis, respectively.

A reproduction study in rats revealed no evidence of harm to the fetus at oral doses up to 30 mg/kg/day, approximately 15-fold and 3-fold the maximum recommended human dose of CONCERTA™ on a mg/kg and mg/m^2 basis, respectively.

Continued on next page

Concerta—Cont.

The approximate plasma exposure to methylphenidate plus its main metabolite PPA in pregnant rats was 2 times that seen in trials in volunteers and patients with the maximum recommended dose of CONCERTA™ based on the AUC. There are no adequate and well-controlled studies in pregnant women. CONCERTA™ should be used during pregnancy only if the potential benefit justifies the potential risk to the fetus.

Nursing Mothers

It is not known whether methylphenidate is excreted in human milk. Because many drugs are excreted in human milk, caution should be exercised if CONCERTA™ is administered to a nursing woman.

Pediatric Use

The safety and efficacy of CONCERTA™ in children under 6 years old have not been established. Long-term effects of methylphenidate in children have not been well established (see WARNINGS).

ADVERSE REACTIONS

The premarketing development program for CONCERTA™ included exposures in a total of 755 participants in clinical trials (469 patients, 286 healthy adult subjects). These participants received CONCERTA™ 18, 36, and/or 54 mg/day. The 469 patients (ages 6 to 13) were evaluated in three controlled clinical studies (Studies 1, 2, and 3), two uncontrolled clinical studies (including a long-term safety study), and one clinical pharmacology study in children with ADHD. Of the 469 patients in this program, 68 CONCERTA™-treated patients in one uncontrolled dose-initiation study were naïve to any pharmacologic therapy for their ADHD. Safety data on all patients are included in the discussion that follows. Adverse reactions were assessed by collecting adverse events, results of physical examinations, vital signs, weights, laboratory analyses, and ECGs.

Adverse events during exposure were obtained primarily by general inquiry and recorded by clinical investigators using terminology of their own choosing. Consequently, it is not possible to provide a meaningful estimate of the proportion of individuals experiencing adverse events without first grouping similar types of events into a smaller number of standardized event categories. In the tables and listings that follow, COSTART terminology has been used to classify reported adverse events.

The stated frequencies of adverse events represent the proportion of individuals who experienced, at least once, a treatment-emergent adverse event of the type listed. An event was considered treatment emergent if it occurred for the first time or worsened while receiving therapy following baseline evaluation.

Adverse Findings in Clinical Trials with CONCERTA™

Adverse Events Associated with Discontinuation of Treatment

In the 4-week placebo-controlled, parallel-group trial one CONCERTA™-treated patient (0.9%; 1/106) and one placebo-treated patient (1.0%; 1/99) discontinued due to an adverse event (sadness and increase in tics, respectively).

In uncontrolled studies up to 12 months with CONCERTA™, 6.6% (29/441) patients discontinued for adverse events. Those events associated with discontinuation of CONCERTA™ in more than one patient included the following: twitching (tics, 1.8%); anorexia (loss of appetite, 0.9%); aggravation reaction (0.7%); hostility (0.7%); insomnia (0.7%); and somnolence (0.5%).

Adverse Events Occurring at an Incidence of 1% or more Among CONCERTA™-Treated Patients

Table 2 enumerates, for a 4-week placebo-controlled, parallel-group trial in children with ADHD at CONCERTA™ doses of 18, 36, or 54 mg/day, the incidence of treatment-emergent adverse events. The table includes only those events that occurred in 1% or more of patients treated with CONCERTA™ where the incidence in patients treated with CONCERTA™ was greater than the incidence in placebo-treated patients.

The prescriber should be aware that these figures cannot be used to predict the incidence of adverse events in the course of usual medical practice where patient characteristics and other factors differ from those which prevailed in the clinical trials. Similarly, the cited frequencies cannot be compared with figures obtained from other clinical investigations involving different treatments, uses, and investigators. The cited figures, however, do provide the prescribing physician with some basis for estimating the relative contribution of drug and non-drug factors to the adverse event incidence rate in the population studied.

[See table below]

Tics

In a long-term uncontrolled study (n=407 children), the cumulative incidence of new onset of tics was 8% after 10 months of treatment with CONCERTA™.

Adverse Events with Other Methylphenidate HCl Products

Nervousness and insomnia are the most common adverse reactions reported with other methylphenidate products. Other reactions include hypersensitivity (including skin rash, urticaria, fever, arthralgia, exfoliative dermatitis, erythema multiforme with histopathological findings of necrotizing vasculitis, and thrombocytopenic purpura); anorexia; nausea; dizziness; palpitations; headache; dyskinesia; drowsiness; blood pressure and pulse changes, both up and down; tachycardia; angina; cardiac arrhythmia; abdominal pain; weight loss during prolonged therapy. There have been rare reports of Tourette's syndrome. Toxic psychosis has been reported. Although a definite causal relationship has not been established, the following have been reported in patients taking this drug: instances of abnormal liver function, ranging from transaminase elevation to hepatic coma; isolated cases of cerebral arteritis and/or occlusion; leukopenia and/or anemia; transient depressed mood; a few instances of scalp hair loss. Very rare reports of neuroleptic malignant syndrome (NMS) have been received, and, in most of these, patients were concurrently receiving therapies associated with NMS. In a single report, a ten year old boy who had been taking methylphenidate for approximately 18 months experienced an NMS-like event within 45 minutes of ingesting his first dose of venlafaxine. It is uncertain whether this case represented a drug-drug interaction, a response to either drug alone, or some other cause.

In children, loss of appetite, abdominal pain, weight loss during prolonged therapy, insomnia, and tachycardia may occur more frequently; however, any of the other adverse reactions listed above may also occur.

DRUG ABUSE AND DEPENDENCE

Controlled Substance Class

CONCERTA™, like other methylphenidate products, is classified as a Schedule II controlled substance by federal regulation.

Abuse, Dependence, and Tolerance

See WARNINGS for boxed warning containing drug abuse and dependence information.

OVERDOSAGE

Signs and Symptoms

Signs and symptoms of acute methylphenidate overdosage, resulting principally from overstimulation of the CNS and from excessive sympathomimetic effects, may include the following: vomiting, agitation, tremors, hyperreflexia, muscle twitching, convulsions (may be followed by coma), euphoria, confusion, hallucinations, delirium, sweating, flushing, headache, hyperpyrexia, tachycardia, palpitations, cardiac arrhythmias, hypertension, mydriasis, and dryness of mucous membranes.

Recommended Treatment

Treatment consists of appropriate supportive measures. The patient must be protected against self-injury and against external stimuli that would aggravate overstimulation already present. Gastric contents may be evacuated by gastric lavage as indicated. Before performing gastric lavage, control agitation and seizures if present and protect the airway. Other measures to detoxify the gut include administration of activated charcoal and a cathartic. Intensive care must be provided to maintain adequate circulation and respiratory exchange; external cooling procedures may be required for hyperpyrexia.

Efficacy of peritoneal dialysis or extracorporeal hemodialysis for CONCERTA™ overdosage has not been established.

The prolonged release of methylphenidate from CONCERTA™ should be considered when treating patients with overdose.

Poison Control Center

As with the management of all overdosage, the possibility of multiple drug ingestion should be considered. The physician may wish to consider contacting a poison control center for up-to-date information on the management of overdosage with methylphenidate.

DOSAGE AND ADMINISTRATION

CONCERTA™ is administered orally once daily in the morning.

CONCERTA™ must be swallowed whole with the aid of liquids, and must not be chewed, divided, or crushed. See PRECAUTIONS: Information for Patients.

CONCERTA™ may be administered with or without food and should be administered once daily in the morning.

Dosage should be individualized according to the needs and responses of the patient.

Patients New to Methylphenidate

The recommended starting dose of CONCERTA™ for patients who are not currently taking methylphenidate, or for patients who are on stimulants other than methylphenidate, is 18 mg once daily.

Dosage may be adjusted in 18 mg increments to a maximum of 54 mg/day taken once daily in the morning. In general, dosage adjustment may proceed at approximately weekly intervals.

Patients Currently Using Methylphenidate

The recommended dose of CONCERTA™ for patients who are currently taking methylphenidate bid, tid, or sustained-release (SR) at doses of 10 to 60 mg/day is provided in Table 3. Dosing recommendations are based on current dose regimen and clinical judgement.

Dosage may be adjusted in 18 mg increments to a maximum of 54 mg/day taken once daily in the morning. In general, dosage adjustment may proceed at approximately weekly intervals.

Table 3
Recommended Dose Conversion from Methylphenidate Regimens to CONCERTA™

Previous Methylphenidate Daily Dose	Recommended CONCERTA™ Dose
5 mg Methylphenidate bid or 5 mg Methylphenidate tid or 20 mg Methylphenidate-SR	18 mg q am
10 mg Methylphenidate bid or 10 mg Methylphenidate tid or 40 mg Methylphenidate-SR	36 mg q am
15 mg Methylphenidate bid or 15 mg Methylphenidate tid or 60 mg Methylphenidate-SR	54 mg q am

Other methylphenidate regimens: Clinical judgement should be used when selecting the starting dose.

Daily dosage above 54 mg is not recommended.

Maintenance/Extended Treatment

There is no body of evidence available from controlled trials to indicate how long the patient with ADHD should be treated with CONCERTA™. It is generally agreed, however, that pharmacological treatment of ADHD may be needed for extended periods. Nevertheless, the physician who elects to use CONCERTA™ for extended periods in patients with ADHD should periodically re-evaluate the long-term usefulness of the drug for the individual patient with trials off medication to assess the patient's functioning without pharmacotherapy. Improvement may be sustained when the drug is either temporarily or permanently discontinued.

Dose Reduction and Discontinuation

If paradoxical aggravation of symptoms or other adverse events occur, the dosage should be reduced, or, if necessary, the drug should be discontinued.

If improvement is not observed after appropriate dosage adjustment over a one-month period, the drug should be discontinued.

HOW SUPPLIED

CONCERTA™ (methylphenidate HCl) Extended-release Tablets are available in 18 mg and 36 mg dosage strengths. The 18 mg tablets are yellow and imprinted with "alza 18". The 36 mg tablets are white and imprinted with "alza 36". Both dosage strengths are supplied in bottles containing 100 tablets.

18 mg	100 count bottle	NDC 17314-5850-2
36 mg	100 count bottle	NDC 17314-5851-2

Storage

Store at 25°C (77°F); excursions permitted to 15–30°C (59–86°F) [see USP Controlled Room Temperature]. Protect from humidity.

REFERENCE

American Psychiatric Association. Diagnosis and Statistical Manual of Mental Disorders. 4th ed. Washington DC: American Psychiatric Association 1994.

Rx Only.

For more information call 1-888-440-7903 or visit www.concerta.net

Manufactured, distributed, and marketed by ALZA Corporation, Mountain View, CA 94043. Marketed by McNeil Consumer Healthcare, Fort Washington, PA 19034.
0009436-4 PI
Edition: 08/2000

Table 2
Incidence of Treatment-Emergent Events[1] in a 4-Week Placebo-Controlled Clinical Trial of CONCERTA™

Body System	Preferred Term	CONCERTA™ (n=106)	Placebo (n=99)
General	Headache	14%	10%
	Abdominal pain (stomach ache)	7%	1%
Digestive	Vomiting	4%	3%
	Anorexia (loss of appetite)	4%	0%
Nervous	Dizziness	2%	0%
	Insomnia	4%	1%
Respiratory	Upper Respiratory Tract Infection	8%	5%
	Cough Increased	4%	2%
	Pharyngitis	4%	3%
	Sinusitis	3%	0%

Events, regardless of causality, for which the incidence for patients treated with CONCERTA™ was at least 1% and greater than the incidence among placebo-treated patients. Incidence greater than 1% has been rounded to the nearest whole number.

INFORMATION FOR PATIENTS TAKING CONCERTA™ OR THEIR PARENTS OR CAREGIVERS
CONCERTA™ (methylphenidate HCl) Extended-release Tablets CII
This information is for patients or their parents or caregivers taking CONCERTA™ Extended-release tablets CII for the treatment of Attention Deficit Hyperactivity Disorder. Please read this before you start taking CONCERTA™. Remember, this information does not take the place of your doctor's instructions. If you have any questions about this information or about CONCERTA™, talk to your doctor or pharmacist.
What is CONCERTA™?
CONCERTA™ is a once-a-day treatment for Attention Deficit Hyperactivity Disorder, or ADHD. CONCERTA™ contains the drug methylphenidate, a central nervous system stimulant that has been used to treat ADHD for more than 30 years. CONCERTA™ is taken by mouth, once each day in the morning.
What is Attention Deficit Hyperactivity Disorder?
ADHD has three main types of symptoms: inattention, hyperactivity, and impulsiveness. Symptoms of inattention include not paying attention, making careless mistakes, not listening, not finishing tasks, not following directions, and being easily distracted. Symptoms of hyperactivity and impulsiveness include fidgeting, talking excessively, running around at inappropriate times, and interrupting others. Some patients have more symptoms of hyperactivity and impulsiveness while others have more symptoms of inattentiveness. Some patients have all three types of symptoms. Many people have symptoms like these from time to time, but patients with ADHD have these symptoms more than others their age. Symptoms must be present for at least 6 months to be certain of the diagnosis.
How does CONCERTA™ work?
Part of the CONCERTA™ tablet dissolves right after you swallow it in the morning, giving you an initial dose of methylphenidate. The remaining drug is slowly released during the day to continue to help lessen the symptoms of ADHD. Methylphenidate, the active ingredient in CONCERTA™, helps increase attention and decrease impulsiveness and hyperactivity in patients with ADHD.
Who should NOT take CONCERTA™?
You should NOT take CONCERTA™ if:
- You have significant anxiety, tension, or agitation since CONCERTA™ may make these conditions worse.
- You are allergic to methylphenidate or any of the other ingredients in CONCERTA™.
- You have glaucoma, an eye disease.
- You have tics or Tourette's Syndrome, or a family history of Tourette's Syndrome.

Talk to your doctor if you believe any of these conditions apply to you.
How should I take CONCERTA™?
Do not chew, crush, or divide the tablets. Swallow CONCERTA™ tablets whole with the help of water or other liquids, such as milk or juice.
Take CONCERTA™ once each day in the morning.
You may take CONCERTA™ before or after you eat.
Take the dose prescribed by your doctor. Your doctor may adjust the amount of drug you take until it is right for you. From time to time, your doctor may interrupt your treatment to check your symptoms while you are not taking the drug.
What are the possible side effects of CONCERTA™?
In the clinical studies with patients using CONCERTA™, the most common side effects were headache, stomach pain, sleeplessness, and decreased appetite. Other side effects seen with methylphenidate, the active ingredient in CONCERTA™, include nausea, vomiting, dizziness, nervousness, tics, allergic reactions, increased blood pressure and psychosis (abnormal thinking or hallucinations).
This is not a complete list of possible side effects. Ask your doctor about other side effects. If you develop any side effect, talk to your doctor.
What must I discuss with my doctor before taking CONCERTA™?
Talk to your doctor ***before*** taking CONCERTA™ if you:
- Are being treated for depression or have symptoms of depression such as feelings of sadness, worthlessness, and hopelessness.
- Have motion tics (hard-to-control, repeated twitching of any parts of your body) or verbal tics (hard-to-control repeating of sounds or words).
- Have someone in your family with motion tics, verbal tics, or Tourette's syndrome.
- Have abnormal thoughts or visions, hear abnormal sounds, or have been diagnosed with psychosis.
- Have had seizures (convulsions, epilepsy) or abnormal EEGs (electroencephalograms).
- Have high blood pressure.
- Have a narrowing or blockage of your gastrointestinal tract (your esophagus, stomach, or small or large intestine).

Tell your doctor ***immediately*** if you develop any of the above conditions or symptoms while taking CONCERTA™.
Can I take CONCERTA™ with other medicines?
Tell your doctor about ***all*** medicines that you are taking. Your doctor should decide whether you can take CONCERTA™ with other medicines. These include:
Other medicines that a doctor has prescribed.
Medicines that you buy yourself without a prescription.
Any herbal remedies that you may be taking.
You should not take CONCERTA™ with monoamine oxidase (MAO) inhibitors.
While on CONCERTA™, do not start taking a new medicine or herbal remedy before checking with your doctor.
CONCERTA™ may change the way your body reacts to certain medicines. These include medicines used to treat depression, prevent seizures, or prevent blood clots (commonly called "blood thinners"). Your doctor may need to change your dose of these medicines if you are taking them with CONCERTA™.
Other Important Safety Information
Abuse of methylphenidate can lead to dependence.
Tell your doctor if you have ever abused or been dependent on alcohol or drugs, or if you are now abusing or dependent on alcohol or drugs.
Before taking CONCERTA™, tell your doctor if you are pregnant or plan on becoming pregnant. If you take methylphenidate, it may be in your breast milk. Tell your doctor if you are nursing a baby.
Tell your doctor if you have blurred vision when taking CONCERTA™.
Slower growth (weight gain and/or height) has been reported with long-term use of methylphenidate in children. Your doctor will be carefully watching your height and weight. If you are not growing or gaining weight as your doctor expects, your doctor may stop your CONCERTA™ treatment.
Call your doctor ***immediately*** if you take more than the amount of CONCERTA™ prescribed by your doctor.
What else should I know about CONCERTA™?
CONCERTA™ has not been studied in children under 6 years of age.
The CONCERTA™ tablet does not dissolve completely after all the drug has been released, and you may sometimes notice it in your stool. This is normal.
CONCERTA™ may be a part of your overall treatment for ADHD. Your doctor may also recommend that you have counseling or other therapy.
As with all medicines, never share CONCERTA™ with anyone else and take only the number of CONCERTA™ tablets prescribed by your doctor.
CONCERTA™ should be stored in a safe place at room temperature (between 59°–86° F). Do not store this medicine in hot, damp, or humid places.
Keep out of the reach of children.
For more information call 1-888-440-7903 or visit www.concerta.net
Manufactured, distributed, and marketed by ALZA Corporation, Mountain View, CA 94043. Marketed by McNeil Consumer Healthcare, Fort Washington, PA 19034.
0009436-4 PPI
Edition: 08/2000
Shown in Product Identification Guide, page 342

Bristol-Myers Squibb Company
P.O. BOX 4500
PRINCETON, NJ 08543-4500

For Medical Information Contact:
Generally:
Bristol-Myers Squibb Drug Information Department
P.O. Box 4500
Princeton, NJ 08543-4500
(800) 321-1335
Adverse Drug Experiences
and Product Defects Reporting call
between 8:30 AM–4:30 PM EST:
(609) 818-3737
Sales and Ordering:
Orders may be placed by:
1. Calling your purchase orders toll-free between 8:30 AM–5:00 PM EST:
(800) 631-5244
2. Mailing your purchase orders to:
Bristol-Myers Squibb U.S. Pharmaceuticals
Attn: Customer Service
P.O. Box 5250
Princeton, NJ 08543-5250
3. Faxing your purchase orders to:
(800) 523-2965
4. Transmitting computer-to-computer on the NWDA and UCS formats through Ordernet Services use: DEA# PE0048579

GLUCOVANCE™ ℞
[glucō-vănce]
(Glyburide and Metformin HCl tablets)
1.25 mg/250 mg
2.5 mg/500 mg
5 mg/500 mg
Rx only

DESCRIPTION
GLUCOVANCE™ (Glyburide and Metformin HCl Tablets) contains two oral antihyperglycemic drugs used in the management of type 2 diabetes, glyburide and metformin hydrochloride.
Glyburide is an oral antihyperglycemic drug of the sulfonylurea class. The chemical name for glyburide is 1-[[p-[2-(5-chloro-o-anisamido) ethyl] phenyl] sulfonyl] -3-cyclohexylurea. Glyburide is a white to off-white crystalline compound with a molecular formula of $C_{23}H_{28}ClN_3O_5S$ and a molecular weight of 494.01. The glyburide used in GLUCOVANCE has a particle size distribution of 25% undersize value not more than 6 µm, 50% undersize value not more than 7–10 µm, and 75% undersize value not more than 21 µm. The structural formula is represented below:

Glyburide

Metformin hydrochloride is an oral antihyperglycemic drug used in the management of type 2 diabetes. Metformin hydrochloride (*N,N*-dimethylimidodicarbonimidic diamide monohydrochloride) is not chemically or pharmacologically related to sulfonylureas, thiazolidinediones, or α-glucosidase inhibitors. It is a white to off-white crystalline compound with a molecular formula of $C_4H_{12}ClN_5$ (monohydrochloride) and a molecular weight of 165.63. Metformin hydrochloride is freely soluble in water and is practically insoluble in acetone, ether, and chloroform. The pKa of metformin is 12.4. The pH of a 1% aqueous solution of metformin hydrochloride is 6.68. The structural formula is as shown:

Metformin Hydrochloride

GLUCOVANCE is available for oral administration in tablets containing 1.25 mg glyburide with 250 mg metformin hydrochloride, 2.5 mg glyburide with 500 mg metformin hydrochloride, and 5 mg glyburide with 500 mg metformin hydrochloride. In addition, each tablet contains the following inactive ingredients: microcrystalline cellulose, povidone, croscarmellose sodium, and magnesium stearate. The tablets are film coated, which provides color differentiation.

CLINICAL PHARMACOLOGY
Mechanism of Action
GLUCOVANCE combines metformin hydrochloride and glyburide, two antihyperglycemic agents with complementary mechanisms of action, to improve glycemic control in patients with type 2 diabetes.
Glyburide appears to lower blood glucose acutely by stimulating the release of insulin from the pancreas, an effect dependent upon functioning beta cells in the pancreatic islets. The mechanism by which glyburide lowers blood glucose during long-term administration has not been clearly established. With chronic administration in patients with type 2 diabetes, the blood glucose lowering effects persists despite a gradual decline in the insulin secretory response to the drug. Extra-pancreatic effects may be involved in the mechanism of action of oral sulfonylulrea hypoglycemic drugs.
Metformin hydrochloride is an antihyperglycemic agent that improves glucose tolerance in patients with type 2 diabetes, lowering both basal and postprandial plasma glucose. Metformin hydrochloride decreases hepatic glucose production, decreases intestinal absorption of glucose, and improves insulin sensitivity by increasing peripheral glucose uptake and utilization.
Pharmacokinetics
Absorption and Bioavailability
GLUCOVANCE
In bioavailability studies of GLUCOVANCE 2.5 mg/500 mg and 5 mg/500 mg, the mean area under the plasma concentration time curve (AUC) for the glyburide component was 18% and 7%, respectively, greater than that of the Micronase® brand of glyburide coadministered with metformin. The glyburide component of GLUCOVANCE, therefore, is not bioequivalent to Micronase®. The metformin component of GLUCOVANCE is bioequivalent to metformin coadministered with glyburide.
Following administration of a single GLUCOVANCE 5 mg/500 mg tablet, with either a 20% glucose solution or a 20% glucose solution with food, there was no effect of food on the C_{max} and a relatively small effect of food on the AUC of the glyburide component. The T_{max} for the glyburide component was shortened from 7.5 hours to 2.75 hours with food compared to the same tablet strength administered fasting with a 20% glucose solution. The clinical significance of an earlier T_{max} for glyburide after food is not known. The effect of food on the pharmacokinetics of the metformin component was indeterminate.
Glyburide
Single-dose studies with Micronase® tablets in normal subjects demonstrate significant absorption of glyburide within one hour, peak drug levels at about four hours, and low but detectable levels at twenty-four hours. Mean serum levels of glyburide, as reflected by areas under the serum concentration-time curve, increase in proportion to corresponding in-

Continued on next page

Glucovance—Cont.

creases in dose. Bioequivalence has not been established between GLUCOVANCE (Glyburide and Metformin HCl tablets) and single ingredient glyburide products.

Metformin hydrochloride

The absolute bioavailability of a 500 mg metformin hydrochloride tablet given under fasting conditions is approximately 50–60%. Studies using single oral doses of metformin tablets of 500 mg and 1500 mg, and 850 mg to 2550 mg, indicate that there is a lack of dose proportionality with increasing doses, which is due to decreased absorption rather than an alteration in elimination. Food decreases the extent of and slightly delays the absorption of metformin, as shown by approximately a 40% lower peak concentration and a 25% lower AUC in plasma and a 35 minute prolongation of time to peak plasma concentration following administration of a single 850 mg tablet of metformin with food, compared to the same tablet strength administered fasting. The clinical relevance of these decreases is unknown.

Distribution

Glyburide

Sulfonylurea drugs are extensively bound to serum proteins. Displacement from protein binding sites by other drugs may lead to enhanced hypoglycemic action. *In vitro*, the protein binding exhibited by glyburide is predominantly non-ionic, whereas that of other sulfonylureas (chlorpropamide, tolbutamide, tolazamide) is predominantly ionic. Acidic drugs such as phenylbutazone, warfarin, and salicylates displace the ionic-binding sulfonylureas from serum proteins to a far greater extent than the non-ionic binding glyburide. It has not been shown that this difference in protein binding results in fewer drug-drug interactions with glyburide tablets in clinical use.

Metformin hydrochloride

The apparent volume of distribution (V/F) of metformin following single oral doses of 850 mg averaged 654±358 L. Metformin is negligibly bound to plasma proteins. Metformin partitions into erythrocytes, most likely as a function of time. At usual clinical doses and dosing schedules of metformin, steady state plasma concentrations of metformin are reached within 24–48 hours and are generally <1 μg/mL. During controlled clinical trials, maximum metformin plasma levels did not exceed 5 μg/mL, even at maximum doses.

Metabolism and Elimination

Glyburide

The decrease of glyburide in the serum of normal healthy individuals is biphasic; the terminal half-life is about 10 hours. The major metabolite of glyburide is the 4-trans-hydroxy derivative. A second metabolite, the 3-cis-hydroxy derivative, also occurs. These metabolites probably contribute no significant hypoglycemic action in humans since they are only weakly active (1/400th and 1/40th as active, respectively, as glyburide) in rabbits. Glyburide is excreted as metabolites in the bile and urine, approximately 50% by each route. This dual excretory pathway is qualitatively different from that of other sulfonylureas, which are excreted primarily in the urine.

Metformin hydrochloride

Intravenous single-dose studies in normal subjects demonstrate that metformin is excreted unchanged in the urine and does not undergo hepatic metabolism (no metabolites have been identified in humans) nor biliary excretion. Renal clearance (see **Table 1**) is approximately 3.5 times greater than creatinine clearance, which indicates that tubular secretion is the major route of metformin elimination. Following oral administration, approximately 90% of the absorbed drug is eliminated via the renal route within the first 24 hours, with a plasma elimination half-life of approximately 6.2 hours. In blood, the elimination half-life is approximately 17.6 hours, suggesting that the erythrocyte mass may be a compartment of distribution.

Special Populations

Patients With Type 2 Diabetes

Multiple-dose studies with glyburide in patients with type 2 diabetes demonstrate drug level concentration-time curves similar to single-dose studies, indicating no buildup of drug in tissue depots.

In the presence of normal renal function, there are no differences between single- or multiple-dose pharmacokinetics of metformin between patients with type 2 diabetes and normal subjects (see **Table 1**), nor is there any accumulation of metformin in either group at usual clinical doses.

Hepatic Insufficiency

No pharmacokinetic studies have been conducted in patients with hepatic insufficiency for either glyburide or metformin.

Renal Insufficiency

No information is available on the pharmacokinetics of glyburide in patients with renal insufficiency.

In patients with decreased renal function (based on creatinine clearance), the plasma and blood half-life of metformin is prolonged and the renal clearance is decreased in proportion to the decrease in creatinine clearance (see **Table 1**; also, see **WARNINGS**).

Geriatrics

There is no information on the pharmacokinetics of glyburide in elderly patients. Limited data from controlled pharmacokinetic studies of metformin in healthy elderly subjects suggest that total plasma clearance is decreased, the half-life is prolonged, and C_{max} is increased, compared to healthy young subjects. From these data, it appears that the change in metformin pharmacokinetics with aging is primarily accounted for by a change in renal function (see **Table 1**). Metformin treatment should not be initiated in patients ≥80 years of age unless measurement of creatinine clearance demonstrates that renal function is not reduced.

[See table 1 above]

Pediatrics

No data from pharmacokinetic studies in pediatric subjects are available for either glyburide or metformin.

Gender

There is no information on the effect of gender on the pharmacokinetics of glyburide. Metformin pharmacokinetic parameters did not differ significantly in subjects with or without type 2 diabetes when analyzed according to gender (males = 19, females = 16). Similarly, in controlled clinical studies in patients with type 2 diabetes, the antihyperglycemic effect of metformin was comparable in males and females.

Race

No information is available on race differences in the pharmacokinetics of glyburide. No studies of metformin pharmacokinetic parameters according to race have been performed. In controlled clinical studies of metformin in patients with type 2 diabetes, the antihyperglycemic effect was comparable in whites (n=249), blacks (n=51), and Hispanics (n=24).

Table 1. Select Mean (±S.D.) Metformin Pharmacokinetic Parameters Following Single or Multiple Oral Doses of Metformin

Subject Groups: Metformin dose[a] (number of subjects)	C_{max}[b] (μg/mL)	T_{max}[c] (hrs)	Renal Clearance (mL/min)
Healthy, nondiabetic adults:			
500 mg SD[d] (24)	1.03 (±0.33)	2.75 (±0.81)	600 (±132)
850 mg SD (74)[e]	1.60 (±0.38)	2.64 (±0.82)	552 (±139)
850 mg t.i.d. for 19 doses[f] (9)	2.01 (±0.42)	1.79 (±0.94)	642 (±173)
Adults with type 2 diabetes:			
850 mg SD (23)	1.48 (±0.5)	3.32 (±1.08)	491 (±138)
850 mg t.i.d. for 19 doses[f] (9)	1.90 (±0.62)	2.01 (±1.22)	550 (±160)
Elderly[g], healthy nondiabetic adults:			
850 mg SD (12)	2.45 (±0.70)	2.71 (±1.05)	412 (±98)
Renal-impaired adults: 850 mg SD			
Mild (CL_{cr}[h] 61–90 mL/min) (5)	1.86 (±0.52)	3.20 (±0.45)	384 (±122)
Moderate (CL_{cr} 31–60 mL/min) (4)	4.12 (±1.83)	3.75 (±0.50)	108 (±57)
Severe (CL_{cr} 10–30 mL/min) (6)	3.93 (±0.92)	4.01 (±1.10)	130 (±90)

[a]-All doses given fasting except the first 18 doses of the multiple-dose studies
[b]-Peak plasma concentration
[c]-Time to peak plasma concentration
[d]-SD = single dose
[e]-Combined results (average means) of five studies: mean age 32 years (range 23–59 years)
[f]-Kinetic study done following dose 19, given fasting
[g]-Elderly subjects, mean age 71 years (range 65–81 years)
[h]-CL_{cr} = creatinine clearance normalized to body surface area of 1.73 m^2

Table 2. Placebo- and Active-Controlled Trial of GLUCOVANCE as Initial Therapy: Summary of Trial Data at 20 Weeks

	Placebo	Glyburide 2.5 mg tablets	Metformin 500 mg tablets	GLUCOVANCE 1.25 mg/250 mg tablets	GLUCOVANCE 2.5 mg/500 mg tablets
Mean Final Dose	0 mg	5.3 mg	1317 mg	2.78 mg/557 mg	4.1 mg/824 mg
Hemoglobin A_{1c}	N=147	N=142	N=141	N=149	N=152
Baseline Mean (%)	8.14	8.14	8.23	8.22	8.20
Mean Change from Baseline	−0.21	−1.24	−1.03	−1.48	−1.53
Difference from Placebo		−1.02	−0.82	−1.26[a]	−1.31[a]
Difference from Glyburide				−0.24[b]	−0.29[b]
Difference from Metformin				−0.44[b]	−0.49[b]
Fasting Plasma Glucose	N=159	N=158	N=156	N=153	N=154
Baseline Mean FPG (mg/dL)	177.2	178.9	175.1	178	176.6
Mean Change from Baseline	4.6	−35.7	−21.2	−41.5	−40.1
Difference from Placebo		−40.3	−25.8	−46.1[a]	−44.7[a]
Difference from Glyburide				−5.8[c]	−4.5[c]
Difference from Metformin				−20.3[c]	−18.9[c]
Body Weight Mean Change from Baseline	−0.7 kg	+1.7 kg	−0.6 kg	+1.4 kg	+1.9 kg
Final HbA_{1c} Distribution (%)	N=147	N=142	N=141	N=149	N=152
< 7%	19.7%	59.9%	50.4%	66.4%	71.7%
≥7% and < 8%	37.4%	26.1%	29.8%	25.5%	19.1%
≥8%	42.9%	14.1%	19.9%	8.1%	9.2%

[a]$p < 0.001$ [b]$p < 0.05$ [c]p = NS

Clinical Studies

Initial Therapy

In a 20-week, double-blind, multicenter U.S. clinical trial, a total of 806 drug-naive patients with type 2 diabetes, whose hyperglycemia was not adequately controlled with diet and exercise alone (baseline fasting plasma glucose [FPG] < 240 mg/dL, baseline hemoglobin A1c [HbA_{1c}] between 7% and 11%), were randomized to receive initial therapy with placebo, 2.5 mg glyburide, 500 mg metformin, GLUCOVANCE 1.25 mg/250 mg, or GLUCOVANCE (Glyburide and Metformin HCl Tablets) 2.5 mg/500 mg. After four weeks, the dose was progressively increased (up to the eight-week visit) to a maximum of four tablets daily as needed to reach a target FPG of 126 mg/dL. Trial data at 20 weeks are summarized in **Table 2**.

[See table 2 above]

Treatment with GLUCOVANCE (Glyburide and Metformin HCl Tablets) resulted in significantly greater reduction in HbA_{1c} and postprandial plasma glucose (PPG) compared to glyburide, metformin, or placebo. Also, GLUCOVANCE therapy resulted in greater reduction in FPG compared to glyburide, metformin, or placebo, but the differences from glyburide and metformin did not reach statistical significance.

Changes in the lipid profile associated with GLUCOVANCE treatment were similar to those seen with glyburide, metformin, and placebo.

Table 3. GLUCOVANCE as Second-Line Therapy: Summary of Trial Data at 16 Weeks

	Glyburide 5 mg tablets	Metformin 500 mg tablets	GLUCOVANCE 2.5 mg/500 mg tablets	GLUCOVANCE 5 mg/500 mg tablets
Mean Final Dose	20 mg	1840 mg	8.8 mg/1760 mg	17 mg/1740 mg
Hemoglobin A_{1c}	N=158	N=142	N=154	N=159
Baseline Mean (%)	9.63	9.51	9.43	9.44
Final Mean	9.61	9.82	7.92	7.91
Difference from Glyburide			−1.69[a]	−1.70[a]
Difference from Metformin			−1.90[a]	−1.91[a]
Fasting Plasma Glucose	N=163	N=152	N=160	N=160
Baseline Mean(mg/dL)	218.4	213.4	212.2	210.2
Final Mean	221.0	233.8	169.6	161.1
Difference from Glyburide			−51.3[a]	−59.9[a]
Difference from Metformin			−64.2[a]	−72.7[a]
Body Weight Mean Change from Baseline	+ 0.43 kg	−2.76 kg	+0.75 kg	+ 0.47 kg
Final HbA_{1c} Distribution (%)	N=158	N=142	N=154	N=159
< 7%	2.5%	2.8%	24.7%	22.6%
≥7% and < 8%	9.5%	11.3%	33.1%	37.1%
≥8%	88%	85.9%	42.2%	40.3%

[a]$p < 0.001$

The double-blind placebo-controlled trial described above restricted enrollment to patients with HbA_{1c} <11% or FPG < 240 mg/dL. Screened patients ineligible for the first trial because of HbA_{1c} and/or FPG exceeding these limits were treated directly with GLUCOVANCE 2.5 mg/500 mg in an open-label uncontrolled protocol. In this study, three out of 173 patients (1.7%) discontinued because of inadequate therapeutic response. Across the group of 144 patients who completed 26 weeks of treatment, mean HbA_{1c} was reduced from a baseline of 10.6% to 7.1%. The mean baseline FPG was 283 mg/dL and was reduced to 164 and 161 mg/dL after 2 and 26 weeks, respectively. The mean final titrated dose of GLUCOVANCE was 7.85 mg/1569 mg (equivalent to approximately three GLUCOVANCE 2.5 mg/500 mg tablets per day).

Second Line Therapy

In a 16-week, double-blind, active-controlled U.S. clinical trial, a total of 639 patients with type 2 diabetes not adequately controlled (mean baseline HbA_{1c} 9.5%, mean baseline FPG 213 mg/dL) while being treated with at least one-half the maximum dose of a sulfonylurea (e.g., glyburide 10 mg, glipizide 20 mg) were randomized to receive glyburide (fixed dose, 20 mg), metformin (500 mg), GLUCOVANCE 2.5 mg/500 mg, or GLUCOVANCE 5 mg/500 mg. The doses of metformin and GLUCOVANCE were titrated to a maximum of four tablets daily as needed to achieve FPG < 140 mg/dL. Trial data at 16 weeks are summarized in **Table 3**.

[See table above]

After 16 weeks, there was no significant change in the mean HbA_{1c} in the patients randomized to glyburide or to metformin therapy. Treatment with GLUCOVANCE at doses up to 20 mg/2000 mg per day resulted in significant lowering of HbA_{1c}, FPG, and PPG from baseline compared to glyburide or metformin alone.

INDICATIONS AND USAGE

GLUCOVANCE is indicated as initial therapy, as an adjunct to diet and exercise, to improve glycemic control in patients with type 2 diabetes whose hyperglycemia cannot be satisfactorily managed with diet and exercise alone.

GLUCOVANCE is indicated as second-line therapy when diet, exercise, and initial treatment with a sulfonylurea or metformin do not result in adequate glycemic control in patients with type 2 diabetes.

CONTRAINDICATIONS

GLUCOVANCE (Glyburide and Metformin HCl Tablets) is contraindicated in patients with:

1. Renal disease or renal dysfunction (e.g., as suggested by serum creatinine levels ≥1.5 mg/dL [males], ≥1.4 mg/dL [females], or abnormal creatinine clearance) which may also result from conditions such as cardiovascular collapse (shock), acute myocardial infarction, and septicemia (see **WARNINGS** and **PRECAUTIONS**).
2. Congestive heart failure requiring pharmacologic treatment.
3. Known hypersensitivity to metformin hydrochloride or glyburide.
4. Acute or chronic metabolic acidosis, including diabetic ketoacidosis, with or without coma. Diabetic ketoacidosis should be treated with insulin.

GLUCOVANCE should be temporarily discontinued in patients undergoing radiologic studies involving intravascular administration of iodinated contrast materials, because use of such products may result in acute alteration of renal function. (See also **PRECAUTIONS**.)

WARNINGS

Metformin Hydrochloride

Lactic Acidosis

Lactic acidosis is a rare, but serious, metabolic complication that can occur due to metformin accumulation during treatment with GLUCOVANCE; when it occurs, it is fatal in approximately 50% of cases. Lactic acidosis may also occur in association with a number of pathophysiologic conditions, including diabetes mellitus, and whenever there is significant tissue hypoperfusion and hypoxemia. Lactic acidosis is characterized by elevated blood lactate levels (>5 mmol/L), decreased blood pH, electrolyte disturbances with an increased anion gap, and an increased lactate/pyruvate ratio. When metformin is implicated as the cause of lactic acidosis, metformin plasma levels >5 µg/mL are generally found.

The reported incidence of lactic acidosis in patients receiving metformin hydrochloride is very low (approximately 0.03 cases/1000 patient-years, with approximately 0.015 fatal cases/1000 patient-years). Reported cases have occurred primarily in diabetic patients with significant renal insufficiency, including both intrinsic renal disease and renal hypoperfusion, often in the setting of multiple concomitant medical/surgical problems and multiple concomitant medications. Patients with congestive heart failure requiring pharmacologic management, in particular those with unstable or acute congestive heart failure who are at risk of hypoperfusion and hypoxemia, are at increased risk of lactic acidosis. The risk of lactic acidosis increases with the degree of renal dysfunction and the patient's age. The risk of lactic acidosis may, therefore, be significantly decreased by regular monitoring of renal function in patients taking metformin and by use of the minimum effective dose of metformin. In particular, treatment of the elderly should be accompanied by careful monitoring of renal function. GLUCOVANCE treatment should not be initiated in patients ≥80 years of age unless measurement of creatinine clearance demonstrates that renal function is not reduced, as these patients are more susceptible to developing lactic acidosis. In addition, GLUCOVANCE should be promptly withheld in the presence of any condition associated with hypoxemia, dehydration, or sepsis. Because impaired hepatic function may significantly limit the ability to clear lactate, GLUCOVANCE should generally be avoided in patients with clinical or laboratory evidence of hepatic disease. Patients should be cautioned against excessive alcohol intake, either acute or chronic, when taking GLUCOVANCE, since alcohol potentiates the effects of metformin hydrochloride on lactate metabolism. In addition, GLUCOVANCE should be temporarily discontinued prior to any intravascular radiocontrast study and for any surgical procedure (see also PRECAUTIONS).

The onset of lactic acidosis often is subtle, and accompanied only by nonspecific symptoms such as malaise, myalgias, respiratory distress, increasing somnolence, and nonspecific abdominal distress. There may be associated hypothermia, hypotension, and resistant bradyarrhythmias with more marked acidosis. The patient and the patient's physician must be aware of the possible importance of such symptoms and the patient should be instructed to notify the physician immediately if they occur (see also PRECAUTIONS). GLUCOVANCE should be withdrawn until the situation is clarified. Serum electrolytes, ketones, blood glucose, and, if indicated, blood pH, lactate levels, and even blood metformin levels may be useful. Once a patient is stabilized on any dose level of GLUCOVANCE, gastrointestinal symptoms, which are common during initiation of therapy with metformin, are unlikely to be drug related. Later occurrence of gastrointestinal symptoms could be due to lactic acidosis or other serious disease.

Levels of fasting venous plasma lactate above the upper limit of normal but less than 5 mmol/L in patients taking GLUCOVANCE do not necessarily indicate impending lactic acidosis and may be explainable by other mechanisms, such as poorly controlled diabetes or obesity, vigorous physical activity, or technical problems in sample handling. (See also PRECAUTIONS.)

Lactic acidosis should be suspected in any diabetic patient with metabolic acidosis lacking evidence of ketoacidosis (ketonuria and ketonemia).

Lactic acidosis is a medical emergency that must be treated in a hospital setting. In a patient with lactic acidosis who is taking GLUCOVANCE, the drug should be discontinued immediately and general supportive measures promptly instituted. Because metformin hydrochloride is dialyzable (with a clearance of up to 170 mL/min under good hemodynamic conditions), prompt hemodialysis is recommended to correct the acidosis and remove the accumulated metformin. Such management often results in prompt reversal of symptoms and recovery. (See also CONTRAINDICATIONS and PRECAUTIONS.)

PRECAUTIONS

General

GLUCOVANCE

Hypoglycemia—GLUCOVANCE (Glyburide and Metformin HCl Tablets) is capable of producing hypoglycemia or hypoglycemic symptoms, therefore, proper patient selection, dosing, and instructions are important to avoid potential hypoglycemic episodes. The risk of hypoglycemia is increased when caloric intake is deficient, when strenuous exercise is not compensated by caloric supplementation, or during concomitant use with other glucose-lowering agents or ethanol. Renal or hepatic insufficiency may cause elevated drug levels of both glyburide and metformin hydrochloride and the hepatic insufficiency may also diminish gluconeogenic capacity, both of which increase the risk of hypoglycemic reactions. Elderly, debilitated, or malnourished patients and those with adrenal or pituitary insufficiency or alcohol intoxication are particularly susceptible to hypoglycemic effects. Hypoglycemia may be difficult to recognize in the elderly, and in people who are taking beta-adrenergic blocking drugs.

Metformin Hydrochloride

Monitoring of renal function—Metformin is known to be substantially excreted by the kidney, and the risk of metformin accumulation and lactic acidosis increases with the degree of impairment of renal function. Thus, patients with serum creatinine levels above the upper limit of normal for their age should not receive GLUCOVANCE. In patients with advanced age, GLUCOVANCE should be carefully titrated to establish the minimum dose for adequate glycemic effect, because aging is associated with reduced renal function. In elderly patients, particularly those ≥80 years of age, renal function should be monitored regularly and, generally, GLUCOVANCE should not be titrated to the maximum dose (see **WARNINGS** and **DOSAGE AND ADMINISTRATION**). Before initiation of GLUCOVANCE therapy and at least annually thereafter, renal function should be assessed and verified as normal. In patients in whom development of renal dysfunction is anticipated, renal function should be assessed more frequently and GLUCOVANCE discontinued if evidence of renal impairment is present.

Use of concomitant medications that may affect renal function or metformin disposition—Concomitant medication(s) that may affect renal function or result in significant hemodynamic change or may interfere with the disposition of metformin, such as cationic drugs that are eliminated by renal tubular secretion (see **PRECAUTIONS: Drug Interactions**), should be used with caution.

Radiologic studies involving the use of intravascular iodinated contrast materials (for example, intravenous urogram, intravenous cholangiography, angiography, and computed tomography (CT) scans with intravascular contrast materials)—Intravascular contrast studies with iodinated materials can lead to acute alteration of renal function and have been associated with lactic acidosis in patients receiving metformin (see **CONTRAINDICATIONS**). Therefore, in patients in whom any such study is planned, GLUCOVANCE should be temporarily discontinued at the time of or prior to the procedure, and withheld for 48 hours subsequent to the procedure and reinstituted only after renal function has been reevaluated and found to be normal.

Hypoxic states—Cardiovascular collapse (shock) from whatever cause, acute congestive heart failure, acute myocardial infarction, and other conditions characterized by hypoxemia have been associated with lactic acidosis and may also cause prerenal azotemia. When such events occur in patients on GLUCOVANCE therapy, the drug should be promptly discontinued.

Continued on next page

Glucovance—Cont.

Surgical procedures—GLUCOVANCE therapy should be temporarily suspended for any surgical procedure (except minor procedures not associated with restricted intake of food and fluids) and should not be restarted until the patient's oral intake has resumed and renal function has been evaluated as normal.
Alcohol intake—Alcohol is known to potentiate the effect of metformin on lactate metabolism. Patients, therefore, should be warned against excessive alcohol intake, acute or chronic, while receiving GLUCOVANCE. Due to its effect on the gluconeogenic capacity of the liver, alcohol may also increase the risk of hypoglycemia.
Impaired hepatic function—Since impaired hepatic function has been associated with some cases of lactic acidosis, GLUCOVANCE should generally be avoided in patients with clinical or laboratory evidence of hepatic disease.
Vitamin B_{12} levels—In controlled clinical trials with metformin of 29 weeks duration, a decrease to subnormal levels of previously normal serum Vitamin B_{12}, without clinical manifestations, was observed in approximately 7% of patients. Such decrease, possibly due to interference with B_{12} absorption from the B_{12}-intrinsic factor complex, is, however, very rarely associated with anemia and appears to be rapidly reversible with discontinuation of metformin or Vitamin B_{12} supplementation. Measurement of hematologic parameters on an annual basis is advised in patients on metformin and any apparent abnormalities should be appropriately investigated and managed (see **PRECAUTIONS: Laboratory Tests**).
Certain individuals (those with inadequate Vitamin B_{12} or calcium intake or absorption) appear to be predisposed to developing subnormal Vitamin B_{12} levels. In these patients, routine serum Vitamin B_{12} measurements at two- to three-year intervals may be useful.
Change in clinical status of patients with previously controlled type 2 diabetes—A patient with type 2 diabetes previously well controlled on metformin who develops laboratory abnormalities or clinical illness (especially vague and poorly defined illness) should be evaluated promptly for evidence of ketoacidosis or lactic acidosis. Evaluation should include serum electrolytes and ketones, blood glucose and, if indicated, blood pH, lactate, pyruvate, and metformin levels. If acidosis of either form occurs, GLUCOVANCE must be stopped immediately and other appropriate corrective measures initiated (see also **WARNINGS**).

Information for Patients

GLUCOVANCE

Patients should be informed of the potential risks and benefits of GLUCOVANCE and of alternative modes of therapy. They should also be informed about the importance of adherence to dietary instructions, of a regular exercise program, and of regular testing of blood glucose, glycosylated hemoglobin, renal function, and hematologic parameters.
The risks of lactic acidosis associated with metformin therapy, its symptoms, and conditions that predispose to its development, as noted in the **WARNINGS** and **PRECAUTIONS** sections, should be explained to patients. Patients should be advised to discontinue GLUCOVANCE (Glyburide and Metformin HCl Tablets) immediately and to promptly notify their health practitioner if unexplained hyperventilation, myalgia, malaise, unusual somnolence, or other nonspecific symptoms occur. Once a patient is stabilized on any dose level of GLUCOVANCE, gastrointestinal symptoms, which are common during initiation of metformin therapy, are unlikely to be drug related. Later occurrence of gastrointestinal symptoms could be due to lactic acidosis or other serious disease.
The risks of hypoglycemia, its symptoms and treatment, and conditions that predispose to its development should be explained to patients and responsible family members.
Patients should be counseled against excessive alcohol intake, either acute or chronic, while receiving GLUCOVANCE.
(See **Patient Information** Printed Below.)

Laboratory Tests

Periodic fasting blood glucose and glycosylated hemoglobin (HbA_{1c}) measurements should be performed to monitor therapeutic response.
Initial and periodic monitoring of hematologic parameters (e.g., hemoglobin/hematocrit and red blood cell indices) and renal function (serum creatinine) should be performed, at least on an annual basis. While megaloblastic anemia has rarely been seen with metformin therapy, if this is suspected, Vitamin B_{12} deficiency should be excluded.

Drug Interactions

GLUCOVANCE

Certain drugs tend to produce hyperglycemia and may lead to loss of blood glucose control. These drugs include the thiazides and other diuretics, corticosteroids, phenothiazines, thyroid products, estrogens, oral contraceptives, phenytoin, nicotinic acid, sympathomimetics, calcium channel blocking drugs, and isoniazid. When such drugs are administered to a patient receiving GLUCOVANCE, the patient should be closely observed for loss of blood glucose control. When such drugs are withdrawn from a patient receiving GLUCOVANCE, the patient should be observed closely for hypoglycemia. Metformin is negligibly bound to plasma proteins and is, therefore, less likely to interact with highly protein-bound drugs such as salicylates, sulfonamides, chloramphenicol, and probenecid as compared to sulfonylureas, which are extensively bound to serum proteins.

Glyburide

The hypoglycemic action of sulfonylureas may be potentiated by certain drugs including nonsteroidal anti-inflammatory agents and other drugs that are highly protein bound, salicylates, sulfonamides, chloramphenicol, probenecid, coumarins, monoamine oxidase inhibitors, and beta adrenergic blocking agents. When such drugs are administered to a patient receiving GLUCOVANCE, the patient should be observed closely for hypoglycemia. When such drugs are withdrawn from a patient receiving GLUCOVANCE, the patient should be observed closely for loss of blood glucose control.
A possible interaction between glyburide and ciprofloxacin, a fluoroquinolone antibiotic, has been reported, resulting in a potentiation of the hypoglycemic action of glyburide. The mechanism for this interaction is not known.
A potential interaction between oral miconazole and oral hypoglycemic agents leading to severe hypoglycemia has been reported. Whether this interaction also occurs with the intravenous, topical, or vaginal preparations of miconazole is not known.

Metformin Hydrochloride

Furosemide—A single-dose, metformin-furosemide drug interaction study in healthy subjects demonstrated that pharmacokinetic parameters of both compounds were affected by co-administration. Furosemide increased the metformin plasma and blood C_{max} by 22% and blood AUC by 15%, without any significant change in metformin renal clearance. When administered with metformin, the C_{max} and AUC of furosemide were 31% and 12% smaller, respectively, than when administered alone, and the terminal half-life was decreased by 32%, without any significant change in furosemide renal clearance. No information is available about the interaction of metformin and furosemide when co-administered chronically.
Nifedipine—A single-dose, metformin-nifedipine drug interaction study in normal healthy volunteers demonstrated that co-administration of nifedipine increased plasma metformin C_{max} and AUC by 20% and 9%, respectively, and increased the amount excreted in the urine. T_{max} and half-life were unaffected. Nifedipine appears to enhance the absorption of metformin. Metformin had minimal effects on nifedipine.
Cationic drugs—Cationic drugs (e.g., amiloride, digoxin, morphine, procainamide, quinidine, quinine, ranitidine, triamterene, trimethoprim, or vancomycin) that are eliminated by renal tubular secretion theoretically have the potential for interaction with metformin by competing for common renal tubular transport systems. Such interaction between metformin and oral cimetidine has been observed in normal healthy volunteers in both single- and multiple-dose, metformin-cimetidine drug interaction studies, with a 60% increase in peak metformin plasma and whole blood concentrations and a 40% increase in plasma and whole blood metformin AUC. There was no change in elimination half-life in the single-dose study. Metformin had no effect on cimetidine pharmacokinetics. Although such interactions remain theoretical (except for cimetidine), careful patient monitoring and dose adjustment of GLUCOVANCE and/or the interfering drug is recommended in patients who are taking cationic medications that are excreted via the proximal renal tubular secretory system.
Other—In healthy volunteers, the pharmacokinetics of metformin and propranolol and metformin and ibuprofen were not affected when co-administered in single-dose interaction studies.

Carcinogenesis, Mutagenesis, Impairment of Fertility

No animal studies have been conducted with the combined products in GLUCOVANCE. The following data are based on findings in studies performed with the individual products.

Glyburide

Studies in rats with glyburide alone at doses up to 300 mg/kg/day (approximately 145 times the maximum recommended human daily dose of 20 mg for the glyburide component of GLUCOVANCE based on body surface area comparisons) for 18 months revealed no carcinogenic effects. In a two-year oncogenicity study of glyburide in mice, there was no evidence of treatment-related tumors.
There was no evidence of mutagenic potential of glyburide alone in the following *in vitro* tests: *Salmonella* microsome test (Ames test) and in the DNA damage/alkaline elution assay.

Metformin Hydrochloride

Long-term carcinogenicity studies were performed with metformin alone in rats (dosing duration of 104 weeks) and mice (dosing duration of 91 weeks) at doses up to and including 900 mg/kg/day and 1500 mg/kg/day, respectively. These doses are both approximately four times the maximum recommended human daily dose of 2000 mg of the metformin component of GLUCOVANCE (Glyburide and Metformin HCl Tablets) based on body surface area comparisons. No evidence of carcinogenicity with metformin alone was found in either male or female mice. Similarly, there was no tumorigenic potential observed with metformin alone in male rats. There was, however, an increased incidence of benign stromal uterine polyps in female rats treated with 900 mg/kg/day of metformin alone.
There was no evidence of a mutagenic potential of metformin alone in the following *in vitro* tests: Ames test (*S. typhimurium*), gene mutation test (mouse lymphoma cells), or chromosomal aberrations test (human lymphocytes). Results in the *in vivo* mouse micronucleus test were also negative.
Fertility of male or female rats was unaffected by metformin alone when administered at doses as high as 600 mg/kg/day, which is approximately three times the maximum recommended human daily dose of the metformin component of GLUCOVANCE based on body surface area comparisons.

Pregnancy

Teratogenic Effects: Pregnancy Category B

Recent information strongly suggests that abnormal blood glucose levels during pregnancy are associated with a higher incidence of congenital abnormalities. Most experts recommend that insulin be used during pregnancy to maintain blood glucose as close to normal as possible. Because animal reproduction studies are not always predictive of human response, GLUCOVANCE should not be used during pregnancy unless clearly needed. (See below.)
There are no adequate and well-controlled studies in pregnant women with GLUCOVANCE or its individual components. No animal studies have been conducted with the combined products in GLUCOVANCE. The following data are based on findings in studies performed with the individual products.

Glyburide

Reproduction studies were performed in rats and rabbits at doses up to 500 times the maximum recommended human daily dose of 20 mg of the glyburide component of GLUCOVANCE based on body surface area comparisons and revealed no evidence of impaired fertility or harm to the fetus due to glyburide.

Metformin hydrochloride

Metformin alone was not teratogenic in rats or rabbits at doses up to 600 mg/kg/day. This represents an exposure of about two and six times the maximum recommended human daily dose of 2000 mg of the metformin component of GLUCOVANCE based on body surface area comparisons for rats and rabbits, respectively. Determination of fetal concentrations demonstrated a partial placental barrier to metformin.

Nonteratogenic Effects

Prolonged severe hypoglycemia (4 to 10 days) has been reported in neonates born to mothers who were receiving a sulfonylurea drug at the time of delivery. This has been reported more frequently with the use of agents with prolonged half-lives. It is not recommended that GLUCOVANCE be used during pregnancy. However, if it is used, GLUCOVANCE should be discontinued at least two weeks before the expected delivery date. (See **Pregnancy**; Teratogenic Effects: Pregnancy Category B.)

Nursing Mothers

Although it is not known whether glyburide is excreted in human milk, some sulfonylurea drugs are known to be excreted in human milk. Studies in lactating rats show that metformin is excreted into milk and reaches levels comparable to those in plasma. Similar studies have not been conducted in nursing mothers. Because the potential for hypoglycemia in nursing infants may exist, a decision should be made whether to discontinue nursing or to discontinue GLUCOVANCE, taking into account the importance of the drug to the mother. If GLUCOVANCE is discontinued, and if diet alone is inadequate for controlling blood glucose, insulin therapy should be considered.

Pediatric Use

Safety and effectiveness of GLUCOVANCE in pediatric patients have not been established.

Geriatric Use

Of the 642 patients who received GLUCOVANCE in double-blind clinical studies, 23.8% were 65 and older while 2.8% were 75 and older. Of the 1302 patients who received GLUCOVANCE in open-label clinical studies, 20.7% were 65 and older while 2.5% were 75 and older. No overall differences in effectiveness or safety were observed between these patients and younger patients, and other reported clinical experience has not identified differences in response between the elderly and younger patients, but greater sensitivity of some older individuals cannot be ruled out.
Metformin hydrochloride is known to be substantially excreted by the kidney and because the risk of serious adverse reactions to the drug is greater in patients with impaired renal function, GLUCOVANCE should only be used in patients with normal renal function (see **CONTRAINDICATIONS, WARNINGS**, and **CLINICAL PHARMACOLOGY: Pharmacokinetics**). Because aging is associated with reduced renal function, GLUCOVANCE should be used with caution as age increases. Care should be taken in dose selection and should be based on careful and regular monitoring of renal function. Generally, elderly patients should not be titrated to the maximum dose of GLUCOVANCE (see also **WARNINGS** and **DOSAGE AND ADMINISTRATION**).

ADVERSE REACTIONS

GLUCOVANCE

In double-blind clinical trials involving GLUCOVANCE, a total of 642 patients received GLUCOVANCE, 312 received metformin therapy, 324 received glyburide therapy, and 161 received placebo. The percent of patients reporting events and types of adverse events reported in clinical trials of GLUCOVANCE (all strengths) as initial therapy and second-line therapy are listed in **Table 4.**
[See table 4 at top of next page]
Disulfiram-like reactions have very rarely been reported in patients treated with glyburide tablets.

Hypoglycemia

In controlled clinical trials of GLUCOVANCE (Glyburide and Metformin HCl Tablets) there were no hypoglycemic episodes requiring medical intervention and/or pharmacologic therapy; all events were managed by the patients. The incidence of reported symptoms of hypoglycemia (such as dizziness, shakiness, sweating, and hunger), in the initial therapy trial of GLUCOVANCE are summarized in **Table 5**. The frequency of hypoglycemic symptoms in patients treated with GLUCOVANCE 1.25 mg/250 mg was highest in patients with a baseline $HbA_{1c} < 7\%$, lower in those with a baseline HbA_{1c} of between 7 and 8%, and was comparable to placebo and metformin in those with a baseline $HbA_{1c} > 8\%$. For patients with a baseline HbA_{1c} of between 8% and 11% treated with GLUCOVANCE 2.5 mg/500 mg as initial therapy, the frequency of hypoglycemic symptoms was 30–35%. As second-line therapy in patients inadequately controlled on sulfonylurea alone, approximately 6.8% of all patients treated with GLUCOVANCE experienced hypoglycemic symptoms. (See **PRECAUTIONS** section.)

Gastrointestinal Reactions

The incidence of GI side effects (diarrhea, nausea/vomiting, and abdominal pain) in the initial therapy trial are summarized in **Table 5**. Across all GLUCOVANCE trials, GI symptoms were the most common adverse events with GLUCOVANCE and were more frequent at higher dose levels. In controlled trials, <2% of patients discontinued GLUCOVANCE therapy due to GI adverse events.

[See table 5 in next column]

OVERDOSAGE

Glyburide

Overdosage of sulfonylureas, including glyburide tablets, can produce hypoglycemia. Mild hypoglycemic symptoms, without loss of consciousness or neurological findings, should be treated aggressively with oral glucose and adjustments in drug dosage and/or meal patterns. Close monitoring should continue until the physician is assured that the patient is out of danger. Severe hypoglycemic reactions with coma, seizure, or other neurological impairment occur infrequently, but constitute medical emergencies requiring immediate hospitalization. If hypoglycemic coma is diagnosed or suspected, the patient should be given a rapid intravenous injection of concentrated (50%) glucose solution. This should be followed by a continuous infusion of a more dilute (10%) glucose solution at a rate that will maintain the blood glucose at a level above 100 mg/dL. Patients should be closely monitored for a minimum of 24 to 48 hours, since hypoglycemia may recur after apparent clinical recovery.

Metformin Hydrochloride

Hypoglycemia has not been seen even with ingestion of up to 85 grams of metformin hydrochloride, although lactic acidosis has occurred in such circumstances (see **WARNINGS**). Metformin is dialyzable with a clearance of up to 170 mL/min under good hemodynamic conditions. Therefore, hemodialysis may be useful for removal of accumulated drug from patients in whom metformin overdosage is suspected.

DOSAGE AND ADMINISTRATION

General Considerations

Dosage of GLUCOVANCE must be individualized on the basis of both effectiveness and tolerance while not exceeding the maximum recommended daily dose of 20 mg glyburide/2000 mg metformin. GLUCOVANCE (Glyburide and Metformin HCl Tablets) should be given with meals and should be initiated at a low dose, with gradual dose escalation as described below, in order to avoid hypoglycemia (largely due to glyburide), to reduce GI side effects (largely due to metformin), and to permit determination of the minimum effective dose for adequate control of blood glucose for the individual patient.

With initial treatment and during dose titration, appropriate blood glucose monitoring should be used to determine the therapeutic response to GLUCOVANCE and to identify the minimum effective dose for the patient. Thereafter, HbA_{1c} should be measured at intervals of approximately 3 months to assess the effectiveness of therapy. The therapeutic goal in all patients with type 2 diabetes is to decrease FPG, PPG, and HbA_{1c} to normal or as near normal as possible. Ideally, the response to therapy should be evaluated using HbA_{1c} (glycosylated hemoglobin), which is a better indicator of long-term glycemic control than FPG alone.

No studies have been performed specifically examining the safety and efficacy of switching to GLUCOVANCE therapy in patients taking concomitant glyburide (or other sulfonylurea) plus metformin. Changes in glycemic control may occur in such patients, with either hyperglycemia or hypoglycemia possible. Any change in therapy of type 2 diabetes should be undertaken with care and appropriate monitoring.

GLUCOVANCE As Initial Therapy

Recommended starting dose: 1.25 mg/250 mg once or twice daily with meals.

For patients with type 2 diabetes whose hyperglycemia cannot be satisfactorily managed with diet and exercise alone, the recommended starting dose of GLUCOVANCE is 1.25 mg/250 mg once a day with a meal. As initial therapy in patients with baseline $HbA_{1c} > 9\%$ or an FPG > 200 mg/dL, a starting dose of GLUCOVANCE 1.25 mg/250 mg twice daily with the morning and evening meals may be used. Dosage increases should be made in increments of 1.25 mg/250 mg per day every two weeks up to the minimum effective dose necessary to achieve adequate control of blood glucose. In clinical trials of GLUCOVANCE as initial therapy, there was no experience with total daily doses greater than 10 mg/2000 mg per day. **GLUCOVANCE 5 mg/500 mg should not be used as initial therapy due to an increased risk of hypoglycemia.**

GLUCOVANCE Use in Previously Treated Patients (Second-Line Therapy)

Recommended starting dose: 2.5 mg/500 mg or 5 mg/500 mg twice daily with meals.

Table 4. GLUCOVANCE's Most Common Clinical Adverse Events (>5%) when Compared to Placebo, by Primary Term, in Double-Blind Clinical Studies

	Number (%) of Patients			
Adverse Event	**Placebo** N = 161	**Glyburide** N = 324	**Metformin** N = 312	**GLUCOVANCE** N = 642
Upper respiratory infection	22 (13.7)	57 (17.6)	51 (16.3)	111 (17.3)
Diarrhea	9 (5.6)	20 (6.2)	64 (20.5)	109 (17.0)
Headache	17 (10.6)	37 (11.4)	29 (9.3)	57 (8.9)
Nausea/vomiting	10 (6.2)	17 (5.2)	38 (12.2)	49 (7.6)
Abdominal pain	6 (3.7)	10 (3.1)	25 (8.0)	44 (6.9)
Dizziness	7 (4.3)	18 (5.6)	12 (3.8)	35 (5.5)

Table 5. Treatment Emergent Symptoms of Hypoglycemia or Gastrointestinal Adverse Events in a Placebo- and Active-Controlled Trial of GLUCOVANCE as Initial Therapy

Variable	**Placebo** N=161	**Glyburide** N=160	**Metformin** N=159	**GLUCOVANCE 1.25 mg/250 mg** N=158	**GLUCOVANCE 2.5 mg/500 mg** N=162
Mean Final Dose	0 mg	5.3 mg	1317 mg	2.78 mg/557 mg	4.1 mg/824 mg
Number (%) of patients with symptoms of hypoglycemia	5 (3.1)	34 (21.3)	5 (3.1)	18 (11.4)	61 (37.7)
Number (%) of patients with gastrointestinal adverse events	39 (24.2)	38 (23.8)	69 (43.3)	50 (31.6)	62 (38.3)

For patients not adequately controlled on either glyburide (or another sulfonylurea) or metformin alone, the recommended starting dose of GLUCOVANCE is 2.5 mg/500 mg or 5 mg/500 mg twice daily with the morning and evening meals. In order to avoid hypoglycemia, the starting dose of GLUCOVANCE should not exceed the daily doses of glyburide or metformin already being taken. The daily dose should be titrated in increments of no more than 5 mg/500 mg up to the minimum effective dose to achieve adequate control of blood glucose or to a maximum dose of 20 mg/2000 mg per day.

For patients previously treated with combination therapy of glyburide (or another sulfonylurea) plus metformin, if switched to GLUCOVANCE, the starting dose should not exceed the daily dose of glyburide (or equivalent dose of another sulfonylurea) and metformin already being taken. Patients should be monitored closely for signs and symptoms of hypoglycemia following such a switch and the dose of GLUCOVANCE should be titrated as described above to achieve adequate control of blood glucose.

Specific Patient Populations

GLUCOVANCE is not recommended for use during pregnancy or for use in pediatric patients. The initial and maintenance dosing of GLUCOVANCE should be conservative in patients with advanced age, due to the potential for decreased renal function in this population. Any dosage adjustment requires a careful assessment of renal function. Generally, elderly, debilitated, and malnourished patients should not be titrated to the maximum dose of GLUCOVANCE to avoid the risk of hypoglycemia. Monitoring of renal function is necessary to aid in prevention of metformin-associated lactic acidosis, particularly in the elderly. (See **WARNINGS**.)

HOW SUPPLIED

GLUCOVANCE®

GLUCOVANCE **1.25 mg/250 mg** tablet is a pale yellow, capsule-shaped, bevel edged, biconvex film-coated tablet with **"BMS"** debossed on one side and **"6072"** debossed on the opposite side.

GLUCOVANCE **2.5 mg/500 mg** tablet is a pale orange, capsule-shaped, bevel edged, biconvex film-coated tablet with **"BMS"** debossed on one side and **"6073"** debossed on the opposite side.

GLUCOVANCE **5 mg/500 mg** tablet is a yellow, capsule-shaped, bevel edged, biconvex film-coated tablet with **"BMS"** debossed on one side and **"6074"** debossed on the opposite side.

GLUCOVANCE		NDC 0087-xxxx-xx for unit dose	
Glyburide (mg)	**Metformin Hydrochloride (mg)**	**Bottle of 100**	**500**
1.25	250	6072-11	6072-12
2.5	500	6073-11	6073-12
5	500	6074-11	

STORAGE

Store at temperatures up to 25° C (77° F). [See USP Controlled Room Temperature.] Dispense in light resistant containers.

PATIENT INFORMATION ABOUT GLUCOVANCE™

(Glyburide and Metformin HCl Tablets)

WARNING: A small number of people who have taken metformin hydrochloride have developed a serious condition called lactic acidosis. Properly functioning kidneys are needed to help prevent lactic acidosis. Most people with kidney problems should not take GLUCOVANCE. (See Question Nos. 9–13.)

Q1. Why do I need to take GLUCOVANCE?

Your doctor has prescribed GLUCOVANCE to treat your type 2 diabetes. This is also known as non-insulin-dependent diabetes mellitus.

Q2. What is type 2 diabetes?

People with diabetes are not able to make enough insulin and/or respond normally to the insulin their body does make. When this happens, sugar (glucose) builds up in the blood. This can lead to serious medical problems including kidney damage, amputations, and blindness. Diabetes is also closely linked to heart disease. The main goal of treating diabetes is to lower your blood sugar to a normal level.

Q3. Why is it important to control type 2 diabetes?

The main goal of treating diabetes is to lower your blood sugar to a normal level. Studies have shown that good control of blood sugar may prevent or delay complications such as heart disease, kidney disease, or blindness.

Q4. How is type 2 diabetes usually controlled?

High blood sugar can be lowered by diet and exercise, by a number of oral medications, and by insulin injections. Before taking GLUCOVANCE you should first try to control your diabetes by exercise and weight loss. Even if you are taking GLUCOVANCE, you should still exercise and follow the diet recommended for your diabetes.

Q5. Does GLUCOVANCE work differently from other glucose-control medications?

Yes it does. GLUCOVANCE combines two glucose lowering drugs, glyburide and metformin. These two drugs work together to improve the different metabolic defects found in type 2 diabetes. Glyburide lowers blood sugar primarily by causing more of the body's own insulin to be released, and metformin lowers blood sugar, in part, by helping your body use your own insulin more effectively. Together, they are efficient in helping you achieve better glucose control.

Q6. What happens if my blood sugar is still too high?

When blood sugar cannot be lowered enough by GLUCOVANCE your doctor may prescribe injectable insulin or take other measures to control your diabetes.

Q7. Can GLUCOVANCE cause side effects?

GLUCOVANCE, like all blood sugar-lowering medications, can cause side effects in some patients. Most of these side effects are minor. However, there are also serious, but rare, side effects related to GLUCOVANCE (see **Q9–Q13**).

Q8. What are the most common side effects of GLUCOVANCE?

The most common side effects of GLUCOVANCE are normally minor ones such as diarrhea, nausea, and up-

Continued on next page

Glucovance—Cont.

set stomach. If these side effects occur, they usually occur during the first few weeks of therapy. Taking your GLUCOVANCE with meals can help reduce these side effects.

Less frequently, symptoms of hypoglycemia (low blood sugar), such as lightheadedness, dizziness, shakiness, or hunger may occur. The risk of hypoglycemic symptoms increases when meals are skipped, too much alcohol is consumed, or heavy exercise occurs without enough food. Following the advice of your doctor can help you to avoid these symptoms.

Q9. Are there any serious side effects that GLUCOVANCE can cause?

GLUCOVANCE rarely causes serious side effects. The most serious side effect that GLUCOVANCE can cause is called lactic acidosis.

Q10. What is lactic acidosis and can it happen to me?

Lactic acidosis is caused by a buildup of lactic acid in the blood. Lactic acidosis associated with metformin is rare and has occurred mostly in people whose kidneys were not working normally. Lactic acidosis has been reported in about one in 33,000 patients taking metformin over the course of a year. Although rare, if lactic acidosis does occur, it can be fatal in up to half the cases.

It's also important for your liver to be working normally when you take GLUCOVANCE. Your liver helps remove lactic acid from your bloodstream.

Your doctor will monitor your diabetes and may perform blood tests on you from time to time to make sure your kidneys and your liver are functioning normally. There is no evidence that GLUCOVANCE causes harm to the kidneys or liver.

Q11. Are there other risk factors for lactic acidosis?

Your risk of developing lactic acidosis from taking GLUCOVANCE (Glyburide and Metformin HCl Tablets) is very low as long as your kidneys and liver are healthy. However, some factors can increase your risk because they can affect kidney and liver function. You should discuss your risk with your physician.

You should not take GLUCOVANCE if:

- You have chronic kidney or liver problems
- You have congestive heart failure which is treated with medications, e.g., digoxin (Lanoxin®) or furosemide (Lasix®)
- You drink alcohol excessively (all the time or short-term "binge" drinking)
- You are seriously dehydrated (have lost a large amount of body fluids)
- You are going to have certain x-ray procedures with injectable contrast agents
- You are going to have surgery
- You develop a serious condition such as a heart attack, severe infection, or a stroke
- You are ≥80 years of age and have NOT had your kidney function tested

Q12. What are the symptoms of lactic acidosis?

Some of the symptoms include: feeling very weak, tired or uncomfortable; unusual muscle pain, trouble breathing, unusual or unexpected stomach discomfort, feeling cold, feeling dizzy or lightheaded, or suddenly developing a slow or irregular heartbeat.

If you notice these symptoms, or if your medical condition has suddenly changed, stop taking GLUCOVANCE tablets and call your doctor right away. Lactic acidosis is a medical emergency that must be treated in a hospital.

Q13. What does my doctor need to know to decrease my risk of lactic acidosis?

Tell your doctor if you have an illness that results in severe vomiting, diarrhea, and/or fever, or if your intake of fluids is significantly reduced. These situations can lead to severe dehydration, and it may be necessary to stop taking GLUCOVANCE temporarily.

You should let your doctor know if you are going to have any surgery or specialized x-ray procedures that require injection of contrast agents. GLUCOVANCE therapy will need to be stopped temporarily in such instances.

Q14. Can I take GLUCOVANCE with other medications?

Remind your doctor that you are taking GLUCOVANCE when any new drug is prescribed or a change is made in how you take a drug already prescribed. GLUCOVANCE may interfere with the way some drugs work and some drugs may interfere with the action of GLUCOVANCE.

Q15. What if I become pregnant while taking GLUCOVANCE?

Tell your doctor if you plan to become pregnant or have become pregnant. As with other oral glucose-control medications, you should not take GLUCOVANCE during pregnancy.

Usually your doctor will prescribe insulin while you are pregnant. As with all medications, you and your doctor should discuss the use of GLUCOVANCE if you are nursing a child.

Q16. How do I take GLUCOVANCE?

Your doctor will tell you how many GLUCOVANCE tablets to take and how often. This should also be printed on the label of your prescription. You will probably be started on a low dose of GLUCOVANCE and your dosage will be increased gradually until your blood sugar is controlled.

Q17. Where can I get more information about GLUCOVANCE?

This leaflet is a summary of the most important information about GLUCOVANCE. If you have any questions or problems, you should talk to your doctor or other healthcare provider about type 2 diabetes as well as GLUCOVANCE and its side effects. There is also a leaflet (package insert) written for health professionals that your pharmacist can let you read.

GLUCOVANCE™ is a trademark of LIPHA s.a. Licensed to Bristol-Myers Squibb Company.

Micronase® is a registered trademark of Pharmacia & Upjohn Company.

Distributed by
Bristol-Myers Squibb Company
Princeton, NJ 08543 USA

F7-B001-08-00 Revised: August 2000
607211DIM-02

Bristol-Myers Squibb Oncology/ Immunology Division

A Bristol-Myers Squibb Company
P.O. BOX 4500
PRINCETON, NJ 08543-4500

For Medical Information Contact:

Generally:
Bristol-Myers Squibb Drug Information Department
P.O. Box 4500
Princeton, NJ 08543-4500
(800) 426-7644

Adverse Drug Experiences
and Product Defects Reporting call
between 8:30 AM–4:30 PM EST:
(609) 818-3737

Sales and Ordering:
Orders may be placed by:

1. Calling the following toll-free number between 8:30 AM–5:00 PM EST:
   Continental U.S.: (800) 631-5244
   Alaska-Hawaii: (800) 631-5244
2. Mail orders and all inquiries should be sent to:
   Bristol-Myers Squibb Oncology Division
   Attn: Customer Service
   P.O. Box 5250
   Princeton, NJ 08543-5250
3. Faxing your purchase orders to:
   (800) 523-2965
4. Transmitting computer-to-computer on the NWDA and UCS formats through Ordernet Services use: DEA #PE0048579

VIDEX® ℞

[vī dex]
(didanosine)
VIDEX® (didanosine) Chewable/Dispersible Buffered Tablets
VIDEX® (didanosine) Buffered Powder for Oral Solution
VIDEX® (didanosine) Pediatric Powder for Oral Solution
(Patient Information Leaflet Included)
Rx ONLY

> **WARNING**
> **FATAL AND NONFATAL PANCREATITIS HAS OCCURRED DURING THERAPY WITH VIDEX USED ALONE OR IN COMBINATION REGIMENS IN BOTH TREATMENT-NAIVE AND TREATMENT-EXPERIENCED PATIENTS, REGARDLESS OF DEGREE OF IMMUNOSUPPRESSION. VIDEX SHOULD BE SUSPENDED IN PATIENTS WITH SUSPECTED PANCREATITIS AND DISCONTINUED IN PATIENTS WITH CONFIRMED PANCREATITIS (SEE WARNINGS).**
> **LACTIC ACIDOSIS AND SEVERE HEPATOMEGALY WITH STEATOSIS, INCLUDING FATAL CASES, HAVE BEEN REPORTED WITH THE USE OF NUCLEOSIDE ANALOGUES ALONE OR IN COMBINATION, INCLUDING DIDANOSINE AND OTHER ANTIRETROVIRALS (SEE WARNINGS).**

DESCRIPTION

VIDEX® (didanosine) is the brand name for didanosine (ddI), a synthetic purine nucleoside analogue active against the Human Immunodeficiency Virus (HIV). VIDEX Chewable/Dispersible Buffered Tablets are available for oral administration in strengths of 25, 50, 100, 150, and 200 mg of didanosine. Each tablet is buffered with calcium carbonate and magnesium hydroxide. VIDEX tablets also contain aspartame, sorbitol, microcrystalline cellulose, polyplasdone, mandarin-orange flavor and magnesium stearate.

VIDEX Buffered Powder for Oral Solution is supplied for oral administration in single-dose packets containing 100, 167, or 250 mg of didanosine. Packets of each product strength also contain a citrate-phosphate buffer (composed of dibasic sodium phosphate, sodium citrate, and citric acid) and sucrose.

VIDEX Pediatric Powder for Oral Solution is supplied for oral administration in 4- or 8-ounce glass bottles containing 2 or 4 grams of didanosine, respectively.

The chemical name for didanosine is 2′,3′-dideoxyinosine. The structural formula is:

Didanosine is a white crystalline powder with the molecular formula $C_{10}H_{12}N_4O_3$ and a molecular weight of 236.2. The aqueous solubility of didanosine at 25°C and pH of approximately 6 is 27.3 mg/mL. Didanosine is unstable in acidic solutions. For example at pH <3 and 37°C, 10% of didanosine decomposes to hypoxanthine in less than 2 minutes.

MICROBIOLOGY

Mechanism of Action: Didanosine is a synthetic nucleoside analogue of the naturally occurring nucleoside deoxyadenosine in which the 3′-hydroxyl group is replaced by hydrogen. Intracellularly, didanosine is converted by cellular enzymes to the active metabolite, dideoxyadenosine 5′-triphosphate. Dideoxyadenosine 5′-triphosphate inhibits the activity of HIV-1 reverse transcriptase both by competing with the natural substrate, deoxyadenosine 5′-triphosphate, and by its incorporation into viral DNA causing termination of viral DNA chain elongation.

***In Vitro* HIV Susceptibility:** The *in vitro* anti-HIV-1 activity of didanosine was evaluated in a variety of HIV-1 infected lymphoblastic cell lines and monocyte/macrophage cell cultures. The concentration of drug necessary to inhibit viral replication by 50% (IC_{50}) ranged from 2.5 to 10 μM (1 μM = 0.24 μg/mL) in lymphoblastic cell lines and 0.01 to 0.1 μM in monocyte/macrophage cell cultures. The relationship between *in vitro* susceptibility of HIV to didanosine and the inhibition of HIV replication in humans has not been established.

Drug Resistance: HIV-1 isolates with reduced sensitivity to didanosine have been selected *in vitro* and were also obtained from patients treated with didanosine. Genetic analysis of isolates from didanosine-treated patients showed mutations in the reverse transcriptase gene that resulted in the amino acid substitutions K65R, L74V, and M184V. The L74V mutation was most frequently observed in clinical isolates. Phenotypic analysis of HIV-1 isolates from 60 patients (some with prior zidovudine treatment) receiving 6 to 24 months of didanosine monotherapy showed that isolates from 10 of 60 patients exhibited an average of a 10-fold decrease in susceptibility to didanosine *in vitro* compared to baseline isolates. Clinical isolates that exhibited a decrease in didanosine susceptibility harbored one or more didanosine-associated mutations. The clinical relevance of genotypic and phenotypic changes associated with didanosine therapy has not been established.

Cross-resistance: HIV-1 isolates from 2 of 39 patients receiving combination therapy for up to 2 years with zidovudine and didanosine exhibited decreased susceptibility to zidovudine, didanosine, zalcitabine, stavudine, and lamivudine *in vitro*. These isolates harbored five mutations (A62V, V751, F77L, F116Y, and Q151M) in the reverse transcriptase gene. The clinical relevance of these observations has not been established.

CLINICAL PHARMACOLOGY

Animal Toxicology: Evidence of a dose-limiting skeletal muscle toxicity has been observed in mice and rats (but not in dogs) following long-term (greater than 90 days) dosing with didanosine at doses that were approximately 1.2 to 12 times the estimated human exposure. The relationship of this finding to the potential of VIDEX to cause myopathy in humans is unclear. However, human myopathy has been associated with administration of VIDEX and other nucleoside analogues.

Pharmacokinetics: The pharmacokinetic parameters of didanosine are summarized in Table 1. Didanosine is rapidly absorbed, with peak plasma concentrations generally observed from 0.25 to 1.50 hours following oral dosing. Increases in plasma didanosine concentrations were dose proportional over the range of 50–400 mg. Steady-state pharmacokinetic parameters did not differ significantly from values obtained after a single dose. Binding of didanosine to plasma proteins *in vitro* was low (<5%). Based on data from *in vitro* and animal studies, it is presumed that the metabolism of didanosine in man occurs by the same pathways responsible for the elimination of endogenous purines.

[See table 1 at top of next page]

Effect of Food on Absorption of Didanosine—Didanosine peak plasma concentrations (C_{max}) and area under the plasma concentration time curve (AUC) were decreased by approximately 55% when VIDEX (didanosine) tablets were administered up to 2 hours after a meal. Administration of VIDEX tablets up to 30 minutes before a meal did not result in any significant changes in bioavailability. VIDEX should be taken on an empty stomach, at least 30 minutes before or 2 hours after eating. (See **DOSAGE AND ADMINISTRATION.**)

Special Populations:

Renal Insufficiency—It is recommended that the VIDEX dose be modified in patients with reduced creatinine clearance and in patients receiving maintenance hemodialysis (see **DOSAGE AND ADMINISTRATION**). Data from two studies indicated that the apparent oral clearance of didanosine decreased and the terminal elimination half-life increased as creatinine clearance decreased (see Table 2). Following oral administration, didanosine was not detectable in peritoneal dialysate fluid (n=6); recovery in hemodialysate (n=5) ranged from 0.6% to 7.4% of the dose over a 3–4 hour dialysis period. The absolute bioavailability of didanosine was not affected in patients requiring dialysis.

[See table 2 in next column]

Pediatric Patients—The pharmacokinetics of didanosine have been evaluated in HIV-infected pediatric patients from 0.7 to 18.9 years of age (see Table 1). Overall, the pharmacokinetics of didanosine in pediatric patients greater than 0.7 years of age are similar to those of didanosine in adults. Didanosine plasma concentrations increased in proportion to oral doses ranging from 80 to 180 mg/m^2. For information on controlled clinical studies in pediatric patients, see **PRECAUTIONS, Pediatric Use** and **Clinical Studies**.

Geriatric Patients—Didanosine pharmacokinetics have not been studied in patients over 65 years of age.

Gender—The effects of gender on didanosine pharmacokinetics have not been studied.

Drug Interactions—Drug interaction studies have demonstrated that there are no clinically significant pharmacokinetic interactions between VIDEX and the following: dapsone, loperamide, metoclopramide, nevirapine, ranitidine, rifabutin, ritonavir, stavudine (see **WARNINGS**), sulfamethoxazole, trimethoprim, and zidovudine. Studies with dapsone, nevirapine, rifabutin, ritonavir, stavudine, and zidovudine were multiple-dose studies. Studies with loperamide, metoclopramide, ranitidine, sulfamethoxazole, and trimethoprim were single-dose studies, and effects on pharmacokinetics at steady-state are not known. (See also **PRECAUTIONS: Drug Interactions.**)

INDICATIONS AND USAGE

VIDEX in combination with other antiretroviral agents is indicated for the treatment of HIV-1 infection (see Clinical Studies).

Clinical Studies:

Combination Therapy—START 2 was a multicenter, randomized, open-label study comparing VIDEX (200 mg BID)/ stavudine/indinavir to zidovudine/lamivudine/indinavir in 205 treatment-naive patients. Both regimens resulted in a similar magnitude of suppression of HIV RNA levels and increases in CD4 cell counts through 48 weeks.

Study A1454-148 was a randomized, open-label, multicenter study comparing treatment with VIDEX (400 mg once daily) plus stavudine (40 mg twice daily) and nelfinavir (750 mg three times daily) versus zidovudine (300 mg twice daily) plus lamivudine (150 mg twice daily) and nelfinavir (750 mg three times daily) in 756 treatment-naive patients, with a median CD4 cell count of 340 cells/mm^3 (range 80 to 1568 cells/mm^3) and a median plasma HIV-1 RNA of 4.69 $\log_{10}$ copies/mL (range 2.6 to 5.9 $\log_{10}$ copies/mL at baseline. Median CD4 cell count increases at 48 weeks were 188 cells/ mm^3 in both treatment groups. Treatment response and outcomes through 48 weeks are shown in Figure 1 and Table 3.

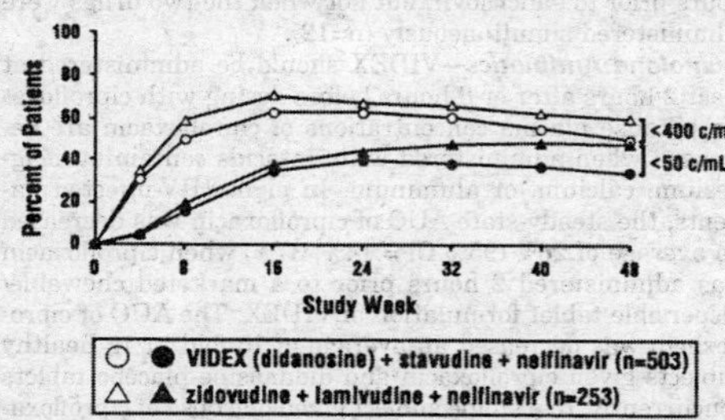

Figure 1. Treatment Response Through Week 48*, AI454-148

* proportion of patients at each time point who have HIV RNA <400 or <50 copies/mL, are on their original study medication (except stavudine-zidovudine switches), and have not experienced an AIDS-defining event.

[See table 3 above]

Monotherapy—The efficacy of VIDEX was demonstrated in two randomized, double-blind studies comparing VIDEX, given on a BID schedule, to zidovudine, given TID, in 617 (ACTG 116A, conducted 1989–1992) and 913 (ACTG 116B/ 117, conducted 1989–1991) patients with symptomatic HIV infection or AIDS who were treated for more than one year. In treatment-naive patients (ACTG 116A), the rate of HIV disease progression or death was similar between the treatment groups; mortality rates were 26% for patients receiving VIDEX and 21% for patients receiving zidovudine. Of the patients who had received previous zidovudine treatment (ACTG 116B/117), those treated with VIDEX had a lower rate of HIV disease progression or death (32%) compared to those treated with zidovudine (41%); however, survival rates were similar between the treatment groups.

Efficacy in pediatric patients was demonstrated in a randomized, double-blind, controlled study (ACTG 152, conducted 1991–1995) involving 831 patients treated for more than 1.5 years with zidovudine (180 mg/m^2 q6h), VIDEX (120 mg/m^2 q12h), or zidovudine (120 mg/m^2 q6h) plus VIDEX (90 mg/m^2 q12h). Patients treated with VIDEX or VIDEX plus zidovudine had lower rates of HIV disease progression or death compared with those treated with zidovudine alone.

Studies have demonstrated that the clinical benefit of monotherapy with antiretrovirals, including VIDEX, was time limited.

Table 1
Mean ± SD Pharmacokinetic Parameters for Didanosine in Adult and Pediatric Patients

Parameter	Adult Patients	n	Pediatric Patients	n
Oral bioavailability	42±12%	6	25±20%	46
Apparent volume of distribution[a]	1.08±0.22 L/kg	6	28±15 L/m^2	49
CSF-plasma ratio[b]	21±0.03%[c]	5	46% (range 12–85%)	7
Systemic clearance[a]	13.0±1.6 mL/min/kg	6	516±184 mL/min/m^2	49
Renal clearance[d]	5.5±2.1 mL/min/kg	6	240±90 mL/min/m^2	15
Elimination half-life[d]	1.5±0.4 hr	6	0.8±0.3 hr	60
Urinary recovery of didanosine[d]	18±8%	6	18±10%	15

CSF = cerebrospinal fluid
[a] following I.V. administration
[b] following I.V. administration in adults and I.V. or oral administration in pediatric patients
[c] mean ± SE
[d] following oral administration

Table 2
Mean ± SD Pharmacokinetic Parameters for Didanosine Following a Single Oral Dose

Parameter	Creatinine Clearance (mL/min)				
	≥ 90 (n=12)	60–90 (n=6)	30–59 (n=6)	10–29 (n=3)	Dialysis Patients (n=11)
CL_{cr}(mL/min)	112±22	68±8	46±8	13±5	ND[a]
CL/F (mL/min)	2164±638	1566±833	1023±378	628±104	543±174
CL_R(mL/min)	485±164	247±153	100±44	20±8	<10
$T_{1/2}$ (h)	1.42±0.33	1.59±0.13	1.75±0.43	2.0±0.3	4.1±1.2

[a]ND = not determined due to anuria
CL_{cr} = creatinine clearance
CL/F = apparent oral clearance
CL_R = renal clearance

Table 3
Outcomes of Randomized Treatment Through Week 48, A1454-148

Week 48 Status	Percent of Patients with HIV RNA <400 copies/mL (<50 copies/mL)	
	VIDEX/ stavudine/ nelfinavir n=503	lamivudine/ zidovudine/ nelfinavir n=253
Responder[a]	50* (34*)	59 (47)
Virologic failure[b]	36 (57)	32 (48)
Death or disease progression	<1 (<1)	1 (<1)
Discontinued due to adverse events	4 (2)	2 (<1)
Discontinued due to other reasons[c]	6 (3)	4 (2)
Never initiated treatment	4 (4)	2 (2)

* $p<0.05$ for the differences between treatment groups, by Cochran-Mantel-Haenszel test.
[a] Patients achieved virologic response [two consecutive viral load <400 (<50) copies/mL] and maintained it to Week 48.
[b] Includes viral rebound and failing to achieve confirmed <400 (<50) copies/mL by Week 48.
[c] Includes lost to follow-up, noncompliance, withdrawal, and pregnancy.

CONTRAINDICATION

VIDEX is contraindicated in patients with previously demonstrated clinically significant hypersensitivity to any of the components of the formulations.

WARNINGS

1. Pancreatitis

FATAL AND NONFATAL PANCREATITIS HAS OCCURRED DURING THERAPY WITH VIDEX USED ALONE OR IN COMBINATION REGIMENS IN BOTH TREATMENT-NAIVE AND TREATMENT-EXPERIENCED PATIENTS, REGARDLESS OF DEGREE OF IMMUNOSUPPRESSION. VIDEX SHOULD BE SUSPENDED IN PATIENTS WITH SIGNS OR SYMPTOMS OF PANCREATITIS AND DISCONTINUED IN PATIENTS WITH CONFIRMED PANCREATITIS. PATIENTS TREATED WITH VIDEX IN COMBINATION WITH STAVUDINE, WITH OR WITHOUT HYDROXYUREA, MAY BE AT INCREASED RISK FOR PANCREATITIS.

When treatment with life-sustaining drugs known to cause pancreatic toxicity is required, suspension of VIDEX therapy is recommended. In patients with risk factors for pancreatitis, VIDEX should be used with extreme caution and only if clearly indicated. Patients with advanced HIV infection, especially the elderly, are at increased risk of pancreatitis and should be followed closely. Patients with renal impairment may be at greater risk for pancreatitis if treated without dose adjustment. The frequency of pancreatitis is dose related. In phase 3 studies, incidence ranged from 1% to 10% with doses higher than are currently recommended and 1% to 7% with recommended dose.

In pediatric studies, pancreatitis occurred in 3% (2/60) of patients treated at entry doses below 300 mg/m^2/day and in 13% (5/38) of patients treated at higher doses. VIDEX use should be suspended in pediatric patients with signs or symptoms of pancreatitis and discontinued in pediatric patients with confirmed pancreatitis.

2. Lactic Acidosis/Severe Hepatomegaly with Steatosis

Lactic acidosis and severe hepatomegaly with steatosis, including fatal cases, have been reported with the use of nucleoside analogues alone or in combination, including didanosine and other antiretrovirals. A majority of these cases have been in women. Obesity and prolonged nucle-

Continued on next page

Videx—Cont.

oside exposure may be risk factors. Particular caution should be exercised when administering VIDEX to any patient with known risk factors for liver disease; however, cases have also been reported in patients with no known risk factors. Treatment with VIDEX should be suspended in any patient who develops clinical or laboratory findings suggestive of lactic acidosis or pronounced hepatotoxicity (which may include hepatomegaly and steatosis even in the absence of marked transaminase elevations).

3. **Retinal Changes and Optic Neuritis**
   Retinal changes and optic neuritis have been reported in adult and pediatric patients. Periodic retinal examinations should be considered for patients receiving VIDEX. (See **ADVERSE REACTIONS**.)

PRECAUTIONS

Frequency of Dosing: The preferred dosing frequency of VIDEX (didanosine) is twice daily because there is more evidence to support the effectiveness of this dosing frequency. Once-daily dosing should be considered only for adult patients whose management requires once-daily dosing of VIDEX (see **Clinical Studies**).

VIDEX should be taken on an empty stomach, at least 30 minutes before or 2 hours after eating.

Peripheral Neuropathy: Peripheral neuropathy, manifested by numbness, tingling, or pain in the hands or feet, has been reported in patients receiving VIDEX therapy. Peripheral neuropathy has occurred more frequently in patients with advanced HIV disease, in patients with a history of neuropathy, or in patients being treated with neurotoxic drug therapy, including stavudine (see **ADVERSE REACTIONS**).

General:

Patients with Phenylketonuria: VIDEX Chewable/Dispersible Buffered Tablets contain the following quantities of phenylalanine:

Table 4

	All Strengths
Phenylalanine per 2-tablet dose	73 mg
Phenylalanine per tablet	36.5 mg

Patients on Sodium-Restricted Diets—VIDEX Buffered Powder for Oral Solution: Each single-dose packet of VIDEX Buffered Powder for Oral Solution contains 1380 mg sodium.

Patients with Renal Impairment—Patients with renal impairment (creatinine clearance <60 mL/min) may be at greater risk of toxicity from VIDEX due to decreased drug clearance (see **CLINICAL PHARMACOLOGY**). A dose reduction is recommended in these patients (see **DOSAGE AND ADMINISTRATION**). The magnesium content of each buffered tablet of VIDEX is 8.6 mEq. This may present an excessive load of magnesium to patients with significant renal impairment, particularly after prolonged dosing.

Patients with Hepatic Impairment—It is unknown if hepatic impairment significantly affects didanosine pharmacokinetics. Therefore, these patients should be monitored closely for evidence of didanosine toxicity.

Hyperuricemia—VIDEX has been associated with asymptomatic hyperuricemia; treatment suspension may be necessary if clinical measures aimed at reducing uric acid levels fail.

***Information for Patients** (see **Patient Information Leaflet**)*—Patients should be informed that a serious toxicity of VIDEX used alone and in combination regimens, is pancreatitis, which may be fatal.

Patients should be informed that the preferred dosing frequency of VIDEX is twice daily because there is more evidence to support the effectiveness of this dosing frequency. Once-daily dosing should be considered only for adult patients whose management requires once-daily dosing of VIDEX.

Patients should also be aware that peripheral neuropathy, manifested by numbness, tingling, or pain in hands or feet, may develop during therapy with VIDEX. Patients should be counseled that peripheral neuropathy occurs with greatest frequency in patients with advanced HIV disease or a history of peripheral neuropathy, and that dose modification and/or discontinuation of VIDEX may be required if toxicity develops.

Patients should be informed that when VIDEX is used in combination with other agents with similar toxicities, the incidence of adverse events may be higher than when VIDEX is used alone. These patients should be followed closely.

Patients should be cautioned about the use of medications or other substances, including alcohol, that may exacerbate VIDEX toxicities.

Patients should be advised that to ensure proper acid neutralization in the stomach they must take at least two of the appropriate strength VIDEX tablets at each dose. To reduce the risk of gastrointestinal side effects from excess antacid, patients should take no more than four VIDEX tablets at each dose.

VIDEX is not a cure for HIV infection, and patients may continue to develop HIV-associated illnesses, including opportunistic infection. Therefore, patients should remain under the care of a physician when using VIDEX. Patients should be advised that VIDEX therapy has not been shown to reduce the risk of transmission of HIV to others through sexual contact or blood contamination. Patients should be informed that the long-term effects of VIDEX are unknown at this time.

Table 5
Selected Clinical Adverse Events from Monotherapy Studies

	Percent of Patients			
	ACTG 116A		ACTG 116B/117	
Adverse Events	VIDEX n=197	zidovudine n=212	VIDEX n=298	zidovudine n=304
Diarrhea	19	15	28	21
Peripheral Neurologic Symptoms/Neuropathy	17	14	20	12
Rash/Pruritus	7	8	9	5
Abdominal Pain	13	8	7	8
Pancreatitis	7	3	6	2

Table 6
Selected Clinical Adverse Events from Combination Studies

	Percent of Patients[a]			
	AI454-148[b]		START 2[b]	
Adverse Events	VIDEX+ stavudine+ nelfinavir n=482	zidovudine+ lamivudine+ nelfinavir n=248	VIDEX+ stavudine+ indinavir n=102	zidovudine+ lamivudine+ indinavir n=103
Diarrhea	70	60	45	39
Nausea	28	40	53	67
Headache	21	30	46	37
Peripheral Neurologic Symptoms/Neuropathy	26	6	21	10
Rash	13	16	30	18
Vomiting	12	14	30	35
Pancreatitis (see below)	1	*	<1	*

[a]Percentages based on treated subjects.
[b] Median duration of treatment 48 weeks.
* This event was not observed in this study arm.

Table 7
Selected Laboratory Abnormalities from Monotherapy Studies

	Percent of Patients			
	ACTG 116A		ACTG 116B/117	
Parameter	VIDEX n=197	zidovudine n=212	VIDEX n=298	zidovudine n=304
SGOT (AST) (>5 × ULN)	9	4	7	6
SGPT (ALT) (>5 × ULN)	9	6	6	6
Alkaline phosphatase (>5 × ULN)	4	1	1	1
Amylase (≥1.4 × ULN)	17	12	15	5
Uric Acid (>12 mg/dL)	3	1	2	1

ULN = upper limit of normal.

Drug Interactions: (see also CLINICAL PHARMACOLOGY, Drug Interactions). Coadministration of VIDEX with drugs that are known to cause pancreatitis may increase the risk of this toxicity (see WARNINGS) and should be done with extreme caution, only if other alternatives are not available, and only if clearly indicated. Neuropathy has occurred more frequently in patients with a history of neuropathy or neurotoxic drug therapy, including stavudine, and these patients may be at increased risk of neuropathy during VIDEX therapy (see **ADVERSE REACTIONS**).

Allopurinol—The AUC of didanosine was increased about 4-fold when allopurinol at 300 mg/day was coadministered with a single 200-mg dose of VIDEX to two patients with renal impairment (Cl_{cr}=15 and 18 mL/min). In 14 healthy volunteers, the mean AUC of didanosine increased approximately 2-fold when a 300-mg dose of allopurinol (daily for 7 days) was given with a single 400-mg dose of VIDEX. Coadministration of didanosine and allopurinol is not recommended.

Antacids—Concomitant administration of antacids containing magnesium or aluminum with VIDEX Chewable/Dispersible Buffered Tablets or Pediatric Powder for Oral Solution may potentiate adverse events associated with the antacid components.

Drugs Whose Absorption Can Be Affected by the Level of Acidity in the Stomach—Drugs such as ketoconazole and itraconazole should be administered at least 2 hours prior to dosing with VIDEX.

Ganciclovir—Administration of VIDEX 2 hours prior to or concurrent with oral ganciclovir was associated with a 111 (±114)% increase in the steady-state AUC of didanosine (n=12). A 21 (±17)% decrease in the steady-state AUC of ganciclovir was observed when VIDEX was administered 2 hours prior to ganciclovir, but not when the two drugs were administered simultaneously (n=12).

Quinolone Antibiotics—VIDEX should be administered at least 2 hours after or 6 hours before dosing with ciprofloxacin because plasma concentrations of ciprofloxacin are decreased when administered with antacids containing magnesium, calcium, or aluminum. In eight HIV-infected patients, the steady-state AUC of ciprofloxacin was decreased an average of 26% (95% CI = 14%, 37%) when ciprofloxacin was administered 2 hours prior to a marketed chewable/dispersible tablet formulation of VIDEX. The AUC of ciprofloxacin was decreased an average of 15-fold in 12 healthy subjects given ciprofloxacin and didanosine-placebo tablets concurrently. In a single subject given one dose of ciprofloxacin 2 hours after a dose of didanosine-placebo tablets, a greater than 50% reduction in the AUC of ciprofloxacin was observed.

Plasma concentrations of quinolone antibiotics are decreased when administered with antacids containing magnesium, calcium, or aluminum. The optimal dosing interval for coadministration with VIDEX should be determined by consulting the appropriate quinolone package insert.

Interactions with Other Antiretroviral Drugs—Significant decreases in the AUC of delavirdine (20%) and indinavir (84%) occurred following simultaneous administration of these agents with VIDEX. To avoid this interaction, delavirdine or indinavir should be given 1 hour prior to dosing with VIDEX. The pharmacokinetics of nelfinavir are not altered to a clinically significant degree when it is administered with a light meal 1 hour after VIDEX.

Carcinogenesis and Mutagenesis: Lifetime carcinogenicity studies were conducted in mice and rats for 22 and 24 months, respectively. In the mouse study, initial doses of 120, 800, and 1200 mg/kg/day for each sex were lowered after 8 months to 120, 210, and 210 mg/kg/day for females and 120, 300, and 600 mg/kg/day for males. The two higher doses exceeded the maximally tolerated dose in females and the high dose exceeded the maximally tolerated dose in males. The low dose in females represented 0.68-fold maximum human exposure and the intermediate dose in males represented 1.7-fold maximum human exposure based on relative AUC comparisons. In the rat study, initial doses were 100, 250, and 1000 mg/kg/day, and the high dose was lowered to 500 mg/kg/day after 18 months. The upper dose in male and female rats represented 3-fold maximum human exposure.

Didanosine induced no significant increase in neoplastic lesions in mice or rats at maximally tolerated doses.

Didanosine was positive in the following genetic toxicology assays: 1) the *Escherichia coli* tester strain WP2 uvrA bacterial mutagenicity assay; 2) the L5178Y/TK+/- mouse lymphoma mammalian cell gene mutation assay; 3) the *in vitro* chromosomal aberrations assay in cultured human peripheral lympocytes; 4) the *in vitro* chromosomal aberrations assay in Chinese Hamster Lung cells; and 5) the BALB/c 3T3 *in vitro* transformation assay. No evidence of mutagenicity was observed in an Ames *Salmonella* bacterial mutagenicity assay or in rat and mouse *in vivo* micronucleus assays.

Pregnancy, Reproduction and Fertility: Pregnancy "Category B". Reproduction studies have been performed in rats and rabbits at doses up to 12 and 14.2 times the estimated human exposure (based upon plasma levels), respectively, and have revealed no evidence of impaired fertility or harm to the fetus due to didanosine. At approximately 12 times the estimated human exposure, didanosine was slightly toxic to female rats and their pups during mid and late lactation. These rats showed reduced food intake and body weight gains but the physical and functional development of the offspring was not impaired and there were no major changes in the F2 generation. A study in rats showed that didanosine and/or its metabolites are transferred to the fetus through the placenta. There are no adequate and well-controlled studies in pregnant women. Because animal reproduction studies are not always predictive of human response, this drug should be used during pregnancy only if clearly needed.

Antiretroviral Pregnancy Registry: To monitor maternal-fetal outcomes of pregnant women exposed to didanosine and other antiretroviral agents, an Antiretroviral Pregnancy Registry has been established. Physicians are encouraged to register patients by calling 1-800-258-4263.

Nursing Mothers: The Centers for Disease Control and Prevention recommend that HIV-infected mothers not breast-feed their infants to avoid risking postnatal transmission of HIV. A study in rats showed that following oral administration, didanosine and/or its metabolites were excreted into the milk of lactating rats. It is not known if didanosine is excreted in human milk. Because of both the potential for HIV transmission and the potential for serious adverse reactions in nursing infants, **mothers should be instructed not to breast-feed if they are receiving VIDEX (didanosine).**

Pediatric Use: Use of VIDEX in pediatric patients is supported by evidence from adequate and well-controlled studies of VIDEX in adults and pediatric patients (see **Clinical Studies, CLINICAL PHARMACOLOGY, ADVERSE REACTIONS,** and **DOSAGE AND ADMINISTRATION**).

Geriatric Use: In an Expanded Access Program for patients with advanced HIV infection, patients aged 65 years and older had a higher frequency of pancreatitis (10%) than younger patients (5%) (see **WARNINGS**). Clinical studies of didanosine did not include sufficient numbers of subjects aged 65 years and over to determine whether they respond differently than younger subjects. Didanosine is known to be substantially excreted by the kidney, and the risk of toxic reactions to this drug may be greater in patients with impaired renal function. Because elderly patients are more likely to have decreased renal function, care should be taken in dose selection. In addition, renal function should be monitored and dosage adjustments should be made accordingly (see **DOSAGE AND ADMINISTRATION: Dose Adjustment**).

ADVERSE REACTIONS

A SERIOUS TOXICITY OF VIDEX IS PANCREATITIS, WHICH MAY BE FATAL (see **WARNINGS**). OTHER IMPORTANT TOXICITIES INCLUDE LACTIC ACIDOSIS/SEVERE HEPATOMEGALY WITH STEATOSIS; RETINAL CHANGES AND OPTIC NEURITIS; AND PERIPHERAL NEUROPATHY (see **WARNINGS** and **PRECAUTIONS**).

When VIDEX is used in combination with other agents with similar toxicities, the incidence of these toxicities may be higher than when VIDEX is used alone. Thus, patients treated with VIDEX in combination with stavudine, with or without hydroxyurea, may be at increased risk for pancreatitis and liver function abnormalities (see WARNINGS). Patients treated with VIDEX in combination with stavudine may also be at increased risk for peripheral neuropathy (see **PRECAUTIONS**).

Adults: Selected clinical adverse events that occurred in adult patients in clinical studies with VIDEX are provided in Table 5 and Table 6.

[See tables 5 & 6 at top of previous page]

Pancreatitis resulting in death was observed in one patient who received VIDEX plus stavudine plus nelfinavir in Study AI454-148 and in one patient who received VIDEX plus stavudine plus indinavir in the START 2 study. In addition, pancreatitis resulting in death was observed in 2 of 68 patients who received VIDEX plus stavudine plus indinavir plus hydroxyurea in an ACTG clinical trial (see WARNINGS).

Selected laboratory abnormalities in clinical studies with VIDEX (didanosine) are shown in Table 7, Table 8, and Table 9.

[See table 7 at top of previous page]
[See tables 8 & 9 above]

Table 8
Selected Laboratory Abnormalities from Combination Studies (Grades 3–4)

	Percent of Patients[a]			
	AI454-148[b]		START 2[b]	
Parameter	VIDEX+ stavudine+ nelfinavir n=482	zidovudine+ lamivudine+ nelfinavir n=248	VIDEX+ stavudine+ indinavir n=102	zidovudine+ lamivudine+ indinavir n=103
Bilirubin (>2.6 × ULN)	<1	<1	16	8
SGOT (AST) (>5 × ULN)	3	2	7	7
SGPT (ALT) (>5 × ULN)	3	3	8	5
GGT (>5 × ULN)	NC	NC	5	2
Lipase (>2 × ULN)	7	2	5	5
Amylase (>2 × ULN)	NC	NC	8	2

ULN = upper limit of normal.
NC = Not Collected
[a]Percentages based on treated subjects.
[b] Median duration of treatment 48 weeks.

Table 9
Selected Laboratory Abnormalities from Combination Studies (All Grades)

	Percent of Patients[a]			
	AI454-148[b]		START 2[b]	
Parameter	VIDEX+ stavudine+ nelfinavir n=482	zidovudine+ lamivudine+ nelfinavir n=248	VIDEX+ stavudine+ indinavir n=102	zidovudine+ lamivudine+ indinavir n=103
Bilirubin	7	3	68	55
SGOT (AST)	42	23	53	20
SGPT (ALT)	37	24	50	18
GGT	NC	NC	28	12
Lipase	17	11	26	19
Amylase	NC	NC	31	17

NC = Not Collected
[a]Percentages based on treated subjects.
[b]Median duration of treatment 48 weeks.

Observed during Clinical Practice: The following events have been identified during postapproval use of VIDEX. Because they are reported voluntarily from a population of unknown size, estimates of frequency cannot be made. These events have been chosen for inclusion due to their seriousness, frequency of reporting, causal connection to VIDEX, or a combination of these factors.

Body as a Whole—alopecia, anaphylactoid reaction, asthenia, chills/fever, and pain.

Digestive Disorders—anorexia, dyspepsia, and flatulence.

Exocrine Gland Disorders—pancreatitis (including fatal cases) (see **WARNINGS**), sialoadenitis, parotid gland enlargement, dry mouth, and dry eyes.

Hematologic Disorders—anemia, leukopenia, and thrombocytopenia.

Liver—lactic acidosis and hepatic steatosis (see **WARNINGS**); hepatitis and liver failure.

Metabolic Disorders—diabetes mellitus, hypoglycemia, and hyperglycemia.

Musculoskeletal Disorders—myalgia (with or without increases in creatinine phosphokinase), rhabdomyolysis including acute renal failure and hemodialysis, arthralgia, and myopathy.

Ophthalmologic Disorders—Retinal depigmentation and optic neuritis (see **WARNINGS**).

Pediatric Patients: Adverse events and laboratory abnormalities reported to occur in the pediatric patients in ACTG 152 were generally similar to adverse events and laboratory abnormalities reported in adult patients.

In pediatric phase 1 studies, pancreatitis occurred in 2 of 60 (3%) patients treated at entry doses below 300 mg/m^2/day and in 5 of 38 (13%) patients treated at higher doses.

Retinal changes and optic neuritis have been reported in pediatric patients.

OVERDOSAGE

There is no known antidote for VIDEX overdosage. In phase 1 studies, in which VIDEX was initially administered at doses ten times the currently recommended dose, toxicities included: pancreatitis, peripheral neuropathy, diarrhea, hyperuricemia and hepatic dysfunction. Didanosine is not dialyzable by peritoneal dialysis, although there is some clearance by hemodialysis (see **CLINICAL PHARMACOLOGY, Pharmacokinetics**).

DOSAGE AND ADMINISTRATION

Dosage: All VIDEX formulations should be administered on an empty stomach, at least 30 minutes before or 2 hours after eating. For either a once-daily or twice-daily regimen, patients must take at least two of the appropriate strength tablets at each dose to provide adequate buffering and prevent gastric acid degradation of didanosine. Because of the need for adequate buffering, the 200-mg strength tablet should only be used as a component of a once-daily regimen. To reduce the risk of gastrointestinal side effects, patients should take no more than four tablets at each dose.

Adults: The preferred dosing frequency of VIDEX is twice daily because there is more evidence to support the effectiveness of this dosing regimen. Once-daily dosing should be considered only for adult patients whose management requires once-daily dosing of VIDEX (see **Clinical Studies**). The daily dose in adult patients in dependent on weight as outlined in Table 10.

Table 10
Adult Dosing

Patient Weight	VIDEX Tablets[a]	VIDEX Buffered Powder[b]
Preferred dosing		
≥60 kg	200 mg BID	250 mg BID
<60 kg	125 mg BID	167 mg BID
Dosing for patients whose management requires once-daily frequency		
≥60 kg	400 mg QD	[b]
<60 kg	250 mg QD	[b]

[a] The 200-mg strength tablet should only be used as a component of a once-daily regimen.
[b] Not suitable for QD dosing except for patients with renal impairment. See Table 11.

Pediatric Patients—The recommended dose of VIDEX (didanosine) in pediatric patients is 120 mg/m^2 BID. There are no data on once-daily dosing of VIDEX in pediatric patients.

Dose Adjustment: Clinical and laboratory signs suggestive of pancreatitis should prompt dose suspension and careful evaluation of the possibility of pancreatitis. VIDEX use should be discontinued in patients with confirmed pancreatitis (see WARNINGS).

Patients with symptoms of peripheral neuropathy may tolerate a reduced dose of VIDEX after resolution of the symptoms of peripheral neuropathy upon drug discontinuation. If neuropathy recurs after resumption of VIDEX, permanent discontinuation of VIDEX should be considered.

In adult patients with impaired renal function, the dose of VIDEX should be adjusted to compensate for the slower rate of elimination. The recommended doses and dosing intervals of VIDEX in adult patients with renal insufficiency are presented in Table 11.

[See table 11 at top of next page]

Urinary excretion is also a major route of elimination of didanosine in pediatric patients; therefore, the clearance of didanosine may be altered in children with renal impairment. Although there are insufficient data to recommend a

Continued on next page

Videx—Cont.

specific dose adjustment of VIDEX in this patient population, a reduction in the dose and/or an increase in the interval between doses should be considered.

Patients Requiring Continuous Ambulatory Peritoneal Dialysis (CAPD) or Hemodialysis—It is recommended that one fourth of the total daily dose of VIDEX be administered once a day (see Table 11, recommended dosage for patients with CL_{CR} <10 mL/min). It is not necessary to administer a supplemental dose of VIDEX following hemodialysis.

Hepatic Impairment—See **WARNINGS** and **PRECAUTIONS**.

Method of Preparation:

VIDEX Chewable/Dispersible Buffered Tablets

Adult Dosing—To provide adequate buffering, at least two of the appropriate strength tablets, but no more than four tablets, should be thoroughly chewed or dispersed in at least 1 ounce of water prior to consumption (see **PRECAUTIONS: Information for Patients**). To disperse tablets, add 2 tablets to at least 1 ounce of drinking water. Stir until a uniform dispersion forms, and drink the entire dispersion immediately. If additional flavoring is desired, the dispersion may be diluted with one ounce of clear apple juice. Stir the further diluted dispersion just prior to consumption. The dispersion with clear apple juice is stable at room temperature, 62° to 73°F (17° to 23°C), for up to one hour.

VIDEX Buffered Powder for Oral Solution

1. Open packet carefully and pour contents into a container with approximately 4 ounces of drinking water. Do not mix with fruit juice or other acid-containing liquid.
2. Stir until the powder completely dissolves (approximately 2 to 3 minutes).
3. Drink the entire solution immediately.

VIDEX Pediatric Powder for Oral Solution

Prior to dispensing, the pharmacist must constitute dry powder with Purified Water, USP, to an initial concentration of 20 mg/mL and immediately mix the resulting solution with antacid to a final concentration of 10 mg/mL as follows:

20 mg/mL Initial Solution—Constitute the product to 20 mg/mL by adding 100 mL or 200 mL of Purified Water, USP, to the 2 g or 4 g of VIDEX powder, respectively, in the product bottle.

10 mg/mL Final Admixture—1. Immediately mix one part of the 20 mg/mL initial solution with one part of either Mylanta® Double Strength Liquid, Extra Strength Maalox® Plus Suspension, or Maalox® TC Suspension for a final dispensing concentration of 10 mg VIDEX per mL. For patient home use, the admixture should be dispensed in appropriately sized, flint-glass or plastic (HDPE, PET, or PETG) bottles with child-resistant closures. This admixture is stable for 30 days under refrigeration, 36° to 46°F (2° to 8°C).
2. Instruct the patient to shake the admixture thoroughly prior to use and to store the tightly closed container in the refrigerator, 36° to 46°F (2° to 8°C), up to 30 days.

Mylanta® is a registered trademark of Johnson & Johnson-Merck Consumer Pharmaceuticals Company.

Maalox® is a registered trademark of Novartis Consumer Health, Inc.

HOW SUPPLIED

VIDEX® (didanosine) Chewable/Dispersible Buffered Tablets are round, off white to light orange/yellow with a mottled appearance, orange-flavored, tablets embossed with "VIDEX" on one side and the product strength on the other. The tablets are available in the following strengths of VIDEX: 25, 50, 100, 150, and 200 mg. Sixty tablets are packaged in bottles with child-resistant closures.

The tablets should be stored in tightly closed bottles at 59° to 86°F (15° to 30°C). If dispersed in water, the dose may be held for up to 1 hour at ambient temperature.

VIDEX® (didanosine) Buffered Powder for Oral Solution is supplied in single-dose, child-resistant foil packets in the following strengths of VIDEX: 100, 167, or 250 mg. Each product strength provides a sweetened, buffered solution of VIDEX.

The packets should be stored at 59° to 86°F (15° to 30°C). After dissolving in water, the solution may be stored at ambient room temperature for up to 4 hours.

VIDEX® (didanosine) Pediatric Powder for Oral Solution is supplied in 4- and 8-ounce glass bottles containing 2 g or 4 g of VIDEX, respectively.

The bottles of powder should be stored at 59° to 86°F (15° to 30°C). The VIDEX admixture may be stored up to 30 days in a refrigerator, 36° to 46°F (2° to 8°C). Discard any unused portion after 30 days.

The NDC numbers for the previously described VIDEX products are:

[See table 12 above]

US Patent Nos.: 4,861,759 and 5,616,566.

HANDLING AND DISPOSAL

Spill, Leak and Disposal Procedure: Avoid generating dust during clean-up of powdered products; use wet mop or damp sponge. Clean surface with soap and water as necessary. Containerize larger spills.

There is no single preferred method of disposal of containerized waste. Disposal options include incineration, landfill, or sewer as dictated by specific circumstances and relevant national, state, and local regulations.

BRISTOL-MYERS SQUIBB IMMUNOLOGY
Bristol-Myers Squibb Company
Princeton, NJ 08543
U.S.A.

Table 11
Recommended Dosage of VIDEX in Renal Impairment

	≥60 kg		<60 kg	
Creatinine Clearance (mL/min)	**Tablet[a] (mg)**	**Buffered Powder[b] (mg)**	**Tablet[a] (mg)**	**Buffered Powder[b] (mg)**
≥60	200 BID[c]	250 BID	125 BID[c]	167 BID
30–59	200 QD or 100 BID	100 BID	150 QD or 75 BID	100 BID
10–29	150 QD	167 QD	100 QD	100 QD
<10	100 QD	100 QD	75 QD	100 QD

[a] VIDEX Chewable/Dispersible Buffered Tablet. Two VIDEX tablets must be taken with each dose; different strengths of tablets may be combined to yield the recommended dose.
[b] VIDEX Buffered Powder for Oral Solution
[c] 400 mg QD (≥60 kg) or 250 mg QD (<60 kg) for patients whose management requires once-daily frequency of administration.

Table 12

NDC No.	Packaging Information	Product Strength
VIDEX® Chewable/Dispersible Buffered Tablets		
0087-6650-01	60 tablets/bottle	25 mg/tablet
0087-6651-01	60 tablets/bottle	50 mg/tablet
0087-6652-01	60 tablets/bottle	100 mg/tablet
0087-6653-01	60 tablets/bottle	150 mg/tablet
0087-6665-15	60 tablets/bottle	200 mg/tablet
VIDEX® Buffered Powder for Oral Solution		
0087-6614-43	One single-dose foil packet*	100 mg/packet
0087-6615-43	One single-dose foil packet*	167 mg/packet
0087-6616-43	One single-dose foil packet*	250 mg/packet
VIDEX® Pediatric Powder for Oral Solution		
0087-6632-41	One bottle per carton	2 g/bottle
0087-6633-41	One bottle per carton	4 g/bottle

* Packaged as 30 packets per carton.

F8-B001-8-00 Revised July 2000
1099814A3

PATIENT INFORMATION

VIDEX®
(generic name =
didanosine also known as ddl)

VIDEX® (didanosine) Chewable/Dispersible Buffered Tablets
VIDEX® (didanosine) Buffered Powder for Oral Solution
VIDEX® (didanosine) Pediatric Powder for Oral Solution

WHAT IS VIDEX?

VIDEX (pronunced VY dex) is a prescription medicine used in combination with other drugs to treat children and adults who are infected with HIV (the human immunodeficiency virus, the virus that causes AIDS). VIDEX belongs to a class of drugs called nucleoside analogues. By reducing the growth of HIV, VIDEX helps your body maintain its supply of CD4 cells, which are important for fighting HIV and other infections.

VIDEX will not cure your HIV infection. At present there is no cure for HIV infection. Even while taking VIDEX, you may continue to have HIV-related illnesses, including infections with other disease-producing organisms. Continue to see your doctor regularly and report any medical problems that occur.

VIDEX does not prevent a patient infected with HIV from passing the virus to other people. To protect others, you must continue to practice safe sex and take precautions to prevent others from coming in contact with your blood and other body fluids.

There is limited information on the effects of long-term use of VIDEX.

WHO SHOULD NOT TAKE VIDEX?

Do not take VIDEX if you are allergic to any of its ingredients, including its active ingredient, didanosine, and the inactive ingredients. (See **Inactive Ingredients** at the end of this leaflet.) Tell your doctor if you think you have had an allergic reaction to any of these ingredients.

HOW SHOULD I TAKE VIDEX? HOW SHOULD I STORE IT?

Your doctor will determine your dose based on your body weight, kidney and liver function, and any side effects that you may have had with other medicines. Take VIDEX **on an empty stomach—that means at least 30 minutes before or 2 hours after eating. Do not take VIDEX with food.** Try not to miss a dose, but if you do, take it as soon as possible. If it is almost time for the next dose, skip the missed dose and continue your regular dosing schedule.

Chewable/Dispersible Tablets: Each VIDEX tablet contains antacid.

Each time you take VIDEX, you must take at least two, but not more than four, tablets. This is because VIDEX tablets contain an antacid to reduce the amount of acid in your stomach. If you have too much acid, the medicine will break down. However, too much antacid may cause stomach problems.

— **DO NOT** swallow VIDEX tablets whole. Chew the tablets well or mix them in water. Many patients drop the tablets in at least one ounce of water and stir well before swallowing. If you choose to mix the tablets in water, you may add one ounce (2 tablespoons) of clear apple juice to the mixture for flavor (do not use any other kind of juice).

— Store tablets in a tightly closed container at room temperature away from heat and out of the reach of children and pets. Do NOT store the tablets in a damp place such as a bathroom medicine cabinet or near the kitchen sink.

Buffered Powder for Oral Solution: Pour the contents of a packet into a glass with 4 ounces (1/2 measuring cup) of water. Stir until completely dissolved. Drink the entire solution right away. Do not mix with fruit juice. Store packets at room temperature before use.

Pediatric Oral Solution: Your pharmacist will prepare the oral solution. Shake the solution well before each use. Store in the refrigerator. Throw away any unused portion after 30 days.

If you have kidney disease: If your kidneys are not working properly, your doctor will need to do regular tests to check how they are working while you take VIDEX. Your doctor may also lower your dosage of VIDEX.

WHAT SHOULD I DO IF SOMEONE TAKES AN OVERDOSE OF VIDEX?

If someone may have taken an overdose of VIDEX, get medical help right away. Contact their doctor or a poison control center.

WHAT SHOULD I AVOID WHILE TAKING VIDEX?

Alcohol. Avoid drinking alcohol while taking VIDEX since alcohol may increase your risk of pancreatitis (pain and inflammation of the pancreas) or liver damage.

Other medicines. Other medicines, including those you can buy without a prescription, may interfere with the actions of VIDEX. **Do not take any medicine, vitamin supplement, or other health preparation without first checking with your doctor.**

Antacids—Since VIDEX (didanosine) contains some of the same ingredients found in antacids, any side effects related to VIDEX's ingredients may get worse if you also take an antacid.

Medicines at the same time as VIDEX—Some medicines should not be taken at the same time of day that you take VIDEX. Check with your doctor.

Pregnancy: It is not known if VIDEX can harm a human fetus, so VIDEX should be used during pregnancy only after discussion with your doctor. **Tell your doctor if you become pregnant or plan to become pregnant while taking VIDEX.**

Nursing: Studies have shown VIDEX is in the breast milk of animals getting the drug. It may also be in human breast milk. The Centers for Disease Control and Prevention (CDC) recommends that HIV-infected mothers **not** breast-feed. This should reduce the risk of passing HIV infection to their babies and the potential for serious adverse reactions in nursing infants. Therefore, do not nurse a baby while taking VIDEX.

WHAT ARE THE POSSIBLE SIDE EFFECTS OF VIDEX?

Pancreatitis: Pancreatitis is a dangerous inflammation of the pancreas that may cause death. ***Tell your doctor right away if you or a child taking VIDEX develops stomach pain, nausea, or vomiting. These can be signs of pancreatitis.*** Before starting VIDEX therapy, let your doctor know if you or a child for whom it has been prescribed has ever had pancreatitis. This condition is more likely to happen in people who have had it before. It is also more likely in people with advanced HIV disease. However, it can occur at any stage of HIV disease. It may be more common in patients with kidney problems, those who drink alcohol, and those who are also treated with ZERIT (stavudine), also known as d4T, or hydroxyurea. If you get pancreatitis, your doctor will tell you to stop taking VIDEX.

Lactic acidosis, severe liver enlargement, and **liver failure,** including deaths, have been reported among patients taking VIDEX. Symptoms that may indicate a liver problem are:

- feeling very weak, tired, or uncomfortable,
- unusual or unexpected stomach discomfort,
- feeling cold,
- feeling dizzy or lightheaded,
- suddenly developing a slow or irregular heartbeat.

Lactic acidosis is a medical emergency that must be treated in a hospital: If you notice any of these symptoms or if your medical condition changes, stop taking VIDEX and **call your doctor right away.** Women, overweight patients, and those who have been treated for a long time with other medicines used to treat HIV infection are more likely to develop lactic acidosis. Your doctor should check your liver function periodically while you are taking VIDEX. You should be especially careful if you have a history of heavy alcohol use or a liver problem.

Vision changes: VIDEX may affect the nerves in your eyes. Because of this, you should have regular eye examinations. You should also report any changes in vision to your doctor right away. This includes, for example, seeing colors abnormally or blurred vision.

Peripheral neuropathy: This is a problem with the nerves in your hands or feet. The nerve problem may be serious. ***Tell your doctor right away if you or a child taking VIDEX has continuing numbness, tingling, or pain in the feet or hands.*** A child may not recognize these symptoms or know to tell you that his or her feet or hands are numb, burning, tingling, or painful. Ask your child's doctor how to find out if your child is developing peripheral neuropathy.

Before starting VIDEX therapy, let your doctor know if you or a child for whom it has been prescribed has ever had peripheral neuropathy. This condition is more likely to happen in people who have had it before. It is also more likely in patients taking the medicines that affect the nerves and in people with advanced HIV disease. However, it can occur at any stage of HIV disease. If you get peripheral neuropathy, your doctor will tell you to stop taking VIDEX. After stopping VIDEX, the symptoms may get worse for a short time and then get better. Once symptoms of peripheral neuropathy go away completely, you and your doctor should decide if starting VIDEX is right for you. If so, you might be started at a lower dose.

Special note about other medicines: If you take VIDEX along with other medicines with similar side effects, you may increase the chance of having these side effects. For example, using VIDEX in combination with other medicines that may cause pancreatitis, peripheral neuropathy, or liver problems (including stavudine and hydroxyurea) may increase your chance of having these side effects.

Other side effects: The most comon side effects in adults taking VIDEX are diarrhea, neuropathy, (nerve disorders), chilld or fever, rash, abdominal pain, weakness, headache, and nausea and vomiting. Children may have similar side effects as adults.

WHAT ELSE SHOULD I KNOW ABOUT VIDEX?

If you should limit sodium (salt) intake: Each single-dose packet of Buffered Powder for Oral Solution contains 1380 mg of sodium. Each Chewable/Dispersible Tablet contains 264.5 mg of sodium.

If you have phenylketonuria: Each Chewable/Dispersible Tablet contains 36.5 mg of phenylalanine.

Inactive Ingredients:

Chewable/Dispersible Tablets—calcium carbonate, magnesium hydroxide, aspartame, sorbitol, mandarin orange flavor, polyplasdone, microcrystalline cellulose, and magnesium stearate.

Buffered Powder for Oral Solution—citrate-phosphate buffer (dibasic sodium phosphate, sodium citrate, and citric acid) and sucrose.

Pediatric Oral Solution—Mylanta® Double Strength Liquid, Extra Strength Maalox® Plus or Maalox® TC Suspension.

This medicine was prescribed for your particular condition. Do not use VIDEX for another condition or give it to others. Keep VIDEX and all medicines out of the reach of children. Throw away VIDEX when it is outdated or no longer needed by flushing it down the toilet or pouring it down the sink.

This summary does not include everything there is to know about VIDEX. Medicines are sometimes prescribed for purposes other than those listed in a Patient Information Leaflet. If you have questions or concerns, or want more information about VIDEX, your physician and pharmacist have the complete prescribing information upon which this leaflet is based. You may want to read it and discuss it with your doctor or other healthcare professional. Remember, no written summary can replace careful discussion with your doctor.

Mylanta® is a registered trademark of Johnson & Johnson-Merck Consumer Pharmaceuticals Company.

Maalox® is a registered trademark of Novartis Consumer Health, Inc.

This Patient Information Leaflet has been approved by the U.S. Food and Drug Administration.

BRISTOL-MYERS SQUIBB IMMUNOLOGY
Bristol-Myers Squibb Company
Princeton, NJ 08543
U.S.A.
F8-B001-8-00 Revised July 2000
Based on 1099814A4(7/00)

Edwards Lifesciences Research Medical, Inc.

ONE EDWARDS WAY
IRVINE, CA 92614

Direct Inquiries to:
Customer Service
(800) 453-8432
FAX: (801) 565-6209
www.edwards.com

RIMSO®-50 ℞
brand of dimethyl sulfoxide irrigation, U.S.P.
PRESCRIBING INFORMATION

DESCRIPTION

RIMSO®-50, brand of dimethyl sulfoxide (DMSO) 50% w/w Aqueous Solution for intravesical instillation.

Each mL contains 0.54 gm dimethyl sulfoxide STERILE AND NON-PYROGENIC

Intravesical instillation for the treatment of interstitial cystitis

NOT FOR I.M. OR I.V. INJECTION.

Rx only.

The active component of RIMSO®-50 is dimethyl sulfoxide which has the empirical formula C_2H_6OS, and is structurally represented as:

$$CH_3-\overset{O}{\overset{\|}{S}}-CH_3$$

Dimethyl sulfoxide is a clear, colorless and essentially odorless liquid which is miscible with water and most organic solvents. Other physical characteristics include: molecular weight 78.13, melting point 18.3° C, and a specific gravity of 1.096.

CLINICAL PHARMACOLOGY

Dimethyl sulfoxide is metabolized in man by oxidation to dimethyl sulfone or by reduction in dimethyl sulfide. Dimethyl sulfoxide and dimethyl sulfone are excreted in the urine and feces. Dimethyl sulfide is eliminated through the breath and skin and is responsible for the characteristic odor from patients on dimethyl sulfoxide medication. Dimethyl sulfone can persist in serum for longer than two weeks after a single intravesical instillation. No residual accumulation of dimethyl sulfoxide has occurred in man or lower animals who have received treatment for protracted periods of time. Following topical application, dimethyl sulfoxide is absorbed and generally distributed in the tissues and body fluids.

INDICATIONS AND USAGE

RIMSO®-50 (dimethyl sulfoxide) is indicated for the symptomatic relief of patients with interstitial cystitis. RIMSO®-50 has not been approved as being safe and effective for any other indication. There is no clinical evidence of effectiveness of dimethyl sulfoxide in the treatment of bacterial infections of the urinary tract.

CONTRAINDICATIONS

None known.

WARNINGS

Dimethyl sulfoxide can initiate the liberation of histamine and there has been occasional hypersensitivity reaction with topical administration of dimethyl sulfoxide. This hypersensitivity has been reported in one patient receiving intravesical RIMSO®-50. The physician should be cognizant of this possibility in prescribing RIMSO®-50. If anaphylactoid symptoms develop, appropriate therapy should be instituted.

PRECAUTIONS

Changes in the refractive index and lens opacities have been seen in monkeys, dogs and rabbits given high doses of dimethyl sulfoxide chronically. Since lens changes were noted in animals, full eye evaluations, including slit lamp examinations, are recommended prior to and periodically during treatment.

Approximately every six months patients receiving dimethyl sulfoxide should have a biogenetical screening, particularly liver and renal function tests, and complete blood count.

Intravesical instillation of RIMSO®-50 may be harmful to patients with urinary tract malignancy because of dimethyl sulfoxide-induced vasodilation.

Some data indicate that dimethyl sulfoxide potentiates other concomitantly administered medications.

Pregnancy Category C. Dimethyl sulfoxide caused teratogenic responses in hamsters, rats and mice when administered intraperitoneally at high doses (2.5 to 12 gm/kg). Oral or topical doses of dimethyl sulfoxide did not cause problems of reproduction in rats, mice and hamsters. Topical doses (5 gm/kg first two days, then 2.5 gm/kg—last eight days) produced lorata in rabbits, but in another study, topical doses of 1.1 gm/kg days 3 through 16 of gestation failed to produce any abnormalities. There are no adequate and well controlled studies in pregnant women. Dimethyl sulfoxide should be used during pregnancy only if the potential benefit justifies the potential risk to the fetus.

It is not known whether this drug is excreted in human milk. Because many drugs are excreted in human milk, caution should be exercised when dimethyl sulfoxide is administered to a nursing woman.

Safety and effectiveness in children have not been established.

ADVERSE REACTIONS

The garlic-like taste may be noted by the patient within a few minutes after instillation of RIMSO®-50 (dimethyl sulfoxide). This taste may last several hours and because of the presence of metabolites, an odor on the breath and skin may remain for 72 hours.

Transient chemical cystitis has been noted following instillation of dimethyl sulfoxide.

The patient may experience moderately severe discomfort on administration. Usually this becomes less prominent with repeated administration.

DRUG ABUSE AND DEPENDENCE

None known.

OVERDOSAGE

The oral LD_{50} of dimethyl sulfoxide in the dog is greater than 10 gm/kg. It is improbable that this dosage level could be obtained with intravesical instillation of RIMSO®-50 in the patient.

In case of accidental oral ingestion, specific measures should be taken to induce emesis. Additional measures which may be considered are gastric lavage, activated charcoal and force diuresis.

DOSAGE AND ADMINISTRATION

Instillation of 50 mL of RIMSO®-50 (dimethyl sulfoxide) directly into the bladder may be accomplished by catheter or aseptic syringe and allow to remain for 15 minutes. Application of an analgesic lubricant gel such as lidocaine jelly to the urethra is suggested prior to insertion of the catheter to avoid spasm. The medication is expelled by spontaneous voiding. It is recommended that the treatment be repeated every two weeks until maximum symptomatic relief is obtained. Thereafter, time intervals between therapy may be increased appropriately.

Administration of oral analgesic medication or suppositories containing belladonna and opium prior to the instillation of RIMSO®-50 can reduce bladder spasm.

In patients with severe interstitial cystitis with very sensitive bladders, the initial treatment, and possibly the second and third (depending on patient response) should be done under anesthesia. (Saddle block has been suggested.)

HOW SUPPLIED

Bottles contain 50 mL of sterile and non-pyrogenic RIMSO®-50 (50% w/w dimethyl sulfoxide aqueous solution). Dimethyl sulfoxide is clear and colorless.

Protect from strong light

Store at room temperature (59° to 86°F) (15° to 30°C)

NDC #0433-0433-05

For additional information concerning RIMSO®-50, contact Edwards Lifesciences Research Medical, Inc., Irvine, CA 92614 (800) 453-8432.

RIMSO®-50 is manufactured by: Ben Venue Laboratories, Inc., Bedford, OH 44146, for Edwards Lifesciences Research Medical, Inc., Irvine, CA 92614.

Ligand Pharmaceuticals Incorporated

10275 SCIENCE CENTER DRIVE
SAN DIEGO, CA 92121

Direct Inquiries to:
(858) 550-7500
Customer Service
(877) 454-4263
Medical Information
(800) 964-5836
Reimbursement Support
(877) 654-4263

TARGRETIN® ℞
[tahr-greh' tən]
(bexarotene)
Capsules, 75 mg
Rx only.

Targretin® capsules are a member of the retinoid class of drugs that is associated with birth defects in humans. Targretin® capsules also caused birth defects

Continued on next page

Targretin—Cont.

when administered orally to pregnant rats. Targretin® capsules must not be administered to a pregnant woman. See CONTRAINDICATIONS.

DESCRIPTION

Targretin® (bexarotene) is a member of a subclass of retinoids that selectively activate retinoid X receptors (RXRs). These retinoid receptors have biologic activity distinct from that of retinoic acid receptors (RARs). Each soft gelatin capsule for oral administration contains 75 mg of bexarotene. The chemical name is 4-[1-(5,6,7,8-tetrahydro-3,5,5,8,8-pentamethyl-2-naphthalenyl) ethenyl] benzoic acid, and the structural formula is as follows:

Bexarotene is an off-white to white powder with a molecular weight of 348.48 and a molecular formula of $C_{24}H_{28}O_2$. It is insoluble in water and slightly soluble in vegetable oils and ethanol, USP.

Each Targretin® (bexarotene) capsule also contains the following inactive ingredients: polyethylene glycol 400, NF, polysorbate 20, NF, povidone, USP, and butylated hydroxyanisol, NF. The capsule shell contains gelatin, NF, sorbitol special-glycerin blend, and titanium dioxide, USP.

CLINICAL PHARMACOLOGY

Mechanism of Action

Bexarotene selectively binds and activates retinoid X receptor subtypes (RXRα, RXRβ, RXRγ). RXRs can form heterodimers with various receptor partners such as retinoic acid receptors (RARs), vitamin D receptor, thyroid receptor, and peroxisome proliferator activator receptors (PPARs). Once activated, these receptors function as transcription factors that regulate the expression of genes that control cellular differentiation and proliferation. Bexarotene inhibits the growth *in vitro* of some tumor cell lines of hematopoietic and squamous cell origin. It also induces tumor regression *in vivo* in some animal models. The exact mechanism of action of bexarotene in the treatment of cutaneous T-cell lymphoma (CTCL) is unknown.

Pharmacokinetics

General

After oral administration of Targretin® capsules, bexarotene is absorbed with a T_{max} of about two hours. Terminal half-life of bexarotene is about seven hours. Studies in patients with advanced malignancies show approximate single dose linearity within the therapeutic range and low accumulation with multiple doses. Plasma bexarotene AUC and C_{max} values resulting from a 75 to 300 mg dose were 35% and 48% higher, respectively, after a fat-containing meal than after a glucose solution (see **PRECAUTIONS: *Drug-Food Interaction*** and **DOSAGE AND ADMINISTRATION**). Bexarotene is highly bound (>99%) to plasma proteins. The plasma proteins to which bexarotene binds have not been elucidated, and the ability of bexarotene to displace drugs bound to plasma proteins and the ability of drugs to displace bexarotene binding have not been studied (see **PRECAUTIONS: Protein Binding**). The uptake of bexarotene by organs or tissues has not been evaluated.

Metabolism

Four bexarotene metabolites have been identified in plasma: 6- and 7-hydroxy-bexarotene and 6- and 7-oxo-bexarotene. *In vitro* studies suggest that cytochrome P450 3A4 is the major cytochrome P450 responsible for formation of the oxidative metabolites and that the oxidative metabolites may be glucuronidated. The oxidative metabolites are active in *in vitro* assays of retinoid receptor activation, but the relative contribution of the parent and any metabolites to the efficacy and safety of Targretin® capsules is unknown.

Elimination

The renal elimination of bexarotene and its metabolites was examined in patients with Type 2 diabetes mellitus. Neither bexarotene nor its metabolites were excreted in urine in appreciable amounts. Bexarotene is thought to be eliminated primarily through the hepatobiliary system.

Special Populations

Elderly: Bexarotene C_{max} and AUC were similar in advanced cancer patients <60 years old and in patients >60 years old, including a subset of patients >70 years old.

Pediatric: Studies to evaluate bexarotene pharmacokinetics in the pediatric population have not been conducted (see **PRECAUTIONS: *Pediatric Use***).

Gender: The pharmacokinetics of bexarotene were similar in male and female patients with advanced cancer.

Ethnic Origin: The effect of ethnic origin on bexarotene pharmacokinetics is unknown.

Renal Insufficiency: No formal studies have been conducted with Targretin® capsules in patients with renal insufficiency. Urinary elimination of bexarotene and its known metabolites is a minor excretory pathway (<1% of administered dose), but because renal insufficiency can result in significant protein binding changes, pharmacokinetics may be altered in patients with renal insufficiency (see **PRECAUTIONS: *Renal Insufficiency***).

Hepatic Insufficiency: No specific studies have been conducted with Targretin® capsules in patients with hepatic insufficiency. Because less than 1% of the dose is excreted in the urine unchanged and there is *in vitro* evidence of extensive hepatic contribution to bexarotene elimination, hepatic impairment would be expected to lead to greatly decreased clearance (see **WARNINGS:** *Hepatic insufficiency*).

Drug-Drug Interactions

No specific studies to evaluate drug interactions with bexarotene have been conducted. Bexarotene oxidative metabolites appear to be formed by cytochrome P450 3A4.

Because bexarotene is metabolized by cytochrome P450 3A4, ketoconazole, itraconazole, erythromycin, gemfibrozil, grapefruit juice, and other inhibitors of cytochrome P450 3A4 would be expected to lead to an increase in plasma bexarotene concentrations. Furthermore, rifampin, phenytoin, phenobarbital and other inducers of cytochrome P450 3A4 may cause a reduction in plasma bexarotene concentrations.

Concomitant administration of Targretin® capsules and gemfibrozil resulted in substantial increases in plasma concentrations of bexarotene, probably at least partially related to cytochrome P450 3A4 inhibition by gemfibrozil. Under similar conditions, bexarotene concentrations were not affected by concomitant atorvastatin administration. Concomitant administration of gemfibrozil with Targretin® capsules is not recommended (see **PRECAUTIONS: *Drug-Drug Interactions***).

Clinical Studies

Targretin® capsules were evaluated in 152 patients with advanced and early stage cutaneous T-cell lymphoma (CTCL) in two multicenter, open-label, historically-controlled clinical studies conducted in the U.S., Canada, Europe, and Australia.

The advanced disease patients had disease refractory to at least one prior systemic therapy (median of two, range one to six prior systemic therapies) and had been treated with a median of five (range 1 to 11) prior systemic, irradiation, and/or topical therapies. Early disease patients were intolerant to, had disease that was refractory to, or had reached a response plateau of six months on, at least two prior therapies. The patients entered had been treated with a median of 3.5 (range 2 to 12) therapies (systemic, irradiation, and/or topical).

The two clinical studies enrolled a total of 152 patients, 102 of whom had disease refractory to at least one prior systemic therapy, 90 with advanced disease and 12 with early disease. This is the patient population for whom Targretin® capsules are indicated.

Patients were initially treated with a starting dose of 650 mg/m²/day with a subsequent reduction of starting dose to 500 mg/m²/day. Neither of these starting doses was tolerated, and the starting dose was then reduced to 300 mg/m²/day. If, however, a patient on 300 mg/m²/day of Targretin® capsules showed no response after eight or more weeks of therapy, the dose could be increased to 400 mg/m²/day.

Tumor response was assessed in both studies by observation of up to five baseline-defined index lesions using a Composite Assessment of Index Lesion Disease Severity (CA). This endpoint was based on a summation of the grades, for all index lesions, of erythema, scaling, plaque elevation, hypopigmentation or hyperpigmentation, and area of involvement. Also considered in response assessment was the presence or absence of cutaneous tumors and extracutaneous disease manifestations.

All tumor responses required confirmation over at least two assessments separated by at least four weeks. A partial response was defined as an improvement of at least 50% in the index lesions without worsening, or development of new cutaneous tumors or non-cutaneous manifestations. A complete clinical response required complete disappearance of all manifestations of disease, but did not require confirmation by biopsy.

At the initial dose of 300 mg/m²/day, 1/62 (1.6%) of patients had a complete clinical tumor response and 19/62 (30%) of patients had a partial tumor response. The rate of relapse (25% increase in CA or worsening of other aspects of disease) in the 20 patients who had a tumor response was 6/20 (30%) over a median duration of observation of 21 weeks, and the median duration of tumor response had not been reached. Responses were seen as early as 4 weeks and new responses continued to be seen at later visits.

INDICATIONS AND USAGE

Targretin® (bexarotene) capsules are indicated for the treatment of cutaneous manifestations of cutaneous T-cell lymphoma in patients who are refractory to at least one prior systemic therapy.

CONTRAINDICATIONS

Targretin® capsules are contraindicated in patients with a known hypersensitivity to bexarotene or other components of the product.

Pregnancy: Category X

Targretin® (bexarotene) capsules may cause fetal harm when administered to a pregnant woman. Targretin® capsules must not be given to a pregnant woman or a woman who intends to become pregnant. If a woman becomes pregnant while taking Targretin® capsules, Targretin® capsules must be stopped immediately and the woman given appropriate counseling.

Bexarotene caused malformations when administered orally to pregnant rats during days 7–17 of gestation. Developmental abnormalities included incomplete ossification at 4 mg/kg/day and cleft palate, depressed eye bulge/microphthalmia, and small ears at 16 mg/kg/day. The plasma AUC of bexarotene in rats at 4 mg/kg/day is approximately one third the AUC in humans at the recommended daily dose. At doses greater than 10 mg/kg/day, bexarotene caused developmental mortality. The no effect dose for fetal effects in rats was 1 mg/kg/day (producing an AUC approximately one sixth of the AUC at the recommended human daily dose).

Women of child-bearing potential should be advised to avoid becoming pregnant when Targretin® capsules are used. The possibility that a woman of child-bearing potential is pregnant at the time therapy is instituted should be considered. A negative pregnancy test (e.g., serum beta-human chorionic gonadotropin, beta-HCG) with a sensitivity of at least 50 mIU/L should be obtained within one week prior to Targretin® capsules therapy, and the pregnancy test must be repeated at monthly intervals while the patient remains on Targretin® capsules. Effective contraception must be used for one month prior to the initiation of therapy, during therapy and for at least one month following discontinuation of therapy; it is recommended that two reliable forms of contraception be used simultaneously unless abstinence is the chosen method. Male patients with sexual partners who are pregnant, possibly pregnant, or who could become pregnant must use condoms during sexual intercourse while taking Targretin® capsules and for at least one month after the last dose of drug. Targretin® capsules therapy should be initiated on the second or third day of a normal menstrual period. No more than a one month supply of Targretin® capsules should be given to the patient so that the results of pregnancy testing can be assessed and counseling regarding avoidance of pregnancy and birth defects can be reinforced.

WARNINGS

Lipid abnormalities: Targretin® capsules induce major lipid abnormalities in most patients. These must be monitored and treated during long-term therapy. About 70% of patients with CTCL who received an initial dose of ≥300 mg/m²/day of Targretin® capsules had fasting triglyceride levels greater than 2.5 times the upper limit of normal. About 55% had values over 800 mg/dL with a median of about 1200 mg/dL in those patients. Cholesterol elevations above 300 mg/dL occurred in approximately 60% and 75% of patients with CTCL who received an initial dose of 300 mg/m²/day or greater than 300 mg/m²/day, respectively. Decreases in high density lipoprotein (HDL) cholesterol to less than 25 mg/dL were seen in about 55% and 90% of patients receiving an initial dose of 300 mg/m²/day or greater than 300 mg/m²/day, respectively, of Targretin® capsules. The effects on triglycerides, HDL cholesterol, and total cholesterol were reversible with cessation of therapy, and could generally be mitigated by dose reduction or concomitant antilipemic therapy.

Fasting blood lipid determinations should be performed before Targretin® capsules therapy is initiated and weekly until the lipid response to Targretin® capsules is established, which usually occurs within two to four weeks, and at eight week intervals thereafter. Fasting triglycerides should be normal or normalized with appropriate intervention prior to initiating Targretin® capsules therapy. Attempts should be made to maintain triglyceride levels below 400 mg/dL to reduce the risk of clinical sequelae (see **WARNINGS:** *Pancreatitis*). If fasting triglycerides are elevated or become elevated during treatment, antilipemic therapy should be instituted, and if necessary, the dose of Targretin® capsules reduced or suspended. In the 300 mg/m²/day initial dose group, 60% of patients were given lipid lowering drugs. Atorvastatin was used in 48% (73/152) of patients with CTCL. Because of a potential drug-drug interaction (see **PRECAUTIONS: *Drug-Drug Interactions***), gemfibrozil is not recommended for use with Targretin® capsules.

Pancreatitis: Acute pancreatitis has been reported in four patients with CTCL and in six patients with non-CTCL cancers treated with Targretin® capsules; the cases were associated with marked elevations of fasting serum triglycerides, the lowest being 770 mg/dL in one patient. One patient with advanced non-CTCL cancer died of pancreatitis. Patients with CTCL who have risk factors for pancreatitis (e.g., prior pancreatitis, uncontrolled hyperlipidemia, excessive alcohol consumption, uncontrolled diabetes mellitus, biliary tract disease, and medications known to increase triglyceride levels or to be associated with pancreatic toxicity) should generally not be treated with Targretin® capsules (see **WARNINGS:** *Lipids abnormalities* and **PRECAUTIONS: *Laboratory Tests***).

Liver function test abnormalities: For patients with CTCL receiving an initial dose of 300 mg/m²/day of Targretin® capsules, elevations in liver function tests (LFTs) have been observed in 5% (SGOT/AST), 2% (SGPT/ALT), and 0% (bilirubin). In contrast, with an initial dose greater than 300 mg/m²/day of Targretin® capsules, the incidence of LFT elevations was higher at 7% (SGOT/AST), 9% (SGPT/ALT), and 6% (bilirubin). Two patients developed cholestasis, including one patient who died of liver failure. In clinical trials, elevation of LFTs resolved within one month in 80% of patients following a decrease in dose or discontinuation of therapy. Baseline LFTs should be obtained, and LFTs should be carefully monitored after one, two and four weeks of treatment initiation, and if stable, at least every eight weeks thereafter during treatment. Consideration should be given to a suspension or discontinuation of Targretin® capsules if test results reach greater than three times the upper limit of normal values for SGOT/AST, SGPT/ALT, or bilirubin.

Hepatic insufficiency: No specific studies have been conducted with Targretin® capsules in patients with hepatic insufficiency. Because less than 1% of the dose is excreted in the urine unchanged and there is *in vitro* evidence of extensive hepatic contribution to bexarotene elimination, hepatic impairment would be expected to lead to greatly decreased clearance. Targretin® capsules should be used only with great caution in this population.

Thyroid axis alterations: Targretin® capsules induce biochemical evidence of or clinical hypothyroidism in about half of all patients treated, causing a reversible reduction in thyroid hormone (total thyroxine [total T4]) and thyroid-stimulating hormone (TSH) levels. The incidence of decreases in TSH and total T4 were about 60% and 45%, respectively, in patients with CTCL receiving an initial dose of 300 mg/m²/day. Hypothyroidism was reported as an adverse event in 29% of patients. Treatment with thyroid hormone supplements should be considered in patients with laboratory evidence of hypothyroidism. In the 300 mg/m²/day initial dose group, 37% of patients were treated with thyroid hormone replacement. Baseline thyroid function tests should be obtained and patients monitored during treatment.

Leukopenia: A total of 18% of patients with CTCL receiving an initial dose of 300 mg/m²/day of Targretin® capsules had reversible leukopenia in the range of 1000 to <3000 WBC/mm³. Patients receiving an initial dose greater than 300 mg/m²/day of Targretin® capsules had an incidence of leukopenia of 43%. No patient with CTCL treated with Targretin® capsules developed leukopenia of less than 1000 WBC/mm³. The time to onset of leukopenia was generally four to eight weeks. The leukopenia observed in most patients was explained by neutropenia. In the 300 mg/m²/day initial dose group, the incidence of NCI Grade 3 and Grade 4 neutropenia, respectively, was 12% and 4%. The leukopenia and neutropenia experienced during Targretin® capsules therapy resolved after dose reduction or discontinuation of treatment, on average within 30 days in 93% of the patients with CTCL and 82% of patients with non-CTCL cancers. Leukopenia and neutropenia were rarely associated with severe sequelae or serious adverse events. Determination of WBC with differential should be obtained at baseline and periodically during treatment.

Cataracts: Posterior subcapsular cataracts were observed in preclinical toxicity studies in rats and dogs administered bexarotene daily for 6 months. In 15 of 79 patients who had serial slit lamp examinations, new cataracts or worsening of previous cataracts were found. Because of the high prevalence and rate of cataract formation in older patient populations, the relationship of Targretin® capsules and cataracts cannot be determined in the absence of an appropriate control group. Patients treated with Targretin® capsules who experience visual difficulties should have an appropriate ophthalmologic evaluation.

PRECAUTIONS

***Pregnancy:* Category X.** See **CONTRAINDICATIONS**.

General: Targretin® capsules should be used with caution in patients with a known hypersensitivity to retinoids. Clinical instances of cross-reactivity have not been noted.

Vitamin A Supplementation: In clinical studies, patients were advised to limit vitamin A intake to ≤15,000 IU/day. Because of the relationship of bexarotene to vitamin A, patients should be advised to limit vitamin A supplements to avoid potential additive toxic effects.

Patients with Diabetes Mellitus: Caution should be used when administering Targretin® capsules in patients using insulin, agents enhancing insulin secretion (e.g., sulfonylureas), or insulin-sensitizers (e.g., troglitazone). Based on the mechanism of action, Targretin® capsules could enhance the action of these agents, resulting in hypoglycemia. Hypoglycemia has not been associated with the use of Targretin® capsules as monotherapy.

Photosensitivity: Retinoids as a class have been associated with photosensitivity. *In vitro* assays indicate that bexarotene is a potential photosensitizing agent. Mild phototoxicity manifested as sunburn and skin sensitivity to sunlight was observed in patients who were exposed to direct sunlight while receiving Targretin® capsules. Patients should be advised to minimize exposure to sunlight and artificial ultraviolet light while receiving Targretin® capsules.

Laboratory Tests

Blood lipid determinations should be performed before Targretin® capsules are given. Fasting triglycerides should be normal or normalized with appropriate intervention prior to therapy. Hyperlipidemia usually occurs within the initial two to four weeks. Therefore, weekly lipid determinations are recommended during this interval. Subsequently, in patients not hyperlipidemic, determinations can be performed less frequently (see **WARNINGS:** *Lipid abnormalities*).

A white blood cell count with differential should be obtained at baseline and periodically during treatment. Baseline liver function tests should be obtained and should be carefully monitored after one, two and four weeks of treatment initiation, and if stable, periodically thereafter during treatment. Baseline thyroid function tests should be obtained and then monitored during treatment as indicated (see **WARNINGS:** *Leukopenia, Liver function test abnormalities*, and *Thyroid axis alterations*).

Drug-Food Interaction

In all clinical trials, patients were instructed to take Targretin® capsules with or immediately following a meal. In one clinical study, plasma bexarotene AUC and C_{max} values were substantially higher following a fat-containing meal versus those following the administration of a glucose solution. Because safety and efficacy data are based upon administration with food, it is recommended that Targretin® capsules be administered with food (see **CLINICAL PHARMACOLOGY: Pharmacokinetics** and **DOSAGE AND ADMINISTRATION**).

Drug-Drug Interactions

No formal studies to evaluate drug interactions with bexarotene have been conducted. Bexarotene oxidative metabolites appear to be formed by cytochrome P450 3A4.

On the basis of the metabolism of bexarotene by cytochrome P450 3A4, ketoconazole, itraconazole, erythromycin, gemfibrozil, grapefruit juice, and other inhibitors of cytochrome P450 3A4 would be expected to lead to an increase in plasma bexarotene concentrations. Furthermore, rifampin, phenytoin, phenobarbital, and other inducers of cytochrome P450 3A4 may cause a reduction in plasma bexarotene concentrations.

Concomitant administration of Targretin® capsules and gemfibrozil resulted in substantial increases in plasma concentrations of bexarotene, probably at least partially related to cytochrome P450 3A4 inhibition by gemfibrozil. Under similar conditions, bexarotene concentrations were not affected by concomitant atorvastatin administration. Concomitant administration of gemfibrozil with Targretin® capsules is not recommended.

Renal Insufficiency

No formal studies have been conducted with Targretin® capsules in patients with renal insufficiency. Urinary elim-

Continued on next page

Table 1. Adverse Events with Incidence ≥10% in CTCL Trials

Body System Adverse Event[1,2]	Initial Assigned Dose Group (mg/m²/day) 300 N=84 N (%)	 >300 N=53 N (%)
METABOLIC AND NUTRITIONAL DISORDERS		
Hyperlipemia	66 (78.6)	42 (79.2)
Hypercholesteremia	27 (32.1)	33 (62.3)
Lactic dehydrogenase increased	6 (7.1)	7 (13.2)
BODY AS A WHOLE		
Headache	25 (29.8)	22 (41.5)
Asthenia	17 (20.2)	24 (45.3)
Infection	11 (13.1)	12 (22.6)
Abdominal pain	9 (10.7)	2 (3.8)
Chills	8 (9.5)	7 (13.2)
Fever	4 (4.8)	9 (17.0)
Flu syndrome	3 (3.6)	7 (13.2)
Back pain	2 (2.4)	6 (11.3)
Infection bacterial	1 (1.2)	7 (13.2)
ENDOCRINE		
Hypothyroidism	24 (28.6)	28 (52.8)
SKIN AND APPENDAGES		
Rash	14 (16.7)	12 (22.6)
Dry skin	9 (10.7)	5 (9.4)
Exfoliative dermatitis	8 (9.5)	15 (28.3)
Alopecia	3 (3.6)	6 (11.3)
HEMIC AND LYMPHATIC SYSTEM		
Leukopenia	14 (16.7)	25 (47.2)
Anemia	5 (6.0)	13 (24.5)
Hypochromic anemia	3 (3.6)	7 (13.2)
DIGESTIVE SYSTEM		
Nausea	13 (15.5)	4 (7.5)
Diarrhea	6 (7.1)	22 (41.5)
Vomiting	3 (3.6)	7 (13.2)
Anorexia	2 (2.4)	12 (22.6)
CARDIOVASCULAR SYSTEM		
Peripheral edema	11 (13.1)	6 (11.3)
NERVOUS SYSTEM		
Insomnia	4 (4.8)	6 (11.3)

[1] Preferred English term coded according to Ligand-modified COSTART 5 Dictionary.
[2] Patients are counted at most once in each AE category.

Table 2. Incidence of Moderately Severe and Severe Adverse Events Reported in at Least Two Patients (CTCL Trials)

	Initial Assigned Dose Group (mg/m²/day)			
	300 (N=84)		>300 (N=53)	
	Mod Sev	Severe	Mod Sev	Severe
Body System Adverse Event[1,2]	N (%)	N (%)	N (%)	N (%)
BODY AS A WHOLE				
Asthenia	1 (1.2)	0 (0.0)	11 (20.8)	0 (0.0)
Headache	3 (3.6)	0 (0.0)	5 (9.4)	1 (1.9)
Infection bacterial	1 (1.2)	0 (0.0)	0 (0.0)	2 (3.8)
CARDIOVASCULAR SYS.				
Peripheral edema	2 (2.4)	1 (1.2)	0 (0.0)	0 (0.0)
DIGESTIVE SYSTEM				
Anorexia	0 (0.0)	0 (0.0)	3 (5.7)	0 (0.0)
Diarrhea	1 (1.2)	1 (1.2)	2 (3.8)	1 (1.9)
Pancreatitis	1 (1.2)	0 (0.0)	3 (5.7)	0 (0.0)
Vomiting	0 (0.0)	0 (0.0)	2 (3.8)	0 (0.0)
ENDOCRINE				
Hypothyroidism	1 (1.2)	1 (1.2)	2 (3.8)	0 (0.0)
HEM. & LYMPH. SYS.				
Leukopenia	3 (3.6)	0 (0.0)	6 (11.3)	1 (1.9)
META. AND NUTR. DIS.				
Bilirubinemia	0 (0.0)	1 (1.2)	2 (3.8)	0 (0.0)
Hypercholesteremia	2 (2.4)	0 (0.0)	5 (9.4)	0 (0.0)
Hyperlipemia	16 (19.0)	6 (7.1)	17 (32.1)	5 (9.4)
SGOT/AST increased	0 (0.0)	0 (0.0)	2 (3.8)	0 (0.0)
SGPT/ALT increased	0 (0.0)	0 (0.0)	2 (3.8)	0 (0.0)
RESPIRATORY SYSTEM				
Pneumonia	0 (0.0)	0 (0.0)	2 (3.8)	2 (3.8)
SKIN AND APPENDAGES				
Exfoliative dermatitis	0 (0.0)	1 (1.2)	3 (5.7)	1 (1.9)
Rash	1 (1.2)	2 (2.4)	1 (1.9)	0 (0.0)

[1] Preferred English term coded according to Ligand-modified COSTART 5 Dictionary.
[2] Patients are counted at most once in each AE category. Patients are classified by the highest severity within each row.

Targretin—Cont.

ination of bexarotene and its known metabolites is a minor excretory pathway for bexarotene (<1% of administered dose), but because renal insufficiency can result in significant protein binding changes, and bexarotene is >99% protein bound, pharmacokinetics may be altered in patients with renal insufficiency.

Protein Binding

Bexarotene is highly bound (>99%) to plasma proteins. The plasma proteins to which bexarotene binds have not been elucidated, and the ability of bexarotene to displace drugs bound to plasma proteins and the ability of drugs to displace bexarotene binding have not been studied.

Drug/Laboratory Test Interactions

CA125 assay values in patients with ovarian cancer may be increased by Targretin® capsule therapy.

Carcinogenesis, Mutagenesis, Impairment of Fertility

Long-term studies in animals to assess the carcinogenic potential of bexarotene have not been conducted. Bexarotene is not mutagenic to bacteria (Ames assay) or mammalian cells (mouse lymphoma assay). Bexarotene was not clastogenic *in vivo* (micronucleus test in mice). No formal fertility studies were conducted with bexarotene. Bexarotene caused testicular degeneration when oral doses of 1.5 mg/kg/day were given to dogs for 91 days (producing an AUC of approximately one fifth the AUC at the recommended human daily dose).

Use in Nursing Mothers

It is not known whether bexarotene is excreted in human milk. Because many drugs are excreted in human milk and because of the potential for serious adverse reactions in nursing infants from bexarotene, a decision should be made whether to discontinue nursing or to discontinue the drug, taking into account the importance of the drug to the mother.

Pediatric Use

Safety and effectiveness in pediatric patients have not been established.

Geriatric Use

Of the total patients with CTCL in clinical studies of Targretin® capsules, 64% were 60 years or older, while 33% were 70 years or older. No overall differences in safety were observed between patients 70 years or older and younger patients, but greater sensitivity of some older individuals to Targretin® capsules cannot be ruled out. Responses to Targretin® capsules were observed across all age group decades, without preference for any individual age group decade.

ADVERSE REACTIONS

The safety of Targretin® capsules has been evaluated in clinical studies of 152 patients with CTCL who received Targretin® capsules for up to 97 weeks and in 352 patients in other studies. The mean duration of therapy for the 152 patients with CTCL was 166 days. The most common adverse events reported with an incidence of at least 10% in patients with CTCL treated at an initial dose of 300 mg/m^2/day of Targretin® capsules are shown in Table 1. The events at least possibly related to treatment are lipid abnormalities (elevated triglycerides, elevated total and LDL cholesterol and decreased HDL cholesterol), hypothyroidism, headache, asthenia, rash, leukopenia, anemia, nausea, infection, peripheral edema, abdominal pain, and dry skin. Most adverse events occurred at a higher incidence in patients treated at starting doses of greater than 300 mg/m^2/day (see Table 1).

Adverse events leading to dose reduction or study drug discontinuation in at least two patients were hyperlipemia, neutropenia/leukopenia, diarrhea, fatigue/lethargy, hypothyroidism, headache, liver function test abnormalities, rash, pancreatitis, nausea, anemia, allergic reaction, muscle spasm, pneumonia, and confusion.

The moderately severe (NCI Grade 3) and severe (NCI Grade 4) adverse events reported in two or more patients with CTCL treated at an initial dose of 300 mg/m^2/day of Targretin® capsules (see Table 2) were hypertriglyceridemia, pruritus, headache, peripheral edema, leukopenia, rash, and hypercholesteremia. Most of these moderately severe or severe adverse events occurred at a higher rate in patients treated at starting doses of greater than 300 mg/m^2/day than in patients treated at a starting dose of 300 mg/m^2/day.

As shown in Table 3, in patients with CTCL receiving an initial dose of 300 mg/m^2/day, the incidence of NCI Grade 3 or 4 elevations in triglycerides and total cholesterol was 28% and 25%, respectively. In contrast, in patients with CTCL receiving greater than 300 mg/m^2/day, the incidence of NCI Grade 3 or 4 elevated triglycerides and total cholesterol was 45% and 45%, respectively. Other Grade 3 and 4 laboratory abnormalities are shown in Table 3.

In addition to the 152 patients enrolled in the two CTCL studies, 352 patients received Targretin® capsules as monotherapy for various advanced malignancies at doses from 5 mg/m^2/day to 1000 mg/m^2/day. The common adverse events (incidence greater than 10%) were similar to those seen in patients with CTCL.

In the 504 patients (CTCL and non-CTCL) who received Targretin® capsules as monotherapy, drug-related serious adverse events that were fatal, in one patient each, were acute pancreatitis, subdural hematoma, and liver failure.

In the patients with CTCL receiving an initial dose of 300 mg/m^2/day of Targretin® capsules, adverse events reported at an incidence of less than 10% and not included in Tables 1–3 or discussed in other parts of labeling and possibly related to treatment were as follows:

Body as a Whole: chills, cellulitis, chest pain, sepsis, and monilia.

Cardiovascular: hemorrhage, hypertension, angina pectoris, right heart failure, syncope, and tachycardia.

Digestive: constipation, dry mouth, flatulence, colitis, dyspepsia, cheilitis, gastroenteritis, gingivitis, liver failure, and melena.

Hemic and Lymphatic: eosinophilia, thrombocythemia, coagulation time increased, lymphocytosis, and thrombocytopenia.

Metabolic and Nutritional: LDH increased, creatinine increased, hypoproteinemia, hyperglycemia, weight decreased, weight increased, and amylase increased.

Musculoskeletal: arthralgia, myalgia, bone pain, myasthenia, and arthrosis.

Nervous: depression, agitation, ataxia, cerebrovascular accident, confusion, dizziness, hyperesthesia, hypesthesia, and neuropathy.

Respiratory: pharyngitis, rhinitis, dyspnea, pleural effusion, bronchitis, cough increased, lung edema, hemoptysis, and hypoxia.

Skin and Appendages: skin ulcer, acne, alopecia, skin nodule, macular papular rash, pustular rash, serous drainage, and vesicular bullous rash.

Special Senses: dry eyes, conjunctivitis, ear pain, blepharitis, corneal lesion, keratitis, otitis externa, and visual field defect.

Urogenital: albuminuria, hematuria, urinary incontinence, urinary tract infection, urinary urgency, dysuria, kidney function abnormal, and breast pain.

[See table 1 & 2 at top of previous page]
[See table 3 below]

Table 3. Treatment-Emergent Abnormal Laboratory Values in CTCL Trials

	Initial Assigned Dose (mg/m^2/day)			
	300		>300	
	N=83[1]		N=53[1]	
Analyte	Grade 3[2] (%)	Grade 4[2] (%)	Grade 3 (%)	Grade 4 (%)
Triglycerides[3]	21.3	6.7	31.8	13.6
Total Cholesterol[3]	18.7	6.7	15.9	29.5
Alkaline Phosphatase	1.2	0.0	0.0	1.9
Hyperglycemia	1.2	0.0	5.7	0.0
Hypocalcemia	1.2	0.0	0.0	0.0
Hyponatremia	1.2	0.0	9.4	0.0
SGPT/ALT	1.2	0.0	1.9	1.9
Hyperkalemia	0.0	0.0	1.9	0.0
Hypernatremia	0.0	1.2	0.0	0.0
SGOT/AST	0.0	0.0	1.9	1.9
Total Bilirubin	0.0	0.0	0.0	1.9
ANC	12.0	3.6	18.9	7.5
ALC	7.2	0.0	15.1	0.0
WBC	3.6	0.0	11.3	0.0
Hemoglobin	0.0	0.0	1.9	0.0

[1] Number of patients with at least one analyte value post-baseline.

[2] Adapted from NCI Common Toxicity Criteria, Grade 3 and 4, Version 2.0. Patients are considered to have had a Grade 3 or 4 value if either of the following occurred: a) Value becomes Grade 3 or 4 during the study; b) Value is abnormal at baseline and worsens to Grade 3 or 4 on study, including all values beyond study drug discontinuation, as defined in data handling conventions.

[3] The denominator used to calculate the incidence rates for fasting Total Cholesterol and Triglycerides were N=75 for the 300 mg/m^2/day initial dose group and N=44 for the >300 mg/m^2/day initial dose group.

OVERDOSAGE

Doses up to 1000 mg/m^2/day of Targretin® capsules have been administered in short-term studies in patients with advanced cancer without acute toxic effects. Single doses of 1500 mg/kg and 720 mg/kg were tolerated without significant toxicity in rats and dogs, respectively. These doses are approximately 30 and 50 times, respectively, the recommended human dose on a mg/m^2 basis.

No clinical experience with an overdose of Targretin® capsules has been reported. Any overdose with Targretin® capsules should be treated with supportive care for the signs and symptoms exhibited by the patient.

DOSAGE AND ADMINISTRATION

The recommended initial dose of Targretin® capsules is 300 mg/m^2/day. (See Table 4.) Targretin® capsules should be taken as a single oral daily dose with a meal. See **CONTRAINDICATIONS**: ***Pregnancy: Category X*** section for precautions to prevent pregnancy and birth defects in women of child-bearing potential.

Table 4.
Targretin® Capsule Initial Dose Calculation According to Body Surface Area

Initial Dose Level (300 mg/m^2/day)		Number of 75 mg Targretin® Capsules
Body Surface Area (m^2)	Total Daily Dose (mg/day)	
0.88 – 1.12	300	4
1.13 – 1.37	375	5
1.38 – 1.62	450	6
1.63 – 1.87	525	7
1.88 – 2.12	600	8
2.13 – 2.37	675	9
2.38 – 2.62	750	10

Dose Modification Guidelines: The 300 mg/m^2/day dose level of Targretin® capsules may be adjusted to 200 mg/m^2/day then to 100 mg/m^2/day, or temporarily suspended, if necessitated by toxicity. When toxicity is controlled, doses may be carefully readjusted upward. If there is no tumor response after eight weeks of treatment and if the initial dose of 300 mg/m^2/day is well tolerated, the dose may be escalated to 400 mg/m^2/day with careful monitoring.

Duration of Therapy: In clinical trials in CTCL, Targretin® capsules were administered for up to 97 weeks.

Targretin® capsules should be continued as long as the patient is deriving benefit.

HOW SUPPLIED

Targretin® capsules are supplied as 75 mg off-white, oblong soft gelatin capsules, imprinted with "Targretin", in high density polyethylene bottles with child-resistant closures.

Bottles of 100 capsules .... NDC 64365-502-01

Store at 2°–25°C (36°–77°F). Avoid exposing to high temperatures and humidity after the bottle is opened. Protect from light.

Manufactured for: Ligand Pharmaceuticals Incorporated
San Diego, CA 92121
by: R.P. Scherer
St. Petersburg, FL 33716

Ligand Part #3000207 (Rev. 1299)
Anderson Part #5422101-1

Sanofi-Synthelabo Inc.

90 PARK AVENUE
NEW YORK, NY 10016

Direct Inquiries to:
(212) 551-4000

For Medical Information Contact:
Product Information Services
(800) 446-6267

Sales and Ordering:
East Coast: (800) 223-1062
West Coast: (800) 223-5511

HYALGAN® ℞
sodium hyaluronate

LABELING

CAUTION

Federal law restricts this device to sale by or on the order of a physician.

DESCRIPTION

Hyalgan® is a viscous solution consisting of a high molecular weight (500,000–730,000 daltons) fraction of purified

TABLE 2. STUDY DESIGN

Routes of Administration	Hyalgan®	Placebo	Naproxen
s.c.	Lidocaine (1%)	Lidocaine (1%)	Lidocaine (1%)
i.a.*	Hyalgan® (20 mg/2 mL)	Phosphate-Buffered Saline (2 mL)	none
p.o./b.i.d.	Placebo for naproxen capsules	Placebo for naproxen capsules	Naproxen capsules (500 mg)
p.o./p.r.n. (not to exceed 4 grams/day)	Acetaminophen	Acetaminophen	Acetaminophen

Legend: s.c. = subcutaneous; i.a. = intra-articular; p.o. = by mouth; b.i.d. = twice a day; p.r.n. = as needed
* Synovial fluid was aspirated (when present) in the Hyalgan® and placebo groups.

TABLE 3
Demographic Characteristics of All Randomized Subjects

DEMOGRAPHIC VARIABLE	TREATMENT			
	Hyalgan® N = 164	Placebo N = 168	Naproxen N = 163	TOTAL N = 495
AGE (years):				
Mean	63.5	64.3	63.2	63.7
SD	10.1	10.0	9.2	9.8
Range	41–90	44–85	40–80	40–90
Gender [N (%)]:				
Female	99 (60.3)	91 (54.1)	99 (60.7)	289 (58.4)
Male	65 (39.6)	77 (45.8)	64 (39.3)	206 (41.6)
Race [N (%)]:				
Caucasian	137 (83.6)	135 (80.4)	133 (81.6)	405 (81.8)
Black	23 (14.0)	32 (19.0)	25 (15.3)	80 (16.2)
Other	4 (4.2)	1 (1.0)	5 (3.1)	10 (2.0)
Height (cm):				
Mean	167.8	168.6	167.6	168.0
SD	8.8	10.7	11.9	10.5
Range	145–190	142–193	102–198	102–198
Weight (kg):				
Mean	88.4	88.1	89.7	88.7
SD	18.0	18.2	18.4	18.2
Range	46–139	49–170	45–150	45–170
NSAIDs Use (N, %)	107 (65.2)	117 (69.6)	113 (69.3)	337 (68.1)
Use of Assistive Devices (N, %)	35 (21.3)	34 (20.2)	32 (19.6)	101 (20.4)
Physical Therapy (N, %)	20 (12.2)	17 (10.1)	25 (15.3)	62 (12.5)

Legend: cm = centimeters; kg = kilograms; SD = standard deviation

natural sodium hyaluronate in buffered physiological sodium chloride, having a pH of 6.8–7.5. The sodium hyaluronate is extracted from rooster combs. Hyaluronic acid is a natural complex sugar of the glycosaminoglycan family and is a long-chain polymer containing repeating disaccharide units of Na-glucuronate-N-acetylglucosamine.

INDICATIONS

Hyalgan® is indicated for the treatment of pain in osteoarthritis (OA) of the knee in patients who have failed to respond adequately to conservative nonpharmacologic therapy, and to simple analgesics, e.g., acetaminophen.

CONTRAINDICATIONS

- Do not administer to patients with known hypersensitivity to hyaluronate preparations.
- Intra-articular injections are contraindicated in cases of past and present infections or skin diseases in the area of the injection site.

WARNINGS

- Do not concomitantly use disinfectants containing quaternary ammonium salts for skin preparation because hyaluronic acid can precipitate in their presence.
- Anaphylactoid and allergic reactions have been reported with this product. See Adverse Events Section for more detail.
- Transient increases in inflammation in the injected knee following Hyalgan® injection in some patients with inflammatory arthritis such as rheumatoid arthritis or gouty arthritis have been reported.

PRECAUTIONS

General

- The effectiveness of a single treatment cycle of less than 3 injections has not been established.
- The safety and effectiveness of the use of Hyalgan® in joints other than the knee have not been established.
- The safety and effectiveness of the use of Hyalgan® concomitantly with other intra-articular injectables have not been established.
- Use caution when injecting Hyalgan® into patients who are allergic to avian proteins, feathers, and egg products.
- Strict aseptic administration technique must be followed.
- **STERILE CONTENTS.** The vial/syringe is intended for single use. The contents of the vial must be used immediately once the container has been opened. Discard any unused Hyalgan®.
- Do not use Hyalgan® if the package is opened or damaged. Store in the original packaging (protected from light) below 77° F (25° C). DO NOT FREEZE.
- Remove joint effusion, if present, before injecting Hyalgan®.

Information for Patients

- Provide patients with a copy of the Patient Information prior to use.
- Transient pain and/or swelling of the injected joint may occur after intra-articular injection of Hyalgan®.
- As with any invasive joint procedure, it is recommended that the patient avoid any strenuous activities or prolonged (i.e., more than 1 hour) weight-bearing activities such as jogging or tennis within 48 hours following the intra-articular injection.

Use in Specific Populations

- **Pregnancy:** *Teratogenic Effects*—Reproductive toxicity studies, including multigeneration studies, have been performed in rats and rabbits at doses up to 11 times the anticipated human dose (1.43 mg/kg per treatment cycle) and have revealed no evidence of impaired fertility or harm to the experimental animal fetus due to intra-articular injections of Hyalgan®. Animal reproduction studies are not always predictive of human response. The safety and effectiveness of Hyalgan® have not been established in pregnant women.
- **Nursing Mothers:** It is not known if Hyalgan® is excreted in human milk. The safety and effectiveness of Hyalgan® have not been established in lactating women.
- **Pediatrics:** The safety and effectiveness of Hyalgan® have not been demonstrated in children.

ADVERSE EVENTS

Hyalgan® was investigated in a pivotal clinical investigation conducted in the United States in which there were three arms (164 subjects treated with Hyalgan®; 168 with placebo; and 163 with naproxen) (refer to Table 1). Common adverse events reported for the Hyalgan®-treated subjects were gastrointestinal complaints, injection site pain, knee swelling/effusion, local skin reactions (rash, ecchymosis), pruritus, and headache. Swelling and effusion, local skin reactions (ecchymosis and rash), and headache occurred at equal frequency in the Hyalgan®- and placebo-treated groups. Hyalgan®-treated subjects had 48/164 (29%) incidents of gastrointestinal complaints that were not statistically different from the placebo-treated group. A statistically significant difference in the occurrence of pain at the injection site was noted in the Hyalgan®-treated subjects: 38/164 (23%) in comparison to 22/168 (13%) in the placebo-treated subjects (p = 0.022). There were 6/164 (4%) premature discontinuations in Hyalgan®-treated subjects due to injection site pain in comparison to 1/168 (<1%) in the placebo-treated subjects. These differences were not statistically significant.

Two (2/164, 1.2%) Hyalgan®-treated subjects and 3/168 (1.8%) placebo-treated subjects were reported to have positive bacterial cultures of effusion aspirated from the treated knee. The two Hyalgan®-treated subjects and two of the placebo-treated subjects did not exhibit evidence of infection clinically or subsequently and were not treated with antibiotics. One of the placebo-treated subjects was hospitalized and received presumptive treatment for septic arthritis.

Hyalgan® has been in clinical use in Europe since 1987. Analysis of the adverse events that have been reported with the use of Hyalgan® in Europe reveals that most of the events are related to local symptoms such as pain, swelling/effusion, and warmth or redness at the injection site. In the two events reported as anaphylactoid reactions, Hyalgan® treatment was discontinued and both had favorable outcomes. Three cases of allergic reactions were reported in which the patients were discontinued from Hyalgan® treatment and the incidents resolved. Seven cases of fever were reported in which three of the cases were reported to be associated with local reactions; pyogenic arthritis was reported to be ruled out in these three cases. All the fever patients were discontinued from Hyalgan® treatment and all incidents resolved. One incident of shock (which was described as a "hypotensive crisis") was reported. The incident resolved and Hyalgan® treatment was continued.

Adverse experience data from the literature contain no evidence of increased risk relating to retreatment with Hyalgan®. The frequency and severity of adverse events occurring during repeat treatment cycles did not increase over that reported for a single treatment cycle. (Carrabba et al., 1995; Carrabba et al., 1991; Kotz and Kolarz, 1999; Scali, 1995).

TABLE 1
Incidence[1] of Adverse Events Occurring in More Than 5% of All Subjects

Adverse Event	Hyalgan® N = 164	Placebo N = 168
Gastrointestinal Complaints[2]	48 (29%)	59 (36%)
Injection site pain[3]	38 (23%)[4]	22 (13%)
Headache	30 (18%)	29 (17%)
Local skin[5]	23 (14%)	17 (10%)
Local joint pain and swelling[6]	21 (13%)	22 (13%)
Pruritus (local)	12 (7%)	7 (4%)

Notes: [1] Number and % of subjects
[2] Severe in 4 Hyalgan®-treated subjects and 4 placebo-treated subjects
[3] Severe in 5 Hyalgan®-treated subjects and 2 placebo-treated subjects
[4] Statistically significant (p=0.02)
[5] Includes ecchymosis and rash
[6] Severe in 2 Hyalgan®-treated subjects (1.2%) and 1 placebo-treated subjects

CLINICAL STUDY

The use of Hyalgan® as a treatment for pain in OA of the knee was investigated in a multicenter clinical trial conducted in the United States.

Study Design

This study was a double-masked, placebo and naproxen-controlled, multicenter prospective clinical trial with three treatment arms, as summarized in Table 2. A total of 495 subjects with moderate to severe pain was randomized (at baseline evaluation) into three treatment groups in a ratio of 1:1:1 Hyalgan®, placebo, or naproxen.

[See table 2 above]

Patient Population and Demographics

The demographics of trial participants were comparable across treatment groups with regard to age, sex, race, height, weight, history of osteoarthritis, prior use of NSAIDs, prior physical therapy, and use of assistive devices (refer to Table 3).

[See table 3 above]

Evaluation Schedule

After meeting initial screening requirements NSAID therapy was discontinued. After 2 weeks, all subjects returned

Continued on next page

This product information was prepared in September 2000. On these and other products of Sanofi-Synthelabo Inc., detailed information may be obtained on a current basis by direct inquiry to Product Information Services, 90 Park Avenue, New York, NY 10016 (toll free 1-800-446-6267).

Hyalgan—Cont.

for baseline evaluations. The baseline evaluation included assessment of three primary effectiveness criteria; measurement of pain during a 50-foot walk test using a 100 mm Visual Analog Scale (VAS), a categorical assessment (0 = none to 5 = disabled) of pain, as assessed by a masked evaluator, during the 48 hours preceding the visit, and a categorical assessment (0 = none to 5 = disabled) of pain, as assessed by the subject, during the 48 hours preceding the visit.

All subjects who completed the NSAID washout period and met all entry requirements received their first injection after randomization. All subjects received subcutaneous lidocaine injections. Intra-articular injections (Hyalgan®, placebo) were administered weekly for a total of 5 injections (Weeks 0–4). The naproxen group received 500 mg of naproxen to be taken b.i.d. for 26 weeks.

Subsequent visits and evaluations took place at Weeks 5, 9, 12, 16, 21, and 26. Safety and effectiveness criteria were assessed and recorded at these time periods.

Clinical Results

For this trial, overall success for effectiveness was defined as meeting all four of the success criteria listed in Table 4 using scores from week 26. The criteria were met (refer to Tables 4 through 8).

[See table 4, 5 & 6 in next column]
[See table 7 & 8 at top of next page]

Additional Analyses

a. An analysis of study completers was performed as follows: Success was defined as 1) achieving a 20 mm decrease in the VAS for the 50-foot walk test by Week 5, and 2) maintaining this improvement through Week 26. In this analysis greater proportions of Hyalgan®-treated subjects (59/105, 56%) than either placebo- (47/115, 41%) or naproxen-treated subjects (51/113, 45%) were successful under this definition. The Hyalgan®-placebo comparison was statistically significant (p = 0.031, Fisher's Exact Test).

Since patients were not followed beyond Week 26, it is unknown how long pain relief continued. There are reports in the literature of some patients experiencing benefit beyond 26 weeks.

b. *Categorical Assessment of Pain—Subjects:* A longitudinal analysis of categorical assessment of pain by the subject, which analyzed the percentage of subjects who attained success revealed that a significantly higher percentage of Hyalgan®-treated subjects as compared to the placebo-treated subjects (55/105, 52% vs 43/115, 37%, p = 0.030, Fisher's Exact Test) achieved success (an improvement of greater than or equal to one point on the five-point scale) and maintained this success from Week 5 until Week 26.

Supplementary Clinical Information

Three randomized, controlled clinical investigations were performed that provide information about a three-injection treatment course of Hyalgan®. In all of the studies the patients were followed for 60 days.

Two studies provided a comparison to placebo. One of the placebo-controlled studies evaluated two treatment doses of Hyalgan®, 20 mg/2 ml and 40 mg/2 ml. The 20 mg/2 ml treatment arm included 19 knees, the 40 mg/2 ml included 20 knees, and the placebo arm included 18 knees. The other placebo study included 20 knees in the treatment group and 18 knees in the placebo-treatment group. The third study provided a comparison between patients treated with three weekly injections of Hyalgan® followed by 2 weekly treatments with arthrocentesis with patients treated with arthrocentesis for five weeks, and arthrocentesis and placebo injections for five weeks. Additional arms of this study assessed additional treatment regimens. Statistical evaluation of the data was performed at day 60. In this study only patients considered to be a success were followed beyond day 60. These patients were followed for 180 days, however, due to the number of dropouts, statistical evaluation was not performed on data gathered at time points beyond day 60. The results of these investigations reported that the three-injection Hyalgan® treated patients experienced pain relief beginning at day 21 and continuing throughout the remaining 60-day observation period.

Safety

In order for the product to be considered safe, the incidence of severe swelling and pain consequent to intra-articular injection should be less than 5%. This criterion was met as indicated in Table 1. See the Adverse Events Section.

DETAILED DEVICE DESCRIPTION

Each vial or syringe contains:

Sodium Hyaluronate	20.0 mg
Sodium chloride	17.0 mg
Monobasic sodium phosphate • $2H_2O$	0.1 mg
Dibasic sodium phosphate • $12H_2O$	1.2 mg
Water for injection	q.s.* to 2.0 mL

*q.s. = up to

HOW SUPPLIED

Hyalgan® is supplied as a sterile, non-pyrogenic solution in 2 mL vials or 2 mL pre-filled syringes.

TABLE 4
Clinical Results

Evaluation	Success Criteria	Results
100 mm VAS for pain during 50- foot walk.	A statistically significant (alpha = 0.05) reduction on mean VAS for Hyalgan® when compared to placebo at Week 26. This difference was also to exceed one fourth of the Standard Deviation of the mean change from baseline.	At Week 26, the difference between the Hyalgan®-treated group and the placebo-treated group adjusted means was 8.85 mm (p = 0.0043), which is a difference of approximately one-third of a standard deviation (Table 5).
Masked Evaluator Categorical Assessment of subject pain (0=none to 5=disabled) during the 48 hours preceding visits.	The number of Hyalgan®-treated subjects showing improvement at Week 26 was to be concordant with the VAS results; however, not required to be independently statistically significant.	At Week 26 the masked evaluator's categorical assessment of pain indicated that the Hyalgan®-treated subjects experienced less pain than the placebo-treated subjects (Table 6).
Subjects' Categorical Assessment of pain (0=none to 5=disabled) during the 48 hours preceding visits.	The number of Hyalgan®-treated subjects showing improvement at Week 26 was to be concordant with the VAS results; however, not required to be independently statistically significant.	At Week 26 the subjects' categorical assessment of pain indicated that the Hyalgan®-treated subjects experienced less pain than the placebo-treated subjects (Table 7).
Magnitude of the observed effect for Hyalgan® versus placebo on both the VAS and the categorical pain assessments.	At Week 26 the magnitude of the observed effect for Hyalgan® versus placebo on both the VAS and the categorical pain assessments were to be at least 50% of those observed for the naproxen group.	The improvement in pain on the VAS exhibited by the Hyalgan®-treated group relative to the placebo-treated group were at least 50% of the benefits exhibited by the naproxen-treated group relative to the placebo-treated group. The results of the categorical assessments by the masked evaluator and the subject indicated that improvement of the Hyalgan®-treated group relative to the placebo-treated group was at least 50% of the benefits exhibited by the naproxen-treated group relative to the placebo-treated group (Table 8).

TABLE 5
ANCOVA of 50-Foot Walk Test (mm) VAS by Week for All Completed Subjects

	Week							
	3	4	5	9	12	16	21	26
Adjusted Means Hyalgan®	27.23	21.54	19.29	20.04	20.26	20.83	18.44	17.88
Placebo	32.35	28.57	25.67	24.28	26.66	25.44	24.77	26.73
Hyalgan® versus Placebo	5.13	7.03	6.39	4.24	6.40	4.61	6.33	8.846
p-value	0.06	0.01	0.01	0.1	0.03	0.1	0.02	0.004

TABLE 6
Masked Evaluators' Categorical Assessments of Pain for Completed Subjects in Prior 48 Hours: Level of Pain by Treatment Group at Baseline and Week 26

	NUMBER (%) OF SUBJECTS IN CATEGORY					
	Hyalgan®		Placebo		Naproxen	
	Baseline	Week 26	Baseline	Week 26	Baseline	Week 26
None (0)	0 (0.0)	27 (25.7)	0 (0.0)	15 (13.0)	0 (0.0)	17 (15.0)
Slight (1)	1 (1.0)	23 (21.9)	0 (0.0)	27 (23.5)	0 (0.0)	32 (28.3)
Mild (2)	2 (1.9)	24 (22.9)	2 (1.7)	29 (25.2)	2 (1.8)	27 (23.9)
Moderate (3)	69 (65.7)	26 (24.8)	85 (73.9)	34 (29.6)	79 (70.5)	28 (24.8)
Marked (4)	33 (31.4)	5 (4.8)	28 (24.3)	10 (8.7)	31 (27.7)	9 (8.0)
TOTAL	105 (100)	105 (100)	115 (100)	115 (100)	112* (100)	113 (100)

*One Naproxen treated subject was missing a Baseline assessment.

DIRECTIONS FOR USE

Hyalgan® is administered by intra-articular injection. A treatment cycle consists of five injections given at weekly intervals. Some patients may experience benefit with three injections given at weekly intervals. This has been noted in studies reported in the literature in which patients treated with three injections were followed for 60 days.

Precaution: Do not use Hyalgan® if the package is opened or damaged. Store in the original packaging (protected from light) below 77° F (25° C). DO NOT FREEZE.

Precaution: Strict aseptic administration technique must be followed.

Warning: Do not concomitantly use disinfectants containing quaternary ammonium salts for skin preparation because hyaluronic acid can precipitate in their presence.

Inject subcutaneous lidocaine or similar local anesthetic prior to injection of Hyalgan®.

Precaution: Remove joint effusion, if present, before injection of Hyalgan®.

Do not use the same syringe for removing joint effusion and for injecting Hyalgan®.

Take care to remove the tip cap of the syringe and needle aseptically.

Inject Hyalgan® into the joint through a 20-gauge needle.

Precaution: The vial/syringe is intended for single use. The contents of the vial must be used immediately once the container has been opened. Discard any unused Hyalgan®. Inject the full 2 mL in one knee only. If treatment is bilateral, a separate vial should be used for each knee.

TABLE 7
Subjects' Categorical Assessments of Pain for Completed Subjects in Prior 48 Hours: Level of Pain by Treatment Group at Baseline and Week 26

	NUMBER (%) OF SUBJECTS IN CATEGORY					
	Hyalgan®		Placebo		Naproxen	
	Baseline	Week 26	Baseline	Week 26	Baseline	Week 26
None (0)	1 (1.0)	23 (21.9)	0 (0.0)	14 (12.2)	0 (0.0)	13 (11.5)
Slight (1)	2 (1.9)	27 (25.7)	0 (0.0)	24 (20.9)	1 (0.9)	31 (27.4)
Mild (2)	6 (5.7)	19 (18.1)	8 (7.0)	24 (20.9)	7 (6.2)	26 (23.0)
Moderate (3)	62 (59.0)	26 (24.8)	78 (67.8)	40 (34.8)	72 (63.7)	31 (27.4)
Marked (4)	34 (32.4)	10 (9.5)	29 (25.2)	13 (11.3)	33 (29.2)	12 (10.6)
TOTAL	105 (100)	105 (100)	115 (100)	115 (100)	113 (100)	113 (100)

TABLE 8
Hyalgan® Effect as a Percentage of the Naproxen-Placebo Difference

Assessment	Hyalgan® (HYL)	Placebo (PLA)	Naproxen (NAP)	HYL-PLA	NAP-HYL	NAP-PLA	(HYL-PLA) % of (NAP-PLA)
VAS for 50 foot Walk Baseline Adjusted Mean Effect Sizes From ANCOVA				−8.85 mm on a 100 mm VAS	4.12 mm on a 100 mm VAS	−4.73* mm on a 100 mm VAS	187%
% of Subjects Improved by Masked Evaluators	78.1	69.6	73.2	8.5	−4.9	3.6	236%
% of Subjects Improved by Subjects	73.3	62.6	67.3	10.7	−6.0	4.7	228%

*Imputed as (NAP-HYL)+(HYL-PLA).

Note that Effectiveness Success Criterion D is satisfied since ((HYL-PLA) % of (NAP-PLA))>50% for all three of the above pain assessments.

MANUFACTURED BY
FIDIA S.p.A.
Via Ponte della Fabbrica 3/A
35031 Abano Terme, Padua (PD), Italy

DISTRIBUTED BY
Sanofi-Synthelabo Inc.
90 Park Avenue
New York, NY 10016

REFERENCES

1. M. Carrabba et al., 1991 Hyaluronic acid sodium salt (Hyalgan®) in the treatment of patients with osteoarthritis of the knee: a controlled trial versus Orgotein, Final Report, April 1991. Data on file.
2. M. Carrabba et al., 1995. Effectiveness and safety of 1, 3 and 5 injections of 20 mg/2 ml Hyalgan® in comparison with a placebo and with arthrocentesis only, in the treatment of knee osteoarthritis. European Journal of Rheumatology and Inflammation 15:25–31.
3. M. Dougados et al., 1993. High molecular weight sodium hyaluronate (hyalectin) in osteoarthritis of the knee: a one-year placebo-controlled trial. Osteoarthritis and Cartilage 1:97–103.
4. R. Kotz and G. Kolarz, 1997 pulished as R. Kotz and G. Kolarz, 1999. Intra-articular hyaluronic acid: duration of effect and results of repeated treatment cycles. The American Journal of Orthopedics, 28:5–7.
5. G. Leardini et al., 1987. Intra-articular sodium hyaluronate (Hyalgan®) in gonarthrosis. Clinical Trials Journal 24(4):341–350.
6. J.J. Scali, 1995. Intra-articular hyaluronic acid in the treatment of osteoarthritis of the knee: a long term study 15(1):57–62.

07240211
Revised August 2000

Shown in Product Identification Guide, page 333

For information on over-the-counter drugs, consult **PDR For Nonprescription Drugs.**

Sepracor Inc.
111 LOCKE DRIVE
MARLBOROUGH, MA 01752

Direct Inquiries to:
Customer Service
1-877-SEPRACOR
FAX (508) 357-7589

XOPENEX® ℞
[zō' pə-neks"]
(levalbuterol HCl) Inhalation Solution,
0.63 mg*, 1.25 mg*
***Potency expressed as levalbuterol**

PRESCRIBING INFORMATION

DESCRIPTION

Xopenex® (levalbuterol HCl) Inhalation Solution is a sterile, clear, colorless, preservative-free solution of the hydrochloride salt of levalbuterol, the (R)-enantiomer of the drug substance racemic albuterol. Levalbuterol HCl is a relatively selective beta$_2$-adrenergic receptor agonist (see **CLINICAL PHARMACOLOGY**). The chemical name for levalbuterol HCl is (R)-α^1-[[(1,1-dimethylethyl)amino] methyl]-4-hydroxy-1,3-benzenedimethanol hydrochloride, and its established chemical structure is as follows:

OH, H, N, CH3, CH3, CH3, •HCl, HO, CH2OH

The molecular weight of levalbuterol HCl is 275.8, and its empirical formula is $C_{13}H_{21}NO_3$•HCl. It is a white to off-white, crystalline solid, with a melting point of approximately 187°C and solubility of approximately 180 mg/mL in water.

Levalbuterol HCl is the USAN modified name for (R)-albuterol HCl in the United States.

Xopenex® (levalbuterol HCl) Inhalation Solution is supplied in unit-dose vials and requires no dilution before administration by nebulization. Each 3 mL unit-dose vial contains either 0.63 mg of levalbuterol (as 0.73 mg of levalbuterol HCl) or 1.25 mg of levalbuterol (as 1.44 mg of levalbuterol HCl), sodium chloride to adjust tonicity, and sulfuric acid to adjust the pH to 4.0 (3.3 to 4.5).

CLINICAL PHARMACOLOGY

Activation of beta$_2$-adrenergic receptors on airway smooth muscle leads to the activation of adenylcyclase and to an increase in the intracellular concentration of cyclic-3′,5′-adenosine monophosphate (cyclic AMP). This increase in cyclic AMP leads to the activation of protein kinase A, which inhibits the phosphorylation of myosin and lowers intracellular ionic calcium concentrations, resulting in relaxation. Levalbuterol relaxes the smooth muscles of all airways, from the trachea to the terminal bronchioles. Levalbuterol acts as a functional antagonist to relax the airway irrespective of the spasmogen involved, thus protecting against all bronchoconstrictor challenges. Increased cyclic AMP concentrations are also associated with the inhibition of release of mediators from mast cells in the airway.

While it is recognized that beta$_2$-adrenergic receptors are the predominant receptors on bronchial smooth muscle, data indicate that there is a population of beta$_2$-receptors in the human heart that comprise between 10% and 50% of cardiac beta-adrenergic receptors. The precise function of these receptors has not been established (see **WARNINGS**). However, all beta-adrenergic agonist drugs can produce a significant cardiovascular effect in some patients, as measured by pulse rate, blood pressure, symptoms, and/or electrocardiographic changes.

Preclinical Studies

Results from an *in vitro* study of binding to human beta-adrenergic receptors demonstrated that levalbuterol has approximately 2-fold greater binding affinity than racemic albuterol and approximately 100-fold greater binding affinity than (S)-albuterol. In guinea pig airways, levalbuterol HCl and racemic albuterol decreased the response to spasmogens (e.g., acetylcholine and histamine), whereas (S)-albuterol was ineffective. These results suggest that most of the bronchodilatory effect of racemic albuterol is due to the (R)-enantiomer.

Intravenous studies in rats with racemic albuterol sulfate have demonstrated that albuterol crosses the blood-brain barrier and reaches brain concentrations amounting to approximately 5.0% of the plasma concentrations. In structures outside the blood-brain barrier (pineal and pituitary glands), albuterol concentrations were found to be 100 times those in the whole brain.

Studies in laboratory animals (minipigs, rodents, and dogs) have demonstrated the occurrence of cardiac arrhythmias and sudden death (with histologic evidence of myocardial necrosis) when beta-agonists and methylxanthines are administered concurrently. The clinical significance of these findings is unknown.

Pharmacokinetics

The inhalation pharmacokinetics of Xopenex® Inhalation Solution were investigated in a randomized cross-over study in 30 healthy adults following administration of a single dose of 1.25 mg and a cumulative dose of 5 mg of Xopenex® Inhalation Solution and a single dose of 2.5 mg and a cumulative dose of 10 mg of racemic albuterol sulfate inhalation solution by nebulization using a PARI LC Jet™ nebulizer with a Dura-Neb® 2000 compressor.

Following administration of a single 1.25 mg dose of Xopenex® Inhalation Solution, exposure, as measured by C_{max} and area under the curve (AUC) of (R)-albuterol, was 1.5 and 2 times greater, respectively, than that following administration of a single 2.5 mg dose of racemic albuterol sulfate inhalation solution (see **Table 1**). Following administration of a cumulative 5 mg dose of Xopenex® Inhalation Solution (1.25 mg given every 30 minutes for a total of four doses) or a cumulative 10 mg dose of racemic albuterol sulfate inhalation solution (2.5 mg given every 30 minutes for a total of four doses), C_{max} and AUC of (R)-albuterol were comparable (see **Table 1**).

[See table at top of next page]

Levalbuterol appears to be stereochemically stable *in vivo* and does not appear to interconvert metabolically to (S)-albuterol.

Pharmacodynamics

In a randomized, double-blind, placebo-controlled, cross-over study, 20 adults with mild-to-moderate asthma received single doses of Xopenex® Inhalation Solution (0.31, 0.63, and 1.25 mg) and racemic albuterol sulfate inhalation solution (2.5 mg). All doses of active treatment produced a significantly greater degree of bronchodilation (as measured by percent change from pre-dose in mean FEV_1) than placebo, and there were no significant differences between any of the active treatment arms. The bronchodilator responses to 1.25 mg of Xopenex® Inhalation Solution and 2.5 mg of racemic albuterol sulfate inhalation solution were clinically comparable over the 6-hour evaluation period, except for a slightly longer duration of action (>15% increase in FEV_1 from baseline) after administration of 1.25 mg of Xopenex® Inhalation Solution. Systemic beta-adrenergic adverse effects were observed with all active doses and were generally dose-related for (R)-albuterol. Xopenex® Inhalation Solution at a dose of 1.25 mg produced a slightly higher rate of systemic beta-adrenergic adverse effects than the 2.5 mg dose of racemic albuterol sulfate inhalation solution.

In a randomized, double-blind, placebo-controlled, cross-over study, 12 adults with mild-to-moderate asthma were challenged with inhaled methacholine chloride 20 and 180 minutes following administration of a single dose of either 2.5 mg of racemic albuterol sulfate, 1.25 mg of Xopenex®, 1.25 mg of (S)-albuterol, or placebo using a PARI LC Jet™

Continued on next page

Xopenex—Cont.

nebulizer. Racemic albuterol sulfate, Xopenex®, and (S)-albuterol had a protective effect against methacholine-induced bronchoconstriction 20 minutes after administration, although the effect of (S)-albuterol was minimal. At 180 minutes after administration, the bronchoprotective effect of 1.25 mg of Xopenex® was comparable to that of 2.5 mg of racemic albuterol sulfate. At 180 minutes after administration, 1.25 mg of (S)-albuterol had no bronchoprotective effect.

In a clinical study in adults with mild-to-moderate asthma, comparable efficacy (as measured by change from baseline in FEV_1) and safety (as measured by heart rate, blood pressure, ECG, serum potassium, and tremor) were demonstrated after a cumulative dose of 5 mg of Xopenex® Inhalation Solution (four consecutive doses of 1.25 mg administered every 30 minutes) and 10 mg of racemic albuterol sulfate inhalation solution (four consecutive doses of 2.5 mg administered every 30 minutes).

Clinical Trials

The safety and efficacy of Xopenex® Inhalation Solution were evaluated in a 4-week, multicenter, randomized, double-blind, placebo-controlled, parallel group study in 362 adult and adolescent patients 12 years of age and older, with mild-to-moderate asthma (mean baseline FEV_1 60% of predicted). Approximately half of the patients were also receiving inhaled corticosteroids. Patients were randomized to receive Xopenex® 0.63 mg, Xopenex® 1.25 mg, racemic albuterol sulfate 1.25 mg, racemic albuterol sulfate 2.5 mg, or placebo three times a day administered via a PARI LC Plus™ nebulizer and a Dura-Neb® portable compressor. Racemic albuterol delivered by a chlorofluorocarbon (CFC) metered dose inhaler (MDI) was used on an as-needed basis as the rescue medication.

Efficacy, as measured by the mean percent change from baseline in FEV_1, was demonstrated for all active treatment regimens compared with placebo on day 1 and day 29. On both day 1 (see **Figure 1**) and day 29 (see **Figure 2**), 1.25 mg of Xopenex® demonstrated the largest mean percent change from baseline in FEV_1 compared to the other active treatments. A dose of 0.63 mg of Xopenex® and 2.5 mg of racemic albuterol sulfate produced a clinically comparable mean percent change from baseline in FEV_1 on both day 1 and day 29.

Figure 1: Mean Percent Change from Baseline in FEV_1 on Day 1, All Patients

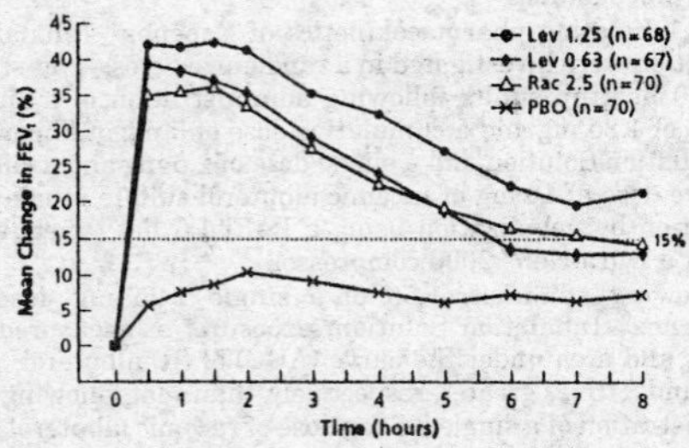

Figure 2: Mean Percent Change from Baseline in FEV_1 on Day 29, All Patients

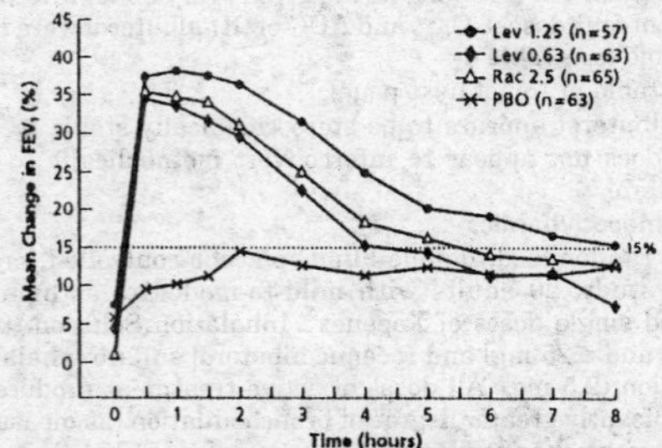

The mean time to onset of a 15% increase in FEV_1 over baseline for levalbuterol at doses of 0.63 mg and 1.25 mg was approximately 17 minutes and 10 minutes, respectively, and the mean time to peak effect for both doses was approximately 1.5 hours after 4 weeks of treatment. The mean duration of effect, as measured by a >15% increase from baseline in FEV_1, was approximately 5 hours after administration of 0.63 mg of levalbuterol and approximately 6 hours after administration of 1.25 mg of levalbuterol after 4 weeks of treatment. In some patients, the duration of effect was as long as 8 hours.

INDICATIONS AND USAGE

Xopenex® (levalbuterol HCl) Inhalation Solution is indicated for the treatment or prevention of bronchospasm in adults and adolescents 12 years of age and older with reversible obstructive airway disease.

CONTRAINDICATIONS

Xopenex® (levalbuterol HCl) Inhalation Solution is contraindicated in patients with a history of hypersensitivity to levalbuterol HCl or racemic albuterol.

Table 1: Mean (SD) Values for Pharmacokinetic Parameters in Healthy Adults

	Single Dose		Cumulative Dose	
	Xopenex® 1.25 mg	Racemic albuterol sulfate 2.5 mg	Xopenex® 5 mg	Racemic albuterol sulfate 10 mg
C_{max} (ng/mL)				
(R)-albuterol	1.1 (0.45)	0.8 (0.41)**	4.5 (2.20)	4.2 (1.51)**
T_{max} (h)$^{\gamma}$				
(R)-albuterol	0.2 (0.17, 0.37)	0.2 (0.17, 1.50)	0.2 (–0.18*, 1.25)	0.2 (–0.28*, 1.00)
AUC (ng•h/mL)				
(R)-albuterol	3.3 (1.58)	1.7 (0.99)**	17.4 (8.56)	16.0 (7.12)**
$T_{1/2}$ (h)				
(R)-albuterol	3.3 (2.48)	1.5 (0.61)	4.0 (1.05)	4.1 (0.97)

$^{\gamma}$Median (Min, Max) reported for T_{max}

*A negative T_{max} indicates C_{max} occurred between first and last nebulizations.

**Values reflect only (R)-albuterol and do not include (S)-albuterol.

WARNINGS

1. Paradoxical Bronchospasm: Like other inhaled beta-adrenergic agonists, Xopenex® Inhalation Solution can produce paradoxical bronchospasm, which may be life threatening. If paradoxical bronchospasm occurs, Xopenex® Inhalation Solution should be discontinued immediately and alternative therapy instituted. It should be recognized that paradoxical bronchospasm, when associated with inhaled formulations, frequently occurs with the first use of a new canister or vial.

2. Deterioration of Asthma: Asthma may deteriorate acutely over a period of hours or chronically over several days or longer. If the patient needs more doses of Xopenex® Inhalation Solution than usual, this may be a marker of destabilization of asthma and requires reevaluation of the patient and treatment regimen, giving special consideration to the possible need for anti-inflammatory treatment, e.g., corticosteroids.

3. Use of Anti-Inflammatory Agents: The use of beta-adrenergic agonist bronchodilators alone may not be adequate to control asthma in many patients. Early consideration should be given to adding anti-inflammatory agents, e.g., corticosteroids, to the therapeutic regimen.

4. Cardiovascular Effects: Xopenex® Inhalation Solution, like all other beta-adrenergic agonists, can produce a clinically significant cardiovascular effect in some patients, as measured by pulse rate, blood pressure, and/or symptoms. Although such effects are uncommon after administration of Xopenex® Inhalation Solution at recommended doses, if they occur, the drug may need to be discontinued. In addition, beta-agonists have been reported to produce ECG changes, such as flattening of the T wave, prolongation of the QTc interval, and ST segment depression. The clinical significance of these findings is unknown. Therefore, Xopenex® Inhalation Solution, like all sympathomimetic amines, should be used with caution in patients with cardiovascular disorders, especially coronary insufficiency, cardiac arrhythmias, and hypertension.

5. Do Not Exceed Recommended Dose: Fatalities have been reported in association with excessive use of inhaled sympathomimetic drugs in patients with asthma. The exact cause of death is unknown, but cardiac arrest following an unexpected development of a severe acute asthmatic crisis and subsequent hypoxia is suspected.

6. Immediate Hypersensitivity Reactions: Immediate hypersensitivity reactions may occur after administration of racemic albuterol, as demonstrated by rare cases of urticaria, angioedema, rash, bronchospasm, anaphylaxis, and oropharyngeal edema. The potential for hypersensitivity must be considered in the clinical evaluation of patients who experience immediate hypersensitivity reactions while receiving Xopenex® Inhalation Solution.

PRECAUTIONS

General

Levalbuterol HCl, like all sympathomimetic amines, should be used with caution in patients with cardiovascular disorders, especially coronary insufficiency, hypertension, and cardiac arrhythmias; in patients with convulsive disorders, hyperthyroidism, or diabetes mellitus; and in patients who are unusually responsive to sympathomimetic amines. Clinically significant changes in systolic and diastolic blood pressure have been seen in individual patients and could be expected to occur in some patients after the use of any beta-adrenergic bronchodilator.

Large doses of intravenous racemic albuterol have been reported to aggravate preexisting diabetes mellitus and ketoacidosis. As with other beta-adrenergic agonist medications, levalbuterol may produce significant hypokalemia in some patients, possibly through intracellular shunting, which has the potential to produce adverse cardiovascular effects. The decrease is usually transient, not requiring supplementation.

Information for Patients

See illustrated Patient's Instructions for Use.

The action of Xopenex® (levalbuterol HCl) Inhalation Solution may last up to 8 hours. Xopenex® Inhalation Solution should not be used more frequently than recommended. Do not increase the dose or frequency of dosing of Xopenex® Inhalation Solution without consulting your physician. If you find that treatment with Xopenex® Inhalation Solution becomes less effective for symptomatic relief, your symptoms become worse, and/or you need to use the product more frequently than usual, you should seek medical attention immediately. While you are taking Xopenex® Inhalation Solution, other inhaled drugs and asthma medications should be taken only as directed by your physician. Common adverse effects include palpitations, chest pain, rapid heart rate, headache, dizziness, and tremor or nervousness. If you are pregnant or nursing, contact your physician about the use of Xopenex® Inhalation Solution.

Effective and safe use of Xopenex® Inhalation Solution requires consideration of the following information in addition to that provided under Patient's Instructions for Use:

Xopenex® Inhalation Solution single-use low-density polyethylene (LDPE) vials should be protected from light and excessive heat. Store in the protective foil pouch between 15°C and 25°C (59°F and 77°F). Do not use after the expiration date stamped on the container. Unused vials should be stored in the protective foil pouch. Once the foil pouch is opened, the vials should be used within two weeks. Vials removed from the pouch, if not used immediately, should be protected from light and used within one week. Discard any vial if the solution is not colorless.

The drug compatibility (physical and chemical), efficacy, and safety of Xopenex® Inhalation Solution when mixed with other drugs in a nebulizer have not been established.

Drug Interactions

Other short-acting sympathomimetic aerosol bronchodilators or epinephrine should be used with caution with levalbuterol. If additional adrenergic drugs are to be administered by any route, they should be used with caution to avoid deleterious cardiovascular effects.

1. Beta-blockers: Beta-adrenergic receptor blocking agents not only block the pulmonary effect of beta-agonists such as Xopenex® (levalbuterol HCl) Inhalation Solution, but may also produce severe bronchospasm in asthmatic patients. Therefore, patients with asthma should not normally be treated with beta-blockers. However, under certain circumstances, e.g., as prophylaxis after myocardial infarction, there may be no acceptable alternatives to the use of beta-adrenergic blocking agents in patients with asthma. In this setting, cardioselective beta-blockers could be considered, although they should be administered with caution.

2. Diuretics: The ECG changes and/or hypokalemia that may result from the administration of non-potassium sparing diuretics (such as loop or thiazide diuretics) can be acutely worsened by beta-agonists, especially when the recommended dose of the beta-agonist is exceeded. Although the clinical significance of these effects is not known, caution is advised in the coadministration of beta-agonists with non-potassium sparing diuretics.

3. Digoxin: Mean decreases of 16% and 22% in serum digoxin levels were demonstrated after single-dose intravenous and oral administration of racemic albuterol, respectively, to normal volunteers who had received digoxin for 10 days. The clinical significance of these findings for patients with obstructive airway disease who are receiving levalbuterol HCl and digoxin on a chronic basis is unclear. Nevertheless, it would be prudent to carefully evaluate the serum digoxin levels in patients who are currently receiving digoxin and Xopenex® Inhalation Solution.

4. Monoamine Oxidase Inhibitors or Tricyclic Antidepressants: Xopenex® Inhalation Solution should be administered with extreme caution to patients being treated with monoamine oxidase inhibitors or tricyclic antidepressants, or within 2 weeks of discontinuation of such agents, because the action of levalbuterol HCl on the vascular system may be potentiated.

Carcinogenesis, Mutagenesis, and Impairment of Fertility

No carcinogenesis or impairment of fertility studies have been carried out with levalbuterol HCl alone. However, racemic albuterol sulfate has been evaluated for its carcinogenic potential and ability to impair fertility.

In a 2-year study in Sprague-Dawley rats, racemic albuterol sulfate caused a significant dose-related increase in the incidence of benign leiomyomas of the mesovarium at and above dietary doses of 2 mg/kg (approximately 2 times the maximum recommended daily inhalation dose of levalbuterol HCl for adults on a mg/m^2 basis). In another study, this effect was blocked by the coadministration of propranolol, a nonselective beta-adrenergic antagonist. In an 18-month study in CD-1 mice, racemic albuterol sulfate showed no evidence of tumorigenicity at dietary doses up to 500 mg/kg (approximately 270 times the maximum recommended daily inhalation dose of levalbuterol HCl for adults on a mg/m^2 basis). In a 22-month study in the Golden hamster, racemic albuterol sulfate showed no evidence of tumorigenicity at dietary doses up to 50 mg/kg (approximately 35 times the maximum recommended daily inhalation dose of levalbuterol HCl for adults on a mg/m^2 basis).

Levalbuterol HCl was not mutagenic in the Ames test or the CHO/HPRT Mammalian Forward Gene Mutation Assay. Although levalbuterol HCl has not been tested for clastogenicity, racemic albuterol sulfate was not clastogenic in a human peripheral lymphocyte assay or in an AH1 strain mouse micronucleus assay. Reproduction studies in rats using racemic albuterol sulfate demonstrated no evidence of impaired fertility at oral doses up to 50 mg/kg (approximately 55 times the maximum recommended daily inhalation dose of levalbuterol HCl for adults on a mg/m^2 basis).

Teratogenic Effects—Pregnancy Category C

A reproduction study in New Zealand White rabbits demonstrated that levalbuterol HCl was not teratogenic when administered orally at doses up to 25 mg/kg (approximately 110 times the maximum recommended daily inhalation dose of levalbuterol HCl for adults on a mg/m^2 basis). However, racemic albuterol sulfate has been shown to be teratogenic in mice and rabbits. A study in CD-1 mice given racemic albuterol sulfate subcutaneously showed cleft palate formation in 5 of 111 (4.5%) fetuses at 0.25 mg/kg (less than the maximum recommended daily inhalation dose of levalbuterol HCl for adults on a mg/m^2 basis) and in 10 of 108 (9.3%) fetuses at 2.5 mg/kg (approximately equal to the maximum recommended daily inhalation dose of levalbuterol HCl for adults on a mg/m^2 basis). The drug did not induce cleft palate formation when administered subcutaneously at a dose of 0.025 mg/kg (less than the maximum recommended daily inhalation dose of levalbuterol HCl for adults on a mg/m^2 basis). Cleft palate also occurred in 22 of 72 (30.5%) fetuses from females treated subcutaneously with 2.5 mg/kg of isoproterenol (positive control).

A reproduction study in Stride Dutch rabbits revealed cranioschisis in 7 of 19 (37%) fetuses when racemic albuterol sulfate was administered orally at a dose of 50 mg/kg (approximately 110 times the maximum recommended daily inhalation dose of levalbuterol HCl for adults on a mg/m^2 basis).

A study in which pregnant rats were dosed with radiolabeled racemic albuterol sulfate demonstrated that drug-related material is transferred from the maternal circulation to the fetus.

There are no adequate and well-controlled studies of Xopenex® Inhalation Solution in pregnant women. Because animal reproduction studies are not always predictive of human response, Xopenex® Inhalation Solution should be used during pregnancy only if the potential benefit justifies the potential risk to the fetus.

During marketing experience of racemic albuterol, various congenital anomalies, including cleft palate and limb defects, have been rarely reported in the offspring of patients being treated with racemic albuterol. Some of the mothers were taking multiple medications during their pregnancies. No consistent pattern of defects can be discerned, and a relationship between racemic albuterol use and congenital anomalies has not been established.

Use in Labor and Delivery

Because of the potential for beta-adrenergic agonists to interfere with uterine contractility, the use of Xopenex® Inhalation Solution for the treatment of bronchospasm during labor should be restricted to those patients in whom the benefits clearly outweigh the risk.

Tocolysis

Levalbuterol HCl has not been approved for the management of preterm labor. The benefit:risk ratio when levalbuterol HCl is administered for tocolysis has not been established. Serious adverse reactions, including maternal pulmonary edema, have been reported during or following treatment of premature labor with beta$_2$-agonists, including racemic albuterol.

Nursing Mothers

Plasma levels of levalbuterol after inhalation of therapeutic doses are very low in humans, but it is not known whether levalbuterol is excreted in human milk.

Because of the potential for tumorigenicity shown for racemic albuterol in animal studies and the lack of experience with the use of Xopenex® Inhalation Solution by nursing mothers, a decision should be made whether to discontinue nursing or to discontinue the drug, taking into account the importance of the drug to the mother. Caution should be exercised when Xopenex® Inhalation Solution is administered to a nursing woman.

Pediatrics

The safety and effectiveness of Xopenex® (levalbuterol HCl) Inhalation Solution in children less than 12 years of age have not been established.

Geriatrics

Data on the use of Xopenex® in patients 65 years of age and older are very limited. A very small number of patients 65 years of age and older were treated with Xopenex® Inhalation Solution in a 4-week clinical study (see **CLINICAL PHARMACOLOGY; Clinical Trials**) (n=2 for 0.63 mg and n=3 for 1.25 mg). In these patients, bronchodilation was observed after the first dose on day 1 and after 4 weeks of treatment. There are insufficient data to determine if the safety and efficacy of Xopenex® Inhalation Solution are different in patients <65 years of age and patients 65 years of age and older. In general, patients 65 years of age and older should be started at a dose of 0.63 mg of Xopenex® Inhalation Solution. If clinically warranted due to insufficient bronchodilator response, the dose of Xopenex® Inhalation Solution may be increased in elderly patients as tolerated, in conjunction with frequent clinical and laboratory monitoring, to the maximum recommended daily dose (See **DOSAGE AND ADMINISTRATION**).

Table 2: Adverse Events Reported in a 4-Week, Controlled Clinical Trial

Body System Preferred Term	Placebo (n=75)	Xopenex® 1.25 mg (n=73)	Xopenex® 0.63 mg (n=72)	Racemic albuterol 2.5 mg (n=74)
	Percent of Patients			
Body as a Whole				
Allergic reaction	1.3	0	0	2.7
Flu syndrome	0	1.4	4.2	2.7
Accidental injury	0	2.7	0	0
Pain	1.3	1.4	2.8	2.7
Back pain	0	0	0	2.7
Cardiovascular System				
Tachycardia	0	2.7	2.8	2.7
Migraine	0	2.7	0	0
Digestive System				
Dyspepsia	1.3	2.7	1.4	1.4
Musculoskeletal System				
Leg cramps	1.3	2.7	0	1.4
Central Nervous System				
Dizziness	1.3	2.7	1.4	0
Hypertonia	0	0	0	2.7
Nervousness	0	9.6	2.8	8.1
Tremor	0	6.8	0	2.7
Anxiety	0	2.7	0	0
Respiratory System				
Cough increased	2.7	4.1	1.4	2.7
Infection viral	9.3	12.3	6.9	12.2
Rhinitis	2.7	2.7	11.1	6.8
Sinusitis	2.7	1.4	4.2	2.7
Turbinate edema	0	1.4	2.8	0

Table 3: Mean Changes from Baseline in Heart Rate at 15 Minutes and in Glucose and Potassium at 1 Hour after First Dose (Day 1)

Treatment	Heart Rate (bpm)	Glucose (mg/dL)	Potassium (mEq/L)
	Mean Changes (day 1)		
Xopenex® 0.63 mg, n=72	2.4	4.6	–0.2
Xopenex® 1.25 mg, n=73	6.9	10.3	–0.3
Racemic albuterol 2.5 mg, n=74	5.7	8.2	–0.3
Placebo, n=75	–2.8	–0.2	–0.2

ADVERSE REACTIONS

Adverse events reported in ≥2% of patients receiving Xopenex® Inhalation Solution or racemic albuterol and more frequently than in patients receiving placebo in a 4-week, controlled clinical trial are listed in **Table 2**.

[See table 2 above]

The incidence of certain systemic beta-adrenergic adverse effects (e.g., tremor, nervousness) was slightly less in the Xopenex® 0.63 mg group as compared to the other active treatment groups. The clinical significance of these small differences is unknown.

Changes in heart rate 15 minutes after drug administration and in plasma glucose and potassium one hour after drug administration on day 1 and day 29 were clinically comparable in the Xopenex® 1.25 mg and the racemic albuterol 2.5 mg groups (see **Table 3**). Changes in heart rate and plasma glucose were slightly less in the Xopenex® 0.63 mg group compared to the other active treatment groups (see **Table 3**). The clinical significance of these small differences is unknown. After 4 weeks, effects on heart rate, plasma glucose, and plasma potassium were generally diminished compared with day 1 in all active treatment groups.

[See table 3 above]

No other clinically relevant laboratory abnormalities related to administration of Xopenex® Inhalation Solution were observed in this study. In the clinical trials, a slightly greater number of serious adverse events, discontinuations due to adverse events, and clinically significant ECG changes were reported in patients who received Xopenex® 1.25 mg compared to the other active treatment groups.

The following adverse events, considered potentially related to Xopenex®, occurred in less than 2% of the 292 subjects who received Xopenex® and more frequently than in patients who received placebo in any clinical trial:

Body as a Whole:	chills, pain, chest pain
Cardiovascular System:	ECG abnormal, ECG change, hypertension, hypotension, syncope
Digestive System:	diarrhea, dry mouth, dry throat, dyspepsia, gastroenteritis, nausea
Hemic and Lymphatic System:	lymphadenopathy
Musculoskeletal System:	leg cramps, myalgia
Nervous System:	anxiety, hypesthesia of the hand, insomnia, paresthesia, tremor
Special Senses:	eye itch

The following events, considered potentially related to Xopenex®, occurred in less than 2% of the treated subjects but a frequency less than in patients who received placebo: asthma exacerbation, cough increased, wheezing, sweating, and vomiting.

OVERDOSAGE

The expected symptoms with overdosage are those of excessive beta-adrenergic receptor stimulation and/or occurrence or exaggeration of any of the symptoms listed under **ADVERSE REACTIONS**, e.g., seizures, angina, hypertension or hypotension, tachycardia with rates up to 200 beats/min., arrhythmias, nervousness, headache, tremor, dry mouth, palpitation, nausea, dizziness, fatigue, malaise, and sleeplessness. Hypokalemia also may occur. As with all sympathomimetic medications, cardiac arrest and even death may be associated with the abuse of Xopenex® Inhalation Solution. Treatment consists of discontinuation of Xopenex® Inhalation Solution together with appropriate symptomatic therapy. The judicious use of a cardioselective beta-receptor blocker may be considered, bearing in mind that such medication can produce bronchospasm. There is insufficient evidence to determine if dialysis is beneficial for overdosage of Xopenex® Inhalation Solution.

The intravenous median lethal dose of levalbuterol HCl in mice is approximately 66 mg/kg (approximately 70 times the maximum recommended daily inhalation dose of levalbuterol HCl for adults on a mg/m^2 basis). The inhalation median lethal dose has not been determined in animals.

DOSAGE AND ADMINISTRATION

The usual starting dosage of Xopenex® (levalbuterol HCl) Inhalation Solution for patients 12 years of age and older is 0.63 mg administered three times a day, every 6 to 8 hours, by nebulization.

Patients 12 years of age and older with more severe asthma or patients who do not respond adequately to a dose of 0.63 mg of Xopenex® Inhalation Solution may benefit from a dosage of 1.25 mg three times a day. Patients receiving the higher dose of Xopenex® Inhalation Solution should be monitored closely for adverse systemic effects, and the risks of such effects should be balanced against the potential for improved efficacy.

The use of Xopenex® Inhalation Solution can be continued as medically indicated to control recurring bouts of bronchospasm. During this time, most patients gain optimal benefit from regular use of the inhalation solution.

If a previously effective dosage regimen fails to provide the expected relief, medical advice should be sought immediately, since this is often a sign of seriously worsening asthma that would require reassessment of therapy.

The drug compatibility (physical and chemical), efficacy, and safety of Xopenex® Inhalation Solution when mixed with other drugs in a nebulizer have not been established.

The safety and efficacy of Xopenex® Inhalation Solution have been established in clinical trials when administered using the PARI LC Jet™ and the PARI LC Plus™ nebulizers, and the PARI Master® and Dura-Neb® 2000 compressors. The safety and efficacy of Xopenex® Inhalation Solution when administered using other nebulizer systems have not been established.

HOW SUPPLIED

Xopenex® (levalbuterol HCl) Inhalation Solution is supplied in 3 mL unit-dose, low-density polyethylene (LDPE) vials as

Continued on next page

Xopenex—Cont.

a clear, colorless, sterile, preservative-free, aqueous solution in two different strengths of levalbuterol (0.63 mg, 1.25 mg). Each strength of Xopenex® Inhalation Solution is available in a shelf-carton containing one or more foil pouches, each containing 12 unit-dose LDPE vials.

Xopenex® (levalbuterol HCl) Inhalation Solution, 0.63 mg *(foil pouch label color yellow)* contains 0.63 mg of levalbuterol (as 0.73 mg of levalbuterol HCl) and is available in cartons of 24 unit-dose LDPE vials (NDC 63402-512-24) and 60 unit-dose LDPE vials (NDC 63402-512-60).

Xopenex® (levalbuterol HCl) Inhalation Solution, 1.25 mg *(foil pouch label color red)* contains 1.25 mg of levalbuterol (as 1.44 mg of levalbuterol HCl) and is available in cartons of 24 unit-dose LDPE vials (NDC 63402-513-24) and 96 unit-dose LDPE vials (NDC 63402-513-96).

CAUTION

Federal law (U.S.) prohibits dispensing without prescription.

Store the Xopenex® (levalbuterol HCl) Inhalation Solution in the protective foil pouch between 15°C and 25°C (59°F and 77°F). Protect from light and excessive heat. Keep unopened vials in the foil pouch. Once the foil pouch is opened, the vials should be used within two weeks. Vials removed from the pouch, if not used immediately, should be protected from light and used within one week. Discard any vial if the solution is not colorless.

Manufactured for: September 1999
Sepracor Inc. 400437-R1
Marlborough, MA 01752 USA
by ALP Inc., Woodstock, IL 60098 USA
1-877-SEPRACOR

Patient's Instructions for Use

Read complete instructions carefully before using.

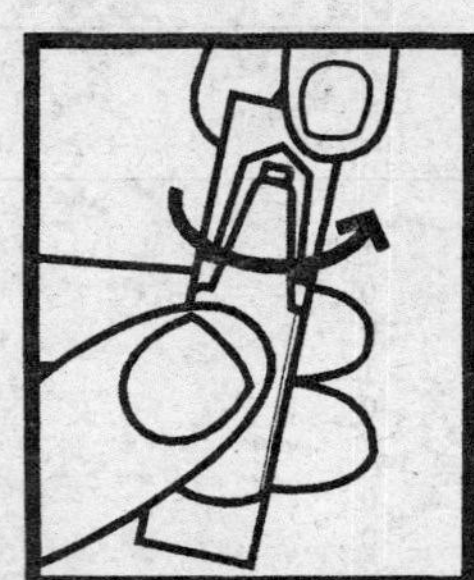

Figure 1

1. Open the foil pouch by tearing on the serrated edge along the seam of the pouch. Remove one unit-dose vial for immediate use. Keep the rest of the unused unit-dose vials in the foil pouch to protect them from light.

2. Carefully twist open the top of one unit-dose vial (**Figure 1**) and squeeze the entire contents into the nebulizer reservoir.

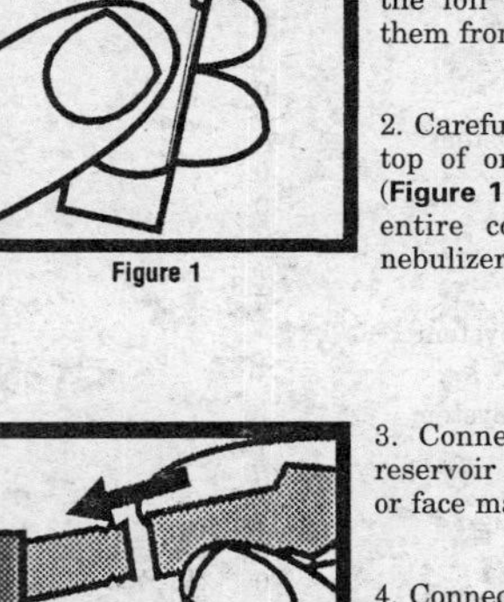

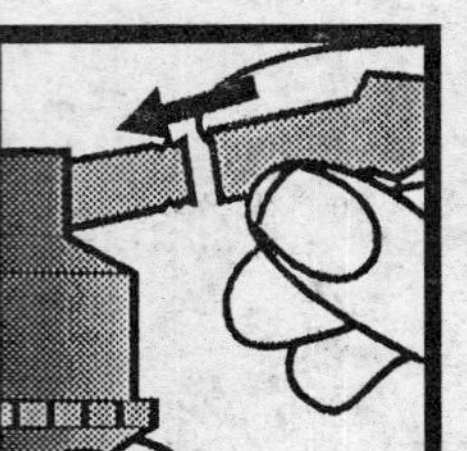

Figure 2

3. Connect the nebulizer reservoir to the mouthpiece or face mask (**Figure 2**).

4. Connect the nebulizer to the compressor.

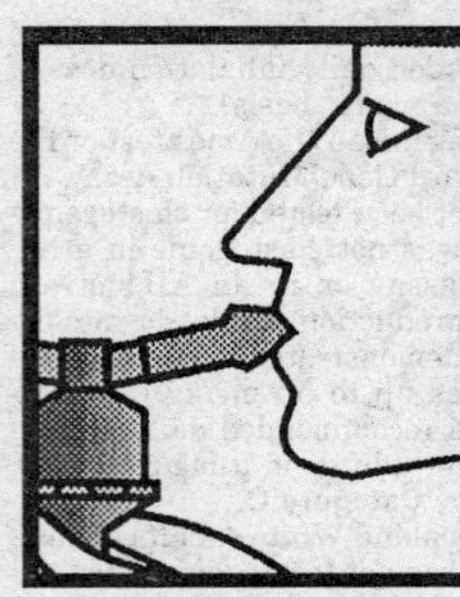

Figure 3

5. Sit in a comfortable, upright position. Place the mouthpiece in your mouth (**Figure 3**) (or put on the face mask) and turn on the compressor.

6. Breathe as calmly, deeply, and evenly as possible until no more mist is formed in the nebulizer reservoir (about 5 to 15 minutes). At this point, the treatment is finished.

7. Clean the nebulizer (see manufacturer's instructions).

Note: Xopenex® (levalbuterol HCl) Inhalation Solution should be used in a nebulizer only under the direction of a physician. More frequent administration or higher doses are not recommended. This solution should not be injected or administered orally. Protect from light and excessive heat. Store in the protective foil pouch between 15°C and 25°C (59°F and 77°F). Keep unopened vials in the foil pouch. Once the foil pouch is opened, the vials should be used within two weeks. Vials removed from the pouch, if not used immediately, should be protected from light and used within one week. Discard any vial if the solution is not colorless.

The safety and effectiveness of Xopenex® Inhalation Solution have not been determined when one or more drugs are mixed with it in a nebulizer. Check with your doctor before mixing any medications in your nebulizer.

Manufactured for: September 1999
Sepracor Inc. 400437-R1
Marlborough, MA 01752 USA
by ALP Inc., Woodstock, IL 60098 USA
1-877-SEPRACOR

SECTION 6

DIAGNOSTIC PRODUCT INFORMATION

This section is made possible through the courtesy of the manufacturers whose products appear on the following pages. The information concerning each product has been prepared, edited, and approved by the medical department, medical director, and/or medical counsel of its manufacturer.

When a product appearing in PHYSICIANS' DESK REFERENCE has an official package circular, its description must be in full compliance with Food and Drug Administration (FDA) regulations pertaining to labeling for prescription drugs. These regulations require that in PDR "indications, effects, dosages, routes, methods, and frequency and duration of administration, and any relevant warnings, hazards, contraindications, side effects, and precautions" must be *"same in language and emphasis"* as the approved labeling for the product. The FDA regards the words *"same in language and emphasis"* as requiring VERBATIM use of the approved labeling providing such information. Furthermore, information that is emphasized in the approved labeling by the use of type set in a box, or in capitals, boldface, or italics, must be given the same emphasis in PDR.

For products that do not have official package circulars, the publisher has emphasized the necessity of describing such products comprehensively, so that physicians can have access to all information essential for intelligent and informed decision-making.

The product descriptions in PHYSICIANS' DESK REFERENCE include all information made available to PDR by the manufacturer. The publisher does not warrant or guarantee any product, and does not perform any independent analysis of the information provided. Inclusion of a product in PDR does not represent an endorsement, and the publisher does not necessarily advocate the use of any product listed.

This edition of PHYSICIANS' DESK REFERENCE contains the latest information available when the book went to press. As new drugs are released and new research data and clinical findings become available throughout the year, the information in the PDR database is revised accordingly. These revisions are published twice annually in the PDR Supplements and are then incorporated in the following edition of the book. To be certain that you have the most current data, always consult the supplements or the latest edition before administering any product described in the following pages.

Aventis Pasteur Inc.
SWIFTWATER PA 18370

For Medical Information Contact:
Generally:
Medical Affairs
(800) VACCINE
(800) 822-2463

Adverse Drug Experiences:
Medical Director
(570) 839-7187
(800) 822-2463

Sales and Ordering:
Aventis Pasteur Inc.
Customer Service
(800) VACCINE
(800) 822-2463
(570) 839-7187

MUMPS SKIN TEST ANTIGEN USP ℞
MSTA®
NOT FOR IMMUNIZATION, DIAGNOSIS, OR TREATMENT
NOT FOR DIAGNOSIS OF IMMUNITY TO MUMPS
Rx only

Caution: Federal (USA) law prohibits dispensing without prescription.

DESCRIPTION

MSTA®, Mumps Skin Test Antigen, is a sterile suspension of killed mumps virus for intradermal use. It is prepared from the extraembryonic fluid of the virus-infected chicken embryo and is concentrated and purified by differential centrifugation. The virus is killed with formaldehyde solution, 1:1000, and is then diluted with isotonic sodium chloride solution. The resultant product contains approximately 0.012 molar glycine and less than 1:8,000 formaldehyde solution. Thimerosal (mercury derivative) 1:10,000 is added as a preservative. The skin test antigen is formulated to contain at least 40 complement fixing units (CFU) per mL, at the time of release, as determined by the Complement-Fixation Test. This product, after shaking, is slightly opalescent in color.

CLINICAL PHARMACOLOGY

Information is available concerning the pharmacologic mode of action of skin test antigens.[1] Skin testing is a widely employed and readily available method of clinically assessing the cellular immune response. A positive skin-test reaction indicates previous antigenic exposure, T-cell competence, an intact inflammatory response, and is an assessment of the cellular integrity of the immune response.
Skin testing with MSTA detects delayed-hypersensitivity.[2] Since most of the population (except for the very young) have had contact or infection with mumps virus,[3] they usually demonstrate a delayed-hypersensitivity reaction to MSTA if an adequate cellular immune system exists.[4]
A single masked placebo-controlled study involving 90 cancer subjects was performed using MSTA, Tetanus Toxoid Fluid, Mixed Respiratory Vaccine, Dermatophyton O. staphage lysate and PPD (Tubersol®). The injection sites were read at 48 and 72 hours. The number of positive reactors to MSTA was greater than the number of positive subjects receiving the other antigens. None of the patients experienced any sloughing, necrosis, abscess formation, or painful lymphadenopathy as a result of the MSTA skin test. This study demonstrated that MSTA evoked a positive delayed-hypersensitivity (DH) reaction in immunocompetent individuals. The frequency of reactions in subjects with an impaired immune system was reduced. The sensitivity of MSTA has been demonstrated by the fact that: 1) in all instances when any of the other test antigens were positive, MSTA was also positive; and 2) several subjects showed a DH reaction to MSTA but did not show a DH reaction to the other antigens.[2]

INDICATIONS AND USAGE

MSTA, Mumps Skin Test Antigen, is indicated when detection of a delayed hypersensitivity (DH) reaction is desired. MSTA has not been tested in persons immunized with live mumps vaccine; therefore, its safety and efficacy in this population group has not been established.
MSTA is not indicated for the immunization, diagnosis, or treatment of mumps virus infection, or determination of immune status to mumps virus.

CONTRAINDICATIONS

MUMPS VIRUS FOR THE PREPARATION OF MUMPS SKIN TEST ANTIGEN IS PROPAGATED IN EGGS. THEREFORE, THIS PRODUCT SHOULD NOT BE ADMINISTERED TO ANYONE WITH A HISTORY OF HYPERSENSITIVITY (ALLERGY), ESPECIALLY ANAPHYLACTIC REACTIONS TO EGGS OR EGG PRODUCTS. IT IS ALSO A CONTRAINDICATION TO ADMINISTER MSTA TO INDIVIDUALS KNOWN TO BE SENSITIVE TO THIMEROSAL. IN ANY CASE, EPINEPHRINE INJECTION (1:1000) MUST BE IMMEDIATELY AVAILABLE TO COMBAT UNEXPECTED ANAPHYLACTIC OR OTHER ALLERGIC REACTIONS.

WARNINGS

This product contains dry natural latex rubber as follows: The stopper to the vial contains dry natural latex rubber.
Neurologic complications, such as encephalopathies or peripheral-nervous systems disorders, or anaphylactic reactions have followed the administration of almost all biologics, although these have not been reported after the injection of MSTA.

PRECAUTIONS

GENERAL
Care is to be taken by the health-care provider for the safe and effective use of this product and to possible sensitivity to dry natural latex rubber.
EPINEPHRINE INJECTION (1:1000) MUST BE IMMEDIATELY AVAILABLE TO COMBAT UNEXPECTED ANAPHYLACTIC OR OTHER ALLERGIC REACTIONS.
A separate, sterile syringe and needle or a sterile disposable unit should be used for each patient to prevent transmission of hepatitis or other infectious agents from person to person. Needles should not be recapped and should be disposed of according to biohazard waste guidelines.
Special care should be taken to ensure the product is not injected into a blood vessel.
The antigen must be given intradermally. If it is injected subcutaneously, no reaction or an unreliable reaction may occur.
DRUG INTERACTIONS
MSTA has not been tested in persons immunized with live mumps vaccine; therefore, its safety and efficacy in this population has not been established.
CARCINOGENESIS, MUTAGENESIS, IMPAIRMENT OF FERTILITY
MSTA has not been evaluated for its carcinogenic, mutagenic potentials or impairment of fertility.
PREGNANCY
REPRODUCTIVE STUDIES—PREGNANCY CATEGORY C
Animal reproduction studies have not been conducted with Mumps Skin Test Antigen. It is not known whether Mumps Skin Test Antigen can cause fetal harm when administered to a pregnant woman or can affect reproduction capacity. Mumps Skin Test Antigen should be given to a pregnant woman only if clearly needed. There are no carefully done studies available on the effect of the drug on later growth, development and functional maturation of the child.
USAGE IN NURSING MOTHERS
It is not known whether this drug is excreted in human milk. Because many drugs are excreted in human milk, caution should be exercised when Mumps Skin Test Antigen is administered to a nursing woman.
PEDIATRIC USE
SAFETY AND EFFECTIVENESS OF MSTA IN CHILDREN HAVE NOT BEEN ESTABLISHED.
USAGE IN YOUNG ADULTS
SAFETY AND EFFECTIVENESS HAVE NOT BEEN ESTABLISHED IN YOUNG ADULTS WHO HAVE BEEN IMMUNIZED WITH MUMPS VACCINE.

ADVERSE REACTIONS

Local reactions may include tenderness, pruritus, vesiculation and rash. Sloughing, necrosis, abscess formation, and/or regional lymphadenopathy may be associated with unusually large DH reactions. Adverse reactions may include nausea, anorexia, headache, unsteadiness, drowsiness, sweating, sensation of warmth and lymphadenopathy. None of these reactions were noted in the clinical study.[2]
Epinephrine Injection (1:1000) must be immediately available to combat unexpected anaphylactic and other allergic reactions.

DOSAGE AND ADMINISTRATION

Parenteral drug products should be inspected visually for extraneous particulate matter and/or discoloration prior to administration. If these conditions exist, Mumps Skin Test Antigen should not be administered.
SHAKE VIAL WELL before withdrawing each dose.
A separate, sterile syringe and needle or a sterile disposable unit should be used for each patient to prevent transmission of hepatitis or other infectious agents from person to person. Needles should not be recapped and should be disposed of according to biohazard waste guidelines.
An injection of 0.1 mL of the antigen is made on the inner surface of the forearm. Before injection, the skin over the site to be injected should be cleansed with a suitable germicide. Care should be taken to inject the test antigen intradermally.
Interpretation of Reactions—The reaction should be examined in 48 to 72 hours. A mean diameter (i.e., the longest width plus the longest length, divided by 2) of induration of 5 mm or more indicates a positive DH reaction to the antigen. A negative reaction, if the test dose has been given correctly, usually indicates either anergy or nonsensitivity. Pseudopositive reactions may develop in persons highly sensitive to egg protein.

HOW SUPPLIED

Vial, 1 mL (10 tests)—Product No. 49281-240-10
STORAGE
Store between 2° – 8°C (35° – 46°F). DO NOT FREEZE.

REFERENCES

1. Holborow EJ, et al. Immunology in Medicine. Second Edition, pp 19 and 121. Grune & Stratton, 1983
2. Unpublished data available from Aventis Pasteur Inc.
3. Petersdorf RG. Mumps. in Harrison's Principles of Internal Medicine, Ed. 7 (edited by M.M. Wintrobe, G.W. Thorn, R.D. Adams, E. Braunwald, K.J. Isselbacher, and R.G. Petersdorf) p 985. New York: McGraw-Hill Book Company, 1974
4. Dempster G. Mumps in Textbook of Virology, Ed. 5 (edited by A.J. Rhodes and C.E. Van Rooyen) p 461 Baltimore: The Williams & Wilkins Co., 1968

Product information
as of February 1997

Manufactured by:
Aventis Pasteur Inc.
Swiftwater PA 18370 USA 4246

TUBERSOL® ℞
[tū ′-bur-sŏl]
Tuberculin Purified Protein Derivative (Mantoux)
Diagnostic Antigen
Rx only

DESCRIPTION

Tuberculin PPD[1] (Mantoux)—Tubersol® for intracutaneous (Mantoux) tuberculin testing is available in stabilized solutions bio-equivalent to 5 US units (TU) PPD-S per test dose (0.1 mL) and stabilized solutions diluted to a calculated bioequivalence of 1 TU and 250 TU strengths per test dose (0.1 mL).
Tubersol® is prepared by the Aventis Pasteur Limited from a large Master Batch, Connaught Tuberculin (CT68), which has been obtained from a human strain of *Mycobacterium tuberculosis* grown on a protein-free synthetic medium. The use of a standard preparation derived from a single batch (CT68) has been recommended[2] in order to eliminate batch to batch variation by the same manufacturer.
Tubersol® is a sterile isotonic solution of Tuberculin in phosphate buffered saline containing Tween 80 (0.0005%) as a stabilizer. Phenol 0.28% is added as a preservative.[3,4,5]
Independent studies conducted by the US Public Health Service in humans have determined the amount of CT68 in stabilized solution necessary to produce bio-equivalency with Tuberculin PPD-S (in phosphate buffer without Tween 80) using 5 US units (TU) Tuberculin PPD-S as the standard.
Prior to release, each successive lot is tested for potency in sensitized guinea pigs in comparison with the US Standard Tuberculin PPD-S distributed by the Office of Biologics, Food and Drug Administration, Bethesda, Maryland, USA[6]

CLINICAL PHARMACOLOGY

Intracutaneous tuberculin testing is an accepted aid in the diagnosis of tuberculosis infection.
The reaction to intracutaneously injected tuberculin is a delayed (cellular) hypersensitivity reaction. The reaction which characteristically shows a delayed course, reaching its peak more than 24 hours after administration, consists of induration due to cell infiltration and occasionally vesiculation and necrosis. Clinically, a delayed hypersensitivity reaction to tuberculin is a manifestation of previous infection with *M. tuberculosis* or a variety of non-tuberculosis bacteria. In most cases sensitization is induced by natural mycobacterial infection or by vaccination with BCG Vaccine.
The sensitization following infection with mycobacteria occurs primarily in the regional lymph nodes. Small lymphocytes (T lymphocytes) proliferate in response to the antigenic stimulus to give rise to specifically sensitized lymphocytes. After several weeks, these lymphocytes enter the blood stream and circulate for long periods of time. Subsequent restimulation of these sensitized lymphocytes with the same or a similar antigen, such as the intradermal injection of tuberculin, evokes a local reaction mediated by these cells.
The tuberculin reaction is characterized by the early predominance of mononuclear cells (small and medium sized lymphocytes and monocytes). Only a small proportion of these cells appear to be lymphocytes sensitized to tuberculin. Most cells are brought into the reaction through the release of biologically active substances by sensitized lymphocytes. An increase in vascular permeability leading to erythema and edema also occurs in tuberculin reactions.
Characteristically, delayed hypersensitivity reactions to tuberculin begin at 5 to 6 hours, are maximal at 48 to 72 hours and subside over a period of days. In those who are elderly or those who are being tested for the first time reactions may develop slowly and may not peak until after 72 hours. Immediate hypersensitivity reactions to tuberculin or to constituents of the diluent can also occur.
Not all infected persons will have a delayed hypersensitivity reaction to a tuberculin test. A large number of factors has been reported to cause a decreased ability to respond to the tuberculin test in the presence of tuberculous infection including viral infections (measles, mumps, chickenpox), live virus vaccinations (measles, mumps, polio), overwhelming tuberculosis, other bacterial infections, drugs (corticosteroids and many other immunosuppressive agents), and malignancy.[7]

INDICATIONS AND USAGE

Tubersol® is indicated as an aid in the detection of infection with *Mycobacterium tuberculosis.*
For the initial intracutaneous (Mantoux) tuberculin test it is customary to use 5 US units (TU) per test dose of 0.1 mL. The 1 TU per test dose (0.1 mL) preparation is used for in-

dividuals suspected of being highly sensitized since larger initial doses may result in severe skin reactions. The preparation containing **250 TU per test dose (0.1 mL), should be used exclusively for the testing of individuals who fail to react to a previous injection of 5 TU and under no circumstances is it to be used for the initial injection.**

CONTRAINDICATIONS

Tubersol® should not be administered to known tuberculin positive reactors because of the severity of reactions (eg. vesiculation, ulceration or necrosis) that may occur at the test site in highly sensitive persons.

WARNINGS

Tubersol® 250 TU per test dose (0.1 mL) is not, under any circumstances, to be used for the initial injection.
Avoid injecting Tubersol® subcutaneously. If this occurs, no local reaction will develop, but a general febrile reaction and/or acute inflammation around old tuberculosis lesions may occur in highly sensitive individuals.

PRECAUTIONS

a) General
A separate **sterile** syringe and needle must be used for each individual injection to prevent the possibility of transmission of viral hepatitis or other infectious agents from one person to another.
The possibility of allergic reactions in individuals sensitive to the components of the product should be borne in mind. Epinephrine Hydrochloride Solution (1:1000) should be readily available for use in case an anaphylactic or acute hypersensitivity reaction occurs.
Failure to store and handle Tubersol® as recommended will result in a loss of potency and inaccurate test results.
b) Information for Patients
Reactivity to the test may be depressed or suppressed for as long as 5 to 6 weeks in individuals who have received concurrent or recent immunization with certain virus vaccines (measles, influenza), who have had viral infections (rubeola, influenza, mumps and probably others) or who are receiving corticosteroids or immunosuppressive agents.
In those who are elderly or being tested for the first time reactions may develop slowly and may not peak until after 72 hours.
Vesiculation, ulceration or necrosis may appear at the test site in highly sensitive persons. Pain, pruritis and discomfort at the site may also occur.
c) Laboratory Tests
Since a positive tuberculin reaction (10 mm or more) does not necessarily indicate the presence of active tuberculous disease, individuals showing such positive tuberculin reactions should be subjected to other diagnostic procedures, such as X-ray examination of the chest and microbiological examination of the sputum.
In the case of the doubtful tuberculin reactions (5 to 9 mm) to 5 TU, the possibility should not be excluded that the skin sensitivity is due to previous contact with atypical mycobacteria or previous BCG vaccination. In the absence of signs of tuberculous disease, differential diagnosis by means of intracutaneous skin tests with PPD's derived from atypical mycobacteria may be indicated.
d) Drug Interactions
Reactivity to the test may be depressed or suppressed in individuals who are receiving corticosteroids or immunosuppressive agents.
Reactivity to PPD may be temporarily depressed by certain live virus vaccines (measles, mumps, rubella). Therefore, if a tuberculin test is to be performed, it should be administered either before or simultaneously with the injection of measles, mumps and rubella vaccines in combined form or as separate antigens.
e) Carcinogenesis, Mutagenesis, Impairment of Fertility
The product is not used for extended treatment over a long period of time.
f) Pregnancy Category C (Tuberculin)
Animal reproduction studies have not been conducted with Tubersol®. It is also not known whether Tubersol® can cause fetal harm when administered to a pregnant woman or can affect reproduction capacity. Tubersol® should be given to a pregnant woman only if clearly needed.
However, the risk of unrecognized tuberculosis and the close post partum contact between a mother with active disease and an infant leaves the infant in grave danger of tuberculosis and complications such as tuberculous meningitis. Therefore, the prescribing physician will want to consider if the potential benefits outweigh the possible risks for performing the tuberculin test on a pregnant woman or a woman of childbearing age, particularly in certain high risk populations.

ADVERSE REACTIONS

In highly sensitized individuals, strongly positive reactions including vesiculation, ulceration or necrosis may occur at the test site. Cold packs or topical steroid preparations may be employed for symptomatic relief of the associated pain, pruritus and discomfort.
Strongly positive reactions may result in scarring at the test site.
Immediate erythematous or other reactions may occur at the injection site. The reason(s) for these infrequent occurrences are presently unknown.

DOSAGE AND ADMINISTRATION

The Test: The Mantoux test is performed by intracutaneously injecting, with a syringe and needle, 0.1 mL of Tubersol®. It is customary to use 5 TU per test dose. The 1 TU per test dose preparation is used for individuals suspected of being highly sensitized since larger initial doses may result in severe skin reactions. **The preparation containing 250 TU per test dose should be used exclusively for the testing of individuals who fail to react to a previous injection of 5 TU and under no circumstances is to be used for the initial injection.**
The result is read 48 to 72 hours after administration and induration only is considered in interpreting the test.
Method of Administration: The following procedure is recommended for performing the Mantoux test:

1. The site of the test is the flexor surface of the forearm about 4 inches below the bend of the elbow.
2. The skin of the forearm is first cleansed with alcohol and allowed to dry.
3. The test dose (0.1 mL) of Tuberculin PPD is administered with a 1 mL syringe calibrated in tenths and fitted with a short, one-half inch, 26 or 27 gauge needle.
4. Disposable sterile syringes and needles may be used. Glass syringes and needles should be sterilized by autoclaving (121°C for 30 minutes), by boiling or by the use of dry heat. Do not sterilize by means of alcohol.
5. The rubber cap of the vial should be wiped with sterile piece of cotton moistened with alcohol and allowed to dry. The needle is then inserted gently through the cap and the required amount of Tuberculin PPD is drawn into the syringe.
6. The point of the needle is inserted into the most superficial layers of the skin with the needle bevel pointing upward. If the intracutaneous injection is performed properly, a definite white bleb will rise at the needle point, about 10 mm ($^3/_8$") in diameter. This will disappear within minutes. No dressing is required.

In the event of a subcutaneous injection (i.e. no bleb formed), the test should be repeated immediately at another site.
Tubersol® is a stabilized solution of Tuberculin PPD. Data indicates that Tubersol® will remain stable for at least four weeks when prefilled into syringes and stored between 2° and 8°C.[4] However, in order to avoid possible contamination of the product this practice is not recommended.
Parenteral drug products should be inspected visually for particulate matter and discoloration prior to administration, whenever solutions and container permit.
Interpretation of the Test: The test should be read 48 to 72 hours after administration of Tubersol®. Sensitivity is indicated by induration, usually accompanied by erythema. The widest diameter of distinctly palpable induration should be recorded in millimeters (mm). Presence of edema and necrosis should also be recorded.
A positive reaction indicates a sensitivity to tuberculin, which may be the result of a previous infection with mycobacteria. This infection, likely due to *Mycobacterium tuberculosis,* may have occurred years ago or may be of recent origin.
Reactions should be interpreted as follows:
Positive Reaction—Any palpable induration measuring 10 mm or more is considered a positive reaction. In the case of tuberculosis suspects or close contacts of individuals with tuberculosis an induration of 5 mm or even smaller should be interpreted as a positive reaction and appropriate additional follow-up measures indicated.
Doubtful Reaction—Induration measuring 5 to 9 mm indicates a doubtful reaction. Retesting is indicated using a different site and 5 TU per test dose.
The possibility should not be excluded that the skin sensitivity is due to previous contact with atypical mycobacteria or previous BCG vaccination.
Negative Reaction—Induration of less than 5 mm is considered negative. An individual who does not show a positive reaction to either 1 TU or 5 TU on the first test may be retested with 5 TU and if still found negative further testing with 0.1 mL containing 250 TU of Tuberculin PPD (Mantoux) is suggested. If the latter test is employed, it may be given in the other forearm.
An individual who does not show a positive reaction to an initial injection of either 1 TU and 5 TU, or 5 TU alone, and to a subsequent injection of 250 TU of Tuberculin PPD may be considered as tuberculin negative.
Booster Effect—Infection of an individual with tubercle bacilli or other mycobacteria results in a delayed hypersensitivity response to tuberculin which is demonstrated by the skin test. The delayed hypersensitivity response may gradually wane over a period of years. If a person receives a tuberculin test at this time (after several years) the response may be a reaction that is not significant. The stimulus of the test may boost or increase the size of the reaction to a second test, sometimes causing an apparent conversion or development of sensitivity. The booster effect can be seen on a second test done as soon as a week after the initial stimulating test and can persist for a year, and perhaps longer. When routine periodic tuberculin testing of adults is done, two stage testing should be used to minimize the likelihood of interpreting a boosted reaction as a conversion.[7,8]
Since a positive tuberculin reaction does not necessarily indicate the presence of active tuberculosis disease, individuals showing a positive tuberculin reaction should be subjected to other diagnostic procedures.
Those individuals giving a positive tuberculin reaction may or may not show evidence of tuberculosis disease. Chest X-ray examination and microbiological examination of the sputum in these cases are recommended as a means of determining the presence or absence of pulmonary tuberculosis.

HOW SUPPLIED

Tubersol® bioequivalent to 5 US units (TU) PPD-S per test dose (0.1 mL) is available in 1 mL and 5 mL vials. Tubersol® 1 TU and 250 TU per test dose (0.1 mL) are available in 1 mL vials. Tubersol® solutions are ready for immediate use without any further dilution.
STORAGE
Tubersol® should be stored between 2° and 8°C (35° and 46°F).[5,9] Tuberculin solutions can be adversely affected by exposure to light. The product should be stored in the dark except when doses are actually being withdrawn from the vial.[10]
A vial of Tuberculin PPD which has been opened and in use for one month should be discarded because oxidation and degradation may have reduced the potency.[11]

REFERENCES

1. Landi, S.: Preparation, purification, and stability of tuberculin. Appl. Microbiol. 11: 408–412.
2. Canadian Tuberculosis and Respiratory Disease Association: Classification and reporting of tuberculosis in Canada. Ottawa, the Association, 1972 p. 42.
3. Landi S., et al.: Adsorption of tuberculin PPD to glass and plastic surfaces. Bull. WHO 1966; 35: 593–602.
4. Landi S., et al.: Disparity of potency between stabilized and nonstabilized dilute tuberculin solutions. Am Rev Respir Dis 1971; 104: 385–393.
5. Landi, S., et al.: Stability of dilute solutions of tuberculin purified protien derivative. Tubercle 1978; 59: 121–133.
6. US Code of Federal Regulations, Title 21, Part 650, Subpart B—tuberculin, 144–146, April 1, 1981.
7. The Tuberculin Skin Test. Am Rev Respir Dis 1981; 124: 356–363.
8. American Thoracic Society: Diagnostic Standards and Classification of Tuberculosis and Other Mycobacterial Diseases (14th ed.), 1980. Am Rev Respir Dis 1981; 123: 343–358.
9. Landi, S., et al.: Stability of dilute solution of tuberculin purified protein derivative at extreme temperatures. J Biol Stand 1981; 9: 195–199.
10. Landi, S., et al.: Effect of light on tuberculin purified protein derivative solutions. Am Rev Respir Dis 1975; 111:52–61.
11. Landi, S., et al.: Effect of oxidation on the stability of tuberculin purified protein derivative (PPD) In: International Symposium on Tuberculins and BCG Vaccine. Basel: International Association of Biological Standardization, 1983. (Developments in Biological Standardization) 1986; 58: 545–552.

Manufactured by:
Aventis Pasteur Limited
Toronto Ontario Canada
Distributed by:
Aventis Pasteur Inc.
Swiftwater PA 18370 USA

R4-0400 USA 4301
D34-95C
20001616

Ferring Pharmaceuticals Inc.

120 WHITE PLAINS ROAD, SUITE # 400
TARRYTOWN, NY 10591

Direct Inquiries to:
Ferring Pharmaceuticals Inc.
Customer Service Department
120 White Plains Road, Suite #400
Tarrytown, NY 10591
1-(888)-FERRING (337-7464)

For Medical Information Contact:
In Emergencies:
Ferring Pharmaceuticals Inc.
Professional Services Department
120 White Plains Road, Suite #400
Tarrytown, NY 10591
(800) 822-8214

ACTHREL® ℞

(corticorelin ovine triflutate for injection)
For intravenous injection only
DIAGNOSTIC USE ONLY

DESCRIPTION

ACTHREL® (corticorelin ovine triflutate for injection) is a sterile, nonpyrogenic, lyophilized white cake powder, containing corticorelin ovine triflutate, a trifluoroacetate salt of a synthetic peptide that is used for the determination of pituitary corticotroph responsiveness. Corticorelin ovine has an amino acid sequence identical to ovine corticotropin-releasing hormone (oCRH). Corticorelin ovine is an analogue of the naturally occurring human CRH (hCRH) peptide. Both peptides are potent stimulators of adrenocorticotropic hormone (ACTH) release from the anterior pituitary. ACTH stimulates cortisol production from the adrenal cor-

Continued on next page

Acthrel—Cont.

tex. The structural formula for corticorelin ovine triflutate is described below:

Ser-Gln-Glu-Pro-Pro-Ile-Ser-Leu-Asp-Leu-Thr-Phe-His-Leu-Leu-Arg-Glu-Val-Leu-Glu-Met-Thr-Lys-Ala-Asp-Gln-Leu-Ala-Gln-Gln-Ala-His-Ser-Asn-Arg-Lys-Leu-Leu-Asp-Ile-Ala-NH_2 • xCF_3COOH

whereas x=4 - 8.

The empirical formula of corticorelin ovine is $C_{205}H_{339}N_{59}O_{63}S$ with a molecular weight of 4670.35 Daltons.

ACTHREL® for injection is available in vials containing 100 mcg corticorelin ovine (as the trifluoroacetate), 0.88 mg ascorbic acid, 10 mg lactose, and 26 mg cysteine hydrochloride monohydrate. Trace amounts of chloride ion may be present from the manufacturing process. The preparation is intended for intravenous administration.

CLINICAL PHARMACOLOGY

Pharmacodynamics: In normal subjects, intravenous administration of corticorelin results in a rapid and sustained increase of plasma ACTH levels and a near parallel increase of plasma cortisol. In addition, intravenous administration of corticorelin to normal subjects causes a concomitant and prolonged release of the related proopiomelanocortin peptides β- and γ-lipotropins (β-and γ-LPH) and β-endorphin (β-END). A number of dose-response studies have been performed on normal subjects using a range of corticorelin doses. In one study, doses of corticorelin ranging from 0.001 to 30 mcg/kg body weight were administered to 29 healthy volunteers. Blood samples were taken over a 2-hour period for determination of plasma ACTH and cortisol concentrations. There was a direct dose-dependent relationship that was more pronounced for ACTH than for cortisol. The threshold dose was 0.03 mcg/kg, the half-maximal dose was 0.3-1.0 mcg/kg and the maximally effective dose was 3-10 mcg/kg.

Plasma ACTH levels in normal subjects increased 2 minutes after injection of corticorelin doses of ≥0.3 mcg/kg and reached peak levels after 10-15 minutes. Plasma cortisol levels increased within 10 minutes and reached peak levels at 30 to 60 minutes. As the dose of corticorelin was increased, the rises in plasma ACTH and cortisol were more sustained, showing a biphasic response with a second lower peak at 2-3 hours after injection. Similar results were found in another study using 0.3, 3.0, and 30 mcg/kg doses. The duration of mean plasma ACTH increase after injection of 0.3, 3.0, and 30 mcg/kg was 4, 7, and 8 hours, respectively. The effect on plasma cortisol was similar, but more prolonged. Because there are differences in basal levels and peak response levels following a.m. or p.m. administration, it is recommended that subsequent evaluations in the same patient using the corticorelin stimulation test be carried out at the same time of day as the original evaluation.

Baseline ACTH and cortisol levels are usually higher in the morning. Pooled ACTH values from normal unstressed subjects (n=119) were 25 ± 7 pg/mL in the a.m. and 10 ± 3 in the p.m.; similar pooled cortisol values (n=170) were 11 ± 3 mcg/dL in the a.m. and 4 ± 2 mcg/dL in the p.m. The normal unstressed person has about seven to ten secretory episodes of ACTH each day. Most of them occur in the early morning hours and are responsible for the morning plasma cortisol surge. The following figure shows the daily circadian rhythm of ACTH and cortisol secretions in a normal unstressed person. Insulin, plasma renin activity, prolactin, and growth hormone release are not affected by corticorelin administration in humans.

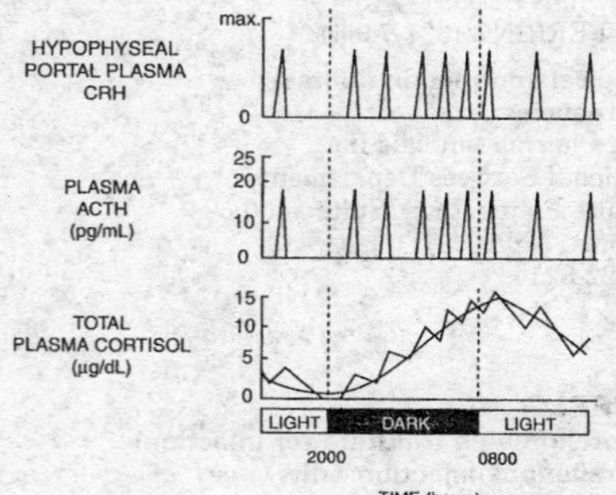

Continuous 24-hour infusion of corticorelin (0.5, 1.0, and 3.0 mcg/kg/hr) increased plasma ACTH concentrations to a plateau of 15-20 pg/mL by the third hour and urinary-free cortisol reaches 173 ± 43 mcg/dL by 24 hours, comparable to those levels observed in patients with major depression, but less than levels noted in Cushing's disease. Continuous infusion did not abolish the circadian rhythm of plasma ACTH and cortisol, but did appear to desensitize the corticotroph. Intermittent doses of corticorelin (25 mcg every 4 hours for 72 hours), however, continued to elicit the expected ACTH and cortisol responses.

Intravenous administration of 1 mcg/kg corticorelin in combination with 10 pressor units intramuscular vasopressin had a synergistic effect on ACTH and a less marked synergistic effect on cortisol secretion.

Basal Concentrations and Peak Responses of ACTH and Cortisol in Normal Subjects after 1 mcg/kg or 100 mcg of ACTHREL®

Time of Day	No. of Subjects	ACTH Concentration mean (range) pg/mL		Cortisol Concentration mean (range) mcg/dL	
		Basal	Peak	Basal	Peak
a.m.	143	28 (16-65)	68 (39-114)	11 (8-13)	21 (17-25)
p.m.	70	9 (8-13)	30 (25-42)	4 (2-6)	16 (15-18)

The basal and peak response levels of ACTH and cortisol to a 1 mcg/kg or 100 mcg dose of corticorelin administered to normal volunteers in the morning and the evening are given below. These values were obtained by combining the results from 9 clinical trials conducted in the a.m. and 4 clinical trials conducted in the p.m.

The following table is to be used only as a general guide. [See table above]

Pharmokinetics: Following a single intravenous injection of 1 mcg/kg of corticorelin to normal men, the disappearance of immunoreactive corticorelin (IR-corticorelin) from plasma follows a biexponential decay curve. Plasma half-lives for IR-corticorelin are 11.6 ±1.5 minutes (mean ± SE) for the fast component and 73 ± 8 minutes for the slow component. The mean volume of distribution for IR-corticorelin is 6.2 ± 0.5 L with an approximate metabolic clearance rate of 95 ± 11 L/m²/day. Graded intravenous doses of corticorelin (0.01, 0.03, 0.1, 0.3, 1, 3, 10, 30 mcg/kg) produced a linear increase in plasma IR-corticorelin. Corticorelin does not appear to be bound specifically by a circulating plasma protein.

INDICATIONS AND USAGE

ACTHREL® is indicated for use in differentiating pituitary and ectopic production of ACTH in patients with ACTH-dependent Cushing's syndrome.

Differential Diagnosis: There are two forms of Cushing's syndrome:

(a) ACTH-dependent (83%), in which hypercortisolism is due either to pituitary hypersecretion of ACTH (Cushing's disease) resulting from an adenoma (40%, usually microadenomas) or nonadenomatous hyperplasia, possibly of hypothalamic origin (28%), or to hypercortisolism that is secondary to ectopic secretion of ACTH (15%) and,

(b) ACTH- independent (17%), in which hypercortisolism is due to autonomous cortisol secretion by an adrenal tumor (9% adenomas, 8% carcinomas),

After the establishment of hypercortisolism consistent with the presence of Cushing's syndrome, and following the elimination of autonomous adrenal hyperfunction as its cause, the corticorelin test is used to aid in establishing the source of excessive ACTH secretion.

The corticorelin stimulation test helps to differentiate between the etiologies of ACTH-dependent hypercortisolism as follows:

1. High basal plasma ACTH plus high basal plasma cortisol (20 - 40 mcg/dL).
   ACTHREL® injection (1 mcg/kg) results in:
   a. Increased plasma ACTH levels
   b. Increased plasma cortisol levels
   Diagnosis: Cushing's disease (ACTH of pituitary origin)
2. High basal plasma ACTH (may be very high) plus high basal plasma cortisol (20 - 40 mcg/dL).
   ACTHREL® injection (1 mcg/kg) results in:
   a. Little or no response of plasma ACTH levels
   b. Little or no response of plasma cortisol levels
   Diagnosis: Ectopic ACTH syndrome

Test Methodology: To evaluate the status of the pituitary-adrenal axis in the differentiation of a pituitary source from an ectopic source of excessive ACTH secretion, a corticorelin test procedure requires a minimum of five blood samples.

Procedure

1. Venous blood samples should be drawn 15 minutes before and immediately prior to ACTHREL® administration. The ACTH baseline is obtained by averaging the values of the two samples.
2. Administer ACTHREL® as an intravenous infusion over a 30- to 60- second interval at a dose of 1 mcg/kg body weight. Higher doses are not recommended (see **PRECAUTIONS** and **ADVERSE REACTIONS**).
3. Draw venous blood samples at 15, 30, and 60 minutes after administration.
4. Blood samples should be handled as recommended by the laboratory that will determine their ACTH content. It is extremely important to recognize that the reliability of the ACTHREL® test is directly related to the inter-assay and intra-assay variability of the laboratory performing the assay.

Cortisol determinations may be performed on the same blood samples for the same time points as outlined above. The blood sample handling precautions noted for ACTH should be followed for cortisol.

Interpretation of Test Results: The interpretation of the ACTH and cortisol responses following ACTHREL® administration requires a knowledge of the clinical status of the individual patient, understanding of hypothalamic-pituitary-adrenal physiology, and familiarity with the normal hormonal ranges and the standards used by the laboratory that performs the ACTH and cortisol assays.

Cushing's Disease

The results of challenge with corticorelin injection have been reported in approximately 300 patients with Cushing's disease. Although the ACTH and cortisol responses were variable, a hyper-response to corticorelin was seen in a majority of patients, despite high basal cortisol levels. This response pattern indicates an impairment of the negative feedback of cortisol on the pituitary. Patients with pituitary-dependent Cushing's disease tested with corticorelin do not show the negative correlation between basal and stimulated levels of ACTH and cortisol that is found in normal subjects. A positive correlation between basal ACTH levels and maximum ACTH increments after corticorelin administration has been found in Cushing's disease patients.

Ectopic ACTH Secretion

Patients with Cushing's syndrome due to ectopic ACTH secretion (N=32) were found to have very high basal levels of ACTH and cortisol, which were not further stimulated by corticorelin. However, there have been rare instances of patients with ectopic sources of ACTH that have responded to the corticorelin test.

SUMMARY OF ACTH RESPONSES IN PATIENTS WITH HIGH BASAL CORTISOL

	High ACTH Response	Low ACTH Response
High Basal ACTH	Cushing's Disease	Ectopic ACTH Secretion

CUSHING'S DISEASE ACTH RESPONSES
(mean of 181 patients)
Basal ACTH 63 ± 72 pg/mL (mean ± SD)
Peak ACTH 189 ± 262 pg/mL (mean ± SD)
Mean of individual change from baseline + 227%

ECTOPIC ACTH SECRETION RESPONSES
(mean for 31 patients)
Basal ACTH 266 ± 464 pg/mL (mean ± SD)
Peak ACTH 276 ± 466 pg/mL (mean ± SD)
Mean of individual change from baseline + 15%

False negative responses to the corticorelin test in Cushing's disease patients occur approximately 5 to 10% of the time, which may lead the clinician to an incorrect diagnosis of ectopic production of ACTH at that frequency. (See **INDICATIONS AND USAGE, Differential Diagnosis**)

PRECAUTIONS

General: The severity of adverse effects to a corticorelin injection appear to be dose-dependent. Dosages above 1 mcg/kg are not recommended. While few adverse effects have been observed at the 1 mcg/kg or 100 mcg dose, higher doses have been associated with transient tachycardia, decreased blood pressure, loss of consciousness, and asystole (see **ADVERSE REACTIONS**). These symptoms can be substantially reduced by administering the drug as a 30-second intravenous infusion instead of a bolus injection. At a dose of 200 mcg corticorelin, 4 of 60 volunteers and patients with disturbances of the hypothalamic-pituitary-adrenal (HPA) axis were reported to have had decreased blood pressures. One patient had a severe hypotensive reaction with asystole. Three other patients had an "absence-like" loss of consciousness lasting approximately 5 minutes. In subsequent investigations by the same researchers over a 3-year period using 100 mcg of corticorelin, one patient in approximately 150 to 200 experienced a severe drop in blood pressure and loss of sinus rhythm after receiving 55 mcg of corticorelin, which may have been due to interaction with heparin. (See **Drug Interactions**)

Drug Interactions: The plasma ACTH response to corticorelin injection is inhibited or blunted in normal subjects pretreated with dexamethasone. The use of a heparin solution to maintain i.v. cannula patency during the corticorelin test is not recommended. A possible interaction between corticorelin and heparin may have been responsible for a major hypotensive reaction that occurred after corticorelin administration. (See **ADVERSE REACTIONS**)

Carcinogenesis, Mutagenesis, Impairment of Fertility: Animal studies have not been conducted with corticorelin to evaluate carcinogenic potential, mutagenicity, or effect on fertility.

Pregnancy (Pregnancy Category C): Animal reproduction studies have not been conducted with corticorelin. It is also not known whether corticorelin can cause fetal harm when administered to a pregnant woman or can affect reproductive capacity. ACTHREL® should be given to a pregnant woman only if clearly needed.

Nursing Mothers: It is not known whether corticorelin is secreted in human milk. Because many drugs are excreted in human milk, caution should be exercised when ACTHREL® is administered to a nursing woman.

PEDIATRIC USE

Only a few tests have been performed on children. Dosages were 1 mcg/kg body weight. Patient studies have involved only children with multiple hypothalamic and/or pituitary hormone deficiencies, or tumors. Only two studies with normal pediatric subjects have been conducted. No differences in response to the corticorelin test have been reported in the children studied.

ADVERSE REACTIONS

Adverse effects reported with 1 mcg/kg or 100 mcg/patient include flushing of the face, neck, and upper chest (16%; 45/276), beginning almost immediately and lasting 3 to 5 minutes. Recipients have also reported an urge to take a deep breath (6%; 3/49), which occurs with a timing similar to, but less frequently than, that of flushing. Higher doses (≥3mcg/kg) are associated with more prolonged flushing, tachycardia, hypotension, dyspnea, and "chest compression" or tightness. In addition, at doses of ≥ 5 mcg/kg, significant increases in heart rate and decreases in blood pressure were observed. The cardiovascular effects occurred 2-3 minutes after injection and lasted for 30-60 minutes. The facial flushing was more prolonged, lasting up to 4 hours in some subjects. All signs and symptoms could be reduced by administering the drug as a 30-second infusion instead of by bolus injection.

Total doses of up to 200 mcg of corticorelin were administered as a bolus injection to 60 men and women, including both healthy normal subjects and patients with endocrine disorders. In most cases, only minor adverse effects, such as transient flushing and feelings of dyspnea, were noted. However, a few patients with disorders of the pituitary-adrenal axis had major symptoms. One patient had a precipitous fall in blood pressure and pulse rate and developed asystole, which required resuscitation. In two patients with Cushing's disease and in one with secondary adrenal insufficiency, an "absence-like" loss of consciousness occurred, which started within a few seconds after injection of corticorelin and lasted from 10 seconds to 5 minutes. This was accompanied by a slight fall in blood pressure. One patient with a well documented seizure diathesis experienced a grand mal epileptic seizure following ACTHREL® administration. The patient had discontinued anti-convulsant therapy the day of the procedure. (See **PRECAUTIONS** and **Drug Interactions**)

OVERDOSAGE

Symptoms of overdose include severe facial flushing, cardiovascular changes, and dyspnea. In the event of toxic overdose (see **ADVERSE REACTIONS**), adverse effects should be treated symptomatically.

DOSAGE AND ADMINISTRATION

Dosage: A single intravenous dose of ACTHREL® at 1 mcg/kg is recommended for the testing of pituitary corticotrophin function. A dose of 1 mcg/kg is the lowest dose that produces maximal cortisol responses and significant (though apparently sub-maximal) ACTH responses. Doses above 1 mcg/kg are not recommended. (See **PRECAUTIONS** and **ADVERSE REACTIONS**)

At a dose of 1 mcg/kg, the ACTH and cortisol responses to ACTHREL® are prolonged and remain elevated for up to 2 hours. The maximum increment in plasma ACTH occurs between 15 and 60 minutes after ACTHREL® administration, whereas the maximum increment in plasma cortisol occurs between 30 and 120 minutes. In a clinical study of 30 normal healthy men, the peak plasma ACTH and cortisol responses to ACTHREL® administration in the early afternoon occurred at 42 ± 29 minutes and 65 ± 26 minutes (average ± SD), respectively. **If a repeated evaluation using the corticorelin stimulation test with ACTHREL® is needed, it is recommended that the repeat test be carried out at the same time of day as the original test because there are differences in basal levels and peak response levels following a.m. or p.m. administration to normal humans.**

Administration: ACTHREL® is to be reconstituted aseptically with 2 mL of Sodium Chloride injection, USP (0.9% sodium chloride), at the time of use by injecting 2 mL of the saline diluent into the lyophilized drug product cake. To avoid bubble formation, DO NOT SHAKE the vial; instead, roll the vial to dissolve the product. The sterile solution containing 50 mcg corticorelin/mL is then ready for injection by the intravenous route. The dosage to be administered is determined by the patient's weight (1 mcg corticorelin/kg). Some of the adverse effects can be reduced by administering the drug as an infusion over 30 seconds instead of as a bolus injection.

Parenteral drug products should be inspected visually for particulate matter and discoloration prior to administration, whenever solution and container permit.

HOW SUPPLIED

ACTHREL® is supplied as a sterile, nonpyrogenic, lyophilized, white cake containing 100 mcg corticorelin ovine (as the trifluoroacetate), 0.88 mg ascorbic acid, 10 mg lactose, and 26 mg cysteine hydrochloride monohydrate. Trace amounts of chloride ion may be present from the manufacturing process. The package provides a single-dose, rubber-capped, 5 mL, brown-glass vial (NDC 55566-0302-1) containing 100 mcg corticorelin ovine (as the trifluoroacetate). ACTHREL® is stable in the lyophilized form when stored refrigerated at 2°C to 8°C (36°F to 45°F) and protected from light. The reconstituted solution is stable up to 8 hours under refrigerated conditions. Discard unused reconstituted solution.

Manufactured for:
Ferring Pharmaceuticals, Inc.
Tarrytown, New York 10591
By:
Ben Venue Laboratories, Inc.
Bedford, OH 44146
Rx only

03/98 6011-01

THYREL® TRH ℞

(protirelin)
Injection
FOR INTRAVENOUS ADMINISTRATION

DESCRIPTION

Chemically, Thyrel® TRH (protirelin) is identified as 5-oxo-L-prolyl-L-histidyl-L-proline amide. It is a synthetic tripeptide that is believed to be structurally identical to the naturally-occurring thyrotropin-releasing hormone produced by the hypothalamus. The CAS Registry Number is 24305-27-9. The structural formula is:

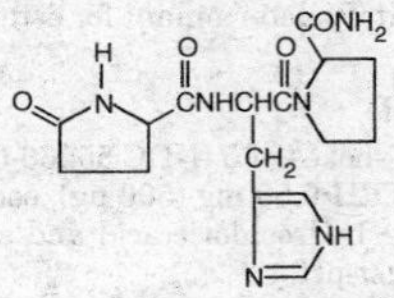

Thyrel TRH is supplied as 1 mL ampuls. Each ampul contains 500 µg protirelin in a sterile nonpyrogenic isotonic saline solution having a pH of approximately 6.5. In addition, each ampul contains sodium chloride 9.0 mg, Water for Injection, hydrochloric acid and sodium hydroxide as needed to adjust pH. Thyrel TRH is intended for intravenous administration.

CLINICAL PHARMACOLOGY

Pharmacologically, Thyrel TRH increases the release of the thyroid stimulating hormone (TSH) from the anterior pituitary. Prolactin release is also increased. It has recently been observed that approximately 65% of acromegalic patients tested respond with a rise in circulating growth hormone levels; the clinical significance is as yet not clear. Following intravenous administration, the mean plasma half-life of protirelin in normal subjects is approximately five minutes. TSH levels rise rapidly and reach a peak at 20 to 30 minutes. The decline in TSH levels takes place more slowly, approaching baseline levels after approximately three hours.

INDICATIONS AND USAGE

Thyrel TRH is indicated as an adjunctive agent in the diagnostic assessment of thyroid function. As an adjunct to other diagnostic procedures, testing with Thyrel® TRH (protirelin) may yield useful information in patients with pituitary or hypothalamic dysfunction.

Thyrel TRH is indicated as an adjunct to evaluate the effectiveness of thyrotropin suppression with a particular dose of T4 in patients with nodular or diffuse goiter. A normal TSH baseline value and a minimal difference between the 30 minute and baseline response to Thyrel TRH injection would indicate adequate suppression of the pituitary secretion of TSH.

Thyrel TRH may be used, adjunctively, for adjustment of thyroid hormone dosage given to patients with primary hypothyroidism. A normal or slightly blunted TSH response, thirty minutes following Thyrel TRH injection, would indicate adequate replacement therapy.

CONTRAINDICATIONS

Thyrel TRH is contraindicated in patients with a known hypersensitivity to the drug.

WARNINGS

Transient changes in blood pressure, either increases or decreases, frequently occur immediately following administration of Thyrel TRH. Blood pressure should therefore be measured before Thyrel TRH is administered and at frequent intervals during the first 15 minutes after its administration.

Increases in systolic pressure (usually less than 30 mm Hg) and/or increases in diastolic pressure (usually less than 20 mm Hg) have been observed more frequently than decreases in pressure. These changes have not ordinarily persisted for more than 15 minutes nor have they required therapy. More severe degrees of hypertension or hypotension with or without syncope have been reported in a few patients. To minimize the incidence and/or severity of hypotension, the patient should be supine before, during, and after Thyrel TRH administration. If a clinically important change in blood pressure occurs, monitoring of blood pressure should be continued until it returns to baseline levels. Thyrel TRH should not be administered to patients in whom marked, rapid changes in blood pressure would be dangerous unless the potential benefit clearly outweighs the potential risk.

PRECAUTIONS

Thyroid hormones reduce the TSH response to Thyrel® TRH. Accordingly, patients in whom Thyrel TRH is to be used diagnostically should be taken off liothyronine (T3) approximately seven days prior to testing and should be taken off thyroid medications containing levothyroxine (T4), e.g., desiccated thyroid, thyroglobulin, or liotrix, at least 14 days before testing. Hormone therapy is NOT to be discontinued when the test is used to evaluate the effectiveness of thyroid suppression with a particular dose of T4 in patients with nodular or diffuse goiter, or for adjustment of thyroid hormone dosage given to patients with primary hypothyroidism.

Chronic administration of levodopa has been reported to inhibit the TSH response to Thyrel TRH.

It is not advisable to withdraw maintenance doses of adrenocortical drugs used in the therapy of known hypopituitarism. Several published reports have shown that prolonged treatment with glucocorticoids at physiologic doses has no significant effect on the TSH response to thyrotropin releasing hormone, but that the administration of pharmacologic doses of steroids reduces the TSH response. Therapeutic doses of acetylsalicylic acid (2 to 3.6 g/day) have been reported to inhibit the TSH response to protirelin. The ingestion of acetylsalicylic acid caused the peak level of TSH to decrease approximately 30% as compared to values obtained without acetylsalicylic acid administration. In both cases, the TSH peak occurred 30 minutes post-administration of protirelin.

Carcinogenesis, Mutagenesis, Impairment of Fertility

Long-term animal studies have not been performed to evaluate the carcinogenic potential of protirelin. Studies to determine potential effects concerning mutagenesis or impairment of fertility have also not been performed.

Pregnancy (Category C)

Protirelin has been shown to increase the number of resorptions in rabbits, but not in rats, when given in doses 1½ and 6 times the human dose. There are no adequate and well-controlled studies in pregnant women. Thyrel TRH should be used during pregnancy only if the potential benefit justifies the potential risk to the fetus.

Nursing Mothers

It is not known whether this drug is excreted in human milk. Because many drugs are excreted in human milk, caution should be exercised when Thyrel® TRH is administered to a nursing woman.

ADVERSE REACTIONS

Side effects have been reported in about 50% of the patients tested with Thyrel TRH. Generally, the side effects are minor, have occurred promptly, and have persisted for only a few minutes following injection.

Cardiovascular reactions:

Marked changes in blood pressure, including both hypertension and hypotension with or without syncope, have been reported in a small number of patients.

Endocrine reaction:

Breast enlargement and leakage in lactating women for up to two or three days.

Other reactions:

Headaches, sometimes severe, and transient amaurosis in patients with pituitary tumors. Rarely, convulsions may occur in patients with predisposing conditions, e.g., epilepsy, brain damage. Nausea; urge to urinate; flushed sensation; lightheadedness; bad taste in mouth; abdominal discomfort; and dry mouth. Less frequently reported were: Anxiety; sweating; tightness in the throat; pressure in the chest; tingling sensation; drowsiness; and allergic reactions.

Pituitary apoplexy requiring acute neurosurgical intervention has been reported infrequently for patients with pituitary macroadenomas following the acute administration of protirelin injection in the setting of combined anterior pituitary function testing in conjunction with LHRH and insulin.

DOSAGE AND ADMINISTRATION

Thyrel TRH is intended for intravenous administration with the patient in the supine position. The drug is administered as a bolus over a period of 15 to 30 seconds, with the patient remaining supine until all scheduled postinjection blood samples have been taken. Blood pressure should be measured before Thyrel TRH is administered and at frequent intervals during the first 15 minutes thereafter (see **WARNINGS**). Have the patient urinate before injecting Thyrel TRH.

Dosage:

Adults: 500 µg. Doses between 200 and 500 µg have been used. 500 µg is considered the optimum dose to give the maximum response in the greatest number of patients. Doses greater than 500 µg are unlikely to elicit a greater TSH response.

Children age 6 to 16 years; 7 µg/kg body weight up to dose of 500 µg.

Infants and children up to 6 years: Experience is limited in this age group; doses of 7 µg/kg have been administered.

One blood sample for TSH assay should be drawn immediately prior to the injection of Thyrel® TRH, and a second sample should be obtained 30 minutes after injection.

The TSH response to Thyrel TRH is reduced by repetitive administration of the drug. Accordingly, if the Thyrel TRH test is repeated, an interval of seven days before testing is recommended.

Elevated serum lipids may interfere with the TSH assay.

Continued on next page

Thyrel TRH—Cont.

Thus, fasting (except in patients with hypopituitarism) or a low-fat meal is recommended prior to the test.

INTERPRETATION OF TEST RESULTS

Interpretation of the TSH response to Thyrel TRH requires an understanding of thyroid-pituitary-hypothalamic physiology and knowledge of the clinical status of the individual patient.

Because the TSH test results may vary with the laboratory, the physician should be familiar with the TSH assay method used and the normal range for the laboratory performing the assay. TSH response 30 minutes after Thyrel TRH administration in normal subjects and in patients with hyperthyroidism and hypothyroidism are presented in Figure 1. The diagnoses were established prior to the administration of Thyrel TRH on the basis of the clinical history, physical examination, and the results of other thyroid and/or pituitary function tests.

Among the normal euthyroid subjects, women and children were found to have higher levels of TSH at 30 minutes than men.

Among the patients with hyperthyroidism or primary (thyroidal), secondary pituitary), or tertiary (hypothalamic) hypothyroidism, no significant differences in TSH levels by age or sex were found.

Normal: Baseline TSH levels of less than 10 microunits/mL (µU/mL) were observed in 97% of euthyroid normal subjects tested. Thirty minutes after Thyrel TRH, the serum TSH increased by 2.0 mµ/mL or more in 95% of euthyroid subjects.

Hyperthyroidism: All hyperthyroid patients tested had baseline TSH levels of less than 10 µU/mL and a rise of less than 2 µU/mL 30 minutes after Thyrel® TRH.

Figure 1

Mean ± One Standard Deviation of TSH Levels (µU/mL) Observed at Baseline and 30 Minutes After Thyrel® TRH (protirelin)

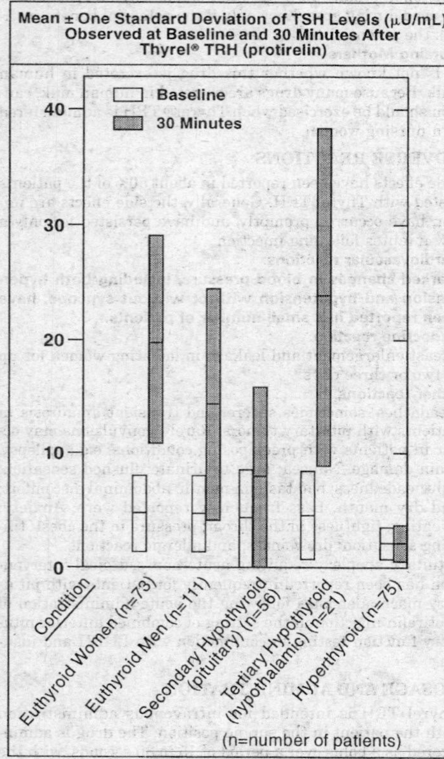

Primary (thyroidal) hypothyroidism: The diagnosis of primary hypothyroidism is frequently supported by finding clearly elevated baseline TSH levels; 93% of patients tested had levels above 10 µU/mL, Thyrel TRH administration to these patients generally would not be expected to yield additional useful information. Ninety-four percent of patients with primary hypothyroidism given Thyrel® TRH in clinical trials responded with a rise in TSH of 2.0 µU/mL or greater. Since this response is also found in normal subjects, Thyrel TRH testing does not differentiate primary hypothyroidism from normal.

Table 1

Characterization Based on Serum TSH Levels at Baseline and 30 Minutes After Thyrel® TRH (protirelin)

	Baseline Serum TSH (µU/mL)	Change of Serum TSH (µU/mL) at 30 minutes
Euthyroidism (normal thyroid function)	10 or less (usually 6 or less; 20% have <1.5 µU/mL)	2 or more (usually 6 to 30)
Hyperthyroidism	10 or less (usually 4 or less)	less than 2
Primary Hypothyroidism (thyroidal)	more than 10 (usually 15 to 100)	2 or more (usually 20 or more)
Secondary Hypothyroidism (pituitary)	10 or less (usually 6 or less)	less than 2 (59%) 2 to 50 (41%)
Tertiary Hypothyroidism (hypothalamic)	10 or less (often less than 2)	2 or more

Secondary (pituitary) and tertiary (hypothalamic) hypothyroidism: In the presence of clinical and other laboratory evidence of hypothyroidism, the finding of a baseline TSH level less than 10 µU/mL should suggest secondary or tertiary hypothyroidism. In this situation, a response to Thyrel TRH of less than 2 µU/mL suggests secondary hypothyroidism since this response was observed in about 60% of patients with secondary hypothyroidism and only approximately 5% of patients with tertiary hypothyroidism. A TSH response to Thyrel TRH greater than 2 µU/mL is not helpful in differentiating between secondary and tertiary hypothyroidism since this response was noted in about 40% of the former and about 95% of the latter.

Establishing the diagnosis of secondary or tertiary hypothyroidism requires a careful history and physical examination along with appropriate tests of anterior pituitary and/or target gland function. The Thyrel TRH test should not be used as the only laboratory determinant for establishing these diagnoses.

HOW SUPPLIED

As 1 mL ampuls—boxes of 5 (NDC 55566-0081-5). Each mL contains Thyrel TRH 0.50 mg (500 µg), sodium chloride 9.0 mg for isotonicity, hydrochloric acid and sodium hydroxide as needed to adjust pH.

Store at controlled room temperature 15° to 30°C (59° to 86°F).

Rx only

Manufactured for:
FERRING PHARMACEUTICALS INC.
Tarrytown, NY 10591
By: Taylor Pharmaceuticals
Decatur, IL 62525
6015-02 (9/99)

LEDERLE PHARMACEUTICAL

Division American Cyanamid Company
PEARL RIVER, NY 10965
US Gov't. License No. 17

For Medical Information Contact:

MARKETED ONCOLOGY PRODUCTS:
Immunex Corporation
Professional Services Department
51 University Street
Seattle, WA 98101
(800) IMMUNEX

OTHER MARKETED DRUG PRODUCTS:
Lederle Pharmaceutical/Wyeth-Ayerst Pharmaceuticals
Medical Affairs Department
P.O. Box 8299
Philadelphia, PA 19101
Day: (800) 934-5556
8:30 AM to 4:30 PM
(Eastern Standard Time),
Weekdays only
Night: (610) 688-4400 (Emergencies only; non-emergencies should wait until the next day)

MARKETED VACCINES AND TINE TESTS:
Lederle Pharmaceutical/Wyeth-Ayerst Pharmaceuticals
Medical Affairs Department
P.O. Box 8299
Philadelphia, PA 19101
Day: (800) 934-5556
8:30 AM to 4:30 PM
(Eastern Standard Time),
Weekdays only
Night: (610) 688-4400 (Emergencies only; non-emergencies should wait until the next day)

Tuberculin, Purified Protein Derivative
Rx only

PPD TINE TEST® ℞

[tine tĕst]

DESCRIPTION

The Tuberculin, Purified Protein Derivative PPD TINE TEST® is a sterile, simple, multiple-puncture, disposable intradermal test device for the detection of tuberculin reactivity. These convenient devices are especially useful in mass tuberculosis screening programs.

Each test unit consists of a stainless steel disk attached to a light blue plastic handle. Projecting from the disk are four triangular-shaped prongs (tines) that are 2 mm long and approximately 4 mm apart. The tines have been mechanically dipped into a concentrated solution of Purified Protein Derivative (PPD). The PPD concentrate used is purified from culture filtrates of human-type strains (C, DT, and PN) of *Mycobacterium tuberculosis* grown in synthetic medium and precipitated with ammonium sulfate according to the Seibert Process.[1,2] It is stabilized with 7% acacia (gum arabic), 30% dextrose, and 5% glycerol as a humectant. The PPD concentrate for dipping is standardized against U.S. Standard Tuberculin, Purified Protein Derivative in sensitized guinea pigs. Following dipping, the tines are capped and the entire unit is sterilized by Cobalt 60 irradiation. No preservative has been added. The device is for single dose, single use.

PPD TINE TEST has been standardized by clinical evaluation in human subjects to elicit at least a 2 mm reaction or more in a person who responds with a 5 mm reaction or more to 5 TU (US tuberculin units) of Tuberculin, PPD administered intradermally in the Mantoux test.[3]

CLINICAL PHARMACOLOGY

Between 1953 and 1985, the number of cases of tuberculosis (TB) reported annually in the U.S. decreased by 74%, from 84,304 to 22,201 cases.[4–7] Between 1985 and 1992, there was a 20% increase in the number of reported TB cases, to 26,673 in 1992. This resurgence was attributed to the emergence of the human immunodeficiency virus (HIV) epidemic, increased immigration from countries with high TB prevalence, social factors such as homelessness and substance abuse, increased numbers of persons in institutionalized settings, and decreased resources allocated to TB control programs.[4–6] Between 1992 and 1995, the reported number of TB cases in the U.S. decreased by 4% to 6% annually.[5] This decline has been attributed to decreased transmission among persons in congregative settings (eg, hospitals, correctional facilities) and improvement in TB control measures. Despite the declining incidence, TB rates remain elevated in certain high-risk groups, such as immigrants, substance abusers, and the homeless.

The classic delayed-type tuberculin skin reaction is elicited in sensitive individuals by intradermal injection of tuberculoprotein antigens (purified protein derivative, old tuberculin).[3] Production of delayed skin reaction involves recognition of antigen by sensitized lymphocytes (T cells), immobilization of lymphocytes at the site, production and release of lymphocyte mediators, and accumulation of macrophages, with eventual destruction of antigen and resolution of the resolution of the reaction.[8] Fixed tissue macrophages and basophilic leukocytes, along with fibrin deposition and vessel permeability, are also found.[9] The result is an inflammatory response in the skin with the induration and erythema characteristic of a "positive" reaction.

Data were obtained from clinical studies with a total of 3,062 volunteer subjects (males and females), ranging in age from 4 to 96 years, of which 47.5% (1,443) were Mantoux positive (induration of 10 mm or larger).

The following test results for the Mantoux test and corresponding measurements of the PPD TINE TEST were considered positive: 5 – 9 mm induration Mantoux was equivalent to 2 mm PPD TINE TEST; 10 – 19 mm Mantoux was equivalent to 3 – 8 mm PPD TINE TEST; >20 mm Mantoux was equivalent to >9 mm PPD TINE TEST.

The PPD TINE TEST demonstrated a sensitivity of 93.8% (95% Cl: 92.7% – 94.9%), which corresponds with a false negative rate of 6.2%, and a specificity of 82.5% (95% Cl: 80.4% – 84.6%), which corresponds with a false positive rate of 17.5%.[10,11] Based on these results, the positive predictive value ranges from 37.2% to 97.9% as the prevalence of positive Mantoux PPD-T (Tween 80) tests varies from 10% to 90% in different populations. In the population studied, the positive accuracy, which correlates with the positive predictive value, was 89.1%.[11] It should be noted that these results are based on the accuracy of the Mantoux test in predicting the presence of TB infection; Mantoux test error rates have been reported to range from 2% to 10%.[11] In studies in which individual lots of PPD TINE TEST are standardized to elicit at least a 22 mm reaction or more in 50 persons who are known to test positive with the Mantoux test, the sensitivity of the PPD TINE TEST was at least 95%.[10]

PPD TINE TEST reactions are measured at 48 to 72 hours.[3,11] Various factors may influence the time to maximum reaction or the possibility of a false-negative reaction, including waning sensitivity in older persons.[12] Among individuals with waning sensitivity to homologous or heterologous mycobacterial antigens, however, the stimulus of a tuberculin test may "boost" or increase the size of the reaction to a second test, even causing an apparent development of sensitivity in some cases.[13]

The recommended frequency of repeated tuberculin tests depends on risk of exposure of the individual and on the prevalence of tuberculosis in the population group. The repeated testing of uninfected individuals does not sensitize to tuberculin.

INDICATIONS AND USAGE

- Tuberculin, Purified Protein Derivative PPD TINE TEST is indicated as an aid in the detection of *M. tuberculosis* infection and not for the treatment of actual infection. Screening methods include the Mantoux test and multiple-puncture-type devices. Persons who are contacts of TB patients or who have clinical evidence of disease should be screened by the Mantoux test or chest radiography, even if they have demonstrated a negative reaction to PPD TINE

TEST. PPD TINE TEST units are also useful in programs to determine priorities for additional testing (eg, chest X-rays) and in epidemiological surveys to identity those areas having high levels of infection.

- Screening for disease with methods such as chest radiography may be preferred when the tuberculin skin test results may be unreliable, when administering and reading the test or following up infected persons for preventive therapy may be impractical, when the risk for disease is high, or when the consequences of an undiagnosed case may be severe.[12]
- PPD TINE TEST is neither 100% sensitive in identifying those persons who have TB nor 100% specific in identifying those persons who do not have TB.[12]
- The positive predictive value, the ability of a positive tuberculin test to identify those persons who have TB, varies with the prevalence of TB infection in the population tested. The prevalence of TB infection among the adult population of the U.S. is 5% to 10%.[12]
- All multiple-puncture-type devices must be regarded as screening tools, and other appropriate diagnostic procedures, such as the Mantoux test, should be utilized for retesting individuals with positive reactions. Multiple-puncture-type devices should not be used to screen high-risk populations.
- The Mantoux test with 5 TU PPD is the preferred method of screening persons who are HIV-infected.[12]

CONTRAINDICATIONS

Highly sensitive persons may respond to skin testing with vesicular or ulcerating local reactions. These reactions are interpreted as positive. Persons who are known to be tuberculin-positive generally should not be tested with PPD TINE TEST (see **WARNINGS**).[14]

There is no reliable method to distinguish a tuberculin reaction caused by vaccination with the bacille Calmette-Guerin (BCG) vaccine from those caused by natural mycobacterial infections. Therefore, a previously vaccinated person with a significant reaction to the PPD TINE TEST should be evaluated for the presence of TB disease and managed accordingly.[14] Previous BCG vaccination is not a contraindication to the use of PPD TINE TEST.

There are case reports of anaphylactic reactions to the PPD TINE TEST. Any individual with a known significant immediate-type hypersensitivity to tuberculin or any component of the PPD TINE TEST, including acacia (gum arabic), should not be tested with the PPD TINE TEST.

WARNINGS

Tuberculin testing generally should not be administered to individuals with known active tuberculosis. Although activation of quiescent lesions is rare, if a patient has a history of occurrence of vesiculation and necrosis with a previous tuberculin test by any method, tuberculin testing should be avoided.

Skin testing is not to be used as the sole diagnostic factor and patients who have a positive reaction to PPD TINE TEST should be evaluated further with additional laboratory tests. Chest radiography is the preferred screening method for persons with current pulmonary TB.[12]

PRECAUTIONS

General

Not all persons infected with *M. tuberculosis* will have a delayed-type hypersensitivity reaction to a tuberculin skin test. Factors which may cause a decreased ability to respond to tuberculin testing include: viral infections (eg, measles, mumps, chicken pox), live virus vaccinations (eg, measles, mumps, rubella, polio), overwhelming tuberculosis or other bacterial infections, drugs (eg, corticosteroids, immunosuppressive agents), metabolic derangements, nutritional factors, age (eg, newborns, elderly), and stress (eg, surgery, burns, mental illness, graft-host reactions).[14–16]

Anything that impairs or attenuates cell-mediated immunity potentially can cause a false negative reaction (eg, viral infections, particularly HIV; live viral vaccines; protein malnutrition; lymphoma; leukemia; sarcoidosis, use of glucocorticoid and other immunosuppressive drugs). Reactivity to the test also may be suppressed in individuals who are anergic.

As with any biological product, allergic reactions including anaphylaxis may occur. Before administration of PPD TINE TEST, the healthcare professional should take all known precautions for prevention of allergic or any other reactions. This includes a review of the patient's history for possible sensitivity to this or similar products or to any component of PPD TINE TEST, including acacia. Epinephrine injection (1:1,000) and other appropriate agents used for control of immediate allergic reactions should be available for immediate use. The healthcare professional should also obtain information about the patient's previous immunization history, including immunization with the BCG vaccination.

The utility of the tuberculin skin test depends on the prevalence of *M. tuberculosis* infection and the relative prevalence of cross-reaction with nontuberculous mycobacteria.

The reactivity of the PPD TINE TEST may be suppressed or depressed in persons who recently received live virus vaccines, who have had a viral infection, or who are receiving corticosteroids or immunosuppressive agents.[14–16]

Antituberculous chemotherapy should not be instituted solely on the basis of a single positive PPD TINE TEST unless vesiculation occurs, in which case management of the patient is the same as that for one classified as positive to the Mantoux test.

Tuberculin, Purified Protein Derivative PPD TINE TEST units must never be reused. The units should be discarded into an impenetrable sharps container with recapping.

Information for Patients

Prior to administration of this product, the healthcare professional should inform the patient, parent, guardian, or other responsible adult, of the benefits and risks of tuberculin skin tests. The healthcare professional should inform the patient that pain, pruritus, and discomfort may occur at the injection site. Patients, parents or guardians should be instructed to report vesiculation, ulceration or necrosis which may appear at the test site in highly sensitive patients, and any adverse experience to their healthcare professional.

The patient should be given oral instructions regarding how to read the test, the importance of reading the skin test reactions at 48 hours, and the importance of returning the induration indicator card to the healthcare professional. The induration indicator card is an important health record.

Drug Interactions

Reactivity to the test may be suppressed in patients who are receiving corticosteroids or immunosuppressive agents, or those who have recently been immunized with live vaccines such as Measles-Mumps-Rubella vaccine (MMR) and oral polio vaccine. If tuberculin skin testing is indicated, it should be done preceding, or at the time of such immunization, and read 48 to 72 hours later. If the test is not administered in the time suggested, an interval of 4 to 6 weeks should be allowed between tuberculin skin testing and immunization with live measles vaccine or MMR to prevent suppression of tuberculin reactivity.[3,6,13,19] The effect of live-virus varicella and yellow-fever vaccines on tuberculin skin testing is not known.[19]

Carcinogenesis, Mutagensis, Impairment of Fertility

PPD TINE TEST has not been evaluated for its carcinogenic or mutagenic potential or its potential to impair fertility.

Pregnancy

Pregnancy Category C.

Animal reproduction studies have not been conducted with Tuberculin, Purified Protein Derivative PPD TINE TEST. It is also not known whether PPD TINE TEST can cause fetal harm when administered to a pregnant woman or affect reproduction capacity.

Pregnancy is known to cause physiologic suppression of cell-medicated immunity.[20] Several studies on tuberculin testing have been conducted during pregnancy.[21–25] Earlier studies suggested that a negative response to tuberculin may occur late in pregnancy while tests prior to pregnancy had been positive.[21–23] However, a well-controlled study and a study in which women who tested positive during pregnancy were retested in the postpartum period showed no indication that pregnancy affected the level of tuberculin sensitivity.[24,25]

The Advisory Council for the Elimination of Tuberculosis of the Centers for Disease Control and Prevention (CDC) considers tuberculin skin testing valid and safe throughout pregnancy.[12]

Because of the possibility that a false negative response may occur during pregnancy, further diagnostic procedures should be considered if tuberculosis is suspected clinically. The clinical judgment of the healthcare professional should prevail at all times.

Pediatric Use

The American Academy of Pediatrics (AAP) and the Advisory Council for the Elimination of Tuberculosis of the CDC recommend focusing tuberculosis skin testing on children who are at increased risk of acquiring TB infection or disease.[12,26] Children without risk factors who reside in low-TB-prevalence areas, including those under 1 year of age, do not require routine TB skin testing. The AAP states that children who have no risk factors, but who reside in high-prevalence regions, and children whose histories for risk factors are incomplete or unreliable should be considered for tuberculin (Mantoux) skin testing at 4 to 6 and 11 to 16 years of age. Family investigation is implicated whenever a tuberculin skin test result of a parent or child converts from negative to positive (indicating recent infection). Children with HIV infection and those living with HIV-infected persons should receive annual tuberculin (Mantoux) skin testing.[26] Healthcare professionals in their own judgement may decide to administer tuberculin skin testing to specific children at earlier ages, if circumstances warrant.

Geriatric Use

Because TB case rates increase with age among all racial and ethnic groups and both sexes, screening for TB in facilities providing long-term care to the elderly is recommended. The incidence of disease is two to seven times higher among nursing home residents in some areas than among demographically similar persons in other settings. Studies indicated that unsuspected transmission of *M. tuberculosis* in nursing homes/facilities presents a risk to residents and workers.[12]

ADVERSE REACTIONS

Data obtained from clinical studies with a total of 3,062 volunteer subjects (males and females), ranging in age from 4 to 96 years, of which 47.5% (1,443) were Mantoux positive clearly demonstrate that PPD TINE TEST, when used as a screening test to determine tuberculin reactivity, is associated with very little, if any, adverse reactivity. Other than the skin test reaction itself, modest or mild vesiculation and ulceration were the only adverse experiences reported. The modest or mild vesiculation was equally divided between the two tests (PPD TINE TEST, 54/3062, 1.78%; and PPD-T Mantoux, 55/3062, 1.81%). The slight ulceration observed with one subject at 72 hours was associated with the PPD TINE TEST site.

Postmarketing, voluntary reports of adverse events temporally associated with PPD TINE TEST have been received for which an association with the product is unknown. The following local reactions have been reported: rash, pain or discomfort, induration, pruritus, transient bleeding at the puncture site, petechiae, cellulitis, and skin necrosis in highly sensitive persons. Systemic reactions have also be reported. These reactions include fever, urticaria, lymphangitis and allergic reactions, including anaphylactoid reactions. However, there is no indication as to the frequency and severity of reaction relating to these reports.

Healthcare professionals should report suspected adverse events after administration of PPD TINE TEST to the Center for Biologics Evaluation and Research of the Food and Drug Administration by submitting a MedWatch form.[27]

DOSAGE AND ADMINISTRATION

The volar surface of the upper one third of the forearm, over the fleshly portion of a muscle is the preferred site. Hairy areas, and areas without adequate subcutaneous tissue, eg, concavities over a tendon or bone, should be avoided.

Alcohol, acetone, ether, or soap and water may be used to cleanse the skin. The area must be clean and thoroughly dry before application of the PPD TINE TEST.

Expose the four coated tines by removing the protective cap while holding the plastic handle. Grasp the patient's forearm firmly, since the sharp momentary sting may cause the patient to jerk his or her arm, resulting in scratching. Stretch the skin of the forearm tightly and apply the disk with the other hand. **Hold at least 1 second. Sufficient pressure should be exerted so that the four puncture sites and circular depression of the skin from the plastic base are visible.** Release tension grip on forearm. Withdraw the PPD TINE TEST unit.

After administration of the test, local care of the skin is not necessary.

Tuberculin, Purified Protein Derivative PPD TINE TEST units *must never be reused.* The units should be discarded into an impenetrable sharps container without recapping.

Reading Reactions: Tests should be read at 48 to 72 hours. Vesiculation or the extent of induration are the determining factors. The size of any erythema or necrosis, if present, should be recorded, although not used in the interpretation of the test. Readings should be made in good light with the forearm slightly flexed. The size of the induration in millimeters should be determined by inspection, measuring, and palpation with gentle finger stroking. Identification of the application site is usually easy because of the distinct four-point pattern. The diameter of the largest single reaction around one of the puncture sites should be measured. With pronounced reactions, the areas of induration around the puncture sites may coalesce.

Interpretation:

Positive Reactions

A. Vesiculation. If vesiculation is present the test may be interpreted as positive, in which case the management of the patient is the same as that for one classified as positive to the Mantoux test.[13]

B. Induration, 2 mm or greater in diameter or similar in appearance to box 2, 3 or 4 of induration indicator card.[11]

With a positive reaction, further diagnostic procedures must be considered. These may include X-ray of the chest, microbiological examination of sputa and other specimens, and confirmation of the positive PPD THE TEST reaction (except vesiculation reactions) using the Mantoux method. In general, the PPD TINE TEST does not need to be repeated. When vesiculation occurs, the reaction is to be interpreted as strongly positive and a repeat test by the Mantoux method is not required.[14,17]

The PPD TINE TEST has been standardized by clinical evaluation in human subjects to elicit at least a 2 mm reaction or more in a person who responds with a 5 mm reaction or more to 5 TU of Tuberculin, PPD administered intradermally in the Mantoux test.[3] However, there are certain high-risk populations in whom this reaction would not be considered positive including:[12]

- Injecting-drug users known to be HIV seronegative;
- Persons who have other medical conditions that have been reported to increase the risk for progressing from latent TB infection to active TB;
- Residents and employees of high-risk congregate settings (eg, prisons, nursing homes, residential healthcare facilities, homeless shelters);
- Foreign-born persons recently arrived (ie, within the last 5 years) from countries having a high prevalence of incidence of TB;
- Some medically underserved, low-income populations;
- High-risk racial or ethnic minority populations;
- Children < 4 years of age or infants, children, and adolescents exposed to adults in high-risk categories.

Appropriate diagnostic procedures, such as the Mantoux test, should be utilized for retesting individuals who display at 2 mm or greater reaction to PPD TINE TEST. For interpretation of the Mantoux test in various population groups,

Continued on next page

PPD Tine Test—Cont.

the healthcare professional should refer to the recommendations of the Advisory Council for the Elimination of Tuberculosis of the CDC.[12]

Negative Reaction

Induration less than 2 mm. Persons who are contacts of TB patients or who have clinical evidence of disease should be screened by the Mantoux test or chest radiography, even if they have demonstrated a negative reaction to PPD TINE TEST.

Induration indicator cards illustrating typical reactions are enclosed and are considered an important health record. They should be used to record reactions, and become a permanent part of the patient's file. Patients should be instructed to complete and return the card to the healthcare professional.

HOW SUPPLIED

Tuberculin, Purified Protein Derivative (PPD) TINE TEST is supplied as follows:
NDC 0005-2720-25 25 individual tests
NDC 0005-2720-28 100 individual tests

STORAGE

STORE AT CONTROLLED ROOM TEMPERATURE 15°C to 30°C (59°F to 86°F). DO NOT REFRIGERATE.

REFERENCES

1. Seibert FB. Isolation and properties of purified protein derivative of tuberculin. Am Rev Tuberc. 1934; 30:713–720.
2. Seibert FB, Glenn JF. Tuberculin purified protein derivative – preparation and analysis of a large quantity for standard. Am Rev Tuberc. 1941; 44:9–25.
3. Code of Federal Regulations, Food and Drugs; 21 CFR. Subpart B – Tuberculin. 1996; 650.10.
4. Daley CL. Current issues in the pathogenesis and management of HIV-related tuberculosis. AIDS Clin Rev. 1997–1998; 289–321.
5. McCray E, et al. The epidemiology of tuberculosis in the United States. Clin Chest Med. 1997; 18(1):99–113.
6. Kaye K, Frieden TR. Tuberculosis control; the relevance of classic principles in an era of acquired immunodeficiency syndrome and multidrug resistance. Epidemiol Rev. 1996; 18(*):52–63.
7. CDC: Tuberculosis morbidity – United States, 1995. MMWR. 1996; 45(18):365–370.
8. Seil S. Immunology, Immunopathology and Immunity. 4th ed. New York, NY: Elseveir. 1987; 476–478.
9. Dvorak HF, Mihm MC, Dvorak AM, et al. Morphology of delayed type hypersensitivity reactions in man. I. Quantitative description of the inflammatory response. Lab Invest. 1974; 31(2):111–130.
10. Wyeth-Ayerst Laboratoies, Data on file.
11. Professional Services Brochure. Lederle Laboratories, Data on File. 1980.
12. Advisory Council for the Elimination of Tuberculosis: Screening for tuberculosis and tuberculosis infection in high-risk populations. MMWR. 1995; 44(RR-11); 19–35.
13. Comstock GW, Daniel TM, Snider DE Jr, et al. The tuberculin skin test. Am Rev Respir Dis. 1981; 124:356–363.
14. Anonymous: Diagnostic standards and classification of tuberculosis. Official statement of the American Thoracic Society. Am Rev Respir Dis. 1990; 142:725–735.
15. Tager IB, et al. Variability in the intradermal and in-vitro lymphocyte responses to PPD in patients receiving isoniazid chemoprophylaxis. Am Rev Respir Dis. 1985; 131:214–220.
16. Brickman HF, et al. The timing of tuberculin tests in relation to immunization with live viral vaccines. Pediatric. 1975; 55:392–396.
17. Huebner RE, et al. The tuberculin skin test. Clin Inf Dis. 1993; 17;968–975.
18. American Academy of Pediatrics. Report of the Committee on Infectious Diseases. 24th ed. Elk Grove Village, IL: American Academy of Pediatrics. 1997; 564.
19. American Academy of Pediatrics. Report of the Committee on Infectious Diseases. 24th ed. Elk Grove Village, IL: American Academy of Pediatrics. 1997; 24, 354.
20. Lederman MM. Cell-mediated immunity and pregnancy. Chest. 1984; 86(3 Suppl):65–95.
21. Rich AR. The pathogenesis of tuberculosis. Springfield, IL. Charles C. Thomas, Publisher, 1944; 513.
22. Lichtenstein MR. Tuberculosis in pregnancy. Am Rev Tuberc. 1942; 46:89.
23. Conn RW. Effect of pregnancy upon tuberculin reactions. Am Rev Tuberc. 1942; 46:350.
24. Present PA, Comstock GW, Tuberculin sensitivity in pregnancy. Am Rev Respir Dis. 1975; 112:413–416.
25. Montgomery WP, et al. The tuberculin test in pregnancy. Am J Obstet Gyne. 1968; 100(6):829–831.
26. American Academy of Pediatrics. Report of the Committee on Infectious Diseases. 24th ed. Elk Grove Village, IL: American Academy of Pediatrics. 1997; 554–547.
27. Code of Federal Regulations, Food and Drugs; 21 CFR Subpart D-Reporting of Adverse Experiences. 1999; 600.80.

Manufactured by:
LEDERLE LABORATORIES
Division American Cyanamid Company
Pearl River, NY 10965 USA
US Govt. License No. 17

Marketed by:
WYETH LEDERLE VACCINES and PEDIATRICS
Philadelphia, PA 19101
Cl 6127-1 Issued March 15, 2000

TUBERCULIN, OLD, TINE TEST® ℞

[too-ber-cu-lĭn]

DESCRIPTION

The Tuberculin, Old, TINE TEST is a sterile, simple, multiple-puncture, disposable intradermal test device for the detection of tuberculin reactivity. These convenient devices are especially useful in mass tuberculosis screening programs.

Each test unit consists of a stainless steel disc attached to a white plastic handle. Projecting from the disc are four triangular-shaped prongs (tines) which are 2 mm long and approximately 4 mm apart. The tines have been mechanically dipped into a solution of Old Tuberculin, containing 7% acacia (gum arabic) and 8.5% lactose as stabilizers, and then dried. The entire unit has been sterilized by Cobalt 60 irradiation. No preservative has been added. The unit is disposable and there is no need for syringes, needles, and other equipment necessary for the standard intradermal tests.

Tuberculin, Old, TINE TEST units have been standardized by clinical evaluation in human subjects to give reactions equivalent to or more potent than 5 TU (US tuberculin units) of standard Old Tuberculin administered intradermally in the Mantoux test. However, all multiple-puncture-type devices must be regarded as screening tools, and other appropriate diagnostic procedures, such as the Mantoux test, should be utilized for retesting individuals with positive reactions.

CLINICAL PHARMACOLOGY

Tuberculin deposited in the skin of tuberculin reactive individuals reacts with sensitized lymphocytes to effect the release of mediators of cellular hypersensitivity. Some of these mediators (eg, skin reactive factor) induce an inflammatory response in the skin causing the induration and erythema characteristic of a "positive" reaction.[1,2]

INDICATIONS AND USAGE

Tuberculin, Old, TINE TEST is indicated to detect tuberculin-sensitive individuals. Tuberculin, Old, TINE TEST units are also useful in programs to determine priorities for additional testing (eg, chest X-rays) and in epidemiological surveys to identify those areas having high levels of infection. In clinical studies covering various geographical areas of the US and all age groups, with a total of 30,588 test subjects, there were 911 (4%) false positive reactors among 26,236 subjects who were Mantoux negative, and 342 (8%) false negative reactors among 4,352 subjects who were Mantoux positive.

The frequency of repeated tuberculin tests depends on risk of exposure of the individual and on the prevalence of tuberculosis in the population group. The repeated testing of uninfected individuals does not sensitize to tuberculin. Among individuals with waning sensitivity to homologous or heterologous mycobacterial antigens, however, the stimulus of a tuberculin test may "boost" or increase the size of the reaction to a second test, even causing an apparent development of sensitivity in some cases.[1]

Tuberculin testing should be done with caution in individuals with active tuberculosis (see **PRECAUTIONS**).

CONTRAINDICATIONS

There are no known contraindications for use of Tuberculin, Old, TINE TEST. See **PRECAUTIONS** for information regarding special care to be exercised for safe and effective use.

WARNINGS

There are no known serious adverse reactions or potential safety hazards associated with the use of Tuberculin, Old, TINE TEST. However, as with the use of any biological product, the possibility of anaphylactic reaction should be considered. See **PRECAUTIONS** for information regarding special care to be exercised for safe and effective use.

PRECAUTIONS

Tuberculin testing should be done with caution in individuals with active tuberculosis. Although activation of quiescent lesions is rare, if a patient has a history of occurrence of vesiculation and necrosis with a previous tuberculin test by any method, tuberculin testing should be avoided.

Although clinical allergy to acacia is very rare, this product contains some acacia as stabilizer and should be used with caution in patients with known allergy to this component. In these instances remedial measures for anaphylactoid reactions, including epinephrine injection (1:1000), must be available for immediate use.

Reactivity to the test may be suppressed in patients who are receiving corticosteroids or immunosuppressive agents, or those who have recently been immunized with live virus vaccines such as measles, mumps, rubella, polio. If tuberculin skin testing is indicated it should be done preceding, or at the time of such immunization, and read 48 to 72 hours later. If the test is not administered in the time suggested, an interval of 4 to 6 weeks should be allowed between tuberculin skin testing and immunization with live virus vaccines to prevent suppression of tuberculin reactivity.[3]

With a positive reaction further diagnostic procedures must be considered. These may include X-ray of the chest, microbiological examinations of sputa and other specimens, and confirmation of the positive TINE TEST reaction (except vesiculation reactions) using the Mantoux method. In general, the TINE TEST does not need to be repeated.

Antituberculous chemotherapy should not be instituted solely on the basis of a single positive TINE TEST.

When vesiculation occurs, the reaction is to be interpreted as strongly positive and a repeat test by the Mantoux method must not be attempted. Similar or more severe vesiculation with or without necrosis is likely to occur.

Pregnancy Category C. Animal reproduction studies have not been conducted with Tuberculin, Old, TINE TEST. It is also not known whether Tuberculin, Old, TINE TEST can cause fetal harm when administered to a pregnant woman or affect reproduction capacity. Tuberculin, Old, TINE TEST should be given to a pregnant woman only if clearly needed. During pregnancy, known positive reactors may demonstrate a negative response to a Tuberculin, Old, TINE TEST.

Tuberculin, Old, TINE TEST units must never be reused. The units should be discarded into an impenetrable sharps container without recapping.

ADVERSE REACTIONS

Vesiculation (positive reaction), ulceration, or necrosis may occur at the test site in highly sensitive persons. Pain, pruritus, and discomfort at the test site may be relieved by cold packs or by topical glucocorticoid ointment or cream. Transient bleeding may be observed at a puncture site and is of no significance.

DOSAGE AND ADMINISTRATION

Tuberculin, Old, TINE TEST units have been standardized by clinical evaluation in human subjects to give reactions equivalent to or more potent than 5 TU (US tuberculin units) of standard Old Tuberculin administered intradermally in the Mantoux test. However, all multiple-puncture-type devices must be regarded as screening tools, and other appropriate diagnostic procedures, such as the Mantoux test, should be utilized for retesting reactors.

The volar surface of the upper one-third of the forearm, over a muscle belly, is the preferred site. Hairy areas, and areas without adequate subcutaneous tissue, eg, concavities over a tendon or bone, should be avoided.

Alcohol, acetone, ether, or soap and water may be used to cleanse the skin. The area must be clean and thoroughly dry before application of the Tuberculin, Old, TINE TEST.

Expose the four coated tines by removing the protective cap while holding the plastic handle. Grasp the patient's forearm firmly, since the sharp momentary sting may cause the patient to jerk his or her arm, resulting in scratching. Stretch the skin of the forearm tightly and apply the disc with the other hand. **Hold at least one second.** Release tension grip on forearm. Withdraw tine unit.

Sufficient pressure should be exerted so that the four puncture sites, and circular depression of the skin from the plastic base are visible.

After administration of the test, local care of the skin is not necessary.

Tuberculin, Old, TINE TEST units *must never be reused.* The units should be discarded into an impenetrable sharps container without recapping.

Reading Reactions. Tests should be read at 48 to 72 hours. Vesiculation or the extent of induration are the determining factors; erythema without induration is of no significance. Readings should be made in good light with the forearm slightly flexed. The size of the induration in millimeters should be determined by inspection, measuring, and palpation with gentle finger stroking. Identification of the application site is usually easy because of the distinct four-point pattern. The diameter of the largest single reaction around one of the puncture sites should be measured. With pronounced reactions, the areas of induration around the puncture sites may coalesce.

INTERPRETATION:

Positive Reactions

A. Vesiculation. If vesiculation is present the test may be interpreted as positive, in which case the management of the patient is the same as that for one classified as positive to the Mantoux test.[1]

B. Induration, 2 mm or greater. The test may be interpreted as positive but further diagnostic procedures must be considered. These may include X-ray of the chest, microbiological examination of sputa and other specimens, and confirmation of the positive TINE TEST reaction using the Mantoux method.

Negative Reaction

Induration less than 2 mm. With a negative reaction there is no need for retesting unless the person is a contact of a patient with tuberculosis or there is clinical evidence suggestive of the disease.[1]

Induration indicator cards illustrating typical reactions are enclosed.

HOW SUPPLIED

Tuberculin, Old, TINE TEST is supplied as follows:

NDC 0005-2722-25	25 individual tests
NDC 0005-2722-28	100 individual tests
NDC 0005-2722-34	250 individual tests

STORAGE

STORE AT CONTROLLED ROOM TEMPERATURE 15°C to 30°C (59°F to 86°F).

DO NOT REFRIGERATE.

REFERENCES

1. Comstock GW, Daniel TM, Snider DE Jr, et al. The tuberculin skin test. *Am Rev Respir Dis.* 1981;124:356–363.
2. Freeman BA. *Burrows Textbook of Microbiology,* 22nd ed. Philadelphia, Pa: W. B. Saunders Company; 1985:295–299.
3. *American Academy of Pediatrics. Report of the Committee on Infectious Diseases.* 21st ed. Elk Grove Village, Ill: American Academy of Pediatrics; 1988:429–447.

Manufactured by:
LEDERLE LABORATORIES
Division American Cyanamid Company
Pearl River, NY 10965
US Gov't. License No. 17
Marketed by:
WYETH-LEDERLE VACCINES
Wyeth-Ayerst Laboratories
Philadelphia, PA 19101
CI 4560–1 Issued October 24, 1995

Shown in Product Identification Guide, page 320

Wyeth-Ayerst Pharmaceuticals

Division of American Home Products Corporation
P.O. BOX 8299
PHILADELPHIA, PA 19101

Direct General Inquiries to:
(610) 688-4400
For Medical Information Contact:
Medical Affairs
Day: (800) 934-5556
8:30 AM to 4:30 PM (Eastern Standard Time), Weekdays only
In Emergencies:
Day: (800) 934-5556
Night: (610) 688-4400
(Emergencies only;
non-emergencies should wait until the next day)

FACTREL® ℞

[*făc 'trel*]
(gonadorelin hydrochloride)
Synthetic Luteinizing Hormone Releasing Hormone (LH-RH)
DIAGNOSTIC USE ONLY

Caution: Federal law prohibits dispensing without prescription.

DESCRIPTION

An agent for use in evaluating hypothalamic-pituitary gonadotropic function. Factrel (gonadorelin hydrochloride) injectable is available as a sterile lyophilized powder for reconstitution and administration by subcutaneous or intravenous routes.

Chemical Name: 5-oxo-L-prolyl-L-histidyl-L-tryptophyl-L-seryl -L- tyrosyl-glycyl -L- leucyl-L-arginyl-L-prolyl glycinamide hydrochloride
[See chemical structure above]

Structural Formula:

Factrel is $C_{55}H_{75}N_{17}O_{13}HCl$, as the mono- or dihydrochloride, or their mixture. The gonadorelin base has a molecular weight of 1182.33. It is a white powder, soluble in alcohol and water, hygroscopic and moisture-sensitive, and stable at room temperature. The synthetic decapeptide, Factrel, has a chemical composition and structure identical to the natural hormone, identified from porcine or ovine hypothalami.

Each Secule® vial of Factrel contains 100 or 500 mcg gonadorelin as the hydrochloride, with 100 mg lactose, USP. Each ampul of sterile diluent contains 2% benzyl alcohol in sterile water.

CLINICAL PHARMACOLOGY

Factrel has been shown to have gonadotropin-releasing effects upon the anterior pituitary. The range for normal baseline LH levels, as determined from the literature, is 5–25 mIU/mL in postpubertal males, and postpubertal and premenopausal females. The standard used is the Second International Reference Preparation—HMC. This range may not correspond in each laboratory performing the assay since the concentration of LH in normal individuals varies with different assay methods. The normal responses to Factrel analyzed from the results of clinical studies included:

(1) LH peak (mIU/mL)
  (highest LH value post-Factrel administration)
(2) Maximum LH increase (mIU/mL)
  (peak LH value—LH baseline value)
(3) LH percent response

$$\frac{\text{peak LH—baseline LH}}{\text{baseline LH}} \times 100\%$$

(4) Time to peak (minutes)
  (time required to reach LH peak value)

Normal adult subjects were shown to have these LH responses following Factrel administration by subcutaneous or intravenous routes.

I. MALE ADULTS:

A) Subcutaneous Administration

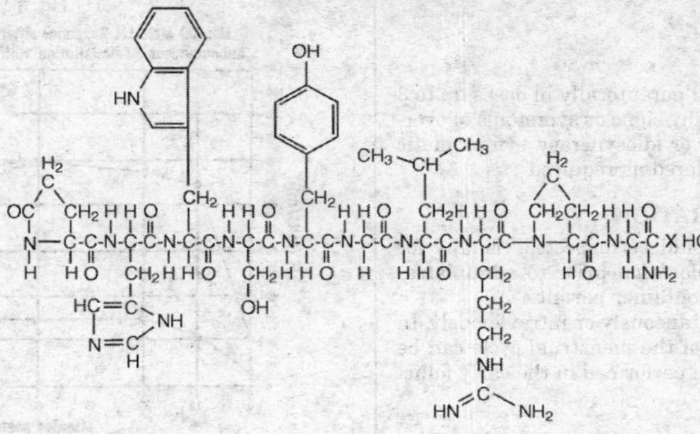

The results are based on 18 tests in males between the ages of 18–42 years, inclusive:
(1) LH peak: mean 60.3 ± 26.2 mIU/mL
 100% ≥ 24.0 mIU/mL
 90% ≥ 32.8 mIU/mL
(2) Maximum LH increase: mean 46.7 ± 20.8 mIU/mL
 100% ≥ 12.3 mIU/mL
 90% ≥ 20.9 mIU/mL
(3) LH percent response: mean 437 ± 243% range: 66–1853%
 90% ≥ 188%
(4) Time to peak: mean 34 ± 13 min

B) Intravenous Administration

The results are based on 26 tests in males between the ages of 19–58 years, inclusive:
(1) LH peak: mean 63.8 ± 40.3 mIU/mL
 100% ≥ 12.6 mIU/mL
 90% ≥ 26.0 mIU/mL
(2) Maximum LH increase: mean 51.3 ± 35.2 mIU/mL
 100% ≥ 7.4 mIU/mL
 90% ≥ 14.8 mIU/mL
(3) LH percent response: mean 481 ± 184% range: 67–2139%
 90% ≥ 142%
(4) Time to peak: mean 27 ± 14 min

In males older than 50 years, the LH baseline and peak levels tend to be higher; however, the maximum LH increases do not differ in regard to age.

II. FEMALE ADULTS:

A) Subcutaneous Administration

The results are based on 38 tests in females between the ages of 19–36 years, inclusive:
(1) LH peak: mean 67.9 ± 27.5 mIU/mL
 100% ≥ 12.5 mIU/mL
 90% ≥ 39.0 mIU/mL
(2) Maximum LH increase: mean 52.8 ± 26.4 mIU/mL
 100% ≥ 7.5 mIU/mL
 90% ≥ 23.8 mIU/mL
(3) LH percent response: mean 374 ± 221% range: 108–981%
 90% ≥ 185%
(4) Time to peak: mean 71.5 ± 49.6 min

B) Intravenous Administration

The results are based on 31 tests in females between the ages of 20–35 years, inclusive:
(1) LH peak: mean 57.6 ± 36.7 mIU/mL
 100% ≥ 20.0 mIU/mL
 90% ≥ 24.6 mIU/mL
(2) Maximum LH increase: mean 44.5 ± 31.8 mIU/mL
 100% ≥ 7.5 mIU/mL
 90% ≥ 16.2 mIU/mL
(3) LH percent response: mean 356 ± 282% range: 60–1300%
 90% ≥ 142%
(4) Time to peak: mean 36 ± 24 min

The Factrel tests on which the normal female responses are based were performed in the early follicular phase of the menstrual cycle (Days 1–7).

In menopausal and postmenopausal females, the baseline LH levels are elevated and the maximum LH increases are exaggerated when compared with the premenopausal levels.

Patients with clinically diagnosed or suspected pituitary and/or hypothalamic dysfunction were often shown to have subnormal or no LH responses following Factrel administration. For example, in clinical tests of 6 patients with known postpubertal panhypopituitarism, and 11 patients with Prader-Willi syndrome, 100% showed subnormal responses or no rise in LH. Subnormal responses to the Factrel test also were observed in 21 (95%) of 22 patients with prepubertal panhypopituitarism. In 19 patients with Sheehan's syndrome, 16 (84%) had a subnormal response. In the Factrel test in 44 patients with Kallmann's syndrome, 33 (77%) had subnormal LH responses.

INDICATIONS AND USAGE

Factrel as a single injection is indicated for evaluating the functional capacity and response of the gonadotropes of the anterior pituitary. This single-injection test does not measure pituitary gonadotropic reserve, for which more prolonged or repeated administration may be required. The LH response is useful in testing patients with suspected gonadotropin deficiency, whether due to the hypothalamus alone or in combination with anterior pituitary failure. Factrel is also indicated for evaluating residual gonadotropic function of the pituitary following removal of a pituitary tumor by surgery and/or irradiation. In clinical studies to date, however, the single-injection test has not been useful in differentiating pituitary disorders from hypothalamic disorders. The Factrel test can be performed concomitantly with other post-treatment evaluations. The results of the Factrel test complement the clinical examination and other laboratory tests used to confirm or substantiate hypogonadotropic hypogonadism.

In cases where there is a normal response, it indicates the presence of functional pituitary gonadotropes. The single-injection test does not measure pituitary gonadotropic reserve.

CONTRAINDICATIONS

Hypersensitivity to gonadorelin hydrochloride or any of the components.

PRECAUTIONS

A. General

Although allergic and hypersensitivity reactions have been observed with other polypeptide hormones, and rarely with multiple doses of Factrel, to date no such reactions have been reported following the administration of a single 100 mcg dose of Factrel.

Antibody formation has been reported rarely after chronic administration of large doses of Factrel.

B. Drug Interactions

The Factrel test should be conducted in the absence of other drugs which directly affect the pituitary secretion of the gonadotropins. These would include a variety of preparations which contain androgens, estrogens, progestins, or glucocorticoids. The gonadotropin levels may be transiently elevated by spironolactone, minimally elevated by levodopa, and suppressed by oral contraceptives and digoxin. The response to Factrel may be blunted by phenothiazines and dopamine antagonists which cause a rise in prolactin.

C. Carcinogenesis, Mutagenesis, Impairment of Fertility

Repetitive, high doses of Factrel may cause luteolysis and inhibition of spermatogenesis. No long-term animal studies have been done to evaluate carcinogenic potential.

D. Pregnancy Category B

Reproduction studies have been performed in mice, rats, and rabbits at doses up to 50 times the human dose, and have revealed no evidence of harm to the fetus due to Factrel. There are, however, no adequate and well-controlled studies in pregnant women. Because animal reproduction studies are not always predictive of human response, this drug should be used during pregnancy only if clearly needed.

Appropriate precautions should be taken because the effects of LH-RH on the fetus and developing offspring have not been adequately evaluated.

Nursing Mothers: It is not known whether this drug is excreted in human milk. Because many drugs are excreted in human milk, caution should be exercised when Factrel is administered to a nursing woman.

Pediatric Use: Safety and effectiveness in pediatric patients have not been established.

ADVERSE REACTIONS

Systemic effects have been reported rarely following administration of 100 mcg of Factrel.

CNS: headache, light-headedness.

GI: nausea, abdominal discomfort.

Dermatologic: local swelling, occasionally with pain and pruritis, at the injection site may occur following subcutaneous administration; local and generalized skin rash have been noted after chronic subcutaneous administration.

Cardiovascular: flushing.

Rare instances of hypersensitivity reaction (bronchospasm, tachycardia, flushing, urticaria, induration at injection site) and anaphylactic reactions have been reported following multiple-dose administration.

There has been a report of pituitary apoplexy and sudden blindness following gonadotropin-releasing hormone administration to a patient with a gonadotropin-secreting adenoma.

Continued on next page

Factrel—Cont.

OVERDOSAGE

Factrel has been administered parenterally in doses up to 3 mg b.i.d. for 28 days without any signs or symptoms of overdosage. In case of overdosage or idiosyncrasy, symptomatic treatment should be administered as required.

DOSAGE AND ADMINISTRATION

Parenteral drug products should be inspected visually for particulate matter and discoloration prior to administration, whenever solution and container permit.
Adults: 100 mcg dose, subcutaneously or intravenously. In females for whom the phase of the menstrual cycle can be established, the test should be performed in the early follicular phase (Days 1–7).

TEST METHODOLOGY

To determine the status of the gonadotropin secretory capacity of the anterior pituitary, a test procedure requiring seven venous blood samples for LH is recommended.

Procedure:

1. Venous blood samples should be drawn at -15 minutes and immediately prior to Factrel administration. The LH baseline is obtained by averaging the LH values of the two samples.
2. Administer a bolus of 100 mcg of Factrel subcutaneously or intravenously.
3. Draw venous blood samples at 15, 30, 45, 60, and 120 minutes after administration.
4. Blood samples should be handled as recommended by the laboratory that will determine the LH content. It must be emphasized that the reliability of the test is directly related to the inter-assay and intra-assay reliability of the laboratory performing the assay.

INTERPRETATION OF TEST RESULTS

Interpretation of the LH response to Factrel requires an understanding of the hypothalamic-pituitary physiology, knowledge of the clinical status of the individual patient, and familiarity with the normal ranges and the standards used in the laboratory performing the LH assays.
Figures 1 through 4 represent the LH response curves after Factrel administration in normal subjects. The normal LH response curves were established between the 10th percentile (B line) and 90th percentile (A line) of all LH responses in normal subjects analyzed from the results of clinical studies. LH values are reported in units of mIU/mL and time is displayed in minutes. Individual patient responses should be plotted on the appropriate curve. A subnormal response in patients is defined as three or more LH values which fall below the B line of the normal LH response curve. In cases where there is a blunted or borderline response, the Factrel test should be repeated.

Fig. 1
Normal Male LH Response After Factrel 100 mcg, Subcutaneous Administration 10th and 90th percentiles.

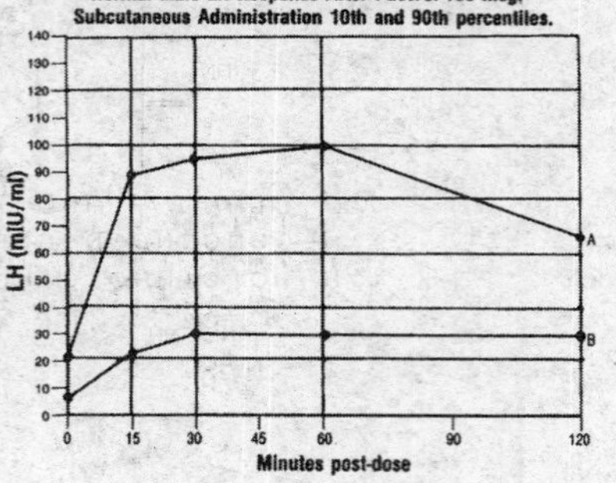

Fig. 2
Normal Male LH Response After Factrel 100 mcg, Intravenous Administration 10th and 90th percentiles.

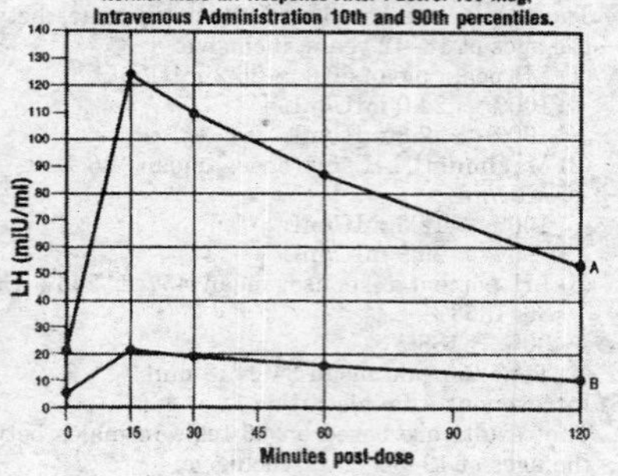

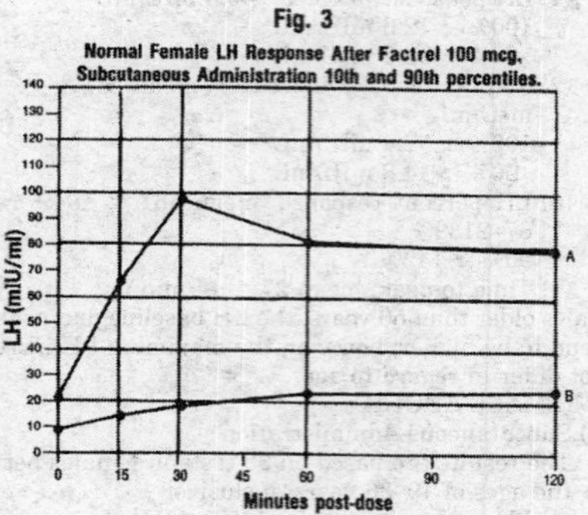

Fig. 3
Normal Female LH Response After Factrel 100 mcg, Subcutaneous Administration 10th and 90th percentiles.

Fig. 4
Normal Female LH Response After Factrel 100 mcg, Intravenous Administration 10th and 90th percentiles.

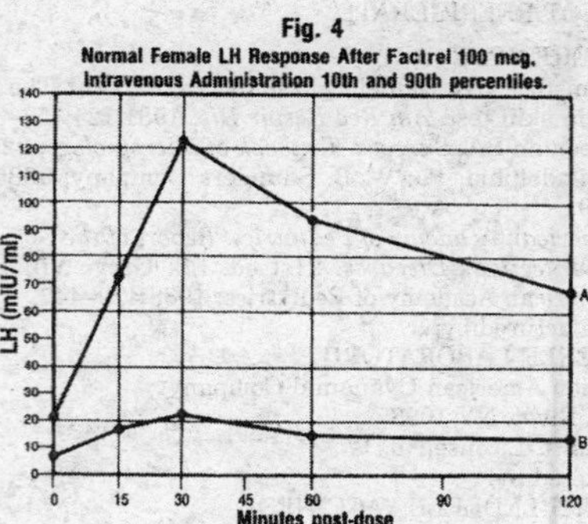

The Factrel test complements the clinical assessment of patients with a variety of endocrine disorders involving the hypothalamic-pituitary axis. In cases where there is a normal response, it indicates the presence of functional pituitary gonadotropes. The single-injection test does not determine the pathophysiological cause for the subnormal response and does not measure pituitary gonadotropic reserve.

HOW SUPPLIED

Lyophilized Powder—in single-dose Secule® vials containing 100 mcg (NDC 0046-0507-05) and 500 mcg (NDC 0046-0509-05) gonadorelin as the hydrochloride with 100 mg lactose, USP. Each Secule vial is accompanied by one ampul containing 2 mL sterile diluent of 2% benzyl alcohol in sterile water.

DIRECTIONS

Store at room temperature (approximately 25°C).
Reconstitute 100 mcg Secule® vial with 1.0 mL of the accompanying sterile diluent.
Reconstitute 500 mcg Secule® vial with 2.0 mL of the accompanying sterile diluent.
Prepare solution immediately before use. After reconstitution, store at room temperature and use within 1 day.
Discard unused reconstituted solution and diluent.
Secule®—Registered trademark to designate a vial containing an injectable preparation in dry form.
Manufactured by:
Ayerst Laboratories Inc.
A Wyeth-Ayerst Company
Philadelphia, PA 19101
CI 4992-1 Issued July 25, 1997

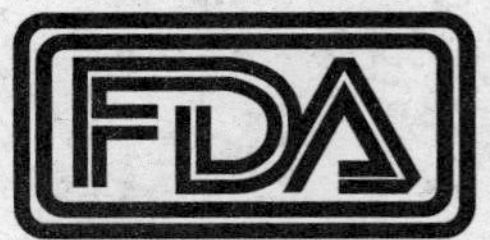

U.S. FOOD AND DRUG ADMINISTRATION

Professional and Consumer Information Numbers

Medical Product Reporting Programs

MedWatch (24-hour service) **800-332-1088**
Reporting of problems with drugs, devices, biologics (except vaccines), medical foods, dietary supplements.

Vaccine Adverse Event Reporting System (24 hour service) **800-822-7967**
Reporting of vaccine-related problems.

Mandatory Medical Device Reporting **301-827-0360**
Reporting required from user-facilities (eg, hospitals, nursing homes) regarding device-related deaths and serious injuries.

Veterinary Adverse Drug Reaction Program **888-332-8387**
Reporting of adverse drug events in animals.

Medical Advertising Information **301-827-2828**
Inquiries from health professionals regarding product promotion.

USP Medication Errors **800-233-7767**
Reporting of medication errors or near-errors to help avoid future problems through improvement in product names and packaging.

Information for Health Professionals

Center for Drugs Information Branch **301-827-4573**
Information on human drugs including hormones.

Center for Biologics Office of Communications **301-827-2000**
Information on biological products including vaccines and blood.

Center for Devices and Radiological Health **301-443-4190**
Automated request for information on medical devices and radiation-emitting products.

Emergency Operations **301-443-1240**
Emergencies involving FDA-regulated products, tampering reports, and after-hours emergency Investigational New Drug requests.

Office of Orphan Products Development **301-827-3666**
Information on products for rare diseases.

General Information

General Consumer Inquiries **888-463-6332**
Consumer information on regulated products/issues.

Freedom of Information **301-827-6500**
Requests for publicly available FDA documents.

Office of Public Affairs **301-827-6250**
Interviews/press inquiries on FDA activities.

Center for Food Safety and Applied Nutrition **888-723-3366**
Information on food safety, seafood, dietary supplements, women's nutrition, and cosmetics.

DRUG INFORMATION CENTERS

ALABAMA

BIRMINGHAM

Drug Information Service
University of Alabama Hospital
619 S. 20th St.
1720 Jefferson Tower
Birmingham, AL 35249-6860
Mon.-Fri. 8 AM-5 PM
205-934-2162
Fax: 205-934-3501

Global Drug Information Center
Samford University
McWhorter School of Pharmacy
800 Lakeshore Dr.
Birmingham, AL 35229-7027
Mon.-Fri. 8 AM-4:30 PM
205-870-2659
Fax: 205-726-4012
samford. edu.schools/pharmacy/dic/index.html

HUNTSVILLE

Huntsville Hospital Drug Information Center
101 Sivley Rd.
Huntsville, AL 35801
Mon.-Fri. 8 AM-5 PM
256-517-8284
Fax: 256-517-6558

ARIZONA

TUCSON

Arizona Poison and Drug Information Center
Arizona Health Sciences Center
University Medical Center
1501 N. Campbell Ave.
Room 1156
Tucson, AZ 85724
7 days/week, 24 hours
520-626-6016
800-362-0101 (AZ)
Fax: 520-626-2720

CALIFORNIA

LOS ANGELES

Los Angeles Regional Drug Information Center
LAC & USC Medical Center
1200 N. State St.
Room 1107 A & B
Los Angeles, CA 90033
Mon.-Fri. 8AM-4:30PM
323-226-7741
Fax: 323-226-4194

SAN DIEGO

Drug Information Center
U.S. Naval Hospital
34800 Bob Wilson Dr.
San Diego, CA 92134-5000
Mon.-Fri. 8 AM-4 PM
619-532-8417
Fax: 619-352-5898

Drug Information Service
University of California San Diego Medical Center
135 Dickinson St.
San Diego, CA 92103-8925
Mon.-Fri. 9 AM-5 PM
900-288-8273
Fax: 858-715-6323

STANFORD

Drug Information Center
University of California Stanford Health
Stanford Campus
300 Pasteur Dr.
Room H-0301
Stanford, CA 94305
Mon.-Fri. 8 AM-4 PM
650-723-6422
Fax: 650-725-5028

COLORADO

DENVER

Rocky Mountain Poison and Drug Consultation Center
1010 Yosemite Circle
Denver, CO 80230
Mon.-Fri. 8 AM-4:30 PM
303-893-3784
(For Denver County residents only)
Fax: 303-739-1119

Drug Information Center
University of Colorado Health Science Center
4200 E. 9th Ave., Box C239
Denver, CO 80262
Mon.-Fri. 8:30 AM-4:30 PM
303-315-8489
Fax: 303-315-3353

CONNECTICUT

FARMINGTON

Drug Information Service
University of Connecticut Health Center
263 Farmington Ave.
Farmington, CT 06030
Mon.-Fri. 7 AM-4 PM
860-679-2783
Fax: 860-679-1231
wnelson@nso.uchc.edu

HARTFORD

Drug Information Center
Hartford Hospital
P.O. Box 5037
80 Seymour St.
Hartford, CT 06102
Mon.-Fri. 8:30 AM-5 PM
860-545-2221
860-545-2961
Fax: 860-545-4371

NEW HAVEN

Drug Information Center
Yale-New Haven Hospital
20 York St.
New Haven, CT 06504
Mon.-Fri. 12 PM-4:30 PM
203-688-2248
Fax: 203-688-3691

DISTRICT OF COLUMBIA

Drug Information Service
Howard University Hospital
Room BB06
2041 Georgia Ave. NW
Washington, DC 20060
7 days/week, 24 hours
202-865-1325
Fax: 202-865-7410

FLORIDA

GAINESVILLE

Drug Information & Pharmacy Resource Center
SHANDS Hospital at University of Florida
P.O. Box 100316
Gainesville, FL 32610-0316
Mon.-Fri. 9 AM-5 PM
352-395-0408
(for healthcare professionals only)
Fax: 352-338-9860

JACKSONVILLE

Drug Information Service
SHANDS Jacksonville
655 W. 8th St.
Jacksonville, FL 32209
Mon.-Fri. 8 AM-5 PM
904-244-4185
Fax: 904-244-4272

MIAMI

Drug Information Center (119)
Miami VA Medical Center
1201 NW 16th St.
Pharmacy 119
Miami, FL 33125
Mon.-Fri. 7:00 AM-3:30 PM
305-324-3237
(for healthcare professionals only)
Fax: 305-324-3394

ORLANDO

Orlando Regional Drug Information Service
Orlando Regional Healthcare System
1414 Kuhl Ave., MP 192
Orlando, FL 32806
Mon.-Fri. 8 AM-5 PM
407-841-5111, ext. 8717
Fax: 407-650-9052

TALLAHASSEE

Drug Information Education Center
Florida Agricultural and Mechanical University College of Pharmacy
Honor House, Room 200
Tallahassee, FL 32307
Mon.-Fri. 9 AM-5 PM
850-488-5239
850-599-3064
800-451-3181
Fax: 850-412-7020

GEORGIA

ATLANTA

Emory University Hospital
Dept. of Pharmaceutical Services-Drug Information
1364 Clifton Rd. NE
Atlanta, GA 30322
Mon.-Fri. 8:30 AM-5 PM
404-712-4640
Fax: 404-712-7577

Drug Information Service
Northside Hospital
1000 Johnson Ferry Rd. NE
Atlanta, GA 30342
Mon.-Fri. 9 AM-4 PM
404-851-8676(GA only)
Fax: 404-851-8682

AUGUSTA

Drug Information Center
University of Georgia Medical College of GA
Room BIW201
1120 15th St.
Augusta, GA 30912-5600
Mon.-Fri. 8:30 AM-5 PM
706-721-2887
Fax: 706-721-3827

IDAHO

POCATELLO

Idaho Drug Information Service
Campus Box 8092
Pocatello, ID 83209
Mon.-Fri. 8 AM-5 PM
208-282-4689
Fax: 208-282-3003

ILLINOIS

CHICAGO

Drug Information Center
Northwestern Memorial Hospital
251 E. Huron
Feinberg LC-700B
Chicago, IL 60611
Mon.-Fri. 8 AM-5 PM
312-926-7573
Fax: 312-926-7956

Saint Joseph Hospital Pharmacy
2900 N. Lake Shore Dr.
Chicago, IL 60657
7 days/week, 24 hours
773-665-3140
Fax: 773-665-3462

Drug Information Services
University of Chicago
5841 S. Maryland Ave.
MC 0010
Chicago, IL 60637
Mon.-Fri. 8 AM-5 PM
773-702-1388
Fax: 773-702-6631

Drug Information Center
University of Illinois at Chicago
833 S. Wood St.
Chicago, IL 60612
Mon.-Fri. 8 AM-4 PM
312-996-0209
Fax: 312-996-0448

HARVEY

Drug Information Center
Ingalls Memorial Hospital
1 Ingalls Dr.
Harvey, IL 60426
Mon.-Fri. 8 AM-4:30 PM
708-915-6413
800-543-6543 (IL only)
Fax: 708-915-4609

HINES

Drug Information Service
Hines Veterans Administration Hospital
Inpatient Pharmacy (119B)
P.O. Box 5000
Hines, IL 60141-5000
Mon.-Fri. 8 AM-4:30 PM
708-202-8387
Fax: 708-202-2201

PARK RIDGE

Drug Information Center
Lutheran General Hospital
1775 Dempster St.
Park Ridge, IL 60068
Mon.-Fri. 7:30 AM-4 PM
847-723-8128
Fax: 847-723-2326

INDIANA

INDIANAPOLIS

Drug Information Center
St. Vincent Hospital and Health Services
2001 W. 86th St.
P.O. Box 40970
Indianapolis, IN 46240
Mon.-Fri. 8 AM-4 PM
317-338-3200
(for healthcare professionals only)
Fax: 317-338-3041

IOWA

DES MOINES

Regional Drug Information Center
Mercy Medical Center-Des Moines
1111 Sixth Ave.
Des Moines, IA 50314
Mon.-Fri. 8 AM-4:30 PM
515-247-3286
(answered 7 days/week, 24 hours)
Fax: 515-247-3966

IOWA CITY

Drug Information Center
University of Iowa Hospitals and Clinics
200 Hawkins Dr.
Iowa City, IA 52242
Mon.-Fri. 8 AM-5 PM
319-356-2600
(for healthcare professionals only)
Fax: 319-384-8840

SIOUX CITY

Iowa Statewide Poison Center
2720 Stone Park Blvd.
Sioux City, IA 51104
7 days/week, 24 hours
712-277-2222
800-352-2222 (IA)
Fax: 712-234-8775

KANSAS

KANSAS CITY

Drug Information Center
University of Kansas Medical Center
3901 Rainbow Blvd.
Kansas City, KS 66160
Mon.-Fri. 8 AM-6 PM
913-588-2328
(for healthcare professionals only)
Fax: 913-588-2350

KENTUCKY

LEXINGTON

Drug Information Center
Chandler Medical Center
College of Pharmacy
University of Kentucky
800 Rose St., C-117
Lexington, KY 40536-0293
Mon.-Fri. 8 AM-5 PM
606-323-5320
Fax: 606-323-2049

LOUISIANA

NEW ORLEANS

Xavier University Drug Information Center
Tulane University Hospital and Clinic
Box HC12
1415 Tulane Ave.
New Orleans, LA 70112
Mon.-Fri. 9 AM-5 PM
504-588-5670
Fax: 504-588-5862
mharris@tulane.edu

MARYLAND

ANDREWS AFB

Drug Information Services
89 MDTS/SGQP
1050 W. Perimeter Rd.
Suite D1-119
Andrews AFB, MD 20762-6660
Mon.-Fri. 7:30 AM-6 PM
240-857-4565
Fax: 240-857-8892

ANNAPOLIS

The Anne Arundel Medical Center
Dept. of Pharmacy
P.O. Box 64
Franklin St.
Annapolis, MD 21401
7 days/week, 24 hours
410-267-1126
410-267-1000
(switchboard)
Fax: 410-267-1628

BALTIMORE

Drug Information Service
Johns Hopkins Hospital
600 N. Wolfe St.,
Halsted 503
Baltimore, MD 21287-6180
Mon.-Fri. 8:30 AM-5 PM
410-955-6348
Fax: 410-955-8283

Drug Information Service
University of Maryland at Baltimore School of Pharmacy
506 W. Fayette, 3rd Floor
Baltimore, MD 21201
Mon.-Fri. 8:30 AM-5 PM
410-706-7568
Fax: 410-706-0897

BETHESDA

Drug Information Center
National Institutes of Health
Building 10, Room 1S-259
10 Center Drive (MSC1196)
Bethesda, MD 20892-1196
Mon.-Fri. 8:30 AM-5 PM
301-496-2407
Fax: 301-496-0210

EASTON

Drug Information
Pharmacy Dept.
Memorial Hospital
219 S. Washington St.
Easton, MD 21601
Mon.-Fri. 7 AM-Midnight
Sat.-Sun. 7 AM-5:30 PM
410-822-1000
Fax: 410-820-9489

MASSACHUSETTS

BOSTON

Drug Information Services
Brigham and Women's Hospital
75 Frances St.
Boston, MA 02115
Mon.-Fri. 7 AM-3:30 PM
617-732-7166
Fax: 617-732-7497

Drug Information Center
New England Medical Center Pharmacy
750 Washington St., Box 420
Boston, MA 02111
Mon.-Fri. 9 AM-5 PM
617-636-8985
Fax: 617-636-4567

WORCESTER

Drug Information Center
U.M.M.H.C. Hospital
55 Lake Ave. North
Worcester, MA 01655
Mon.-Fri. 8:30 AM-5 PM
508-856-3456
508-856-2775
Fax: 508-856-1850

MICHIGAN

ANN ARBOR

Drug Information and Pharmacy Services
University of Michigan Medical Center
1500 East Medical
Center Dr.
UHB2 D301 Box 0008
Ann Arbor, MI 48109/0008
Mon.-Fri. 8 AM-5 PM
734-936-8200
734-936-8251
Fax: 734-936-7027

DETROIT

Drug Information Services
Harper Hospital
3990 John R. St.
Detroit, MI 48201
Mon.-Fri. 8 AM-5 PM
313-745-4556
313-745-2006
Fax: 313-745-1628

PONTIAC

Drug Information Center
St. Joseph Mercy Hospital
900 Woodward
Pontiac, MI 48341
Mon.-Fri. 8 AM-4:30 PM
248-858-3055
Fax: 248-858-3010

ROYAL OAK

Drug Information Services
William Beaumont Hospital
3601 West 13 Mile Rd.
Royal Oak, MI 48073-6769
Mon.-Fri. 8 AM-4:30 PM
248-551-4077
Fax: 248-551-3301

SOUTHFIELD

Drug Information Service
Providence Hospital
16001 West 9 Mile Rd.
Southfield, MI 48075
Mon.-Fri. 8 AM-4 PM
248-424-3125
Fax: 248-424-5364

MISSISSIPPI

JACKSON

Drug Information Center
University of Mississippi Medical Center
2500 N. State St.
Jackson, MS 39216
Mon.-Fri. 8 AM-4:30 PM
601-984-2060
Fax: 601-984-2064

MISSOURI

KANSAS CITY

University of Missouri-Kansas City
Drug Information Center
2411 Holmes St., MG-200
Kansas City, MO 64108-2792
Mon.-Fri. 8 AM-5 PM
816-235-5490
Fax: 816-235-5491

SPRINGFIELD

Drug Information
St. Johns Regional Health Center
1235 E. Cherokee
Springfield, MO 65804
Mon.-Fri. 7:30 AM-4:30 PM
417-885-3488
Fax: 417-888-7788

ST. JOSEPH

Drug Information Service
Heartland Hospital West
801 Faraon St.
St. Joseph, MO 64501
Mon.-Fri. 9 AM-5:30 PM
816-271-7582
Fax: 816-271-7590

NEBRASKA

OMAHA

Drug Information Service
School of Pharmacy
Creighton University
2500 California Plaza
Omaha, NE 68178
Mon.-Fri. 8:30 AM-5:00 PM
402-280-5101
Fax: 402-280-5149

NEW MEXICO

ALBUQUERQUE

New Mexico Poison & Drug Information Center
University of New Mexico
Albuquerque, NM 87131
7 days/week, 24 hours
505-272-2222
800-432-6866 (NM only)
Fax: 505-272-5892

NEW YORK

BROOKLYN

International Drug Information Center
Long Island University
Arnold & Marie Schwartz College of Pharmacy & Health Sciences
1 University Plaza
RM-HS509
75 Dekalb Ave.
Brooklyn, NY 11201
Mon.-Fri. 9 AM-5 PM
718-488-1064
Fax: 718-780-4056

Drug Information Center
Brookdale University Hospital and Medical Center
1 Brookdale Plaza
Brooklyn, NY 11212
Mon.-Fri. 8 AM-4:30 PM
718-240-5983
Fax: 718-240-5987

COOPERSTOWN

Drug Information Center
Bassett Healthcare
1 Atwell Rd.
Cooperstown, NY 13326
Mon.-Fri. 8:30 AM-5 PM
607-547-3686
Fax: 607-547-3629

JAMAICA

Drug Information Center
St. John's University College of Pharmacy and Allied Health Professions
8000 Utopia Pkwy.
Jamaica, NY 11439
Mon.-Fri. 8:30 AM-3:30 PM
718-990-2149
Fax: 718-990-2151

NEW YORK CITY

Drug Information Center
Bellevue Hospital Center
462 1st Ave.
New York, NY 10016
7 days/week, 24 hours
212-562-6501
Fax: 212-562-2949

Drug Information Center
Memorial Sloan-Kettering Cancer Center
1275 York Ave.
RM S-712
New York, NY 10021
Mon.-Fri. 9 AM-5 PM
212-639-7552
Fax: 212-639-2171

Drug Information Center
Mount Sinai Medical Center
1 Gustave Levy Pl.
New York, NY 10029
Mon.-Fri. 9 AM-5 PM
212-241-6619
Fax: 212-348-7927

Drug Information Service
New York Presbyterian Hospital
Room K04
525 E. 68th St.
New York, NY 10021
Mon.-Fri. 9 AM-5 PM
212-746-0741
Fax: 212-746-8506

ROCHESTER

Poison and Drug Information Center
University of Rochester
601 Elmwood Ave.
Rochester, NY 14642
7 days/week, 24 hours
716-275-3718
716-275-3232
(after 5 PM)
Fax: 716-244-1677

STONY BROOK

Suffolk Drug Information Center
University Hospital
S.U.N.Y. - Stony Brook
Stony Brook, NY 11794-7310
Mon.-Fri. 8 AM-3:00 PM
631-444-2675
631-444-2680 (after hours)
Fax: 631-444-7935

NORTH CAROLINA

BUIES CREEK

Drug Information Center
School of Pharmacy
Campbell University
P.O. Box 1090
Buies Creek, NC 27506
Mon.-Fri. 8:30 AM-4:30 PM
910-893-1478
800-327-5467 (NC only)
Fax: 910-893-1476

CHAPEL HILL

Drug Information Center
University of North Carolina Hospitals
101 Manning Dr.
Chapel Hill, NC 27514
Mon.-Fri. 8 AM-4:30 PM
919-966-2373
Fax: 919-966-1791

GREENVILLE

Eastern Carolina Drug Information Center
Pitt County Memorial Hospital
Dept. of Pharmacy Service
2100 Stantonsburg Rd.
Greenville, NC 27834
Mon.-Fri. 8 AM-5 PM
252-816-4257
Fax: 252-816-7425

WINSTON-SALEM

Drug Information Service Center
Wake-Forest University Baptist Medical Center
Medical Center Blvd.
Winston-Salem, NC 27157
Mon.-Fri. 8 AM-5 PM
336-716-2037
Fax: 336-716-2186

OHIO

ADA

Drug Information Center
Raabe College of Pharmacy
Ohio Northern University
Ada, OH 45810
Mon.-Fri. 9 AM-5 PM
419-772-2307
Fax: 419-772-2289

CLEVELAND

Drug Information Center
Cleveland Clinic Foundation
9500 Euclid Ave.
Cleveland, OH 44195
Mon.-Fri. 8:30 AM-4:30 PM
216-444-6456
Fax: 216-444-6157

COLUMBUS

Drug Information Center
Ohio State University Hospital
Dept. of Pharmacy
Doan Hall 368
410 W. 10th Ave.
Columbus, OH 43210-1228
Mon.-Fri. 8 AM-4 PM
614-293-8679
Fax: 614-293-3264

Drug Information Center
Riverside Methodist Hospital
3535 Olentangy River Road
Columbus, OH 43214
Mon.-Fri. 8 AM-5 PM
614-566-5425
Fax: 614-566-5447

TOLEDO

Drug Information Services
St. Vincent Mercy Medical Center
2213 Cherry St.
Toledo, Ohio 43608-2691
Mon.-Fri. 8 AM-4 PM
419-251-4227
Fax: 419-251-3662

OKLAHOMA

OKLAHOMA CITY

Drug Information Service
Integris Health
3300 Northwest Expressway
Oklahoma City, OK 73112
Mon.-Fri. 8 AM-4:30 PM
405-949-3660
Fax: 405-951-8274

Drug Information Center
Presbyterian Hospital
700 NE 13th St.
Oklahoma City, OK 73104
Mon.-Fri. 8 AM-4:30 PM
405-271-6226
Fax: 405-271-6281

TULSA

Drug Information Service
St. Francis Hospital
6161 S. Yale Ave.
Tulsa, OK 74136
Mon.-Fri. 7 AM-4:30 PM
918-494-6339
(for healthcare professionals only)
Fax: 918-494-1893

PENNSYLVANIA

PHILADELPHIA

Drug Information Center
Temple University Hospital
Dept. of Pharmacy
3401 N. Broad St.
Philadelphia, PA 19140
Mon.-Fri. 8 AM-4:30 PM
215-707-4644
Fax: 215-707-3463

Drug Information Service
Dept. of Pharmacy
Thomas Jefferson University Hospital
111 S. 11th St.
Philadelphia, PA 19107-5098
Mon.-Fri. 8 AM-5 PM
215-955-8877
Fax: 215-923-3316

PITTSBURGH

The Christopher and Nicole Browett Pharmaceutical Information Center
Mylan School of Pharmacy
Duquesne University
431 Mellon Hall
Pittsburgh, PA 15282
Mon.-Fri. 8 AM-4 PM
412-396-4600
Fax: 412-396-4488

Drug Information and Pharmacoepidemiology Center
University of Pittsburgh Medical Center
137 Victoria Hall
Pittsburgh, PA 15261
Mon.-Fri. 8:30 AM-4:30 PM
412-624-3784
Fax: 412-624-6350

UPLAND

Drug Information Center
Crozer-Chester Medical Center
Dept. of Pharmacy
1 Medical Center Blvd.
Upland, PA 19013
Mon.-Fri. 8 AM-4:30 PM
610-447-2851
610-447-2862
(after hours)
(both numbers are for healthcare professionals only)
Fax: 610-447-2820

WILKES-BARRE

Drug Information Center
Nesbitt School of Pharmacy
Wilkes University
150-180 S. River St.
Stark Learning Center, Room 1060
Wilkes-Barre, PA 18766
Mon.-Fri. 9 AM- 3 PM
570-408-3295
Fax: 570-408-7828
dicenter@wilkes.edu

WILLIAMSPORT

Drug Information
Pharmacy Dept.
Susquehanna Health System
Rural Avenue Campus
Williamsport, PA 17701
24 hours/7 days a week
570-321-3083
Fax: 570-321-3230

PUERTO RICO

PONCE

Centro Informacion Medicamentos
Escuela de Medicina de Ponce
P.O. Box 7004
Ponce, PR 00732
Mon.-Fri. 8 AM-4:30 PM
787-259-7085
(Spanish and English)
787-840-2575
(switchboard)
Fax: 787-259-7085

SOUTH CAROLINA

CHARLESTON

Drug Information Service
Medical University of South Carolina
150 Ashley Ave.
Rutledge Tower
Annex, Room 604
P.O. Box 25058
Charleston, SC 29425-0810
Mon.-Fri. 9 AM-5:30 PM
843-792-3896
800-922-5250
Fax: 843-792-5532

SPARTANBURG

Drug Information Center
Spartanburg Regional Medical Center
101 E. Wood St.
Spartanburg, SC 29303
Mon.-Fri. 8 AM-5 PM
864-560-6910
Fax: 864-560-7323

TENNESSEE

MEMPHIS

South East Regional Drug Information Center
VA Medical Center
1030 Jefferson Ave.
Memphis, TN 38104
Mon.-Fri. 7:30 AM-4 PM
901-523-8990, ext. 6720
Fax: 901-577-7306

Drug Information Center
University of Tennessee
875 Monroe Ave.
Suite 116
Memphis, TN 38163
Mon.-Fri. 8 AM-5 PM
901-448-5555
Fax: 901-448-5419

TEXAS

GALVESTON

Drug Information Center
University of Texas Medical Branch
301 University Blvd. - G01
Galveston, TX 77555-0701
Mon.-Fri. 8 AM-5 PM
409-772-2734
Fax: 409-747-5222

HOUSTON

Drug Information Center
Ben Taub General Hospital
Texas Southern University/HCHD
1504 Taub Loop
Houston, TX 77030
Mon.-Fri. 8 AM-5 PM
713-793-2917
Fax: 713-793-2998

Drug Information Center
Methodist Hospital
6565 Fannin (MSDB109)
Houston, TX 77030
Mon.-Fri. 8 AM-5 PM
713-790-4190
Fax: 713-793-1224

LACKLAND A.F.B.

Drug Information Center
Dept. of Pharmacy
Wilford Hall Medical Center
2200 Berquist Dr., Suite 1
Lackland A.F.B., TX 78236
7 days/week, 24 hours
210-292-5418
Fax: 210-292-3722

LUBBOCK

Drug Information and Consultation Service
Covenant Medical Center
3615 19th St.
Lubbock, TX 79410
Mon.-Fri. 8 AM-5 PM
806-725-0419
Fax: 806-725-0305

TEMPLE

Drug Information Center
Scott and White Memorial Hospital
2401 S. 31st St.
Temple, TX 76508
Mon.-Fri. 8 AM-6 PM
254-724-4636
Fax: 254-724-1731

UTAH

SALT LAKE CITY

Drug Information Service
University of Utah Hospital
Dept. of Pharmacy Services
Room A-050
50 N. Medical Dr.
Salt Lake City, UT 84132
Mon.-Fri. 8:30 AM-4:30 PM
801-581-2073
Fax: 801-585-6688

WEST VIRGINIA

MORGANTOWN

West Virginia Drug Information Center
WV University-
Robert C. Byrd Health Sciences Center
1124 HSN, P.O. Box 9550
Morgantown, WV 26506
Mon.-Fri. 8:30 AM-5 PM
304-293-6640
800-352-2501 (WV)
Fax: 304-293-7672

WISCONSIN

MADISON

University of Wisconsin Hospital & Clinics
Poison Control Center
600 Highland Ave.
Madison, WI 53792
800-815-8855 (WI only)
drug.info@hosp.wisc.edu
(for healthcare professionals only)

WYOMING

LARAMIE

Drug Information Center
University of Wyoming
P.O. Box 3375
Laramie, WY 82071
Mon.-Fri. 8 AM-5 PM
307-766-6988
Fax: 307-766-2953

LOOK-ALIKE, SOUND-ALIKE DRUG NAMES

Confusion over the similarity of drug names, either written or spoken, accounts for approximately one-quarter of all reports to the USP Medications Errors Reporting Program. This naming issue involves confusion between similar brand names, between generic names, and between brand and generic names. Such confusion is compounded by illegible handwriting, incomplete knowledge of drug names, newly available products, similar packaging or labeling, and incorrect selection of a similar name from a computerized list.

Below is the list of similar drug names reported to the USP Medication Errors Reporting Program. Remember that these names may not sound alike as you read them or look alike in print, but when handwritten or communicated verbally, these names have caused or could cause a mix-up.

Accupril	Accutane
Accupril	Monopril
Accutane	Accupril
Acetazolamide	Acetohexamide
Acetohexamide	Acetazolamide
Acular	Ocular
Adderall	Inderal
Adenosine	Adenosine Phosphate
Adenosine Phosphate	Adenosine
Adriamycin	Aredia
Adriamycin	Idamycin
Akarpine	Atropine
Aldara	Alora
Allegra	Viagra
Allopurinol	Apresoline
Alora	Aldara
Alprazolam	Lorazepam
Altace	Amaryl
Altace	Artane
Alupent	Atrovent
Amantadine	Ranitidine, Rimantadine
Amaryl	Altace
Ambien	Amen
Amen	Ambien
Amicar	Amikin
Amikin	Amicar
Amiloride	Amlodipine
Amiodarone	Amrinone
Amlodipine	Amiloride
Amoxicillin	Amoxil
Amoxicillin	Atarax
Amoxil	Amoxicillin
Amrinone	Amiodarone
Anaspaz	Antispas
Ansaid	Asacol
Antispas	Anaspaz
Anusol	Anusol-HC
Anusol-HC	Anusol
Apresoline	Allopurinol
Aredia	Adriamycin
Artane	Altace
Asacol	Ansaid
Asacol	Os-Cal

Asparaginase	Pegaspargase
Atarax	Amoxicillin
Atarax	Ativan
Ativan	Atarax
Atropine	Akarpine
Atrovent	Alupent
Attenuvax	Meruvax
Azithromycin	Erythromycin
Benadryl	Benylin
Benylin	Benadryl
Benylin	Ventolin
Bepridil	Prepidil
Betagan	Betagen
Betagan	Betoptic
Betagen	Betagan
Betoptic	Betagan
Betoptic	Betoptic S
Betoptic S	Betoptic
Brevibloc	Brevital
Brevital	Brevibloc
Bumex	Buprenex
Bumex	Permax
Buprenex	Bumex
Buspirone	Bupropion
Bupropion	Buspirone
Cafergot	Carafate
Calan	Colace
Calciferol	Calcitriol
Calcitriol	Calciferol
Captopril	Carvedilol
Carafate	Cafergot
Carboplatin	Cisplatin
Cardene	Cardizem
Cardene	Cardura
Cardene	Codeine
Cardene SR	Cardizem SR
Cardiem	Cardizem
Cardizem	Cardene
Cardizem	Cardiem
Cardizem CD	Cardizem SR
Cardizem SR	Cardene SR
Cardizem SR	Cardizem CD
Cardura	Cardene
Cardura	Coumadin
Cardura	Ridaura

Carteolol	Carvedilol
Carvedilol	Captopril
Carvedilol	Carteolol
Cataflam	Catapres
Catapres	Cataflam
Cefaclor	Cephalexin
Cefazolin	Cefprozil
Cefol	Cefzil
Cefotan	Ceftin
Cefotaxime	Cefuroxime
Cefprozil	Cefazolin
Cefprozil	Cefuroxime
Ceftazidime	Ceftizoxime
Ceftin	Cefotan
Ceftin	Cefzil
Ceftin	Cipro
Ceftizoxime	Ceftazidime
Cefuroxime	Cefotaxime
Cefuroxime	Cefprozil
Cefuroxime	Deferoxamine
Cefzil	Cefol
Cefzil	Ceftin
Cefzil	Kefzol
Celebrex	Celexa, Cerebyx
Celexa	Cerebyx, Celebrex
Celexa	Zyprexa
Centoxin	Cytoxan
Cephalexin	Cefaclor
Cephalexin	Ciprofloxacin
Cerebyx	Celebrex, Celexa
Chlorpromazine	Chlorpropamide
Chlorpromazine	Prochlorperazine
Chlorpropamide	Chlorpromazine
Cipro	Ceftin
Ciprofloxacin	Cephalexin
Cisplatin	Carboplatin
Claritin-D	Claritin-D 24-hour
Claritin-D 24-hour	Claritin-D
Clinoril	Clozaril
Clinoril	Oruvail
Clomiphene	Clomipramine
Clomipramine	Clomiphene
Clomipramine	Desipramine

Clonazepam	Clonidine, Klonopin
Clonazepam	Clorazepate
Clonidine	Klonopin
Clonidine	Klonopin, Clonazepam
Clorazepate	Clonazepam
Clozaril	Clinoril
Codeine	Cardene
Codeine	Iodine
Codeine	Lodine
Cognex	Corgard
Colace	Calan
Corgard	Cognex
Cortef	Lortab
Coumadin	Cardura
Covera	Provera
Cozaar	Zocor
Cyclobenzaprine	Cyproheptadine
Cyclophosphamide	Cyclosporine
Cycloserine	Cyclosporine
Cyclosporine	Cyclophosphamide
Cyclosporine	Cycloserine
Cyproheptadine	Cyclobenzaprine
Cytarabine	Cytosar, Cytoxan
CytoGam	Gamimune N
Cytosar	Cytovene
Cytosar	Cytoxan, Cytarabine
Cytosar-U	Neosar
Cytotec	Cytoxan
Cytovene	Cytosar
Cytoxan	Centoxin
Cytoxan	Cytotec
Cytoxan	Cytosar, Cytarabine
Danazol	Dantrium
Dantrium	Danazol
Darvon	Diovan
Daunorubicin	Doxorubicin
Daypro	Diupres
Deferoxamine	Cefuroxime
Demerol	Desyrel
Denavir	Indinavir

Depakote	Senokot
Depo-Estradiol	Depo-Testadiol
Depo-Testadiol	Depo-Estradiol
Desferal	DexFerrum
Desipramine	Clomipramine
Desipramine	Imipramine
Desipramine	Nortriptyline
Desyrel	Demerol
DexFerrum	Desferal
DiaBeta	Zebeta
Diamox	Dobutrex
Diazepam	Ditropan
Diazepam	Lorazepam
Dicyclomine	Diphenhydramine
Diflucan	Diprivan
Diovan	Darvon
Diovan	Dioval
Diovan	Zyban
Dioval	Diovan
Diphenatol	Diphenidol
Diphenhydramine	Dicyclomine
Diphenidol	Diphenatol
Diprivan	Diflucan
Ditropan	Diazepam
Diupres	Daypro
Dobutamine	Dopamine
Dobutrex	Diamox
Dolobid	Slo-bid
Dopamine	Dobutamine
Doxepin	Doxycycline
Doxorubicin	Daunorubicin
Doxorubicin	Doxorubicin Liposomal
Doxorubicin	Idarubicin
Doxorubicin Liposomal	Doxorubicin
Doxycycline	Doxepin
Dynabac	DynaCirc
Dynacin	DynaCirc
DynaCirc	Dynabac
DynaCirc	Dynacin
Edecrin	Eulexin
Efudex	Eurax
Elavil	Oruvail
Elavil	Plavix
Eldepryl	Enalapril
Elmiron	Imuran
Enalapril	Eldepryl
Equagesic	EquiGesic
EquiGesic	Equagesic
Erex	Urex
Erythrocin	Ethmozine
Erythromycin	Azithromycin
Eskalith	Estratest
Estraderm	Testoderm
Estratab	Estratest
Estratest	Eskalith
Estratest	Estratab
Estratest	Estratest HS
Estratest HS	Estratest
Ethmozine	Erythrocin
Etidronate	Etomidate
Etidronate	Etretinate
Etomidate	Etidronate
Etretinate	Etidronate
Eulexin	Edecrin
Eurax	Efudex
Fam-Pren Forte	Parafon Forte
Fentanyl Citrate	Sufentanil Citrate
Fioricet	Fiorinal
Fiorinal	Fioricet
Flomax	Fosamax
Flomax	Volmax
Flucytosine	Fluorouracil
Fludara	FUDR
Fludarabine	Flumadine
Flumadine	Fludarabine
Fluorouracil	Flucytosine
Flurazepam	Temazepam
Folic Acid	Folinic Acid
Folinic Acid	Folic Acid
Fosamax	Flomax
FUDR	Fludara
Furosemide	Torsemide
Gamimune N	CytoGam
Gemzar	Zinecard
Glipizide	Glyburide
Glucophage	Glutofac
Glucotrol	Glucotrol XL
Glucotrol	Glyburide
Glucotrol XL	Glucotrol
Glutofac	Glucophage
Glyburide	Glipizide
Glyburide	Glucotrol
Granulex	Regranex
Haldol	Stadol
Haloperidol	Halotestin
Halotestin	Haloperidol
Hemoccult	Seracult
Heparin	Hespan
Hespan	Heparin
Humalog	Humulin
Humulin	Humalog
Hydralazine	Hydroxyzine
Hydrocodone	Hydrocortisone
Hydrocortisone	Hydrocodone
Hydromorphone	Morphine
Hydroxyzine	Hydralazine
Idamycin	Adriamycin
Idarubicin	Doxorubicin
IMDUR	Imuran
IMDUR	Inderal LA
IMDUR	K-Dur
Imipenem	Omnipen
Imipramine	Desipramine
Imovax	Imovax I.D.
Imovax I.D.	Imovax
Imuran	Elmiron
Imuran	IMDUR
Imuran	Tenormin
Inderal	Adderall
Inderal	Isordil
Inderal	Toradol
Inderal LA	IMDUR
Indinavir	Denavir
Iodine	Codeine
Iodine	Lodine
Isordil	Inderal
K-Dur	IMDUR
K-Phos Neutral	Neutra-Phos-K
Kefzol	Cefzil
Klonopin	Clonidine, Clonazepam
Lamictal	Lamisil
Lamictal	Lomotil
Lamictal	Ludiomil
Lamisil	Lamictal
Lamisil	Lomotil
Lamivudine	Lamotrigine
Lamotrigine	Lamivudine
Lanoxin	Lasix, Lomotil
Lanoxin	Levoxine, Levoxyl
Lanoxin	Lonox
Lanoxin	Xanax
Lasix	Lomotil, Lanoxin
Lasix	Luvox
L-Dopa	Levodopa, Methyldopa
Leucovorin	Leukine, Leukeran
Leukeran	Leucovorin, Leukine
Leukine	Leukeran, Leucovorin
Levbid	Lithobid
Levbid	Lopid
Levbid	Lorabid
Levobunolol	Levocabastine
Levocabastine	Levobunolol
Levodopa	L-Dopa, Methyldopa
Levoxine	Lanoxin, Levoxyl
Levoxine	Levsin
Levoxyl	Lanoxin, Levoxine
Levoxyl	Luvox
Levsin	Levoxine
Librax	Librium
Librium	Librax
Lioresal	Lotensin
Lisinopril	Risperdal
Lithobid	Lithostat
Lithobid	Levbid
Lithostat	Lithobid
Lodine	Codeine
Lodine	Iodine
Lomotil	Lamictal
Lomotil	Lamisil
Lomotil	Lanoxin, Lasix
Loniten	Lotensin
Lonox	Lanoxin
Lopid	Levbid
Lopid	Lorabid, Slo-bid
Lorabid	Levbid
Lorabid	Lortab
Lorabid	Slo-bid, Lopid
Lorazepam	Alprazolam
Lorazepam	Diazepam
Lortab	Cortef
Lortab	Lorabid
Lortab	Luride
Losartan	Valsartan
Lotensin	Lioresal
Lotensin	Loniten
Lotensin	Lovastatin
Lotrimin	Lotrisone
Lotrisone	Lotrimin
Lovastatin	Lotensin
Loxitane	Soriatane
Ludiomil	Lamictal
Luride	Lortab
Luvox	Lasix
Luvox	Levoxyl
Medi-Gesic	Medigesic
Medigesic	Medi-Gesic
Medrol ADT	Medrol Dosepak
Medrol Dosepak	Medrol ADT
Medroxyprogesterone	Methylprednisolone
Megace	Reglan
Mepron (Atovaquone in U.S.)	Mepron (Meprobamate in Australia)
Meruvax	Attenuvax
Methadone	Methylphenidate
Methotrexate	Metolazone

Methyldopa	L-Dopa, Levodopa
Methylphenidate	Methadone
Methyl-prednisolone	Medroxy-progesterone
Methylprednisolone	Prednisone
Metoclopramide	Metolazone
Metolazone	Methotrexate
Metolazone	Metoclopramide
Metoprolol	Misoprostol
Micro-K	Micronase
Micronase	Micro-K
Minoxidil	Monopril
Misoprostol	Metoprolol
Mitomycin	Mitoxantrone
Mitoxantrone	Mitomycin
Monoket	Monopril
Monopril	Accupril
Monopril	Minoxidil
Monopril	Monoket
Morphine	Hydromorphone
Murocel	Murocoll-2
Murocoll-2	Murocel
Naprelan	Naprosyn
Naprosyn	Naprelan
Narcan	Norcuron
Nasalcrom	Nasalide
Nasalide	Nasalcrom
Nasarel	Nizoral
Navane	Norvasc
Nebcin	Nubain
Nelfinavir	Nevirapine
Neocare	Neocate
Neocate	Neocare
Neoral	Nizoral
Neosar	Cytosar-U
Nephrox	Niferex
Neumega	Neupogen
Neupogen	Neumega
Neurontin	Noroxin
Neutra-Phos-K	K-Phos Neutral
Nevirapine	Nelfinavir
Niacin	Nispan
Nicardipine	Nifedipine, Nimodipine
Nicoderm	Nitroderm
Nifedipine	Nicardipine, Nimodipine
Niferex	Nephrox
Nimodipine	Nicardipine, Nifedipine
Nispan	Niacin
Nitroderm	Nicoderm
Nimbex	Revex
Nizoral	Nasarel
Nizoral	Neoral
Norcuron	Narcan
Norflex	Noroxin, Norfloxacin
Norfloxacin	Norflex, Noroxin
Noroxin	Neurontin
Noroxin	Norflex, Norfloxacin
Norpramin	Nortriptyline
Nortriptyline	Desipramine
Nortriptyline	Norpramin
Norvasc	Navane
Nubain	Nebcin
Ocufen	Ocuflox
Ocufen	Ocupress
Ocuflox	Ocufen
Ocular	Acular
Ocu-Mycin	Ocumycin
Ocumycin	Ocu-Mycin
Ocupress	Ocufen
Omnipen	Imipenem
Ortho-Cept	Ortho-Cyclen
Ortho-Cyclen	Ortho-Cept
Oruvail	Clinoril
Oruvail	Elavil
Os-Cal	Asacol
Oxycodone	OxyContin
OxyContin	Oxycodone
Paclitaxel	Paroxetine
Paclitaxel	Paxil
Parafon Forte	Fam-Pren Forte
Paraplatin	Platinol
Parlodel	Pindolol
Paroxetine	Paclitaxel
Paxil	Paclitaxel
Paxil	Taxol
Pediapred	Pediazole
Pediazole	Pediapred
Pegaspargase	Asparaginase
Penicillamine	Penicillin
Penicillin	Penicillamine
Penicillin G Potassium	Penicillin G Procaine
Penicillin G Procaine	Penicillin G Potassium
Pentobarbital	Phenobarbital
Perative	Periactin
Periactin	Perative
Percocet	Percodan
Percodan	Percocet
Permax	Bumex
Phenobarbital	Pentobarbital
Pindolol	Parlodel
Pindolol	Plendil
Pitocin	Pitressin
Pitressin	Pitocin
Platinol	Paraplatin
Plavix	Elavil
Plendil	Pindolol
Plendil	Prilosec
Plendil	Prinivil
Pondimin	Prednisone
Potassium Phosphates	Sodium Phosphates
Pravachol	Prevacid
Pravachol	Propranolol
Precare	Precose
Precose	Precare
Prednisone	Methyl-prednisolone
Prednisone	Pondimin
Prednisone	Prilosec
Prednisone	Primidone
Premarin	Primaxin
Premarin	Provera
Prepidil	Bepridil
Prevacid	Pravachol
Prevacid	Prinivil
Prilosec	Plendil
Prilosec	Prednisone
Prilosec	Prinivil
Prilosec	Prozac
Primaxin	Premarin
Primidone	Prednisone
Prinivil	Plendil
Prinivil	Prevacid
Prinivil	Prilosec
Prinivil	Proventil
Prochlorperazine	Chlorpromazine
Proctocort	Proctocream HC
Proctocream HC	Proctocort
Profen	Profen II, Profen LA
Profen II	Profen, Profen LA
Profen LA	Profen, Profen II
Promethazine	Promethazine w/ Codeine
Promethazine w/ Codeine	Promethazine
Propranolol	Pravachol
Propranolol	Propulsid
Propulsid	Propranolol
Proscar	ProSom, Prozac
ProSom	Prozac, Proscar
Proventil	Prinivil
Provera	Covera
Provera	Premarin
Prozac	Prilosec
Prozac	Proscar, ProSom
Quinidine	Quinine
Quinine	Quinidine
Ranitidine	Amantadine, Rimantadine
ReFresh (breath drops)	ReFresh (lubricant eye drops)
ReFresh (lubricant eye drops)	ReFresh (breath drops)
Reglan	Megace
Regranex	Granulex
Relafen	Rezulin
Remeron	Zemuron
Reno-M-60	Renografin-60
Renografin-60	Reno-M-60
Reserpine	Risperdal, Risperidone
Retrovir	Ritonavir
Revex	Nimbex
Revex	ReVia
ReVia	Revex
Rezulin	Relafen
Ridaura	Cardura
Rifabutin	Rifampin
Rifampin	Rifabutin
Rimantadine	Amantadine, Ranitidine
Risperdal	Lisinopril
Risperdal	Reserpine, Risperidone
Risperidone	Reserpine, Risperdal
Ritonavir	Retrovir
Roxanol	Roxicet
Roxicet	Roxanol
Rynatan	Rynatuss
Rynatuss	Rynatan
Salbutamol	Salmeterol
Salmeterol	Salbutamol
Selegiline	Serentil, Sertraline Serzone
Selegiline	Sertraline
Senokot	Depakote
Seracult	Hemoccult
Serentil	Selegiline, Sertraline, Serzone
Serentil	Serzone
Serentil	Sinequan
Seroquel	Serzone
Serzone	Sertraline, Selegiline, Serentil
Serzone	Seroquel
Sinequan	Serentil
Slo-bid	Lopid, Lorabid

Slo-bid	Dolobid
Sodium Phosphates	Potassium Phosphates
Solu-Medrol	Depo-Medrol
Soma	Soma Compound
Soma Compound	Soma
Soriatane	Loxitane
Stadol	Haldol
Sufentanil Citrate	Fentanyl Citrate
Sulfadiazine	Sulfasalazine
Sulfasalazine	Sulfadiazine
Sulfasalazine	Sulfisoxazole
Sulfisoxazole	Sulfasalazine
Sumatriptan	Zolmitriptan
Symmetrel	Synthroid
Synagis	Synvisc
Synthroid	Symmetrel
Synvisc	Synagis
Taxol	Paxil
Tegretol	Toradol
Temazepam	Flurazepam
Tenormin	Imuran
Tenormin	Thiamine
Tenormin	Trovan
Testoderm	Estraderm
Tetracycline	Tetradecyl Sulfate
Tetradecyl Sulfate	Tetracycline
Thiamine	Tenormin

Tiagabine	Tizanidine
Tiazac	Ziac
Tizanidine	Tiagabine
Tobradex	Tobrex
Tobrex	Tobradex
Tolazamide	Tolbutamide
Tolbutamide	Tolazamide
Toradol	Inderal
Toradol	Tegretol
Toradol	Torecan
Toradol	Tramadol
Torecan	Toradol
Torsemide	Furosemide
Tramadol	Toradol
Tramadol	Voltaren
Trandate	Tridrate
Triad (Butalbital/ Acetaminophen/ Caffeine)	Triad (topical)
Tridrate	Trandate
Trifluoperazine	Trihexyphenidyl
Trihexyphenidyl	Trifluoperazine
Tri-Norinyl	Triphasil
Triphasil	Tri-Norinyl
Trovan	Tenormin
Ultane	Ultram
Ultram	Ultane
Ultram	Voltaren
Urex	Erex
Uricit-K	Urised

Uridon	Vicodin
Urised	Uricit-K
Valsartan	Losartan
Vancenase	Vanceril
Vanceril	Vancenase
Vancomycin	Vecuronium
Vantin	Ventolin
Vecuronium	Vancomycin
Ventolin	Benylin
Ventolin	Vantin
Vepesid	Versed
Verapamil	Verelan
Verelan	Verapamil
Verelan	Virilon
Versed	Vepesid
Versed	Vistaril
Vexol	VoSol
Viagra	Allegra
Vicodin	Uridon
Vinblastine	Vincristine
Vincristine	Vinblastine
Viracept	Viramune
Viramune	Viracept
Virilon	Verelan
Vistaril	Versed
Vistaril	Zestril
Volmax	Flomax
Voltaren	Tramadol
Voltaren	Ultram
VoSol	Vexol

Xanax	Lanoxin
Xanax	Zantac, Zyrtec
Yocon	Zocor
Zagam	Zyban
Zantac	Zofran
Zantac	Xanax, Zyrtec
Zebeta	DiaBeta
Zemuron	Remeron
Zestril	Vistaril
Ziac	Tiazac
Zinacef	Zithromax
Zinecard	Gemzar
Zithromax	Zinacef
Zocor	Cozaar
Zocor	Yocon
Zocor	Zoloft
Zofran	Zantac
Zofran	Zosyn
Zoloft	Zocor
Zolomitriptan	Sumatriptan
Zonalon	Zone A Forte
Zone A Forte	Zonalon
Zosyn	Zofran
Zyban	Zagam
Zyrtec	Xanax, Zantac
Zyprexa	Celexa
Zyprexa	Zyrtec
Zyrtec	Zyprex
Zyrtec	Zyprexa

VACCINE ADVERSE EVENT REPORTING SYSTEM

VAERS

24 Hour Toll-free information line 1-800-822-7967
P.O. Box 1100, Rockville, MD 20849-1100
PATIENT IDENTITY KEPT CONFIDENTIAL

For CDC/FDA Use Only

VAERS Number ______

Date Received ______

Patient Name:

____
Last First M.I.

Address

City State Zip

Telephone no. (____) ______

Vaccine administered by (Name):

Responsible Physician ______

Facility Name/Address

City State Zip

Telephone no. (____) ______

Form completed by (Name):

Relation to Patient ☐ Vaccine Provider ☐ Patient/Parent ☐ Manufacturer ☐ Other

Address *(if different from patient or provider)*

City State Zip

Telephone no. (____) ______

1. State

2. County where administered

3. Date of birth __/__/__ mm dd yy

4. Patient age

5. Sex ☐ M ☐ F

6. Date form completed __/__/__ mm dd yy

7. Describe adverse event(s) (symptoms, signs, time course) and treatment, if any

8. Check all appropriate:
- ☐ Patient died (date __/__/__ mm dd yy)
- ☐ Life threatening illness
- ☐ Required emergency room/doctor visit
- ☐ Required hospitalization (____days)
- ☐ Resulted in prolongation of hospitalization
- ☐ Resulted in permanent disability
- ☐ None of the above

9. Patient recovered ☐ YES ☐ NO ☐ UNKNOWN

10. Date of vaccination __/__/__ mm dd yy Time ____ AM PM

11. Adverse event onset __/__/__ mm dd yy Time ____ AM PM

12. Relevant diagnostic tests/laboratory data

13. Enter all vaccines given on date listed in no. 10

	Vaccine (type)	Manufacturer	Lot number	Route/Site	No. Previous Doses
a.					
b.					
c.					
d.					

14. Any other vaccinations within 4 weeks prior to the date listed in no. 10

	Vaccine (type)	Manufacturer	Lot number	Route/Site	No. Previous doses	Date given
a.						
b.						

15. Vaccinated at:
- ☐ Private doctor's office/hospital
- ☐ Public health clinic/hospital
- ☐ Military clinic/hospital
- ☐ Other/unknown

16. Vaccine purchased with:
- ☐ Private funds
- ☐ Public funds
- ☐ Military funds
- ☐ Other/unknown

17. Other medications

18. Illness at time of vaccination (specify)

19. Pre-existing physician-diagnosed allergies, birth defects, medical conditions(specify)

20. Have you reported this adverse event previously? ☐ No ☐ To doctor ☐ To health department ☐ To manufacturer

21. Adverse event following prior vaccination (check all applicable, specify)

	Adverse Event	Onset Age	Type Vaccine	Dose no. in series
☐ In patient				
☐ In brother or sister				

Only for children 5 and under

22. Birth weight ____ lb. ____ oz.

23. No. of brothers and sisters

Only for reports submitted by manufacturer/Immunization project

24. Mfr./imm. proj. report no.

25. Date received by mfr./imm.proj.

26. 15 day report? ☐ Yes ☐ No

27. Report type ☐ Initial ☐ Follow-Up

Health care providers and manufacturers are required by law (42 USC 300aa-25) to report reactions to vaccines listed in the Table of Reportable Events Following Immunization Reports for reactions to other vaccines are voluntary except when required as a condition of immunization grant awards.

orm VAERS-1

Vaccine Adverse Event Reporting System

Health care providers and manufacturers are required by law (42 USC 300aa-25) to report reactions to vaccines listed in the Vaccine Injury Table. Reports for reactions to other vaccines are voluntary except when required as a condition of immunization grant awards.

The form appears overleaf and may be photocopied for submission, or can be downloaded from www.vaers.org.

DIRECTIONS FOR COMPLETING FORM

(Additional pages may be attached if more space is needed.)

GENERAL

- Use a separate form for each patient. Complete the form to the best of your abilities. Items 3, 4, 7, 8, 10, 11, and 13 are considered essential and should be completed whenever possible. Parents/Guardians may need to consult the facility where the vaccine was administered for some of the information (such as manufacturer, lot number or laboratory data.)
- Refer to the Reportable Events Table (RET) for events mandated for reporting by law. Reporting for other serious events felt to be related but not on the RET is encouraged.
- Health care providers other than the vaccine administrator (VA) treating a patient for a suspected adverse event should notify the VA and provide the information about the adverse event to allow the VA to complete the form to meet the VA's legal responsibility.
- These data will be used to increase understanding of adverse events following vaccination and will become part of CDC Privacy Act System 09-20-0136, "Epidemiologic Studies and Surveillance of Disease Problems". Information identifying the person who received the vaccine or that person's legal representative will not be made available to the public, but may be available to the vaccinee or legal representative.
- Postage will be paid by addressee. Forms may be photocopied (must be front & back on same sheet).

SPECIFIC INSTRUCTIONS

Form Completed By: To be used by parents/guardians, vaccine manufacturers/distributors, vaccine administrators, and/or the person completing the form on behalf of the patient or the health professional who administered the vaccine.

Item 7: Describe the suspected adverse event. Such things as temperature, local and general signs and symptoms, time course, duration of symptoms diagnosis, treatment and recovery should be noted.

Item 9: Check "YES" if the patient's health condition is the same as it was prior to the vaccine, "NO" if the patient has not returned to the pre-vaccination state of health, or "UNKNOWN" if the patient's condition is not known.

Item 10: and 11: Give dates and times as specifically as you can remember. If you do not know the exact time, please indicate "AM" or "PM" when possible if this information is known. If more than one adverse event, give the onset date and time for the most serious event.

Item 12: Include "negative" or "normal" results of any relevant tests performed as well as abnormal findings.

Item 13: List ONLY those vaccines given on the day listed in Item 10.

Item 14: List any other vaccines that the patient received within 4 weeks prior to the date listed in Item 10.

Item 16: This section refers to how the person who gave the vaccine purchased it, not to the patient's insurance.

Item 17: List any prescription or non-prescription medications the patient was taking when the vaccine(s) was given.

Item 18: List any short term illnesses the patient had on the date the vaccine(s) was given (i.e., cold, flu, ear infection).

Item 19: List any pre-existing physician-diagnosed allergies, birth defects, medical conditions (including developmental and/or neurologic disorders) for the patient.

Item 21: List any suspected adverse events the patient, or the patient's brothers or sisters, may have had to previous vaccinations. If more than one brother or sister, or if the patient has reacted to more than one prior vaccine, use additional pages to explain completely. For the onset age of a patient, provide the age in months if less than two years old.

Item 26: This space is for manufacturers' use only.

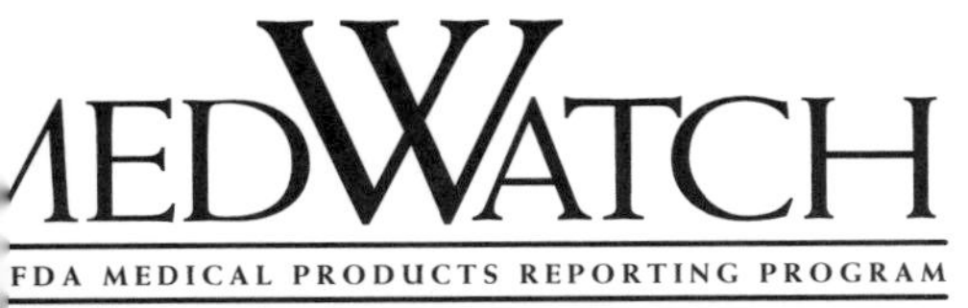

FDA MEDICAL PRODUCTS REPORTING PROGRAM

For VOLUNTARY reporting by health professionals of adverse events and product problems

Page ____ of ____

Form Approved: OMB No. 0910-0291 Expires: 11/30/00
See OMB statement on reverse

FDA Use Only

Triage unit sequence #

Patient information

tient identifier | 2. Age at time of event: or Date of birth: | 3. Sex ☐ female ☐ male | 4. Weight ____ lbs or ____ kgs

confidence

Adverse event or product problem

☐ Adverse event and/or ☐ Product problem (e.g., defects/malfunctions)

utcomes attributed to adverse event
neck all that apply)

☐ death ____________ (mo/day/yr)
☐ life-threatening
☐ hospitalization – initial or prolonged
☐ disability
☐ congenital anomaly
☐ required intervention to prevent permanent impairment/damage
☐ other: ____________

te of ent /day/yr) | 4. Date of this report (mo/day/yr)

escribe event or problem

elevant tests/laboratory data, including dates

Other relevant history, including preexisting medical conditions (e.g., allergies, race, pregnancy, smoking and alcohol use, hepatic/renal dysfunction, etc.)

C. Suspect medication(s)

1. Name (give labeled strength & mfr/labeler, if known)
#1
#2

2. Dose, frequency & route used
#1
#2

3. Therapy dates (if unknown, give duration) from/to (or best estimate)
#1
#2

4. Diagnosis for use (indication)
#1
#2

5. Event abated after use stopped or dose reduced
#1 ☐ yes ☐ no ☐ doesn't apply
#2 ☐ yes ☐ no ☐ doesn't apply

6. Lot # (if known)
#1
#2

7. Exp. date (if known)
#1
#2

8. Event reappeared after reintroduction
#1 ☐ yes ☐ no ☐ doesn't apply
#2 ☐ yes ☐ no ☐ doesn't apply

9. NDC # (for product problems only)
– –

10. Concomitant medical products and therapy dates (exclude treatment of event)

D. Suspect medical device

1. Brand name

2. Type of device

3. Manufacturer name & address

4. Operator of device
☐ health professional
☐ lay user/patient
☐ other: ____________

5. Expiration date (mo/day/yr)

6.
model # ____________
catalog # ____________
serial # ____________
lot # ____________
other #

7. If implanted, give date (mo/day/yr)

8. If explanted, give date (mo/day/yr)

9. Device available for evaluation? (Do not send to FDA)
☐ yes ☐ no ☐ returned to manufacturer on ____________ (mo/day/yr)

10. Concomitant medical products and therapy dates (exclude treatment of event)

E. Reporter (see confidentiality section on back)

1. Name & address | phone #

2. Health professional? ☐ yes ☐ no

3. Occupation

4. Also reported to
☐ manufacturer
☐ user facility
☐ distributor

5. If you do NOT want your identity disclosed to the manufacturer, place an " X " in this box. ☐

FDA

Mail to: MEDWATCH
5600 Fishers Lane
Rockville, MD 20852-9787

or FAX to:
1-800-FDA-0178

Form 3500

Submission of a report does not constitute an admission that medical personnel or the product caused or contributed to the event.

ADVICE ABOUT VOLUNTARY REPORTING

Report experiences with:

- medications (drugs or biologics)
- medical devices (including in-vitro diagnostics)
- special nutritional products (dietary supplements, medical foods, infant formulas)
- other products regulated by FDA

Report SERIOUS adverse events. An event is serious when the patient outcome is:

- death
- life-threatening (real risk of dying)
- hospitalization (initial or prolonged)
- disability (significant, persistent or permanent)
- congenital anomaly
- required intervention to prevent permanent impairment or damage

Report even if:

- you're not certain the product caused the event
- you don't have all the details

Report product problems – quality, performance or safety concerns such as:

- suspected contamination
- questionable stability
- defective components
- poor packaging or labeling
- therapeutic failures

How to report:

- just fill in the sections that apply to your report
- use section C for all products except medical devices
- attach additional blank pages if needed
- use a separate form for each patient
- report either to FDA or the manufacturer (or both)

Important numbers:

- 1-800-FDA-0178 to FAX report
- 1-800-FDA-7737 to report by modem
- 1-800-FDA-1088 to report by phone or for more information
- 1-800-822-7967 for a VAERS form for vaccines

If your report involves a serious adverse event with a device and it occurred in a facility outside a doctor's office, that facility may be legally required to report to FDA and/or the manufacturer. Please notify the person in that facility who would handle such reporting.

Confidentiality: The patient's identity is held in strict confidence by FDA and protected to the fullest extent of the law. The reporter's identity, including the identity of a self-reporter, may be shared with the manufacturer unless requested otherwise. However, FDA will not disclose the reporter's identity in response to a request from the public, pursuant to the Freedom of Information Act.

The public reporting burden for this collection of information has been estimated to average 30 minutes per response, including the time for reviewing instructions, searching existing data sources, gathering and maintaining the data needed, and completing and reviewing the collection of information. Send comments regarding this burden estimate or any other aspect of this collection of information, including suggestions for reducing this burden to:

DHHS Reports Clearance Office
Paperwork Reduction Project (0910-0291)
Hubert H. Humphrey Building, Room 531-H
200 Independence Avenue, S.W.
Washington, DC 20201

"An agency may not conduct or sponsor, and a person is not required to respond to, a collection of information unless it displays a currently valid OMB control number."

Please DO NOT RETURN this form to this address.

U.S. DEPARTMENT OF HEALTH AND HUMAN SERVICES
Public Health Service • Food and Drug Administration

FDA Form 3500-back

Please Use Address Provided Below – Just Fold In Thirds, Tape and Mail

Department of Health and Human Services
Public Health Service
Food and Drug Administration
Rockville, MD 20857

Official Business
Penalty for Private Use $300

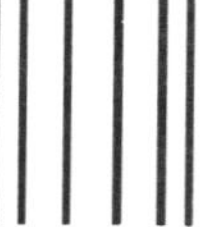

BUSINESS REPLY MAIL

FIRST CLASS MAIL PERMIT NO. 946 ROCKVILLE, MD

POSTAGE WILL BE PAID BY FOOD AND DRUG ADMINISTRATION

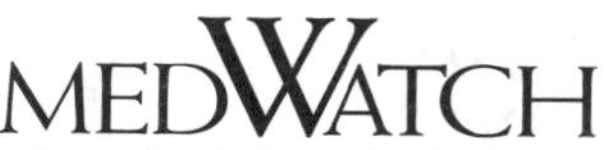

The FDA Medical Products Reporting Program
Food and Drug Administration
5600 Fishers Lane
Rockville, MD 20852-9787